STEDMAN'S

PRONUNCIATION

You can use this dictionary to learn how to pronounce medical terms. The pronunciation appears in parentheses between the term and the beginning of its definition. The pronunciation of terms defined in this dictionary is indicated with letters of the English alphabet rather than with phonetic symbols. The following key shows the sounds represented by these letters.

VOWELS

ā day, care, trait, gauge
a mat, damage, far
ă about, hepatitis, data, tartar
ah father, what
aw raw, fall, cause
ē ego, here, bead, beet, artery
e bed, head, therapy, teratoma
ĕ erythrocyte, genesis, system, lower
ī isle, lie, pyre, bacilli
i igloo, hip, irritate
ĭ pencil, circus
ō oval, form, go
o got, bought
ŏ oven, bottom, motor
ow cow, hour
oy boy, oil
ū prune, fruit, genu, food
yū cube, urine, beauty, value
u put, wool
ŭ upset, putt, murmur, tough

CONSONANTS

b bad, tab
ch child, itch
d dog, bad
dh this, smooth (cf. th)
f fit, defect; phase, hyphen; tough
g got, bag
h hit, behold
[h] Denotes an approximation of a tone used in French words whereby the sound is pulled to the back of the tongue. The closest equivalent in English is found in the word 'zone' wherein the ending of that word is pronounced as if swallowed.
j jade; gender, rigid, edge (cf. g)
k cut, tic; tachycardia (cf. ch)
ks extra, tax
kw quick, aqua
l law, kill
m me, timid, bum
n no, tender, run
ng ring
p pan, upset, top
r rot, atropy, tar
s so, distill, mess (cf z); center, council (cf k)
sh show, wish; social
t ten, batter, put
th thin, with (cf dh)
v vote, oven, nerve
w we, awake, tow
y yes, payload
z zero; disease, faces (cf s); xiphoid (cf ks)
zh azure, vision, measure

BUILDING BLOCKS OF MEDICAL LANGUAGE

The most common medical word parts can be found in the appendix section of this dictionary. These are prefixes, suffixes, and combining forms that make up 90 to 95 percent of medical vocabulary.

Throughout the A–Z section these terms are marked with the ♲ symbol.

♲ **a-** not, without, less
♲ **ab-** from, away from, off
♲ **abs-** from, away from, off
♲ **ad-** increase, adherence, motion toward; very
♲ **-ad** toward, in the direction of; -ward
♲ **alge-** pain
♲ **cardi-** **1** heart; **2** esophageal opening of stomach
♲ **cardio-** **1** heart; **2** esophageal opening of stomach
♲ **cata-** down
♲ **cephal-** the head
♲ **cephaol-** the head
♲ **chem-** **1** chemistry, **2** drug
♲ **chemo-** **1** chemistry, **2** drug
♲ **cyst-** **1** bladder; **2** cyst; **3** cystic duct
♲ **cysti-** **1** bladder; **2** cyst; **3** cystic duct
♲ **cysto-** **1** bladder; **2** cyst; **3** cystic duct
♲ **cyt-** cell
♲ **-cyte** cell
♲ **cyto-** cell
♲ **dactyl-** finger, toe

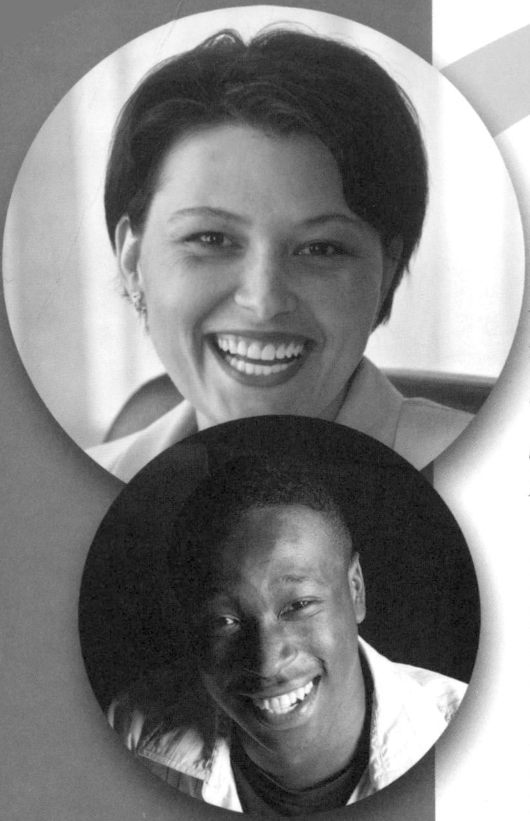

thePoint

Where Teaching, Learning, & Technology Click

Provides flexible learning solutions and resources for students and faculty using ***Stedman's Medical Dictionary for the Health Professions and Nursing, Illustrated, Sixth Edition***

Resources for instructors*:

- Image Bank
- LifeART™ Images
- Appendices

Resources for students:

- LifeART™ Images
- Appendices
- Macintosh compatible download of CD-content

**The faculty resources are restricted to adopters of the text. Adopters have to be approved before accessing the faculty resources.*

http://thepoint.lww.com/hpnd6e

Scratch Off Below

Stedman

Note: Book cannot be returned once panel is scratched off.

Log on today!

Visit **http://thepoint.lww.com/hpnd6e** to learn more about **thePoint™** and the resources available. Use the code on this page to access the student resources.

Wolters Kluwer Health | Lippincott Williams & Wilkins

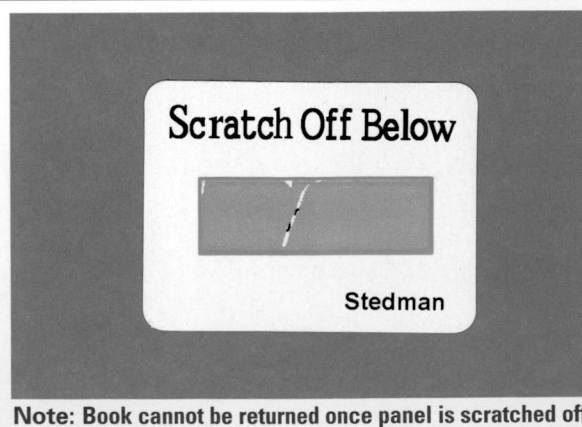

STEDMAN'S

Medical Dictionary for the Health Professions and Nursing

ILLUSTRATED

SIXTH EDITION

Wolters Kluwer | Lippincott Williams & Wilkins
Health
Philadelphia • Baltimore • New York • London
Buenos Aires • Hong Kong • Sydney • Tokyo

Publisher: Julie K. Stegman
Senior Product Manager: Eric Branger
Managing Editor: Tiffany Piper
Chief Copyeditor: Raymond Lukens
General Editor: John H. Dirckx, M.D.
On-Line Editor: Kathryn J. Cadle
Proofreaders: Raymond Lukens, Kristi Lukens
Graphic Artist: Susan Caldwell
Typographic Design: Parkton Art Studio, Inc.
Senior Software Development Manager: David Horne
Manufacturing Coordinator: Margie Orzech

DISCLAIMER
Care has been taken to confirm the accuracy of the information present and to describe generally accepted practices. However, the authors, editors, and publisher are not responsible for errors or omissions or for any consequences from application of the information in this book and make no warranty, expressed or implied, with respect to the currency, completeness, or accuracy of the contents of the publication. Application of this information in a particular situation remains the professional responsibility of the practitioner; the clinical treatments described and recommended may not be considered absolute and universal recommendations.

The authors, editors, and publishers have exerted every effort to ensure that drug selection and dosage set forth in this text are in accordance with current recommendations and practice at the time of publication. However, in view of ongoing research, changes in government regulations, and the constant flow of information relating to drug therapy and drug reactions, the reader is urged to check the package insert for each drug for any change in indications and dosage and for added warnings and precautions. This is particularly important when the recommended agent is a new or infrequently employed drug.

Some drugs and medical devices presented in this publication have Food and Drug Administration (FDA) clearance for limited use in restricted research settings. It is the responsibility of the health care provider to ascertain the FDA status of each drug or device planned for use in their clinical practice.

Database design by Lexi-Comp Inc. Hudson, OH
Printed in China

Library of Congress Cataloging-in-Publication Data

Stedman's medical dictionary for the health professions and nursing : illustrated.—6th ed.
p. ; cm.
Includes index.
ISBN 978-0-7817-7618-9—ISBN 978-0-7817-7616-5
1. Medicine—Dictionaries. I. Stedman, Thomas Lathrop, 1853-1938. II. Title: Medical dictionary for the health professions and nursing.
[DNLM: 1. Medicine—Dictionary—English. W 13 S814 2008]
R121.S8 2008
610.3—dc22

2007031761

RRS1010

Contents

A Message from the Publisher

Stedman's, first produced as Dunglison's *New Dictionary of Medical Science and Literature* in 1833, has a long standing tradition of excellence. With this new edition of *Stedman's Medical Dictionary for the Health Professions and Nursing, Illustrated*, we strove to continue this reputation of excellence, providing our readers with our most comprehensive dictionary to date, delivered in both the print and electronic mediums.

With our last edition of *Stedman's Medical Dictionary for the Health Professions and Nursing*, we removed the word "Concise" from our title. This was done in the hopes of dispelling the misconception that the dictionary was a smaller, scaled-down version of the larger *Stedman's Medical Dictionary*. While this dictionary is built upon the foundation terminology of the Stedman's Medical Dictionary Series as a whole, *Stedman's Medical Dictionary for the Health Professions and Nursing* has numerous terms, images, and appendices that are entirely unique to this edition.

Starting with the previous edition, readers may have also noticed that we added the word "Nursing" to the title. Whereas we have no intention of steering away from our readership of health professionals (of which we assuredly consider nursing a part), we believed that collaborating with and extending our consultant board to include a diverse group of nursing consultants would ensure that we provide even more well-rounded definitions for the core medical terminology encountered by all health professionals. Thus, "Nursing" was added to the title separately from "Health Professions" simply as a means of highlighting the fact that the core medical terminology was newly reviewed and enhanced by our expert team of nursing consultants.

This new edition features more than 4,000 new entries, 54,000 terms overall, and over 900 illustrations, all of which have been reviewed by consultants and revised as necessary. *Stedman's Medical Dictionary for the Health Professions and Nursing, Illustrated 6th Edition*, provides students, educators, and practitioners access to the core language of medicine, health professions, and nursing. With particular emphasis on and coverage of Athletic Training, Embryology, Exercise Science, Health Information Management, Massage Therapy, Medical Assisting, Medical Transcription, Occupational Therapy, Nursing, Pharmacy/Pharmacy Technology, and Weapons of Mass Destruction/Mass Casualty Weapons/Bioterrorism, this new edition meets the needs of our readers throughout the health professions and nursing.

Our revision process includes a significant collaboration with our readers. We have again increased our representation in the health professions and nursing fields, working with over 45 consultants to ensure that our content is of the utmost quality, currency, and accuracy. A full listing of our consultants can be found in our front matter material. Our consultants worked tirelessly to review and enhance our terminology, as well as our robust art program, including two full inserts and our substantial Appendices section. This section now features three new appendices: Commonly Used Herbs and Their Side Effects/or Drug Interactions; General Cancer Classification, Staging, and Grouping Systems; Pain Assessment Tools. We have also continued our efforts to recognize our readers in other parts of the world. As with the previous edition, the sixth edition includes consultants from outside the United States, international content in our appendices, and provides British spellings for appropriate terms.

Exciting Electronic Additions

In addition to the revision of our print version of *Stedman's Medical Dictionary for the Health Professions and Nursing, Illustrated, 6th Edition*, readers will also recognize the substantial revision of our Bonus CD-ROM. This CD-ROM features the entire content of the dictionary in an easy-to-use, searchable interface. To enhance this content, we have included all of the images that are in the print product with the ability to copy and paste the images to the reader's computer and to reuse them in presentations and documentation. We have increased our audio pronunciations to include over 48,000 terms, enabling readers to not only read the written pronunciation but hear how the term is pronounced. To further our goals of making the most comprehensive dictionary possible, we have also included videos for key terms to aid in comprehension. These videos come from *Acland's DVD Atlas of Human Anatomy*, and we are proud to have them as a featured component of our electronic dictionary.

Brand new to the Bonus CD-ROM of this new edition is the addition of our *Stedman's Plus Medical/Pharmaceutical Spellchecker*. *Stedman's Plus Spellchecker* has been providing medical, pharmaceutical, and bioscience terms to medical language specialists for nearly 15 years. Since *Stedman's Plus Spellchecker* provides authoritative content and up-to-date medical **AND** pharmaceutical terminology, it's no wonder healthcare professionals rely on *Stedman's Plus Spellchecker* for the most comprehensive and cutting-edge medical spellchecking available. *Stedman's Plus Spellchecker* will seamlessly load into your word processor of choice and you'll have the confidence of knowing that nearly half a million Stedman's terms are working behind the scenes to spellcheck all of your documentation. Sold traditionally for $99.95, it is included **FREE** on our Bonus CD-ROM—a real value to our readers.

Finally, we have also several resources for our readers on our thePoint site, thePoint.lww.com/hpnd6e. Instructors will find a comprehensive image bank, appendices available as PDFs, an additional 300 LifeART™ images, and How to Use the Dictionary demos (for both the print dictionary and the electronic version on the Bonus CD-ROM) to ensure students are getting the full benefit of the features of our product. Students and other readers will also be able to access the appendices and How to Use the Dictionary demos.

Acknowledgments

As always, we at Lippincott Williams & Wilkins are grateful to all of our consultants from the medical, nursing, and health professions disciplines for their help in reviewing, writing, and revising the thousands of entries in this dictionary. Without them, none of the terminology presented here would be relevant or useful. We are also indebted to the many reviewers who assisted us in making critical decisions about the presentation of the dictionary, the actual dictionary entries themselves, and the content presented in this new edition. Finally, we continue to be thankful to have Dr. John H. Dirckx as a long-standing member of our dictionary team. His expertise, love of language, and consistent availability to consult with us cannot be replaced.

The development of this new edition, *Stedman's Medical Dictionary for the Health Professions and Nursing, Illustrated, 6th Edition*, has greatly benefited from the experience and expertise of Raymond Lukens, Chief Copyeditor, whose patience, dedication, and hard work have given this edition an unparallel level of quality. Our thanks must also go out to Kathryn Cadle, who worked countless hours to ensure that all of the content corrections made by our consultants, copyeditors, and in-house editorial team were made accurately and in a timely fashion. We would also like to thank Susan Caldwell for her assistance and quality work in helping us prepare the art program for this edition. A key ingredient to making sure we are successful is making sure we listen to our customers. Representing our customers are the Publishing Representatives who worked with us to ensure we were meeting our customers' needs in all aspects of development. We are indebted to our colleagues at Lippincott Williams & Wilkins, including Tiffany Piper, Managing Editor; Margie Orzech, Manufacturing Coordinator; Jennifer Clements, Art Program Consultant; Zhan Caplan, Senior Marketing Manager; and David Horne, Senior Software Development Manager. Without the Lippincott Williams & Wilkins team's commitment to our readers and to the quality expected of Stedman's publications, this new edition would not have been possible. Finally, we must thank you, the reader. We have appreciated all of the input we have received from previous editions and thank you for your continued support of our dictionary.

Your Medical Word Resource Publisher

We strive to provide our readers of students, educators, and practitioners with the most up-to-date and accurate medical language references. We, as always, welcome any suggestions you may have for improvements, changes, corrections, and additions—whatever makes it possible for this Stedman's product to serve you better.

Julie K. Stegman
Senior Publisher

Eric Branger
Senior Product Manager

Stedman's Medical Dictionary for the Health Professions and Nursing, Illustrated, 6th Edition
Lippincott Williams & Wilkins
Baltimore, Maryland

Consultants in the Health Professions and Nursing

Naomi Adams, RN, BN, CLNC — ESL
CEO, Adams Medical-Legal Consulting, Woodbridge, VA USA;
Instructor, Practical Nursing Program MCI@ECPI College of Technology,
Manassas, VA, USA

Amy S. Alfriend, RN, MPH, COHN-S/CM — Nursing
Assistant Director, Division of Occupational and Environmental Medicine,
Johns Hopkins University, School of Medicine, Baltimore, MD, USA

Debra Kay Arver, RDH, BSDH, Masters Candidate — Dental Hygiene
Dental Hygiene Instructor, Argosy University Health Sciences,
Department of Dental Hygiene, Eagan, MN, USA

Tricia Berry, OTR/L, MATL — Medical Assisting
Director of Clinical Placement, Kaplan University, Johnston, IA, USA

Dolores Bertoti, MS, PT — Physical Therapy
Associate Professor and Department Chair, Alvernia College,
Reading, PA, USA

Mary Ellen Camire, PhD — Nutrition
Professor, Department of Food Science and Human Nutrition,
University of Maine, Orono, ME, USA

Philip Docking, EdD, MSc, Cert Ed, RN MFPHC — Nursing
Associate Director, Education and Development, HMI Institute
of Health Sciences, Singapore

Mark Drnach, PT, DPT, MBA, PCS — Physical Therapy
Clinical Associate Professor, Department of Physical Therapy,
Wheeling Jesuit University, Wheeling, WV, USA

Michelle R. Easton, PharmD — Pharmacy
Assistant Dean, Professional and Student Affairs and Associate Professor,
School of Pharmacy, University of Charleston, Charleston, WV, USA

Nancy L. Evans, RN, MS — Nursing
Professor of Nursing, Bristol Community College, Fall River, MA, USA

Mary Kaye Griffin, BSH RT(R)(M) Radiology Program Director, Spencerian College, Louisville, KY, USA	**Radiology Technology**
Joyce P. Griffin-Sobel, PhD, RN, AOCN, APRN.BC, CNE Director, Undergraduate Programs, Bellevue School of Nursing, Hunter College, New York, NY, USA	**Nursing Oncology**
Kerri Hines, RN, BSN San Jacinto College, Houston, TX, USA	**Nursing**
Nicholas M. Hipskind, PhD, CCC-A Professor Emeritus, Department of Speech and Hearing Sciences, Indiana University, Bloomington, IN, USA	**Audiology**
Nancy Hislop, RN, BSN Online Instructor, Globe University/Minnesota School of Business, Richfield, MN, USA	**Medical Terminology**
Marian Kovatchitch, MS, RN Dean of Academic Affairs, St. Elizabeth College of Nursing, Utica, NY, USA	**Nursing**
Kathy A. Locke, BA, CMA, RMA Program Coordinator, School of Health Science, Northwestern Business College, Bridgeview, IL, USA	**Medical Assisting**
James M. Madsen, MD, MPH, FCAP, FACOEM COL, MC-FS, USA Scientific Advisor, Chemical Casualty Care Division, U.S. Army Medical Research Institute of Chemical Defense (USAMRICD), APG-EA, MD; Associate Professor of Preventive Medicine and Biometrics; Assistant Professor of Pathology; Assistant Professor of Military and Emergency Medicine; Assistant Professor of Emerging Infectious Diseases, Uniformed Services University of the Health Sciences, Bethesda, MD, USA	**Weapons of Mass Destruction/ Bioterrorism**
Connie R. Mahon, MS, CLS Microbiologist, Center for Drug Evaluation and Research, U.S. Food and Drug Administration, Rockville, MD, USA	**Clinical Lab Sciences, Bacteriology and Mycology**
Gail Metzger, MS, OTR/L Assistant Professor, Department of Occupational Therapy, Alvernia College, Reading, PA, USA	**Occupational Therapy**

Laurie Milliken, PhD — **Exercise Science**
Associate Professor, Department of Exercise and Health Sciences,
University of Massachusetts, Boston, MA, USA

Keith L. Moore, MSc, PhD, FIAC, FRSM — **Embryology and British Medical Terminology**
Professor Emeritus, Division of Anatomy, Department of Surgery,
Faculty of Medicine, University of Toronto, Toronto, Ontario, Canada;
Recipient of the 2007 Henry Gray/Elsevier Distinguished Educator Award,
awarded by the American Association of Anatomists

Marilyn H. Oermann, PhD, RN, FAAN — **Nursing**
Professor and Division Chair, School of Nursing; Editor, Journal of
Nursing Care Quality; The University of North Carolina at Chapel Hill,
Chapel Hill, NC, USA

Kathleen M. O'Malley, CPhT — **Pharm Tech**
American Medical Careers, Flint, MI, USA

Wanda Pierson, RN, MSN, PhD — **Nursing**
Chair, Nursing Department, Langara College, Vancouver, BC, Canada

Susan Polasek, MA, RD, LD — **Nutrition**
Austin, TX, USA

Lisa Radak, RT(R)(T)(CT) — **Radiation Therapy**
Academic Clinical Coordinator, Radiation Therapy Program,
Baker College of Jackson, Jackson, MI, USA

Deneen Raysor, BS, CPT — **Physiology**
Exercise Physiologist, Aquatic and Fitness Center, Philadelphia, PA, USA

Jo Ann Runewicz, RN.C, MSN, EdD — **Nursing**
Drexel University, Philadelphia, PA, USA

Georgina Sampson, RHIA — **Health Information Technology**
Professor, Rasmussen College, Brooklyn Park, MN, USA

Susan Slajus, MBA, RHIA — **Health Information Technology**
Davenport University, Grand Rapids, MI, USA

Carlotta South, AAS, ADN, RN — Nursing
San Jacinto College North, Houston, TX, USA

Linda Spang, EMT-P, RMA, JD — Emergency Medical Services
Department Coordinator Allied Health, MA Program Director,
Davenport University, Lansing, MI, USA

Margaret M. Spieth, MAEd, CMT — Medical Transcription
Faculty, Medical Transcription Program, Moraine Park Technical College,
West Bend, WI, USA

Scott Stanley, EdD, RRT, FAARC — Respiration Therapy
Assistant Dean for Undergraduate Affairs, Health and Liberal Arts
Director of the Respiratory Care Programs School of Professional and
Continuing Studies Northeastern University Boston, MA, USA

Erin K. Stauder, MS, CCC/SLP — Speech-Language Pathology
Speech-Language Pathologist, Loyola College in Maryland,
Baltimore, MD, USA

Nona K. Stinemetz, LPN — Medical Terminology
Vatterott College, Des Moines, IA, USA

Robin Sylvis, RDH, MS — Dental Hygiene
Director, International Business Development,
The CoreMedical Group, Salem, NH, USA

Geoffrey Tabin, MD — Ophthalmology and Optometry
Professor of Ophthalmology and Visual Sciences, Moran Eye Center,
University of Utah, Salt Lake City, UT, USA

Nina Thierer, CMA, BS, CPC, CCAT — Medical Assisting
Ivy Tech Community College Northeast, Fort Wayne, IN, USA

Walter R. Thompson, PhD, FACSM, FAACVPR — Exercise Science
Professor, Department of Kinesiology and Health,
College of Education; Professor, Division of Nutrition,
School of Health Professions, College of Health and Human Sciences,
Georgia State University, Atlanta, GA, USA

Kelly S. Ullmer, ND, LDHS, OTR
Sheboygan, WI, USA
Alternative/Holistic Medicine

Amy Carson VonKadich, MEd, RTT
Radiation Therapy Program Director, New Hampshire Technical Institute, Concord, NH, USA
Radiology Technology

Bruce J. Walz, PhD
Professor and Chair, Department of Emergency Health Services, University of Maryland, Baltimore County, Baltimore, MD, USA
Emergency Medical Services

Marsha Wamsley, RN, MS
Associate Professor of Nursing, Sinclair Community College, Dayton, OH, USA
Nursing

Ruth Werner, LMP, NCTMB
Faculty, Myotherapy College of Utah, Layton, UT, USA
Massage Therapy

Barry M. Westling, MS, RRT-NPS, RPFT
Administrative Director, Respiratory Care Education, San Joaquin Valley College, Visalia, CA, USA
Respiratory Therapy

Reviewers

Kellie Bassell, MSN, RN
Associate Professor, Nursing, Palm Beach Community College, Lake Worth, FL, USA

Brian Baumgardner
Johnson County Community College, Overland Park, KS, USA

Barbara J. Blake, RN, PhD, ACRN
Kennesaw State University, Kennesaw, GA, USA

Julie E. Boles, MS, RHIA
Assistant Professor, Ithaca College, Ithaca, NY, USA

Brenda Boyer, RN, BSN
Ivy Tech Community College, Terre Haute, IN, USA

Barbara A. Broome, PhD, RN
Associate Dean and Chair, College of Nursing, Community/Mental Health University of South Alabama, Mobile, AL, USA

Susan Buchholz, RN, MSN
Associate Professor of Nursing, Georgia Perimeter College, Lawrenceville, GA, USA

Monica Cauley, RN, MSN, GCNP/GCNS
Chair Health Science, Lurleen B. Wallace Community College, Opp, AL, USA

Alexander M. Clark
Associate Professor, University of Alberta, Edmonton, Alberta, Canada

Bobby M. Collins, DDS, MS
Associate Professor, Department of Diagnostic Sciences, University of Pittsburgh School of Dental Medicine, Pittsburgh, PA, USA

Kozy Corsaut, MT(ASCP), CLS(NCA)
Associate Professor, Stark State College, North Canton, OH, USA

Wanda C. Dubuisson, RN, PhD (c)
Associate Professor and Director MSN Program, Joseph and Nancy Fail School of Nursing, William Carey University, Hattiesburg, MS, USA

Marianne Durling
Medical Coding Instructor, Vance-Granville Community College, Henderson, NC, USA

Susan S. Erue, RN, BSN, MS, PhD
Professor and Chair of the Division of Nursing, Iowa Wesleyan College, Mount Pleasant, IA, USA

Mary Fabick, MSN, MEd, RN, CEN
Associate Professor of Nursing, Milligan College, Milligan College, TN, USA

Tammy T. Gant, RHIT, CMA, CPC, CAHI
Surry Community College, Dobson, NC, USA

Robin Gardenhire, MS, ATC, CSCS
Faculty, Georgia State University, Atlanta, GA, USA

Barbara E. Geary, MA
Adjunct Faculty, North Seattle Community College, Seattle, WA, USA

Diana Girdley, RN, MS
Clinical Associate Professor, School of Nursing, University of Wisconsin-Madison, Madison, WI, USA

Tamra Greco, BS
Health Professions Writing and Editing Consultant, Las Cruces, NM, USA

Kay A. Hanna, BS, MT(ASCP)
Clinical Coordinator, MLT Program, Stark State College of Technology, North Canton, OH, USA

William J. Horton
Part-Time Faculty, Health Information Technology, Hutchinson Community College, Hutchinson, KS, USA

Darcy Johnson
San Diego, CA, USA

Carrie M. Keller, CMA
EHOVE Ghrist Adult Career Center; Milan, OH, USA

Jacki King, CMT, CCA
Instructor, Mid-State Technical College, Marshfield, WI, USA

Lori J. Knight, CHIM
Health Information Management Program, SIAST Wascana Campus, Regina, SK, Canada

Rhonda Lansdell, PhD, RN
Northeast Mississippi Community College, Booneville, MS, USA

W. Greg Leader, PharmD
Associate Dean, Academic Affairs; Professor, Clinical Pharmacy Practice, College of Pharmacy, University of Louisiana Monroe, Monroe, LA, USA

Judith Lichtenberger, CMT, FAAMT, RHIT
Adjunct Professor, Northampton Community College, Bethlehem, PA, USA

Dimitra Loukissa, PhD, RN
College of Nursing, Rush University, Chicago, IL USA

Ngina Lynch, CPC
Computer Career Institute, Johns Hopkins University, Columbia, MD, USA

Claire E. Maday-Travis, MA MBA CPHQ
Program Director, Allied Health, The Salter School, West Boylston, MA, USA

B. Gail Marshall, RN, MSN, MEd
Associate Professor, Luzerne County Community College, Nanticoke, PA, USA

Randy Meador, MS, ATC
Athletic Trainer, West Virginia University, Morgantown, WV, USA

Patricia Neafsey
Professor, School of Nursing, University of Connecticut, Storrs, CT, USA

Nichole Oocumma, RDH, BS, MA, CHES
Department Chair, Dental Programs, Stark State College of Technology, North Canton, OH, USA

Brian K. Paulson, PhD
California University of Pennsylvania, California, PA, USA

Donna Pyne
Nurse Educator, Centre for Nursing Studies, St. John's, Newfoundland & Labrador, Canada

Kaye Roberson, BA, CMA
Program Director/Instructor, Medical Assisting Technology, Northeast Mississippi Community College, Booneville, MS, USA

Heather R. Roberts, PhD
Professor of Human Anatomy, Sierra College,
Rocklin, CA, USA

Linda Servidio, MSN, APRN, BC, CNE
Professor, Nursing, Brookdale Community
College, Lincroft, NJ, USA

Gloria Jean Shover, RN, BSN, AHI
Practical Nurse Program Administrator,
Erie Business Center, Erie, PA, USA

Rose M. Skaife, MEd
Instructor, Health Sciences, National Park
Community College, Hot Springs, AR, USA

Nora F. Steele, DNS, RN.C, PNP
Professor, Charity/Delgado School of Nursing,
New Orleans, LA, USA

Marilyn Smith-Stoner, RN, PhD, CHPN
Associate Professor of Nursing, California
State University San Bernardino,
San Bernardino, CA, USA

Brenda J. Stutsky, RN, BN, MScN
Director, Nursing Education, Health Sciences
Centre Winnipeg, Winnipeg, Manitoba,
Canada

Reynell Y. Turner, MBA, CHI, CMAA
Senior Medical Administrative Instructor,
Computer Career Institute, Johns Hopkins
University, Baltimore, MD, USA

Denise H. Woodson, MA, MT(ASCP)SC
Academic Coordinator of Health Professions
and Nursing, Smarthinking, Inc., Washington,
DC, USA

Mary Young
Training Coordinator, TransHealth Medical
Transcription Services, Brentwood, TN, USA

Stedman's Publishing Representatives

Heidi Alexander

Director of Corporate & Government Sales

John Antosz

Senior Sales Representative: MA, NY, CT, RI

Matthew Bruns

Publisher's Representative: Eastern MO, Southern IL

Melanie Harrison

Midwest Instructional Services Consultant: OH, MI, KY, IN, IL, MO, NE, KS

Garry Huff

Senior Publisher's Representative: Upstate NY, Erie, PA

Shirley Jones

Publisher's Representative: TX, WI, KS, VA, SC, ME

Gregory Kinsky

Senior Educational Sales Representative: MA, NH, ME

Keith Pyle

Educational Sales Representative: Central and North FL

Kristin Slavin

Executive Director of Educational Sales

Malcolm Ward

Senior Publisher's Representative: AZ, NM, El Paso, TX

Steve White

Senior Educational Sales Representative: TN, AR

Consultants to the Stedman's Dictionaries

Steven Ades, MD, FRCPC — **Oncology**

Associate Professor of Medicine and Oncology,
McGill University Health Center, Montreal, Quebec, Canada

R. Donald Allison, PhD — **Biochemistry**

Associate Scientist, Department of Biochemistry and Molecular Biology,
University of Florida College of Medicine, Gainesville, FL, USA

David A. Bloom, MD — **Genitourinary Surgery**

The Jack Lapides Professor of Urology,
University of Michigan, Ann Arbor, MI, USA

Jane Bruner, PhD — **Bacteriology**

Chair, Department of Biological Sciences,
California State University, Stanislaus, Turlock, CA, USA

Kathleen E. Cavanagh, BSC, DVM — **Veterinary Medicine**

Fonthill, ON, Canada

Mitchell Charap, MD, FACP — **Internal Medicine**

The Abraham Sunshine Associate Professor of Clinical Medicine,
Associate Chair for Postgraduate Programs, Program Director,
Department of Medicine, NYU School of Medicine, New York, NY, USA

George P. Chrousos, MD, FAAP, MACP, MACE — **Endocrinology**

Professor and Chairman, First Department of Pediatrics, Athens University
Medical School, Aghia Sophia Children's Hospital, Athens, Greece

Mark B. Constantian, MD — **Plastic/Reconstructive Surgery**

St. Joseph Hospital, Southern New Hampshire Medical Center,
Nashua, NH, USA

Arthur F. Dalley, II, PhD — **Gross Anatomy**

Professor of Cell and Developmental Biology and Director,
Gross Anatomy Program, Department of Cell and Developmental
Biology, Vanderbilt University School of Medicine, Nashville, TN, USA;
Adjunct Professor for Anatomy, Belmont University School of Physical Therapy,
Nashville, TN, USA

Ivan Damjanov, MD, PhD — **Pathology/Anatomy**
Professor of Pathology, University of Kansas School of Medicine,
Kansas City, KS, USA

John A. Day, Jr., MD, FCCP — **Pulmonary Diseases**
Assistant Professor of Medicine, University of Massachusetts
Medical School, Worcester, MA, USA

John H. Dirckx, MD — **Etymologies and High Profile Terms**
Dayton, Ohio, USA

Thomas W. Filardo, MD — **Chief Lexicographer and New Terms Editor**
Physician-Consultant, Evendale, OH, USA

Benjamin K. Fisher, MD, FRCP(C) — **Dermatology**
Professor Emeritus, University of Toronto Medical School,
Toronto, Ontario, Canada

Lee A. Fleisher, MD — **Anesthesiology**
Robert D. Dripps Professor and Chair of Anesthesiology and Critical Care,
Professor of Medicine, University of Pennsylvania School of Medicine,
Philadelphia, PA, USA

Robert J. Fontana, MD — **Gastroenterology**
Associate Professor of Medicine, University of Michigan,
Ann Arbor, MI, USA

Paul J. Friedman, MD — **Radiology**
Professor Emeritus, Department of Radiology, University of California,
San Diego, CA, USA

Leslie P. Gartner, PhD — **Histology**
Professor of Anatomy, Department of Biomedical Sciences,
Dental School, University of Maryland at Baltimore, Baltimore, MD, USA

Douglas J. Gould, PhD — **Gross Anatomy**
Associate Professor, University of Kentucky College of Medicine,
Lexington, KY, USA

Steven Gutman, MD, MBA — **Stains/Procedures**
Director, Office of In Vitro Diagnostics, Center for Devices and
Radiological Health, Food and Drug Administration, Rockville, MD, USA

Duane E. Haines, PhD — **Neuroanatomy**

Professor and Chairman of Anatomy, Professor of Neurosurgery and of Neurology, University of Mississippi Medical Center, Jackson, MS, USA

Nicola C. Y. Ho, MD — **Genetics**

Assistant Professor of Pediatrics and Active Staff of Johns Hopkins Medical Institutions, Baltimore, MD, USA

Iain H. Kalfas MD, FACS — **Neurosurgery**

Chairman, Department of Neurosurgery, Cleveland Clinic Foundation, Cleveland, OH, USA

John B. Kerrison, MD — **Ophthalmology**

Assistant Professor of Ophthalmology, Neurology, and Neurosurgery, Wilmer Eye Institute, Johns Hopkins Hospital, Baltimore, MD, USA

Jeffrey L. Kishiyama — **Immunology**

Associate Clinical Professor of Medicine, University of California, San Francisco, CA, USA

John M. Last, MD, FRACP, FRCPC, FFPH(UK) — **Medical Statistics/Epidemiology**

Professor Emeritus, Department of Epidemiology and Community Medicine, University of Ottawa, Ottawa, Ontario, Canada

James L. Lear, MD — **Nuclear Medicine**

Founder, Scientific Imaging, Inc., Larkspur, CO, USA; Professor and Director, Division of Nuclear Medicine, University of Colorado Health Sciences Center, Denver, CO, USA

Joseph LoCicero, III, MD — **Thoracic Surgery**

Professor and Chair, Department of Surgery, University of South Alabama, Mobile, AL, USA

Lisa Marcucci, MD — **Biography/Eponyms**

Fellow, Division of Critical Care, Department of Surgery, Johns Hopkins University, Baltimore, MD, USA

Keith L. Moore, PhD, FIAC, FRSM — **Embryology**

Professor Emeritus in Division of Anatomy, Department of Surgery, Faculty of Medicine, University of Toronto, Toronto, Ontario, Canada; Member of Federative International Committee on Anatomical Terminology of the International Federation of Associations of Anatomists

Marianna M. Newkirk, MSc, PhD Rheumatology
Associated Professor of Medicine, Physiology, Microbiology and Immunology, McGill University, Montreal, Quebec, Canada

J. Patrick O'Leary, MD General Surgery
Associate Dean for Clinical Affairs, The Isidore Cohn, Jr. Professor and Chairman of Surgery, LSU Health Sciences Center, New Orleans, LA, USA

Stephen J. Peroutka, MD, PhD Biotechnology
Consultant, Hillsborough, CA, USA

Sharon T. Phelan, MD, FACOG Obstetrics/Gynecology
Professor, Department of Obstetrics and Gynecology, University of New Mexico, Albuquerque, NM, USA

Richard A. Prayson, MD Neuropathology
Section Head of Neuropathology, Department of Anatomic Pathology, Cleveland Clinic Foundation, Cleveland, OH, USA

William Reichel, MD Geriatrics
Affiliated Scholar, Center for Clinical Bioethics, Georgetown University, School of Medicine, Washington, DC, USA

George S. Schuster, DDS, MS, PhD Dentistry
Ione and Arthur Merritt Professor, Chair, Department of Oral Biology and Maxillofacial Pathology, Medical College of Georgia, School of Dentistry, Augusta, GA, USA

Linda N. Sevier, MD Pediatrics
Pediatric Faculty, The Children's Hospital at Sinai, Baltimore, MD, USA

James B. Snow, Jr., MD, FACS Otorhinolaryngology
Former Director, National Institute on Deafness and Other Communication Disorders, National Institutes of Health, Bethesda, MD, USA; Professor Emeritus of Otorhinolaryngology, University of Pennsylvania, Philadelphia, PA, USA

Roger M. Stone, MD, MS, FAAEM, FACEP Emergency Medicine
Clinical Assistant Professor, Emergency Medicine Residency, University of Maryland School of Medicine, Baltimore, MD, USA; EMS Medical Director, Montgomery and Caroline Counties, MD, USA

Janet L. Stringer, MD, PhD — **Pharmacology/Toxicology**
Associate Professor of Pharmacology and Neuroscience,
Baylor College of Medicine, Houston, TX, USA

Deanna A. Sutton, PhD, MT, SM(ASCP), RM, SM(NRM) — **Medical Mycology**
Assistant Professor, Department of Pathology, Administrative Director,
Fungus Testing Laboratory, University of Texas Health Science Center at
San Antonio, San Antonio, TX, USA

Alexandra Valsamakis, MD, PhD — **Virology**
Assistant Professor of Pathology, Johns Hopkins School of Medicine,
Baltimore, MD, USA

Galen S. Wagner, MD — **Cardiology**
Duke University Medical Center, Durham, NC, USA

Dr. Brian J. Ward — **Parasitology/Tropical Medicine**
Chief, McGill University Division of Infectious Diseases,
Departments of Medicine & Microbiology, McGill University,
Montreal, Quebec, Canada

Asa J. Wilbourn, MD — **Neurology**
Director, EMG Laboratory, Cleveland Clinic; Clinical Professor
of Neurology, Case University School of Medicine, Cleveland, OH, USA

Helaine R. Wolpert, MD — **Clinical Pathology/Hematology/Laboratory Medicine**
Anatomic and Clinical Pathologist, Newton, MA, USA

Douglas B. Woodruff, MD — **Psychiatry/Psychology**
Private Practice, Baltimore, MD, USA

David B. Young, PhD — **Physiology**
Professor, Physiology and Biophysics, University of Mississippi
Medical Center, Jackson, MS, USA

Joseph D. Zuckerman, MD — **Orthopaedics**
Professor & Chairman, Department of Orthopaedic Surgery,
NYU – Hospital for Joint Diseases, New York, NY, USA

Illustrations Index

The Illustrations Index provides a quick way to find any image in *Stedman's Health Professions & Nursing Dictionary*. The page number accompanying each term listed below tells you where an illustration related to that term is found. A page number preceded by the letter *A* indicates that the image can be found in the first color insert, the 40-page anatomic atlas. A page number preceded by the letter *B* indicates that the image can be found in the second color insert, a 32-page section dedicated to diagnostic medicine, imaging techniques, and condition images. When you look up a word in the A to Z section, you can tell it is illustrated—either at the word itself or in the inserts or appendices—if it is accompanied by this symbol: i.

Illustration Sources

Courtesy of Acuson Corporation, Mountain View, CA (Doppler ultrasonography).

Jennifer Anderson @ USDA-NRCS PLANTS Database (poison ivy).

From Anderson SC, Poulson K. *Anderson's Atlas of Hematology*. Baltimore, MD: Lippincott Williams & Wilkins; 2003 (bacteria: spirochetes; keratocyte; beta-thalassemia major; chronic lymphocytic leukemia; Heinz bodies; Hodgkin disease; lymphocyte; microcytosis; non-Hodgkin lymphoma).

Courtesy of Benjamin Barankin, MD, Edmonton, Alberta, Canada (elephantiasis; nodulocystic acne of the back; acrodermatitis; actinic granuloma; hypertropic actinic keratoses; amyloidosis; atopic dermatitis; Becker nevus; bullous pemphigoid; calcinosis; cellulitis surrounding ulcer; chemotherapy; cherry angiomas; cold urticaria; congenital nevus; contact dermatitis; cutis rhomboidalis nuchae; dermatitis; pigmented dermatofibroma; dermatomyositis on the knee; discoid lupus erythematosus; dry gangrene; dystrophia unguium; epidermolysis bullosa; erysipelas; erythema caloricum; erythema nodosum; erythroderma; erythromelalgia; ganglion; gouty tophus; graft-versus-host disease; granuloma; herpes zoster; herpetic whitlow; hyperpigmentation; hyperplasia; hypopigmentation; ichthyosis vulgaris; keratosis follicularis; Langerhans cell histiocytosis; lichen planus; livedo reticularis; Marfan syndrome; Mycobacterium marinum infection; mycosis fungoides; necrosis; nevus; nummular eczema; chronic paronychia; pemphigus vulgaris; pilomatrixoma; plantar warts; pneumonia; pseudopelade; psoriasis; psoriatic arthritis; pyoderma gangrenosum; aphthous ulcer; scabies; seborrheic dermatitis; seborrheic keratoses; secondary syphilis; skin tag; squamous cell carcinoma; stasis dermatitis; thromboangiitis obliterans; tinea; verruca; vitiligo; xanthogranuloma; xerosis; herpes simplex infection; rheumatoid nodules: elbow; impetigo: forearms, hands; subcutaneous hematoma; arachnid bite; birthmark: strawberry hemangioma; cheilitis; comedones; contact dermatitis; cradle cap; cutaneous lymphoma; Darier disease: nails; geographic tongue; metastatic lymphoma; molluscum contagiosum; onycholysis: nails; onychomycosis: nails; psoriasis; rheumatoid arthritis; scleroderma; seborrheic dermatitis; seborrheic keratosis; shingles; trichotillomania: hair).

From Barker LR, Burton JR, Zieve PD. *Principles of Ambulatory Medicine.* 4th ed. Baltimore, MD: Williams & Wilkins; 1995 (gout).

Courtesy of Baschat A, MD, Center for Advanced Fetal Care, University of Maryland School of Medicine, Baltimore, MD (Doppler flow sonogram).

From Bear MF, Connors BW, and Parasido, MA. *Neuroscience: Exploring the Brain.* 2nd ed. Baltimore, PA: Lippincott Williams & Wilkins; 2001 (alarm reaction; mitochondrion & cellular respiration).

From Bear MF, Connors BW, Paradiso MA. *Neuroscience: Exploring the Brain.* 3rd ed. Baltimore, MD: Lippincott Williams & Wilkins; 2006 (placement of eeg electrodes; Brodmann areas).

From Beckmann CRB, Ling FW, Laube DW, Smith RP, Barzansky BM, Herbert WN. *Obstetrics and Gynecology.* 4th ed. Baltimore, MD: Lippincott Williams & Wilkins; 2002 (multifocal duct carcinoma; scirrhous carcinoma).

Courtesy of Bennett J, PhD, National Institutes of Health, Bethesda, MD (brain MRI).

From Berg D, Worzala K. *Atlas of Adult Physical Diagnosis.* Philadelphia, PA: Lippincott Williams & Wilkins; 2005 (wheal; tongue; nodular malignant melanoma).

From Bickley LS, Szilagyi P. *Bates' Guide to Physical Examination and History Taking.* 8th ed. Philadelphia: Lippincott Williams & Wilkins; 2003 (sounds in recording blood pressure; carotid pulse; milestones in normal child development; ecchymosis; macules; pustules; vesicles).

From Blackbourne LH. *Advanced Surgical Recall.* 2nd ed. Baltimore, MD: Lippincott Williams & Wilkins; 2004 (jack-knife prone position; kidney position).

From Brant WE, Helms CA. *Fundamentals of Diagnostic Radiology.* 2nd ed. Baltimore: Lippincott Williams & Wilkins; 1998 (upper gastrointestinal series; breast cancer; mammography; normal breast).

From Brant WE, Helmes CA. *Fundamentals of Diagnostic Radiology.* 3rd ed. Philadelphia, PA: Lippincott Williams & Wilkins; 2007 (bladder stones, fused PET-CT image of physiologic colon activity; rheumatoid arthritis: shoulder).

From Bucholz RW, Heckman JD. *Rockwood & Green's Fractures in Adults.* 5th ed. Philadelphia, PA: Lippincott Williams & Wilkins; 2001 (dislocations; Klippel-Feil deformity; avulsion fracture, compression fracture, fatigue fracture, hangman's fracture, MR angiography, spiral fracture).

Courtesy of Center for Disease Control and Prevention, Atlanta, GA (bacteria: bacilli; chickenpox; measles; mumps; rubella).

From Chung EK. Visual Diagnosis in Pediatrics. Philadelphia, PA: Lippincott Williams & Wilkins; 2006 (mastioditis).

From Clay JH, Pounds DM. *Basic Clinical Massage Therapy: Integrating Anatomy and Treatment.* Baltimore: Lippincott Williams & Wilkins; 2003 (achilles tendon; adductor hallucis muscle; adductor magnus muscle; ankle joint; anterior border of the tibia; arm; atlas; axial skeleton; brachial plexus; calcaneus; carpal bones; cervical vertebrae; crura of the diaphragm; deltoid muscle; diaphragm; elbow joint; erector spinae muscles; extensor digitorum brevis muscle; extensor digitorum longus muscle; extensor digitorum muscle, extensor retinaculum; external oblique muscle; facial bones; plantar fascia; femur; flexor digiti minimi brevis muscle of hand; flexor digitorum brevis muscle; flexor digitorum profundus muscle; flexor digitorum superficialis muscle; forearm; glenohumeral joint; gluteus maximus muscle; gluteus medius muscle; hamstring; humerus; hypothenar eminence; iliac crest; iliotibial tract; ilium; infraspinatus muscle; inguinal ligament; inguinal region; internal oblique muscle; latissimus dorsi muscle; lumbrical muscles of hand; maxilla; median nerve; metacarpophalangeal joint; multifidus muscles; muscles of the head; nasal cavity; obturator externus muscle; obturator internus muscle; occipital bone; orbicularis oris muscle; palmar interosseous muscle; pectoral region; pelvic diaphragm; pelvic girdle; platysma muscle; popliteal fossa; popliteus muscle; pronator quadratus muscle; pubic bone; quadratus lumborum muscle; quadratus plantae muscle; quadriceps; rectus abdominis muscle; rib (II-XI); rotatores muscles; sacral foramen; sacrum; scapula; sciatic nerve; serratus anterior muscle; shoulder girdle; shoulder joint; soft palate; soleus muscle; splenius capitis muscle; subscapularis muscle; supinator muscle; temporalis muscle; thoracic cage; thoracolumbar fascia; thyroid; tibialis anterior muscle; transversus abdominis muscle; trapezius muscle; triceps brachii muscle; vastus lateralis muscle; vertebral column; zygomaticus major muscle).

From Cohen BJ. *Medical Terminology.* 4th ed. Philadelphia: Lippincott Williams & Wilkins; 2003 (osteoarthritis; volvulus of the sigmoid colon; greenstick fracture; percutaneous endoscopic gastrostomy tube).

From Cohen BJ, Wood DL. *Memmler's The Human Body in Health and Disease.* 9th ed. Philadelphia: Lippincott Williams & Wilkins; 2000 (erythrocyte).

From Cormack DH. *Essential Histology.* Philadelphia: Lippincott–Raven; 1997 (microtubule).

From Crapo JD, Glassroth J, Karlinsky JB, King TE Jr. *Baum's Textbook of Pulmonary Diseases.* 7th ed. Philadelphia: Lippincott Williams & Wilkins; 2004 (arteriography: arteriovenous fistula; rheumatoid nodules: lower lung zones; ankylosing spondylitis; *Aspergillus fumigatus* infection; bony blastomycosis; lung collapse; thoracoscopes).

From Daffner RH. *Clinical Radiology: The Essentials.* 2nd ed. Baltimore: Williams & Wilkins; 1998 (rheumatoid arthritis; spondylosis; multiple sclerosis; radiography).

From Dart RC. *Medical Toxicology.* 3rd ed. Philadelphia, PA: Lippincott Williams & Wilkins; 2004 (right index bleb: snakebite).

Courtesy of Day JA, MD, University of Massachusetts Medical School, Worcester, MA (adult respiratory distress syndrome; interstitial lung disease).

From Dean D, Herbener TE. *Cross-Sectional Human Anatomy.* Baltimore, MD: Lippincott Williams & Wilkins; 2000 (3D CT; carpal tunnel syndrome; Pott fracture).

Courtesy of Dr. Philip Docking, Eatons Hill, QLD, Australia (laryngeal mask; nebulizer; Yankauer suction catheter).

From Effeney DJ, Stoney RJ. *Wylie's Atlas of Vascular Surgery: Disorders of the Extremities.* Philadelphia, PA: Lippincott Williams & Wilkins; 1993 (Raynaud phenomenon).

From Eisenberg RL. *Clinical Imaging: An Atlas of Differential Diagnosis.* 4th ed. Philadelphia: Lippincott Williams & Wilkins; 2003 (arteriography: Marfan syndrome; *Pneumocystis jiroveci* pneumonia).

From Engleberg NC, Demody T, DiRita V. *Schaechter's Mechanisms of Microbial Disease.* 4th ed. Philadelphia, PA: Lippincott Williams & Wilkins; 2006 (congenital cytomegalovirus).

From Erkonen WE, Smith WL. *Radiology 101: Basics and Fundamentals of Imaging.* Philadelphia: Lippincott Williams & Wilkins, 1998 (intravenous urogram).

From Eroschenko VP PhD. *di Fiore's Atlas of Histology with Functional Correlations.* 9th ed. Baltimore: Lippincott Williams & Wilkins; 2000 (bone).

From Fleisher GR, Ludwig S, Baskin MN. *Atlas of Pediatric Emergency Medicine.* Philadelphia, PA: Lippincott Williams & Wilkins; 2004 (Legg-Calvé-Perthes disease; gonorrhea infection; herpes zoster; pyogenic granuloma; scabies; scabies mite; *Staphylococcus aureus* infection; tick bite; tinea corporis; wheal).

From Farhi DC, et al. *Pathology of Bone Marrow and Blood Cells.* Philadelphia: Lippincott Williams & Wilkins; 2004 (dacryocytes; elliptocytes).

From Feigenbaum H, Armstrong WF, Ryan T. *Feigenbaum's Echocardiography.* 6th ed. Philadelphia, PA: Lippincott Williams & Wilkins; 2004 (two-dimensional echocardiography).

From Feinsilver SH, Fein A. *A Textbook on Bronchoscopy.* Baltimore, MD: Lippincott Williams & Wilkins; 1995 (bronchus; carina; trachea; vocal folds).

From Gartner LW, Hiatt JL. *Color Atlas of Histology.* 3rd ed. Baltimore, MD: Lippincott Williams & Wilkins; 1999 (neutrophil; eosinophil; basophil; myocyte).

From Gartner LP, Hiatt JL. *Color Atlas of Histology.* 4th ed. Baltimore, MD: Lippincott Williams & Wilkins; 2006 (spiral organ of Corti).

Courtesy of General Electric Medical Systems, Milwaukee, WI (meniscal tear; nuclear lung scan, gamma camera).

From Gladwin M, Bagby M. *Clinical Aspects of Dental Materials.* 2nd ed. Baltimore, MD: Lippincott Williams & Wilkins; 2004 (restoration).

From Gold DH, Weingeist TA. *Color Atlas of the Eye in Systemic Disease.* Baltimore, MD: Lippincott Williams & Wilkins; 2001 (chronic tophaceous gout; Chédiak-Higashi syndrome; orbital tumor; plaque).

From Goodheart HP. *A Photo Guide of Common Skin Disorders: Diagnosis and Management.* Baltimore, MD: Lippincott Williams & Wilkins; 1999 (morpheaform, nodular, and ulcerated basal cell carcinoma).

From Goodheart HP. *Goodheart's Photoguide of Common Skin Disorders.* 2nd ed. Philadelphia, PA: Lippincott Williams & Wilkins; 2003 (superficial basal cell carcinoma; alopecia areata; angioedema due to bee sting; sarcoidosis; scleroderma; melasma; bulla; burrows; chronic paronychia: nails; cryptococcosis; excoriation; fissure; furuncle; head lice; hirsutism; jellyfish sting; lichenification; linea nigra and striae gravidarum; Lyme disease; onychoschizia: nails; petechiae; purpura; spider angioma; telangiectasis; tinea capitis; tinea pedis; warts; hot tub foliculitis).

From Haines DE PhD. *Neuroanatomy: An Atlas of Structures, Sections, and Systems.* 6th ed. Baltimore, MD: Lippincott Williams & Wilkins; 2004 (filum terminale; CT myelogram).

Courtesy of Hawke M, MD, Toronto, Canada (acute otitis media; cholesteatoma; normal tympanic membrane; otitis externa; tympanosclerosis).

From Hall JC. *Sauer's Manual of Skin Diseases.* 8th ed. Philadelphia, PA: Lippincott Williams & Wilkins; 2000 (papules).

From Hall JC. *Sauer's Manual of Skin Diseases.* 9th ed. Philadelphia, PA: Lippincott Williams & Wilkins; 2006 (exfoliative dermatitis; xanthelasma palpebrarum).

From Harris JH Jr, Harris WH. *The Radiology of Emergency Medicine.* 3rd ed. Philadelphia, PA: Lippincott-Raven; 2000 (Barton fracture; Galeazzi fracture; Smith fracture).

From Harwood-Nuss A, Wolfson AB, et al. *The Clinical Practice of Emergency Medicine.* 3rd ed. Philadelphia, PA: Lippincott Williams & Wilkins; 2001 (croup; direct trauma injury; osteosarcoma; Monteggia fracture).

Reprinted with permission from Hertig AT, Rock J, Adams EC. A description of a 34 human ova within the first 17 days of development. *American Journal of Anatomy* 98:435, 1956. Courtesy of Carnegie Institution of Washington, Washington, DC (human blasocyst).

Reprinted with permission from Heuser CH. A presomite embryo with a definate chorda canal. *Contributions in Embryology* 23:253, 1932. Courtesy of Carnegie Institution of Washington, Washington, DC (18 day human embryo).

Courtesy of Hoag Memorial Presbyterian Hospital, Bloomington, IN (bone scan).

From Hosley JB, Molle-Matthews E. *Lippincott's Pocket Guide to Medical Assisting.* Philadelphia, PA: Lippincott Williams & Wilkins; 1998 (dorsal recumbent position; Fowler position; lithotomy position; prone position; high Fowler position; Sims position; sitting position; standing position; supine position).

Courtesy of Dr. Norman Jacobs. From Center for Disease Control and Prevention, Atlanta, GA (bacteria: diplococci).

From Kelsen DP, Daly JM, Kern SE, Lebin B, Tepper JE. *Gastroinstestinal Oncology: Principles and Practice.* Philadelphia, PA: Lippincott Williams & Wilkins; 2002 (barium enema study; endoscopy: adenocarcinoma; gallbladder carcinoma; endoscopy: non-Hodgkin lymphoma).

From Koneman EW, Allen SD, Janda WM, Schreckenberger PC, Winn WC Jr. *Color Atlas and Textbook of Diagnostic Microbiology.* 5th ed. Philadelphia, PA: Lippincott; 1997 (Enterobius vermicularis).

From Koval KJ, Zuckerman JD. Atlas of Orthopaedic Surgery: *A Multimedial Reference.* Philadelphia, PA: Lippincott Williams & Wilkins; 2004 (beach chair position; knee-chest position; lateral decubitus position).

Reprinted with permission from Krumlauf R. Hox genes and pattern formation in the branchial region of the vertebrate head. *Trends in Genetics* 9:106-112, 1993 (human embryo).

From Langlais RP, Miller CS. *Color Atlas of Common Oral Diseases.* 3rd ed. Baltimore, MD: Lippincott Williams & Wilkins; 2003 (angular cheilosis; ameloblastoma; attrition; bilateral cleft lip; cleft palate; cold sores; dental caries, class II and III; dentigerous cyst; erosion; hypohidrotic ectodermal dysplasia; thrush).

From Langland OE, Langlais RP. *Principles of Dental Imaging.* Baltimore, MD: Williams & Wilkins; 1997 (apical granuloma; apical periodontal cyst).

From *LifeART Emergency 3* (CD-ROM). Baltimore, MD: Lippincott Williams & Wilkins; 2000 (rule of nines; adult vs. pediatric airway).

From *LifeART Emergency 4* (CD-ROM). Baltimore, MD: Lippincott Williams & Wilkins; 2001 (oropharyngeal tube; jaw thrust).

From *LifeART Nursing 1* (CD-ROM). Baltimore, MD: Lippincott Williams & Wilkins; 2000 (Brudzinski sign; central venous pressure catheterization; intracranial pressure monitoring; venipuncture).

From *LifeART Nursing 2* (CD-ROM). Baltimore, MD: Lippincott Williams & Wilkins; 2000 (rigidity).

From *LifeART Nursing 3* (CD-ROM). Baltimore, MD: Lippincott Williams & Wilkins; 2000 (cricothyrotomy; tympanic thermometer; vasectomy).

From *LifeART Super Anatomy 1* (CD-ROM). Baltimore, MD: Lippincott Williams & Wilkins; 2002 (surgical incisions).

From *LWW's Organism Central* (CD_ROM). Baltimore, MD: Lippincott Williams & Wilkins; 2001 (*Entamoeba histolytica*).

From Marks R. *Skin Disease in Old Age.* Philadelphia, PA: JB Lippincott; 1987 (ulcer).

From McClatchey KD. *Clinical Laboratory Medicine.* 2nd ed. Philadelphia: Lippincott Williams & Wilkins; 2002 (staphylococci; streptococci; *Aspergillus fumigatus; Borrelia; Candida albicans; Cryptococcus neoformans; Fusarium solani; Haemophilus influenzae; Microsporum canis; Neisseria gonorrhoeae; Pneumocystis carinii; Staphylococcus aureus; Trichophyton tonsurans;* Zygomycetes; zygomycosis).

From McConnell TH. *The Nature of Disease, Pathology for Health Professions.* Baltimore, MD: Lippincott Williams & Wilkins; 2007 (congestive splenomegaly in cirrhosis).

From McKenzie SB, Clare N, Burns C, Larson L, Metz J. *Textbook of Hematology.* 2nd ed. Baltimore, MD: Williams & Wilkins; 1996 (Philadelphia chromosome translocation; hemolytic anemia; anisocytosis; macrocytosis; microcytic, hypochromic anemia; poikilocytosis; rouleaux; sickle cell anemia).

Courtesy of Mission Hospital Regional Medical Center, Mission Viejo, CA (breech fetus; colon polypectomy; esophageal varices).

Robert H. Mohlenbrock @ USDA-NRCS PLANTS Database / USDA SCS. 1991. *Southern wetland flora: Field office guide to plant species.* South National Technical Center, Fort Worth, TX (poison oak and sumac).

From Moore KL, Dalley AF. *Clinical Oriented Anatomy.* 4th ed. Baltimore, MD: Lippincott Williams & Wilkins; 1999 (swallowing; tracheostomy).

Courtesy of Dr. P. Motta. From Sadler T. *Langman's Medical Embryology.* 9th ed [image bank]. Baltimore, MD: Lippincott Williams & Wilkins; 2003 (zona pellucida).

From the National Pressure Ulcer Advisory Panel. Reston, VA (ulcers).

From Nettina, SM. *The Lippincott Manual of Nursing Practice.* 7th ed. Philadelphia, PA: Lippincott Williams & Wilkins; 2001 (Gardner-Wells traction tongs; Venturi mask; lentigo maligna melanoma).

From Neville BW, Damm DD, White DK. *Color Atlas of Clinical Oral Pathology.* 2nd ed. Baltimore, MD: Williams & Wilkins, 1998 (leukoplakia; hairy tongue).

Courtesy of Newport Diagnostic Center, Newport Beach, CA (Alzheimer disease).

From *Nursing Procedures.* 4th ed. Ambler, PA: Lippincott Williams & Wilkins; 2004 (electrocardiography photo; flow rates for IV drips; nasopharyngeal airway; oropharyngeal airway).

From Oatis CA. *Kinesiology: The Mechanics and Pathomechanics of Human Movement.* Baltimore, MD: Lippincott Williams & Wilkins; 2003 (articular cartilage; medial meniscus: top image; pinch patterns; scoliosis).

Courtesy of Olympus Corporation of Tokyo (colonoscope).

Courtesy of Philips Ultrasound, Bothell, WA (obstetrical sonography).

From Pillitteri A. *Maternal and Child Nursing.* 4th ed. Philadelphia, PA: Lippincott Williams & Wilkins; 2003 (Ambu bag; male and female condom drawings; meninges; multiple gestation; ventriculoperitoneal shunt; common sites of endometriosis formation).

From Pizzo PA, Poplack DG. *Principles and Practice of Pediatric Oncology.* 5th ed. Philadelphia, PA: Lippincott Williams & Wilkins; 2006 (astrocytoma).

Courtesy of Potter B, DDS. School of Dentistry, Medical College of Georgia, Augusta, GA (bitewing radiograph; cephalometry; dentition; endosteal implants; molar tooth; radiolucent area; panoramic radiograph).

From Pray WS. *Nonprescription Product Therapeutics.* Baltimore, MD: Lippincott Williams & Wilkins; 1999 (androgenic alopecia: female & male pattern).

From Premkumar K. *The Massage Connection: Anatomy and Physiology.* Baltimore, MD. Lippincott Williams & Wilkins; 2003 (wound healing).

From Premkumar K. *The Massage Connection, Anatomy and Physiology.* 2nd ed. Baltimore, MD: Lippincott Williams and Wilkins; 2004 (Golgi tendon organ).

From Riordan CL, McDonough M, Davidson JM, et al. Noncontact laser Doppler imaging in burn depth analysis of the extremities. *Journal of Burn Care & Rehabilitation* 24:177-86, 2003 (burns).

From Robinson HBG, Miller AS. *Colby, Kerr, and Robinson's Color Atlas of Oral Pathology.* Philadelphia, PA: JB Lippincott; 1990 (candidiasis).

From Rosdahl DB. *Textbook of Basic Nursing.* 7th ed. Philadelphia, PA: Lippincott Williams & Wilkins; 1999 (auscultation of the lungs).

From Rubin E, Farber JL. *Pathology.* 3rd ed. Philadelphia, PA: Lippincott Williams & Wilkins; 1999 (*Ascaris*; berry aneurysm; cholelithiasis; budding of virions from the plasma membrane of HIV-infected cell; spina bifida with meningomyelocele; adenocarcinoma; adenovirus: bronchiolitis; crust; Cytomegalovirus vs. normal respiratory tract; bancroftian filariasis infestation; fibroadenoma; *Haemophilus influenzae* meningitis; Hepatitis A virus; Hepatitis B virus; keloid).

From Rubin E, et al. *Rubin's Pathology: Clinicopathologic Foundations of Medicine.* 4th ed. Philadelphia, PA: Lippincott Williams & Wilkins; 2005 (bronchiolar carcinoma; diabetic retinopathy).

From Rubin R, Strayer DS, et al. *Rubin's Pathology: Clinicopathologic Foundations of Medicine.* 5th ed. Baltimore, MD: Lippincott Williams & Wilkins; 2008 (endometriosis nodules; subdural hematoma; cerebral hemorrhage; anthracosilicosis; centrilobular emphysema; alcoholic cirrhosis; Crohn disease; panacinar emphysema; gastric ulcer; acute hemorrhagic cystitis; hydronephrosis; hyperplastic polyp; interstitial cystitis; jaundice; Meckel diverticulum; multiple myeloma; Paget disease; chronic pyelonephritis; staghorn calculi; development of subdural hematoma; arterial thrombus; trichobezoar; ulcerative colitis; gallbladder carcinoma; myocardial hypertrophy; cataract).

From Sadler TW, PhD. *Langman's Medical Embryology.* 8th ed. Philadelphia, PA: Lippincott Williams & Wilkins; 2000 (histologic development of the lung; liver development in the embryo; metanephric diverticulum; stages in development of the pancreas; respiratory diverticulum).

From Sadler T. *Langman's Medical Embryology.* 9th ed [image bank]. Baltimore, MD: Lippincott Williams & Wilkins; 2003 (human blastocyst; fetus; dwarfism; 22/23 day human embryo; fetus; human embryo: 3rd week; zygote and morula).

From Salter RD. *Textbook of Disorders and Injuries of the Musculoskeletal System.* 2nd ed. Baltimore, MD: Williams & Wilkins; 1983 (bursitis).

From Sanders CV, Nesbitt LT Jr. *The Skin and Infection: A Color Atlas and Text.* Baltimore, MD: Williams & Wilkins; 1995 (Kaposi sarcoma; AIDS; tinea capitis: trichophyton tonsurans infection; toxic epidermal necrolysis).

From Sauer GC, Hall JC. Manual of Skin Diseases. 7th ed. Philadelphia, PA: Lippincott-Raven Publishers; 1996 (acne).

Courtesy of Scheie Eye Institute, Philadelphia, PA (normal retina; retinal detachment). Reprinted with permission from The Skin Cancer Foundation, New York, NY (squamous cell carcinoma).

Reprinted with permission from The Skin Cancer Foundation, New York, NY. *Basal Bell Carcinoma: The Most Common Skin Cancer.* Copyright © 1986, Revised 1999 (basal cell carcinoma).

From Smeltzer SC, Bare BG. *Brunner & Suddarth's Textbook of Medical-Surgical Nursing.* 9th ed. Philadelphia, PA: Lippincott Williams & Wilkins; 2000 (arterial aneurysm; progression of atherosclerosis; breast self-examination; hives; wounds; gangrene of the toes; securing nasogastric and nasoenteric tubes; Trousseau sign; tuberculin test; thoracoscopy; esophagogastroduodenoscopy; colonoscopy).

From Smeltzer SC, Bare BG, Hinkle JL, Cheever KH. *Brunner & Suddarth's Textbook of Medical-Surgical Nursing.* 11th ed. Philadelphia, PA: Lippincott Williams & Wilkins; 2008 (anesthetic delivery methods; anatomy of autonomic nervous system; cardiomyopathies that lead to congestive heart failure; implantable cardioverter defibrillator; cochlear implant; injection sites for spinal and epidural anesthesia; insulin pump; intravenous cannulation sites; knee joint; laproscopic cholecystectomy; knee ligaments, tendons, and menisci; osteophytes; pannus; deep peptic ulcer; common GI causes of peritonitis; pharyngitis; oral structures; pitting edema; shingles; anatomic structures of skin; Kaposi sarcoma; electrocardiography strip; impetigo: nostril; color flow duplex image: popliteal artery).

From Snell R. *Clinical Anatomy.* 7th ed. Philadelphia, PA: Lippincott Williams & Wilkins; 2003 (mature placenta; medial meniscus: bottom image; umbilical cord).

Courtesy of Larry Staugger, Oregon State Public Health Laboratory. From Center for Disease Control and Prevention, Atlanta, GA (bacteria: bacilli).

Courtesy of Stoelting Co., Wood Dale, IL (Adson forceps).

Reprinted with permission from Streeter GL. Developmental horizons in human embryos: age groups XV, XVl, XVll, and XVlll [the third issue of a survey of the Carnegie Collection]. *Contributions in Embryology* 32:133, 1948. Courtesy of Carnegie Institution of Washington, Washington, DC (28-somite human embryo; yolk sac).

From Sun T. *Parasitic Disorders: Pathology, Diagnosis, and Management.* 2nd ed. Baltimore, MD: Lippincott Williams & Wilkins; 1999 (*Entamoeba coli; Giardia lamblia;* hookworm; *Isospora belli*; nematode; cestode; trematode; *Taenia saginata; Trichinella spiralis; Wuchereria bancrofti*).

From Swischuk LE. *Imaging of the Newborn, Infant, and Young Child.* 4th ed. Philadelphia, PA: Lippincott Williams & Wilkins; 1997 (Wilms tumor; neuroblastoma).

From Tasman W, Jaeger E. *The Wills Eye Hospital Atlas of Clinical Ophthalmology.* 2 ed. Baltimore, MD: Lippincott Williams & Wilkins; 2001 (mature cataract with complete opacification of lens; Goldenhar syndrome; blepharitis; drusen; *Candida albicans* infection; conjunctivitis; corneal foreign body; corneal ulcer; cotton wool spots; endophthalmitis; episcleritis; *Fusarium* infection; hyphema; keratoacanthoma; milia; normal angiogram; normal macula; orbital cellulites; *Phthiriasis pubis* infestation; retinoblastoma causing glaucoma; retinoblastoma; rhabdomyosarcoma; tumor).

From Taylor C, Lillis C, LeMone P. *Fundamentals of Nursing: The Art and Science of Nursing Care.* 4th ed. Philadelphia, PA: Lippincott Williams & Wilkins; 2001 (nasal cannula; lumbar puncture).

From Taylor C, Lillis C, LeMone P, Lynn P. *Fundamentals of Nursing: The Art and Science of Nursing Care.* 6th ed. Philadelphia, PA: Lippincott Williams & Wilkins; 2008 (stoma; injections; apical pulse; lateral view of female breast; location of lymph nodes of the neck; sphygmomanometer; parts of needle and syringe; transcutaneous electrical nerve stimulation; Z-track method).

Courtesy of Wang F, MD, Orange, CA (perfusion scan, ventilation scan).

From Weber J, Kelley J. *Health Assessment in Nursing.* 2nd ed. Philadelphia, PA: Lippincott Williams & Wilkins; 2003 (Hegar sign; pain scales; cerumen; bunion; cherry angiomas; patches; scar).

Courtesy of Welch Allyn, Inc., Skaneateles Falls, NY (exostosis; glaucoma; ophthalmoscope; otomycosis; otoscope; otoscopy; perforation).

From Westheimer R, Lopater S. *Human Sexuality: A Psychosocial Perspective.* Baltimore, MD: Lippincott Williams & Wilkins; 2002 (female condom photograph).

From Willis MC. *Medical Terminology: A Programmed Learning Approach to the Language of Health Care.* Baltimore, MD: Lippincott Williams & Wilkins; 2002 (atherectomy devices; incentive spirometer; 8-week embryo).

From Willis MC. *Medical Terminology: The Language of Health Care.* Baltimore, MD: Williams & Wilkins; 1996 (lesions; rhythm).

From Winn WC Jr, et al. *Koneman's Color Atlas and Textbook of Diagnostic Microbiology.* 6th ed. Philadelphia, PA: Lippincott; 2005 (*Plasmodium vivax*).

Courtesy of World Health Organization, Washington, DC (polio).

From Yamada T, et al. *Atlas of Gastroenterology.* 3rd ed. Philadelphia, PA: Lippincott Williams & Wilkins; 2003 (diverticulosis; ulcerative colitis).

From Yochum TR, Rowe LJ. *Essentials of Skeletal Radiology.* 2nd ed. Baltimore, MD: Lippincott Williams & Wilkins; 1996 (myositis ossificans).

Artwork Credits

Artwork in this edition of *Stedman's Medical Dictionary for the Health Professions and Nursing* was created or adapted by the following individuals (see Illustration Sources for sources of adaptions):

Anatomical Chart Company: umbilical cord prolapse, tooth anatomy, left kidney and adrenal gland, malignant melanoma, nephrolithiasis, bony orbit, conception, respiration, Lund-Browder chart, blood cell development, all artwork in the anatomy insert, all rights reserved.

Mary Anna Barratt-Dimes, Parkton, MD: tympanogram

Susan Caldwell, Parsonsburg, MD: apgar score, arterial blood gases, normal body temperature by age

Jonathon Clements, Baltimore, MD: hearing aids, male condom photograph

Neil O. Hardy, Westport, CT: ectopic pregnancy, eye, facial nerves, Foley catheter, types of fractures, gastric bypass, glaucoma, gestation, antibody, arteriole, asthma, auditory ossicles, biopsy, segmental bronchi, capillary bed, dental caries, cerebral cortex, coronary arteries, frontal section of ear, embolism, enterostomy tubes, types of epithelium, Heimleich maneuver, invertebral disc herniation, hyperopia, hyphema, ileostomy, indirect ingiunal hernia, innervation of the hand and wrist, intestines, pancreas, joints, laryngeal cartilages, Le Fort classification of facial fractures, lungs and respiratory anatomy, metered dose inhaler, mouth, myopia, neuroglia, typical efferent neurons, nutrient absorption, nystagmus, olfaction, otitis externa, otitis media, pancreas, percussion, percutaneous transluminal angioplasty, permanent dentition, polyps, postural drainage, pulmonary circulation, peripheral pulses, quadrants of abdomen, layers of the retina, scoliosis, skeletal muscle, spirometry, spondylolosthesis, vascular stent, talipes cavus and talipes planus, temporomandibular joint, vertical banded gastroplasty, digital clubbing, cochlea, cranial nerves, deciduous dentition, decubitus ulcer, dental implant, dermatomes, DNA, abdominal regions, alveolar abscess, amniocentesis, palpation technique, varicosis, venous valves, ventricles of the brain, vision, electrocardiography, colostomy, heart valves, bronchoscopy, computed tomography, MRI machine, computer monitors

Siri Mills, Munich, Germany: human heart, sympathetic trunk

Barbara Proud, Wilmington, DE: female condom photograph

Michael Schenk, Jackson, MS: bomb calorimeter, carpal tunnel syndrome, finger deformities and fractures, grasp patterns, sliding esophageal and paraesophageal hernias, muscles of mastication, skinfold measurement sites

Mikki Senkarik, San Antonio, TX: thoracoscopy, esophagogastroduodenoscopy, colonoscopy

A

α (al′fa) SEE alpha.

A **1.** Abbreviation for adenine; alanine. **2.** As a subscript, refers to alveolar gas. **3.** Symbol (usually capitalized italic, i.e., *A*), for absorbance. **4.** Symbol for adenosine or adenylic acid in polynucleotides; alanine in polypeptides; first substrate in a multisubstrate enzyme-catalyzed reaction.

°A Abbreviation for degree absolute; replaced by K (kelvin).

Å Abbreviation for angstrom.

A⁻ Abbreviation for anion.

A Abbreviation for absorbance.

a **1.** Abbreviation for ante; area; asymmetric; artery; auris; atto-. **2.** As a subscript, refers to systemic arterial blood.

a Abbreviation for specific absorption coefficient; absorptivity.

a-, an- Prefix denoting not, without, -less; equivalent to L. *in-* and E. *un-*. [G. not, un-; usually *an-* before a vowel]

AA, aa Abbreviation for amino acid; aminoacyl; Alcoholics Anonymous.

AAA Abbreviation for abdominal aortic aneurysm; commonly, procedure for surgical correction of an abdominal aortic aneurysm; area agency on aging.

AAAI Abbreviation for American Academy of Allergy and Immunology

AAC Abbreviation for augmentative and alternative communication.

AACN Abbreviation for American Association of Colleges of Nursing.

AAD Abbreviation for antibiotic-associated diarrhea.

AAHAM Abbreviation for American Association of Healthcare Administrative Management.

AAI Abbreviation for ankle-arm index.

AAMA Abbreviation for American Association of Medical Assistants.

AAMC Abbreviation for Association of American Medical Colleges.

AAMT Abbreviation for American Association for Medical Transcription.

AAN Abbreviation for American Academy of Nursing.

AANA Abbreviation for American Association of Nurse Anesthetists.

AANN Abbreviation for American Association of Neurological Nurses; American Association of Neuroscience Nurses.

A-aO₂ dif•fer•ence (dif′ĕr-ĕns) The difference or gradient between the partial pressure of oxygen in the alveolar spaces and that in arterial blood. Normally less than 10 mmHg, it is increased with large right-to-left cardiac or vascular shunts. SEE alveolar air equation. SYN alveolar-arterial oxygen tension difference.

AAOHN Abbreviation for American Association of Occupational Health Nurses.

AAOP Abbreviation for American Academy of Orthotists and Prosthetists.

AAPA Abbreviation for American Academy of Physician Assistants.

AAPB Abbreviation for American Association of Pathologists and Bacteriologists.

AAPC Abbreviation for American Academy of Professional Coders.

AAPMR Abbreviation for American Academy of Physical Medicine and Rehabilitation.

Aar•on sign (ar′ŏn sīn) In acute appendicitis, a diagnostic sign, indicating referred pain or feeling of distress in the epigastrium or precordial region on continuous firm pressure over the McBurney point.

AARP Abbreviation for American Association of Retired Persons.

AART Abbreviation for American Academy of Respiratory Therapy

AASH Abbreviation for adrenal androgen-stimulating hormone.

AAUP Abbreviation for American Association of University Professors.

Ab Abbreviation for antibody.

ab-, abs- **1.** Combining forms meaning from, away from, off. **2.** Combining forms applied to electrical units in the CGS-electromagnetic system to distinguish them from units in the CGS-electrostatic system (prefix stat-) and those in the metric system or SI (no prefix). [L. *ab,* from; usually *abs-* before c, q, and t; often *a-* before m, p, or v]

a•bac•te•ri•al (ā′bak-tēr′ē-ăl) Not caused by or characterized by the presence of bacteria.

A•bad•ie sign of ta•bes dor•sa•lis (ah-bah-dē′ sīn tā′bēz dōr-sā′lis) Insensibility to pressure over the Achilles tendon.

ab•am•pere (ab-am′pēr) Electromagnetic unit of current equal to 10 absolute amperes; a current that exerts a force of 2π dynes on a unit magnetic pole at the center of a circle of wire 1 cm in radius.

A band (band) Muscle striation containing myosin filaments; appears dark under light microscope and light in polarized light.

a•bap•i•cal (ă-bap′i-kăl) Opposite the apex.

a•bar•og•no•sis (ā-bar′ŏg-nō′sis) Loss of ability to appreciate the weight of objects held in the hand, or to differentiate objects of different weights. When the primary senses are intact, abarognosis is caused by a lesion of the contralateral parietal lobe. [G. *a-* priv. + *baros,* weight, + *gnōsis,* knowledge]

a•ba•si•a (ă-bā′zē-ă) Inability to walk. SEE gait. [G. *a-* priv. + *basis,* step]

a•ba•si•a-a•sta•si•a (ă-bā′zē-ă-ă-stā′zē-ă) SEE astasia-abasia.

a•ba•si•a tre•pi•dans (ă-bā′zē-ă trep′i-danz) Abasia due to trembling of the lower limbs.

a•ba•sic, **a•ba•tic** (ă-bā′sik, ă-bat′ik) **1.** Affected by, or associated with, abasia. **2.** Refers to loss of pyrimidine sites in DNA.

ab•ax•i•al, **ab•ax•ile** (ab-ak′sē-ăl, -ak′sīl) **1.** Lying outside the axis of any body or part. **2.** Situated at the opposite extremity of the axis of a part.

Ab•be-Est•lan•der op•er•a•tion (ab′ē-āst′lahn-der op′ĕr-ā′shŭn) Involving graft of flap of tissue from one lip of the oral cavity to the other lip to correct a defect.

Ab•be flap (ab′ē flap) Colloquially called a "pedicle flap," this regional full-thickness flap (including skin and labial mucosa) is used to reconstruct medial defects of the opposing lip, especially bilateral cleft.

Ab•bott ar•ter•y (ab′ŏt ahr′tĕr-ē) An anomalous artery arising from the posteromedial proximal descending aorta, important during coarctation repair.

Ab•bott meth•od (ab′ŏt meth′ŏd) A method of treatment of scoliosis by use of a series of plaster jackets applied after partial correction of the curvature by external force.

Ab•bott stain for spores (ab′ŏt stān spōrz) Spores are stained blue with alkaline methylene blue; bodies of the bacilli become pink with eosin counterstain.

Ab•bott tube (ab′ŏt tūb) SYN Miller-Abbott tube.

ab•bre•vi•a•ted new drug ap•pli•ca•tion (ă-brē′vē-ā-tĕd nū drŭg ap′li-kā′shŭn) A request by a pharmaceutical company to market and sell a pharmaceutical that is essentially the same as another, which has already been granted such approval.

ABC 1. Abbreviation used in both basic and advanced cardiac life support to ensure continued attention to airway, breathing, and circulation. **2.** Abbreviation for American Board for Certification in Orthotics and Prosthetics.

ABCDE Abbreviation used in advanced trauma life support to ensure continued attention to airway, breathing, circulation and cervical spine, disability, and exposure.

ab•do•men (ab′dŏ-mĕn) [TA] The part of the trunk that lies between the thorax and the pelvis; considered by some anatomists to include the pelvis (abdominopelvic cavity). It includes the greater part of the abdominal cavity (cavitas abdominis [TA]), and is divided by arbitrary planes into nine regions. SEE ALSO abdominal regions. SYN venter (1). [L. *abdomen,* etym. uncertain]

ab•dom•i•nal (ab-dom′ĭ-năl) Relating to the abdomen.

ab•dom•i•nal an•gi•na, **an•gi•na ab•do•mi•nis** (ab-dom′i-năl an′ji-nă, an′ji-nă ab-dō′mi-nis) Intermittent abdominal pain, frequently occurring at a fixed time after eating, caused by inadequacy of the mesenteric circulation resulting from arteriosclerosis or other arterial disease, with associated significant weight loss. SYN intestinal angina.

ab•dom•i•nal a•or•ta (ab-dom′i-năl ā-ōr′tă) The part of the descending aorta that supplies structures below the diaphragm. SYN abdominal part of aorta, aorta abdominalis, pars abdominalis aortae.

ab•dom•i•nal as•sess•ment (ab-dom′i-năl ă-ses′mĕnt) The appraisal of the abdomen by a health care provider. The assessment is conducted in a predetermined order: inspection, auscultation, and palpation.

ab•dom•i•nal au•ra (ab-dom′i-năl awr′ă) Epileptic aura characterized by abdominal discomfort; it involves nausea, malaise, pain, and hunger. Some phenomena reflect ictal autonomic dysfunction. SEE ALSO aura (1).

ab•dom•i•nal cav•i•ty (ab-dom′i-năl kav′i-tē) The space bounded by the abdominal walls, the diaphragm, and the pelvis; it usually is arbitrarily separated from the pelvic cavity by a plane across the superior aperture of the pelvis; however, it may include the pelvis with the abdomen (SEE abdominopelvic cavity); within the cavity lie the greater part of the organs of digestion, spleen, kidneys, and suprarenal glands. SYN enterocele (2).

ab•dom•i•nal ges•ta•tion (ab-dom′i-năl jes-tā′shŭn) An extrauterine pregnancy in which the embryo develops in the peritoneal cavity.

ab•dom•i•nal guard•ing (ab-dom′i-năl gahrd′ing) A spasm of abdominal wall muscles, detected on palpation, to protect inflamed abdominal viscera from pressure; usually results from inflammation of the peritoneal surface as seen in appendicitis, diverticulitis, or generalized peritonitis.

ab•dom•i•nal her•ni•a (ab-dom′i-năl hĕr′nē-ă) A hernia protruding through or into any part of the abdominal wall. SYN laparocele.

ab·dom·i·nal hys·ter·ec·to·my (ab-dom′i-năl his′tĕr-ek′tŏ-mē) Removal of the uterus through an incision in the abdominal wall. SYN abdominohysterectomy.

ab·dom·i·nal hys·ter·ot·o·my (ab-dom′i-năl his′tĕr-ot′ŏ-mē) Transabdominal incision into the uterus; also called abdominohysterotomy, celiohysterotomy, laparohysterotomy, and laparouterotomy. SYN abdominohysterotomy.

ab·dom·i·nal os·ti·um of u·ter·ine tube (ab-dom′i-năl os′tē-ŭm yū′tĕr-in tūb) The fimbriated or ovarian extremity of an oviduct.

ab·dom·i·nal pad (ab-dom′i-năl pad) SYN laparotomy pad.

ab·dom·i·nal part of a·or·ta (ab-dom′i-năl pahrt ā-ōr′tă) SYN abdominal aorta.

ab·dom·i·nal preg·nan·cy (ab-dom′i-năl preg′năn-sē) Implantation and development of a fertilized oocyte in the peritoneal cavity, usually after early rupture of a tubal pregnancy; very rarely, primary implantation may occur in the peritoneal cavity. SYN abdominocyesis (1).

ab·dom·i·nal pres·sure (ab-dom′i-năl presh′ŭr) Pressure surrounding the bladder; estimated from rectal, gastric, or intraperitoneal pressure.

ab·dom·i·nal quad·rant (ab-dom′i-năl kwahd′rănt) Any of the four segments into which the abdomen is divided by vertical and horizontal partitioning through the midpoint.

ab·dom·i·nal re·flex (ab-dom′i-năl rē′fleks) Abdominal wall muscle contraction in response to stimulation of abdominal skin.

ab·dom·i·nal re·gions (ab-dom′i-năl rē′jŭnz) The topographic subdivisions of the abdomen; based on subdividing the abdomen by the transpyloric, transtubercular, and midinguinal planes; including the right and left hypochondriac, right and left lateral, right and left inguinal, and the unpaired epigastric, umbilical, and pubic regions. See this page.

ab·dom·i·nal res·pi·ra·tion (ab-dom′i-năl res′pir-ā′shŭn) Breathing produced mainly by action of the diaphragm.

ab·dom·i·nal sec·tion (ab-dom′i-năl sek′shŭn) SYN celiotomy.

ab·dom·i·nal tes·tis (ab-dom′i-năl tes′tis) A testis that has never descended from its retroperitoneal-abdominal origin through the internal inguinal ring.

abdomino-, abdomin- Combining forms meaning the abdomen, abdominal. [L. *abdomen, abdominis*]

ab·dom·i·no·cen·te·sis (ab-dom′i-nō-sen-tē′sis) Paracentesis of the abdomen. [abdomino- + G. *kentēsis,* puncture]

ab·dom·i·no·cy·e·sis (ab-dom′i-nō-sī-ē′sis)

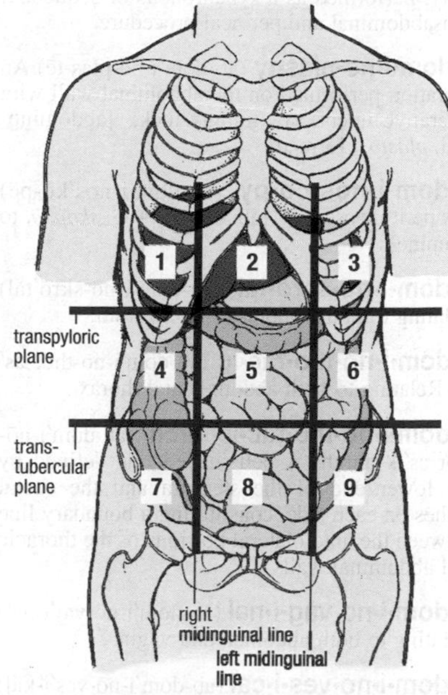

abdominal regions: (1) right hypochondriac, (2) epigastric, (3) left hypochondriac, (4) right lateral (lumbar), (5) umbilical, (6) left lateral (lumbar), (7) right iliac, (8) hypogastric (suprapubic), (9) left iliac

1. SYN abdominal pregnancy. **2.** SYN secondary abdominal pregnancy. [abdomino- + G. *kyēsis,* pregnancy]

ab·dom·i·no·cys·tic (ab-dom′i-nō-sis′tik) SYN abdominovesical. [abdomino- + G. *kystis,* bladder]

ab·dom·i·no·gen·i·tal (ab-dom′i-nō-gen′i-tăl) Relating to the abdomen and the genital organs.

ab·dom·i·no·hys·ter·ec·to·my (ab-dom′i-nō-his′tŏr-ek′tŏ-mē) SYN abdominal hysterectomy.

ab·dom·i·no·hys·ter·ot·o·my (ab-dom′i-nō-his-ter-ot′ō-mē) SYN abdominal hysterotomy.

ab·dom·i·no·pel·vic (ab-dom′i-nō-pel′vik) Relating to the abdomen and pelvis, especially the abdominal and pelvic cavities in combination.

ab·dom·i·no·pel·vic cav·i·ty (ab-dom′i-nō-pel′vik kav′i-tē) The combined and continuous abdominal and pelvic cavities. SEE ALSO abdominal cavity.

ab·dom·i·no·per·i·ne·al (ab-dom′i-nō-per-i-nē′ăl) Relating to both abdomen and perineum.

ab·dom·i·no·per·i·ne·al re·sec·tion (ab-dom′i-nō-per-i-nē′ăl rē-sek′shŭn) A surgical treatment for cancer involving resection of the lower sigmoid colon, rectum, anus, and surrounding skin, and formation of a sigmoid colostomy; performed as a synchronous or sequential transabdominal and perineal procedure.

ab•dom•i•no•plas•ty (ab-dom′i-nō-plas-tē) An operation performed on the abdominal wall with reparative intent. SYN tummy tuck. [abdomino- + G. *plastos,* formed]

ab•dom•i•nos•co•py (ab-dom′i-nos′kŏ-pē) SYN peritoneoscopy. [abdomino- + G. *skopeō,* to examine]

ab•dom•i•no•scro•tal (ab-dom′i-nō-skrō′tăl) Relating to both abdomen and scrotum.

ab•dom•i•no•tho•rac•ic (ab-dom′i-nō-thŏr-as′ik) Relating to both abdomen and thorax.

ab•dom•i•no•tho•rac•ic arch (ab-dom′i-nō-thŏr-as′ik ahrch) A bell-shaped line defined by the lower end of the sternum and the costal arches on each side, constituting a boundary line between the anterolateral portions of the thoracic and abdominal walls.

ab•dom•i•no•vag•i•nal (ab-dom′i-nō-vaj′i-năl) Relating to both abdomen and vagina.

ab•dom•i•no•ves•i•cal (ab-dom′i-nō-ves′i-kăl) Relating to both abdomen and urinary bladder, or to abdomen and gallbladder. SYN abdominocystic.

ab•duce (ab-dūs′) SYN abduct.

ab•du•cens (ab-dū′senz) SYN abducent (1). [L.]

ab•du•cens nerve (ab-dū′senz nĕrv) SYN abducent nerve [CN VI].

ab•du•cens oc•u•li (ab-dū′senz ok′yū-lī) SYN lateral rectus muscle.

ab•du•cent (ab-dū′sĕnt) **1.** Abducting; drawing away, especially away from the median plane. SYN abducens. **2.** SYN abducent nerve [CN VI]. [L. *abducens*]

ab•du•cent nerve [CN VI] (ab-dū′sĕnt nĕrv) A small motor nerve supplying the lateral rectus muscle of the eye; its origin is in the dorsal part of the tegmentum of the pons just below the surface of the rhomboid fossa, and it emerges from the brain in the fissure between the medulla oblongata and the posterior border of the pons (medullopontine sulcus); it enters the dura of the clivus and passes through the cavernous sinus, entering the orbit through the superior orbital fissure. SYN nervus abducens [CN VI] [TA], abducens nerve, abducent (2), sixth cranial nerve [CN VI].

ab•duct (ab-dŭkt′) To move away from the median plane. SYN abduce.

ab•duc•tion (ab-dŭk′shŭn) **1.** Movement of a body part away from the median plane (of the body, in the case of limbs; of the hand or foot, in the case of digits). **2.** Monocular rotation (duction) of the eye toward the temple. **3.** A position resulting from such movement. Cf. adduction. [L. *abductio*]

ab•duc•tor (ab-dŭk′tŏr) A muscle that draws a part away from the median plane, or, in the case of the digits, away from the normal axis of the middle finger or the second toe.

ab•duc•tor di•gi•ti mi•ni•mi mus•cle of foot (ab-dŭk′tŏr dij′i-tī mi′ni-mī mŭs′ĕl fut) *Origin*, lateral and medial processes of calcaneal tuberosity; *insertion*, lateral side of proximal phalanx of the fifth toe; *action*, abducts and flexes little toe; *nerve supply*, lateral plantar nerve.

ab•duc•tor di•gi•ti mi•ni•mi mus•cle of hand (ab-dŭk′tŏr dij′i-tī mi′ni-mī mŭs′ĕl hand) *Origin*, pisiform bone and pisohamate ligament; *insertion*, medial side of base of proximal phalanx of the little finger; *action*, abducts and flexes little finger; *nerve supply*, ulnar.

ab•duc•tor hal•lu•cis mus•cle (ab-dŭk′tŏr hal′ū-sis mŭs′ĕl) *Origin*, medial process of calcaneal tuberosity, flexor retinaculum, and plantar aponeurosis; *insertion*, medial side of proximal phalanx of great toe; *action*, abducts great toe; *nerve supply*, medial plantar. SYN musculus abductor hallucis [TA].

ab•duc•tor pol•li•cis brev•is mus•cle (ab-dŭk′tŏr pol′li-sis brev′is mŭs′ĕl) Superficial thenar muscle; *origin*, tubercle of trapezium and flexor retinaculum; *insertion*, lateral side of proximal phalanx of thumb; *action*, abducts thumb; *nerve supply*, median. SYN musculus abductor pollicis brevis, short abductor muscle of thumb.

ab•duc•tor pol•li•cis long•us mus•cle (ab-dŭk′tŏr pol′li-sis long′gus mŭs′ĕl) Outcropping muscle of posterior compartment of forearm; *origin*, interosseous membrane and posterior surfaces of radius and ulna; *insertion*, lateral side of base of first metacarpal bone; *action*, abducts and assists in extending thumb; *nerve supply*, radial. SYN long abductor muscle of thumb, musculus abductor pollicis longus, musculus extensor ossis metacarpi pollicis.

ab•duc•tor spas•mod•ic dys•pho•ni•a (ab-dŭk′tŏr spaz-mod′ik dis-fōn-ē-ă) A breathy form of spasmodic dysphonia caused by excessive and long vocal cord opening for voiceless phonemes extending into vowels.

Ab•egg rule (ah′beg rūl) The tendency of the sum of the maximum positive and maximum negative valences of a particular element to equal 8 (e.g., C may have a valence of +4 and –4, O of +6 and –2).

A•bell-Ken•dall meth•od (ā′bel ken′dăl meth′ŏd) A methodology for determining total serum cholesterol that avoids interference by bilirubin, protein, and hemoglobin.

ab•em•bry•on•ic (ab′em-brē-on′ik) Remote

from the embryo, referring to the pole of the blastocyst opposite the embryonic pole.

ab·em·bry·on·ic pole (ab′em-brē-on′ik pōl) The area of the blastocyst opposite the embryonic pole where the embryoblast is located.

ab·er·rant (ab-er′ănt) **1.** Wandering off; said of certain ducts, vessels, or nerves deviating from the normal course or pattern. **2.** Differing from the normal; in botany or zoology, said of certain atypical individuals in a species. **3.** SYN ectopic (1). [L. *aberrans*]

ab·er·rant goi·ter (ab-er′ănt goy′tĕr) Enlargement of a supernumerary thyroid gland. SYN aberrant goitre.

aberrant goitre [Br.] SYN aberrant goiter.

ab·er·ra·tion (ab′ĕr-ā′shŭn) **1.** Deviation from the usual or normal course or pattern. **2.** Deviant development or growth. SEE ALSO chromosome aberration. [L. *aberratio*]

abetalipoproteinaemia [Br.] SYN abetalipoproteinemia.

a·be·ta·lip·o·pro·tein·e·mi·a (ā-bā′tă-lip′ō-prō′tēn-ē′mē-ă) A disorder characterized by an absence from plasma of low density lipoproteins that migrate electrophoretically as beta globulins, the presence of acanthocytes in the blood, retinal pigmentary degeneration, malabsorption, engorgement of upper intestinal absorptive cells with dietary triglycerides, and neuromuscular abnormalities; autosomal recessive inheritance. SYN abetalipoproteinaemia, Bassen-Kornzweig syndrome. [G. *a-*, priv., + β, + lipoprotein + *-emia*, blood]

ab·frac·tion (ab-frak′shŭn) Pathologic loss of hard tooth substance caused by biomechanical loading forces. [ab- + L. *fractio*, a breaking, Fr. *frango, fractum*, to break]

ABG Abbreviation for arterial blood gas; air-bone gap.

ABI Abbreviation for acquired brain injury; ankle-brachial index.

ab·i·ent (ab′ē-ĕnt) Characterized by avoidance or withdrawal. [L. *abeo*, to go away]

a·bil·i·ties (ă-bil′i-tēz) Enduring traits that are primarily genetically predetermined and underlie a person's skilled motor performance (e.g., visual acuity, body configuration, numeric reasoning). [L. *habilitas*, capacity, aptitude]

a·bi·o·gen·e·sis (ā′bī-ō-jen′ĕ-sis) Spontaneous origination of living organ directly from lifeless matter. SEE ALSO spontaneous generation. [G. *a-*, without, + *bios*, life, + *genesis*, formation]

a·bi·ot·ic (ā-bī-ot′ik) **1.** Incompatible with life. **2.** Without life.

Ab·i·o·tro·phi·a (ab′ē-ō-trō′fē-a) A bacterial genus originally referred to as "nutritionally variant or nutritionally deficient" streptococci, associated with various infections, particularly subacute bacterial endocarditis.

ab·i·ot·ro·phy (ab′ē-ot′trŏ-fē) An age-dependent manifestation of a genetically determined trait that has been latent from the time of conception. [G. *a-* priv. + *bios*, life, + *trophē*, nourishment]

abl An oncogene found in the Abelson strain of mouse leukemia virus and involved in the Philadelphia chromosome translocation in chronic granulocytic leukemia.

a·blas·te·mic (ā′blas-tē′mik) Incapable of blastema formation.

ab·late (ab-lāt′) To remove, or to destroy the function of. [L. *au- fero*, pp. *ab-latus*, to take away]

ab·la·tion (ab-lā′shŭn) Removal of a body part or the destruction of its function, as by a surgical procedure, morbid process, or noxious substance. [L. see ablate]

ab·lu·ted (ă-blū′tĕd) Washed clean. [L. *abluo, ablutum*, to wash off]

a·blu·tion (ă-blū′shŭn) Washing of one's body or part of it. [L. *ab-luo, ab-lutus*, to wash off]

ABN Abbreviation for advance beneficiary notice.

ab·ner·val, **ab·neu·ral** (ab-nĕr′văl, ab-nūr′ăl) **1.** Away from a nerve or neural axis. **2.** Denoting specifically a current of electricity passing through a muscular fiber in a direction away from the point of entrance of the nerve fiber.

ab·nor·mal·i·ty (ab′nōr-mal′i-tē) **1.** The state or quality of being abnormal; that which deviates from the norm. **2.** An anomaly, deformity, malformation, impairment, or dysfunction.

ab·nor·mal oc·clu·sion (ab-nōr′măl ŏ-klū′zhŭn) An arrangement of the teeth that is not considered to be within the normal range of variation.

ab·nor·mal ST seg·ment (ab-nōr′măl seg′mĕnt) SYN isoelectric period.

ab·nor·mal tone (ab-nōr′măl tōn) Any increase or decrease of muscle tone that results in functional impairment.

ABO haemolytic disease of the newborn [Br.] SYN ABO hemolytic disease of the newborn.

ABO he·mo·lyt·ic dis·ease of the new·born (HDN) (hē′mō-lit′ik di-zēz′ nū′bōrn) Erythroblastosis fetalis due to maternal-fetal incompatibility with respect to an antigen of the ABO blood group; the fetus possesses A or B antigen that is lacking in the mother, and the mother produces immune antibody that causes hemolysis of fetal erythrocytes. SYN ABO haemolytic disease of the newborn.

ab•o•rad, ab•o•ral (ab-ōr′ad, -ăl) In a direction away from the mouth; opposite of orad. [L. *ab,* from, + *os* (*or-*), mouth]

a•bort (ă-bōrt) **1.** To give birth to an embryo or fetus before it is viable. **2.** To arrest a disease in its earliest stages. **3.** To arrest growth or development; to cause to remain rudimentary. **4.** To remove products of conception before viability. [L. *aborior,* to fail at onset]

a•bort•ed sys•to•le (ă-bōrt′ĕd sis′tŏ-lē) A loss of the systolic beat in the radial pulse through weakness of the ventricular contraction.

a•bor•ti•fa•cient (ă-bōr′ti-fā′shĕnt) **1.** Producing abortion. SYN abortive (3). **2.** Any agent (usually a drug or pharmacotherapeutic) that produces abortion. [L. *abortus,* abortion, + *facio,* to make]

a•bor•tion (ă-bōr′shŭn) **1.** Expulsion from the uterus of an embryo or fetus before the stage of viability (20 weeks' gestation [18 weeks after gestation] or fetal weight less than 500 g). A distinction is made between abortion and premature birth: premature infants are those born after the stage of viability but before 37 weeks' gestation. Abortion may be either spontaneous (occurring from natural causes) or induced (artificial or therapeutic). **2.** The arrest of any action or process before its normal completion.

a•bor•tion•ist (ă-bōr′shŭn-ist) One who interrupts a pregnancy.

a•bor•tion pill (ă-bōr′shŭn pil) A means of expelling an embryo or fetus during the first 7 weeks of pregnancy with a combination of a progesterone antagonist and prostaglandins.

a•bor•tive (ă-bōr′tiv) **1.** Not reaching completion; said of a disease subsiding before it has completed its course. **2.** SYN rudimentary. **3.** SYN abortifacient (1). [L. *abortivus*]

a•bor•tive trans•duc•tion (ă-bōr′tiv tranz-dŭk′shŭn) Process in which the genetic fragment from the donor bacterium is not integrated in the genome of the recipient bacterium and, when the latter divides, is transmitted to only one of the daughter cells.

a•bor•tus (ă-bōr′tŭs) **1.** An embryo or fetus and membranes. 2. Any product (or all products) of an abortion. [L.]

ABP Abbreviation for androgen binding protein.

ABR Abbreviation for auditory brainstem response.

a•bra•chi•a (ă-brā′kē-ă) Congenital absence of upper limbs. SEE amelia. [G. *a-* priv. + *brachiōn,* arm]

a•bra•chi•o•ceph•a•ly, a•bra•chi•o•ce•pha•li•a (ă-brā′kē-ō-sef′ă-lē, -se-fā′lē-ă) Congenital absence of upper limbs and head. [G. *a-* priv. + *brachiōn,* arm, + *kephalē,* head]

a•brade (ă-brād′) **1.** To wear away by mechanical action. **2.** To scrape away the surface layer from a part. [L. *ab-rado,* pp. *-rasus,* to scrape off]

a•brad•ed wound (ă-brād′ĕd wūnd) SYN abrasion (1).

A•brams heart re•flex (ā′brămz hahrt rē′fleks) A contraction of the myocardium when the skin of the precordial region is irritated.

a•bra•sion (ă-brā′zhŭn) **1.** An excoriation, or circumscribed removal of the superficial layers of skin or mucous membrane. SYN abraded wound. **2.** A scraping away of a portion of the surface. **3.** In dentistry, the pathologic grinding or wearing away of tooth substance by incorrect tooth-brushing methods, the presence of foreign objects, bruxism, or similar causes. SYN grinding. SEE ALSO bruxism, abrade. Cf. attrition. SEE abrade.

a•bra•sive (ă-brā′siv) **1.** Causing abrasion. **2.** Any material used to produce abrasions. **3.** A substance used in dentistry for abrading, grinding, or polishing.

a•bra•sive•ness (ă-brā′siv-nes) **1.** The property of a substance that causes surface wear by friction. **2.** The capacity of one material to scratch or wear away another material.

ab•re•ac•tion (ab-rē-ak′shŭn) FREUDIAN PSYCHOANALYSIS an emotional release or catharsis associated with the recollection of previously repressed unpleasant experiences.

a•bro•si•a (ă-brō′zē-ă) Abstinence from food. [G. *abrōsia,* fasting]

ab•rup•tion (ab-rŭp′shŭn) A breaking away. [L. *abruptio,* Fr. *abrumpo,* to break off]

ab•rup•ti•o pla•cen•tae (ăb-rŭp′shē-ō plă-sen′tē) Premature detachment of a normally situated placenta.

ab•scess (ab′ses) **1.** A circumscribed collection of purulent exudate appearing in an acute or chronic localized infection, caused by tissue destruction and frequently associated with swelling, pain, and other signs of inflammation. **2.** A cavity formed by liquefactive necrosis within solid tissue; healing may be promoted by excision and drainage. [L. *abscessus,* a going away]

ab•scis•sion (ab-sĭ′zhŭn) Cutting away. [L. *abscindo,* pp. *-scissus,* to cut away from]

ab•sco•pal (ab-skō′păl) Denoting the effect that irradiation of a tissue has on remote nonirradiated tissue. [ab- + G. *skopos,* target, + -al]

ab•sco•pal ef•fect (ab-skō′păl e-fekt′) A reaction produced following irradiation but occurring outside the zone of actual radiation absorption.

ab•sence (ab′sĕns) Paroxysmal attacks of impaired consciousness, occasionally accompanied by spasm or twitching of cephalic muscles, which usually can be brought on by hyperventilation. [L. *absentia*]

ab•sence sei•zure (ab′sĕns sē′zhŭr) A brief seizure characterized by arrest of activity and occasionally clonic movements. There is loss of consciousness or slowing of thought. The EEG typically shows generalized spike wave discharges greater than 2.5 Hz. More prolonged absence seizures may have automatisms.

Ab•sid•i•a (ab-sid′ē-ă) A genus of fungi commonly found in nature. Thermophilic species survive in compost piles at temperatures exceeding 45°C and may cause zygomycosis in humans. A zygomycete, *Absidia* is differentiated from other members by the presence of rhizoids that are produced between sporangiophores.

ab•sinthe (ab′sinth) **1.** A woody European herb (*Artemisia absinthium*) formerly used as a flavoring agent, tonic, and vermifuge. The active principle is thujone (q.v.). **2.** A liquor consisting of 60–75% ethanol flavored with absinthium, anise, fennel, and other herbs, long banned in the U.S. and some other countries because of its toxic effects and addictiveness. SYN wormwood.

ab•so•lute en•dur•ance (ab′sō-lūt′ en-dūr′ăns) Muscular endurance that exists when the force of the tested contraction does not include or take into account interpersonal variance in strength.

ab•so•lute hu•mid•i•ty (ab-sŏ-lūt′ hyū-mid′i-tē) The mass of water vapor actually present per unit volume of gas or air.

ab•so•lute hy•per•o•pi•a (ab-sŏ-lūt′ hī′pĕr-ō′pē-ă) Manifest hyperopia that cannot be overcome by an effort of accommodation.

ab•so•lute rate ox•y•gen up•take (ab′sŏ-lūt′ rāt ok′si-jen ŭp′tāk) Rate of VO_2 conversion to energy expenditure or kilocalorie.

ab•so•lute re•frac•to•ry pe•ri•od (ab′sō-lūt′ rē-frak′tŏr-ē pēr′ē-ŏd) Period after the firing of a nerve fiber during which it cannot be induced to fire again by any stimulus, no matter how strong.

ab•so•lute scale (ab-sŏ-lūt′ skāl) SYN Kelvin scale.

ab•so•lute tem•per•a•ture (*T*) (ab-sŏ-lūt′ tem′pĕr-ă-chŭr) Temperature reckoned in the Kelvin scale from absolute zero.

ab•so•lute u•nit (ab-sŏ-lūt′ yū′nit) A unit the value of which remains constant regardless of place or time and not dependent on gravitation.

ab•so•lute ze•ro (ab-sŏ-lūt′ zēr′ō) The lowest possible temperature; the temperature at which the form of translational motion constituting heat is assumed no longer to exist, determined as −273.15°C or 0° Kelvin.

ab•sorb (ăb-sōr′b) **1.** To take in by absorption. **2.** To reduce the intensity of transmitted light. [L. *ab-sorbeo,* pp. *-sorptus,* to suck in]

ab•sorb•a•ble gel•a•tin film (ăb-sōr′bă-bĕl jel′ă-tin film) A sterile, nonantigenic, water-insoluble sheet of gelatin prepared by drying a gelatin-formaldehyde solution on plates; used in the closure and repair of defects in membranes such as the dura mater or the pleura; it undergoes absorption over a period of 1–6 months.

ab•sorb•a•ble su•ture (ăb-sōr′bă-bĕl sū′chŭr) Suture material dissolved by the body's enzymes during the healing process; used when deep tissue requires inner layers of suture to close a wound.

ab•sor•bance (*A*, A), ab•sor•ban•cy, ab•sorb•en•cy (ăb-sōr′băns, ăb-sōr′băn-sē, ăb-sōr′băn-sē) SPECTROPHOTOMETRY 2 minus the log of the percentage transmittance of light. SYN extinction (2), optic density.

ab•sorb•an•cy in•dex (ăb-sōr′băn-sē in′deks) **1.** SYN specific absorption coefficient. **2.** SYN molar absorption coefficient.

ab•sorbed dose (ăb-sōrbd′ dōs) **1.** The amount of a substance that is absorbed by the body by penetrating an epithelial barrier such as the skin, eyes, respiratory tract, or gastrointestinal tract. **2.** The amount of energy absorbed per unit mass of irradiated material at the target site. **3.** RADIATION THERAPY The former unit for absorbed dose is the rad; the current (SI) unit is the gray.

ab•sor•bent (ăb-sōr′bĕnt) **1.** Having the power to soak up or take into itself a gas, liquid, light rays, or heat. SYN absorptive. **2.** Any substance possessing such power. **3.** Material (usually caustic) to remove carbon dioxide from circuits in which rebreathing occurs (e.g., anesthesia equipment).

ab•sorb•ent gauze (ăb-sōr′bĕnt gawz) White cotton cloth in folds or rolls used for surgical or wound dressings.

ab•sorp•ti•om•etry (ăb-sōrp′shē-om′ĕ-trē) A measure of the absorption of one thing by another. [absorption + -metry]

ab•sorp•tion (ăb-sōrp′shŭn) **1.** The taking in, incorporation, or reception of gases, liquids, light, or heat. Cf. adsorption. **2.** RADIOLOGY the uptake of energy from radiation by the tissue or medium through which it passes. **3.** MEDICAL PHYSICS the number of disintegrations per second of a radionuclide. Radioactivity. Unit (SI): becquerel. **4.** NUTRITION uptake of nutrients and nonnutrients by cells in the GI tract. **5.** The process by which a compound penetrates an epithelial barrier such as the skin, eyes, respiratory tract, or gastrointestinal tract to reach the interior of the body. SEE ALSO absorbed dose, internal dose. [L. *absorptio*, fr. *absorbeo*, to swallow]

ab•sorp•tion chro•ma•tog•ra•phy (ăb-sōrp′shŭn krō′mă-tog′ră-fē) SYN chromatography.

ab·sorp·tion co·ef·fi·cient (ăb-sōrp′shŭn kō-ĕ-fish′ĕnt) **1.** The milliliters of a gas at standard temperature and pressure that will saturate 100 mL of liquid. **2.** The amount of light absorbed in passing through 1 cm of a 1 molar solution of a given substance, expressed as a constant in Beer-Lambert law. **3.** RADIOLOGY a measure of the rate of decrease of intensity of a beam in its passage through matter, resulting from a combination of scattering and conversion to other forms of energy. SEE ALSO attenuation.

ab·sorp·tion lines (ăb-sōrp′shŭn līnz) Dark lines in the solar spectrum due to absorption by the solar and the earth's atmosphere.

ab·sorp·tion spec·trum (ăb-sōrp′shŭn spek′trŭm) The spectrum observed after light has passed through, and been partially absorbed by, a solution or translucent substance. Many molecular groupings have characteristic light absorption patterns, which can be used for detection and quantitative assay.

ab·sorp·tive (ăb-sōrp′tiv) SYN absorbent (1).

ab·sorp·tiv·i·ty (*a*) (ab-sōrp-tiv′i-tē) **1.** SYN specific absorption coefficient. **2.** SYN molar absorption coefficient.

ab·sti·nence (ab′sti-nĕns) Refraining from the use of certain articles of diet, alcoholic beverages, illegal drugs, or from sexual intercourse. [L. *abs-tineo,* to hold back, fr. *teneo,* to hold]

ab·stract (ab′strakt) **1.** A condensation, summary, or brief description of a scientific or literary article or the results of a study. **2.** A preparation made by evaporating a fluid extract to a powder and triturating it with milk sugar. **3.** To collect information from the medical record for research, billing, or statistical purposes. [L. *abs-traho,* pp. *-tractus,* to draw away]

ab·strac·tion (ăb-strak′shŭn) **1.** Distillation or separation of the volatile constituents of a substance. **2.** Exclusive mental concentration. **3.** The making of an abstract from a crude drug. **4.** Malocclusion in which the teeth or associated structures are lower than their normal occlusal plane. **5.** The process of selecting a certain aspect of a concept from the whole. [L. *abs-traho,* pp. *-tractus,* to draw away]

ab·stract think·ing (ab′strakt thingk′ing) Consideration in terms of concepts and general principles (e.g., perceiving a table and a chair as furniture), as contrasted with concrete thinking.

ab·ter·mi·nal (ab-ter′mi-năl) In a direction away from the end and toward the center; denoting the course of an electrical current in a muscle. [L. *ab,* from, + *terminus,* end]

a·bu·li·a (ā-bū′lē-ă) **1.** Loss or impairment of the ability to perform voluntary actions or to make decisions. **2.** Reduction in speech, movement, thought, and emotional reaction; a common result of bilateral frontal lobe disease. [G. *a-* priv. + *boulē,* will]

a·bu·lic (ā-bū′lĭk) Relating to, or suffering from, abulia.

a·buse (ă-byūs′) **1.** Misuse, wrong use, especially excessive use, of anything, intentionally or unintentionally. **2.** Injurious, harmful, or offensive treatment, as in child abuse or sexual abuse

a·but·ment (ă-bŭt′mĕnt) DENTISTRY a natural tooth or implanted tooth substitute, used to support or anchor a fixed or removable prosthesis.

AC, ac, a.c. **1.** Abbreviation for alternating current; ante cibum. **2.** NATO code for hydrogen cyanide.

Ac Abbreviation for actinium; acetyl.

AC:A Abbreviation for accommodative convergence accommodation ratio.

A·ca·ci·a (ă-kā′shē-ă) **1.** A tree or shrub with distribution in arid geographic regions. **2.** Gum arabic, the dried gummy exudation from *Acacia senegal* and other species of *Acacia* (family Leguminosae), prepared as a and syrup; used as an emollient, demulcent, excipient, and suspending agent in pharmaceuticals and foods; formerly used as a transfusion fluid. SYN gum arabic. [G. *akakia*]

A·cad·e·my of Cer·ti·fied So·cial Work·ers (ACSW) (ă-kad′ĕ-mē sĕr′ti-fīd sō′shăl wŏrk-ĕrz) A professional organization, established in 1960, which offers credentials to social workers to certify that they have attained and have maintained a measurable level of expertise in their discipline.

a·cal·cu·li·a (ā-kal′kyū-lē-ă) A form of aphasia characterized by the inability to perform simple mathematical problems; found with lesions of the cerebral hemispheres, and often an early sign of dementia. [G. *a-* priv. + L. *calculo,* to reckon]

a·can·tha (ă-kan′thă) **1.** A spine or spinous process. **2.** The spinous process of a vertebra. [G. *akantha,* a thorn]

acanthaesthesia [Br.] SYN acanthesthesia.

a·can·tha·me·bi·a·sis (ă-kan′thă-mē-bī′ă-sis) Infection by free-living soil amebae of the genus *Acanthamoeba* that may result in a necrotizing dermal or tissue invasion, or a fulminating and usually fatal primary amebic meningoencephalitis. SYN acanthamoebiasis.

***A·can·tha·moe·ba* me·di·um** (ă-kan-thă-mē′bă mē′dē-ŭm) Nonnutrient agar plates with an *Escherichia coli* overlay used to detect the presence of *Acanthamoeba* or *Naegleria* in tissue or soil samples.

acanthamoebiasis [Br.] SYN acanthamebiasis.

a·can·thes·the·si·a (ă-kan′thes-thē′zē-ă) Paresthesia in which there is the sensation of a pinprick. SYN acanthaesthesia. [G. *akantha,* thorn, + *aisthēsis,* sensation]

a•can•thi•on (ă-kan′thē-on) The tip of the anterior nasal spine. [G. *akantha,* thorn]

♻**acantho-** Prefix meaning a spinous process; spiny, thorny. [G. *akantha,* a thorn, the backbone, the spine, fr. *akē,* a point, + *anthos,* a flower]

a•can•tho•cyte (ă-kan′thō-sīt) **1.** Erythrocytes characterized by spiny cytoplasmic projections. SYN acanthrocytes. **2.** Sharp thornlike projections on their outer edges; inherited abnormality may be seen in retinitis pigmentosa. [acantho- + G. *kytos,* cell]

a•can•tho•cy•to•sis (ă-kan′thō-sī-tō′sis) A rare condition in which most erythrocytes are acanthocytes; a regular finding in abetalipoproteinemia. SYN acanthrocytosis.

a•can•thoid (ă-kan′thoyd) Spine shaped.

ac•an•thol•y•sis (ak′an-thol′i-sis) Separation of individual epidermal keratinocytes from their neighbors, as in conditions such as pemphigus vulgaris and Darier disease. [acantho- + G. *lysis,* loosening]

ac•an•tho•ma (ak′an-thō′mă) A tumor formed by proliferation of epithelial squamous cells. SEE ALSO keratoacanthoma. [acantho- + G. *-oma,* tumor]

a•can•tho•me•a•tal line (ă-kan′thō-mē-ā′tăl līn) An imaginary line between the acanthion and the external auditory meatus; used for radiographic positioning of the skull.

a•can•thor•rhex•is (ă-kan-thŏ-rek′sis) Rupture of the intercellular bridges of the prickle cell layer of the epidermis, as in contact-type dermatitis. SEE spongiosis. [acantho + G. *rhexis,* rupture]

ac•an•tho•sis (ak-an-thō′sis) An increase in the thickness of the stratum spinosum of the epidermis. [acantho- + G. *-osis,* condition]

ac•an•tho•sis ni•gri•cans (ak-an-thō′sis nī′gri-kanz) An eruption of velvet warty benign growths and hyperpigmentation occurring in the skin of the axillae, neck, anogenital area, and groins; in adults, may be associated with internal malignancy, endocrine disorders, or obesity; a benign (juvenile) type occurs in children. [L. fr. *niger,* black]

ac•an•thot•ic (ak-an-thot′ik) Pertaining to or characteristic of acanthosis.

a•can•thro•cytes (ă-kan′thrŏ-sīts) SYN acanthocyte (1).

a•can•thro•cy•to•sis (ă-kan′thrō-sī-tō′sis) SYN acanthocytosis.

a•cap•ni•a (ă-kap′nē-ă) Absence of carbon dioxide in the blood. USAGE NOTE sometimes used erroneously for hypocapnia. [G. *a-* priv. + *kapnos,* smoke]

a•car•di•a (ā-kahr′dē-ă) Congenital absence of the heart; a condition sometimes occurring in monozygotic twins or in the smaller of conjoined twins when its partner monopolizes the placental blood supply. [G. *a-* priv. + *kardia,* heart]

ac•a•ri•a•sis (ak′ăr-ī′ă-sĭs) Any disease caused by mites, usually a skin infestation. SEE mange. SYN acaridiasis, acarinosis.

a•car•i•cide (ă-kar′i-sīd) An agent that kills acarines; commonly used to denote chemicals that kill ticks. [Mod. L. *acarus,* a mite, fr. G. *akari* + L. *caedo,* to cut, kill]

ac•a•rid (ak′ă-rid) A general term for a member of the family Acaridae or for a mite. [G. *akari,* mite]

A•car•i•dae (ă-kar′i-dē) A family of the order Acarina, a large group of exceptionally small mites, usually 0.5 mm or less, abundant in dried fruits and meats, grain, meal, and flour; frequently a cause of severe dermatitis among people hypersensitized by frequent handling of infested products.

ac•ar•i•di•a•sis (ak-ăr-i-dī′ă-sis) SYN acariasis.

Ac•a•ri•na (ak-ă-rī′nă) An order of Arachnida that includes mites and ticks. [G. *akari,* a mite]

ac•a•rine (ak′ă-rīn) A member of the order Acarina.

ac•ar•i•no•sis (ak′ă-ri-nō′sis) SYN acariasis.

ac•a•ro•der•ma•ti•tis (ak′ă-rō-dĕr-mă-tī′tis) A skin inflammation or eruption produced by a mite. [G. *akari,* mite, + *derma* (*dermat-*), skin]

ac•a•ro•pho•bi•a (ak′ă-rō-fō′bē-ă) Morbid fear of small parasites, small particles, or itching. [G. *akari,* mite, + *phobos,* fear]

Ac•a•rus (ak′ă-rŭs) A genus of mites of the family Acaridae. [G. *akari,* mite]

Ac•a•rus sca•bi•e•i (ak′ăr-ŭs skā′bē-ī) Former term for *Sarcoptes scabiei.*

a•car•y•ote (ă-kar′ē-ōt) SYN akaryocyte.

ACBE Abbreviation for air contrast barium enema.

ac•cel•er•ant (ak-sel′ĕr-ănt) SYN accelerator (3).

ac•cel•er•at•ed hy•per•ten•sion (ak-sel′ĕr-ā-tĕd hī′pĕr-ten′shŭn) Hypertension advancing rapidly with increasing blood pressure and associated with acute and rapidly worsening signs and symptoms.

ac•cel•er•at•ed id•i•o•ven•tric•u•lar rhythm (ak-sel′ĕr-ā-tĕd id′ē-ō-ven-trik′yū-lăr ridh′ŭm) Tachycardia originating from a ventricular pacemaker.

ac•cel•er•a•ted junc•tion•al rhythm (ak-sel′ĕr-ā-tĕd jŭngk′shŭn-ăl ridh′ĕm) Cardiac activation arising from the atrioventricular junction at a rate between 60 and 100 beats per minute.

ac·cel·er·a·tion-de·cel·er·a·tion in·ju·ry (ak-sel-ĕr-ā′shŭn-dē′sel-ĕr-ā′shŭn in′jŭr-ē) SYN whiplash injury.

ac·cel·er·a·tion in·ju·ry (ak-sel′ĕr-ā′shŭn in′jŭr-ē) Injury sustained when the body is abruptly set in motion from a position of rest, referring especially to injuries of the head or neck in rear-end automobile collisions.

ac·cel·er·a·tor (ak-sel′ĕr-ā-tŏr) **1.** Anything that increases rapidity of action or function. **2.** PHYSIOLOGY a nerve, muscle, or substance that quickens movement or response. **3.** A catalytic agent used to hasten a chemical reaction. SYN accelerant. **4.** NUCLEAR PHYSICS a device that accelerates charged particles (e.g., protons) to high speed to produce nuclear reactions in a target, often for the production of radionuclides or for radiation therapy. [L. *accelerans,* pres. p. of *ac-celero,* to hasten, fr. *celer,* swift]

ac·cel·er·a·tor fac·tor (ak-sel′ĕ-rā-tŏr fak′tŏr) SYN factor V.

ac·cel·er·a·tor fi·bers (ak-sel′ĕr-ā-tŏr fī′bĕrz) Postganglionic sympathetic nerve fibers originating in the superior, middle, and inferior cervical ganglia of the sympathetic trunk, conveying nervous impulses to the heart that increase the rapidity and force of the cardiac pulsations. SYN accelerator fibres.

accelerator fibres [Br.] SYN accelerator fibers.

ac·cel·er·a·tor glob·u·lin (AcG, ac-g) (ak-sel′ĕr-ā-tŏr glob′yū-lin) Blood protein in serum that promotes the conversion of prothrombin to thrombin in the presence of thromboplastin and ionized calcium. SEE factor V, serum accelerator globulin.

ac·cel·er·a·tor nerves (ak-sel′ĕr-ā-tŏr nĕrvz) Certain of the cardiopulmonary splanchnic nerves establishing sympathetic innervation of the heart; originating from ganglion cells of the superior, middle, and inferior cervical ganglion of the sympathetic trunk, the unmyelinated efferent fibers of the accelerator nerves stimulate an increase in the heart rate.

ac·cen·tu·a·tor (ak-sen′chū-ā-tŏr) A substance (e.g., aniline) the presence of which allows a combination between a tissue or histologic element and a stain that might otherwise be impossible. [L. *accentus,* accent, fr. *cano,* to sing]

ac·cep·ta·ble dai·ly in·take (ADI) (ak-sep′tă-bĕl dā′lē in′tāk) SEE acceptable intake.

ac·cept·a·ble in·take (AI) (ak-sep′tă-bĕl in′tāk) Value for suggested daily intake of a nutrient in cases in which data are insufficient to determine an estimated average requirement (EAR) and thus a recommended dietary allowance (RDA). The issuance of an AI indicates that more research is needed to determine the mean and distribution of requirements for that specific nutrient. SEE ALSO Dietary Reference Intake.

ac·cept·a·ble mac·ro·nu·tri·ent dis·tri·bu·tion range (AMDR) (ak-sep′tă-bĕl mak′rō-nū′trē-ĕnt dis′tri-byū′shŭn rānj) A range of intakes for a particular energy source that is associated with reduced risk of chronic disease while providing adequate intakes of essential nutrients. Expressed as a percentage of total energy intake, AMDR have been established for protein, carbohydrate, fat, and linoleic (n-6) and alpha-linolenic (n-3) polyunsaturated fatty acids.

ac·cep·tor (ak-sept′ŏr) A compound that will take up a chemical group (e.g., an amine group, a methyl group, a carbamoyl group) from another compound (the donor). [L. *ac-cipio,* pp. *-ceptus,* to accept]

ac·cess (ak′ses) **1.** A way or means of approach or admittance. **2.** The space required for visualization and for manipulation of instruments to remove decay and prepare a tooth for restoration. **3.** The opening in the crown of a tooth required to allow adequate admittance to the pulp space to clean, shape, and seal the root canal(s) during endodontic or root canal therapy. **4.** A patient's entry into health care process; admittance and ability to get care. [L. *accessus*]

ac·ces·si·bil·i·ty (ak-ses′ă-bil′i-tē) The degree to which someone can use something in his or her environment or society; has a common application in regard to people with disabilities and access to a service or a physical space. SEE ALSO health-related quality of life, Americans with Disabilities Act.

ac·ces·so·ry (ak-ses′ŏr-ē) ANATOMY denoting a muscle, nerve, gland, or similar, which is auxiliary or supernumerary to some other, generally more important structure. [L. *accessorius,* fr. *ac-cedo,* pp. *-cessus,* to move toward]

ac·ces·so·ry cell (ak-ses′ŏr-ē sel) SYN antigen-presenting cell.

ac·ces·so·ry ce·phal·ic vein (ak-ses′ŏr-ē sĕ-fal′ik vān) A variable vein that passes along the radial border of the forearm to join the cephalic vein near the elbow. SYN vena cephalica accessoria [TA].

ac·ces·so·ry gland (ak-ses′ŏr-ē gland) A small mass of glandular structure, detached from but lying near another and larger gland, to which it is similar in structure and probably in function.

ac·ces·so·ry hem·i·a·zy·gos vein (ak-ses′ŏr-ē hem′ē-ā-zī′gos vān) Formed by the union of the fourth to seventh left posterior intercostal veins, passes along the side of the bodies of the fifth, sixth, and seventh thoracic vertebrae, then crosses the midline behind the aorta, esophagus, and thoracic duct, and empties into the azygos vein, sometimes in common with the hemiazygos vein. SYN vena hemiazygos accessoria [TA].

ac·ces·so·ry lig·a·ments (ak-ses′ŏr-ē lig′ă-mĕnts) Ligaments about a joint that are in addition to the articular capsule. They may lie within or on the outside of the latter.

ac•ces•so•ry mol•e•cules (ak-ses′ŏr-ē mol′ĕ-kyūlz) Cell surface adhesion molecules on T cells that are involved in binding of one cell to another cell or in signal transduction.

ac•ces•so•ry nerve [CN XI] (ak-ses′ŏr-ē nĕrv) Arises by two sets of roots: the presumed cranial, emerging from the side of the medulla, and spinal, emerging from the ventrolateral part of the first five cervical segments of the spinal cord; these roots unite to form the accessory nerve trunk, which divides into two branches, internal and external; the internal branch, carrying fibers of the cranial root, unites with the vagus in the jugular foramen and supplies the muscles of the pharynx, larynx, and soft palate; the external branch continues independently through the jugular foramen to supply the sternocleidomastoid and trapezius muscles. Although the accessory nerve was originally believed to have cranial and spinal roots, it is now the general view that the so-called cranial root is actually a portion of the vagus nerve. SYN nervus accessorius [CN XI] [TA], eleventh cranial nerve [CN XI].

ac•ces•so•ry nip•ple (ak-ses′ŏr-ē nip′ĕl) A supernumerary nipple occurring on the mammary crest or line.

ac•ces•so•ry ob•tu•ra•tor ar•ter•y (ak-ses′ŏr-ē ob′tū-rā-tŏr ahr′tĕr-ē) Term applied to the anastomosis of the pubic branch of the inferior epigastric artery with the pubic branch of the obturator artery when it contributes a significant supply through the obturator canal. SYN arteria obturatoria accessoria [TA].

ac•ces•so•ry or•gans of the eye (ak-ses′ŏr-ē ōr′gănz ī) The eyelids, with lashes and eyebrows, lacrimal apparatus, conjunctival sac, and extrinsic muscles of the eyeball.

ac•ces•so•ry pan•cre•at•ic duct (ak-ses′ŏr-ē pan-krē-at′ik dŭkt) The excretory duct of the head of the pancreas, one branch of which joins the pancreatic duct, the other opening independently into the duodenum at the lesser duodenal papilla. SYN ductus pancreaticus accessorius [TA], Bernard duct, Santorini canal, Santorini duct.

ac•ces•so•ry phren•ic nerves (ak-ses′ŏr-ē fren′ik nĕrvz) Accessory nerve strands that arise from the fifth cervical nerve, often as branches of the nerve to the subclavius, passing downward to join the phrenic nerve. SYN nervi phrenici accessorii [TA].

ac•ces•so•ry spleen (ak-ses′ŏr-ē splēn) One of the small globular masses of splenic tissue occasionally found in the region of the spleen, in one of the peritoneal folds, or elsewhere. SYN lien accessorius.

ac•ces•so•ry su•pra•re•nal (ak-ses′ŏr-ē sū′pră-rē′năl) An island of cortical tissue separate from the suprarenal gland, usually found in the retroperitoneal tissues, kidney, or genital organs. SYN adrenal rest.

ac•ces•so•ry symp•tom (ak-ses′ŏr-ē simp′tŏm) A symptom that usually but not always accompanies a certain disease, as distinguished from a pathognomonic symptom. SYN concomitant symptom.

ac•ces•so•ry ver•te•bral vein (ak-ses′ŏr-ē vĕr′tĕ-brăl vān) A vein that accompanies the vertebral vein but passes through the foramen of the transverse process of the seventh cervical vertebra and opens independently into the brachiocephalic vein. SYN vena vertebralis accessoria [TA].

ac•ci•dent (ak′si-dĕnt) An unanticipated but often predictable event leading to injury (e.g., in traffic, industry, or a domestic setting) or such an event that develops in the course of a disease. [L. *ac-cido,* to happen]

ac•ci•den•tal hy•po•ther•mi•a (ak-si-den′tăl hī′pō-thĕr′mē-ă) Unintentional decrease in body temperature, especially in the newborn, infants, and elderly, particularly during operations. Also associated with exposure to wet and cold environments, rather than to diseases.

ac•ci•den•tal my•i•a•sis (ak-si-den′tăl mī-ī′ă-sis) Gastrointestinal myiasis from ingestion of contaminated food.

ac•ci•den•tal par•a•site (ak-si-den′tăl par′ă-sīt) SYN incidental parasite.

ac•ci•dent-prone (ak′si-dĕnt-prōn) Term denoting one who suffers a greater number of accidents than an average person.

acclimatisation [Br.] SYN acclimatization.

ac•cli•ma•ti•za•tion, ac•cli•ma•tion (ă-klī′mă-tī-zā′shŭn, ak-li-mā′shŭn) Physiologic adaptation to a variation in environmental factors such as temperature, climate, or altitude. SYN acclimatisation.

ac•com•mo•dat•ing re•sis•tance (ă-kom′ŏ-dā-ting rĕ-zis′tăns) In isokinetic testing or training, application of a counterforce to muscle action to regulate the speed of contraction.

ac•com•mo•da•tion (ă-kom′ŏ-dā′shŭn) **1.** The act or state of adjustment or adaptation; especially change in the shape of the ocular lens for various focal distances. **2.** SENSORIMOTOR THEORY the alteration of schemata or cognitive expectations to conform with experience. **3.** The ability of the ciliary muscle to adjust the curvature of the lens, increasing it for near vision and decreasing it for distant vision. [L. *ac-commodo,* pp. *-atus,* to adapt, fr. *modus,* a measure]

ac•com•mo•da•tion re•flex (ă-kom′ŏ-dā′shŭn rē′fleks) Increased convexity of the lens, due to contraction of the ciliary muscle and relaxation of the suspensory ligament, to maintain a distinct retinal image.

ac·com·mo·da·tive (ă-kom′ŏ-dā-tiv) Relating to accommodation.

ac·com·mo·da·tive as·the·no·pi·a (ă-kom′ŏ-dā-tiv as′thĕ-nō′pē-ă) Ocular discomfort, headache, and other symptoms of eyestrain resulting from refractive error and excessive contraction of ciliary muscle.

ac·com·mo·da·tive con·ver·gence ac·com·mo·da·tion ra·ti·o (AC:A) (ă-kom′ŏ-dā′tiv kŏn-vĕr′jĕns ă-kom′ŏ-dā′shŭn rā′shē-ō) The amount of convergence (measured in prism diopters of convergence) divided by the amount of accommodation (measured in diopters) required to direct both eyes on an object.

ac·com·mo·da·tive in·suf·fi·cien·cy (ă-kom′ŏ-dā-tiv in′sŭ-fish′ĕn-sē) A lack of appropriate accommodation for near focus.

ac·cor·di·on graft (ă-kōr′dē-ŏn graft) A skin graft in which multiple slits have been made, so it can be stretched to cover a large area.

ac·cou·cheur's hand (ah-kū-shĕrz′ hand) Position of the hand in tetany or in muscular dystrophy; the fingers are flexed at the metacarpophalangeal joints and extended at the phalangeal joints, with the thumb flexed and adducted into the palm; in resemblance to the position of the physician's hand in making a vaginal examination. SYN obstetric hand.

ac·counts pay·a·ble (AP, A/P) (ă-kownts′ pā′ă-bĕl) The aggregate of money owed by the health care practice or hospital to its suppliers and employees.

ac·counts re·ceiv·a·ble (AR, A/R) (ă-kownts′ rē-sē′vă-bĕl) The aggregate of money owed to the health care practice by all patients and/or insurers.

ac·cred·i·ta·tion (ă-kred′i-tā′shŭn) Approval, certification, or endorsement by an authority. [F. *accréditation*, fr. L. *ad-*, to, + *credo, creditum*, to believe, trust]

ac·cre·ti·o cor·dis (ă-krē′shē-ō kōr′dis) Pericarditis involving adhesion extending from the pericardium to the mediastinum, pleura, diaphragm, and chest wall.

ac·cre·tion (ă-krē′shŭn) **1.** Increase by addition to the periphery of material of the same nature as that already present; e.g., the manner of growth of crystals. **2.** DENTISTRY foreign material (usually plaque or calculus) collecting on the surface of a tooth or in a cavity. **3.** A growing together of parts normally separate. [L. *accretio*, fr. *ad*, to, + *crescere,* to grow]

ac·cre·tion·ar·y growth (ă-krē′shŭn-ar-ē grōth) Growth by an increase of intercellular material.

ac·cul·tur·a·tion (ă-kŭl′chŭr-ā′shŭn) Adaptation by a person or group to customs, values, beliefs, and behaviors of a new country or culture.

ac·cur·a·cy (ak′kyūr-ă-sē) The degree to which a measurement represents the true value of the attribute that is being measured; refers to the closeness of an analytic result to an actual result. In the laboratory, accuracy of a test is determined when possible by comparing results from the test in question with results generated from an established reference method.

ACE Abbreviation for angiotensin-converting enzyme.

a·cel·lu·lar (ā-sel′yū-lăr) **1.** Devoid of cells. **2.** A term applied to unicellular organisms that do not become multicellular and are complete within a single cell unit. [G. *a-* priv. + L. *cellula,* a small chamber]

a·cen·tric (ā-sen′trik) **1.** Lacking a center. **2.** CYTOGENETICS denoting a chromosome fragment without a centromere. [G. *a-* priv. + *kentron,* center]

a·ce·phal·gic mi·graine (ā-se-fal′jik mī′grān) A classic migraine episode in which the teichopsia is not followed by a headache.

a·ce·pha·li·a, **a·ceph·a·lism** (ā-sĕ-fā′lē-ă, ā-sef′ă-lizm) SYN acephaly.

a·ceph·a·lo·car·di·a (ā-sef′ă-lō-kahr′dē-ă) Absence of head and heart in a parasitic twin. [G. *a-* priv. + *kephalē,* head, + *kardia,* heart]

a·ceph·a·lo·chei·ri·a, **a·ceph·a·lo·chi·ri·a** (ā-sef′ă-lō-kī′rē-ă) Congenital absence of head and hands. [G. *a-* priv. + *kephalē,* head, + *cheir,* hand]

a·ceph·a·lo·gas·ter·i·a (ā-sef′ă-lō-gas-tĕr′ē-ă) Congenital absence of head, thorax, and abdomen in a parasitic twin with pelvis and lower limbs only.

a·ceph·a·lo·po·di·a (ā-sef′ă-lō-pō′dē-ă) Congenital absence of head and feet. [G. *a-* priv. + *kephalē,* head, + *pous,* foot]

a·ceph·a·lo·sto·mi·a (ă-sef′ă-lō-stō′mē-ă) Congenital absence of most of the head with, however, the presence of a mouthlike opening. [G. *a-* priv. + *kephalē,* head, + *stoma,* mouth]

a·ceph·a·lo·tho·ra·ci·a (ā-sef′ă-lō-thōr-ā′sē-ă) Congenital absence of head and thorax. [G. *a-* priv. + *kephalē,* head, + *thorax,* chest]

a·ceph·a·lous (ā-sef′ă-lŭs) Headless.

a·ceph·a·lus (ā-sef′ă-lŭs) A headless fetus. [G. *a-* priv. + *kephalē,* head]

a·ceph·a·ly (ā-sef′ă-lē) Congenital absence of the head. SYN acephalia, acephalism. [G. *a-* priv. + *kephalē,* head]

♻**acet-, aceto-** Combining forms denoting the two-carbon fragment of acetic acid.

ac•e•tab•u•la (as-ĕ-tab′yū-lă) Plural of acetabulum.

ac•e•tab•u•lar (as-ĕ-ta′byū-lăr) Relating to the acetabulum.

ac•e•tab•u•lar fos•sa (as-ĕ-ta′byū-lăr fos′ă) A depressed area in the floor of the acetabulum superior to the acetabular notch. SYN fossa acetabuli [TA].

ac•e•tab•u•lec•to•my (as′ĕ-ta-byū-lek-tŏ-mē) Excision of the acetabulum. [acetabulum + G. *ektomē,* excision]

ac•e•tab•u•lo•plas•ty (as-ĕ-ta-byū-lō-plas-tē) Any operation aimed at restoring the acetabulum to as near a normal state as possible. [acetabulum + G. *plastos,* formed]

ac•e•tab•u•lum, pl. **ac•e•tab•u•la** (as-ĕ-tab′yū-lŭm, -lă) [TA] A cup-shaped depression on the external surface of the hip bone, with which the head of the femur articulates. SYN cotyloid cavity. [L. vinegar cup]

ac•e•tal (as′ĕ-tăl) Product of the addition of 2 mol alcohol to 1 mol of an aldehyde. SEE ALSO hemiacetal, hemiketal, ketal.

ac•et•al•de•hyde (as′ĕ-tal′dĕ-hīd) An intermediary product in the metabolism of alcohol.

ac•e•tate (as′ĕ-tāt) A salt or ester of acetic acid.

ac•e•tate-CoA li•gase (as′ĕ-tāt lī′gās) SYN acetyl-CoA ligase.

ac•e•tate thi•o•ki•nase (as′ĕ-tāt thī-ō-kī′nās) SYN acetyl-CoA ligase.

ac•e•to•ac•e•tate (as′ĕ-tō-as′ĕ-tāt) A salt or ion of acetoacetic acid. A ketone body formed in ketogenesis.

ac•e•to•a•ce•tic ac•id (as′ĕ-tō-ă-sē′tik) One of the ketone bodies, formed in excess and appearing in the urine in starvation or in diabetic acidosis. SYN diacetic acid.

ac•e•to•a•ce•tyl-CoA (as′ĕ-tō-ă-sē′til) Intermediate in the oxidation of fatty acids and in the formation of ketone bodies; also formed from two molecules of acetyl-CoA; major role is condensation with acetyl-CoA to form the important β-hydroxy-β-methylglutaryl-CoA. SYN acetyl-coenzyme A, active acetate.

ac•e•to•a•ce•tyl-CoA thi•o•lase (as′ĕ-tō-ă-sē′til thī′ō-lās) SYN acetyl-CoA acetyltransferase.

acetonaemia [Br.] SYN acetonemia.

ac•e•tone (as′ĕ-tōn) A colorless, volatile, inflammable liquid; small amounts are found in normal urine, but larger quantities occur in urine and blood of diabetic patients; sometimes imparts an ethereal odor to the urine and breath as a result of starvation or excessive vomiting. Used as a solvent in some pharmaceutical and commercial preparations.

ac•e•tone bod•y (as′ĕ-tōn bod′ē) SYN ketone body.

ac•e•ton•e•mi•a (as′ĕ-tŏ-nē′mē-ă) The presence of acetone or acetone bodies in relatively large amounts in the blood. SYN acetonaemia. [acetone + G. *haima,* blood]

ac•e•to•nu•ri•a (as′e-tō-nyūr′ē-ă) Excretion in the urine of large amounts of acetone. [acetone + G. *ouron,* urine]

ace•to•whit•en•ing (ă-sē′tō-wīt′ĕn-ing) Blanching of skin or mucous membranes after application of 3–5% acetic acid solution, a sign of increased cellular protein and increased nuclear density; used particularly on genital skin and mucous membranes, including the uterine cervix, to identify zones of squamous cell change for biopsy and condyloma acuminatum for treatment. SYN cervicoscopy, visual inspection with acetic acid. [acetic acid + whitening]

a•ce•tyl (Ac) (as′ĕ-til) An acetic acid molecule from which the hydroxyl group has been removed.

a•ce•tyl-ac•ti•vat•ing en•zyme (as′ĕ-til-ak′ti-vāt-ing en′zīm) SYN acetyl-CoA ligase.

a•cet•y•lase (a-set′il-ās) Any enzyme catalyzing acetylation or deacetylation, as in the formation of *N*-acetylglutamate from glutamate plus acetyl-CoA, or the reverse; acetylases are usually called acetyltransferases.

a•cet•y•la•tion (a-set′i-lā′shŭn) Formation of an acetyl derivative.

a•ce•tyl•cho•line (ACh) A neurotransmitter that stimulates nicotinic receptors in autonomic ganglia, at the motor endplates of skeletal muscle, and in the central nervous system as well as muscarinic receptors in smooth muscle, in exocrine glands, and in the central nervous system.

ac•e•tyl•cho•lin•est•er•ase (AChE) (as′ĕ-til-kō′lin-es′tĕr-ās) One of a family of enzymes capable of catalyzing the hydrolysis of acetylcholine.

a•ce•tyl-CoA (as′ĕ-til) Condensation product of coenzyme A and acetic acid, symbolized as $CoAS{\sim}COCH_3$; intermediate in transfer of two-carbon fragment, notably in its entrance into the tricarboxylic acid cycle and in fatty acid synthesis.

a•ce•tyl-CoA a•ce•tyl•trans•fer•ase (as′ĕ-til as′e-til-trans′fĕr-ās) An acetyltransferase forming acetoacetyl-CoA from two molecules of acetyl-CoA, releasing one CoA. A key step in ketogenesis and sterol synthesis. SYN acetoacetyl-CoA thiolase, acetyl-CoA thiolase.

a•ce•tyl-CoA li•gase (as′ĕ-til lī′gās) A ligase that catalyzes the reaction of acetate and CoA and ATP to form AMP, pyrophosphate, and acetyl-CoA. A key step in the activation of acetate. SYN acetate thiokinase, acetate-CoA ligase, acetyl-activating enzyme, acetyl-CoA synthetase.

a•ce•tyl-CoA syn•the•tase (as′ĕ-til sin′thĕ-tās) SYN acetyl-CoA ligase.

a•ce•tyl-CoA thi•o•lase (as′ĕ-til thī-ō-lāz) SYN acetyl-CoA acetyltransferase.

a•ce•tyl-co•en•zyme A (as′ĕ-til-kō-en′zīm) SYN acetoacetyl-CoA.

a•ce•tyl•sal•i•cy•lic ac•id (ASA) (as′e-til-sal-i-sil′ik as′id) Generic name of aspirin; this term is used in Canada and other countries where Aspirin remains a proprietary term.

a•ce•tyl•trans•fer•ase (as′e-til-trans′fĕr-ās) Any enzyme transferring acetyl groups from one compound to another. SEE ALSO choline acetyltransferase. SYN transacetylase.

AcG, ac-g Abbreviation for accelerator globulin.

ACh Abbreviation for acetylcholine.

a•cha•la•si•a (ak-ă-lā′zē-ă) Failure to relax; referring especially to visceral openings such as the pylorus, cardia, or any other sphincter muscles. [G. *a-* priv. + *chalasis,* a slackening]

ach•a•la•si•a of the car•di•a (ak-ă-lā′zē-ă kahr′dē-ă) SYN esophageal achalasia.

ach•a•la•si•a of the up•per sphinc•ter (ak-ă-lā′zē-ă ŭp′ĕr sfingk′tĕr) SYN cricopharyngeal achalasia.

AChE Abbreviation for acetylcholinesterase; anticholinesterase.

ache (āk) A dull or generalized localized pain, usually one of less than severe intensity.

a•chei•ri•a (ă-kī′rē-ă) **1.** Congenital absence of one or both hands. **2.** Anesthesia in, with loss of the sense of possession of, one or both hands. **3.** A form of dyscheiria in which the patient is unable to tell which side of the body has received a stimulus. [G. *a-* priv. + *cheir,* hand]

a•chei•rop•o•dy, a•chi•rop•o•dy (ă-kī-rop′ŏ-dē, ă-kī-rop′ŏ-dē) Congenital absence of the hands and feet; autosomal recessive inheritance. [G. *a-* priv. + *cheir,* hand, + *podos,* foot]

a•chei•rous, a•chi•rous (ă-kī′rŭs, ă-kī′rŭs) Characterized by or relating to acheiria (1).

a•chene (ă-kēn′) A small one-seeded fruit. [G. *a* priv. + *chainō,* to yawn]

a•chieve•ment age (ă-chēv′mĕnt āj) The relationship between the chronologic age and the age of achievement, as established by standard achievement tests.

a•chieve•ment quo•tient (ă-chēv′mĕnt kwō′shĕnt) A ratio, percentile rating, or related quotient denoting the amount a child has learned in relation to peers of the same age or level of education.

a•chieve•ment test (ă-chēv′mĕnt test) A standardized test used to measure acquired learning, in contrast to an intelligence test, which is an index of potential learning ability.

A•chil•les re•flex, A•chil•les ten•don re•flex (ă-kil′ēz rē′fleks, ă-kil′ēz ten′dŏn rē′fleks) A contraction of the calf muscles when the tendo calcaneus is sharply struck. SYN ankle reflex, triceps surae reflex.

A•chil•les squeeze test (ah-kil′ēz skwēz test) This test result is considered positive if plantar flexion does not occur when the calf is squeezed.

A•chil•les ten•don (ă-kil′ēz ten′dŏn) SYN tendo calcaneus. See page 15.

a•chil•lo•bur•si•tis (ă-kil′ō-bŭr-sī′tis) Inflammation of a bursa in proximity to the tendo calcaneus. SYN retrocalcaneobursitis.

a•chil•lo•dyn•i•a (ă-kil′ō-din′ē-ă) Pain due to inflammation of the bursa between the calcaneus and the tendo calcaneus (achilloburisitis). [Achilles (tendon) + G. *odynē,* pain]

a•chil•lor•rha•phy (ak′il-ōr′ă-fē) Suture of the tendo calcaneus. [Achilles (tendon) + G. *rhaphē,* a sewing]

a•chil•lot•o•my (ak′il-ot′ŏ-mē) Division of the tendo calcaneus. [Achilles (tendon) + G. *tomē,* incision]

ach•ing (āk′ing) A dull continuous pain. [O.E. *acan,* to ache]

a•chlor•hy•dri•a (ā-klōr-hī′drē-ă) Absence of hydrochloric acid from the gastric juice. [G. *a-* priv. + chlorhydric (acid)]

a•chlor•o•phyl•lous (ā-klōr-of′i-lŭs) Without chlorophyll, as in fungi.

a•cho•li•a (ā-kō′lē-ă) Suppressed or absent secretion of bile. [G. *a-* priv. + *cholē,* bile]

a•chol•ic (ā-kol′ik) Without bile, as in acholic (pale) stools.

a•chol•u•ri•a (ā-kō-lyūr′ē-ă) Absence of bile pigments from the urine in certain cases of jaundice. [G. *a-* priv. + *cholē,* bile, + *ouron,* urine]

a•chol•u•ric (ā-kō-lyūr′ik) Without bile in the urine.

a•chol•u•ric jaun•dice (ā-kō-lyūr′ik jawn′dis) Hepatic disorder with excessive amounts of unconjugated bilirubin in the plasma but without bile pigments in the urine.

a•chon•dro•gen•e•sis (ā-kon-drō-jen′ĕ-sis) Dwarfism accompanied by various bone aplasias of all four limbs, a normal or enlarged cranium, and a short trunk with delayed ossification of the lower vertebral column and pelvic bones. [G. *a-* priv. + *chondros,* cartilage, + *genesis,* origin]

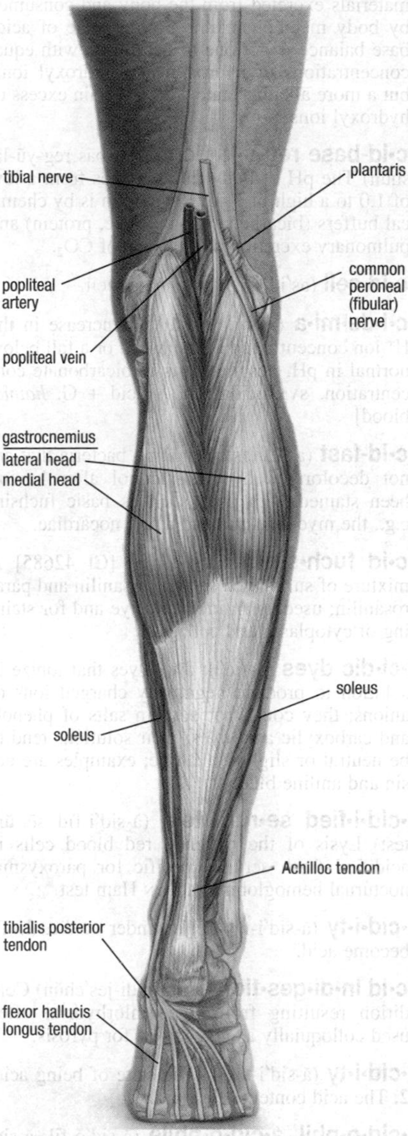

Achilles tendon

a•chon•dro•gen•e•sis type IA (ā-kon-drō-jen′ĕ-sis tīp) The condition as seen with hypervascular cartilage and hypercellular bone; uncertain inheritance pattern. SYN Houston-Harris syndrome.

a•chon•dro•gen•e•sis type IB (ā-kon-drō-jen′ĕ-sis tīp) Achondrogenesis with severely disorganized intracartilaginous ossification; autosomal recessive inheritance, caused by mutation in the diastrophic dysplasia sulfate transporter gene (DTDST) on chromosome 5q. SYN Parenti-Fraccaro syndrome.

a•chon•dro•gen•e•sis type II (ā-kon-drō-jen′ĕ-sis tīp) Achondrogenesis with autosomal dominant inheritance, caused by mutation in the collagen type II gene (COL2A1) on chromosome 12q. SYN Langer-Saldino syndrome.

a•chon•dro•pla•si•a (ā-kon-drō-plā′zē-ă) A hereditary type of chondrodystrophy characterized by an abnormality in conversion of cartilage into bone, predominantly affecting long bones, in which epiphysial growth is retarded and ceases early, resulting in dwarfism apparent at birth, with short limbs but normal trunk. See page B30. SYN achondroplastic dwarfism. [G. *a*- priv. + *chondros,* cartilage, + *plasis,* a molding]

a•chon•dro•plas•tic (ā-kon-drō-plas′tik) Relating to or characterized by achondroplasia.

a•chon•dro•plas•tic dwarf•ism (ā-kon-drō-plas′tik dwōrf′izm) SYN achondroplasia.

achrestic anaemia [Br.] SYN achrestic anemia.

a•chres•tic a•ne•mi•a (ă-kres′tik ă-nē′mē-ă) A potentially fatal form of chronic progressive macrocytic anemia in which the changes in bone marrow and circulating blood closely resemble those of pernicious anemia, but there is only transient or no response to therapy with vitamin B12; glossitis, gastrointestinal disturbances, central nervous system disease, and pyrexia are not observed; there is little bleeding or hemolysis. SYN achrestic anaemia. [G. *a*- priv. + *chrēsis,* a using]

a•chro•ma•cyte (ā-krō′mă-sīt) SYN achromocyte.

a•chro•mat•ic (ā′krō-mat′ik) **1.** Without hue; of black, white or gray color. **2.** Not staining readily. **3.** Refracting light without chromatic aberration. [G. *a,* without, + *chrōma,* color]

a•ch•ro•mat•ic lens (ā-krō-mat′ik lenz) A compound lens made of two or more lenses having different indices of refraction, so correlated as to minimize chromatic aberration.

a•ch•ro•mat•ic ob•jec•tive (ā-krō-mat′ik ŏb-jek′tiv) An objective that is corrected for two colors chromatically, and one color spherically.

a•ch•ro•mat•ic vi•sion (ā-krō-mat′ik vizh′ŭn) SYN achromatopsia.

a•chro•ma•tism (ă-krō′mă-tizm) **1.** The quality of being achromatic. **2.** The annulment of chromatic aberration by combining glasses of different refractive indices and different dispersion.

a•chro•mat•o•cyte (ā-krō-mat′ō-sīt) SYN achromocyte.

a•chro•mat•o•phil (ă-krō-mat′ō-fil) **1.** Not being colored by histologic or bacteriologic stains. SYN achromophilic, achromophilous. **2.** A cell or tissue that cannot be stained in the usual way. SYN achromophil. [G. *a*- priv. + *chrōma,* color, + *philos,* fond]

a•chro•ma•top•si•a, **a•chro•ma•top•sy** (ă-krō-mă-top′sē-ă, ă-krō′mă-top-sē) A severe congenital deficiency in color perception, often associated with nystagmus and reduced visual acuity. SYN achromatic vision, monochromatism (2). [G. *a-* priv. + *chrōma,* color, + *opsis,* vision]

a•chro•ma•tous (ă-krō′mă-tŭs) Colorless.

a•chro•ma•tu•ri•a (ă-krō-mă-tyūr′ē-ă) The passage of colorless or very pale urine. [G. *a-* priv. + *chrōma,* color, + *ouron,* urine]

a•chro•mi•a (ā-krō′mē-ă) **1.** Depigmentation (q.v.); absence or loss of natural pigmentation of the skin and iris. **2.** Inability of a cell or tissue to be colored by one or more biologic stains [G. *a-* priv. + *chrōma,* color]

a•chro•mic (ā-krō′mik) Colorless.

A•chro•mo•bac•ter (a′krō-mō-bak′tĕr) A gram-negative bacterial genus of uncertain clinical significance, closely related to members of the *Alcaligenes* and *Ochrobactrum* species.

a•chro•mo•cyte (ă-krō′mō-sīt) A hypochromic, crescent-shaped erythrocyte, probably resulting from artifactual rupture of a red blood cell. SYN achromacyte, achromatocyte, crescent bodies, ghost corpuscle, phantom corpuscle, Ponfick shadow, selenoid bodies, semilunar bodies, shadow (3), Traube corpuscle. [G. *a-* priv. + *chrōma,* color, + *kytos,* hollow (cell)]

a•chro•mo•phil (ă-krō′mŏ-fil) SYN achromatophil.

a•chro•mo•phil•ic, **a•chro•moph•i•lous** (ā-krō-mŏ-fil′ik, ā-krō-mŏ′fi-lŭs) SYN achromatophil (1).

a•chy•li•a (ă-kī′lē-ă) **1.** Absence of gastric juice or other digestive secretions. **2.** Absence of chyle. [G. *a-* priv. + *chylos,* juice]

a•chy•lous (ă-kī′lŭs) **1.** Lacking in gastric juice or other digestive secretions. **2.** Having no chyle. [G. *achylos,* without juice]

ac•id (as′id) **1.** A compound yielding a hydrogen ion in a polar solvent (e.g., in water); acids form salts by replacing all or part of the ionizable hydrogen with an electropositive element or radical. **2.** In popular language, any chemical compound that has a sharp or sour taste (given by the hydrogen ion). **3.** Relating to acid; giving an acidic reaction. [L. *acidus,* sour]

acidaemia [Br.] SYN acidemia.

ac•id-ash di•et (as′id-ash dī′ĕt) SYN alkaline-ash diet.

ac•id-base bal•ance (as′id-bās bal′ăns) The normal balance between acid and base in the blood plasma, expressed in the hydrogen ion concentration or pH, resulting from the relative amounts of acidic and basic materials ingested and produced by body metabolism, compared with the relative amounts of acidic and basic materials excreted from the body and consumed by body metabolism; the normal state of acid-base balance is not one of neutrality, with equal concentrations of hydrogen and hydroxyl ions, but a more alkaline state with a certain excess of hydroxyl ions.

ac•id-base reg•u•la•tion (as′id-bās reg-yū-lā′shŭn) The pH of body fluids ranges from a low of 1.0 to a high of 7.45. Regulation is by chemical buffers (bicarbonate, phosphate, protein) and pulmonary excretion or retention of CO_2.

ac•id cell (as′id sel) SYN parietal cell.

ac•i•de•mi•a (as-i-dē′mē-ă) An increase in the H^+ ion concentration of the blood or a fall below normal in pH, despite shifts in bicarbonate concentration. SYN acidaemia. [acid + G. *haima,* blood]

ac•id-fast (as′id-fast) Denoting bacteria that are not decolorized by acid-alcohol after having been stained with dyes such as basic fuchsin; e.g., the mycobacteria and a few nocardiae.

ac•id fuch•sin (as′id fūk′sin) [CI 42685] A mixture of sulfonated salts of rosanilin and pararosanilin; used as an indicator dye and for staining of cytoplasm and collagen.

a•ci•dic dyes (ă-sid′ik dīz) Dyes that ionize in solution to produce negatively charged ions or anions; they consist of sodium salts of phenols and carboxylic acid dyes; their solutions tend to be neutral or slightly alkaline; examples are eosin and aniline blue.

a•cid•i•fied se•rum test (ă-sid′i-fīd sēr′ŭm test) Lysis of the patient's red blood cells in acidified fresh serum, specific for paroxysmal nocturnal hemoglobinuria. SYN Ham test.

a•cid•i•fy (ă-sid′i-fī) **1.** To render acidic. **2.** To become acid.

ac•id in•di•ges•tion (as′id in′di-jes′chŭn) Condition resulting from hyperchlorhydria; often used colloquially as a synonym for pyrosis.

a•cid•i•ty (ă-sid′i-tē) **1.** The state of being acid. **2.** The acid content of a fluid.

a•cid•o•phil, **a•cid•o•phile** (ă-sid′ŏ-fil, ă-sid′ŏ-fīl) **1.** SYN acidophilic. **2.** One of the acid-staining cells of the anterior pituitary. **3.** A microorganism that grows well in a highly acid medium. [acid + G. *philos,* fond]

a•cid•o•phil ad•e•no•ma (ă-sid′ŏ-fil ad′ĕ-nō′mă) A tumor of the adenohypophysis in which cell cytoplasm stains with acid dyes; often growth-hormone producing. SYN eosinophil adenoma.

ac•i•do•phil•ic (as′i-dŏ-fil′ik) Having an affinity for acid dyes; denoting a cell or tissue element that stains with an acid dye, such as eosin. SYN acidophil (1), acidophile, oxychromatic.

ac•i•do•sis (as-i-dō′sis) A pathologic state characterized by an increase in the concentration of hydrogen ions in the arterial blood below the normal range of pH 7.35 to 7.45; the condition may be caused by an accumulation of carbon dioxide or acidic products of metabolism (respiratory acidosis), or by a decrease in the concentration of alkaline compounds (metabolic acidosis). Various forms include metabolic and respiratory. [acid + G. *-ōsis,* condition]

ac•id per•fu•sion test (as′id pĕr-fyū′zhŭn test) SYN Bernstein test.

ac•id phos•pha•tase (as′id fos′fă-tās) A phosphatase with an optimal pH of less than 7.0, notably present in the prostate gland.

ac•id stain (as′id stān) A dye in which the anion is the colored component of the dye molecule, e.g., sodium eosinate (eosin).

ac•id sul•fate (as′id sŭl′fāt) SYN bisulfate. SYN acid sulphate.

acid sulphate [Br.] SYN acid sulfate.

ac•id tide (as′id tīd) A temporary increase in the acidity of the urine that occurs during fasting.

a•cid•u•lous (a-sid′yŭ-lŭs) Acid or sour.

ac•i•du•ri•a (as′i-dyūr′ē-ă) **1.** Excretion of acidic urine. **2.** Excretion of an abnormal amount of any specified acid. Individual types of aciduria are prefixed by the specific acid, e.g., aminoaciduria, ketoaciduria. [acid + G. *ouron,* urine]

ac•i•du•ric (as′i-dyūr′ik) Pertaining to bacteria that tolerate an acid environment. [acid + L. *duro,* to endure]

ac•i•nar (as′i-năr) Pertaining to an acinus. SYN acinic.

ac•i•nar cell (as′i-năr sel) Any secreting cell lining an acinus, especially applied to the cells of the pancreas that furnish pancreatic juice and enzymes to distinguish them from the cells of ducts and the islets of Langerhans. SYN acinous cell.

Ac•i•ne•to•bac•ter (as-i-nē′tō-bak′tĕr) A genus of nonmotile, aerobic bacteria (family Moraxellaceae), frequently a cause of nosocomial infections; often resistant to antibiotics, can also cause severe primary infections in immunocompromised patients. SYN *Lingelsheimia.* [*a-,* priv. + *cineto-,* fr. G. *kineō,* to move, + bacter]

ac•i•ni (as′i-nī) Plural of acinus.

a•cin•ic (ă-sin′ik) SYN acinar.

a•cin•ic cell ad•e•no•car•ci•no•ma (ă-sin′ik sel ad′ĕ-nō-kahr-si-nō′mă) An adenocarcinoma arising from secreting cells of a racemose gland, particularly the salivary glands.

a•cin•i•form (ă-sin′i-fōrm) SYN acinous. [L. *acinus,* grape, + *forma,* shape]

ac•i•ni•tis (as-in-ī′tis) Inflammation of an acinus.

ac•i•nose (as′i-nōs) SYN acinous.

ac•i•no•tu•bu•lar gland (as′i-nō-tū′byŭ-lăr gland) SYN tubuloacinar gland.

ac•i•nous (as′i-nŭs) Resembling an acinus or grape-shaped structure. SYN aciniform, acinose.

ac•i•nous cell (as′i-nŭs sel) SYN acinar cell.

ac•i•nous gland (as′i-nŭs gland) A gland in which the secretory unit(s) has a grapelike shape and a very small lumen; e.g., the exocrine part of the pancreas.

a-c interval (in′tĕr-văl) The interval between the onset of the a wave and that of the c wave of the jugular pulse.

ac•i•nus, gen. and pl. **ac•i•ni** (as′i-nŭs, as′i-nī) [TA] One of the minute grape-shaped secretory portions of an acinous gland. Some authorities use the terms acinus and alveolus interchangeably, whereas others differentiate them by the constricted openings of the acinus into the excretory duct. [L. berry, grape]

AC joint (joynt) Abbreviation for acromioclavicular joint.

Ac•knowl•edg•ment of Re•ceipt of No•tice of Pri•va•cy Prac•ti•ces (ak-nol′ĕj-mĕnt rē-sēt′ nō′tis prī′vă-sē prak′tis-ĕz) A form that patients sign to show they received a notice about privacy from an HIPAA-compliant health care supplier.

ac•la•sis (ak′lă-sis) A state of continuity between normal and abnormal tissue. [G. *a-* priv. + *klasis,* a breaking away, a fragment]

ACLS Abbreviation for advanced cardiac life support.

ac•mes•the•si•a (ak′mes-thē′zē-ă) **1.** Sensitivity to pinprick. **2.** A cutaneous sensation of a sharp point. [G. *acmē,* point, + *aisthēsis,* sensation]

ac•ne (ak′nē) Inflammatory disease of sebaceous follicles marked by papules and pustules. Typically begins during puberty; affects chest, back, and face, but sometimes other areas. Cause remains unknown. Predisposing factors include heredity and androgen-estrogen imbalance. See page 18, B9. [probably a corruption (or copyist's error) of G. *akmē,* point of efflorescence]

ac•ne con•glo•ba•ta (ak′nē kon-glō-bā′tă) Severe cystic acne, characterized by cystic lesions, abscesses, communicating sinuses, and thickened, nodular scars; usually spares the face.

ac•ne cos•me•ti•ca (ak′nē koz-mē′tik-ă) Low-grade, noninflammatory acne lesions due to repeated application of comedogenic agents in cosmetics.

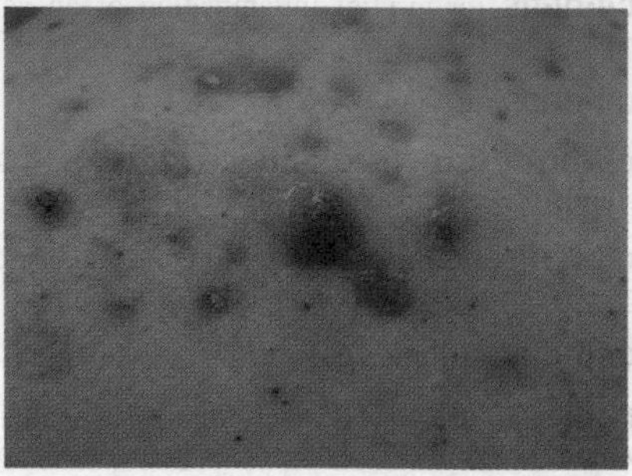

nodulocystic acne of the back

ac•ne er•y•the•ma•to•sa (ak′nē ĕ-rith′ĕ-mă-tō′să) SYN rosacea.

ac•ne•form, **ac•ne•i•form** (ak′nē-fōrm, ak-nē′i-fōrm) Resembling acne.

ac•ne ful•mi•nans (ak′nē ful′mi-nanz) Severe scarring acne in male teenagers, which may be associated with fever, polyarthralgia, crusted ulcerative lesions, weight loss, and anemia. [L. *fulmen, fulminis*, thunder, lightning]

ac•ne•gen•ic (ak′nē-jen′ik) Inducing acne or increasing its severity.

ac•ne in•du•ra•ta (ak′nē in-dū-rā′tă) Deeply seated acne, with large papules and pustules, large scars, and hypertrophic scars.

ac•ne ke•loid (ak′nē kē′loyd) A chronic eruption of fibrous papules that develop at the site of follicular lesions, usually on the back of the neck at the hairline. SYN dermatitis papillaris capillitii, folliculitis keloidalis.

ac•ne ke•ra•to•sa (ak′nē ker-ă-tō′să) An eruption of papules consisting of horny plugs projecting from the hair follicles, accompanied by inflammation.

ac•ne me•di•ca•men•to•sa (ak′nē med-i-kă-men-tō′să) Acne caused or exacerbated by drugs.

ac•ne ne•crot•i•ca mil•i•ar•is (ak′nē ne-krot′i-kă mil-ē-ā′ris) SYN acne varioliformis.

ac•ne pa•pu•lo•sa (ak′nē pap-yū-lō′să) Dermatologic condition in which papular lesions predominate.

ac•ne punc•ta•ta (ak′nē pŭngk-tā′tă) Dermatologic condition with black comedones.

ac•ne pus•tu•lo•sa (ak′nē pus-tū-lō′să) State of acne vulgaris in which pustular lesions predominate.

ac•ne ro•sa•ce•a (ak′nē rō-sā′shē-ă) SYN rosacea.

ac•ne va•ri•o•li•for•mis (ak′nē vā-rē-ō-li-fōr′mis) A pyogenic infection involving follicles occurring chiefly on the forehead and temples, followed by scar formation. SYN acne necrotica miliaris.

ac•ne vul•ga•ris (ak′nē vŭl-gā′ris) An eruption, predominantly of the face, upper back, and chest, composed of comedones, cysts, papules, and pustules on an inflammatory base; the condition usually develops during puberty and adolescence, due to androgenic stimulation of sebum secretion, with plugging of follicles by keratinization, associated with proliferation of *Propionibacterium acnes*.

ACOEM (ā′com) Acronym for American College of Occupational and Environmental Medicine

ac•o•nite (ak′ŏ-nīt) The dried root of *Aconitum napellus* (family Ranuculaceae), commonly known as monkshood or wolfsbane; a powerful and rapid-acting poison formerly used as an antipyretic, diuretic, diaphoretic, anodyne, cardiac and respiratory depressant, and externally as an analgesic. SYN fu tzu, monkshood. [L. *aconitum*, fr. G. *akoniton*]

***cis*-ac•o•nit•ic ac•id** (ak-ō-nit′ik as′id) Dehydration product of citric acid; an intermediate in the tricarboxylic acid cycle.

a•co•re•a (ă-kōr′ē-ă) Congenital absence of the pupil of the eye. [G. *a-* priv. + *korē*, pupil]

a•corn (ā′kōrn) SEE oak. [O.E.]

A•cos•ta dis•ease (ah-cōs′tah di-zēz′) SYN altitude sickness.

-acousis, **-acusis** **1.** Suffix referring to hearing and the ability to hear. **2.** SYN hearing. SEE audio-, audition.

a•cous•ma (ă-kūs′mă) Auditory hallucination of a simple nonverbal sound (buzzing or ringing). [G. *akousma*, that which is heard]

a•cous•tic, **a•cous•ti•cal** (ă-kūs′tik, -tik-al) Pertaining to hearing and the perception of sound. [Gr. *akoustikos*]

a•cous•tic me•a•tus (ă-kūs′tik mē-ā′tŭs) **1.** External: auditory canal; the passage leading inward through the tympanic portion of the temporal bone, from the auricle to the membrana tympani; **2.** Internal: a canal running through the petrous portion of the temporal bone, giving passage to the facial and vestibulocochlear nerves and to the labyrinthine artery and veins. SYN meatus acusticus.

a•cous•tic nerve (ă-kūs′tik nĕrv) SYN vestibulocochlear nerve [CN VIII].

a•cous•tic neu•ro•ma, **a•cous•tic neu•ri•le•mo•ma** (ă-kūs′tik nūr-ō′mă, ă-kūs′tik nūr′i-lē-mō′mă) A benign tumor arising from Schwann cells of the auditory nerve (CN VIII). Symptoms may include dizziness, unsteady gait, and papilledema.

a•cous•tic ra•di•a•tion (ă-kūs′tik rā′dē-ā′

shŭn) The fibers that pass from the medial geniculate body to the transverse temporal gyri of the cerebral cortex by way of the sublentiform part of the internal capsule. SYN radiatio acustica [TA].

a•cous•tic re•flex (ă-kūs′tik rē′fleks) Contraction of the stapedius muscle in response to intense sound, increasing impedance of the middle ear and thereby protecting the inner ear from the sound. SYN stapedial reflex.

a•cous•tic re•flex thres•hold (ART) (ă-kūs′tik rē′fleks thresh′ōld) Lowest sound intensity required to elicit contraction of the stapedius muscle in the middle ear.

a•cous•tics (ă-kūs′tiks) The science concerned with sounds and their perception. [G. *akoustikos,* relating to hearing]

a•cous•tic stim•u•la•tion test (ă-kūs′tik stim′yū-lā′shŭn test) A test for fetal well-being through use of an acoustic device to stimulate the fetus and cause acceleration of fetal heart rate.

a•cous•tic sur•round (ă-kūs′tik sŭr-ownd′) SYN sound field.

a•cous•tic trau•ma•tic hear•ing loss (ă-kūs′tik traw′mat′ik hēr′ing laws) Sensory hearing loss due to exposure to high-intensity noise.

ACP Abbreviation for acyl carrier protein.

ac•quired (ă-kwīrd′) Denoting a disease, condition, or abnormality that is not inherited. [L. *acquiro* (*adq-*), to obtain, fr. *quaero,* to seek]

ac•quired brain in•ju•ry (ABI) (ă-kwīrd′ brān in′jŭr-ē) SYN traumatic brain injury.

ac•quired cen•tric (ă-kwīrd sen′trik) SYN centric occlusion.

ac•quired char•ac•ter (ă-kwīrd′ kar′ăk-tĕr) A character developed in a plant or animal as a result of environmental influences during the individual's life.

ac•quired drives (ă-kwīrd′ drīvz) SYN secondary drives.

ac•quired ep•i•lep•tic a•pha•si•a (ă-kwīrd′ ep′i-lep′tik ă-fā′zē-ă) SYN Landau-Kleffner syndrome.

acquired hyperlipoproteinaemia [Br.] SYN acquired hyperlipoproteinemia.

ac•quired hy•per•lip•o•pro•tein•e•mi•a (ă-kwīrd′ hī′pĕr-lip′ō-prō′tē-nē′mē-ă) Nonfamilial hyperlipoproteinemia that develops as a consequence of some primary disease, such as thyroid deficiency. SYN acquired hyperlipoproteinaemia.

ac•quired im•mu•ni•ty (ă-kwīrd′ i-myū′ni-tē) Resistance resulting from previous exposure of the individual in question to an infectious agent or antigen; it may be active, as a result of naturally acquired infection or vaccination; or passive, being acquired from transfer of antibodies from another person or from an animal, either from mother to fetus or by inoculation.

ac•quired im•mu•no•de•fi•cien•cy syn•drome (ă-kwīrd′ im′yū-nō-dĕ-fish′ĕn-sē sin′drōm) SYN AIDS.

acquired naevus [Br.] SYN acquired nevus.

ac•quired ne•vus (ă-kwīrd′ nē′vŭs) A melanocytic nevus that is not visible at birth, but appears in childhood or adult life. SYN acquired naevus.

ac•quired tox•o•plas•mo•sis in a•dults (ă-kwīrd′ tok′sō-plaz-mō′sis ă-dŭlts′) A form of toxoplasmosis that may result in fever, encephalomyelitis, chorioretinopathy, maculopapular rash, arthralgia, myalgia, myocarditis, and pneumonitis; a lymphadenopathic form seems to be more prevalent in adults, who may manifest fever, lymphadenopathy, malaise, and headache; a form frequently found in patients with AIDS (q.v.).

ac•qui•si•tion (ak-wĭ-zish′ŭn) PSYCHOLOGY the empiric demonstration of an increase in the strength of the conditioned response in successive trials of pairing the conditioned and unconditioned stimuli.

ac•ral (ak′răl) Relating to or affecting the peripheral parts, e.g., limbs, fingers, ears, and other body parts. [G. *akron,* extremity]

A•cra•ni•a (ă-krā′nē-ă) A group of the phylum Chordata the members of which possess a notochord, gill slits, and nerve cord but no vertebrae, ribs, or skull; e.g., *Amphioxus,* tunicates, and acorn worms. [G. *a-* priv. + *kranion,* skull]

a•cra•ni•a (ă-krā′nē-ă) Complete or partial absence of a cranium; associated with meroencephaly. [G. *a-* priv. + *kranion,* skull]

a•cra•ni•al (ă-krā′nē-ăl) Having no cranium; relating to acrania or an acranius.

Ac•re•mo•ni•um (ak′rĕ-mō′nē-ŭm) A genus of fungi that occurs in soil and decaying plant matter; causes onychomycosis, corneal ulcers, eumycotic mycetoma, and endophthalmitis.

ac•ri•dine orange (ak′ri-dēn awr′ănj) [CI 46005] A basic fluorescent dye useful as a metachromatic stain for nucleic acids; also used in screening cervical smears for abnormal and malignant cells.

♻ **acro-** Combining form meaning extremity, tip, end, peak, topmost; extreme. [G. *akron,* highest point, extremity; *akros,* topmost, outermost, inmost, extreme, tip]

acroaesthesia [Br.] SYN acroesthesia.

ac•ro•ag•no•sis (ak′rō-ag-nō′sis) Loss or impairment of the sensory recognition of a limb. Absence of acrognosis.

acroanaesthesia [Br.] SYN acroanesthesia.

ac•ro•an•es•the•si•a (ak′rō-an-es-thē′zē-ă) Anesthesia of one or more of the extremities. SYN acroanaesthesia. [acro- + G. *an-* priv. + *aisthēsis* sensation]

ac•ro•a•tax•i•a (ak′rō-ă-tak′sē-ă) Ataxia affecting the distal portion of the extremities, i.e., hands, fingers, feet, and toes. Cf. proximoataxia. [acro- + ataxia]

ac•ro•blast (ak′rō-blast) Component of the developing spermatid composed of numerous Golgi elements; it contains the proacrosomal granules. [acro- + G. *blastos,* germ]

ac•ro•brach•y•ceph•a•ly (ak′rō-brak-i-sef′ă-lē) Type of craniosynostosis with premature closure of the coronal suture, resulting in an abnormally short anteroposterior diameter of the cranium. [acro- + G. *brachys,* short, + *kephalē,* head]

ac•ro•cen•tric (ak′rō-sen′trik) Having the centromere close to one end; said of a normal chromosome. [acro- + G. *kentron,* center]

ac•ro•cen•tric chro•mo•some (ak′rō-sen′trik krō′mō-sōm) A chromosome with the centromere placed very close to one end so that the short arm is very small, often with a satellite.

ac•ro•ce•phal•ic (ak′rō-sĕ-fal′ik) SYN oxycephalic.

ac•ro•ceph•a•lo•syn•dac•ty•ly (ak′rō-sef′ă-lō-sin-dak′ti-lē) A group of congenital syndromes characterized by peaking of the cranium and fusion or webbing of fingers or digits. [acrocephaly + G. *syn,* together, + *daktylos,* finger]

ac•ro•ceph•a•lous (ak′rō-sef′ă-lŭs) SYN oxycephalic.

ac•ro•ceph•a•ly, **ac•ro•ce•pha•li•a** (ak′rō-sef′ă-lē, ak′rō-sĕ-fā′lē-ă) SYN oxycephaly. [acro- + G. *kephalē,* head]

ac•ro•chor•don (ak′rō-kōr′dŏn) SYN skin tag. [acro- + G. *chordē,* cord]

ac•ro•cy•a•no•sis (ak′rō-sī-ă-nō′sis) A circulatory disorder in which the hands, and less commonly the feet, are persistently cold and blue; some forms are related to the Raynaud phenomenon. SYN Crocq disease, Raynaud sign. [acro- + G. *kyanos,* blue, + *-osis,* condition]

ac•ro•cy•a•not•ic (ak′rō-sī-ă-not′ik) Characterized by acrocyanosis.

ac•ro•der•ma•ti•tis (ak′rō-dĕr-mă-tī′tis) Inflammation of the skin of the extremities. See this page. [acro- + G. *derma,* skin, + *-itis,* inflammation]

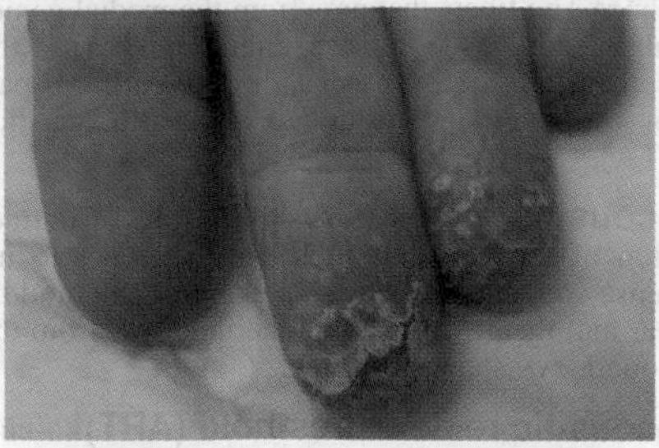

acrodermatitis

ac•ro•der•ma•ti•tis chron•i•ca a•troph•i•cans (ak′rō-dĕr-mă-tī′tis kron′i-kă ă-trō-fi-kanz) A late dermal manifestation of Lyme disease, appearing first on the feet, hands, elbows, or knees, and composed of indurated, erythematous plaques that become atrophic.

ac•ro•der•ma•ti•tis con•tin•u•a (ak′rō-dĕr′mă-tī′tis kŏn-tin′yū-ă) SYN pustulosis palmaris et plantaris.

ac•ro•der•ma•ti•tis en•ter•o•path•i•ca (ak′rō-dĕr′mă-tī′tis en′tĕr-ō-path′i-kă) A progressive hereditary defect of zinc metabolism in young children (onset, 3 weeks–18 months); often manifests first as a blistering, oozing, and crusting eruption on an extremity or around one of the orifices of the body, followed by loss of hair and by diarrhea or other gastrointestinal disturbances; relieved by lifelong oral zinc supplementation; autosomal recessive trait. [Aspergillus flavus + toxin]

ac•ro•der•ma•ti•tis per•stans (ak′rō-dĕr′mă-tī′tis pĕr′stanz) SYN pustulosis palmaris et plantaris.

ac•ro•der•ma•to•sis (ak′rō-dĕr′mă-tō′sis) Any cutaneous affection involving the more distal portions of the extremities. [acro- + G. *derma,* skin, + *-osis,* condition]

ac•ro•dyn•i•a (ak′rō-din′ē-ă) **1.** Pain in peripheral or acral parts of the body. **2.** A syndrome caused almost exclusively by mercury poisoning: in children, characterized by erythema of the extremities, chest, and nose, polyneuritis, and gastrointestinal symptoms; in adults, by anorexia, photophobia, sweating, and tachycardia. SYN dermatopolyneuritis, erythredema, erythroedema, Feer disease, pink disease, polyneuropathy (3), Swift disease. [acro- + G. *odynē,* pain]

ac•ro•es•the•si•a (ak′rō-es-thē′zē-ă) **1.** An extreme degree of hyperesthesia. **2.** Hyperesthesia of one or more of the extremities. SYN acroaesthesia. [acro- + G. *aisthēsis,* sensation]

ac•rog•no•sis (ak′rog-nō′sis) Cenesthesia, or normal sensory perception, of the extremities. [acro- + G. *gnōsis,* knowledge]

ac•ro•ker•a•to•sis (ak′rō-ker-ă-tō′sis) Nodular overgrowth of the horny layer of the skin on the fingers and toes, and occasionally on the ears and nose. [acro- + G. *keras,* horn, + *-osis,* condition]

ac·ro·me·gal·ic (ak′rō-mĕ-gal′ik) Pertaining to or characterized by acromegaly.

ac·ro·meg·a·ly (ak′rō-meg′ă-lē) A disorder marked by progressive enlargement of the head, face, hands, and feet, due to excessive secretion of somatotropin; organomegaly and metabolic disorders occur; diabetes mellitus may develop. [acro- + G. *megas,* large]

ac·ro·mel·al·gi·a (ak′rō-mĕ-lal′jē-ă) SEE erythromelalgia. [acro- + G. *melos,* limb, + *algos,* pain]

ac·ro·me·li·a (ak′rō-mē′lē-ă) SYN acromesomelia.

ac·ro·mel·ic (ak′rō-mē′lik) Affecting the terminal part of a limb. [acro- + G. *melos,* limb]

ac·ro·mes·o·me·li·a (ak′rō-mez′ō-mē′lē-ă) A form of dwarfism in which shortening is striking in the most distal segment of the limbs; autosomal recessive inheritance. SYN acromelia. [acro- + G. *melos,* limb, + *ia,* condition]

ac·ro·mes·o·mel·ic dwarf·ism (ak′rō-mez′ō-mē′lik dwōrf′izm) A form of short-limb dwarfism characterized by pug-nose and shortening particularly striking in the distal segment of the limbs, i.e., the forearms, lower legs, fingers, and toes; autosomal recessive inheritance.

ac·ro·met·a·gen·e·sis (ak′rō-met-ă-jen′ĕ-sis) Abnormal growth of the limbs resulting in deformity. [acro- + G. *meta,* beyond, + *genesis,* origin]

a·cro·mi·al (ă-krō′mē-ăl) Relating to the acromion.

a·cro·mi·al an·gle (ă-krō′mē-ăl ang′gĕl) The prominent angle at the junction of the posterior and lateral borders of the acromion. SYN angulus acromii [TA].

a·cro·mi·al pro·cess (ă-kro′me-ăl pros′es) SYN acromion.

a·cro·mi·o·cla·vic·u·lar (ă-krō′mē-ō-klă-vik′yū-lăr) Relating to the acromion and the clavicle; denoting the articulation and ligaments between the clavicle and the acromion of the scapula. SYN scapuloclavicular (1).

a·cro·mi·o·cla·vic·u·lar joint (AC joint) (ă-krō′mē-ō-klă-vik′yū-lăr joynt) A plane synovial joint between the acromial end of the clavicle and the medial margin of the acromion.

a·cro·mi·o·cor·a·coid (ă-krō′mē-ō-kōr′ă-koyd) SYN coracoacromial.

a·cro·mi·o·hu·mer·al (ă-krō′mē-ō-hyū′mĕr-ăl) Relating to the acromion and the humerus.

a·cro·mi·on (ă-krō′mē-on) The lateral end of the spine of the scapula, which projects as a broad flattened process overhanging the glenoid fossa; it articulates with the clavicle and gives attachment to part of the deltoid and trapezius muscles. SYN acromial process. [G. *akrōmion,* fr. *akron,* tip, + *ōmos,* shoulder]

a·cro·mi·o·scap·u·lar (ă-krō′mē-ō-skap′yū-lăr) Relating to both the acromion and body of the scapula.

a·cro·mi·o·tho·rac·ic (ă-krō′mē-ō-thōr-as′ik) SYN thoracoacromial.

a·cro·mi·o·tho·rac·ic ar·ter·y (ă-krō′mē-ō-thōr-as′ik ahr′tĕr-ē) SYN thoracoacromial artery.

ac·ro·my·o·to·ni·a, ac·ro·my·ot·o·nus (ak′rō-mī-ō-tō′nē-ă, ak-rō-mī-ot′ō-nŭs) Myotonia affecting the extremities only, resulting in spastic deformity of the hand or foot. [acro- + G. *mys,* muscle, + *tonos,* tension]

ac·ro·nym (ak′rō-nim) A pronounceable word formed from the initial letters of each word or selected words in a phrase (e.g., AIDS).

ac·ro·os·te·ol·y·sis (ak′rō-os-tē-ol′i-sis) Congenital condition manifested by palmar and plantar ulcerating lesions with osteolysis involving distal phalanges of the fingers and toes. [acro- + G. *osteon,* bone, + *lysis,* loosening]

acroparesthaesia [Br.] SYN acroparesthesia.

ac·ro·par·es·the·si·a (ak′rō-par-es-thē′zē-ă) **1.** Paresthesia of one or more of the extremities. **2.** Nocturnal paresthesia involving the hands, most often of middle-aged women; formerly attributed to a lesion in the thoracic outlet, but now known to be a classic symptom of carpal tunnel syndrome. SYN acroparesthaesia. [acro- + paresthesia]

a·crop·e·tal (ă-krop′ĕ-tăl) Developing from the base toward the apex. [G. *akron,* extremity, + L. *peto,* to seek]

ac·ro·pho·bi·a (ak′rŏ-fō′bē-ă) Morbid fear of heights. [acro- + G. *phobos,* fear]

ac·ro·pus·tu·lo·sis (ak′rō-pŭs-chū-lō′sis) Pustular eruptions of the hands and feet, often a form of psoriasis. [acro- + pustulosis]

ac·ro·scle·ro·sis, ac·ro·scle·ro·der·ma (ak′rō-skler-ō′sis, ak′rō-skler-ō-dĕr′mă) Stiffness and tightness of the skin of the fingers, with atrophy of the soft tissue and osteoporosis of the distal phalanges of the hands and feet; a limited form of progressive systemic sclerosis occurring with Raynaud phenomenon. SEE CREST syndrome. SYN sclerodactyly, sclerodactylia.

ac·ro·sin (ak′rō-sin) A serine proteinase in spermatozoa similar in specificity to trypsin.

ac·ro·so·mal cap (ak′rō-sō′măl kap) A collapsed caplike membranous vesicle that covers the anterior part of the nucleus of a spermatid, derived from the acrosomal granule.

ac·ro·so·mal gran·ule (ak′rō-sō′măl gran′yūl) The single glycoprotein-rich granule within an acrosomal vesicle, which results from the coalescence of proacrosomal granules.

ac•ro•so•mal ves•i•cle (ak′rō-sō′măl ves′i-kĕl) A vesicle derived from the Golgi apparatus during spermiogenesis; together with the acrosomal granule within, it spreads in a thin layer over the pole of the nucleus to form the acrosome.

ac•ro•some (ak′rō-sōm) A caplike organelle that surrounds the anterior two thirds of the nucleus of a sperm. Within this cap are enzymes that are thought to facilitate entry of the sperm into the oocyte. [acro- + G. *soma,* body]

a•crot•ic (ă-krot′ik) Marked by weakness or absence of pulse; pulseless. [G. *a-* priv. + *krotos,* a striking]

ac•ro•tism (ak′rō-tizm) Absence or imperceptibility of the pulse. [G. *a-* priv. + *krotos,* a striking]

a•cryl•ic res•in base (ă-kril′ik rez′in bās) Material used for cast and molded parts or as coatings and adhesives.

ACS Abbreviation for acute coronary syndrome.

ACSW Abbreviation for Academy of Certified Social Workers.

ACT (akt) Acronym for activated clotting time.

ACTH Abbreviation for adrenocorticotropic hormone.

ACTH-pro•duc•ing ad•e•no•ma (prŏ-dūs′ing ad′ĕ-nō′mă) A pituitary tumor composed of corticotrophs that produce ACTH, often a basophilic adenoma; may give rise to Cushing disease or Nelson syndrome.

ac•tig•ra•phy (ak-tig′ră-fē) Monitoring of movement, especially during testing to assess sleep disorders. SEE ALSO wheeze. [L. *actus,* action, + -graphy]

ac•tin (ak′tin) One of the protein components into which actomyosin can be split; it can exist in a fibrous form (F-actin) or a globular form (G-actin).

ac•tin fil•a•ment (ak′tin fil′ă-mĕnt) One of the contractile elements in muscular fibers and other cells; in skeletal muscle, the actin filaments are about 5 nm wide and 100 mcm long; they attach to the transverse Z filaments.

act•ing out (akt′ing owt) An overt act or set of actions that provides an emotional outlet for the expression of emotional conflicts (usually unconscious).

ac•tin•ic (ak-tin′ik) Relating to the chemically active rays of the electromagnetic spectrum, particularly to sunlight. [G. *aktis* (*aktin-*), a ray]

ac•tin•ic der•ma•ti•tis (ak-tin′ik dĕr′mă-tī′tis) SYN photodermatitis.

ac•tin•ic gran•u•lo•ma (ak-tin′ik gran′yū-lō′mă) An anular eruption on sun-exposed skin that microscopically shows phagocytosis of dermal elastic fibers by giant cells and histiocytes. See this page. SYN Miescher granuloma.

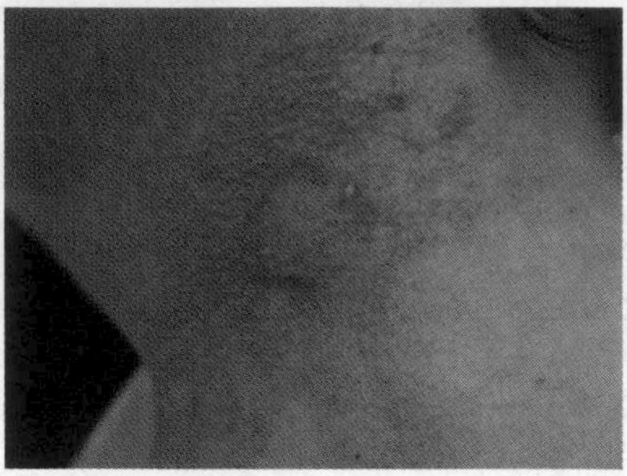

actinic granuloma: neck

ac•tin•ic ker•a•to•sis (ak-tin′ik ker′ă-tō′sis) A premalignant warty lesion occurring on the sun-exposed skin of the face or hands in aged light-skinned people; hyperkeratosis may form a cutaneous horn, and squamous cell carcinoma of low-grade malignancy may develop in a small proportion of untreated patients. Treatment includes cryotherapy, surgical excision, or topical chemotherapy. See this page.

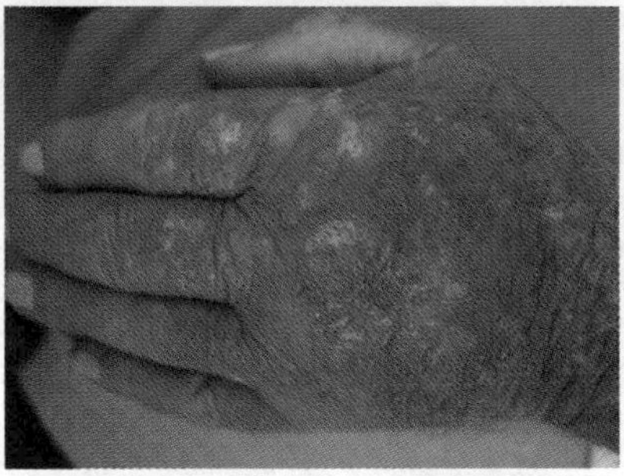

actinic keratoses: hand

ac•tin•ides (ak′tin-īdz) Those elements with atomic numbers 89–103, corresponding to the lanthanides in the Periodic Table. [*actinium,* first element of the series]

ac•tin•i•um (Ac) (ak-tin′ē-ŭm) An element, atomic no. 89, atomic wt. 227.05; it possesses no stable isotopes and exists in nature only as a disintegration product of uranium and thorium. [G. *aktis,* a ray]

actino- Combining form meaning a ray, as of light; applied to any form of radiation or to any structure with radiating parts. SEE ALSO radio-. [G. *aktis*, *aktinos*, a ray of light, a beam.]

Ac•ti•no•ba•cil•lus (ak′tin-ō-bă-sil′lŭs) A genus of nonmotile, non-spore-forming, aerobic, facultatively anaerobic bacteria (family Brucellaceae) containing gram-negative rods interspersed with coccal elements. The metabolism of these bacteria is fermentative. They are pathogenic to animals. The type species is *A. lignieresii*. [actino- + L. *bacillus*, a little rod]

ac•ti•no•der•ma•ti•tis (ak′ti-nō-dĕr′mă-tī′tis) SYN photodermatitis.

Ac•ti•no•ma•du•ra (ak′ti-nō-mă-dūr′ă) A genus of aerobic, gram-positive, non-acid-fast fungi with filaments that fragment into spores. *A. pelletieri* is an agent of mycetoma. [actino- + *Madura*, India]

Ac•ti•no•ma•du•ra la•ti•na (ak′ti-nō-ma-dūr′ă lă-tē′nă) A species of bacteria associated with mycetoma in South America.

Ac•ti•no•ma•du•ra ma•du•rae (ak′ti-nō-mad-ū′ră mă-dū′rē) An aerobic gram-positive filamentous bacillus that causes actinomycotic mycetoma, similar to those caused by *Nocardia* species.

Ac•ti•no•ma•du•ra pel•le•ti•e•ri (ak′ti-nō-mă-dūr′ă pel-ĕ-tyār′ē) SEE *Actinomadura latina.*

Ac•ti•no•my•ces (ak′ti-nō-mī′sēz) A genus of slow-growing, nonmotile, non-spore-forming, anaerobic to facultatively anaerobic bacteria (family Actinomycetaceae) containing gram-positive, irregularly staining filaments. These organisms can cause chronic suppurative infection in humans. The type species is *A. bovis*. [actino- + G. *mykēs*, fungus]

Ac•ti•no•my•ces bo•vis (ak′ti-nō-mī′sēz bō′vis) A species of bacteria causing actinomycosis in cattle; infection in humans is not established. It is the type species of its genus.

Ac•ti•no•my•ces is•ra•el•i•i (ak′ti-nō-mī′sēz iz-rā-el′ē-i) A species of bacteria causing human actinomycosis and, occasionally, infections in cattle.

Ac•ti•no•my•ce•ta•ce•ae (ak′ti-nō-mī-sē-tā′shē-ē) A family of non-spore-forming, nonmotile, facultatively anaerobic bacteria (order Actinomycetales) containing gram-positive, non-acid-fast, predominantly diphtheroid cells that tend to form branched filaments. This family contains the genera *Actinomyces* (type genus), *Arachnia*, *Bacterionema*, *Bifidobacterium*, and *Rothia*.

Ac•ti•no•my•ce•ta•les (ak′ti-nō-mī-sē-tā′lēs) An order of bacteria consisting of moldlike, rod-shaped, clubbed, or filamentous forms with tendency to branching. It includes the families Mycobacteriaceae, Actinomycetaceae, Streptomycetaceae, and Nocardiaceae.

ac•ti•no•my•ce•tes (ak′ti-nō-mī′sē-tēz) A term used to refer to members of the genus *Actinomyces;* USAGE NOTE sometimes improperly used to refer to any member of the family Actinomycetaceae or order Actinomycetales.

ac•ti•no•my•ce•to•ma (ak′tin-ō-mī′sĕ-tō′mă) Mycetoma caused by higher bacteria. Cf. eumycetoma.

ac•ti•no•my•co•ma (ak′ti-nō-mī-kō′mă) A swelling caused by an actinomycete. SEE mycetoma. [actino- + G. *mykēs*, fungus, + *-oma*, tumor]

ac•ti•no•my•co•sis (ak′ti-nō-mī-kō′sis) A disease primarily of cattle and humans caused by *Actinomyces bovis* in cattle and by *Actinomyces israelii* and *Arachnia propionica* in humans. These actinomycetes are part of the normal bacterial flora of the mouth and pharynx, but they may produce chronic destructive abscesses or granulomas that eventually discharge a viscid pus containing minute yellowish granules (sulfur granules). In humans, the disease commonly affects the cervicofacial area, abdomen, or thorax. [actino- + G. *mykēs*, fungus, + *-osis*, condition]

ac•ti•no•my•cot•ic (ak′ti-nō-mī-kot′ik) Relating to actinomycosis.

ac•ti•no•ther•a•py (ak′ti-nō-thār′ă-pē) DERMATOLOGY ultraviolet light therapy.

ac•tion (ak′shŭn) **1.** Performance of any function, the manner of such performance, or its result. **2.** Exertion of any force or power: physical, chemical, or mental. [L. *actio*, from *ago*, pp. *actus*, to do]

ac•tion cur•rent (ak′shŭn kŭr′rĕnt) An electrical current induced in muscle fibers when they are effectively stimulated; normally it is followed by contraction.

ac•tion po•ten•tial (ak′shŭn pŏ-ten′shăl) The change in membrane potential occurring in nerve, muscle, or other excitable tissue when excitation occurs.

ac•ti•vat•ed char•coal (ak′ti-vā-tĕd chahr′kōl) An agent administered orally to prevent intestinal absorption of ingested poisons or drugs taken in excessive dose.

ac•ti•vat•ed clot•ting time (ACT) (ak′ti-vā-tĕd klot′ing tīm) The most common test used for coagulation time in cardiovascular surgery.

ac•ti•vat•ed par•tial throm•bo•plas•tin time (aPTT) (ak′ti-vā-tĕd pahr′shăl throm-bō-plas′tin tīm) The time needed for plasma to form a fibrin clot following the addition of calcium and a phospholipid reagent; used to evaluate the intrinsic clotting system.

ac•ti•va•tion (ak′ti-vā′shŭn) **1.** The act of rendering active. **2.** An increase in the energy content of an atom or molecule, through the raising of temperature, absorption of light photons, or other means. **3.** Techniques of stimulating the brain by light, sound, electricity, or chemical agents, to elicit abnormal activity in the electroencephalogram. **4.** Stimulation of peripheral nerve fibers to the point that action potentials are initiated. **5.** Stimulation of cell division in an oocyte by fertilization or by artificial means. **6.** The act of making radioactive.

ac·ti·va·tion en·er·gy (ak′ti-vā′shŭn en′ĕr-jē) Minimum amount of energy to convert a stable molecule to a reactive molecule.

ac·ti·va·tor (ak′ti-vā-tŏr) **1.** A substance that renders another substance active, or one that accelerates a process or reaction. **2.** The fragment, produced by chemical cleavage of a proactivator, that induces the enzymatic activity of another substance. **3.** An apparatus for making substances radioactive. **4.** A removable type of myofunctional orthodontic appliance that acts as a passive transmitter of force, which is produced by the function of the activated muscles, to the teeth and alveolar process that are in contact with it. **5.** A protein that binds to a DNA sequence before DNA polymerase transcription. **6.** Manually assisted thrust instrument that activates mechanoreceptors; used by many chiropractors. [activate + *-or*, agent suffix]

ac·tive ac·e·tate (ak′tiv as′ĕ-tāt) SYN acetoacetyl-CoA.

ac·tive an·a·phy·lax·is (ak′tiv an′ă-fi-lak′sis) Reaction following inoculation of antigen in a subject previously sensitized to the specific antigen, in contrast to passive anaphylaxis.

ac·tive chron·ic hep·a·ti·tis (ak′tiv kron′ik hep′ă-tī′tis) Liver disease with chronic portal inflammation and progressive hepatic degeneration; an autoimmune sequela to hepatitis B or C. SYN posthepatitic cirrhosis.

ac·tive con·ges·tion (ak′tiv kŏn-jes′chŭn) Congestion due to an increased flow of arterial blood to a part of the body or organ.

ac·tive cool-down (ak′tiv kūl′down) SYN active recovery.

active hyperaemia [Br.] SYN active hyperemia.

ac·tive hy·per·e·mi·a (ak′tiv hī′pĕr-ē′mē-ă) Hyperemia due to an increased afflux of arterial blood into dilated capillaries. SYN active hyperaemia, fluxionary hyperemia.

ac·tive im·mu·ni·ty (ak′tiv i-myū′ni-tē) SEE acquired immunity.

ac·tive in·gre·di·ent (ak′tiv in-grē′dē-ĕnt) Any component of a pharmaceutical product that exerts pharmacologic activity. SYN active pharmaceutical ingredient.

ac·tive la·bor (ak′tiv lā′bŏr) Contractions resulting in progressive effacement and dilation of the cervix. Cf. prodromal labor.

ac·tive meth·yl (ak′tiv meth′il) A methyl group attached to a quaternary ammonium ion or a tertiary sulfonium ion that can take part in transmethylation reactions.

ac·tive pharm·a·ceu·ti·cal in·gre·di·ent (API) (ak′tiv fahr′mă-sū′ti-kăl in-grē′dē-ĕnt) SYN active ingredient.

ac·tive prin·ci·ple (ak′tiv prin′si-pĕl) A constituent of a drug, usually an alkaloid or glycoside, on which the characteristic therapeutic action of the substance largely depends.

ac·tive range of mo·tion (AROM) (ak′tiv rānj mō′shŭn) Amount of motion at a given joint when the subject moves the part voluntarily.

ac·tive re·cov·er·y (ak′tiv rĕ-kŭv′ĕr-ē) Exercising with gradually diminishing intensity immediately after a bout of vigorous exercise; facilitates lactate and metabolic waste removal by maintaining blood flow in muscles during recovery. SYN active cool-down, tapering-off.

ac·tive re·pres·sor (ak′tiv rĕ-pres′ŏr) A repressor that combines directly with an operator gene to repress the operator and its structural genes, thus repressing protein synthesis; may be repressed by an inducer, with resulting protein synthesis; a homeostatic mechanism for regulation of inducible enzyme systems.

ac·tive site (ak′tiv sīt) That portion of an enzyme molecule at which the actual reaction proceeds; one or more residues or atoms in a spatial arrangement that permits interaction with the substrate.

ac·tive splint (ak′tiv splint) SYN dynamic splint.

ac·tive trans·port (ak′tiv trans′pōrt) The passage of ions or molecules across a cell membrane, not by passive diffusion but by an energy-consuming process against an electrochemical gradient.

ac·tiv·in (ak′ti-vin) Placental hormone that reaches maximum levels in maternal serum during labor. [active + -in]

ac·tiv·i·ties of dai·ly liv·ing (ADL) (ak-tiv′i-tēz dā′lē liv′ing) Everyday routines generally involving functional mobility and personal care, such as bathing, dressing, toileting, and meal preparation. An inability to perform these renders one dependent on others, resulting in a self-care deficit. A major goal of occupational therapy is to enable the client to perform activities of daily living.

ac·tiv·i·ties of dai·ly liv·ing scale (ak-tiv′i-tēz dā′lē liv′ing skāl) A measurement to score physical activity and its limitations, based on answers to simple questions about mobility, self-care, and grooming; widely used in health care professions (e.g., rehabilitation therapy, occupational therapy, and nursing).

ac·tiv·i·ty (ak-tiv′i-tē) **1.** ELECTROENCEPHALOGRAPHY the presence of neurogenic electrical energy. **2.** PHYSICAL CHEMISTRY an ideal concentration for which the law of mass action will apply perfectly; the ratio of the activity to the true concentration is the activity coefficient (γ), which becomes 1.00 at infinite dilution. **3.** For enzymes, the amount of substrate consumed (or product formed) in a given time under given conditions; turnover number. **4.** The number of nuclear transformations (disintegrations) in a given quantity of a material per unit time. Units: curie (Ci), millicurie (mCi), becquerel (Bq), megabecquerel (MBq). SEE ALSO radioactivity. **5.** Producing movement. **6.** A class of goal-directed human actions.

ac•tiv•i•ty ad•ap•ta•tion (ak-tiv′i-tē ad′ap-tā′shŭn) The change in an aspect of an activity to make successful performance possible.

ac•tiv•i•ty a•nal•y•sis (ak-tiv′i-tē ă-nal′i-sis) **1.** The process of examining an activity or movement pattern to distinguish its component parts. **2.** Any method of determining the type, amount, and organization of activity that occupies the lives of people on a recurring basis. SYN biomechanical analysis.

ac•tiv•i•ty co•ef•fi•cient (γ) (ak-tiv′i-tē kō-ĕ-fish′ĕnt) SEE activity (2).

ac•tiv•i•ty de•mands (ak-tiv′i-tē dĕ-mandz′) Elements of an activity that must be present if it is to be executed successfully. These include the appropriate objects, space, social components, sequencing or timing, actions, underlying body functions, and body structure.

ac•tiv•i•ty grad•ing (ak-tiv′i-tē grād′ing) Incrementally changing the process, tools, materials, or environment of a given activity to increase or decrease performance demands gradually, and ultimately to ensure best performance. SYN sport-specific training.

ac•tiv•i•ty group (ak-tiv′i-tē grūp) A treatment modality in which a group of clients is assembled to share common concerns or problems related to the acquisition or maintenance of performance components and occupational skills.

ac•tiv•i•ty in•tol•er•ance (ak-tiv′i-tē in-tol′ĕr-ăns) Inability to perform daily activities because of decreased energy for any reason.

ac•tiv•i•ty pat•tern a•nal•y•sis (ak-tiv′i-tē pat′ĕrn ă-nal′i-sis) SYN activity analysis (2).

ac•tiv•i•ty syn•the•sis (ak-tiv′i-tē sin′thĕ-sis) The process of combining components of the human and nonhuman environment so as to design an activity suitable for evaluation or intervention.

ac•to•my•o•sin (ak′tō-mī′ō-sin) A protein complex composed of actin and myosin; the essential contractile substance of muscle fiber.

ac•tu•al cau•ter•y (ak′chū-ăl kaw′tĕr-ē) A cautery acting directly through heat and not by chemical means.

a•cu•i•ty (ă-kyū′i-tē) **1.** Sharpness, clearness, distinctness. **2.** Severity. [thr. Fr., fr. L. *acuo,* pp. *acutus,* sharpen]

a•cu•le•ate (ă-kyū′lē-āt) Pointed; covered with sharp spines. [L. *aculeatus,* pointed, fr. *acus,* needle]

ac•u•men•tin (ak′yū-men′tin) A neutrophil and macrophage motility protein that links to the actin molecule to control filament length.

a•cu•mi•nate (ă-kyū′mi-nāt) Tapering to a point. [L. *acumino,* pp. *-atus,* to sharpen]

a•cu•pres•sure (ak′yū-presh-ŭr) Application of pressure in sites used for acupuncture with therapeutic intent.

ac•u•punc•ture (ak′yū-pungk′shŭr) **1.** An ancient Asian system of healing that uses long fine needles. **2.** More recently, acupuncture anesthesia or analgesia. [L. *acus,* needle, + puncture]

ac•u•punc•ture an•es•the•si•a (ak′yū-pungk′shŭr an′es-thē′zē-ă) Percutaneous insertion of, and stimulation by, needles placed in critical areas of the body to produce loss of sensation in another area.

ac•u•punc•ture points (ak′yū-pungk′shŭr poynts) Points on the body surface at which acupuncture is believed to correct disturbances of energy flow associated with disease.

a•cute (ă-kyūt′) **1.** Referring to a disease of sudden onset and brief course, not chronic, sometimes loosely used to mean severe. **2.** Referring to treatment or exposure: brief, intense, short-term; sometimes specifically referring to brief exposure of high intensity. [L. *acutus,* sharp]

a•cute ab•do•men (ă-kyūt′ ab′dŏ-mĕn) Any serious sudden intraabdominal condition (such as appendicitis) attended by pain, tenderness, and muscular rigidity, and for which emergency surgery must be considered. SYN surgical abdomen.

a•cute a•dre•no•cor•ti•cal in•suf•fi•cien•cy (ă-kyūt′ ă-drē′nō-kōr′ti-kăl in′sŭ-fish′ĕn-sē) Sudden worsening of signs and symptoms of corticosteroid deficiency when trauma or illness causes increased demand in a patient with impaired adrenal insufficiency. SYN addisonian crisis, adrenal crisis.

a•cute Af•ri•can sleep•ing sick•ness (ă-kyūt′ af′ri-kăn slēp′ing sik′nĕs) SYN Rhodesian trypanosomiasis.

a•cute an•te•ri•or po•li•o•my•e•li•tis (ă-kyūt′ an-tēr′ē-ŏr pō′lē-ō-mī-ĕ-lī′tis) Inflammation of the anterior cornua of the spinal cord; an acute infectious disease caused by the poliomyelitis virus and marked by fever, pains, and gastroenteric disturbances, followed by a flaccid paralysis of one or more muscular groups, and later by atrophy.

a•cute as•cend•ing pa•ral•y•sis (ă-kyūt′ ă-send′ing păr-al′i-sis) A paralysis of rapid course beginning in the legs and involving progressively the trunk, arms, and neck, ending sometimes in death in from 1 to 3 weeks.

a•cute bul•bar po•li•o•my•e•li•tis (ă-kyūt′ bŭl′bahr pō′lē-ō-mī-ĕ-lī′tis) Poliomyelitis virus infection affecting nerve cells in the medulla oblongata that paralyzes the lower motor cranial nerves.

a•cute care (ă-kyūt′ kār) Short-term care for serious diseases or trauma.

a•cute care hos•pi•tal (ă-kyūt′ kār hos′pi-tăl) An inpatient medical facility providing therapy for individual episodes of severe illness or injury; average length of stay of 30 days or fewer.

a•cute com•pres•sion tri•ad (ă-kyūt′ kŏm-presh′ŭn trī′ad) The rising venous pressure, falling arterial pressure, and decreased heart sounds of pericardial tamponade. SYN Beck triad.

a•cute cor•o•nar•y syn•drome (ACS) (ă-kyūt′ kōr′ŏ-nār-ē sin′drōm) A general term for clinical syndromes due to reduction of blood flow in coronary arteries (e.g., unstable angina, acute myocardial infarction). SYN acute myocardial infarction, preinfarction angina, unstable angina.

a•cute dis•ease (ă-kyūt′ di-zēz′) Disorder with sudden onset and short duration of symptoms.

a•cute dis•sem•i•nat•ed en•ceph•a•lo•my•e•li•tis (ă-kyūt′ di-sem′i-nā-tĕd en-sef′a-lō-mī′ĕ-lī′tis) An acute demyelinating disorder of the central nervous system in which focal demyelination is present throughout the brain and spinal cord. This process is common to postinfectious, postexanthem, and postvaccinal encephalomyelitis.

a•cute ef•fects (ă-kyūt′ e-fekts′) Short-term signs and symptoms of a disorder or condition.

a•cute ep•i•dem•ic leu•ko•en•ceph•a•li•tis (ă-kyūt′ ep′i-dem′ik lū′kō-en-sef′ă-lī′tis) A disease characterized by acute onset of fever, followed by convulsions, delirium, and coma, and associated with perivascular demyelination and hemorrhagic foci in the central nervous system. SYN Strümpell disease (2).

a•cute ful•mi•nat•ing me•nin•go•coc•ce•mi•a (ă-kyūt′ ful′mi-nā′ting mĕ-ning′gō-kok-sē′mē-ă) Rapidly systemic infection with *Neisseria meningitidis*, usually without meningitis, characterized by rash, usually petechial or purpuric, high fever, and hypotension. May lead to death within hours.

a•cute gran•u•lo•cyt•ic leu•ke•mi•a (ă-kyūt′ gran′yū-lō-sit′ik lū-kē′mē-ă) SYN myeloblastic leukemia.

acute haemorrhagic conjunctivitis [Br.] SYN acute hemorrhagic conjunctivitis.

acute haemorrhagic pancreatitis [Br.] SYN acute hemorrhagic pancreatitis.

a•cute hem•or•rhag•ic con•junc•ti•vi•tis (ă-kyūt′ hem′ŏr-aj′ik kŏn-jŭngk′ti-vī′tis) Specific acute endemic conjunctivitis with eyelid swelling, tearing, conjunctival hemorrhages, and follicles; usually caused by enterovirus type 70. SYN acute haemorrhagic conjunctivitis.

a•cute hem•or•rhag•ic pan•cre•a•ti•tis (ă-kyūt′ hem′ŏr-aj′ik pan′krē-ă-tī′tis) An acute inflammation of the pancreas accompanied by the formation of necrotic areas and hemorrhages into the substance of the gland; clinically marked by sudden severe abdominal pain, nausea, fever, and leukocytosis; areas of fat necrosis are present on the surface of the pancreas and in the omentum due to the action of escaped pancreatic enzyme (trypsin and lipase). SYN acute haemorrhagic pancreatitis.

a•cute id•i•o•path•ic pol•y•neu•ri•tis (ă-kyūt′ id′ē-ō-path′ik pol′ē-nūr-ī′tis) A neurologic syndrome, probably an immune-mediated disorder, often a sequela of certain virus infections, marked by paresthesia of the limbs and muscular weakness or a flaccid paralysis; the characteristic laboratory finding is increased protein in the cerebrospinal fluid without increase in cell count.

a•cute in•fec•tion (ă-kyūt in-fek′shŭn) A long- or short-lived severe infection of sudden onset.

a•cute in•flam•ma•tion (ă-kyūt′ in′flă-mā′shŭn) Any inflammation that has a fairly rapid onset, quickly becomes severe, and is usually manifested for only a few days; characterized histopathologically by edema, hyperemia, and infiltrates of polymorphonuclear leukocytes.

a•cute in•flam•ma•tor•y de•my•e•li•nat•ing pol•y•ra•dic•u•lo•neu•rop•a•thy (ă-kyūt′ in-flam′ă-tōr-ē dē-mī′ĕ-lin-āt-ing pol′ē-ră-dik′yū-lō-nūr-op′ă-thē) Classic Guillain-Barré syndrome (q.v.) in which the predominant type of underlying nerve fiber pathology is demyelination. SEE ALSO acute motor axonal neuropathy.

a•cute in•ter•mit•tent por•phyr•i•a, a•cute por•phyr•i•a (ă-kyūt′ in′tĕr-mit′ĕnt pōr-fir′ē-ă, ă-kyūt′ pōr-fir′ē-ă) SYN intermittent acute porphyria.

a•cute is•che•mic stroke (AIS) (ă-kyūt′ is-kē′mik strōk) Circulatory cerebral occlusion that produces varying degrees of neurologic deficits. Ischemic strokes account for 85% of all attacks; most are caused by thrombus formation or embolus due to atherosclerosis. Cardiogenic embolic stroke, usually caused by atrial fibrillation, is the second major cause of acute ischemic stroke. SYN brain attack, cerebral vascular attack.

a•cute i•so•lat•ed my•o•car•di•tis (ă-kyūt′ ī′sō-lā-tĕd mī′ō-kahr-dī′tis) An acute interstitial myocarditis of unknown cause, the endocardium and pericardium being unaffected. SYN Fiedler myocarditis.

a•cute lung in•ju•ry (ă-kyūt′ lŭng in′jŭr-ē) Any acute decline in lung function of sudden onset, whether traumatic or related to disease state; may be life threatening.

acute lymphocytic leukaemia [Br.] SYN acute lymphocytic leukemia.

a•cute lym•pho•cy•tic leu•ke•mi•a (ALL) (ă-kyūt′ lim′fō-sit′ik lū-kē′mē-ă) SYN acute lymphocytic leukaemia. SEE lymphocytic leukemia.

a•cute ma•lar•i•a (ă-kyūt′ mă-lar′ē-ă) A form of the disease consisting of a chill accompanied by and followed by fever with its attendant general symptoms and terminating in a sweating stage; the paroxysms, caused by release of merozoites from infected cells, recur after becoming synchronized every 48 hours in tertian (vivax or ovale) malaria, every 72 hours in quartan (malariae) malaria, and at indefinite but frequent intervals, usually about 48 hours, in malignant tertian (falciparum) malaria.

a•cute mas•sive liv•er ne•cro•sis (ă-kyūt′ mas′iv liv′ĕr nĕ-krō′sis) A lesion in which there is extensive and rapid death of parenchymal cells of the liver, sometimes with fatty degeneration; the necrosis may result from fulminant viral infection or chemical poisoning; associated with jaundice.

a•cute mo•tor ax•o•nal neu•rop•a•thy (ă-kyūt′ mō′tŏr ak-sō′năl nūr-op′ă-thē) An acute, pure motor axon-degenerating type of polyradiculoneuropathy, a variant of Guillain-Barré syndrome; seen principally in a seasonal pattern (spring or summer) among children in rural China following epidemics of diarrhea caused by *Campylobacter jejuni*.

a•cute pos•ter•i•or mul•ti•fo•cal plac•oid pig•ment ep•i•the•li•op•a•thy (APMPPE) (ă-kyūt′ pos-tēr′ē-ŏr mŭl-tē-fō′kăl plak′oyd pig′mĕnt ep′i-thē-lē-op′ă-thē) An acute, inflammatory, self-limited disease manifested by decreased vision and multifocal, cream-colored placoid lesions of the retinal pigment epithelium; resolves with restoration of vision.

a•cute my•e•lo•blas•tic leu•ke•mi•a (AML) (ă-kyūt′ mī′ĕ-lō-blas′tik lū-kē′mē-ă) SYN myeloblastic leukemia.

a•cute my•o•car•di•al in•farc•tion (AMI) (ă-kyūt′ mī′ō-kahr′dē-ăl in-fahrk′shŭn) SYN acute coronary syndrome.

a•cute nec•ro•tiz•ing en•ceph•a•li•tis (ă-kyūt′ nek′rō-tīz-ing en-sef′ă-lī′tis) An acute form of encephalitis, characterized by destruction of brain parenchyma.

a•cute nec•ro•tiz•ing hem•or•rhag•ic en•ceph•a•lo•my•e•li•tis (ă-kyūt′ nek′rō-tīz-ing hem′ŏr-aj′ik en-sef′a-lō-mī′ĕ-lī′tis) A fulminating demyelinating disorder of the central nervous system that affects mainly children and young adults. Almost always preceded by a respiratory infection, characterized by the abrupt onset of fever, headache, confusion, and nuchal rigidity, soon followed by focal seizures, hemiplegia, or quadriplegia, brainstem findings, and coma. SYN Hurst disease.

a•cute nec•ro•tiz•ing ul•cer•a•tive gin•gi•vi•tis (ANUG) (ă-kyūt′ nek′rō-tīz-ing ŭl′sĕr-ă-tiv jin′ji-vī′tis) SEE necrotizing ulcerative gingivitis.

a•cute pan•cre•a•ti•tis (ă-kyūt′ pan′krē-ă-tī′tis) Inflammation of the pancreas, frequently involving destruction of tissue by pancreatic enzymes. When severe, may lead to local necrosis, hemorrhage, and shock.

a•cute phase re•ac•tion (ă-kyūt′ fāz rē-ak′shŭn) Refers to the changes in synthesis on certain proteins within the serum during an inflammatory response; this response provides rapid protection for the host against microorganisms via nonspecific defense mechanisms. SYN acute phase response.

a•cute phase re•sponse (ă-kyūt′ fāz rē-spons′) SYN acute phase reaction.

acute promyelocytic leukaemia [Br.] SYN acute promyelocytic leukemia.

a•cute pro•my•e•lo•cyt•ic leu•ke•mi•a (ă-kyūt′ prō′mī-ĕ-lō-sit′ik lū-kē′mē-ă) The disorder presenting as a severe bleeding disorder, with infiltration of the bone marrow by abnormal promyelocytes and myelocytes, low plasma fibrinogen, and defective coagulation. SYN acute promyelocytic leukaemia.

a•cute pul•mo•nar•y al•ve•o•li•tis (ă-kyūt′ pul′mŏ-nār-ē al′vē-ō-lī′tis) Acute inflammation involving formation of exudate in pulmonary alveoli and impaired gas exchange; may result in necrosis with hemorrhage into the lungs; occurs in Goodpasture syndrome, in association with glomerulonephritis.

a•cute re•nal fail•ure (ARF) (ă-kyūt′ rē′năl fāl′yŭr) A rapid decline of kidney function due to tubular injury. Signs are azotemia, fluid and electrolyte imbalance, and metabolic acidosis. Commonly caused by ischemia or nephrotoxins.

a•cute res•pi•ra•to•ry dis•tress syn•drome (ARDS) (ă-kyūt′ res′pir-ă-tōr-ē dis-tres′ sin′drōm) SYN adult respiratory distress syndrome.

a•cute res•pi•ra•to•ry fail•ure (ARF) (ă-kyūt′ res′pir-ă-tōr-ē fāl′yŭr) Loss of pulmonary function either acute or chronic that results in hypoxemia or hypercarbia.

a•cute ret•i•nal ne•cro•sis (ARN) (ă-kyūt′ ret′i-năl nĕ-krō′sis) A viral syndrome occurring in immunocompetent patients, characterized by peripheral retinal destruction that becomes circumferential and often eads to retinal detachment.

a•cute rhi•ni•tis (ă-kyūt′ rī-nī′tis) Sudden onset catarrhal inflammation of the mucous membrane of the nose, marked by sneezing, lacrimation, and a profuse secretion of watery mucus; usually associated with infection by one of the common cold viruses. SYN coryza.

a·cute sen·sor·y-mo·tor ax·o·nal neu·rop·a·thy (ă-kyūt′ sen′sŏr-ē-mō′tŏr ak-sō′năl nūr-op′ă-thē) An acute axon-degenerating polyradiculoneuropathy that affects both motor and sensory fibers; a variant of Guillain-Barré syndrome.

a·cute sit·u·a·tion·al re·ac·tion (ă-kyūt′ sich′ū-ā′shŭn-ăl rē-ak′shŭn) SYN stress reaction.

a·cute try·pan·o·so·mi·a·sis (ă-kyūt′ trī-pan′ō-sō-mī′ă-sis) SYN Rhodesian trypanosomiasis.

a·cute tu·ber·cu·lo·sis (ă-kyūt′ tū-bĕr′kyū-lō′sis) A rapidly fatal disease due to the general dissemination of acid-fast bacilli in the blood, resulting in the formation of miliary tubercles in various organs and tissues, and producing symptoms of profound toxemia. SYN disseminated tuberculosis.

a·cute vi·ral con·junc·ti·vi·tis (ă-kyūt′ vī′răl kŏn-jŭngk′ti-vī′tis) Acute conjunctivitis marked by intense hyperemia and a watery discharge; usually caused by adenovirus types 8 and 19; considered highly contagious. SYN pinkeye (1).

a·cute yel·low at·ro·phy of the liv·er (ă-kyūt′ yel′ō at′rō-fē liv′ĕr) A lesion in which there is extensive and rapid death of parenchymal cells of the liver, sometimes with fatty degeneration; may result from fulminant viral infection or chemical poisoning; associated with jaundice. SYN Rokitansky disease.

a·cy·a·not·ic (ā-sī′ă-not′ik) Characterized by absence of cyanosis.

a·cy·clic com·pound (ā-sik′lik kom′pownd) An organic compound in which the chain does not form a ring. SYN open chain compound.

ac·yl (as′il) An organic radical derived from an organic acid by the removal of the carboxylic hydroxyl group.

ac·yl·am·i·dase (as′il-am′i-dās) SYN amidase.

ac·yl car·ri·er pro·tein (ACP) (as′il kar′ē-ĕr prō′tēn) One of the proteins of the complex in cytoplasm that contains all the enzymes required to convert acetyl-CoA (and, in certain cases, butyryl-CoA or propionyl-CoA) and malonyl-CoA to palmitic acid. This complex is tightly bound together in mammalian tissues and in yeast, but that taken from *Escherichia coli* is readily dissociated. The ACP thus isolated is a heat-stable protein with a molecular weight of about 10,000. It contains a free –SH that binds the acyl intermediates in the synthesis of fatty acids as thioesters. This –SH group is part of a 4′-phosphopantetheine, added to the apoprotein by ACP phosphodiesterase, which thus plays the same role that it does in coenzyme A. ACP is involved in every step of the fatty acid synthetic process.

ac·yl-CoA (as′il-kō-ā) Condensation product of a carboxylic acid and coenzyme A; metabolic intermediate of importance, notably in the oxidation and synthesis of fat.

ac·yl-CoA de·hy·dro·ge·nase (NADPH) (as′il-kō-ā dē-hī-droj′ĕ-nās) Enzyme catalyzing the reversible reduction of enoyl-CoA derivatives of chain length 4–16, with NADPH as the hydrogen donor, forming acyl-CoA and $NADP^+$.

ac·yl·trans·fer·ase (as′il-trans′fĕr-ās) [EC class 2.3] An enzyme catalyzing the transfer of an acyl group from an acyl-CoA to any of various acceptors. SYN transacylase.

a·cys·ti·a (ā-sis′tē-ă) Congenital absence of urinary bladder. [G. *a-* priv. + *kystis,* bladder]

A.D. Abbreviation for *auris dextra* [L.], right ear. USAGE NOTE The JCAHO directs that *right ear* be written in full to avoid confusion with similar abbreviations.

♻ **ad-** Prefix denoting increase, adherence, to, toward; near; very. [L. *ad,* to, toward;]

♻ **-ad** Suffix used in anatomic nomenclature meaning -ward; toward or in the direction of the part indicated by the main portion of the word. [L. *ad,* to]

ADA Abbreviation for U.S. Americans with Disabilities Act; American Dental Association; American Diabetes Association; American Dietetic Association.

a·dac·ty·lous (ā-dak′ti-lŭs) Without fingers or toes.

a·dac·ty·ly (ā-dak′ti-lē) Congenital absence of digits (fingers or toes). [G. *a-* priv. + *daktylos,* digit]

ad·a·man·ti·no·ma (ad′ă-man′ti-nō′mă) SEE ameloblastoma.

ad·a·man·to·blas·to·ma (ad′ă-man′tō-blas-tō′mă) SEE ameloblastoma.

Ad·am's ap·ple (ad′ămz ap′ĕl) Colloquial name for the laryngeal prominence formed by the ventral edges of the thyroid cartilage.

Ad·ams·ite (DM) (ad′ămz-īt) A vomiting agent, diphenylaminearsine (NATO code DM). SEE ALSO riot-control agent, vomiting agent.

Ad·ams-Stokes dis·ease (ad′ămz-stōks di-zēz′) SYN Adams-Stokes syndrome.

Ad·ams-Stokes syn·drome (ad′ămz-stōks sin′drōm) A disorder characterized by slow or absent pulse, vertigo, syncope, convulsions, and sometimes Cheyne-Stokes respiration; usually as a result of advanced A-V block or sick sinus syndrome. SYN Adams-Stokes disease, Morgagni disease, Spens syndrome, Stokes-Adams syndrome.

ad·an·so·ni·an clas·si·fi·ca·tion (ad′ăn-sō′nē-ăn klas′i-fi-kā′shŭn) The classification of organisms based on giving equal weight to every character of the organism; this principle has its greatest application in numeric taxonomy.

ad•ap•ta•tion (ad′ap-tā′shŭn) **1.** Preferential survival of members of a species because of a phenotype that gives them an enhanced capacity to withstand the environment. **2.** An advantageous change in function or constitution of an organ or tissue to meet new conditions. **3.** Adjustment of the sensitivity of the retina to light intensity. **4.** A property of certain sensory receptors that modifies the response to repeated or continued stimuli at constant intensity. **5.** DENTISTRY The fitting, condensing, or contouring of a restorative material, foil, or shell to a tooth or cast so as to ensure close contact. **6.** The dynamic process wherein the thoughts, feelings, behavior, and biophysiologic mechanisms of a person continually change to adjust to a constantly changing environment. **7.** A homeostatic response. **8.** OCCUPATIONAL THERAPY The ability to anticipate, correct for, and benefit by learning from the consquences of errors that arise during task performances. [L. *ad-apto,* pp. *-atus,* to adjust]

a•dapt•er, a•dap•tor (ă-dap′tĕr, ă-dap′tŏr) **1.** A connecting part, joining two pieces of apparatus. **2.** A converter of electric current to a desired form.

a•dap•tive be•hav•ior scales (ă-dap′tiv bē-hāv′yŏr skālz) A behavioral assessment device to quantify the levels of skills of mentally retarded and developmentally delayed people in interacting with the environment; consists of three developmentally related factors: 1) personal self-sufficiency, e.g., eating, dressing; 2) community self-sufficiency, e.g., shopping, communicating; 3) personal and social responsibility, e.g., use of leisure time, job performance. SEE intelligence.

a•dap•tive hy•per•tro•phy (ă-dap′tiv hī-pĕr′trō-fē) Thickening of the walls of a hollow organ (e.g., urinary bladder) when there is obstruction to outflow.

a•dap•tive ther•mo•gen•e•sis (ă-dap′tiv thĕr′mō-jen′ĕ-sis) Regulated production of heat, which is influenced by environmental temperature and diet.

ad•ap•tom•e•ter (ad′ap-tom′ĕ-tĕr) A device for determining the course of retinal dark adaptation and for measuring the minimum light threshold.

ADAT Abbreviation for advance diet as tolerated.

ADD Abbreviation for attention deficit disorder.

ad•der•wort (ad′ĕr-wōrt) SYN bistort.

ad•dict (ad′ikt) A person who is physiologically or psychologically habituated to a substance or practice.

ad•dic•tion (ă-dik′shŭn) Habitual psychological and physiologic dependence on a substance or practice that is beyond voluntary control. Commonly abused substances include alcohol and drugs, although gasoline intoxication has been widely found among Aboriginal youth in Nunavit and elsewhere in northern Canada. [L. *ad-dico,* pp. *-dictus,* consent, fr. *ad-* + *dico,* to say]

ad•dic•tion se•ver•i•ty in•dex (ASI) (ă-dik′shŭn sĕ-ver′i-tē in′deks) A measurement instrument used to assess a patient's level of substance abuse or dependency.

Addison anaemia [Br.] SYN Addison anemia.

Ad•di•son a•ne•mi•a (ad′i-sŏn ă-nē′mē-ă) SYN pernicious anemia. SYN Addison anaemia.

Ad•di•son dis•ease (ad′ĭ-sŏn di-zēz′) SYN chronic adrenocortical insufficiency.

ad•di•so•ni•an cri•sis (ad′i-sōn′ē-ăn krī′sis) SYN acute adrenocortical insufficiency.

ad•di•tive (ad′i-tiv) **1.** A substance not naturally a part of a material (e.g., food) but deliberately added to fulfill some specific purpose (e.g., preservation). **2.** Tending to add or be added; denoting addition. **3.** In quantitative studies (e.g., genetics, epidemiology, physiology, statistics), having the property that the total combined effect of two or more factors equals the sum of their individual effects in isolation. Cf. synergism.

ad•di•tive ef•fect (ad′i-tiv e-fekt′) An effect wherein two or more substances or actions used in combination produce a total effect the same as the arithmetic sum of the individual effects.

ad•dres•sin (ă-dres′in) A molecule on the surface of a cell that serves as a homing device to direct another molecule to a specific location. [address, fr. O.Fr. *adresser,* to direct, fr. L.L. *addirectiare,* fr. L. *ad,* to, + *directus,* straight, direct, + -in]

ad•dress•in li•gands (ă-dres′in lī′gandz) Ligands on cells for specific homing receptors on lymphocytes.

ad•duct (ă-dŭkt′) To draw toward the median plane. [L. *ad-duco,* pp. *-ductus,* to bring toward]

ad•duc•tion (ă-dŭk′shŭn) **1.** Movement of a body part toward the median plane (of the body, in the case of limbs; of the hand or foot, in the case of digits) or midline of the body. **2.** Monocular rotation (duction) of the eye toward the nose. **3.** A position resulting from such movement. Cf. abduction.

ad•duc•tor (ă-dŭk′tŏr) A muscle that draws a part toward the median plane; or, in the case of the digits, toward the normal axis of the middle finger or the second toe.

ad•duc•tor brev•is mus•cle (ă-dŭk′tŏr brev′is mŭs′ĕl) *Origin,* superior ramus of pubis; *insertion,* upper third of medial lip of linea aspera; *action,* adducts thigh; *nerve supply,* obturator. SYN musculus adductor brevis [TA], short adductor muscle.

ad•duc•tor ca•nal (ă-dŭk′tŏr kă-nal′) The space in the middle third of the thigh between the vastus medialis and adductor muscles, converted into a canal by the overlying sartorius muscle. It gives passage to the femoral vessels and saphenous nerve, ending at the adductor hiatus. SYN canalis adductorius [TA], Hunter canal.

ad•duc•tor hal•lu•cis mus•cle (ă-dŭk′tŏr hal′ū-sis mŭs′ĕl) *Origin*, by two heads, the transverse head from the capsules of the lateral four metatarsophalangeal joints and the oblique head from the lateral cuneiform and bases of the third and fourth metatarsal bones; *insertion*, lateral side of base of proximal phalanx of great toe; *action*, adducts great toe; *nerve supply*, lateral plantar. See this page. SYN musculus adductor hallucis [TA].

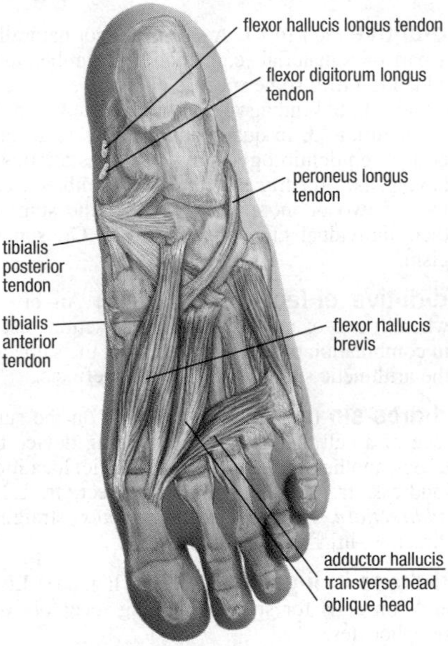

adductor hallucis muscle

ad•duc•tor lon•gus mus•cle (ă-dŭk′tŏr long′gus mŭs′ĕl) *Origin*, symphysis and crest of pubis; *insertion*, middle third of medial lip of linea aspera; *action*, adducts thigh; *nerve supply*, obturator. SYN musculus adductor longus [TA], long adductor muscle.

ad•duc•tor mag•nus mus•cle (ă-dŭk′tŏr mag′nŭs mŭs′ĕl) *Origin*, ischial tuberosity and ischiopubic ramus; *insertion*, linea aspera and adductor tubercle of femur; *action*, adducts and extends thigh; *nerve supply*, obturator and sciatic. See this page. SYN musculus adductor magnus [TA], great adductor muscle.

ad•duc•tor min•i•mus mus•cle (ad-dŭk′tŏr min′ē-mus mŭs′ĕl) A small flat muscle of the medial (adductor) compartment of the thigh; forms upper portion of adductor magnus, *insertion*, space above linea aspera. SYN musculus adductor minimus.

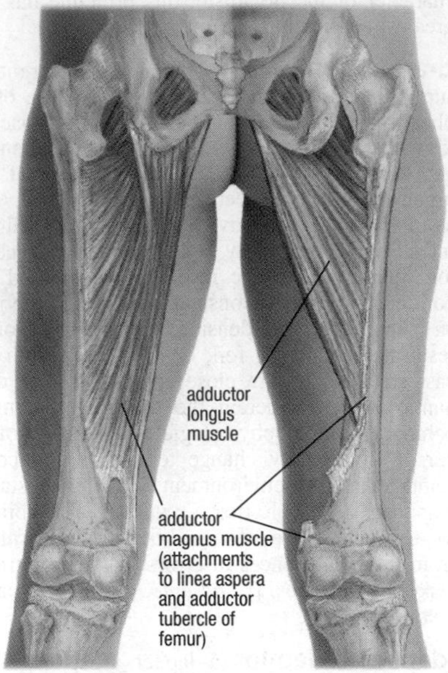

adductor magnus muscle

ad•duc•tor pol•li•cis mus•cle (ă-dŭk′tŏr pol′li-sis mŭs′ĕl) *Origin*, by two heads, the transverse head from the shaft of the third metacarpal and the oblique head from the front of the base of the second metacarpal, the trapezoid and capitate bones; *insertion*, medial side of base of proximal phalanx of thumb; *action*, adducts thumb; *nerve supply*, ulnar. SYN musculus adductor pollicis [TA].

ad•duc•tor spas•mod•ic dys•pho•ni•a (ă-dŭk′tŏr spaz-mod′ik dis-fō′nē-ă) A form of spasmodic dysphonia in which excessive closure of the vocal cords affects the initiation and maintenance of phonation.

ad•duc•tor tu•ber•cle of fe•mur (ă-dŭk′tŏr tū′bĕr-kĕl fē′mŭr) The prominence above the medial epicondyle of the femur to which the tendon of the adductor magnus attaches.

ADE Abbreviation for adverse drug effect.

Ade Abbreviation for adenine.

a•den•drit•ic, a•den•dric (ā-den-drit′ik, ā-den′drik) Without dendrites. [G., *a-* priv. + *dendron,* tree]

ad•e•nec•to•my (ad′ĕ-nek′tŏ-mē) Excision of a gland. [aden- + G. *ektomē,* excision]

ad•e•nec•to•pi•a (ad′ĕ-nek-tō′pē-ă) Presence of a gland in other than its normal anatomic position. [aden- + G. *ek,* out of, + *topos,* place]

a•den•i•form (ă-den′i-fōrm) SYN adenoid (1).

ad•e•nine (A, Ade) (ad′ĕ-nēn) One of the two major purines (the other being guanine) found in both RNA and DNA, and also in various free nucleotides.

ad•e•nine de•ox•y•ri•bo•nu•cle•o•tide (ad′ĕ-nēn dē-oks′ē-rī-bō-nū′klē-ō-tīd) SYN deoxyadenylic acid.

ad•e•nine nu•cle•o•tide (ad′ĕ-nēn nū′klē-ō-tīd) SYN adenylic acid.

ad•e•ni•tis (ad′ĕ-nī′tis) Inflammation of a lymph node or of a gland. [aden- + G. *-itis,* inflammation]

ad•e•ni•za•tion (ad′ĕ-nī-zā′shŭn) Conversion into a glandlike structure.

♻**adeno-, aden-** Combining forms denoting gland, glandular; corresponds to L. *glandul-, glandi-*. [G. *adēn, adenos,* a gland]

ad•e•no•ac•an•tho•ma (ad′ĕ-nō-ak′an-thō′mă) A malignant neoplasm consisting chiefly of glandular epithelium (adenocarcinoma), usually well differentiated, with foci of metaplasia to squamous (or epidermoid) neoplastic cells. SYN adenoid squamous cell carcinoma.

ad•e•no•blast (ad′ĕ-nō-blast) A proliferating embryonic cell with the potential to form glandular parenchyma. [adeno- + G. *blastos,* germ]

ℹ**ad•e•no•car•ci•no•ma** (ad′ĕ-nō-kahr′si-nō′mă) A malignant neoplasm of epithelial cells in glandular or glandlike pattern. See page B14, B16.

ad•e•no•car•ci•no•ma in Bar•rett e•soph•a•gus (ad′ĕ-nō-kahr′si-nō′mă bar′ĕt ĕ-sof′ă-gŭs) An adenocarcinoma arising in the esophagus, which has become lined with columnar cells (Barrett mucosa).

ad•e•no•car•ci•no•ma•tous (ad′ĕ-nō-kahr′si-nō′mă-tŭs) Pertaining to a malignant tumor originating in glandular epithelium.

ad•e•no•cel•lu•li•tis (ad′ĕ-nō-sel′yū-lī′tis) Inflammation of a gland, usually a lymph node, and of the adjacent connective tissue.

ad•e•no•chon•dro•ma (ad′ĕ-nō-kon-drō′mă) SYN pulmonary hamartoma. [adeno- + G. *chondros,* cartilage, + *-oma,* tumor]

ad•e•no•cys•to•ma (ad′ĕ-nō-sis-tō′mă) Adenoma in which the neoplastic glandular epithelium forms cysts.

ad•e•no•cyte (ad′ĕ-nō-sīt) A secretory cell of a gland. [adeno- + G. *kytos,* a hollow (cell)]

ad•e•no•fi•bro•ma (ad′ĕ-nō-fī-brō′mă) A benign neoplasm composed of glandular and fibrous tissues.

ad•e•no•fi•bro•my•o•ma (ad′ĕ-nō-fī′brō-mī-ō′mă) SYN adenomatoid tumor.

ad•e•no•fi•bro•sis (ad′ĕ-nō-fī-brō′sis) SYN sclerosing adenosis.

ad•e•nog•en•ous (ad′ĕ-noj′en-ŭs) Having an origin from glandular tissue.

ad•e•no•hy•po•phy•si•al (ad′ĕ-nō-hī-pō-fiz′ē-ăl) Relating to the adenohypophysis.

a•de•no•hy•po•phy•si•al pouch (ad′ĕ-nō-hī-pō-fiz′ē-ăl powch) SYN hypophysial diverticulum.

ad•e•no•hy•poph•y•sis (ad′ĕ-nō-hī-pof′i-sis) The anterior pituitary gland. It consists of the distal part, intermediate part, and infundibular part. SEE ALSO hypophysis. SYN lobus anterior hypophyseos [TA], anterior lobe of hypophysis.

ad•e•no•hy•poph•y•si•tis (ad′ĕ-nō-hī-pof-i-sī′tis) Inflammatory reaction or sepsis affecting the anterior pituitary gland, often related to pregnancy.

ad•e•noid (ad′ĕ-noyd) **1.** Glandlike; of glandular appearance. SYN adeniform, lymphoid (2). **2.** SEE adenoids. [adeno- + G. *eidos,* appearance]

ad•e•noi•dal-pha•ryn•ge•al-con•junc•ti•val vi•rus (ad-ĕ-noy′dăl-făr-in′jē-ăl- kŏn-jŭngk′ti-văl vī′rŭs) SYN adenovirus.

ad•e•noid cys•tic car•ci•no•ma (ad′ĕ-noyd sis′tik kahr′si-nō′mă) A histologic type of carcinoma characterized by round, glandlike spaces or cysts bordered by layers of epithelial cells without intervening stroma, forming a pattern like a slice of Swiss cheese; perineural invasion and hematogenous metastasis are common; occurs most commonly in salivary glands. SYN cylindromatous carcinoma.

ad•e•noid•ec•to•my (ad′ĕ-noyd-ek′tŏ-mē) An operation for the removal of adenoid growths in the nasopharynx. [adenoid + G. *ektomē,* excision]

ad•e•noid fa•ci•es (ad′ĕ-noyd fā′shē-ēz) The open-mouthed and often dull appearance in children with adenoid hypertrophy, associated with a pinched nose.

ad•e•noid•i•tis (ad′ĕ-noyd-ī′tis) Inflammation of nasopharyngeal lymphoid tissue.

ad•e•noids (ad′ĕ-noydz) **1.** A normal collection of unencapsulated lymphoid tissue in the nasopharynx. Also called pharyngeal tonsils. **2.** Common terminology for the large (normal) pharyngeal tonsils of children. [G. *adēn,* gland, + *-eidos,* resemblance]

ad•e•noid squa•mous cell car•ci•no•ma (ad′ĕ-noyd skwā′mŭs sel kahr′si-nō′mă) SYN adenoacanthoma.

ad•e•noid tis•sue (ad′ĕ-noyd tish′ū) SYN lymphatic tissue.

ad•e•no•li•po•ma (ad′ĕ-nō-li-pō′mă) A benign neoplasm composed of glandular and adipose tissues. [G. *adēn,* gland, + *lipos,* fat, + *-oma,* tumor]

ad•e•no•lip•o•ma•to•sis (ad′ĕ-nō-lip′ō-mă-tō′sis) A condition characterized by development of multiple adenolipomas.

ad•e•no•ma (ad′ĕ-nō′mă) An ordinarily benign neoplasm of epithelial tissue in which the tumor cells form glands or glandlike structures in the stroma; usually well circumscribed, tending to compress rather than infiltrate or invade adjacent tissue. [adeno- + G. *-oma,* tumor]

a•de•no•ma•la•ci•a (ad′ĕ-nō-mă-lā′shē-ă) Abnormal softening of a gland.

ad•e•no•ma•toid (ad′ĕ-nō′mă-toyd) Resembling an adenoma.

ad•e•no•ma•toid o•don•to•gen•ic tu•mor (ad′ĕ-nō′mă-toyd ō-don′tō-jen′ik tū′mŏr) A benign epithelial odontogenic tumor appearing radiographically as a well-circumscribed, radiolucent-radiopaque lesion usually surrounding the crown of an impacted tooth in an adolescent or young adult; characterized histologically by columnar cells organized in a ductlike configuration interspersed with spindle-shaped cells and amyloidlike deposition that gradually undergoes dystrophic calcification. SYN ameloblastic adenomatoid tumor.

ad•e•no•ma•toid tu•mor (ad′ĕ-nō′mă-toyd tū′mŏr) A small benign neoplasm of the epididymis or female genital tract, consisting of fibrous tissue enclosing glandlike spaces lined by mesothelial cells. SYN adenofibromyoma, Recklinghausen tumor.

ad•e•no•ma•to•sis (ad′ĕ-nō′mă-tō′sis) A condition characterized by numerous overgrowths of glandular tissue.

ad•e•no•ma•tous (ad′ĕ-nō′mă-tŭs) Relating to an adenoma, and to some types of glandular hyperplasia.

ad•e•no•ma•tous goi•ter (ad′ĕ-nō′mă-tŭs goy′tĕr) An enlargement of the thyroid gland due to the growth of one or more encapsulated adenomas or multiple nonencapsulated colloid nodules within its substance. SYN adenomatous goitre.

adenomatous goitre [Br.] SYN adenomatous goiter.

ad•e•no•ma•tous hy•per•pla•si•a (ad′ĕ-nō′mă-tŭs hī′pĕr-plā′zē-ă) SYN complex endometrial hyperplasia.

ad•e•no•ma•tous pol•yp (ad′ĕ-nō′mă-tŭs pol′ip) A polyp that consists of benign neoplastic tissue derived from glandular epithelium.

ad•e•no•ma•tous pol•y•po•sis co•li (ad′ĕ-nō′mă-tŭs pol′i-pō′sis kō′lī) SYN familial adenomatous polyposis.

a•de•no•meg•a•ly (ad′ĕ-nō-meg′ă-lē) Enlargement of a gland.

ad•e•no•mere (ad′ĕ-nō-mēr) Structural unit in the parenchyma of a developing gland that becomes the functional portion of the organ. [adeno- + G. *meros,* part]

ad•e•no•my•o•ma (ad′ĕ-nō-mī-ō′mă) A benign neoplasm of muscle (usually smooth muscle) with glandular elements; occurs most frequently in uterus and uterine ligaments. [G. *adēn*, gland, + *mys*, muscle, + *-oma*, tumor]

ad•e•no•my•o•sis (ad′ĕ-nō-mī-ō′sis) The ectopic occurrence or diffuse implantation of adenomatous tissue in muscle (usually smooth muscle). [G. *adēn*, gland, + *mys*, muscle, + *-osis* condition]

ad•e•nop•a•thy (ad′ĕ-nop′ă-thē) Swelling or morbid enlargement of the lymph nodes. [adeno- + G. *pathos,* suffering]

ad•e•no•sal•pin•gi•tis (ad′ĕ-nō-sal′pin-jī′tis) SYN salpingitis isthmica nodosa.

ad•e•no•sar•co•ma (ad′ĕ-nō-sahr-kō′mă) A malignant neoplasm arising simultaneously or consecutively in mesodermal tissue and glandular epithelium of the same part.

a•den•o•sine (Ado) (ă-den′ō-sēn) **1.** A condensation product of adenine and D-ribose; a nucleoside found among the hydrolysis products of all nucleic acids and of the various adenine nucleotides. **2.** A potent coronary vasodilator used in place of exercise for radionuclide myocardial perfusion studies. SYN gamma (γ)-beta (β)-D-ribofuranosyladenine.

a•den•o•sine 3′,5′-cy•clic mon•o•phos•phate (cAMP) (ă-den′ō-sēn sik′lik mon′ō-fos′fāt) An activator of phosphorylase kinase and an effector of other enzymes, formed in muscle from ATP by adenylate cyclase and broken down to 5′-AMP by a phosphodiesterase; sometimes referred to as the "second messenger." A related compound (2′,3′) is also known. SYN cyclic AMP.

a•den•o•sine 5′-di•phos•phate (ADP) (ă-den′ō-sēn dī-fos′fāt) A condensation product of adenosine with pyrophosphoric acid, formed from ATP by the hydrolysis of the terminal phosphate group of the latter compound.

a•den•o•sine di•phos•phate (ă-den′ō-sēn dī-fos′fāt) SEE adenosine 5′-diphosphate.

a•den•o•sine mon•o•phos•phate (AMP) (ă-den′ō-sēn mon′ō-fos′fāt) Adenosine-5′-monophosphate. SEE adenylic acid.

a•den•o•sine phos•phate (ă-den′ō-sēn fos′fāt) Specifically, adenosine 3′- or 5′-phosphate. SEE adenylic acid.

a•den•o•sine 5′-phos•pho•sul•fate (APS) (ă-den′ō-sēn fos′fō-sŭl′fāt) An intermediate in the formation of PAPS (active sulfate). SYN adenosine 5′-phosphosulphate.

adenosine 5′-phosphosulphate [Br.] SYN adenosine 5′-phosphosulfate.

a·den·o·sine tri·phos·pha·tase (ATPase) (ă-den′ō-sēn trī-fos′fă-tās) An enzyme in muscle (myosin) and elsewhere that catalyzes the release of the terminal phosphate group of adenosine 5′-triphosphate.

a·den·o·sine 5′-tri·phos·phate (ATP) (ă-den′ō-sēn trī-fos′fāt) Adenosine (5) pyrophosphate; adenosine with triphosphoric acid esterfied at its 5′ position; immediate precursor of adenine nucleotides in RNA. The primary energy currency of a cell.

ad·e·no·sis (ad′ĕ-nō′sis) **1.** A more-or-less generalized glandular disease. **2.** Glandular tissue in one or more sites in which it is not usually found.

ad·e·not·o·my (ad′ĕ-not′ŏ-mē) Incision of a gland. [adeno- + G. *tomē,* a cutting]

ad·e·no·ton·sil·lec·to·my (ad′ĕ-nō-ton′si-lek′tŏ-mē) Operative removal of tonsils and adenoids.

Ad·e·no·vi·ri·dae (ad′ĕ-nō-vir′i-dē) A family of double-stranded DNA viruses, commonly known as adenoviruses, which develop in the nuclei of infected cells in mammals and birds.

i **ad·e·no·vi·rus** (ad′ĕ-nō-vī′rŭs) Adenoidal-pharyngeal-conjunctival (A-P-C) virus; any virus of the family Adenoviridae. More than 40 types are known to infect humans, causing upper respiratory symptoms, acute respiratory disease, conjunctivitis, gastroenteritis, hemorrhagic cystitis, and serous infections in neonates. See page B6. SYN adenoidal-pharyngeal-conjunctival virus. [G. *adēn,* gland, + virus]

ad·e·nyl (ad′ĕ-nil) The radical or ion of adenine.

a·den·y·late (ă-den′i-lāt) Salt or ester of adenylic acid.

a·den·y·late cy·clase (ă-den′i-lāt sī′klās) An enzyme acting on ATP to form 3′,5′-cyclic AMP plus pyrophosphate. A crucial step in the regulation and formation of second messengers. SYN 3′,5′-cyclic AMP synthetase.

a·den·y·late ki·nase (ă-den′i-lāt kī′nās) Adenylic acid kinase; a phosphotransferase that catalyzes the reversible phosphorylation of a molecule of ADP by MgADP, yielding MgATP and AMP.

ad·e·nyl·ic ac·id (ad′ĕ-nil′ik as′id) A condensation product of adenosine and phosphoric acid; a nucleotide found among the hydrolysis products of all nucleic acids. SEE ALSO AMP. SYN adenine nucleotide.

ad·eps, gen. **ad·i·pis** (ad′eps, ad′i-pis) Denoting fat or adipose tissue. [L. lard, fat]

ad·eps la·nae (ad′eps lā′nē) The greasy substance obtained from the wool of the sheep *Ovis aries* (family Bovidae); used as an emollient base for creams and ointments. SYN lanolin. [L. fat of wool]

ad·e·quate in·take (AI) (ad′ĕ-kwăt in′tāk) A recommended intake value based on observed or experimentally determined approximations or estimates of nutrient intake by a group (or groups) of healthy people, which are assumed to be adequate—used when an RDA cannot be determined.

ad·e·quate stim·u·lus (ad′ĕ-kwăt stim′yū-lŭs) A stimulus to which a particular receptor responds effectively and that gives rise to a characteristic sensation (e.g., light and sound waves that stimulate, respectively, visual and auditory receptors).

a·der·mi·a (ā-dĕr′mē-ă) Congenital defect or absence of skin. [G. *a-* priv. + *derma,* skin]

a·der·mo·gen·e·sis (ă-dĕr′mō-jen′ĕ-sis) Failure or imperfection in the regeneration of the skin, especially the imperfect repair of a cutaneous defect. [G. *a-* priv. + *derma,* skin, + *genesis,* origin]

ADH Abbreviation for alcohol dehydrogenase; antidiuretic hormone.

ADHA Abbreviation for American Dental Hygienists Association.

ADHD Abbreviation for attention deficit hyperactivity disorder.

ad·her·ence (ad-hēr′ĕns) **1.** The act or quality of sticking to something. SEE ALSO adhesion. **2.** The extent to which a patient continues treatment under limited supervision. Cf. compliance (2), maintenance. [L. *adhaereo,* to stick to]

ad·hes·i·ol·y·sis (ad-hē′zē-ol′i-sis) Severing of adhesive band(s); done by laparoscopy or laparotomy. [adhesion + lysis]

ad·he·sion (ad-hē′zhŭn) **1.** The adhering or uniting of two surfaces or parts, especially the union of the opposing surfaces of a wound or adjacent layers of fascia. SYN conglutination (1). **2.** In the pleural or peritoneal cavity, inflammatory bands that connect opposing serous surfaces. **3.** Mutual attraction of unlike molecules. [L. *adhaesio,* fr. *adhaereo,* to stick to]

ad·he·sion mol·e·cules (ad-hē′zhŭn mol′ĕ-kyūlz) Molecules that are involved in T-helper accessory cell, T-helper B cell, and T-cytotoxic target cell interactions.

ad·he·si·ot·o·my (ad-hē′zē-ot′ŏ-mē) Surgical section or lysis of adhesions.

ad·he·sive (ad-hē′siv) **1.** Relating to, or having the characteristics of, an adhesion. **2.** Any material that adheres to a surface or causes adherence between surfaces.

ad·he·sive ab·sor·bent dress·ing (ad-hē′siv ab-sōr′bĕnt dres′ing) A sterile individual dressing consisting of a plain absorbent compress affixed to a film of fabric coated with a pressure-sensitive adhesive. SYN adhesive bandage.

ad•he•sive ban•dage (ad-hē′siv ban′dăj) SYN adhesive absorbent dressing.

ad•he•sive cap•su•li•tis (ad-hē′siv kap′sŭ-lī′tis) A condition with limitation of motion in a joint due to inflammatory thickening of the capsule, a common cause of stiffness in the shoulder.

ad•he•sive in•flam•ma•tion (ad-hē′siv in′flă-mā′shŭn) Inflammation in which the amount of fibrin in the exudate is sufficient to result in a slight or moderate degree of adherence of adjacent tissues, as in healing by first intention.

ad•he•sive o•ti•tis (ad-hē′siv ō-tī′tis) Inflammation of the middle ear caused by prolonged auditory tube dysfunction resulting in permanent retraction of the eardrum and obliteration of the middle ear space.

ad•he•sive per•i•car•di•tis (ad-hē′siv per′ē-kahr-dī′tis) Pericarditis with adhesions between the two pericardial layers, between the pericardium and heart, or between the pericardium and neighboring structures.

ad•he•sive per•i•to•ni•tis (ad-hē′siv per′i-tō-nī′tis) A form of peritonitis in which a fibrinous exudate occurs, matting together the intestines and various other organs.

ad•he•sive pleu•ri•sy (ad-hē′siv plūr′i-sē) SYN dry pleurisy.

ad•he•sive vag•i•ni•tis (ad-hē′siv vaj′i-nī′tis) Inflammation of vaginal mucosa with adhesions of the vaginal walls to each other.

ADI Abbreviation for acceptable daily intake.

a•di•a•ba•tic (ā′dē-ă-bat′ik) Referring to a thermodynamic process in which there is no gain or loss of heat between the system and its surroundings. [G. *adiabatos,* impassable, fr. *a* priv. + *diabainō,* to go through]

ad•i•ad•o•cho•ki•ne•si•a (ă-dī′ă-dō-kō-kin-ē′zē-ă) SYN adiadochokinesis.

ad•i•ad•o•cho•ki•ne•sis (ă-dī′ă-dō-kō-kin-ē′sis) Inability to perform rapid alternating movements, a sign of cerebellar dysfunction. Cf. diadochokinesia. SYN adiadochokinesia. [G. *a-* priv. + *diadochos,* successive, + *kinēsis,* movement]

a•di•a•pho•re•sis (ā′dī-ă-fōr-ē′sis) SYN anhidrosis. [G. *a-* priv. + *diaphorēsis,* perspiration]

a•di•a•pho•ri•a (ă-dī′ă-fōr′ē-ă) Failure to respond to stimulation after a series of previously applied stimuli. [G. *a-* priv. + *dia,* through, + *phoros,* bearing]

A•die syn•drome, **A•die pu•pil** (a′dē sin′drōm, a′dē pyū′pil) An idiopathic postganglionic denervation of the parasympathetically innervated intraocular muscles, usually complicated by signs of aberrant regeneration of these nerves: a weak light reaction with segmental palsy of iris sphincter, a strong, slow near response. Deep tendon reflexes are often asymmetrically reduced. SEE ALSO tonic pupil. SYN Holmes-Adie pupil, Holmes-Adie syndrome, pupillotonic pseudostrabismus.

♲ **adip-**, **adipo-** Combining forms meaning fat, fatty. Corresponds to G. lip-, lipo-. SEE ALSO lipo-. [L. *adeps, adipis,* soft animal fat, lard, grease]

ad•i•pis (ad′i-pis) Genitive form of adeps.

ad•i•po•cel•lu•lar (ad′i-pō-sel′yū-lăr) Relating to both fatty and cellular tissues, or to connective tissue with many fat cells.

ad•i•po•cer•a•tous (ad′i-pō-ser′ă-tŭs) Relating to adipocere. SYN lipoceratous.

ad•i•po•cere (ad′i-pō-sēr) A fatty substance of waxy consistency into which dead animal tissues (e.g., those of a corpse) are sometimes converted when kept from the air under certain conditions of temperature. SYN lipocere. [adipo- + L. *cera,* wax]

ad•i•po•cyte (ad′i-pō-sīt) SYN fat cell.

ad•i•po•cy•to•kines (ad′i-pō-sī′tō-kēnz) SYN adipokines.

ad•i•po•gen•e•sis (ad′i-pō-jen′ĕ-sis) SYN lipogenesis.

ad•i•po•gen•ic, **ad•i•pog•e•nous** (ad′i-pō-jen′ik, ad′i-poj′ĕ-nŭs) SYN lipogenic.

ad•i•poid (ad′i-poyd) SYN lipoid. [adipo- + G. *eidos,* resemblance]

ad•i•po•kines (ad′i-pō′kēnz) Autocrine and paracrine factors released from human adipose tissue, in particular the visceral depots; including cytokines, acute phase reactants, growth factors, and other inflammatory mediators. Many are involved in the pathogenesis of hypertension, insulin resistance, and atherosclerosis. SYN adipocytokines. [adipo- + G. *kineō* to set in motion]

ad•i•po•ki•net•ic (ad′i-pō-ki-net′ik) Denoting a substance or factor that causes mobilization of stored lipid. [adipo- + G. *kinēsis,* movement]

ad•i•po•ki•nin, **ad•i•po•ki•net•ic hor•mone** (ad′i-pō-kī′nin, ad′i-pō-ki-net′ik hōr′mōn) An anterior pituitary hormone that causes mobilization of fat from adipose tissue.

ad•i•po•nec•tin (ad′i-pō-nek′tin) Protective adipokine that reduces lipid accumulation and endothelial adhesion resulting from vascular injury; increases skeletal muscle oxidation of free fatty acids; reduces hepatic glucose output; increases peripheral insulin sensitivity. [adipo- + L. *necto,* to join together, + -in]

ad•i•pose (ad′i-pōs) Denoting fat.

ad•i•pose cell (ad′i-pōs sel) SYN fat cell.

ad•i•pose de•gen•er•a•tion (ad′i-pōs dĕ-jen′ĕr-ā′shŭn) SYN fatty degeneration.

ad•i•pose fos•sae (ad′i-pōs fos′ē) Subcutaneous spaces containing accumulations of fat in the breast.

ad•i•pose in•fil•tra•tion (ad′i-pōs in′fil-trā′shŭn) Growth of normal adult fat cells in sites where they are not usually present.

ad•i•pose tis•sue (AT) (ad′i-pōs tish′ū) A connective tissue consisting chiefly of fat cells surrounded by reticular fibers and arranged in lobular groups or along the course of one of the smaller blood vessels. SYN fat (1).

ad•i•po•sis (ad′i-pō′sis) Excessive local or general accumulation of fat in the body. SYN lipomatosis, liposis (1), steatosis (1). [adipo- + G. *-osis,* condition]

ad•i•po•sis car•di•ac•a (ad′i-pō′sis kahr-dē-ā′kă) SYN fatty heart (2).

ad•i•pos•i•ty (ad′i-pos′i-tē) **1.** SYN obesity. **2.** Excessive accumulation of lipids in a site or organ.

ad•i•po•so•gen•i•tal dys•tro•phy (ad′i-pō-sō-jen′i-tăl dis′trŏ-fē) SYN dystrophia adiposogenitalis.

ad•i•po•su•ri•a (ad′i-pō-syūr′ē-ă) SYN lipuria. [adipo- + G. *ouron,* urine]

ad•i•tus, pl. **ad•i•tus** (ad′i-tŭs, ad′i-tūs) [TA] SYN aperture, inlet. [L. access, fr. *ad-eo,* pp. *-itus,* go to]

ad•junc•tive ther•a•py (ad-jungk′tiv thār′ă-pē) Any accessory treatment used in combination to enhance to primary treatment.

ad•just•ment (ă-jŭst′mĕnt) **1.** SYN spinal adjustment. **2.** SYN occlusal adjustment. **3.** In health care accounting, any addition or deletion in a patient's record that will alter the balance due.

ad•just•ment dis•or•der (ă-jŭst′mĕnt dis-ōr′dĕr) **1.** A class of mental and behavioral disorders in which the development of symptoms is related to the presence of some environmental stressor or life event and is expected to remit when the stress ceases. **2.** A disorder the essential feature of which is a maladaptive reaction to an identifiable psychological stress, or stressors, which occurs within weeks of the onset of the stressors and persists for up to 6 months.

ad•ju•vant (ad′jū-vănt) **1.** A substance added to a drug product formulation that affects the action of the active ingredient in a predictable way. **2.** IMMUNOLOGY a vehicle used to enhance antigenicity. **3.** Additional therapy given to enhance or extend primary therapy's effect, such as in chemotherapy in addition to a surgical regimen. **4.** A treatment added to a curative treatment to prevent recurrence of clinical cancer from microscopic residual disease. [L. *ad-juvo,* pres. p. *-juvans,* to give aid to]

ADL Abbreviation for activities of daily living. SEE ALSO activities of daily living scale.

ad•ler•i•an psy•chol•o•gy (ad-ler′ē-ĕn sī-kŏl′ŏ-jē) Psychotherapeutic technique based on the theory that the major issues to be resolved during life involve social adjustments, occupations, and love. Major distinguishing tenet is that neurosis results from a feeling of inferiority that arises when the drive for superiority is frustrated. SYN individual psychology.

ad lib. Abbreviation for L. *ad libitum,* freely, as desired.

ad•min•i•stra•tion (ad-min′ĭ-strā′shŭn) **1.** The management of the affairs and activities of a group or entity. **2.** Persons charged with executive functions. **3.** The giving of a medicine or other treatment. [L. *administro,* to manage]

ad•mit•tance (ad-mit′ăns) SYN immittance.

ad•mit•ting di•ag•nosis (ad-mit′ing dī′ăg-nō′sis) Probable determination of a patient's condition or disorder used when a patient is admitted to a health care facility.

ad•mit•ting phys•i•cian (ad-mit′ing fi-zish′ŭn) A physician who is formally and legally responsible for admitting a patient to a health care facility.

ad•mix•ture (ad′miks-chŭr) A product of mixing.

ADN Abbreviation for Associate Degree in Nursing.

ad•neu•ral, ad•ner•val (ad-nūr′ăl, ad-nĕr′văl) **1.** Lying near a nerve. **2.** In the direction of a nerve; said of an electric current passing through muscular tissue toward the point of entrance of the nerve.

ad•nex•a, sing. **ad•nex•um** (ad-nek′să, ad-nek′sŭm) Parts accessory to an organ or structure, especially the uterus. SEE ALSO appendage. SYN annexa. [L. connected parts]

ad•nex•al (ad-nek′săl) Relating to the adnexa. SYN annexal.

ad•nex•al ad•e•no•ma (ad-nek′săl ad′ĕ-nō′mă) An adenoma arising in, or forming structures resembling, skin appendages.

ad•nex•um (ad-nek′sŭm) Singular of adnexa.

Ado Symbol for adenosine.

ad•o•les•cence (ad′ŏ-les′ĕns) The period of life beginning with puberty and ending with physical maturity. [L. *adolescentia*]

ad•o•les•cent (ad′ŏ-les′ĕnt) **1.** Pertaining to adolescence. **2.** A person in that stage of development.

ad•o•les•cent med•i•cine (ad′ŏ-les′ĕnt med′i-sin) The branch of medicine concerned with the treatment of youth in the approximate age range of 13–21 years. SYN hebiatrics.

a•don•is (ă-don′is) Flowering plant (*Adonis ver-*

nalis) thought to have medicinal qualities similar to those of *Digitalis* (q.v.); may cause serious drug interactions. [G. *Adonis,* handsome young man of myth, loved by Aphrodite]

a•dop•tive im•mu•no•ther•a•py (ă-dop′tiv im′yū-nō-thār′ă-pē) Passive transfer of immunity from an immune donor through inoculation of sensitized lymphocytes, transfer factor, immune RNA, or antibodies in serum or gamma globulin.

ADP Abbreviation for adenosine 5′-diphosphate.

ADR Abbreviation for adverse drug reaction.

ad•re•nal (ă-drē′năl) **1.** Near or on the kidney; denoting the suprarenal (adrenal) gland. **2.** A suprarenal gland or separate tissue or product thereof. SEE ALSO suprarenal. [L. *ad,* to, + *ren,* kidney]

ad•re•nal an•dro•gen-stim•u•lat•ing hor•mone (AASH) (ă-drē′năl an′drŏ-jen-stim′yū-lāt-ing hōr′mōn) A putative pituitary hormone that may be responsible for increased secretion of adrenal androgens at the time of puberty.

ad•re•nal cor•ti•cal car•ci•no•ma (ă-drē′năl kōr′ti-kăl kahr′si-nō′mă) A carcinoma arising in the cortex of the suprarenal gland that may cause virilism or Cushing syndrome.

ad•re•nal cri•sis (ă-drē′năl krī′sis) SYN acute adrenocortical insufficiency.

ad•re•nal•ec•to•my (ă-drē′năl-ek′tŏ-mē) Removal of one or both suprarenal glands, may be total or partial. Preoperative steroid replacement therapy may be required. [adrenal + G. *ektomē,* excision]

ad•re•nal gland (ă-drē′năl gland) SYN suprarenal gland.

ad•re•nal hy•per•ten•sion (ă-drē′năl hī′pĕr-ten′shŭn) Hypertension due to an adrenal medullary pheochromocytoma or to hyperactivity or functioning tumor of the cortex of suprarenal gland.

ad•ren•a•line (ă-dren′ă-lin) SYN epinephrine.

a•dre•nal•i•tis (ă-drē′năl-ī′tis) Inflammation of the suprarenal gland.

a•dre•na•lop•a•thy (ă-drē′nă-lop′ă-thē) Any pathologic condition of the suprarenal glands. SYN adrenopathy. [adrenal + G. *pathos,* suffering]

ad•re•nal rest (ă-drē′năl rest) SYN accessory suprarenal.

ad•ren•ar•che (ad′rĕ-nahr-kē) Increase in the production of androgens by the cortex of suprarenal gland that occurs at the age of 8–9 years old. [adrenal + G. *archē,* beginning]

ad•re•ner•gic (ad′rĕ-nĕr′jik) **1.** Relating to nerve cells or fibers of the autonomic nervous system that employ norepinephrine as their neurotransmitter. Cf. cholinergic. **2.** Relating to drugs that mimic the actions of the sympathetic nervous system. SEE alpha (α)-adrenergic receptors, beta (β)-adrenergic receptors. [adren- + G. *ergon,* work]

ad•re•ner•gic block•ade (ad′rĕ-nĕr′jik blok-ād′) Selective inhibition by a drug of the responses of effector cells to adrenergic sympathetic nerve impulses (sympatholytic) and to epinephrine and related amines (adrenolytic).

ad•re•ner•gic block•ing a•gent (ad′rĕ-nĕr′jik blok′ing ā′jĕnt) A compound that selectively blocks or inhibits responses to sympathetic adrenergic nerve activity (sympatholytic agent) and to epinephrine, norepinephrine, and other adrenergic amines (adrenolytic agent); two distinct classes exist, alpha- and beta-adrenergic receptor blocking agents.

ad•re•ner•gic bron•cho•di•la•tors (ad′rĕ-nĕr′jik brong′kō-dī′lā-tŏrz) A class of sympathomimetic drugs that act by stimulating receptors in the bronchi and other organs, producing smooth muscle relaxation. They are classified into three groups: alpha-adrenergic, $beta_1$-adrenergic, and $beta_2$-adrenergic bronchodilators.

ad•re•ner•gic fi•bers (ad′rĕ-nĕr′jik fī′bĕrz) Nerve fibers that transmit nervous impulses to other nerve cells (or smooth muscle or gland cells) by the medium of the adrenalinelike transmitter substance norepinephrine (noradrenaline). SYN adrenergic fibres.

adrenergic fibres [Br.] SYN adrenergic fibers.

ad•re•ner•gic neu•ro•nal block•ing a•gent (ad′rĕ-nĕr′jik nūr-ō′năl blok′ing ā′jĕnt) A drug that prevents the release of norepinephrine from sympathetic nerve terminals.

ad•re•ner•gic re•cep•tors (ad′rĕ-nĕr′jik rĕ-sep′tŏrz) Reactive components of effector tissues, most of which are innervated by the sympathetic nervous system. Such receptors can be activated by norepinephrine, epinephrine, and adrenergic drugs; receptor activation results in a change in effector tissue function, such as contraction of arteriolar muscles or relaxation of bronchial muscles. SYN adrenoreceptor.

a•dren•ic (ă-drē′nik) Relating to the suprarenal gland.

♻ **adreno-, adrenal-, adren-** Combining forms meaning related to the suprarenal gland. [L. *ad,* to, near, + *renes,* the kidneys, + -o- + *-alis,* pertaining to]

ad•re•no•cep•tive (ă-drē′nō-sep′tiv) Referring to chemical sites in effectors with which the adrenergic mediator unites. Cf. cholinoceptive.

ad•re•no•cor•ti•cal (ă-drē′nō-kōr′ti-kăl) Pertaining to the cortex of the suprarenal gland.

ad•re•no•cor•ti•cal in•suf•fi•cien•cy (ă-drē′nō-kōr′ti-kăl in′sŭ-fish′ĕn-sē) Loss, to varying degrees, of adrenocortical function. SYN hypocorticoidism.

ad•re•no•cor•ti•co•mi•met•ic (ă-drē′nō-kōr′ti-kō-mi-met′ik) Mimicking or producing effects similar to adrenocortical function. [adrenal + cortex + G. *mimētikos*, imitating]

ad•re•no•cor•ti•co•tro•pic hor•mone (ACTH) (ă-drē′nō-kōr′ti-kō-trō′pik hōr′mōn) The hormone of the anterior lobe of the hypophysis that governs the nutrition and growth of the cortex of suprarenal gland and stimulates it to functional activity; also possesses extraadrenal adipokinetic activity. SYN adrenotropin, corticotropin.

ad•re•no•cor•ti•co•tro•pic re•leas•ing fac•tor (ă-drē′nō-kōr′ti-kō-trō′pik rĕ-lēs′ing fak′tŏr) Hormone produced by the hypothalamus that causes the pituitary to secrete adrenocorticotropic hormone.

ad•re•no•cor•ti•co•tro•pin (ă-drē′nō-kōr′ti-kō-trō′pin) Protein hormone of the anterior pituitary gland that stimulates the cortex of the suprarenal gland.

ad•re•no•gen•ic, **ad•re•nog•e•nous** (ă-drē′nō-jen′ik, ad′rĕ-noj′ĕ-nŭs) Of adrenal origin. [adreno- + G. *-gen*, producing]

ad•re•no•gen•i•tal syn•drome (ă-drē′nō-jen′i-tal sin′drōm) Generic designation for a group of disorders caused by adrenocortical hyperplasia or malignant tumors and characterized by masculinization of women, feminization of men, or precocious sexual development of children; representative of excessive or abnormal secretory patterns of adrenocortical steroids, especially those with androgenic or estrogenic effects.

ad•re•no•leu•ko•dys•tro•phy (ALD) (ă-drē′nō-lū′kō-dis′trŏ-fē) Rare disease of the central nervous system characterized by progressive blindness, deafness, tonic spasms, mental retardation, and atrophy of the suprarenal gland; inherited as an X-linked recessive trait primarily affecting males.

ad•re•no•lyt•ic (ă-drē′nō-lit′ik) Denoting antagonism to or inhibition or blockade of the action of epinephrine, norepinephrine, and related sympathomimetics. SEE ALSO adrenergic blocking agent. [adreno- + G. *lysis*, loosening, dissolution]

a•dre•no•med•ul•lary hor•mones (ă-drē′nō-med′ŭ-lar-ē′ hōr′mōnz) Those produced by the medulla of the suprarenal gland, particularly the catecholamines epinephrine and norepinephrine.

ad•re•no•meg•a•ly (ă-drē′nō-meg′ă-lē) Enlargement of the suprarenal gland. [adreno- + G. *megas*, big]

ad•re•no•mi•met•ic (ă-drē′nō-mi-met′ik) Having an action similar to that of the compounds epinephrine and norepinephrine; a term intended to supplant a less accurate term, sympathomimetic. Cf. adrenergic, cholinomimetic. [adreno- + G. *mimētikos*, imitative]

ad•re•no•mi•met•ic a•mine (ă-drē′nō-mi-met′ik ă-mēn′) SYN sympathomimetic amine.

ad•re•no•my•e•lo•neu•rop•a•thy (ă-drē′nō-mī′ĕ-lō-nūr-op′ă-thē) A disorder of men, consisting of long-standing adrenal insufficiency, hypogonadism, progressive myelopathy, peripheral neuropathy, and sphincter disturbances; considered a variant of adrenoleukodystrophy. [adreno- + G. *myelos*, medulla, + *neuron*, nerve, + *pathos*, suffering]

ad•re•nop•a•thy (ad′ren-op′ă-thē) SYN adrenalopathy.

ad•re•no•pause (ă-drē′nō-pawz) Decrease in function of the suprarenal glands with increasing age, analogous to menopause.

ad•re•no•re•cep•tor (ă-drē′nō-rĕ-sep′tŏr) SYN adrenergic receptors.

ad•re•no•tro•pin (ă-drē′nō-trō′pin) SYN adrenocorticotropic hormone.

Ad•son for•ceps (ad′sŏn fōr′seps) A thumb forceps with serrated tip used to pick up tissue or grasp gauze dressings. See this page.

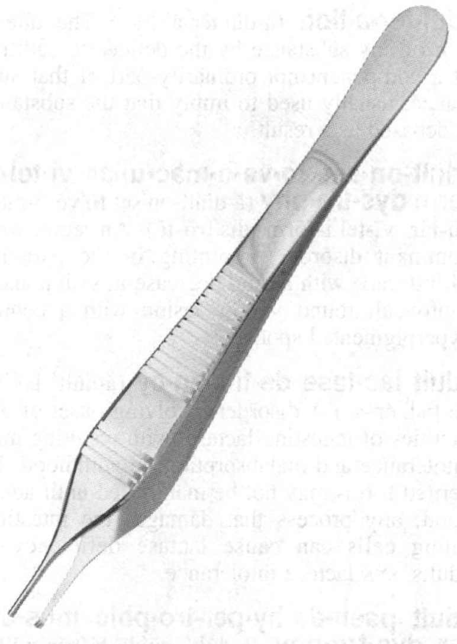

Adson forceps with teeth

Ad•son test (ad′sŏn test) A measurement of thoracic outlet syndrome; the patient is seated, with head extended and turned to the side of the lesion; with deep inspiration, there is a diminution or total loss of radial pulse on the affected side. Not all patients with a positive Adson test result have thoracic outlet syndrome.

ad·sorb (ad-sōrb′) To gather on or attract to a surface in a layer of condensation; to attach without covalent bonding. Cf. absorb. [L. *ad,* to, + *sorbeo,* to suck in]

ad·sorb·ent (ad-sōr′bĕnt) **1.** A solid substance with the property of attaching other substances to its surface without covalent bonding. **2.** An antigen or antibody used in immune adsorption.

ad·sorp·tion (ad-sōrp′shŭn) The property of a solid substance to attract and hold to its surface a gas, liquid, or a substance in solution or in suspension. Cf. absorption. [L. *ad,* to, + *sorbeo,* to suck up]

ad·sorp·tion the·o·ry of nar·co·sis (ad-sōrp′shŭn thē′ŏr-ē nahr-kō′sis) That a drug becomes concentrated at the surface of the cell as a result of adsorption, and thus alters permeability and metabolism.

ad·ter·mi·nal (ad-tĕr′mi-năl) In a direction toward the nerve endings, muscular insertions, or the extremity of any structure.

a·dult (ă-dŭlt′) Fully grown and physically mature. [L. *adultus*, grown up fr. *adolesco*, to grow up]

a·dul·ter·ant (ă-dŭl′tĕr-ănt) An impurity; an additive that is considered to have an undesirable effect or to dilute the active material so as to reduce its therapeutic or monetary value.

a·dul·ter·a·tion (ă-dŭl′tĕr-ā′shŭn) The alteration of any substance by the deliberate addition of a component not ordinarily part of that substance; usually used to imply that the substance is debased as a result.

a·dult-on·set fo·ve·o·mac·u·lar vi·tel·li·form dys·tro·phy (ă-dŭlt′-on′set fō′vē-ō-mak′yū-lăr vī-tel′i-fōrm dis′trŏ-fē) An autosomal dominant disorder presenting in the patients' fifth decade with a mild decrease in vision and a subfoveal, round yellow lesion with a central hyperpigmented spot.

a·dult lac·tase de·fi·cien·cy (ă-dŭlt′ lak′tās dĕ-fish′ĕn-sē) A disorder involving onset of difficulties of ingesting lactase, with resulting milk intolerance and malabsorption, in adulthood. Inherited forms may not be manifested until adulthood; any process that damages the intestinal lining cells can cause lactase deficiency in adults. SYN lactose intolerance.

a·dult pseu·do·hy·per·tro·phic mus·cu·lar dys·tro·phy (ă-dŭlt′ sū′dō-hī′pĕr-trō′fik mŭs′kyū-lăr dis′trŏ-fē) Muscular dystrophy of late onset, often in the second or third decade, with relatively mild course.

a·dult res·pi·ra·to·ry dis·tress syn·drome (ARDS) (ă-dŭlt′ res′pir-ă-tōr-ē dis-tres′ sin′drōm) Disorder with rapid onset of progressive malfunction of the lungs usually associated with malfunction of other organs attributable to inability to take in oxygen. Condition is associated with extensive injury to the alveolar capillary membrane, lung inflammation, and small blood vessel injury in affected organs. See page B18. SYN acute respiratory distress syndrome, wet lung (2), white lung.

a·dult rick·ets (ă-dŭlt′ rik′ĕts) SYN osteomalacia.

a·dult T-cell leu·ke·mi·a (ATL) (ă-dŭlt′ sel lū-kē′mē-ă) SYN adult T-cell lymphoma.

a·dult T-cell lym·pho·ma (ATL) (ă-dŭlt′ sel lim-fō′mă) An acute or subacute disease associated with a human T-cell virus, with lymphadenopathy, hepatosplenomegaly, skin lesions, peripheral blood involvement, and hypercalcemia. SYN adult T-cell leukemia.

a·dust (ă-dŭst′) Dried or burnt by excessive heat. [L. *aduro, adustum,* to set fire to]

ad·vance ben·e·fic·i·ar·y no·tice (ABN) (ăd-vans′ ben′ĕ-fish′ē-ar-ē nō′tis) A document signed by or on behalf of a patient that authorizes a care provider to bill the patient for services that Medicare may consider not medically necessary and may thereby decline to cover. SYN notice of noncoverage.

ad·vanced car·di·ac life sup·port (ACLS) (ăd-vanst′ kahr′dē-ak līf sŭ-pōrt′) Definitive emergency medical care that includes defibrillation, airway management, and use of drugs and medications. Usually begun by EMTs who do intubation and defibrillation at the direction of a doctor or nurse. Continues through various modalities until the patient arrives at the trauma center. Cf. basic life support.

ad·vance dir·ec·tive (ăd-vans′ dĭr-ek′tiv) A legal document with written instructions signed by the patient (or the patient's designee if the patient cannot sign) stating the type of care measures and services that are or are not to be provided to prolong life in the event of a life-threatening illness. SYN durable power of attorney (1).

ad·vanced mul·ti·ple-beam e·qual·i·za·tion ra·di·og·ra·phy (AMBER) (ăd-vanst′ mŭl′ti-pĕl-bēm′ ē′kwăl-ī-zā′shŭn rā′dē-og′ră-fē) A variant of scanning equalization radiography using several x-ray beams.

ad·vanced prac·tice nurse (ăd-vanst′ prak′tis nŭrs) Registered nurse with specialized knowledge and skills acquired through graduate study in nursing; category includes nurse practitioner, clinical nurse specialist, nurse midwife, and nurse anesthetist.

Ad·vanced Trau·ma Life Sup·port (ATLS) (ăd-vanst′ traw′mă līf sŭ-pōrt′) Educational course addressing acute care for trauma patients.

ad·vance·ment (ăd-vans′mĕnt) Surgical procedure in which a ligamentous or partially tendinous insertion or a skin flap is partially severed or released from its attachment and sutured to a more distal point.

ad•vance•ment flap (ăd-vans′mĕnt flap) SYN bipedicle flap.

ad•ven•ti•ti•a (ad′vĕn-tish′ă) The outermost connective tissue covering of any organ, vessel, or other structure not covered by a serosa. SYN tunica adventitia [TA]. [L. *adventicius,* coming from abroad, foreign, fr. *ad,* to + *venio,* to come]

ad•ven•ti•tial (ad′vĕn-tish′ăl) Relating to the outer coat or adventitia of a blood vessel or other structure. SYN adventitious (3).

ad•ven•ti•tial cell (ad′vĕn-tish′ăl sel) SYN pericyte.

ad•ven•ti•tial neu•ri•tis (ad′vĕn-tish′ăl nūr-ī′tis) Inflammation of the sheath of a nerve. SEE ALSO perineuritis.

ad•ven•ti•tious (ad′vĕn-tish′ŭs) **1.** Arising from an external source or occurring in an unusual place or manner. SEE ALSO extrinsic. **2.** Occurring accidentally or spontaneously, as opposed to natural causes or hereditary. **3.** SYN adventitial.

ad•ven•ti•tious cyst (ad′vĕn-tish′ŭs sist) SYN pseudocyst (1).

ad•ven•ti•tious lung sounds (ad′vĕn-tish′ŭs lŭng sowndz) Breath sounds that are not normally heard or are heard in an inappropriate place that fall into one of two categories: (1) continuous: musical sounds with a persistent pitch (e.g., wheezes, rhonchi); (2) discontinuous: nonmusical, intermittent, crackling, or bubbling sounds (rales).

ad•verse drug ef•fect (ADE) (ad-vĕrs′ drŭg e-fekt′) SYN adverse drug reaction.

ad•verse drug re•ac•tion (ADR), ad•verse drug e•vent (ad-vĕrs′ drŭg rē-ak′shŭn, ad-vĕrs′ drŭg ĕ-vent′) Any noxious, unintended, and undesired effect of a drug after its administration for prophylaxis, diagnosis, or therapy. SYN adverse drug effect.

ad•verse e•vent (ad-vĕrs′ ĕ-vent′) In nursing usage, an injury resulting from a patient's medical management rather than from the underlying condition itself.

ad•verse re•ac•tion (ad-vĕrs′ rē-ak′shŭn) Any undesirable or unwanted consequence of a preventive, diagnostic, or therapeutic procedure or regimen.

ad•vo•cate (ad′vŏ-kăt) NURSING a person who speaks on behalf of another. [L. *advocatus,* counsel, supporter, fr. *advoco,* to consult]

a•dy•nam•ic il•e•us (ā′dī-nam′ik il′ē-ŭs) Obstruction of the bowel due to paralysis of the bowel wall, usually as a result of localized or generalized peritonitis or shock. SYN paralytic ileus.

♻ **ae-** For words so beginning and not found here, see under e-.

A-E am•pu•ta•tion (amp′yū-tā′shŭn) Abbreviation for *a*bove-the-*e*lbow amputation.

AED Abbreviation for automatic external defibrillator; automated external defibrillator.

A•e•des (ā-ē′dēz) A widespread genus of small mosquitoes frequently found in tropic and subtropic regions; various species are vectors for yellow fever, dengue, and other human diseases. [G. *aēdēs,* unpleasant, unfriendly]

A•e•des at•lan•ti•cus (ā-ē′dēz at-lan′ti-kus) Mosquito species in the family Culicidae known to transmit viruses that cause dengue, yellow fever, and encephalitis.

A•e•des dor•sa•lis (ā-ē′dēz dōr-sā′lis) Mosquito species that is a secondary or suspected vector of Western equine encephalitis.

A•e•des mel•an•im•on (ā-ē′dēz mē-lan′i-mon) Mosquito species that is a vector of Western equine encephalitis and California group encephalitis.

A•e•des mitch•el•lae (ā-ē′dēz mĭ-chel′ē) Mosquito species that is a secondary or suspected vector of Eastern equine encephalitis.

A•e•des ni•gro•mac•u•lis (ā-ē′dēz nī-grō-mak′yū-lis) Mosquito species that is a secondary or suspected vector of Western equine encephalitis and California group encephalitis.

A•e•des tae•ni•o•rhyn•chus (ā-ē′dēz tē-nē-ō-ringk′us) Mosquito species that is a vector of Venezuelan equine encephalitis and a secondary or suspected vector of California group encephalitis.

A•e•des tri•se•ri•a•tus (ā-ē′dēz trī-ser-ē-ā′tŭs) Mosquito species that is a vector of California group encephalitis.

A•e•des tri•vit•ta•tus (ā-ē′dēz trī-vi-tā′tŭs) Mosquito species that is a vector of California group encephalitis.

A•e•des vex•ans (ā-ē′dēz veks′anz) Mosquito species that is a vector of California group encephalitis and a secondary or suspected vector of Eastern equine encephalitis.

-aemia [Br.] SYN -emia.

ae•quor•in (ē-kwōr′in) A luminescent protein isolated from the jellyfish *Aequorea,* which emits blue light in the presence of even minute amounts of calcium ion; injected intracellularly, it is used to measure free calcium ion transients within cells. SEE ALSO fura-2.

♻ **aer-, aero-** Combining forms meaning the air, a gas; aerial, gassy. [G. *aēr* (L. *aer*), air]

aer•ate (ār′āt) **1.** To supply (blood) with oxygen. **2.** To expose to the circulation of air for purification. **3.** To supply or charge (liquid) with a gas, especially carbon dioxide.

aer•a•tion (ār-ā′shŭn) The process of charging a liquid with air or gas; especially the transfer of oxygen to the blood in the lungs.

aer•i•al sick•ness (ār′ē-ăl sik′nĕs) SYN altitude sickness.

aer•obe (ār′ōb) **1.** An organism that can live and grow in the presence of oxygen. **2.** An organism that can use oxygen as a final electron acceptor in a respiratory chain. [aero- + G. *bios,* life]

aer•o•bic (ār-ō′bik) **1.** Living in air. **2.** Relating to an aerobe. **3.** Oxygen consumed to produce energy. SYN aerophilic, aerophilous.

aer•o•bic cap•ac•i•ty (ār-ō′bik kă-pas′i-tē) SYN maximal oxygen consumption.

aer•o•bic pow•er (ār-ō′bik pow′ĕr) SYN maximal oxygen consumption.

aer•o•bic res•pi•ra•tion (ār-ō′bik res′pir-ā′shŭn) A form of respiration in which molecular oxygen is consumed and carbon dioxide and water are produced.

aer•o•bics (ār-ō′biks) A program of physical conditioning based on sustained strenuous exercise intended to improve cardiovascular and respiratory fitness.

aer•o•bic sys•tem (ār-ō′bik sis′tĕm) The combination of oxygen-consuming physiologic (i.e., pulmonary, cardiovascular, muscular) and biochemical (i.e., aerobic glycolysis, citric acid cycle, electron transport chain) functions normally used in performing physical work.

aer•o•bi•o•sis (ār′ō-bī-ō′sis) Existence in an atmosphere containing oxygen. [aero- + G. *biōsis,* mode of living]

aer•o•bi•ot•ic (ār′ō-bī-ot′ik) Relating to aerobiosis.

aer•o•cele (ār′ō-sēl) Distention of a small natural cavity with gas. [aero- + G. *kēlē,* tumor]

aer•o•col•pos (ār′ō-kōl′pōs) Distention of the vagina with gas. [aero- + G. *kolpos,* lap, hollow]

aer•o•don•tal•gi•a (ār′ō-don-tal′jē-ă) Dental pain caused by a change in atmospheric pressure. [aero- + G. *odous,* tooth, + *algos,* pain]

aer•o•dy•nam•ics (ār′ō-dī-nam′iks) The study of air and other gases in motion, the forces that set them in motion, and the results of such motion. [aero- + G. *dynamis,* force]

aer•o•dy•nam•ic the•o•ry (ār′ō-dī-nam′ik thē′ŏr-ē) Generally accepted proposition that the vibration of the vocal folds in phonation is produced by the flow of exhaled air past lightly approximated vocal folds; opposed to the now untenable concept that vocal fold motion in phonation results from contraction of the intrinsic muscles of the larynx at the frequency of the vocal fold vibration.

aer•o•gas•tral•gi•a (ār′ō-gas-tral′jē-ă) Pain due to distention of the stomach by swallowed air. [aero- + G. *gastēr,* stomach, + *algos,* pain]

aer•o•gen•ic, aer•og•e•nous (ār′ō-jen′ik, ăr-oj′ĕ-nŭs) Gas-forming.

aer•o•med•i•cine (ār′ō-med′i-sin) SYN aviation medicine.

aer•o•mo•nad (ār′ō-mō′nad) Any of a group of bacterial species that belong to the genus *Aeromonas.*

Aer•o•mon•as (ār-ō-mō′năs) A genus of aerobic, facultatively anaerobic bacteria (family Vibrionaceae) containing gram-negative, rod-shaped coccoid cells that occur singly or in pairs or in clumps of chains; motile cells ordinarily possess a single, polar flagellum; some species are nonmotile. The metabolism of these organisms is both respiratory and fermentative. These bacteria are found in water and sewage; some are pathogenic to fresh water and marine animals. The type species is *A. hydrophila.*

aer•o•pha•gi•a, aer•oph•a•gy (ār′ō-fā′jē-ă, -of′ă-jē) **1.** Excessive swallowing of air due to anxiety, hunger, improper eating habits, or other causes; can lead to abdominal distress, belching, and flatulence. **2.** VETERINARY MEDICINE Wind-sucking, a behavioral disorder of horses sometimes associated with crib-biting. [aero- + G. *phagō,* to eat]

aer•o•phil, aer•o•phile (ār′ō-fil, -fīl) **1.** Air-loving. **2.** An aerobic organism (aerobe), especially an obligate aerobe. [aero- + G. *philos,* fond]

aer•o•phil•ic, aer•oph•i•lous (ār′ō-fil′ik, ār-of′i-lŭs) SYN aerobic.

aer•o•pho•bi•a (ār′ō-fō′bē-ă) Morbid dread of fresh air or of air in motion. [aero- + G. *phobos,* fear]

aer•o•pi•e•so•ther•a•py (ār′ō-pī-ē′sō-thār′ă-pē) Treatment of disease by compressed (or rarified) air. [aero- + G. *piesis,* pressure, + *therapeia,* medical treatment]

aeroplane splint [Br.] SYN airplane splint.

aer•o•si•nus•i•tis (ār′ō-sī′nŭ-sī′tis) Inflammation of the paranasal sinuses caused by pressure differences within the sinus relative to ambient pressure, secondary to obstruction of the sinus orifice, sometimes due to high altitude flying or by descent from high altitude. SYN barosinusitis.

aer•o•sol (ār′ō-sol) **1.** Liquid or particulate matter in the form of a stable suspension for therapeutic, insecticidal, or other purposes, including bioterrorism and bioweapons; forms include dusts, smokes, mists, clouds, fumes, and fogs. **2.** A product that is packaged under pressure and contains therapeutically or chemically active ingredients intended for topical application, inhalation, or introduction into body orifices. [aero- + solution]

aer•o•sol gen•er•a•tor (ār′ō-sol jen′ĕr-ā-tŏr) A device for producing airborne suspensions of small particles for inhalation therapy or experimental work.

aer•o•space med•i•cine (ār′ō-spās med′i-sin) Medical specialty focusing on health and medical problems of air and space flight personnel.

aer•o•sphere (ār′ō-sfēr) The lower portion of the earth's atmosphere, containing sufficient oxygen to support life. [aero- + sphere]

aer•o•tax•is (ār′ō-tak′sis) Movement of an organism with respect to a supply of air or oxygen. [aero- + G. *taxis,* orderly arrangement]

aer•o•ther•a•py (ār′ō-thār′ă-pē) Treatment of disease by changing pressure or composition of air.

aer•o•ti•tis me•di•a (ār′ō-tī′tis mē′dē-ă) An acute or chronic inflammation of the middle ear caused by a reduction in pressure in the tympanic cavity relative to ambient pressure, secondary to auditory tube obstruction; often occurs on descent from high altitude. SYN barotitis media. [aero- + G. *ous,* ear, + *-itis,* inflammation]

aer•o•tol•er•ant (ār′ō-tol′ĕr-ănt) Able to survive in the presence of oxygen; said of some anaerobic microorganisms. [aero- + tolerant]

aer•o•trop•ism (ār′o-trō′pizm) Movement of an organism with respect to a supply of air or oxygen. [aero- + tropism]

aes•cu•la•pi•an (es′kyū-lā′pē-ăn) Relating to Aesculapius, the art of medicine, or a medical practitioner. [L. *Aesculapius,* G. *Asklēpios,* the god of medicine]

aesthesia [Br.] SYN esthesia.

aesthesio- SYN esthesio-.

aesthesiogenesis [Br.] SYN esthesiogenesis.

aesthesiogenic [Br.] SYN esthesiogenic.

aesthesiometer [Br.] SYN esthesiometer.

aesthesiometry [Br.] SYN esthesiometry.

aesthesioneurosis [Br.] SYN esthesioneurosis.

aesthesiophysiology [Br.] SYN esthesiophysiology.

aesthesodic [Br.] SYN esthesiodic.

aesthetic [Br.] SYN esthetic.

aesthetics [Br.] SYN esthetics.

aestival [Br.] SYN estival.

aestivation [Br.] SYN estivation.

aestivoautumnal [Br.] SYN estivoautumnal.

aetiologic [Br.] SYN etiologic.

aetiological [Br.] SYN etiologic.

aetiology [Br.] SYN etiology.

AFB Abbreviation for acid-fast bacillus.

a•fe•brile (ā-feb′ril) SYN apyretic.

a•fe•tal (ā-fē′tăl) Without relation to a fetus or intrauterine life.

af•fect (a′fekt) The emotional feeling, tone, and mood attached to a thought, including its external manifestations; especially as demonstrated by postural and facial expressions. [L. *affectus,* state of mind, fr. *afficio,* to have influence on]

af•fec•tion (ă-fek′shŭn) **1.** A moderate feeling of tenderness, caring, or love. **2.** An abnormal condition of body or mind. [L. *affectio*, fr. *afficio*, to affect, influence]

af•fec•tive (a-fek′tiv) Pertaining to mood, emotion, feeling, sensibility, or mental state.

af•fec•tive dis•or•der (a-fek′tiv dis-ōr′dĕr) A mental condition characterized by a disturbance in mood.

af•fec•tive per•son•al•i•ty (a-fek′tiv pĕr-sŏn-al′i-tē) A chronic behavioral pattern in an enduring disturbance of feelings or mood expressed as a form of depression and related emotional features that color the whole of the psychic life.

af•fec•tive psy•cho•sis (a-fek′tiv sī-kō′sis) Psychosis with predominant affective features.

af•fer•ent (af′ĕr-ĕnt) Inflowing; conducting toward a center, denoting certain arteries, veins, lymphatics, and nerves. Opposite of efferent. SYN centripetal (1). [L. *afferens,* fr. *af-fero,* to bring to]

af•fer•ent fi•bers (af′ĕr-ĕnt fī′bĕrz) Those that convey impulses to a ganglion or to a nerve center in the brain or spinal cord.

af•fer•ent glo•mer•u•lar ar•te•ri•ole (af′ĕr-ĕnt glō-mer′yū-lăr ahr-tēr′ē-ōl) A branch of an interlobular artery of the kidney that conveys blood to the glomerulus. SYN arteriola glomerularis afferens [TA].

af•fer•ent lym•phat•ic (af′ĕr-ĕnt lim-fat′ik) A lymphatic vessel entering, or bringing lymph to, a node.

af•fer•ent nerve (af′ĕr-ĕnt nĕrv) A nerve conveying impulses from the periphery to the central nervous system. SYN centripetal nerve.

af•fer•ent ves•sel (af′ĕr-ĕnt ves′ĕl) Any artery conveying blood to a part.

af•fin•i•ty (ă-fin′i-tē) **1.** CHEMISTRY the force that impels certain atoms to unite with certain others. **2.** Selective staining of a tissue by a dye. **3.** The strength of binding between a Fab site of an antibody and an antigenic determinant. **4.** In a general sense, an attraction. [L. *affinis,* neighboring, fr. *ad,* to, + *finis,* end, boundary]

af•flux (af′lŭks) Flowing to or toward a body part. [L. *af-fluo, af-fluxus,* to flow toward]

af•ford•ance (ă-fōr′dăns) The relationship that exists between the individual and the environment that will facilitate a certain type of movement (e.g., a sliding board affords a child with the opportunity to climb up, sit, and slide down). [afford + -ance, noun suffix]

a•fi•bril•lar (ā-fī′bri-lăr) Denoting a biologic structure that does not contain fibrils.

afibrinogenaemia [Br.] SYN afibrinogenemia.

a•fi•brin•o•gen•e•mi•a (ā-fī′brin-ō-jĕ-nē′mē-ă) The absence of fibrinogen in the plasma. SEE ALSO hypofibrinogenemia. SYN afibrinogenaemia.

A•fip•i•a (ă-fip′ē-ă) A genus of gram-negative, oxidase-positive, motile, nonfermenting bacteria that have been placed in the class Proteobacteria. They are morphologically variable, appearing as rods or filaments that may stain poorly. More than 10 species have been identified, one of which was formerly thought to be the cause of catscratch disease. Their current pathogenic role is uncertain. The type strain is *A. felis.*

AFO Abbreviation for ankle-foot orthotic.

AFORMED phe•nom•e•non (ă-fōr′med fĕ-nom′ĕ-non) As induced pulsus alternans progresses, a state in which alternating heart depolarizations fail to eject any blood, thus allowing longer diastolic filling; the subsequent beat is then able to produce a significant ejection; at high rates the cardiac minute volume and blood pressure may appear normal. [Acronym for alternating failure of response, mechanical to electrical depolarization]

AFP Abbreviation for alpha (α)-fetoprotein.

Af•ri•can sleep•ing sick•ness (af′ri-kăn slēp′ing sik′nĕs) SEE Gambian trypanosomiasis, Rhodesian trypanosomiasis.

Af•ri•can tick-bite fe•ver (af′ri-kăn tik′bīt fē′vĕr) A febrile disease caused by the bacterium *Rickettsia africae* in southern Africa and characterized by taches noires at the sites of bites by infected *Amblyomma* ticks and lymphadenopathy.

Af•ri•can try•pan•o•so•mi•a•sis (af′ri-kăn trī-pan′ō-sō-mī′ă-sis) A serious endemic disease in tropic Africa, of two types: Gambian or West African trypanosomiasis and Rhodesian or East African trypanosomiasis.

af•ter•birth (af′tĕr-bĕrth) The placenta and membranes that are extruded from the uterus after birth of a baby. SYN secundines.

af•ter•im•age (af′tĕr-im′ăj) Persistence of a visual response after cessation of the stimulus.

af•ter•im•pres•sion (af′tĕr-im-presh′ŭn) SYN aftersensation.

af•ter•load (af′tĕr-lōd) **1.** The arrangement of a muscle so that, in shortening, it creates a force from an adjustable support or otherwise does work against a constant opposing force to which it is not exposed at rest. **2.** The load or force thus encountered in shortening. **3.** That resistance against which the left ventricle must eject its volume of blood during contraction.

af•ter•load•ing ra•di•a•tion (af′tĕr-lōd′ing rā′dē-ā′shŭn) Method of administering radiation that involves initial placement of local catheters during an operative procedure. Installation of the radiation source is performed later in a controlled environment that includes protective equipment for personnel.

af•ter•pains (af′tĕr-pānz) Painful cramplike contractions of the uterus occurring after childbirth.

af•ter•per•cep•tion (af′tĕr-pĕr-sep′shŭn) Subjective persistence of a stimulus after its cessation. Cf. palinopsia.

af•ter•po•ten•tial (af′tĕr-pŏ-ten′shăl) The small change in electrical potential in a stimulated nerve that follows the main, or spike, potential; it consists of an initial negative deflection followed by a positive deflection in the oscillograph record.

af•ter•sen•sa•tion (af′tĕr-sen-sā′shŭn) Subjective persistence of sensation after cessation of stimulus. SYN afterimpression.

af•ter•sound (af′tĕr-sownd) Subjective persistence of an auditory stimulus after cessation of the stimulus.

af•ter•taste (af′tĕr-tāst) Subjective persistence of a gustatory stimulus after contact with the stimulating substance has ceased.

a•func•tion•al oc•clu•sion (ā-fŭngk′shŭn-ăl ŏ-klū′zhŭn) A malocclusion that does not permit normal function of the dentition.

Ag **1.** Symbol for silver (argentum). **2.** Abbreviation for antigen.

AGA Abbreviation for appropriate for gestational age.

a•ga•lac•ti•a, a•ga•lac•to•sis (ā′gal-ak′shē-ă, ā′gal-ak-tō′sis) Absence of milk in the breasts after childbirth. [G. *a-* priv. + *gala* (*galakt-*), milk]

a•ga•lac•tor•rhe•a (ā′gal-ak′tō-rē′ă) Absence of the secretion or flow of breast milk. SYN agalactorrhoea. [G. *a-* priv. + *gala,* milk, + *rhoia,* a flow]

agalactorrhoea [Br.] SYN agalactorrhea.

a•ga•lac•tous (ā′gal-ak′tŭs) Relating to agalactia, or to the diminution or absence of breast milk.

a•ga•mete (ā′gam′ēt) A cell produced by asexual reproduction (fission). [G. *a-*, without, + *gametēs,* spouse]

a•gam•ic, a•ga•mous (ā-gam′ik, ag′ă-mŭs) Denoting nonsexual reproduction, as by fission or budding.

agammaglobulinaemia [Br.] SYN agammaglobulinemia.

a•gam•ma•glob•u•lin•e•mi•a (ā-gam′ă-glob′yū-li-nē′mē-ă) Absence of, or extremely low levels of, the gamma fraction of serum globulin; sometimes used loosely to denote absence of immunoglobulins in general. SEE ALSO hypogammaglobulinemia. SYN agammaglobulinaemia.

a•gan•gli•on•ic (ā′gang-glē-on′ik) Without ganglia.

a•gan•gli•o•no•sis (ā-gang′glē-ŏ-nō′sis) The state of being without ganglia; e.g., absence of ganglion cells from the myenteric plexus as a characteristic of congenital megacolon. [G. *a-* priv. + ganglion + *-osis,* condition]

a•gar (ā′gahr) A complex polysaccharide (a sulfated galactan) derived from seaweed (various red algae); used as a solidifying agent in culture media. It has the valuable property of melting at 100°C but not solidifying until 49°C. [Malay *agar-agar*]

a•gas•ta•che (ă-gas′tă-kē) *Agastache rugosa,* a botanical sometimes used as a flavoring agent; purported value as useful in pregnancy disorders in traditional Chinese medicine. SYN Korean mint. [G. *agastachē,* fr. *agan,* much, + *stachys,* spike, ear of corn]

a•gas•tric (ā-gas′trik) Without stomach or alimentary (digestive) tract. [G. *a-* priv. + *gastēr,* belly]

AGC Abbreviation for automatic gain control.

AGCUS Abbreviation for atypical glandular cells of undetermined significance.

age (āj) **1.** The period elapsed since birth. **2.** One of the periods into which human life is divided, distinguished by physical evolution, equilibrium, and involution; e.g., the seven human ages are: infancy, childhood, adolescence, maturity, middle life, senescence, and senility. **3.** To grow old; to gradually develop changes in structure that are not due to preventable disease or trauma and that are associated with decreased functional capacity and an increased probability of death. **4.** To cause artificially the appearance characteristic of one who has lived long or of a thing that has existed for a long time. **5.** To render the bond between a nerve agent and acetylcholinesterase refractory to disruption by an oxime antidote. [F. *âge,* L. *aetas*]

age•ism (āj′izm) Actions and attitudes that place different values on, or create unequal opportunities for, people or groups because of their age.

A•gen•cy for Health•care Re•search and Qual•i•ty (AHRQ) (ā′jĕn-sē helth′kār rĕ-sĕrch′ kwahl′i-tē) A group that supports research designed to improve outcomes and quality of health care, reduce costs, address patient safety and medical errors, and broaden access to effective services; translates research findings into improved patient care; formerly called the Agency for Health Care Policy and Research.

a•gen•e•sis (ā-jen′ĕ-sis) Absence or failure of formation of any part. [G. *a-* priv. + *genesis,* production]

a•gen•i•tal•ism (ā-jen′i-tăl-izm) **1.** Congenital absence of genitalia. **2.** Any condition caused by lack of sex hormones.

a•gen•o•so•mi•a (ā′jen-ō-sō′mē-ă) Markedly defective formation or absence of the genitalia; usually accompanied by protrusion of the abdominal viscera through an incomplete abdominal wall. [G. *a-* priv. + *genos,* sex, + *soma,* body]

A•gent 15 (ā′jĕnt) An incapacitating chemical-warfare agent purportedly developed by Iraq in the 1980s; thought to be similar or identical to QNB.

a•gent (ā′jĕnt) **1.** An active force or substance capable of producing an effect. **2.** A factor such as a microorganism, chemical substance, or a form of radiation the presence or absence of which (as in deficiency diseases) results in disease or more advanced disease. [L. *ago,* pres. p. *agens* (*agent-*), to perform]

a•gen•tic (a-jen′tik) Denotes self-directed actions aimed at personal development or personally chosen goals.

age-re•lat•ed mac•u•lar de•gen•er•a•tion (āj-rē-lāt′ĕd mak′yū-lăr dĕ-jen′ĕr-ā′shŭn) SYN macular degeneration.

a•geu•si•a (ă-gū′sē-ă) Loss of the sense of taste. [G. *a-* priv. + *geusis,* taste]

ag•ger (aj′ĕr) Any anatomic prominence. [L. rampart]

ag•glom•er•ate (ă-glom′ĕr-āt) To gather into a mass. [L. *agglomero,* fr. ad *to,* + glomus (glomer-) mass, ball of yarn]

ag•glu•ti•nant (ă-glū′ti-nănt) A substance that holds parts together or causes agglutination. [L. *ad,* to + *gluten,* glue]

ag•glu•ti•na•tion (ă-glū′ti-nā′shŭn) **1.** The process by which suspended bacteria, cells, or other particles are caused to adhere and form clumps; similar to precipitation, but the particles are larger and are in suspension rather than being in solution. **2.** Adhesion of the surfaces of a wound. **3.** The process of adhering. [L. *ad,* to, + *gluten,* glue]

ag•glu•ti•na•tive (ă-glū′ti-nă-tiv) Causing, or able to cause, agglutination.

ag•glu•ti•nin (ă-glū′ti-nin) **1.** An antibody that causes clumping or agglutination of the bacteria or other cells that either stimulated the formation of the agglutinin, or contain immunologically similar, reactive antigen. **2.** A substance, other than a specific agglutinating antibody, that causes organic particles to agglutinate.

ag•glu•tin•o•gen (ă-glū-tin′ō-jen) An antigenic substance that stimulates the formation of specific agglutinin, which, under certain conditions, causes agglutination of cells that contain the antigen or particles coated with the antigen. SYN agglutogen. [agglutinin + G. *-gen,* production]

ag•glu•tin•o•gen•ic (ă-glū′tin-ō-jen′ik) Capable of causing the production of an agglutinin. SYN agglutogenic.

ag•glu•tin•o•phil•ic (ă-glū′tin-ō-fil′ik) Readily undergoing agglutination. [agglutination + G. *phileō,* to love]

ag•glu•to•gen (ă-glū′tō-jen) SYN agglutinogen.

ag•glu•to•gen•ic (ă-glū′tō-jen′ik) SYN agglutinogenic.

ag•gra•va•tion (ag′ră-vā′shŭn) Intensification of severity. [L. *aggravatio,* fr. *ag-gravo, aggravatus,* to make serious]

ag•gre•can (ag′rĕ-kan) Candidate gene for otosclerosis located at 15q25-q26.

ag•gre•gate (ag′rĕ-gāt) **1.** To unite or come together in a mass or cluster. **2.** (ag′grĕ-găt) The total of individual units making up a mass or cluster. [L. *ag-grego,* pp. *-atus,* to add to, fr. *grex* (*greg-*), a flock]

ag•gre•gat•ed fol•li•cle (ag′rĕ-gā-tĕd fol′i-kĕl) SEE Peyer patches.

ag•gre•ga•tion (ag′rĕ-gā′shŭn) A crowded mass of independent but similar units; a cluster.

ag•gres•sion (ă-gresh′ŭn) A domineering, forceful, or assaultive verbal or physical action toward another person as the motor component of anger, hostility, or rage. [L. *aggressio,* fr. *aggredior,* to accost, attack]

ag•gres•sive (ă-gres′iv) **1.** Denoting aggression. **2.** Denoting a competitive forcefulness or invasiveness, as of a behavioral pattern, a pathogenic organism, or a disease process.

ag•gres•sive an•gi•o•myx•o•ma (ă-gres′iv an′jē-ō-miks-ō′mă) Locally invasive, but nonmetastasizing tumor of genital organs in young women.

a•gil•i•ty (ă-jil′i-tē) The ability to accelerate, decelerate, stabilize, and change directions quickly while maintaining proper body posture.

ag•ing (ā′jing) **1.** The process of growing old, especially by failure of replacement of cells in sufficient number to maintain full functional capacity; particularly affects cells (e.g., neurons) incapable of mitotic division. **2.** The gradual deterioration of a mature organism resulting from time-dependent, irreversible changes in structure. **3.** In the cardiovascular system, the progressive replacement of functional cell types by fibrous connective tissue. **4.** DEMOGRAPHY an increase over time in the proportion of older people in the population. **5.** The process, analogous to the setting of glue, by which the bond between a nerve agent and acetylcholinesterase becomes refractory to disruption by an oxime antidote.

ag•ing re•port (āj′ing rē-pōrt′) In health care billing, a review, usually done with a computer program, of any monies owed the health care provider and any reasons for lack of payment; used to keep track of delayed receivables.

ag•i•tat•ed de•pres•sion (aj′i-tāt-ĕd dĕ-presh′ŭn) Depression with excitement and restlessness.

ag•i•to•pha•si•a (aj′i-tō-fā′zē-ă) Rapid speech with deletion and distortion of sounds and words. [L. *agitatus,* excited, + G. *phasis,* speech]

a•glos•so•sto•mi•a (ā′glos-ō-stō′mē-ă) Congenital absence of the tongue, with a malformed (usually closed) mouth. [G. *a-* priv. + *glōssa,* tongue, + *stoma,* mouth]

a•glu•ti•tion (ā′glū-tish′ŭn) SYN dysphagia.

a•gly•cos•u•ri•a (ā′glī-kō-syūr′ē-ă) Absence of glucose in the urine.

a•gly•cos•u•ric (ā′glī-kō-syūr′ik) Relating to aglycosuria.

ag•mi•nat•ed fol•li•cle (ag′mi-nā-tĕd fol′i-kĕl) SEE Peyer patches.

ag•na•thi•a (āg-nā′thē-ă) Congenital absence of the mandible, usually accompanied by approximation of the ears. SEE ALSO otocephaly, synotia. [G. *a-* priv. + *gnathos,* jaw]

ag•na•thous (āg′nā-thŭs) Relating to agnathia.

ag•no•gen•ic (ag′nō-jen′ik) SYN idiopathic. [G. *a-* priv. + *gnosis,* knowledge, + *genesis,* origin]

ag•no•si•a (ag-nō′zē-ă) Impairment of ability to recognize, or comprehend the meaning of, various sensory stimuli, not attributable to disorders of the primary receptors or general intellect; receptive defects caused by lesions in various portions of the cerebrum. [G. ignorance; from *a-* priv. + *gnōsis,* knowledge]

-agogue, -agog Suffixes meaning leading, promoting, stimulating; a promoter or stimulant of. [G. *agōgos,* leading forth, fr. *agō,* to lead]

a•gom•pho•sis, a•gom•phi•a•sis (ā′gom-fō′sis, ā′gom-fī′ă-sis) SYN anodontia. [G. *a-* priv. + *gomphos,* peg, bolt]

a•go•nad•al (ā′gō-nad′ăl) Denoting the absence of gonads (testes or ovaries).

ag•o•nal (ag′ŏ-năl) Relating to struggles preceding death. [G. *agōn,* contest, struggle]

ag•o•nist (ag′ŏn-ist) **1.** Denoting a muscle in a state of contraction, with reference to its opposing muscle, or antagonist. **2.** A drug capable of combining with receptors to initiate drug actions; it possesses affinity and intrinsic activity. [G. *agōn,* a contest]

ag•o•ny (ag′ŏ-nē) Intense pain or anguish of body or mind. [G. *agōn,* a struggle, trial]

ag•o•ra•pho•bi•a (ag′ŏr-ă-fō′bē-ă) A mental disorder characterized by an irrational fear of leaving the familiar setting of home, or venturing into the open; often associated with panic attacks. [G. *agora,* marketplace, + *phobos,* fear]

ag•or•a•pho•bic (ag′ŏr-ă-fō′bik) Relating to or characteristic of agoraphobia.

♻ **-agra** Combining form meaning sudden onslaught of acute pain. [G. *agra,* a hunting, a catching, a trap]

a•gram•ma•tism (ā-gram′ă-tizm) A form of aphasia characterized by a reduced ability to understand or produce most grammatical markers, usually related to severe expressive aphasia.

a•gran•u•lar en•do•plas•mic re•tic•u•lum (ā-gran′yŭ-lăr en′dō-plaz′mik rĕ-tik′yŭ-lŭm) Endoplasmic reticulum that is lacking in ribosomal granules; involved in synthesis of complex lipids and fatty acids, detoxification of drugs, carbohydrate synthesis, and sequestering of Ca^{++}.

a•gran•u•lo•cyte (ā-grăn′ŭ-lō-sīt) White blood cell without granules (e.g., monocytes and lymphocytes). [G. *a-* priv. + L. *granulum,* granule, + G. *kytos,* cell]

a•gran•u•lo•cy•to•sis (ā′gran′yŭ-lō-sī-tō′sis) An acute condition characterized by pronounced leukopenia; infected ulcers are likely to develop in the throat, intestinal tract, and other mucous membranes, as well as in the skin. Condition is an immunocompromised state.

a•gran•u•lo•plas•tic (ā′gran′yŭ-lō-plas′tik) Capable of forming nongranular cells, and incapable of forming granular cells. [G. *a-* priv. + L. *granulum,* granule, + G. *plastikos,* formative]

a•graph•i•a (ă-graf′ē-ă) Inability to write properly in the absence of abnormalities of the limb; often accompanies aphasia and alexia; caused by lesions in various portions of the cerebrum. SYN anorthography, logagraphia. [G. *a-* priv. + *graphō,* to write]

a•graph•ic (ă-graf′ik) Relating to or marked by agraphia.

a•gree•ment (ă-grē′mĕnt) The act or result of concurring in a belief, opinion, or plan of action. [O.Fr. *agreer,* fr. L.L. *aggrato,* to make onself pleasing]

ag•re•tope (ag′rĕ-tōp) That part of a processed antigen that binds to the major histocompatibility complex molecule. [*a*ntigen + *re*striction + -tope]

ag•ri•mo•ny (ag′ri-mō-nē) A perennial herb (*Agrimonia eupatoria, A. herba*) used in desiccated form in tablets and infusions, as well as topically (wound healing, astringent). SYN cocklebur (1), sticklewort. [L. *agrimonia,* fr. G. *argemōnē*]

a•gryp•ni•a (ă-grip′nē-ă) Difficulty obtaining sleep for a prolonged period of time. [G., sleeplessness]

a•gue (ā′gyū) An intermittent fever. [Fr. *aiguK,* acute, fr. L. *acutus*]

a•gue•weed (ā′gyū-wēd) SYN boneset.

AGUS Abbreviation for atypical glandular cells of undetermined significance. SEE ALSO Bethesda system.

a•gy•ri•a (ā-jī′rē-ă) Congenital lack or underdevelopment of the convolutional pattern of the cerebral cortex. SYN lissencephalia. [G. *a-* priv. + *gyros,* circle]

AHA Abbreviation for American Hospital Association.

AH con•duc•tion time (kŏn-dŭk′shŭn tīm) SEE atrioventricular conduction.

AHF Abbreviation for antihemophilic factor A.

AHI Abbreviation for apnea-hypopnea index.

AHIMA Abbreviation for American Health Information Management Association.

AH in•ter•val (in′tĕr-văl) The time from the initial rapid deflection of the atrial wave to the initial rapid deflection of the His bundle (H) potential; it approximates the conduction time through the AV node (normally 50–120 msec).

AHRQ Abbreviation for Agency for Healthcare Research and Quality.

A•hu•ma•da-del Cas•ti•llo syn•drome (ī-ū-mah′dah-del kahs-tē′yō sin′drōm) Unphysiologic lactation and amenorrhea not following pregnancy characterized by hyperprolactinemia and a pituitary adenoma.

AI Abbreviation for acceptable intake; adequate intake.

Ai•car•di syn•drome (ī-kahr′dē sin′drōm) An X-linked dominant disorder with lethality in hemizygous males; characterized by agenesis of corpus callosum, chorioretinal abnormality with "holes," cleft lip with or without cleft palate, seizures, and characteristic EEG changes.

AID Abbreviation for artificial insemination donor.

AIDS (ādz) Acronym for acquired immune deficiency (or immunodeficiency) syndrome; disorder of the immune system characterized by opportunistic diseases, including candidiasis, *Pneumocystis jiroveci* pneumonia, oral hairy leukoplakia, herpes zoster, Kaposi sarcoma, toxoplasmosis, isosporiasis, cryptococcosis, non-Hodgkin lymphoma, and tuberculosis. The syndrome is caused by the human immunodeficiency virus (HIV-1, groups M and O, and HIV-2), which is transmitted in body fluids (notably breast milk, blood, and semen) through sexual contact, sharing of contaminated needles (by IV drug abusers), accidental needle sticks, contact with contaminated blood, or transfusion of contaminated blood or blood products. Hallmark of the immunodeficiency is depletion of $T4^+$ or $CD4^+$ helper/inducer lymphocytes, primarily the result of selective tropism of the virus for the lymphocytes. SYN acquired immunodeficiency syndrome.

AIDS quack·er·y (ādz kwak′ĕr-ē) Unvalidated therapy that suggests—among other things—that HIV does not cause AIDS and that antiretroviral drugs are poison; some believers assert that HIV/AIDS results from poverty, racism, or political policy.

AIDS-re·lat·ed com·plex (ARC) (ādz-rē-lāt′ĕd kom′pleks) Manifestations of AIDS in patients who have not yet developed major deficient immune function, characterized by fever with generalized lymphadenopathy, diarrhea, weight loss, minor opportunistic infections, and cytopenias.

AIH Abbreviation for artificial insemination (homologous).

ai·lu·ro·pho·bi·a (ī′lūr-ō-fō′bē-ă) Morbid fear of or aversion to cats. [G. *ailouros,* cat, + *phobos,* fear]

ai·nhum (ī-nyum′) An acquired, slowly progressive painful fibrous constriction that develops in the digitoplantar fold, usually of the little toe, gradually resulting in spontaneous amputation of the toe; most commonly affects black males in the tropics. [Pg., fr. Yoruba *eyun,* to saw]

AIR Abbreviation for 5-aminoimidazole ribose 5-phosphate; 5-aminoimidazole ribotide.

air (ār) **1.** A mixture of odorless gases found in the atmosphere in the following approximate percentages: oxygen, 20.95; nitrogen, 78.08; argon 0.93; carbon dioxide, 0.03; other gases, 0.01. **2.** SYN ventilate. [G. *aēr;* L. *aer*]

air a·bra·sion (ār ă-brā′zhŭn) The use of abrasive particles such as aluminum oxide under high pressure to abrade and sometimes remove dentin and enamel.

air-bone gap (ABG) (ār-bōn gap) An abnormal condition in which the auditory threshold for an air-conducted test tone is higher than that for a bone-conducted test tone of the same frequency. SEE ALSO conductive hearing loss.

air·borne in·fec·tion (ār′bōrn in-fek′shŭn) A mechanism of transmission of an infectious agent by particles, dust, or droplet nuclei suspended in the air.

air·borne pre·cau·tions (ār′bōrn prĕ-kaw′shŭnz) Measures taken to prevent transmission of infectious agents by airborne droplet spray. Airborne precautions include use of masks and air filtration systems.

air·bras·ive (ār-brā′siv) A dental device designed for polishing and removing stains from teeth, powered by air and water pressure, which delivers a stream of processed sodium bicarbonate slurry mixture through a handpiece nozzle.

air bron·cho·gram (ār brong′kō-gram) Radiographic appearance of an air-filled bronchus surrounded by fluid-filled airspaces.

air cells (ār selz) **1.** SYN pulmonary alveoli. **2.** Air-containing spaces in the skull.

air-con·di·tion·er lung (ār′kŏn-dish′ŭn-ĕr lŭng) An extrinsic allergic alveolitis caused by forced air contaminated with thermophilic actinomycetes and other organisms.

air con·duc·tion (ār kŏn-dŭk′shŭn) In relation to hearing, the transmission of sound to the inner ear through the external auditory canal and the structures of the middle ear.

air con·trast bar·i·um en·e·ma (ACBE) (ār kon′trast bar′ē-ŭm en′ĕ-mă) SYN air contrast enema.

air con·trast en·e·ma (ār kon′trast en′ĕ-mă) A double contrast enema in which air is introduced after coating of the colon with a dense barium suspension for radiographic study. SYN air contrast barium enema, double contrast enema.

air em·bo·lism (ār em′bŏ-lizm) Embolism that occurs when air enters a blood vessel, usually a vein, as a result of trauma, surgery, or deliberate injection; a large air embolism can cause lethal derangement of cardiac function.

air-flu·i·dized bed (ār-flū′i-dīzd bed) Type of bed intended to promote skin integrity and prevent skin breakdown. Within the mattress, small ceramic spheres are constantly blown by temperature-controlled airflow to distribute the client's weight evenly keeping pressure off bony prominences.

air hun·ger (ār hŭng′ĕr) Extremely deep ventilation such as occurs in patients with acidosis who are attempting to increase ventilation of alveoli and thus exhale more carbon dioxide. SEE ALSO Kussmaul respiration.

air med·i·cal trans·port (ār med′i-kăl trans′pōrt) The transport of patients by aircraft, either from the scene of a medical or trauma incident or from one facility to another using aircraft, most often helicopters.

air·plane splint (ār′plān splint) A complicated splint that holds the arm in abduction at about shoulder level with the forearm midway in flexion, generally with an axillary strut for support. SYN aeroplane splint.

air pol·lu·tion (ār pŏ-lū'shŭn) Contamination of air by smoke, particulate matter, and harmful gases, mainly oxides of carbon, sulfur, and nitrogen, as from automobile exhausts, industrial emissions, and burning rubbish. SEE ALSO smog.

air·port ma·lar·i·a (ār'pōrt mă-lar'ē-ă) The disease inadvertently imported by transport of an infected anopheline mosquito on an airplane.

air-pu·ri·fy·ing res·pi·ra·tor (ār-pyūr'i-fī-ing res'pir-ā-tŏr) An air-filtering respirator using filters designed to remove a specific substance from ambient air.

air sick·ness (ār sik'nĕs) A form of motion sickness caused by flying in an airplane. SEE ALSO motion sickness.

air splint (ār splint) A plastic splint inflated by air used to immobilize part or all of an extremity.

air·trap·ping (ār'trap-ing) Slow or incomplete emptying of air from all or part of a lung on expiration; implies obstruction of regional airways or emphysema.

air ves·i·cles (ār ves'i-kĕlz) SYN pulmonary alveoli.

air·way (ār'wā) **1.** Any part of the respiratory tract through which air passes during breathing. **2.** ANESTHESIA during resuscitation, a type of device to correct obstruction to breathing, especially an oropharyngeal, nasopharyngeal, or endotracheal airway, or tracheotomy tube. See page B32.

air·way a·nat·o·my (ār'wā ă-nat'ŏ-mē) The tracheobronchial structure, similar in shape to that of an inverted tree, containing three types of airways: cartilaginous airways (trachea, main stem bronchi, and approximately five generations of small bronchi); membranous bronchioles (approximately eight generations of noncartilaginous airways); and respiratory bronchioles (approximately five generations of gas-exchange or alveolar ducts).

air·way man·age·ment (ār'wā man'ăj-mĕnt) Assistance given a patient to maintain a patent airway, with or without intubation.

air·way ob·struc·tion (ār'wā ŏb-strŭk'shŭn) A type of respiratory dysfunction that produces reduced airflow, usually on expiration; the obstruction can be localized (e.g., tumor, stricture, foreign body) or generalized (e.g., emphysema, asthma).

air·way pres·sure re·lease ven·ti·la·tion (APRV) (ār'wā presh'ŭr rĕ-lēs' ven'ti-lā'shŭn) A mode of mechanical ventilation.

air·way re·sis·tance (ār'wā rĕ-zis'tăns) PHYSIOLOGY resistance to flow of gases during ventilation due to obstruction or turbulent flow in the upper and lower airways; to be differentiated during inhalation from resistance to inflation due to decreases in pulmonary or thoracic compliance.

Air·y disc (ār'ē disk) The image of a circular blur formed by a distant point source of light on the retina because of diffraction by the edge of the pupillary aperture where the diameter of the image decreases as the aperture increases.

AIS Abbreviation for acute ischemic stroke.

AIT (āt) Acronym for auditory integration training.

A-K am·pu·ta·tion (amp'yū-tā'shŭn) Abbreviation for above-the-knee amputation.

ak·a·mu·shi dis·ease (ah-kah-mū'shē di-zēz') SYN tsutsugamushi disease.

a·kar·y·o·cyte, **a·kar·y·ote** (ā-kar'ē-ō-sīt, ā-kar'ē-ōt) A cell without a nucleus, such as the erythrocyte. SYN acaryote. [G. *a-* priv. + *karyon,* kernel, + *kytos,* a hollow (cell)]

a·ka·thi·si·a (ak-ă-thiz'ē-ă) A syndrome characterized by an inability to remain in a sitting posture, with motor restlessness and a feeling of muscular quivering; may appear as a side effect of antipsychotic and neuroleptic medication. [G. *a-* priv. + *kathisis,* a sitting]

a·ker·a·to·sis (ă-ker-ă-tō'sis) Deficiency or absence of the horny layer of the epidermis.

Ak·er·lund de·for·mi·ty (ā'kĕr-lŭnd dĕ-fōrm'i-tē) Indentation (incisura) with niche of duodenal cap as seen radiologically.

akinaesthesia [Br.] SYN akinesthesia.

a·ki·ne·si·a, **a·ki·ne·sis** (ā'ki-nē'sē-ă, ā'ki-nē'sis) Absence or loss of the power of voluntary movement due to an extrapyramidal disorder. [G. *a-* priv. + *kinēsis,* movement]

a·kin·es·the·si·a (ā-kin'es-thē'zē-ă) Inability to perceive movement or position. SYN akinaesthesia. [G. *a-* priv. + *kinēsis,* motion, + *aisthēsis,* sensation]

a·ki·net·ic, **a·ki·ne·sic** (ā'ki-net'ik, ā'ki-nē'sik) Relating to or suffering from akinesia.

a·ki·net·ic mu·tism (ā'ki-net'ik myū'tizm) Subacute or chronic state of altered consciousness, in which the patient appears alert intermittently but is not responsive, although the descending motor pathways appear intact; due to lesions of various cerebral structures.

Al Symbol for aluminum.

ALA Abbreviation for delta (δ)-aminolevulinic acid. Cf. Ala.

Ala Abbreviation for alanine or its monoradical or diradical.

a·la, gen. and pl. **a·lae** (ā'lă, ā'lē) **1.** [TA] A

winglike anatomic structure. **2.** Pronounced, longitudinal cuticular ridges in nematodes, usually found in larval stages (*Ascaris lumbricoides*), although occasionally present in adult worms (*Enterobius vermicularis*). [L. wing]

Al•a•gille syn•drome (ah-lah-zhēl′ sin′drōm) An autosomal dominant syndrome that becomes apparent in childhood and is associated with jaundice due to a paucity of intrahepatic bile ducts; characteristics include a narrow face and pointed chin, broad forehead, long, straight nose, deep-set eyes, posterior embryotoxon in the eye, cardiovascular abnormalities, vertebral defects, and nephropathy.

a•la•li•a (ă-lā′lē-ă) Mutism; inability to speak. SEE aphonia. [G. *a-* priv. + *lalia,* talking]

a•la mi•nor os•sis sphe•noi•da•lis (ā′lă mī′nŏr os′is sfē-noyd-dā′lis) [TA] SYN lesser wing of sphenoid bone.

a•la na•si (ā′lă nā′sī) The lateral wall of each naris.

A•land Is•land al•bi•nism (ā′lahnd ī′lănd al′bin-izm) SYN ocular albinism.

al•a•nine (A, Ala) (al′ă-nēn) 2-Aminopropionic acid; α-aminopropionic acid; one of the amino acids widely occurring in proteins.

al•a•nine a•mi•no•trans•fer•ase (ALT) (al′ă-nēn ă-mē′nō-trans′fĕr-ās) An enzyme transferring amino groups from L-alanine to 2-ketoglutarate, or the reverse (from L-glutamate to pyruvate); serum concentration is increased in viral hepatitis and myocardial infarction. SYN glutamic-pyruvic transaminase, serum glutamic-pyruvic transaminase.

al•a•nine-glu•cose cy•cle (al′ă-nēn-glū′kōs sī′kĕl) Alanine, synthesized in muscle from glucose-derived pyruvate, travels from the blood to the liver, which converts the alanine to glucose and urea. The liver releases glucose back into the blood to transport to muscle as an energy substrate, thereby completing the cycle.

a•la of nose (ā′lă nōz) The outer wall of each nostril. SYN wing of nose.

Al•an•son am•pu•ta•tion (al′ăn-sŏn amp′yū-tā′shŭn) A circular amputation, with the stump shaped like a cone.

al•a•nyl (al′ă-nil) The acyl radical of alanine.

a•lar (ā′lăr) **1.** Relating to a wing; winged. **2.** SYN axillary. **3.** Relating to the wings (alae) of such structures as the nose, sphenoid, or sacrum.

ALARA (ă-lahr′ă) Acronym for a philosophy of use of radiation based on using dosages as low as reasonably achievable to attain the desired diagnostic, therapeutic, or other goal.

a•lar lam•i•na of neu•ral tube (ā′lăr lam′i-nă nūr′ăl tūb) SYN alar plate of neural tube.

a•larm re•ac•tion (ă-lahrm′ rē-ak′shŭn) The various phenomena (e.g., stimulated endocrine activity) the body exhibits as an adaptive response to injury or stress; first phase of the general adaptation syndrome. See this page.

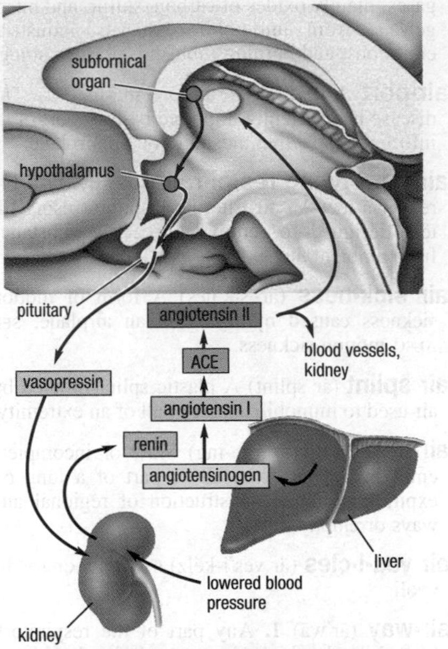

communication between kidneys and brain (alarm reaction): when blood volume or pressure is low, the kidney secretes renin into the bloodstream; renin in the blood promotes synthesis of the peptide angiotensin II, which excites the neurons in the subfornical organ; the subfornical neurons stimulate the hypothalamus, thus increasing production of antidiuretic hormone (vasopressin)

a•lar plate of neu•ral tube (ā′lăr plāt nūr′ăl tūb) The dorsal division of the lateral walls of the neural tube. SYN alar lamina of neural tube.

a•lar spine (ā′lăr spīn) SYN sphenoidal spine.

a•lar•yn•ge•al speech (ā-lăr-in′jē-ăl spēch) Production of speech using a sound source other than the larynx, as in esophageal speech or use of a tracheoesophageal voice prosthesis or an artificial larynx. SEE esophageal speech. SEE ALSO artificial larynx, tracheoesophageal puncture.

al•ba (al′bă) SYN white matter. [fem. of L. *albus,* white]

Al•bar•ran test (ahl-bah-rahn′ test) A procedure involving renal insufficiency wherein the drinking of large quantities of water will cause a proportionate increase in the volume of urine if the kidneys are sound, but not if the epithelium of the secreting tubules is damaged.

Al•bers-Schön•berg dis•ease (ahl′berz-shern′bĕrg di-zēz′) SYN osteopetrosis.

Al•bert dis•ease (ahl′bert di-zēz′) Bursitis of the Achilles tendon, sometimes seen in association with calcification. May result from either trauma or poorly fitted shoes. SYN Schantz disease.

Al•bert su•ture (ahl′bert sū′chŭr) A modified Czerny suture, the first row of stitches passing through the entire thickness of the wall of the gut.

al•bi•cans, pl. **al•bi•can•ti•a** (al′bi-kanz, -kan′shē-ă) **1.** SYN white. **2.** SYN corpus albicans. [L.]

al•bi•du•ri•a (al-bi-dyūr′ē-ă) The passing of pale or white urine of low specific gravity, as in chyluria. SYN albinuria. [L. *albidus,* whitish, + G. *ouron,* urine]

Al•bi•ni nod•ules (ahl-bē′nē nod′yūlz) Any of several minute fibrous nodules on the margins of the mitral and tricuspid valves of the heart, sometimes present in the neonate and representing fetal tissue rests (remnants of embryonic tissue).

al•bi•nism (al′bi-nizm) A group of inherited (usually autosomal recessive) disorders with deficiency or absence of pigment in the skin, hair, and eyes, or eyes only, due to an abnormality in production of melanin. SEE ocular albinism, piebaldism. [albino + ism]

al•bi•no (al-bī′nō) An individual with albinism. [Pg., little white one, fr. *albo*, white, fr. L. *albus* + *-ino*, dim. suffix]

al•bi•no rats (al-bī′nō rats) Rats with white fur and pink eyes, used extensively in laboratory experiments.

al•bi•not•ic (al-bi-not′ik) Pertaining to albinism.

al•bi•nu•ri•a (al-bi-nyūr′ē-ă) SYN albiduria.

Al•bright dis•ease (awl′brīt di-zēz′) SYN McCune-Albright syndrome.

Al•bright he•red•i•tar•y os•te•o•dys•tro•phy (awl′brīt hĕr-ed′i-tar-ē os′tē-ō-dis′trŏ-fē) An inherited form of hyperparathyroidism associated with ectopic calcification and ossification and skeletal defects, notably small fourth metacarpals; intelligence may be normal or subnormal. Inheritance is heterogeneous; the autosomal form is caused by mutation in the guanine nucleotide-binding protein gene (GNAS1) on 20q. There are also the recessive and X-linked forms. SEE ALSO pseudohypoparathyroidism. SYN Albright syndrome (2).

Al•bright syn•drome (awl′brīt sin′drōm) **1.** SYN McCune-Albright syndrome. **2.** SYN Albright hereditary osteodystrophy.

al•bu•gin•e•a (al-bū-jin′ē-ă) A white fibrous tissue layer, such as the tunica albuginea (q.v.). [L. *albugineus,* fr. *albugo,* white spot]

al•bu•men (al-bū′mĕn) SYN ovalbumin. SEE ALSO albumin.

al•bu•min (al-bū′min) A type of simple protein, varieties of which are widely distributed throughout the tissues and fluids of plants and animals; albumin is soluble in pure water, precipitable from solution by strong acids, and coagulable by heat in acid or neutral solution. [L. *albumen* (*-min-*), the white of egg]

al•bu•min:glob•u•lin ra•ti•o (al-bū′min-ō-glob′yū-lin rā′shē-ō) The ratio of albumin to globulin in serum plasma or urine; the normal ratio in the serum is approximately 1.55.

al•bu•mi•noid (al-bū′min-oyd) **1.** Resembling albumin. **2.** Any protein. **3.** A simple type of protein, insoluble in neutral solvents, present in horny and cartilaginous tissues and in the lens of the eye; e.g., keratin, elastin, collagen. SYN scleroprotein.

al•bu•min•ous (al-bū′min-ŭs) Relating to, containing, or consisting of albumin.

al•bu•min•ur•i•a (al-bū′mi-nyūr′ē-ă) Presence of protein in urine, chiefly albumin but also globulin; usually indicative of disease, but sometimes resulting from a temporary or transient dysfunction. SYN proteinuria (2). [albumin + G. *ouron,* urine]

al•bu•min•ur•ic (al-bū′mi-nyūr′ik) Relating to or characterized by albuminuria.

Al•ca•lig•e•nes fae•ca•lis (al-kă-lij′ĕ-nēz fē-kā′lis) A genus of gram-negative, rod-shaped, nonfermenting bacteria (family Achromobacteraceae) that are either motile and peritrichous or nonmotile. They are strictly aerobic; some strains are capable of anaerobic respiration in the presence of nitrate or nitrite; their metabolism is respiratory, never fermentative; they do not use carbohydrates. Found mostly in the intestinal canal, decaying materials, dairy products, water, and soil; they can be isolated from human respiratory and gastrointestinal tracts and wounds in hospitalized patients with compromised immune systems; occasionally the cause of opportunistic infections, including nosocomial septicemia. [alkali + G. *-gen,* producing]

al•cap•ton (al-kap′tŏn) SYN homogentisic acid.

al•cap•ton•u•ri•a, al•kap•ton•u•ri•a (al-kap′tŏ-nyūr′ē-ă, al-kap′tŏ-nyūr′ē-ă) Excretion of homogentisic acid (alkapton) in the urine due to congenital lack of the enzyme homogentisate 1,2-dioxygenase; urine turns dark if allowed to stand; may recur and subside at irregular intervals; arthritis and ochronosis are late complications. [alkapton + G. *ouron,* urine]

al•co•hol (al′kŏ-hol) **1.** One of a series of organic chemical compounds in which a hydrogen (H) attached to carbon is replaced by a hydroxyl (OH); alcohols react with acids to form esters and with alkali metals to form alcoholates. **2.** Ethanol, C_2H_5OH, made from carbohydrates by fermentation and synthetically from ethylene or acetylene. It has been used in beverages and as a solvent, vehicle, and preservative; medicinally, it is used externally as a rubefacient, coolant, and disinfectant, and internally as an analgesic, stomachic, and sedative. SYN ethanol, ethyl alcohol. **3.** The azeotropic mixture of CH_3CH_2OH and water (92.3% by weight of ethanol). [Ar. *al,* the, + *kohl,* fine antimonial powder, the term being applied first to a fine powder, then to anything impalpable (spirit)]

al•co•hol am•nes•tic syn•drome (al′kŏ-hol am-nes′tik sin′drōm) An amnestic syndrome resulting from alcoholism; alcoholic "blackouts." Cf. Korsakoff syndrome.

al•co•hol de•hy•dro•gen•ase (ADH) (al′kŏ-hol dē-hī-droj′en-ās) An oxidoreductase that reversibly converts an alcohol to an aldehyde (or ketone) with NAD^+ as the H acceptor. For example, ethanol + NAD^+ ↔ acetaldehyde + NADH. Plays an important role in alcoholism.

al•co•hol, for•ma•lin, and a•ce•tic a•cid (AFA) fix•a•tive (al′kŏ-hol fōr′mă-lin ă-sē′tik as′id fik′să-tiv) A combination used for the fixation of nematodes, trematodes, and cestodes.

al•co•hol-gly•cer•in fix•a•tive (al′kŏ-hol-glis′ĕr-in fik′să-tiv) Alcohol (70%) with 5% glycerin; suitable for fixing most nematodes.

al•co•hol•ic (al′kŏ-hol′ik) **1.** Relating to, containing, or produced by alcohol. **2.** One who suffers from alcoholism. **3.** One who abuses or depends on alcohol.

al•co•hol•ic cir•rho•sis (al′kŏ-hol′ik sir-ō′sis) Hepatic condition that frequently develops in chronic alcoholism, characterized in an early stage by enlargement of the liver due to fatty change with mild fibrosis, and later by Laënnec cirrhosis with contraction of the liver.

al•co•hol•ic hep•a•ti•tis (al′kŏ-hol′ik hep′ă-tī′tis) Inflammation of the liver due to abuse of alcohol.

Al•co•hol•ics A•non•y•mous (AA, aa) (al′kŏ-hol′iks ă-non′i-mŭs) Mutual support group that helps its members remain sober.

al•co•hol•ism (al′kŏ-hol-ism) A chronic, progressive behavioral disorder characterized by a strong urge to consume ethanol and an inability to limit the amount of drinking despite adverse consequences, which may include social or occupational impairment and deterioration of physical health. Both physical dependence (withdrawal symptoms such as nausea, sweating, tremors, and delirium resulting from abstinence) and tolerance (the need to increase alcohol intake to achieve the desired effect) occur.

al•co•hol•y•sis (al′kŏ-hol′i-sis) Splitting of a chemical bond with the addition of the elements of alcohol at the point of splitting. [alcohol + G. *lysis,* dissolution]

ALD Abbreviation for assistive listening device; adrenoleukodystrophy.

al•de•hyde (al′dĕ-hīd) A compound containing the radical —CH=O, reducible to an alcohol (—CH_2OH), oxidizable to a carboxylic acid (—COOH); e.g., acetaldehyde.

Al•der a•nom•a•ly (ahl′der ă-nom′ă-lē) Coarse azurophilic granulation of leukocytes, especially granulocytes in both the nucleus and cytoplasm, which may be associated with gargoylism and Morquio disease.

al•do•pen•tose (al-dō-pen′tōs) A monosaccharide with five carbon atoms, of which one is a (potential) aldehyde group; e.g., ribose.

al•dose (al′dōs) A monosaccharide potentially containing the characteristic group of the aldehydes, —CHO; a polyhydroxyaldehyde.

al•dos•ter•one (al-dos′tĕr-ōn) A hormone produced by the cortex of suprarenal gland; its major action is to facilitate potassium exchange for sodium in the distal renal tubule, causing sodium reabsorption and potassium and hydrogen loss; the principal mineralocorticoid.

al•dos•ter•one an•tag•o•nist (al-dos′tĕr-ōn an-tag′ŏ-nist) An agent that opposes the action of the adrenal hormone aldosterone on renal tubular mineralocorticoid retention; these agents (e.g., spironolactone) are useful in treating the hypertension of primary hyperaldosteronism, or the sodium retention of secondary hyperaldosteronism.

al•do•ste•ron•ism (al-dos′tĕr-ŏn-izm) A disorder caused by excessive secretion of aldosterone. SYN hyperaldosteronism.

a•lec•i•thal (ā-les′i-thal) Without a yolk; denoting oocytes (ova) with little or no deutoplasm. [G. *a-* priv. + *lekithos,* yolk]

A•lep•po boil (ă-lep′ō boyl) The lesion occurring in cutaneous leishmaniasis. SEE cutaneous leishmaniasis. SYN Baghdad boil, bouton de Baghdad.

aleukaemia [Br.] SYN aleukemia.

aleukaemic [Br.] SYN aleukemic.

aleukaemic leukaemia [Br.] SYN aleukemic leukemia.

aleukaemoid [Br.] SYN aleukemoid.

a•leu•ke•mi•a (ā-lū-kē′mē-ă) **1.** Literally, a lack of leukocytes in the blood. Generally used to indicate varieties of leukemic disease in which the leukocyte count in circulating blood is normal or even subnormal (i.e., no leukocytosis), but a few young leukocytes are observed; sometimes used more restrictedly for unusual instances of leukemia with no leukocytosis and no young forms in the blood. **2.** Leukemic changes in bone marrow associated with a subnormal number of leukocytes in the blood. SEE ALSO subleukemic leukemia. SYN aleukaemia. [G. *a-* priv. + *leukos,* white, + *haima,* blood]

a•leu•ke•mic (ā′lū-kē′mik) Pertaining to aleukemia. SYN aleukaemic.

a•leu•ke•mic leu•ke•mi•a (ā′lū-kē′mik lū-kē′mē-ă) Disorder in which abnormal (or leukemic) cells are absent in the peripheral blood. SYN aleukaemic leukaemia.

a•leu•ke•moid (ā′lū-kē′moyd) Resembling aleukemia symptomatically. SYN aleukaemoid.

a•leu•ki•a (ā-lū′kē-ă) Absence or extremely decreased number of leukocytes in the circulating blood; sometimes also termed aleukemic myelosis. [G. *a-* priv. + *leukos,* white]

a•leu•ko•cyt•ic (ā′lū-kō-sit′ik) Manifesting absence or extremely reduced numbers of leukocytes in blood or lesions.

a•leu•ko•cy•to•sis (ā′lū-kō-sī-tō′sis) Absence or great reduction of white blood cells in the circulating blood, or the lack of leukocytes in an anatomic lesion. [G. *a-* priv. + *leukos,* white, + *kytos,* a hollow (cell)]

Al•ex•an•der dis•ease (al-ĕg-zan′dĕr di-zēz′) A rare, fatal central nervous system degenerative disease of infants, characterized by psychomotor retardation, seizures, and paralysis; megaloencephaly is associated with widespread leukodystrophic changes, especially in the frontal lobes.

Al•ex•an•der hear•ing im•pair•ment (al-ĕg-zan′dĕr hēr′ing im-pār′mĕnt) High frequency deafness due to membranous cochlear dysplasia.

Al•ex•an•der law (al-ĕg-zan′dĕr law) States that a jerk nystagmus becomes worse when gazing in the direction of the fast component.

Al•ex•an•der tech•nique (al-ĕg-zan′dĕr tek-nēk′) The use of movement and exercise to improve posture, breathing, and other functions.

a•lex•i•a (ă-lek′sē-ă) An inability to comprehend the meaning of written or printed words and sentences, caused by a cerebral lesion. Also called optic alexia, sensory alexia, or visual alexia, in distinction to motor alexia (anarthria), in which there is loss of the power to read aloud although the significance of what is written or printed is understood. SYN text blindness, word blindness, visual aphasia (1). [G. *a-* priv. + *lexis,* a word or phrase]

a•lex•ic (ă-lek′sik) Pertaining to alexia.

a•lex•i•thy•mi•a (ă-lek′si-thī′mē-ă) Difficulty in recognizing and describing one's emotions, defining them in terms of somatic sensations or behavioral reactions. [G. *a-* priv. + *lexis,* word, + *-thymia,* feelings, passion]

al•fa fe•ta•pro•tein test (AFP) (al′fă fē′tō-prō′tēn test) Fetal blood protein found abnormally in adults with some forms of cancer; low levels in amniotic fluid are associated with Down syndrome; high levels with neural tube defects.

al•fal•fa (al-fal′fă) (*Medicago sativa*) A form of ground cover used as animal feed and as a nutritional supplement in humans. Sometimes eaten in salads. Many drug interactions are reported. SYN lucerne, purple medick. [Sp., fr. Ar. *al-fasfasah*]

al•gae (al′jē) A division of eukaryotic, photosynthetic, nonflowering organisms that includes many seaweeds. [pl. of L. *alga,* seaweed]

algaesthesia [Br.] SYN algesthesia.

al•gal (al′găl) Resembling or pertaining to algae.

♻ **alge-, algesi-, algio-, algo-** Combining forms meaning pain; correspond to L. dolor-. [G. *algos,* a pain]

al•ge•si•a (al-jē′zē-ă) SYN algesthesia. [G. *algēsis,* a sense of pain]

al•ge•sic (al-jē′zik) **1.** Painful; related to or causing pain. **2.** Relating to hypersensitivity to pain. SYN algetic.

al•ge•sim•e•ter (al′jĕ-sim′ĕ-ter) SYN algesiometer.

al•ge•si•o•gen•ic (al′jē′zē-ō-jen′ik) Pain-producing. SYN algogenic. [G. *algēsis,* sense of pain, + *-gen,* production]

al•ge•si•om•e•ter (al′jĕ-zē-om′ĕ-tĕr) An instrument for measuring the degree of sensitivity to a painful stimulus. SYN algesimeter, algometer, odynometer. [G. *algēsis,* sense of pain, + *metron,* measure]

al•ges•the•si•a, al•ges•the•sis (al′jes-thē′zē-ă, al′jes-thē′sis) **1.** The appreciation of pain. **2.** Hypersensitivity to pain. SYN algaesthesia, algesia. [G. *algos,* pain, + *aisthēsis,* sensation]

al•get•ic (al-jet′ik) SYN algesic.

♻ **-algia** Suffix meaning pain, painful condition. [G. *algos,* a pain]

al•gid (al′jid) Characterized by prostration, cold, clammy skin, and hypotension. [L. *algidus,* cold]

al•gid stage (al′jid stāj) The stage of collapse in cholera.

al•go•gen•ic (al′gō-jen′ik) SYN algesiogenic.

al•go•lag•ni•a (al′gō-lag′nē-ă) Form of sexual perversion in which the infliction or the experiencing of pain increases the pleasure of the sexual act or causes sexual pleasure independent of the act; includes both sadism (active algolagnia) and masochism (passive algolagnia). SYN algophilia (2). [algo- + G. *lagneia,* lust]

al•gom•e•ter (al-gom′ĕ-tĕr) SYN algesiometer. [algo- + G. *metron,* measure]

al•go•phil•i•a (al′gō-fil′ē-ă) **1.** Pleasure experienced in the thought of pain in others or in oneself. **2.** SYN algolagnia. [algo- + G. *phileō,* to love]

al•go•pho•bi•a (al′gō-fō′bē-ă) Abnormal fear of or sensitiveness to pain. [algo- + G. *phobos,* fear]

al•go•rithm (al′gŏr-idhm) **1.** A process consisting of steps, each depending on the outcome of the previous one. **2.** CLINICAL MEDICINE a step-by-step protocol for management of a health care problem. **3.** COMPUTED TOMOGRAPHY the formulas used for calculation of the final image from the x-ray transmission data. [Mediev. L. *algorismus,* after Muhammad ibn-Musa *al-Khwarizmi,* Arabian mathematician, + G. *arithmos,* number]

al•go•vas•cu•lar (al′gō-vas′kyū-lăr) Relating to changes in the lumen of the blood vessels occurring under the influence of pain. [G. *algos,* pain]

ALI Abbreviation for acute lung injury.

a•li•as•ing (āl′ē-ăs-ing) Magnetic resonance imaging artifact produced when anatomy outside the field of view is mismapped inside it.

Al•ice in Won•der•land syn•drome (al′is wŭn′dĕr-land sin′drōm) Syndrome of disturbed space, time, and body image associated with visual hallucinations.

a•li•en•a•tion (ā′lē-ĕn-ā′shŭn) A condition characterized by lack of meaningful relationships with others, sometimes resulting in depersonalization and estrangement from others. [L. *alieno,* pp. *-atus,* to make strange]

a•li•e•ni•a (ā′li-ē′nē-ă) Congenital absence of the spleen. [G. *a-* priv. + L. *lien,* spleen]

al•i•form (al′i-fōrm) Wing-shaped. [L. *ala,* + *forma,* shape]

a•lign•ment (ă-līn′mĕnt) **1.** The longitudinal position of a bone or limb. **2.** DENTISTRY the arrangement of the teeth in relation to the supporting structures and the adjacent and opposing dentitions.

a•lign•ment curve (ă-līn′mĕnt kŭrv) The line passing through the center of the teeth laterally in the direction of the curve of the dental arch.

al•i•men•ta•ry (al′i-men′tăr-ē) Relating to food or nutrition. [L. *alimentarius,* fr. *alimentum,* nourishment]

al•i•men•ta•ry ca•nal (al′i-men′tăr-ē kă-nal′) SYN digestive tract.

al•i•men•ta•ry gly•cos•ur•i•a (al′i-men′tăr-ē glī-kō-syūr′ē-ă) Condition that develops after the ingestion of a moderate amount of sugar or starch because the rate of intestinal absorption exceeds the capacity of the liver and the other tissues to remove the glucose, thus allowing blood glucose levels to become high enough for renal excretion to occur.

al•i•men•ta•ry hy•per•in•su•lin•ism (al′i-men′tăr-ē hī′pĕr-in′sŭ-lin-izm) Elevated levels of insulin in the plasma following ingestion of meals by people with abnormally rapid gastric emptying.

al•i•men•ta•ry li•pe•mi•a (al′i-men′tăr-ē li-pē′mē-ă) Relatively transient lipemia occurring after ingestion of foods with a higher fat content.

al•i•men•ta•ry pen•to•su•ri•a (al′i-men′tăr-ē pen-tō-syūr′ē-ă) The urinary excretion of L-arabinose and L-xylose as the result of the excessive ingestion of fruits containing these pentoses (e.g., grapes, plums, cherries).

al•i•men•ta•ry tox•ic a•leu•ki•a (ATA) tox•i•co•sis (al′i-men′tăr-ē tok′sik ā-lū′kē-ă tok′si-kō′sis) A form of toxicosis caused by ingestion of grain contaminated with any of several kinds of trichothecene mycotoxins; characterized by nausea, vomiting, diarrhea, leukopenia (aleukia), hemorrhaging, skin inflammation, and, in severe cases, death.

al•i•men•ta•ry tract (al′i-men′tăr-ē trakt) SYN digestive tract.

al•i•men•ta•tion (al′i-mĕn-tā′shŭn) Providing nourishment. SEE ALSO feeding.

al•i•na•sal (al′i-nā′zăl) Relating to the wings of the nose (alae nasi), or flaring portions of the nostrils. [L. *ala,* + *nasus,* nose]

al•i•phat•ic (al′i-fat′ik) Denoting the acyclic carbon compounds, most of which belong to the fatty acid series. [G. *aleiphar* (*aleiphat-*), fat, oil]

al•i•phat•ic ac•ids (al′i-fat′ik as′idz) The acids of nonaromatic hydrocarbons (e.g., acetic, propionic, butyric acids); the so-called fatty acids of the formula R–COOH, where R is a nonaromatic (aliphatic) hydrocarbon.

al•i•quant (al′i-kwahnt) CHEMISTRY, IMMUNOLOGY a portion that results from dividing the whole in a manner that some is left after the aliquants (equal in volume or weight) have been apportioned.

al•i•quot (al′i-kwot) A sample the mass of volume of which is a known fraction of that of the whole. [L. a few, several]

a•lis•ma (ă-liz′mă) (*Alisma plantago-aquatica*) A water-loving plant used in traditional Chinese medicine for many purposes; purported value also in treating dermatologic disorders. SYN maddog weed, marsh drain, water plantain. [L., G.]

al•i•sphe•noid (al′i-sfē′noyd) Relating to the greater wing of the sphenoid bone. [L. *ala,* + *sphēn,* wedge]

a•live (ă-līv′) Living; perceptive mentally. [M.E.]

a•live and well (A/W) (ă-līv′ wel) Notation made, as appropriate, with respect to the health status of blood relatives in the family history. SYN living and well.

a•liz•a•rin (ă-liz′ă-rin) [CI 58000] A red dye that occurs in the root of madder as orange needles, slightly soluble in water; used by the ancients as a dye. Now made synthetically from anthracene and used in the manufacture of dyes, e.g., alizarin blue, alizarin orange, "Turkey red." As an indicator, it is yellow below pH 5.5 and red above pH 6.8; other modified alizarins have other colors and change color at other pH values.

alkalaemia [Br.] SYN alkalemia.

al•ka•le•mi•a (al′kă-lē′mē-ă) A decrease in H-ion concentration of the blood or a rise in pH, irrespective of alterations in the level of bicarbonate ion. SYN alkalaemia. [alkali + G. *haima,* blood]

al•ka•les•cent (al′kă-les′ĕnt) **1.** Slightly alkaline. **2.** Becoming alkaline.

al•ka•li, pl. **al•ka•lis, al•ka•lies** (al′kă-lī, -līz, al′kă-līz) **1.** A strongly basic substance yielding hydroxide ions (OH^-) in solution; e.g., sodium hydroxide, potassium hydroxide. **2.** SYN base (3). **3.** SYN alkali metal. [Ar. *al,* the, + *qalīy,* soda ash]

al•ka•li met•al (al′kă-lī met′ăl) An alkali of the family Li, Na, K, Rb, Cs, and Fr, all of which have highly ionized hydroxides. SYN alkali (3).

al•ka•line (al′kă-lin) Relating to or having the reaction of an alkali.

al•ka•line-ash di•et (al′kă-lin-ash dī′ĕt) A diet consisting mainly of fruits, vegetables, and milk that, when catabolized, leaves an alkaline residue to be excreted in the urine. SYN acid-ash diet.

al•ka•line earth el•e•ments (al′kă-lin ĕrth el′ĕ-mĕnts) Those elements in the family Be, Mg, Ca, Sr, Ba, and Ra, the hydroxides of which are highly ionized and hence alkaline in water solution.

al•ka•line earths (al′kă-lin ĕrths) SEE alkaline earth elements.

al•ka•line phos•pha•tase (al′kă-lin fos′fă-tās) A phosphatase with an optimal pH of above 7.0 present in many tissues; low levels of this enzyme are seen in cases of hypophosphatasia.

al•ka•line tide (al′kă-lin tīd) A period of urinary neutrality or even alkalinity after meals due to withdrawal of hydrogen ions for the purpose of secretion of highly acid gastric juices.

al•ka•lin•i•ty (al′kă-lin′i-tē) The state of being alkaline.

al•ka•li•nu•ri•a (al′kă-li-nyūr′ē-ă) The passage of alkaline urine. SYN alkaluria. [alkaline + G. *ouron,* urine]

al•ka•li re•serve (al′kă-lī rē-zĕrv′) The sum total of the basic ions (mainly bicarbonates) of the blood and other body fluids that, acting as buffers, maintain the normal pH of the blood.

al•ka•loid (al′kă-loyd) Originally, any one of hundreds of plant products distinguished by alkaline (basic) reactions, but now restricted to heterocyclic nitrogen-containing and often complex structures possessing pharmacologic activity; their trivial names usually end in -ine (e.g., morphine, atropine, colchicine). Alkaloids are synthesized by plants and are found in the leaf, bark, seed, or other parts, usually constituting the active principle of the crude drug; they are a loosely defined group but may be classified according to the chemical structure of their main nucleus. For medicinal purposes, due to improved water solubility, the salts of alkaloids are typically used. SEE ALSO individual alkaloid or alkaloid class.

al•ka•lo•sis (al-kă-lō′sis) A state characterized by a decrease in the hydrogen ion concentration of arterial blood below the normal level, 40 nmol/L N pH 7.2. The condition may be caused by H-ion loss or base excess in body fluids (metabolic alkalosis), or caused by CO_2 loss due to hyperventilation (respiratory alkalosis).

al•ka•lot•ic (al-kă-lot′ik) Relating to alkalosis.

al•ka•lu•ri•a (al-kă-lyūr′ē-ă) SYN alkalinuria.

al•kane (al′kān) The general term for a saturated acyclic hydrocarbon (e.g., propane, butane).

al•ka•net (al′kă-net) *Alkanna tinctoria;* roots of this herb are prepared for purported value as a topical astringent. [Sp. *alcaneta*]

al•kap•ton (al-kap′tŏn) SYN homogentisic acid. [alkali + G. *kaptō,* to suck up greedily]

al•kene (al′kēn) An acyclic hydrocarbon containing one or more double bonds; e.g., ethene, propene. SYN olefin.

al•ke•nyl (al′kĕ-nil) The radical of an alkene.

al•kide (al′kīd) SYN alkyl (2).

al•kyl (al′kil) **1.** A hydrocarbon radical of the general formula C_nH_{2n+1}. **2.** A compound, such as tetraethyl lead, in which a metal is combined with alkyl radicals. SYN alkide.

al•kyl•a•tion (al′ki-lā′shŭn) Substitution of an alkyl radical for a hydrogen atom; e.g., introduction of a side chain into an aromatic compound.

ALL Abbreviation for acute lymphocytic leukemia.

allachaesthesia [Br.] SYN allachesthesia.

al•la•ches•the•si•a (al′ă-kes-thē′zē-ă) A condition in which a tactile sensation is referred to a point other than that to which the stimulus is applied. SYN allachaesthesia. [G. *allachē,* elsewhere, + *aisthēsis,* sensation]

allaesthesia [Br.] SYN allesthesia.

♻ **allanto-, allant-** Combining forms meaning allantois; allantoid; sausagelike. [G. *allas, allantos,* sausage]

al·lan·to·cho·ri·on (ă-lan′tō-kōr′ē-on) Extra-embryonic membrane formed by fusion of the allantois and chorion.

al·lan·to·ic (al′an-tō′ik) Relating to the allantois.

al·lan·to·ic flu·id (al′an-tō′ik flū′id) The liquid within the allantoic cavity.

al·lan·to·ic stalk (al′an-tō′ik stawk) The narrow connection between the intraembryonic portion of the allantois and the extraembryonic allantoic vesicle.

al·lan·to·ic ves·i·cle (al′an-tō′ik ves′i-kĕl) The hollow portion of the allantois.

al·lan·toid (ă-lan′toyd) **1.** Sausage-shaped. **2.** Relating to, or resembling, the allantois. [allanto- + G. *eidos,* appearance]

al·lan·toid mem·brane (ă-lan′toyd mem′brān) SYN allantois.

al·lan·toid·o·an·gi·op·a·gous twins (ă-lan-toyd′ō-an-jē-op′ă-gŭs twinz) Unequal monochorial twins with fusion of their allantoic vessels within the placenta; the lesser twin is essentially a parasite on the placental circulation of the larger twin.

al·lan·to·in·u·ri·a (ă-lan′tō-i-nyūr′ē-ă) The urinary excretion of allantoin; normal in most mammals, but abnormal in humans. [allantoin + G. *ouron,* urine]

al·lan·to·is (ă-lan′tō-is) A fetal membrane developing from the hindgut (or umbilical vesicle, in humans). Also in humans it becomes a fibrous cord, the urachus; externally, in mammals, it contributes to the formation of the umbilical cord and placenta. SYN allantoid membrane. [allanto- + G. *eidos,* appearance]

al·lele (ă-lēl′) Any one of a series of two or more different genes that may occupy the same locus on a specific chromosome. As autosomal chromosomes are paired, each autosomal gene is represented twice in normal somatic cells. If the same allele occupies both units of the locus, the individual or cell is homozygous for this allele. If the alleles are different, the individual or cell is heterozygous for both alleles. SEE ALSO DNA markers. SYN allelomorph. [G. *allēlōn,* reciprocally]

al·le·lic (ă-lē′lik) Relating to an allele.

al·le·lic gene (ă-lē′lik jēn) SEE allele, dominance of traits.

al·le·lo·morph (ă-lē′lō-mōrf) SYN allele. [G. *allēlōn,* reciprocally, + *morphē,* shape]

al·le·lo·tax·is, al·le·lo·tax·y (ă-lē′lō-taks′is, -taks′ē) Development of an organ from a number of embryonal structures or tissues. [G. *allēlōn,* reciprocally, + *taxis,* an arranging]

Al·len Cog·ni·tive Lev·el Screen (al′ĕn kog′ni-tiv lev′ĕl skrēn) OCCUPATIONAL THERAPY a tool for assessing the ability to perform visual-motor tasks through the application of cognitive skills such as deduction, planning, and problem solving; consists of three leather-lacing exercises.

Al·len test (al′ĕn test) A measurement of radial or ulnar patency; either the radial or ulnar artery is digitally compressed by the examiner after blood has been forced out of the hand by clenching it into a fist; failure of the blood to diffuse into the hand when opened indicates that the artery not compressed is occluded.

al·ler·gen (al′ĕr-jĕn) An incitant of altered reactivity (allergy), an antigenic substance. [allergy + G. *-gen,* producing]

al·ler·gen·ic (al′ĕr-jen′ik) SYN antigenic.

al·ler·gen·ic ex·tract (al′ĕr-jen′ik eks′trakt) Extract (usually containing protein) from various sources (e.g., food, bacteria, pollen) suspected of stimulating manifestations of allergy; may be used for skin testing or desensitization. SYN allergic extract.

al·ler·gic (ă-lĕr′jik) Relating to any response stimulated by an allergen.

al·ler·gic con·junc·ti·vi·tis (ă-lĕr′jik kŏn-jŭngk′ti-vī′tis) Acute conjunctivitis characterized by itching and watery discharge; typically with bilateral involvement.

al·ler·gic con·tact der·ma·ti·tis (ă-lĕr′jik kon′takt dĕr′mă-tī′tis) A delayed type IV allergic reaction of the skin with varying degrees of erythema, edema, and vesiculation resulting from cutaneous contact with a specific allergen. SYN contact allergy.

al·ler·gic ec·ze·ma (ă-lĕr′jik ek′zĕ-mă) Macular, papular, or vesicular eruption due to an allergic reaction.

al·ler·gic ex·tract (ă-lĕr′jik eks′trakt) SYN allergenic extract.

al·ler·gic pur·pu·ra (ă-lĕr′jik pŭr′pyŭr-ă) Nonthrombocytopenic purpura due to sensitization to foods, drugs, and insect bites. SYN anaphylactoid purpura (1).

al·ler·gic re·ac·tion (ă-lĕr′jik rē-ak′shŭn) A local or general reaction of an organism following contact with a specific allergen to which it has been previously exposed and sensitized.

al·ler·gic rhi·ni·tis (ă-lĕr′jik rī-nī′tis) Rhinitis associated with hay fever.

al·ler·gic sa·lute (ă-lĕr′jik să-lūt′) A characteristic wiping or rubbing of the nose with a transverse or upward movement of the hand, as seen in children with allergic rhinitis.

al·ler·gist (al′ĕr-jist) A health care specialist in the treatment of allergies.

al•ler•gol•o•gy (al′ĕr-gol′ŏ-jē) The science concerned with allergic conditions.

al•ler•gy (al′ĕr-jē) **1.** Hypersensitivity caused by exposure to a particular antigen (allergen) resulting in a marked increase in reactivity to that antigen on subsequent exposure, sometimes resulting in harmful consequences. SEE ALSO allergic reaction, anaphylaxis, immune. **2.** That branch of medicine concerned with the study, diagnosis, and treatment of allergic manifestations. **3.** An acquired hypersensitivity to certain drugs and biologic materials. [G. *allos,* other, + *ergon,* work]

all•es•the•si•a (al′es-thē′zē-ă) SYN allocheiria. SYN allaesthesia.

al•lied health pro•fes•sion•al (al′īd helth prŏ-fesh′ŭn-ăl) A person trained to provide patient services in specialties that include dental hygiene, clinical laboratory science, and physical therapy, among many others.

al•li•ga•tor for•ceps (al′i-gā-tŏr fōr′seps) A long forceps with a small hinged jaw on the end.

Al•lis for•ceps (ăl′is fōr′seps) A ring-handled tissue forceps with fine teeth on the tips.

all or none law (awl nŏn law) SYN Bowditch law.

♻ **allo-** **1.** Prefix meaning other; differing from the normal or usual. **2.** Chemical prefix formerly used with amino acids whenever their side chain contained an asymmetric carbon; for example, the alloisoleucines and allothreonines. [G. *allos,* other]

al•lo•an•ti•bod•y (al′o-an′ti-bud-ē) An antibody specific for an alloantigen. Isoantibody is sometimes used in this sense.

al•lo•an•ti•gen (al′ō-an′ti-jĕn) An antigen that occurs in some, but not in other members of the same species. Isoantigen is sometimes used in this sense.

al•lo•chei•ri•a, **al•lo•chi•ri•a** (al′ō-kī′rē-ă, al′ō-kī′rē-ă) A form of allachesthesia in which the sensation of a stimulus in one limb is referred to the contralateral limb. SYN allesthesia, Bamberger sign (2). [allo- + G. *cheir,* hand]

al•lo•cor•tex (al′ō-kōr′teks) O. Vogt's term denoting several regions of the cerebral cortex, in particular the olfactory cortex and the hippocampus, characterized by fewer cell layers than the isocortex. SEE ALSO cerebral cortex. SYN heterotypic cortex. [allo- + L. *cortex,* bark (cortex)]

al•lo•dip•loid (al′ō-dip′loyd) SEE alloploid.

al•lo•dyn•i•a (al′ō-din′ē-ă) Condition in which ordinarily nonpainful stimuli evoke pain. [allo- + G. *odynē,* pain]

al•lo•e•rot•ic (al′ō-ĕr-ot′ik) Pertaining to or characterized by alloerotism. SYN heteroerotic.

al•lo•er•o•tism (al′ō-ār′ō-tizm) Sexual attraction toward another person. Cf. autoerotism. SYN heteroerotism. [allo- + G. *erōs,* love]

al•lo•ge•ne•ic graft (al′ō-jen′ik graft) SYN allograft.

al•lo•graft (al′ō-graft) A graft transplanted between genetically nonidentical individuals of the same species. SYN allogeneic graft, homologous graft, homoplastic graft.

al•lo•graft re•jec•tion (al′lō-graft rĕ-jek′shŭn) The rejection of tissue transplanted between two genetically different individuals of the same species. Rejection is caused by T lymphocytes responding to the foreign major histocompatibility complex of the graft.

al•lo•ker•a•to•plas•ty (al′ō-ker′ă-tō-plas-tē) Replacement of opaque corneal tissue with a transparent prosthesis, usually plastic.

al•lo•la•li•a (al′ō-lā′lē-ă) Any speech defect, especially one caused by a cerebral disorder. [allo- + G. *lalia,* talking]

al•lom•er•ism (ă-lom′ĕr-izm) The state of differing in chemical composition but having the same crystalline form. [allo- + G. *meros,* part]

al•lo•mor•phism (al′ō-mōr′fizm) **1.** Change of shape in cells due to mechanical causes, such as flattening from pressure, or to progressive metaplasia, such as the change of bile duct cells into liver cells. **2.** The state of being similar in chemical composition but differing in form (especially crystalline). [allo- + G. *morphē,* form]

al•lo•path•ic (al′ō-path′ik) Relating to allopathy.

al•lop•a•thy (al-op′ă-thē) A therapeutic system in which a disease is treated by producing a second condition that is incompatible with or antagonistic to the first. Cf. homeopathy. SYN heteropathy (2). [allo- + G. *pathos,* suffering]

al•lo•plast (al′ō-plast) **1.** A graft of an inert metal or plastic material. **2.** A relatively inert foreign body used for implantation into tissues. [allo- + G. *plastos,* formed]

al•lo•plas•ty (al′ō-plas-tē) Repair of defects by allotransplantation.

al•lo•ploid (al′ō-ployd) Relating to a hybrid individual or cell with two or more sets of chromosomes derived from two different ancestral species. [allo- + -ploid]

al•lo•ploi•dy (al′ō-ploy′dē) The condition of being alloploid.

al•lo•pol•y•ploid (al′ō-pol′i-ployd) An alloploid having three or more haploid sets of chromosomes. [allo- + polyploid]

al•lo•pol•y•ploi•dy (al′ō-pol′i-ploy′dē) The condition of being allopolyploid.

al•lo•psy•chic (al′ō-sī′kik) Denoting the mental

processes in their relation to the outer world. [allo- + G. *psychē,* mind]

al·lo·rhyth·mi·a (al′ō-ridh′mē-ă) An irregularity in the cardiac rhythm that repeats itself any number of times. [allo- + G. *rhythmos,* rhythm]

al·lo·rhyth·mic (al′ō-ridh′mik) Relating to or characterized by allorhythmia.

al·lo·some (al′ō-sōm) One of the chromosomes differing in appearance or behavior from the autosomes and sometimes unequally distributed among the germ cells. SYN heterochromosome, heterotypical chromosome. [allo- + G. *sōma,* body]

al·lo·ste·ric (al′ō-ster′ik) Pertaining to or characterized by allosterism.

al·lo·ste·ric site (al′ō-ster′ik sīt) Postulated as the place on an enzyme, other than the active site, where a compound, which may be the ultimate product of the biosynthetic pathway involving the enzyme, may bind and influence the activity of the enzyme by changing the enzyme's conformation.

al·lo·ster·ism, **al·lo·ste·ry** (al′ō-ster′izm, al′ō-ster′ē) The influencing of an enzyme activity, or the binding of a ligand to a protein, by a change in the conformation of the protein, brought about by the binding of a substrate or other effector at a site (allosteric site) other than the active site of the protein. Cf. hysteresis.

al·lo·tope (al′ō-tōp) The antigenic determinant of an allotype. [allo- + -tope]

al·lo·trans·plan·ta·tion (al′ō-trans′plan-tā′shŭn) Transplantation of an allograft.

al·lo·trope (al′ō-trōp) An element in one of the allotropic forms that it may assume. [allo- + G. *tropos,* a turning]

al·lo·tro·pic (al′ō-trō′pik) **1.** Relating to allotropism. **2.** Denoting a type of personality characterized by a preoccupation with the reactions of others.

al·lot·ro·pism, **al·lot·ro·py** (ă-lot′rō-pizm, -lot′rō-pē) The existence of certain elements, in several forms differing in physical properties; e.g., carbon black, graphite, and diamonds are all pure carbon. [allo- + G. *tropos,* a turning]

al·lo·type (al′ō-tīp) Any one of the genetically determined antigenic differences within a given class of immunoglobulin that occur among members of the same species. SEE ALSO antibody. [allo- + G. *typos,* model]

al·lo·typ·ic (al′ō-tip′ik) Pertaining to an allotype.

al·low·ance (a′low-ans) **1.** Permission. **2.** A portion allotted.

alloxuraemia [Br.] SYN alloxuremia.

al·lox·u·re·mi·a (al′oks-yūr-ē′mē-ă) The presence of purine bases in the blood. SYN alloxuraemia. [alloxan + G. *haima,* blood]

al·lox·u·ri·a (al′oks-yūr′ē-ă) The presence of purine bodies in the urine. [alloxan + G. *ouron,* urine]

al·loy (al′oy) A substance composed of a mixture of two or more metals.

all·spice (awl′spīs) *Pimenta officinalis;* the dried fruit is used as a carminative and flavoring agent; of purported value as a topical anesthetic. SYN Jamaica pepper.

Al·mei·da dis·ease (ahl-mā′dah di-zēz′) SYN paracoccidioidomycosis.

Al·oe ve·ra (English, a′lō vē′ră; Latin, al′ō-ē vē′ră) A botanical used topically in wound care; used internally as a stimulant laxative (long-term use may elicit blood disorders). Other interstitial remediation has been reported but not confirmed clinically. SYN first aid plant, hsiang-dan, kumari, lu-hui. [L., fr. G. *aloē*]

a·lo·gi·a (ă-lō′jē-ă) **1.** SYN aphasia. **2.** Inability to speak due to mental deficiency or an episode of dementia. [G. *a-* priv. + *logos,* speech]

al·o·pe·ci·a (al-ō-pē′shē-ă) Complete or partial absence or loss of hair. Results from normal aging, endocrine disorders, skin disease, or drug reactions (especially various forms of chemotherapy). SYN baldness. [G. *alōpekia,* a disease like fox mange, fr. *alōpēx,* a fox]

al·o·pe·ci·a ad·na·ta (al-ō-pē′shē-ă ad-nā′tă) Underdevelopment of the eyelashes. SEE ALSO alopecia congenitalis. SYN madarosis.

i **al·o·pe·ci·a ar·e·a·ta** (al-ō-pē′shē-ă ā-rē-ā′tă) A condition of undetermined etiology characterized by circumscribed, nonscarring, usually asymmetric areas of baldness on the scalp, eyebrows, and beard area. See page 57. SYN alopecia circumscripta, Cazenove vitiligo, Jonston alopecia.

al·o·pe·ci·a ca·pi·tis to·ta·lis (al-ō-pē′shē-ă kap′i-tis tō-tā′lis) SYN alopecia totalis.

al·o·pe·ci·a cir·cum·scrip·ta (al-ō-pē′shē-ă sĭr-kŭm-skrip′tă) SYN alopecia areata.

al·o·pe·ci·a con·ge·ni·ta·lis (al-ō-pē′shē-ă kon-jen-i-tā′lis) Absence of all hair at birth, associated with psychomotor epilepsy.

al·o·pe·ci·a he·re·di·ta·ri·a (al-ō-pē′shē-ă hĕ-red-i-tā′rē-ă) SYN androgenic alopecia.

al·o·pe·ci·a mar·gi·na·lis (al-ō-pē′shē-ă mar-jī-nā′lis) Hair loss at the hair line, a condition most commonly seen in blacks; commonly transient and caused by chronic traction, although long-continued traction may cause permanent alopecia.

al·o·pe·ci·a me·di·ca·men·to·sa (al-ō-pē′shē-ă med-i-kă-men-tō′să) Diffuse hair loss,

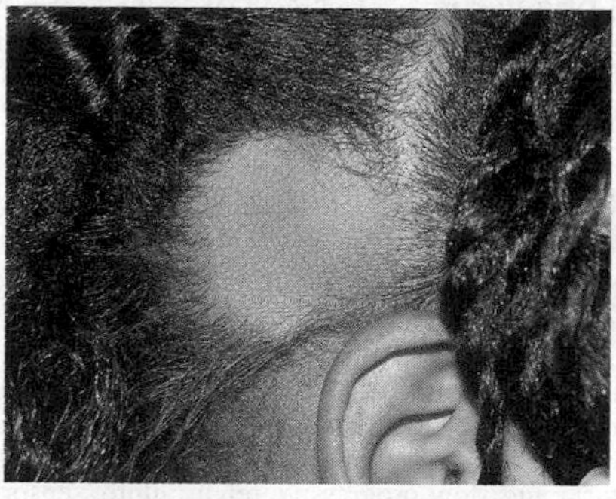

alopecia areata: area of hair loss is a round patch (note the absence of scales or inflammation)

most notably of the scalp, attributable to prescribed drugs.

al·o·pe·ci·a pit·y·ro·des (al-ō-pē′shē-ă pit-i-rō′dēz) A loss of hair, of the body as well as of the scalp, accompanied by an abundant branlike desquamation.

al·o·pe·ci·a symp·to·ma·ti·ca (al-ō-pē′shē-ă sim-tō-mat′i-kă) A loss of hair occurring in the course of various constitutional or local diseases, or following prolonged febrile illness.

al·o·pe·ci·a to·ta·lis (al-ō-pē′shē-ă tō-tā′lis) Total loss of hair of the scalp either within a very short period of time or from progression of localized alopecia, especially alopecia areata. Cf. alopecia universalis. SYN alopecia capitis totalis.

al·o·pe·ci·a u·ni·ver·sa·lis (al-ō-pē′shē-ă yū′ni-vĕr-sā′lis) Total loss of hair from all parts of the body. Cf. alopecia totalis.

al·o·pe·cic (al′ō-pē′sik) Relating to alopecia.

al·pha (α) (al′fă) **1.** First letter of the Greek alphabet; used as a classifier in the nomenclature of many sciences. **2.** Bunsen solubility coefficient. **3.** CHEMISTRY denotes the first in a series, a position immediately adjacent to a carboxyl group, the first of a series of closely related compounds, an aromatic substituent on an aliphatic chain, or the direction of a chemical bond away from the viewer. **4.** Alpha (α) particle. **5.** CHEMISTRY symbol for angle of optic rotation; degree of dissociation. For terms with the prefix α, see the specific term.

al·pha (α)-ad·re·ner·gic block·ing a·gent (al′fă ad′rĕ-nĕr′jik blok′ing ā′jĕnt) An agent that competitively blocks α-adrenergic receptors; used in the treatment of hypertension. SYN alpha (α)-adrenoceptor antagonist.

al·pha (α)-ad·re·ner·gic re·cep·tors (al′fă ad′rĕ-nĕr′jik rĕ-sep′tŏrz) Adrenergic receptors in effector tissues capable of selective activation by methoxamine and blockade by phenoxybenzamine. Their activation results in physiologic responses (e.g., increased peripheral vascular resistance, mydriasis, and contraction of pilomotor muscles).

al·pha (α)-adre·no·cep·tor an·tag·o·nist (al′fă ă-drē′nō-sep′tŏr an-tag′ŏ-nist) SYN alpha (α)-adrenergic blocking agent.

al·pha (α)-a·mi·no ac·id (al′fă ă-mē′nō as′id) Typically, an amino acid of the general formula R-CHNH$_2$-COOH (i.e., the NH$_2$ in the α position); the L forms of these are the hydrolysis products of proteins.

al·pha (α)-a·mi·no·suc·cin·ic ac·id (al′fă a-mē′nō-sŭk-sin′ik as′id) SYN aspartic acid.

al·pha (α) an·gle (al′fă ang′gĕl) **1.** The angle between the visual and optic axes as they cross at the nodal point of the eye. **2.** The angle between the visual line and the major axis of the corneal ellipse.

al·pha (α)$_1$-an·ti·chy·mo·tryp·sin (al′fă an′tē-kī′mō-trip-sin) A protein inhibitor of the digestive protease chymotrypsin.

al·pha (α)$_2$ an·ti·plas·min (al′fă an′tē-plaz′min) A major protease inhibitor of plasmin and plasminogen, key components of the fibrinolytic system. Also inhibits other serine proteases, including the coagulation contact factors, factor Xa, and thrombin.

al·pha (α)$_1$-an·ti·tryp·sin de·fi·cien·cy (al′fă an′tē-trip′sin dĕ-fish′ĕn-sē) Absence of a serum proteinase inhibitor, which may cause relapsing nodular nonsuppurative panniculitis.

al·pha (α)$_1$ an·ti·tryp·sin de·fi·cien·cy pan·nic·u·li·tis (al′fă an′tē-trip′sin dĕ-fish′ĕn-sē pan-ik yū lī′tis) Painful subcutaneous nodules in severe antitrypsin deficiency.

al·pha (α) bands (al′fă banz) The dark-staining anisotropic cross striations in the myofibrils of muscle fibers, comprising regions of overlapping thick (myosin) and thin (actin) filaments.

al·pha (α) cells (al′fă selz) **1.** Acidophil cells that constitute about 35% of the cells of the anterior lobe of the hypophysis; there are two varieties: one elaborates somatotropic hormone, the other mammotropic hormone. **2.** Cells of the islets of Langerhans that secrete glucagon. **3.** The alpha cells of the pancreas or the anterior lobe of the hypophysis.

al·pha (α) chain (al′fă chān) **1.** A polypeptide component of insulin containing 21 amino acyl residues. **2.** In general, one of the polypeptides in a multiprotein complex.

al·pha (α)-dex·trin en·do-1,6-α-glu·co·si·dase (al′fă deks′trin en′dō-al′fă-glū-kō′si-dās) An enzyme with action similar to that of isoamylase; it cleaves 1,6-α-glucosidic linkages in pullalan, amylopectin, and glycogen, and in α- and β-amylase limit-dextrins of amylopectin and glycogen. Cf. isoamylase.

al•pha (α) er•ror (al′fă er′ŏr) SYN error of the first kind.

al•pha (α) fi•bers (al′fă fī′bĕrz) Large myelinated somatic motor or proprioceptive nerve fibers conducting impulses at rates near 100 m/sec.

al•pha (α)-D-ga•lac•to•sid•ase (al′fă gă-lak′tō-sī′dās) An enzyme catalyzing the hydrolysis of α-D-galactosides to release free D-galactose. A deficiency of type A α-D-galactosidase is associated with Fabry disease.

al•pha (α) gran•ule (al′fă gran′yūl) A granule of an alpha cell that was named as the first of several kinds or because it was acidophilic.

al•pha (α)-he•mo•lyt•ic strep•to•coc•ci (al′fă-hē′mō-lit′ik strep-tŏ-kok′sī) Streptococci that form a green zone around the colony on a blood-agar medium due to incomplete hemolysis of erythrocytes. SEE ALSO *Streptococcus viridans.*

Al•pha•her•pes•vir•i•nae (al′fă-hĕr′pēz-vir′i-nē) A subfamily of herpesviridae containing herpes simplex virus and varicellavirus.

al•pha (α)-li•no•le•nic ac•id (al′fă lin′ō-lē′nik as′id) One of the omega-3 fatty acids, having the chemical designation: all-*cis*-9,12,15-octadecatrienoic acid or 18:3 (n-3).

al•pha-1 (α_1)-lip•o•pro•tein (al′fă lip′ō-prō′tēn) A lipoprotein fraction of relatively low molecular weight and high density, rich in phospholipids, and found in the α_1-globulin fraction of human plasma.

al•pha (α) low•er mo•tor neu•ron (al′fă lō′ĕr mō′tŏr nūr′on) SYN alpha (α) motor neuron.

al•pha (α) mo•tor neu•ron (al′fă mō′tŏr nūr′on) Motor neuron that terminates in skeletal muscle; sends messages from the central nervous system to initiate and sustain voluntary, conscious movement. Cf. gamma motor neuron. SYN alpha (α) lower motor neuron.

al•pha (α) par•ti•cle (al′fă pahr′ti-kĕl) A particle consisting of two neutrons and two protons, with a positive charge ($2e^+$); emitted energetically from the nuclei of unstable isotopes of high atomic number (elements of mass number from 82 up); identical to the helium nucleus.

al•pha (α) rhythm (al′fă ridh′ŭm) **1.** A wave pattern in the encephalogram in the frequency band of 8–13 Hz. **2.** The posterior dominant 8–13 Hz rhythm in the awake, relaxed person with closed eyes. SYN alpha (α) wave.

al•pha (α)-strep•to•coc•ci (al′fă strep-tŏ-kok′sī) Streptococci that form a green variety of reduced hemoglobin in the area of the colony on a blood agar medium.

al•pha (α) thal•as•se•mi•a (al′fă thal′ă-sē′mē-ă) Hematologic disorder due to one of two or more genes that depress synthesis of α-globin chains.

al•pha•vi•rus (al′fă-vī′rŭs) One of the genera of the family Togaviridae that was formerly classified as part of the "group A" arboviruses and includes the viruses that cause eastern equine, western equine, and Venezuelan encephalitis.

al•pha (α) wave (al′fă wāv) SYN alpha (α) rhythm.

Al•pin•i•a car•da•mom (al-pin′ē-ă kahr′dă-mŏm) SYN cardamom.

Al•port syn•drome (al′pōrt sin′drōm) A genetically heterogeneous disorder characterized by nephritis associated with microscopic hematuria and slow progressive renal failure, sensorineural hearing loss, and ocular abnormalities such as lenticonus and maculopathy; autosomal dominant, autosomal recessive, and X-linked recessive forms exist. The X-linked form is caused by mutation in the collagen type IV alpha-5 gene (COL4A5) on chromosome Xq; the autosomal recessive form is due to mutation in the collagen type IV alpha-3 gene (COL4A3) or alpha-4 gene (COL4A4) on 2q.

ALS Abbreviation for amyotrophic lateral sclerosis; antilymphocyte serum.

Al•ström syn•drome (ahl′strem sin′drōm) Retinal degeneration with nystagmus and loss of central vision, associated with obesity in childhood; sensorineural hearing loss and diabetes mellitus usually occur after age 10 years; autosomal recessive inheritance.

ALT Abbreviation for alanine aminotransferase.

ALT:AST ra•ti•o (rā′shē-ō) The ratio of serum alanine aminotransferase to serum aspartate aminotransferase; elevated serum levels of both enzymes characterize hepatic disease; when both levels are abnormally elevated and the ALT:AST ratio is greater than 1.0, severe hepatic necrosis or alcoholic hepatic disease is likely; when the ratio is less than 1.0, an acute nonalcoholic hepatic condition is favored.

ALTE Abbreviation for apparent life-threatening episode; apparent life-threatening event.

Al•te•mei•er op•er•a•tion (ahl′tĕ-mī-ĕr op-ĕr-ā′shŭn) An operation for rectal prolapse that involves a sleeve resection of the prolapsed rectum and colon with a primary anastomosis performed transanally.

al•ter•nans (awl-ter′nanz) Alternating; used as a noun in the sense of pulsus alternans. [L.]

Al•ter•na•ri•a (awl-tĕr-nā′rē-ă) A rapidly growing dematiaceous fungal genus, ubiquitous in nature, associated with subcutaneous infections such as phaeohyphomycosis, sinusitis, erosion of the nasal septum, and infections of skin and nails. This fungus is also a common cause of allergic rhinitis and asthma.

al•ter•nate cov•er test (awl-tĕr′năt kŏv′ĕr test) A test to detect phoria or strabismus; attention is directed to a small fixation object, and one eye is covered for several seconds; then the cover is moved quickly to the other eye; if the eye moves when it is uncovered, a strabismus or phoria is present.

al·ter·nate lev·el of care (awl′tĕr-năt lev′ĕl kār) Therapy provided to patients whose disability fails to rise to the acute standard. This degree of therapy includes many options (e.g., long-term care facility, respite care, in-home care).

al·ter·nat·ing cur·rent (AC, ac, a.c.) (awl′tĕr-nāt-ing kŭr′rĕnt) Electric current that reverses direction (positive-negative polarity) many times each second (with each rotation of the armature of the dynamo generating the current).

al·ter·nat·ing pres·sure air mat·tress (awl′tĕr-nā-ting presh′ŭr ār mat′trĕs) Air mattress that is placed on top of a regular bed mattress; used to promote skin integrity and prevent skin breakdown, has air-filled channels that alternately fill and empty to keep bearing weight off bony prominences of immobilized or weak patients who are unable to shift their weight frequently.

al·ter·nat·ing pulse (awl′tĕr-nāt-ing pŭls) Mechanical alternation, a pulse regular in time but with alternate beats stronger and weaker, often detectable only with the sphygmomanometer and usually indicating serious myocardial disease. SYN pulsus alternans.

al·ter·nat·ing trem·or (awl′tĕr-nāt-ing trem′ŏr) A form of hyperkinesia characterized by regular, symmetric, to-and-fro movements (at about 4 per second) that are produced by patterned, alternating contraction of muscles and their antagonists.

al·ter·na·tion (awl′tĕr-nā′shŭn) The occurrence of two things or phases in succession and recurrently; used interchangeably with alternans.

al·ter·na·tive med·i·cine (awl-tĕr′nă-tiv med′i-sin) A term used by some practitioners of Western medicine for methods of healing, some ancient and widely practiced, which may not be firmly based on accepted scientific principles and may thereby be of limited known effectiveness. Examples of alternative practices include acupuncture and acupressure, homeopathy, osteopathy, chiropractic, massage, hypnosis, megavitamin therapy, pulse diagnosis, tongue diagnosis, iridology, rolfing, faith healing, and prayer. SEE ALSO complementary medicine.

al·ter·na·tive splic·ing (awl-tĕr′nă-tiv splīs′ing) Different ways of assembling exons to produce different mature mRNAs.

al·the·a (al-thē′ă) *Althaea officinalis*, a perennial herb found wild in moist places in Europe. Contains high proportions of starches, pectin, and sugars; used as a flavoring and demulcent agent. SYN hollyhock, marshmallow root. [L., fr. G. *althaia*, marshmallow]

al·ti·tude sick·ness (al′ti-tūd sik′nĕs) A syndrome caused by low inspired oxygen pressure (as at high altitude) and characterized by nausea, headache, dyspnea, malaise, and insomnia; in severe instances, pulmonary edema and adult respiratory distress syndrome can occur. SYN Acosta disease, aerial sickness, mountain sickness.

Alt·mann an·i·lin-ac·id fuch·sin stain (ahlt′mahn an′i-lin-ik as′id fūk′sin stān) A mixture of picric acid, anilin, and acid fuchsin that stains mitochondria crimson against a yellow background.

Alt·mann fix·a·tive (ahlt′mahn fiks′ă-tiv) A bichromate-osmic acid fixative.

a·lu·mi·no·sis (ă-lū′min-ō′sis) A pneumoconiosis caused by inhalation of aluminum particles.

a·lu·mi·num (Al) (ă-lū′min-ŭm) A white silvery metal of very light weight; atomic no. 13, atomic wt. 26.981539. Many salts and compounds are used in medicine and dentistry. [L. *alumen*, alum]

al·um·root (al′ŭm-rūt) SYN cranesbill.

al·ve·i (al′vē-ī) Plural of alveus.

al·ve·o·al·gi·a (al-vē′ō-al′jē-ă) A postoperative complication of tooth extraction in which the blood clot in the socket disintegrates, resulting in focal osteomyelitis and severe pain. SYN alveolalgia. [alveolus + G. *algos*, pain]

al·ve·o·lal·gia (al-vē′ō-lal′jē-ă) SYN alveoalgia.

al·ve·o·lar (al-vē′ŏ-lăr) Relating to an alveolus.

al·ve·o·lar ab·scess (al-vē′ŏ-lăr ab′ses) An abscess situated within the alveolar process of the jaws, most often caused by extension of infection from an adjacent nonvital tooth. See page 60. SYN dental abscess, dentoalveolar abscess.

al·ve·o·lar air (al-vē′ŏ-lăr ār) SYN alveolar gas.

al·ve·o·lar air e·qua·tion (al-vē′ŏ-lăr ār ē-kwā′zhŭn) An equation that calculates an approximation of alveolar oxygen tension if the fractional concentration of inspired oxygen, arterial carbon dioxide tension, and respiratory exchange ratio (i.e., carbon dioxide production divided by oxygen consumption) are known.

al·ve·o·lar-ar·te·ri·al ox·y·gen dif·fer·ence (al-vē′ŏ-lăr-ahr-tēr′ē-ăl ok′si-jĕn dif′ĕr-ĕns) The gradient between the partial pressure of oxygen in the alveolar spaces and the arterial blood: $P_{(A-a)}O_2$. Normally, in young adults this value is less than 20 mmHg.

al·ve·o·lar-ar·te·ri·al ox·y·gen ten·sion dif·fer·ence (al-vē′ŏ-lăr-ahr-tēr′ē-ăl ok′si-jĕn ten′shŭn dif′ĕr-ĕns) SYN A-aO_2 difference.

al·ve·o·lar ca·nals of max·il·la (al-vē′ŏ-lăr kă-nalz′ mak-sil′ă) Canals in the body of the

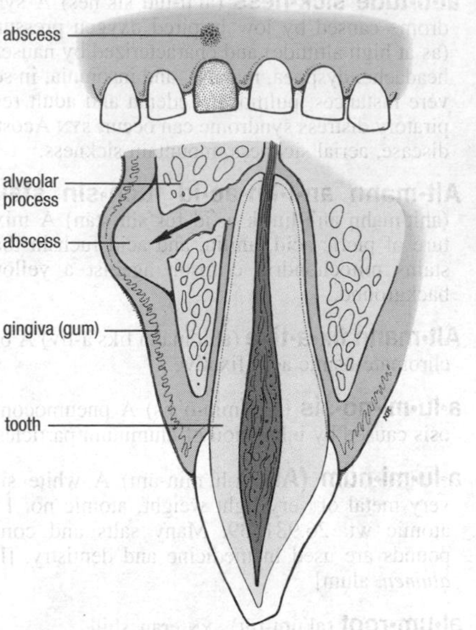

alveolar abscess: sagittal section

maxilla that transmit nerves and vessels from the alveolar foramina to the maxillary teeth.

al•ve•o•lar-cap•il•lar•y mem•brane (al-vē′ŏ-lăr-kap′i-lar-ē mem′brān) The alveolar epithelium, interstitial space, and the capillary endothelium barrier that gases must cross in respiration; it is approximately 1 mcm thick in healthy people and normally represents only a minimal obstacle to gas diffusion.

al•ve•o•lar cell (al-vē′ŏ-lăr sel) Any of the cells lining the alveoli of the lung, including the squamous alveolar cells, the great alveolar cells, and the alveolar macrophages.

al•ve•o•lar cell car•ci•no•ma (al-vē′ŏ-lăr sel kahr′si-nō′mă) SYN bronchiolar carcinoma.

al•ve•o•lar con•so•nant (al-vē′ŏ-lăr kon′sŏ-nănt) A speech sound involving contact between the tongue and the alveolar ridge (/t/ and /d/).

al•ve•o•lar dead space (al-vē′ŏ-lăr ded spās) The difference between physiologic dead space and anatomic dead space; it represents that part of the physiologic dead space resulting from ventilation of relatively underperfused or nonperfused alveoli; it differs specifically in being placed so as to fill and empty in parallel with functional alveoli, rather than being interposed in the conducting tubes between functional alveoli and the external environment.

al•ve•o•lar duct (al-vē′ŏ-lăr dŭkt) **1.** The part of the respiratory passages distal to the respiratory bronchiole; from it arise alveolar sacs and alveoli. **2.** The smallest of the intralobular ducts in the mammary gland, into which the secretory alveoli open. SYN ductulus alveolaris.

al•ve•o•lar gas (al-vē′ŏ-lăr gas) Gas symbol subscript A; the gas in the pulmonary alveoli, where O_2-CO_2 exchange with pulmonary capillary blood occurs. SYN alveolar air.

al•ve•o•lar gin•gi•va (al-vē′ŏ-lăr jin′ji-vă) Gingival tissue attached to the alveolar bone.

al•ve•o•lar gland (al-vē′ŏ-lăr gland) A gland in which the secretory unit(s) has a saclike form and an obvious lumen; e.g., the active mammary gland.

al•ve•o•lar in•dex (al-vē′ŏ-lăr in′deks) SYN basilar index.

al•ve•o•lar mac•ro•phage (al-vē′ŏ-lăr mak′rō-fāj) A vigorously phagocytic macrophage on the epithelial surface of lung alveoli where it ingests inhaled particulate matter. SYN coniophage, dust cell.

al•ve•o•lar pe•ri•od of lung de•vel•op•ment (al-vē′ŏ-lăr pēr′ē-ŏd lŭng dĕ-vel′ŏp-mĕnt) The period (32 weeks–8 years) when alveoli develop; characteristic mature alveoli do not form until after birth.

al•ve•o•lar point (al-vē′ŏ-lăr poynt) SYN prosthion.

al•ve•o•lar pores (al-vē′ŏ-lăr pōrz) Openings in the interalveolar septa of the lung that permit air flow between adjacent alveoli.

al•ve•o•lar pro•cess (al-vē′ŏ-lăr pros′es) That portion of bone in either the maxilla or the mandible that surrounds and supports the teeth.

al•ve•olar ridge (al-vē′ŏ-lăr rij) That portion of bone in the maxilla that surrounds and supports teeth. SEE ALSO alveolar process.

al•ve•o•lar sac (al-vē′ŏ-lăr sak) Terminal dilation of the alveolar ducts that give rise to alveoli in the lung; a small air chamber in the pulmonary tissue from which the pulmonary alveoli project like bays and into which an alveolar duct opens. SYN sacculus alveolaris [TA].

al•ve•o•lar soft part sar•co•ma (al-vē′ŏ-lăr sawft pahrt sahr-kō′mă) A malignant tumor formed of a reticular stroma of connective tissue enclosing aggregates of large round or polygonal cells; occurs in subcutaneous and fibromuscular tissues.

al•ve•o•lar ven•ti•la•tion ($\mathring{V}_A$) (al-vē′ŏ-lăr ven′ti-lā′shŭn) The volume of gas per minute expired from the alveoli to the atmosphere and the product of the respiratory frequency (f) multiplied by the difference between tidal volume and the dead space ($V_T - V_D$); units: mL/min BTPS.

al•ve•o•lec•to•my (al′vē-ō-lek′tŏ-mē) Surgical excision of a portion of the dentoalveolar process at the time of tooth removal to facilitate placement of a dental prosthesis. [alveolus + G. *ektomē*, excision]

al•ve•o•li (al-vē′ō-lī) Plural of alveolus.

al•ve•o•lin•gual (al-vē′ō-ling′gwăl) SYN alveololingual.

al•ve•o•li pul•mo•nis (al-vi′ō-lī pul-mō′nis) SYN pulmonary alveoli.

al•ve•o•li•tis (al′vē-ō-lī′tis) **1.** Inflammation of lung alveoli. **2.** Inflammation of a tooth socket.

♻**alveolo-** Combining form indicating an alveolus, the alveolar process; alveolar. [L. *alveolus*, a concave vessel, a bowl, a basin, fr. *alveus*, a trough, + *-olus*, small, little; akin to *alvus*, the belly, the womb]

al•ve•o•lo•cap•il•lar•y block (al-vē′ŏ-lō-kap′i-lar-ē blok) The presence of material that impairs the diffusion of gases between the air in the alveolar spaces and the blood in alveolar capillaries; block can be caused by edema, cellular infiltration, fibrosis, or tumor, and results in undersaturation of peripheral arterial blood with oxygen.

al•ve•o•lo•cap•il•lar•y mem•brane (al-vē′ŏ-lō-kap′i-lar-ē mem′brān) The pulmonary diffusion barrier.

al•ve•o•lo•cla•si•a (al-vē′ŏ-lō-klā′zē-ă) Destruction of the alveolus. [alveolo- + G. *klasis*, breaking]

al•ve•o•lo•den•tal (al-vē′ŏ-lō-den′tăl) Relating to the alveoli and the teeth.

al•ve•o•lo•den•tal lig•a•ment (al-vē′ŏ-lō-den′tăl lig′ă-mĕnt) SYN periodontal ligament.

al•ve•o•lo•den•tal mem•brane (al-vē′ŏ-lō-den′tăl mem′brān) SYN periodontal ligament.

al•ve•o•lo•la•bi•al (al-vē′ŏ-lō-lā′bē-ăl) Relating to the labial or vestibular (outer) surface of the alveolar process of the upper or lower jaw.

al•ve•o•lo•lin•gual (al-vē′ŏ-lō-ling′gwăl) Relating to the lingual (inner) surface of the alveolar process of the lower jaw. SYN alveolingual.

al•ve•o•lo•pal•a•tal (al-vē′ŏ-lō-pal′ă-tăl) Relating to the palatal surface of the alveolar process of the upper jaw.

al•ve•o•lo•plas•ty (al-vē′ŏ-lō-plas-tē) Surgical preparation of the alveolar ridges for the reception of dentures; shaping and smoothing of socket margins after extraction of teeth with subsequent suturing to ensure optimal healing. SYN alveoplasty. [alveolo- + G. *plassō*, to form]

al•ve•o•lot•o•my (al-vē-ŏ-lot′ŏ-mē) Surgical opening into a dental alveolus to allow drainage of pus from a periapical or other intraosseous abscess. [alveolo- + G. *tomē*, incision]

al•ve•o•lus, gen. and pl. **al•ve•o•li** (al-vē′ō-lŭs, al-vē′ō-lī) [TA] **1.** SYN pulmonary alveoli. **2.** One of the terminal secretory portions of an alveolar or racemose gland. **3.** One of the honeycomb pits in the wall of the stomach. **4.** SYN tooth socket. [L. dim. of *alveus*, trough, hollow sac, cavity]

al•ve•o•plas•ty (al-vē′ŏ-plas′tē) SYN alveoloplasty.

al•ve•us, pl. **al•ve•i** (al′vē-ŭs, al′vē-ī) A channel or trough. [L. tray, trough, cavity, fr. *alvus*, belly]

a•lym•pho•cy•to•sis (ā-lim′fō-sī-tō′sis) Absence or great reduction of lymphocytes.

a•lym•pho•pla•si•a (ā-lim′fō-plā′zē-ă) Aplasia or hypoplasia of lymphoid tissue.

🅸 **Alz•heim•er dis•ease, Alz•heim•er de•men•ti•a** (awlts′hī-mĕr di-zēz′, awlts′hī-mĕr dĕ-men′shē-ă) Progressive mental deterioration manifested by loss of memory, ability to calculate, and visual-spatial orientation; confusion; and disorientation. Begins in late middle life and usually results in death in 5–10 years. The brain is atrophic; histologically, there is distortion of the intracellular neurofibrils (neurofibrillary tangles) and senile plaques composed of granular or filamentous argentophilic masses with an amyloid core; the most common degenerative brain disorder. See page B23. SYN presenile dementia (2), dementia presenilis, primary senile dementia.

Alz•heim•er scle•ro•sis (awlts′hī-mĕr skler-ō′sis) Hyaline degeneration of the medium and smaller blood vessels of the brain.

al•zyme (al′zīm) Union of antibody and enzyme to form a hybrid catalytic molecule.

Am Symbol for americium.

am Abbreviation for ammeter.

AMA Abbreviation for American Medical Association.

am•a•crine (am′ă-krēn) **1.** A cell or structure lacking a long, fibrous process. **2.** Denoting such a cell or structure. [G. *a-* priv. + *makros*, long, + *is* (*in-*), fiber]

am•al•gam (ă-mal′găm) An alloy of an element or a metal with mercury. In dentistry, primarily of two types: silver-tin alloy, containing small amounts of copper, zinc, and perhaps other metals, and a second type containing more copper (12–30% by weight); they are used in restoring teeth. [G. *malagma*, a soft mass]

am•al•gam tat•too (ă-mal′găm ta-tū′) A bluish-black or gray macular lesion of the oral mucous membrane caused by accidental implantation of particles of silver amalgam into the tissue during tooth restoration or extraction. The condition is asymptomatic. SYN tattoo (3).

Am•a•ni•ta (am′ă-nī′tă) A genus of fungi, many members of which are highly poisonous. [G. *amanitai*, fungi]

Am•a•ni•ta mus•ca•ri•a (am′ă-nī′tă mŭs-kā′

rē-ă) A toxic species of mushroom with yellow to red pileus and white gills; contains muscarine, which produces psychosislike states and other symptoms.

Am•a•ni•ta phal•loi•des (am′ă-nī′tă fă-loy′dēz) A species of mushroom containing poisonous principles (including phalloidin and amanitin) that cause gastroenteritis, hepatic necrosis, and renal necrosis.

am•a•ranth (am′ă-ranth) A weed (*Amaranthus*) of widespread geographic distribution; some species are consumed as a foodstuff; its prolific ability to produce seed allows its use as a flour. Purported value both internally and externally (e.g., astringent). SYN love-lies-bleeding, red cockscomb. [G. *amaranton,* immortal, incorruptible, infl. by *anthos,* flower]

a•mas•ti•a (ā-mas′tē-ă) Absence of breasts. SYN amazia. [G. *a-* priv. + *mastos,* breast]

a•mas•ti•gote (ă-mas′ti-gōt) SYN Leishman-Donovan body. [G. *a-* priv. + *mastix,* whip]

am•au•ro•sis (am′aw-rō′sis) Blindness, especially that occurring without apparent change in the eye itself, as from a brain lesion. [G. *amauros,* dark, obscure, + *-osis,* condition]

am•au•ro•sis fu•gax (am′aw-rō′sis fū′gaks) Transient blindness that may result from carotid artery insufficiency, retinal artery embolus, or centrifugal force (visual blackout in flight).

am•au•rot•ic (am′aw-rot′ik) Relating to or suffering from amaurosis.

am•au•rot•ic cat eye (am′aw-rot′ik kat ī) A yellow reflex from the pupil in cases of retinoblastoma or pseudoglioma.

am•au•rot•ic fa•mil•i•al id•i•o•cy (am′aw-rot′ik fă-mil′ē-ăl id′ē-ŏ-sē) Family of recessive genetic diseases marked by accumulation of lipid containing cells in viscera and nervous system, mental retardation, and impaired vision.

am•au•rot•ic pu•pil (am′aw-rot′ik pyū′pil) Pupil in an eye that is blind because of ocular or optic nerve disease; this pupil will not contract to light except when the normal fellow eye is stimulated with light.

a•ma•zi•a (ă-mā′zē-ă) SYN amastia.

am•ba•geu•sia (am′bă-gū′sē-ă) Loss of taste from both sides of the tongue. [L. *ambo,* both, + G. *a-* priv. + *geusis,* taste]

AMBER (am′bĕr) Acronym for advanced multiple-beam equalization radiography.

am•ber co•don (am′bĕr kō′don) The termination codon UAG.

♻ **ambi-** Prefix meaning around; on all (both) sides; both, double; corresponds to G. *amphi-*. [L., around, about, akin to *ambo,* both]

am•bi•dex•ter•i•ty (am′bi-deks-ter′i-tē) The ability to use both hands with equal ease.

am•bi•dex•trous (am′bi-deks′trŭs) Having equal facility in the use of both hands.

am•bi•ent (am′bē-ĕnt) Surrounding, encompassing; pertaining to the environment in which an organism or apparatus functions. [L. *ambiens,* going around]

am•bi•gu•i•ty (am′bi-gyū′i-tē) Condition of being ambiguous; uncertainty.

am•big•u•ous ex•ter•nal gen•i•ta•li•a (am-big′yū-ŭs eks-tĕr′năl jen′i-tā′lē-ă) External genitalia not clearly of either sex; most commonly designates external genitalia that are incompletely masculinized. SEE ALSO genital ambiguity.

am•bi•lat•er•al (am′bi-lat′ĕr-ăl) Relating to both sides. [ambi- + L. *latus,* side]

am•bi•le•vous (am′bi-lē′vŭs) Awkwardness in the use of both hands. [ambi- + L. *laevus,* left]

am•bi•o•pi•a (am′bē-ō′pē-ă) Double vision. [ambi + G. *ōps,* eye, vision]

am•bi•sex•u•al (am′bi-sek′shū-ăl) **1.** Denoting sexual characteristics found in both sexes (e.g., breasts, pubic hair). **2.** Slang term for bisexual.

am•biv•a•lence (am-biv′ă-lĕns) The coexistence of conflicting or oppositional attitudes or emotions toward a given person, thing, or idea, as in the simultaneous feeling and expression of love and hate toward the same person. [ambi- + L. *valentia,* strength]

am•biv•a•lent (am-biv′ă-lĕnt) Relating to or characterized by ambivalence.

am•bi•vert (am′bi-vĕrt) Person with characteristics of both extrovert and introvert qualities. [ambi + L. *verto,* to turn]

♻ **ambly-** Combining form meaning dullness, dimness; blunt, dull, dim, dimmed. [G. *amblys,* blunt, dulled; faint, dim]

am•bly•a•phi•a (am′blē-ā′fē-ă) Diminution in tactile sensibility. [ambly- + G. *haphē,* touch]

am•bly•geus•ti•a (am′blē-gū′stē-ă) A diminution in the sense of taste. [ambly- + G. *geusis,* taste]

am•bly•o•gen•ic (am′blē-ō-jen′ik) Inducing amblyopia. [amblyopia + -genic]

am•bly•o•gen•ic per•i•od (am′blē-ō-jen′ik pēr′ē-ŏd) Period during early visual development when the visual neurosensory system is vulnerable to developing amblyopia from blurred retinal image formation, bilateral cortical suppression (as in strabismic amblyopia), or both.

Am•bly•om•ma (am′blē-ō′mă) A genus of male hard ticks characterized by eyes, festoons, and deeply imbedded ventral plates near these festoons. [ambly- + G. *omma*, eye, vision]

am•bly•o•pi•a (am′blē-ō′pē-ă) Visual impairment not due to an ocular lesion and not fully correctable by an artificial lens. Possibly caused by abnormal visual experience during early life. [G. *amblyōpia*, dimness of vision, fr. *amblys*, dull, + *ōps*, eye]

am•bly•o•pi•a SYN lazy eye. SEE ALSO extroversion.

am•bly•o•pic (am′blē-op′ik) Relating to, or suffering from, amblyopia.

am•bly•o•scope (am′blē-ō-skōp) A reflecting stereoscope used to evaluate or simulate binocular vision. SEE ALSO haploscope. [amblyopia + G. *skopeō*, to view]

am•bo•cep•tor (am′bō-sep-tŏr) Complement-fixing antibody; now used chiefly to denote the anti-sheep erythrocyte antibody used in the hemolytic system of complement-fixation tests. [ambo- + L. *capio*, to take]

Am•bu bag (am′byū bag) Respiration device with a nonrebreathing valve to provide positive pressure for manual ventilation needed when a patient lacks respiratory drive during resuscitation involving oxygen or air. [NOTE: This name is a registered trademark of Ambu, Inc. of Glen Burnie, MD, USA and Ambu A/S of Ballerup, Denmark. Although it is sometimes incorrectly and improperly used as a generic product name by some health care practitioners, all rights and privileges attached to the product remain those of the proprietors.] See this page.

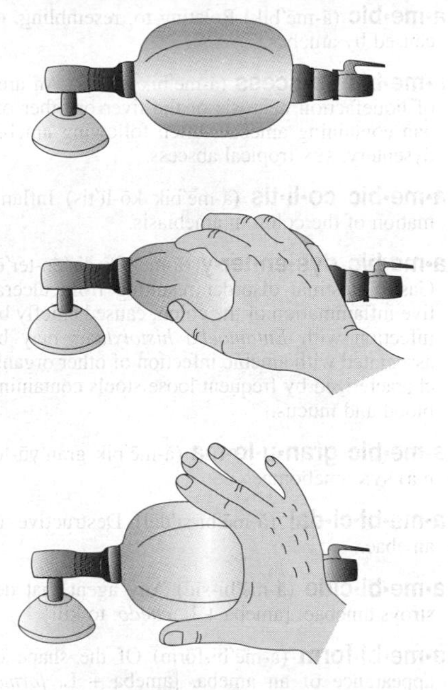

Ambu bag: the self-inflating bag refills after each manual compression and does not require a source of compressed gas

am•bu•lance (am′byū-lăns) A vehicle used to transport sick or injured people to a treatment facility. [Fr., fr. *hôpital, ambulant*, mobile hospital]

am•bu•lance ser•vice (am′byū-lăns sĕr′vis) SYN emergency medical services.

am•bu•la•tion (am′byū-lā′shŭn) The activity of walking about. [L. *ambulo*, to walk]

am•bu•la•to•ry, am•bu•lant (am′byū-lă-tōr-ē, am′byū-lănt) Walking about or able to walk about; denoting a patient who is not confined to bed or hospital as a result of disease or surgery. [L. *ambulans*, walking]

am•bu•la•to•ry care (am′byū-lă-tōr-ē kār) Medical or surgical health treatment provided during an episode of care that does not require an overnight stay in a medical facility and from which the patient goes home; outpatient rather than inpatient care.

Am•bu•la•to•ry Pa•tient Group (am′byū-lă-tōr-ē pā′shĕnt grūp) A payment system replaced by the Ambulatory Payment Classification (q.v.).

Am•bu•la•to•ry Pay•ment Clas•si•fi•ca•tion (APC) (am′byū-lă-tōr-ē pā′mĕnt klas′i-fi-kā′shŭn) In U.S. medical care, a system for grouping outpatient services provided by hospitals on the basis of similarity of costs and clinical indications; used by the Centers for Medicare and Medicaid Services to set the rates at which it will reimburse hospitals for outpatient care; replaced the Ambulatory Patient Group (APG) classification system in 2000.

am•bu•la•to•ry phle•bec•to•my (am′byū-lă-tōr-ē flĕ-bek′tō-mē) A minimally invasive procedure in which subcutaneous varices are excised through small punctures.

am•bu•la•to•ry set•ting (am′byū-lă-tōr-ē set′ing) An environment in which health care services are provided to nonhospitalized patients.

am•bu•la•to•ry sur•ger•y (am′byū-lă-tōr-ē sŭr′jĕr-ē) Operative procedures performed on patients who are admitted to and discharged from a hospital on the same day. SEE ALSO ambulatory care. SYN outpatient surgery, same-day surgery.

AMDR Abbreviation for acceptable macronutrient distribution range. SEE ALSO Dietary Reference Intake.

a•me•ba, pl. **a•me•bae, a•me•bas** (ă-mē′bă, -bē, -băz) Common name for *Amoeba* and similar naked, lobose, sarcodine protozoa. SYN amoeba.

a•me•bi•a•sis (am′ē-bī′ă-sis) Infection with *Entamoeba histolytica* or other pathogenic amebae. [ameba + G. *-iasis*, condition]

a•me•bic (ă-mē′bik) Relating to, resembling, or caused by amebas.

a•me•bic ab•scess (ă-mē′bik ab′ses) An area of liquefaction necrosis of the liver or other organ containing amebae, often following amebic dysentery. SYN tropical abscess.

a•me•bic co•li•tis (ă-mē′bik kō-lī′tis) Inflammation of the colon in amebiasis.

a•me•bic dys•en•ter•y (ă-mē′bik dis′ĕn-ter′ē) Gastrointestinal disorder resulting from ulcerative inflammation of the colon, caused chiefly by infection with *Entamoeba histolytica;* may be associated with amebic infection of other organs; characterized by frequent loose stools containing blood and mucus.

a•me•bic gran•u•lo•ma (ă-mē′bik gran′yū-lō′mă) SYN ameboma.

a•me•bi•ci•dal (ă-mē′bi-sī′dăl) Destructive to amebae.

a•me•bi•cide (ă-mē′bi-sīd) Any agent that destroys amebae. [ameba + L. *caedo,* to kill]

a•me•bi•form (ă-mē′bi-fōrm) Of the shape or appearance of an ameba. [ameba + L. *forma,* shape]

a•me•bo•cyte (ă-mē′bō-sīt) **1.** A wandering cell found in invertebrates. **2.** An in vitro tissue culture leukocyte. SYN amoebocyte. [ameba, + *kytos,* cell]

a•me•boid (ă-mē′boyd) **1.** Resembling an ameba in appearance or characteristics. **2.** Of irregular outline with peripheral projections; denoting the outline of a form of colony in plate culture. SYN amoeboid. [ameba + G. *eidos,* appearance]

a•me•boid cell (ă-mē′boyd sel) A cell such as a leukocyte, having ameboid movements, with a power of locomotion. SYN wandering cell.

a•me•boid move•ment (ă-mē′boyd mūv′mĕnt) The form of motion characteristic of the protoplasm of leukocytes, amebae, and other unicellular organisms; involves the massing of the protoplasm at a point where surface pressure is lowest where it extrudes in the form of a pseudopod; the protoplasm may return to the body of the cell, resulting in the retraction of the pseudopod, or the entire mass may flow into the cell body, resulting in locomotion of the cell.

a•me•bo•ma (am′ē-bō′mă) A nodular, tumorlike focus of proliferative inflammation sometimes developing in chronic amebiasis, especially in the wall of the colon. SYN amebic granuloma. [ameba + G. *-oma,* tumor]

am•e•bu•ri•a (am′ē-byūr′ē-ă) The presence of amebas in the urine. [ameba + G. *ouron,* urine]

a•mel•a•not•ic (ā-mel′ă-not′ik) Containing little to no melanin. [G. *a,* without, + *melas,* black]

a•me•li•a (ă-mē′lē-ă) Congenital absence of a limb or limbs. [G. *a-* priv. + *melos,* a limb]

am•e•lo•blast (ă-mel′ō-blast) One of the columnar epithelial cells of the inner layer of the enamel organ of a developing tooth, concerned with the formation of enamel. [Early E. *amel,* enamel, + G. *blastos,* germ]

am•e•lo•blas•tic ad•e•no•ma•toid tu•mor (ă-mel′ō-blas′tik ad′ĕ-nō′mă-toyd tū′mŏr) SYN adenomatoid odontogenic tumor.

am•e•lo•blas•tic fi•bro•ma (ă-mel′ō-blas′tik fī-brō′mă) A benign mixed odontogenic tumor characterized by neoplastic proliferation of both epithelial and mesenchymal components of the tooth bud without the production of dental hard tissue; presents clinically as a slowly growing painless radiolucency; occurs most commonly in the mandibles of children and adolescents.

am•e•lo•blas•tic fi•bro•sar•co•ma (ă-mel′ō-blas′tik fī′brō-sahr-kō′mă) A rapidly growing, painful, destructive, radiolucent odontogenic tumor that usually arises through malignant change in the mesenchymal and epithelial tissue component of a preexisting ameloblastic fibroma; occurs without formation of dentin or enamel. SYN ameloblastic sarcoma.

am•e•lo•blas•tic lay•er (ă-mel′ō-blas′tik lā′ĕr) The internal layer of the enamel organ. SYN enamel layer.

am•e•lo•blas•tic o•don•to•ma (ă-mel′ō-blas′tik ō′don-tō′mă) A benign mixed odontogenic tumor composed of an undifferentiated component histologically identical to an ameloblastoma and a well-differentiated component identical to an odontoma.

am•e•lo•blas•tic sar•co•ma (ă-mel′ō-blas′tik sahr-kō′mă) SYN ameloblastic fibrosarcoma.

am•e•lo•blas•to•ma (ă-mel′ō-blas-tō′mă) A benign odontogenic epithelial neoplasm; it behaves as a slowly growing expansile radiolucent tumor, occurs most commonly in the posterior regions of the mandible, and has a marked tendency to recur if inadequately excised. See page B15. [ameloblast + G. *-oma,* tumor]

am•e•lo•den•tin•al (am′ĕ-lō-den′ti-năl) SYN dentinoenamel.

am•e•lo•gen•e•sis (am′ĕ-lō-jen′ĕ-sis) The deposition and maturation of enamel. SYN enamelogenesis.

a•mel•o•gen•in (am′el-ō-jen′in) A class of proteins that form much of the organic matrix during the early development of tooth enamel. [amelogenesis + -in]

a•men•or•rhe•a (ā-men-ŏr-ē′ă) Absence or abnormal cessation of the menses. SYN amenorrhoea. [G. *a-* priv. + *mēn,* month, + *rhoia,* flow]

a•men•or•rhe•a-ga•lac•tor•rhe•a syn•

drome (ā-men-ŏr-ē′ă-gă-lak′tōr-ē′ă sin′drōm) Unphysiologic lactation from endocrinologic causes or from a pituitary tumor. SYN amenorrhoea-galactorrhoea syndrome.

a•men•or•rhe•al, **a•men•or•rhe•ic** (ā′men-or-ē′ăl, -rē′ik) Relating to, accompanied by, or due to amenorrhea. SYN amenorrhoeal.

amenorrhoea [Br.] SYN amenorrhea.

amenorrhoea-galactorrhoea syndrome [Br.] SYN amenorrhea-galactorrhea syndrome.

amenorrhoeal [Br.] SYN amenorrheal.

amenorrhoeic [Br.] SYN amenorrheic.

a•men•ti•a (ā-men′shē-ă) SYN dementia. [L. madness, fr. *ab,* from, + *mens,* mind]

a•men•ti•al (ā-men′sh ē- ăl) Pertaining to amentia.

A•mer•i•can A•cad•e•my of Al•ler•gy and Im•mu•nol•o•gy (ă-mer′i-kăn ă-kad′ĕ-mē al′lĕr-gē im′yū-nol′ŏ-jē) Organized professional group of specialists in the field of allergy and immunology.

A•mer•i•can A•cad•e•my of Nurs•ing (AAN) (ă-mer′i-kăn ă-kad′ĕ-mē nŭrs′ing) A professional group composed of about 1500 nursing leaders who address national and international issues of health care and policy; nursing leaders are selected as Fellows in recognition of their accomplishments within the nursing profession.

A•mer•i•can A•cad•e•my of Or•thot•ists and Pros•the•tists (AAOP) (ă-mer′i-kăn ă-kad′ĕ mē ōr-thot′ists pros′thĕ-tists) An allied health organization; its members are trained constructors of orthotics and prosthetics. These medical professionals provide orthotic and prosthetic services in every state of the nation. The association seeks to sustain education and therapy through research and provision of established standards of care.

A•mer•i•can A•cad•e•my of Phy•si•cian As•sis•tants (AAPA) (ă-mer′i-kăn ă-kad′ĕ-mē fi-zish′ŭn ă-sis′tănts) Organized professional group of physician assistants.

A•mer•i•can A•cad•e•my of Pro•fes•sion•al Co•ders (AAPC) (ă-mer′i-kăn ă-kad′ĕ-mē prō-fesh′ŭn-ăl kō′dĕrz) A national organization that offers three specialized certifications for medical coders: that for coders in a physician's office is guaranteed by Certified Professional Coder (CPC), for coding billing for outpatients in a hospital Certified Professional Coder-Hospital (CPC-H), and for payer perspective coding, Certified Professional Coder-Payer (CPC-P).

A•mer•i•can As•so•ci•a•tion of Col•leges of Nurs•ing (ă-mer′i-kăn ă-sō′sē-ā′shŭn kol′ĕj-ĕz nŭrs′ing) A national organization of U.S. educational programs offering baccalaureate and higher degrees in nursing.

A•mer•i•can As•so•ci•a•tion of Med•i•cal As•sis•tants (AAMA) (ă-mer′i-kăn ă-sō′sē-ā′shŭn med′i-kăl ă-sis′tănts) A professional organization comprising over 350 chapters nationally. The group awards a certificate verifying that the holder has met the standards of knowledge for the discipline and maintains them on a regular basis.

A•mer•i•can As•so•ci•a•tion for Med•i•cal Tran•scrip•tion (AAMT) (ă-mer′i-kăn ă-sō′sē-ā′shŭn med′i-kăl trans-krip′shŭn) Former name of Association for Healthcare Documentation Integrity (AHDI), national association for professional medical transcriptionists.

A•mer•i•can As•so•ci•a•tion of Neu•ro•log•i•cal Nurs•es (AANN) (ă-mer′i-kăn ă-sō′sē-ā′shŭn nūr′ŏ-loj′i-kăl nŭrs′ĕz) Organized professional group of nurses specializing in the neurological field.

A•mer•i•can As•so•ci•a•tion of Neu•ro•science Nurs•es (AANN) (ă-mer′i-kăn ă-sō′sē-ā′shŭn nūr′ō-sī′ĕns nŭrs′ĕz) Organized professional group of nurses specializing in the field of neuroscience.

A•mer•i•can As•so•ci•a•tion of Nurse An•es•the•tists (AANA) (ă-mer′i-kăn ă-sō′sē-ā′shŭn nŭrs ă-nes′thĕ-tists) Organized professional group of nurse anesthetists.

A•mer•i•can As•so•ci•a•tion of Oc•cu•pa•tion•al Health Nurs•es (AAOHN) (ă-mer′i-kăn ă-sō′sē-ā′shŭn ok′yū-pā′shŭn-ăl helth nŭr′sĕz) National organization of registered nurses practicing in the specialty of occupational health.

A•mer•i•can As•so•ci•a•tion of Re•tired Per•sons (AARP) (ă-mer′i-kăn ă-sō′sē-ā′shŭn rē-tīrd′ pĕr′sŏnz) A nonprofit, nonpartisan organization providing information, advocacy, benefits, and services for people aged 50 and older.

A•mer•i•can Board for Cer•ti•fi•ca•tion in Or•thot•ics and Pros•thet•ics (ABC) (ă-mer′i-kăn bōrd sĕr′ti-fi-kā′shŭn ōr-thot′iks pros-thet′iks) A national organization that evaluates the training and standards for makers of orthotics and prosthetics. Among its many functions, it offers testing and continuing education programs to its members.

A•mer•i•can Col•lege of Oc•cu•pa•tion•al and En•vi•ron•men•tal Med•i•cine (ACOEM) (ă-mer′i-kăn kol′ĕj ok′yū-pā′shŭn-ăl en-vī′rŏn-men′tăl med′ĭ-sin) National organization of clinicians practicing in the specialty of occupational and environmental medicine.

A•mer•i•can Health In•for•ma•tion Man•age•ment As•so•ci•a•tion (AHIMA) (ă-mer′i-kăn helth in′fōr-mā′shŭn man′āj-mĕnt ă-sō′sē-ā′shŭn) Organization that offers various forms of certification for supervisors and medical coders (e.g., registered health information administrator [RHIA], registered health information technician [RHIT], certified coding associate [CCA], and certified coding specialist [CCS]), although there are many other levels of certification available from this organization

A·mer·i·can Law In·sti·tute rule (ă-mer′i-kăn law in′sti-tūt rūl) A test of criminal responsibility (1962): "a person is not responsible for criminal conduct if at the time of such conduct as a result of mental disease or defect he lacks substantial capacity either to appreciate the wrongfulness of his conduct or to conform his conduct to the requirements of law."

A·mer·i·can leish·man·i·a·sis (ă-mer′i-kăn lēsh′mă-nī′ă-sis) SYN mucocutaneous leishmaniasis.

A·mer·i·can Man·u·al Al·pha·bet (ă-mer′i-kăn man′yū-ăl al′fă-bet) Specific hand and finger positions used to represent each letter of the alphabet, used in conjunction with American Sign Language and other sign languages. SEE ALSO augmentative and alternative communication, fingerspelling, sign language.

A·mer·i·can Med·i·cal As·so·ci·a·tion (AMA) (ă-mer′i-kăn med′i-kăl ă-sō′sē-ā′shŭn) Professional organization for physicians.

A·mer·i·can mis·tle·toe (ă-mer′i-kăn mis′ĕl-tō) *Phoradendron leucarpum*, a plant most often encountered as a Christmas decoration; purported medicinal value in treating internal disorders and as an anticarcinogenic.

A·mer·i·can Na·tion·al Stand·ards In·sti·tute (ANSI) (ă-mer′i-kan nash′ŭn-ăl stand′ărdz in′sti-tūt) Organization that sets standards for physical measures in the United States.

A·mer·i·can Nurs·es As·so·ci·a·tion (ANA) (ă-mer′i-kăn nŭrs′ĕz ă-sō′sē-ā′shŭn) A full-service professional organization representing the U.S.'s 2.7 million registered nurses through its 54 constituent state associations. ANA advances the nursing profession by fostering high standards of nursing practice, promoting the economic and general welfare of nurses in the workplace, projecting a positive and realistic view of nursing, and by lobbying the U.S. Congress and regulatory agencies on health care issues affecting nurses and the public.

A·mer·i·can Nurs·es Cre·den·tial·ing Cen·ter (ANCC) (ă-mer′i-kăn nŭrs′ĕz krē-den′shăl-ling sen′tĕr) The mission of the ANCC is to promote excellence in nursing and health care globally through credentialing programs and related services; certifies health care providers; accredits educational providers, approvers, and programs; recognizes excellence in nursing and health care services; educates the public; collaborates with organizations to advance the understanding of credentialing services; and supports credentialing through research, education, and consultative services.

A·mer·i·can Sign Lan·guage (ASL) (ă-mer′i-kăn sīn lang′gwăj) The manual sign and gesture language used by the deaf community in the United States. It is a language distinct from English, with its own grammar and syntax, but no written form.

A·mer·i·can sloe (ă-mer′i-kăn slō) SYN black haw.

A·mer·i·can So·ci·e·ty of An·es·the·si·ol·o·gists (ASA) Pa·tient Clas·si·fi·ca·tion Sta·tus (ă-mer′i-kăn sŏ-sī′ĕ-tē an′ĕs-thē′zē-ol′ŏ-jists pā′shĕnt klas′i-fi-kā′shŭn stat′ŭs) A five-level thumbnail assessment of patients' condition: I, healthy; II, mild systemic disorder; III, severe systemic disorder; IV, severe systemic disorder with threat to life; and V, state of illness sufficiently dire so as to indicate death within 24 hours without surgical intervention.

A·mer·i·cans with Dis·a·bil·i·ties Act (ADA) (ă-mer′i-kănz dis′ă-bil′i-tēz akt) U.S. federal legislation (Public Law 101-336, enacted in 1990) prohibiting discrimination against those with disabilities and ensuring equal access to employment, education, public accommodations, transportation, telecommunications, and government services at all levels.

A·mer·i·can wild yam (ă-mer′i-kăn wīld yam) SYN colic root.

A·mer·i·can worm·seed (ă-mer′i-kăn wŏrm′sēd) SYN epizote.

am·er·i·ci·um (Am) (am′ĕ-rish′ē-ŭm) An element obtained by the bombardment of uranium with neutrons or beta decay of plutoniums 241, 242, and 243; atomic no. 95; atomic weight 243.06. ^{241}Am (half-life of 432.2 years) has been used in the diagnosis of bone disorders. ^{243}Am has a half-life of 7370 years. [the Americas]

Ames test (āmz test) A screening procedure for possible carcinogens using strains of *Salmonella typhimurium* that are unable to synthesize histidine; if the test substance produces mutations that regain the ability to synthesize histidine, the substance is carcinogenic.

a·me·tri·a (ā-mē′trē-ă) Congenital absence of the uterus. [G. *a-* priv. + *mētra,* uterus]

am·e·tro·pi·a (am′ĕ-trō′pē-ă) The optic condition in which there is an error of refraction so that with the eye at rest the retina is not in conjugate focus with light rays from distant objects, i.e., only less distant objects are focused on the retina. [G. *ametros,* disproportionate, fr. *a-* priv. + *metron,* measure, + *ōps,* eye]

am·e·tro·pic (am′ĕ-trō′pik) Relating to, or suffering from, ametropia.

AMI Abbreviation for acute myocardial infarction.

♻ **-amic** Chemical suffix denoting the replacement of one COOH group of a dicarboxylic acid by a carboxamide group (—$CONH_2$); applied only to trivial names (e.g., succinamic acid).

a·mi·cro·bic (ā′mī-krō′bik) Not microbic; not related to or caused by microorganisms.

am·i·dase (am′i-dās) An enzyme that catalyzes the hydrolysis of monocarboxylic amides to free acid plus NH_3; ω-amidase acts on amides such as α-ketoglutaramic acid and α-ketosuccinamic acid. SYN acylamidase.

am·i·das·es (am′i-dās′ĕz) SYN amidohydrolase.

am·ide (am′īd) A substance formally derived from ammonia through the substitution of one or more of the hydrogen atoms by acyl groups, R—CO—NH_2, or from a carboxylic acid by replacement of a carboxylic OH by NH_2. Replacement of one hydrogen atom constitutes a primary amide; that of two hydrogen atoms, a secondary amide; and that of three atoms, a tertiary amide.

am·i·dine (am′i-dēn) The monovalent radical —C(NH)-NH_2.

♻**amido-** Prefix denoting the amide radical, R-CO-NH- or R-SO_2-NH-. [am(monia) + -id(e) + -o-]

am·i·do·hy·dro·lase (am′i-dō-hī′drō-lās) [EC class 3.5.1 and 3.5.2] An enzyme hydrolyzing C—N bonds of amides and cyclic amides; e.g., asparaginase, barbiturase, urease, amidase. SYN amidases, deamidase, deamidizing enzyme.

a·mim·i·a (ā-mim′ē-a) **1.** Inability to express ideas by nonverbal communication, such as gestures or signs. **2.** Asymbolia; the inability to comprehend the meaning of gestures, signs, symbols, or pantomime. [G. *a-* priv. + *minos*, a mimic]

am·i·nate (am′i-nāt) To combine with ammonia.

a·mine (ă-mēn′) A substance derived from ammonia by the replacement of one or more of the hydrogen atoms by hydrocarbon or other radicals. The substitution of one hydrogen atom constitutes a primary amine, e.g., NH_2CH_3; that of two atoms, a secondary amine, e.g., $NH(CH_3)_2$; that of three atoms, a tertiary amine, e.g., $N(CH_3)_3$; and that of four atoms, a quaternary ammonium ion, e.g., $^+N(CH_3)_4$, a positively charged ion isolated only in association with a negative ion. The amines form salts with acids.

a·mine ox·i·dase (fla·vin-con·tain·ing) (ă-mēn′ oks′i-dās flā′vin-kŏn-tān′ing) An oxidoreductase containing flavin and oxidizing amines with the aid of O_2 and water to aldehydes or ketones with the release of NH_3 and H_2O_2. Acted upon by antidepressants.

♻**amino-** Combining form denoting a compound containing the radical, —NH_2. [am(monia) + in(e) + -o-]

a·mi·no ac·id (AA, aa) (ă-mē′nō as′id) An organic acid in which one of the hydrogen atoms on a carbon atom have been replaced by NH_2. Usually refers to an aminocarboxylic acid. However, taurine is also an amino acid. SEE ALSO alpha (α)-amino acid.

aminoacidaemia [Br.] SYN aminoacidemia.

a·mi·no ac·id de·hy·dro·gen·ase (ă-mē′nō as′id dē-hī-droj′ĕn-ās) Enzyme catalyzing the oxidative deamination of amino acids to the corresponding oxo (keto) acids. Cf. amino acid oxidase.

a·mi·no·ac·i·de·mi·a (ă-mē′nō-as′i-dē′mē-ă, am′i-nō-) The presence of excessive amounts of specific amino acids in the blood. SYN aminoacidaemia. [amino acid + G. *haima*, blood]

a·mi·no ac·id ox·i·dase (ă-mē′nō as′id oks′-i-dās) Flavoenzyme oxidizing, with O_2 and H_2O, either L- or D-amino acids specifically, to the corresponding 2-keto acids, NH_3 and H_2O_2. Cf. amino acid dehydrogenase.

a·mi·no·ac·i·du·ri·a (ă-mē′-nō-as′i-dyūr′ē-ă) Excretion of amino acids in the urine, especially in excessive amounts. [amino acid + G. *ouron*, urine]

a·mi·no·ac·yl (AA, aa) (ă-mē′nō-as′il) The radical formed from an amino acid by removal of OH from a COOH group.

a·mi·no·ac·yl·ase (ă-mē′nō-as′i-lās) An enzyme catalyzing hydrolysis of a wide variety of *N*-acyl amino acids to the corresponding amino acid and an acid anion.

5-a·mi·no·im·id·az·ole ri·bose 5-phos·phate (AIR) (a-mē′nō-im-id-āz′ōl rī-bōs fos-fāt) An intermediate in the biosynthesis of purines. SYN 5-aminoimidazole ribotide.

5-a·mi·no·im·id·a·zole ri·bo·tide (AIR) (ă-mē′no-im-id-āz′ōl) SYN 5-aminoimidazole ribose 5-phosphate.

am·i·nol·y·sis (am′i-nol′i-sis) Replacement of a halogen in an alkyl or aryl molecule by an amine radical, with elimination of hydrogen halide.

a·mi·no·pep·ti·dase (ă-mē′nō-pep′ti-dās) [EC sub-group 3.4.11] Enzyme catalyzing the breakdown of a peptide, removing the amino acid at the amino end of the chain (i.e., an exopeptidase); found in intestinal secretions.

a·mi·no·pep·ti·dase (cy·to·sol) (ă-mē′nō-pep′ti-dās sī′tŏ-sol) An enzyme of broad specificity, containing zinc, and catalyzing the hydrolysis of the *N*-terminal amino acid of a peptide (i.e., an exopeptidase).

a·mi·no·pep·ti·dase (mi·cro·som·al) (ă-mē′nō-pep′ti-dās′ mī′krŏ-sō′măl) An aminopeptidase of broad specificity, but preferring alanine and discriminating against proline.

am·i·noph·er·ase (am′i-nof′ĕr-ās) SYN aminotransferase.

a·mi·no-ter·mi·nal (ă-mē′nō-tĕr′mi-năl) The

α-NH_2 group or the aminoacyl residue containing it at one end of a peptide or protein (usually at left as written).

a•mi•no•trans•fer•ase (ă-mē′nō-trans′fĕr-ās) [EC sub-group 2.6.1] Enzyme transferring amino groups between an amino acid to (usually) a 2-keto acid. SYN aminopherase, transaminase.

am•i•nu•ri•a (am′i-nyūr′ē-ă) Excretion of amines in the urine. [amine + G. *ouron,* urine]

am•i•to•sis (am′i-tō′sis) Direct division of the nucleus and cell, without the complicated changes in the nucleus that occur in the ordinary process of cell reproduction. SYN direct nuclear division, Remak nuclear division. [G. *a-* priv. + mitosis]

am•i•tot•ic (am′i-tot′ik) Relating to or marked by amitosis.

AML Abbreviation for acute myeloblastic leukemia.

am•me•ter (am) (am′ē-tĕr) An instrument for measuring strength of electric current in amperes.

am•mo•ne•mi•a, **am•mo•ni•e•mi•a** (ă-mō-nē′mē-ă, ă-mō′nē-ē′mē-ă) The presence of ammonia or some of its compounds in the blood, thought to be formed from the decomposition of urea; it usually results in subnormal temperature, weak pulse, gastroenteric symptoms, and coma. [ammonia + G. *haima,* blood]

Am•mon horn (am′ŏn hōrn) One of the two interlocking gyri comprising the hippocampus, the other being the dentate gyrus. Based on cytoarchitectural features, Ammon horn can be divided into region I (regio I cornus ammonis [TA]), region II (regio II cornus ammonis [TA]), region III (regio III cornus ammonis [TA]), and region IV (regio IV cornus ammonis [TA]). SYN cornu ammonis [TA]. [G. *Ammōn,* the Egyptian deity *Amūn*]

ammoniaemia [Br.] SYN ammoniemia.

am•mo•ni•a-ly•ase (ă-mō′nē-ă-lī′ās) Enzyme removing ammonia or an amino compound nonhydrolytically by rupture of a C—N bond leaving a double bond.

ammonio- Combining form indicating an ammonium group.

am•mo•ni•um (ă-mō′nē-ŭm) The ion, NH_4^+, formed by combination of NH_3 and H^+; behaves as a univalent metal in forming compounds.

am•mo•ni•u•ri•a (ă-mō-nē-yūr′ē-ă) Excretion of urine that contains an excessive amount of ammonia. [ammonia + G. *ouron,* urine]

am•mo•nol•y•sis (am′ō-nol′i-sis) The breaking of a chemical bond with the addition of the elements of ammonia (NH_2 and H) at the point of breakage. [ammonia + G. *lysis,* dissolution]

am•ne•si•a (am-nē′zē-ă) A disturbance in the memory of information stored in long-term memory, in contrast to short-term memory, manifested by total or partial inability to recall past experiences. [G. *amnēsia,* forgetfulness]

am•ne•si•ac (am-nē′sē-ak) One suffering from amnesia.

am•ne•sic (am-nē′sik) Relating to or characterized by amnesia. SYN amnestic (1).

am•nes•tic (am-nes′tik) **1.** SYN amnesic. **2.** An agent causing amnesia. **3.** A disorder in which the essential feature is an impairment of the memory function.

am•nes•tic a•pha•si•a, **am•ne•sic a•pha•si•a, am•nes•tic a•no•mi•a** (am-nes′tik ă-fā′zē-ă, am-nē′sik ă-fā′zē-ă, ā-nō′mē-ă) SYN anomic aphasia.

am•nes•tic syn•drome (am-nes′tik sin′drōm) **1.** SYN Korsakoff syndrome. **2.** An organic brain syndrome with short-term (but not immediate) memory disturbance, regardless of the etiology.

amnio- Prefix meaning the amnion. [G. *amnion*]

am•ni•o•cen•te•sis (am′nē-ō-sen-tē′sis) Transabdominal aspiration of fluid from the amniotic sac for diagnostic purposes. See this page. [amnio- + G. *kentēsis,* puncture]

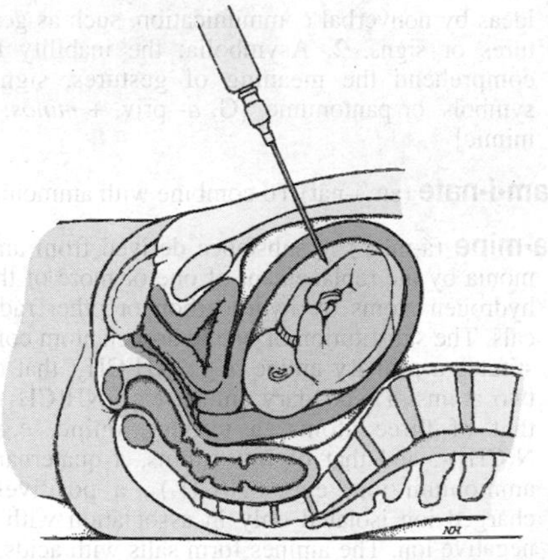

amniocentesis: procedure is usually performed at 15–17 weeks' gestation; amnionic fluid contains fetal cells, which can be examined for chromosomal abnormalities, and may contain biochemical markers of inherited disease

am•ni•o•cho•ri•al, **am•ni•o•cho•ri•on•ic** (am′nē-ō-kōr′ē-ăl, -kōr′ē-on′ik) Relating to both amnion and chorion.

am•ni•o•gen•e•sis (am′nē-ō-jen′ĕ-sis) Formation of the amnion. [amnio- + G. *genesis,* production]

am•ni•og•ra•phy (am′nē-og′ră-fē) X-ray imaging of the amniotic cavity and fetus with contrast medium injected into the amniotic fluid.

am·ni·o·hook (am′nē-ō-huk) Instrument designed to tear a hole in the amnion without injuring the fetus.

am·ni·o·in·fu·sion (am′nē-ō-in-fyū′zhŭn) Infusion of warmed saline through an intrauterine catheter during labor, for umbilical cord compromise due to low volume of amnionic fluid, or for thick meconium in labor.

am·ni·o·ma (am′nē-ō′mă) Broad flat tumor of the skin resulting from antenatal adhesion of the amnion. [amnio- + G. *-oma,* tumor]

am·ni·on (am′nē-on) Innermost of the extraembryonic membranes enveloping the embryo and later the fetus, containing the amniotic fluid; it consists of an internal embryonic layer with its ectodermal component, and an external somatic mesodermal component; in the later stages of pregnancy, the amnion expands and partially fuses to the inner wall of the chorionic sac; derived from the trophoblast cells. See page B1. SYN amnionic sac. [G. the membrane around the fetus, fr. *amnios,* lamb]

am·ni·on·ic, am·ni·ot·ic (am′nē-on′ik, am′nē-ot′ik) Relating to the amnion.

am·ni·on·ic am·pu·ta·tion (am′nē-on′ik amp′yū-tā′shŭn) SYN congenital amputation.

am·ni·on·ic band, am·ni·ot·ic band (am′nē-on′ik band, am′nē-ot′ik band) Strand of amnionic tissue adherent to the embryo or fetus, which constricts the embryonic limbs. SEE ALSO congenital amputation. SYN amnionic band syndrome, anular band, constriction ring (2), Simonart bands (1), Simonart ligaments.

am·ni·on·ic band syn·drome (am′nē-on′ik band sin′drōm) SYN amnionic band.

am·ni·on·ic cav·i·ty (am′nē-on′ik kav′i-tē) The fluid-filled cavity inside the amnion that contains amniotic fluid and the embryo.

am·ni·on·ic cor·pus·cle (am′nē-on′ik kōr′pŭs-ĕl) SYN corpus amylaceum.

am·ni·on·ic flu·id, am·ni·ot·ic flu·id (am′nē-on′ik flū′id, am′nē-ot′ik flū′id) A liquid within the amniotic sac that surrounds embryo, and later, the fetus and protects it from mechanical injury. SYN liquor amnii.

am·ni·on·ic flu·id em·bo·lism (am′nē-on′ik flū′id em′bŏ-lizm) Obstruction and constriction of pulmonary blood vessels by amnionic fluid entering the maternal circulation, causing obstetric shock. SEE ALSO amnionic fluid syndrome.

am·ni·on·ic flu·id in·dex (am′nē-on′ik flū′id in′deks) The sum of the diameters of the largest vertical pocket of amnionic fluid in each of the four quadrants of the uterus as obtained by ultrasound; a measure of fluid volume during pregnancy.

am·ni·on·ic flu·id syn·drome (am′nē-on′ik flū′id sin′drōm) Pulmonary embolic phenomena thought to be due to infusion of amnionic fluid containing epithelial squama into maternal blood vessels; shock ensues and sudden death may occur. SEE amnionic fluid embolism.

am·ni·on·ic sac (am′nē-on′ik sak) SYN amnion.

am·ni·o·ni·tis (am′nē-ō-nī′tis) Inflammation resulting from infection of the amnion, which, in turn, usually results from premature rupture of the membranes (a condition often associated with neonatal infection). [amnion + G. *-itis,* inflammation]

am·ni·on no·do·sum (am′nē-on nō-dō′sŭm) Nodules in the amnion that consist of typical stratified squamous epithelium. SYN squamous metaplasia of amnion.

am·ni·or·rhe·a (am′nē-ō-rē′ă) Escape of amniotic fluid. [amnio- + G. *rhoia,* flow]

am·ni·or·rhex·is (am′nē-ō-rek′sis) Rupture of the amniotic membrane. [amnio- + G. *rhēxis,* rupture]

am·ni·o·scope (am′nē-ō-skōp) An endoscope for studying amniotic fluid through the intact amniotic sac.

am·ni·os·co·py (am′nē-os′kŏ-pē) Examination of the amniotic fluid in the lowest part of the amniotic sac by means of an endoscope introduced through the cervical canal. [amnio- + G. *skopeō,* to view]

am·ni·o·tome (am′nē-ō-tōm) An instrument for puncturing the fetal membranes. [amnio- + G. *tomē,* cutting]

am·ni·ot·o·my (am′nē-ot′ŏ-mē) Artificial rupture of the fetal membranes as a means of inducing or expediting labor.

A-mode (mōd) DIAGNOSTIC ULTRASOUND a one-dimensional presentation of a reflected sound wave in which echo amplitude (A) is displayed along the vertical axis and time of rebound (depth) along the horizontal axis; the echo information is presented from interfaces along a single line in the direction of the sound beam.

A·moe·ba (ă-mē′bă) A genus of naked, lobose, pseudopod-forming protozoa of the class Sarcodina (or Rhizopoda), which are abundant soil-dwellers, especially in rich organic debris, and are also commonly found as parasites. The typical amebic parasites in humans are placed in the genera *Entamoeba*, *Endolimax*, and *Iodamoeba*. [Mod. L. fr. G. *amoibē* change]

amoeba [Br.] SYN ameba.

a·moe·ba·pore (ă-mē′bă-pōr) An active peptide released from *Entamoeba histolytica* that can insert ion channels into liposomes and possesses cytolytic and bactericidal activities. [amoeba + G. *poros,* passageway]

A•moe•bi•da (ă-mē′bi-dă) An order of ameboid protozoa, distinguished by possession of mitochondria and lack of a flagellate phase; most species are free living, but some are parasites of humans or animals; *Entamoeba* is an important human pathogen.

amoebocyte [Br.] SYN amebocyte.

amoeboid [Br.] SYN ameboid.

a•mo•mum (ă-mō′mŭm) *Amomum villosum,* a plant rather similar to cardamom; used as a flavoring agent and in traditional Chinese medicine, where it is allegedly useful in gastrointestinal disorders. SYN grains of paradise. [G. *amōmon*]

a•morph (ā′mōrf) An allele that has no phenotypically recognizable product and therefore its existence can be inferred on molecular evidence only. [G. *a-* neg. + *morphē,* form, shape]

a•mor•phi•a, a•mor•phism (ā-mōr′fē-ă, -fizm) Condition of being amorphous (1). [G. *a-* priv. + *morphē,* form]

a•mor•phous (ā-mōr′fŭs) **1.** Without definite form or visible differentiation in structure. **2.** Not crystallized.

a•mor•phous se•le•ni•um plate (ā-mōr′fŭs sĕ-lē′nē-ŭm plāt) SYN selenium plate.

a•mor•phous sil•i•con (ā-mōr′fŭs sil′i-kon) Light-sensitive material used in digital radiography and fluoroscopy.

AMP Abbreviation for adenosine monophosphate; specifically, the 5′-monophosphate, unless modified by a numeric prefix. SEE adenylic acid.

am•pere (A) (am′pēr) **1.** The practical unit of electrical current; the absolute, practical ampere originally was defined as having the value of 1/10 of the electromagnetic unit (see abampere and coulomb). **2.** Legal definition: the current that, flowing for 1 second, will deposit 1.118 mg of silver from silver nitrate solution. **3.** Scientific (SI) definition: the current that, if maintained in two straight parallel conductors of infinite length and of negligible circular cross-sections and placed 1 m apart in a vacuum, produces between them a force of 2×10^{-7} N/m of length. [A. M. Ampère]

Am•père pos•tu•late (am′pēr pos′chū-lăt) SYN Avogadro law.

♻ **amph-** SEE amphi-, ampho-.

♻ **amphi-** Combining form meaning on both sides, surrounding, double; corresponds to L. *ambi-*. [G. *amphi, amphi-,* on both sides, about, around]

am•phi•ar•thro•di•al (am′fē-ahrth-rō′dē-ăl) Relating to a symphysis (1) (amphiarthrosis).

am•phi•as•ter (am′fē-as′tĕr) The double-star figure formed by the two astrospheres and their connecting spindle fibers during mitosis. [amphi- + G. *astēr,* star]

am•phi•bol•ic fis•tu•la, am•phib•o•lous fis•tu•la (am′fi-bol′ik fis′chū-lă, am-fib′ŏ-lŭs fis′chū-lă) A complete anal fistula with both external and internal openings.

am•phi•cen•tric (am′fi-sen′trik) Centering at both ends, said of a rete mirabile that begins when a vessel breaks up into a number of branches and ends as the branches join again to reconstitute the vessel. [amphi- + G. *kentron,* center]

am•phid (am′fid) In the nervous system of nematodes, a pair of laterally placed minute receptor organs in the cephalic or cervical region. [amphi- + -id]

♻ **ampho-** Combining form meaning on both sides, surrounding, double. [G. *amphō,* both]

am•pho•cyte (am′fō-sīt) SYN amphophil (2).

am•pho•phil, am•pho•phile (am′fō-fil, -fīl) **1.** Having an affinity for both acid and basic dyes. SYN amphophilic, amphophilous. **2.** A cell that stains readily with either acidic or basic dyes. SYN amphocyte. [ampho- + G. *philos,* fond]

am•pho•phil•ic, am•phoph•i•lous (am′fō-fil′ik, am-fof′i-lŭs) SYN amphophil (1).

am•phor•ic (am-fōr′ik) Denoting a hollow sound heard on percussion and auscultation of the thorax over a pulmonary cavity or pneumothorax. [G. *amphora,* a jar]

am•phor•ic rale (am-fōr′ik rahl) Sound heard through the stethoscope associated with the movement of fluid in a lung cavity communicating with a bronchus.

am•phor•ic res•o•nance (am-fōr′ik rez′ŏ-năns) A hollow sound produced by percussing over a pulmonary cavity or pneumothorax.

am•pho•ter•ic (am-fō-ter′ik) Having two opposite characteristics, especially having the capacity of reacting as either an acid or a base. [G. *amphoteroi* (pl.), both, fr. *amphō,* both]

am•pho•ter•ism (am-fō′ter-izm) The property of being amphoteric.

am•pho•tro•pic vi•rus (am′fō-trō′pik vī′rŭs) An oncornavirus that does not produce disease in its natural host but does replicate in tissue culture cells of the host species and also in cells from other species.

am•pli•fi•ca•tion (am′pli-fi-kā′shŭn) **1.** The process of making larger, as in increasing an auditory or visual stimulus to enhance its perception. **2.** MOLECULAR BIOLOGY process of increasing the number of nucleic acid copies in a sample to millions within a short period. [L. *amplificatio,* an enlarging]

am•pli•fi•er (am′pli-fī′ĕr) **1.** A device that increases the magnification of a microscope. **2.** An electronic apparatus that increases the strength of input signals. SEE ALSO klystron, magnetron.

am·pli·tude of ac·com·mo·da·tion (am′pli-tūd ă-kom′ŏ-dā′shŭn) The difference in refractivity of the eye at rest and when fully accommodated.

ampoule [Br.] SYN ampule.

am·pule (am′pyūl) A hermetically sealed container, usually made of glass, containing a sterile medicinal solution, or powder to be made up in solution, to be used for subcutaneous, intramuscular, or intravenous injection. Sometimes spelled ampul in the United States. SYN ampoule.

am·pul·la, gen. and pl. **am·pul·lae** (am-pul′ă, -ē) [TA] A saccular dilation of a canal or duct. [L. a two-handled bottle]

am·pul·la of duc·tus def·er·ens (am-pul′ă dŭk′tŭs def′ĕr-enz) The dilation of the ductus deferens where it approaches its contralateral partner just before it is joined by the duct of the seminal vesicle. SYN ampulla ductus deferentis [TA].

am·pul·la duc·tus de·fe·ren·tis (am-pul′ă dŭk′tŭs def-ĕr-en′tis) [TA] SYN ampulla of ductus deferens.

am·pul·la mem·bra·na·ce·a (am-pul′ă mem-bră-nā′shē-ă) SYN membranous ampullae of the semicircular ducts.

am·pul·lar (am-pul′ăr) Relating in any sense to an ampulla.

am·pul·lar preg·nan·cy (am-pul′ăr preg′năn-sē) Tubal pregnancy situated near the midportion of the oviduct.

am·pul·la·ry crest (am′pul-ar-ē krest) An elevation on the inner surface of the ampulla of each semicircular duct; filaments of the vestibular nerve pass through the crista to reach hair cells on its surface; the hair cells are capped by the cupula, a gelatinous protein-polysaccharide mass.

am·pul·la of the sem·i·cir·cu·lar ducts (am-pul′ă sem′ē-sĕr′kyū-lăr dŭkts) A nearly spheric enlargement of one end of each of the three semicircular ducts, anterior, posterior, and lateral, where they connect with the utricle. Each contains a neuroepithelial crista ampullaris.

am·pul·la tu·bae u·ter·in·ae (am-pul′ă tū′bē yū-ter′i-nē) [TA] SYN ampulla of uterine tube.

am·pul·la of u·ter·ine tube (am-pul′ă yū′tĕr-in tūb) The wide portion of the uterine (fallopian) tube near the fimbriated extremity; it has a complexly folded mucosa with a columnar epithelium of mostly ciliated cells among which are secretory cells. SYN ampulla tubae uterinae [TA].

am·pul·la of Va·ter (am-pul′ă vah′tĕr) The dilation at the junction of the common bile duct and pancreatic ducts before they enter the duodenum.

am·pul·li·tis (am′pul-ī′tis) Inflammation of any ampulla, especially of the dilated extremity of the vas deferens or of the ampulla of Vater. [ampulla + G. *itis,* inflammation]

am·pu·ta·tion (amp′yū-tā′shŭn) **1.** The severing of a limb or part of a limb, the breast, or other projecting part. SEE ALSO congenital amputation. **2.** DENTISTRY removal of the root of a tooth, or of the pulp, or of a nerve root or ganglion; a modifying adjective is therefore used (e.g., pulp amputation; root amputation). [L. *amputatio,* fr. *am-puto,* pp. *-atus,* to cut around, prune]

am·pu·ta·tion in con·ti·nu·i·ty (amp′yū-tā′shŭn kon′ti-nū′i-tē) Surgical removal through a segment of a limb rather than at a joint.

am·pu·ta·tion neu·ro·ma (amp′yū-tā′shŭn nūr-ō′mă) SYN traumatic neuroma.

am·pu·tee (amp′yū-tē′) A person with an amputated limb or part of limb.

Am·sel cri·ter·i·a (am′sel krī-tēr′ē-ă) Findings necessary for clinical diagnosis of bacterial vaginosis; the diagnosis is made if three of the following four criteria are positive: homogeneous discharge, 4.8 pH or higher, presence of clue cells, and amine odor with the application of potassium hydroxide to the discharge.

Ams·ler chart (ahmz′ler chahrt) A 10-cm square divided into 5-mm squares on which a person may project a defect in the central visual field.

AMT Abbreviation for American Medical Technologists.

amu Abbreviation for atomic mass unit.

a·mu·si·a (ā-mū′zē-ă) A form of aphasia characterized by an inability to produce or recognize music. [G. *a-* priv. + *mousa,* music]

A·mus·sat val·vu·la (ah-mū-sat′ val′vyū-lă) SYN posterior urethral valves.

a·my·e·li·a (ā′mī-ē′lē-ă) Congenital absence of the spinal cord, found in association with meroencephaly. [G. *a-* priv. + *myelos,* marrow]

a·my·el·ic (ā′mī-ē′lik) SYN amyelous.

a·my·e·li·nat·ed (ā-mī′ĕ-li-nā′ted) SYN unmyelinated.

a·my·e·li·na·tion (ā-mī′ĕ-li-nā′shŭn) Failure of formation of myelin sheath of a nerve.

a·my·e·lin·ic (ā-mī′ĕ-lin′ik) SYN unmyelinated.

a·my·e·lo·ic, a·my·e·lon·ic (ā-mī′ĕ-lō′ik, ā-mī-ĕ-lon′ik) **1.** SYN amyelous. **2.** HEMATOLOGY term sometimes used to indicate the absence of bone marrow or the lack of functional participation of bone marrow in hemopoiesis. [G. *a-* priv. + *myelos,* marrow]

a•my•e•lous (ā-mī′ĕ-lŭs) Without a spinal cord. SYN amyelic, amyeloic (1), amyelonic.

a•myg•da•la, gen. and pl. **a•myg•da•lae** (ă-mig′dă-lă, -lē) Denoting the cerebellar tonsil, as well as the lymphatic tonsils (pharyngeal, palatine, lingual, laryngeal, and tubal). [L. fr. G. *amygdalē,* almond; in Mediev. & Mod. L., a tonsil]

a•myg•da•lin (ă-mig′dă-lin) A cyanogenic glucoside present in almonds and seeds of other plants of the family Rosaceae; the principal component of laetrile. Emulsin splits amygdalin into benzaldehyde, D-glucose, and hydrocyanic acid. [G. *amygdala,* almond, + -in]

a•myg•da•loid (ă-mig′dă-loyd) Resembling an almond or a tonsil. [amygdala + G. *eidos,* appearance]

a•myg•da•loid bod•y (ă-mig′dă-loyd bod′ē) A rounded mass of gray matter in the temporal lobe internal to the cortex of the uncus and immediately anterior to the inferior horn of the lateral ventricle; its major afferents are olfactory and its efferent connections are with the hypothalamus and mediodorsal nucleus of the thalamus and it is also reciprocally associated with the cortex of the temporal lobe; it is subdivided into two major nuclear groups, basolateral and corticomedial.

a•myg•dal•ose (ā-mig′dăl-ōs) SYN gentiobiose.

am•yl (am′il) The radical formed from a pentane, C_5H_{12}, by removal of one H. Several isomeric forms exist. SYN pentyl (1).

amyl- 1. SEE amylo-. 2. Pentyl-. SEE amyl.

am•y•la•ce•ous (am′i-lā′shē-ŭs) Starchy.

am•y•lase (am′il-ās) One of a group of amylolytic enzymes that cleave starch, glycogen, and related 1,4-α-glucans.

am•y•lase:cre•at•i•nine clear•ance ra•ti•o (am′i-lās-krē-at′i-nēn klēr′ăns rā′shē-ō) A test for the diagnosis of acute pancreatitis; it is determined by measuring amylase and creatinine in serum and urine.

am•y•la•su•ri•a (am′i-lā-syūr′ē-ă) The excretion of amylase (sometimes termed diastase) in the urine, especially increased amounts in acute pancreatitis. SYN diastasuria.

am•y•lin (am′i-lin) The cellulose of starch; the insoluble envelope of starch grains.

am•yl ni•trite (ă′mil nīt′rīt) An inhalable compound used in the United States as the first step in the antidotal treatment of cyanide poisoning. SEE ALSO sodium nitrite, sodium thiosulfate, hydroxycobalamin.

amylo- Combining form meaning starch, of polysaccharide nature or origin. [G. *amylon,* unmilled; starch, fr. *a-* + *mylē,* a mill]

am•y•lo•gen•e•sis (am′i-lō-jen′ĕ-sis) Biosynthesis of starch. [amylo- + G. *genesis,* production]

am•y•lo•gen•ic (am′i-lō-jen′ik) Relating to amylogenesis.

am•y•loid (am′i-loyd) **1.** Any of a group of chemically diverse proteins that appears microscopically homogeneous but is composed of linear nonbranching aggregated fibrils arranged in sheets when seen under the electron microscope; it stains dark brown with iodine, produces a characteristic green color in polarized light after staining with Congo red, is metachromatic with either methyl violet (pink-red) or crystal violet (purple-red), and fluoresces yellow after thioflavine T staining; amyloid occurs characteristically as pathologic extracellular deposits (amyloidosis), especially in association with reticuloendothelial tissue; the chemical nature of the proteinaceous fibrils is dependent on the underlying disease process. **2.** Resembling or containing starch. [amylo- + G. *eidos,* resemblance]

am•y•loid de•gen•er•a•tion (am′i-loyd dĕ-jen′ĕr-ā′shŭn) Infiltration of amyloid between cells and fibers of tissues and organs. SYN waxy degeneration (1).

am•y•loid kid•ney (am′i-loyd kid′nē) A kidney in which amyloidosis has occurred, usually in association with some chronic illness such as multiple myeloma, tuberculosis, osteomyelitis, or other chronic suppurative inflammation. SYN waxy kidney.

am•y•loid ne•phro•sis (am′i-loyd nef-rō′sis) **1.** SYN renal amyloidosis. **2.** Nephrotic syndrome due to deposition of amyloid in the kidney.

am•y•loi•do•sis (am′i-loy-dō′sis) **1.** A disease characterized by extracellular accumulation of amyloid in various organs and tissues of the body; may be primary or secondary. **2.** The process of deposition of amyloid protein. See page 73. [amyloid + G. *-osis,* condition]

am•y•loi•do•sis of ag•ing (am′i-loy-dō′sis āj′ing) A process characterized by deposition of Congo-red–staining material, derived from a variety of proteins, especially in nervous tissue, myocardium, and pancreas; associated with Alzheimer disease; intractable congestive heart failure may result.

am•y•loid tu•mor (am′i-loyd tū′mŏr) SYN nodular amyloidosis.

am•y•lol•y•sis (am′i-lol′i-sis) Hydrolysis of starch into soluble products. [amylo- + G. *lysis,* dissolution]

am•y•lo•lyt•ic (am′i-lō-lit′ik) Relating to amylolysis.

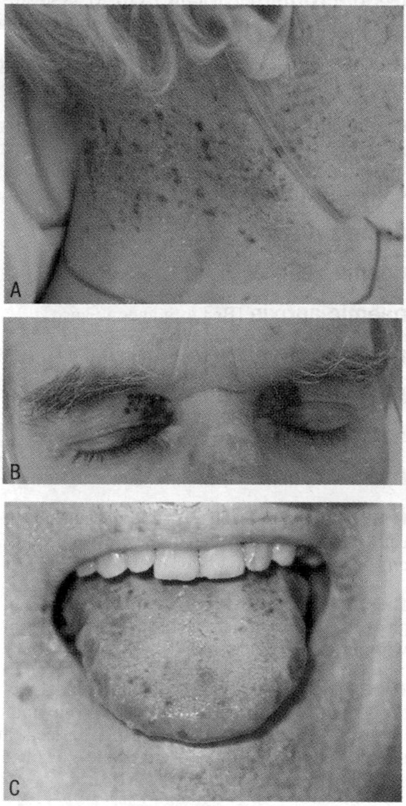

amyloidosis: (A) neck; (B) pinch purpura of eyelids; (C) tongue

am·y·lo·pec·tin (am′i-lō-pek′tin) A branched-chain polyglucose (glucan) in starch containing both 1,4 and 1,6 linkages. Cf. amylose.

am·y·lor·rhe·a (am′i-lō-rē′ă) Passage of undigested starch in the stools, implying a deficiency of amylase activity in the intestine. SYN amylorrhoea. [amylo- + G. *rhoia,* flow]

amylorrhoea [Br.] SYN amylorrhea.

am·y·lose (am′i-lōs) An unbranched polyglucose (glucan) in starch, similar to cellulose, containing α(1→4) linkages. Cf. amylopectin.

am·y·lo·su·ri·a, **am·y·lu·ri·a** (am′i-lō-syūr′ē-ă, am′i-lyūr′ē-a) Excretion of starch in the urine.

amyoaesthesia [Br.] SYN amyoesthesia.

amyoaesthesis [Br.] SYN amyoesthesis.

a·my·o·es·the·si·a, **a·my·o·es·the·sis** (ă-mī′ō-es-thē′zē-ă, -thē′sis) Absence of muscle sensation. SYN amyoaesthesia. [G. *a-* priv. + *mys,* muscle, + *aisthēsis,* perception]

a·my·o·pla·si·a (ă-mī′ō-plā′zē-ă) Deficient formation of muscle and muscle growth. [G. *a-* priv. + *mys,* muscle, + *plasis,* a molding]

a·my·o·sta·si·a (ă-mī′ō-stā′zē-ă) Difficulty in standing, due to muscular tremor or incoordination. [G. *a-* priv. + *mys,* muscle, + *stasis,* standing]

a·my·o·stat·ic (ă-mī′ō-stat′ik) Showing muscular tremors.

a·my·os·the·ni·a (ă-mī′os-thē′nē-ă) Muscular weakness. [G. *a-* priv. + *mys,* muscle, + *sthenos,* strength]

a·my·os·then·ic (ă-mī′os-then′ik) Relating to or causing muscular weakness.

a·my·o·tax·y, **a·my·o·tax·i·a** (ă-mī′ō-tak-sē, ă-mī′ō-tak′sē-ă) Muscular ataxia. [G. *a-* priv. + *mys,* muscle, + *taxis,* order]

a·my·o·to·ni·a (ă-mī′ō-tō′nē-ă) Generalized absence of muscle tone, usually associated with flabby musculature and an increased range of passive movement at joints. [G. *a-* priv. + *mys,* muscle, + *tonos,* tone]

a·my·o·to·ni·a con·gen·i·ta (ă-mī′ō-tō′nē-ă kon-jen′i-tă) **1.** Atonic pseudoparalysis of congenital origin (neither familial nor hereditary), observed especially in infants and characterized by absence of tone in muscles innervated by the spinal nerves. **2.** An indefinite term for a number of congenital neuromuscular disorders that cause generalized myotonia in young children and have a benign course. SYN Oppenheim disease.

a·my·o·tro·phic (ă-mī′ō-trō′fik) Relating to muscular atrophy.

a·my·o·tro·phic lat·er·al scle·ro·sis (ALS) (ă-mī′ō-trō′fik lat′ĕr-ăl skler-ō′sis) A disease of the motor tracts of the lateral columns and anterior horns of the spinal cord, causing progressive muscular atrophy, increased reflexes, fibrillary twitching, and spastic irritability of muscles; associated with a defect in superoxide dismutase. SYN Aran-Duchenne disease, Charcot disease, Cruveilhier disease, Duchenne-Aran disease, Lou Gehrig disease, progressive muscular atrophy.

a·my·ot·ro·phy (ă′mī-ot′rō-fē) Muscular wasting or atrophy. [G. *a-* priv. + *mys,* muscle, + *trophē,* nourishment]

a·myx·or·rhe·a (ă-mik′sōr-ē′ă) Absence of the normal secretion of mucus. [G. *a-* priv. + *myxa,* mucus, + *rhoia,* flow]

ANA Abbreviation for antinuclear antibody; American Nurses Association.

♻ **ana-** Prefix meaning up, toward, apart. USAGE NOTE not to be confused with *an-* (a form of the prefix *a-*, without, used before a vowel). [G. *ana,* up]

an·a·bi·o·sis (an′ă-bī-ō′sis) Resuscitation after

apparent death. [G. a reviving, fr. *ana,* again, + *biōsis,* life]

an•a•bi•ot•ic cell (an′ă-bī-ot′ik sel) Cell that is capable of resuscitation after apparent death; the existence of anabiotic tumor cells is postulated to explain the recurrence of a cancer after a very long symptomless period following operation.

an•a•bol•ic (an′ă-bol′ik) Relating to or promoting anabolism.

an•a•bol•ic ste•roid (an′ă-bol′ik ster′oyd) Prescription drug abused by some athletes to increase muscle mass; functions in a manner similar to that of the chief male hormone, testosterone. Masculinizing effects are minimized by synthetically manipulating chemical structure to emphasize tissue-building, nitrogen-retaining processes. SEE ALSO ergogenic aid. SYN androgenic steroid.

an•ab•o•lism (ă-nab′ō-lizm) **1.** The building up in the body of complex chemical compounds from simpler compounds (e.g., proteins from amino acids), usually with the use of energy. Cf. catabolism, metabolism. **2.** The sum of synthetic metabolic reactions. [G. *anabolē,* a raising up]

an•ab•o•lite (ă-nab′ō-līt) Any substance formed as a result of anabolic processes.

an•a•cid•i•ty (an′ă-sid′i-tē) Absence of acidity; used especially to denote absence of hydrochloric acid in the gastric juice.

an•ac•la•sis (ă-nak′lă-sis) **1.** Reflection of light or sound. **2.** Refraction of the ocular media. [G. a bending back, reflection]

an•a•clit•ic (an′ă-klit′ik) Leaning or depending on; in psychoanalysis, relating to the dependence of the infant on the mother or mother substitute. SEE anaclitic depression. [G. *ana,* toward, + *klinō,* to lean]

an•a•clit•ic de•pres•sion (an′ă-klit′ik dĕ-presh′ŭn) Impairment of an infant's physical, social, and intellectual development following separation from its mother or from a mothering surrogate; characterized by listlessness, withdrawal, and anorexia.

an•a•crot•ic, an•a•di•crot•ic (an′ă-krot′ik, an′ă-dī-krot′ik) Referring to the upstroke or ascending limb of the arterial pulse tracing.

an•a•crot•ic pulse, an•a•di•crot•ic pulse (an′ă-krot′ik pŭls, an′ă-dī-krot′ik pŭls) A pulse wave showing one or more notches or indentations on its rising limb that are sometimes detectable by palpation.

an•ac•ro•tism (ă-nak′rŏ-tizm) Peculiarity of the pulse wave. SEE anacrotic pulse. SYN anadicrotism. [G. *ana,* up, + *krotos,* a beat]

an•a•cu•sis (an′ă-kyū′sis) Absence of the ability to perceive sound. SYN anakusis. [G. *an-* priv. + *akousis,* hearing]

an•a•di•cro•tism (an′ă-dik′rŏ-tizm) SYN anacrotism. [G. *ana,* up, + *di-krotos,* double beating]

an•ad•re•nal•ism (an′ă-drē′năl-izm) Complete lack of adrenal function.

an•a•dro•mous (an′a-drō′mŭs) Denotes fish that migrate from ocean water to fresh water to spawn; some such fish harbor human pathogens. SEE ALSO catadromous.

anaemia [Br.] SYN anemia.

anaemic [Br.] SYN anemic.

anaemic anoxia [Br.] SYN anemic anoxia.

anaemic halo [Br.] SYN anemic halo.

anaemic hypoxia [Br.] SYN anemic hypoxia.

anaemic infarct [Br.] SYN anemic infarct.

anaemic murmur [Br.] SYN anemic murmur.

an•aer•obe (an-ār′ōb) A microorganism that can live and grow in the absence of oxygen. [G. *an-* priv. + *aēr,* air, + *bios,* life]

an•aer•o•bic, an•aer•o•bi•ot•ic (an′ār-ō′bik, an′ār-ō-bī-ot′ik) Relating to an anaerobe; living without oxygen.

an•aer•o•bic ca•pa•ci•ty (an′ār-ō′bik kă-pas′i-tē) Maximal work performed during maximum-intensity short-term physical effort; reflects the energy output capacity of anaerobic glycolysis. SEE ALSO Wingate test.

an•aer•o•bic pow•er (an′ār-ō′bik pow′ĕr) Maximal power (work per unit time) developed during all-out, short-term physical effort; reflects energy-output capacity of intramuscular high-energy phosphates (ATP and PCr).

an•aer•o•bic res•pi•ra•tion (an′ār-ō′bik res′pir-ā′shŭn) A form of respiration in which molecular oxygen is not consumed (e.g., nitrate respiration, sulfate respiration).

an•aer•o•bic thresh•old (an′ār-ō′bik thresh′ōld) A hybrid term to describe the onset of blood lactate accumulation estimated by using either ventilatory measures (ventilatory threshold) or blood lactate measures (lactate threshold).

an•aer•o•bic ven•ti•la•to•ry thresh•old (an′ār-ō′bik ven′ti-lă-tōr-ē thresh′ōld) The onset of metabolic acidosis during exercise signifying the peak work rate of oxygen consumption (VO_{2max}) in which energy demands exceed circulatory ability to sustain aerobic metabolism.

an•aer•o•bi•o•sis (an′ār-ō-bī-ō′sis) Existence in an oxygen-free atmosphere. [G. *an-* priv. + *aēr,* air, + *biōsis,* way of living]

An•aer•o•bo•plas•ma (an′ār-ō′bō-plaz′mă) An order in the class Molicutes that is oxygen sensitive. A role in human disease has not been defined.

an•aer•o•gen•ic (an′ār-ō-jen′ik) Not producing gas. [G. *an-* priv. + *aēr,* air, + *-gen,* producing]

anaesthekinesia [Br.] SYN anesthekinesia.

anaesthesia [Br.] SYN anesthesia.

anaesthesia dolorosa [Br.] SYN anesthesia dolorosa.

anaesthesia record [Br.] SYN anesthesia record.

anaesthesiologist [Br.] SYN anesthesiologist.

anaesthesiology [Br.] SYN anesthesiology.

anaesthetic [Br.] SYN anesthetic.

anaesthetist [Br.] SYN anesthetist.

an•a•gen (an′ă-jen) Growth phase of the hair cycle, lasting about 3–6 years in human scalp hair. [G. *ana,* up, + *-gen,* producing]

an•a•gen ef•flu•vi•um (an′ă-jen ĕ-flū′vē-ŭm) Sudden diffuse hair shedding with cancer chemotherapy or radiation, usually reversible when treatment ends. SEE ALSO telogen effluvium.

an•a•ku•sis (an′ă-kyū′sis) SYN anacusis.

a•nal (ā′năl) Relating to the anus.

a•nal a•tre•si•a, **a•tre•si•a a•ni** (ā′năl ă-trē′zē-ă, ă-trē′zē-ă′ ā′nī) Congenital absence of an anal opening due to the presence of a membranous septum (persistence of the cloacal membrane) or a complete absence of the anal canal. SYN imperforate anus (1), proctatresia.

analbuminaemia [Br.] SYN analbuminemia.

an•al•bu•mi•ne•mi•a (an′al-bū′mi-nē′mē-ă) Absence of albumin from the serum. SYN analbuminaemia. [G. *an-* priv. + albumin + G. *haima,* blood]

a•nal ca•nal (ā′năl kă-nal′) The terminal portion of the alimentary canal; it extends from the pelvic diaphragm to the anal orifice. SYN canalis analis [TA].

a•nal col•umns (ā′năl kol′ŭmz) Vertical ridges in the mucous membrane of the upper half of the anal canal that are formed as the caliber of the canal is sharply reduced from that of the rectal ampulla. SYN columnae anales [TA], Morgagni columns, rectal columns.

a•nal ducts (ā′năl dŭkts) Short ducts lined with simple columnar to stratified columnar epithelium that extend from the valvulae anales to the sinus anales.

an•a•lep•tic (an′ă-lep′tik) **1.** Strengthening, stimulating, or invigorating. **2.** A restorative remedy. **3.** A central nervous system stimulant, particularly used to denote agents that reverse depressed central nervous system function. [G. *analēptikos,* restorative]

an•a•lep•tic en•e•ma (an′ă-lep′tik en′ĕ-mă) An enema comprising a pint of lukewarm water with one-half teaspoonful of table salt.

a•nal fis•sure (ā′năl fish′ŭr) A crack or slit in the mucous membrane of the anus.

a•nal fis•tu•la (ā′năl fis′chū-lă) A fistula opening at or near the anus; usually, but not always, opening into the rectum above the internal sphincter.

an•al•ge•si•a (an′ăl-jē′zē-ă) **1.** A neurologic or pharmacologic state in which painful stimuli are so moderated that, although still perceptible, they are no longer painful. Cf. anesthesia. **2.** Denotes process of relieving pain. [G. insensibility, fr. *an-* priv. + *algēsis,* sensation of pain]

an•al•ge•si•a al•ge•ra (an′ăl-jē′zē-ă al-jē′ră) SYN analgesia dolorosa.

an•al•ge•si•a do•lo•ro•sa (an′ăl-jē′zē-ă dō-lō-rō′să) Spontaneous pain in a body area that lacks sensation. SYN analgesia algera.

an•al•ge•sic (an′ăl-jē′zik) **1.** A compound capable of producing analgesia, i.e., one that relieves pain by altering perception of nociceptive stimuli without producing anesthesia or loss of consciousness. **2.** Characterized by reduced response to painful stimuli.

a•nal•i•ty (ā-nal′i-tē) Referring to the psychic organization derived from, and characteristic of, the freudian anal period of psychosexual development.

an•al•ler•gic (an′ă-ler′jik) Not allergic.

an•a•log (an′ă-lawg) SYN analogue.

a•nal•o•gous (ă-nal′ŏ-gŭs) Possessing a functional resemblance, but having a different origin or structure.

an•a•logue (an′ă-lawg) **1.** One of two organs or parts in different species of animals or plants that differ in structure or development but are similar in function. **2.** A compound that resembles another in structure but is not necessarily an isomer; analogues are often used to block enzymatic reactions by combining with enzymes. SYN analog. [G. *analogos,* proportionate]

an•a•logue dic•ta•tion (an′ă-lawg dik-tā′shŭn) System in which health care professionals' dictation is recorded on cassette tapes.

a•nal pec•ten (ā′năl pek′ten) The middle third of the anal canal. SYN pecten analis, pecten (2).

analphalipoproteinaemia [Br.] SYN analphalipoproteinemia.

an•al•pha•lip•o•pro•tein•e•mi•a (an′al′fă-lip′ō-prō′tēn-ē′mē-ă) Familial high density lipoprotein deficiency; an inheritable disorder of lipid metabolism characterized by an almost complete absence from plasma of high density lipoproteins, and by storage of cholesterol esters in foam cells, tonsillar enlargement, an orange or yellow-gray color of the pharyngeal and rectal mucosa, hepatosplenomegaly, lymph node enlargement, corneal opacity, and peripheral neuropathy; autosomal recessive inheritance. SYN analphalipoproteinaemia. [G. *an-*, priv., + *alpha*, α, + lipoprotein + *-emia*, blood]

a•nal phase (ā′năl fāz) In psychoanalytic personality theory, the stage of psychosexual development, occurring when a child is 1–3 years old, during which activities, interests, and concerns center on the anal zone.

a•nal pit (ā′năl pit) **1.** An ectodermally lined depression under the taillike caudal eminence adjacent to the terminal part of the embryonic hindgut; at its bottom, proctodeal ectoderm and cloacal endoderm form the cloacal plate. When this epithelial plate ruptures, the anal and urogenital external orifices are established. SYN proctodeum. **2.** Terminal portion of the insect alimentary canal.

a•nal plate (ā′năl plāt) The anal portion of the cloacal membrane.

a•nal re•flex (ā′năl rē′fleks) Contraction of the internal sphincter gripping the finger passed into the rectum.

a•nal si•nus•es (ā′năl sī′nŭs-ĕz) **1.** The grooves between the anal columns; SYN Morgagni sinus (1). **2.** Pockets or crypts in the columnar zone of the anal canal between the anocutaneous line and the anorectal line; the sinuses give the mucosa a scalloped appearance.

a•nal verge (ā′năl vĕrj) The transitional zone between the moist, hairless, modified skin of the anal canal and the perianal skin.

a•nal•y•sand (ă-nal′i-sand) Individual who is undergoing psychoanalysis.

a•nal•y•sis, pl. **a•nal•y•ses** (ă-nal′i-sis, -sēz) **1.** The disaggregation of a compound or mixture into simpler elements; a process by which the composition of a substance is determined. Cf. synthesis (1). **2.** The study of a whole in terms of its parts. **3.** SEE psychoanalysis. **4.** NURSING the process of organizing and synthesizing data so as to address research questions or to make a clinical judgment related to care. **5.** In occupational therapy, the process of studying an activity or occupation-related activities so as to break down its components or constituent parts. [G. a breaking up, fr. *ana*, up, + *lysis*, a loosening]

a•nal•y•sis of var•i•ance (ANOVA) (ă-nal′i-sis var′ē-ăns) A statistical technique that isolates and assesses the contribution of categoric independent variables to variation in the mean of a continuous dependent variable.

an•a•lyst (an′ă-list) **1.** One who makes analytic determinations. **2.** Psychoanalyst.

an•a•lyte (an′ă-līt) A material or substance the presence or concentration of which in a specimen is determined by analysis.

an•a•lyt•ic, **an•a•lyt•i•cal** (an′ă-lit′-ik, -i-kăl) **1.** Relating to analysis. **2.** Relating to psychoanalysis.

an•a•lyt•ic psy•chol•o•gy (an′ă-lit′ik sī-kol′ŏ-jē) SYN jungian psychoanalysis.

an•a•lyt•ic sen•si•tiv•i•ty (an′a-lit′ik sen′si-tiv′i-tē) The ability of a test to detect a particular analyte or substance or a minimal change in the concentration of the substance.

an•a•lyt•ic spec•i•fic•i•ty (an′a-lit′ik spes′i-fis′i-tē) The ability of a test to react only to the substance of interest and no other.

an•a•lyz•er, **an•a•lyz•or** (an′ă-līz-er, -ŏr) **1.** Any instrument that performs an analysis. **2.** The prism in a polariscope used to examine polarized light. **3.** The neural basis of the conditioned reflex; includes all the sensory side of the reflex arc and its central connections. **4.** A device that electronically determines the frequency and amplitude of a particular channel of an electroencephalogram.

an•am•ne•sis (an′am-nē′sis) **1.** The act of remembering. **2.** The medical or developmental history of a patient. [G. *anamnēsis*, recollection]

an•am•nes•tic (an′am-nes′tik) **1.** Assisting the memory. SYN mnemonic. **2.** Relating to the medical history of a patient.

an•am•nes•tic re•ac•tion (an′am-nes′tik rē-ak′shŭn) Augmented production of an antibody due to previous response of the subject to stimulus by the same antigen.

an•a•phase (an′ă-fāz) The stage of mitosis or meiosis in which the chromosomes move from the equatorial plate toward the poles of the cell. In mitosis a full set of daughter chromosomes (46 in humans) moves toward each pole. In the first division of meiosis, one member of each homologous pair (23 in humans), consisting of two chromatids united at the centromere, moves toward each pole. In the second division of meiosis, the centromere divides, and the two chromatids separate, with one moving to each pole. [G. *ana*, up, + *phasis*, appearance]

an•a•phi•a (ă-nā′fē-ă) Absence of the sense of touch. [G. *an-* priv. + *haphē*, touch]

an•aph•ro•di•si•ac (an′af-rō-diz′ē-ak) **1.** Repressing or destroying sexual desire. **2.** An agent that lessens or abolishes sexual desire. [G. *an-* priv. + *aphrodisia*, sexual pleasure]

an•a•phy•lac•tic (an′ă-fi-lak′tik) Relating to anaphylaxis; manifesting extremely great sensitivity to foreign protein or other material.

an•a•phy•lac•tic an•ti•bod•y (an′ă-fi-lak′tik an′ti-bod-ē) SYN cytotropic antibody.

an•a•phy•lac•tic shock (an′ă-fi-lak′tik shok) A severe, often fatal form of shock characterized by smooth muscle contraction and capillary dilation initiated by cytotropic (IgE class) antibodies. SEE ALSO anaphylaxis, serum sickness.

an·a·phy·lac·to·gen (an′ă-fi-lak′tō-jen) A substance (antigen) capable of rendering a person susceptible to anaphylaxis; a substance (antigen) that will cause an anaphylactic reaction in such a sensitized person.

an·a·phy·lac·to·gen·e·sis (an′ă-fi-lak′tō-jen′ĕ-sis) The production of anaphylaxis.

an·a·phy·lac·to·gen·ic (an′ă-fi-lak′tō-jen′ik) Producing anaphylaxis; pertaining to substances (antigens) that result in a person's becoming susceptible to anaphylaxis.

an·a·phy·lac·toid (an′ă-fi-lak′toyd) Resembling anaphylaxis. [anaphylaxis + G. *eidos,* resemblance]

an·a·phy·lac·toid pur·pu·ra (an′ă-fi-lak′toyd pŭr′pyŭr-ă) **1.** SYN allergic purpura. **2.** SYN Henoch-Schönlein purpura.

an·a·phy·lac·toid shock (an′ă-fi-lak′toyd shok) A reaction that is similar to anaphylactic shock, but that does not require the incubation period characteristic of induced sensitivity (anaphylaxis); it is unrelated to antigen-antibody reactions.

an·a·phyl·a·tox·in, an·a·phyl·o·tox·in (an′ă-fil′ă-tok′sin, an′ă-fil′ō-tok′sin) **1.** A substance postulated to be the immediate cause of anaphylactic shock and that is assumed to result from the in vivo combination of specific antibody and the specific sensitizing material. **2.** The small fragment (C3a) split from the third component (C3) of complement, which produces a local wheal following intracutaneous injection. [anaphylaxis + toxin]

an·a·phy·lax·is (an′ă-fi-lak′sis) The immediate, transient kind of immunologic (allergic) reaction characterized by contraction of smooth muscle and dilation of capillaries due to release of pharmacologically active substances (histamine, bradykinin, serotonin, and slow-reacting substance), classically initiated by the combination of antigen (allergen) with mast-cell–fixed, cytophilic antibody (chiefly IgE); the reaction can be initiated, also, by relatively large quantities of serum aggregates (antigen-antibody complexes, and others) that seemingly activate complement leading to production of anaphylatoxin, a reaction sometimes termed "aggregate anaphylaxis." [G. *ana,* away from, back from, + *phylaxis,* protection]

an·a·pla·si·a (an′ă-plā′zē-ă) Loss of structural differentiation, especially as seen in most, but not all, malignant neoplasms. SYN dedifferentiation (2). [G. *ana,* again, + *plasis,* a molding]

A·na·plas·ma pha·go·cy·to·phil·um (an′ă-plaz′mă fā′gō-sī′tō-fil′ŭm) A bacterial species that causes human granulocytic ehrlichiosis; also causes tick-borne fever in cattle; spread by ticks (*Ixodes*), it occurs in the United States in the Middle Atlantic states, southern New England, and the lower Midwest.

an·a·plas·tic (an′ă-plas′tik) **1.** Relating to anaplasty. **2.** Characterized by or pertaining to anaplasia. **3.** Growing without form or structure, as in loss of cellular differentiation in association with malignancies.

an·a·plas·tic cell (an′ă-plas′tik sel) **1.** A cell that has reverted to an embryonal state. **2.** An undifferentiated cell, characteristic of malignant neoplasms.

an·a·plas·tol·o·gy (an′ă-plas-tol′ŏ-jē) Application of prosthetic materials for construction and/or reconstruction of a missing body part. [G. *ana,* again, + *plastos,* formed]

an·a·poph·y·sis (an′ă-pof′i-sis) An accessory spinal process of a vertebra, found especially in the thoracic or lumbar vertebrae. [G. *ana,* back, + *apophysis,* offshoot]

a·nap·tic (ă-nap′tik) Relating to anaphia.

an·a·rith·mi·a (an′ă-ridh′mē-ă) Aphasia characterized by an inability to count or use numbers. [G. *an-* priv. + *arithmos,* number]

an·ar·thri·a (an-ahrth′rē-a) Loss of the power of articulate speech. SEE ALSO aphasia, alexia, dysarthria. [G. *anarthros,* without joints; (of sound) inarticulate]

an·a·sar·ca (an′ah-sahr′kă) A generalized infiltration of edema fluid into subcutaneous connective tissue. [G. *ana,* through, + *sarx* (*sark-*), flesh]

an·a·sar·cous (an′ah-sahr′kŭs) Characterized by anasarca.

an·as·tig·mats (an′ă-stig′mats) **1.** Lenses with which astigmatism is corrected. **2.** Lenses in which both astigmatism and field curvature are corrected.

a·nas·to·mose (ă-nas′tŏ-mōs) **1.** To form one or more open communications with another structure; said of blood vessels and tubular and hollow viscera. USAGE NOTE Not correctly said of nerves. **2.** To unite surgically by means of an anastomosis; to make a communication between formerly separate structures.

a·nas·to·mo·sis, pl. **a·nas·to·mo·ses** (ă-nas′tŏ-mō′sis, mō′sēz) **1.** A natural communication, direct or indirect, between two blood vessels or other tubular structures. USAGE NOTE Not correctly applied to nerves. SEE communication. **2.** An operative union of two hollow or tubular structures. **3.** An opening created by surgery, trauma, or disease between two or more normally separate spaces or organs. [G. *anastomōsis,* from *anastomoō,* to furnish with a mouth]

a·nas·to·mot·ic (ă-nas′tŏ-mot′ik) Pertaining to an anastomosis.

a·nas·to·mot·ic branch (ă-nas′tŏ-mot′ik

branch) A blood vessel that interconnects two neighboring vessels. USAGE NOTE Not correctly applied to nerves.

a•nas•to•mot•ic ul•cer (ă-nas′tō-mot′ik ŭl′sĕr) An ulcer of the jejunum, after gastroenterostomy.

an•a•tom•ic (an′ă-tom′ik) **1.** Relating to anatomy. **2.** SYN structural. **3.** Denoting a strictly morphologic feature distinct from its physiologic or surgical considerations, e.g., anatomic neck of humerus, anatomic dead space, anatomic lobulation of the liver.

an•a•tom•ic con•ju•gate (an′ă-tom′ik kon′jŭ-găt) Measure of pelvic dimension describing the distance between the sacral promontory and the inferior border of the pubic symphysis, measured manually per vaginam or by ultrasonography. It is used to extrapolate the true conjugate.

an•a•tom•ic crown (an′ă-tom′ik krown) The portion of a tooth covered by enamel.

an•a•tom•i•c dead space (an′ă-tom′ik ded spās) The volume of the conducting airways from the external environment (at the nose and mouth) down to the level at which inspired gas exchanges oxygen and carbon dioxide with pulmonary capillary blood; formerly presumed to extend down to the beginning of alveolar epithelium in the respiratory bronchioles, but more recent evidence indicates that effective gas exchange extends some distance up the thicker-walled conducting airways because of rapid longitudinal mixing. Cf. alveolar dead space, physiologic dead space.

an•a•tom•ic im•po•tence (an′ă-tom′ik im′pŏ-tĕns) Inability of a male to achieve an erection or ejaculate due to physical defect. SEE erectile dysfunction.

an•a•tom•ic pa•thol•o•gy (an′ă-tom′ik pă-thol′ŏ-jē) The subspecialty of pathology that pertains to the gross and microscopic study of organs and tissues removed for biopsy or during postmortem examination, and also the interpretation of the results of such study. SYN pathologic anatomy.

an•a•tom•ic po•si•tion (an′ă-tŏm′ik pŏ-zish′ŏn) Standing erect, arms at the sides, with palms facing forward.

an•a•tom•ic snuff•box (an′ă-tom′ik snŭf′boks) A hollow seen on the radial aspect of the wrist when the thumb is extended fully; it is bounded by the tendon of the extensor pollicis longus posteriorly and of the tendons of the extensor pollicis brevis and abductor pollicis longus anteriorly. The radial artery crosses the floor that is formed by the scaphoid and the trapezium bones.

an•a•tom•ic tooth (an′ă-tom′ik tūth) An artificial tooth that duplicates the anatomic form of a natural tooth.

an•a•tom•ic wart (an′ă-tom′ik wōrt) SYN postmortem wart.

a•nat•o•mist (ă-nat′ŏ-mist) A specialist in the science of anatomy.

a•nat•o•my (ă-nat′ŏ-mē) **1.** The morphologic structure of an organism. **2.** The science of the morphology or structure of organisms. **3.** SYN dissection. **4.** A work describing the form and structure of an organism and its various parts. [G. *anatomē,* dissection, from *ana,* apart, + *tomē,* a cutting]

an•a•tox•in (an′ă-toks′in) A weakened bacterial toxin. [ana- + toxin]

an•a•tri•crot•ic (an′ă-trī-krot′ik) Characterized by anatricrotism; denoting a sphygmographic tracing with three waves on the ascending limb.

an•a•tric•ro•tism (an′ă-trik′rō-tizm) A condition of the pulse manifested by a triple beat on the ascending limb of the sphygmographic tracing. [G. *ana,* up, + *tri-,* thrice, + *krotos,* beating]

ANCA (an′să) Acronym for antineutrophil cytoplasmic antibody.

ANCC Abbreviation for American Nurses Credentialing Center.

an•chor•age (ang′kŏr-ăj) **1.** Operative fixation of loose or prolapsed abdominal or pelvic organs. **2.** The part to which anything is fastened. **3.** DENTISTRY a tooth or an implanted tooth substitute with which a fixed or removable partial denture, crown, or restoration is retained. **4.** The nature and degree of resistance to displacement offered by an anatomic unit when used for the purpose of effecting tooth movement. [L. *ancora,* fr. G. *ankyra,* anchor]

an•chor•ing fi•brils (ang′kŏr-ing fī′brilz) Collagen fibrils that insert into the basal lamina of the epidermis and bind it down to the underlying dermis.

an•chor splint (ang′kŏr splint) An apparatus used to support and immobilize a fractured jaw; wire loops are fitted around the teeth and an external rod is used to hold the device in place.

an•cil•la•ry (an′sil-ar-ē) Auxiliary, accessory, or secondary. [L. *ancillaris,* relating to a maidservant]

an•cil•la•ry ports (an′sil-ar-ē pōrts) A supplemental entry site to allow insertion of instruments other than the endoscope during endoscopic surgery.

an•cil•la•ry ser•vic•es (an′sil-ar-ē sĕr′vi-sĕz) Diagnostic or therapeutic services provided by a professional health care provider for clients on an outpatient basis as an adjunct to basic medical or surgical services.

an•cip•i•tal, an•cip•i•tate, an•cip•i•tous (an-sip′i-tăl, -i-tāt, -i-tŭs) Two-headed; two-edged. [L. *anceps,* two-headed]

an·co·nad (an′kō-nad) Toward the elbow. [G. *ankōn,* elbow, + L. *ad,* to]

an·co·nal, an·co·ne·al (an′kō-năl, an-kō′nē-ăl) **1.** Relating to the elbow (ancon). **2.** Relating to the anconeus muscle.

an·co·ne·us mus·cle (an-kō′nē-ŭs mŭs′ĕl) *Origin,* back of lateral condyle of humerus; *insertion,* olecranon process and posterior surface of ulna; *action,* extends forearm and abducts ulna in pronation of wrist; *nerve supply,* radial. SYN musculus anconeus [TA].

ancylo- SEE ankylo-.

An·cy·lo·sto·ma (an′ki-lo-stō′mă) A genus of Nematoda, the Old World hookworm, the members of which are parasitic in the duodenum. They attach themselves to the mucous membrane, suck blood, and may cause anemia. The eggs are passed with the feces, and the larvae develop in moist soil to become infectious third-stage (filariform) larvae that enter the human body through the skin and possibly in drinking water; they migrate by the bloodstream to lung alveoli, are carried to bronchi and trachea, swallowed, and passed to the intestine, where they mature. SEE ALSO ancylostomiasis, *Necator.* [G. *ankylos,* curved, hooked, + *stoma,* mouth]

An·cy·lo·sto·ma bra·zi·li·en·se (an′ki-lo-stō′mă bră-zil-ē-en′sē) A nematode species characterized by one pair of ventral buccal teeth, normally an intestinal parasite of dogs and cats but also found in humans as a cause of human cutaneous larva migrans.

An·cy·lo·sto·ma ca·ni·num (an′ki-lo-stō′mă kā-nī′nŭm) A nematode species possessing three pairs of ventral teeth in the oral cavity; common in dogs, but also occurring in human skin as a cause of cutaneous larva migrans.

An·cy·lo·sto·ma du·o·de·na·le (an′ki-lo-stō′mă dū-ō′dē-nālē) The Old World hookworm of humans, a species widespread in temperate areas, in contrast to the New World hookworm, *Necator americanus,* which has a more tropical distribution. It is the only hookworm found in the United States.

An·cy·lo·sto·ma tu·bae·for·me (an′ki-lo-stō′mă tū′bē-fōr′mē) A nematode species found in cats; cutaneous larva migrans worms are seen in humans.

an·cy·lo·sto·mi·a·sis (an′ki-lō-stō-mī′ă-sis) Hookworm disease caused by *Ancylostoma duodenale* and characterized by eosinophilia, anemia, emaciation, dyspepsia, and, in children with severe chronic infections, swelling of the abdomen and mental and physical maldevelopment.

an·cy·roid (an-kīr′oyd) Shaped like the fluke of an anchor; denoting the cornua of the lateral ventricles of the brain and the coracoid process of the scapula. [G. *ankyra,* anchor, + *eidos,* resemblance]

An·dersch nerve (ahn′dersh nĕrv) SYN tympanic nerve.

An·der·sen dis·ease (an′dĕr-sĕn di-zēz′) SYN glycogenosis type 4.

An·der·son-Fa·bry dis·ease (an′dĕr-sŏn-fah′brē di-zēz′) SYN Fabry disease.

An·der·son splint (an′dĕr-sŏn splint) A skeletal traction splint with pins inserted into proximal and distal ends of a fracture; reduction is obtained by an external plate attached to the pins.

An·des vi·rus (an′dēz vī′rŭs) A species of hantavirus in Argentina causing hantavirus pulmonary syndrome.

An·drews ma·neu·ver (an′drūz mă-nū′vĕr) SYN Brandt-Andrews maneuver.

andro- Masculine. [G. *anēr, andros,* a male human being]

an·dro·blas·to·ma (an′drō-blas-tō′mă) **1.** A testicular tumor microscopically resembling fetal testis, with varying proportions of tubular and stromal elements; the tubules contain Sertoli cells, which may cause feminization. **2.** SYN arrhenoblastoma. [G. *anēr (andro-),* man, + *blastos,* germ, + *-oma,* tumor]

an·dro·gen (an′drŏ-jen) Generic term for an agent, usually a hormone (e.g., androsterone, testosterone), that stimulates activity of the accessory male sex organs, promotes development of male sex characteristics, or prevents changes in the latter that follow castration; natural androgens are steroids, derivatives of androstane.

an·dro·gen bind·ing pro·tein (ABP) (an′drŏ-jen bīnd′ing prō′tēn) A protein secreted by testicular Sertoli cells along with inhibin and müllerian inhibiting substance. Androgen binding protein probably maintains a high concentration of androgen in the seminiferous tubules.

an·dro·gen·ic al·o·pe·ci·a (an′drō-jen′ik al′ō-pē′shē-ă) Gradual decrease of scalp hair density in adults as a result of familial increased susceptibility of hair follicles to androgen secretion following puberty. SEE ALSO female pattern alopecia, male pattern alopecia. See page 80. SYN alopecia hereditaria, patterned alopecia.

an·dro·gen·ic ste·roid (an′drō-jen′ik ster′oyd) SYN anabolic steroid.

an·dro·gen in·sen·si·tiv·i·ty syn·drome (an′drŏ-jen in-sen′si-tiv′i-tē sin′drōm) SYN androgen resistance syndromes.

an·dro·gen re·sis·tance syn·dromes (an′drŏ-jen rĕ-zis′tăns sin′drōmz) A class of disorders associated with 5α-steroid reductase deficiency, testicular feminization, and related disorders. Cf. Reifenstein syndrome, testicular feminization syndrome. SYN androgen insensitivity syndrome.

an•dro•graph•is (an-drō-graf′is) An Indian herb (*Andrographis paniculata*) that is alleged to be of value in treating cardiovascular disease and disorders of the GI system. Some studies have suggested it may be useful as an anticarcinogenic agent. [G. *aner, andros,* man, + *graphis,* stylus, pencil]

an•drog•y•nous (an-droj′i-nŭs) Pertaining to androgyny.

an•drog•y•ny (an-droj′i-nē) **1.** SYN female pseudohermaphroditism. **2.** Having both masculine and feminine characteristics, as in attitudes and behaviors that contain features of stereotyped, culturally sanctioned sexual roles of both male and female. [andro- + G. *gynē,* woman]

an•droid o•be•si•ty (an′droyd ō-bē′si-tē) Central obesity (apple shape) with fat excess primarily in abdominal wall and visceral mesentery; associated with glucose intolerance, diabetes, decreased sex hormone–binding globulin, increased levels of free testosterone, and increased cardiovascular risk.

an•droid pel•vis (an′droyd pel′vis) A masculine or funnel-shaped pelvis.

an•drol•o•gy (an-drol′ŏ-jē) Branch of medicine concerned with male diseases especially with those affecting the reproductive system. [G. *aner, andros,* man, + *logos,* study,discourse]

an•dro•mor•phous (an′drō-mōr′fŭs) Having a male form or habitus. [andro- + G. *morphē,* form]

an•drop•a•thy (an-drop′ă-thē) A disease or disorder peculiar to males.

an•dro•pause (an′drō-pawz) A postulated decrease in function of male gonads with increasing age, analogous to menopause.

an•dro•pho•bi•a (an′drō-fō′bē-ă) Morbid fear of men, or of the male sex, resulting in avoidance of situations where men are present. [andro- + G. *phobos,* fear]

an•dro•stane (an′drō-stān) The parent hydrocarbon of the androgenic steroids.

an•dro•stane•di•ol (an′drō-stān′dī-ol) 5α-androstane-3β,17β-diol; A steroid metabolite, of which 5β isomers are also known.

an•dro•stane•di•one (an′drō-stān′dī-ōn) A steroid metabolite, of which the 5β isomer is also known.

an•dro•stene (an′drō-stēn) Androstane with an unsaturated (i.e., —CH=CH—) bond in the molecule.

an•dro•stene•di•ol (an′drō-stēn′dī-ol) A steroid metabolite differing from androstanediol by possessing a double bond between C-5 and C-6.

an•dro•stene•di•one (an′drō-stēn′dī-ōn) An androgenic steroid of weaker biologic potency than testosterone; secreted by the testis, ovary, and adrenal cortex.

an•dro•ste•nol (an′drō-stē′nol) A substance that is a postulated pheromone; it is found in male human sweat where it is oxidized to androstenone. In tests, women like the dry, musky smell of androstenol, but find androstenone to have a chemical, urinelike odor that is unpleasant; however, ovulating women react neutrally.

an•dros•ter•one (an-dros′tĕr-ōn) A steroid metabolite, found in male urine, having weak androgenic potency. Formed in testes from progesterone.

an•e•cho•ic (an′ĕ-kō′ik) The property of appearing echo free on a sonographic image; a clear cyst appears anechoic. [G. *an-* priv. + echo + ic]

an•e•cho•ic cham•ber (an′ĕ-kō′ik chām′bĕr) A soundproof environment in which reverbera-

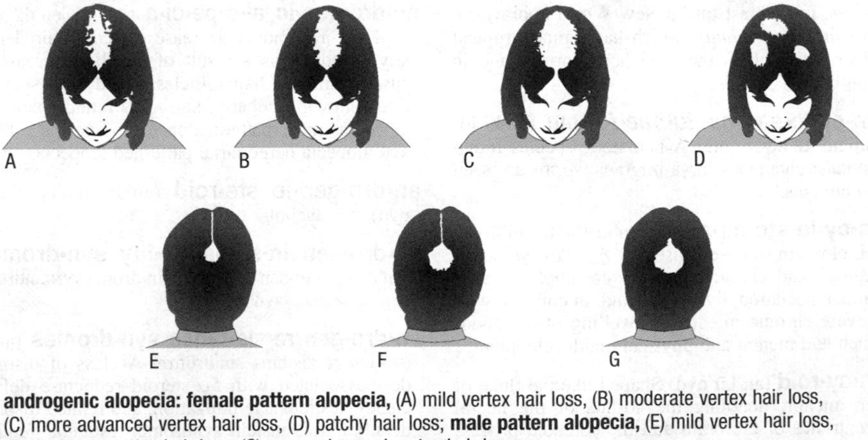

androgenic alopecia: female pattern alopecia, (A) mild vertex hair loss, (B) moderate vertex hair loss, (C) more advanced vertex hair loss, (D) patchy hair loss; **male pattern alopecia,** (E) mild vertex hair loss, (F) moderate vertex hair loss, (G) more advanced vertex hair loss

tion is largely eliminated, for the performance of audiologic testing and research.

A•nel meth•od (ah′nel meth′ŏd) Ligation of an artery immediately above (on the proximal side of) an aneurysm.

A•nem•ar•rhe•na (ă-nem′ă-rē′nă) *A. asphodeloides*, an herb used in traditional Chinese medicine where it is purportedly of value in treating fever, bowel and urinary disorders, and some infectious diseases.

a•ne•mi•a (ă-nē′mē-ă) Any condition in which the number of red blood cells per mm^3, the amount of hemoglobin in 100 mL of blood, or the volume of packed red blood cells per 100 mL of blood is less than normal; clinically, generally pertaining to the concentration of oxygen-transporting material in a designated volume of blood, in contrast to total quantities as in oligocythemia, oligochromemia, and oligemia. Anemia is frequently manifested by pallor of the skin and mucous membranes, shortness of breath, palpitations of the heart, soft systolic murmurs, lethargy, and fatigability. SYN anaemia. [G. *anaimia,* fr. *an-* priv. + *haima,* blood]

a•ne•mic (ă-nē′mik) Pertaining to or manifesting the various features of anemia. SYN anaemic.

a•ne•mic an•ox•i•a (ă-nē′mik an-ok′sē-ă) Anemic hypoxia in which oxygen is almost completely lacking. SYN anaemic anoxia.

a•ne•mic ha•lo (ă-nē′mik hā′lō) Pale, relatively avascular areas in the skin seen around vascular spiders, cherry angiomas, and sometimes in acute macular eruptions. SYN anaemic halo.

a•ne•mic hy•pox•i•a (ă-nē′mik hī-pok′sē-ă) Hypoxia resulting from a decreased concentration of functional hemoglobin or a reduced number of erythrocytes. SYN anaemic hypoxia.

a•ne•mic in•farct (ă-nē′mik in′fahrkt) An infarct in which little or no bleeding into tissue spaces occurs when the blood supply is obstructed. SYN anaemic infarct, white infarct (1).

a•ne•mic mur•mur (ă-nē′mik mŭr′mŭr) A nonvalvular murmur heard on auscultation of the heart and large blood vessels in cases of profound anemia associated mainly with turbulent blood flow due to decreased blood viscosity. SYN anaemic murmur, hemic murmur.

an•e•mo•pho•bi•a (an′ĕ-mō-fō′bē-ă) Morbid fear of wind. [G. *anemos,* wind, + *phobos,* fear]

an•en•ce•phal•ic (an′en-sĕ-fal′ik) Relating to meroencephaly.

an•en•ceph•a•lus (an′en-sef′ă-lŭs) A fetus lacking all or most of the brain. [G. *an,* without, + *enkephalos,* brain]

an•en•ceph•a•ly (an′en-sef′ă-lē) SYN meroencephaly. [G. *an-* priv. + *enkephalos,* brain]

a•neph•ric (ā-nef′rik) Lacking kidneys. [*a-* priv. + G. *nephros,* kidney]

an•er•ga•si•a (an′ĕr-gā′zē-ă) Absence of psychic activity as the result of organic brain disease. [G. *an-* priv. + *ergasia,* work]

an•er•gas•tic (an′ĕr-gas′tik) Pertaining to or characterized by anergasia.

an•er•gic (an-ĕr′jik) Relating to, or marked by, anergy.

an•er•gy (an′ĕr-jē) **1.** Absence of ability to generate a sensitivity reaction in a subject to substances expected to be antigenic (immunogenic, allergenic) in that individual. **2.** Lack of energy. [G. *an-* priv. + *energeia,* energy, from *ergon,* work]

an•er•oid (an′ĕr-oyd) Not containing liquid (e.g., a sphygmomanometer that does not contain a column of liquid mercury).

an•e•ryth•ro•pla•si•a (an′ĕ-rith′rō-plā′zē-ă) A condition in which red blood cells do not form. [G. *an-* priv. + erythro(cyte) + G. *plasis,* a molding]

an•e•ryth•ro•plas•tic (an′ĕ-rith′rō-plas′tik) Pertaining to or characterized by anerythroplasia.

an•es•the•ki•ne•si•a (an-es′thē-ki-nē′zē-ă) Combined sensory and motor paralysis. SYN anaesthekinesia. [G. *an-* priv. + *aisthēsis,* sensation, + *kinēsis,* movement]

an•es•the•si•a (an′es-thē′zē-ă) **1.** Loss of sensation resulting from pharmacologic depression of nerve function or from neurologic dysfunction; may be local, topical, general, or regional, depending on the affected area. **2.** Broad term for anesthesiology as a clinical specialty. SYN anaesthesia. [G. *anaisthēsia,* fr. *an-* priv. + *aisthēsis,* sensation]

an•es•the•si•a do•lo•ro•sa (an′es-thē′zē-ă dō-lō-rō′să) Severe spontaneous pain occurring in an anesthetized area. SYN anaesthesia dolorosa.

an•es•the•si•a rec•ord (an′es-thē′zē-ă rek′ŏrd) A written account of drug(s) administered, treatment, procedures, and physiologic responses observed during the course of anesthesia. SYN anaesthesia record.

an•es•the•si•ol•o•gist (an′es-thē′zē-ol′ŏ-jist) **1.** A physician specializing in anesthesiology. **2.** A person with a doctoral degree who is certified and legally qualified to administer anesthetics and related techniques. Cf. anesthetist. SYN anaesthesiologist.

an•es•the•si•ol•o•gy (an′es-thē′zē-ol′ŏ-jē) The medical specialty concerned with the pharmacologic, physiologic, and clinical basis of anesthesia and related fields, including resuscitation, intensive respiratory care, and the management of acute and chronic pain. SYN anaesthesiology. [anesthesia + G. *logos,* treatise]

an·es·thet·ic (an′es-thet′ik) **1.** A compound that depresses neuronal function, producing loss of ability to perceive pain and/or other sensations. **2.** Collective designation for anesthetizing agents administered to a person at a particular time. **3.** Characterized by loss of sensation or capable of producing loss of sensation. **4.** Associated with or due to the state of anesthesia. See this page. SYN anaesthetic.

an·es·thet·ic depth (an′es-thet′ik depth) The degree of central nervous system depression produced by a general anesthetic agent; a function of potency of the anesthetic and the concentration in which it is administered.

an·es·thet·ic gas (an′es-thet′ik gas) SEE inhalation anesthetic.

an·es·thet·ic in·dex (an′es-thet′ik in′deks) Ratio of the number of units of anesthetic required for anesthesia to the number of units of anesthetic required to produce respiratory or cardiovascular failure.

an·es·thet·ic lep·ro·sy (an′es-thet′ik lep′rŏ-sē) A form of leprosy chiefly affecting the nerves, marked by hyperesthesia succeeded by anesthesia, and by paralysis, ulceration, and various trophic disturbances, terminating in gangrene and mutilation. SYN Danielssen disease, trophoneurotic leprosy.

a·nes·the·tist (ă-nes′thĕ-tist) One who administers an anesthetic, whether an anesthesiologist, a physician who is not an anesthesiologist, a nurse anesthetist, or an anesthesia assistant. SYN anaesthetist.

a·nes·the·ti·za·tion (ă-nes′thĕ-tī-ză′shun) The act of producing loss of sensation.

a·nes·the·tize (ă-nes′thĕ-tīz) To produce loss of sensation.

an·es·trus (an-es′trŭs) The period between two estrus (heat) cycles. SYN anoestrus. [G. *an-* priv. + *oistros,* estrus]

an·e·to·der·ma (an′ĕ-tō-dĕr′mă) Atrophoderma in which the skin becomes baglike and wrinkled. [G. *anetos,* relaxed, + *derma,* skin]

an·eu·ploid (an′yū-ployd) Having an abnormal number of chromosomes not an exact multiple of the haploid number, as contrasted with abnormal numbers of complete haploid sets of chromosomes, such as diploid, triploid. [G. *an-* priv. + euploid]

an·eu·ploi·dy (an′yū-ploy′dē) State of being aneuploid.

an·eu·rysm (an′yūr-izm) **1.** Circumscribed dilation of an artery in direct communication with the lumen, usually due to an acquired or congenital weakness of the wall of the artery. **2.** Circumscribed dilation of a cardiac chamber usually due to an acquired or congenital weakness of the wall of the heart. See page 83. [G. *aneurysma* (*-mat-*), a dilation, fr. *eurys,* wide]

an·eu·rys·mal, an·eu·rys·mat·ic (an′yūr-iz′măl, iz-mat′ik) Relating to an aneurysm.

an·eu·rys·mal bone cyst (an′yūr-iz′măl bōn sist) A solitary benign osteolytic lesion expanding a long bone or within a vertebra, consisting of blood-filled spaces, and separated by fibrous tissue containing multinucleated giant cells; such cysts cause swelling, pain, and tenderness.

an·eu·rys·mal bru·it (an′yūr-iz′măl brū-ē′) Blowing murmur heard over an aneurysm.

an·eu·rys·mal var·ix (an′yūr-iz′măl var′iks) Dilation and tortuosity of a vein resulting from an acquired communication with an adjacent artery. SYN Pott aneurysm.

an·eu·rys·mec·to·my (an′yūr-iz-mek′tŏ-mē) Excision of an aneurysm. [aneurysm + G. *ektomē,* excision]

an·eu·rys·mo·graph (an′yūr-iz′mō-graf) Demonstration of an aneurysm, usually by means of x-rays and a contrast medium. [aneurysm + G. *graphō,* to write]

an·eu·rys·mo·plas·ty (an′yūr-iz′mō-plas-tē) Repair of an aneurysm by opening the sac and suturing its walls. SEE ALSO aneurysmorrhaphy. SYN endoaneurysmoplasty, endoaneurysmorrhaphy. [aneurysm + G. *plastos,* formed]

an·eu·rys·mor·rha·phy (an′yūr-iz-mōr′ă-fē) Closure by suture of the sac of an aneurysm to restore the normal lumen dimensions. [aneurysm + G. *rhaphē,* suture]

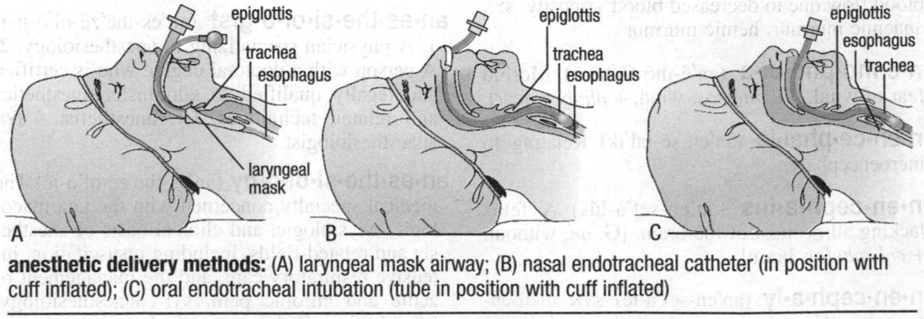

anesthetic delivery methods: (A) laryngeal mask airway; (B) nasal endotracheal catheter (in position with cuff inflated); (C) oral endotracheal intubation (tube in position with cuff inflated)

an•eu•rys•mot•o•my (an′yūr-iz-mot′ŏ-mē) Incision into the sac of an aneurysm. [aneurysm + G. *tomē,* incision]

ANF **1.** Abbreviation for antinuclear factor; Australian Nurses Association; American Nurses Foundation. **2.** Abbreviation of atrial natriuretic factor also known as ANP (i.e., atrial natriuretic peptide); a hormone produced by cardiac atria in response to increased fluid volume or pressure.

an•gel•i•ca (an-jel′i-kă) An Asian herb (*A. sinensis*) that is used in many forms (dried root preparations, oils, tinctures) against myriad complaints; adverse reactions have been widely reported with use of this agent. SYN dong quai. [L., angelic]

An•gel•man syn•drome (an′jĕl-măn sin′drōm) Genetic condition characterized by mental retardation, seizures, ataxic gait, jerky movements, lack of speech, and frequent smiling or laughing.

An•ge•luc•ci syn•drome (ahn-jĕ-lū′chē sin′drōm) Extreme excitability, vasomotor disturbances, and palpitation associated with vernal conjunctivitis.

an•gel wing (ān′jĕl wing) A deformity in which both scapulae project conspicuously. SEE ALSO winged scapula.

an•gi•ec•ta•si•a, **an•gi•ec•ta•sis** (an′jē-ek-tā′zē-ă, -ek′tă-sis) Dilation of a lymphatic or blood vessel. [angio- + G. *ektasis,* a stretching]

an•gi•ec•tat•ic (an′jē-ek-tat′ik) Marked by the presence of dilated blood vessels. [angio- + G. *ektatos,* capable of extension]

an•gi•ec•to•pi•a (an′jē-ek-tō′pē-ă) Abnormal location of a blood vessel. [angio- + G. *ektopos,* out of place]

an•gi•i•tis, **an•gi•tis** (an′jē-ī′tis, an-jī′tis) Inflammation of a blood vessel (arteritis, phlebitis) or lymphatic vessel (lymphangitis). SYN vasculitis. [angio- + G. *-itis,* inflammation]

an•gi•na (an′ji-nă) A severe, often constricting pain; caused by reduced arterial blood to the myocardium, which reduces oxygen supplied to the myocardial cells; causes injury and ischemia and the sharp precordial pain directly related to cardiac ischemia; usually refers to angina pectoris. [L. quinsy]

an•gi•na cru•ris (an′ji-nă krū′ris) Intermittent claudication of the leg.

an•gi•na in•ver•sa (an′ji-nă in-vĕr′să) SYN Prinzmetal angina.

an•gi•nal (an′ji-năl) Relating to angina in any sense.

an•gi•na pec•to•ris (an′ji-nă pek′tō′ris) Paroxysmal severe constricting pain or pressure in the chest due to myocardial ischemia; typically radiates from the precordium to one or both shoulders, neck, or jaw; often precipitated by exertion, exposure to cold, or emotional excitement. SYN stenocardia.

an•gi•na scale (an′ji-nă skāl) A four-part scale used to describe the severity of angina (1+ = mild, to 4+ = severe).

an•gi•noid (an′jin-oid) Resembling angina, especially angina pectoris; term rarely used.

an•gi•nose, **an•gi•nous** (an′ji-nōs, -ji-nŭs) Relating to angina; term rarely used.

an•gi•nose scar•la•ti•na, **scar•la•ti•na an•gi•no•sa** (an′ji-nōs skahr′lă-tē′nă, skahr′lă-tē′nă an-jē-nō′să) A form of scarlatina in which the throat affliction is unusually severe. SYN Fothergill disease (2).

♻**angio-**, **angi-** Combining forms meaning blood or lymph vessels; a covering, an enclosure; corresponds to L. *vas*, *vaso-*, *vasculo-*. [G. *angeion,* a vessel or cavity of the body, fr. *angos*, a vessel, vat, bucket, + *-eion*, small, little]

an•gi•o•blast (an′jē-ō-blast) **1.** A cell taking part in blood vessel formation. SYN vasoformative cell. **2.** Primordial mesenchymal tissue from which embryonic blood cells and vascular endothelium are differentiated. [angio- + G. *blastos,* germ]

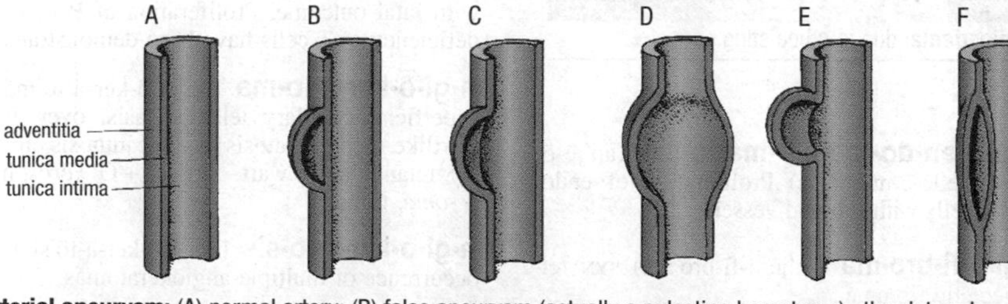

arterial aneurysm: (A) normal artery; (B) false aneurysm (actually a pulsating hematoma)–the clot and connective tissue are outside the arterial wall; (C) true aneurysm–one, two, or all three layers may be involved; (D) fusiform aneurysm–symmetric, spindle-shaped expansion of entire circumference of involved vessel; (E) saccular aneurysm–a bulbous protrusion of one side of the arterial wall; (F) dissecting aneurysm–this usually is an expanding hematoma that splits the layers of the arterial wall

an·gi·o·blas·to·ma (an′jē-ō-blas-tō′mă) SYN hemangioblastoma.

an·gi·o·car·di·og·ra·phy (an′jē-ō-kahr-dē-og′ră-fē) Diagnostic x-ray imaging of the heart and great vessels made visible by injection of a radiopaque solution. SEE coronary angiography. [angio- + G. *kardia,* heart, + *graphō,* to write]

an·gi·o·car·di·o·ki·net·ic, **an·gi·o·car·di·o·ci·net·ic** (an′jē-ō-kahr′dē-ō-ki-net′ik, an′jē-ō-kahr′dē-ō-si-net′ik) Causing dilation or contraction in the heart and blood vessels. [angio- + G. *kardia,* heart, + *kinēsis,* movement]

an·gi·o·car·di·op·a·thy (an′jē-ō-kahr′dē-op′ă-thē) Disease affecting both heart and blood vessels. [angio- + G. *kardia,* heart, + *pathos,* disease]

an·gi·o·dys·pla·si·a (an′jē-ō-dis-plā′zē-ă) Degenerative or congenital structural abnormality of the normally distributed vasculature.

an·gi·o·dys·tro·phy, **an·gi·o·dys·tro·phi·a** (an′jē-ō-dis′trŏ-fē, -dis-trō′fē-ă) Defective formation or growth associated with marked vascular changes. [angio- + G. *dys-,* bad, + *trophē,* nourishment]

an·gi·o·e·de·ma (an′jē-ō-ĕ-dē′mă) **1.** Recurrent large circumscribed areas of subcutaneous edema of sudden onset, usually disappearing within 24 hours; seen mainly in young women, frequently as an allergic reaction to foods or drugs. See this page. SYN angio-oedema, angioneurotic edema (1), Bannister disease, giant urticaria. **2.** SYN Quincke disease.

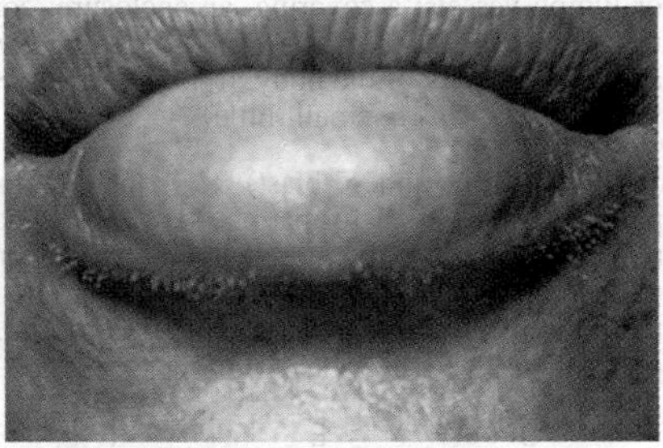

angioedema: due to a bee sting

an·gi·o·en·do·the·li·o·ma·to·sis (an′jē-ō-en-dō-thē′lē-ō-mă-tō′sis) Proliferation of endothelial cells within blood vessels.

an·gi·o·fi·bro·ma (an′jē-ō-fī-brō′mă) SYN telangiectatic fibroma.

an·gi·o·fi·bro·sis (an′jē-ō-fī-brō′sis) Fibrosis of the walls of blood vessels.

an·gi·o·gen·e·sis (an′jē-ō-jen′ĕ-sis) 1. Development of blood vessels in the embryo. 2. Any formation of new blood vessels. [angio- + G. *genesis,* birth, formation]

an·gi·o·gen·e·sis fac·tor (an′jē-ō-jen′ĕ-sis fak′tŏr) A substance of 2000–20,000 MW that is secreted by macrophages and stimulates neovascularization in healing wounds or in the stroma of tumors.

an·gi·o·gen·ic (an′jē-ō-jen′ik) **1.** Relating to angiogenesis. **2.** Of vascular origin.

an·gi·o·gli·o·ma (an′jē-ō-glī-ō′mă) A mixed glioma and angioma.

an·gi·o·gram (an′jē-ō-gram) Radiograph obtained by angiography. See page B22, B26. [angio- + G. *gramma,* a writing]

an·gi·o·graph·ic (an′jē-ō-graf′ik) Relating to or using angiography.

an·gi·og·ra·phy (an′jē-og′ră-fē) Radiography of vessels after the injection of a radiopaque contrast material; usually requires percutaneous insertion of a radiopaque catheter and positioning under fluoroscopic control. SEE ALSO arteriography, venography. See page B22. [angio- + G. *graphō,* to write]

an·gi·og·ra·phy cath·e·ter (an′jē-og′ră-fē kath′ĕ-tĕr) A thin-walled tube suitable for percutaneous puncture and injection of contrast media for radiography.

an·gi·oid (an′jē-oyd) Resembling blood vessels; in a branching pattern. [angio- + G. *eidos,* resemblance]

an·gi·oid streaks (an′jē-oyd strēks) Breaks in Bruch membrane visible in the peripapillary fundus oculi, and sometimes mistaken for choroidal vessels. SYN Knapp streaks, Knapp striae.

an·gi·o·im·mu·no·blas·tic lym·phad·e·nop·a·thy with dys·pro·tein·e·mi·a (an′jē-ō-im′yū-nō-blas′tik limf′ad-ĕ-nŏp′ă-thē dis′prō-tēn-ē′mē-ă) A lymphoproliferative disorder characterized by generalized lymphadenopathy, hepatosplenomegaly, fever, sweats, weight loss, skin lesions, and pruritus with hypergammaglobulinemia; occurs primarily in older adults, often with fatal outcome. Proliferation of B cells and deficiency of T cells have been demonstrated.

an·gi·o·ker·a·to·ma (an′jē-ō-ker-ă-tō′mă) A superficial capillary telangiectasis, over which wartlike hyperkeratosis and acanthosis appear. SYN telangiectatic wart. [angio- + G. *keras,* horn, + *-ōma,* tumor]

an·gi·o·ker·a·to·sis (an′jē-ō-ker-ă-tō′sis) The occurrence of multiple angiokeratomas.

an·gi·o·ki·ne·sis (an′jē-ō-ki-nē′sis) SYN vasomotion. [angio- + G. *kinēsis,* movement]

an·gi·o·ki·net·ic (an′jē-ō-ki-net′ik) SYN vasomotor. [angio- + G. *kinētikos,* pertaining to movement]

an·gi·o·lith (an′jē-ō-lith) An arteriolith or a phlebolith. [angio- + G. *lithos,* stone]

an·gi·o·lith·ic (an′jē-ō-lith′ik) Relating to an angiolith.

an·gi·ol·o·gy (an-jē-ol′ŏ-jē) The science concerned with the blood vessels and lymphatics in all their relations. [angio- + G. *logos,* treatise, discourse]

an·gi·o·lu·poid (an′jē-ō-lū′poyd) A sarcoidlike eruption of the skin in which the granulomatous telangiectatic papules are distributed over the nose and cheeks. [angio- + L. *lupus,* wolf, + G. *eidos,* resemblance]

an·gi·ol·y·sis (an′jē-ol′i-sis) Obliteration of a blood vessel, such as occurs in the newborn infant after tying of the umbilical cord. [angio- + G. *lysis,* destruction]

an·gi·o·ma (an′jē-ō′mă) A swelling or benign tumor due to proliferation, with or without dilation, of the blood vessels (hemangioma) or lymphatics (lymphangioma). [angio- + G. *-ōma,* tumor]

an·gi·o·ma ser·pi·gi·no·sum (an′jē-ō′mă sĕr-pij-i-nō′sŭm) The presence of rings of red dots on the skin (especially in female children) that tend to widen peripherally, due to dilatation of superficial capillaries. SYN essential telangiectasia (2).

an·gi·o·ma·toid (an′jē-ō′mă-toyd) Resembling a tumor of vascular origin.

an·gi·o·ma·to·sis (an′jē-ō-mă-tō′sis) A condition characterized by multiple angiomas.

an·gi·o·ma·tous (an′jē-ō′mă-tŭs) Relating to or resembling an angioma.

an·gi·o·myx·o·ma (an′jē-ō-miks-ō′mă) A myxoma in which there is an unusually large number of vascular structures.

an·gi·o·neu·rec·to·my (an′jē-ō-nūr-ek′tō-mē) **1.** Excision of the vessels and nerves of a part. **2.** Excision of a segment of the spermatic cord to produce sterility. [angio- + G. *neuron,* nerve, + *ektomē,* excision]

an·gi·o·neu·rot·ic e·de·ma (an′jē-ō-nūr-ot′ik ĕ-dē′mă) **1.** SYN angioedema. **2.** SYN Quincke disease.

angio-oedema [Br.] SYN angioedema.

an·gi·op·a·thy (an′jē-op′ă-thē) Any disease of the blood vessels or lymphatics. SYN angiosis. [angio- + G. *pathos,* suffering]

an·gi·o·phac·o·ma·to·sis, an·gi·o·phak·o·ma·to·sis (an′jē-ō-fak′ō-mă-tō′sis, an′jē-ō′fak′ō-mă-tō′sis) The angiomatous phacomatoses: von Hippel-Lindau disease and Sturge-Weber syndrome.

an·gi·o·plas·ty (an′jē-ō-plas-tē) Reconstitution or recanalization of a blood vessel; may involve balloon dilation, mechanical stripping of intima, forceful injection of fibrinolytics, or placement of a stent. SEE percutaneous coronary intervention. [angio- + G. *plastos,* formed, shaped]

an·gi·o·plas·ty bal·loon (an′jē-ō-plas-tē bă-lūn′) A balloon near the tip of an angiographic catheter, designed to distend narrowed vessels. SEE balloon-tip catheter.

an·gi·o·poi·e·sis (an′jē-ō-poy-ē′sis) Formation of blood or lymphatic vessels. SYN vasifaction, vasoformation. [angio- + G. *poiesis,* making]

an·gi·o·poi·et·ic (an′jē-ō-poy-et′ik) Relating to angiopoiesis. SYN vasifactive, vasoformative.

an·gi·or·rha·phy (an′jē-ōr′ă-fē) Suture repair of any vessel, especially of a blood vessel. [angio- + G. *rhaphē,* a seam]

an·gi·o·sar·co·ma (an′jē-ō-sahr-kō′mă) A rare malignant neoplasm occurring most often in the breast and skin, and believed to originate from the endothelial and fibroblastic cells of blood vessels; microscopically composed of closely packed round or spindle-shaped cells, some of which line small spaces resembling vascular clefts.

an·gi·os·co·py (an′jē-os′kŏ-pē) **1.** Visualization with a microscope of the passage of substances (e.g., contrast media, radiopaque agents) through capillaries after intravenous injection. **2.** Visualization of the interior of blood vessels, especially the pulmonary arteries, using a fiberoptic catheter inserted through a peripheral artery. [angio- + G. *skopeō,* to view]

an·gi·o·sco·to·ma (an′jē-ō-skō-tō′mă) Ribbon-shaped defect of the visual fields caused by the retinal vessels overlying photoreceptors. [angio- + G. *skotōma,* dizziness, vertigo]

an·gi·o·sco·tom·e·try (an′jē-ō-skō-tom′ĕ-trē) The measurement or projection of the angioscotoma pattern.

an·gi·o·sis (an-jē-ō′sis) SYN angiopathy.

an·gi·o·some (an′je-ō-sōm) Composite anatomic vascular territories of skin and underlying muscles, tendons, nerves, and bones, based on segmental or distributing arteries.

an·gi·o·spasm (an′jē-ō-spazm) SYN vasospasm.

an·gi·o·spas·tic (an′jē-ō-spas′tik) SYN vasospastic.

an·gi·o·ste·no·sis (an′jē-ō-stĕ-nō′sis) Narrowing of one or more blood vessels. [angio- + G. *stenōsis,* a narrowing]

an·gi·o·ten·sin (an′jē-ō-ten′sin) A family of peptides with vasoconstrictive activity, produced by action of renin on angiotensinogen.

an·gi·o·ten·sin-con·vert·ing en·zyme (ACE) (an′jē-ō-ten′sin-kŏn-vĕrt′ing en′zīm) A hydrolase responsible for the conversion of angiotensin I to the vasoactive angiotensin II by removal of a dipeptide (histidylleucine) from angiotensin I. Drugs that inhibit ACE are used to treat hypertension and congestive heart failure.

an•gi•o•ten•sin-con•vert•ing en•zyme (ACE) in•hib•i•tor (an′jē-ō-ten′sin-kŏn-vĕrt′ing en′zīm in-hib′i-tŏr) A class of drugs used in the treatment of hypertension; they produce a reduction of peripheral arterial resistance, although the exact mechanism of action has not been fully determined; they block the conversion of angiotensin I to angiotensin II, a powerful vasoconstrictor.

an•gi•o•ten•sin II (an′jē-ō-ten′sin) A vasoactive octapeptide produced by the action of angiotensin-converting enzyme on angiotensin I; produces stimulation of vascular smooth muscle, promotes aldosterone production, and stimulates the sympathetic nervous system.

an•gi•o•ten•sin III am•ide (an′jē-ō-tēn′sin am′īd) A synthetic substance closely related to naturally occurring angiotensin II; it is a potent vasopressor useful in certain types of shock and circulatory collapse.

an•gi•o•ten•sin II re•cep•tor block•er (ARB) (an′jē-ō-ten′sin rĕ-sep′tŏr blok′ĕr) A drug that binds with angiotensin receptors, preventing endogenous angiotensin II from acting on them and thus reducing the vasoconstriction and sodium retention usually induced by that agonist; used to treat hypertension.

an•gi•o•ten•sin•o•gen (an′jē-ō-ten-sin′ō-jen) The substrate for renin whereon through enzymatic action angiotensin I is liberated; an abundant α_2-globulin that circulates in the blood plasma.

an•gi•o•ten•sin•o•gen•ase (an′jē-ō-ten-si-noj′ĕn-ās) SYN renin.

an•gi•o•ten•sin re•cep•tor block•er (an′jē-ō-ten′sin rĕ-sep′tŏr blok′ĕr) An agent (e.g., losartan) that binds with angiotensin receptors, thus preventing access of angiotensin II to the receptor and consequently reducing the vasoconstriction produced by this agonist; used in the treatment of hypertension.

an•gi•o•ten•sin re•cep•tors (an′jē-ō-ten′sin rē-sep′tŏrz) Cell-surface G-protein–coupled receptors that mediate the effects of angiotensin II. Two types are recognized: AT_1 and AT_2; the former mediates the powerful vascular smooth-muscle contraction responsible for the hypertensive response produced by angiotensin II; the latter is not sufficiently understood to be assigned any physiologic function.

an•gi•ot•o•my (an′jē-ot′ŏ-mē) Sectioning of a blood vessel, or the creation of an opening into a vessel before it undergoes repair. [angio- + G. *tomē,* cutting]

an•gi•o•to•ni•a (an′jē-ō-tō′nē-ă) SYN vasotonia.

an•gi•o•tro•phic (an′jē-ō-trō′fik) Rarely used term for vasotrophic. [angio- + G. *trophē,* nourishment]

an•gle (ang′gĕl) The figure formed by the junction of two lines or planes; the space bounded on two sides by lines or planes that meet. For specific angles, see the descriptive term, e.g., axioincisal, distobuccal, labiogingival, linguogingival (2), mesiogingival, proximobuccal. SYN angulus [TA]. [L. *angulus*]

An•gle clas•si•fi•ca•tion of mal•oc•clu•sion (ang′gĕl klas′i-fi-kā′shŭn mal′ŏ-klū′zhŭn) A classification of different types of malocclusion, based primarily on the mesiodistal relationship of the permanent molars on their eruption and locking, and composed of three classes; *Class I,* normal relationship of the jaws, wherein the mesiobuccal cusp of the maxillary first molar occludes in the buccal groove of the mandibular first permanent molar but with crowding and rotation of teeth elsewhere; *Class II,* distal relationship of the mandible, wherein the distobuccal cusp of the maxillary first permanent molar occludes in the buccal groove of the mandibular first molar, and further classified as Division 1, labioversion of maxillary incisor teeth, and Division 2, linguoversion of maxillary central incisors, both of which may be unilateral conditions; *Class III,* mesial relationship of the mandible, wherein the mesiobuccal cusp of the maxillary first molar occludes in the embrasure between the mandibular first and second permanent molars, and further classified as a unilateral condition.

an•gle-clo•sure glau•co•ma (ang′gĕl-klō′zhŭr glaw-kō′mă) Primary glaucoma in which contact of the iris with the peripheral cornea excludes aqueous humor from the trabecular drainage meshwork; may develop in either eye or both. SYN narrow-angle glaucoma.

an•gle of con•ver•gence (ang′gĕl kŏn-vĕr′jĕns) The angle that the visual axis forms with the median line when a near object is viewed.

an•gle of ec•cen•tric•i•ty (ang′gĕl ek′sen-tris′i-tē) In strabismus, the angle between the line of fixation and the line of normal foveal fixation.

an•gle of i•ris (ang′gĕl ī′ris) SYN iridocorneal angle.

an•gle of jaw (ang′gĕl jaw) SYN angle of mandible.

an•gle of man•di•ble (ang′gĕl man′di-bĕl) The angle formed by the lower margin of the body and the posterior margin of the ramus of the mandible. SYN angulus mandibulae [TA], angle of jaw.

an•gle re•ces•sion (ang′gĕl rĕ-sesh′ŭn) Tearing of the iris root between the longitudinal and circular ciliary muscles; often leading to glaucoma.

an•gle of re•tro•ver•sion (ang′gĕl ret′rō-vĕr′

zhŭn) The angle formed by a line drawn through the center of the longitudinal axis of the neck and head of the humerus meeting a line drawn along the transverse axis of the condyles, when the base is viewed from above, looking straight down from above the head of the humerus; the normal angle of retroversion of the humerus is 20 to 40 degrees.

an•gle of tor•sion (ang′gĕl tōr′shŭn) The amount of rotation of a long bone along its axis or between two axes, measured in degrees.

ang•strom (Å) (ang′strŏm) A unit of wavelength, 10^{-10} m, roughly the diameter of an atom; equivalent to 0.1 nm.

Ång•ström law (eng′strŏm law) A substance absorbs light of the same wavelength as it emits when luminous.

Ång•ström u•nit (Å) (eng′strŏm yū′nit) SEE angstrom.

an•gu•lar ar•ter•y (ang′gyŭ-lăr ahr′tĕr-ē) The terminal branch of the facial artery; *distribution*, muscles and skin of side of nose; *anastomoses*, lateral nasal, and dorsal artery of nose and palpebrals from the ophthalmic artery, thereby providing an external-internal carotid arterial anastomosis. SYN arteria angularis [TA].

an•gu•lar chei•li•tis (ang′gyŭ-lăr kī-lī′tis) SYN angular cheilosis.

an•gu•lar chei•lo•sis (ang′gyŭ-lăr kī-lō′sis) Reddish inflammation of the lip or lips and production of fissures that radiate from the angles of the mouth. See this page. SYN angular cheilitis, angular stomatitis.

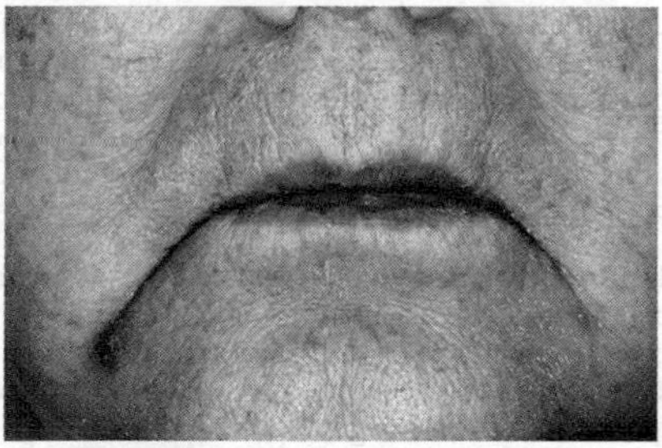

angular cheilosis: flaccid perioral folds

an•gu•lar cur•va•ture (ang′gyŭ-lăr kŭr′vă-chŭr) A gibbous deformity, i.e., a sharp angulation of the spine, occurring in Pott disease. SYN Pott curvature.

an•gu•lar gy•rus (ang′gyŭ-lăr jī′rŭs) A folded convolution in the inferior parietal lobule formed by the union of the posterior ends of the superior and middle temporal gyri.

an•gu•lar mo•men•tum (ang′gyŭ-lăr mō-men′tŭm) The spin of MR active nuclei, which depends on the balance between the number of protons and neutrons in the nucleus.

an•gu•lar spine (ang′gyŭ-lăr spīn) SYN sphenoidal spine.

an•gu•lar sto•ma•ti•tis (ang′gyŭ-lăr stō′mă-tī′tis) SYN angular cheilosis.

an•gu•lar vein (ang′gyŭ-lăr vān) A short vein at the medial angle of the eye, formed by the supraorbital and supratrochlear veins and continuing as the facial vein.

an•gu•la•tion (ang′gyū-lā′shŭn) **1.** Formation of an angle; an abnormal angle or bend in an organ. **2.** In orthopedics, a method of describing the alignment of long bones that have been affected by injury or disease; can be described in both anteroposterior and lateral planes.

an•gu•lus, gen. and pl. **an•gu•li** (ang′gyū-lŭs, -lī) [TA] SYN angle. [L.]

an•gu•lus ac•ro•mi•i (ang′gyū-lŭs ak-rō′mē-ī) [TA] SYN acromial angle.

an•gu•lus cos•tae (ang′gyū-lŭs kos′tē) [TA] SYN costal angle.

an•gu•lus ir•i•do•cor•ne•a•lis (ang′gyū-lŭs ir′i-dō-kōr-nē-ā′lis) [TA] SYN iridocorneal angle.

an•gu•lus man•dib•u•lae (ang′gyū-lŭs man-dib′yū-lē) [TA] SYN angle of mandible.

an•gu•lus pon•to•cer•e•bel•la•ris (ang′gyū-lŭs pon′tō-ser-ĕ-bel-ā′ris) [TA] SYN cerebellopontine angle.

an•gu•lus ster•ni (ang′gyū-lŭs stĕr′nī) [TA] SYN sternal angle.

an•gu•lus sub•pu•bi•cus (ang′gyū-lŭs sŭb-pyū′bi-kŭs) [TA] SYN subpubic angle.

an•he•do•ni•a (an′hē-dō′nē-ă) Absence of pleasure from the performance of acts that would ordinarily be pleasurable. [G. *an-* priv. + *hedonē*, pleasure]

an•hi•dro•sis (an′hī-drō′sis) Inability to tolerate heat; reduction or complete absence of sweating. SYN adiaphoresis. [G. *an-* priv. + *hidrōs*, sweat]

an•hi•drot•ic (an′hī-drot′ik) **1.** Relating to, or characterized by, anhidrosis. **2.** Denoting a reduction or absence of sweat glands, characteristic of congenital ectodermal defect and anhidrotic ectodermal dysplasia.

an•hy•dram•ni•os (an-hī-dram′nē-os) A lack of amniotic fluid. [*an- priv.* + hydramnios]

an•hy•drase (an-hī′drās) An enzyme that catalyzes the removal of water from a compound; most such enzymes are now known as hydrases, hydrolyases, or dehydratases.

an•hy•dra•tion (an′hī-drā′shŭn) SYN dehydration (1).

an•hy•dride (an-hī′drīd) An oxide that can combine with water to form an acid or that is derived from an acid by the abstraction of water.

♻**anhydro-** Chemical prefix denoting the removal of water. Cf. pyro- (2). [G. *an-* priv., + *hydōr,* water]

an•hy•drous (an-hī′drŭs) Containing no water, especially water of crystallization.

an•ic•ter•ic vi•ral hep•a•ti•tis (an′ik-ter′ik vī′răl hep′ă-tī′tis) A relatively mild hepatitis, without jaundice.

an•i•lide (an′i-līd) An *N*-acyl aniline; e.g., acetanilide.

an•i•linc•tion, **an•i•linc•tus** (a′nĭ-lingk′shŭn, -lingk′tŭs) SYN anilingus.

an•i•line (an′i-lin) An oily, colorless or brownish liquid, of aromatic odor and acrid taste, which is the parent substance of many synthetic dyes. Aniline is highly toxic and may cause industrial poisoning. [Ar. *an-nil,* indigo]

an•i•lin•gus (ā-nĭ-ling′gŭs) Sexual stimulation by licking or kissing the anus. SYN anilinction, anilinctus. [L. *anus,* + *lingo,* to lick]

an•il•ism (an′ĭ-lizm) Chronic aniline poisoning, characterized by nausea, vertigo, muscular weakness, cyanosis, and respiratory and circulatory failure.

an•i•ma (an′i-mă) **1.** The soul or spirit. SEE animus (4). **2.** In jungian psychology, the inner self, in contrast to persona; a female archetype in a man. Cf. animus (5). [L. breath, soul]

an•i•mal (an′i-măl) **1.** A living, sentient organism that has membranous cell walls, requires oxygen and organic foods, and is capable of voluntary movement, as distinguished from a plant or mineral. **2.** One of the lower animal organisms as distinguished from humans. [L.]

an•i•mal mod•el (an′i-măl mod′ĕl) Study in a population of laboratory animals that uses conditions of animals analogous to conditions of humans to simulate processes comparable with those that occur in human populations.

an•i•mal pole (an′i-măl pōl) The point in a telolecithal egg opposite the yolk, it is the site of the nucleus and most of the protoplasm; from this region, polar bodies are extruded during maturation. SYN germinal pole.

an•i•mal starch (an′i-măl stahrch) SYN glycogen.

an•i•ma•tion (an′i-mā′shŭn) **1.** The state of being alive. **2.** Liveliness; high spirits. [L. *animo,* pp. *-atus,* to make alive; *anima,* breath, soul]

an•i•mus (an′i-mŭs) **1.** An animating or energizing spirit. **2.** Intention to do something; disposition. **3.** PSYCHIATRY a spirit of active hostility or grudge. **4.** The ideal image toward which a person strives. **5.** PSYCHOLOGY a male archetype in a woman in Jung's theory. Cf. anima (2). [L. *animus,* breath, rational soul in man, will]

AN in•ter•val (in′tĕr-văl) The time between onset of the atrial deflection and the nodal potential (normally 40–100 msec).

an•i•on (A^-) (an′ī-on) An ion that carries a negative charge, going therefore to the positively charged anode; in salts, acid radicals are anions.

an•i•on ex•change (an′ī-on eks-chānj′) The process by which an anion in a mobile (liquid) phase exchanges with another anion previously bound to a solid, positively charged phase, the latter being an anion exchanger. Anion exchange may also be used chromatographically, to separate anions, and medicinally, to remove an anion (e.g., Cl^-) from gastric contents or bile acids in the intestine.

an•i•on-ex•change res•in (an′ī-on-eks-chānj′ rez′in) SEE anion exchange.

an•i•on gap (an′ī-on gap) The arithmetic difference between the concentrations of routinely measured cations (Na^+ + K^+) and of routinely measured anions (Cl^- + HCO_3^-) in plasma or serum; unmeasured anions (phosphate, sulfate, protein, other organic ions) account for the gap, which is increased in metabolic acidosis due to diabetic ketosis, renal failure, or extraneous substances (methanol, salicylate).

an•i•on•ic neu•tro•phil-ac•ti•vat•ing pep•tide (an′i-on′ik nū′trō-fil-ak′ti-vāt-ing pep′tīd) SYN interleukin-8.

an•i•rid•i•a (an′i-rid′ē-ă) Absence of the iris. Cf. irideremia. [G. *an-* priv. + irid- + -ia]

an•ise (an′is) (*Pimpinella anisum*) An herbal extract that is marketed in many different forms. Unconfirmed uses include as a therapeutic agent in asthma, gastrointestinal disorders, and some forms of neurologic disease. Dangerous reactions have been reported. [L. *anisum,* fr. G. *anēson,*]

an•is•ei•ko•ni•a (an′i-sī-kō′nē-ă) An ocular condition in which the image of an object in one eye differs in size or shape from the image of the same object in the fellow eye. [G. *anisos,* unequal, + *eikōn,* an image]

♻**aniso-** Combining form meaning unequal, dissimilar, unlike. [G. *anisos,* unequal, fr. an-, not, + *isos,* equal]

an•i•so•ac•com•mo•da•tion (an-ī′sō-ă-kom-ŏ-dā′shŭn) Variation between the two eyes in accommodation capacity. [aniso- + L. *accommodo,* to adapt]

an•i•so•chro•mat•ic (an-ī′sō-krŏ-mat′ik) Not uniformly of one color.

an•i•so•co•ri•a (an-ī′sō-kōr′ē-ă) A condition in which the two pupils are not of equal size. [aniso- + G. *korē,* pupil]

an•i•so•cy•to•sis (an-ī′sō-sī-tō′sis) Variation in the size of cells that are normally uniform, especially red blood cells. See page B3. [aniso- + G. *kytos,* cell, + *-osis,* condition]

an•i•so•dac•ty•lous (an-ī′sō-dak′ti-lŭs) Relating to anisodactyly.

an•i•so•dac•ty•ly (an-ī′sō-dak′ti-lē) Unequal length in corresponding fingers. [aniso- + G. *daktylos,* finger]

an•i•sog•a•my (an′-i-sog′ă-mē) Fusion of two gametes unequal in size or form; fertilization as distinguished from isogamy or conjugation. [aniso- + G. *gamos,* marriage]

an•i•sog•na•thous (an′i-sog′nă-thŭs) Having jaws of unequal size, the upper being wider than the lower. Mandibular and maxillary arches are of significantly different sizes (and often in an abnormal relation). [aniso- + G. *gnathos,* jaw]

an•i•so•kar•y•o•sis (an-ī′sō-kar-ē-ō′sis) Variation in size of nuclei, greater than the normal range for a tissue. [aniso- + G. *karyon,* nut (nucleus), + *-osis,* condition]

an•i•so•mas•ti•a (an-ī′sō-mas′tē-ă) Inequality in the size of the breasts. [aniso- + G. *mastos,* breast]

an•i•so•me•li•a (an-ī′sō-mē′lē-ă) A condition of inequality between two paired limbs. [aniso- + G. *melos,* limb]

an•i•so•me•tro•pi•a (an-ī′sō-mĕ-trō′pē-ă) SYN heterometropia. [aniso- + G. *metron,* measure, + *ōps,* sight]

an•i•so•me•tro•pic (an-ī′sō-mĕ-trō′pik) **1.** Relating to anisometropia. **2.** Having eyes of unequal refractive power.

an•i•so•pi•e•sis (an-ī′sō-pī-ē′sis) Unequal arterial blood pressure on the two sides of the body. [aniso- + G. *piesis,* pressure]

an•i•so•sphyg•mi•a (an-ī′sō-sfig′mē-ă) Difference in volume, force, or time of the pulse in the corresponding arteries on two sides of the body, e.g., the two radials, or femorals. [aniso- + G. *sphygmos,* pulse]

an•i•sos•then•ic (an-ī′sos-then′ik) Of unequal strength; denoting two muscles or groups of muscles that are either paired or are antagonists. [aniso- + G. *sthenos,* strength]

an•i•so•ton•ic (an-ī′sō-ton′ik) Not having equal tension; having unequal osmotic pressure. [aniso- + G. *tonus,* tension]

A•nitsch•kow cell (ah-nich′kov sel) SYN cardiac histiocyte.

A•nitsch•kow my•o•cyte (ah-nich′kov mī′ō-sīt) SYN cardiac histiocyte.

an•kle (ang′kĕl) **1.** SYN ankle joint. **2.** The region of the ankle joint. **3.** SYN talus. See page A16.

an•kle-arm in•dex (AAI) (ang′kĕl-ahrm in′deks) SYN ankle-brachial index.

an•kle bone (ang′kĕl bōn) SYN talus.

an•kle-bra•chi•al in•dex (ABI) (angk′el-brā′kē-ăl in′deks) Objective measurement of arterial insufficiency based on the ratio of ankle systolic pressure to brachial systolic pressure. An ABI of 1.0 indicates absence of arterial insufficiency; an ABI of less than 0.50 indicates severe arterial insufficiency. SYN ankle-arm index.

an•kle-foot or•thot•ic (AFO) (ang′kĕl-fut ōr-thot′ik) A device that encompasses the ankle and foot to provide ankle stability and assist knee extension control during ambulation.

an•kle joint (ang′kĕl joynt) A hinge synovial joint that is placed between the tibia and fibula above and with the talus below. See this page. SYN ankle (1), mortise joint, talocrural joint.

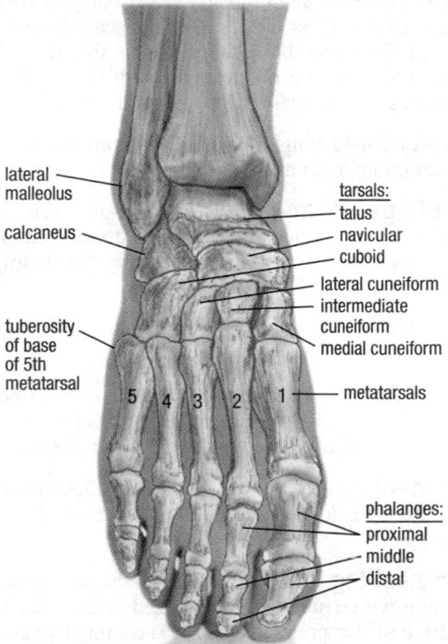

ankle joint: dorsal view

an•kle re•flex (ang′kĕl rē′fleks) SYN Achilles reflex.

ankylo- Combining form meaning bent, crooked, stiff, fused, fixed, closed. SEE ALSO ancylo-. [G. *ankylos,* bent, crooked; *ankylōsis,* stiffening of the joints, fr. *ankos*, a bend, a hollow]

an•ky•lo•bleph•a•ron (ang′ki-lō-blef′ă-ron) Adhesion between upper and lower eyelids; seen most commonly in ocular inflammatory disease or in injuries related to burns. [ankylo- + blepharon]

an•ky•lo•glos•si•a (ang′ki-lō-glos′ē-ă) Partial

or complete fusion of the tongue to the floor of the mouth; abnormal shortness of the frenulum linguae. SYN tongue-tie. [ankylo- + G. *glōssa,* tongue]

an•ky•lo•poi•et•ic (ang′ki-lō-poy-et′ik) Forming ankylosis.

an•ky•losed (ang′ki-lōst) Stiffened; bound by adhesions; denoting a joint in a state of ankylosis.

an•ky•los•ing spon•dy•li•tis (ang′ki-lōs-ing spon′di-lī′tis) Arthritis of the spine, resembling rheumatoid arthritis, which may progress to bony ankylosis with lipping of vertebral margins; the disease is more common in the male, often with the rheumatoid factor absent and the HLA antigen present. There is a striking association with the B27 tissue type and the strong familial aggregation suggests an important genetic factor. See page B24. SYN rheumatoid spondylitis.

an•ky•lo•sis (ang′ki-lō′sis) **1.** Stiffening or fixation of a joint as the result of a disease process, with fibrous or bony union across the joint. **2.** DENTISTRY fusion of the tooth with the alveolar process. [G. *ankylōsis,* stiffening of a joint]

an•ky•lot•ic (ang′ki-lot′ik) Characterized by or pertaining to an ankylosis.

an•la•ge, pl. **an•la•gen** (ahn′lah-ge, -gen) **1.** SYN primordium. **2.** PSYCHOANALYSIS genetic predisposition to a given trait or personality characteristic. [Ger. plan, outline]

ANNA Abbreviation for American Nephrology Nurses' Association

Ann Ar•bor stag•ing sys•tem (an ahr′bŏr stāg′ing sis′tĕm) A system used for classifying Hodgkin disease and non-Hodgkin lymphoma.

an•neal (ă-nēl′) Process by which oligonucleotides affix to targeted DNA sequences. [M.E. *anelen*]

an•neal•ing lamp (ă-nēl′ing lamp) An alcohol lamp with a soot-free flame used in dentistry to drive off the protective NH_3 gas coating from the surface of cohesive gold foil.

an•nec•tent (ă-nek′tĕnt) Connected with; joined. [L. *an-necto,* pres. p. *an-nectens,* to join to]

an•nex•a (ă-nek′să) SYN adnexa.

an•nex•al (ă-neks-ăl) SYN adnexal.

an•nu•al de•duc•ti•ble (an′yū-ăl dĕ-dŭk′ti-bel) SYN deductible.

a•no•coc•cy•ge•al (ā′nō-kok-sij′ē-ăl) Relating to both anus and coccyx.

a•no•coc•cy•ge•al bod•y (ā′nō-kok-sij′ē-ăl bod′ē) A musculofibrous band that passes between the anus and the coccyx.

a•no•coc•cy•ge•al nerve (ā′nō-kok-sij′ē-ăl nĕrv) One of several small nerves arising from the coccygeal plexus, supplying the skin over the coccyx. SYN nervus anococcygeus [TA].

an•ode (an′ōd) **1.** The positive pole of a galvanic battery or the electrode connected with it; an electrode toward which negatively charged ions (anions) migrate; a positively charged electrode. **2.** The portion, usually made of tungsten, of an x-ray tube from which x-rays are released by bombardment by cathode rays (electrons). [G. *anodos,* a way up, fr. *ana,* up, + *hodos,* a way]

an•o•derm (ā′nō-dĕrm) Lining of the anal canal, extending from the dentate line to the anal verge; it is devoid of hair and sebaceous and sweat glands but is richly supplied with tactile and nociceptive (pain, itch) endings innervated by the inferior rectal (pudendal) nerve.

an•o•don•ti•a (an′ō-don′shē-ă) Complete absence of teeth. SYN agomphosis, agomphiasis. [G. *an-* priv. + *odous,* tooth]

an•o•dyne (an′ō-dīn) A substance that soothes or relieves pain.

anoestrus [Br.] SYN anestrus.

a•no•gen•i•tal (ā′nō-jen′i-tăl) Relating to both the anal and the genital regions.

a•no•gen•i•tal ra•phe (ā′nō-jen′i-tăl rā′fē) In the male embryo, the line of closure of the urogenital folds and labioscrotal swellings extending from the anus to the tip of the penis; it is differentiated in the adult into three regions: perineal raphe, scrotal raphe, and penile raphe.

a•nom•a•lad (ă-nom′ă-lad) A malformation together with its subsequently derived structural changes. SEE anomaly.

a•nom•a•lous (ă-nom′ă-lŭs) Of abnormal quality. [G. *anōmalos,* irregular]

a•nom•a•lous com•plex (ă-nom′ă-lŭs kom′pleks) A complex in the electrocardiogram differing significantly from the physiologic type in the same lead.

a•nom•a•lous pul•mo•nar•y ve•nous con•nec•tions, to•tal or par•tial (ă-nom′ă-lŭs pul′mŏ-nar-ē vē′nŭs kŏ-nek′shŭnz, tō′tăl pahr′shăl) Connections in which some or all of the pulmonary veins connect to the right atrium or one of its tributaries.

a•nom•a•lous ret•i•nal cor•re•spon•dence (ă-nom′ă-lŭs ret′i-năl kōr′ĕ-spon′dĕns) A condition, frequent in strabismus, in which corresponding retinal points do not have the same visual direction; the fovea of one eye corresponds to an extrafoveal area of the fellow eye.

a•nom•a•ly (ă-nom′ă-lē) A birth defect caused by a structural abnormality or a marked deviation from the average or normal standard; anything that is structurally unusual, irregular, or contrary to a general rule, especially a congenital defect. [G. *anōmalia,* irregularity]

an·o·mer (an′ō-mĕr) One of two sugar molecules that are epimeric at the hemiacetal or hemiketal carbon atom. SEE ALSO sugars. Cf. epimer.

a·no·mi·a (ă-nō′mē-ă) SYN anomic aphasia. [G. *a-* priv. + *ōnoma,* name]

a·nom·ic a·pha·si·a (ă-nom′ik ă-fā′zē-ă) Aphasia in which the patient cannot name people and objects seen, heard, or felt because of a lesion in the left temporal lobe. SYN amnestic aphasia, amnesic aphasia, amnestic anomia, anomia, nominal aphasia.

a·no·mie (an′ō-mē) Social instability as a result of a loss of accepted standards and values. [F., fr. G. *anomia,* lawlessness]

an·o·nych·i·a, **an·o·ny·cho·sis** (an′ō-nik′ē-ă, an′ō-ni-kō′sis) Absence of the nails. [G. *an-* priv. + *onyx* (*onych-*), nail]

a·non·y·ma (ă-non′i-mă) Without name; a term formerly applied to the large vessels in the thorax (now called the brachiocephalic trunk and vein) and the hip bone. SYN innominate. [G. *an-* priv. + *onyma,* name]

a·no·nym·i·ty (an′ŏ-nim′i-tē) Protection of participants in a study or report so that even the researchers or authors cannot link specific respondents with the information provided.

A·noph·e·les (ă-nof′ĕ-lēz) A genus of mosquitoes (family Culicidae, subfamily Anophelinae). The sporogenous cycle of the malarial parasite is passed in the body cavity of female mosquitoes of certain species of this genus. [G. *anōphelēs,* useless, harmful, fr. *an-* priv. + *ōpheleō,* to be of use]

a·noph·e·line (ă-nof′ĕ-lēn) Referring to the *Anopheles* mosquito.

an·oph·thal·mi·a (an′of-thal′mē-ă) Congenital absence of all tissues of the eyes. [G. *an-* priv. + *ophthalmos,* eye]

a·no·plas·ty (ā′nō-plas-tē) Plastic surgery of the anus. [L. *anus* + G. *plastos,* formed]

an·op·si·a (an-op′sē-ă) Defect of vision. [G. *an,* without, + *ōps,* eye, vision]

an·or·chi·a (an-ōr′kē-ă) SYN anorchism.

an·or·chid·ism (an-ōr′kid-izm) SYN anorchism.

an·or·chism (an-ōr′kizm) Absence of the testes; may be congenital or acquired. SYN anorchia, anorchidism. [G. *an-* priv. + *orchis,* testicle]

a·no·rec·tal (ā′nō-rek′tăl) Relating to both anus and rectum.

an·o·rec·tic (an′ŏ-rek′tic) **1.** Relating to, characteristic of, or suffering from anorexia, especially anorexia nervosa. **2.** An agent that causes anorexia. SYN anorexic.

an·o·rex·i·a (an′ŏ-rek′sē-ă) Diminished appetite; aversion to food. [G. fr. *an-* priv. + *orexis,* appetite]

an·o·rex·i·a ath·let·i·ca (an′ŏ-rek′sē-ă ath-let′i-kă) Continuum of subclinical eating behaviors of athletes who do not meet the criteria for a true eating disorder, but who practice at least one unhealthful method of weight control (e.g., fasting, vomiting, or use of diet pills, laxatives, or diuretics).

an·o·rex·i·a ner·vo·sa (an′ŏ-rek′sē-ă nĕr-vō′să) A personality disorder manifested by extreme fear of becoming obese and an aversion to eating, usually occurring in young women and often resulting in life-threatening weight loss, accompanied by a disturbance in body image, hyperactivity, and amenorrhea.

an·o·rex·i·ant (an′ŏ-rek′sē-ănt) A drug (e.g., so-called diet pills), process, or event that leads to anorexia.

an·o·rex·ic (an′ŏ-rek′sik) SYN anorectic.

an·or·gas·my, **an·or·gas·mi·a** (an′ōr-gaz′mē, -gaz′mē-ă) Failure to experience an orgasm; may be biogenic (secondary to a physical disorder or medication), psychogenic (secondary to psychological or situational factors), or a combination of the two. [G. *an-* priv. + orgasm + -ia]

an·or·thog·ra·phy (an′ōr-thog′ră-fē) SYN agraphia. [G. *an-* priv. + *orthos,* straight, + *graphō,* to write]

a·no·scope (ā′nō-skōp) A short speculum for examining the anal canal and lower rectum. Cf. proctoscope.

a·no·sig·moid·os·co·py (ā′nō-sig′moy-dos′kŏ-pē) Endoscopy of the anus, rectum, and sigmoid colon.

an·os·mi·a (an-oz′mē-ă) Loss of the sense of smell. It may be due to lesion of the olfactory nerve, obstruction of the nasal fossae, or functional, without any apparent causative lesion. [G. *an-* priv. + *osmē,* sense of smell]

an·os·mic (an-oz′mik) Relating to anosmia.

a·no·sog·no·si·a (ă-nō′sō-nō′sē-ă) Ignorance of the presence of disease, specifically of paralysis. Most often seen in patients with nondominant parietal lobe lesions, who deny their hemiparesis. [G. *a-* priv. + *nosos,* disease, + *gnōsis,* knowledge]

a·no·sog·no·sic (ă-nō′sō-nō′sik) Relating to anosognosia.

a·no·sog·no·sic ep·i·lep·sy (ă-nō′sō-nō′sik ep′i-lep′sē) Epilepsy characterized by attacks of which the person is unaware.

a·no·spi·nal (ā′nō-spī′năl) Relating to the anus and the spinal cord.

an·os·to·sis (an′os-tō′sis) Failure of ossification. [G. *an-* priv. + *osteon,* bone]

an·o·ti·a (an-ō′shē-ă) Congenital absence of one or both external ears. [G. *an-* priv. + *ous,* ear]

ANOVA (ă-nō′vă) Acronym for analysis of variance.

a·no·ves·i·cal (ā′nō-ves′i-kăl) Relating in any way to both anus and urinary bladder.

an·ov·u·lar (an-ov′yū-lăr) Absence of discharge of an ovum from the ovary during an ovarian cycle.

an·ov·u·lar men·stru·a·tion (an-ov′yū-lăr men′strū-ā′shŭn) Menstrual bleeding without recent ovulation; also occurs in subhuman primates.

an·ov·u·la·tion (an′ov-yū-lā′shŭn) Suspension or cessation of ovulation.

anoxaemia [Br.] SYN anoxemia.

an·ox·e·mi·a (an′ok-sē′mē-ă) Absence of oxygen in arterial blood; formerly used to include the moderate decrease in oxygen, now properly distinguished as hypoxemia. SYN anoxaemia. [G. *an-* priv. + oxygen + G. *haima,* blood]

an·ox·i·a (an-ok′sē-ă) Absence or almost complete absence of oxygen from inspired gases, arterial blood, or tissues; to be differentiated from hypoxia. [G. *an-* priv. + oxygen]

an·ox·ic (an-ok′sik) Denoting or characteristic of anoxia.

an·ox·ic an·ox·i·a (an-ok′sik an-ok′sē-ă) Hypoxic hypoxia in which oxygen is almost completely lacking.

An·rep phe·nom·e·non (ahn′rep fĕ-nom′ĕ-non) Homeometric autoregulation of the heart whereby cardiac performance improves as the afterload (aortic pressure) is increased.

ANS Abbreviation for autonomic nervous system.

an·sa, gen. and pl. **an·sae** (an′să, -sē) [TA] Any anatomic structure in the form of a loop or an arc. SEE ALSO loop. [L. loop, handle]

an·sa cer·vi·ca·lis (an′să sĕr-vi-kā′lis) [TA] A loop in the cervical plexus consisting of fibers from the first three cervical nerves. Fibers from a loop between the C1 and C2 spinal nerves accompany the hypoglossal nerve for a short distance, leaving it as the superior root of the ansa cervicalis. Fibers from a loop between the C2 and C3 spinal nerves form the inferior root of the ansa cervicalis. Most commonly, the roots merge, forming the ansa cervicalis, which gives rise to branches innervating infrahyoid muscles. SYN cervical loop.

an·sae ner·vo·rum spi·na·li·um (an′sē nĕr-vō′rŭm spī-nā′lē-ŭm) SYN loops of spinal nerves.

an·sa pe·dun·cu·la·ris (an′să pe-dŭnk-yū-lā′ris) [TA] A complex fiber bundle curving around the medial edge of the internal capsule and connecting the anterior part of the temporal lobe (temporal cortex), amygdala, and olfactory cortex with the mediodorsal nucleus of the thalamus; it enters the thalamus as a component of the inferior thalamic peduncle, which also contains a major part of the fibers connecting the mediodorsal nucleus to the orbitofrontal cortex.

an·sa sub·cla·vi·a (an′să sŭb-klā′vē-ă) [TA] A nerve cord connecting the middle cervical and stellate sympathetic ganglia, forming a loop around the subclavian artery.

an·sate (an′sāt) SYN ansiform.

an·ser·ine bur·sa (an′sĕr-īn bŭr′să) The bursa between the tibial collateral ligament of the knee joint and the tendons of the sartorius, gracilis, and semitendinosus muscles.

an·se·rine bur·si·tis (an′sĕr-īn bŭr-sī′tis) Inflammation of the anserine bursa lying between the pes anserinus and the upper medial surface of the tibia.

ANSI Abbreviation for American National Standards Institute.

an·si·form (an′si-fōrm) In the shape of a loop or arc. SYN ansate. [L. *ansa,* handle, + *forma,* shape]

an·so·par·a·me·di·an fis·sure (an′sō-par-ă-mē′dē-ăn fish′ŭr) The fissure separating lobule HVIIA, crus II of the ansiform lobule, from lobule HVIIB, the paramedian lobule, of the posterior lobe of the cerebellum.

ant (ant) One of the most numerous insects (order Hymenoptera), characterized by an extraordinary development of colonial dwelling and caste specialization.

♻ **ant-** SEE anti-.

ant·ac·id (ant-as′id) **1.** Neutralizing an acid. **2.** Any agent that reduces or neutralizes acidity, as of the gastric juice or any other secretion.

an·tag·o·nism (an-tag′ŏ-nizm) **1.** Denoting mutual opposition in action between structures, agents, diseases, or physiologic processes. Cf. synergism. **2.** The situation in which the combined effect of two or more factors is smaller than the solitary effect of any one of the factors. SYN mutual resistance. [G. *antagōnisma,* from *anti,* against, + *agōnizomai,* to fight, fr. *agōn,* a contest]

an·tag·o·nist (an-tag′ŏ-nist) Something opposing or resisting the action of another; any structure, agent, disease, or physiologic process that tends to neutralize or impede some action or effect. Cf. synergist.

an·tag·o·nis·tic mus·cles (an-tag′ŏ-nist′ik mŭs′ĕlz) Those having opposite functions, the contraction of one tending to "neutralize" that of the other.

an·tal·gic gait (ant-al′jik gāt) Ambulation pattern characterized by a shortened stance phase on the affected side. [G. *anti*, against, + *algos*, pain]

ante- Prefix meaning before, in front of (in time or place or order). SEE ALSO pre-, pro- (1). [L. *ante*, before, in front of]

an·te·bra·chi·al (an′tē-brā′kē-ăl) Relating to the forearm.

an·te·bra·chi·um (an′tē-brā′kē-ŭm) [TA] SYN forearm. [ante- + L. *brachium*, arm]

an·te·ced·ent (an′tĕ-sē′dĕnt) A precursor. [L. *antecedo*, to go before]

an·te ci·bum (AC, ac, a.c.) (an′tē sī′bŭm) Before a meal. The plural is *ante cibos*, before meals. [L.]

an·te·cu·bi·tal (an′tē-kyū′bi-tăl) In front of the elbow. [ante- + L. *cubitum*, elbow]

an·te·flex·ion (an′tē-flek′shŭn) A bending forward; a sharp forward curve or angulation; denoting especially the normal forward bend in the uterus at the junction of corpus and cervix uteri.

an·te·gon·i·al notch (an′tĕ-gō′nē-ăl noch) The highest point of the notch or concavity of the lower border of the ramus where it joins the body of the mandible.

an·te·grade (an′tĕ-grād) In the direction of normal movement, as in blood flow or peristalsis. [ante- + L. *gradior*, to walk]

an·te·grade block (an′tĕ-grād blok) SYN anterograde block.

an·te·grade ur·og·ra·phy (an′tĕ-grād yūr-og′ră-fē) Radiography following percutaneous injection of contrast agent with a needle or catheter into the renal calyces or pelvis (antegrade pyelography), or into the urinary bladder (antegrade cystography).

an·te·mor·tem (an′tē-mōr′tĕm) Before death. Cf. postmortem. [ante- + L. *mors* (*mort-*), death]

an·te·na·tal (an′tē-nā′tăl) SYN prenatal. [ante- + L. *natus*, birth]

anteorbital [Br.] SYN antorbital.

an·te·par·tum (an′tē-pahr′tŭm) Before labor or childbirth. Cf. intrapartum, postpartum. [ante- + L. *pario*, pp. *partus*, to bring forth]

antepileptic [Br.] SYN antiepileptic.

an·te·py·ret·ic (an′tē-pī-ret′ik) Before the occurrence of fever; before the period of reaction following shock. [ante- + G. *pyretos*, fever]

an·te·ri·or (an-tēr′ē-ōr) **1.** HUMAN ANATOMY denoting the front surface of the body; often used to indicate the position of one structure relative to another, i.e., situated nearer the front part of the body. SYN ventral (2). **2.** Near the head or rostral end of certain embryos. **3.** Before, in relation to time or space. [L.]

an·te·ri·or a·myg·da·loid ar·e·a (an-tēr′ē-ōr ă-mig′dă-loyd ār′ē-ă) The most rostral portion of the amygdaloid complex composed of scattered cells representing a transition into the more distinctly organized divisions of the amygdala. SYN area amygdaloidea anterior [TA].

an·te·ri·or ap·pre·hen·sion test (an-tēr′ē-ōr ap′rē-hen′shŭn test) **1.** SYN shoulder apprehension sign. **2.** A test of shoulder stability; apprehension with abduction and external rotation of the joint suggests anterior instability. SYN crank test.

an·te·ri·or au·ric·u·lar mus·cle (an-tēr′ē-ōr awr-ik′yū-lăr mŭs′ĕl) *Origin*, galea aponeurotica; *insertion*, cartilage of auricle; *action*, draws pinna of ear upward and forward; *nerve supply*, facial. Considered by some to be the anterior part of the temporoparietal muscle. SYN auricularis anterior muscle, musculus attrahens aurem, musculus attrahens auriculam.

an·te·ri·or au·ric·u·lar nerves (an-tēr′ē-ōr awr-ik′yū-lăr nĕrvz) Branches of the auriculotemporal nerve that supply the tragus and upper part of the auricle. SYN nervi auriculares anteriores [TA].

an·te·ri·or ax·il·lar·y line (an-tēr′ē-ōr ak′sil-ar-ē līn) A vertical line extending inferiorly from the anterior axillary fold.

an·te·ri·or ba·sal seg·men·tal ar·ter·y (an-tēr′ē-ōr bā′săl seg-men′tăl ahr′tĕr-ē) Anterior basal branch of superior basal veins of the lower right and left lobes of left and right lungs.

an·te·ri·or bor·der of tib·i·a (an-tēr′ē-ōr bōr′dĕr tib′ē-ă) The sharp subcutaneous ridge of the tibia that extends from the tuberosity to the anterior part of the medial malleolus. See page 94 SYN shin (2).

an·te·ri·or car·di·nal veins (an-tēr′ē-ōr kahr′di-năl vānz) SEE cardinal veins.

an·te·ri·or cer·e·bral ar·ter·y (an-tēr′ē-ōr ser′ĕ-brăl ahr′tĕr-ē) One of two terminal branches (with middle cerebral artery) of internal carotid; passes anteriorly, loops around genu of corpus callosum, then passes posteriorly in interhemispheric fissure along with its fellow of opposite side, the two being joined by the anterior communicating artery. SYN arteria cerebri anterior.

an·te·ri·or ce·re·bral vein (an-tēr′ē-ōr ser′ĕ-brăl vān) A small vein that parallels the anterior cerebral artery and drains into the basal vein.

an·te·ri·or cham·ber of eye·ball (an-tēr′ē-ōr chām′bĕr ī′bawl) The space between the cornea anteriorly and the iris posteriorly, filled with a watery fluid (aqueous humor) and communicating through the pupil with the posterior chamber. SYN camera anterior bulbi oculi [TA].

an·te·ri·or cil·i·ar·y ar·ter·y (an-tēr′ē-ōr sil′ē-ar-ē ahr′tĕr-ē) One of several arteries derived

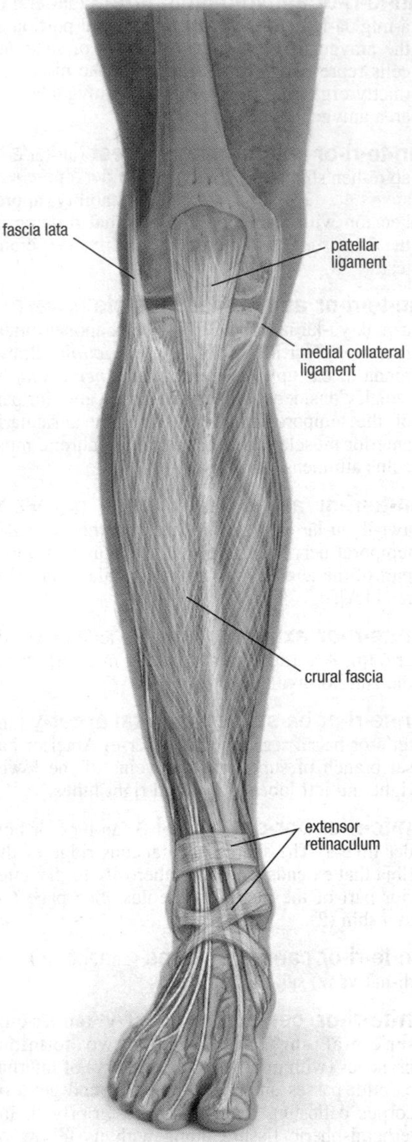

anterior border of the tibia

from muscular branches of the ophthalmic that perforate the anterior part of the sclera and anastomose with posterior ciliary arteries.

an•te•ri•or cir•cum•flex hu•mer•al ar•ter•y (an-tēr′ē-ŏr sĭr′kŭm-fleks hyū′mĕr-ăl ahr′tĕr-ē) *Origin*, axillary; *distribution*, shoulder joint and biceps muscle; *anastomoses*, posterior circumflex humeral artery. SYN anterior humeral circumflex artery, arteria circumflexa humeri anterior.

an•te•ri•or clin•oid pro•cess (an-tēr′ē-ŏr klin′oyd pros′es) The posteriorly directed projection that is the medial end of the sphenoidal ridge (lesser wing of sphenoid); it provides attachment for the free edge of the tentorium cerebelli. SYN processus clinoideus anterior [TA].

an•te•ri•or col•umn (an-tēr′ē-ŏr kol′ŭm) The pronounced, ventrally oriented ridge of gray matter in each half of the spinal cord; it corresponds to the anterior or ventral horn appearing in transverse sections of the cord and contains the motor neurons innervating the skeletal musculature of the trunk, neck, and extremities. SEE ALSO gray columns.

an•te•ri•or com•mis•sure (an-tēr′ē-ŏr kō-mish′ŭr) A round bundle of nerve fibers that crosses the midline of the brain near the anterior limit of the third ventricle. It consists of a smaller anterior part, the fibers of which pass in part to the olfactory bulbs, and a larger posterior part, which interconnects the left and right temporal lobes. SYN precommissure.

an•te•ri•or com•mis•sure of lar•ynx (an-tēr′ē-ŏr kō-mish′ŭr lar′ingks) The junction of the vocal cords anteriorly in the larynx.

an•te•ri•or com•mu•ni•cat•ing ar•ter•y (an-tēr′ē-ŏr kŏm-yū′ni-kāt-ing ahr′tĕr-ē) A short vessel joining the two anterior cerebral arteries and completing the cerebral arterial circle (i.e., circle of Willis) anteriorly. SYN arteria communicans anterior.

an•te•ri•or con•dy•loid fo•ra•men (an-tēr′ē-ŏr kon′di-loyd fōr-ā′mĕn) SYN hypoglossal canal.

an•te•ri•or cor•ne•al dy•stro•phy (an-tēr′ē-ŏr kōr′nē-ăl dis′trŏ-fē) Bilateral corneal abnormality involving the epithelium, basement membrane, or Bowman membrane of the cornea.

an•te•ri•or cru•ci•ate lig•a•ment (an-tēr′ē-ŏr krū′shē-ăt lig′ă-mĕnt) The ligament that extends from the anterior intercondylar area of the tibia to the posterior part of the medial surface of the lateral condyle of the femur. SYN ligamentum cruciatum anterius [TA].

an•te•ri•or cu•ta•ne•ous branch•es of fe•mor•al nerve (an-tēr′ē-ŏr kyū-tā′nē-ŭs branch′ĕz fem′ŏr-ăl nĕrv) Cutaneous branches of the femoral nerve distributed to the anterior and medial aspects of the thigh; they convey general sensation. SYN anterior femoral cutaneous nerves, rami cutanei anteriores nervi femoralis.

an•te•ri•or draw•er test (an-tēr′ē-ŏr drōr test) Assessment tool used to asses the integrity of the anterior cruciate ligament at the knee or the anterior talofibular ligament at the ankle.

an•te•ri•or e•las•tic lam•i•na of cor•ne•a (an-tēr′ē-ŏr ĕ-las′tik lam′in-ă kōr′nē-ă) A homogeneous, acellular tissue layer just beneath the epithelium of the cornea. SYN Bowman membrane, Bowman layer, lamina limitans anterior corneae.

an•te•ri•or em•bry•o•tox•on (an-tēr′ē-ōr em′brē-ō-tok′son) SYN arcus senilis.

an•te•ri•or eth•moi•dal ar•ter•y (an-tēr′ē-ŏr eth-moyd′ăl ahr′tĕr-ē) *Origin*, ophthalmic; *distribution*, cerebral membranes in anterior cranial fossa, anterior ethmoidal cells, frontal sinus, anterior upper part of nasal mucous membrane, skin of dorsum of nose. SYN arteria ethmoidalis anterior.

an•te•ri•or eth•moi•dal nerve (an-tēr′ē-ŏr eth-moyd′ăl nĕrv) A branch of the nasociliary nerve; passes through the anterior ethmoidal foramen on the superomedial wall of orbit into the cranial cavity, giving rise to anterior meningeal nerves, then passes through the cribriform plate into the nasal cavity, supplying the anterosuperior nasal mucosa. SYN nervus ethmoidalis anterior.

an•te•ri•or fem•or•al cu•ta•ne•ous nerves (an-tēr′ē-ŏr fem′ŏr-ăl kyū-tān′ē-ŭs nĕrvz) SYN anterior cutaneous branches of femoral nerve.

an•te•ri•or fo•cal point (an-tēr′ē-ŏr fō′kăl poynt) The point where parallel rays from the retina are focused.

an•te•ri•or fu•nic•u•lus (an-tēr′ē-ŏr fyū-nik′yū-lŭs) Anterior white column of spinal cord, a column or bundle of white matter on either side of the anterior median fissure, between that and the anterolateral sulcus.

an•te•ri•or horn (an-tēr′ē-ŏr hōrn) **1.** The anterior or frontal division of the lateral ventricle of the brain, extending forward from Monro interventricular foramen. SEE lateral ventricle. **2.** The anterior or ventral gray column of the spinal cord as appearing in cross-section. SEE ALSO gray columns. SYN cornu anterius [TA], precornu, ventral horn.

an•te•ri•or hu•mer•al cir•cum•flex ar•ter•y (an-tēr′ē-ŏr hyū′mĕr-ăl sĭr′kŭm-fleks ahr′tĕr-ē) SYN anterior circumflex humeral artery.

an•te•ri•or in•fe•ri•or ce•re•bel•lar ar•ter•y (an-tēr′ē-ŏr in-fēr′ē-ŏr ser′ĕ-bĕl′ăr ahr′tĕr-ē) *Origin*, basilar artery; *distribution*, lower surface of lateral lobes of cerebellum, choroid plexus in cerebellopontine angle; *anastomoses*, posterior inferior cerebellar; usual source of labyrinthine artery. SYN arteria inferior anterior cerebelli.

an•te•ri•or in•fe•ri•or il•i•ac spine (an-tēr′ē-ŏr in-fēr′ē-ŏr il′ē-ak spīn) The landmark on the anterior aspect of the ilium, inferior to the anterior superior iliac spine.

an•te•ri•or in•ter•cos•tal ar•ter•ies (an-tēr′ē-ŏr in′tĕr-kos′tăl ahr′tĕr-ēz) SYN anterior intercostal branches of internal thoracic artery.

an•te•ri•or in•ter•cos•tal branch•es of in•ter•nal thor•a•cic ar•ter•y (an-tēr′ē-ŏr in′tĕr-kost′ăl branch′ĕz in-ter′năl thōr-as′ik ahr′tĕr-ē) An artery supplying anterior portions of intercostal spaces of thoracic wall. Anterior intercostal arteries 1–6 arise as branches of the internal thoracic artery; 7–11 arise as branches of the musculophrenic artery. SYN anterior intercostal arteries, rami intercostales anteriores arteriae thoracicae internae, rami intercostales anteriores.

an•te•ri•or in•ter•cos•tal veins (an-tēr′ē-ŏr in′tĕr-kost′ăl vānz) Tributaries to the musculophrenic or internal thoracic veins from the anterior portions of intercostal spaces.

an•te•ri•or in•ter•os•se•ous ar•ter•y (an-tēr′ē-ŏr in′tĕr-os′ē-ŭs ahr′tĕr-ē) *Origin*, common interosseous; *distribution*, deep parts of the forearm anteriorly; *anastomoses*, posterior interosseous. SYN arteria interossea anterior, arteria interossea volaris, volar interosseous artery.

an•te•ri•or in•ter•os•se•ous nerve (an-tēr′ē-ŏr in′tĕr-os′ē-ŭs nĕrv) A branch of the median nerve arising in the elbow region, running on interosseous membrane, supplying the flexor pollicis longus, part of flexor digitorum profundus, and the pronator quadratus muscles, as well as radiocarpal and intercarpal joints. SYN nervus interosseus antebrachii anterior [TA].

an•te•ri•or in•ter•ven•tric•u•lar ar•ter•y (an-tēr′ē-ŏr in′tĕr-ven-trik′yū-lăr ahr′tĕr-ē) SYN anterior interventricular branch of left coronary artery.

an•te•ri•or in•ter•ven•tric•u•lar branch of left cor•o•na•ry ar•ter•y (an-tēr′ē-ŏr in′tĕr-ven-trik′yū-lăr branch left kōr′ŏ-nar-ē ahr′tĕr-ē) Terminal branch (with circumflex coronary artery of left coronary artery); descends in anterior interventricular groove to apex, anastomosing with posterior interventricular artery. Supplies most of sternal aspect of ventricles and anterior two thirds of interventricular septum, including atrioventricular bundle of conducting tissue. SYN anterior interventricular artery, left anterior descending artery, ramus interventricularis anterior arteriae coronariae sinistrae.

an•te•ri•or la•bi•al veins (an-tēr′ē-ŏr lā′bē-ăl vānz) Tributaries of the femoral or external pudendal veins draining the mons pubis and anterior labia majora.

an•te•ri•or lac•ri•mal crest (an-tēr′ē-ŏr lak′ri-măl krest) A vertical ridge on the lateral surface of the frontal process of the maxilla that forms part of the medial rim of the orbit.

an•te•ri•or lay•er of thor•a•co•lum•bar fas•ci•a (an-tēr′ē-ŏr lā′ĕr thōr′ă-kō-lŭm′bahr fash′ē-ă) Fascial membrane extending from transverse processes of lumbar vertebrae. SYN fascia musculi quadrati lumborum.

an•te•ri•or lim•it•ing lay•er of cor•ne•a (an-tēr′ē-ŏr lim′it-ing lā′ĕr kōr′nē-ă) A transparent homogeneous acellular layer, 6–9 mcm thick, lying between the basal lamina of the outer layer of stratified epithelium and the substantia propria of the cornea; considered to be a basement membrane.

an·te·ri·or lim·it·ing ring (an-tēr′ē-ŏr lim′it-ing ring) The periphery of the cornea marking the termination of Descemet membrane and the anterior border of the trabecular meshwork; an important landmark in gonioscopy. SYN Schwalbe ring.

an·te·ri·or lin·gual gland (an-tēr′ē-ŏr ling′gwăl gland) One of the small mixed glands deeply placed near the apex of the tongue on each side of the frenulum. SYN apical gland.

an·te·ri·or lobe of hy·poph·y·sis (an-tēr′ē-ŏr lōb hī-pof′i-sis) SYN adenohypophysis.

an·te·ri·or me·di·as·ti·nos·co·py (an-tēr′ē-ŏr mē′dē-as-ti-nos′kŏ-pē) Modification of the Chamberlain procedure in which a mediastinoscope is used for exploration of the anterior mediastinum and subaortic regions.

an·te·ri·or me·nin·ge·al branch of an·ter·i·or eth·moid·al ar·ter·y (an-tēr′ē-ŏr mĕ-nin′jē-ăl branch an-tēr′ē-ŏr eth-moy′dăl ahr′tĕr-ē) *Origin*, anterior ethmoidal; *distribution*, meninges in anterior cranial fossa; *anastomoses*, branches of middle meningeal and meningeal branches of internal carotid and lacrimal.

an·te·ri·or na·sal spine (an-tēr′ē-ŏr nā′zăl spīn) A pointed projection at the anterior extremity of the intermaxillary suture; the tip, as seen on a lateral cephalometric radiograph, is used as a cephalometric landmark.

an·te·ri·or nu·cle·i of thal·a·mus (an-tēr′ē-ŏr nū′klē-ī thal′ă-mŭs) Collective term for three groups of nerve cells that together form the anterior thalamic tubercle; the anteroventral nerve, a relatively large nerve; the anteromedial nerve; and the anterodorsal nerve, a small (but large-celled) nerve. These nuclei receive the mammillothalamic tract from the mammillary body, and additional afferents by way of the fornix; they project collectively to the cortex of the cingulate and parahippocampal gyrus. SYN nuclei anteriores thalami [TA].

an·te·ri·or nu·cle·us (an-tēr′ē-ŏr nū′klē-ŭs) SEE anterior horn.

an·te·ri·or oc·u·lar seg·ment (an-tēr′ē-ŏr ok′yū-lăr seg′mĕnt) That portion of the eye comprising the cornea, iris, lens, and their associated chambers and adnexa.

an·te·ri·or per·fo·rat·ing ar·ter·ies (an-tēr′ē-ŏr pĕr′fŏr-āt-ing ahr′tĕr-ēz) *Origin:* as part of the anteromedial central arteries arising from the precommunicating part (A1 segment) of the anterior cerebral artery; enters the anterior perforated substance of the cranial base.

an·te·ri·or pi·tu·i·tar·y go·nad·o·tro·pin (an-tēr′ē-ŏr pi-tū′i-tār-ē gō-nad′ō-trō′pin) Any gonadotropin of hypophysial origin. SYN pituitary gonadotropic hormone.

an·te·ri·or pi·tu·i·tar·y-like hor·mone (an-tēr′ē-ŏr pi-tū′i-tār-ē-līk hōr′mōn) SYN chorionic gonadotropin.

an·te·ri·or and pos·te·ri·or ra·dic·u·lar ar·ter·ies (an-tēr′ē-ŏr pos-tēr′ē-ŏr ră-dik′yū-lăr ahr′tĕr-ēz) Branches of spinal arteries that are distributed to the dorsal and ventral roots of spinal nerves and their coverings. SYN arteriae radiculares anterior et posterior.

an·te·ri·or and pos·te·ri·or su·pe·ri·or pan·cre·at·i·co·du·o·de·nal ar·ter·y (an-tēr′ē-ŏr pos-tēr′ē-ŏr sŭ-pēr′ē-ŏr pan′krē-at′ik-ō-dū′ō-dē′năl ahr′tĕr-ē) *Origin*, gastroduodenal; one of two arteries, anterior and superior; *distribution*, head of pancreas, duodenum, common bile duct; *anastomoses*, inferior pancreaticoduodenal, splenic. SYN arteria pancreaticoduodenalis superior anterior et posterior.

an·te·ri·or pyr·a·mid (an-tēr′ē-ŏr pir′ă-mid) SYN pyramid of medulla oblongata.

an·te·ri·or rhi·nos·co·py (an-tēr′ē-ŏr rī-nos′kŏ-pē) Inspection of the anterior portion of the nasal cavity with or without the aid of a nasal speculum.

an·te·ri·or sca·lene mus·cle (an-tēr′ē-ŏr skā′lēn mŭs′ĕl) SYN scalenus anterior muscle.

an·te·ri·or scle·ri·tis (an-tēr′ē-ŏr skler-ī′tis) Inflammation of the sclera adjacent to the cornea.

an·te·ri·or seg·men·tal ar·ter·y (an-tēr′ē-ŏr seg-men′tăl ahr′tĕr-ē) SEE left pulmonary artery, right pulmonary artery.

an·te·ri·or spi·nal ar·ter·y (an-tēr′ē-ŏr spī′năl ahr′tĕr-ē) *Origin*, intracranial part of vertebral artery; *distribution*, anteromedial spinal cord and adjacent pia mater; *anastomoses*, spinal branches of intercostal and lumbar arteries. SYN arteria spinalis anterior.

an·te·ri·or spi·no·cer·e·bel·lar tract (an-tēr′ē-ŏr spī′nō-ser′ĕ-bel′ăr trakt) A bundle of fibers originating in the base of the posterior horn and zona intermedia throughout lumbosacral segments of the spinal cord, crossing to the opposite side and ascending in a peripheral position in the ventral half of the lateral funiculus. In its ascent through the rhombencephalon, the tract curves sharply dorsad along the rostral border of the trigeminal motor nucleus, entering the cerebellum in a caudal direction over the dorsal surface of the superior cerebellar peduncle, and terminating as mossy fibers in the granular layer of the cortex of the cerebellar vermis. The bundle conveys proprioceptive and exteroceptive information largely from the opposite lower extremity. SYN Gowers tract.

an·te·ri·or staph·y·lo·ma (an-tēr′ē-ŏr staf′i-lō′mă) A bulging near the anterior pole of the eye. SYN corneal staphyloma.

an·te·ri·or su·pe·ri·or al·ve·o·lar ar·te·ry (an-tēr′ē-ŏr sŭ-pēr′ē-ŏr al-vē′ŏ-lăr ahr′tĕr-ē) *Ori-*

gin, infraorbital artery within intraorbital canal; *distribution,* through anterior alveolar canals to upper incisors and canine teeth, mucous membrane of maxillary sinus. SYN anterior superior dental arteries, arteriae alveolares superiores anteriores.

an·te·ri·or su·pe·ri·or den·tal ar·ter·ies (an-tēr′ē-ŏr sŭ-pēr′ē-ŏr den′tăl ahr′tĕr-ēz) SYN anterior superior alveolar artery.

an·te·ri·or su·pe·ri·or il·i·ac spine (ASIS) (an-tēr′ē-ŏr sŭ-pēr′ē-ŏr il′ē-ak spīn) The prominence at the anterior projection of the iliac crest.

an·te·ri·or su·pra·cla·vic·u·lar nerve (an-tēr′ē-ŏr sū′pra-klă-vik′yū-lăr nĕrv) SYN medial supraclavicular nerve.

an·te·ri·or thor·a·cot·o·my (an-tēr′ē-ŏr thōr′ă-kot′ŏ-mē) Anterior incision into the chest, usually submammary.

an·te·ri·or ti·bi·al ar·ter·y (an-tēr′ē-ŏr tib′ē-ăl ahr′tĕr-ē) *Origin,* popliteal; *branches,* posterior and anterior tibial recurrent, lateral and medial anterior malleolar, dorsalis pedis, lateral tarsal, medial tarsal, arcuate, dorsal metatarsal, and dorsal digital. SYN arteria tibialis anterior.

an·te·ri·or tib·i·al com·part·ment syn·drome (an-tēr′ē-ŏr tib′ē-ăl kŏm-pahrt′mĕnt sin′drōm) Ischemic necrosis of the muscles of the anterior tibial compartment of the leg, presumed due to compression of arteries by swollen muscles following unaccustomed exertion.

an·te·ri·or ti·bi·al nerve (an-tēr′ē-ŏr tib′ē-ăl nĕrv) SYN deep fibular nerve.

an·te·ri·or tib·i·o·fas·ci·al mus·cle (an-tēr′ē-ŏr tib′ē-ō-fash′ē-ăl mŭs′ĕl) Separate fibers of the tibialis anterior inserted into the fascia of the dorsum of the foot. SYN musculus tibiofascialis anterior, musculus tibiofascialis anticus.

an·te·ri·or tooth (an-tēr′ē-ŏr tūth) Any of the incisor and canine teeth on the mandible or maxillae located at the front of the oral cavity.

an·te·ri·or ver·te·bral vein (an-tēr′ē-ŏr vĕr′tĕ-brăl vān) The small vein that accompanies the ascending cervical artery; it opens below into the vertebral vein.

an·te·ri·or ves·ti·bu·lar ar·ter·y (an-tēr′ē-ŏr ves-tib′yū-lăr ahr′tĕr-ē) *Origin:* as a terminal branch, with the common cochlear artery, of the labyrinthine artery; *branch:* vestibulocochlear artery; *distribution:* to vestibular ganglion, utricle and (especially the ampullae of the) lateral and posterior semicircular ducts.

♻ **antero-** Prefix meaning anterior. [L. *anterior,* more before, earlier, fr. *ante,* before, + -r- + *-ior,* more]

an·ter·o·grade (an′tĕr-ō-grād) **1.** Moving forward. Cf. antegrade. **2.** Extending forward from a particular timepoint; used in reference to amnesia. [L. *gradior,* pp. *gressus,* to step, go]

an·ter·o·grade am·ne·si·a (an′tĕr-ō-grād am-nē′zē-ă) Amnesia in reference to events occurring after the trauma or disease that caused the condition.

an·ter·o·grade block (an′tĕr-ō-grād blok) Conduction block of an impulse traveling in its ordinary direction, for example, from the sinuatrial node toward the ventricular myocardium. SYN antegrade block.

an·ter·o·in·fe·ri·or (an′tĕr-ō-in-fēr′ē-ŏr) In front and below.

an·ter·o·lat·er·al (an′tĕr-ō-lat′ĕr-ăl) In front and away from the middle line.

an·te·ro·lis·the·sis (an′tĕr-ō-lis′thĕ-sis) Forward displacement of a vertebral body with respect to the vertebral body immediately below it, due to congenital anomaly, degenerative change, or trauma. SYN spondylolisthesis. [antero- + G. *olisthēsis,* a slipping]

an·ter·o·me·di·al (an′tĕr-ō-mē′dē-ăl) In front and toward the middle line.

an·ter·o·me·di·an (an′tĕr-ō-mē′dē-ăn) In front and in the central line.

an·ter·o·pos·te·ri·or (AP, A/P) (an′tĕr-ō-pos-tēr′ē-ŏr) **1.** Relating to both front and rear. **2.** In x-ray imaging, describing the direction of the beam through the patient from anterior to posterior.

an·ter·o·pos·te·ri·or pro·jec·tion (an′tĕr-ō-pos-tēr′ē-ŏr prŏ-jek′shŭn) SYN AP projection.

an·ter·o·su·pe·ri·or (an′tĕr-ō-sū-pēr′ē-ŏr) In front and above.

an·ter·o·ven·tral nu·cle·i of thal·a·mus (an′tĕr-ō-ven′trăl nū′klē-ī thal′ă-mŭs) SEE anterior nuclei of thalamus.

an·te·sys·to·le (an′tĕ-sis′tō-lē) Premature activation of the ventricle, responsible for the preexcitation syndrome of the Wolff-Parkinson-White or Lown-Ganong-Levine types.

an·te·ver·sion (an′tĕ-vĕr′zhŭn) Forward displacement or turning forward of a body segment. [L. *ante,* before, forward, + *verto, versus,* to turn]

an·te·vert·ed (an′tĕ-vĕrt′ĕd) Tilted forward; in a position of anteversion.

ant·he·lix (ant′hē-liks) SYN antihelix. [anti- + G. *helix,* coil]

an·thel·min·tic (ant′hĕl-min′tik) **1.** An agent that destroys or expels intestinal worms. SYN helminthagogue. **2.** Having the power to destroy or expel intestinal worms. [anti- + G. *helmins,* worm]

an·thrac·ic (an-thras′ik) Relating to anthrax.

an·thra·coid (an′thră-koyd) Resembling a carbuncle or cutaneous anthrax. [G. *anthrax,* carbuncle, + *eidos,* resemblance]

an•thra•co•sil•i•co•sis (an′thră-kō-sil′i-kō′sis) Pneumonoconiosis from accumulation of carbon and silica in the lungs from inhaled coal dust; the silica content produces fibrous nodules. See this page. SYN coal worker's pneumoconiosis. [anthraco- + silicosis]

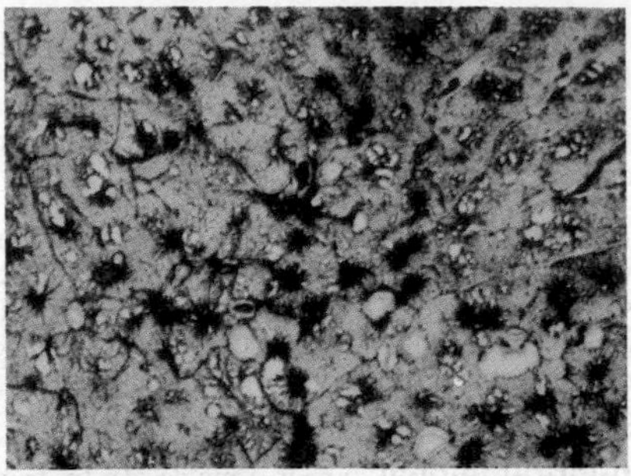

anthracosilicosis: lung of coal miner with scattered, irregular, pigmented nodules throughout parenchyma

an•thra•co•sis (an′thră-kō′sis) Pneumonoconiosis from accumulation of carbon from inhaled smoke or coal dust in the lungs. SYN collier's lung, melanedema, miner's lung (1). [anthraco- + G. *-osis,* condition]

an•thrax (an′thraks) A disease in humans caused by infection with *Bacillus anthracis;* marked by hemorrhage and serous effusions in various organs and body cavities and by symptoms of extreme prostration. [G. *anthrax* (*anthrak-*), charcoal, coal, a carbuncle]

anthropo- Prefix meaning human. [G. *anthrōpos,* a human being (of either sex)]

an•thro•po•cen•tric (an′thrō-pō-sen′trik) With a human bias, under the assumption that humankind is the central fact of the universe. [anthropo- + G. *kentron,* center]

an•thro•poid (an′thrŏ-poyd) **1.** Resembling a human in structure and form. **2.** One of the monkeys resembling humans; an ape. [G. *anthrōpo-eidēs,* man-like]

an•thro•poid pel•vis (an′thrŏ-poyd pel′vis) An apelike pelvis, with a long anteroposterior diameter and a narrow transverse diameter.

an•thro•pol•o•gy (an′thrŏ-pol′ŏ-jē) The scientific study of human beings with respect to physical features, classification, distribution, and social and cultural relationships. [anthropo- + G. *logos,* treatise]

an•thro•po•met•ric (an′thrŏ-pō-met′rik) Relating to anthropometry.

an•thro•po•met•rics (an′thrō-pō-met′riks) A measurement or description of the physical dimensions and properties of the body; typically, used on upper and lower limbs, neck, and trunk. SEE ALSO ergonomics.

an•thro•pom•e•try (an′thrŏ-pom′ĕ-trē) The branch of anthropology concerned with comparative measurements of the human body. [anthropo- + G. *metron,* measure]

an•thro•po•mor•phism (an′thrŏ-pō-mōr′fizm) Assignment of human shape or qualities to nonhuman creatures or inanimate objects. [anthropo- + G. *morphē,* form]

an•thro•po•phil•ic (an′thrŏ-pō-fil′ik) Human-seeking or human-preferring, especially with reference to: 1) bloodsucking arthropods, denoting the preference of a parasite for the human host as a source of blood or tissues over an animal host; and 2) dermatophytic fungi that grow preferentially on humans rather than other animals. [anthropo- + G. *phileō,* to love]

an•thro•po•zo•o•no•sis (an′thrŏ-pō-zō′ō-nō′sis) A zoonosis maintained in nature by animals and transmissible to humans (e.g., rabies, brucellosis). [anthropo- + G. *zōon,* animal, + *nosos,* disease]

anti- **1.** Combining form meaning against, opposing, or, in relation to symptoms and diseases, curative. **2.** Combining form meaning an antibody (immunoglobulin) specific for the thing indicated (e.g., antitoxin, as in antibody specific for a toxin). [G. *anti,* against, opposite, instead of]

an•ti•ad•ren•er•gic (an′tē-ad-rĕ-nĕr′jik) Antagonistic to the action of sympathetic or other adrenergic nerve fibers. SEE ALSO sympatholytic.

an•ti•ag•glu•ti•nin (an′tē-ă-glū′ti-nin) A specific antibody that inhibits or destroys the action of an agglutinin.

antianaemic [Br.] SYN antianemic.

an•ti•an•a•phy•lax•is (an′tē-an′ă-fi-lak′sis) SYN desensitization (1).

an•ti•a•ne•mic (an′tē-ă-nē′mik) Pertaining to factors or substances that prevent or correct anemic conditions. SYN antianaemic.

an•ti•an•ti•bod•y (an′tē-an′ti-bod-ē) Antibody specific for another antibody.

an•ti•an•ti•tox•in (an′tē-an-tē-tok′sin) An anti-antibody that inhibits or counteracts the effects of an antitoxin.

an•ti•anx•i•e•ty a•gent (an′tē-ang-zī′ĕ-tē ā′jĕnt) A functional category of drugs useful in the treatment of anxiety and able to reduce anxiety at dosage that does not cause excessive sedation (e.g., diazepam). SYN anxiolytic (1).

an•ti•bac•te•ri•al (an′tē-bak-tēr′ē-ăl) Destructive to or preventing the growth of bacteria.

an•ti-base•ment mem•brane an•ti•bod•y (an′tē-bās′mĕnt mem′brān an′ti-bod-ē) Autoantibodies to renal glomerular basement membrane antigens.

an•ti-base•ment mem•brane glo•mer•u•lo•ne•phri•tis (an′tē-bās′mĕnt mem′brān glō-mer′yū-lō-nĕ-frī′tis) Condition resulting from anti-basement membrane antibodies, characterized by smooth linear deposits of IgG and C3 along glomerular capillary walls; includes rapidly progressive glomerulonephritis and glomerulonephritis in Goodpasture syndrome.

an•ti-base•ment mem•brane ne•phri•tis (an′tē-bās′mĕnt mem′brān nĕ-frī′tis) Glomerulonephritis produced by autologous or heterologous antibodies to the glomerular capillary basement membranes, the latter known as anti-kidney serum nephritis.

an•ti•bi•o•gram (an′tē-bī′ō-gram) A profile of the antimicrobial resistance and susceptibility of a particular microorganism.

an•ti•bi•o•sis (an′tē-bī-ō′sis) **1.** An association of two organisms that is detrimental to one of them, in contrast to probiosis. **2.** Production of an antibiotic by bacteria or other organisms inhibitory to other living things, especially among soil microbes. [anti- + G. *biōsis,* life]

an•ti•bi•ot•ic (an′tē-bī-ot′ik) **1.** Relating to antibiosis. **2.** Prejudicial to life. **3.** Denotes any substance that acts against susceptible microorganisms. **4.** Relating to such an action.

an•ti•bi•ot•ic-as•so•ci•at•ed en•ter•o•co•li•tis (an′tē-bī-ot′ik ă-sō′sē-āt-ĕd en′tĕr-ō-kŏ-lī′tis) Enterocolitis following oral administration of broad-spectrum antibiotics and caused by suppression of normal intestinal bacterial flora, with overgrowth of resistant organisms, resulting in diarrhea or pseudomembranous disease.

an•ti•bi•ot•ic bond•ing (an′tē-bī-ot′ik bond′ing) Coating of an indwelling tube or catheter with a complex of surfactant and antibiotic to reduce the risk of infection.

an•ti•bi•ot•ic re•mov•al de•vice (ARD), an•ti•mi•cro•bi•al re•mov•al de•vice (an′tē-bī-ot′ik rē-mūv′ăl dĕ-vīs′, an′tē-mī-krō′bē-ăl rē-mūv′ăl dĕ-vīs′) A blood culture bottle containing a resin that removes antimicrobials (antibiotics) from the specimen.

an•ti•bi•ot•ic sus•cep•ti•bil•i•ty (an′tē-bī-ot′ik sŭs-sep′ti-bil′i-tē) Vulnerability of a specific microorganism to inhibition or destruction by an antibiotic.

i an•ti•bod•y (Ab) (an′ti-bod-ē) An immunoglobulin molecule with a specific amino acid sequence evoked in humans or other animals by an antigen and characterized by reacting specifically with the antigen in some demonstrable way, produced by B lymphocytes in response to an antigen. It is believed that antibodies also may exist naturally, without being present as a result of the stimulus provided by the introduction of an antigen. SEE ALSO immunoglobulin. See this page.

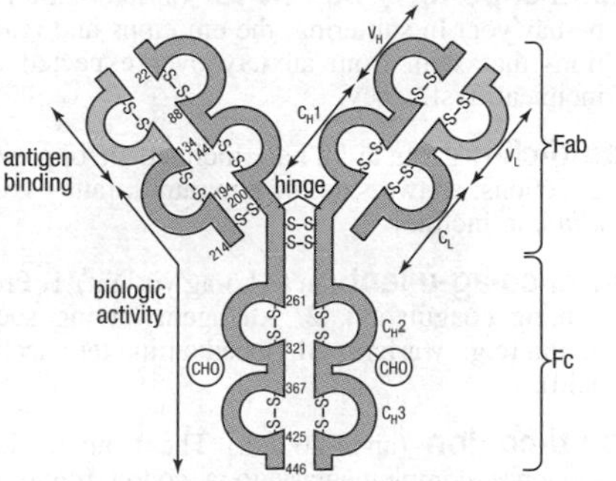

antibody: schematic view of an immunoglobulin molecule

an•ti•bod•y-com•bin•ing site (an′ti-bod-ē-kŏm-bīn′ing sīt) SYN paratope.

an•ti•bod•y ex•cess (an′ti-bod-ē eks′es) In a precipitation test, the presence of antibody in an amount greater than that required to combine with all of the antigen present.

an•ti•bod•y screen (an′ti-bod-ē skrēn) Screening for antibodies in the blood. Used in immunohematology to assess compatibility for blood transfusion.

an•ti•car•ci•no•gen•ic (an′tē-kahr′si-nō-jen′ik) Tending to inhibit or prevent the activity of a carcinogen.

an•ti•cho•lin•er•gic (an′tē-kō′li-nĕr′jik) **1.** Antagonistic to the action of parasympathetic or other cholinergic nerve fibers (e.g., atropine). **2.** Any of a class of compounds exerting anticholinergic effects. Some of these compounds (e.g., atropine) are used medicinally; one, QNB, was developed as an incapacitating chemical-warfare agent.

an•ti•cho•li•ner•gic tox•i•drome (an′tē-kō′li-nĕr′jik tok′si-drōm) The constellation of clinical effects (i.e., signs and symptoms) characteristic of poisoning caused by an anticholinergic agent; conveniently remembered as "blind as a bat, dry as a bone, hot as a hare, red as a beet, and mad as a hatter." SEE ALSO Mad Hatter syndrome (2), toxidrome.

an•ti•cho•lin•es•ter•ase (AChE) (an′tē-kō-lin-es′tĕr-ās) Any compound that inhibits or inactivates acetylcholinesterase, either reversibly (as e.g., physostigmine and other carbamates) or irreversibly (e.g., tetraethyl pyrophosphate and other organophosphorous compounds, including nerve agents).

an•ti•ci•pa•tion (ăn-tis′i-pā′shŭn) Foreknowledge or expectation. [L. *anticipatio,* fr. *anticipo,* to take before]

an•ti•ci•pa•tor•y be•hav•ior (an-tis′i-pă-tōr-ē bē-hāv′yŏr) In stuttering, the emotions and reactions that stem from anxiety over expected or incipient dysfluency.

an•ti•cli•nal (an′tē-klī′năl) Inclined in opposite directions, as two sides of a pyramid. [anti- + G. *klinō,* to incline]

an•ti•co•ag•u•lant (an′tē-kō-ag′yŭ-lănt) **1.** Preventing coagulation. **2.** An agent having such action (e.g., warfarin ethylenediamine tetraacetic acid).

an•ti•co•don (an′tē-kō′don) The trinucleotide sequence complementary to a codon found in one loop of a tRNA molecule; e.g., if a codon is A-G-C, its anticodon is U (or T)-C-G. The complementarity principle arises from Watson-Crick base-pairing, in which A is complementary to U (or T) and G is complementary to C. Sometimes called "nodoc."

an•ti•com•ple•ment (an′tē-kom′plĕ-mĕnt) A substance that combines with a complement and neutralizes its action by preventing its union with an antibody.

an•ti•con•vul•sant (an′tē-kŏn-vŭl′sănt) **1.** Preventing or arresting seizures. **2.** An agent having such action.

an•ti•de•pres•sant (an′tē-dĕ-pres′ănt) **1.** Counteracting depression. **2.** An agent or medication used in treating depression.

an•ti•di•ar•rhe•al (an′tē-dī-ă-rē′ăl) Counteracting diarrhea. SYN antidiarrhoeal.

antidiarrhoeal [Br.] SYN antidiarrheal.

an•ti•di•u•re•sis (an′tē-dī-yŭr-ē′sis) Reduction of urinary volume.

an•ti•di•u•ret•ic (an′tē-dī-yŭr-et′ik) A drug or hormone that reduces urine production by the kidneys.

an•ti•di•u•ret•ic hor•mone (ADH) (an′tē-dī-yŭr-et′ik hōr′mōn) SYN vasopressin.

an•ti•dot•al (an′ti-dō′tăl) Relating to or acting as an antidote.

an•ti•dote (an′ti-dōt) An agent that neutralizes a poison or counteracts its effects. [G. *antidotos,* fr. *anti,* against, + *dotos,* what is given, fr. *didōmi,* to give]

an•ti•drom•ic (an′tē-drom′ik) Moving in the direction opposite to normal; said of impulses in nerves and in the conduction system of the heart.

an•ti•dump•ing law (an′tē-dŭmp′ing law) Governmental regulation that may vary by jurisdiction, but which, in general, mandates that a hospital or care facility must either provide therapy regardless of ability to pay or transfer the penurious or destitute patient to another facility; such laws generally forbid health care facilities from refusing care to such patients or 'dumping' them on another care provider (or city street).

an•ti•dys•ki•net•ic a•gent (an′tē-dis-ki-net′ik ā′jĕnt) A functional category of drugs with anticholinergic action, used to treat Parkinson disease and some acute movement disorders that may be caused by antipsychotic agents.

an•ti•em•bo•lism hose (an′tē-em′bŏ-lizm hōz) SYN antiembolism stockings. SEE ALSO TED hose.

an•ti•em•bo•lism stock•ings (an′tē-ĕm′bŏ-lizm stok′ingz) Specially fitted elastic stockings used to compress lower extremities, reduce blood pooling, and promote venous return, thus reducing risk of thrombus formation. Stockings must be correctly fitted and reapplied for optimal effectiveness. SYN antiembolism hose.

an•ti•e•met•ic (an′tē-ĕ-met′ik) **1.** Preventing or arresting vomiting. **2.** A remedy that tends to control nausea and vomiting. [anti- + G. *emetikos,* emetic]

an•ti•en•zyme (an′tē-en′zīm) An agent or principle that retards, inhibits, or destroys the activity of an enzyme; may be an inhibitory enzyme or an antibody to an enzyme.

an•ti•ep•i•lep•tic (an′tē-ep-i-lep′tik) **1.** Preventing or arresting epilepsy. **2.** An agent having such action. SYN antepileptic.

an•ti•es•tro•gen (an′tē-es′trō-jĕn) Any substance capable of preventing full expression of the biologic effects of estrogenic hormones on responsive tissues. SYN antioestrogen.

an•ti•es•tro•gen•ic (an′tē-es-trō-jen′ik) Counteracting or suppressing estrogenic activity. SYN antioestrogenic.

an•ti•fe•brile (an′tē-feb′ril) SYN antipyretic (1). [anti- + L. *febris,* fever]

an•ti•fi•bri•nol•y•sin (an′tē-fī-bri-nol′i-sin) SYN antiplasmin.

an•ti•fi•bri•no•lyt•ic (an′tē-fī-brin-ō-lit′ik) Denoting a substance that decreases the breakdown of fibrin (e.g., aminocaproic acid).

an•ti•gen (Ag) (an′ti-jen) Any substance that, as a result of coming in contact with target cells, induces a state of sensitivity or immune responsiveness after a latent period (days to weeks) and that reacts in a demonstrable way with antibodies or immune cells of the sensitized subject in vivo or in vitro. Modern usage tends to retain the broad meaning of antigen, employing the terms "antigenic determinant" or "determinant group" for the particular chemical group of a molecule that confers antigenic specificity. SEE ALSO hapten. SYN immunogen. [anti(body) + G. *-gen,* producing]

antigenaemia [Br.] SYN antigenemia.

an•ti•gen-an•ti•bod•y re•ac•tion (an′ti-jen-an′ti-bod-ē rē-ak′shŭn) The phenomenon, occurring in vitro or in vivo, of antibody combining with antigen of the type that stimulated the formation of the antibody, thereby resulting in agglutination, precipitation, complement fixation, greater susceptibility to ingestion and destruction by phagocytes, or neutralization of exotoxin. SEE ALSO skin test.

an·ti·ge·ne·mi·a (an′ti-jĕ-nē′mē-ă) Persistence of antigen in circulating blood, such as HB_s-antigenemia (presence of hepatitis B virus surface antigen in serum). SYN antigenaemia. [antigen + G. *haima,* blood]

an·ti·gen ex·cess (an′ti-jen eks′es) **1.** In a precipitation test, the presence of uncombined antigen above that required to combine with all of the antibody. **2.** In vivo the resultant antigen-antibody interaction in such an antigen excess may give rise to immune complexes, which have a potential to induce cellular damage.

an·ti·gen·ic (an′ti-jen′ik) Having the properties of an antigen (allergen). SYN allergenic, immunogenic.

an·ti·gen·ic de·ter·mi·nant (an′ti-jen′ik dĕ-tĕr′mi-nănt) The particular chemical group of a molecule that determines immunologic specificity.

an·ti·gen·ic drift (an′ti-jen′ik drift) The process of "evolutionary" changes in molecular structure of DNA/RNA in microorganisms during their passage from one host to another; it may be due to recombination, deletion, or insertion of genes, point mutations, or combinations of these events; it leads to alteration (usually slow and progressive) in the antigenic composition, and therefore in the immunologic responses of individual people and populations to exposure to the microorganism concerned.

an·ti·ge·nic·i·ty (an′ti-jĕ-nis′i-tē) The state or property of being antigenic. SYN immunogenicity.

an·ti·gen·ic shift (an′ti-jen′ik shift) Mutation, i.e., sudden change in molecular structure of RNA/DNA in microorganisms, especially viruses, which produces new strains of the microorganism; hosts previously exposed to other strains have little or no acquired immunity to the new strain.

an·ti·gen·ome (an′tē-jē′nōm) The complementary positive RNA strand on which the negative-strand genome of a virus is made.

an·ti·gen pep·tides (an′ti-jen pep′tīdz) The protein fragments that bind to MHC molecules.

an·ti·gen-pre·sent·ing cell (APC) (an′ti-jen-prē-zent′ing sel) Cells that process protein antigens into peptides and present them on their surface in a form that can be recognized by lymphocytes. APCs include Langerhans cells, dendritic cells, macrophages, B cells, and in humans, activated T cells. SYN accessory cell.

an·ti·gen-sen·si·tive cell (an′ti-jen-sen′si-tiv sel) A small lymphocyte that, although not itself an immunologically activated cell, responds to antigenic (immunogenic) stimulus by a process of division and differentiation that results in the production of immunologically activated cells.

an·ti·gen u·nit (an′ti-jen yū′nit) The smallest amount of antigen that, in the presence of specific antiserum, will fix one complement unit.

an·ti·glob·u·lin (an′tē-glob′yū-lin) Antibody that combines with and precipitates globulin.

an·ti·glob·u·lin test (an′tē-glob′yū-lin test) Laboratory assessment to detect red blood cell antibodies in patient serum (indirect) or immunoglobulin bound to the surface of the red blood cell (direct).

an·ti·gly·co·ly·tic a·gent (an′tē-glī-kō-lit′ik ā′jĕnt) A substance that inhibits the metabolism of glucose by cells in a specimen of blood. The most common antiglycolytic agents are sodium fluoride and lithium iodoacetate.

an·ti G suit (an′tē sūt) For *antigravity.* Clothing outfit designed to counteract the physiologic effects of acceleration on an aviator or astronaut.

antihaemaglutinin [Br.] SYN antihemagglutinin.

antihaemolysin [Br.] SYN antihemolysin.

antihaemophilic [Br.] SYN antihemophilic.

antihaemophilic factor a [Br.] SYN antihemophilic factor A.

antihaemophilic globulin a [Br.] SYN antihemophilic globulin A.

antihaemophilic globulin b [Br.] SYN antihemophilic globulin B.

antihaemorrhagic [Br.] SYN antihemorrhagic.

an·ti-HB$_c$ (an′tē) Antibody to the hepatitis B core antigen (HB_cAg).

an·ti-HB$_s$ (an′tē) Antibody to the hepatitis B surface antigen (HB_sAg).

an·ti·he·lix (an′tē-hē′liks) An elevated ridge of cartilage anterior and roughly parallel to the posterior portion of the helix of the auricle. SYN anthelix.

an·ti·hem·ag·glu·ti·nin (an′tē-hē-mă-glū′ti-nin) A substance (including antibody) that inhibits or prevents hemagglutination. SYN antihaemaglutinin.

an·ti·he·mo·ly·sin (an′tē-hē-mol′i-sin) A substance (including antibody) that inhibits or prevents the effects of hemolysin. SYN antihaemolysin.

an·ti·he·mo·lyt·ic (an′tē-hē-mō-lit′ik) Preventing hemolysis.

an·ti·he·mo·phil·ic (an′tē-hē-mō-fil′ik)

Correcting or counteracting the hemorrhagic tendency in hemophilia. SYN antihaemophilic. [anti- + hemophilic]

an·ti·he·mo·phil·ic fac·tor A (AHF) (an′tē-hē-mō-fil′ik fak′tŏr) SYN factor VIII. SYN antihaemophilic factor a.

an·ti·he·mo·phil·ic glob·u·lin A (an′tē-hē-mō-fil′ik glob′yū-lin) SYN factor VIII. SYN antihaemophilic globulin a.

an·ti·he·mo·phil·ic glob·u·lin B (an′tē-hē-mō-fil′ik glob′yū-lin) SYN factor IX. SYN antihaemophilic globulin b.

an·ti·hem·or·rhag·ic (an′tē-hem-ō-raj′ik) Arresting hemorrhage. SYN antihaemorrhagic, hemostatic (2).

an·ti·his·ta·mines (an′tē-his′tă-mēnz) Drugs with an action antagonistic to that of histamine; used to treat allergic symptoms.

an·ti·his·ta·min·ic (an′tē-his-tă-min′ik) **1.** Tending to neutralize or antagonize the action of histamine or to inhibit its production in the body. **2.** An agent having such an effect, used to relieve allergy symptoms.

an·ti·hor·mone (an′tē-hōr′mōn) Any substance demonstrable in serum that inhibits or prevents the usual effects of certain hormones, e.g., specific antibodies.

an·ti·hu·man glob·u·lin (an′tē-hyū′măn glob′yū-lin) Serum from a rabbit or other animal previously immunized with purified human globulin to prepare antibodies directed against IgG and complement; used in the direct and indirect Coombs tests. SYN Coombs serum.

an·ti·hy·per·lip·i·de·mic (an′tē-hī′pĕr-lip′i-dē′mik) Acting to prevent or counteract the buildup of lipids in the blood.

an·ti·hy·per·ten·sive (an′tē-hī-pĕr-ten′siv) Indicating a drug or mode of treatment that reduces the blood pressure of people with hypertension.

an·ti·id·i·o·type an·ti·bod·y, an·ti·id·i·o·type au·to·an·ti·bod·y (an′tē-id′ē-ō-tīp an′ti-bod-ē, an′tē-id′ē-ō-tīp aw′tō-an′ti-bod-ē) An antiantibody, the activity of which is directed specifically against the antigenic determinants (idiotope) of a particular immunoglobulin (antibody) molecule.

an·ti·in·flam·ma·to·ry (an′tē-in-flam′ă-tōr-ē) Reducing inflammation by acting on body responses, without directly antagonizing the causative agent; denoting agents such as glucocorticoids and aspirin.

an·ti·leu·ko·tri·ene (an′tē-lū-ko-trī′ēn) A drug that prevents or alleviates bronchoconstriction in asthma by blocking the production or action of naturally occurring leukotrienes; may also be useful in psoriasis.

an·ti·li·pe·mics (an′tē-li-pē′miks) Drugs used to reduce lipid levels in blood in patients with a history of coronary heart disease or diabetes mellitus. Proven effectiveness in reducing incidence of nonfatal myocardial infarction and coronary death. [anti- + lipemia + -ic]

an·ti·lith·ic (an′tē-lith′ik) **1.** Preventing the formation of calculi or promoting their dissolution. **2.** An agent so acting. [anti- + G. *lithos,* stone]

an·ti·lym·pho·cyte se·rum (ALS) (an′tē-lim′fō-sīt sēr′ŭm) Antiserum against lymphocytes; used to suppress rejection of grafts or organ transplants.

an·ti·ly·sin (an′tē-lī′sin) An antibody that inhibits or prevents the effects of lysin.

an·ti-MAG an·ti·bod·y (an′tē-mag an′ti-bod-ē) A specific antibody against myelin-associated glycoprotein; the most important of the specific antibodies against myelin so far identified, present in the majority of patients with IgM-associated polyneuropathies.

an·ti·ma·lar·i·als (an′tē-mă-lar′ē-ălz) Drugs that are used to prevent or treat malaria.

an·ti·mere (an′ti-mēr) **1.** A segment of an animal body formed by planes cutting the axis of the body at right angles. **2.** One of the symmetric parts of a bilateral organism. **3.** The right or left half of the body. [anti- + G. *meros,* a part]

an·ti·me·tab·o·lite (an′tē-mĕ-tab′ō-līt) A substance that competes with, replaces, or antagonizes a particular metabolite; e.g., ethionine is an antimetabolite of methionine.

an·ti·mi·cro·bi·al (an′tē-mī-krō′bē-ăl) Tending to destroy microbes, to prevent their multiplication or growth, or to prevent their pathogenic action.

an·ti·mi·cro·bi·al break·point (an′tē-mī-krō′bē-ăl brāk′poynt) The concentration of an antimicrobial agent that can be achieved in the body fluids or target site(s) during optimal therapy.

an·ti·mi·tot·ic (an′tē-mī-tot′ik) Inhibiting the process of mitosis.

an·ti·mon·gol·oid (an′tē-mong′ŏ-loyd) The condition in which the lateral portion of the palpebral fissure is lower than the medial portion.

an·ti·mo·ny (Sb) (an′ti-mō-nē) A metallic element; atomic no. 51, atomic wt. 121.757; valences 0, −3, +3, +5; used in alloys; toxic and irritating to the skin and mucous membranes. [G. *anti* + *monos*, not found alone]

an·ti·mu·ta·gen (an′tē-myū′tă-jen) A factor that reduces or interferes with the mutagenic actions of effects of a substance.

an·ti·my·cot·ic (an′tē-mī-kot′ik) Antagonistic to fungi. [anti- + G. *mykēs,* fungus]

an·ti·ne·o·plas·tic (an′tē-nē′ō-plas′tik) Preventing the development, maturation, or spread of neoplastic cells.

an·ti·ne·o·plas·tic an·ti·bi·ot·ic (an′tē-nē′ō-plas′tik an′tē-bī-ot′ik) An antibiotic that inhibits the growth and spread of neoplasms or malignant cells.

an·ti·neu·rit·ic vi·ta·min (an′tē-nūr-it′ik vī′tă-min) Agent used to prevent or relieve neuritis.

an·ti·neu·tro·phil cy·to·plas·mic an·ti·bod·y (ANCA) (an′tē-nū′trō-fil sī′tō-plaz′mik an′ti-bod-ē) An autoantibody to cytoplasmic constituents of monocytes and neutrophils found in patients with vasculitis.

an·tin·i·on (an-tin′ē-on) The space between the eyebrows; the point on the skull opposite the inion. SEE ALSO glabella. [anti- + G. *inion,* nape of the neck]

an·ti·nu·cle·ar an·ti·bod·y (ANA), an·ti·nu·cle·ar fac·tor (ANF) (an′tē-nū′klē-ăr an′ti-bod-ē, an′tē-nū′klē-ăr fak′tŏr) An antibody showing an affinity for cell nuclei, demonstrated by exposing a cell substrate to the serum to be tested, followed by exposure to an antihuman-globulin serum; found in the serum of a high proportion of patients with systemic lupus erythematosus, rheumatoid arthritis, and certain collagen diseases, in some of their healthy relatives, and in about 1% of unaffected people.

antioestrogen [Br.] SYN antiestrogen.

antioestrogenic [Br.] SYN antiestrogenic.

an·ti·on·co·gene (an′tē-ong′kō-jēn) A tumor-suppressing gene involved in controlling cellular growth; inactivation of this type of gene leads to deregulated cellular proliferation, as in cancer. SYN tumor suppressor gene (2).

an·ti·ox·i·dant (an′tē-ŏks-i-dănt) Any substance that may prevent organ damage by scavenging free radicals, including catalase, glutathione, peroxidase, superoxide dismutase, vitamins A, C, and E. SEE ALSO angina, free radical.

an·ti·par·a·sit·ic (an′tē-par-ă-sit′ik) Destructive to parasites.

an·tip·a·thy (an-tip′ă-thē) Aversion, repugnance, intolerance. [G. *antipatheia*]

an·ti·per·i·stal·sis (an′tē-per-i-stal′sis) SYN reversed peristalsis.

an·ti·per·i·stal·tic (an′tē-per-i-stal′tik) **1.** Relating to antiperistalsis. **2.** Impeding or arresting peristalsis.

an·ti·per·spi·rant (an′tē-pĕr′spir-ănt) An agent that has an inhibitory action on the secretion of sweat (e.g., aluminum chloride).

an·ti·phlo·gis·tic (an′tē-flō-jis′tik) **1.** Older term denoting the capacity to prevent or relieve inflammation. **2.** An agent that reduces inflammation and fever. [anti- + G. *phogistos,* burnt up]

an·ti·phos·pho·lip·id an·ti·bod·y syn·drome (aPLS, APS) (an′tē-fos-fō-lip′id an′ti-bod-ē sin′drōm) A tendency for recurrent thrombosis together with recurrent abortion, thrombocytopenia, and neurologic disease, and elevated blood counts of antibodies against certain negatively charged phospholipids (e.g., cardiolipin, phosphatidylserine, and phosphatidylethanolamine).

an·ti·plas·min (an′tē-plaz′min) A substance that inhibits or prevents the effects of plasmin; found in plasma and some tissues, especially the spleen and liver. SYN antifibrinolysin.

an·ti·plate·let a·gent (an′tē-plāt′lĕt ā′jĕnt) Agent that inhibits platelet aggregation and thus reduces the risk of thrombus formation.

an·ti·pode (an′ti-pōd) That which is diametrically opposite. [G. *antipous,* with the feet opposite]

an·ti·port (an′ti-pōrt) The coupled transport of two different molecules or ions through a membrane in opposite directions by a common carrier mechanism (antiporter). Cf. symport, uniport. [anti- + L. *porto,* to carry]

an·ti·pro·te·ase (an′tē-prō′tē-ās) Substance that inhibits the activity of a protease.

an·ti·pro·throm·bin (an′tē-prō-throm′bin) An anticoagulant that inhibits or prevents the conversion of prothrombin into thrombin (e.g., heparin, which is present in various tissues, especially in liver, and dicoumarin, which is isolated from partially decomposed sweet clover).

an·ti·pru·rit·ic (an′tē-prūr-it′ik) **1.** Preventing or relieving itching. **2.** An agent that relieves itching.

an·ti·psy·chot·ic (an′tē-sī-kot′ik) **1.** SYN antipsychotic agent. **2.** Denoting the actions of such an agent.

an·ti·psy·chot·ic a·gent (an′tē-sī-kot′ik ā′jĕnt) A functional category of neuroleptic drugs that are helpful in the treatment of psychosis and have a capacity to decrease symptoms of thought disorders (e.g., chlorpromazine, haloperidol); generally classified as typical or atypical. SYN antipsychotic (1).

an·ti·py·ret·ic (an′tē-pī-ret′ik) **1.** Reducing fever. SYN antifebrile. **2.** An agent that reduces fever (e.g., acetaminophen, aspirin). [anti- + G. *pyretos,* fever]

an·ti·py·ret·ic bath (an′tē-pī-ret′ik bath) Sponging or soaking to reduce fever. [anti- + G. *pyretos,* fever]

an·ti·ra·chit·ic (an′tē-ră-kit′ik) Agent used to prevent the development of rickets. [anti + G. *rachitis,* disease of the spine]

an·ti·ra·chit·ic bath (an′tē-ră-kit′ik bath) Sponging or soaking to reduce fever. [anti + G. *pyretos,* fever]

an·ti·scor·bu·tic (an′tē-skōr-byū′tik) **1.** Preventive or curative of scurvy (scorbutus). **2.** A treatment for scurvy (e.g., vitamin C).

an·ti·se·cre·to·ry (an′tē-sĕ-krē′tōr-ē) Inhibitory to secretion, said of certain drugs that reduce or suppress gastric secretion (e.g., ranitidine, omeprazole).

an·ti·sense (an′tē-sens) Pertaining to the strand of a double stranded DNA or RNA molecule that is complementary to the sense strand.

an·ti·sep·sis (an′ti-sep′sis) Prevention of infection by inhibiting the growth of infectious agents. SEE ALSO disinfection. [anti- + G. *sēpsis,* putrefaction]

an·ti·sep·tic (an′ti-sep′tik) **1.** Relating to antisepsis. **2.** An agent or substance capable of effecting antisepsis.

an·ti·sep·tic dress·ing (an′ti-sep′tik dres′ing) A sterile dressing of gauze impregnated with an antiseptic.

an·ti·sep·tic gauze (an′ti-sep′tik gawz) Surgical or wound dressing treated with a substance that inhibits growth of infectious agents.

an·ti·se·rum (an′tē-sēr′ŭm) Serum that contains demonstrable antibody or antibodies specific for one or more antigens; may be prepared from the blood of animals inoculated with an antigenic material or from the blood of animals and people who have been stimulated by natural contact with an antigen (as by an attack of disease). SYN immune serum.

an·ti·se·rum an·a·phy·lax·is (an′tē-sēr′ŭm an′ă-fi-lak′sis) SYN passive anaphylaxis.

an·ti·so·cial (an′tē-sō′shăl) Opposed to the rights of people or to the legal norms of society. Cf. asocial.

an·ti·so·cial per·son·al·i·ty dis·or·der (an′tē-sō′shăl pĕr-sŏn-al′i-tē dis-ōr′dĕr) A personality disorder characterized by a history of continuous and chronic antisocial behavior with disregard for and violation of the rights of others, beginning before the age of 15 years; early childhood signs include chronic lying, stealing, fighting, and truancy; in adolescence there may be unusually early or aggressive sexual behavior, excessive drinking, and use of illicit drugs. Such behavior continues to adulthood.

an·ti·spas·mod·ic (an′tē-spaz-mod′ik) **1.** Preventing or alleviating muscle spasms (cramps). **2.** An agent that quiets spasm.

an·ti·strep·to·coc·cic (an′tē-strep-tō-kok′sik) Destructive to streptococci or antagonistic to their toxins.

an·ti·tac (an′tē-tak) Monoclonal antibody that recognizes the alpha chain of the IL-2 receptor.

an·ti·ter·min·a·tion (an′tē-tĕr-mi-nā′shŭn) A state of bacterial RNA polymerase wherein it is resistant to pause, arrest, or termination signals. SEE ALSO hesitant, overdrive.

an·ti·tox·ic (an′tē-tok′sik) Neutralizing the action of a poison; specifically, relating to an antitoxin. SEE ALSO antidotal.

an·ti·tox·in (an′tē-tok′sin) Antibody formed in response to antigenic poisonous substances of biologic origin (e.g., bacterial exotoxins, phytotoxins, and zootoxins); in general usage, serum from humans or animals (usually horses) immunized by injections of the specific toxoid. Antitoxin neutralizes the pharmacologic effects of its specific toxin. [anti- + G. *toxikon,* poison]

an·ti·tox·in u·nit (an′tē-tok′sin yū′nit) A unit expressing the strength or activity of an antitoxin; in general, determined with reference to a preserved standard preparation of antitoxin. SEE ALSO L doses.

an·ti·trag·i·cus mus·cle (an′tē-trā′ji-kŭs mŭs′ĕl) A band of transverse muscular fibers on the outer surface of the antitragus, arising from the border of the intertragic notch and inserted into the anthelix and cauda helicis. SYN musculus antitragicus [TA].

an·ti·tra·gus (an-tē-trā′gŭs) [TA] A projection of the cartilage of the auricle, in front of the tail of the helix, just above the lobule, and posterior to the tragus from which it is separated by the intertragic notch. [G. *anti-tragos,* the eminence of the external ear, fr. *anti,* opposite, + *tragos,* a goat, the tragus]

an·ti·trep·o·ne·mal (an′tē-trep-ō-nē′măl) SYN treponemicidal.

an·ti·tro·pic (an′tē-trō′pik) Similar, bilaterally symmetric, but in an opposite location (as in a mirror image), e.g., the right thumb in relation to the left thumb.

an·ti·tryp·sic (an′tē-trip′sik) SYN antitryptic.

an·ti·tryp·sin (an′tē-trip′sin) A substance that blocks the action of trypsin.

an·ti·tryp·tic (an′tē-trip′tik) Possessing properties of antitrypsin. SYN antitrypsic.

an·ti·tus·sive (an′tē-tŭs′iv) **1.** Relieving cough. **2.** A cough remedy (e.g., codeine). [anti- + L. *tussis,* cough]

an·ti·ven·in (an′tē-ven′in) An antitoxin specific for an animal or insect venom. [anti- + L. *venenum,* poison]

an·ti·vi·ral (an′tē-vī′răl) Opposing a virus; interfering with its replication; weakening or abolishing its action.

an·ti·vi·ral pro·tein (AVP) (an′tē-vī′răl

prō′tēn) A human or animal factor, induced by interferon in virus-infected cells, which mediates interferon inhibition of virus replication.

an·ti·vi·ta·min (an′tē-vī′tă-min) A substance that prevents a vitamin from exerting its typical biologic effects. Most antivitamins have chemical structures like those of vitamins and appear to function as competitive antagonists.

An·ton syn·drome (ahn′ton sin′drōm) In cortical blindness, lack of awareness of being blind.

ant·orb·i·tal (ant-ōr′bi-tăl) Situated in front of an orbit. SYN anteorbital.

an·tra (an′tră) Plural of antrum.

an·tral (an′trăl) Relating to an antrum.

an·tral fol·li·cle (an′trăl fol′i-kĕl) SYN vesicular ovarian follicle.

an·tral la·vage (an′trăl lă-vahzh′) Irrigation of the maxillary sinus through its natural ostium or through a puncture of the inferior meatus.

an·trec·to·my (an-trek′tŏ-mē) **1.** Removal of the walls of an antrum. **2.** Removal of the antrum (distal half) of the stomach. [antrum + G. *ektomē,* excision]

♻**antro-** Prefix meaning an antrum. [L. *antrum,* from G. *antron,* a cave]

an·tro·du·o·de·nec·to·my (an′trō-dū′ŏ-dĕ-nek′tŏ-mē) Surgical removal of the antrum of the stomach and the ulcer-bearing part of the duodenum.

an·tro·na·sal (an′trō-nā′zăl) Relating to a maxillary sinus and the corresponding nasal cavity.

an·tro·scope (an′trō-skōp) An instrument to aid in the visual examination of any cavity, particularly the maxillary sinus. [antro- + G. *skopeō,* to view]

an·tros·co·py (an-tros′kŏ-pē) Examination of any cavity, especially of the maxillary sinus, by means of an antroscope.

an·tros·to·my (an-tros′tŏ-mē) Formation of a permanent opening into any antrum. [antro- + G. *stoma,* mouth]

an·trot·o·my (an-trot′ŏ-mē) Incision through the wall of any antrum. [antro- + G. *tomē,* incision]

an·tro·tym·pan·ic (an′trō-tim-pan′ik) Relating to the mastoid antrum and the tympanic cavity.

an·trum, pl. **an·tra** (an′trŭm, an′tră) **1.** Any nearly closed cavity, particularly one with bony walls. **2.** SYN pyloric antrum. [L. fr. G. *antron,* a cave]

an·trum of High·more (an′trŭm hī′mōr) SYN maxillary sinus.

An·tyl·lus meth·od (an-til′ŭs meth′ŏd) Ligation of the artery above and below an aneurysm, followed by incision into and emptying of the sac.

ANUG Abbreviation for acute necrotizing ulcerative gingivitis.

a·nu·lar (an′yŭ-lăr) Ring-shaped.

an·u·lar band (an′yŭ-lăr band) SYN amnionic band.

an·u·lar cat·a·ract (an′yŭ-lăr kat′ăr-akt) Congenital cataract in which a central white membrane replaces the nucleus.

an·u·lar lig·a·ment (an′yŭ-lăr lig′ă-mĕnt) Circular band of tissue surrounding a part. [L. *anulus,* ring]

an·u·lar lip·id (an′yŭ-lăr lip′id) The layer(s) of lipid bound to and/or surrounding an integral membrane protein.

an·u·lar pla·cen·ta (an′yŭ-lăr plă-sen′tă) A placenta in the form of a band encircling the interior of the uterus.

an·u·lar scle·ri·tis (an′yŭ-lăr skler-ī′tis) An often protracted inflammation of the anterior portion of the sclera, forming a ring around the corneoscleral limbus.

an·u·lar sco·to·ma (an′yŭ-lăr skō-tō′mă) A circular scotoma surrounding the center of the field of vision. SEE ring scotoma.

an·u·lar staph·y·lo·ma (an′yŭ-lăr staf′i-lō′mă) A staphyloma extending around the periphery of the cornea.

an·u·lar stric·ture (an′yŭ-lăr strik′shŭr) A ringlike constriction encircling the wall of a canal.

an·u·lar syn·ech·i·a (an′yŭ-lăr si-nek′ē-ă) Adhesion of the entire pupillary margin of the iris to the capsule of the lens.

an·u·lo·a·or·tic ec·ta·si·a (an′yŭ-lō-ā-ōr′tik ek-tā′zē-ă) Supravalvular dilation of the aorta involving both its wall and the valve ring, whose diameter however, remains smaller diameter than that of the more distal ectatic wall; many cases are related to Marfan syndrome.

a·nu·lo·plas·ty (an′yŭ-lō-plas-tē) Reconstruction of the ring (or anulus) of an incompetent cardiac valve. [L. *anulus,* ring, + G. *plastos,* formed]

a·nu·lor·rha·phy (an′yŭ-lōr′ă-fē) Closure of a hernial ring by suture. [L. *anulus,* ring, + G. *rhaphē,* seam]

an·u·lus (an′yū-lŭs) [TA] SYN ring (1). [L.]

an·u·lus fi·bro·sus (an′yū-lŭs fī-brō′sŭs) [TA] **1.** SYN right and left fibrous rings of heart. **2.** SYN anulus fibrosus of intervertebral disc.

an·u·lus fi·bro·sus dis·ci in·ter·ver·te·bra·lis (an′yū-lŭs fī-brō′sŭs dis′kī in-tĕr-vĕr′tĕ-brā′lis) [TA] SYN anulus fibrosus of intervertebral disc.

an·u·lus fi·bro·sus of in·ter·ver·te·bral disc (an′yū-lŭs fī-brō-sŭs in-tĕr-vĕr′tĕ-brăl disk) The ring of fibrocartilage and fibrous tissue forming the circumference of the intervertebral disc; surrounds the nucleus pulposus, which can herniate when the anulus is diseased or injured. SYN anulus fibrosus disci intervertebralis [TA], anulus fibrosus (2) [TA].

an·u·lus in·gui·na·lis su·per·fi·ci·a·lis (an′yū′lŭs ing-gwin-ā′lis sū′pĕr-fish′ē-ā′lis) [TA] SYN superficial inguinal ring.

an·u·lus tym·pa·ni·cus (an′yū-lŭs tim-pan′ik-ŭs) [TA] SYN tympanic ring.

an·u·lus um·bi·li·ca·lis (an′yū-lŭs ŭm-bil-i-kā′lis) [TA] SYN umbilical ring.

an·u·lus of Zinn (an′yū-lŭs tsin) SYN common tendinous ring of extraocular muscles.

an·u·re·sis (an′yūr-ē′sis) Inability to urinate. [G. *an,* without, + *ourēsis,* urination]

an·u·ri·a (ă-nyūr′ē-ă) Absence of urine formation.

an·u·ric (ă-nyūr′ik) Relating to anuria.

a·nus, gen. and pl. **a·ni** (ā′nŭs, ā′nī) [TA] The lower opening of the alimentary (digestive) tract, lying in the intergluteal cleft between the buttocks, through which feces or excrement is discharged. [L.]

an·vil (an′vil) SYN incus.

anx·i·e·ty (ang-zī′ĕ-tē) **1.** Apprehension of danger and dread accompanied by restlessness, tension, tachycardia, and dyspnea unattached to a clearly identifiable stimulus. **2.** EXPERIMENTAL PSYCHOLOGY a drive or motivational state learned from and thereafter associated with previously neutral cues. [L. *anxietas,* anxiety, fr. *anxius,* distressed, fr. *ango,* to press tight, to torment]

anx·i·e·ty dis·or·ders (ang-zī′ĕ-tē dis-ōr′dĕrz) A category of interrelated mental illnesses involving anxiety reactions in response to stress. The types include: 1) generalized anxiety, by far the most prevalent condition, which strikes slightly more females than males, mostly in the 20–35-year-old age group; 2) panic disorder, in which a person suffers repeated panic attacks. Some 2–5% of U.S. residents are subject to this ailment, about twice as many women as men; 3) obsessive-compulsive disorder, afflicting 2–3% of the U.S. population. About two thirds of these patients go on to experience a major depressive episode; 4) posttraumatic stress disorder, most frequent among combat veterans or survivors of major physical trauma; and 5) the phobias (e.g., fear of snakes, crowds, confinement, heights, and many other things), which on a minor scale affect about 1 in 8 people in the U.S. Drugs that have proven effective against anxiety disorders are beta-blockers, which act on adrenaline receptors; anxiolytics; antidepressants; and serotonergic drugs. Regular exercise has also proved beneficial.

anx·i·e·ty hys·te·ri·a (ang-zī′ĕ-tē his-ter′ē-ă) Hysteria characterized by manifest anxiety.

anx·i·e·ty neu·ro·sis (ang-zī′ĕ-tē nūr-ō′sis) Chronic abnormal distress and worry to the point of panic followed by a tendency to avoid or run from the feared situation, associated with overaction of the sympathetic nervous system.

anx·i·e·ty re·ac·tion (ang-zī′ĕ-tē rē-ak′shŭn) A psychological reaction or experience involving the apprehension of danger accompanied by a feeling of dread and such physical symptoms as an increase in the rate of breathing, sweating, and tachycardia, in the absence of a clearly identifiable fear stimulus; when chronic, it is called generalized anxiety disorder. SEE ALSO panic attack.

anx·i·o·lyt·ic (ang′zē-ō-lit′ik) **1.** SYN antianxiety agent. **2.** Denoting the actions of such an agent or medication. [anxiety + G. *lysis,* a dissolution or loosening]

A·on·cho·the·ca (ā-on-kō-thē′kă) One of three trichurid nematode genera, commonly referred to as *Capillaria.*

AOPA Abbreviation for American Board for Certification of the Orthotic and Prosthetic Association.

AORN Abbreviation for Association of Perioperative Registered Nurses.

a·or·ta, gen. and pl. **a·or·tae** (ā-ōr′tă, tē) [TA] A large artery that is the main trunk of the systemic arterial system, arising from the left ventricle and ending at the left side of the body of the fourth lumbar vertebra by dividing to form the right and left common iliac arteries. The aorta is made up of the ascending aorta, aortic arch, and descending aorta, which is divided into the thoracic aorta and the abdominal aorta. [Mod. L. fr. G. *aortē,* from *aeirō,* to lift up]

a·or·ta ab·dom·i·na·lis (ā-ōr′tă ab-dom-i-nā′lis) SYN abdominal aorta.

a·or·ta as·cen·dens (ā-ōr′tă ă-sen′denz) SYN ascending aorta.

a·or·tal (ā-ōr′tăl) SYN aortic.

a·or·tal·gi·a (ā-ōr-tal′jē-ă) Pain assumed to be due to aneurysm or other pathologic conditions of the aorta. [aorta + G. *algos,* pain]

a·or·ta tho·ra·ci·ca (ā-ōr′tă thō-ras′i-kă) SYN thoracic aorta.

a·or·tic (ā-ōr′tik) Relating to the aorta or the aortic orifice of the left ventricle of the heart. SYN aortal.

a·or·tic arch (ā-ōr′tik ahrch) **1.** The curved portion of the aorta between its ascending and descending parts; SYN arch of aorta. **2.** Any member of the several pairs of arterial channels encircling the embryonic pharynx in the mesenchyme of the branchial arches.

a•or•tic arch syn•drome (ā-ōr′tik ahrch sin′drōm) SYN Takayasu arteritis.

a•or•tic a•tre•si•a (ā-ōr′tik ă-trē′zē-ă) Congenital absence of the normal valvular orifice into the aorta.

a•or•tic bulb (ā-ōr′tik bŭlb) The dilated first part of the aorta containing the aortic semilunar valves and the aortic sinuses. SYN bulbus aortae [TA].

a•or•tic co•arc•ta•tion (ā-ōr′tik kō-ahrk-tā′shŭn) Congenital narrowing of the aorta, usually located just distal to the left subclavian artery, causing upper extremity hypertension, excess left ventricular workload, and diminished blood flow to the lower extremities and abdominal viscera.

a•or•tic dis•sec•tion (ā-ōr′tik di-sek′shŭn) A pathologic process, characterized by splitting of the media layer of the aorta, which leads to formation of a dissecting aneurysm.

a•or•tic hi•a•tus (ā-ōr′tik hī-ā′tŭs) The opening in the diaphragm bounded by the two crura, the vertebral column, and the median arcuate ligament, through which pass the aorta and thoracic duct.

a•or•tic in•suf•fi•cien•cy (ā-ōr′tik in′sŭ-fish′ĕn-sē) SYN aortic regurgitation.

a•or•tic mur•mur (ā-ōr′tik mŭr′mŭr) A murmur produced at the aortic orifice, either obstructive or regurgitant.

a•or•tic nip•ple (ā-ōr′tik nip′ĕl) A colloquial term for the radiographic appearance of the left superior intercostal or accessory hemiazygos vein as a bump on the aortic knob.

a•or•tic notch (ā-ōr′tik noch) The notch in a sphygmographic tracing caused by rebound following closure of the aortic valves.

a•or•tic or•i•fice (ā-ōr′tik ōr′i-fis) The opening from the left ventricle into the ascending aorta; it is guarded by the aortic valve.

a•or•tic re•gur•gi•ta•tion (ā-ōr′tik rē-gŭr′ji-tā′shŭn) Reflux of blood through an incompetent aortic valve into the left ventricle during ventricular diastole. SYN aortic insufficiency, Corrigan disease.

a•or•tic si•nus (ā-ōr′tik sī′nŭs) The space between the superior aspect of each cusp of the aortic valve and the dilated portion of the wall of the ascending aorta, immediately above each cusp.

a•or•tic ste•no•sis (ā-ōr′tik stĕ-nō′sis) Pathologic narrowing of the aortic valve orifice, blocking blood flow from the left ventricle, thus decreasing cardiac output.

a•or•tic valve (ā-ōr′tik valv) The valve between the left ventricle and the ascending aorta, consisting of three fibrous semilunar cusps (valvules). They are named in accordance with their embryonic derivation: the anteriorly located cusp is the right cusp (above which the right coronary artery arises), the left posteriorly positioned cusp is the left cusp (above which the left coronary artery arises), and the right posteriorly positioned cusp is the posterior or noncoronary cusp. See page 108.

a•or•tic ves•ti•bule (ā-ōr′tik ves′ti-byūl) The anterosuperior portion of the left ventricle of the heart immediately below the aortic orifice, having fibrous walls and affording room for the segments of the closed aortic valve.

a•or•ti•tis (ā-ōr-tī′tis) Inflammation of the aorta.

a•or•to•cor•o•na•ry (ā-ōr′tō-kōr′ō-nar-ē) Relating to the aorta and the coronary arteries.

a•or•to•gram (ā-ōr′tō-gram) The image or set of images resulting from aortography.

a•or•tog•ra•phy (ā-ōr-tog′ră-fē) **1.** Radiographic imaging of the aorta and its branches by injection of contrast medium. **2.** Imaging of the aorta by ultrasound or magnetic resonance. [aorta + G. *graphō,* to write]

a•or•to•il•i•ac by•pass (ā-ōr′tō-il′ē-ak bī′pas) An operation in which a vascular prosthesis is united with the aorta and iliac artery to relieve obstruction of the lower abdominal aorta, its bifurcation, and the proximal iliac branches.

a•or•to•il•i•ac oc•clu•sive dis•ease (ā-ōr′tō-il′ē-ak ŏ-klū′siv di-zēz′) Obstruction of the abdominal aorta and its main branches by atherosclerosis.

a•or•top•a•thy (ā-ōr-top′ă-thē) Disease affecting the aorta. [aorta + G. *pathos,* suffering]

a•or•to•plas•ty (ā-ōr′tō-plas′tē) A procedure for surgical repair of the aorta.

a•or•to•re•nal by•pass (ā-ōr′tō-rē′năl bī′pas) Insertion of a graft of autogenous artery, saphenous vein, or synthetic material between the aorta and the distal renal artery, to circumvent an obstruction of the renal artery.

a•or•tor•rha•phy (ā-ōr-tōr′ă-fē) Suture of the aorta. [aorta + G. *rhaphē,* seam]

a•or•to•scle•ro•sis (ā-ōr′tō-skler-ō′sis) Arteriosclerosis of the aorta.

a•or•tot•o•my (ā-ōr-tot′ŏ-mē) Incision of the aorta. [aorta + G. *tomē,* a cutting]

AP, **A/P** Abbreviation for anteroposterior; accounts payable.

apallaesthesia [Br.] SYN apallesthesia.

a•pal•les•the•si•a (ă-pal-es-thē′zē-ă) SYN pallanesthesia. SYN apallaesthesia. [G. *a-* priv. + *pallo,* to tremble, quiver, + *aisthēsis,* feeling]

APAP Abbreviation for acetaminophen *N*-acetyl-*P*-aminophenol.

a•par•a•lyt•ic (ā-par′ă-lit′ik) Without paralysis; not causing paralysis.

ap•a•thet•ic (ap-ă-thet′ik) PSYCHOLOGY denotes a patient exhibiting lack of emotion; indifferent.

ap•a•thism (ap′ă-thizm) A sluggishness of reaction. Cf. erethism.

ap•a•thy (ap′ă-thē) Indifference; absence of interest in the environment. Often one of the earliest signs of cerebral disease or depression. [G. *apatheia,* fr. *a-* priv. + *pathos,* suffering]

ap•a•tite (ap′ă-tīt) A class of naturally occurring crystalline minerals containing calcium and phosphorus; hydroxyapatite is a component of bones and teeth. SEE ALSO fluorapatite, hydroxyapatite.

ap•a•tite cal•cu•lus (ap′ă-tīt kal′kyū-lŭs) A calculus in which the crystalloid component consists of calcium fluorophosphate.

A-pat•tern es•o•tro•pi•a (pat′ĕrn es′ō-trō′pē-ă) Convergent strabismus greater in upward than in downward gaze.

A-pat•tern ex•o•tro•pi•a (pat′ĕrn ek′sō-trō′pē-ă) Divergent strabismus greater in downward than in upward gaze.

APC Abbreviation for Ambulatory Payment Classification; antigen-presenting cell.

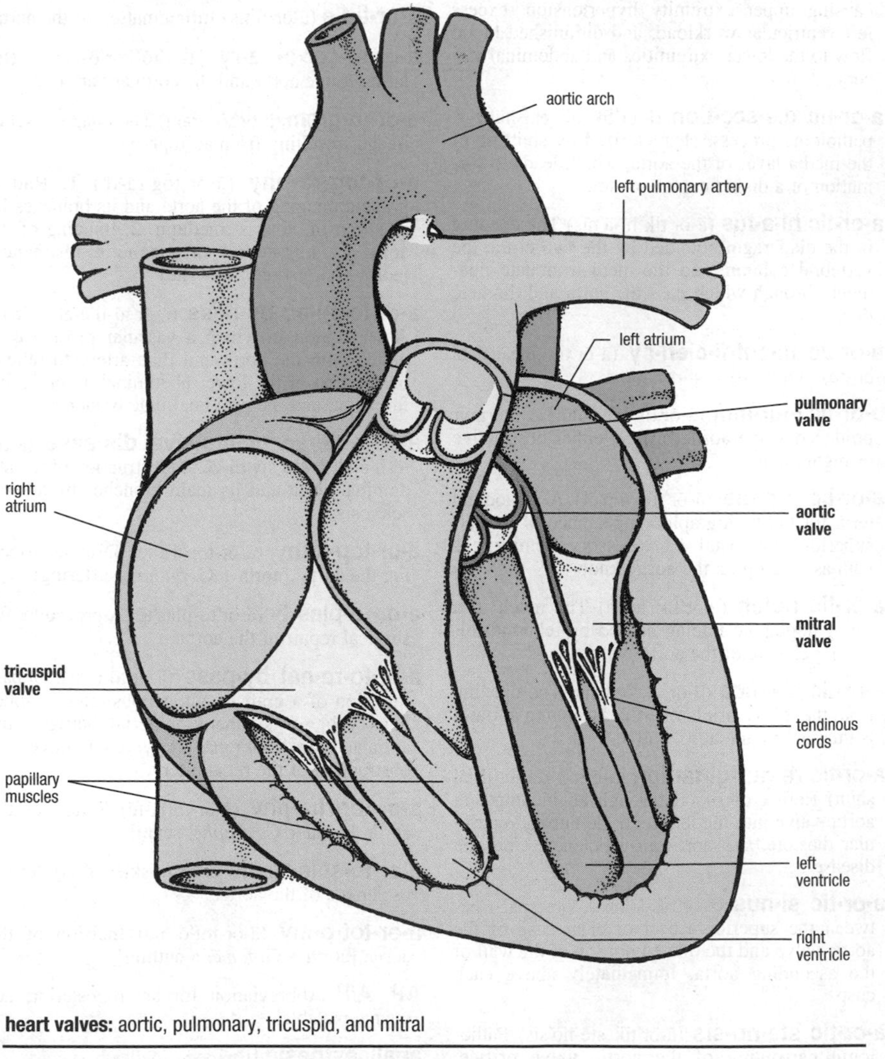

heart valves: aortic, pulmonary, tricuspid, and mitral

a·pel·lous (ă-pel′ŭs) **1.** Without skin. **2.** Without foreskin; circumcised. [G. *a-* not + L. *pellis,* skin]

a·pe·ri·ent (ah-pēr′ē-ĕnt) SYN laxative.

a·pe·ri·od·ic (ā′pēr-ē-od′ik) Not occurring periodically.

a·per·i·stal·sis (ā′per-i-stal′sis) Absence of peristalsis.

a·per·i·tive (ă-per′i-tiv) Stimulating the appetite. [M.L. *aperitivus,* fr. L. *aperio,* to open]

a·per·to·gnath·i·a (a-per′tog-nā′thē-ă) An open bite deformity, a type of malocclusion characterized by premature posterior occlusion and absence of anterior occlusion. [L. *apertus,* open, + G. *gnathos,* jaw]

A·pert syn·drome (ah-pār′ sin′drōm) Disorder characterized by craniosynostosis and syndactyly; associated with hearing loss; mental retardation is a variable feature. SEE ALSO acrocephalosyndactyly.

ap·er·tu·ra, pl. **ap·er·tu·rae** (ap-ĕr-tū′ră, -rē) [TA] SYN aperture. [L. fr. *aperio,* pp. *apertus,* to open]

ap·er·tu·ra la·te·ra·lis ven·tric·u·li quar·ti (ap-ĕr-tū′ră lat-ĕr-ā′lis ven-trik′yū-lī kwōr′tī) [TA] SYN lateral aperture of fourth ventricle.

ap·er·tu·ra me·di·a·na ven·tric·u·li quar·ti (ap-ĕr-tū′ră mē-dē-ā′nă ven-trik′yū-lī kwōr′tī) [TA] SYN median aperture of fourth ventricle.

ap·er·ture (ap′ĕr-chŭr) **1.** An inlet or entrance to a cavity or channel; in anatomy, an open gap or hole. **2.** The diameter of the objective of a microscope. SYN aditus [TA], apertura [TA]. [L. *apertura,* an opening]

a·pex, gen. **ap·i·cis**, pl. **ap·i·ces** (ā′peks, ap′i-sis, ap′i-sēz) [TA] The extremity of a conic or pyramidal structure, such as the heart or the lung. [L. summit or tip]

a·pex an·te·ri·or an·gu·la·tion (ā′peks an-tēr′ē-ŏr ang′gyū-lā′shŭn) Angulation in the lateral plane in which the apex of the angle is directed anteriorly.

a·pex beat (ā′peks bēt) The visible and/or palpable pulsation made by the apex of the left ventricle as it strikes the chest wall in systole; normally in the fifth intercostal space, about 10 cm to the left of the median line. SYN ictus cordis.

a·pex·car·di·og·ra·phy (ā′peks-kahr′dē-og′ră-fē) Noninvasive graphic recording of cardiac pulsations from the region of the apex, usually of the left ventricle, and resembling the ventricular pressure curve.

a·pex·i·fi·ca·tion (ā-pek′si-fi-kā′shŭn) Induced tooth root development or closure of the root apex by hard tissue deposition.

a·pex·o·gen·e·sis (ā-pek′sō-jen′i-sis) Normal development of the apex of the root of a tooth. [apex- + G. *genesis,* origin, birth]

a·pex pneu·mo·ni·a, **ap·i·cal pneu·mo·ni·a** (ā′peks nū-mō′nē-ă, ap′i-kăl nū-mō′nē-ă) An infiltrative process confined to the apex of one or both lungs; typical of tuberculosis and *Pneumocystis jiroveci* pneumonia.

a·pex pos·ter·i·or an·gu·la·tion (ā′peks pos-tēr′ē-ŏr ang′gyū-lā′shŭn) Angulation in the lateral plane in which the apex of the angle is directed posteriorly.

i **Ap·gar score** (ap′gahr skōr) Evaluation of a newborn infant's physical status by assigning numeric values (0–2) to each of 5 criteria: 1) heart rate, 2) respiratory effort, 3) muscle tone, 4) response to stimulation, and 5) skin color; a score of 8–10 indicates the best possible condition. See this page.

Apgar score

after 60 seconds	score	0	1	2
heart rate	......	absent	under 100	over 100
respiratory effort	......	absent	slow, irregular	good (screams)
muscle tone	......	limp	good in limbs	active movement
reaction to nasal catheter	......	none	makes grimaces	coughing or sneezing
skin color	......	pale	rosy trunk, blue extremities	rosy
score	____	(total points: 8–10 is normal)		

a·pha·gi·a (ă-fā′jē-ă) Inability to eat. [G. *a-* priv. + *phagō,* to eat]

a·pha·ki·a (ă-fā′kē-ă) Absence of the lens of the eye. [G. *a-* priv. + *phakos,* lentil, anything shaped like a lentil]

a·pha·kic eye (ă-fā′kik ī) The eye from which the lens is absent.

a·pha·lan·gi·a (ā-fă-lan′jē-ă) Congenital absence of a digit, or more specifically, absence of one or more of the long bones (phalanges) of a finger or toe. [G. *a-* priv. + phalanx]

a·pha·si·a (ă-fā′zē-ă) Impaired or absent comprehension or production of, or communication by, speech, writing, or signs; due to an acquired lesion of or injury to a language center of the brain; may be transient if cerebral swelling subsides. SYN alogia (1), dysphasia, dysphrasia, logagnosia, logamnesia, logasthenia. [G. speechlessness, fr. *a-* priv. + *phasis,* speech]

a·pha·si·ac, **a·pha·sic** (ă-fā′zē-ak, ă-fā′zik)

Relating to or suffering from aphasia. SYN dysphasic.

a•pha•si•ol•o•gist (ă-fā′zē-ol′ŏ-jist) A specialist who deals with speech disorders caused by dysfunction of the language areas of the brain.

a•pha•si•ol•o•gy (ă-fā′zē-ol′ŏ-jē) The science of language disorders caused by dysfunction of the cerebral language areas.

a•phe•mi•a (ă-fē′mē-ă) Motor aphasia. [G. *a,* without, + *phēmē,* speech]

a•pher•e•sis (ā-fĕr-ē′sis) Extraction of certain fluid or cellular elements from withdrawn blood, which is then reinfused into the donor or patient; performed therapeutically to remove harmful elements from the blood, and also to obtain immune globulins. [G. *aphairesis,* withdrawal]

a•pho•ni•a (ă-fō′nē-ă) Loss of the voice as a result of disease or injury to the larynx. [G. *a-* priv. + *phōnē,* voice]

a•phon•ic (ă-fon′ik) Relating to aphonia.

a•phra•si•a (ă-frā′zē-ă) Inability to speak, due to any cause. [G. *a-* priv. + *phrasis,* speaking]

aph•ro•di•si•ac (af-rō-diz′ē-ak) **1.** Increasing sexual desire. **2.** Anything that arouses or increases sexual desire.

aph•tha, pl. **aph•thae** (af′thă, af′thē) **1.** In the singular, a small ulcer on a mucous membrane. **2.** In the plural, stomatitis characterized by episodes of painful oral ulcers of unknown etiology that are covered by gray exudate, are surrounded by an erythematous halo, and that heal spontaneously in 1–2 weeks. SYN aphthae minor, aphthous stomatitis, canker sores, recurrent aphthous ulcers, recurrent ulcerative stomatitis, ulcerative stomatitis. [G. ulceration]

aph•thae (af′thē) Plural of aphtha.

aph•thae ma•jor (af′thē mā′jŏr) A severe form of aphthae characterized by unusually numerous, large, deep, and frequent ulcers; healing may take as long as 6 weeks and results in scarring. SYN Mikulicz aphthae, periadenitis mucosa necrotica recurrens, Sutton disease.

aph•thae mi•nor (af′thē mī′nŏr) SYN aphtha (2).

aph•thoid (af′thoyd) Resembling aphthae.

aph•tho•sis (af-thō′sis) Any condition characterized by the presence of aphthae.

aph•thous (af′thŭs) Characterized by or relating to aphthae or aphthosis.

aph•thous sto•ma•ti•tis (af′thŭs stō′mă-tī′tis) SYN aphtha (2).

Aph•tho•vi•rus (af′thō-vī′rus) A genus in the family Picornaviridae associated with foot and mouth disease of cattle.

API Abbreviation for active pharmaceutical ingredient.

ap•i•cal (ap′i-kăl) **1.** Relating to the apex or tip of a pyramidal or pointed structure. **2.** Situated nearer to the apex of a structure in relation to a specific reference point; opposite of basal. **3.** SYN point of maximal impulse.

ap•i•cal cap (ap′i-kăl kap) A curved shadow at the apex of one or both hemithoraces on chest x-ray; caused by pleural and pulmonary fibrosis.

ap•i•cal fo•ra•men of tooth (ap′i-kăl fōr-ā′mĕn tūth) The opening at the apex of the root of a tooth that gives passage to the nerve and blood vessels.

ap•i•cal gland (ap′i-kăl gland) SYN anterior lingual gland.

ap•i•cal gran•u•lo•ma (ap′i-kăl gran′yū-lō′mă) SYN periapical granuloma. See this page.

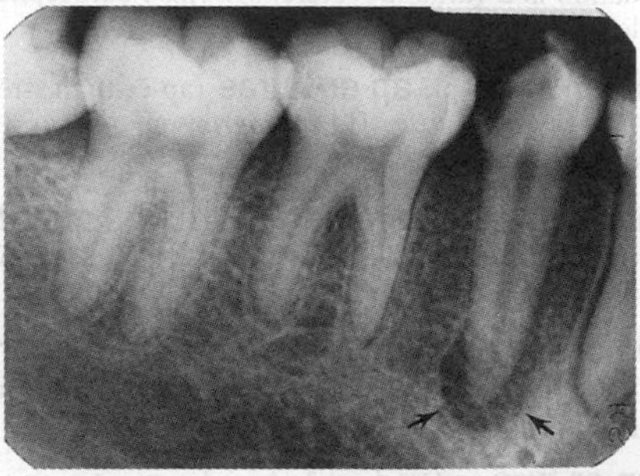

apical granuloma (arrows) of nonvital mandibular second premolar

ap•i•cal in•fec•tion (ā′pi-kăl in-fek′shŭn) Implantation of microorganisms at the apex of a tooth, usually the result of the migration of microorganisms from the pulp canal through the apical foramen.

ap•i•cal per•i•o•don•tal cyst (ap′i-kăl per′ē-ō-don′tăl sist) An inflammatory odontogenic cyst derived histogenetically from Malassez epithelial rests surrounding the root apex of a nonvital tooth. See page 111.

ap•i•cal pulse (ap′i-kăl pŭls) A heart sound heard directly over the apex of the heart by means of clinical use of a stethoscope. See page 111.

ap•i•cal seg•men•tal ar•ter•y (ap′i-kăl seg-men′tăl ahr′tĕr-ē) SEE left pulmonary artery, right pulmonary artery.

ap•i•cal seg•men•tal ar•ter•y of su•per•i•or lo•bar ar•ter•y of right lung (ap′i-kăl seg-men′tăl ahr′tĕr-ē sŭ-pēr′ē-ŏr lō′bahr ahr′tĕr-ē rīt lŭng) Branch (of the inferior lobar branch) of the right pulmonary artery serving the apical segment of the inferior lobe of the right lung.

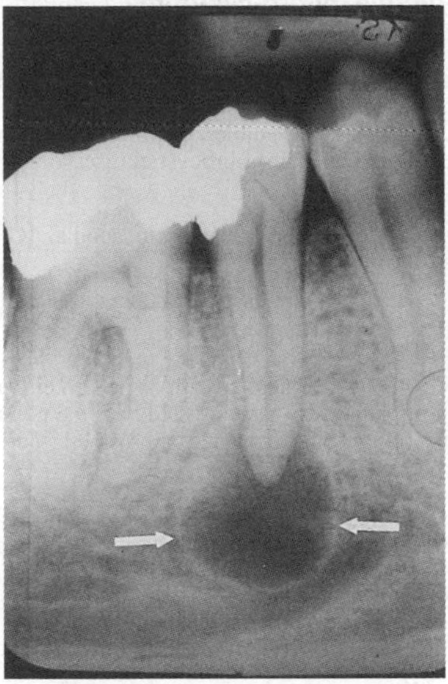

apical periodontal cyst (arrows) at roots of mandibular second premolar

ap·i·cal space (ap′i-kăl spās) The space between the alveolar wall and the apex of the root of a tooth where an alveolar abscess usually has its origin.

ap·i·cec·to·my (ap-i-sek′tŏ-mē) **1.** Opening and exenteration of air cells in the apex of the petrous part of the temporal bone. **2.** DENTAL SURGERY an obsolete synonym for apicoectomy. [L. *apex,* summit or tip, + G. *ektomē,* excision]

ap·i·ces (ap′i-sēz) Plural of apex.

ap·i·ci·tis (ap-i-sī′tis) Inflammation of the apex of a structure or organ.

♻**apico-** Prefix meaning an apex; apical. [L. *apex, apicis,* a summit or a tip + -o-]

ap·i·co·ec·to·my (ap′i-kō-ek′tŏ-mē) Surgical removal of a dental root apex. SYN root resection. [apico- + G. *ektomē,* excision]

ap·i·col·y·sis (ap-i-kol′i-sis) Surgical collapse of the upper portion of the lung by the operative detachment of the parietal pleura allowing a medial displacement of the pulmonary apex. [apico- + G. *lysis,* destruction]

ap·i·cot·o·my (ap-i-kot′ŏ-mē) Incision into an apical structure. [apico- + G. *tomē,* a cutting]

a·pi·o·ther·a·py (ā′pē-ō-thār′ă-pē) The medicinal use of honeybee venom to treat inflammatory and degenerative diseases. [L. *apis,* bee, + therapy]

ap·la·nat·ic (ap-lă-nat′ik) Pertaining to aplanatism, or to an aplanatic lens.

ap·la·nat·ic lens (ap-lă-nat′ik lenz) A lens designed to correct spheric aberration and coma.

a·pla·si·a (ă-plā′zē-ă) **1.** Defective development or congenital absence of an organ or tissue. **2.** HEMATOLOGY incomplete, retarded, or defective development, or cessation of the usual regenerative process. [G. *a-* priv. + *plasis,* a molding]

a·plas·tic (ā-plas′tik) Pertaining to aplasia, or conditions characterized by defective regeneration, as in aplastic anemia.

a·plas·tic a·ne·mi·a (ā-plas′tik ă-nē′mē-ă) Disorder characterized by a greatly decreased formation of erythrocytes and hemoglobin, usually associated with pronounced granulocytopenia and thrombocytopenia, as a result of hypoplastic or aplastic bone marrow. SYN Ehrlich anemia.

a·plas·tic lymph (ā-plas′tik limf) Fluid containing a relatively large number of leukocytes, but comparatively little fibrinogen; does not form a good clot and manifests only a slight tendency to become organized.

aPLS Abbreviation for antiphospholipid antibody syndrome.

APMPPE Abbreviation for acute posterior multifocal placoid pigment epitheliopathy.

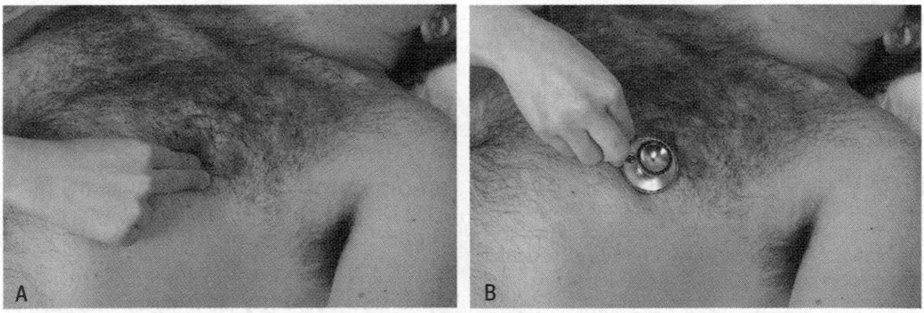

apical pulse: usually found at (A) fifth intercostal space just inside the midclavicular line and can be heard (B) over the apex of the heart

ap•ne•a (ap′nē-ă) Absence of spontaneous breathing. SYN apnoea. [G. *apnoia,* want of breath]

ap•ne•a-hy•pop•ne•a in•dex (AHI) (ap′nē-ă-hī-pop′nē-ă in′deks) The number of apneic and hypopneic episodes combined per hour of sleep. SYN apnoea-hypopnoea index.

ap•ne•ic (ap′nē-ik) Related to or suffering from apnea. SYN apnoeic.

ap•ne•ic pause (ap′nē-ik pawz) Cessation of air flow for longer than 10 seconds. SEE sleep apnea. SYN apnoeic pause.

ap•neu•mi•a (ap-nū′mē-ă) Congenital absence of the lungs. [G. *a-* priv. + *pneumōn,* lung]

ap•neu•sis, ap•neus•tic breath•ing (ap-nū′sis, ap-nūs′tik brēdh′ing) An abnormal respiratory pattern consisting of a pause at full inspiration; cramp caused by a lesion at the mid or caudal pontine level of the brainstem. [G. *a-* priv. + *pneusis,* a breathing, fr. *pneō,* to breathe]

apnoea [Br.] SYN apnea.

apnoea-hypopnoea index [Br.] SYN apnea-hypopnea index.

apnoeic [Br.] SYN apneic.

apnoeic pause [Br.] SYN apneic pause.

♻ **apo-** Combining form meaning, usually, separated from or derived from. [G. *apo,* away from, off; *apo-* becomes *ap-*, especially before a vowel or h]

ap•o•chro•mat•ic ob•jec•tive (ap′ō-krō-mat′ik ŏb-jek′tiv) An objective in which chromatic aberration is corrected for three colors and spheric aberration is corrected for two.

ap•o•crine (ap′ō-krin) Denoting a mechanism of glandular secretion in which the apical portion of secretory cells is shed and incorporated into the secretion. SEE ALSO apocrine gland. [G. *apo-krinō,* to separate]

ap•o•crine ad•e•no•ma (ap′ō-krin ad′ĕ-nō′mă) SYN papillary hidradenoma.

ap•o•crine car•ci•no•ma (ap′ō-krin kahr′si-nō′mă) **1.** A carcinoma composed predominantly of secretory cells with abundant eosinophilic granular cytoplasm, occurring in the breast. **2.** A carcinoma of the apocrine glands, especially those found in the groin and axilla.

ap•o•crine chrom•hi•dro•sis (ap′ō-krin krōm-hī-drō′sis) Excretion of colored sweat, usually black, from apocrine glands of the face; attributable to an abnormal lipochrome content of the secretion.

ap•o•crine gland (ap′ō-krin gland) A gland the secretory product of which includes an apical portion of the secretory cell such as the secretion of lipid droplets in lactation.

ap•o•crine hi•dro•cys•to•ma (ap′ō-krin hī′drō-sis-tō′mă) SYN sudoriferous cyst.

ap•o•crine met•a•pla•si•a (ap′ō-krin met-ă-plā′zē-ă) Alteration of acinar epithelium of breast tissue to resemble apocrine sweat glands; seen commonly in fibrocystic disease of the breasts.

a•po•dal (ā-pō′dal) Relating to apodia. [G. *a-* priv. + *pous,* foot]

a•po•di•a (ā-pō′dē-ă) Congenital absence of feet. [G. *a-* priv. + *pous,* foot]

ap•o•en•zyme (ap′ō-en-zīm) The protein portion of an enzyme as contrasted with the nonprotein portion, or coenzyme, or prosthetic portion (if present).

ap•o•fer•ri•tin (ap-ō-fer′i-tin) A protein in the intestinal wall that combines with a ferric hydroxide-phosphate compound to form ferritin, the first stage in the absorption of iron.

a•po-2L (ap′ō) SYN TRAIL.

a•po•lip•o•pro•tein (ap′ō-lip-ō-prō′tēn) The protein component of lipoprotein complexes that is a normal constituent of plasma chylomicrons, HDL, LDL, and VLDL in humans.

ap•o•neu•rec•to•my (ap′ō-nūr-ek′tŏ-mē) Excision of an aponeurosis. [aponeurosis + G. *ektomē,* excision]

ap•o•neu•ror•rha•phy (ap′ō-nūr-ōr′ă-fē) SYN fasciorrhaphy. [aponeurosis + G. *rhaphē,* suture]

ap•o•neu•ro•sis, pl. **ap•o•neu•ro•ses** (ap′ō-nūr-ō′sis, -sēz) A fibrous sheet or flat, expanded tendon, giving attachment to muscular fibers and serving as the means of origin or insertion of a flat muscle; it sometimes also performs the functions of a fascia for other muscles. [G. the end of the muscle where it becomes tendon, fr. *apo,* from, + *neuron,* sinew]

ap•o•neu•ro•si•tis (ap′ō-nūr′ō-sī′tis) Inflammation of an aponeurosis.

ap•o•neu•rot•ic (ap′ō-nūr-ot′ik) Relating to an aponeurosis.

ap•o•neu•rot•ic fi•bro•ma (ap′ō-nūr-ot′ik fī-brō′mă) A calcifying recurrent nonmetastasizing but infiltrating fibroma seen most frequently on the palms of young people as a small firm nodule not attached to the overlying skin.

ap•o•neu•rot•ic pto•sis (ap′ō-nūr-ō-jen′ik tō′sis) Drooping of the eyelid caused by dehiscence of the tendon of the levator muscle. SYN involutional ptosis.

ap•o•neu•rot•o•my (ap′ō-nūr-ot′ŏ-mē) Incision of an aponeurosis.

ap•o•phys•i•al frac•ture (ap′ō-fiz′ē-ăl frak′shŭr) Separation of apophysis from bone.

a•poph•y•sis, pl. **a•poph•y•ses** (ă-pof′i-sis, -sēz) An outgrowth or projection, especially one from a bone. A bony process or outgrowth that lacks an independent center of ossification. [G. an offshoot]

a•poph•y•si•tis (ă-pof-i-sī′tis) Inflammation of any apophysis.

Ap•o•phy•so•my•ces (ap-ō-fiz-ō-mī′sēz) A genus of fungi in the family Mucoraceae; a cause of zygomycosis, including necrotizing fasciitis and osteomyelitis. Infections occur after fungals are implanted in traumatic wounds.

ap•o•plex•y (ap′ō-pleks-ē) SYN stroke.

ap•o•pro•tein (ap′ō-prō′tēn) A polypeptide chain (protein) not yet complexed with the prosthetic group that is necessary to form the active holoprotein.

ap•o•pto•sis (ap′ō-tō′sis) Programmed cell death; deletion of individual cells by fragmentation into membrane-bound particles, which are phagocytized by other cells. SYN programmed cell death. [G. a falling or dropping off, fr. *apo,* off, + *ptosis*, a falling]

ap•o•re•pres•sor (ap′ō-rĕ-pres′ŏr) SYN inactive repressor.

ap•o•stax•is (ap′ō-staks′is) Slight hemorrhage, or bleeding by drops. [G. a trickling down]

a•pos•thi•a (ă-pos′thē-ă) Congenital absence of the prepuce of the penis or clitoris. [G. *a-* priv. + *posthē,* foreskin]

a•poth•e•car•ies' weight (ă-poth′ĕ-kar-ēz wāt) A system of weights based on the weight of a grain of wheat; superseded by the metric system (based on grams). One grain is the equivalent of 64.8 mg. One scruple contains 20 grains; 1 dram contains 60 grains; 1 apothecary ounce contains 8 drams (480 grains); apothecary pound contains 12 ounces (5760 grains).

ap•pa•ra•tus (ap′ă-rat′ŭs) **1.** A collection of instruments adapted for a special purpose. **2.** An instrument made up of several parts. **3.** A group or system of glands, ducts, blood vessels, muscles, or other anatomic structures involved in the performance of some function. SEE ALSO system. [L. equipment. fr. *ap-paro,* pp. *-atus,* to prepare]

ap•par•ent life-threat•en•ing e•vent (ALTE) (ă-par′ĕnt līf-thret′ĕn-ing ĕ-vent′) An ill-defined condition that occurs in infants; involves a change in breathing and either cyanosis, muscle weakness, choking/gagging, or apnea; causes the patient's caregiver to seek immediate medical assistance.

ap•peal (ă-pēl′) In health care accounting, denotes a request from a physician or clerical worker in a health care facility for a third-party payer to reconsider a decision about a disallowed claim for compensation.

ap•pend•age (ă-pen′dăj) Any part, subordinate in function or size, attached to a main structure. SEE ALSO adnexa. SYN appendix (1). [L. *appendix*]

ap•pend•ag•es of skin (ă-pend′dăj-ĕz skin) Hair, fingernails, toenails, and sweat, sebaceous, and mammary glands.

ap•pen•dec•to•my (ap′pĕn-dek′tŏ-mē) Surgical removal of the vermiform appendix. SYN appendicectomy. [appendix + G. *ektomē,* excision]

ap•pen•dic•e•al, ap•pen•di•cal (ap′ĕn-dis′ē-ăl, ă-pen′di-kăl) Relating to an appendix.

ap•pen•dic•e•al ab•scess (ap′ĕn-dis′ē-ăl ab′ses) An intraperitoneal abscess, usually in the right iliac fossa, resulting from extension of infection in acute appendicitis, especially with perforation of the appendix. SYN periappendiceal abscess.

ap•pen•di•cec•to•my (ap-pen′di-sek′tŏ-mē) SYN appendectomy.

ap•pen•di•ces o•men•ta•les (ă-pen′di-sēz ō-men-tā′lēz) [TA] SYN omental appendices.

ap•pen•di•ci•tis (ă-pen′di-sī′tis) Inflammation of the vermiform appendix. [appendix + G. *-itis,* inflammation]

♻**appendico-** Combining form meaning an appendix, usually the vermiform appendix. [L. *appendix, appendicis* an appendage, fr. *appendo*, to hang something onto something, fr. *ad-, ap-*, to, onto, + *pendo*, to hang, + -o-]

ap•pen•di•co•lith (ă-pen′di-kō-lith) A calcified concretion in the appendix visible on an abdominal radiograph. [appendico- + G. *lithos*, stone]

ap•pen•di•co•li•thi•a•sis (ă-pen′di-kō-li-thī′ă-sis) The presence of concretions in the vermiform appendix. [appendico- + G. *lithos,* stone]

ap•pen•di•col•y•sis (ă-pen′di-kol′i-sis) An operation for freeing the appendix from adhesions. [appendico- + G. *lysis,* a loosening]

ap•pen•di•cos•to•my (ă-pen′di-kos′tō-mē) An operation for opening into the intestine through the tip of the vermiform appendix, previously attached to the anterior abdominal wall. [appendico- + G. *stoma,* mouth]

ap•pen•dic•u•lar (ap′ĕn-dik′yŭ-lăr) **1.** Relating to an appendix or appendage. **2.** Relating to the limbs, as opposed to axial, which refers to the trunk and head.

ap•pen•dic•u•lar ar•ter•y (ap′ĕn-dik′yŭ-lăr ahr′tĕr-ē) The branch of the ileocolic artery that descends posterior to the terminal ileum in the mesoappendix to supply the vermiform appendix. SYN arteria appendicularis [TA].

ap•pen•dic•u•lar mus•cle (ap′ĕn-dik′yŭ-lăr mŭs′ĕl) One of the skeletal muscles of the limbs.

ap•pen•dic•u•lar skel•e•ton (ap′ĕn-dik′yŭ-lăr

skel′ĕ-tŏn) The bones of the limbs including the shoulder and pelvic girdles.

ap·pen·dic·u·lar vein (ap′ĕn-dik′yŭ-lăr vān) The tributary of the ileocolic vein that accompanies the appendicular artery.

ap·pen·dix, gen. **ap·pen·di·cis**, pl. **ap·pen·di·ces** (ă-pen′diks, -di-sis, -di-sēz) **1.** SYN appendage. **2.** A wormlike intestinal diverticulum extending from the blind end of the cecum; it varies in length and ends in a blind extremity. [L. appendage, fr. *ap-pendo,* to hang something on]

ap·pen·dix ep·i·plo·i·ca, pl. **ap·pen·di·ces ep·i·plo·i·cae** (ă-pen′diks ep-i-plō′i-kă, ă-pen′di-sēz ep-i-plō′i-sē) One of a number of little processes or sacs of peritoneum filled with adipose tissue and projecting from the serous coat of the large intestine, except the rectum; they are most evident on the transverse and sigmoid colon, being most numerous along the free tenia.

ap·pen·dix of tes·tis (ă-pen′diks tes′tis) A vesicular structure attached to the cephalic pole of the testis; a vestige of the paramesonephric (müllerian) duct.

ap·pen·dix ver·mi·for·mis (ă-pen′diks ver-mi-fōr′mis) [TA] SYN vermiform appendix.

ap·per·cep·tion (ap′ĕr-sep′shŭn) **1.** The final stage of attentive perception in which something is clearly apprehended and thus is relatively prominent in awareness; the full apprehension of any psychic content. **2.** The process of referring the perception of ideas to one's own personality. [L. *ad,* to, + *per- cipio,* pp. *-ceptus,* to take wholly, perceive]

ap·per·cep·tive (ap′ĕr-sep′tiv) Relating to, involved in, or capable of apperception.

ap·pe·tite (ap′ĕ-tīt) A desire or motive derived from a biologic or psychological need for food, water, sex, or affection; a desire or longing to satisfy any conscious physical or mental need. [L. *ad-peto,* pp. *-petitus,* to seek after, desire]

ap·pla·na·tion (ap′lă-nā′shŭn) TONOMETRY the flattening of the cornea by pressure. Intraocular pressure is directly proportional to external pressure, and inversely proportional to the area flattened. SEE ALSO applanation tonometer. [L. *ad,* toward, + *planum,* plane]

ap·pla·na·tion to·nom·e·ter (ap′lă-nā′shŭn tō-nom′ĕ-tĕr) An instrument for determining ocular tension by application of a small, flat disc to the cornea.

ap·pla·nom·e·try (ap′lăn-om′ĕ-trē) Use of an applanation tonometer.

ap·ple (ap′ĕl) The edible, roughly spheric fruit of trees of the genus *Malus.* [O.E. *aeppel*]

ap·ple jel·ly nod·ules (ap′ĕl jel′ē nod′yūlz) Descriptive term for the papular lesions of lupus vulgaris, as they appear on diascopy.

ap·pli·ance (ă-plī′ăns) A device used to provide function to a part, or for therapeutic purposes. [fr, O. Fr. *aplier,* to apply, fr. L. *applico,* to fold together]

ap·pli·ca·tion (ap′li-kā′shŭn) **1.** The act of applying, as in bringing a medicine, dressing, or device into contact with the body surface. **2.** The act of putting to a specific use, or the capacity of being so used. **3.** A formal request, usually in writing.

ap·pli·ca·tor (ap′li-kā-tŏr) A slender rod of wood, flexible metal, or synthetic material, at one end of which is attached a pledget of cotton or other substance for making local applications to any accessible surface. [L. *ap-plico,* to attach to]

ap·plied ki·ne·si·ol·o·gy (ă-plīd′ kin-ē′sē-ol′ŏ-jē) An approach to diagnosis and treatment based on the tenet that a dysfunction in a body organ or area will be reflected in muscle groups. By testing the strength and weakness of muscles, clinicians can determine the nature of the patient's illness and identify which nutritional supplements will help palliate the condition.

ap·po·si·tion (ap′ō-zish′ŭn) **1.** The placing in contact of two substances. **2.** The condition of being placed or fitted together. **3.** The relationship of fracture fragments to one another. **4.** The process of thickening of the cell wall. **5.** The deposition of the matrix of the hard dental structures; enamel, dentin, and cementum. [L. *ap-pono,* pp. *-positus,* to place at or to]

ap·po·si·tion·al growth (ap′ō-zish′ŭn-ăl grōth) Growth accomplished by the addition of new layers on those previously formed; e.g., the addition of lamellae in the formation of bone; it is the characteristic mode of growth when rigid materials are involved.

ap·po·si·tion su·ture (ap′ō-zish′ŭn sū′chŭr) A suture that holds together margins of a skin only. SYN coaptation suture.

ap·pos·i·tive (ă-poz′i-tiv) Word or phrase preceding or following a noun that identifies or explains the noun. [L. *appono, appositum,* to place next to]

ap·proach (ă-prōch′) **1.** PSYCHIATRY a term used to describe how interpersonal relationships are negotiated. **2.** The path or method used to expose the operative field during an operation. [M.E., fr. O. Fr., fr L.L. *appropio,* to come nearer, fr. *ad,* to + *propius,* nearer]

AP pro·jec·tion (prŏ-jek′shŭn) A radiographic study in which x-rays travel from anterior to posterior. SYN anteroposterior projection.

ap·pro·pri·ate for ges·ta·tion·al age (AGA) (ă-prō′prē-ăt jes-tā′shŭn-ăl āj) Referring to an infant whose birth weight is appropriate for its gestational age.

ap·prox·i·mate (ă-prok′si-māt) **1.** To bring

close together. DENTISTRY 2. (ă-prok′sĭ-măt) Proximate, denoting the contact surfaces, either mesial or distal, of two adjacent teeth. 3. Close together; denoting the teeth in the human jaw, as distinguished from the separated teeth in certain of the lower animals. [L. *ad,* to, + *proximus,* nearest]

ap•prox•i•ma•tion (ă-prok′si-mā′shŭn) In surgery, bringing tissue edges into desired apposition for suturing.

ap•prox•i•ma•tion su•ture (ă-prok′si-mā′shŭn sū′chŭr) A suture that pulls together the deep tissues.

a•prac•tic (ă-prak′tik) SYN apraxic.

a•prax•i•a (ă-prak′sē-ă) 1. A disorder of voluntary movement, consisting of impairment in the performance of skilled or purposeful movements, notwithstanding the preservation of comprehension, muscular power, sensibility, and coordination in general; due to congenital or otherwise acquired cerebral disease. 2. A psychomotor defect in which the proper use of an object cannot be carried out although the object can be named and its uses described correctly. [G. *a-* priv. + *prattō,* to do]

a•prax•i•a of speech (ă-prak′sē-ă spēch) Speech disorder due to cortical sensorimotor damage that impairs the ability to program speech musculature for volitional production of sequenced phonemes. Often accompanies motor aphasia. SEE apraxia, oral apraxia, developmental apraxia of speech. SYN articulatory apraxia, dyspraxia of speech, verbal apraxia, verbal dyspraxia.

a•prax•ic (ă-prak′sik) Marked by or pertaining to apraxia. SYN apractic.

a•proc•ti•a (ă-prok′shē-ă) Congenital absence or imperforation of the anus. [G. *a-* priv. + *prōktos,* anus]

a•pron•ec•to•my (ap′rō-nek′tŏ-mē) Surgical excision of a redundant and dependent panniculus adiposus of the abdominal wall, which is commonly called an apron.

a•pro•so•dy, a•pro•so•di•a (ā-pros′ŏ-dē, ā-prō-zō′dē-ă) Complete loss of speech intonation patterns, usually due to a neurologic disorder. SEE ALSO dysprosody. [G. *a-* priv. + prosody]

ap•ro•so•pi•a (ap′rō-sō′pē-ă) Congenital absence of most or all of the face, usually associated with other malformations. [G. *a-* priv. + *prosōpon,* face]

APRV Abbreviation for airway pressure release ventilation.

APS Abbreviation for adenosine 5′-phosphosulfate; antiphospholipid antibody syndrome.

ap•ti•tude test (ap′ti-tūd test) An occupation-oriented intelligence test used to evaluate a person's abilities, talents, and skills; particularly valuable in vocational counseling.

aPTT Abbreviation for activated partial thromboplastin time.

APUD, APUD cells (ap′ŭd, ap′ŭd selz) Designation for cells in various organs secreting polypeptide hormones. Cells in this group have certain biochemical characteristics in common: they contain amines, such as catecholamine and 5-hydroxytryptamine; take up precursors of these amines in vivo; and contain amino acid decarboxylase. [*a*mine *p*recursor *u*ptake, *d*ecarboxylase]

a•py•ret•ic (ā-pī-ret′ik) Without fever, denoting apyrexia; having a normal body temperature. SYN afebrile.

a•py•rex•i•a (ā-pī-rek′sē-ă) Absence of fever. [G. *a-* priv. + *pyrexis,* fever]

aq. Abbreviation for water. [L. *aqua*]

aq. dest. Abbreviation for distilled water. [L. *aqua destillata*]

aq•ua•gen•ic pru•ri•tus (ahk′wă-jen′ik prū-rī′tŭs) Intense itching produced by brief contact with water at any temperature without visible changes in the skin.

aq•ua•pho•bi•a (ahk′wă-fō′bē-ă) Morbid fear of water. [L. *aqua,* water, + G. *phobos,* fear]

aq•ue•duct (ahk′wă-dŭkt) A conduit or canal. SYN aqueductus [TA]. [L. *aquaeductus*]

aq•ue•duc•tus, pl. **aq•ue•duc•tus** (ahk′wĕ-dŭk′tŭs, ahk′wĕ-dŭk′tŭs) [TA] SYN aqueduct. [L. fr. *aqua,* water, + *ductus,* a leading, fr. *duco,* pp. *ductus,* to lead]

aq•ue•duc•tus co•chle•ae (ahk′wĕ-dŭk′tŭs kō′lē-ē) [TA] SYN perilymphatic duct.

aq•ue•ous (ā′kwē-ŭs) Watery; of, like, or containing water.

aq•ue•ous cham•bers (ā′kwē-ŭs chām′bĕrz) The combined anterior and posterior chambers of the eye containing the aqueous humor.

aq•ue•ous hu•mor (ā′kwē-ŭs hyū′mŏr) The watery fluid that fills the anterior chamber of the eye. It is secreted by the ciliary processes within the posterior chamber and passes through the pupil into the anterior chamber where it filters through the trabecular meshwork and is reabsorbed into the venous system at the iridocorneal angle by way of the sinus venosus of the sclera.

aq•ue•ous phase (ā′kwē-ŭs fāz) The water portion of a system consisting of two liquid phases, one mainly water, the other a liquid immiscible with water (e.g., benzene, ether).

AR, A/R Abbreviation for accounts receivable.

Ar Symbol for argon.

♻ **arab-** Combining form meaning gum arabic or similar gummy substances. [G. *Araps, Arabos,* an Arab]

ar·a·chi·don·ic ac·id (ar′ă-ki-don′ik as′id) Liquid unsaturated fatty acid that occurs in most animal fats; considered essential in animal nutrition.

a·rach·nase (ă-rak′nās) A positive control plasma for the monitoring of clotting-endpoint coagulation tests used in the detection of circulating lupus anticoagulants. It is a normal plasma that contains a venom extract from the brown recluse spider, *Loxosceles reclusa,* which mimics the presence of a lupus anticoagulant in several clotting-endpoint tests.

a·rach·ne·pho·bi·a (ă-rak′nĕ-fō′bē-ă) Morbid fear of spiders. SYN arachnophobia. [G. *arachnē,* spider, + *phobos,* fear]

A·rach·ni·da (ă-rak′ni-dă) A class of arthropods in the subphylum Chelicerata, consisting of spiders, scorpions, harvestmen, mites, ticks, and allies. See page B8. [G. *arachnē,* spider]

a·rach·nid·ism (ă-rak′ni-dizm) Systemic poisoning following the bite of a venomous spider (especially the black widow).

ar·ach·ni·tis (ar′ak-nī′tis) Inflammation of the arachnoid membrane.

a·rach·no·dac·ty·ly (ă-rak′nō-dak′ti-lē) A condition in which the hands and fingers, and often the feet and toes, are abnormally long and slender; a characteristic of Marfan syndrome and kindred hereditary disorders of connective tissue. [G. *arachnē,* spider, + *daktylos,* finger]

a·rach·noid (ă-rak′noyd) A delicate fibrous membrane forming the middle of the three coverings (i.e., meninges) of the central nervous system. Its external surface is closely applied (but not attached) to the internal surface of the dura mater, with only a potential space (subdural space) intervening. Thus, in a spinal puncture, dura mater and arachnoid are penetrated simultaneously as if a single layer. SEE ALSO leptomeninges, arachnoid mater. SYN arachnoidea mater [TA], arachnoid membrane, arachnoidea, arachnoides. [G. *arachnē,* spider, cobweb, + *eidos,* resemblance]

a·rach·noid of brain (ă-rak′noyd brān) SYN cranial arachnoid mater.

a·rach·noid cyst (ă-rak′noyd sist) A fluid-filled cyst lined with arachnoid mater, frequently situated near the lateral aspect of the lateral sulcus; usually congenital in origin.

a·rach·noi·de·a, a·rach·noi·des (ă-rak-noyd′ē-ă, noy′dēz) SYN arachnoid. [Mod. L. *arachnoideus* fr. G. *arachnē,* spider, + *eidos,* resemblance]

a·rach·noi·de·a ma·ter (ă-rak-noyd′ē-ă mā′tĕr) [TA] SYN arachnoid.

a·rach·noi·de·a ma·ter cra·ni·a·lis (ă-rak′noyd mā′ter krā-nē-ā′lis) [TA] SYN cranial arachnoid mater.

a·rach·noi·de·a ma·ter en·ceph·a·li (ă-rak′noyd mā′ter en-sef′ă-lī) SYN cranial arachnoid mater.

a·rach·noid gran·u·la·tions (ă-rak′noyd gran-yū-lā′shŭnz) Tufted prolongations of pia-arachnoid, composed of numerous arachnoid villi that penetrate the dural venous sinuses and effect transfer of cerebrospinal fluid to the venous system. SYN granulationes arachnoideales [TA], pacchionian bodies.

a·rach·noid·i·tis (ă-rak′noy-dī′tis) Inflammation of the arachnoid membrane often with involvement of the subjacent subarachnoid space. SEE ALSO leptomeningitis. [arachnoidea + *-itis,* inflammation]

a·rach·noid ma·ter (ă-rak′noyd mā′tĕr) A delicate fibrous membrane forming the middle of the three coverings of the central nervous system. In life the arachnoid (specifically the arachnoid barrier cell layer) is tenuously attached to the externally adjacent dura mater (specifically the dural border cells) and there is no naturally occurring space at the dura-arachnoid interface. Thus, in a spinal puncture, dura mater and arachnoid are penetrated simultaneously as if a single layer. Separation of the arachnoid mater from the dura mater (usually through the dural border cell layer) may result from traumatic or pathologic processes creating what is commonly, but quite incorrectly, called a subdural hematoma. The arachnoid mater is named for the delicate, spiderweblike filaments that extend from its deep surface, through the cerebrospinal fluid of the subarachnoid space, to the pia mater.

a·rach·noid mem·brane (ă-rak′noyd mem′brān) SYN arachnoid.

a·rach·noid vil·li (ă-rak′noyd vil′ī) Tufted prolongations of pia-arachnoid that protrude through the meningeal layer of the dura mater and have a thin limiting membrane; collections of arachnoid villi form arachnoid granulations that lie in venous lacunae at the margin of the superior sagittal sinus; the spongy tissue of the arachnoid villus contains tubules that serve as one-way valves for transfer of cerebrospinal fluid from the subarachnoid space to the venous system. Both arachnoid villi and the granulations formed from them are major sites of fluid transfer. SEE ALSO arachnoid granulations.

a·rach·no·pho·bi·a (ă-rak′nŏ-fō′bē-ă) SYN arachnephobia.

A·ran-Du·chenne dis·ease (ah-rahn′ dū-shen′ di-zēz′) SYN amyotrophic lateral sclerosis.

ARB Abbreviation for angiotensin II receptor blocker.

ar·bor, pl. **ar·bo·res** (ahr′bŏr, ahr-bōr′ēz)

ANATOMY any treelike structure with branchings. [L. tree]

ar•bo•res•cent (ahr′bŏr-es′ĕnt) SYN dendriform.

ar•bo•ri•za•tion (ahr′bŏr-ī-zā′shŭn) **1.** The terminal branching of nerve fibers or blood vessels in a treelike pattern. **2.** The branched pattern formed by a dried smear of cervical mucus, indicating the effect of estrogen unopposed by progesterone.

ar•bo•rize (ahr′bŏr-īz) To spread in a treelike branching pattern.

ar•bo•vi•rus (ahr′bō-vī′rŭs) A large, heterogeneous group of RNA viruses. There are more than 500 species, which have been recovered from arthropods, bats, and rodents. These taxonomically diverse viruses are unified by an epidemiologic concept, i.e., transmission between vertebrate hosts by blood-feeding arthropod vectors, such as mosquitoes, ticks, sandflies, and midges. In most instances diseases produced by these viruses are mild and difficult to distinguish from illnesses caused by viruses of other taxonomic groups. Infections may be separated into several clinical syndromes: undifferentiated type fevers (systemic febrile disease), hepatitis, hemorrhagic fevers, and encephalitides. [*ar,* arthropod, + *bo,* borne, + virus]

ARC Acronym for AIDS-related complex.

arc (ahrk) **1.** A curved line or segment of a circle. **2.** Continuous luminous passage of an electric current in a gas or vacuum between two or more separated carbon or other electrodes. [L. *arcus,* a bow]

ar•cade (ahr-kād′) An anatomic structure or structures (especially a blood vessel) taking the form of a series of arches. [L. *arcus,* arc, bow]

Ar•can•o•bac•te•ri•um (ahr-kă′nō-bac-tēr′ē-ŭm) A genus of nonmotile, facultatively anaerobic bacteria containing gram-positive slender irregular rods, sometimes showing clubbed ends. These organisms are obligate parasites of the pharynx in farm animals and humans, occasionally causing lesions on the pharynx or skin. The type species is *A. haemolyticum.*

arch (ahrch) Any structure resembling a bent bow or an arch; an arc. ANATOMY any vaulted or archlike structure. SYN arcus [TA]. [thru O. Fr. fr. L. *arcus,* bow]

♻**arch-, arche-, archi-, ar•cho-** **1.** Combining forms meaning primordial, ancestral, first, chief, or extreme. **2.** DENTISTRY denoting the maxillary or mandibular arch. [G. *archē,* origin, beginning, + -o-]

ar•chae•bac•te•ri•a (ahr′kē-bak-tēr′ē-ā) A group of microorganisms that thrive in the absence of oxygen, produce methane, and live only in bodies of highly concentrated salt water, or in the acidic waters of sulfur springs, at temperatures near 80° Celsius and pH levels as low as 2.

arch of a•or•ta (ahrch ā-ōr′tă) SYN aortic arch (1).

ar•che•o•ki•net•ic (ahrk′ē-ō-ki-net′ik) Denoting a low and primordial type of motor nerve mechanism, such as is found in the peripheral and the ganglionic nervous systems. Cf. neokinetic, paleokinetic. [G. *archaios,* ancient, + *kinētikos,* relating to movement]

ar•che•type (ahr′kĕ-tīp) **1.** A primordial structural plan from which various modifications have evolved. **2.** PSYCHOLOGY C.G. Jung's term for structural manifestation of the collective unconscious. SYN imago (2). [G. *archetypos,* pattern, model, fr. *archē,* beginning, + *typtō,* to stamp out]

arch of foot (ahrch fut) **1.** Longitudinal: consisting of a medial longitudinal arch, including the calcaneus, talus, navicular, three cuneiform bones, and the three medial metatarsals, and a lateral longitudinal arch formed by calcaneus, cuboid and two lateral metatarsals. **2.** Transverse: formed by the proximal parts of the metatarsal bones, the three cuneiform bones, and the cuboid. SYN arcus pedis.

Ar•chi•me•des prin•ci•ple (ahr-ki-mē′dēz prin′si-pĕl) Tenet that a body placed in liquid is buoyed up by a force equal to the weight of the liquid displaced.

arch of tho•rac•ic duct (ahrch thōr-as′ik dŭkt) SEE thoracic duct.

arch•wire (arch′wīr) A device consisting of various types of wires from which the dental arch will take its shape, conforming to the alveolar or dental arch, used as an anchorage in correcting irregularities in the position of the teeth.

ar•ci•form (ahr′si-fōrm) SYN arcuate.

Ar•co•bac•ter (ahr′kō-bak′tĕr) A genus of bacteria in the family Campylobacteraceae that is gram negative, aerotolerant, and able to grow at 15°C. The type strain is *A. butzleri.*

Ar•co•bac•ter butz•ler•i (ahr′kō-bak′tĕr būts-lē-rī) Formerly, *Campylobacter butzleri;* a bacterial species associated with diarrheal disease in humans; may cause recurring gastrointestinal illness in children.

arc•ta•tion (ahrk-tā′shŭn) A narrowing, contraction, stricture, or coarctation. [L. *arto* (improp. *arcto*), pp. *-atus,* to tighten]

ar•cu•ate (ahrk′yū-ăt) Denoting a form that is arched or has the shape of a bow. SYN arciform. [L. *arcuatus,* bowed]

ar•cu•ate ar•ter•ies of kid•ney (ahrk′yū-ăt ahr′tĕr-ēz kid′nē) Curved arteries at the corticomedullary border, arising from interlobar arteries and giving rise to interlobular arteries. SYN arteriae arcuatae renis [TA].

ar·cu·ate ar·ter·y of foot (in·con·stant) (ahrk′yū-ăt ahr′tĕr-ē fut in-kon′stănt) *Origin*, dorsalis pedis; *branches*, passes laterally dorsal to the bases of the metatarsals, giving rise to the second, third, and fourth dorsal metatarsal arteries at the level of the medial cuneiform bone. SYN arteria arcuata [TA].

ar·cu·ate fi·bers (ahrk′yū-ăt fī′bĕrz) Nervous or tendinous fibers passing in the form of an arch from one part to another.

ar·cu·ate ker·a·tot·o·my (ahrk′yū-ăt ker′ă-tot′ŏ-mē) Surgical procedure used to remodel the cornea in the management of astigmatism; peripheral incisions are made parallel to the corneal limbus in the steep meridian.

ar·cu·ate nu·cle·i (ahrk′yū-ăt nū′klē-ī) A variable assembly of small cell groups, probably outlying components of the pontine nuclei, on the ventral and medial aspects of the pyramid in the medulla oblongata.

ar·cu·ate veins of kid·ney (ahrk′yū-ăt vānz kid′nē) Veins that parallel the arcuate arteries, receive blood from interlobular veins and straight venules, and terminate in interlobar veins.

ar·cu·ate zone (ahrk′yū-ăt zōn) The inner third of the basilar membrane of the cochlear duct extending from the tympanic lip of the osseous spiral lamina to the outer pillar cell of the spiral organ (organ of Corti). SYN zona arcuata, zona tecta.

ar·cu·a·tion (ahr′kyū-ā′shŭn) A bending or curvature.

ar·cus (ar′kŭs) [TA] SYN arch. [L. a bow]

ar·cus cor·ne·a·lis (ar′kŭs kōr-nē-ā′lis) SYN arcus senilis.

ar·cus mar·gi·nal·is co·li (ahr′kūs mahr-ji-nā′lis kō′lī) SYN marginal artery of colon.

ar·cus pal·mar·is (ar′kŭs pal-mā′ris) SYN palmar arch.

ar·cus pal·ma·ris pro·fun·dus (ahr′kŭs pal-mā′ris prō-fun′dŭs) [TA] SYN palmar arch (1).

ar·cus pal·ma·ris su·per·fi·ci·a·les (ahr′kŭs pal-mā′ris sū′pĕr-fish-ē-ā′lēz) [TA] SYN palmar arch (2).

ar·cus pe·dis (ar′kŭs pĕd′is) SYN arch of foot.

ar·cus se·nil·is (ahr′kŭs sē-nil′is) An opaque, grayish ring at the periphery of the cornea just within the sclerocorneal junction; frequent occurrence in old people; it results from a deposit of fatty granules in, or hyaline degeneration of, the lamellae and cells of the cornea. SYN anterior embryotoxon, arcus cornealis, gerontoxon.

ar·cus vo·lar·is su·per·fi·ci·a·lis (ahr′kŭs vō-lā′ris sū′pĕr-fish′ē-ā′lis) SYN superficial palmar arterial arch.

ARD Abbreviation for antibiotic removal device.

ARDS (ahrdz) Acronym for acute respiratory distress syndrome; adult respiratory distress syndrome.

ar·e·a (a), pl. **ar·e·ae** (ār′ē-ă, -ē) **1.** Any circumscribed surface or space. **2.** All of the part supplied by a given artery or nerve. **3.** A part of an organ having a special function, as the motor area of the brain. SEE ALSO regio, region, space, spatium, zone. [L. a courtyard]

ar·e·a a·gen·cy on ag·ing (AAA) (ār′ē-ă ā′jĕn-sē ā′jing) State and local programs that help older adults plan and coordinate for their lifelong needs. Services include adult day care, skilled nursing care/therapy, transportation, personal care, respite care, and meals.

ar·e·a a·myg·da·loi·de·a an·te·ri·or (ār′ē-ă ă-mig-dă-loyd′ē-ă an-tēr′ē-ŏr) [TA] SYN anterior amygdaloid area.

ar·e·a of car·di·ac dull·ness (ār′ē-ă kahr′dē-ak dŭl′nĕs) A triangular delimit determined by percussion of the front of the chest; it corresponds to the part of the heart that is not covered by lung tissue.

ar·e·a coch·le·ae (ār′ē-ă kok′lē-ē) [TA] SYN cochlear area.

a·re·a of oc·cu·pa·tion (ār′ē-ă ok-yū-pā′shŭn) Various kinds of activities of life in which people take part (e.g., activities of daily living, education, work, play, leisure, and social participation).

ar·e·a-spe·cif·ic cu·rettes (ār′ē-ă spĕ-sif′ik kyūr-ets′) Periodontal instruments used to remove calculus deposits from the crowns and roots of teeth. Each area-specific curette is designed for use only on certain teeth and certain surfaces. These curettes have long functional shanks; one working cutting edge is used for calculus removal. SYN Gracey curettes.

a·re·ca nut (ă-rē′kă nŭt) SYN betel palm (nut). [Pg., betel palm, fr. Malayalam *atekka*]

a·re·flex·i·a (ā-rĕ-flek′sē-ă) Absence of reflexes.

A·re·na·vi·ri·dae (ă-rē-nă-vir′i-dē) A family of RNA viruses, many of which are parasites of rodents, which includes lymphocytic choriomeningitis virus, Lassa virus, and the Tacaribe virus complex. [L. *arena* (*harena*), sand]

A·re·na·vi·rus (ă-rē′nă-vī′rŭs) A genus in the family Arenaviridae that is associated with lymphocytic choriomeningitis and a number of hemorrhagic fevers.

a·re·o·la, pl. **a·re·o·lae** (ă-rē′ō-lă, -lē) **1.** Any small area. **2.** One of the spaces or interstices in areolar tissue. **3.** SYN areola of breast. **4.** A pigmented, depigmented, or erythematous zone surrounding a papule, pustule, wheal, or cutaneous neoplasm. SYN halo (3). [L. dim. of *area*]

a•re•o•la of breast (ă-rē′ō-lă brest) A circular pigmented area surrounding the nipple or papilla mammae; its surface is dotted with little projections corresponding to the areolar glands beneath. SYN areola mammae [TA], areola papillaris, areola (3).

a•re•o•la mam•mae (ă-rē′ō-lă mam′ē) [TA] SYN areola of breast.

a•re•o•la pa•pil•la•ris (ă-rē′ō-lă pa-pi-lā′ris) SYN areola of breast.

a•re•o•lar (ă-rē′ō-lăr) Relating to an areola.

a•re•o•lar glands (ă-rē′ō-lăr glandz) A number of small mammary glands forming small rounded projections from the surface of the areola of the breast; they enlarge with pregnancy and during lactation secrete a substance presumed to resist chapping. SYN Montgomery follicles.

a•re•o•lar tis•sue (ă-rē′ō-lăr tish′ū) Loose, irregularly arranged connective tissue that consists of collagenous and elastic fibers, a protein polysaccharide ground substance, and connective tissue cells (fibroblasts, macrophages, mast cells, and sometimes fat cells, plasma cells, leukocytes, and pigment cells).

a•re•o•lar ve•nous plex•us (ă-rē′ō-lăr vē′nŭs plek′sŭs) A venous plexus in the areola surrounding the nipple, formed by the mammary veins, and sending its blood to the lateral thoracic vein. SYN Haller circle (2).

a•re•o•la um•bil•i•ci (ă-rē′ō-lă ŭm-bil′i-sī) A pigmented ring around the umbilicus in the pregnant woman.

ARF Abbreviation for acute respiratory failure; acute renal failure.

ar•gas•id (ahr-gas′id) Common name for members of the family Argasidae.

Ar•gas•i•dae (ahr-gas′i-dē) Family of soft ticks, so called because of their wrinkled appearance, which fills out when the tick is engorged with blood. Argasid ticks, chiefly species of *Ornithodoros*, harbor and transmit spirochetes of the genus *Borrelia* that cause relapsing fever in birds and mammals. [G. *argas,* idle, nonproductive, useless]

ar•gen•taf•fin, **ar•gen•taf•fine** (ahr-jen′tă-fin, -fēn) Pertaining to cells or tissue elements that reduce silver ions in solution, thereby becoming stained brown or black. [L. *argentum,* silver, + *affinitas,* affinity]

ar•gen•taf•fin cell (ahr-jen′tă-fin sel) Cell containing granules that precipitate silver from an ammoniac silver nitrate solution. SEE ALSO enteroendocrine cells.

ar•gen•taf•fi•no•ma (ar′jen-tă-fi-nō′mă) SYN carcinoid tumor.

ar•gen•to•phil, **ar•gen•to•phile** (ar-jen′tō-fil, -fīl) SYN argyrophil.

ar•gi•nase (ahr′ji-nās) An enzyme of the liver that catalyzes the hydrolysis of L-arginine to L-ornithine and urea; a key enzyme of the urea cycle.

ar•gi•nine (ahr′ji-nēn) One of the amino acids occurring among the hydrolysis products of proteins, particularly abundant in the basic proteins such as histones and protamines. A dibasic amino acid.

ar•gi•nine va•so•pres•sin (AVP) (ahr′ji-nēn vā′sō-pres′in) This agent contains an arginyl residue in position 8 (as in chickens and most mammals, including humans); porcine vasopressin has a lysyl residue at position 8. All are vasopressors.

ar•gi•ni•no•suc•cin•ic ac•id (ahr′ji-ni-nō-sŭk-sin′ik as′id) Formed as an intermediate in the conversion of L-citrulline to L-arginine in the urea cycle.

ar•gi•ni•no•suc•cin•ic ac•i•du•ri•a (ahr′ji-nī′nō-sŭk-sin′ik-as-i-dyūr′ē-ă) An autosomal recessive disorder characterized by excessive urinary excretion of argininosuccinic acid, epilepsy, ataxia, mental retardation, liver disease, and friable, tufted hair; presumed to be the consequence of a deficiency of an enzyme responsible for splitting argininosuccinic acid to arginine and fumaric acid.

ar•gon (Ar) (ahr′gon) A gaseous element; atomic no. 18, atomic wt. 39.948; present in the dry atmosphere in the proportion of about 0.94%; one of the noble gases. [G. ntr. of *argos,* lazy, inactive, fr. *a-* priv. + *ergon,* work]

ar•gon la•ser (ahr′gon lā′zĕr) Laser used for ophthalmic procedures, including retinal photocoagulation and trabeculoplasty, consisting of photons in the blue (488 nm) or green (514 nm) spectrum.

Ar•gyll Ro•bert•son pu•pil (ahr′gīl rob′ĕrt-sŏn pyū′pil) A form of reflex iridoplegia characterized by miosis, irregular shape, and a loss of the direct and consensual pupillary reflex to light, with normal pupillary constriction to a near vision effort (light-near dissociation); often present in tabetic neurosyphilis.

ar•gyr•i•a, **ar•gy•rism** (ahr-jir′ē-ă, ahr′ji-rizm) A slate-gray or bluish discoloration of the skin and deep tissues due to the deposit of silver, occurring after medicinal administration of a soluble silver salt. [G. *argyros,* silver]

ar•gyr•ic (ahr-jir′ik) Relating to argyria.

ar•gyr•o•phil, **ar•gyr•o•phile** (ahr-jir′ō-fil, -fīl) Pertaining to tissue elements that are capable of impregnation with silver ions and being made visible after an external reducing agent is used. SYN argentophil, argentophile. [G. *argyros,* silver, + *philos,* fond]

a·rhin·i·a (ā-rī'nē-ă) Congenital absence of the nose. SYN arrhinia.

a·ri·bo·fla·vin·o·sis (ă-rī'bō-flā-vi-nō'sis) A commonly used term for hyporiboflavinosis.

A·ris·to·lo·chi·a fang·chi (ă-ris'tō-lō'kē-ă fahng'kē) An extremely toxic preparation (aristolochic acid is the active ingredient) that causes cancer and hepatic disease; appears in some Chinese traditional medicines and compounds; reported one of the most dangerous of all herbal agents. SYN birthwort. [G. *aristolochia,* easy birth, fr. *aristos,* best, + *locheia,* childbirth]

ar·is·to·te·li·an meth·od (ă-ris-tŏ-tē'lē-ăn meth'ŏd) A method of reasoning based on the teachings of the Greek philosopher Aristotle (384–322 BCE). It posits that we form universal ideas (e.g., tree, beauty) by abstracting from reality and universal propositions (e.g., all men are mortal) by induction. True and certain knowledge can be attained by deduction through the vigorous applications of logical principles.

A·ris·tot·le a·nom·a·ly (ar'is-tot'ĕl ă-nom'ă-lē) When a small object is held between the first and second fingers crossed in such a way that it touches or presses upon skin surfaces that ordinarily are not pressed upon simultaneously by a single object, it is perceived falsely as two.

a·rith·me·tic mean (ar'ith-met'ik mēn) The mean calculated by adding a set of values and then dividing the sum by the number of values. SYN average (2).

Arlt op·er·a·tion (ahrlt op-ĕr-ā'shŭn) Transplantation of the eyelashes back from the edge of the lid in trichiasis.

i **arm** (ahrm) **1.** The segment of the upper limb between the shoulder and the elbow; colloquially, the whole upper limb. SYN brachium (1) [TA], brachio- (1). **2.** An anatomic extension resembling an arm. **3.** A specifically shaped and positioned extension of a removable partial denture framework. See this page. [L. *armus,* forequarter of an animal; G. *harmos,* a shoulder joint]

ar·ma·men·tar·i·um (ahrm'ă-men-tar'ē-ŭm) All therapeutic means available to the health care practitioner for professional practice. [L. an arsenal, fr. *armamenta,* implements, tackle, fr. *arma,* armor, arms]

arm-crank er·gom·e·ter (ahrm'krangk ĕr-gom'ĕ-tĕr) Device used for graded exercise of the upper limbs for stress testing of amputees and others who cannot use a treadmill.

Arm·i·tage-Doll mod·el (ahrm'i-tazh-dol mod'ĕl) A model of carcinogenesis with the premise that the main variable determining change in risk is not age but time.

ARN Abbreviation for acute retinal necrosis.

Ar·neth count (ahr-net' kownt) The percentage distribution of polymorphonuclear neutrophils, based on the number of lobes in the nuclei (from one to five). SEE ALSO Arneth index.

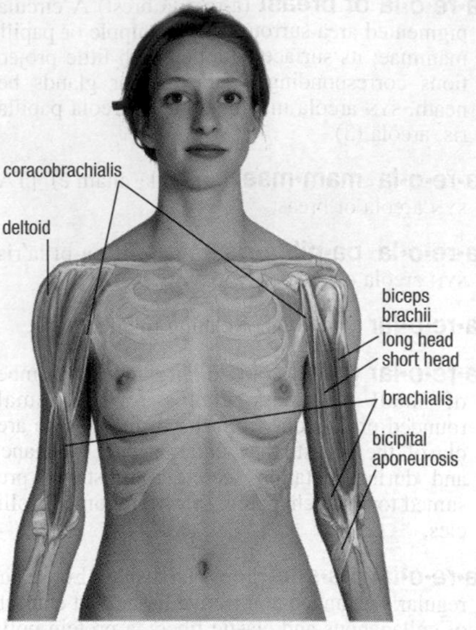

muscles of the anterior arm

Ar·neth in·dex (ahr-net' in'deks) An expression based on adding the percentages of polymorphonuclear neutrophils with one or two lobes in their nuclei, plus one-half the percentage with three lobes; the normal value is 60%. SEE ALSO Arneth count.

ar·ni·ca (ahr'ni-kă) (*A. montana*) Herbal agent of purported value in therapy for muscular pain and in wound healing. Serious reactions in children reported after overingestion. Some compounds containing arnica also include more dangerous agents. SYN leopard bane, mountain daisy, wolf bane.

Ar·nold bod·y (ahr'nŏld bod'ē) A minute fragment or "ghost" resulting from degeneration of an erythrocyte (sometimes mistakenly referred to as a blood platelet).

Ar·nold-Chi·a·ri mal·for·ma·tion (ahr'nŏld kē-ah'rē mal'fōr-mā'shŭn) Deformity of posterior cranial fossa structures caused by tethering of the spinal cord with caudad traction and displacement of the rhombencephalon; may be accompanied by spina bifida and associated anomalies such as meningomyelocele; weak evidence of autosomal recessive inheritance.

Ar·nold re·flex (ahr'nŏld rē'fleks) Coughing or discomfort resulting from touching the external auditory meatus during cerumen extraction or the insertion of earplugs, earmolds, or hearing aids. The Arnold nerve is a branch of the vagus nerve (cranial nerve X).

AROM (ar'om) Acronym for active range of motion. SEE ALSO range of motion, passive range of motion.

a·ro·ma·ther·a·py (ă-rō′mă-thār′ă-pē) Use of essential oils through inhalation or direct application to promote healing and well-being.

ar·o·mat·ic (ār′ō-mat′ik) **1.** Having an agreeable, somewhat pungent, spicy odor. **2.** One of a group of vegetable drugs having a fragrant odor and slightly stimulant properties. **3.** SEE cyclic compound. [G. *arōmatikos,* fr. *arōma,* spice, sweet herb]

ar·o·mat·ic D-a·mi·no ac·id de·car·box·yl·ase (ār′ō-mat′ik ă-mē′nō as′id dē′kahr-bok′sil-ās) An enzyme that catalyzes the decarboxylation of L-dopa to dopamine, of L-tryptophan to tryptamine, and of L-hydroxytryptophan to serotonin; important in the biosynthetic pathway of catecholamines and melanin.

ar·o·mat·ic am·mo·ni·a spir·it (ār′ō-mat′ik ă-mōn′yă spir′it) A hydroalcoholic solution containing approximately 2% ammonia, 4% ammonium carbonate, and the aromatics: lemon oil, lavender oil, and myristica oil. Used mainly by inhalation to produce reflex stimulation in people who have fainted or are at risk of syncope.

ar·o·mat·ic com·pound (ār′ō-mat′ik kom′pownd) SEE cyclic compound.

ar·o·mat·ic se·ries (ār′ō-mat′ik sēr′ēz) All the compounds derived from benzene, or similar cyclic compounds that obey the Hückel rule.

aromatisation [Br.] SYN aromatization.

aromatise [Br.] SYN aromatize.

a·ro·ma·ti·za·tion (ă-rō′mă-tī-zā′shŭn) Conversion of a nonaromatic compound to an aromatic compound. SYN aromatisation.

a·ro·ma·tize (ă-rō′mă-tīz) To convert a nonaromatic compound to an aromatic compound. SYN aromatise.

a·rous·al dis·or·der (ă-row′zăl dis-ōr′dĕr) **1.** A broad term for parasomnia disorders that range from sleepwalking to sleep terrors; involves a state of being between sleep and wakefulness. **2.** A condition or disorder in which normal response is impaired or lacking (e.g., physiologic vaginal lubrication, maintenance of male erection).

a·rous·al in·dex (ă-row′zăl in′deks) A measurement calculated from sleep disruptions observed during a sleep study.

ar·rec·tor, pl. **ar·rec·to·res** (ă-rek′tōr, ă-rek-tō′rēz) SYN erector. [L. that which raises, fr. *arrigo,* pp. *-rectus,* to raise up]

ar·rec·tor mus·cle of hair, ar·rec·tor pi·li mus·cles (ă-rek′tŏr mŭs′ĕl hār, ă-rek′tŏr pī′lī mŭs′ĕlz) Bundles of smooth muscle fibers, attached to the deep part of the hair follicles, passing outward alongside the sebaceous glands to the papillary layer of the corium; they act to pull the hairs erect, causing "goose bumps" or "goose flesh" (cutis anserina). SYN musculi arrectores pilorum [TA], erector muscles of hairs.

ar·rest (ă-rest′) **1.** To stop, check, or restrain. **2.** A stoppage; interference with, or checking of, the regular course of a disease, a symptom, or the performance of a function. **3.** Inhibition of a developmental process, usually at the ultimate stage of development; premature arrest may lead to a congenital abnormality. [O. Fr. *arester,* fr. LL. *adresto,* to stop behind]

ar·rest of ac·tive phase dys·to·ci·a (ă-rest′ ak′tiv fāz dis-tō′sē-ă) Stoppage of further cervical dilation for longer than 2 hours after labor has entered active phase (generally defined as active contraction with at least 4 cm of cervical dilatation); causes include inadequate uterine contractions and cephalopelvic disproportion.

ar·rest of des·cent dys·to·ci·a (ă-rest′ dĕ-sent′ dis-tō′sē-ă) Failure of fetus to descend after an hour in second stage despite maternal effort; typically due to inadequate maternal effort, fetal malposition, or fetal size.

ar·rest·ed la·bor (ă-res′tĕd lā′bŏr) A cessation in the birth process, of varying duration, especially one caused by weakened, diminished, or absent contractions.

ar·rest of la·bor (ă-rest′ lā′bŏr) Absence of progress of active labor (as defined by cervical dilation and descent of the presenting part) for 2 hours or longer.

ar·rest sig·nal (ă-rest′ sig′năl) A DNA sequence that causes arrest of RNA polymerase transcription.

Ar·rhe·ni·us-Mad·sen the·o·ry (ă-rē′nē-ŭs mad′sĕn thē′ŏr-ē) That the reaction of an antigen with its antibody is a reversible reaction, the equilibrium is determined according to the law of mass action by the concentrations of the reacting substances.

ar·rhe·no·blas·to·ma (ă-rē′nō-blas-tō′mă) A rare ovarian tumor that produces masculinization and often contains tubules and luteinized cells. SYN androblastoma (2), gynandroblastoma (1). [G. *arrhēn,* male, + *blastos,* germ, + *-ōma,* tumor]

ar·rhin·i·a (ā-rī′nē-ă) SYN arhinia. [G. *a-* priv. + *rhis* (*rhin-*), nose]

ar·rhyth·mi·a (ā-ridh′mē-ă) Loss of rhythm; denoting especially an irregularity of the heartbeat. SEE ALSO dysrhythmia. [G. *a-* priv. + *rhythmos,* rhythm]

ar·rhyth·mic (ā-ridh′mik) Marked by loss of rhythm; pertaining to arrhythmia.

ar·rhyth·mo·gen·ic (ă-rith′mō-jen′ik) Capable of inducing cardiac arrhythmias. SYN dysrhythmogenic. [G. *a-* priv. + *rhythmos,* rhythm, + *-gen,* production]

Ar•ru•ga for•ceps (ah-rū′gah fōr′seps) Forceps for the intracapsular extraction of a cataract.

ar•se•nic (As) (ahr′sĕ-nik) A metallic element, atomic no. 33, atomic wt. 74.92159; forms a number of poisonous compounds, some of which are used in medicine. [L. *arsenicum,* G. *arsenikon,* fr. Pers. *zarnik*]

ar•sen•i•cal (ahr-sen′i-kăl) **1.** Denoting or containing arsenic. **2.** A drug or agent, the effect of which depends on its arsenic content. **3.** A class of chemical agents that contain arsenic.

ART Abbreviation for acoustic reflex threshold.

ar•te•fact (ahr′tĕ-fakt) SYN artifact.

ar•te•ri•a, gen. and pl. **ar•te•ri•ae** (ahr-tēr′ē-ă, -ē) [TA] SYN artery. SEE ALSO branch. [L. from G. *artēria,* the windpipe, later an artery as distinct from a vein]

ar•ter•i•a al•ve•o•la•ris su•pe•ri•or pos•te•ri•or (ahr-tēr′ē-ă al-vē-ō-lā′ris sŭ-pē-rē-ōr pos-tēr′ē-ōr) SYN posterior superior alveolar artery.

ar•te•ri•a an•as•to•mo•ti•ca mag•na (ahr-tēr′ē-ă an-as-tō′mō′tik-ă mag′nă) SYN inferior ulnar collateral artery.

ar•te•ri•a an•gu•la•ris (ahr-tēr′ē-ă ang-gyū-lā′ris) [TA] SYN angular artery.

ar•te•ri•a ap•pen•di•cu•la•ris (ahr-tēr′ē-ă ă-pen-dik-yū-lā′ris) [TA] SYN appendicular artery.

ar•te•ri•a ar•cu•a•ta (ahr-tēr′ē-ă ar-kyū-ā′tă) [TA] SYN arcuate artery of foot (inconstant).

ar•te•ri•a as•cen•dens (ahr-tēr′ē-ă ă-sen′denz) [TA] SYN ascending artery.

ar•te•ri•a au•ri•cu•la•ris pos•te•ri•or (ahr-tēr′ē-ă aw-rik′yū-lā′ris pos-tēr′ē-ōr) SYN posterior auricular artery.

ar•te•ri•a au•ri•cu•la•ris pro•fun•da (ahr-tēr′ē-ă aw-rik′yū-lā′ris prō-fun′dă) SYN deep auricular artery.

ar•te•ri•a ax•il•la•ris (ahr-tēr′ē-ă ak-si-lā′ris) [TA] SYN axillary artery.

ar•te•ri•a bas•i•la•ris (ahr-tēr′ē-ă bas-i-lā′ris) [TA] SYN basilar artery.

ar•te•ri•a bra•chi•a•lis (ahr-tēr′ē-ă brā-kē-ā′lis) [TA] SYN brachial artery.

ar•te•ri•a buc•ca•lis (ahr-tēr′ē-ă bŭ-kā′lis) [TA] SYN buccal artery.

ar•te•ri•a bul•bi pe•nis (ahr-tēr′ē-ă bŭl′bī pē′nis) [TA] SYN artery of bulb of penis.

ar•te•ri•a bul•bi ves•tib•u•li (ahr-tēr′ē-ă bŭl′bī ves-tib′yū-lī) [TA] SYN artery of bulb of vestibule.

ar•te•ri•a ca•na•lis pte•ry•goi•de•i (ahr-tēr′ē-ă kă-nā′lis ter-i-goy′dē-ī) [TA] SYN artery of pterygoid canal.

ar•te•ri•a ca•rot•is com•mu•nis (ahr-tēr′ē-ă kă-rot′is ko-myū′nis) SYN common carotid artery.

ar•te•ri•a ca•rot•is ex•ter•na (ahr-tēr′ē-ă kă-rot′is eks-ter′nă) SYN external carotid artery.

ar•te•ri•a ca•rot•is in•ter•na (ahr-tēr′ē-ă kă-rot′is in-ter′nă) SYN internal carotid artery.

ar•te•ri•a ce•li•a•ca (ahr-tēr′ē-ă sel-ē-ā′kă) SYN celiac trunk.

ar•te•ri•a cen•tra•lis ret•i•nae (ahr-tēr′ē-ă sen-trā′lis ret′i-nē) [TA] SYN central retinal artery.

ar•te•ri•a cer•e•bri an•te•ri•or (ahr-tēr′ē-ă ser′ĕ-brī an-tēr′ē-ōr) SYN anterior cerebral artery.

ar•te•ri•a cer•e•bri me•di•a (ahr-tēr′ē-ă ser′ĕ-brī mē′dē-ă) SYN middle cerebral artery.

ar•te•ri•a cer•e•bri pos•te•ri•or (ahr-tēr′ē-ă ser′ĕ-brī pos-tēr′ē-ōr) SYN posterior cerebral artery.

ar•te•ri•a cer•vi•ca•lis as•cen•dens (ahr-tēr′ē-ă ser-vi-kā′lis a-sen′denz) SYN ascending cervical artery.

ar•te•ri•a ci•li•ar•is pos•te•ri•or brev•is (ahr-tēr′ē-ă si-lē-ā′ris pos-tēr′ē-ōr brev′is) SYN short posterior ciliary artery.

ar•te•ri•a cir•cum•flex•a fe•mor•is la•ter•a•lis (ahr-tēr′ē-ă ser-kŭm-fleks′ă fem′ō-ris lat-ĕr-ā′lis) SYN lateral circumflex femoral artery.

ar•te•ri•a cir•cum•flex•a fe•mor•is me•di•a•lis (ahr-tēr′ē-ă ser-kŭm-fleks′ă fem′ō-ris mē-dē-ā′lis) SYN medial circumflex femoral artery.

ar•te•ri•a cir•cum•flex•a hu•mer•i an•te•ri•or (ahr-tēr′ē-ă ser-kŭm-fleks′ă hyū′mĕr-ī an-tēr′ē-ōr) SYN anterior circumflex humeral artery.

ar•te•ri•a cir•cum•flex•a hu•mer•i pos•te•ri•or (ahr-tēr′ē-ă ser-kŭm-fleks′ă hyū-mĕr′ī pos-tēr′ē-ōr) SYN posterior circumflex humeral artery.

ar•te•ri•a cir•cum•flex•a il•i•ac•a pro•fun•da (ahr-tēr′ē-ă ser-kŭm-fleks′ă il-ē-ā′kă prō-fŭn′dă) SYN deep circumflex iliac artery.

ar•te•ri•a cir•cum•flex•a i•li•ac•a su•per•fi•ci•al•is (ahr-tēr′ē-ă ser-kŭm-fleks′ă il-ē-ā′kă sū-pĕr-fish′ē-ā′lis) SYN superficial circumflex iliac artery.

ar•te•ri•a coch•le•a•ris com•mu•nis (ah-tēr′ē-ă kok-lē-ā′ris kom′yū-nis) [TA] SYN common cochlear artery.

ar•te•ri•a col•i•ca dex•tra (ahr-tēr′ē-ă kol′i-kă deks′tră) SYN right colic artery.

ar·te·ri·a col·i·ca si·ni·stra (ahr-tēr′ē-ă kol′i-kă sin′is-tră) SYN left colic artery.

ar·te·ri·a col·la·te·ra·lis me·di·a (ahr-tēr′ē-ă kō-lat-ĕr-ā′lis mē′dē-ă) SYN middle collateral artery.

ar·te·ri·a col·la·te·ra·lis ul·na·ris in·fe·ri·or (ahr-tēr′ē-ă kō-lat-ĕr-ā′lis ul-nā′ris in-fēr′ē-ŏr) SYN inferior ulnar collateral artery.

ar·te·ri·a col·la·te·ra·lis ul·na·ris su·pe·ri·or (ahr-tēr′ē-ă kō-lat-ĕr-ā′lis ul-nar′is sŭ-pēr′ē-ŏr) SYN superior ulnar collateral artery.

ar·te·ri·a com·mu·ni·cans an·te·ri·or (ahr-tēr′ē-ă kom-yūn′i-kanz an-tēr′ē-ŏr) SYN anterior communicating artery.

ar·te·ri·a com·mu·ni·cans pos·te·ri·or (ahr-tēr′ē-ă kom-yūn′i-kanz pos-tēr′ē-ŏr) SYN posterior communicating artery.

ar·te·ri·a co·ro·na·ri·a dex·tra (ahr-tēr′ē-ă kōr-ō-nā′rē-ă deks′tră) SYN right coronary artery.

ar·te·ri·a co·ro·na·ri·a si·nis·tra (ahr-tēr′ē-ă kōr-ō-nā′rē-ă sin′is-tră) SYN left coronary artery.

ar·te·ri·a cre·ma·ste·ri·ca (ahr-tēr′ē-ă krē-mas-ter′i-kă) [TA] SYN cremasteric artery.

ar·te·ri·a cys·ti·ca (ahr-tēr′ē-ă sis′ti-kă) [TA] SYN cystic artery.

ar·te·ri·a def·er·en·ti·al·is (ahr-tēr′ē-ă de-fĕr-en-shē-ā′lis) SYN artery to ductus deferens.

ar·te·ri·a des·cen·dens ge·nus (ahr-tēr′ē-ă dē-sen′denz jē′nŭs) [TA] SYN descending genicular artery.

ar·te·ri·a di·gi·tal·is pal·ma·ris com·mu·nis (ahr-tēr′ē-ă di-ji-tā′lis pahl-mā′ris kom-myūn′is) SYN common palmar digital artery.

ar·te·ri·a di·gi·ta·lis pal·ma·ris pro·pri·a (ahr-tēr′ē-ă di-ji-tā′lis pahl-mā′ris prō′prē-ă) SYN proper palmar digital artery.

ar·te·ri·a dor·sa·lis cli·to·ri·dis (ahr-tēr′ē-ă dōr-sā′lis kli-tō′ri-dis) [TA] SYN dorsal artery of clitoris.

ar·te·ri·a dor·sa·lis pe·nis (ahr-tēr′ē-ă dōr-sā′lis pē′nis) [TA] SYN dorsal artery of penis.

ar·te·ri·a duc·tus de·fe·ren·tis (ahr-tēr′ē-ă dŭk′tŭs def-ĕr-en′tis) [TA] SYN artery to ductus deferens.

ar·te·ri·ae al·ve·o·la·res su·pe·ri·or·es an·te·ri·o·res (ahr-tēr′ē-ē al-vē-ō-lā′rēz sū-pēr′ē-ōr′ēz an-tēr-ē-ōr′ēz) SYN anterior superior alveolar artery.

ar·te·ri·ae ar·cu·a·tae re·nis (ahr-tēr′ē-ē ahr-kyū-ā′tē rē′nis) [TA] SYN arcuate arteries of kidney.

ar·te·ri·ae a·tri·a·les (ahr-tēr′ē-ē ā-trē-ā′lēz) SYN atrial arteries.

ar·te·ri·ae ci·li·ar·es pos·te·ri·or·es lon·gae (ahr-tēr′ē-ē sil-ī-ā′rēz pos-tē-rē-ō′rēz long′gē) SYN long posterior ciliary arteries.

ar·te·ri·ae il·e·a·les (ahr-tēr′ē-ē il-ē-ā′lēz) [TA] SYN ileal arteries.

ar·te·ri·ae in·ter·cos·tal·es pos·te·ri·or·es III–XI (ahr-tēr′ē-ē in-tĕr-kos-tā′lēz pos-tēr-ē-ōr′ēz) SYN posterior intercostal arteries 3–11.

ar·te·ri·ae in·ter·cos·tal·es pos·te·ri·or·es I et II (ahr-tēr′ē-ē in-tĕr-kos-tā′lēz pos-tēr-ē-ōr′ēz) SYN first and second posterior intercostal arteries.

ar·te·ri·ae in·ter·lo·bu·la·res (ahr-tēr′ē-ē in′tĕr-lob-yū-lā′rēz) [TA] SYN interlobular arteries.

ar·te·ri·ae je·ju·na·les (ahr-tēr′ē-ē jē-jū-nā′lēz) [TA] SYN jejunal arteries.

ar·te·ri·ae lum·ba·les (ahr-tēr′ē-ē lŭm-bā′lēz) [TA] SYN lumbar artery.

ar·te·ri·ae me·dul·lar·es seg·men·tal·es (ahr-tēr′ē-ē me-dū-lā′rēz seg-men-tā′lēz) SYN segmental medullary arteries.

ar·te·ri·ae na·sa·les pos·te·ri·or·es lat·er·al·es (ahr-tēr′ē-ē nā-zā′lēz pos-tēr-ē-ōr′ēz lat-ĕr-ā′lēz) SYN posterior lateral nasal arteries.

ar·te·ri·ae pal·pe·bra·les (ahr-tēr′ē-ē pal-pē-brā′lēz) [TA] SYN palpebral arteries.

ar·te·ri·ae per·fo·ran·tes (ahr-tēr′ē-ē per-fō-ran′tēz) [TA] SYN perforating arteries.

ar·te·ri·a ep·i·gas·tri·ca su·per·fi·ci·al·is (ahr-tēr′ē-ă ep-i-gas′tri-kă sū′pĕr-fish′ē-ā′lis) SYN superficial epigastric artery.

ar·te·ri·a ep·i·gas·tri·ca su·pe·ri·or (ahr-tēr′ē-ă ep-i-gas′tri-kă sŭ-pēr′ē-ŏr) SYN superior epigastric artery.

ar·te·ri·a ep·i·scle·ra·lis (ahr-tēr′ē-ă ep′i-skler-ā′lis) [TA] SYN episcleral artery.

ar·te·ri·ae pu·den·dae ex·ter·nae (ahr-tēr′ē-ē pū-den′dē eks-tĕr′nē) [TA] SYN external pudendal arteries.

ar·te·ri·ae ra·di·cu·lar·es an·te·ri·or et pos·te·ri·or (ahr-tēr′ē-ē ra-dik′yū-lā′rēz an-tēr′ē-ŏr et pos-tēr′ē-ŏr) SYN anterior and posterior radicular arteries.

ar·te·ri·ae sa·cra·les la·ter·al·es (ahr-tēr′ē-ē sā-krā′lez lat-ĕr-ā′lēz) SYN lateral sacral arteries.

ar·te·ri·ae sig·moi·de·ae (ahr-tēr′ē-ē sig-moy′dē-ē) [TA] SYN sigmoid arteries.

ar·te·ri·ae su·pra·re·nal·es su·p·er·i·or·es (ahr-tēr′ē-ē sū-pră-rē-nā′lēz sū-pēr-ē-ōr′ēz) SYN superior suprarenal arteries.

ar·te·ri·a eth·moi·dal·is an·te·ri·or (ahr-tēr′ē-ă eth-moy-dā′lis an-tēr′ē-ŏr) SYN anterior ethmoidal artery.

ar•te•ri•a eth•moi•dal•is pos•te•ri•or (ahr-tēr′ē-ă eht-moy-dā′lis pos-tēr′ē-ŏr) SYN posterior ethmoidal artery.

ar•te•ri•ae ven•tri•cu•lar•es (ahr-tēr′ē-ē ven-trik-yū-lā′rēz) [TA] SYN ventricular arteries.

ar•te•ri•a fa•ci•a•lis (ahr-tēr′ē-ă fā-shē-ā′lis) [TA] SYN facial artery.

ar•te•ri•a fe•mo•ra•lis (ahr-tēr′ē-ă fem-ō-rā′lis) [TA] SYN femoral artery.

ar•te•ri•a gas•tri•ca pos•te•ri•or (ahr-tēr′ē-ă gas-trik′tă pos-tēr′ē-ŏr) SYN posterior gastric artery.

ar•te•ri•a gas•tro•du•o•de•na•lis (ahr-tēr′ē-ă gas′trō-dū′ō-dē-nā′lis) [TA] SYN gastroduodenal artery.

ar•te•ri•a gas•tro•ep•i•plo•i•ca si•nis•tra (ahr-tēr′ē-ă gas-trō-ep-i-plō′ik-ă sin′is-tră) SYN left gastroomental artery.

ar•te•ri•a gas•tro•o•men•ta•lis si•nis•tra (ahr-tēr′ē-ă gas-trō-men-tā′lis sin′is-tră) SYN left gastroomental artery.

ar•te•ri•a glu•te•a in•fe•ri•or (ahr-tēr′ē-ă glū′tē-ă in-fēr′ē-ŏr) SYN inferior gluteal artery.

ar•te•ri•a glu•te•a su•pe•ri•or (ahr-tēr′ē-ă glū′tē-ă sŭ-pēr′ē-ŏr) SYN superior gluteal artery.

ar•te•ri•a he•pa•ti•ca com•mu•nis (ahr-tēr′ē-ă he-pat′ik-ă kom-yū′nis) SYN common hepatic artery.

ar•te•ri•a he•pa•ti•ca pro•pri•a (ahr-tēr′ē-ă he-pat′ik-ă prō′prē-ă) SYN hepatic artery proper.

ar•te•ri•a hy•a•loi•de•a (ahr-tēr′ē-ă hī-ă-loy′dē-ă) [TA] SYN hyaloid artery.

ar•te•ri•a hy•po•gas•tri•ca (ahr-tēr′ē-ă hī-po-gas′trik-ă) SYN internal iliac artery.

ar•te•ri•a il•e•o•co•li•ca (ahr-tēr′ē-ă il-ē-ō-kol′i-kă) [TA] SYN ileocolic artery.

ar•te•ri•a il•i•a•ca com•mu•nis (ahr-tēr′ē-ă il-ē-ā′kă kom-yū′nis) SYN common iliac artery.

ar•te•ri•a il•i•a•ca in•ter•na (ahr-tēr′ē-ă il-ē-ā′kă in-ter′nă) SYN internal iliac artery.

ar•te•ri•a il•i•o•lum•ba•lis (ahr-tēr′ē-ă il′ē-ō-lŭm-bā′lis) [TA] SYN iliolumbar artery.

ar•te•ri•a in•fe•ri•or an•te•ri•or ce•re•bel•li (ahr-tēr′ē-ă in-fēr′ē-ŏr an-tēr′ē-ŏr ser-ĕ-bel′ī) SYN anterior inferior cerebellar artery.

ar•te•ri•a in•fe•ri•or pos•te•ri•or ce•re•bel•li (ahr-tēr′ē-ă in-fēr′ē-ŏr pos-tēr′ē-ŏr ser-ĕ-bel′ī) SYN posterior inferior cerebellar artery.

ar•te•ri•a in•fra•or•bi•ta•lis (ahr-tēr′ē-ă in′fră-ōr-bi-tā′lis) [TA] SYN infraorbital artery.

ar•te•ri•a in•ter•cos•ta•lis su•pre•ma (ahr-tēr′ē-ă in-tĕr-kos-tā′lis sū-prē′mă) SYN supreme intercostal artery.

ar•te•ri•a in•ter•os•se•a an•te•ri•or (ahr-tēr′ē-ă in-tĕr-os′ē-ă an-tēr′ē-ŏr) SYN anterior interosseous artery.

ar•te•ri•a in•ter•os•se•a com•mu•nis (ahr-tēr′ē-ă in-tĕr-os′ē-ă kom-yū′nis) SYN common interosseous artery.

ar•te•ri•a in•ter•os•se•a pos•te•ri•or (ahr-tēr′ē-ă in-tĕr-os′ē-ă pos-tēr′ē-ŏr) SYN posterior interosseous artery.

ar•te•ri•a in•ter•os•se•a vo•lar•is (ahr-tēr′ē-ă in-tĕr-os′ē-ă vō-lā′ris) SYN anterior interosseous artery.

ar•te•ri•a isch•i•a•di•ca (ahr-tēr′ē-ă is-kē-ad′i-kă) SYN inferior gluteal artery.

ar•te•ri•a jux•ta•co•li•ca (ahr-tēr′ē-ă jŭks-tă-kol′ik-ă) SYN marginal artery of colon.

ar•te•ri•al (ahr-tēr′ē-ăl) Relating to one or more arteries or to the entire system of arteries.

ar•te•ri•a la•bi•al•is in•fe•ri•or (ahr-tēr′ē-ă lā-bē-ā′lis in-fēr′ē-ŏr) SYN inferior labial branch of facial artery.

ar•te•ri•a la•bi•al•is su•pe•ri•or (ahr-tēr′ē-ă lā-bē-ā′lis sŭ-pēr′ē-ŏr) SYN superior labial branch of facial artery.

ar•te•ri•a la•cri•ma•lis (ahr-tēr′ē-ă lak′ri-mā′lis) [TA] SYN lacrimal artery.

ar•te•ri•a la•ryn•ge•a su•pe•ri•or (ahr-tēr′ē-ă lă-rin′jē-ă sŭ-pēr′ē-ŏr) SYN superior laryngeal artery.

ar•te•ri•al blood (ahr-tēr′ē-ăl blŭd) Blood that has been oxygenated in the lungs; found in the left chambers of the heart and in the arteries, and relatively bright red. See page 125.

ar•te•ri•al ca•nal (ahr-tēr′ē-ăl kă-nal′) SYN ductus arteriosus.

ar•te•ri•al cap•il•lar•y (ahr-tēr′ē-ăl kap′i-lar-ē) A capillary opening from an arteriole or metarteriole.

ar•te•ri•al cir•cle of cer•e•brum (ahr-tēr′ē-ăl sĭr′kĕl ser′ĕ-brŭm) An anastomotic "circle" of arteries (roughly pentagonal in outline) at the base of the brain, formed, sequentially and in anterior to posterior direction, by the anterior communicating artery, the two anterior cerebral, the two internal carotid, the two posterior communicating, and the two posterior cerebral arteries.

ar•te•ri•al cone (ahr-tēr′ē-ăl kōn) The left or anterosuperior, smooth-walled portion of the cavity of the right ventricle of the heart, which begins at the supraventricular crest and terminates in the pulmonary trunk. SYN conus arteriosus [TA], infundibulum (4).

ar•te•ri•al duct (ahr-tēr′ē-ăl dŭkt) SYN ductus arteriosus.

ar•te•ri•al for•ceps (ahr-tēr′ē-ăl fōr′seps) A locking forceps with sloping blades for grasping the end of a blood vessel until a ligature is applied.

ar•te•ri•a li•e•na•lis (ahr-tēr′ē-ă lī-en-ā′lis) [TA] SYN splenic artery.

ar•te•ri•a lig•a•men•ti ter•e•tis u•ter•i (ahr-tēr′ē-ă lig-ă-men′tī ter′ĕ-tis yū′tĕr-ī) [TA] SYN artery of round ligament of uterus.

ar•te•ria lin•gu•lar•is (ahr-tēr′ē-ă ling-gyū-lā′ris) [TA] SEE left pulmonary artery.

ar•te•ri•a lin•gu•lar•is in•fe•ri•or (ahr-tēr′ē-ă ling-gyū-lā′ris in-fēr′ē-ŏr) SYN inferior lingular artery.

ar•te•ri•a lin•gu•lar•is su•pe•ri•or (ahr-tēr′ē-ă ling-gyū-lā′ris sŭ-pēr′ē-ŏr) SYN superior lingular artery.

ar•te•ri•al line (ahr-tēr′ē-ăl līn) An intraarterial catheter usually connected to a monitoring system consisting of pressure tubing, a transducer, and a monitor that permits continuous monitoring of blood pressure and access to arterial blood for sample analysis.

ar•te•ri•al neph•ro•scle•ro•sis (ahr-tēr′ē-ăl nef′rō-skler-ō′sis) Patchy atrophic scarring of the kidney due to arteriosclerotic narrowing of the lumens of large branches of the renal artery, occurring in old or hypertensive people and occasionally causing hypertension. SYN arterionephrosclerosis.

ar•te•ri•al oc•clu•sive dis•ease (ahr-tēr′ē-ăl ŏ-klū′siv di-zēz′) Obstruction of a major artery, resulting in ischemia distal to the obstruction. Usually refers to the femoral, popliteal, or innominate arteries. Signs include mottling, pallor, coolness, paralysis/paresthesia of the affected limb, pulselessness, and sudden pain of affected limb. May also affect internal, external carotid arteries, subclavian artery, vertebral and basilar arteries. Causes include atherosclerosis, emboli, thrombosis, trauma, and fracture.

ar•te•ri•al scle•ro•sis (ahr-tēr′ē-ăl skler-ō′sis) SYN arteriosclerosis.

ar•te•ri•al spi•der (ahr-tēr′ē-ăl spī′dĕr) SYN spider angioma.

ar•te•ri•al ten•sion (ahr-tēr′ē-ăl ten′shŭn) The blood pressure within an artery.

ar•te•ri•a lu•so•ri•a (ahr-tēr′ē-ă lū-sōr′ē-ă) An aberrant right subclavian artery arising from the descending aorta; it passes posterior to the esophagus, often producing dysphagia.

ar•te•ri•a mar•gi•nal•is co•li (ahr-tēr′ē-ă mahr-ji-nā′lis kō′lī) SYN marginal artery of colon.

ar•te•ri•a mas•se•te•ri•ca (ahr-tēr′ē-ă mas-ĕ-ter′i-kă) [TA] SYN masseteric artery.

ar•te•ri•a max•il•la•ris (ahr-tēr′ē-ă mak-si-lā′ris) [TA] SYN maxillary artery.

ar•te•ri•a me•di•a•na (ahr-tēr′ē-ă mē-dē-ā′nă) SYN median artery.

ar•te•ri•a men•ta•lis (ahr-tēr′ē-ă men-tā′lis) [TA] SYN mental artery.

ar•te•ri•a mes•en•te•ri•ca in•fe•ri•or (ahr-

Arterial blood gases

Gases	Normal values	Abnormal values
Partial pressure of oxygen (PaO_2)	70–100 millimeters of mercury (mmHg)	High PaO_2 may indicate rapid breathing. Low PaO_2 may indicate hypoventilation, pneumonia, chronic obstructive pulmonary disease (COPD), or certain heart disorders
Partial pressure of carbon dioxide ($PaCO_2$)	35–45 mmHg	High $PaCO_2$ may indicate COPD, severe head injury, obesity hypoventilation syndrome, hypoventilation, and disturbed sleep Low $PaCO_2$ may be caused by hyperventilation, pulmonary embolism, or pregnancy
pH	7.35–7.44	High pH with low $PaCO_2$ and normal or low HCO_3 is called respiratory alkalosis Low pH with high $PaCO_2$ and normal HCO_3 is called respiratory acidosis. Low pH with normal or low $PaCO_2$ and concurrent low HCO_3 is called metabolic acidosis
Bicarbonate (HCO_3^-)	21–28 milliequivalents per liter (mEq/L)	
Oxygen content (O_2CT)	15–23%	
Oxygen saturation (O_2Sat)	95–100%	

tēr′ē-ă mez-en-ter′ik-ă in-fēr′ē-ōr) SYN inferior mesenteric artery.

ar·te·ri·a mes·en·te·ri·ca su·pe·ri·or (ahr-tēr′ē-ă mez-en-ter′ik-ă sŭ-pēr′ē-ŏr) SYN superior mesenteric artery.

ar·te·ri·a met·a·car·pal·is dor·sal·is (ahr-tēr′ē-ă met′ă-kahr-pā′lis dor-sā′lis) SYN dorsal metacarpal artery.

ar·te·ri·a met·a·car·pal·is pal·mar·is (ahr-tēr′ē-ă met′ă-kahr-pā′lis pahl-mā′ris) SYN palmar metacarpal artery.

ar·te·ri·a met·a·tar·sal·is dor·sal·is (ahr-tēr′ē-ă met′ă-tahr-sā′lis dor-sā′lis) SYN dorsal metatarsal artery.

ar·te·ri·a me·ta·tar·sal·is plan·tar·is (ahr-tēr′ē-ă met′ă-tahr-sā′lis plan-tā′ris) [TA] SYN plantar metatarsal artery.

ar·te·ri·a mus·cu·lo·phre·ni·ca (ahr-tēr′ē-ă mŭs′kyū-lō-fren′i-kă) [TA] SYN musculophrenic artery.

ar·te·ri·a na·sal·is pos·te·ri·or sep·ti (ahr-tēr′ē-ă nā-sā′lis pos-tēr′ē-ŏr sep′tī) SYN posterior septal branch of nose.

ar·te·ri·a nu·tri·ci·a (ahr-tēr′ē-ă nū-trish′ē-ă) [TA] SYN nutrient artery.

ar·te·ri·a nu·tri·ci·a fe·mo·ris (ahr-tēr′ē-ă nū-trish′ē-ă fem′ŏr-is) [TA] SYN nutrient artery of femur.

ar·te·ria nu·tri·ci·a fi·bu·lae (ahr-tēr′ē-ă nū-trish′ē-ă fib′yū-lē) [TA] SYN nutrient artery of fibula.

ar·te·ri·a ob·tu·ra·to·ri·a (ahr-tēr′ē-ă ob′tū-rā-tō′rē-ă) [TA] SYN obturator artery.

ar·te·ri·a ob·tu·ra·to·ri·a ac·ces·so·ri·a (ahr-tēr′ē-ă ob′tū-ră-tō′rē-ă ak-ses-sō′rē-ă) [TA] SYN accessory obturator artery.

ar·te·ri·a oc·ci·pi·ta·lis (ahr-tēr′ē-ă ok′sip-i-tā′lis) [TA] SYN occipital artery.

ar·te·ri·a oph·thal·mi·ca (ahr-tēr′ē-ă of-thal′mi-kă) [TA] SYN ophthalmic artery.

ar·te·ri·a o·va·ri·ca (ahr-tēr′ē-ă ō-vā′ri-kă) [TA] SYN ovarian artery.

ar·te·ri·a pal·a·ti·na as·cen·dens (ahr-tēr′ē-ă pal-ă-tī′nă ă-sen′denz) SYN ascending palatine artery.

ar·te·ri·a pal·a·ti·na des·cen·dens (ahr-tēr′ē-ă pal-ă-tī′nă de-sen′denz) SYN descending palatine artery.

ar·te·ri·a pal·a·ti·na mi·nor (ahr-tēr′ē-ă pal-ă-tī′nă mī′nŏr) SYN lesser palatine artery.

ar·te·ri·a pan·cre·at·ic·a mag·na (ahr-tēr′ē-ă pan-krē-at′ik-ă mag′nă) SYN greater pancreatic artery.

ar·te·ri·a pan·cre·at·i·co·du·od·e·nal·is in·fe·ri·or (ahr-tēr′ē-ă pan-krē-at-ik-ō-dū-ō-dē-nā′lis in-fēr′ē-ŏr) SYN inferior pancreaticoduodenal artery.

ar·te·ri·a pan·cre·at·i·co·du·od·e·nal·is su·pe·ri·or an·te·ri·or et pos·te·ri·or (ahr-tē′ē-ă pan-krē-at-ik-ō-dū-ō-dē-nā′lis sŭ-pēr′ē-ŏr an-tēr′ē-ŏr pos-tēr′ē-ŏr) SYN anterior and posterior superior pancreaticoduodenal artery.

ar·te·ri·a pe·ri·car·di·a·co·phre·ni·ca (ahr-tēr′ē-ă per-i-kahr′dē-ă-kō-fren′i-kă) [TA] SYN pericardiacophrenic artery.

ar·te·ri·a pe·ri·ne·al·is (ahr-tēr′ē-ă pĕ-rin-ē-ā′lis) [TA] SYN perineal artery.

ar·te·ri·a pe·ro·ne·a (ahr-tēr′ē-ă per-ō-nē′ă) [TA] SYN peroneal artery.

ar·te·ri·a pha·ryn·ge·a as·cen·dens (ahr-tēr′ē-ă fă-rin′jē-ă ă-sen′denz) [TA] SYN ascending pharyngeal artery.

ar·te·ri·a phre·ni·ca in·fe·ri·or (ahr-tēr′ē-ă frē′ni-kă in-fēr′ē-ŏr) SYN inferior phrenic artery.

ar·te·ri·a phre·ni·ca su·pe·ri·or (ahr-tēr′ē-ă frē′ni-kă sŭ-pēr′ē-ŏr) SYN superior phrenic artery.

ar·te·ri·a plan·tar·is la·ter·al·is (ahr-tēr′ē-ă plan-tā′ris la-tĕr-ā′lis) SYN lateral plantar artery.

ar·te·ri·a plan·tar·is me·di·al·is (ahr-tēr′ē-ă plan-tā′ris mē-dē-ā′lis) SYN medial plantar artery.

ar·te·ri·a plan·tar·is pro·fun·da (ahr-tēr′ē-ă plan-tā′ris prō-fŭn′dă) [TA] SYN deep plantar artery.

ar·te·ri·a po·lar·is tem·po·ral·is (ahr-tēr′ē-ă pō-lā′ris tem-pōr-ā′lis) [TA] SYN polar temporal artery.

ar·te·ri·a pop·lit·e·a (ahr-tēr′ē-ă pop-lit′ē-ă) [TA] SYN popliteal artery.

ar·te·ria pre·pan·cre·a·ti·ca (ahr-tēr′ē-ă prē′pan-krē-at′i-kă) [TA] SYN prepancreatic artery.

ar·te·ri·a pro·fun·da cli·to·ri·dis (ahr-tēr′ē-ă prō-fŭn′dă kli-tōr′id-is) [TA] SYN deep artery of clitoris.

ar·te·ri·a pro·fun·da fe·mo·ris (ahr-tēr′ē-ă prō-fŭn′dă fem′ŏr-is) SYN deep artery of thigh.

ar·te·ri·a pro·fun·da pe·nis (ahr-tēr′ē-ă prō-fŭn′dă pē′nis) [TA] SYN deep artery of penis.

ar·te·ri·a pte·ry·go·men·in·ge·a·lis (ahr-tēr′ē-ă ter′i-gō-mĕ-nin-jē-ā′lis) [TA] SYN pterygomeningeal artery.

ar·te·ri·a pul·mo·na·lis (ahr-tēr′ē-ă pŭl-mō-nā′lis) SYN pulmonary trunk.

ar·te·ri·a qua·dri·gem·in·a·lis (ahr-tēr′ē-ă kwah′dri-jem-i-nā′lis) SYN collicular artery.

ar·te·ri·a ra·di·a·lis (ahr-tēr′ē-ă rā-dē-ā′lis) [TA] SYN radial artery.

ar•te•ri•a ra•di•al•is in•di•cis (ahr-tēr′ē-ă rā-dē-ā′lis in′di-sis) SYN radialis indicis artery.

ar•te•ri•a rec•tal•is in•fe•ri•or (ahr-tēr′ē-ă rek-tā′lis in-fēr′ē-ŏr) SYN inferior rectal artery.

ar•te•ri•a rec•tal•is me•di•a (ahr-tēr′ē-ă rek-tā′lis mē′dē-ă) SYN middle rectal artery.

ar•te•ri•a rec•tal•is su•pe•ri•or (ahr-tēr′ē-ă rek-tā′lis sŭ-pēr′ē-ŏr) SYN superior rectal artery.

ar•te•ria re•cur•rens ul•na•ris (ahr-tēr′ē-ă rē-kŭr′enz ŭl-nā′ris) [TA] SYN recurrent ulnar artery.

ar•te•ri•a re•na•lis (ahr-tēr′ē-ă rē-nā′lis) [TA] SYN renal artery.

ar•te•ri•a re•tro•du•od•e•nal•is (ahr-tēr′ē-ă rē′trō-dū-od-ĕ-nā′lis) SYN retroduodenal artery.

ar•te•ri•a sphe•no•pa•la•ti•na (ahr-tēr′ē-ă sfē′nō-pal-ă-tī-nă) [TA] SYN sphenopalatine artery.

ar•te•ri•a spi•nal•is an•te•ri•or (ahr-tēr′ē-ă spī-nā′lis an-tēr′ē-ŏr) SYN anterior spinal artery.

ar•te•ri•a spi•nal•is pos•te•ri•or (ahr-tēr′ē-ă spī-nā′lis pos-tēr′ē-ŏr) SYN posterior spinal artery.

ar•te•ri•a sty•lo•mas•toi•de•a (ahr-tēr′ē-ă stī′lō-mas-toy′dē-ă) [TA] SYN stylomastoid artery.

ar•te•ri•a sub•cla•vi•a (ahr-tēr′ē-ă sŭb-klā′vē-ă) [TA] SYN subclavian artery.

ar•te•ri•a sub•cos•ta•lis (ahr-tēr′ē-ă sŭb-kos-tā′lis) [TA] SYN subcostal artery.

ar•te•ri•a sub•lin•gua•lis (ahr-tēr′ē-ă sŭb ling-gwā′lis) [TA] SYN sublingual artery.

ar•te•ri•a sub•men•ta•lis (ahr-tēr′ē-ă sŭb-men-tā′lis) [TA] SYN submental artery.

ar•te•ri•a sub•scap•u•la•ris (ahr-tēr′ē-ă sŭb′skap-yū-lā′ris) [TA] SYN subscapular artery.

ar•te•ri•a su•pra•du•od•e•nal•is (ahr-tēr′ē-ă sū′pră-dū-od-en-ā′lis) SYN supraduodenal artery.

ar•te•ri•a su•pra•or•bi•ta•lis (ahr-tēr′ē-ă sū′pră-ōr-bi-tā′lis) [TA] SYN supraorbital artery.

ar•te•ri•a su•pra•re•nal•is in•fe•ri•or (ahr-tēr′ē-ă sū′pră-re-nā′lis in-fēr′ē-ŏr) SYN inferior suprarenal artery.

ar•te•ri•a su•pra•re•nal•is me•di•a (ahr-tēr′ē-ă sū′pră-rē-nā′lis mē′dē-ă) SYN middle suprarenal artery.

ar•te•ri•a su•pra•scap•u•la•ris (ahr-tēr′ē-ă sū′pră-skap-yū-lā′lis) [TA] SYN suprascapular artery.

ar•te•ri•a su•pra•troch•le•a•ris (ahr-tēr′ē-ă sū′pră-trok-lē-ā′ris) [TA] SYN supratrochlear artery.

ar•te•ri•a su•ra•lis (ahr-tēr′ē-ă sū-rā′lis) [TA] SYN sural artery.

ar•te•ri•a tem•po•ral•is pro•fun•da (ahr-tēr′ē-ă tem-pō-rā′lis prō-fŭn′dă) SYN deep temporal artery.

ar•te•ri•a tem•po•ral•is su•per•fi•ci•al•is (ahr-tēr′ē-ă tem-pō-rā′lis sū′pĕr-fish′ē-ā′lis) SYN superficial temporal artery.

ar•te•ri•a tes•ti•cu•la•ris (ahr-tēr′ē-ă tes-tik-yū-lā′ris) [TA] SYN testicular artery.

ar•te•ri•a tho•ra•ci•ca la•ter•al•is (ahr-tēr′ē-ă tho-ras′i-kă lat-ĕr-ā′lis) SYN lateral thoracic artery.

ar•te•ri•a tho•ra•ci•ca su•pe•ri•or (ahr-tēr′ē-ă tho-ras′i-kă sŭ-pēr′ē-ŏr) SYN superior thoracic artery.

ar•te•ri•a tho•ra•co•a•cro•mi•a•lis (ahr-tēr′ē-ă thō′ră-kō-ă-krō-mē-ā′lis) [TA] SYN thoracoacromial artery.

ar•te•ri•a tho•ra•co•dor•sa•lis (ahr-tēr′ē-ă thōr′ă-kō-dōr-sā′lis) [TA] SYN thoracodorsal artery.

ar•te•ri•a thy•roi•de•a i•ma (ahr-tēr′ē-ă thī-roy′dē-ă ī′mă) SYN thyroid ima artery.

ar•te•ri•a thy•roi•de•a in•fe•ri•or (ahr-tēr′ē-ă thī-roy′dē-ă in-fēr′ē-ŏr) SYN inferior thyroid artery.

ar•te•ri•a thy•roi•de•a su•pe•ri•or (ahr-tēr′ē-ă thī-roy′dē-ă sŭ-pēr′ē-ŏr) SYN superior thyroid artery.

ar•te•ri•a ti•bi•al•is an•te•ri•or (ahr-tēr′ē-ă ti-bē′ā′lis an-tēr′ē-ŏr) SYN anterior tibial artery.

ar•te•ri•a ti•bi•al•is pos•te•ri•or (ahr-tēr′ē-ă ti-bē-ā′lis pos-tēr′ē-ŏr) SYN posterior superior alveolar artery.

ar•te•ri•a trans•ver•sa col•li (ahr-tēr′ē-ă tranz-vĕr′să kol′ī) [TA] SYN transverse cervical artery.

ar•te•ri•a trans•ver•sa fa•ci•e•i (ahr-tēr′ē-ă tranz-vĕr′să fā′shē-ī) [TA] SYN transverse facial artery.

ar•te•ri•a ul•na•ris (ahr-tēr′ē-ă ŭl-nā′ris) [TA] SYN ulnar artery.

ar•te•ri•a um•bi•li•ca•lis (ahr-tēr′ē-ă ŭm-bil-i-kā′lis) [TA] SYN umbilical artery.

ar•te•ri•a u•re•thra•lis (ahr-tēr′ē-ă yū-rē-thrā′lis) [TA] SYN urethral artery.

ar•te•ri•a u•te•ri•na (ahr-tēr′ē-ă yū-tĕr-ī′nă) [TA] SYN uterine artery.

ar•te•ri•a va•gi•na•lis (ahr-tēr′ē-ă va-ji-nā′lis) [TA] SYN vaginal artery.

ar•te•ri•a ver•te•bra•lis (ahr-tēr′ē-ă vĕr-tĕ-brā′lis) [TA] SYN vertebral artery.

ar•te•ri•a ves•i•cal•is in•fe•ri•or (ahr-tēr′ē-ă ves-ik-ā′lis in-fēr′ē-ŏr) SYN inferior vesical artery.

ar•te•ri•a ves•i•cal•is su•pe•ri•or (ahr-tēr′ē-ă ves-ik-ā′lis sŭ-pēr′ē-ŏr) SYN superior vesical artery.

ar•te•ri•a vo•lar•is in•di•cis ra•di•al•is (ahr-tēr′ē-ă vō-lār′is in-di′shis rā-dē-ā′lis) SYN radialis indicis artery.

ar•te•ri•a zy•go•mat•i•co•or•bi•ta•lis (ahr-tēr′ē-ă zī-gō-mat′i-kō-ōr-bi-tā′lis) [TA] SYN zygomaticoorbital artery.

ar•te•ri•ec•to•my (ar-tēr-ē-ek′tō-mē) Excision of part of an artery. [L. *arteria,* artery, + G. *ektomē,* excision]

ar•te•ries of brain (ahr′tĕr-ēz brān) Arteries and arterial branches supplying the brain; they are derived from the cerebral arterial circle and the anterior choroidal artery.

ar•te•ries of pe•nis (ahr′tĕr-ēz pē′nis) SEE dorsal artery of penis, deep artery of penis.

arterio-, arteri- Combining forms denoting artery. [L. *arteria,* fr. G. *artēria,* a windpipe, an artery]

ar•te•ri•o•cap•il•lar•y (ahr-tēr′ē-ō-cap′i-lār-ē) Relating to both arteries and capillaries.

ar•te•ri•o•gram (ahr-tēr′ē-ō-gram) Radiographic demonstration of an artery after injection of contrast medium. [arterio- + G. *gramma,* something written]

ar•te•ri•o•graph•ic (ahr-tēr′ē-ō-graf′ik) Relating to or using arteriography.

ar•te•ri•og•ra•phy (ahr-ter′ē-og′ră-fē) Visualization of an artery or arteries by x-ray imaging after injection of a radiopaque contrast medium. See this page. [arterio- + G. *graphō,* to write]

ar•te•ri•o•la, pl. **ar•te•ri•o•lae** (ahr-tēr-ē-ō′lă, ahr-tēr-ē-ō′lē) [TA] SYN arteriole. [Mod. L. dim. of *arteria,* artery]

ar•ter•i•o•la glo•mer•u•lar•is af•fer•ens (ahr-tēr-ē-ō′lă glō′mer-yū-lā′ris af′ĕr-enz) [TA] SYN afferent glomerular arteriole.

ar•ter•i•o•la glo•mer•u•la•ris ef•fer•ens (ahr-tēr-ē-ō′lă glō′mer-yū-lā′ris ef′ĕr-enz) [TA] SYN ductus deferens.

ar•te•ri•o•la ma•cu•la•ris in•fe•ri•or (ahr-tēr-ē-ō′lă mak-yū-lā′ris in-fēr′ē-ŏr) [TA] SYN inferior macular arteriole.

ar•te•ri•o•la ma•cu•la•ris su•pe•ri•or (ahr-tēr-ē-ō′lă mak-yū-lā′ris sŭ-pēr′ē-ŏr) [TA] SYN superior macular arteriole.

ar•te•ri•o•lar (ahr-tēr′ē-ō′lăr) Of or pertaining to an arteriole or the arterioles collectively.

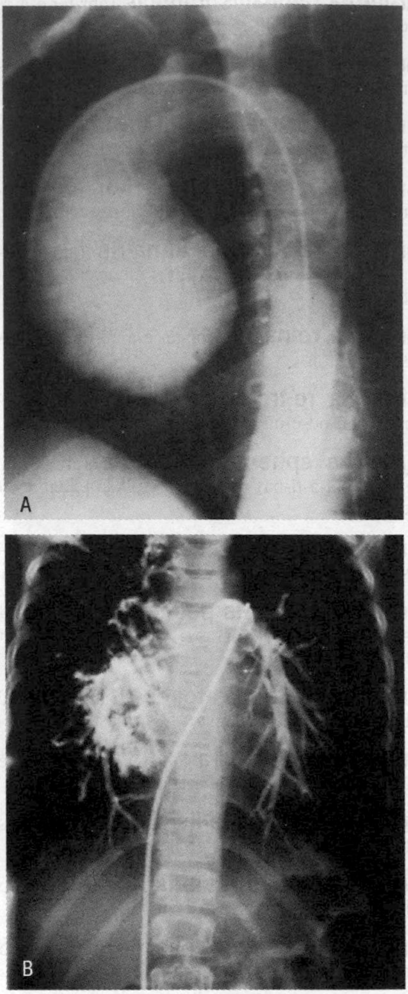

arteriography: (A) cardiovascular findings associated with Marfan syndrome; (B) single pulmonary arteriovenous fistula allows passage of contrast medium directly into the pulmonary venous system

ar•te•ri•o•lar neph•ro•scle•ro•sis (ahr-tēr′ē-ō′lăr nef′rō-skler-ō′sis) Renal scarring due to arteriolar sclerosis resulting from long-standing hypertension; chronic renal failure develops infrequently. SYN arteriolonephrosclerosis.

ar•te•ri•o•lar net•work (ahr-tēr′ē-ō′lăr net′wŏrk) A vascular network formed by anastomoses between minute arteries just before they become capillaries.

ar•te•ri•ole (ahr-tēr′ē-ōl) A minute artery with a tunica media comprising only one or two layers of smooth muscle cells; a terminal artery continuous with the capillary network. See page 129. SYN arteriola [TA].

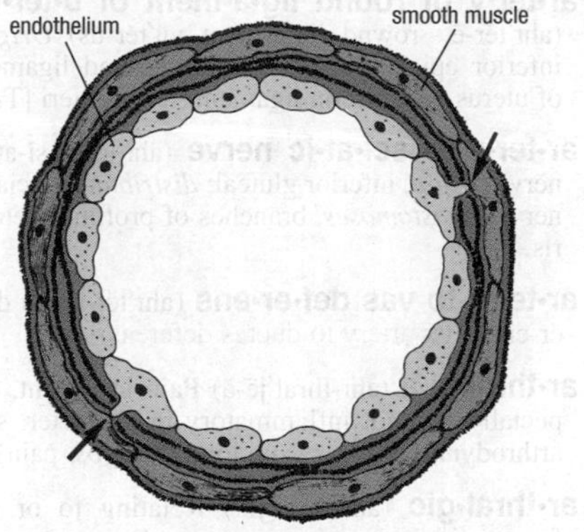

arteriole: arrows show points of contact between endothelium and smooth muscle

ar·te·ri·o·lith (ahr-tēr′ē-ō-lith) A calcareous deposit in an arterial wall or thrombus. [L. *arteria,* artery, + G. *lithos,* a stone]

ar·ter·i·o·li·tis (ahr-tēr′ē-ō-lī′tis) Inflammation of the wall of the arterioles. [L. *arteriola,* arteriole, + G. *-itis,* inflammation]

♻**arteriolo-** Combining form indicating the arterioles. [Modern L. *arteriola,* arteriole]

ar·te·ri·o·lo·ne·cro·sis (ahr-tēr-ē-ō′lō-nĕ-krō′sis) SYN necrotizing arteriolitis. [L. *arteriola,* arteriole, + G. *nekrōsis,* a killing]

ar·te·ri·o·lo·neph·ro·scle·ro·sis (ar-tēr-ē-ō′lō-nef′rō-skler-ō′sis) SYN arteriolar nephrosclerosis.

ar·te·ri·o·lo·scle·ro·sis (ahr-tēr-ē-ō′lō-skler-ō′sis) Arteriosclerosis affecting mainly the arterioles, seen especially in chronic hypertension.

ar·te·ri·o·mo·tor (ahr-tēr′ē-ō-mō′tŏr) Causing changes in the caliber of an artery; vasomotor with special reference to the arteries.

ar·te·ri·o·neph·ro·scle·ro·sis (ahr-tēr′ē-ō-nef′rō-skler-ō′sis) SYN arterial nephrosclerosis.

ar·te·ri·op·a·thy (ahr-tēr′ē-op′ă-thē) Any disease of the arteries. [arterio- + G. *pathos,* suffering]

ar·te·ri·o·plas·ty (ahr-tēr′ē-ō-plas-tē) Any operation for the reconstruction of the wall of an artery. [arterio- + G. *plastos,* formed]

ar·te·ri·o·pres·sor (ahr-tēr′ē-ō-pres′sŏr) Causing increased arterial blood pressure.

ar·te·ri·or·rha·phy (ahr-tēr′ē-ōr′ă-fē) Suture of an artery. [arterio- + G. *rhaphē,* seam]

ar·te·ri·or·rhex·is (ahr-tēr′ē-ō-rek′sis) Rupture of an artery. [arterio- + G. *rhēxis,* rupture]

ar·te·ri·o·scle·ro·sis (ahr-tēr′ē-ō-skler-ō′sis) Hardening of the arteries; types generally recognized are: atherosclerosis, Mönckeberg arteriosclerosis, and arteriolosclerosis. SYN arterial sclerosis. [arterio- + G. *sklērōsis,* hardness]

ar·te·ri·o·scle·ro·sis ob·lit·er·ans (ahr-tēr′ē-ō-skler-ō′sis ob-lit′ĕr-anz) Arteriosclerosis producing narrowing and occlusion of the arterial lumen.

ar·te·ri·o·scle·rot·ic (ahr-tēr′ē-ō-skler-ot′ik) Relating to or affected by arteriosclerosis.

ar·te·ri·o·scle·rot·ic an·eu·rysm (ahr-tēr′ē-ō-skler-ot′ik an′yūr-izm) The most common type of aneurysm, occurring in the abdominal aorta and other large arteries, primarily in the elderly.

ar·te·ri·o·spasm (ahr-tēr′ē-ō-spazm) Spasm of an artery or arteries.

ar·te·ri·o·ste·no·sis (ahr-tēr′ē-ō-stĕ-nō′sis) Narrowing of the caliber of an artery, either temporary, through vasoconstriction, or permanent, through arteriosclerosis. [arterio- + G. *stenōsis,* a narrowing]

ar·te·ri·o·sus (ar-tēr′ē-ō′sŭs) Pertaining to or of the nature of an artery. [L.]

ar·te·ri·ot·o·my (ahr-tēr′ē-ot′ŏ-mē) Any surgical incision into the lumen of an artery, e.g., to remove an embolus. [arterio- + G. *tomē,* incision]

ar·te·ri·o·ve·nous (A-V, AV) (ahr-tēr′ē-ō-vē′nŭs) Relating to both an artery and a vein or to both arteries and veins in general; both arterial and venous, as an "arteriovenous (A-V) anastomosis."

ar·te·ri·o·ve·nous a·nas·to·mo·sis (ava) (ahr-tēr′ē-ō-vē′nŭs ă-nas′tŏ-mō′sis) Vessels through which blood is shunted from arterioles to venules without passing through the capillaries.

ar·te·ri·o·ve·nous an·eu·rysm (ahr-tēr′ē-ō-vē′nŭs an′yūr-izm) **1.** A dilated arteriovenous shunt. **2.** Communication between an artery and a vein, sometimes congenital.

ar·te·ri·o·ve·nous car·bon di·ox·ide dif·fer·ence (ahr-tēr′ē-ō-vē′nŭs kahr′bŏn dī-oks′īd dif′ĕr-ĕns) The difference in carbon dioxide content (in milliliters per 100 mL blood) between arterial and venous blood.

ar·te·ri·o·ve·nous fis·tu·la (ahr-tēr′ē-ō-vē′nŭs fis′chū-lă) An abnormal communication between an artery and a vein, usually resulting in the formation of an arteriovenous aneurysm.

ar·te·ri·o·ve·nous ox·y·gen dif·fer·ence (ahr-tēr′ē-ō-vē′nŭs ok′si-jĕn dif′ĕr-ĕns) The difference in the oxygen content (in milliliters per 100 mL blood) between arterial and venous blood.

ar·te·ri·o·ve·nous shunt (ahr-tēr′ē-ō-vē′nŭs shŭnt) The passage of blood directly from arteries to veins, without going through the capillary network.

ar•ter•i•tis (ahr′tĕr-ī′tis) Inflammation or infection involving an artery or arteries. [L. *arteria,* artery, + G. *-itis,* inflammation]

ar•ter•i•tis ob•li•te•rans, ob•lit•er•at•ing ar•ter•i•tis (ahr′tĕr-ī′tis ob-lit′ĕr-anz, ob-lit′ĕr-āt-ing ahr′tĕr-ī′tis) SYN endarteritis obliterans.

ar•ter•y (ar′tĕr-ē) A relatively thick-walled, muscular blood vessel conveying blood away from the heart and pulsating with each heartbeat. With the exception of the pulmonary and umbilical arteries, the arteries convey red or oxygenated blood. SYN arteria [TA]. [L. *arteria,* fr. G. *artēria*]

ar•ter•y of an•gu•lar gy•rus (ahr′tĕr-ē ang′gyū-lăr jī′rŭs) The last branch of the terminal part of the middle cerebral artery distributed to parts of the temporal, parietal, and occipital lobes.

ar•ter•y to a•tri•o•ven•tric•u•lar node (ahr′tĕr-ē ā′trē-ō-ven-trik′yū-lăr nōd) SYN atrioventricular nodal branches.

ar•ter•y of bulb of pe•nis (ahr′tĕr-ē bŭlb pē′nis) A branch of the internal pudendal artery that supplies the bulb of the penis including the bulbar urethra. SYN arteria bulbi penis [TA].

ar•ter•y of bulb of ves•ti•bule (ahr′tĕr-ē bŭlb ves′ti-byūl) The branch of the internal pudendal artery in the female that supplies the bulb of the vestibule. SYN arteria bulbi vestibuli [TA].

ar•ter•y of Drum•mond (ahr′tĕr-ē drŭm′ŏnd) SYN marginal artery of colon.

ar•ter•y to duc•tus def•er•ens (ahr′tĕr-ē dŭk′tŭs def′er-enz) *Origin*, anterior division of internal iliac, or sometimes superior vesical; *distribution*, ductus deferens, seminal vesicles, testicle, ureter; *anastomoses*, testicular, cremasteric arteries. SYN arteria ductus deferentis [TA], arteria deferentialis, artery to vas deferens, deferential artery.

ar•ter•y for•ceps (ahr′tĕr-ē fōr′seps) SYN hemostatic forceps.

ar•ter•y of the pan•cre•at•ic tail (ahr′tĕr-ē pan-krē-at′ik tāl) *Origin*, splenic artery near the left gastroepiploic; *distribution*, the tail of the pancreas; *anastomoses*, with other pancreatic arteries.

ar•ter•y of pter•y•goid ca•nal (ahr′tĕr-ē ter′i-goyd kă-nal′) *Origin*, usually arises from the third part of the maxillary artery, but frequently from the greater palatine artery, within the pterygopalatine fossa. Passes posteriorly to run through the pterygoid canal with the corresponding nerve, supplying the contents and wall of the canal, the mucous membrane of the upper pharynx, the auditory tube, and the tympanic cavity. SYN arteria canalis pterygoidei [TA].

ar•ter•y of round lig•a•ment of u•ter•us (ahr′tĕr-ē rownd lig′ă-mĕnt yū′tĕr-ŭs) *Origin*, inferior epigastric; *distribution*, round ligament of uterus. SYN arteria ligamenti teretis uteri [TA].

ar•ter•y to sci•at•ic nerve (ahr′tĕr-ē sī-at′ik nĕrv) *Origin*, inferior gluteal; *distribution*, sciatic nerve; *anastomoses*, branches of profunda femoris.

ar•te•ry to vas def•er•ens (ahr′tĕr-ē vas def′ĕr-enz) SYN artery to ductus deferens.

ar•thral•gi•a (ahr-thral′jē-ă) Pain in a joint, especially one not inflammatory in character. SYN arthrodynia. [G. *arthron,* joint, + *algos,* pain]

ar•thral•gic (ahr-thral′jik) Relating to or affected with arthralgia. SYN arthrodynic.

ar•threc•to•my (ahr-threk′tŏ-mē) Excision of a joint. [G. *arthron,* joint, + *ektomē,* excision]

ar•thrit•ic (ahr-thrit′ik) Relating to arthritis.

ar•thrit•ic gen•er•al pseu•do•pa•ral•y•sis (ahr-thrit′ik jen′ĕr-ăl sū′dō-păr-al′i-sis) A disease, occurring in arthritic patients, having symptoms resembling those of general paresis, the lesions of which consist of diffuse changes of a degenerative and noninflammatory character due to intracranial atheroma.

ar•thri•tis, pl. **ar•thrit•i•des** (ahr-thrī′tis, ahr-thrit′i-dēz) Inflammation of a joint or a state characterized by inflammation of joints. SYN articular rheumatism. [G. fr. *arthron,* joint, + *-itis,* inflammation]

ar•thri•tis de•for•mans (ahr-thrī′tis dē-fōr′manz) SYN rheumatoid arthritis.

♻ **arthro-, arthr-** Combining forms meaning a joint, an articulation; corresponds to L. *articul-*. [G. *arthron,* a joint, fr. *arariskō,* to join, to fit together]

ar•thro•cele (ahr′thrō-sēl) **1.** Hernia of the synovial membrane through the capsule of a joint. **2.** Any swelling of a joint. [arthro- + G. *kēlē,* hernia, tumor]

ar•thro•cen•te•sis (ahr′thrō-sen-tē′sis) Aspiration of fluid from a joint through a needle. [arthro- + G. *kentēsis,* puncture]

ar•thro•chon•dri•tis (ahr′thrō-kon-drī′tis) Inflammation of an articular cartilage. [arthro- + G. *chondros,* cartilage, + *-itis,* inflammation]

ar•thro•cla•si•a (ahr′thrō-klā′zē-ă) Forcible breaking up of adhesions in ankylosis. [arthro- + G. *klasis,* a breaking]

Arth•ro•der•ma (ahr′thrō-dĕr′mă) A genus of ascomycetous fungi composed of the anamorph genera *Microsporium* and *Trichoderma* species.

ar•throd•e•sis (ahr-throd′ĕ-sis) The stiffening of a joint by operative means. SYN artificial ankylosis, syndesis. [arthro- + G. *desis,* a binding together]

ar·thro·di·a (ahr-thrō′dē-ă) SYN plane joint. [G. *arthrōdia,* a gliding joint, fr. *arthron,* joint, + *eidos,* form]

ar·thro·di·al (ahr-thrō′dē-ăl) Relating to arthrodia.

ar·thro·di·al joint (ahr-thrō′dē-ăl joynt) SYN plane joint.

ar·thro·dyn·i·a (ahr′thrō-din′ē-ă) SYN arthralgia. [arthro- + G. *odynē,* pain]

ar·thro·dyn·ic (ahr′thrō-din′ik) SYN arthralgic.

ar·thro·dys·pla·si·a (ahr′thrō-dis-plā′zē-ă) Hereditary congenital defect of joint development. [arthro- + G. *dys,* bad, + *plasis,* a molding]

ar·thro·en·dos·co·py (ahr′thrō-en-dos′kŏ-pē) SYN arthroscopy.

ar·thro·gram (ahr′thrō-gram) Radiograph of a joint; usually implies the introduction of a contrast agent into the joint capsule. [arthro- + G. *gramma,* a writing]

ar·throg·ra·phy (ahr-throg′ră-fē) Radiography of a joint after injecting one or more contrast media into the joint. [arthro- + G. *graphō,* to describe]

ar·thro·gry·po·sis (ahr′thrō-gri-pō′sis) Congenital defect of the limbs characterized by contractures of multiple joints. [arthro- + G. *gryphōsis,* a crooking]

ar·thro·gry·po·sis mul·ti·plex con·gen·i·ta (ahr′thrō-gri-pō′sis mŭl′ti-pleks kon-jen′i-tă) Limitation of range of joint motion and contractures present at birth, usually involving multiple joints; a syndrome probably of diverse etiology that may result from changes in spinal cord, muscle, or connective tissue.

ar·thro·kin·e·mat·ics (ahr′thrō-kin′ĕ-mat′iks) The study of movements between adjoining articular (joint) surfaces. [arthro- + G. *kinēma, kinēmatos,* movement, + -ics]

ar·throl·y·sis (ahr-throl′i-sis) Restoration of mobility in stiff and ankylosed joints. [arthro- + G. *lysis,* a loosening]

ar·throm·e·ter (ahr-throm′ĕ-ter) SYN goniometer (3).

ar·throm·e·try (ahr-throm′ĕ-trē) Measurement of the range of movement in a joint. [arthro- + G. *metron,* measure]

ar·thro·my·o·neu·rop·a·thy syn·drome (ahrth′rō-mī′ō-nŭr-op′ă-thē sin′drōm) A subset of symptoms of Gulf War Syndrome that includes joint and muscle pains, muscle fatigue, and difficulty with lifting objects, as well as prickling, tingling, or crawling sensation in the extremities.

ar·thro·oph·thal·mop·a·thy (ahr′thrō-of′thal-mop′ă-thē) Disease affecting joints and eyes. [arthro- + ophthalmo- + G. *pathos,* suffering]

ar·thro·path·i·a pso·ri·a·ti·ca (ăr′thrō-pā′thē-ă sōr-ē-at′ĭk-ă) SYN psoriatic arthritis.

ar·throp·a·thy (ahr-throp′ă-thē) Any disease affecting a joint. [arthro- + G. *pathos,* suffering]

ar·thro·plas·ty (ahr′thrō-plas-tē) **1.** Creation of an artificial joint to correct ankylosis. **2.** An operation to restore as far as possible the integrity and functional power of a joint. [arthro- + G. *plastos,* formed]

ar·thro·pneu·mo·ra·di·og·ra·phy (ahr′thrō-nū′mō-rā-dē-og′ră-fē) Radiographic examination of a joint after it has been injected with air. [arthro- + pneumo- + radiography]

ar·thro·pod (ahr′thrō-pod) A member of the phylum Arthropoda. [arthro- + G. *pous,* foot]

Ar·throp·o·da (ahr-throp′ŏ-dă) A phylum of the Metazoa that includes the classes Crustacea (crabs, shrimp, crayfish, lobsters), Insecta, Arachnida (spiders, scorpions, mites, ticks), Chilopoda (centipedes), Diplopoda (millipedes), Merostomata (horseshoe crabs), and various other extinct or lesser known groups. Arthropoda forms the largest assemblage of living organisms, 75% insects, of which more than a million species are known. [arthro- + G. *pous,* foot]

ar·thro·po·di·a·sis (ahr′thrō-pŏ-dī′ă-sis) Direct effects of arthropods on vertebrates, including acariasis, allergy, dermatosis, entomophobia, and actions of contact toxins.

ar·thro·py·o·sis (ahr′thrō-pī-ō′sis) Suppuration in a joint. [arthro- + G. *pyōsis,* suppuration]

ar·thro·scle·ro·sis (ahr′thrō-skler-ō′sis) Stiffness of the joints, especially in the aged. [arthro- + G. *sklērōsis,* hardening]

ar·thro·scope (ahr′thrŏ-skōp) An endoscope for examining the interior of a joint.

ar·thros·co·py (ahr-thros′kŏ-pē) Endoscopic examination of the interior of a joint. SYN arthroendoscopy. [arthro- + G. *skopeō,* to view]

ar·thro·sis (ahr-thrō′sis) **1.** SYN joint. [G. *arthrōsis,* a jointing] **2.** A degenerative disorder of a joint. [arthro- + G. *-osis,* condition]

ar·thros·to·my (ahr-thros′tŏ-mē) Establishment of a temporary opening into a joint cavity. [arthro- + G. *stoma,* mouth]

ar·thro·sy·no·vi·tis (ahr′thrō-sin-ō-vī′tis) Inflammation of the synovial membrane of a joint.

ar·throt·o·my (ahr-throt′ŏ-mē) Cutting into a joint. [arthro- + G. *tomē,* a cutting]

ar·throx·e·sis (ahr-throk′sĕ-sis) Removal of diseased tissue from a joint by means of a sharp spoon or other scraping instrument. [arthro- + G. *xesis,* a scraping]

ar·ti·choke (ahr′ti-chōk) A vegetable (*Cynara scolymus*) that has purported medicinal value in treating high cholesterol, snakebite, and sundry intestinal disorders. [It. *articiocco,* fr. Ar. *al-khurshuf*]

ar·tic·u·lar (ahr-tik′yū-lăr) Relating to a joint.

ar·tic·u·lar cap·sule (ahr-tik′yū-lăr kap′sŭl) A sac enclosing a joint, formed by an outer fibrous articular capsule and an inner synovial membrane. SYN capsula articularis [TA], joint capsule.

ar·tic·u·lar car·ti·lage (ahr-tik′yū-lăr kahr′ti-lăj) The cartilage covering the articular surfaces of the bones participating in a synovial joint.

ar·tic·u·lar cor·pus·cles (ahr-tik′yū-lăr kōr′pŭs-ĕlz) Encapsulated nerve terminations within joint capsules. SYN corpuscula articularia [TA].

ar·tic·u·lar crest (ahr-tik′yū-lăr krest) SYN intermediate sacral crest.

ar·tic·u·lar disc (ahr-tik′yū-lăr disk) A plate or ring of fibrocartilage attached to the joint capsule and separating the articular surfaces of the bones for a varying distance, sometimes completely; it serves to adapt two articular surfaces that are not entirely congruent.

ar·tic·u·la·ris cu·bi·ti mus·cle (ahr-tik-ū-lā′ris kyū′bi-tī mŭs′ĕl) The name applied to a small slip of the medial head of the triceps that inserts into the capsule of the elbow joint. SYN musculus articularis cubiti [TA].

ar·ti·cu·la·ris gen·us mus·cle (ahr-tik-ū-lā′ris jē′nŭs mŭs′ĕl) *Origin,* lower fourth of anterior surface of shaft of femur; *insertion,* suprapatellar bursa of knee joint; *action,* retracts suprapatellar bursa, during extension of knee; *nerve supply,* femoral. SYN musculus articularis genus [TA].

ar·tic·u·lar la·mel·la (ahr-tik′yū-lăr lă-mel′ă) The compact layer of bone on its articular surface that is firmly attached to the overlying articular cartilage.

ar·tic·u·lar mus·cle (ahr-tik′yū-lăr mŭs′ĕl) A muscle that inserts directly onto the capsule of a joint, acting to retract the capsule in certain movements.

ar·tic·u·lar nerve (ahr-tik′yū-lăr nĕrv) A branch of a nerve supplying a joint.

ar·ti·cu·lar pro·cess (ahr-tik′yū-lăr pros′es) One of the bilateral small flat projections on the surfaces of the arches of the vertebae, at the point where the pedicles and laminae join, forming the zygapophysial joint surfaces. SYN processus articularis [TA], zygapophysis, zygapophyses.

ar·tic·u·lar rheu·ma·tism (ahr-tik′yū-lăr rū′mă-tizm) SYN arthritis.

ar·tic·u·lar vas·cu·lar net·work of el·bow (ahr-tik′yū-lăr vas′kyū-lăr net′wŏrk el′bō) Vascular networks in the region of the elbow, composed of anastomoses between branches of the radial and middle collateral, superior and inferior ulnar collateral, radial recurrent, interosseous recurrent, and recurrent ulnar arteries.

ar·tic·u·late **1.** (ahr-tik′yŭ-lăt) SYN articulated. **2.** Capable of distinct and connected speech. **3.** (ahr-tik′yū-lāt) To join or connect together loosely to allow motion between the parts. **4.** To speak distinctly and connectedly. [L. *articulo,* pp. *-atus,* to articulate]

ar·tic·u·lat·ed (ahr-tik′yŭ-lāt-ĕd) Jointed. SYN articulate (1).

ar·tic·u·la·ti·o, pl. **ar·tic·u·la·ti·o·nes** (ahr-tik-ū-lā′shē-ō, ahr-tik-ū-lā-shē-ō′nēz) [TA] SYN synovial joint. [L. a forming of vines]

ar·tic·u·la·tion (ahr-tik′yū-lā′shŭn) **1.** SYN joint. **2.** A loose juncture or connection that permits motion between parts. **3.** The process of moving and coordinating oral, laryngeal, and pharyngeal structures to produce speech. **4.** DENTISTRY the contact relationship of the occlusal surfaces of the teeth during jaw movement. SEE ALSO synovial joint.

ar·tic·u·la·tion dis·or·der (ahr-tik′yū-lā′shŭn dis-ōr′dĕr) Any error in pronunciation including phoneme omissions, substitutions, distortions, and additions.

ar·tic·u·la·tor (ahr-tik′yū-lā-tŏr) A mechanical device that represents the temporomandibular joints and jaw members to which maxillary and mandibular casts may be attached; used in the fabrication and testing of dentures.

ar·tic·u·la·tors (ahr-tik′yŭ-lā-tŏrz) Organs of the speech mechanism that form the configurations required for production of meaningful speech sounds, i.e., the teeth, lips, mandible, tongue, velum, and pharynx. SEE ALSO speech mechanism.

ar·tic·u·la·to·ry a·prax·i·a (ahr-tik′yū-lă-tōr-ē ă-prak′sē-ă) SYN apraxia of speech.

ar·ti·fact (ahr′ti-fakt) **1.** Anything (especially in a histologic specimen or a graphic record) that is caused by the technique used or is not a natural occurrence but is merely incidental. **2.** A skin lesion produced or perpetuated by self-inflicted action, such as scratching in dermatitis artefacta. SYN artefact. [L. *ars,* art, + *facio,* pp. *factus,* to make]

ar·ti·fac·tu·al, **ar·ti·fac·ti·tious** (ahr′ti-fak′chū-ăl, ahr′ti-fak-tish′ŭs) Produced or caused by an artifact.

ar·ti·fi·cial an·ky·lo·sis (ahr′ti-fish′ăl ang′ki-lō′sis) SYN arthrodesis.

ar·ti·fi·cial heart (ahr′ti-fish′ăl hahrt) A mechanical pump used to replace the function of a damaged heart, either temporarily or as a permanent prosthesis.

ar·ti·fi·cial in·sem·i·na·tion (ahr′ti-fish′ăl in-sem′i-nā′shŭn) The introduction of semen into the vagina other than by coitus.

ar•ti•fi•cial kid•ney (ahr′ti-fish′ăl kid′nē) SYN hemodialyzer.

ar•ti•fi•cial la•bor (ahr′ti-fish′ăl lā′bŏr) Induced labor.

ar•ti•fi•cial lar•ynx (ahr′ti-fish′ăl lar′ingks) Mechanical device used to create alaryngeal speech. The most common types are battery powered and provide a buzzing sound source; the vibrating source is placed against the neck or in the oral cavity through a tube, and speech is articulated normally. Pneumatic assistive listening devices use expired air from the trachea to create vibration, which is relayed to the oral cavity by a tube. SYN electrolarynx.

ar•ti•fi•cial mem•brane rup•ture (ahr′ti-fish′ ăl mem′brān rŭp′chŭr) Rupture of the membranes induced by use of an amniohook or similar device.

ar•ti•fi•cial nose (ahr′ti-fish′ăl nōz) SYN hygroscopic condenser humidifier.

ar•ti•fi•cial pace•mak•er (ahr′ti-fish′ăl pās′ mā-kĕr) Any device that substitutes for the normal pacemaker and controls the rhythm of the organ; especially an electronic cardiac pacemaker, which may be implanted in the chest, with electrodes attached to the external cardiac surface, or passed through the venous circulation into the right side of the heart (pervenous pacemaker).

ar•ti•fi•cial pneu•mo•tho•rax (ahr′ti-fish′ăl nū′mō-thōr′aks) Pneumothorax produced by the injection of air, or a more slowly absorbed gas such as nitrogen, into the pleural space to collapse the lung.

ar•ti•fi•cial ra•di•o•ac•tiv•i•ty (ahr′ti-fish′ăl rā′dē-ō-ak-tiv′i-tē) The radioactivity of isotopes created by the bombardment of naturally occurring isotopes by subatomic particles, or high levels of x- or gamma radiation.

ar•ti•fi•cial res•pi•ra•tion (ahr′ti-fish′ăl res′ pir-ā′shŭn) SYN artificial ventilation.

ar•ti•fi•cial sa•li•va (ahr′ti-fish′ăl să-lī′vă) SYN saliva substitute.

ar•ti•fi•cial se•lec•tion (ahr′ti-fish′ăl sĕ-lek′ shŭn) Interference with natural selection by purposeful breeding of animals or plants of specific genotype or phenotype to produce a strain with desired characteristics.

ar•ti•fi•cial ven•ti•la•tion (ahr′ti-fish′ăl ven′ti-lā′shŭn) The process of supporting breathing by application of mechanical or manual means, when normal breathing is inefficient or has stopped. SYN artificial respiration.

ar•y•ep•i•glot•tic fold, ar•y•te•no•ep•i•glot•tid•e•an fold (ar′ē-ep-i-glot′ik fōld, ar-it′ ĕ-nō-ep′i-glot-id′ē-ăn fōld) A prominent fold of mucous membrane stretching between the lateral margin of the epiglottis and the arytenoid cartilage on either side; it encloses the aryepiglottic muscle. SYN plica aryepiglottica [TA].

ar•y•ep•i•glot•tic mus•cle (ar′ē-ep-i-glot′ik mŭs′ĕl) The fibers of the oblique arytenoid muscle that extend from the summit of the arytenoid cartilage to the side of the epiglottis; *action*, constricts the laryngeal aperture. SYN musculus aryepiglotticus [TA].

ar•yl (ar′il) An organic radical derived from an aromatic compound by removing a hydrogen atom.

ar•yl•sul•fa•tase (ar′il-sŭl′fă-tās) An enzyme that cleaves phenol sulfates, including cerebroside sulfates (i.e., a phenol sulfate + $H_2O \rightarrow$ a phenol + sulfate anion). Some arylsulfatases are inhibited by sulfate (type II) and some are not (type I). SYN arylsulphatase, sulfatase (2).

arylsulphatase [Br.] SYN arylsulfatase.

ar•y•te•noid (ar-i-tē′noyd) Denoting a cartilage (arytenoid cartilage) and muscles (oblique and transverse arytenoid muscles) of the larynx.

ar•y•te•noid car•ti•lage (ar-i-tē′noyd kahr′ti-lăj) One of a pair of small triangular pyramidal laryngeal cartilages that articulate with the lamina of the cricoid cartilage. It gives attachment at its anteriorly directed vocal process to the posterior part of the corresponding vocal ligament and to several muscles at its laterally directed muscular process. SYN cartilago arytenoidea [TA].

ar•y•te•noid dis•lo•ca•tion (ar-i-tē′noyd dis-lō-kā′shŭn) Separation of the cricoarytenoid joint with subluxation of the arytenoid cartilage.

ar•y•te•noi•dec•to•my (ar′i-tē-noy-dek′tŏ-mē) Excision of an arytenoid cartilage, usually in bilateral vocal fold paralysis, to improve breathing. [arytenoid + G. *ektomē,* excision]

ar•y•te•noi•di•tis (ar′i-tē-noy-dī′tis) Inflammation of an arytenoid cartilage or its mucosal cover.

ar•y•te•noi•do•pexy (ar′i-tē-noy′dō-pek′sē) Excision of an arytenoid cartilage, usually in bilateral vocal fold paralysis, to improve breathing. [arytenoid + G. *pēxis,* fixation]

A.S. Abbreviation for left ear. USAGE NOTE The JCAHO directs that *left ear* be written in full to avoid confusion with similar abbreviations. [L. *auris sinistra*]

As Symbol for arsenic.

ASA Abbreviation for acetylsalicylic acid; American Society of Anesthesiologists.

a•sac•cha•ro•lyt•ic (ă-sak′ă-rō-lit′ik) A microorganism unable to metabolize carbohydrates in the presence or absence of oxygen and that must rely on other carbon sources for energy.

ASA clas·si·fi·ca·tion (klas′i-fi-kā′shŭn) SYN Dripps classification.

as·a·foet·i·da (as′ă-fet′i-dă) A gum resin, the inspissated exudate from the root of *Ferula foetida* (family Umbelliferae); malodorous material used as a repellant against dogs, cats, and rabbits, and formerly used as an antispasmodic; in Asia, used as a condiment and flavoring agent. SYN devil's dung. [Pers. *aza,* mastic, + L. *foetidus,* fetid]

ASBESTOS (as-bes′tŏs) Acronym used in assessing casualties from chemical (and radiologic) agents. The components of the acronym are *A* for agent (type of chemical or radiation); *S* for state (e.g., solid, liquid, gas, vapor, aerosol); *B* for body site, or route of exposure (e.g., inhalational, percutaneous, ocular, enteral, parenteral); *E* for effects (local vs. systemic); *S* for severity of effects and of exposure; *T* for time course (e.g., time from exposure, length of latent period, prognosis); *O* for other diagnoses (both instead of and in addition to the agent originally considered); and *S* for synergism (interaction among multiple diagnoses).

as·bes·tos (as-bes′tŏs) Product obtained from fibrous hydrated silicates divided into amphiboles and serpentines; it is insoluble and is used to provide tensile strength and moldability,. thermal insulation, and resistance to fire, heat, and corrosion; inhalation of asbestos particles can cause asbestosis and cancer of the lung and pleura. [G. unquenchable; so called in the erroneous belief that when heated, it could not be quenched]

as·bes·tos bod·ies (as-bes′tŏs bod′ēz) Ferruginous bodies with asbestos fibers as a core; a histologic hallmark of exposure to asbestos.

as·bes·to·sis (as-bes-tō′sis) Pneumoconiosis due to inhalation of asbestos fibers suspended in the ambient air; sometimes complicated by pleural mesothelioma or bronchogenic carcinoma.

as·ca·ri·a·sis (as-kă-rī′ă-sis) A disease caused by infection with *Ascaris* or related ascarid nematodes. [G. *askaris,* an intestinal worm, + *-iasis,* condition]

as·car·i·cide (as-kar′i-sīd) **1.** Causing the death of ascarid nematodes. **2.** An agent having such properties. [ascarid + L. *caedo,* to kill]

As·car·is (as′kă-ris) A genus of large, heavy-bodied roundworms parasitic in the small intestine; abundant in humans and many other vertebrates. See this page. [G. *askaris,* an intestinal worm]

As·car·is lum·bri·coi·des (as′kă-ris lŭm-bri-koy′dēz) A large roundworm of humans, one of the commonest human parasites; various symptoms such as restlessness, fever, and diarrhea are attributed to its presence, but usually it causes no definite symptoms.

as·cend·ing a·or·ta (ă-send′ing ā-ōr′tă) The part of the aorta proximal to the aortic arch, from which the coronary arteries arise. SYN aorta ascendens, ascending part of aorta, pars ascendens aortae.

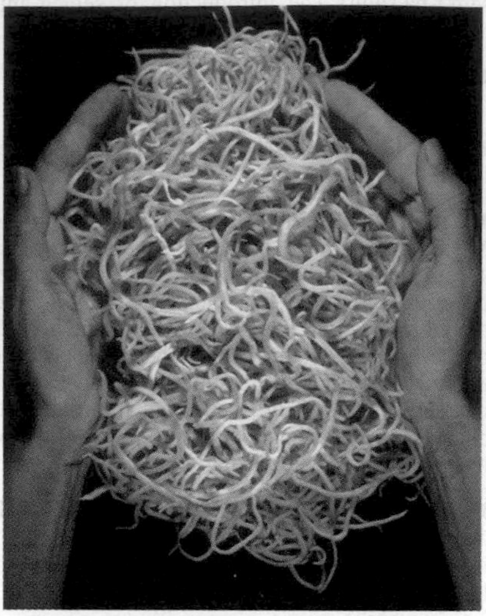

Ascaris: this mass of over 800 worms of *A. lumbricoides* obstructed and impacted the ileum of a 2-year-old girl in South Africa

as·cend·ing ar·ter·y (ă-send′ing ahr′tĕr-ē) The portion of the inferior branch of the ileocolic artery that passes superiorly along the ascending colon to communicate with a branch of the right colic artery to supply the ascending colon. SYN arteria ascendens [TA].

as·cend·ing branch of in·fe·ri·or mes·en·ter·ic ar·ter·y (ă-send′ing branch in-fēr′ē-ŏr mez-en-ter′ik ahr′tĕr-ē) Branch of the left colic artery (from inferior mesenteric artery) that passes anteriorly to the left kidney into the transverse mesocolon, where it anastomoses with the middle colic artery. It thus forms an anastomosis between superior and inferior mesenteric arteries, and is a component of the marginal artery (Drummond) of the colon.

as·cen·ding cer·vi·cal ar·ter·y (ă-send′ing sĕr′vi-kăl ahr′tĕr-ē) *Origin,* usually a terminal branch of the thyrocervical trunk (along with interior thyroid artery); *distribution,* muscles of neck and spinal cord; *anastomoses,* branches of vertebral, occipital, ascending pharyngeal, and deep cervical. SYN arteria cervicalis ascendens.

as·cend·ing co·lon (ă-send′ing kō′lŏn) The portion of the colon between the ileocecal orifice and the right colic flexure.

as·cend·ing de·gen·er·a·tion (ă-send′ing dĕ-jen′ĕr-ā′shŭn) **1.** Retrograde degeneration of an injured nerve fiber; i.e., toward the nerve cell of the fiber. **2.** Degeneration cephalad to a spinal cord lesion.

as·cend·ing lum·bar vein (ă-send′ing lŭm′bahr vān) A paired, vertical vein of the posterior abdominal wall, adjacent and parallel to the vertebral column, posterior to the origin of the psoas major muscle; it connects the common iliac, iliolumbar, and lumbar veins in the paravertebral line, the right vein joining the right subcostal vein to form the azygos vein, the left vein uniting with the left subcostal vein to form the hemiazygos vein.

as·cend·ing pal·a·tine ar·ter·y (ă-send′ing pal′ă-tīn ahr′tĕr-ē) *Origin*, facial; *distribution*, lateral walls of pharynx, tonsils, auditory tubes, and soft palate; *anastomoses*, tonsillar branch of facial, dorsal lingual, and descending palatine. SYN arteria palatina ascendens.

as·cend·ing part of a·or·ta (ă-send′ing pahrt ā-ōr′tă) SYN ascending aorta.

as·cend·ing pha·ryn·ge·al ar·ter·y (ă-send′ing făr-in′jē-ăl ahr′tĕr-ē) *Origin*, external carotid; *distribution*, wall of pharynx and soft palate, posterior cranial fossa. SYN arteria pharyngea ascendens [TA].

as·cer·tain·ment bi·as (as-ĕr-tān′mĕnt bī′ăs) Systematic failure to represent equally all classes of cases or people supposed to be represented in a sample.

Asch·er syn·drome (ahsh′ĕr sin′drōm) A condition in which a congenital double lip is associated with blepharochalasis and nontoxic thyroid gland enlargement.

Asch·off bod·ies (ahsh′of bod′ēz) A form of granulomatous inflammation observed in acute rheumatic carditis.

Asch·off node (ahsh′of nōd) Atrioventricular node located in the right atrium between the coronary sinus opening and the tricuspid valve; composed of Purkinje fibers that receive electrical impulses from the sinuatrial node before distributing them to the ventricles. SYN Aschoff-Tarawa node.

Asch·off-Ta·ra·wa node (ahsh′of tahr-ah′wă nōd) SYN Aschoff node.

as·ci·tes (ă-sī′tēz) Accumulation of serous fluid in the peritoneal cavity. May be a complication of cirrhosis, congestive heart failure, malignancy, peritonitis, or paralytic disease. SYN hydroperitoneum, hydroperitonia. [L. fr. G. *askos,* a bag, + *-ites*]

as·cit·ic (ă-sit′ik) Relating to ascites.

As·co·li re·ac·tion (as-kō′lē rē-ak′shŭn) SYN Ascoli test.

As·co·li test (as-kōl′ē test) Method to detect anthrax that uses a precipitin test with antiserum and tissue extract. SYN Ascoli reaction.

As·co·my·ce·tes (as′kō-mī-sē′tēz) A class of fungi characterized by the presence of asci and ascospores. Such fungi have generally two distinct reproductive phases, the sexual or perfect stage and the asexual or imperfect stage. *Ajellomyces capsulatum* and *A. dermatitidis* are pathogenic members of this class. [G. *askos,* a bag, + *mykēs,* mushroom]

as·cor·bate (ă-skōr′bāt) A salt or ester of ascorbic acid.

as·cor·bate ox·i·dase (ă-skōr′bāt ok′si-dās) A copper-containing enzyme that catalyzes the oxidation of L-ascorbic acid with O_2 to L-dehydroascorbic acid. Some forms of ascorbate oxidase use $NADP^+$ as well. Used as an antitumor enzyme.

as·cor·bic ac·id (ă-skōr′bik as′id) Agent used in preventing scurvy, as a strong reducing agent, and as an antioxidant. SYN vitamin C. [G. *a-* priv. + Mod.L. *scorbutus,* scurvy, fr. Germanic]

ASCUS (as′kŭs) Acronym for atypical squamous cells of undetermined significance.

ASD Abbreviation for atrial septal defect.

♻ **-ase** A suffix denoting an enzyme; attached to the end of the name of the substance (substrate) on which the enzyme acts; e.g., phosphatase, lipase, proteinase. May also indicate the reaction catalyzed, e.g., decarboxylase, oxidase. [Fr. *(diast)ase,* an amylase that converts starch to maltose, fr. G. *diastasis,* separation, fr. *dia-,* through, apart, + *stasis,* a standing]

A·sel·li gland (ă-sel′ē gland) A single large lymph node ventral to the abdominal aorta that receives all the lymph from the intestines in many smaller mammals.

as·e·ma·si·a, a·se·mi·a (as-ĕ-mā′zē-ă, ā-sē′mē-ă) SYN asymbolia. [G. *a-* priv. + *sēmasia,* the giving of a signal, fr. *sēma,* sign]

a·sep·sis (ā-sep′sis) A condition in which living pathogenic organisms are absent; a state of sterility (q.v.). [G. *a-* priv. + *sēpsis,* putrefaction]

a·sep·tic (ā-sep′tik) Marked by or relating to asepsis.

a·sep·tic gauze (ā-sep′tik gawz) Sterilized gauze.

a·sep·tic ne·cro·sis (ā-sep′tik nĕ-krō′sis) Death or decay of tissue due to local ischemia in the absence of infection. SYN avascular necrosis.

a·sep·tic sur·ger·y (ā-sep′tik sŭr′jĕr-ē) The performance of an operation with sterilized hands, instruments, and environment, taking precautions against the introduction of infectious microorganisms from without.

a·sep·tic tech·nique (ā-sep′tik tek-nēk′) Health care procedures designed to reduce the risk of transmission of pathogenic microorganisms to patients.

a·sex·u·al (ā-sek′shū-ăl) **1.** Referring to reproduction without nuclear fusion in an organism. **2.**

Having no sexual desire or interest. [G. *a-* priv. + sexual]

a•sex•u•al dwarf•ism (ā-sek′shū-ăl dwōrf′izm) Dwarfism in which adult sexual development is deficient.

a•sex•u•al gen•er•a•tion (ā-sek′shū-ăl jen-ĕr-ā′shŭn) Reproduction by fission, gemmation, or in any other way without union of the male and female cells, or conjugation. SEE ALSO parthenogenesis. SYN heterogenesis (2), nonsexual generation.

a•sex•u•al•i•ty (ā′sek′shū-al′i-tē) Lacking sex or sexually functioning organs; without sexual orientation.

a•sex•u•al re•pro•duc•tion (ā-sek′shū-ăl rē′prō-dŭk′shŭn) Reproduction other than by union of male and female sex cells.

ash (ash) Nostrums made from the leaves and bark of the tree (*Fraxinus excelsior*) are alleged to have value in therapy of GI disease; clinical tests are ongoing.

ASHA Abbreviation for American Speech Language and Hearing Association.

Ash•er•man syn•drome (ash′ĕr-măn sin′drōm) SYN traumatic amenorrhea.

Ash•hurst clas•si•fi•ca•tion (ash-hŭrst′ klas′i-fi-kā′shŭn) Method used to delineate and describe fractures and sprains about the ankle.

ash-leaf mac•ule (ash′lēf mak′yūl) A hypopigmented, often ash-leaf–shaped macule that is present at birth in many patients with tuberous sclerosis.

Ash•man phe•nom•e•non (ash′măn fĕ-nom′ĕ-non) Aberrant ventricular conduction of a beat ending a short cycle that is preceded by a longer cycle most commonly during atrial fibrillation.

ash•wa•gan•dha (ahsh-wă-gahn′dă) An Indian herb (*Withania somnifera*), available in many forms; purported use in inflammation, tumors; has been suggested for use as an antidepressant. Clinical studies ongoing into its efficacy. SYN Indian ginseng. [Sansk., horse smell]

Ash•worth scale (ash′wŏrth skāl) An ordinal scale used to apply a grade to increased muscle tone. A grade of 0 corresponds to no increase in muscle tone; a 4 corresponds to the presence of rigidity in the tested body part.

ASI Abbreviation for addiction severity index.

a•si•a•lism (ā-sī′ă-lizm) Absence of saliva. [G. *a-* priv. + *sialon* saliva + -ism]

A•sian flu (ā′zhăn flū) Influenza caused by H_2N_2 influenza A that was responsible for over 60,000 deaths in the United States during the 1957 to 1958 influenza pandemic.

ASIS Abbreviation for anterior superior iliac spine.

ASL Abbreviation for American Sign Language.

a•so•cial (ā-sō′shăl) Not social; withdrawn from society; indifferent to social rules or customs; e.g., a recluse, a regressed schizophrenic person, a schizoid personality. Cf. antisocial.

Asp Abbreviation for aspartic acid or its radical forms.

As•par•a•gus (ă-spar′ă-gŭs) A genus of plants of the family Liliaceae. *A. officinalis* is an edible vegetable, the rhizome and roots of which, together with the young edible shoots, were used as a diuretic. SYN sparrowgrass. [L. fr. G. *asparagus*]

as•par•tate (as-pahr′tāt) A salt or ester of aspartic acid.

as•par•tate a•mi•no•trans•fer•ase (AST) (as-pahr′tāt ă-mē′nō-trans′fĕr-ās) An enzyme catalyzing the reversible transfer of an amine group from L-glutamic acid to oxaloacetic acid, forming α-ketoglutaric acid and L-aspartic acid; a diagnostic aid in viral hepatitis and in myocardial infarction. SYN glutamic-oxaloacetic transaminase, serum glutamic-oxaloacetic transaminase.

as•par•tic ac•id (Asp) (as-pahr′tik as′id) The L-isomer is one of the amino acids occurring in proteins. SYN alpha (α)-aminosuccinic acid.

as•pect (as′pekt) **1.** The manner of appearance; looks. **2.** The side of an object that is exposed to a view from a designated direction. [L. *aspectus,* fr. *a-spicio,* pp. *-spectus,* to look at]

As•per•ger dis•or•der (ahs′per-ger dis-ōr′dĕr) A pervasive developmental disorder characterized by severe and enduring impairment in social skills and restrictive and repetitive behaviors and interests, leading to impaired social and occupational functioning but without significant delays in language development.

as•per•gil•lo•ma (as′pĕr-ji-lō′mă) **1.** An infectious granuloma caused by *Aspergillus.* **2.** A variety of bronchopulmonary aspergillosis; a ball-like mass of *Aspergillus fumigatus* colonizing an existing cavity in the lung. [aspergillus + *-oma,* tumor]

as•per•gil•lo•sis (as′pĕr-ji-lō′sis) The presence of *Aspergillus* in the tissues or on a mucous surface of humans and animals, and the symptoms produced thereby.

As•per•gil•lus (as-pĕr-jil′ŭs) A genus of fungi that contains many species, a number of them with black, brown, or green spores. A few species are pathogenic for man. [Med. L. a sprinkler, fr. L. *aspergo,* to sprinkle]

As•per•gil•lus fla•vus (as-pĕr-jil′ŭs flā′vŭs) A hyaline septate fungal species found widespread in soil and decaying matter. Associated with respiratory infections and hypersensitivity pneumonitis. Produces aflatoxins responsible for mycotoxicoses; may produce invasive disease in the granulocytopenic patient.

As·per·gil·lus fu·mi·ga·tus (as′pĕr-jil′ŭs fy-ūm′i-gā′tŭs) Widely spread in the environment, a fungal species found in the soil or decaying vegetation; most common cause of aspergillosis in humans, particularly in the immunocompromised patient. Associated with pulmonary, bone, ocular, nasal, and deep organ disease; extremely angioinvasive. See page B5.

a·sper·mi·a (ā-spĕr′mē-ă) Inability to produce or ejaculate semen.

as·phyx·i·a (as-fik′sē-ă) Impairment of ventilatory exchange of oxygen and carbon dioxide; combined hypercapnia, hypoxia, or anoxia; causes death if not corrected. [G. *a-* priv. + *sphyzō,* to throb]

as·phyx·i·al (as-fik′sē-ăl) Relating to asphyxia.

as·phyx·i·a li·vi·da (as-fik′sē-ă liv′i-dă) A form of asphyxia neonatorum in which the skin is cyanotic, but the heart remains strong and the reflexes preserved.

as·phyx·i·a ne·o·na·to·rum (as-fik′sē-ă nē-ō-nā-to′rum) Asphyxia occurring in the newborn.

as·phyx·i·ate (as-fik′sē-āt) To induce asphyxia.

as·phyx·i·at·ing tho·rac·ic dy·stro·phy (as-fik′sē-āt-ing thōr-as′ik dis′trŏ-fē) Hereditary hypoplasia of the thorax, associated with pelvic skeletal abnormality. SYN Jeune syndrome.

as·phyx·i·a·tion (as-fik′sē-ā′shŭn) The production of, or the state of, asphyxia.

as·pi·rate (as′pir′āt) **1.** (as′pi-rāt) To remove by aspiration. **2.** (as′pi-rit) The substance removed by aspiration. [L. *a-spiro,* pp. *-atus,* to breathe on, give the H sound]

as·pi·ra·tion (as-pir-ā′shŭn) **1.** Removal, by suction, of a gas or fluid from a body cavity, from unusual accumulations, or from a container. **2.** Inhalation into the airways of fluid or foreign body (e.g., vomitus, food, fluid). **3.** A surgical technique for treatment of cataract, requiring a small corneal incision, severance of the lens capsule, fragmentation of the lens material, and removal with a needle. [L. *aspiratio*, fr. *aspiro*, to breathe on]

as·pi·ra·tion bi·op·sy (as-pir-ā′shŭn bī′op-sē) SYN needle biopsy.

as·pi·ra·tion pneu·mo·ni·a (as-pir-ā′shŭn nū-mō′nē-ă) Bronchopneumonia resulting from the inhalation of foreign material, usually food particles or vomit, into the bronchi; pneumonia developing secondary to the presence in the airways of fluid, blood, saliva, or gastric contents.

as·pi·ra·tor (as′pir-ā-tŏr) An apparatus for removing fluid by aspiration from any of the body cavities; it consists usually of a hollow needle or trocar and cannula, connected by tubing with a container vacuumized by a syringe or reversed air (suction) pump.

a·sple·ni·a (ā-splē′nē-ă) Congenital or surgical absence of the spleen (e.g., after surgical removal).

a·splen·ic (ā-splen′ik) Having no spleen.

as·sas·sin bug (ă-sas′in bŭg) An insect of the family Reduviidae that inflicts irritating, painful bites in animals and humans; related to the cone-nosed bugs (triatomines), a vector of American trypanosomiasis. [Fr., fr. It. *assassino,* fr. Ar. *hashshāshin,* those addicted to hashish]

as·say (as′ā) **1.** Test of purity; trial. **2.** To examine; to subject to analysis. **3.** The quantitative or qualitative evaluation of a substance for impurities, toxicity, or other attributes; the results of such an evaluation. [M.E., fr. O.Fr. *essaier,* fr. L.L. *exagium,* a weighing]

as·sess·ment (ă-ses′mĕnt) **1.** SYN evaluation. **2.** An ongoing study that captures changes over time and is useful in program planning. [assess, fr. O.Fr. *assesser*, fr. L. *adsideo, adsessum*, to sit by (as an assistant judge), + -ment]

As·séz·at tri·an·gle (ah-sā-zah′ trī′ang-gĕl) An area formed by lines connecting the nasion with the alveolar and nasal point; used to indicate prognathism in comparative craniology.

as·sign·ment (ă-sīn′mĕnt) A doctor "accepts assignment" when the insurance fee is considered as payment in full. SEE ALSO par. [assign, fr. O.Fr. *assigner*, fr. L. *adsigno*, to mark, label, + -ment]

as·sign·ment of ben·e·fits (ă-sīn′mĕnt ben′ĕ-fits) Authorization from an insured to allow any payment to go directly to the physician.

as·sim·i·la·tion (ă-sim′i-lā′shŭn) **1.** Incorporation of digested materials from food into the tissues. **2.** Integration of newly perceived information and experiences into the existing cognitive structure. [L. *as-similo,* pp. *-atus,* to make alike]

as·sim·i·la·tion pel·vis (ă-sim′i-lā′shŭn pel′vis) A deformity in which the transverse processes of the last lumbar vertebra are fused with the sacrum, or the last sacral with the first coccygeal body.

as·sis·tant (ă-sis′tănt) Provider of subordinate support services to patients under the guidance of a health care professional.

as·sist-con·trol ven·ti·la·tion (ă-sist′ kŏn-trōl′ ven′ti-lā′shŭn) **1.** Continuous mandatory ventilation. **2.** A mode of mechanical ventilation in which all breaths are mandatory and are either patient or machine triggered, and machine cycled; a minimum breathing rate is set but the patient can trigger breaths at a higher frequency.

as·sis·ted liv·ing (ă-sis′tĕd liv′ing) Type of living arrangement or accommodation in which personal care services (e.g., meals, housekeeping, and assistance with activities of daily living) are available to residents as needed; residents live on their own in the facility.

as·sis·ted liv·ing fa·cil·i·ty (ă-sis′tĕd liv′ing fă-sil′i-tē) SYN nursing facility.

as·sist·ed re·pro·duc·tion (ă-sis′tĕd rē′prō-dŭk′shŭn) SEE surrogate mother, in vitro fertilization.

as·sist·ed res·pi·ra·tion (ă-sis′tĕd res′pir-ā′shŭn) SYN assisted ventilation.

as·sist·ed ven·ti·la·tion (ă-sis′tĕd ven′ti-lā′shŭn) Application of mechanically or manually generated positive pressure to gas(es) in or about the airway during inhalation as a means of augmenting movement of gases into the lungs. SYN assisted respiration.

as·sis·tive lis·ten·ing de·vice (ALD) (ă-sis′tiv lis′ĕn-ing dĕ-vīs′) Any device that improves sound perception for listeners with hearing impairments; usually applied to devices such as closed-loop FM systems used in addition to or instead of hearing aids.

as·sis·tive tech·nol·o·gy (ă-sis′tiv tek-nol′ŏ-jē) Any piece of equipment or device used to maintain or promote function in someone with a disability. Can range from low (e.g., cane) to high (e.g., computerized communication device).

As·so·ci·ate De·gree in Nurs·ing (ADN) (ă-sō′sē-ăt dĕ-grē′ nŭrs′ing) A professional nursing degree conferred after a period of training (e.g., 2–3 years) shorter than that needed for the bachelor's degree.

as·so·ci·a·ted move·ment (ă-sō′sē-āt-ĕd mūv′mĕnt) A motion seen in the contralateral limb when increased concentration, muscle tone, or effort is exerted, as in increased elbow flexion seen in one arm while the other arm engages in a movement.

as·so·ci·a·ted re·ac·tion (ăs-ō′sē-ā-tĕd rē-ak′shŭn) An involuntary movement of a body part associated with the resisted movement of another body part. Associated reactions are typically seen in children until the age of 8 years of age, but are also seen in people who have sustained a CNS injury.

as·so·ci·a·tion (ă-sō′sē-ā′shŭn) **1.** A connection of people, things, or ideas by some common factor. **2.** A movement seen in the opposite limb when increased concentration, tone, or effort is exerted (e.g., increased elbow flexion in one arm while the other moves). **3.** A functional connection of two ideas, events, or psychological phenomena established through learning or experience. SEE ALSO conditioning. **4.** Statistical dependence between two or more events, characteristics, or other variables. **5.** GENETICS a grouping of congenital anomalies found together more frequently than otherwise expected; the use of this term implies that the cause is unknown. [L. *as-socio,* pp. *-sociatus,* to join to; *ad* + *socius,* companion]

As·so·ci·a·tion of A·mer·i·can Med·i·cal Col·leges (AAMC) (ă-sō′sē-ā′shŭn ă-mer′i-kăn med′i-kăl kol′ĕj-ĕz) A nonprofit organization of U.S. medical schools, teaching hospitals, and academic societies.

as·so·ci·a·tion cor·tex, as·so·ci·a·tion ar·e·as (ă-sō′sē-ā′shŭn kōr′teks, ă-sō′sē-ā′shŭn ār′ē-ăz) Generic term denoting the large expanses of the cerebral cortex that are not sensory or motor in the customary sense, but are involved in advanced stages of sensory information processing, multisensory integration, or sensorimotor integration. SEE ALSO cerebral cortex.

as·so·ci·a·tion fi·bers (ă-sō′sē-ā′shŭn fī′bĕrz) Nerve fibers interconnecting subdivisions of the cerebral cortex of the same hemisphere or different segments of the spinal cord on the same side.

As·so·ci·a·tion for Health·care Doc·u·men ta·tion In·teg·ri·ty (AHDI) (ă-sō′sē-ā′shŭn helth′kār dok′yū-mĕn-ta′shŭn in-teg′ri-tē) Association for professional medical transcriptionists, formerly American Association for Medical Transcription (AAMT).

as·so·ci·a·tion test (ă-sō′sē-ā′shŭn test) A word (i.e., stimulus word) is spoken to the subject, who is to reply immediately with another word (reaction word) suggested by the first; used as a diagnostic aid in psychiatry and psychology.

as·so·ci·a·tive a·pha·si·a (ă-sō′sē-ă-tiv ă-fā′zē-ă) SYN conduction aphasia.

as·so·ci·a·tive play (ă-sō′sē-ă-tiv plā) Play in which each child participates in a separate activity, but with the cooperation and assistance of the others.

as·sort·a·tive mat·ing (ă-sōrt′ă-tiv māt′ing) Selection of a mate with preference for (or aversion to) a particular genotype, i.e., nonrandom mating.

as·sort·ment (ă-sōrt′mĕnt) In genetics, the relationship between nonallelic genetic traits that are transmitted from parent to child more or less independently in accordance with the degree of linkage between the respective loci.

as·sump·tion (ă-sŭmp′shŭn) A basic principle that is accepted as being true on the basis of logic or reason but without proof or verification. [L. *adsumptio,* fr. *assumo,* to adopt]

AST Abbreviation for aspartate aminotransferase.

a·sta·si·a (ă-stā′zē-ă) Inability, through muscular incoordination, to stand. [G. unsteadiness, from *a-* priv. + *stasis,* standing]

a·sta·si·a-a·ba·si·a (ă-stā′zē-ă-ă-bā′zē-ă) Inability to stand or walk in a normal manner; the gait is bizarre and often the patient sways and nearly falls, but recovers at the last moment; a symptom of hysteria-conversion reaction. SYN Blocq disease.

a·stat·ic (ā-stat′ik) Pertaining to astasia.

a·stat·ic sei·zure (ā-stat′ik sē′zhŭr) Seizure causing loss of erect posture.

as·ta·tine (At) (as′tă-tēn) An artificial radioactive element of the halogen series; atomic no. 85, atomic wt. 211. [G. *astatos,* unstable]

a·ste·a·to·sis (as′tē-ă-tō′sis) Diminished or arrested secretion of the sebaceous glands. [G. *a-* priv. + *stear* (*steat-*), fat]

as·ter (as′tĕr) SYN astrosphere. [Mod. L. fr. G. *astēr,* a star]

a·ste·re·og·no·sis (ă-stĕr′ē-og-nō′sis) SYN tactile agnosia. [G. *a-* priv. + *stereos,* solid + *gnōsis,* knowledge]

as·te·ri·on (as-tē′rē-on) A craniometric point at the junction of the lambdoid, occipitomastoid, and parietomastoid sutures. [G. *asterios,* starry]

as·ter·ix·is (as-tĕr-ik′sis) Involuntary jerking movements, especially in the hands, due to arrhythmic lapses of sustained posture; seen primarily with metabolic and toxic encephalopathies, especially hepatic encephalopathy. SYN flapping tremor. [G. *a-* priv. + *stērixis,* fixed position]

a·ster·nal (ā-stĕr′năl) **1.** Not related to or connected with the sternum, e.g., asternal rib. **2.** Without a sternum. [G. *a-* priv. + *sternon,* chest]

a·ster·ni·a (ā-stĕr′nē-ă) Congenital absence of the sternum.

as·ter·oid bod·y (as′tĕr-oyd bod′ē) **1.** An eosinophilic inclusion resembling a star with delicate radiating lines, occurring in a vacuolated area of cytoplasm of a multinucleated giant cell. **2.** A structure that is characteristic of sporotrichosis when found in the skin or secondary lesions of this mycosis; in tissue, it surrounds the 3- to 5-mcm (diameter) ovoid yeast of *Sporothrix schenkii.*

as·ter·oid hy·a·lo·sis (as′tĕr-oyd hī′ă-lō′sis) Numerous small refractive spheric bodies in the vitreous (composed of calcium soaps), visible ophthalmoscopically; an age change, usually unilateral, and not affecting vision.

as·the·ni·a (as-thē′nē-ă) Weakness or debility. [G. *astheneia,* weakness, fr. *a-* priv. + *sthenos,* strength]

as·then·ic (as-then′ik) **1.** Relating to asthenia. **2.** Denoting a thin, delicate body habitus.

as·the·no·pi·a (as′thĕ-nō′pē-ă) Subjective symptoms of ocular fatigue, discomfort, lacrimation, and headaches arising from use of the eyes. SYN eyestrain. [G. *astheneia,* weakness, + *ōps,* eye]

as·the·nop·ic (as′thĕ-nop′ik) Relating to or suffering from asthenopia.

as·the·no·sper·mi·a (as′thĕ-nō-spĕr′mē-ă) SYN asthenozoospermia. [G. *astheneia,* weakness, + *sperma,* seed, semen]

as·the·no·zo·o·sper·mi·a (as′thĕ-nō-zō-ō-spĕrm′ē-ă) Loss or reduction of mobility of sperms, frequently associated with infertility. SYN asthenospermia. [G. *astheneia,* weakness + *zōos,* living, + *sperma,* seed, semen, + -ia]

asth·ma (az′mă) An inflammatory disease of the lungs characterized by reversible (in most cases) inflammation and narrowing of the airway. Originally, a term used to mean "difficult breathing"; now used to denote bronchial asthma. See this page. SYN reactive airways disease. [G.]

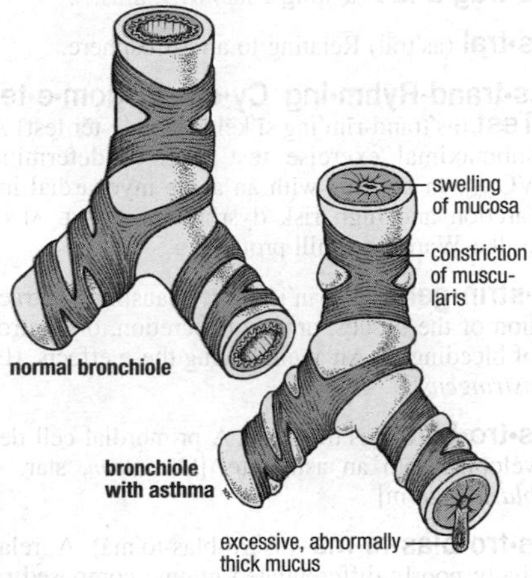

asthma: changes in bronchiole during asthma attack

asth·mat·ic (az-mat′ik) Relating to or suffering from asthma.

as·tig·mat·ic (as′tig-mat′ik) Relating to or suffering from astigmatism.

as·tig·mat·ic lens (as′tig-mat′ik lenz) SYN cylindric lens.

a·stig·ma·tism (ă-stig′mă-tizm) **1.** A lens or optic system having different refractivity in different meridians. **2.** A condition of unequal curvatures along the different meridians in one or more of the refractive surfaces (cornea, anterior or posterior surface of the lens) of the eye, in consequence of which the rays from a luminous point are not focused at a single point on the retina. SYN astigmia. [G. *a-* priv. + *stigma* (*stigmat-*), a point]

a·stig·ma·tom·e·try, **as·tig·mom·e·try** (ă-stig′mă-tom′ĕ-trē, as′tig-mom′ĕ-trē) Determination of the form and measurement of the degree of astigmatism.

a·stig·mi·a (ă-stig′mē-ă) SYN astigmatism.

a·sto·mi·a (ă-stō′mē-ă) Congenital absence of the mouth. [G. *a-* priv. + *stoma,* mouth]

as·trag·a·lar (as-trag′ă-lăr) Relating to the astragalus or talus.

as·trag·a·lec·to·my (as-trag′ă-lek′tŏ-mē) Removal of the astragalus or talus. [astragalus, + G. *ektomē,* excision]

As·trag·a·lus (ă-strag′ă-lŭs) A genus of plants (e.g., locoweed) on the range lands of western North America, capable of taking selenium from the soil and poisoning sheep, cattle, and horses. *A. gummifer* is a source of tragacanth. SYN goat thorn, huang chi, milk vetch root, yellow leader. [L., fr. G. *astragalos,* ankle bone]

as·trag·a·lus (ă-strag′ă-lŭs) SYN talus.

as·tral (as′trăl) Relating to an astrosphere.

As·trand-Ryhm·ing Cy·cle Er·gom·e·ter Test (as′trand-rīm′ing sī′kĕl ĕr-gom′ĕ-tĕr test) A submaximal exercise test used to determine VO_{2max} in patients with an acute myocardial infarction and high risk dysrhythmias. SEE ALSO Balke-Ware treadmill protocol.

a·strin·gent (ă-strin′jĕnt) **1.** Causing contraction of the tissues, arrest of secretion, or control of bleeding. **2.** An agent having these effects. [L. *astringens*]

as·tro·blast (as′trō-blast) A primordial cell developing into an astrocyte. [G. *astron,* star, + *blastos,* germ]

as·tro·blas·to·ma (as′trō-blas-tō′mă) A relatively poorly differentiated glioma composed of young, immature, neoplastic cells of the astrocytic series, frequently arranged radially with short fibrils terminating on small blood vessels. [astro- + G. *blastos,* germ, + *-oma,* tumor]

as·tro·cyte (as′trō-sīt) One of the large neuroglia cells of nervous tissue. SEE ALSO neuroglia. SYN astroglia, macroglia. [G. *astron,* star, + *kytos,* hollow (cell)]

as·tro·cy·to·ma (as′trō-sī-tō′mă) A glioma derived from astrocytes; in people younger than 20 years of age, astrocytomas usually arise in a cerebellar hemisphere; in adults, astrocytoma usually occur in the cerebrum, sometimes growing rapidly and invading extensively. See page B31. [G. *astron,* star, + *kytos,* cell, + *-oma,* tumor]

as·trog·li·a (as-trog′lē-ă) SYN astrocyte. [G. *astron,* star, + neuroglia]

as·tro·sphere (as′trō-sfēr) A set of radiating microtubules extending outward from the cytocentrum and centrosphere of a dividing cell. SYN aster, attraction sphere. [G. *astron,* star, + *sphaira,* ball]

as·tro·vi·rus (as′trō-vī′rŭs) A small RNA virus and the only genus in the family Astroviridae; it is associated with diarrhea and is detected in the feces of numerous animals.

a·sy·lum (ă-sī′lŭm) Facility dedicated for the relief of care of the destitute or sick, especially those with mental illness. [G. *asylon,* refuge]

a·sym·bo·li·a (ā-sim-bō′lē-ă) A form of aphasia in which the significance of signs and symbols is not appreciated. SYN asemasia, asemia. [G. *a-* priv. + *symbolon,* an outward sign]

a·sym·met·ric (a) (ā-si-met′rik) Not symmetric; denoting a lack of symmetry between two or more like parts.

a·sym·met·ric col·li·ma·tion (ā′si-met′rik kol′i-mā′shŭn) The process of restricting an x-ray beam to a given area by the use of collimators that are capable of independent movement.

a·sym·met·ric fe·tal growth re·stric·tion (ā-si-met′rik fē′tăl grōth rĕ-strik′shŭn) Normal fetal head size as a result of preferential shunting of blood to brain, and decreased abdominal circumference from decreased adipose tissue and liver size; probably caused by placental insufficiency.

a·sym·me·try (ā-sim′ĕ-trē) **1.** Lack of symmetry; disproportion between two normally similar parts. **2.** Significant difference in amplitude or frequency of EEG activity recorded simultaneously from the two sides of the brain.

a·symp·tom·at·ic (ā′simp-tŏ-mat′ik) Without symptoms, or producing no symptoms.

a·symp·tot·ic (ā′simp-tot′ik) Pertaining to a limiting value (e.g., a dependent variable) when the independent variable approaches zero or infinity.

a·syn·cli·tism (ă-sin′kli-tizm) Absence of synclitism or parallelism; may be used, e.g., to refer to the axis of the presenting part of the child and the pelvic planes in childbirth, to the dental arches, or to the planes of the skull. SYN obliquity. [G. *a-* priv. + *syn-klinō,* to incline together]

a·syn·cli·tism of the skull (ă-sin′kli-tizm skŭl) SYN plagiocephaly.

a·syn·de·sis (ă-sin′dĕ-sis) **1.** Rarely used term for a mental defect in which separate ideas or thoughts cannot be joined into a coherent concept. **2.** A breaking up of the connecting links in language, said to be characteristic of the language disturbance of schizophrenics. [G. *a-* priv. + *syn,* together, + *desis,* binding]

a·syn·ech·i·a (ă-si-nek′ē-ă) Discontinuity of structure. [G. *a-* priv. + *synecheia,* continuity]

a·syn·er·gic (ā′sin-ĕr′jik) Characterized by asynergia.

a·syn·er·gy (ā-sin′ĕr-jē) Lack of coordination among various muscle groups during the performance of complex movements, resulting in loss of skill and speed. When severe, results in decomposition of movement, wherein complex motor acts are performed in a series of isolated movements; caused by cerebellar disorders.

a·sys·tem·at·ic (ā′sis-tĕ-mat′ik) Not systematic; not relating to one system or set of organs.

a·sys·to·le (ā-sis′tŏ-lē) Absence of contractions

of the heart. SYN cardiac standstill. [G. *a-* priv, + *systolē,* a contracting]

a•sys•tol•ic (ā′sis-tol′ik) **1.** Relating to asystole. **2.** Not systolic.

AT Abbreviation for an adenine-thymine hydrogen-bonded base pair observed in double-stranded polynucleotides; adipose tissue.

At Abbreviation for astatine.

a•tac•tic a•ba•si•a, a•tax•ic a•ba•si•a (ă-tak′tik ă-bā′zē-ă, ă-tak′sik ă-bā′zē-ă) Difficulty in walking due to ataxia of the legs.

at•a•rac•tic (at′ăr-ak′tik) Tending to tranquilize. [G. *a,* without, + *taraxis,* excitement, confusion]

at•a•vism (at′ă-vizm) The appearance in an individual of characteristics presumed to have been present in some remote ancestor; reversion to an earlier biologic type; a throwback. [L. *atavus,* a remote ancestor]

at•a•vis•tic (at-ă-vis′tik) Relating to atavism.

a•tax•i•a (ă-tak′sē-ă) An inability to coordinate muscle activity, causing jerkiness, incoordination, and inefficiency of voluntary movement. Most often due to disorders of the cerebellum or the posterior columns of the spinal cord; may involve limbs, head, or trunk. SYN incoordination. [G. *a-* priv. + *taxis,* order]

a•tax•i•a•pha•si•a (ă-tak′sē-ă-fā′zē-ă) Inability to form connected sentences, although single words may be used intelligibly. [G. *a-* priv. + *taxis,* order, + *phasis,* an affirmation, speech]

a•tax•i•a tel•an•gi•ec•ta•si•a, a•tax•i•a-tel•an•gi•ec•ta•si•a (ă-tak′sē-ă tel-an′jē-ek-tā′zē-ă, ă-taks′ē-ă-tel-an-jē′ek-tā′zē-ă) A slowly progressive multisystem disorder with ataxia appearing with the onset of walking; telangiectases of the conjunctiva and skin; athetosis and nystagmus; and recurrent infections of the respiratory system caused by immunoglobulin deficiencies. Approximately 70% of affected patients have an IgA deficiency concomitant with decreased T helper cell function.

a•tax•ic (ă-tak′sik) Relating to, marked by, or suffering from ataxia.

a•tax•ic dys•ar•thri•a (ă-tak′sik dis-ahr′thrē-ă) Dysarthria associated with damage to the cerebellar system, characterized by imprecise consonants, excess and equal stress, inconsistent articulatory errors, and monotony of pitch and volume. SEE ataxia.

a•tax•ic gait (ă-tak′sik gāt) SYN cerebellar gait.

a•tax•i•o•phe•mi•a (ă-tak′sē-ō-fē′mē-ă) Incoordination of the muscles concerned in speech production. [G. *a-* priv. + *taxis,* order, + *phēmē,* voice, speech]

ATC Abbreviation for "around the clock."

A/T clon•ing (klōn′ing) Cloning of fragments where the only overhanging (or uncomplemented) ends are the A or T bases; occurs often in use of specific enzymes to cut or make DNA fragments.

-ate Suffix used as a replacement for "-ic acid" when the acid is neutralized (e.g., sodium acetate) or esterified (e.g., ethyl acetate).

at•el•ec•ta•sis (at-ĕ-lek′tă-sis) Reduction or absence of air in part or all of a lung, with resulting loss of lung volume. SEE ALSO pulmonary collapse. [G. *atelēs,* incomplete, + *ektasis,* extension]

at•e•lec•ta•sis of mid•dle ear (at-ĕ-lek′tă-sis mid′ĕl ēr) Reduction in the volume of the middle ear because of obstruction of the pharyngotympanic (auditory) tube followed by absorption of the oxygen in the middle ear and subsequent retraction of the tympanic membrane medially.

at•e•lec•tat•ic (at-ĕ-lek-tat′ik) Relating to atelectasis.

a•te•li•a (ă-tē′lē-ă) SYN ateliosis.

a•te•li•o•sis (ă-tē′lē-ō′sis) Incomplete development of the body or any of its parts, as in infantilism and dwarfism. SYN atelia. [G. *atelēs,* incomplete, + *-osis,* condition]

a•te•li•ot•ic (ă-tē′lē-ot′ik) Marked by ateliosis.

a•the•li•a (ă-thē′lē-ă) Congenital absence of the nipples. [G. *a-* priv. + *thēlē,* nipple]

ath•er•ec•to•my (ath-ĕr-ek′tŏ-mē) Invasive removal of an atheroma or plaque from an artery. See page 142.

athero- Combining form meaning gruellike, soft, pasty materials; atheroma, atheromatous. [G. *athērē,* gruel, porridge]

ath•er•o•em•bo•lism (ath′ĕr-ō-em′bŏ-lizm) Cholesterol embolism, with or without calcific matter, originating from an atheroma of the aorta or other diseased artery.

ath•er•o•gen•e•sis (ath′ĕr-ō-jen′ĕ-sis) Formation of atheroma, important in the pathogenesis of arteriosclerosis.

ath•er•o•gen•ic (ath′ĕr-ō-jen′ik) Having the capacity to initiate, increase, or accelerate the process of atherogenesis.

ath•er•o•ma (ath′ĕr-ō′mă) The lipid deposits in the intima of arteries, producing a yellow swelling on the endothelial surface; a characteristic of atherosclerosis. [G. *athērē,* gruel, + *-ōma,* tumor]

ath•er•o•ma•to•sis (ath′ĕr-ō-mă-tō′sis) Disease characterized by atheromatous degeneration of the arteries.

ath•er•om•a•tous (ath′ĕr-ō′mă-tŭs) Relating to or affected by atheroma.

ath•er•om•a•tous de•gen•er•a•tion (ath′ĕr-ō′mă-tŭs dĕ-jen′ĕr-ā′shŭn) Focal accumulation of lipid material (atheroma) in the intima and subintimal portion of arteries, eventually resulting in fibrous thickening or calcification.

ath•er•o•matous em•bo•lism (ath′ĕr-ō′mă-tŭs em′bŏ-lizm) SYN cholesterol embolism.

ath•er•o•scle•ro•sis (ath′ĕr-ō-skler-ō′sis) Arteriosclerosis characterized by irregularly distributed lipid deposits in the intima of large and medium arteries; such deposits provoke fibrosis and calcification. Atherosclerosis is set in motion when cells lining the arteries are damaged as a result of high blood pressure, smoking, toxic substances in the environment, and other agents. Plaques develop when low density lipoproteins accumulate at the site of arterial damage and platelets act to form a fibrous cap over this fatty core. Deposits impede or eventually shut off blood flow. See page 143.

ath•er•o•scle•rot•ic (ath′ĕr-ō-skler-ot′ik) Relating to or characterized by atherosclerosis.

ath•e•toid (ath′ĕ-toyd) Resembling athetosis.

ath•e•to•sic, ath•e•tot•ic (ath′ĕ-tō′sik, ath′ĕ-tot′ik) Pertaining to, or marked by, athetosis.

ath•e•to•sis (ath′ĕ-tō′sis) Slow, writhing, snakelike involuntary movements involving flexion, extension, pronation, and supination of the fingers and hands, and sometimes of the toes and feet as well. Usually caused by an extrapyramidal lesion. SYN Hammond disease. [G. *athetos,* without position or place]

ath•lete's foot (ath′lēts fut) SYN tinea pedis.

ath•lete's heart (ath′lēts hahrt) Nonpathologic enlarged heart in athletes reflecting specific adaptation to prolonged training. Manifestations in response to resistance training are thickened left ventricular wall and concentric hypertrophy, and in response to endurance training are enlarged left ventricular cavity and eccentric hypertrophy. SEE hypertrophy.

ath•let•ic a•men•or•rhe•a (ath-let′ik ā-men′ŏr-ē′ă) Irregularities in the menstrual cycle presenting as either oligomenorrhea (35–90 days between menses) or secondary amenorrhea (cessation of menstrual cycles for at least 3 months) caused by intense athletic training or disordered eating behavior.

ath•le•tic train•er (ath-let′ik trān′ĕr) One who is skilled in the prevention, evaluation, treatment, and rehabilitation of athletic injuries.

ath•le•tic train•ing (ath-let′ik trān′ing) Provision of comprehensive health care services to athletes, including prevent preparation, evaluation of illnesses and injuries, first aid and emergency care, rehabilitation, and other related services.

a•thy•mi•a (ā-thī′mē-ă) **1.** PSYCHOLOGY absence of affect or emotion; morbid impassivity. **2.** Congenital absence of the thymus, often with associated immunodeficiency. SYN athymism. [G. *a-* priv. + *thymos,* mind, also thymus]

a•thy•mism (ā-thī′mizm) SYN athymia (2).

a•thy•roid•ism (ā-thī′royd-izm) Congenital absence of the thyroid gland or suppression or absence of its hormonal secretion. SEE hypothyroidism.

a•thy•rot•ic (ā′thī-rot′ik) Relating to athyroidism.

At•kins di•et (at′kinz dī′ĕt) Controversial weight loss program developed in the early 1970s by Dr. Robert Atkins, in which carbohydrate consumption is severely restricted to attain significant weight loss.

ATL Abbreviation for adult T-cell leukemia; adult T-cell lymphoma.

at•lan•tad (at-lan′tad) In a direction toward the atlas.

at•lan•tal (at-lan′tăl) Relating to the atlas.

atlanto-, atlo- Combining forms denoting the atlas (the bone that supports the head). [G. *Atlas, Atlantos,* Atlas, the Titan who supported the heavens on his shoulders in Greek myth]

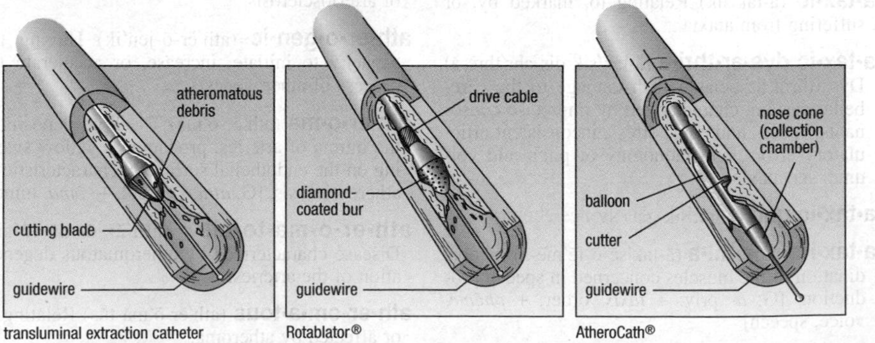

atherectomy devices

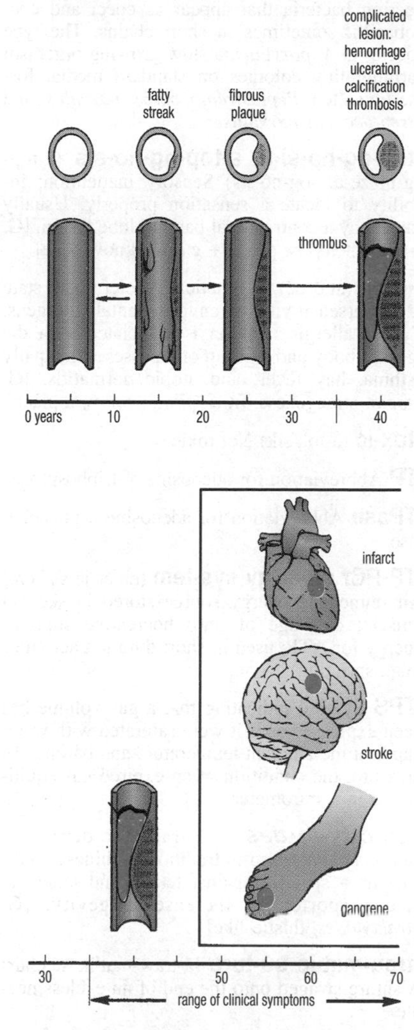

progression of atherosclerosis: fatty streaks constitute one of the earliest lesions of atherosclerosis; many regress, whereas others progress to fibrous plaques and eventually to atheroma, which may be complicated by hemorrhage, ulceration, calcification, or thrombosis. It also may produce myocardial infarction, stroke, or gangrene

at·lan·to·ax·i·al (at-lan′tō-ak′sē-ăl) Pertaining to the atlas and the axis; denoting the joint between the first two cervical vertebrae. SYN atloaxoid.

at·las (at′lăs) First cervical vertebra, articulating with the occipital bone and rotating around the dens of the axis. See this page. SYN vertebra C1. [G. *Atlas,* the Titan who supported the heavens on his shoulders in Greek myth]

at·lo·ax·oid (at′lō-ak′soyd) SYN atlantoaxial.

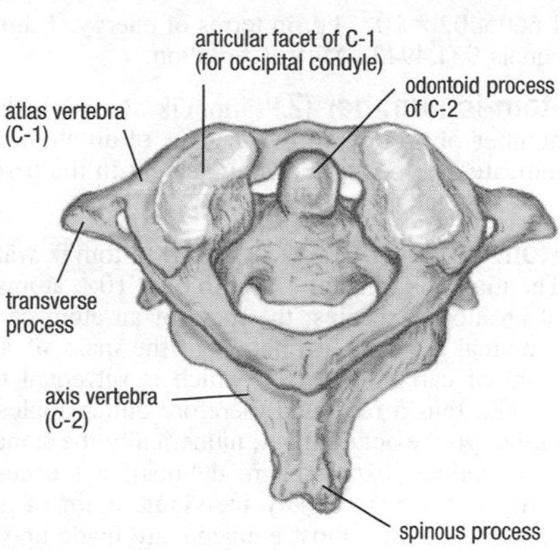

atlas

ATLS Abbreviation for Advanced Trauma Life Support.

atm Abbreviation for standard atmosphere.

atmo- Prefix denoting steam or vapor; or derived by action of steam or vapor. [G. *atmos,* steam, vapor]

at·mos·phere (at′mŏs-fēr) **1.** Any gas surrounding a given body; a gaseous medium. **2.** A unit of air pressure equal to 101.325 kPa. SEE ALSO standard atmosphere. [atmo- + G. *sphaira,* sphere]

at·om (at′ŏm) Formerly considered the ultimate particle of an element, believed to be as indivisible as its name indicates. Discovery of radioactivity demonstrated the existence of subatomic particles, notably protons, neutrons, and electrons, the first two comprising most of the mass of the atomic nucleus. We now know that subatomic particles are further divisible ino hadrons, leptons, and quarks. [G. *atomos,* indivisible, uncut]

a·tom·ic (ă-tom′ik) Relating to an atom.

a·tom·ic ab·sorp·tion spec·tro·pho·tom·e·try (ă-tom′ik ab-sōrp′shŭn spek′trō-fō-tom′ĕ-trē) Determination of concentration by the ability of atoms to absorb radiant energy of specific wavelengths.

a·tom·ic mass num·ber (ă-tom′ik mas nŭm′bĕr) The mass of the atom of a particular isotope relative to hydrogen-1 (or to one twelfth the mass of carbon-12), generally very close to the whole number represented by the sum of the protons and neutrons in the atomic nucleus of the isotope; it is not to be confused with the atomic weight of an element, which may include a number of isotopes in natural proportion.

a·tom·ic mass u·nit (amu) (ă-tom′ik mas yū′nit) A unit of mass by definition equal to $\frac{1}{12}$ of the mass of an atom of carbon-12, which equals

$1.6605402 \times 10^{-27}$ kg; in terms of energy, 1 amu equals 931.49432 MeV. Cf. dalton.

a•tom•ic num•ber (Z) (ă-tom′ik nŭm′bĕr) The number of protons in the nucleus of an atom; it indicates the position of the element in the periodic system.

a•tom•ic weight (AW, at. wt.) (ă-tom′ik wāt) The mass in grams of 1 mol (6.02×10^{23}, atoms) of an atomic species; the mass of an atom of a chemical element in relation to the mass of an atom of carbon-12 (^{12}C), which is set equal to 12.000, thus a ratio and therefore dimensionless (although the actual mass, numerically the same, is sometimes expressed in daltons); not necessarily the weight of any individual atom of an element, because most elements are made up of several isotopes of different masses. SEE ALSO molecular weight.

at•om•iz•er (at′ŏm-ī-zĕr) A device used to reduce liquid medication to fine particles in the form of a spray or aerosol; useful in delivering medication to the nose and throat. SEE ALSO nebulizer, vaporizer. [G. *atomos*, indivisible particle]

a•to•ni•a (ā-tō′nē-ă) SYN atony.

a•ton•ic (ā-ton′ik) Relaxed; without normal tone or tension.

a•ton•ic blad•der (ā-ton′ik blad′ĕr) A large, dilated, and nonemptying urinary bladder; usually due to disturbance of innervation or to chronic obstruction.

a•ton•ic im•po•tence (ā-ton′ik im′pŏ-tĕns) Physiologic dysfunction that makes male erection impossible due to neurologic or muscular conditions, rather than psychological factors.

at•o•ny (at′ŏ-nē) Relaxation, flaccidity, or lack of tone or tension. SYN atonia. [G. *atonia*, languor]

at•o•pen (at′ŏ-pen) The excitant causing any form of atopy.

a•top•ic (ā-top′ik) Relating to or marked by atopy; allergic. [G. *atopos*, out of place; strange]

a•top•ic al•ler•gy (ā-top′ik al′ĕr-jē) SEE atopy.

a•top•ic cat•a•ract (ā-top′ik kat′ăr-akt) A cataract associated with atopic dermatitis.

i **a•top•ic der•ma•ti•tis** (ā-top′ik dĕr′mă-tī′tis) Skin disorder characterized by the distinctive phenomena of atopy, including infantile and flexural eczema. See page 145.

a•top•ic ker•a•to•con•junc•ti•vi•tis (ā-top′ik ker′ă-tō-kŏn-jŭngk′ti-vī′tis) A chronic papillary inflammation of the conjunctiva showing Trantas dots in a patient with a history of hypersensitivity.

At•o•po•bi•um (at-ō-pō′bē-um) An obligately anaerobic genus of gram-positive, non-spore-bearing bacteria that appear as cocci and coccobacilli, sometimes in short chains. The type species is *A. parvulus*, a slow-growing organism forming tiny colonies on standard media, formerly called *Peptostreptococcus parvulus* and *Streptococcus parvulus*.

a•top•og•no•si•a, a•top•og•no•sis (ā-top-og-nō′zē-ă, -og-nō′sis) Sensory inattention; inability to locate a sensation properly. Usually caused by a contralateral parietal lobe lesion. [G. *a-* priv. + *topos*, place, + *gnōsis*, knowledge]

at•o•py (at′ŏ-pē) A genetically determined state of hypersensitivity to environmental allergens. Type I allergic reaction is associated with the IgE antibody and a group of diseases, principally asthma, hay fever, and atopic dermatitis. [G. *atopia*, strangeness, fr. *a-* priv. + *topos*, a place]

a•tox•ic (ā-tok′sik) Not toxic.

ATP Abbreviation for adenosine 5′-triphosphate.

ATPase Abbreviation for adenosine triphosphatase.

ATP-PCr en•er•gy sys•tem (en′ĕr-jē sĭs′tĕm) An immediate energy source stored in skeletal muscle; cleavage of phosphocreatine supplies energy for ATP; used in short duration activities (e.g., sprinting).

ATPS Symbol indicating that a gas volume has been expressed as if it were saturated with water vapor at the ambient temperature and barometric pressure; the condition of an expired gas equilibrated in a spirometer.

A•trac•ty•lo•des (ă-trak′ti-lō′dēz) *A. macrocephala*, used in traditional Chinese medicine as a specific against tetany and jaundice; also purported to increase longevity. [G. *atraktylōdes*, thistle-like]

a•trau•mat•ic su•ture (ā-traw-mat′ik sū′chŭr) A suture swaged onto the end of an eyeless needle.

a•tre•si•a (ă-trē′zē-ă′) Congenital absence of a normal opening or normally patent lumen. [G. *a-* priv. + *trēsis*, a hole]

a•tret•ic (ă-tret′ik) Relating to atresia. SYN imperforate.

a•tre•tic fol•li•cle (ă-tret′ik fol′i-kĕl) A follicle that degenerates before coming to maturity; many atretic follicles occur in the ovary before puberty; in the sexually mature woman, several are formed each month. SYN corpus atreticum.

atreto- Prefix meaning lack of an opening. [G. *atrētos*, imperforate fr. *a-*, not + *trētos*, perforated, fr. *tetrainō, titrēmi*, to bore through, to pierce.]

a•tri•a (ā′trē-ă) Plural of atrium.

a•tri•al (ā′trē-ăl) Relating to an atrium.

a•tri•al ar•ter•ies (ā′trē-ăl ahr′tĕr-ēz) Branches

of the right and left coronary arteries distributed to the muscle of the atria. SYN arteriae atriales.

a·tri·al au·ri·cle (ā′trē-ăl awr′i-kĕl) SYN auricle of atrium.

a·tri·al cap·ture beat (ā′trē-ăl kap′shŭr bēt) The cardiac cycle resulting when, after a period of A-V dissociation, the atria regain control of the ventricles; atrial depolarization due to retrograde transmission from a ventricular ectopic beat or an electronically paced ventricular impulse.

a·tri·al cha·ot·ic tach·y·car·di·a (ā′trē-ăl kā-ot′ik tak′i-kahr′dē-ă) Multifocal origin of tachycardia within the atrium; often confused with atrial fibrillation during physical examination. SYN multifocal atrial tachycardia.

a·tri·al com·plex (ā′trē-ăl kom′pleks) P wave in the electrocardiogram.

a·tri·al dis·so·ci·a·tion (ā′trē-ăl di-sō′sē-ā′shŭn) Mutually independent beating of the two atria or of parts of the atria.

a·tri·al ex·tra·sys·to·le (ā′trē-ăl eks′tră-sis′tō-

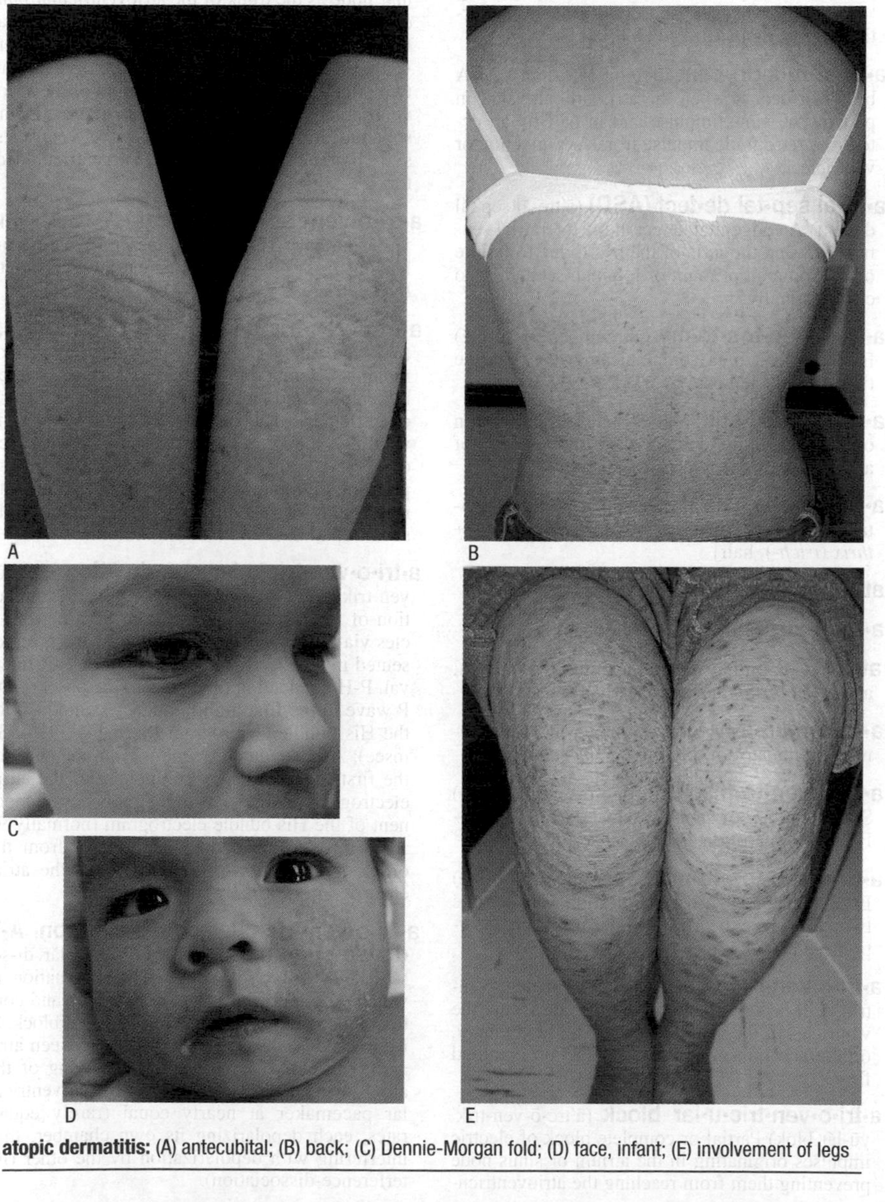

A B C D E

atopic dermatitis: (A) antecubital; (B) back; (C) Dennie-Morgan fold; (D) face, infant; (E) involvement of legs

lē) A premature contraction of the heart arising from an ectopic atrial focus.

a·tri·al fi·bril·la·tion, au·ric·u·lar fi·bril·la·tion (ā′trē-ăl fib′ri-lā′shŭn, awr-ik′yū-lăr fib′ri-lā′shŭn) Fibrillation in which the normal rhythmic contractions of the cardiac atria are replaced by rapid irregular twitchings of the muscular wall; the ventricles respond irregularly to the dysrhythmic bombardment from the atria.

a·tri·al flut·ter, au·ric·u·lar flut·ter (ā′trē-ăl flŭt′ĕr, awr-ik′yū-lăr flŭt′ĕr) Rapid regular atrial contractions occurring usually at rates between 250 and 350 per minute and often producing "saw-tooth" waves in the electrocardiogram, particularly leads II, III, and aVF.

a·tri·al fu·sion beat (ā′trē-ăl fyū′zhŭn bēt) A beat that occurs when the atria are activated in part by the sinus impulse and in part by an ectopic or retrograde impulse from A-V junction or ventricle.

a·tri·al sep·tal de·fect (ASD) (ā′trē-ăl sep′tăl dē′fekt) A congenital defect in the interatrial septum between the atria of the heart, due to failure of the foramen primum or foramen secundum to close normally.

a·tri·al sep·tos·to·my (ā′trē-ăl sep-tos′tŏ-mē) Establishment of a communication between the two atria of the heart.

a·tri·al stand·still (ā′trē-ăl stand′stil) Cessation of atrial contractions, marked by absence of atrial waves in the electrocardiogram.

a·trich·i·a (ă-trik′ē-ă) Absence of hair, congenital or acquired. SYN atrichosis. [G. *a-* priv. + *thrix* (*trich-*), hair]

at·ri·cho·sis (at-ri-kō′sis) SYN atrichia.

a·trich·ous (ă-trik′ŭs) Without hair.

♻ **atrio-** Combining form meaning the atrium; atrial. [L. *atrium*, an entrance hall]

a·tri·o·meg·a·ly (ā′trē-ō-meg′ă-lē) Enlargement of the atrium. [atrio- + G. *megas*, great]

a·tri·o·sep·to·plas·ty (ā′trē-ō-sep′tō-plas-tē) Surgical repair of an atrial septal defect. [atrio- + L. *septum*, partition, + G. *plastos*, formed]

a·tri·o·sep·tos·to·my (ā′trē-ō-sep-tos′tŏ-mē) Establishment of a communication between the two atria of the heart. [atrio- + L. *septum*, partition, + G. *stoma*, mouth]

a·tri·o·ven·tric·u·lar (A-V, AV) (ā′trē-ō-ven-trik′yū-lăr) Relating to both the atria and the ventricles of the heart, especially to the ordinary, orthograde transmission of conduction or blood flow.

a·tri·o·ven·tric·u·lar block (ā′trē-ō-ven-trik′yū-lăr blok) Partial or complete block of electric impulses originating in the atrium or sinus node preventing them from reaching the atrioventricular node and ventricles. In first degree A-V block, there is prolongation of A-V conduction time (P-R interval); in second degree A-V block, some but not all atrial impulses fail to reach the ventricles, thus some ventricular beats are dropped; in complete A-V block, complete atrioventricular dissociation (2) occurs; no impulses can reach the ventricles despite even a slow ventricular rate (under 45 per minute); atria and ventricles beat independently. SYN block (4).

a·tri·o·ven·tric·u·lar bun·dle (ā′trē-ō-ven-trik′yū-lăr bŭn′dĕl) The bundle of modified cardiac muscle fibers that begins at the atrioventricular node as the trunk of the atrioventricular bundle and passes through the right atrioventricular fibrous ring to the membranous part of the interventricular septum where the trunk divides into two branches, the right and left crura of the atrioventricular bundle; the two crura ramify in the subendocardium of their respective ventricles. SYN His bundle, Kent bundle (1), ventriculonector.

a·tri·o·ven·tric·u·lar ca·nal (ā′trē-ō-ven-trik′yū-lăr kă-nal′) The canal in the embryonic heart leading from the common sinuatrial chamber to the ventricle.

a·tri·o·ven·tric·u·lar ca·nal cush·ions (ā′trē-ō-ven-trik′yū-lăr kă-nal′ ku′shŏnz) A pair of mounds of embryonic connective tissue covered by endothelium, bulging into the embryonic atrioventricular canal; one located dorsally and one ventrally, they grow together and fuse with each other and with the lower edge of the septum primum, dividing the originally single canal into right and left atrioventricular orifices. Frequently seen in patients with Down syndrome.

a·tri·o·ven·tric·u·lar con·duc·tion (ā′trē-ō-ven-trik′yū-lăr kŏn-dŭk′shŭn) Forward conduction of the cardiac impulse from atria to ventricles via the A-V node or any bypass tract, represented in the electrocardiogram by the P-R interval. P-H conduction time is from the onset of the P wave to the first high frequency component of the His bundle electrogram (normally 119 ± 38 msec); A-H conduction time is from the onset of the first high frequency component of the atrial electrogram to the first high frequency component of the His bundle electrogram (normally 92 ± 38 msec); P-A conduction time is from the onset of the P wave to the onset of the atrial electrogram (normally 27 ± 18 msec).

a·tri·o·ven·tric·u·lar dis·so·ci·a·tion, A-V dis·so·ci·a·tion (ā′trē-ō-ven-trik′yū-lăr di-sō′sē-ā′shŭn, dis-sō′sē-ā′shŭn) **1.** Any situation in which atria and ventricles are activated and contract independently, as in complete A-V block. **2.** More specifically, the dissociation between atria and ventricles that results from slowing of the atrial pacemaker or acceleration of the ventricular pacemaker at nearly equal (rarely equal) rates, each depolarizing its own chamber, thus interfering with depolarization by the other (interference-dissociation).

a•tri•o•ven•tric•u•lar ex•tra•sys•to•le, A-V ex•tra•sys•to•le (ā′trē-ō-ven-trik′yū-lăr eks′trā-sis′tō-lē, eks′trā-sis′tō-lē) An extrasystole arising from the "junctional" tissues, either the A-V node or A-V bundle.

a•tri•o•ven•tric•u•lar junc•tion•al bi•gem•i•ny (ā′trē-ō-ven-trik′yū-lăr jungk′shŭn-ăl bī-jem′i-nē) Paired beats, each pair consisting of an A-V nodal extrasystole coupled to a beat of the dominant, usually sinus, rhythm.

a•tri•o•ven•tric•u•lar junc•tion•al rhythm (ā′trē-ō-ven-trik′yū-lăr jungk′shŭn-ăl ridh′ŭm) The cardiac rhythm when the heart is controlled by the A-V junction (including node); arising in the A-V junction, the impulse ascends to the atria and descends to the ventricles, each at varying speeds depending on site of the pacemaker. SYN AV junctional rhythm.

a•tri•o•ven•tric•u•lar no•dal branch•es (ā′trē-ō-ven-trik′yū-lăr nō′dăl branch′ĕz) Small arteries supplying the atrioventricular node; usually arise from the right coronary artery as it starts to descend the posterior interventricular sulcus. SYN artery to atrioventricular node, branch to atrioventricular node, ramus nodi atrioventricularis.

a•tri•o•ven•tric•u•lar no•dal ex•tra•sys•to•le, A-V no•dal ex•tra•sys•to•le (ā′trē-ō-ven-trik′yū-lăr nō′dăl eks′trā-sis′tō-lē, nō′dăl eks′trā-sis′tō-lē) A premature beat arising from the A-V junction and leading to a simultaneous or almost simultaneous contraction of atria and ventricles.

a•tri•o•ven•tric•u•lar node (AV node) (ā′trē-ō-ven-trik′yū-lăr nōd) A small node of modified cardiac muscle fibers located near the ostium of the coronary sinus; it gives rise to the atrioventricular bundle of the conduction system of the heart.

a•tri•o•ven•tric•u•lar sep•tum (ā′trē-ō-ven-trik′yū-lăr sep′tŭm) The small part of the membranous septum of the heart just above the septal cusp of the tricuspid valve that separates the right atrium from the left ventricle.

a•tri•o•ven•tric•u•lar valves (ā′trē-ō-ven-trik′yū-lăr valvz) SEE tricuspid valve, mitral valve.

a•tri•um, pl. **a•tri•a** (ā′trē-ŭm, ā′trē-ă) [TA] **1.** A chamber or cavity to which are connected several chambers or passageways. **2.** SYN atrium of heart. **3.** That part of the tympanic cavity that lies immediately deep to the tympanic membrane (eardrum). **4.** In the lung, a subdivision of the alveolar duct from which alveolar sacs open. [L. entrance hall]

a•tri•um cor•dis (ā′trē-ŭm kōr′dis) [TA] SYN atrium of heart.

a•tri•um cor•dis dex•trum (ā′trē-ŭm kōr′dis deks′trŭm) [TA] SYN right atrium of heart.

a•tri•um cor•dis si•nis•trum (ā′trē-ŭm kōr′dis sin-is′trŭm) [TA] SYN left atrium of heart.

a•tri•um dex•trum cor•dis (ā′trē-ŭm deks′trŭm kōr′dis) SYN right atrium of heart.

a•tri•um of heart (ā′trē-ŭm hahrt) The upper chamber of each half of the heart. SYN atrium cordis [TA], atrium (2) [TA].

a•tri•um pul•mo•na•le (ā′trē-ŭm pul-mō-nā′lē) SYN left atrium of heart.

a•tri•um si•nis•trum cor•dis (ā′trē-ŭm sin-is′trŭm kōr′dis) SYN left atrium of heart.

A•tro•pa bel•la•don•na (ā-trō′pă bel′ă-don′ă) A perennial herb with dark purple flowers and berries. Originally used as source of atropine.

a•tro•phi•a (ă-trō′fē-ă) SYN atrophy. [G. fr. *a-* priv. + *trophē*, nourishment]

a•troph•ic (ā-trō′fik) Denoting atrophy.

a•troph•ic ex•ca•va•tion (ā-trō′fik eks′kă-vā′shŭn) An exaggeration of the normal or physiologic cupping of the optic disc caused by atrophy of the optic nerve.

a•troph•ic gas•tri•tis (ā-trō′fik gas-trī′tis) Chronic gastritis with atrophy of the mucous membrane and destruction of the peptic glands, sometimes associated with pernicious anemia or gastric carcinoma; also applied to gastric atrophy without inflammatory changes.

a•troph•ic rhi•ni•tis (ā-trō′fik rī-nī′tis) Chronic rhinitis with thinning of the mucous membrane; often associated with crusts and foul-smelling discharge.

a•troph•ic vag•i•ni•tis (ā-trō′fik vaj′i-nī′tis) Thinning and atrophy of the vaginal epithelium usually resulting from diminished estrogen stimulation; a common occurrence in postmenopausal women.

at•ro•phied (at′rŏ-fēd) Characterized by atrophy.

at•ro•pho•der•ma (at′rō-fō-dĕr′mă) Atrophy of the skin that may occur either in discrete localized areas or in widespread areas. SEE ALSO anetoderma.

at•ro•pho•der•ma•to•sis (at′rō-fō-dĕr′mă-tō′sis) Any cutaneous disorder in which a prominent symptom is skin atrophy.

at•ro•phy (at′rŏ-fē) A wasting of tissues, organs, or the entire body, as from death and reabsorption of cells, diminished cellular proliferation, decreased cellular volume, pressure, ischemia, malnutrition, lessened function, or hormonal changes. SYN atrophia. [G. *atrophia,* fr. *a-* priv. + *trophē,* nourishment]

at•tached gin•gi•va (ă-tacht′ jin′ji-vă) That part of the oral mucosa that is firmly bound to the tooth and alveolar process.

at•tach•ment (ă-tach′mĕnt) **1.** A connection of one part with another. **2.** DENTISTRY a mechanical device for the fixation and stabilization of a dental prosthesis.

at·tack (ă-tak′) A sudden illness or an episode or exacerbation of chronic or recurrent illness.

at·tack rate (ă-tak′ rāt) A cumulative incidence rate used for particular groups observed for limited periods under special circumstances, such as during an epidemic.

at·tend·ing phys·i·cian (ă-tend′ing fi-zish′ŭn) The physician formally and legally responsible for primary care and treatment throughout stay in a health care facility.

at·tend·ing staff (ă-tend′ing staf) Physicians and surgeons who are members of a hospital staff and regularly see their patients at the hospital; may also supervise and teach house staff, fellows, and medical students.

at·ten·tion def·i·cit dis·or·der (ADD) (ă-ten′shŭn def′i-sit dis-ōr′dĕr) A disorder of attention and impulse control with specific DSM criteria, appearing in childhood and sometimes persisting to adulthood. Hyperactivity may be a feature but is not necessary for the diagnosis. SEE ALSO attention deficit hyperactivity disorder.

at·ten·tion def·i·cit hy·per·ac·tiv·i·ty dis·or·der (ADHD) (ă-ten′shŭn def′i-sit hī′pĕr-ak-tiv′i-tē dis-ōr′dĕr) A disorder of childhood and adolescence manifested at home, in school, and in social situations by developmentally inappropriate degrees of inattention, impulsiveness, and hyperactivity; also called hyperactivity or hyperactive child syndrome. SEE ALSO attention deficit disorder.

at·ten·tion span (ă-ten′shŭn span) The length of time a person can concentrate on a subject.

at·ten·u·at·ed vi·rus (ă-ten′yū-ā′tĕd vī′rŭs) A variant strain of a pathogenic virus, so modified as to excite the production of protective antibodies, yet not producing the specific disease.

at·ten·u·a·tion (ă-ten′yū-ā′shŭn) **1.** The act of attenuating. **2.** Diminution of virulence in a strain of an organism, obtained through selection of variants that occur naturally or through experimental means. **3.** Loss of energy of a beam of radiant energy due to absorption, scattering, beam divergence, and other causes as the beam propagates through a medium. **4.** Regulation of termination of transcription; involved in the control of gene expression in specific tissues.

at·ti·cot·o·my (at′i-kot′ŏ-mē) Operative opening into the tympanic attic. [attic + G. *tomē,* incision]

at·ti·tude (at′i-tūd) **1.** Position of the body and limbs. **2.** Manner of acting. **3.** PSYCHOLOGY a predisposition to behave or react in a certain way toward people, objects, institutions, or issues. [Mediev. L. *aptitudo,* fr. L. *aptus,* fit]

atto- (a) Prefix used in the SI and in the metric system to signify one quintillionth (10^{-18}). [Danish *atten,* eighteen]

at·trac·tin (ă-trak′tin) A glycoprotein of T-cell origin involved in T-cell clustering and monocyte movement.

at·trac·tion (ă-trak′shŭn) A property or force by which anything tends to cause something else to approach it. [L. *at-traho,* pp. *-tractus,* to draw toward]

at·trac·tion sphere (ă-trak′shŭn sfēr) SYN astrosphere.

at·tri·tion (ă-trish′ŭn) **1.** Wearing away by friction or rubbing. **2.** In dentistry, physiologic loss of tooth structure caused by normal wear inherent in the aging process, as well as by the abrasive character of food or by bruxism. Cf. abrasion. **3.** The loss of participants over the course of a study, which can create bias and threaten the internal validity of the study. See page B15. [L. *at-tero,* pp. *-tritus,* to rub against, rub away]

at. wt. Abbreviation for atomic weight.

a·typ·i·a (ā-tip′ē-ă) Uncharacteristic or not uniform. [G. *a,* without, + *typos,* type, form]

a·typ·i·cal (ā-tip′i-kăl) Denotes the unexpected or unanticipated; not corresponding to the normal form or type. [G. *a-* priv. + *typikos,* conformed to a type]

a·typ·i·cal an·ti·psy·chot·ic a·gent (ā-tip′i-kăl an′tē-sī-kot′ik ā′jĕnt) A functional category of newer antipsychotic drugs (e.g., olanzapine, clozapine) thought to exert their action predominantly through serotonergic blockade.

a·typ·i·cal en·do·me·tri·al hy·per·pla·si·a (ā-tip′i-kăl en′dō-mē′trē-ăl hī′pĕr-plā′zē-ă) Increase in the number of endometrial glands, which have little, if any, stroma separating them but retain an orderly architecture distinguishing them from adenocarcinoma.

a·typ·i·cal gland·u·lar cells of un·de·ter·mined sig·nif·i·cance (AGUS, AGCUS) (ā-tip′i-kăl glan′dyū-lăr selz ŭn-dĕ-tĕr′mind sig-nif′i-kăns) The term in the Bethesda system for reporting cervical or vaginal cytologic diagnosis describing cells that show either endometrial or endocervical differentiation and display nuclear atypia that exceeds reactive or reparative changes but lacks definite features of invasive adenocarcinoma. SEE ALSO Bethesda system.

a·typ·i·cal li·po·ma (ā-tip′i-kăl li-pō′mă) Lipoma, occurring primarily in older men on the posterior neck, shoulders, and back, which is benign but microscopically atypical, containing giant cells with multiple overlapping nuclei forming a circle. SYN pleomorphic lipoma.

a·typ·i·cal mea·sles (ā-tip′i-kăl mē′zĕlz) Unusual clinical manifestation of natural measles infection in people with waning vaccination immunity, particularly in those who had received formaldehyde-inactivated vaccine; an accelerated allergic reaction characterized by high fever, absence of Koplik spots, a shortened prodromal period, atypical rash, and pneumonia.

a·typ·i·cal my·co·bac·te·ri·a (ā-tip′i-kăl mī′kō-bak-tēr′ē-ă) Species of mycobacteria other than *M. tuberculosis* or *M. bovis* that can cause disease in immunocompromised humans.

a·typ·i·cal pneu·mo·ni·a (ā-tip′i-kăl nū-mō′nē-ă) SYN primary atypical pneumonia.

a·typ·i·cal squa·mous cells of un·de·ter·mined sig·nif·i·cance (ASCUS) (ā-tip′i-kăl skwā′mŭs selz ŭn-dĕ-tĕr′mind sig-nif′i-kăns) The term in the Bethesda system for reporting cervical-vaginal cytologic diagnosis describing cellular abnormalities that are more marked than those attributable to reactive changes but that quantitatively or qualitatively fall short of a definitive diagnosis of squamous intraepithelial lesion (SIL); may reflect a benign or a potentially serious lesion. SEE ALSO Bethesda system, reactive changes.

a·typ·i·cal ver·ru·cous en·do·car·di·tis (ā-tip′i-kăl ver-ū′kŭs en′dō-kahr-dī′tis) SYN Libman-Sacks endocarditis.

A.U. Abbreviation for *auris utraque* [L.], each ear or both ears. USAGE NOTE The ungrammatical expansion of this abbreviation, *aures unitas*, given in many reference works, is entirely without historical foundation. The JCAHO directs that *each ear* or *both ears* be written in full to avoid confusion with similar abbreviations.

Au Symbol for gold (aurum).

Au·ber·ger blood group (ō-ber-zher′ blŭd grūp) A group defined by the presence of a serum protein in 80% of whites.

Au·bert phe·nom·e·non (ow′bert fĕ-nom′ĕ-non) A phenomenon in which a bright perpendicular line appears to incline to one side when the observer turns the head to the opposite side in a dark room.

au·dile (awd′īl) **1.** Relating to ability to hear. **2.** Denoting the type of mental imagery in which one recalls most readily that which has been heard rather than seen or read. Cf. motile. **3.** SYN auditive.

♲ **audio-** The sense of hearing. [L. *audio,* to hear]

au·di·o·an·al·ge·si·a (aw′dē-ō-an-ăl-jē′zē-ă) Use of music or sound delivered through earphones to enhance relaxation and distract a patient from feeling pain during dental or surgical procedures.

au·di·o·gen·ic (aw′dē-ō-jen′ik) **1.** Caused by sound, especially a loud noise. **2.** Sound-producing. [audio- + G. *genesis,* production]

au·di·o·gram (aw′dē-ō-gram) The graphic record drawn from the results of hearing tests with the audiometer; charts the threshold of hearing at various frequencies against sound intensity in decibels. [audio- + G. *gramma,* a drawing]

au·di·ol·o·gist (aw′dē-ol′ŏ-jist) A specialist in evaluation and rehabilitation of those whose communication disorders center in whole or in part in the hearing function.

au·di·ol·o·gy (aw′dē-ol′ŏ-jē) The study of hearing disorders through the identification and measurement of hearing function loss as well as the rehabilitation of persons with hearing impairments.

au·di·om·e·ter (aw′dē-om′ĕ-tĕr) An electrical instrument for measuring the threshold of hearing for pure tones of frequencies generally varying from 128–8000 Hz (recorded in decibels). [audio- + G. *metron,* measure]

au·di·o·met·ric (aw′dē-ō-met′rik) Related to measurement of hearing levels.

au·di·om·e·try (aw′dē-om′ĕ-trē) **1.** The measurement of hearing. **2.** The use of an audiometer. **3.** Rapid measurement of the hearing of an individual or a group against a predetermined limit of normality; auditory responses to different frequencies presented at a constant intensity level are tested.

au·di·o·vi·su·al (aw′dē-ō-vizh′ū-ăl) Pertaining to a communication or teaching technique that combines both audible and visible symbols.

au·dit (aw′dit) **1.** A formal review or analysis of a body of data, particularly fiscal accounts. **2.** To perform an audit. **3.** Detailed retrospective evaluation of medical records to assess quality of health care given. [L. *auditus,* a hearing, fr. *audio,* to hear]

au·di·tion (aw-dish′ŭn) SYN hearing. [L. *auditio,* a hearing, fr. *audio,* to hear]

au·di·tive (aw′di-tiv) One who recalls most readily that which has been heard. SYN audile (3).

au·di·to·ry (aw′di-tōr-ē) Pertaining to the sense of hearing or to the organs of hearing. [L. *audio,* pp. *auditus,* to hear]

au·di·to·ry ag·no·si·a (aw′di-tōr-ē ag-nō′zē-ă) Inability to recognize sounds, words, or music; caused by a lesion of the auditory cortex of the temporal lobe.

au·di·to·ry a·pha·si·a (aw′di-tōr-ē ă-fā′zē-ă) An impairment in comprehension of the auditory forms of language and communication, including the ability to write from dictation in the presence of normal hearing. Spontaneous speech, reading, and writing are not affected. SYN word deafness.

au·di·to·ry ar·e·a (aw′di-tōr-ē ār′ē-ă) SYN auditory cortex.

au·di·to·ry au·ra (aw′di-tōr-ē awr′ă) Epileptic aura characterized by illusions or hallucinations of sounds. SEE ALSO aura (1).

au·di·to·ry brain·stem re·sponse (ABR) (aw′di-tōr-ē brān′stem rĕ-spons′) A response produced by the auditory nerve and the brainstem to repetitive acoustic stimuli. SYN brainstem evoked response.

au·di·to·ry brain·stem re·sponse au·di·om·e·try, ABR au·di·om·e·try (aw′di-tōr-ē brān′stem rĕ-spons′ aw′dē-om′ĕ-trē, aw′dē-om′ĕ-trē) An electrophysiologic measure of auditory function using responses produced by the auditory nerve and the brainstem to repetitive acoustic stimuli. SYN brainstem evoked response audiometry, BSER audiometry.

au·di·to·ry cap·sule (aw′di-tōr-ē kap′sŭl) SYN otic capsule.

au·di·to·ry cor·tex (aw′di-tōr-ē kōr′teks) The region of the cerebral cortex that receives the auditory radiation from the medial geniculate body, a thalamic cell group receiving auditory input from the cochlear nuclei in the rhombencephalon. SYN auditory area.

au·di·to·ry de·fen·sive·ness (aw′di-tōr-ē dĕ-fen′siv-nĕs) Excessive reaction to sound (e.g., because of its volume or novelty).

au·di·to·ry feed·back (aw′di-tōr-ē fēd′bak) The unwanted sound that occurs in an amplification system when the microphone picks up the sound from the speaker; a major problem in the use of hearing aids.

au·di·to·ry field (aw′di-tōr-ē fēld) The space included within the limits of hearing of a definite sound, as of a tuning fork.

au·di·to·ry hairs (aw′di-tōr-ē hārz) Cilia on the free surface of the auditory cells.

au·di·to·ry in·te·gra·tion train·ing (AIT) (aw′di-tōr-ē in-tĕ-grā′shŭn trān′ing) A series of exercises in listening designed to help people who have difficulty processing complex acoustic signals (e.g., rapid speech).

au·di·tor·y mas·sage (aw′di-tōr-ē mă-sahzh′) Palpation of eardrum for diagnostic or therapeutic purposes.

au·di·to·ry nerve (aw′di-tōr-ē nĕrv) SYN cochlear nerve.

au·di·to·ry neu·rop·a·thy (aw′di-tōr-ē nūr-op′ă-thē) A distinctive type of hearing deficit that seemingly is due to a malfunction of the eighth cranial nerve. Previously referred to as auditory neural synchrony disorder. Speech comprehension in quiet surroundings is out of proportion to the pure tone threshold elevation.

au·di·to·ry os·si·cles (aw′di-tōr-ē os′i-kŭlz) The small bones of the middle ear; they are articulated to form a chain for the transmission of sound from the tympanic membrane to the oval window. See this page. SYN ossicula auditus [TA], ear bones.

au·di·to·ry pits (aw′di-tōr-ē pits) Paired depressions, one on either side of the head of the embryo, marking the location of the otic placodes, the future auditory vesicles.

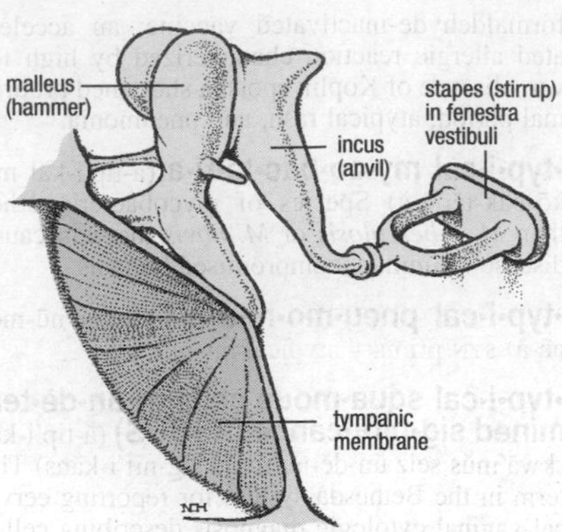

auditory ossicles: bones of the middle ear

au·di·to·ry pro·cess·ing dis·or·der (aw′di-tōr-ē pros′es-sing dis-ōr′dĕr) Impaired ability to attend to or comprehend auditory information despite normal hearing and intellect; a type of receptive language disorder.

au·di·to·ry pros·the·sis (aw′di-tōr-ē pros-thē′sis) Generic term for implantable devices to restore sound perception to the deaf, the most common of which is the cochlear implant; a brainstem implant to stimulate the neurons of the cochlear nucleus is under development.

au·di·to·ry re·cep·tor cells (aw′di-tōr-ē rĕ-sep′tŏr selz) Columnar cells in the epithelium of the organ of Corti, having hairs (stereocilia) on their apical ends.

au·di·to·ry re·flex (aw′di-tōr-ē rē′fleks) Any reflex occurring in response to a sound (e.g., cochleopalpebral reflex).

au·di·to·ry tube (aw′di-tōr-ē tūb) SYN pharyngotympanic (auditory) tube.

au·di·to·ry ver·ti·go (aw′di-tōr-ē vĕr′ti-gō) SYN Ménière disease.

au·dit trail (aw′dit trāl) SYN documentation trail.

Au·dou·in mi·cro·spor·um (ō-dwahn′ mī-krō-spōr′ŭm) SYN *Microsporum audouini.*

Au·en·brug·ger sign (ow′en-brūg-er sīn) An epigastric prominence seen in cases of marked pericardial effusion.

Au·er bod·ies, Au·er rods (ow′ĕr bod′ēz, rodz) Rod-shaped structures of uncertain nature in the cytoplasm of immature myeloid cells, especially myeloblasts, in acute myelocytic leukemia.

aug·men·ta·tion (awg′men-tā′shŭn) Process of increasing in size, amount, degree, or severity. [L. *augmentum,* growth, increase]

aug•men•ta•tion mam•ma•plas•ty (awg′men-tā′shŭn mam′ă-plas-tē) Plastic surgery to enlarge the breast, often by insertion of an implant.

aug•men•ta•tive and al•ter•na•tive com•mun•i•ca•tion (AAC) (awg-men′tă-tiv awl-tĕr′nă-tiv kă-myūn′i-kā′shŭn) **1.** Any type of compensation for impaired use of verbal language, including techniques such as gesture systems and devices such as voice amplifiers, picture boards, and computerized instrumentation; SEE ALSO communication board. **2.** The clinical practice of determining appropriate compensatory techniques for inadequate verbal communication and providing training in the use of those techniques. SYN nonoral communication, nonverbal communication.

aug•ment•ed la•bor (awg-men′tĕd lā′bŏr) Induced labor.

au•ra, pl. **au•rae** (awr′ă, awr′ē) **1.** Subjective symptoms occurring at the onset of a partial epileptic seizure; often characteristic for the brain region involved in the seizure, e.g., visual aura, occipital lobe auditory aura, temporal lobe. **2.** Subjective symptoms at the onset of a migraine headache. [L. breeze, odor, gleam of light]

au•ral (awr′ăl) **1.** Relating to the ear (auris). **2.** Relating to an aura.

au•ral•ly (awr′ă-lē) Related to the ear or sense of hearing. [L. *auris,* ear]

au•ral re•ha•bil•i•ta•tion (awr′ăl rē′hă-bil′i-tā′shŭn) Procedures to enhance the communication capacity of people with hearing impairments, such as auditory training, lip reading, and hearing aid orientation.

♻ **auri-** Combining form denoting the ear. SEE ALSO ot-, oto-. [L. *auris,* an ear.]

au•ri•cle (awr′i-kĕl) **1.** The projecting shell-like structure on the side of the head, constituting, with the external acoustic meatus, the external ear. SYN auricula (1), pinna (1). **2.** SYN auricle of atrium.

au•ri•cle of a•tri•um (awr′i-kĕl ā′trē-ŭm) A small conic ("ear-shaped") pouch projecting from the upper anterior portion of each atrium of the heart, increasing slightly the atrial volume. SYN atrial auricle, auricle (2), auricula (2).

au•ri•cle he•ma•to•ma (awr′i-kĕl hē′mă-tō′mă) Hematoma between the perichondrium and cartilage of the outer ear.

au•ri•cles of a•tri•a (aw′rik-ĕlz ā′trē-ă) SYN auricula atrii.

au•ric•u•la, pl. **au•ric•u•lae** (aw-rik′ū-lă, -lē) **1.** SYN auricle (1). **2.** SYN auricle of atrium. [L. the external ear, dim. of *auris,* ear]

au•ric•u•la a•tri•i (aw-rik′yū-lă ā′trē-ī) [TA] A small conic ("ear-shaped") pouch projecting from the upper anterior portion of each atrium of the heart, increasing slightly the atrial volume. SEE left atrium of heart, right atrium of heart. SYN auricles of atria.

au•ric•u•lar (awr-ik′yū-lăr) Relating to the ear, or to an auricle in any sense.

au•ric•u•lar car•ti•lage (awr-ik′yū-lăr kahr′ti-lăj) The cartilage of the auricle. SYN cartilago auriculae [TA].

au•ric•u•la•re (aw-rik-ū-lā′rē) A craniometric point at the center of the opening of the external auditory meatus or, in certain cases, the middle of the upper edge of this opening. SYN auricular point. [L. *auricularis,* pertaining to the ear]

au•ric•u•la•ris an•te•ri•or mus•cle (aw-rik-yū′lar′is an-tēr′ē-ŏr mŭs′ĕl) SYN anterior auricular muscle. SYN musculus auricularis anterior, zygomaticoauricularis.

au•ric•u•la•ris pos•te•ri•or mus•cle (aw-rik-yū′lar′is pos-tēr′ē-ŏr mŭs′ĕl) Facial muscle of external ear; *origin*, mastoid process; *insertion*, posterior portion of root of auricle; *action*, draws back the pinna; *nerve supply*, facial. SYN musculus auricularis posterior, musculus retrahens aurem, posterior auricular muscle.

au•ric•u•la•ris su•pe•ri•or mus•cle (aw-rik-yū′lar′is sŭ-pēr′ē-ŏr mŭs′ĕl) Facial muscle associated with external ear; *origin*, galea aponeurotica; *insertion*, cartilage of auricle; *action*, draws pinna of ear upward and backward; *nerve supply*, facial. SYN musculus attollens aurem, musculus attollens auriculam, musculus auricularis superior, superior auricular muscle.

au•ric•u•lar point (awr-ik′yū-lăr poynt) SYN auriculare.

au•ric•u•lar tu•ber•cle (awr-ik′yū-lăr tū′bĕr-kĕl) A small projection from the upper end of the posterior portion of the incurved free margin of the helix. SYN darwinian tubercle.

au•ric•u•lo•pres•sor re•flex (awr-ik′yū-lō-pres′ŏr rē′fleks) Peripheral vasoconstriction and a rise in blood pressure in response to a fall in pressure in the great veins. SYN Pavlov reflex.

au•ric•u•lo•tem•po•ral (awr-ik′yū-lō-tem′pŏr-ăl) Relating to the auricle or pinna of the ear and the temporal region.

au•ric•u•lo•tem•po•ral nerve (awr-ik′yū-lō-tem′pŏr-ăl nĕrv) A branch of the mandibular, usually arising by two roots embracing the middle meningeal artery; it passes through the parotid gland conveying postsynaptic parasympathetic secretomotor fibers from the otic ganglion, and terminating in the skin of the temple and scalp; also sends branches to the external acoustic meatus, tympanic membrane, and auricle as well as a communicating branch to the facial nerve. SYN nervus auriculotemporalis [TA].

au•ris, pl. **au•res** (awr′is, awr′ēz) [TA] SYN ear. [L.]

au•ro•pal•pe•bral re•flex (awr′ō-pal′pĕ-brăl rē′fleks) Brisk closure of the eyes in reaction to sudden presentation of a loud noise.

au•ro•thi•o•glu•cose (awr′ō-thī′ō-glū′kōs) Organic compound of gold injected intramuscularly in the treatment of rheumatoid arthritis and lupus erythematosus.

au•rum (awr′ŭm) SYN gold. [L.]

aus•cul•tate, **aus•cult** (aws′kŭl-tāt, aws-kŭlt′) To perform auscultation.

aus•cul•ta•tion (aws′kŭl-tā′shŭn) Listening to the sounds made by various body structures and functions as a diagnostic method, usually with a stethoscope. See this page. [L. *ausculto,* pp. *-atus,* to listen to]

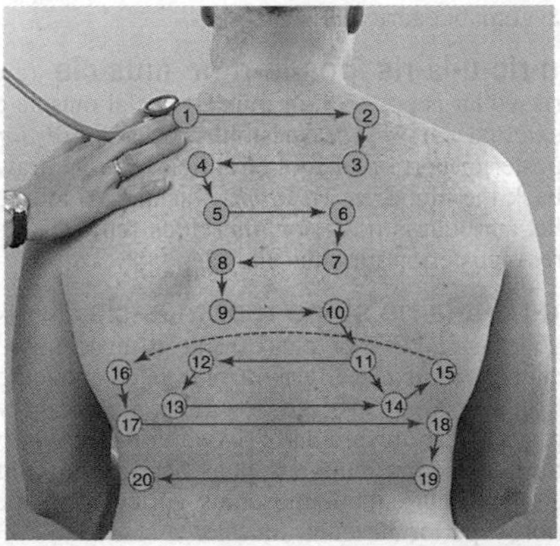

auscultation of the lungs: the examiner places the chest-piece of the stethoscope at selected sites on the surface of the thorax while the subject breathes deeply in and out through the mouth

aus•cul•ta•to•ry (aws-kŭl′tă-tōr-ē) Relating to auscultation.

aus•cul•ta•to•ry al•ter•nans (aws-kŭl′tă-tōr-ē awl-tĕr′nanz) Alternation in the intensity of heart sounds or murmurs in the presence of a regular cardiac rhythm.

aus•cul•ta•to•ry gap (aws-kŭl′tă-tōr-ē gap) The period during which Korotkoff sounds indicating true systolic pressure fade away and reappear at a lower pressure point; responsible for errors made in recording falsely low systolic blood pressure, especially in hypertensive patients, of up to 25 mmHg, and avoided by pumping the cuff 30 mmHg above palpable systolic pressure.

aus•cul•ta•to•ry per•cus•sion (aws-kŭl′tă-tōr-ē pĕr-kŭsh′ŭn) Auscultation of the chest or other part at the same time that percussion is made, to facilitate hearing the sound made by percussion.

Au•spitz sign (ow′spits sīn) A finding typical of psoriasis, in which removal of a scale leads to pinpoint bleeding.

Aus•tin Flint phe•nom•e•non, **Aus•tin Flint mur•mur** (aw′stin flint fĕ-nom′ĕ-non, mŭr′mŭr) The murmur of relative mitral stenosis during significant aortic regurgitation owing to narrowing of the mitral orifice by pressure of the aortic regurgitant flow on the anterior mitral leaflet. The low-pitched murmur is evident at the left ventricular apex; may be either middiastolic or presystolic.

Aus•tin Moore pros•the•sis (aw′stin mōr pros-thē′sis) Introduced in 1940, this metal hip prosthesis replaces the upper portion of the femur. It is the most commonly used type of uncemented hemiarthroplasty in treatment of displaced femoral neck fractures. [Austin Moore, 1899–1963, American orthopedist]

Aus•tra•li•an X dis•ease (aw-strā′lē-ăn di-zēz′) SYN Murray Valley encephalitis.

au•thor (aw′thŏr) MEDICAL TRANSCRIPTION person who orally creates a report to be transcribed. SYN dictator, originator.

au•thor•i•tar•i•an per•son•al•i•ty (aw-thōr′i-tār′ē-ăn pĕr-sŏn-al′i-tē) A cluster of personality traits reflecting a desire for security and order (e.g., rigidity, unquestioning obedience, scapegoating, desire for structured lines of authority).

au•thor•i•ty fig•ure (aw-thōr′i-tē fig′yŭr) A real or projected person in a position of power; parents, police, and bosses are authority figures to some people; during the transference phase of psychoanalysis, the psychoanalyst becomes an authority figure.

au•tho•ri•za•tion (aw′thŏr-ī-zā′shŭn) **1.** In health care accounting, guaranteed acceptance of a procedure or therapy and payment thereof by a third-party payer. **2.** An agreement or acknowledgement, generally written, from a patient or caregiver that records and documents may be shared among other health care providers. SEE ALSO gatekeeper.

au•tism (aw′tizm) A mental disorder characterized by severely abnormal development of social interaction and of verbal and nonverbal communication skills. Affected people may adhere to inflexible, nonfunctional rituals or routines. They may become upset with even trivial changes in their environment. They often have a limited range of interests but may become preoccupied with a narrow range of subjects or activities. They appear unable to understand others' feelings and often have poor eye contact with others. Unpredictable mood swings may occur. Many affected patients demonstrate stereotypical motor mannerisms such as hand or finger flapping, body rocking, or dipping. The disorder is probably caused by organically based central nervous system dysfunction, especially in the ability to process social or emotional information or language. [G. *autos,* self]

au·tis·tic (aw-tis′tik) Pertaining to or characterized by autism.

au·tis·tic spec·trum dis·or·der (aw-tis′tik spek′trŭm dis-ōr′dĕr) A nonspecific diagnosis of any developmental disorder characterized by poor social abilities and impaired communication.

auto-, aut- Prefixes meaning self, same. [G. *autos,* self]

au·to·ag·glu·ti·na·tion (aw′to-ă-glū′ti-nā′shŭn) **1.** Nonspecific agglutination or clumping together of cells (e.g., bacteria, erythrocytes) due to physical-chemical factors. **2.** The agglutination of red blood cells by specific autoantibody present in one's own serum.

au·to·ag·glu·ti·nin (aw′tō-ă-glū′ti-nin) An agglutinating autoantibody.

au·to·al·ler·gic (aw′tō-ă-lĕr′jik) Pertaining to autoallergy.

au·to·al·ler·gy (aw′tō-al′ĕr-jē) An altered reactivity in which antibodies (autoantibodies) are produced against an individual's own tissues, causing a destructive rather than a protective effect. SYN autoimmunity.

au·to·an·ti·body (aw′tō-an′ti-bod-ē) Antibody occurring in response to antigenic constituents of the host's tissue, and which reacts with the inciting tissue component.

au·to·an·ti·gen (aw′to-an′ti-jĕn) A "self" antigen; any tissue constituent that evokes an immune response by the host.

au·to·ca·tal·y·sis (aw′tō-kă-tal′i-sis) A reaction in which one or more of the products formed acts to catalyze the reaction; beginning slowly, the rate of such a reaction rapidly increases. Cf. chain reaction.

au·to·cat·a·lyt·ic (aw′tō-kat-ă-lit′ik) Relating to autocatalysis.

au·toch·tho·nous (aw-tok′thŏn-ŭs) **1.** Native to the place inhabited; aboriginal. **2.** Originating in the place where found; said of a disease originating in the part of the body where found, or of a disease acquired in the place where the patient is. [auto- + G. *chthon,* land, ground, country]

au·toch·tho·nous i·de·as (aw-tok′thŏn-ŭs ī-dē′ă) Thoughts that suddenly burst into awareness as if they are vitally important, often as if they have come from an outside source.

au·toch·tho·nous in·fec·tion (aw-tok′thŏ-nŭs in-fek′shŭn) Infection that has originated in the place where found; acquired in a location in which a person is located.

au·toc·la·sis, au·to·cla·si·a (aw-tok′lă-sis, aw′tō-klā′zē-ă) **1.** A breaking up or rupturing from intrinsic or internal causes. **2.** Progressive immunologically induced tissue destruction. [auto- + G. *klasis,* breaking]

au·to·clave (aw′tō-klāv) **1.** An apparatus for sterilization by steam under pressure. **2.** To sterilize in an autoclave. [auto- + L. *clavis,* a key, in the sense of self-locking]

au·to·coid (aw′tō-koyd) A chemical substance produced by one type of cell that affects the function of different types of cells in the same region, thus functioning as a local hormone or messenger. [G. *autos,* self, + *eidos,* form]

au·to·crat·ic (aw′tō-krat′ik) Exercising unlimited authority or control over the actions of a group. [G. *autokratēs,* ruling absolutely, fr. *autos* self, + krateō, to rule]

au·to·crine (aw′tō-krin) Denoting self-stimulation through cellular production of a factor and a specific receptor for it. [auto- + G. *krinō,* to separate]

au·to·crine hy·poth·e·sis (aw′tō-krin hī-poth′ĕ-sis) That tumor cells containing viral oncogenes may have encoded a growth factor, normally produced by other cell types, and thereby produce the factor autonomously, leading to uncontrolled proliferation.

au·to·cy·to·ly·sin (aw′tō-sī-tol′i-sin) SYN autolysin.

au·to·cy·tol·y·sis (aw′tō-sī-tol′i-sis) SYN autolysis.

au·to·cy·to·tox·in (aw′tō-sī-tō-toks′in) A cytotoxic autoantibody.

au·to·der·mic graft (aw′tō-dĕr′mik graft) A skin autograft.

au·to·di·ges·tion (aw′tō-di-jes′chŭn) SYN autolysis.

au·to·ech·o·la·li·a (aw′tō-ek-ō-lā′lē-ă) A morbid repetition of another person's or one's own words. [auto- + echolalia]

au·to·e·rot·ic (aw′tō-ĕr-ot′ik) Pertaining to autoerotism.

au·to·e·rot·ic death (aw′tō-ĕr-ot′ik deth) Death as a result of strangulation with a rope or cord affixed to the neck during the course of masturbation, based on the premise that the strength of the orgasm is increased somewhat by hypoxia.

au·to·er·o·tism (aw′tō-er′ō-tizm) **1.** Sexual arousal or gratification using one's own body, as in masturbation. **2.** Sexual self-love. SEE ALSO narcissism (1). Cf. alloerotism. [auto- + G. *erōtikos,* relating to love]

au·to·e·ryth·ro·cyte sen·si·ti·za·tion syn·drome (aw′tō-ĕ-rith′rō-sīt sen′si-tī-zā′shŭn sin′drōm) A condition that usually occurs primarily in women, in which the person bruises easily (purpura simplex). These bruises tend to enlarge and involve adjacent tissues, resulting in pain in the affected parts; thought to be a form of localized autosensitization. SYN Gardner-Diamond syndrome.

au·tog·a·my (aw-tog′ă-mē) A form of self-fertilization in which fission of the cell nucleus occurs without division of the cell, the two pronuclei so formed reuniting to form the synkaryon; in other cases, the cell body also divides, but the two daughter cells immediately conjugate. [auto- + G. *gamos,* marriage]

au·to·ge·ne·ic graft (aw′tō-jen-ē′ik graft) SYN autograft.

au·to·gen·ic in·hi·bi·tion (aw′tō-jen′ik in′hi-bish′ŭn) A protective mechanism of the Golgi tendon organ, whereby a sudden stretch in a muscle causes a reflexive activation of the antagonist muscle and relaxation of the agonist.

au·tog·e·nous vac·cine (aw-toj′ĕ-nŭs vak-sēn′) A vaccine made from a culture of the patient's own bacteria.

au·to·graft (aw′tō-graft) A tissue or an organ transferred by grafting into a new position in the body of the same individual. SYN autogeneic graft, autologous graft, autoplastic graft, autotransplant. [auto- + A.S. *graef*]

autohaemagglutination [Br.] SYN autohemagglutination.

autohaemolysin [Br.] SYN autohemolysin.

autohaemolysis [Br.] SYN autohemolysis.

au·to·hem·ag·glu·ti·na·tion (aw′tō-hē′mă-glū-ti-nā′shŭn) Autoagglutination of erythrocytes. SYN autohaemagglutination.

au·to·he·mo·ly·sin (aw′tō-hē-mol′i-sin) An autoantibody that causes lysis of erythrocytes in the same person in whose body the lysin is formed. SYN autohaemolysin.

au·to·he·mol·y·sis (aw′tō-hē-mol′i-sis) Hemolysis occurring in certain diseases as a result of an autohemolysin. SYN autohaemolysis.

au·to·im·mune (aw′tō-i-myūn′) Arising from and directed against the person's own tissues, as in autoimmune disease.

au·to·im·mune dis·ease (aw′tō-i-myūn′ di-zēz′) Any disorder in which loss of function or destruction of normal tissue arises from humoral or cellular immune responses of the person to her or his own tissue constituents; may be systemic, as systemic lupus erythematosus, or organ specific, as thyroiditis.

au·to·im·mune he·mo·lyt·ic a·ne·mi·a (aw′tō-i-myūn′ hē′mō-lit′ik ă-nē′mē-ă) **1.** Disorder caused by severe hemolysis in cold hemagglutinin disease. **2.** Warm antibody type: acquired hemolytic anemia due to serum autoantibodies that react with the patient's red blood cells, antigenic specificity being chiefly in the Rh complex; may be idiopathic or secondary to neoplastic, autoimmune, among others.

au·to·im·mu·ni·ty (aw′tō-i-myū′ni-tē) IMMUNOLOGY the condition in which one's own tissues are subject to deleterious effects of the immune system, as in autoallergy and in autoimmune disease; immune response against the body's own tissues. SYN autoallergy.

au·to·im·mu·ni·za·tion (aw′tō-im′yū-nī-zā′shŭn) Induction of autoimmunity.

au·to·im·mu·no·cy·to·pe·ni·a (aw′tō-im′yū-nō-sī-tō-pē′nē-ă) Anemia, thrombocytopenia, and leukopenia resulting from cytotoxic autoimmune reactions.

au·to·in·fec·tion (aw′tō-in-fek′shŭn) **1.** Reinfection by microbes or parasitic organisms on or within the body that have already passed through an infective cycle, such as a succession of boils, or a new infective cycle with production of a new generation of larvae and adults. **2.** Self-infection by direct contagion as with parasite eggs passed in the infectious state transmitted by fingernails (anal-oral route). SYN autoreinfection.

au·to·in·fu·sion (aw′tō-in-fyū′zhŭn) Forcing the blood from the extremities or other areas such as the spleen, as by the application of a bandage or pressure device, to raise the blood pressure and fill the vessels in the vital centers; resorted to after excessive loss of blood or other body fluids. Cf. autotransfusion.

au·to·in·oc·u·la·tion (aw′tō-in-ok-yū-lā′shŭn) A secondary infection originating from a focus of infection already present in the body.

au·to·in·tox·i·cant (aw′tō-in-toks′i-kănt) An endogenous toxic agent that causes autointoxication.

au·to·in·tox·i·ca·tion (aw′tō-in-toks-i-kā′shŭn) A disorder resulting from absorption of the waste products of metabolism, decomposed matter from the intestine, or the products of dead and infected tissue, as in gangrene. SYN endogenic toxicosis.

au·to·i·sol·y·sin (aw′tō-ī-sol′i-sin) An antibody that in the presence of complement causes lysis of cells in the person in whose body the lysin is formed, as well as in others of the same species.

au·to·ker·a·to·plas·ty (aw′tō-ker′ă-tō-plas-tē) Grafting of corneal tissue from one eye of a patient to the fellow eye. [auto- + G. *keras,* horn, + *plastos,* formed]

au·to·ki·ne·si·a, au·to·ki·ne·sis (aw′tō-ki-ne′sē-ă, aw′tō-ki-nē′sis) Voluntary movement. [auto- + G. *kinēsis,* movement]

au·to·ki·net·ic (aw′tō-ki-net′ik) Relating to autokinesis.

au·tol·o·gous (aw-tol′ŏ-gŭs) **1.** Occurring naturally and normally in a certain type of tissue or in a specific structure of the body. **2.** Sometimes used to denote a neoplasm derived from cells that occur normally at that site, e.g., a squamous cell carcinoma in the upper esophagus. **3.** TRANSPLANTATION referring to a graft in which the donor and recipient areas are in the same person. [auto- + G. *logos,* relation]

au·tol·o·gous do·na·tion (aw-tol′ŏ-gŭs dō-nā′shŭn) A blood transfusion or tissue graft involving one person as both donor and recipient.

au·tol·o·gous graft (aw-tol′ŏ-gŭs graft) SYN autograft.

au·tol·o·gous trans·fu·sion (aw-tol′ŏ-gŭs trans-fyū′zhŭn) Transfusion of the patient's own blood, previously drawn and stored.

au·tol·o·gous trans·plan·ta·tion (aw-tol′ŏ-gŭs trans′plan-tā′shŭn) Transplant involving one person as both donor and recipient.

au·tol·y·sate (aw-tol′i-sāt) The mixture of substances resulting from autolysis.

au·tol·y·sin (aw-tol′i-sin) An antibody that causes lysis of the cells and tissues in the body of the individual in whom the lysin is formed. SYN autocytolysin.

au·tol·y·sis (aw-tol′i-sis) **1.** Enzymatic digestion of cells (especially dead or degenerate) by enzymes present within them (autogenous). **2.** Destruction of cells as a result of a lysin formed in those cells or others in the same organism. SYN autocytolysis, autodigestion, isophagy. [auto- + G. *lysis,* dissolution]

au·to·lyt·ic (aw′tō-lit′ik) Pertaining to or causing autolysis.

au·to·lyt·ic en·zyme (aw′tō-lit′ik en′zīm) An enzyme capable of causing lysis of the cell forming it.

au·to·mat·ed de·pos·it (aw′tō-mā′tĕd dē-poz′it) SYN electronic funds transfer.

au·to·mat·ed dif·fer·en·tial leu·ko·cyte count·er (aw′tō-māt-ĕd dif′ĕr-en′shăl lū′kō-sīt kown′tĕr) An instrument using digital imaging or cytochemical techniques to differentiate leukocytes.

au·to·ma·ted dis·pens·ing ma·chine (aw′tō-māt-ĕd dis-pens′ing mă-shēn′) A device from which nursing staff can retrieve medications for patients after pharmacist review at the nursing unit.

au·to·mat·ed ex·ter·nal de·fib·ril·la·tor (AED) (aw′tō-mā-tĕd eks-tĕr′năl dē-fib′ri-lā-tŏr) Device that automatically analyzes the heart rhythm and if a problem is detected that may respond to an electric shock, permits a shock to be delivered to restore a normal heart rhythm.

au·to·mat·ed la·mel·lar ker·a·tec·to·my (aw′tō-māt-ĕd lă-mel′ăr ker-ă-tek′tō-mē) Resection of a disc of corneal tissue using a precise machine to alter the refractive power of the eye.

au·to·mat·ic au·di·to·ry brain·stem re·sponse (ABR) (aw′tō-mat′ik aw′di-tōr-ē brān′stem rĕ-spons′) A technique of ABR in which the stimulus modification is programmed based on the electrical responses recorded. The device automatically determines whether predetermined thresholds have been achieved. It is useful in screening the hearing capacity in newborns.

au·to·mat·ic beat (aw′tō-mat′ik bēt) In contrast to forced beat, an ectopic beat that arises de novo and is not precipitated by the preceding beat; thus escaped and parasystolic beats are automatic.

au·to·mat·ic ex·ter·nal de·fib·ril·la·tor (AED) (aw′tō-mat′ik eks-tĕr′năl dē-fib′ri-lā-tŏr) Device used to administer electric shock to arrest fibrillation of the atria or ventricles and restore normal heart rhythm; can be used by technicians without medical training.

au·to·mat·ic gain con·trol (AGC) (aw′tō-mat′ik gān kŏn-trōl′) A feature of some hearing aids that reduces amplification at high-input intensity levels.

au·to·mat·ic speech (aw′tō-mat′ik spēch) Overlearned or low-content language that can be produced with little awareness of meaning, such as consecutive numbers, days of the week, verses, prayers, expletives, or other common expressions. SYN nonpropositional speech.

au·to·mat·ic trans·port ven·til·a·tor (aw′tō-mat′ik trans′pōrt ven′ti-lā-tŏr) A positive-pressure ventilator that supports respiration automatically and with less need for adjustment than a standard hospital ventilator; designed for use in an ambulance to ventilate an intubated patient. SEE ALSO ventilator.

au·tom·a·tism (aw-tom′ă-tizm) **1.** The state of being independent of the will or of central innervation; applicable, for example, to the heart's action. **2.** An epileptic attack consisting of stereotyped psychic, sensory, or motor phenomena carried out in a state of impaired consciousness and of which the person usually has no knowledge. **3.** A condition in which a person is consciously or unconsciously, but involuntarily, compelled to the performance of certain motor or verbal acts, often purposeless and sometimes foolish or harmful. SYN telergy. [G. *automatos,* self-moving, + -in]

au·to·mo·tor sei·zure (aw′tō-mō′tŏr sē′zhŭr) Seizure characterized by an automatism predominantly involving the distal limbs.

au·to·nom·ic (aw′tō-nom′ik) Relating to the autonomic nervous system.

au·to·no·mic di·vi·sion of ner·vous sys·tem (aw′tō-nom′ik di-vizh′ŭn nĕr′vŭs sis′tĕm) That part of the nervous system that represents the motor innervation of smooth muscle, cardiac muscle, and gland cells. It consists of two physiologically and anatomically distinct, mutually antagonistic components: the sympathetic and parasympathetic parts. In both of these parts the pathway of innervation consists of a synaptic sequence of two motor neurons, one of which lies in the spinal cord or brainstem as the presynaptic (preganglionic) neuron, the thin but myelinated axon of which (preganglionic [presynaptic] or B fiber) emerges with an outgoing spinal or cranial nerve and synapses with one or more of the postsynaptic (postganglionic or, more strictly, ganglionic) neurons comprising the autonomic ganglia; the unmyelinated postsynaptic fibers in turn innervate the smooth muscle, cardiac muscle, or gland cells. The presynaptic neurons of the sympathetic part lie in the intermediolateral cell column of the thoracic and upper two lumbar segments of the spinal gray matter; those of the parasympathetic part comprise the visceral motor (visceral efferent) nuclei of the brainstem as well as the lateral column of the second to fourth sacral segments of the spinal cord. The ganglia of the sympathetic part are the paravertebral ganglia of the sympathetic trunk and the lumbar and sacral prevertebral or collateral ganglia; those of the parasympathetic part lie either near the organ to be innervated or as intramural ganglia within the organ itself except in the head, where there are four discrete parasympathetic ganglia (ciliary, otic, pterygopalatine, and submandibular). Impulse transmission from presynaptic to postsynaptic neuron is mediated by acetylcholine in both the sympathetic and parasympathetic parts; transmission from the postsynaptic fiber to the visceral effector tissues is classically said to be by acetylcholine in the parasympathetic part and by noradrenalin in the sympathetic part; recent evidence suggests the existence of further noncholinergic, nonadrenergic classes of postsynaptic fibers. See this page. SYN divisio autonomica systematis nervosi peripherici [TA], autonomic nervous system.

au·to·no·mic dys·re·flex·i·a (aw′tō-nom′ik

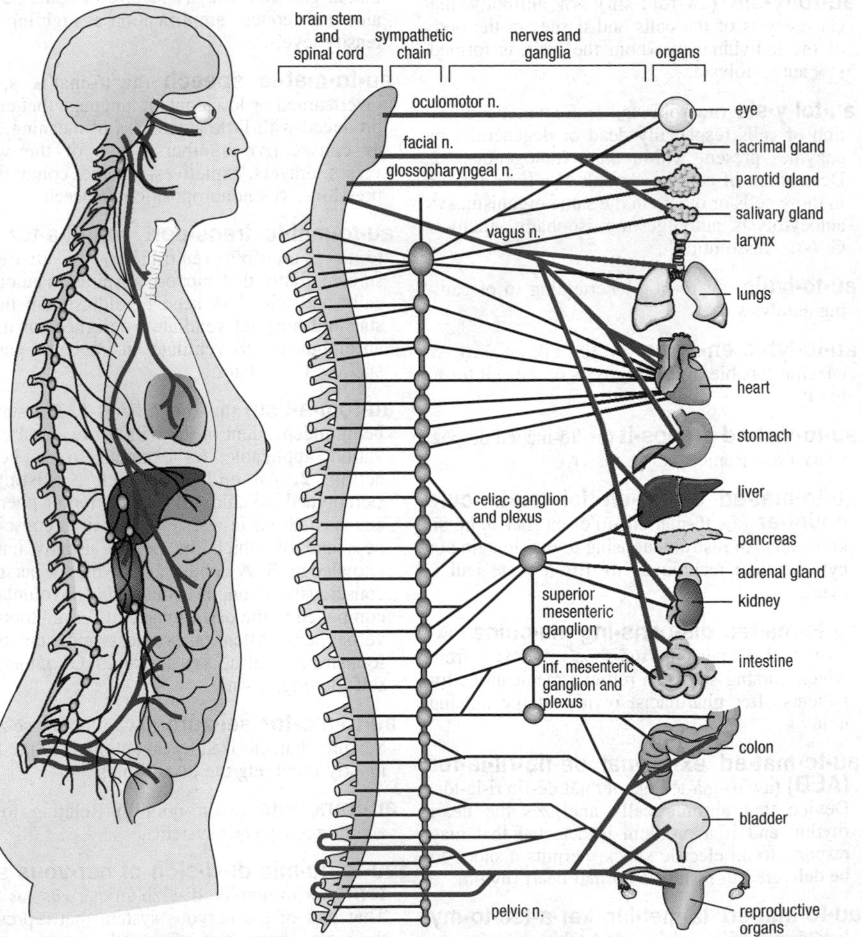

anatomy of autonomic nervous system

dis-rē-flek′sē-ă) A syndrome occurring in some people with spinal cord lesions and resulting from functional impairment of the autonomic nervous system. Symptoms include hypertension, bradycardia, severe headaches, pallor below and flushing above the cord lesion, and convulsions. SYN autonomic hyperreflexia.

au•to•nom•ic gan•gli•a (aw′tō-nom′ik gang′glē-a) Visceral ganglia. SEE autonomic division of nervous system.

au•to•nom•ic hy•per•re•flex•i•a (aw′tō-nom′ik hī′pĕr-rē-flek′sē-ă) SYN autonomic dysreflexia.

au•to•nom•ic im•bal•ance (aw′tō-nom′ik im-bal′ăns) A lack of balance between sympathetic and parasympathetic nervous systems, especially in relation to vasomotor disturbances. SYN vasomotor imbalance.

au•to•nom•ic ner•vous sys•tem (ANS) (aw′tō-nom′ik nĕr′vŭs sis′tĕm) SYN autonomic division of nervous system.

au•to•nom•ic neu•ro•gen•ic blad•der (aw′tō-nom′ik nūr-ō-jen′ik blad′ĕr) Malfunctioning urinary bladder, secondary to low spinal cord lesions.

au•to•nom•ic plex•us•es (aw′tō-nom′ik plek′sŭs-ĕz) Plexuses of nerves in relation to blood vessels and viscera, the component fibers of which are sympathetic, parasympathetic, and sensory.

au•to•nom•ic sei•zure (aw′tō-nom′ik sē′zhŭr) Seizure characterized by objectively documented dysfunction of the autonomic nervous system, usually involving cardiovascular, gastrointestinal, or sudomotor functions.

au•to•nom•ic vis•cer•al mo•tor nu•cle•i (aw′tō-nom′ik vis′ĕr-ăl mō′tŏr nū′klē-ī) Nuclei located in the spinal cord (T1–L2, S2–S4) and in the brainstem (Edinger-Westphal nucleus, superior and inferior salivatory nuclei, dorsal vagal nucleus, and parts of the ambiguus nucleus) from which general visceral efferent preganglionic fibers arise; may be sympathetic (T1–L2) or parasympathetic (craniosacral); hypothalamic nuclei (areas) function in concert with autonomic nuclei.

au•to•nom•o•tro•pic (aw′tō-nom-ō-trō′pik) Acting on the autonomic nervous system. [autonomic + G. *trepō,* to turn]

au•ton•o•my (aw-ton′ă-mē) NURSING a patient's personal independence; of being self-governing. [auto- + G. *nomos*

au•to•ox•i•da•tion (aw′tō-oks-i-dā′shŭn) The direct combination of a substance with molecular oxygen at ordinary temperatures. SYN autoxidation.

au•to-PEEP (aw′tō-pēp) Acronym for auto-positive-end-expiratory-pressure. SYN extrinsic PEEP.

au•to•pha•gi•a (aw′tō-fā′jē-ă) **1.** Biting one's own flesh; e.g., as a symptom of Lesch-Nyhan syndrome. **2.** Maintenance of the nutrition of the whole body by metabolic consumption of some of the body tissues. **3.** SYN autophagy. [auto- + G. *phagō,* to eat]

au•to•pha•gic (aw′tō-fā′jik) Relating to or characterized by autophagia.

au•toph•a•gy (aw-tof′ă-jē) Segregation and disposal of damaged organelles within a cell. SYN autophagia (3). [auto- + G. *phagō,* to eat]

au•toph•o•ny (au-tof′ŏ-nē) Undue accentuation of the sound produced by one's own voice, usually caused by a middle-ear disorder; produces the "head-in-the-barrel" sensation. [auto- + G. *phonē,* sound, voice]

au•to•plas•tic (aw′tō-plas′tik) Relating to autoplasty.

au•to•plas•tic graft (aw′tō-plas′tik graft) SYN autograft.

au•to•plas•ty (aw′tō-plas-tē) Repair of defects by autotransplantation.

au•to•pol•y•mer res•in, au•to•po•ly•mer•iz•ing res•in (aw′to-pol′i-mĕr rez′in, aw′tō-pol′i-mĕr-īz-ing rez′in) Any resin that can be polymerized by chemical catalysis rather than by the application of heat; in dentistry used in making dental restorations, denture repairs, and impression trays. SYN cold cure resin, cold-curing resin.

au•to-pos•i•tive-end-ex•pi•ra•to•ry-pres•sure (au•to-PEEP) (aw′tō-pos′i-tiv-end-eks-pīr′ă-tōr-ē presh′ŭr) The difference between expiratory alveolar pressure and end expiratory pressure at the airway opening: the pressure is associated with the trapped gas when dynamic hyperinflation occurs in the lungs. SYN intrinsic PEEP, occult PEEP.

au•top•sy (aw′top-sē) An examination of a corpse and the organs of a dead body to determine the cause of death or to study the pathologic changes present. (Colloquially called postmortem.) SYN necropsy. [G. *autopsia,* seeing with one's own eyes]

au•to•ra•di•o•graph (aw′tō-rā′dē-ō-graf) Image of the distribution and concentration of radioactivity in a tissue or other substance made by placing a photographic emulsion on the surface of, or in close proximity to, the substance.

au•to•ra•di•og•ra•phy (aw′tō-rā-dē-og′ră-fē) The process of producing an autoradiograph. SYN radioautography.

au•to•re•cep•tor (aw′tō-rĕ-sep′tŏr) A site on a neuron that binds the neurotransmitter released by that neuron, which then regulates the neuron's activity. [auto- + receptor]

au•to•reg•u•la•tion (aw′tō-reg-yū-lā′shŭn) **1.** The tendency of the blood flow to an organ or part to remain at or return to the same level despite changes in the pressure in the artery which conveys blood to it. **2.** In general, any biologic system equipped with inhibitory feedback systems such that a given change tends to be largely or completely counteracted; e.g., baroreceptor reflexes form a basis for autoregulation of the systemic arterial blood pressure.

au·to·re·in·fec·tion (aw′tō-rē-in-fek′shŭn) SYN autoinfection.

au·to·re·pro·duc·tion (aw′tō-rē-prŏ-dŭk′shŭn) The ability of a gene or virus, or nucleoprotein molecule generally, to bring about the synthesis of another molecule like itself from smaller molecules within the cell.

au·to·se·rum (aw′tō-sēr′ŭm) Serum obtained from the patient's own blood and used in autoserotherapy.

au·to·site (aw′tō-sīt) That member of abnormal, unequal conjoined twins that is able to live independently and nourish the other member (parasite) of the pair. [auto- + G. *sitos,* food]

au·to·so·mal (aw′tō-sō′măl) Pertaining to an autosome.

au·to·so·mal gene (aw′tō-sō′măl jēn) A gene located on any chromosome other than the sex chromosomes (X or Y).

au·to·some (aw′tō-sōm) Any chromosome other than a sex chromosome; autosomes normally occur in pairs in somatic cells and singly in gametes. [auto- + G. *sōma,* body]

au·to·sug·ges·tion (aw′tō-sŭg-jes′chŭn) **1.** Constant dwelling on an idea or concept, thereby inducing some change in the mental or bodily functions. **2.** Reproduction in the brain of impressions previously received which become then the starting point of new acts or ideas.

au·to·top·ag·no·si·a (aw′tō-top′ag-nō′zē-ă) Inability to recognize or to orient any part of one's own body; caused by a parietal lobe lesion. Cf. somatotopagnosis. [auto- + G. *topos,* place, + G. *a-* priv. + gnōsis]

au·to·tox·ic (aw′tō-toks′ik) Relating to autointoxication.

au·to·trans·fu·sion (aw′tō-trans-fyū′zhŭn) Withdrawal and reinjection-transfusion of the patient's own blood. Cf. autoinfusion.

au·to·trans·plant (aw′tō-trans′plant) SYN autograft.

au·to·trans·plan·ta·tion (aw′tō-trans-plan-tā′shŭn) The performance of an autograft.

au·to·troph (aw′tō-trōf) A microorganism that uses only inorganic materials as its source of nutrients; carbon dioxide serves as the sole carbon source. [auto- + G. *trophē,* nourishment]

au·to·tro·phic (aw′tō-trō′fik) **1.** Self-nourishing; the ability of an organism to produce food from inorganic compounds. **2.** Pertaining to an autotroph.

au·tox·i·da·tion (aw′tok-si-dā′shŭn) SYN autoxidation.

♻ **auxano-, auxo-, aux-** Combining forms meaning increase (e.g., in size, intensity, speed). [G. *auxanō,* to increase]

aux·an·o·gram (awk-san′ŏ-gram) A plate culture of bacteria in which variable conditions are provided to determine the effect of these conditions on the growth of the bacteria. [auxano- + G. *gramma,* something written]

aux·an·o·graph·ic (awk-san′ŏ-graf′ik) Pertaining to auxanogram or auxanography.

aux·a·nog·ra·phy (awk′să-nog′ră-fē) The study, using auxanograms, of the effects of different conditions on the growth of bacteria.

aux·e·sis (awk-sē′sis) Increase in size, especially as in hypertrophy. [G. increase]

aux·il·ia·ry (awg-zil′yă-rē) **1.** Functioning in an augmenting capacity; supplementary. **2.** Functioning as a subordinate; secondary.

aux·il·ia·ry nurse (awg-zil′yăr-ē nŭrs) SYN enrolled nurse.

aux·i·lyt·ic (awk′si-lit′ik) Increasing the destructive power of a lysin, or favoring lysis. [G. *auxō,* to increase, + *lysis,* dissolution]

aux·o·chrome (awk′sō-krōm) The chemical group within a dye molecule by which the dye is bound to reactive end groups in tissues. [auxo- + G. *chrōma,* color]

aux·o·ton·ic (awk′sō-ton′ik) Denoting the condition in which a contracting muscle shortens against an increasing load. Cf. isometric (2), isotonic (3).

aux·o·troph (awk′sō-trōf) A mutant microorganism that requires some nutrient that is not required by the organism (prototroph) from which the mutant was derived. [auxo- + G. *trophē,* nourishment]

aux·o·tro·phic (awk′sō-trō′fik) Pertaining to an auxotroph.

A-V, AV Abbreviation for arteriovenous; atrioventricular.

ava Abbreviation for arteriovenous anastomosis.

a·val·vu·lar (ā-val′vyū-lăr) Without valves; not affecting valves.

a·vas·cu·lar (ā-vas′kyū-lăr) Without blood or lymphatic vessels.

a·vas·cu·lar·i·za·tion (ā-vas′kyū-lar-ī-zā′shŭn) **1.** Expulsion of blood from a part, as by means of an Esmarch tourniquet or arterial compression. **2.** Loss of vascularity, as by scarring.

a•vas•cu•lar ne•cro•sis (ā-vas′kyū-lăr nĕ-krō′sis) SYN aseptic necrosis.

AV dif•fer•ence (dif′ĕr-ĕns) Arteriovenous (AV) difference of concentration of a substance.

A•vel•lis syn•drome (ah-vel′is sin′drōm) Unilateral paralysis of the larynx and velum palati, with contralateral loss of pain and temperature sensibility in the parts below.

av•er•age (av′răj) **1.** A value that represents or summarizes the relevant features of a set of values; it is usually computed by a mathematical manipulation of the individual values in a set. **2.** SYN arithmetic mean. [M.E. *averays*, loss from damage to ship or cargo, fr. It. *avaris*, fr. Ar. *'awariya*, damaged goods, + damage]

av•er•age life (av′ĕr-ăj līf) SYN mean life.

a•ver•sion ther•a•py (ă-vĕr′zhŭn thār′ă-pē) A form of behavior therapy that pairs an unpleasant stimulus with undesirable behavior(s) so that the patient learns to avoid the latter.

aVF, aVL, aVR Augmented electrocardiographic leads from the foot (left), left arm, and right arm, respectively.

a•vi•an (ā′vē-ăn) Pertaining to birds. [L. *avis*, bird]

a•vi•an in•flu•en•za (ā′vē-ăn in′flū-en′ză) A disease of birds due to strains of influenza A virus. Although wild birds, the natural hosts, seldom become sick when infected, avian influenza viruses can cause disease in domestic poultry and, rarely, in human beings. Transmission of the virus occurs through direct contact with an infected bird. The consequences of human infection vary from conjunctivitis and respiratory symptoms to severe systemic illness with fatal outcome. SYN bird flu.

a•vi•an leu•ko•sis-sar•co•ma com•plex, a•vi•an leu•ke•mi•a-sar•co•ma com•plex (ā′vē-ăn lū-kō′sis-sahr-kō′mă kom′pleks, lū-kē′mē-ă-sahr-kō′mă) **1.** A group of transmissible virus-induced diseases of chickens; the agents are closely related viruses (avian leukosis-sarcoma virus) causing proliferation of immature erythroid, myeloid, or lymphoid cells. **2.** A division of the RNA tumor viruses causing the avian leukosis-sarcoma complex of diseases. SYN avian leukosis-sarcoma virus.

a•vi•an leu•ko•sis-sar•co•ma vi•rus (ā′vē-ăn lū-kō′sis-sahr-kō′mă vī′rŭs) SYN avian leukosis-sarcoma complex (2).

a•vi•an neu•ro•lym•pho•ma•to•sis vi•rus (ă′vē-ăn nūr′ō-lim-fō′mă-tō′sis vī′rŭs) The herpesvirus that causes avian lymphomatosis (Marek disease); is distinct from those causing other forms of leukosis. SYN Marek disease virus.

a•vi•a•tion med•i•cine (ā′vē-ā′shŭn med′i-sin) The study and practice of medicine as it applies to physiologic problems peculiar to aviation. SYN aeromedicine.

a•vid•i•ty (ă-vid′i-tē) A measure of the binding strength of a multivalent antibody to a multivalent antigen. SEE ALSO affinity.

AV in•ter•val (in′tĕr-văl) The time from the beginning of atrial systole to the beginning of ventricular systole as measured from pressure pulses or cardiac volume curves in animals, or from the electrocardiogram in humans.

a•vir•u•lent (ā-vir′yū-lĕnt) Not virulent.

a•vi•ta•min•o•sis (ā-vī′tă-min-ō′sis) Properly, hypovitaminosis.

AV junc•tion (jŭngk′shŭn) Imprecisely defined zone surrounding and including the AV node and the adjacent atrial and ventricular myocardium.

AV junc•tion•al rhythm (jŭngk′shŭn-ăl ridh′ŭm) SYN atrioventricular junctional rhythm.

AV node (nōd) Abbreviation for atrioventricular node.

Avo•gad•ro con•stant (ah-vō-gahd′rō kon′stănt) SYN Avogadro number.

Avo•gad•ro hy•poth•e•sis (ah-vō-gahd′rō hī-poth′ĕ-sis) SYN Avogadro law.

Avo•gad•ro law (ah-vō-gahd′rō law) Equal volumes of gases contain equal numbers of molecules, the conditions of pressure and temperature being the same. SYN Ampère postulate, Avogadro hypothesis, Avogadro postulate.

Avo•gad•ro num•ber (N_A, lamb•da) (ah-vō-gahd′rō nŭm′bĕr) The number of molecules in 1 gram-molecular weight (1 mol) of any compound; defined as the number of atoms in 0.0120 kg of pure carbon-12; equivalent to 6.0221367×10^{23}. SYN Avogadro constant.

Avo•gad•ro pos•tu•late (ah-vō-gahd′rō pos′chū-lāt) SYN Avogadro law.

avoid•ant per•son•al•i•ty (ă-voyd′ănt pĕr-sŏn-al′i-tē) A personality characterized by a hypersensitivity to potential rejection, humiliation, or shame, an unwillingness to enter into relationships without unusually strong guarantees of uncritical acceptance, social withdrawal in spite of a desire for affection and acceptance, and low self-esteem.

av•oir•du•pois (av′wahr-dyū-pwah′) A system of weights in which 16 oz make a pound, equivalent of 453.59237 g. See Weights and Measures appendix. [Fr. to have weight, corrupted fr. O. Fr. *avoir*, property, + *de*, of, + *pois*, weight]

AVP Abbreviation for antiviral protein; arginine vasopressin.

AVPU Abbreviation and mnemonic for prehospital assessment of mental status. Refers to assessments: alert; responsive to verbal stimuli; responsive to painful stimuli; and unresponsive.

a•vulse (ă-vŭls′) To separate or tear away a body part as from an accident or surgery. [L. *a vello, pp. a vulsus,* to tear away]

a•vulsed tooth (ă-vŭlst′ tūth) A tooth that has been separated from the alveolus, generally by traumatic action.

a•vulsed wound (ă-vŭlst′ wūnd) A wound caused by or resulting from avulsion.

a•vul•sion (ă-vŭl′shŭn) A tearing away or forcible separation. Cf. evulsion. [L. *a-vello,* pp. *-vulsus,* to tear away]

a•vul•sion frac•ture (ă-vŭl′shŭn frak′shŭr) A fracture that occurs when a joint capsule, ligament, or muscle insertion of origin is pulled from the bone as a result of a sprain, dislocation, or strong contracture of the muscle against resistance; as the soft tissue is pulled away from the bone, a fragment or fragments of the bone may come away with it. See page B25.

AW Abbreviation for atomic weight.

A/W Abbreviation for alive and well.

AWHONN Abbreviation for Association of Women's Health, Obstetric, and Neonatal Nurses.

ax Abbreviation for axis.

A•xen•feld a•nom•a•ly (ahks′en-felt ă-nom′ă-lē) SYN embryotoxon.

a•xe•nic (ā-zen′ik) Sterile, denoting especially a pure culture (e.g., a protozoan culture uncontaminated by bacteria). Also used to denote "germ-free" animals born and raised in a sterile environment. [G. *a-* priv. + *xenos,* foreign]

ax•es (ak′sēz) Plural of axis.

ax•es of Fick (ak′sēz fik) Three axes that pass through the center of the eye vertically (Z), horizontally in the coronal plane (X), and horizontally in the sagittal plane (Y). All ocular rotations can be described by rotation along one of these axes.

ax•i•al (ak′sē-ăl) **1.** Relating to an axis. SYN axialis, axile. **2.** Relating to or situated in the central part of the body, in the head and trunk as distinguished from the limbs, e.g., axial skeleton. **3.** DENTISTRY relating to or parallel with the long axis of a tooth.

ax•i•al an•gle (ak′sē-ăl ang′gĕl) An angle formed by two surfaces of a body, the line of union of which is parallel with its axis; the axial angles of a tooth are the distobuccal, distolabial, distolingual, mesiobuccal, mesiolabial, and mesiolingual.

ax•i•al cur•rent (ak′sē-ăl kŭr′rĕnt) The central rapidly moving portion of the bloodstream in an artery.

ax•i•al fil•a•ment (ak′sē-ăl fil′ă-mĕnt) The central filament of a flagellum or cilium; with the electron microscope it is seen as a complex of nine peripheral diplomicrotubules and a central pair of microtubules. SYN axoneme (2).

ax•i•al hy•per•o•pi•a (ak′sē-ăl hī′pĕr-ō′pē-ă) Hyperopia due to shortening of the anteroposterior diameter of the globe of the eye.

ax•i•al im•age (ak′sē-ăl im′ăj) RADIOLOGY a view obtained by rotating around the axis of the body, producing a transverse planar image, i.e., a section transverse to the axis.

ax•i•a•lis (ak′sē-ā′lis) SYN axial (1).

ax•i•al load•ing (ak′sē-ăl lōd′ing) Application of weight or force along the course of the long axis of the body.

ax•i•al mus•cle (ak′sē-ăl mŭs′ĕl) One of the skeletal muscles of the trunk or head.

ax•i•al pat•tern flap (ak′sē-ăl pat′ĕrn flap) A flap that includes a direct specific artery within its longitudinal axis.

ax•i•al plate (ak′sē-ăl plāt) The primitive streak of an embryo.

ax•i•al point (ak′sē-ăl poynt) SYN nodal point.

ax•i•al skel•e•ton (ak′sē-ăl skel′ĕ-tŏn) Articulated bones of head and vertebral column, i.e., head and trunk, as opposed to the appendicular skeleton, the articulated bones of the upper and lower limbs. See this page.

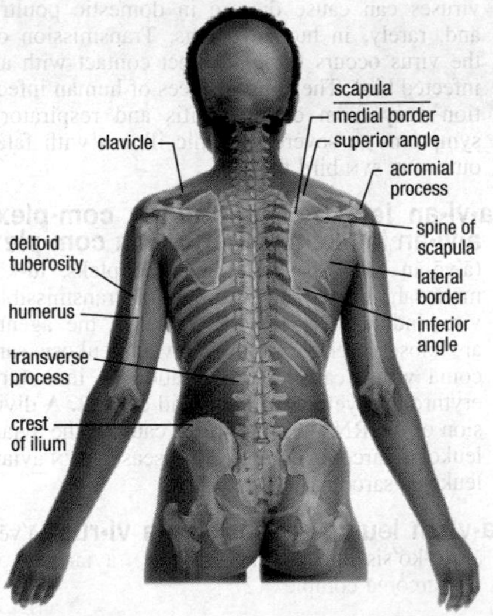

axial skeleton

ax•if•u•gal (ak-sif′yū-găl) Extending away from an axis or axon. SYN axofugal. [L. *axis* + *fugio,* to flee from]

ax•ile (ak′sīl) SYN axial (1).

ax·il·la, gen. and pl. **ax·il·lae** (ak-sil'ă, ak-sil'ē) The space below the shoulder joint, bounded by the pectoralis major anteriorly, the latissimus dorsi posteriorly, the serratus anterior medially, and the humerus laterally; it has a superior opening between the clavicle, scapula, and first rib (cervicoaxillary canal), and an inferior opening covered by the axillary fascia; it contains the axillary artery and vein, the infraclavicular part of the brachial plexus, axillary lymph nodes and vessels, and areolar tissue. SYN axillary cavity. [L.]

ax·il·lar·y (ak'sil-ār-ē) Relating to the axilla. SYN alar (2).

ax·il·lar·y ar·ter·y (ak'sil-ār-ē ahr'tĕr-ē) The continuation of the subclavian artery after crossing the first rib to enter the axilla; becomes the brachial artery upon passing the inferior border of the teres major muscle. It is accompanied by the cords of the brachial plexus, and is enclosed with them and the axillary vein in the axillary sheath as it traverses the axilla. Three parts of the axillary artery are described: proximal, posterior, and distal to the pectoralis minor muscle. *Branches:* 1st part—superior thoracic artery; 2nd part—thoracoacromial arterial trunk, lateral thoracic artery; 3rd part—subscapular artery, anterior and posterior humeral circumflex arteries. SYN arteria axillaris [TA].

ax·il·lar·y cav·i·ty (ak'sil-ār-ē kav'i-tē) SYN axilla.

ax·il·lar·y hair (ak'sil-ār-ē hār) Hair of the armpit.

ax·il·lar·y lymph nodes (ak'si-lār-rē limf nōdz) Numerous nodes around the axillary veins that receive the lymphatic drainage from the upper limb, scapular region, and pectoral region (including mammary glands); they drain into the subclavian trunk.

ax·il·lar·y nerve (ak'sil-ār-ē nĕrv) Arises from the posterior cord of the brachial plexus in the axilla, passes laterally and posteriorly through quadrangular space with the posterior circumflex artery, winding round the surgical neck of the humerus to supply the deltoid and teres minor muscles, terminating as the superior lateral brachial cutaneous nerve. SYN nervus axillaris [TA].

ax·il·lar·y thor·a·cot·o·my (ak'sil-ār-ē thōr'ă-kot'ŏ-mē) Lateral thoracotomy placed below the axillary hairline; may be transverse or vertical.

ax·il·lar·y vein (ak'sil-ār-ē vān) A continuation of the basilic and brachial veins running from the lower border of the teres major muscle to the outer border of the first rib where it becomes the subclavian vein.

♻ **axio-** Prefix meaning an axis. SEE ALSO axo-. [L. *axis*]

ax·i·o·plasm (ak'sē-ō-plazm) SYN axoplasm.

ax·i·o·pul·pal (ak'sē-ō-pŭl'păl) Referring to the line angle formed by the junction of an axial and pulpal wall of a tooth cavity.

ax·i·o·ver·sion (ak'sē-ō-vĕr'zhŭn) Abnormal inclination of the long axis of a tooth.

ax·ip·e·tal (ak-sip'ĕ-tăl) SYN centripetal (2). [L. *axis* + *peto,* to seek]

ax·is (ax), pl. **ax·es** (ak'sis, ak'sēz) **1.** A straight line joining two opposing poles of a spheric body, about which the body may revolve. **2.** The central line of the body or any of its parts. **3.** The vertebral column. **4.** The central nervous system. **5.** The second cervical vertebra. SYN epistropheus, vertebra C2, vertebra dentata. **6.** An artery that divides, immediately on its origin, into a number of branches, e.g., celiac axis. SEE trunk. [L. axle, axis]

ax·is de·vi·a·tion (ak'sis dē-vē-ā'shŭn) Deflection of the electrical axis of the heart to the right or left of the normal. SEE ALSO axis. SYN axis shift.

ax·is shift (ak'sis shift) SYN axis deviation.

ax·is-trac·tion for·ceps (aks'is-trak'shŭn fōr'seps) Obstetric forceps provided with a second handle so attached that traction can be made in the line in which the head must move in the axis of the pelvis.

♻ **axo-** Prefix meaning axis; axion. [G. *axōn,* axis]

ax·o·ax·on·ic (ak'sō-ak-son'ik) Relating to synaptic contact between the axon of one nerve cell and that of another. SEE synapse.

ax·o·den·drit·ic (ak'sō-den-drit'ik) Pertaining to the synaptic relationship of an axon with a dendrite of another neuron. SEE synapse.

ax·of·u·gal (ak-sof'yū-găl) SYN axifugal. [axo- + L. *fugio,* to flee]

ax·o·lem·ma (ak'sō-lem'ă) The plasma membrane of the axon. SYN Mauthner sheath. [axo- + G. *lemma,* husk]

ax·ol·y·sis (ak-sol'i-sis) Destruction or dissolution of a nerve axon. [axo- + G. *lysis,* dissolution]

ax·on (ak'son) The single process of a nerve cell that under normal conditions conducts nervous impulses away from the cell body and its remaining processes (dendrites). Axons 0.5 mcm thick or thicker are generally enveloped by a segmented myelin sheath provided by oligodendroglia cells (in brain and spinal cord) or Schwann cells (in peripheral nerves). Nerve cells synaptically transmit impulses to other nerve cells or to effector cells (muscle cells, gland cells) exclusively by way of the synaptic terminals of their axons. [G. *axōn,* axis]

ax·o·nal (ak'sō-năl) Pertaining to an axon.

ax·o·neme (ak'sō-nēm) **1.** The central thread

running in the axis of the chromosome. **2.** SYN axial filament. **3.** The distinctive array of microtubules in the core of eukaryotic cilia and flagella comprising a central pair surrounded by a sheaf of nine doublet microtubules. [axo- + G. *nēma,* a thread]

ax•on hil•lock (ak′son hil′lok) The conic area of origin of the axon from the nerve cell body; it contains parallel arrays of microtubules and is devoid of Nissl substance.

ax•on•og•ra•phy (ak′sŏ-nog′ră-fē) The recording of electrical changes in axons.

ax•on•ot•me•sis (ak′son-ot-mē′sis) Interruption of the axons of a nerve followed by complete degeneration of the peripheral segment, without severance of the supporting structure of the nerve; such a lesion may result from pinching, crushing, or prolonged pressure. SEE ALSO neurapraxia, neurotmesis. [axon + G. *tmēsis,* a cutting]

ax•on ter•mi•nals (ak′son tĕr′mi-nălz) The somewhat enlarged, often club-shaped endings by which axons make synaptic contacts with other nerve cells or with effector cells (muscle or gland cells). Axon terminals contain neurotransmitters of various kinds, sometimes more than one. SEE ALSO synapse. SYN end-feet, neuropodia, terminal boutons, boutons terminaux.

ax•op•e•tal (ak-sop′ĕ-tăl) Extending in a direction toward an axon. [axo- + L. *peto,* to seek]

ax•o•plasm (ak′sō-plazm) Neuroplasm of the axon. SYN axioplasm.

ax•o•plas•mic trans•port (ak′sō-plaz′mik trans′pōrt) Transport by way of flow of axoplasm toward cell soma (retrograde) or toward axon terminal (anterograde).

ax•o•so•mat•ic (ak′sō-sō-mat′ik) Relating to the synaptic relationship of an axon with a nerve cell body. SEE synapse. [axo- + G. *sōma,* body]

A•yer•za syn•drome (ah-yer′sah sin′drōm) Sclerosis of the pulmonary arteries in chronic cor pulmonale; associated with severe cyanosis, it is a condition resembling polycythemia vera but resulting from primary pulmonary arteriosclerosis or primary pulmonary hypertension and characterized by plexiform lesions of arterioles.

A•yur•ve•dic med•i•cine (ī′yŭr-ved′ik med′ĭ-sin) A system of alternative medicine that uses herbs, aromatherapy, music therapy, massage, yoga, and other measures; places equal emphasis on mind, body, and spirit. [Sansk. *āyurveda,* science of life, fr. *āyur,* life, + *veda,* knowledge]

a•ze•o•trope (ā′zē-ō-trōp) A mixture of two or more liquids that boils without change in proportion of the liquids, either in the liquid or the vapor phase. [G. *a-* priv. + *zeō,* to boil, + *tropos,* a turning]

a•ze•o•tro•pic (ā′zē-ō-trō′pik) Denoting or characteristic of an azeotrope.

az•i•do•thy•mi•dine (az′i-dō-thī′mi-dēn) SEE zidovudine.

az•i•muth re•so•lu•tion (az′i-mūth rez′ŏ-lū′shŭn) Ability to determine spatial distance between two objects that emit or reflect sound; important in the description of ability of ultrasound beam to differentiate two objects closely placed. SYN elevation resolution. [Ar. *as-samt,* compass bearing, fr. L. *semita,* path]

♻ **azo-** Prefix denoting the presence in a molecule of the group ≡C–N=N–C≡. Cf. diazo-. [Fr. *azote,* nitrogen]

az•ole (az′ōl) SYN pyrrole.

a•zo•o•sper•mi•a (ā′zō-ō-spĕr′mē-ă) Absence of living sperms in the semen; failure of spermatogenesis. [G. *a-* priv. + *zōon,* animal, + *sperma,* seed]

az•o•pro•tein (ā′zō-prō′tēn) Any of the modified proteins produced by treatment with diazonium derivatives of various aromatic amines; used to elicit antibody formation and demonstrate antibody specificity.

azotaemia [Br.] SYN azotemia.

azotaemic [Br.] SYN azotemic.

az•o•te•mi•a (ā′zō-tē′mē-ă) SYN uremia. SYN azotaemia. [azo- (azote) + G. *haima,* blood]

az•o•tem•ic (ā′zō-tēm′ik) Relating to azotemia. SYN azotaemic.

a•zo•tu•ri•a (az′ō-tyūr′ē-ă) An increased elimination of urea in the urine. [azo- (azote) + G. *ouron,* urine]

az•ure (azh′ŭr) A term for a group of basic blue methylthionine or phenothiazine dyes; used as biologic stains, especially in blood and nuclear stains.

az•ure lu•nules of nails (azh′ŭr lūn′yūlz nālz) Bluish, nonblanching discoloration of the lunules of all the fingernails, in hepatolenticular degeneration.

az•u•res•in (azh′ū-rez′in) A complex of azure A and carbacrylic resin; used as an indicator for the detection of gastric achlorhydria without intubation.

az•u•ro•phil, az•u•ro•phile (azh′ŭr-ō-fil, -fīl) Staining readily with an azure dye, denoting especially the hyperchromatin and reddish-purple granules (i.e., azurophilic granules) of certain blood cells. [azure + G. *philos,* fond]

az•y•go•gram (az′i-gō-gram) Radiographic demonstration of the azygos venous system after injection of contrast medium. [azygos + G. *gramma,* a writing]

az•y•gog•ra•phy (az′i-gog′ră-fē) Radiography

of the azygos venous system after injection of contrast medium.

az·y·gos (az′i-gŏs) **1.** An unpaired (azygous) anatomic structure. **2.** SYN azygos vein. [G. *a*- priv. + *zygon,* a yoke]

az·y·gos lobe of right lung (az′i-gŏs lōb rīt lŭng) A small accessory lobe sometimes formed superior to the hilum of the right lung; separated from the rest of the upper lobe by a deep groove lodging the azygos vein.

az·y·gos vein (az′i-gŏs vān) Arises from the merger of the right ascending lumbar vein with the right subcostal vein and often a communication with the inferior vena cava; ascends through the aortic hiatus of the diaphragm or its right crus; it runs along the right side of the thoracic vertebral bodies in the posterior mediastinum, and terminates by arching anteriorly over the root of the right lung to enter the posterior aspect of the superior vena cava. SYN azygos (2).

az·y·gous (az′i-gŭs) Unpaired; single. [G. *azygos*]

β– Symbol for electron.

β (bā′tă) SEE beta.

β+ Symbol for positron.

B **1.** Abbreviation for boron; aspartic acid; bromouridine; second substrate in a multisubstrate enzyme-catalyzed reaction. **2.** As a subscript, refers to barometric pressure.

b **1.** Abbreviation used as a subscript to refer to blood. **2.** Abbreviation for twice. [L. *bis*]

Ba Symbol for barium.

bab•bit (bab′it) Metal alloy material used in preparing dental fillings.

Ba•be•si•a (bă-bē′zē-ă) The most important genus of the family Babesiidae; characterized by multiplication in host red blood cells to form pairs and tetrads. It causes babesiosis (piroplasmosis) in most types of domestic animals, and two species cause disease in splenectomized or normal people. Vectors are ixodid or argasid ticks.

Ba•be•si•a mi•cro•ti (bă-bē′zē-ă mī′krō-tī) A malarialike protozoan naturally parasitizing certain rodents; several human cases have been reported from the islands of Nantucket and Martha's Vineyard and nearby coastal New England. The local tick vector is *Ixodes scapularis*, the numbers and infection levels of which have greatly increased in parallel with the increase in the deer population, which serves as an abundant blood source for *I. scapularis*. SEE ALSO *Borrelia burgdorferi*.

ba•be•si•o•sis (bă-bē′zē-ō′sis) An infectious disease caused by a species of *Babesia*, transmitted by ticks. Animal hosts include cattle, sheep, deer, and dogs. Subclinical human infection may be common but symptomatic disease occurs only sporadically and in limited geographic distribution. Immunodeficient and asplenic people are at higher risk of infection. Clinical features of the disease include fever, chills, and hemolysis with hemoglobinuria and jaundice. Severe disease may be complicated by cardiac and renal failure, respiratory distress syndrome, and CNS involvement. As in animals, human morbidity and mortality increase with age.

Ba•bès nodes (bah′besh nōdz) Collections of lymphocytes in the central nervous system found in rabies.

Ba•bin•ski phe•nom•e•non (bă-bin′skē fe-nom′ĕ-non) SYN Babinski sign (1).

Ba•bin•ski sign (bă-bin′skē sīn) **1.** Extension of the great toe and abduction of the other toes instead of the normal flexion reflex to plantar stimulation, considered indicative of pyramidal tract involvement ("positive" Babinski); SYN Babinski phenomenon, paradoxic extensor reflex. **2.** In hemiplegia, weakness of the platysma muscle on the affected side, as is evident in such actions as blowing or opening the mouth. **3.** When the patient is lying supine with arms crossed on the front of the chest, and attempts to assume the sitting posture, the thigh on the side of an *organic* paralysis is flexed and the heel raised, whereas the limb on the sound side remains flat. **4.** In hemiplegia, the forearm on the affected side turns to a pronated position when placed in a position of supination.

Ba•bin•ski syn•drome (bă-bin′skē sin′drōm) The combination of cardiac, arterial, and central nervous system manifestations of late syphilis.

ba•by (bā′bē) **1.** An infant; a newborn child. **2.** Colloquially, in some usages, the younger child.

Ba•by Doe law (bā′bē dō law) General term for those regulations intended to protect children with handicaps or disability from mistreatment related to withholding of nourishment, warmth, and medical care.

ba•by fat (bā′bē fat) **1.** Colloquial term for obesity in children or young adolescents that presumably will disappear with age. **2.** Obesity in postpartum women.

ba•by tooth (bā′bē tūth) SYN deciduous tooth.

bac•cate (bak′āt) Berrylike. [L. *bacca,* berry]

bac•ci•form (bak′si-fōrm) Berry-shaped. [L. *bacca,* berry]

Bach•e•lor of Phar•ma•cy (Phar.B.) (bach′ĕ-lŏr fahr′mă-sē) An undergraduate academic degree in the field of pharmacy that has now largely been supplanted in the U.S. by the Pharm.D (q.v.).

bach•e•lor's but•ton (bach′ĕ-lŏrz but′ŏn) SYN feverfew.

Bach•e•lor of Sci•ence de•gree in Nurs•ing (BSN) (bach′ĕ-lŏr sī′ĕns dĕ-grē′ nŭrs′ing) A degree conferred at completion of a full academic course (usually 8 semesters) of professional training in nursing.

Bach flow•er rem•e•dies (bahk flow′ĕr rem′ĕ-dēz) Developed by the English physician Edward Bach, these modalities are thought useful by some practitioners to rebalance one's emotional state to reduce stress on the body.

Ba•cil•la•ce•ae (bă-si-lā′sē-ē) A family of aerobic or facultatively anaerobic, sporeforming, ordinarily motile bacteria (order Eubacteriales) containing gram-positive rods. Some species are pathogenic. Ordinarily two genera, *Bacillus* and *Clostridium*, are included. The type genus is *Bacillus*.

bacillaemia [Br.] SYN bacillemia.

ba•cil•lar, **bac•il•la•ry** (bas′i-lăr, bas′i-lār-ē) Shaped like a rod; consisting of rods or rodlike elements.

bac•il•la•ry an•gi•o•ma•to•sis (bas′i-lār-ē an′

jē-ō-mă-tō′sis) An infection of immunocompromised patients by the rickettsial species *Bartonella henselae*, characterized by fever and granulomatous cutaneous nodules, and peliosis hepatis in some cases. Skin biopsy shows vascular proliferation and infiltration of vessel walls by neutrophils and clumps of organisms seen with Warthin-Starry silver staining.

bac•il•la•ry dys•en•ter•y (bas′i-lār-ē dis′ĕn-ter′ē) Infection with *Shigella dysenteriae, S. flexneri*, or other organisms.

ba•cil•le Cal•mette-Gué•rin (BCG) (bah-sēl′ kahl-met′gā-rin[h]′) An attenuated strain of *Mycobacterium bovis* used in the preparation of BCG vaccine, which is used for immunization against tuberculosis and leprosy and in cancer chemotherapy. SYN Calmette-Guérin bacillus. [Fr.]

bac•il•le•mi•a (bas-i-lē′mē-ă) The presence of gram-negative or gram-positive rod-shaped bacteria in the circulating blood. SYN bacillaemia. [bacillus + G. *haima,* blood]

ba•cil•li (bă-sil′ī) Plural of bacillus.

ba•cil•li•form (ba-sil′i-fōrm) Rod-shaped. [L. *bacillus,* a rod, + *forma,* form]

ba•cil•lin (ba-sil′in) An antibiotic substance produced by *Bacillus subtilis*.

bac•il•lo•sis (bas-i-lō′sis) A general infection with bacilli.

bac•il•lu•ri•a (bas-il-yūr′ē-ă) The presence of gram-negative or gram-positive bacilli in the urine. [bacillus + G. *ouron,* urine]

Ba•cil•lus (bă-sil′ŭs) A genus of aerobic or facultatively anaerobic, spore-forming, ordinarily motile bacteria (family Bacillaceae) containing gram-positive rods. Motile cells are peritrichous; spores are thick-walled and stain poorly with Gram stain; these organisms are chemoheterotrophic and are found primarily in soil. A few species are animal pathogens; some species evoke antibody production. The type species is *Bacillus subtilis*. [L. dim. of *baculus,* rod, staff]

ba•cil•lus, pl. **ba•cil•li** (bă-sil′ŭs, bă-sil′ī) **1.** A term used to refer to any member of the genus *Bacillus*. **2.** Term used to refer to any rod-shaped bacterium. [L. dim. of *baculus,* a rod, staff]

Ba•cil•lus ce•re•us (bă-sil′ŭs sĕr-ē′ŭs) A species that causes an emetic type and a diarrheal type of food poisoning in humans and can cause infections in humans and other mammals.

Ba•cil•lus cir•cu•lans (bă-sil′ŭs sĕr-kyū′lanz) A bacterial species found in soil that has been incriminated in human infections including septicemia, mixed abscess infections, and wound infections.

Ba•cil•lus pu•mil•is (bă-sil′ŭs pū-mil′is) A usually saprophytic species of bacteria that has been associated with food poisoning and rarely with abscess or bowel fistula formation.

Ba•cil•lus sphae•ri•cus (bă-sil′ŭs sfē-rik′ŭs) A bacterial species that is an insect pathogen and has been associated with human and other mammalian infections, especially in compromised hosts.

back•ache (bak′āk) Nonspecific term used to describe back pain; generally refers to pain below the cervical level.

back•board splint (bak′bōrd splint) A long, wide splint with slots for fixation by straps to immobilize a supine patient; most often used to stabilize suspected spinal injury.

back•bone (bak′bōn) SYN vertebral column.

back•cross (bak′kraws) Mating of an individual heterozygous at one or more loci to an individual homozygous at the same loci.

back-ex•trap•o•la•tion (bak′eks-trap′ō-lā′ shŭn) A process to determine the onset of exhalation during the forced expiratory vital capacity maneuver; excessive back extrapolation volume (usually expressed as a percentage of the forced vital capacity) is an indication of hesitation or false starting.

back•flow (bak′flō) The reversal of the normal flow of a current. SEE ALSO regurgitation.

back•ground ra•di•a•tion (bak′grownd rā′dē-ā′shŭn) Irradiation from environmental sources, including the earth's crust, the atmosphere, cosmic rays, and ingested radionuclides in the body.

back la•bor (bak lā′bŏr) A condition of pregnancy related to the malpresentation of the fetal head against the maternal sacrum, which causes acute back pain in the mother. SYN posterior presentation.

back pres•sure (bak presh′ŭr) Pressure exerted upstream in the circulation as a result of obstruction to forward flow, as when congestion in the pulmonary circulation results from stenosis of the mitral valve or failure of the left ventricle.

back•pro•jec•tion (bak′prŏ-jek′shŭn) In computed tomography or other imaging techniques requiring reconstruction from multiple projections, an algorithm for calculating the contribution of each voxel of the structure to the measured ray data, to generate an image; the oldest and simplest method of image reconstruction.

back•scat•ter (bak′skat-ĕr) Deflection of diagnostic radiation at angles exceeding 90 degrees to the direction of the beam.

back ta•ble pro•ce•dure (bak tā′bĕl prŏ-sē′ jŭr) Operation performed on an organ that has been removed from a patient before it is replaced.

back•track•ing (bak′trak-ing) The backward movement of RNA polymerase along the DNA template to a state more stable than that encountered when some base pairs disrupt the attachment of the 3′ end from the active transcription site.

back•ward heart fail•ure (bak′wărd hahrt fāl′yūr) A concept that maintains that the phenomena of congestive heart failure result from passive engorgement of the veins caused by a "backward" rise in pressure proximal to the failing cardiac chambers. Cf. forward heart failure.

Ba•con a•no•scope (bā′kŏn ā′nō-skōp) An instrument resembling a rectal speculum, with a long slit on one side and a light source opposite.

bacteraemia [Br.] SYN bacteremia.

bac•te•re•mi•a (bak′tĕr-ē′mē-ă) The presence of viable bacteria in the circulating blood; may be transient following trauma such as dental or other iatrogenic manipulation or may be persistent or recurrent as a result of infection. SYN bacteraemia, bacteriemia. [bacteria + G. *haima*, blood]

bac•te•ri•a (bak-tēr′ē-ă) Plural of bacterium. See this page.

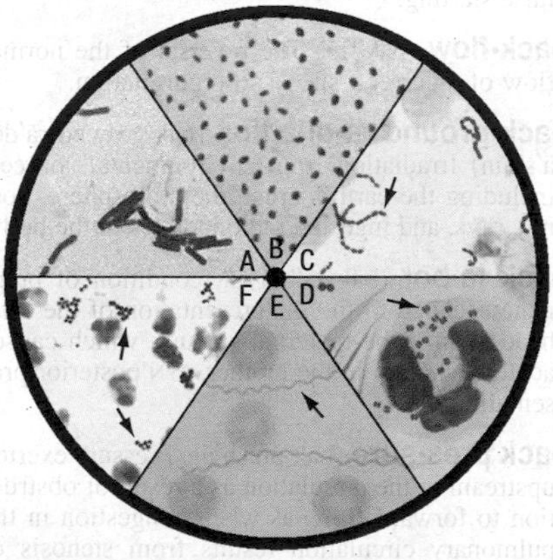

bacteria: (A) ***Bacillus sp.,*** malachite green spore stain; (B) ***Brucella melitensis***, short gram-negative bacilli in a broth culture; (C) **streptococci**, gram-positive cocci in chains, blood culture broth; (D) **diplococci**, smear of urethral exudate showing intracellular gram-negative diplococci *(Neisseria gonorrhoeae)*; (E) **spirochetes**, *Borrelia recurrentis* in a peripheral blood smear; (F) ***Staphylococcus aureus***, gram-positive cocci in clusters with neutrophils, smear of pus

bacteriaemia [Br.] SYN bacteriemia.

bac•te•ri•al (bak-tēr′ē-ăl) Relating to bacteria.

bac•te•ri•al cap•sule (bak-tēr′ē-ăl kap′sūl) A layer of slime of variable composition that covers the surface of some bacteria; capsulated cells of pathogenic bacteria are usually more virulent than cells without capsules because the former are more resistant to phagocytic action.

bac•te•ri•al end•ar•ter•i•tis (bak-tēr′ē-ăl end′ahr-tĕr-ī′tis) Implantation and growth of bacteria with formation of vegetations on the arterial wall, such as may occur in a patent ductus arteriosus or arteriovenous fistula.

bac•te•ri•al en•do•car•di•tis (bak-tēr′ē-ăl en′dō-kahr-dī′tis) Condition caused by the direct invasion of bacteria and leading to deformity and destruction of the valve leaflets. Two types are acute bacterial endocarditis and subacute bacterial endocarditis.

bac•te•ri•al food poi•son•ing (bak-tēr′ē-ăl fūd poy′zŏn-ing) A term commonly used to refer to conditions limited to enteritis or gastroenteritis (excluding the enteric fevers and the dysenteries) caused by bacterial multiplication itself or by a soluble bacterial exotoxin.

bac•te•ri•al in•fec•tion (bak-tēr′ē-ăl in-fek′shŭn) Generalized term for any internal or external disorder resulting from any bacterium.

bac•te•ri•al plaque (bak-tēr′ē-ăl plak) DENTISTRY a mass of filamentous microorganisms and large variety of smaller forms attached to the surface of a tooth that, depending on bacterial activity and environmental factors, may give rise to caries, calculus, or inflammatory changes in adjacent tissue. SYN dental plaque (2).

bac•te•ri•al trans•lo•ca•tion (bak-tēr′ē-ăl tranz-lō-kā′shŭn) The movement of bacteria or bacterial products across the intestinal membrane to emerge either in the lymphatics or the visceral circulation.

bac•te•ri•al vag•in•o•sis (bak-tēr′ē-ăl vaj′i-nō′sis) Infection of the vagina apparently caused by *Gardnerella vaginalis* and other anaerobes. Characterized by excessive, sometimes malodorous, discharge.

bac•te•ri•al vi•rus (bak-tēr′ē-ăl vī′rŭs) A virus that "infects" bacteria; a bacteriophage.

bac•te•ri•cid•al (bak-tēr′i-sī′dăl) Causing the death of bacteria. Cf. bacteriostatic.

bac•te•ri•cide (bak-tēr′i-sīd) An agent that destroys bacteria. [bacteria + L. *caedo,* to kill]

bac•te•ri•cid•in (bak-tēr′i-sī′din) An antibody that kills bacteria in the presence of complement.

bac•ter•id (bak′tĕr-id) **1.** A recurrent or persistent eruption of discrete sterile pustules of the palms and soles, thought to be an allergic response to bacterial infection at a remote site. **2.** A dissemination of a previously localized bacterial skin infection. [bacteria + *-id* (1)]

bac•te•ri•e•mi•a (bak′tēr-ē-ē′mē-ă) SYN bacteremia. SYN bacteriaemia.

bacterio-, bacteri- Combining forms meaning bacteria. SEE bacterium.

bac•te•ri•o•ci•din (bak-tēr′ē-ō-sī′din) Antibody with bactericidal activity.

bac•te•ri•o•cin•o•gen•ic plas•mids (bak-tēr′ē-ō-sin′ō-jen′ĭk plaz′midz) Bacterial plasmids responsible for the elaboration of bacteriocins. SYN bacteriocinogens.

bac•te•ri•o•cin•o•gens (bak-tēr′ē-ō-sin′ō-jĕnz) SYN bacteriocinogenic plasmids.

bac•te•ri•o•cins (bak-tēr′ē-ō-sinz) Proteins produced by certain bacteria that exert a lethal effect on closely related bacteria; in general, bacteriocins have a narrower range of activity than antibiotics and are more potent.

bac•te•ri•o•gen•ic (bak-tēr′ē-ŏ-jen′ik) Caused by bacteria.

bac•te•ri•o•gen•ic ag•glu•ti•na•tion (bak-tēr′ē-ŏ-jen′ik ă-glū′ti-nā′shŭn) The clumping of erythrocytes as a result of effects of bacteria or their products.

bac•te•ri•o•log•ic, **bac•te•ri•o•log•i•cal** (bak′tēr-ē-ŏ-loj′ik, -i-kăl) Relating to bacteria or to bacteriology.

bac•te•ri•ol•o•gist (bak-tēr′ē-ol′ŏ-jist) One who primarily studies or works with bacteria.

bac•te•ri•ol•o•gy (bak-tēr′ē-ol′ŏ-jē) The branch of science concerned with the study of bacteria. [bacterio- + G. *logos,* study]

bac•te•ri•ol•y•sin (bak-tēr′ē-ol′i-sin) Specific antibody that combines with bacterial cells (i.e., antigen) and, in the presence of complement, causes lysis or dissolution of the cells.

bac•te•ri•ol•y•sis (bak-tēr′ē-ol′i-sis) The dissolution of bacteria, e.g., by means of hypotonic solutions or by specific antibody and complement. [bacterio- + G. *lysis,* dissolution]

bac•te•ri•o•lyt•ic (bak-tēr′ē-ō-lit′ik) Pertaining to lytic destruction of bacteria; manifesting the ability to cause dissolution of bacterial cells.

bac•te•ri•o•pex•y (bak-tēr′ē-ō-pek-sē) Immobilization of bacteria by phagocytic cells. [bacterio- + G. *pēxis,* fixation]

bac•te•ri•o•phage (bak-tēr′ē-ō-fāj) A virus with specific affinity for bacteria. Bacteriophages have been found in essentially all groups of bacteria; like other viruses they contain either RNA or DNA (but never both) and vary in structure from simple to complex; their relationships to host bacteria are specific and may be genetically intimate. Bacteriophages are named after the bacterial species, group, or strain for which they are specific, e.g., corynebacteriophage, coliphage. SEE ALSO coliphage. SYN phage. [bacterio- + G. *phagō,* to eat]

bac•te•ri•op•so•nin (bak-tēr′ē-op′sō-nin) An opsonin that acts on bacteria.

bac•te•ri•o•sis (bak-tēr′ē-ō′sis) A localized or generalized bacterial infection.

bac•te•ri•o•stat•ic (bak-tēr′ē-ō-stat′ik) Inhibiting or retarding the growth of bacteria.

bac•te•ri•um, pl. **bac•te•ri•a** (bak-tēr′ē-ŭm, -ă) A unicellular prokaryotic microorganism that usually multiplies by cell division and has a cell wall that provides a constancy of form; may be aerobic or anaerobic, motile or nonmotile, and free-living, saprophytic, parasitic, or pathogenic. SEE ALSO Cyanobacteria. [Mod. L. fr. G. *baktērion,* dim. of *baktron,* a staff]

bac•te•ri•u•ri•a (bak-tēr′ē-yūr′ē-ă) The presence of bacteria in the urine.

Bac•te•roi•des (bak-ter-oy′dēz) A genus that includes species of obligate anaerobic, nonspore-forming bacteria (family Bacteroidaceae) containing gram-negative rods. Both motile and nonmotile species occur; motile cells are peritrichous. Some species ferment carbohydrates and produce combinations of succinic, lactic, acetic, formic, or propionic acids, sometimes with short-chained alcohols; butyric acid is not a major product. Those species that do not ferment carbohydrates produce from peptone either trace to moderate amounts of succinic, formic, acetic, and lactic acids or major amounts of acetic and butyric acids with moderate amounts of alcohols and isovaleric, propionic, and isobutyric acids. They are part of the normal flora of the intestinal tract and, to a lesser degree, the respiratory, and urogenital cavities of humans and animals. A number of *Bacteroides* species have been reclassified as belonging to the genus *Prevotella.* Many species can be pathogenic. The type species is *B. fragilis.* [G. *bacterion* + *eidos,* form]

Bac•te•roi•des ca•pil•lo•sus (bak-tēr oy′dēz kap-i-lō′sŭs) A bacterial species isolated from human cysts, wounds, mouths, and feces.

Bac•te•roi•des dis•i•ens (bak-tēr-oy′dēz dis′ē-enz) A bacterial species isolated from abdominal and urogenital infections and from the mouth.

Bac•te•roi•des dis•ta•so•nis (bak-tēr-oy′dēz dis-tă-sō′nis) A bacterial species that is part of the normal human fecal flora; an occasional cause of intraabdominal infections.

Bac•te•roi•des frag•il•is (bak-tēr-oy′dēz fraj′i-lis) A species that is one of the predominant organisms in the lower intestinal tract of humans and other animals; also found in specimens from appendicitis, peritonitis, rectal abscesses, pilonidal cysts, surgical wounds, and lesions of the urogenital tract. It is the type species of the genus *Bacteroides.*

Bac•te•roi•des mel•an•in•o•gen•i•cus (bak-tēr-oy′dēz mel′ă-nin-ō-jen′i-kŭs) SEE *Prevotella melaninogenica.*

Bac•te•roi•des o•ris (bak-tēr-oy′dēz ō′ris) A species isolated from the gingival crevice; systemic infections; face, neck, and chest abscesses; wound drainages; and blood and various body fluids.

Bac·te·roi·des splanch·ni·cus (bak-tēr-oy′dēz splangk′ni-kŭs) A species in the indole positive group, found in normal human colonic flora, and occasionally in human specimens with unique metabolic properties that include production of large amounts of *N*-butyric acid. It appears to be closely related to the genus *Porphyromonas*.

Bac·te·roi·des the·ta·i·o·ta·mi·cron (bak-tēr-oy′dēz thā′tă-ī-ō′tă-mī′kron) A species implicated in intraabdominal infections.

bad cho·les·ter·ol (bad kŏ-les′tĕr-ol) Colloquial term for cholesterol bound to low density lipoproteins; generally thought that elevated levels increase threat of stroke and coronary disease.

BADL Abbreviation for basic activities of daily living.

BAER (bār) Abbreviation for brainstem auditory evoked response. SEE evoked response.

Baer law (bā′er law) The general organ characteristics found in all members of a group appear earlier in embryogenesis than the special organ characteristics that distinguish specific members of the group; this law is the predecessor of the recapitulation theory.

Baer·mann con·cen·tra·tion (bā′er-mahn kon-sĕn-trā′shŭn) Preparation that relies on the principle that active nematode larvae will migrate from a fresh fecal specimen through several layers of gauze into tap water, from which the larvae can be recovered by centrifugation.

Bae·yer the·o·ry (bā′er thē′ŏr-ē) Theory that carbon bonds are set at fixed angles (109° 28′) and that those carbon rings are most stable that least distort those angles; for this reason, planar rings composed of five or six carbon atoms (e.g., cyclopentane, benzene) are more common than rings containing less than five or more than six carbon atoms.

bag (bag) A pouch, sac, or receptacle. [A.S. *baelg*]

bag·as·so·sis (bag′ă-sō′sis) Extrinsic allergic alveolitis following exposure to sugar cane fiber (bagasse); variously attributed to inhalation of spores of soil fungi and, more particularly, thermophilic actinomycetes.

Bagh·dad boil (bag′dad boyl) SYN Aleppo boil. [Baghdad, capital of Iraq]

bag-valve-mask de·vice, bag-mask de·vice (bag-valv-mask dĕ-vīs′, bag′mask dĕ-vīs′) A hand-powered, positive-pressure, ventilation device consisting of a mask, one-way valve, and self-inflating bag; may be attached to an endotracheal or tracheostomy tube or a face mask.

bag of wa·ters (bag waw′tĕrs) Colloquialism for the amniotic sac and contained amniotic fluid.

Bail·lar·ger lines, Bail·lar·ger bands (bī-yahr-zhā′ līnz, bī-yahr-zhā′ bandz) Two laminae of white fibers that course parallel to the surface of the cerebral cortex and are visible as the stria of the internal pyramidal layer in cortical layer V (outer line) and the stria of the internal granular layer in cortical layer IV (inner line); the line of Gennari in the calcarine cortex represents the outer of these lines

Bail·li·art oph·thal·mo·dy·na·mom·e·ter (bī-yē-ahr′ of-thal′mō-dī-nă-mom′ĕ-tĕr) An instrument used to measure the blood pressure of the central retinal artery; of value in diagnosing occlusion of the proximal carotid artery.

Bain·bridge re·flex (bān′brij rē′fleks) Reflex mechanism causing accleration of the heart rate following the stimulation of local muscle spindles when blood pressure in the venae cavae and right atrium is increased.

Ba·ker ac·id he·ma·tein (bā′kĕr as′id hē′mă-tēn) An acidic solution of oxidized hematoxylin used on frozen sections for staining phospholipids.

Ba·ker cyst (bā′kĕr sist) A collection of synovial fluid that has escaped from the knee joint or a bursa and formed a new synovial-fluid–lined sac in the popliteal space; seen in degenerative or other joint diseases that produce increased amounts of synovial fluid.

Ba·ker pyr·i·dine ex·trac·tion (bā′kĕr pir′i-dēn eks-trak′shŭn) Hot pyridine treatment, used to extract phospholipids from tissues in histochemical staining of this material.

bak·er's itch (bā′kĕrz ich) An eruption on the hands and arms of bakers due to an allergic reaction to flour or other substances handled, or to the grain itch mite. SYN grocer's itch.

BAL Abbreviation for bronchoalveolar lavage, British anti-Lewisite.

Bal·a·muth a·que·ous egg yolk in·fu·sion me·di·um (bal′ă-mūt ā′kwē-ŭs eg yōk in-fyū′zhŭn mē′dē-ŭm) Used to detect the presence of intestinal amebae, primarily *Entamoeba histolytica*.

Ba·la·mu·thi·a (bal-ă-mū′thē-ă) A genus of free-living amebae that causes granulomatous amebic encephalitis.

bal·ance (bal′ăns) **1.** An apparatus for weighing (e.g., scales). **2.** The normal state of action and reaction between two or more parts or organs of the body. **3.** Quantities, concentrations, and proportionate amounts of bodily constituents. **4.** The difference between intake and use, storage, or excretion of a substance by the body. SEE ALSO equilibrium. **5.** The act of maintaining an upright posture in standing or locomotion. **6.** The system that depends on vestibular function, vision, and proprioception to maintain posture, navigate in one's surroundings, coordinate motion of body parts, modulate fine motor control, and initiate the vestibulo-oculomotor reflexes. [L. *bi-,* twice, + *lanx,* dish, scale]

bal•ance bil•ling (bal′ăns bil′ing) Sending a financial statement to the patient for the remainder of the amount charged and remaining unpaid after the third-party payer has submitted their financial contribution.

bal•anced an•es•the•si•a (bal′ănst an′es-thē′zē-ă) A technique of general anesthesia based on the concept that administration of a mixture of small amounts of several neuronal depressants summates the advantages, but not the disadvantages, of the individual components of the mixture.

bal•anced di•et (bal′ănst dī′ĕt) A diet containing the essential nutrients, with a reasonable ration of all major food groups.

bal•anced oc•clu•sion (bal′ănst ŏ-klū′zhŭn) The simultaneous contacting of the upper and lower teeth on the right and left and in the anterior and posterior occlusal areas in centric and eccentric positions within the functional range.

bal•anced pol•y•mor•phism (bal′ănst pol′ē-mōr′fizm) A unilocal trait in which two alleles are maintained at stable frequencies because the heterozygote is more fit than either of the homozygotes. SEE ALSO overdominance.

bal•anced trans•lo•ca•tion (bal′ănst tranz-lō-kā′shŭn) Translocation of the long arm of an acrocentric chromosome to another chromosome; a person with a balanced translocation has a normal diploid genome and is clinically normal but has a chromosome count of 45 and as a result of asymmetric meiosis may have children lacking the genes on the translocated segment or having them in trisomy.

bal•anc•ing side (bal′ăns-ing sīd) The segment of the dentition that is opposite the direction in which the lower jaw is being moved. Cf. working side.

bal•anc•ing side con•dyle (bal′ăns-ing sīd kon′dīl) DENTISTRY the mandibular condyle on the side away from which the mandible moves in a lateral excursion.

ba•lan•ic (bă-lan′ik) Relating to the glans penis or glans clitoridis. [G. *balanos,* acorn, glans]

bal•a•ni•tis (bal′ă-nī′tis) Inflammation of the glans penis or clitoris. [G. *balanos,* acorn, glans, + *-itis,* inflammation]

♻ **balano-, balan-** Combining forms denoting glans penis. [G. *balanos,* acorn, glans]

bal•a•no•plas•ty (bal′ă-nō-plas-tē) Surgical reconstruction of the glans penis to improve its appearance or correct a congenital defect. [balano- + G. *plastos,* formed]

bal•a•no•pos•thi•tis (bal′ă-nō-pos-thī′tis) Inflammation of the glans penis and overlying prepuce. [balano- + G. *posthē,* prepuce, + *-itis,* inflammation]

bal•an•ti•di•a•sis (bal′an-ti-dī′ă-sis) A disease caused by the presence of *Balantidium coli* in the large intestine; characterized by diarrhea, vomiting, weight loss, dysentery, and occasionally ulceration.

Bal•an•tid•i•um (bal-an-tid′ē-ŭm) A genus of ciliates (family Balantidiidae) found in the digestive tract of vertebrates and invertebrates. [G. *balantidion,* dim of *ballantion,* a bag]

Ba•lan•tid•i•um co•li (bal-an-tid′ē-ŭm kō′lī) A very large parasitic ciliate species, usually 50–80 mcm in length (to 200 mcm in pigs) found in the cecum or large intestine, swimming actively in the lumen; usually harmless in humans but may invade and ulcerate the intestinal wall, producing a colitis resembling amebic dysentery.

bald•ness (bawld′nĕs) SYN alopecia.

Ba•lint syn•drome (bah-lēnt′ sin′drōm) An entity characterized by optic ataxia and simultanagnosia. This difficulty in applying the visual system to a visual task is usually due to damage to the superior temporal-occipital areas in both hemispheres.

Bal•kan frame, Bal•kan splint (bawl′kăn frām, bawl′kăn splint) An overhead frame, supported on uprights attached to the bedposts or to a separate stand, from which a splinted limb is slung in the treatment of fracture or joint disease.

Balke-Ware tread•mill pro•to•col (bawlk-wār tred′mil prō′tŏ-kawl) A submaximal exercise test performed on a treadmill to evaluate patients with acute myocardial infarction and high risk dysrhythmias. SEE ALSO Astrand-Ryhming Cycle Ergometer Test.

ball (bawl) **1.** A round mass. SEE ALSO bezoar. **2.** In veterinary medicine, a large pill or bolus.

Bal•lance sign (bal′ăns sīn) The presence of a dull percussion note in both flanks, constant on the left side but shifting with change of position on the right, said to indicate ruptured spleen; the dullness is due to the presence of fluid blood on the right side but coagulated blood on the left.

ball-and-sock•et a•but•ment (bawl-and-sok′ĕt ă-bŭt′mĕnt) An abutment connected to a fixed partial denture by a ball-and-socket–shaped nonrigid connector.

ball-and-sock•et joint (bawl-and-sok′ĕt joynt) A multiaxial synovial joint in which a more or less extensive sphere on the head of one bone fits into a rounded cavity in the other bone. SYN cotyloid joint, enarthrodial joint, enarthrosis, spheroid joint.

Bal•lan•tyne dis•ease (bal′ăn-tīn di-zēz′) Disorder of newborns marked by prolonged gestation (i.e., longer than 39 weeks), decreased alertness, low birth weight, and increased respiratory distress. Skin, nails, and cord often have a greenish tint. Cause is likely placental insufficiency. SYN Clifford disease, dysmaturity syndrome, Runge disease.

bal•lis•mus (bă-liz′mŭs) A type of involuntary movement affecting the proximal limb musculature, manifested as jerking, flinging movements of the extremity; caused by a lesion of or near the contralateral subthalamic nucleus. Usually only one side of the body is involved, resulting in hemiballismus. [G. *ballismos,* a jumping about]

bal•lis•tic re•sis•tance train•ing (bă-lis′tĭk rĕ-zis′tăns trān′ing) A form of resistance training in which an object or weight is moved quickly with maximal force, then immediately released.

bal•loon (bă-lūn′) **1.** An inflatable spheric or ovoid device used to retain tubes or catheters in, or provide support to, various body structures. **2.** A distensible device used to stretch or occlude a stenotic viscus or blood vessel. **3.** To distend a body cavity with a gas or fluid to facilitate its examination, dilate a structure, or occlude its lumen. [Fr. *ballon,* fr. It. *ballone,* fr. *balla,* ball, fr. Germanic]

bal•loon an•gi•o•plas•ty (bă-lūn′ an′jē-ō-plas′tē) Dilation of an obstructed atherosclerotic artery by passage of a balloon catheter through the vessel to the area of disease where the plaque is compressed against the vessel wall.

bal•loon sep•tos•to•my (bă-lūn′ sep-tos′tŏ-mē) Creation of an artificial interatrial septal defect by cardiac catheterization during which an inflated balloon is pulled across the interatrial septum through the foramen ovale; used in cases of transposition of the great vessels and tricuspid atresia.

bal•loon-tip cath•e•ter (bă-lūn′tip kath′ĕ-tĕr) **1.** A single- or double-lumen tube with a balloon at its tip that can be inflated or deflated without removal after installation; the balloon may be inflated to facilitate the passage of the tube through a blood vessel (propelled by the bloodstream) or to occlude the vessel in which the tube alone would allow free flow; such catheters are used to enter the pulmonary artery to facilitate hemodynamic measurements. SEE ALSO Swan-Ganz catheter. **2.** A tube with an inflatable balloon at its tip used to enter arteries and then removed while inflated to withdraw clots (embolectomy catheter) **3.** SYN Fogarty catheter.

Ball op•er•a•tion (bawl op-ĕr-ā′shŭn) Division of the sensory nerve trunks supplying the anus, for relief of pruritus ani.

bal•lot•a•ble pa•tel•la (bă-lot′ă-bĕl pă-tel′ă) A condition in which the patella can be balloted because of an effusion of blood or fluid in the capsule of the knee joint. SYN floating patella.

bal•lotte•ment (bal-ot-mōn[h]′) **1.** Maneuver used in physical examination to estimate the size, shape, or consistency of an organ not near the surface, particularly when there is ascites, by a rhythmic, thrusting motion of the hand or fingers similar to that involved in bouncing a ball. **2.** A diagnostic measure in pregnancy. [Fr. *balloter,* to toss up]

ball valve (bawl valv) Any of a variety of prosthetic cardiac valves consisting of a ball within a retaining cage affixed to the orifice; when appropriately sized, used in aortic, mitral, or tricuspid position.

balm (bawlm) **1.** An ointment, especially a fragrant one. **2.** A soothing application. [L. *balsamum,* fr. G. *balsamon,* the balsam tree]

bal•ne•ol•o•gy (bal′nē-ol′ŏ-jē) The science of the therapeutic use of baths. [L. *balneum,* bath, + G. *logos,* study, discourse]

bal•ne•o•ther•a•py (bal′nē-ō-thār′ă-pē) Treatment of disease by baths.

bal•sam of Pe•ru (bawl′sŭm pĕr-ū′) A liquid extracted from the bark of *Myroxylon balsamum;* has mildly astringent properties; other purported uses include as an antineoplastic, anthelminthic, stimulant, and as an adjunct during dental procedures. Adverse effects have been widely reported. SYN *Toluifera pereirae.*

BALT (bawlt) Abbreviation and acronym for bronchus-associated lymphoid tissue.

Bam•ber•ger dis•ease (bahm′ber-ger di-zēz′) **1.** SYN saltatory spasm. **2.** SYN polyserositis.

Bam•ber•ger-Ma•rie dis•ease (bahm′ber-ger mah-rē′ di-zēz′) SYN hypertrophic pulmonary osteoarthropathy.

Bam•ber•ger-Pins-Ew•art sign (bahm′ber-ger-pinz-yū′ărt sīn) SYN Bamberger sign.

Bam•ber•ger sign (bahm′ber-ger sīn) **1.** Jugular pulse in tricuspid insufficiency. **2.** SYN allocheiria. **3.** Dullness on percussion at the angle of the scapula, clearing up as the patient leans forward, indicating pericarditis with effusion. SYN Bamberger-Pins-Ewart sign.

bam•boo hair (bam-bū′ hār) Hair with regularly spaced nodules along the shaft caused by intermittent fractures with invagination of the distal hair into the proximal portion, with intervening lengths of normal hair, giving the appearance of bamboo; seen in Netherton syndrome. SYN trichorrhexis invaginata.

bam•boo spine (bam-bū′ spīn) RADIOLOGY the appearance of the thoracic or lumbar spine with ankylosing spondylitis.

BAMDI Abbreviation for breath activated metered dose inhaler.

ba•na•na sign (bă-nan′ă sīn) The abnormal curvature of the cerebellum noted on ultrasound imaging in a fetus with Arnold-Chiari malformation.

Ban•croft sign (ban′krawft sīn) Finding that indicates thrombosis in veins in the deep calf; tenderness with anterior but not lateral compression of calf. Positive in roughly one third of cases. [Frederic w. Bancroft, 1880–, American surgeon]

band (band) **1.** Any appliance or part of an apparatus that encircles or binds a part of the body. SEE ALSO zone. **2.** Any ribbon-shaped or cordlike anatomic structure that encircles or binds another structure or that connects two or more parts. SEE fascia, line, linea, stria, tenia. **3.** A narrow strip containing one or more macromolecules (on occasion, small molecules) detected in electrophoresis or certain types of chromatography. **4.** DENTISTRY a strip of metal that fits around a tooth and serves as an attachment for orthodontic components. **5.** ORTHODONTICS part of an appliance used to align teeth. **6.** A nonfilamentous neutrophil.

ban•dage (ban′dăj) **1.** A piece of cloth or other material, of varying shape and size, applied to a body part to provide compression, protect from external contamination, prevent drying, absorb drainage, prevent motion, and retain surgical dressings. **2.** To cover a body part by application of a bandage.

ban•dage con•tact lens (ban′dăj kon′takt lenz) A contact lens placed on the cornea to cover a defect.

band cell (band sel) Any cell of the granulocytic (leukocytic) series that has a nucleus that could be described as a curved or coiled band, no matter how marked the indentation, if it does not completely segment the nucleus into lobes connected by a filament. SYN stab cell, staff cell.

band•ing (band′ing) The process of differential staining of chromosomes to reveal characteristic patterns of bands that permit identification of individual chromosomes and recognition of missing segments; each of the 22 pairs of human chromosomes and the X and Y chromosomes has an identifying banding pattern.

Ban•dl ring (bahn′dĕl ring) SYN pathologic retraction ring.

band-shaped ker•a•top•a•thy (band-shāpt′ ker′ă-top′ă-thē) A horizontal, gray, interpalpebral opacity of the cornea from calcium deposits at the Bowman layer. It is seen in hypercalcemia, chronic iridocyclitis, and Still disease.

band•width (band′width) The arithmetic difference between the upper and lower frequencies of a band of electromagnetic radiation.

bane•ber•ry (bān′ber-ē) SYN black cohosh.

Bang ba•cil•lus (bahng bă-sil′ŭs) SYN *Brucella abortus.*

Ban•kart le•sion (bangk′ărt lē′zhŭn) Avulsion or damage to the anterior lip of the glenoid fossa when the humerus slides forward in an anterior dislocation.

Ban•nis•ter dis•ease (ban′is-tĕr di-zēz′) SYN angioedema.

Bann•warth syn•drome (bahn′vahrt sin′drōm) Neurologic manifestations of Lyme disease, also called chronic lymphocytic meningitis and tick-borne meningopolyneuritis.

bar (bahr) **1.** A unit of pressure equal to 1 megadyne (10^6 dyne) per cm^2 in the CGS system, 0.9869233 atmosphere, or 10^5 Pa (N/m^2) in the SI system. **2.** A metal segment of greater length than width that serves to connect two or more parts of a removable partial denture. SYN beam (2). **3.** A segment of tissue or bone that unites two or more similar structures.

baraesthesia [Br.] SYN baresthesia.

baraesthesiometer [Br.] SYN baresthesiometer.

bar•ag•no•sis (bar-ag-nō′sis) Loss of ability to appreciate the weight of objects held in the hand, or to differentiate objects of different weights. When the primary senses are intact, caused by a lesion of the contralateral parietal lobe. [G. *baros,* weight + *a-* priv., + *gnōsis,* a knowing]

Bá•rá•ny ca•lo•ric test (bah′rah-nē kă-lōr′ik test) A test for vestibular function, made by irrigating the external auditory meatus with either hot or cold water; this normally stimulates the vestibular apparatus, resulting in nystagmus and past-pointing; in vestibular disease, the response may be reduced or absent. SYN caloric test.

Bá•rá•ny sign (bah′rah-nē sīn) In cases of ear disease, in which the vestibule is healthy, injection into the external auditory canal of water below the body temperature will cause rotatory nystagmus toward the opposite side; when the injected fluid is above the body temperature the nystagmus will be toward the injected side; if the labyrinth is diseased or nonfunctional there may be diminished or absent nystagmus.

bar•ber•ry (bahr′ber-ē) (*Mahonia vulgaris, Berberis aquifolium*) Available in many forms (e.g., extract, infusion); purported uses include as an antidiarrheal, antipyretic, and as a cough suppressant. Potential toxicity in pregnancy. SYN jaundice berry, Oregon grape, sowberry, wood sour.

bar•ber's itch (bahr′bĕrz ich) SYN tinea barbae.

bar•ber's pi•lo•ni•dal si•nus (bahr′bĕrz pī′lō-nī′dăl sī′nŭs) Pilonidal sinus occurring in barbers, usually in the web between the fingers, due to the burying of exogenous hairs by the alternate loosening and tightening of tissues of the hand by the manipulation of scissors.

bar•bi•tu•rate (bahr-bich′ŭr-ăt) Any of various derivatives of barbituric acid used as sedatives, hypnotics, and anticonvulsants.

bar•bi•tu•rism (bahr-bich′ŭr-izm) Chronic poisoning by any of the derivatives of barbituric acid; symptoms include cutaneous eruption, chills, fever, and headache.

bar•bo•tage (bahr-bō-tahzh′) A method of spinal anesthesia in which a portion of the anesthetic solution is injected into the cerebrospinal fluid, which is then aspirated back into the syringe and reinjected. [Fr. *barboter,* to dabble]

bar code (bahr kōd) A code consisting of a group of printed, variably patterned bars and spaces scanned by lasers into a computer to identify the object it labels.

Bard-Pic dis•ease (bahrd-pik di-zēz′) SYN Courvoisier gallbladder.

bare lym•pho•cyte syn•drome (bār lim′fō-sīt sin′drōm) Absence of human leukocyte antigens on peripheral mononuclear cells, which may result in immunodeficiency.

bar•es•the•si•a (bar′es-thē′zē-ă) SYN pressure sense. SYN baraesthesia. [G. *baros,* weight, + *aisthēsis,* sensation]

bar•es•the•si•om•e•ter (bar′es-thē′zē-om′ĕ-tĕr) An instrument for measuring the pressure sense. SYN baraesthesiometer. [G. *baros,* weight, + *aisthēsis,* sensation, + *metron,* measure]

barf (bahrf) Colloquial, to vomit; vomitus.

bar•i•at•ric (bar′ē-at′rik) Relating to bariatrics.

bar•i•at•rics (bar′ē-at′riks) That branch of medicine concerned with the management of obesity. [G. *baros,* weight, + *iatreia,* medical treatment]

bar•i•at•ric sur•ger•y (bar′ē-at′rik sŭr′jĕr-ē) Operation performed for the management of obesity.

bar•i•um (Ba) (bar′ē-ŭm) A metallic, alkaline, divalent earth element; atomic no. 56, atomic wt. 137.327. Salts are often used in diagnosis. [G. *barys,* heavy]

bar•i•um en•e•ma (BE) (bar′ē-ŭm en′ĕ-mă) A type of contrast enema; administration of barium, a radiopaque medium, for radiographic and fluoroscopic study of the lower intestinal tract. For maximal effectiveness, the colon is usually cleared of fecal material with a cathartic before the procedure. See this page.

bar•i•um swal•low (bar′ē-ŭm swahl′ō) Oral administration of barium sulfate suspension for radiographic investigation of the hypopharynx and esophagus.

Bar•kan mem•brane (bahr′kăn mem′brān) A theoretic tissue covering the trabecular meshwork; thought to obstruct aqueous humor outflow and be responsible for congenital glaucoma.

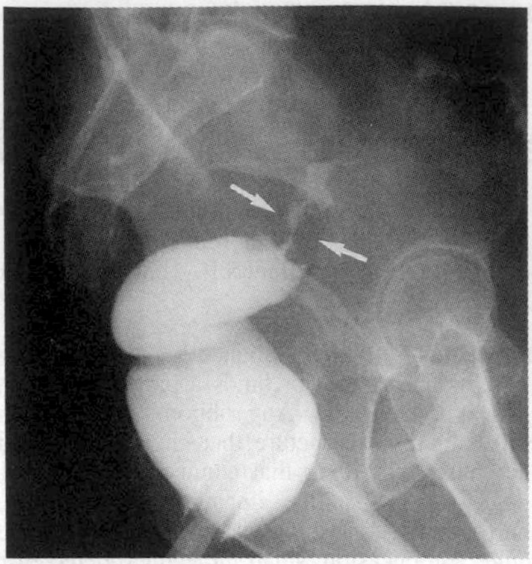

barium enema study demonstrating a circumferential mass (arrows): adenocarcinoma of the colon presenting as an apple-core-shaped lesion

Bar•kan op•er•a•tion (bahr′kăn op-ĕr-ā′shŭn) Goniotomy to open the Barkan membrane for congenital glaucoma under direct observation of the anterior chamber angle.

Bark•man re•flex (bahrk′mahn rē′-fleks) Contraction of the ipsilateral rectus muscle in response to a stimulus applied to the skin below a nipple.

bar•ley (bahr′lē) (*Hordeum*) A foodstuff commonly found in breakfast cereal and soup; reports allege benefit in lowering cholesterol levels, against diabetes, and in the prevention of cancer. SYN foxtail grass, pearl barley.

Bar•low dis•ease (bahr′lō di-zēz′) SYN infantile scurvy.

Bar•low ma•neu•ver (bahr′lō mă-nū′vĕr) Test for hip instability, with dislocation occurring with flexion, adduction, and posterior force.

Bar•mah For•est virus (bahr′mă fōr′ĕst vī′rus) A species of Alphavirus that has caused outbreaks of polyarthritis in humans in Australia; transmitted by mosquitoes. [the virus was first isolated from mosquitoes collected in the Barmah Forest in southeastern Australia in 1974]

Barnes curve (bahrnz kŭrv) A curve corresponding in general with Carus curve, being the segment of a circle the center of which is the promontory of the sacrum.

Barnes zone (bahrnz zōn) The lower fourth of the pregnant uterus, attachment of the placenta to any part of which may cause dangerous hemorrhage.

baro- Prefix meaning weight, pressure. [G. *baros,* weight]

bar•o•cep•tor (bar′ō-sep-tŏr) SYN baroreceptor.

bar•og•no•sis (bar′og-nō′sis) Ability to appreciate the weight of objects, or to differentiate objects of different weights. [G. *baros*, weight, + *gnōsis*, knowledge]

ba•rom•e•ter (bă-rom′ĕ-tĕr) Instrument used to measure atmospheric pressure. [G. *baros,* weight, + *metron,* measure]

bar•o•met•ric pres•sure (P_b) (bar′ō-met′rik presh′ŭr) The absolute pressure of the ambient atmosphere, varying with weather, altitude, or other factors; expressed in millibars (meteorology) or mmHg or torr (respiratory physiology); at sea level, one atmosphere (atm, 760 mmHg or torr) is equivalent to 14.69595 lb/in^2, 1013.25 millibars, 1013.25 $\times$ 10^6 dynes/cm^2, and, in SI units, 101,325 pascals (Pa).

bar•o•phil•ic (bar′ō-fil′ik) Thriving under high environmental pressure; applied to microorganisms. [G. *baros,* weight, + *phileō,* to love]

bar•o•re•cep•tor (bar′ō-rĕ-sep′tŏr) **1.** In general, any sensor of pressure changes. **2.** Sensory nerve ending in the cardiac atria, vena cava, aortic arch, and carotid sinus, sensitive to stretching of the wall resulting from increased pressure from within, and functioning as the receptor of central reflex mechanisms that tend to reduce that pressure. SYN baroceptor, pressoreceptor. [G. *baros,* weight, + receptor]

bar•o•re•flex (bar′ō-rē′fleks) A reflex triggered by stimulation of a baroreceptor.

bar•o•si•nus•i•tis (bar′ō-sī-nŭs-ī′tis) SYN aerosinusitis. [G. *baros,* weight, pressure, + sinusitis]

bar•o•stat (bar′ō-stat) A pressure-regulating device or structure. [G., *baros*, weight, pressure, + *statos*, made to stand]

bar•o•tax•is (bar′ō-tak′sis) Reaction of living tissue to changes in pressure. [G. *baros,* weight, + *taxis,* order]

bar•o•ti•tis me•di•a (bar′ō-tī′tis mē′dē-ă) SYN aerotitis media.

bar•o•trau•ma (bar′ō-traw′mă) **1.** Injury to the middle ear or paranasal sinuses, resulting from imbalance between ambient pressure and that within the affected cavity. **2.** Lung injury that occurs when a patient is on a ventilator and is subjected to excessive airway pressure (pulmonary barotrauma). [G. *baros,* weight, + trauma]

Bar•ra•quer meth•od (bah-rah-kār′ meth′ŏd) SYN zonulolysis.

Barr chro•ma•tin bod•y (bahr krō′mă-tin bod′ē) SYN sex chromatin.

bar•rel chest (bar′ĕl chest) A chest with increased anteroposterior diameter, seen in emphysema.

bar•rel dis•tor•tion (bar′ĕl dis-tōr′shŭn) Irregular image produced when peripheral magnification is greater than axial magnification. SEE Petzval surface.

Bar•ré sign (bah-rā′ sīn) A hemiplegic patient placed in the prone position with the limbs flexed at the knees is unable to maintain the flexed position on the side of the lesion but extends the leg.

Bar•rett ep•i•the•li•um (bar′ĕt ep′i-thē′lē-ŭm) Columnar esophageal epithelium seen in Barrett syndrome.

Bar•rett syn•drome, Bar•rett e•soph•a•gus, Bar•rett met•a•pla•si•a (bar′ĕt sin′drōm, bar′ĕt ĕ-sof′ă-gŭs, bar′ĕt met-ă-plā′zē-ă) Chronic peptic ulceration of the lower esophagus, which is lined by columnar epithelium, resembling the mucosa of the gastric cardia, acquired as a result of long-standing chronic esophagitis; esophageal stricture with reflux, and adenocarcinoma, also have been reported.

bar•ri•er (bar′ē-ĕr) **1.** An obstacle or impediment. **2.** PSYCHIATRY a conflictual agent that blocks behavior that could help resolve a personal struggle. [M.E., fr. O.Fr. *barriere*, fr. L.L. *barraria*]

bar•ri•er con•tra•cep•tive (bar′ē-ĕr kon-tră-sep′tiv) A mechanical device designed to prevent sperms from penetrating the cervical os; usually used in combination with a spermicidal agent.

bar•ri•er pro•tec•tion (bar′ē-ĕr prō-tek′shŭn) A physical obstacle protecting the health care provider from contact with potentially infective fluids from a patient such as blood, mucus, or saliva.

Bar•thel Self-Care In•dex (bahr′tel self-kār in′dĕks) A screening scale used in geriatric patients to measure ten self-care tasks (e.g., ADLs, IADLs) on a scale from 1–10.

Barth her•ni•a (bahrt hĕr-nē′ă) A loop of intestine between a persistent vitelline duct and the abdominal wall.

Bar•tho•lin ab•scess (bahr′tō-lin ab′ses) An abscess of the vulvovaginal gland.

Bar•tho•lin cyst (bahr′tō-lin sist) A cyst arising from the major vestibular gland or its ducts.

Bar•tho•lin cys•tec•to•my (bahr′tō-lin sis-tek′tŏ-mē) Removal of a cyst of a major vestibular gland.

Bar•tho•lin duct (bahr′tō-lin dŭkt) Large duct draining the sublingual gland and opening into the Wharton duct or near it.

Bar•tho•lin gland (bahr′tō-lin gland) SYN greater vestibular gland.

bar·tho·lin·i·tis (bar′tō-lin-ī′tis) Inflammation of a vulvovaginal (Bartholin) gland.

Bar·thol·o·mew's tea (bahr-thol′ō-myūz tē) SYN yerba maté.

Barth syn·drome (bahrt sin′drōm) An X-linked syndrome characterized by poor growth, neutropenia, cardiomyopathy, and excess excretion of 3-methylglutaconic acid in the urine; some patients also show skeletal muscle weakness.

Bar·ton ban·dage (bahr′tŏn ban′dăj) A figure-of-8 bandage supporting the mandible below and anteriorly; used in mandibular fracture.

Bar·to·nel·la (bahr-tō-nel′ă) A genus of bacteria closely resembling *Rickettsia* in staining properties, morphology, and mode of transmission between hosts. Organisms usually reside extracellularly in arthropod hosts and intracellularly in mammalian hosts.

Bar·to·nel·la ba·cil·li·for·mis (bahr-tō-nel′ă ba-sil-i-fōr′mis) A species found in the blood, lymph nodes, spleen, and liver in Oroya fever and in blood and eruptive elements in verruga peruana.

Bar·to·nel·la·ce·ae (bahr-ton-el-ā′sē-ē) A family of bacteria that currently includes the genus *Bartonella*. On the basis of S16 rRNA studies, the former genera of *Rochalimaea* and *Grahamella* have been merged with the genus *Bartonella*, retaining their species names.

Bar·to·nel·la hen·se·lae (bahr-tō-nel′ă hen′sĕ-lē) A species formerly classified as a riskettsialike organism in the genus *Rochalimaea;* causes bacillary angiomatosis, particularly in immunocompromised people, and a form of catscratch disease.

Bar·to·nel·la quin·ta·na (bahr-tō-nel′ă kwin-tan′ă) A bacterial species closely resembling *Rickettsia* in staining properties, morphology, and mode of transmission between hosts. Organisms usually reside extracellularly in arthropod hosts and intracellularly in mammalian hosts. Type species of the genus *Bartonella*.

bar·ton·el·lo·sis (bahr-tō-nĕ-lō′sis) A disease, endemic in certain valleys of the Andes in Peru, Chile, Ecuador, Bolivia, and Colombia, caused by *Bartonella bacilliformis;* transmitted by the bite of the nocturnally biting sandfly, *Phlebotomus verrucarum;* occurs in three forms: 1) Oroya fever; 2) verruga peruana; 3) a combination or sequence of these.

Bar·ton for·ceps (bahr′tŏn fōr′seps) OBSTETRICS obstetric forceps with a sliding lock that is useful when the infant's head is in the occiput transverse position during delivery.

Bar·ton frac·ture (bahr′tŏn frak′shŭr) Break in the distal radius with volar subluxation or dislocation of the radiocarpal joint. See page B25.

Bart syn·drome (bahrt sin′drōm) A form of epidermolysis bullosa with blistering of the extremities and intertriginous areas, congenital localized absence of skin, erosions of the mouth, and dystrophic nails; there is often spontaneous improvement with no residual scarring; autosomal dominant inheritance, caused by mutation in the collagen type VII gene (COL7A1) on chromosome 3p.

Bart·ter syn·drome (bahr′tĕr sin′drōm) A disorder due to a defect in active chloride reabsorption in the loop of Henle; characterized by primary juxtaglomerular cell hyperplasia with secondary hyperaldosteronism, hypokalemic alkalosis, hypercalciuria, elevated renin or angiotensin levels, normal or low blood pressure, and growth retardation; edema is absent. Autosomal recessive inheritance, caused by mutation in either the Na-K-2Cl cotransporter gene (SLC12A1) on chromosome 15q or the K(+) channel gene (KCNJ1) on 11q.

bar·y·o·pho·bi·a (bar′ē-ō-fō′bē-ă) An irrational fear of becoming overweight.

baryto- Prefix indicating the presence of barium in a mineral.

ba·sad (bā′sad) In a direction toward the base of any object or structure.

ba·sal (bā′săl) **1.** Situated nearer the base of a pyramidal organ in relation to a specific reference point; opposite of apical. **2.** DENTISTRY Denoting the floor of a cavity in the grinding surface of a tooth. **3.** Denoting a standard or reference state of a function, as a basis for comparison.

ba·sal an·es·the·si·a (bā′săl an′es-thē′zē-ă) Parenteral administration of one or more sedatives to produce a state of depressed consciousness short of a general anesthesia.

ba·sal bod·y (bā′săl bod′ē) An elongated centriolar structure situated at the base of each cilium at the apical margin of a cell. SYN basal granule.

ba·sal cell (bā′săl sel) A cell of the deepest layer of stratified epithelium.

ba·sal cell car·ci·no·ma, ba·sal cell ep·i·the·li·o·ma (bā′săl sel kahr′si-nō′mă, bā′săl sel ep′i-thē-lē-ō′mă) A slow-growing, malignant, but usually nonmetastasizing epithelial neoplasm of the epidermis or hair follicles, most commonly arising in sun-damaged skin of the elderly and fair-skinned. Cryotherapy is the primary treatment to eradicate the lesion. See page 175, B14.

ba·sal cell ne·vus (bā′săl sel nē′vŭs) A hereditary disease noted in infancy or adolescence, characterized by lesions of the eyelids, nose, cheeks, neck, and axillae, appearing as flesh-colored papules histologically indistinguishable from basal cell epithelioma; the lesions usually remain benign, but in some cases malignant change occurs.

ba•sal cell ne•vus syn•drome (bā′săl sel nē′vŭs sin′drōm) A syndrome of myriad basal cell nevi with development of basal cell carcinomas in adult life, odontogenic keratocysts, erythematous pitting of the palms and soles, calcification of the cerebral falx, and frequently skeletal anomalies, particularly ribs that are bifid or broadened anteriorly; autosomal dominant inheritance. SYN Gorlin syndrome.

ba•sal en•ceph•a•lo•cele (bā′săl en-sef′ă-lō-sēl) A defect in the skull floor with the herniation of brain tissue sometimes associated with coloboma of optic nerve.

ba•sal gan•gli•a (bā′săl gang′glē-ă) Large masses of gray matter at the base of the cerebral hemisphere: the striate body (caudate and lentiform nuclei) and cell groups associated with the striate body, such as the subthalamic nucleus and substantia nigra.

ba•sal gran•ule (bā′săl gran′yūl) SYN basal body.

ba•sal joint re•flex (bā′săl joynt rē′fleks) Opposition and adduction of the thumb with flexion at its metacarpophalangeal joint and extension at its interphalangeal joint, when firm passive flexion of the third, fourth, or fifth finger is made; the reflex is present normally but is absent in pyramidal lesions. SYN finger-thumb reflex, Mayer reflex.

ba•sal lam•i•na of cil•i•ar•y bod•y (bā′săl lam′i-nă sil′ē-ar-ē bod′ē) The inner layer of the ciliary body, continuous with the basal layer of the choroid and supporting the pigment epithelium of the ciliary retina.

ba•sal lam•i•na of neu•ral tube (bā′săl lam′i-nă nūr′ăl tūb) SYN basal plate of neural tube.

ba•sal lam•i•nar dru•sen (bā′săl lam′i-năr drū′sĕn) Small, round, translucent lesions measuring 25–75 mcm in diameter, which represent nodular thickening of the basement membrane of the retinal pigment eplithelium, often with an overlying focal detachment of the retinal pigment epithelium from Bruch membrane. SYN cuticular drusen.

ba•sal lay•er (bā′săl lā′ĕr) SYN stratum basale (1).

ba•sal lay•er of cho•roid (bā′săl lā′ĕr kōr′oyd) SYN lamina basalis choroideae.

ba•sal lin•e•ar dru•sen (bā′săl lin′ē-ăr drū′sĕn) Deposits of long-spaced collagen located between the plasma membrane and basement membrane of the retinal pigment epithelium.

ba•sal met•a•bol•ic rate (BMR) (bā′săl met′

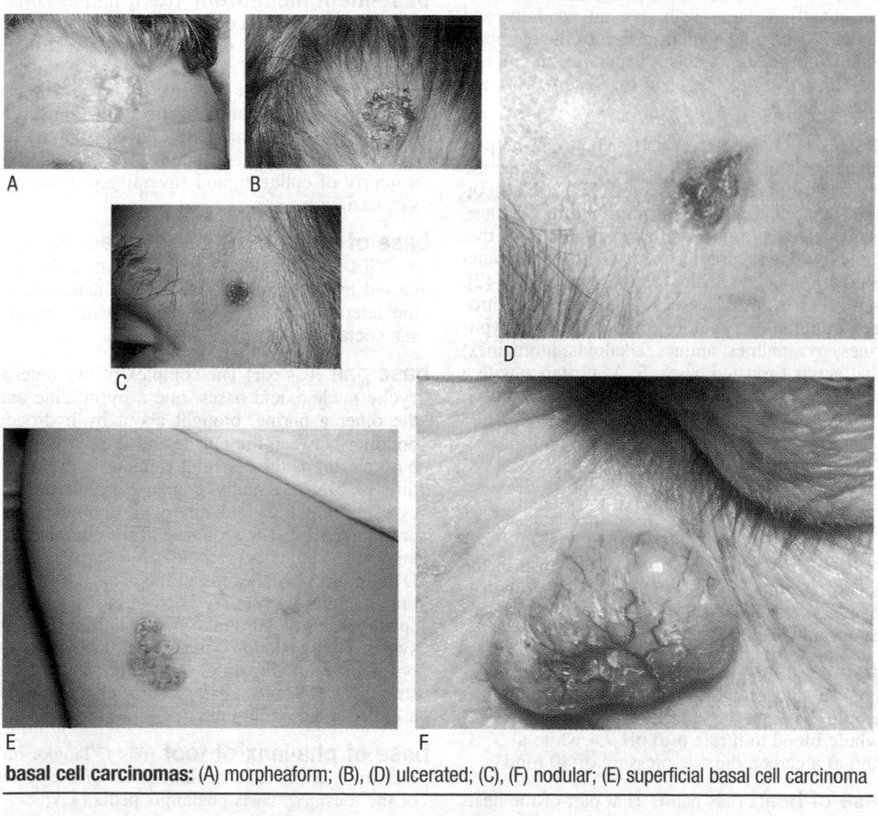

basal cell carcinomas: (A) morpheaform; (B), (D) ulcerated; (C), (F) nodular; (E) superficial basal cell carcinoma

ă-bol-′ik rāt) The minimal amount of energy required to sustain life in the waking state. SEE ALSO resting energy expenditure.

ba•sal plate of neu•ral tube (bā′săl plāt nūr′ ăl tūb) The ventral division of the lateral walls of the neural tube in the embryo; it contains neuroblasts giving rise to somatic and visceral motor neurons. SYN basal lamina of neural tube.

ba•sal rod (bā′săl rod) SYN costa (2).

ba•sal state (bā′săl stāt) A resting metabolic state early in the morning after a minimum of 12 hours of fasting. Used for laboratory tests.

ba•sal sub•stan•ti•a (bā′săl sŭb-stan′shē-ă) Basal structures associated with the amygdaloid complex and its connections; includes the basal nucleus (nucleus basalis [TA]) also called the nucleus of Gansser, the sublenticular extended nucleus (pars sublenticularis amygdalae [TA]), and bed nucleus of the stria terminalis (nucleus striae terminalis [TA]). SYN substantia basalis [TA].

ba•sal ten•to•ri•al branch of in•ter•nal ca•rot•id ar•ter•y (bā′săl ten-tōr′ē-ăl branch in-tĕr′năl kă-rot′id ahr′tĕr-ē) A small branch from the cavernous part of the internal carotid artery to the base of the tentorium.

ba•sal vein of Ro•sen•thal (bā′săl vān rō′ zĕn-thawl) A large vein passing caudally and dorsally along the medial surface of the temporal lobe from which it receives tributaries; it empties into the great cerebral vein (of Galen) from the lateral side.

base (bās) **1.** The lower part or bottom; the part of a pyramidal or conic structure opposite the apex; the foundation. SYN basis [TA]. **2.** PHARMACY the chief ingredient of a mixture. **3.** CHEMISTRY an electropositive element (cation) that unites with an anion to form a salt; a compound ionizing to yield hydroxyl ion. SYN alkali (2). SEE ALSO Brønsted base, Lewis base. **4.** Nitrogen-containing organic compounds (e.g., purines, pyrimidines, amines, alkaloids, ptomaines) that act as Brønsted bases. **5.** A substance with a pH over 7.0, in contrast to an acid. [L. and G. *basis*]

base•ball fin•ger (bās′bawl fing′gĕr) An avulsion, partial or complete, of the long finger extensor from the base of the distal phalanx. SYN mallet finger (2).

base def•i•cit (bās def′i-sit) A decrease in the total concentration of blood buffer base, indicative of metabolic acidosis or compensated respiratory alkalosis.

base ex•cess (bās eks′es) A measure of metabolic alkalosis; the amount of strong acid that would have to be added per unit volume of whole blood to titrate it to pH 7.4 while at 37°C and at a carbon dioxide pressure of 40 mmHg.

base of heart (bās hahrt) That part of the heart that lies opposite the apex, formed mainly by the left atrium but to a small extent by the posterior part of the right atrium; it is directed backward and to the right and is separated from the vertebral column by the esophagus and aorta. SYN basis cordis [TA].

base in•crease at low lev•els (bās in′krēs lō lev′ĕlz) A hearing aid signal-processing strategy to increase gradually the amplification of low frequencies at low-intensity levels.

BASE jump•ing (bās jŭmp′ing) A sport in which participants use a parachute and jump from four types of fixed man-made or natural objects: *b*uilding or skyscraper, *a*ntenna or tower, *s*pan (bridge arch or deck), and *e*arth (cliff).

base•line (bās′līn) **1.** A line approximating the base of the skull, passing from the infraorbital ridge to the midline of the occiput, intersecting the superior margin of the external auditory meatus; the skull is in the anatomic position when the baseline lies in the horizontal plane. **2.** Level of performance or aggregate findings before initiation of therapy. SYN orbitomeatal line.

base of lung (bās lŭng) The lower concave part of the lung that rests on the convexity of the diaphragm. SYN basis pulmonis [TA].

base•ment mem•brane (bās′mĕnt mem′brān) An amorphous extracellular layer closely applied to the basal surface of epithelium and also investing muscle cells, fat cells, and Schwann cells; thought to be a selective filter and to serve both structural and morphogenetic functions. It is composed of three successive layers (lamina lucida, lamina densa, and lamina fibroreticularis), a matrix of collagen, and several glycoproteins. SYN basilemma.

base of mo•di•o•lus of co•chle•a (bās mō-dē-ō′lŭs kok′lē-ă) The part of the modiolus enclosed by the basal turn of the cochlea; it faces the lateral end of the internal acoustic meatus. SEE cochlear area.

base pair (bās pār) The complex of two heterocyclic nucleic acid bases, one a pyrimidine and the other a purine, brought about by hydrogen bonding between the purine and the pyrimidine; base pairing is the essential element in the structure of DNA. Usually guanine is paired with cytosine (G·C), and adenine with thymine (A·T) or uracil (A·U). The sequence of the complementary bases in either strand of a two-stranded DNA molecule codes for amino acids used in the manufacture of proteins. Trios of bases (codons) specify each of 20 amino acids. During protein synthesis (translation), messenger RNA and ribosomes read the order of amino acids from strings of DNA to create protein chains, which are then released into the cell.

base of pha•lanx of foot (bās fā′langks fut) Proximal, concave, articulating end of the bones of the toes. SYN basis phalangis pedis [TA].

base of pha•lanx of hand (bās fā′langks hand) Proximal, concave, articulating end of the bones of the fingers. SYN basis phalangis manus [TA].

base•plate (bās′plāt) A temporary form representing the base of a denture; used for making maxillomandibular (jaw) relation records or for arranging artificial trial placement in the mouth to ensure exact fit of a denture.

base of skull (bās skŭl) The sloping floor of the cranial cavity. It comprises both the external base of skull (external view) and the internal base of skull (internal view). SYN basis cranii [TA].

base of sta•pes (bās stā′pēz) The flat portion of the stapes that fits in the oval window. SYN basis stapedis [TA], footplate (1), foot-plate.

base sta•tion (bās stā′shŭn) **1.** General term used for the emergency medical service radio console in a hospital emergency department. Also used to refer to a hospital that provides direct medical control to prehospital providers. **2.** A hospital that provides direct medical control to prehospital providers.

base of sup•port (BOS) (bās sŭ-pōrt′) Area defined by the parts of the body and assistive devices that are in contact with the supporting surface. SEE repetitive lifting test.

base u•nits (bās yū′nits) The fundamental measurements of length, mass, time, electric current, thermodynamic temperature, amount of substance, and luminous intensity in the International System of Units (SI); the names and symbols of the units for these quantities are meter (m), kilogram (kg), second (s), ampere (A), kelvin (K), mole (mol), and candela (cd). SEE ALSO International System of Units.

♻**basi-, baso-, basio-** Combining forms meaning base; basis. [G. and L. *basis*]

ba•si•breg•mat•ic ax•is (bā′si-breg-mat′ik ak′sis) A line extending from the basion to the bregma.

ba•sic (bā′sik) Relating to a base.

ba•sic ac•tiv•i•ties of dai•ly liv•ing (BADL) (bā′sik ak-tiv′i-tēz dā′lē liv′ing) Those activities that concern personal care (e.g., brushing one's teeth, bathing, other forms of self-care).

ba•sic dyes (bā′sik dīz) Dyes that ionize in solution to give positively charged ions or cations; the auxochrome group is an amine that can form a salt with an acid; solutions are usually slightly acidic.

ba•sic fuch•sin (bā′sik fūk′sin) [CI 42500] A triphenylmethane dye the dominant component of which is pararosanilin; an important stain in histology, histochemistry, and bacteriology.

ba•sic fuch•sin-meth•y•lene blue stain (bā′sik fūk′sin-meth′i-lēn blū stān) A stain for intact epoxy sections; semithick sections of plastic-embedded tissues have nuclei stained purple; collagen, elastic lamina, and connective tissue are stained blue; mitochondria, myelin, and lipid droplets are stained red; cytoplasm, smooth muscle cells, axoplasm, and chondroblast are stained pink.

ba•sic•i•ty (bā-sis′i-tē) **1.** The valence or combining power of an acid, or the number of replaceable atoms of hydrogen in its molecule. **2.** The characteristic(s) of being a chemical base.

ba•sic life sup•port (bā′sik līf sŭ-pōrt′) Provision of resuscitation and management and assessment of life-threatening conditions.

ba•sic per•son•al•i•ty type (bā′sik pĕr-sŏn-al′i-tē tīp) **1.** A person's unique, covert, or underlying personality propensities, whether behaviorally manifest or overt. **2.** Personality characteristics of a person that are also shared by a majority of the members of a social group.

ba•si•cra•ni•al ax•is (bā′si-krā′nē-ăl ak′sis) A line drawn from the basion to the midpoint of the sphenoethmoidal suture.

ba•si•cra•ni•al flex•ure (bā′si-krā′nē-ăl flek′shŭr) SYN pontine flexure.

ba•sic stain (bā′sik stān) A dye in which the cation is the colored component of the dye molecule that binds to anionic groups of nucleic acids ($PO_4\equiv$) or acidic mucopolysaccharides.

Ba•sid•i•ob•o•lus (bă-sid′ē-ob′ō-lŭs) A genus of fungi. *B. subcutaneous ranarum* has been isolated from cases of zygomycosis; usually it affects the trunk and limbs of children in tropical environments. [Mod. L. *basidium,* dim. of G. *basis,* base, + L. *bolus,* fr. G. *bolos,* lump or clod]

Ba•sid•i•o•my•co•ta (bă-sid′ē-ō-mī-kō′tă) A phylum of fungi characterized by a spore-bearing organ, the basidium, that is usually a clavate cell that bears basidiospores after karyogamy and meiosis. As found in the environment, basidiomycetes are generally plant pathogens and only rarely cause disease in humans.

ba•sid•i•um, pl. **ba•sid•i•a** (bă-sid′ē-ŭm, -ă) A cell or spore-bearing organ, usually club-shaped, that is characteristic of the Basidiomycota. It bears basidiospores externally after karyogamy and meiosis. It is composed of a swollen terminal cell situated on a slender stalk, and gives rise to slender filaments (sterigmata), usually four in number, from the ends of which the basidiospores are developed. [L., fr G. *basis,* base]

ba•si•fa•cial (bā′si-fā′shăl) Relating to the lower portion of the face.

ba•si•fa•cial ax•is (bā′si-fā′shăl ak′sis) A line drawn from the subnasal point to the midpoint of the sphenoethmoidal suture. SYN facial axis.

bas•il (bā′zil) (*Ocimum basilicum, O. sanctum*) Herb widely used in Meditarranean cuisine (e.g., pesto). Studies confirm utility in lowering glucose levels; also purported of value as an analgesic, antioxidant, and antiulcerative. [L. *basilicum,* fr. G. *basilikon,* royal]

bas•i•lar, **bas•i•la•ris** (bas′i-lăr, bas-i-lā′ris) Relating to the base of a pyramidal or broad structure.

bas•i•lar ar•ter•y (bas′i-lăr ahr′tĕr-ē) Formed by union of the intracranial portions of the two vertebral arteries; runs along the clivus in the pontine cistern of the subarachnoid space from the lower to the upper border of the pons, where it bifurcates into the two posterior cerebral arteries; *branches*, anterior, inferior, cerebellar, labyrinthine, pontine, mesencephalic, and superior cerebellar. SYN arteria basilaris [TA].

bas•i•lar in•dex (bas′i-lăr in′deks) Ratio between the basialveolar line and the maximum length of the cranium, according to the formula: (basialveolar line × 100)/length of cranium. SYN alveolar index.

bas•i•lar lam•i•na (bas′i-lăr lam′i-nă) SYN basilar membrane.

bas•i•lar mem•brane (bas′i-lăr mem′brān) The membrane extending from the bony spiral membrane to the basilar crest of the cochlea; it forms the greater part of the floor of the cochlear duct separating the latter from the scala tympani and it supports the spiral organ. SYN basilar lamina.

bas•i•lar men•in•gi•tis (bas′i-lăr men′in-jī′tis) Meningitis at the base of the brain, due usually to tuberculosis, syphilis, or any low-grade chronic granulomatous process; may result in an internal hydrocephalus.

bas•i•lar pa•pil•la (bas′i-lăr pă-pil′ă) The auditory sense organ of birds, amphibians, and reptiles; homologous to the spiral organ in mammals.

bas•i•lar ver•te•bra (bas′i-lăr vĕr′tĕ-bră) The lowest lumbar vertebra.

ba•si•lat•er•al (bā′si-lat′ĕr-ăl) Relating to the base and one or more sides of any part.

ba•si•lem•ma (bā′si-lem′ă) SYN basement membrane. [basi- + G. *lemma,* rind]

ba•sil•ic vein (bă-sil′ik vān) Arises from the ulnar side of the dorsal venous network of the hand; it curves around the medial side of the forearm, communicates with the cephalic vein through the median cubital vein, and passes up the medial side of the arm to join the axillary vein.

ba•si•on (bā′sē-on) The middle point on the anterior margin of the foramen magnum, opposite the opisthion. [G. *basis,* a base]

ba•sip•e•tal (bā-sip′ĕ-tăl) **1.** In a direction toward the base. **2.** Pertaining to asexual conidial production in fungi, in which successive budding of the basal conidium forms an unbranched chain with the youngest at the base. [basi- + L. *peto,* to seek]

bas•i•pho•bi•a (bās-i-fō′bē-ă) Morbid fear of walking. [G. *basis,* a stepping, + *phobos,* fear]

ba•sis (bā′sis) [TA] SYN base (1). [L. and G.]

ba•sis cor•dis (bā′sis kōr′dis) [TA] SYN base of heart.

ba•sis cra•ni•i (bā′sis krā′nē-ī) [TA] SYN base of skull.

ba•sis pha•lan•gis ma•nus (bā′sis fă-lan′jis mā′nŭs) [TA] SYN base of phalanx of hand.

ba•sis pha•lan•gis pe•dis (bā′sis fă-lan′jis pē′dis) [TA] SYN base of phalanx of foot.

ba•si•sphe•noid (bā′si-sfē′noyd) Relating to the base or body of the sphenoid bone.

ba•sis pul•mo•nis (bā′sis pul-mō′nis) [TA] SYN base of lung.

ba•sis sta•pe•dis (bā′sis stā-pē′dis) [TA] SYN base of stapes.

bas•ket cell (bas′kĕt sel) **1.** A neuron enmeshing the cell body of another neuron with its terminal axon ramifications. **2.** SYN smudge cells. **3.** A myoepithelial cell with branching processes that occurs basal to the secretory cells of certain salivary gland and lacrimal gland alveoli.

bas•ket nu•cle•us (bas′kĕt nū′klē-ŭs) Nuclear structure that may be seen in *Iodamoeba bütschlii* cysts and occasionally in trophozoites; in stained preparations, fibrils may be seen running between the karyosome and the chromatin granules.

ba•so•e•ryth•ro•cyte (bā′sō-ĕ-rith′rō-sīt) A red blood cell that manifests changes of basophilic degeneration, such as basophilic stippling, punctate basophilia, or basophilic granules.

ba•so•e•ryth•ro•cy•to•sis (bā′sō-ĕ-rith′rō-sī-tō′sis) An increase of red blood cells with basophilic degenerative changes, frequently observed in hypochromic anemia.

ba•so•lat•er•al (bā′sō-lat′ĕr-ăl) Basal and lateral; specifically used to refer to one of the two major cytologic divisions of the amygdaloid complex.

ba•so•phil, **ba•so•phile** (bā′sō-fil, -fīl) **1.** A cell with granules that stain specifically with basic dyes. **2.** SYN basophilic. **3.** A phagocytic leukocyte of the blood characterized by basophilic granules containing heparin and histamine; except for its segmented nucleus, it is morphologically and physiologically similar to the mast cell, although the two cell types originate from different stem cells in the bone marrow. See page B2. [baso- + G. *phileō,* to love]

ba•so•phil ad•e•no•ma (bā′sō-fil ad′ĕ-nō′mă) A tumor of the adenohypophysis in which the cell cytoplasm stains with basic dyes, often producing ACTH.

ba•so•phil•i•a (bā′sō-fil′ē-ă) **1.** A condition in which there are more than the usual number of basophilic leukocytes in the circulating blood (basophilic leukocytosis) or an increase in the proportion of parenchymatous basophilic cells in an organ (in the bone marrow, basophilic hyperplasia). **2.** A condition in which basophilic erythrocytes are found in circulating blood, as in certain instances of leukemia, advanced anemia, malaria, and lead poisoning. **3.** The reaction of immature erythrocytes to basic dyes whereby the cells appear blue or contain bluish granules. SYN basophilism.

ba•so•phil•ic (bā′sō-fil′ik) Denoting tissue components having an affinity for basic dyes. SYN basophil (2), basophile.

basophilic leukaemia [Br.] SYN basophilic leukemia.

ba•so•phil•ic leu•ke•mi•a, ba•so•phil•o•cyt•ic leu•ke•mi•a (bā′sō-fil′ik lū-kē′mē-ă, bā′sō-fil-ō-sit′ik) A form of granulocytic leukemia in which there are unusually great numbers of basophilic granulocytes in the tissues and circulating blood. SYN basophilic leukaemia, mast cell leukemia.

ba•so•phil•ic leu•ko•cyte (bā′sō-fil′ik lū′kō-sīt) A polymorphonuclear leukocyte characterized by many large, coarse, metachromatic granules (dark purple or blue-black with Wright stain) that usually fill the cytoplasm and may almost mask the nucleus; they usually do not occur in increased numbers as the result of acute infectious disease; the granules, which contain heparin and histamine, may degranulate in response to hypersensitivity reactions and can be of significance in general inflammation. SYN mast leukocyte.

ba•so•phil•ic leu•ko•pe•ni•a (bā′sō-fil′ik lū-kō-pē′nē-ă) A decrease in the number of basophilic granulocytes in the circulating blood.

ba•soph•i•lism (bā-sof′i-lizm) SYN basophilia.

basophilocytic leukaemia [Br.] SYN basophilocytic leukemia.

ba•so•squa•mous car•ci•no•ma, ba•si•squa•mous car•ci•no•ma (bā′sō-skwā′mŭs kahr′si-nō′mă, bā′si-skwā′mŭs) A carcinoma of the skin which in structure and behavior is considered transitional between basal cell and squamous cell carcinoma.

Bas•sen-Korn•zweig syn•drome (bas′en kōrn′zwīg sin′drōm) SYN abetalipoproteinemia.

Bas•si•ni her•ni•or•rha•phy (bă-sē′nē hĕr′nē-ōr′ă-fē) An operation for indirect inguinal hernia repair; after reduction of the hernia, the sac is twisted, ligated, and cut off, then a new inguinal floor is made by uniting the edge of the internal oblique muscle to the inguinal ligament, placing on this the cord, and covering the latter by the external oblique muscle.

bas•to•ki•nin (bas′tō-kin′in) SYN uteroglobin.

BAT Abbreviation for breath alcohol technician.

batch an•a•ly•zer (bach an′ă-līz-ĕr) A discrete automated chemical analyzer in which the instrument system sequentially performs a single test on each of a group of samples.

bath (bath) **1.** Immersion of the body or any of its parts in water or any other yielding or fluid medium, or application of such medium in any form to the body or any of its parts. May be used for cleansing or therapy. **2.** Apparatus used in giving a bath of any form. **3.** Fluid used for maintenance of metabolic activities or growth of living organisms, e.g., cells derived from body tissue. [A.S. *baeth*]

bath•ing trunk ne•vus (bādh′ing trŭngk nē′vŭs) A large hairy congenital pigmented nevus with a predilection for the entire lower trunk; malignant melanoma may develop in childhood.

bath itch (bath ich) SYN bath pruritus.

bath•mo•tro•pic (bath′mō-trō′pik) Influencing nervous and muscular irritability in response to stimuli. [G. *bathmos,* threshold, + *tropē,* a turning]

♻**batho-, bathy-** Combining forms meaning depth. [G. *bathos,* depth]

bath•o•pho•bi•a (bath′ō-fō′bē-ă) Morbid fear of deep places or of looking into them. [G. *bathos,* depth, + *phobos,* fear]

bath pru•ri•tus (bath prū-rī′tŭs) Itching produced by inadequate rinsing off of soap or by overdrying of skin from excessive bathing. SYN bath itch.

bathyaesthesia [Br.] SYN bathyesthesia.

bathyanaesthesia [Br.] SYN bathyanesthesia.

bath•y•an•es•the•si•a (bath′ē-an′es-thē′zē-ă) Loss of deep sensibility, i.e., from muscles, ligaments, tendons, bones, and joints. SYN bathyanaesthesia. [G. *bathys,* deep, + *an-* priv. + *aisthēsis,* sensation]

bath•y•es•the•si•a (bath′ē-es-thē′zē-ă) General term for all sensation from the tissues beneath the skin, i.e., muscles, ligaments, tendons, bones, and joints. SEE ALSO myesthesia. SYN bathyaesthesia. [G. *bathys,* deep, + *aisthēsis,* sensation]

bathyhypaesthesia [Br.] SYN bathyhypesthesia.

bathyhyperaesthesia [Br.] SYN bathyhyperesthesia.

bath•y•hy•per•es•the•si•a (bath′ē-hī′pĕr-es-thē′zē-ă) Exaggerated sensitiveness of deep structures, e.g., muscular tissue. SYN bathyhyperaesthesia. [G. *bathys,* deep, + *hyper,* above, + *aisthēsis,* sensation]

bath•y•hyp•es•the•si•a (bath′ē-hip′es-thē′zē-ă) Impairment of sensation in the structures beneath the skin, e.g., muscle tissue. SYN bathyhypaesthesia. [G. *bathys,* deep, + *hypo,* under, + *aisthēsis,* sensation]

Bat•ten dis•ease (bat′ĕn di-zēz′) Fatal autosomal recessive trait with onset between 5–9 years of age, marked by early symptoms, which progress to blindness, paralysis, and dementia.

bat•ter•y (bat′ĕr-ē) **1.** A group or series of tests administered for analytic or diagnostic purposes. **2.** Device that turns chemical energy into electrical. **3.** Unlawful touching of another person. **4.** Any form of physical violence against another person. [M.E. *batri,* beaten metal, fr. O.Fr. *batre,* to beat]

Bat•tis•ta op•er•a•tion (bah-tēs′tă op-ĕr-ā′shŭn) SYN left ventricular volume reduction surgery.

Bat•tis•ta pro•ce•dure (bah-tēs′tah prŏ-sē′jŭr) SYN left ventricular volume reduction surgery.

bat•tle•dore pla•cen•ta (bat′ĕl-dōr plă-sen′tă) A placenta in which the umbilical cord is attached at the border; so-called because of the fancied resemblance to the racquet used in battledore, a precursor to badminton.

bat•tle fa•tigue (bat′ĕl fă-tēg′) A term used to denote psychiatric illness consequent to the stresses of battle. SEE ALSO war neurosis. SYN shell shock.

Bat•tle in•ci•sion (bat′ĕl in-sizh′ŭn) A paramedian abdominal incision traversing the anterior and posterior rectus sheaths but with medial retraction of the rectus muscle.

bat•tle neu•ro•sis (bat′ĕl nūr-ō′sis) SYN war neurosis.

Bat•tle sign (bat′ĕl sīn) Postauricular ecchymosis in cases of fracture of the base of the skull.

Bau•de•locque op•er•a•tion (bō-dĕ-lōk′ op-ĕr-ā′shŭn) An incision through the posterior cul-de-sac of the vagina for the removal of the ovum, in extrauterine pregnancy.

Bau•er chro•mic ac•id leu•co•fuch•sin stain (bow′ĕr krō′mik as′id lū′kō-fūk′sin stān) A stain for glycogen and fungi using chromic acid as an oxidizing agent of polysaccharides, followed by Schiff reagent; glycogen and fungi cell walls appear deep red.

Bau•er-Kir•by test (bow′ĕr kĕr′bē test) A standardized procedure for microbiologic susceptibility performed by transferring a standardized pure culture of the organism of interest onto a sensitivity plate (Petri dish with Mueller-Hinton agar) and observing the amount of growth in the presence of discs containing antibiotics.

Bau•er syn•drome (bow′ĕr sin′drōm) Aortitis and aortic endocarditis as a little-recognized manifestation of rheumatoid arthritis.

Bau•mé scale (bō-mā′ skāl) Measurement allowing calculation of specific gravity of fluids at a baseline temperature of 60°F.

Baum•gar•ten glands (bowm′gahr-ten glandz) Lacrimal glands in the palpebral conjunctiva.

Baum•gar•ten veins (bowm′gahr-ten vānz) Nonobliterated remnants of the umbilical veins.

bawl (bawl) To cry uncontrollably.

bay (bā) (*Laurus nobilis*) Available as a berry, leaves, oils, and extract; clinical studies suggest value as an antiulcerative in laboratory animals and in GI disease; purported uses include as an antirheumatic, diuretic, and antiseptic. SYN sweet bay.

bay•ber•ry (bā′ber-ē) A fragrant shrub (*Myrica pensylvanica, M. cerifera*) native to North America with leaves that are prepared in various medicinal formulations. SYN candleberry, southern wax myrtle, waxberry.

baye•si•an a•nal•y•sis (bā′zē-ăn ă-nal′i-sis) SYN Bayes theorem.

Bayes the•o•rem (bāyz thē′ŏr-ĕm) A method of calculating statistical probability that combines a prior estimate of probability with statistics derived from subsequent events or experiments. Although it lacks mathematical rigor, it is often used to infer degree of risk in various medical settings. SYN bayesian analysis.

Bayle dis•ease (bāl di-zēz′) SYN paresis (2).

Bay•ley scale of in•fant de•vel•op•ment (bā′lē skāl in′fănt dĕ-vĕl′ŏp-mĕnt) Screen for mental and motor skills from birth to 30 months. Use is discouraged in children with physical handicaps.

bay•o•net ap•po•si•tion (bā-ŏ-net′ ap-ŏ-zish′ŭn) Relationship of two fracture fragments that lie next to each other, rather than in end-to-end contact.

ba•y•o•net for•ceps (bā-ŏ-net′ fōr′seps) Device with offset blades, such as those for use through an otoscope.

bay•o•net hair (bā-ŏ-net′ hār) A spindle-shaped developmental defect occurring at the tapered end of a hair.

Bay•ou vi•rus (bī′yu vī′rŭs) A species of hantavirus in the U.S. causing hantavirus pulmonary syndrome; transmitted by the rice rat.

Ba•zett for•mu•la (bă-zet′ fōrm′yū-lă) A formula for correcting the observed QT interval in the electrocardiogram for cardiac rate (R-R interval): corrected QT = Q-T sec/$\sqrt{RR}$ sec.

Ba•zin dis•ease (bah-zin[h]′ di-zēz′) SYN erythema induratum.

BBB Abbreviation for blood-brain barrier.

BBOT Abbreviation for 2,5-bis(5-*t*-butylbenzoxazol-2-yl)thiophene, a liquid scintillator.

BBP Abbreviation for bloodborne pathogens.

BBS Abbreviation for Berg Balance Scale.

bc, **bcc** Abbreviation meaning blind copy(ies).

BCBS Abbreviation for Blue Cross-Blue Shield.

B-cell co•re•cep•tor (sel kō′rĕ-sĕp′tŏr) A complex of three proteins associated with the B-cell receptor (CR2, CD19, and TAPA-1).

B-cell dif•fer•en•ti•at•ing fac•tor (sel dif′ĕr-en′shē-āt-ing fak′tŏr) SYN interleukin-4.

B-cell re•cep•tors (sel rĕ-sep′tŏrz) A complex comprising a membrane-bound immunoglobulin molecule and two associated signal-transducing α and β chains.

B cells (selz) SYN beta (β) cells (1).

B-cell stim•u•la•to•ry fac•tor 2 (sel stim′yŭ-lă-tōr′ē fak′tŏr) SYN interleukin-6.

BCG Abbreviation for bacille Calmette-Guérin.

B chain (chān) A polypeptide component of insulin containing 30 amino acyl residues; insulin is formed by the linkage of a B chain to an A chain.

BCL-2 An oncogene that inhibits apoptosis.

BCR/ABL gene (jēn) A fusion gene produced when a segment of the Abelson protooncogene, ABL, from chromosome 9, translocates to the major breakpoint cluster region (M-BCR) on chromosome 22. The fusion gene produces a specific protein, P210. This fusion gene is found in chronic myelocytic leukemia (CML).

Bdel•lo•vib•ri•o bac•ter•i•o•vo•rus (del′ō-vib′rē-ō bak-tēr-ē-ō-vōr′ŭs) An unusual species of obligatory aerobic, gram-negative, comma-shaped bacteria that penetrates the cell walls and infects other gram-negative species of bacteria. It is used extensively for research purposes, primarily in genetic recombinant studies; not known to be a human pathogen.

BDI Abbreviation for Beck Depression Inventory.

BE Abbreviation for barium enema; below elbow (amputation).

Be Symbol for beryllium.

bead•ed (bēd′ĕd) **1.** Marked by numerous small rounded projections, often arranged in a row like a string of beads. **2.** Applied to a series of noncontinuous bacterial colonies along the line of inoculation in a stab culture. **3.** Denoting stained bacteria in which more deeply stained granules occur at regular intervals in the organism.

bead•ed hair (bēd′ĕd hār) SYN monilethrix.

bead•ing (bēd′ing) **1.** Rounded elevation along the border of the tissue surface of the major connectors of a maxillary dental prosthesis. **2.** Protection of the formed borders of final impressions for a dental prosthesis done by placement of wax sticks or a plaster-pumice combination adjacent to the borders prior to forming the master cast. **3.** Numerous small rounded projections, often in a row like a string of beads.

beaked pel•vis (bēkt pel′vis) SYN osteomalacic pelvis.

beak•er cell (bē′kĕr sel) SYN goblet cell.

beam (bēm) **1.** Any bar with a curvature that changes under load. **2.** DENTISTRY SYN bar (2). **3.** A collimated emission of light or other radiation, such as an x-ray beam. [O.H.G. *boum*]

beam•let (bēm′lĕt) Also referred to as a bixel; a small photon intensity element used to subdivide an IMRT beam for the purpose of treatment calculation for radiation therapy. SYN bixel. [*beam* + *-let,* dim. suffix]

bear•ber•ry (bār′ber-ē) A shrub (*Arctostaphylos uva-ursi*) whose dried leaves are used in various formulations; studies suggest value in diabetes and weight loss; purported value as a diuretic; use has been known to discolor urine. SYN crowberry, foxberry, uva-ursi.

bear•ing down (bār′ing down) Expulsive effort of a parturient woman in the second stage of labor.

bear•ing-down pain (bār′ing-down pān) A uterine contraction accompanied by straining and tenesmus; usually appearing in the second stage of labor.

beat (bēt) **1.** To strike; to throb or pulsate. **2.** A stroke, impulse, or pulsation, as of the heart or pulse. **3.** Mechanical activity of a cardiac chamber produced by catching a stimulus generated elsewhere in the heart. [A.S. *beatan*]

Beau lines (bō līnz) Transverse grooves on the fingernails following fever, malnutrition, trauma, myocardial infarction, or other severe or systemic illness.

Bea•ver meth•od (bē′vĕr meth′ŏd) Technique used to count *Ascaris* or *Trichuris* egg infestation in feces. Fecal samples are diluted with saline and viewed using a photoelectric light meter.

Bech•te•rew dis•ease (bek-ter′yev di-zēz′) SYN spondylitis deformans.

Bech•te•rew-Men•del re•flex (bek-ter′yev men′dĕl rē′fleks) Percussion of the dorsum of the foot causes flexion of the toes; present in a pyramidal lesion. SYN Mendel-Bechterew reflex.

Bech•te•rew sign (bek-ter′yev sīn) Paralysis of automatic facial movements, the power of voluntary movement being retained.

Beck De•pres•sion In•ven•to•ry (BDI) (bek dĕ-presh′ŭn in′vĕn-tōr-ē) Standardized psychiatric questionnaire in which the subject rates statements on a sliding scale; used in the diagnosis of depression.

Beck•er dis•ease (bek′ĕr di-zēz′) An obscure South African cardiomyopathy leading to rapidly fatal congestive heart failure and idiopathic mural endomyocardial disease. SYN dilated cardiomyopathy.

Beck•er mus•cu•lar dys•tro•phy (bek′er mŭs′kyū-lăr dis′trŏ-fē) A hereditary muscle disorder of late onset, usually in the second or third decade, affecting the proximal muscles with characteristic pseudohypertrophy of the calves; clinical features similar to Duchenne muscular dystrophy but much milder and not a genetic lethal; X-linked recessive inheritance, with both Becker and Duchenne dystrophies caused by mutation in the dystrophin gene on Xp. Cf. Duchenne dystrophy.

Beck•er ne•vus (bek′ĕr nē′vŭs) A nevus first seen as an irregular pigmentation of the shoulders, upper chest, or scapular area, gradually enlarging irregularly and becoming thickened and hairy. See this page.

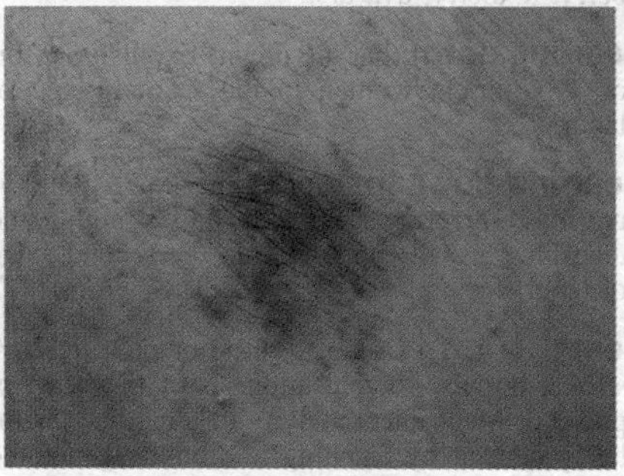

Becker nevus: upper back

Beck•er stain for spi•ro•chetes (bek′ĕr stān spī′rō-kēts) A stain applied to thin films fixed in formaldehyde-acetic acid; preparations are treated successively with tannin, carbolic acid, and carbol fuchsin.

Beck•mann ap•pa•ra•tus (bek′mahn a′păr-a′tŭs) Device for the accurate measurement of melting points and boiling points in connection with molecular weight determinations.

Beck meth•od (bek meth′ŏd) A permanent opening into the stomach made from its greater curvature.

Beck tri•ad (bek trī′ad) SYN acute compression triad.

Beck•with-Wie•de•mann syn•drome (bek′with vē′de-mahn sin′drōm) Exomphalos, macroglossia, and gigantism, often with neonatal hypoglycemia; autosomal recessive inheritance.

Bé•clard her•ni•a (bā-klahr′ hĕr′nē-a) A hernia through the opening for the saphenous vein.

bec•que•rel (bek-ă-rel′) The SI unit of measurement of radioactivity, equal to 1 disintegration per second; 1 Bq = 0.027 × 10^{-9} Ci. SEE ALSO absorption. [*Antoine Henri Becquerel*]

BED Abbreviation for biologically effective dose.

bed (bed) **1.** ANATOMY a base or structure that supports another structure. **2.** A piece of furniture used for rest, recuperation, or treatment.

bed bath (bed bath) Washing of a bed-restricted patient's body.

bed•bug (bed′bŭg) SYN *Cimex.*

Bed•nar aph•thae (bed′nahr af′thē) Traumatic ulcers located on the posterior portion of the hard palate in infants who place infected objects in the mouth, bilaterally on either side of the midpalatal raphe in infants.

bed rest (bed rest) Maintenance of the recumbent position, in bed, to minimize activity and facilitate recovery from disease.

bed•side man•ner (bed′sīd man′ĕr) Behavior of a health care professional toward a patient, client, or resident of a facility.

bed•side test•ing (bed′sīd test′ing) SYN point of care testing.

bed•sore, bed sore (bed′sōr, bed sōr) SYN decubitus ulcer.

bed-wet•ting (bed′wet-ing) SYN nocturnal enuresis.

bee•bread (bē′bred) SYN borage.

bee pol•len (bē pol′ĕn) Plant pollen collected by bees; alleged value against prostatitis and inflammatory disorders; studies suggest value in eliminating acetaminophen toxicity; may vary widely in strength because of vast geographic distribution of the bees themselves.

Beer law (bēr law) The intensity of a color or of a light ray is inversely proportional to the depth of liquid through which it is transmitted; it is concluded that the absorption depends on the number of molecules in the path of the ray.

Bee•vor sign (bē′vŏr sīn) With paralysis of the lower portions of the recti abdominis muscles the umbilicus moves, upward.

beg•gar's but•tons (beg′ărz bŭt′ŏnz) SYN burdock.

be•hav•ior (bē-hāv′yŏr) **1.** Any response emitted by or elicited from an organism. **2.** Any mental or motor act or activity. **3.** Parts of a total response pattern. SYN behaviour. [M.E., fr. O. Fr. *avoir*, to have]

be•hav•ior•al (bē-hāv′yŏr-ăl) Pertaining to behavior. SYN behavioural.

be•hav•ior•al ep•i•dem•ic (bē-hāv′yŏr-ăl ep′i-dem′ik) An epidemic originating in behavioral patterns (as opposed to invading microorganisms); examples include medieval dancing mania and episodes of crowd panic.

be•hav•ior•al ge•net•ics (bē-hāv′yŏr-ăl jĕ-net′iks) The study of heritable factors in behavioral patterns, as by pedigree analysis, biochemical abnormality, or karyotypic analysis.

be•hav•ior•al im•mu•no•gen (bē-hāv′yŏr-ăl im′yū-nō-jĕn) Not smoking, getting regular exercise, and maintaining related health-enhancing personal habits and lifestyle of a person that are associated with a decreased risk of physical illness and dysfunction, and with greater longevity.

be•hav•ior•al in•at•ten•tion test (BIT) (bē-hāv′yŏr-ăl in′ă-ten′shŭn test) An assessment of safety used to determine areas of negligence in daily living. Subsets include eating a meal, sorting coins, copying an address, and following a map for directions.

be•hav•ior•al ob•ser•va•tion au•di•o•me•try (bē-hāv′yŏr-ăl ob′sĕr-vā′shŭn aw′dē-om′ĕ-trē) A method of observing the motor responses of young children to test sound intensities to determine the hearing threshold.

be•hav•ior•al path•o•gen (bē-hāv′yŏr-ăl path′ŏ-jĕn) The personal habits and lifestyle behaviors of a person that are associated with an increased risk of physical illness and dysfunction. Cf. behavioral immunogen.

be•hav•ior•al psy•chol•o•gy (bē-hāv′yŏr-ăl sī-kol′ŏ-jē) SYN behaviorism.

be•hav•ior•al sci•enc•es (bē-hāv′yŏr-ăl sī′ĕns-ĕz) A collective term for those disciplines or branches of science, such as psychology, sociology, and anthropology, that derive their theories and methods from the study of the behavior of living organisms.

be•hav•ior dis•or•der (bē-hāv′yŏr dis-ōr′dĕr) General term used to denote mental illness or psychological dysfunction, specifically those mental, emotional, or behavioral subclasses for which organic correlates do not exist. SEE ALSO antisocial personality disorder.

be•hav•ior•ism (bē-hāv′yŏr-izm) A branch of psychology that formulates, through systematic observation and experimentation, the laws and principles that underlie the behavior of humans and animals; its major contributions have been made in the areas of conditioning and learning. SYN behavioral psychology, behaviourism.

be•hav•ior•ist (bē-hāv′yŏr-ist) A person who supports or practices behaviorism.

be•hav•ior mod•i•fi•ca•tion (bē-hāv′yŏr mod′i-fi-kā′shŭn) **1.** A systematic treatment technique that attempts to change a person's habitual maladaptive response by creating rewards for a new, desired response or unrewarding outcomes for the habitual response; intended to teach certain skills or to extinguish undesirable behaviors, attitudes, or phobias. **2.** A psychological theory based on observation of behavior and operant principles of behavior change.

be•hav•ior ther•a•py (bē-hāv′yŏr thār′ă-pē) An offshoot of psychotherapy involving the use of procedures and techniques associated with conditioning and learning for the treatment of a variety of psychological conditions.

behaviour [Br.] SYN behavior.

behavioural [Br.] SYN behavioral.

behaviourism [Br.] SYN behaviorism.

Beh•çet syn•drome, Beh•çet dis•ease (beh-chet′ sin′drōm, beh-chet′ di-zēz′) A syndrome characterized by simultaneously or successively occurring recurrent attacks of genital and oral ulcerations (aphthae) and uveitis or iridocyclitis with hypopyon, often with arthritis; a phase of a generalized disorder, occurring more often in men than in women, with variable manifestations, including dermatitis, erythema nodosum, thrombophlebitis, and cerebral involvement. SYN uveoencephalitic syndrome.

be•hind-the-ear hear•ing aid (bē-hīnd′ ēr hēr′ing ād) Hearing aid that rests on the medial aspect of the pinna.

Beh•ring law (bā′ring law) Parenteral administration of serum from an immunized person provides a relative, passive immunity to that disease (i.e., prevents it, or favorably modifies its course) in a previously susceptible person.

Behr syn•drome (bār sin′drōm) Characterized by bilateral optic atrophy with temporal field defects, nystagmus, ataxia, spasticity, and mental retardation; probably autosomal recessive inheritance.

bel (bel) Unit expressing the relative intensity of a sound. The intensity in bels is the logarithm (to the base 10) of the ratio of the power of the sound to that of a reference sound. Ordinarily, the reference sound is assumed to be one with a power of 10^{-16} watts per sq cm, approximately the threshold of a normal human ear at 1000 Hz.

belch•ing (belch′ing) SYN eructation. [A.S. *baelcian*]

bel•la•don•na (bel′ă-don′ă) *Atropa belladonna;* a perennial herb with dark purple flowers and berries. Originally used as a source of atropine. SYN deadly nightshade.

belle in·dif·fér·ence (bĕl in′dēf-ār-ahns) SEE la belle indifference.

Bel·li·ni ducts (bel-lē′nē dŭkts) SYN papillary ducts.

Bell law (bel law) The ventral spinal roots are motor, the dorsal are sensory. SYN Magendie law.

Bell pal·sy (bel pawl′zē) Paresis or paralysis, usually unilateral, of the facial muscles, caused by dysfunction of the seventh cranial nerve; probably due to a viral infection; usually demyelinating in type. SYN peripheral facial paralysis.

Bell phe·nom·e·non (bel fē-nom′ĕ-non) Reflex upper deviation of the eye on attempted eye closure; seen with several disorders, including facial mononeuropathies, Guillain-Barré syndrome, and myasthenia gravis.

bell-shap·ed curve (bel′shāpt kŭrv) SYN gaussian distribution.

Bell spasm (bel spazm) SYN facial tic.

bel·ly (bel′ē) **1.** The abdomen. **2.** The wide swelling part of a muscle. SYN venter (2). **3.** Popularly, the stomach or womb. [O.E. *belig,* bag]

bel·o·ne·pho·bi·a (bel′ō-nē-fō′bē-ă) Morbid fear of needles, pins, and other sharp-pointed objects. [G. *belonē,* needle, + *phobos,* fear]

be·low el·bow (BE) am·pu·ta·tion (bĕ-lō′ el′bō amp′yū-tā′shŭn) Removal of the forearm with preservation of the elbow joint.

Bel·sey fun·do·pli·ca·tion (bel′sē fun′dō-pli-kā′shŭn) Partial (270°) fundoplication performed through thoracotomy.

Bence Jones pro·teins (bens jōnz prō′tēnz) Light-chain protein fragments with molecular weights of 25–50 kD; seen in urine in cases of multiple myeloma and Waldenström macroglobinemia.

Bence Jones pro·tein·u·ri·a (bens jōnz prō′tē-nūr′ē-ă) Presence of Bence Jones protein in the urine, indicative of multiple myeloma, amyloidosis, or Waldenström macroglobulinemia.

Bence Jones re·ac·tion (bens jōnz rē-ak′shŭn) The classic means of identifying Bence Jones protein, which precipitates when urine containing it is gradually warmed to 45–70°C, and redissolves as the urine is heated to near boiling.

bench·mark·ing (bench′mahrk-ing) Use of the sustained superior performance of a department or an organization as a standard of comparison; a reference tool to rate quality of care.

Ben·der ge·stalt test (ben′dĕr gesh-tahlt′ test) A psychological test used by neurologists and clinical psychologists to measure a person's ability to copy visually a set of geometric designs; useful for measuring visuospatial and visuomotor coordination to detect brain damage.

bend frac·ture (bend frak′shŭr) An injury in which a long bone or bones, usually the radius and ulna, are bent (i.e., angulated) due to multiple microfractures, none of which can be seen by x-ray imaging.

bend·ing frac·ture (bend′ing frak′shŭr) An injury in which a long bone or bones, usually the radius and ulna, are bent due to multiple microfractures, none of which can be seen by x-ray imaging.

bends (bendz) Colloquialism for caisson sickness; decompression sickness. [fr. convulsive posture of those so afflicted]

Be·ne·dek re·flex (ben′ĕ-dek rē′fleks) Plantar flexion of the foot caused by tapping the anterior margin of the lower part of the fibula while the foot is slightly dorsiflexed.

Ben·e·dict-Roth spi·rom·e·ter (bĕn′ĕ-dikt-rawth spī-rom′ĕ-tĕr) Closed-circuit instrument used to determine oxygen consumption over time and to calculate basal metabolic rate. Each liter of oxygen consumed represents 4.825 calories.

Ben·e·dict test (ben′ĕ-dikt test) A copper-reduction test for glucose in urine; a red or orange precipitate indicates a sugar content exceeding 2%.

Ben·e·dikt syn·drome (ben′ĕ-dikt sin′drōm) Hemiplegia with clonic spasm or tremor and oculomotor paralysis on the opposite side.

ben·e·fi·cence (bĕ-nif′i-sĕns) The habit, intention, or practice of doing good. [L. *beneficencia,* fr. *bene,* well, + *facio,* to do]

ben·e·fi·ci·ar·y (ben′ĕ-fish′ē-ār-ē) A person with health care insurance coverage, usually through the Medicare program. SYN insured, recipient. [Med.L. *beneficiarius,* fr. *beneficium,* benefit]

ben·e·fit (ben′ĕ-fit) The payment or services provided by an insurance policy or health care plan.

be·nign (bĕ-nīn′) Denoting the mild character of an illness or the nonmalignant character of a neoplasm. [through O. Fr., fr. L. *benignus,* kind]

be·nign co·i·tal ceph·a·lal·gi·a (bĕ-nīn′ kō′i-tăl sef′ă-lal′jē-ă) SYN coital headache.

be·nign ex·er·tion·al head·ache (bĕ-nīn′ eg-zĕr′shŭn-ăl hed′āk) Headache occurring with exertion or straining in the absence of any intracranial disease.

be·nign hy·per·ten·sion (bĕ-nīn′ hī′pĕr-ten′shŭn) Hypertension that runs a relatively long and symptomless course.

be·nign in·fan·tile my·oc·lo·nus (bĕ-nīn′

in′făn-tĭl mī-ok′lō-nŭs) A seizure disorder of infancy in which myoclonic movements occur in the neck, trunk, and extremities; the EEG is normal, and seizures do not persist in patients older than 2 years of age.

be•nign in•oc•u•la•tion lym•pho•re•tic•u•lo•sis, be•nign in•oc•u•la•tion re•tic•u•lo•sis (bĕ-nīn′ i-nok′yū-lā′shŭn lim′fō-rĕ-tik′yū-lō′sis, bĕ-nīn′ i-nok′yū-lā′shŭn rĕ-tik′yū-lō′sis) SYN catscratch disease.

be•nign in•tra•cra•ni•al hy•per•ten•sion (bĕ-nīn′ in′tră-krā′nē-ăl hī′pĕr-ten′shŭn) SEE pseudotumor cerebri.

be•nign lym•pho•cy•to•ma cu•tis (bĕ-nīn′ lim′fō-sī-tō′mă kū′tis) A soft red to violaceous skin nodule caused by dense infiltration of the dermis by lymphocytes and histiocytes. SYN cutaneous pseudolymphoma.

be•nign mon•o•clo•nal gam•mop•a•thy (bĕ-nīn′ mon-ō-klōn′ăl gam-op′ă-thē) SYN monoclonal gammopathy of unknown significance.

be•nign my•al•gic en•ceph•a•lo•my•e•li•tis (bĕ-nīn′ mī-al′jik en-sef′a-lō-mī′ĕ-lī′tis) SYN epidemic neuromyasthenia.

be•nign par•ox•ys•mal po•si•tion•al ver•ti•go (bĕ-nīn′ păr-ok-siz′măl pŏ-zish′ŭn-ăl vĕr′ti-gō) A recurrent, brief form of positional vertigo occurring in clusters; believed to result from displaced remnants of utricular otoconia.

be•nign po•si•tion•al ver•ti•go (bĕ-nīn′ pŏ-zish′ŭn-ăl vĕr′ti-gō) Brief attacks of paroxysmal vertigo and nystagmus that occur solely with certain head movements or positions, e.g., with neck extension; due to labyrinthine dysfunction. SYN postural vertigo (1).

be•nign pros•tat•ic hy•per•pla•si•a (BPH) (bĕ-nīn′ pros-tat′ik hī′pĕr-plā′zē-ă) Progressive enlargement of the prostate due to hyperplasia of both glandular and stromal components, typically beginning in the fifth decade and sometimes causing obstructive or irritative symptoms or both; does not evolve into cancer.

be•nign ter•tian fe•ver (bĕ-nīn′ tĕr′shăn fē′vĕr) SYN vivax malaria.

be•nign tet•a•nus (bĕ-nīn′ tet′ă-nŭs) A disorder marked by intermittent tonic muscular contractions of the extremities, especially the hands and feet (carpopedal spasm), accompanied by paresthesias and, when severe, by crowing respirations due to laryngospasm and seizures; results from hypocalcemia, caused by various disorders, including gastrointestinal abnormalities. SYN intermittent cramp (2).

be•nign tu•mor (bĕ-nīn′ tū′mŏr) A tumor that does not form metastases and does not invade and destroy adjacent normal tissue.

Ben•ja•min tree (ben′jă-min trē) SYN benzoin.

Ben•nett frac•ture (ben′ĕt frak′shŭr) Dislocation and break of the first metacarpal bone at the carpal-metacarpal joint.

Ben•nett move•ment (ben′ĕt mūv′mĕnt) A lateral, bodily shift of the condyles of the lower jaw during lateral excursions.

Benn•hold Con•go red stain (ben′hōld kong′gō red stān) An amyloid stain useful for amyloid detection in pathologic tissue; gives red staining of amyloid; also induces green birefringence to amyloid under polarized light.

Ben•son dis•ease (bens′sŏn di-zēz′) Disorder marked by presence of crystals of calcium stearate or polynitrile precipitating as irregularly shaped bodies in the vitreous of the eye. Common in elderly persons, impairment of vision is negligible. [Alfred H. Benson, 1852–1912, Irish ophthalmologist]

ben•tir•o•mide test (bĕn-tēr′ō-mīd test) A measurement of pancreatic exocrine function that does not require duodenal intubation: orally administered bentiromide is cleaved by chymotrypsin within the lumen of the small intestine, releasing *p*-aminobenzoic acid that is absorbed and excreted in the urine; diminished urinary excretion of *p*-aminobenzoic acid suggests pancreatic insufficiency.

ben•ton•ite floc•cu•la•tion test (ben′tŏn-īt flok′yū-lā′shŭn test) A procedure measuring rheumatoid arthritis in which sensitized bentonite particles are added to inactivated serum; the test result is positive if half of the particles are clumped while the other half remain in suspension.

♻ **benz-** Combining form denoting benzene.

ben•zene ring (ben′zen ring) The closed-chain arrangement of the carbon and hydrogen atoms in the benzene molecule. SEE ALSO cyclic compound.

ben•zo•in (ben′zō-in) A resin from the tree *Styrax benzoin;* alleged efficacy in treating URI, in antisepsis, and in wound healing; use as a healing agent confirmed in dental procedures; severe adverse effects (e.g., hemorrhage) have been reported. SYN Benjamin tree. [Ar. *lubān,* incense, + *jāwi,* of Java]

ben•zo•thi•a•di•a•zides (ben′zō-thī′ă-dī′ă-zīdz) A class of diuretics that increase the excretion of sodium and chloride and an accompanying volume of water, independent of alterations in acid-base balance; most of the compounds in this group are analogues of 1,2,4-benzothiadiazine-1,1-dioxide.

ben•zo•yl (ben′zoyl) The benzoic acid radical, C_6H_5CO—, forming benzoyl compounds.

benz•thi•a•zide (benz-thī′ă-zīd) A diuretic and antihypertensive agent.

ben•zyl•i•dene (ben-zil′i-dēn) The hydrocarbon radical, C_6H_5CH=.

ben·zyl·ox·y·car·bon·yl (Z) (ben′zil-ok′sē-kahr′bon-il) Amino-protecting radical used (as the chloride) in peptide synthesis, yielding $PhCH_2OCO$—NHR. SYN carbobenzoxy.

Bé·rard an·eu·rysm (bā-rahr′ an′yūr-izm) An arteriovenous aneurysm in the tissues outside the injured vein.

Ber·ar·di·nel·li syn·drome (bĕr-ahr′di-nel′ē sin′drōm) SYN congenital total lipodystrophy.

be·reave·ment (bĕr-ēv′mĕnt) An acute state of intense psychological sadness and suffering experienced after the tragic loss of a loved one or some highly valued possession. [M.E., *bireven*, to deprive, + -ment]

Berg Bal·ance Scale (BBS) (bĕrg bal′ăns skāl) An assessment of balance to determine risk of falling in older and neurologically impaired patients; comprises 14 tasks that are rated from 0 (cannot perform) to 4 (normal performance) for a total of 56 points.

Ber·ger dis·ease, **Ber·ger fo·cal glo·mer·u·lo·ne·phri·tis** (bār-zhār′ di-zēz′, bār-zhār′ fō′kăl glō-mer′yū-lō-nĕ-frī′tis) SYN focal glomerulonephritis.

Ber·ger space (ber′gĕr spās) The space between the patellar fossa of the vitreous and the lens.

Ber·gey clas·si·fi·ca·tion (bĕr′gē klas′i-fi-kā′shŭn) System for categorization of bacteria based on findings on Gram stain, morphology, order, family, genus, and species.

Berg·man sign (bĕrg′măn sīn) A radiographic finding in which 1) the ureter is dilated distal to a ureteral obstruction and 2) a catheter, passed retrograde, coils in the dilated ureter. SYN catheter coiling sign.

Berg stain (berg stān) A method for staining spermatozoa, using a carbol-fuchsin solution followed by dilute acetic acid and methylene blue; spermatozoa are stained a brilliant red and most other structures appear blue to purple.

ber·i·beri, **ber·i ber·i** (ber′ē-ber′ē) A nutritional deficiency syndrome occurring in endemic form in eastern and southern Asia, sporadically in other parts of the world, and sometimes in alcoholic patients, resulting mainly from a dietary deficiency of thiamine; characterized by painful polyneuritis, diarrhea, weight loss, fatigue, poor memory, and edema resulting from a high-output form of heart failure. SYN endemic neuritis. [Singhalese, extreme weakness]

berke·li·um (Bk) (bĕrk′lē-ŭm) An artificial transuranium radioactive element; atomic no. 97, atomic wt. 247.07. [*Berkeley*, Calif., city where first prepared]

Ber·lin blue (bĕr-lin′ blū) [CI 77510] A ferric ferrocyanide dye used to color injection masses for blood vessels and lymphatics, and in staining of siderocytes. SYN Prussian blue.

Ber·lin blue re·ac·tion (bĕr-lin′ blū rē-ak′shŭn) Bichromic stain; uses nuclear fast red to stain nuclei red and calcium ferrocyanide to stain hemosiderin and iron blue.

Ber·lin e·de·ma (ber-lēn′ ĕ-dē′mă) Focal retinal whitening of the macula after blunt trauma to the globe; thought due to photoreceptor disruption. SEE ALSO commotio retinae.

ber·loque der·ma·ti·tis, **ber·lock der·ma·ti·tis** (bĕr-lōk′ dĕr′mă-tī′tis, bĕr′lok dĕr′mă-tī′tis) A type of photosensitization resulting in deep brown pigmentation on exposure to sunlight after application of bergamot oil and other essential oils in perfume.

Ber·nard-Can·non ho·me·o·sta·sis (bār-nahd′ kan′ŏn hō-mē-ō-stā′sis) The set of mechanisms responsible for the cybernetic adjustment of physiologic and biochemical states in postnatal life. SYN physiologic homeostasis.

Ber·nard duct (bār-nahd′ dŭkt) SYN accessory pancreatic duct.

Ber·nays sponge (bĕr-nāz′ spŏnj) A compressed disc of aseptic cotton that swells when moistened; used in packing cavities.

Bern·hardt dis·ease (bern′hahrt di-zēz′) SYN meralgia paraesthetica.

Bern·hardt-Roth sign (bĕrn-hahrt′rawth sīn) SYN Bernhardt sign.

Bern·hardt sign (bern-hahrt′sīn) Pain on anterior lateral thigh; caused by injury to external cutaneous nerve. SYN Bernhardt-Roth sign, Roth sign.

Bern·heim syn·drome (bārn′hīm sin′drōm) Systemic congestion resembling the consequences of right heart failure (enlarged liver, distended neck veins, and edema) without pulmonary congestion in subjects with left ventricular enlargement from any cause; reduction in the size of the right ventricular cavity is found by contrast imaging or echocardiography or at postmortem due to encroachment by the hypertrophied or aneurysmal ventricular septum.

Ber·noul·li dis·tri·bu·tion (ber-nū′lē dis′tri-byū′shŭn) Probability distribution that describes likelihood of various combinations of two alternate outcomes in a series of independent trials. SYN binomial distribution.

Ber·noul·li law (bĕr-nū′lē law) When friction is negligible, the velocity of flow of a gas or fluid through a tube is inversely related to its pressure against the side of the tube; i.e., velocity is greatest and pressure lowest at a point of constriction.

Bern·stein test (bĕrn′stēn test) A test to establish that substernal pain is due to reflux esophagitis, performed by instillation of a weak hydrochloric acid solution directly into the lower esophagus. SYN acid perfusion test.

ber·ry an·eu·rysm (ber′ē an′yūr-izm) A small saccular aneurysm of a cerebral artery that resembles a berry. Such aneurysms frequently rupture, causing subarachnoid hemorrhage. See this page.

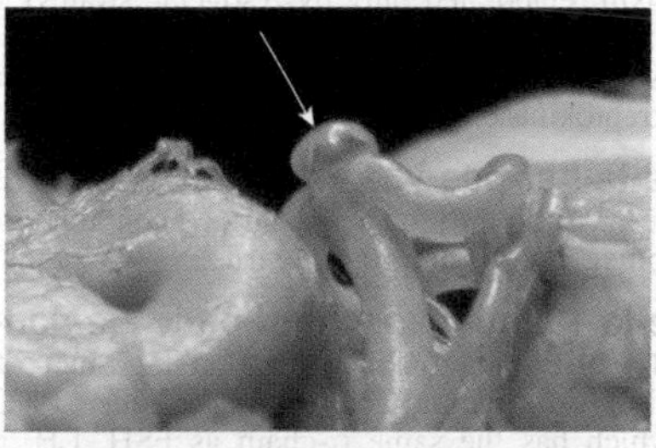

berry aneurysm: a thin-walled aneurysm protrudes from an arterial bifurcation in the circle of Willis

Ber·thol·let law (ber-tō-lā′ law) Salts in solution always react with each other so as to form a less soluble salt, if possible.

Ber·ti·el·la stu·de·ri (bĕr-tē-el′ă stūd-er′ē) Common tapeworm found in lower primates; incidental zoonotic infections in humans in the tropics have been reported.

Ber·tin col·umns (bār-tan[h]′ kol′ŭmz) SYN renal columns.

be·ryl·li·o·sis (bĕ-ril′ē-ō′sis) Beryllium poisoning characterized by granulomatous fibrosis of the lungs from chronic inhalation of beryllium.

be·ryl·li·um (Be) (bĕ-ril′ē-ŭm) A toxic white metal element belonging to the alkaline earths; atomic no. 4, atomic wt. 9.012182; widely used in dentistry as a hardening agent in alloys. [G. *beryllos*, beryl]

Bes·nier-Boeck-Schau·mann dis·ease (bā-nyā′ bĕrk show′mahn di-zēz′) SYN sarcoidosis.

Bes·nier pru·ri·go (bā-nyā′ prū-rī′gō) European term for prurigo, possibly atopic.

Best car·mine stain (best kahr′mīn stān) A method for the demonstration of glycogen in tissues.

Best dis·ease (best di-zēz′) Autosomal dominant macular degeneration beginning during the first years of life. SYN vitelliform retinal dystrophy.

best fre·quen·cy (best frē′kwĕn-sē) SYN characteristic frequency.

bes·ti·al·i·ty (bes-tē-al′i-tē) Sexual relations between a human and an animal. SYN zooerastia. [L. *bestia*, beast]

be·ta (β) (bā′tă) **1.** Second letter of the Greek alphabet. **2.** CHEMISTRY denotes the second in a series, the second carbon from a functional (e.g., carboxylic) group, or the direction of a chemical bond toward the viewer. For terms with the prefix β, see the specific term.

be·ta (β)-ad·re·ner·gic block·ing a·gent (bā′tă ad′rĕ-nĕr′jik blok′ing ā′jĕnt) A class of drugs that competes with β-adrenergic agonists for available receptor sites; some compete for both β_1 and β_2 receptors (e.g., propranolol), whereas others are primarily either β_1 (e.g., metoprolol) or β_2 blockers; used in the treatment of a variety of cardiovascular diseases and related conditions, for which β-adrenergic blockade is desirable. SYN beta (β)-blocker.

be·ta (β)-ad·re·ner·gic re·cep·tors (bā′tă ad′rĕ-nĕr′jik rē-sep′tŏrz) Adrenergic receptors in effector tissues capable of selective activation by isoproterenol and blockade by propranolol. Their activation results in physiologic responses such as increases in cardiac rate and force of contraction (β_1), and relaxation of bronchial and vascular smooth muscle (β_2).

be·ta (β)-as·par·tyl(a·ce·tyl·glu·co·sa·mine) (bā′tă as-pahr′til-as′e-til-glū-kō′să-mēn) A compound of *N*-acetylglucosamine and asparagine, linked through the amide nitrogen of the latter and carbon-1 of the former. An important structural linkage in many glycoproteins.

be·ta (β)-block·er (bā′tă-blok′ĕr) SYN beta (β)-adrenergic blocking agent.

be·ta (β) car·o·tene (bā′tă kar′ŏ-tēn) Isomer of carotene found in dark green and yellow vegetables and fruits.

be·ta (β)-car·o·tene-cleav·age en·zyme (bā′tă kar′ō-tēn-klē′văj en′zīm) SYN beta (β) carotene 15,15′-dioxygenase.

be·ta (β)-car·o·tene 15,15′-di·ox·y·gen·ase (bā′tă-kar′ŏ-tēn dī-oks′ē-jĕn-āz) An enzyme catalyzing the reaction of β-carotene plus O_2 producing two retinals. SYN beta (β)-carotene-cleavage enzyme.

be·ta (β) cells (bā′tă selz) **1.** Basophil cells of the anterior lobe of the hypophysis that contain basophil granules and are believed to produce gonadotropic hormones. SYN B cells. **2.** The predominant cells of the islets of Langerhans, which produce insulin.

be·ta·cism (bā′tă-sizm) A defect in speech in which the sound of *b* is given to other consonants. [G. *bēta*, the second letter of the alphabet]

be·ta-del·ta (β-δ) thal·as·se·mi·a (bā′tă-del′tă thal′ă-sē′mē-ă) Hematologic disorder due to a gene that depresses synthesis of both β- and δ-globin chains.

beta (β) error (bā′tă er′ŏr) SYN error of the second kind.

be·ta (β) fi·bers (bā′tă fī′bĕrz) Nerve fibers

having conduction velocities of about 40 milliseconds. SYN beta fibres.

beta fibres [Br.] SYN beta (β) fibers.

beta (β)-fruc•to•fu•ran•o•sid•ase (bā′tă fruk′tō-fūr-ă-nō-sīd′ās) Beta-*H*-fructosidase; An enzyme hydrolyzing beta-D-fructofuranosides and releasing free D-fructose; if the substrate is sucrose, the product is D-glucose plus D-fructose (invert sugar); invert sugar is more easily digestible than sucrose.

be•ta (β)-ga•lac•to•sid•ase (bā′tă-ga-lak-tō′si-dās) An enzyme that hydrolyzes the β-galactoside linkage in lactose-producing glucose and galactose; also hydrolyzes the chromogenic substrate IPTG (isopropylthiogalactoside) and thus is used as an indicator of fused genes and gene expression.

be•ta (β)-D-ga•lac•to•sid•ase (bā′tă gă-lak-tō′si-dās) A sugar-splitting enzyme that catalyzes the hydrolysis of lactose into D-glucose and D-galactose, and that of other β-D-galactosides; it also catalyzes galactotransferase reactions; a deficiency of β-D-galactosidase leads to problems in the intestinal digestion of lactose; used in the production of milk products for adults who do not have the intestinal enzyme; a defect of one isozyme of β-D-galactosidase is associated with Morquio syndrome type B. SYN lactase.

be•ta (β)$_{1C}$ glob•u•lin (bā′tă glob′yū-lin) The third component (C3) of complement. SEE component of complement.

be•ta (β)$_{1E}$ glob•u•lin (bā′tă glob′yū-lin) The fourth component (C4) of complement. SEE component of complement.

be•ta (β)$_{1F}$ glob•u•lin (bā′tă glob′yū-lin) The fifth component (C5) of complement. SEE component of complement.

be•ta (β)-D-glu•cu•ron•i•dase (bā′tă glū-kyū-ron′i-dās) An enzyme catalyzing the hydrolysis of various β-D-glucuronides, liberating free D-glucuronic acid and an alcohol; a deficiency of this enzyme is associated with Sly syndrome.

be•ta (β)-*d*-glu•cu•ron•i•dase de•fi•cien•cy (bā′tă glū-kyū-ron′i-dās dĕ-fish′ĕn-sē) A rare deficiency of β-*d*-glucuronidase; an autosomal recessive disorder with several allelic forms, characterized by abnormal mucopolysaccharide metabolism, and leading to progressive mental deterioration, splenic and hepatic enlargement, and dysostosis multiplex.

be•ta gran•ule (bā′tă gran′yūl) A granule of a beta cell.

be•ta (β)-he•mo•lyt•ic strep•to•coc•ci (bā′tă hē′mō-lit′ik strep-tō-kok′sī) Those that produce active hemolysins (O and S) that cause a zone in the blood agar medium in the area of the colony; β-hemolytic streptococci are divided into groups (A to O) on the basis of cell wall C carbohydrate (see Lancefield classification); Group A includes strains that cause human infections such as streptococcal pharyngitis, impetigo, erysipelas, otitis media, and wound infections and can stimulate production of autoimmune globulins that cause acute rheumatic fever and acute glomerulonephritis. Induced are more than 20 extracellular substances elaborated by strains of beta-hemolytic streptococci are erythrogenic toxin (elaborated only by lysogenic strains), deoxyribonuclease (streptodornase), hemolysins (streptolysins O and S), hyaluronidase, and streptokinase.

Be•ta•her•pes•vir•i•nae (bā′tă-hĕr′pēz-vir′ĭ-nē) A subfamily of herpesviridae containing cytomegalovirus and roseolovirus.

be•ta (β)-hu•man cho•ri•on•ic go•nad•o•tro•pin (bā′tă hyū′măn kōr′ē-on′ik gō-nad′ō-trō′pin) A 145-amino acid subunit unique to HCG, which has the same α-chain as FSH, LH, and TSH. Pregnancy tests specific for β-HCG are more sensitive because there is no confusion with other gonadotropins secreted by the pituitary.

3-be•ta (β)-hy•drox•y•ste•roid sul•fa•tase (bā′tă-hī-drok′sē-ster′ōid sŭl-fă-tāse) An enzyme, found in most mammalian tissues, which is capable of hydrolyzing the sulfate ester bonds of a variety of sulfated sterols; a deficiency of this enzyme will result in X-linked ichthyosis.

be•ta•ine (bā′tă-ēn) An oxidation product of choline and a transmethylating intermediate in metabolism.

be•ta (β)-lac•tam (bā′tă-lak′tam) A cyclic unit found in the molecular structure of penicillins and cephalosporins.

be•ta (β)-lac•tam an•ti•bi•ot•ics (bā′tă-lak′tam an′tē-bī-ot′iks) A group of natural and semisynthetic agents that inhibit the final stage of cell wall synthesis by binding with transpeptidases essential in the formation of peptide bonds. These antibiotics have a common chemical structure called the beta-lactam ring. (See figure). Beta-lactam antibiotics include the penicillins and cephalosporins.

be•ta (β)-lac•ta•mase (bā′tă-lak′tă-mās) An enzyme that brings about the hydrolysis of a β-lactam (such as penicillin to penicilloic acid); found in most staphylococcus strains that are naturally resistant to penicillin.

be•ta (β)-lac•tam•ase in•hib•i•tors (bā′tă-lak′tă-mās in-hib′i-tŏrz) Drugs such as clavulanic acid that are used to inhibit bacterial β-lactamases; often used with a penicillin or cephalosporin to overcome drug resistance.

be•ta-one (β$_1$)-lip•o•pro•tein (bā′tă--lip′ō-prō′tēn) A lipoprotein fraction of relatively high molecular weight and low density, rich in cholesterol, and found in the β-globulin fraction of human plasma.

be•ta (β)-ox•i•da•tion (bā′tă-oks-i-dā′shŭn)

Metabolic breakdown of free fatty acids to the 2-carbon acetyl coenzyme A, which is then used in the production of energy. SEE ALSO fatty acid.

be·ta (β) par·ti·cle (bā′tă-pahr′ti-kĕl) An electron, either positively (positron, β^+) or negatively (negatron, β^-) charged, emitted during beta decay of a radionuclide. SYN beta ray.

be·ta ray (bā′tă rā) SYN beta (β) particle.

be·ta (β) rhythm (bā′tă ridh′ŭm) A wave pattern in the electroencephalogram in the frequency band of 18–30 Hz. SYN beta (β) wave.

be·ta test·ing (bā′tă test′ing) In health care, assessment of a product (e.g., software) in the manner it will, in fact, be used in clinical practice, so as to discover and remove any difficulties before such product is put onto the general market.

beta-thalassaemia [Br.] SYN beta (β) thalassemia.

be·ta (β) thal·as·se·mi·a (bā′tă thal′ă-sē′mē-ă) Hematologic disorder due to one of two or more genes that depress (partially or completely) synthesis of β-globin chains. SYN beta-thalassaemia.

be·ta·tron (bā′tă-tron) A circular electron accelerator that is a source of either high energy electrons or x-rays.

be·ta (β) wave (bā′tă wāv) SYN beta (β) rhythm.

be·tel palm (nut) (bē′tăl pawlm nŭt) (*Areca catechu*) Widely used agent to induce general stimulation (the active ingredient is arecoline); can elicit disorders of the oral cavity; causes severely unattractive discoloration of gums and teeth; suggested link with induction of Type 2 diabetes. SYN areca nut, paan.

Be·thes·da sys·tem, Be·thes·da class·i·fi·ca·tion (bĕ-thez′dă sis′tĕm, bĕ-thez′dă klas′i-fi-kā′shŭn) A comprehensive system for reporting findings on cervical Papanicolaou smears; includes observations on the adequacy of the specimen, benign cellular changes (inflammation, infection), changes in squamous or glandular epithelial cells reflecting atypia or malignancy, and hormonal status. [*Bethesda*, MD, site of NIH]

Be·thes·da u·nit (bĕ-thez′dă yū′nit) A measure of inhibitor activity: the amount of inhibitor that will inactivate 50% or 0.5 unit of a coagulation factor during the incubation period. [*Bethesda*, MD]

beth root (beth rūt) SYN trillium.

Bet·ke-Klei·hau·er test (bet′kĕ klī′how-ĕr test) A slide-based procedure for the presence of fetal red blood cells among maternal cells. The test is performed if a fetal-maternal hemorrhage is possible.

bet·o·ny (bet′ŏ-nē) Agent derived from *Stachys officinalis;* suggested ability to lower blood pressure; completely unsubstantiated claims as valuable in therapy for asthma, bronchitis, toothache, and many more disorders. SYN bishop's wort. [L. *betonicus, vettonicus,* pertaining to the Vettones, an ancient people]

Betz cells (bets selz) Large pyramidal cells in the motor area of the precentral gyrus of the cerebral cortex.

Beu·ren syn·drome (būr′en sin′drōm) Supravalvular aortic stenosis with multiple areas of peripheral pulmonary arterial stenosis, mental retardation, and dental anomalies.

bev·el (bev′ĕl) **1.** The line of intersection of two surfaces that meet at any angle other than a right angle. **2.** The angled point of an injection needle. [O.Fr.]

be·zoar (bē′zōr) A concretion formed in the alimentary canal of animals, and occasionally humans; formerly considered to be a useful medicine with magical properties and apparently still used for this purpose in some places; according to the substance forming the ball, may be termed trichobezoar (hairball), trichophytobezoar (hair and vegetable fiber mixed), or phytobezoar (foodball). [Pers. *padzahr,* antidote]

B fi·bers (fī′bĕrz) Myelinated fibers autonomic nerves, with a diameter of 2 mcm or less, conducting at a rate of 3–15 m/sec. SYN B fibres.

B fibres [Br.] SYN B fibers.

Bh Symbol for bohrium.

BHC Any of several chlorine derivatives in which the chlorine atoms are all attached to carbon atoms.

Bi Symbol for bismuth.

♻ **bi-** **1.** Prefix meaning twice or double, referring to double structures, dual actions, for example . **2.** CHEMISTRY used to denote a partially neutralized acid (an acid salt); e.g., bisulfate. Cf. bis-, di-. [L.]

BIA Abbreviation for bioelectrical impedance analysis.

Bi an·ti·gen (an′ti-jen) SYN bile antigen. SYN bile antigen.

bi·ar·tic·u·lar (bī′ahr-tik′yū-lăr) SYN diarthric.

bi·as (bī′ăs) **1.** Systematic discrepancy between a measurement and the true value; may be constant or proportionate and may adversely affect test results. **2.** Any trend in the collection, analysis, interpretation, publication, or review of data that can lead to conclusions that differ systematically from the truth; deviation of results or inferences from the truth, or processes leading to deviation. [Fr. *biais*, obliquity, perh. fr. L. *bifax*, two-faced]

bi·au·ric·u·lar (bī′awr-ik′yū-lăr) Pertaining to both ears.

bi•au•ric•u•lar ax•is (bī-aw-rik′yū-lăr ak′sis) A straight line joining the two auricles.

bi•ax•i•al joint (bī-ak′sē-ăl joynt) One in which there are two principal axes of movement situated at right angles to each other; e.g., saddle joints.

bi bi re•ac•tion, bi-bi re•ac•tion (bē bē rē-ak′shŭn, bē′bē rē-ak′shŭn) A reaction catalyzed by a single enzyme in which two substrates and two products are involved; the ping-pong mechanism may be involved in such a reaction. Cf. mechanism.

bib•li•o•ther•a•py (bib′lē-ō-thār′ă-pē) Use of specific reading materials as therapeutic treatment in medicine and psychiatry.

bib•u•lous (bib′yū-lŭs) Absorbent; in medical terms, refers to materials used to soak up fluids, such as saliva during dental procedures.

bi•cam•er•al (bī-kam′ĕr-ăl) Having two chambers; denoting especially an abscess divided by a more or less complete septum. [bi- + L. *camera,* chamber]

BICAP cau•ter•y (bī-kap kaw′tĕr-ē) A form of bipolar electrocoagulation frequently used to arrest gastrointestinal bleeding.

bi•cap•su•lar (bī-kap′sŭ-lăr) Having a double capsule.

bi•car•bon•ate (bī-kahr′bŏn-āt) The ion remaining after the first dissociation of carbonic acid; a central buffering agent in blood.

bi•car•di•o•gram (bī-kahr′dē-ō-gram) The composite curve of an electrocardiogram representing the combined effects of the right and left ventricles.

bi•cel•lu•lar (bī-sel′yū-lăr) Having two cells or subdivisions.

bi•ceps (bī′seps) A muscle with two origins or heads. Commonly used to refer to the biceps brachii muscle. [bi- + L. *caput,* head]

bi•ceps bra•chi•i mus•cle (bī′seps brā′kē-ī mŭs′ĕl) *Origin*, long head from supraglenoidal tuberosity of scapula, short head from coracoid process; *insertion*, tuberosity of radius; *action*, flexes and supinates forearm (it is the primary supinator of the forearm); *nerve supply*, musculocutaneous. SYN musculus biceps brachii [TA].

bi•ceps fe•mo•ris mus•cle (bī′seps fem′ŏr-is mŭs′ĕl) *Origin*, long head (caput longum) from tuberosity of ischium, short head (caput breve) from lower half of lateral lip of linea aspera; *insertion*, head of fibula; *action*, flexes knee and rotates leg laterally; *nerve supply*, long head, tibial, short head, peroneal. SYN musculus biceps femoris [TA].

bi•ceps re•flex (bī′seps rē′fleks) Contraction of the biceps brachii muscle when its tendon of insertion is struck.

Bi•chat fis•sure (bē-shah′ fish′ŭr) The nearly circular fissure corresponding to the medial margin of the cerebral (pallial) mantle, marking the hilus of the cerebral hemisphere, consisting of the callosomarginal fissure and choroidal fissure along the hippocampus, both of which are continuous with the stem of the fissure of Sylvius at the anterior extremity of the temporal lobe.

Bi•chat mem•brane (bē-shah′ mem′brān) The inner elastic membrane of arteries.

bi•chlor•ide (bī-klōr′īd) A compound containing two chlorine atoms.

bi•cip•i•tal (bī-sip′i-tăl) **1.** Two-headed. **2.** Relating to a biceps muscle. [bi- + L. *caput,* head]

bi•cip•i•tal rib (bī-sip′i-tăl rib) Fusion of first thoracic rib with cervical vertebra.

bi•clo•nal (bī-klō′năl) Pertaining to or characterized by biclonality.

bi•clon•al•i•ty (bī-klŏn-al′i-tē) A condition in which some cells have markers of one cell line and other cells have markers of another cell line, as in biclonal leukemias.

bi•con•cave (bī-kon′kāv) Concave on two sides; denoting especially a form of lens. SYN concavoconcave.

bi•con•cave lens (bī-kon′kāv lenz) A lens that is concave on two opposing surfaces. SYN concavoconcave lens.

bi•con•dy•lar joint (bī-kon′di-lăr joynt) A synovial joint in which two distinct rounded surfaces of one bone articulate with shallow depressions on another bone.

bi•con•vex (bī-kon′veks) Convex on two sides; denoting especially a form of lens. SYN convexoconvex.

bi•con•vex lens (bī-kon′veks lenz) A lens with both surfaces convex. SYN convexoconvex lens.

bi•cor•nate (bī-kōr′nāt) SYN bicornuate.

bi•cor•nate u•ter•us (bī-kōr′nāt yū′tĕr-ŭs) A uterus that is more or less completely divided into two lateral horns as a result of imperfect fusion of the paramesonephric ducts during embryonic development; it differs from septate uterus, in which there is no external mark of separation; in bicornate uterus (uterus bicornis), the cervix may be single (uterus bicornis unicollis) or double (uterus bicornis bicollis).

bi•cor•nous, bi•cor•nu•ate, bi•cor•nate (bī-kōr′nŭs, -nū-āt, -nāt) Two-horned; having two processes or projections. [bi- + L. *cornu,* horn]

♻ **bicro-** SYN pico- (2).

bi•cron (bī′kron) SYN picometer.

bi•cus•pid (bī-kŭs′pid) Having two points, prongs, or cusps. [bi- + L. *cuspis,* point]

bi•cus•pid mur•mur (bī-kŭs′pid mŭr′mŭr) SYN Flint murmur.

bi•cus•pid tooth (bī-kŭs′pid tūth) SYN premolar tooth.

bi•cus•pid valve (bī-kŭs′pid valv) SYN mitral valve.

bi•dac•ty•ly (bī-dak′ti-lē) Abnormality in which the medial fingers are lacking, with only the first and fifth represented. SEE ALSO ectrodactyly. [bi- + G. *daktylos,* finger]

bi•det (bē-dā) Bathroom fixture similar to a toilet used for washing the perineal and perianal regions. [F.]

bi•di•rec•tion•al ven•tric•u•lar tach•y•car•di•a (bī-dir-ek′shŭn-ăl ven-trik′yū-lăr tak′i-kahr′dē-ă) Ventricular tachycardia in which the QRS complexes in the electrocardiogram are alternately mainly positive and mainly negative; many such cases may represent ventricular tachycardia with alternating forms of aberrant ventricular conduction.

bi•dis•coi•dal pla•cen•ta (bī-dis-koy′dăl plă-sen′tă) A placenta with two separate disc-shaped portions attached to opposite walls of the uterus, normal for certain monkeys and shrews, and occasionally found in humans.

BIDS (bidz) Acronym for condition involving brittle hair, impaired intelligence, decreased fertility, and short stature; usually manifested as an inherited deficiency of a high-sulfur protein.

Biel•schow•sky dis•ease (byels-chov′skē di-zēz′) Early childhood type of lipofuscinosis.

Biel•schow•sky sign (byels-chov′skē sīn) In paralysis of a superior oblique muscle, tilting the head to the side of the involved eye causes that eye to rotate upward.

Biel•schow•sky stain (byels-chov′skē stān) A method of treating tissues with silver nitrate to demonstrate reticular fibers, neurofibrils, axons, and dendrites.

Biel•schow•sky test (byels-chov′skē test) A measurement of vertical strabismus in which the angle of ocular deviation is measured with changes in turning the head and angle of gaze to allow the clinician to isolate the paralytic muscle in vertical diplopia. This procedure is most useful in diagnosing palsies of the superior oblique muscle.

Bier am•pu•ta•tion (bēr amp′yū-tā′shŭn) Osteoplastic amputation of tibia and fibula.

Bier block an•es•the•si•a (bēr blok an′ĕs-thē′zē-ă) Regional limb anesthesia produced by intravenous injection of local anesthesia; used in conjunction with extremity tourniquet. [August Bier, 1861–1949, German surgeon]

Bier hy•per•e•mi•a (bēr hī′pĕr-ē′mē-ă) Obsolete term for hyperemia produced by Bier method (2).

Bier meth•od (bēr meth′ŏd) **1.** SYN intravenous regional anesthesia. **2.** Treatment of various surgical conditions by reactive hyperemia.

Bier•nac•ki sign (byer-naht′skē sīn) Analgesia to percussion of the ulnar nerve in tabes dorsalis and dementia paralytica.

bi•fid (bī′fid) Split or cleft; separated into two parts. [L. *bifidus,* cleft in two parts]

bi•fid ep•i•glot•tis (bī′fid ep′i-glot′is) Congenital malformation in which the right and left sides of the epiglottis are not joined; associated with stridor and aspiration in the newborn due to the rotation of the two sides of the epiglottis into the glottis.

Bi•fi•do•bac•te•ri•um (bī′fī-dō-bak-tēr′ē-ŭm) A genus of anaerobic bacteria (family Actinomycetaceae) containing gram-positive rods of highly variable appearance; freshly isolated strains characteristically show true and false branching, with bifurcated V and Y forms that are uniform or branched, and club or spatulate forms. It frequently stains irregularly; two or more granules may stain with methylene blue, whereas the remainder of the cell is unstained. It is not acid fast, is nonmotile, and does not produce spores; acetic and lactic acids are produced from glucose. Pathogenicity in humans is rare, although the bacterium has been found in the feces and alimentary tract of infants, some older people, and animals. The type species is *Bifidobacterium bifidum.* [L. *bifidus,* cleft in two parts, + bacterium]

Bi•fi•do•bac•te•ri•um den•ti•um (bī′fī-dō-bak-tēr′e-ŭm den′shē-ŭm) A bacterial species recovered in association with dental caries and periodontal disease. It is also an opportunistic pathogen, recovered in mixed infections associated with abscess formation.

bi•fid tongue (bī′fid tŭng) A congenital structural defect of the tongue in which its anterior part is divided longitudinally for a greater or lesser distance. SEE ALSO diglossia. SYN cleft tongue.

bi•fo•cal (bī-fō′kăl) Having two foci.

bi•fo•cal lens (bī-fō′kăl lenz) A lens used in cases of presbyopia, in which one portion is suited for distant vision, the other for reading and close work in general.

bi•fo•rate (bī-fōr′āt) Having two openings. [bi- + L. *foro,* pp. *-atus,* to bore, pierce]

bi•fur•cate, bi•fur•cat•ed (bī-fŭr′kāt, -kā-ted) Forked; two-pronged; having two branches. [bi- + L. *furca,* fork]

bi•fur•ca•tion (bī′fŭr-kā′shŭn) A forking; a division into two branches.

big a•dre•no•cor•ti•co•tro•pic hor•mone

(ACTH) (big ă-drē′nō-kōr-ti-kō-trō′pik hōr′mōn) A form of ACTH, produced by certain tumors, not immunochemically distinguishable from little ACTH, but not exerting any of the biologic effects characteristic of ACTH.

bi•gem•i•nal (bī-jem′i-năl) Characterized by two beats close together with a pause following each pair of beats. [bi- + L. *geminus,* double, paired]

bi•gem•i•nal pulse (bī-jem′i-năl pŭls) A pulse in which the beats occur in pairs. SYN coupled pulse, pulsus bigeminus.

bi•gem•i•nal rhythm (bī-jem′i-năl ridh′ŭm) Cardiac rhythm in which each beat of the dominant rhythm (sinus or other) is followed by a premature beat, with the result that the heartbeats occur in pairs (bigeminy). SYN coupled rhythm.

bi•gem•i•ny (bī-jem′i-nē) Pairing; especially, the occurrence of heartbeats in pairs. [bi- + L. *geminus,* twin]

bi•la•bi•al (bī-lā′bē-ăl) **1.** Pertaining to both lips. **2.** Speech sounds formed by contact or controlled airflow between the two lips, as in the sounds /b/ and /p/. [bi + L. *labium,* lip]

bi•lat•er•al (bī-lat′ĕr-ăl) Relating to, or having, two sides. [bi- + L. *latus,* side]

bi•lat•er•al co•or•din•a•tion (bī-lat′ĕr-ăl kō-ōr′di-nā′shŭn) The synchronization of movement of the sides of the body.

bi•lat•er•al her•maph•ro•dit•ism (bī-lat′ĕr-ăl hĕr-maf′rō-dīt-izm) True hermaphroditism with an ovotestis on each side.

bi•lat•er•al reach (bī-lat′ĕr-al rēch) Simultaneous use of both hands in a reaching activity.

bil•ber•ry (bil′ber-ē) Agent derived from dried fruit of *Vaccinum myrtillus;* studies suggest value in cardiovascular disease; also used to treat optic disorders; anecdotal reports claim use improved vision. SYN European blueberry, huckleberry, whortleberry.

bile (bīl) The yellowish-brown or greenish fluid secreted by the liver and discharged into the duodenum, where it aids in the emulsification of fats, increases peristalsis, and retards putrefaction; contains sodium glycocholate and sodium taurocholate, cholesterol, biliverdin and bilirubin, mucus, fat, lecithin, cells, and cellular debris. [L. *bilis*]

bile ac•ids (bīl as′idz) Steroid acids found in bile (e.g., taurocholic and glycocholic acids), used therapeutically when biliary secretion is inadequate and for biliary colic. Their physiologic roles include fat emulsification.

bile an•ti•gen (bīl an′ti-jen) SYN Bi antigen. SYN Bi antigen.

bile duct (bīl dŭkt) Any of the ducts conveying bile between the liver and the intestine, including hepatic, cystic, and common bile duct. SYN biliary duct.

bile pig•ments (bīl pig′mĕnts) Coloring matter in the bile derived from porphyrins by rupture of a methane bridge (e.g., bilirubin, biliverdin).

bi•le•vel pos•i•tive air•way pres•sure (BiPAP) (bī-lev′ĕl poz′i-tiv ār′wā presh′ŭr) A term applied to several pressure-controlled modes of mechanical ventilation. The sequence can be continuous mandatory ventilation (CMV), intermittent mandatory ventilation (IMV), or continuous spontaneous ventilation. Inspiration is either machine or patient triggered, pressure limited, or machine and patient cycled. The distinguishing feature of these modes is that the ventilator allows spontaneous breaths to occur during as well as between mandatory breaths. SEE ALSO mandatory breath, spontaneous breath, mode of ventilation.

bil•har•zi•al dys•en•ter•y (bil-hahr′zē-ăl dis′ĕn-ter′ē) Dysentery due to infection with *Schistosoma mansoni, S. haematobium,* or *S. japonicum.*

♻**bili-** Combining form denoting bile. [L. *bilis,* bile]

bil•i•ar•y (bil′ē-ār-ē) Relating to bile or the biliary tract.

bil•i•ar•y a•tre•si•a (bil′ē-ār-ē ă-trē′zē-ă) Atresia of the major bile ducts, causing cholestasis and jaundice, which does not become apparent until several days after birth; periportal fibrosis develops and leads to cirrhosis, with proliferation of small bile ducts and giant cell transformation of hepatic cells. Cf. neonatal hepatitis.

bil•i•ar•y can•a•lic•u•lus (bil′ē-ār-ē kan-ă-lik′yŭ-lŭs) One of the intercellular channels, 1 mcm or smaller in diameter, which occur between liver cells forming the first portion of the bile system.

bil•i•ar•y cir•rho•sis (bil′ē-ār-ē sir-ō′sis) Hepatic disorder due to biliary obstruction, which may be a primary intrahepatic disease or secondary to obstruction of extrahepatic bile ducts; the latter may lead to cholestasis and proliferation in small bile ducts with fibrosis, but marked disturbance of the lobular pattern is infrequent.

bil•i•ar•y col•ic (bil′ē-ār-ē kol′ik) Steady, ill-defined epigastric or right upper quadrant pain generally resulting from impaction of a gallstone in the cystic duct or ampulla of Vater with resulting distention of the gallbladder or biliary tract.

bil•i•ar•y duct (bil′ē-ār-ē dŭkt) SYN bile duct.

bil•i•ar•y duc•tules (bil′ē-ār-ē dŭk′tyūlz) The excretory ducts of the liver that connect the interlobular ductules to the right or left hepatic duct. SYN ductuli biliferi.

bil•i•gen•e•sis (bil′i-jen′ĕ-sis) Bile production. [bili- + G. *genesis,* production]

bil•i•gen•ic (bil′i-jen′ik) Producing bile.

bil•i•ous (bil′yŭs) **1.** Relating to or characteristic of biliousness. **2.** Formerly, denoting a temperament characterized by a quick, irritable temper. SYN choleric.

bil•i•ra•chi•a (bil′i-rā′kē-ă) Occurrence of bile pigments in the spinal fluid. [bili- + G. *rhachis,* spine]

bil•i•ru•bin (bil′i-rū′bin) A yellow bile pigment found as sodium bilirubinate (soluble), or as an insoluble calcium salt in gallstones, formed from hemoglobin during normal and abnormal destruction of erythrocytes by the reticuloendothelial system. Excess levels of bilirubin are associated with jaundice. [bili- + L. *ruber,* red]

bilirubinaemia [Br.] SYN bilirubinemia.

bil•i•ru•bi•ne•mi•a (bil′i-rū-bin-ē′mē-ă) The presence of increased amounts of bilirubin in the blood, where it is normally present in only relatively small amounts; usually used to describe various pathologic conditions in which there is excessive destruction of erythrocytes or interference with the mechanism of excretion in the bile. Determination of the quantity of bilirubin in the blood serum reveals two fractions, namely direct reacting (conjugated) and indirect reacting (nonconjugated) bilirubin; determination of direct bilirubin and total bilirubin in serum is an important and frequently used clinical laboratory test. SYN bilirubinaemia. [bilirubin + G. *haima,* blood]

bil•i•ru•bin en•ceph•a•lop•a•thy (bil′i-rū′bin en-sef′a-lop′ă-thē) SYN kernicterus.

bil•i•ru•bin•oids (bil′i-rū′bin-oydz) Generic term denoting intermediates in the conversion of bilirubin to stercobilin by reductive enzymes in intestinal bacteria; most are found in normal urine and feces.

bil•i•ru•bi•nu•ri•a (bil′i-rū-bi-nyūr′ē-ă) The presence of bilirubin in the urine. [bilirubin + G. *ouron,* urine]

bil•i•u•ri•a (bil′ē-yūr′ē-ă) The presence of various bile salts, or bile, in the urine. SYN choleuria, choluria. [bili- + G. *ouron,* urine]

bil•i•ver•din (bil′i-vĕr-din) Green pigment that occurs in bile.

bil•la•ble (bil′ă-bĕl) Denotes those procedures or therapies for which the health care professional or facility may expect compensation from the party legally responsible.

Bil•lings meth•od (bil′ingz meth′ŏd) A contraceptive method that involves periods of abstinence determined by changes in cervical mucus.

Bill ma•neu•ver (bil mă-nū′vĕr) Forceps rotation of the fetal head at mid-pelvis before extraction of the head. SYN Bill manoeuvre.

Bill manoeuvre [Br.] SYN Bill maneuver.

Bill•roth dis•ease (bil′rōt di-zēz′) **1.** Bladder cancer caused by chronic infection by *Schistosoma haematobium.* **2.** Fluid accumulation under scalp caused by skull fracture and arachnoid tear.

Bill•roth op•er•a•tion I (bil′rōt op-ĕr-ā′shŭn) Excision of the pylorus and antrum and partial closure of the gastric end with end-to-end anastomosis of stomach and duodenum.

Bill•roth op•er•a•tion II (bil′rōt op-ĕr-ā′shŭn) Excision of the pylorus and antrum with closure of the cut ends of the duodenum and stomach, followed by a gastrojejunostomy.

Bill•roth-von Wi•ni•war•ter dis•ease (bil′rōt-fōn vē-nē′vahr-ter di-zēz′) SYN Buerger disease.

bi•lo•bate, bi•lobed (bī-lō′bāt, bī′lōbd) Having two lobes.

bi•lo•bate pla•cen•ta (bī-lō′bāt plă-sen′tă) Placenta divided into two lobes.

bi•lob•u•lar (bī-lob′yū-lăr) Having two lobules.

bi•loc•u•lar, bi•loc•u•late (bī-lok′yū-lăr, -yū-lāt) Having two compartments or spaces. [bi- + L. *loculus,* dim. of *locus,* a place]

bi•loc•u•lar joint (bī-lok′yū-lăr joynt) One in which the intraarticular disc is complete, dividing the joint into two distinct cavities.

bi•mal•le•o•lar frac•ture (bī-mă-lē′ō-lăr frak′shŭr) Breakage of both medial and lateral malleoli. SEE ALSO malleolus.

bi•man•u•al (bī-man′yū-ăl) Relating to, or performed by, both hands. [bi- + L. *manus,* hand]

bi•man•u•al ver•sion (bī-man′yū-ăl vĕr′zhŭn) Turning of the baby in utero, performed by the hands acting on both extremities of the fetus; it may be the external or combined version.

bi•mas•toid (bī-mas′toyd) Relating to both mastoid processes.

bi•max•il•lar•y (bī-mak′si-lar-ē) Relating to both right and left maxillae; sometimes used to describe something affecting both halves of the upper jaw.

bi•na•ry (bī′nar-ē) **1.** Comprising two components, elements, molecules, or other. **2.** Denoting a choice of two mutually exclusive outcomes for one event (e.g., male or female, heads or tails, affected or unaffected). [L. *binarius,* consisting of two, fr. *bini,* two at a time]

bi•na•ry dig•it (bī′nar-ē dij′it) **1.** The smallest unit of digital information expressed in the binary system of notation (either 0 or 1). **2.** The signal in computing.

bi•na•ry fis•sion (bī′nar-ē fish′ŭn) Simple fission in which the two new cells are approximately equal in size.

bi•nau•ral (bī-naw′răl) Relating to both ears. SYN binotic. [L. *bini,* a pair, + *auris,* ear]

bi·nau·ral dip·la·cu·sis (bī-naw′răl dip′lă-kū′sis) A diplacusis in which the same sound is heard differently by the two ears.

bind·er (bīnd′ĕr) **1.** A broad bandage, especially one encircling the abdomen. **2.** Anything that binds.

bind·ing en·er·gy (bīnd′ing en′ĕr-jē) The force of attraction that holds an electron in its corresponding orbital shell.

Bi·net age (bi-nā′ āj) Mental age as determined by the Binet Simon scale.

Bi·net scale, Bi·net test (bi-nā′ skāl, bi-nā′ test) SYN Stanford-Binet intelligence scale.

binge, bing·ing (binj, binj′ing) Consumption of a foodstuff or alcoholic beverage in a compulsive manner in a short time.

Bing re·flex (bing rē′fleks) When the foot is passively dorsiflexed, plantar flexion occurs if any point on the ankle between the two malleoli is tapped.

bin·oc·u·lar (bin-ok′yū-lăr) Adapted to the use of both eyes; said of an optic instrument. [L. *bini,* paired, + *oculus,* eye]

bin·oc·u·lar mi·cro·scope (bin-ok′yū-lăr mī′krŏ-skōp) A microscope having two eyepieces; it may be a compound microscope or a stereoscopic microscope.

bin·oc·u·lar vi·sion (bin-ok′yū-lăr vizh′ŭn) vision with a single image, by both eyes simultaneously.

bi·no·mi·al (bī-nō′mē-ăl) A set of two terms or names; in the probabilistic or statistical sense it corresponds to a Bernoulli trial. [bi- + G. *nomos,* name]

bi·no·mi·al dis·tri·bu·tion (bī-nō′mē-ăl dis′tri-byū′shŭn) SYN Bernoulli distribution.

bi·no·mi·al no·men·cla·ture (bī-nō′mē-ăl nō′mĕn-klā′chŭr) Naming system in which each species of animal or plant has a name composed of two terms, one identifying the genus to which it belongs and the second the species.

bin·ot·ic (bin-ot′ik) SYN binaural. [L. *bini,* a pair, + G. *ous* (*ōt-*), ear]

bin·ov·u·lar (bin-ov′yū-lăr) Derived from two ova; of fraternal twins.

Bins·wan·ger dis·ease (bin′swahng-er di-zēz′) One of the causes of multiinfarct dementia, in which there are many infarcts and lacunae in the white matter, with relative sparing of the cortex and basal ganglia.

bi·nu·cle·ar, bi·nu·cle·ate (bī-nū′klē-ăr, -klē-āt) Having two nuclei.

bi·nu·cle·o·late (bī-nū′klē-ō-lāt) Having two nucleoli.

♲ **bio-** Combining form denoting life. [G. *bios,* life]

bi·o·a·cous·tics (bī′ō-ă-kūs′tiks) The science dealing with the effects of sound or vibration on living organisms.

bi·o·ac·tive non·nu·tri·ent (bī′ō-ak′tiv non-nū′trē-ĕnt) SYN phytochemical.

bi·o·ac·tiv·i·ty (bī′ō-ak-tiv′i-tē) Having an effect on a living organism.

bi·o·as·say (bī′ō-as′ā) Determination of the potency or concentration of a compound by its effect on animals, isolated tissues, or microorganisms, as contrasted with analysis of its chemical or physical properties. SYN biologic assay, biotest.

bi·o·a·vail·a·bil·i·ty (bī′ō-ă-vāl′ă-bil′i-tē) The physiologic availability of a given amount of a drug, as distinct from its chemical potency; proportion of the administered dose that is absorbed into the bloodstream.

bi·o·bur·den (bī′ō-bŭr′dĕn) Degree of microbial contamination or microbial load; the number of microorganisms contaminating an object.

bi·o·chem·i·cal (bī′ō-kem′i-kăl) Relating to biochemistry.

bi·o·chem·i·cal mod·u·la·tion (bī′ō-kem′i-kăl mod-yū-lā′shŭn) Modification (either enhancement of activity or reduction of toxicity) of a chemotherapeutic agent by another agent, which may or may not have antineoplastic activity of its own.

bi·o·chem·i·cal pro·file (bī′ō-kem′i-kăl prō′fīl) A combination of biochemical tests usually performed with automated instrumentation.

bi·o·chem·is·try (bī′ō-kem′is-trē) The chemistry of living organisms and of the chemical, molecular, and physical changes occurring therein. SYN biologic chemistry, physiologic chemistry.

bi·o·cid·al (bī′ō-sī′dăl) Destructive of life; particularly pertaining to microorganisms. [bio- + L. *caedo,* to kill]

bi·o·cide (bī′ō-sīd) A compound capable of killing something living. [bio- + -cide]

bi·o·com·pa·ti·bil·i·ty (bī′ō-kŏm-pat′i-bil′i-tē) The relative ability of a material to interact favorably with a biologic system. [bio- + compatibility]

bi·o·con·ver·sion (bī′ō-kŏn-vĕr′zhŭn) Transformation of organic matter into energy. [bio- + conversion]

bi·o·cy·ber·net·ics (bī′ō-sī′bĕr-net′iks) The science of communication and control within a living organism, particularly on a molecular basis.

bi·o·cy·tin (bī′ō-sī′tin) A complex molecule of biotin and lysine released from digested protein to act as a catalyst in the tricarboxylic acid cycle.

bi•o•de•grad•a•ble (bī′ō-dĕ-grād′ă-bĕl) Denoting a substance that can be chemically degraded or decomposed by natural effectors (e.g., weather, soil bacteria, plants, animals).

bi•o•deg•ra•da•tion (bī′ō-deg-rĕ-dā′shŭn) SYN biotransformation.

bi•o•dy•nam•ics (bī′ō-dī-nam′iks) The dynamic relationship existing between organisms, their physiology, and their environment.

bi•o•e•lec•tri•cal im•pe•dance a•nal•y•sis (BIA) (bī′ō-ē-lek′tri-kăl im-pē′dăns ă-nal′i-sis) Method of determining body fat, fat-free body mass, and total body water by measuring resistance to the flow of a small electrical current passed through the body.

bi•o•e•lec•tric•i•ty (bī′ō-ē-lek-tris′i-tē) Of or relating to electric phenomena in living organisms.

bi•o•en•er•get•ics (bī′ō-en′ĕr-jet′iks) **1.** The study of energy changes involved in the chemical reactions within living tissue. **2.** The study of energy exchanges between living organisms and their environments.

bi•o•eth•ics (bī′ō-eth′iks) Branch of ethics dealing with the use of the human body or body tissue in medical procedures (i.e., organ and fetal tissue transplant). [bio- + ethics]

bi•o•feed•back (bī′ō-fēd′bak) A training technique that enables a person to gain some element of voluntary control over autonomic body functions; based on the learning principle that a desired response is learned when received information such as a recorded increase in skin temperature (feedback) indicates that a specific thought complex or action has produced the desired physiologic response.

bi•o•field med•i•cine (bī′ō-fēld med′i-sin) Purported therapy involving analysis of energy fields around a patient's body; an unproved procedure.

bi•o•film (bī′ō-film) Thin coating of microorganisms that forms on a body surface, especially the surface of a tooth.

bi•o•fla•vo•noid (vit•a•min P) (bī′ō-flā′vŏ-noyd) A group of over 4000 types of colored, mostly water soluble, compounds found in vascular plants. They are essential for the absorption of ascorbic acid.

bi•o•gen•e•sis (bī′ō-jen′ĕ-sis) **1.** Term given by T.H. Huxley to the principle that life originates from only preexisting life and never from nonliving material. SEE spontaneous generation, recapitulation theory. **2.** SYN biosynthesis. [bio- + G. *genesis*, origin]

bi•o•ge•net•ic (bī′ō-jĕ-net′ik) Relating to biogenesis.

bi•o•haz•ard (bī′ō-haz′ărd) Contaminated or infective waste such as blood and body fluids. [bio- + hazard]

bi•o•in•for•mat•ics (bī′ō-in′fŏr-mat′iks) A scientific discipline encompassing all aspects of biologic information acquisition, processing, storage, distribution, analysis, and interpretation; it combines the tools and techniques of mathematics, computer science, and biology with the aim of understanding the biologic significance of a variety of data.

bi•o•in•stru•ment (bī′ō-in′strŭ-mĕnt) A sensor or device attached to or embedded in the body to record and transmit physiologic data to a receiving station.

bi•o•ki•net•ics (bī′ō-ki-net′iks) The study of the growth changes and movements that developing organisms undergo. [bio- + G. *kinēsis,* motion]

bi•o•log•ic, bi•o•log•i•cal (bī′ŏ-loj′ik, -loj′i-kăl) Relating to biology.

bi•o•log•i•cal (bī′ŏ-loj′i-kăl) A compound or medicine derived from living products, rather than chemicals (e.g., serum, antivenin).

bi•o•log•ic•al•ly ef•fec•tive dose (BED) (bī′ō-loj′ik-ă-lē e-fek′tiv dōs) The amount of an absorbed compound that reaches targets or sites of action within the body to cause a biologic effect.

bi•o•log•ic as•say (bī′ŏ-loj′ik as′ā) SYN bioassay.

bi•o•log•ic chem•is•try (bī′ŏ-loj′ik kem′is-trē) SYN biochemistry.

bi•o•log•ic con•trol (bī′ŏ-loj′ik kŏn-trōl′) Control of living organisms, including vectors and reservoirs of disease, by means of their natural enemies (i.e., predators, parasites, competitors).

bi•o•log•ic ev•o•lu•tion (bī′ŏ-loj′ik ev′ŏ-lū′shŭn) The doctrine that all forms of animal or plant life have been derived by gradual changes from simpler forms and ultimately unicellular organisms. SYN organic evolution.

bi•o•log•ic half-life (bī′ŏ-loj′ik haf′līf) The time required for one half of an amount of a substance to be lost through biologic processes.

bi•o•log•ic im•mu•no•ther•a•py (bī′ŏ-loj′ik im′yū-nō-thār′ă-pē) SYN immunotherapy.

bi•o•log•ic in•di•ca•tor (bī′ŏ-loj′ik in′di-kā-tŏr) A preparation of nonpathogenic microorganisms, usually bacterial spores, carried by an ampule or specially impregnated paper enclosed within a package during sterilization and subsequently incubated to verify that the spores were killed by the sterilization process.

bi•o•log•ic psy•chi•a•try (bī′ŏ-loj′ik sī-kī′ă-trē) A branch of the medical discipline that emphasizes molecular, genetic, and pharmacologic methods in the diagnosis and treatment of mental disorders.

bi•o•log•ic re•sponse mod•i•fi•er (bī′ō-loj′ik rĕ-spons′ mod′i-fī-ĕr) Agent that modifies host responses to neoplasms by enhancing immune systems or reconstituting impaired immune mechanisms.

bi•o•log•ic safe•ty hood (bī′ō-loj′ik sāf′tē hud) Protective cabinet used for handling potentially dangerous aerosols. Airflow draws particles away from the laboratory worker.

bi•o•log•ic sam•pling (bī′ō-loj′ik samp′ling) Denotes sampling that can be taken without jeopardy to the whole organism (e.g., for hematologic or biochemical study).

bi•o•log•ic vec•tor (bī′ō-loj′ik vek′tŏr) A vector, such as the *Anopheles* mosquito for malarial agents or the tsetse fly for agents of African sleeping sickness, in which the agent multiplies before transmission to another host.

bi•o•log•ic-war•fare (BW) a•gent (bī′ō-loj′ik wōr′fār ā′jĕnt) **1.** Living organisms (e.g., bacteria, viruses, fungi) used for military purposes. **2.** Living organisms or products (e.g., toxins) of living organisms used for military purposes.

bi•ol•o•gist (bī-ol′ŏ-jist) A specialist or expert in biology.

bi•ol•o•gy (bī-ol′ŏ-jē) The science concerned with the phenomena of life and living organisms. [bio- + G. *logos,* study]

bi•ol•y•sis (bī-ol′i-sis) Decomposition by living organisms of sewage and other complex materials. [bio + lysis]

bi•o•mass (bī′ō-mas) The total weight of all living things in a given area, biotic community, species population, or habitat; a measure of total biotic productivity.

bi•o•ma•te•ri•al (bī′ō-mă-tēr′ē-ăl) A synthetic or semisynthetic material chosen for its biocompatibility and used in a biologic system to construct an implantable prosthesis. [bio- + material]

bi•ome (bī′ōm) The total complex of biotic communities occupying and characterizing a particular geographic area or zone. [bio- + -ome]

bi•o•me•chan•i•cal a•nal•y•sis (bī′ō-mĕ-kan′i-kăl ă-nal′i-sis) SYN activity analysis.

bi•o•me•chan•i•cal frame of ref•er•ence (bī′ō-mĕ-kan′i-kăl frām ref′ĕr-rĕns) **1.** An intervention approach used when a person cannot maintain posture through appropriate involuntary muscle activity because of neuromuscular or musculoskeletal dysfunction; artificial supports are provided, temporarily or permanently. **2.** A therapeutic technique in which strength, endurance, and range of motion are increased in patients who have dysfunction in the nervous system or the musculoskeletal, integumentary, or cardiopulmonary systems.

bi•o•me•chan•ics (bī′ō-mĕ-kan′iks) The science concerned with the action of forces, internal or external, on the living body.

bi•o•med•i•cal (bī′ō-med′i-kăl) **1.** Pertaining to aspects of the biologic sciences that relate to or underlie medicine and medical technology. **2.** Biologic and medical, i.e., encompassing both the science(s) and the art of medicine.

bi•o•med•i•cal en•gi•neer•ing (bī′ō-med′i-kăl en′ji-nēr′ing) Biologic or medical application of engineering principles.

bi•o•med•i•cal mod•el (bī′ō-med′i-kăl mod′ĕl) A conceptual model of illness that excludes psychological and social factors.

bi•o•mem•brane (bī′ō-mem′brān) A structure bounding a cell or cell organelle; it contains lipids, proteins, glycolipids, and steroids. SYN membrana [TA], membrane (2).

bi•o•me•tri•cian (bī′ō-mĕ-trish′ăn) One who specializes in the science of biometry.

bi•om•e•try (bī-om′ĕ-trē) The application of statistical methods to the study of numeric data based on biologic observations and phenomena. [bio- + G. *metron,* measure]

bi•o•mi•cro•scope (bī′ō-mī′krŏ-skōp) SYN slitlamp.

bi•o•mi•cros•co•py (bī′ō-mī-kros′kŏ-pē) **1.** Microscopic examination of living tissue in the body. **2.** Examination of the cornea, aqueous humor, lens, vitreous humor, and retina by use of a slitlamp combined with a binocular microscope.

bi•o•ne•cro•sis (bī′ō-nĕ-krō′sis) SYN necrobiosis.

bi•on•ic (bī-on′ik) Relating to or developed from bionics.

bi•on•ics (bī-on′iks) **1.** The science of biologic functions and mechanisms as applied to electronic technology. **2.** The science of applying the knowledge gained by studying the characteristics of living organisms to the formulation of nonorganic devices and techniques. [bio- + electronics]

bi•o•ox•i•da•tive ther•a•py (bī-ok′si-dātiv thār′ă-pē) SYN oxygen therapy.

bi•o•phar•ma•ceu•tics (bī′ō-fahr′mă-sū′tiks) The study of the physical and chemical properties of a drug, and its dosage form, as related to the onset, duration, and intensity of drug action.

bi•o•phys•ics (bī′ō-fiz′iks) **1.** The study of biologic processes and materials by means of the theories and tools of physics. **2.** The study of physical processes (e.g., electricity, luminescence) occurring in organisms.

bi•o•po•ten•ti•al•i•ty (bī′ō-pŏ-ten′shē-al′i-tē) Capacity to develop in either of two mutually exclusive directions (i.e., male or female).

bi•op•sy (bī′op-sē) **1.** Process of removing tissue

from living patients for macroscopic diagnostic examination. **2.** A specimen obtained by brush or needle and syringe aspiration for biopsy. See page 198. [bio- + G. *opsis,* vision]

bi•o•psy•cho•so•cial mod•el (bī′ō-sī′kō-sō′ shăl mod′ĕl) A conceptual model that assumes that psychological and social factors must also be included along with the biologic in understanding a person's medical illness or disorder.

bi•op•tome (bī′op-tōm) A biopsy instrument passed through a catheter into the heart to obtain tissue for diagnosis. [*biop*sy + G. *tomē,* a cutting]

bi•o•reg•u•la•tor (bī′ō-reg-yŭ′lā-tŏr) Any endogenous substance that modifies the rate or intensity of a biologic process so as to maintain homeostasis or meet changing needs of the organism. Cf. bioregulator. SYN melanocyte-stimulating hormone.

bi•o•rhythm (bī′ō-ridh-ĕm) A biologically inherent cyclic variation or recurrence of an event or state, such as the sleep cycle, circadian rhythms, or periodic diseases. [bio- + G. *rhythmos,* rhythm]

bi•o•safe•ty (bī′ō-sāf′tē) Safety measures applied to the handling of biologic materials or organisms with a known potential to cause disease in humans.

bi•o•so•cial (bī′ō-sō′shăl) Involving the interplay of biologic and social influences.

bi•o•spec•trom•e•try (bī′ō-spek-trom′ĕ-trē) Spectroscopic determination of the types and amounts of various substances in living tissue or fluid from a living body. [bio- + L. *spectrum,* an image, + G. *metron,* measure]

bi•o•spec•tros•co•py (bī′ō-spek-tros′kŏ-pē) Spectroscopic examination of specimens of living tissue, including fluids removed therefrom. [bio- + L. *spectrum,* image, + G. *skopeō,* to examine]

bi•o•sphere (bī′ō-sfēr) All the regions in the world where living organisms are found. [bio- + G. *sphaira,* sphere]

bi•o•sta•tis•tics (bī′ō-stă-tis′tiks) The science of statistics applied to biologic or medical data.

bi•o•syn•the•sis (bī′ō-sin′thĕ-sis) Formation of a chemical compound by enzymes, either in the organism (in vivo) or by fragments or extracts of cells (in vitro). SYN biogenesis (2).

bi•o•syn•thet•ic (bī′ō-sin-thet′ik) Relating to or produced by biosynthesis.

bi•o•sys•tem (bī′ō-sis′tĕm) A living organism or any complete system of living things that can, directly or indirectly, interact with others.

bi•o•ta (bī-ō′tă) The collective flora and fauna of a region. [Mod. L., fr. G. *bios,* life]

Bi•ot breath•ing sign (bē-ō′ brēdh′ing sīn) Irregular periods of apnea alternating with four or five deep breaths; seen with increased intracranial pressure.

bi•o•te•lem•e•try (bī′ō-tĕ-lem′ĕ-trē) The technique of monitoring vital processes and transmitting data without wires to a point remote from the subject.

bi•o•ter•ror•ism (bī′ō-ter′ŏr-izm) **1.** The use of biologic organisms (e.g., bacteria, viruses, or fungi) or their products (e.g., toxins) in terrorist activities. **2.** A common but incorrect designation for the use of chemical, biologic, or radiologic agents in terrorism.

bi•o•test (bī′ō-test) SYN bioassay.

bi•ot•ic (bī-ot′ik) Pertaining to life.

bi•o•tin (bī′ō-tin) The D-isomer component of the vitamin B2 complex occurring in or required by most organisms and inactivated by avidin; participates in biologic carboxylations.

bi•ot•i•nides (bī-ot′i-nīdz) Compounds of biotin; e.g., biocytin.

bi•o•tope (bī′ō-tōp) The smallest geographic area providing uniform conditions for life; the physical part of an ecosystem. [G. *bios,* life, + *topos,* place]

bi•o•tox•i•col•o•gy (bī′ō-tok′si-kol′ŏ-jē) The study of poisons produced by living organisms.

bi•o•tox•in (bī′ō-tok′sin) A common misnomer for toxin (q.v.) (by definition, a toxin is of biologic origin).

bi•o•trans•for•ma•tion (bī′ō-trans′fōr-mā′ shŭn) The conversion of molecules from one form to another within an organism, often associated with change in pharmacologic activity; refers especially to drugs and other xenobiotics. SYN biodegradation.

Bi•ot res•pi•ra•tion (bē-ō′ res′pir-ā′shŭn) Completely irregular breathing pattern, with continually variable rate and depth of breathing; results from lesions in the respiratory centers in the brainstem, extending from the dorsomedial medulla caudally to the obex.

bi•o•type (bī′ō-tīp) **1.** A population or group of individuals composed of the same genotype. **2.** SYN biovar. SYN biovar (2). [bio- + G. *typos,* model]

bi•o•var (bī′ō-vahr) **1.** A group of bacterial strains distinguishable from other strains of the same species on the basis of physiologic characters. **2.** BACTERIOLOGY SYN biotype. SYN biotype (2). [bio- + *variant*]

bi•o•vu•lar (bī-ov′yū-l′ar) SYN diovular.

bi•o•war•fare (bī′ō-wōr′fār) **1.** The use of biologic organisms (e.g., bacteria, viruses, or fungi) or their products (e.g., toxins) in warfare. **2.** A

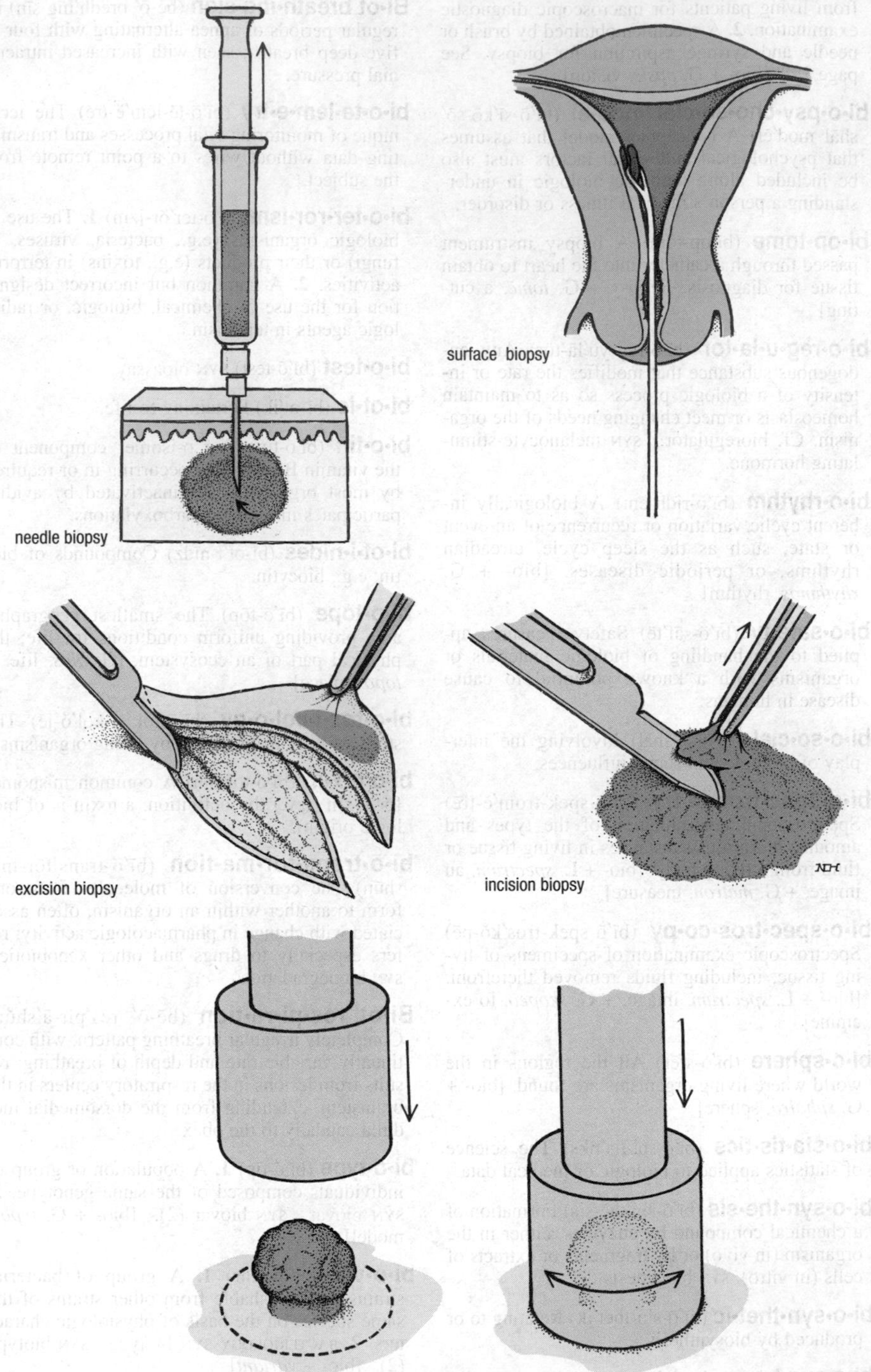
surface biopsy
needle biopsy
excision biopsy
incision biopsy
punch biopsy

biopsy

common but incorrect designation for the use of chemical, biologic, or radiologic agents in warfare.

BiPAP (bī′pap) Acronym for bilevel positive airway pressure.

bi•pa•ren•tal (bī′păr-ent′ăl) Having two parents, male and female.

bi•pa•ri•e•tal (bī′păr-ī′ĕ-tăl) Relating to both parietal bones, especially to the greatest diameter measured externally from one parietal bone to the other.

bi•pa•ri•e•tal di•am•e•ter (bī′pă-rī′ĕ-tăl dī-am′ĕ-tĕr) The diameter of the fetal head between the two parietal eminences.

bip•a•rous (bip′ă-rŭs) Bearing two young. [bi- + L. *pario,* to give birth]

bi•par•tite (bī-par′tīt) Consisting of two parts or divisions.

bi•ped•i•cle flap (bī-ped′i-kĕl flap) A flap with two pedicles, one at each end. SYN advancement flap.

bi•pen•nate, **bi•pen•ni•form** (bī-pen′āt, bī-pen′i-fōrm) Pertaining to a muscle with a central tendon toward which the fibers converge on either side like the barbs of a feather. [bi- + L. *penna,* feather]

bi•pha•sic trans•tho•rac•ic de•fib•ril•la•tion (bī-fā′zik tranz′thōr-as′ik dē-fib′ri-lā′shŭn) Transthoracic defibrillation that delivers a calibrated fixed low-energy waveform.

bi•phe•no•typ•ic (bī′fē-nō-tip′ik) Pertaining to or characterized by biphenotypy.

bi•phe•no•typ•y (bī-fē′nō-tī′pē) The expression of markers of more than one cell type by the same cell, as in certain leukemias.

bi•phen•yl (bī-fen′il) SYN diphenyl.

bi•po•lar (bī-pō′lăr) **1.** Having two poles, ends, or extremes. **2.** Pertaining to a mood disorder involving alternating mania and depression.

bi•po•lar cau•ter•y (bī-pō′lăr kaw′tĕr-ē) Electrocautery by high frequency electrical current passed through tissue from an active to a passive electrode; used for hemostasis.

bi•po•lar cell (bī-pō′lăr sel) A neuron having two processes, such as those of the retina or the spiral and vestibular ganglia of the eighth cranial nerve.

bi•po•lar dis•or•der (bī-pō′lăr dis-ōr′dĕr) An affective disorder characterized by the occurrence of alternating periods of euphoria (mania) and depression. SYN manic-depressive psychosis.

Bi•po•lar•is (bī-pō-la′ris) Genus of dematiaceous fungi that is among the causes of phaeohyphomycosis.

Bi•po•lar•is au•stra•li•en•sis (bī-pō-la′ris aws-trā′lē-en′sis) Species of dematiaceous fungi that is among the causes of phaeohyphomycosis; may cause fungal sinusitis.

Bi•po•lar•is ha•wai•i•en•sis (bī-pō-la′ris hă-wah-ē-en′sis) Species of dematiaceous fungi that is among the causes of phaeohyphomycosis.

Bi•po•lar•is spi•ci•fe•ra (bī-pō-la′ris spi-sif′ĕr-ă) Species of dematiaceous fungi that is among the causes of phaeohyphomycosis; common cause of fungal sinusitis. Cases of disease involving pulmonary and cerebral disorders have been reported.

bi•po•lar lead (bī-pō′lăr lēd) A record obtained with two electrodes placed on different regions of the body, each electrode contributing significantly to the record; e.g., a standard limb lead.

bi•po•lar neu•ron (bī-pō′lăr nūr′on) A neuron that has two processes arising from opposite poles of the cell body.

bi•po•ten•ti•al•i•ty (bī′pŏ-ten′shē-al′i-tē) Capability of differentiating along either of two developmental pathways. An example is the capacity of the primordial gonad to develop into either an ovary or a testis.

bi•ra•mous (bī-rā′mŭs) Having two branches. [bi- + L. *ramus,* branch]

birch (bĭrch) (*Betula alba*) Often consumed as a tea; the oil preparation is of alleged value in bladder disorders; sometimes used topically, although its toxicity makes it unsuitable for pediatric patients. SYN white birch.

bird-breed•er's lung, **bird-fan•ci•er's lung** (bĭrd′brēd-ĕrz lŭng, bĭrd′fan′sē-ĕrz lŭng) Extrinsic allergic alveolitis caused by inhalation of particulate avian emanations.

bird flu (bĭrd flū) SYN avian influenza.

bird shot ret•i•no•cho•roid•i•tis (bĭrd shot ret′i-nō-kōr′oyd-ī′tis) Bilateral diffuse retinal vasculitis with depigmentation of multiple areas of the choroid and retinal pigment epithelium posterior to the ocular equator, often with an associated papillitis or optic atrophy; vitiligo occurs occasionally. SYN vitiliginous choroiditis.

bi•re•frin•gence (bī-rĕ-frin′jĕns) SYN double refraction.

bi•re•frin•gent (bī-rĕ-frin′jĕnt) Refracting twice; splitting a ray of light in two.

birth (bĭrth) **1.** Passage of the fetus from the uterus to the outside world; the act of being born. **2.** Specifically, complete expulsion or extraction of a fetus from its mother.

birth am•pu•ta•tion (bĭrth amp′yū-tā′shŭn) SYN congenital amputation.

birth ca•nal (bĭrth kă-nal′) Cavity of the uterus

and vagina through which the fetus passes. SYN parturient canal.

birth con·trol (bĭrth kŏn-trōl′) **1.** Restriction of the number of offspring by means of contraceptive measures. **2.** Projects, programs, or methods to control reproduction, by either improving or diminishing fertility.

birth con·trol pill (bĭrth kŏn-trōl′ pil) Oral medication containing estrogen alone or combined with progesterone; used to prevent conception.

birth·day rule (bĭrth′dā rūl) A principle involving coordination of benefits of health insurance plans to determine which insurance plan should cover costs of health care for dependent children; states that the insurance of the parent whose birth month is first in the calendar year is primary. (If both are in the same month, then coverage derives from the plan carried by the parent born earlier in the month. If both are the same month and day, coverage comes from the parent who has been covered for a longer period.)

birth de·fect (bĭrth dē-fekt′) Any structural or biochemical abnormality present at birth; may be due to genetic or developmental factors. Cf. congenital anomaly.

birth·ing (bĭrth′ing) Parturition; the act of giving birth.

birth·ing cen·ter (bĭrth′ing sen′tĕr) A facility, usually in a hospital, which provides labor and delivery services in a comfortable, homelike setting.

birth in·ju·ry (bĭrth in′jŭr-ē) SYN birth trauma (1).

birth·mark (bĭrth′mahrk) A persistent congenital visible lesion, usually on the skin, identified at or near birth; commonly due to nevus or hemangioma. SEE nevus (1).

birth pal·sy (bĭrth pawl′zē) Any motor abnormality in the infant caused by or attributed to the birthing process (e.g., includes obstetric paralysis, infantile hemiplegia).

birth·rate (bĭrth′rāt) A summary rate based on the number of live births in a population over a given period, usually 1 year; the numerator is the number of live births, the denominator is the midyear population.

birth trau·ma (bĭrth traw′mă) **1.** Physical injury to an infant during its delivery. SYN birth injury. **2.** The supposed emotional injury, inflicted by events incident to birth, on an infant which allegedly appears in symbolic form in patients with mental illness.

birth weight (bĭrth wāt) In humans, the first weight of an infant obtained within less than the first 60 completed minutes after birth; a full-size infant weighs 2500 g or more; low birth weight is less than 2500 g.

birth·wort (bĭrth′wōrt) SYN *Aristolochia fangchi.*

♻ **bis-** **1.** Prefix signifying two or twice. **2.** CHEMISTRY used to denote the presence of two identical but separated complex groups in one molecule. Cf. bi-, di-. [L.]

2,5-bis(5-*t*-bu·tyl·ben·zox·a·zol-2-yl)thi·o·phene (BBOT) (bis byū′til-ben-zoks′ă-zol thī′ō-fēn) A scintillator used in radioactivity measurements by scintillation counting.

Bisch·of my·e·lot·o·my (bish′of mī′ĕ-lot′ŏ-mē) Longitudinal incision of the spinal cord through the lateral column for treatment of spasticity of the lower extremities.

bis in die, bid (bis in dē′ā) Twice a day. [L.]

bi·sex·u·al (bī-sek′shū-ăl) **1.** Having gonads of both sexes. SEE ALSO hermaphroditism. **2.** Denoting a person attracted to members of both sexes.

bis·fer·i·ous pulse (bis-fer′ē-ŭs pŭls) Having two beats; an arterial pulse with peaks that may be palpable. SYN pulsus bisferiens.

BIS-GMA The abbreviation for bisphenol A-glycidal methyl methacrylate, a resin material used in dentistry.

Bish·op score (bish′ŏp skōr) System to determine the inducibility of the cervix in a pregnant patient, based on dilation, effacement, station, and cervical consistency and position.

Bish·op sphyg·mo·scope (bish′ŏp sfig′mō-skōp) An instrument for measuring the blood pressure, with special reference to diastolic pressure; the tube is filled with a solution of cadmium borotungstate, and the scale is the reverse of that of a mercurial manometer, the pressure being made directly by the weight of the liquid and not by compressed air.

bish·op's wort (bish′ŭps wōrt) SYN betony.

bis·il·i·ac (bis-il′ē-ak) Relating to any two corresponding iliac parts or structures, as the iliac bones or iliac fossae.

bis·muth (Bi) (biz′mŭth) A trivalent metallic element; atomic no. 83, atomic wt. 20.98037. Several of its salts are used in medicine. [Ger. *Wismut, weisse Masse*, white mass]

bis·muth line (biz′mŭth līn) A black zone on the free marginal gingiva, often the first sign of poisoning from prolonged parenteral administration of bismuth.

bis·mu·tho·sis (biz′mŭ-thō′sis) Chronic bismuth poisoning.

bis·muth·yl (biz′mŭ-thil) The group, BiO^+, that behaves chemically as the ion of a univalent metal; its salts are subsalts of bismuth.

bi·spec·tral in·dex (bī-spek′trăl in′deks) A measure derived from the domain of time; the frequency and bispectral analysis of the encephalogram that correlates with depth of sedation and anesthesia in clinical medicine.

1,3-bis•phos•pho•glyc•er•ate (bis-fos′fō-glis′ĕr-āt) An intermediate in glycolysis which enzymatically reacts with ADP to generate ATP and 3-phosphoglycerate.

2,3-bis•phos•pho•glyc•er•ate (bis′fos-fō-glis′ĕr-āt) An intermediate in the Rapoport-Luebering shunt, formed between 1,3-bisphosphoglycerate and 3-phosphoglycerate; an important regulator of the affinity of hemoglobin for oxygen; an intermediate of phosphoglycerate mutase.

bis•phos•pho•nates (bis-fos′fō-nāts) Class of medications to treat osteoporosis.

bis•tort (bis′tōrt) (*Polygonum bistorta*) A strongly astringent botanical with purported medicinal properties that is used both internally and externally. Scientific trials have been limited. SYN adderwort, dragonwort, snakeweed, twice writhen. [L. *bis,* twice, + *tortus,* twisted]

bis•tou•ry (bis′tū-rē) A long, narrow-bladed knife, with a straight or curved edge and sharp or blunt point (probe-point); used for opening or slitting cavities or hollow structures. [Fr. *bistouri,* fr. It. dialect *bistori,* perh. fr. *Pistoia,* Italy]

bi•sul•fate (bī-sŭl′fāt) A salt containing HSO_4^-. SYN acid sulfate, bisulphate.

bi•sul•fide (bī-sŭl′fīd) A compound of the anion HS^-; an acid sulfide. SYN bisulphide.

bi•sul•fite (bī-sŭl′fīt) A salt or ion of HSO_3^-. SYN bisulphite.

bisulphate [Br.] SYN bisulfate.

bisulphide [Br.] SYN bisulfide.

bisulphite [Br.] SYN bisulfite.

BIT (bit) Abbreviation for behavioral inattention test.

bite (bīt) **1.** To incise or seize with the teeth. **2.** The act of incision or seizure with the teeth. **3.** A morsel of food held between the teeth. **4.** Term used to denote the amount of pressure developed in closing the jaws. **5.** Colloquial usage for terms such as interocclusal record, maxillomandibular registration, denture space, and interarch distance. **6.** A wound or puncture of the skin made by animal or insect. SEE ALSO bites. [A.S. *bītan*]

bite a•nal•y•sis (bīt ă-nal′i-sis) SYN occlusal analysis.

bite block (bīt blok) Device used in dentistry for recording the spatial relation of the jaws in respect to the occlusion of teeth.

bi•tem•po•ral (bī-tem′pŏr′ăl) Relating to both temporal bones, especially to the greatest diameter measured externally from one temporal bone to the other.

bite•plate, bite•plane (bīt′plāt, bīt′plān) A removable appliance that incorporates a plane of acrylic designed to occlude with the opposing teeth.

bites (bīts) Multiple penetrations of the skin (puncture or laceration) causing reactions that result from 1) mechanical injury; 2) injection of toxic material such as snake or scorpion venom; 3) injection of antigenic substances, especially by insect or arthropod bites, capable of inducing and eliciting allergic sensitization; 4) introduction of otherwise indigenous mouth flora in the instance of human bites; 5) invasion of the tissue as in myiasis; 6) transmission of diseases such as typhus and rabies. SEE ALSO bite.

bite•wing film (bīt′wing film) A special packaging of radiographic film that allows an appendage of the film package to be held between the occlusal surfaces of the teeth.

bite•wing ra•di•o•graph, bite•wing (bīt′wing rā′dē-ō-graf, bīt′wing) Intraoral dental film adapted to show the coronal portion and cervical third of the root of the teeth in near occlusion; especially useful in detecting interproximal caries and determining alveolar septal height. See this page.

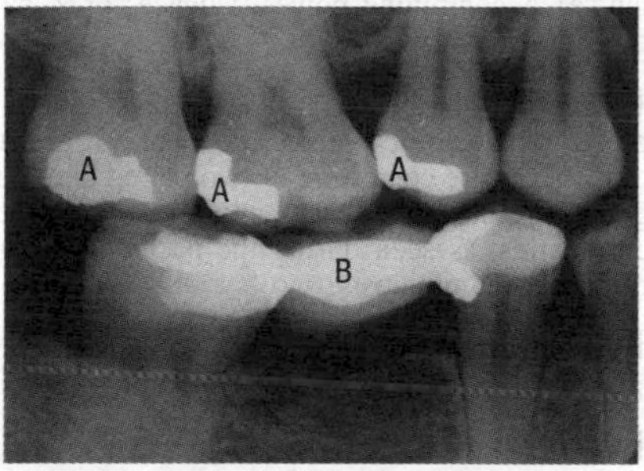

bitewing radiograph: (A) amalgam restorations; (B) fixed partial denture

bi•ther•mal ca•lo•ric test (bī-thĕr′măl kă-lōr′ik test) A test of vestibular function in which each ear canal is alternately or simultaneously irrigated with water at 7°C above or below body temperature; the nystagmus produced may be monitored for direction, amplitude, speed of the slow component, and duration. SEE ALSO Bárány sign.

Bi•tot spots (bē-tō′ spotz) Any of numerous small, circumscribed, lusterless, grayish white, foamy, greasy, triangular deposits on the bulbar conjunctiva adjacent to the cornea in the area of the palpebral fissure of both eyes; occurs in vitamin A deficiency.

bi•tro•chan•ter•ic (bī′trō-kan-ter′ik) Relating to two trochanters, either to the two trochanters of one femur or to both greater trochanters.

bit•ter mel•on (bit′ĕr mel′ŏn) *Momordica*

charantia, tropical fruit that is typically consumed as a juice, although sometimes eaten. Limited studies suggest use in Type 2 diabetes; also purportedly of value as an antiinfective.

bit·ter or·ange (bit′ĕr ōr′ănj) The fruit of *Citrus aurantium;* clinical reports suggest use as an antiviral, in treating GI and dermatologic disorders. Some have used it as an appetite suppressant (after the ban on ephedra), but severe and frequent adverse effects have been reported (seizure, cardiovascular disorders).

Bit·torf re·ac·tion (bit′orf rē-ak′shŭn) In cases of renal colic, pain radiating to the kidney when a testicle is squeeze or an ovary is pressed.

bi·u·ret (bī′yŭr-ĕt) Obtained by eliminating one NH_3 between two urea molecules. Used in protein determinations. SYN carbamoylurea.

bi·u·ret re·ac·tion, **bi·u·ret test** (bī′yŭr-ĕt rē-ak′shŭn, bī′yŭr-ĕt test) The formation of biuret, which gives a violet color because of the reaction of a polypeptide of more than three amino acids with $CuSO_4$ in strongly alkaline solution; used for the detection and quantitation of polypeptides or protein in biologic fluids.

bi·va·lence, **bi·va·len·cy** (bī-vā′lĕns, bī-vā′lĕn-sē) A combining power (valence) of 2. SYN divalence, divalency.

bi·va·lent (bī-vā′lĕnt) **1.** Having a combining power (valence) of two. SYN divalent. **2.** CYTOLOGY a structure consisting of two paired homologous chromosomes, each split into two sister chromatids, as seen during the pachytene stage of prophase in meiosis.

bi·va·lent chro·mo·some (bī-vā′lĕnt krō′mŏ-sōm) A pair of chromosomes temporarily united.

bi·ven·tral (bī-ven′trăl) SYN digastric (1).

bi·ven·tric·u·la·re (bī-ven-trik′yū-lar′ē) Having two ventricles. [L.]

bix·el (bik′sĕl) SYN beamlet.

Biz·zo·ze·ro red cells (bits′sō-zār′ō red selz) Nucleated red blood cells in human blood.

Bjer·rum sco·to·ma (byer′ŭm skă-tō′mă) A scotoma shaped like a comet's tail; occurs in glaucoma, attached at the temporal end to the blind spot or separated from it by a narrow gap; the defect widens as it extends above and nasally curves around the fixation spot, and then extends downward to end exactly at the nasal horizontal meridian.

Björn·stad syn·drome (byōrn′stahd sin′drōm) Pili torti associated with sensorineural hearing loss; the severity of distortion and brittleness of the hair are correlated with the degree of hearing impairment; autosomal dominant inheritance.

Bk Symbol for berkelium.

B-K am·pu·ta·tion (amp′yū-tā′shŭn) Abbreviation for below-the-knee amputation.

Black·ber·ry Thumb (blak′ber-ē thŭm) A general term used to describe the clinical signs and symptoms of a repetitive motion injury of the hand, thumb, or fingers caused by overuse of a personal digital assistant type device. SEE ALSO tendinitis.

black blood im·ag·ing (blak blŭd im′ăj-ing) Magnetic resonance imaging modality in which blood vessels appear black.

black cat·a·ract (blak kat′ăr-akt) SYN brunnescent cataract.

Black clas·si·fi·ca·tion (blak klas′i-fi-kā′shŭn) A classification of cavities of the teeth based on the tooth surface(s) involved.

black co·hosh (blak kō′hosh) A herbal made from *Cimifuga racemosa* and other *Cimifuga* spp.; widely used for its purported value in treating disorders of the female reproductive system, GI disease, insect bite, and other uses; because of its effect on hormonal states, its use in pregnant women must be monitored very carefully. SYN baneberry, black snake root, rattleweed, squaw root (1).

Black Creek Ca·nal vi·rus (blak crēk kă-nal′ vī′rŭs) A species of Hantavirus in the U.S. causing hantavirus pulmonary syndrome; transmitted by the cotton rat. [Black Creek Canal in Florida, where the cotton rats were captured from which the virus was first isolated]

black death (blak deth) Term applied to the worldwide epidemic of the 14th century, during which some 60 million people are said to have died; the descriptions indicate that it was caused by *Yersinia pestis*. SEE ALSO plague (2).

black eye (blak ī) Ecchymosis of the lids and their surroundings.

black fire ant (blak fīr ant) SYN *Solenopsis richteri*.

black globe ther·mom·e·ter (blak glōb thĕr-mom′ĕ-tĕr) Ambient air thermometer, the bulb of which is enclosed in a black metal sphere that absorbs radiant energy from the surroundings to measure heat gained from this source.

black hair·y tongue (blak hār′ē tŭng) SYN black tongue.

black haw (blak haw) A small tree (*Viburnum prunifolium*), the leaves of which are of purported value as an aid to gynecologic disorders, as a therapeutic in pregnancy, and as a topical astringent. SYN American sloe, cramp bark, nannyberry, sheepberry, shonny.

black·head (blak′hed) **1.** SYN open comedo. **2.** SYN histomoniasis.

black lung (blak lŭng) A form of pneumoconiosis, common in coal miners, characterized by deposit of carbon particles in the lung. SYN miner's lung (2).

black•out (blak′owt) **1.** Temporary loss of consciousness due to decreased blood flow to the brain. SEE ALSO syncope. **2.** Momentary loss of consciousness as in an absence. **3.** Temporary loss of vision, without alteration of consciousness, due to positive (above normal) g (gravity) forces; caused by temporary decreased blood flow in the central retinal artery, and seen mostly in aviators. **4.** A transient episode that occurs during a state of intense intoxication (alcoholic blackout) for which the person has no recall, although not unconscious (as observed by others).

black Pi•e•dra (blak pē-ā′drā) A fungal infection that affects the hair shaft; hard, gritty, brown-to-black crusts composed of hyphal elements are characteristic features; common in tropic areas. *Piedraia hortae* is the causative agent.

black root (blak rūt) Herbal made from *Veronicastrum virginicum;* foul-tasting, used as an emetic and cathartic; purported value in therapy for hepatic and biliary disorders. Hepatotoxicity reported. SYN Culver's root, high veronica, physic root, tall speedwell, veronica.

black snake root (blak snāk rūt) SYN black cohosh.

i **black tongue** (blak tŭng) Black to yellowish-brown discoloration of the dorsum of the tongue due to staining by exogenous material such as the components of tobacco or the use of broad spectrum antibiotics; usually superimposed on hairy tongue. See this page. SYN black hairy tongue, lingua nigra, melanoglossia.

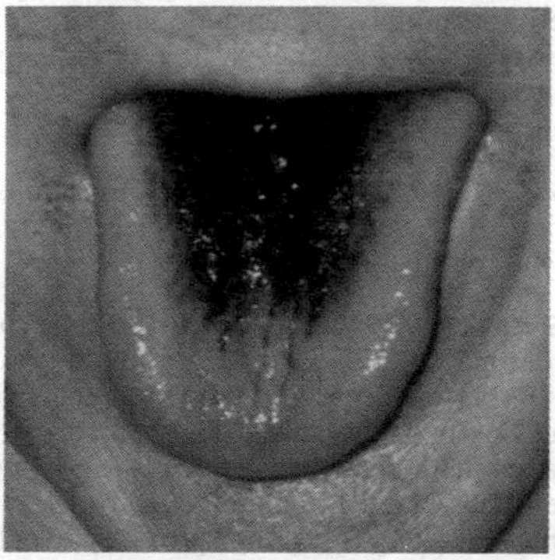

black tongue

black-top tube (blak-top tūb) An evacuated blood collection tube with a black stopper indicating that it contains sodium citrate as anticoagulant; used for determination of the Westergren erythrocyte sedimentation rate.

black•wa•ter fe•ver (blak′waw′tĕr fē′vĕr) Hemoglobinuria resulting from severe hemolysis occurring in falciparum malaria.

black wid•ow spi•der (blak wid′ō spī′dĕr) A venomous arachnid, attacks always come from female (*Latrodectus mactans*); reported throughout the United States, but more common in the South; marked on underside with a white 'hourglass' shape. Only small children and immunocompromised patients are likely to die from her bite, although the acute form of the paralysis can cause severe pain.

blad•der (blad′ĕr) **1.** A distensible musculomembranous organ serving as a receptacle for fluid, as the gallbladder or urinary bladder. SEE detrusor. **2.** SYN urinary bladder. SYN vesica (1). [A.S. *blaedre*]

blad•der ear (blad′ĕr ēr) Protrusion of a portion of the bladder into proximal inguinal canal; often seen in pediatric voiding cystourethrogram and rarely of clinical significance.

blad•der train•ing (blad′ĕr trān′ing) A predetermined schedule of voiding and toileting to maintain or improve bladder functioning.

Blag•den law (blahg′dĕn law) The depression of the freezing point of dilute solutions is proportional to the amount of the dissolved substance.

Blain•ville ears (blăn-vēl′ ērz) Asymmetry in size or shape of the auricles.

Blair-Brown graft (blār-brown graft) A split-thickness graft of intermediate thickness.

Bla•lock-Taus•sig op•er•a•tion (blā′lok taw′sig op-ĕr-ā′shŭn) An operation for congenital malformations of the heart, in which an abnormally small volume of blood passes through the pulmonary circuit; blood from the systemic circulation is directed to the lungs by anastomosing the right or left subclavian artery to the right or left pulmonary artery.

Bla•lock-Taus•sig shunt (blā′lok taw′sig shŭnt) A palliative subclavian artery to pulmonary artery anastomosis.

blanch (blanch) **1.** To become white or pale, as skin or mucous membrane affected by vasoconstriction. **2.** To whiten or bleach a surface or substance. [O.Fr. *blanchir*, fr. *blanc*, white]

bland di•et (bland dī′ĕt) A regular diet omitting foods that mechanically or chemically irritate the gastrointestinal tract.

blank (blangk) A solution consisting of all the analytic components except the compound to be measured; used to establish a baseline of measurement intensity with which the compound of interest is compared. [M.E. white, fr. O.Fr. *blanc*, fr. Germanic]

blan•ket (blangk′ĕt) Any covering.

blan•ket su•ture (blangk′ĕt sū′chŭr) A continuous lock-stitch used to approximate the skin of a wound.

blast (blast) General term for immature or precursor cell. [G. *blastos,* germ]

-blast A suffix meaning an immature precursor cell of the type indicated by the preceding word. [G. *blastos,* germ]

blast cell (blast sel) An immature precursor cell; e.g., erythroblast, lymphoblast, neuroblast. SEE ALSO -blast.

blas•te•ma (blas-tē′mă) **1.** The primordial cellular mass (precursor) from which an organ or part is formed. **2.** A cluster of cells competent to initiate the regeneration of a damaged or ablated structure. [G. a sprout]

blas•tem•ic (blas-tem′ik) Relating to the blastema.

blast in•ju•ry (blast in′jŭr-ē) Tearing of lung tissue or rupture of abdominal viscera without external injury, as by the force of an explosion.

blasto- Prefix pertaining to the process of budding by cells or tissue. [G. *blastos,* germ]

blas•to•cele (blas′tō-sēl) The cavity in the blastula of a developing embryo, such as in amphibians, reptiles, and birds. SYN blastocoele, cleavage cavity, segmentation cavity. [blasto- + G. *koilos,* hollow]

blas•to•cel•ic (blas′tō-sē′lik) Relating to the blastocele. SYN blastocoelic.

blastocoele [Br.] SYN blastocele.

blastocoelic [Br.] SYN blastocelic.

Blas•to•co•nid•i•um (blas′tō-kŏ-nid′ē-ŭm) A holoblastic conidium that is produced singly or in chains, and detached at maturity leaving a bud scar, as in the budding of a yeast cell. [blasto- + conidium]

blas•to•cyst (blas′tō-sist) The modified blastula stage of mammalian embryos (including human), consisting of the embryoblast (inner cell mass) and a thin trophoblast layer enclosing the blastocystic cavity. See this page, B1. SYN blastodermic vesicle. [blasto- + G. *kystis,* bladder]

blas•to•cyte (blas′tō-sīt) An undifferentiated blastomere of the morula, blastula, or blastocyst stage of an embryo. [blasto- + G. *kytos,* cell]

blas•to•cy•to•ma (blas′tō-sī-tō′mă) SYN blastoma.

blas•to•derm, **blas•to•der•ma** (blas′tō-dĕrm, -tō-dĕr′mă) The thin, disc-shaped cell mass of young embryos (e.g., reptiles, birds), and its extraembryonic extensions over the surface of the yolk; when fully formed, all three primary germ layers (ectoderm, endoderm, and mesoderm) are present. SYN germ membrane, germinal membrane. [blasto- + G. *derma,* skin]

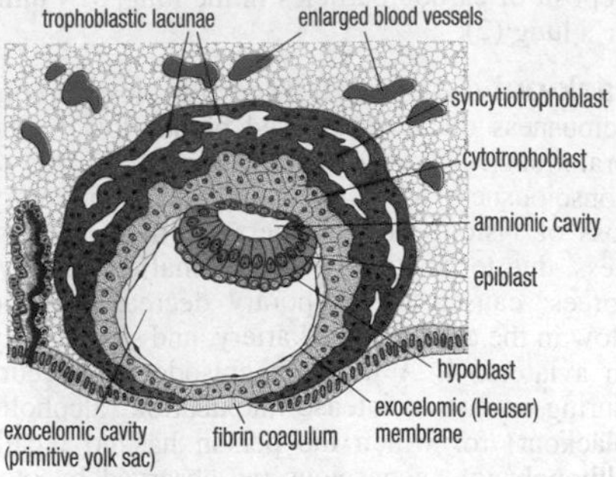

human blastocyst: at 9 days' development

blas•to•der•mal, **blas•to•der•mic** (blas′tō-dĕr′măl, blas′tō-dĕr′mik) Relating to the blastoderm.

blas•to•der•mic ves•i•cle (blas′tō-dĕr′mik ves′i-kĕl) SYN blastocyst.

blas•to•disc (blas′tō-disk) **1.** The disc of active cytoplasm at the animal pole of a telolecithal egg. **2.** The blastoderm, especially in very young stages when it is small. [blasto- + disc]

blas•to•gen•e•sis (blas′tō-jen′ĕ-sis) **1.** Reproduction of unicellular organisms by budding. **2.** Development of an embryo during cleavage and germ layer formation. **3.** Transformation of small lymphocytes of human peripheral blood in tissue culture into large, morphologically primordial blastlike cells capable of undergoing mitosis. [blasto- + G. *genesis,* origin]

blas•to•ge•net•ic, **blas•to•gen•ic** (blas′tō-jĕ-net′ik, -tō-jen′ik) Relating to blastogenesis.

blas•to•ma (blas-tō′mă) A neoplasm composed chiefly or entirely of immature undifferentiated cells (i.e., blast forms), with little or virtually no stroma. SYN blastocytoma. [blasto- + G. *-oma,* tumor]

blas•to•mere (blas′tō-mēr) One of the cells resulting from cleavage of a zygote or fertilized oocyte. [blasto- + G. *meros,* part]

Blas•to•my•ces der•ma•tit•i•dis (blas′tō-mī′sēz dĕr-mă-tit′i-dis) A dimorphic soil fungus that causes blastomycosis. It grows in mammalian tissues as budding cells, with a broad junction between mother and daughter cells (thus "broad-based buds") and in culture as a white or buff filamentous fungus bearing spheric or ovoid conidia. [blasto- + G. *mykēs,* fungus]

blas•to•my•co•sis (blas′tō-mī-kō′sis) A chronic granulomatous and suppurative disease caused by *Blastomyces dermatitidis;* originates as a respiratory infection and disseminates, usually with pulmonary, osseous, and cutaneous involvement predominating. Formerly called North American blastomycosis, the disease now has been found in African countries as well as in

Canada and the U.S. See page B20. SYN Gilchrist disease.

blas•to•pore (blas′tō-pōr) The opening into the archenteron formed by invagination of the blastula (e.g., amphibians) to form a gastrula. [blasto- + G. *poros,* opening]

Blas•to•schiz•o•my•ces (blas′tō-skiz-ō-mī′sēz) A genus of yeastlike fungi; species found in indigenous flora of the skin, and of the respiratory and digestive tracts of humans, and also found in soil.

Blas•to•schiz•o•my•ces cap•i•ta•tus (blas′tō-skiz-ō-mī′sēz kap-ē-tā′tŭs) Fungal species that causes severe disseminated infection in immunosuppressed patients; formerly classified as a species of *Geotrichum.*

blas•tu•la (blas′chū-lă) An early stage of an embryo formed by the rearrangement of the blastomeres of the morula to form a hollow sphere. [G. *blastos,* germ]

blas•tu•lar (blas′chŭ-lăr) Pertaining to the blastula.

blas•tu•la•tion (blas′chŭ-lā′shŭn) Formation of the blastula or blastocyst from the morula.

blast wave (blast wāv) A supersonic pressure front generated by a high-grade explosive.

blast wind (blast wind) A subsonic pressure front generated by both high explosives and also low-grade explosives.

Bla•tin syn•drome (blă-tahn[h]′ sin′drōm) SYN hydatid thrill.

bleb (bleb) **1.** A large, flaccid vesicle. **2.** An acquired lung cyst, usually smaller than 1 cm in diameter, similar to but smaller than a bulla, which is thought to be the most common cause of spontaneous pneumothorax. Blebs occur mainly in the apex of the lung. See page B8.

bleed (blēd) To lose blood as a result of rupture or severance of blood vessels.

bleed•er (blē′dĕr) **1.** A person with a hemorrhagic disease. **2.** A blood vessel severed during surgery.

bleed•ing time (blēd′ing tīm) A screening procedure to detect congenital and acquired platelet disorders. Test is performed at bedside and usually lasts 1–3 minutes but prolonged in cases of thrombocytopenia, diminished prothrombin, phosphorus or chloroform poisoning, and in some liver diseases; it is normal in hemophilia.

blem•ish (blem′ish) **1.** A small circumscribed alteration of the skin considered to be unesthetic but insignificant. **2.** To alter the skin, rendering an unesthetic appearance.

blend•ed fam•i•ly (blend′ĕd fam′i-lē) Family group that includes children from past and present relationships.

blenno-, **blenn-** Combining forms indicating mucus. [G. *blenna, blennos*]

blen•noid (blen′oyd) SYN muciform. [blenno- + G. *eidos,* resemblance]

blen•nor•rhe•a (blen′ŏr-ē′ă) Excessive secretion and discharge of mucus. [G. *blenna,* mucus, + *rhoia,* flow]

blephar- Combining for denoting eyelid.

bleph•ar•ad•e•ni•tis, **bleph•a•ro•ad•e•ni•tis** (blef′ăr-ad′ĕ-nī′tis, blef′ă-rō-ad′ĕ-nī′tis) Inflammation of the meibomian glands or the marginal glands of Moll or Zeis. SYN posterior blepharitis. [blephar- + G. *adēn,* gland, + *-itis,* inflammation]

bleph•a•ral (blef′ă-răl) Relating to the eyelid. [G. *blepharon,* eyelid]

bleph•a•rec•to•my (blef′ă-rek′tŏ-mē) Excision of all or part of an eyelid. [blepharo- + G. *ektomē,* excision]

bleph•ar•e•de•ma (blef′ăr-ĕ-dē′mă) Edema of the eyelids, causing swelling and often a baggy appearance. SYN blepharoedema.

bleph•a•ri•tis (blef′ă-rī′tis) Inflammation of the eyelids. See page B27. [blepharo- + G. *-itis,* inflammation]

blepharo-, **blephar-** Prefix meaning eyelid. [G. *blepharon,* an eyelid]

bleph•a•ro•ad•e•no•ma (blef′ă-rō-ad′ĕ-nō′mă) A tumor or adenoma of a gland of the eyelid. [blepharo- + G. *adēn,* gland, + *-oma,* tumor]

bleph•a•ro•chal•a•sis (blef′ă-rō-kal′ă-sis) SYN dermatochalasis. [blepharo- + G. *chalasis,* relaxation]

bleph•a•ro•col•o•bo•ma (blef′ă-rō-kol′ō-bō′mă) A defect of the eyelid; may be congenital or acquired. [blepharo- + coloboma]

bleph•a•ro•con•junc•ti•vi•tis (blef′ă-rō-kŏn-jungk′ti-vī′tis) Inflammation of the palpebral conjunctiva.

blepharoedema [Br.] SYN blepharedema.

bleph•a•ro•ker•a•to•con•junc•ti•vi•tis (blef′ă-rō-ker′ă-tō-kŏn-jungk′ti-vī′tis) An inflammation involving the eyelids, cornea, and conjunctiva.

bleph•a•ron (blef′ă-ron) SYN eyelid.

bleph•a•ro•phi•mo•sis (blef′ă-rō-fi-mō′sis) Decrease in the size of the palpebral aperture without fusion of lid margins. SYN blepharostenosis. [blepharo- + G. *phimōsis,* an obstruction]

bleph•a•ro•plas•tic (blef′ă-rō-plas′tik) Relating to blepharoplasty.

bleph•a•ro•plas•ty (blef′ă-rō-plast-tē) Any operation for the correction of a defect in the eyelids. [blepharo- + G. *plassō,* to form]

bleph•a•ro•ple•gi•a (blef′ă-rō-plē′jē-ă) Paralysis of an eyelid. [blepharo- + G. *plēgē,* stroke]

bleph•a•rop•to•sis (blef′ă-rop-tō′sis) Drooping of the upper eyelid. SYN ptosis (2). [blepharo- + G. *ptōsis,* a falling]

bleph•a•rop•to•sis a•di•po•sa (blef′ă-rop-tō′sis ad-i-pō′să) Blepharoptosis causing skin to hang over the free border of the eyelid.

bleph•a•ro•spasm, bleph•a•ro•spas•mus (blef′ă-rō-spazm, -spaz′mŭs) Involuntary spasmodic contraction of the orbicularis oculi muscle.

bleph•a•ro•stat (blef′ă-rō-stat) SYN eye speculum. [blepharo- + G. *statos,* fixed]

bleph•a•ro•ste•no•sis (blef′ă-rō-stĕ-nō′sis) SYN blepharophimosis. [blepharo- + G. *stenōsis,* a narrowing]

bleph•a•ro•syn•ech•i•a (blef′ă-rō-si-nek′ē-ă) Adhesion of the eyelids to each other or to the eyeball. SEE ALSO symblepharon. [blepharo- + G. *synecheia,* continuity, fr. *syn-echō,* to hold together]

bleph•a•rot•o•my (blef-ă-rot′ŏ-mē) A cutting operation on an eyelid. [blepharo- + G. *tomē,* incision]

bles•sed this•tle (bles′ĕd this′ĕl) An herbal made from the leaves and flowers of *Cnicus benedictus;* purported therapeutic effect on many internal organs; alleged value in improving memory. This agent has a long history with mentions of its use during the Middle Ages, where it was used as a specific against the Black Death. Approved for use as a medicine in Germany. SYN cardo santo, holy thistle, spotted thistle, St. Benedict thistle.

blind (blīnd) Unable to see; without useful sight. SEE blindness.

blind fis•tu•la (blīnd fis′chū-lă) A fistula that ends in a cul-de-sac, thus open at only one extremity. SYN incomplete fistula.

blind in•tu•ba•tion (blīnd in-tū-bā′shŭn) Placement of an endotracheal tube without direct visualization of the glottic opening. The hand and fingers may be used to guide placement of the endotracheal tube.

blind loop syn•drome (blīnd lūp sin′drōm) A group of symptoms that result from the overgrowth of bacteria (primarily anaerobic) in a surgically bypassed or disconnected segment of intestine: local or systemic infection, fat malabsorption, and vitamin B_{12} and folate deficiencies.

blind•ness (blīnd′nĕs) **1.** Loss of the sense of sight; absolute blindness connotes no light perception. SEE ALSO amblyopia, amaurosis. **2.** Loss of visual appreciation of objects although visual acuity is normal. **3.** Absence of the appreciation of sensation, e.g., taste blindness. SYN typhlosis.

blind spot (blīnd spot) **1.** SYN physiologic scotoma. **2.** SYN mental scotoma. **3.** SYN optic disc.

blink (blingk) To close and open the eyes rapidly; an involuntary act by which the tears are spread over the cornea and conjunctiva, keeping it moist.

blink re•sponse, blink re•flex (blingk rē-spons′, blingk rē′fleks) A response elicited during nerve conduction studies, consisting of muscle action potentials evoked from orbicularis oculi muscles after brief electric or mechanical stimuli to the cutaneous area supplied by the ophthalmic branch of the trigeminal nerve. Characteristically, there is an early response (approximately 10 msec after stimulus) ipsilateral to the stimulation site (labeled R1) and bilateral late responses (approximately 30 msec after stimulus; labeled R2); the latter are responsible for the visible twitch of the orbicularis oculi muscles.

blis•ter (blis′tĕr) **1.** A fluid-filled thin-walled structure under the epidermis or within the epidermis (subepidermal or intradermal). **2.** To form a blister with heat or some other vesiculating agent.

blis•ter•ing (blis′tĕr-ing) SYN vesiculation (1).

blis•ter•ing dis•tal dac•ty•li•tis (blis′tĕr-ing dis′tăl dak′ti-lī′tis) Infection of the volar fat pad of the distal phalanx of the finger by group A β-hemolytic streptococci.

bloat, bloat•ing (blōt, blōt′ing) Abdominal distention due to swallowed air or intestinal gas.

Bloch-Sulz•ber•ger syn•drome (blok-sults′ber-ger sin′drōm) Variously patterned hyperpigmented lesions after development of bullous verrucous skin lesions; associated with many conditions and has onset at birth or during early infancy. Death usually follows while patient is very young; X-linked inheritance.

block (blok) **1.** To obstruct; to arrest passage. **2.** A condition in which the passage of an electrical impulse is arrested, wholly or in part, temporarily or permanently. **3.** Regional anesthesia. **4.** SYN atrioventricular block. [Fr. *bloquer*]

block•ade (blok-ād′) **1.** Isolation of an organ, tissue, or system from communication with or influence by external forces or events. **2.** Receptor blockade, blocking the effect of a hormone at the cell surface. **3.** Arrest of peripheral nerve conduction or transmission at autonomic synaptic junctions, autonomic receptor sites, or myoneural junctions by a drug. **4.** The occupation of receptors by an antagonist so that usual agonists are relatively ineffective.

block an•es•the•si•a (blok an′es-thē′zē-ă) SYN conduction anesthesia.

block•er (blok′ĕr) **1.** An instrument used to obstruct a passage. **2.** SEE blocking agent.

block·ing ac·tiv·i·ty (blok′ing ak-tiv′i-tē) Repression or elimination of electrical activity in the brain by the arrival of a sensory stimulus.

block·ing a·gent (blok′ing ā′jĕnt) A class of drugs that inhibit (block) a biologic activity or process; frequently called "blockers."

block·ing an·ti·bod·y (blok′ing an′ti-bod-ē) **1.** Antibody that, in certain concentrations, does not cause precipitation after combining with specific antigen, and which, in this combined state, "blocks" activity of additional antibody added to increase the concentration to a level at which precipitation would ordinarily occur. **2.** The IgG class of immunoglobulin that combines specifically with an atopic allergen but does not elicit a type I allergic reaction, the combined IgG antibody "blocking" available IgE class (reaginic) antibody activity.

Blocq dis·ease (blawk di-zēz′) SYN astasia-abasia.

Blom-Sing·er valve (blom-sing′ĕr valv) A prosthesis for maintaining the patency of a tracheoesophageal puncture for vocal rehabilitation after laryngectomy.

blood (blŭd) The fluid and its suspended formed elements that are circulated through the heart, arteries, capillaries, and veins; the means by which oxygen and nutritive materials are transported to the tissues, and carbon dioxide and various metabolic products are removed for excretion. The blood consists of a pale yellow or gray-yellow fluid, plasma, in which red blood cells (erythrocytes), white blood cells (leukocytes), and platelets are suspended. SEE ALSO arterial blood, venous blood. See page B2. [A.S. blōd]

blood a·gent (blŭd ā′jĕnt) Military name for cyanide compounds used as chemical agents. The name was applied because these agents are systemically distributed in the blood, but the term is no longer specific to cyanide compounds and also mistakenly implies that the site of action of these compounds is the blood. In fact, these compounds are cellular poisons.

blood-air bar·ri·er (blŭd-ār bar′ē-ĕr) The material intervening between alveolar air and the blood; it consists of a nonstructural film or surfactant, alveolar epithelium, basement lamina, and endothelium.

blood al·bu·min (blŭd al-bū′min) SYN serum albumin.

blood-a·que·ous bar·ri·er (blŭd-ā′kwē-ŭs bar′ē-ĕr) A selectively permeable barrier between the capillary bed in the ciliary body and the aqueous humor.

blood bank (blŭd bank) A place, usually a separate part or division of a hospital laboratory or a free-standing facility, in which blood is collected from donors, typed, tested, separated into several components, stored, and/or prepared for transfusion to recipients.

blood blis·ter (blŭd blis′tĕr) A blister containing blood; resulting from a pinch or crushing injury.

blood boost·ing (blŭd būst′ing) SYN blood doping.

blood-borne (blŭd′bōrn) Capable of being transported in blood.

blood-borne in·fec·tion (blŭd′bōrn in-fek′shŭn) Infection transmitted through blood or blood products (e.g., hepatitis virus, HIV-1).

blood·borne path·o·gens (BBP) (blŭd′bōrn path′ō-jĕnz) Disease-producing microorganisms transmitted by means of blood, tissue, and body fluids containing blood.

blood-brain bar·ri·er (BBB) (blŭd-brān bar′ē-ĕr) A selective mechanism opposing the passage of most ions and large-molecular weight compounds from the blood to brain tissue.

blood cap·il·lar·y (blŭd kap′i-lar-ē) (symbol c, is shown as a subscript) A vessel the wall of which consists of endothelium and its basement membrane; its diameter, when the capillary is open, is about 8 mcm; with the electron microscope, fenestrated capillaries and continuous capillaries are distinguished.

blood-ce·re·bro·spi·nal flu·id bar·ri·er, blood-CSF bar·ri·er (blŭd-ser′ă-brō-spī′năl flū′id bar′ē-ĕr, blŭd bar′ē-ĕr) A barrier located at the tight junctions that surround and connect the cuboidal epithelial cells on the surface of the choroid plexus; capillaries and connective tissue stroma of the choroid do not represent a barrier to protein tracers or dyes.

blood clot (blŭd klot) SYN thrombus.

blood count (blŭd kownt) A determination of the number of red blood cells (RBCs) or white blood cells (WBCs) in a cubic millimeter of blood; calculated by counting the cells in an accurate volume of diluted blood.

blood cul·ture (blŭd kŭl′chŭr) Microbiologic culture of a blood specimen.

blood cyst (blŭd sist) SYN hemorrhagic cyst.

blood disc (blŭd disk) SYN platelet.

blood dop·ing (blŭd dōp′ing) Infusion of red blood cells, usually freeze-preserved autologous packed red blood cells, to increase hematocrit and hemoglobin levels; used by endurance athletes to increase blood's oxygen-carrying capacity and thus enhance endurance performance. SYN blood boosting, induced erythrocythemia.

blood dys·cra·si·a (blŭd dis-krā′zē-ă) A diseased state of the blood; usually refers to abnormal cellular elements of a permanent character.

blood gas a·nal·y·sis (blŭd gas ă-nal′i-sis) The direct electrode measurement of the partial pressure of oxygen and carbon dioxide in the blood.

blood gas·es (blŭd gas′ĕz) A clinical expression for the determination of the partial pressures of oxygen and carbon dioxide in blood.

blood group (blŭd grūp) A system of genetically determined antigens or agglutinogens located on the surface of the erythrocyte. Because of the antigen differences existing in different people, blood groups are significant in blood transfusions, maternal-fetal incompatibilities (erythroblastosis fetalis), tissue and organ transplantation, disputed paternity cases, and in genetic and anthropologic studies; certain blood groups have been supposed to be related to susceptibility or resistance to certain diseases. Often used as synonymous with blood type. SEE ALSO blood type.

blood group an·ti·gen (blŭd grūp an′ti-jen) Generic term for any inherited antigen found on the surface of erythrocytes that determines a blood grouping reaction with specific antiserum; antigens of the ABO and Lewis blood groups may be found also in saliva and other body fluids.

blood group·ing (blŭd grūp′ing) The classification of blood samples by means of laboratory tests of their agglutination reactions with respect to one or more blood groups.

blood group–spe·cif·ic sub·stanc·es A and B (blŭd grūp-spĕ-sif′ik sŭb′stăns-ĕz) Solution of complexes of polysaccharides and amino acids that reduces the titer of anti-A and anti-B isoagglutinins in serum from people in group O; used to render group O blood reasonably safe for transfusion into people in groups A, B, or AB, without affecting any incompatibility that results from various other factors, such as Rh.

blood·less op·er·a·tion (blŭd′lĕs op-ĕr-ā′shŭn) An operation performed with negligible loss of blood.

blood·let·ting (blŭd′let-ing) Removing blood, usually from a vein; used in congestive heart failure and polycythemia.

blood ox·y·gen lev·el de·pen·dent (BOLD) (blŭd ok′si-jĕn lev′ĕl dĕ-pen′dĕnt) A functional MRI technique that utilizes the differences in magnetic susceptibility between oxyhemoglobin and deoxyhemoglobin to image areas activated cerebral cortex.

blood plas·ma (blŭd plaz′mă) SYN plasma (1).

blood plas·ma frac·tions (blŭd plaz′mă frak′shŭnz) Portions of the blood plasma as separated by electrophoresis or other techniques.

blood poi·son·ing (blŭd poy′zŏn-ing) SEE septicemia, pyemia.

blood pool im·ag·ing (blŭd pūl im′ăj-ing) Nuclear medicine study using a radionuclide that is confined to the vascular compartment.

blood pres·sure (blŭd presh′ŭr) The pressure or tension of the blood within the systemic arteries, maintained by the contraction of the left ventricle, the resistance of the arterioles and capillaries, the elasticity of the arterial walls, as well as the viscosity and volume of the blood; expressed as relative to the ambient atmospheric pressure. See this page.

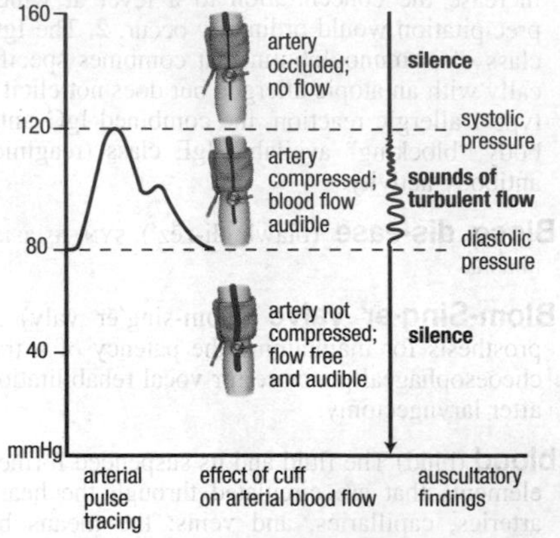

sounds in recording blood pressure

blood re·la·tion·ship (blŭd rĕ-lā′shŭn-ship) SYN consanguinity.

blood root (blŭd rūt) *Sanguinaria canadensis;* purported uses include as an expectorant and carminative. Although used in therapy for skin cancers, horrific adverse effects have been reported (e.g., sudden complete destruction of healthy tissue). Although use in periodontal care has been reported, blood root is toxic if swallowed. The FDA has listed it as unsafe in ingested substances. SYN Indian paint, red puccoon, redroot, tetterwort.

blood·shot (blŭd′shot) Denoting locally congested smaller blood vessels of a part (e.g., the conjunctiva) that are dilated and visible.

blood·stream (blŭd′strēm) The flowing blood as it is encountered in the circulatory system as distinguished from blood that has been removed from the circulatory system or sequestered in a part.

blood sug·ar (blŭd shug′ăr) Amount of glucose in blood; measured regularly by patients with diabetes. SEE ALSO glucose.

blood-thy·mus bar·ri·er (blŭd-thī′mŭs bar′ē-ĕr) A sheath of pericytes and epithelial reticular cells around thymic capillaries that prevents the developing T lymphocytes of the thymus from being exposed to circulating antigens.

blood type (blŭd tīp) The specific reaction pattern of erythrocytes of a person to the antisera of one blood group; e.g., the ABO blood group consists of four major blood types: O, A, B, and AB. This classification depends on the presence or absence of two major antigens: A or B. Type O occurs when neither is present and type AB when both are present. See Blood Groups Appendix. SEE ALSO blood group.

blood u•re•a ni•tro•gen (BUN) (blŭd yūr-ē′ă nī′trŏ-jĕn) Nitrogen, in the form of urea, in the blood; the most prevalent of the nonprotein nitrogenous compounds in blood, which normally contains 10–15 mg of urea/100 mL. Canadian clinicians often use the shortened form urea nitrogen. SEE ALSO urea nitrogen.

blood ves•sel (blŭd ves′ĕl) Any vessel conveying blood: arteries, arterioles, capillaries, venules, veins.

blood work (blŭd wŏrk) Colloquial term for any clinical laboratory study performed on a specimen of blood.

Bloom syn•drome (blūm sin′drōm) Congenital telangiectatic erythema, primarily in butterfly distribution, of the face and occasionally of the hands and forearms, with sun sensitivity of skin lesions and dwarfism with normal body proportions except for a narrow face and dolichocephalic skull; chromosomes are excessively unstable and there is a predisposition to malignancy; autosomal recessive inheritance, caused by mutation in the Bloom syndrome gene (BLM) on chromosome 15q.

blot (blot) SEE Northern blot analysis, Southern blot analysis, Western blot analysis, zoo blot analysis.

blotch (bloch) A skin lesion characterized by irregularly shaped spots. SEE ALSO spot.

Blount dis•ease (blownt di-zēz′) Tibia vara; nonrachitic bowlegs in children.

blow-bot•tles (blō bot′ĕlz) A device consisting of two 1-L bottles connected to a tube used to prevent atelectasis and maintain lung expansion in postsurgical patients. The patient forces water from one bottle to another with a series of slow exhalations, each preceded by a deep inhalation. SEE ALSO incentive spirometer.

blow-out frac•ture (blō′owt frak′shŭr) A fracture of the floor or medial wall of the orbit, without a fracture of the rim, produced by a blow on the globe with the force being transmitted via the globe to the orbital floor.

BLS Abbreviation for basic life support.

blue (blū) A range of hues in the visible spectrum lying between green and indigo. [M.E. fr. Germanic]

blue ba•by (blū bā′bē) **1.** A child born cyanotic because of a congenital cardiac or pulmonary defect causing incomplete oxygenation of the blood. **2.** A neonate with cyanosis of any etiology.

blue•ber•ry muf•fin ba•by (blū-ber′ē mŭf′in bā′bē) Jaundice and purpura, especially of the face in the newborn, which may result from intrauterine viral infection.

blue cat•a•ract (blū kat′ăr-akt) Coronary cataract of bluish color. SYN cerulean cataract.

blue co•hosh (blū kō′hosh) Herbal agent extracted from *Caulophyllum thalictroides;* long in use, purported value includes tonic in pregnancy and as an anticonvulsant, however, use in pregnant women is contraindicated. SYN blue ginseng, papoose root, squaw root (2), yellow ginseng.

Blue Cross-Blue Shield (BCBS) (blū kraws blū shēld) Blue Cross, covering hospital care, and Blue Shield, covering physician's services, is a national U.S. health care benefit company..

Blue Cross and Blue Shield As•so•ci•a•tion (blū kraws blū shēld ă-sō′sē-ā′shŭn) A national U.S. agency that represents the Blue Cross Blue Shield health plans. This body helps maintain the HCPCS level II codes.

blue dome cyst (blū dōm sist) **1.** One of a number of small dark blue nodules or cysts in the vaginal fornix due to retained menstrual blood in endometriosis affecting this region. **2.** A benign retention cyst of the mammary gland in fibrocystic disease, containing a pale slightly yellow fluid that gives a blue color to the cyst when seen through the surrounding fibrous tissue.

blue flag (blū flag) Herbal derived from *Iris versicolor;* purported value as an antiinflammatory, laxative, diuretic; human poisoning reported and use contraindicated. SYN dagger flower, fleur-de-lis, liver lily, poison flag.

blue gin•seng (blū jin′seng) SYN blue cohosh.

blue-green bac•te•ri•a (blū-grēn bak-tēr′ē-ă) SEE Cyanobacteria.

blue line (blū līn) A bluish striation along the free border of the gingiva, occurring in chronic heavy metal poisoning. SEE ALSO Burton line.

blue ne•vus (blū nē′vŭs) A dark blue or blue-black nevus covered by smooth skin and formed by heavily pigmented spindle-shaped or dendritic melanocytes in the reticular dermis.

blue pus (blū pŭs) An inflammatory fluid tinged with pyocyanin, a product of *Pseudomonas aeruginosa.*

blue rub•ber-bleb ne•vi (blū rŭb′ĕr-bleb nē′vī) A syndrome characterized by erectile, easily compressible, thin-walled hemangiomatous nodules, widely distributed in the skin and in the alimentary canal; lesions in the gut may perforate or cause hemorrhage.

blues (blūz) State of depression or sadness. [slang, fr. *blue devils*]

blue spot (blū spot) **1.** SYN macula cerulea. **2.** SYN mongolian spot.

Blum•berg sign (blūm′berg sīn) Pain felt on sudden release of steadily applied pressure on a suspected area of the abdomen, indicative of peritonitis. SYN rebound tenderness.

blunt•ed af•fect (blŭnt′ĕd af′ekt) A disturbance in mood manifested by a severe reduction in the expression of feeling.

blunt-end•ed DNA, **blunt-end** (blŭnt-en′dĕd, blŭnt-end) Double-stranded DNA in which at least one of the ends has no unpaired bases.

blush (blŭsh) **1.** A sudden and brief redness of the face and neck due to emotion. **2.** In angiography, used metaphorically to describe neovascularity or, in some cases, extravasation. [M.E., fr. O.E. *blyscan*,]

B lym•pho•cyte (lim′fŏ-sīt) A lymphocyte that resembles the bursa-derived lymphocyte of birds in that it is responsible for the production of immunoglobulins, i.e., it is the precursor of the plasma cell and expresses immunoglobulins on its surface but does not release them. It does not play a direct role in cell-mediated immunity. SEE ALSO T lymphocyte.

BMD Abbreviation for bone mineral density.

BMI Abbreviation for body mass index.

B-mode (mōd) A two-dimensional diagnostic ultrasound presentation of echo-producing interfaces in a single plane; the intensity of the echo is represented by modulation of the brightness (B) of the spot, and the position of the echo is determined from the position of the transducer and the transit time of the acoustical pulse.

BMR Abbreviation for basal metabolic rate.

BMT Abbreviation for bone and marrow transplantation.

BNP Abbreviation for β-type natriuretic peptide or brain natriuretic peptide; a hormone produced by cardiac ventricles in response to increased fluid volume or pressure.

Bo (bō) The main magnetic field measured in teslas.

board cer•ti•fi•ca•tion (bōrd sĕr′ti-fi-kā′shŭn) A specialty designation typically obtained by the successful completion of an examination signifying the possession of expert knowledge in a field; eligibility requires completion of prerequisites.

board cer•ti•fied (bōrd sĕr′ti-fīd) Referring to someone certified in a specialty area signifying the possession of expert knowledge in the field.

board el•i•gi•ble (bōrd el′i-ji-bĕl) Referring to someone who is not yet certified in a specialty but who has met the requirements to sit for the examination.

Bo•bath meth•od of ex•er•cise (bō′baht meth′ŏd eks′ĕr-sīz) Theory of exercise and muscular training for patients with cerebral palsy and stroke; stresses need for inhibition of hypertonia and for neurodevelopmental sequence training. SEE ALSO neurodevelopmental treatment.

Bo•bath tech•nique (bō′baht tek-nēk′) Series of procedures to provide rehabilitation for the neurologically impaired patient by improving voluntary muscle tone and movement (e.g., weight-bearing, use of the affected hand as an assist) and to control strength.

Boch•da•lek duct (bok′di-lĕk dŭkt) SYN His canal.

Boch•da•lek her•ni•a (bok′di-lĕk hĕr′nē-ă) SYN congenital diaphragmatic hernia.

Bock nerve (bok nĕrv) SYN pharyngeal nerve.

Bo•dan•sky u•nit (bō-dan′skē yū′nit) The amount of phosphatase that liberates 1 mg of phosphorus as inorganic phosphate during the first hour of incubation with a buffered substrate containing sodium β-glycerophosphate.

bod•y (bod′ē) **1.** The head, neck, trunk, and limbs; the human body, consisting of head (caput), neck (collum), trunk (truncus), and limbs (membra). **2.** The material part of a human, as distinguished from the mind and spirit. **3.** The principal mass of any structure. **4.** A thing; a substance. SEE ALSO soma. SYN corpus (1) [TA]. [A.S. *bodig*]

bod•y bur•den (bod′ē bŭr′dĕn) The amount of a harmful substance that is permanently present in a person's body.

bod•y cav•i•ty (bod′ē kav′i-tē) The collective visceral cavity of the trunk (thoracic cavity plus abdominopelvic cavity), bounded by the superior thoracic aperture above, the pelvic floor below, and the body walls (parietes) in between. SYN celom (2), celoma.

bod•y com•po•si•tion (bod′ē kom-pŏ-zish′ŭn) An estimate of the proportions of major components of a living body, as water, nitrogen, sodium; more specifically, the proportion of lean body mass to fat.

bod•y den•si•ty (bod′ē den′si-tē) The quotient of mass divided by volume, used in the calculation of body composition.

bod•y dys•mor•phic dis•or•der (bod′ē dis-mōr′fik dis-ōr′dĕr) **1.** A psychosomatic (somatoform) disorder characterized by preoccupation with some imagined defect in appearance in a person who looks normal. **2.** A DSM diagnosis that is established when the specified criteria are met. SYN dysmorphophobia.

bod•y fat (bod′ē fat) The percentage of adipose tissue compared with muscle estimated by underwater weighing, calculating the ratio of weight in kilograms to height in meters, and/or estimating bioelectrical impedance of the body.

bod•y hab•i•tus (bod′ē hab′i-tŭs) Common variations in the general shape and form of the human body.

bod•y of hy•oid bone (bod′ē hī′oyd bōn) The body of the hyoid bone, from which the greater and lesser horns extend.

bod•y im•age (bod′ē im′ăj) **1.** The cerebral representation of all body sensation organized in the parietal cortex. **2.** Personal conception of one's own body as distinct from one's actual body or the conception other persons have of it.

bod•y im•age dis•tur•bance (bod′ē im′ăj dis-tŭr′băns) Distortion of one's mental picture of oneself; NANDA-approved diagnosis.

bod•y jack•et (bod′ē jak′ĕt) SYN clam-shell brace.

bod•y lan•guage (bod′ē lang′gwăj) A form of communication using body movements or gestures instead of or in addition to the sounds of verbal language or other forms of communication.

bod•y mass in•dex (BMI) (bod′ē mas in′deks) A rough method of assessing weight status; correlates with risk of disease and death due to causes associated with obesity; because it does not distinguish excess adiposity from excess lean body mass, it is not useful in competitive athletes, body builders, pregnant women, or children. BMI = weight (kg) ÷ height (m^2). Also see Appendices.

bod•y me•chan•ics (bod′ē mĕ-kan′iks) The application of physical principles to achieve maximum efficiency and to limit risk of physical stress or injury to the practitioner of physical therapy, massage therapy, or chiropractic or osteopathic manipulation. SEE ALSO ergonomics.

bod•y pierc•ing (bod′ē pērs′ing) Inserting a foreign object of diverse shape (e.g., femur, anchor, dumbbell) generally metal, into a bodily appendage or orifice (e.g., tongue, earlobe) for cosmetic purposes.

bod•y scheme (bod′ē skēm) A kinesthetic awareness of body parts and the relationship of those parts to one another and to objects in the environment. SYN kinesthetic awareness.

bod•y of stom•ach (bod′ē stŏm′ăk) The part of the stomach that lies between the fundus above and the pyloric antrum below; its boundaries are poorly defined.

bod•y sub•stance i•so•la•tion (bod′ē sub′stăns ī′sŏ-lā′shŭn) Precautions taken by health care providers and others to avoid contact with blood and other body fluids.

bod•y sur•face ar•e•a (BSA) (bod′ē sŭr′fās ār′ē-ă) The area of the external surface of the body, expressed in square meters (m^2); used to calculate metabolic, electrolyte, nutritional requirements, drug dosage, and expected pulmonary function measurements.

bod•y•work (bo′dē-wŏrk) Any technique involving touch, massage, manipulation, and/or energetic principles for the improvement or restoration of health. SEE ALSO massage therapy.

Boeck dis•ease (bĕrk di-zēz′) SYN sarcoidosis.

Boeck and Dr•boh•lav Locke-egg-se•rum me•di•um (bĕrk dĕr-bō′lăf lok-eg sēr′ŭm mē′dē-ŭm) A composition of whole eggs, human serum, and rice powder used to detect the presence of intestinal amebae, primarily *Entamoeba histolytica*.

Boeh•mer he•ma•tox•y•lin (bĕr′mer hē′mă-toks′i-lin) An alum type of hematoxylin in which natural ripening occurs in about 8–10 days, and the solution is good for many months.

Boer•haa•ve syn•drome (būr′hah-vē sin′drōm) Spontaneous rupture of the lower esophagus, a variant of Mallory-Weiss syndrome.

bog bean (bog bēn) Herbal derived from *Menyanthes trifoliata;* unproven uses include as an antiscorbutic, antipyretic, antirheumatic, and as a purgative laxative. Safety not proven. SYN marsh trefoil, water shamrock.

Bohn nod•ule (bun nod′yūl) Tiny buccal and palatal cysts in newborns derived from epithelial remnants of mucous gland tissue.

Bohr at•om (bōr at′ŏm) A concept or model of the atom in which the negatively charged electrons move in circular or elliptic orbits around the positively charged nucleus, energy being emitted or absorbed when electrons change from one orbit to another.

Bohr ef•fect (bōr e-fekt′) The product of H^+ concentration on the affinity of hemoglobin for oxygen. As the H^+ concentration increases, the oxygen affinity decreases, causing a release of more oxygen to the tissue. One of the most important buffer systems in the body.

Bohr e•qua•tion (bōr ĕ-kwā′zhŭn) An equation to calculate the respiratory dead space from the fact that gas expired from the lungs is a mixture of gas from the dead space and gas from the alveoli, i.e., the dead space volume divided by the tidal volume equals the difference between alveolar and mixed expired gas composition, divided by the difference between alveolar and inspired gas composition; gas composition can be expressed in any consistent units of concentration or partial pressure of oxygen or carbon dioxide.

Bohr the•o•ry (bōr thē′ŏr-ē) Theory that spectrum lines are produced 1) by the quantized emission of radiant energy when electrons drop from an orbit of a higher to one of a lower energy level, or 2) by absorption of radiation when an electron rises from a lower to a higher energy level.

boil (boyl) SYN furuncle. [A.S. *byl,* a swelling]

boil•er•mak•er's hear•ing loss (boy'lĕr-mā'kĕrz hēr'ing laws) SYN noise-induced hearing loss.

BOLD (bōld) Acronym for blood oxygen level dependent.

Bo•ley gauge (bō'lē gāj) A vernier, metric caliper used in dentistry to measure tooth, arch, and facial dimensions.

bo•lus (bō'lŭs) **1.** A single, relatively large quantity of a substance, usually one intended for therapeutic use (e.g., bolus dose of an intravenously injected drug) generally followed by smaller doses. **2.** A masticated morsel of food or another substance ready to be swallowed (e.g., a bolus of barium for x-ray studies). **3.** In high-energy radiation therapy, a quantity of tissue-equivalent material placed next to the irradiated region to increase the dose of secondary radiation to the superficial tissues. [L. fr. G. *bōlos,* lump, clod]

Bom•bay blood type (bom-bā' blŭd tīp) Blood type of those who possess the genes for A and B antigens but are unable to express the genes because they lack the gene for H antigen, a required precursor of A and B. People with this blood type frequently have anti-H in their blood.

bomb cal•o•rim•e•ter (bom kal'ŏr-im'ĕ-tĕr) An instrument for determining the potential energy of organic substances, including those in foods. It consists of a hollow steel container, lined with platinum and filled with pure oxygen, into which a weighed quantity of substance is placed and ignited with an electric fuse; the heat produced is absorbed by water surrounding the bomb and, from the rise in temperature, the calories liberated are calculated. See this page.

bond (bond) CHEMISTRY the force holding two neighboring atoms in place and resisting their separation; a bond is electrovalent if it consists of the attraction between oppositely charged groups, or covalent if it results from the sharing of one, two, or three pairs of electrons by the bonded atoms.

bond•ing (bond'ing) Formation of a close and enduring emotional attachment, such as between parent and child, lovers, or husband and wife.

bone (bōn) **1.** A hard connective tissue consisting of cells embedded in a matrix of mineralized ground substance and collagen fibers. The fibers are impregnated with a form of calcium phosphate similar to hydroxyapatite as well as with substantial quantities of carbonate, citrate, sodium, and magnesium; by weight, bone is composed of 75% inorganic material and 25% organic material. **2.** A portion of osseous tissue of definite shape and size, forming a part of the animal skeleton; in human adults there are approximately 200 distinct bones in the skeleton, not including the auditory ossicles of the tympanic cavity or the sesamoid bones other than the two patellae. A bone is enveloped by a fibrous membrane, periosteum, that covers the bone's entire surface except for the articular cartilage. Beneath the periosteum is a dense layer, compact bone, and beneath that a cancellous layer, spongy bone. The core of a long bone is filled with marrow. See this page. SYN os [TA]. [A.S. *bān*]

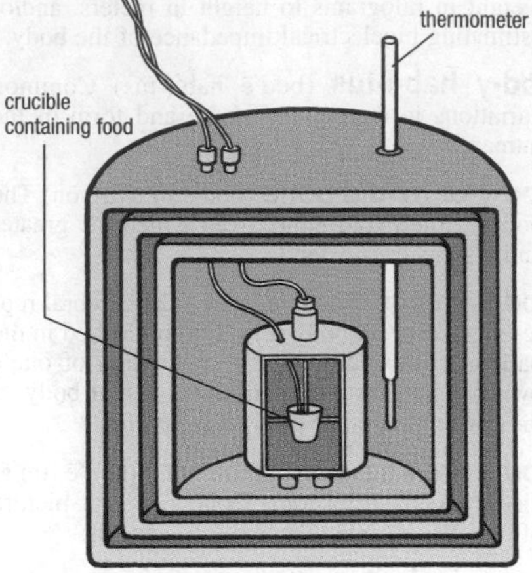

bomb calorimeter: measures heat produced by complete combustion of food sample

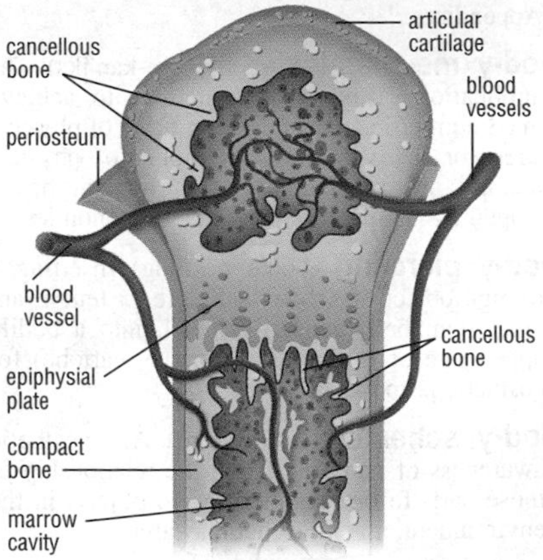

bone

bone block (bōn blok) A surgical procedure in which the bone adjacent to the joint is modified to limit the motion of the joint mechanically.

bone block fu•sion (bōn blok fyū'zhŭn) A method of fusing two bones in which a block of bone graft is placed between the two surfaces to obtain fusion and correct preexisting deformity.

bone can•a•lic•u•lus (bōn kan′ă-lik′yū-lŭs) Canaliculus connecting bone lacunae with one another or with a haversian canal; contains the interconnecting cytoplasmic processes of osteocytes.

bone con•duc•tion (bōn kŏn-dŭk′shŭn) AUDIOLOGY the transmission of sound to the inner ear through vibrations applied to the bones of the skull.

bone den•si•tom•e•try (bōn den′si-tom′ĕ-trē) SYN bone mineral density.

bone den•si•ty (bōn den′si-tē) Quantitative measurement of the mineral content of bone, used as an indicator of the structural strength of the bone and as a screen for osteoporosis.

bone flap (bōn flap) Portion of cranium removed but left attached to overlying muscle-fascial blood supply; term is often used incorrectly for a completely detached cranial section, i.e., a bone graft.

bone for•ceps (bōn fōr′seps) A strong forceps used for seizing or removing fragments of bone.

bone im•plant (bōn im′plant) Use of natural or artificial materials for osseous reconstruction.

bone•let (bōn′lĕt) SYN ossicle.

bone mar•row (bōn mar′ō) The tissue filling the cavities of bones, having a stroma of reticular fibers and cells.

bone mar•row har•vest (bōn mar′ō hahr′vĕst) First step in bone marrow transplantation; blood-producing stem cells are collected that will be used later for transplant. These stem cells can be harvested from either blood or bone marrow.

bone and mar•row trans•plan•ta•tion (BMT) (bōn mar′ō trans′plan-tā′shŭn) Grafting of bone marrow tissue; of value in aplastic anemia, primary immunodeficiency, and acute leukemia (following total body irradiation).

bone ma•trix (bōn mā′triks) The intercellular substance of bone tissue consisting of collagen fibers, ground substance, and inorganic bone salts.

bone min•er•al den•si•ty (BMD) (bōn min′ĕr-al den′si-tē) Measurement of the amount of calcium in bone. Most methods for measuring BMD (also called bone densitometry) are fast, noninvasive, painless, and available on an outpatient basis. Bone densitometry can also be used to estimate a patient's risk of fracture. BMD methods involve taking dual energy x-rays (DEXA) or CT scans of bones in the spinal column, wrist, arm, or leg. These methods compare the numeric density of the bone (calculated from the image) with empiric (historical) databases of bone density to determine whether a patient has osteoporosis, and, to what degree. SYN bone densitometry.

bone scan (bōn skan) Examination involving nuclear medicine of bone after injection of radioactive material, to identify areas of injury, disease, or regeneration, using a gamma camera. See page B23.

bones of cra•ni•um, bones of skull (bōnz krā′nē-ŭm, bōnz skŭl) The paired inferior nasal concha, lacrimal, maxilla, nasal, palatine, parietal, temporal, and zygomatic; and the unpaired ethmoid, frontal, occipital, sphenoid, and vomer. SYN ossa cranii [TA], cranial bones.

bones of dig•its (bōnz dij′its) The phalanges and sesamoid bones of the fingers and toes.

bone•set (bōn′set) Herbal made from leaves of *Eupatorium perfoliatum;* long history of use; purported value as antiinflammatory and antipyretic; used in treatment of URI; employed in Native American medicine as an antimalarial in the 17th century. SYN agueweed, crosswort, feverwort, vegetable antimony.

bone spur (bōn spŭr) An osseus projection arising from a bone. SEE ALSO heel spur.

bone tis•sue (bōn tish′ū) SYN osseous tissue.

Bon•fer•ro•ni meth•od (bōn-fer-rō′nē meth′ŏd) Multiple comparison method used in studies involving analysis of variants.

Bon•fer•ro•ni *t*-test (bōn-fer-rō′nē test) Statistical technique using Bonferroni inequality to isolate differences between comparisons; describes error rate for all comparisons taken as a group.

Bon•hoef•fer sign (bon′hĕrf-ĕr sīn) Loss of normal muscle tone in chorea.

Bon•net cap•sule (bon′ĕt kap′sūl) The anterior part of the vagina bulbi.

Bon•nier syn•drome (bōn-yā′ sin′drōm) A disorder due to a lesion of Deiters nucleus and its connection; the symptoms include ocular disturbances (e.g., paralysis of accommodation, nystagmus, diplopia), as well as deafness, nausea, thirst, anorexia, and symptoms referable to the involvement of the vagus centers.

bon•y am•pul•lae of sem•i•cir•cu•lar ca•nals (bō′nē am-pul′ē sem′ē-sĕr′kyū-lăr kă-nalz′) A circumscribed dilation of one extremity of each of the three bony semicircular canals, anterior, posterior, and lateral; each contains a membranous ampulla of the semicircular ducts.

bon•y an•ky•lo•sis (bō′nē ang′ki-lō′sis) SYN synostosis.

bon•y lab•y•rinth (bō′nē lab′i-rinth) A series of cavities (cochlea, vestibule, and semicircular canals) contained within the otic capsule of the petrous portion of the temporal bone; the bony labyrinth is filled with perilymph, in which the delicate, endolymph-filled membranous labyrinth is suspended.

bon•y pal•ate (bō′nē pal′ăt) A concave elliptic

bony plate, constituting the roof of the oral cavity, formed of the palatine process of the maxilla and the horizontal plate of the palatine bone on either side.

bon•y sem•i•cir•cu•lar ca•nals (bō′nē sem′ē-sĕr′kyū-lăr kă-nalz′) The three bony tubes in the labyrinth of the ear within which the membranous semicircular ducts are located; they lie in planes at right angles to each other and are known as anterior semicircular canal, posterior semicircular canal, and lateral semicircular canal.

BOOP (būp) Acronym for bronchiolitis obliterans with organizing pneumonia, an idiopathic form of bronchiolitis obliterans.

boost•er, **boost•er dose** (būs′tĕr, būs′tĕr dōs) A dose given at some time after an initial dose to enhance the effect, said usually of antigens for the production of antibodies.

boot (būt) A boot-shaped appliance. [M.E. *bote*, fr. O.Fr.]

bor•age (bōr′ăj) A herbal prepared from the plant parts and seeds of *Borago officinalis*. Value as antiinflammatory and tonic. Clinically studied for its value in dermatology; possible use in hepatic and GI disorders. Plant contains toxic pyrrolizidine alkaloids. SYN beebread, ox's tongue, starflower. [L.L. *burrago,* fr. *burra,* shaggy cloth]

bor•bo•ryg•mus, pl. **bor•bo•ryg•mi** (bōr-bō-rig′mŭs, -rig′mī) Rumbling or gurgling noises produced by movement of gas, fluid, or both in the alimentary canal, and audible at a distance. [G. *borborygmos,* rumbling in the bowels]

bor•der (bōr′dĕr) The part of a surface that forms its outer boundary. SEE ALSO margin. SYN margo [TA].

bor•der•line o•var•i•an tu•mor (bōr′dĕr-līn ō-var′ē-ăn tū′mŏr) An ovarian surface epithelial tumor in which the growth pattern is intermediate between benign and malignant; includes mucinous, serous, endometrioid, and Brenner tumors of the ovary; highly curable but may recur after surgical removal.

bor•der•line per•son•al•i•ty dis•or•der (bōr′dĕr-līn pĕr-sŏn-al′i-tē dis-ōr′dĕr) A mental disorder in which the symptoms are not continually psychotic yet are not strictly neurotic: may include impulsivity and unpredictability, unstable interpersonal relationships, inappropriate or uncontrolled anger, identity disturbances, rapid shifts of mood, suicidal acts, self-mutilations, job and marital instability, chronic feelings of emptiness or boredom, and intolerance of being alone.

bor•der move•ment (bōr′dĕr mūv′mĕnt) The limit of movement of the lower jaw as recorded in the sagittal and horizontal planes; often referred to as the envelope of motion.

Bor•de•tel•la (bōr-dĕ-tel′ă) A genus of strictly aerobic bacteria (family Brucellaceae) containing minute gram-negative coccobacilli. Motile and nonmotile species occur; motile cells are peritrichous. The metabolism of these organisms is respiratory. They require nicotinic acid, cysteine, and methionine; hemin (X factor) and coenzyme I (V factor) are not required by some species. They are parasites and pathogens of the mammalian respiratory tract. The type species is *B. pertussis*.

Bor•de•tel•la bron•chi•sep•ti•ca (bōr-dĕ-tel′ă brong-kē-sep′ti-kă) A bacterial species found in a broad range of animal species, causing atrophic rhinitis of swine, bronchopneumonia in rodents, and a highly contagious bronchopneumonia in dogs. It is a rare cause of opportunistic respiratory tract infection in immunocompromised patients.

Bor•de•tel•la hin•zi•i (bōr-dĕ-tel′ă hĭn′zē-ī) A bacterial species isolated from a few human blood cultures and respiratory secretions, as well as from poultry respiratory secretions.

Bor•de•tel•la hol•mi•e•si•i (bōr-dĕ-tel′ă hol-mī-ē′sē-ī) A bacterial species isolated from human blood cultures, primarily from immunocompromised patients.

Bor•de•tel•la per•tus•sis (bōr-dĕ-tel′ă pĕr-tŭs′is) A bacterial species that causes whooping cough; it produces cell-destroying toxins and causes thick mucus to collect in the airway. The type species of the *Bordetella* genus.

Borg scale (bōrg skāl) SYN rating of perceived exertion.

Born•holm dis•ease (bōrn′hōlm di-zēz′) SYN epidemic pleurodynia. [*Bornholm,* Danish island in the Baltic where the d. was first described]

Born•holm dis•ease vi•rus (bōrn′hōlm di-zēz′ vī′rŭs) SYN epidemic pleurodynia virus.

bo•ron (B) (bōr′on) A nonmetallic trivalent element, atomic no. 5, atomic wt. 10.811; occurs as a hard crystalline mass or as a brown powder, and forms borates and boric acid. A nutritional need has been reported in pregnant women. [Pers. *Burah*]

Bor•rel blue stain (bōr-el′ blū stān) A stain for demonstrating spirochetes, treponemes, and Borrelia organisms, using silver oxide (prepared by means of mixing solutions of silver nitrate and sodium bicarbonate) and methylene blue.

i ***Bor•rel•i•a*** (bŏ-rel′ē-ă) A genus of bacteria (family Treponemataceae) containing cells 8 to 16 mcm in length, with coarse, shallow, irregular spirals and tapered, finely filamented ends. These organisms are parasitic on many forms of animal life, are generally hematophytic, or are found on mucous membranes; most are transmitted to animals or humans by the bites of arthropods. The type species is *B. anserina.* See page B4.

Bor·rel·i·a af·zel·i·i (bŏ-rel′ē-ă af-zel′ē-ī) A bacterial genospecies of *B. burgdorferi sensu lato* causing Lyme disease in Europe and Asia; transmitted by the tick *Ixodes ricinus* in central and western Europe and by the tick *I. persulcatus* in Eurasia from the Baltic Sea to the Pacific Ocean. SEE ALSO *Borrelia burgdorferi sensu stricto.*

Bor·rel·i·a burg·dor·fe·ri (bŏ-rel′ē-ă bŭrg-dōr′fĕr-ī) A bacterial species causing Lyme disease. The vector transmitting this spirochete to humans is the tick, *Ixodes scapularis.*

Bor·rel·i·a burg·dor·fe·ri sen·su la·to (bŏ-rel′ē-ă bŭrg-dōr′fĕr-ī sen′sū lā′tō) A bacterial complex causing Lyme disease that is composed of several genospecies including *B. burgdorferi sensu stricto, B. garinii,* and *B. afzelii.*

Bor·rel·i·a burg·dor·fe·ri sen·su strict·o (bŏ-rel′ē-ă bŭrg-dōr′fĕr-ī sen′sū strik′tō) A bacterial genospecies of *B. burgdorferi sensu lato* that causes Lyme disease in North America and Europe; transmitted by the tick *Ixodes scapularis* in the eastern and central U.S., by the tick *I. pacificus* in the western U.S., and by the tick *I. ricinus* in Europe. SEE ALSO *Borrelia garinii.*

Bor·rel·i·a ga·ri·ni·i (bŏ-rel′ē-ă gă-rin′ē-ī) A bacterial genospecies of *B. burgdorferi sensu lato* causing Lyme disease in Europe and Asia; transmitted by the tick *Ixodes ricinus* in central and western Europe and by the tick *Ixodes persulcatus* in Eurasia from the Baltic Sea to the Pacific Ocean. SEE ALSO *Borrelia burgdorferi sensu stricto.*

bor·re·li·o·sis (bŏ-rel′ē-ō′sis) Disease caused by bacteria of the genus *Borrelia.*

BOS Abbreviation for base of support.

Bo·sin dis·ease (bō′sin di-zēz′) SYN subacute sclerosing panencephalitis.

boss (baws) **1.** A protuberance; a circumscribed rounded swelling. **2.** The prominence of a kyphosis. [M. E. *boce*, fr. O. Fr.]

bos·se·lat·ed (baws′ĕ-lā-ted) Marked by numerous bosses or rounded protuberances. [Fr. *bosseler,* to emboss]

Bo·tal·lo duct (bō-tah′lō dŭkt) SYN ductus arteriosus.

Bo·tal·lo fo·ra·men (bō-tah′lō fōr-ā′mĕn) SYN foramen ovale.

bot·ry·oid (bot′rē-oyd) Having numerous rounded protuberances resembling a bunch of grapes. SYN staphyline, uviform. [G. *botryoeidēs,* like a bunch of grapes (*botrys*)]

bot·ry·oid sar·co·ma (bot′rē-oyd sahr-kō′mă) A polypoid form of embryonal rhabdomyosarcoma that occurs in children, most frequently in the urogenital tract, characterized by the formation of grossly apparent grapelike clusters of neoplastic tissue; neoplasms of this type grow relatively rapidly and are highly malignant.

Böt·tcher cells (bĕrt′shĕr selz) Cells of the basilar membrane of the cochlea.

Böt·tcher crys·tals (bĕrt′shĕr kris′tălz) Small crystals observed microscopically in prostatic fluid that has been treated with a drop or two of 1% solution of ammonium phosphate.

Böt·tcher space (bĕrt′shĕr spās) SYN endolymphatic sac.

bot·tle (bot′tĕl) A container for liquids.

bot·u·li·num tox·in (bot-yū-lī′nŭm tok′sin) An extremely potent neurotoxin produced by *Clostridium botulinum,* a gram-positive, strictly anaerobic bacillus; causes botulism when the preformed toxin is ingested in previously contaminated food products. The toxin inhibits release of acetylcholine, a neurotransmitter.

bot·u·li·num tox·in type A (boy′yū-lī′nŭm tok′sin tīp) A biological used as an anesthetic and in cosmesis (with sometimes unsettling results).

bot·u·lism (boch′ŭ-lizm) Food poisoning caused by the ingestion of the neurotoxin produced by *Clostridium botulinum* and related bacteria, usually in improperly canned or preserved food; causes paralysis and can be fatal; can also result from inhalation of preformed botulinum toxin. SEE ALSO *Clostridium botulinum.* [L. *botulus,* sausage]

bou·bas (bū′băz) SYN yaws. [native Brazilian]

Bou·chard dis·ease (bū-shahr′ di-zēz′) Myopathic dilation of the stomach.

Bou·chard node (bū-shahr′ nōd) Bony enlargement of the proximal interphalangeal joints, often associated with osteoarthritis.

Bou·chut tube (bū-shū′ tūb) A short cylindric tube used in intubation of the larynx.

bou·gie (bū-zhē′) A cylindric instrument, usually somewhat flexible and yielding, used for calibrating, examining, measuring, or dilating constricted areas in tubular organs, such as the urethra or esophagus; sometimes containing a medication for local application. [Fr. candle]

bou·gie·nage (boo-zhē-nahz[h]′) Examination or treatment of the interior of any canal by the passage of a bougie or cannula.

Bou·in fix·a·tive (bū′ahn[h] fiks′ă-tiv) A solution of glacial acetic acid, formalin, and picric acid, useful for soft and delicate tissues (as those of embryos) and small pieces of tissues; it preserves glycogen and nuclei and permits brilliant staining, but penetrates slowly, distorts kidney tissue and mitochondria, and does not permit Feulgen stain for DNA.

boun·da·ries (bown′dăr-ēz) The limits of one's

personal space, including physical, psychosocial, and interpersonal domains.

bou·quet (bū-kā′) A cluster or bunch of structures, especially of blood vessels, suggesting a bouquet. [Fr.]

Bour·don gauge (bŭr′dŏn gāj) A type of measuring device used with compressed medical gas. It consists of a coiled metal tube connected to gears and an indicator needle. The tube is straightened and the needle moves in proportion to the gas pressure. The device may also be calibrated to measure flow.

bou·ton (bū-tōn[h]′) A button, pustule, or knoblike swelling. [Fr. button]

bou·ton de Bagh·dad (bū-tōn[h]′ dĕ bahg-dahd′) SYN Aleppo boil.

bou·ton·neuse fe·ver (bu-tō-nuz′ fē′vĕr) Tick-borne infection with *Rickettsia conorii* seen in Africa, Europe, the Middle East, and India. SYN tick typhus.

bou·ton·nière de·form·it·y (bū′tō-nyer′ dĕ-fōrm′i-tē) Rupture of the central slip of a digital extensor tendon at the middle phalanx, marked by extension of the metacarpophalangeal and distal interphalangeal joints and flexion of the proximal interphalangeal joint. [Fr., buttonhole]

Bo·vie (bō′vē) An instrument used for electrosurgical dissection and hemostasis. USAGE NOTE Frequently used as a verb, i.e., to Bovie something is to dissect or cauterize it with the Bovie instrument. [Bovie Medical Corporation]

Bo·vie cau·ter·y (bō′vē kaw′tĕr-ē) SEE Bovie. [Bovie Medical Corporation]

bo·vine (bō′vīn) Relating to cattle. [L. *bos* (*bov-*), ox]

bo·vine ba·be·si·o·sis (bō′vīn bă-bē′sē-ō′sis) An infectious disease of cattle caused by *Babesia* species and transmitted by ticks. SYN tick fever (3).

bo·vine se·rum al·bu·min (BSA) (bō′vīn sēr′ŭm al-bū′min) A source of albumin commonly used in in vitro biologic studies.

bo·vine spon·gi·form en·ceph·a·lop·a·thy (bō′vīn spŭn′ji-fōrm en-sef′a-lop′ă-thē) A disease of cattle first reported in 1986 in Great Britain; characterized clinically by apprehensive behavior, hyperesthesia, and ataxia, and histologically by spongiform changes in the gray matter of the brainstem; caused by a prion, like spongiform encephalopathies of other animals (e.g., scrapie) and human beings (Creutzfeldt-Jakob disease). SEE Creutzfeldt-Jakob disease.

bow (bō) Any device bent in a simple curve or semicircle and possessing flexibility. [A.S. boga]

Bow·ditch law (bō′dich law) Consistently total response to any effective stimulus. SYN all or none law.

bow·el (bow′ĕl) SYN intestine. [through the Fr. from L. *botulus,* sausage]

bow·el by·pass (bow′ĕl bī′pas) SYN jejunoileal bypass.

bow·el sounds (bow′ĕl sowndz) Relatively high-pitched abdominal sounds caused by propulsion of intestinal contents through the lower alimentary tract.

bow·el train·ing (bow′ĕl trān′ing) A method of establishing or reestablishing regularity of fecal elimination. May be accomplished by dietary, pharmacological and /or mechanical (enemas, digital stimulation) interventions.

Bow·en dis·ease (bō′en di-zēz′) A form of intraepidermal carcinoma characterized by the development of slowly enlarging pinkish or brownish papules or eroded plaques covered with a thickened horny layer; microscopically, there is dyskeratosis with large round epidermal cells with large nuclei and pale-staining cytoplasm that are scattered through all levels of the epidermis. Primary treatment includes curettage and electrodesiccation.

bow·en·oid pap·u·lo·sis (bō′ĕn-oyd pap′yū-lō′sis) Condition associated with variant of the human papillomavirus; characterized by pigmented papules in the anal/genital area that are typically benign.

Bow·ie stain (bō′ē stān) A stain for juxtaglomerular granules in which the kidney sections are stained in a mixture of Biebrich scarlet red and ethyl violet; juxtaglomerular granules and elastic fibers are stained a deep purple, erythrocytes are amber, and background tissue appears in shades of red.

bow·ing frac·ture (bō′ing frak′shŭr) Osseous breakage due to impact that ruptures a bone along the longitudinal axis.

bow·leg, bow-leg (bō′leg, bō′leg) SYN genu varum.

bowl·er's thumb (bō′lĕrz thŭmb) Compression of the digital nerve on the medial aspect of the thumb, leading to paresthesia in the thumb.

Bow·man cap·sule (bō′măn kap′sŭl) SYN glomerulus.

Bow·man mem·brane, Bow·man lay·er (bō′măn mem′brān, bō′măn fē′vĕr) SYN anterior elastic lamina of cornea.

Bow·man probe (bō′măn prōb) A double-ended probe for the lacrimal duct.

box·er's frac·ture (boks′ĕrz frak′shŭr) Fracture of the neck of a metacarpal bone (most often the fifth) with volar displacement of the head of the bone. SYN fracture of fifth metacarpal.

box hol·ly (boks hol′ē) SYN butcher's broom.

box jel•ly (boks jel′ē) SYN *Chiropsalmus quadrumanus.*

Boyd com•mu•ni•cat•ing per•fo•ra•tion vein (boyd kŏ-myūn′i-kāt-ing pĕr-fōr-ā′shŭn vān) A vein connecting the superficial and deep venous systems in the anteromedial calf.

Boy•er cyst (bwah-yā′ sist) A subhyoid cyst.

Boyle law (boyl law) At constant temperature, the volume of a given quantity of gas varies inversely with its absolute pressure. SYN Mariotte law.

Boze•man-Fritsch cath•e•ter (bōz′măn frich kath′ĕ-tĕr) A slightly curved double-channel uterine catheter with several openings at the tip.

Boze•man op•er•a•tion (bōz′măn op-ĕr-ā′shŭn) A surgical procedure for uterovaginal fistula, the cervix uteri being attached to the bladder and opening into its cavity.

Boze•man po•si•tion (bōz′măn pŏ-zish′ŏn) Knee-elbow position, the patient being strapped to supports.

Boz•zo•lo sign (bōts′sō-lō sīn) Pulsating vessels in the nasal mucous membrane, noted occasionally in thoracic aneurysm.

BP Abbreviation for blood pressure, birth place.

BPC Abbreviation for bulk pharmaceutical chemicals.

BPF Abbreviation for bronchopleural fistula.

BP fis•tu•la (fis′chū-lă) SYN bronchopleural fistula.

BPH Abbreviation for benign prostatic hyperplasia.

Br Symbol for bromine.

brace (brās) An orthosis or orthopedic appliance that supports or holds in correct position any movable part of the body and that allows motion of the part, in contrast to a splint, which prevents motion of the part. [M. E., fr. O. Fr., fr. L. *bracchium*, arm, fr. G. *brachion*]

brac•es (brās′ĕz) Colloquialism for orthodontic appliances.

bra•chi•a (brā′kē-ă) Plural of brachium.

bra•chi•al (brā′kē-ăl) Relating to the arm.

bra•chi•al ar•ter•y (brā′kē-ăl ahr′tĕr-ē) *Origin*, a continuation of the axillary artery beginning at the inferior border of the teres major muscle; *branches*, deep brachial, superior ulnar collateral, inferior ulnar collateral, muscular, and nutrient; terminates in the cubital fossa by bifurcating into radial and ulnar arteries. SYN arteria brachialis [TA].

bra•chi•al•gi•a (brā′kē-al′jē-ă) Pain in the arm. [L. *brachium*, arm, + *algos*, pain]

bra•chi•a•lis mus•cle (brā-kē-ā′lis mŭs′ĕl) *Origin*, lower two thirds of anterior surface of humerus; *insertion*, coronoid process of ulna; *action*, flexes elbow; *nerve supply*, musculocutaneous, usually with a minor contribution from the radial. SYN musculus brachialis [TA].

bra•chi•al plex•us (brā′kē-ăl plek′sŭs) A complex web of spinal nerves arising from the cervical spine; innervate the upper extremities. See this page.

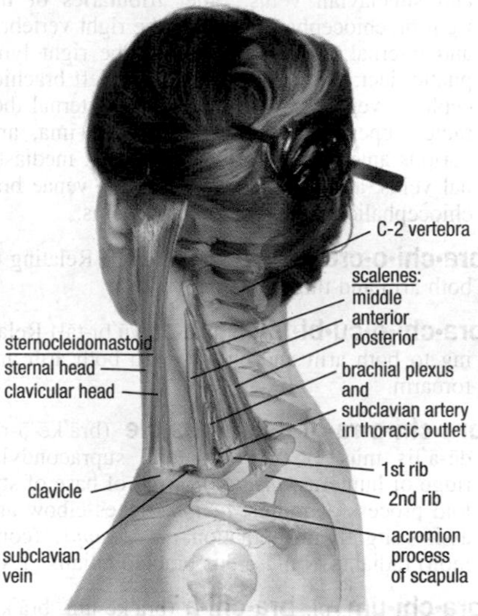

brachial plexus

bra•chi•al plex•us in•ju•ry (brā′kē-ăl plek′sŭs in′jŭr-ē) Damage to the brachial plexus related to delivery; associated with excessive lateral stretching of the head, typically in cases of shoulder dystocia or breech deliveries.

bra•chi•al pulse (brā′kē-ăl pŭls) A palpable rhythmic expansion of the brachial artery in the antecubital space.

bra•chi•al veins (brā′kē-ăl vānz) Venae comitantes of the brachial artery which empty into the axillary vein.

brachio- Combining form denoting **1.** SYN arm (1). **2.** SYN radial. [L. *brachium*]

bra•chi•o•ce•phal•ic (brā′kē-ō-se-fal′ik) Relating to both arm and head.

bra•chi•o•ce•phal•ic ar•te•ri•al trunk (brā′kē-ō-se-fal′ik ahr-tēr′ē-ăl trŭngk) *Origin*, arch of aorta; *branches*, right subclavian and right common carotid; occasionally it gives off the thyroidea ima.

bra•chi•o•ce•phal•ic ar•ter•i•tis (brā′kē-ō-se-fal′ik ahr′tĕr-ī′tis) Giant-cell arteritis seen in older adults; characterized by inflammatory lesions in medium-size arteries, most commonly in the head, neck, or shoulder girdle area. The erythrocyte sedimentation rate is elevated; vision can be damaged or lost.

bra•chi•o•ce•phal•ic trunk (brā′kē-ō-se-fal′ik trŭngk) *Origin*, arch of aorta; *branches*, right subclavian and right common carotid; occasionally it gives off the thyroidea ima. SYN truncus brachiocephalicus [TA].

bra•chi•o•ce•phal•ic veins (brā′kē-ō-se-fal′ik vān) Formed by the union of the internal jugular and subclavian veins; other tributaries of the right brachiocephalic vein are the right vertebral and internal thoracic veins, and the right lymphatic duct; other tributaries of the left brachiocephalic vein are the left vertebral, internal thoracic, superior intercostal, thyroidea ima, and various anterior pericardial, bronchial, mediastinal veins, and the thoracic duct. SYN venae brachiocephalicae [TA], innominate veins.

bra•chi•o•cru•ral (brā′kē-ō-krūr′ăl) Relating to both arm and thigh.

bra•chi•o•cu•bi•tal (brā′kē-ō-kyū′bi-tăl) Relating to both arm and elbow or to both arm and forearm.

bra•chi•o•ra•di•a•lis mus•cle (brā′kē-ō-rā-dē-ā′lis mŭs′ĕl) *Origin*, lateral supracondylar ridge of humerus; *insertion*, front of base of styloid process of radius; *action*, flexes elbow and assists slightly in supination; *nerve supply*, (common) radial. SYN musculus brachioradialis [TA].

bra•chi•um, pl. **bra•chi•a** (brā′kē-ŭm, brā′kē-ă) [TA] **1.** SYN arm (1). **2.** An anatomic structure resembling an arm. [L. arm, prob. akin to G. *brachiōn*]

bra•chi•um of in•fe•ri•or col•lic•u•lus (brā′kē-ŭm in-fēr′ē-ŏr kŏ-lik′yū-lŭs) A fiber bundle passing from the inferior colliculus on either side of the brainstem along the lateral border of the superior colliculus to the posterior part of the thalamus where it enters the medial geniculate body. It forms part of the major ascending auditory pathway.

bra•chi•um of su•pe•ri•or col•lic•u•lus (brā′kē-ŭm sŭ-pēr′ē-ŏr kŏ-lik′yū-lŭs) A band of fibers of the optic tract bypassing the lateral geniculate body to terminate in the superior colliculus and pretectal region.

Bracht ma•neu•ver (brahkt mă-nū′vĕr) Delivery of a fetus in breech position by extension of the legs and trunk of the fetus over the symphysis pubis and abdomen of the mother; the fetal head is born spontaneously as the legs and trunk are lifted above the maternal pelvis, and as the body of the infant is extended by the operator.

♻**brachy-** Combining form meaning short. [G. *brachys*, short]

brach•y•ba•si•a (brak′ē-bā′sē-ă) The shuffling gait of pyramidal tract disease. [brachy- + G. *basis*, a stepping]

brach•y•ba•so•camp•to•dac•ty•ly (brak′ē-bā′sō-kamp-tō-dak′ti-lē) Disproportionate shortness and crookedness of the fingers. [brachy- + G. *basis*, base, + *campylos*, curved, + *daktylos*, finger]

brach•y•ba•so•pha•lan•gi•a (brak′ē-bā′sō-fă-lan′jē-ă) Abnormal shortness of the proximal phalanges. [brachy- + G. *basis*, base, + phalanx]

brach•y•car•di•a (brak′ē-kahr′dē-ă) SYN bradycardia.

brach•y•ceph•a•ly (brak′ē-sef′ă-lē) Shortness or broadness of the head. [G. *brachys*, short, + *kephalē*, head]

brach•y•chei•li•a, brach•y•chi•li•a (brak′ē-kī′lē-ă, brak′ē-kī′lē-ă) Abnormal shortness of the lips. [brachy- + G. *cheilos*, lip]

brach•y•dac•ty•ly (brak′ē-dak′ti-lē) Abnormal shortness of the fingers. [brachy- + G. *daktylos*, finger]

brach•y•gna•thi•a (brak′ig-nā′thē-ă) Abnormal shortness or recession of the mandible. SEE ALSO micrognathia. [brachy- + G. *gnathos*, jaw]

brach•y•me•li•a (brak′ē-mē′lē-ă) Disproportionate shortness of the limbs. [brachy- + G. *melos*, limb]

brach•y•me•so•pha•lan•gi•a (brak′ē-mez′ō-fă-lan′jē-ă) Abnormal shortness of the middle phalanges. [brachy- + G. *mesos*, middle, + phalanx]

brach•y•met•a•car•pi•a (brak′ē-met-ă-kahr′pē-ă) Abnormal shortness of the metacarpals, especially the fourth and fifth.

brach•y•met•a•tar•si•a (brak′ē-met-ă-tahr′sē-ă) Abnormal shortness of the metatarsals.

brach•y•o•dont (brak′ē-ō-dont) A tooth in which the root length exceeds that of the crown. [brachy- + G. *odous*, tooth]

brach•y•o•nych•i•a (brak′ē-ō-nik′ē-ă) Short nails, in which the width of the nail plate and nail bed is greater than the length. [G. *brachys*, short + *onyx, onychos*, nail, + suffix *-ia*, condition]

brach•y•pel•lic pel•vis (brak′ē-pel′ik pel′vis) A pelvis in which the transverse diameter is more than 1 cm longer but less than 3 cm longer than the anteroposterior diameter.

brach•y•pha•lan•gi•a (brak′ē-fă-lan′jē-ă) Abnormal shortness of the phalanges. [brachy- + phalanx]

brach•y•syn•dac•ty•ly (brak′ē-sin-dak′ti-lē) Abnormal shortness of the digits (i.e., fingers, toes) combined with a webbing between the adjacent digits. [brachy- + syndactyly]

brach•y•te•le•pha•lan•gi•a (brak′ē-tel′ĕ-fă-lan′jē-ă) Abnormal shortness of the distal phalanges. [brachy- + G. *telos*, end, + phalanx]

brach•y•ther•a•py (brak′ē-thār′ă-pē) Radiotherapy in which the source of irradiation is placed close to the surface of the body or implanted in the tissues to be treated (e.g., application of radium to the cervix). Treatment targets specific tissues without harm to the surrounding normal tissue.

Brad•bu•ry-Eg•gle•ston syn•drome (brad′bŭr-ē eg′ĕl-stŏn sin′drōm) SYN pure autonomic failure.

Brad•ford frame (brad′fŏrd frām) An oblong rectangular frame made of pipe, over which are stretched transversely two strips of canvas; permits trunk and lower extremities of a bed-ridden patient to move as a unit.

♲ **brady-** Combining form meaning slow. [G. *bradys,* slow]

bradyaesthesia [Br.] SYN bradyesthesia.

bra•dy•ar•rhyth•mi•a (brad′ē-ă-ridh′mē-ă) Any disturbance of the heart's rhythm resulting in a rate less than 60 beats per minute. [brady- + G. *a-* priv. + *rhythmos,* rhythm]

bra•dy•arth•ri•a (brad′ē-ahrth′rē-ă) A form of dysarthria characterized by an abnormal slowness or deliberateness of speech. SYN bradyglossia (2), bradylalia, bradylogia. [brady- + G. *arthroō,* to utter distinctly, fr. *arthron,* a joint]

bra•dy•car•di•a (brad′ē-kahr′dē-ă) Slowness of the heartbeat, usually a rate less than 60 beats per minute. SYN brachycardia. [brady- + G. *kardia,* heart]

bra•dy•car•di•ac, bra•dy•car•dic (brad′ē-kahr′dē-ak, brad′ē-kahr′dik) Relating to or characterized by bradycardia.

bra•dy•di•as•to•le (brad′ē-dī-as′tŏ-lē) Prolongation of the diastole of the heart.

bra•dy•es•the•si•a (brad′ē-es-thē′zē-ă) Slow sensory perception. SYN bradyaesthesia. [brady- + G. *aisthēsis,* sensation]

bra•dy•glos•si•a (brad′ē-glaws′ē-ă) **1.** Slow or difficult tongue movement. **2.** SYN bradyarthria. [brady- + G. *glōssa,* tongue]

bra•dy•ki•ne•si•a (brad′ē-kin-ē′sē-ă) A decrease in spontaneity and movement. One of the features of extrapyramidal disorders, such as Parkinson disease. [brady- + G. *kinēsis,* movement]

bra•dy•ki•net•ic (brad′ē-ki-net′ik) Characterized by or pertaining to slow movement.

bra•dy•ki•nin (brad′ē-kī′nin) The nonapeptide Arg-Pro-Pro-Gly-Phe-Ser-Pro-Phe-Arg, normally present in blood in an inactive form; one of the plasma kinins, a potent vasodilator and mediator of anaphylaxis. [brady- + G. *kineō,* to move]

bra•dy•la•li•a (brad′ē-lā′lē-ă) SYN bradyarthria. [brady- + G. *lalia,* speech]

bra•dy•lex•i•a (brad′ē-lek′sē-ă) Abnormal slowness in reading. [brady- + G. *lexis,* word]

bra•dy•lo•gi•a (brad′ē-lō′jē-ă) SYN bradyarthria. [brady- + G. *logos,* word]

bra•dyp•ne•a (brad′ip-nē′ă) Abnormal slowness of respiration, specifically a low respiratory frequency. [brady- + G. *pnoē,* breathing]

bra•dy•sper•ma•tism (brad′ē-spĕr′mă-tizm) Absence of ejaculatory force, so that the semen trickles away slowly. [brady, + G. *sperma* (*spermat-*), seed, + ism]

bra•dy•sphyg•mi•a (brad′ē-sfig′mē-ă) Slowness of the pulse; can occur without bradycardia, as in ventricular bigeminy when every other beat may fail to produce a peripheral pulse. [brady- + G. *sphygmos,* pulse]

bra•dy•stal•sis (brad′ē-stal′sis) Slow bowel motion. [G. *bradys,* slow, + (*peri*) *stalsis,* contracting around]

bra•dy•to•ci•a (brad′ē-tō′sē-ă) Tedious labor; slow delivery. [brady- + G. *tokos,* childbirth]

bra•dy•u•ri•a (brad′ē-yūr′ē-ă) Slow micturition. [brady- + G. *ouron,* urine]

brad•y•zo•ite (brad′ē-zō′īt) *Toxoplasma gondii* life-cycle stage that forms within a cystlike structure. The organisms multiply slowly but may be transformed into tachyzoites when the host's immune system is impaired.

Brag•ard sign (brah′gahrt sīn) Procedure used to determine whether source of lower back pain is nervous or muscular; leg is kept straight as if flexed at hip. If pain increases during dorsiflexion, pain is likely nervous in origin, whereas with no increase, the source is presumed muscular. SYN stretch test.

i **brain** (brān) That part of the central nervous system contained within the cranium. SEE ALSO encephalon. Cf. cerebrum, cerebellum. See page 220. [A.S. *braegen*]

brain at•tack (brān ă-tak′) SYN acute ischemic stroke.

brain box (brān boks) SYN neurocranium.

brain•case (brān′kās) SYN neurocranium.

brain con•cus•sion (brān kŏn-kŭsh′ŭn) A clinical syndrome due to mechanical, usually traumatic, forces; characterized by immediate and transient impairment of neural function (e.g., alteration of consciousness, disturbance of vision and equilibrium).

brain death (brān deth) Loss of brain function.

brain-gut ax•is (brān-gŭt ak′sis) The continuous feedback loop between sensory neurons in the gastrointestinal tract and motor response generated in the central nervous system. Hypersensitivity in the brain-gut axis contributes to functional GI disorders, including irritable bowel syndrome.

brain im•plant (brān im′plant) Any substance or structure that is placed surgically intracranially.

Brain re•flex (brān rē′fleks) SYN quadripedal extensor reflex.

brain•stem, **brain stem** (brān′stem, brān stem) Originally, the entire unpaired subdivision of the brain, composed of the rhombencephalon, mesencephalon, and diencephalon as distinguished from the brain's only paired subdivision, the telencephalon. More recently, the connotation of the term has undergone several arbitrary modifications: some use it to denote no more than rhombencephalon plus mesencephalon, distinguishing that complex from the prosencepha-

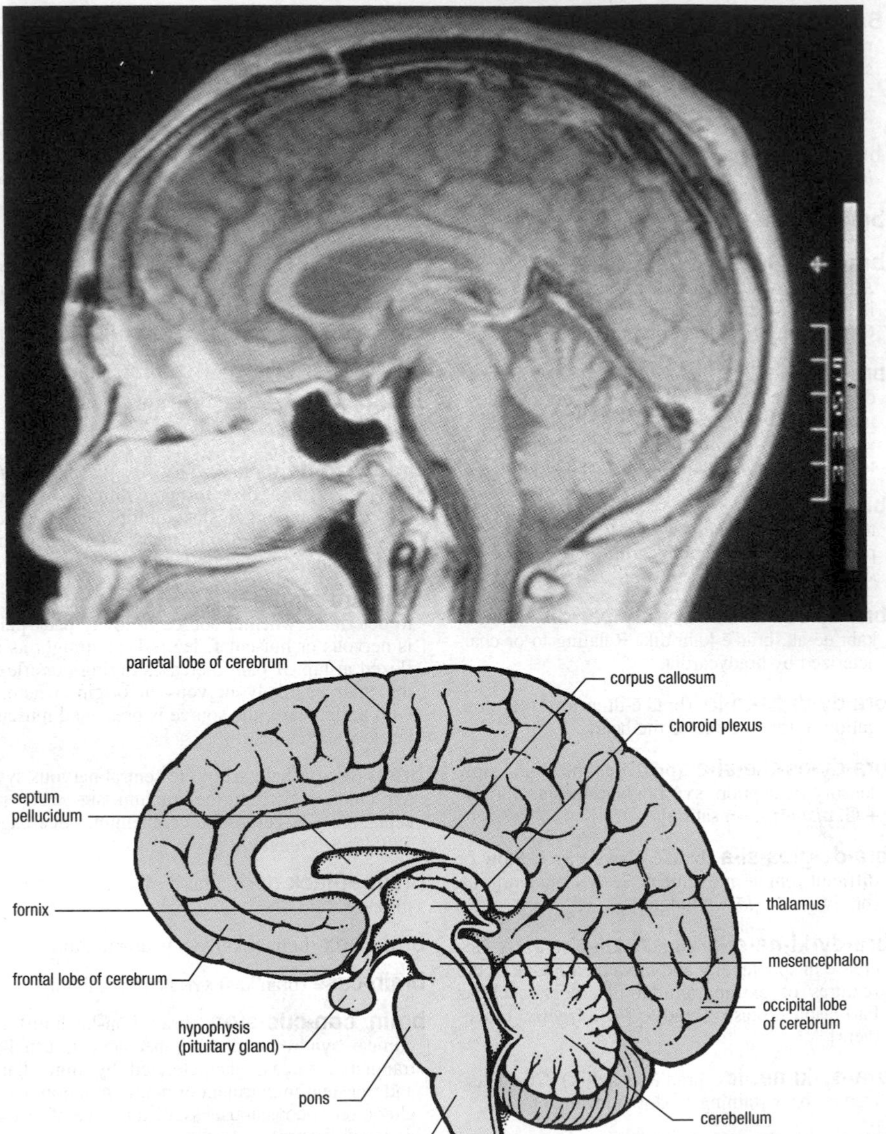

brain: (top) magnetic resonance image of a normal brain; (bottom) illustration of the same midsagittal view

lon (diencephalon plus telencephalon); others restrict it even further to refer exclusively to the rhombencephalon. From both developmental and architectural viewpoints, the original interpretation seems preferable.

brain•stem au•di•tor•y e•voked po•ten•tial (brān′stem aw′di-tōr-ē ē-vōkt′ pŏ-ten′shăl) Responses triggered by click stimuli, which are generated in the acoustic nerve and brainstem auditory pathways; recorded over the scalp.

brain•stem e•voked re•sponse (BSER) (brān′stem ē-vōkt′ rĕ-spons′) SYN auditory brainstem response.

brain•stem e•voked re•sponse au•di•om•e•try, BSER au•di•om•e•try (brān′stem ē-vōkt′ rĕ-spons′ aw′dē-om′ĕ-trē, aw′dē-om′ĕ-trē) SYN auditory brainstem response audiometry.

brain•stem im•plant (brān′stem im′plant) A nonphysiologic structure used to improve or restore audition by stimulation of the cochlear area.

brain sug•ar (brān shug′ăr) D-galactose. SEE galactose.

brain swell•ing (brān swel′ing) A pathologic entity, localized or generalized, characterized by an increase in bulk of brain tissue, due to expansion of the intravascular (congestion) or extravascular (edema) compartments that may coexist or may occur separately and be clinically indistinguishable; clinical manifestations depend on disturbed neuronal function due to local swelling, shifting of intracranial structures, and the effects of intracranial hypertension or circulatory disturbance.

brain•wash•ing (brān′wawsh′ing) Inducing a person to modify his attitudes and behavior in certain directions through various forms of psychological pressure or torture.

brain wave (brān wāv) Colloquialism for electroencephalogram.

brake drug (brāk drŭg) A colloquial and imprecise term for any drug or agent that either accelerates growth or impedes it.

brak•ing ra•di•a•tion (brāk′ing rā′dē-ā′shŭn) SYN Bremsstrahlung radiation.

bran (bran) The outer coatings of grains, which are rich in nutrients and fiber.

branch (branch) An offshoot; in anatomy, one of the primary divisions of a nerve or blood vessel. A branch. SEE ramus, artery, nerve, vein. SYN ramus (1). [Fr. *branche,* related to L. *brachium,* arm]

branch to a•tri•o•ven•tric•u•lar node (branch ā′trē-ō-ven-trik′yū-lăr nōd) SYN atrioventricular nodal branches.

branch•er gly•co•gen stor•age dis•ease (branch′ĕr glī′kō-jen stōr′ăj di-zēz′) Type of glycogen storage disease, due to deficiency of amylo-1,4-1,6-transglucosidase (brancher enzyme).

bran•chi•al ap•par•at•us (brang′kē-ăl ap′ă-rat′ŭs) SYN pharyngeal apparatus.

bran•chi•al arch (brang′kē-ăl ahrch) SYN pharyngeal arch.

bran•chi•al cleft (brang′kē-ăl kleft) SYN pharyngeal groove.

branch•ing (branch′ing) Dividing into parts; sending out offshoots; bifurcating.

bran•chi•o•mo•tor nu•cle•i (brang-kē-ō′mō′tŏr nū′klē-ī) Collective term for those motoneuronal nuclei of the brainstem that develop from the branchiomotor column of the embryo and innervate striated muscle fibers.

bran•chi•o•o•to•re•nal syn•drome (brang′kē-ō-ō′tō-rē′năl sin′drōm) An autosomal dominant disorder characterized by anomalies of the pharyngeal arch (branchial arch) derivatives, sensory hearing impairment, and renal abnormalities.

Brandt-An•drews ma•neu•ver (brahnt an′drūz mă-nū′vĕr) The expression of the placenta by grasping the umbilical cord with one hand and placing the other hand on the abdomen, with the fingers over the anterior surface of the uterus at the junction of the lower uterine segment and the corpus uteri. SYN Andrews maneuver.

Bran•ha•mel•la (bran-hă-mel′ă) A subgenus of aerobic, nonmotile, non-spore-forming bacteria containing gram-negative cocci that occur in pairs with adjacent sides flattened. They are found in the mucous membranes of the upper respiratory tract and occasionally cause respiratory infections and otitis media.

Bran•ham sign (bran′ăm sīn) Bradycardia following compression or excision of an arteriovenous fistula.

bran•ny (bran′ē) Denoting desquamation of small husklike scales. [M.E. *bran,* broken coat of cereal grain]

Bras•dor meth•od (brah-dōr′ meth′ŏd) Treatment of aneurysm by ligation of the artery immediately below (i.e., on the distal side of) the tumor.

brass found•er's fe•ver (bras fown′dĕrz fē′vĕr) An occupational disease, characterized by influenzalike symptoms, due to inhalation of particles and fumes of metallic oxides.

Braun a•nas•to•mo•sis (brown an-as-tŏ′mō′sis) After a loop gastroenterostomy, anastomosis between afferent and efferent loops of jejunum.

brawn•y (brawn′ē) Thickened (lichenified) and dusky (a darkened hue), as of a swelling. [M.E. fleshy]

brawn•y e•de•ma (brawn'ē ĕ-dē'mă) SYN nonpitting edema.

Brax•ton Hicks sign (braks'tŏn-hiks sīn) Irregular uterine contractions occurring after the third month of pregnancy.

Bra•zel•ton Ne•o•na•tal Be•hav•ior•al Assess•ment Scale (brā'zĕl-tŏn nē-ō-nā'tăl bē-hāv'yŏr-ăl ă-ses'mĕnt skāl) A scale used by obstetricians, pediatricians, and pediatric psychologists to assess the sensory, motor, emotional, and physical development of the neonate, usually beginning at birth or in the first month of life.

BRCA1 gene (jēn) A tumor suppressor gene on chromosome 17 at locus 17q21, isolated in 1994; encodes p53 protein, which prevents cells with damaged DNA from dividing; carriers of germline mutations in BRCA1 are predisposed to develop both breast and ovarian cancer. SEE ALSO BRCA2 gene, carcinoma of the breast.

BRCA2 gene (jēn) A tumor suppressor gene identified in 1995 on chromosome 13 at locus 13q12–q13; a large gene consisting of 27 exons distributed over 70 kb, encoding a protein of 3418 amino acids; carriers of germline mutations in BRCA2 have an increased risk, similar to that of those with BRCA1 mutations, of developing breast cancer and a moderately increased risk of ovarian cancer; BRCA2 families also exhibit an increased incidence of male breast, pancreatic, prostate, laryngeal, and ocular cancers. SEE ALSO BRCA1 gene, carcinoma of the breast.

break-e•ven point (brāk-ē'vĕn poynt) The point in sales volume at which total revenue equals total costs; indicating a balance. Sales volume below the break-even point will cause a negative cash flow (loss); sales volume above the break-even point will result in a profit. This point is calculated to help determine whether a new test, procedure, or service should be offered by a health care provider based on projected sales volume.

break•point (brāk'poynt) **1.** In helminth epidemiology, the critical mean wormload in a community, below which the helminth mating frequency is too low to maintain reproduction. Below this level, helminth infection in the community will progressively decline, ultimately to zero. **2.** A point in any continuous process or function at which an interruption, cessation, or change occurs. **3.** In antimicrobial therapy, concentration of an antibiotic that can be achieved in body fluids or target sites during optimal therapy.

break test (brāk test) A form of manual muscle procedure in which the therapist opposes the force exerted by a muscle that is isometrically contracted at its greatest mechanical advantage, so as to grade its strength.

break•through pain (brāk'thrū pān) Discomfort, usually acute and severe, which is experienced by patients between the normal doses of a medication that generally controls or palliates such pain.

breast (brest) **1.** The pectoral surface of the thorax. **2.** The organ of milk secretion; one of two hemispheric projections situated in the subcutaneous tissue anterior to the pectoralis major muscle on either side of the thorax or chest of the mature female; it is rudimentary in the male. See this page, B19. SYN mamma [TA], teat (2). [A.S. *brēost*]

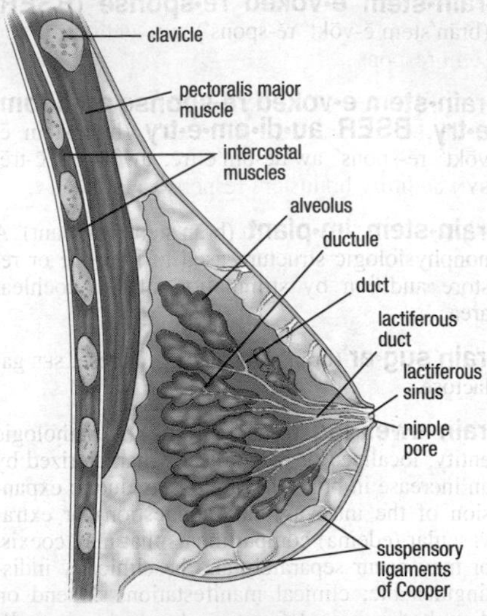

lateral view of female breast

breast bone (brest bōn) SYN sternum.

breast en•gorge•ment (brest en-gōrj'mĕnt) Condition in which maternal breasts become tensely swollen. This usually occurs on the third or fourth day postpartum. Management includes easing maternal discomfort and ensuring that baby feeds effectively. [Fr. *engorger*, to fill to excess]

breast im•plant (brest im'plant) A form of mammillaplasty (q.v.) generally involving insertion of a nonphysiologic substance to enlarge the female breast for putative cosmetic purposes or in reconstruction of a breast that suffered surgical scarring during mastectomy.

breast pump (brest pŭmp) A suction instrument for withdrawing milk from the breast.

breast self-ex•am•i•na•tion (BSE) (brest self'eg-zam'i-nā'shŭn) Procedure by which breasts and accessory anatomic structures are observed and palpated to detect changes or abnormalities that may indicate the presence of malignancy. It is recommended that women undertake breast self-examination once a month. Nurses and other health care professionals play an important role in teaching women to perform this procedure correctly. See page 223.

breath (breth) **1.** The respired air. **2.** An inspiration. **3.** A single cycle of inhalation followed by exhalation. [A.S. *braeth*]

breath ac·ti·va·ted me·tered dose in·ha·ler (BAMDI) (breth ak′ti-vā-tĕd mē′tĕrd dōs in-āl′ĕr) Device that responds to a patient's respiratory activity to provide appropriate dosage of medications in treatment of asthma and other respiratory disease.

breath al·co·hol tech·ni·cian (BAT) (breth al′kŏ-hol tek-nish′ăn) Someone trained and certified to conduct breath alcohol testing.

breath-hold·ing test (breth-hold′ing test) A rough index of cardiopulmonary reserve measured by the length of time that a person can voluntarily stop breathing; normal duration is 30 seconds or longer; diminished cardiac or pulmonary reserve is indicated by a duration of 20 seconds or less.

breath·ing (brēdh′ing) Inhalation and exhalation of air or gaseous mixtures. SEE ALSO respiration.

breath·ing bag (brēdh′ing bag) A collapsible reservoir from which gases are inhaled and into which gases may be exhaled during general anesthesia or artificial ventilation. SYN reservoir bag.

breath·ing re·serve (brēdh′ing rē-zĕrv′) The difference between the pulmonary ventilation (i.e., the volume of air breathed under ordinary resting conditions) and the maximum breathing capacity.

breath sounds (breth sowndz) A murmur, bruit, fremitus, rhonchus, or rale heard on auscultation over the lungs or any part of the respiratory tract. See page 224. SYN respiratory sounds.

breath test (breth test) Any diagnostic procedure in which endogenous or exogenous materials are measured in samples of breath as a means of identifying pathologic processes (e.g., hydrogen breath testing for lactose intolerance, urea breath testing to detect gastric colonization with *Helicobacter pylori*). **2.** A test to measure alcohol consumption.

Bre·da dis·ease (brā′dah di-zēz′) SYN espundia.

breech (brēch) SYN buttocks. See page B21. [A.S. *brēc*]

breech pre·sen·ta·tion (brēch prez′ĕn-tā′shŭn) Presentation of any part of the pelvic extremity of the fetus, the nates, knees, or feet; more properly only of the nates; frank breech presentation occurs when the fetus presents by the pelvic extremity; the thighs may be flexed and the legs extended over the anterior surfaces of the body; in full breech presentation, the thighs may be flexed on the abdomen and the legs on the thighs, in footling presentation, the feet may be the lowest part; in incomplete foot presentation, incomplete knee presentation, one leg may retain the position which is typical of one of the above-mentioned presentations, whereas the other foot or knee may present.

breg·ma (breg′mă) The point on the skull corre-

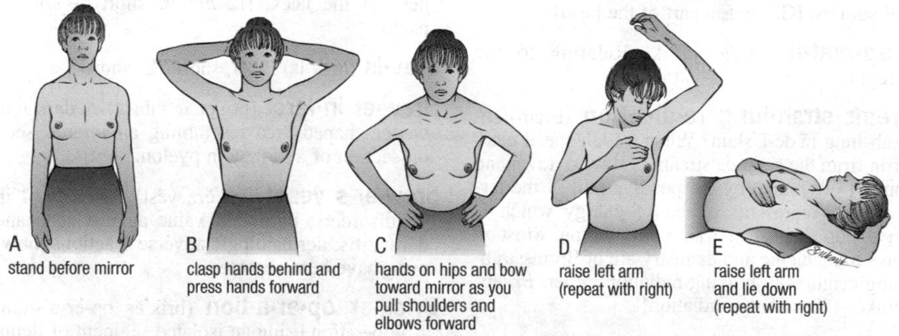
A
stand before mirror
B
clasp hands behind and press hands forward
C
hands on hips and bow toward mirror as you pull shoulders and elbows forward
D
raise left arm (repeat with right)
E
raise left arm and lie down (repeat with right)

breast self-examination: standing before a mirror, (A) check both breasts for anything unusual, (B, C); while in the shower, (D) massage breast in circular pattern feeling for any unusual lumps or masses under the skin and squeeze nipple to look for discharge; (E) using the same circular motion in panel D, check again for any unusual lumps or masses while lying down

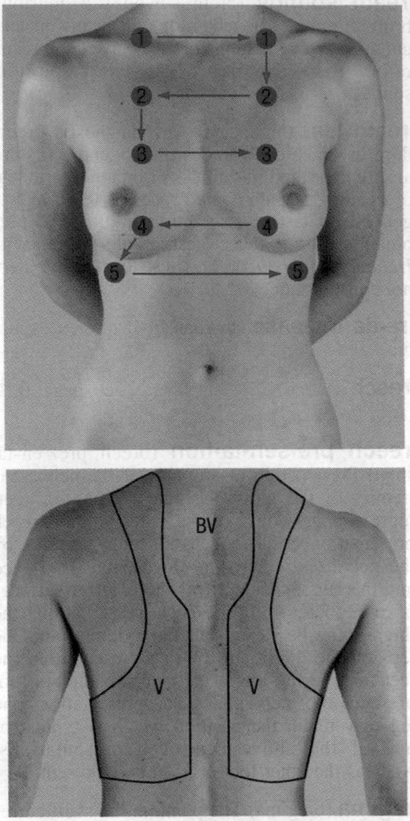

auscultating for breath sounds: BV, bronchovesicular sounds; V, vesicular sounds

sponding to the junction of the coronal and sagittal sutures. [G. the forepart of the head]

breg•mat•ic (breg-mat′ik) Relating to the bregma.

Brems•strah•lung ra•di•a•tion (bremz′sh-trah-lung rā′dē-ā′shŭn) When a high-speed electron from the cathode stream is slowed down and pulled off course by the positive pull of the target, this represents a loss of energy which is given up as heat and an x-ray photon. Most x-rays in medicine and dentistry are of Bremsstrahlung origin. SYN braking radiation. [Ger. *Brems,* brake, + *Strahlung,* radiation]

Bren•ner tu•mor (bren′er tū′mŏr) A benign neoplasm of the ovary, consisting chiefly of fibrous tissue that contains nests of cells resembling transitional type epithelium, as well as glandlike structures that contain mucin; origin is controversial, but it may arise from Walthard cell rest; ordinarily found incidentally in ovaries removed for other reasons, especially in postmenopausal women.

Bres•low meth•od (brez′lō meth′ŏd) Procedure for staging melanoma based on depth of skin penetration, taken from top of granular layer to level of deepest penetration, or from base in ulcerated lesions.

Bres•low thick•ness (brez′lō thik′nĕs) Maximal thickness of a primary cutaneous melanoma measured in tissue sections from the top of the epidermal granular layer, or from the ulcer base (if the tumor is ulcerated), to the bottom of the tumor; metastatic rates correlate closely with tumor thickness.

Breus mole (broys mōl) An aborted oocyte in which the fetal surface of the placenta presents numerous hematomata with an absence of blood vessels in the chorion and an oocyte much smaller in size than normal in relation to the duration of the pregnancy.

bre•ve•tox•in (brev-ĕ-tok′sin) A structurally unique neurotoxin produced by the "red tide" dinoflagellate *Ptychodiscus brevis Davis* (*Gymnodinium brevis Davis*), a species of algae responsible for large fish kills and mollusk and human food poisoning in the Gulf of Mexico and along the Florida coast. Unlike previously isolated dinoflagellate toxins, such as saxitoxin, which are water-soluble sodium channel blockers, the brevotoxins are lipid-soluble sodium channel activators; used in neurobiologic research.

Brev•i•bac•te•ri•um (brev-i-bak-tēr′ē-ŭm) A bacterial genus of nonmotile, non-spore-forming, gram-positive rods found as normal human skin flora, in raw milk, and on the surface of cheeses; some species, recovered from patients with septicemia and from the peritoneum of patients undergoing peritoneal dialysis, appear to be opportunistic human pathogens.

brev•i•col•lis (brev-ē-kol′is) Abnormal shortness of the neck. [L. *brevis,* short, + *collum,* neck]

brev•is (brev′is) Brief, short. [L. short]

Brew•er in•farct (brū′ĕr in′fahrkt) A dark-red, wedge-shaped area resembling an infarct, seen on section of a kidney in pyelonephritis.

brew•er's yeast (brū′ĕrz yēst) Agent used in GI disorders; purported value against acne and dermatitis; dermatologic adverse reactions, however, have been reported.

Brick•er op•er•a•tion (brik′ĕr op-ĕr-ā′shŭn) An operation using an isolated segment of ileum to collect urine from the ureters and conduct it to the skin surface.

bridge (brij) **1.** The upper part of the ridge of the nose formed by the nasal bones. **2.** One of the threads of protoplasm that appear to pass from one cell to another. **3.** SYN fixed partial denture.

bridge•work (brij′wŏrk) SYN partial denture.

brief form (brēf fōrm) Shortened form of a

word; commonly used in medical reports (e.g., "exam" for "examination").

Brigg test (brig test) A test using the reduction of molybdate to follow the excretion of homogentisic acid.

bright blood im•ag•ing (brīt blŭd im′ăj-ing) Magnetic resonance acquisitions in which blood vessels are bright.

Brill dis•ease (bril di-zēz′) SYN Brill-Zinsser disease.

Brill-Zins•ser dis•ease (bril-zin′sĕr di-zēz′) An endogenous reinfection in people who previously had epidemic typhus fever; it is mild and may be mistaken for endemic (murine) typhus. SYN Brill disease, recrudescent typhus.

brim (brim) The upper edge or rim of a hollow structure.

Bri•quet a•tax•i•a (brē-kā′ ă-tak′sē-ă) Weakening of the muscle sense and increased sensibility of the skin, in hysteria.

Bri•quet dis•ease (brē-kā′ di-zēz′) Hysteric neurosis, conversion type.

Bri•quet syn•drome (brē-kā′ sin′drōm) A chronic but fluctuating mental disorder, usually of young women, characterized by frequent complaints of physical illness involving multiple organ systems simultaneously.

brise•ment for•cé (brēs-mōn[h]′ fōr-sā′) Procedure infrequently used to treat frozen shoulder in which a forceful manipulation is performed to restore range of motion that usually results in torn adhesions and adjacent joint capsule. [Fr. forcible breaking]

Bris•saud dis•ease (brē-sō′ di-zēz′) SYN tic.

Bris•saud re•flex (brē-sō′ rē′fleks) Tickling the sole causes a contraction of the tensor fasciae latae muscle, even when there is no responsive movement of the toes.

Bri•tish an•ti-Lew•is•ite (BAL) (brit′ish an′tē-lū′is-īt) A chelating agent used in heavy-metal poisoning and against the chemical-warfare agent Lewisite.

Brit•ish ther•mal u•nit (BTU) (brit′ish thĕr′măl yū′nit) The quantity of heat required to raise 1 pound of water from 3.9–4.4°C; equal to 251.996 calories or to 1055.056 joules.

brit•tle bones (brit′ĕl bōnz) SYN osteogenesis imperfecta.

brit•tle di•a•be•tes (brit′ĕl dī-ă-bē′tēz) Diabetes mellitus in which there are marked fluctuations in blood glucose concentrations that are difficult to control.

broach (brōch) A dental instrument for removing the pulp of a tooth or exploring the dentinal canal.

Broad•bent law (brod′bent law) Lesions of the upper segment of the motor tract cause less marked paralysis of muscles that habitually produce bilateral movements than of those that commonly act independently of the opposite side.

Broad•bent sign (brod′bent sīn) A retraction of the thoracic wall, synchronous with cardiac systole, visible anywhere, but particularly in the left posterior axillary line near the 11th and 12th ribs; a sign of adherent pericardium.

Broad•bent test (brod′bent test) Procedure to determine which cerebral hemisphere is dominant for language. Different words are presented in each ear at the same time; right-handed patients hear the words at the right ear first.

broad lig•a•ment of the u•ter•us (brawd lig′ă-mĕnt yū′tĕr-ŭs) The peritoneal fold passing from the lateral margin of the uterus to the wall of the pelvis on either side and ensheathing the ovaries and uterine tubes. SYN ligamentum latum uteri [TA].

broad spec•trum (brawd spek′trŭm) A term indicating activity of an antibiotic against a wide variety of microorganisms.

broad-spec•trum an•ti•bi•ot•ic (brawd-spek′trŭm an′tē-bī-ot′ik) An antibiotic having a wide range of activity against both gram-positive and gram-negative organisms.

Bro•ca an•gle (brō′kă ang′gĕl) Intersection formed by imaginary lines drawn from the auricular point and glabella to the anterior nasal spine.

Bro•ca a•pha•si•a (brō′kă ă-fā′zē-ă) **1.** SYN motor aphasia. **2.** SYN expressive aphasia.

Bro•ca cen•ter (brō′kă sen′tĕr) The posterior part of the inferior frontal gyrus of the left or dominant hemisphere, corresponding approximately to Brodmann area 44; Broca identified this region as an essential component of the motor mechanisms governing articulated speech. SYN motor speech center.

Bro•ca mo•tor ar•e•as (brō′kă mō′tŏr ār′ē-ăz) Opercular and triangular parts of inferior frontal gyrus and surrounding prefrontal cortex; transforms neural representations to auticulatory sentences. Lesions in this area may cause motor aphasia.

Bro•ca vi•su•al plane (brō′kă vizh′ū-ăl plān) A plane drawn through the visual axes of each eye.

Bro•die ab•scess (brō′dē ab′ses) A chronic abscess of bone surrounded by dense fibrous tissue and sclerotic bone.

Bro•die dis•ease (brō′dē di-zēz′) **1.** SYN Brodie knee. **2.** Hysteric spinal neuralgia, simulating Pott disease, following a trauma.

Bro•die knee (brō′dē nē) Chronic hypertrophic synovitis of the knee. SYN Brodie disease (1).

Brod·mann ar·e·as (brod′mahn ār-ē′ăz) Regions of the cerebral cortex distinguished on the basis of histologic differences and presumed differences in function. See this page.

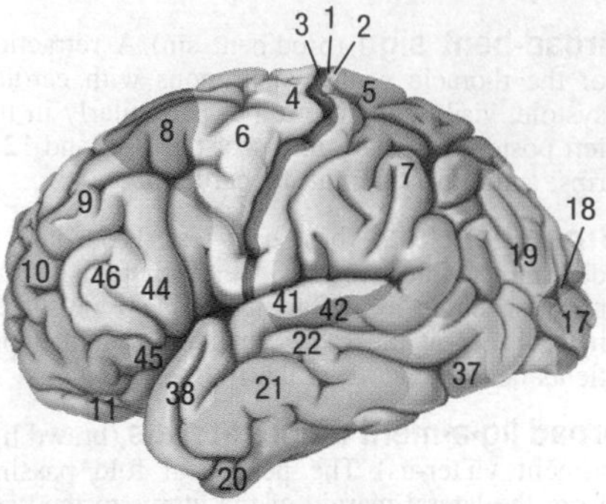

Brodmann areas: zones of the cerebral cortex determined on the basis of histology (i.e., cell type, size, density, lamination) and neural function; lateral aspect of the left cerebral hemisphere is shown here; (1–3) primary somatosensory cortex, (4) primary motor cortex, (5) somatosensory association cortex, (6) premotor and supplementary motor cortices, (7) somatosensory association cortex, (8) frontal eye field, (9) dorsolateral prefrontal cortex, (10) frontopolar area, (11) orbitofrontal area, (17–19) visual cortex, (21) middle temporal gyrus, (22) superior temporal gyrus, (37) fusiform gyrus, (38) temporopolar area, (41, 42) primary and auditory association cortices, (44, 45) Broca motor speech area, (46) dorsolateral prefrontal cortex

brom-, bromo- Prefixes that indicate bromine or a foul odor. [G. *brōmos,* a stench]

bro·mate (brō′māt) Salt or anion of bromic acid.

bro·mat·ed (brō′māt-ĕd) Combined or saturated with bromine or any of its compounds. SYN brominated.

bro·mide (brō′mīd) The anion Br^-; salt of hydrogen bromide (HBr); several salts formerly used as sedatives, hypnotics, and anticonvulsants.

bro·mi·dro·sis, brom·hi·dro·sis (brō′mi-drō′sis, brōm′hī-drō′sis) Fetid or foul-smelling perspiration. SYN osmidrosis. [G. *brōmos,* a stench, + *hidrōs,* perspiration]

bro·min·at·ed (brō′min-āt-ĕd) SYN bromated.

bro·mine (Br) (brō′mēn) A nonmetallic, reddish, volatile, liquid element; atomic no. 35, atomic wt. 79.904; valences 1–7, inclusive; it unites with hydrogen to form hydrobromic acid, and this reacts with many metals to form bromides, some of which are used in medicine. [Fr. *brome,* bromine, fr. G. *bromos,* stench]

bro·mism, bro·min·ism (brō′mizm, -min-izm) Chronic bromide intoxication, characterized by headache, drowsiness, confusion, and occasionally violent delirium, muscular weakness, cardiac depression, an acneform eruption, foul breath, anorexia, and gastric distress.

brom·o·ben·zyl·cy·a·nide (brō′mō-benz′il-sī′ă-nīd) A riot-control agent used by Allied forces during World War I but now essentially obsolete; NATO code is CA. SEE ALSO hydrogen cyanide, cyanogen chloride.

bro·mo·der·ma (brō′mō-dĕr′mă) An acneform or granulomatous eruption due to hypersensitivity to bromide. [bromide + G. *derma,* skin]

bro·mo·sul·fo·phthal·e·in (brō′mō-sŭl′fō-thal′ē-in) SYN sulfobromophthalein sodium. SYN bromosulphophthalein.

bromosulphophthalein [Br.] SYN bromosulfophthalein.

brom·phe·nol test (brōm-fē′nol test) A colorimetric measurement of protein, albumin, and globulin in the urine by use of reagent strips.

Bromp·ton cock·tail (bromp′tŏn kok′tāl) A cocktail of morphine and cocaine usually used for analgesia in terminal cancer patients; formulations vary but typically contain 15 mg of morphine hydrochoride and 10 mg of cocaine hydrochloride per 10 mL of the cocktail. [*Brompton* Chest Hospital, London, England, where developed]

brom·sul·fo·phthal·e·in (brom-sŭl′fō-thal′ē-in) SYN sulfobromophthalein sodium. SYN bromsulphophthalein.

bromsulphophthalein [Br.] SYN bromsulfophthalein.

bronch, bronch·ing (brongk, brongk′ing) Jargonistic verb for use of a bronchoscope during examination.

bron·chi (brong′kī) Plural of bronchus.

bron·chi·a (brong′kē-ă) The smaller divisions of the bronchi. SEE ALSO bronchus, bronchiole. [G. pl. of *bronchion,* dim. of *bronchos,* trachea]

bron·chi·al (brong′kē-ăl) Relating to the bronchi.

bron·chi·al ad·e·no·ma (brong′kē-ăl ad′ē-nō′mă) A benign or malignant polypoid epithelial tumor of bronchial mucosa, arising deep to the surface epithelium, possibly from mucous glands or their ducts.

bron·chi·al ar·te·ri·og·ra·phy (brong′kē-ăl ahr-tēr′ē-og′ră-fē) Radiography of bronchial arteries by selective injection of the intercostal arteries from which they arise.

bron·chi·al asth·ma (brong′kē-ăl az′mă) A condition of the lungs with extensive narrowing of the airways, varying over short periods either spontaneously or as a result of treatment, due in varying degrees to contraction (spasm) of smooth muscle, edema of the mucosa, chronic or recurrent local inflammation of the submucosa with eventual fibrosis, and excessive mucus in the lumen of the bronchi and bronchioles; these changes are caused by the local release of spasmogens and vasoactive substances (e.g., histamine, or certain leukotrienes or prostaglandins) in the course of an allergic process.

bron•chi•al buds (brong'kē-ăl bŭdz) Two lateral outpouchings of the tracheal bud that are the primordia of the bronchi.

bron•chi•al glands (brong'kē-ăl glandz) **1.** SYN bronchopulmonary lymph nodes. **2.** Mucous and seromucous glands with secretory units that lie outside the muscle of the bronchi.

bron•chi•al hy•giene (brong'kē-ăl hī'jēn) Those activities contributing to the removal of bronchial secretions and the maintenance of open airways.

bron•chi•al mu•cous gland ad•e•no•ma (brong'kē-ăl myū'kŭs gland ad'ĕ-nō'mă) A rare benign tumor arising from the mucous glands of bronchial mucosa.

bron•chi•al pneu•mo•ni•a (brong'kē-ăl nū-mō'nē-ă) SYN bronchopneumonia.

bron•chi•al prov•o•ca•tion (brong'kē-ăl prov-ō-kā'shŭn) A procedure for identifying and characterizing hyperresponsive airways by having the subject inhale an agent known to cause (or suspected of causing) a decrease in pulmonary function.

bron•chi•al ste•no•sis (brong'kē-ăl stĕ-nō'sis) Narrowing of the lumen of a bronchial tube.

bron•chi•al veins (brong'kē-ăl vānz) Many veins running in front of and behind the bronchi and uniting into two main trunks that empty on the right side into the azygos vein, on the left into the accessory hemiazygos or the left superior intercostal vein.

bron•chic cell (brong'kik sel) SYN pulmonary alveoli.

bron•chi•ec•ta•sis (brong'kē-ek'tă-sis) Chronic dilation of bronchi or bronchioles as a sequel of inflammatory disease or obstruction. See page B5. [bronchi- + G. *ektasis,* a stretching]

bron•chi•ec•tat•ic (brong'kē-ek-tat'ik) Relating to bronchiectasis.

bron•chi in•tra•seg•men•ta•les (brong'kī intră-seg-men-tā'lēz) SYN intrasegmental bronchi.

bron•chil•o•quy (brong-kil'ō-kwē) Rarely used term for bronchophony [bronchi- + L. *loquor,* to speak]

bron•chi•o•gen•ic (brong'kē-ō-jen'ik) SYN bronchogenic.

bron•chi•o•lar a•de•no•car•ci•no•ma (brong'kē-ō'lăr ad'ĕ-nō-kahr-si-nō'mă) SYN bronchiolar carcinoma.

bron•chi•o•lar car•ci•no•ma (brong'kē-ō'lăr kahr'si-nō'mă) A carcinoma, thought to be derived from epithelium of terminal bronchioles, in which the neoplastic tissue extends along the alveolar walls and grows in small masses within the alveoli; may be diffuse, nodular, or lobular; the neoplastic cells are cuboidal or columnar and form papillary structures; metastases are infrequent. See this page. SYN alveolar cell carcinoma, bronchiolar adenocarcinoma, bronchioloalveolar carcinoma, bronchoalveolar carcinoma.

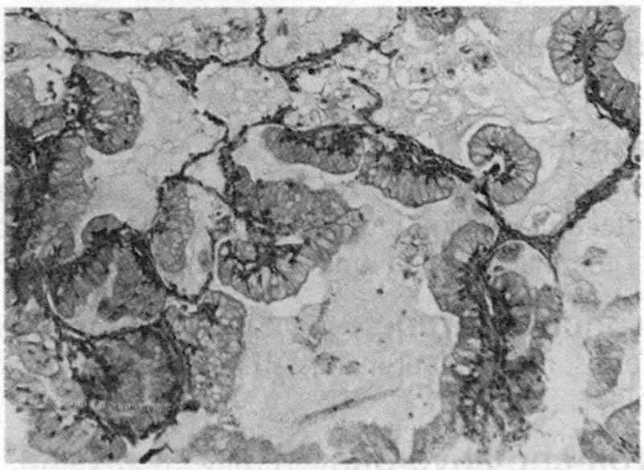

bronchiolar carcinoma: columnar cells hold atypical cytoplasmic mucin and thereby adhere to alveolar walls

bron•chi•ole (brong'kē-ōl) One of approximately six generations of increasingly finer subdivisions of the bronchi, each smaller than 1 mm in diameter, and having no cartilage in its wall, but relatively abundant smooth muscle and elastic fibers. SYN bronchiolus [TA].

bron•chi•o•lec•ta•sis (brong'kē-ō-lek'tă-sis) Bronchiectasis involving the bronchioles. [bronchiole + G. *ektasis,* a stretching]

bron•chi•o•li (brong-kī'ō-lī) Plural of bronchiolus.

bron•chi•ol•i•tis (brong'kē-ō-lī'tis) Acute viral illness common in children younger than 2 years old. Common course is respiratory syncytial virus; findings include inflammation of the bronchioles, often associated with bronchopneumonia. [bronchiole + *-itis,* inflammation]

bron•chi•ol•i•tis fi•bro•sa ob•li•te•rans, bron•chi•ol•i•tis ob•lit•e•rans (brong'kē-ō-lī'tis fī-brō'să ob-lit'ĕr-anz, brong'kē-ō-lī'tis ob-lit'ĕr-anz) Obstruction of bronchioles and alveolar ducts by fibrous granulation tissue induced by mucosal ulceration; the condition may follow inhalation of irritant gases (i.e., silo-filler's lung) or may complicate pneumonia (i.e., BOOP); associated with obstructive findings (i.e., unilateral hyperlucent lung, Swyer-James syndrome).

bron•chi•ol•i•tis ob•li•te•rans with or•ga•niz•ing pneu•mo•ni•a (BOOP) (brong'kē-ō-lī′tis ob-lit′ĕr-anz ōr′gă-nīz′ing nū-mō′nē-ă) Bronchiolitis fibrosa obliterans complicated by pneumonia with organization.

♻ **bronchiolo-** Combining form meaning bronchiole. [L. *bronchiolus*]

bron•chi•o•lo•al•ve•o•lar car•ci•no•ma (brong′kē′ō-lō-al-vē′ō-lăr kahr′si-nō′mă) SYN bronchiolar carcinoma.

bron•chi•o•lus, pl. **bron•chi•o•li** (brong-kī′ō-lŭs, brong-kī′ō-lī) [TA] SYN bronchiole. [Mod. L. dim. of *bronchus*]

bron•chi•o•ste•no•sis (brong′kē-ō-stĕ-nō′sis) Narrowing of the lumen of a bronchial tube.

bron•chit•ic (brong-kit′ik) Relating to bronchitis.

bron•chi•tis (brong-kī′tis) Acute (e.g., caused by recent infection) or chronic (e.g., long-term infection, smoking, cystic fibrosis) inflammation of the mucous membrane of the bronchial tubes.

♻ **broncho-, bronch-, bronchi-** Combining forms meaning bronchus. [G. *bronchos,* windpipe]

bron•cho•al•ve•o•lar (brong′kō-al-vē′ō-lăr) SYN bronchovesicular.

bron•cho•al•ve•o•lar car•ci•no•ma (brong′kō-al-vē′ō-lăr kahr′si-nō′mă) SYN bronchiolar carcinoma.

bron•cho•al•ve•o•lar flu•id (brong′kō-al-vē′ō-lăr flū′id) A liquid (containing several lytic enzymes) that serves to remove inspired particulates from the pulmonary airways.

bron•cho•al•ve•o•lar la•vage (BAL) (brong′kō-al-vē′ō-lăr lă-vahzh′) A procedure performed using fiberoptic bronchoscopy, during which a distal airway is occluded and liquid is then introduced into the airway and recovered for examination of cell types and microorganisms.

bron•cho•cav•ern•ous (brong′kō-kav′ĕr-nŭs) Relating to a bronchus or bronchial tube and a pathologic pulmonary cavity.

bron•cho•cele (brong′kō-sēl) A circumscribed dilation of a bronchus. [broncho- + G. *kēlē,* hernia]

bron•cho•cen•tric gran•u•lo•ma•to•sis (brong′kō-sen′trik gran′yū-lō′mă-tō′sis) A severe form of allergic bronchopulmonary aspergillosis.

bron•cho•con•stric•tion (brong′kō-kŏn-strik′shŭn) Constriction of the bronchi.

bron•cho•con•stric•tor (brong′kō-kŏn-strik′tŏr) **1.** Causing a reduction in caliber of a bronchus or bronchial tube. **2.** An agent that possesses this action (e.g., histamine).

bron•cho•di•la•tion (brong′kō-dī-lā′shŭn) Increase in caliber of the bronchi and bronchioles in response to pharmacologically active substances or autonomic nervous activity.

bron•cho•di•la•tor (brong′kō-dī′lā-tŏr) **1.** Causing an increase in caliber of a bronchus. **2.** An agent that possesses this power (e.g., epinephrine).

bron•cho•e•soph•a•gol•o•gy (brong′kō-ē-sof-ă-gol′ŏ-jē) The specialty concerned with the diagnosis and treatment of diseases of the tracheobronchial tree and esophagus by endoscope and other means. SYN broncho-oesophagology. [broncho- + G. *oisophagos,* esophagus, + *logos,* study]

bron•cho•e•soph•a•gos•co•py (brong′kō-ē-sof-ă-gos′kŏ-pē) Examination of the tracheobronchial tree and esophagus with appropriate endoscopes. SYN broncho-oesophagoscopy.

bron•cho•fi•ber•scope (brong′kō-fī′bĕr-skōp) A fiberoptic endoscope adapted for visualization of the trachea and bronchi. SYN bronchofibrescope.

bronchofibrescope [Br.] SYN bronchofiberscope.

bron•cho•gen•ic (brong′kō-jen′ik) Of bronchial origin; emanating from the bronchi. SYN bronchiogenic.

bron•cho•gen•ic car•ci•no•ma (brong′kō-jen′ik kahr′si-nō′mă) Squamous cell or oat cell carcinoma that arises in the mucosa of the large bronchi; local growth causes bronchial obstruction and is observed radiologically as an enlarging lung mass; malignant tumor cells can be detected in the sputum, and they metastasize early to the thoracic lymph nodes and to the brain, suprarenal glands, and other organs through the bloodstream. Cause usually related to cigarette smoking or exposure to chemical carcinogens.

bron•cho•gen•ic cyst (brong′kō-jen′ik sist) A cyst lined by ciliated columnar epithelium believed to represent bronchial differentiation; smooth muscle and mucous glands may be present.

bron•cho•gram (brong′kō-gram) A radiograph obtained by bronchography; radiographic visualization of a bronchus. [broncho- + G. *gramma,* a writing]

bron•chog•ra•phy (brong-kog′ră-fē) Radiographic visualization of the bronchi using a contrast agent. [broncho- + -graphy]

bron•cho•lith (brong′kō-lith) A hard concretion in a bronchus or bronchial tube. [broncho- + G. *lithos,* stone]

bron•cho•li•thi•a•sis (brong′kō-li-thī′ă-sis) Bronchial inflammation or obstruction caused by broncholiths.

bron•cho•ma•la•ci•a (brong′kō-mă-lā′shē-ă) Degeneration of elastic and connective tissue of bronchi and trachea. [broncho- + G. *malakia,* a softening]

bron·cho·my·co·sis (brong′kō-mī-kō′sis) Any fungal disease of the bronchial tubes or bronchi. [broncho- + G. *mykēs,* fungus]

broncho-oesophagology [Br.] SYN bronchoesophagology.

broncho-oesophagoscopy [Br.] SYN bronchoesophagoscopy.

bron·choph·o·ny (brong-kof′ŏ-nē) Increased intensity and clarity of voice sounds heard over a bronchus surrounded by consolidated lung tissue. SEE ALSO tracheophony. [broncho- + G. *phōnē,* voice]

bron·cho·plas·ty (brong′kō-plas-tē) Surgical repair of the configuration of a bronchus. [broncho- + G. *plastos,* formed]

bron·cho·pleu·ral fis·tu·la (BPF) (brong′kō-plūr′ăl fis′chū-lă) Communication between a bronchus and the pleural cavity; usually caused by necrotizing pneumonia or empyema; also may follow pulmonary surgery or irradiation. SYN BP fistula.

bron·cho·pneu·mo·ni·a (brong′ko-nū-mō′nē-ă) Acute inflammation of the walls of the smaller bronchial tubes, with varying amounts of pulmonary consolidation due to the spread of the inflammation into peribronchiolar alveoli and the alveolar ducts; may become confluent or may be hemorrhagic. SYN bronchial pneumonia.

bron·cho·pul·mo·nar·y (brong′kō-pul′mŏ-nār-ē) Relating to the bronchi and the lungs.

bron·cho·pul·mo·nar·y dys·pla·si·a (brong′kō-pul′mŏ-nār-ē dis-plā′zē-ă) Chronic pulmonary insufficiency arising from long-term artificial pulmonary ventilation; seen more frequently in premature than in mature infants.

bron·cho·pul·mo·nar·y lymph nodes (brong′kō-pul′mŏ-nār-ē limf nōdz) Lymph nodes in the hilum of the lung that receive lymph from the pulmonary nodes and drain to the tracheobronchial nodes. SYN bronchial glands (1).

bron·cho·pul·mo·nar·y seg·ment (brong′kō-pul′mŏ-nār-ē seg′mĕnt) The largest subdivision of a lobe of the lung; it is supplied by a direct tertiary (lobular) bronchus and a tertiary branch of the pulmonary artery; it is separated from adjacent segments by connective tissue septa.

bron·cho·pul·mo·nar·y se·ques·tra·tion (brong′kō-pul′mŏ-nār-ē sē′kwes-trā′shŭn) A congenital anomaly in which a mass of lung tissue becomes isolated during development from the rest of the lung; the bronchi in the mass are usually dilated or cystic and are not connected with the bronchial tree; it is supplied by a branch of the aorta.

bron·chor·rha·phy (brong-kōr′ă-fē) Suture of a wound of the bronchus. [broncho- + G. *rhaphē,* a seam]

bron·chor·rhe·a (brong′kŏ-rē′ă) Excessive secretion of mucus from the bronchial mucous membrane. SYN bronchorrhoea. [broncho- + G. *rhoia,* a flow]

bronchorrhoea [Br.] SYN bronchorrhea.

bron·cho·scope (brong′kō-skōp) An endoscope for inspecting the interior of the tracheobronchial tree. [broncho- + G. *skopeō,* to view]

bron·chos·co·py (brong-kos′kŏ-pē) Inspection of the interior of the tracheobronchial tree through a bronchoscope. See page B16.

bron·cho·spasm (brong′kō-spazm) Contraction of smooth muscle in the walls of the bronchi and bronchioles, causing narrowing of the lumen and obstructing breathing.

bron·cho·spi·rog·ra·phy (brong′kō-spī-rog′ră-fē) Use of a single-lumen endobronchial tube for measurement of ventilatory function of one lung. [broncho- + L. *spiro,* to breathe, + G. *graphō,* to write]

bron·cho·spi·rom·e·ter (brong′kō-spī-rom′ĕ-tĕr) A device for measurement of rates and volumes of airflow into each lung separately, using a double-lumen endobronchial tube. [broncho- + L. *spiro,* to breathe, + G. *metron,* measure]

bron·cho·spi·rom·e·try (brong′kō-spī-rom′ĕ-trē) Use of a bronchospirometer to measure ventilatory function of each lung separately.

bron·cho·stax·is (brong′kō-stak′sis) Hemorrhage from the bronchi. [broncho- + G. *staxis,* a dripping]

bron·cho·ste·no·sis (brong′kō-stĕ-nō′sis) Chronic narrowing of a bronchus.

bron·chos·to·my (brong-kos′tŏ-mē) Surgical formation of a new opening into a bronchus. [broncho- + G. *stoma,* mouth]

bron·chot·o·my (brong-kot′ŏ-mē) Incision of a bronchus.

bron·cho·tra·che·al (brong′kō-trā′kē-ăl) Relating to the trachea and bronchi.

bron·cho·ve·sic·u·lar (brong′kō-vĕ-sik′yū-lăr) Relating to the bronchioles and alveoli in the lungs. SYN bronchoalveolar.

bron·chus, pl. **bron·chi** (brong′kŭs, brong′kī) One of the two subdivisions of the trachea serving to convey air to and from the lungs. The trachea divides into right and left main bronchi, which in turn form lobar, segmental, and subsegmental bronchi. The intrapulmonary bronchi have a lining of pseudostratified ciliated columnar epithelium and a lamina propria with abundant longitudinal networks of elastic fibers; there are spirally arranged bundles of smooth muscle, abundant mucoserous glands, and, in the outer part of the wall, irregular plates of hyaline cartilage. See this page, B16. [Mod. L., fr. G. *bronchos,* windpipe]

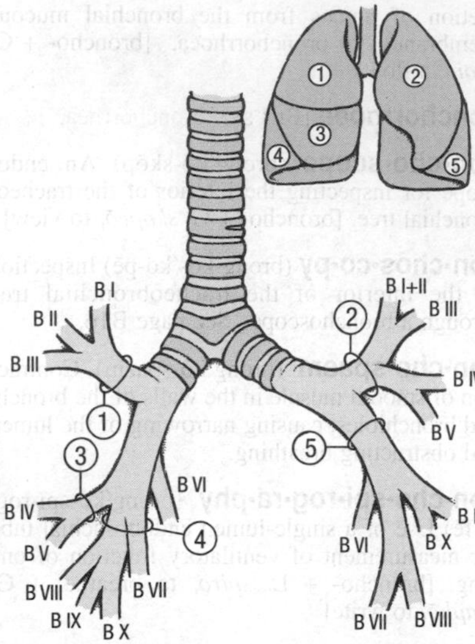

segmental bronchi: right lung: (B I) apical, (B II) posterior, (B III) anterior, (B IV) lateral, (B V) medial, (B VI) apical, (B VII) medial basal, (B VIII) anterior basal, (B IX) lateral basal, (B X) posterior basal; left lung: (B I+II) apicoposterior, (B III) anterior, (B IV) superior lingular, (B V) inferior lingular, (B VI) apical, (B VII) medial basal, (B VIII) anterior basal, (B IX) lateral basal, (B X) posterior basal; lobes of lungs supplied: (1) right superior, (2) left superior, (3) right middle, (4) right inferior, (5) left inferior

bron·chus-as·so·ci·at·ed lym·phoid tis·sue (BALT) (brong′kŭs-ă-sō′sē-ā-tĕd lim′foyd tish′ū) Patches of lymphoid tissues composed mainly of B and T lymphocytes and extending throughout the bronchial airways of the lung.

Brøn·sted ac·id (brŭn′shtet as′id) An acid that is a proton donor.

Brøn·sted base (brŭn′shtet bās) Any molecule or ion that combines with a proton; e.g., OH^-, CN^-, NH_3; this definition replaces the older and more limited concepts of base (3).

Brøn·sted the·o·ry (brŭn′shtet thē′ŏr-ē) That an acid is a substance, charged or uncharged, liberating hydrogen ions in solution, and that a base is a substance that removes them from solution; useful in the concept of weak electrolytes and buffers. Cf. Brønsted acid, Brønsted base.

bron·to·pho·bi·a (bron′tō-fō′bē-ă) Fear of thunder. [G. *brontē,* thunder, + phobia]

bronze di·a·be·tes, bronzed dis·ease (bronz dī-ă-bē′tēz, bronzd di-zēz′) Diabetes mellitus associated with hemochromatosis, with iron deposits in the skin, liver, pancreas, and other viscera, often with severe liver damage and glycosuria. SEE ALSO hemochromatosis.

Brooke tu·mor (bruk tū′mŏr) SYN trichoepithelioma.

broom (brūm) Herbal made from *Cytisus scoparius;* purported value as cathartic, diuretic, and emetic. Known to cause abortion. Poisoning possible with overdose. Not approved for any therapeutic purpose. SYN broomtop, hogweed, Irish tops, Scotch broom.

broom·top (brūm′top) SYN broom.

brow (brow) **1.** The eyebrow. SEE eyebrow. **2.** SYN forehead. [A.S. *brū*]

brow·lift (brow′lift) Operation to elevate the eyebrows.

brown ad·i·pose (brown ad′i-pōs) SYN brown fat.

brown ad·i·pose tis·sue (brown ad′i-pōs tish′ū) SYN brown fat.

brown fat (brown fat) Adipose tissue located near major vessels that occurs primarily in the full-term newborn, aiding in temperature regulation until shivering is established; it turns white as the infant ages. SYN brown adipose tissue, brown adipose, hibernating gland, interscapular gland, interscapular hibernoma, multilocular adipose tissue, multilocular fat.

brown·i·an move·ment (brown′ē-ăn mūv′mĕnt) Erratic, nondirectional, zigzag movement observed by microscope in suspensions of particles in fluid, resulting from the jostling or bumping of the larger particles by the molecules in the suspending medium. SYN molecular movement, pedesis.

brown in·du·ra·tion of the lung (brown in-dūr-ā′shŭn lŭng) Fibrosis and hemosiderin pigmentation of the lungs due to long-standing pulmonary congestion.

brown rec·luse spi·der (brown rek′lūs spī′dĕr) SYN recluse spider.

Brown-Sé·quard syn·drome (brown sā-kahr′ sin′drōm) Syndrome with unilateral spinal cord lesions; proprioception loss and weakness occur ipsilateral to the lesion, whereas pain and temperature loss occur contralaterally.

brow pre·sen·ta·tion (brow prez′ĕn-tā′shŭn) SEE cephalic presentation.

Bru·cel·la (brū-sel′lă) A genus of encapsulated, nonmotile bacteria containing short, rod-shaped to coccoid, gram-negative cells. These organisms are parasitic, invading all animal tissues and causing infection of the genital organs, the mammary gland, and the respiratory and intestinal tracts, and are pathogenic for humans and various species of domestic animals.

Bru·cel·la a·bor·tus (brū-sel′lă ā-bōr′tŭs) A bacterial species that causes undulant fever. SYN Bang bacillus.

Bru·cel·la·ce·ae (brū-sel-ā′sē-ē) A family of bacteria containing small, coccoid to rod-shaped, gram-negative cells that occur singly, in pairs, in short chains, or in groups. The cells may not show bipolar staining. Motile and nonmotile species occur. These organisms are parasites and pathogens that affect warm-blooded animals, including humans. The type genus is *Brucella*.

Bru·cel·la me·li·ten·sis (brū-sel′ă mel-i-ten′sis) A bacterial species that causes brucellosis in humans. It is the type species of the genus *Brucella*.

Bru·cel·la su·is (brū-sel′lă sū′is) A bacterial species causing brucellosis in humans; may also infect horses, dogs, cows, monkeys, goats, and laboratory animals.

bru·cel·lo·sis (brū-sel-ō′sis) An infectious disease caused by *Brucella*, characterized by fever, sweating, weakness, and aching, and transmitted to humans by direct contact with diseased animals or through ingestion of infected meat or milk. SYN undulant fever.

Bruce pro·to·col (brūs prō′tŏ-kawl) A standardized procedure for electrocardiogram-monitored exercise using increasing speeds and elevations of the treadmill; a test for ischemia usually due to coronary artery disease. SEE ALSO stress test.

Bruch mem·brane (bruk mem′brān) SYN lamina basalis choroideae.

Bruck dis·ease (bruk di-zēz′) A disorder marked by osteogenesis imperfecta, ankylosis of the joints, and muscular atrophy.

Brud·zin·ski sign (brū-jin′skē sīn) **1.** In meningitis, on passive flexion of the leg on one side, a similar movement occurs in the opposite leg. **2.** In meningitis, involuntary flexion of the knees and hips following flexion of the neck while supine. See this page.

Brug fil·a·ri·a·sis (brūg fil-ă-rī′ă-sis) Infection with the filarial organism *Brugia malayi*, which causes adenitis, fever, lymphangitis, and sometimes elephantiasis; occurs primarily in Southeast Asia, India, Indonesia, China, Japan, Korea, and the Philippines.

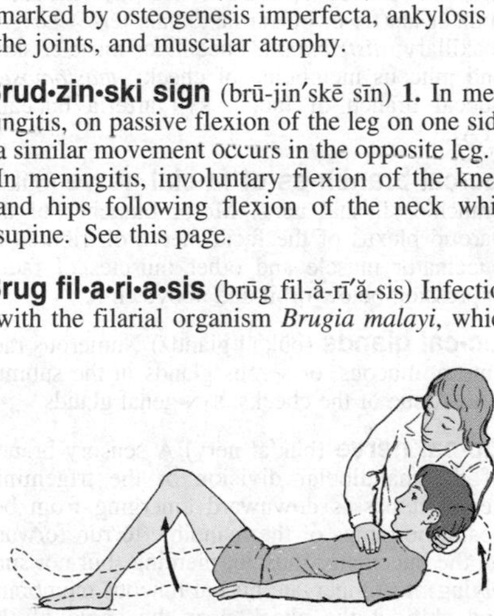

Brudzinski sign: nurse eliciting a positive Brudzinski sign by placing the patient supine and flexing the neck; resulting flexion of hips and knees indicates meningeal irritation

bruise (brūz) **1.** An injury producing a hematoma or diffuse extravasation of blood without rupture of the skin. **2.** SYN contuse. [M.E. *bruisen*, fr. O.Fr., fr. Germanic]

bru·it (brū-ē′) An abnormal swishing, blowing, or murmuring sound. [Fr.]

bru·it de tam·bour (brū-ē′ dĕ tam-būr′) Reverberating, musical tone heard as the second heart sound over the aortic area, associated with syphilitic aortic valvular disease. [Fr. sound of drum]

Brun·ner glands (brūn′er glandz) SYN duodenal glands.

brun·nes·cent cat·a·ract (brŭn′ĕ-sĕnt kat′ă-rakt) A cataract in which the lens is hardened and of a dark brown color. SYN black cataract.

Brunn mem·brane (brūn mem′brān) The epithelium of the olfactory region of the nose.

Brunn·strom meth·od (brŭn′strŏm meth′ŏd) Occupational or physical therapy treatment approach based on synergy patterns of limb and trunk movement. Six categories or levels of recovery of a neurologically impaired patient. SEE ALSO proprioceptive neuromuscular facilitation.

Brunn·strom move·ment ther·a·py (brŭn′strŏm mūv′mĕnt thār′a-pē) A treatment approach in which the physical therapist or occupational therapist uses movement based on synergy patterns of the limb and trunk; consists of six categories or levels of recovery in the neurologically impaired patient.

Bruns a·tax·i·a (brunz ă-taks′ē-ă) An ataxia manifested as a difficulty in initiation of forward movement of the feet when they are in contact with the ground, although leg strength, coordination, and forward movement is normal when the person is supine; due to frontal lobe disease. SYN glue-footed gait, magnetic gait (1), magnetic gait (2).

Bruns nys·tag·mus (brūnz nis-tag′mŭs) A fine, jerking (vestibular) nystagmus on horizontal gaze in one direction, together with a slower, larger amplitude (gaze, paretic) nystagmus on looking in the opposite direction; due to lateral brainstem compression, usually by a cerebellar-pontine angle mass such as an acoustic neuroma.

brush (brŭsh) An instrument consisting of flexible bristles attached to a handle or to the tip of a catheter. [A.S. *byrst,* bristle]

brush bi·op·sy (brŭsh bī′op-sē) Obtained by abrading the surface of a lesion with a brush to obtain cells and tissue for microscopic examination.

brush bor·der (brŭsh bōr′dĕr) An epithelial surface bearing closely packed microvilli about 2 mcm long, such as occurs in the proximal tubule of the nephron.

brush cath•e•ter (brŭsh kath′ĕ-tĕr) A ureteral catheter with a finely bristled brush tip that is endoscopically passed into the ureter or renal pelvis and by gentle to-and-fro movement brushes cells from the surface of suspected tumors.

Brush•field spots (brush′fēld spotz) Light-colored condensations of the surface of the mid-iris; seen in Down syndrome.

Bru•ton a•gam•ma•glob•u•li•ne•mi•a (brū′tŏn ā-gam-mă-glob′yū-lin-ē′mē-ă) An X-linked condition, with hypo- or agammaglobulinemia; the immune deficiency becomes apparent as maternally transmitted immunoglobulin levels decline in early infancy.

brux•ism (brŭk′sizm) A clenching of the teeth, associated with forceful lateral or protrusive jaw movements, resulting in rubbing, gritting, or grinding together of the teeth, usually during sleep; sometimes a pathologic condition. SEE ALSO parafunction. [G. *bruchō*, to grind the teeth]

Bry•ant line (brī′ănt līn) Vertical border of the iliofemoral triangle.

Bry•ant sign (brī′ănt sīn) Lowering of axillary skin folds; seen in association with dislocation of shoulder.

Bry•ant trac•tion (brī′ănt trak′shŭn) Traction on the lower limb placed vertically, employed especially in fractures of the femur in children.

Bry•ant tri•an•gle (brī′ănt trī′ang-gĕl) In fracture of the neck of the femur, to determine upward displacement of the trochanter, lines are drawn on the body to form a triangle: line *a* is drawn around the body at the level of the anterior superior iliac spines; line *b*, perpendicular to line *a*, is drawn to the greater trochanter of the femur; line *c* is drawn from the trochanter to the iliac spine; upward displacement is measured along line *b*. SYN iliofemoral triangle.

BSA Abbreviation for bovine serum albumin; body surface area.

BSE Abbreviation for breast self-examination.

BSER Abbreviation for brainstem evoked response.

BSN Abbreviation for Bachelor of Science degree in Nursing.

BTPS Abbreviation that indicates a gas volume has been expressed as if it were saturated with water vapor at body temperature (37°C) and at the ambient barometric pressure; used for measurements of lung volumes.

BTU Abbreviation for British thermal unit.

bu•ba mad•re (bū′bă mah′drē) SYN mother yaw.

bu•bas (bū′băhs) SYN yaws.

bub•ble gum der•ma•ti•tis (bŭb′ĕl gŭm dĕr′mă-tī′tis) Allergic contact dermatitis developing about the lips in children who chew bubble gum; caused by plastics in the gum.

bub•ble-through hu•mid•i•fi•er (bŭb′ĕl-thrū hyū-mid′i-fī-ĕr) A device that humidifies therapeutic gas (e.g., oxygen) by bubbling the gas through water.

bu•bo (bū′bō) Inflammatory swelling of one or more lymph nodes, usually (but not necessarily) in the groin. [G. *boubōn*, the groin, a swelling in the groin]

bu•bon•al•gi•a (bū′bŏn-al′jē-ă) Rarely used term for pain in the groin. [G. *boubōn*, groin, + *algos*, pain]

bu•bon•ic (bū-bon′ik) Relating in any way to a bubo.

bu•bon•ic plague (bū-bon′ik plāg) The most common form of plague (infection by *Yersinia pestis*), characterized by fever, cutaneous and visceral hemorrhages, and buboes (inflammatory enlargements of lymph nodes draining the bites of infected fleas). Clinical manifestations are caused by the flea-transmitted *Yersinia pestis*.

buc•ca, gen. and pl. **buc•cae** (bŭk′ă, bŭk′ē) SYN cheek. [L.]

buc•cal (bŭk′ăl) Pertaining to, adjacent to, or in the direction of the cheek.

buc•cal ar•ter•y, **buc•ci•na•tor ar•ter•y** (bŭk′ăl ahr′tĕr-ē, bŭk′si-nā′tŏr ahr′tĕr-ē) *Origin*, maxillary; *distribution*, buccinator muscle, skin, and mucous membrane of cheek; *anastomoses*, buccal branch of facial. SYN arteria buccalis [TA].

buc•cal branch•es of fa•cial nerve (bŭk′ăl branch′ĕz fā′shăl nĕrv) Motor branches of the parotid plexus of the facial nerve distributed to buccinator muscle and other muscles of facial expression below orbit and above chin.

buc•cal glands (bŭk′ăl glandz) Numerous racemose, mucous, or serous glands in the submucous tissue of the cheeks. SYN genal glands.

buc•cal nerve (bŭk′ăl nĕrv) A sensory branch of the mandibular division of the trigeminal nerve; it passes downward emerging from beneath the ramus of the mandible to run forward on the buccinator muscle, piercing (but not supplying) it to innervate buccal mucous membrane and skin of the cheek near the angle of the mouth. SYN nervus buccalis [TA].

buc•cal speech (buk′ăl spēch) A way to produce a sound source for speech by trapping air between the cheek and teeth and squeezing it out while articulating; sometimes used when the larynx is absent or nonfunctional for speech.

buc·ci·na·tor mus·cle (bŭk′si-nā′tŏr mŭs′ĕl) *Origin*, posterior portion of alveolar portion of maxilla and mandible and pterygomandibular raphe; *insertion*, orbicularis oris at angle of mouth; *action*, flattens cheek, retracts angle of mouth; *nerve supply*, facial. Plays an important role in mastication, working with tongue to keep food between teeth; when it is paralyzed, food accumulates in the oral vestibule. SYN musculus buccinator [TA].

♻**bucco-** Combining form denoting cheek. [L. *bucca*]

buc·co·gin·gi·val (bŭk′ō-jin′ji-văl) Relating to the cheek and the gum.

buc·co·la·bi·al (bŭk′ō-lā′bē-ăl) **1.** Relating to both cheek and lip. **2.** DENTISTRY referring to that aspect of the dental arch or those surfaces of the teeth in contact with the mucosa of lip and cheek.

buc·co·lin·gual (bŭk′ō-ling′gwăl) **1.** Pertaining to the cheek and the tongue. **2.** DENTISTRY referring to that aspect of the dental arch or those surfaces of the teeth in contact with the mucosa of the lip or cheek and the tongue.

buc·co·pha·ryn·ge·al (bŭk′ō-făr-in′jē-ăl) Relating to both cheek or mouth and pharynx.

buc·co·ver·sion (bŭk′ō-vĕr-zhŭn) Malposition of a posterior tooth from the normal line of occlusion toward the cheek.

buc·cu·la (buk′yū-lă) Excess skin and fat under the chin. SYN double chin. [L. *bucca,* cheek, + *ula,* dim suffix]

bu·chu (bū′kū) Herbal derived from oil in leaves of *Barosma betulina;* unconfirmed claims of value as antirheumatic and diuretic and in treating infection in urogenital tract; may cause spontaneous abortion. [Zulu *bucu*]

Buch·wald at·ro·phy (būk′vold at′rŏ-fē) A progressive form of cutaneous atrophy.

buck·et-han·dle tear (bŭk′ĕt han′dĕl tār) **1.** A tear in the central part of a semilunar cartilage. **2.** A tear in one of the menisci of a knee joint, near the rim and following its curvature, which can allow a flap of cartilage to impede movement of the joint.

Buck ex·ten·sion (buk eks-ten′shŭn) Apparatus for applying longitudinal skin traction on the leg through contact between the skin and adhesive tape.

buck·led in·nom·i·nate ar·ter·y (bŭk′ĕld i-nom′i-năt ahr′tĕr-ē) Elongation of the innominate artery manifest as a pulsating mass in the right supraclavicular space and as a radiographic appearance mimicking an aneurysm or tumor of the apex of the right lung or superior mediastinum.

buck·le frac·ture (bŭk′ĕl frak′shŭr) SYN torus fracture.

buck·thorn (bŭk′thōrn) Shrub or tree of family Rhamnaceae, *Karwinskia humboldtiana*, commonly called coyotillo or tullidora. Found in arid southwestern U.S. environments; contains a highly potent neurotoxin. SEE ALSO polyneuropathy. SYN common buckthorn, waythorn.

buck tooth (bŭk tūth) Colloquialism for an anterior tooth in labioversion.

Buck·y di·a·phragm (bŭk′ē dī′ă-fram) In radiography, a diaphragm with a moving grid that avoids grid shadows. SYN Potter-Bucky diaphragm.

bud (bŭd) **1.** An outgrowth that resembles the bud of a plant, usually pluripotential, and capable of differentiating and growing into a definitive structure. **2.** To give rise to such an outgrowth. SEE ALSO gemmation. **3.** A small outgrowth from a parent cell; a form of asexual reproduction.

Budd-Chi·a·ri syn·drome (bŭd kē-ahr′ē sin′drōm) Hepatic vein obstruction; usually caused by thrombosis in inferior vena cava secondary to hypercoagulable states, vena caval webs, tumors, trauma, and bone marrow transplantation procedures. Can be idiopathic; most often associated with hepatomegaly and ascites. SYN Rokitansky syndrome.

bud·ding (bŭd′ing) SYN gemmation.

Budd syn·drome (bud sin′drōm) SYN Chiari syndrome.

Buer·ger dis·ease (bĕr′gĕr di-zēz′) Pain in extremities similar to those caused by intermittent claudication in association with medial arterial sclerosis. Also affects small veins and the lymphatic system. Almost wholly male preponderance; related to tobacco use, cold, malnutrition, and vascular collagen disorders. SYN Billroth-von Winiwarter disease, endoarteritis obliterans, Winiwarter-Manteuffel-Buerger disease.

Buer·ger sign (bĕr′gĕr sīn) Pallor in extremities on elevation and rubor on dependency; indicates advanced ischemia. Condition caused by significantly restricted arterial inflow and chronic dilatation of peripheral vascular beds, especially those of the postcapillary venules.

buf·fa·lo hump (bŭf′ă-lō hŭmp) SYN buffalo neck.

buf·fa·lo neck (bŭf′ă-lō nek) Combination of moderate kyphosis with a thick heavy fat pad on the neck, seen especially in people with Cushing disease or syndrome. SYN buffalo hump.

buff·er (bŭf′ĕr) **1.** A mixture of an acid and its conjugate base (salt), such as H_2CO_3/HCO_3^-; $H_2PO_4^-/ HPO_4^{2-}$, which, when present in a solution, resists changes in pH that would otherwise occur in the solution when acid or alkali is added to it. SEE ALSO conjugate acid-base pair. **2.** To add a buffer to a solution and thus give it the property of resisting a change in pH.

buff•er val•ue (bŭf′ĕr val′yū) The power of a substance in solution to absorb acid or alkali without change in pH; this is highest at a pH value equal to the pK_a value of the acid of the buffer pair.

buf•fy coat (bŭf′ē kōt) The light-colored layer of blood that is seen when anticoagulated blood is centrifuged or allowed to stand. It appears as a layer between the plasma and eythrocytes and is composed of leukocytes and platelets.

buf•fy coat con•cen•tra•tion (bŭf′ē kōt kon-sĕn-trā′shŭn) Centrifugation of whole blood containing anticoagulant to obtain a buffy coat layer containing white blood cells; blood films for staining can be prepared from this layer of cells and examined for the presence of parasites (trypanosomes and intracellular leishmaniae).

bug (bŭg) **1.** Any insect of the order Hemiptera. **2.** More colloquially, any insect or arachnid. **3.** (slang) An acute febrile illness such as influenza or the common cold. [of unknown origin]

bu•gle•weed (byū′gĕl-wēd) Herbal derived from *Lycopus virginicus*, used in various forms; mild astringent and narcotic, used in treatment of Graves disease; some clinical studies have been completed. SYN carpenter's herb, gypsy weed, menta de lobo, sicklewort.

bulb (bŭlb) **1.** Any rounded, globular, or fusiform structure. SYN bulbus [TA]. **2.** A short, vertical, underground stem of plants, such as onions and garlic. [L. *bulbus*, a bulbous root]

bul•bar (bŭl′bahr) **1.** Relating to a bulb. **2.** Relating to the rhombencephalon (hindbrain). **3.** Bulb-shaped; resembling a bulb.

bul•bar my•e•li•tis (bŭl′bahr mī-ĕ-lī′tis) Inflammation of the medulla oblongata.

bul•bar pal•sy (bŭl′bahr pawl′zē) Flaccid paralysis of the motor units of any or all cranial nerves. Bulbar palsies may also be identifed by the specific nerve affected, such as facial palsy or hypoglossal palsy. SEE ALSO cranial nerves.

bul•bar pa•ral•y•sis (bŭl′bahr păr-al′i-sis) SYN progressive bulbar paralysis.

bulb of cor•pus spon•gi•o•sum (bŭlb kōr′pŭs spŏn-jē-ō′sŭm) SYN bulb of penis.

bulb of eye (bŭlb ī) SYN eyeball.

bulb of hair (bŭlb hār) Hair bulb, the lower expanded extremity of the hair follicle that fits like a cap over the papilla pili.

bul•bi (bŭl′bī) Plural of bulbus.

bul•bi•tis (bŭl-bī′tis) Inflammation of the bulbous portion of the urethra.

♻**bulbo-** Combining form denoting a bulb; bulbus [L. *bulbus*]

bul•bo•cav•er•no•sus mus•cle (bŭl-bō-kav-ĕr-nō′sŭs mŭs′ĕl) SYN bulbospongiosus muscle.

bul•boid (bŭl′boyd) Bulb-shaped. [bulbo- + G. *eidos*, resemblance]

bul•bo•spi•nal (bŭl′bō-spī′năl) Relating to the medulla oblongata and spinal cord, particularly to nerve fibers interconnecting the two. SYN spinobulbar.

bul•bo•spon•gi•o•sus mus•cle (bŭl′bō-spon-jē-ō′sŭs mŭs′ĕl) Perineal muscle; in male: *origin*, perineal membrane fascia on the dorsum of bulb of penis; *insertion*, central tendon of perineum and median raphe on free surface of the bulb; *action*, voluntarily constricts bulbous urethra when attempting to expel last drops after urination, or spasmodically with, and following, ejaculation to expel semen. In female: *origin*, dorsum of the clitoris, the corpus cavernosum, and the perineal membrane; *insertion*, central tendon of the perineum; *action*, acts as a weak sphincter of the vagina; *nerve supply*, pudendal (deep perineal branch). SYN bulbocavernosus muscle, musculus bulbocavernosus, musculus bulbospongiosus, musculus ejaculator seminis, musculus sphincter vaginae, sphincter vaginae.

bul•bo•u•re•thral (bŭl′bō-yūr-ē′thrăl) Relating to the bulbus penis and the urethra. SYN urethrobulbar.

bul•bo•u•re•thral gland (bŭl′bō-yūr-ē′thrăl gland) One of two small compound racemose glands, which produce a mucoid secretion, lying side by side along the membranous urethra just above the bulb of the corpus spongiosum; they discharge through a small duct into the spongy portion of the urethra. SYN Cowper gland.

bul•bous bou•gie (bŭl′bŭs bū-zhē′) A bougie with a bulb-shaped tip, sometimes shaped like an acorn or an olive.

bulb of pe•nis (bŭlb pē′nis) The expanded posterior part of the corpus spongiosum of the penis lying in the interval between the crura of the penis. SYN bulbus penis [TA], bulb of corpus spongiosum, bulb of urethra.

bulb ther•mom•e•ter (bŭlb thĕr-mom′ĕ-tĕr) Standard thermometer used to record ambient air temperature.

bulb of u•re•thra (bŭlb yūr-ē′thră) SYN bulb of penis.

bul•bus, gen. and pl. **bul•bi** (bŭl′bŭs, -bī) [TA] SYN bulb (1). [L. a plant bulb]

bul•bus a•or•tae (bŭl′bŭs ā-ōr′tē) [TA] SYN aortic bulb.

bul•bus oc•u•li (bŭl′bŭs ok′ū-lī) [TA] SYN eyeball.

bul•bus ol•fac•to•ri•us (bŭl′bŭs ōl-fak-tō′rē-ŭs) [TA] SYN olfactory bulb.

bul•bus pe•nis (bŭl′bŭs pē′nis) [TA] SYN bulb of penis.

bulb of ves•ti•bule (bŭlb ves′ti-byūl) A mass of erectile tissue on either side of the vagina united anterior to the urethra by the commissura bulborum.

bu•lim•i•a (bŭ-lē′mē-ă) SYN bulimia nervosa. [G. *bous,* ox, + *limos,* hunger]

bu•lim•i•a ner•vo•sa (bŭ-lē′mē-ă nĕr-vō′să) A chronic morbid disorder involving repeated and secretive episodic bouts of eating characterized by uncontrolled rapid ingestion of large quantities of food over a short period of time (binge eating), followed by self-induced vomiting, use of laxatives or diuretics, fasting, or vigorous exercise to prevent weight gain; often accompanied by feelings of guilt, depression, or self-disgust. SYN bulimia.

bu•lim•ic (bŭ-lē′mik) Relating to, or suffering from, bulimia nervosa.

bul•la, gen. and pl. **bul•lae** (bul′ă, -ē) **1.** A large blister appearing as a circumscribed area of separation of the epidermis from subepidermal structures or as a circumscribed area of separation of epidermal cells caused by the presence of serum, or an injected substance. **2.** A bubblelike structure. See page B10. [L. bubble]

bull•dog for•ceps (bul′dawg fōr′seps) A forceps for occluding a blood vessel.

bul•lec•to•my (bul-ek′tŏ-mē) Resection of a bulla; helpful in treating some forms of bullous emphysema, in which giant bullae compress functioning lung tissue.

bul•let for•ceps (bul′ĕt fōr′seps) A forceps with thin curved blades with serrated grasping surfaces, for extracting a bullet from tissues.

bull neck (bul nek) A heavy thick neck caused by hypertrophied muscles or enlarged cervical lymph nodes.

bul•lous (bul′ŭs) Relating to, of the nature of, or marked by, bullae.

bul•lous con•gen•i•tal ich•thy•o•si•form e•ryth•ro•der•ma (bul′ŭs kŏn-jen′i-tăl ik′thē-ō′si-fōrm ĕ-rith′rō-dĕr′mă) Diffusely red, eroded skin at birth, with subsequent scaling, tending to improve in later life, characterized by generalized epidermolytic hyperkeratosis.

bul•lous em•phy•se•ma (bul′ŭs em′fi-sē′mă) Emphysema in which the enlarged airspaces are up to several cm in diameter, often visible on chest radiographs. Thin-walled air sacs under tension compress pulmonary tissue, either single or multiple.

bul•lous im•pe•ti•go of new•born (bul′ŭs im-pĕ-tī′gō nū′bōrn) Disseminated bullous lesions appearing soon after birth, caused by infection with *Staphylococcus aureus*. See page B4. SYN impetigo neonatorum (2), pemphigus gangrenosus (2).

bul•lous ker•a•top•a•thy (bul′ŭs ker′ă-top′ă-thē) Edema of the corneal stroma and epithelium resulting in formation of bullae on the corneal surface. It occurs in Fuchs epithelial dystrophy, advanced glaucoma and iridocyclitis, endothelial failure, and sometimes after intraocular lens implantation.

bul•lous pem•phi•goid (bul′ŭs pem′fi-goyd) A chronic, generally benign disease, most commonly of old age, characterized by tense nonacantholytic bullae in which serum antibodies are localized to the epidermal basement membrane, causing detachment of the entire thickness of the epidermis. See this page.

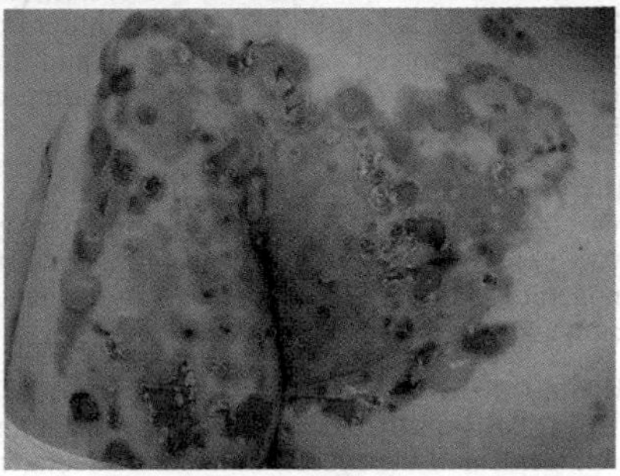

bullous pemphigoid: chest and arm

bull's eye rash (bulz ī rash) A cutaneous eruption consisting of two or more concentric erythematous rings.

Bum•ke pu•pil (bum′ke pyū′pil) Dilation of the pupil in response to anxiety or other psychic stimuli.

BUN (bŭn) Acronym or abbreviation for blood urea nitrogen; use of term is diminishing in Canada.

bun•dle (bŭn′dĕl) [TA] A structure composed of a group of fibers, muscular or nervous. SYN fasciculus (3) [TA].

bun•dle-branch block (bŭn′dĕl-branch blok) Intraventricular block due to interruption of conduction in one of the two main branches of the bundle of His and manifested in the electrocardiogram by marked prolongation of the QRS complex. Block to each branch has distinctive QRS morphology.

bund•led code (bŭn′dĕld kōd) When health care services that are usually discrete are considered as a single entity for purposes of classification and payment.

bun•ion (bŭn′yŏn) A localized swelling at either the medial or dorsal aspect of the first metatarsophalangeal joint, caused by bursal inflammation and fibrosis; a medial bunion is usually associated with hallux valgus. See page B24. [O.F. *buigne,* bump on the head]

bun•ion•ec•to•my (bŭn-yŏn-ek′tŏ-mē) Excision of a bunion.

Bun•nell su•ture (bŭ-nel′ sū′chŭr) A method of tenorrhaphy using a pull-out wire affixed to buttons.

bun•o•dont (bū′nō-dont) A tooth having low, rounded cusps. [G. *bounos,* mound, + *odous* (*odont-*), tooth]

Bun•sen burn•er (bŭn′sĕn bŭr′nĕr) A gas lamp supplied with openings admitting sufficient air that carbon is completely burned, giving a hot but only slightly luminous flame.

Bun•sen sol•u•bil•i•ty co•ef•fi•cient (al•pha) (bŭn′sĕn sol′yū-bil′i-tē) The milliliters of gas STPD dissolved per milliliter of liquid and per atmosphere (760 mmHg) partial pressure of the gas at any given temperature.

bun•ya•vi•rus en•ceph•a•li•tis (bŭn′yă-vī-rŭs en-sef′ă-lī′tis) Encephalitis of abrupt onset, with severe frontal headache and low-grade to moderate fever, caused by members of the genus Bunyavirus.

buph•thal•mi•a, **buph•thal•mus, buph•thal•mos** (būf-thal′mē-ă, -thal′mŭs, -thal′mŏs) Enlargement of the eyeball as a result of congenital glaucoma. [G. *bous,* ox, + *ophthalmos,* eye]

bur (bŭr) A rotary cutting instrument, used in dentistry, consisting of a small metal shaft and a head designed in various shapes; used at various rotational velocities to excavate decay, shape cavity forms, and reduce tooth structure. Cf. burr.

bur•dock (bŭr′dok) Herbal agent made from *Arctium lappa* or *A. minus;* produced in several forms (e.g., cream, tonic, liquid); used against a huge range of disorders (e.g., arthritis, pain syndromes, rash); has been involved in poisoning; safety and efficacy not established. SYN beggar's buttons, cocklebur (2), wild gobo.

Bur•ger tri•an•gle (bĕr′gĕr trī′ang-gĕl) A scalene triangle representing the frontal plane electrocardiographic leads comparable with, but more accurate than, the Einthoven triangle. SEE Einthoven triangle.

bur hole (bŭr hōl) Opening in bone created by a small surgical cutting tool.

bur•ied flap (ber′ēd flap) A flap denuded of both surface epithelium and superficial dermis and transferred into the subcutaneous tissues.

bur•ied su•ture (ber′ēd sū′chŭr) Any suture placed entirely below the surface of the skin.

Burk•hol•der•i•a (bŭrk-hol-der′ē-ă) A genus of motile, nonfermentative, non-spore-forming gram-negative rods, containing significant species of human pathogens; formerly classified as in the genus *Pseudomonas.*

Burk•hol•der•i•a cep•a•ci•a (bŭrk-hol-der′ē-ă sē-pā′shē-ă) A bacterial species found in rotted onions and in clinical specimens; commonly found in respiratory secretions in patients with cystic fibrosis, it is frequently resistant to many antibiotics. Formerly known as *Pseudomonas cepacia.*

Burk•hol•der•i•a mal•le•i (bŭrk-hol-der′ē-ă mal′ē-ī) A bacterial species infectious to horses and donkeys, causing glanders and farcy. SYN *Pseudomonas mallei.*

Burk•hol•der•i•a pseu•do•mal•le•i (bŭrk-hol-der′ē-ă sū-dō-mal′ē-ī) A bacterial species found in cases of melioidosis in humans and other animals and in soil and water in tropical regions.

Bur•kitt lym•pho•ma (bŭr′kit lim-fō′mă) A form of malignant lymphoma reported in African children, frequently involving the jaw and abdominal lymph nodes. Geographic distribution of Burkitt lymphoma suggests that it is found in areas with endemic malaria. It is primarily a B-cell neoplasm and is believed to be caused by Epstein-Barr virus, a member of the family Herpesviridae, which can be isolated from tumor cells in culture; occasional cases of lymphoma with similar features have been reported in the United States.

i **burn** (bŭrn) **1.** To cause a lesion by means of heat or a similar lesion by other means. **2.** A sensation of pain caused by excessive heat, or similar pain from another cause. **3.** A lesion caused by heat or any cauterizing agent, including friction, caustic agents, electricity, or electromagnetic energy. Types of burns resulting from different agents are relatively specific and diagnostic. The division of burns into three types (e.g., superficial, partial thickness, and full thickness) reflects the severity of skin damage (e.g., erythema, blisters, and charring, respectively). SEE ALSO rule of nines. See page 237. [A.S. *baernan*]

Bur•nett syn•drome (bŭr-net′ sin′drōm) SYN milk-alkali syndrome.

burn•ing mouth syn•drome (bŭrn′ing mowth sin′drōm) A clinical condition in which the patient complains of a burning sensation in the oral cavity, although the appearance of the oral mucosa is normal; the cause has not been determined. SYN burning tongue syndrome.

burn•ing tongue (bŭrn′ing tŭng) SYN glossodynia.

burn•ing tongue syn•drome (bŭrn′ing tŭng sin′drōm) SYN burning mouth syndrome.

bur•nish•er (bŭr′nish-ĕr) An instrument for smoothing and polishing the surface or edge of a dental restoration. [O. F. *burnir,* to polish]

bur•nish•ing (bŭr′nish-ing) Smoothing the surface of a dental amalgam after initial carving, or adapting margins of gold restorations by rubbing with a broad-surfaced metal instrument. This term also refers to the rubbing of a medication into the dentinal tubules. [O.Fr. *burnir*, to polish]

burn•out (bŭrn′owt) SYN overtraining syndrome.

Bu•row op•er•a•tion (būr′ov op-ĕr-ā′shŭn) SYN Burow triangle.

Bu•row so•lu•tion (būr′ov sŏ-lū′shŭn) A preparation of aluminium subacetate and glacial acetic acid, used for its antiseptic and astringent action on the skin.

Bu•row tri•an•gle (būr′ov trī′ang-gĕl) A triangle of skin and subcutaneous fat excised so that a flap can be advanced without buckling the adjacent tissue. SYN Burow operation.

burr (bŭr) A drilling tool for enlarging a trephine hole in the cranium. Cf. bur.

bur•sa, pl. **bur•sae** (bŭr′să, -sē) [TA] A closed sac or envelope lined with synovial membrane and containing synovial fluid, usually located or formed in areas subject to friction (e.g., over an exposed or prominent part or where a tendon passes over a bone). [Mediev. L. a purse]

bur•sae (bŭr′sē) Plural of bursa.

bur•sal (bŭr′săl) Relating to a bursa.

bur•sal syn•o•vi•tis (bŭr′săl sin′ō-vī′tis) SYN bursitis.

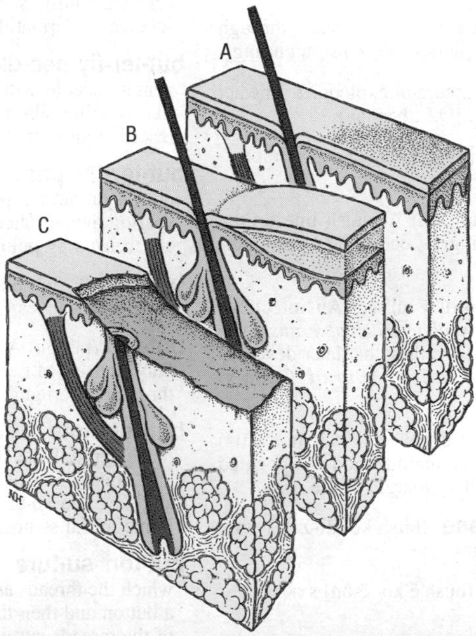

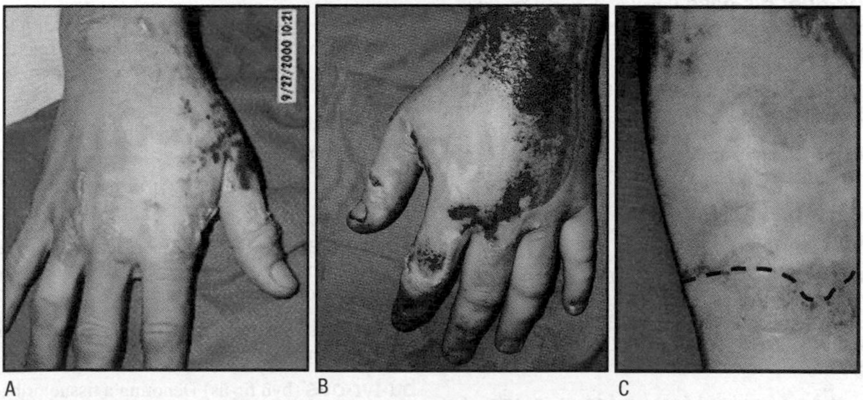

burns: (A) superficial; (B) partial thickness; (C) full thickness

bur•sa of pi•ri•for•mis (bŭr′să pir-i-fōrm′is) A small bursa located between the tendons of the piriformis and superior gemellus and the femur.

bur•sa of ten•do cal•ca•ne•us (bŭr′să ten′dō kal-kā′nē-ŭs) Bursa between the tendo calcaneus and the upper part of the posterior surface of the calcaneum. SYN retrocalcaneal bursa.

bur•sec•to•my (bŭr-sek′tŏ-mē) Surgical removal of a bursa. [bursa + G. *ektomē,* excision]

bur•si•tis (bŭr-sī′tis) Inflammation of a bursa. See page B24. SYN bursal synovitis.

bur•so•lith (bŭr′sō-lith) A calculus formed in a bursa. [bursa + G. *lithos,* stone]

bur•sop•a•thy (bŭr-sop′ă-thē) Any disease of a bursa.

bur•sot•o•my (bŭr-sot′ŏ-mē) Incision through the wall of a bursa. [bursa + G. *tomē,* a cutting]

burst (bŭrst) **1.** To rupture or explode. **2.** The act or result of bursting. [O.E. berstan]

burst frac•ture (bŭrst frak′shŭr) SYN compression fracture.

Bur•ton line (bŭr′tŏn līn) A bluish line on the free border of the gingiva, occurring in lead poisoning.

Bu•ru•li ul•cer (bū-rū′lē ŭl′sĕr) An infectious disease caused by *Mycobacterium ulcerans* characterized by painless swelling that later develops into an ulcerative lesion. [*Buruli* County, Uganda]

Bu•sac•ca nod•ules (bū-sahk′kah nod′yūlz) Inflammatory, granulomatous nodules located away from the pupillary margin of the iris.

Busch•ke dis•ease (būsh′ke di-zēz′) SYN scleredema adultorum.

bush•y cho•ri•on (bush′ē kōr′ē-on) SYN villous chorion.

Bus•quet dis•ease (būs-kā′ di-zēz′) An osteoperiostitis of the metatarsal bones, leading to exostoses on the dorsum of the foot.

Bus•se-Busch•ke dis•ease (bus′e-būsh′ke di-zēz′) SYN cryptococcosis.

bu•tane (byū′tān) A gaseous hydrocarbon present in natural gas.

bu•tan•o•yl (bū′tan-ō′il) The radical of butanoic acid. SYN butyryl.

butch•er's broom (bu′chĕrz brūm) Herbal remedy extracted from *Ruscus aculeatus;* of purported use in treating swelling, as a diuretic, and as a laxative. SYN box holly, pettigree, sweet broom.

bu•thi•o•nine sul•fox•i•mine (byū-thī′ō-nēn sŭl-fox′i-mēn) A compound that decreases intracellular glutathione by inhibition of its synthesis.

but•ter (bŭt′ĕr) **1.** A coherent mass of milk fat, obtained by churning or shaking cream until the separate fat globules run together, leaving a liquid residue, buttermilk. **2.** A soft solid having the consistency of butter. [L. *butyrum,* G. *boutyros,* prob. fr. *bous,* cow, + *tyros,* cheese]

but•ter•bur (bŭt′ĕr-bŭr) Herbal remedy made from *Petasites hybridus;* purported uses in therapy for GI tract, GU tract, and in skin disease. Hepatotoxicity noted; as with most herbals, levels of active agent in formulation vary by manufacturer and batch. SYN sweet coltsfoot, Western coltsfoot.

but•ter•fly (bŭt′ĕr-flī) **1.** Any structure or apparatus resembling in shape a butterfly with outstretched wings. **2.** A scaling erythematous lesion on each cheek, joined by a narrow band across the nose; seen in lupus erythematosus and seborrheic dermatitis.

but•ter•fly nee•dle (bŭt′ĕr-flī nē′dĕl) An intravenous needle with a hub equipped with winglike flexible tabs that serve as a handle during insertion and for skin attachment afterward.

but•ter•fly pat•tern (bŭt′ĕr-flī pat′ĕrn) Bilateral, symmetric, pulmonary alveolar opacities sparing the periphery, on chest radiographs; usually caused by pulmonary edema.

but•tocks (bŭt′ŏks) The two gluteal prominences. SYN nates [TA], breech, clunes.

but•ton (bŭt′ŏn) A structure, lesion, or device of knob shape. [M.E., fr. O.Fr. *bouton,* fr. *bouter,* to thrust, fr. Germanic]

but•ton•hole (bŭt′ŏn-hōl) **1.** A short straight cut made through the wall of a cavity or canal. **2.** The contraction of an orifice down to a narrow slit; i.e., the so-called mitral buttonhole in extreme mitral stenosis.

but•ton su•ture (bŭt′ŏn sū′chŭr) A suture in which the threads are passed through the holes of a button and then tied; used to reduce the danger of the threads cutting through the flesh.

but•tress plate (bŭt′trĕs plāt) A metal plate used to support the internal fixation of a fracture.

bu•tyl (byū′til) A radical of *N*-butane.

bu•ty•ra•ce•ous (byū′tir-ā′shē-ŭs) Buttery in consistency.

bu•ty•rate (byū′ti-rāt) A salt or ester of butyric acid.

bu•tyr•ic ac•id (byū-tir′ik) An acid of unpleasant odor occurring in butter, cod liver oil, sweat, and many other substances.

bu•ty•roid (byū′ti-royd) **1.** Buttery. **2.** Resembling butter.

bu•tyr•ous (byū′tir-ŭs) Denoting a tissue or bacterial growth of butterlike consistency.

bu•tyr•yl (byū′tir-il) SYN butanoyl.

bu·ty·ryl·cho·lin·es·ter·ase (byū′tir-il-kō′lin-es′tĕr-ās) SYN plasma cholinesterase.

Buz·zard ma·neu·ver (bŭz′ărd mă-nū′vĕr) Testing the patellar reflex while the sitting patient makes firm pressure on the floor with his or her toes.

B19 vi·rus (vī′rŭs) A human parvovirus associated with arthritis and arthralgia and a number of specific clinical entities, including erythema infectiosum and aplastic crisis in the presence of hemolytic anemia.

BVM Abbreviation for bag-valve-mask device.

By·ars flap (bī′ărz flap) Skin flap made of dorsal prepuce to resurface the ventral penis in patients with chordee and/or hypospadias.

by·pass (bī′pas) **1.** A shunt or auxiliary flow. **2.** To create new flow from one structure to another through a diversionary channel. SEE ALSO shunt.

bys·si·no·sis (bis′i-nō′sis) Obstructive airway disease in people who work with unprocessed cotton, flax, or hemp; caused by reaction to material in the dust. [G. *byssos,* flax, + *-osis,* condition]

by·stand·er ly·sis (bī′stand-ĕr lī′sis) Complement-mediated lysis of nearby cells in the vicinity of a complement activation site.

BZ NATO code for 3-quinuclidinyl benzilate (QNB), an incapacitating chemical-warfare agent that exists as a crystalline solid that is soluble in certain organic solvents. BZ is an anticholinergic glycolate that causes typical anticholinergic effects and a distinct kind of hallucinations and illusions.

BZ NATO code for 3-quinuclidinyl benzilate (QNB).

C

C **1.** Abbreviation for large calorie; carbon; cathodal; cathode; Celsius; cervical vertebra (C1–C7); closure (of an electrical circuit); congius (gallon); contraction; coulomb; curie; cylinder; cylindric lens; cytidine; cysteine; cytosine; component of complement (C1 1/N C9); third substrate in a multisubstrate enzyme-catalyzed reaction. **2.** When followed by subscript letters, e.g., C_{In}, indicates renal clearance of a substance (e.g., inulin). When followed by subscript numbers, e.g., C_{19}, indicates the number of carbon atoms in a molecule.

c **1.** Abbreviation for centi-; small calorie; centum; concentration; speed of light in a vacuum; circumference; curie. **2.** As a subscript, refers to blood capillary.

CA Abbreviation for carcinoma, cardiac arrest, cancer, chronologic age, and cytosine arabinoside; NATO code for the riot-control agent bromobenzylcyanide.

CA-125 Abbreviation for cancer antigen 125 (CA-125) test.

Ca An alternate abbrevation for cancer or carcinoma; symbol for the element calcium.

CA-125 an•ti•gen (an′ti-jen) Tumor marker elevated in 85% of women with advanced ovarian cancer. SEE ALSO cancer antigen 125 (CA-125) test.

CA-15-3 an•ti•gen (an′ti-jen) Antigen present in some patients with breast cancer.

CA-19-9 an•ti•gen (an′ti-jen) Tumor antigen present in cholangiocarcinomas and pancreatic carcinomas.

cab•bage (kab′ăj) The common foodstuff (*Brassica*); limited animal studies suggest possible value as cancer preventive.

CABG Abbreviation for coronary artery bypass graft.

ca•ble graft (kā′bĕl graft) A multiple strand nerve graft arranged as a pathway for regeneration of axons.

Cab•ot ring bod•ies (kab′ŏt ring bod′ēz) Ring-shaped or figure-8-shaped structures that stain red with Wright stain, found in red blood cells in severe anemias, possibly a remnant of the nuclear membrane; a form of basophilic degenerative process.

ca•chec•tic (kă-kek′tik) Relating to or suffering from cachexia.

ca•chex•i•a (kă-kek′sē-ă) A general weight loss and wasting occurring in the course of a chronic disease or emotional disturbance. [G. *kakos,* bad, + *hexis,* condition of body]

ca•chex•i•a hy•po•phys•e•o•pri•va (kă-kek′sē-ă hī′pō-fiz′ē-ō-prē′vă) A condition following total removal of the hypophysis cerebri resulting in panhypopituitarism marked by a fall of body temperature, electrolyte imbalance, and hypoglycemia, followed by coma and death.

ca•chex•i•a stru•mi•pri•va (kă-kek′sē-ă strū-mi-prē′vă) SYN cachexia thyropriva.

ca•chex•i•a thy•ro•pri•va (kă-kek′sē-ă thī-rō-prē′vă) Signs and symptoms of hypothyroidism (with or without myxedema) resulting from the loss of thyroid tissue, either from surgery, radiotherapy, or disease. SYN cachexia strumipriva.

cach•in•na•tion (kak′i-nā′shŭn) Laughter without apparent cause, often observed in schizophrenia. [L. *cachinno,* to laugh immoderately and loudly]

caco-, cac-, caci- Combining forms meaning bad; ill. Cf. mal-. [G. *kakos*]

cac•o•de•mo•no•ma•ni•a (kak′ŏ-dē-mŏ-nō-mā′nē-ă) Psychiatric condition in which the patient has the delusion of being possessed by an evil spirit. [G. *kakodaimōn,* possessed by evil, + mania]

cac•o•geu•si•a (kak′ō-gū′sē-ă) A bad taste. [caco- + G. *geusis,* taste]

ca•co•gra•phy (kak-og′ră-fē) Poor handwriting. [G. *kakos,* bad + *graphē,* writing]

cac•o•me•li•a (kak′ō-mē′lē-ă) Congenital deformity of one or more limbs. [caco- + G. *melos,* limb]

ca•cos•mi•a (kă-koz′mē-ă) A subjective perception of nonexistent disagreeable odors. [G. *kakosmia,* a bad smell, fr. *kakos,* bad, + *osmē,* the sense of smell]

cac•u•men, pl. **cac•u•mi•na** (kak-ū′men, -mi-nă) The top or apex of a plant or an anatomic structure. [L. summit]

CAD Abbreviation for coronary artery disease.

ca•dav•er (kă-dav′ĕr) A dead body. SYN corpse. [L. fr. *cado,* to fall]

ca•dav•er•ic (kă-dav′ĕr-ik) Relating to a dead body.

ca•dav•er•ine (kă-dav′ĕr-in) A foul-smelling diamine formed by bacterial decarboxylation of lysine; poisonous and irritating to the skin.

ca•dav•er•ous (kă-dav′ĕr-ŭs) Having the pallor and appearance of a corpse.

cad•her•in (kad-hēr′in) One of a class of integral-membrane glycoproteins that has a role in cell-to-cell adhesion and is important in morphogenesis and differentiation; *E*-cadherin (also known as uvomorulin) is concentrated in the belt desmosome in epithelial cells; *N*-cadherin is found in nerve, muscle, and lens cells and helps maintain the integrity of neuronal aggregates; *P*-cadherin is expressed in placental and epidermal cells. [cell + adhere + -in]

cad•mi•um (Cd) (kad′mē-ŭm) A metallic element, atomic no. 48, atomic wt. 112.411; its salts are poisonous and little used in medicine. Various compounds of cadmium are used commercially in fields such as metallurgy, photography, and electrochemistry; a few have been used as ascaricides, antiseptics, and fungicides. [L. *cadmia,* fr. G. *kadmeia* or *kadmia,* an ore of zinc, calamine]

ca•du•ce•us (kă-dū′sē-ŭs) A staff with two oppositely twined serpents and surmounted by two wings; emblem of the U.S. Army Medical Corps. SEE ALSO staff of Aesculapius. [L. the staff of Mercury; G. *kēryx* herald, the staff of Hermes]

♻ **cae-** For words so beginning, see under ce-.

caec- [Br.] SYN cec-.

caeca [Br.] SYN ceca.

caecal [Br.] SYN cecal.

caecectomy [Br.] SYN cecectomy.

caecitis [Br.] SYN cecitis.

caeco- [Br.] SYN ceco-.

caecocentral scotom [Br.] SYN cecocentral scotoma.

caecocolostomy [Br.] SYN cecocolostomy.

caecoileostomy [Br.] SYN -stomy.

caecopexy [Br.] SYN cecopexy.

caecoplication [Br.] SYN cecoplication.

caecorrhaphy [Br.] SYN cecorrhaphy.

caecosigmoidostomy [Br.] SYN cecosigmoidostomy.

caecostomy [Br.] SYN cecostomy.

caecotomy [Br.] SYN cecotomy.

caecoureterocele [Br.] SYN cecoureterocele.

caecum [Br.] SYN cecum.

Caesarean hysterectomy [Br.] SYN cesarean hysterectomy.

Caesarean section [Br.] SYN cesarean section.

caesium [Br.] SYN cesium.

caf•é au lait spot (kaf-ā′ ō lā′ spot) Medium brown spots on the trunk, pelvis, and creases of the elbow and knees that are often seen in neurofibromatosis. See page B10. [F., coffee with milk]

ca•fé cor•o•nar•y (kaf-ā′ kōr′ŏ-nār′ē) Sudden collapse while eating due to food impaction closing the glottis; often erroneously thought to stem from coronary artery disease.

caf•feine (kaf′ēn) An alkaloid obtained from the dried leaves of *Thea sinensis*, tea, or the dried seeds of *Coffea arabica*, coffee; used as a central nervous system stimulant, diuretic, circulatory and respiratory stimulant, and adjunct in the treatment of headaches.

caf•fein•ism (kaf′ēn-izm) Caffeine intoxication characterized by restlessness, tremulousness, excitement, tachycardia, dysrhythmia, insomnia, flushed face, diuresis, and gastrointestinal complaints, brought on by the ingestion of substances containing caffeine.

cage (kāj) [TA] **1.** An enclosure made partly or completely of open work and commonly used to house animals. **2.** A structure resembling such an enclosure. SYN cavea. [M.E., fr. O.Fr., fr. L. *cavea*, hollow, stall]

Ca•got ear (kah′zhō ēr) An auricle having no lobulus. [a people in the Pyrenees among whom physical stigmata are common]

Cain com•plex (kān kom′pleks) Extreme envy or jealousy of a brother, degenerating into hatred. [*Cain,* biblical personage]

cais•son dis•ease (kā′son di-zēz′) SYN decompression sickness. [Fr. *caisson* (fr. *caisse*, a chest) a water-tight box or cylinder containing air under high pressure used in sinking structural pilings underwater]

Ca•jal as•tro•cyte stain (kah-hahl′ as′trŏ-sīt stān) A method for demonstrating astrocytes by impregnation in a solution containing gold chloride and mercuric chloride.

Ca•jal nu•cle•us (kah-hahl′ nū′klē-ŭs) Collection of nerve cells lying at the rostral end of the medial longitudinal fasciculus; has reciprocal projections to the vestibular nuclei and also connects to the spinal cord. SYN interstitial nucleus.

cake kid•ney (kāk kid′nē) A solid, irregularly lobed organ of bizarre shape, usually situated in the pelvis toward the midline, produced by fusion of the primordia of the kidneys.

cal Abbreviation for small calorie.

cal•a•mus (kal′ă-mŭs) A reed-shaped structure. [L. reed, a pen]

cal•a•mus scrip•to•ri•us (kal′ă-mŭs skrip-tō′rē-ŭs) Inferior part of the rhomboid fossa; the narrow lower end of the fourth ventricle between the two clavae. [L. writing pen]

calcaemia [Br.] SYN calcemia.

cal•ca•ne•al, cal•ca•ne•an (kal-kā′nē-ăl, kal-kā′nē-ăn) Relating to the calcaneus or heel bone.

cal•ca•ne•al a•poph•y•si•tis (kal-kā′nē-ăl ă-pof′i-sī′tis) SYN Sever disease.

cal•ca•ne•al ar•ter•ies (kal-kā′nē-ăl ahr′tĕr-ēz) SYN calcaneal branches.

cal•ca•ne•al branch•es (kal-kā′nē-ăl branch′ĕz) The calcaneal branches or arteries, branches to the structures in the calcaneal region from 1) the posterior tibial artery and 2) the fibular artery. SYN calcaneal arteries, rami calcanei.

cal•ca•ne•al pe•te•chi•ae (kal-kā′nē-ăl pe-tē′kē-ē) Traumatic hemorrhage into the stratum corneum of the heel that may persist for several weeks as centrally confluent black dots.

cal•ca•ne•al spur (kal-kā′nē-ăl spŭr) SYN heel spur.

cal•ca•ne•al tu•ber•os•i•ty (kal-kā′nē-ăl tū′bĕr-os′i-tē) The posterior extremity of the calcaneus, or os calcis, forming the projection of the heel.

♻ **calcaneo-** Combining form denoting the calcaneus. [L. *calcaneum*, heel]

cal•ca•ne•o•a•poph•y•si•tis (kal-kā′nē-ō-ă-pof′i-sī′tis) Inflammation at the posterior part of the os calcis, at the insertion of the Achilles tendon.

cal•ca•ne•o•as•trag•a•loid (kal-kā′nē-ō-as-trag′ă-loyd) Relating to the calcaneus, or os calcis, and the talus, or astragalus.

cal•ca•ne•o•cu•boid (kal-kā′nē-ō-kyū′boyd) Relating to the calcaneus and the cuboid bone.

cal•ca•ne•o•dyn•i•a (kal-kā′nē-ō-din′ē-ă) SYN painful heel. [calcaneo- + G. *odynē*, pain]

cal•ca•ne•o•na•vic•u•lar (kal-kā′nē-ō-nă-vik′yŭ-lăr) Relating to the calcaneus and the navicular bone.

cal•ca•ne•o•tib•i•al (kal-kā′nē-ō-tib′ē-ăl) Relating to the calcaneus and the tibia.

cal•ca•ne•um (kal-kā′nē-ŭm) SYN calcaneus (1). [L. the heel]

🅸 **cal•ca•ne•us**, gen. and pl. **cal•ca•ne•i** (kal-kā′nē-ŭs, -kā′nē-ī) **1.** [TA] The largest of the tarsal bones; it forms the heel and articulates with the cuboid anteriorly and the talus above. SYN calcaneum, heel bone. **2.** SYN talipes calcaneus. See this page. [L. the heel (another form of *calcaneum*)]

cal•car (kal′kahr) [TA] **1.** A small projection from any structure; internal spurs (septa) at the level of division of arteries and confluence of veins when branches or roots form an acute angle. **2.** A spine or projection from a bone. SYN spur. [L. spur, cock's spur]

cal•car•e•ous (kal-kār′ē-ŭs) Chalky; relating to or containing lime or calcium, or calcific material. [L. *calcarius*, pertaining to lime, fr. *calx*, lime]

cal•car•e•ous cor•pus•cles (kal-kār′ē-ŭs kōr′pŭs-ĕlz) Rounded masses composed of concentric layers of calcium carbonate, characteristic of tapeworm tissue.

cal•car•e•ous de•gen•er•a•tion (kal-kār′ē-ŭs dĕ-jen′ĕr-ā′shŭn) In a precise sense, not itself a degenerative process, but the deposition of insoluble calcium salts in tissue that has degenerated and become necrotic, as in dystrophic calcification.

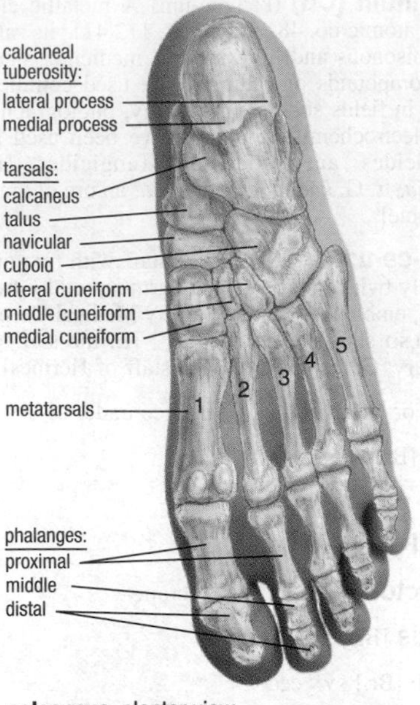

calcaneus: plantar view

cal•car•e•ous in•fil•tra•tion (kal-kār′ē-ŭs in′fil-trā′shŭn) SYN calcification.

cal•ca•rine (kal′kă-rēn) **1.** Relating to a calcar. **2.** Spur-shaped.

cal•ca•rine sul•cus (kal′kă-rēn sŭl′kŭs) A deep fissure on the medial aspect of the cerebral cortex, extending on an arched line from the isthmus of the fornicate gyrus back to the occipital pole, marking the border between the lingual gyrus below and the cuneus above it. The cortex in the depth of the sulcus corresponds to the horizontal meridian of the contralateral half of the visual field.

cal•car•i•u•ri•a (kal-kar-ē-yūr′ē-ă) Excretion of calcium (lime) salts in the urine. [L. *calcarius*, of lime, + G. *ouron*, urine]

cal•ce•mi•a (kal-sē′mē-ă) SYN hypercalcemia. SYN calcaemia.

cal•ces (kal′sēz) Plural of calx.

cal•ci•co•sis (kal-si-kō′sis) Pneumoconiosis from the inhalation of limestone dust.

cal•ci•di•ol (kal-si-dī′ol) The first step in the biologic conversion of vitamin D3 to the more active form, calcitriol; it is more potent than vitamin D3.

cal•cif•er•ol (kal-sif′ĕr-ol) SYN ergocalciferol.

cal·cif·ic (kal-sif′ik) Involving or caused by calcification.

cal·ci·fi·ca·tion (kal′si-fi-kā′shŭn) **1.** Deposition of lime or other insoluble calcium salts. **2.** A process in which tissue or noncellular material in the body becomes hardened as the result of precipitates or larger deposits of insoluble salts of calcium (and also magnesium), especially calcium carbonate and phosphate (hydroxyapatite) normally occurring only in the formation of bone and teeth. SYN calcareous infiltration. [L. *calx,* lime, + *facio,* to make]

cal·cif·ic bur·si·tis (kal-sif′ik bŭr-sī′tis) Inflammation of a bursa that results in the deposition of calcium salts; most commonly associated with subdeltoid bursitis.

cal·cif·ic ten·din·i·tis (kal-sif′ik ten′dŏn-ī′tis) Chronic tendinitis with formation of mineral deposits in and around the tendon.

cal·ci·fy (kal′si-fī) To deposit or lay down calcium salts, as in the formation of bone.

cal·ci·fy·ing o·don·to·gen·ic cyst, cal·ci·fy·ing and ker·a·tin·iz·ing o·don·to·gen·ic cyst (kal′si-fī-ing ō-don-tō-jen′ik sist, kal′si-fī-ing ker′ă-ti-nī′zing ō-don-tō-jen′ik sist) A mixed radiolucent-radiopaque lesion of the jaws with features of both a cyst and a solid neoplasm; characterized by ghost cell keratinization, dentinoid, and calcification.

cal·ci·neu·rin (kal-sē-nūr′in) A calcium-dependent serine-threonine phosphatase involved in T-cell signaling transcription; the reaction cascade in which it resides is referred to as the calcineurin pathway. [calcium + G. *neuron,* nerve, + -in]

cal·ci·no·sis (kal-si-nō′sis) A condition characterized by the deposition of calcium salts in nodular foci in various tissues. See this page. [calcium + *-osis,* condition]

cal·ci·no·sis cir·cum·scrip·ta (kal-si-nō′sis sĭr-kŭm-skrip′tă) Localized deposits of calcium salts in the skin and subcutaneous tissues, usually surrounded by a zone of granulomatous inflammation; clinically, the lesions resemble the tophi of gout.

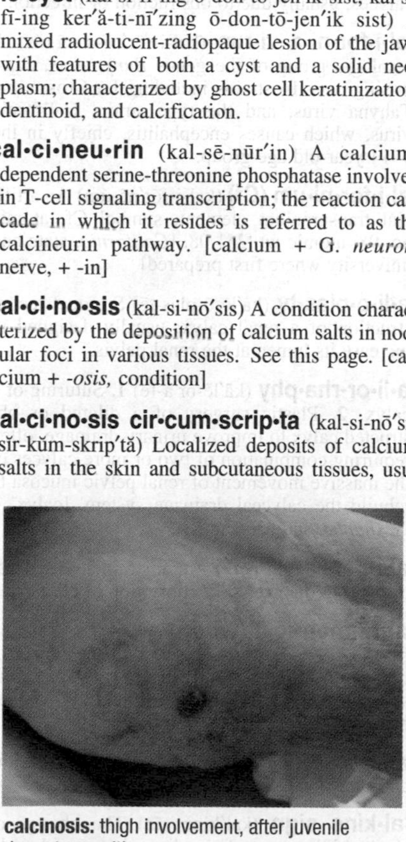
calcinosis: thigh involvement, after juvenile dermatomyositis

cal·ci·no·sis u·ni·ver·sa·lis (kal-si-nō′sis yū-ni-vĕr-sā′lis) Diffuse deposits of calcium salts in the skin and subcutaneous tissues, connective tissue, and other sites; may be associated with dermatomyositis, occurs more frequently in young people, and is often fatal; serum levels of calcium and phosphorus are generally within normal limits.

cal·ci·phil·i·a (kal-si-fil′ē-ă) A condition in which the tissues manifest an unusual affinity for calcium salts. [calcium + G. *phileō,* to love]

cal·ci·phy·lax·is (kal-si-fī-lak′sis) A condition of induced systemic hypersensitivity in which tissues respond to appropriate challenging agents with a sudden, but sometimes evanescent, local calcification.

cal·ci·priv·ic (kal-si-priv′ik) Deprived of calcium.

cal·ci·to·nin (kal-si-tō′nin) A peptide hormone, of which eight forms are known; produced by the parathyroid, thyroid, and thymus glands; its action is opposite to that of parathyroid hormone in that calcitonin increases deposition of calcium and phosphate in bone and lowers the level of calcium in the blood. [calci- + G. *tonos*, stretching, + -in]

cal·ci·to·nin gene–re·lat·ed pep·tide (CGRP) (kal-si-tō′nin jēn-rĕ-lāt′ĕd pep′tīd) A second product transcribed from the calcitonin gene. CGRP is found in a number of tissues including nervous tissue. It is a vasodilator that may participate in the cutaneous triple response.

cal·ci·um (Ca), gen. **cal·ci·i** (kal′sē-ŭm, -sē-ī) A metallic bivalent element; atomic no. 20, atomic wt. 40.078, density 1.55, melting point 842°C. Many calcium salts have crucial uses in metabolism and in medicine. Calcium salts are responsible for the radiopacity of bone, calcified cartilage, and arteriosclerotic plaques in arteries. [Mod. L. fr. L. *calx,* lime]

cal·ci·um 47 (kal′sē-ŭm) A radioisotope of calcium with a half-life of 4.54 days, used in the diagnosis of disorders of calcium metabolism.

cal·ci·um chan·nel block·er (kal′sē-ŭm chan′ĕl blok′ĕr) A class of cardiovascular drugs with the capacity to prevent calcium ions from passing through biologic membranes (e.g., cardiac muscles and blood vessels). These agents are used to treat hypertension, angina pectoris, and cardiac arrhythmias; examples include nifedipine, diltiazem, and verapamil. SYN slow channel-blocking agent.

cal·ci·um group (kal′sē-ŭm grūp) The metals of the alkaline earths: beryllium, magnesium, calcium, strontium, barium, and radium.

cal·ci·um pump (kal′sē-ŭm pŭmp) A membranal protein that can transport calcium ions across the membrane using energy from ATP.

cal•ci•u•ri•a (kal-sē-yūr′ē-ă) The urinary excretion of calcium; sometimes used as a synonym for hypercalciuria.

cal•co•dyn•i•a (kal-kō-din′ē-ă) SYN painful heel. [L. *calx,* heel, + G. *odynē,* pain]

cal•co•sphe•rite (kal-kō-sfēr′īt) A tiny, spheroidal, concentrically laminated body containing deposits of calcium salts; found in papillary carcinoma of the thyroid and ovary and in meningioma. SYN psammoma bodies (3). [L. *calx,* lime, + G. *sphaira,* sphere]

cal•cu•li (kal′kyū-lī) Plural of calculus.

cal•cu•lo•gen•e•sis (kal′kyū-lō-jen′ĕ-sis) Formation of dental calculus. [L. *calculus,* small stone, + G. *genesis,* formation]

cal•cu•lo•sis (kal-kyū-lō′sis) The tendency or disposition to form calculi or stones. [L. *calculus,* small stone, + G. *-osis,* condition]

cal•cu•lus, gen. and pl. **cal•cu•li** (kal′kyū-lŭs, -lī) A concretion formed in any part of the body, most commonly in the passages of the biliary and urinary tracts; usually composed of salts of inorganic or organic acids, or of other material such as cholesterol. SEE ALSO dental calculus. SYN stone (1). [L. a pebble, a calculus]

Cald•well-Luc op•er•a•tion (kawld′wel lūk op-ĕr-ā′shŭn) An intraoral procedure for opening into the maxillary antrum through the supradental (canine) fossa above the maxillary premolar teeth. Usually done to remove tooth roots or abnormal tissue from the sinus. SYN Luc operation.

Cald•well-Mo•loy clas•si•fi•ca•tion (kawld′wel mŏl-oy′ klas′i-fi-kā′shŭn) A classification of the variations in the female pelvis; namely gynecoid, android, anthropoid, and platypelloid pelvis, based on the type of the posterior and anterior segments of the inlet.

cal•e•fa•cient (kal-ĕ-fā′shĕnt) **1.** Making warm or hot. **2.** An agent causing a sense of warmth in the part to which it is applied. [L. *calefacio,* fr. *caleo,* to be warm, + *facio,* to make]

calf, pl. **calves** (kaf, kavz) SYN sural region. [Gael. *kalpa*]

calf bone (kaf bōn) SYN fibula. [O.N. *kalfi,* fibula]

cal•i•ber (kal′i-bĕr) The diameter of a hollow tubular structure. [Fr. *calibre,* of uncert. etym.]

cal•i•brate (kal′i-brāt) **1.** To graduate or standardize any measuring instrument. **2.** To measure the diameter of a tubular structure.

cal•i•bra•tion curve (kal-i-brā′shŭn kŭrv) The graphic or mathematic relationship between the readings obtained in an analytic process and the quantity of analyte in a calibration. The relationship is often a straight line rather than a curve.

cal•i•bra•tion in•ter•val (kal-i-brā′shŭn in′tĕr-văl) The period of time or series of measurements during which calibration can be expected to remain stable within specified and documented limits.

cal•i•bra•tor (kal′i-brā-tŏr) A standard or reference material or substance with a known value that is used to standardize or calibrate an instrument or laboratory procedure.

Cal•i•ci•vi•ri•dae (kal′i-sē-vir′i-dē) A family of RNA viruses associated with epidemic viral gastroenteritis and certain forms of hepatitis.

cal•i•cot•o•my, **cal•i•cec•to•my** (kal-i-kot′ŏ-mē, kal-i-kek′tŏ-mē) Incision into a calyx, usually for removal of a calculus. [calix, + G. *tomē,* a cutting]

ca•lic•u•lus, pl. **ca•lic•u•li** (kă-lik′yŭ-lŭs, -lī) A bud-shaped or cup-shaped structure, resembling the closed calyx of a flower. [L. dim. fr. G. *kalyx,* the cup of a flower]

ca•li•ec•ta•sis (kā-lē-ek′tă-sis) Dilation of the calyces, usually due to obstruction or infection.

Cal•i•for•ni•a vi•rus (kal-i-fōr′nē-ă vī′rŭs) A serologic group of the genus *Bunyavirus,* comprising over 14 strains including La Crosse and Tahyna virus, and the type strain, California virus, which causes encephalitis, chiefly in the 4–14 year-old age group.

cal•i•for•ni•um (Cf) (kal-i-fōr′nē-ŭm) An artificial transuranium element, symbol Cf, atomic no. 98, atomic wt. 251.08. [*California,* state and university where first prepared]

ca•li•o•plas•ty (kā′lē-ō-plas-tē) Surgical reconstruction of a renal calyx, usually designed to increase its lumen at the renal pelvis.

ca•li•or•rha•phy (kā′lē-ōr′ă-fē) **1.** Suturing of a calyx. **2.** Plastic surgery of a dilated or obstructed calyx to improve urinary drainage, often requiring combination of two or more calyces or the massive movement of renal pelvic mucosa to rebuild the calyceal drainage system. [calyx, + G. *rhaphē,* suture, seam]

cal•i•pers (kal′i-pĕrz) An instrument used for measuring diameters. [a corruption of *caliber*]

cal•is•then•ics (kal-is-then′iks) Systematic practice of various exercises with the object of preserving health and increasing physical strength and cardiovascular fitness. [G. *kalos,* beautiful, + *sthenos,* strength]

ca•lix (kā′liks) SYN calyx. [L. fr. G. *kalyx,* the cup of a flower]

Cal•kins sign (kal′kinz sīn) The change of shape of the uterus from discoid to ovoid, indicating placental separation from the uterine wall.

Cal·la·han meth·od (kal'a-han meth'ŏd) SYN chloropercha method.

Cal·lan·der am·pu·ta·tion (kal'ăn-dĕr amp' yū-tā'shŭn) Tenontoplastic amputation through the femur at the knee. SYN knee disarticulation amputation.

Call-Ex·ner bod·ies (kawl eks'nĕr bod'ēz) Small fluid-filled spaces between granulosal cells in ovarian follicles and in ovarian tumors of granulosal origin; they may form a rosettelike structure.

cal·lo·sal (kă-lō'săl) Relating to the corpus callosum.

cal·los·i·ty (kă-los'i-tē) A circumscribed thickening of the keratin layer of the epidermis as a result of repeated friction or intermittent pressure. SYN callus (1), keratoma (1), poroma (1), tyloma. [L. fr. *callosus,* thick-skinned]

cal·lous (kal'ŭs) Relating to a callus or callosity.

cal·lus (kal'ŭs) **1.** SYN callosity. **2.** A composite mass of tissue that forms at a fracture site to establish continuity between the bone ends; it is composed initially of uncallused fibrous tissue and cartilage, and ultimately of bone. [L. hard skin]

calm·a·tive (kawl'mă-tiv) A substance that produces a sedative or tranquilizing effect.

Cal·mette-Guér·in ba·cil·lus (kahl-mĕt'ger-rin[h]' bă-sil'ŭs) SYN bacille Calmette-Guérin.

cal·mod·u·lin (kal-mod'yū-lin) A protein that binds calcium ions, thereby becoming the agent for many of the cellular effects long ascribed to calcium ions. [*calc*ium + *modul*ate]

Ca·lo·di·um (kal-ō'dē-ŭm) One of three trichurid nematode genera, commonly referred to as *Capillaria.*

ca·lor (kā'lōr) Heat, as one of the four signs of inflammation (the others are rubor, tumor, dolor) enunciated by Celsus. [L.]

Ca·lo·ri bur·sa (kah-lō'rē bŭr'să) A bursa between the arch of the aorta and the trachea.

ca·lor·ic (kă-lōr'ik) **1.** Relating to a calorie. **2.** Relating to heat. [L. *calor,* heat]

ca·lor·ic nys·tag·mus (kă-lōr'ik nis-tag'mŭs) Jerky nystagmus induced by labyrinthine stimulation with hot or cold water in the ear.

ca·lor·ic stim·u·la·tion (kă-lōr'ik stim'yŭ-lā' shŭn) In treatment of swallowing disorders, the use of cold (but sometimes hot) temperature to increase awareness of the bolus in the mouth and pharynx; e.g., the use of ice slush rather than a room temperature food of similar consistency. SEE ALSO tactile stimulation. SYN thermal stimulation.

ca·lor·ic test (kă-lōr'ik test) SYN Bárány caloric test.

cal·o·rie (kal'ŏr-ē) A unit of heat content or energy. The amount of heat necessary to raise 1 g of water from 14.5–15.5°C (small calorie). Calorie is being replaced by joule, the SI unit equal to 0.239 calorie. SEE ALSO British thermal unit. [L. *calor,* heat]

ca·lor·i·gen·ic (kă-lōr-i-jen'ik) **1.** Capable of generating heat. **2.** Stimulating metabolic production of heat. SYN thermogenetic (2), thermogenic. [L. *calor,* heat, + G. *genesis,* production]

cal·o·rim·e·ter (kal-ŏr-im'ĕ-tĕr) An apparatus for measuring the amount of heat liberated in a chemical reaction. SEE ALSO human calorimeter. [L. *calor,* heat, + G. *metron,* measure]

cal·o·ri·met·ric (kal-ŏr-i-met'rik) Relating to calorimetry.

cal·o·rim·e·try (kal-ŏr-im'ĕ-trē) Measurement of the amount of heat given off by a reaction or group of reactions (as by an organism).

ca·lum·ba (kă-lŭm'bă) Herbal prepared from dried roots of *Jatrorrhiza palmata;* allegedly useful in treating diarrhea and other GI disorders. [Hausa *kalumbo*]

cal·var·i·a, pl. **cal·var·i·ae** (kal-vā'rē-ă, -ē) [TA] The upper domelike portion of the skull. SYN skullcap. [L. a skull]

cal·var·i·um (kal-vār'ē-ŭm) USAGE NOTE incorrectly used term for calvaria.

cal·vi·ti·es (kal-vish'ē-ēz) Condition of being bald. [L., baldness]

calx, gen. **cal·cis**, pl. **cal·ces** (kalks, kal'sis, kal'sēz) **1.** SYN lime (1). [L. limestone] **2.** The posterior rounded extremity of the foot. SYN heel (1). [L. heel]

cal·y·ce·al (kal'i-sē'ăl) Relating to the calyx.

cal·y·ce·al di·ver·tic·u·lum (kal-i-sē'ăl dī' vĕr-tik'yū-lŭm) A congenital or acquired distention of a kidney calyx that renders it susceptible to calculus formation.

Ca·lym·ma·to·bac·te·ri·um (kă-lim'mă-tō-bak-tēr'ē-ŭm) A genus of nonmotile bacteria containing gram-negative, pleomorphic rods with single or bipolar condensations of chromatin; cells occur singly and in clusters. The organisms are pathogenic only for humans. The type species is *C. granulomatis;* this species causes granuloma inguinale. [G. *kalymma,* hood, veil, + *baktērion,* rod]

ca·lyx, pl. **ca·ly·ces** (kā'liks, kal'i-sēz) A flower-shaped or funnel-shaped structure; specifically one of the branches or recesses of the pelvis of the kidney into which the orifices of the malpighian renal pyramids project. SYN calix. [G. cup of a flower]

CAM (kam) Acronym for complementary and alternative medicine; cell adhesion molecule.

cam·er·a, pl. **cam·er·ae** (kam′er-ă, -ē) **1.** A closed box; one containing a lens, shutter, and light-sensitive film or digital medium for photography. **2.** ANATOMY any chamber or cavity, such as one of the chambers of the heart or eye. [L. a vault]

cam·er·a an·te·ri·or bul·bi oc·u·li (kam′ĕr-ă an-tēr′ē-ōr bŭl′bī ok′yū-lī) [TA] SYN anterior chamber of eyeball.

cam·er·ae bul·bi (kam′ĕr-ē bŭl′bī) [TA] SYN chambers of eyeball.

cam·er·a oc·u·li (kam′ĕr-ă ok′yū-lī) SEE anterior chamber of eyeball, posterior chamber of eyeball.

cam·er·a pos·tre·ma (kam′er-ă pos-trē′mă) SYN postremal chamber of eyeball.

cam·er·a vit·re·a (kam′er-ă vit′rē-ă) SYN postremal chamber of eyeball.

cAMP Abbreviation for adenosine 3′,5′-cyclic monophosphate (cyclic AMP).

Camp·bell de Mor·gan spots (kam′bĕl dĕ mōr′găn spots) SYN senile hemangioma.

camp fe·ver (kamp fē′vĕr) **1.** SYN typhus. **2.** Any epidemic febrile illness affecting overcrowded populations with inadequate sanitary standards.

cam·pim·e·ter (kam-pim′ĕ-tĕr) A small tangent screen used to measure central visual field. [L. *campus,* field, + G. *metron,* measure]

cAMP re·cep·tor pro·tein (CRP) (sē′amp rĕ-sep′tŏr prō′tēn) SYN catabolite (gene) activator protein.

Camp stock·ings (kamp stok′ingz) Graduated compression stockings. [Camp Healthcare is the manufacturer.]

camp·to·cor·mi·a (kamp-tō-kōr′mē-ă) Static, often marked forward flexion of the trunk; usually manifestation of conversion reaction. SYN camptospasm. [G. *kamptos,* bent, + *kormos,* trunk of a tree]

camp·to·dac·ty·ly, **camp·to·dac·tyl·i·a** (kamp-tō-dak′ti-lē, -dak-til′ē-ă) Permanent flexion of one or both interphalangeal joints of one or more fingers, usually the little finger; often congenital in origin. [G. *kamptos,* bent, + *daktylos,* finger]

camp·to·me·li·a (kamp-tō-mē′lē-ă) A skeletal dysplasia characterized by a bending of the long bones of the limbs, resulting in a permanent bowing or curvature of the affected part. [G. *kamptos,* bent, + *melos,* limb]

camp·to·mel·ic (kamp-tō-mel′ik) Denoting or characteristic of camptomelia.

camp·to·mel·ic dwarf·ism (kamp-tō-mel′ik dwōrf′izm) Dwarfism with shortening of the lower limbs due to anterior bending of the femur and tibia.

camp·to·spasm (kamp′tō-spazm) SYN camptocormia.

camp·to·thec·in (kamp-tō-thek′in) Plant alkaloids consisting of a pentacyclic structure with a lactone ring; inhibitors of topoisomerase I, i.e., topotecan and irinotecan (CPT-11). [Camptotheca, genus name of botanic source]

Cam·py·lo·bac·ter (kam′pi-lō-bak′tĕr) A genus of bacteria containing gram-negative, non-spore-forming, curved spiral rods with a single polar flagellum at one or both ends of the cell; they are motile with a characteristic corkscrew-like motion. [G. *campylos,* curved, + *baktron,* staff or rod]

Cam·py·lo·bac·ter co·li (kam′pi-lō-bak′tĕr kō′lī) A thermophilic bacterial species that causes first watery, then inflammatory, diarrheal disease in humans, dogs, and piglets. Pathogen is the second most common cause of human campylobacteriosis.

Cam·py·lo·bac·ter con·cis·us (kam′pi-lō-bak′tĕr kon-sī′sŭs) A catalase-negative bacterial species isolated from normal human fecal flora, gingival crevices in periodontal disease, and occasionally blood.

Cam·py·lo·bac·ter fe·tus (kam′pi-lō-bak′tĕr fē′tŭs) A species that contains various subspecies, particularly *C. jejuni,* which can cause acute bacterial gastroenteritis in humans, as well as abortion in sheep and cattle; it is the type species of the genus *Campylobacter.*

Cam·py·lo·bac·ter hy·o·in·tes·ti·na·lis (kam′pi-lō-bak′tĕr hī′ō-int-tes-ti-nā′lis) A bacterial species that causes an enteropathy in pigs; has been recovered from fecal specimens in humans with diarrhea and proctitis, but its pathogenic role has not been defined.

cam·py·lo·bac·ter·i·o·sis (kam′pi-lō-bak-tēr′ē-ō′sis) Infection caused by microaerophilic bacteria of the genus *Campylobacter.*

Cam·py·lo·bac·ter je·ju·ni (kam′pi-lō-bak′tĕr je-jū′nī) A bacterial species that causes an acute gastroenteritis of sudden onset with constitutional symptoms (malaise, myalgia, arthralgia, and headache) and cramping abdominal pain; potential sources of human infection include poultry, cattle, sheep, pigs, and dogs. Pathogen is the most frequent cause of campylobacteriosis.

Cam·py·lo·bac·ter la·ri (kam′pi-lō-bak′tĕr lā′rī) A bacterial species primarily carried in birds, but associated with water-borne enteritis and occasionally septicemia in humans.

Ca·na·di·an clas·si·fi·ca·tion (kă-nā′dē-ăn klas′i-fi-kā′shŭn) System for description of angina pectoris developed by the Canadian Cardiovascular Society.

ca•nal (kă-nal′) A duct or channel; a tubular structure. SYN canalis [TA]. [L. *canalis*]

ca•na•les (kă-nā′lēz) Plural of canalis.

can•a•lic•u•lar (kan-ă-lik′yū-lăr) Relating to a canaliculus. [L. *canaliculus*, small channel, dim. fr. *canalis*, canal, + suffix *-ar*, pertaining to]

can•a•lic•u•lar stage of lung de•vel•op•ment (kan-ă-lik′yŭ-lar stāj lŭng dĕ-vel′ŏp-mĕnt) The period (16–26 weeks) when lumina of the bronchi and terminal bronchioles enlarge and the lung tissue becomes highly vascular; respiration is possible at the end of this period because some thin-walled terminal saccules have developed at the ends of the respiratory bronchioles. A fetus born at the end of this period may survive if it receives intensive care. See this page.

can•a•lic•u•li (kan-ă-lik′yū-lī) Plural of canaliculus.

can•a•lic•u•li den•ta•les (kan-ă-lik′yū-lī den-tā′lēs) [TA] Minute, wavy, branching tubes or canals in the dentin; they contain the long cytoplasmic processes of odontoblasts and extend radially from the pulp to the dentoenamel junction. SYN dentinal canals, dentinal tubules.

can•a•lic•u•li•tis (kan-ă-lik-yŭ-lī′tis) Inflammation of the lacrimal canaliculus. [canaliculus + G. *-itis*, inflammation]

can•a•lic•u•li•za•tion (kan-ă-lik′yŭ-lī-zā′shŭn) The formation of canaliculi, or small canals, in any tissue.

can•a•lic•u•lus, pl. **can•a•lic•u•li** (kan-ă-lik′yū-lŭs, -lī) [TA] A small canal or channel. SEE ALSO iter. [L. dim. fr. *canalis*, canal]

ca•na•lis, pl. **ca•na•les** (kă-nā′lis, -lēz) [TA] SYN canal. [L.]

ca•na•lis ad•duc•to•ri•us (kă-nā′lis a-dŭk-tō′rē-ŭs) [TA] SYN adductor canal.

ca•na•lis an•a•lis (kă-nā′lis ā-nā′lis) [TA] SYN anal canal.

ca•na•lis ca•ro•ti•cus (kă-nā′lis kă-rot′i-kŭs) [TA] SYN carotid canal.

ca•na•lis car•pi (kă-nā′lis kahr′pī) [TA] SYN carpal tunnel.

ca•na•lis cer•vi•cis u•ter•i (kă-nā′lis sĕr-vī′sis yū′tĕr-ī) [TA] SYN cervical canal.

ca•na•lis fe•mo•ra•lis (kă-nā′lis fem-ō-rā′lis) [TA] SYN femoral canal.

ca•na•lis hy•po•glos•sa•lis (kă-nā′lis hī′pō-glos-ā′lis) [TA] SYN hypoglossal canal.

ca•na•lis in•ci•si•vus (kă-nā′lis in-si-sī′vŭs) [TA] SYN incisive canal.

ca•na•lis in•fra•or•bi•ta•lis (kă-nā′lis in-fră-ōr-bi-tā′lis) [TA] SYN infraorbital canal.

ca•na•lis in•gui•na•lis (kă-nā′lis ing-gwi-nā′lis) [TA] SYN inguinal canal.

ca•na•lis mus•cu•lo•tu•ba•ri•us (kă-nā′lis mŭs′kyū-lō-tū-bā′rē-ŭs) [TA] SYN musculotubal canal.

ca•na•lis na•so•lac•ri•ma•lis (kă-nā′lis nā′sō-lak-ri-mā′lis) [TA] SYN nasolacrimal canal.

ca•na•lis nu•tri•ci•us (kă-nā′lis nū′tri-sī′ŭs) [TA] SYN nutrient canal.

ca•na•lis ob•tu•ra•to•ri•us (kă-nā′lis ob-tū-ră-tō′rē-ŭs) [TA] SYN obturator canal.

ca•na•lis op•ti•cus (kă-nā′lis op′ti-kŭs) [TA] SYN optic canal.

ca•na•lis pte•ry•goi•de•us (kă-nā′lis ter-i-goy′de-ŭs) [TA] SYN pterygoid canal.

ca•na•lis pu•den•da•lis (kă-nā′lis pū-den-dā′lis) [TA] SYN pudendal canal.

ca•na•lis py•lo•ri•cus (kă-nā′lis pī-lō′ri-kŭs) [TA] SYN pyloric canal.

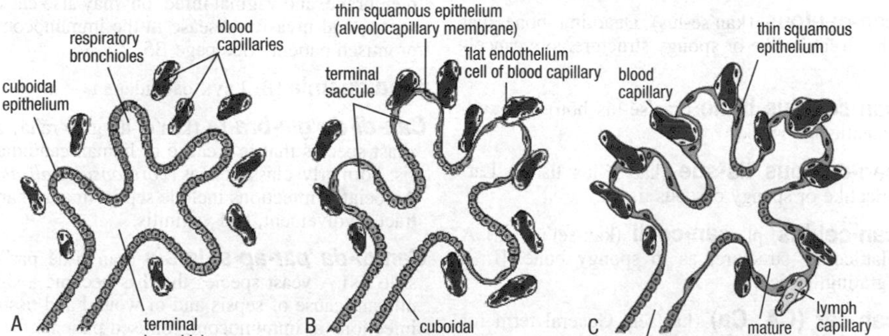

histologic development of the lung: (A) canalicular period, 16th–26th week; (B) terminal sac period, 6th–7th month; (C) alveolar period of lung development, showing full histologic maturation in the newborn

ca•na•lis ra•di•cis den•tis (ka-nā′lis răd′i-sis den′tis) [TA] SYN root canal of tooth.

ca•na•lis sa•cra•lis (kă-nā′lis sak-rā′lis) [TA] SYN sacral canal.

ca•na•lis spi•ra•lis co•chle•ae (ka-nā′lis spī-rā′lis kok′lē-ē) [TA] SYN cochlear canal.

ca•na•lis spi•ra•lis mo•di•o•li (ka-nā′lis spī-rā′lis mō-dī′-ō-lī) [TA] SYN spiral canal of modiolus.

ca•na•lis ver•te•bra•lis (kă-nā′lis vĕr-tē-brā′lis) [TA] SYN vertebral canal.

can•a•li•za•tion (kan-ă-lī-zā′shŭn) The formation of canals or channels in a tissue.

ca•nal for phar•yn•go•tym•pan•ic tube (kă-nal′ far-ing′gō-tim-pan′ik tūb) The inferior division of the musculotubular canal that forms the bony part of the pharyngotympanic (auditory) tube. SYN semicanalis tubae auditoriae.

ca•nals for les•ser pal•a•tine nerves (kă-nalz′ les′ĕr pal′ă-tīn nĕrvz) Canals located in the posterior part of the palatine bone.

Can•a•van dis•ease (kan′ă-van di-zēz′) Progressive degenerative disease of infancy; mostly affecting Ashkenazi Jewish babies; onset typically within the first 3–4 months of birth; characterized by megalencephaly, optic atrophy, blindness, psychomotor regression, hypotonia, and spasticity; increased urinary excretion of *N*-acetylaspartic acid occurs. MRI shows enlarged brain, decreased attenuation of cerebral and cerebellar white matter, and normal ventricles; pathologically, there is increased brain volume and weight, spongy degeneration, as well as in the subcortical white matter. Autosomal recessive inheritance, caused by mutation in the aspartoacyclase A gene (ASPA) on chromosome 17p in afflicted Jewish and Gentile people. SEE ALSO leukodystrophy.

can•cel•lat•ed (kan′sĕ-lā-tĕd) SYN cancellous. [L. *cancello,* to make a lattice work]

can•cel•lous (kan′sĕ-lŭs) Denoting bone that has a latticelike or spongy structure. SYN cancellated.

can•cel•lous bone (kan′sĕ-lŭs bōn) SYN substantia spongiosa.

can•cel•lous tis•sue (kan′sĕ-lŭs tish′ū) Latticelike or spongy osseous tissue.

can•cel•lus, pl. **can•cel•li** (kan-sel′ŭs, -lī) A latticelike structure, as in spongy bone. [L. a grating, lattice]

can•cer (CA, Ca) (kan′sĕr) General term for malignant neoplasms; carcinoma or sarcoma, especially the former. [L. a crab, a cancer]

can•cer an•ti•gen 125 (CA-125) test (kan′sĕr an′ti-jen test) Test for cell-surface antigen found on derivatives of celomic epithelium. Elevated levels of this antigen are associated with ovarian malignancy and benign pelvic disease such as endometriosis.

can•cer cord (kan′sĕr kōrd) A specific pattern of cells found in bronchial carcinoma, characterized by an outer ring of viable cells with a central region of necrosis.

can•cer fam•i•ly (kan′sĕr fam′i-lē) A group of blood relatives of whom several have had cancer.

can•cer•o•pho•bi•a (kan′sĕr-ō-fō′bē-ă) A morbid fear of acquiring a malignant growth. SYN carcinophobia. [cancer + G. *phobos,* fear]

can•cer•ous (kan′sĕr-ŭs) Relating to or pertaining to a malignant neoplasm, or being afflicted with such a process.

can•cra (kang′kră) Plural of cancrum.

can•cri•form (kang′kri-fōrm) Resembling cancer.

can•croid (kang′kroyd) Of or relating to squamous cell carcinoma.

can•crum, pl. **can•cra** (kang′krŭm, -kră) A gangrenous, ulcerative, inflammatory lesion. [Mod. L., fr. L. *cancer,* crab]

can•de•la (kan-dē′lă) The SI unit of luminous intensity, 1 lumen per m^2; the luminous intensity, in a given direction, of a source that emits monochromatic radiation of frequency 540×10^{12} hertz and that has a radiant intensity in that direction of 1/683 watt per steradian (solid angle). [L.]

Can•di•da (kan′di-dă) A genus of yeast fungi found in nature; a few species are isolated from the skin, feces, and vaginal and pharyngeal tissue, but the gastrointestinal tract is the primary source of the single most important species, *C. albicans.* [L. *candidus,* dazzling white]

i ***Can•di•da al•bi•cans*** (kan′di-dă al′bi-kanz) A yeast species; a common cause of skin, mucous membrane, and vaginal infection; may also cause sepsis, and invasive disease in the immunocompromised patient. See page B5.

candidaemia [Br.] SYN candidemia.

Can•di•da gla•bra•ta (kan′di-dă glab-rā′tă) A yeast species that is a cause of human candidiasis; formerly classified as *Torulopsis glabrata.* Associated infections include septicemia, urinary tract involvement, and vaginitis.

Can•di•da par•ap•si•lo•sis (kan′di-dă par′ă-si-lō′sis) A yeast species that has become a significant cause of sepsis and of wound and tissue infections in immunocompromised patients.

Can•di•da tro•pi•ca•lis (kan′di-dă trop-i-kā′lis) A yeast species occasionally associated with candidiasis.

can•di•de•mi•a (kan-di-dē′mē-ă) Presence of

cells of *Candida* species in the peripheral blood. SYN candidaemia. [*Candida* + G. *haima,* blood]

can·di·di·a·sis (kan-di-dī′ă-sis) Infection with, or disease caused by, *Candida*, especially *C. albicans*. This disease usually results from debilitation (as in immunosuppression and especially AIDS), physiologic change, prolonged administration of antibiotics, and barrier breakage. Commonly affected areas include the skin, oral mucous membranes, respiratory tract, and vagina. See this page. SYN candidosis, moniliasis.

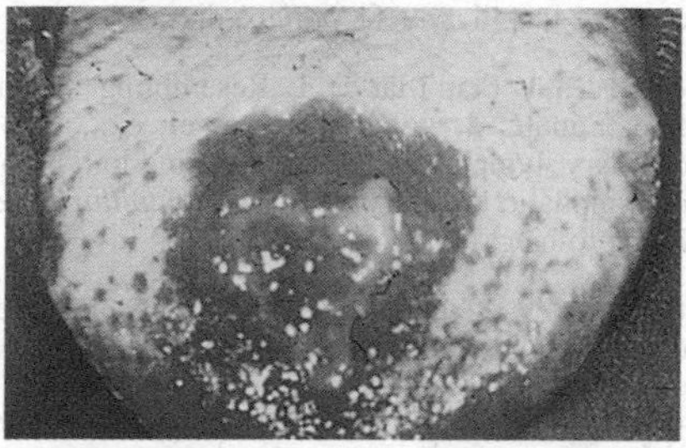

candidiasis: the thick white coat on this tongue is due to *Candida* infection. A raw red surface is left where the coat was scraped off; this infection may also cause redness of the tongue without the white coat; AIDS, among other factors, predisposes patients to this condition

can·di·do·sis (kan-di-dō′sis) SYN candidiasis.

can·dle·ber·ry (kan′dĕl-ber-ē) SYN bayberry.

can·dle-me·ter (kan′dĕl-mē′tĕr) SYN lux.

ca·nine (kā′nīn) **1.** Relating to the dog. **2.** Relating to the canine teeth. **3.** SYN canine tooth. **4.** Referring to the cuspid tooth. [L. *caninus*]

ca·nine tooth (kā′nīn tūth) A tooth having a crown of thick conic shape and a long, slightly flattened conic root; there are two canine teeth in each jaw, one on either side adjacent to the distal surface of the lateral incisors, in both the deciduous and the permanent dentition. SYN dens caninus [TA], canine (3), cuspid (2), eye tooth.

ca·ni·ti·es (kă-nish′ē-ēz) Graying of hair. [L., fr. *canus,* hoary, gray]

can·ker (kang′kĕr) **1.** In cats and dogs, acute inflammation of the external ear and auditory canal. SEE aphtha. **2.** An outmoded term for aphthae. [L. *cancer*, crab, malignant growth]

can·ker sores (kang′kĕr sōrz) SYN aphtha (2).

can·nab·i·noids (kă-nab′i-noydz) Organic substances present in *Cannabis sativa*, having a variety of pharmacologic properties.

can·na·bis (kan′ă-bis) The dried flowering tops of the pistillate plants of *Cannabis sativa* (family Moraceae) containing isomeric tetrahydrocannabinols, cannabinol, and cannabidiol. Preparations of cannabis are smoked or ingested to induce psychotomimetic effects such as euphoria, hallucinations, drowsiness, and other mental changes. Cannabis was formerly used as a sedative and analgesic; now available for restricted use in management of iatrogenic anorexia, especially that associated with oncologic chemotherapy and radiation therapy. Known by many colloquial or slang terms such as marijuana, marihuana, pot, grass, bhang, charas, ganja, and hashish. [L., fr. G. *kannabis,* hemp]

can·na·bism (kan′ă-bizm) Poisoning by preparations of cannabis.

Can·niz·za·ro re·ac·tion (kah′nēts-tsah′rō rē-ak′shŭn) Formation of an acid and an alcohol by the simultaneous oxidation of one aldehyde molecule and reduction of another; a dismutation: $2RCHO \rightarrow RCOOH + RCH_2OH$; when the aldehydes are not identical, this is referred to as a crossed Cannizzaro reaction.

can·non·ball pulse (kan′ŏn-bawl pŭls) SYN water-hammer pulse.

Can·non point (kan′ŏn poynt) The location in the midtransverse colon at which innervation by superior and inferior mesenteric plexuses overlap at the junction of the primitive midgut and hindgut, frequently resulting in narrowing evident on barium enema. SYN Cannon ring.

Can·non ring (kan′ŏn ring) SYN Cannon point.

can·nu·la (kan′yū-lă) A tube that can be inserted into a cavity or vein, usually by means of a trocar filling its lumen; after insertion of the cannula, the trocar is withdrawn and the cannula remains as a channel for the transport of fluid. Intravenous cannulas should be changed regularly to prevent thrombophlebitis. [L. dim. of *canna,* reed]

can·nu·la·tion, can·nu·li·za·tion (kan-yū-lā′shŭn, -yū-lī-zā′shŭn) Insertion of a cannula.

CANS (kanz) Acronym for central auditory nervous system.

Can·tel·li sign (kahn-tel′lē sīn) SEE doll's eye sign.

can·ter·ing rhythm (kan′tĕr-ing ridh′ŭm) SYN gallop.

can·thal (kan′thăl) Relating to a canthus.

can·thec·to·my (kan-thek′tŏ-mē) Excision of a palpebral canthus. [G. *kanthos,* canthus, + *ektomē,* excision]

can·thi (kan′thī) Plural of canthus.

can·thi·tis (kan-thī′tis) Inflammation of a canthus.

can·thol·y·sis (kan-thol′i-sis) SYN canthoplasty (1). [G. *kanthos,* canthus, + *lysis,* loosening]

can·tho·me·a·tal plane (kan′thō-mē-ā′tăl plān) Plane passing through the two lateral angles of the eye and the center of the external acoustic meatus; this plane lies approximately midway between the Frankfort and the supraorbitomeatal planes.

can•tho•plas•ty (kan′thō-plas-tē) **1.** Disruption of canthal tendon insertion; often performed surgically. SYN cantholysis. **2.** An operation for restoration of the canthus. [G. *kanthos,* canthus, + *plassō,* to form]

can•thor•rha•phy (kan-thōr′ă-fē) Suture of the eyelids at either canthus. [G. *kanthos,* canthus, + *rhaphē,* suture]

can•thot•o•my (kan-thot′ŏ-mē) Slitting of the canthus. [G. *kanthos,* canthus, + *tomē,* incision]

can•thus, pl. **can•thi** (kan′thŭs, kan′thī) The angle of the eye. [G. *kanthos,* corner of the eye]

can•ti•le•ver bridge (kan′ti-lē-vĕr brij) A fixed partial bridge denture in which the pontic is retained only on one side by an abutment tooth.

CAP Abbreviation for catabolite (gene) activator protein.

cap (kap) **1.** Any anatomic structure that resembles a cap or cover. **2.** A protective covering for an incomplete tooth. **3.** Colloquialism for restoration of the coronal part of a natural tooth by means of an artificial crown. **4.** The nucleotide structure found at the 5′ terminus of many eukaryotic messenger RNAs.

ca•pac•i•ta•tion (kă-pas′i-tā′shŭn) A conditioning process whereby the glycoprotein coat and seminal proteins are removed from the acrosome of a sperm. After capacitation has occurred, perforations develop in the acrosome. [L. *capacitas,* fr. *capax,* capable of]

ca•pac•i•tor (kă-pas′i-tĕr) A device for holding a charge of electricity. SYN condenser (4).

ca•pac•i•ty (kă-pas′i-tē) **1.** The potential cubic contents of a cavity or receptacle. **2.** Ability to do. SEE ALSO volume. [L. *capax,* able to contain; fr. *capio,* to take]

cap•ac•tins (kap-ak′tinz) A class of proteins capping the ends of actin filaments.

CAPD Abbreviation for continuous ambulatory peritoneal dialysis.

cap•e•line ban•dage (kap′ĕ-līn ban′dăj) A bandage covering the head or an amputation stump like a cap. [L. *capella,* a cap]

Cap•gras syn•drome (kahp′grah sin′drōm) The delusional belief that a person (or people) close to the schizophrenic patient has been substituted for by one or more impostors; may have an organic etiology.

cap•il•la•ri•a gran•u•lo•ma (kap′i-lā′rē-ă gran′yū-lō′mă) Granulomatous lesions found in the liver and lung are a tissue response at the site of eggs or worms.

cap•il•lar•i•o•mo•tor (kap′i-lār′ē-ō-mō′tŏr) Vasomotor, with special reference to the capillaries.

cap•il•lar•i•tis (kap′i-lar-ī′tis) Inflammation of a capillary or capillaries.

cap•il•lar•i•ty (kap′i-lar′i-tē) The rise of liquids in narrow tubes or through the pores of a loose material, as a result of capillary action.

cap•il•la•rop•a•thy (kap′i-lă-rop′ă-thē) Any disease of the capillaries, often applied to vascular changes in diabetes mellitus. SYN microangiopathy. [capillary + G. *pathos,* disease]

cap•il•lar•y (kap′i-lār-ē) **1.** Resembling a hair; fine; minute. **2.** A capillary vessel; e.g., blood capillary, lymph capillary. **3.** Relating to a blood or lymphatic capillary vessel. [L. *capillaris,* relating to hair]

cap•il•lar•y ar•te•ri•ole (kap′i-lār-ē ahr-tēr′ē-ōl) A minute artery that terminates in a capillary.

cap•il•lar•y at•trac•tion (kap′i-lār-ē ă-trak′shŭn) The force that causes fluids to rise up very fine tubes or pass through the pores of a loose material.

cap•il•lar•y bed (kap′i-lār-ē bed) The capillaries considered collectively and their volume capacity for blood. See this page.

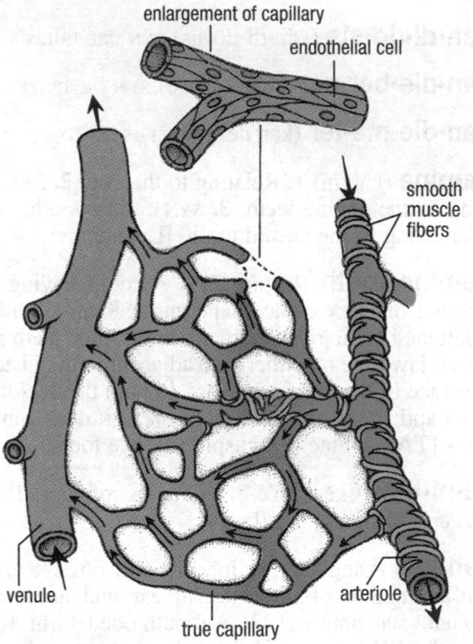

capillary bed

cap•il•lar•y drain•age (kap′i-lār-ē drān′ăj) Drainage by means of a wick of gauze or other material.

cap•il•lar•y fil•ling (kap′i-lār-ē fil′ing) The return of normal color to an area of skin, or a nail bed, after cutaneous capillaries have been emptied of blood by firm digital pressure; the promptness of return is a rough measure of general and vascular competence.

cap·il·lar·y frac·ture (kap′i-lār-ē frak′shŭr) SYN hairline fracture.

cap·il·lar·y fra·gil·i·ty (kap′i-lār-ē fră-jil′i-tē) The susceptibility of capillaries to breakage and extravasation of red blood cells under conditions of increased stress.

cap·il·lar·y he·man·gi·o·ma (kap′i-lār-ē hē-man′jē-ō′mă) An overgrowth of capillary blood vessels, seen most commonly in the skin, at or soon after birth, as a soft bright red to purple nodule or plaque that usually disappears by the fifth year. The most common type of hemangioma. SYN nevus vascularis, nevus vasculosus.

cap·il·lar·y lake (kap′i-lār-ē lāk) The total mass of blood contained in capillary vessels.

cap·il·lar·y vein (kap′i-lār-ē vān) SYN venule.

ca·pi·ta (kap′i-tă) Plural of caput.

cap·i·tate (kap′i-tāt) **1.** The largest of the carpal bones; located in the distal row. SYN capitate bone. **2.** Head-shaped; having a rounded extremity. [L. *caput* (*capit-*), head]

cap·i·tate bone (kap′i-tāt bōn) SYN capitate (1).

cap·i·ta·tion (kap′i-tā′shŭn) A system of medical reimbursement wherein the provider is paid an annual fee per covered patient by an insurer or other financial source; the aggregate fees are intended to reimburse all provided services. SEE ALSO managed care. [L.L. *capitatio,* fr. *caput,* head]

cap·i·tel·lum (kap-i-tel′ŭm) **1.** SYN capitulum (1). **2.** SYN capitulum of humerus. [L. dim. of *caput,* head]

ca·pit·u·la (kă-pit′yū-lă) Plural of capitulum.

ca·pit·u·lar (kă-pit′yū-lăr) Relating to a capitulum.

ca·pit·u·lum, pl. **ca·pit·u·la** (kă-pit′yū-lŭm, -lă) **1.** [TA] A small head or rounded articular extremity of a bone. SYN capitellum (1). SEE ALSO caput. **2.** The bloodsucking, probing, sensing, and holdfast mouthparts of a tick, including the basal supporting structure; relative size and shape of mouthparts forming the capitulum are characteristic for the genera of hard ticks. [L. dim. of *caput,* head]

ca·pit·u·lum of hu·mer·us (kă-pit′yū-lŭm hyū′mĕr-ŭs) The small rounded eminence on the lateral half of the distal end of the humerus for articulation with the radius. SYN capitellum (2).

Cap·lan syn·drome (kap′lăn sin′drōm) Intrapulmonary nodules, histologically similar to subcutaneous rheumatoid nodules, associated with rheumatoid arthritis and pneumoconiosis in coal workers.

Cap·no·cy·to·pha·ga (kap′nō-sī-tof′ă-gă) A genus of gram-negative, fusiform bacteria associated with human periodontal disease.

cap·no·gram (kap′nō-gram) A continuous record of the carbon dioxide content of expired air. [G. *kapnos,* smoke, + *gramma,* something written]

cap·no·graph (kap′nō-graf) Instrument by which a continuous graph of the carbon dioxide content of expired air is obtained.

cap·nom·e·ter (kap-nom′ĕ-tĕr) An instrument that measures the carbon dioxide concentration of exhaled air. SYN CO_2 analyzer. [G. *kapnos,* smoke, + *metron,* a measure]

cap·nom·e·try (kap′nom-ĕ-trē) The process of measuring and recording the carbon dioxide concentration of exhaled air at the patient's airway using a capnometer.

cap·rate (kap′rāt) A salt or ester of capric acid.

***N*-cap·ric ac·id** (kap′rik as′id) A fatty acid found among the hydrolysis products of fat in goat's milk, cow's milk, and other substances. Cf. *N*-caproic acid, caprylic acid.

***N*-ca·pro·ic ac·id** (kap-rō′ik as′id) A fatty acid found among the hydrolysis products of fat in butter, coconut oil, and some other substances.

cap·ro·yl (kap′rō-il) The acyl radical of caproic acid.

cap·ro·y·late (kap-rō′i-lāt) A salt or ester of caproic acid.

cap·ry·late (kap′ri-lāt) A salt or ester of caprylic acid.

ca·pryl·ic ac·id (kă-pril′ik as′id) A fatty acid found among the hydrolysis products of fat in butter, coconut oil, and other substances.

cap·sa·i·cin (kap-sā′i-sin) SYN capsicum. [Irreg. fr. *capsicum,* + *-in*]

cap·si·cum (kap′si-kŭm) Dried herbal remedy (and spice) made from *Capsicum frutescens* and other *Capsicum* spp.; both internal and external medicinal uses have been described (e.g., analgesic, therapy for GU problems). SYN capsaicin, cayenne, hot pepper, red pepper. [L., fr. *capsa,* box, case]

cap·sid (kap′sid) SEE virion.

cap·su·la, gen. and pl. **cap·su·lae** (kap′sū-lă, -lē) [TA] **1.** A membranous structure, usually dense collagenous connective tissue, that envelops an organ, a joint, or any other part. **2.** An anatomic structure resembling a capsule or envelope. SYN capsule (1). [L. dim. of *capsa,* a chest or box]

cap·su·la ar·ti·cu·la·ris (kap′sū-lă ahr-tik-yū-lā′ris) [TA] SYN articular capsule.

cap·su·la ex·ter·na (kap′sū-lă eks-ter′nă) [TA] SYN external capsule.

cap·su·la fi·bro·sa pe·ri·vas·cu·la·ris he·pa·tis (kap′sū-lă fī-brō′să per′ē-vas-kyū-lā′ris hē-pā′tis) [TA] SYN fibrous capsule of liver.

cap·su·la in·ter·na (kap′sū-lă in-ter′nă) [TA] SYN internal capsule.

cap·su·lar (kap′sū-lăr) Relating to any capsule.

cap·su·lar an·ti·gen (kap′sū-lăr an′ti-jen) That found only in the capsules of certain microorganisms; e.g., the specific polysaccharides of various types of pneumococci.

cap·su·lar cat·a·ract (kap′sū-lăr kat′ăr-akt) A cataract in which the opacity affects the capsule.

cap·su·lar lig·a·ment (kap′sū-lăr lig′ă-mĕnt) Thickened portions of the fibrous membrane of an articular capsule.

cap·su·lar pat·tern (kap′sū-lăr pat′ĕrn) The pattern of limitation in range of motion exhibited by specific joints when inflamed; for example, the glenohumeral joint shows more limitation in external rotation than in internal rotation whereas the knee joint shows more limitation in flexion than in extension.

cap·su·lar space (kap′sū-lăr spās) The slitlike space between the visceral and parietal layers of the capsule of the renal corpuscle; it opens into the proximal tubule of the nephron at the neck of the tubule.

cap·su·lar ten·sion ring (kap′sū-lăr ten′shŭn ring) A device that is inserted into the capsular bag to aid in cataract surgery in which loose zonules are involved.

cap·sule (kap′sŭl) **1.** SYN capsula. **2.** A fibrous tissue layer enveloping an organ, joint, or a neoplasm. **3.** A solid dosage form in which a drug is enclosed in either a hard or soft shell of soluble material. **4.** A hyaline polysaccharide coating around a fungal or bacterial wall of a cell. Bacteria may also have a polypeptide capsule or slime layer around the cell. [L. *capsula*, dim. of *capsa*, box]

cap·sule for·ceps (kap′sŭl fōr′seps) Forceps used for grasping the capsule of the lens in extracapsular extraction of a cataract.

cap·sule of lens (kap′sŭl lenz) The capsule enclosing the lens of the eye.

cap·su·li·tis (kap′sū-lī′tis) Inflammation of the capsule of an organ or part, as of the liver or the lens of the eye.

cap·su·lize (kap′sū-līz) To enclose.

cap·su·lo·len·tic·u·lar (kap′sū-lō-len-tik′yū-lăr) Referring to the lens of the eye and its capsule.

cap·su·lo·len·tic·u·lar cat·a·ract (kap′sū-lō-len-tik′yū-lăr kat′ăr-akt) A cataract in which both the lens and its capsule are involved. SEE ALSO membranous cataract.

cap·su·lo·plas·ty (kap′sū-lō-plas-tē) Plastic surgery of a capsule; more specifically, the capsule of a joint. [L. *capsula,* capsule, + G. *plastos,* formed]

cap·su·lor·rha·phy (kap′sū-lōr′ă-fē) Suture of a tear in any capsule; specifically, suture of a joint capsule to prevent recurring dislocation of the articulation. [L. *capsula,* capsule, + *rhaphē,* suture]

cap·su·lor·rhex·is (kap′sū-lō-reks′sis) Technique used in cataract surgery by which a continuous circular tear is made in the anterior lens capsule. [L. *capsula,* capsule, + G. *rhēxis,* rupture]

cap·su·lot·o·my (kap′sū-lot′ŏ-mē) **1.** Division of a capsule as around a breast implant. **2.** Creation of an opening through a capsule; e.g., of a scar around a foreign body. **3.** Incision of the capsule of the lens in the extracapsular cataract operation. [L. *capsula,* capsule, + G. *tomē,* a cutting]

cap·tain of the ship doc·trine (kap′tăn ship dok′trin) The legal principle that the responsibility and accountability for patient care lies with the supervising physician, regardless whether that clinician has performed the procedure in question.

cap·ture (kap′shŭr) Catching and holding a particle or an electrical impulse originating elsewhere. [L. *capio,* pp. *-tus,* to take, seize]

ca·put, gen. **ca·pi·tis**, pl. **ca·pi·ta** (kap′ŭt, -i-tis, -i-tă) [TA] **1.** Head: the superior extremity of the human body, comprising the cranium and face, and containing the brain and organs of sight, hearing, taste, and smell. **2.** The superior, anterior, or larger extremity, expanded or rounded, of any body, organ, or other anatomic structure. **3.** The rounded extremity of a bone. **4.** The end of a muscle that is attached to the less movable part of the skeleton. [L.]

ca·put me·du·sae (kap′ŭt me-dū′sē) **1.** Varicose veins radiating from the umbilicus, seen in Cruveilhier-Baumgarten syndrome. **2.** Dilated ciliary arteries girdling the corneoscleral limbus in rubeosis iridis. SYN Medusa's head. [*Medusa,* G. mythical character]

ca·put suc·ce·da·ne·um (kap′ŭt sŭk-sĕ-dā′nē-ŭm) An edematous swelling formed on the presenting portion of the scalp of an infant during birth.

ca·put zy·go·mat·i·cum quad·ra·ti la·bi·i su·pe·ri·or·is (kap′ŭt zi-go-măt′i-kŭm kwahd′rā′tī lā′bē-ī sū-pēr-ē-ōr′is) SYN zygomaticus minor muscle.

Ca·ra·bel·li cusp (kah-rĕ-bel′lē kŭsp) A cusp found on the lingual surface of the mesiolingual cusp of upper first molars, ranging in size from a pit to a large cusp.

car•a•way (kar′ă-wā) An agent with purported value in reading GI complaints; has been studied for its laxative properties; noted as an antiflatulent. SYN carvi fructus, kümmel, oleum cari.

carb-, carbo- Prefixes indicating carbon, especially the attachment of a group containing a carbon atom. [L. *carbo*, charcoal]

car•ba•mate (kahr′bă-māt) **1.** A salt or ester of carbamic acid, forming the basis of urethane hypnotics. SEE ALSO physostigmine. **2.** A class of compounds that reversibly inhibit the enzyme acetylcholinesterase. Some are used as insecticides, others as medicines. One, pyridostigmine, is a preexposure antidotal enhancer (often incorrectly called "pretreatment") against the nerve agent soman; another, physostigmine, is used as an antidote to anticholinergic incapacitating agents. SYN carbamoate.

car•bam•ic ac•id (kahr-bam′ik as′id) A hypothetical acid, NH_2-COOH, forming carbamates; the acyl radical is carbamoyl.

car•ba•mi•no com•pound (kahr-bam′i-nō kom′pownd) Any carbamic acid derivative formed by the combination of carbon dioxide with a free amino group to form an *N*-carboxyl group.

carbaminohaemoglobin [Br.] SYN carbaminohemoglobin.

car•ba•mi•no•he•mo•glo•bin (kahr-bam′i-nō-hē′mō-glō′bin) Carbon dioxide bound to hemoglobin by means of a reactive amino group on the latter; approximately 20% of the total carbon dioxide in blood is combined with hemoglobin in this manner. SYN carbaminohaemoglobin.

car•ba•moate (kahr′bă-mōt) SYN carbamate.

car•bam•o•yl (kar′bă-mō-il) The acyl radical, NH_2-CO-, the transfer of which plays an important role in certain biochemical reactions. SYN carbamyl.

***N*-car•bam•o•yl•as•par•tic acid** (kahr′bă-mō-il-as-pahr′tik as′id) SYN ureidosuccinic acid.

car•bam•o•yl•trans•fer•as•es (kahr′bă-mō-il-trans′fĕr-ās-ĕz) [EC group 2.1.3] Enzymes transferring carbamoyl groups from one compound to another. SYN transcarbamoylases.

car•bam•o•yl•u•re•a (kahr′bă-mō-il-yūr′ē-ă) SYN biuret.

car•ba•myl (kahr′bă-mil) SYN carbamoyl.

car•bo•ben•zox•y (kahr′bō-ben-zok′sē) SYN benzyloxycarbonyl.

car•bo•gen (kahr′bō-jen) A mixture of 10% carbon dioxide and 90% oxygen used for inhalation therapy to produce vasodilation. [*carbo*n dioxide + oxy*gen*]

car•bo•hy•drate load•ing (kahr-bō-hī′drāt lōd′ing) Manipulation of diet and exercise to significantly increase muscle and liver glycogen content. Frequently used by endurance athletes to enhance performance. SYN glycogen loading, glycogen supercompensation.

car•bo•hy•drates (CHO) (kahr-bō-hī′drāts) Class name for the aldehydic or ketonic derivatives of polyhydric alcohols. Most such compounds have formulas that may be written $C_n(H_2O)_n$, although they are not true hydrates. The group includes simple sugars (monosaccharides, disaccharides), as well as macromolecular (polymeric) substances such as starch, glycogen, and cellulose polysaccharides. SEE ALSO saccharides.

car•bo•hy•drat•u•ri•a (kahr-bō-hī-dră-tyūr′ē-ă) Excretion of one or more carbohydrates in the urine.

car•bo•lu•ri•a (kahr-bō-lyūr′ē-ă) The presence of phenol (carbolic acid) in the urine. [carbolic acid + G. *ouron,* urine]

car•bon (C) (kahr′bŏn) A nonmetallic tetravalent element, atomic no. 6, atomic wt. 12.011; the major bioelement. It has two natural isotopes, ^{12}C and ^{13}C (the former, set at 12.00000, being the standard for all molecular weights), and two artificial, radioactive isotopes of interest, ^{11}C and ^{14}C. The element occurs in diamond, graphite, charcoal, coke, and soot, and in the atmosphere as CO_2. Its compounds are found in all living tissues, and the study of its vast number of compounds constitutes most of organic chemistry. [L. *carbo,* coal]

car•bo•na•ceous (kahr-bŏ-nā′shŭs) Containing or yielding carbon.

car•bon•ate (kahr′bŏn-āt) **1.** A salt of carbonic acid. **2.** The ion $CO_3^{=}$.

car•bon di•ox•ide (CO_2) (kahr′bŏn dī-oks′īd) The product of the combustion of carbon with an excess of air; in concentrations not less than 99.0% by volume of CO_2, used as a respiratory stimulant.

car•bon di•ox•ide com•bin•ing pow•er (kahr′bŏn dī-oks′īd kŏm-bīn′ing pow′ĕr) A measurement of the total CO_2 that can be bound as HCO_2 at a P_{CO_2} of 40 mmHg at 25°C by serum, plasma, or whole blood.

car•bon di•ox•ide cy•cle, car•bon cy•cle (kahr′bŏn dī-oks′īd sī′kĕl, kahr′bŏn sī′kĕl) The circulation of carbon as CO_2 from the expired air of animals and decaying organic matter to plant life where it is synthesized (through photosynthesis) to carbohydrate material, from which, as a result of catabolic processes in all life, it is again ultimately released to the atmosphere as carbon dioxide.

car•bon di•ox•ide pro•duc•tion ($\dot{V}CO_2$) (kahr-bŏn dī-oks′īd prō-duk′shŭn) The volume of carbon dioxide produced by the body, per minute; it is reported in liters or mL per minute at STPD.

car·bon mon·ox·ide (CO) (kahr′bŏn mŏ-noks′īd) A colorless, practically odorless, poisonous gas formed by the incomplete combustion of carbon; its toxic action is due to its strong affinity for hemoglobin, myoglobin, and the cytochromes, reducing oxygen transport and blocking oxygen use.

car·bon mon·ox·ide he·mo·glo·bin (kahr′bŏn mŏ-noks′īd hē′mō-glō-bin) SYN carboxyhemoglobin.

car·bon mon·ox·ide poi·son·ing (kahr′bŏn mŏ-noks′īd poy′zŏn-ing) A potentially fatal acute or chronic intoxication caused by inhalation of carbon monoxide gas that competes favorably with oxygen for binding with hemoglobin (carboxyhemoglobinemia) and thus interferes with the transportation of oxygen and carbon dioxide by the blood.

car·bon·yl (kahr′bŏn-il) The characteristic group, —CO—, of the ketones, aldehydes, and organic acids.

carboxy- Combining form indicating addition of CO or CO_2.

carboxyhaemoglobin [Br.] SYN carboxyhemoglobin.

carboxyhaemoglobinaemia [Br.] SYN carboxyhemoglobinemia.

car·box·y·he·mo·glo·bin (kahr-bok′sē-hē′mŏ-glō′bin) A stable union of carbon monoxide with hemoglobin. The formation of carboxyhemoglobin prevents the normal transfer of carbon dioxide and oxygen during the circulation of blood; thus, increasing levels of carboxyhemoglobin result in various degrees of asphyxiation, including death. SYN carbon monoxide hemoglobin, carboxyhaemoglobin.

car·box·y·he·mo·glo·bi·ne·mi·a (kahr-bok′sē-hē′mŏ-glō-bi-nē′mē-ă) Presence of carboxyhemoglobin in the blood, as in carbon monoxide poisoning. SYN carboxyhaemoglobinaemia.

car·box·yl (kahr-bok′sil) The characterizing group (—COOH) of organic acids.

car·box·yl·ase (kahr-bok′sil-ās) One of several carboxylyases catalyzing the addition of CO_2 to another molecule to create an additional—COOH group.

car·box·yl·a·tion (kahr-bok′si-lā′shŭn) Addition of CO_2 to an organic acceptor to yield a —COOH group; catalyzed by carboxylases.

car·box·yl·trans·fer·as·es (kahr-bok′sil-trans′fĕr-ās-ēz) [EC group 2.1.3] Enzymes transferring carboxyl groups from one compound to another. SYN transcarboxylases.

car·box·y·pep·ti·dase (kahr-bok′sē-pep′ti-dās) A hydrolase that removes the amino acid at the free carboxyl end of a polypeptide chain; an exopeptidase.

car·bun·cle (kahr′bŭng-kĕl) Deep-seated pyogenic infection of the skin and subcutaneous tissues, usually arising in several contiguous hair follicles, with formation of connecting sinuses. [L. *carbunculus,* dim. of *carbo,* a live coal, a carbuncle]

car·bun·cu·lar (kahr-bŭng′kyū-lăr) Relating to a carbuncle.

car·bun·cu·lo·sis (kahr-bŭng′kyū-lō′sis) A condition marked by the occurrence of several carbuncles simultaneously or within a short period of time.

carcinaemia [Br.] SYN carcinemia.

car·ci·ne·mi·a (kahr′si-nē′mē-ă) The presence of malignant cells in the blood. SYN carcinaemia. [carcin- + G. *haima,* blood]

carcino-, carcin- Combining forms meaning cancer; crab. [G. *karkinos,* crab, cancer]

car·ci·no·em·bry·on·ic (kahr′si-nō-em-brē-on′ik) Pertaining to a substance found in embryonic tissue but absent from adult tissue except in certain carcinomas of the lung, digestive tract, and pancreas.

car·ci·no·em·bry·on·ic an·ti·gen (CEA) (kahr′si-nō-em-brē-on′ik an′ti-jen) A glycoprotein constituent of the glycocalyx of embryonic endodermal epithelium, generally absent from adult cells with the exception of some carcinomas. It may also be detected in the serum of patients with colon cancer.

car·cin·o·gen (kahr-sin′ŏ-jen) Any cancer-producing substance or organism, such as polycyclic aromatic hydrocarbons, or agents such as certain types of irradiation. [carcino- + G, *-gen,* producing]

car·ci·no·gen·e·sis (kahr′si-nō-jen′ĕ-sis) The origin, production, or development of cancer, including carcinomas and other malignant neoplasms. [carcino- + G. *genesis,* generation]

car·ci·no·gen·ic (kahr′si-nō-jen′ik) Causing cancer.

car·ci·noid syn·drome (kahr′si-noyd sin′drōm) A combination of symptoms and lesions usually produced by the release of serotonin from carcinoid tumors of the gastrointestinal tract that have metastasized to the liver; consists of irregular mottled blushing, flat angiomas of the skin, acquired tricuspid and pulmonary stenosis often with regurgitation, diarrhea, bronchial spasm, mental aberration, and excretion of large quantities of 5-hydroxyindoleacetic acid. Surgical excision is performed when feasible. Treatment may include chemotherapy and radiation therapy.

car·ci·noid tu·mor (kahr′si-noyd tū′mŏr) A neoplasm composed of cells of medium size, with moderately small vesicular nuclei; neoplastic cells are frequently palisaded at the periphery of small groups. Such neoplasms occur in the gastrointestinal tract, the lungs, and other sites, with approximately 90% in the appendix. SEE ALSO carcinoid syndrome. SYN argentaffinoma.

car·ci·no·lyt·ic (kahr′si-nō-lit′ik) Destructive to the cells of carcinoma. [carcino- + G. *lytikos,* causing a solution]

car·ci·no·ma (CA, Ca), pl. **car·ci·no·mas, car·cin·o·ma·ta** (kahr′si-nō′mă, -măz, -mă-tă) Any of the various types of malignant neoplasm derived from epithelial tissue, occurring more frequently in the skin and large intestine in both sexes, the lung and prostate gland in men, and the lung and breast in women. Carcinomas are identified histologically on the basis of invasiveness and the changes that indicate anaplasia, i.e., loss of polarity of nuclei, loss of orderly maturation of cells (especially in squamous cell type), variation in the size and shape of cells, hyperchromatism of nuclei (with clumping of chromatin), and increase in the nuclear-cytoplasmic ratio. Carcinomas may be undifferentiated, or the neoplastic tissue may resemble (to varying degrees) one of the types of normal epithelium. See this page, B14. [G. *karkinōma,* fr. *karkinos,* cancer, + *-oma,* tumor]

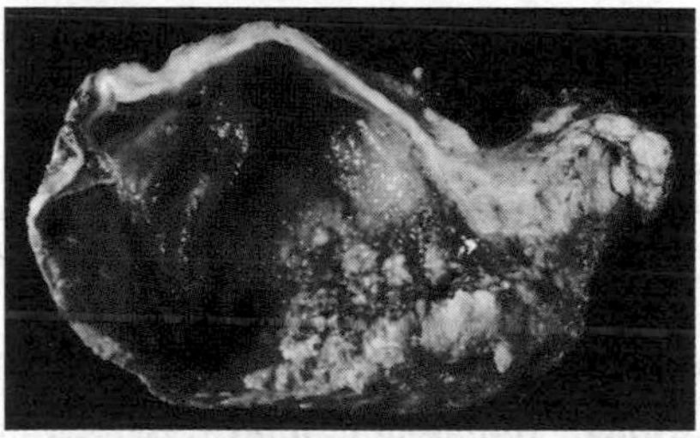

carcinoma of the gallbladder

car·ci·no·ma of the breast (kahr′si-nō′mă brest) A malignant tumor arising from epithelial cells of the female (and occasionally the male) breast, usually adenocarcinoma arising from ductal epithelium. See page B19.

car·ci·no·ma of the pros·tate (kahr′si-nō′mă pros′tāt) A malignant neoplasm arising from glandular epithelial cells of the prostate gland.

car·ci·no·ma in si·tu (CIS) (kahr′si-nō′mă in sī′tū) A lesion characterized by cytologic changes of the type associated with invasive carcinoma, but with the pathologic process limited to the lining epithelium and without histologic evidence of extension to adjacent structures. The lesion is presumed to be the precursor of invasive carcinoma, i.e., a localized and curable phase of carcinoma.

car·ci·no·ma·ta (kahr′si-nō′mă-tă) Alternative plural of carcinoma.

car·ci·no·ma·to·sis (kahr′si-nō-mă-tō′sis) Widespread dissemination of carcinoma in various organs or tissues of the body. SYN carcinosis.

car·ci·no·ma·tous (kahr′si-nō′mă-tŭs) Pertaining to or manifesting the properties of carcinoma.

car·ci·no·pho·bi·a (kahr′sin-ō-fō′bē-ă) SYN cancerophobia.

car·ci·no·sar·co·ma (kahr′si-nō-sahr-kō′mă) A malignant neoplasm that contains elements of carcinoma and sarcoma so extensively intermixed as to indicate neoplasia of epithelial and mesenchymal tissue.

car·ci·no·sis (kahr′si-nō′sis) SYN carcinomatosis.

car·da·mom (kahr′dă-mŏm) Herbal agent derived from *Elettaria cardamomum;* purportedly useful against flatulence; widely used as a cooking spice. SYN *Alpinia cardamom,* Malabar cardamom. [L. *cardamomum,* fr. G. *kardamōmon*]

Car·den am·pu·ta·tion (kahr′dĕn amp′yū-tā′shŭn) Transcondylar amputation of the leg; the femur is sawed through the condyles just above the articular surface.

car·di·a (kahr′dē-ă) Opening of the esophagus into the stomach.

car·di·ac ar·rest (CA) (kahr′dē-ak ă-rest′) Complete cessation of cardiac activity either electric, mechanical, or both; may be purposely induced for therapeutic reasons.

car·di·ac ar·rhyth·mi·a (kahr′dē-ak ā-ridh′mē-ă) SEE cardiac dysrhythmia.

car·di·ac as·sess·ment (kahr′dē-ak ă-ses′mĕnt) The appraisal of the cardiovascular system by a health care provider. See page 256.

car·di·ac asth·ma (kahr′dē-ak az′mă) An asthmatic attack due to the pulmonary congestion and edema caused by left ventricular failure.

car·di·ac care tech·ni·cian (kahr′dē-ak kār tek-nish′ŭn) SYN emergency medical technician–intermediate.

car·di·ac cath·e·ter (kahr′dē-ak kath′ĕ-tĕr) SYN intracardiac catheter.

car·di·ac cir·rho·sis (kahr′dē-ak sir-ō′sis) An extensive fibrotic reaction within the liver as a result of chronic constrictive pericarditis or prolonged congestive heart failure; true cirrhosis with fibrous bridging of lobules is unusual.

car·di·ac cy·cle (kahr′dē-ak sī′kĕl) The complete round of cardiac systole and diastole with the intervals between, commencing with any event in the heart's action and ending when same event is repeated.

car·di·ac de·com·pres·sion (kahr′dē-ak dē-kŏm-presh′ŭn) Incision into the pericardium or aspiration of fluid from pericardium to relieve

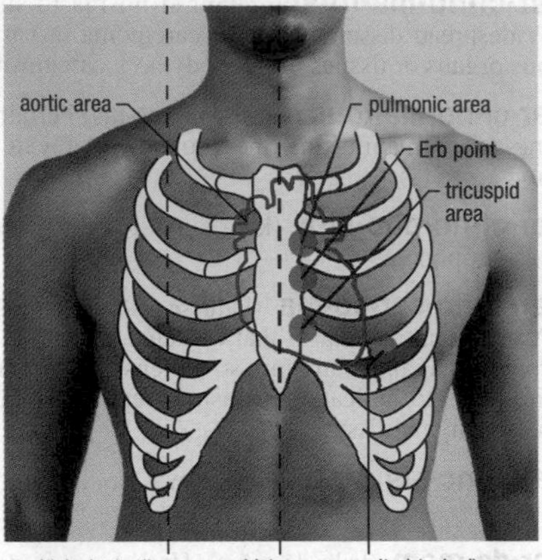

cardiac assessment: areas for auscultating heart sounds

pressure due to blood or other fluid in the pericardial sac. SYN pericardial decompression.

car·di·ac dys·rhyth·mi·a (kahr′dē-ak dis-ridh′mē-ă) Any abnormality in the rate, regularity, or sequence of cardiac activation.

car·di·ac e·de·ma (kahr′dē-ak ĕ-dē′mă) Edema resulting from congestive heart failure. SYN cardiacoedema.

car·di·ac gan·gli·a (kahr′dē-ak gang′glē-ă) Parasympathetic ganglia of the cardiac plexus lying between the arch of the aorta and the bifurcation of the pulmonary artery.

car·di·ac gat·ing (kahr′dē-ak gāt′ing) Using an electronic signal from the cardiac cycle to trigger an event, such as in imaging separate phases of cardiac contraction.

car·di·ac gland (kahr′dē-ak gland) A coiled tubular gland located in the cardiac region of the stomach; secretes primarily mucus.

car·di·ac his·ti·o·cyte (kahr′dē-ak his′tē-ō-sīt) A large mononuclear cell found in connective tissue of the heart wall in inflammatory conditions, especially in the Aschoff body. SYN Anitschkow cell, Anitschkow myocyte.

car·di·ac in·dex (kahr′dē-ak in′deks) The amount of blood ejected by the heart in a unit of time divided by the body surface area; usually expressed in liters per minute per square meter. The normal average is 2.8 L.

car·di·ac in·suf·fi·cien·cy (kahr′dē-ak in′sŭ-fish′ĕn-sē) SYN heart failure (1).

car·di·ac jel·ly (kahr′dē-ak jel′ē) The gelatinous, noncellular material between the endothelial lining and the myocardial layer of the heart in very early embryos; later in development it serves as a substratum for cardiac mesenchyme (i.e., embryonic connective tissue).

car·di·ac mas·sage (kahr′dē-ak mă-sahzh′) SYN heart massage.

car·di·ac mur·mur (kahr′dē-ak mŭr′mŭr) A sound generated by blood flow through the heart, at one of its valvular orifices or across ventricular septal defects.

car·di·ac mus·cle (kahr′dē-ak mŭs′ĕl) The muscle forming the myocardium, consisting of anastomosing transversely striated muscle fibers formed of cells united at intercalated discs. SYN muscle of heart.

car·di·ac neu·ro·sis (kahr′dē-ak nūr-ō′sis) Anxiety concerning the state of the heart, as a result of palpitation, chest pain, or other symptoms not due to heart disease; a form of hypochondriasis. SYN cardioneurosis.

car·di·ac notch (kahr′dē-ak noch) A deep notch between the esophagus and fundus of the stomach.

cardiacoedema [Br.] SYN cardiac edema.

car·di·ac or·i·fice (kahr′dē-ak ōr′i-fis) The trumpet-shaped opening of the esophagus into the stomach.

car·di·ac out·put (CO) (kahr′dē-ak owt′put) The product of heart rate and stroke volume, measured in liters per minute; the amount of blood that is pumped by the heart in 1 minute.

car·di·ac plex·us (kahr′dē-ak pleks′ŭs) A wide-meshed network of cardiopulmonary and splanchnic nerves arising from the afferent and autonomic nerve fibers (sympathetic) and vagus (parasympathetic) nerves, surrounding the arch of the aorta, the pulmonary artery, and continuing to the atria, ventricles, and coronary vessels.

car·di·ac re·ha·bil·i·ta·tion (kahr′dē-ak rē′hă-bil′i-tā′shŭn) A systematic program of exercise and nutritional, behavioral, and vocational counseling to optimize the recovery and physiologic capacity of the patient with cardiovascular disease.

car·di·ac res·cue tech·ni·cian (kahr′dē-ak res′kyū tek-nish′ŭn) SYN emergency medical technician–intermediate.

car·di·ac re·serve (kahr′dē-ak rē-zĕrv′) The work the heart is able to perform beyond that required under the ordinary circumstances of daily life, depending on the state of the myocardium and the degree to which, within physiologic limits, the cardiac muscle fibers can be stretched by the volume of blood reaching the heart during diastole.

car·di·ac souf·fle (kahr′dē-ak sū′fĕl) A soft, puffing heart murmur.

car·di·ac sphinc·ter (kahr′dē-ak sfingk′tĕr) A physiologic sphincter at the esophagogastric junction.

car·di·ac stand·still (kahr′dē-ak stand′stil) SYN asystole.

car·di·ac tam·pon·ade (kahr′dē-ak tam′pŏ-nahd′) Compression of the heart due to critically increased volume of fluid in the pericardium.

car·di·ac val·vu·lar in·com·pe·tence (kahr′dē-ak val′vyū-lăr in-kom′pĕ-tĕns) Failure of a valve to close its aperture completely and prevent regurgitation of blood.

car·di·ec·ta·si·a (kahr′dē-ek-tā′zē-ă) SYN ectasia cordis. [cardi- + G. *ektasis,* a stretching]

car·di·nal lig·a·ment (kahr′di-năl lig′ă-mĕnt) A fibrous band attached to the uterine cervix and the vault of the lateral fornix of the vagina; continuous with the tissue ensheathing the pelvic vessels.

car·di·nal points (kahr′di-năl poynts) **1.** The four points in the pelvic inlet toward one of which the occiput of the baby is usually directed in case of head presentation: two sacroiliac articulations and the two iliopectineal eminences corresponding to the acetabula. **2.** Six points of a compound optic system: the anterior focal point, the posterior focal point, the two principal points, and the two nodal points.

car·di·nal symp·tom (kahr′di-năl simp′tŏm) The primary or major symptom of diagnostic importance.

car·di·nal veins (kahr′di-năl vānz) The major systemic venous channels in adult primitive vertebrates and in the embryos of higher vertebrates; the **anterior cardinal veins** are the major drainage channels from the cephalic part of the body, and the **posterior cardinal veins**, from the caudal part; the **common cardinal veins**, formed by the anastomosis of the anterior and posterior cardinal veins, are the main systemic return channels to the heart.

♲ **cardio-**, **cardi-** Combining forms indicating the heart. [G. *kardia,* heart]

car·di·o·ac·cel·er·a·tor (kahr′dē-ō-ak-sel′ĕr-ā-tŏr) Accelerator of the heart beat.

car·di·o·ac·tive (kahr′dē-ō-ak′tiv) Influencing the heart.

car·di·o·a·or·tic (kahr′dē-ō-ā-ōr′tik) Relating to the heart and the aorta.

car·di·o·ar·te·ri·al (kahr′dē-ō-ahr-tēr′ē-ăl) Relating to the heart and the arteries.

Car·di·o·bac·te·ri·um (kahr′dē-ō-bak-tē′rē-ŭm) A genus of nonmotile, pleomorphic, gram-negative, facultatively anaerobic, rod-shaped bacteria found in the nasal flora and associated with endocarditis in humans. The type species is *C. hominis.*

Car·di·o·bac·te·ri·um hom·i·nis (kahr′dē-ō-bak-tē′rē-ŭm hom′i-nis) A species found as normal flora of the human upper respiratory tract that causes endocarditis. The type species of *Cardiobacterium.* SEE HACEK group.

car·di·o·cele (kahr′dē-ō-sēl) A herniation or protrusion of the heart through an opening in the diaphragm, or through a wound. [cardio- + G. *kēlē,* hernia]

car·di·o·cha·la·si·a (kahr′dē-ō-kă-lā′zē-ă) **1.** Achalasia of the cardia. **2.** Relaxation or incompetence of the cardiac orifice of the stomach.

car·di·o·dy·nam·ics (kahr′dē-ō-dī-nam′iks) The mechanics of the heart's action, including its movement and the forces generated thereby.

car·di·o·dyn·i·a (kahr′dē-ō-din′ē-ă) Pain in the heart. [cardio- + G. *odynē,* pain]

car·di·o·e·soph·a·ge·al (kahr′dē-ō-ē-sō-fā′jē-ăl) Denoting the junction of the esophagus and cardiac part of the stomach. SYN cardio-oesophageal.

car·di·o·e·soph·a·ge·al junc·tion (kahr′dē-ō-ē-sō-fā′jē-ăl jŭngk′shŭn) The abrupt transition from esophageal mucosa to that of the cardiac portion of stomach, demarcated internally in the living by the z-line, and approximated externally by the cardiac notch. SYN cardio-oesophageal junction.

car·di·o·gen·ic (kahr′dē-ō-jen′ik) Of cardiac origin.

car·di·o·gen·ic shock (kahr′dē-ō-jen′ik shok) Condition resulting from decline in cardiac output secondary to serious heart disease, usually myocardial infarction.

car·di·o·gram (kahr′dē-ō-gram) **1.** The graphic tracing made by the stylet of a cardiograph. **2.** Any recording derived from the heart, with such prefixes as apex-, echo-, electro-, phono-, or vector- being understood. [cardio- + G. *gramma,* a diagram]

car·di·o·graph (kahr′dē-ō-graf) An instrument for recording graphically the movements of the heart, constructed on the principle of the sphygmograph. [cardio- + G. *graphō,* to write]

car·di·og·ra·phy (kahr′dē-og′ră-fē) The use of the cardiograph.

car·di·o·he·pat·ic (kahr′dē-ō-hĕ-pat′ik) Relating to the heart and the liver.

car·di·o·ky·mo·gram (kahr′dē-ō-kī′mō-gram) Record made by a cardiokymograph.

car·di·o·ky·mo·graph (kahr′dē-ō-kī′mō-graf) Device placed on the chest to record anterior left ventricle segmental wall motion; consists of a plate transducer with recording probe; changes in wall motion affect the magnetic field and thus the oscillatory frequency, which is recorded on a waveform polygraph.

car·di·o·ky·mog·ra·phy (kahr′dē-ō-kī-mog′ră-fē) Use of a cardiokymograph.

car·di·o·lip·in (kahr′dē-ō-lip′in) A 1,3-bis-(phosphatidyl)glycerol found in many biomembranes with immunologic properties; used in serologic diagnosis of syphilis.

car·di·ol·o·gist (kahr′dē-ol′ŏ-jist) Physician specializing in cardiology.

car·di·ol·o·gy (kahr′dē-ol′ŏ-jē) The medical specialty concerned with the diagnosis and treatment of heart disease. [cardio- + G. *logos,* study]

car·di·o·ma·la·ci·a (kahr′dē-ō-mă-lā′shē-ă) Softening of the walls of the heart. [cardio- + G. *malakia,* softness]

car·di·o·meg·a·ly (kahr′dē-ō-meg′ă-lē) Enlargement of the heart. SYN macrocardia, megalocardia. [cardio- + G. *megas,* large]

car·di·o·mo·til·i·ty (kahr′dē-ō-mō-til′i-tē) Movements of the heart.

car·di·o·mus·cu·lar (kahr′dē-ō-mŭs′kyū-lăr) Pertaining to the cardiac musculature.

car·di·o·my·o·li·po·sis (kahr′dē-ō-mī′ō-li-pō′sis) Fatty degeneration of the myocardium. [cardio- + G. *mys,* muscle, + *lipos,* fat, + *-osis,* condition]

car·di·o·my·op·a·thy (kahr′dē-ō-mī-op′ă-thē) Disease of the myocardium; a primary disease of heart muscle in the absence of a known underlying etiology. See this page. SYN myocardiopathy. [cardio- + G. *mys,* muscle, + *pathos,* disease]

car·di·o·my·o·plas·ty (kahr′dē-ō-mī′ō-plas-tē) An operation that uses latissimus dorsi muscle to assist cardiac function. The muscle is moved into the thorax through the bed of the resected second or third rib, wrapped around the left and right ventricles, and stimulated to contract during cardiac systole by means of an implanted burst-stimulator.

car·di·o·neph·ric (kahr′dē-ō-nef′rik) SYN cardiorenal.

car·di·o·neu·ral (kahr′dē-ō-nūr′ăl) Relating to the nervous control of the heart. [cardio- + G. *neuron,* nerve]

car·di·o·neu·ro·sis (kahr′dē-ō-nūr-ō′sis) SYN cardiac neurosis.

cardio-oesophageal [Br.] SYN cardioesophageal.

cardio-oesophageal junction [Br.] SYN cardioesophageal junction.

car·di·o·o·men·to·pex·y (kahr′dē-ō-ō-men′tō-pek-sē) Operation for the attachment of omentum to the heart with the object of improving its blood supply. [cardio- + omentum, + G. *pēxis,* fixation]

car·di·op·a·thy (kahr′dē-op′ă-thē) Any disease of the heart. [cardio- + G. *pathos,* disease]

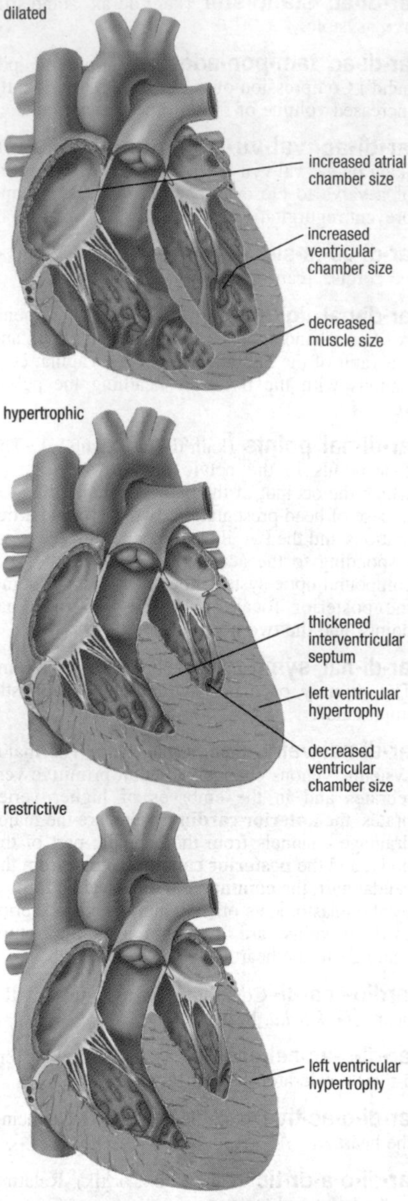

cardiomyopathies that lead to congestive heart failure

car·di·o·per·i·car·di·o·pex·y (kahr′dē-ō-per-i-kahr′dē-ō-pek-sē) An operation to increase the blood supply to the myocardium; magnesium silicate is spread within the pericardial sac, or the sac is mechanically abraded, to cause an adhesive pericarditis and an increase in blood supply to develop through stimulation of intraarterial coronary anastomoses and pericardial collaterals. [cardio- + pericardium, + G. *pēxis,* fixation]

car·di·o·pho·bi·a (kahr′dē-ō-fō′bē-ă) Morbid fear of heart disease.

car·di·o·phren·ic an·gle (kahr′dē-ō-fren′ik ang′gĕl) The angle between the heart and the diaphragm at either side of the cardiac projection, usually as seen in a posteroanterior chest x-ray.

car·di·o·plas·ty (kahr′dē-ō-plas-tē) An operation on the cardia of the stomach. SYN esophagogastroplasty. [cardio- (2) + G. *plastos,* formed]

car·di·o·ple·gi·a (kahr′dē-ō-plē′jē-ă) **1.** Paralysis of the heart. **2.** An elective temporary cessation of cardiac activity by injection of chemicals, selective hypothermia, or electrical stimuli and used to perform surgery on the heart. [cardio- + G. *plēgē,* stroke]

car·di·o·ple·gic (kahr′dē-ō-plē′jik) Relating to cardioplegia.

car·di·o·ple·gic ar·rest (kahr′dē-ō-plē′jik ă-rest′) Stoppage of electrical and mechanical cardiac activity, used by surgeons when operating on the heart.

car·di·op·to·si·a, car·di·op·to·sis (kahr′dē-op-tō′sē-ă, kahr′dē-op′tō-sis) A condition in which the heart is unduly movable and displaced downward, as distinguished from bathycardia. [cardio- + G. *ptōsis,* a falling]

car·di·o·pul·mo·nar·y (kahr′dē-ō-pul′mŏ-nār-ē) Relating to the heart and lungs. SYN pneumocardial.

car·di·o·pul·mo·nar·y by·pass (kahr′dē-ō-pul′mŏ-nār-ē bī′pas) Diversion of the blood flow returning to the heart through a pump oxygenator (heart-lung machine) and then returning it to the arterial side of the circulation; used in operations on the heart to maintain extracorporeal circulation.

car·di·o·pul·mo·na·ry ex·er·cise test (CPX) (kahr′dē-ō-pul′mŏ-nār-ē eks′ĕr-sīz test) Assessment of heart disease involving patient's use of a treadmill or cycling machine while attached to an ECG machine; measures oxygen use and evaluates electrical cardiac patterns.

car·di·o·pul·mo·nar·y mur·mur (kahr′dē-ō-pul′mŏ-nār-ē mŭr′mŭr) An innocent extracardiac murmur, synchronous with the heart's beat but disappearing when the breath is held, believed due to movement of air in a segment of lung compressed by the contracting heart.

car·di·o·pul·mo·nar·y re·sus·ci·ta·tion (CPR) (kahr′dē-ō-pul′mŏ-nār-ē rē-sŭs′i-tā′shŭn) Restoration of cardiac output and pulmonary ventilation following cardiac arrest and apnea, using artificial respiration and manual or mechanical closed chest compression or open chest cardiac massage.

car·di·o·pul·mo·nar·y splanch·nic nerves (kahr′dē-ō-pul′mŏ-nār-ē splăngk′nik nĕrvz) Visceral branches of the sympathetic trunks conveying postsynaptic sympathetic fibers to and visceral afferent fibers from viscera located above the diaphragm, mainly through the cardiac, pulmonary, and esophageal plexuses. The cervical and upper thoracic splanchnic nerves are part of this group.

car·di·o·py·lo·ric (kahr′dē-ō-pī-lōr′ik) Relating to the cardiac and pyloric extremities of the stomach.

car·di·o·re·nal (kahr′dē-ō-rē′năl) Relating to the heart and the kidney. SYN cardionephric, nephrocardiac.

car·di·o·res·pi·ra·tory train·ing (kahr′dē-ō-res′pir-ă-tōr-ē trān′ing) SYN endurance phase.

car·di·or·rha·phy (kahr′dē-ōr′ă-fē) Suture of the heart wall. [cardio- + G. *rhaphē,* suture]

car·di·or·rhex·is (kahr′dē-ō-rek′sis) Rupture of the heart wall. [cardio- + G. *rhēxis,* rupture]

car·di·o·se·lec·tive (kahr′dē-ō-sĕ-lek′tiv) Denoting or having the properties of cardioselectivity.

car·di·o·se·lec·tiv·i·ty (kahr′dē-ō-sĕ-lek-tiv′i-tē) The relatively predominant cardiovascular pharmacologic effect of a drug with multipharmacologic effects; used especially when describing beta-blocking agents.

car·di·o·spasm (kahr′dē-ō-spazm) SYN esophageal achalasia.

car·di·o·sphyg·mo·graph (kahr′dē-ō-sfig′mō-graf) An instrument for recording graphically the movements of the heart and the radial pulse. [cardio- + G. *sphygmos,* pulse, + *graphō,* to write]

car·di·o·ta·chom·e·ter (kahr′dē-ō-tă-kom′ĕ-tĕr) An instrument for measuring heart rate over long periods. [cardio- + G. *tachos,* rapidity, + *metron,* measure]

car·di·o·tho·rac·ic ra·ti·o (kahr′dē-ō-thōr-as′ik rā′shē-ō) The ratio of the horizontal diameter of the heart to the inner diameter of the rib cage at its widest point as determined on a chest roentgenogram.

car·di·o·to·cog·ra·phy (CTG) (kahr′de-ō-tō-kog′ră-fē) Method of monitoring and recording fetal heart rate and uterine contractions during pregnancy and labor, allowing for assessment of fetal response and well-being. [cardio- + G. *tokos*, childbirth, + *graphē*, writing]

car·di·ot·o·my (kahr′dē-ot′ŏ-mē) **1.** Incision of a heart wall. **2.** Incision of the cardiac part of the stomach. [cardio- + G. *tomē,* incision]

car·di·o·ton·ic (kahr′dē-ō-ton′ik) Exerting a favorable, so-called tonic effect on the action of the heart; usually intended to indicate increased force of contraction. [cardio- + G. *tonos,* tension]

car•di•o•tox•ic (kahr′dē-ō-tok′sik) Having a deleterious effect on the action of the heart, due to poisoning of the cardiac muscle or of its conducting system. [cardio- + G. *toxikon,* poison]

car•di•o•val•vu•li•tis (kahr′dē-ō-val-vyū-lī′tis) Inflammation of the heart valves.

car•di•o•vas•cu•lar (kahr′dē-ō-vas′kyū-lăr) Relating to the heart and the blood vessels or the circulation. SYN cardiovasculare. [cardio- + L. *vasculum,* vessel]

car•di•o•vas•cu•lar drift (kahr′dē-ō-vas′kyū-lăr drift) The gradual time-dependent "drift" in several cardiovascular responses, most notably decreased stroke volume (with concomitant heart rate increase), during prolonged steady-rate exercise. The progressive increase in heart rate with cardiovascular drift during exercise decreases end-diastolic volume and hence stroke volume.

car•di•o•vas•cu•la•re (kahr-dē-ō-vas-kyū-lahr′rā) SYN cardiovascular.

car•di•o•ver•sion (kahr′dē-ō-vĕr′zhŭn) Restoration of the heart's rhythm to normal by electrical countershock. [cardio- + con*version*]

car•di•o•vert (kahr′dē-ō-vĕrt) To subject to cardioversion.

car•di•o•ver•ter (kahr′dē-ō-vĕr′tĕr) A machine used to perform cardioversion. See this page.

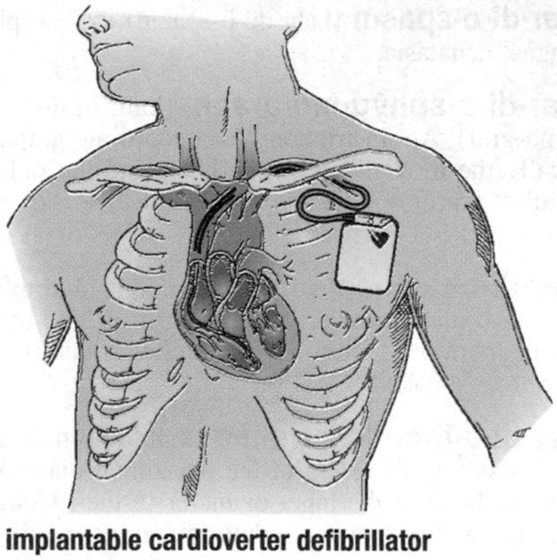

implantable cardioverter defibrillator

car•di•tis (kahr-dī′tis) Inflammation of the heart.

car•do san•to (kahr′dō sahn′tō) SYN blessed thistle. [Sp., holy thistle]

care (kār) **1.** MEDICINE, PUBLIC HEALTH a general term for the application of knowledge to benefit a person, family, or a community. **2.** To provide a medical or health care–related service to a patient.

Care Co•or•di•na•tor (kār kō-ōr′di-nā-tŏr) A health care provider who has been assigned a caseload of clients and has the responsibility of organizing the care provided. Generally responsible for organizing home care and insurance validation.

care•giv•er (kār′giv-ĕr) **1.** General term for a physician, nurse, or other health care practitioner who cares for patients. **2.** Any person, including a family member, who provides care or assistance to one who is ill.

care plan (kār plan) A carefully prepared outline of nursing care showing all of the patient's needs and the ways of meeting them; a dynamic document initiated at admission and subject to continuous reassessment and change by the nursing staff caring for the patient; typically includes nursing diagnoses, nursing interventions, and outcomes; ensures consistency of care; may be standardized or preprinted. SYN plan of care.

Car•ey Coombs mur•mur (kār′ē kūmz mŭr′mŭr) A blubbering apical middiastolic murmur occurring in the acute stage of rheumatic mitral valvulitis and disappearing as the valvulitis subsides.

C.A.R.F. Abbreviation for Commission on Accreditation of Rehabilitation Facilities.

Car•hart notch (kahr′hahrt noch) Isolated depression around 2000 Hz in the bone-conduction audiogram of patients with otosclerosis. SEE air-bone gap. SEE ALSO otosclerosis.

car•ies, pl. **car•ies** (kar′ēz, kar′ēz) Microbial destruction or necrosis of teeth. See page 261, B15. [L. dry rot]

ca•ri•na, pl. **ca•ri•nae** (kă-rī′nă, -nē) A term applied to anatomic structures forming a projecting central ridge. See page B16. [L. the keel of a boat]

car•i•nate (kar′i-nāt) Shaped like a ship's keel; relating to or resembling a carina.

car•i•nate ab•do•men (kar′i-nāt ab′dŏ-mĕn) A sloping of the sides with prominence of the central line of the abdomen.

cario- Prefix meaning caries. [L. *caries*]

car•i•o•gen•e•sis (kar′ē-ō-jen′ĕ-sis) The process of producing caries; the mechanism of caries production.

car•i•o•gen•ic (kar′ē-ō-jen′ik) Producing caries; usually said of diets.

car•i•o•ge•nic•i•ty (kar′ē-ō-jĕ-nis′i-tē) Potential for caries production.

car•i•ol•o•gy (kar′ē-ol′ŏ-jē) The study of dental caries and cariogenesis.

car•i•o•stat•ic (kar′ē-ō-stat′ik) Referring to a material or procedure that prevents or retards the formation and progression of dental caries. [L. *caries,* decay, + G. *statikos,* bringing to a stop]

car•i•ous (kar′ē-ŭs) Relating to or affected with caries.

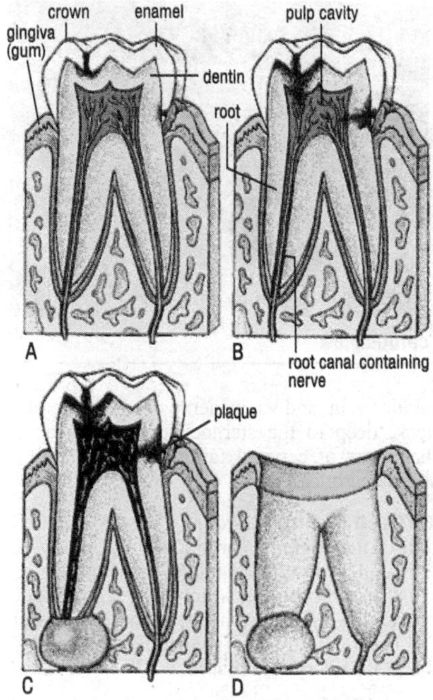

caries (zones of dental caries shown in black): (A) acid, enzymes, or both produced by oral bacteria break down enamel to form cavities; (B) bacteria penetrate dentin to invade pulp cavity; (C) infection destroys pulp and extends through left root canal to cause periapical disease; (D) tooth has been lost, leaving periapical cyst on lower left

Car•len tube (kahr′lĕn tūb) A double-lumen, flexible endobronchial tube used for bronchospirometry, for isolation of one lung to prevent contamination or secretions from the contralateral lung, or for ventilation of one lung.

car•line this•tle (kahr′lēn this′ĕl) Herbal made from *Carlina acaulis;* of purported therapeutic value in antisepsis and in treating menstrual disorders; seizures in users have been reported. SYN felon herb, mugwort.

Car•man sign (kahr′măn sīn) In gastric radiology, the appearance of a contrast-filled malignant ulcer, which does not extend beyond the line of the gastric wall as a benign ulcer would; also has a thick overhanging rim of tumor tissue.

car•min•a•tive (kahr-min′ă-tiv) An agent such as peppermint oil that is taken after a meal to facilitate belching through relaxation of the lower esophageal sphincter, thereby averting passage of swallowed air into the intestine as flatus. [L. *carmino,* pp. *-atus,* to card wool; special Mod. L. usage, to expel wind]

car•mine (kahr′mēn) [CI 75470] Red coloring matter used as a histology stain, derived from cochineal. [Mediev. L. *carminus,* contr. fr. *carmisinus,* fr. Ar. *qirmizē,* the cochineal insect]

car•min•o•phil, car•min•o•phile (kahr-min′ō-fil, -fīl) Staining readily with carmine dyes. [G. *phileō,* to love]

car•nas•si•al tooth (kahr-nas′ē-ăl tūth) A long-bladed premolar or molar of the Carnivora that has a cutting or shearing action, as in dogs or cats. SYN sectorial tooth.

Car•nett sign (kahr-net′ sīn) Disappearance of abdominal tenderness to palpation when the anterior abdominal muscles are contracted, indicating pain of intraabdominal origin; persistence of tenderness suggests a source in the abdominal wall, which is also indicated when tenderness is caused by gently pinching a fold of skin and fat between the thumb and forefinger.

car•ni•tine (kahr′ni-tēn) A trimethylammonium (betaine) derivative of gamma-amino-beta-hydroxybutyric acid, formed from N^E,N^E,N^E-trimethyllsine and from gamma-butyrobetaine; the L-isomer is a thyroid inhibitor found in muscle, liver, and meat extracts; L-carnitine is an acyl carrier with respect to the mitochondrial membrane; it thus stimulates fatty acid oxidation. [L. *caro, carn-*, flesh, + ine]

car•niv•o•rous (kahr-niv′ŏr-ŭs) Flesh-eating; having a diet composed largely of animal food. Cf. herbivorous.

Car•noy fix•a•tive (kahr′noy fik′să-tiv) Ethanol, chloroform, and acetic acid (6:3:1) or ethanol and acetic acid (3:1), an extremely rapid fixative used for glycogen preservation and as a nuclear fixative.

Ca•ro•li dis•ease, Ca•ro•li syn•drome (kah-rō-lē′ di-zēz′, kah-rō-lē′ sin′drōm) Congenital cystic dilation of the intrahepatic bile ducts, sometimes associated with intrahepatic stones and biliary obstruction.

carotenaemia [Br.] SYN carotenemia.

car•o•tene (kar′ō-tēn) Yellow-red pigments (lipochromes) widely distributed in plants and animals, notably in carrots, and closely related in structure to the xanthophylls and lycopenes and to the open-chain squalene; they include precursors of vitamin A (provitamin A carotenoids).

car•o•ten•e•mi•a (kar′ŏ-tĕ-nē′mē-ă) Carotene in the blood, especially pertaining to increased quantities, which sometimes cause a pale yellow-red pigmentation of the skin that may resemble icterus. SYN carotenaemia, xanthemia.

ca•rot•en•o•der•ma (kă-rot′ĕ-nō-dĕr′mă) SYN carotenosis cutis. [carotene + G. *derma*, skin]

ca•rot•e•noid (kă-rot′ĕ-noyd) **1.** Resembling carotene; having a yellow color. **2.** One of the carotenoids.

ca•rot•e•noids (kă-rot′ĕ-noydz) Generic term for a class of carotenes and their oxygenated derivatives (xanthophylls). Many carotenoids have anticancer activities.

car·o·te·no·sis cu·tis (kar′ŏ-tē-nō′sis kū′tis) A harmless reversible yellow coloration of the skin caused by an increase in carotene content. SYN carotenoderma.

ca·rot·i·co·cav·er·nous fis·tu·la (kă-rot′i-kō-kav′ĕr-nŭs fis′chū-lă) SYN carotid-cavernous fistula.

ca·rot·i·co·tym·pan·ic (kă-rot′i-kō-tim-pan′ik) Relating to the carotid canal and the tympanum.

ca·rot·i·co·tym·pan·ic ar·ter·ies (of in·ter·nal ca·rot·id ar·ter·y) (kă-rot′i-kō-tim-pan′ik ahr′tĕr-ēz in-tĕr′năl kă-rot′id ahr′tĕr-ē) Small branches from the petrous part of the internal carotid artery supplying the tympanic cavity; anastomose with the anterior tympanic and maxillary arteries.

ca·rot·id (kă-rot′id) Pertaining to any carotid structure. [G. *karōtides,* the carotid arteries, fr. *karoō,* to put to sleep (because compression of the c. artery results in unconsciousness)]

ca·rot·id bod·y (kă-rot′id bod′ē) A small epithelioid structure located just above the bifurcation of the common carotid artery on each side. It serves as a chemoreceptor organ responsive to oxygen lack, carbon dioxide excess, and increased hydrogen ion concentration. SYN intercarotid body.

ca·rot·id bru·it (kă-rot′id brū-ē′) A systolic murmur heard in the neck but not at the aortic area; any bruit produced by blood flow in a carotid artery.

ca·rot·id ca·nal (kă-rot′id kă-nal′) A passage through the petrous part of the temporal bone from its inferior surface upward, medially, and forward to the apex where it opens into the foramen lacerum. It transmits the internal carotid artery and plexuses of veins and autonomic nerves. SYN canalis caroticus [TA].

ca·rot·id-cav·ern·ous fis·tu·la (kă-rot′id-kav′ĕr-nŭs fis′chū-lă) A fistulous communication between the cavernous sinus and the traversing internal carotid artery, of spontaneous or traumatic origin; common manifestations are a pulsating unilateral exophthalmos and a detectable cranial bruit. SYN caroticocavernous fistula.

ca·rot·id gan·gli·on (kă-rot′id gang′glē-ŏn) A small ganglionic swelling on filaments from the internal carotid plexus, lying on the undersurface of the carotid artery in the cavernous sinus.

ca·rot·id pulse (kă-rot′id pŭls) A palpable rhythmic expansion of the common carotid artery in the neck; palpated during adult CPR. See this page.

ca·rot·id sheath (kă-rot′id shēth) The dense fibrous investment of the carotid artery, internal jugular vein, and vagus nerve on each side of the neck, deep to the sternocleidomastoid muscle; the layers of cervical fascia blend with it. SYN vagina carotica [TA].

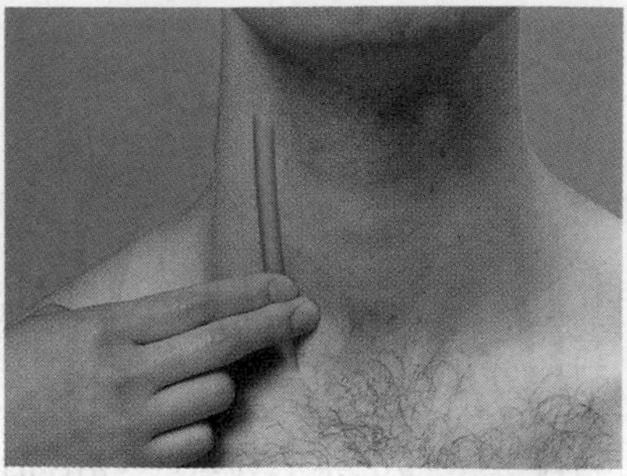
carotid pulse

ca·rot·id si·nus (kă-rot′id sī′nŭs) A slight dilation of the common carotid artery at its bifurcation into external and internal carotids; it contains baroreceptors, which, when stimulated, cause slowing of the heart, vasodilation, and a fall in blood pressure; is innervated primarily by the glossopharyngeal nerve.

ca·rot·id si·nus mas·sage (kă-rot′id sī′nŭs mă-sahzh′) Therapeutic manipulation of the carotid sinus in treatment of supraventricular tachycardia.

ca·rot·id si·nus re·flex (kă-rot′id sī′nus rē′fleks) A normal reflex relating to the carotid sinus syndrome, which results from hypersensitivity or hyperactivation of the carotid sinus.

ca·rot·id si·nus syn·co·pe (kă-rot′id sī′nŭs sing′kŏ-pē) Syncope resulting from overactivity of the carotid sinus; attacks may be spontaneous or produced by pressure on a sensitive carotid sinus.

ca·rot·id si·nus syn·drome (kă-rot′id sī′nŭs sin′drōm) Stimulation of a hyperactive carotid sinus, causing a marked fall in blood pressure due to vasodilation, cardiac slowing, or both; syncope with or without convulsions or A-V block may occur.

ca·rot·id tri·an·gle (kă-rot′id trī′ang-gĕl) A space bounded by the superior belly of the omohyoid muscle, anterior border of the sternocleidomastoid, and posterior belly of the digastric; it contains the bifurcation of the common carotid artery.

ca·rot·o·dyn·i·a (kă-rot′ō-din′ē-ă) Pain caused by pressure on the carotid artery. [G. *odynē,* pain]

car·pal (kahr′păl) Relating to the carpus.

car·pal bones (kahr′păl bōnz) Eight bones arranged in two rows that articulate proximally with the radius and indirectly with the ulna, and

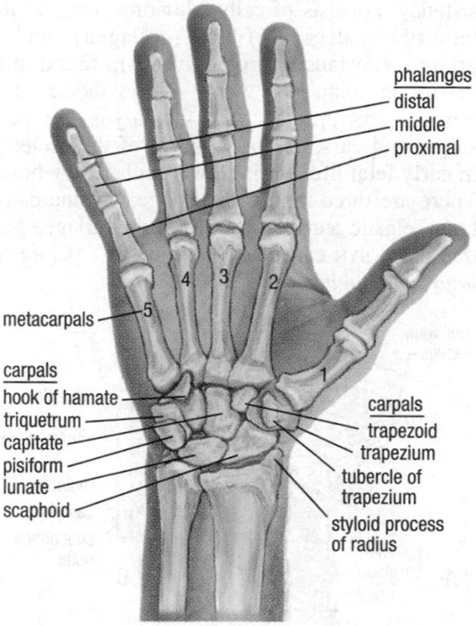

carpal bones

distally with the five metacarpal bones. See this page. SYN carpus (2) [TA].

car·pal joints (kahr′păl joynts) **1.** SYN intercarpal joints. **2.** SYN wrist joint.

car·pal tun·nel (kahr′păl tŭn′ĕl) The passageway deep to the transverse carpal ligament between tubercles of the scaphoid and trapezoid bones on the radial side and the pisiform and hook of the hamate on the ulnar side, through which the median nerve and the flexor tendons of the fingers and thumb pass. SYN canalis carpi [TA].

i **car·pal tun·nel syn·drome** (kahr′păl tŭn′ĕl sin′drōm) A common nerve entrapment syndrome, characterized by nocturnal hand paresthesia and pain, and sometimes sensory loss and wasting of muscle in the median nerve distribution; caused by entrapment of the median nerve at the wrist, within the carpal tunnel. See page B24.

car·pec·to·my (kahr-pek′tŏ-mē) Excision of a portion or all of the carpus. [G. *karpos,* wrist, + *ektomē,* excision]

car·pen·ter's herb (kahr′pĕn-tĕrz ĕrb) SYN bugleweed.

Car·pen·ter syn·drome (kahr′pĕn-tĕr sin′drōm) The association of primary hypothyroidism, primary adrenocortical insufficiency, and diabetes mellitus.

carp mouth (kahrp mowth) A mouth like that of the carp, with downturning of the corners; observed in Cornelia de Lange syndrome and Silver-Russell dwarfism.

Car·po·gly·phus (kahr-pō-glif′ŭs) A genus of mites including *Carpoglyphus passularum,* the fruit mite, which causes a form of dermatitis among handlers of dried fruit. [G. *karpos,* fruit, + *glyphō,* to carve]

car·po·met·a·car·pal (kahr′pō-met′ă-kahr′păl) Relating to both carpus and metacarpus.

car·po·met·a·car·pal joints (kahr′pō-met′ă-kahr′păl joynts) The synovial joints between the carpal and metacarpal bones; these are all plane joints except that of the thumb, which is saddle-shaped.

car·po·ped·al (kahr′pō-ped′ăl) Relating to the wrist and the foot, or the hands and feet; denoting especially carpopedal spasm. [G. *karpos,* wrist, + L. *pes* (*ped-*), foot]

car·po·ped·al con·trac·tion (kahr′pō-ped′ăl kŏn-trak′shŭn) SYN carpopedal spasm.

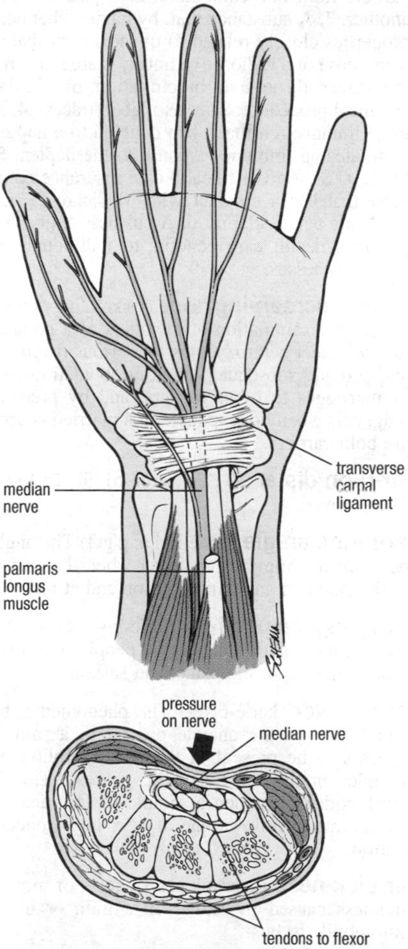

carpal tunnel syndrome

car•po•ped•al spasm (kahr′pō-ped′ăl spazm) Spasm of the feet and hands observed in hyperventilation, calcium deprivation, and tetany: flexion of the hands at the wrists and of the fingers at the metacarpophalangeal joints and extension of the fingers at the phalangeal joints; the feet are dorsiflexed at the ankles and the toes plantar flexed. SYN carpopedal contraction.

car•pus, gen. and pl. **car•pi** (kahr′pŭs, -pī) [TA] **1.** SYN wrist. **2.** SYN carpal bones. [Mod. L. fr. Gr. *karpos*]

Car•rel treat•ment (kah-rel′ trēt′mĕnt) Treatment of wound surfaces by intermittent flushing with Dakin solution (sodium hypochlorite and boric acid in a dilute, neutral solution).

car•ri•er (kar′ē-ĕr) **1.** A person or animal harboring a specific infectious agent in the absence of clinical disease symptoms and serving as a potential source of infection. **2.** Any chemical capable of accepting an atom, radical, or subatomic particle from one compound, then passing it to another. **3.** A substance that, by having chemical properties closely related to or indistinguishable from those of a radioactive tracer, is able to carry the tracer through a precipitation or similar chemical procedure. SEE ALSO label, tracer. **4.** A large immunogen that when coupled to a hapten facilitates an immune response to the hapten. **5.** In the U.S., a private health care insurance company that has a contract with Medicare to pay Medicare part B claims. **6.** A business entity that provides health care benefits to individuals or other businesses.

car•ri•er screen•ing (kar′ē-ĕr skrēn′ing) Indiscriminate examination of members of a population to detect heterozygotes for serious disorders and provide subsequent counsel about the risks of marriages to other carriers, and by prenatal diagnosis when both spouses in a married couple are both carriers.

Car•ri•ón dis•ease (kah-rē-ōn[h]′ di-zēz′) SYN Oroya fever.

car•ry•ing an•gle (kar′ē-ing ang′gĕl) The angle between the humerus and ulna when the arm is in the standard anatomic position and at rest.

car•ry•ing ca•pac•i•ty (kar′ē-ing kă-pas′i-tē) An estimate of the number of people that a region, a nation, or the planet can sustain.

car•ry-o•ver (kar′ē-ō′vĕr) The phenomenon by which part of the analyte present in a sample appears to be present in the next or following samples in the same analytic process. This is most noticeable when a sample of low analyte concentration follows one of very high concentration.

car sick•ness (kahr sik′nĕs) A form of motion sickness caused by riding on a train or in an automobile or bus.

i **car•ti•lage** (kahr′ti-lăj) A connective tissue characterized by its nonvascularity and firm consistency; consists of cells (chondrocytes), an interstitial matrix of fibers (collagen), and a ground substance (proteoglycans); found primarily in joints, the walls of the thorax, and tubular structures such as the larynx, air passages, and ears; comprises most of the skeleton in early fetal life, but is slowly replaced by bone. There are three kinds of cartilage: hyaline cartilage, elastic cartilage, and fibrocartilage. See this page. SYN cartilago [TA], gristle. [L. *cartilago* (*cartilagin-*), gristle]

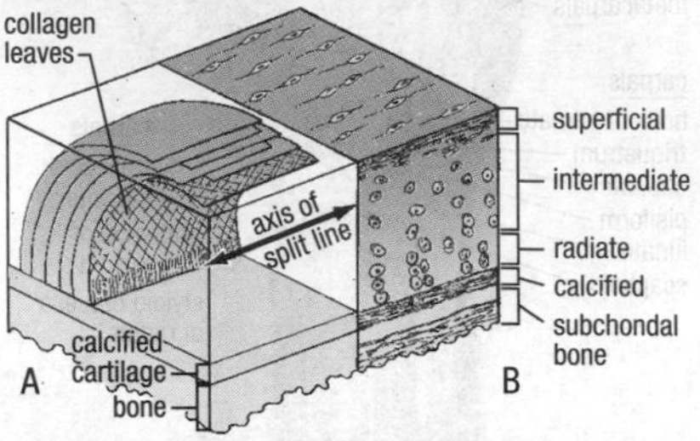

articular cartilage: (A) the organization of collagen fibers into "leaves" with varying structure and organization through the thickness of the cartilage (the leaves of collagen are connected by small fibers not shown in the figure); (B) the four zones of the cartilage: superficial, intermediate, radiate and calcified

car•ti•lage bone (kahr′ti-lăj bōn) SYN endochondral bone.

car•ti•lage cap•sule (kahr′ti-lăj kap′sŭl) The more intensely basophilic matrix in hyaline cartilage surrounding the lacunae in which the cartilage cells lie. SYN territorial matrix.

car•ti•lage-hair hy•po•pla•si•a (kahr′ti-lăj-hār hī′pō-plā′zē-ă) A skeletal dysplasia prevalent among the Amish, characterized by short-limb dwarfism; sparse, light-colored hair; T-cell immunologic defects rendering them susceptible to infections; and radiographic findings of metaphyseal dysplasia. Autosomal recessive inheritance, the gene maps to 9p. SYN McKusick metaphysial dysplasia.

car•ti•lage la•cu•na (kahr′ti-lăj lă-kū′nă) A cavity within the matrix of cartilage, occupied by a chondrocyte. SYN cartilage space.

car•ti•lage ma•trix (kahr′ti-lăj mā′triks) The intercellular substance of cartilage consisting of fibers and ground substance.

car•ti•lage space (kahr′ti-lăj spās) SYN cartilage lacuna.

car•ti•la•gi•nes (kahr-ti-laj′i-nēz) Plural of cartilago.

car•ti•la•gi•nes tra•che•a•les (kahr-ti-laj′i-nēz trā-kē-ā′lēz) [TA] SYN tracheal cartilages.

car•ti•lag•i•noid (kahr-ti-laj′i-noyd) SYN chondroid (1).

car•ti•lag•i•nous (kahr-ti-laj′i-nŭs) Relating to or consisting of cartilage. SYN chondral.

car•ti•lag•i•nous joint (kahr-ti-laj′i-nŭs joynt) A joint in which the apposed bony surfaces are united by cartilage. SYN synarthrodial joint (2).

car•ti•la•go, pl. **car•ti•la•gi•nes** (kahr-ti-lā′gō, kahr-ti-laj′i-nēz) [TA] SYN cartilage. [L. gristle]

car•ti•la•go ar•y•te•noi•de•a (kahr-ti-lā′gō ar′i-tē-noy′dē-ă) [TA] SYN arytenoid cartilage.

car•ti•la•go au•ric•u•lae (kahr-ti-lā′gō aw-rik′yū-lē) [TA] SYN auricular cartilage.

car•ti•la•go cor•ni•cu•la•ta (kahr-ti-lā′gō kōr-nik-yū-lā′tă) [TA] SYN corniculate cartilage.

car•ti•la•go cos•ta•lis (kahr-ti-lā′gō kos-tā′lis) [TA] SYN costal cartilage.

car•ti•la•go cri•coi•de•a (kahr-ti-lā′gō krī-koy′dē-ă) [TA] SYN cricoid cartilage.

car•ti•la•go cu•ne•i•for•mis (kahr-ti-lā′gō kyū′nē-i-fōr′mis) [TA] SYN cuneiform cartilage.

car•ti•la•go ep•i•glot•ti•ca (kahr-ti-lā′gō ep-i-glot′i-kă) [TA] SYN epiglottic cartilage.

car•ti•la•go ep•i•phy•si•a•lis (kahr-ti-lā′gō ep′i-fis-ē-ā′lis) [TA] SYN epiphysial plate.

car•ti•la•go na•si la•te•ra•lis (kahr-ti-lā′gō nā′sī lat-ĕr-ā′lis) [TA] SYN lateral cartilage of nose.

car•ti•la•go thy•roi•de•a (kahr-ti-lā′gō thi-roy′dē-ă) [TA] SYN thyroid cartilage.

car•ti•la•go vo•me•ro•na•sa•lis (kahr-ti-lā′gō vō′mĕr-ō-nā-sā′lis) [TA] SYN vomeronasal cartilage.

ca•run•cle (kar′ŭng-kĕl) SYN caruncula.

ca•run•cu•la, pl. **ca•run•cu•lae** (kă-rŭng′kyū-lă, -lē) A small, fleshy protuberance, or similarly shaped structure. SYN caruncle. [L. a small fleshy mass, fr. *caro,* flesh]

Ca•rus curve, **Ca•rus cir•cle** (kahr′ŭs kŭrv, kahr′ŭs sĭr′kĕl) An imaginary curved line obtained from a mathematical formula, supposed to indicate the outlet of the pelvic canal.

Car•val•lo sign (kahr-vah′yō sīn) An increase in the intensity of the pansystolic murmur of tricuspid regurgitation during or at the end of inspiration, which distinguishes tricuspid from mitral involvement.

carv•i fruc•tus (kahr′vī fruk′tŭs) SYN caraway. [M.L. *carvi,* fr. Ar. *karawyā,* fr. G. *karon,* + L. *fructus,* fruit]

♻ **caryo-** Combining form meaning nucleus. SEE karyo-. [G. *karyon,* nut, kernel]

CAS Abbreviation for Chemical Abstracts Service.

Ca•sal neck•lace (kah-sahl′ nek′lăs) A dermatitis partly or completely encircling the lower part of the neck in pellagra.

cas•cade (kas-kād′) **1.** A series of sequential interactions, as of a physiologic process, which after being initiated continues to the final one; each interaction is activated by the preceding one, sometimes with cumulative effect. **2.** To spill over, especially rapidly. [Fr., fr. It. *cascare,* to fall]

cas•cade stom•ach (kas-kād′ stŏm′ăk) A radiographic description: when contrast material is swallowed while the patient is in the upright position, the gastric fundus acts as a reservoir until contrast overflows (cascades) into the antrum; a normal variant in a horizontal stomach.

cas•car•a sa•gra•da (kas-kar′ă să-grā′dă) An herbal remedy made from the bark of *Rhamnus purshiana;* a strong purgative laxative. SYN sacred bark. [Sp. *cascara,* rind, peel, + *sagrada,* sacred]

case (kās) **1.** An instance of disease. Cf. patient. **2.** A box or container. [L. *casus,* an occurrence]

ca•se•a•tion (kā-sē-ā′shŭn) A form of coagulation necrosis in which the necrotic tissue resembles cheese and contains a mixture of protein and fat that is absorbed very slowly; occurs particularly in tuberculosis. SEE ALSO caseous necrosis. [L. *caseus,* cheese]

case def•i•ni•tion (kās def′i-nish′ŭn) Established parameters that define a case in an outbreak investigation.

case fa•tal•i•ty rate (kās fă-tal′i-tē rāt) The proportion of people contracting a disease who die of that disease.

case his•to•ry (kās his′tŏr-ē) Detailed recension, generally written, of all particulars of a patient's familial, medical, and social involvements related to a condition or disease process.

ca•sein (kā′sēn) The principal protein of cow's milk and the chief constituent of cheese.

case man•age•ment (kās man′ăj-mĕnt) A process in the U.S. whereby covered people with specific health care needs are identified and an efficient treatment plan is formulated and implemented to produce the most cost-effective outcomes; usually done in reference to participants in a managed care program.

case mix (kās miks) The relative numbers of various types of patients being treated as categorized by disease-related groups, severity of illness, rate of consumption of resources, and other indicators; used as a tool for managing and planning health care services.

ca•se•ous (kā′sē-ŭs) Pertaining to or manifesting the features of tissue affected by caseation.

ca•se•ous de•gen•er•a•tion (kā′sē-ŭs dĕ-jen′ĕr-ā′shŭn) SYN caseous necrosis.

ca•se•ous ne•cro•sis, ca•se•a•tion ne•cro•sis (kā′sē-ŭs nĕ-krō′sis, kā-sē-ā′shŭn nĕ-krō′sis) Necrosis characteristic of certain inflammations (e.g., tuberculosis, histoplasmosis); affected tissue manifests the friable, crumbly consistency and dull, opaque quality observed in cheese. SYN caseous degeneration.

ca•se•ous os•te•i•tis (kā′sē-ŭs os-tē-ī′tis) Tuberculous caries in bone.

case re•serve (kās rē-zĕrv′) The dollar amount stated in health care claims file that represents an estimate of the unpaid balance.

Ca•so•ni an•ti•gen (kah-sō′nē an′ti-jen) Skin-test antigen composed of sterile hydatid fluid; used in test for hydatid disease.

cas•sette (kă-set′) **1.** A plate, film, or tape holder for use in photography or radiography. A radiographic cassette contains one or two intensifying screens and a sheet of x-ray film. **2.** A perforated holder in which tissue blocks are placed for paraffin embedding. [Fr., dim. of *casse,* box]

cast (kast) **1.** An object formed by solidification of a liquid poured into a mold. **2.** Rigid encasement of a part, as with plaster, fiberglass, or plastic, to immobilize (e.g., long-leg cast, short-leg cast) a fractured bone. **3.** An elongated or cylindric mold formed in a tubular structure (e.g., renal tubule, bronchiole) that may be observed in histologic sections or in material such as urine or sputum; results from inspissation of fluid material secreted or excreted in the tubular structures. **4.** Restraint of a large animal, usually a horse, with ropes and harnesses in a recumbent position. **5.** DENTISTRY a positive reproduction of the form of the tissues of the upper or lower jaw, formed by pouring gypsum or metal into an impression of the tissues, allowing it to set, and then removing the impression. Resulting structure provides a base on which dental restorations may be fabricated. [M.E. *kasten,* fr. O.Norse *kasta*]

cast brace (kast brās) A specially designed plaster or plastic cast incorporating hinges and other brace components; used in the treatment of fractures to promote early activity and early joint motion.

cas•tor bean (kast′ŏr bēn) Herbal agent made from the seed of *Ricinus communis;* widely used as a cathartic laxative; overdosage can produce gastrointestinal problems. SYN Mexico seed, peima.

cas•tor oil (kas′tŏr oyl) Fatty oil from castor beans used as a cathartic or lubricant.

cas•trate (kas′trāt) To remove the testicles or the ovaries. [L. *castro,* pp. *-atus,* to deprive of generative power (male or female)]

cas•tra•tion (kas-trā′shŭn) **1.** Removal of the testicles or ovaries. **2.** SEE castration complex, castrate.

cas•tra•tion cells (kas-trā′shŭn selz) Altered basophilic cells of the anterior lobe of the pituitary that develop following castration; the body of the cell is occupied by a large vacuole that displaces the nucleus to the periphery, giving the cell a resemblance to a signet ring. SYN signet ring cells.

cas•tra•tion com•plex (kas-trā′shŭn kom′pleks) **1.** A child's fear of injury to the genitals by the parent of the same sex as punishment for unconscious guilt over oedipal feelings. **2.** Fantasied loss of the penis by a female or fear of its actual loss by a male. **3.** Unconscious fear of injury from those in authority.

ca•su•al•ty (kazh′ū-ăl-tē) Injury or death from accident. [L. *casus,* a falling, accident]

CAT (kat) Acronym and abbreviation for computed axial tomography (usage obsolete); chloramphenicol acetyl transferase.

♻ **cata-** Combining form meaning down; opposite of ana-. SEE ALSO kata-. Cf. de-. [G. *kata,* down]

cat•a•bi•ot•ic (kat′ă-bī-ot′ik) Used up in the carrying on of the vital processes other than growth, or in the performance of function, referring to the energy derived from food. [cata- + G. *biōtikos,* relating to life]

cat•a•bol•ic (kat′ă-bol′ik) Relating to or promoting catabolism.

ca•tab•o•lism (kă-tab′ō-lizm) **1.** The breaking down in the body of complex chemical compounds into simpler ones, often accompanied by the liberation of energy. **2.** The sum of all degradative processes. Cf. anabolism, metabolism. [G. *katabolē,* a casting down]

ca•tab•o•lite (kă-tab′ō-līt) Any product of catabolism.

ca•tab•o•lite (gene) ac•ti•va•tor pro•tein (CAP) (kă-tab′ō-līt jēn ak′ti-vā-tŏr prō′tēn) A protein that can be activated by cAMP, whereon it affects the action of RNA polymerase by binding with it or near it on the DNA to be transcribed. SYN cAMP receptor protein.

cat•a•chron•o•bi•ol•o•gy (kat′ă-kron′ō-bī-ol′ŏ-jē) The study of the deleterious effects of time on a living system. [cata- + G. *chronos,* time, + biology]

cat•a•crot•ic (kat′ă-krot′ik) Relating to or characterized by catacrotism.

ca•tac•ro•tism (kă-tak′rō-tizm) An anomaly of the pulse with one or more secondary expansions of the artery following the main beat, producing secondary upward waves on the downstroke of the pulse tracing. [cata- + G. *krotos,* beat]

cat•a•di•crot•ic (kat′ă-dī-krot′ik) Relating to or characterized by catadicrotism.

cat•a•di•cro•tism (kat′ă-dī′krō-tizm) An anomaly of the pulse marked by two minor expansions of the artery following the main beat, producing two secondary upward waves on the downstroke of the pulse tracing. [cata + G. *di-*, two, + *krotos*, beat]

cat•a•dro•mous (kat′ă-drō′mus) Migrating from fresh water to the ocean to spawn. SEE ALSO anadromous.

cat•a•gen (kat′ă-jen) A regressing phase of the hair growth cycle during which cell proliferation ceases, the hair follicle shortens, and an anchored club hair is produced.

cat•a•gen•e•sis (kat′ă-jen′ĕ-sis) SYN involution. [cata- + G. *genesis*, origin]

cat•a•lase (kat′ă-lās) A hemoprotein catalyzing the decomposition of hydrogen peroxide to water and oxygen ($2H_2O_2 \rightarrow O_2 + 2H_2O$).

cat•a•lep•sy (kat′ă-lep-sē) A morbid condition characterized by waxy rigidity of the limbs, lack of response to stimuli, mutism, and inactivity; occurs with some psychoses, especially catatonic schizophrenia. [G. *katalēpsis*, a seizing, catalepsy, fr. *kata*, down, + *lēpsis*, a seizure]

cat•a•lep•tic (kat′ă-lep′tik) Relating to, or suffering from, catalepsy.

cat•a•lep•toid (kat′ă-lep′toyd) Simulating or resembling catalepsy.

ca•tal•y•sis (kă-tal′i-sis) The effect that a catalyst exerts on a chemical reaction. [G. *katalysis*, dissolution]

cat•a•lyst (kat′ă-list) A substance that accelerates a chemical reaction but is not consumed or changed permanently thereby.

cat•a•lyt•ic (kat′ă-lit′ik) Relating to or effecting catalysis.

cat•a•lyze (kat′ă-līz) To act as a catalyst.

cat•a•me•ni•al pneu•mo•tho•rax (kat′ă-mē′nē-ăl nū′mō-thōr′aks) Pneumothorax occurring in young women during menstruation, usually on the right side.

cat•am•ne•sis (kat′am-nē′sis) The medical history of a patient after an illness; the follow-up history. [cata- + G *mnēmē*, memory]

cat•am•nes•tic (kat′am-nes′tik) Related to catamnesis.

cat•a•pha•si•a (kat′ă-fā′zē-ă) SYN verbigeration. [cata- + G. *phasis*, a saying]

ca•taph•o•ra (kă-taf′ŏr-ă) Semicoma or somnolence interrupted by intervals of partial consciousness. [G. a falling down]

cat•a•pla•si•a, cat•a•pla•sis (kat′ă-plā′zē-ă, -plā′sis) A degenerative change in cells or tissues that is the reverse of constructive or developmental change; a return to an earlier or embryonic stage. SYN retrogression. [cata- + G. *plasis*, a molding]

cat•a•plec•tic (kat′ă-plek′tik) **1.** Developing suddenly. **2.** Pertaining to cataplexy.

cat•a•plex•y (kat′ă-plek-sē) A transient attack of extreme generalized muscular weakness, often precipitated by an emotional state such as laughing, surprise, fear, or anger. [cata- + G. *plēxis*, a blow, stroke]

cat•a•ract (kat′ăr-akt) Complete or partial opacity of the ocular lens. See this page, B27 . [L. *cataracta* fr. G. *katarrhaktes*, a downrushing, a waterfall, fr. *katarrhegnymi*, to break down, rush down]

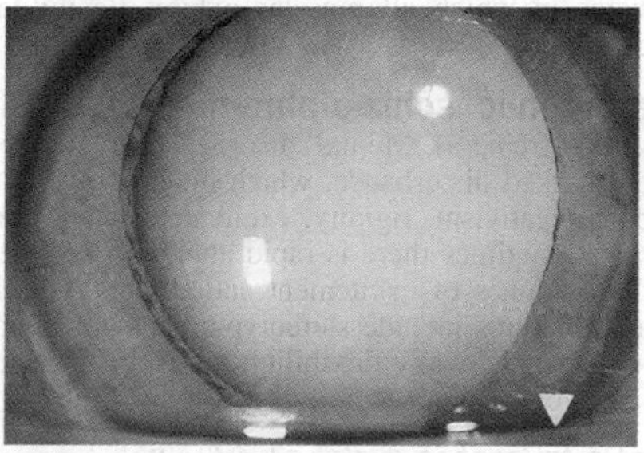

mature cataract with complete opacification of lens

cat•a•rac•to•gen•ic (kat′ă-rak-tō-jen′ik) Cataract-producing.

cat•a•rac•tous (kat′ă-rak′tŭs) Relating to a cataract.

ca•tarrh (kă-tahr′) Inflammation of a mucous membrane with increased flow of mucus or exudate. [G. *katarrheō*, to flow down]

ca•tarrh•al (kă-tahr′ăl) Relating to or affected by catarrh.

ca•tarrh•al gas•tri•tis (kă-tahr′ăl gas-trī′tis) Stomach inflammation with excessive secretion of mucus.

ca•tarrh•al in•flam•ma•tion (kă-tahr′ăl in′flă-mā′shŭn) An inflammatory process that may occur in any mucous membrane, characterized by hyperemia of the mucosal vessels, edema of the interstitial tissue, enlargement of the secretory epithelial cells, and an irregular layer of viscous, mucinous material on the surface.

cat•a•stal•sis (kat′ă-stal′sis) A contraction wave resembling ordinary peristalsis but not preceded by a zone of inhibition. [G. *kata-stellō*, to put in order, check]

cat•a•stal•tic (kat′ă-stal′tik) **1.** Inhibitory, restricting, or restraining. **2.** An inhibitory or checking agent, such as an astringent or antispasmodic. [cata- + G. *staltos*, contracted, fr. *stellō*, to contract]

cat•a•stroph•ic re•ac•tion (kat′ă-strof′ik rē-ak′shŭn) The disorganized behavior that is the response to a severe shock or threatening situation with which the person cannot cope.

cat•a•to•ni•a (kat′ă-tō′nē-ă) A syndrome of psychomotor disturbances characterized by periods of physical rigidity, negativism, or stupor; may occur in schizophrenia, mood disorders, or organic mental disorders. [G. *katatonos*, stretching down, depressed, fr. *kata*, down, + *tonos*, tone]

cat•a•ton•ic, cat•a•to•ni•ac (kat′ă-ton′ik, -tō′nē-ak) Relating to, or characterized by, catatonia.

cat•a•ton•ic ri•gid•i•ty (kat′ă-ton′ik ri-jid′i-tē) Rigidity associated with catatonic psychotic states in which all muscles exhibit flexibilitas cerea.

cat•a•ton•ic schiz•o•phre•ni•a (kat′ă-ton′ik skits′ō-frē′nē-ă) Mental disorder characterized by marked disturbance, which may involve stupor, negativism, rigidity, excitement, or posturing; sometimes there is rapid alteration between the extremes of excitement and stupor. Associated features include stereotypic behavior, mannerisms, and waxy flexibility; mutism is particularly common.

cat•a•tri•crot•ic (kat′ă-trī-krot′ik) Relating to or characterized by catatricrotism.

cat•a•tri•cro•tism (kat′ă-trī′krō-tizm) An anomaly or condition of the pulse marked by three minor expansions of the artery following the main beat, producing three secondary upward waves on the downstroke of the pulse tracing. [cata- + G. *tri-*, three, + *krotos*, beat]

catch (kach) **1.** To capture or seize. **2.** The act of catching, or that which is caught. [O.Fr. *cachier*, to chase, fr. L. *capto*, to seize]

cat•e•chol•a•mines (kat′ĕ-kol′ă-mēnz) Pyrocatechols with an alkylamine side chain; examples of biochemical interest are epinephrine, norepinephrine, and L-dopa. Catecholamines are major elements in responses to stress.

cat•e•chol ox•i•dase (di•mer•iz•ing) (kat′ĕ-kol ok′si-dās dī′mĕr-īz-ing) An enzyme oxidizing a catechol, with O_2, to a diphenylenedioxide quinone (e.g., 4 catechol + $3O_2 \rightarrow 2$ dibenzo[1,4]-2,3-dione + $6H_2O$).

cat•e•gor•ic trait (kat′ĕ-gōr′ik trāt) GENETICS a feature that can conveniently and effectively be analyzed by sorting into classes either because there is no satisfactory way of measuring it or because it falls into natural classes so that the variation among classes far exceeds that within classes; existence of categories suggests but does not prove the operation of a major, simple, underlying cause.

cat•e•gor•i•za•tion (kat′ĕ-gōr-ī-zā′shŭn) A process by which a hospital self-designates providing a specialized service; criteria may be internal or based on national standards. Differs from designation, which is a legal process with external review.

cat•en•ate (kat′ĕn-āt) To connect in a series of links like a chain. [L. *catenatus*, chained together, fr. *catena*, chain]

cat•en•in (kă-tē′nin) Cytoplasmic molecule that serves as a link between cadherins and the cytoskeleton of cells, allowing the formation of adherent junctions. There are two types: beta-catenin, which is linked to the cadherin itself, and alpha-catenin, which associates with actin microfilaments. [L. *catena*, chain, + -in]

cat•er•pil•lar (kat′ĕr-pil-ĕr) The wormlike larval stage of a butterfly or a moth. [M.E. *catirpeller*, fr. O.Fr. *cate*, cat, + *pelose*, hairy]

cat•er•pil•lar flap (kat′ĕr-pil-ĕr flap) A tubed flap transferred end-over-end (in stages) from the donor area to a distant recipient area. SYN waltzed flap.

cat•gut (kat′gŭt) An absorbable surgical suture material made from the collagenous fibers of the submucosa of certain animals, usually sheep or cows. [probably from *kit*, a small violin, through confusion with *kit*, a small cat]

ca•thar•sis (kă-thahr′sis) **1.** SYN purgation. **2.** The release or discharge of emotional tension or anxiety by psychoanalytically guided emotional reliving of past, especially repressed, events. [G. *katharsis*, purification, fr. *katharos*, pure]

ca•thar•tic (kă-thahr′tik) **1.** Relating to catharsis. **2.** An agent having purgative action (i.e., of the bowel).

ca•thec•tic (kă-thek′tik) Pertaining to cathexis.

cath•e•ter (kath′ĕ-tĕr) **1.** A flexible tube that enables passage of fluid from or into a body cavity or blood vessel. SEE ALSO line (3). **2.** A tube designed to be passed through the urethra into the bladder to drain it of urine; usually composed of latex, silicone, or soft plastic. [G. *kathetēr*, fr. *kathiēmi*, to send down]

cath•e•ter coil•ing sign (kath′ĕ-tĕr koyl′ing sīn) SYN Bergman sign.

cath•e•ter em•bo•lus (kath′ĕ-tĕr em′bō-lŭs) Coiled worm-shaped platelet and fibrin aggregates produced during vascular catheterization, originating on the catheter or its guide wire; embolization of the catheter itself.

catheterisation [Br.] SYN catheterization.

cath•e•ter•i•za•tion (kath′ĕ-tĕr-ī-zā′shŭn) Passage of a catheter. SYN catheterisation.

cath•e•ter spec•i•men of ur•ine (CSU) (kath′ĕ-tĕr spes′i-mĕn yūr′in) Specimen collected from an indwelling urinary catheter under clean conditions for testing.

ca•thex•is (kă-thek′sis) A conscious or unconscious attachment of psychic energy to an idea, object, or person. [G. *kathexis,* a holding in, retention]

cath•o•dal (C) (kath′ō-dăl) Of, pertaining to, or emanating from a cathode.

cath•ode (C) (kath′ōd) **1.** The negative pole of a galvanic battery or the electrode connected with it; the electrode to which positively charged ions (cations) migrate. Cf. anode. **2.** Negatively charged part of the x-ray tube head; it contains the tungsten filament. SYN negative electrode. [G. *kathodos,* a way down, fr. *kata,* down, + *hodos,* a way]

cat•i•on (kat′ī-on) An ion carrying a charge of positive electricity, therefore going to the negatively charged cathode. [G. *katiōn,* going down]

cat•i•on ex•change (kat′ī-on eks-chānj′) The process by which a cation in a liquid phase exchanges with another cation present as the counter-ion of a negatively charged solid polymer (cation exchanger). Cation exchange may be used chromatographically, to separate cations, and medicinally, to remove a cation. SEE ALSO anion exchange.

cat•i•on-ex•change res•in (kat′ī-on eks-chānj′ rez′in) SEE cation exchange.

cat•nip (kat′nip) Herbal made from *Nepeta cataria;* aside from its value in amusing cats (and their owners), the agent has been used in humans for its suggested value in treating GI problems, headache, urticaria, and as a sleep aid. SYN field balm.

cat's claw (kats klaw) Herbal prepared from fibers of *Uncaria tomentosa* and other *Uncaria* spp. Value suggested as therapy for inflammatory diseases and GI disorders; South American folk medicine uses it as a contraceptive. SYN samento.

cat•scratch dis•ease (CSD), cat•scratch fe•ver (kat′skrach di-zēz′, kat′skrach fē′vĕr) An infection that causes chronic benign adenopathy in most cases, especially in children and young adults, usually associated with a cat scratch or bite. In most cases it is caused by the bacterium *Bartonella henselae*. The lymphadenopathy usually resolves spontaneously within a period of several months. The infection may cause other clinical symptoms such as fever of unknown origin, encephalitis, microabscess in the liver and spleen, and osteomyelitis. SYN benign inoculation lymphoreticulosis, benign inoculation reticulosis, regional granulomatous lymphadenitis.

cau•da, pl. **cau•dae** (kaw′dă, -dē) [TA] SYN tail. [L. a tail]

cau•dad (kaw′dad) **1.** In a direction toward the tail. **2.** Situated nearer the tail in relation to a specific reference point; opposite of craniad. SEE ALSO inferior.

cau•da e•qui•na (kaw′dă ē-kwī′nă) [TA] The bundle of spinal nerve roots arising from the lumbosacral enlargement and medullary cone and running through the lumbar cistern (subarachnoid space) within the vertebral canal below the first lumbar vertebra; it comprises the roots of all the spinal nerves below the first lumbar. [L. horse tail]

cau•da e•qui•na syn•drome (kaw′dă ē-kwī′ nă sin′drōm) Dull pain in upper sacral region, with anesthesia or analgesia in buttocks, genitalia, or thigh; accompanied by disturbed bowel and bladder function. Indicative of pressure on the cauda equina, as from a tumor or degenerative disc disease. [L. horse tail]

cau•dal (kaw′dăl) **1.** Pertaining to the tail. **2.** VETERINARY ANATOMY denoting a position nearer to the tail. [Mod. L. *caudalis*]

cau•dal an•es•the•si•a (kaw′dăl an′es-thē′zē-ă) Regional anesthesia by injection of local anesthetic solution into the epidural space through the sacral hiatus.

cau•dal em•i•nence (kaw′dăl em′ī-nĕns) The taillike caudal end of the embryo; it does not, however, form a tail in human embryos. SYN end bud, tail bud.

cau•dal flex•ure (kaw′dăl flek′shŭr) The bend in the lumbosacral region of the embryo. SYN sacral flexure.

cau•dal trans•verse fis•sure (kaw′dăl trans-vĕrs′ fish′ŭr) SYN porta hepatis.

cau•date lobe (kaw′dāt lōb) SYN lobus caudatus.

cau•date nu•cle•us (kaw′dāt nū′klē-ŭs) An elongated curved mass of gray matter, consisting of an anterior thick portion, the caput or head, which protrudes into the anterior horn of the lateral ventricle, a portion extending along the floor of the body of the lateral ventricle, known as the corpus or body, and an elongated curved thin portion, the cauda or tail, which curves downward, backward, and forward in the temporal lobe in the wall of the lateral ventricle.

cau•date pro•cess (kaw′dāt pros′es) A narrow band of hepatic tissue connecting the caudate and right lobes of the liver posterior to the porta hepatis.

caul, cowl (kawl, kowl) **1.** The amnion, either as a piece of membrane capping the baby's head at birth or the whole membrane when delivered unruptured with the baby. SYN galea (4), veil (2), velum (2). **2.** SYN greater omentum. [Gaelic, *call,* a veil]

cau•li•flow•er ear (kawl′i-flow-ĕr ēr) Thickening and induration of the pinna and external ear with distortion of contours following extravasation of blood within its tissues; a chronic deformity following (usually) repeated trauma. Plastic or reconstructive surgery will generally improve appearance.

caumaesthesia [Br.] SYN caumesthesia.

cau·mes·the·si·a (kaw-mes-thē′zē-ă) Subjective heat sensation of uncomfortably high temperature; a type of thermal dysesthesia. SYN caumaesthesia. [G. *kauma,* heat, + *aisthēsis,* sensation]

cau·sal·gi·a (kaw-zal′jē-ă) Persistent severe burning sensation, usually following partial injury of a peripheral nerve, accompanied by trophic changes (thinning of skin, loss of sweat glands and hair follicles). [G. *kausis,* burning, + *algos,* pain]

caus·tic (kaws′tik) **1.** Exerting an effect resembling a burn. **2.** An agent producing this effect. **3.** Denoting a solution of a strong alkali (e.g., caustic soda, NaOH). [G. *kaustikos,* fr. *kaiō,* to burn]

cauterisation [Br.] SYN cauterization.

cauterise [Br.] SYN cauterize.

cau·ter·i·za·tion (kaw-tĕr-ī-zā′shŭn)The act of cauterizing. SEE ALSO cautery. SYN cauterisation.

cau·ter·ize (kaw′tĕr-īz) To apply a cautery; to burn with a cautery. SYN cauterise.

cau·ter·y (kaw′tĕr-ē) **1.** An agent or device used for scarring, burning, or cutting the skin or other tissues by means of heat, cold, electric current, or caustic chemicals. **2.** Use of a cautery. [G. *kautērion,* a branding iron]

ca·va (kā′vă) SEE inferior vena cava, superior vena cava.

ca·va·gram (kā′vă-gram) SYN cavogram.

ca·val (kā′văl) Relating to a vena cava.

cave (kāv) Any hollow or enclosed space or cavity. SEE ALSO cavern, cavity. SYN cavum.

ca·ve·a (kā′vē-ă) SYN cage.

ca·ve·a tho·ra·cis (kā′vē-ă thō-rā′sis) [TA] SYN thoracic cage.

ca·ve·o·la, pl. **ca·ve·o·lae** (kā-vē-ō′lă, -lē) A small pocket, vesicle, cave, or recess communicating with the outside of a cell and extending inward, indenting the cytoplasm and the cell membrane. Caveolae are considered to be sites of uptake of materials into the cell, expulsion of materials from the cell, or addition or removal of cell (unit) membrane to or from the cell surface. [L.]

cav·ern (kav′ĕrn) An anatomic cavity with many interconnecting chambers. SEE ALSO cave, cavity.

cav·er·nil·o·quy (kav′ĕr-nil′ō-kwē) Low-pitched resonant pectoriloquy heard over a lung cavity. [L. *caverna,* cavern, + *loquor,* to talk]

cav·er·ni·tis, **cav·er·no·si·tis** (kav′ĕr-nī′tis, kav′ĕr-nō-sī′tis) Inflammation of the corpus cavernosum penis.

cav·er·no·ma (kav′ĕr-ō′mă) A cavernous vascular tumor. [L. *caverna,* cave, hollow place, + *oma,* neoplasm]

cav·ern·ous (kav′ĕr-nŭs) Relating to a cavern or a cavity; containing many cavities.

cav·ern·ous an·gi·o·ma (kav′ĕr-nŭs an′jē-ō′mă) Vascular malformation composed of sinusoidal vessels without a large feeding artery.

cav·ern·ous bod·y (kav′ĕr-nŭs bod′ē) SEE corpus cavernosum clitoridis, corpus cavernosum penis.

cav·ern·ous he·man·gi·o·ma (kav′ĕr-nŭs hē-man′jē-ō′mă) A vascular malformation containing large blood-filled spaces, due apparently to dilation and thickening of the walls of the capillary loops; in the skin, extends more deeply than a capillary hemangioma and is less likely to regress spontaneously.

cav·ern·ous nerves of clit·o·ris (kav′ĕr-nŭs nĕrvz klit′ŏr-is) Nerves corresponding to the cavernous nerves of penis in the male, arising from the vesicular portion of the pelvic plexus. SYN nervi cavernosi clitoridis [TA].

cav·ern·ous nerves of pe·nis (kav′ĕr-nŭs nĕrvz pē′nis) Two nerves, major and minor, derived from the prostatic portion of the pelvic plexus supplying sympathetic and parasympathetic fibers to the helicine arteries and arteriovenous anastomoses of the corpus cavernosum stimulating erection. SYN nervi cavernosi penis [TA].

cav·ern·ous plex·us of con·chae (kav′ĕr-nŭs plek′sŭs kong′kē) Erectile tissue in the mucous membrane covering the conchae of the nasal cavity.

cav·ern·ous rale (kav′ĕr-nŭs rahl) A resonating, bubbling sound caused by air entering a cavity partly filled with fluid.

cav·ern·ous si·nus (kav′ĕr-nŭs sī′nŭs) A paired dural venous sinus on either side of the sella turcica, the two being connected by anastomoses, the anterior and posterior intercavernous sinus, in front of and behind the hypophysis, respectively, making thus the circular sinus; the cavernous sinus is unique among dural venous sinuses in being trabeculated; coursing within the sinus are the internal carotid artery and the abducent nerve. SYN sinus cavernosus [TA].

cav·ern·ous si·nus branch of in·ter·nal ca·rot·id ar·ter·y (kav′ĕr-nŭs sī′nŭs branch in-tĕr′năl kă-rot′id ahr′tĕr-ē) A number of small branches of the cavernous part of the internal carotid artery. SEE ganglionic branch of internal carotid artery, basal tentorial branch of internal carotid artery, marginal tentorial branch of internal carotid artery.

cav•ern•ous space (kav'ĕr-nŭs spās) An anatomic cavity with many interconnecting chambers.

cav•ern•ous trans•for•ma•tion of por•tal vein (kav'ĕr-nŭs trans-fōr-mā'shŭn pōr'tăl vān) Replacement of the portal vein by a number of collateral channels, a consequence of thrombosis.

cav•ern•ous veins of pe•nis (kav'ĕr-nŭs vānz pē'nis) The cavernous venous spaces in the erectile tissue of the penis.

CAVH Abbreviation for continuous arteriovenous hemofiltration.

cav•i•tar•y (kav'i-tār-ē) Relating to a cavity or having a cavity or cavities.

cav•i•tas, pl. **cav•i•ta•tes** (kav'i-tahs, -tā'tēs) SYN cavity. [Mod. L.]

cav•i•tate (kav'i-tāt) To form cavities in an organ or tissue.

cav•i•ta•tion (kav-i-tā'shŭn) **1.** Formation of a cavity, as in the lung in tuberculosis. **2.** The production of small, vapor-containing bubbles or cavities in a liquid by ultrasound.

ca•vi•tis (kā-vī'tis) SYN celophlebitis.

cav•i•ty (kav'i-tē) **1.** A hollow space; hole. SEE cave, cavitas, cavernous space. **2.** Lay term for the loss of tooth structure due to dental caries. SYN cavitas. [L. *cavus,* hollow]

cav•i•ty of sep•tum pel•lu•ci•dum (kav'i-tē sep'tŭm pe-lū'si-dŭm) A slitlike, fluid-filled space of variable width between the left and right transparent septum, which occurs in fewer than 10% of human brains and may communicate with the third ventricle.

cav•i•ty of tooth (kav'i-tē tūth) SYN root canal of tooth.

ca•vo•gram (kā'vō-gram) An angiogram of a vena cava. SYN cavagram. [(vena) cava + G. *gramma,* a writing]

ca•vog•ra•phy (kā-vog'ră-fē) SYN venacavography.

ca•vo•pul•mo•nar•y a•nas•to•mo•sis (kā-vō-pul'mŏ-nār-ē ă-nas'tŏ-mō'sis) A means of palliating cyanotic heart disease by anastomosing the right pulmonary artery to the superior vena cava.

ca•vo•sur•face (kā-vō-sŭr'făs) Relating to a cavity and the surface of a tooth.

ca•vo•sur•face an•gle (kā-vō-sŭr'făs ang'gĕl) The angle formed by the junction of a cavity wall and the external surface of the tooth.

ca•vum, pl. **ca•va** (kah'vŭm, -vă) SYN cave. [L. ntr. of adj. *cavus,* hollow]

cay•enne (kī-en') SYN capsicum. [*Cayenne,* French Guiana]

Ca•ze•nove vi•til•i•go (kah-zĕ-nōv' vit'i-lī'gō) SYN alopecia areata.

C-band•ing stain (band'ing stān) A selective chromosome banding stain used in human cytogenetics, employing Giemsa stain after most of the DNA is denatured or extracted by treatment with alkali, acid, salt, or heat; only heterochromatic regions close to the centromeres and rich in satellite DNA stain, with the exception of the Y chromosome, the long arm of which usually stains throughout.

CBC Abbreviation for complete blood count.

CBG Abbreviation for corticosteroid-binding globulin.

CBN Abbreviation for collected by nurse.

CBP Abbreviation for community-based practice.

CBR Abbreviation for chemical, biologic, and radiologic, as types of mass-casualty weapons. SEE ALSO CBRNE, mass-casualty weapons, MCW, NBC, weapons of mass destruction, WMD.

CBRNE Abbreviation for chemical, biologic, radiologic, nuclear, explosive, as types of unconventional weapons. SEE ALSO CBR, mass-casualty weapons, MCW, NBC, weapons of mass destruction, WMD.

CBRNI Abbreviation for chemical, biological, radiological, nuclear, and incendiary (types of weapons of mass destruction [WMD]) used in terrorist attacks.

CBT Abbreviation for cognitive behavioral therapy.

CC Abbreviation for chief complaint.

cc, c.c. Abbreviation for cubic centimeter; chief complaint. USAGE NOTE Although the SI unit of volume is the cubic meter and, by extension, the cubic centimeter (1 cm^3 = 0.000 001 m^3), the liter and its submultiples are preferred to the cubic meter and its submultiples for the expression of volumes and substance or mass concentrations in clinical chemistry, for practical purposes, 1 cm^3 = 1 mL. The JCAHO directs that this abbreviation not be used because, when handwritten, it can easily be mistaken for *U,* units, or the numeral *4.*

CCAT Abbreviation for Certified Clinical Account Technician.

CCDM Abbreviation for *Control of Communicable Diseases Manual.*

CCK Abbreviation for cholecystokinin.

CCP Abbreviation for critical control point.

CCPD Abbreviation for continuous cyclic peritoneal dialysis.

CCU Abbreviation for coronary care unit; critical care unit.

CD Abbreviation for curative dose; circular dichroism; cluster of differentiation; controlled diffusion.

Cd Symbol for cadmium.

CDC Abbreviation for U.S. Centers for Disease Control and Prevention; formerly known as the Communicable Disease Center.

CDC cat•e•gor•ies of bi•o•log•ic a•gents (kat′ĕ-gōr-ēz bī-ŏ-loj′ik ā′jĕnts) Three categories (Category A, the highest risk; Category B, the next highest risk; and Category C) used by the U.S. Centers for Disease Control and Prevention (CDC) to rank biologic warfare agents (and toxins) according to perceived threat.

CDC Cat•e•gor•y A bi•o•log•ic a•gents (kat′ĕ-gōr-ē bī-ŏ-loj′ik ā′jĕnts) Those biologic agents and toxins considered by the CDC to represent the highest-priority agents because of their ease of dissemination or transmission from person to person, their potential for producing high mortality rates and a major impact on public health, their capacity for causing public panic and social disruption, and special actions required for public-health preparedness. The Category A agents are *Bacillus anthracis* (causing anthrax); botulinum toxin from *Clostridium botulinum; Yersinia pestis* (causing plague); smallpox virus (causing smallpox, or *variola major*); *Francisella tularensis* (causing tularemia); and filoviruses (e.g., Ebola and Marburg viruses) and arenavirus (e.g., Lassa and Machupo viruses, causing viral hemorrhagic fevers).

CDC Cat•e•gor•y B bi•o•log•ic a•gents (kat′ĕ-gōr′ē bī-ŏ-loj′ik ā′jĕnts) Those biologic agents and toxins considered by the CDC to represent the second highest-priority agents by reason of their moderate ease of dissemination, their potential for producing moderate morbidity rates and low mortality rates, and their requiring specific enhancements of CDC's diagnostic capacity and enhanced disease surveillance. The Category B agents are *Brucella* sp. (causing brucellosis); epsilon toxin *Clostridium perfringens; Salmonella* sp., *Escherichia coli* 0157:H7, *Shigella*, and other food-safety threats leading to food poisoning; *Burkholderia mallei* (causing glanders); *Burkholderia pseudomallei* (causing melioidosis); *Chlamydia psittaci* (causing psittacosis); *Coxiella burnetii* (causing Q fever); ricin toxin; staphylococcal enterotoxin B (SEB); *Rickettsia prowazekii* (causing typhus fever); alphaviruses (e.g., Venezuelan equine encephalitis, Eastern equine encephalitis, and Western equine encephalitis viruses) that cause equine encephatilides; and *Vibrio cholerae*, *Cryptosporidium parvum*, and other water-safety threats causing waterborne infections.

CDC Cat•e•gor•y C bi•o•log•ic a•gents (kat′ĕ-gōr-ē bī-ŏ-loj′ik ā′jĕnts) Those biologic agents and toxins considered by the CDC to represent the third highest-priority agents because of their availability, ease of production and dissemination, and potential for producing high morbidity and mortality rates and for a major impact on health. They include emerging pathogens such as Nipah virus and Hantavirus that are not currently used as weapons but could be engineered for mass dissemination in the future.

CD4:CD8 count (kownt) The ratio of the number of helper-inducer T lymphocytes to cytotoxic-suppressor T lymphocytes, as measured by monoclonal antibodies to the CD4 surface antigen found on helper-inducer T cells, and the CD8 surface antigen found on cytotoxic-suppressor T cells. In healthy people, the H:S ratio ranges between 1.6 and 2.2. The CD4:CD8 count is used to monitor for signs of organ rejection after transplants, and to assess the degree of immunocompromise in patients with HIV.

C-Diff (dif) SYN *Clostridium difficile.* [Colloquial, slang]

cDNA Abbreviation for complementary DNA.

CDP Abbreviation for cytidine 5′-diphosphate.

CDT SYN *Clostridium difficile.*

Ce Symbol for cerium.

CEA Abbreviation for carcinoembryonic antigen.

ce•ca (sē′kă) Plural of cecum. SYN caeca.

ce•cal (sē′kăl) **1.** Relating to the cecum. **2.** Ending blindly or in a cul-de-sac. SYN caecal.

ce•cec•to•my (sē-sek′tŏ-mē) Excision of the cecum. SYN caecectomy, typhlectomy. [ceco- + G. *ektomē,* excision]

Ce•cil op•er•a•tion (sē′sil op-ĕr-ā′shŭn) Three-stage repair of urethral stricture; consists of excision of strictured segment through a venal approach, construction of a new urethral segment buried in the scrotum, and separation of the new segment from the scrotum.

ce•ci•tis (sē-sī′tis) Inflammation of the cecum. SYN caecitis, typhlenteritis, typhlitis, typhloenteritis.

♻ **ceco-, cec-** Combining forms denoting the cecum. SEE ALSO typhlo- (1). Cf. typhlo-. SYN caeco-. [L. *caecum,* cecum, blind]

ce•co•cen•tral sco•to•ma (sē-kō-sen′trăl skō-tō′mă) A scotoma involving the optic disc area (blind spot) and the papillomacular fibers; there are three forms: 1) the cecocentral defect that extends from the blind spot toward or into the fixation area; 2) angioscotoma; 3) glaucomatous nerve-fiber bundle scotoma, due to involvement of nerve-fiber bundles at the edge of the optic disc. SYN caecocentral scotom.

ce•co•co•los•to•my (sē′kō-kō-los′tŏ-mē) Formation of an anastomosis between cecum and colon. SYN caecocolostomy.

ce•co•il•e•os•to•my (sē′kō-il-ē-os′tŏ-mē) SYN ileocecostomy.

ce•co•pex•y (sē′kō-pek-sē) Operative anchoring of a movable cecum. SYN caecopexy, typhlopexy, typhlopexia. [ceco- + G. *pexis,* fixation]

ce•co•pli•ca•tion (sē′kō-pli-kā′shŭn) Operative reduction in size of a dilated cecum by the formation of folds or tucks in its wall. SYN caecoplication. [ceco- + L. *plico,* pp. *-atus,* to fold]

ce•cor•rha•phy (sē-kōr′ă-fē) Suture of the cecum. SYN caecorrhaphy, typhlorrhaphy. [ceco- + G. *rhaphē,* suture]

ce•co•sig•moid•os•to•my (sē′kō-sig-moy-dos′tŏ-mē) Formation of a communication between the cecum and the sigmoid colon. SYN caecosigmoidostomy.

ce•cos•to•my (sē-kos′tŏ-mē) Operative formation of a cecal fistula. SYN caecostomy, typhlostomy. [ceco- + G. *stoma,* mouth]

ce•cot•o•my (sē-kot′ŏ-mē) Incision into the cecum. SYN caecotomy, typhlotomy. [ceco- + G. *tomē,* incision]

ce•co•u•re•ter•o•cele (sē′kō-yūr-ē′tĕr-ō-sēl) A ureterocele that extends far along the urethra, sometimes even through the urethral meatus. SYN caecoureterocele.

ce•cro•pins (sē′krō-pinz) Antibacterial peptides consisting of two amphipathic α-helix components.

ce•cum, pl. **ce•ca** (sē′kŭm, -kă) **1.** The cul-de-sac, about 6 cm in depth, lying below the terminal ileum forming the first part of the large intestine. **2.** Any similar structure ending in a cul-de-sac. SYN caecum. [L. ntr. of *caecus,* blind]

Ced•e•ce•a (sed-ē′sē-ă) A genus in the Enterobacteriaceae group that includes the species *Cedecea davisae* (the type strain), *C. lapagei,* and *C. neteri;* they have been recovered from the human respiratory tract, but their role in disease has not yet been delineated.

CEJ Abbreviation for cementoenamel junction.

cel•an•dine (sel′ăn-dēn) (*Chelidonium majus*) Herbal recommended for use against GI disorders and palliation of dermatologic problems; clinical studies suggest possible use as an antineoplastic; hepatitis reported as adverse effect; ought be considered toxic; not approved in U.S. markets as a drug, but is often found combined with other ingredients in herbal compounds. SYN felonwort, rock poppy. [L. *chelidonia,* fr. G. *chelidōn,* swallow]

♻**-cele** Suffix meaning swelling; hernia. [G. *kēlē,* tumor]

ce•li•ac (sē′lē-ak) Relating to the abdominal cavity. SYN coeliac. [G. *koilia,* belly]

ce•li•ac ar•ter•y (sē′lē-ak ahr′tĕr-ē) SYN celiac trunk. SYN coeliac artery.

ce•li•ac dis•ease (sē′lē-ak di-zēz′) A disease occurring in children and adults characterized by sensitivity to gluten, with chronic inflammation and atrophy of the mucosa of the upper small intestine; manifestations include diarrhea, malabsorption, steatorrhea, and nutritional and vitamin deficiencies. SYN coeliac disease, gluten enteropathy.

ce•li•ac gan•gli•a (sē′lē-ak gang′glē-ă) The largest and highest group of prevertebral sympathetic ganglia, located on the superior part of the abdominal aorta, on either side of the origin of the celiac artery; contains sympathetic neurons with unmyelinated postganglionic axons that innervate the stomach, liver, gallbladder, spleen, kidney, small intestine, and ascending and transverse colon. SYN coeliac ganglia.

ce•li•ac lymph nodes (sē′lē-ak limf nōdz) Nodes located along the celiac trunk that drain lymph from the stomach, duodenum, pancreas, spleen, and biliary tract and drain to the cisterna chyli through the right and left intestinal lymphatic trunks. SYN coeliac lymph nodes.

ce•li•ac (nerve) plex•us (sē′lē-ak nĕrv pleks′ŭs) The most substantial, superior portion of the abdominal aortic plexus lying anterior to the aorta at the level of origin of the celiac trunk (vertebral level T-12); the celiac ganglia lie within the plexus; it is formed by contributions from the greater splanchnic and vagus (especially the posterior or right vagus) nerves and communicating branches to and from the superior mesenteric and renal plexuses and ganglia; most sympathetic, parasympathetic and visceral afferent fibers serving the abdominal viscera pass through this plexus. SYN solar plexus.

ce•li•ac plex•us (sē′lē-ak pleks′ŭs) The most substantial, superior portion of the abdominal aortic plexus lying anterior to the aorta at the level of origin of the celiac trunk (vertebral level T-12); the celiac ganglia lie within the plexus; it is formed by contributions from the greater splanchnic and vagus (especially the posterior or right vagus) nerves and communicating branches to and from the superior mesenteric and renal plexuses and ganglia; most sympathetic, parasympathetic and visceral afferent fibers serving the abdominal viscera pass through this plexus. SYN plexus celiacus [TA], coeliac plexus.

ce•li•ac plex•us re•flex (sē′lē-ak pleks′ŭs rē′fleks) Arterial hypotension coincident with surgical manipulations in the upper abdomen during general anesthesia. SYN coeliac plexus reflex.

ce•li•ac trunk (sē′lē-ak trŭngk) *Origin,* abdominal aorta just below diaphragm; *branches,* left gastric, common hepatic, splenic. SYN truncus celiacus [TA], arteria celiaca, celiac artery, coeliac trunk.

♻ **celio-** Prefix meaning the abdomen. SYN coelio-. [G. *koilia,* belly]

ce·li·o·cen·te·sis (sē′lē-ō-sen-tē′sis) Rarely used term for paracentesis of the abdomen. SYN coeliocentesis. [celio- + G. *kentēsis,* puncture]

ce·li·or·rha·phy (sē′lē-ōr′ă-fē) Suture of a wound in the abdominal wall. SYN coeliorrhaphy, laparorrhaphy. [celio- + G. *rhaphē,* seam]

ce·li·os·co·py (sē′lē-os′kŏ-pē) SYN peritoneoscopy. SYN coelioscopy. [celio- + G. *skopeō,* to view]

ce·li·ot·o·my (sē′lē-ot′ŏ-mē) Transabdominal incision into the peritoneal cavity. SYN abdominal section, coeliotomy, laparotomy (2), ventrotomy. [celio- + G. *tomē,* incision]

ce·li·tis (sē-lī′tis) Any inflammation of the abdomen. SYN coelitis. [G. *koilia,* belly, + *-itis,* inflammation]

cell (sel) **1.** The smallest unit of living structure capable of independent existence, composed of a membrane-enclosed mass of protoplasm and containing a nucleus or nucleoid. Cells are highly variable and specialized in both structure and function, although all must at some stage replicate proteins and nucleic acids, use energy, and reproduce themselves. **2.** A small closed or partly closed cavity; a compartment or hollow receptacle. **3.** A container of glass, ceramic, or other solid material within which chemical reactions that generate electricity occur. [L. *cella,* a storeroom, a chamber]

cell ad·he·sion mol·e·cule (CAM) (sel ad-hē′zhŭn mol′ĕ-kyūl) Proteins that hold cells together, e.g., uvomorulin, and hold them to their substrates, e.g., laminin.

cell bod·y (sel bod′ē) The part of the cell containing the nucleus.

cell bridg·es (sel brij′ĕz) SYN intercellular bridges.

cell of Cor·ti (sel kōr′tē) A hair cell in the organ of Corti.

cell cul·ture (sel kŭl′chŭr) The maintenance or growth of dispersed cells after removal from the body, commonly on a glass surface immersed in nutrient fluid.

cell cy·cle (sel sī′kĕl) The periodic biochemical and structural events occurring during proliferation of cells such as in tissue culture.

cell fu·sion (sel fyū′zhŭn) The merging of the contents of two cells by artificial means without the destruction of either, resulting in a heterokaryon that, for at least a few generations, will reproduce its kind; an important method in assignment of loci to chromosomes.

cell in·clu·sions (sel in-klū′zhŭnz) **1.** The residual elements of the cytoplasm that are metabolic products of the cell (e.g., pigment granules or crystals). SYN metaplasm. **2.** Storage materials such as glycogen or fat. **3.** Engulfed material such as carbon or other foreign substances. SEE ALSO inclusion bodies.

cell line (sel līn) **1.** In tissue culture, the cells growing in the first or later subculture from a primary culture. **2.** A clone of cultured cells derived from an identified parental cell type.

cell-me·di·at·ed im·mu·ni·ty (CMI), cel·lu·lar im·mu·ni·ty (sel′mē′dē-āt-ĕd i-myū′ni-tē, sel′yū-lăr i-myū′ni-tē) Immune responses that are initiated by T lymphocytes and mediated by T lymphocytes, macrophages, or both (e.g., graft rejection, delayed-type hypersensitivity).

cell-me·di·at·ed re·ac·tion (sel′mē′dē-āt-ĕd rē-ak′shŭn) Immunologic reaction of the delayed type, involving chiefly T lymphocytes; important in host defense against infection, in autoimmune diseases, and in organ transplant rejection. SEE ALSO skin test.

cell mem·brane (sel mem′brān) The protoplasmic boundary of all cells that controls permeability and may serve other functions through surface specializations (e.g., active ion transport, absorption by formation of pinocytotic vesicles, and antigen recognition). Its fine structure is trilaminar and consists of the electron-dense lamina externa and lamina interna with an electron-lucent lamina intermedia. SYN plasma membrane, plasmalemma, Wachendorf membrane (2).

cell nest (sel nest) A small focus or accumulation of one type of cell that is different from the other cells in the tissue.

cel·lu·la, gen. and pl. **cel·lu·lae** (sel′yū-lă, -lē) **1.** GROSS ANATOMY a small but macroscopic compartment. SYN cellule. **2.** IN HISTOLOGY a cell. [L. a small chamber, dim. of *cella*]

cel·lu·lar (sel′yū-lăr) **1.** Relating to, derived from, or composed of cells. **2.** Having numerous compartments or interstices. [L. *cellula,* dim. of *cella,* storeroom]

cel·lu·lar bi·ol·o·gy (sel′yū-lăr bī-ol′ŏ-jē) SYN cytology.

cel·lu·lar im·mu·no·de·fi·cien·cy with ab·nor·mal im·mu·no·glob·u·lin syn·the·sis (sel′yū-lăr im′yū-nō-dĕ-fish′ĕn-sē ab-nōr′măl im′yū-nō-glob′yū-lin sin′thĕ-sis) A group of disorders of unknown cause, associated with recurrent bacterial, fungal, protozoal, and viral infections; there is thymic hypoplasia with depressed cellular (T-lymphocyte) immunity combined with defective humoral (B-lymphocyte) immunity.

cel·lu·lar in·fil·tra·tion (sel′yū-lăr in′fil-trā′shŭn) Migration of cells from their sources of origin, or direct extension of cells as a result of unusual growth and multiplication; used especially with reference to such changes associated with inflammations and certain types of malignant neoplasms.

cel•lu•lar•i•ty (sel′yū-lar′i-tē) The degree, quality, or condition of cells that are present.

cel•lu•lar pa•thol•o•gy (sel′yū-lăr pă-thol′ŏ-jē) **1.** The interpretation of diseases in terms of cellular alterations. **2.** Sometimes used as a synonym for cytopathology (1).

cel•lu•lase (sel′yū-lās) An enzyme catalyzing the hydrolysis of 1,4-β-glucoside links in cellulose. Used to produce digestive tablets and in the removal of cellulose from foods for special diets.

cel•lule (sel′yūl) SYN cellula (1).

cel•lu•li•ci•dal (sel′yū-li-sī′dăl) Destructive to cells. [cellula + L. *caedo,* to kill]

cel•lu•lif•u•gal (sel′yū-lif′ŭ-găl) Moving from, or extending in a direction away from, a cell or cell body. [cellula + L. *fugio,* to flee]

cel•lu•lip•e•tal (sel′yū-lip′ĕ-tăl) Moving toward, or extending in a direction toward, a cell or cell body. [cellula + L. *peto,* to seek]

cel•lu•lite (sel′yū-līt) **1.** Colloquial term for deposits of fat and fibrous tissue causing dimpling of the overlying skin. **2.** SYN lipoedema.

cel•lu•li•tis (sel′yū-lī′tis) Inflammation of subcutaneous, loose connective tissue (formerly called cellular tissue). See this page, B9.

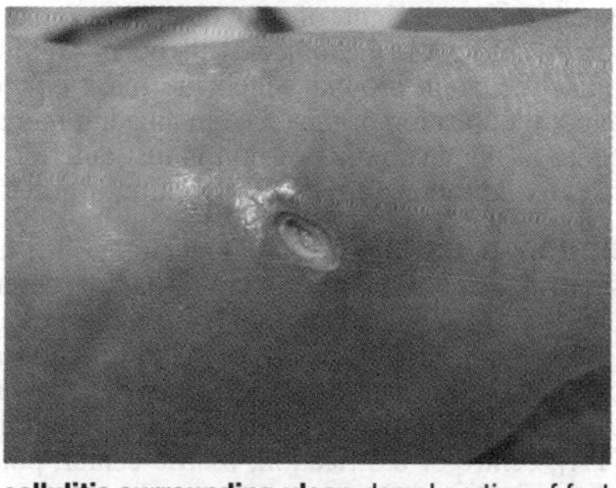

cellulitis surrounding ulcer: dorsal portion of foot

cel•lu•lose (sel′yū-lōs) An indigestible carbohydrate found in plants.

cell wall (sel wawl) The outer layer or membrane of some animal and plant cells; in the latter, it is mainly cellulose.

cell wall–de•fec•tive bac•te•ri•a (sel wawl-dĕ-fek′tiv bak-tēr′ē-ă) Bacteria with absent or damaged cell walls; morphologically, they may become spheroplasts, round structures with little or no cell wall, or they may develop filamentous forms, with or without bulbous, extruded portions.

celo- Combining form denoting (1) the celom [G. *koilōma,* hollow (celom)]; (2) hernia [G. *kēlē,* hernia]; (3) abdomen [G. *koilia,* belly]. SEE ALSO celio-. SYN coelo-.

ce•lom, ce•lo•ma (sē′lŏm, sē-lō′mă) **1.** The cavity between the splanchnic and somatic mesoderm in the embryo. SYN coelom. **2.** SYN intraembryonic celom. **3.** SYN body cavity. [G. *koilōma,* a hollow]

ce•lom•ic (se-lom′ik) Relating to the body cavity. SYN coelomic.

ce•lo•phle•bi•tis (sē′lō-flĕ-bī′tis) Inflammation of a vena cava. SYN cavitis. [G. *koilos,* hollow, + phlebitis]

CELO vi•rus (vī′rŭs) A virus with characteristics of adenovirus, and similar to quail bronchitis virus.

Cel•si•us (C) (sel′sē-ŭs) SEE Celsius scale.

Cel•si•us scale (sel′sē-ŭs skāl) A temperature scale that is based on the triple point of water (defined to be 273.16°K) and assigned the value of 0.01°C; has replaced the centigrade scale because the triple point of water can be more accurately measured than the ice point; for most practical purposes, however, the two scales are equivalent.

ce•ment (sĕ-ment′) DENTISTRY a nonmetallic material used for luting, filling, or permanent or temporary restoration, or as an adherent sealer in attaching various dental restorations in or on the tooth made by mixing components into a plastic mass that sets.

ce•ment dis•ease (sĕ-ment′ di-zēz′) The osteolysis that frequently occurs in association with loosening of cemented total hip replacements; microscopic particles of polymethylmethacrylate cement induce a biologic reaction by osteoclasts leading to bone resorption and progressive bone loss.

ce•ment•i•cle (sĕ-men′ti-kel) A calcified spherical body, composed of cementum lying free within the periodontal membrane, attached to the cementum or imbedded within it.

ce•ment line (sĕ-ment′ līn) The refractile boundary of an osteon or interstitial lamellar system in compact bone.

ce•ment•o•blast (sĕ-men′tō-blast) One of the cells concerned with the formation of the layer of cementum on the roots of teeth. [L. *cementum,* cement, + G. *blastos,* germ]

ce•ment•o•blas•to•ma (sĕ-men′tō-blas-tō′mă) A benign odontogenic tumor of functional cementoblasts; appears as a mixed radiolucent-radiopaque lesion attached to a tooth root.

ce•ment•o•cla•si•a (sĕ-ment′ō-klā′zē-ă) Destruction of cementum by cementoclasts. [L. *cementum,* cement, + G. *klasis,* fracture]

ce•ment•o•clast (sĕ-men′tō-klast) One of the

multinucleated giant cells, identical with osteoclasts, that are associated with the resorption of cementum. [L. *cementum,* cement, + G. *klastos,* broken]

ce•ment•o•cyte (sĕ-men′tō-sīt) An osteocyte-like cell with numerous processes, trapped in a lacuna in the cementum of the tooth. [L. *cementum,* cement, + G. *kytos,* cell]

ce•ment•o•den•tin•al junc•tion (sĕ-ment′ō-den′ti-năl jŭngk′shŭn) The surface at which the cementum and dentin of the root of a tooth are joined.

ce•men•to•e•nam•el junc•tion (CEJ) (sĕ-men′tō-ĕ-nam′ĕl jŭngk′shŭn) The surface at which the enamel of the crown and the cementum of the root of a tooth are joined. SEE ALSO cervical line.

ce•men•to•ma (sē′mĕn-tō′mă) Any benign cementum-producing tumor; four types are recognized: 1) periapical cemental dysplasia, 2) central ossifying fibroma, 3) cementoblastoma, 4) sclerotic cemental mass; when type not specified, usually refers to periapical cemental dysplasia. [L. *cementum,* cement, + G. *-ōma,* tumor]

ce•men•to•os•si•fy•ing fi•bro•ma (sĕ-men′tō-os′i-fī-ing fī-brō′mă) A form of fibroma with cementicles and bone rimmed with osteoblasts in moderately cellular stroma.

ce•men•tum (sĕ-men′tŭm) A layer of bonelike mineralized tissue covering the dentin of the root and neck of a tooth that blends with the fibers of the periodontal ligament. [L. *caementum,* rough quarry stone, fr. *caedo,* to cut]

cenaesthesia [Br.] SYN cenesthesia.

cenaesthesic [Br.] SYN cenesthesic.

cenaesthetic [Br.] SYN cenesthetic.

ce•nes•the•si•a (sē′nes-thē′zē-ă) The general sense of bodily existence; the sensation caused by the functioning of the internal organs. SYN cenaesthesia. [G. *koinos,* common, + *aisthēsis,* sensation]

ce•nes•the•sic, **ce•nes•thet•ic** (sē′nes-thē′zik, -sik; -thet′ik) Relating to cenesthesia. SYN cenaesthesic.

♻ **ceno-** Combining form denoting (1) shared in common [G. *koinos,* common]; (2) [G. *kainos,* new]; (3) emptiness (rare) [G. *kenos,* empty]. SEE ALSO coeno-.

ce•no•cyte (sē′nō-sīt) A multinucleate cell or hyphae without cross walls, characteristic of the hyphae of zygomycetes. SYN coenocyte. [G. *koinos,* common, + *kytos,* cell]

cen•o•site (sē′nō-sīt) A facultative commensal organism that can sustain itself apart from its usual host. SYN coinosite. [G. *koinos,* common, + *sitos,* food]

cen•sor (sen′sŏr) PSYCHOANALYTIC THEORY the psychic barrier that prevents certain unconscious thoughts and wishes from coming to consciousness. [L. a judge, critic, fr. *censeo,* to value, judge]

cen•sor•ing (sen′sŏr-ing) **1.** EPIDEMIOLOGY loss of subjects from a follow-up study for unknown reasons. **2.** Observations with unknown values from one end of a frequency distribution, beyond a measurement threshold.

cen•sus (sen′sŭs) An enumeration of a population, originally for taxation and military purposes, now with many other purposes; basic facts about all persons (e.g., age, sex, occupation, nature of residence) are recorded in the census, which often also includes some information about health status. [L., fr. *censeo,* to count]

cen•ter (sen′tĕr) **1.** The middle point of a body; loosely, the interior of a body. A center of any kind, especially an anatomic center. SYN centrum [TA]. **2.** A group of nerve cells governing a specific function. **3.** A health care or therapeutic facility performing a particular function or service for people in the surrounding area. SYN centre. [L. *centrum;* G. *kentron*]

cen•ter of ex•cel•lence (sen′tĕr ek′sĕ-lens) A colloquial, jargonistic, and vastly overused term for any health care facility that is reputed, by means of public survey or in the opinion of the facility itself, to be superior in one or more ways to other such care facilities.

cen•ter of grav•i•ty (COG) (sen′tĕr grav′i-tē) The point on a body or system where, if pressure equal to the weight of the object is applied, forces acting on the object will be in equilibrium; the point around which the mass is centered; the location of the COG in an adult human being in the anatomic position is just anterior to the second sacral vertebra. SYN centre of gravity.

cen•ter of os•si•fi•ca•tion (sen′tĕr os′i-fi-kā′shŭn) A site of bone formation through accumulation of osteoblasts within connective tissue (membranous ossification), or of destruction of cartilage before onset of ossification (endochondral ossification). SYN centrum ossificationis [TA], centre of ossification, ossific center, point of ossification.

Cen•ters for Dis•ease Con•trol and Pre•ven•tion (CDC) (sen′tĕrz di-zēz′ kŏn-trōl′ prē-ven′shŭn) The U.S. federal facility for disease eradication, epidemiology, and education headquartered in Atlanta, Georgia, which encompasses the Center for Infectious Diseases, Center for Environmental Health, Center for Health Promotion and Education, Center for Prevention Services, Center for Professional Development and Training, and Center for Occupational Safety and Health. It maintains several coding sets included in HIPAA standards (e.g., ICD-9-CM codes). Formerly named the Center for Disease Control (1970) and the Communicable Disease Center (1946).

Cen·ters for Med·i·care and Med·i·caid Ser·vic·es (CMS) (sen′tĕrz med′i-kār med′i-kād sĕr′vi-sĕz) An agency of the U.S. Department of Health and Human Services that manages the federal health care programs of Medicare and Medicaid; before July 2001, known as the Health Care Financing Administration (HCFA).

cen·te·sis (sen-tē′sis) Puncture, especially when used as a suffix, as in paracentesis. [G. *kentēsis,* puncture, fr. *kenteō,* to prick, pierce]

♻**centi- (c)** Prefix used in the SI and metric system to signify one hundredth (10^{-2}). [L. *centum,* one hundred]

cen·ti·grade (C) (sen′ti-grād) **1.** Basis of an earlier temperature scale in which 100° separates the melting and boiling points of water. SEE Celsius scale. **2.** One hundredth of a circle, equal to 3.6 degrees of the astronomic circle. [L. *centum,* one hundred, + *gradus,* step, degree]

cen·ti·gram (sen′ti-gram) One hundredth of a gram.

cen·tile (sen′tīl) One hundredth. [L. *centum,* one hundred, + *-ilis,* adj. suffix]

cen·ti·li·ter (cL) (sen′ti-lē-tĕr) Ten milliliters; one hundredth of a liter; 162.3073 minims (U.S.). SYN centilitre.

centilitre [Br.] SYN centiliter.

cen·ti·me·ter (cm) (sen′ti-mē-tĕr) One hundredth of a meter; 0.3937008 inch. SYN centimetre.

cen·ti·me·ter-gram-sec·ond sys·tem (CGS, cgs) (sen′ti-mē-tĕr-gram-sek′ŏnd sis′tĕm) The scientific system of expressing the fundamental physical units of length, mass, and time, and those units derived from them, in centimeters, grams, and seconds; is being replaced by the International System of Units based on the meter, kilogram, and second.

cen·ti·me·ter-gram-sec·ond u·nit (CGS, cgs), cgs u·nit (sen′ti-mē-tĕr-gram-sek′ŏnd yū′nit) An absolute unit of the centimeter-gram-second system.

centimetre [Br.] SYN centimeter.

cen·ti·mor·gan (cM) (sen′ti-mōr-găn) SEE morgan.

Cen·ti·nel·a test (sen′ti-nel′ă test) Maneuver used to determine the integrity of the supraspinatus muscle or tendon. While the patient has both arms in 90 degrees of abduction and 30 degrees of horizontal adduction with the humerus internally rotated (thumbs down), the clinician applies downward pressure, noting pain and weakness. [Centinela Hospital Medical Center, Tenet, California]

cen·ti·nor·mal (sen′ti-nōr′măl) One-hundredth normal; denoting the concentration of a solution.

cen·ti·poise (sen′ti-poyz) One hundredth of a poise.

cen·tra (sen′tră) Plural of centrum.

cen·trad (sen′trad) **1.** Toward the center. **2.** A unit of measurement of the refracting strength of a prism; it corresponds to the deviation of a ray of light, the arc of which is 1/100 of the radius of the circle, or 0.57°.

cen·tral am·pu·ta·tion (sen′trăl amp′yū-tā′shŭn) Amputation in which the flaps are so united that the cicatrix runs across the end of the stump.

cen·tral ap·ne·a (sen′trăl ap′nē-ă) Apnea as the result of medullary depression, which inhibits respiratory movement.

cen·tral a·re·o·lar cho·roi·dal dys·tro·phy (sen′trăl ă-rē′ō-lăr kōr-oyd′ăl dis′trŏ-fē) An autosomal dominant progressive disorder of vision loss with well-demarcated areas of atrophy of the pigmented layer of the retina and choriocapillaris.

cen·tral ar·ter·y of ret·i·na (sen′trăl ahr′tĕr-ē ret′i-nă) A branch of the ophthalmic artery that penetrates the optic nerve 1 cm behind the eye to enter the eye at the optic papilla in the retina; it divides into superior and inferior temporal and nasal branches.

cen·tral au·di·tor·y ner·vous sys·tem (CANS) (sen′trăl aw′di-tōr-ē nĕr′vŭs sis′tĕm) Auditory neural pathway from the cochleae to the auditory cortex. SEE vestibulocochlear nerve [CN VIII].

cen·tral cloud·y cor·ne·al dys·tro·phy of Fran·çois (sen′tral klow′dē kōr′nē-ăl dis′trŏ-fē frahn-swah′) An autosomal dominant opacification of the central corneal stroma consisting of cloudy polygonal areas.

cen·tral cord syn·drome (sen′trăl kōrd sin′drōm) Quadriparesis most severely involving the distal upper extremities, with or without sensory loss and bladder dysfunction, usually due to ischemia from osteophytic or traumatic compression of the central part of the cervical spinal cord and/or artery.

cen·tral cry·stal·line cor·ne·al dys·tro·phy of Sny·der (sen′trăl kris′tăl-lēn kōr′nē-ăl dis′trŏ-fē snī′dĕr) An autosomal dominant opacification of the central corneal stroma by needle-shaped polychromatic crystals.

cen·tral deaf·ness (sen′trăl def′nĕs) Deafness due to disorder of the auditory system of the brainstem or cerebral cortex.

cen·tral gan·gli·o·neu·ro·ma (sen′trăl gang′glē-ō-nūr-ō′mă) SYN gangliocytoma.

cen·tral gy·ri (sen′trăl jī′rē) The precentral and postcentral gyri.

cen·tra·li·za·tion phe·nom·e·non (sen-trăl-ī-zā′shŭn fĕ-nom′ĕ-non) The relatively rapid change in the perceived location of pain, from more peripheral, or distal, to a more proximal, or central, location; commonly occurs during initial evaluation of patients with low back and radiating limb pain; helpful in determining the type and prognosis of physical therapy.

cen·tral ne·cro·sis (sen′trăl nĕ-krō′sis) Necrosis involving the deeper or inner portions of a tissue, or an organ or its units.

cen·tral ner·vous sys·tem (CNS) (sen′trăl nĕr′vŭs sis′tĕm) The brain and the spinal cord.

cen·tral os·si·fy·ing fi·bro·ma (sen′trăl os′i-fī-ing fī-brō′mă) A painless, slowly expansile, sharply circumscribed benign fibroosseus tumor of the jaws that is derived from cells of the periodontal ligament; presents initially as a radiolucency that becomes progressively more opaque as it matures.

cen·tral os·te·i·tis (sen′trăl os-tē-ī′tis) **1.** SYN osteomyelitis. **2.** SYN endosteitis.

cen·tral pal·mar space (sen′trăl pahl′măr spās) The more medial of the central palmar spaces, bounded medially by the hypothenar compartment; related distally to the synovial tendon sheaths of digits 3 and 4 and proximally to the common flexor sheath.

cen·tral pa·ral·y·sis (sen′trăl păr-al′i-sis) Paralysis caused by a lesion in the brain or spinal cord.

cen·tral pat·tern gen·er·a·tor (sen′trăl pat′ĕrn jen′ĕr-ā-tŏr) Theoretic network of neurons in the brain or spinal cord that are involved in the activation and use of a group of muscles during a patterned movement.

cen·tral ret·i·nal ar·ter·y (sen′trăl ret′i-năl ahr′tĕr-ē) A branch of the ophthalmic artery that penetrates the optic nerve 1 cm behind the eye (extraocular part) to enter the eye (intraocular part) at the optic papilla in the retina; it divides into superior and inferior temporal and nasal branches. SYN arteria centralis retinae [TA].

cen·tral ret·i·nal fo·ve·a (sen′trăl ret′i-năl fō′vē-ă) A depression in the center of the macula retinae containing only cones and lacking blood vessels. SYN fovea centralis maculae luteae [TA].

cen·tral sco·to·ma (sen′trăl skō-tō′mă) A scotoma involving the fixation point.

cen·tral spin·dle (sen′trăl spin′dĕl) In mitosis, a central group of microtubules (continuous fibers) that course uninterrupted, between the asters, in contrast to the microtubules attached to the individual chromosomes (spindle fibers).

cen·tral sul·cus (sen′trăl sŭl′kŭs) A double-S–shaped fissure extending obliquely upward and backward on the lateral surface of each cerebral hemisphere at the boundary between frontal and parietal lobes.

cen·tral vein of ret·i·na (sen′trăl vān ret′i-nă) Formed by union of the retinal veins and accompanies the artery of the same name in the optic nerve. SYN vena centralis retinae [TA].

cen·tral veins of liv·er (sen′trăl vānz liv′ĕr) Initial vein of the hepatic venous system, located in the center of the conceptual hepatic lobule, receiving blood from sinuses and draining into collecting veins that become hepatic veins. SYN Krukenberg veins.

cen·tral vein of su·pra·re·nal gland (sen′trăl vān sū′pră-rē′năl gland) The single draining vein of the gland; it receives a number of medullary veins; on the right side it empties directly into the inferior vena cava and on the left into the left renal vein. SYN vena centralis glandulae suprarenalis [TA].

cen·tral ve·nous cath·e·ter (sen′trăl vē′nŭs kath′ĕ-tĕr) Tube surgically inserted into a vein in the central circulation (usually the superior vena cava). Commonly used for long-term IV therapy, nutritional support, or chemotherapy.

cen·tral ve·nous pres·sure (CVP) (sen′trăl vē′nŭs presh′ŭr) The pressure of the blood within the venous system in the superior and inferior vena cava, normally between 4 and 10 cm of water (1–3 mmHg); it is depressed in circulatory shock and deficiencies of circulating blood volume and increased with cardiac failure and congestion of the venous circulation. See this page.

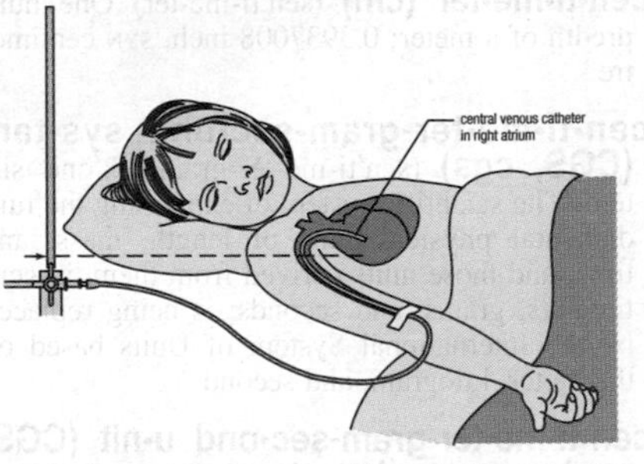

central venous pressure catheterization: child in supine position with central venous catheter inserted into right atrium

cen·tral vi·sion (sen′trăl vizh′ŭn) Vision stimulated by an object imaged on the fovea centralis. SYN direct vision.

centre [Br.] SYN center.

centre of gravity [Br.] SYN center of gravity.

cen·tren·ce·phal·ic (sen′tren-sĕ-fal′ik) Relating to the center of the encephalon.

centre of ossification [Br.] SYN center of ossification.

cen·tri·ac·i·nar em·phy·se·ma (sen′tri-as′i-năr em′fi-sē′mă) SYN centrilobular emphysema.

cen•tric (sen′trik) DENTISTRY pertaining to ideally centered occlusion, with optimal contact and intercuspation. [G. *kentron,* center]

-centric Combining form meaning having a center (of a specific kind or number) or having a specific thing as its center (of interest, focus).

cen•tric fu•sion (sen′trik fyū′zhŭn) SYN robertsonian translocation.

cen•tric•i•put (sen-tris′i-put) The central portion of the upper surface of the skull, between the occiput and the sinciput. [L. *centrum,* center, + *caput,* head]

cen•tric oc•clu•sion (sen′trik ŏ-klū′zhŭn) **1.** The relation of opposing occlusal surfaces that provides the maximum contact and intercuspation. **2.** The occlusion of the teeth when the mandible is in centric relation to the maxillae. SYN acquired centric, habitual centric, intercuspal position.

cen•tric re•la•tion (sen′trik rĕ-lā′shŭn) The relation of the lower to the upper jaw when the condyles are in their most posterior and superior position in the mandibular (glenoid) fossae. SYN terminal hinge position.

cen•trif•u•gal (sen-trif′ŭ-găl) **1.** Denoting the direction of the force pulling an object outward (away) from an axis of rotation. **2.** Sometimes, by analogy, extended to describe any movement away from a center. Cf. eccentric (2). [L. *centrum,* center, + *fugio,* to flee]

cen•trif•u•gal nerve (sen-trif′ŭ-găl nĕrv) SYN efferent nerve.

cen•trif•u•ga•tion (sen-trif′ŭ-gā′shŭn) Sedimentation, by means of a centrifuge, of solids suspended in a fluid. After the process, supernatant fluid and sediment are separated.

cen•tri•fuge (sen′tri-fyūzh) **1.** An apparatus by means of which particles in suspension in a fluid are separated by spinning the fluid, the centrifugal force throwing the particles to the periphery of the rotated vessel. **2.** To submit to rapid rotary action, as in a centrifuge.

cen•tri•lob•u•lar (sen′tri-lob′yū-lăr) At or near the center of a lobule, e.g., of the liver.

cen•tri•lob•u•lar em•phy•se•ma (sen′tri-lob′yū-lăr em′fi-sē′mă) Emphysema affecting the lobules around their central bronchioles, causally related to bronchiolitis, and seen in coal-miner's pneumoconiosis. See this page. SYN centriacinar emphysema.

cen•tri•ole (sen′trē-ōl) Tubular structures usually seen as paired organelles lying in the cyto-

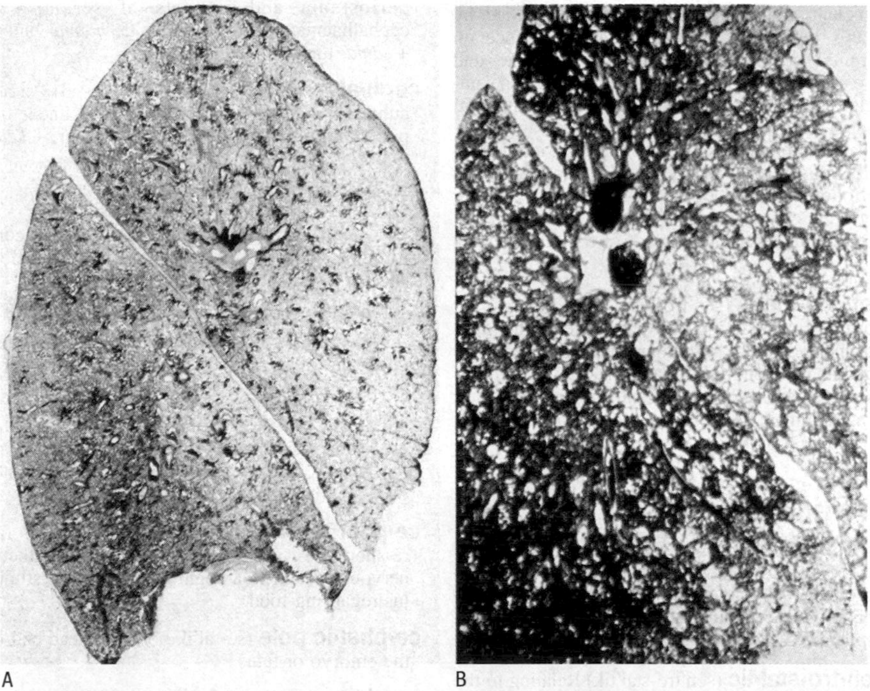

A B

centrilobular emphysema: (A) lung of smoker with mild emphysema shows enlarged air spaces scattered throughout both lobes; (B) in a more advanced case, destruction of lung has progressed to produce large, irregular air spaces

centrum; centrioles may be multiple and numerous in some cells, such as the giant cells of bone marrow. [G. *kentron,* a point, center]

cen•trip•e•tal (sĕn-trip′ĕ-tăl) **1.** SYN afferent. **2.** Denoting the direction of the force pulling an object toward an axis of rotation. SYN axipetal. [L. *centrum,* center, + *peto,* to seek]

cen•trip•e•tal nerve (sĕn-trip′ĕ-tăl nĕrv) SYN afferent nerve.

♻**centro-** Combining form denoting center. [G. *kentron*]

cen•tro•ac•i•nar cell (sen′trō-as′i-năr sel) A cell of the pancreatic ductule that occupies the lumen of an acinus; it secretes bicarbonate and water, providing an alkaline pH necessary for enzyme activity in the intestine.

cen•tro•ki•ne•si•a (sen′trō-ki-nē′sē-ă) Movement excited by a stimulus of central origin. [centro- + G. *kinēsis,* movement]

cen•tro•ki•net•ic (sen′trō-ki-net′ik) **1.** Relating to centrokinesia. **2.** SYN excitomotor.

cen•tro•me•di•an nu•cle•us (sen′trō-mē′dē-ăn nū′klē-ŭs) A large, lentil-shaped cell group, the largest and most caudal of the intralaminar nuclei, located within the lamina medullaris interna of the thalamus between the mediodorsal nucleus and ventrobasal nucleus; so called by Luys because of its prominent appearance on frontal sections midway between the anterior and posterior pole of the human thalamus. The nucleus receives numerous fibers from the internal segment of the globus pallidus by way of the thalamic fasciculus, ansa lenticularis, and lenticular fasciculus as well as projections from Brodmann area 4 of the motor cortex; its major efferent connection is with the putamen although collaterals reach broad areas of the cerebral cortex.

cen•tro•mere (sen′trō-mēr) The nonstaining primary constriction of a chromosome; the centromere divides the chromosome into two arms and its position is constant for a specific chromosome: near one end (acrocentric), near the center (metacentric), or between (submetacentric). [centro- + G. *meros,* part]

cen•tro•some (sen′trō-sōm) SYN cytocentrum. [centro- + G. *sōma,* body]

cen•tro•sphere (sen′trō-sfēr) The specialized cytoplasm of the cytocentrum. Contains the centrioles from which the astral fibers (microtubules) extend during mitosis. [centro- + G. *sphaira,* a ball, sphere]

cen•tro•stal•tic (sen′trō-stal′tik) Relating to the center of motion. [centro- + G. *stallein,* set forth, fetch]

cen•trum, pl. **cen•tra** (sen′trŭm, -tră) [TA] SYN center (1). [L. fr. G. *kentron*]

cen•trum os•si•fi•ca•ti•o•nis (sen′trŭm os-i-fi-kā′shē-ō′nis) [TA] SYN center of ossification.

cen•tum (c) (sen′tŭm) L. hundred [L. one hundred]

ceph•a•lad (sef′ă-lad) In a direction toward the head. SEE ALSO cranial (1).

ceph•a•lal•gi•a (sef′ă-lal′jē-ă) SYN headache. [cephal- + G. *algos,* pain]

ceph•al•e•de•ma (sef′al-ĕ-dē′mă) Edema of the head. SYN cephaloedema.

cephalhaematocoele [Br.] SYN cephalhematocele.

cephalhaematoma [Br.] SYN cephalhematoma.

ceph•al•he•ma•to•cele, **ceph•a•lo•he•ma•to•cele** (sef′ăl-hē-mat′ō-sēl, sef′ă-lō-hē-mat′ō-sēl) A cephalhematoma under the periosteum of the skull communicating with the dural sinuses. SYN cephalhaematocoele. [cephal- + G. *haima,* blood, + *kēlē,* tumor]

ceph•al•he•ma•to•ma, **ceph•a•lo•he•ma•to•ma** (sef′ăl-hē-mă-tō′mă, sef′ă-lō-hē-mă-tō′mă) An effusion of blood beneath the periosteum of a cranial bone, seen frequently in a newborn as a result of birth trauma; contrasted with caput succedaneum, in which the effusion overlies the periosteum and consists of serum. SYN cephalhaematoma. [cephal- + G. *haima,* blood, + *-ōma,* tumor]

ceph•al•hy•dro•cele (sef-ăl-hī′drō-sēl) An accumulation of serous or watery fluid under the pericranium. [cephal- + G. *hydōr,* water, + *kēlē,* tumor]

ce•phal•ic (sĕ-fal′ik) SYN cranial (1).

ce•pha•lic curve (sĕ-fal′ik kŭrv) Curve conforming to that of the fetal head, used in reference to the shape of obstetric forceps.

ce•phal•ic flex•ure (sĕ-fal′ik flek′shŭr) The sharp, ventrally concave bend in the developing midbrain of the embryo. SYN cranial flexure, mesencephalic flexure.

ce•phal•ic in•dex (se-fal′ik in′deks) The ratio of the maximal breadth to the maximal length of the head, obtained by the formula: (breadth × 100)/length. SYN length-breadth index.

ce•phal•ic phase re•sponse (sĕ-fal′ik fāz rē-spons′) A response of the parasympathetic nervous system to a cognitive or sensory stimulus regarding food.

ce•phal•ic pole (sĕ-fal′ik pōl) The head end of the embryo or fetus.

ce•phal•ic pre•sen•ta•tion (sĕ-fal′ik prez′ĕn-tā′shŭn) Presentation of any part of the fetal head, usually the upper and back part as a result of flexion such that the chin is in contact with the thorax in vertex presentation; there may be degrees of flexion so that the presenting part is the large fontanelle in sincipital presentation, the brow in brow presentation, or the face in face presentation.

ceph•a•lic re•place•ment (sě-fal′ik rē-plās′ mĕnt) In cases of shoulder dystocia when vaginal delivery cannot be effected, the fetal head is flexed and reinserted into the vagina to reestablish umbilical cord blood flow and delivery performed through cesarean section. SYN Zavanelli maneuver.

ce•phal•ic tet•a•nus (sě-fal′ik tet′ă-nŭs) A type of local tetanus that follows wounds to the face and head; after a brief incubation (1–2 days) the facial and ocular muscles become paretic yet undergo repeated tetanic spasms. The throat and tongue muscles may also be affected.

ce•phal•ic vein (sě-fal′ik vān) Arises at the radial border of the dorsal venous rete of the hand, passes upward in front of the elbow and along the lateral side of the arm; it empties into the upper part of the axillary vein.

ce•phal•ic ver•sion (sě-fal′ik vĕr′zhŭn) Placement in which the fetus is turned so that the head presents; can be external cephalic version or internal cephalic version. SEE ALSO external cephalic version, internal cephalic version.

ceph•a•li•tis (sef′ă-lī′tis) SYN encephalitis.

cephalo-, cephal- Combining forms meaning the head. [G. *kephalē*]

ceph•a•lo•cau•dal ax•is (sef′ă-lō-kaw′dăl ak′sis) Long axis of the body; the imaginary straight line in the median plane that runs from the apex of the skull through the center of the perineum and continuing between the lower limbs.

ceph•a•lo•cele (sef′ă-lō-sēl) Protrusion of part of the cranial contents, e.g., meningocele, encephalocele. SEE ALSO encephalocele.

ceph•a•lo•cen•te•sis (sef′ă-lō-sen-tē′sis) Passage of a hollow needle or trocar into the brain to drain or aspirate an abscess or the fluid of a hydrocephalus. [cephalo- + G. *kentēsis*, puncture]

ceph•a•lo•dyn•i•a (sef′ă-lō-din′ē-ă) Headache. [cephalo- + G. *odynē*, pain]

cephaloedema [Br.] SYN cephaledema.

ceph•a•lo•gy•ric (sef′ă-lō-jī′rik) Relating to rotation of the head. [cephalo- + G. *gyros*, a circle]

cephalohaematocoele [Br.] SYN cephalohematocele.

cephalohaematoma [Br.] SYN cephalohematoma.

ceph•a•lo•meg•a•ly (sef′ă-lō-meg′ă-lē) Enlargement of the head. [cephalo- + G. *megas*, great]

ceph•a•lom•e•ter (sef′ă-lom′ĕ-tĕr) An instrument used to position the head to produce oriented, reproducible lateral and posterior-anterior head films. SYN cephalostat. [cephalo- + G. *metron*, measure]

ceph•a•lo•met•rics (sef′ă-lō-met′riks) **1.** ORAL SURGERY, ORTHODONTICS the scientific measurement of the bones of the cranium and face, using a fixed, reproducible position for lateral radiographic exposure of skull and facial bones. **2.** A scientific study of the measurements of the head with relation to specific reference points; used for evaluation of facial growth and development, including soft tissue profile. [cephalo- + G. *metron*, measure]

ceph•a•lom•e•try (sef′ă-lom′ĕ-trē) Measurements on the living head, or head without removal of the soft parts. SEE ALSO cephalometrics. See this page. [cephalo- + G. *metron*, measure]

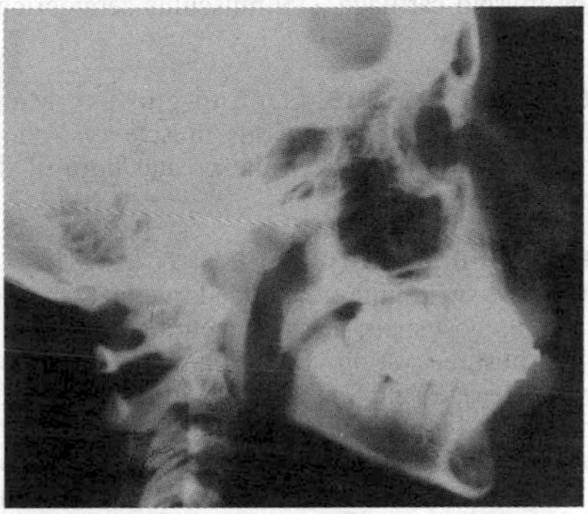

cephalometry: radiograph reveals bony structures and overlying soft tissues

ceph•a•lo•mo•tor (sef′ă-lō-mō′tŏr) Relating to movements of the head.

ceph•a•lop•a•thy (sef′ă-lop′ă-thē) SYN encephalopathy. [cephalo- + G. *pathos*, suffering]

ceph•a•lo•pel•vic (sef′ă-lō-pel′vik) Pertaining to the size of the fetal head in relation to the maternal pelvis.

ceph•a•lo•pel•vic dis•pro•por•tion (CPT) (sef′ă-lō-pel′vik dis′prō-pōr′shŭn) A condition in which the fetal head is too large to traverse the maternal pelvis, causing arrest of labor.

ceph•a•lo•pel•vim•e•try (sef′ă-lō-pel-vim′ĕ-trē) Roentgenographic measurement of the dimensions of the pelvis and the fetal head. [cephalo- + pelvimetry]

ceph•a•lo•stat (sef′ă-lō-stat) SYN cephalometer. [cephalo- + G. *statos*, stationary]

ce•phal•o•tho•rac•ic (sef′ă-lō-thōr-as′ik) Relating to the head and the chest.

-cephaly Suffix indicating an anomalous condition of the head.

-ceptor Combining form denoting taker, receiver. [L. *capio,* pp. *captus,* to take]

cer·am·i·dase (sĕr-am′i-dās) An enzyme that hydrolyzes ceramides into sphingosine and a fatty acid. A deficiency of this enzyme is associated with Farber disease.

cer·a·mide (ser′ă-mīd) Generic term for a class of sphingolipid, *N*-acyl (fatty acid) derivatives of a long chain base or sphingoid such as sphingenine or sphingosine. Ceramides accumulate in people with Farber disease.

cerat- SEE kerat-.

cerato- SEE kerato-.

cer·a·to·cri·coid mus·cle (ser′ă-tō-krī′koyd mŭs′ĕl) A fasciculus from the posterior cricoarytenoid muscle inserted into the inferior horn of the thyroid cartilage. SYN musculus ceratocricoideus [TA].

cer·a·to·glos·sus (ser′ă-tō-glos′ŭs) Main, posterior part of hyoglossus muscle (vs. chondroglossus) arising from the greater horn of the hyoid bone.

cer·car·i·a, pl. **cer·car·i·ae** (sĕr-kar′ē-ă, -ē-ē) The free-swimming trematode larva that emerges from its host snail; it may penetrate the skin of a final host, encyst on vegetation, or in or on fish, or penetrate and encyst in various arthropod hosts. Body and tail are greatly varied in form, and specialized functions are adapted to the particular life-cycle demands of each species. SEE ALSO sporocyst (1). [G. *kerkos,* tail]

cer·ci (ser′sī) Plural of cercus.

cer·clage (ser-klazh′) **1.** Bringing into close opposition and binding together the ends of an obliquely fractured bone or the fragments of a broken patella by a ring or by an encircling, tightly drawn wire loop. **2.** Operation for retinal detachment in which the choroid and retinal pigment epithelia are brought in contact with the detached sensory retina by a band encircling the sclera posterior. **3.** The placing of a nonabsorbable suture around an incompetent cervical os. SYN tiring. [Fr. an encircling, hooping, banding]

cer·co·cys·tis (ser′kō-sis′tis) A form of tapeworm larva that develops within a vertebrate host villus rather than in an invertebrate host's. SEE ALSO cysticercus. [G. *kerkos,* tail, + *kystis,* bladder]

cer·co·pith·e·crine her·pes·vi·rus (ser′kō-pith′ĕ-krēn hĕr′pēz-vī-rŭs) A herpesvirus, in the family Herpesviridae, affecting Old World monkeys, which is very similar morphologically to herpes simplex virus; fatal infection may occur in humans following the bite of an infected monkey, although other modes of transmission have also been documented.

cer·cus, gen. and pl. **cer·ci** (ser′kŭs, ser′sī) A stiff hairlike structure. [Mod. L., fr. G. *kerkos,* tail]

ce·re·a flex·i·bil·i·tas (sē′rē-ă flek-si-bil′i-tas) So-called waxy flexibility, in which the limb remains where placed; often seen in patients with catatonia. [L.]

cer·e·bel·lar (ser-ĕ-bel′ăr) Relating to the cerebellum.

cer·e·bel·lar cor·tex (ser-ĕ-bel′ăr kōr′teks) The thin gray surface layer of the cerebellum, consisting of an outer molecular layer or stratum moleculare, a single layer of Purkinje cells (the ganglionic layer), and an inner granular layer or stratum granulosum.

cer·e·bel·lar fis·sure (ser-ĕ-bel′ăr fish′ŭr) The deep furrows that divide the lobules of the cerebellum. SYN fissurae cerebelli [TA].

cer·e·bel·lar gait (ser-ĕ-bel′ăr gāt) Wide-based gait with lateral veering, unsteadiness, and irregularity of steps; often with a tendency to fall to one side, forward, or backward. SYN ataxic gait.

cer·e·bel·lar hem·i·sphere (ser-ĕ-bel′ăr hem′is-fēr) The large part of the cerebellum lateral to the vermis cerebelli.

cer·e·bel·lar pe·dun·cle (ser-ĕ-bel′ăr pĕ-dŭngk′ĕl) Pedunculus cerebellaris inferior, medius, and superior.

cer·e·bel·li·tis (ser′ĕ-bel-ī′tis) Inflammation of the cerebellum.

cerebello- Prefix meaning the cerebellum. [L. *cerebrum,* brain, + *-ellum,* dim. suff.]

cer·e·bel·lo·pon·tine ang·le (ser-ĕ-bel′ō-pon′tēn ang′gĕl) The recess at the junction of the cerebellum, pons, and medulla. SYN angulus pontocerebellaris [TA].

cer·e·bel·lum, pl. **ce·re·bel·la** (ser-ĕ-bel′ŭm, -bel′ă) [TA] The large posterior brain mass lying dorsal to the pons and medulla and ventral to the posterior portion of the cerebrum; it consists of two lateral hemispheres united by a narrow middle portion, the vermis. [L. dim. of *cerebrum,* brain]

cer·e·bra (sĕ-rē′bră) Plural of cerebrum.

ce·re·bral (ser′ĕ-brăl) Relating to the cerebrum.

ce·re·bral am·y·loid an·gi·op·a·thy (ser′ĕ-brăl am′i-loyd an′jē-op′ă-thē) A pathologic condition of small cerebral vessels characterized by deposits of amyloid in the vessel walls, which may lead to infarcts or hemorrhage; may also occur in Alzheimer disease. SEE ALSO congophilic angiopathy.

ce·re·bral aq·ue·duct (ser′ĕ-brăl ahk′wĕ-dŭkt) An ependyma-lined canal in the mesencephalon about 20 mm long, connecting the third to the fourth ventricle.

ce•re•bral cor•tex (ser′ĕ-brăl kōr′teks) The gray cellular mantle (1–4 mm thick) covering the entire surface of the cerebral hemisphere of mammals; characterized by a laminar organization of cellular and fibrous components such that its nerve cells are stacked in defined layers varying in number from one, as in the archicortex of the hippocampus, to five or six in the larger neocortex; the outermost (molecular or plexiform) layer contains very few cell bodies and is composed largely of the distal ramifications of the long apical dendrites issued perpendicularly to the surface by pyramidal and fusiform cells in deeper layers. From the surface inward, the layers as classified in K. Brodmann's parcellation are: 1) molecular or plexiform layer; 2) outer granular layer; 3) pyramidal cell layer; 4) inner granular layer; 5) inner pyramidal layer (ganglionic layer); and 6) multiform cell layer, many of which are fusiform. This multilaminate organization is typical of the neocortex (homotypic cortex; isocortex in O. Vogt's terminology), which in humans covers the largest part by far of the cerebral hemisphere. The more primordial heterotypic cortex or allocortex (Vogt) has fewer cell layers. A form of cortex intermediate between isocortex and allocortex, called juxtallocortex (Vogt), covers the ventral part of the cingulate gyrus and the entorhinal area of the parahippocampal gyrus.

On the basis of local differences in the arrangement of nerve cells (cytoarchitecture), Brodmann outlined 47 areas in the cerebral cortex that, in functional terms, can be classified into three categories: motor cortex (Brodmann areas 4 and 6), characterized by a poorly developed inner granular layer (agranular cortex) and prominent pyramidal cell layers; sensory cortex, characterized by a prominent inner granular layer (granular cortex or koniocortex) and comprising the somatic sensory cortex (Brodmann areas 1–3), the auditory cortex (Brodmann areas 41 and 42), and the visual cortex (Brodmann areas 17–19); and association cortex, the vast remaining expanses of the cerebral cortex. SEE ALSO Brodmann areas. See this page.

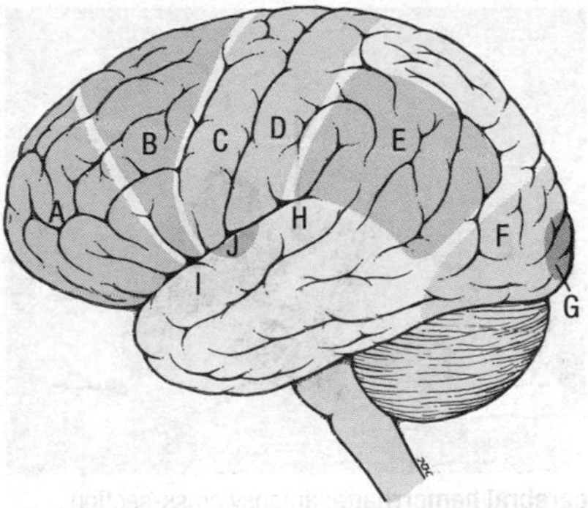

cerebral cortex: major functional areas: (A) biological intelligence, (B) premotor, (C) somatomotor, (D) somatosensory, (E) bodily awareness, (F) visual psychic, (G) visual sensory, (H) speech understanding, (I) auditory psychic, (J) auditory sensory

ce•re•bral death (ser′ĕ-brăl deth) A clinical syndrome characterized by the permanent loss of cerebral and brain stem function, manifested by absence of responsiveness to external stimuli, absence of cephalic reflexes, and apnea. Findings on an isoelectric electroencephalogram for at least 30 minutes in the absence of hypothermia and poisoning by central nervous system depressants supports the diagnosis.

ce•re•bral de•com•pres•sion (ser′ĕ-brăl dē-kŏm-presh′ŭn) Removal of a piece of the cranium, usually in the subtemporal region, with incision of the dura, to relieve intracranial pressure.

ce•re•bral dom•i•nance (ser′ĕ-brăl dom′i-năns) The fact that one hemisphere is dominant over the other and exercises greater influence over certain functions; the left cerebral hemisphere is usually dominant in the control of speech, language and analytical processing, and mathematics, whereas the right hemisphere (usually nondominant) processes spatial concepts and language as related to certain types of visual images; handedness (right-handed people have left cerebral dominance) is considered a general example of cerebral dominance.

ce•re•bral dys•pla•si•a (ser′ĕ-brăl dis-plā′zē-ă) Abnormal development of the telencephalon.

ce•re•bral e•de•ma (ser′ĕ-brăl ĕ-dē′mă) Brain swelling due to increased volume of the extravascular compartment from the uptake of water in the neuropile and white matter. SEE ALSO brain swelling.

ce•re•bral gi•gan•tism (ser′ĕ-brăl jī-gant′izm) A syndrome characterized by increased birth weight and length (above the 90th percentile), an accelerated growth rate for the first 4 or 5 years without elevation of serum growth hormone levels, then reversion to normal growth rate; characteristic facies include prognathism, hypertelorism, antimongoloid slant, and dolichocephalic cranium; moderate mental retardation and impaired coordination are also associated.

ce•re•bral hem•i•sphere (ser′ĕ-brăl hem′is-fēr′) **1.** SYN hemisphere. **2.** The large mass of the telencephalon, on either side of the midline, consisting of the cerebral cortex and its associated fiber systems, together with the deeper-lying subcortical telencephalic nuclei (i.e., basal ganglia [nuclei]). See page A5. SYN hemispherium (1).

ce•re•bral hem•or•rhage (ser′ĕ-brăl hem′ŏr-ăj) Hemorrhage into the substance of the cerebrum, usually in the region of the internal capsule by the rupture of the lenticulostriate artery. See page 284. SYN hematencephalon.

ce•re•bral her•ni•a (ser′ĕ-brăl hĕr′nē-ă) Protru-

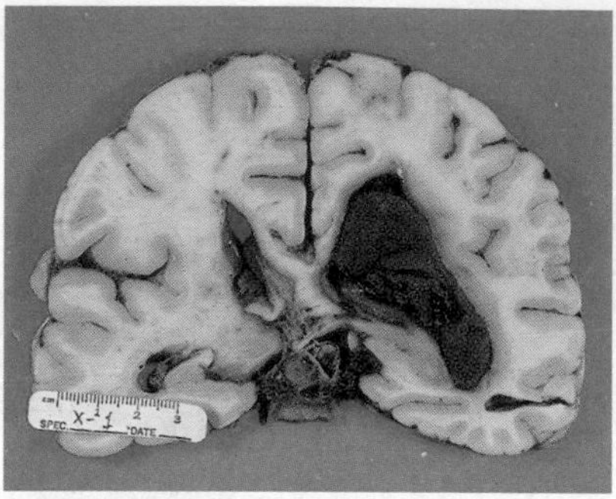

cerebral hemorrhage: autopsy cross-section (coronal) of patient who suffered arteriovenous malformation with associated right ventricle hemorrhage

sion of brain substance through a defect in the skull.

ce•re•bral in•dex (ser′ĕ-brăl in′deks) The ratio of the transverse to the anteroposterior diameter of the cranial cavity multiplied by 100.

ce•re•bral lo•cal•i•za•tion (ser′ĕ-brăl lō′kăl-ī-zā′shŭn) The mapping of the cerebral cortex into areas and the correlation of the various areas with cerebral function, or determining the site of a brain lesion, based on the signs and symptoms manifested by the patient or by neuroimaging.

ce•re•bral pal•sy (ser′ĕ-brăl pawl′zē) Defect of motor power and coordination related to damage to the brain that occurred prenatally, perinatally, or in the first 3 years of life.

ce•re•bral pe•dun•cle (ser′ĕ-brăl pĕ-dŭngk′ĕl) Large bundles of corticofugal fibers forming the crus cerebri, plus the midbrain tegmentum; the substantia nigra, although a part of the base of the peduncle (basis pedunculi), is considered a structure separating the midbrain tegmentum from the crus cerebri. SEE ALSO crus cerebri.

ce•re•bral re•vas•cu•lar•i•za•tion (ser′ĕ-brăl rē-vas′kyū-lăr-ī-zā′shŭn) Restoration of blood flow to the brain by surgical intervention.

ce•re•bral vas•cu•lar at•tack (CVA) (ser′ĕ-bral vas-kyū′lăr ă-tak′) SYN acute ischemic stroke.

ce•re•bral ves•i•cle (ser′ĕ-brăl ves′i-kĕl) Each of the three divisions of the early embryonic brain (prosencephalon, mesencephalon, and rhombencephalon). SYN primary brain vesicle.

cer•e•bra•tion (ser′ĕ-brā′shŭn) Activity of the mental processes; thinking. SEE ALSO cognition.

cer•e•bri•form (se-rē′bri-fōrm) Resembling the external fissures and convolutions of the brain. [cerebri- + L. *forma,* shape, appearance, nature]

cer•e•bri•tis (ser′ĕ-brī′tis) Focal inflammatory infiltrates in the brain parenchyma.

♻ **cerebro-, cerebr-, cerebri-** Combining forms meaning the cerebrum. SEE ALSO encephalo-. [L. *cerebrum,* brain]

cer•e•broid (ser′ĕ-broyd) Resembling the cerebrum.

cer•e•bro•ma (ser′ĕ-brō′mă) SYN encephaloma.

cer•e•bro•ma•la•ci•a (ser′ĕ-brō-mă-lā′shē-ă) SYN encephalomalacia.

cer•e•bro•men•in•gi•tis (ser′ĕ-brō-men-in-jī′tis) SYN meningoencephalitis.

cer•e•brop•a•thy (ser′ĕ-brop′ă-thē) SYN encephalopathy.

cer•e•bro•scle•ro•sis (ser′ĕ-brō-skler-ō′sis) Encephalosclerosis, hardening of the cerebral hemispheres. [cerebro- + G. *sklērōsis,* hardening]

cer•e•bro•side (ser′ĕ-brō-sīd) A class of glycosphingolipid; cerebrosides are found in the myelin sheath of nerve tissue.

cer•e•bro•spi•nal (ser′ĕ-brō-spī′năl) Relating to the brain and the spinal cord.

cer•e•bro•spi•nal ax•is (ser′ĕ-brō-spī′năl ak′sis) The central nervous system; the brain and spinal cord.

cer•e•bro•spi•nal flu•id (CSF) (ser′ĕ-brō-spī′năl flū′id) A fluid largely secreted by the choroid plexuses of the ventricles of the brain, filling the ventricles and the subarachnoid cavities of the brain and spinal cord.

cer•e•bro•spi•nal flu•id rhi•nor•rhe•a (ser′ĕ-brō-spī′năl flū′id rī-nōr-ē′ă) A discharge of cerebrospinal fluid from the nose. Basal skull fracture may cause tears in the dura, thus allowing cerebrospinal fluid to leak through the nose.

cer•e•bro•spi•nal men•in•gi•tis (ser′ĕ-brō-spī′năl men-in-jī′tis) SYN meningitis.

cer•e•bro•spi•nal pres•sure (ser′ĕ-brō-spī′năl presh′ŭr) The pressure of the cerebrospinal fluid, normally 100–150 mm of water, relative to the ambient atmospheric pressure.

cer•e•brot•o•my (ser′ĕ-brot′ŏ-mē) Incision of the brain. [cerebro- + G. *tomē,* incision]

cer•e•bro•vas•cu•lar (ser′ĕ-brō-vas′kyū-lăr) Relating to the blood supply to the brain, particularly with reference to pathologic changes.

cer•e•bro•vas•cu•lar ac•ci•dent (CVA) (ser′ĕ-brō-vas′kyū-lăr ak′si-dĕnt) An imprecise term for cerebral stroke.

cer•e•brum, pl. **cer•e•bra**, **cer•e•brums** (ser′ĕ-brŭm, -bră, -brŭmz) [TA] Originally referred to the largest portion of the brain; it now usually refers only to the parts derived from the telencephalon and includes mainly the cerebral hemispheres (cerebral cortex and basal ganglia). [L., brain]

ce•ri•um (Ce) (sēr′ē-ŭm) A metallic element, atomic no. 58, atomic wt. 140.115. [fr. *Ceres,* the planetoid]

cer•ti•fi•a•ble (sĕr′ti-fī′ă-bĕl) Denoting a person showing disordered behavior of sufficient gravity to justify involuntary mental hospitalization.

cer•ti•fi•ca•tion (sĕr′ti-fi-kā′shŭn) **1.** The attainment of board certification in a specialty. **2.** The court procedure by which a patient is committed to a mental institution. **3.** Involuntary mental hospitalization.

cer•ti•fied hand ther•a•pist (CHT) (sĕr′ti-fīd hand thār′ă-pĭst) An occupational therapist who has been awarded a specialty certification in the area of hand rehabilitation.

cer•ti•fied milk (sĕr′ti-fīd milk) Cow's milk that does not have more than the maximal permissible limit of 10,000 bacteria per mL at any time before delivery to the consumer; must be cooled to 10°C or cooler and maintained at that temperature until delivery.

cer•ti•fied nurse-mid•wife (sĕr′ti-fīd nŭrs mid′wīf) A registered nurse who holds at least a master's degree in nursing and advanced levels of education in the management of maternity. Certification is achieved through an organized program of study and national testing by the American College of Nurse-Midwives.

Cer•ti•fied Oc•cu•pa•tion•al Health Nurse (COHN) (sĕr′ti-fīd ok-yū-pā′shŭn-ăl helth nŭrs) Specialty designation signifying the successful completion of an examination concentrating on occupational health.

cer•ti•fied or•thot•ist (CO) (sĕr′ti-fīd ōr-thot′ist) A maker and fitter of orthotic devices who has passed certification according to the standards of one of the several national licensing bodies.

cer•ti•fied pas•teur•ized milk (sĕr′ti-fīd pas′chŭr-īzd milk) Cow's milk in which the maximum permissible limit is 10,000 bacteria per mL before pasteurization and 500 bacteria per mL after pasteurization; it must be cooled to 7.2°C or less and maintained at that temperature until delivery.

Cer•ti•fied Phar•ma•cy Tech•ni•cian (CPhT) (sĕr′ti-fīd fahr′mă-sē tek-ni′shŭn) A pharmacy technician who has successfully passed the Pharmacy Technician Certification Board (PTCB) examination.

cer•ti•fied pros•the•tist (CP) (sĕr′ti-fīd pros′thĕ-tist) A maker and fitter of prosthetic devices who has passed certification according to the standards of one of the several licensing bodies.

cer•ti•fied pros•the•tist/or•thot•ist (CPO) (sĕr′ti-fīd pros′thĕ-tist ōr-thot′ist) A maker and fitter of prosthetic and orthotic devices who has passed certification according to the standards of one of the several licensing bodies.

cer•ti•fied ref•er•ence ma•ter•i•al (CRM) (sĕr′ti-fīd ref′rĕns mă-tēr′ē-ăl) A reference material documented by or traceable to a certificate or publication from a reputable source and stating the values of the properties concerned.

Cer•ti•fied Res•pi•ra•tor•y Ther•a•pist (CRT) (sĕr′tĭ-fīd res′pir-ă-tōr-ē thār′ă-pist) A health care professional, generally holding an associate's degree, who is licensed at the state level to treat patients with various lung disorders using modalities that include mechanical devices and is also trained in the use of associated testing apparatus.

cer•u•le•an cat•a•ract (sĕ-rū′lē-ăn kat′ăr-akt) SYN blue cataract.

ce•ru•le•in (sĕ-rū′lē-in) A decapeptide with hypotensive activity, which stimulates smooth muscle and increases digestive secretions. It is similar in structure to cholecystokinin and the gastrins, but much more potent as a stimulant to gallbladder contraction; also stimulates release of insulin. [Fr. *Hyla caerulea,* from which isolated]

ce•ru•lo•plas•min (sĕ-rū′lō-plaz-min) A blue, copper-containing alpha-globulin of blood plasma; involved in copper transport and regulation, and can reduce O_2 directly without known intermediates. Ceruloplasmin is absent in congenital Wilson disease. [L. *caeruleus,* dark blue]

ce•ru•men (sĕ-rū′mĕn) The soft, brownish yellow, waxy secretion (a modified sebum) of the ceruminous glands of the external auditory meatus. See page B28. [L. *cera,* wax]

ce•ru•mi•nal (sĕ-rū′mi-năl) Relating to cerumen.

ce•ru•mi•no•lyt•ic (sĕ-rū′mi-nō-lit′ik) Any substance instilled into the external auditory canal to soften wax. [cerumen, + G. *lysis,* a loosening]

ce•ru•mi•no•sis (se-rū′mi-nō′sis) Excessive formation of cerumen.

ce•ru•mi•nous (sĕ-rū′mi-nŭs) Relating to cerumen.

ce•ru•mi•nous glands (sĕ-rū′mi-nŭs glandz) Apocrine sudoriferous glands in the external acoustic meatus. SYN glandulae ceruminosae (1) [TA].

cer•vi•cal (sĕr′vi-kăl) Relating to a neck, or cervix, in any sense. [L. *cervix (cervic-),* neck]

cer•vi•cal ca•nal (sĕr′vi-kăl kă-nal′) A fusiform canal extending from the isthmus of the uterus to the opening of the uterus into the vagina. SYN canalis cervicis uteri [TA].

cer•vi•cal col•lar (sĕr′vi-kăl kol′ăr) Splinting device used to stabilize the neck.

cer•vi•cal com•pres•sion test (sĕr′vi-kăl kŏm-presh′ŭn test) Maneuver in which the examiner exerts downward pressure on the subject's head. Increased pain or altered sensation indicates pressure on a nerve root.

cer•vi•cal disc syn•drome (sĕr′vi-kăl disk sin′drōm) Pain, paresthesias, and sometimes weakness in the area of the distribution of one or more cervical roots, due to pressure of a protruded cervical intervertebral disc.

cer•vi•cal flex•ure (sĕr′vi-kăl flek′shŭr) The ventrally concave bend at the juncture of the brainstem and spinal cord in the embryo.

cer•vi•cal glands (sĕr′vi-kăl glandz) Branched mucus-secreting glands in the mucosa of the cervix.

cer•vi•cal in•tra•ep•i•the•li•al ne•o•pla•si•a (CIN) (sĕr′vi-kăl in′tră-ep-i-thē′lē-ăl nē-ō-plā′zē-ă) Dysplastic changes beginning at the squamocolumnar junction in the uterine cervix that may be precursors of squamous cell carcinoma: Grade 1, mild dysplasia involving the lower one third or less of the epithelial thickness; Grade 2, moderate dysplasia with one third to two thirds involvement; Grade 3, severe dysplasia or carcinoma in situ, with two thirds to full-thickness involvement.

cer•vi•cal line (sĕr′vi-kăl līn) A continuous anatomic irregular curved line marking the junction of the crown and the root of a tooth. SEE ALSO cementoenamel junction.

cer•vi•cal loop (sĕr′vi-kăl lūp) SYN ansa cervicalis.

cer•vi•cal lor•do•sis (sĕr′vi-kăl lōr-dō′sis) The normal, anteriorly convex curvature of the cervical segment of the vertebral column; a secondary curvature, acquired postnatally as the infant lifts its head. SYN lordosis cervicis [TA], lordosis colli.

cer•vi•cal or•tho•sis (sĕr′vi-kăl ōr-thō′sis) An orthosis designed to limit cervical spine motion to varying degrees (e.g., a soft cervical collar).

cer•vi•cal plex•us (sĕr′vi-kăl pleks′ŭs) Formed by loops joining the adjacent ventral primary rami of the first four cervical nerves and receiving gray communicating rami from the superior cervical ganglion; it lies deep to the sternocleidomastoid muscle, and sends out numerous cutaneous, muscular, and communicating rami.

cer•vi•cal preg•nan•cy (sĕr′vi-kăl preg′năn-sē) The implantation and development of the impregnated ovum in the cervical canal.

cer•vi•cal rib (sĕr′vi-kăl rib) A supernumerary rib articulating with a cervical vertebra, usually the seventh, but not reaching the sternum anteriorly. SEE ALSO cervical rib syndrome. SYN costa cervicalis [TA].

cer•vi•cal rib syn•drome (sĕr′vi-kăl rib sin′drōm) **1.** Arterial thoracic outlet syndrome, in which the subclavian artery is compromised by a fully formed cervical rib. **2.** True neurogenic thoracic outlet syndrome, in which the proximal lower trunk of the brachial plexus is compromised by a radiolucent band extending from a rudimentary cervical rib to the first rib.

cer•vi•cal ver•te•brae [C1–C7] (sĕr′vi-kăl vĕr′tĕ-brē) The seven segments of the vertebral column located in the neck. See this page. SYN vertebrae cervicales [C1–C7] [TA].

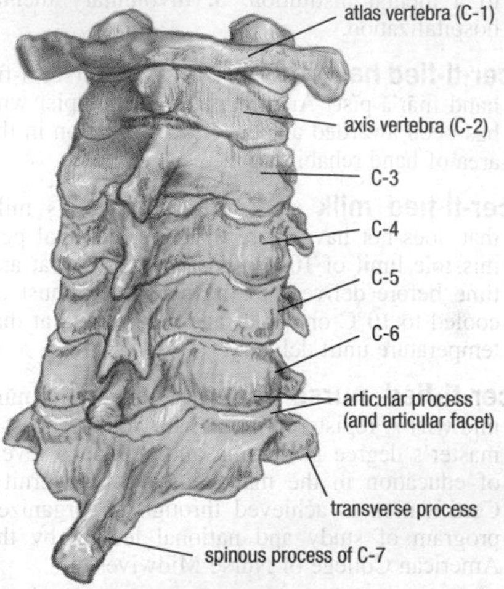

cervical vertebrae [C1-C7]

cer•vi•cec•to•my (sĕr′vi-sek′tŏ-mē) Excision of the cervix uteri. SYN trachelectomy. [cervix + G. *ektomē,* excision]

cer•vi•ces (sĕr′vi-sēz) Plural of cervix.

cer•vi•cis (sĕr-vī′sis) Genitive of cervix.

cer•vi•ci•tis (sĕr′vi-sī′tis) Inflammation of the mucous membrane, frequently involving also the deeper structures, of the cervix uteri. SYN trachelitis.

cervico- Prefix meaning a cervix, or neck, in any sense. [L. *cervix,* neck]

cer•vi•co•brach•i•al (ser′vi-kō-brā′kē-ăl) Relating to the neck and the arm.

cer•vi•co•dyn•i•a (sĕr′vi-kō-din′ē-ă) Neck pain. SYN trachelodynia. [cervico- + G. *odynē,* pain]

cer•vi•co•fa•cial (sĕr′vi-kō-fā′shăl) Relating to the neck and the face.

cer•vi•cog•ra•phy (sĕr′vi-kog′ră-fē) Technique, equivalent to colposcopy, for photographing all or part of the uterine cervix. [cervix + G. *graphō,* to write]

cer•vi•co•oc•cip•i•tal (sĕr′vi-kō-ok-sip′i-tăl) Relating to the neck and the occiput.

cer•vi•co•oc•u•lo•a•cous•tic syn•drome (sĕr′vi-kō-ok′yū-lō-ă-kū′stik sin′drōm) A disorder characterized by a congenitally short neck with fused cervical vertebrae (Klippel-Feil anomaly), sixth cranial nerve paralysis with retraction of the eye globe and narrowing of the palpebral fissure on adduction (Duane palsy), and sensorineural deafness; inheritance is thought to be multifactorial with limitation to females.

cer•vi•co•plas•ty (sĕr′vi-kō-plas-tē) Surgical repair on the cervix uteri or on the neck.

cer•vi•cos•co•py (sĕr-vi-kos′kŏ-pē) SYN acetowhitening.

cer•vi•co•tho•rac•ic (sĕr′vi-kō-thōr-as′ik) Term describing: 1) the neck and thorax; 2) the transition between the neck and thorax; 3) the fusion of the cervical and thoracic vertebrae.

cer•vi•co•tho•rac•ic gan•gli•on (sĕr′vi-kō-thōr-as′ik gang′glē-ŏn) A sympathetic trunk ganglion lying behind the subclavian artery near the origin of the vertebral artery, it is formed by the fusion of the inferior cervical ganglion, at the level of the seventh cervical vertebra, with the first thoracic ganglion. SYN ganglion cervicothoracicum [TA].

cer•vi•co•tho•rac•ic or•tho•sis (sĕr′vi-kō-thōr-as′ik ōr-thō′sis) A device designed to limit cervical spine motion by extending to cover more of the upper torso than a standard cervical orthosis.

cer•vi•cot•o•my (sĕr-vi-kot′ŏ-mē) Incision into the cervix uteri. SYN trachelotomy. [cervico- + G. *tomē,* incision]

cer•vi•co•ves•i•cal (sĕr′vi-kō-ves′i-kăl) Relating to the cervix of the uterus and the bladder.

cer•vix, gen. **cer•vi•cis**, pl. **cer•vi•ces** (sĕr′viks, sĕr-vī′sis, sĕr′vi-sēz) [TA] **1.** SYN neck. **2.** Any necklike structure. **3.** SYN cervix of uterus. [L. neck]

cer•vix of u•ter•us (sĕr′viks yū′tĕr-ŭs) The lower part of the uterus extending from the isthmus of the uterus into the vagina. It is divided into supravaginal and vaginal parts by its passage through the vaginal wall. SYN cervix (3) [TA].

ce•sar•e•an hys•ter•ec•to•my (se-zār′ē-ăn his′tĕr-ek′tŏ-mē) Cesarean section followed by hysterectomy. SYN Caesarean hysterectomy.

ce•sar•e•an sec•tion (se-zār′ē-ăn sek′shŭn) Incision through the abdominal wall and the uterus (abdominal hysterotomy) for extraction of the fetus. SYN Caesarean section.

ce•si•um (Cs) (sē′zē-ŭm) A metallic element, atomic no. 55, atomic wt. 132.90543; a member of the alkali metal group. ^{137}Cs (half-life equal to 30.1 years) is used in treatment of certain malignancies. SYN caesium. [L. *caesius,* bluish gray]

Ces•tan-Che•nais syn•drome (ses-tahn[h]′ shĕ-nā′ sin′drōm) Contralateral hemiplegia, hemianesthesia, and loss of pain and temperature sensibility, with ipsilateral hemiasynergia and lateropulsion, paralysis of the larynx and soft palate, enophthalmia, miosis, and ptosis, due to lesions of the brainstem.

Ces•to•da (ses-tō′dă) A class of the flatworm phylum Platyhelminthes. There are two subclasses, Cestodaria and Eucestoda. The latter are the segmented tapeworms that parasitize humans and domestic animals. [G. *kestos,* girdle]

Ces•to•dar•i•a (ses-tō-dā′rē-ă) A subclass of the class Cestoidea. Cestodarians are intestinal and celomic parasites of elasmobranchs and primitive telost fish. They are trematodelike but are classified with cestodes because they lack an intestine.

i **ces•tode**, **ces•toid** (ses′tōd, -toyd) Common name for tapeworms of the subclass Eucestoda. See page B7.

Ces•toi•de•a (ses-toy′dē-ă) The tapeworms, a class of platyhelminth flatworms characterized by lack of an alimentary canal and a segmented body with a scolex or holdfast organ at one end; adult worms are vertebrate parasites, usually found in the small intestine. [G. *kestos,* girdle, + *eidos,* form]

ce•tyl (sē′til) The univalent radical $C_{16}H_{33}-$ of cetyl alcohol.

CF Abbreviation for citrovorum factor; coupling factor.

Cf Symbol for californium.

C fi•bers (fī′bĕrz) Unmyelinated fibers, 0.4–1.2 mcm in diameter, conducting nerve impulses at a velocity of 0.7–2.3 m/sec. SYN C fibres.

C fibres [Br.] SYN C fibers.

CFIDS Abbreviation for chronic fatigue and immune dysfunction syndrome.

CFR Abbreviation for Code of Federal Regulations Title 21.

CFTR Abbreviation for cystic fibrosis transmembrane regulator.

CFU Abbreviation for colony-forming unit.

CG NATO code for phosgene oxime.

CGRP Abbreviation for calcitonin gene–related peptide.

CGS, **cgs** Abbreviation for centimeter-gram-second. SEE centimeter-gram-second system.

Chad•dock sign, **Chad•dock re•flex** (chad′ ŏk sīn, chad′ŏk rē′fleks) When the external malleolar skin area is irritated, extension of the great toe occurs in cases of organic disease of the corticospinal reflex paths.

Chad•wick sign (chad′wik sīn) A bluish discoloration of the cervix and vagina; a sign of pregnancy.

chafe (chāf) To cause irritation of the skin by friction. [Fr. *chauffer,* to heat, fr. L. *calefacio,* to make warm]

Cha•gas dis•ease, Cha•gas-Cruz dis•ease (shah′găs di-zēz′, shah′găs krūz di-zēz′) SYN South American trypanosomiasis.

cha•go•ma (chă-gō′mă) The skin lesion produced by acute Chagas disease.

chain (chān) **1.** CHEMISTRY a series of atoms held together by one or more covalent bonds. **2.** BACTERIOLOGY a linear arrangement of living cells that have divided in one plane and remain attached to each other. **3.** A series of reactions. **4.** ANATOMY a linked series of structures, e.g., ossicular chain, chain ganglia. SEE ALSO sympathetic trunk. [L. *catena*]

chain of cus•to•dy (chān kŭs′tŏ-dē) A procedure that makes certain that a biologic specimen is always in the custody of a person legally responsible for maintaining the integrity of the sample. The chain begins with patient identification, continues during collection, processing, and testing. Every step in the process is monitored and documented (e.g., date, time, and identification of the handler). Additional documentation includes special containers, sealing material, and forms.

chain re•ac•tion (chān rē-ak′shŭn) A self-perpetuating reaction in which a product of one step in the reaction itself serves to bring about the next step in the reaction, and so on. Cf. autocatalysis.

chain re•flex (chān rē′fleks) A series of reflexes, each serving as a stimulus for the next.

chain of sur•vi•val (chān sŭr-vī′văl) The American Heart Association's term for four major interventions designed to reduce sudden cardiac death—early access, early cardiopulmonary resuscitation (CPR), early defibrillation, and early advanced life support (ALS).

chak•ra (shahk′rah) An ancient Indian tradition of understanding human energy in a system of seven major vortices that activate and energize surrounding areas. Chakras are said to be accessed through the practice of polarity therapy, Reiki, and yoga. SEE ALSO polarity therapy, Reiki.

cha•la•si•a, cha•la•sis (kă-lā′zē-ă, -lā′sis) Inhibition and relaxation of any previously sustained contraction of muscle, usually of a synergic group of muscles. [G. *chalaō,* to loosen]

cha•la•zi•on, pl. **cha•la•zi•a** (kă-lā′zē-on, -zē-ă) A chronic inflammatory granuloma of a meibomian gland; sometimes related to blockage. SYN meibomian cyst, tarsal cyst. [G. dim. of *chalaza,* a sty]

chal•i•co•sis (kal-i-kō′sis) Pneumoconiosis caused by the inhalation of dust incident to the occupation of stone cutting. [G. *chalix,* gravel]

chal•lenge di•et (chal′ĕnj dī′ĕt) A diet in which one or more specific substances are included for the purpose of determining whether an abnormal reaction occurs.

cha•lone (kal′ōn) Any of a number of mitotic inhibitors elaborated by a tissue and active only on that type of tissue, regardless of species; a reversible tissue-specific mitotic inhibitor. [G. + *chalaō,* to relax, + -one]

cham•ber (chām′bĕr) **1.** A compartment or enclosed space. **2.** Divisions of a hemocytometer. SEE ALSO camera. [L. *camera*]

Cham•ber•lain line (chām′bĕr-lăn līn) Imaginary delimit at base of skull running between the dorsal tip of the foramen magnum and the dorsal margin of the hard palate; normally lies above the tip of the odontoid process of this axis.

Cham•ber•len for•ceps (chām′bĕr-lĕn fōr′seps) The original obstetric forceps, without a curvature.

cham•bers of eye•ball (chām′bĕrz ī′bawl) The cavities within the eyeball: anterior and posterior chambers, filled with aqueous, and the postremal (vitreous) chamber, occupied by the vitreous. SEE ALSO anterior chamber of eyeball, posterior chamber of eyeball, postremal chamber of eyeball. SYN camerae bulbi [TA].

cham•o•mile (kam′ŏ-mīl) (*Matricaria*) Herbal agent used in infusions for stomach disorders; alleged to induce sleep; some topical use reported; danger in pregnant women due to abortifacient properties. [L.L. *chamomilla,* fr. G. *chamaimēlon*]

CHAMPUS (champ′ŭs) Acronym (obsolete) for Civilian Health and Medical Program of the Uniformed Services. SEE TRICARE.

CHAMPVA (champ′vă) Acronym (obsolete) for Civilian Health and Medical Program of the Veterans' Administration. SEE TRICARE.

Cham•py fix•a•tive (shahm-pē′ fiks′ă-tiv) A mixture of potassium bichromate, chromic acid, and osmic acid, considered an excellent cytologic fixative with advantages and disadvantages similar to those of Flemming fixative; it differs from Flemming fixative in substituting bichromate for acetic acid.

chan•cre (shang′kĕr) The primary lesion of syphilis, which begins at the site of infection after an interval of 10–30 days as a papule or area of infiltration, of dull red color, hard, and insensitive; the center usually becomes eroded or breaks down into an ulcer that heals slowly after 4–6 weeks. SYN hard chancre, hard ulcer. [Fr. indirectly from L. *cancer*]

chan•cri•form (shang′kri-fōrm) Resembling chancre.

chan•croid (shang′kroyd) An infectious, painful, ragged venereal ulcer at the site of infection by *Haemophilus ducreyi,* beginning after an incubation period of 3–5 days; seen more commonly in men. SYN soft chancre, soft ulcer, venereal ulcer. [chancre + G. *eidos,* resemblance]

chan•croi•dal (shang-kroy′dăl) Relating to or of the nature of chancroid.

chan•crous (shang′krŭs) Characterized by having a chancre.

chan•de•lier sign (shan′dĕ-lēr′ sīn) Colloquial term referring to severe pain elicited during pelvic examination of patients with pelvic inflammatory disease, in which the patient responds by reaching upward toward the ceiling for relief.

Chand•ler syn•drome (chand′lĕr sin′drōm) Iris atrophy with corneal edema.

change (chānj) An alteration; in pathology, structural alteration of which the cause and significance is uncertain. SYN shift (1).

change blind•ness (chānj blīnd′nĕs) Failure to observe large changes in the vision field that occur simultaneously with brief disturbances.

chan•nel•op•a•thies (chan-ĕ-lop′ă-thēz) SYN ion channel disorders. [channel + G. *pathos,* disease]

cha•ot•ic rhythm (kā-ot′ik ridh′ŭm) Completely irregular cardiac rhythm at varying rates. SEE ALSO arrhythmia.

chap•pa•ral (shap-ă-ral′) Herbal prepared from *Larrea tridentata* and *L. divaricata;* used by Native American shamans in bronchitis and dermatologic disorders; hepatotoxicity widely reported. SYN creosote bush. [Sp. *chaparral,* thicket of evergreen oak, fr. *chaparra,* dwarf evergreen oak, fr. Basque *txapar*]

chapped (chapt) Having or pertaining to skin, especially of the hands, which is dry, scaly, and fissured, owing to the action of cold or to the excess rate of evaporation of moisture from the skin surface. [M.E. *chap,* to chop, split]

Cha•put tu•ber•cle (sha′pū tū′bĕr-kĕl) Anterior tubercle of the distal tibia; attachment site of the anterior tibiofibular ligament.

char•ac•ter (kar′ăk-tĕr) An attribute in people that is amenable to formal and logical analysis and may be used as the basis of generalizations about classes and other statements that transcend individuality. SYN characteristic (1). [G. *charakter,* stamp, mark, fr. *charassō,* to engrave]

char•ac•ter dis•or•der (kar′ăk-tĕr dis-ōr′dĕr) A term referring to a group of behavioral disorders, now replaced by a more general term, personality disorder, of which character disorders are now a subclass.

char•ac•ter•is•tic (kar′ăk-tĕr-is′tik) **1.** SYN character. **2.** Typical or distinctive of a particular disorder.

char•ac•ter•is•tic fre•quen•cy (kar′ăk-tĕr-is′tik frē′kwĕn-sē) Frequency at which a given neuron responds to the least sound intensity. SYN best frequency.

char•ac•ter•is•tic ra•di•a•tion (kar′ăk-tĕr-is′tik rā′dē-ā′shŭn) When an incoming electron from the cathode stream that has enough energy to overcome the binding energy of electrons in the inner shells of the target material knocks the electron out of its shell, the outer electrons fall into the inner shell, giving up energy in the form of x-radiation. Produced at levels of greater than 69.5 kV. This process leaves the atom ionized.

char•ac•ter•iz•ing group (kar′ăk-tĕr-īz′ing grūp) A group of atoms in a molecule that distinguishes the class of substances in which it occurs from all other classes; thus carbonyl (CO) is the characterizing group of ketones; COOH, of organic acids, among other examples.

char•ac•ter neu•ro•sis (kar′ăk-tĕr nūr-ō′sis) A subclass of personality disorders.

char•coal (chahr′kōl) Carbon obtained by heating or burning wood with restricted access of air.

Char•cot an•gi•na (shahr-kō′ an′ji-nă) Global insufficiency of blood flow to supply metabolic tissue demand during exertion; marked by cold extremities, weakness, cramps, and pain. Rest ameliorates condition.

Char•cot dis•ease (shahr-kō′ di-zēz′) SYN amyotrophic lateral sclerosis.

Char•cot gait (shahr-kō′ gāt) The gait of hereditary ataxia.

Char•cot in•ter•mit•tent fe•ver (shahr-kō′ in′tĕr-mit′ĕnt fē′vĕr) Fever, chills, right upper quadrant pain, and jaundice associated with intermittently obstructing common duct stones.

Char•cot joint (shahr-kō′ joynt) SYN neuropathic joint.

Char•cot-Ley•den crys•tals (shahr-kō′ lī′dĕn kris′tălz) Crystals in the shape of elongated double pyramids, formed from eosinophils, found in the sputum in bronchial asthma.

Char•cot-Ma•rie-Tooth dis•ease (shahr-kō′ mah-rē′ tūth di-zēz′) SYN peroneal muscular atrophy.

Char•cot syn•drome (shahr-kō′ sin′drōm) SYN intermittent claudication.

Char•cot tri•ad (shahr-kō′ trī′ad) **1.** In multiple (disseminated) sclerosis, the three symptoms: nystagmus, tremor, and scanning speech. **2.** Combination of jaundice, fever, and upper abdominal pain that occurs as a result of cholangitis.

Char•cot ver•ti•go (shahr-kō′ vĕr′ti-gō) SYN tussive syncope.

Char•gaff rule (shahr′gahf rūl) In DNA the number of adenine units equals the number of thymine units; likewise, the number of guanine units equals the number of cytosine units.

CHARGE com•plex (chahrj kom′pleks) A complex diagnosed in infants with four of the seven components of the CHARGE acronym: coloboma, heart defects, atresia of the nasal choanae, retarded growth and development, genital hypoplasia, ear anomalies, and/or deafness.

charge nurse (chahrj nŭrs) The nurse who supervises patient care during a shift in a hospital unit.

char•la•tan (shahr′lă-tăn) A medical fraud claiming to cure disease by useless procedures, secret remedies, and worthless diagnostic and therapeutic machines. SYN quack. [Fr., fr. It. *ciarlare*, to prattle]

char•la•tan•ism (shahr′lă-tăn-izm) A fraudulent claim to medical knowledge; treating the sick without knowledge of medicine or authority to practice medicine.

Charles law (shahrlz law) All gases expand equally on heating, namely, 1/273.16 of their volume at 0°C for every degree Celsius. SYN Gay-Lussac law.

char•ley horse (chahr′lē hōrs) Localized pain or muscle stiffness following a strain or contusion of a muscle. [slang]

chart (chahrt) **1.** A record, hand written or on computer, of clinical data relating to a patient's case. **2.** SYN curve (2). **3.** OPHTHALMOLOGY symbols of graduated size for measuring visual acuity, or test types for determining far or near vision. **4.** To record clinical data relating to a patient's care. SEE ALSO Snellen test type, chart war. [L. *charta*, sheet of papyrus]

Char•ter meth•od (chahr′tĕr meth′ŏd) A method of toothbrushing using a restricted circular motion with the bristles inclined coronally at a 45-degree angle.

chart•ing by ex•cep•tion (chahrt′ing ek-sep′shŭn) A method of documentation based on established standards of practice, for which reason only exceptions to these standards are documented.

chart war (chahrt wōr) Disagreements or criticisms over patient treatment expressed by medical professionals as they keep written patient records; usually indicates that such professionals have not met to resolve such disputes.

chauf•feur's frac•ture (shō-fŭrz′ frak′shŭr) SYN Hutchinson fracture.

Chaus•si•er sign (shō-sē-ā′ sīn) Severe pain in the epigastrium, a prodrome of eclampsia; may be of central origin or caused by distention of the capsule of liver by hemorrhage.

Chayes meth•od (chāyz meth′ŏd) A method of replacing lost teeth using a mechanical device for the fixation and stabilization of the dental prosthesis, which allows "movement in function" of the abutment teeth.

ChE Abbreviation for cholinesterase.

check (chek) **1.** To stop or obstruct. **2.** To examine or test. **3.** The act or result of checking. [O.Fr. *eschec*, to checkmate, fr. Persian *shāh*, king]

Ché•di•ak-Hi•ga•shi syn•drome (chā′dē-ahk-hē-gah′shē sin′drōm) A genetic disorder associated with abnormalities of granulation and nuclear structure of all types of leukocytes and with the presence of peroxidase-positive granules, cytoplasmic inclusions, and Dohle bodies; characterized by hepatosplenomegaly, lymphadenopathy, anemia, neutropenia, partial albinism, nystagmus, photophobia, and susceptibilities to infection and lymphoma; death usually occurs in childhood; occurs in mink, cattle, mice, killer whales, and humans; autosomal recessive inheritance, caused by mutation in the Chediak-Higashi gene (CHS) on chromosome 1q. See page B12.

cheek (chēk) The side of the face forming the lateral wall of the mouth. SYN bucca, gena, mala (1). [A. S. *ceáce*]

cheek tooth (chēk tūth) Colloqualism for a posterior tooth, specifically a premolar or molar.

cheese work•er's lung (chēz wŏrk′ĕrz lŭng) Extrinsic allergic alveolitis caused by inhalation of spores of *Penicillium casei* from moldy cheese.

chei•lec•to•my, chi•lec•to•my (kī-lek′tŏ-mē, kī-lĕk′tŏ-mē) **1.** Excision of a portion of the lip. **2.** Chiseling away bony irregularities at osteochondral margin of a joint cavity that interfere with movements of the joint. [cheil- + G. *ektomē*, excision]

cheil•ec•tro•pi•on, chil•ec•tro•pi•on (kī-lek-trō′pē-on, kī-lek-trō′pē-on) Eversion of the lips or a lip. [cheil- + G. *ektropos*, a turning out]

chei•li•tis, chi•li•tis (kī-lī′tis, kī-lī′tĭs) Inflammation of the lips or of a lip. SEE ALSO cheilosis. See page B15. [cheil- + G. *-itis*, inflammation]

chei•li•tis gland•u•lar•is (kī-lī′tis gland′yū-lā′ris) An acquired disorder, of unknown etiology, of the lower lip characterized by swelling, ulceration, crusting, mucous gland hyperplasia, and abscesses. SYN Volkmann cheilitis.

chei•li•tis gran•u•lo•ma•to•sa (kī-lī′tis gran′yū-lō-mă-tō′să) Chronic, diffuse, soft swelling of the lips, of unknown etiology, microscopically characterized by noncaseating granulomatous inflammation. SYN Meischer syndrome.

♻ **cheilo-, cheil-** Combining forms meaning lips. SEE ALSO chilo-, labio-. [G. *cheilos*, lip]

chei•lo•plas•ty, chi•lo•plas•ty (kī′lō-plas-tē, kī′lō-plas-tē) Surgical repair of the lips. [cheilo- + G. *plastos*, formed]

chei•lor•rha•phy, chi•lor•rha•phy (kī-lōr′ă-fē, kī-lōr′ă-fē) Suturing of the lip. [cheilo- + G. *rhaphē*, suture]

chei•lo•sis, chi•lo•sis (kī-lō′sis, kī-lō′sis) A condition characterized by dry scaling and fissuring of the lips and angle of the mouth caused by riboflavin deficiency. SEE ALSO cheilitis. Cf. rhagades. [cheil- + G. *-osis*, condition]

chei•lot•o•my, chi•lot•o•my (kī-lot′ō-mē, kī-lot′ō-mē) Incision into the lip. [cheilo- + G. *tomē*, incision]

chei•ral•gi•a (kī-ral′jē-ă) Pain and paresthesia in the hand.

chei•ral•gi•a pa•res•thet•i•ca (kī-ral′jē-ă pares-thet′i-kă) Compression neuropathy of the superficial branch of the radial nerve, marked by pain and paresthesia over the course of the nerve.

♻ **cheiro-, cheir-** Combining forms meaning hand. SEE ALSO chiro-. [G. *cheir*, a hand]

chei•rog•nos•tic, chi•rog•nos•tic (kī′rog-nos′tik, kī-rog-nos′tik) Able to distinguish between right and left, as of the hands or of which side of the body is touched. [cheiro- + G. *gnostikos*, perceptive]

cheirokinaesthesia [Br.] SYN cheirokinesthesia.

cheirokinaesthetic [Br.] SYN cheirokinesthetic.

chei•ro•kin•es•the•si•a (kī′rō-kin-es-thē′zē-ă) The subjective sensation of movement of the hands. SYN cheirokinaesthesia. [cheiro- + G. *kinēsis*, movement, + *aisthēsis*, sensation]

chei•ro•kin•es•thet•ic (kī′rō-kin-ĕs-thet′ik) Relating to cheirokinesthesia. SYN cheirokinaesthetic.

chei•ro•plas•ty, chi•ro•plas•ty (kī′rō-plas-tē, kī′rō-plas-tē) Rarely used term for surgical repair of the hand. [cheiro- + G. *plastos*, formed]

chei•ro•po•dal•gi•a, chi•ro•po•dal•gi•a (kī′rō-pō-dal′jē-ă, kī′rō-pō-dal′jē-ă) Pain in the hands and in the feet. [cheiro- + G. *pous*, foot, + *algos*, pain]

chei•ro•pom•pho•lyx, chi•ro•pom•pho•lyx (kī′rō-pom′fō-liks, kī′rō-pom′fō-liks) SYN dyshidrosis. [cheiro- + G. *pompholyx*, a bubble, fr. *pomphos*, a blister]

chei•ro•spasm, chi•ro•spasm (kī′rō-spazm, kī′rō-spazm) Spasm of the muscles of the hand, as in writer's cramp. [cheiro- + G. *spasmos*, spasm]

che•late (kē′lāt) **1.** To effect chelation. **2.** Pertaining to chelation. **3.** A complex formed through chelation.

che•la•tion (kē-lā′shŭn) Complex formation involving a metal ion and two or more polar groupings of a single molecule; can be used to remove an ion from participation in biologic reactions, as in the chelation of Ca^{2+} of blood by ethylenediaminetetraacetic acid, which thus acts as an anticoagulant in vitro. [G. *chēlē*, claw]

chem•ex•fo•li•a•tion (kem′eks-fō-lē-ā′shŭn) A chemosurgical technique to remove acne scars or treat chronic skin changes caused by sunlight.

chem•i•cal (kem′i-kăl) Relating to chemistry.

Chem•i•cal Ab•stracts Ser•vice (CAS) (kem′i-kăl ab′strakts sĕr′vis) This service assigns a unique CAS number to each chemical for identification. The service also provides a physical and chemical description of the chemical.

chem•i•cal an•ti•dote (kem′i-kăl an′ti-dōt) A substance that unites with a poison to form an innocuous chemical compound.

chem•i•cal at•trac•tion (kem′i-kăl ă-trak′shŭn) The force impelling atoms of different elements or molecules to unite to form new substances or compounds.

chem•i•cal der•ma•ti•tis (kem′i-kăl dĕr′mă-tī′tis) Allergic contact dermatitis or primary irritation dermatitis due to application of chemicals; usually characterized by erythema, edema, and vesiculation.

chem•i•cal dot ther•mom•e•ter (kem′i-kal dot thĕr-mom′ĕ-tĕr) Thermometer that indicates changes in temperature by color changes in chemical dots bonded to a plastic strip.

chem•i•cal en•er•gy (kem′i-kăl en′ĕr-jē) Energy liberated or absorbed by a chemical reaction (e.g., oxidation of carbon) or absorbed in the formation of a chemical compound.

chem•i•cal hy•giene plan (kem′i-kăl hī′jēn plan) All safety procedures, special precautions, and emergency procedures used when working with chemicals. All personnel must receive training in the particulars of the plan.

chem•i•cal per•i•to•ni•tis (kem′i-kăl per′i-tō-nī′tis) Peritonitis due to the escape of bile, contents of the gastrointestinal tract, or pancreatic juice into the peritoneal cavity; the contents of the fluid causes chemical injury, shock, and peritoneal exudation.

chem•i•cal po•ten•tial (kem′i-kăl pŏ-ten′shăl) A measurement of how the free energy of a phase depends on any change in the composition of that phase.

chem•i•cal preg•nan•cy (kem′i-kăl preg′năn-sē) Slight, unsustained rise in levels of human chorionic gonadotropin.

chem•i•cal re•pair (kem′i-kăl rē-pār′) Conversion of a free radical to a stable molecule.

chem•i•cal sen•ses (kem′i-kăl sens′ĕz) The senses of smell and taste.

chem•i•cal shift (kĕm-i′kăl shift) Magnetic resonance artifact along the frequency axis caused by the difference in frequency between fat and water.

chem•i•cal-war•fare (CW) a•gent (kem′i-kăl-wōr′fā ā′jĕnt) **1.** In U.S. military parlance, any chemical compound developed for battlefield use either to kill or seriously injure (i.e., toxic chemical agents) or else to incapacitate (i.e., incapacitating agents) humans or animals by means of its toxicologic effects. Within the United States, regulation specifically excludes riot-control agents, herbicides, smoke, and flame. **2.** A chemical poison synthesized or of natural (including plant) origin and intended for military use. This definition includes toxins as chemical-warfare agents. **3.** A precursor compound used in the synthesis of a chemical-warfare agent.

chem•i•lu•mi•nes•cence (kem′ē-lū-mi-nes′ĕns) Light produced by chemical action usually at, or below, room temperature.

chem•i•lu•mi•nes•cence im•mu•no•as•say (kem′ē-lū-mi-nes′ĕns im′yū-nō-as′ā) An immunoassay technique in which the antigen or antibody is labeled with a molecule capable of emitting light during a chemical reaction; this light is used to measure the formation of the antigen-antibody complex.

chem•ist (kem′ist) **1.** A specialist or expert in chemistry. **2.** Pharmacist (U.K. and some areas of Canada).

chem•is•try (kem′is-trē) **1.** The science concerned with the atomic composition of substances, the elements and their interreactions, and the formation, decomposition, and properties of molecules. **2.** The chemical properties of a substance. **3.** Chemical processes. [G. *chēmeia,* alchemy]

♻ **chemo-**, **chem-** Combining forms denoting chemistry. [G. *chēmeia,* alchemy]

che•mo•at•tract•ant (kē′mō-ă-trak′tănt) A chemical substance that influences the migration of cells. [chem- + attract + -i]

che•mo•au•to•troph (kē′mō-aw′tō-trōf) An organism that depends on inorganic chemicals for its energy and principally on carbon dioxide for its carbon. SYN chemolithotroph. [chemo- + G. *autos,* self, + *trophikos,* nourishing]

che•mo•au•to•tro•phic (kē′mō-aw-tō-trō′fik) Pertaining to a chemoautotroph. SYN chemolithotrophic.

che•mo•cau•ter•y (kē′mō-kaw′tĕr-ē) Destruction of tissue by application of a chemical substance.

che•mo•dec•to•ma (kē′mō-dek-tō′mă) A relatively rare, usually benign neoplasm originating in the chemoreceptor tissue of the carotid body, glomus jugulare, and aortic bodies. Cf. paraganglioma. SYN glomus jugulare tumor. [chemo- + G. *dektēs*, receiver, fr. *dechomai*, to receive, + -*oma*, tumor]

che•mo•dec•to•ma•to•sis (kē′mō-dek-tō-mă-tō′sis) Multiple tumors of perivascular tissue of chemoreceptor type, which have been reported in the lungs as minute neoplasms.

che•mo•kines (kē′mō-kīnz) Several groups composed of usually 8–10 kD polypepytide cytokines that are chemokinetic and chemotactic stimulating leukocyte movement and attraction. SYN intercrines.

che•mo•ki•ne•sis (kē′mō-ki-nē′sis) Stimulation of an organism by a chemical. [chemo- + G. *kinēsis,* movement]

che•mo•ki•net•ic (kē′mō-ki-net′ik) Referring to chemokinesis.

che•mo•lith•o•troph (kē′mō-lith′ō-trōf) SYN chemoautotroph.

che•mo•lith•o•tro•phic (kē′mō-lith-ō-trō′fik) SYN chemoautotrophic.

che•mo•nu•cle•ol•y•sis (kē′mō-nū-klē-ol′i-sis) Injection of chymopapain (an enzyme) into the herniated nucleus pulposus of an intervertebral disc.

che•mo•or•ga•no•troph (kē′mō-ōr′gă-nō-trōf) An organism that depends on organic chemicals for its energy and carbon. [chemo- + G. *organon,* organ, + *trophē,* nourishment]

che•mo•or•ga•no•tro•phic (kē′mō-ōr′gă-nō-trō′fik) Pertaining to a chemoorganotroph.

che•mo•pro•phy•lax•is (kē′mō-pro′fi-lak′sis) Prevention of disease by the use of chemicals or drugs.

che•mo•ra•di•o•ther•a•py (kē′mō-rā′dē-ō-thār′ă-pē) A treatment plan that combines chemotherapy and radiotherapy.

che•mo•re•cep•tion (kē′mō-rĕ-sep′shŭn) The ability to perceive chemicals in the environment that are odorants or tastants. SYN chemosensation.

che•mo•re•cep•tive (kē′mō-rĕ-sep′tiv) Relating to chemoreception.

che•mo•re•cep•tor (kē′mō-rĕ-sep′tŏr) Any cell that responds to a change in its chemical milieu with a nerve impulse. Such cells can be either "transducer" cells innervated by sensory nerve fibers (e.g., the gustatory cells of the taste buds) or nerve cells proper, such as the olfactory receptor cells of the olfactory mucosa.

che•mo•re•sist•ance (kē′mō-rē-zis′tăns) The state of being resistant to a chemical.

che•mo•re•sponse (kē′mō-rĕ-spons′) A reaction to chemical stimulation.

che•mo•sen•sa•tion (kē′mō-sen-sā′shŭn) SYN chemoreception.

che•mo•sen•si•tive (kē′mō-sen′si-tiv) Capable of perceiving changes in the chemical composition of the environment.

che•mo•sis (kē-mō′sis) Edema of the bulbar conjunctiva, forming a swelling around the cornea. [G. *chēmē,* a yawning, the cockle (from its gaping shell)]

che•mo•sur•ger•y (kē′mō-sŭr′jĕr-ē) Excision of diseased tissue after it has been fixed in situ by chemical means.

che•mo•tac•tic (kē′mō-tak′tik) Relating to chemotaxis.

che•mo•tax•is (kē′mō-tak′sis) Movement of cells or organisms in response to chemicals. SYN chemotropism. [chemo- + G. *taxis,* orderly arrangement]

che•mo•ther•a•peu•tic (kē′mō-thār-ă-pyū′tik) Relating to chemotherapy.

che•mo•ther•a•peu•tic in•dex (kē′mō-thār′ă-pyū′tik in′deks) The ratio of the minimal effective dose of a chemotherapeutic agent to the maximal tolerated dose. Originally used by Ehrlich to express the relative toxicity of a chemotherapeutic agent to a parasite and to its host.

che•mo•ther•a•py (kē′mō-thār′ă-pē) Treatment of disease by means of chemical substances or drugs; usually used in reference to neoplastic disease. SEE ALSO pharmacotherapy. See this page.

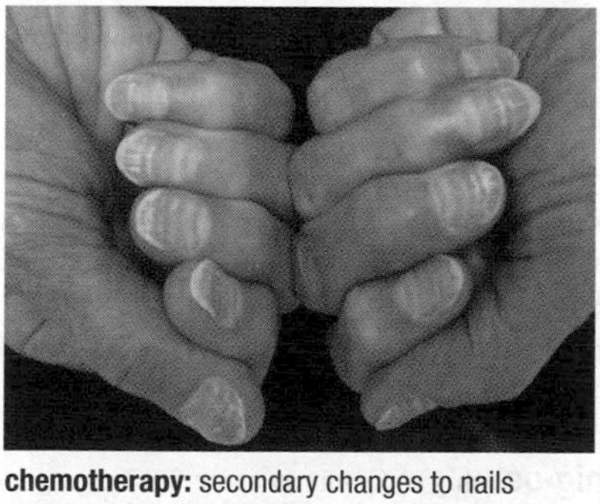

chemotherapy: secondary changes to nails

che•mot•ic (kē-mot′ic) Relating to chemosis.

che•mot•ro•pism (kē-mot′rō-pizm) SYN chemotaxis. [chemo- + G. *tropos,* direction, turn]

CHEMTREC (kem′trek) Acronym for Chemical Transportation Emergency Center, a service of the Chemical Manufacturers Association that provides round-the-clock advice on handling emergencies related to transport of hazardous material.

cher•ry an•gi•o•ma (cher′ē an′jē-ō′mă) SYN senile hemangioma. See this page, B13.

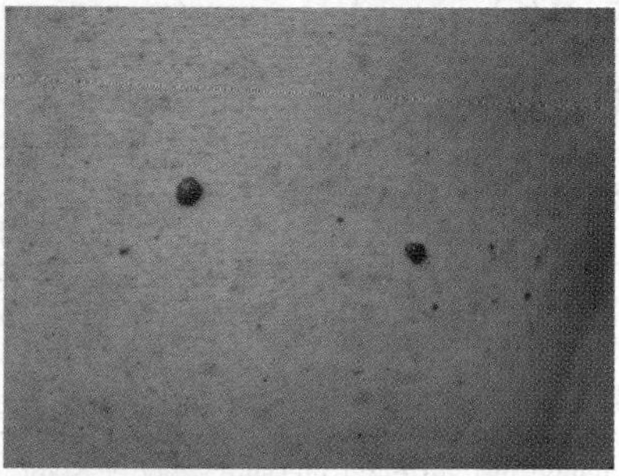

cherry angiomas: back

cher•ry-red spot (cher′ē-red spot) The ophthalmoscopic appearance of the normal choroid beneath the fovea centralis, appearing as a red spot surrounded by white retinal edema in central artery closure or lipid infiltration in sphingolipidosis. SYN Tay cherry-red spot.

cher•ry-red spot my•oc•lo•nus syn•drome (cher′ē-red spot mī-ok′lō-nŭs sin′drōm) A neuronal storage disorder in children characterized by a cherry-red spot at the macula, progressive myoclonus, and easily controlled seizures; the result of sialidase deficiency. SYN sialidosis.

che•rub•ism (cher′ŭb-izm) Progressive symmetric, painless swelling of the jaws beginning in early childhood and due to hereditary giant cell lesions manifested radiographically as multilocular radiolucencies. Condition tends to regress during adulthood. [Hebr. *kerubh,* cherub]

chest (chest) The anterior wall of the thorax. SEE ALSO thorax. SYN pectus [TA]. [A.S. *cest,* a box]

chest film (chest film) Colloquial usage for the most common radiographic views of the thorax and contiguous areas (i.e., posteroanterior and lateral chest radiographs).

chest leads (chest lēdz) A unipolar electrocardiographic lead the exploring electrode of which is on the chest overlying the heart or its vicinity; there are six standard chest leads, designated as V_1–V_6. SYN precordial leads.

chest phys•i•cal ther•a•py (CPT, chest P.T.) (chest fiz′i-kăl thār′ă-pē) A type of respiratory care performed to promote coughing and the removal of lung secretions through percussion (clapping) and vibration on the affected areas, postural drainage, and breathing exercises; usually contraindicated in persons with bleeding abnormalities, anticoagulant therapy, chest and/or head/neck trauma, recent myocardial infarctions, or pacemaker insertion. SYN chest physiotherapy, pulmonary rehabilitation, pulmonary toileting.

chest phy•si•o•ther•a•py (chest fiz′ē-ō-thār′ă-pē) SYN chest physical therapy.

chest P.T. (chest) Abbreviation for chest physical therapy.

chest tube (chest tūb) A tube introduced into the intrapleural space to evacuate gas or liquid.

chest wall (chest wawl) RESPIRATORY PHYSIOLOGY the total system of structures outside the lungs that move as a part of breathing; it comprises the rib cage, diaphragm, abdominal wall, and abdominal contents. SYN thoracic wall.

chest wall com•pli•ance (chest wawl kŏm-plī′ăns) The change in chest wall volume per unit change in transmural pressure; may be static or dynamic.

chew•ing (chū′ing) The act of grinding or crushing with the teeth; mastication. [O.E. cēowan]

Cheyne-Stokes res•pi•ra•tion (chān stōks res′pir-ā′shŭn) The pattern of breathing with gradual increase in depth and sometimes in rate to a maximum, followed by a decrease resulting in apnea; the cycles ordinarily are 30 seconds to 2 minutes in duration, with 5 to 30 seconds of apnea; seen with bilateral deep febrile hemispheric lesions, with metabolic encephalopathy, and, characteristically, in coma from disorders of the nervous centers of respiration.

CHF Abbreviation for congestive heart failure.

CHI Abbreviation for closed head injury.

chi (kī; chē) **1.** The 22nd letter of the Greek alphabet, χ. **2.** In chemistry, denotes the 22nd in a series. **3.** Symbol for the dihedral angle between the α-carbon and the side-chains of amino acids in peptides and proteins. **4.** In Asian medical traditions, the force of energy existing in all life forms. Chi manifests as five different elements; these are labeled according to either the Asian or Ayurvedic tradition. SYN qi. SEE ALSO five-element theory. SYN ki.

Chi•a•ri-From•mel syn•drome (kē-ahr′ē-from′ĕl sin′drōm) A condition usually occurring postpartum characterized by amenorrhea, galactorrhea, obesity, and atrophy of the uterus and ovaries.

Chi•a•ri net (kē-ah′rē net) Abnormal fibrous or lacelike strands in the right atrium, extending from the margins of the coronary or caval valves and attaching to the atrial wall along the line of the crista terminalis; results when resorption of the septum spurium is markedly less than normal.

Chi•a•ri syn•drome (kē-ah′rē sin′drōm) Thrombosis of the hepatic vein with great enlargement of the liver and extensive development of collateral vessels, intractable ascites, and severe portal hypertension. SYN Budd syndrome.

chi•asm (kī′azm) **1.** An intersection or crossing of two lines. **2.** ANATOMY a decussation or crossing of two fibrous bundles, such as tendons, nerves, or tracts. **3.** CYTOGENETICS the site at which two homologous chromosomes make contact (thus appearing to be crossed), enabling the exchange of genetic material during the prophase stage of meiosis. [G. *chiasma*]

chi•as•ma, pl. **chi•as•ma•ta** (kī-az′mă, -mă-tă) **1.** A decussation or crossing of two tracts, such as tendons or nerves. **2.** A site at which two homologous chromosomes appear to have exchanged material during meiosis. [G. *chiasma,* two crossing lines, fr. the letter *chi,* 3]

chick•en breast (chik′ĕn brest) SYN pectus carinatum.

chick•en fat clot (chik′ĕn fat klot) Clot formed in vitro or postmortem from leukocytes and plasma of sedimented blood.

chick•en•pox (chik′ĕn-poks) SYN varicella. See page B30.

chick•en•pox vi•rus (chik′ĕn-poks vī′rŭs) SYN varicella-zoster virus.

chick•weed (chik′wēd) (*Stellaria media*) This herbal preparation is widely used as a specific against inflammation. SYN star chickweed.

chi•cle (chik′el) **1.** The partially evaporated viscous, milky juice from *Manilkara zapotilla* (family Sapotaceae), which is native to the West Indies, Mexico, and Central America. **2.** A mixture of gutta with triterpene alcohols. Used in the manufacture of chewing gum. [Sp., from Nahuatl *chictli*]

CHID Abbreviation for Combined Health Information Database.

chief ag•glu•ti•nin (chēf ă-glū′ti-nin) SYN major agglutinin.

chief cell (chēf sel) The predominant cell type of a gland.

chief com•plaint (cc, c.c., CC) (chēf kŏm-plānt′) The primary symptom that a patient states as the reason for seeking medical care.

chig•ger (chig′ĕr) The six-legged larva of *Trombicula* species; a bloodsucking stage of mites that includes the vectors of scrub typhus.

chig•oe (chig′ō) Common name for *Tunga penetrans.*

chik•un•gun•ya (chik′ŭn-gŭn′yă) A febrile viral disease resembling dengue, transmitted by mosquitoes. [Swahili, that which bends]

Chi•lai•di•ti syn•drome (kī-lā′dē-tē sin′drōm) Interposition of the colon between the liver and the diaphragm.

chil·blain (chil′blān) Erythema, itching, and burning, especially of the dorsa of the fingers and toes, and of the heels, nose, and ears caused by vascular constriction on exposure to extreme cold (usually associated with high humidity); lesions can be single or multiple, and can become blistered and ulcerated. SYN erythema pernio. [chill + A.S. *blegen,* a blain]

child a·buse (chīld ă-byūs′) The psychological, emotional, and sexual abuse of a child. SEE domestic violence.

child-bear·ing (chīld′bār-ing) Pregnancy and parturition.

child·bed fe·ver (chīld′bed fē′vĕr) SYN puerperal fever.

child·birth (chīld′bĭrth) The process of labor and delivery in the birth of a child. SEE ALSO birth. SYN parturition.

child·hood (chīld′hud) The period of life between infancy and puberty.

child·hood ab·sence ep·i·lep·sy (chīld′hud ab′sĕns ep′i-lep-sē) A generalized epilepsy syndrome characterized by the onset of absence seizures in childhood, typically at age 6 or 7 years. There is a strong genetic predisposition and girls are affected more often than boys. EEG reveals generalized 3-Hz spike-wave activity on a normal background. Prognosis for remission is good if the patient does not also have generalized tonic-clonic seizures. SEE ALSO absence.

child·hood a·prax·i·a (chīld′hud ă-prak′sē-ă) SYN developmental apraxia of speech.

child·proof (chīld′prūf) Denotes packaging designed to prevent injury to children, refers particularly to medicines and household chemicals.

child psy·chi·a·try (chīld sī-kī′ă-trē) The branch of psychiatry that deals with the emotional and mental disorders of children.

chill (chil) **1.** A sensation of cold. **2.** A feeling of cold with shivering and pallor, accompanied by an elevation of temperature in the interior of the body; usually a prodromal symptom of an infectious disease due to the presence in the blood of foreign protein or toxins. SYN rigor (2). [A.S. *cele,* cold]

chilo-, chil- Combining forms meaning lips. SEE ALSO cheilo-. [G. *cheilos,* lip]

chi·me·ra (kī-mēr′ă) **1.** The individual produced by grafting an embryonic part of one animal onto the embryo of another, either of the same or of another species. **2.** An organism that has received a transplant of genetically and immunologically different tissue, such as bone marrow. **3.** Dizygotic twins that have immunologically distinct types of erythrocytes. **4.** A protein fusion in which two different proteins, usually from different species, are linked through peptide bonds; usually genetically engineered. Chimeric antibodies may have the Fab fragment from one species fused with the Fc fragment from another. **5.** Any macromolecule fusion formed by two or more macromolecules from different species or from different genes. [L. *Chimaera,* G. *Chimaira,* mythic monster (lit. a she-goat)]

chi·mer·ic (kī-mēr′ik) **1.** Relating to a chimera. Cf. chimera (5). **2.** Composed of parts that are of different origin and are seemingly incompatible.

chin (chin) The prominence formed by the anterior projection of the mandible, or lower jaw. SYN mentum. [A.S. *cin*]

Chi·nese an·gel·i·ca (chī-nēz′ an-jel′i-kă) Herbal prepared from *Angelica polymorpha* var. *sinensis;* widely used for alleged value against gynecologic disorders; composed of a wide range of ingredients, some of which are thought carcinogenic. SYN tang-kuei.

Chi·nese ham·ster o·va·ry cells (chī-nēz′ ham′stĕr ō′văr-ē selz) Well-established experimental strain of fibroblasts used in biomedical research.

Chi·nese res·tau·rant syn·drome (chī-nēz′ rest′ă-rahnt sin′drōm) Colloquial usage for development of chest pain, feelings of facial pressure, and a sensation of burning over variable portions of the body surface after ingestion of food that contains monosodium L-glutamate (MSG) by people sensitive to this food additive.

Chi·nese rhu·barb (chī-nēz′ rū′bahrb) (*Rheum palmatum*) Used in traditional Chinese medicine as a purgative and therapy for other GI diseases; possibly dangerous because of the presence of oxalic acid in the plant itself. SYN da-huang.

chip graft (chip graft) A graft consisting of small pieces of cartilage or bone which are packed into a bone defect.

chip sy·ringe (chip sĭr-inj′) A tapered metal tube through which air is forced from a rubber bulb or pressure tank to blow debris from, or to dry, a cavity in preparing teeth for restoration.

chi·ral·i·ty (kī-ral′i-tē) The property of nonidentity of an object with its mirror image; used in chemistry with respect to stereochemical isomers. [G. *cheir,* hand]

chiro-, chir- Combining forms meaning the hand. SEE ALSO cheiro-. [G. *cheir,* hand]

chi·rop·o·dist (kī-rop′ŏ-dist) SYN podiatrist. [chiro- + G. *pous,* foot]

chi·rop·o·dy (kī-rop′ŏ-dē) SYN podiatry.

chi·ro·prac·tic (kī′rō-prak′tik) Chiropractic is a health care discipline that emphasizes the inherent recuperative powers of the body to heal itself without drugs or surgery. The practice of chiropractic focuses on the relationship between structure (primarily the spine) and function (as coordinated by the nervous system) and how that relationship affects both preservation and restoration of health. [chiro- + G. *praktikos,* efficient]

chi·ro·prac·tic tech·nique (kī′rō-prak′tik tek-nēk′) Manual treatment, prescription of preventive and rehabilitative exercises, and patient education on matters such as posture, ergonomics, nutrition and diet, and healthy lifestyle.

chi·ro·prac·tor (kī′rō-prak′tŏr) One who is licensed to practice the art and science of chiropractic.

Chi·rop·sal·mus (kī-rop′sal-mŭs) A genus of the invertebrate phylum Cnidaria, which includes the sea wasp.

Chi·rop·sal·mus qua·dru·ma·nus (kī-rō-sal′mŭs kwahd-rū-mā′nŭs) The sea wasp, the most venomous jellyfish inhabiting the waters surrounding the United States. SEE ALSO jellyfish. SYN box jelly, sea wasp.

chi-square (χ^2) test (kī′skwār test) A statistical method of assessing the significance of a difference, as when the data from two or more samples are represented by a discrete number such as the numbers of females and males attending each of two colleges.

chi·tin (kī′tin) A polymer of *N*-acetyl-D-glucosamine similar in structure to cellulose and the second most abundant polysaccharide in nature, comprising the horny substance in the exoskeleton of beetles, crabs, certain microorganisms, and other life forms.

chi·tin·ous (kī′tin-ŭs) Of or relating to chitin.

CHL Abbreviation for crown-heel length.

Chla·myd·i·a (klă-mid′ē-ă) One of three genera in the family Chlamydiaceae; includes *Chlamydia muridarum*, the cause of pneumonitis in mice, *C. suis*, and *C. trachomatis*, the type species. Chlamydiae are obligatory intracellular spheric or avoid bacteria with a complex intracellular life cycle; the infective form is the elementary body, which penetrates the host cell, replicating as the reticulate body by binary fission. Replication occurs in a vacuole called the inclusion body. Chlamydiae lack peptidoglycan in their cell walls. Formerly called *Bedsonia*. [G. *chlamys,* cloak]

chla·myd·i·a, pl. **chla·myd·i·ae** (klă-mid′ē-ă, -ē-ē) A vernacular term used to refer to any member of the genus *Chlamydia*.

Chla·myd·i·a·ce·ae (klă-mid′ē-ā′shē-ē) A family of the order Chlamydiales (formerly included in the order Rickettsiales) that includes the agents of the psittacosis-lymphogranuloma-trachoma group. The family contains small, coccoid, gram-negative bacteria that resemble rickettsiae but differ from them by possessing a unique, obligately intracellular developmental cycle. Intracytoplasmic microcolonies give rise to infectious forms by division.

chla·myd·i·al (kla-mid′ē-ăl) Relating to or caused by any bacterium of the genus *Chlamydia*.

Chla·myd·i·a pneu·mo·ni·ae (klă-mi′dē-a nū-mō′nē-ē) A species that causes pneumonia and upper and lower respiratory disease. SYN TWAR.

Chla·myd·i·a psit·ta·ci (klă-mi′dē-a sē-tā′shē) Organisms that resemble *C. trachomatis* but do not produce glycogen and are not susceptible to sulfadiazine therapy. Various strains of this species cause psittacosis in humans and ornithosis in birds.

Chla·myd·i·a tra·cho·ma·tis (klă-mi′dē-a trak-ō′mă-tis) Spheric nonmotile organisms that accumulate glycogen and are susceptible to sulfadiazine and tetracycline; various strains of this species cause trachoma, inclusion and neonatal conjunctivitis, lymphogranuloma venereum, nonspecific urethritis, epididymitis, cervicitis, salpingitis, proctitis, and pneumonia; chief agent of bacterial sexually transmitted diseases in the U.S. The type species of the genus *Chlamydia*.

chla·myd·i·o·sis (klă-mid′ē-ō′sis) General term for diseases caused by *Chlamydia* species. SEE ALSO ornithosis, psittacosis.

chlo·as·ma (klō-az′mă) Melanoderma or melasma characterized by brown patches of irregular shape and size on the face and elsewhere; if confluent, facial patches are called the mask of pregnancy and are associated most commonly with pregnancy and use of oral contraceptives. [G. *chloazō*, to become green]

♻ **chlor-**, **chloro-** Combining forms meaning (1) green, (2) chlorine. [G. *chloros*, green]

chlor·a·cet·o·phe·none (klōr′as-ē-tō-fē′nōn) SYN chloroacetophenone. SEE ALSO biologic-warfare (BW) agent, mid-spectrum agent.

chlor·ac·ne, **chlo·rine ac·ne** (klōr-ak′nē, klōr′ēn ak′nē) An occupational acnelike eruption due to prolonged contact with certain chlorinated compounds.

chlor·am·phen·i·col (klōr′am-fen′i-kol) An antibiotic originally obtained from *Streptomyces venezuelae*. It is effective against a number of pathogenic microorganisms, including *Staphylococcus aureus*, *Brucella abortus*, Friedländer bacillus, and the organisms of typhoid, typhus, and Rocky Mountain spotted fever; active by mouth. A serious reaction resulting in marrow damage with agranulocytosis or aplastic anemia may occur.

chlor·am·phen·i·col a·ce·tyl trans·fer·ase (CAT) (klōr′am-fen′i-kol as′ē-til trans′fĕr-ās) A bacterial enzyme often used as a marker for examining the control of eucaryotic gene expression.

chlo·rate (klōr′āt) A salt of chloric acid.

chlor•hy•dri•a (klōr-hī′drē-ă) SYN hyperchlorhydria.

chlo•ride (klōr′īd) A compound containing chlorine, at a valence of −1, as in the salts of hydrochloric acid.

chlo•ride shift (klōr′īd shift) When CO_2 enters the blood from the tissues, it passes into the red blood cell and is converted by carbonate dehydratase to bicarbonate (HCO_3-); HCO_3- ion passes out into the plasma, whereas Cl^- migrates into the red blood cell. Reverse changes occur in the lungs when CO_2 is eliminated from the blood. SYN Hamburger phenomenon.

chlor•i•du•ria (klōr′i-dyūr′ē-ă) SYN chloruresis.

chlo•ri•nat•ed (klōr′in-āt-ĕd) Having been treated with chlorine.

chlo•ri•na•tion (klōr′i-nā′shŭn) Treatment with chlorine or a chlorine compound.

chlo•rine (Cl) (klōr′ēn) **1.** A greenish, toxic, gaseous element, atomic no. 17, atomic wt. 35.4527; a halogen used as a disinfectant and bleaching agent in the form of hypochlorite or chlorine water, because of its oxidizing power; also used as a chemical warfare agent. **2.** The molecular form of chlorine (1), Cl_2. [G. *chloros*, greenish yellow]

chlo•rine group (klōr′ēn grūp) The halogens.

chlo•rite (klōr′īt) A salt of chlorous acid; the radical ClO_2-.

chlo•ro•a•ce•to•phe•none (klōr′ō-ă-sē′tē-fē′nōn) A compound (NATO code CN) used as a lacrimator in World War I, as a riot control agent in law enforcement, and in sprays for personal protection. SEE cesium. SYN chloracetophenone.

chlo•ro•form•ism (klōr′ŏ-fōrm-izm) Habitual chloroform inhalation, or the symptoms caused thereby.

chloroleukaemia [Br.] SYN chloroleukemia.

chlo•ro•ma, **chlo•ro•leu•ke•mi•a** (klōr-ō′mă, klōr′ō-lū-kē′mē-ă) A condition characterized by green masses of abnormal cells (in most instances, myeloblasts), especially in relation to the periosteum of the skull, spine, and ribs; the clinical course is similar to that of acute myeloid leukemia. SEE ALSO granulocytic sarcoma. SYN chloromyeloma. [chloro- + G. *-ōma,* tumor]

chlo•ro•my•e•lo•ma (klōr′ō-mī-ĕ-lō′mă) SYN chloroma. [chloro- + G. *myelos,* marrow, + *-ōma,* tumor]

chlo•ro•per•cha meth•od (klōr′ō-pĕr′chă meth′ŏd) A method of filling the root canals of teeth by dissolving gutta-percha cones in a chloroform-rosin medium within the root canal. SYN Callahan method, Johnson method.

chlo•ro•phyll (klōr′ō-fil) A complex of light-absorbing green pigments that, in living plants, convert light energy into oxidizing and reducing power, thus fixing CO_2 and evolving O_2; the naturally occurring forms are chlorophyll *a*, *b*, *c*, and *d*.

chlo•rop•si•a (klōr-op′sē-ă) A condition in which objects appear to be colored green, as may occur in digitalis intoxication. [chloro- + G. *opsis,* eyesight]

chlo•rot•ic (klōr-ot′ik) Pertaining to or having the characteristic features of chlorosis.

chlor•u•re•sis, **chlor•u•ri•a** (klōr-yū-rē′sis, klōr-yūr′ē-ă) The excretion of chloride in the urine. SYN chloriduria.

chlor•u•ret•ic (klōr′yū-ret′ik) Increasing the excretion of chloride in the urine.

CHO Abbreviation for carbohydrates.

cho•a•na, pl. **cho•a•nae** (kō′ă-nă, -nē) The opening into the nasopharynx of the nasal cavity on either side. USAGE NOTE often incorrectly called posterior choana(e). [Mod. L. fr. G. *choanē,* a funnel]

choc•o•late cyst (chawk′lăt sist) Cyst of the ovary with intracavitary hemorrhage and formation of a hematoma containing old brown blood; often seen with endometriosis of the ovary but occasionally with other types of cysts.

Chodz•ko re•flex (hōts′kō rē′fleks) Contractions of several muscles of the shoulder girdle and arm when the manubrium sterni is percussed.

choke (chōk) To prevent respiration by compression or obstruction of the larynx or trachea. [M.E. *choken,* fr. O.E. *āceōcian*]

choked disc (chōkt disk) SYN papilledema.

chokes (chōks) A manifestation of decompression sickness or altitude sickness characterized by dyspnea, coughing, and choking.

chok•ing (chōk′ing) Upper airway obstruction resulting from a foreign object in the trachea or oropharynx, laryngeal spasm or edema, or external compression of the neck. A life-threatening situation such as asphyxia, hypoxia, and death may occur if the victim is unable to clear the airway by coughing. The inability to speak indicates a complete airway obstruction. The universal sign for choking is the grasping of the throat by the person choking. SEE ALSO Heimlich maneuver.

cholaemia [Br.] SYN cholemia.

cholaemic [Br.] SYN cholemic.

cho•la•gog•ic (kō-lă-goj′ik) SYN cholagogue (2).

cho•la•gogue (kō′lă-gog) **1.** An agent that promotes the flow of bile into the intestine, especially as a result of contraction of the gallbladder. **2.** Relating to such an agent or effect. SYN cholagogic. [chol- + G. *agōgos,* drawing forth]

chol•an•gi•ec•ta•sis (kō-lan′jē-ek′tă-sis) Dilation of the bile ducts, usually as a sequel to obstruction. [chol- + G. *angeion,* vessel, + *ektasis,* a stretching]

chol•an•gi•o•car•ci•no•ma (kō-lan′jē-ō-kahr-si-nō′mă) An adenocarcinoma, primarily in intrahepatic bile ducts, composed of ducts lined by cuboidal or columnar cells that do not contain bile, with abundant fibrous stroma.

chol•an•gi•o•en•ter•os•to•my (kō-lan′jē-ō-en-tĕr-os′tŏ-mē) Surgical anastomosis of bile duct to intestine.

chol•an•gi•o•fi•bro•sis (kō-lan′jē-ō-fī-brō′sis) Fibrosis of the bile ducts. [chol- + G. *angeion,* vessel, + fibrosis]

chol•an•gi•o•gas•tros•to•my (kō-lan′jē-ō-gas-tros′tŏ-mē) Formation of a communication between a bile duct and the stomach. [chol- + G. *angeion,* vessel, + *gastēr,* belly, + *stoma,* mouth]

chol•an•gi•o•gram (kō-lan′jē-ō-gram) The radiographic record of the bile ducts obtained by cholangiography.

chol•an•gi•og•ra•phy (kō-lan′jē-og′ră-fē) Radiographic examination of the bile ducts using a contrast medium. [chol- + G. *angeion,* vessel, + *graphō,* to write]

chol•an•gi•ole (kō-lan′jē-ōl) A ductule occurring between a bile canaliculus and an interlobular bile duct. [chol- + G. *angeion,* vessel, + *-ole,* small]

chol•an•gi•o•lit•ic cir•rho•sis (kō-lan′jē-ō-lit′ik sir-ō′sis) Liver disease in which there is diffuse inflammation of the cholangioles, with inflammation, fibrosis, and regeneration; characterized by chronicity, relapses, and febrile episodes.

chol•an•gi•o•lit•ic hep•a•ti•tis (kō-lan′jē-ō-lit′ik hep′ă-tī′tis) Liver disease with inflammatory changes around small bile ducts, producing mainly obstructive jaundice; may be due to viral infection or bacterial infection.

chol•an•gi•o•li•tis (kō-lan′jē-ō-lī′tis) Inflammation of the small bile radicles or cholangioles.

chol•an•gi•o•ma (kō-lan′jē-ō′mă) A neoplasm of bile duct origin, especially within the liver; may be either benign or malignant (cholangiocarcinoma). [chol- + G. *angeion,* vessel, + *-oma,* tumor]

chol•an•gi•o•pan•cre•a•tog•ra•phy (kō-lan′jē-ō-pan′krē-ă-tog′ră-fē) Radiographic examination of the bile and pancreatic ducts with contrast medium.

chol•an•gi•os•co•py (kō-lan′jē-os′kŏ-pē) Visual examination of bile ducts using a fiberoptic endoscope. [chol- + G. *angeion,* vessel, + *skopeō,* to examine]

chol•an•gi•os•to•my (kō-lan′jē-os′tŏ-mē) Formation of a fistula into a bile duct. [chol- + G. *angeion,* vessel, + *stoma,* mouth]

chol•an•gi•ot•o•my (kō-lan′jē-ot′ŏ-mē) Incision into a bile duct. [chol- + G. *angeion,* vessel, + *tomē,* incision]

chol•an•gi•tis, cho•lan•gi•i•tis (kō′lan-jī′tis, kō′lan-jē-ī′tis) Inflammation of a bile duct or the entire biliary tree. [chol- + G. *angeion,* vessel, + *-itis,* inflammation]

cho•lan•o•poi•e•sis (kō′lă-nō-poy-ē′sis) Synthesis by the liver of cholic acid or its conjugates, or of natural bile salts. [chol- + G. *anō,* upward, + *poiēsis,* making]

cho•lan•o•poi•et•ic (kō′lă-nō-poy-et′ik) Pertaining to or promoting cholanopoiesis.

cho•late (kō′lāt) A salt or ester of a cholic acid.

♻ **chole-, chol-, cholo-** Combining forms indicating bile. Cf. bili-. [G. *cholē*]

cho•le•cal•cif•er•ol (kō′lĕ-kal-sif′ĕr-ol) The vitamin D of animal origin found in the skin, fur, and feathers of animals and birds exposed to sunlight, and also in butter, brain, fish oils, and egg yolk. SYN vitamin D3.

cho•le•cyst (kō′lĕ-sist) SYN gallbladder.

cho•le•cys•ta•gog•ic (kō′lĕ-sis′tă-goj′ik) Stimulating activity of the gallbladder.

cho•le•cys•ta•gogue (kō′lĕ-sis′tă-gog) A substance that stimulates activity of the gallbladder. [chole- + G. *kystis,* bladder, + *agōgos,* leader]

cho•le•cys•tec•ta•si•a (kō′lĕ-sis′tek-tā′zē-ă) Rarely used term for dilation of the gallbladder. [chole- + G. *kystis,* bladder, + *ektasis,* extension]

cho•le•cys•tec•to•my (kō′lĕ-sis-tek′tŏ-mē) Surgical removal of the gallbladder. [chole- + G. *kystis,* bladder, + *ektomē,* excision]

cho•le•cyst•en•ter•os•to•my (kō′lĕ-sist-en′tĕr-os′tō-mē) Formation of a direct communication between the gallbladder and the intestine. [chole- + G. *kystis,* bladder, + *enteron,* intestine, + *stoma,* mouth]

cho•le•cys•tic (kō′lĕ-sis′tik) Relating to the cholecyst, or gallbladder.

cho•le•cys•tis (kō′lĕ-sis′tis) SYN gallbladder. [chole- + G. *kystis,* bladder]

cho•le•cys•ti•tis (kō′lĕ-sis-tī′tis) Inflammation of the gallbladder. [chole- + G. *kystis,* bladder, + *-itis,* inflammation]

cho•le•cys•to•co•los•to•my (kō′lĕ-sis′tō-kō-los′tŏ-mē) Establishment of a communication between the gallbladder and the colon. SYN colocholecystostomy. [chole- + G. *kystis,* bladder, + *kōlon,* colon, + *stoma,* mouth]

cho•le•cys•to•du•o•de•nos•to•my (kō′lĕ-sis′tō-dū′ō-dē-nos′tŏ-mē) Establishment of a direct communication between the gallbladder and the duodenum. SYN duodenocholecystostomy, duodenocystostomy (1). [chole- + G. *kystis,* bladder, + L. *duodenum* + G. *stoma,* mouth]

cho•le•cys•to•gas•tros•to•my (kō′lĕ-sis′tō-gas-tros′tŏ-mē) Establishment of a communication between the gallbladder and the stomach. [chole- + G. *kystis,* bladder, + *gastēr,* stomach, + *stoma,* mouth]

cho•le•cys•to•gram (kō′lĕ-sis′tŏ-gram) The radiographic record of the gallbladder obtained by cholecystography.

cho•le•cys•tog•ra•phy (kō′lĕ-sis-tog′ră-fē) Radiographic study of the gallbladder after oral administration of a cholecystopaque or scintigraphic imaging of the gallbladder and central bile ducts after administration of a radiopharmaceutical secreted by the liver. [chole- + G. *kystis,* bladder, + *grapho,* to write]

cho•le•cys•to•il•e•os•to•my (kō′lĕ-sis′tō-il-ē-os′tŏ-mē) Establishment of a communication between the gallbladder and the ileum. [chole- + G. *kystis,* bladder, + ileum + G. *stoma,* mouth]

cho•le•cys•to•je•ju•nos•to•my (kō′lĕ-sis′tō-jē-jū-nos′tŏ-mē) Establishment of a communication between the gallbladder and the jejunum. [chole- + G. *kystis,* bladder, + jejunum, + G. *stoma,* mouth]

cho•le•cys•to•ki•net•ic (kō′lĕ-sis′tō-ki-net′ik) Promoting emptying of the gallbladder.

cho•le•cys•to•ki•nin (CCK) (kō′lĕ-sis′tō-kī′nin) A polypeptide hormone liberated by the upper intestinal mucosa on contact with gastric contents; stimulates contraction of the gallbladder and secretion of pancreatic juice.

cho•le•cys•to•li•thi•a•sis (kō′lĕ-sis′tō-li-thī′ă-sis) Presence of one or more gallstones in the gallbladder. [chole- + G. *kystis,* bladder, + *lithos,* stone]

cho•le•cys•top•a•thy (kō′lĕ-sis-top′ă-thē) Disease of the gallbladder.

cho•le•cys•to•pexy (kō′lĕ-sis′tō-pek-sē) Suture of the gallbladder to the abdominal wall. [chole- + G. *kystis,* bladder, + *pēxis,* fixation]

cho•le•cys•tor•rha•phy (kō′lĕ-sis-tōr′ă-fē) Suture of an incised or ruptured gallbladder. [chole- + G. *kystis,* bladder, + *rhaphē,* sewing]

cho•le•cys•to•so•nog•ra•phy (kō′lĕ-sis′tō-sŏ-nog′ră-fē) Ultrasonic examination of the gallbladder. [cholecysto- + sonography]

cho•le•cys•tos•to•my (kō′lĕ-sis-tos′tŏ-mē) Establishment of a fistula into the gallbladder. [chole- + G. *kystis,* bladder, + *stoma,* mouth]

cho•le•cys•tot•o•my (kō′lĕ-sis-tot′ŏ-mē) Incision into the gallbladder. [chole- + G. *kystis,* bladder, + *tomē,* incision]

cho•le•doch•al (kō-led′ŏ-kăl) Relating to the common bile duct.

cho•le•doch•al cyst (kō-led′ŏ-kăl sist) Cyst originating from common bile duct; usually becomes apparent early in life as a right upper abdominal mass in association with jaundice.

cho•led•o•chec•to•my (kol′ĕ-dō-kek′tŏ-mē) Surgical removal of a portion of the common bile duct. [choledoch- + G. *ektomē,* excision]

cho•led•o•chi•tis (kol′ĕ-dō-kī′tis) Inflammation of the common bile duct. [choledoch- + G. *-itis,* inflammation]

♻ **choledocho-, choledoch-** Combining forms meaning the ductus choledochus (the common bile duct). [G. *cholēdochos,* containing bile, fr. *cholē,* bile, + *dechomai,* to receive]

cho•led•o•cho•du•o•de•nos•to•my (kol′ĕ-dō-kō-dū′ō-dē-nos′tŏ-mē) Formation of a communication, other than the natural one, between the common bile duct and the duodenum. [choledocho- + duodenum + G. *stoma,* mouth]

cho•led•o•cho•en•ter•os•to•my (ko′led′ŏ-kō-en′tĕr-os′t ŏ-mē) Establishment of a communication, other than the natural one, between the common bile duct and any part of the intestine. [choledocho- + G. *enteron,* intestine, + *stoma,* mouth]

cho•led•o•cho•je•ju•nos•to•my (kō-led′ō-kō-jĕ-jū-nos′tŏ-mē) Anastomosis between the common bile duct and the jejunum. [choledocho- + jejuno- + G. *stoma,* mouth]

cho•led•o•cho•li•thi•a•sis (kol′ĕ-dō-kō-lith-ī′ă-sis) Presence of a gallstone in the common bile duct.

cho•led•o•cho•li•thot•o•my (kol′ĕ-dō-kō-li-thot′ŏ-mē) Incision of the common bile duct for the extraction of an impacted gallstone. [choledocho- + G. *lithos,* stone, + *tomē,* incision]

cho•led•o•cho•plas•ty (kol′ĕ-dō-kō-plas-tē) Plastic surgery of the common bile duct. [choledocho- + G. *plastos,* formed]

cho•led•o•chor•rha•phy (kol′ĕ-dō-kōr′ră-fē) Suturing together the divided ends of the common bile duct. [choledocho- + G. *rhaphē,* suture]

cho•led•o•chos•to•my (kol′ĕ-dō-kos′tŏ-mē) Establishment of a fistula into the common bile duct. [choledocho- + G. *stoma,* mouth]

cho•led•o•chot•o•my (kol′ĕ-dō-kot′ŏ-mē) Incision into the common bile duct. [choledocho- + G. *tomē,* incision]

cho•led•o•chous (kō-led′ŏ-kŭs) Containing or conveying bile.

cho•le•ic (kō-lē′ik) SYN cholic.

cho•le•ic ac•ids (kō-lē′ik as′idz) Compounds of bile acids and sterols.

cho•le•lith (kō′lĕ-lith) SYN gallstone. [chole- + G. *lithos,* stone]

cho•le•li•thi•a•sis (kō′lĕ-li-thī′ă-sis) Presence of gallstones in the gallbladder or bile ducts. See this page.

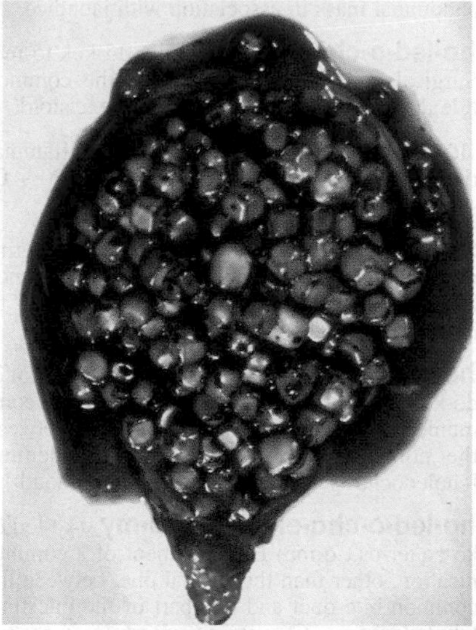

cholelithiasis: the gallbladder has been opened to reveal numerous yellow cholesterol gallstones

cho•le•li•thot•o•my (kō′lĕ-li-thot′ŏ-mē) Operative removal of a gallstone. [chole- + G. *lithos,* stone, + *tomē,* incision]

cho•le•lith•o•trip•sy (kō′lĕ-lith′ō-trip-sē) The crushing of a gallstone. [chole- + G. *lithos,* stone, + *tripsis,* a rubbing]

cho•lem•e•sis (kō-lem′ĕ-sis) Vomiting bile. [chole- + G. *emesis,* vomiting]

cho•le•mi•a (kō-lē′mē-ă) The presence of bile salts in the circulating blood. SYN cholaemia. [chole- + G. *haima,* blood]

cho•lem•ic (kō-lē′mik) Relating to cholemia. SYN cholaemic.

cho•le•per•i•to•ne•um (kō′lĕ-per′i-tŏ-nē′ŭm) Bile in the peritoneum, which may lead to bile peritonitis.

cho•le•poi•e•sis (kō′lĕ-poy-ē′sis) Formation of bile. [chole- + G. *poiēsis,* making]

cho•le•poi•et•ic (kō′lĕ-poy-et′ik) Relating to the formation of bile.

chol•er•a (kol′ĕr-ă) An acute epidemic infectious disease caused by the bacterium *Vibrio cholerae*, occurring primarily in Asia. A toxin elaborated by the bacterium activates the adenylate cyclase of the mucosa, causing active secretion of an isotonic fluid resulting in watery diarrhea, loss of fluid and electrolytes, and dehydration and collapse, but no gross morphologic change in the intestinal mucosa. [L. a bilious disease, fr. G. *cholē,* bile]

chol•er•a•ic (kol′ĕr-ā′ik) Relating to cholera.

chol•er•a•ic di•ar•rhe•a (kol′ĕr-ā′ik dī′ă-rē′ă) SYN summer diarrhea.

cho•le•re•sis (kō′lĕr-ē′sis) The secretion, as opposed to the expulsion, of bile by the gallbladder. [chole- + G. *hairesis,* a taking]

cho•le•ret•ic (kō′lĕr-et′ik) **1.** Relating to choleresis. **2.** An agent, usually a drug, that stimulates the liver to increase bile output.

chol•er•ic (kol′ĕr-ik) SYN bilious (2).

chol•er•i•form (kō-ler′i-fōrm) Resembling cholera. SYN choleroid.

chol•er•ine (kol′ĕr-ēn) A mild form of diarrhea seen during epidemics of Asiatic cholera.

chol•er•oid (kol′ĕr-oyd) SYN choleriform.

cho•ler•rha•gic (kol′ĕr-aj′ik) Referring to the flow of bile.

cho•le•sta•si•a, cho•le•sta•sis (kō-lĕ-stā′sē-ă, -sis) An arrest in the flow of bile. [chole- + G. *stasis,* a standing still]

cho•les•ta•sis of preg•nan•cy (kō′lĕ-stā′sis preg′năn-sē) SYN intrahepatic cholestasis of pregnancy.

cho•le•stat•ic (kō′lĕ-stat′ik) Tending to diminish or stop the flow of bile.

cho•le•stat•ic jaun•dice (kō′lĕ-stat′ik jawn′dis) Liver disorder produced by inspissated bile or bile plugs in small biliary passages in the liver.

cho•les•te•a•to•ma (kō′lĕ-stē′ă-tō′mă) **1.** A mass of keratinizing squamous epithelium and cholesterol in the middle ear, usually caused by chronic otitis media, with squamous metaplasia or extension of squamous epithelium inward to line an expanding cystic cavity that may involve the mastoid and erode surrounding bone. **2.** An epidermoid cyst arising in the central nervous system in man or animals. See page B28. [cholesterol + G. *stear (steat-),* tallow, + *-ōma,* tumor]

cholesteraemia [Br.] SYN cholesteremia.

cho•les•ter•e•mi•a, cho•les•ter•ol•e•mi•a (kō-les′tĕr-ē′mē-ă, kō-les′tĕr-ol-ē′mē-ă) The presence of excessive cholesterol in the blood. SYN cholesteraemia. [cholesterol + G. *haima,* blood]

cho•les•ter•in•ized an•ti•gen (kō-les′tĕr-in-īzd an′ti-jen) Cardiolipin to which cholesterol has been added.

cho•les•ter•ol (kŏ-les′tĕr-ol) The most abundant steroid in animal tissues; circulates in the plasma complexed to proteins of various densities; plays an important role in the pathogenesis of atheroma formation in arteries.

cholesterolaemia [Br.] SYN cholesterolemia.

cho•les•ter•ol em•bo•lism (kŏ-les′tĕr-ol em′bŏ-lizm) Embolism of lipid debris from an ulcerated atheromatous deposit, generally from a large artery to small arterial branches; it is usually small and rarely causes infarction. SYN atheromatous embolism.

cho•les•ter•ol•e•mi•a (kō-les′tĕr-ol-ē′mē-ă) The presence of excessive cholesterol in the blood.

cho•les•ter•ol es•ter stor•age dis•ease (kŏ-les′tĕr-ol es′tĕr stōr′ăj di-zēz′) A lipidosis caused by a deficiency of lysosomal acid lipase activity resulting in widespread accumulation of cholesterol esters and triglycerides in viscera with xanthomatosis, adrenal calcification, hepatosplenomegaly, foam cells in bone marrow and other tissues, and vacuolated lymphocytes in peripheral blood; autosomal recessive inheritance, caused by mutation in the lysosomal and lipase gene (LIPA) on chromosome 10q. SYN Wolman disease, Wolman xanthomatosis.

cho•les•ter•ol-free (kŏ-les′tĕr-ol-frē′) A product so labeled contains, by F.D.A. order, less than 2 mg cholesterol per serving and 2 g saturated fat per serving.

cho•les•ter•ol gran•u•lo•ma (kŏ-les′tĕr-ol gran′yū-lō′mă) Granuloma with prominent clefts of cholesterol surrounded by foreign-body giant cells found in chronic otitis media and sinusitis.

cho•les•ter•ol•o•sis, cho•les•ter•o•sis (kō-les′ter-ol′ō-sis, kō′les-tĕr-ō′sis) **1.** A condition resulting from a disturbance in metabolism of lipids, characterized by deposits of cholesterol in tissue. **2.** Cholesterol crystals in the anterior chamber of the eye.

cho•les•ter•ol•u•ri•a (kō-les′ter-ol-yūr′ē-ă) The excretion of cholesterol in the urine.

cho•le•u•ri•a (kō′lē-yūr′ē-ă) SYN biliuria.

cho•lic (kō′lik) Relating to the bile. SYN choleic.

cho•lic ac•id (kō′lik as′id) A family of steroids comprising the bile acids (or salts), generally in conjugated form (e.g., glycocholic and taurocholic acids); cholic acids are derived from cholesterol.

cho•line (kō′lēn) An amine found in most animal tissues. It is included in the vitamin B complex; as acetylcholine, it is essential for synaptic transmission. Several salts of choline are used in medicine.

cho•line a•ce•tyl•trans•fer•ase (kō′lēn ă-sē′til-trans′fĕr-ās) An enzyme catalyzing the condensation of choline and acetyl-coenzyme A, forming *O*-acetylcholine and coenzyme A.

cho•line ki•nase (kō′lēn kī′nās) An enzyme that catalyzes the formation of *O*-phosphocholine and ADP from choline and ATP.

cho•lin•er•gic (kō′lin-ĕr′jik) Relating to nerve cells or fibers that employ acetylcholine as their neurotransmitter. Cf. adrenergic. [choline + G. *ergon,* work]

cho•lin•er•gic block•ade (kō′lin-ĕr′jik blok-ād′) **1.** Inhibition by a drug of nerve impulse transmission at autonomic ganglionic synapses (ganglionic blockade), at postganglionic parasympathetic effector cells (e.g., by atropine), and at myoneural junctions (myoneural blockade). **2.** The inhibition of a cholinergic agent.

cho•lin•er•gic fi•bers (kō′lin-ĕr′jik fī′bĕrz) Nerve fibers that transmit impulses to other nerve cells, muscle fibers, or gland cells by the medium of the transmitter substance acetylcholine.

cho•lin•er•gic re•cep•tors (kō′lin-ĕr′jik rĕ-sep′tŏrz) Chemical sites in effector cells or at synapses through which acetylcholine exerts its action.

cho•lin•er•gic tox•i•drome (kō′lin-ĕr′jik tok′si-drōm) The constellation of clinical effects (i.e., signs and symptoms) characteristic of poisoning by a cholinergic agent such as an anticholinesterase compound and caused by overstimulation and eventually fatigue and failure of cholinergically innervated target organs; typical effects involve skeletal muscle (e.g., twitching, fasciculations, weakness, paresis, paralysis), smooth muscle (e.g., miosis, bronchospasm due to overstimulation of bronchial smooth muscle, and nausea, vomiting, and diarrhea due to hyperperistalsis), exocrine glands (e.g., lacrimation, rhinorrhea, hypersalivation, bronchorrhea, diaphoresis), and neurons in the central nervous system (e.g., seizures, convulsions, central apnea).

cho•lin•er•gic ur•ti•car•i•a (kō′lin-ĕr′jik ŭr′ti-kar′ē-ă) A form of physical or nonallergic urticaria initiated by heat (e.g., hot baths, physical exercise, pyrexia, exposure to sun or to a warm room) or by excitement; the rather distinctive lesions consist of pruritic areas 1–2 mm in diameter surrounded by bright red macules. SYN heat urticaria.

cho•lin•es•ter•ase (ChE) (kō′lin-es′tĕr-ās) One of a family of enzymes capable of catalyzing the hydrolysis of acylcholines and a few other compounds. Found in cobra venom.

cho•lin•es•ter•ase in•hib•i•tor (kō′lin-es′tĕr-ās in-hib′i-tŏr) A drug, such as neostigmine, which, by inhibiting biodegradation of acetylcholine, restores myoneural function in myasthenia gravis or after nondepolarizing neuromuscular relaxants have been administered.

cho•lin•o•cep•tive (kō′lin-ō-sep′tiv) Referring to chemical sites in effector cells with which acetylcholine unites to exert its actions. Cf. adrenoceptive. [acetylcholine + L. *capio*, to take]

cho•li•no•lyt•ic (kō′lin-ō-lit′ik) Preventing the action of acetylcholine. [acetylcholine + G. *lysis*, loosening]

chol•i•no•mi•met•ic (kō′lin-ō-mi-met′ik) Having an action similar to that of acetylcholine; replaces the less specific term parasympathomimetic. Cf. adrenomimetic. SYN parasympathomimetic. [acetylcholine + G. *mimētikos*, imitating]

cho•lin•o•re•ac•tive (kō′lin-ō-rē-ak′tiv) Responding to acetylcholine and related compounds.

chol•i•no•re•cep•tors (kol′i-nō-rē-sep′tŏrz) SEE cholinergic receptors.

cho•lo•yl (kō′lō-il) The radical of cholic acid or cholate.

chol•ur•i•a (kō-lyūr′ē-ă) SYN biliuria. [G. *cholē*, bile, + *ouron*, urine]

chon•dral (kon′drăl) SYN cartilaginous. [G. *chondros*, cartilage]

chon•dral frac•ture (kon′drăl frak′shŭr) Fracture involving the articular cartilage of a joint. SEE ALSO articular cartilage.

chon•dral•gi•a (kon-dral′jē-ă) SYN chondrodynia. [G. *chondros*, cartilage, + *algos*, pain]

chon•drec•to•my (kon-drek′tō-mē) Excision of cartilage. [G. *chondros*, cartilage, + *ektomē*, excision]

chon•dri•fi•ca•tion (kon′dri-fi-kā′shŭn) Conversion into cartilage. [G. *chondros*, cartilage, + L. *facio*, to make]

chon•dri•fi•ca•tion cen•ter (kon′dri-fi-kā′shŭn sen′tĕr) Site of earliest cartilage formation in the fetus.

chon•dri•tis (kon-drī′tis) Inflammation of cartilage. [G. *chondros*, cartilage, + *-itis*, inflammation]

♻**chondro-, chondrio-** Combining forms meaning (1) cartilage or cartilaginous, (2) granular or gritty substance. [G. *chondrion*, dim. of *chondros*, groats (coarsely ground grain), grit, gristle, cartilage]

chon•dro•blast (kon′drō-blast) A dividing cell of growing cartilage tissue. SYN chondroplast. [chondro- + G. *blastos*, germ]

chon•dro•blas•to•ma (kon′drō-blas-tō′mă) A benign tumor arising in the epiphyses of long bones, consisting of highly cellular tissue resembling fetal cartilage.

chon•dro•cal•ci•no•sis (kon′drō-kal-si-nō′sis) Calcification of cartilage. [chondro- + calcium + G. *-osis*, condition]

chon•dro•clast (kon′drō-klast) A multinucleated giant cell involved in the resorption of calcified cartilage; morphologically identical to osteoblasts. [chondro- + G. *klastos*, broken in pieces]

chon•dro•cos•tal (kon′drō-kaws′tăl) SYN costochondral. [chondro- + L. *costa*, rib]

chon•dro•cra•ni•um (kon′drō-krā′nē-ŭm) A cartilaginous cranium; the cartilaginous parts of the developing cranium. [chondro- + G. *kranion*, skull]

chon•dro•cyte (kon′drō-sīt) A nondividing cartilage cell; occupies a lacuna within the cartilage matrix. [chondro- + G. *kytos*, a hollow (cell)]

chon•dro•dyn•i•a (kon′drō-din′ē-ă) Pain in cartilage. SYN chondralgia. [chondro- + G. *odynē*, pain]

chon•dro•dys•pla•si•a (kon′drō-dis-plā′zē-ă) SYN chondrodystrophy. [chondro- + G. *dys*, bad, + *plasis*, a molding]

chon•dro•dys•pla•si•a cal•cif•i•cans con•gen•i•ta (kon′drō-dis-plā′zē-ă kal-sif′i-kanz kon-jen′i-tă) A form of hereditary chondrodysplasia characterized by asymmetric calcifications, dysplastic skeletal changes, and relatively good prognosis. SYN Conradi disease.

chon•dro•dys•tro•phic dwarf•ism (kon′drō-dis-trō′fik dwōrf′izm) SEE chondrodystrophy.

chon•dro•dys•tro•phy, chon•dro•dys•tro•phi•a (kon′drō-dis′trŏ-fē, kon′drō-dis-trō′fē-ă) A disturbance in the development of the cartilage of the long bones, especially of the epiphysial plates, resulting in arrested growth and dwarfism in which the limbs are abnormally short, but the head and trunk are essentially normal. SYN chondrodysplasia. [chondro- + G. *dys*, bad, + *trophē* nourishment]

chon•dro•dys•tro•phy with sen•sor•i•neu•ral deaf•ness (kon′drō-dis′trŏ-fē sen′sŏr-ē-nūr′ăl def′nĕs) A skeletal dysplasia characterized by dwarfism, flat nasal bridge, cleft palate, sensorineural deafness, large epiphyses, and flattening of the vertebral bodies; autosomal recessive inheritance, caused by mutation in the type XI collagen gene (COL11A2) on chromosome 6p; dominant forms exist. SYN Nance-Insley syndrome, Nance-Sweeney chondrodysplasia, otospondylomegaepiphysial dysplasia.

chon•dro•ec•to•der•mal dys•pla•si•a (kon′drō-ek-tō-dĕr′măl dis-plā′zē-ă) Triad of chondrodysplasia, ectodermal dysplasia, and polydactyly, with congenital heart defects in over half of patients; autosomal recessive inheritance.

chon•dro•fi•bro•ma (kon′drō-fī-brō′mă) SYN chondromyxoid fibroma.

chon•dro•gen•e•sis (kon′drō-jen′ĕ-sis) Formation of cartilage. SYN chondrosis. [chondro- + G. *genesis,* origin]

chon•droid (kon′droyd) **1.** Resembling cartilage. SYN cartilaginoid. **2.** Uncharacteristically developed cartilage, primarily cellular with a basophilic matrix and thin or nonexistent capsules. [chondro- + G. *eidos,* resemblance]

chon•droid tis•sue (kon′droyd tish′ū) **1.** In an adult, tissue resembling cartilage; SYN pseudocartilage. **2.** In an embryo, an early stage in cartilage formation.

chon•dro•i•tin (kon-drō′i-tin) Dietary supplement made from bovine cartilage; widely used for its purported efficacy against osteoarthritis; some clinical studies suggest its value, others make no such confirmation. Association with spontaneous internal bleeding. [*chondroit-* fr. *chondroitic acid,* + -in]

chon•drol•y•sis (kon-drol′i-sis) Disappearance of articular cartilage as the result of disintegration or dissolution of the cartilage matrix and cells.

chon•dro•ma (kon-drō′mă) A benign neoplasm derived from mesodermal cells that form cartilage. [chondro- + G. *-ōma,* tumor]

chon•dro•ma•la•ci•a (kon′drō-mă-lā′shē-ă) Softening of any cartilage. [chondro- + G. *malakia,* softness]

chon•dro•ma•la•ci•a pa•tel•lae (kon′drō-mă-lā′shē-ă pă-tel′ē) Degenerative condition in the articular cartilage of the patella caused by abnormal compression or shearing forces at the knee joint; may cause patellalgia. SEE ALSO patellofemoral syndrome.

chon•dro•ma•to•sis (kon′drō-mă-tō′sis) Presence of multiple tumorlike foci of cartilage.

chon•dro•ma•tous (kon-drō′mă-tŭs) Pertaining to or manifesting the features of a chondroma.

chon•dro•mere (kon′drō-mēr) A cartilage unit of the fetal axial skeleton; a primordial cartilaginous vertebra together with its costal component. [chondro- + G. *meros,* part]

chon•dro•myx•oid fi•bro•ma, chon•dro•myx•o•ma (kon′drō-miks′oyd fī-brō′mă, kon′drō-mik-sō′mă) An uncommon benign bone tumor, occurring most frequently in the tibia of adolescents and young adults, composed of lobulated myxoid tissue with scanty chondroid foci. SYN chondrofibroma.

chon•dro•nec•tin (kon′drō-nek′tin) A glycoprotein of cartilage matrix that mediates the adhesion of chondrocytes to type II collagen. [chondro- + L. *necto,* to bind, + -in]

chon•dro•os•se•ous (kon′drō-os′ē-ŭs) Relating to cartilage and bone. [chondro- + osseous]

chon•dro•os•te•o•dys•tro•phy (kon′drō-os′tē-ō-dis′trŏ-fē) Term used for a group of disorders of bone and cartilage that includes Morquio syndrome and similar conditions. SYN osteochondrodystrophy.

chon•drop•a•thy (kon-drop′ă-thē) Any disease of cartilage. [chondro- + G. *pathos,* suffering]

chon•dro•phyte (kon′drō-fīt) An abnormal cartilaginous mass that develops at the articular surface of a bone. [chondro- + G. *phytos,* a growth]

chon•dro•plast (kon′drō-plast) SYN chondroblast. [chondro- + G. *plastos,* formed]

chon•dro•plas•ty (kon′drō-plas-tē) Reparative or plastic surgery of cartilage. [chondro- + G. *plastos,* formed]

chon•dro•po•ro•sis (kon′drō-pōr-ō′sis) Condition of cartilage in which spaces appear, either normal (in the process of ossification) or pathologic. [chondro- + L. *porosus,* porous]

chon•dro•sar•co•ma (kon′drō-sahr-kō′mă) A malignant neoplasm derived from cartilage cells.

chon•dro•sis (kon-drō′sis) SYN chondrogenesis.

chon•dro•ster•nal (kon′drō-stĕr′năl) **1.** Relating to a sternal cartilage. **2.** Relating to the costal cartilages and the sternum.

chon•dro•ster•no•plas•ty (kon′drō-stĕr′nō-plas-tē) Surgical correction of malformations of the sternum.

chon•drot•o•my (kon-drot′ŏ-mē) Division of cartilage. [chondro- + G. *tomē,* a cutting]

chon•dro•xi•phoid (kon′drō-zī′foyd) Relating to the xiphoid or ensiform cartilage. [chondro- + G. *xiphos,* sword, + *eidos,* appearance]

Cho•part am•pu•ta•tion (shō-pahr′ amp′yū-tā′shŭn) Amputation through the midtarsal joint; i.e., between the tarsal navicular and the calcaneocuboid joints. SYN mediotarsal amputation.

♻ **chord-** Combining form for cord. SEE ALSO cord-. [G. *chordē*]

chor•da, pl. **chor•dae** (kōr′dă, -dē) [TA] A tendinous or a cordlike structure. SEE ALSO cord. [L. cord]

chor•dae ten•di•ne•ae cor•dis (kōr′dē ten-din′ē-ē kōr′dis) [TA] SYN chordae tendineae of heart.

chor•dae ten•di•ne•ae fal•sae (kōr′dē ten-din′ē-ē fal′sē) [TA] SYN false chordae tendineae.

chor•dae ten•din•e•ae of heart (kōr′dē ten-din′ē-ē hahrt) The tendinous strands running from the papillary muscles to the leaflets of the atrioventricular (mitral and tricuspid) valves. Based on their shape, position, or specific area of attachment to the leaflets, several varieties have been described: fan-shaped chordae, rough zone chordae, free-edge chordae, deep chordae, and basal chordae. SYN chordae tendineae cordis [TA], tendinous cords.

chor·dae ten·din·e·ae spur·i·ae (kōr′dē ten-din′ē-ē spūr′ē-ē) SYN false chordae tendineae.

chord·al (kōr′dăl) Relating to any chorda or cord, especially the notochord.

Chor·da·ta (kōr-dā′tă) The phylum that includes the vertebrates, defined by possession of 1) a single dorsal nerve cord (the brain and spinal cord of mammals); 2) a cartilaginous rod, the notochord, which forms dorsal to the primitive gut in the early embryo and is surrounded and replaced by the vertebral column in the subphylum vertebrata; 3) the presence at some stage in development of gill slits in the pharynx or throat. [L. *chorda,* fr. G. *chordē,* a string]

chor·date (kōr′dāt) An animal of the phylum *Chordata.*

chor·da tym·pa·ni (kōr′dă tim′pan-ī) [TA] A nerve given off from the facial nerve in the facial canal that passes through the posterior canaliculus of the chorda tympani into the tympanic cavity, crosses over the tympanic membrane and handle of the malleus, and passes out through the anterior canaliculus of the chorda tympani in the petrotympanic fissure to join the lingual branch of the mandibular nerve in the infratemporal fossa; it conveys taste sensation from the anterior two thirds of the tongue and carries parasympathetic preganglionic fibers to the submandibular ganglion, for innervation of the submandibular and sublingual salivary glands.

chor·dee (kōr-dē′) **1.** Painful erection of the penis in association with gonorrhea or Peyronie disease, with curvature resulting from lack of distensibility of the corpora cavernosa of the urethra. **2.** Ventral curvature of the penis, most apparent on erection, as seen in hypospadias due to congenital shortness of the ventral skin and, on rare occasions, in patients with a normally situated meatus. [Fr. corded]

chor·di·tis (kōr-dī′tis) Inflammation of a cord; usually a vocal cord. [G. *chordē,* cord, + *-itis,* inflammation]

chor·do·ma (kōr-dō′mă) A rare neoplasm of skeletal tissue in adults, derived from persistent portions of the notochord. [(noto)chord + G. *-oma,* tumor]

chor·do·skel·e·ton (kōr′dō-skel′ĕ-tŏn) The part of the embryonic skeleton that develops in conjunction with the notochord.

chor·dot·o·my (kōr-dot′ŏ-mē) SYN cordotomy.

cho·re·a (kōr-ē′ă) Irregular, spasmodic, involuntary movements of the limbs or facial muscles, often accompanied by hypotonia. The location of the responsible cerebral lesion is not known. SEE ALSO Huntington chorea, Sydenham chorea. [L. fr. G. *choreia,* a choral dance, fr. *choros,* a dance]

cho·re·al (kōr-ē′ăl) Relating to involuntary writhing of the limbs or facial muscles.

cho·re·ic (kōr-ē′ik) Relating to or of the nature of chorea.

cho·re·ic a·ba·si·a (kōr-ē′ik ă-bā′zē-ă) Abasia related to choreiform movements of the legs.

cho·re·ic move·ment (kōr-ē′ik mūv′mĕnt) An involuntary spasmodic twitching or jerking in groups of muscles not associated in the production of definite purposeful movements.

cho·re·i·form (kōr-ē′i-fōrm) SYN choreoid.

♻ **choreo-** Combining form denoting chorea.

cho·re·o·ath·e·toid (kōr′ē-ō-ath′ĕ-toyd) Pertaining to or characterized by choreoathetosis.

cho·re·o·ath·e·to·sis (kōr′ē-ō-ath-ĕ-tō′sis) Abnormal movements of body of combined choreic and athetoid pattern. [choreo- + G. *athētos,* unfixed, + *-ōsis,* condition]

cho·re·oid (kōr′ē-oyd) Resembling chorea. SYN choreiform.

cho·re·o·phra·si·a (kōr′ē-ō-frā′zē-ă) Continual repetition of meaningless phrases. [choreo- + G. *phrasis,* speaking]

♻ **chorio-** Combining form denoting any membrane, but especially that enclosing the embryo, and later, fetus. [G. *chorion,* membrane]

cho·ri·o·ad·e·no·ma (kōr′ē-ō-ad-ĕ-nō′mă) A benign neoplasm of chorion, especially with hydatidiform mole formation.

cho·ri·o·ad·e·no·ma des·tru·ens (kōr′ē-ō-ad′ĕ-nō′mă des′trūenz) Hydatidiform mole in which there is an unusual degree of invasion of the myometrium or its blood vessels, causing hemorrhage, necrosis, and occasionally rupture of the uterus or embolism of molar tissue to the lungs; there is marked proliferation of the trophoblast, but avascular villi may also be found. SYN invasive mole.

cho·ri·o·al·lan·to·ic (kōr′ē-ō-al′an-tō′ik) Pertaining to the chorioallantois.

cho·ri·o·al·lan·to·is (kōr′ē-ō-ă-lan′tō-is) Extraembryonic membrane formed by the fusion of the allantois with the serosa or false chorion. In mammals it forms the fetal portion of the placenta; in avian embryos it is fused with the shell.

cho·ri·o·am·ni·o·ni·tis (kōr′ē-ō-am′nē-ō-nī′tis) Infection involving the chorion, amnion, and amniotic fluid; usually the placental villi and decidua are also involved.

cho·ri·o·an·gi·o·ma (kōr′ē-ō-an-jē-ō′mă) Benign tumor of placental blood vessels, usually of no clinical significance. SEE ALSO chorioangiosis. [chorion + angioma]

cho•ri•o•an•gi•o•sis (kōr′ē-ō-an-jē-ō′sis) An abnormal increase in the number of vascular channels in placental villi; severe chorioangiosis is associated with a high incidence of neonatal death and major congenital malformations. [chorio- + G. *angeion,* vessel, + *-osis,* condition]

cho•ri•o•cap•il•la•ris (kōr′ē-ō-kap-i-lā′ris) SYN choriocapillary layer.

cho•ri•o•cap•il•la•ry lay•er (kōr′ē-ō-kap′i-lar-ē lā′ĕr) The internal layer of the choroidea of the eye, composed of a very close capillary network. SYN lamina choroidocapillaris [TA], choriocapillaris, entochoroidea, Ruysch membrane.

cho•ri•o•car•ci•no•ma (kō′rē-ō-kahr-si-nō′mă) A highly malignant neoplasm derived from placental syncytial trophoblasts and cytotrophoblasts; villi are not formed; neoplastic cells invade blood vessels. Hemorrhagic metastases are found in the lungs, liver, brain, and vagina; choriocarcinoma may follow any type of pregnancy, especially hydatidiform mole, and occasionally originates in teratoid neoplasms of the ovaries or testes. SYN chorioepithelioma.

cho•ri•o•cele (kō′rē-ō-sēl) A hernia of the choroid coat of the eye through a defect in the sclera. [chorio- + G. *kēlē,* hernia]

cho•ri•o•ep•i•the•li•o•ma (kōr′ē-ō-ep-i-thē′lē-ō′mă) SYN choriocarcinoma.

cho•ri•o•men•in•gi•tis (kōr′ē-ō-men-in-jī′tis) A cerebral meningitis with a more or less marked cellular infiltration of the meninges, often with a lymphocytic infiltration of the choroid plexuses.

cho•ri•on (kōr′ē-on) The multilayered, outermost fetal membrane consisting of extraembryonic somatic mesoderm, trophoblast, and, on the maternal surface, its villi are bathed by maternal blood; as pregnancy progresses, part of the villous chorion becomes the fetal part of placenta. SYN membrana serosa (1). [G. *chorion,* membrane enclosing the fetus]

cho•ri•on fron•do•sum (kōr′ē-on fron-dō′sŭm) SYN villous chorion.

cho•ri•on•ic (kōr′ē-on′ik) Relating to the chorion.

chor•i•on•ic cav•i•ty (kōr′ē-on′ik cav′i-tē) The space surrounding the umbilical vesicle (primary yolk sac) and amniotic sac, except where the connecting stalk attaches to the cytotrophoblast of the blastocyst. SYN extraembryonic celom.

cho•ri•on•ic ep•i•the•li•o•ma (kōr′ē-on′ik ep′i-thē′lē-ō′mă) Obsolete term for choriocarcinoma.

cho•ri•on•ic go•nad•o•tro•pic hor•mone, cho•ri•on•ic go•nad•o•tro•phic hor•mone (kōr′ē-on′ik gō-nad′ō-trō′pik hōr′mōn, kōr′ē-on′ik gō-nad′o-trō′fik hōr′mōn) SYN chorionic gonadotropin.

cho•ri•on•ic go•nad•o•tro•pin (kōr′ē-on′ik gō-nad′ō-trō′pin) A glycoprotein with a carbohydrate fraction composed of D-galactose and hexosamine, produced by the placental trophoblastic cells; its most important role appears to be stimulation (during the first trimester) of ovarian secretion of the estrogen and progesterone required for the integrity of the conceptus; it appears to play no significant role in the last two trimesters of pregnancy, as the estrogen and progesterone are then formed by the placenta. Testing for the beta fraction of human chorionic gonadotropin is the basis for most serum and urine pregnancy tests. SYN anterior pituitarylike hormone, chorionic gonadotropic hormone, chorionic gonadotrophic hormone.

cho•ri•on•ic growth hor•mone-pro•lac•tin (kōr′ē-on′ik grōth hōr′mōn-prō-lak′tin) SYN human placental lactogen.

cho•ri•on•ic vil•li (kōr′ē-on′ik vil′ī) Vascular processes of the chorion of the embryo entering into the formation of the placenta.

cho•ri•on•ic vil•lus bi•op•sy (kōr′ē-on′ik vil′ŭs bī′op-sē) Transcervical or transabdominal sampling of the chorionic villi for genetic analysis.

cho•ri•on•ic vil•lus sam•pling (CVS) (kōr′ē-on′ik vil′ŭs samp′ling) A biopsy of the chorion frondosum through the abdominal wall or through the endocervical canal at 6–12 weeks' gestation to obtain fetal cells for diagnosis of chromosomal abnormalities.

cho•ri•o•ret•i•nal (kōr′ē-ō-ret′i-năl) Relating to the choroid coat of the eye and the retina. SYN retinochoroid.

cho•ri•o•ret•i•ni•tis (kōr′ē-ō-ret′i-nī′tis) Inflammation in the choroid and retina with its origin in the choroid.

cho•ri•o•ret•i•nop•a•thy (kōr′ē-ō-ret′i-nop′ă-thē) A primary abnormality of the choroid with extension to the retina. SEE ALSO choroidopathy.

cho•ris•ta (kōr′is-tă) A focus of tissue that is itself histologically normal, but not normally found in the organ or structure in which it is located. Cf. choristoma. [G. *chōristos,* separated]

cho•ris•to•ma (kōr′is-tō′mă) A mass formed by maldevelopment of tissue of a type not normally found at that site. [G. *chōristos,* separated, + *-ōma*]

cho•roid (kōr′oyd) The middle vascular tunic of the eye lying between the retina and the sclera. SYN choroidea [TA]. [G. *choroeidēs,* a false reading for *chorioeidēs,* like a membrane]

cho•roi•dal (kōr-oyd′ăl) Relating to the choroid (choroidea).

cho•roi•dal ne•o•vas•cu•lar•i•za•tion (kōr-oyd′ăl nē-ō-vas′kyū-lar-ī-zā′shŭn) Ingrowth of new vessels from the choriocapillaris into the subretinal pigment epithelial space; associated with damage to the outer retina.

cho•roid cap•il•lar•y lay•er (kōr′oyd kap′i-lar-ē lā′ĕr) SEE choriocapillary layer.

cho•roi•de•a (kōr-oyd′ē-ă) [TA] SYN choroid.

choroideraemia [Br.] SYN choroideremia.

cho•roid•er•e•mi•a (kōr′oyd-ĕr-ē′mē-ă) Progressive degeneration of the choroid in males, occasionally in females, beginning with peripheral pigmentary retinopathy, followed by atrophy of the retinal pigment epithelium and of the choriocapillaris, night blindness, progressive constriction of visual fields, and finally complete blindness; X-linked inheritance; heterozygous females show a pigmentary retinopathy but without visual defect or peripheral progression. SYN choroideraemia, progressive choroidal atrophy, progressive tapetochoroidal dystrophy. [choroid + G. *erēmia,* absence]

cho•roid fis•sure (kōr′oyd fish′ŭr) SYN retinal fissure.

cho•roid glo•mus (kōr′oyd glō′mŭs) A marked enlargement of the choroid plexus of the lateral ventricle at the junction of the central part with the inferior horn.

cho•roid•i•tis (kōr′oyd-ī′tis) Inflammation of the choroid. Cf. choroidopathy, chorioretinopathy.

♻**choroido-** Combining form meaning the choroid.

cho•roid•o•cy•cli•tis (kōr-oyd′ō-sik-lī′tis) Inflammation of the choroid coat and the ciliary body. [choroido- + G. *kyklos,* circle]

cho•roid•op•a•thy (kōr′oyd-op′ă-thē) Noninflammatory degeneration of the choroid.

cho•roid•o•ret•i•ni•tis (kōr-oyd′ō-ret-i-nī′tis) Inflammation of the choroid and retina with the primary process in the choroid.

cho•roid plex•us (kōr′oyd pleks′ŭs) A vascular proliferation or fringe of the tela choroidea in the third, fourth, and lateral cerebral ventricles; it secretes cerebrospinal fluid thereby regulating to some degree the intraventricular pressure.

cho•roid te•la of third ven•tri•cle (kōr′oyd tē′lă thĕrd ven′tri-kĕl) A double fold of pia mater, enclosing subarachnoid trabeculae, between the fornix above and the epithelial roof of the third ventricle and the thalami below; at each lateral margin is a vascular fringe projecting into the choroidal fissure of the lateral ventricle; on its undersurface are several small vascular projections filling the folds of the ependymal roof of the third ventricle. SYN tela choroidea ventriculi tertii [TA].

cho•ro•pleth•ic map (kōr′ō-pleth-ik map) A method of mapping to display quantitative information such as death rates in defined jurisdictions (states, counties) by color coding or shading. [G. *chōros,* district, + *plēthos,* multitude, + -ic]

Chris•tian dis•ease, **Chris•tian syn•drome** (kris′chĕn di-zēz′, kris′chĕn sin′drōm) **1.** SYN Hand-Schüller-Christian disease. **2.** SYN relapsing febrile nodular nonsuppurative panniculitis.

Christ•mas dis•ease (kris′măs di-zēz′) SYN hemophilia B.

Christ•mas fac•tor (kris′măs fak′tŏr) SYN factor IX.

♻**chrom-**, **chromat-**, **chromato-**, **chromo-** Combining forms denoting color. [G. *chrōma*]

chromaesthesia [Br.] SYN chromesthesia.

chro•maf•fin (krō-maf′in) Giving a brownish yellow reaction with chromic salts; denoting certain cells in the medulla of the suprarenal glands and in paraganglia. SYN chromatophil (3), chromophil (3), chromophile, pheochrome (1). [chrom- + L. *affinis,* affinity]

chro•maf•fin bod•y (krō-maf′in bod′ē) SYN paraganglion.

chro•maf•fin cell (krō-maf′in sel) A cell that stains with chromic salts, in medulla of suprarenal gland and paraganglia of the sympathetic nervous system.

chro•maf•fin•o•ma (krō-maf′in-ō′mă) A neoplasm composed of chromaffin cells occurring in the medulla of suprarenal gland, the organs of Zuckerkandl, or the paraganglia of the thoracolumbar sympathetic chain; some chromaffinomas secrete catecholamines. SEE ALSO pheochromocytoma. SYN chromaffin tumor.

chro•maf•fin•op•a•thy (krō-maf′in-op′ă-thē) Any pathologic condition of chromaffin tissue, as in the medulla of suprarenal gland or the organs of Zuckerkandl. [chromaffin + G. *pathos,* suffering]

chro•maf•fin tis•sue (krō-maf′in tish′ū) A cellular tissue, vascular and well supplied with nerves, made up chiefly of chromaffin cells; it is found in the medulla of the suprarenal glands and, in smaller collections, in the paraganglia.

chro•maf•fin tu•mor (krō-maf′in tū′mŏr) SYN chromaffinoma.

chro•mat•ic (krō-mat′ik) Of or pertaining to color or colors; produced by, or made in, a color or colors.

chro•mat•ic ab•er•ra•tion (krō-mat′ik ab-ĕr-ā′shŭn) The difference in focus or magnification of an image arising because of a difference in the refraction of different wavelengths composing white light. SYN chromatism (2).

chro·ma·tic chart (krō-mat′ik chahrt) SYN color chart.

chro·ma·tic vi·sion (krō-mat′ik vizh′ŭn) SYN chromatopsia.

chro·ma·tid (krō′mă-tid) Each of the two strands formed by longitudinal duplication of a chromosome that becomes visible during prophase of mitosis or meiosis; the two chromatids are joined by the still undivided centromere; after the centromere has divided at metaphase and the two chromatids have separated, each chromatid becomes a chromosome. [G. *chrōma,* color, + *-id*]

chro·ma·tin (krō′mă-tin) The genetic material of the nucleus, consisting of deoxyribonucleoprotein. During mitotic division the chromatin condenses into chromosomes. [G. *chrōma,* color]

chro·ma·tin bod·y (krō′mă-tin bod′ē) The genetic apparatus of bacteria. SEE nucleus (2).

chro·ma·tism (krō′mă-tizm) **1.** Abnormal pigmentation. **2.** SYN chromatic aberration. [G. *chrōma,* color]

chro·ma·tog·e·nous (krō′mă-toj′ĕ-nŭs) Producing color; causing pigmentation. [chromato- + *-gen,* producing]

chro·mat·o·gram (krō-mat′ō-gram) A graphic record produced by chromatography.

chro·mat·o·graph·ic (krō′mă-tō-graf′ik) Pertaining to chromatography.

chro·ma·tog·ra·phy (krō′mă-tog′ră-fē) The separation of chemical substances and particles by differential movement through a two-phase system. SYN absorption chromatography. [chromato- + G. *graphō,* to write]

chro·ma·tol·y·sis (krō′mă-tol′i-sis) The disintegration of the granules of chromophil substance (Nissl bodies) in a nerve cell body that may occur after exhaustion of the cell or damage to its peripheral process. SYN chromolysis. [chromato- + G. *lysis,* dissolution]

chro·mat·o·lyt·ic (krō-mat′ō-lit′ik) Relating to chromatolysis.

chro·mat·o·phil (krō-mat′ō-fil) **1.** SYN chromophilic. **2.** SYN chromophil (2). **3.** SYN chromaffin.

chro·mat·o·phil·i·a (krō′mă-tō-fil′ē-ă) SYN chromophilia.

chro·mat·o·phil·ic, chro·ma·toph·i·lous (krō′mă-tō-fil′ik, -tof′i-lŭs) SYN chromophilic.

chro·mat·o·pho·bi·a (krō′mă-tō-fō′bē-ă) SYN chromophobia.

chro·mat·o·phore (krō-mat′ō-fōr) **1.** A plastid, colored because of the presence of chlorophyll or other pigments, found in certain forms of protozoa. **2.** Melanophage; a pigment-bearing phagocyte found chiefly in the skin, mucous membrane, and choroid coat of the eye, and also in melanomas. **3.** SYN chromophore. **4.** A colored plastid in plants (e.g., chloroplasts, leukoplasts). [chromato- + G. *phoros,* bearing]

chro·ma·top·si·a (krō′mă-top′sē-ă) A condition in which objects appear to be abnormally colored or tinged with color. SYN chromatic vision, colored vision. Cf. dyschromatopsia. [chromato- + G. *opsis,* vision]

chro·ma·tu·ri·a (krō′mă-tyūr′ē-ă) Abnormal coloration of the urine. [chromato- + G. *ouron,* urine]

chrome (krōm) Chromium, especially as a source of pigment.

-chrome A suffix indicating relationship to color. [G. *chrŏma* color]

chro·mes·the·si·a (krō′mes-thē′zē-ă) **1.** The color sense. **2.** A condition in which nonvisual stimuli, such as taste or smell, cause the perception of color. SYN chromaesthesia. [G. *chrōma,* color, + *aisthēsis,* sensation]

chrom·hi·dro·sis (krōm′hī-drō′sis) A rare condition characterized by the excretion of sweat containing pigment. SEE ALSO apocrine chromhidrosis. [chrom- + G. *hidros,* sweat]

chro·mic phos·phate ^{32}P col·loi·dal sus·pen·sion (krō′mik fos′făt kŏ-loyd′ăl sŭs-pen′shŭn) A pure beta-emitting colloidal, nonabsorbable radiopharmaceutical administered into body cavities such as the pleural or peritoneal spaces to control malignant effusions. SEE ALSO sodium phosphate ^{32}P.

chro·mi·um (Cr) (krō′mē-ŭm) A metallic element, atomic no. 24, atomic wt. 51.9961. A dietary essential bioelement, ^{51}Cr (half-life of 27.70 days) is used as a diagnostic aid in many disorders (e.g., gastrointestinal protein loss). [G. *chroma,* color]

chro·mi·um pic·o·lin·ate (krō′mē-ŭm pik-ō′lin-āt) A chromium salt taken by many athletes with the unsubstantiated belief that additional chromium promotes muscle growth, curbs appetite, and fosters body fat loss.

Chro·mo·bac·te·ri·um vi·o·la·ce·um (krō′mō-bak-tē′rē-ŭm vī-ō-lā′sē-ŭm) A motile, gram-negative, non-spore-bearing rod found in soil in tropic and subtropic environments. A cause of human infections including septicemia, pneumonia, wound infections, and abscesses; infection can be rapidly fatal and may relapse after cessation of antibiotic therapy.

chro·mo·blast (krō′mō-blast) An embryonic cell with the potential of developing into a pigment cell. [chromo- + G. *blastos,* germ]

chro·mo·blas·to·my·co·sis (krō′mō-blas′tō-mī-kō′sis) A localized chronic mycosis of the skin and subcutaneous tissues characterized by skin lesions so rough and irregular as to present a cauliflowerlike appearance; caused by dematiaceous fungi such as *Phialophora verrucosa, P. dermatitidis, Fonsecaea pedrosoi, F. compacta,* and *Cladophialophora carrionii;* fungal cells resembling pennies form rounded sclerotic bodies in tissue, with epidermal hyperplasia and intraepidermal microabscesses. SYN chromomycosis. [chromo- + G. *blastos,* germ, + *mykē,* fungus, + *-osis,* condition]

chro·mo·cys·tos·co·py (krō′mō-sis-tos′kŏ-pē) SYN cystochromoscopy. [chromo- + G. *kystis,* bladder, + *skopeō,* to view]

chro·mo·cyte (krō′mō-sīt) Any pigmented cell, such as a red blood corpuscle. [chromo- + G. *kytos,* cell]

chro·mo·gen (krō′mō-jen) **1.** A substance, itself without definite color, that may be transformed into a pigment. **2.** A microorganism that produces pigment.

chro·mo·gen·e·sis (krō′mō-jen′ĕ-sis) Production of coloring matter or pigment. [chromo- + G. *genesis,* production]

chro·mo·gen·ic (krō′mō-jen′ik) **1.** Denoting a chromogen. **2.** Relating to chromogenesis.

chro·mol·y·sis (krō-mol′i-sis) SYN chromatolysis.

chro·mo·mere (krō′mō-mēr) **1.** A condensed segment of a chromonema; densely staining bands visible in chromosomes under certain conditions. **2.** SYN granulomere. [chromo- + G. *meros,* a part]

chro·mo·my·co·sis (krō′mō-mī-kō′sis) SYN chromoblastomycosis. [chromo- + G. *mykēs,* fungus, + *-osis,* condition]

chro·mo·ne·ma, pl. **chro·mo·ne·ma·ta** (krō′mō-nē′mă, -mă-tă) The coiled filament in which the genes are located, which extends the entire length of a chromosome. [chromo- + G. *nēma,* thread]

chro·mo·phil, **chro·mo·phile** (krō′mō-fil, krō′mō-fīl) **1.** SYN chromophilic. **2.** A cell or any histologic element that stains readily. SYN chromatophil (2). **3.** SYN chromaffin. [chromo- + G. *phileō,* to love]

chro·mo·phil ad·e·no·ma (krō′mō-fil ad′ĕ-nō′mă) Any adenoma composed of cells that stain readily.

chro·mo·phil·i·a (krō′mō-fil′ē-ă) The property possessed by most cells of staining readily with appropriate dyes. SYN chromatophilia. [chromo- + G. *phileō,* to love]

chro·mo·phil·ic, **chro·moph·i·lous** (krō′mō-fil′ik, -mof′i-lŭs) Staining readily; denoting certain cells and histologic structures. SYN chromatophil (1), chromatophilic, chromatophilous, chromophil (1), chromophile.

chro·mo·phobe (krō′mō-fōb) Resistant to stains, staining with difficulty or not at all; denoting certain degranulated cells in the anterior lobe of the pituitary gland. SYN chromophobic. [chromo- + G. *phobos,* fear]

chro·mo·phobe ad·e·no·ma, **chro·mo·pho·bic ad·e·no·ma** (krō′mō-fōb ad′ĕ-nō′mă, krō′mō-fō′bik ad′ĕ-nō′mă) A tumor of the adenohypophysis with cells that do not stain with either acid or basic dyes.

chro·mo·phobe cell (krō′mō-fōb sel) A cell in the adenohypophysis without stainable cytoplasmic granules.

chro·mo·pho·bi·a (krō′mō-fō′bē-ă) **1.** Resistance to stains on the part of cells and tissues. **2.** A morbid dislike of color. SYN chromatophobia. [chromo- + G. *phobos,* fear]

chro·mo·pho·bic (krō′mō-fō′bik) SYN chromophobe. [chromo- + *phobos,* fear]

chro·mo·phore (krō′mō-fōr) The atomic grouping on which the color of a substance depends. SYN chromatophore (3). [chromo- + G. *phoros,* bearing]

chro·mo·phor·ic, **chro·moph·o·rous** (krō′mō-fōr′ik, -mof′ŏr-ŭs) **1.** Relating to a chromophore. **2.** Producing or carrying color; denoting certain microorganisms.

chro·mo·som·al (krō′mō-sō′măl) Pertaining to chromosomes.

chro·mo·som·al de·le·tion (krō′mō-sō′măl dĕ-lē′shŭn) A microscopically evident loss of part of a chromosome. SEE ALSO monosomy.

chro·mo·som·al in·sta·bil·i·ty syn·dromes, **chro·mo·som·al break·age syn·dromes** (krō′mō-sō′măl in′stă-bil′i-tē sin′drōm, krō′mō-sō′măl brāk′ăj sin′drōm) A group of mendelian conditions associated with chromosomal instability and breakage in vitro, they often manifest an increased tendency to certain types of malignancies. SEE fragile X chromosome, xeroderma pigmentosum.

chro·mo·som·al map (krō′mō-sō′măl map) A formal, stylized representation of the karyotype and of the positioning and ordering on it of those loci that have been localized by any of several mapping methods.

chro·mo·som·al re·gion (krō′mō-sō′măl rē′jŭn) That part of a chromosome defined either by anatomic details, notably banding, or by its linkages (linkage group).

chro·mo·som·al syn·drome (krō′mō-sō′măl sin′drōm) General designation for syndromes due to chromosomal aberrations; typically associated with mental retardation and multiple congenital anomalies.

chro·mo·som·al trait (krō′mō-sō′măl trāt) A trait dependent on a recurrent chromosomal aberration.

chro•mo•some (krō′mŏ-sōm) A body in the cell nucleus (of which there are normally 46 in humans) that is a bearer of genes, has the form of a delicate chromatin filament during interphase, contracts to form a compact cylinder segmented into two arms by the centromere during metaphase and anaphase stages of cell divison, and is capable of reproducing its physical and chemical structure through successive cell divisons. [chromo- + G. *sōma,* body]

chro•mo•some ab•er•ra•tion (krō′mŏ-sōm ab-ĕr-ā′shŭn) Any deviation from the normal number or morphology of chromosomes; also the phenotypic consequences thereof.

chro•mo•some band (krō′mŏ-sōm band) A region of darker or contrasting staining across the width of a chromosome; the pattern of bands is characteristic for most chromosomes. SEE banding.

chro•mo•some map•ping (krō′mŏ-sōm map′ing) The process of determining the position of loci on specific chromosomes and constructing a diagram of each chromosome showing the relative positions of loci; techniques include family studies with linkage analysis, somatic cell hybridization, and chromosome deletion mapping.

chro•mo•some sat•el•lite (krō′mŏ-sōm sat′ĕ-līt) A small chromosomal segment separated from the main body of the chromosome by a secondary constriction; in humans it is usually associated with the short arm of an acrocentric chromosome.

chro•mo•some walk•ing (krō′mŏ-sōm wawk′ing) A process of extending a genetic map by successive hybridization steps.

chro•mo•ther•a•py (krō′mō-thār′ă-pē) Treatment of disease by colored light.

chro•nax•ie (krō′nak-sē) A measurement of excitability of nervous or muscular tissue; the shortest duration of an effective electrical stimulus having a strength equal to twice the minimum strength required for excitation. [G. *chronos,* time, + *axia,* value]

chron•ic (kron′ik) **1.** Term used to describe persistent disease or illness. **2.** Referring to exposure, prolonged or long-term, sometimes meaning also low intensity. **3.** The U.S. National Center for Health Statistics defines a chronic condition as one of 3 months' duration or longer. [G. *chronos,* time]

chron•ic a•dre•no•cor•ti•cal in•suf•fi•cien•cy (kron′ik ă-drē′nō-kōr′ti-kăl in′sŭ-fish′ĕn-sē) Adrenocortical insufficiency usually as the result of idiopathic atrophy or destruction of both suprarenal glands by tuberculosis, an autoimmune process, or other diseases. SYN Addison disease.

chron•ic a•tro•phic thy•roid•i•tis (kron′ik ā-trō′fik thī-roy-dī′tis) Replacement of the thyroid gland by fibrous tissue, the commonest cause of myxedema in older people.

chron•ic bron•chi•tis (kron′ik brong-kī′tis) A condition of the bronchial tree characterized by cough, hypersecretion of mucus, and expectoration of sputum over a long period, associated with frequent bronchial infections; usually due to smoking.

chron•ic care (kron′ik kār) Therapy provided for long-term health problems.

chron•ic des•qua•ma•tive gin•gi•vi•tis (kron′ik des-kwahm′ă-tiv jin′ji-vī′tis) A gingival condition of unknown etiology in middle-aged and older women, characterized by erythema, mucosal atrophy, and desquamation, and usually accompanied by a burning sensation and pain; diagnosis is usually made by biopsy and direct immunofluorescence. SYN gingivosis.

chron•ic dis•ease (kron′ik di-zēz′) Disease of long duration.

chron•ic er•y•thre•mic my•e•lo•sis (kron′ik er′i-thrē′mik mī-ĕ-lō′sis) SYN myelodysplastic syndrome.

chron•ic fa•tigue and im•mune dys•func•tion syn•drome (CFIDS) (kron′ik fă-tēg′ i-myūn′ dis-fŭngk′shŭn sin′drōm) SYN chronic fatigue syndrome.

chron•ic fa•tigue syn•drome (kron′ik fă-tēg′ sin′drōm) Clinically evaluated new onset debilitating fatigue not substantially relieved by rest and concurrent four of eight symptoms persisting or occurring during 6 or more consecutive months and not predating the fatigue: substantial short-term memory impairment or concentration; sore throat; tender lymph nodes; muscle and multijoint pain; unusual headache; unrefreshing sleep; postexertional malaise lasting more than 24 hours; of unknown etiology. SYN chronic fatigue and immune dysfunction syndrome, myalgic encephalomyelitis.

chron•ic fi•bros•ing pan•cre•a•ti•tis (kron′ik fī-brōs′ing pan′krē-ă-tī′tis) Inflammation of the pancreas consisting of fibrosis, acinar atrophy, and calcification. Clinically, it follows a protracted course with relapses and remissions, and is usually due to alcohol abuse or malnutrition.

chron•ic gran•u•lo•cyt•ic leu•ke•mi•a (kron′ik gran′yū-lō-sit′ik lū-kē′mē-ă) SYN chronic myelocytic leukemia.

chron•ic gran•u•lom•a•tous dis•ease (kron′ik gran′yū-lom′ă-tŭs di-zēz′) A congenital defect in the killing of phagocytosed bacteria by polymorphonuclear leukocytes; results in increased susceptibility to severe infection.

chron•ic in•fec•tion (kron′ik in-fek′shŭn) Any prolonged or persistent invasion of the body by pathogens.

chron•ic in•flam•ma•tion (kron′ik in′flă-mā′shŭn) An inflammation that may begin with a relatively rapid onset or in a slow, insidious, and even unnoticed manner, tends to persist for several weeks, months, or years and has a vague and indefinite termination; characterized histopathologically by infiltrates of small, round cells (lymphocytes), fibrosis, and granuloma formation.

chron•ic in•ter•sti•tial sal•pin•gi•tis (kron′ik in′tĕr-stish′ăl sal′pin-jī′tis) Salpingitis in which fibrosis or mononuclear cell infiltration involves all layers of the uterine or eustachian tube. SYN pachysalpingitis.

chro•nic•i•ty (kron-is′i-tē) The quality of being chronic, referring to diseases.

chron•ic ma•lar•i•a (kron′ik mă-lar′ē-ă) Form of the disease that develops after frequently repeated attacks of one of the acute forms, usually falciparum malaria; it is characterized by profound anemia, enlargement of the spleen, emaciation, mental depression, sallow complexion, edema of the ankles, feeble digestion, and muscular weakness.

chron•ic moun•tain sick•ness (kron′ik mown′tăn sik′nĕs) Loss of high altitude tolerance after prolonged exposure (e.g., by residence), characterized by extreme polycythemia, exaggerated hypoxemia, and reduced mental and physical capacity; relieved by descent. SYN Monge disease.

chron•ic mye•lo•cy•tic leu•ke•mi•a (kron′ik mī′ĕ-lō-sit′ik lū-kē′mē-ă) A heterogeneous group of myeloproliferative disorders that may evolve into acute leukemia in late stages (i.e., blast crisis). Slow onset, usually in older adults. SYN chronic granulocytic leukemia, chronic myelogenous leukemia, chronic myeloid leukemia.

chron•ic my•e•log•e•nous leu•ke•mi•a (kron′ik mī′ĕ-loj′ĕ-nŭs lū-kē′mē-ă) SYN chronic myelocytic leukemia.

chron•ic my•e•loid leu•ke•mi•a (kron′ik mī′ĕ-loyd lū-kē′mē-ă) SYN chronic myelocytic leukemia.

chron•ic ob•struc•tive pul•mo•nar•y dis•ease (COPD) (kron′ik ŏb-strŭk′tiv pul′mŏ-nar-ē di-zēz′) General term used for those diseases with permanent or temporary narrowing of small bronchi, in which forced expiratory flow is slowed, especially when no etiologic or other more specific term can be applied.

chron•ic pos•te•ri•or lar•yn•gi•tis (kron′ik pos-tēr′ē-ŏr lar-in-jī′tis) A form of laryngitis involving principally the interarytenoid area; thought to be caused by regurgitation of gastric contents.

chron•ic pro•gress•ive ex•ter•nal oph•thal•mo•ple•gi•a (kron′ik prŏ-gres′iv eks-tĕr′năl of-thal-mō-plē′jē-ă) A specific type of slowly worsening weakness of the ocular muscles, usually associated with a pigmentary retinopathy. SEE Kearns-Sayre syndrome, oculopharyngeal dystrophy.

chron•ic re•laps•ing pan•cre•a•ti•tis (kron′ik rē-lap′sing pan′krē-ă-tī′tis) Repeated exacerbations of pancreatitis in patients with chronic inflammation of that organ.

chron•ic shock (kron′ik shok) The state of peripheral circulatory insufficiency developing in old people with a debilitating disease, e.g., carcinoma; a subnormal blood volume makes the patient susceptible to hemorrhagic shock as a result of even a moderate blood loss such as may occur during an operation.

chron•ic try•pan•o•so•mi•a•sis (kron′ik trī-pan′ō-sō-mī′ă-sis) SYN Gambian trypanosomiasis.

chron•ic ul•cer (kron′ik ŭl′sĕr) A long-standing ulcer with fibrous scar tissue in the floor of the ulcer.

♻**chrono-** Combining form referring to time. [G. *chronos*]

chro•no•bi•ol•o•gy (kron′ō-bī-ol′ŏ-jē) That aspect of biology concerned with the timing of biologic events, especially repetitive or cyclic phenomena. [chrono- + G. *bios*, life, + *logos*, study]

chro•no•log•ic age (CA) (kron′ŏ-loj′ik āj) Age expressed in years and months; used as a measurement against which to evaluate a child's mental age in computing the Stanford-Binet intelligence quotient.

chron•o•on•col•o•gy (kron′ō-on-kol′ŏ-jē) The study of the influence of biologic rhythms on neoplastic growth. [G. *chronos*, time, + oncology]

chro•no•tro•pic (kron′ō-trō′pik) Affecting the rate of rhythmic movements such as the heartbeat.

chro•not•ro•pism (krō-not′rō-pizm) Modification of the rate of a periodic movement, e.g., the heartbeat, through some external influence. [chrono- + G. *tropē*, turn, change]

♻**chrys-, chryso-** Combining forms denoting gold; corresponds to L. *auro-*. [G. *chrysos*]

Chrys•a•or•a (kris-ā-ōr′ă) A genus of the invertebrate phylum Cnidaria that includes the sea nettle.

Chrys•a•or•a quin•que•cir•rha (kris-ā-ōr′ă kwin-kwĕ-sir′ă) The sea nettle, a jellyfish that can inflict moderate to severe stings. SEE ALSO jellyfish. SYN sea nettle.

Chrys•e•o•bac•te•ri•um me•nin•go•sep•ti•cum (kris′ē-ō-bak-tē′rē-yŭm mĕ-nin′gō-sep-tē′kŭm) Among the normal flora of the human respiratory tract, this bacterial species occasionally causes nosocomial infection, including neonatal meningitis. Formerly called *Flavobacterium meningosepticum*.

chry•si•a•sis (kris-ī′ă-sis) A permanent slate-gray discoloration of the skin and sclera resulting from deposition of gold in the connective tissue of the skin and eye together with increased melanin formation after administration of gold. SYN chrysoderma. [G. *chrysos,* gold]

chrys•o•der•ma (kris-ō-dĕr′mă) SYN chrysiasis. [G. *chrysos,* gold, + *derma,* skin]

Chrys•ops (kris′ops) The deerfly (or mangefly), a genus of biting flies with about 80 North American species; *C. discalis* is a vector of *Francisella tularensis* in the U.S.; *C. dimidiatus* and *C. silaceus* are the principal vectors of *Loa loa* in West Africa. [G. *chrysos,* gold, + *ōps,* eye]

chrys•o•ther•a•py (kris′ō-thār′ă-pē) Treatment of disease by the administration of gold salts. [G. *chrysos,* gold]

CHT Abbreviation for certified hand therapist.

chuck (chŭk) A clamp or fastener that secures a moving part of a tool, or the object being worked on.

Churg-Strauss dis•ease (chŭrg-strows di-zēz′) Allergic vasculitis marked by involvement of small and medium-sized arteries (e.g., in lungs), fever, weight loss, myalgia, headache, and respiratory distress. Usually determined by cutaneous biopsy revealing eosinophilic vasculitis.

Chvos•tek sign (kvos′tek sīn) Facial irritability in tetany, unilateral spasm of the orbicularis oculi or orbicularis oris muscle being excited by a slight tap over the facial nerve just anterior to the external auditory meatus. SYN Weiss sign.

♻ **chyl-** SEE chylo-, chyle. [G. *chylos,* juice, chyle]

♻ **-chyl** SEE chyl-.

chylaemia [Br.] SYN chylemia.

chy•lan•gi•o•ma (kī-lan′jē-ō′mă) A mass of prominent, dilated lacteals and larger intestinal lymphatic vessels. [chyl- + G. *angeion,* vessel, + *-ōma,* tumor]

chyle (kīl) A turbid white or pale yellow fluid taken up by the lacteals from the intestine during digestion and carried by the lymphatic system through the thoracic duct into the circulation. [G. *chylos,* juice]

chyle fis•tu•la (kīl fis′chū-lă) A leak of chyle from a lymph vessel to the skin surface; a complication of radical neck dissection when the thoracic duct is injured.

chy•le•mi•a (kī-lē′mē-ă) The presence of chyle in the circulating blood. SYN chylaemia. [chyl- + G. *haima,* blood]

chyle ves•sel (kīl ves′ĕl) SYN lacteal (2).

♻ **chyli-** SEE chyl-.

chy•li•fac•tion (kī′li-fak′shŭn) SYN chylopoiesis. [chyl- + L. *facio,* to make]

chy•li•fac•tive (kī′li-fak′tiv) SYN chylopoietic.

chy•lif•er•ous (kī-lif′er-ŭs) Conveying chyle. SYN chylophoric. [chyl- + L. *fero,* to carry]

chy•li•fi•ca•tion (kī′li-fi-kā′shŭn) SYN chylopoiesis.

chy•li•form (kī′li-fōrm) Resembling chyle.

♻ **chylo-** Prefix meaning chyle. [G. *chylos,* juice]

chy•lo•cele (kī′lō-sēl) A cystlike lesion resulting from the effusion of chyle into the tunica vaginalis propria and cavity of the tunica vaginalis testis. [chylo- + G. *kēlē,* tumor]

chy•lo•der•ma (kī′lō-dĕr′mă) SYN elephantiasis scroti. [chylo- + G. *derma,* skin]

chy•lo•me•di•as•ti•num (kī′lō-mē-dē-as-tī′nŭm) Abnormal presence of chyle in the mediastinum.

chy•lo•mi•cron, pl. **chy•lo•mi•cra**, **chy•lo•mi•crons** (kī′lō-mī′kron, -kră, -kronz) A droplet of reprocessed lipid synthesized in epithelial cells of the small intestine; the least dense of the plasma lipoproteins. [chylo- + G. *micros,* small]

chylomicronaemia [Br.] SYN chylomicronemia.

chy•lo•mi•cro•ne•mi•a (kī′lō-mī-krō-nē′mē-ă) The presence of chylomicrons, especially an increased number, in the circulating blood, as in type I familial hyperlipoproteinemia. SYN chylomicronaemia.

chy•lo•per•i•car•di•um (kī′lō-per′i-kahr′dē-ŭm) A milky pericardial effusion resulting from obstruction of the thoracic duct, from trauma, or of idiopathic origin.

chy•lo•per•i•to•ne•um (kī′lō-per′i-tō-nē′ŭm) SYN chylous ascites.

chy•lo•phor•ic (kī′lō-fōr′ik) SYN chyliferous. [chylo- + G. *phoros,* bearing]

chy•lo•pneu•mo•tho•rax (kī′lō-nū-mō-thōr′aks) Free chyle and air in the pleural space.

chy•lo•poi•e•sis (kī′lō-poy-ē′sis) Formation of chyle in the intestine. SYN chylifaction, chylification. [chylo- + G. *poiesis,* a making]

chy•lo•poi•et•ic (kī′lō-poy-et′ik) Relating to chylopoiesis. SYN chylifactive.

chy•lo•sis (kī-lō′sis) The formation of chyle from the food in the intestine, its digestion and absorption by the intestinal mucosa, and its mixture with the blood and conveyance to the tissues.

chy•lo•tho•rax (kī′lō-thōr′aks) An accumulation of milky chylous fluid in the pleural space, usually on the left.

chy•lous (kī′lŭs) Relating to chyle.

chy•lous as•ci•tes, as•ci•tes chy•lo•sus (kī′lŭs ă-sī′tēz, ă-sī′tēz kī-lō′sŭs) Presence in the peritoneal cavity of a milky fluid containing suspended fat, ordinarily caused by an obstruction or injury of the thoracic duct or cisterna. SYN chyloperitoneum.

chy•lu•ri•a (kī-lyūr′ē-ă) The passage of chyle in the urine; a form of albiduria. [chyl- + G. *ouron,* urine]

chyme (kīm) The semifluid mass of partly digested food passed from the stomach into the duodenum. SYN pulp (3). [G. *chymos,* juice]

chy•mi•fi•ca•tion (kī′mi-fi-kā′shŭn) SYN chymopoiesis. [G. *chymos,* juice, + L. *facio,* to make]

chy•mo•poi•e•sis (kī′mō-poy-ē′sis) The production of chyme; the physical state of food (semifluid) brought about by digestion in the stomach. SYN chymification. [G. *chymos,* juice, chyme, + *poiesis,* a making]

chy•mo•sin (kī′mō-sin) A proteinase structurally homologous with pepsin; the milk-curdling enzyme obtained from the stomach of the calf. SYN rennin.

chy•mo•tryp•sin (kī′mō-trip′sin) A serine proteinase of the gastrointestinal tract, synthesized in the pancreas as chymotrypsinogen; used in the treatment of inflammation and edema associated with trauma and to facilitate intracapsular cataract extraction.

chy•mo•tryp•sin•o•gen (kī′mō-trip-sin′ō-jen) The precursor of chymotrypsin. Converted to π-chymotrypsin by the action of trypsin.

CI Abbreviation for Colour Index.

Ci Abbreviation for curie.

Ci•ac•ci•o stain (chē-ah′chē-ō stān) A method for demonstrating complex insoluble intracellular lipids using fixation in a formalin-dichromate solution, embedding in paraffin, staining with Sudan III or IV, and examination in aqueous mountant.

Ci•an•ca syn•drome (chē-ahn′kă sin′drōm) A severe form of infantile esotropia characterized by cross-fixation, tight medial rectus muscles, and nystagmus with abduction of the fixating eye.

CIC Abbreviation for completely in the canal (hearing aid).

cic•a•trec•to•my (sik′ă-trek′tō-mē) Excision of a scar. [L. *cicatrix,* scar, + G. *ektomē,* excision]

cic•a•tri•ces (sik′ă-trī′sēz) Plural of cicatrix.

cic•a•tri•cial (sik′ă-trish′ăl) Relating to a scar.

cic•a•tri•cial al•o•pe•ci•a (sik′ă-trish′ăl al-ō-pē′shē-ă) SYN scarring alopecia. [L. *cicatrix, cicatricis,* scar + suffix *-al,* characterized by]

cic•a•tri•cial pem•phi•goid (sik′ă-trish′ăl pem′fi-goyd) A chronic disease that produces adhesions and progressive cicatrization and shrinkage of the conjunctival, oral, and vaginal mucous membranes.

cic•a•trix, pl. **cic•a•tri•ces** (sik′ă-triks, si-kā′triks; -sēz) A scar. [L.]

cic•a•tri•za•tion (sik′ă-trī-zā′shŭn) **1.** The process of scar formation. **2.** The healing of a wound otherwise than by first intention.

ci•clo•pir•ox•ol•a•mine (sī′klō-pir′oks-ōl′ă-mēn) A broad-spectrum antifungal agent used to treat a variety of fungus and yeast skin infections.

♻**-cidal** SEE -cide.

♻**-cide, -cido** Combining forms denoting an agent that kills (e.g., insecticide), or the act of killing (e.g., suicide). [L. *-cida, -cidium,* fr. *caedo,* to kill]

cig•a•rette drain (sig′ă-ret′ drān) A wick of gauze wrapped in rubber tissue, providing capillary drainage.

cil•i•a (sil′ē-ă) Plural of cilium.

cil•i•ar•y (sil′ē-ar-ē) **1.** Relating to any cilia or hairlike processes, specifically, the eyelashes. **2.** Relating to certain of the structures of the eyeball. [Mod. L. *ciliaris,* relating to or resembling an eyelid, or eyelash, fr. L. *cilium,* eyelid]

cil•i•ar•y bod•y (sil′ē-ar-ē bod′ē) A thickened portion of the vascular tunic of the eye between the choroid and the iris; it consists of three parts or zones: orbiculus ciliaris, corona ciliaris, and ciliary muscle. SYN corpus ciliare [TA].

cil•i•ar•y disc (sil′ē-ar-ē disk) SYN orbiculus ciliaris.

cil•i•ar•y dys•ci•ne•sis (sil′ē-ar-ē dis′ki-nē′sis) Absent or impaired motion of the cilia, occurring as a primary or secondary disorder; associated with recurrent infections in the respiratory tract. [dys- + G. *kinēsis,* movement]

cil•i•ar•y gan•gli•on (sil′ē-ar-ē gang′glē-ŏn) A small parasympathetic ganglion lying in the orbit between the optic nerve and the lateral rectus muscle; it receives preganglionic innervation from the Edinger-Westphal nucleus by way of the oculomotor nerve, and in turn gives rise to postganglionic fibers that innervate the ciliary muscle and the sphincter of the iris (sphincter pupillae muscle).

cil•i•ar•y glands (sil′ē-ar-ē glandz) A number of modified apocrine sudoriferous glands in the eyelids, with ducts that usually open into the follicles of the eyelashes. SYN Moll glands.

cil·i·ar·y move·ment (sil′ē-ar-ē mūv′mĕnt) The rhythmic, sweeping movement of epithelial cell cilia, of ciliate protozoans, or the sculling movement of flagella, possibly resulting from the alternate contraction and relaxation of contractile threads (myoids) on one side of the cilium or flagellum.

cil·i·ar·y mus·cle (sil′ē-ar-ē mŭs′ĕl) The smooth muscle of the ciliary body; it consists of circular fibers (Müller muscle) and radiating fibers (meridional fibers, or Brücke muscle); *action*, in contracting, its diameter is reduced (like a sphincter), reducing tensile (stretching) forces on lens, allowing it to thicken for near vision (accommodation). SYN musculus ciliaris [TA].

cil·i·ar·y pro·cess (sil′ē-ar-ē pros′es) One of the radiating pigmented ridges, usually 70 in number, on the inner surface of the ciliary body, increasing in thickness as they advance from the orbiculus ciliaris to the external border of the iris; these, together with the folds (plicae) in the furrows between them, constitute the corona ciliaris.

cil·i·ar·y ring (sil′ē-ar-ē ring) SYN orbiculus ciliaris.

cil·i·ar·y veins (sil′ē-ar-ē vānz) Several small veins, anterior and posterior, coming from the ciliary body and emptying into the superior and inferior ophthalmic veins.

cil·i·ar·y zone (sil′ē-ar-ē zōn) The outer, wider zone of the anterior surface of the iris, separated from the pupillary zone by the collarette.

cil·i·ar·y zon·ule (sil′ē-ar-ē zōn′yūl) A series of delicate meridional fibers arising from the inner surface of the orbiculus ciliaris that run in bundles between, and in a very thin layer over, the ciliary processes; at the inner border of the corona, the fibers diverge into two groups that are attached to the capsule on the anterior and posterior surfaces of the lens close to the equator; the spaces between these two layers of fibers are filled with aqueous humor. SYN zonula ciliaris [TA], suspensory ligament of lens, Zinn zonule.

Ci·li·a·ta (sil-ē-ā′tă) A class within the protozoal phylum Ciliophora. Typical members, such as *Paramecium* or *Balantidium coli* (a parasite of humans), possess two distinctive nuclei, a macronucleus and a micronucleus; only the latter bears the hereditary material exchanged in conjugation, a form of sexual reproduction found only in the Ciliata. [L. *cilium,* eyelid]

cil·i·at·ed (sil′ē-ā-tĕd) Having cilia.

cil·i·at·ed ep·i·the·li·um (sil′ē-ā-tĕd ep′i-thē′lē-ŭm) Any epithelium having motile cilia on the free surface (e.g., bronchial epithelium).

cil·i·ates (sil′ē-āts) Common name for members of the Ciliata.

cil·i·ec·to·my (sil′ē-ek′tŏ-mē) SYN cyclectomy.

♻**cilio-**, **cili-** Combining forms meaning cilia or ciliary, in any sense; eyelashes. [L. *cilium,* eyelid (eyelash)]

cil·i·o·cy·toph·thor·i·a (sil′ē-ō-sī-tof-thōr′ē-ă) A detached ciliary tuft (a remnant of ciliated epithelium) that can be seen in a variety of body fluids, especially peritoneal, amnionic, and respiratory specimens; they are motile and can be confused with ciliated or flagellated protozoa. [fr. cilio- + cyto- + G. *phthora* corruption, decay, + *-ium,* noun suffix]

cil·i·o·ret·i·nal (sil′ē-ō-ret′i-năl) Pertaining to the ciliary body and the retina.

cil·i·o·scle·ral (sil′ē-ō-skler′ăl) Relating to the ciliary body and the sclera.

cil·i·o·spi·nal (sil′ē-ō-spī′năl) Relating to the ciliary body and the spinal cord; denoting in particular the ciliospinal center.

cil·i·o·spi·nal cen·ter (sil′ē-ō-spī′năl sen′tĕr) The preganglionic motor neurons in the first thoracic segment of the spinal cord that give rise to the sympathetic innervation of the dilator muscle of the pupil.

cil·i·o·spi·nal re·flex (sil′ē-ō-spī′năl rē′fleks) SYN pupillary-skin reflex.

cil·i·um, pl. **cil·i·a** (sil′ē-ŭm, -ă) **1.** SYN eyelash. **2.** A motile extension of a cell surface, e.g., of certain epithelial cells, containing nine longitudinal double microtubules arranged in a peripheral ring, together with a central pair. [L. an eyelid]

Ci·mex (sī′meks) A genus of bedbugs of the family Cimicidae in the order Hemiptera, with flat, reddish-brown, wingless bodies, prominent lateral eyes, a three-jointed beak, and a characteristic odor from thoracic stink glands; an abundant pest in human abodes. Although its bite produces characteristic linear groups of pruritic wheals with a central hemorrhagic punctum, the bedbug is not a proven vector of human disease, with the possible exception of hepatitis B. SYN bedbug. [L. *cimex,* bug]

CIN Abbreviation for cervical intraepithelial neoplasia.

CINAHL Abbreviation for Cumulative Index to Nursing and Allied Health Literature.

Cin·cin·nat·i Pre·hos·pi·tal Stroke Scale (sin′si-nat′ē prē-hos′pi-tăl strōk skāl) SYN Cincinnati stroke scale.

Cin·cin·nat·i stroke scale (sin′si-nat′ē strōk skāl) Measurement for diagnosis of possible stroke; assesses three areas for abnormal findings: facial droop, arm drift, and speech. SYN Cincinnati Prehospital Stroke Scale.

♻**cine-**, **cin-** Combining forms denoting movement, usually relating to motion pictures. [G. *kineō,* to move]

cin·e·an·gi·o·car·di·og·ra·phy (sin′ē-an′jē-ō-kahr-dē-og′ră-fē) Motion pictures of the passage of a contrast medium through chambers of the heart and great vessels.

cin•e•fluo•rog•ra•phy (sin′ĕ-flōr-og′ră-fē) SYN cineradiography.

cin•e•plas•tic am•pu•ta•tion, **cin•e•plas•tics** (sin′ĕ-plas′tik amp′yū-tā′shŭn, sin′ĕ-plas′tiks) A method of amputation of an extremity whereby the muscles and tendons are so arranged in the stump that they are able to execute independent movements and to communicate motion to a specially constructed prosthetic apparatus. SYN kineplastics.

cin•e•ra•di•og•ra•phy (sin′ĕ-rā-dē-og′ră-fē) Radiography of an organ in motion, e.g., the heart, the gastrointestinal tract. SYN cinefluorography.

ci•ne•re•a (si-nēr′ē-ă) The gray matter of the brain and other parts of the nervous system. [L. fem. of *cinereus,* ashy, fr. *cinis,* ashes]

ci•ne•re•al (si-nēr′ē-ăl) Relating to the gray matter of the nervous system.

cin•gu•late (sing′yū-lāt) Relating to a cingulum.

cin•gu•late gy•rus (sing′yū-lāt jī′rŭs) A long, curved convolution of the medial surface of the cortical hemisphere, arched over the corpus callosum from which it is separated by the deep sulcus of corpus callosum; together with the parahippocampal gyrus, with which it is continuous behind the corpus callosum, it forms the fornicate gyrus.

cin•gu•late sul•cus (sing′yū-lāt sŭl′kŭs) A fissure on the mesial surface of the cerebral hemisphere, bounding the upper surface of the cingulate gyrus (callosal convolution); the anterior portion is called the pars subfrontalis; the posterior portion which curves up to the superomedial margin of the hemisphere and borders the paracentral lobule posteriorly, the pars marginalis.

cin•gu•lot•o•my, **cin•gu•lec•to•my** (sing′gyū-lot′ŏ-mē, sin-gyū-lek′tŏ-mē) Electrolytic destruction of the anterior cingulate gyrus and callosum. [cingulum + G. *tomē,* a cutting]

cin•gu•lum, gen. **cin•gu•li**, pl. **cin•gu•la** (sing′yū-lŭm, -lē, -lă) [TA] **1.** SYN girdle. **2.** A well-marked fiber bundle passing longitudinally in the white matter of the cingulate gyrus; the bundle extends from the region of the anterior perforated substance back over the dorsal surface of the corpus callosum; behind the splenium of the latter it curves down and then forward in the white matter of the parahippocampal gyrus; composed largely of fibers from the anterior thalamic nucleus to the cingulate and parahippocampal gyri, it also contains association fibers connecting these gyri with the frontal cortex, and their various subdivisions with each other. **3.** The lingual portion of an incisor or canine tooth, which forms a convexity on the cervical third of the crown. **4.** The cervical third of the crown of a molar, which is the source of the developing cusps. [L. girdle, fr. *cingo,* to surround]

cir•ca•di•an (sĭr-kā′dē-ăn) Relating to biologic variations or rhythms with a cycle of about 24 hours. Cf. infradian, ultradian. [L. *circa,* about, + *dies,* day]

cir•ci•nate (sĭr′si-nāt) Circular; ring-shaped, anular. [L. *circinatus,* made round, pp. of *circino,* to make round, fr. *circinus,* a pair of compasses]

cir•cle (sĭr′kĕl) **1.** A ring-shaped structure or group of structures. SYN circulus (1) [TA]. **2.** A line or process with every point equidistant from the center. [L. *circulus*]

cir•cle ab•sorp•tion an•es•the•si•a (sĭr′kĕl ab-sōrp′shŭn an′es-thē′zē-ă) Inhalation anesthesia in which a circuit with carbon dioxide absorbent is used for complete (closed) or partial (semiclosed) rebreathing of exhaled gases.

cir•cle of Wil•lis (sĭr′kĕl wil′is) A ring of arteries at the base of the brain formed by anastomoses of the internal carotid arteries and the basilar artery.

cir•cling the drain (CTD) (sĕr′kling drān) Jargonistic and grossly inhumane term for a patient who is in the final days or weeks before death.

cir•cuit (sĭr′kŭt) The path or course of flow of electric or other currents. [L. *circuitus,* a going round, fr. *circum,* around, + *eo,* pp. *itus,* to go]

cir•cuit re•sis•tance train•ing (CRT) (sĭr′kŭt rĕ-zis′tăns trān′ing) Modification of standard strength training emphasizing relatively light load (40–60% of maximum strength) and continuous exercise to provide a more general conditioning to improve body composition, muscular strength and endurance, and cardiovascular fitness. SYN circuit training, circuit weight training.

cir•cuit train•ing, **cir•cuit weight train•ing** (sĭr′kŭt trān′ing, sĭr′kŭt wāt trān′ing) SYN circuit resistance training.

cir•cu•lar am•pu•ta•tion (sĭr′kyū-lăr amp′yū-tā′shŭn) Surgical removal performed by a circular incision through the skin, the muscles being similarly divided higher up, and the bone higher still.

cir•cu•lar di•chro•ism (CD) (sĭr′kyū-lăr dī′krō-izm) The change from circular polarization to elliptic polarization of monochromatic, circularly polarized light in the immediate vicinity of the absorption band of the substance through which the light passes.

cir•cu•lar folds of small in•tes•tine (sĭr′kyū-lăr fōldz smawl in-tes′tin) The numerous folds of the mucous membrane of the small intestine, running transversely for about two thirds of the circumference of the gut. SYN plicae circulares intestini tenuis [TA], Kerckring folds, Kerckring valves.

cir·cu·lar si·nus (sĭr′kyū-lăr sī′nŭs) **1.** Dural venous formation that surrounds the hypophysis, composed of right and left cavernous sinuses and the intercavernous sinuses; **2.** A venous sinus at the periphery of the placenta; **3.** SYN sinus venosus sclerae.

cir·cu·la·tion (sĭr′kyū-lā′shŭn) Movements in a circle, or through a circular course, or through a course that leads back to the same point; usually referring to blood circulation through the network of arteries and veins unless otherwise specified. [L. *circulatio*]

cir·cu·la·to·ry (sĭr′kū-lă-tōr-ē) **1.** Relating to the circulation. **2.** SYN sanguiferous.

cir·cu·la·to·ry o·ver·load (sĭr′kyū-lă-tōr-ē ō′vĕr-lōd) SYN hypervolemia.

cir·cu·lus, gen. and pl. **cir·cu·li** (sĭr′kū-lŭs, -lī) [TA] **1.** SYN circle (1). **2.** A circle formed by connecting arteries, veins, or nerves. [L. dim. of *circus,* circle]

♻**circum-** Combining form indicating a circular movement, or a position surrounding the part indicated by the word to which it is joined. SEE ALSO peri-. [L. around]

cir·cum·a·nal glands (sĭr′kŭm-ā′năl glandz) Large apocrine sweat glands surrounding the anus.

cir·cum·ar·tic·u·lar (sĭr′kŭm-ahr-tik′yū-lăr) Surrounding a joint. [circum- + L. *articulus,* joint]

cir·cum·ax·il·lary (sĭr′kŭm-ak′si-lar-ē) Around the axilla.

cir·cum·cise (sĭr′kŭm-sīz) To perform circumcision, especially of the prepuce.

cir·cum·ci·sion (sĭr′kŭm-sizh′ŭn) **1.** Operation to remove part or all of the prepuce. SYN peritomy (2). **2.** Cutting around an anatomic part (e.g., the areola of the breast). SYN peritectomy (2). [L. *circumcido,* to cut around, fr. *circum,* around, + *caedo,* to cut]

cir·cum·duc·ti·o (sĭr′kŭm-dŭk′shē-ō) [TA] SYN circumduction.

cir·cum·duc·tion (sĭr′kŭm-dŭk′shŭn) **1.** Movement of a part, e.g., an extremity, in a circular direction. **2.** SYN cycloduction. SYN circumductio [TA]. [circum- + L. *duco,* pp. *ductus,* to draw]

cir·cum·fer·ence (c) (sĭr-kŭm′fĕr-ĕns) The outer boundary, especially of a circular area. SYN circumferentia [TA]. [L. *circumferentia,* a bearing around]

cir·cum·fer·en·ti·a (sĭr′kŭm-fĕr-en′shē-ă) [TA] SYN circumference. [L. a bearing around]

cir·cum·fer·en·tial fi·bro·car·ti·lage (sĭr′kŭm-fĕr-en′shăl fī′brō-kahr′ti-lăj) A ring of fibrocartilage around the articular end of a bone, serving to deepen the joint cavity.

cir·cum·fer·en·tial la·mel·la (sĭr′kŭm-fĕr-en′shăl lă-mel′ă) A bony lamella that encircles the outer or inner surface of a bone.

cir·cum·flex (sĭr′kŭm-fleks) Describing an arc of a circle or that which winds around something; denotes several anatomic structures: arteries, veins, nerves, and muscles. [circum- + L. *flexus,* to bend]

cir·cum·flex branch of left co·ro·nar·y ar·ter·y (sĭr′kŭm′fleks branch left kōr′ŏ-nar-ē ahr′tĕr-ē) Terminal branch (with anterior interventricular artery) of left coronary artery that runs leftward and then posteriorly in the coronary groove supplying atrial and ventricular branches. SYN ramus circumflexus arteriae coronariae sinistrae.

cir·cum·flex scap·u·lar ar·ter·y (sĭr′kŭm-fleks skap′yū-lăr ahr′tĕr-ē) *Origin,* subscapular; *distribution,* muscles of shoulder and scapular region; *anastomoses,* branches of suprascapular and transverse cervical.

cir·cum·lo·cu·tion (sĭr′kŭm-lō-kyū′shŭn) Indirect, roundabout, wordy, or evasive speech, noted in Alzheimer disease and other dementias.

cir·cum·or·bit·al (sĭr′kŭm-ōr′bi-tăl) Around the orbit. SYN periorbital (2).

cir·cum·scribed (sĭr′kŭm-skrībd) Bounded by a line; limited or confined. [circum- + L. *scribo,* to write]

cir·cum·scribed myx·e·de·ma (sĭr′kŭm-skrībd mik′sĕ-dē′mă) Nodules and plaques of mucoid edema of the skin, usually in the pretibial region, occurring in some patients with hyperthyroidism. SYN pretibial myxedema.

cir·cum·scribed pos·te·ri·or ker·a·to·co·nus (sĭr′kŭm-skrībd pos-tēr′ē-ŏr ker′ă-tō-kō′nŭs) Congenital corneal defect characterized by a craterlike defect on the posterior corneal surface.

cir·cum·spor·o·zo·ite pro·tein (sĭr′kŭm-spōr-ō-zō′īt prō′tēn) One of two proteins (the other is thrombospondin-related adhesive protein) involved in sporozoite recognition of host cells in malaria.

cir·cum·stan·ti·al ho·mo·sex·u·al·i·ty (sĕr′kŭm-stan′shăl hō′mō-seks′shū-al′i-tē) Sexual contact between members of the same sex due to absence of the opposite sex (e.g., military, prison) rather than desire or predisposition. SYN situational homosexuality, transient homosexuality.

cir·cum·stan·ti·al·i·ty (sĭr′kŭm-stan-shē-al′i-tē) A disturbance in the thought process in which one gives an excessive amount of detail that is often tangential, elaborate, and irrelevant, to avoid making a direct statement or answer to a question; observed in schizophrenia and in obsessional disorders. Cf. tangentiality. [L. *circum-sto,* pr. p. *-stans,* to stand around]

cir·cum·val·late (sĭr′kŭm-val′āt) Denoting a structure surrounded by a wall, as the circumvallate (vallate) papillae of the tongue. [circum- + L. *vallum,* wall]

cir·cum·val·late pa·pil·lae (sĭr′kŭm-val′āt pă-pil′ē) SYN vallate papilla.

cir·cum·ven·tric·u·lar or·gans (sĭr′kŭm-ven-trik′yū-lăr ōr′gănz) Four small areas at the base of the brain that are outside the blood-brain barrier. They are neurohypophysis, area postrema, organum vasculosum of the lamina terminalis, and subfornical organ (SFO).

cir·cum·vo·lute (sĭr′kŭm-vol′yūt) Twisted around; rolled about. [L. *circum-volvo,* pp. *-volutus,* to roll around]

cir·cum·zy·go·mat·ic wir·ing (sĭr′kŭm-zī-gō-mat′ik wīr′ing) A means of fixation for mandibular fractures in which the mandible is fastened to the zygomatic arches with wire.

cir·rho·sis (sir-ō′sis) Liver disease characterized by diffuse damage to hepatic parenchymal cells, with nodular regeneration, fibrosis, and disturbance of normal architecture; associated with failure in the function of hepatic cells and interference with blood flow in the liver, frequently resulting in jaundice, portal hypertension, ascites, and ultimately biochemical and functional signs of hepatic failure. See this page. [G. *kirrhos,* yellow (liver), + *-osis,* condition]

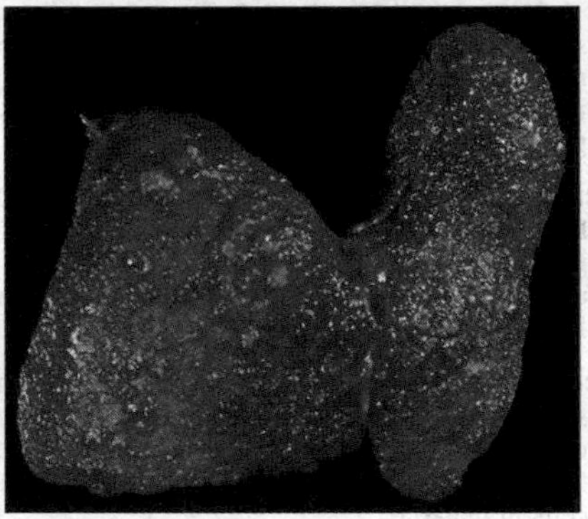

alcoholic cirrhosis: surface of liver displays innumerable small, regular nodules

cir·rhot·ic (sir-rot′ik) Relating to or affected with cirrhosis or advanced fibrosis.

cir·soid an·eu·rysm (sir′soyd an′yūr-izm) Dilation of a group of blood vessels owing to congenital malformation with arteriovenous shunting. SYN racemose aneurysm.

CIS Abbreviation for carcinoma in situ.

cis- **1.** Prefix meaning on this side, on the near side; opposite of trans-. **2.** GENETICS a prefix denoting the location of two or more genes on the same chromosome of a homologous pair, in coupling. **3.** ORGANIC CHEMISTRY a prefix denoting a form of geometric isomerism in which similar functional groups are attached on the same side of the plane that includes two adjacent, fixed carbon atoms in a ring structure. **4.** ORGANIC CHEMISTRY a prefix denoting a form of geometric isomerism with regard to carbon-carbon double bonds. Identical functional groups on the same side of the double bond are cis-. When the four moieties attached to the carbons of the double bond are all different, then the E/Z nomenclature has to be followed. [L.]

cis·tern (sis′tĕrn) **1.** Any cavity or enclosed space serving as a reservoir, especially for chyle, lymph, or cerebrospinal fluid. **2.** An ultramicroscopic space occurring between the membranes of the flattened sacs of the endoplasmic reticulum, the Golgi complex, or the two membranes of the nuclear envelope. SYN cisterna [TA]. [L. *cisterna*]

cis·ter·na, gen. and pl. **cis·ter·nae** (sis-tĕr′nă, -nē) [TA] SYN cistern. [L. an underground cistern for water, fr. *cista,* a box]

cis·ter·nal (sis-tĕr′năl) Relating to a cisterna.

cis·ter·nal punc·ture (sis-tĕr′năl pungk′shŭr) Passage of a hollow needle through the posterior atlantooccipital membrane into the cisterna cerebellomedullaris.

cis·tern·og·ra·phy (sis′tĕrn-og′ră-fē) The radiographic study of the basal cisterns of the brain after the subarachnoid introduction of contrast medium, or a radiopharmaceutical with a suitable detector. [cisterna + G. *graphō,* to write]

cis·tron (sis′tron) **1.** The smallest functional unit of heritability; a length of chromosomal DNA associated with a single biochemical function. In modern molecular biology, the cistron is essentially equivalent to the structural gene. **2.** The genetic unit defined by the *cis/trans* test. [*cis tr*-ans + -on]

cit·rate (sit′rāt) A salt or ester of citric acid; used as an anticoagulant because it binds calcium ions.

cit·ric ac·id (sit′rik as′id) The acid of citrus fruits, widely distributed in nature and a key intermediate in intermediary metabolism.

ci·tro·vo·rum fac·tor (CF) (sī′trō-vōr′ŭm fak′tŏr) SYN folinic acid.

ci·trul·line (sit′rŭ-lēn) An amino acid formed from L-ornithine in the course of the urea cycle as well as a product in nitric oxide biosynthesis; also found in watermelon (*Citrullus vulgaris*) and in casein. Elevated in people with a deficiency of argininosuccinate synthetase or argininosuccinate lyase.

cit·rul·li·nu·ri·a (sit′rŭ-li-nyūr′ē-ă) Enhanced urinary excretion of citrulline; a manifestation of citrullinemia.

Ci·vil·ian Health and Med·i·cal Pro·gram of the U·ni·formed Ser·vic·es (CHAMPUS) (si-vil′yăn helth med′i-kăl prō′gram yū′ni-fōrmd sĕr′vi-sĕz) SEE TRICARE.

Ci·vil·ian Health and Med·i·cal Pro·gram of the Vet·er·ans' Ad·min·is·tra·tion (CHAMPVA) (si-vil′yăn helth med′i-kăl prō′gram vet′rănz ad-min′i-strā′shŭn) SEE TRICARE.

CJD Abbreviation for Creutzfeldt-Jakob disease.

CK Abbreviation for creatine kinase; cyanogen chloride; NATO code for cyanogen chloride.

Cl Abbreviation for chlorine.

cL Abbreviation for centiliter.

Clad·o·ph·i·a·lo·phor·a ban·ti·an·a (klad-ō-fī-ă-lof′ō-ră ban-shē-ā′nă) A species of fungi that causes cerebral phaeohyphomycosis. Formerly known as *Cladosporium bantianum.*

Clad·o·ph·i·a·lo·phor·a ca·ro·ni·i (klad-ō-fī-ă-lof′ō-ră kā-rō′nē-ī) A fungus associated with olive-to-black chromomycosis; primarily found in tropic and subtropic areas. Infections are acquired through trauma, usually to the lower extremities.

Cla·do point (klah-dō′ poynt) A point at the junction of the interspinous and right semilunar lines, at the lateral border of the rectus abdominis muscle, where marked tenderness on pressure is felt in some cases of appendicitis.

Clad·o·spo·ri·um (klad-ō-spō′rē-ŭm) A genus of fungi having dematiaceous or dark-colored conidiophores with long chains of oval or round spores, commonly isolated in soil or plant residues. [G. *klados,* a branch, + *sporos,* seed]

claim (clām) A statement from a patient of health care provider presented to an insurance company or HMO for payment for services performed.

claim scrub·ber (clām skrŭb′ĕr) Software platform that reviews claims for key components before the claims are presented to an insurance company.

clair·voy·ance (klār-voy′ăns) Perception of objective events (past, present, or future) not ordinarily discernible by the senses; a type of extrasensory perception. [Fr.]

clamp (klamp) An instrument for compression of a structure. Cf. forceps. [M.E., fr. Middle Dutch *klampe*]

clamp for·ceps (klamp fōr′seps) A forceps with pronged jaws designed to engage the jaws of a rubber dam clamp so that they may be separated to pass over the widest buccolingual contour of a tooth. SYN rubber dam clamp forceps.

clam-shell brace (clam-shel brās) An orthopedic cast that encloses the trunk between anterior and posterior foam-lined rigid plastic components; permits ambulation of patients with injuries of the vertebral column and neck. SYN body jacket, Risser cast.

clam·shell in·ci·sion, clam·shell thor·a·cot·o·my (klam′shel in-sizh′ŭn, klam′shel thōr-ă-kot′ō-mē) Incision made up of bilateral submammary anterior thoracotomies connected by a transverse sternotomy and providing access similar to that of a standard sternotomy. SEE ALSO transverse thoracosternotomy.

clang as·so·ci·a·tion (klang ă-sō′sē-ā′shŭn) Psychic associations resulting from sounds; often encountered in the manic phase of manic-depressive psychosis.

Clap·ton line (klap′tŏn līn) A greenish discoloration of the marginal gingiva in cases of chronic copper poisoning.

cla·rif·i·cant (klar-if′i-kănt) An agent that makes a turbid liquid clear. [L. *clarus,* clear, + *facio,* to make]

Clarke sign (klahrk sīn) Maneuver used to determine chondromalacia patellae, whereby the patient sits with legs extended on a table and the clinician places the web of a hand proximal to the superior pole of the patella. The person examined is asked to contract the quadriceps while the clinician pushes gently downward on the patella. A positive sign is indicated if pain is experienced during this maneuver or if it is not possible to hold the contraction.

Clark lev·el (klahrk lev′ĕl) The level of invasion of primary malignant melanoma of the skin; limited to the epidermis, I; into the underlying papillary dermis, II; to the junction of the papillary and reticular dermis, III; into the reticular dermis, IV; into the subcutaneous fat, V. The prognosis is worse with each successively deeper level of invasion.

Clark ne·vus (klahrk nē′vŭs) Dysplastic melanotic nevi with notched, irregular borders on lesions; considered premalignant and marker for increased risk of melanoma. Seen in 5% of whites.

clasp (klasp) **1.** A part of a removable partial denture that acts as a direct retainer or stabilizer for the denture by partially surrounding or contacting an abutment tooth. **2.** A direct retainer of a removable partial denture, usually consisting of two arms joined by a body that connects with an occlusal rest; at least one arm of a clasp usually terminates in the infrabulge (gingival convergence) area of the tooth enclosed. **3.** Any device for holding tissues together.

clasp-knife spas·tic·i·ty, clasp-knife ri·gid·i·ty (klasp-nīf′ spas-tis′i-tē, klasp-nīf′ ri-jid′i-tē) Initial increased resistance to stretch of the extensor muscles of a joint that give way rather suddenly, allowing the joint then to be easily flexed; the rigidity is due to an exaggeration of the stretch reflex.

class (klas) In biologic classification, the next division below the phylum (or subphylum) and above the order. [L. *classis,* a class, division]

class I an•ti•gens (klas an′ti-jenz) Cell-membrane-bound glycoproteins that are coded by genes of the major histocompatibility complex.

class I mol•e•cule (klas mol′ĕ-kyūl) A major histocompatibility complex antigen made up of two noncovalently bonded polypeptide chains, one glycosylated, heavy, and variable with antigen specificity; the other chain is β_2-microglobulin.

class II an•ti•gens (klas an′ti-jenz) A cell-membrane glycoprotein encoded by genes of the major histocompatibility complex. These antigens are distributed on antigen-presenting cells such as macrophages, B cells, and dendritic cells.

class II mol•e•cule (klas mol′ĕ-kyūl) A major histocompatibility complex membrane-piercing antigen made up of two noncovalently bonded polypeptide chains designated α and β.

class III an•ti•gens (klas an′ti-jenz) Non-cell-membrane molecules that are encoded by the S region of the major histocompatibility complex. These antigens are not involved in determining histocompatibility and include the complement proteins.

clas•sic cho•roi•dal neo•vas•cu•lar•i•za•tion (klas′ik kōr-oy′dăl nē-ō-vas′kyū-lar-ī-zā′shŭn) Well-demarcated areas of hyperfluorescence observed in the early phases of a retinal angiogram; caused by blood vessels from the choroid breakup in the subretinal space.

classic haemophilia [Br.] SYN classic hemophilia.

clas•sic he•mo•phil•i•a (klas′ik hē′mō-fil′ē-ă) SYN hemophilia A. SYN classic haemophilia.

clas•sic mi•graine (klas′ik mī′grān) A form of hemicrania migraine preceded by a scintillating scotoma (teichopsia).

clas•si•fi•ca•tion (klas′i-fi-kā′shŭn) A systematic arrangement into classes or groups based on perceived common characteristics; a means of giving order to a group of disconnected facts.

class re•call (klas rē′kawl) A legal term that, in health care, mandates that all patients who have received a given form of implant be examined for possible malfunction of the implant.

clas•tic (klas′tik) Breaking up into pieces, or exhibiting a tendency so to break or divide. [G. *klastos,* broken]

clas•to•gen•ic (klas-tō-jen′ik) Relating to the action of a clastogen.

clas•to•thrix (klas′tō-thriks) SYN trichorrhexis nodosa. [G. *klastos,* broken, + *thrix,* hair]

clath•rate (klath′rāt) A type of inclusion compound in which small molecules are trapped in the cagelike lattice of macromolecules. [L. *clathrare,* pp. *-atus,* to furnish with a lattice]

Claude syn•drome (klōd sin′drōm) Midbrain syndrome with oculomotor palsy on the side of the lesion and incoordination on the opposite side.

clau•di•ca•tion (klaw′di-kā′shŭn) Limping, usually referring to intermittent claudication. [L. *claudicatio,* fr. *claudico,* to limp]

clau•di•ca•tor•y (klaw′di-kă-tōr-ē) Relating to claudication, especially intermittent claudication.

Clau•di•us cells (klaw′dē-ŭs selz) Columnar cells on the floor of the ductus cochlearis external to the organ of Corti.

claus•tral (klaws′trăl) Relating to the claustrum.

claus•tro•pho•bi•a (klaw′strŏ-fō′bē-ă) A morbid fear of being in a confined place. [L. *claustrum,* an enclosed space, + G. *phobos,* fear]

claus•tro•pho•bic (klaw′strŏ-fō′bik) Relating to or suffering from claustrophobia.

claus•trum, pl. **claus•tra** (klaws′trŭm, -tră) **1.** One of several anatomic structures bearing a resemblance to a barrier. **2.** [TA] A thin, vertically placed lamina of gray matter lying close to the putamen, from which it is separated by the external capsule. Cells of the claustrum have reciprocal connections with sensory areas of the cerebral cortex. [L. barrier]

cla•vi (klā′vī) Plural of clavus.

clav•i•cle (klav′i-kĕl) A doubly curved long bone that forms part of the shoulder girdle. Its medial end articulates with the manubrium sterni at the sternoclavicular joint, its lateral end with the acromion of the scapula at the acromioclavicular joint. SYN clavicula [TA], collar bone.

cla•vic•u•la, pl. **cla•vic•u•lae** (klă-vik′yū-lă, -lī) [TA] SYN clavicle. [L. *clavicula,* a small key, fr. *clavis,* key]

cla•vic•u•lar (klă-vik′yū-lăr) Relating to the clavicle.

cla•vic•u•lar res•pi•ra•tion (klă-vik′yū-lăr res′pir-ā′shŭn) An effortful method of respiration that uses neck strap muscles to raise the shoulders and thus enlarge the thorax so inhalation can take place. This method is inefficient compared with diaphragmatic respiration.

cla•vus, pl. **cla•vi** (klā′vŭs, klā′vī) A small conic callosity caused by pressure over a bony prominence, usually on a toe. SYN heloma. [L. a nail, wart, corn]

claw•foot, **claw foot** (klaw′fut, klaw fut) SYN pes cavus.

claw•hand, claw hand (klaw′hand, klaw hand) Atrophy of the interosseous muscles of the hand with hyperextension of the metacarpophalangeal joints and flexion of the interphalangeal joints.

clay shov•el•er's frac•ture (klā shŭv′ĕl-ĕrz frak′shŭr) An avulsion fracture of the base of spinous processes of C-7, C-6, or T-1 (in order of prevalence).

CLB Abbreviation for *Cyanobacteria*-like, *Coccidia*-like, or *Cryptosporidium*-like organisms that have now been identified as coccidia in the genus *Cyclospora* (*C. cayetanensis*).

clean catch (klēn kach) Method of collecting a urine specimen to avoid artifacts in the specimen; the patient cleanses the external urinary opening before collecting the urine specimen.

clean in•ter•mit•tent blad•der cath•e•ter•i•za•tion (klēn in′tĕr-mit′ĕnt blad′ĕr kath′ĕ-tĕr-ī-zā′shŭn) A common way for patients with neurogenic bladders that do not empty normally to empty their bladders on a routine schedule.

clear•ance (klēr′ăns) **1.** Indicated as *C* with a subscript to show the substance removed: removal of a substance from the blood, e.g., by renal excretion, expressed in terms of the volume flow of arterial blood or plasma that would contain the amount of substance removed per unit time; measured in mL per minute; normal values in humans are commonly expressed per 1.73 m^2 body surface area. **2.** A condition in which bodies may pass each other without hindrance, or the distance between bodies. **3.** Removal of something from some place; e.g., "esophageal acid clearance" refers to removal from the esophagus of some acid that has refluxed into it from the stomach, evaluated by the time taken for restoration of a normal pH in the esophagus.

clear cell (klēr sel) **1.** A cell in which the cytoplasm appears empty with the light microscope, as occurs in certain secretory cells of eccrine sweat glands and in the parathyroid glands when the glycogen is unstained; **2.** Any cell, particularly a neoplastic one, containing abundant glycogen or other material that is not stained by hematoxylin or eosin, so that the cell cytoplasm is very pale in routinely stained sections.

clear cell car•ci•no•ma (klēr sel kahr′si-nō′mă) SYN mesonephroma.

clear cell car•ci•no•ma of sal•i•var•y glands (klēr sel kahr′si-nō′mă sal′i-var-ē glandz) A malignant tumor, comprising several subtypes such as clear cell oncocytoma, hyalinizing clear cell carcinoma, and epithelial-myoepithelial (intercalated duct) carcinoma.

clear•ing fac•tors (klēr′ing fak′tŏrz) Lipoprotein lipases that appear in plasma during lipemia and catalyze hydrolysis of triglycerides only when the latter are bound to protein and when an acceptor (e.g., serum albumin) is present, thus "clearing" the plasma.

clear lay•er of ep•i•der•mis (klēr lā′ĕr ep′i-dĕrm′is) SYN stratum lucidum.

cleav•age (klēv′ăj) **1.** Series of mitotic cell divisions occurring in the oocyte immediately after its fertilization. SEE ALSO cleavage division. **2.** Splitting of a complex molecule into two or more simpler molecules. SYN scission (2). **3.** Linear clefts in the skin indicating the direction of the fibers in the dermis. SEE ALSO cleavage lines.

cleav•age cav•i•ty (klēv′ăj kav′i-tē) SYN blastocele.

cleav•age di•vi•sion (klēv′ăj di-vizh′ŭn) The rapid mitotic division of the zygote with decrease in size of individual cells or blastomeres and the formation of a morula. SEE ALSO cleavage (1).

cleav•age lines (klēv′ăj līnz) Lines that can be extrapolated by connecting linear openings made when a round pin is driven into the skin of a cadaver, resulting from the principal axis of orientation of the subcutaneous connective tissue (collagen) fibers of the dermis; they vary in direction with the region of the body surface.

cleav•age prod•uct (klēv′ăj prod′ŭkt) A substance resulting from the splitting of a molecule into two or more simpler molecules.

cleav•age site (klēv′ăj sīt) SYN restriction site.

cleav•age spin•dle (klēv′ăj spin′dĕl) The spindle formed during the cleavage of a zygote or its blastomeres.

Cleaves po•si•tion (klēvz pŏ-zish′ŏn) Radiographic film technique using rolled film axial projection to visualize shoulder joint of patients who cannot abduct arm; provides images of the scapulohumeral joint, humeral head tuberosities, bicipital groove, and coracoid process.

cleav•ing zy•gote (klēv′ing zī′gōt) A zygote that is undergoing mitotic division to form blastomeres.

cleft (kleft) A fissure or groove.

cleft hand (kleft hand) A congenital deformity in which the division between the fingers, especially between the third and fourth, extends into the metacarpal region. SYN split hand.

cleft lip (kleft lip) A congenital facial defect of the lip (usually the upper lip) due to failure of fusion of the medial and lateral nasal prominences and maxillary prominence; frequently associated with cleft alveolus and cleft palate. See page B30. SYN harelip.

cleft pal•ate (kleft pal′ăt) A congenital fissure in the median line of the palate, often associated with cleft lip; often occurs as a feature of a syndrome or generalized condition (e.g., diastrophic dwarfism or spondyloepiphysial dysplasia congenita); its general genetic behavior resembles that of cleft lip. Care of the affected child requires a team approach involving a plastic surgeon, orthodontist, dentist, nurse, speech and hearing specialists, and social workers. See page B30. SYN palatoschisis.

cleft spine (kleft spīn) SEE spina bifida.

cleft tongue (kleft tŭng) SYN bifid tongue.

clei•dal (klī′dăl) Relating to the clavicle. SYN clidal.

♻ **cleido-, cleid-** Combining forms indicating the clavicle; also spelled clido-, clid-. [G. *kleis,* bar, bolt]

clei•do•cos•tal (klī′dō-kos′tăl) Relating to the clavicle and a rib. SYN clidocostal. [cleido- + L. *costa,* rib]

clei•do•cra•ni•al (klī′dō-krā′nē-ăl) Relating to the clavicle and the cranium. SYN clidocranial. [G. *kleis,* clavicle, + *kranion,* cranium]

clei•dot•o•my (klī-dot′ŏ-mē) Cutting the clavicle of a dead fetus to effect a vaginal delivery. [cleido- + -tomy]

♻ **-cleisis** Suffix indicating closure. [G. *kleisis,* a closing]

clenched fist sign (klencht fist sīn) In angina pectoris, pressing of the clenched fist against the chest to indicate the constricting, pressing quality of the pain.

CLIA Abbreviation for Clinical Laboratory Improvement Act.

CLIA ’67 Abbreviation for Clinical Laboratory Improvement Act of 1967.

CLIA ’88 Abbreviation for Clinical Laboratory Improvement Act Amendments of 1988.

click (klik) A slight, sharp sound.

cli•dal (klī′dăl) SYN cleidal.

♻ **clido-, clid-** Combining forms denoting the clavicle. SEE ALSO cleido-. [G. *kleis,* bar, bolt]

cli•do•cos•tal (klī′dō-kos′tăl) SYN cleidocostal.

cli•do•cra•ni•al (klī′dō-krā′nē-ăl) SYN cleidocranial.

cli•ent (klī′ĕnt) A patron or customer; one who receives a professional service from another; one who seeks or receives advice or therapy from a health care professional. Cf. patient. [L. *cliens,* protégé, dependent]

cli•ent-cen•tered ap•proach (klī′ĕnt-sen′tĕrd ă-prōch′) Honoring the desires, interests, priorities, and motivations of a client and/or client’s family/significant others in conducting evaluations and designing interventions (also called patient-centered approach).

cli•ent-cen•tered ther•a•py (klī′ĕnt-sen′tĕrd thār′ă-pē) A system of nondirective psychotherapy based on the assumption that the client (or patient) both has the internal resources to improve and is in the best position to resolve personality dysfunction.

client-centred therapy [Br.] SEE client-centered therapy.

Cliff•ord dis•ease (clif′ŏrd di-zēz′) SYN Ballantyne disease.

cli•mac•ter•ic (klī-mak′tĕr-ik) **1.** The period of endocrinal, somatic, and transitory psychological changes occurring in the menopause. **2.** A critical period of life. [G. *klimaktēr,* the rung of a ladder]

cli•max (klī′maks) **1.** The height or acme of a disease; its stage of greatest severity. **2.** SYN orgasm. [G. *klimax,* staircase]

clin•i•cal (klin′i-kăl) **1.** Relating to the bedside of a patient. **2.** Denoting the symptoms and course of a disease, as distinguished from the laboratory findings of anatomic changes. **3.** Relating to a clinic.

clin•i•cal a•nat•o•my (klin′i-kĕl ă-nat′ŏ-mē) The practical application of anatomic knowledge to diagnosis and treatment.

clin•i•cal at•tach•ment lev•el (klin′i-kăl ă-tach′mĕnt lev′ĕl) The estimated position of structures that support the tooth as measured with a periodontal probe; provides an estimate of a tooth’s stability and of loss of bone support.

clin•i•cal at•tach•ment loss (klin′i-kăl ă-tach′mĕnt laws) The extent of periodontal support that has been destroyed around a tooth.

clin•i•cal crown (klin′i-kăl krown) That portion of the anatomic crown of a tooth that is covered with enamel and visible in the oral cavity.

clin•i•cal di•ag•no•sis (klin′i-kăl dī-ăg-nō′sis) A diagnosis made from a study of the signs and symptoms of a disease.

clin•i•cal drug tri•al (clin′i-kăl drŭg trī′ăl) SYN drug use review.

clin•i•cal end point (klin′i-kăl end poynt) Traditional medical measures of a diagnostic or therapeutic impact that may or may not be perceived by the patient.

clin•i•cal fit•ness (klin′i-kăl fit′nĕs) Absence of frank disease or of subclinical precursors.

clin•i•cal ge•net•ics (klin′i-kăl jĕ-net′iks) Genetics applied to the diagnosis, prognosis, management, and prevention of genetic diseases. Cf. medical genetics.

clin•i•cal in•di•ca•tor (klin′i-kăl in′di-kā-tŏr) A measure, process, or outcome used to judge a particular clinical situation and indicate whether the care delivered was appropriate.

clin·i·cal judg·ment (klin′i-kăl jŭj′mĕnt) Cognitive or thinking process used for analyzing data, deriving diagnoses, deciding on interventions, and evaluating care.

Clin·i·cal Lab·o·ra·to·ry Im·prove·ment Act (CLIA) (klin′i-kăl lab′ră-tōr-ē im-prūv′mĕnt akt) U.S. federal legislation, and the personnel and procedures established by it under the aegis of the Commission on Medicare and Medicaid Services (CMS), for the surveillance and regulation of all clinical laboratory procedures in the U.S.

Clin·i·cal Lab·o·ra·to·ry Im·prove·ment Act of 1967 (CLIA '67) (klin′i-kăl lab′ră-tōr-ē im-prūv′mĕnt akt) U.S. federal law (Public Law 90-174) regulating medical laboratories that process more than 100 specimens per year in interstate commerce. Usually applied to only large, independent laboratories. SEE ALSO Clinical Laboratory Improvement Act Amendments of 1988.

Clin·i·cal Lab·o·ra·to·ry Im·prove·ment Act A·mend·ments of 1988 (CLIA '88) (klin′i-kăl lab′ră-tōr-ē im-prūv′mĕnt akt ă-mend′mĕnts) Amendments enacted by the U.S. Congress in 1988 (Public Law 100-578) to revise and expand the Clinical Laboratory Improvement Act of 1967 and Medicare and Medicaid provisions. The amendments classify and regulate laboratories based on the complexity of procedures being performed and establish personnel qualifications. These rules apply to all testing sites, but several procedures and tests have waivers from these regulations. SEE ALSO Clinical Laboratory Improvement Act of 1967.

clin·i·cal le·thal (klin′i-kăl lē′thăl) A term describing a disorder that culminates in premature death.

clin·i·cal·ly com·pe·tent (klin′i-kăl-ē kom′pĕ-tĕnt) Performing within the legal scope of defined practice, following standards or principles that satisfy the demands of the given situation.

clin·i·cal med·i·cine (klin′i-kăl med′i-sin) The study and practice of medicine in relation to the care of patients; the art of medicine as distinguished from laboratory science.

clin·i·cal nurse spe·cial·ist (klin′i-kăl nŭrs spesh′ăl-ist) A registered nurse with at least a master's degree in nursing who has advanced education in a particular area of clinical practice, such as oncology or psychiatry.

clin·i·cal path (klin′i-kăl path) A map that outlines the entire track or path a patient is expected to follow throughout the course of treatment and beyond. SEE ALSO clinical pathway.

clin·i·cal pa·thol·o·gy (klin′i-kăl pă-thol′ŏ-jē) **1.** Any part of the medical practice of pathology as it pertains to the care of patients. **2.** PATHOLOGY subspecialty concerned with the theoretic and technical aspects of chemistry, immunohematology, microbiology, parasitology, immunology, hematology, and other fields as they pertain to the diagnosis of disease.

clin·i·cal path·way (klin′i-kăl path′wā) Standardized interdisplinary care map for a specific diagnosis from the diagnosis-related group. Clinical pathways guide a patient's plan of care through attainment of specific clinical outcomes by the patient from admission to discharge. Benefits for the pathway include increased communication between members of the healthcare team, standardization of care, documentation and evaluation tools, decreased cost and length of stay, and increased patient and family satisfaction. SYN critical path.

clin·i·cal phar·ma·cist (klin-i′kăl fahr′mă-sist) A registered pharmacist trained in clinical aspects of patient care.

clin·i·cal prac·tice guide·lines (klin′i-kăl prak′tis gīd′līnz) A formal statement about a defined task or function in clinical practice, such as desirable diagnostic tests or the optimal treatment regimen for a specific diagnosis; generally based on the best available evidence (e.g., randomized controlled trials that have been assessed by a Cochrane collaborating group). SEE ALSO Cochrane collaboration.

clin·i·cal psy·chol·o·gy (klin′i-kăl sī-kol′ŏ-jē) A branch of psychology that specializes in both discovering new knowledge and in applying the art and science of psychology to persons with emotional or behavioral disorders; subspecialities include clinical child psychology and pediatric psychology.

clin·i·cal root of tooth (klin′i-kăl rūt tūth) That portion of a tooth embedded in the investing structures; the portion of a tooth not visible in the oral cavity. SYN radix clinica dentis [TA].

clin·i·cal sen·si·tiv·i·ty (klin′i-kăl sen′si-tiv′i-tē) The frequency of positive test results in patients with the disease (true-positive results). SYN diagnostic sensitivity.

clin·i·cal spec·i·fic·i·ty (klin′i-kăl spes′i-fis′i-tē) The frequency of negative results in patients without the disease (true-negative results).

clin·i·cal sus·pi·cion (klin′i-kăl sŭs-pi′shŭn) A strong presumption that, absent a diagnostic or algorithmic certainty, a patient is suffering from a given disorder or state (e.g., AIDS, TB, pregnancy).

clin·i·cal ther·mom·e·ter (klin′i-kăl thĕr-mom′ĕ-tĕr) A device for measuring the temperature of the human body.

cli·ni·cian (klin-ish′ŭn) A health care professional engaged in the care of patients, as distinguished from one working in other areas.

clin·i·co·path·o·log·ic (klin′i-kō-path-ŏ-loj′

ik) Pertaining to the signs and symptoms manifested by a patient, and also the results of laboratory studies, as they relate to the findings in the gross and histologic examination of tissue by means of biopsy or autopsy, or both.

♲ **clino-** Prefix meaning a slope (inclination or declination) or bend. [G. *klinō,* to slope, incline, or bend]

cli•no•ceph•a•ly (klī′nō-sef′ă-lē) Craniosynostosis in which the superior surface of the cranium is concave, presenting a saddle-shaped appearance in profile. SYN saddle head. [clino- + G. *kephalē,* head]

cli•no•dac•ty•ly (klī′nō-dak′ti-lē) Permanent deflection of one or more fingers. [clino- + G. *daktylos,* finger]

cli•noid pro•cess (klin′ōyd pros′es) One of three pairs of bony projections from the sphenoid bone: anterior clinoid process, the recurved posterior angle of the lesser wing; middle clinoid process, a little spur of bone on the body of the sphenoid, posterolateral to the tuberculum sellae; posterior clinoid process, a spur of bone at each superior angle of the dorsum sellae.

CLIP (klip) Acronym for corticotropinlike intermediate-lobe peptide.

clip (klip) **1.** A fastener used to hold a part or thing together with another. **2.** A fastener used to close off a small vessel.

clip for•ceps (klip fōr′seps) A small forceps with spring catch to hold a bleeding vessel.

clipped sen•tence (klipt sen′tĕns) A common method of dictating and transcribing in which the subject of a sentence is omitted (e.g., "Presents today for annual exam").

clith•ro•pho•bi•a (klīth′rō-fō′bē-ă) Morbid fear of being locked in. [G. *kleithron,* a bolt, + *phobos,* fear]

clit•o•ri•dec•to•my (klit′ōr-i-dek′tŏ-mē) Removal of the clitoris. [clitoris + G. *ektomē,* excision]

clit•o•ri•di•tis (klit′ōr-i-dī′tis) Inflammation of the clitoris. SYN clitoritis. [clitoris + G. *-itis,* inflammation]

clit•o•ris, pl. **cli•to•ri•des** (klit′ŏr-is, kli-tōr′i-dēz; klī′tō-ri-dēz) [TA] A cylindric, erectile body, rarely exceeding 2 cm in length, situated at the most anterior portion of the vulva and projecting between the branched limbs or laminae of the labia minora, which form its prepuce and frenulum. It consists of a glans, a corpus, and two crura. [G. *kleitoris*]

clit•o•rism (klit′ōr-ism) Prolonged and usually painful erection of the clitoris; the analogue of priapism.

clit•o•ri•tis (klit′ōr-ī′tis) SYN clitoriditis.

clit•or•o•meg•a•ly (klit′ōr-ō-meg′ă-lē) An enlarged clitoris. [clitoris + G. *megas,* great]

cli•vus, pl. **cli•vi** (klī′vŭs, -vē) [TA] **1.** A downward sloping surface. **2.** The sloping surface from the dorsum sellae to the foramen magnum composed of part of the body of the sphenoid and part of the basal part of the occipital bone. [L. slope]

clo•a•ca (klō-ā′kă) **1.** In early embryos, the endodermally lined chamber into which the hindgut and allantois empty. **2.** In birds and monotremes, the common chamber into which the hindgut, bladder, and genital ducts empty. [L. sewer]

clo•a•cal (klō-ā′kăl) Pertaining to the cloaca.

clo•a•cal mem•brane (klō-ā′kăl mem′brān) A transitory membrane in the caudal area of the ventral wall of the embryo, separating the endodermal from the ectodermal cloaca; it is divided into anal and genitourinary membranes that break down during the eighth to ninth weeks to establish the external opening for the alimentary and genitourinary tracts.

clo•a•co•gen•ic car•ci•no•ma (klō′ā-kō-jen′ik kahr′si-nō′mă) **1.** A type of squamous cell carcinoma of the anus originating in tissues arising from, or in remnants of, the cloaca. **2.** In oncology, anal cancer arising proximal to the pectinate line. SYN cuboidal carcinoma. [cloaca + -genic]

clo•nal (klō′năl) Pertaining to a clone.

clo•nal se•lec•tion the•o•ry (klō′năl sĕ-lek′shŭn thē′ŏr-ē) A theory that states that each lymphocyte has membrane-bound immunoglobulin receptors specific for a particular antigen and after the receptor is engaged, proliferation of the cell occurs such that a clone of antibody producing cells (plasma cell) is produced.

clone (klōn) **1.** A colony of organisms or cells derived from a single organism or cell by asexual reproduction, all having identical genetic constitutions. **2.** To produce such a colony or individual. **3.** A short section of DNA that has been copied by means of gene cloning. SEE cloning. [G. *klōn,* slip, cutting used for propagation]

clo•nic (klon′ik) Relating to or characterized by clonus.

clo•nic con•vul•sion (klon′ik kŏn-vŭl′shŭn) A convulsion in which the contractions are intermittent, the muscles alternately contracting and relaxing.

clon•ic•i•ty (klon-is′i-tē) The state of being clonic.

clon•i•co•ton•ic (klon′i-kō-ton′ik) Both clonic and tonic; said of certain forms of muscular spasm.

clo•nic spasm (klon′ik spazm) Alternate involuntary contraction and relaxation of a muscle.

clo•nic state (klon′ik stāt) Movement marked by repetitive muscle contractions and relaxations in rapid succession.

clon•ing (klōn′ing) **1.** Growing a colony of genetically identical cells or organisms in vitro. **2.** Transplantation of a nucleus from a somatic cell to an oocyte or ovum, which then develops into an embryo; many identical embryos can thus be generated by asexual reproduction. **3.** Replication of genetically identical embryos by microsurgical division of a blastocyst and implantation of resulting cells in animal wombs for gestation. **4.** Therapeutic cloning: growth of somatic stem cells in an embryo that has been produced by in vitro fertilization and modified by replacement of its nuclear material with DNA from a host with deficient or diseased tissue (e.g., heart, liver, pancreas); subsequent harvesting of the stem cells for implantation in the host subject destroys the embryo. **5.** A recombinant DNA technique used to produce millions of copies of a DNA fragment. The fragment is spliced into a cloning vehicle (i.e., plasmid, bacteriophage, or animal virus). The cloning vehicle penetrates a bacterial cell or yeast (the host), which is then grown in vitro or in an animal host. In some cases, as in the production of genetically engineered drugs, the inserted DNA becomes activated and alters the chemical functioning of the host cell.

clon•ing vec•tor (klōn′ing vek′tŏr) An autonomously replicating plasmid or phage with regions that are not essential for its propagation in bacteria and into which foreign DNA can be inserted; this foreign DNA is replicated and propagated as if it were a normal component of the vector.

clo•nism (klō′nizm) A long continued state of clonic spasms.

clo•no•gen•ic (klō-nō-jen′ik) Arising from or consisting of a clone.

clo•nor•chi•a•sis (klō′nōr-kī′ă-sis) A disease caused by the fluke *Clonorchis sinensis*, affecting the distal bile ducts after ingestion of raw, smoked, or undercooked fish or raw crayfish; repeated or chronic infection induces an intense proliferative and granulomatous condition.

Clo•nor•chis si•nen•sis (klō-nōr′kis sī-nen′sis) The Chinese liver fluke, a species of trematodes that in East Asia infects the bile passages; fish serve as second intermediate hosts and snails as first intermediate hosts.

clon•o•spasm (klon′ō-spazm) SYN clonus.

clo•nus (klō′nŭs) A form of movement marked by contractions and relaxations of a muscle, occurring in rapid succession seen with, among other conditions, spasticity, and some seizure disorders. SEE ALSO contraction. SYN clonospasm. [G. *klonos,* a tumult]

Clo•quet her•ni•a (klō-kā′ hĕr′nē-ă) A femoral hernia perforating the aponeurosis of the pectineus and insinuating itself between this aponeurosis and the muscle, lying therefore behind the femoral vessels.

closed an•es•the•si•a (klōzd an′es-thē′zē-ă) Inhalation anesthesia in which there is total rebreathing of all exhaled gases, except carbon dioxide, which is absorbed; gas flow into the anesthetic circuit consists only of oxygen, in amounts equal to the patient's metabolic consumption, plus small amounts of other gases (e.g., nitrous oxide) which undergo continued uptake by and distribution in the patient.

closed chain com•pound (klōzd chān kom′pownd) SYN cyclic compound.

closed-chain move•ment (klōzd-chān mūv′mĕnt) Kinematic chain movement in which the distal end of the body part is fixed and the proximal body part moves.

closed chest mas•sage (klōzd chest mă-sahzh′) Rhythmic compression of the heart between sternum and spine by depressing the lower sternum with the heels of the hands, the patient lying supine.

closed-cir•cuit he•li•um di•lu•tion (klōzd-sĭr′kŭt hē′lē-ŭm di-lū′shŭn) A gas dilution technique for measuring functional residual capacity (FRC); the patient rebreathes helium from a spirometer while oxygen is added and carbon dioxide is removed to maintain a constant system volume.

closed-cir•cuit meth•od (klōzd-sĭr′kŭt meth′ŏd) A method for measuring oxygen consumption in which the patient rebreathes an initial quantity of oxygen through a carbon dioxide absorber and the decrease in the volume of oxygen being rebreathed is noted.

closed-cir•cuit spi•rom•e•try (klōzd-sĭr′kŭt spī-rom′ĕ-trē) Measurement of CO_2 and O_2 in inspired and expired air by means of a device that, along with the patient's respiratory tract, forms a closed circuit.

closed com•e•do (klōzd kom′ĕ-dō) A comedo with a narrow or obstructed opening on the skin surface; closed comedos may rupture, producing a low-grade dermal inflammatory reaction. SYN whitehead (2).

closed dis•lo•ca•tion (klōzd dis-lō-kā′shŭn) A dislocation not complicated by an external wound. SYN simple dislocation.

closed drain•age (klōzd drān′ăj) Drainage of a body cavity through a water- or air-tight system.

closed frac•ture (klōzd frak′shŭr) A fracture in which skin is intact at site of fracture. SYN simple fracture.

closed head in•ju•ry (klōzd hed in′jŭr-ē) A head injury in which continuity of the scalp and mucous membranes is maintained.

closed hos•pi•tal (klōzd hos′pi-tăl) A hospital that restricts membership on its attending or consulting staff and thereby limits who may admit and treat patients.

closed loop ob•struc•tion (klōzd lūp ŏb-strŭk′shŭn) Obstruction of a segment of intestine either rotated on a fixed point (volvulus) or herniated through a fibrous opening (as under an adhesion or into a hernia); frequently associated with impaired perfusion ultimately resulting in gangrene.

closed re•duc•tion of frac•tures (klōzd rē-dŭk′shŭn frak′shŭrz) Reduction by manipulation of bone, without incision in the skin.

closed skill (klōzd skil) One of a series of movement patterns performed in a predictable, nonchanging environment so that movements can be planned in advance (e.g., keyboarding).

closed sur•ger•y (klōzd sŭr′jĕr-ē) Surgery without incision into skin, e.g., reduction of a fracture or dislocation.

close-packed po•si•tion (klōs′pakt pŏ-zish′ŏn) Joint position in which contact between the articulation structures is maximal. SYN joint extension.

clos•ing snap (klōz′ing snap) The accentuated first heart sound of mitral stenosis, related to closure of the abnormal valve.

clos•ing vol•ume (klōz′ing vol′yūm) The lung volume at which the flow from the lower parts of the lungs becomes severely reduced or stops during expiration, presumably because of airway closure; measured by the sharp rise in expiratory concentration of a tracer gas that had been inspired at the beginning of a breath that started from residual volume.

clos•trid•i•al (klos-trid′ē-ăl) Relating to any bacterium of the genus *Clostridium.*

Clos•trid•i•um (klos-trid′ē-ŭm) A genus of anaerobic (or anaerobic, aerotolerant), spore-forming, motile (occasionally nonmotile) bacteria containing gram-positive rods. Exotoxins are sometimes produced by these organisms. They may cause disease in humans and other animals. They are generally found in soil and in the intestinal tract of humans and other animals. The type species is *C. butyricum.* [G. *klōstēr,* a spindle]

clos•trid•i•um, pl. **clos•trid•i•a** (klos-trid′ē-ŭm, -ă) A vernacular term used to refer to any member of the genus *Clostridium.*

Clos•tri•di•um bi•fer•men•tans (klos-trid′ē-ŭm bī-fĕr-men′tanz) A bacterial species found in putrid meat and gaseous gangrene; also commonly in soil, feces, and sewage. Its pathogenicity varies from strain to strain.

Clos•tri•di•um bot•u•li•num (klos-trid′ē-ŭm bot-chū-lī′nŭm) A bacterial species that occurs widely in nature and is a frequent cause of food poisoning (botulism) from preserved meats, fruits, or vegetables that have not been properly sterilized before canning.

Clos•tri•di•um dif•fi•ci•le (klos-trid′ē-ŭm dif-ē-sē′lā) Gram-positive obligate anaerobic or microaerophilic, rod-shaped bacterium; causes antibiotic-associated colitis. SYN C-Diff, CDT.

Clos•tri•di•um his•to•lyt•i•cum (klos-trid′ē-ŭm his-tō-lit′i-kŭm) A bacterial species found in war wounds, where it induces necrosis of tissue; it produces a cytolytic exotoxin that causes local necrosis and sloughing on injection; it is not toxic on feeding; it is pathogenic for small laboratory animals.

Clos•tri•di•um no•vy•i (klos-trid′ē-ŭm nō′vī-ē) A bacterial species that causes gas gangrene and necrotic hepatitis.

Clos•tri•di•um per•frin•gens (klos-trid′ē-ŭm pĕr-frin′jenz) A bacterial species that causes gas gangrene; it also may be involved in causing enteritis, appendicitis, and puerperal fever. It is one of the most common causes of food poisoning in the U.S. SYN gas bacillus, Welch bacillus.

***Clos•tri•di•um per•frin•gens* al•pha tox•in** (klos-trid′ē-ŭm pĕr-frin′jenz al′fă tok′sin) A phospholipase produced by *C. perfringens* that increases vascular permeability and produces necrosis.

***Clos•tri•di•um per•frin•gens* be•ta tox•in** (klos-trid′ē-ŭm pĕr-frin′jenz bā′tă tok′sin) A substance produced by *C. perfringens* that causes necrosis and induces hypertension by causing release of catecholamine.

***Clos•tri•di•um per•frin•gens* en•ter•o•tox•in** (klos-trid′ē-ŭm pĕr-frin′jenz en-ter′ō-tok′sin) A toxin produced by *C. perfringens* that alters membrane permeability.

***Clos•tri•di•um per•frin•gens* ep•si•lon tox•in** (klos-trid′ē-ŭm pĕr-frin′jenz ep′si-lon tok′sin) A toxin produced by *C. perfringens* that increases the permeability of the gastrointestinal wall.

***Clos•tri•di•um per•frin•gens* i•o•ta tox•in** (klos-trid′ē-ŭm pĕr-frin′jenz ī-ō′tă tok′sin) A binary toxin produced by *C. perfringens* that is responsible for necrosis and increased vascular permeability.

Clos•tri•di•um sep•ti•cum (klos-trid′ē-ŭm sep′ti-kŭm) Gram-positive, anaerobic bacillus associated with gas gangrene or myonecrosis; infection occurs when the organism contaminates wounds through trauma or surgery.

Clos•tri•di•um sor•del•li•i (klos-trid′ē-ŭm sōr-del′ē-ī) A bacterial species that produces multiple toxins including a lecithinase, hemolysin, and a fibrinolysin, which results in edema and potentially fatal hypotension, and necrotic infections in humans. It is especially associated with abdominal and gynecologic posttraumatic and postoperative wound infection; also causes big head in rams.

Clos•tri•di•um te•ta•ni (klos-trid′ē-ŭm tet′ă-nī) A bacterial species that causes tetanus; it produces a potent exotoxin (neurotoxin) that is intensely toxic for humans and other animals when formed in tissues or injected, but not when ingested.

clo•sure (klō′zhŭr) **1.** The completion of a reflex pathway. **2.** The place of coupling between stimuli in the establishment of conditioned learning. **3.** To achieve or experience a sense of completion in a mental task. **4.** Definitive repair of an open wound, traumatic or surgical. **5.** Pertaining to the manner of fastening a garment, shoe, or appliance.

clo•sure prin•ci•ple (klō′zhŭr prin′si-pĕl) PSYCHOLOGY the principle that when one views fragmentary stimuli forming a nearly complete figure (e.g., an incomplete rectangle) one tends to ignore the missing parts and perceive the figure as whole. SEE gestalt.

clot (klot) **1.** To coagulate, said especially of blood. **2.** A soft, nonrigid, insoluble mass formed when a liquid (e.g., blood or lymph) gels. [O.E. *klott,* lump]

clot•ting fac•tor (klot′ing fak′tŏr) Any of the various plasma components involved in the clotting process.

cloud•y swell•ing (klow′dē swel′ing) Swelling of cells due to injury to the membranes affecting ionic transfer; causes an accumulation of intracellular water. SYN hydropic degeneration, parenchymatous degeneration.

clubbed dig•it (klŭbd dij′it) SEE clubbing.

clubbed fin•gers (klŭbd fing′gĕrz) SEE clubbing.

club•bing (klŭb′ing) A condition affecting the fingers and toes in which proliferation of distal tissues, especially the nail beds, results in thickening and widening of the extremities of the digits; the nails are abnormally curved and shiny. See this page.

club drug (klŭb drŭg) A drug of abuse (e.g., ecstasy) that is typically used by most or all members of a social gathering rather than in solitude.

club•foot, club foot (klŭb′fut, klŭb fut) SYN talipes equinovarus.

club hair (klŭb hār) A hair in resting state, before shedding, in which the bulb has become a club-shaped mass.

club•hand, club hand (klŭb′hand, klŭb hand) Congenital or acquired angulation deformity of the hand associated with partial or complete absence of the radius or ulna; usually with intrinsic deformities in the hand in congenital variants.

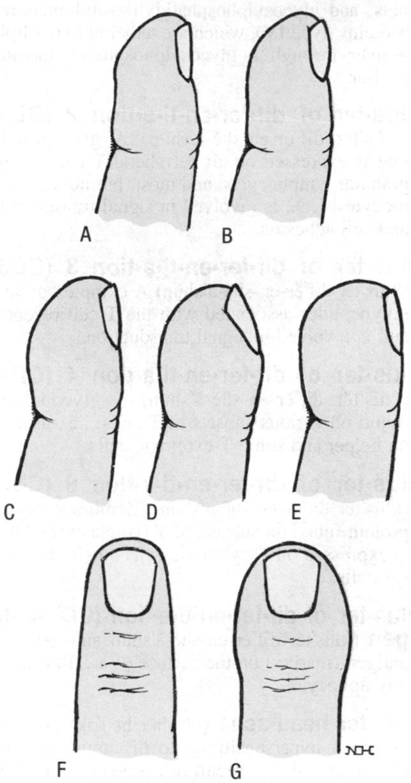

varieties of digital clubbing: (A) normal, (B) increased curvature on nail, (C) mild clubbing, (D) parrot's beak type, (E) watch glass type, (F) normal, (G) drumstick type

clue cell (klū sel) A type of vaginal epithelial cell that appears granular and is coated with coccobacillary organisms; seen in bacterial vaginosis.

clump•ing (klŭmp′ing) The massing together of bacteria or other cells or particles suspended in a fluid.

clu•ne•al (klū′nē-ăl) Pertaining to the clunes.

clu•nes (klū′nēz) SYN buttocks. [pl. of L. *clunis,* buttock]

clus•ter of dif•fer•en•ti•a•tion (CD) (klŭs′tĕr dif′ĕr-en-shē-ā′shŭn) Cell membrane molecules that are used to classify leukocytes into subsets. CD molecules are classified by monoclonal antibodies. There are four general types: type I transmembrane proteins have their COOH-termini in the cytoplasm and their NH_2-termini outside the cell; type II transmembrane proteins have their NH_2-termini in the cytoplasm and their COOH-termini outside the cell; type III transmembrane proteins cross the plasma membrane more than once and hence may form transmembrane channels; and glycosylphosphatidylinositol-anchored proteins (type IV), which are tethered to the lipid bilayer through a glycosylphosphatidylinositol anchor.

clus·ter of dif·fer·en·ti·a·tion 2 (CD2) (klŭs′tĕr dif′ĕr-en-shē-ā′shŭn) A glycoprotein that is expressed on all peripheral T cells, large granular lymphocytes, and most, but not all, thymocytes. CD2 is involved in signal transduction and cell adhesion.

clus·ter of dif·fer·en·ti·a·tion 3 (CD3) (klŭs′tĕr dif′ĕr-en-shē-ā′shŭn) A complex of five polypeptides associated with the T-cell receptor and is involved in signal transduction.

clus·ter of dif·fer·en·ti·a·tion 4 (CD4) (klŭs′tĕr dif′ĕr-en-shē-ā′shŭn) A glycoprotein found on various subsets of T cells, i.e., usually on helper and some T-cytotoxic cells.

clus·ter of dif·fer·en·ti·a·tion 8 (CD8) (klŭs′tĕr dif′ĕr-en-shē-ā′shŭn) Membrane glycoprotein found on subsets of T lymphocytes. CD8 is expressed on T-cytotoxic cells and T-suppressor cells.

clus·ter of dif·fer·en·ti·a·tion (CD) an·ti·gen (klŭs′tĕr dif′ĕr-en-shē-ā′shŭn an′ti-jen) An antigen (marker) on the surface of a cell, usually a lymphocyte.

clus·ter head·ache (klŭs′tĕr hed′āk) Possibly due to a hypersensitivity to histamine; usually characterized by recurrent, severe, unilateral orbitotemporal headaches associated with ipsilateral photophobia, lacrimation, and nasal congestion. SYN histaminic headache, Horton headache.

clut·ter·ing (klŭt′ĕr-ing) Speech disorder characterized by rapid, jerky utterances with many omissions and transpositions of speech sounds; sometimes confused with stuttering. SEE stuttering.

cly·sis (klī′sis) **1.** An infusion of fluid, usually subcutaneously, for therapeutic purposes. **2.** Formerly, a fluid enema; later, the washing out of material from any body space or cavity by fluids. [G. *klysis,* a drenching by a clyster]

Cm Symbol for curium.

cM Abbreviation for centimorgan.

cm Abbreviation for centimeter; cm^2 for square centimeter; cm^3 for cubic centimeter.

CMA Abbreviation for Certified Medical Assistant.

cmc Abbreviation for critical micelle concentration.

CMI Abbreviation for cell-mediated immunity.

CML Abbreviation for cell-mediated lymphocytotoxicity.

CMP Abbreviation for cytidine 5′-monophosphate (secondarily, any cytidine monophosphate).

CMS Abbreviation for U.S. Centers for Medicare and Medicaid Services.

CMS-1450 The uniform institutional health care insurance claim form in the U.S. Previously known as the HCFA-1450 claim form or UB-92. SYN HCFA-1450, UB-92.

CMS-1500 The uniform professional health care insurance claim form in the U.S. Previously known as the HCFA-1500 claim form. SYN HCFA-1500, Health Insurance Claim Form.

CMT Abbreviation for certified medical transcriptionist; certified massage therapist. SEE medical transcriptionist.

CMV Abbreviation for cytomegalovirus; a cancer drug combination treatment consisting of cisplatin, methotrexate, and vinblastine, used in the treatment of bladder and other malignancies; and continuous mandatory ventilation.

CN 1. NATO code for a riot-control agent, L-chloroacetophenone, which was previously widely used by military and law-enforcement agencies but that now is more typically found as a component of personal-defense spray. SEE cesium. **2.** Chemical symbol for the cyanide radical. SEE ALSO cyanide.

CNS 1. Abbreviation for central nervous system. **2.** Symbol for the thiocyanate radical, CNS^- or —CNS.

CO Abbrevation for certified orthotist; carbon monoxide; cardiac output.

CO_2 Abbreviation for carbon dioxide.

Co Symbol for cobalt; abbreviation for coccygeal.

♻ **co-** SEE con-.

CoA Abbreviation for coenzyme A.

co·ad·ap·ta·tion (kō′ad-ap-tā′shŭn) GENETICS the operation of selection jointly on two or more loci.

co·ag·glu·ti·nin (kō′ă-glū′ti-nin) A substance that does not agglutinate an antigen but does result in agglutination of antigen that is coated with univalent antibody. SEE ALSO conglutination.

co·ag·u·la (kō-ag′yū-lă) Plural of coagulum.

co·ag·u·la·ble (kō-ag′yū-lă-bĕl) Capable of being coagulated or clotted.

co·ag·u·lant (kō-ag′yū-lant) **1.** An agent that causes, stimulates, or accelerates coagulation, especially with reference to blood. **2.** SYN coagulative.

co·ag·u·late (kō-ag′yū-lāt) **1.** To convert a fluid or a substance in solution into a solid or gel. **2.**

To clot; to curdle; to change from a liquid to a solid or gel. [L. *coagulo,* pp. *-atus,* to curdle]

co·ag·u·la·tion (kō-ag′yū-lā′shŭn) **1.** Clotting; the process by which a liquid, especially blood, changes from a liquid to a solid. **2.** A clot or coagulum. **3.** Transformation of a solution into a gel or semisolid mass.

co·ag·u·la·tion ne·cro·sis (kō-ag′yū-lā′shŭn nĕ-krō′sis) A type of necrosis in which the affected cells or tissue are converted into a dry, dull, homogeneous eosinophilic mass without nuclei, as a result of the coagulation of protein as occurs in an infarct.

co·ag·u·la·tion time (kō-ag′yū-lā′shŭn tīm) The time required for blood to coagulate; prolonged in hemophilia and in the presence of obstructive jaundice, some anemias and leukemias, and some of the infectious diseases; also prolonged by some medications.

co·ag·u·la·tive (kō-ag′yū-lă-tiv) Causing coagulation. SYN coagulant (2).

co·ag·u·lop·a·thy (kō-ag′yū-lop′ă-thē) A disease affecting the coagulability of the blood.

co·ag·u·lum, pl. **co·ag·u·la** (kō-ag′yū-lŭm, -lă) A clot or a curd; a soft, nonrigid, insoluble mass formed when a solution undergoes coagulation. [L. a means of coagulating, rennet]

co·al·co·hol·ic (kō-al′kŏ-hol′ik) **1.** The person who enables an alcoholic person by assuming responsibilities on the alcoholic's behalf, minimizing or denying the problem drinking, or making amends for the alcoholic's behavior. SEE ALSO codependent. **2.** Pertaining to the coalcoholic or to coalcoholism.

co·al·co·hol·ism (kō-al′kŏ-hol-izm) The constellation of attitudes, attributes, and behaviors of the person who enables the alcoholic, which are necessary for the attainment of a symbiotic balance between alcoholic and coalcoholic. SEE ALSO symbiosis.

co·a·les·cence (kō′ă-les′ĕns) Fusion of originally separate parts. SYN concrescence (1).

coal gas (kōl gas) A synthetic gas produced from coal and used for heating and in the production of methanol and ammonia; contains carbon monoxide, carbon dioxide, and hydrogen; can cause death through asphyxiation as well as fire and explosion.

coal work·er's pneu·mo·co·ni·o·sis (kōl wŏrk′ĕrz nū′mō-kō-nē-ō′sis) SYN anthracosilicosis.

CO_2 an·a·ly·zer (an′ă-lī-zĕr) SYN capnometer.

co·ap·ta·tion (kō′ap-tā′shŭn) Joining or fitting together of two surfaces; e.g., the lips of a wound or the ends of a broken bone. [L. *co-apto,* pp. *-aptatus,* to fit together]

co·ap·ta·tion splint (kō′ap-tā′shŭn splint) A short splint designed to prevent overriding of the ends of a fractured bone, usually supplemented by a longer splint to fix the entire limb.

co·ap·ta·tion su·ture (kō′ap-tā′shŭn sū′chŭr) SYN apposition suture.

co·arct (kō-ahrkt′) To restrict or press together. SYN coarctate (1). [L. *co-arcto,* pp. *-arctatus,* to press together]

co·arc·tate (kō-ahrk′tāt) **1.** SYN coarct. **2.** Pressed together.

co·arc·ta·tion (kō′ahrk-tā′shŭn) A constriction, stricture, or stenosis, particularly of the aorta.

CoAS–, CoASH Symbols for the coenzyme A radical and reduced coenzyme A, respectively.

coat (kōt) **1.** The outer covering or envelope of an organ or part. **2.** One of the layers of membranous or other tissues forming the wall of a canal or hollow organ. SEE tunic.

coat·ed tongue (kōt′ĕd tŭng) A tongue with a whitish layer on its upper surface, composed of epithelial debris, food particles, and bacteria; often an indication of indigestion or of fever.

Coats dis·ease (kōts di-zēz′) A condition with findings that include yellow subretinal exudates and telangiectactic retinal vessels; typically unilateral and often associated with serous retinal detachment.

COB Abbreviation for Coordination of Benefits.

co·bal·a·min (kō-bal′ă-min) General term for compounds containing the dimethylbenzimidazolylcobamide nucleus of vitamin B_{12}.

co·balt (Co) (kō′bawlt) A steel-gray metallic element, atomic no. 27, atomic wt. 58.93320; a bioelement and a constituent of vitamin B_{12}; certain of its compounds are pigments, e.g., cobalt blue. [Ger. *kobalt*, goblin or evil spirit]

co·balt 60 (kō′bawlt) Radioactive isotope created by irradiating stable ^{59}Co with neutrons in a reactor; has a mass number of 60; half-life 5.3 years; used in teletherapy and brachytherapy; emits beta particles and gamma-rays.

cob·bler's su·ture (kob′lĕrz sū′chŭr) SYN doubly armed suture.

Cobb meth·od (kob meth′ŏd) A technique to determine the degree of curvature of the spine. The measurement is made by drawing a line perpendicular to a second line drawn across the superior endplate of the upper-end (most tilted) vertebra and the inferior endplate of the lower-end vertebra; the angle formed by the intersection of the two perpendicular lines is the Cobb angle, which is the measure of the magnitude of the curve.

Cobb syn·drome (kob sin′drōm) Cutaneous angiomas, usually in a dermatomal distribution on the trunk, associated with vascular abnormality of the spinal cord and resulting neurologic symptoms.

COBRA (kō′bră) Acronym for U.S. federal Consolidated Omnibus Budget Reconciliation Act.

co·caine (kō-kān′) A crystalline alkaloid obtained from the leaves of *Erythroxylon coca* (family Erythroxylaceae) and other species of *Erythroxylon*, or by synthesis from ecgonine or its derivatives; a potent central nervous system stimulant, vasoconstrictor, and topical anesthetic, widely abused as a euphoriant and associated with the risk of severe adverse physical and mental effects.

co·caine ba·by (kō-kān′ bā′bē) An infant who displays disabilities from the after-effects of cocaine experienced in utero; such children may also experience disabilities related to intercurrent addictive or compulsive behavior by both parents.

co·caine hy·dro·chlor·ide (kō-kān′ hī′drō-klōr′īd) A water-soluble salt used for local anesthesia of the eye or mucous membranes.

co·caine nose (kō-kān′ nōz) A constellation of findings in chronic intranasal abusers of cocaine, including damage to the mucous membrane of the nose, nasal collapse with saddle-nose deformity, palatal retraction and perforation, pharyngeal wall ulceration, sinusitis, and turbinate necrosis.

co·car·cin·o·gen (kō′kahr-sin′ō-jen) A substance that works symbiotically with a carcinogen in the production of cancer.

coc·cal (kok′ăl) Relating to cocci.

coc·ci (kok′kī) Plural of coccus.

Coc·cid·i·a (kok-sid′ē-ă) A subclass of protozoa in which mature trophozoites are small and typically intracellular. [Mod. L., fr. G. *kokkos,* berry]

coc·cid·i·al (kok-sid′ē-ăl) Relating to coccidia.

coc·cid·i·oi·dal (kok-sid′ē-oy′dăl) Referring to the disease or to the infecting organism of coccidioidomycosis.

Coc·cid·i·oi·des (kok-sid′ē-oy′dēz) A genus of fungi found in the soil of the semiarid areas of the southwestern U.S. and smaller areas throughout Central and South America. The only pathogenic species, *Coccidioides immitis*, causes coccidioidomycosis. [coccidium + G. *eidos,* resemblance]

Coc·cid·i·oi·des im·mit·is (kok-sid′ē-oy′dēz i-mī′tis) A dimorphic fungus widely distributed in desert and semiarid areas of the Southwestern U.S., Mexico, and South and Central America; causes coccidioidomycosis, the clinical manifestations of which range from self-limited primary pulmonary infection to a disseminated fatal disease.

coc·cid·i·oi·do·ma (kok-sid′ē-oy-dō′mă) A benign localized residual granulomatous lesion or scar in a lung following primary coccidioidomycosis.

coc·cid·i·oi·do·my·co·sis (kok-sid′ē-oy′dō-mī-kō′sis) A variable, sometimes fatal systemic fungal disease due to inhalation of arthroconidia of *Coccidioides immitis*. In benign forms of the infection, the lesions are limited to the upper respiratory tract, lungs, and near lymph nodes; in a small percentage of cases, the disease disseminates to other organs, meninges, bones, joints, skin, and subcutaneous tissues. [*Coccidioides* + G. *mykēs,* fungus, + *-osis,* condition]

coc·cid·i·o·sis (kok-sid′ē-ō′sis) Group name for diseases attributable to any species of coccidia; a common disease of many species of domestic animals and birds; both intestinal and pulmonary coccidiosis have been reported in patients with AIDS.

coc·cid·i·um, pl. **coc·cid·i·a** (kok-sid′ē-ŭm, kok-sid′ē-ă) Common name given to protozoan parasites in which schizogony occurs within epithelial cells, generally in the intestine; parasitic in domestic and wild birds and mammals, and occasionally in humans; most are nonpathogenic. SEE *Isospora.* [Mod. L. dim. of G. *kokkos,* berry]

coc·co·bac·il·lar·y (kok′ō-bas′i-lar-ē) Relating to a coccobacillus.

coc·co·ba·cil·lus (kok′ō-bă-sil′ŭs) A short, thick bacterial rod of the shape of an oval or slightly elongated coccus. [G. *kokkos,* berry]

coc·coid (kok′oyd) Resembling a coccus. [G. *kokkos,* berry, + *eidos,* resemblance]

coc·cus, pl. **coc·ci** (kok′ŭs, kok′sī) **1.** A bacterium of round, spheroid, or ovoid form. **2.** SYN cochineal. [G. *kokkos,* berry]

coc·cy·al·gi·a (kok′sē-al′jē-ă) SYN coccygodynia. [coccyx + G. *algos,* pain]

coc·cy·dyn·i·a (kok′sē-din′ē-ă) SYN coccygodynia. [coccyx + G. *ōdyne, pain*]

coc·cy·ge·al (Co) (kok-sij′ē-ăl) Relating to the coccyx.

coc·cy·ge·al bod·y (kok-sij′ē-ăl bod′ē) An arteriovenous (arteriolovenular) anastomosis supplied by the middle sacral artery and located on the pelvic surface of the coccyx.

coc·cy·ge·al gan·gli·on (kok-sij′ē-ăl gang′glē-ŏn) SYN ganglion impar.

coc·cy·ge·al mus·cle (kok-sij′ē-ăl mŭs′ĕl) SYN coccygeus muscle.

coc·cy·ge·al nerve [Co] (kok-sij′ē-ăl nĕrv) A small nerve, the lowest of the spinal nerves, entering into the formation of the coccygeal plexus. SYN nervus coccygeus [TA].

coc·cy·ge·al plex·us (kok-sij′ē-ăl plek′sŭs) A small plexus formed by the fifth sacral and the coccygeal nerves; it gives origin to the anococcygeal nerves.

coc·cy·ge·al si·nus (kok-sij′ē-ăl sī′nŭs) A fistula or channel opening just posterior or near to the tip of the coccyx, being the result of incomplete closure of the caudal end of the neurenteric canal. SEE ALSO pilonidal sinus.

coc·cy·ge·al ver·te·brae Co1–Co4 (kok-sij′ē-ăl vĕr′tĕ-brē) The four terminal segments of the vertebral column, usually fused to form the coccyx. SYN vertebrae coccygeae [Co1–Co4] [TA].

coc·cy·gec·to·my (kok′si-jek′tŏ-mē) Removal of the coccyx. [coccyx + G. *ektomē,* excision]

coc·cy·ge·us mus·cle (kok-sij-ē′ŭs mŭs′ĕl) *Origin,* spine of ischium and sacrospinous ligament; *insertion,* sides of lower part of sacrum and upper part of coccyx; *action,* assists in support of pelvic floor, especially when intraabdominal pressures increase; *nerve supply,* third and fourth sacral. SYN musculus coccygeus [TA], coccygeal muscle, ischiococcygeus, musculus ischiococcygeus.

coc·cy·go·dyn·i·a (kok′si-gō-din′ē-ă) Pain in the coccygeal region. SYN coccygalgia, coccydynia, coccyodynia. [coccyx + G. *odynē,* pain]

coc·cy·got·o·my (kok′si-got′ŏ-mē) Operation for freeing the coccyx from its attachments. [coccyx + G. *tomē,* a cutting]

coc·cy·o·dyn·i·a (kok′sē-ō-din′ē-ă) SYN coccygodynia.

coc·cyx, gen. **coc·cy·gis**, pl. **coc·cy·ges** (kok′siks, -si-jis, -si-jēz) [TA] The small bone at the end of the vertebral column in humans, formed by the fusion of four rudimentary vertebrae; it articulates above with the sacrum. [G. *kokkyx,* a cuckoo, the coccyx]

coch·i·neal (kotch′i-nēl) [CI 75470] The dried female insects, *Coccus cacti*, enclosing the young larvae, or the dried female insect, *Dactylopius coccus*, containing eggs and larvae, from which coccinellin is obtained; used as a red coloring agent and a stain. SEE carmine. SYN coccus (2). [O.Sp. *cochinilla,* wood louse, fr. G. *kokkinos*, berry]

co·chle·a, pl. **co·chle·ae** (kok′lē-ă, -ē) [TA] A conic cavity in the petrous portion of the temporal bone, forming one of the divisions of the labyrinth or internal ear. It consists of a spiral canal making two and a half turns around a central core of spongy bone, the modiolus; this spiral canal of the cochlea contains the membranous cochlea, or cochlear duct, in which is the spiral organ (Corti organ). See this page. [L. snail shell]

co·chle·ar (kok′lē-ăr) Relating to the cochlea.

coch·le·ar ar·e·a (kok′lē-ăr ār′ē-ă) The area inferior to the transverse crest of the fundus of the internal acoustic meatus through which the filaments of the cochlear nerve pass to enter the cochlea; forms the base of the conic modiolus about which the cochlear canal spirals. SEE base of modiolus of cochlea. SYN area cochleae [TA].

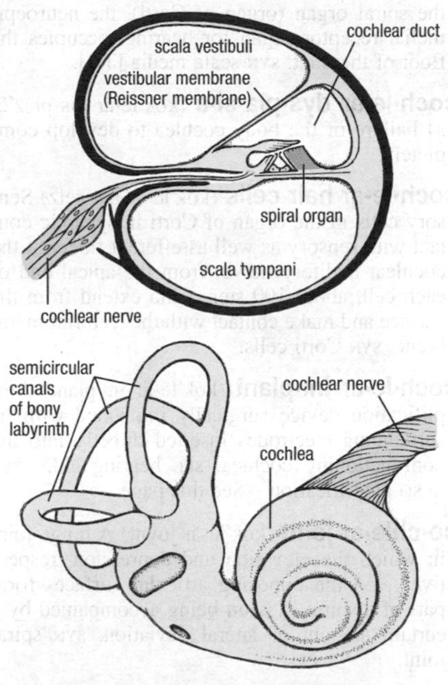

cochlea (inner ear): with cross-section

co·chle·ar ca·nal (kok′lē-ăr kă-nal′) The winding tube of the bony labyrinth that makes two-and-a-half turns about the modiolus of the cochlea; it is divided incompletely into two compartments by a winding shelf of bone, the bony spiral lamina. SYN canalis spiralis cochleae [TA].

co·chle·ar can·a·lic·u·lus (kok′lē-ăr kan′ă-lik′yŭ-lŭs) A minute canal in the temporal bone that passes from the cochlea inferiorly to open in front of the medial side of the jugular fossa. It contains the perilymphatic duct.

coch·le·ar drill-out (kok′lē-ăr dril′owt) Implantation of electrodes in a cochlea in which the lumen of the scala tympani has been obliterated by the deposition of new bone due to the inflammatory process in labyrinthitis; the cochlear wall and new bone are drilled away so that the electrodes can be placed close to the remaining neurons of the auditory division of the eighth cranial nerve.

co·chle·ar duct (kok′lē-ăr dŭkt) A spirally arranged membranous tube suspended within the cochlea, occupying the lower portion of the scala vestibuli; it begins by a blind extremity, the vestibular cecum, in the cochlear recess of the vestibule, and ends in another blind extremity, the cecum cupulare or lagena, at the cupola of the cochlea; it contains endolymph and communicates with the sacculus by the ductus reuniens;

the spiral organ (organ of Corti), the neuroepithelial receptor organ for hearing, occupies the floor of the duct. SYN scala media [TA].

coch•le•ar dys•pla•si•a (kok′lē-ăr dis-plāz′ē-ă) Failure of the bony cochlea to develop completely.

coch•le•ar hair cells (kok′lē-ăr hār selz) Sensory cells in the organ of Corti in synaptic contact with sensory as well as efferent fibers of the cochlear auditory nerve; from the apical end of each cell, about 100 stereocilia extend from the surface and make contact with the tectorial membrane. SYN Corti cells.

coch•le•ar im•plant (kok′lē-ăr im′plant) Amplification device surgically implanted with its stimulating electrodes inserted directly into the nonfunctioning cochlea. SEE hearing aid. SEE ALSO amplification. See this page.

co•chle•ar joint (kok′lē-ăr joynt) A hinge joint in which the elevation and depression, respectively, on the opposing articular surfaces form part of a spiral, flexion being accompanied by a certain amount of lateral deviation. SYN spiral joint.

coch•le•ar mic•ro•phon•ic (kok′lē-ar mī′krō-fon′ik) Bioelectric potentials produced by the hair cells of the spiral organ (organ of Corti) in response to sound that faithfully represent the frequency and intensity of the acoustic stimulation.

co•chle•ar nerve (kok′lē-ăr nĕrv) The part of the vestibulocochlear nerve peripheral to the cochlear root. It is composed of fibers with central nerve processes that arise from the bipolar neurons of the spiral ganglion and that have their peripheral processes on the four rows of neuroepithelial cells (hair cells) of the spiral organ. SYN auditory nerve.

coch•le•i•tis (kok′lē-ī′tis) Inflammation of the cochlea. [cochlea + G. *-itis,* inflammation]

co•chle•o•pal•pe•bral re•flex (kok′lē-ō-pal′pĕ-bral rē′fleks) A form of the wink reflex in which there is a contraction, sometimes very slight, of the orbicularis palpebrarum muscle when a sudden noise is made close to the ear. It is absent in labyrinthine disease with total deafness. SYN startle reflex (2).

coch•le•o•top•ic (kok′lē-ō-top′ik) Referring to the frequency-responsive organization of the central auditory pathways in the brain. [cochlea + G. *topos,* place, + -ic]

co•chle•o•ves•tib•u•lar (kok′lē-ō-ves-tib′yū-lăr) Relating to the cochlea and the vestibule of the ear.

Coch•rane col•lab•o•ra•tion (kok′răn kŏ-lab′ŏr-ā′shŭn) A worldwide network of clinical epidemiologists who review and publish results of randomized controlled trials. The aim is to provide improved data for use in evidence-based medicine and for setting clinical practice guidelines. SEE ALSO evidence-based medicine, clinical practice guidelines.

Cock•ayne syn•drome (kok-ān′ sin′drōm) Dwarfism, precociously senile appearance, pig-

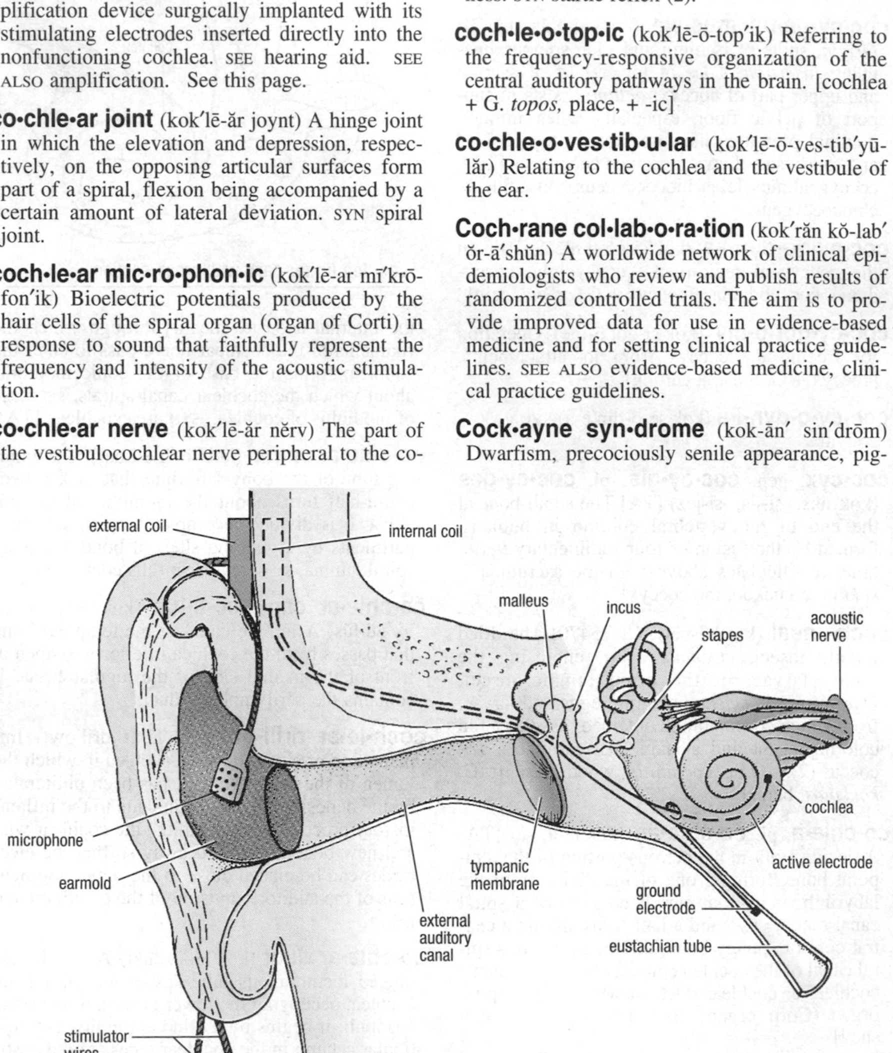

cochlear implant

mentary degeneration of the retina, optic atrophy, deafness, sensitivity to sunlight, microcephaly, and mental retardation; autosomal recessive inheritance associated with defective excision repair of DNA. There are various complementation groups.

cock·le·bur (kok'ĕl-bŭr) **1.** SYN agrimony. **2.** SYN burdock.

cock·tail (kok'tāl) A mixture that includes several ingredients or drugs.

co·con·trac·tion (kō'kŏn-trak'shŭn) Simultaneous contraction of both the agonist and the antagonist around a joint to hold a stable position.

code (kōd) **1.** A set of rules, principles, or ethics. **2.** Any system devised to convey information or facilitate communication. **3.** Term used in hospitals to describe an emergency situation requiring trained members of the staff, such as a cardiopulmonary resuscitation team, or the signal to summon such a team. **4.** A numeric system for ordering and classifying information (e.g., about diagnostic categories). **5.** To assign an alphanumeric combination to a diagnosis or procedure. SEE ALSO NATO code. [L. *codex*, book]

code black (kōd blak) A vague term that means different things in different areas. **1.** A patient in ER intake is dead on arrival. **2.** Warning indicating an explosive device may be present in a health care facility. **3.** Warning that a mass casualty incident has occurred.

code blue (kōd blū) In some health care facilities, oral announcement concerning a patient whose state of cardiac arrest is such as to require urgent use of CPR.

code link·age (kōd lingk'ăj) In health care accounting, verification that the diagnosis code and procedure code match up to support medical necessity for therapy.

code or·ange (kōd awr'ănj) A vague term for an oral directive that varies in meaning from one health care facility to another; in Australia, indicates need for immediate evacuation of a health care premises.

co·de·pen·dent (kō'dĕ-pen'dĕnt) Someone who supports the addiction of another person by excusing, denying, or concealing behavior. SEE ALSO coalcoholic.

code pur·ple (kōd pŭr'pĕl) A vague term for an oral directive that varies in meaning from one health care facility to another; in Australia, indicates need for explosive device alert.

code red (kōd red) A vague term for an oral directive that indicates immediate danger (e.g., fire, inclement weather, overcrowding of ER areas).

cod·ing (kōd'ing) Assigning a number to a disease process, surgical procedure, or other type of health care service for the purpose of reimbursement, health care planning, and research.

cod·ing se·quence (kōd'ing sē'kwĕns) The portion of DNA that codes for transcription of messenger RNA. SEE exon.

Cod·man tri·an·gle (kod'măn trī'ang-gĕl) RADIOLOGY the interface between growing bone tumor and normal bone, presenting as an incomplete triangle formed by periosteum.

Cod·man tu·mor (kod'măn tū'mŏr) Chondroblastoma of the proximal humerus.

co·do·cyte (kō'dō-sīt) SYN target cell.

co·dom·i·nant (kō-dom'i-nănt) GENETICS denoting an equal degree of dominance of two genes, both being expressed in the phenotype of the individual (e.g., genes A and B of the ABO blood group are codominant); individuals with both are type AB.

co·dom·i·nant in·her·i·tance (kō-dom'i-nănt in-her'i-tăns) Mode by which two alleles are individually expressed in the presence of each other.

co·dom·i·nant trait (kō-dom'i-nănt trāt) SEE codominant.

co·don (kō'don) A set of three consecutive nucleotides in a strand of DNA or RNA that provides the genetic information to code for a specific amino acid that will be incorporated into a protein chain or that serves as a termination signal. SYN triplet (3). [code + -on]

♻ **coe-** For words so beginning, and not found here, see entries beginning ce-.

co·ef·fi·cient (kō'ĕ-fish'ĕnt) **1.** The expression of the amount or degree of any quality possessed by a substance, or of the degree of physical or chemical change normally occurring in that substance under stated conditions. **2.** The ratio or factor that relates a quantity observed under one set of conditions to that observed under standard conditions, usually when all variables are either 1 or a simple power of 10. [L. *co-* + *efficio* (*exfacio*), to accomplish]

co·ef·fi·cient of var·i·a·tion (CV) (kō'ĕ-fish'ĕnt var'ē-ā'shŭn) A unitless number used to describe dispersion of data. It allows comparison of standard deviations of test results expressed in different units. It is calculated from the standard deviation (s) and mean (x). CV = 100s ÷ x.

Coe·len·ter·a·ta (sē-len-tĕ-rā'tă) One of the major phyla of invertebrates, to which forms such as jellyfish belong.

coe·len·ter·ate (sē-len'tĕr-āt) Common name for members of the Coelenterata.

coeliac [Br.] SYN celiac.

coeliac artery [Br.] SYN celiac artery.

coeliac disease [Br.] SYN celiac disease.

coeliac ganglia [Br.] SYN celiac ganglia.

coeliac lymph nodes [Br.] SYN celiac lymph nodes.

coeliac plexus [Br.] SYN celiac plexus.

coeliac plexus reflex [Br.] SYN celiac plexus reflex.

coeliac trunk [Br.] SYN celiac trunk.

coelio- [Br.] SYN celio-.

coeliocentesis [Br.] SYN celiocentesis.

coeliorrhaphy [Br.] SYN celiorrhaphy.

coelioscopy [Br.] SYN celioscopy.

coeliotomy [Br.] SYN celiotomy.

coelitis [Br.] SYN celitis.

coelo- [Br.] SYN celo-.

coelom, pl. **coeloma [Br.]** SYN celom.

coeloma [Br.] SYN celoma.

coelomic [Br.] SYN celomic.

♻**coeno-** Combining form meaning shared in common. SEE ALSO ceno-. [G. *koinos,* common]

coenocyte [Br.] SYN cenocyte.

co•en•zyme (kō-en′zīm) A substance (excluding solo metal ions) that enhances or is necessary for the action of enzymes; coenzymes are of smaller molecular size than the enzymes themselves; several vitamins are coenzyme precursors. SYN cofactor (1).

co•en•zyme A (CoA) (kō-en′zīm) A coenzyme containing pantothenic acid, adenosine 3′-phosphate 5′-pyrophosphate, and cysteamine; involved in the transfer of acyl groups, notably in transacetylations.

co•en•zyme Q (Q) (kō-en′zīm) Quinones with isoprenoid side chains (specifically, ubiquinones) that mediate electron transfer between cytochrome *b* and cytochrome *c*.

coeur (kur) SYN heart. [Fr.]

coeur en sa•bot (kur awn[h] sah-bo′) The radiographic configuration of the heart in the tetralogy of Fallot; the elevated apex gives a silhouette like that of a wooden shoe.

Coe vi•rus (kō vī′rŭs) A virus serologically identical with the A-21 strain of Coxsackievirus; the cause of a common-cold–like disease in military recruits.

co•fac•tor (kō′fak′tŏr) **1.** SYN coenzyme. **2.** An atom or molecule essential for the action of a large molecule; e.g., heme in hemoglobin, magnesium in chlorophyll.

COG Abbreviation for center of gravity.

Co•gan oc•u•lo•mo•tor a•prax•i•a (kō′găn ok′yū-lō-mō′tŏr ă-praks′ē-ă) Inability to move eyes in one or both directions, horizontally; patient must turn head to view an object in periphery. Condition more prevalent in males and is especially noticeable in children.

Co•gan-Reese syn•drome (kō′găn rēs sin′drōm) SYN iridocorneal endothelial syndrome.

cog•ni•tion (kog-ni′shŭn) **1.** The mental activities associated with thinking, learning, and memory. **2.** Any process whereby one acquires knowledge. [L. *cognitio*]

cog•ni•tive (kog′ni-tiv) Pertaining to cognition.

cog•ni•tive be•hav•i•or•al ther•a•py (CBT) (kog′ni-tiv bē-hāv′yŏr-ăl thār′ă-pē) A form of psychotherapy that emphasizes the role of thoughts and attitudes in one's feelings and behavior.

cog•ni•tive de•vel•op•ment (kog′ni-tiv dĕ-vel′ŏp-mĕnt) Process of acquiring more complex ways of thinking as a person grows from infancy through adulthood.

cog•ni•tive dis•so•nance (kog′ni-tiv dis′ŏ-năns) A motivational state that exists when a person's attitudes, perceptions, and related cognitive state are inconsistent with each other, e.g., hating African Americans as a group but admiring Martin Luther King, Jr.

cog•ni•tive lat•er•al•i•ty quo•tient (kog′ni-tiv lat′ĕr-al′i-tē kwō′shĕnt) Test for difference in cognitive performance of left and right sides of the brain.

cog•ni•tive ther•a•py (kog′ni-tiv thār′ă-pē) Any one of a variety of techniques in psychotherapy that uses guided self-discovery, imaging, self-instruction, symbolic modeling, and related forms of explicitly elicited cognitions as the principal mode of treatment.

cog•wheel res•pi•ra•tion (kog′wēl res′pir-ā′shŭn) The inspiratory sound being broken into two or three by silent intervals.

cog•wheel ri•gid•i•ty (kog′wēl ri-jid′i-tē) A type of rigidity seen in parkinsonism in which the muscles respond with cogwheellike jerks to the use of constant force in bending the limb.

co•he•rin (kō-hēr′in) A posterior pituitary hormone that regulates peristaltic activity in intestinal smooth muscle. [cohere + -in]

co•he•sion (kō-hē′zhŭn) The attraction between molecules or masses that holds them together. [L. *co-haereo,* pp. *-haesus,* to stick together]

COHN Abbreviation for Certified Occupational Health Nurse.

co•hort (kō′hōrt) **1.** Component of the population born during a particular period and identified by period of birth so that its characteristics can be ascertained as it enters successive time and age periods. **2.** Any designated group followed or traced over a period, as in an epidemiological cohort study. [L. *cohors,* retinue, military unit]

coil (koyl) **1.** A spiral or series of loops. **2.** An object made of wire wound in a spiral configuration, used in electronic applications, or a loop of wire used as an antenna.

co•in•fec•tion (kō′in-fek′shŭn) Concurrent infection by two or more pathogens.

coi•no•site (koyn′ō-sīt) SYN cenosite.

co•in•sur•ance (kō-in-shŭr′ăns) The amount or percentage the insured is responsible for after the deductible has been met. SEE ALSO copayment, cost sharing.

co•i•tal (kō′i-tăl) Pertaining to coitus.

co•i•tal head•ache (kō′i-tăl hed′āk) A form of benign exertional headache occurring during sexual activity. SYN benign coital cephalalgia.

co•i•tion (kō-ish′ŭn) SYN coitus. [L. *co-eo,* pp. *-itus,* to come together]

co•i•tus (kō′i-tŭs) Sexual union. SYN coition, copulation (1), pareunia, sexual intercourse. [L.]

co•i•tus in•ter•rup•tus (kō′i-tŭs in-tĕr-rŭp′tŭs) Sexual intercourse that is interrupted before the male ejaculates. SYN withdrawal (5).

co•i•tus re•ser•va•tus (kō′i-tŭs rez-ĕr-vā′tŭs) Sexual intercourse in which ejaculation is postponed or suppressed.

coke bugs (kōk bŭgz) SYN Magnan sign.

Co•ker•o•my•ces re•cur•va•tus (kō′ker-ō-mī′sēz rē-kŭr-vā′tŭs) A fungal genus in the order Mucorales; a rare cause of disease in humans, but isolation from pleural and peritoneal fluid has been reported.

col (kol) A craterlike area of the interproximal oral mucosa joining the lingual and buccal interdental papillae.

cold (kōld) **1.** A low temperature; the sensation produced by a temperature notably below an accustomed norm or a comfortable level. **2.** Popular term for a virus infection involving the upper respiratory tract and characterized by congestion of the mucosa, watery nasal discharge, and general malaise, with a duration of 3–5 days. SEE ALSO rhinitis. SYN common cold, frigid (1), upper respiratory infection, upper respiratory tract infection.

cold ab•scess (kōld ab′ses) **1.** An abscess without heat or other usual signs of inflammation. **2.** SYN tuberculous abscess.

cold ag•glu•ti•na•tion (kōld ă-glū′ti-nā′shŭn) Clumping of red blood cells by their own serum, or by any other serum when the blood is cooled below body temperature; seen occasionally in the blood of normal people or as a pathologic finding in mycoplasmal pneumonia, infectious mononucleosis, certain protozoan infections, or lymphoproliferative neoplasms. SEE autoagglutination.

cold ag•glu•ti•nin (kōld ă-glū′ti-nin) An antibody that reacts more efficiently at temperatures below 37°C.

cold cure res•in, cold-cur•ing res•in (kōld kyūr rez′in, kōld-kyūr′ing rez′in) SYN autopolymer resin.

cold-in•duced ur•ti•car•i•a (kōld′in-dūst′ ŭr′ti-kar′ē-ă) Hives resulting from exposure to cold.

cold-in•duced vas•o•di•la•tion (kōld′in-dūst′ vā′zō-dī-lā′shŭn) Application of cold to increase the cross-sectional diameter of blood vessels.

cold knife con•i•za•tion (kōld nīf kon′i-zā′shŭn) Obtaining a cone of endocervical tissue with a cold knife blade so as to preserve histologic characteristics and avoid desiccating tissue.

cold nod•ule (kōld nod′yūl) A thyroid nodule with a much lower uptake of radioactive iodine than the surrounding parenchyma; about one in four proves to be malignant.

cold press•ing (kōld pres′ing) A method used to process oils from food without heat, so as to preserve the nutrients.

cold-sen•si•tive en•zyme (kōld-sen′si-tiv en′zīm) An enzyme that loses its stability as the temperature is lowered.

cold sore (kōld sōr) Colloquialism for herpes simplex. See page B15.

cold stage (kōld stāj) The stage of chill in a malarial paroxysm.

cold ther•a•py (kōld thār′ă-pē) A type of care in which ice or cold water is applied to a body part. SYN cryotherapy.

cold ul•cer (kōld ŭl′sĕr) A small, gangrenous ulcer on the extremities due to defective circulation.

cold ur•ti•ca•ri•a (kōld ŭr′ti-kar′ē-ă) Hypersensitivity to cold leading to superficial vascular reaction manifested by transient itching, erythema, and hives. SEE ALSO hypothermia. See page 334.

col•ec•to•my (kŏ-lek′tŏ-mē) Excision of a segment or all of the colon. [G. *kolon,* colon, + *ektomē,* excision]

co•li•bac•il•lo•sis (kō′li-bas-i-lō′sis) Diarrheal disease caused by the bacterium *Escherichia coli.* Often called enteric colibacillosis.

col•ic (kol′ik) **1.** Relating to the colon. **2.** Spasmodic pains in the abdomen. **3.** In young infants, paroxysms of gastrointestinal pain, with crying and irritability, due to a variety of causes, such as swallowing of air, emotional upset, or overfeeding. [G. *kōlikos,* relating to the colon]

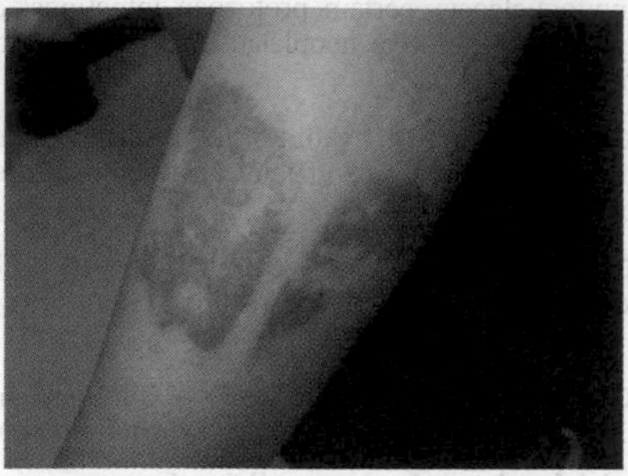

cold urticaria: leg, after overuse of ice pack

col·i·cin (kol′i-sin) Bacteriocin produced by strains of *Escherichia coli* and other enterobacteria. [(*Escherichia*) *coli* + bacteriocin]

col·ick·y (kol′ik-ē) Denoting or resembling the pain of colic.

col·ic root (kol′ik rūt) A common weed of the eastern United States (*Aletris farinosa*) with purported value as a specific against stomach ache (as the common name suggests) and allegedly of value in treating menstrual disorders. SYN American wild yam.

col·i·form ba·cil·li (kō′li-fōrm bă-sil′ī) Common name for *Escherichia coli* that is used as an indicator of fecal contamination of water, measured in terms of coliform count. Occasionally used to refer to all lactose-fermenting enteric bacteria.

co·lin·e·ar·i·ty (kō′lin-ē-ar′i-tē) **1.** Lying in a straight line. **2.** The phenomenon that the orderings of the corresponding elements of DNA, the RNA transcribed from it, and the amino acid sequence translated from the RNA are identical. [L. *collineo,* to direct in a straight line]

co·lip·ase (kō′lip-ās) A small protein in pancreatic juice that is essential for the efficient action of pancreatic lipase. [co- + lipase]

co·li·phage (kol′i-fāj) A bacteriophage with an affinity for one or another strain of *Escherichia coli.* [(*Escherichia*) *coli* + bacteriophage]

i **co·li·tis** (kō-lī′tis) Inflammation of the colon. See page B17. [G. *kōlon,* colon, + *-itis,* inflammation]

col·la (kol′ă) Plural of collum.

col·lab·or·a·tive ac·tions (kŏ-lab′ŏr-ă-tiv ak′shŭnz) Interdependent actions performed by the members of the health care team.

col·la·gen (kol′ă-jen) The major protein of the white fibers of connective tissue, cartilage, and bone; insoluble in water but can be altered to easily digestible, soluble gelatins by boiling in water, dilute acids, or alkalies. SEE ALSO collagen fiber. SYN ossein, osseine, ostein, osteine. [G. *koila,* glue, + *-gen,* producing]

col·lag·e·nase (kŏ-laj′ĕ-nās) A proteolytic enzyme that acts on one or more of the collagens.

col·la·gen dis·ease, col·la·gen-vas·cu·lar dis·ease (kol′ă-jen di-zēz′, kol′ă-jen-vas′kyū-lăr di-zēz′) A group of generalized diseases affecting connective tissue and frequently characterized by fibrinoid necrosis or vasculitis; in some collagen diseases, autoimmunization, particularly antinuclear antibodies, has been shown and circulating immune complexes are found. The term is not entirely acceptable because there is no evidence that collagen is primarily involved; "collagen" was once synonymous with "connective tissue" rather than describing a specific protein in that tissue. SEE ALSO connective-tissue disease.

col·la·gen fi·ber, col·lag·e·nous fi·ber (kol′ă-jen fī′bĕr, kŏ-laj′ĕ-nŭs fī′bĕr) An individual fiber that varies in diameter from less than 1 mcm to about 12 mcm and is composed of fibrils. The fibers, which are usually arranged in bundles, undergo some branching and are of indefinite length; chemically the fiber is a glycoprotein, collagen, which yields gelatin on boiling; they make up the principal element of irregular connective tissue, tendons, aponeuroses, and most ligaments, and occur in the matrix of cartilage and osseous tissue. SYN collagen fibre, white fiber (2).

collagen fibre [Br.] SYN collagen fiber.

col·la·gen·ic (kol′ă-jen′ik) SYN collagenous.

col·la·gen im·plan·ta·tion (kol′ă-jen im′plan-tā′shŭn) SYN collagen injection.

col·la·gen in·jec·tion (kol′ă-jen in-jek′shŭn) Correction of superficial soft tissue deformities, acne scars, or age-related skin changes by injection (implantation) of collagen; bovine collagen preparations are commonly used. Prior intradermal testing is necessary to exclude hypersensitivity. SYN collagen implantation.

col·lag·e·ni·za·tion (kŏ-laj′ĕ-nī-zā′shŭn) **1.** Replacement of tissues or fibrin by collagen. **2.** Synthesis of collagen by fibroblasts.

col·lag·e·no·lyt·ic (kŏ-laj′ĕ-nō-lit′ik) Causing the lysis of collagen, gelatin, and other proteins containing proline. [collagen + G. *lysis,* dissolving]

col·lag·e·nous (kŏ-laj′ĕ-nŭs) Producing or containing collagen. SYN collagenic.

col·lag·e·nous co·li·tis (kŏ-laj′ĕ-nŭs kō-lī′tis) The disorder as it occurs mostly in middle-aged women and characterized by persistent watery diarrhea and a deposit of a band of collagen beneath the basement membrane of the surface epithelium of the colon.

collagenous fibre [Br.] SYN collagenous fiber.

col·lapse (kŏ-laps′) **1.** A condition of extreme prostration. **2.** A state of profound physical depression. **3.** A falling together of the walls of a structure or the failure of a physiologic system. [L. *col-labor,* pp. *-lapsus,* to fall together]

col·lar (kol′ăr) **1.** A garment or part of a garment surrounding the neck. **2.** Any encircling band. [L. *collare,* fr. *collum,* neck]

col·lar bone (kol′ăr bōn) SYN clavicle.

col·lar-but·ton ab·scess (kol′ăr-bŭt′ŏn ab′ses) An abscess consisting of two cavities connected by a narrow channel, usually formed by rupture of an abscess through an overlying fascia. SYN shirt-stud abscess.

col·lat·er·al (kŏ-lat′ĕr-ăl) **1.** Indirect, subsidiary, or accessory to the main thing; side by side. **2.** A side branch of a nerve axon or blood vessel.

col·lat·er·al ar·ter·y (kŏ-lat′ĕr-ăl ahr′tĕr-ē) **1.** One that runs parallel with a nerve or other structure. **2.** One through which a collateral circulation is established.

col·lat·er·al cir·cu·la·tion (kŏ-lat′ĕr-ăl sĭr′kyū-lā′shŭn) Circulation maintained in small anastomosing vessels when the main vessel is obstructed.

col·lat·er·al dig·i·tal ar·ter·y (kŏ-lat′ĕr-ăl dij′i-tăl ahr′tĕr-ē) SYN proper palmar digital artery.

col·lat·er·al hy·per·e·mi·a (kŏ-lat′ĕr-ăl hī′pĕr-ē′mē-ă) Increased blood flow through abundant collateral channels when the circulation through the main artery to a part is arrested.

col·lat·er·al in·her·i·tance (kŏ-lat′ĕr-ăl in-her′i-tăns) The appearance of characters in collateral members of a family group, as when an uncle and a niece show the same character inherited from a common ancestor.

col·lat·er·al sul·cus (kŏ-lat′ĕr-ăl sŭl′kŭs) A long, deep sagittal fissure on the undersurface of the temporal lobe, marking the border between the fusiform gyrus laterally and the hippocampal and lingual gyri medially; the great depth of the collateral sulcus results in a bulging of the floor of the occipital and temporal horn of the lateral ventricle, the collateral eminence.

col·lat·er·al ves·sel (kŏ-lat′ĕr-ăl ves′ĕl) **1.** A branch of an artery running parallel with the parent trunk. **2.** A vessel that runs in parallel with another vessel, nerve, or other long structure.

col·lec·tion (kŏ-lek′shŭn) Procurement of a biologic specimen.

col·lec·tive un·con·scious (kŏ-lek′tiv ŭn-kon′shŭs) PSYCHOLOGY the combined engrams or memory potentials inherited from a person's phylogenetic past in C.G. Jung's theory.

Col·les fas·ci·a (kol′ēz fash′ē-ă) Superficial perineal fascia covering the external genitalia; attaches on each side to lower margin of ischiopubic ramus and to ischial tuberosity.

Col·les frac·ture (kol′ēz frak′shŭr) A fracture of the distal radius with displacement and/or angulation of the distal fragment dorsally.

col·lic·u·lar ar·ter·y (kŏ-lik′yū-lăr ahr′tĕr-ē) *Origin,* precommunicating part (P1 segment) of posterior cerebral artery; *distribution,* to superior and inferior colliculi (corpora quadrigemina) of tectum of midbrain. SYN arteria quadrigeminalis.

col·lic·u·lec·to·my (kŏ-lik′yū-lek′tŏ-mē) Excision of the colliculus seminalis.

col·lic·u·li·tis (kŏ-lik′yū-lī′tis) Inflammation of the urethra in the region of the colliculus seminalis.

col·lic·u·lus, pl. **col·lic·u·li** (kŏ-lik′yū-lŭs, -lī) A small elevation above the surrounding parts. [L. mound, dim. of *collis,* hill]

Col·lier sign (kol′yĕr sīn) Unilateral or bilateral lid retraction due to midbrain lesion; occurring at any age. SEE setting sun sign, Epstein sign.

col·lier's lung (kol′yĕrz lŭng) SYN anthracosis.

col·li·mate (kol′i-māt) To make parallel.

col·li·ma·tion (kol′i-mā′shŭn) **1.** RADIOLOGY the process of restricting and confining the x-ray beam to a given area. **2.** NUCLEAR MEDICINE restricting the detection of emitted radiations from a given area of interest. [L. *collineo,* to direct in a straight line]

col·li·ma·tor (kol′i-mā-tŏr) An appliance with blocks or jaws that restrict a beam of emitted radiation to a given area; composed of a high-absorption coefficient material such as lead or tungsten.

col·li·qua·tion (kol′i-kwā′zhŭn) **1.** Excessive discharge of fluid. **2.** Liquefaction in the process of necrosis. [L. *col-,* together, + *liquo,* pp. *liquatus,* to cause to melt]

col·liq·ua·tive (kŏ-lik′wă-tiv) Denoting or characteristic of colliquation.

Col·lis-Bel·sey fun·do·pli·ca·tion (kol′is-bel′sē fun′dō-pli-kā′shŭn) SYN Collis-Nissen fundoplication.

Col·lis-Nis·sen fun·do·pli·ca·tion (kol′is-nis′en fun′dō-pli-kā′shŭn) Operation for fundoplication in the presence of a shortened esophagus; the esophagus is lengthened by tubular stapling of the gastric cardia, and the fundoplication is then performed around this neoesophagus. SYN Collis-Belsey fundoplication.

col·loid (kol′oyd) **1.** Aggregates of atoms or molecules in a finely divided state (submicroscopic), dispersed in a gaseous, liquid, or solid medium, and resisting sedimentation, diffusion, and filtration, thus differing from precipitates. SEE ALSO hydrocolloid. **2.** Gluelike. **3.** A translucent, yellowish, homogeneous material of the consistency of glue, less fluid than mucoid or mucinoid, found in the cells and tissues in a state of colloid degeneration. SYN colloidin. **4.** The stored secretion within follicles of the thyroid gland. [G. *kolla,* glue, + *eidos,* appearance]

col·loid ac·ne (kol′oyd ak′nē) SYN colloid milium.

col·loi·dal (kol-oyd′ăl) Denoting or characteristic of a colloid.

col·loi·dal gel (kol-oyd′ăl jel) A colloid that has developed resistance to flow because of chemical or thermal change.

col·loi·dal so·lu·tion (kol-oyd′ăl sŏ-lū′shŭn) A dispersoid, emulsoid, or suspensoid.

col·loid bath (kol′oyd bath) A bath prepared by adding soothing agents such as sodium bicarbonate or oatmeal to the bath water to relieve skin irritation and pruritus.

col·loid car·ci·no·ma (kol′oyd kahr′si-nō′mă) SYN mucinous carcinoma.

col·loid de·gen·er·a·tion (kol′oyd dĕ-jen′ĕr-ā′shŭn) A degeneration similar to mucoid degeneration, in which the material is inspissated.

col·loid goi·ter (kol′oyd goy′tĕr) A form of goiter in which the contents of the follicles increase greatly, causing pressure atrophy of the epithelium so that the gelatinous matter predominates in the tumor.

col·loi·din (kol-oy′din) SYN colloid (3).

col·loid mil·i·um (kol′oyd mil′ē-ŭm) Yellow papules developing in sun-damaged skin of the head and backs of the hands, composed of colloid material in the dermis resembling amyloid but with a different ultrastructure. SYN colloid acne, colloid pseudomilium. [L. *milium,* millet]

col·loid pseu·do·mil·i·um (kol′oyd sū′dō-mil′ē-ŭm) SYN colloid milium.

col·lum, pl. **col·la** (kol′ŭm, -ă) SYN neck. [L.]

col·lum pan·cre·at·is (kol′ŭm pan-krē-ă′tis) [TA] SYN neck of pancreas.

col·lyr·i·um (kŏ-lir′ē-ŭm) An eyewash; originally, any preparation for the eye. [G. *kollyrion,* poultice, eye salve]

♻ **colo-** Combining form denoting the colon. [G. *kolon*]

col·o·bo·ma (kol′ō-bō′mă) Any defect, congenital, pathologic, or artificial, especially of the eye due to incomplete closure of the optic fissure. [G. *kolobōma,* lit., the part taken away in mutilation, fr. *koloboō,* to dock, mutilate]

col·o·bo·ma·tous mi·croph·thal·mi·a (kol′ō-bō′mă-tŭs mī′krof-thal′mē-ă) A congenital defect occurring along an embryonic fissure in a small eye, sometimes associated with cysts.

co·lo·cen·te·sis (kō′lō-sen-tē′sis) Puncture of the colon with a trochar or scalpel to relieve distention. SYN colopuncture. [colo- + G. *kentēsis,* a puncture]

co·lo·cho·le·cys·tos·to·my (kō′lō-kō-lĕ-sis-tos′tŏ-mē) SYN cholecystocolostomy.

co·lo·co·los·to·my (kō′lō-kō-los′tŏ-mē) Establishment of a communication between two noncontinuous segments of the colon. [colo- + colo- + G. *stoma,* mouth]

co·lo·en·ter·i·tis (kō′lō-en-tĕr-ī′tis) SYN enterocolitis.

co·lon (kō′lŏn) The division of the large intestine extending from the cecum to the rectum. [G. *kolon*]

co·lon·ic (kō-lon′ik) Relating to the colon.

co·lon·op·a·thy, **co·lop·a·thy** (kō′lŏn-op′ă-thē, kō-lop′ă-thē) Rarely used term for any disordered condition of the colon.

ℹ **co·lon·o·scope** (kō-lon′ō-skōp) An elongated endoscope, usually fiberoptic, used to examine the colon. See page B17.

ℹ **co·lon·os·co·py**, **co·los·co·py** (kō′lŏn-os′kŏ-pē, kō-los′kŏ-pē) Visual examination of the inner surface of the colon by means of a colonoscope. See page B17. [colon + G. *skopeō,* to view]

co·lon sig·moid·e·um (kō′lŏn sig-moy′dē-ŭm) [TA] SYN sigmoid colon.

col·o·ny (kol′ŏ-nē) **1.** A group of cells growing on a solid nutrient surface, each arising from the multiplication of an individual cell; a clone. **2.** A group of people with similar interests, living in a particular location or area. [L. *colonia,* a colony]

col·o·ny count (kol′ŏ-nē kownt) Enumeration of individual colonies in a bacterial culture.

col·o·ny-form·ing u·nit (CFU) (kol′ŏ-nē-fōrm′ing yū′nit) A stem cell in culture capable of proliferating and differentiating into more mature cells. If the CFU is committed to a specific cell line, it is designated by an additional letter to indicate its commitment; e.g., CFU-E is committed to erythroid maturation; CFU-GM is committed to granulocyte-monocyte maturation.

col·o·ny-stim·u·lat·ing fac·tors (CSF) (kol′ŏ-nē-stim′yū-lāt-ing fak′tŏrz) A group of glycoprotein growth factors regulating differentiation in myeloid cell lines.

col·o·pex·y (ko′lō-pek-sē) Attachment of a portion of the colon to the abdominal wall. [colo- + G. *pēxis,* fixation]

co·lo·pli·ca·tion (kō′lō-pli-kā′shŭn) Reduction of the lumen of a dilated colon by making folds or tucks in its walls. [colo- + Mod. L. *plica,* fold]

co·lo·proc·ti·tis (kō′lō-prok-tī′tis) Inflammation of both colon and rectum. SYN colorectitis.

[colo- + G. *prōktos,* anus (rectum), + *-itis,* inflammation]

co•lo•proc•tos•to•my (kō′lō-prok-tos′tŏ-mē) Establishment of a communication between the rectum and a discontinuous segment of the colon. SYN colorectostomy. [colo- + G. *prōktos,* anus (rectum), + *stoma,* mouth]

co•lop•to•sis, **co•lop•to•si•a** (kō′lop-tō′sis, -tō′sē-ă) Downward displacement, or prolapse, of the colon, especially of the transverse portion. [colo- + G. *ptōsis,* a falling]

co•lo•punc•ture (kō′lō-pŭngk′shŭr) SYN colocentesis.

col•or (kŏl′ŏr) **1.** That aspect of the appearance of objects and light sources that may be specified as to hue, lightness (brightness), and saturation. **2.** That portion of the visible (370–760 nm) electromagnetic spectrum specified as to wavelength, luminosity, and purity. SYN colour. [L.]

Col•o•ra•do tick fe•ver (kol′ŏr-ah′dō tik fē′vĕr) An infection caused by Colorado tick fever virus and transmitted to humans by *Dermacentor andersoni;* the symptoms are mild, there is no rash, fever is not excessive, and the disease is rarely fatal. SYN tick fever (5).

Col•o•ra•do tick fe•ver vi•rus (kol′ŏr-ah′dō tik fē′vĕr vī′rŭs) A virus of the genus *Orbivirus,* found in the Rocky Mountain region of the United States and transmitted by the tick *Dermacentor andersoni;* causes Colorado tick fever.

col•or ag•no•si•a (kŏl′ŏr ag-nō′zē-ă) Inability to name or identify colors; caused by lesions of the dominant occipital and temporal lobes. SYN colour agnosia.

col•or blind•ness (kŏl′ŏr blīnd′nĕs) Misleading term for anomalous or deficient color vision; complete color blindness is the absence of one of the primary cone pigments of the retina. SEE protanopia, deuteranopia, tritanopia. SYN colour blindness.

col•or chart (kŏl′ŏr chahrt) An assembly of chromatic samples used in checking color vision. SYN chromatic chart, colour chart.

co•lo•rec•tal (kō′lō-rek′tăl) Relating to the colon and rectum, or to the entire large bowel.

co•lo•rec•ti•tis (kō′lō-rek-tī′tis) SYN coloproctitis.

co•lo•rec•tos•to•my (kō′lō-rek-tos′tŏ-mē) SYN coloproctostomy.

col•ored vi•sion (VC) (kŏl′ĕrd vizh′ŭn) SYN chromatopsia. SYN coloured vision.

col•or hear•ing (kŏl′ŏr hēr′ing) A subjective perception of color produced by certain sounds. SYN colour hearing, pseudochromesthesia (2).

col•or•im•e•ter (kŏl′ŏr-im′ĕ-tĕr) An optic device for determining the color and/or intensity of the color of a liquid. SYN colourimeter.

col•or•i•met•ric (kŏl′ŏr-i-met′rik) Relating to colorimetry. SYN colourimetric.

col•or•im•e•try (kŏl′ŏr-im′ĕ-trē) A procedure for quantitative chemical analysis, based on comparison of the color developed in a solution of the test material with that in a standard solution; the two solutions are observed simultaneously in a colorimeter, and quantitated on the basis of the absorption of light. SYN colourimetry.

co•lor•rha•gi•a (kō′lō-rā′jē-ă) An abnormal discharge from the colon. [colo- + G. *rhēgnymi,* to burst forth]

co•lor•rha•phy (kō-lōr′ă-fē) Suture of the colon. [colo- + G. *rhaphē,* suture]

col•or sco•to•ma (kŏl′ŏr skō-tō′mă) An area of depressed color vision in the visual field. SYN colour scotoma.

col•or taste (kŏl′ŏr tāst) A form of synesthesia in which the color sense and taste are associated, with stimulation of either sense inducing a subjective sensation in the associated sense. SYN colour taste, pseudogeusesthesia.

co•lo•sig•moi•dos•to•my (kō′lō-sig-moy-dos′tŏ-mē) Establishment of an anastomosis between any other part of the colon and the sigmoid colon.

i **co•los•to•my** (kō-los′tŏ-mē) Establishment of an artificial cutaneous opening into the colon. See page 338. [colo- + G. *stoma,* mouth]

co•los•to•my bag (kō-los′tŏ-mē bag) A bag worn over an artificial anus to collect feces.

co•los•tric (kō-los′trik) Relating to the colostrum.

co•los•tror•rhe•a (kō′los-trōr-ē′ă) Abnormally profuse secretion of colostrum. SYN colostrorrhoea. [colostrum, + G. *rhoia,* flow]

colostrorrhoea [Br.] SYN colostrorrhea.

co•los•trum (kō-los′trŭm) A thin white opalescent fluid, the first milk secreted at the termination of pregnancy; it differs from the milk secreted later by containing more lactalbumin and lactoprotein; colostrum is also rich in antibodies which confer passive immunity to the newborn. SYN foremilk. [L.]

co•lot•o•my (kō-lot′ŏ-mē) Incision into the colon. [colo- + G. *tomē,* incision]

colour [Br.] SYN color.

colour agnosia [Br.] SYN color agnosia.

colour blindness [Br.] SYN color blindness.

colour chart [Br.] SYN color chart.

coloured vision [Br.] SYN colored vision.

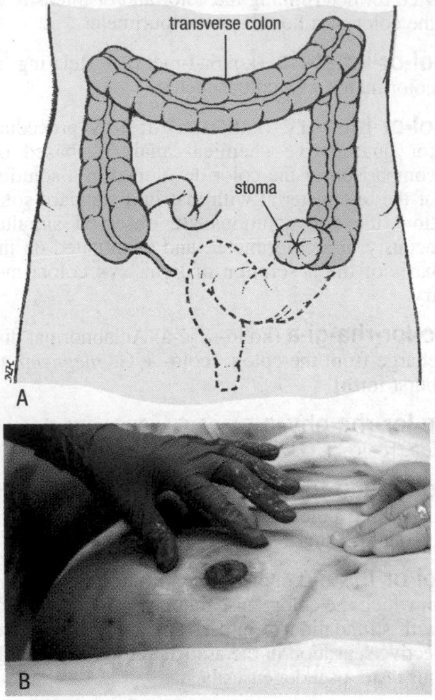

colostomy: (A) stoma opens on anterior abdominal wall; (B) stoma and peristomal skin

colour hearing [Br.] SYN color hearing.

colourimeter [Br.] SYN colorimeter.

colourimetric [Br.] SYN colorimetric.

colourimetry [Br.] SYN colorimetry.

Col·our In·dex (CI) (kŏl′ŏr in′deks) A publication concerned with the chemistry of dyes, with each listed dye identified by a five-digit Colour Index number, e.g., methylene blue is Colour Index 52015.

colour scotoma [Br.] SYN color scotoma.

colour taste [Br.] SYN color taste.

col·pa·tre·si·a (kol′pă-trē′zē-ă) SYN vaginal atresia. [colp- + G. *atrētos,* imperforate]

col·pec·ta·sis, **col·pec·ta·si·a** (kol-pek′tă-sis, -pek-tā′zē-ă) Distention of the vagina. [colp- + G. *aktasis,* stretching]

col·pec·to·my (kol-pek′tŏ-mē) SYN vaginectomy. [colp- + G. *ektomē,* excision]

colpo-, **colp-** Combining forms meaning the vagina. SEE ALSO vagino-. [G. *kolpos,* fold or hollow]

col·po·cele (kol′pō-sēl) **1.** A hernia projecting into the vagina. SYN vaginocele. **2.** SYN colpoptosis. [colpo- + G. *kēlē,* hernia]

col·po·clei·sis (kol′pō-klī′sis) Operation for obliterating the lumen of the vagina. [colpo- + G. *kleisis,* closure]

col·po·cys·to·cele (kol′pō-sis′tō-sēl) SYN cystocele. [colpo- + G. *kystis,* bladder, + *kēlē,* hernia]

col·po·cys·to·plas·ty (kol′pō-sis′tō-plas-tē) Plastic surgery to repair the vesicovaginal wall. [colpo- + G. *kystis,* bladder, + *plastos,* formed]

col·po·dyn·i·a (kol′pō-din′ē-ă) SYN vaginodynia. [colpo- + G. *odynē,* pain]

col·po·mi·cros·co·py (kol′pō-mī-kros′kŏ-pē) Direct observation and study of cells in the vagina and cervix magnified in vivo, in the undisturbed tissue, by means of a colpomicroscope.

col·po·per·i·ne·o·plas·ty (kol′pō-par-i-nē′ō-plas-tē) SYN vaginoperineoplasty. [colpo- + perineum, + G. *plastos,* formed]

col·po·per·i·ne·or·rha·phy (kol′pō-per-i-nē-ōr′ă-fē) SYN vaginoperineorrhaphy. [colpo- + perineum, + G. *rhaphē,* sewing]

col·po·pexy (kol′pō-pek-sē) SYN vaginofixation. [colpo- + G. *pēxis,* fixation]

col·po·plas·ty (kol′pō-plas-tē) SYN vaginoplasty. [colpo- + G. *plastos,* formed]

col·po·poi·e·sis (kol′pō-poy-ē′sis) Surgical construction of a vagina. [colpo- + G. *poiēsis,* a making]

col·po·pto·sis, **col·po·pto·si·a** (kol′pō-tō′sis, kol′pō-tō′sē-ă) Prolapse of the vaginal walls. SYN colpocele (2). [colpo- + G. *ptōsis,* a falling]

col·por·rha·gi·a (kol′pōr-ā′jē-ă) A vaginal hemorrhage. [colpo-+ G. *rhēgnymi,* to burst forth]

col·por·rha·phy (kol-pōr′ă-fē) Repair of a rupture of the vagina by excision and suturing of the edges of the tear. [colpo- + G. *rhaphē,* suture]

col·por·rhex·is (kol′pō-rek′sis) Tearing of the vaginal wall. [colpo- + G. *rhēxis,* rupture]

col·po·scope (kol′pō-skōp) Endoscopic instrument that magnifies cells of the vagina and cervix in vivo to allow direct observation and study of these tissues.

col·pos·co·py (kol-pos′kŏ-pē) Examination of vagina and cervix by means of an endoscope. [colpo- + G. *skopeō,* to view]

col·po·spasm (kol′pō-spazm) Spasmodic contraction of the vagina.

col·po·stats (kōl′pō-stats) SYN ovoids.

col·po·ste·no·sis (kol′pō-stĕ-nō′sis) Narrowing of the lumen of the vagina. [colpo- + G. *stenōsis,* narrowing]

col·po·ste·not·o·my (kol′pō-stĕ-not′ō-mē)

Surgical correction of a colpostenosis. [colpo- + G. *stenōsis,* narrowing, + *tomē,* incision]

col·po·sus·pen·sion (kol′pō-sŭs-pen′shŭn) Suture fixation of the lateral vaginal fornix to Cooper ligament on each side, as a modification and enhancement of the standard Marshall-Marchetti-Kranz urethrovesical suspension for stress urinary incontinence due to cystocele. [colpo- + suspension]

col·pot·o·my (kol-pot′ŏ-mē) SYN vaginotomy. [colpo- + G. *tomē,* incision]

col·po·xe·ro·sis (kol′pō-zē-rō′sis) Abnormal dryness of the vaginal mucous membrane. [colpo- + G. *xērōsis,* dryness]

col·ti·vi·rus (kol′tē-vī-rus) A genus in the family Reoviridae that causes Colorado tick fever. [*Col*orado *ti*ck fever + virus]

colts·foot (kōlts′fut) (*Tussilago farfara*) Purportedly useful in infections of upper respiratory tract. Plant contains toxic pyrrolizidine alkaloids.

col·u·mel·la, pl. **col·u·mel·lae** (kol′yū-mel′ă, -mel′ē) **1.** A small column. SYN columnella. **2.** In fungi, a sterile invagination of a sporangium, as in Zygomycetes. [L. dim. of *columna,* column]

col·umn (kol′ŭm) **1.** An anatomic part or structure in the form of a pillar or cylindric funiculus. SYN columna [TA]. SEE ALSO fascicle. **2.** A vertical object (usually cylindric), mass, or formation. [L. *columna*]

co·lum·na, gen. and pl. **co·lum·nae** (kō-lŭm′nă, -nē) [TA] SYN column (1). [L.]

co·lum·nae a·na·les (kō-lŭm′nē a-nā′lēz) [TA] SYN anal columns.

co·lum·nae gri·se·ae (kō-lŭm′nē gris′ē-ē) [TA] SYN gray columns.

co·lum·nae re·na·les (kō-lŭm′nē rē-nā′lēz) [TA] SYN renal columns.

co·lum·nar ep·i·the·li·um (kō-lŭm′năr ep′i-thē′lē-ŭm) Epithelium formed of a single layer of prismatic cells taller than they are wide.

co·lum·na ver·te·bra·lis (kō-lŭm′nă vĕr-tē-brā′lis) [TA] SYN vertebral column.

col·umn chro·ma·tog·ra·phy (kol′ŭm krō′mă-tog′ră-fē) A form of partition, adsorption, ion exchange, or affinity chromatography in which one phase is liquid (aqueous) flowing down a column packed with the second phase, a solid.

co·lum·nel·la, pl. **col·um·nel·lae** (kō′lŭm-nel′ă, -nel′ē) SYN columella (1). [L. dim. of *columna,* a column; another form of *columella*]

col·umn of for·nix (kol′ŭm fōr′niks) That part of the fornix that curves down in front of the thalamus and the interventricular foramen of Monro, then continues through the hypothalamus to the mammillary body; consisting primarily of fibers originating in the hippocampus and subiculum, the column of fornix is the direct continuation of the body of the fornix.

♻ **com-** SEE con-.

co·ma (kō′mă) **1.** A state of profound unconsciousness from which one cannot be roused; may result from trauma, disease, or the action of an ingested toxic substance or of one formed in the body. [G. *kōma,* deep sleep, trance] **2.** An aberration of spheric lenses; occurring in cases of oblique incidence (e.g., the image of a point becomes comet-shaped). [G. *kome,* hair] **3.** SYN coma aberration.

co·ma ab·er·ra·tion (kō′mă ab-ĕr-ā′shŭn) The distortion of image formation created when a bundle of light rays enters an optic system not parallel to the optic axis. SYN coma (3). [G. *komē*, hair, foliage]

co·ma scale (kō′mă skāl) A clinical scale to assess impaired consciousness; assessment may include motor responsiveness, verbal performance, and eye opening, as in the Glasgow (Scotland) coma scale, or the same three items and dysfunction of cranial nerves, as in the Maryland (U.S.) coma scale.

co·ma·tose (kō′mă-tōs) In a state of coma.

comb flow·er (kōm flow′ĕr) SYN echinacea.

com·bined glau·co·ma (kŏm-bīnd′ glaw-kō′mă) Glaucoma with angle-closure and open-angle mechanisms in the same eye.

Com·bined Health In·for·ma·tion Da·ta·base (CHID) (kŏm-bīnd′ helth in′fōr-mā′shŭn dā′tă-bās) Bibliographic database produced by health-related agencies of U.S. federal government; database provides titles, abstracts, and availability information for health information and health education resources.

com·bined im·mu·no·de·fi·cien·cy (kŏm-bīnd′ im′yū-nō-dĕ-fish′ĕn-sē) Immunodeficiency of both the B-lymphocytes and T-lymphocytes.

com·bined meth·ods (kŏm-bīnd′ meth′ŏdz) Varying combinations of the oral auditory method and the manual visual method of education of deaf children. SEE ALSO oral auditory method, manual visual method, total communication.

com·bined preg·nan·cy (kŏm-bīnd′ preg′năn-sē) Coexisting uterine and ectopic pregnancy.

com·bus·ti·ble (kŏm-bŭs′ti-bĕl) Capable of combustion.

com·bus·tion (kŏm-bŭs′chŭn) Burning; rapid oxidation of any substance accompanied by the production of heat and light. [L. *comburo,* pp. *-bustus,* to burn up]

Com·by sign (kom′bē sīn) An early sign of

measles, consisting of thin, whitish patches on the gums and buccal mucous membrane, formed of desquamating epithelial cells.

com•e•do, pl. **com•e•dos**, **com•e•do•nes** (kom′ĕ-dō, -dōz, -dō′nēz) A dilated hair follicle infundibulum filled with keratin squamae, bacteria, particularly *Propionibacterium acnes*, and sebum; the primary lesion of acne vulgaris. See page B13. [L. a glutton, fr. *com-edo,* to eat up]

com•e•do•car•ci•no•ma (kom′ĕ-dō-kahr-si-nō′mă) Form of carcinoma of the breast or other organ in which plugs of necrotic malignant cells may be expressed from the ducts.

com•e•do•gen•ic (kom′ĕ-dō-jen′ik) Tending to promote the formation of comedones. [comedo + G. *genesis,* production]

co•mes, pl. **com•i•tes** (kō′mēz, kom′i-tēz) A blood vessel accompanying another vessel or a nerve; the veins accompanying an artery, often two in number, are called venae comitantes or venae comites. [L. a companion, fr. *com-,* together, + *eo,* pp. *itus,* to go]

com•fort mea•sures on•ly (kŏm′fŏrt mezh′ ūrz ōn′lē) An order that supports a dignified and comfortable natural death without life-sustaining intervention.

com•fort zone (kŏm′fŏrt zōn) The temperature range between 28–30°C at which the naked body is able to maintain the heat balance without either shivering or sweating; in the clothed body, the range is from 13–21°C.

com•i•tant ar•ter•y of me•di•an nerve (kom′i-tănt ahr′tĕr-ē mē′dē-ăn nĕrv) SYN median artery.

com•i•tant stra•bis•mus (kom′i-tănt stră-biz′ mŭs) A condition in which the degree of strabismus is the same in all directions of gaze.

com•ma ba•cil•lus (kom′ă bă-sil′ŭs) SYN *Vibrio cholerae.*

com•mand hal•lu•ci•na•tion (kŏ-mand′ hă-lū′si-nā′shŭn) A symptom, usually auditory but sometimes visual, consisting of a message, from no external source, to do something.

com•man•do pro•ce•dure (kŏ-man′dō prŏ-sē′jŭr) An operation for malignant tumors of the floor of the oral cavity, involving resection of portions of the mandible in continuity with the oral lesion and radical neck dissection.

com•men•sal (kŏ-men′săl) **1.** Pertaining to or characterized by commensalism. **2.** An organism participating in commensalism.

com•men•sal•ism (kŏ-men′săl-izm) A symbiotic relationship in which one species derives benefit and the other is unharmed. Cf. metabiosis, mutualism, parasitism. [L. *con-,* with, together, + *mensa,* table]

com•mi•nut•ed (kom′i-nū′tĕd) Broken into several pieces; denoting especially a fractured bone. [L. *com-minuo,* pp. *-minutus,* to make smaller, break into pieces, fr. *minor,* less]

com•mi•nut•ed frac•ture (kom′i-nū′tĕd frak′ shŭr) A fracture in which the bone is broken into pieces.

com•mi•nu•tion (kom′i-nū′shŭn) A breaking into several pieces.

Com•mis•sion E (kŏ-mish′ŭn) A German federal study set up to analyze and make consistent the contents of herbals and to analyze and approve the use of these herbals medicinally. No such research has been done on anything like a similar scale in the United States. The monographs of this commission have been translated into English, providing clinical proof about the efficacy and safety (or lack thereof) of the herbals and botanicals that were considered.

Com•mis•sion on Ac•cred•i•ta•tion of Re•ha•bil•i•ta•tion Fa•cil•i•ties (C.A.R.F.) (kŏ-mish′ŏn ă-kred′i-tā′shŭn rē′hă-bil′i-tā′shŭn fă-sil′i-tēz) A voluntary association dedicated to maintaining standards for rehabilitation facilities. SEE ALSO accreditation.

com•mis•sur•a, gen. and pl. **com•mis•sur•ae** (kom-i-syūr′ă, -syūr′ē) [TA] SYN commissure. [L. a joining together, seam, fr. *com- mitto,* to send together, combine]

com•mis•sur•ae su•pra•op•ti•cae (kom-i-syūr′ē sū-pră-op′ti-sē) [TA] The commissural fibers that lie above and behind the optic chiasm. SYN supraoptic commissures.

com•mis•sur•al (kom-i-shŭr′ăl) Relating to a commissure.

com•mis•sur•al fi•bers (kom-i-shŭr′ăl fī′bĕrz) Nerve fibers crossing the midline and connecting two corresponding parts or regions of the nervous system.

com•mis•sur•a pos•te•ri•or ce•re•bri (kom-i-syūr′ă pos-tēr′ē-ŏr ser′ĕ-brī) [TA] SYN posterior cerebral commissure.

com•mis•sure (kom′i-shŭr) **1.** Angle or corner of the eye, lips, or labia. **2.** A bundle of nerve fibers passing from one side to the other in the brain or spinal cord. SYN commissura [TA].

com•mis•sur•ot•o•my (kom′i-shŭr-ot′ŏ-mē) **1.** Surgical division of any commissure, fibrous band, or ring using surgery or a balloon catheter technique. **2.** SYN midline myelotomy.

com•mon an•ti•gen (kom′ŏn an′ti-jen) Cross-reacting antigen (epitope), a common antigen that occurs in two or more different molecules or organisms. SYN heterogenic enterobacterial antigen.

com•mon a•tri•um (kom′ŏn ā′trē-ŭm) A single abnormal atrium in a three-chambered heart in which the interatrial septum is absent. SYN cor triloculare biventriculare.

com•mon ba•sal vein (kom′ŏn bā′săl vān) The tributary to the inferior pulmonary vein (right and left) that receives blood from the superior and inferior basal veins.

com•mon bile duct (kom′ŏn bīl dŭkt) A duct formed by the union of the hepatic and cystic ducts; it discharges at the duodenal papilla.

com•mon buck•thorn (kom′ŏn bŭk′thōrn) SYN buckthorn.

com•mon ca•rot•id ar•ter•y (kom′ŏn kă-rot′id ahr′tĕr-ē) *Origin*, right from brachiocephalic, left from arch of aorta; runs upward in the neck and divides opposite upper border of thyroid cartilage (C-4 vertebral level) into *terminal branches*, external and internal carotid. SYN arteria carotis communis.

com•mon co•chle•ar ar•ter•y (kom′ŏn kok′lē-ăr ahr′tĕr-ē) *Origin*, as a terminal branch, with the anterior vestibular artery, of the labyrinthine artery; *distribution*, runs in the cochlear axis of modiolus serving the spiral ganglia; sends the proper cochlear artery to the cochlear duct and supplies the apical two turns of the spiral modiolar artery. SYN arteria cochlearis communis [TA].

com•mon cold (kom′ŏn kōld) SYN cold.

com•mon fa•cial vein (kom′ŏn fā′shăl vān) A short vessel formed by the union of the facial vein and the retromandibular vein, emptying into the jugular vein; considered to be a continuation of the facial vein in the NA.

com•mon fib•u•lar nerve (kom′ŏn fib′yū-lăr nĕrv) Terminal division of the sciatic nerve, diverging from the tibial nerve at the upper end of the popliteal fossa, then coursing with the biceps tendon along the lateral portion of the popliteal space to wind around the neck of the fibula where it divides into the superficial and deep peroneal nerves. The common peroneal nerve, or its deep branch, is the most commonly injured nerve, being located in a lateral subcutaneous position at the fibular neck; a lesion causes a loss of ability to dorsiflex the foot ("foot drop"). SYN common peroneal nerve, nervus fibularis communis, nervus peroneus communis.

com•mon he•pat•ic ar•ter•y (kom′ŏn hĕ-pat′ik ahr′tĕr-ē) *Origin*, celiac; *branches*, right gastric, gastroduodenal, and proper hepatic. SYN arteria hepatica communis.

com•mon he•pat•ic duct (kom′ŏn hĕ-pat′ik dŭkt) The part of the biliary duct system that is formed by the confluence of the right and left hepatic ducts. At the porta hepatis it is joined by the cystic duct to become the bile duct.

com•mon il•i•ac ar•ter•y (kom′ŏn il′ē-ak ahr′tĕr-ē) One of two terminal branches of the abdominal aorta; anterior to the sacroiliac joint at the level of the sacral promontory, it bifurcates to form the internal iliac and the external iliac. SYN arteria iliaca communis.

com•mon in•ter•os•se•ous ar•ter•y (kom′ŏn in′tĕr-os′ē-ŭs ahr′tĕr-ē) *Origin*, ulnar; *branches*, anterior and posterior interosseous. SYN arteria interossea communis.

com•mon mi•graine (kom′ŏn mī′grān) A form of migraine headache without the visual prodrome, which is not limited on one side of the head but nevertheless is recognizable as migraine because of the stereotyped course; the tendency to nausea, photophobia, and phonophobia; and the relief produced by sleep.

com•mon pal•mar dig•i•tal ar•ter•y (kom′ŏn pahl′măr dij′i-tăl ahr′tĕr-ē) One of three arteries arising from the superficial palmar arch and running to the interdigital clefts where each divides into two proper palmar digital arteries. SYN arteria digitalis palmaris communis.

com•mon pal•mar dig•i•tal nerve (kom′ŏn pahl′măr dij′i-tăl nĕrv) Four nerves in the palm that send branches (proper palmar digital nerves) to adjacent sides of two digits; three are branches of the median nerve, the other the ulnar nerve. SYN nervi digitales palmares communes.

com•mon path•way of co•ag•u•la•tion (kom′ŏn path′wā kō-ag′yū-lā′shŭn) A part of the coagulation system where the intrinsic and extrinsic pathways converge to activate factor X. Coagulation factors X, V, II, and fibrinogen are part of this pathway; both the APTT and PT measure the integrity of this system.

com•mon per•o•ne•al nerve (kom′ŏn per′ō-nē′ăl nĕrv) SYN common fibular nerve.

com•mon plan•tar dig•i•tal nerves (kom′ŏn plan′tahr dij′i-tăl nĕrvz) Three nerves derived from the medial plantar nerve and the other the lateral plantar nerve that supply the skin overlying the metatarsals and terminate as proper plantar digital nerves to the side of each toe. SYN nervi digitales plantares communes.

com•mon ten•di•nous ring of ex•tra•oc•u•lar mus•cles (kom′ŏn ten′di-nŭs ring eks-tră-ok′yū-lăr mŭs′ĕlz) A fibrous ring that surrounds the optic canal and the medial part of the superior orbital fissure. It gives origin to the four rectus muscles of the eye and is partially fused with the sheath of the optic nerve. SYN anulus of Zinn.

com•mo•ti•o cor•dis (kō-mō′shē-ō kōr′dis) A disturbance in the electrical activity of the heart induced by blunt trauma to the anterior chest (as in athletic injuries, steering wheel injuries, and criminal assaults) without demonstrable structural damage. It can lead to ventricular fibrillation or other fatal arrhythmias and is among the more frequent causes of sudden death in athletes. [L. agitation of the heart]

com•mo•ti•o ret•i•nae (kō-mō′shē-ō ret′in-ē) Disruption or disorganization of photoreceptors caused by edema resulting from blunt trauma.

SEE ALSO Berlin edema. [L., agitation of the retina]

com•mu•ni•ca•bil•i•ty (kŏ-myū′ni-kă-bil′i-tē) The ability of a disease to be transmitted from one host to another.

com•mu•ni•ca•ble (kŏ-myūn′i-kă-bĕl) Capable of being communicated or transmitted; said especially of disease.

com•mu•ni•ca•ble dis•ease (kŏ-myūn′i-kă-bĕl di-zēz′) Any disorder that is transmissible by infection or contagion directly or indirectly or through the agency of a vector.

com•mu•ni•cat•ing ar•ter•y (kŏ-myūn′i-kāt-ing ahr′tĕr-ē) An artery that connects two larger arteries.

com•mu•ni•cat•ing branch (kŏ-myū′n-i-kāt-ing branch) A bundle of nerve fibers passing from one named nerve to join another.

com•mu•ni•cat•ing branch of fib•u•lar ar•ter•y (kŏ-myūn′i-kāt-ing branch fib′yū-lăr ahr′tĕr-ē) The communicating branch of the fibular (peroneal) artery.

com•mu•ni•cat•ing branch of in•ter•nal la•ryn•ge•al nerve with re•cur•rent lar•yn•ge•al nerve (kŏ-myūn′i-kāt-ing branch in-tĕr′năl lă-rin′jē-ăl nĕrv rē-kŭr′ĕnt lă-rin′jē-ăl nĕrv) Branch of internal branch of superior laryngeal nerve communicating with the recurrent laryngeal nerve in the wall of the laryngopharynx supplying sensory fibers to the latter.

com•mu•ni•cat•ing hy•dro•ceph•a•lus (kŏ-myūn′i-kāt-ing hī′drō-sef′ă-lŭs) Type of hydrocephalus in which there is an abnormality in cerebrospinal fluid absorption; there is no obstruction to cerebrospinal fluid flow in the ventricular system or where the cerebrospinal fluid passes into the vertebral canal.

com•mu•ni•ca•tion (kŏ-myūn′i-kā′shŭn) **1.** An opening or connecting passage between two structures. **2.** ANATOMY a joining or connecting; said of fibrous, solid structures, e.g., tendons and nerves. **3.** The exchange of information between individuals using symbol systems such as spoken language or writing but also including elements such as icons, gestures, tone of voice, and facial expression. [L. *communicatio*]

com•mu•ni•ca•tion board (kŏ-myūn′i-kā′shŭn bōrd) Any arrangement of letters, words, symbols, or pictures designed to aid a person whose expressive language ability is inadequate. SEE augmentative and alternative communication. SYN conversation board, language board.

com•mu•ni•ca•tion dis•or•der (kŏ-myūn′i-kā′shŭn dis-ōr′dĕr) Any impairment of hearing, language, or speech that interferes with the ability to transmit or receive linguistic information. SYN communicative disorder.

com•mu•ni•ca•tion-in•ter•ac•tions skills (kŏ-myūn′i-kā′shŭn in-tĕr-ak′shŭnz skilz) The ability to convey intentions and needs and to socially interact with other people.

com•mu•ni•ca•tive dis•or•der (kŏ-myūn′i-kă-tiv dis-ōr′dĕr) SYN communication disorder.

com•mu•ni•ty (kŏ-myūn′i-tē) A group of people united by some common feature or shared interest; the social context in which professional services are provided. A community may be united by physical or geographic factors, by one or more common characteristics such as age, gender, developmental level, culture, or health or disability status, or by a shared perspective. SEE ALSO community-based practice. [L. *communitas,* fellowship, fr. *communis,* common]

com•mu•ni•ty-based prac•tice (CBP) (kŏ-myūn′i-tē-bāst prak′tis) Provision of skilled therapy services within a client's own home or community, with the requirement that the therapist take into consideration the lifestyle of the client and the cultural and social characteristics of the client's community. Typically such a practice provides expert knowledge that is not otherwise available to the client and ends when the needs calling it into existence have been met.

com•mu•ni•ty health nurs•ing (kŏ-myūn′i-tē helth nŭrs′ing) Health care divided into public health and home care nursing; home care nursing provides intravenous therapy and wound care; public health nursing focuses on health promotion and illness prevention. Programs such as administration of flu vaccine in shopping centers are carried out by public health nurses; allows nurses a more independent practice than offered in a hospital.

com•mu•ni•ty med•i•cine (kŏ-myū-ni-tē med′i-sin) The study of health and disease in a defined community; the practice of medicine in such a setting.

com•mu•ni•ty men•tal health cen•ter (kŏ-myūn′i-tē men′tăl helth sen′tĕr) A mental health treatment center located in a neighborhood catchment area close to the homes of patients, introduced in the 1960s under new U.S. federal legislation designed to replace the large state hospitals, which usually were located in remote rural areas; features include offering a series of comprehensive services by one or more members of the four mental health care professions, provision of continuity of care, participation of consumers in the centers, community location to provide accessibility, a combination of indirect or preventive and direct services, the use of program-centered as well as case-centered consultation, a requirement for program evaluation, and various linkages to a variety of health and human services.

Com•mu•ni•ty Pe•ri•o•don•tal In•dex of Treat•ment Needs (CPITN) (kŏ-myūn′i-tē per′ē-ō-don′tăl in′deks trēt′mĕnt nēdz) An assessment of periodontal treatment needs that divides the mouth into sextants and uses a standard probe for examinations.

com•mu•ni•ty psy•chi•a•try (kŏ-myūn′i-tē sī-kī′ă-trē) Psychiatry focusing on the detection, prevention, early treatment, and rehabilitation of patients with emotional disorders and social deviance as they develop in the community.

com•mu•ni•ty psy•chol•o•gy (kŏ-myūn′i-tē sī-kol′ŏ-jē) The application of psychology to community programs, e.g., in the schools, correctional and welfare systems, and community mental health care centers.

Co•mol•li sign (kō-mōl′lē sīn) In cases of fracture of the scapula, a typical triangular cushion-like swelling appears, corresponding to the outline of the scapula.

co•mor•bid•i•ty (kō-mōr-bid′i-tē) **1.** A concomitant but unrelated pathologic or disease process. **2.** EPIDEMIOLOGY coexistence of two or more disease processes. [co- + L. *morbidus,* diseased]

com•pact bone (kŏm-pakt′ bōn) The compact, noncancellous portion of bone that consists largely of concentric lamellar osteons and interstitial lamellae. SYN substantia compacta [TA], compact substance.

com•pact sub•stance (kŏm-pakt′ sub′stăns) SYN compact bone.

com•par•a•tive a•nat•o•my (kŏm-par′ă-tiv ă-nat′ŏ-mē) The comparative study of animal structure with regard to homologous organs or parts.

com•par•a•tive pa•thol•o•gy (kŏm-par′ă-tiv pă-thol′ŏ-jē) The pathology of diseases of animals, especially in relation to human pathology.

com•par•ti•men•tum (kom-pahr-ti-men′tŭm) [TA] SYN compartment (1).

com•part•ment (kŏm-pahrt′mĕnt) **1.** Partitioned off portion of a larger bound space; a separate section or chamber; the compartments of the limbs are bound deeply by bones and intermuscular septa and superficially by deep fascia and generally are not in communication with one another, and thus infection or increased pathologic pressure may be limited to a compartment; muscles contained within the compartments of the limbs share similar functions and innervation. SYN compartimentum [TA]. **2.** A separate division; specifically, a structural or biochemical portion of a cell that is separated from the rest of the cell.

com•part•ment syn•drome (kŏm-pahrt′mĕnt sin′drōm) Condition in which increased intramuscular pressure in a confined anatomic space brought on by overactivity or trauma impedes blood flow and function of tissues within that space. SYN compression syndrome (2).

com•pen•sat•ed ac•i•do•sis (kom′pĕn-sāt-ĕd as′i-dō′sis) An acidosis in which the pH of body fluids is normal; compensation is achieved by respiratory or renal mechanisms.

com•pen•sat•ed al•ka•lo•sis (kom′pĕn-sāt-ĕd al′hă-lō′sis) Disorder in which there is a change in bicarbonate but the pH of body fluids approaches normal; respiratory alkalosis may be compensated by increased production of metabolic acids or increased renal excretion of bicarbonate; metabolic alkalosis is rarely compensated by hypoventilation.

com•pen•sat•ing curve (kom′pĕn-sāt′ing kŭrv) The curve of Spee applied to dentures. SEE ALSO curve of Spee.

com•pen•sa•tion (kom′pĕn-sā′shŭn) **1.** A process in which a tendency for a change in a given direction is counteracted by another change so that the original change is not evident. **2.** An unconscious mechanism by which one tries to make up for fancied or real deficiencies. [L. *com-penso,* pp. *-atus,* to weigh together, counterbalance]

com•pen•sa•tion neu•ro•sis (kom′pĕn-sā′shŭn nūr-ō′sis) The development of symptoms of neurosis believed to be motivated by the desire for, and hope of, monetary or interpersonal gain.

com•pen•sa•to•ry (kŏm-pen′să-tōr-ē) Providing compensation; making up for a deficiency or loss.

com•pen•sa•to•ry cir•cu•la•tion (kŏm-pen′să-tōr-ē sĭr′kyū-lā′shŭn) Circulation established in dilated collateral vessels when the main vessel of the part is obstructed.

com•pen•sa•to•ry hy•per•tro•phy (kŏm-pen′să-tōr-ē hī-pĕr′trō-fē) Increase in size of an organ or part of an organ or tissue, when called on to do additional work or perform the work of destroyed tissue or of a paired organ. SYN complementary hypertrophy.

com•pen•sa•to•ry move•ment (kŏm-pen′să-tōr-ē mūv′mĕnt) Movement used habitually to achieve functional motor skills when a normal movement pattern has not been established or is unavailable (e.g., lateral trunk flexion and exaggerated weight shift to substitute for incomplete shoulder flexion while reaching above shoulder level or external rotation of the shoulder that extends the elbow if the triceps muscle is insufficient).

com•pen•sa•to•ry pause (kŏm-pen′să-tōr-ē pawz) The pause following an extrasystole, when the pause is long enough to compensate for the prematurity of the extrasystole; the short cycle ending with the extrasystole plus the pause following the extrasystole together equal two of the regular cycles.

com•pen•sa•to•ry pol•y•cy•the•mi•a (kŏm-pen′să-tōr-ē pol′ē-sī-thē′mē-ă) A secondary increase in red blood cell count resulting from anoxia (e.g., in congenital heart disease, pulmonary emphysema, or prolonged residence at a high elevation).

com·pe·tence (kom′pĕ-tĕns) **1.** The quality of being skilled or capable of performing an allotted function. **2.** The normal tight closure of a cardiac valve. **3.** The ability of a group of embryonic cells to respond to an inducer. **4.** The ability of a (bacterial) cell to take up free DNA, which may lead to transformation. **5.** PSYCHIATRY the mental ability to distinguish right from wrong and to manage one's own affairs, or to assist one's counsel in a legal proceeding. **6.** The state of reactivity of a cell, tissue, or organism that allows it to respond to certain stimuli. [Fr. *competence,* fr. L.L. *competentia,* congruity]

com·pe·tence test·ing (kom′pĕ-tĕns test′ing) SYN skills validation.

com·pe·tent (kom′pĕ-tĕnt) Capable or qualified; able to perform a task or function. [L. *competo,* to be suitable]

com·pet·i·tive bind·ing as·say (kŏm-pet′i-tive bīnd′ing as′ā) An assay in which a binder competes for labeled versus unlabeled ligand; following separation of free and bound ligand, the ligand is quantitated by relating bound and unbound ratios to known standards. SEE ALSO enzyme-linked immunosorbent assay, immunoassay, enzyme-multiplied immunoassay technique, radioimmunoassay.

com·pet·i·tive in·hi·bi·tion (kŏm-pet′i-tiv in′hi-bish′ŭn) Blocking of the action of an enzyme by a compound that binds to the free enzyme, preventing the substrate from binding and thus preventing the enzyme from acting on that substrate. SYN selective inhibition.

com·plaint (kŏm-plānt′) A disorder, disease, or symptom, or the description of it. [O. Fr. *complainte,* fr. L. *complango,* to lament]

com·ple·ment (kom′plĕ-mĕnt) The thermolabile substance, normally present in serum, which is destructive to certain bacteria and other cells sensitized by a specific complement-fixing antibody. Complement is a group of at least 20 distinct serum proteins, the activity of which is affected by a series of interactions resulting in enzymatic cleavages and which can follow one or the other of at least two pathways. In the case of immune hemolysis (classical pathway), the complex comprises nine components (designated C1–C9) that react in a definite sequence and the activation of which is usually effected by the antigen-antibody complex; only the first seven components are involved in chemotaxis, and only the first four are involved in immune adherence or phagocytosis or are fixed by conglutinins. An alternative pathway (see properdin system) may be activated by factors other than antigen-antibody complexes and involves components other than C1, C4, and C2 in the activation of C3. SEE ALSO component of complement. [L. *complementum,* that which completes, fr. *com-pleo,* to fill up]

com·ple·men·tal air (kom′plĕ-ment′ăl ār) SYN inspiratory reserve volume.

com·ple·men·tar·i·ty (kom′plĕ-men-tār′i-tē) **1.** The degree of base-pairing between two sequences of DNA and/or RNA molecules. **2.** The degree of affinity, or fit, of antigen and antibody combining sites.

com·ple·men·ta·ry air (kom′plĕ-ment′tăr-ē ār) SYN inspiratory capacity.

com·ple·men·ta·ry DNA (cDNA) (kom′plĕ-men′tăr-ē) **1.** Single-stranded DNA that is complementary to messenger RNA. **2.** DNA that has been synthesized from mRNA by the action of reverse transcriptase.

com·ple·men·ta·ry hy·per·tro·phy (kom′plĕ-men′tăr-ē hī-pĕr′trō-fē) SYN compensatory hypertrophy.

com·ple·men·ta·ry med·i·cine (kom′plĕ-men′tăr-ē med′i-sin) A general term for therapeutic methods, some ancient and widely practiced, to treat nonemergency conditions from a holistic and noninvasive approach. Increasingly used in conjunction with standard allopathic methods, examples of complementary practices include acupuncture and acupressure, homeopathy, osteopathy, chiropractic, massage therapy, pulse diagnosis, Reiki, tongue diagnosis, iridology, faith healing, and prayer. SEE ALSO alternative medicine. Cf. allopathy. [L. *compleo,* to fill out]

com·ple·men·ta·tion (kom′plĕ-men-tā′shŭn) **1.** Interaction between two defective viruses permitting replication under conditions inhibitory to the single virus. **2.** Interaction between two genetic units, one or both of which are defective, permitting the organism containing these units to function normally, whereas it could not do so if either unit were absent.

com·ple·ment bind·ing as·say (kom′plĕ-mĕnt bīnd′ing as′ā) A test for the detection of immune complexes.

com·ple·ment che·mo·tac·tic fac·tor (kom′plĕ-mĕnt kē′mō-tak′tik fak′tŏr) The activated complex of the fifth, sixth, and seventh components of complement (C567), which induces chemotaxis of polymorphonuclear leukocytes.

com·ple·ment fix·a·tion (kom′plĕ-mĕnt fik-sā′shŭn) A process in serum whereby an antigen-antibody combination is rendered unavailable to complete a reaction in a second antigen-antibody combination for which complement is necessary; the second system usually serves as an indicator (red blood cells plus specific hemolysin); if complement is fixed with the first antigen-antibody union, hemolysis does not occur, but, if complement is not so removed, it causes hemolysis in the second system.

com·ple·ment-fix·a·tion test (kom′plĕ-mĕnt-fik-sā′shŭn test) An immunologic test for determining the presence of a particular antigen or antibody when one of the two is known to be present, based on the fact that complement is "fixed" in the presence of antigen and its specific antibody.

com·ple·ment-fix·ing an·ti·bod·y (kom′plĕ-mĕnt-fiks′ing an′ti-bod-ē) Antibody that combines with and sensitizes antigen leading to the activation of complement, which may result in cell lysis.

com·ple·ment path·ways (kom′plĕ-mĕnt path′wāz) **1.** The classical complement pathway (initiated usually by binding of C1 to IgG or IgM antibody to C1) is a complex of three subunits: C1q, C1r, and C1s. After C1q is bound, C$\overline{1r}$ (an overbar indicates enzymatic activity) cleaves C1s to C$\overline{1s}$. C$\overline{1s}$ cleaves both C4 into C4a and C4b as well as C2 into C2a and C2b. C2b combines with C4b to form C$\overline{4b2b}$, which is a C3 convertase. C3 convertase cleaves C3 into C3a and C3b. C3b joins C4bC2b to form a C5 convertase (also known as C$\overline{4b2b3b}$), which cleaves C5 into C5a and C5b. After C5b is bound to the cell surface the remainder of the complement components (C6–C9) as well as C5b form the membrane attack complex (MAC). MAC causes a hole in the cell membrane. **2.** In the alternative complement pathway, surface-bound C3b binds Factor B, which is cleaved by Factor D into Ba and Bb. C$\overline{3bBb}$ is an unstable C3 convertase unless properdin (P) binds to it to form C$\overline{3bBbP}$. The stable C3 convertase generates more C3b. When a complex of C$\overline{3bBbC3b}$ is formed, this is the alternative pathway C5 convertase. From C5b through C9, the classical and alternative pathways are the same. **3.** In the lectin-binding pathway, mannose-binding protein (MBP) initiates the pathway, which then uses components of the classical complement pathway. Some of the "a" components of both pathways have various biologic activities, i.e., C3a is an anaphylatoxin.

com·ple·ment u·nit (kom′plĕ-mĕnt yū′nit) The smallest amount (highest dilution) of complement that will cause hemolysis of a unit of red blood cells in the presence of a hemolysin unit.

com·plete an·dro·gen in·sen·si·tiv·i·ty syn·drome (kŏm-plēt′ an′drō-jen in-sen′si-tiv′i-tē sin′drōm) SYN testicular feminization syndrome.

com·plete an·ti·bod·y (kŏm-plēt′ an′ti-bod-ē) SYN saline agglutinin.

com·plete an·ti·gen (kŏm-plēt′ an′ti-jen) Any antigen capable of stimulating the formation of antibody with which it reacts in vivo or in vitro, as distinguished from incomplete antigen (hapten).

com·plete A-V block, com·plete AV block (kŏm-plēt′ blok, kŏm-plēt′ blok) SEE atrioventricular block.

com·plete blood count (CBC) (kŏm-plēt′ blŭd kownt) A combination of the following determinations: red blood cell indices and count, white blood cell count, hematocrit, hemoglobin, platelets, and differential blood count.

com·plete car·cin·o·gen (kŏm-plēt′ kahr-sin′ō-jen) A chemical carcinogen that is able to induce cancer without provocation by a tumor-promoting agent introduced during therapy.

com·plete den·ture (kom′plēt den′shŭr) Dental prosthesis that is a substitute for the lost natural dentition and associated structures of the maxillae or mandible. SYN full denture.

com·plete fis·tu·la (kŏm-plēt′ fis′chū-lă) A fistula that is open at both ends.

com·plete frac·ture (kŏm-plēt′ frak′shŭr) A break in a bone with total separation of the fragments.

com·plete her·ni·a (kŏm-plēt′ hĕr′nē-ă) An indirect inguinal hernia in which the contents extend into the tunica vaginalis.

com·plete·ly in the ca·nal (CIC) hear·ing aid (kŏm-plēt′lē kă-nal′ hēr′ing ād) A hearing aid that fits entirely in the external auditory canal and is not visible at the surface of the body.

com·plete mas·toi·dec·to·my (kŏm-plēt′ mas′toy-dek′tŏ-mē) An operation to exenterate the air-cell system from the mastoid process of the temporal bone for the drainage of the suppuration in acute mastoiditis.

com·plete pos·te·ri·or la·ryn·ge·al cleft (kŏm-plēt′ pos-tēr′ē-ŏr lă-rin′jē-ăl kleft) SEE laryngotracheoesophageal cleft.

com·plete trans·duc·tion (kŏm-plēt′ trans-dŭk′shŭn) Transduction in which the transferred genetic fragment is fully integrated in the genome of the recipient bacterium.

com·plex (kom′pleks) **1.** PSYCHIATRY an organized constellation of feelings, thoughts, perceptions, and memories that may be in part unconscious and may strongly influence associations and attitudes. **2.** CHEMISTRY the relatively stable combination of two or more compounds into a larger molecule without covalent binding. **3.** A composite of chemical or immunologic structures. **4.** An anatomic structure made up of three or more interrelated parts. **5.** An informal term used to denote a group of individual structures known or believed to be anatomically, embryologically, or physiologically related. **6.** Atrial or ventricular systole as it appears on an electrocardiographic tracing. [L. *complexus,* woven together]

com·plex en·do·me·tri·al hy·per·pla·si·a (kom′pleks en′dō-mē′trē-ăl hī′pĕr-plā′zē-ă) Closely packed endometrial glands, with a single layer of cells with slightly enlarged nuclei that are generally basally located. SYN adenomatous hyperplasia.

com•plex frac•ture (kom′pleks frak′shŭr) A fracture with significant soft tissue injury.

com•plex•ion (kŏm-plek′shŭn) The color, texture, and general appearance of the skin of the face. [L. *complexio,* a combination, (later) physical condition]

com•plex learn•ing pro•cess•es (kom′pleks lĕrn′ing pro′ses-ĕz) Those thought patterns that require the use of symbolic manipulations, as in reasoning.

com•plex mo•tor sei•zure (kom′pleks mō′tŏr sē′zhŭr) Seizure characterized by muscles of each limb contracting asynchronously and sequentially to produce a movement that may resemble voluntary activity.

com•plex o•don•to•ma (kom′pleks ō-don-tō′mă) An odontoma in which the various odontogenic tissues are organized in a haphazard arrangement with no resemblance to teeth.

com•plex par•tial sei•zure (kom′pleks pahr′shăl sē′zhŭr) A partial seizure with impairment of consciousness without features of a generalized seizure. Complex partial seizures are commonly associated with automatisms.

com•plex pleu•ral ef•fu•sion (kom′pleks plūr′ăl ĕ-fyū′zhŭn) A pleural effusion without actual infection but with signs of a high degree of inflammation (e.g., low pH, low glucose, high lactate dehydrogenase, many white blood cells).

com•plex pre•cip•i•tat•ed ep•i•lep•sy (kom′pleks prĕ-sip′i-tā-tĕd ep′i-lep′sē) A form of reflex epilepsy initiated by specialized sensory stimuli, e.g., certain visual patterns.

com•plex sound (kom′pleks sownd) A sound composed of a number of sounds of different frequencies.

com•plex•us stim•u•lans cor•dis (kom-plek′sŭs stim′yū-lanz kōr′dis) [TA] SYN conducting system of heart.

com•pli•ance (kŏm-plī′ăns) **1.** A measure of the distensibility of a chamber expressed as a change in volume per unit change in pressure. **2.** The consistency and accuracy with which a patient follows the regimen prescribed by a physician or other health care professional. Cf. adherence (2), maintenance. **3.** PHYSIOLOGY a measure of the ease with which a hollow viscus (e.g., lung, urinary bladder, gallbladder) may be distended, i.e., the volume change resulting from the application of a unit pressure differential between the inside and outside of the organ or sac; the reciprocal of elastance. **4.** Observance of rules or guidelines, such as those governing provision of medical services and billing for them; fulfillment of a requirement. **5.** A term considered prejudicial in distinguishing more or less aggressive patients. [M.E. fr. O. Fr., fr. L. *compleo,* to fulfill]

com•pli•ance plan (kŏm-plī′ăns plan) A program set up by a health care provider to ensure compliance with regulations regarding coding and billing to prevent fraud and abuse.

com•pli•cat•ed frac•ture (kom′pli-kāt-ĕd frak′shŭr) Breakage in an osseous structure such that the sharp edges of the bone have pierced an organ or bodily structure.

com•pli•cat•ed la•bor (kom′pli-kāt-ĕd lā′bŏr) Any process of birth that is exacerbated by disorder or state (e.g., intercurrent illness, morbid obesity, death).

com•pli•ca•tion (kom′pli-kā′shŭn) A morbid process or event occurring during a disease that is not an essential part of the disease, although it may result from it or from independent causes.

com•po•mer (kom′pŏ-mĕr) Material used for cementation of fixed crowns and bridges and also for some dental restorations. Combines the benefits of composite materials with glass ionomer cements. [*compo*site + poly*mer*]

com•po•nent (kŏm-pō′nĕnt) An element forming a part of the whole. [L. *com-pono,* pp. *-positus,* to place together]

com•po•nent of com•ple•ment (C) (kŏm-pō′nĕnt kom′plĕ-mĕnt) Any one of the nine distinct protein units (designated C1–C9) that effect the immunologic activities associated with complement.

com•po•nent man•age•ment (kŏm-pō′nĕnt man′ăj-mĕnt) The approach to health care cost containment that involves trying to control individual components (e.g., drug, hospitalization, or laboratory testing costs). SEE ALSO managed care.

com•po•nent ther•a•py (kŏm-pō′nĕnt thār′ă-pē) A means of providing patients with a specific blood component.

com•pos•ite flap, com•pound flap (kŏm-poz′it flap, kom′pownd flap) A flap of two or more elements incorporating underlying muscle, bone, or cartilage.

com•pos•ite graft (kŏm-poz′it graft) A graft made up of several structures, such as skin and cartilage or a full-thickness segment of the ear.

com•pos men•tis (kom′pos men′tis) Of sound mind; usually used in its opposite form, non compos mentis. [L. possessed of one's mind; *compos,* having control, + *mens* (*ment-*), mind]

com•pound (kom′pownd) **1.** CHEMISTRY a substance formed by the covalent or electrostatic union of two or more elements, generally differing entirely in physical characteristics from any of its components. **2.** PHARMACY a preparation containing several ingredients. [through O.Fr., fr. L. *compono*]

com•pound ac•tion po•ten•tial (kom′pownd ak′shŭn pŏ-ten′shăl) The combined potentials resulting from activation of the auditory division of the eighth cranial nerve.

com•pound an•eu•rysm (kom′pownd an′yūr-izm) An aneurysm in which some of the coats of the artery are ruptured, others intact.

com•pound dis•lo•ca•tion (kom′pownd dis-lō-kā′shŭn) SYN open dislocation.

com•pound frac•ture (kom′pownd frak′shŭr) SYN open fracture.

com•pound gland (kom′pownd gland) A gland with larger excretory ducts that branch repeatedly into smaller ducts, which ultimately drain secretory units.

com•pound het•er•o•zy•gote (kom′pownd het′ĕr-ō-zī′gōt) MEDICAL GENETICS the presence of two different mutant alleles at the same loci.

com•pound hy•per•o•pic a•stig•ma•tism (kom′pownd hī′pĕr-ō′pik ă-stig′mă-tizm) Astigmatism in which all meridians are hyperopic but to different degrees.

com•pound•ing (kom′pownd-ing) The act of combining parts to form a whole. [L. *compono*, to put together]

com•pound joint (kom′pownd joynt) A joint made up of three or more skeletal elements, or in which two anatomically separate joints function as a unit.

com•pound mi•cro•scope (kom′pownd mī′krŏ-skōp) A microscope having two or more magnifying lenses.

com•pound my•op•ic a•stig•ma•tism (kom′pownd mī-op′ik ă-stig′mă-tizm) Astigmatism in which all meridians are myopic but to different degrees.

com•pound o•don•to•ma (kom′pownd ō-don-tō′mă) An odontoma in which the odontogenic tissues are organized and resemble anomalous teeth.

com•pound pre•sen•ta•tion (kom′pownd prez′ĕn-tā′shŭn) Prolapse of an extremity, usually a hand, along with the presenting part during the second stage of labor, with both in the pelvis simultaneously.

com•pre•hen•sion (kom′prē-hen′shŭn) Knowledge or understanding of an object, situation, event, or verbal statement.

com•press (kom′pres) A pad of gauze or other material applied for local pressure. [L. *comprimo*, pp. *-pressus*, to press together]

com•pres•si•ble vol•ume (kŏm-pres′ă-bĕl vol′yūm) The volume of gas compressed (and therefore lost) in the mechanical ventilator circuit per delivered pressure; most systems have compressible volume loss factors of 3–5 mL/cm H_2O; some newer mechanical ventilators calculate the loss factor and monitor gas delivery so that the set volume is the volume that actually enters the patient's airway.

com•pres•sion (kŏm-presh′ŭn) A squeezing together; the exertion of pressure on a body to tend to increase its density; the decrease in a dimension of a body under the action of two external forces directed toward one another.

com•pres•sion cy•a•no•sis (kŏm-presh′ŭn sī-ă-nō′sis) Cyanosis accompanied by edema and petechial hemorrhages over the head, neck, and upper part of the chest, as a venous reflex resulting from severe compression of the thorax or abdomen; the conjunctiva and retinas are similarly affected.

i **com•pres•sion frac•ture** (kŏm-presh′ŭn frak′shŭr) Breakage causing loss of height of the vertebral body either by trauma or by pathology. It occurs most commonly in thoracic and lumbar spines. A common sequela of osteoporosis. See page B20. SYN burst fracture.

com•pres•sion lim•it•ing (kŏm-presh′ŭn lim′it-ing) A hearing aid circuit in which amplification is reduced at high input levels.

com•pres•sion neu•rop•a•thy (kŏm-presh′ŭn nūr-op′ă-thē) A focal nerve lesion produced when sustained pressure is applied to a localized portion of the nerve, either from an external or internal source.

com•pres•sion pa•ral•y•sis (kŏm-presh′ŭn păr-al′i-sis) Paralysis due to external pressure on a nerve.

com•pres•sion plate (kŏm-presh′ŭn plāt) A plate for internal fracture fixation with screw holes so designed that insertion of screws draws bone fragments more firmly together.

com•pres•sion syn•drome (kŏm-presh′ŭn sin′drōm) **1.** SYN crush syndrome. **2.** SYN compartment syndrome.

com•pres•sion ther•a•py (kŏm-presh′ŭn thār′ă-pē) Use of circumferential elastic tubing, gloves, bandages, or a custom garment to apply pressure in the treatment of conditions such as burns, lymphedema, edema, and venous stasis, and formation of scar tissue.

com•pres•sor (kŏm-pres′ŏr) **1.** A muscle, contraction of which causes compression of any structure. **2.** An instrument for applying pressure on a part, especially on an artery to prevent loss of blood.

Comp•ton ef•fect, **Comp•ton scat•ter•ing** (kom′tŏn e-fekt′, kom′tŏn skă-tĕr′ing) Change in wavelength of x-rays or gamma rays due to interaction of electron orbiting nucleus and incidental photon, resulting in scattered photons of lower energy and recoil electrons.

com•pul•sion (kŏm-pŭl′shŭn) Uncontrollable impulses to perform an act, often repetitively, as an unconscious mechanism to avoid unacceptable ideas and desires which, by themselves, arouse anxiety; the anxiety becomes fully manifest if performance of the compulsive act is prevented; may be associated with obsessive thoughts. [L. *com-pello* pp. *-pulsus,* to drive together, compel]

com•pul•sive (kŏm-pŭl′siv) Influenced by compulsion; of a compelling and irresistible nature.

com•pul•sive i•de•a (kŏm-pŭl′siv ī-dē′ă) A fixed and repetitively recurring idea.

com•pul•sive per•son•al•i•ty (kŏm-pŭl′siv pĕr-sŏn-al′i-tē) A personality characterized by rigidity, extreme inhibition, perfectionism, and excessive concern with conformity and adherence to standards of conscience either for the individual person or for others.

com•pul•so•ry li•cens•ing (kŏm-pŭl′sŏr-ē lī′sĕns-ing) An imprecise term intended to denote any occupation or business that requires the participant or professional to gain or acquire approval from a regulatory body before such person may pursue such occupation within any given jurisdiction.

com•put•ed ax•i•al to•mog•ra•phy (CAT) (kŏm-pyū′tĕd ak′sē-ăl tŏ-mog′ră-fē) Obsolete. SYN computed tomography.

i **com•put•ed to•mog•ra•phy (CT)** (kŏm-pyū′tĕd tŏ-mog′ră-fē) Imaging anatomic information from a cross-sectional plane of the body, each image generated by a computer synthesis of x-ray transmission data obtained in many different directions in a given plane. See page B20. SYN computed axial tomography.

com•pu•ter-based pa•tient re•cord (CPR) (kŏm-pyū′tĕr-bāst pā′shŭnt rek′ŏrd) Electronic health care record that integrates patient information into a database for accessibility; the CPR supports patient care, decision making, and research.

com•pu•ter phy•si•cian or•der en•try (kŏm-pyū′tĕr fi-zish′ŭn ōr′dĕr en′trē) An electronic prescribing system that allows physicians to enter orders into a computer.

♻ **con-** Prefix meaning with, together, in association; appears as com- before p, b, or m; as col- before l; and as co- before a vowel; corresponds to G. *syn-*. [L. *cum,* with, together]

conA, con A Abbreviation for concanavalin A.

co•na•tion (kō-nā′shŭn) The conscious tendency to act, usually an aspect of mental process; historically aligned with cognition and affection, but more recently used in the wider sense of impulse, desire, purposeful striving. [L. *conātio,* an undertaking, effort]

co•na•tive (kon′ă-tiv) Pertaining to, or characterized by, conation.

con•ca•nav•a•lin A (conA, con A) (kon-kă-nav′ă-lin) A phytomitogen, extracted from the jack bean (*Canavalia ensiformis*), which agglutinates the blood of mammals and reacts with glucosans; like other phytohemagglutinins, conA stimulates T lymphocytes more vigorously than it does B lymphocytes.

Con•ca•to dis•ease (kon-kah′tō di-zēz′) SYN polyserositis.

con•cave (kon-kāv′) Having a depressed or hollowed surface. [L. *concavus,* arched or vaulted]

con•cave lens (kon-kāv′ lenz) A diverging minus power lens.

con•cav•i•ty (kŏn-kav′i-tē) A hollow or depression, with more or less evenly curved sides, on any surface.

con•ca•vo•con•cave (kŏn-kā′vō-kon′kāv) SYN biconcave.

con•ca•vo•con•cave lens (kŏn-kā′vō-kon′kāv lenz) SYN biconcave lens.

con•ca•vo•con•vex (kŏn-kā′vō-kon′veks) Concave on one surface and convex on the opposite surface.

con•ca•vo•con•vex lens (kŏn-kā′vō-kon′veks lenz) A converging meniscus lens that is concave on one surface and convex on the opposite surface.

con•cealed hem•or•rhage (kŏn-sēld′ hem′ŏr-ăj) SYN internal hemorrhage.

con•ceal•ment (kŏn-sēl′mĕnt) The collection of research data or the provision of an intervention without participant's knowledge or consent.

con•cen•tra•tion (c) (kon′sĕn-trā′shŭn) **1.** A preparation made by extracting a crude drug, precipitating from the solution, and drying. **2.** Increasing the amount of solute in a given volume of solution by evaporation of the solvent. **3.** The quantity of a substance per unit volume or weight. **4.** PHYSIOLOGY symbol U for urinary concentration, P for plasma concentration. **5.** RESPIRATORY PHYSIOLOGY symbol C for amount per unit volume in blood, F for fractional concentration (mole fraction or volume per volume) in dried gas. **6.** Subscripts indicate location and chemical species. [L. *con-,* together, + *centrum,* center]

con•cen•tra•tion-time prod•uct (Ct) (kon′sĕn-trā′shŭn-tīme prod′ŭkt) A measure, obtained by multiplying concentration of agent by duration of exposure; used to approximate the external dose of a chemical agent existing as a vapor or a gas. SYN CT product, Ct product.

con•cen•tra•tor (kon′sĕn-trā-tŏr) A device for making a substance stronger or purer.

con•cen•tric (kŏn-sen′trik) Having a common center; said of two or more circles or spheres having a common center.

con·cen·tric con·trac·tion (kŏn-sen′trik kŏn-trak′shŭn) A shortening contraction in which a muscle's attachments are drawn toward one another as the muscle contracts and overcomes an external resistance.

con·cen·tric hy·per·tro·phy (kŏn-sen′trik hī-pĕr′trō-fē) Thickening of the walls of the heart or any cavity with apparent diminution of the capacity of the cavity.

con·cen·tric la·mel·la (kŏn-sen′trik lă-mel′ă) One of the concentric tubular layers of bone surrounding the central canal in an osteon. SYN haversian lamella.

con·cept (kon′sept) **1.** An abstract idea or notion. **2.** An explanatory variable or principle in a scientific system. SYN conception (1). [L. *conceptum,* something understood, pp. ntr. of *concipio,* to receive, apprehend]

con·cept for·ma·tion (kon′sept fōr-mā′shŭn) PSYCHOLOGY learning to conceive and respond in terms of abstract ideas based on an action or object.

con·cep·tion (kŏn-sep′shŭn) **1.** SYN concept. **2.** Act of forming a general idea or notion. **3.** Act of conceiving, or becoming pregnant; fertilization of the oocyte by a sperm to form a zygote. [L. *conceptio;* see concept]

con·cep·tu·al (kŏn-sep′shū-ăl) Relating to the formation of ideas, usually higher order abstractions, mental conceptions.

con·cep·tu·al age (kŏn-sep′shū-ăl āj) SYN fertilization age.

con·cep·tus, pl. **con·cep·tus** (kŏn-sep′tŭs, kŏn-sep′tŭs) The products of conception (i.e., fetus, placenta, embryo, and fetal membranes).

con·cha, pl. **con·chae** (kong′kă, -kē) ANATOMY a structure similar to a shell in shape, as the auricle or pinna of the ear or a turbinate bone in the nose. [L. a shell]

con·cha of ear (kong′kă ēr) The large hollow, or floor of the auricle, between the anterior portion of the helix and the antihelix. It is divided by the crus of the helix into the cymba above and the cavum below.

con·cha san·to·ri·ni (kong′kă sahn-tō-rē′nē) SYN supreme nasal concha.

con·com·i·tant symp·tom (kŏn-kom′i-tănt simp′tŏm) SYN accessory symptom.

con·cor·dance (kŏn-kōr′dăns) Agreement in the types of data that occur in natural pairs. [L. *concordia,* agreeing, harmony]

con·cor·dance rate (kŏn-kōr′dăns rāt) The rate of occurrence of a trait, behavior, or action in members of a specified group as compared with the occurrence of a trait of interest. Broadly, it is taken as evidence of causal connection.

con·cor·dant (kŏn-kōr′dănt) Denoting or exhibiting concordance.

con·cor·dant al·ter·nans (kŏn-kōr′dănt awl-tĕr′nanz) Simultaneous occurrence of right ventricular and pulmonary artery alternans with left ventricular and peripheral pulsus alternans.

con·cor·dant al·ter·na·tion (kŏn-kōr′dănt awl′tĕr-nā′shŭn) Alternation in either the mechanical or electrical activity of the heart, occurring in both systemic and pulmonary circulations.

con·cor·dant chan·ges e·lec·tro·car·di·o·gram (kŏn-kōr′dănt chān′jĕz ĕ-lek′trō-kahr′dē-ō-gram) The presence of more than one waveform change, each in the same direction (polarity).

con·cres·cence (kŏn-kres′ĕns) **1.** SYN coalescence. **2.** DENTISTRY the union of the roots of two adjacent teeth by cementum.

con·crete think·ing (kon′krēt thingk′ing) Consideration of objects or ideas as specific items rather than as an abstract representation of a more general concept, as contrasted with abstract thinking (e.g., perceiving a chair and a table as individual useful items and not as members of the general class, furniture).

con·cre·ti·o cor·dis (kon-krē′shē-ō kōr′dis) Extensive adhesion between parietal and visceral layers of the pericardium with partial or complete obliteration of the pericardial cavity. SYN internal adhesive pericarditis.

con·cre·tion (kŏn-krē′shŭn) Formation of solid material by the aggregation of discrete units or particles. [L. *cum,* together, + *crescere,* to grow]

con·cur·rent dis·in·fec·tion (kon-kŭr′ĕnt dis-in-fek′shŭn) Application of disinfective measures as soon as possible after discharge of infectious material from the body of an infected person, or after soiling of articles with such infectious discharges.

con·cur·rent in·fec·tion (kŏn-kŭr′ĕnt in-fek′shŭn) SEE superinfection.

con·cus·sion (kŏn-kŭsh′ŭn) **1.** A violent shaking or jarring. **2.** An injury of a soft structure, as the brain, resulting from a blow or violent shaking; with partial to complete loss of function. [L. *concussio,* fr. *con- cutio,* pp. *-cussus,* to shake violently]

con·den·sa·tion (kon′dĕn-sā′shŭn) **1.** Making more solid or dense. **2.** The change of a gas to a liquid, or of a liquid to a solid. **3.** PSYCHOANALYSIS an unconscious mental process in which one symbol stands for a number of others. **4.** DENTISTRY the process of packing a filling material into a cavity, using such force and direction that no voids result. [L. *con- denso,* pp. *-atus,* to make thick, condense]

con·dens·er (kŏn-den′sĕr) **1.** An apparatus for

cooling a gas to a liquid or a liquid to a solid. **2.** DENTISTRY a manual or powered instrument used for packing a plastic or unset material into a prepared tooth cavity; variation in size and shape permit conformation of the mass to the cavity outline. **3.** The simple or compound lens on a microscope that is used to supply sufficient illumination necessary to view the specimen under observation. **4.** SYN capacitor.

con·di·tion (kŏn-dish′ŭn) **1.** To train; to undergo conditioning. **2.** BEHAVIORAL PSYCHOLOGY a certain response elicited by a specifiable stimulus or emitted in the presence of certain stimuli with reward of the response during prior occurrence. **3.** Referring to several classes of learning in the behavioristic branch of psychology. [L. *conditio*, fr. *condico*, to agree]

con·di·tioned re·flex (Cr) (kŏn-dish′ŭnd rē′fleks) A reflex that is gradually developed by training and association through the frequent repetition of a definite stimulus. SEE conditioning.

con·di·tioned re·sponse (kŏn-dish′ŭnd rē-spons′) A response already in a person's repertoire but through repeated pairings with its natural stimulus, has been acquired or conditioned anew to a previously neutral or conditioned stimulus. SEE conditioning. Cf. unconditioned response.

con·di·tioned stim·u·lus (kŏn-dish′ŭnd stim′yū-lŭs) **1.** A stimulus applied to one of the sense organs that are an essential and integral part of the neural mechanism underlying a conditioned reflex. **2.** A neutral stimulus, when paired with the unconditioned stimulus in simultaneous presentation to an organism, capable of eliciting a given response.

con·di·tion·ing (kŏn-dish′ŭn-ing) The process of acquiring, developing, educating, establishing, learning, or training new responses in a person; a change in the frequency or form of behavior as a result of the influence of the environment.

con·dom (kŏn′dom) Sheath or cover for the penis or vagina, for use in the prevention of conception or infection during coitus. See this page.

con·duc·tance (kŏn-dŭk′tăns) **1.** A measure of conductivity; the ratio of the current flowing through a conductor to the difference in potential between the ends of the conductor; the conductance of a circuit is the reciprocal of its resistance. **2.** The ease with which a fluid or gas enters and flows through a conduit, air passage, or respiratory tract; the flow per unit pressure difference.

con·duct dis·or·der (kon′dŭkt dis-ōr′dĕr) A mental disorder of childhood or adolescence characterized by a persistent pattern of violating societal norms and the rights of others; children with the disorder may exhibit physical aggression, cruelty to animals, vandalism, and robbery,

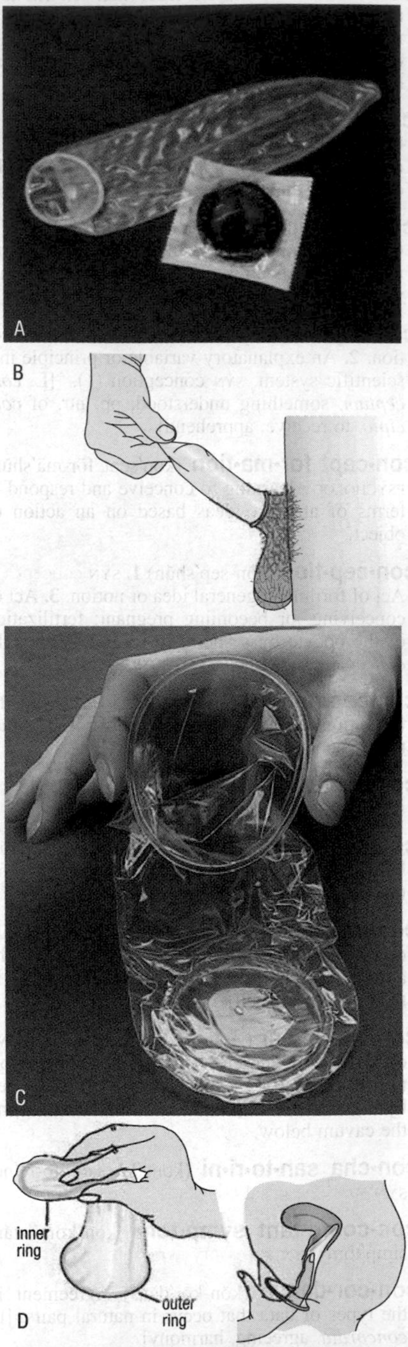

condoms: (A) male condoms; (B) external view of male genitalia with condom in place on penis: right hand allows slack at end of condom; (C) female condom; (D) correct insertion technique of female condom

along with truancy, cheating, and lying. SEE borderline personality disorder.

con·duct·ing sys·tem of heart (kŏn-dŭkt′ ing sis′tĕm hahrt) The system of atypical cardiac muscle fibers comprising the sinuatrial node, internodal tracts, atrioventricular node and bundle, the bundle branches, and their terminal ramifications into the Purkinje network; sometimes also called cardionector. SYN complexus stimulans cordis [TA].

con·duc·tion (kŏn-dŭk′shŭn) **1.** The act of transmitting or conveying certain forms of energy, such as heat, sound, or electricity, from one point to another, without evident movement in the conducting body. **2.** The transmission of stimuli of various sorts by living protoplasm. **3.** The process by which a nerve impulse is transmitted. [L. *con- duco,* pp. *ductus,* to lead, conduct]

con·duc·tion an·al·ge·si·a (kŏn-dŭk′shŭn an′ăl-jē′zē-ă) SYN regional anesthesia.

con·duc·tion an·es·the·si·a (kŏn-dŭk′shŭn an′es-thē′zē-ă) Regional anesthesia in which local anesthetic solution is injected about nerves to inhibit nerve transmission; includes spinal, epidural, nerve block, and field block anesthesia, but not local or topical anesthesia. SYN block anesthesia.

con·duc·tion a·pha·si·a (kŏn-dŭk′shŭn ă-fā′zē-ă) A form of aphasia in which the patient understands spoken and written words, is aware of his deficit, and can speak and write, but skips or repeats words, or substitutes one word for another (paraphasia); word repetition is severely impaired. The responsible lesion is in the associate tracts connecting the various language centers. SYN associative aphasia.

con·duc·tive deaf·ness (kŏn-dŭk′tiv def′nĕs) Hearing impairment caused by interference with sound or transmission through the external canal, middle ear, or ossicles.

con·duc·tive hear·ing im·pair·ment (kŏn-dŭk′tiv hēr′ing im-păr′mĕnt) A form of hearing impairment due to a lesion in the external auditory canal or middle ear.

con·duc·tive hear·ing loss (kŏn-dŭk′tiv hēr′ing laws) Hearing loss caused by an obstruction or lesion in the outer ear, middle ear, or both. SEE ALSO air-bone gap.

con·duc·tive heat (kŏn-dŭk′tiv hēt) A rise in temperature conveyed from one structure or appliance to another in which the warmer affects the cooler by conduction. SEE superinfection.

con·duc·tiv·i·ty (kon′dŭk-tiv′i-tē) **1.** The power of transmission or conveyance of certain forms of energy, such as heat, sound, and electricity, without perceptible motion in the conducting body. **2.** The property, inherent in living protoplasm, of transmitting a state of excitation; e.g., in muscle or nerve.

con·duc·tor (kŏn-dŭk′ter) **1.** A probe or sound with a groove along which a knife is passed in slitting open a sinus or fistula; a grooved director. **2.** Any substance possessing conductivity.

con·du·it (kon′dū-it) A channel.

con·du·pli·cate (kon-dū′pli-kăt) Folded in on itself lengthwise. [L. *con-,* with, + *duplico,* pp. *-atus*]

con·dy·lar (kon′di-lăr) Relating to a condyle.

con·dy·lar ca·nal (kon′di-lăr kă-nal′) The inconstant opening through the occipital bone posterior to the condyle on each side that transmits the occipital emissary vein.

con·dy·lar fos·sa (kon′di-lăr fos′ă) A depression behind the condyle of the occipital bone in which the posterior margin of the superior facet of the atlas lies in extension.

con·dy·lar joint (kon′di-lăr joynt) SYN ellipsoid joint.

con·dy·lar pro·cess of man·di·ble (kon′di-lăr pros′es man′di-bĕl) The articular process of the ramus of the mandible; it includes the head of the mandible, the neck of the mandible and pterygoid fovea.

con·dy·lar·thro·sis (kon′dil-ahr-thrō′sis) A joint, like that of the knee, formed by condylar surfaces. [G. *kondylos,* condyle, + *arthrōsis,* a jointing]

con·dyle (kon′dīl) A rounded articular surface at the extremity of a bone. SYN condylus.

con·dy·lec·to·my (kon′di-lek′tŏ-mē) Excision of a condyle. [G. *kondylos,* condyle, + *ektomē,* excision]

con·dy·loid (kon′di-loyd) Relating to or resembling a condyle. [G. *kondylōdēs,* like a knuckle, fr. *kondylos,* condyle, + *eidos,* resemblance]

con·dy·lo·ma, pl. **con·dy·lo·ma·ta** (kon-di-lō′mă, -mah′tă) A wartlike excrescence on the skin of the genitals, perineum, or anus, usually sexually transmitted. [G. *kondylōma,* a knob]

con·dy·lo·ma a·cu·mi·na·tum (kon-di-lō′mă ă-kū-mi-nā′tŭm) A warty growth on the external genitals or at the anus, consisting of fibrous overgrowths covered by thickened epithelium showing koilocytosis, due to sexually transmitted infection with human papillomavirus; malignant change is associated with particular types of the virus. SYN genital wart, venereal wart.

con·dy·lo·ma la·tum (kon-di-lō′mă lā′tŭm) A secondary syphilitic eruption of flat-topped papules, found at the anus and wherever contiguous folds of skin produce heat and moisture. SYN flat condyloma (1).

con·dy·lom·a·tous (kon′di-lō′mă-tŭs) Relating to a condyloma.

con·dy·lot·o·my (kon′di-lot′ŏ-mē) Division,

without removal, of a condyle. [G. *kondylos,* condyle, + *tomē,* incision]

con·dy·lus (kon′di-lŭs) SYN condyle. [L. fr. G. *kondylos,* knuckle, the knuckle of any joint]

cone (kōn) **1.** A surface joining a circle to a point above the plane containing the circle. **2.** The photosensitive, outward-directed, conical process of a cone cell essential for sharp vision and color vision; cones are the only photoreceptor in the fovea centralis and become interspersed with increasing numbers of rods toward the periphery of the retina. **3.** Metallic cylinder or truncated cone, either circular or square in cross-section, used to confine a beam of x-rays. SYN conus (1). [G. *kōnos,* cone]

-cone Suffix indicating the cusp of a tooth in the upper jaw.

cone cell (kōn sel) One of the two types of visual receptor cells of the retina, essential for visual acuity and color vision; the second type is the rod cell.

cone down (kōn down) **1.** To narrow a beam of x-rays to a region of interest using a collimator or cone (3). **2.** Colloquialism, to delimit one's attention or activities.

cone gran·ule (kōn gran′yūl) Nucleus of a retinal cell connecting with one of the cones.

cone of light (kōn līt) SYN red reflex.

cone-rod re·ti·nal dys·tro·phy (kōn-rod ret′i-năl dis′trŏ-fē) A disorder affecting the retinal cones more than the rods, characterized by diminished central vision and color vision.

con·fab·u·la·tion (kŏn-fab′yū-lā′shŭn) The making of bizarre and incorrect responses, and a readiness to give a fluent but tangential answer, with no regard whatever to facts, to any question put; seen in amnesia, presbyophrenia, and Wernicke-Korsakoff syndrome. [L. *con-fabulor,* pp. *-fabulatus,* to talk together, fr. *fabula,* narrative]

con·fec·tion (kŏn-fek′shŭn) A pharmaceutical preparation consisting of a drug mixed with honey or syrup; a soft solid, sometimes used as an excipient for pill masses. [L. *confectio*]

con·fi·den·ti·al·i·ty (kon′fi-den-shē-al′i-tē) The statutorily protected right and duty of health professionals not to disclose information acquired during consultation with a patient. [L. *con-fido,* to trust, be assured]

con·fig·u·ra·tion (kŏn-fig′yūr-ā′shŭn) **1.** The general form of a body and its parts. **2.** CHEMISTRY the spatial arrangement of atoms in a molecule. The configuration of a compound (e.g., a sugar) is the unique spatial arrangement of its atoms, on which no other arrangement of these atoms can be superimposed with complete correspondence. Cf. conformation.

con·fine·ment (kŏn-fīn′mĕnt) Lying-in; giving birth to a child. [L. *confine* {ntr.}, a boundary, confine, fr. *con-* + *finis,* boundary]

con·flict (kon′flikt) Tension or stress experienced by an organism when satisfaction of a need, drive, motive, or wish is thwarted by the presence of other attractive or unattractive needs, drives, or motives.

con·flict of in·ter·est (kon′flik in′tĕr-ĕst) A conflict between the personal interests and professional responsibilities of a health care provider toward a patient or other consumer.

con·flu·ence (kon′flū-ĕns) A flowing together; a joining of two or more streams. [L. *confluens*]

con·flu·ent (kon′flū-ĕnt) **1.** Joining; running together; denoting certain skin lesions which become merged, forming a patch; denoting a disease characterized by lesions which are not discrete, or distinct one from the other. **2.** Denoting a bone formed by the blending together of two originally distinct bones. [L. *con-fluo,* to flow together]

con·fo·cal mi·cro·scope (kon-fō′kăl mī′krŏ-skōp) A microscope that allows the observer to visualize objects in a single plane of focus, thereby creating a sharper image (usually the objects are fluorescent molecules); a refinement of this microscope uses optic sectioning and a computer to record serial sections. This permits three-dimensional reconstruction.

con·for·ma·tion (kon′fōr-mā′shŭn) The spatial arrangement of a molecule achieved by rotation of groups about single covalent bonds, without breaking any covalent bonds. Cf. configuration.

con·found·ing (kŏn-fown′ding) **1.** A situation in which the effects of two or more processes are not separated; the distortion of the apparent effect of an exposure on risk, brought about by the association with other factors that can influence the outcome. **2.** A relationship between the effects of two or more causal factors observed in a set of data, such that it is not logically possible to separate the contribution of any single causal factor to the observed effects.

con·fron·ta·tion test (kon′frŭn-tā′shŭn test) A rough assessment of the visual fields in which the examiner and subject look into one another's eyes while objects are brought into view from each side, above, and below. SYN visual confrontation.

con·fu·sion (kŏn-fyū′zhŭn) A mental state in which reactions to environmental stimuli are inappropriate because the subject is bewildered, perplexed, or disoriented. [L. *confusio,* a confounding]

con·fu·sion-a·tax·i·a syn·drome (kŏn-fyū′zhŭn-ă-tak′sē-ă sin′drōm) Second of three identified types of Gulf War syndrome (q.v.).

con·ge·ner (kon′jĕ-nĕr) **1.** One of two or more things of the same kind, as of animal or plant with respect to classification. **2.** One of two or more muscles with the same function. [L. *con-*, with, + *genus,* race]

con•gen•i•tal (kŏn-jen′i-tăl) Existing at birth, referring to mental or physical traits, anomalies, malformations, or diseases, which may be either hereditary or due to an influence occurring during gestation up to the moment of birth. USAGE NOTE often misused as a synonym of hereditary. [L. *congenitus,* born with]

con•gen•i•tal a•fi•brin•o•gen•e•mi•a (kŏn-jen′i-tăl ā-fī′brin-ō-jĕ-nē′mē-ă) A rare disorder of blood coagulation in which little or no fibrinogen can be detected in plasma.

con•gen•i•tal am•pu•ta•tion (kŏn-jen′i-tăl amp′yū-tā′shŭn) Amputation, usually a limb or part of a limb, produced in utero; usually attributed to the pressure of constricting amniotic bands. SYN amnionic amputation, birth amputation, intrauterine amputation, spontaneous amputation (1).

con•gen•i•tal a•ne•mi•a (kŏn-jen′i-tăl ă-nē′mē-ă) SYN erythroblastosis fetalis.

con•gen•i•tal a•nom•a•ly (kŏn-jen′i-tăl ă-nom′ă-lē) A structural abnormality present at birth. SEE ALSO birth defect.

con•gen•i•tal di•a•phrag•mat•ic her•ni•a (kŏn-jen′i-tăl dī′ă-frag-mat′ik hĕr′nē-ă) Defective development of the pleuroperitoneal membrane (usually on the left) results in a posterolateral defect in the diaphragm and allows the abdominal viscera to protrude into the thorax. SYN Bochdalek hernia.

con•gen•i•tal ec•to•der•mal de•fect, **con•gen•i•tal ec•to•der•mal dys•pla•si•a** (kŏn-jen′i-tăl ek-tō-dĕr′măl dē-fekt′, kŏn-jen′i-tăl ek-tō-dĕr′măl dis-plā′zē-ă) Incomplete development of the epidermis and skin appendages; the skin is smooth and hairless, the face is abnormal, and the teeth and nails may be affected; sweating may be deficient.

con•gen•i•tal e•ryth•ro•poi•et•ic por•phyr•i•a (kŏn-jen′i-tăl ĕ-rith′rō-poy-et′ik pōr-fir′ē-ă) Enhanced porphyrin formation by erythroid cells in bone marrow, leading to severe porphyrinuria, often with hemolytic anemia and persistent cutaneous photosensitivity; caused by a deficiency of uroporphyrinogen III cosynthetase.

con•gen•i•tal Heinz bod•y he•mo•ly•tic a•ne•mi•a (kŏn-jen′i-tăl hīnz bod′ē hē′mō-lit′ik ă-nē′mē-ă) Any of several inherited disorders of hemoglobin synthesis in which an amino acid substitution results in faulty molecular configuration, with defective binding of heme to globin. Denatured hemoglobin forms Heinz bodies, which damage the erythrocyte membrane and promote premature hemolysis.

con•gen•i•tal he•mo•lyt•ic a•ne•mi•a (kŏn-jen′i-tăl hē′mō-lit′ik ă-nē′mē-ă) Accelerated destruction of red blood cells due to an inherited defect, such as in the membrane in hereditary spherocytosis.

con•gen•i•tal he•red•i•tary en•do•the•li•al dys•tro•phy (kŏn-jen′i-tăl hĕr-ed′i-tar-ē en′dō-thē′lē-ăl dis′trŏ-fē) A dominantly or recessively inherited condition characterized by bilateral cloudy, thickened corneas at birth or in the neonatal period.

con•gen•i•tal hip dys•pla•si•a (kŏn-jen′i-tăl hip dis-plā′zē-ă) A developmental abnormality in which a neonate's hips easily become dislocated; etiology is complex, with mechanical, familial, hormonal, and obstetric factors all contributing; female predominance is 9:1. SYN developmental hip dysplasia.

con•gen•i•tal hy•po•plas•tic a•ne•mi•a (kŏn-jen′i-tăl hī′pō-plas′tik ă-nē′mē-ă) Congenital nonregenerative, familial hypoplastic, or pure red blood cell anemia; erythrogenesis imperfecta; Diamond-Blackfan syndrome; anemia resulting from congenital hypoplasia of the bone marrow, which is grossly deficient in erythroid precursors whereas other elements are normal; anemia is progressive and severe, but leukocyte and platelet counts are normal or slightly reduced; survival of transfused erythrocytes is normal. SYN Diamond-Blackfan syndrome.

con•gen•i•tal hy•po•thy•roid•ism (kŏn-jen′i-tăl hī′pō-thī′royd-izm) Lack of thyroid secretion. SEE infantile hypothyroidism.

con•gen•i•tal ich•thy•o•si•form e•ryth•ro•der•ma (kŏn-jen′i-tăl ik′thē-ō′si-fōrm ĕ-rith′rō-dĕr′mă) A genodermatosis characterized by diffuse chronic erythema and scale formation, which occurs in bullous and nonbullous forms. SYN ichthyosiform erythroderma.

con•gen•i•tal meg•a•co•lon, **meg•a•co•lon con•gen•i•tum** (kŏn-jen′i-tăl meg′ă-kō-lŏn, meg-ă-kō′lon kon-jen′i-tŭm) Congenital dilation and hypertrophy of the colon due to absence (aganglionosis) or marked reduction (hypoganglionosis) in the number of ganglion cells of the myenteric plexus of the rectum and a varying but continuous length of colon above the rectum. SYN Hirschsprung disease.

con•gen•i•tal ne•vus (kŏn-jen′i-tăl nē′vŭs) A melanocytic nevus that is visible at birth, is often larger than an acquired nevus, and more frequently involves deeper structures. See page 354.

con•gen•i•tal nys•tag•mus (kŏn-jen′i-tăl nis-tag′mŭs) **1.** Nystagmus present at birth or caused by lesions sustained in utero or at birth; **2.** Inherited nystagmus, usually X-linked, without associated neurologic lesions and nonprogressive. **3.** The nystagmus associated with albinism, achromatopsia, and hypoplasia of the macula.

con•gen•i•tal par•a•my•o•to•ni•a, **pa•ra•my•o•to•ni•a con•gen•i•ta** (kŏn-jen′i-tăl par-

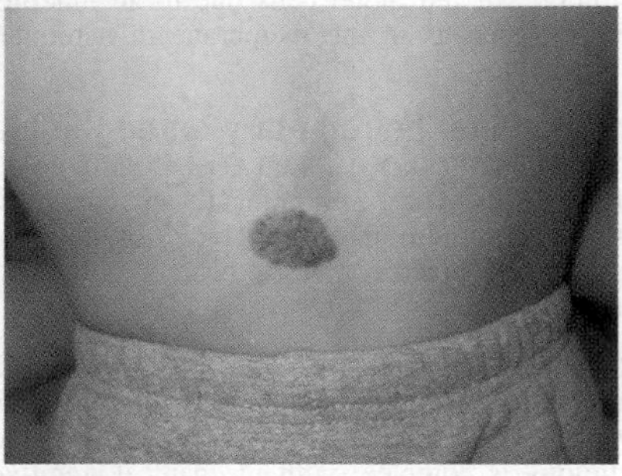

congenital nevus: lower back, child

ă-mī-ō-tō′nē-ă, par′ă-mī-ō-tō′nē-ă kon-jen′i-tă) A nonprogressive myotonia induced by exposure of muscles to cold; there are episodes of intermittent flaccid paralysis, but no atrophy or hypertrophy of muscles; autosomal dominant inheritance. There is a variant autosomal dominant form in which cold is not a provoking factor. SYN Eulenburg disease.

con•gen•i•tal py•lor•ic ste•no•sis (kŏn-jen′i-tăl pī-lōr′ik stĕ-nō′sis) SYN hypertrophic pyloric stenosis.

con•gen•i•tal stri•dor (kŏn-jen′i-tăl strī′dōr) Crowing inspiration occurring at birth or within the first few months of life; sometimes without apparent cause and sometimes due to abnormal flaccidity of epiglottis or arytenoids.

con•gen•i•tal syph•i•lis (kŏn-jen′i-tăl sif′i-lis) Venereal disease acquired by the fetus in utero, thus present at birth.

con•gen•i•tal to•tal li•po•dys•tro•phy (kŏn-jen′i-tăl tō′tăl lip′ō-dis′trŏ-fē) Characterized by almost complete lack of subcutaneous fat, accelerated rate of growth and skeletal development during the first 3–4 years of life, muscular hypertrophy, cardiac enlargement, hepatosplenomegaly, acanthosis nigricans, hypertrichosis, renal enlargement, hypertriglyceridemia, and hypermetabolism; autosomal recessive inheritance. SYN Berardinelli syndrome, Seip syndrome.

con•gen•i•tal tox•o•plas•mo•sis (kŏn-jen′i-tăl tok′sō-plaz-mō′sis) A disease caused by the protozoan parasite *Toxoplasma gondii*, which is transmitted in utero to the fetus, observed as three syndromes: 1) acute: most of the organs contain foci of necrosis in association with fever, jaundice, hydrocephaly, encephalomyelitis, pneumonitis, rash, ophthalmic lesions, hepatomegaly, and splenomegaly; 2) subacute: most of these lesions are partly healed or calcified, but those in the brain and eye seem to remain active, inasmuch as chorioretinitis is observed in more than 80% of diseased infants; and 3) chronic: usually not recognized during the newborn period, but chorioretinitis and cerebral lesions may be detected weeks to years later.

con•gen•i•tal valve (kŏn-jen′i-tăl valv) An abnormal lining fold obstructing a passage.

con•gen•i•tal vir•il•iz•ing ad•re•nal hy•per•pla•si•a (kŏn-jen′i-tăl vir′i-līz-ing ă-drē′năl hī′pĕr-plā′zē-ă) Any inborn error of metabolism causing hyperplasia of the cortex of suprarenal gland and overproduction of virilizing hormones. Most forms are due to partial or complete 21-hydroxylase deficiency, leading to increased ACTH production by the pituitary, stimulating adrenal growth and function. Clinical features include ambiguous genitalia, virilization, and salt-wasting.

con•gest•ed (kŏn-jes′tĕd) Containing an abnormal amount of blood or tissue fluid; in a state of congestion.

con•ges•tion (kŏn-jes′chŭn) Presence of an abnormal amount of fluid in the vessels or passages of a part or organ; especially, of blood due either to increased influx or to an obstruction to the return flow. SEE ALSO hyperemia. [L. *congestio,* a bringing together, a heap, fr. *con-gero,* pp. *-gestus,* to bring together]

con•ges•tive (kŏn-jes′tiv) Relating to congestion.

con•ges•tive heart fail•ure (CHF) (kŏn-jes′tiv hahrt fāl′yŭr) SYN heart failure (1).

con•ges•tive sple•no•meg•a•ly (kŏn-jes′tiv splē-nō-meg′ă-lē) Enlargement of the spleen due to passive congestion; sometimes used as a synonym for Banti syndrome.

con•glo•bate (kon′glō-bāt) Formed in a single rounded mass. [L. *con-globo,* pp. *-atus,* to gather into a *globus,* ball]

con•glom•er•ate (kŏn-glom′ĕr-ăt) Composed of several parts aggregated into one mass. [L. *con- glomero,* pp. *-atus,* to roll together, fr. *glomus,* a ball]

con•glu•ti•nant (kŏn-glū′ti-nănt) Adhesive, promoting the union of a wound. [L. *con-glutino,* pp. *-atus,* to glue together, fr. *gluten,* glue]

con•glu•ti•na•tion (kŏn-glū′ti-nā′shŭn) **1.** SYN adhesion (1). **2.** Agglutination of antigen-(erythrocyte)-antibody-complement complex by normal bovine serum (and certain other colloidal materials); the procedure provides a means of detecting the presence of nonagglutinating antibody.

Con•go blue (kong′gō blū) Sodium salt used to stain and identify protozoa. SYN Niagara blue, trypan blue.

con•go•phil•ic (kong′gō-fil′ik) Denoting any substance that takes a Congo red stain.

con•go•phil•ic an•gi•op•a•thy (kong′gō-fil′ik an′jē-op′ă-thē) A condition of blood vessels characterized by deposits in the vessel walls of a substance, usually amyloid, that takes a Congo red stain. SEE ALSO cerebral amyloid angiopathy.

Con·go red (kong′gō red) [CI 22120] An acid direct cotton dye, used as an indicator (pH 3.0, blue-violet, to pH 5.0, red) in testing for free hydrochloric acid in gastric contents; the dye is absorbed by amyloid and induces green fluorescence to amyloid in polarized light; used as a laboratory aid in the diagnosis of amyloidosis and as a histologic stain.

co·ni (kō′nī) Plural of conus.

con·ic cor·ne·a (kon′ik kōr′nē-ă) SYN keratoconus.

con·ic pa·pil·lae (kon′ik pă-pil′ē) Numerous projections on the dorsum of the tongue, scattered among the filiform papillae and similar to them, but shorter.

♻ **-conid** Suffix indicating the cusp of a tooth in the lower jaw.

Co·nid·i·o·bo·lus (kō-nid′ē-ō-bō′lŭs) A fungal genus in the family Entomophthoraceae, widely distributed in soil and among plants, insects, and amphibians. *C. coronatus* causes conidiobolomycosis, a chronic granulomatous disease of submucosal and subcutaneous tissues. Formerly *Entomopthora* and *E. coronata*.

co·ni·o·fi·bro·sis (kō′nē-ō-fī-brō′sis) Fibrosis produced by dust, especially of the lungs by inhaled dust. [G. *konis,* dust, + fibrosis]

co·ni·o·phage (kō′nē-ō-fāj) SYN alveolar macrophage. [G. *konis,* dust, + *phagō,* to eat]

co·ni·o·sis (kō′nē-ō′sis) Any disease or morbid condition caused by inhalation of dust. [G. *konis,* dust]

con·i·za·tion (kon′i-zā′shŭn) Excision of a cone of tissue, e.g., mucosa of the cervix uteri.

con·joined a·nas·to·mo·sis (kŏn-joynd′ ă-nas′tō-mō′sis) The joining together of two small blood vessels by side-to-side elliptic anastomosis to create a single larger stoma for subsequent end-to-end anastomosis.

con·joined twins (kon-joynd′ twinz) Monozygotic twins with varying extent of union and different degrees of residual duplication. The various types of union are named by the use of a prefix designating the region that is united and adding the suffix *-pagus*, meaning fused (e.g., craniopagus, thoracopagus); the various types of residual duplication are named by designating the parts duplicated and adding the suffix *-didymus*, or *-dymus*, meaning twin (e.g., cephalodidymus, cephalodymus).

con·ju·gant (kon′jū-gănt) A member of a mating pair of organisms or gametes undergoing conjugation. [L. *con-jugo,* to join]

con·ju·ga·ta (kon-jū-gā′tă) Any conjugate diameter of the pelvis. SEE conjugate. [L. fem. of *conjugatus,* pp. of *conjugo,* to join together]

con·ju·gate (kon′jŭ-găt) **1.** Joined or paired. SYN conjugated. **2.** A conjugate diameter of the pelvis. The distance between any two specified points on the periphery of the pelvic canal. SEE conjugata. [L. *conjugatus,* joined together.]

con·ju·gate ac·id-base pair (kon′jŭ-găt as′id-bās pār) In prototonic solvents (e.g., H_2O, NH_3, acetic acid), two molecular species differing only in the presence or absence of a hydrogen ion (e.g., carbonic acid/bicarbonate ion or ammonium ion/ammonia); the basis of buffer action.

con·ju·gat·ed (kon′jŭ-gā-tĕd) SYN conjugate (1).

con·ju·gat·ed an·ti·gen (kon′jŭ-gā-tĕd an′ti-jen) SYN conjugated hapten.

con·ju·gat·ed dou·ble bonds (kon′jŭ-gā-tĕd dŭb′ĕl bondz) Two or more double bonds separated by each single bond.

con·ju·gate de·vi·a·tion of the eyes (kon′jŭ-găt dē-vē-a′shŭn īz) **1.** Rotation of the eyes equally and simultaneously in the same direction, as occurs normally. **2.** A condition in which both eyes are turned to the same side as a result of either paralysis or muscular spasm.

con·ju·gat·ed hap·ten (kon′jŭ-gā-tĕd hap′ten) A hapten that may cause the production of antibodies when it has been covalently linked to protein. SYN conjugated antigen.

con·ju·gat·ed pro·tein (kon′jŭ-gā-tĕd prō′tēn) Protein attached to some other molecule or molecules (not amino acid in nature) other than as a salt. SEE ALSO prosthetic group. Cf. simple protein.

con·ju·gate fo·ra·men (kon′jŭ-găt fōr-ā′mĕn) A foramen formed by the notches of two bones in apposition.

con·ju·gate nys·tag·mus (kon′jŭ-găt nis-tag′mŭs) A nystagmus in which the two eyes move simultaneously in the same direction.

con·ju·gate of pel·vic in·let (kon′jŭ-găt pel′vik in′lĕt) Distance from the promontory of the sacrum to the upper posterior edge of the pubic symphysis.

con·ju·gate point (kon′jŭ-găt poynt) A point so related to another that an object at one is imaged at the other.

con·ju·ga·tion (kon′jŭ-gā′shŭn) **1.** Union of two unicellular organisms or of the male and female gametes of multicellular forms followed by partition of the chromatin and the production of two new cells. **2.** Bacterial conjugation, effected by simple contact, through which transfer genes and other genes of the plasmid are transferred to recipient bacteria through pili. **3.** Sexual reproduction among protozoan ciliates, during which two individuals of appropriate mating types fuse along part of their lengths; their macronuclei degenerate and the micronuclei in each macronucleus divide several times (including a meiotic division); one of the resulting haploid pronuclei passes from each conjugant into the other and fuses with the remaining haploid nucleus in each conjugant; the organisms then separate (becoming exconjugants), undergo nuclear reorganization, and subsequently divide by asexual mitosis. **4.** The combination, especially in the liver, of certain toxic substances formed in the intestine, drugs, or steroid hormones with glucuronic or sulfuric acid; a means by which the biologic activity of certain chemical substances is terminated and the substances made ready for excretion. **5.** The formation of glycyl or tauryl derivatives of the bile acids. [L. *conjugo,* pp. *-jugatus,* to join together]

con•ju•ga•tive plas•mid (kon′jŭ-gā-tiv plaz′mid) A plasmid that can effect its own intercellular transfer by means of conjugation; this transfer is accomplished by a bacterium being rendered a donor, usually with specialized pili.

con•junc•ti•va, pl. **con•junc•ti•vae** (kŏn-jŭngk′tiv-ă, -vē) The mucous membrane investing the anterior surface of the eyeball and the posterior surface of the lids. [L. fem. of *conjunctivus,* from *conjungo,* pp. *-junctus,* to bind together]

con•junc•ti•val (kŏn-jŭngk′ti-văl) Relating to the conjunctiva.

con•junc•ti•val re•flex (kŏn-jŭngk′ti-văl rē′fleks) Closure of the eyes in response to irritation of the conjunctiva.

con•junc•ti•val ring (kŏn-jŭngk′ti-văl ring) A narrow ring at the junction of the periphery of the cornea with the conjunctiva.

con•junc•ti•val sac (kŏn-jŭngk′ti-văl sak) The space bound by the conjunctival membrane between the palpebral and bulbar conjunctivae, into which the lacrimal fluid is secreted; it opens anteriorly between the eyelids. SYN saccus conjunctivalis [TA].

con•junc•ti•val veins (kŏn-jŭngk′ti-văl vānz) The veins of the conjunctiva that drain primarily to the ophthalmic veins.

i **con•junc•ti•vi•tis** (kŏn-jŭngk′ti-vī′tis) Disorder in which the conjunctivae are reddened. The eyes tear and produce exudate along the eyelid; may progress to drooping of the eyelid such that abnormal tissue may form. Therapy may involve instillation of antibiotic eyedrops. See page B27.

con•junc•ti•vo•chal•a•sis (kŏn-jŭngk′ti-vō-kă-lă′sis) Condition in which redundant bulbar conjunctiva billows over the eyelid margin or covers the lower punctum. [conjunctiva + G. *chalasis,* a loosening]

con•junc•ti•vo•plas•ty (kŏn-jŭngk′ti-vō-plas-tē) Plastic surgery on the conjunctiva.

con•nect•ing car•ti•lage (kŏ-nek′ting kahr′ti-lăj) The cartilage in a cartilaginous joint such as the symphysis pubis. SYN interosseous cartilage.

con•nec•tion (kŏ-nek′shŭn) A union of elements or things; a connecting structure. SYN connexus.

con•nec•tive tis•sue (kŏ-nek′tiv tish′ū) The supporting or framework tissue of the animal body, formed of fibrous and ground substance with more or less numerous cells of various kinds. It is derived from the mesenchyme, and this in turn from the mesoderm. The varieties of connective tissue are: areolar or loose; adipose; dense, regular or irregular, white fibrous; elastic; mucous; lymphoid tissue; cartilage; and bone. Blood and lymph may be regarded as connective tissues, the ground substance of which is a liquid. SYN interstitial tissue.

con•nec•tive-tis•sue dis•ease (kŏ-nek′tiv-tish′ū di-zēz′) A group of generalized disorders affecting connective tissue, especially those not inherited as mendelian characteristics; rheumatic fever and rheumatoid arthritis were first proposed as such diseases, and other so-called collagen diseases have been added. SEE ALSO collagen disease.

con•nec•tive tu•mor (kŏ-nek′tiv tū′mŏr) Any tumor of the connective tissue group, such as osteoma, fibroma, sarcoma.

con•nec•tor (kŏ-nek′-tŏr) DENTISTRY a part of a partial denture that unites its components.

Con•nell su•ture (kon′ĕl sū′chŭr) A continuous suture used for inverting the gastric or intestinal walls in performing an anastomosis.

con•nex•in 26 (kon-eks′in) The gap junction protein, the gene for which (Cx26) when mutated, accounts for a major portion of recessive nonsyndromic hearing impairment.

con•nex•us (ko-nek′sŭs) SYN connection. [L.]

Conn syn•drome (kon sin′drōm) SYN primary aldosteronism.

co•noid (kō′noyd) **1.** A cone-shaped structure. **2.** Part of the apical complex characteristic of the protozoan subphylum Apicomplexa; seen in sporozoites, merozoites, or other developmental stages of sporozoans, less developed in the piroplasms (families Babesiidae and Theileriidae). The function of the conoid is unknown, but it is thought to be an organelle of penetration into the host cell, possibly aided by a protrusible form of the conoid. [G. *kōnoeidēs,* cone-shaped]

co•noid tu•ber•cle (kō′noyd tū′bĕr-kĕl) The prominence near the lateral end of the inferior surface of the clavicle that gives attachment to the conoid ligament.

Con•ra•di dis•ease (kon-rah′dē di-zēz′) SYN chondrodysplasia calcificans congenita.

Con•ra•di-Hü•ner•mann syn•drome (kon-rah′dē hyū′nĕr-mahn sin′drōm) One of the syndromes of chondrodysplasia punctata, autosomal dominant, with variable skin keratinization disorders and facial, cardiac, optic, and central nervous system abnormalities; epiphyseal stippling is also present.

Con•ra•di line (kon-rah′dē līn) A line extending from the base of the ensiform cartilage to the apex beat of the heart, corresponding approximately to the lower edge of the cardiac area.

con•san•guin•e•ous (kon-sang-gwin′ē-ŭs) Denoting consanguinity. [L. *cum,* with, + *sanguis,* blood: *consanguineus*]

con•san•guin•i•ty (kon-sang-gwin′i-tē) Kinship because of common ancestry. SYN blood relationship. [L. *consanguinitas,* blood relationship]

con•scious (kon′shŭs) **1.** Aware; having present knowledge or perception of oneself, one's acts and surroundings. **2.** Denoting something occurring with the perceptive attention of the individual, as a conscious act or idea, distinguished from automatic or instinctive. [L. *conscius,* knowing]

con•scious•ness (kon′shŭs-nĕs) The state of being aware, or perceiving physical facts or mental concepts; a state of general wakefulness and responsiveness to environment; a functioning sensorium. [L. *con-scio,* to know, to be aware of]

con•scious se•da•tion (kon′shŭs sĕ-dā′shŭn) A medically controlled state of depressed consciousness in which airway patency, protective reflexes, and the ability to respond to stimulation or verbal commands are preserved.

con•sec•u•tive am•pu•ta•tion (kŏn-sek′yū-tiv amp′yū-tā′shŭn) A revision or secondary amputation of a limb.

con•sen•su•al (kŏn-sen′shū-ăl) **1.** The fact of agreement among the perceptions of several people. **2.** Denotes the act of agreeing with or to any behavior, action, or thought. [L. *con-,* with, + *sensus,* sensation]

con•sen•su•al light re•flex (kŏn-sen′shū-ăl līt rē′fleks) Constriction of both pupils when only one is exposed to bright light; indicates integrity of optic nerve on exposed side and of oculomotor nerves on both sides.

con•ser•va•tive (kŏn-sĕr′vă-tiv) Denoting treatment by gradual, limited, or well-established procedures, as opposed to radical.

con•sis•ten•cy prin•ci•ple (kŏn-sis′tĕn-sē prin′si-pĕl) PSYCHOLOGY the desire of human beings to be consistent, especially in their attitudes and beliefs; theories of attitude formation and change based on the consistency principle include balance theory, which suggests that people seek to avoid incongruity in their various attitudes.

Con•sol•i•dat•ed Om•ni•bus Bud•get Re•con•ci•li•a•tion Act (COBRA) (kŏn-sol′i-dā-tĕd om′ni-bŭs bŭj′ĕt rek′ŏn-sil-ē-ā′shŭn akt) U.S. federal law that allows an employee to remain covered under employer's group health insurance plan for a given period of time after death of a spouse, divorce, termination, or having work hours reduced.

con•sol•i•da•tion (kŏn-sol′i-dā′shŭn) Solidification into a firm dense mass; applied especially to inflammatory induration of a normally aerated lung due to the presence of cellular exudate in the pulmonary alveoli. [L. *consolido,* to make thick, condense, fr. *solidus,* solid]

con•so•nant (kon′sŏ-nănt) A speech sound produced by partial or complete obstruction to the flow of air at any point in the vocal apparatus. [L. *consono,* to sound together]

con•spi•cu•i•ty (kon′spi-kyū′i-tē) The visibility of a structure of interest on a radiograph, a function of the inherent contrast of the structure and the complexity (noise) of the surrounding image.

con•stan•cy (kon′stăn-sē) The quality of being constant. [L. *constantia,* fr. *consto,* to stand still]

con•stant (kon′stănt) A quantity that, under stated conditions, does not vary with changes in the environment.

con•sti•pate (kon′sti-pāt) To cause constipation.

con•sti•pat•ed (kon′sti-pāt-ĕd) Suffering from constipation.

con•sti•pa•tion (kon′sti-pā′shŭn) A condition in which bowel movements are infrequent or incomplete. [L. *con-stipo,* pp. *-atus,* to press together]

con•sti•tu•tion (kon′sti-tū′shŭn) **1.** The physical makeup of a body, including the mode of performance of its functions, the activity of its metabolic processes, the manner and degree of its reactions to stimuli, and its power of resistance to the attack of pathogenic organisms. **2.** CHEMISTRY the number and kind of atoms in the molecule and the relation they bear to each other. [L. *constitutio,* constitution, disposition, fr. *constituo,* pp. *-stitutus,* to establish, fr. *statuo,* to set up]

con•sti•tu•tion•al (kon′sti-tū′shŭn-ăl) **1.** Relating to a body's constitution. **2.** General; relating to the system as a whole; not local.

con•sti•tu•tion•al re•ac•tion (kon′sti-tū′shŭn-ăl rē-ak′shŭn) A generalized reaction in contrast to a focal or local reaction; in allergy, the immediate or delayed response, following the introduction of an allergen, occurring at sites remote from that of injection.

con•sti•tu•tion•al symp•tom (kon′sti-tū′shŭn-ăl simp′tŏm) A symptom indicating a systemic effect of a disease; e.g., weight loss.

con·stric·ti·o (kon-strik′shē-ō) [TA] SYN constriction (1).

con·stric·tion (kŏn-strik′shŭn) **1.** A normally or pathologically constricted or narrowed portion of a luminal structure. SYN constrictio [TA]. SEE ALSO stricture, stenosis. **2.** The act or process of binding or contracting, becoming narrowed; the condition of being constricted or squeezed. **3.** A subjective sensation of pressure or tightness, as if the body or any part were tightly bound or squeezed. [L. *con-stringo,* pp. *-strictus,* to draw together]

con·stric·tion ring (kŏn-strik′shŭn ring) **1.** Spastic stricture of the uterine cavity resulting when a zone of muscle goes into local tetanic contraction and forms a tight constriction of some part of the fetus; **2.** SYN amnionic band.

con·stric·tive bron·chi·ol·i·tis (kŏn-strik′tiv brong′kē-ō-lī′tis) Obliteration of bronchioles by scarring following bronchiolitis obliterans.

con·stric·tive per·i·car·di·tis (kŏn-strik′tiv per′i-kahr-dī′tis) Postinflammatory thickening and scarring of the membrane producing constriction of the cardiac chambers; may be acute, subacute, or chronic. Formerly called chronic constrictive pericarditis.

con·stric·tor (kŏn-strik′tŏr) **1.** Anything that binds or squeezes a part. **2.** A muscle, the action of which is to narrow a canal; a sphincter. [L. fr. *constringo,* to draw together]

con·struc·tion·al a·prax·i·a (kŏn-strŭkt′shŭn-ăl ă-praks′ē-ă) Patient's inability to reproduce geometric designs and figures.

con·sul·tant (kŏn-sŭl′tănt) **1.** A physician or surgeon who does not take full responsibility for a patient, but acts in an advisory capacity, deliberating with and counseling the attending physician or surgeon. **2.** A member of a hospital staff who has no active service but stands ready to advise in any case, at the request of the attending physician or surgeon. [L. *consulto,* pp. *-atus,* to deliberate, ask advice]

con·sul·ta·tion (kon′sŭl-tā′shŭn) Meeting of two or more physicians or surgeons to evaluate the nature and progress of disease in a particular patient and to establish diagnosis, prognosis, and/or therapy.

con·sult·ing staff (kŏn-sul′ting staf) Specialists affiliated with a hospital who serve in an advisory capacity to the attending staff.

con·sump·tion (kŏn-sŭmp′shŭn) **1.** The using up of something, especially the rate at which it is used. **2.** Older term for tuberculosis. [L. *con-sumo,* pp. *-sumptus,* to take up wholly, use up, waste]

con·sump·tion co·ag·u·lop·a·thy (kŏn-sŭmp′shŭn kō-ag′yū-lop′ă-thē) A disorder in which marked reductions develop in blood concentrations of platelets with exhaustion of the coagulation factors in the peripheral blood as a result of disseminated intravascular coagulation.

con·tact (kon′takt) **1.** The touching or apposition of two surfaces. **2.** A person who has been exposed to a contagious disease. **3.** DENTISTRY the area of two teeth in an arch where mesial and distal surfaces touch. [L. *con- tingo,* pp. *-tactus,* to touch, seize, fr. *tango,* to touch]

con·tact al·ler·gy (kon′takt al′ĕr-jē) SYN allergic contact dermatitis.

con·tac·tant (kŏn-tak′tănt) Any allergen that elicits manifestations of hypersensitivity by direct contact with skin or mucosa.

con·tact chei·li·tis (kon′takt kī-lī′tis) Inflammation of the lips resulting from contact with a primary irritant or specific allergen, including ingredients of lipsticks.

con·tact der·ma·ti·tis (kon′takt dĕr′mă-tī′tis) Inflammatory rash marked by itching and redness resulting from cutaneous contact with a specific allergen (allergic contact dermatitis) or irritant (irritant contact dermatitis). See this page, B9.

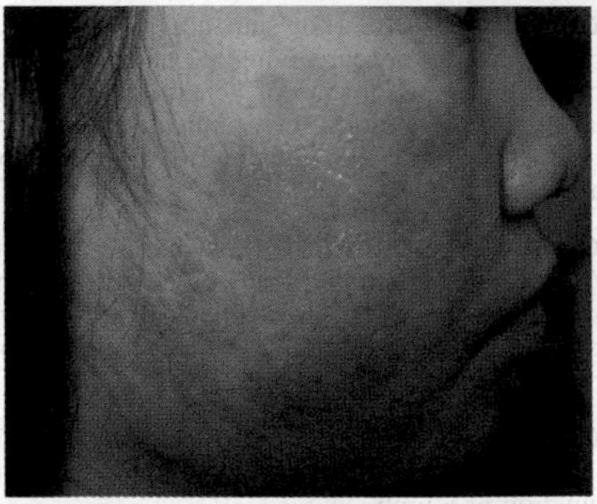

A

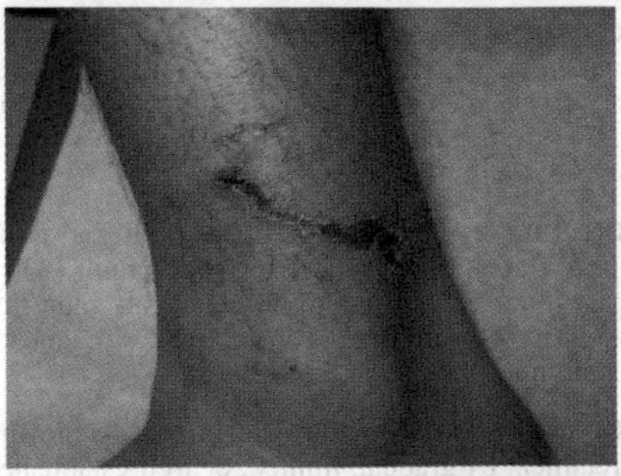

B

contact dermatitis: (A) allergic, cheek; (B) jellyfish sting, leg

con·tact hy·ster·o·scope (kon′takt his′tĕr-ō-skōp) Hysteroscope with a graded refractive index rod lens. It does not require distension for visualization and affords very short focal length views; suitable for localizing hemorrhages.

con•tact in•hi•bi•tion (kon′takt in′hi-bish′ŭn) Cessation of replication of dividing cells that come into contact, as in the center of a healing wound.

con•tact i•so•la•tion (kon′takt ī′sō-lā′shŭn) Form of isolation in which anyone entering the patient's room and having direct contact with the patient wears gloves and a gown.

con•tact lens (kon′takt lenz) A lens that fits over the cornea and sclera or cornea only; used to correct refractive errors.

con•tact pre•cau•tions (kon′takt prĕ-kaw′shŭnz) Procedures that reduce the risk of spread of infections through direct or indirect contact. Transmission occurs with physical contact of the infected patient or handling of a contaminated object in the infected patient's room. Masks, gowns, and gloves as well as standard precautions (q.v.) must be used by health care providers when in the infected patient's room.

con•tact splint (kon′takt splint) A slotted plate, held by screws, used in the treatment of fracture of long bones.

con•tact-type der•ma•ti•tis (kon′takt-tīp dĕr′mă-tī′tis) Dermatitis resembling contact dermatitis or eczema, but caused by an ingested or injected allergen, usually a drug, and with a widespread or generalized distribution.

con•tact ul•cer (kon′takt ŭl′sĕr) Ulceration of the vocal folds along their posterior borders, overlying the vocal processes of the arytenoid cartilages. Usually caused by vocal fold abuse; results in hoarse voice.

con•tact with re•al•i•ty (kon′takt rē-al′i-tē) Correctly interpreting external phenomena in relation to the norms of one's social or cultural milieu.

con•ta•gion (kŏn-tā′jŭn) **1.** SYN contagium. **2.** Transmission of infection by direct contact, droplet spread, or contaminated fomites. **3.** Production through suggestion or imitation of a neurosis or psychosis in several or more members of a group. SYN infectious (2). [L. *contagio;* fr. *contingo,* to touch closely]

con•ta•gious (kŏn-tā′jŭs) Relating to contagion; communicable or transmissible by contact with the sick or their fresh secretions or excretions. SYN infectious (2).

con•ta•gious dis•ease (kŏn-tā′jŭs di-zēz′) An infectious disease transmissible by direct or indirect contact; now used synonymously with communicable disease.

con•ta•gious•ness (kŏn-tā′jŭs-nĕs) The quality of being contagious.

con•ta•gi•um (kon-tā′jē-ŭm) The agent of an infectious disease. SYN contagion (1). [L. a touching]

con•tained disc her•ni•a•tion (kŏn-tānd′ disk hĕr′nē-ā′shŭn) Herniated disc material that remains covered by a thin layer of posterior anulus fibrosus or posterior longitudinal ligament; a disc protrusion is an example of a contained disc herniation.

con•tain•er (kŏn-tā′nĕr) A receptacle in which anything is confined. [L. *contineo,* to hold togethr]

con•tam•i•nant (kŏn-tam′i-nănt) An impurity; any extraneous material associated with a chemical, a pharmaceutical preparation, a physiologic principle, or an infectious agent.

con•tam•i•nate (kŏn-tam′i-nāt) **1.** To cause or result in contamination. **2.** Introduction of pathogens or infectious material into or on clean or sterile surfaces. [L. *con-tamino,* to mingle, corrupt]

con•tam•i•na•tion (kŏn-tam′i-nā′shŭn) **1.** The presence of an infectious agent on a body surface or on or in clothes, bedding, toys, surgical instruments or dressings, or other inanimate articles or substances including water, milk, and food, or that infectious agent itself. **2.** That portion of a chemical, biologic, or radiologic agent that remains on (external contamination) or in (internal contamination) a victim or inanimate object, especially, but not necessarily, after evaporation and absorption. **3.** EPIDEMIOLOGY the situation that exists when a population being studied for one condition or factor also possesses other conditions or factors that modify results of the study. **4.** PSYCHOLOGY/PSYCHIATRY freudian term for a fusion and condensation of words. SEE ALSO residual dose contamination. [L. *contamino,* pp. *-atus,* to stain, defile]

con•tent (kon′tent) **1.** That which is contained within something else, usually in this sense in the plural form, contents. **2.** PSYCHOLOGY the form of a dream as presented to consciousness. **3.** Ambiguous usage for concentration (3); e.g., blood hemoglobin content could mean either its concentration or the product of its concentration and the blood volume. **4.** BIOWARFARE a biologic agent within a delivery device. [L. *contentus,* fr. *con-tineo,* pp. *-tentus,* to hold together, contain]

con•tent a•nal•y•sis (kon′tent ă-nal′i-sis) Any of a variety of techniques for classification and study of the verbal products of normal or of psychologically impaired people.

con•tig map (kon-tig′ map) A physical map of a chromosome or stretch of DNA constructed from sets of overlapping and order clones (contig).

con•ti•gu•i•ty (kon′ti-gyū′i-tē) **1.** Contact without structural continuity, e.g., the contact of the bones entering into the formation of a cranial suture. Cf. continuity. **2.** Occurrence of two or more objects, events, or mental impressions together in space or time. [L. *contiguus,* touching, fr. *contingo,* to touch]

con·tig·u·ous (kon-tig′yū-ŭs) Adjacent or in actual contact.

con·ti·nence (kon′ti-nĕns) **1.** Moderation, temperance, or self-restraint in respect to the appetites, especially to sexual intercourse. **2.** The ability to retain urine and/or feces until a proper time for their discharge. [L. *continentia,* fr. *contineo,* to hold back]

con·ti·nent (kon′ti-nĕnt) **1.** Able to retain urine or stool. **2.** Referring to an enterostomy with sphincterlike control. SEE ALSO continence.

con·tin·u·ing ed·u·ca·tion (kon-tin′yū-ing ej′ū-kā′shŭn) Systematic professional learning experiences designed to augment knowledge and skills of health care professionals; education completed after the initial educational program; required for relicensure in some fields.

con·tin·u·ing ed·u·ca·tion u·nits (kon-tin′yū-ing ej′ū-kā′shŭn yū′nits) Credit given to a participant after completing a designated program (workshop or seminar), to upgrade skills and knowledge.

con·ti·nu·i·ty (kon′ti-nū′i-tē) Absence of interruption, a succession of parts intimately united, e.g., the unbroken conjunction of cells and structures that make up a single bone of the skull. Cf. contiguity. [L. *continuus,* continued]

con·tin·u·ous am·bu·la·to·ry per·i·to·ne·al di·al·y·sis (CAPD) (kŏn-tin′yū-ŭs am′byū-lă-tōr-ē per′i-tō-nē′ăl dī-al′i-sis) Method of peritoneal dialysis performed in ambulatory patients with influx and efflux of dialysate during normal activities.

con·tin·u·ous ar·ter·i·o·ve·nous he·mo·fil·tra·tion (CAVH) (kŏn-tin′yū-ŭs ahr-tēr′ē-ō-vē′nŭs hē′mō-fil-trā′shŭn) Removal of fluid and uremic solutes from the circulation in acute and chronic renal failure by continuous pressure- or vacuum-assisted, convection-based filtration across a membrane.

con·tin·u·ous bar re·tain·er (kŏn-tin′yū-ŭs bahr rĕ-tān′ĕr) A metal bar, usually resting on the lingual surfaces of teeth that aids in their stabilization and acts as an indirect retainer.

con·tin·u·ous cap·il·lar·y (kŏn-tin′yū-ŭs kap′i-lar-ē) A capillary in which small vesicles (caveolae) are numerous and pores are absent.

con·tin·u·ous cyc·lic per·i·to·ne·al di·al·y·sis (CCPD) (kŏn-tin′yū-ŭs sik′lik per′i-tō-nē′ăl dī-al′i-sis) Intermittent peritoneal dialysis infused overnight with a prolonged equilibrating time during the day.

con·tin·u·ous flow an·a·lyz·er (kŏn-tin′yū-ŭs flō an′ă-līz-ĕr) An automated chemical analyzer in which the samples and reagents are pumped continuously through a system of modules interconnected by tubing.

con·tin·u·ous in·ter·leaved sam·pling (kŏn-tin′yū-ŭs in′tĕr-lēvd sam′pling) A strategy in speech processing for cochlear implants in which brief pulses are presented to each electrode in a nonoverlapping sequence.

con·tin·u·ous man·da·tor·y ven·ti·la·tion (CMV) (kŏn-tin′yū-ŭs man′dă-tōr-ē ven′ti-lā′shŭn) SYN controlled mechanical ventilation.

con·tin·u·ous mur·mur (kŏn-tin′yū-ŭs mŭr′mŭr) A murmur that is heard without interruption throughout systole and into diastole.

con·tin·u·ous o·to·a·cou·stic e·mis·sion (kŏn-tin′yū-ŭs ō′tō-ă-kū′stik ē-mish′ŭn) A form of evoked otoacoustic emission in which the emission is of the same frequency as the stimulus and persists as long as the stimulus.

con·ti·nu·ous pas·sive mo·tion ma·chine (CPM ma·chine) (kŏn-tin-yū′ŭs pas′iv mō′shŭn mă′shēn) Device used to promote normal movement, prevent stiffness, and relieve pain after surgery or injury to major joints of upper and lower extremities.

con·tin·u·ous pos·i·tive air·way pres·sure (CPAP) (kŏn-tin′yū-ŭs poz′i-tiv ār′wā presh′ŭr) A technique of respiratory therapy, in either spontaneously breathing or mechanically ventilated patients, in which the mean airway pressure is maintained above atmospheric pressure throughout the respiratory cycle by pressurization of the ventilatory circuit.

con·tin·u·ous pos·i·tive pres·sure ven·ti·la·tion (CPPV) (kŏn-tin′yū-ŭs poz′i-tiv presh′chŭr ven′ti-lā′shŭn) SYN controlled mechanical ventilation.

con·tin·u·ous qual·i·ty im·prove·ment (kŏn-tin′yū-ŭs kwahl′i-tē im-prūv′mĕnt) Structured process to improve all aspects of care and service continually; ongoing study to improve performance.

con·tin·u·ous skill (kŏn-tin′yū-ŭs skil) A skill or pattern of movement that does not appear to have a distinct beginning or end; the motor patterns usually form a repetitive or ongoing process (e.g., swimming, steering a car).

con·tin·u·ous spon·ta·ne·ous ven·til·a·tion (CSV) (kŏn-tin′yū-ŭs spon-tā′nē-ŭs ven′ti-lā′shŭn) A mode of mechanical ventilation in which every breath is spontaneous.

con·tin·u·ous su·ture (kŏn-tin′yū-ŭs sū′chŭr) An uninterrupted series of stitches using one suture; the stitching is fastened at each end by a knot. SYN uninterrupted suture.

con·tin·u·ous train·ing (kŏn-tin′yū-ŭs trān′ing) Use of steady-state exercise to overload the aerobic system of energy transfer. Because of its submaximal nature, exercise continues for considerable time in relative comfort; ideal exercise for weight loss and improved health. SYN long slow distance training.

con·tin·u·ous ve·no·ve·nous he·mo·di·a·fil·tra·tion (CVVHD) (kŏn-tin′yū-us vē-no-vē′nŭs hē′mō-dī′ă-fil-trā′shŭn) A form of therapy that uses a diffusion solution clearance as a modality.

con·tin·u·ous ve·no·ve·nous he·mo·di·al·y·sis (CVVHD) (kŏn-tin′yū-ŭs vē-nō-vē′nŭs hē′mō-dī-al′i-sis) Continuous hemodialysis in which blood is pumped from a vein to the dialyzing unit and treated blood is returned to the venous circulation.

con·tin·u·ous ve·no·ve·nous he·mo·fil·tra·tion (CVVH) (kŏn-tin′yū-ŭs vē-nō-vē′nŭs hē′mō-fil-trā′shŭn) Continuous hemofiltration in which blood is pumped from a vein to the filtration unit and filtred blood is returned to the venous circulation.

con·tin·u·ous wave la·ser (kŏn-tin′yū-ŭs wāv lā′zĕr) A laser in which energy output is constant.

con·tour (kon′tūr) **1.** The outline of a part; the surface configuration. **2.** DENTISTRY to restore the normal outlines of a broken or otherwise misshapen tooth, or to create the external shape or form of a prosthesis. [L. *con-* (intens.), + *torno,* to turn (in a lathe), fr. *tornus,* a lathe]

contra- Prefix meaning opposed, against. SEE ALSO counter-. Cf. anti-. [L.]

con·tra·an·gle (kon′tră-ang′el) **1.** One of the double or triple angles in the shank of an instrument by means of which the cutting edge or point is brought into the axis of the handle. **2.** An extension piece added to the end of a dental handpiece which, through a set of bevel gears, changes the angle of the axis of rotation of the bur in relation to the axis of the handpiece.

con·tra·ap·er·ture (kon′tră-ap′ĕr-chŭr) SYN counteropening.

con·tra·cep·tion (kon′tră-sep′shŭn) Prevention of conception or impregnation.

con·tra·cep·tive (kon′tră-sep′tiv) **1.** An agent that prevents conception. **2.** Relating to any measure or agent designed to prevent conception. [L. *contra,* against, + conceptive]

con·tra·cep·tive de·vice (kon′tră-sep′tiv dĕ-vīs′) A device used to prevent pregnancy (e.g., occlusive diaphragm, condom, intrauterine device).

con·tra·cep·tive sponge (kon′tră-sep′tiv spŭnj) A pliable hydrophilic piece of polyurethane foam infused with spermicide that is inserted into the vagina before coitus; used as a nonprescription contraceptive device.

con·tract (kon-trakt′) **1.** To shorten; to become reduced in size; in the case of muscle, either to shorten or to undergo an increase in tension. **2.** To acquire by contagion or infection. **3.** (kon′trakt) An explicit bilateral commitment by psychotherapist and patient to a defined course of action to attain the goal of the psychotherapy. [L. *con-traho,* pp. *-tractus,* to draw together]

con·tract·ed dis·count (kŏn-trak′tĕd dis′kownt) The amount a health care provider writes off or adjusts from a patient's balance in accordance with agreement with the insurer covering that patient.

con·tract·ed kid·ney (kŏn-trakt′ĕd kid′nē) A diffusely scarred kidney in which fibrous tissue and ischemic atrophy lead to reduction in the size of the organ.

con·tract·ed pel·vis (kŏn-trakt′ĕd pel′vis) A pelvis with less than normal measurements in any diameter.

con·trac·tile (kon-trak′tīl) Having the property of contracting.

con·trac·til·i·ty (kon′trak-til′i-tē) The ability or property of a substance, especially of muscle, of shortening, or becoming reduced in size, or developing increased tension.

con·trac·tion (C) (kŏn-trak′shŭn) **1.** A shortening or increase in tension; denoting the normal function of muscle. **2.** A shrinkage or reduction in size. **3.** Heart beat, as in premature contraction. [L. *contractus,* drawn together]

con·trac·tion stress test (kŏn-trak′shŭn stres test) SYN oxytocin challenge test.

con·trac·tu·al psy·chi·a·try (kŏn-trak′shū-ăl sī-kī′ă-trē) Psychiatric intervention voluntarily assumed by the patient, who is prompted by his personal difficulties or suffering and who retains control over his participation with the psychiatrist.

con·trac·ture (kŏn-trak′shŭr) Static muscle shortening due to tonic spasm or fibrosis, to loss of muscular balance (the antagonists are paralyzed), or to a loss of motion of the adjacent joint. [L. *contractura,* fr. *con-traho,* to draw together]

con·tra·fis·sur·a (kon′tră-fi-shū′ră) Fracture of a bone, as in the skull, at a point opposite that where the blow was received. [L. *contra,* against, counter, + *fissura,* fissure]

con·tra·in·di·ca·tion (kon′tră-in-di-kā′shŭn) Any special symptom or circumstance that renders the use of a remedy or the carrying out of a procedure inadvisable, usually because of risk.

con·tra·lat·er·al (kon′tră-lat′ĕr-ăl) Relating to the opposite side, as when pain is felt or paralysis occurs on the side opposite to that of the lesion. SYN heterolateral. [L. *contra,* opposite, + *latus,* side]

con·tra·lat·er·al hem·i·ple·gi·a (kon′tră-lat′ĕr-ăl hem′ē-plē′jē-ă) Paralysis occurring on the side opposite to the causal central lesion.

con·tra·lat·er·al rout·ing of sig·nals (kon′

tră-lat′ĕr-ăl rowt′ing sig′nălz) A hearing aid configuration for greater hearing loss in one ear than the other in which sound is picked up by the microphone at the worse hearing ear and delivered to the better hearing ear.

con•trast (kon′trast) **1.** A comparison in which differences are demonstrated or enhanced. **2.** RADIOLOGY the difference between the image densities of two areas. [L. *contra,* against, + *sto,* pp. *status,* to stand]

con•trast bath (kon′trast bath) A bath in which a body part is immersed in hot water for a period of a few minutes and then in cold, the hot and cold periods alternated regularly at intervals; used to increase the blood flow to the body part.

con•trast me•di•um (kon′trast mē′dē-ŭm) Any internally administered substance that has a different opacity from soft tissue on radiography or computed tomography; used to opacify parts of the gastrointestinal tract, blood vessels, or the genitourinary tract.

con•trast sen•si•tiv•it•y test•ing (kon′trast sen′si-tiv′i-tē test′ing) Examination of the visual recognition of the variation in brightness of an object.

con•trast stain (kon′trast stān) A dye used to color one portion of a tissue or cell that remained unaffected when the other part was stained by a dye of different color.

con•tre•coup (kōn′trĕ-kū′) Denoting the manner of a contrafissura, as in the skull, at a point opposite that at which the blow was received. SEE ALSO contrecoup injury of brain. [Fr. counter-blow]

con•tre•coup frac•ture (kōn′trĕ-kū′ frak′shŭr) A fracture of the cranial vault occurring at a site approximately opposite the point of impact. [Fr. counter-blow]

con•tre•coup in•ju•ry of brain (kōn′trĕ-kū′ in′jŭr-ē brān) Concussion, contusion, or laceration due to propulsion of the brain in its fluid medium against the inner surface of the skull at a site approximately opposite the point of external impact. [Fr. counter-blow]

con•trol (kŏn-trōl′) **1.** (v.) To regulate, restrain, correct, restore to normal. **2.** (n.) Ongoing operations or programs aimed at reducing a disease. **3.** (n.) Members of a comparison group who differ in disease experience or allocation to a regimen from the subjects of a study. **4.** (v). STATISTICS to adjust or take into account extraneous influences. [Mediev. L. *contrarotulum,* a counterroll for checking accounts, fr. L. *rotula,* dim. of *rota,* a wheel]

***Con•trol of Com•mun•i•ca•ble Dis•eas•es Man•u•al* (CCDM)** (kŏn-trōl′ kŏ-myūn′i-kă-bĕl di-zēz′ĕz man′yū-ăl) The internationally recognized authoritative manual (17th edition in 2000), published by the American Public Health Association.

con•trol ex•per•i•ment (kŏn-trōl′ eks-per′i-mĕnt) An experiment used to check another, to verify the result, or to demonstrate what would have occurred had the factor under study been omitted. SEE ALSO control.

con•trol group (kŏn-trōl′ grūp) A group of subjects participating in the same experiment as another group of subjects, but not exposed to the variable under investigation. SEE ALSO experimental group.

con•trolled me•chan•i•cal ven•ti•la•tion (kŏn-trōld′ mĕ-kan′i-kăl ven′ti-lā′shŭn) A term sometimes applied to a mode of mechanical ventilation that provides a breath sequence independent of the patient's inspiratory effort. SYN continuous mandatory ventilation, continuous positive pressure ventilation, intermittent positive pressure breathing.

con•trolled sub•stance (kŏn-trōld′ sub′stăns) A substance subject to the U.S. federal Controlled Substances Act (1970), which regulates the prescribing and dispensing, as well as the manufacturing, storage, sale, or distribution, of substances assigned to five schedules according to their: 1) potential for or evidence of abuse; 2) potential for psychic or physiologic dependence; 3) role in putting the health of the public at risk; 4) harmful pharmacologic effect; or 5) role as a precursor of other controlled substances.

con•trol sy•ringe (kŏn-trōl′ sir-inj′) A type of Luer-Lok syringe with thumb and finger rings attached to the proximal end of the barrel and to the tip of the plunger, allowing operation of the syringe with one hand. SYN ring syringe.

con•tuse (kŏn-tūz′) To injure a tissue without laceration. SYN bruise (2). [L. *con tundo, con tusus,* to strike, beat]

con•tu•sion (kŏn-tū′zhŭn) Any mechanical injury (usually caused by a blow) resulting in hemorrhage beneath unbroken skin. SEE ALSO bruise. [L. *contusio,* a bruising]

Co•nus (kō′nŭs) A genus of shellfish that inhabits the shores of some South Pacific islands. Several species are poisonous, their sting or spine causing acute pain, edema, numbness, spreading paralysis, and sometimes coma and death.

co•nus, pl. **co•ni** (kō′nŭs, -nī) **1.** SYN cone. **2.** Posterior staphyloma in myopic choroidopathy. [L. fr. G. *kōnos,* cone]

co•nus ar•te•ri•o•sus (kō′nŭs ar-tē-rē-ō′sŭs) [TA] SYN arterial cone.

co•nus me•dul•la•ris (kō′nŭs mĕd-ū-lā′ris) [TA] SYN medullary cone.

con•va•les•cence (kon′vă-les′ĕns) A period between the end of a disease and the patient's restoration to complete health. [L. *con-valesco,* to grow strong, fr. *valeo,* to be strong]

con•va•les•cent (kon′vă-les′ĕnt) **1.** Getting

well or one who is getting well. **2.** Denoting the period of convalescence.

con•vec•tion (kŏn-vek′shŭn) Conveyance of heat in liquids or gases by movement of the heated particles, as when the layer of water at the bottom of a heated pot rises or the warm air of a room ascends to the ceiling. [L. *con-veho,* pp. *-vectus,* to carry or bring together]

con•vec•tive heat (kŏn-vek′tive hēt) A rise in temperature conveyed from one structure or appliance to another in which the warmer affects the cooler by convection.

con•ven•tion•al signs (kŏn-ven′shŭn-ăl sīnz) Signs that acquire their function through social (linguistic) custom (e.g., words, mathematical symbols).

con•ven•tion•al thor•a•co•plas•ty (kŏn-ven′shŭn-ăl thōr′ă-kō-plas-tē) Resection of ribs to allow inward retraction of the chest wall to reduce size of the pleural space; may be used in the treatment of empyema.

con•ver•gence (kŏn-vĕr′jĕns) **1.** The tending of two or more objects toward a common point. **2.** The direction of the visual lines to a near point. [L. *con-vergere,* to incline together]

con•ver•gence ex•cess (kŏn-vĕr′jĕns eks′es) That condition in which an esophoria or esotropia is greater for near vision than for far vision.

con•ver•gence in•suf•fi•cien•cy (kŏn-vĕr′jĕns in′sŭ-fish′ĕn-sē) That condition in which an esophoria or esotropia is more marked for far vision than for near vision.

con•ver•gent (kŏn-vĕr′jĕnt) Tending toward a common point.

con•ver•gent ev•o•lu•tion (kŏn-vĕr′jĕnt ev′ŏ-lū′shŭn) The evolutionary development of similar structures in two or more species, often widely separated phylogenetically, in response to similarities of environment; for example, the wings in insects, birds, and flying mammals.

con•ver•gent stra•bis•mus (kŏn-vĕr′jĕnt stră-biz′mŭs) SYN esotropia.

con•ver•sa•tion board (kon-vĕr-sā′shŭn bōrd) SYN communication board.

con•ver•sion (kŏn-vĕr′zhŭn) **1.** SYN transmutation. **2.** An unconscious defense mechanism by which the anxiety that stems from an unconscious conflict is converted and expressed symbolically as a physical symptom; transformation of an emotion into a physical manifestation, as in conversion hysteria. SEE conversion hysteria. **3.** VIROLOGY the acquisition by bacteria of a new property associated with presence of a prophage. SEE ALSO lysogeny. [L. *con-verto,* pp. *-versus,* to turn around, to change]

con•ver•sion cho•re•a (kŏn-vĕr′zhŭn kōr-ē′ă) A conversion disorder in which involuntary, quick, and purposeless (choreiform) movement constitute the chief feature.

con•ver•sion dis•or•der (kŏn-vĕr′zhŭn dis-ōr′dĕr) A mental disorder in which an unconscious emotional conflict is expressed as an alteration or loss of physical functioning, usually controlled by the voluntary nervous system.

con•ver•sion hys•te•ri•a (kŏn-vĕr′zhŭn his-ter′ē-ă) Hysteria characterized by the substitution of physical signs or symptoms (e.g., blindness, deafness, and paralysis) for anxiety. SYN conversion hysteria neurosis, conversion reaction.

con•ver•sion hys•te•ri•a neu•ro•sis (kŏn-vĕr′zhŭn his-ter′ē-ă nūr-ō′sis) SYN conversion hysteria.

con•ver•sion re•ac•tion (kŏn-vĕr′zhŭn rē-ak′shŭn) SYN conversion hysteria.

con•ver•sive heat (kŏn-vĕr′siv hēt) Heat produced in a body by the absorption of waves that are not in themselves hot, such as the sun's rays or infrared radiation.

con•ver•tase (kon′vĕr-tās) Proteases of complement that convert one component into another. SEE component of complement.

con•ver•tin (kon-vĕr′tin) Active form of factor VII designated VIIa.

con•vex (kon′veks) Applied to a surface that is evenly curved outward, as the segment of a sphere. [L. *convexus,* vaulted, arched, convex, fr. *con-veho,* to bring together]

con•vex lens (kon′veks lenz) A converging lens.

con•vex•o•con•cave (kon-vek′sō-kon′kāv) Convex on one surface and concave on the opposite surface.

con•vex•o•con•cave lens (kon-vek′sō-kon′kāv lenz) A minus power lens having one surface convex and the opposite surface concave, with the latter having the greater curvature.

con•vex•o•con•vex (kon-vek′sō-kon′veks) SYN biconvex.

con•vex•o•con•vex lens (kon-vek′sō-kon′veks lenz) SYN biconvex lens.

con•vo•lut•ed part of kid•ney lob•ule (kon′vŏ-lūt′ĕd pahrt kid′nē lob′yūl) Proximal and distal convoluted tubules and the associated renal corpuscles supplied by branches of the interlobular arteries. SYN renal labyrinth.

con•vo•lu•ted sem•i•nif•er•ous tu•bule (kon′vŏ-lūt′ĕd sem′i-nif′ĕr-ŭs tū′byūl) SYN seminiferous tubule.

con•vo•lu•ted tu•bule (kon′vŏ-lūt′ĕd tū′byūl) Either of the two intricately coiled segments of the renal tubule; the proximal convoluted tubule leads from the capsule of the kidney to the straight portion of the proximal tubule; the distal convoluted tubule is formed from the ascending limb of the loop of Henle and ends in a collecting tubule. SYN tubuli contorti (1).

con•vo•lu•tion (kon-vŏ-lū′shŭn) **1.** A coiling or rolling of an organ. **2.** Specifically, a gyrus of the cerebral or cerebellar cortex. [L. *convolutio*]

con•vul•sion (kŏn-vŭl′shŭn) **1.** A violent spasm or series of jerkings of the face, trunk, or extremities. **2.** SYN seizure (2). [L. *convulsio,* fr. *con-vello,* pp. *-vulsus,* to tear up]

con•vul•sive (kŏn-vŭl′siv) Relating to convulsions; marked by or producing convulsions.

cook•book med•i•cine (kuk′buk med′i-sin) SEE evidence-based medicine.

Cooke spec•u•lum (kuk spek′yŭ-lŭm) A three-pronged speculum for rectal examinations and operations.

cool down (kūl down) A gradual decrease in blood pressure, temperature, and heart rate returning to baseline after exercise. SEE endurance phase, endurance training.

Coo•ley a•ne•mi•a (koo′lē ă-nē′mē-ă) SYN thalassemia major.

Coombs di•rect test (kūmz dĭr-ekt′ test) Laboratory test using erythrocytes to detect antibodies to them or to complement. Positive findings in leukemia, lymphoma, systemic lupus erythematosa and other conditions. SEE Coombs test.

Coombs in•di•rect test (kūmz in′dĭr-ekt′ test) Laboratory test using serum that contains an antibody that may be used for erythrocyte typing; positive (i.e., abnormal) finding in isoimmunization from previous transfusions of incorrect cross-matching. SEE Coombs test. SYN indirect Coombs test.

Coombs se•rum (kūmz sēr′ŭm) SYN antihuman globulin.

Coombs test (kūmz test) A procedure for measuring antibodies, the so-called anti-human globulin test, using either the direct or indirect Coombs tests.

Coo•per her•ni•a (kū′pĕr hĕr′nē-ă) A femoral hernia with two sacs, the first being in the femoral canal, and the second passing through a defect in the superficial fascia and appearing immediately beneath the skin. SYN Hey hernia.

Coo•per her•ni•o•tome (kū′pĕr hĕr′nē-ō-tōm) A slender bistoury with short cutting edge for dividing the constricting tissues at the neck of a hernial sac.

Coo•per-Rand art•i•fi•cial lar•ynx (kū′pĕr-rand ahr-ti-fish′ăl lar′ingks) An electronic device for vocal rehabilitation after laryngectomy that produces an intraoral sound articulated into speech with the pharynx, palate, tongue, lips, and teeth.

Coo•per tes•tis (kū′pĕr tĕs′tis) Pain in testicles resulting from neuralgia.

co•or•di•na•tion (kō-ōr′di-nā′shun) The harmonious function of interrelated structures, especially of several muscles or muscle groups in the execution of complicated movements. [L. *co-,* together, + *ordino,* pp. *-atus,* to arrange, fr. *ordo* (*ordin-*), arrangement, order]

Co•or•di•na•tion of Ben•e•fits (COB) (kō-ōr′di-nā′shŭn ben′ĕ-fits) A clause in insurance policies for patients with more than one carrier to provide a maximum of 100% benefits. One carrier is designated as primary carrier; a second carrier covers any remaining costs not covered by the primary carrier.

co•or•di•na•tor (kō-ōr′di-nā-tŏr) One who arranges, organizes, or harmonizes. [L. *coordino,* to put in order]

co•ox•im•e•ter (kō-oks-im′ĕ-tĕr) SYN oximeter.

co•pay•ment (kō′pā-mĕnt) A fixed or set amount paid for each health care or medical service; the remainder is paid by the health insurance plan. In common parlance, copay is the term used. SEE ALSO coinsurance, cost sharing. SYN out-of-pocket costs, out-of-pocket expenses.

COPD Abbreviation for chronic obstructive pulmonary disease.

cope (kōp) **1.** The upper half of a flask in the casting art; hence applicable to the upper or cavity side of a denture flask. **2.** An act that enables one to adjust to the environmental circumstances.

Cope clamp (kōp klamp) A clamp used in excision of colon and rectum.

co•pol•y•mer (kō′pol′i-mĕr) A polymer in which two or more monomers or base units are combined.

co•pol•y•mer-1 (kō′pol′i-mĕr) Acetate salt of a mixture of synthetic polypeptides composed of four amino acids; used to reduce the relapse rate with relapsing-remitting multiple sclerosis.

cop•per (Cu) (kop′ĕr) A metallic element, atomic no. 29, atomic wt. 63.546; several of its salts are used in medicine. A bioelement found in a number of proteins. [L. *cuprum,* orig. *Cyprium,* fr. Cyprus, where it was mined]

Cop•pet law (kop-e′ law) Solutions having the same freezing point have equal concentrations of dissolved substances.

cop•rem•e•sis (kop-rem′ĕ-sis) SYN fecal vomiting. [G. *kopros,* dung, + emesis]

♻ **copro-** Prefix meaning filth, dung, usually used in referring to feces. SEE ALSO scato-, sterco-. [G. *kopros,* dung]

cop•ro•an•ti•bod•ies (kop′rō-an′ti-bod-ēz) Antibodies found in the intestine and in feces;

they probably are formed by plasma cells in the intestinal mucosa and consist chiefly of the IgA class.

cop·ro·lag·ni·a (kop′rō-lag′nē-ă) A form of sexual perversion in which the thought or sight of excrement causes pleasurable sensation. [copro- + G. *lagneia,* lust]

cop·ro·la·li·a (kop′rō-lā′lē-ă) Involuntary utterances of vulgar or obscene words; seen in Tourette syndrome. [copro- + G. *lalia,* talk]

cop·ro·lith (kop′rō-lith) A hard mass consisting of inspissated feces. SYN fecalith, stercolith. [copro- + G. *lithos,* stone]

co·prol·o·gy (kop-rol′ŏ-jē) SYN scatology (1). [copro- + G. *logos,* study]

cop·ro·ma (kop-rō′mă) An accumulation of inspissated feces in the colon or rectum giving the appearance of an abdominal tumor. SYN fecaloma, stercoroma. [copro- + G. *-ōma,* tumor]

cop·ro·pha·gi·a (kop′rō-fā′jē-ă) The eating of excrement.

cop·ro·phil, **cop·ro·phil·ic** (kop′rō-fil, -fil′ik) **1.** Denoting microorganisms occurring in fecal matter. **2.** Relating to coprophilia. SEE coprophilia.

cop·ro·phil·i·a (kop′rō-fil′ē-ă) **1.** Attraction of microorganisms to fecal matter. **2.** PSYCHIATRY a morbid attraction to, and interest in (with a sexual element), fecal matter. [copro- + G. *philos,* fond]

cop·ro·pho·bi·a (kop′rō-fō′bē-ă) Morbid fear of defecation and feces. [copro- + G. *phobos,* fear]

cop·ro·por·phy·ri·a (kop′rō-pōr-fir′ē-ă) Presence of coproporphyrins in the urine, as in variegate porphyria.

cop·ro·por·phy·rin (kop′rō-pōr′fir-in) One of two porphyrin compounds found normally in feces as a decomposition product of bilirubin (hence, from hemoglobin); certain corproporphyrins are elevated in certain porphyrias. SEE ALSO porphyrinogens.

cop·ros·ta·sis (kop-ros′tă-sis) Impaction of feces in the colon and sometimes the small intestine. [copro- + G. *stasis,* a standing]

cop·u·la (kop′yū-lă) **1.** ANATOMY a narrow part connecting two structures (e.g., the body of the hyoid bone). **2.** A swelling that is formed during the early development of the tongue by the medial portion of the second pharyngeal arch; it is overgrown by the hypobranchial eminence and is not present in the adult tongue. [L. a bond, tie]

cop·u·la·tion (kop′yū-lā′shŭn) **1.** SYN coitus. **2.** PROTOZOOLOGY conjugation between two cells that do not fuse but separate after mutual fertilization; observed in the ciliophora, as in *Paramecium.* [L. *copulatio,* a joining]

cop·u·line (kop′yū-līn) Any of several pheromones that occur in vaginal secretions; men who were exposed to copulines rated women as more attractive, especially those women considered less attractive by controls tested with water. Copulines from ovulatory (but not menstrual or premenstrual) women caused a rise in salivary testosterone in men.

cor, gen. **cor·dis** (kōr, kōr′dis) [TA] SYN heart. [L.]

cor·a·co·a·cro·mi·al (kōr′ă-kō-ă-krō′mē-ăl) Relating to the coracoid and acromial processes. SYN acromiocoracoid.

cor·a·co·a·cro·mi·al lig·a·ment (kōr′ă-kō-ă-krō′mē-ăl lig′ă-mĕnt) The heavy arched fibrous band that passes between the coracoid process and the acromion above the shoulder joint; the osseofibrous arch thus formed prevents upward dislocation of the shoulder (glenohumeral) joint. SYN ligamentum coracoacromiale [TA].

cor·a·co·bra·chi·a·lis mus·cle (kōr′ă-kō-brā-kē-ā′lis mŭs′ĕl) *Origin*, coracoid process of scapula; *insertion*, middle of medial border of humerus; *action*, adducts and flexes the arm; resists downward dislocation of shoulder joint; *nerve supply*, musculocutaneous. SYN musculus coracobrachialis [TA].

cor·a·co·cla·vic·u·lar (kōr′ă-kō-klă-vik′yū-lăr) Relating to the coracoid process and the clavicle. SYN scapuloclavicular (2).

cor·a·co·cla·vic·u·lar lig·a·ment (kōr′ă-kō-klă-vik′yū-lăr lig′ă-mĕnt) The strong ligament that unites the clavicle to the coracoid process; it is subdivided into the conoid ligament and the trapezoid ligament. The free upper limb is passively suspended from the clavicular “strut” by the coracoclavicular ligament; the ligament also plays an important role in preventing dislocation of the acromioclavicular joint. SYN ligamentum coracoclaviculare [TA].

cor·a·co·hu·mer·al (kōr′ă-kō-hyū′mĕr-ăl) Relating to the coracoid process and the humerus.

cor·a·coid (kōr′ă-koyd) Shaped like a crow’s beak; denoting a process of the scapula. [G. *korakōdēs,* like a crow’s beak, fr. *korax,* raven, + *eidos,* appearance]

cor·a·coid pro·cess (kōr′ă-koyd pros′es) A long curved projection from the neck of the scapula overhanging the glenoid cavity. It gives attachment to the short head of the biceps, the coracobrachialis, and the pectoralis minor muscles, and the conoid and coracoacromial ligaments.

cor a·di·po·sum (kōr a-di-pō′sŭm) SYN fatty heart (2).

cor bi·loc·u·la·re (kōr bī-lok-yū-lā′rē) A heart in which the interatrial and interventricular septa are absent or incomplete.

cor bo•vi•num (kōr bō-vī′nŭm) SYN ox heart.

cord (kōrd) **1.** ANATOMY any long, ropelike structure. A small, cordlike structure composed of several to many longitudinally oriented fibers, vessels, ducts, or combinations thereof. SYN fasciculus (2) [TA], funiculus [TA], funicle. SEE ALSO chorda. **2.** HISTOPATHOLOGY a line of tumor cells only one cell in width. [L. *chorda,* a string]

cord- SEE chord-.

cor•date (kōr′dāt) Heart-shaped.

cor•date pel•vis, **cor•di•form pel•vis** (kōr′dāt pel′vis, kōr′di-fōrm pel′vis) A pelvis with the sacrum projecting forward between the ilia, giving the brim a heart shape.

cord blood (kōrd blŭd) Blood present in the umbilical vessels at the time of delivery.

cor•dec•to•my (kōr-dek′tŏ-mē) Excision of a part or whole of a cord. [G. *chordē,* cord, + *ektomē,* excision]

cor•di•form (kōr′di-fōrm) Heart-shaped. [L. *cor* (*cord-*), heart, + *forma,* shape]

cor•di•form u•ter•us (kōr′di-fōrm yū′tĕr-ŭs) An incomplete uterus bicornis with a wedge-shaped depression at the fundus.

cor•do•cen•te•sis (kōr′dō-sen-tē′sis) Transabdominal blood sampling of the fetal umbilical cord, performed under ultrasound guidance. SYN funipuncture. [cord + G. *kentēsis,* puncture]

cor•do•pex•y (kōr′dō-pek-sē) **1.** Operative fixation of any displaced anatomic cord. **2.** Lateral fixation of one or both vocal cords to correct glottic stenosis. [G. *chordē,* cord, + *pēxis,* fixation]

cor•dot•o•my (kōr-dot′ŏ-mē) **1.** Any operation on the spinal cord. **2.** Division of tracts of the spinal cord, which may be performed percutaneously (stereotactic cordotomy) or after laminectomy (open cordotomy) by various techniques such as incision or radio frequency coagulation. **3.** Incision through the membranous vocal fold to widen the posterior glottis in bilateral vocal paralysis. SYN chordotomy. [G. *chordē,* cord, + *tomē,* a cutting]

core (kōr) Made up of the rectus abdominis, transversus abdominis, internal and external oblique muscles. The muscles are used to stabilize the upper torso during movement.

core-, **coreo-**, **coro-** Combining forms denoting the pupil (of the eye). [G. *korē,* pupil]

co•re•cep•tor (kō-rĕ-sep′tŏr) A cell surface protein that increases the sensitivity of the antigen receptor to antigen by binding to other ligands.

cor•ec•to•pi•a (kōr′ek-tō′pē-ă) Eccentric location of the pupil so that it is not in the center of the iris. [G. *korē,* pupil, + *ektopos,* out of place]

co•rel•y•sis (kō-rē-lī′sis) A rarely used term for freeing of adhesions between lens capsule and the iris. [G. *korē,* pupil, + *lysis,* a loosening]

cor•e•o•plas•ty (kōr′ē-ō-plas-tē) The procedure to correct a misshapen, miotic, or occluded pupil. [G. *korē,* pupil, + *plassō,* to form]

cor•e•pex•y (kōr′ē-pek-sē) A suturing of the iris to modify the shape or size of the pupil.

cor•e•prax•y (kōr′ē-prak′sē) A procedure designed to widen a small pupil. [G. *korē,* pupil, + *praxis,* action]

co•re•pres•sor (kō-rĕ-pres′ŏr) A molecule, usually a product of a specific metabolic pathway, which combines with and activates a repressor produced by a regulator gene. The repressor then attaches to an operator gene site and inhibits activity of the structural genes. This homeostatic mechanism regulates enzyme production in repressible enzyme systems.

core tem•per•a•ture (kōr tem′pĕr-ă-chŭr) The temperature of the interior of the body.

CORF Abbreviation for comprehensive outpatient rehabilitation facility.

Co•ri cy•cle (kō′rē sī′kĕl) The phases in the metabolism of carbohydrate: 1) glycogenolysis in the liver; 2) passage of glucose into the circulation; 3) deposition of glucose in the muscles as glycogen; and 4) glycogenolysis during muscular activity and conversion to lactate, which is converted to glycogen in the liver.

Co•ri dis•ease (kō′rē di-zēz′) SYN glycogenosis type 3.

co•ri•um, pl. **co•ri•a** (kō′rē-ŭm, -ă) SYN dermis. [L. skin, hide, leather]

cork•screw ves•sels (kōrk′scrū vĕs′ĕlz) SYN hairpin vessels.

corn (kōrn) **1.** The foodstuff, *Zea mays*. **2.** A hard or soft hyperkeratosis of the sole of the foot due to friction and pressure. [L. *cornu,* horn, hoof]

cor•ne•a (kōr′nē-ă) [TA] The transparent tissue constituting the anterior sixth of the outer wall of the eye, with a 7.7-mm radius of curvature as contrasted with the 13.5-mm of the sclera. It consists of stratified squamous epithelium continuous with that of the conjunctiva, a substantia propria, regularly arranged collagen imbedded in mucopolysaccharide, and an inner layer of endothelium. It is the chief refractory structure of the eye. See page B5, B27. [L. fem. of *corneus,* horny]

cor•ne•al (kōr′nē-ăl) Relating to the cornea.

cor•ne•al a•stig•ma•tism (kōr′nē-ăl ă-stig′mă-tizm) Astigmatism due to a defect in the curvature of the corneal surface.

cor•ne•al cor•pus•cles (kōr′nē-ăl kōr′pŭs-ĕlz)

Connective tissue cells found between the laminae of fibrous tissue in the cornea.

cor·ne·al graft (kōr′nē-ăl graft) SYN keratoplasty.

cor·ne·al lay·er (kōr′nē-ăl lā′ĕr) SYN stratum corneum epidermidis.

cor·ne·al pan·nus (kōr′nē-ăl pan′ŭs) Fibrovascular connective tissue that proliferates in the anterior layers of the peripheral cornea in inflammatory corneal disease, particularly trachoma in which the pannus involves the superior cornea.

cor·ne·al re·flex (kōr′nē-ăl rē′fleks) **1.** A contraction of the eyelids when the cornea is lightly touched. **2.** Reflection of light from the surface of the cornea.

cor·ne·al space (kōr′nē-ăl spās) One of the stellate spaces between the lamellae of the cornea, each of which contains a cell or corneal corpuscle. SYN lacuna (4).

cor·ne·al staph·y·lo·ma (kōr′nē-ăl staf′i-lō′mă) SYN anterior staphyloma.

cor·ne·a pla·na (kōr′nē-ă plā′nă) A congenital disorder in which the arc of curvature of the cornea is flatter than normal, leaving the eye hyperopic.

cor·ne·o·cyte en·ve·lope (kōr′nē-ō-sīt en′vĕ-lōp) An electron-dense layer of highly cross-linked protein on the cytoplasmic surface of the cell membrane of epidermal corneocytes.

cor·ne·o·scle·ra (kōr′nē-ō-skler′ă) The combined cornea and sclera when considered as forming the external coat of the eyeball.

cor·ne·o·scle·ral (kōr′nē-ō-skler′ăl) Pertaining to the cornea and sclera.

cor·ne·ous (kōr′nē-ŭs) SYN horny. [L. *corneus,* fr. *cornu,* horn]

Cor·ner tam·pon (kōr′nĕr tam′pon) A plug of omentum stuffed into a wound of the stomach or intestine as a temporary tampon.

corn·flow·er (kōrn′flow-ĕr) SYN echinacea.

cor·nic·u·late (kōr-nik′yū-lăt) **1.** Resembling a horn. **2.** Having horns or horn-shaped appendages. [L. *corniculatus,* horned]

cor·nic·u·late car·ti·lage (kōr-nik′yū-lăt kahr′ti-lăj) A conic nodule of elastic cartilage surmounting the apex of each arytenoid cartilage. SYN cartilago corniculata [TA].

cor·nic·u·lum (kōr-nik′yū-lŭm) A cornu of small size. [L. dim. of *cornu,* horn]

cor·ni·fi·ca·tion (kōr′ni-fi-kā′shŭn) SYN keratinization. [L. *cornu,* horn, + *facio,* to make]

cor·nu, gen. **cor·nus**, pl. **cor·nu·a** (kōr′nū, -nŭs, -nū-ă) **1.** SYN horn. **2.** Any structure composed of horny substance. **3.** One of the coronal extensions of the dental pulp underlying a cusp or lobe. **4.** The major subdivisions of the lateral ventricle in the cerebral hemisphere (the frontal horn, occipital horn, and temporal horn). SEE ALSO lateral ventricle. **5.** The major divisions of the gray columns of the spinal cord (anterior horn, lateral horn, posterior horn). [L. horn]

cor·nu·al (kōr′nū-ăl) Relating to a cornu.

cor·nu·al preg·nan·cy (kōr′nū-ăl preg′năn-sē) The implantation and development of the impregnated oocyte in one of the cornua of the uterus.

cor·nu am·mo·nis (kōr′nū a-mō′nis) [TA] SYN Ammon horn.

cor·nu an·te·ri·us (kōr′nū an-tē′rē-ŭs) [TA] SYN anterior horn.

cor·nu pos·te·ri·us (kōr′nū pos-tē′rē-ŭs) SYN posterior horn.

co·ro·na, pl. **co·ro·nae** (kŏ-rō′nă, -nē) [TA] SYN crown. [L. garland, crown, fr. G. *korōnē*]

cor·o·nad (kōr′ŏ-nad) In a direction toward any corona.

co·ro·na of glans pe·nis (kŏ-rō′nă glanz pē′nis) The prominent posterior border of the glans penis.

cor·o·nal (kōr′ŏ-năl) Relating to a corona or the coronal plane.

cor·o·nal plane (kōr′ŏ-năl plān) A vertical plane at right angles to a sagittal plane, dividing the body into anterior and posterior portions. SYN frontal plane.

cor·o·nal su·ture (kōr′ŏ-năl sū′chŭr) The line of junction of the frontal with the two parietal bones of the skull.

co·ro·na ra·di·a·ta (kŏ-rō′nă rā-dē-ā′tă) [TA] **1.** A fan-shaped fiber mass on the white matter of the cerebral cortex, composed of the widely radiating fibers of the internal capsule. **2.** A single layer of columnar cells derived from the cumulus oophorus, which anchor on the pellucid zone of the oocyte in a secondary follicle. SYN radiate crown.

cor·o·na·ri·tis (kōr′ō-nă-rī′tis) Inflammation of coronary artery or arteries.

cor·o·nar·y (kōr′ŏ-nār-ē) **1.** Relating to or resembling a crown. **2.** Encircling; denoting various anatomic structures, e.g., nerves, blood vessels, ligaments. **3.** Specifically, denoting the coronary blood vessels of the heart; colloquially, myocardial infarction or coronary thrombosis. [L. *coronarius;* fr. *corona,* a crown]

cor·o·nar·y an·gi·og·ra·phy (kōr′ŏ-nār-ē an′jē-og′ră-fē) Imaging of the circulation of the myocardium by injection of contrast medium, usually by selective catheterization of each coronary artery, formerly by injection at the root of the aorta.

cor•o•nar•y ar•ter•ies (kōr′ŏ-nār-ē ahr′tĕr-ēz) A pair of arteries that branch from the aorta and supply blood to the myocardium. 1) Right coronary artery: *origin,* right aortic sinus; *distribution,* it passes around the right side of the heart in the coronary sulcus, giving branches to the right atrium and ventricle, including the atrioventricular branches and the posterior interventricular branch. 2) Left coronary artery: *origin,* left aortic sinus; *distribution,* divides into two major branches, anterior interventricular, which descends in anterior interventricular sulcus, and circumflex branch which passes to the diaphragmatic surface of left ventricle; it gives atrial, ventricular, and atrioventricular branches. See this page.

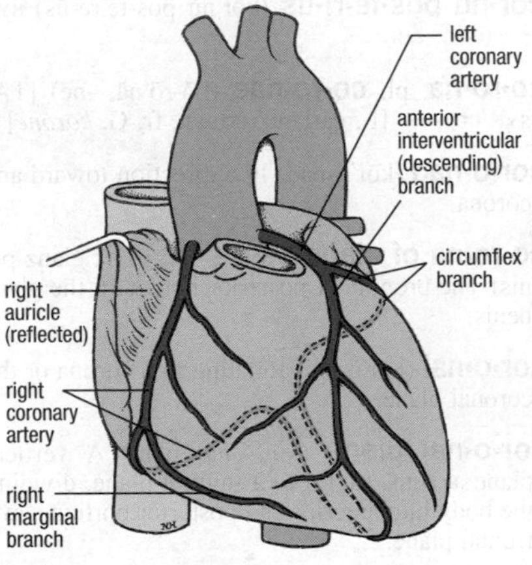

coronary arteries

cor•o•nar•y ar•ter•y by•pass (kōr′ŏ-nār-ē ahr′tĕr-ē bī′pas) Conduit, usually a vein graft or internal mammary artery, surgically interposed between the aorta and a coronary artery branch to coronary shunt blood beyond an obstruction.

cor•o•nar•y ar•ter•y by•pass graft (CABG) (kōr′ŏ-nār-ē ahr′tĕr-ē bī′pās graft) A surgical procedure in which damaged sections of the coronary arteries are replaced with new articular or venous graftings to increase rate of cardiac blood flow. Sometimes colloquially known as a 'cabbage procedure.'

cor•o•nar•y ar•ter•y dis•ease (CAD) (kōr′ŏ-nār-ē ahr′tĕr-ē di-zēz′) Narrowing of the lumen of one or more of the coronary arteries, usually due to atherosclerosis; myocardial ischemia; can cause congestive heart failure, angina pectoris, or myocardial infarction.

cor•o•nar•y by•pass (kōr′ŏ-nār-ē bī′pas) Vein grafts or other conduits shunting blood from the aorta to branches of the coronary arteries, to increase the flow beyond the local obstruction.

cor•o•nar•y care u•nit (CCU) (kōr′ŏ-nār-ē kār yū′nit) A group of beds within a hospital set aside for the care of patients having or suspected of having acute cardiac episodes.

cor•o•nar•y cat•a•ract (kōr′ŏ-nār-ē kat′ăr-akt) Peripheral cortical developmental cataract occurring just after puberty; transmitted as a hereditary dominant characteristic.

cor•o•nar•y fail•ure (kōr′ŏ-nār-ē fāl′yŭr) Acute coronary insufficiency.

cor•o•nar•y groove (kōr′ŏ-nār-ē grūv) A groove on the outer surface of the heart marking the division between the atria and the ventricles.

cor•o•nar•y in•suf•fi•cien•cy (kōr′ŏ-nār-ē in′sŭ-fish′ĕn-sē) Inadequate coronary circulation leading to anginal pain.

cor•o•nar•y oc•clu•sion (kōr′ŏ-nār-ē ŏ-klū′zhŭn) Blockage of a coronary vessel, usually by thrombosis or atheroma, often leading to myocardial infarction.

cor•o•nar•y si•nus (kōr′ŏ-nār-ē sī′nŭs) A short trunk receiving most of the cardiac veins, beginning at the junction of the great cardiac vein and the oblique vein of the left atrium, running in the posterior part of the coronary sulcus and emptying into the right atrium between the inferior vena cava and the atrioventricular orifice.

cor•o•nar•y throm•bo•sis (kōr′ŏ-nār-ē throm-bō′sis) Coronary occlusion by thrombus formation, usually the result of atheromatous changes in the arterial wall and usually leading to myocardial infarction.

Co•ro•na•vir•i•dae (kō-rō′nă-vir′i-dē) A family of single-stranded RNA-containing viruses, some of which cause upper respiratory tract infections in humans similar to the "common cold." [L. *corona,* garland, crown]

co•ro•na•vi•rus (kō-rō′nă-vī′rŭs) A genus in the family Coronaviridae that is associated with upper respiratory tract infections and possibly gastroenteritis in humans.

cor•o•ner (kŏr′ŏ-nĕr) An official whose duty is to investigate sudden, suspicious, or violent death to determine its cause. In some communities, the office has been replaced by that of medical examiner. [L. *corona,* a crown]

cor•o•noi•dec•to•my (kōr′ŏ-noyd-ek′tŏ-mē) Surgical removal of the coronoid process of the mandible. [coronoid + G. *ektomē,* excision]

cor•o•noid pro•cess (kōr′ŏ-noyd pros′es) A sharp triangular projection from a bone; coronoid process of the mandible, the triangular anterior process of the mandibular ramus, giving attachment to the temporal muscle; coronoid process of the ulna, a bracketlike projection from the anterior portion of the proximal extremity of the ulna; its anterior surface gives attachment to the brachialis, its proximal surface enters into the formation of the trochlear notch.

cor•o•noid pro•cess of ul•na (kōr′ō-noyd pros′es ŭl′nă) A bracketlike projection from the anterior portion of the proximal extremity of the ulna; its anterior surface gives attachment to the brachialis, and its proximal surface enters into the formation of the trochlear notch.

cor•po•ra (kōr-pōr′ă) Plural of corpus.

cor•po•ra ar•e•na•ce•a (kŏr-pōr′ă ahr-ĕ-nā′shē-ă) Small calcareous concretions in the stroma of the pineal and other central nervous system tissues. SYN psammoma bodies (2).

cor•po•ra par•a•a•or•ti•ca (kōr-pōr′ă par′ă-ā-ōr′ti-kă) [TA] SYN paraaortic bodies.

cor•po•re•al (kōr-pōr′ē-ăl) Pertaining to the body, or to a corpus.

corpse (kōrps) SYN cadaver. [L. *corpus,* body]

cor•pu•lence, **cor•pu•len•cy** (kōr′pyū-lĕns, -lĕn-sē) SYN obesity. [L. *corpulentia,* magnification of *corpus,* body]

cor•pu•lent (kōr′pyū-lĕnt) SYN obese.

cor pul•mo•na•le (kōr pul-mō-nā′lē) Chronic cor pulmonale is characterized by hypertrophy of the right ventricle resulting from disease of the lungs; acute cor pulmonale is characterized by dilation and failure of the right side of the heart due to pulmonary embolism. In both types, characteristic electrocardiogram changes occur, and in later stages there is usually right-sided cardiac failure.

cor•pus, gen. **cor•po•ris**, pl. **cor•po•ra** (kōr′pŭs, kōr--pōr′is, -pōr′ă) [TA] **1.** SYN body. **2.** Any body or mass. **3.** The main part of an organ or other anatomic structure, as distinguished from the head or caudal region. SEE ALSO body, shaft, soma. [L. body]

cor•pus al•bi•cans (kōr′pŭs al′bi-kanz) [TA] A retrogressed corpus luteum, characterized by a shrinking cicatricial core surrounded by an amorphous, convoluted, completely hyalinized lutein zone. SYN albicans (2).

cor•pus am•y•la•ce•um, pl. **cor•po•ra am•y•la•ce•a** (kōr′pŭs am-i-lā′shē-ŭm, kōr-pōr′ă am′i-lā′shē-ă) One of a number of small ovoid or rounded, sometimes laminated, bodies resembling a grain of starch and found in nervous tissue, in the prostate, and in pulmonary alveoli. SYN amnionic corpuscle.

cor•pus a•tre•ti•cum (kōr′pŭs ă-trē′ti-kŭm) SYN atretic follicle.

cor•pus cal•lo•sum (kōr′pŭs ka-lō′sŭm) [TA] The great commissural plate of nerve fibers interconnecting the cortical hemispheres (with the exception of most of the temporal lobes, which are interconnected by the anterior commissure). Lying at the floor of the longitudinal fissure, and covered on each side by the cingulate gyrus, it is arched from behind forward and is thick at each extremity (splenium and genu) but thinner in its long central portion (truncus); it curves back underneath itself at the genu to form the rostrum of the corpus callosum.

cor•pus ca•ver•no•sum cli•to•ri•dis (kōr′pŭs ka-vĕr-nō′sŭm klit′ōr-i-dis) [TA] One of the two parallel columns of erectile tissue forming the body of the clitoris; they diverge at the root to form the crura of the clitoris.

cor•pus ca•ver•no•sum pe•nis (kōr′pŭs ka-vĕr-nō′sŭm pē′nis) [TA] One of two parallel columns of erectile tissue forming the dorsal part of the body of the penis; they are separated posteriorly, forming the crura of the penis.

cor•pus ci•li•a•re (kōr′pŭs si-lī-ā′rē) [TA] SYN ciliary body.

cor•pus•cle (kōr′pŭs-ĕl) **1.** A small mass or body. **2.** A blood cell. SYN corpusculum. [L. *corpusculum,* dim. of *corpus,* body]

cor•pus•cu•la ar•tic•u•la•ri•a (kōr-pŭs′kyū-lă ar-tik-yū-lā′rē-ă) [TA] SYN articular corpuscles.

cor•pus•cu•la gen•i•ta•li•a (kōr-pŭs′kyū-lă jen′i-tā′lē-ă) [TA] SYN genital corpuscles.

cor•pus•cu•la la•mel•lo•sa (kōr-pŭs-kyū′lă lam-ĕl-ō′să) [TA] SYN lamellated corpuscles.

cor•pus•cu•lar (kōr-pŭs′kyū-lăr) Relating to a corpuscle.

cor•pus•cu•lar ra•di•a•tion (kōr-pŭs′kyū-lăr rā′dē-ā′shŭn) Radiation consisting of streams of subatomic particles such as protons, electrons, and neutrons.

cor•pus•cu•lum, pl. **cor•pus•cu•la** (kōr-pŭs′kyū-lŭm, -lă) SYN corpuscle.

cor•pus•cu•lum re•nis, pl. **cor•pus•cu•la re•nis** (kōr-pŭs′kyū-lŭm rē′nis, kōr-pus′kyū-lă rē′nis) SYN renal corpuscle.

cor•pus fim•bri•a•tum (kōr′pŭs fim-brē-ā′tŭm) **1.** SYN fimbria hippocampi. **2.** The outer, ovarian end of the uterine tube.

cor•pus ge•nic•u•la•tum la•te•ra•le (kōr′pŭs jen′ik-yū-lā′tŭm lat′ĕr-ā′lē) [TA] SYN lateral geniculate body.

cor•pus he•mor•rha•gi•cum (kōr′pŭs hem-ŏ-raj′i-kŭm) A hematoma within an ovarian follicle; gradual resorption of the blood elements leaves a cavity filled with a clear fluid, i.e., a corpus luteum cyst.

cor•pus lu•te•um (kōr′pŭs lū′tē-ŭm) [TA] The yellow endocrine body formed in the ovary at the site of a ruptured ovarian follicle; a stage of proliferation and vascularization precedes full maturity; later, a bright yellow lutein zone is traversed by trabeculae of theca interna containing numerous blood vessels; the corpus luteum secretes estrogen, as did the follicle, and also secretes progesterone. If pregnancy does not occur, it is called a corpus luteum spurium, which undergoes progressive retrogression to become a corpus albicans. If pregnancy does occur, it is called a corpus luteum verum, which grows, persisting to the fifth or sixth month of pregnancy before retrogression.

cor•pus lu•te•um cyst (kōr′pŭs lū′tē-ŭm sist) Persistent corpus luteum with cyst formation.

cor•pus mam•mil•la•re (kōr′pŭs ma-mi-lā′rē) [TA] SYN mammillary body.

cor•pus o•li•va•re (kōr′pŭs ol-i-vā′rē) [TA] SYN oliva.

cor•pus pi•ne•a•le (kōr′pŭs pi-nē-ā′lē) [TA] SYN pineal gland.

cor•pus spon•gi•o•sum pe•nis (kōr′pŭs spŏn-jē-ō′sŭm pē′nis) [TA] The median column of erectile tissue located between and ventral to the two corpora cavernosa penis; posteriorly it expands into the bulbus penis and anteriorly it terminates as the enlarged glans penis. It is traversed by the urethra.

cor•pus spon•gi•o•sum u•re•thrae mu•li•e•bris (kōr′pŭs spŏn-jē-ō′sŭm yū-rē′thrē mū-lē-ē′bris) The submucous coat of the female urethra, containing a venous network that insinuates itself between the muscular layers, giving to them an erectile nature.

cor•pus stri•a•tum (kōr′pŭs strī-ā′tŭm) [TA] SYN striate body.

cor•pus vit•re•um (kōr′pŭs vit′rē-ŭm) [TA] SYN vitreous body. SEE ALSO vitreous.

Cor•rect Cod•ing In•i•ti•a•tive (kŏr-ekt′ kōd′ing i-nish′ă-tiv) Computerized editing system for health insurance claims to avoid overpayments on covered procedures. SEE ALSO National Correct Coding Initiative.

cor•rec•tion•al med•i•cine (kōr-ek′shŭn-ăl med′i-sin) SYN desmoteric medicine.

cor•rec•tive (kŏr-ek′tiv) **1.** Counteracting, modifying, or changing what is injurious. **2.** A drug that modifies or corrects an undesirable or injurious effect of another drug. [L. *cor-rigo* (*conr-*), pp. *-rectus,* to set right, fr. *rego,* to keep straight]

Cor•rer•a line (kōr-rār′ă līn) Outline of lung fields seen on plain film radiograph of thorax.

cor•re•spon•dence (kōr′ĕ-spon′dĕns) OPTICS the points on each retina that have the same visual direction.

Cor•ri•gan dis•ease (kōr′i-găn di-zēz′) SYN aortic regurgitation.

Cor•ri•gan line (kōr′i-găn līn) SYN Corrigan sign (1).

Cor•ri•gan pulse (kōr′i-găn pŭls) A pulse marked by a sharp rise to full expansion followed by collapse; seen in aortic insufficiency.

Cor•ri•gan sign (kōr′i-găn sīn) **1.** A purple line at the junction of teeth and gingiva in chronic copper poisoning. SYN Corrigan line. **2.** Expanding pulsatile mass seen in abdominal aortic aneurysm.

cor•rin (kōr′in) The cyclic system of four pyrrole rings forming corrinoids, which are the central structure of the vitamins B12 and related compounds. [fr. *core* (of vitamin B12 molecule)]

cor•ro•sive (kŏr-ō′siv) **1.** Causing corrosion. **2.** An agent that produces corrosion (e.g., a strong acid or alkali).

cor•ru•ga•tor (kōr′ŭ-gā′tŏr) A muscle that draws together the skin, causing it to wrinkle. [L. *cor-rugo* (*conr-*), pp. *-atus,* to wrinkle, fr. *ruga,* a wrinkle]

cor•ru•ga•tor su•per•ci•li•i mus•cle (kōr′ŭ-gā′tŏr sū′pĕr-sil′ē-ī mŭs′ĕl) *Origin,* from orbital portion of musculus orbicularis oculi and nasal prominence; *insertion,* skin of eyebrow; *action,* draws medial end of eyebrow downward and wrinkles forehead vertically; *nerve supply,* facial. SYN musculus corrugator supercilii [TA].

cor•tex, gen. **cor•ti•cis**, pl. **cor•ti•ces** (kōr′teks, -ti-sis, -ti-sēz) The outer portion of an organ, such as the kidney, as distinguished from the inner, or medullary, portion. [L. bark]

cor•tex of o•va•ry (kōr′teks ō′vă-rē) The layer of the ovarian stroma lying immediately beneath the tunica albuginea, composed of connective tissue cells and fibers, among which are scattered primary and secondary (antral) follicles in various stages of development; the cortex varies in thickness according to the age of the individual, becoming thinner with advancing years.

Cor•ti arch (kōr′tē ahrch) That formed by the junction of the heads of Corti's inner and outer pillar cells, in the inner ear.

cor•ti•cal (kōr′ti-kăl) Relating to a cortex.

cor•ti•cal ar•ter•ies (kōr′ti-kăl ahr′tĕr-ēz) Branches of the anterior, middle, and posterior cerebral arteries that supply the cerebral cortex.

cor•ti•cal au•di•om•e•try (kōr′ti-kăl aw′dē-om′ĕ-trē) Measurement of the potentials that arise in the auditory system above the level of the brainstem.

cor•ti•cal blind•ness (kōr′ti-kăl blīnd′nĕs) Loss of sight due to an organic lesion in the visual cortex.

cor•ti•cal bone (kōr′ti-kăl bōn) The superficial thin layer of compact bone. SYN substantia corticalis [TA], cortical substance.

cor•ti•cal cat•a•ract (kōr′ti-kăl kat′ăr-akt) A cataract in which the opacity affects the cortex of the lens.

cor•ti•cal cords (kōr′ti-kal kōrdz) The cellular cords arising from the surface epithelium of the embryonic ovaries; the primordial germ cells in the cords differentiate into oogonia.

cor•ti•cal deaf•ness (kōr′ti-kăl def′nĕs) Deafness resulting from bilateral lesions of the primary receptive area of the temporal lobe.

cor•ti•cal hor•mones (kōr′ti-kăl hōr′mōnz) Steroid hormones produced by the cortex of the suprarenal gland, chiefly cortisol, a glucocorticoid; aldosterone, a mineralocorticoid; and dehydroepiandrosterone, an androgen.

cor•ti•cal lob•ules of kid•ney (kōr′ti-kăl lob′yūlz kid′nē) One of the subdivisions of the kidney, consisting of a medullary ray and that portion of the convoluted port (renal corpuscles and convoluted tubules) associated with its collecting duct.

cor•ti•cal ra•di•ate ar•ter•ies (kōr′ti-kăl rā′dē-āt ahr′tĕr-ēz) The branches of the arcuate arteries of the kidney radiating outward through the renal columns and cortex and supplying the glomeruli.

cor•ti•cal sub•stance (kōr′ti-kăl sub′stăns) SYN cortical bone.

Cor•ti ca•nal (kōr′tē kă-nal′) SYN spiral canal of cochlea.

Cor•ti cells (kōr′tē selz) SYN cochlear hair cells.

cor•ti•ces (kōr′ti-sēz) Plural of cortex.

cor•ti•cif•u•gal, **cor•ti•cof•u•gal** (kōr-ti-sif′yū-găl, kōr′ti-kof′yū′găl) Passing in a direction away from the outer surface; denoting especially nerve fibers conveying impulses away from the cerebral cortex. [L. *cortex,* rind, bark, + *fugio,* to flee]

cor•ti•cip•e•tal (kōr′ti-sip′ĕ-tăl) Passing in a direction toward the outer surface; denoting nerve fibers conveying impulses toward the cerebral cortex. [L. *cortex,* rind, bark, + *peto,* to seek]

cor•ti•co•ba•sal de•gen•er•a•tion (kōr′ti-kō-bā′săl dĕ-jen′ĕr-ā′shŭn) A rare, progressive disease involving both cerebral cortex and extrapyramidal structures; clinically manifested as disturbances of voluntary movements and rigidity; pathologic characteristics include degeneration of the cerebral cortex with balloon neurons and degeneration of the substantia nigra.

cor•ti•co•bul•bar (kōr′ti-kō-bŭl′bahr) Pertaining to corticofugal fibers projecting to the rhombencephalon that terminate 1) directly on some motor cranial nerve nuclei, 2) in the reticular formation, or 3) on sensory relay nuclei, such as the cuneate, gracile, and spinal trigeminal nucleus.

cor•ti•coid (kōr′ti-koyd) **1.** Having an action similar to that of a hormone of the cortex of the suprarenal gland. **2.** Any substance exhibiting this action. **3.** SYN corticosteroid.

cor•ti•co•lib•er•in (kōr′ti-kō-lib′ĕr-in) SYN corticotropin-releasing hormone. [corticosteroid + L. *libero,* to free, + -in]

cor•ti•co•ste•roid (kōr′ti-kō-ster′oyd) A steroid produced by the cortex of the suprarenal gland (i.e., adrenal corticoid); a corticoid containing a steroid. SYN corticoid (3).

cor•ti•co•ste•roid-bind•ing glob•u•lin (CBG) (kōr′ti-kō-ster′oyd-bīnd′ing glob′yū-lin) SYN transcortin.

cor•ti•co•troph (kōr′ti-kō-trōf) A cell of the adenohypophysis that produces adrenocorticotropic hormone.

cor•ti•co•tro•pin (kōr′ti-kō-trō′pin) SYN adrenocorticotropic hormone. [G. *tropē,* a turning]

cor•ti•co•trop•in•like in•ter•me•di•ate-lobe pep•tide (CLIP) (kōr′ti-kō-trō′pin-līk in′tĕr-mē′dē-ăt-lōb pep′tīd) Product of propiomelanocortin with unknown function.

cor•ti•co•tro•pin-re•leas•ing fac•tor (CRF) (kōr′ti-kō-trō′pin-rĕ-lēs′ing fak′tŏr) SYN corticotropin-releasing hormone.

cor•ti•co•tro•pin-re•leas•ing hor•mone (CRH) (kōr′ti-kō-trō′pin-rĕ-lēs′ing hōr′mōn) A factor secreted by the hypothalamus that stimulates the pituitary to release adrenocorticotropic hormone. SYN corticoliberin, corticotropin-releasing factor.

Cor•ti•co•vi•rus (kōr′ti-kō-vī′rŭs) Only genus in family of Corticoviridae.

cor•ti•lymph (kōr′ti-limf) The fluid in the Corti tunnel.

Cor•ti mem•brane (kor′tē mem′brān) SYN tectorial membrane of cochlear duct.

Cor•ti or•gan (kōr′tē ōr′găn) SYN spiral organ.

cor•ti•sol (kōr′ti-sol) SYN hydrocortisone.

cor•ti•sone (kōr′ti-sōn) A glucocorticoid not normally secreted in significant quantities by the human cortex of the suprarenal gland. It exhibits no biologic activity until converted to hydrocortisone (cortisol); it acts on carbohydrate metabolism and influences the nutrition and growth of connective (collagenous) tissues.

Cor•ti tun•nel (kōr′tē tŭn′ĕl) The spiral canal in the organ of Corti, formed by the outer and inner pillar cells or rods of Corti. It is filled with fluid and occasionally crossed by nonmedullated nerve fibers.

cor tri•at•ri•a•tum (kōr trī-at-rī-ā′tŭm) A congenital anomaly characterized by a heart with three atrial chambers, the left atrium being subdivided by a transverse septum with a single small opening which separates the openings of the pulmonary veins from the mitral valve.

cor tri•lo•cu•la•re (kōr trī-lok-yū-lā′rē) Three-chambered heart due to absence of the interatrial or the interventricular septum.

cor tri·lo·cu·la·re bi·ven·tric·u·la·re (kōr trī-lok-yū-lā′rē bi-ven-trik′yu-lā-rē) SYN common atrium.

Cor·vi·sart fa·ci·es (kōr′vē-sahr′ fash′ē-ēz) The characteristic facies seen in cardiac insufficiency or aortic regurgitation; a swollen, purplish, cyanotic face with shiny eyes and puffy eyelids; nonspecific.

co·rym·bi·form (kŏr-im′bi-fōrm) Denoting the flowerlike clustering configuration of skin lesions in granulomatous diseases (e.g., syphilis, tuberculosis). [L. *corymbus,* cluster, garland]

Cor·y·ne·bac·te·ri·um (kŏ-rī′nē-bak-tēr′ē-ŭm) A genus of nonmotile (except for some plant pathogens), aerobic to facultatively anaerobic bacteria (family Corynebacteriaceae) containing irregularly staining, gram-positive, straight to slightly curved, often club-shaped rods that, as a result of snapping division, show a picket fence arrangement. These organisms are widely distributed in nature. The best known species are parasites and pathogens of humans and domestic animals. The type species is *C. diphtheriae*. [G. *coryne,* a club, + *bacterium,* a small rod]

cor·y·ne·bac·te·ri·um, pl. **cor·y·ne·bac·te·ri·a** (kŏ-rī′nē-bak-tēr′ē-ŭm, -ă) A vernacular term used to refer to any member of the genus *Corynebacterium*.

Cor·y·ne·bac·te·ri·um am·y·co·la·tum (kŏ-rī′nē-bak-tēr′ē-ŭm am-i-kō-lā′tŭm) A species found as normal skin flora that causes septicemia; frequently associated with use of venous access devices; has been recovered from urinary tract infections and mixed flora abscesses.

Cor·y·ne·bac·te·ri·um diph·the·ri·ae (kŏ-rī′nē-bak-tēr′ē-ŭm dip′thēr-ē-ē) Type species of the genus *Corynebacterium,* the cause of diphtheria. It induces a severe membranous pharyngitis and produces an exotoxin that damages myocardium and other tissues; may also infect superficial wounds; an asymptomatic carrier state is common. SYN Löffler bacillus.

Cor·y·ne·bac·te·ri·um glu·cu·ron·o·ly·ti·cum (kŏ-rī′nē-bak-tēr′ē-ŭm glū-kū-ron-ō-lit′i-kŭm) A species isolated from patients with urinary tract infections.

Cor·y·ne·bac·te·ri·um jei·kei·um (kŏ-rī′nē-bak-tēr′ē-ŭm jī-kī′ŭm) Species associated with septicemia and skin lesions in immunocompromised patients; especially associated with venous access devices.

Cor·y·ne·bac·te·ri·um ma·tru·cho·ti·i (kŏ-rī′nē-bak-tēr′ē-ŭm mat-rū-kosh′ē-ē) A species recovered in mixed infections from human eye specimens.

co·ry·za (kō-rī′ză) SYN acute rhinitis. [G.]

co·ry·za·vi·rus (kŏ-rī′ză-vī′rŭs) Former name for rhinovirus.

co·sleep·ing (kō′slēp-ing) An increasingly common activity in which one or more children sleep with one or both parents. Clinical opinion is widely divergent on the benefits or harm related to such behavior (e.g., nurturing, long-term psychological trauma for both children and parents).

cos·me·sis (koz-mē′sis) A concern in therapeutics, especially in surgical operations, for the appearance of the patient. [G. *kosmēsis,* an adorning, fr. *kosmeō,* to order, arrange, adorn, fr. *kosmos,* order]

cos·met·ic (koz-met′ik) **1.** Relating to cosmesis. **2.** Relating to the use of cosmetics.

cos·met·ics (koz-met′iks) Composite term for a variety of adornments and camouflages applied to the skin, lips, hair, and nails in accordance with cultural dictates.

cos·met·ic sur·ger·y (koz-met′ik sŭr′jĕr-ē) Operative procedure in which the principal purpose is to improve the appearance, usually with the connotation that the improvement sought is beyond the normal appearance, and its acceptable variations, for the age and the ethnic origin of the patient.

cos·mo·pol·i·tan (koz′mō-pol′i-tăn) BIOLOGIC SCIENCES a term denoting worldwide distribution. [G. *kosmos,* universe, + *polis,* city-state]

cost (kawst) That amount of money, time, labor, or other expense required to gain possession of something or to attain a goal. [L. *consto,* to be fixed]

cos·ta, gen. and pl. **cos·tae** (kos′tă, -tē) [TA] **1.** SYN rib [I–XII]. **2.** A rodlike internal supporting organelle that runs along the base of the undulating membrane of certain flagellate parasites such as *Trichomonas*. SYN basal rod. [L.]

cos·ta cer·vi·ca·lis (kos′tă sĕr-vi-kā′lis) [TA] SYN cervical rib.

cos·tae fluc·tu·an·tes [XI–XII] (kos′tē flŭk-tyū-an′tēz) [TA] SYN floating ribs [XI–XII].

cos·tae spu·ri·ae (kos′tē spū′rē-ē) [TA] SYN false ribs.

cos·tae ve·rae (kos′tē vē′rē) [TA] SYN true ribs [I–VII].

cos·tal (kos′tăl) Relating to a rib.

cos·tal an·gle (kos′tăl ang′gĕl) The rather abrupt change in curvature of the body of a rib posteriorly, such that the neck and head of the rib are directed upward. SYN angulus costae [TA].

cos·tal arch (kos′tăl ahrch) That portion of the inferior aperture of the thorax formed by the articulated cartilages of the seventh to tenth (false) ribs.

cos·tal car·ti·lage (kos′tăl kahr′ti-lăj) The cartilage forming the anterior continuation of a rib, providing the means by which it reaches and articulates with the sternum. SYN cartilago costalis [TA].

cos·tal·gi·a (kos-tal′jē-ă) SYN pleurodynia. [L. *costa,* rib, + G. *algos,* pain]

cos·tec·to·my (kos-tek′tŏ-mē) Excision of a rib. [L. *costa,* rib, + G. *ektomē,* excision]

cost-ef·fec·tive·ness (kawst-e-fekt′iv-nĕs) The proportion between expense and the goods and services received for them.

co·stim·u·la·tor·y mol·e·cule (kō-stim′yū-lă-tōr′ē mol′ĕ-kyūl) Membrane-bound or secreted product of accessory cells that is required for signal transduction.

♻ **costo-** Prefix meaning the ribs. [L. *costa,* rib]

cos·to·ax·il·lar·y vein (kos′tō-aks′i-lar-ē vān) One of a number of anastomotic veins connecting the intercostal veins of the first to seventh intercostal spaces with the lateral thoracic or the thoracoepigastric vein.

cos·to·cer·vi·cal trunk, **cos·to·cer·vi·cal ar·ter·y** (kos′tō-sĕr′vi-kăl trŭngk, kos′tō-sĕr′vi-kăl ahr′tĕr-ē) A short artery that arises from the subclavian artery on each side and divides into deep cervical and superior intercostal branches, the latter dividing usually to form the first and second posterior intercostal arteries. SYN truncus costocervicalis [TA].

cos·to·chon·dral (kos′tō-kon′drăl) Relating to the costal cartilages. SYN chondrocostal.

cos·to·chon·dri·tis (kos′tō-kŏn-drī′tis) Inflammation of one or more costal cartilages, characterized by local tenderness and pain of the anterior chest wall that may radiate, but without the local swelling typical of Tietze syndrome. [costo- + G. *chondros,* cartilage, + *-itis,* inflammation]

cos·to·cla·vic·u·lar (kos′tō-klă-vik′yū-lăr) Relating to the ribs and the clavicle.

cos·to·cla·vic·u·lar lig·a·ment (kos′tō-klă-vik′yū-lăr lig′ă-mĕnt) The ligament that connects the first rib and the clavicle near its sternal end; limits elevation of shoulder (at sternoclavicular joint). SYN ligamentum costoclaviculare [TA], rhomboid ligament.

cos·to·cla·vic·u·lar syn·drome (kos′tō-klă-vik′yū-lăr sin′drōm) SYN thoracic outlet syndrome.

cos·to·cor·a·coid (kos′tō-kōr′ă-koyd) Relating to the ribs and the coracoid process of the scapula.

cos·to·gen·ic (kos′tō-jen′ik) Arising from a rib.

cos·to·phren·ic an·gle (kos′tō-fren′ik ang′gĕl) The angle between the costal and diaphragmatic parietal pleura as they meet at the costodiaphragmatic line of pleura reflection. Used as a synonym in radiology to identify the costodiaphragmatic recess.

cos·to·scap·u·lar (kos′tō-skap′yū-lăr) Relating to the ribs and the scapula.

cos·to·ster·nal (kos′tō-stĕr′năl) Pertaining to the ribs and the sternum.

cos·to·ster·no·plas·ty (kos′tō-stĕr′nō-plas-tē) Surgery to correct a malformation of the anterior chest wall. [costo- + G. *sternon,* chest, + *plastos,* formed]

cos·tot·o·my (kos-tot′ŏ-mē) Division of a rib. [costo- + G. *tomē,* a cutting]

cos·to·trans·verse (kos′tō-trans-vĕrs′) Relating to the ribs and the transverse processes of the vertebrae articulating with them.

cos·to·trans·ver·sec·to·my (kos′tō-trans-vĕrs-ek′tŏ-mē) Excision of a proximal portion of a rib and the articulating transverse process.

cos·to·trans·verse lig·a·ment (kos′tō-trans-vĕrs′ lig′ă-mĕnt) The ligament that connects the dorsal aspect of the neck of a rib to the ventral aspect of the corresponding transverse process. SYN ligamentum costotransversarium [TA].

cos·to·ver·te·bral (kos′tō-vĕr′tĕ-brăl) Relating to the ribs and the bodies of the thoracic vertebrae with which they articulate. SYN vertebrocostal (1).

cos·to·ver·te·bral an·gle (kos′tō-vĕr′tĕ-brăl ang′gĕl) The acute angle formed between either twelfth rib and the vertebral column.

cos·to·xi·phoid (kos′tō-zī′foyd) Relating to the ribs and the xiphoid cartilage of the sternum.

cost shar·ing (kawst shār′ing) The amount paid for medical services including coinsurance, copay, or deductible.

Co·tard syn·drome (kō-tahr′ sin′drōm) Psychotic depression involving delusion of the existence of one's body, along with ideas of negation and suicidal impulses.

Côte-d'I·voire virus (kōt dē′vwahr vī′rus) A variant of Ebola virus. SYN Ebola virus Côte-d'Ivoire.

co·throm·bo·plas·tin (kō′throm′bō-plas′tin) SYN factor VII.

co·trans·port (kō′trans′pōrt) The transport of one substance across a membrane, coupled with the simultaneous transport of another substance across the same membrane in the same direction.

Cotte op·er·a·tion (kut′ē op-ĕr-ā′shŭn) SYN presacral neurectomy.

cot·ton (kot′ŏn) SYN gossypol.

cot·ton-fi·ber em·bo·lism (kot′ŏn-fī′bĕr em′bŏ-lizm) Embolism by cotton fibers from sterile gauze used in intravenous medication or transfusion; may form as foreign body granulomas in small pulmonary arteries.

cot·ton-wool patch·es (kot′ŏn-wul pach′ĕz) White, fuzzy areas on the surface of the retina (accumulations of cellular organelles) caused by damage (usually infarction) of the retinal fiber layer. See page B26.

Co·tun·ni·us nerve (kō-tŭn′ē-ŭs nĕrv) SYN nasopalatine nerve.

cot·y·le·don (kot′i-lē′dŏn) **1.** In plants, a seed leaf, the first leaf to grow from a seed. **2.** Irregular convex area of the fetal part of the placenta composed of stem villi. [G. *kotylēdon,* any cup-shaped hollow]

cot·y·loid (kot′i-loyd) **1.** Cup-shaped; cuplike. **2.** Relating to the cotyloid cavity or acetabulum. [G. *kotylē,* a small cup, + *eidos,* appearance]

cot·y·loid cav·i·ty (kot′i-loyd kav′i-tē) SYN acetabulum.

cot·y·loid joint (kot′i-loyd joynt) SYN ball-and-socket joint.

cough (kawf) **1.** A sudden expulsion of air through the glottis, occurring immediately on opening the previously closed glottis, and excited by mechanical or chemical irritation of the trachea or bronchi, or by pressure from adjacent structures. **2.** To force air through the glottis by a series of expiratory efforts. [echoic]

cough re·flex (kawf rē′fleks) The reflex that mediates coughing in response to irritation of the larynx or tracheobronchial tree.

cough·root (kawf′rūt) SYN trillium.

cou·lomb (C, Q) (kū′lom) The SI unit of electrical charge, equal to 3×10^9 electrostatic units; the quantity of electricity delivered by a current of 1 ampere in 1 sec; equal to 1/96,485 faraday; also used to measure radiation. SEE ALSO roentgen.

Cou·lomb law (kū′lom law) The principle that opposite charges attract and like charges repel each other.

cou·lom·e·try (kū-lom′ĕ-trē) A titration technique in which the titrant is electrochemically generated. The Ag^+ titrant in the chloridometer is commonly used to determine the concentration of chloride in the sample. [coulomb + -metry]

Cou·mel tach·y·car·di·a (kū′mel tak′i-kahr′dē-ă) A persistent junctional reciprocating tachycardia that usually uses a slowly conducting posteroseptal pathway for the retrograde journey.

coun·sel·ing (kown′sĕ-ling) A professional relationship and activity in which one person endeavors to help another to understand and to solve his or her adjustment problems; the giving of advice, opinion, and instruction to direct the judgment or conduct of another. SEE psychotherapy. SYN counselling. [L. *consilium,* deliberation]

counselling [Br.] SYN counseling.

count (kownt) **1.** A reckoning, enumeration, or accounting. **2.** To enumerate or score. **3.** A tally of instruments and materials performed at the beginning of a surgical operation and again before the incision is closed, to ensure that no foreign object remains in the patient.

count·er (kown′tĕr) A device that counts.

counter- Combining form meaning opposite, opposed, against. SEE ALSO contra-. [L. *contra,* against]

count·er·con·di·tion·ing (kown′tĕr-kon-dish′ŭn-ing) Any behavior therapy in which a second conditioned response (e.g., approaching or even touching a snake) is introduced for the purpose of counteracting or nullifying a previously conditioned or learned response (e.g., fear and avoidance of snakes).

coun·ter·cur·rent flow (kownt′ĕr-kŭr′ĕnt flō) Flow in the opposite direction to slice excitation during magnetic resonance imaging.

count·er·cur·rent mech·a·nism (kownt′ĕr-kŭr′ĕnt mek′ă-nizm) A system in the renal medulla that facilitates concentration of the urine as it passes through the renal tubules.

count·er·ex·ten·sion (kown′tĕr-eks-ten′shŭn) SYN countertraction.

count·er·im·mu·no·e·lec·tro·pho·re·sis (kown′tĕr-im′yū-nō-ĕ-lek′trō-fŏr-ē′sis) Immunoelectrophoresis in which antigen is placed in wells cut in the sheet of agar gel toward the cathode, and antiserum is placed in wells toward the anode; antigen and antibody, moving in opposite directions, form precipitates in the area between the cells where they meet in concentrations of optimal proportions.

count·er·in·ci·sion (kown′tĕr-in-sizh′ŭn) A second incision adjacent to a primary incision.

count·er·ir·ri·tant (kown′tĕr-ir′i-tănt) **1.** An agent that causes irritation or a mild inflammation of the skin to relieve symptoms of a deep-seated inflammatory process. **2.** Relating to or producing counterirritation.

count·er·ir·ri·ta·tion (kown′ter-ir-i-tā′shŭn) Irritation or mild inflammation (redness, vesication, or pustulation) of the skin excited for the purpose of relieving symptoms of an inflammation of the deeper structures. SYN revulsion (1).

coun·ter·mea·sure (kown′tĕr-mezh′ŭr) SYN intervention (2).

coun·ter·nu·ta·tion (kown′tĕr-nū-tā′shŭn) Anterior rotation of the sacrum against the left and right ilia. Cf. nutation. [counter- + *nutation,* fr. L. *nuto,* to nod]

count·er·o·pen·ing (kown′tĕr-ō′pĕn-ing) A second opening made at the dependent part of an abscess or other cavity containing fluid, which is not draining satisfactorily through an opening previously made. SYN contraaperture, counterpuncture.

count·er·pul·sa·tion (kown′tĕr-pŭl-sā′shŭn) A means of assisting the failing heart by automatically removing arterial blood just before and during ventricular ejection and returning it to the circulation during diastole; a balloon catheter is inserted into the aorta and activated by an automatic mechanism triggered by the ECG.

count·er·punc·ture (kown′tĕr-pŭngk′shŭr) SYN counteropening.

count·er·shock (kown′tĕr-shok) An electric shock applied to the heart to terminate a disturbance of its rhythm.

count·er·stain (kown′tĕr-stān) A second stain of a different color, having affinity for tissues, cells, or parts of cells other than those taking the primary stain, used to render more distinct the parts taking the first stain.

count·er·trac·tion (kown′tĕr-trak′shŭn) The resistance, or back-pull, made to traction or pulling on a limb; e.g., in the case of traction made on the leg, countertraction may be effected by raising the foot of the bed so that the weight of the body pulls against the weight attached to the limb. SYN counterextension.

count·er·trans·fer·ence (kown′tĕr-trans-fer′ĕns) PSYCHOANALYSIS the analyst's transference (often unconscious) toward the patient of his or her emotional needs and feelings, with personal involvement to the detriment of the desired objective analyst-patient relationship.

count·er·trans·port (kown′tĕr-trans′pōrt) The transport of one substance across a membrane, coupled with the simultaneous transport of another substance across the same membrane in the opposite direction.

count·ing cham·ber (kown′ting chām′bĕr) A standardized ruled-glass slide used for counting cells (especially erythrocytes and leukocytes) and other particulate material in a measured volume of fluid. Such slides are frequently known as hemocytometers.

coup in·ju·ry of brain (kū in′jŭr-ē brān) An injury occurring directly beneath the skull at the area of impact.

cou·ple (kŭp′ĕl) To copulate; to perform coitus; said especially of the lower animals.

cou·pled pulse (kŭp′ĕld pŭls) SYN bigeminal pulse.

cou·pled rhythm (kŭp′ĕld ridh′ŭm) SYN bigeminal rhythm.

cou·plet (kŭp′lĕt) A series of two consecutive premature ventricular contractions.

cou·pling (kŭp′ling) **1.** The repeated pairing of a normal sinus beat with a ventricular extrasystole. **2.** A condition in which one or more products of a reaction are the subsequent reactants (or substrates) of a second reaction.

cou·pling a·gent (kŭp′ling ā′jĕnt) A gel or lotion used to improve contact and reduce friction between transducer and skin during ultrasound examinations and treatmnts.

cou·pling fac·tors (kŭp′ling fak′tŏrz) Proteins that restore phosphorylating ability to mitochondria.

Cour·nand dip (kūr-nahn′ dip) In constrictive pericarditis, rapid early diastolic fall and reascent of the ventricular pressure curve to an elevated plateau (square root configuration).

Cour·voi·si·er gall·blad·der (kūr-vwah′zē-ā′ gawl′blad-ĕr) An enlarged, often palpable gallbladder in a patient with carcinoma of the head of the pancreas. It is associated with jaundice due to obstruction of the common bile duct. SEE Courvoisier law. SYN Bard-Pic disease, Courvoisier sign.

Cour·voi·si·er law (kūr-vwah′zē-ā′ law) Painless enlargement of the gallbladder with jaundice is likely to result from carcinoma of the head of the pancreas and not from a stone in the common duct, because in the latter the gallbladder is usually scarred from infection and does not distend.

Cour·voi·si·er sign (kūr-vwah′zē-ā′ sīn) SYN Courvoisier gallbladder.

cou·vade (kū-vahd′) A primitive custom in certain cultures in which a man develops labor pains while his wife is in labor and then submits to the same postpartum purification rites and taboos. [Fr. *couver,* to hatch]

Cou·ve·laire u·ter·us (kū-vĕ-lār′ yū′tĕr-us) Extravasation of blood into the uterine musculature and beneath the uterine peritoneum in association with severe forms of abruptio placentae.

co·va·lent (kō-vā′lĕnt) Denoting an interatomic bond characterized by the sharing of two, four, or six electrons.

cov·er·age (kŏv′ĕr-ăj) A measure of the extent to which the services rendered cover the potential need for these services in a community; applied specifically to such services as immunization in developing countries.

cov·ered en·ti·ty (kŭv′ĕrd en′ti-tē) Any health care plan, provider, or service that transmits health care information in an electronic form and is thereby governed by laws and regulations in the handling of such data.

cov·er·ing (kŭv′ĕr-ing) In health care, agreement by one doctor to attend the patients of another when the first physician is unavailable due to unexpected absence or prior commitment.

cov·ert sen·si·ti·za·tion (kō-vĕrt′ sen′si-tī-zā′shŭn) Aversive conditioning or training to abolish an unwanted behavior, during which the patient is taught to imagine unpleasant and related aversive consequences while engaging in the unwanted habit.

cov·er-un·cov·er test (kŏv′ĕr-ŭn′kŏv-ĕr test) A test to detect strabismus. The patient's attention is directed to a small fixation object, one eye is covered and after a few seconds, uncovered; if the uncovered eye moves to see the picture, strabismus is present.

Cow·den dis·ease (kow′dĕn di-zēz′) Hypertrichosis and gingival fibromatosis from infancy, accompanied by postpubertal fibroadenomatous breast enlargement; papules of the face are characteristic of multiple trichilemmomas.

Cow·dry type A in·clu·sion bod·ies (kow′drē tīp in-klū′zhŭn bod′ēz) Dropletlike masses of acidophilic material surrounded by clear halos within nuclei, with margination of chromatin on the nuclear membrane as seen in human herpesvirus–infected cells.

Cow·dry type B in·clu·sion bod·ies (kow′drē tīp in-klū′zhŭn bod′ēz) Obsolete term for dropletlike masses of acidophilic material surrounded by clear halos within nuclei, without other nuclear changes during early stages of development of the inclusion, as seen in poliomyelitis.

Cow·per cyst (kow′pĕr sist) A retention cyst of a Cowper (bulbourethral) gland.

Cow·per gland (kow′pĕr gland) SYN bulbourethral gland.

cow·per·i·tis (kow′pĕr-ī′tis) Inflammation of a bulbourethral or Cowper gland.

cox·a, gen. and pl. **cox·ae** (kok′să, -sē) **1.** SYN hip bone. **2.** SYN hip joint. [L]

cox·al·gia (koks-al′jē-ă) SYN coxodynia. [L. *coxa,* hip, + G. *algos,* pain]

cox·a mag·na (kok′să mag′nă) Enlargement, and often deformation of the femoral head; usually refers to a sequela of Legg-Calvé-Perthes disease or osteoarthritis.

cox·a pla·na (kok′să plā′nă) SYN Legg-Calvé-Perthes disease.

cox·a val·ga (kok′să val′gă) Alteration of the angle made by the axis of the femoral neck to the axis of the femoral shaft, so that the angle exceeds 135°; the femoral neck is in more of a straight-line relationship to the shaft of the femur.

cox·a va·ra (kok′să vā′ră) Alteration of the angle made by the axis of the femoral neck to the axis of the femoral shaft so that the angle is less than 135 degrees; the femoral neck becomes more horizontal.

Cox·i·el·la (kok-sē-el′ă) A genus of filterable bacteria (order Rickettsiales) containing small, pleomorphic, rod-shaped or coccoid, gram-negative cells that occur intracellularly in the cytoplasm of infected cells and possibly extracellularly in infected ticks. These organisms have not been cultivated in cell-free media; they are parasitic on humans and other animals. The type species is *C. burnetii.*

Cox·i·el·la bur·ne·ti·i (kok-sē-el′ă bŭr-nē′shē-ē) A species that causes Q fever in humans. It is more resistant than other rickettsiae and may be passed in aerosols as well as living vectors. Acute pneumonia and chronic endocarditis are also associated with this species. The type species of the genus *Coxiella.*

cox·o·dyn·i·a (kok′sō-din′ē-ă) Pain in the hip joint. SYN coxalgia. [L. *coxa,* hip, + G. *odynē,* pain]

cox·o·fem·o·ral (kok′sō-fem′ŏ-răl) Relating to the hip bone and the femur.

cox·o·tu·ber·cu·lo·sis (kok′sō-tū-bĕr-kyū-lō′sis) Tuberculous hip-joint disease.

Cox·sack·ie en·ceph·a·li·tis (kok-sak′ē en-sef′ă-lī′tis) A viral encephalitis, seen mainly in infants and involving principally the gray matter of the medulla and cord, caused by Enterovirus Coxsackie B.

cox·sack·ie·vi·rus, Cox·sack·ie vi·rus (kok-sak′ē-vī′rŭs) A group of picornaviruses causing myositis, paralysis, and death in young mice, and responsible for a variety of diseases in humans, although inapparent infections are common. They are divided antigenically into two groups, A and B, each of which includes a number of serologic types. Type A viruses cause herpangina and hand-foot-and-mouth disease; type B viruses cause epidemic pleurodynia; both type viruses may cause aseptic meningitis, myocarditis and pericarditis, and acute onset juvenile diabetes. [*Coxsackie,* N.Y., where virus first isolated]

CP Abbreviation for certified prosthetist.

CPAP Abbreviation for continuous positive airway pressure.

CPAT Abbreviation for Certified Patient Account Technician.

CPhT Abbreviation for Certified Pharmacy Technician. SEE ALSO pharmacy technician.

CPITN Abbreviation for Community Periodontal Index of Treatment Needs.

CPM ma·chine (mă-shēn′) Abbreviation for continuous passive motion machine.

CPO Abbreviation for certified prosthetist/orthotist.

CPOE Abbreviation for computer physician order entry.

CPPV Abbreviation for continuous positive pressure ventilation.

CPR Abbreviation for cardiopulmonary resuscitation; computer-based patient record.

cps Abbreviation for cycles per second.

CPT Abbreviation for Current Procedural Terminology; chest physical therapy.

CPX Abbreviation for cardiopulmonary exercise test.

CR **1.** NATO code for a riot-control agent, dibenz(*b,f*)-1:4-oxazepine, which is more potent than CS and has a higher safety margin. **2.** Abbreviation for controlled release.

Cr **1.** Abbreviation for conditioned reflex; creatinine. **2.** Symbol for chromium.

crack (krak) **1.** A fissure. **2.** SEE crack cocaine. [slang]

crack ba•by (krak bā′bē) An infant who was exposed to rock cocaine in utero; symptoms and findings vary across a very wide spectrum.

crack co•caine (krak kō-kān′) A derivative of cocaine, usually smoked, producing brief, intense euphoria. Crack cocaine is relatively inexpensive and extremely addictive; dependency can develop in less than 2 weeks. Like snorted or injected cocaine, it has both acute and chronic adverse effects, including heart and nasopharyngeal damage, seizures, sudden death, and psychosis. SEE ALSO street drug.

cracked heel (krakt hēl) SYN keratoderma plantare sulcatum.

cracked tooth syn•drome (krakt tūth sin′drōm) Transient acute pain that is difficult to locate and experienced occasionally while chewing. Usually a vertical crack or split in the tooth extends across a marginal ridge through the crown and into the root, involving the pulp. Cracked teeth may be identified using transilluminated light or disclosing dyes.

crac•kle (krak′ĕl) Short, sharp, or rough sounds heard with a stethoscope over the chest. Abnormal breath sounds caused by excessive fluid within the airways. [echoic]

cra•dle (krā′dĕl) A frame used to keep bedclothes from coming in contact with a patient. [M.E. *cradel*]

cra•dle cap (krā′dĕl kap) Colloquialism for seborrheic dermatitis of the scalp of the newborn. See page B30.

Craig test (krāg test) Technique to assess forward torsion of femur or femoral anteversion.

cramp (kramp) **1.** A painful muscle spasm caused by prolonged tetanic contraction. **2.** A localized muscle spasm related to occupational use, qualified according to the occupation of the sufferer (e.g., writer's cramp). [M.E. *crampe*, fr. O. Fr., fr. Germanic]

cramp bark (kramp bahrk) SYN black haw.

Cramp•ton test (kramp′tŏn test) A test for physical condition and resistance; a record is made of the pulse and the blood pressure in the recumbent and in the standing positions, and the difference is graded from the theoretic perfection of 100 (seldom attained) downward (a reading of 75 is considered excellent, 65 poor).

Cran•dall syn•drome (kran′dăl sin′drōm) Characterized by pili torti, sensorineural deafness, and hypogonadism; a familial trait in which there is a deficiency of luteinizing and growth hormones. SEE ALSO Björnstad syndrome.

cranes•bill, A•mer•i•can cranes•bill (ă-mer′i-kăn krānz′bil, ă-mer′i-kăn krānz′bil) (*Geranium maculatum*) The dried roots and leaves of this plant are used in decoctions and tinctures as a purported specific against cancer, cholera, plague, and numerous other disorders and diseases. Hepatotoxicity has been confirmed in studies SYN alumroot.

cra•ni•a (krā′nē-ă) Plural of cranium.

cra•ni•ad (krā′nē-ad) Situated nearer the head in relation to a specific reference point; opposite of caudad. SEE ALSO superior.

cra•ni•al (krā′nē-ăl) **1.** Relating to the cranium or head. SYN cephalic. SEE ALSO cephalad. **2.** SYN superior (2).

cra•ni•al a•rach•noid ma•ter (krā′nē ăl ă-rak′noyd mā′tĕr) That portion of the arachnoid that lies within the cranial cavity and surrounds the brain and the cranial portion of the subarachnoid space. In several sites it is relatively widely separated from the pia mater, creating the cranial subarachnoid cisterns. SYN arachnoidea mater cranialis [TA], arachnoid of brain, arachnoidea mater encephali.

cra•ni•al ar•te•ri•tis (krā′nē-ăl ahr′tĕr-ī′tis) SYN temporal arteritis.

cra•ni•al bones (krā′nē-ăl bōnz) SYN bones of cranium.

cra•ni•al cav•i•ty (krā′nē-ăl kav′i-tē) The space within the skull occupied by the brain, its coverings, and cerebrospinal fluid. SYN intracranial cavity.

cra•ni•al flex•ure (krā′nē-ăl flek′shŭr) SYN cephalic flexure.

cra•ni•al nerves (krā′nē-ăl nĕrvz) Those nerves that emerge from, or enter, the cranium or skull, in contrast to the spinal nerves, which emerge from the spine or vertebral column. The twelve paired cranial nerves are the olfactory, optic, oculomotor, trochlear, trigeminal, abducent, facial, vestibulocochlear, glossopharyngeal, vagal, accessory, and hypoglossal nerves. SEE ALSO Brodmann areas. See this page. SYN nervi craniales [TA].

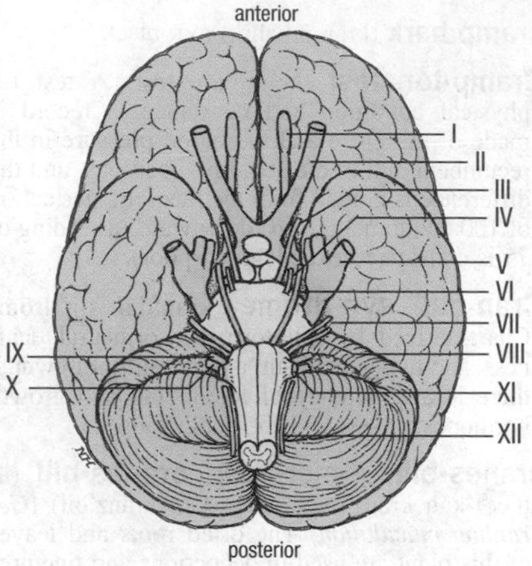

cranial nerves: (inferior view): (I) olfactory, (II) optic, (III) oculomotor, (IV) trochlear, (V) trigeminal, (VI) abducens, (VII) facial, (VIII) vestibulocochlear, (IX) glossopharyngeal, (X) vagus, (XI) accessory, (XII) hypoglossal

cra·ni·al pi·a ma·ter (krā′nē-ăl pē′ă mā′tĕr) The pia mater found specifically around the brain; contiguous with the arachnoid mater through the arachnoid trabeculae. SEE ALSO pia mater. SYN pia mater encephali [TA].

cra·ni·al root of ac·ces·so·ry nerve (krā′nē-ăl rūt ak-ses′ŏr-ē nĕrv) The roots of the accessory nerve that arise from the medulla; the nerve fibers of the cranial root join the intracranial portion of the vagus nerve and are distributed to the pharyngeal plexus, providing the motor innervation of the soft palate (except the tensor veli palati) and the pharynx.

cra·ni·al su·tures (krā′nē-ăl sū′chŭrz) The sutures between the bones of the skull.

cra·ni·al ver·te·bra (krā′nē-ăl vĕr′tĕ-bră) A segment of the skull regarded as homologous with a segment of the vertebral column.

cra·ni·ec·to·my (krā′nē-ek′tŏ-mē) Excision of a portion of the skull. [G. *kranion,* skull, + *ektomē,* excision]

♻ **cranio-, crani-** Combining forms meaning the cranium. Cf. cerebro-. [G. *kranion,* skull]

cra·ni·o·cele (krā′nē-ō-sēl) SYN encephalocele. [cranio- + G. *kēlē,* hernia]

cra·ni·o·ce·re·bral (krā′nē-ō-ser′ĕ-brăl) Relating to the skull and the brain.

cra·ni·o·fa·cial (krā′nē-ō-fā′shăl) Relating to both the face and the cranium.

cra·ni·o·fa·cial dys·junc·tion frac·ture (krā′nē-ō-fā′shăl dis-jŭngk′shŭn frak′shŭr) A complex fracture in which the facial bones are separated from the cranial bones. SYN Le Fort III fracture.

cra·ni·o·fe·nes·tri·a (krā′nē-ō-fĕ-nes′trē-ă) SYN craniolacunia. [cranio- + L. *fenestra,* window]

cra·ni·o·la·cu·ni·a (krā′nē-ō-lă-kū′nē-ă) Incomplete formation of the bones of the domelike calvaria of the fetal cranium so that there are nonossified areas in the calvaria. SYN craniofenestria. [cranio- + L. *lacuna,* cleft]

cra·ni·o·ma·la·ci·a (krā′nē-ō-mă-lā′shē-ă) Softening of the bones of the cranium. [cranio- + G. *malakia,* softness]

cra·ni·o·met·ric points (krā′nē-ō-met′rik poynts) Fixed points on the skull used as landmarks in craniometry.

cra·ni·op·a·thy (krā′nē-op′ă-thē) Any pathologic condition of the cranial bones. [cranio- + G. *pathos,* suffering]

cra·ni·o·pha·ryn·ge·al (krā′nē-ō-făr-in′jē-ăl) Relating to the skull and to the pharynx.

cra·ni·o·pha·ryn·gi·o·ma (krā′nē-ō-făr-in′jē-ō′mă) A suprasellar neoplasm that develops from Rathke pouch; the histologic pattern consists of nesting of squamous epithelium bordered by radially arranged cells. SYN Rathke pouch tumor. [cranio- + pharyngio- + -oma]

cra·ni·o·plas·ty (krā′nē-ō-plas-tē) Plastic surgery of the skull; a surgical correction of a skull defect. [cranio- + G. *plastos,* formed]

cra·ni·o·punc·ture (krā′nē-ō-pŭngk′shŭr) Puncture of the brain for exploratory purposes.

cra·ni·or·rha·chis·chi·sis (krā′nē-ō-ră-kis′ki-sis) Severe congenital malformation in which there is incomplete closure of the cranium and vertebral column. [cranio- + G. *rhachis,* spine, + *schisis,* a cleaving]

cra·ni·o·sa·cral (krā′nē-ō-sā′krăl) Denoting the cranial and sacral origins of the parasympathetic division of the autonomic nervous system.

cra·ni·o·sa·cral ther·a·py (CST) (krā′nē-ō-sā′krăl thār′ă-pē) A bodywork modality that focuses on identifying and resolving restrictions in the dural sheath that are said to cause restrictions in fascia throughout the body. Practitioners perform therapy by means of palpating and influencing the rhythmic movements of cerebrospinal fluid.

cra·ni·os·chi·sis (krā′nē-os′ki-sis) Congenital malformation in which there is incomplete closure of the cranium. Usually accompanied by grossly defective development of the brain. [cranio- + G. *schisis,* a cleavage]

cra•ni•o•scle•ro•sis (krā′nē-ō-skler-ō′sis) Thickening of the skull. [cranio- + G. *sklēros,* hard, + *-osis,* condition]

cra•ni•o•spi•nal (krā′nē-ō-spī′năl) Relating to the cranium and spinal column.

cra•ni•o•spi•nal sen•so•ry gan•gli•a (krā′nē-ō-spī′năl sen′sŏr-ē gang′glē-ă) A term collectively designating the sensory ganglia on the dorsal (posterior) roots of spinal nerves and on those cranial nerves that contain general sensory and taste fibers; also called encephalospinal ganglia.

cra•ni•o•ste•no•sis (krā′nē-ō-stĕ-nō′sis) Premature closure of cranial sutures resulting in malformation of the cranium. [cranio- + G. *stenōsis,* a narrowing]

cra•ni•o•syn•os•to•sis (krā′nē-ō-sin′os-tō′sis) Premature ossification of the cranium and obliteration of the sutures.

cra•ni•o•ta•bes (krā′nē-ō-tā′bēz) A disease marked by areas of thinning and softening in the bones of the skull and widening of the sutures and fontanelles. Usually of syphilitic or rachitic origin. [cranio- + L. *tabes,* a wasting]

cra•ni•ot•o•my (krā′nē-ot′ŏ-mē) Opening into the skull, either by attached or detached craniotomy or by trephination. [cranio- + G. *tomē,* incision]

cra•ni•o•tym•pan•ic (krā′nē-ō-tim-pan′ik) Relating to the skull and the middle ear.

cra•ni•um, pl. **cra•ni•a** (krā′nē-ŭm, krā′nē-ă) [TA] The bones of the head collectively. SEE skull. [mediev. L. fr. Gr. *kranion*]

crank test (krangk test) SYN anterior apprehension test.

crash cart (krash kahrt) A movable collection of emergency equipment and supplies meant to be readily available for resuscitative effort. It includes medication as well as the equipment for defibrillation, intubation, intravenous medication, and passage of central lines.

cra•vat ban•dage (kră′vat ban′dăj) A bandage made by bringing the point of a triangular bandage to the middle of the base and then folding lengthwise to the desired width.

C-re•ac•tive pro•tein (CRP) (rē-ak′tiv prō′tēn) A β-globulin found in the serum of various people with certain inflammatory, degenerative, and neoplastic diseases; although the protein is not a specific antibody, it precipitates in vitro the C polysaccharide present in all types of pneumococci.

cream (krēm) **1.** The upper fatty layer that forms in milk on standing or is separated from it by centrifugation; it contains about the same amount of sugar and protein as milk, but 12–40% more fat. **2.** Any whitish viscid fluid resembling cream. **3.** A semisolid emulsion of either the oil-in-water or the water-in-oil type, ordinarily intended for topical use. [L. *cremor,* thick juice, broth]

crease (krēs) A line or linear depression as produced by a fold. SEE ALSO fold, groove, line.

creatinaemia [Br.] SYN creatinemia.

cre•a•ti•nase (krē-at′i-nās) An enzyme catalyzing the hydrolysis of creatine to sarcosine and urea.

cre•a•tine (krē′ă-tin) *N*-(aminoiminomethyl) -*N*-methylglycine; occurs in urine, sometimes as such, but generally as creatinine, and in muscle, generally as phosphocreatine; elevated in urine in muscular dystrophy; synthesized in liver and pancreas from amino acids; absorbed in bloodstream, it is deposited in tissue (e.g., muscles, brain).

cre•a•tine ki•nase (CK) (krē′ă-tin kī′nās) An enzyme catalyzing the reversible transfer of phosphate from phosphocreatine to ADP, forming creatine and ATP; of importance in muscle contraction. Certain isozymes are elevated in plasma following myocardial infarctions.

cre•a•tine ki•nase i•so•en•zymes (krē′ă-tin kī′nās ī′sō-en′zīmz) CK-MM, the predominant form, is found primarily in skeletal muscle; CK-MB, is found in cardiac muscle, tongue, diaphragm, and in small amounts in skeletal muscle; and CK-BB found in the brain, smooth muscle, thyroid, lungs, and prostate. Elevations can help in the differential diagnosis of a variety of states, with CK-MB elevations as an important marker following myocardial infarctions, elevations in CK-MM an indicator of muscle disease, and elevations in CK-BB an occasional finding following brain infarcts, bowel infarcts, or in the presence of certain malignancies.

cre•a•ti•ne•mi•a (krē′ă-ti-nē′mē-ă) The presence of abnormal concentrations of creatine in peripheral blood. SYN creatinaemia. [creatine + G. *haima,* blood]

cre•a•tine mon•o•hy•drate (krē′ă-tēn mon′ō-hī′drāt) A physiologic amino acid that is taken as a supplement by athletes to improve performance; GI complaints common; suggested cause of impaired renal function.

cre•a•tine phos•phate (krē′ă-tin fos′fāt) SYN phosphocreatine.

cre•at•i•nin•ase (krē-at′i-nin-ās) An amidohydrolase catalyzing the conversion of creatine to creatinine.

cre•at•i•nine (Cr) (krē-at′i-nin) A component of urine and the final product of creatine catabolism; formed by the nonenzymatic dephosphorylative cyclization of phosphocreatine to form the internal anhydride of creatine.

cre•at•i•nine clear•ance (krē-at′i-nin klēr′ăns) A mathematical calculation of the total amount of creatinine excreted in the urine over a period of time, usually 24 hours to test renal function. The calculation is: creatinine clearance (mL/minute) = urine creatinine concentration (mL/dL) × volume of urine (mL/24 hour) ÷ plasma creatinine concentration (mg/dL) × 1440 minute/24 hour.

cre•a•tin•u•ri•a (krē′ă-ti-nūr′ē-ă) The urinary excretion of increased amounts of creatine. [creatine + G. *ouron,* urine]

Cre•dé meth•od (krĕ-dā′ meth′ŏd) **1.** Instillation of one drop of a 2% solution of silver nitrate into each eye of the newborn infant, to prevent ophthalmia neonatorum. **2.** Resting the hand on the fundus uteri from the moment of the expulsion of the fetus, and gently rubbing in case of hemorrhage or failing contraction; then, when the afterbirth is loosened it is expelled by firm compression or squeezing of the fundus by the hand. **3.** Use of manual pressure on a bladder, particularly a paralyzed bladder, to express urine.

cre•den•tial•ing (krĕ-den′shăl-ing) A formal review of the qualifications of a provider who has applied to participate in a health care system or plan. SYN credentialling. [*credential,* proof of authenticity, fr. Med. L. *credentialis,* fr. *credo,* to believe, + -ing]

credentialling [Br.] SYN credentialing.

cre•mas•ter (krē-mas′tĕr) SEE cremaster muscle. [G. *kremastēr,* a suspender, fr. *kremannymi,* to hang]

crem•as•ter•ic (krem′as-ter′ik) Relating to the cremaster.

crem•as•ter•ic ar•ter•y (krem′as-ter′ik ahr′tĕr-ē) *Origin*, inferior epigastric; *distribution*, coverings of spermatic cord; *anastomoses*, external pudendal, spermatic, and perineal arteries. SYN arteria cremasterica [TA].

crem•as•ter•ic re•flex (krem′as-ter′ik rē′fleks) A drawing up of the scrotum and testicle of the same side when the skin over the Scarpa triangle or on the inner side of the thigh is scratched.

cre•mas•ter mus•cle (krē-mas′tĕr mŭs′ĕl) *Origin*, from internal oblique muscle and inguinal ligament; *insertion*, cremasteric fascia (spermatic cord); *action*, raises testicle; *nerve supply*, genital branch of genitofemoral; in the male the muscle envelops the spermatic cord and testis; in the female, the round ligament of the uterus. SYN musculus cremaster [TA].

crem•no•cele (krem′nō-sēl) A protrusion of intestine into the labium majus. [G. *krēmnos,* overhanging cliff, labium pudendi, + *kēlē,* hernia]

cre•na, pl. **cre•nae** (krē′nă, -nē) A V-shaped cut or the space created by such a cut; one of the notches into which the opposing projections fit in the cranial sutures. [L. a notch]

cre•nate, **cre•nat•ed** (krē′nāt, -nā-ted) Indented; denoting the outline of a shriveled red blood cell, as observed in a hypertonic solution. [L. *crena,* a notch]

cre•no•cyte (krē′nō-sīt) A red blood cell with serrated edges. [L. *crena,* a notch, + G. *kytos,* a hollow (cell)]

cre•o•sote bush (krē′ō-sōt bush) SYN chapparal.

crep•i•tant (krep′i-tănt) **1.** Relating to or characterized by crepitation. **2.** Denoting a fine bubbling noise (rale) produced by air entering fluid in lung tissue; heard in pneumonia and in certain other conditions. **3.** The sensation imparted to the palpating finger by gas or air in the subcutaneous tissues.

crep•i•tant rale (krep′i-tănt rahl) A fine bubbling or crackling sound produced by air mixing with very thin secretions in the smaller bronchial tubes.

crep•i•ta•tion (krep′i-tā′shŭn) **1.** Crackling; the quality of a fine bubbling sound (rale) that resembles noise heard on rubbing hair between the fingers. **2.** The sensation felt on placing the hand over the seat of a fracture when the broken ends of the bone are moved, or over tissue, in which gas gangrene is present. **3.** Noise or vibration produced by rubbing bone or irregular cartilage surfaces together as by movement of patella against femoral condyles in arthritis and other conditions. SYN crepitus (1). [see crepitus]

crep•i•tus (krep′i-tŭs) **1.** SYN crepitation. **2.** A noisy discharge of gas from the intestine. **3.** The grating of a joint, often in association with osteoarthritis. [L. fr. *crepo,* to rattle]

cre•scen•do an•gi•na (krĕ-shen′dō an′ji-nă) Angina pectoris that occurs with increasing frequency, intensity, or duration.

cre•scen•do mur•mur (krĕ-shen′dō mŭr′mŭr) A murmur that increases in intensity and suddenly ceases; the presystolic murmur of mitral stenosis is a common example.

cres•cent (kres′ĕnt) **1.** Any figure in the shape of the moon in its first quarter. **2.** The figure made by the gray columns or cornua on cross-section of the spinal cord. **3.** SYN malarial crescent. [L. *cresco,* pr. p. *crescens,* to grow]

cres•cent bod•ies (kres′ĕnt bod′ēz) SYN achromocyte.

cres•cent cell a•ne•mi•a (kres′ĕnt sel ă-nē′mē-ă) SYN sickle cell anemia.

cres•cen•tic (krĕ-sen′tik) Shaped like a crescent.

cres•cent sign (kres′ĕnt sīn) **1.** RADIOGRAPHY in the lung, a crescent of gas near the top of a mass lesion, signifying cavitation with a space above the debris; seen in aspergilloma, hydatidoma. **2.** COMPUTED TOMOGRAPHY a high attenuating layer of new blood in an aneurysm; indicates a ruptured abdominal aortic aneurysm. **3.** DIAGNOSTIC ULTRASOUND a sonolucent crescentic layer in a tumor mass, typically necrosis in stromal tumors of the small bowel. **4.** DIAGNOSTIC ULTRASOUND a hyperechoic crescent, representing the entering limb of an intussusception; also known as crescent-in-a-doughnut. **5.** OSTEORADIOLOGY a subcortical lucent crescent in the femoral head, signifying osteonecrosis. SYN meniscus sign.

cre•sol red (kre′sōl red) An acid-base indicator with a pK value of 8.3; yellow at pH values below 7.4, red above 9.0.

CREST (krest) SEE CREST syndrome.

crest (krest) A ridge, especially a bony ridge. SYN crista [TA]. [L. *crista*]

crest of head of rib (krest hed rib) The ridge that separates the superior and inferior articular surfaces of the head of a rib.

crest of pal•a•tine bone, pal•a•tine crest (krest pal′ă-tīn bōn, pal′ă-tīn krest) A transverse ridge near the posterior border of the bony palate, located on the inferior surface of the horizontal plate of the palatine bone.

crests of nail ma•trix (krests nāl mā′triks) The numerous longitudinal ridges of the nail bed distal to the lunula.

CREST syn•drome (krest sin′drōm) An acronymic designation for a variant of scleroderma characterized by calcinosis, Raynaud phenomenon, esophageal motility disorders, sclerodactyly, and telangiectasia.

cres•yl echt vi•o•let stain (kres′il ekt vī′ŏ-lĕt stān) A stain used for identification of *Pneumocystis jiroveci*.

cre•tin (kret′in) An obsolete term for a person exhibiting cretinism caused by congenital severe hypothyroidism. [Fr. *crétin*]

cre•tin•ism (kret′in-izm) Obsolete term for congenital hypothyroidism. SEE ALSO infantile hypothyroidism.

cre•tin•oid (kret′in-oyd) An obsolete term for resembling a cretin; presenting symptoms similar to those of congenital hypothyroidism.

cre•tin•ous (kret′in-ŭs) An obsolete term for relating to cretinism or a cretin; affected with congenital hypothyroidism.

Creutz•feldt-Jak•ob dis•ease (CJD) (kroyts′felt-yah′kōp di-zēz′) A progressive neurologic disorder, one of the subacute spongiform encephalopathies caused by prions. Clinical features of CJD include a progressive cerebellar syndrome, including ataxia, abnormalities of gait and speech, and dementia. In most patients, these symptoms are followed by involuntary movements (myoclonus) and the appearance of a typical diagnostic electroencephalogram tracing (burst suppression, consisting of intermittent sharp and slow wave complexes on a flat background). The average survival is less than 1 year after onset of symptoms. SEE ALSO bovine spongiform encephalopathy.

crev•ice (krev′is) A crack or small fissure, especially in a solid substance. [Fr. *crevasse*]

cre•vic•u•lar (krĕ-vik′yū-lăr) **1.** Relating to any crevice. **2.** DENTISTRY relating especially to the gingival crevice or sulcus.

CRF Abbreviation for corticotropin-releasing factor.

CRH Abbreviation for corticotropin-releasing hormone.

crib-bit•ing (krib′bīt-ing) A behavior disorder of horses in which the animal grasps the edge of a convenient fixture and presses down, raising the floor of its mouth, forcing the soft palate open, and sometimes swallowing air. SEE aerophagia. SEE ALSO wind-sucking.

crib death (krib deth) SYN sudden infant death syndrome.

cri•bra (krib′ră) Plural of cribrum.

crib•rate (krib′rāt) SYN cribriform.

cri•bra•tion (kri-brā′shŭn) **1.** Sifting; passing through a sieve. **2.** The condition of being cribrate or numerously pitted or punctured.

crib•ri•form (krib′ri-fōrm) Sievelike; containing many perforations. SYN cribrate, polyporous. [L. *cribrum,* a sieve, + *forma,* form]

crib•ri•form plate of eth•moid bone (krib′ri-fōrm plāt eth′moyd bōn) A horizontal lamina from which are suspended the labyrinth, on either side, and the lamina perpendicularis in the center. It fits into the ethmoidal notch of the frontal bone and supports the olfactory lobes of the cerebrum, being pierced with numerous openings for the passage of the olfactory nerves. SYN lamina cribrosa ossis ethmoidalis [TA], cribrum.

cri•brum, pl. **cri•bra** (krib′rŭm, -ră) SYN cribriform plate of ethmoid bone. [L. a sieve]

cri•co•ar•y•te•noid (krī′kō-ar-i-tē′noyd) Relating to the cricoid and arytenoid cartilages.

cri•coid (krī′koyd) Ring-shaped; denoting the cricoid cartilage. [L. *cricoideus,* fr. G. *krikos,* a ring, + *eidos,* form]

cri•coid car•ti•lage (krī′koyd kahr′ti-lăj) The lowermost of the laryngeal cartilages. It is shaped like a signet ring, being expanded into a nearly quadrilateral plate (lamina) posteriorly; the anterior portion is called the arch (arcus). SYN cartilago cricoidea [TA].

cri•coid split op•er•a•tion (krī′koyd split op-ĕr-ā′shŭn) An operation to repair subglottic stenosis by transecting the anterior and posterior aspects of the ring of the cricoid cartilage, with or without the insertion of grafts to reconstruct the subglottic lumen.

cri·co·pha·ryn·ge·al (krī′kō-făr-in′jē-ăl) Relating to the cricoid cartilage and the pharynx; a part of the inferior constrictor muscle of the pharynx. SEE inferior constrictor muscle of pharynx.

cri·co·pha·ryn·ge·al ach·a·la·si·a (krī′kō-făr-in′jē-ăl ak-ă-lā′zē-ă) Functional obstruction at the level of the upper esophageal sphincter due to failure of relaxation of the cricopharyngeal muscles; often associated with a pharyngoesophageal diverticulum. SYN achalasia of the upper sphincter, hypertensive upper esophageal sphincter.

cri·co·pha·ryn·ge·al part of in·fe·ri·or con·stric·tor mus·cle of phar·ynx (krī-kō′făr-in′jē-ăl pahrt in-fēr′ē-ŏr kŏn-strik′tĕr mŭs′ĕl far′ingks) SYN cricopharyngeus muscle. SEE inferior constrictor muscle of pharynx.

cri·co·pha·ryn·ge·us mus·cle (krī-kō′făr-in′jē-yŭs mŭs′ĕl) SYN cricopharyngeal part of inferior constrictor muscle of pharynx.

cri·co·thy·roid (krī′kō-thī′royd) Relating to the cricoid and thyroid cartilages.

cri·co·thy·roid mus·cle (krī′kō-thī′royd mŭs′ĕl) *Origin*, anterior surface of arch of cricoid; *insertion*, the anterior or straight part passes upward to ala of thyroid; the posterior or oblique part passes more outward to inferior horn of thyroid; *action*, makes vocal folds tense, increasing the pitch of voice tone; *nerve supply*, external laryngeal branch of superior laryngeal nerve (from vagus). SYN musculus cricothyroideus [TA].

i **cri·co·thy·rot·o·my** (krī′kō-thī-rot′ŏ-mē) Incision through the skin and cricothyroid membrane for relief of respiratory obstruction; used before or in place of tracheotomy in certain emergency respiratory obstructions. See this page. SYN intercricothyrotomy. [cricoid + thyroid + G. *tomē*, incision]

cri·cot·o·my (krī-kot′ŏ-mē) Division of the cricoid cartilage, as in cricoid split, to enlarge the subglottic airway. [cricoid + G. *tomē*, incision]

cri-du-chat syn·drome, cat-cry syn·drome (krē-dū-shah′ sin′drōm, kat′krī sin′drōm) A disorder due to deletion of the short arm of chromosome 5, characterized by microcephaly, hypertelorism, antimongoloid palpebral fissures, epicanthal folds, micrognathia, strabismus, mental and physical retardation, and a characteristic high-pitched catlike whine.

Crig·ler-Naj·jar syn·drome (krig′lĕr nah′jahr sin′drōm) A defect in ability to form bilirubin glucuronide due to deficiency of bilirubin-glucuronide glucuronosyltransferase; characterized by familial nonhemolytic jaundice and, in its severe form, by irreversible brain damage in infancy that resembles kernicterus and may be fatal.

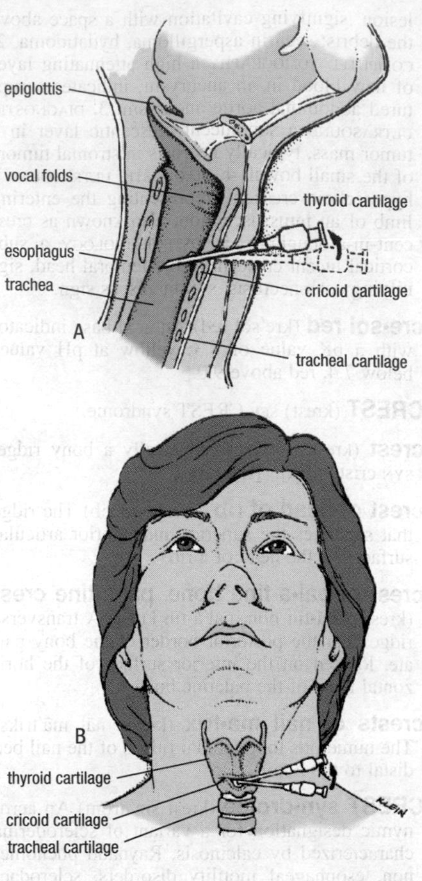

cricothyrotomy: (A) procedure; (B) cricothyroid membrane puncture

Crile clamp (krīl klamp) A clamp for temporary stoppage of blood flow. SYN Crile hemostatic forceps.

Crile he·mo·stat·ic for·ceps (krīl hē′mō-stat′ik fōr′seps) SYN Crile clamp.

crim·i·nal a·bor·tion (krim′i-năl ă-bōr′shŭn) Termination of pregnancy without legal justification.

crim·i·nal psy·chol·o·gy (krim′i-năl sī-kol′ŏ-jē) The study of the mind and its workings in relation to crime. SEE forensic psychology.

crin·o·gen·ic (krin′ō-jen′ik) Causing secretion; stimulating a gland to increased function. [G. *krinō*, to separate, + *-gen*, to produce]

crin·oph·a·gy (krin-of′ă-jē) Disposal of excess secretory granules by lysosomes.

cri•sis, pl. **cri•ses** (krī′sis, -sēz) **1.** A sudden change, usually for the better, in the course of an acute disease, in contrast to gradual improvement by lysis. **2.** A paroxysmal pain in an organ or circumscribed region of the body occurring in the course of tabetic neurosyphilis. **3.** A convulsive attack. [G. *krisis,* a separation, crisis]

cris•ta, pl. **cris•tae** (kris′tă, -tē) [TA] SYN crest. [L. crest]

cris•ta gal•li (kris′tă gal′ē) [TA] The triangular midline process of the ethmoid bone extending superiorly from the cribriform plate; it gives anterior attachment to the falx cerebri.

cri•te•ri•a (krī-tēr′ē-ă) Plural of criterion.

cri•te•ri•on, pl. **cri•te•ri•a** (krī-tēr′ē-ŏn, -ă) **1.** A standard or rule for judging; usually plural (criteria) denoting a set of standards or rules. **2.** PSYCHOLOGY a standard such as school grades against which test scores on intelligence tests or other measured behaviors are validated. **3.** A list of manifestations of a disease or disorder, a certain number of which must be present to warrant diagnosis in a given patient. [G. *kritērion,* a standard]

cri•te•ri•on-re•fer•enced (krī-tēr′ē-ŏn ref′ĕr-ĕnst) A psychometric property of a standardized test that compares a person's performance against a set of standard criteria.

crit•i•cal ap•prai•sal (krit′i-kăl ă-prā′zăl) The systematic process used to locate evidence and evaluate for validity and usefulness; an integral part of evidence-based practice. SEE ALSO evidence-based practice.

crit•i•cal care u•nit (CCU) (krit′i-kăl kār yū′nit) SYN intensive care unit.

crit•i•cal con•trol point (krit′i-kăl kŏn-trōl′ poynt) A point, step, or procedure in cooking at which controls can be applied and a food safety hazard can be prevented, eliminated, or reduced to acceptable levels.

crit•i•cal in•ci•dent stress man•age•ment (krit′i-kăl in′si-dĕnt stres man′ăj-mĕnt) A process of providing mental health management and support to providers who have experienced a critical stress incident.

crit•i•cal lim•it (krit′i-kăl lim′it) The upper or lower boundary of a laboratory test result that indicates a life-threatening value.

crit•i•cal mi•celle con•cen•tra•tion (cmc) (krit′i-kăl mi-sel′ kon′sĕn-trā′shŭn) The concentration at which an amphipathic molecule (e.g., a phospholipid) will form a micelle.

crit•i•cal or•gan (krit′i-kăl ōr′găn) The organ or physiologic system that for a given source of radiation would first reach its legally defined maximum permissible radiation exposure as the dose of radiopharmaceutical is increased.

crit•i•cal path (krit′i-kăl path) SYN clinical pathway.

crit•i•cal path•way (krit′i-kăl path′wā) A schedule of medical and nursing procedures, including diagnostic tests, medications, and consultations, designed to provide practice guidelines for the efficient, coordinated treatment of a specific condition.

crit•i•cal point of de•vel•op•ment (krit′i-kăl poynt dĕ-vel′ŏp-mĕnt) A period of time in the developing embryo that may present irreversible effects for developmental stages due to nutritional deficiencies. Some clinicians suggest the action of other external factors.

crit•i•cal tem•per•a•ture (krit′i-kăl tem′pĕr-ă-chŭr) The temperature of a gas above which it is no longer possible by use of any pressure, however great, to convert it into a liquid.

crit•i•cal think•ing (krit′i-kăl thingk′ing) **1.** The practice of considering all aspects of a situation when deciding what to believe or what to do. **2.** NURSING reflective and reasoned thinking, leading to judgments about what to believe or actions to take in any given situation.

CRL Abbreviation for crown-rump length.

CRM Abbreviation for certified reference material.

cRNA Abbreviation for complementary ribonucleic acid.

croc•o•dile tears syn•drome (krok′ŏ-dīl tērz sin′drōm) A flow of tears, usually unilateral, on eating or the anticipation of eating; this happens when nerve fibers originally destined for a salivary gland are damaged and regrow, aberrantly, into the lacrimal gland.

Crocq dis•ease (krok di-zēz′) SYN acrocyanosis.

i **Crohn dis•ease** (krōn di-zēz′) SYN regional enteritis. See page 384.

cro•mone (krō′mōn) Class of drugs that prevents release of histamine from mast cells; useful in prophylaxis of respiratory allergies and asthma but lacking in antiinflammatory effect.

Crooke gran•ules (kruk gran′yūlz) Lumpy masses of basophilic material in the basophil cells of the anterior lobe of the pituitary, associated with Cushing disease, or following the administration of ACTH.

Crooke hy•a•line change (kruk hī′ŏ-lēn chānj) Replacement of cytoplasmic granules of basophil cells of the anterior pituitary by homogeneous hyaline material; a characteristic finding in Cushing syndrome, but usually not present in the cells of a basophil adenoma.

Crookes glass (kruks glas) A spectacle lens combined with metallic oxides to absorb ultraviolet or infrared rays.

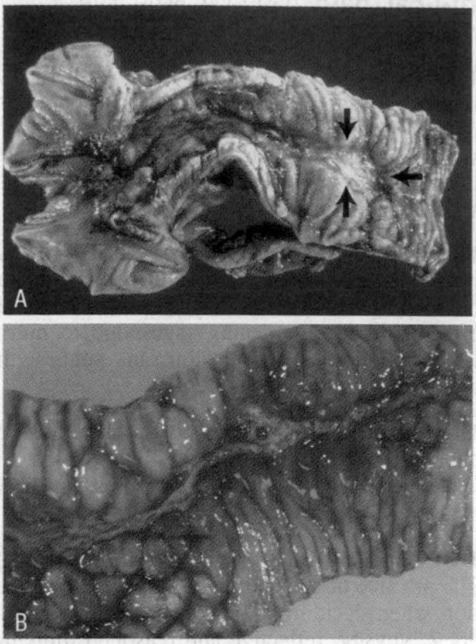

Crohn disease: (A) terminal ileum shows striking thickening of wall of distal portion with distortion of ileal papilla, longitudinal ulcer is present (arrows); (B) longitudinal ulcer is seen in this segment of ileum; large rounded areas of edematous damaged mucosa give "cobblestone" appearance to involved mucosa; portion of the mucosa to the lower right is uninvolved

cross (kraws) **1.** Any figure or structure characterized by the intersection of two lines. SYN crux. **2.** A method of hybridization or the hybrid so produced. [F. *croix,* L. *crux*]

cross-bite (kraws′bīt) An abnormal relation of one or more teeth of one arch to the opposing tooth or teeth of the other arch due to labial, buccal, or lingual deviation of tooth position, or to abnormal jaw position.

cross-bite tooth (kraws′bīt tūth) A posterior tooth designed to permit the modified cusp of the upper tooth to be positioned in the fossae of the lower tooth.

cross-dress•ing (kraws′dres′ing) Clothing oneself in attire generally associated with the opposite sex. SEE transvestism.

crossed di•plo•pi•a (krawst dip-lō′pē-ă) Diplopia in which the image seen by the right eye is to the left of the image seen by the left eye.

crossed em•bo•lism (krawst em′bŏ-lizm) **1.** Obstruction of a systemic artery by an embolus originating in the venous system that passes through a septal defect, patent foramen ovale, or other shunt to the arterial system. **2.** Obstruction by a minute embolism that passes through the pulmonary capillaries from the venous to the arterial system.

crossed ex•ten•sion re•flex (krawst eks-ten′shŭn rē′fleks) A spinal level reflex elicited by application of a noxious stimulus, distally, to an extremity fixed in extension (commonly, the foot) with the patient supine. The response is for the opposing extremity to flex, then adduct and extend.

crossed eyes, cross-eye (krawst īz, kraws′ī) SYN strabismus.

crossed re•flex (krawst rē′fleks) A reflex movement on one side of the body in response to a stimulus applied to the opposite side.

crossed re•nal ec•to•pi•a (krawst rē′năl ek-tō′pē-ă) Ectopic kidney located on opposite (contralateral) side of midline from its ureteral insertion into bladder. In most instances, the two renal moieties are fused (crossed fused ectopia).

cross-ex•ci•ta•tion (kraws′ek′sī-tā′shŭn) MAGNETIC RESONANCE IMAGING an artifact created when energy is given to nuclei in adjacent anatomy by the radiofrequency pulse.

cross-flap (kraws flap) A skin flap transferred from one part of the body to a corresponding part, as from one arm to the other.

cross-hybridisation [Br.] SYN cross-hybridization.

cross-hy•brid•i•za•tion (kraws-hī′brid-ī-zā′shŭn) Annealing of a DNA probe to an imperfectly matching DNA molecule. SYN cross-hybridisation.

cross-in•fec•tion (kraws in-fek′shŭn) Infection spread from one source to another; person to person, animal to person, person to animal, animal to animal.

cross•ing-o•ver, cross•o•ver (kraws′ing-ō′vĕr, kraws′ō-vĕr) **1.** Reciprocal exchange of material between two paired chromosomes during meiosis, resulting in the transfer of a block of genes from each chromosome to its homologue. **2.** The phenomenon that sound presented to one ear may be perceived in the other ear by passing around the head by air conduction or through the head by bone conduction.

cross-le•vel bi•as (kraws′lev′ĕl bī′ăs) A bias due to aggregation at the population level of causes and effects that are unlike at the individual level; can occur in ecologic studies.

cross-match•ing (kraws′mach-ing) **1.** A test for incompatibility between donor and recipient blood, carried out before transfusion to avoid hemolytic reactions between the donor's red blood cells and antibodies in the recipient's plasma, or the reverse; performed by mixing a sample of red blood cells of the donor with plasma of the recipient (major crossmatch) and the red blood cells of the recipient with the plasma of the donor (minor crossmatch). Incompatibility is indicated by clumping of red blood cells and contraindicates use of the donor's blood. **2.** In allotransplantation of solid organs (e.g., kidney), a test for identification of antibody in the serum of potential allograft recipients that reacts directly with the lymphocytes or other cells of a potential allograft donor; presence of these antibodies usually, if not always, contraindicates the performance of the transplantation because virtually all such grafts will be subject to a hyperacute type of rejection.

cross-o•ver claim (kraws′ō-vĕr klām) Claim in which the primary insurer sends patient information on to the secondary insurer (e.g., Medicare/Medicaid claims).

cross-o•ver stud•y (kraws′ō′vĕr stŭd′ē) A study in which the subject is switched from the experimental to the control procedure (or vice versa).

cross-re•act•ing ag•glu•ti•nin (kraws′rē-ak′ting ă-glū′ti-nin) SYN group agglutinin.

cross-re•act•ing an•ti•bod•y (kraws′rē-ak′ting an′ti-bod-ē) **1.** Antibody specific for group antigens, i.e., those with identical functional groups. **2.** Antibody for antigens that have functional groups of closely similar, but not identical, chemical structure.

cross-re•ac•tion (kraws′rē-ak′shŭn) A specific reaction between an antiserum and an antigen complex other than the antigen complex that evoked the various specific antibodies of the antiserum. It is due to at least one antigenic determinant that is included among the determinants of the other complex.

cross-sec•tion (kraws′sek′shŭn) **1.** A planar or two-dimensional view, diagram, or image of the internal structure of the body, part of the body, or any anatomic structure afforded by slicing, actually or through imaging (radiographic, magnetic, or microscopic) techniques, the body or structure along a particular plane. **2.** The slice or section of a given thickness created by actual serial parallel cuts through a structure or by the application of imaging technique.

cross-sec•tion•al stud•y (kraws′sek′shŭn-ăl stŭd′ē) A study in which groups of individuals of different types are composed into one large sample and studied at only a single point in time (e.g., a survey in which all voters, regardless of age, religion, gender, or geographic location, are sampled in 1 day). SYN synchronic study.

cross-ta•ble lat•er•al pro•jec•tion (kraws-tā′bĕl lat′ĕr-ăl prō-jek′shŭn) Lateral projection radiography of a supine subject using a horizontal x-ray beam.

cross-ta•per (kraws tā′per) PHARMACOTHERAPY the practice of lowering the dosage of one medication while simultaneously increasing the dosage of another medication.

cross-tol•er•ance (kraws tol′ĕr-ăns) The resistance to one or more effects of a compound as a result of tolerance developed to a pharmacologically similar compound.

cross•wort (kraws′wōrt) SYN boneset.

crouch gait (krowch gāt) Gait pattern seen in patients with cerebral palsy in which the patient walks in a stooped posture due to nonphysiologic tightening of certain ligaments and muscles.

croup (krūp) **1.** Laryngotracheobronchitis in infants and young children caused by parainfluenza viruses 1 and 2. **2.** Any infection of the larynx in children, characterized by difficult and noisy respiration and a hoarse cough. See page B30. [Scots, probably from A.S. *kropan,* to cry aloud]

croup-as•so•ci•at•ed vi•rus (krūp-ă-sō′sē-āt-ĕd vī′rŭs) Parainfluenza virus type 2. SEE parainfluenza viruses.

croup•ous (krū′pŭs) Relating to croup; marked by a fibrinous exudation.

croup•ous mem•brane (krū′pŭs mem′brān) SYN false membrane.

Crou•zon syn•drome (krū-zōn[h]′ sin′drōm) Craniosynostosis with broad forehead, ocular hypertelorism, exophthalmos, beaked nose, and hypoplasia of the maxilla; associated with hearing loss.

crow•ber•ry (krō′ber-ē) SYN bearberry.

crowd•ing (krowd′ing) A condition in which the teeth are crowded, assuming altered positions (e.g., bunching, overlapping, displacement in various directions, torsiversion).

crowd•ing phe•nom•e•non (krowd′ing fĕ-nom′ĕ-non) A characteristic of amblyopic vision in which vision is better for single optotype presentation than multiple, simultaneous optotype presentation.

Crowe-Da•vis mouth gag (krō-dā′vis mowth gag) Instrument used for opening the mouth, depressing the tongue, maintaining the airway, and transmitting volatile anesthetics during tonsillectomy or other oropharyngeal surgery.

crown (krown) **1.** Any structure, normal or pathologic, resembling or suggesting a crown or a wreath. **2.** DENTISTRY that part of a tooth that is covered with enamel, or an artificial substitute for that part. SYN corona [TA]. [L. *corona*]

crown-heel length (CHL) (krown-hēl length) Length of an outstretched 8-week embryo or fetus from the vertex of the cranium to the heel. SEE ALSO crown-rump length.

crown•ing (krown′ing) **1.** Preparation of the natural crown of a tooth and covering the prepared crown with a veneer of suitable dental material (gold or nonprecious metal casting, porcelain, plastic, or combinations). **2.** That stage of childbirth when the fetal head has negotiated the pelvic outlet and the largest diameter of the head is encircled by the vulvar ring.

crown-rump length (Cr, CRL) (krown-rŭmp length) A measurement from the vertex of the cranium to the midpoint between the apices of the buttocks of an embryo or fetus, which permits approximation of embryonic or fetal age. SEE ALSO crown-heel length.

CRP Abbreviation for cAMP receptor protein; C-reactive protein.

CRT Abbreviation for circuit resistance training; Certified Respiratory Therapist.

cru•ces (krū'sēz) Plural of crux.

cru•ces pi•lo•rum (krū'sĕz pī-lō'rŭm) Crosslike figures formed by hairs growing from two directions that meet and then separate in a direction perpendicular to the original orientation.

cru•ci•ate (krū'shē-āt) Shaped like, or resembling, a cross. [L. *cruciatus*]

cru•ci•ate a•nas•to•mo•sis, **cru•cial a•nas•to•mo•sis** (krū'shē-āt ă-nas'tŏ-mō'sis, krū'shăl ă-nas'tŏ-mō'sis) A four-way anastomosis between branches of the first perforating branch of the deep femoral, inferior gluteal, and medial and lateral circumflex femoral arteries, located posterior to the upper part of the femur.

cru•ci•ate lig•a•ments (krū'shē-āt lig'ă-mĕnts) Major ligaments that crisscross the knee in the anteroposterior direction, providing stability in that plane. SEE ALSO Lachman test.

cru•ci•ate mus•cle (krū'shē-āt mŭs'ĕl) A general type of muscle in which the muscles or bundles of muscle fibers cross in an X-shaped configuration; e.g., the oblique arytenoid muscles.

crunch test (krŭnch test) SYN curl-up test.

cru•ra (krū'ră) Plural of crus.

cru•ra of the di•a•phragm (krūr'ă dī'ă-fram) The muscular origins of the diaphragm from the bodies of the upper lumbar vertebrae that pass the aorta upward to the central tendon. See this page. SYN crura diaphragmatis [TA].

cru•ra di•a•phrag•ma•tis (krū'ră dī-ă-frag-mā'tis) [TA] SYN crura of the diaphragm.

cru•ral (krūr'ăl) Relating to the leg or thigh, or to any crus.

cru•ral her•ni•a (krūr'ăl hĕr'nē-ă) SYN femoral hernia.

cru•ral in•ter•os•se•ous nerve (krūr'ăl in'tĕr-os'ē-ŭs nĕrv) A nerve given off from one of the muscular branches of the tibial nerve that passes down over the posterior surface of the interosseous membrane supplying it and the two bones of the leg. SYN nervus interosseus cruris [TA].

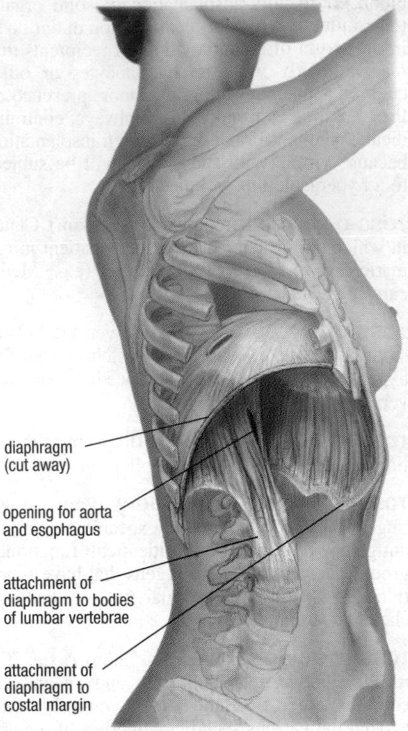

crura of the diaphragm

cru•ral sheath (krūr'ăl shēth) SYN femoral sheath.

cru•ris (krūr'is) Genitive form of crus.

crus, gen. **cru•ris**, pl. **cru•ra** (krūs, krūr'is, krūr'ă) [TA] **1.** SYN leg. **2.** Any anatomic structure resembling a leg; usually (in the plural) a pair of diverging bands or elongated masses. SEE ALSO limb. [L.]

crus ce•re•bri (krūs sĕ-rē'brē) [TA] Specifically, the massive bundle of corticofugal nerve fibers passing longitudinally on the ventral surface of the midbrain on each side of the midline. It consists of fibers descending from the cortex to the tegmentum of the brainstem, pontine gray matter, and spinal cord. SEE ALSO cerebral peduncle.

crus cli•to•ris (krūs klit'ŏr-is) [TA] SYN crus of clitoris.

crus of cli•to•ris (krūs klit'ŏr-is) The continuation on each side of the corpus cavernosum of the clitoris that diverges from the body posteriorly and is attached to the pubic arch. SYN crus clitoris [TA].

crus for•ni•cis (krūs for'ni-sis) [TA] That part of the fornix that rises in a forward curve behind the thalamus to continue forward as the body for fornix ventral to the corpus callosum.

crush syn·drome (krŭsh sin′drōm) The shock-like state that follows release of a limb or limbs or the trunk and pelvis after a prolonged period of compression, as by a heavy weight; characterized by suppression of urine, probably the result of damage to the renal tubules by myoglobin from the damaged muscles. SYN compression syndrome (1).

crus pe·nis (krūs pē′nis) [TA] SYN crus of penis.

crus of pe·nis (krūs pē′nis) The posterior, tapering portion of the corpus cavernosum penis that diverges from its contralateral partner to be attached to the ischiopubic ramus. SYN crus penis [TA].

crust (krŭst) **1.** A hard outer layer or covering; cutaneous crusts are often formed by dried serum or pus on the surface of a ruptured blister or pustule. **2.** A scab. See page B11. SYN crusta. [L. *crusta*]

crus·ta, pl. **crus·tae** (krŭs′tă, -tē) SYN crust. [L.]

crus·ta lac·te·a (krŭs′tă lak′shē-ă) Seborrhea of the scalp in an infant. SYN milk crust.

crutch (krŭch) A device used singly or in pairs to assist in walking when the act is impaired by a lower extremity (or trunk) disability. It transfers all or part of weight bearing to the upper extremity. [A. S. *cryce*]

Crutch·field tongs (krŭch′fēld tawngz) Instrument to provide skull traction by immobilizing the cervical spine.

Cru·veil·hier-Baum·gar·ten sign, **Cru·veil·hier-Baum·gar·ten mur·mur** (krū-vāl-yā′ bahm′gahr-ten sīn, krū-vāl-yā′ bahm′gahr-ten mŭr′mŭr) A murmur over the umbilicus often in the presence of caput medusae, resulting from portal hypertension, usually with hepatic cirrhosis; recanalization of the umbilical vein with reverse blood flow from the liver into the abdominal wall veins creates the murmur.

Cru·veil·hier dis·ease (krū-vāl-yā′ di-zēz′) SYN amyotrophic lateral sclerosis.

Cru·veil·hier ul·cer (krū-vāl-yā′ ul′sĕr) SYN gastric ulcer.

crux, pl. **cru·ces** (krŭks, krū′sēz) A junction or crossing. SYN cross (1). [L.]

Cruz try·pan·o·so·mi·a·sis (krūz trī-pan′ō-sō-mī′ă-sis) SYN South American trypanosomiasis.

cryaesthesia [Br.] SYN cryesthesia.

cry·al·ge·si·a (krī′al-jē′zē-ă) Pain caused by cold. SYN crymodynia. [G. *kryos,* cold, + *algos,* pain]

cryanaesthesia [Br.] SYN cryanesthesia.

cry·an·es·the·si·a (krī′an-es-thē′zē-ă) Inability to perceive cold. SYN cryanaesthesia. [G. *kryos,* cold, + *an-* priv. + *aisthēsis,* sensation]

cry·es·the·si·a (krī′es-thē′zē-ă) **1.** A subjective sensation of cold. **2.** Sensitiveness to cold. SYN cryaesthesia. [G. *kryos,* cold, + *aisthēsis,* sensation]

cry for help (krī help) Telephone calls, notes left in conspicuous places, and other behaviors that communicate extreme distress and possible consideration of suicide.

crymo- Prefix meaning cold. SEE ALSO cryo-, psychro-. [G. *krymos,*]

cry·mo·dyn·i·a (krī′mō-din′ē-ă) SYN cryalgesia. [crymo- + G. *odynē,* pain]

cry·mo·phil·ic (krī′mō-fil′ik) Preferring cold; denoting microorganisms that thrive best at low temperatures. SYN cryophilic. [crymo- + G. *philos,* fond]

cry·mo·phy·lac·tic (krī′mō-fi-lak′tik) Resistant to cold, said of certain microorganisms that are not destroyed even by freezing temperatures. SYN cryophylactic. [crymo- + G. *phylaxis,* a guarding against]

cryo-, **cry-** Combining forms meaning cold. SEE ALSO crymo-, psychro-. [G. *kryos,*]

cry·o·an·es·the·si·a (krī′ō-an-es-thē′zē-ă) Localized application of cold as a means of producing regional anesthesia. SYN refrigeration anesthesia.

cry·o·cau·ter·y (krī′ō-kaw′tĕr-ē) Any substance, such as liquid air or carbon dioxide snow, or a low temperature instrument, the application of which causes destruction of tissue by freezing.

cry·o·ex·trac·tion (krī′ō-ek-strak′shŭn) Removal of cataracts by the adhesion of a freezing probe to the lens; now rarely done.

cry·o·fi·brin·o·gen (krī′ō-fī-brin′ō-jen) An abnormal type of fibrinogen very rarely found in human plasma; precipitated on cooling, but redissolves when warmed to room temperature.

cryofibrinogenaemia [Br.] SYN cryofibrinogenemia.

cry·o·fi·brin·o·gen·e·mi·a (krī′ō-fī-brin′ō-jĕ-nē′mē-ă) The presence in the blood of cryofibrinogens. SYN cryofibrinogenaemia.

cry·o·frac·ture (kri′ō-frak′shŭr) SYN freeze fracture. [cryo- + fracture]

cry·o·gen (krī′ō-jen) A substance used to obtain low temperatures. [G. *kryos,* cold, + -gen]

cry·o·gen·ic (krī′ō-jen′ik) **1.** Denoting or characteristic of a cryogen. **2.** Relating to cryogenics.

cryoglobulinaemia [Br.] SYN cryoglobulinemia.

cry•o•glob•u•lin•e•mi•a (krī′ō-glob′yū-li-nē′mē-ă) The presence of abnormal quantities of cryoglobulin in blood plasma. SYN cryoglobulinaemia.

cry•o•glob•u•lins (krī′ō-glob′yū-linz) Abnormal plasma proteins characterized by precipitating, gelling, or crystallizing when serum or solutions containing them are cooled; may appear in patients with multiple myeloma.

cry•o•ki•net•ics (krī′ō-ki-net′iks) The combination of cryotherapy with exercise. SEE ALSO cryotherapy. [cryo- + kinetics]

cry•ol•y•sis (krī-ol′i-sis) Destruction by cold. [cryo- + G. *lysis,* dissolution]

cry•op•a•thy (krī-op′ă-thē) A morbid condition in which exposure to cold is an important factor. [cryo- + G. *pathos,* suffering]

cry•o•pex•y (krī′ō-pek-sē) In retinal detachment surgery, sealing the sensory retina to the pigment epithelium and choroid by a freezing probe applied to the sclera. [cryo- + G. *pēxis,* a fixing in place]

cry•o•phil•ic (krī′ō-fil′ik) SYN crymophilic. [cryo- + G. *philos,* fond]

cry•o•phy•lac•tic (krī′ō-fi-lak′tik) SYN crymophylactic.

cry•o•pre•cip•i•tate (krī′ō-prē-sip′i-tāt) Precipitate that forms when soluble material is cooled, especially with reference to the precipitate that forms in normal blood plasma that has been subjected to cold precipitation and is rich in factor VIII.

cry•o•pres•er•va•tion (krī′ō-prez-ĕr-vā′shŭn) Maintenance of the viability of excised tissues or organs at extremely low temperatures.

cry•o•probe (krī′ō-prōb) An instrument used in cryosurgery to apply extreme cold to a selected area. [cryo- + L. *probo,* to test]

cry•o•pro•tein (krī′ō-prō′tēn) A protein that precipitates from solution when cooled and redissolves on warming.

cry•os•co•py (krī′os′kŏ-pē) The determination of the freezing point of a fluid, usually blood or urine, compared with that of distilled water. [cryo- + G. *skopeō,* to examine]

cry•o•sur•ger•y (krī′ō-sŭr′jĕr-ē) An operation using freezing temperature (achieved by liquid nitrogen or carbon dioxide) to destroy tissue.

cry•o•ther•a•py (krī′ō-thār′ă-pē) SYN cold therapy.

cry•o•tol•er•ant (krī′ō-tol′ĕr-ănt) Tolerant of very low temperatures.

crypt (kript) A pitlike depression or tubular recess.

crypt ab•scess•es (kript ab′ses-ĕz) Abscesses in the intestinal glands, a characteristic feature of ulcerative colitis.

cryp•tec•to•my (krip-tek′tŏ-mē) Excision of a tonsillar or other crypt. [crypt + G. *ektomē,* excision]

cryp•tic (krip′tik) Hidden; occult; larvate. [G. *kryptikos*]

cryp•ti•tis (krip-tī′tis) Inflammation of a follicle or glandular tubule, particularly in the rectum.

crypto-, crypt- Combining forms meaning hidden, obscure; without apparent cause. [G. *kryptos,* hidden, concealed]

cryp•to•chrome (krip′tō-krōm) Flavoprotein ultraviolet-A receptor involved in circadian rhythm entrainment in plants, insects, and mammals.

cryp•to•coc•co•sis (krip′tō-kok-ō′sis) Infection by *Cryptococcus neoformans,* causing a pulmonary, disseminated, or meningeal mycosis. The most familiar and readily recognized form involves the central nervous system, with subacute or chronic meningitis. See page B5. SYN Busse-Buschke disease.

Cryp•to•coc•cus (krip′tō-kok′ŭs) A genus of yeastlike fungi that reproduce by budding. See page B5. [crypto- + G. *kokkos,* berry]

cryp•to•gen•ic (krip′tō-jen′ik) Of obscure, indeterminate etiology or origin, in contrast to phanerogenic. [crypto- + G. *genesis,* origin]

cryp•to•gen•ic fi•bros•ing al•ve•o•li•tis (krip′tō-jen′ik fī-brōs′ing al-vē′ō-lī′tis) SYN idiopathic pulmonary fibrosis.

cryp•to•gen•ic in•fec•tion (krip′tō-jen′ik in-fek′shŭn) Bacterial, viral, or other infection, the source of which is unknown.

cryp•to•gen•ic sep•ti•ce•mi•a (krip′tō-jen′ik sep′ti-sē′mē-ă) A form of septicemia in which no primary focus of infection can be found.

cryp•to•lith (krip′tō-lith) A concretion in a gland follicle. [crypto- + G. *lithos,* stone]

cryp•to•men•or•rhe•a (krip′tō-men-ŏr-ē′ă) Occurrence each month of the general symptoms of the menses without any flow of blood, as in cases of imperforate hymen. SYN cryptomenorrhoea. [crypto- + G. *mēn,* month, + *rhoia,* flow]

cryptomenorrhoea [Br.] SYN cryptomenorrhea.

cryp•to•po•di•a (krip′tō-pō′dē-ă) A swelling of the lower part of the leg and the foot, in such a manner that there is great distortion and the sole seems to be a flattened pad. [crypto- + G. *pous,* foot]

cryp•tor•chi•dism (kript-ōr′ki-dizm) SYN cryptorchism.

cryp•tor•chi•do•pex•y (kript-ōr′ki-dō-pek-sē) SYN orchiopexy. [crypto- + G. *orchis,* testis, + *pēxis,* fixation]

cryp•tor•chism (kript-ōr′kizm) Failure of one or both testes to descend. SYN cryptorchidism.

cryp•to•spo•rid•i•o•sis (krip′tō-spōr-i-dē-ō′sis) An enteric disease caused by waterborne protozoan parasites of the genus *Cryptosporidium;* disease in immunocompetent people is seen as a self-limiting diarrhea, whereas in immunocompromised people it is manifest as a prolonged severe diarrhea that can be fatal.

Cryp•to•spo•rid•i•um (krip′tō-spō-rid′ē-ŭm) A genus of coccidian sporozoans (family Cryptosporidiidae, suborder Eimeriina) that are important pathogens of calves and other domestic animals, and common opportunistic parasites of humans; they flourish under conditions of compromised immune function; can cause self-limiting diarrhea in immunocompetent people.

Cryp•to•spo•rid•i•um par•vum (krip′tō-spō-rid′ē-ŭm pahr′vŭm) A sporozoan species that is an important cause of neonatal diarrhea in calves and lambs; causes mild, self-limiting to severe, chronic diarrhea in humans.

cryp•to•zy•gous (krip-toz′i-gŭs) Having a narrow face compared with the width of the cranium, so that, when the skull is viewed from above, the zygomatic arches are not visible. [crypto- + G. *zygon,* yoke]

crys•tal (kris′tăl) A solid of regular shape and, for any given compound, characteristic angles, formed when an element or compound solidifies slowly enough, as a result either of freezing from the liquid form or of precipitating out of solution, to allow the individual molecules to take up regular positions with respect to one another; can be seen in body fluids. [G. *krystallos,* clear ice, crystal]

crys•tal•lin (kris′tă-lin) A type of protein found in the lens of the eye.

crys•tal•line (kris′tă-lēn) **1.** Clear; transparent. **2.** Relating to a crystal or crystals.

crys•tal•li•za•tion (kris′tăl-ī-zā′shŭn) Assumption of a crystalline form when a vapor or liquid becomes solidified, or a solute precipitates from solution.

crys•tal•loid (kris′tăl-oyd) **1.** Resembling a crystal, or being such. **2.** A body that in solution can pass through a semipermeable membrane, as distinguished from a colloid, which cannot do so.

crys•tal•lu•ri•a (kris-tăl-yūr′ē-ă) The excretion of crystalline materials in the urine.

CS NATO code for a riot-control agent, *o*-chlorobenzylidene malononitrile, which is more effective than its predecessor, CN, and is used widely by military forces and in law-enforcement agencies.

Cs Abbreviation for cesium.

CSD Abbreviation for catscratch disease.

C-sec•tion (sek′shŭn) SEE cesarean section.

CSF Abbreviation for cerebrospinal fluid; colony-stimulating factors.

CST Abbreviation for craniosacral therapy.

CSU Abbreviation for catheter specimen of urine.

CSV Abbreviation for continuous spontaneous ventilation.

CT Abbreviation for computed tomography.

Ct Abbreviation for concentration-time product.

CTD Abbreviation for cumulative trauma disorder; circling the drain.

Cteno•ce•phal•i•des (tē-nō-se-fal′i-dēz) A genus of fleas; *C. canis* (dog flea) and *C. felis* (cat flea) are nearly universal ectoparasites of household pets; in the absence of pets, they will attack humans when starving. [G. *ktenōdēs,* like a cockle, + *kephalē,* head]

C ter•mi•nus (tĕr′mi-nŭs) The end of a peptide or protein having a free carboxyl (–COOH) group.

CTG Abbreviation for cardiotocography.

CTP Abbreviation for cytidine 5′-triphosphate.

CT pel•vim•e•try (pel-vim′ĕ-trē) Procedure for measurement of the bony pelvis and fetal head through use of CT images; currently the more accurate imaging technique.

CT prod•uct, **Ct prod•uct** (prod′ŭkt, prod′ŭkt) SYN concentration-time product.

Cu Symbol for copper.

cu•bic cen•ti•me•ter (cc, c.c.) (kyū′bik sen′ti-mē-tĕr) One thousandth of a liter; 1 milliliter. SYN cubic centimetre.

cubic centimetre [Br.] SYN cubic centimeter.

cu•bi•tal (kyū′bi-tăl) Relating to the elbow or to the ulna.

cu•bi•tal joint (kyū′bi-tăl joynt) SYN elbow joint.

cu•bi•tal nerve (kyū′bi-tăl nĕrv) SYN ulnar nerve.

cu•bi•tal tun•nel syn•drome (kyū′bi-tăl tŭn′ĕl sin′drōm) A group of symptoms that develop from compression of the ulnar nerve within the cubital tunnel at the elbow; can include paresthesia into the fourth and fifth digits and weakness of the intrinsic muscles of the hand.

cu•bi•tus, gen. and pl. **cu•bi•ti** (kyū′bi-tŭs, -tī) [TA] **1.** SYN elbow (2). **2.** SYN ulna. [L. elbow]

cu•bi•tus val•gus (kyū′bi-tŭs val′gŭs) Deviation of the extended forearm to the outer (radial) side of the axis of the limb.

cu•bi•tus var•us (kyū′bi-tŭs var′ŭs) Deviation of the extended forearm to the inward (ulnar) side of the axis of the limb.

cu•boid, **cu•boi•dal** (kyū′boyd, kyū-boy′dăl) **1.** Resembling a cube in shape. **2.** Relating to the os cuboideum. [G. *kybos,* cube, + *eidos,* resemblance]

cu•boi•dal car•ci•no•ma (kyū-boy′dăl kahr′si-nō′mă) SYN cloacogenic carcinoma.

cu•boi•dal ep•i•the•li•um (kyū-boy′dăl ep′i-thē′lē-ŭm) Simple epithelium with cells appearing as cubes in a vertical section but as polyhedra in surface view.

cu•boid bone (kyū′boyd bōn) The lateral bone of the distal row of the tarsus, articulating with the calcaneus, lateral cuneiform, navicular (occasionally), and fourth and fifth metatarsal bones.

cued speech (kyūd spēch) A system of communication with a person with profound hearing impairment in which handshapes are used to cue sounds to supplement spoken language.

cuff-in•fla•tion hy•per•ten•sion (kŭf′in-flā′shŭn hī′pĕr-ten′shŭn) A rise in blood pressure that results from the application of the sphygomomanometer cuff itself.

cul-de-sac, pl. **culs-de-sac** (kul-dĕ-sahk′) **1.** A blind pouch or tubular cavity closed at one end; e.g., diverticulum; cecum. **2.** SYN rectouterine pouch. [Fr. bottom of a sack]

cul•do•cen•te•sis (kŭl′dō-sen-tē′sis) Aspiration of fluid from the cul-de-sac by puncture of the vaginal vault near the midline between the uterosacral ligaments. [cul-de-sac + G. *kentēsis,* puncture]

cul•do•plas•ty (kŭl′dō-plas-tē) Plastic surgery to remedy relaxation of the posterior fornix of the vagina. [cul-de-sac + G. *plastos,* formed]

cul•do•scope (kŭl′dŏ-skōp) Endoscopic instrument used in culdoscopy.

cul•dos•co•py (kŭl-dos′kŏ-pē) Introduction of an endoscope through the posterior vaginal wall for viewing the rectovaginal pouch and pelvic viscera. [cul-de-sac + G. *skopeō,* to view]

Cu•lex (kū′leks) A genus of mosquitoes including over 2000 species. Largely tropical but worldwide in distribution; they are vectors for a number of diseases of humans and of domestic and wild animals and birds. [L. gnat]

Cu•lex ni•gri•pal•pus (kū′leks nī-gri-pal′pŭs) Mosquito species that is a vector of St. Louis encephalitis within the U.S.

Cu•lex res•tu•ans (kū′leks res′tū-anz) Mosquito species that is a secondary or suspected vector of Eastern equine encephalitis and Western equine encephalitis within the U.S.

Cu•lex sa•li•na•ri•us (kū′leks sal-i-nā′rē-ŭs) Mosquito species that is a secondary or suspected vector of Eastern equine encephalitis within the U.S.

cu•li•ci•dal (kū-li-sī′dăl) Destructive to mosquitoes. [L. *culex,* gnat, + *caedo,* to kill]

cu•li•cide (kū′li-sīd) An agent that destroys mosquitoes.

Cu•li•coi•des (kū′li-koy′dēz) A genus of biting midges; among the most abundant of the hematophagous insects that transmit numerous pathogens of humans and animals; they transmit the minimally pathogenic *Mansonella streptocerca* to humans, but their primary importance is as a vector of arboviruses to livestock. [L. *culex,* gnat]

Cu•li•se•ta (kū-li-sē′tă) A genus of mosquitoes (family Culicidae); vectors for several diseases of humans, domestic and wild animals, and birds.

Cu•li•se•ta in•or•na•ta (kū-li-sē′tă in-ōr-nā′tă) Mosquito species that is a secondary or suspected vector of Western equine encephalitis and California group encephalitis within the U.S.

Cul•len sign (kŭ′lĕn sīn) Periumbilical darkening of the skin from blood, a sign of intraperitoneal hemorrhage, especially in ruptured ectopic pregnancy.

cul•ti•va•tion (kŭl-ti-vā′shŭn) SYN culture. [Mediev. L. *cultivo,* pp. *-atus,* fr. L. *colo,* pp. *cultus,* to till]

cul•tur•al com•pe•tence (kŭl′chŭr-ăl kom′pĕ-tĕns) NURSING knowledge and understanding of another person's culture; adapting interventions and approaches to health care adjusted to the specific culture of the patient, family, and social group.

cul•tur•al di•ver•si•ty (kŭl′chŭ-răl di-vĕr′si-tē) The inevitable variety in customs, attitudes, practices, and behavior that exists among groups of people from different ethnic, racial, or national backgrounds who come into contact.

cul•tur•al shock (kŭl-chŭr-ăl shok) A form of stress associated with the beginning of a person's assimilation into a new and vastly different culture.

cul•ture (kŭl′chŭr) **1.** The propagation of microorganisms on or in various media. **2.** A mass of microorganisms on or in a medium. **3.** The propagation of mammalian cells, i.e., cell culture. SEE cell culture. **4.** A set of beliefs, values, artistic, historical, and religious characteristics; customs common to a community or nation. SYN cultivation. [L. *cultura,* tillage, fr. *colo,* pp. *cultus,* to till]

cul·ture me·di·um (kŭl′chŭr mē′dē-ŭm) A substance, either solid or liquid, used for the cultivation, isolation, identification, or storage of microorganisms. SYN medium (3).

Cul·ver's root (kŭl′vĕrz rūt) SYN black root.

Cum·mer clas·si·fi·ca·tion (kŭm′ĕr klas′i-fi-kā′shŭn) A listing of several types of removable partial dentures in accordance with the distribution of direct retainers.

cu·mu·la·tive (kyūm′yŭ-lă-tiv) Tending to accumulate or pile up, as with certain drugs that may have a cumulative effect.

cu·mu·la·tive ac·tion (kyūm′yŭ-lă-tiv ak′shŭn) SYN cumulative effect.

cu·mu·la·tive ef·fect (kyūm′yŭ-lă-tiv e-fekt′) The condition in which repeated administration of a drug may produce effects that are more pronounced than those produced by the first dose. SYN cumulative action.

Cu·mu·la·tive In·dex Med·i·cus (kyūm′yū-lă-tiv in′deks med′i-kŭs) Collection of medical literature, published annually, which began in the U.S. Army Surgeon General's office at the end of the U.S. Civil War in 1865. It has been taken over by the National Library of Medicine and has evolved into a database called MEDLINE.

Cu·mu·la·tive In·dex to Nurs·ing and Al·lied Health Li·ter·a·ture (CINAHL) (kyūm′yŭ-lă-tiv in′deks nŭrs′ing al′īd helth lit′ĕr-ă-chŭr) Database of major English language nursing journal publications from the American Nursing Association and the National League for Nursing as well as other professional journals including occupational and physical therapy citations.

cu·mu·la·tive trau·ma dis·or·der (CTD) (kyūm′yŭ-lă-tiv traw′mă dis-ōr′dĕr) Any of the chronic disorders involving tendon, muscle, joint, and nerve damage, often resulting from work-related physical activities. CTDs, including repetitive motion disorders and carpal tunnel syndrome, result when the body is subjected to direct pressure, vibration, or repetitive movements for prolonged periods. SYN microtrauma, repetitive strain disorder.

cu·ne·ate (kyū′nē-āt) Wedge-shaped. [L. *cuneus,* wedge]

cu·ne·ate fas·cic·u·lus, cu·ne·ate fu·nic·u·lus (kyū′nē-āt fă-sik′kyū-lŭs, kyū′nē-āt fyū-nik′yū-lŭs) The larger lateral subdivision of the posterior funiculus.

cu·ne·ate nu·cle·us (kyū′nē-āt nū′klē-ŭs) The larger Burdach nucleus; one of the three nuclei of the posterior column of the spinal cord; located near the dorsal surface of the medulla oblongata at and below the level of the obex, the nucleus receives posterior root fibers corresponding to the sensory innervation of the arm and hand of the same side; together with its medial companion, the gracile nucleus, it is the major source of origin of the medial lemniscus.

cu·ne·i·form bone (kyū-nē′i-fōrm bōn) SEE triquetral bone.

cu·ne·i·form car·ti·lage (kyū-nē′i-fōrm kahr′ti-lăj) A small nonarticulating rod of elastic cartilage in the aryepiglottic fold anterolateral and somewhat superior to the corniculate cartilage. SYN cartilago cuneiformis [TA].

cu·ne·o·cu·boid (kyū′nē-ō-kyū′boyd) Relating to the lateral cuneiform and the cuboid bones.

cu·ne·o·na·vic·u·lar (kyū′nē-ō-nă-vik′yū-lăr) Relating to the cuneiform and the navicular bones.

cu·ne·us, pl. **cu·ne·i** (kyū′nē-ŭs, -ī) That region of the medial aspect of the occipital lobe of each cerebral hemisphere bounded by the parietooccipital fissure and the calcarine fissure. [L. wedge]

cu·nic·u·lus, pl. **cu·nic·u·li** (kū-nik′yū-lŭs, -lī) The burrow of the scabies mite in the epidermis. [L. a rabbit; an underground passage]

cun·ni·lin·gus (kŭn′i-ling′gŭs) Oral stimulation of the vulva or clitoris; contrasted with fellatio, which is the oral stimulation of the penis. [L. *cunnus,* pudendum, + *lingo,* to lick]

cup (kŭp) An excavated or cup-shaped structure, either anatomic or pathologic. [A.S. *cuppe*]

cup bi·op·sy for·ceps (kŭp bī′op-sē fōr′seps) A slender flexible forceps with movable cup-shaped jaws, used to obtain biopsy specimens through an endoscope.

cup:disc ra·ti·o (kŭp disk rā′shē-ō) The ratio between the diameter of the cupped or depressed central zone of the optic disc and the diameter of the entire disc; normally lower than 1:3, it is increased in glaucoma.

Cu·pid's bow (kyū′pidz bō) The contour of the superior margin of the upper lip.

cu·po·la (kyū′pō-lă) SYN cupula.

cup·ping (kŭp′ing) **1.** Formation of a hollow, or cup-shaped excavation. **2.** Application of a cupping glass. SEE ALSO cup.

cup·ping glass (kŭp′ing glas) A glass vessel, from which the air has been exhausted by heat or a special suction apparatus, formerly applied to the skin in order to draw blood to the surface. SEE ALSO cupping, cup.

cu·pu·la, pl. **cu·pu·lae** (kŭ′pū-lă, -lē) [TA] A cup-shaped or domelike structure. SYN cupola. [L. dim. of *cupa,* a tub]

cu·pu·lar ce·cum of the co·chle·ar duct (kyū′pyū-lăr sē′kŭm of the kok′lē-ăr dŭkt) The upper blind extremity of the cochlear duct. SYN lagena (1).

cu•pu•lo•gram (kyū′pyū-lō-gram) A graphic representation of vestibular function relative to normal performance.

cur•a•tive (kyūr′ă-tiv) **1.** That which heals or cures. **2.** Tending to heal or cure.

cur•a•tive dose (CD) (kyūr′ă-tiv dōs) **1.** The quantity of any substance required to effect the cure of a disease or that will correct the manifestations of a deficiency of a particular factor in the diet. **2.** Effective dose used with therapeutically applied compounds.

curb•stone frac•ture (kŭrb′stōn frak′shŭr) SEE Lisfranc injury.

cure (kyūr) **1.** To heal; to make well. **2.** A restoration to health. **3.** A special method or course of treatment. **4.** Hardening of certain materials with time or by the application of heat, light, or chemical agents, e.g., polymerization of acrylic denture-based material. [L. *curo,* to care for]

cu•ret•ment (kyūr-et-mōn[h]′) SYN curettage.

cu•ret•tage (kūr′ĕ-tahzh′) A scraping, usually of the interior of a cavity or tract, for the removal of new growths or other abnormal tissues, or to obtain material for tissue diagnosis. SYN curetment, curettement.

cu•rette, **cu•ret** (kyūr-et′) Instrument in the form of a loop, ring, or scoop with sharpened edges attached to a rod-shaped handle, used for curettage. [Fr.]

cu•rette•ment (kyūr-et-mōn[h]′) SYN curettage.

cu•rie (c, C, Ci) (kyūr′ē) A unit of measurement of radioactivity, 3.70 × 10^{10} disintegrations per second; superseded by the S.I. unit, the becquerel (1 disintegration per second). [Marie (1867–1934) and Pierre (1859–1906) *Curie,* French chemists and physicists and Nobel laureates]

cu•ri•um (Cm) (kyūr′ē-ŭm) An element, atomic no. 96, atomic wt. 247.07, not occurring naturally on earth, but first formed artificially in 1944 by bombarding ^{239}Pu with alpha particles; the most stable of the curium isotopes is ^{247}Cm, with a half-life of 15.6 million years. [see curie]

Curl•ing ul•cer (kŭr′ling ŭl′sĕr) SYN stress ulcer.

curl-up test (kŭrl′ŭp test) An assessment for abdominal muscular endurance. SYN crunch test.

cur•rant jel•ly clot (kŭr′ănt jel′ē klot) A jelly-like mass of red blood cells and fibrin formed by the in vitro or postmortem clotting of whole or sedimented blood.

cur•rent (kŭr′rĕnt) A stream or flow of fluid, air, or electricity. [L. *currens,* pr. p. of *curro,* to run]

Cur•rent Pro•ce•du•ral Ter•min•o•lo•gy (CPT) (kŭr′rĕnt prō-sē′jŭr-ăl tĕr-mi-nol′ŏ-jē) A coding system for professional medical procedures and services, published by the American Medical Association (as *Current Procedural Terminology*) and revised annually.

Cursch•mann spi•ral (kūrsh′mahn spī′răl) A spirally twisted mass of mucus occurring in the sputum in bronchial asthma.

curse (kŭrs) An affliction thought to be invoked by a malevolent spirit.

cur•va•tu•ra, pl. **cur•va•tu•rae** (kŭr′vă-tū′ră, -rē) SYN curvature. [L.]

cur•va•ture (kŭr′vă-chŭr) A bending or flexure. SEE angulation. SYN curvatura. [L. *curvatura,* fr. *curvo,* pp. *-atus,* to bend, curve]

cur•va•ture ab•er•ra•tion (kŭr′vă-chŭr ab-ĕr-ā′shŭn) Lack of spatial correspondence causing the image of a straight extended object to appear curved.

cur•va•ture hy•per•o•pi•a (kŭr′vă-chŭr hī′pĕr-ō′pē-ă) Hyperopia due to decreased refraction of the anterior ocular segment.

cur•va•ture my•o•pi•a (kŭr′vă-chŭr mī-ō′pē-ă) Myopia due to refractive errors resulting from excessive corneal curvature.

curve (kŭrv) **1.** A nonangular continuous bend or line. **2.** A chart or graphic representation, by means of a continuous line connecting individual observations of the course of a physiologic activity, of the number of cases of a disease in a given period, or of any entity that might be otherwise presented by a table of figures. SYN chart (2). [L. *curvo,* to bend]

curve of oc•clu•sion (kŭrv ŏ-klū′zhŭn) **1.** A curved surface that makes simultaneous contact with the major portion of the incisal and occlusal prominences of the existing teeth; **2.** The curve of a dentition on which the occlusal surfaces lie.

curve of Spee (kŭrv shpā) An anatomic curvature determined by the occlusal surfaces of the teeth following the anterior mandibular cusp tips to the buccal cusp tips of the mandibular posterior teeth. SYN von Spee curve.

curve of Wil•son (kŭrv wil′sŏn) The curvature in a frontal plane through the cusp tips of both the right and left molars.

Cur•vu•la•ri•a (kŭr-vyū-lār′ē-ă) An opportunistic fungus widely spread in nature; plant pathogen known to cause leaf spots, seedling blight, and failure of seeds to germinate. In humans, this fungus has been associated with sinusitis, keratitis, pulmonary infections, and in the immunocompromised patient, occasionally, disseminated disease.

Cush•ing ba•soph•i•lism (kush′ing bā-sof′i-lizm) SYN Cushing syndrome.

Cush•ing dis•ease (kush′ing di-zēz′) Adrenal

hyperplasia (Cushing syndrome) caused by an ACTH-secreting basophil adenoma of the pituitary.

Cush·ing dis·ease of the o·men·tum (kush′ing di-zēz′ ō-men′tŭm) Central obesity in association with glucocorticoid excess, in which adipose stromal cells of the omental fat, but not subcutaneous tissue, can generate active cortisol from inactive cortisone. Patients have increased cortisol production and urinary cortisol excretion but no abnormality in the hypothalamicopituitary-adrenal axis.

Cush·ing neu·ro·ma (kush′ing nūr-ō′mă) An acoustic lesion with a 3:1 female predilection. Therapy is usually surgical removal.

cush·ing·oid (kush′ing-oyd) Resembling the signs and symptoms of Cushing disease or syndrome: buffalo hump obesity, striations, adiposity, hypertension, diabetes, and osteoporosis, usually due to exogenous corticosteroids.

Cush·ing su·ture (kush′ing sū′chŭr) A running horizontal mattress suture used to approximate two adjacent surfaces.

Cush·ing syn·drome (kush′ing sin′drōm) A disorder resulting from increased adrenocortical secretion of cortisol (giving a clinical picture of Cushing disease), due to any one of several sources: ACTH-dependent adrenocortical hyperplasia or tumor, ectopic ACTH-secreting tumor, or excessive administration of steroids; characterized by truncal obesity, moon face, acne, abdominal striae, hypertension, decreased carbohydrate tolerance, protein catabolism, psychiatric disturbances, and osteoporosis, amenorrhea, and hirsutism in females; when associated with an ACTH-producing adenoma, called Cushing disease. SYN Cushing basophilism.

Cush·ing ul·cer (kush′ing ŭl′sĕr) Peptic ulcer occurring after severe head injury or with other CNS lesions.

cush·ion (kush′ŭn) ANATOMY any structure resembling a pad or cushion.

cusp (kŭsp) **1.** DENTISTRY a conic elevation arising on the surface of a tooth from an independent calcification center. **2.** A leaflet of a cardiac valve. SYN cuspis [TA]. [L. *cuspis,* point]

cus·pal (kŭs′păl) Pertaining to a cusp.

cusp and groove pat·tern (kŭsp grūv pat′ĕrn) The arrangement of the cusps and grooves on molars; in the lower molars there are four principal ones, Y-5, Y-4, +5, and +4

cusp height (kŭsp hīt) **1.** The shortest distance between the tip of a cusp and its base plane. **2.** The shortest distance between the deepest part of the central fossa of a posterior tooth and a line connecting the points of the cusps of the tooth.

cus·pid (kŭs′pid) **1.** Having but one cusp. **2.** SYN canine tooth. [L. *cuspis,* point]

cus·pi·date (kŭs′pi-dāt) Having a cusp or cusps.

cus·pis, pl. **cus·pi·des** (kŭs′pis, kŭs′pi-dēz) [TA] SYN cusp. [L. a point]

cusp ridge (kŭsp rij) An elevation extending both mesially and distally from the cusp tip of molars and premolars, thus forming the lingual and buccal boundaries of the occlusal surface.

cus·to·di·al care (kŭs-tō′dē-ăl kār) Nonskilled personal care to assist with ADLs.

cus·to·dy (kŭs′tŏ-dē) Care, guardianship, or control of a person or thing exercised by one in authority. [L. *custodia*]

cu·ta·ne·ous (kyū-tā′nē-ŭs) Relating to the skin. [L. *cutis,* skin]

cu·ta·ne·ous an·cy·lo·sto·mi·a·sis (kyū-tā′nē-ŭs an′ki-lō-stō-mī′ă-sis) Cutaneous larva migrans caused by larvae of hookworms. SYN swimmer's itch (1), water itch (1).

cu·ta·ne·ous branch of an·te·ri·or branch of ob·tu·ra·tor nerve (kyū-tā′nē-ŭs branch an-tēr′ē-ŏr ob′tŭr-ā-tŏr nĕrv) Branch of the anterior branch of obturator nerve supplying skin of medial thigh above knee.

cu·ta·ne·ous branch of mixed nerve (kyū-tā′nē-ŭs branch mikst nĕrv) Branch of a mixed spinal nerve (or its derivatives) innervating skin; such branches would convey mostly somatic sensory but also visceral motor fibers (postsynaptic sympathetic fibers for vasomotion and pilomotion).

cu·ta·ne·ous horn (kyū-tā′nē-ŭs hōrn) A protruding keratotic growth of the skin; the base may show changes of actinic keratosis or carcinoma.

cu·ta·ne·ous lar·va mi·grans (kyū-tā′nē-ŭs lahr′vă mī′granz) An advancing serpiginous or netlike tunneling in the skin, with marked pruritus, caused by wandering hookworm larvae not adapted to intestinal maturation in humans; especially common in the eastern and southern coastal U.S. and other tropical and subtropical coastal areas; various hookworms of dogs and cats have been implicated, chiefly *Ancylostoma braziliense* in the U.S., but also *A. caninum* of dogs, *Uncinaria stenocephalia*, the European dog hookworm, and *Bunostomum phlebotomum*, the cattle hookworm; *Strongyloides* species of animal origin may also contribute to human cutaneous larva migrans. See page B7.

cu·ta·ne·ous leish·man·i·a·sis (kyū-tā′nē-ŭs lēsh′mă-nī′ă-sis) Infection with promastigotes (leptomonads) of *Leishmania tropica* and of *L. major* inoculated into the skin by the bite of an infected sandfly, *Phlebotomus* (commonly *P. papatasi*); it is endemic in parts of Turkey, northern Africa, and India. The ulcer begins as a papule that enlarges to a nodule and then breaks down into an ulcer. Two distinctive clinical and epidemiologic diseases are recognized, the more common and widespread zoonotic rural disease with a moist acute form, caused by *L. major*, with reservoir rodent hosts, and an urban, anthroponotic, dry, chronic form of leishmaniasis caused by *L. tropica*, without a reservoir host, and now largely controlled. SEE zoonotic cutaneous leishmaniasis. SYN Old World leishmaniasis, tropical sore.

cu•ta•ne•ous leish•man•i•a•sis gran•u•lo•ma (kyū-tā′nē-ŭs lēsh′mă-nī′ă-sis gran′yū-lō′mă) Lymphocytic granuloma with a necrotic center found during the healing process.

cu•ta•ne•ous mus•cle (kyū-tā′nē-ŭs mŭs′ĕl) A muscle that lies in the subcutaneous tissue and attaches to the skin; it may or may not have a bony attachment. The muscles of expression are the chief examples of cutaneous muscles in the human.

cu•ta•ne•ous nerve (kyū-tā′nē-ŭs nĕrv) A mixed nerve supplying a region of the skin, including its sensory endings, blood vessels, smooth muscle, and glands.

cu•ta•ne•ous pseu•do•lym•pho•ma (kyū-tā′nē-ŭs sū′dō-lim-fō′mă) SYN benign lymphocytoma cutis.

cu•ta•ne•ous tu•ber•cu•lo•sis (kyū-tā′nē-ŭs tū-bĕr′kyū-lō′sis) Pathologic lesions of the skin caused by *Mycobacterium tuberculosis*.

cu•ta•ne•ous vas•cu•li•tis (kyū-tā′nē-ŭs vas′kyū-lī′tis) An acute form of vasculitis that may affect the skin only, but also may involve other organs, with a polymorphonuclear infiltrate in the walls of and surrounding small (dermal) vessels. Nuclear fragments are formed by karyorrhexis of the neutrophils. SEE ALSO leukocytoclastic vasculitis.

cut•down (kŭt′down) Dissection of a vein for insertion of a cannula or needle for the administration of intravenous fluids or medication. SYN venostomy.

cu•ti•cle (kyū′ti-kĕl) **1.** An outer thin layer, usually of a horny composition. SYN cuticula (1). **2.** The layer, chitinous in some invertebrates, which occurs on the surface of epithelial cells. **3.** SYN epidermis. [L. *cuticula,* dim. of *cutis,* skin]

cu•tic•u•la, pl. **cu•tic•u•lae** (kyū-tik′yū-lă, -lē) **1.** SYN cuticle (1). **2.** SYN epidermis. [L. cuticle]

cu•tic•u•lar dru•sen (kyū-tik′yū′lăr drū′sĕn) SYN basal laminar drusen.

cu•ti•re•ac•tion (kyū′ti-rē-ak′shŭn) The inflammatory reaction to a skin test in a sensitive (allergic) subject. [L. *cutis,* skin, + reaction]

cu•tis (kyū′tis) [TA] SYN skin. [L.]

cu•tis an•se•ri•na (kyū′tis an-sĕ-rē′nă) Contraction of the arrectores pilorum produced by cold, fear, or other stimulus, causing the follicular orifices to become prominent. SYN gooseflesh.

cu•tis lax•a (kyū′tis lak′să) [TA] SYN dermatochalasis.

cu•tis mar•mo•ra•ta (kyū′tis mar-mō-rā′tă) A normal, physiologic, pink, marblelike mottling of the skin in infants, persisting abnormally in some children on exposure to cold.

cu•tis mar•mo•ra•ta tel•an•gi•ec•tat•i•ca con•gen•i•ta (kyū′tis mar-mō-rā′tă tel-an′jē-ek-tat′i-kă kon-jen′i-tă) Capillary-venous cutaneous malformation with "marbled" appearance. SYN Van Lohuizen syndrome.

cu•tis plate (kyū′tis plāt) SYN dermatome (2).

cu•tis rhom•boi•da•lis nu•chae (kyū′tis rom-boy-dā′lis nū′kē) Geometric furrowed configurations of the skin of the back of the neck as a result of prolonged exposure to sunlight with solar elastosis. See this page.

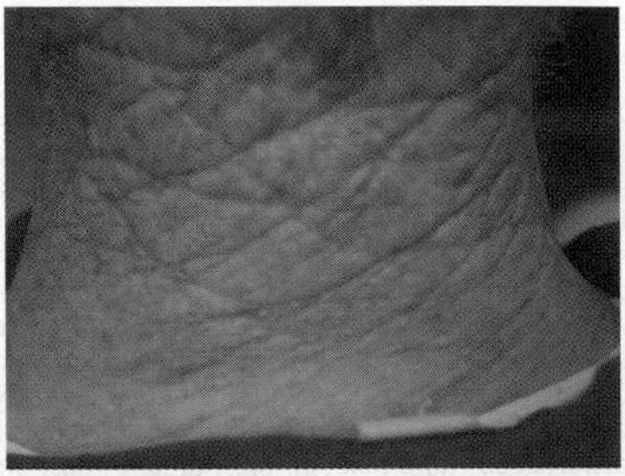

cutis rhomboidalis nuchae

cu•tis ve•ra (kyū′tis vē′ră) SYN dermis.

cut•point (kŭt′poynt) Arbitrary value on an ordinal scale such as blood pressure, beyond which values are regarded as clinically abnormal.

Cu•vi•er ducts (kū-vyā′ dŭkts) Obsolete term for the common cardinal veins.

Cu•vi•er veins (kū-vyā′ vānz) Obsolete term for the common cardinal veins of the embryo. SEE cardinal veins.

CV Abbreviation for coefficient of variation.

CVA Abbreviation for cerebral vascular attack; cerebrovascular accident.

CVC Abbreviation for central venous catheter.

CVP Abbreviation for central venous pressure.

CVS Abbreviation for chorionic villus sampling.

CVVH Abbreviation for continuous venovenous hemofiltration.

CVVHD Abbreviation for continuous venovenous hemodialysis; continuous venovenous hemodiafiltration.

CW a•gent (ā′jĕnt) Abbreviation for chemical-warfare agent.

CX NATO code for phosgene oxime.

CXR Abbreviation for chest x-ray. SEE radiograph.

cy•a•nide (sī′ăn-īd) **1.** The radical -CN or ion (CN-). The ion is extremely poisonous, forming hydrocyanic acid in water; inhibits respiratory enzymes. 2. A salt of HCN. 3. A molecule containing a cyanide group. 4. A class of toxic chemical-warfare agents. see also blood agent, hydrogen cyanide, and cyanogen chloride. **2.** A salt of HCN. **3.** A molecule containing a cyanide group. **4.** A class of toxic chemical-warfare agents. SEE ALSO blood agent, hydrogen cyanide, cyanogen chloride.

cyanmethaemoglobin [Br.] SYN cyanmethemoglobin.

cy•an•met•he•mo•glo•bin (sī′an-met-hē′mō-glō-bin) A relatively nontoxic compound of cyanide with methemoglobin, which is formed when methylene blue is administered in cases of cyanide poisoning. SYN cyanmethaemoglobin.

♻**cyano-**, **cyan-** **1.** Combining forms meaning blue. **2.** Chemical prefixes frequently used in naming compounds that contain the cyanide group, CN. [G. *kyanos,* a dark blue substance]

Cy•a•no•bac•te•ri•a (sī′ă-nō-bak-tēr′ē-ă) A division of the kingdom Prokaryotae consisting of unicellular or filamentous bacteria that are either nonmotile or possess a gliding motility, reproduce by binary fission, and perform photosynthesis with the production of oxygen. SYN Cyanophyceae.

cy•an•o•bac•te•ri•um•like bod•ies (sī′ă-nō-bak-tēr′ē-ŭm-līk bod′ēz) SYN *Cyclospora.*

cy•a•no•co•bal•a•min (sī′ă-nō-kō-bal′ă-min) A complex of cyanide and cobalamin, as in vitamin B_{12}.

cy•an•o•gen (sī-an′ō-jen) **1.** SYN ethanedinitrile. **2.** A term used to refer to the cyanide radical in compounds, such as cyanogen chloride ($CNCl_2$) and cyanogen bromide ($CNBr_2$), in which the cyanide moiety is bound to one or more halide atoms.

cy•an•o•gen chlo•ride (CK) (si-an′ō-jen klōr′īd) A highly toxic poison, $CNCl_2$, which as a chemical-warfare agent, has been assigned the NATO code CK.

cy•an•o•phil, **cy•an•o•phile** (sī-an′ō-fil, -fīl) A cell or element that is colored blue by a staining procedure differentially. [cyano- + G. *philos,* fond]

cy•a•noph•i•lous (sī′ă-nof′i-lŭs) Readily stainable with a blue dye.

Cy•a•no•phy•ce•ae (sī′ă-nō-fī′shē-ē) SYN Cyanobacteria. [cyano- + G. *phykos,* seaweed]

cy•a•nop•si•a (sī′ă-nop′sē-ă) A condition in which all objects appear blue; may temporarily follow cataract extraction. [cyano- + G. *opsis,* vision]

cy•a•nosed (sī′ă-nōst) SYN cyanotic.

cy•a•nose tar•dive (sī′ă-nōs tahr′div) Cyanosis developing in congenital heart disease only after the heart begins to fail. SYN tardive cyanosis. [F. delayed cyanosis]

cy•a•no•sis (sī′ă-nō′sis) A dark blue or purple discoloration of the skin, nail beds, lips, or mucous membranes seen with sulfmethemoglobin concentrations of 0.5 g per 100 mL or greater, methemoglobin concentrations of 1.5 g per 100 mL or greater, or deoxyhemoglobin concentrations of 5.0 g per 100 mL or greater. [G. dark blue color, fr. *kyanos,* blue substance]

cy•a•not•ic (sī′ă-not′ik) Relating to or marked by cyanosis. SYN cyanosed.

cy•a•not•ic in•du•ra•tion (sī′ă-not′ik in-dūr-ā′shŭn) Induration related to persistent, chronic venous congestion in an organ or tissue, frequently resulting in fibrous thickening of the walls of the veins and eventual fibrosis of adjacent tissue.

cy•ber•net•ics (sī′bĕr-net′iks) **1.** The comparative study of computers and the human nervous system, with intent to explain the functioning of the brain. **2.** The science of control and communication in both living and nonliving systems; characteristically, control is governed by feedback, that is, by communication within the system concerning the difference between the actual and the desired result, action then being modified so as to minimize this difference. SEE ALSO feedback. [G. *kybernētica,* things pertaining to control or piloting]

cy•clar•thro•di•al (sī′klahr-thrō′dē-ăl) Relating to a cyclarthrosis.

cy•clar•thro•sis (sī′klahr-thrō′sis) A joint capable of rotation. [cyclo- + G. *arthrōsis,* articulation]

cy•clase (sī′klās) Descriptive name applied to an enzyme that forms a cyclic compound; e.g., adenylate cyclase.

cy•cle (sī′kĕl) **1.** A recurrent series of events. **2.** A recurring period of time. **3.** One successive compression and rarefaction of a wave, as of a sound wave. [G. *kyklos,* circle]

cy•clec•to•my (sī-klek′tŏ-mē) Excision of a portion of the ciliary body. SYN ciliectomy. [cyclo- + G. *ektomē,* excision]

cy•cle length al•ter•nans (sī′kĕl length awl-tĕr′nanz) A succession of alternately long and short diastolic intervals.

cy•clen•ceph•a•ly, **cy•clen•ce•pha•li•a** (sīklen-sef′ă-lē, -se-fā′lē-ă) Condition in a malformed fetus characterized by poor development and a varying degree of fusion of the two cerebral hemispheres. SYN cyclocephaly, cyclocephalia. [cyclo- + G. *enkephalos,* brain]

cy·cles per sec·ond (cps) (sī′kĕlz pĕr sek′ŏnd) The number of successive compressions and rarefactions per second of a sound wave. The preferred designation for this unit of frequency is hertz.

cy·clic (sik′lik) **1.** Pertaining to, or characteristic of, a cycle; occurring periodically, denoting the course of the symptoms in certain diseases or disorders. **2.** CHEMISTRY pertaining to a molecule containing a ring of atoms; denoting a cyclic compound.

cy·clic AMP (sik′lik) SYN adenosine 3′,5′-cyclic monophosphate.

3′,5′-cy·clic AMP syn·the·tase (sik′lik sin′thĕ-tās) SYN adenylate cyclase.

cy·clic com·pound (sik′lik kom′pownd) Any compound in which the constituent atoms, or any part of them, form a ring. Used mainly in organic chemistry. SYN closed chain compound.

cy·clin D (sik′lin) Protein involved in progression to cell division.

cy·clist's nip·ples (sī′klists nip′ĕlz) Nipple irritation due to the combined effects of perspiration and wind-chill producing a cold, painful sensation.

cy·clist's pal·sy (sī′klists pawl′zē) Paresthesia of the ulnar nerve in cyclists resulting from leaning on the handlebars for an extended period. SYN ulnar nerve compression syndrome.

cy·cli·tis (sik-lī′tis) Inflammation of the ciliary body. [G. *kyklos,* circle (ciliary body), + *-itis,* inflammation]

♻ **cyclo-, cycl-** **1.** Combining forms meaning a circle or cycle; the ciliary body. **2.** CHEMISTRY prefix meaning a molecule consisting of atoms in a ring. [G. *kyklos,* circle]

cy·clo·ceph·a·ly, cy·clo·ce·pha·li·a (sī′klō-sef′ă-lē, -sĕ-fā′lē-ă) SYN cyclencephaly. [cyclo- + G. *kephalē,* head]

cy·clo·cho·roid·i·tis (sī′klō-kōr′oyd-ī′tis) Inflammation of the ciliary body and the choroid.

cy·clo·cry·o·ther·a·py (sī′klō-krī′ō-thār′ă-pē) Transscleral freezing of the ciliary body in the treatment of glaucoma.

cy·clo·di·al·y·sis (sī′klō-dī-al′i-sis) Establishment of a communication between the anterior chamber and the suprachoroidal space in order to reduce intraocular pressure in glaucoma. [cyclo- + G. *dialysis,* separation]

cy·clo·di·a·ther·my (sī′klō-dī′ă-thĕr-mē) Diathermy applied to the sclera adjacent to the ciliary body in the treatment of glaucoma.

cy·clo·duc·tion (sī′klō-dŭk′shŭn) Rotation of the eye around its visual axis. SYN circumduction (2). [cyclo- + L. *duco,* pp. *ductus,* to draw]

cy·clo·pep·tide (sī′klō-pep′tīd) A polypeptide lacking terminal —NH_2 and —COOH groups by virtue of their combination to form another peptide link, forming a ring.

cy·clo·pho·ras·es (sī′klō-fōr′ās-ĕz) The group of enzymes in mitochondria that catalyze the complete oxidation of pyruvic acid to carbon dioxide and water; essentially, those enzymes and coenzymes involved in the tricarboxylic acid cycle.

cy·clo·pho·ri·a (sī′klō-fōr′ē-ă) Abnormal tendency for each eye to rotate around its anteroposterior axis, the rotation being prevented by visual fusional impulses. [cyclo- + G. *phora,* movement]

cy·clo·pho·to·co·ag·u·la·tion (sī′klō-fō′tō-kō-ag′yŭ-lā′shŭn) Photocoagulation of the ciliary processes to reduce the secretion of aqueous humor in glaucoma. [cyclo- + photocoagulation]

cy·clo·pi·a (sī-klō′pē-ă) A congenital defect in which the two orbits are united to form a single cavity containing one eye, its origin evidenced by fusion of the right and left optic primordia, and in which the nose is absent; usually combined with cyclencephaly. SYN synophthalmia. [G. *Kyklōps,* mythic one-eyed giant, fr. *kyklos,* circle, + *ōps,* eye]

cy·clo·pi·an (sī-klō′pē-ăn) Denoting or relating to cyclopia.

cy·clo·ple·gi·a (sī′klō-plē′jē-ă) Loss of power in the ciliary muscle of the eye; may be by denervation or by pharmacologic action. [cyclo- + G. *plēgē,* stroke]

cy·clo·ple·gic (sī′klō-plē′jik) **1.** Relating to cycloplegia. **2.** A drug that paralyzes the ciliary muscle and thus the power of accommodation.

cy·clo·sar·in (sī′klō-sar′in) A nonpersistent nerve agent. Its NATO code is GF.

Cy·clo·spor·a (sī′klō-spōr′ă) A *Cryptosporidium*-like genus of coccidian parasites reported from millipedes, reptiles, insectivores, and one rodent species; characterized by acid-fast oocysts with two sporocysts, each with two sporozoites; implicated as the cause of a widespread, prolonged, but self-limited human diarrhea in patients in the Americas, Caribbean countries, Southeast Asia, and eastern Europe previously reported as caused by cyanobacteriumlike bodies. SYN cyanobacteriumlike bodies.

Cy·clo·spor·a cay·e·ta·nen·sis (sī′klō-spōr′ă kā-ĕ-tă-nen′sis) A parasitic species causing enteritis with persistent diarrhea; usually acquired by ingestion of contaminated water or food.

cy·clo·thy·mi·a (sī′klō-thī′mē-ă) A mental disorder characterized by marked swings of mood from depression to hypomania but not to the degree that occurs in bipolar disorder. [cyclo- + G. *thymos,* rage]

cy·clo·thy·mic dis·or·der (sī′klō-thī′mik dis-ōr′dĕr) An affective disorder characterized by mood swings including periods of hypomania and depression; a form of depressive disorder.

cy·clo·thy·mic per·son·al·i·ty (sī′klō-thī′ mik pĕr-sŏn-al′i-tē) A personality disorder in which a person experiences regularly alternating periods of elation and depression, usually not related to external circumstances.

cy·clot·o·my (sī-klot′ŏ-mē) Operation of cutting the ciliary muscle. [cyclo- + G. *tomē,* incision]

cy·clo·tron (sī′klō-tron) A particle accelerator that speeds up particles in a spiral pattern to produce protons for nuclear research or radiation treatment.

cy·clo·tro·pi·a (sī′klō-trō′pē-a) A disparity of ocular position in which one eye is rotated around its visual axis, with respect to the other eye. [cyclo- + G. *tropē,* a turn, turning]

Cyd Abbreviation for cytidine.

cyl·in·der (C) (sil′in-dĕr) **1.** A cylindric lens. **2.** A cylindric or rodlike renal cast. **3.** A cylindric metal container for gases stored under high pressure. [G. *kylindros,* a roll]

cy·lin·dric lens (C) (si-lin′drik lenz) A lens in which one of the surfaces is curved in one meridian and less curved in the opposite meridian; commonly used to correct the visual distortion resulting from astigmatism. SYN astigmatic lens.

cyl·in·dro·ad·e·no·ma (sil′in-drō-ad′ĕ-nō′mă) SYN cylindroma.

cyl·in·dro·ma (sil′in-drō′mă) A histologic type of epithelial neoplasm, frequently malignant, characterized by islands of neoplastic cells embedded in a hyalinized stroma; may form from ducts of glands, especially in salivary glands, skin, and bronchi. SYN cylindroadenoma. [G. *kylindros,* cylinder, *-oma,* tumor]

cyl·in·drom·a·tous car·ci·no·ma (sil′in-drō′mă-tŭs kahr′si-nō′mă) SYN adenoid cystic carcinoma.

cyl·in·dru·ri·a (sil′in-drūr′ē-ă) The presence of renal cylinders or casts in the urine.

cym·bo·ce·phal·ic, cym·bo·ceph·a·lous (sim′bō-sĕ-fal′ik, -sef′ă-lŭs) Relating to cymbocephaly.

cym·bo·ceph·a·ly (sim′bō-sef′ă-lē) SYN scaphocephaly. [G. *kymbē,* the hollow of a vessel, a boat-shaped structure, + *kephalē,* head]

cyn·ic spasm (sī′nik spazm) SYN risus caninus.

cy·no·ceph·a·ly (sī′nō-sef′ă-lē) Craniostenosis in which the skull slopes back from the orbits, producing a resemblance to the head of a dog. [G. *kyōn,* dog, + *kephalē,* head]

cy·no·pho·bi·a (sī′nō-fō′bē-ă) Morbid fear of dogs. [G. *kyōn,* dog, + *phobos,* fear]

CYP Abbreviation for cytochrome P450 enzymes; usually followed by an arabic numeral, a letter, and another arabic numeral (e.g., CYP 2D6). These enzymes are found in and on the smooth endoplasmic reticulum of liver and other cells and are responsible for a large number of drug biotransformation reactions.

CYP 1A2 A microsomal enzyme, the substrates of which include theophylline, antidepressants, and tacrine. It is inhibited by grapefruit juice and quinolones, and induced by smoking, phenobarbital, phenytoin, rifampin, and omeprazole.

CYP 2C19 Abbreviation for a microsomal enzyme partially responsible for the oxidation of clomipramine, diazepam, propranolol, imipramine, and omeprazole. Inhibited by fluoxetine, sertraline, omeprazole, and ritonavir.

CYP 2C9 Abbreviation for a microsomal enzyme responsible for the oxidation of S-warfarin, phenytoin, and numerous NSAIDs. Inhibitors include azole antifungals (e.g., ketoconazole, itraconazole, metronidazole); induced by rifampin.

CYP 2D6 Abbreviation for an isoenzyme that metabolizes many antidepressants, antipsychotic agents, beta-adrenergic blockers, and codeine. It is inhibited by cimetidine and several antidepressants and antipsychotics.

CYP 2E1 Abbreviation for a microsomal enzyme that participates in the oxidation of ethanol and acetaminophen. Inhibited by disulfiram and induced by ethanol and isoniazid (INH). Believed to be responsible for the hepatotoxic metabolite of acetaminophen.

CYP 3A Abbreviation for a cytochrome P450 isoform found in the gastrointestinal tract as well as hepatic and other cells; substrates include benzodiazepines, calcium channel blockers, antihistamines, steroid hormones, and protease inhibitors. Inhibited by antidepressants, azole antifungals, cimetidine, and erythromycin. Induced by phenobarbital, phenytoin, rifampin, and carbamazepine.

Cys Abbreviation for cysteine (half-cystine) or its mono- or diradical.

cyst (sist) **1.** An abnormal sac containing gas, fluid, or a semisolid material, with a membranous lining. SEE ALSO pseudocyst. **2.** Larval stage of some cestodes. See page B7. [G. *kystis,* bladder]

cyst·ad·e·no·car·ci·no·ma (sist-ad′ĕ-nō-kahr′si-nō′mă) A malignant neoplasm derived from glandular epithelium, in which cystic accumulations of retained secretions are formed; the neoplastic cells manifest varying degrees of anaplasia and invasiveness, and local extension and metastases occur; cystadenocarcinomas develop frequently in the ovaries, where pseudomucinous and serous types are recognized.

cyst•ad•e•no•ma (sist′ad-ĕ-nō′mă) A histologically benign neoplasm derived from glandular epithelium, in which cystic accumulations of retained secretions are formed. SYN cystoadenoma.

cyst•al•gi•a (sist-al′jē-ă) Pain in a bladder, especially the urinary bladder. [cyst- + G. *algos,* pain]

cys•ta•thi•o•nase (sis′tă-thī′ō-nās) SYN cystathionine gamma (γ)-lyase.

cys•ta•thi•o•nine (sis′tă-thī′ō-nēn) An intermediate in the conversion of L-methionine to L-cysteine; cleaved by cystathionases.

cys•ta•thi•o•nine gamma (γ)-ly•ase (sis′tă-thī′ō-nēn lī′ās) A liver enzyme that catalyzes the hydrolysis of L-cystathionine to L-cysteine and 2-ketobutyrate. A deficiency of this enzyme results in cystathioninuria. A step in methionine catabolism and in cysteine biosynthesis. SYN cystathionase.

cys•tec•ta•si•a, **cys•tec•ta•sy** (sis′tek-tā′zē-ă, sis-tek′tă-sē) Dilation of the bladder. [cyst- + G. *ektasis,* a stretching]

cys•tec•to•my (sis-tek′tŏ-mē) **1.** Excision of the the urinary bladder. **2.** Excision of the gallbladder (cholecystectomy). **3.** Removal of a cyst. [cyst- + G. *ektomē,* excision]

cys•te•ic ac•id (sis-tē′ik as′id) An oxidation product of cysteine, and a precursor of taurine and isethionic acid.

cys•te•ine (C, Cys) (sis-tē′in) An amino acid found in most proteins; especially abundant in keratin.

cys•tic (sis′tik) **1.** Relating to the urinary bladder or gallbladder. **2.** Relating to a cyst. **3.** Containing cysts.

cys•tic ac•ne (sis′tik ak′nē) Severe acne in which the predominant lesions are follicular cysts that rupture and scar.

cys•tic ar•ter•y (sis′tik ahr′tĕr-ē) *Origin,* right branch of hepatic; *distribution,* gall bladder and visceral surface of the liver. SYN arteria cystica [TA].

cys•tic dis•ease of the breast (sis′tik di-zēz′ brest) Fibrocystic condition of the breasts.

cys•tic duct, **cys•tic gall duct** (sis′tik dŭkt, sis′tik gawl dŭkt) The ductus leading from the gallbladder; it joins the hepatic duct to form the common bile duct.

cys•ti•cer•co•sis (sis′ti-sĕr-kō′sis) **1.** Disease caused by encystment of cysticercus larvae (e.g., *Taenia solium* or *T. saginata*) in subcutaneous, muscle, or central nervous system tissues; cysticercosis typically develops in swine and cattle, producing measly pork and beef. In humans, it results from the hatching of the eggs of *T. solium* in the intestines or by accidental ingestion of eggs from human feces; encystment in the brain may cause serious nervous damage, and encystment in the eye (usually the rear chamber) may cause ophthalmic damage. **2.** Larval infections in animals with other taeniid tapeworm larvae.

Cys•ti•cer•cus (sis′ti-sĕr′kŭs) The encysted larva of taenioid tapeworms. SEE cysticercus. [G. *kystis,* bladder, + *kerkos,* tail]

cys•ti•cer•cus, pl. **cys•ti•cer•ci** (sis′ti-sĕr′kŭs, -sĕr′sī) The larval form of certain *Taenia* species, typically found in muscles of mammalian intermediate hosts; it consists of a fluid-filled bladder in which the invaginated cestode scolex develops. SEE ALSO *Taenia saginata, Taenia solium.* [G. *kystis,* bladder, + *kerkos,* tail]

cys•tic fi•bro•sis, **cys•tic fi•bro•sis of the pan•cre•as** (sis′tik fī-brō′sis, sis′tik fī-brō′sis pan′krē-ăs) A congenital metabolic disorder, inherited as an autosomal trait, in which secretions of exocrine glands are abnormal; excessively viscid mucus causes obstruction of passageways (including pancreatic and bile ducts, intestines, and bronchi), and the sodium and chloride content of sweat are increased throughout the patient's life; symptoms usually appear in childhood and include meconium ileus, poor growth despite good appetite, malabsorption and foul bulky stools, chronic bronchitis with cough, recurrent pneumonia, bronchiectasis, emphysema, clubbing of the fingers, and salt depletion in hot weather. Detailed genetic mapping and molecular biology have been accomplished by the methods of reverse genetics.

cys•tic fi•bro•sis trans•mem•brane reg•u•la•tor (CFTR) (sis′tik fī-brō′sis trans-mem′brān reg′yŭ-lā-tŏr) Mutation in the CF gene.

cys•tic goi•ter (sis′tik goy′tĕr) An enlargement in the thyroid region due to the presence of one or more cysts within the gland.

cys•tic lymph node (sis′tik limf nōd) A lymph node at the neck of the gallbladder draining lymph into the hepatic nodes.

cys•tic veins (sis′tik vānz) Veins, usually anterior and posterior, which drain the neck of the gallbladder and cystic duct, along which they pass to enter the right branch of the portal vein; they communicate extensively with surrounding veins of the stomach, duodenum, and pancreas.

cys•ti•form (sis′ti-fōrm) SYN cystoid (1).

cystinaemia [Br.] SYN cystinemia.

cys•tine (sis′tēn) The disulfide product of two cysteines in which two –SH groups become one –S–S– group; sometimes occurs as a deposit in the urine, or forming a vesical calculus.

cys•tine cal•cu•lus (sis′tēn kal′kyū-lŭs) A soft and faintly radiopaque urinary tract stone composed of cystine.

cys•ti•ne•mi•a (sis′ti-nē′mē-ă) The presence of cystine in the blood. SYN cystinaemia. [cystine + G. *haima,* blood]

cys•ti•nu•ri•a (sis′ti-nyūr′ē-ă) Excessive urinary excretion of cystine, along with lysine, arginine, and ornithine, arising from defective transport systems for these acids in the kidney and intestine; renal function is sometimes compromised by cystine crystalluria and nephrolithiasis; occurs in certain heritable diseases, such as Fanconi syndrome (cystinosis) and hepatolenticular degeneration. [cystine + G. *ouron,* urine]

cys•ti•tis (sis-tī′tis) Inflammation of the urinary bladder. [cyst- + G. *-itis,* inflammation]

cys•ti•tis cys•ti•ca (sis-tī′tis sis′ti-kă) Cystitis glandularis with the formation of cysts.

cys•ti•tis glan•du•la•ris (sis-tī′tis glan-dyū-lā′ris) Chronic cystitis with glandlike metaplasia of transitional epithelium.

♻ **cysto-, cysti-, cyst-** Combining forms relating to the bladder; the cystic duct; a cyst. Cf. vesico-. [G. *kystis,* bladder, pouch]

cys•to•ad•e•no•ma (sis′tō-ad-ĕ-nō′mă) SYN cystadenoma.

cys•to•car•ci•no•ma (sis′tō-kahr-si-nō′mă) A carcinoma in which cystic degeneration has occurred; sometimes used incorrectly as a term for cystadenocarcinoma. SYN cystoepithelioma.

cys•to•cele (sis′tō-sēl) Hernia of the bladder usually into the vagina and introitus. SYN colpocystocele, vesicocele. [cysto- + G. *kēlē,* hernia]

cys•to•chro•mos•co•py (sis′tō-krō-mos′kŏ-pē) Examination of the interior of the bladder after administration of a dye to aid in the identification or study of the function of the ureteral orifices. SYN chromocystoscopy. [cysto- + G. *chrōma,* color + *skopeō,* to view]

cys•to•du•o•de•nal lig•a•ment (sis′tō-dū-ō-dē′năl lig′ă-mĕnt) A peritoneal fold that sometimes passes from the gallbladder to the first part of the duodenum.

cys•to•du•o•de•nos•to•my (sis′tō-dū′ō-dē-nos′tŏ-mē) Drainage of a cyst, usually a pancreatic pseudocyst, into the duodenum. SYN duodenocystostomy (2). [cysto- + duodenum, + G. *stoma,* mouth]

cys•to•ep•i•the•li•o•ma (sis′tō-ep-i-thē′lē-ō′mă) SYN cystocarcinoma.

cys•to•fi•bro•ma (sis′tō-fī-brō′mă) A fibroma in which cysts or cystlike foci have formed.

cys•to•gram (sis′tō-gram) Radiographic demonstration of the bladder filled with contrast medium.

cys•tog•ra•phy (sis-tog′ră-fē) Radiography of the bladder following injection of a radiopaque substance. [cysto- + G. *graphō,* to write]

cys•toid (sis′toyd) **1.** Bladderlike, resembling a cyst. SYN cystiform, cystomorphous. **2.** A tumor resembling a cyst, with fluid, granular, or pulpy contents, but without a capsule. [cysto- + G. *eidos,* appearance]

cys•toid mac•u•lop•a•thy (sis′toyd mak′yū-lop′ă-thē) Cystic degeneration of the central retina that may occur after cataract extraction, in senile macular degeneration, and in other retinal abnormalities.

cys•to•li•thi•a•sis (sis′tō-li-thī′ă-sis) The presence of a vesical calculus. [cysto- + G. *lithos,* stone, + *-iasis,* condition]

cys•to•lith•ic (sis′tō-lith′ik) Relating to a vesical calculus.

cy•sto•lith•o•la•pax•y (sis′tō-lith′ō-lā-paks-ē) Removal of bladder calculi by intravesical crushing and then irrigating to remove fragments. [cysto- + G. *lithos*, stone, + *lapaxis*, an emptying out]

cys•to•li•thot•o•my (sis′tō-li-thot′ŏ-mē) Removal of a stone from the bladder through an incision in its wall. [cysto- + G. *lithos,* stone, + *tomē,* incision]

cys•to•ma (sis-tō′mă) A cystic tumor; a new growth containing cysts. [cyst- + G. *-oma,* tumor]

cys•tom•e•ter (sis-tom′ĕ-tĕr) A device for studying bladder function by measuring capacity, sensation, intravesical pressure, and residual urine. [cysto- + G. *metron,* measure]

cys•to•met•ro•gram (sis′tō-met′rō-gram) A graphic recording of urinary bladder pressure at various volumes. [cysto- + G. *metron,* measure, + *gramma,* a writing]

cys•tom•e•try, cys•to•me•trog•ra•phy (sis-tom′ĕ-trē, sis′tō-mĕ-trog′ră-fē) A method for measurement of the pressure/volume relationship of the bladder. SEE cystometer.

cys•to•mor•phous (sis′tō-mōr′fŭs) SYN cystoid (1). [cysto- + G. *morphē,* form]

cys•to•pan•en•dos•co•py (sis′tō-pan-en-dos′kŏ-pē) Inspection of the interior of the bladder and urethra by means of specially designed endoscopes introduced in retrograde fashion through the urethra and into the bladder. [cysto- + panendoscope]

cys•to•pa•ral•y•sis (sis′tō-păr-al′i-sis) SYN cystoplegia.

cys•to•pex•y (sis′tō-pek-sē) Surgical attachment of the gallbladder or of the urinary bladder to the abdominal wall or to other supporting structures. [cysto- + G. *pēxis,* fixation]

cys·to·plas·ty (sis′tō-plas-tē) Any reconstructive surgery on the urinary bladder. Cf. ileocystoplasty. [cysto- + G. *plastos,* formed]

cys·to·ple·gi·a (sis′tō-plē′jē-ă) Paralysis of the bladder. SYN cystoparalysis. [cysto- + G. *plēgē,* a stroke]

cys·top·to·sis, **cys·to·pto·si·a** (sis′tō-tō′sis -tō-tō′sis, sis-top-tō′sē-ă) Prolapse of the vesical mucous membrane into the urethra. [cysto- + G. *ptosis,* a falling]

cys·to·py·e·li·tis (sis′tō-pī-ĕl-ī′tis) Inflammation of both the bladder and the pelvis of the kidney. [cysto- + G. *pyelos,* trough (pelvis), + *-itis,* inflammation]

cys·to·py·e·lo·ne·phri·tis (sis′tō-pī′ĕl-ō-nef-rī′tis) Inflammation of the bladder, the pelvis of the kidney, and the kidney parenchyma. [cysto- + G. *pyelos,* trough (pelvis), + *nephros,* kidney, + *-itis,* inflammation]

cys·to·rec·tos·to·my (sis′tō-rek-tos′tō-mē) SYN vesicorectostomy. [cysto + rectum + G. *stoma,* mouth]

cys·tor·rha·phy (sis-tōr′ă-fē) Suture of a wound or defect in the urinary bladder. [cysto- + G. *rhaphē,* a sewing]

cys·tor·rhe·a (sis′tōr-ē′ă) A mucous discharge from the bladder. SYN cystorrhoea. [cysto- + G. *rhoia,* a flow]

cystorrhoea [Br.] SYN cystorrhea.

cys·to·sar·co·ma (sis′tō-sahr-kō′mă) A sarcoma in which the formation of cysts or cystlike foci has occurred.

cys·to·scope (sis′tŏ-skōp) A lighted tubular endoscope for examining the interior of the bladder. [cysto- + G. *skopeō,* to examine]

cys·to·scop·ic ur·og·ra·phy (sis′tŏ-skop′ik yūr-og′ră-fē) SYN retrograde urography.

cys·tos·co·py (sis-tos′kŏ-pē) The inspection of the interior of the bladder by means of a cystoscope.

cys·tos·to·my (sis-tos′tŏ-mē) Creation of an opening into the urinary bladder. SYN vesicostomy. [cysto- + G. *stoma,* mouth]

cys·to·tome (sis′tō-tōm) **1.** An instrument for incising the urinary bladder or gallbladder. **2.** A surgical instrument used for incising the capsule of a lens.

cys·tot·o·my (sis-tot′ŏ-mē) Incision into urinary bladder or gallbladder. SYN vesicotomy. [cysto- + G. *tomē,* incision]

cys·to·u·re·ter·i·tis (sis′tō-yūr′ĕ-tĕr-ī′tis) Inflammation of the bladder and of one or both ureters.

cys·to·u·re·ter·o·gram (sis′tō-yūr-ē′tĕr-ō-gram) Radiographic demonstration of the bladder and ureters.

cys·to·u·re·ter·og·ra·phy (sis′tō-yūr′ĕ-tĕr-og′ră-fē) Radiography of the bladder and ureters.

cys·to·u·re·thri·tis (sis′tō-yūr′ĕ-thrī′tis) Inflammation of the bladder and of the urethra.

cys·to·u·re·thro·gram (sis′tō-yūr-ē′thrō-gram) An x-ray image made during voiding and with the bladder and urethra filled with contrast medium to demonstrate the urethra. SYN voiding cystogram.

cys·to·u·re·throg·ra·phy (sis′tō-yūr′ĕ-throg′ră-fē) Radiography of the bladder and urethra during voiding, after the bladder has been filled with a radiopaque contrast medium either by intravenous injection or retrograde catheterization.

cys·to·u·re·thro·scope (sis′tō-yūr-ē′thrŏ-skōp) An instrument combining the uses of a cystoscope and a urethroscope, whereby both the bladder and urethra can be visually inspected.

Cyt Abbreviation for cytosine.

cy·ta·pher·e·sis (sī′tă-fĕr-ē′sis) A procedure in which various cells can be separated from the withdrawn blood and retained, with the plasma and other formed elements retransfused into the donor. [cyt- + G. *aphairesis,* a withdrawal]

♻ **-cyte** Suffix meaning cell. [G. *kyton,* a hollow (cell)]

cyt·i·dine (C, Cyd) (sī′ti-dēn) A major component of ribonucleic acids. SYN cytosine ribonucleoside.

cyt·i·dine 5′-di·phos·phate (CDP) (sī′ti-dēn dī-fos′fāt) An ester, at the 5′ position, between cytidine and diphosphoric acid.

cyt·i·dine 5′-tri·phos·phate (CTP) (sī′ti-dēn trī-fos′fāt) An ester, at the 5′ position, between cytidine and triphosphoric acid.

cyt·i·dyl·ic ac·id (sī-ti-dil′ik as′id) Cytidine monophosphate (five are possible, depending on the site of attachment of the phosphate to the ribosyl OHs); a constituent of ribonucleic acids.

♻ **cyto-**, **cyt-** Combining forms meaning a cell. [G. *kytos,* a hollow (cell)]

cy·to·ar·chi·tec·ture (sī′tō-ahr′ki-tek-shŭr) The arrangement of cells in a tissue; the term commonly refers to the arrangement of nerve-cell bodies in the brain, especially the cerebral cortex.

cy·to·cen·trum (sī′tō-sen′trŭm) A zone of cytoplasm containing one or two centrioles but devoid of other organelles; usually located near the nucleus of a cell. SYN centrosome, microcentrum. [cyto- + G. *kentron,* center]

cy·to·chem·is·try (sī′tō-kem′is-trē) The study of intracellular distribution of chemicals, reaction sites, and enzymes, often by means of staining reactions, radioactive isotope uptake, selective metal distribution in electron microscopy, or other methods. SYN histochemistry.

cy•to•chrome (sī′tō-krōm) A class of hemoprotein the principal biologic function of which is electron or hydrogen transport by virtue of a reversible valency change of the heme iron. Many variants exist, particularly among bacteria and in green plants and algae, one being a variant of the *c* type cytochrome called cytochrome *f*. The mitochondrial system of cytochromes provides electron transport through cytochrome *c* oxidase to molecular oxygen as the terminal electron acceptor (respiration). [cyto- + G. *chrōma,* color]

cy•to•chrome P-450 sys•tem (sī′tō-krōm sis′tĕm) A heterogeneous group of enzymes that catalyze various oxidative reactions in the human liver, intestine, kidney, lung, and central nervous system; these enzymes are involved in the metabolism of many endogenous and exogenous substrates, including drugs, toxins, hormones, and natural plant products. Cytochrome P-450 enzymes are classified on the basis of chemical structure (amino acid sequencing). The designation of each enzyme is CYP followed by a numeral for the family to which it has been assigned, a letter for its subfamily, and sometimes a second numeral for the individual enzyme.

cy•to•ci•dal (sī′tō-sī′dăl) Causing the death of cells. [cyto- + L. *caedo,* to kill]

cy•to•cide (sī′tō-sīd) An agent that destroys cells. [cyto- + L. *caedo,* to kill]

cy•toc•la•sis (sī-tok′lă-sis) Fragmentation of cells. [cyto- + G. *klasis,* a breaking]

cy•to•clas•tic (sī′tō-klas′tik) Relating to cytoclasis.

cy•to•di•ag•no•sis (sī′tō-dī-ăg-nō′sis) Diagnosis of a pathologic process by means of microscopic study of cells.

cy•to•gen•e•sis (sī′tō-jen′ĕ-sis) The origin and development of cells. [cyto- + G. *genesis,* origin]

cy•to•ge•net•i•cist (sī′tō-jĕ-net′i-sist) A specialist in cytogenetics.

cy•to•ge•net•ics (sī′tō-jĕ-net′iks) The branch of genetics concerned with the structure and function of the cell, especially the chromosomes. Modern molecular cytogenetics involves the microscopic study of chromosomes that have been arranged as karyotypes. Individuals can be classified according to characteristic banding patterns that appear when the karyotypes are exposed to certain dyes. In addition, DNA probes may be applied to locate specific gene sequences. Cytogenetic techniques are used to test for inborn errors of metabolism, for disorders such as Down syndrome, and to determine sex in cases where anatomy is inconclusive.

cy•to•gen•ic (sī′tō-jen′ik) Relating to cytogenesis.

cy•to•gen•ic re•pro•duc•tion (sī′tō-jen′ik rē′prō-dŭk′shŭn) Reproduction by means of unicellular germ cells; includes both sexual reproduction and asexual reproduction by means of spores.

cy•tog•e•nous (sī-toj′ĕ-nŭs) Cell-forming.

cy•to•glu•co•pe•ni•a (sī′tō-glū-kō-pē′nē-ă) An intracellular deficiency of glucose. [cyto- + glucose + G. *penia,* poverty]

cy•toid (sī′toyd) Resembling a cell. [cyto- + G. *eidos,* resemblance]

cy•to•ker•a•tin (sī′tō-ker′a-tin) SYN keratin.

cy•to•kine (sī′tō-kīn) Hormonelike proteins, secreted by many cell types, which regulate the intensity and duration of immune responses and are involved in cell-to-cell communication. SEE ALSO interferon, interleukin, lymphokine. [cyto- + G. *kinēsis,* movement]

cy•to•ki•ne•sis (sī′tō-ki-nē′sis) Changes occurring in the protoplasm of the cell outside the nucleus during cell division. [cyto- + G. *kinēsis,* movement]

cy•to•log•ic (sī′tō-loj′ik) Relating to cytology.

cy•to•log•ic smear (sī′tō-loj′ik smēr) A type of cytologic specimen made by smearing a sample (obtained by a variety of methods from a number of sites), then fixing it and staining it, usually with 95% ethyl alcohol and Papanicolaou stain.

cy•tol•o•gist (sī-tol′ŏ-jist) One who specializes in cytology.

cy•tol•o•gy (sī-tol′ŏ-jē) The study of the anatomy, physiology, pathology, and chemistry of the cell. SYN cellular biology. [cyto- + G. *logos,* study]

cy•tol•y•sin (sī-tol′i-sin) A substance, i.e., an antibody, that effects partial or complete destruction of an animal cell; may require complement. SEE ALSO perforin.

cy•tol•y•sis (sī-tol′i-sis) The dissolution of a cell. [cyto- + G. *lysis,* loosening]

cy•to•ly•so•some (sī′tō-lī′sō-sōm) A variety of secondary lysosome that contains the remnants of mitochondria, ribosomes, or other organelles.

cy•to•lyt•ic (sī′tō-lit′ik) Pertaining to cytolysis; possessing a solvent or destructive action on cells.

cy•to•me•ga•lic in•clu•sion dis•ease (sī′tō-me-gal′ik in-klū′zhŭn di-zēz′) The presence of inclusion bodies within the cytoplasm and nuclei of enlarged cells of various organs of newborn infants dying with jaundice, hepatomegaly, splenomegaly, purpura, thrombocytopenia, and fever; the condition also occurs, at all ages, as a complication of other diseases in which immune mechanisms are severely depressed, and has been found incidentally in salivary gland epithelium, apparently as a localized or mild infection (salivary gland virus disease). SYN inclusion body disease.

cy·to·meg·a·lo·vi·rus (CMV) (sī′tō-meg′ă-lō-vī′rŭs) A group of herpesviruses infecting humans and other animals, many having special affinity for salivary glands, and causing development of characteristic inclusions in the cytoplasm or nucleus. Most infections are asymptomatic, but if symptoms are present, they manifest as mononucleosislike illness. Congenital infection may cause malformation or fetal death; infection in immunocompromised persons may be life-threatening. See page B6. SYN human herpesvirus 5. [cyto- + G. *megas,* big]

cy·to·met·a·pla·si·a (sī′tō-met-ă-plā′zē-ă) Change of form or function of a cell, other than that related to neoplasia. [cyto- + G. *metaplasis,* transformation]

cy·tom·e·ter (sī-tom′ĕ-ter) A device used to count and measure cells, especially blood cells, either visually (with a microscope) or automatically (as in flow cytometry). [cyto- + G. *metron,* measure]

cy·tom·e·try (sī-tom′ĕ-trē) The counting of cells, especially blood cells, using a cytometer or hemocytometer.

cy·to·mor·phol·o·gy (sī′tō-mōr-fol′ŏ-jē) The study of the structure of cells.

cy·to·mor·pho·sis (sī′tō-mōr-fō′sis) Changes that the cell undergoes during the various stages of its existence. SEE ALSO prosoplasia. [cyto- + G. *morphōsis,* a shaping]

cy·to·path·ic (sī′tō-path′ik) Pertaining to or exhibiting cytopathy.

cy·to·path·o·gen·ic (sī′tō-path-ŏ-jen′ik) Pertaining to an agent or substance that causes a diseased condition in cells, in contrast to histologic changes; used especially with reference to effects observed in cells in tissue cultures.

cy·to·path·o·gen·ic vi·rus (sī′tō-path-ŏ-jen′ik vī′rŭs) A virus the multiplication of which leads to degenerative changes in the host cell.

cy·to·path·o·log·ic, **cy·to·path·o·log·i·cal** (sī′tō-path-ŏ-loj′ik, -loj′i-kăl) **1.** Denoting cellular changes in disease. **2.** Relating to cytopathology.

cy·to·pa·thol·o·gist (sī′tō-pă-thol′ŏ-jist) A physician specially trained and experienced in cytopathology.

cy·to·pa·thol·o·gy (sī′tō-pă-thol′ŏ-jē) **1.** The study of disease changes within individual cells or cell types. **2.** SYN exfoliative cytology.

cy·top·a·thy (sī-top′ă-thē) Any disorder of a cell or anomaly of any of its constituents. [cyto- + G. *pathos,* disease]

cy·to·pe·ni·a (sī′tō-pē′nē-ă) A reduction, i.e., hypocytosis, or a lack of cellular elements in the circulating blood. [cyto- + G. *penia,* poverty]

cy·toph·a·gous (sī-tof′ă-gŭs) Devouring, or destructive to, cells.

cy·toph·a·gy (sī-tof′ă-jē) Devouring of other cells by phagocytes. [cyto- + G. *phagō,* to devour]

cy·to·phil·ic (sī′tō-fil′ik) SYN cytotropic. [cyto- + G. *philos,* fond]

cy·to·phil·ic an·ti·bod·y (sī′tō-fil′ik an′ti-bod-ē) SYN cytotropic antibody.

cy·to·pho·tom·e·try (sī′tō-fō-tom′ĕ-trē) A method of measuring the absorption of monochromatic light by stained microscopic structures (e.g., chromosomes, nuclei, whole cells) with the aid of a photoelectric cell; also used to measure emitted light from such objects by fluorescence in combination with selected fluorochrome dyes. [cyto- + G. *phōs,* light + *metron,* measure]

cy·to·phy·lac·tic (sī′tō-fi-lak′tik) Relating to cytophylaxis.

cy·to·phy·lax·is (sī′tō-fī-lak′sis) Protection of cells against lytic agents. [cyto- + G. *phylaxis,* a guarding]

cy·to·plasm (sī′tō-plazm) The substance of a cell, exclusive of the nucleus, that contains various organelles and inclusions within a colloidal protoplasm. SEE ALSO protoplasm, hyaloplasm, cytosol. [cyto- + G. *plasma,* thing formed]

cy·to·plas·mic (sī′tō-plaz′mik) Relating to the cytoplasm.

cy·to·plas·mic bridg·es (sī′tō-plaz′mik brij′ĕz) SYN intercellular bridges.

cy·to·plas·mic in·clu·sion bod·ies (sī′tō-plaz′mik in-klū′zhŭn bod′ēz) SEE inclusion bodies.

cy·to·plas·mic in·her·i·tance (sī′tō-plaz′mik in-her′i-tăns) Transmission of characters dependent on self-perpetuating elements not nuclear in origin (e.g., mitochondrial DNA).

cy·to·plast (sī′tō-plast) The living intact cytoplasm that remains following cell enucleation. [cyto- + G. *plastos,* formed]

cy·to·re·duc·tive ther·a·py (sī′tō-rĕ-dŭk′tiv thār′ă-pē) Care intended to reduce the number of cells in a lesion, usually a malignancy.

cy·to·screen·er (sī′tō-skrēn′ĕr) SYN cytotechnologist.

cy·to·sine (Cyt) (sī′tō-sēn) A pyrimidine found in nucleic acids.

cy·to·sine ar·a·bin·o·side (CA) (sī′tō-sēn

ar′ă-bin′ō-sīd) **1.** A synthetic nucleoside used as an antimetabolite in the treatment of neoplasms. **2.** Incorrect term for arabinosylcytosine.

cy·to·sine ri·bo·nu·cle·o·side (sī′tō-sēn rī′bō-nū′klē-ō-sīd) SYN cytidine.

cy·to·sis (sī-tō′sis) **1.** A condition with more than the usual number of cells present, as in the spinal fluid in meningitis. **2.** Frequently used with a prefixed combining form as a means of describing certain features pertaining to cells; e.g., isocytosis, equality in size; polycytosis, abnormal increase in number. [cyto- + G. *-osis,* condition]

cy·to·skel·e·ton (sī′tō-skel′ĕ-tŏn) The tonofilaments, keratin, desmin, neurofilaments, or other intermediate filaments serving as supportive cytoplasmic elements to stiffen cells or to organize intracellular organelles.

cy·to·sol (sī′tō-sol) Cytoplasm exclusive of the mitochondria, endoplasmic reticulum, and other membranous components. [cyto- + "sol," abbrev. of soluble]

cy·to·sol·ic (sī-tō-sol′ik) Relating to or contained in the cytosol.

cy·to·some (sī′tō-sōm) **1.** The cell body exclusive of the nucleus. **2.** One of the osmiophilic bodies that are 1 mcm or less in diameter, have concentric lamellae, and occur in the great alveolar cells of the lung. SYN multilamellar body. [cyto- + G. *sōma,* body]

cy·tos·ta·sis (sī-tos′tă-sis) The slowing of movement and accumulation of blood cells, especially polymorphonuclear leukocytes, in the capillaries, as in a region of inflammation; obstruction of a capillary as the result of accumulated leukocytes. [cyto- + G. *stasis,* standing]

cy·to·stat·ic (sī′tō-stat′ik) Characterized by cytostasis.

cy·to·tac·tic (sī′tō-tak′tik) Relating to cytotaxis.

cy·to·tax·is, **cy·to·tax·i·a** (sī′tō-tak′sis, -sē-ă) The attraction (positive cytotaxis) or repulsion (negative cytotaxis) of cells for one another. [cyto- + G. *taxis,* arrangement]

cy·to·tech·nol·o·gist (sī′tō-tek-nol′ŏ-jist) A person with special training in cytopathology who is responsible for screening Papanicolaou smears and determining which results are negative and which require further review by a pathologist. SEE ALSO Papanicolaou (Pap) smear, Papanicolaou (Pap) test. SYN cytoscreener.

cy·toth·e·sis (sī-toth′ĕ-sis) The repair of injury in a cell; the restoration of cells. [cyto- + G. *thesis,* a placing]

cy·to·tox·ic (sī′tō-tok′sik) Detrimental or destructive to cells; pertaining to the effect of noncytophilic antibody on specific antigen, frequently, but not always, mediating the action of complement.

cy·to·tox·ic·i·ty (sī′tō-tok-sis′i-tē) The quality or state of being cytotoxic.

cy·to·tox·ic re·ac·tion (sī′tō-tok′sik rē-ak′shŭn) An immunologic (allergic) reaction in which noncytotropic IgG or IgM antibody combines with a specific antigen on cell surfaces; the resulting complex initiates the activation of complement which causes cell lysis or other damage, or, in the absence of complement, may lead to phagocytosis or may enhance T-lymphocyte involvement.

cy·to·tox·in (sī′tō-tok′sin) A specific substance, which may or may not be an antibody, that inhibits or prevents the functions of cells, causes destruction of cells, or both. [cyto- + G. *toxikon,* poison]

cy·to·tro·pho·blast (sī′tō-trof′ō-blast) The inner cellular layer of the trophoblast.

cy·to·tro·pho·blas·tic cells (sī′tō-trof′ō-blast′ik selz) Stem cells that fuse to form the overlying syncytiotrophoblast of placental villi. SYN Langhans cells (2).

cy·to·tro·pic (sī′tō-trō′pik) Having an affinity for cells. SYN cytophilic.

cy·to·tro·pic an·ti·bod·y (sī′tō-trō′pik an′ti-bod-ē) Antibody that has an affinity for certain kinds of cells, in addition to and unrelated to its specific affinity for the antigen that induced it, because of the properties of the Fc portion of the heavy chain. SEE ALSO heterocytotropic antibody, homocytotropic antibody. SYN anaphylactic antibody, cytophilic antibody.

cy·tot·ro·pism (sī-tot′rō-pizm) **1.** Affinity for cells. **2.** Affinity for specific cells, especially the ability of viruses to localize in and damage specific cells. [cyto- + G. *tropos,* a turning]

cy·tu·ri·a (sī-tyūr′ē-ă) The passage of cells in unusual numbers in the urine. [G. *kytos,* cell, + *ouron,* urine]

Cza·pek so·lu·tion a·gar (chah′pek sŏ-lū′shŭn ā′gahr) A culture medium used for the cultivation of fungus species and for identification of *Aspergillus* and *Penicillium* species.

Czer·ny-Lem·bert su·ture (sher′nē lem-bār′ sū′chŭr) An intestinal suture in two rows combining the Czerny suture (first) and the Lembert suture (second).

Czer·ny su·ture (cher′nē sū′chŭr) The first row of Czerny-Lembert intestinal sutures; the needle enters the serosa and passes out through the submucosa or muscularis, and then enters the submucosa or muscularis of the opposite side and emerges from the serosa.

D

Δ, δ Delta. SEE delta.

D Abbreviation meaning date dictated; dictated; diopter; dalton.

d Abbreviation meaning deci-; *dexter* [L], right; diameter; day.

d- Prefix indicating a chemical compound to be dextrorotatory; should be avoided when (+) or (–) could be used. Cf. L-.

D- Prefix indicating that a chemical compound is sterically related to D-glyceraldehyde, the basis of stereochemical nomenclature. Cf. lambda.

-d Suffix indicating the presence of deuterium in a compound in concentrations above normal, thus labeling the compound; subscripts (d_2, d_3, etc.) indicate the number of such atoms so fortified.

DA Abbreviation for developmental age.

Da Abbreviation for dalton.

dA, **dAdo** Abbreviation for deoxyadenosine.

da Abbreviation for deca-.

Da•ae dis•ease (dah′ĕ di-zēz′) SYN epidemic pleurodynia. SEE ALSO hand-foot-and-mouth disease.

d'A•cos•ta syn•drome (dah-kōs′tă sin′drōm) Onset of nausea, vomiting, headache, mood changes, and insomnia occurring several hours to days after ascent to a higher altitude, with pulmonary and cerebral edema; death ensues in severe cases. Caused by hypoxia with increased ventilation rate and resulting respiratory alkalosis.

dacryo-, **dacry-** Combining forms meaning tears; lacrimal sac or duct. [G. *dakryon,* tear]

dac•ry•o•ad•e•ni•tis (dak′rē-ō-ad-ĕ-nī′tis) Inflammation of the lacrimal gland. [dacryo- + G. *adēn,* gland, + *-itis,* inflammation]

dac•ry•o•blen•nor•rhe•a (dak′rē-ō-blen-ŏr-ē′ă) A chronic discharge of mucus from a lacrimal sac. SYN dacryoblennorrhoea. [dacryo- + G. *blenna,* mucus, + *rhoia,* flow]

dacryoblennorrhoea [Br.] SYN dacryoblennorrhea.

dac•ry•o•cele (dak′rē-ō-sēl) SYN dacryocystocele.

dac•ry•o•cyst (dak′rē-ō-sist) SYN lacrimal sac. [dacryo- + G. *kystis,* sac]

dac•ry•o•cys•tal•gi•a (dak′rē-ō-sis-tal′jē-ă) Pain in the lacrimal sac. [dacryocyst + G. *algos,* pain]

dac•ry•o•cys•tec•to•my (dak′rē-ō-sis-tek′tŏ-mē) Surgical removal of the lacrimal sac. [dacryocyst + G. *ektomē,* excision]

dac•ry•o•cys•to•cele (dak′rē-ō-sis′tō-sēl) Enlargement of the lacrimal sac with fluid. SYN dacryocele. [dacryocyst + G. *kēlē,* hernia]

dac•ry•o•cys•to•rhi•nos•to•my (dak′rē-ō-sis′tō-rī-nos′tŏ-mē) An operation providing an anastomosis between the lacrimal sac and the nasal mucosa through an opening in the lacrimal bone. [dacryocyst + G. *rhis* (*rhin-*), nose, + *stoma,* mouth]

dac•ry•o•cys•tot•o•my (dak′rē-ō-sis-tot′ŏ-mē) Incision of the lacrimal sac. [dacryocyst + G. *tomē,* incision]

dac•ry•o•cyte (dak′rē-ō-sīt) An abnormally shaped red blood cell with a single point or elongation; also called a teardrop. This form of poikilocyte is associated with myelofibrosis with myeloid metaplasia. See page B3. SYN teardrop cell. [dacryo- + -cyte]

dacryohaemorrhoea [Br.] SYN dacryohemorrhea.

dac•ry•o•hem•or•rhe•a (dak′rē-ō-hem-ŏr-ē′ă) Bloody tears. SYN dacryohaemorrhoea. [dacryo- + G. *haima,* blood, + *rhoia,* flow]

dac•ry•o•lith (dak′rē-ō-lith) A concretion in the lacrimal apparatus. SYN ophthalmolith, tear stone. [dacryo- + G. *lithos,* stone]

dac•ry•o•li•thi•a•sis (dak′rē-ō-li-thī′ă-sis) The formation and presence of dacryoliths.

dac•ry•ops (dak′rē-ops) **1.** Excess of tears in the eye. **2.** A cyst of a duct of the lacrimal gland. [dacryo- + G. *ōps,* eye]

dac•ry•o•py•or•rhe•a (dak′rē-ō-pī′ŏr-ē′ă) The discharge of tears containing leukocytes. SYN dacryopyorrhoea. [dacryo- + G. *pyon,* pus, + *rhoia,* flow]

dacryopyorrhoea [Br.] SYN dacryopyorrhea.

dac•ry•or•rhe•a (dak′rē-ō-rē′ă) An excessive secretion of tears. SYN dacryorrhoea. [dacryo- + G. *rhoia,* flow]

dacryorrhoea [Br.] SYN dacryorrhea.

dac•ry•o•ste•no•sis (dak′rē-ō-stĕ-nō′sis) Stricture of a lacrimal or nasal duct. [dacryo- + G. *stenōsis,* narrowing]

dac•tyl (dak′til) SYN digit. [G. *daktylos*]

dac•ty•li•tis (dak′ti-lī′tis) Inflammation of one or more fingers.

dactylo-, **dactyl-** Combining forms meaning the fingers, and (less often) toes. See entries under digit. [G. *daktylos,* finger]

dac•ty•lo•camp•sis (dak′ti-lō-kamp′sis) Permanent flexion of the fingers. [dactylo- + G. *kampsis,* bending]

dac•ty•lo•gry•po•sis (dak′ti-lō-gri-pō′sis) Permanent curvature or deformity of the fingers. [dactylo- + G. *grypōsis,* a crooking]

dac•ty•lol•y•sis (dak′ti-lol′i-sis) Spontaneous loss of digits, seen in leprosy, ainhum, and in utero when hair firmly wraps around the finger or toe, resulting in an amputation. [dactylo- + lysis]

dac•tyl•o•meg•a•ly (dak′til-ō-meg′ă-lē) SYN megadactyly. [dactylo- + G. *megas,* large]

dac•ty•lus, pl. **dac•ty•li** (dak′ti-lŭs, -lī) SYN digit. [G. *daktylos*]

DAF (dăf) Acronym for delayed auditory feedback.

Da Fa•no stain (dă fah′nō stān) A silver stain that produces a blackening of Golgi elements after tissues are fixed in a mixture of nitrate and formalin.

dag•ger flow•er (dag′ĕr flow′ĕr) SYN blue flag.

da-huang (dah-hwahng) SYN Chinese rhubarb.

dail•y val•ue (DV) (dā′lē val′yū) Standard values for daily nutrient intake developed for use on food labels in Canada and the U.S.

Dal•rym•ple sign (dal′rim-pĕl sīn) Retraction of the upper eyelid in Graves disease; abnormal wideness of the palpebral fissure present.

dal•ton (Da, D) (dawl′tŏn) Term unofficially used to indicate a unit of mass equal to 1/12 the mass of a carbon-12 atom, 1.0000 in the atomic mass scale; numerically, but not dimensionally, equal to molecular or particle weight (atomic mass units).

dal•ton•ism (dawl′tŏn-izm) Red green color blindness, transmitted as an X-linked trait.

Dal•ton law (dawl′tŏn law) Each gas in a mixture of gases exerts a pressure proportionate to the percentage of the gas and independent of the presence of the other gases present. SYN law of partial pressures.

DALYs (dā′lēz) Acronym and abbreviation for disability-adjusted life years.

dam (dam) **1.** Any barrier to the flow of fluid. **2.** SURGERY, DENTISTRY a sheet of thin rubber arranged so as to shut off the part operated upon from the access of fluid. [A.S. *fordemman,* to stop up]

dam•age risk cri•te•ri•a (dam′ăj risk krī-tēr′ē-ă) The maximum safe or allowable noise levels for various frequencies. The risk of suffering a hearing loss as a result of a specified noise exposure. Provides a method for determining the acceptable limits of noise exposure.

dam•i•an•a (dah-mē-ah′nah) Herbal made from *Turnera diffusa;* purported value as an aphrodisiac and weight-loss supplement; tetanic seizures reported. SYN herba de la pastora, miziboc. [Sp.]

dAMP Abbreviation for deoxyadenylic acid.

damp (damp) **1.** Humid; moist. **2.** Atmospheric moisture. **3.** Foul air in a mine; air charged with carbon oxides (black or choke damp) or with various explosive hydrocarbon vapors (firedamp).

Da•na op•er•a•tion (dā′nă op-ĕr-ā′shŭn) SYN posterior rhizotomy.

dance (dans) Rhythmic or patterned movement, particularly involuntary movements due to a CNS-related disorder.

Dance sign (dans sīn) A slight retraction in the neighborhood of the right iliac fossa in some cases of intussusception.

dan•der (dan′dĕr) **1.** A fine scaling of the skin and scalp. SEE ALSO dandruff. **2.** A normal effluvium of animal hair or coat capable of causing allergic responses in atopic people.

dan•druff (dan′drŭf) The presence, in varying amounts, of white or gray scales in the hair of the scalp, due to exfoliation of the epidermis. SEE ALSO seborrheic dermatitis. SYN scurf, seborrhea sicca (2).

Dan•dy op•er•a•tion (dan′dē op-ĕr-ā′shŭn) SEE third ventriculostomy, trigeminal rhizotomy.

Dan•dy-Walk•er syn•drome (dan′dē waw′kĕr sin′drōm) Developmental anomaly of the fourth ventricle associated with atresia of the foramina of Luschka and Magendie that results in cerebellar hypoplasia, hydrocephalus, and posterior fossa cyst formation.

Dane par•ti•cles (dān pahr′ti-kĕlz) The larger spheric forms of hepatitis-associated antigens; they comprise the virion of hepatitis B virus. See page B6.

Dane stain (dān stān) A stain for prekeratin, keratin, and mucin that employs hemalum, phloxine, Alcian blue, and orange G; nuclei appear orange to brown, acid mucopolysaccharides pale blue, and keratins orange to red-orange.

Dan•forth sign (dan′fōrth sīn) Shoulder pain on inspiration, due to irritation of the diaphragm by a hemoperitoneum in ruptured ectopic pregnancy.

Dan•iels•sen dis•ease (dan′yĕl′sen di-zēz′) SYN anesthetic leprosy.

DANS (dans) Acronym for 1-dimethylaminonaphthalene-5-sulfonic acid; a green fluorescing compound used in immunohistochemistry to detect antigens.

dan•syl (dns, DNS) (dan′sil) The 5-dimethylaminonaphthalene-1-sulfonyl radical; a blocking agent for NH_2 groups, used in peptide synthesis.

d'Ar•cet met•al (dahr-sā′ met′ăl) An alloy of lead, bismuth, and tin; used in dentistry.

Da•ri•er dis•ease (dah-rē-ā′ di-zēz′) SYN keratosis follicularis. See page B12.

Da•ri•er sign (dah-rē-ā′ sīn) Urtication on stroking of cutaneous lesions of urticaria pigmentosa (mastocytosis).

dark ad•ap•ta•tion (dahrk ad′ap-tā′shŭn) The visual adjustment occurring under reduced illumination in which the retinal sensitivity to light is increased. SEE ALSO dark-adapted eye. SYN scotopic adaptation.

dark-a•dapt•ed eye (dahrk-ă-dap′tĕd ī) An eye that has been in darkness or semidarkness and has undergone regeneration of rhodopsin (visual purple), which renders it more sensitive to reduced illumination. SYN scotopic eye.

dark cells (dahrk selz) Inner ear pigmented cells that secrete endolymph.

dark-field mi•cro•scope (dahrk-fēld mī′krō-skōp) A microscope that has a special condenser and objective with a diaphragm or stop that scatters light from the object observed, with the result that the object appears bright on a dark background.

dark green top tube (dahrk grēn-top tūb) Color denoting that the attached tube contains sodium heparin; used for the collection of heparinized plasma or whole blood for more specialized tests.

Dar•row red (dar′ō red) A basic oxazin dye, $C_{18}H_{14}N_3O_2Cl$, used as a substitute for cresyl violet acetate in the staining of Nissl substance.

dar•win•i•an (dahr-win′ē-ăn) Relating to or ascribed to Charles Darwin.

dar•win•i•an ev•o•lu•tion (dahr-win′ē-ăn ev-ō-lū′shŭn) The proposition that the phylogeny of all species is wholly ascribable to random variation (mutation) in genotypes and the operation of preferential survival of those resulting phenotypes most suited to survive in the contemporary environment.

dar•win•i•an re•flex (dahr-win′ē-ăn rē′fleks) The tendency of young infants to grasp a bar and hang suspended. Cf. grasping reflex.

dar•win•i•an tu•ber•cle (dahr-win′ē-ăn tū′bĕr-kĕl) SYN auricular tubercle.

DAS Abbreviation for developmental apraxia of speech.

da•ta (dā′tă) **1.** Facts (usually established by observation, measurement, or experiment) used as a basis for inference, testing, or models. **2.** Information collected about a patient, family, or community, often during intake of nursing history. USAGE NOTE the word is plural and takes a plural verb.

da•ta•base (dā′tă-bās) A collection of information on a given topic, stored digitally for rapid search and retrieval.

da•ta dic•tion•a•ry (dā′tă dik′shŭn-ār-ē) A set of standardized definitions of all data elements collected in a given health care facility.

date (dāt) A particular day of a particular month and year. [L. *data*, (document) issued]

date of birth (DOB) (dāt bĭrth) The day of birth of a patient or the insured party; often essential in determining eligibility, especially during coordination of benefits.

date boil, Del•hi boil, Jer•i•cho boil (dāt boyl, del′ē, jer′i-kō) The lesion occurring in cutaneous leishmaniasis.

date of ser•vice (DOS) (dāt sĕr′vis) In health care finance, the day when a therapy was initially provided; often of great importance in verifying charges covered with a third-party payer.

da•tum (dā′tŭm) An individual piece of information used in a scholarly field. The plural form is data. [L., *given*, fr. *do*, pp. *datum*, to give]

da•tum plane (dā′tŭm plān) An arbitrary plane used as a base from which to make craniometric measurements.

daugh•ter (daw′tĕr) In nuclear medicine, an isotope that is the disintegration product of a radionuclide. SEE daughter isotope, radionuclide generator. [O.E. *dohtor*]

daugh•ter cell (daw′tĕr sel) One of the two or more cells formed in the division of a parent cell.

daugh•ter cyst (daw′tĕr sist) A secondary cyst, usually multiple, derived from a mother cyst.

daugh•ter i•so•tope (daw′tĕr ī′sŏ-tōp) An element produced by radioactive decay of another. SEE ALSO radionuclide generator.

daugh•ter star (daw′tĕr stahr) One of the figures forming the diaster. SYN polar star.

dau•no•ru•bi•cin (daw′nō-rū′bi-sin) SYN rubidomycin.

Da•vis bat•ter•y mod•el of trans•duc•tion (dā′vis mod′ĕl trans-dŭk′shŭn) A concept in which the positive endocochlear potential and the negative intracellular potential of the hair cells provide the electromotive force to pass current through the reticular lamina of the organ of Corti.

Da•vis graft (dā′vis graft) "Pinch grafts," i.e., small pieces (2–3 mm) of full-thickness skin grafts.

DAW Abbreviation for dispense as written.

dawn phe•nom•e•non (dawn fĕ-nom′ĕ-non) Abrupt increases in fasting levels of plasma glucose concentrations between 5–9 AM in the absence of antecedent hypoglycemia; occurs in diabetic patients receiving insulin therapy.

Daw•son en•ceph•a•li•tis (daw′sŏn en-sef′ă-lī′tis) SYN subacute sclerosing panencephalitis.

day blind·ness (dā blīnd′nĕs) SYN hemeralopia.

day·sheet (dā′shēt) A page that lists all health care procedures, payments, and adjustments for a single day; used in some accounting systems.

dB Abbreviation for decibel.

DC Abbreviation for diphenylcyanoarsine; direct current; discharge; discontinue; Dental Corps; Doctor of Chiropractic.

D & C Abbreviation for dilation and curettage.

DCA Abbreviation for directional atherectomy.

dCMP Abbreviation for deoxycytidylic acid.

DD Abbreviation meaning date dictated, dictated; developmental disability.

D-di·mer (dī′mer) A covalently cross-linked degradation product released from the cross-linked fibrin polymer during plasmin-mediated fibrinolysis. Laboratory measurements of this product are made using latex bead assay, or enzyme-linked immunosorbent assay can be used to identify the presence of fibrinolysis; helpful in diagnosis of deep vein thrombosis.

DDS **1.** Abbreviation for Denver Developmental Screening Test. **2.** Abbreviation for Doctor of Dental Surgery.

DDT Abbreviation for dichloro-diphenyl-trichloroethane.

D & E Abbreviation for dilation and evacuation.

♻ **de-** Prefix meaning away from, cessation, without; sometimes has an intensive force. [L. *de*, from, away]

DEA Abbreviation for U.S. Drug Enforcement Administration.

de·ac·yl·ase (dē-as′il-ās) **1.** A member of the subclass of hydrolases (EC class 3), especially of that subclass of esterases, lipases, lactonases, and hydrolases (EC subclass 3.1). **2.** Any enzyme catalyzing the hydrolytic cleavage of an acyl group (R-CO-) in an ester linkage; also includes enzymes cleaving amide linkages (EC subclass 3.5) and similar acyl compounds.

dead arm syn·drome (ded ahrm sin′drōm) Sensory diminution or loss in an arm after anterior shoulder dislocation or subluxation.

dead-end host (ded-end hōst) A host from which infectious agents are not transmitted to other susceptible hosts.

dead-in-bed syn·drome (ded′in-bed′ sin′drōm) The finding of young, insulin-dependent diabetic patients without previous illness or abnormal glucose control dead in bed in the morning. Assumed to be due to hypoglycemia but it has been difficult to confirm that postmortem. Usually occurs in diabetic patients taking three daily doses of insulin, suggesting inadvertent administration of an erroneous dose, with lack of awareness of hypoglycemia during sleep.

dead·ly night·shade (ded′lē nīt′shād) SYN belladonna.

dead pulp (ded pŭlp) SYN necrotic pulp.

dead space (ded spās) A cavity, potential or real, remaining after the closure of a wound that is not obliterated by the operative technique. SEE anatomic dead space, physiologic dead space.

deaf (def) Unable to hear; hearing indistinctly; hard of hearing. [A.S. *deáf*]

deaf cul·ture (def kŭl′chŭr) Deafness perceived as a culture (rather than as a disability), which is characterized by having its own language, American Sign Language (ASL).

de·af·fer·en·ta·tion (dē-af′ĕr-ĕn-tā′shŭn) A loss of the sensory input from a portion of the body, usually caused by interruption of the peripheral sensory fibers. [L. *de*, from, + afferent]

deaf·mut·ism (def-myū′tizm) Inability to speak, due to congenital or early acquired profound deafness.

deaf·ness (def′nĕs) General term for loss of the ability to hear, without designation of the degree or cause of the loss.

de·al·co·hol·i·za·tion (dē-al′kŏ-hol-ī-zā′shŭn) The removal of alcohol from a fluid; in histologic technique, the removal of alcohol from a specimen that has been previously immersed in this fluid.

de·am·i·dase (dē-am′i-dās) SYN amidohydrolase.

de·am·i·da·tion, de·am·i·di·za·tion (dē-am′i-dā′shŭn, dē-am′i-dī-zā′shŭn) The hydrolytic removal of an amide group.

de·am·i·diz·ing en·zyme (dē-am′i-dīz-ing en′zīm) SYN amidohydrolase.

de·am·i·nas·es (dē-am′i-nā-sĕz) [EC group 3.5.4] Enzymes catalyzing simple hydrolysis of C—NH_2 bonds of purines, pyrimidines, and pterins. SYN deaminating enzymes.

de·am·i·nat·ing en·zymes (dē-am′i-nā′ting en′zīmz) SYN deaminases.

de·am·i·na·tion, de·am·i·ni·za·tion (dē′am-i-nā′shŭn, dē-am′i-nī-zā′shŭn) Removal, usually by hydrolysis, of the NH_2 group from an amino compound.

Dean fluo·ro·sis in·dex (dēn flūr-ō′sis in′deks) A measure of the degree of mottled enamel (fluorosis) in teeth; used most often in epidemiologic field studies.

de·ar·te·ri·al·i·za·tion (dē′ahr-tēr′ē-ăl-ī-zā′shŭn) Changing the character of arterial blood to that of venous blood; i.e., deoxygenation of blood.

death (deth) The irreversible cessation of life. In lower multicellular organisms, death is a gradual process at the cellular level, because tissues vary in their ability to withstand deprivation of oxygen; in higher organisms, a cessation of integrated tissue and organ functions; in humans, manifested by the loss of heartbeat, absence of spontaneous breathing, and cerebral death. SYN mors. [A.S. *dēath*]

death in•stinct (deth in′stingkt) The instinct of all living creatures toward self-destruction, death, or a return to the inorganic lifelessness from which they arose.

death rate (deth rāt) An estimate of the proportion of the population that dies during a specified period, usually a year; the numerator is the number of people dying, the denominator is the number in the population, usually an estimate of the number at the midperiod. SYN mortality rate, mortality (2).

death rat•tle (deth rat′ĕl) A respiratory noise from the pharynx or trachea of a dying person, caused by the loss of the cough reflex and accumulation of mucus.

death with dig•ni•ty (deth dig′ni-tē) An option chosen by a competent individual or one having power of attorney when he/she is incompetent to make an informed choice about actions to be taken when that individual is dying. Death with dignity often includes the implementation or withholding of various treatments as defined by the competent person and/or person with power of attorney. These treatments may range from the implementation of comfort measures, including pain control, antibiotic therapy, blood administration, cardiovascular medications, and palliative measures to life sustaining devices. Other treatments may include the withdrawal of life sustaining measures such as enteral feedings and resuscitative interventions, including CPR and medications.

Dea•ver in•ci•sion (dē′vĕr in-si′zhŭn) An incision in the right lower abdominal quadrant, with medial displacement of the rectus muscle.

De•Bak•ey clas•si•fi•ca•tion of a•or•tic dis•sec•tion (dĕ-bā′kē klas′i-fi-kā′shŭn ā-ōr′tik di-sek′shŭn) Consists of three types: type I extends into the transverse arch and distal aorta and type II is confined to the ascending aorta; type III dissections begin in the descending aorta, with type IIIA extending toward the diaphragm and type IIIB extending below it.

de•band•ing (dē-band′ing) The removal of fixed orthodontic appliances.

de•bil•i•tat•ing (dĕ-bil′i-tāt-ing) Denoting or characteristic of a morbid process that causes weakness.

de•bond (dē-bond′) To separate a dental appliance such as an orthodontic band from the tooth to which it has been attached or bonded by a resin cement. [de- + bond]

de•branch•ing en•zymes (dē-bran′ching en′zīmz) Enzymes that bring about destruction of branches in glycogen; a mixture of transferases and hydrolases.

dé•bride•ment (dā-brēd-mōn[h]′) **1.** Removal of foreign materials, necrotic matter, and devitalized tissue from a wound or burn. **2.** DENTISTRY involves scaling, root planing, and ultrasonic instrumentation of the root surfaces of teeth subgingivally to attain healthy periodontal tissue.

de•bris (dĕ-brē′) A useless accumulation of miscellaneous particles; waste in the form of fragments. [Fr. *débris,* fr. O.Fr. *desbrisier,* to break apart, (fr. *des-* down, away + *brisier* to break) rubble, rubbish]

debt (det) A deficit; a liability. [L. *debitum,* debt]

de•bulk•ing op•er•a•tion (dē-bŭlk′ing op-ĕr-ā′shŭn) Excision of a major part of a malignant tumor that cannot be completely removed, so as to enhance the effectiveness of subsequent radio- or chemotherapy.

♻ **deca- (da)** Prefix used in the S.I. and metric system to signify 10. Also spelled deka-. [G. *deka,* ten]

de•cal•ci•fi•ca•tion (dē-kal′si-fi-kā′shŭn) **1.** Removal of calcium salts from bones and teeth, either in vitro or as a result of a pathologic process. **2.** Precipitation of calcium from blood as by oxalate or fluoride, or the conversion of blood calcium to an un-ionized form as by citrate, thus preventing or delaying coagulation. [L. *de-,* away, + *calx* (*calc-*), lime, + *facio,* to make]

de•cal•ci•fy•ing (dē-kal′si-fī-ing) Denoting an agent, measure, or process that causes decalcification.

de•can•nul•a•tion (de-kan′yū-lā′shŭn) Planned or accidental removal of a tracheostomy tube.

de•ca•pac•i•ta•tion (dē′kă-pas-i-tā′shŭn) Prevention of sperms from undergoing capacitation and thus from becoming able to fertilize oocytes.

de•cap•i•ta•tion (dē′kap-i-tā′shŭn) Removal of a head.

de•cap•su•la•tion (dē′kap-sū-lā′shŭn) Incision and removal of a capsule or enveloping membrane.

de•car•box•yl•ase (dē′kahr-bok′sil-ās) Any enzyme (EC subclass 4.1.1) that removes a molecule of carbon dioxide from a carboxylic group.

de•car•box•yl•a•tion (dē′kahr-bok-sil-ā′shŭn) A reaction involving the removal of a molecule of carbon dioxide from a carboxylic acid.

de•cay (dĕ-kā′) **1.** Destruction of an organic substance by slow combustion or gradual oxidation. **2.** SYN putrefaction. **3.** To deteriorate; to undergo slow combustion or putrefaction. **4.** DENTISTRY caries. **5.** PSYCHOLOGY loss of information registered by the senses and processed into short-term memory. SEE ALSO memory. **6.** Loss of radioactivity over time; spontaneous emission of radiation or charged particles or both from an unstable nucleus. **7.** SYN disintegration. [L. *de,* down, + *cado,* to fall]

de•cay con•stant (dĕ-kā′ kon′stănt) The fractional change in the number of atoms of a radionuclide that occurs in a unit of time; the constant l in the equation for the fraction (DN/N) of the number of atoms (N) of a radionuclide disintegrating in time *Dt, DN/N* = – *lDt.* SYN radioactive constant.

de•cay the•o•ry (dĕ-kā′ thē′ŏr-ē) A theory of forgetting based on the premise that an engram or memory trace dissipates progressively with time during the interval when it is not activated.

de•cel•er•a•tion (dē-sel′ĕr-ā′shŭn) **1.** A slowing of contractions during the first stage of labor. **2.** A slowing of the fetal heart rate during uterine contractions. [de- + as*celeration*]

de•cer•e•brate (dē-ser′ĕ-brāt) **1.** To cause decerebration. **2.** Denoting an animal so prepared, or a patient whose brain has suffered an injury causing neurologic impairment comparable with that of a decerebrate animal.

de•cer•e•brate ri•gid•i•ty (dē-ser′ĕ-brāt ri-jid′i-tē) A postural change that occurs in some comatose patients, consisting of episodes of opisthotonos, rigid extension of the limbs, internal rotation of the upper extremities, and marked plantar flexion of the feet; produced by a variety of metabolic and structural brain disorders. SEE ALSO decorticate rigidity.

de•cer•e•bra•tion (dē-ser′ĕ-brā′shŭn) Removal of the brain above the lower border of the corpora quadrigemina, or a complete section of the brain at this level or somewhat below.

de•cho•les•ter•ol•i•za•tion (dē′kō-les′tĕr-ol-ī-zā′shŭn) Therapeutic reduction of the cholesterol concentration of the blood.

deci- (d) Prefix used in the SI and metric system to signify one tenth (10^{-}). [L. *decimus,* tenth]

dec•i•bel (dB) (des′i-bĕl) One tenth of a bel; unit for expressing the relative loudness of sound on a logarithmic scale. [L. *decimus,* tenth, + bel]

de•cid•u•a (dē-sij′ū-ă) The endometrium of the pregnant uterus that has undergone changes, under the influence of hormones produced by the ovarian (ovulation) cycle, to prepare it for the implantation and nutrition of the blastocyst; so-called because the membrane is cast off after labor. SYN deciduous membrane, membrana decidua. [L. falling off (qualifying *membrana,* membrane, understood)]

de•cid•u•a ba•sa•lis (dē-sij′ū-ă bā-sā′lis) [TA] The area of endometrium between the implanted chorionic sac and the myometrium, which develops into the maternal part of the placenta. SYN decidua serotina.

de•cid•u•a cap•su•lar•is (dē-sij′ū-ă kap-sū-lā′ris) [TA] The layer of endometrium overlying the implanted chorionic sac; it becomes progressively attenuated as the chorionic sac enlarges and, by the fourth month, is squeezed against the decidua parietalis and thereafter undergoes rapid regression. SYN decidua reflexa, membrana adventitia.

de•cid•u•al (dĕ-sij′ū-ăl) Relating to the decidua.

de•cid•u•al cell (dĕ-sij′ū-ăl sel) An enlarged, ovoid connective tissue cell appearing in the endometrium of pregnancy.

de•cid•u•a men•stru•a•lis (dē-sij′ū-ă men-strū-ā′lis) The succulent mucous membrane of the nonpregnant uterus at the menstrual period.

de•cid•u•a pa•ri•e•tal•is (dē-sij′ū-ă pă-rī-ĕ-tā′lis) The altered endometrium lining the main cavity of the pregnant uterus other than at the site of attachment of the chorionic sac. SYN decidua vera.

de•cid•u•a po•ly•po•sa (dē-sij′ū-ă pol-i-pō′să) Decidua parietalis showing polypoid projections of the endometrial surface.

de•cid•u•a re•flex•a (dē-sij′ū-ă rē-fleks′ă) SYN decidua capsularis.

de•cid•u•a ser•o•ti•na (dē-sij′ū-ă ser-ō-tī′nă) SYN decidua basalis.

de•cid•u•a spon•gi•o•sa (dē-sij′ū-ă spŏn-jē-ō′să) The portion of the decidua basalis attached to the myometrium.

de•cid•u•a•tion (dĕ-sij′ū-ā′shŭn) Shedding of endometrial tissue during menstruation. [L. *deciduus,* falling off]

de•cid•u•a ve•ra (dē-sij′ū-ă vēr′ă) SYN decidua parietalis.

de•cid•u•i•tis (dē-sij′ū-ī′tis) Inflammation of the decidua.

de•cid•u•o•ma (dĕ-sij′ū-ō′mă) An intrauterine mass of decidual tissue, probably the result of hyperplasia of decidual cells retained in the uterus. SYN placentoma.

de•cid•u•ous (dĕ-sij′ū-ŭs) **1.** Not permanent; denoting that which eventually falls off. **2.** DENTISTRY referring to the first or primary dentition. SEE deciduous tooth. [L. *deciduus,* falling off]

de•cid•u•ous den•ti•tion (dĕ-sij′ū-ŭs den-tish′ŭn) SYN deciduous tooth. See page 410.

de•cid•u•ous mem•brane (dĕ-sij′ū-ŭs mem′brān) SYN decidua.

de•cid•u•ous tooth (dĕ-sij′ū-ŭs tūth) One of the first set of teeth, comprising 20 in all, that erupts between the mean ages of 6 and 28

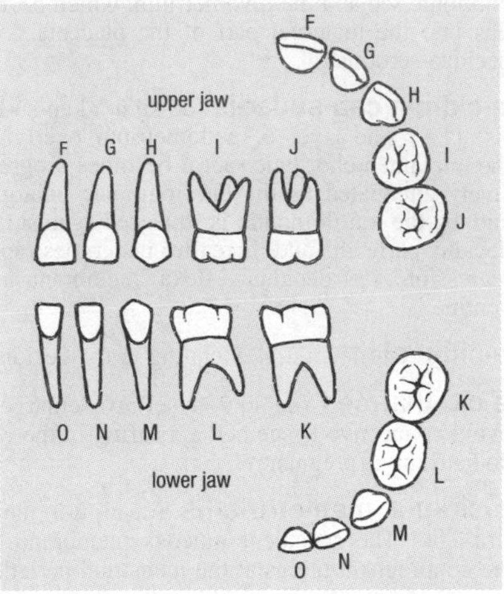

deciduous dentition, half view, left side (lettering code, universal system of deciduous teeth): central incisor F, O; lateral incisor G, N; canine H, M; first molar I, L; second molar J, K

months of life. SYN dens deciduus [TA], baby tooth, deciduous dentition, milk dentition, milk tooth, primary dentition, primary tooth, temporary tooth.

dec·i·me·ter (des′i-mē-tĕr) One tenth of a meter. SYN decimetre.

decimetre [Br.] SYN decimeter.

de·ci·sion (dĕ-sizh′ŭn) A conclusion or judgment reached after consideration of an issue or proposal. [L. *decido*, to cut off, decide]

de·ci·sion tree (dĕ-sizh′ŭn trē) A graphic construct showing available choices at each decision node of managing a clinical problem along with probabilities (if known) of possible outcomes for patient's freedom from disability, life expectancy, and mortality.

de·clamp·ing phe·nom·e·non (dē-klamp′ing fĕ-nom′ĕ-non) Shock or hypotension following abrupt release of clamps from a large portion of the vascular bed, as from the aorta; apparently caused by transient pooling of blood in a previously ischemic area. SYN declamping shock.

de·clamp·ing shock (dē-klamp′ing shok) SYN declamping phenomenon.

dec·li·na·tion (dek′li-nā′shŭn) A bending, sloping, or other deviation from a normal vertical position. [L. *declinatio*, a bending aside]

de·clive (dē-klīv′) [TA] The posterior sloping portion of the monticulus of the vermis of the cerebellum; vermal lobule caudal to the primary fissure. SYN declivis. [L. *declivis*, sloping downward, fr. *clivus*, a slope]

de·cli·vis (dē-klī′vis) SYN declive.

de·com·pen·sa·tion (dē-kom′pĕn-sā′shŭn) **1.** A failure of compensation in heart disease. **2.** The appearance or exacerbation of a mental disorder due to failure of defense mechanisms.

de·com·po·si·tion (dē-kŏm′pŏ-zish′ŭn) SYN putrefaction.

de·com·pres·sion (dē-kŏm-presh′ŭn) Removal of pressure. [L. *de-*, from, down, + *comprimo*, pp. *-pressus*, to press together]

de·com·pres·sion sick·ness (dē-kŏm-presh′ŭn sik′nĕs) A symptom complex caused by the escape from solution in the body fluids of nitrogen bubbles absorbed originally at high atmospheric pressure, as a result of abrupt reduction in atmospheric pressure (either rapid ascent to high altitude or return from a compressed-air environment); it is characterized by headache; pain in the arms, legs, joints, and epigastrium; itching of the skin; vertigo; dyspnea; coughing; choking; vomiting; weakness; sometimes paralysis; and severe peripheral circulatory collapse. SYN caisson disease.

de·con·ges·tant (dē-kŏn-jes′tănt) **1.** Having the property of reducing congestion. **2.** An agent that reduces congestion.

de·con·tam·i·na·tion (dē-kŏn-tam′i-nā′shŭn) Removal or neutralization of poisonous gas or other injurious agents from the environment, or from victims of such agents.

de·cor·ti·cate ri·gid·i·ty (dĕ-kōr′ti-kāt ri-jid′i-tē) A unilateral or bilateral postural change, in which the upper extremities are flexed and adducted and the lower extremities are held in rigid extension; due to structural lesions of the thalamus, internal capsule, or cerebral white matter.

de·cor·ti·ca·tion (dē-kōr′ti-kā′shŭn) **1.** Removal of the cortex, or external layer, beneath the capsule from any organ or structure. **2.** An operation to remove a clot and scar tissue that formed after a hemothorax or neglected empyema. [L. *decortico*, pp. *-atus*, to deprive of bark, fr. *de*, from, + *cortex*, rind, bark]

de·coy cell (dē′koy sel) Benign exfoliated epithelial cell with pyknotic nucleus seen in urinary infections; may be mistaken for a malignant cell.

de·cru·des·cence (dē-krū-des′ĕns) Abatement of the symptoms of disease. [L. *de*, from, + *crudesco*, to become worse, fr. *crudus*, crude]

de·cu·bi·tal (dē-kyū′bi-tăl) Relating to a decubitus ulcer.

de·cu·bi·tus (dē-kyū′bi-tŭs) **1.** The position of the patient in bed; e.g., dorsal decubitus, lateral decubitus. SEE ALSO decubitus film. **2.** Sometimes used in referring to a decubitus ulcer. See page B29. [L. *decumbo*, to lie down]

de·cu·bi·tus film (dē-kyū′bi-tŭs film) A radiograph exposed with the subject in the decubitus position; named for the side that is dependent.

de·cu·bi·tus pro·jec·tion (dē-kyū′bi-tŭs prŏ-jek′shŭn) RADIOLOGY procedure in which a patient to be x-rayed is placed in a decubitus position, with the x-ray beam directed horizontally.

de·cu·bi·tus ul·cer (dē-kyū′bi-tŭs ŭl′sĕr) Focal ischemic necrosis of skin and underlying tissues at sites of constant pressure or recurring friction in patients confined to bed or immobilized by illness; malnutrition worsens the prognosis. SEE decubitus. See this page. SYN bedsore, bed sore, pressure sore, pressure ulcer.

de·cus·sate (dē-kŭs′āt) **1.** To cross. **2.** Crossed like the arms of an X. [L. *decusso,* pp. *-atus,* to make in the form of an X, fr. *decussis,* a large, bronze Roman coin marked with an X to indicate its denomination]

de·cus·sa·ti·o, pl. **de·cus·sa·ti·o·nes** (dē′kŭ-sā′shē-ō, ōnēz) **1.** In general, any crossing over or intersection of parts. **2.** The intercrossing of two homonymous fiber bundles as each crosses over to the opposite side of the brain in the course of its ascent or descent through the brainstem or spinal cord. SYN decussation. [L. (see decussate)]

de·cus·sa·ti·o lem·ni·sco·rum (dē′kŭ-sā′shē-ō lem-ni-skō′rŭm) SYN decussation of medial lemniscus.

de·cus·sa·tion (dē-kŭs-ā′shŭn) SYN decussatio. [L. *decussatio*]

de·cus·sa·ti·o·nes teg·men·ti (dē′kŭ-sā′shē-ō′nēz teg-men′tī) SYN tegmental decussations.

de·cus·sa·tion of me·di·al lem·nis·cus (dē-kŭs-ā′shŭn mē′dē-ăl lem-nis′kŭs) The intercrossing of the fibers of the left and right medial lemniscus ascending from the gracile and cuneate nuclei, immediately rostral to the level of the decussation of the pyramidal tracts in the medulla oblongata. SYN decussatio lemniscorum.

de·cus·sa·tion of su·pe·ri·or cer·e·bel·lar pe·dun·cles (dē-kŭs-ā′shŭn sŭ-pēr′ē-ŏr ser′ĕ-bel′ăr pĕ-dŭng′kĕlz) The decussation of the left and right superior cerebellar peduncles in the tegmentum of the caudal mesencephalon.

de·cus·sa·ti·o py·ra·mi·dum (dē′kŭ-sā′shē-ō pir-ă-mid′ŭm) [TA] SYN pyramidal decussation.

de·dif·fer·en·ti·a·tion (dē-dif′ĕr-en′shē-ā′shŭn) **1.** The return of parts to a more homogeneous state. **2.** SYN anaplasia.

de·duc·ti·ble (dĕ-dŭk′ti-bĕl) The amount for which the insured is responsible before the health care plan pays; amount usually set on an annual basis. SYN annual deductible.

de·duc·tion (dĕ-dŭk′shŭn) The logical derivation of a conclusion based on certain premises. The conclusion will be true if the premises are true and the deductive argument is valid. Cf. induction (9).

deep ar·ter·y of arm (dēp ahr′tĕr-ē ahrm) SYN profunda brachii artery.

deep ar·ter·y of clit·o·ris (dēp ahr′tĕr-ē klit′ŏr-is) The deep terminal branch of the internal pudendal artery in the female; it supplies the crus of the clitoris. SYN arteria profunda clitoridis [TA].

deep ar·ter·y of pe·nis (dēp ahr′tĕr-ē pē′nis) *Origin,* terminal branch (with dorsal artery of penis) of the internal pudendal artery; *distribution,* corpus cavernosum of the penis through capillary beds and through helicine arteries and arteriovenous anastomoses to produce erection. SYN arteria profunda penis [TA].

deep ar·ter·y of thigh (dēp ahr′tĕr-ē thī) *Origin,* femoral; *branches,* lateral circumflex femoral, medial circumflex femoral, terminating in three or four perforating arteries. SYN arteria profunda femoris, profunda femoris artery.

deep au·ri·cu·lar ar·ter·y (dēp awr-ik′yū-lar ahr′tĕr-ē) *Origin,* first part of maxillary; *distribution,* articulation of jaw, parotid gland, and external acoustic meatus and external tympanic membrane; *anastomoses,* auricular branches of superficial temporal and posterior auricular. SYN arteria auricularis profunda.

deep branch of ra·di·al nerve (dēp branch rā′dē-al nĕrv) Originates in cubital fossa (with superficial branch) as termination of (common) radial nerve; pierces supinator, supplying it and other extensors of forearm. Its terminal portion is the posterior interosseous nerve, which runs on

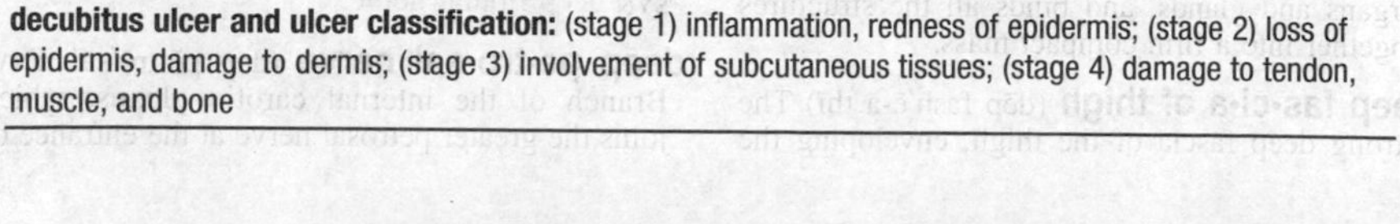

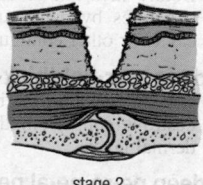

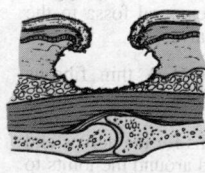

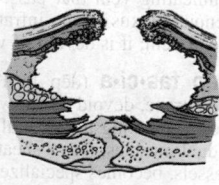

decubitus ulcer and ulcer classification: (stage 1) inflammation, redness of epidermis; (stage 2) loss of epidermis, damage to dermis; (stage 3) involvement of subcutaneous tissues; (stage 4) damage to tendon, muscle, and bone

the interosseous membrane in the distal third of the forearm. SYN ramus profundus nervi radialis.

deep branch of ul•nar nerve (dēp branch ŭl′năr nĕrv) Accompanies deep palmar branch of ulnar artery and deep palmar arch to supply wrist joint, lumbricals 3 and 4, palmar and dorsal interossei, adductor pollicis, and deep head of flexor pollicis brevis muscles. SYN ramus profundus nervi ulnaris.

deep ce•re•bral veins (dēp ser′ĕ-brăl vānz) The numerous veins draining the deep structures of the cerebral hemispheres; they empty into the tributaries of the great cerebral vein. SYN venae profundae cerebri [TA].

(deep) cer•vi•cal fas•ci•a (dēp sĕr′vi-kăl fash′ē-ă) Fascia of the neck; it is divided into an external or investing layer (superficial lamina) that surrounds the neck and encloses the trapezius and sternocleidomastoid muscles, a middle or pretracheal layer in relation to the infrahyoid muscles and cervical viscera, and a deep or prevertebral layer applied to the vertebrae and axial muscles.

deep cer•vi•cal vein (dēp sĕr′vi-kăl vān) Large vein running with the artery of the same name between the semispinalis capitis and semispinalis cervicis, draining the deep muscles at the back of the neck and emptying into the brachiocephalic or the vertebral vein.

deep cir•cum•flex il•i•ac ar•ter•y (dēp sir′kŭm-fleks il′ē-ak ahr′tĕr-ē) *Origin*, external iliac; *distribution*, muscles and skin of lower abdomen, sartorius, and tensor fasciae latae; *anastomoses*, lumbar, inferior epigastric, superior gluteal, iliolumbar, and superficial circumflex iliac. SYN arteria circumflexa iliaca profunda.

deep dor•sal vein of clit•o•ris (dēp dōr′săl vān klit′ŏr-is) A tributary of the vesical venous plexus; it runs a course deep to the fascia on the dorsum of the clitoris. SYN vena dorsalis profunda clitoridis [TA].

deep dor•sal vein of pe•nis (dēp dōr′săl vān pē′nis) A vein on the dorsum of the penis deep to the fascia of the penis; it is a tributary to the prostatic venous plexus. SYN vena dorsalis profunda penis [TA].

deep fa•cial vein (dēp fā′shăl vān) The communicating vein that passes from the pterygoid venous plexus of the infratemporal fossa to the facial vein; it is devoid of valves.

deep fas•ci•a (dēp fash′ē-ă) A thin fibrous membrane, devoid of fat, which invests the muscles, separating the several groups and the individual muscles, forms sheaths for the nerves and vessels, becomes specialized around the joints to form or strengthen ligaments, envelops various organs and glands, and binds all the structures together into a firm compact mass.

deep fas•ci•a of thigh (dēp fash′ē-ă thī) The strong deep fascia of the thigh, enveloping the muscles of the thigh and thickened laterally as the iliotibial tract.

deep fem•o•ral vein (dēp fem′ŏr-ăl vān) Accompanies the deep femoral artery, receiving perforating veins from the lateral and posterior aspects of the thigh. It joins the femoral vein in the femoral triangle, usually in common with the medial and lateral circumflex femoral veins.

deep fi•bu•lar nerve (dēp fib′yū-lăr nĕrv) A terminal branch of the common peroneal nerve, arising at the fibular neck and passing into the anterior compartment of the leg; it supplies the tibialis anterior, extensor hallucis longus, extensor digitorum longus, and peroneus tertius muscles in the leg, then crosses the ankle joint to supply the muscles on the dorsum of the foot (extensor hallucis and digitorum brevis), becoming cutaneous to innervate adjacent sides of the great and second toes. SYN anterior tibial nerve, deep peroneal nerve, nervus fibularis profundus, nervus peroneus profundus.

deep in•gui•nal ring (dēp ing′gwi-năl ring) The opening in the transversalis fascia through which the ductus deferens (or round ligament in the female) and gonadal vessels enter the inguinal canal. Located midway between anterior superior iliac spine and pubic tubercle; bounded medially by the lateral umbilical ligament (inferior epigastric vessels) and inferiorly by the inguinal ligament; indirect inguinal hernias exit the abdominal cavity through the deep inguinal ring.

deep la•mel•lar en•do•the•li•al ker•a•to•plas•ty (DLEK) (dēp lă-mel′ăr en′dō-thē′lē-ăl ker′ă-tō-plas-tē) A surgical procedure whereby only the inner retinal layers are subject to transplantation.

deep lin•gual ar•ter•y (dēp ling′gwăl ahr′tĕr-ē) Termination of lingual artery; *distribution*, muscles and mucous membrane of under surface of tongue.

deep lin•gual vein (dēp ling′gwăl vān) The principal vein of the tongue that accompanies the deep lingual artery and joins the lingual vein; drains the body and apex of the tongue, running posteriorly near the median plane; often visible through the mucosa on the underside of the tongue, to each side of the frenulum.

deep neck in•fec•tion (dēp nek in-fek′shŭn) Bodily invasion of tissues and cavity of neck structures by pathogens originating in the oral cavity or other contiguous area.

deep par•tial-thick•ness burn (dēp pahr′shăl-thik′nĕs bŭrn) A burn or thermal injury that destroys cells from the epidermis to the deep dermal layer.

deep pe•ro•ne•al nerve (dēp per′ō-nē′ăl nĕrv) SYN deep fibular nerve.

deep pe•tro•sal nerve (dēp pĕ-trō′săl nĕrv) Branch of the internal carotid plexus, which joins the greater petrosal nerve at the entrance of the pterygoid canal forming the nerve of the pterygoid canal and thus provides postsynaptic fibers to the pterygopalatine ganglion. SYN nervus petrosus profundus, radix sympathica ganglii pterygopalatini, sympathetic root of pterygopalatine ganglion.

deep plan·tar (ar·te·ri·al) arch (dēp plan′tahr ahr-tēr′ē-ăl ahrch) **1.** The arterial arch formed by the lateral plantar artery running across the bases of the metatarsal bones and anastomosing with the dorsalis pedis artery via the deep plantar artery. **2.** Either of two bony arches of the foot, longitudinal arch or transverse arch.

deep plan·tar ar·ter·y (dēp plan′tahr ahr′tĕr-ē) Deep plantar branch of arcuate artery or its first metatarsal artery branch that penetrates the foot between first and second metatarsal bones to anastomose with the termination of the plantar arterial arch. SYN arteria plantaris profunda [TA].

deep re·flex (dēp rē′fleks) An involuntary muscular contraction following percussion of a tendon or bone. SYN jerk (2).

deep tem·po·ral ar·ter·y (dēp tem′pŏr-ăl ahr′tĕr-ē) Anterior and posterior branches; *origin*, maxillary; *distribution*, temporal muscle and periosteum, bone and diploe of temporal fossa; *anastomoses*, branches of superficial temporal, lacrimal, and middle meningeal. SYN arteria temporalis profunda.

deep tem·po·ral nerves (dēp tem′pŏr-ăl nĕrvz) Two branches, anterior and posterior, from the mandibular nerve, supplying the temporalis muscle and periosteum of the temporal fossa. SYN nervi temporales profundi [TA].

deep ten·don re·flex (dēp ten′dŏn rē′fleks) SYN myotactic reflex.

deep tis·sue mas·sage (dēp tish′ū mă-sahzh′) A group of massage techniques designed to access deep layers of muscle and fascia to improve alignment, reduce levels of resting tension, and create more efficient postural and movement patterns. Includes rolfing, myofascial release, and structural integration.

deep trans·verse per·i·ne·al mus·cle (dēp trans-vĕrs′ per′i-nē′ăl mŭs′ĕl) *Origin*, ramus of ischium; *insertion*, with its fellow in a median raphe; *action*, assists sphincter urethrae with some sphincteric action on vagina in female; *nerve supply*, pudendal (dorsal nerve of penis/clitoris). SYN musculus transversus perinei profundus [TA].

deep vein of pe·nis (dēp vān pē′nis) The vein to the deep fascia on the dorsum of the penis; it enters the prostatic plexus by passing through a gap between the arcuate pubic ligament and the transverse perineal ligament.

deep veins of clit·o·ris (dēp vānz klit′ŏr-is) The veins that pass from the dorsum of the clitoris to join the vesical plexus.

deep ve·nous throm·bo·sis (DVT) (dēp vē′nŭs throm-bō′sis) Formation of one or more thrombi in the deep veins, usually of the lower extremity or in the pelvis; carries a high risk of pulmonary embolism. SEE ALSO thrombophlebitis.

deer·fly fe·ver (dēr′flī fē′vĕr) SYN tularemia.

DEERS Abbreviation for Defense Enrollment Eligibility Record System.

def, DEF Abbreviation for decayed, extracted, or filled tooth.

defaecation [Br.] SYN defecation.

DEF car·ies in·dex (def kār′ēz in′deks) An index of past caries experience that includes decayed, extracted, and filled deciduous teeth; sometimes the extracted portion (e) is not included.

def·e·cate (def′ĕ-kāt) To perform defecation.

def·e·ca·tion (def-ĕ-kā′shŭn) The discharge of feces from the rectum. SYN defaecation, movement (3). [L. *defaeco*, pp. *-atus*, to remove the dregs, purify]

de·fe·cog·ra·phy (def′ĕ-kog′ră-fē) Radiographic examination of the act of defecation of a radiopaque stool. [defecation + G. *graphō*, to write]

de·fect (dē-fekt′) An imperfection, anomaly, malformation, dysfunction, or absence; a qualitative departure from what is expected. USAGE NOTE often confused with deficiency, which is a quantitative shortcoming. [L. *deficio*, pp. *-fectus*, to fail, to lack]

de·fec·tive (dĕ-fek′tiv) Denoting or exhibiting a defect; imperfect; a failure of quality.

de·fec·tive bac·te·ri·o·phage (dĕ-fek′tiv bak-tēr′ē-ō-fāj) A temperate bacteriophage mutant the genome of which does not contain all of the normal components and cannot become a fully infectious virus, yet it can replicate indefinitely in the bacterial genome as a defective probacteriophage; many defective bacteriophages are mediators of transduction.

de·fec·tive vi·rus (dĕ-fek′tiv vī′rŭs) A virus particle that contains insufficient nucleic acid to provide for production of all essential viral components.

defence [Br.] SYN defense.

defence mechanism [Br.] SYN defense mechanism.

de·fense (dĕ-fens′) **1.** The psychological mechanisms used to control anxiety, e.g., rationalization, projection. **2.** Any protective posture, drug, or device. SYN defence. [L. *defendo*, to ward off]

De·fense En·roll·ment El·i·gi·bil·i·ty Re·cord Sys·tem (DEERS) (dĕ-fens′ en-rōl′mĕnt el′i-ji-bil′i-tē rek′ŏrd sis′tĕm) The system used by the U.S. military to determine coverage for insurance benefits.

de·fense mech·a·nism (dĕ-fens′ mek′ă-nizm) **1.** A psychological means of coping with conflict or anxiety (e.g., conversion, denial, dissociation, rationalization, repression, sublimation). **2.** The psychic structure underlying a coping strategy. **3.** Immunologic mechanism versus nonspecific defense mechanism. SYN defence mechanism.

de·fen·sins (dē-fen′sinz) A class of basic antibiotic peptides, found in neutrophils, which apparently kill bacteria by causing membrane damage. [L. *de-fendo,* pp. *de-fensum,* to repel, avert, + -in]

de·fen·sive med·i·cine (dĕ-fen′siv med′i-sin) Diagnostic or therapeutic measures conducted primarily as a safeguard against possible subsequent malpractice liability.

de·fen·sive·ness (dē-fen′siv-nĕs) Excessive reaction to nonnoxious stimuli, across one or more sensory systems. SEE ALSO tactile defensiveness.

def·er·ent (def′ĕr-ĕnt) Carrying away. [L. *deferens,* pres. p. of *defero,* to carry away]

def·er·ent duct (def′ĕr-ĕnt dŭkt) SYN ductus deferens.

def·er·en·tec·to·my (def′ĕr-en-tek′tō-mē) SYN vasectomy. [(ductus) deferens, + G. *ektomē,* excision]

def·er·en·tial (def′ĕr-en′shăl) Relating to the ductus deferens.

def·er·en·tial ar·ter·y (def′ĕr-en′shăl ahr′tĕr-ē) SYN artery to ductus deferens.

def·er·en·ti·tis (def′ĕr-en-tī′tis) Inflammation of the ductus deferens. SYN vasitis.

de·fer·ves·cence (def′ĕr-ves′ĕns) Falling of an elevated temperature; abatement of fever. [L. *defervesco,* to cease boiling, fr. *de-* neg. + *fervesco,* to begin to boil]

de·fi·bril·la·tion (dē-fib′ri-lā′shŭn) The arrest of fibrillation of the cardiac muscle (atrial or ventricular) with restoration of the normal rhythm.

de·fi·bril·la·tor (dē-fib′ri-lā-tōr) **1.** Any agent or measure (e.g., an electric shock) that arrests fibrillation of the atria or ventricles and restores the normal rhythm. **2.** The machine designed to administer a defibrillating electric shock.

de·fi·bri·na·tion (dē-fī′bri-nā′shŭn) Removal of fibrin from the blood, usually by means of constant agitation while the blood is collected in a container with glass beads or chips.

de·fi·cien·cy (dĕ-fish′ĕn-sē) An insufficient quantity of some substance (as in dietary deficiency, hemoglobin deficiency as in marrow aplasia), organization (as in mental deficiency), activity (as in enzyme deficiency or reduced oxygen-carrying capacity of the blood), or other process or component of which the amount present is of decreased quantity. SEE ALSO deficiency disease. [L. *deficio,* to fail, fr. *facio,* to do]

de·fi·cien·cy dis·ease (dĕ-fish′ĕn-sē di-zēz′) Any disorder resulting from undernutrition or an inadequacy of calories, proteins, essential amino acids, fatty acids, vitamins, or trace minerals.

de·fi·cien·cy symp·tom (dĕ-fish′ĕn-sē simp′tŏm) Manifestation of a lack, in varying degrees, of some substance (e.g., hormone, enzyme, vitamin) necessary for normal structure and/or function of an organism.

def·i·cit (def′i-sit) The result of consuming or losing something faster than it is replenished or replaced. [L. *deficio,* to fail]

de·fi·ning char·ac·ter·is·tics (dĕ-fīn′ing kar′ăk-tĕr-is′tiks) NURSING signs and symptoms associated with a specific nursing diagnosis.

def·i·ni·tion (def′i-nish′ŭn) In optics, the power of a lens to give a distinct image. SEE ALSO resolving power. [L. *de-finio,* pp. *-finitus,* to bound, fr. *finis,* limit]

de·fin·i·tive (dĕ-fin′i-tiv) Fully differentiated or developed.

de·fin·i·tive host (dĕ-fin′i-tiv hōst) One in which a parasite reaches the adult or sexually mature stage.

de·flec·tion (dĕ-flek′shŭn) **1.** A moving to one side. **2.** In the electrocardiogram, a deviation of the curve from the isoelectric base line; any wave or complex of the electrocardiogram. [L. *de-flecto,* pp. *-flexus,* to bend aside]

de·flex·ion (dĕ-flek′shŭn) Term used to describe the position of the fetal head in relation to the maternal pelvis in which the head is descending in a nonflexed or extended attitude. [de- + L. *flexio,* a bending, fr. *flecto,* pp. *flexum,* to bend]

de·flu·vi·um (dē-flū′vē-ŭm) SYN defluxion (2). [L. fr. *de-fluo,* pp. *-fluxus,* to flow down]

de·flux·ion (dē-flŭk′shŭn) **1.** A falling down or out, as of the hair. SEE ALSO effluvium. **2.** A flowing down or discharge of fluid. SYN defluvium. [L. *defluxio, de-fluo,* pp. *-fluxus,* to flow down]

de·for·ma·tion (dē-fōr-mā′shŭn) **1.** Deviation of form from normal; specifically, an alteration in shape or structure of a previously normally formed part. It occurs after organogenesis and often involves the musculoskeletal system (e.g., clubfoot). **2.** SYN deformity. **3.** RHEOLOGY the change in the physical shape of a mass by applied stress. [L. *de-formo,* pp. *-atus,* to deform, fr. *forma,* form]

de·for·mi·ty (dĕ-fōrm′i-tē) A permanent structural deviation from the normal shape or size, resulting in disfigurement; may be congenital or acquired. SYN deformation (2).

defs, DMFS Abbreviation for decayed, missing, or filled tooth surfaces.

deft, DMFT Abbreviation for decayed, missing, or filled teeth.

de Ga·lan·tha stain (dā gă-lanth'ă stān) Stain used to demonstrate sodium urate monohydrate crystals in gout.

de·gen·er·ate 1. (dē-jen'ĕr-āt) To pass to a lower level of mental, physical, or moral state; to fall below the normal or acceptable type or state. **2.** (dē-jen'ĕr-ăt) Below the normal or acceptable; that which has passed to a lower level.

de·gen·er·a·tion (dĕ-jen'ĕr-ā'shŭn) **1.** Deterioration; passing from a higher to a lower level or type. **2.** A worsening of mental, physical, or moral qualities. **3.** A retrogressive pathologic change in cells or tissues, in consequence of which their functions are often impaired or destroyed; sometimes reversible; in the early stages, necrosis results. [L. *degeneratio*]

de·gen·er·a·tive (dĕ-jen'ĕr-ă-tiv) Relating to degeneration.

de·gen·e·ra·tive disc dis·ease (dĕ-jen'ĕr-ă-tiv disk di-zēz') Protrusion, herniation, or fragmentation of an intervertebral disc beyond its borders with potential compression of a nerve root, the cauda equina in the lumbar region, or the spinal cord at higher levels.

de·gen·er·a·tive joint dis·ease (dĕ-jen'ĕr-ă-tiv joynt di-zēz') SYN osteoarthritis.

de·glov·ing (dē-glŏv'ing) **1.** Intraoral surgical exposure of the anterior mandible used in various orthognathic surgical operations such as genioplasty or mandibular alveolar surgery. **2.** SEE degloving injury.

de·glov·ing in·ju·ry (dē-glŏv'ing in'jŭr-ē) Avulsion of the skin of the hand (or foot) in which the part is skeletonized by removal of most or all of the skin and subcutaneous tissue.

de·glu·ti·tion (dē-glū-tish'ŭn) The act of swallowing. [L. *de-glutio*, to swallow]

de·glu·ti·tion syn·co·pe (dē-glū-tish'ŭn sing'kŏ-pē) Faintness or unconsciousness on swallowing. This is nearly always due to excessive vagal effect on a heart that may already have bradycardia or atrioventricular block.

deg·ra·da·tion (deg'ră-dā'shŭn) The change of a chemical compound into a less complex compound. [L. *degradatus*, degrade]

de·gree (dĕ-grē') **1.** One of the divisions on the scale of a measuring instrument such as a thermometer or barometer. SEE Comparative Temperature Scales appendix; scale. **2.** The 360th part of the circumference of a circle. **3.** A position or rank within a graded series. **4.** A measure of damage to tissue. [Fr. *degré;* L. *gradus*, a step]

de·grees of free·dom (dĕ-grēz' frē'dŏm) **1.** The number of planes (e.g., one, two, or three) within which a joint can move. **2.** The variety of possible movement combinations that can occur within a segment of the human body.

de·gus·ta·tion (dē-gŭs-tā'shŭn) **1.** The act of tasting. **2.** The sense of taste. [L. *degustatio*, fr. *de-gusto*, pp. *-atus*, to taste]

De·hi·o test (dĕ-hē'ō test) If an injection of atropine relieves bradycardia, the condition is due to action of the vagus; if it does not, the condition may be due to an affliction of the heart itself.

de·his·cence (dē-his'ĕns) A bursting open, splitting, or gaping along natural or sutured lines. See this page. [L. *dehisco*, to split apart or open]

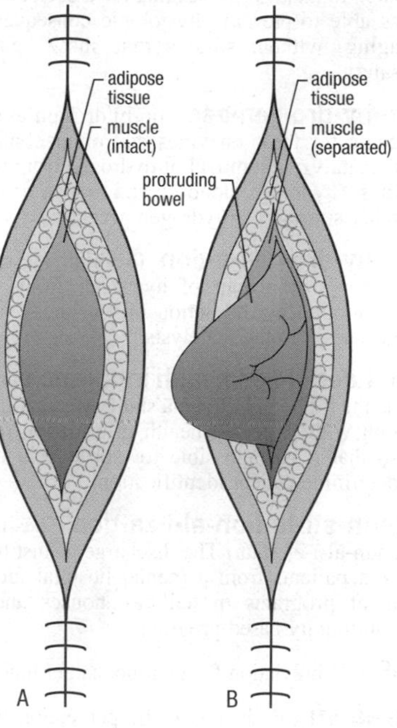

wounds: (A) dehiscence; (B) evisceration

de·hu·mid·i·fi·er (dē'hyū-mid'i-fī-ĕr) Equipment used to remove moisture from air.

de·hy·drase (dē-hī'drās) Former name for dehydratase.

de·hy·dra·tase (dē-hī'dră-tās) A subclass (EC 4.2.1) of lyases (hydrolyases) that remove H and OH as H_2O from a substrate, leaving a double bond, or add a group to a double bond by the elimination of water from two substances to form a third.

de·hy·dra·tion (dē-hī-drā′shŭn) **1.** Deprivation of water. SYN anhydration. **2.** Process of losing body water, progressing either from the hyperhydrated state to euhydration or from euhydration downward to hypohydration. **3.** SYN excision (2). **4.** SYN desiccation.

♻**dehydro-** Prefix used in the names of chemical compounds that differ from more familiar compounds in the absence of two hydrogen atoms; e.g., dehydroascorbic acid, which resembles ascorbic acid in all structural features except for its lack of two hydrogen atoms that are present in the ascorbic acid molecule. In systematic nomenclature, didehydro- is preferred as being more exact.

11-de·hy·dro·cor·ti·cos·ter·one (dē-hī′drō-kōr-ti-kos′tĕr-ōn) A metabolite of corticosterone, found in the cortex of suprarenal gland.

de·hy·dro·ep·i·and·ros·ter·one (DHEA) (dē-hī′drō-ep-ē-an-dros′tĕr-ōn) Steroid agent related to male hormones that have been advocated as able to prevent physiologic consequences of aging, without studies that show benefit or safety.

de·hy·dro·gen·ase (dē-hī′drō-jen-ās) Class name for those enzymes that oxidize substrates by catalyzing removal of hydrogen from metabolites (hydrogen donors) and transferring it to other substances (hydrogen acceptors).

de·hy·dro·gen·a·tion (dē-hī′drō-jĕ-nā′shŭn) Removal of a pair of hydrogen atoms from a compound by the action of enzymes (dehydrogenases) or other catalysts.

de·i·den·ti·fied health in·for·ma·tion (dē′ī-den′ti-fīd helth in′fŏr-mā′shŭn) Medical information with protected health information removed so that it is impossible for subsequent users to determine patient identification.

de·in·sti·tu·tion·al·i·za·tion (dē-in′sti-tū′shŭn-ăl-ī-zā′shŭn) The discharge of institutionalized patients from a mental hospital into treatment programs in halfway houses and other community-based programs.

DEJ Abbreviation for dentinoenamel junction.

dé·jà vu (dā-zhah vū) The perception that one has previously experienced a new experience. SEE ALSO jamais vu. [Fr., already seen]

de·jec·tion (dĕ-jek′shŭn) SYN depression (4). [L. *dejectio,* fr. *de- jicio,* pp. *-jectus,* to cast down]

De·je·rine dis·ease (dĕ-zhĕ-rēn′ di-zēz′) SYN Dejerine-Sottas disease.

De·je·rine hand phe·nom·e·non (dĕ-zhĕ-rēn′ hand fĕ-nom′ĕ-non) Clonic contractions of the flexors of the hand (wrist) on tapping the dorsum of the hand or the volar side of the forearm near the wrist; occurs in normal people but is exaggerated in pyramidal tract lesions.

De·je·rine-Klump·ke syn·drome (dĕ-zhĕ-rēn′ klump′ke sin′drōm) Injury or lesion of the inner cord of the brachial plexus; marked by numbness, hyperesthesia, pain on the ulnar side of the arm, and atrophy of hand muscles with eventual paralysis. Also associated with vision defects and Horner syndrome

De·je·rine sign (dĕ-zhĕ-rēn′ sīn) Aggravation of symptoms of root irritation by the acts of coughing, sneezing, or straining to defecate.

De·je·rine-Sot·tas dis·ease (dĕ-zhĕ-rēn′-sō-tahz′ di-zēz′) A familial type of demyelinating sensorimotor polyneuropathy that begins in early childhood and is slowly progressive; clinically characterized by foot pain and paresthesias, followed by symmetric weakness and wasting of the distal limbs; one of the causes of stork legs; patients are nonambulatory at an early age; peripheral nerves are palpably enlarged and nontender; pathologically, onion bulb formation is seen in the nerves: whorls of overlapping, intertwined Schwann cell processes that encircle bare axons; usually autosomal recessive inheritance. SYN Dejerine disease, progressive hypertrophic polyneuropathy.

♻**deka-** SEE deca-.

Del·a·field flu·id (dĕl′ă-fēld flū′id) Histologic fixative; contains alcohol and acetic, osmic, and chromic acids.

Del·a·field he·ma·tox·y·lin (del′ă-fēld hē′mă-toks′i-lin) An alum type of hematoxylin used in histology; natural ripening takes about 2 months and the solution is good for years.

de·lam·i·na·tion (dē-lam′i-nā′shŭn) Division into separate layers. [L. *de,* from, + *lamina,* a thin plate]

de·lay (dĕ-lā′) Postponement or deferral to a later time. [O.Fr. *deslaier,* fr. Germanic]

de·layed al·ler·gy (dĕ-lād′ al′ĕr-jē) A type IV allergic reaction; so called because in a sensitized subject the reaction becomes evident hours after contact with the allergen (antigen), reaches its peak after 36–48 hours, then recedes slowly. Associated with cell-mediated responses. SEE ALSO delayed reaction. Cf. immediate allergy.

de·layed au·di·tor·y feed·back (DAF) (dĕ-lād′ aw′di-tōr-ē fēd′bak) **1.** A time-lapsed auditory signal that is recorded and then played back with a delay of a set number of milliseconds. **2.** A system used for speech and stuttering treatment in which the subject's voice is recorded and played back, through an earpiece, with a time delay. The distraction caused by the altered feedback enhances fluency and slows speech rate for some users.

de·layed den·ti·tion (dĕ-lād′ den-tish′ŭn) Delayed eruption of the teeth.

de·layed flap (dĕ-lād′ flap) A flap raised in its

donor area in two or more stages to increase its chances of survival after transfer.

de·layed graft (dĕ-lād′ graft) Application of a skin graft after waiting several days for healthy granulations to form.

de·layed on·set mus·cle sore·ness (DOMS) (dĕ-lād on′set mus′ĕl sōr′nĕs) A state of muscular pain and discomfort that begins several hours after a period of intense exercise, particularly with eccentric muscle actions; state usually persists from 24 to 48 hours; thought to be due to microtrauma to muscle fibers.

de·layed pu·ber·ty (dĕ-lād′ pyū′bĕr-tē) Lack of any signs of puberty by age 14 years in either sex.

de·layed re·ac·tion (dĕ-lād′ rē-ak′shŭn) A local or generalized immune response that begins 24–48 hours after exposure to an antigen. SEE cell-mediated reaction.

de·layed u·nion (dĕ-lād′ yū′nyŭn) Healing of a fracture that takes longer than expected.

Del·bet sign (del-bā′ sīn) In aneurysm of a main artery, maintenance of nutrition in distal tissues indicates efficient collateral circulation even when the pulse has disappeared.

de-lead (dē-led′) To cause the mobilization and excretion of lead deposited in the bones and other tissues, as by the administration of a chelating agent.

del·e·te·ri·ous (del′ĕ-tēr′ē-ŭs) Injurious; noxious; harmful. [G. *dēlētērios,* fr. *dēleomai,* to injure]

de·le·tion (dĕ-lē′shŭn) GENETICS any spontaneous elimination of part of the normal genetic complement, whether cytogenetically visible (chromosomal deletion) or inferred from phenotypic evidence (point deletion). [L. *deletio,* destruction]

Delf·ti·a a·cid·o·vor·ans (delf′shē-ă as′id-ō-vōr′anz) Formerly classified as *Comamonas acidovorans.* Aerobic, non-spore-forming, gram-negative bacilli found in the environment (e.g., as in soil, water) and on plants including fruits and vegetables. *D. acidovorans* has been reported as agent of bacteremia, intravenous drug use–related endocarditis, and acute suppurative otitis.

del·i·ques·cence (del′i-kwes′ĕns) Becoming damp or liquid by absorption of water from the atmosphere; a property of certain salts, such as $CaCl_2$. [L. *de-liquesco,* to melt or become liquid]

de·lir·i·ous (dĕ-lir′ē-ŭs) In a state of delirium.

de·lir·i·um, pl. **de·li·ri·a** (dĕ-lir′ē-ŭm, -ă) An altered state of consciousness, consisting of confusion, distractibility, disorientation, disordered thinking and memory, defective perception (illusions and hallucinations), prominent hyperactivity, agitation, and autonomic nervous system overactivity; caused by a number of toxic structural and metabolic disorders. [L. fr. *deliro,* to be crazy, fr. *de-* + *lira,* a furrow (*i.e.,* go out of the furrow)]

de·lir·i·um tre·mens (DTs) (dĕ-lir′ē-ŭm trĕ′mĕnz) A severe, sometimes fatal, form of delirium due to alcoholic withdrawal after a period of sustained intoxication. SYN oenomania. [L. pres. p. of *tremo,* to tremble]

de·liv·er (dĕ-liv′ĕr) **1.** To assist a woman in childbirth. **2.** To extract from an enclosed place, as the fetus from the womb, an object or foreign body, e.g., a tumor from its capsule or surroundings, or the lens of the eye in cases of cataract. [fr. O. Fr. fr. L. *de-* + *liber,* free]

de·liv·er·y (dĕ-liv′ĕr-ē) Passage of the fetus and the placenta from the genital canal into the external world.

del·le (del′ĕ) The central lighter-colored portion of the erythrocyte, as observed in a stained film of blood. [Ger. *Delle,* low ground, pit]

del·len (del′ĕn) Shallow, saucerlike, clearly defined excavations at the margin of the cornea, about 1.5 by 2 mm, due to localized dehydration; also called Fuchs dellen. [Ger. pl. of *Delle,* low ground, pit]

De·lorme op·er·a·tion (dĕ-lōrm′ op-ĕr-ā′shŭn) Surgical correction of rectal prolapse by plicaton of redundant mucosa rather than resection.

del·phi·an node (del′fē-ăn nōd) A midline prelaryngeal lymph node, adjacent to the thyroid gland, enlargement of which is indicative of thyroid disease or early metastasis from the subglottic larynx.

del·ta (Δ, δ) (del′tă) **1.** Fourth letter of the Greek alphabet. **2.** CHEMISTRY a double bond, usually with a superscript to indicate position in a chain (Δ^5); application of heat in a reaction ($A \xrightarrow{\Delta} B$); absence of heat treatment ($\not\Delta$); distance between two atoms in a molecule, or position of a substituent located on the fourth atom from the carboxyl or other primary functional group (δ); change (Δ); thickness (δ); chemical shift in NMR (δ). **3.** ANATOMY a triangular surface.

del·ta a·gent (del′tă ā′jĕnt) SYN hepatitis D virus.

del·ta (δ)-a·mi·no·bu·tyr·ic ac·id a·mi·no·trans·fer·ase (del′tă ă-mē′nō-byū-tir′ik as′id ă-mē′nō-trans′fĕr-ās) An enzyme catalyzing the reversible transfer of an amino group from δ-aminobutyric acid to 2-oxoglutarate, thus forming an L-glutamic acid and succinate semialdehyde. An important step in the catabolism of δ-aminobutyric acid.

del·ta (δ)-a·mi·no·lev·u·lin·ic ac·id (ALA) (del′tă ă-mē′nō-lev-yū-lin′ik as′id) An acid formed by δ-aminolevulinate synthase from glycine and succinyl-coenzyme A; a precursor of porphobilinogen, hence an important intermediate in the biosynthesis of hematin. ALA levels are elevated in cases of lead poisoning.

del•ta bil•i•ru•bin (del′tă bil′i-rū′bin) The fraction of bilirubin covalently bound to albumin.

del•ta cell (del′tă sel) **1.** A variety of cell in the anterior lobe of the hypophysis that has basophilic granules. **2.** A cell of the islets of Langerhans, with fine granules that stain with aniline blue; secretes somatostatin.

del•ta check (del′tă chek) A comparison of consecutive values for a given test in a patient's laboratory file used to detect abrupt changes, usually generated as a part of computer-based quality control programs.

del•ta fi•bers (del′tă fī′bĕrz) Nerve fibers with conduction velocities in the range of 8–30 m/sec.

del•ta gran•ule (del′tă gran′yūl) A granule of a delta cell.

del•ta hep•a•ti•tis (del′tă hep′ă-tī′tis) SYN viral hepatitis type D.

del•ta rhythm (del′tă ridh′ŭm) A wave pattern in the electroencephalogram in the frequency band of 1.5–4.0 Hz. SYN delta wave (2).

del•ta test (del′tă test) Comparison between the current results of a laboratory test and the previous test results for the same patient. [δ(delta), math. symbol for change in a variable]

del•ta wave (del′tă wāv) **1.** A premature upstroke of the QRS complex due to an atrioventricular bypass tract as in Wolff-Parkinson-White syndrome. **2.** SYN delta rhythm.

del•toid (del′toyd) **1.** Resembling the Greek letter delta (Δ); triangular. **2.** SYN deltoid muscle. [G. *deltoeidēs,* shaped like the letter *delta*]

del•toid lig•a•ment (del′toyd lig′ă-mĕnt) Compound ligament consisting of four component ligaments that pass downward from the medial malleolus of the tibia to the tarsal bones: 1) tibionavicular ligament (pars tibionavicularis [TA]), 2) tibiocalcaneal ligament (pars tibiocalcanea [TA]), 3) anterior tibiotalar ligament (pars tibiotalaris anterior), and 4) posterior tibiotalar ligament (pars tibiotalaris posterior). SYN ligamentum deltoideum.

i **del•toid mus•cle** (del′toyd mŭs′ĕl) *Origin*, lateral third of clavicle, lateral border of acromion process, lower border of spine of scapula; *insertion*, lateral side of shaft of humerus a little above its middle (deltoid tuberosity); *action*, abduction, flexion, extension, and rotation of arm; *nerve supply*, axillary from fifth and sixth cervical spinal cord segments through brachial plexus. See this page. SYN musculus deltoideus [TA], deltoid (2).

del•toid tu•ber•os•i•ty (del′toyd tū′bĕr-os′i-tē) The prominence at the middle section of the lateral humerus that marks the point of attachment for the deltoid muscle.

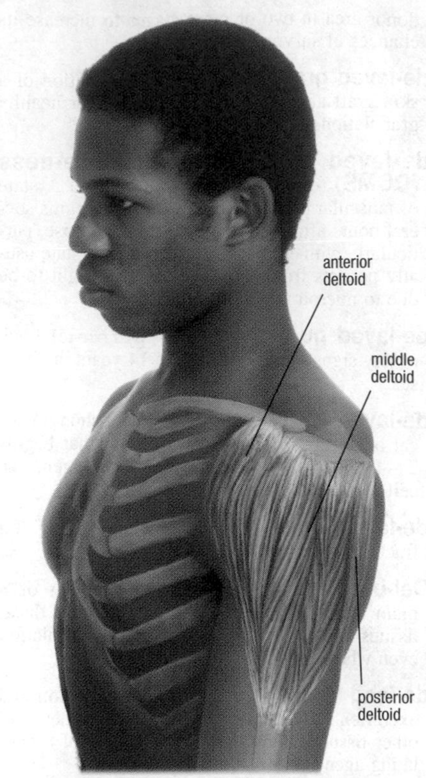

deltoid muscle

de•lu•sion (dĕ-lū′zhŭn) A false belief or wrong judgment held with conviction despite incontrovertible evidence to the contrary. [L. *de-ludo,* pp. *-lusus,* to play false, deceive, fr. *ludo,* to play]

de•lu•sion•al (dĕ-lū′zhŭn-ăl) Relating to a delusion.

de•lu•sion of gran•deur (dĕ-lū′zhŭn gran′dyŭr) A mental disorder in which one believes oneself possessed of great wealth, intellect, importance, or power.

de•lu•sion of ne•ga•tion (dĕ-lū′zhŭn nĕ-gā′shŭn) A delusion in which one imagines that the world and all that relates to it have ceased to exist.

de•lu•sion of per•se•cu•tion, per•se•cu•to•ry de•lu•sion (dĕ-lū′zhŭn pĕr′sĕ-kyū′shŭn, pĕr′sĕ-kyū-tōr-ē dĕ-lū′zhŭn) A false notion that one is being persecuted; characteristic symptom of paranoid schizophrenia.

de•mand (dĕ-mand′) **1.** To ask, claim, or require with urgency or authority. **2.** The act or result of demanding. [Med.L. *demandare*]

de•mand ox•y•gen de•li•ver•y de•vice (dĕ-mand′ ok′si-jĕn dĕ-liv′ĕr-ē dĕ-vīs′) Apparatus that conserves oxygen by sensing the initiation of an inspiratory effort and then delivering oxygen only during the inspiratory phase. Usually attached to a nasal cannula.

de•mand pace•mak•er (dĕ-mand′ pās′mā-kĕr) A form of artificial pacemaker usually implanted into cardiac tissue because its output of electrical stimuli can be inhibited by endogenous cardiac electrical activity; stimulates heart when that organ's impulses are not sufficient.

de•mat•i•a•ceous (dē-mat′ē-ā′shŭs) Denoting dark conidia and/or hyphae, usually brown or black; used frequently to denote dark-colored fungi.

de•mat•i•a•ceous fun•gi (dē-mat′ē-ā′shŭs fŭng′gī) Dark fungi that form melanin. [Mod. L. *Dematium* (genus name), fr. G. *demation,* fine strand, fr. *dema,* band, fr. *deō,* to bind + suffix *-aceous,* characterized by]

de•men•ti•a (dĕ-men′shē-ă) The loss, usually progressive, of cognitive and intellectual functions, without impairment of perception or consciousness; caused by a variety of disorders including severe infections and toxins, but most commonly associated with structural brain disease. Characterized by disorientation, impaired memory, judgment, and intellect, and a shallow labile affect. SYN amentia. [L. fr. *de-* priv. + *mens,* mind]

♲**demi-** Prefix meaning half, lesser. SEE ALSO hemi-, semi-. [Fr. fr. L. *dimidius,* half]

dem•i•gaunt•let ban•dage (dem′ē-găwnt′lĕt ban′dăj) A gauntlet bandage that covers only the hand, leaving the fingers exposed.

dem•i•lune (dem′ē-lūn) **1.** A small body with a form similar to that of a half-moon or a crescent. **2.** Term frequently applied to the gametocyte of *Plasmodium falciparum.* [Fr. half-moon]

de•min•er•al•i•za•tion (dē-min′ĕr-ăl-ī-zā′shŭn) A loss or decrease of the mineral constituents of the body or individual tissues, especially of bone.

Dem•o•dex (dem′ō-deks) A genus of minute mites that inhabit the skin and are usually found in the sebaceous glands and hair follicles. [G. *dēmos,* tallow, + *dēx,* a woodworm]

dem•o•di•co•sis (dem′ō-di-kō′sis) Infestation by mites of the species *Demodex,* chiefly involving hair follicles and characterized by varying degrees of local inflammation and immune response.

de•mog•ra•phy (dĕ-mog′ră-fē) The study of populations, especially with reference to size, density, fertility, mortality, growth rate, age distribution, migration, and vital statistics. [G. *demos,* people, + *graphō,* to write]

De Mor•gan spot (dĕ mōr′găn spot) SYN senile hemangioma.

de Mor•si•er syn•drome (dĕ mōr′sē-ā sin′drōm) SYN septooptic dysplasia.

de•mul•cent (dĕ-mŭl′sĕnt) **1.** Soothing; relieving irritation. **2.** An agent, such as a mucilage or oil, that soothes and relieves irritation, especially of the mucous surfaces. [L. *de-mulceo,* pp. *-mulctus,* to stroke lightly, to soften]

de Mus•set sign (dĕ mū-sā′ sīn) SYN Musset sign.

de•my•e•li•nat•ing dis•ease (dē-mī′ĕ-li-nāt-ing di-zēz′) Generic term for a group of diseases, of unknown cause, in which there is extensive loss of the myelin in the central nervous system, as in multiple sclerosis.

de•my•e•li•na•tion, **de•my•e•lin•i•za•tion** (dē-mī′e-lin-ā′shŭn, dē-mī′ĕ-lin-ī-zā′shŭn) Loss of myelin with preservation of the axons or fiber tracts. Central demyelination occurs within the central nervous system (e.g., the demyelination seen with multiple sclerosis); peripheral demyelination affects the peripheral nervous system (e.g., the demyelination seen with Guillain-Barré syndrome).

demyelinisation [Br.] SYN demyelinization.

de•na•tur•a•tion (dē-nā′chŭr-ā′shŭn) The process of becoming denatured.

de•na•tured (dē-nā′chŭrd) **1.** Made unnatural or changed from the normal; often applied to proteins or nucleic acids heated or otherwise treated to the point where tertiary structural characteristics are altered. **2.** Adulterated, as by addition of methanol to ethanol.

den•dri•form (den′dri-fōrm) Tree-shaped, or branching. SYN arborescent, dendritic (1), dendroid. [G. *dendron,* tree, + L. *forma,* form]

den•dri•form ker•a•ti•tis, den•drit•ic ker•a•ti•tis (den′dri-fōrm ker′ă-tī′tis, den-drit′ik) A form of herpetic keratitis.

den•drite (den′drīt) **1.** One of the two types of branching protoplasmic processes of the nerve cell (the other being the axon). SYN dendritic process, dendron, neurodendrite. **2.** A crystalline treelike structure formed during the freezing of an alloy. [G. *dendritēs,* relating to a tree]

den•drit•ic (den-drit′ik) **1.** SYN dendriform. **2.** Relating to the dendrites of nerve cells.

den•drit•ic cell (den-drit′ik sel) Cell of neural crest origin with extensive processes; they develop melanin early.

den•drit•ic cor•ne•al ul•cer (den-drit′ik kōr′nē-ăl ŭl′sĕr) Keratitis caused by herpes simplex virus.

den•drit•ic pro•cess (den-drit′ik pros′es) SYN dendrite (1).

den•drit•ic spines (den-drit′ik spīnz) Variably long excrescences of nerve cell dendrites, varying in shape from small knobs to thornlike or filamentous processes, usually more numerous on distal dendrite arborizations than on the proximal part of dendritic trunks; they are a preferential site of synaptic axodendritic contact; sparse or absent in some types of nerve cells (motor neurons, the large cells of the globus pallidus, stellate cells of the cerebral cortex), exceedingly numerous in others such as the pyramidal cells of the cerebral cortex and the Purkinje cells of the cerebellar cortex. SYN gemmule (2).

den•droid (den′droyd) SYN dendriform. [G. *dendron,* tree, + *eidos,* appearance]

den•dron (den′dron) SYN dendrite (1). [G. a tree]

de•ner•vate (dē′nĕr-vāt) To cause loss of neural supply.

de•ner•va•tion (dē′nĕr-vā′shŭn) Loss of nerve supply.

den•gue, **den•gue hem•or•rhag•ic fe•ver, den•gue fe•ver** (den-gā′, den-gā′ hem′ŏr-aj′ik fē′vĕr, den-gā′ fē′vĕr) A disease of tropic and subtropic regions, caused by dengue virus and transmitted by a mosquito of the genus *Aedes.* Four grades of severity are recognized: grade I, fever and constitutional symptoms; grade II, spontaneous bleeding (of skin, gums, or gastrointestinal tract); grade III, agitation and circulatory failure; and grade IV, profound shock. [Sp. corruption of "dandy" fever]

den•gue vi•rus (den-gā′ vī′rŭs) A virus of the genus flavivirus; the etiologic agent of dengue in humans and also occurring in monkeys and chimpanzees, usually as an inapparent infection; four serotypes are recognized; transmission is effected by mosquitoes of the genus *Aedes.*

de•ni•al (dĕ-nī′ăl) An unconscious defense mechanism used to allay anxiety by denying the existence of important conflicts or troublesome impulses. SYN negation. [M.E., fr, O. Fr., fr. L. *denegare,* to say no]

de•ni•al man•age•ment (dĕ-nī′ăl man′ăj-mĕnt) A possibly criminal procedure whereby insurers employ subsidiary firms to find reasons to deny payment on legitimate claims.

den•i•da•tion (den′i-dā′shŭn) Exfoliation of the superficial portion of the mucous membrane of the uterus; stripping off of the menstrual decidua. [L. *de,* from, + *nidus,* nest]

de•nied claim (dē-nīd′ klām) A statement from a third-party payer that a claim (i.e., a bill) sent for reimbursement has not been paid for some reason (e.g., clerical error, patient's lack of coverage).

Den•is Browne pouch (den′is brown powch) A pocket formed between scarpa and external oblique fascia adjacent to external inguinal ring; a common lodging site for an undescended testis (as in cryptorchism).

Den•is Browne splint (den′is brown splint) A light aluminum splint applied to the lateral aspect of the leg and foot; used for clubfoot.

Den•nie-Mor•gan fold, **Den•nie line** (den′ē mōr′găn fold, den′ē līn) A fold or line below each lower eyelid caused by edema in atopic dermatitis.

De•non•vill•iers fas•ci•a (dĕ-nōn[h]-vē-ā′ fash′ē-ă) Extension of endopelvic fascia covering anterior extraperitoneal rectum and lying between prostate and rectum; important landmark in radical prostatectomy.

dens, pl. **den•tes** (denz, den′tēz) [TA] **1.** SYN tooth. **2.** A strong toothlike process projecting superiorly from the body of the axis (second cervical vertebra), around which the atlas rotates. SYN odontoid process of epistropheus. [L.]

dens ca•ni•nus, pl. **den•tes ca•ni•ni** (denz kā-nī′nŭs, den′tēz kā-nī′nē) [TA] SYN canine tooth.

dens de•ci•du•us, pl. **den•tes de•ci•du•i** (denz dē-sid′yū-ŭs, den′tēz dē-sid′yū-ī) [TA] SYN deciduous tooth.

dens in den•te (denz den′tē) A developmental disturbance in tooth formation resulting from invagination of the epithelium associated with crown development into the area destined to become pulp space; after calcification there is an invagination of enamel and dentin into the pulp space, giving the radiographic appearance of a "tooth within a tooth."

dense bod•ies (dens bŏd′ēz) **1.** Granules in the central granulomere of blood platelets that take up and store serotonin from plasma. **2.** Electron-dense bodies containing α-actinin in the cytoplasm of smooth muscle cells, believed to be homologous to the Z-lines of striated muscle.

den•sim•e•ter (den-sim′ĕ-tĕr) SYN densitometer (1). [L. *densitas,* density, + G. *metron,* measure]

dens in•ci•si•vus, pl. **den•tes in•ci•si•vi** (denz in-si-sī′vŭs, den′tēz in-si-sī′vī) [TA] SYN incisor tooth.

den•si•tom•e•ter (dens′i-tom′ĕ-tĕr) **1.** An instrument for measuring the density of a fluid. SYN densimeter. **2.** An instrument for measuring, by virtue of relative turbidity, the growth of bacteria in broth; useful in microbiologic assay of nutrients and antibiotics and phage studies. **3.** An instrument for measuring the density of components (e.g., protein fractions) separated by electrophoresis or chromatography, using light absorption or reflection. **4.** An electronic instrument for measuring the blackening of radiographic film by x-ray exposure; used for film densitometry, bone densitometry, measurement of line spread function (microdensitometer). [L. *densitas,* density, + G. *metron,* measure]

den·si·tom·e·try (dens′i-tom′ĕ-trē) SYN underwater weighing.

den·si·ty (dens′i-tē) **1.** The compactness of a substance; the ratio of mass to unit volume, usually expressed as $g:cm^3$ ($kg:m^3$ in the SI system). **2.** The quantity of electricity on a given surface or in a given time per unit of volume. **3.** RADIOLOGIC PHYSICS the opacity to light of an exposed radiographic or photographic film; the darker the film, the greater the measured density. **4.** CLINICAL RADIOLOGY a less-exposed area on a film, corresponding to a region of greater x-ray attenuation (radiopacity) in the subject; the more light transmitted by the film, the greater the density of the subject; this is not actually the opposite of the sense 3 definition, because one concerns film density and the other subject density. [L. *densitas,* fr. *densus,* thick]

dens mo·la·ris, pl. **den·tes mo·la·res** (denz mō-lā′ris, den′tēz mō-lā′rēz) [TA] SYN molar tooth. SEE ALSO molar.

dens per·ma·nens, pl. **den·tes per·ma·nen·tes** (denz pĕr′mă-nenz, den-tēz′ pĕr-mă-nen′tēz) [TA] SYN permanent tooth.

dens pre·mo·la·ris, pl. **den·tes pre·mo·la·res** (denz prē-mō-lā′ris, den-tez′ prē-mō-lā′rēz) [TA] SYN premolar tooth.

dens se·ro·ti·nus (denz sē-rō-tī′nŭs) [TA] SYN third molar tooth.

♲**dent-**, **denti-**, **dento-** Combining forms meaning teeth; dental. SEE ALSO odonto-. [L. *dens,* tooth]

den·tal (den′tăl) Relating to the teeth. [L. *dens,* tooth]

den·tal ab·scess, **den·to·al·ve·o·lar ab·scess** (den′tăl ab′ses, den′to-al-vē′ō-lăr ab′ses) SYN alveolar abscess.

den·tal ac·quired pel·li·cle (den′tăl ă-kwīrd′ pel′i-kĕl) A thin membranous layer, amorphous, acellular, and organic, which forms on exposed tooth surfaces, dental restorations, and dental calculus deposits.

den·tal a·nat·o·my (den′tăl ă-nat′ŏ-mē) That branch of gross anatomy concerned with the morphology of teeth and their location, position, and relationships.

den·tal an·ky·lo·sis (den′tăl ang′ki-lō′sis) Rigid fixation of a tooth to the surrounding alveolus as a result of ossification of the ligament; prevents eruption and orthodontic movement.

den·tal an·thro·po·lo·gy (den′tăl an′thrŏ-pol′ŏ-jē) A branch of physical anthropology concerned with the origin, evolution, and development of the dentitions of primates, especially humans, and to the relationship between primates' dentition and their physical, social, and cultural relationships.

den·tal arch (den′tăl ahrch) The curved structure formed by the natural dentition and the residual ridge, which remains after the loss of some or all of the natural teeth.

den·tal as·sis·tant (den′tăl ă-sis′tănt) A person trained to provide support to a dentist with general tasks ranging from clerical work and assistance at chairside to laboratory, infection control, dental laboratory, and exposure of radiographic images.

den·tal bulb (den′tăl bŭlb) The papilla, derived from mesenchyme, which forms the part of the primordium of a tooth that is situated within the cup-shaped enamel organ.

den·tal cal·cu·lus (den′tăl kal′kyū-lŭs) **1.** Calcified deposits formed around the teeth; may appear as subgingival or supragingival calculus. **2.** SYN tartar (1).

den·tal crypt (den′tăl kript) The space filled by the dental follicle.

den·tal cur·ette (den′tăl kyūr-et′) A curved dental instrument used for scaling, root planing, and gingival curettage.

den·tal en·do·scope (den′tăl en′dō-skōp) An illuminated optic instrument that is inserted into the periodontal pocket to provide the clinician with direct vision of subgingival root conditions.

den·tal fol·li·cle (den′tăl fol′i-kĕl) The dental sac with its enclosed odontogenic organ and developing tooth.

den·tal for·ceps (den′tăl fōr′seps) Device used to luxate teeth and to remove them from the alveolus. SYN extracting forceps.

den·tal for·mu·la (den′tăl fōrm′yū-lă) A statement in tabular form of the number of each kind of teeth in the jaw.

den·tal ger·i·at·rics (den′tăl jer′ē-at′riks) Treatment of dental problems peculiar to advanced age. SYN gerodontics, gerodontology.

den·tal·gi·a (den-tal′jē-ă) SYN toothache. [L. *dens,* tooth, + G. *algos,* pain]

den·tal gran·u·lo·ma (den′tăl gran′yū-lō′mă) SYN periapical granuloma.

den·tal his·to·ry (den′tăl his′tŏr-ē) A written documentation of a patient's oral health covering all particulars of disease and therapy.

den·tal hy·gien·ist (den′tăl hī-jē′nist) A licensed, professional auxiliary in dentistry who is both an oral health educator and a clinician, and who uses preventive, therapeutic, and educational methods for the control of oral diseases.

den·tal im·plants (den′tăl im′plants) Various types of metal anchors attaching crowns, bridges, or dentures to the jaw permanently. See page 422.

den·tal med·i·cine (den′tăl med′i-sin) SYN dentistry.

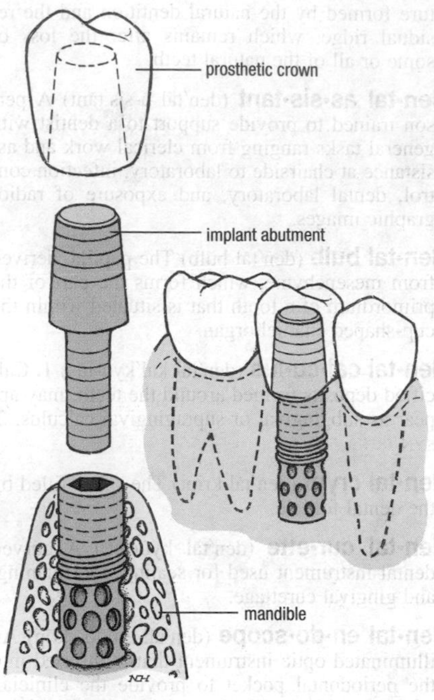

dental implant

den·tal or·gan (den′tăl ōr′găn) SYN enamel organ.

den·tal pa·pil·la (den′tăl pă-pil′ă) A projection of the mesenchymal tissue of the developing jaw into the cup of the enamel organ; its outer layer becomes a layer of specialized columnar cells, the odontoblasts, which form the dentin of the tooth.

den·tal plaque (den′tăl plak) **1.** The noncalcified accumulation, mainly of oral microorganisms and their products, which adheres tenaciously to the teeth and is not readily dislodged. **2.** SYN bacterial plaque.

den·tal proph·y·lax·is (den′tăl prō′fi-lak′sis) Measures to promote the health and prevent disease of the teeth and gums that include scaling and polishing procedures performed to remove plaque, calculus, and stains.

den·tal pub·lic health (den′tăl pŭb′lik helth) The science and art of preventing and controlling dental diseases and promoting dental health through organized community efforts. One of the dental specialties.

den·tal pulp, den·ti·nal pulp (den′tăl pŭlp, den′ti-năl pŭlp) The soft tissue within the pulp cavity, consisting of connective tissue containing blood vessels, nerves, and lymphatics, and at the periphery a layer of odontoblasts capable of internal repair of the dentin. SYN pulp (2), tooth pulp.

den·tal ridge (den′tăl rij) The prominent border of a cusp or margin of a tooth.

den·tal sac (den′tăl sak) The outer connective tissue envelope surrounding a developing tooth; also applied to the mesenchymal concentration that is the primordium of the sac. SEE ALSO dental follicle.

den·tal sur·geon (den′tăl sŭr′jŏn) A general practitioner of dentistry. SYN oral surgeon.

den·tal sy·ringe (den′tăl sir-inj′) A breech-loading metal cartridge syringe into which fits a hermetically sealed glass cartridge containing anesthetic solution.

den·tal var·nish (den′tăl vahr′nish) Solutions of natural resins and gums in a suitable solvent; a thin coating is applied over the surfaces of the cavity preparations before placement of restorations; used to protect tooth against the constituents of restorative materials. SYN vernix.

den·tate (den′tāt) Notched; toothed; cogged. [L. *dentatus,* toothed]

den·tate gy·rus (den′tāt jī′rŭs) One of the two interlocking gyri composing the hippocampus, the other one being the Ammon horn.

den·tate nu·cle·us of cer·e·bel·lum (den′tāt nū′klē-ŭs ser′ĕ-bel′ŭm) The most lateral and largest of the cerebellar nuclei; it receives the axons of the Purkinje cells of the neocerebellum (lateral areas of cerebellar cortex); together with the more medially located globosus and emboliform nuclei it is the major source of fibers composing the massive superior cerebellar peduncle or brachium conjunctivum. SYN nucleus dentatus [TA].

den·tate su·ture (den′tāt sū′chŭr) SYN serrate suture.

den·tes (den′tēz) Plural of dens. [L.]

den·ti·cle (den′ti-kĕl) **1.** SYN endolith. **2.** A toothlike projection from a hard surface. [L. *denticulus,* a small tooth]

den·ti·frice (den′ti-fris) Any preparation used in the cleansing of the teeth, e.g., a tooth powder, toothpaste, or tooth wash. [L. *dentifricium,* fr. *dens,* tooth, + *frico,* pp. *frictus,* to rub]

den·tig·er·ous (den-tij′ĕr-ŭs) Arising from or associated with teeth, as a dentigerous cyst. [denti- + L. *gero,* to bear]

den·tig·er·ous cyst (den-tij′ĕr-ŭs sist) An odontogenic cyst derived from the reduced enamel epithelium surrounding the crown of an impacted, unerupted, or embedded tooth. See page B15. SYN follicular cyst (2).

den·ti·la·bi·al (den′ti-lā′bē-ăl) Relating to the teeth and lips. [denti- + L. *labium,* lip]

den·ti·lin·gual (den′ti-ling′gwăl) Relating to the teeth and tongue. [denti- + L. *lingua,* tongue]

den·tin (den′tin) The ivory forming the mass of the tooth. Calcified tissue that is not as hard as enamel but harder than cementum. About 20% is organic matrix, mostly a fibrous protein collagen, with some elastin and a small amount of mucopolysaccharide; the inorganic fraction (70%) is mainly hydroxyapatite, with some carbonate, magnesium, and fluoride. The dentine is traversed by closely packed tubules running from the pulp cavity outward; within the tubules are processes from the odontoblasts. SYN dentinum. [L. *dens,* tooth]

den·ti·nal (den′ti-năl) Relating to dentin.

den·ti·nal ca·nals (den′ti-năl kă-nalz′) SYN canaliculi dentales.

den·ti·nal·gi·a (den′ti-nal′jē-ă) Dentinal sensitivity or pain. [dentin + G. *algos,* pain]

den·ti·nal la·mi·na cyst (den′ti-năl lam′i-nă sist) A small keratin-filled cyst, usually multiple, on the alveolar ridge of newborn infants; it is derived from remnants of the dental lamina.

den·ti·nal sheath (den′ti-năl shēth) A layer of tissue relatively resistant to the action of acids, which forms the walls of the dentinal tubules.

den·ti·nal tu·bules (den′ti-năl tū′byūlz) SYN canaliculi dentales.

den·tin dys·pla·si·a (den′tin dis-plā′zē-ă) A hereditary disorder of the teeth, involving both primary and permanent dentition, in which the clinical morphology and color of the teeth are normal, but the teeth radiographically exhibit short roots, obliteration of the pulp chambers and canals, mobility, and premature exfoliation.

den·tine bridge (den′tēn brij) A deposit of reparative dentine or other calcific substances that forms across and reseals exposed tooth pulp tissue.

den·tin·o·ce·ment·al (den′ti-nō-sĕ-men′tăl) Relating to the dentine and cementum of teeth.

den·tin·o·e·nam·el (den′ti-nō-ĕ-nam′ĕl) Relating to the dentine and enamel of teeth. SYN amelodentinal.

den·tin·o·e·nam·el junc·tion (DEJ) (den′ti-nō-ĕ-nam′ĕl jŭngk′shŭn) The surface at which the enamel and the dentine of the crown of a tooth are joined.

den·tin·o·gen·e·sis (den′ti-nō-jen′ĕ-sis) The process of dentine formation in the development of teeth. [dentin + G. *genesis,* production]

den·tin·o·gen·e·sis im·per·fec·ta (den′ti-nō-jen′ĕ-sis im-pĕr-fek′tă) A hereditary disorder of the teeth characterized by translucent gray to yellow-brown teeth involving both primary and permanent dentition; the enamel fractures easily, leaving exposed dentine that undergoes rapid attrition; radiographically, the pulp chambers and canals appear obliterated and the roots are short and blunted; sometimes occurs in association with osteogenesis imperfecta.

den·ti·noid (den′ti-noyd) **1.** Resembling dentine. **2.** SYN dentinoma. [dentin + G. *eidos,* resembling]

den·ti·no·ma (den′ti-nō′mă) A rare benign odontogenic tumor consisting microscopically of dysplastic dentine and strands of epithelium within a fibrous stroma. SYN dentinoid (2). [dentin + G. *-oma,* tumor]

den·ti·num (den′ti-nŭm) SYN dentin. [L. *dens,* tooth]

den·tip·a·rous (den-tip′ă-rŭs) Tooth-bearing. [denti- + L. *pario,* to bear]

den·tist (den′tist) A legally qualified practitioner of dentistry.

den·tis·try (den′tis-trē) The healing science and art concerned with the embryology, anatomy, physiology, and pathology of the oral-facial complex, and with the prevention, diagnosis, and treatment of deformities, diseases, and injuries thereof. SYN dental medicine.

den·ti·tion (den-tish′ŭn) The natural teeth, as considered collectively, in the dental arch; may be deciduous, permanent, or mixed. See this page. [L. *dentitio,* teething]

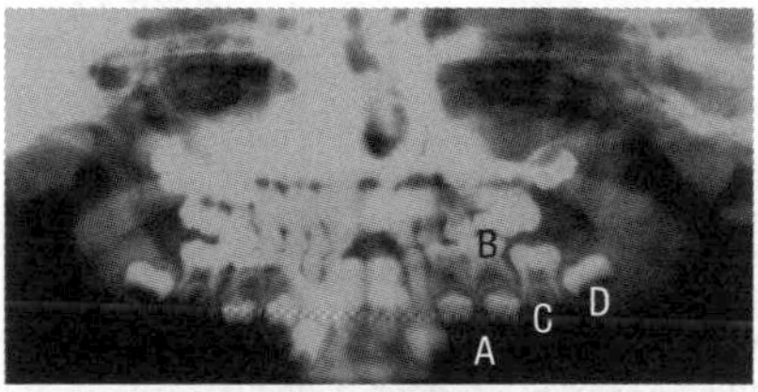

dentition: mixed findings reveal (A) partially formed permanent mandibular molars erupting below (B) deciduous molars; (C) erupted permanent first molar with incompletely formed roots; (D) crown of incompletely formed, unerupted, second permanent molar

den·to·al·ve·o·lar (den′tō-al-vē′ō-lăr) Usually, denoting that portion of the alveolar bone immediately about the teeth; used also to denote the functional unity of teeth and alveolar bone.

den·to·fa·cial (den′tō-fā′shăl) Of or relating to the dentition and face.

den·tu·lous (den′tyū-lŭs) Having natural teeth present in the mouth.

den·ture (den′chŭr) An artificial substitute for missing natural teeth and adjacent tissues; sometimes used to denote the dentition of animals.

den·ture base (den′chŭr bās) **1.** That part of a denture that rests on the oral mucosa and to which teeth are attached. **2.** That part of a complete or partial denture that rests on the basal seat and to which teeth are attached. SYN saddle (2).

den·ture bor·der (den′chŭr bōr′dĕr) **1.** The limit, boundary, or circumferential margin of a denture base. **2.** The margin of the denture base at the junction of the polished surface with the impression (tissue) surface. **3.** The extreme edges of a denture base at the buccolabial, lingual, and posterior limits. SYN periphery (2).

den·ture foun·da·tion (den′chŭr fown-dā′shŭn) That portion of the oral structures that is available to support a denture.

den·ture sta·bil·i·ty (den′chŭr stă-bil′i-tē) The capacity of a denture to be firm, steady, constant, and resist change of position when functional forces are applied. SYN stabilization (2).

de·nu·cle·at·ed (dē-nū′klē-ā-tĕd) Deprived of a nucleus.

de·nu·da·tion (den′yū-dā′shŭn) Depriving of a covering or protecting layer; the act of laying bare, as in the removal of the epithelium from an underlying surface. [L. *de-nudo,* to lay bare, fr. *de,* from, + *nudus,* naked]

de·nude (dē-nūd′) To perform denudation.

Den·ver De·vel·op·men·tal Screen·ing Test (DDS) (den′vĕr dĕ-vel′ŏp-men′tăl skrēn′ing test) A scale used by psychologists and pediatricians to assess the developmental, intellectual, motor, and social maturity of children from birth to age 6 years.

de·o·dor·ant (dē-ō′dŏr-ănt) **1.** Eliminating or masking a smell, especially an unpleasant one. **2.** An agent having such an action, especially a cosmetic combined with an antiperspirant. SYN deodorizer. [L. *de-* priv. + *odoro,* pp. *-atus,* to give an odor to, fr. *odor,* a smell]

de·o·dor·iz·er (dē-ō′dăr-īz-ĕr) SYN deodorant (2).

de·os·si·fi·ca·tion (dē-os′i-fi-kā′shŭn) Removal of the mineral constituents of bone. [L. *de,* from, + *os,* bone, + *facio,* to make]

de·ox·y·a·den·o·sine (dA, dAdo) (dē-oks′ē-ă-den′ō-sēn) One of the four major nucleosides of DNA (the others being deoxycytidine, deoxyguanosine, and thymidine). The 5′ derivative is also an important component of one form of vitamin B_{12}. Deoxyadenosine accumulates in individuals with severe combined immunodeficiency disease.

de·ox·y·ad·e·nyl·ic ac·id (dAMP) (dē-oks′ē-ad-ĕ-nil′ik as′id) Deoxyadenosine monophosphate, a hydrolysis product of DNA, differing from adenylic acid in containing deoxyribose in place of ribose. SYN adenine deoxyribonucleotide.

de·ox·y·cho·late (dē-oks′ē-kō′lāt) A salt or ester of deoxycholic acid.

de·ox·y·cho·lic ac·id (dē-oks′ē-kō′lik as′id) A bile acid and choleretic; used in biochemical preparations as a detergent.

de·ox·y·cor·ti·cos·ter·one (dē-oks′ē-kōr-ti-kos′tĕr-ōn) An adrenocortical steroid, principally a biosynthetic precursor of corticosterone and possibly aldosterone, which rarely appears in adrenocortical secretions; a potent mineralocorticoid with no appreciable glucocorticoid activity. Cf. bioregulator. SYN 21-hydroxyprogesterone.

de·ox·y·cyt·i·dine (dē-oks′ē-sī′ti-dēn) One of the four major nucleosides of DNA (the others being deoxyadenosine, deoxyguanosine, and thymidine).

de·ox·y·cyt·i·dyl·ic ac·id (dCMP) (dē-oks′ē-sī-ti-dil′ik as′id) Deoxycytidine monophosphate, a hydrolysis product of DNA.

de·ox·y·gua·no·sine (dē-oks′ē-gwahn′ō-sēn) One of the four major nucleosides of DNA (the others being deoxyadenosine, deoxycytidine, and thymidine). Found to accumulate in patients with purine nucleoside phosphorylase deficiency.

de·ox·y·gua·nyl·ic ac·id (dGMP) (dē-oks′ē-gwahn-il′ik as′id) Deoxyguanosine monophosphate, a hydrolysis product of DNA. SYN guanine deoxyribonucleotide.

deoxyhaemoglobin [Br.] SYN deoxyhemoglobin.

de·ox·y·he·mo·glo·bin (dē-oks′ē-hē′mŏ-glō-bin) The reduced form of hemoglobin, resulting when oxyhemoglobin loses its oxygen. SYN deoxyhaemoglobin. [de- + oxy- + hemoglobin]

de·ox·y·ri·bo·nu·cle·ase (DNase) (de-oks′ē-rī′bō-nū′klē-ās) Any enzyme (phosphodiesterase) hydrolyzing phosphodiester bonds in DNA. SEE ALSO endonuclease, nuclease.

de·ox·y·ri·bo·nu·cle·ic ac·id (DNA) (dē-oks′ē-rī′bō-nū-klē′ik as′id) The type of nucleic acid containing deoxyribose as the sugar component and found principally in the nuclei (chromatin, chromosomes) and mitochondria of animal and plant cells, usually loosely bound to protein (hence the term deoxyribonucleoprotein); considered to be the autoreproducing component of chromosomes and of many viruses, and the repository of hereditary characteristics. Its linear macromolecular chain consists of deoxyribose molecules esterified with phosphate groups between the 3′ and 5′-hydroxyl groups; linked to this structure are the purines adenine (A) and guanine (G) and the pyrimidines cytosine (C) and thymine (T). DNA may be open ended or circular, single or double stranded, and many forms are known, the most commonly described of which is double-stranded, wherein the pyrimidines and purines cross-link through hydrogen bonding in the schema A-T and C-G, bringing two antiparallel strands into a double helix. Chromosomes are composed of double-stranded DNA; mitochondrial DNA is circular.

de•ox•y•ri•bo•nu•cle•o•pro•tein (dē-oks′ē-rī′bō-nū′klē-ō-prō′tēn) The complex of DNA and protein in which DNA is usually found upon cell disruption and isolation.

de•ox•y•ri•bo•nu•cle•o•side (dē-oks′ē-rī-bō-nū′klē-ō-sīd) A nucleoside component of DNA containing 2-deoxy-D-ribose; the condensation product of deoxy-D-ribose with purines or pyrimidines.

de•ox•y•ri•bo•nu•cle•o•tide (dē-oks′ē-rī′bō-nū′klē-ō-tīd) A nucleotide component of DNA containing 2-deoxy-D-ribose; the phosphoric ester of deoxyribonucleoside; formed in nucleotide biosynthesis.

de•ox•y•ri•bose (dē-oks′ē-rī′bōs) A deoxypentose, 2-deoxy-D-ribose being the most common example, occurring in DNA and responsible for its name.

de•ox•y•ri•bo•vi•rus (dē-ok′sē-rī′bō-vī-rŭs) SYN DNA virus.

de•ox•y sug•ar (dē-oks′ē shug′ăr) A sugar containing fewer oxygen atoms than carbon atoms and in which, consequently, one or more carbons in the molecule lack an attached hydroxyl group.

de•ox•y•thy•mi•dine (dT) (dē-oks′ē-thī′mi-dēn) SYN thymidine.

de•ox•y•thy•mi•dyl•ic ac•id (dTMP) (dē-oks′ē-thī-mi-dil′ik as′id) A component of DNA; originally and properly called thymidylic acid, but use of deoxy- is less ambiguous, because ribothymidylic acid is now known to exist.

de•pen•dence (dĕ-pen′dĕns) The quality or condition of relying on, being influenced by, or being subservient to a person or object reflecting a particular need. [L. *dependeo,* to hang from]

de•pen•dent (dĕ-pen′dĕnt) In health care finance, a patient, other than the insured, who is entitled to coverage under the insured's policy; such designation varies widely according to insurer or geographic or legal jurisdiction.

de•pen•dent drain•age (dĕ-pen′dĕnt drān′ăj) Drainage from the lowest part and into a receptacle at a level lower than the structure being drained.

de•pen•dent e•de•ma (dĕ-pen′dĕnt ĕ-dē′mă) A clinically detectable increase in extracellular fluid volume localized in a dependent area, as of a limb, characterized by swelling or pitting.

de•pen•dent nurs•ing ac•tions (dĕ-pen′dĕnt nŭrs′ing ak′shŭnz) NURSING actions prescribed by physician or by operational protocol in a health care facility; physician-initiated interventions carried out by nurses for patient care.

de•pen•dent per•son•al•i•ty (dĕ-pen′dĕnt pĕr-sŏn-al′i-tē) A personality disorder in which a person passively allows others to assume responsibility for making decisions.

depersonalisation [Br.] SYN depersonalization.

de•per•son•al•i•za•tion (dē-pĕr′sŏn-ăl-ī-zā′shŭn) A state in which someone loses the feeling of his own identity in relation to others in his family or peer group, or loses the feeling of his own reality. SYN depersonalisation.

de•phas•ing (dē-fāz′ing) MAGNETIC RESONANCE the gradual loss of orientation of the magnetic atomic nuclei due to random molecular energy transfer or relaxation following alignment by a radiofrequency pulse.

de•pig•men•ta•tion (dē-pig′men-tā′shŭn) Loss of pigment which may be partial or complete. SEE ALSO achromia (1).

dep•i•late (dep′i-lāt) To remove hair by any means. Cf. epilate. [L. *de-pilo,* pp. *-atus,* to deprive of hair, fr. *de-* neg. + *pilo,* to grow hair]

dep•i•la•tion (dep′i-lā′shŭn) SYN epilation.

de•pil•a•to•ry (dĕ-pil′ă-tŏr-ē) **1.** Pertaining to removal of hair at the surface of the skin by shaving or applying alkaline chemical hair removal products. **2.** An agent having this action. Cf. epilatory.

de•po•lar•i•za•tion (dē-pō′lăr-ī-zā′shŭn) The destruction, neutralization, or change in direction of polarity.

de•po•lar•iz•ing block (dē-pōl′ăr-īz-ing blok) Skeletal muscle paralysis associated with loss of polarity of the motor endplate, as occurs following administration of succinylcholine.

de•pol•y•mer•ase (dē-pol′i-mĕr-ās) An enzyme catalyzing the hydrolysis of a macromolecule to simpler components. SEE nuclease.

depolymerisation [Br.] SYN depolymerization.

de•po•lym•er•i•za•tion (dē-pol′i-mĕr-ī-zā′shŭn) The dismantling of a polymer into individual monomers. SYN depolymerisation.

dep•o•si•tion (dep′ŏ-zish′ŭn) A sworn pretrial testimony given by a witness in response to oral and written questions and cross examination. The deposition is transcribed and may be used for further pretrial investigation. It may also be presented at the trial if the witness cannot be present; often used in the case of workers' compensation adjudication.

de•pot in•jec•tion (dē′pō in-jek′shŭn) An injection of a substance in a vehicle that tends to keep it at the site of injection so that absorption occurs over a prolonged period.

de•pres•sant (dĕ-pres′ănt) **1.** Diminishing functional tone or activity. **2.** An agent that reduces nervous or functional activity, such as a sedative or anesthetic. [L. *de-primo,* pp. *-pressus,* to press down]

de•pressed (dĕ-prest′) **1.** Flattened from above

downward. **2.** Below the normal level or the level of the surrounding parts. **3.** Below the normal functional level. **4.** Dejected; low in spirits.

de·pressed skull frac·ture (dĕ-prest′ skŭl frak′shŭr) A fracture with inward displacement of a part of the calvarium; may or may not be associated with disruption of the underlying dura or cerebral cortex.

de·pres·sion (dĕ-presh′ŭn) **1.** Reduction of the level of functioning. **2.** A hollow or sunken area. **3.** Displacement of a part downward or inward. **4.** A temporary mental state or chronic mental disorder characterized by feelings of sadness, loneliness, despair, low self-esteem, and self-reproach; accompanying signs include psychomotor retardation or less frequently agitation, withdrawal from social contact, and vegetative states such as loss of appetite and insomnia. SYN dejection. [L. *depressio*, fr. *deprimo*, to press down]

de·pres·sor (dĕ-pres′ŏr) **1.** A muscle that flattens or lowers a part. **2.** Anything that depresses or retards functional activity. **3.** An instrument or device used to push certain structures out of the way during an operation or examination. **4.** An agent that decreases blood pressure. [L. *deprimo*, pp. *-pressus*, to press down]

de·pres·sor an·gu·li o·ris mus·cle (dĕ-pres′ŏr ang′yū-lī ōr′is mŭs′ĕl) *Origin*, lower border of mandible anteriorly; *insertion*, blends with other muscles in lower lip near angle of mouth; *action*, pulls down corners of mouth; *nerve supply*, facial. SYN musculus depressor anguli oris [TA], triangular muscle (2).

de·pres·sor fi·bers (dĕ-pres′ŏr fī′bĕrz) Sensory nerve fibers having pressure-sensitive endings; situated in the walls of certain arteries; capable of activating brainstem mechanisms to lower blood pressure when stimulated by an increase in intraarterial pressure.

de·pres·sor la·bi·i in·fe·ri·o·ris mus·cle (dĕ-pres′ŏr lā′bē-ī in-fēr′ē-ōr′is mŭs′ĕl) *Origin*, anterior portion of lower border of mandible; *insertion*, orbicularis oris musculus and skin of lower lip; *action*, depresses lower lip; *nerve supply*, facial. SYN musculus depressor labii inferioris [TA].

de·pres·sor mus·cle of sep·tum (dĕ-prĕs′ ŏr mŭs′ĕl sĕp′tŭm) SYN depressor septi nasi muscle.

de·pres·sor sep·ti na·si mus·cle (dĕ-prĕs′ ŏr sep′tī nā′sī mŭs′ĕl) *Origin*, facial muscle of nose; a vertical fasciculus from maxilla superior to central incisor passing upward along median line of upper lip to insert into mobile part of nasal septum; *action*, works with alar (dilator) part of nasalis muscle to widen the nares during deep inspiration; depresses septum; *nerve supply*, buccal branch of facial. SYN musculus depressor septi [TA], depressor muscle of septum.

de·pres·sor su·per·ci·li·i mus·cle (dĕ-pres′ ŏr sū′pĕr-sil′ē-ī mŭs′ĕl) Fibers of the orbital part of the orbicularis oculi musculus insert in the eyebrow; *action*, depresses eyebrow; *nerve supply*, facial. SYN musculus depressor supercilii [TA].

dep·ri·va·tion (dep′ri-vā′shŭn) Absence, loss, or withholding of something needed.

depth (depth) Distance from the surface downward.

depth per·cep·tion (depth pĕr-sep′shŭn) The visual ability to judge depth or distance.

de Quer·vain dis·ease (dĕ-kār′vahn[h]′ di-zēz′) Fibrosis of the sheath of a tendon of the thumb.

de Quer·vain frac·ture (dĕ kār′vahn[h]′ frak′ shŭr) Break of the scaphoid bone of the wrist with volar subluxation of fragments and lunate. [Fritz de Qurvain, 1868–1940, Swiss physician]

de Quer·vain ten·o·syn·o·vi·tis (dĕ kār′ vahn[h]′ ten′ō-sin-ō-vī′tis) Inflammation of the tendons of the first dorsal compartment of the wrist, which includes the abductor pollicis longus and extensor pollicis brevis; diagnosed by a specific provocative test (Finkelstein test).

de Quer·vain thy·roid·i·tis (dĕ kār-vahn[h]′ thī′royd-ī′tis) SYN subacute granulomatous thyroiditis.

de·range·ment (dĕ-rānj′mĕnt) **1.** A disturbance of the regular order or arrangement. **2.** Rarely used term for a mental disturbance or disorder. [Fr.]

de·re·al·i·za·tion (dē-rē′ă-lī-zā′shŭn) An alteration in one's perception of the environment such that things that are ordinarily familiar seem strange, unreal, or two dimensional.

de·re·ism (dē-rē′izm) Mental activity in fantasy in contrast to reality. [L. *de*, away, + *res*, thing]

de·re·is·tic (dē′rē-is′tik) Living in imagination or fantasy with thoughts that are incongruent with logic or experience.

der·en·ceph·a·ly (der′en-sef′ă-lē) Cervical rachischisis and meroencephaly; a malformation involving an open neurocranium with a rudimentary brain usually crowded back toward bifid cervical vertebrae. [G. *derē*, neck, + *enkephalos*, brain]

de·re·pres·sion (dē-rĕ-presh′ŭn) A homeostatic mechanism for regulating enzyme production in an inducible enzyme system: an inducer, usually a substrate of a specific enzyme pathway, by combining with an active repressor (produced by a regulator gene) deactivates it.

der·i·va·tion (der′i-vā′shŭn) The source, origin, or evolutionary course of a structure or process. SYN revulsion (2). [L. *derivatio*, fr. *derivo*, pp. *-atus*, to draw off, fr. *rivus*, a stream]

de•riv•a•tive (dĕ-riv′ă-tiv) **1.** Relating to or producing derivation. **2.** Something produced by modification of something preexisting. **3.** Specifically, a chemical compound produced from another compound in one or more steps, as in replacement of H by an alkyl, acyl, or amino group.

derm-, **derma-** Combining forms meaning the skin; corresponds to the L. *cut-*. See entries under cut. [G. *derma*]

der•ma•brad•er (dĕrm′ă-brād-ĕr) A motor-driven device used in dermabrasion.

der•ma•bra•sion (dĕrm′ă-brā′zhŭn) Operative procedure used to remove acne scars or pits performed with sandpaper, rotating wire brushes, or other abrasive materials. SYN planing.

Der•ma•cen•tor (dĕr-mă-sen′tōr) An ornate, characteristically marked genus of hard ticks (family Ixodidae) that possess eyes and 11 festoons; it consists of some 20 species with members that commonly attack dogs, humans, and other mammals. [derm- + G. *kentōr,* a goader]

Der•ma•cen•tor an•der•son•i (dĕr-mă-sen′tōr an-dĕr-sō′nī) The wood tick; vector of Rocky Mountain spotted fever; also transmits tularemia and causes tick paralysis.

Der•ma•cen•tor mar•gi•na•tus (dĕr-mă-sen′tōr mar-ji-nā-tus) A tick species found across Europe and the vector of a human rickettsiosis caused by *Rickettsia slovaca*.

Der•ma•cen•tor va•ri•a•bil•is (dĕr-mă-sen′tōr vā-rē-ă-bil′is) The American dog tick, a common pest of dogs along the eastern seaboard of the U.S., a vector of tularemia, and a principal vector of *Rickettsia rickettsii,* which causes Rocky Mountain spotted fever in the central and eastern U.S.; may also cause tick paralysis.

Der•ma•coc•cus (dĕr-mă-kok′ŭs) A genus of gram-positive, aerobic cocci found on human skin.

der•mal (dĕr′măl) Relating to the skin. SYN dermatic, dermatoid (2), dermic.

der•mal graft (dĕr′măl graft) A graft of dermis, made from skin by cutting away a thin split-thickness graft.

der•mal pa•pil•lae (dĕr′măl pă-pil′ē) SYN papilla of dermis.

der•mal si•nus (dĕr′măl sī′nŭs) A sinus lined with epidermis and skin appendages extending from the skin to some deeper-lying structure, most frequently the spinal cord.

dermat- Prefix meaning the skin. SEE ALSO derm-, dermato-, dermo-. [G. *derma*]

der•mat•ic (dĕr-mat′ik) SYN dermal.

der•ma•ti•tis, pl. **der•ma•tit•i•des** (dĕr′mă-tī′tis, -tit′i-dēz) Inflammation of the skin. See this page, B9. [derm- + G. *-itis,* inflammation]

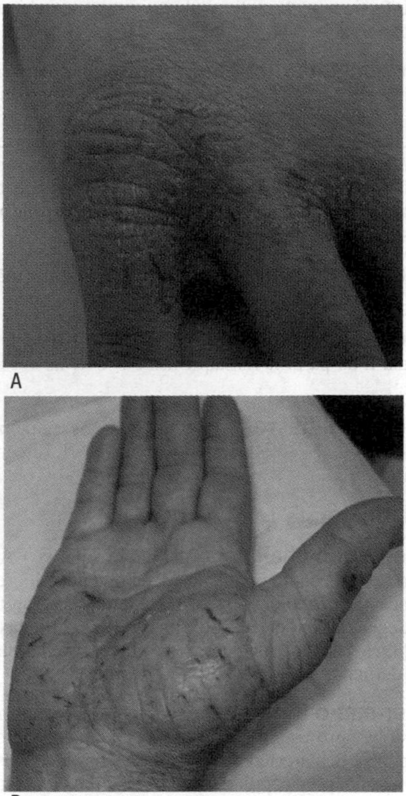

dermatitis: (A) hand, fissuring; (B) palmar

der•ma•ti•tis-caus•ing cat•er•pil•lar (dĕr′mă-tī′tis-kawz′ing kat′ĕr-pil-ăr) One of several species with hairs that can cause an allergic dermatitis; the saddleback caterpillar (*Sibine stimulea*) and the brown-tail moth (*Euproctis chrysorrhoea*) are common examples.

der•ma•ti•tis ex•fo•li•a•ti•va in•fan•tum, **der•ma•ti•tis ex•fo•li•a•ti•va ne•o•na•to•rum** (dĕr′mă-tī′tis eks-fō-lē-a-tī′vă in-fan′tŭm, dĕr′mă-tī′tis eks-fō-lē-a-tī′vă nē-ō-nā-tō′rŭm) A generalized pyoderma accompanied by exfoliative dermatitis, with constitutional symptoms, affecting young infants; may result from atopic dermatitis, Leiner disease, or staphylococcal scalded skin syndrome. SYN impetigo neonatorum (1).

der•ma•ti•tis gan•gre•no•sa in•fan•tum (dĕr′mă-tī′tis gang-grē-nō′să in-fan′tŭm) A bullous or pustular eruption, of uncertain origin, followed by necrotic ulcers or extensive gangrene in children younger than 2 years of age; if untreated, death may result from hematogenous infection, such as liver abscess. SYN pemphigus gangrenosus (1).

der•ma•ti•tis her•pet•i•for•mis (dĕr′mă-tī′tis hĕr-pet-i-fōr′mis) A chronic disease of the skin marked by a symmetric itching eruption of vesicles and papules that occur in groups; relapses are common; associated with gluten-sensitive enteropathy and IgA immune complexes beneath the epidermis of lesioned and normal-appearing skin. SYN Duhring disease.

der•ma•ti•tis me•di•ca•men•to•sa (dĕr′mă-tī′tis med-i-kă-men-tō′să) SYN drug eruption.

der•ma•ti•tis pa•pil•la•ris ca•pil•li•ti•i (dĕr′mă-tī′tis pa-pi-lā′ris kap-i-lish′ē-ī) SYN acne keloid.

der•ma•ti•tis re•pens (dĕr′mă-tī′tis rē′penz) SYN pustulosis palmaris et plantaris. [L. creeping]

dermato- SEE derm-. [G. *derma,* skin]

der•mat•o•cha•la•sis (der′mă-tō-kal′ă-sis) An acquired condition characterized by undue looseness or pendulousness of the eyelid skin due to degeneration of elastic fibers. SYN cutis laxa [TA], pachydermatocele. SYN blepharochalasis. [dermato- + G. *chalasis,* a loosening]

der•mat•o•fi•bro•ma (dĕr′mă-tō-fī-brō′mă) A slowly growing benign skin nodule consisting of poorly demarcated cellular fibrous tissue enclosing collapsed capillaries, with scattered hemosiderin-pigmented and lipid macrophages. The following terms are considered by some to be synonymous with, and by others to be varieties of, dermatofibroma: sclerosing hemangioma, fibrous histiocytoma, nodular subepidermal fibrosis. See this page.

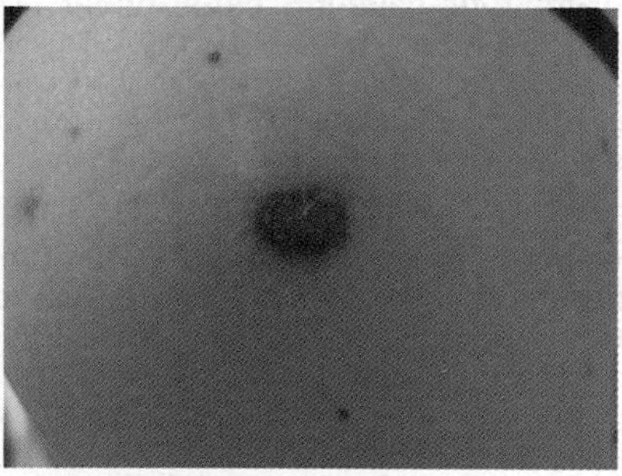

pigmented dermatofibroma: shoulder

der•mat•o•glyph•ics (dĕr′mă-tō-glif′iks) **1.** The configurations of the characteristic ridge patterns of the volar surfaces of the skin; in the human hand, the distal segment of each digit has three types of configurations: whorl, loop, and arch. SEE ALSO fingerprint. **2.** The science or study of these configurations or patterns. [dermato- + *glyphē,* carved work]

der•ma•tog•ra•phism (dĕ′-mă-tog′ră-fizm) A form of urticaria in which whealing occurs in the site and in the configuration of application of stroking (pressure, friction) of the skin. SYN dermographia, dermographism. [dermato- + G. *graphō,* to write]

der•ma•toid (dĕr′mă-toyd) **1.** Resembling skin. SYN dermoid (1). **2.** SYN dermal.

der•ma•tol•o•gist (dĕr′mă-tol′ŏ-jist) A physician who specializes in diagnosing and treating cutaneous and related systemic diseases.

der•ma•tol•o•gy (dĕr′mă-tol′ŏ-jē) The branch of medicine concerned with the study of the skin, diseases of the skin, and the relationship of cutaneous lesions to systemic disease. [dermato- + G. *logos,* study]

der•ma•tol•y•sis (dĕr′mă-tol′i-sis) Loosening of the skin or atrophy of the skin by disease; erroneously used as a synonym for cutis laxa. [dermato- + G. *lysis,* a loosening]

der•ma•to•ma (dĕr′mă-tō′mă) A circumscribed thickening or hypertrophy of the skin. [dermato- + G. *-oma,* tumor]

der•ma•tome (dĕr′mă-tōm) **1.** An instrument for cutting thin slices of skin for grafting, or excising small lesions. **2.** The dorsolateral part of an embryonic somite. SYN cutis plate. **3.** The area of skin supplied by cutaneous branches from a single spinal nerve; neighboring dermatomes may overlap. See page 429. [dermato- + G. *tomē,* a cutting]

der•mat•o•meg•a•ly (dĕr′mă-tō-meg′ă-lē) Congenital or acquired defect in which the skin hangs in folds. [dermato- + G. *megas,* large]

der•mat•o•mere (dĕr′mă-tō-mēr) A metameric area of the embryonic integument. [dermato- + G. *meros,* part]

der•mat•o•my•co•sis (dĕr′mă-tō-mī-kō′sis) Fungus infection of the skin caused by dermatophytes, yeasts, and other fungi. Cf. dermatophytosis.

der•mat•o•my•o•ma (dĕr′mă-tō-mī-ō′mă) SYN leiomyoma cutis. [dermato- + G. *mys,* muscle, + *-oma,* tumor]

der•mat•o•my•o•si•tis (der′mă-tō-mī′ō-sī′tis) A progressive condition characterized by symmetric proximal muscular weakness with elevated muscle enzyme levels and a rash, typically a purplish-red or heliotrope erythema on the face, and edema of the eyelids and periorbital tissue; affected muscle tissue shows degeneration of fibers with a chronic inflammatory reaction; occurs in children and adults, and in the latter may be associated with visceral cancer. See page 429. [dermato- + G. *mys,* muscle, + *-itis,* inflammation]

der•mat•o•neu•ro•sis (dĕr′mă-tō-nūr-ŏ′sis)

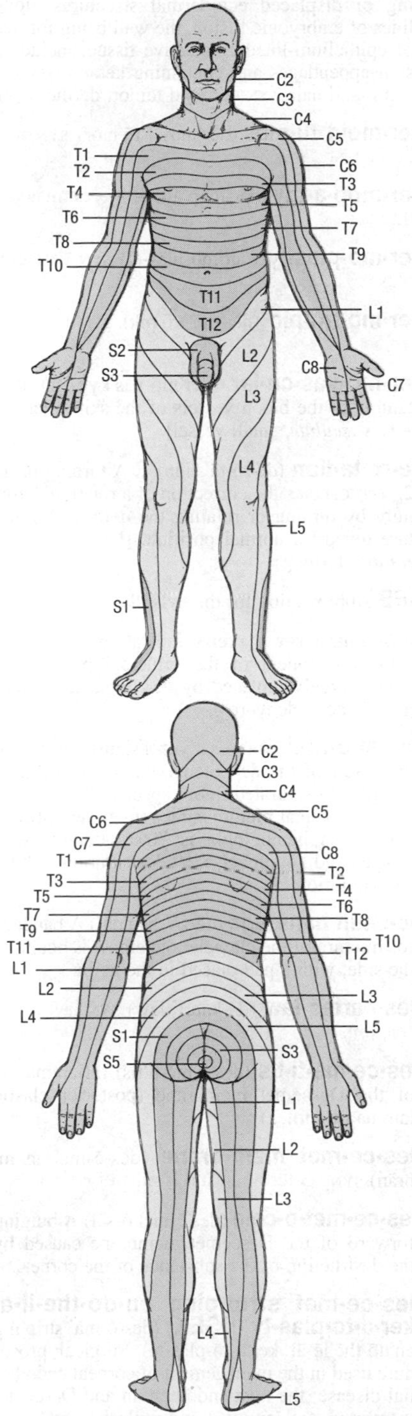

dermatomes: areas of skin supplied by cutaneous branches of spinal nerves

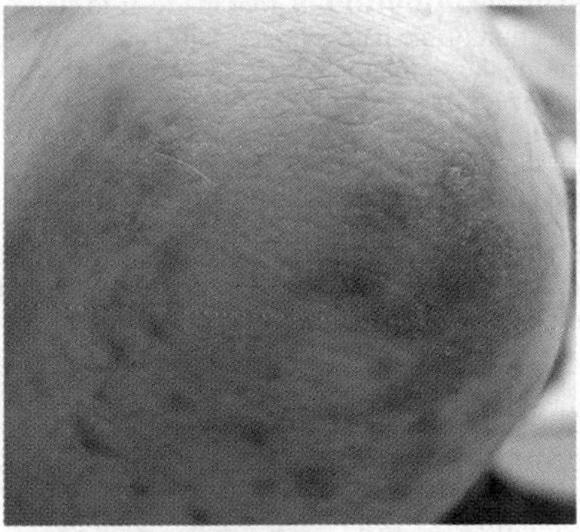

dermatomyositis on the knee

Any cutaneous eruption due to emotional stimuli.

der•mat•o•pa•thol•o•gy (dĕr′mă-tō-pă-thol′ō-jē) Histopathology of the skin and subcutis, and study of the causes of skin disease.

der•ma•top•a•thy (dĕr′mă-top′ă-thē) Any disease of the skin. SYN dermopathy. [dermato- + G. *pathos,* suffering]

Der•ma•toph•a•goi•des pter•o•nys•si•nus (dĕr′mă-tof-ă-goy′dēz ter-ō-ni-sī′nŭs) A species of mites found in house dust and a common cause of atopic asthma. [dermato- + G. *phagō,* to eat; ptero- + G. *nyssō,* to prick, stab]

der•mat•o•phi•lo•sis (der′mă-tō-fī-lō′sis) An exudative, pustular dermatitis affecting a wide range of animals, including, occasionally, humans; particularly severe in ruminants. The etiologic agent is a gram-positive bacterium, *Dermatophilus congolensis.* SYN proliferative dermatitis, streptothrichosis, streptotrichiasis, streptotrichosis.

der•mat•o•phy•lax•is (dĕr′mă-tō-fi-lak′sis) Protection of the skin against potentially harmful agents (e.g., infection, excessive sunlight, noxious agents). [dermato- + G. *phylaxis,* protection]

der•mat•o•phyte (dĕr′mă-tō-fīt) A fungus that causes superficial infections of the skin, hair, and nails, i.e., keratinized tissues. Species of *Epidermophyton*, *Microsporum*, and *Trichophyton* are regarded as dermatophytes, but causative agents of tinea versicolor, tinea nigra, and cutaneous candidiasis are not so classified. [dermato- + G. *phyton,* plant]

der•mat•o•phy•tid (dĕr′mă-tof′i-tid) An allergic manifestation of dermatophytosis at a site distant from that of the primary fungal infection. The lesions, usually small vesicles on the hands and arms, are devoid of the fungus and may become extensive, covering wide areas of the body and causing extreme discomfort to the patient. SEE ALSO -id (1), id reaction.

der•mat•o•phy•to•sis (dĕr′mă-tō-fī-tō′sis) An infection of the hair, skin, or nails caused by any one of the dermatophytes. The lesions are characterized by erythema, small papular vesicles, fissures, and scaling. Common sites of infection are the feet (tinea pedis), nails (onychomycosis), and scalp (tinea capitis). Cf. dermatomycosis.

der•mat•o•plas•ty (dĕr′mă-tō-plas-tē) Surgical repair of the skin, as by skin grafting. SYN dermoplasty. [dermato- + G. *plastos,* formed]

der•mat•o•pol•y•neu•ri•tis (dĕr′mă-tō-pol′ē-nūr-ī′tis) SYN acrodynia (2).

der•mat•o•scle•ro•sis (dĕr′mă-tō-skler-ō′sis) SYN scleroderma. [dermato- + G. *sklēroō,* to harden]

der•ma•to•sis, pl. **der•ma•to•ses** (dĕr′mă-tō′sis, -sēz) Nonspecific term used to denote any cutaneous abnormality or eruption. [dermato- + G. *-osis,* condition]

der•ma•to•sis me•di•ca•men•to•sa (dĕr-mă-tō′sis med-i-kă-men-tō′să) SYN drug eruption.

der•mat•o•ther•a•py (dĕr′mă-tō-thār′ă-pē) Treatment of skin diseases.

der•mat•o•tro•pic (dĕr′mă-tō-trō′pik) Having an affinity for the skin. SYN dermotropic. [dermato- + G. *trōpe,* a turning]

der•mic (dĕr′mik) SYN dermal.

der•mis (dĕr′mis) A layer of skin composed of a superficial thin layer that interdigitates with the epidermis, the stratum papillare, and the stratum reticulare; it contains blood and lymphatic vessels, nerves and nerve endings, glands, and, except for glabrous skin, hair follicles. SYN corium, cutis vera. [G. *derma,* skin]

♻ **dermo-** SEE derm-. [G. *derma,* skin]

Der•mo•bac•ter (dĕr′mō-bak′tĕr) A bacterial genus of nonmotile, non-spore-bearing gram-positive rods, recovered from human skin. *Dermobacter hominis* has been found in blood cultures.

der•mo•blast (dĕr′mō-blast) One of the mesodermal cells from which the corium is developed. [dermo- + G. *blastos,* germ]

der•mo•graph•i•a, **der•mog•ra•phism** (dĕr′mō-graf′ē-ă, dĕr-mog′ră-fizm) SYN dermatographism.

dermohaemal [Br.] SYN dermohemal.

der•mo•he•mal (dĕr′mō-hē′măl) Possessing both dermal and hemal structures, as in certain fishes. SYN dermohaemal.

der•moid (dĕr′moyd) **1.** SYN dermatoid (1). **2.** SYN dermoid cyst. [dermo- + G. *eidos,* resemblance]

der•moid cyst (dĕr′moyd sist) A tumor consisting of displaced ectodermal structures along lines of embryonic fusion, the wall being formed of epithelium-lined connective tissue, including skin appendages and containing keratin, sebum, teeth, and hair. SYN dermoid tumor, dermoid (2).

der•moid tu•mor (dĕr′moyd tū′mŏr) SYN dermoid cyst.

der•mop•a•thy (dĕr-mop′ă-thē) SYN dermatopathy.

der•mo•plas•ty (dĕr′mō-plas-tē) SYN dermatoplasty.

der•mo•tro•pic (dĕr′mō-trō′pik) SYN dermatotropic.

der•mo•vas•cu•lar (dĕr′mō-vas′kyū-lăr) Pertaining to the blood vessels of the skin. [dermo- + L. *vasculum,* small vessel]

de•ro•ta•tion (dē-rō-tā′shŭn) **1.** A turning back. **2.** ORTHOPEDICS the correction of a rotation deformity by turning or rotating the deformed structure toward a normal position. [L. *de,* away, + *rotatio,* turning]

DES Abbreviation for diethylstilbestrol.

♻ **des-** CHEMISTRY a prefix indicating absence of some component of the principal part of the name; largely replaced by de- (e.g., deoxyribonucleic acid, dehydro-).

de•sat•u•ra•tion (dē-sat′yūr-ā′shŭn) The act, or the result of the act, of making something less completely saturated; more specifically, the percentage of total binding sites remaining unfilled, e.g., when hemoglobin is 70% saturated with oxygen and nothing else, its desaturation is 30%. Cf. saturation (5).

De•sault ban•dage (dĕ-sō′ ban′dăj) A bandage for fracture of the clavicle; the elbow is bound to the side, with a pad placed in the axilla.

Des•cartes law (dā-kahrt′ law) SYN law of refraction.

des•ce•me•ti•tis (des′ĕ-mĕ-tī′tis) Inflammation of the Descemet membrane (posterior elastic lamina of cornea).

Des•ce•met mem•brane (des-ĕ-mā′ mem′brān) SYN posterior elastic lamina of cornea.

des•ce•met•o•cele (des′ĕ-met′ō-sēl) A bulging forward of the Descemet membrane caused by the destruction of the substance of the cornea.

Des•ce•met strip•ping en•do•the•li•al ker•a•to•plas•ty (DSEK) (des-ĕ-mā′ strip′ing en′dō-thē′lē-ăl ker′ă-tō-plas-tē) Surgical procedure used in the management of corneal endothelial disease; the host endothelium and Descemet membrane are removed and replaced with a cadaveric donor transplant of endothelium and Descemet membrane.

des•cend•ing co•lon (dĕ-send′ing kō′lŏn) The

part of the colon extending from the left colic flexure to the pelvic brim.

des·cend·ing de·gen·er·a·tion (dĕ-send′ing dĕ-jen′ĕr-ā′shŭn) **1.** Orthograde (wallerian) degeneration of an injured nerve fiber; i.e., distal to the lesion. **2.** Degeneration caudal to the level of a spinal cord lesion.

des·cend·ing ge·nic·u·lar ar·ter·y (dĕ-send′ing je-nik′yū-lăr ahr′tĕr-ē) *Origin*, femoral, in adductor canal; *distribution*, penetrates vasoadductor fascia to supply knee joint and adjacent parts; *anastomoses*, medial superior genicular, medial inferior genicular, lateral superior genicular, lateral inferior genicular, and anterior tibial recurrent arteries, i.e., articular network of knee. SYN arteria descendens genus [TA].

des·cend·ing pal·a·tine ar·ter·y (dĕ-send′ing pal′ă-tīn ahr′tĕr-ē) *Origin*, maxillary; *distribution*, soft palate, gums, and bones and mucous membrane of hard palate; *anastomoses*, sphenopalatine, ascending palatine, ascending pharyngeal, and tonsillar branches of facial. SYN arteria palatina descendens.

de·scen·sus (dē-sen′sŭs) SYN descensus testis. [L.]

de·scen·sus tes·tis (dē-sen′sŭs tes′tis) [TA] Descent of the testis from the abdomen into the scrotum during the seventh and eighth months of intrauterine life. SEE ALSO ptosis, procidentia. SYN descensus, descent (1).

de·scent (dĕ-sent′) **1.** SYN descensus testis. **2.** OBSTETRICS the passage of the presenting part of the fetus into and through the birth canal. [L. descensus]

DES daugh·ter (daw′tĕr) The daughter of a woman who received diethylstilbestrol (DES) during pregnancy; DES daughters are at risk of deformity, adenosis, and other epithelial changes of the vagina and cervix, including clear cell adenocarcinoma.

desensitisation [Br.] SYN desensitization.

de·sen·si·ti·za·tion (dē-sen′si-tī-zā′shŭn) **1.** The reduction or abolition of allergic sensitivity or reactions to the specific antigen (allergen). SYN antianaphylaxis. **2.** The act of removing an emotional complex. SYN desensitisation.

de·sen·si·tize (dē-sen′si-tīz) **1.** To reduce or remove any form of sensitivity. **2.** To effect desensitization (1). **3.** DENTISTRY to eliminate or subdue the painful response of exposed, vital dentine to irritative agents or thermal changes.

des·e·tope (des′ĕ-tōp) That part of the Class II major histocompatibility molecule that interacts with the antigen. [*de*terminant *se*lection + -tope]

des·flu·rane (des-flūr′ān) An inhalation anesthetic with physical characteristics that provide rapid induction of and recovery from anesthesia.

des·ic·cant (des′i-kănt) **1.** Drying; causing or promoting dryness. SYN desiccative. **2.** An agent that absorbs moisture; a drying agent. SYN exsiccant. [L. *de-sicco,* pp. *-siccatus,* to dry up]

des·ic·cate (des′i-kāt) To dry thoroughly; to render free from moisture. SYN exsiccate.

des·ic·ca·tion (des′i-kā′shŭn) The process of being desiccated. SYN dehydration (4), exsiccation (1).

des·ic·ca·tive (des′i-kā′tiv) SYN desiccant (1).

de·sign (dĕ-zīn′) **1.** To devise, plan, or contrive. **2.** the act or result of designing. [L. *designo,* to appoint, designate]

de·sig·na·tion (dez′ig-nā′shŭn) A legal process by which a hospital is formally designated to provide a specialized service. Usually requires meeting set standards and an external review (e.g., trauma center).

Des·mar·res re·trac·tor (dē-mahr′ rē-trak′tŏr) An instrument used to withdraw an eyelid.

des·min (dez′min) Any of various proteins found in intermediate filaments that copolymerize with vimentin to form constituents of connective tissue, cell walls, and filaments. Found in Z disc of skeletal and cardiac muscle cells.

des·mi·tis (dez-mī′tis) Inflammation of a ligament. [desm- + G. *-itis,* inflammation]

desmo-, desm- Combining forms meaning fibrous connection; ligament. [G. *desmos,* a band]

des·mo·cra·ni·um (dez′mō-krā′nē-ŭm) The mesenchymal primordium of the cranium.

des·mo·den·ti·um, des·mo·don·ti·um (dez′mō-den′tē ŭm, don′tē-ŭm) The collagen fibers, running from the cementum to the alveolar bone, that suspend a tooth in its socket; they include apical, oblique, horizontal, and alveolar crest fibers, indicating that the orientation of the fibers varies at different levels.

des·mog·e·nous (dez-moj′ĕ-nŭs) Of connective tissue or ligamentous origin or causation; e.g., denoting a deformity due to contraction of ligaments, fascia, or a scar. [desmo- + G. *-gen,* producing]

des·moid (dez′moyd) **1.** Fibrous or ligamentous. **2.** A nodule or mass of firm scarlike connective tissue resulting from active proliferation of fibroblasts, occurring most frequently in the abdominal muscles of women who have borne children. SYN desmoid tumor. [desmo- + G. *eidos,* appearance, form]

des·moid tu·mor (dez′moyd tū′mŏr) SYN desmoid (2).

des·mo·las·es (dez′mō-lā′sēz) Enzymes catalyzing reactions other than those involving hydrolysis; e.g., those involving oxidation and reduction, isomerization, the breaking of carbon-carbon bonds.

des•mop•a•thy (dez-mop′ă-thē) Any disease of the ligaments. [desmo- + G. *pathos,* suffering]

des•mo•pla•si•a (dez′mō-plā′zē-ă) Hyperplasia of fibroblasts and disproportionate formation of fibrous connective tissue, especially in the stroma of a carcinoma. [desmo- + G. *plasis,* a molding]

des•mo•plas•tic (dez′mō-plas′tik) **1.** Causing or forming adhesions. **2.** Causing fibrosis in the vascular stroma of a neoplasm.

des•mo•plas•tic fi•bro•ma (dez′mō-plas′tik fī-brō′mă) A benign fibrous tumor of bone affecting children and young adults; cortical destruction may result.

des•mo•plas•tic small cell tu•mor (dez′mō-plas′tik smawl sel tū′mŏr) A high-grade malignant tumor found most often in the abdomen of adolescent males; typically tumor cells contain both desmin and keratin, i.e., show hybrid features like fetal mesothelial cells; the exact nature of these cells remains unknown.

des•mo•plas•tic trich•o•ep•i•the•li•o•ma (dez′mō-plas′tik trik′ō-ep-i-thē′lē-ō′mă) A solitary, hard, anular, centrally depressed papule, occurring usually in women on the face, consisting of dermal strands of basaloid cells and small keratinous cysts within sclerotic desmoplastic stroma.

des•mo•pres•sin (dez′mō-pres′in) An analogue of vasopressin (antidiuretic hormone, ADH) possessing powerful antidiuretic activity.

des•mo•some (dez′mō-sōm) A site of adhesion between two epithelial cells, consisting of a dense attachment plaque separated from a similar structure in the other cell by a thin layer of extracellular material. SYN macula adherens. [desmo- + G. *sōma,* body]

des•mo•ter•ic med•i•cine (des′mō-ter′ik med′i-sin) The branch of medical practice that deals with health problems in prison inmates. SYN correctional medicine. [G. *desmōtērion,* prison, fr. *deō,* to bind, + -ic]

de•spe•ci•a•tion (dē-spē′shē-ā′shŭn) **1.** Alteration or loss of species characteristics. **2.** Removal of species-specific antigenic properties from a foreign protein.

des•qua•ma•tion (des′kwă-mā′shŭn) The shedding of the cuticle in scales or of the outer layer of any surface.

des•qua•ma•tive (des-kwahm′ă-tiv) Relating to or marked by desquamation.

de•sulf•hy•dras•es (dē-sŭlf-hī′drā-sĕz) Enzymes or groups of enzymes catalyzing the removal of a molecule of H_2S or substituted H_2S from a compound, as in the conversion of cysteine to pyruvic acid by cysteine desulfhydrase (cystathionine γ-lyase).

desulphurisation [Br.] SYN desulphurization.

de•sul•phur•i•za•tion (dē-sul′fŭr-ī-zā′shŭn) The process of removing sulfur from a molecule. SYN desulphurisation.

de•tach•ment (dĕ-tach′mĕnt) **1.** A voluntary or involuntary feeling or emotion that accompanies a sense of separation from normal associations or environment. **2.** Lack of connection to other people or the environment. **3.** Separation of a structure from its support.

de•tailed phy•si•cal ex•am•i•na•tion (dē′tāld fiz′i-kăl eg-zam′i-nā′shŭn) A head-to-toe patient assessment that follows the focused history and physical examination and is more thorough than the rapid trauma assessment or rapid medical assessment.

de•tec•tor (dĕ-tek′tŏr) The component of a laboratory instrument that detects the chemical or physical signal indicating the presence or quantity of the substance of interest.

de•tec•tor coil (dĕ-tek′tŏr koyl) A coil used in magnetic resonance imaging as an antenna to record radiofrequency emissions of stimulated nuclei, e.g., body coil, head coil.

de•ter•gent (dĕ-tĕr′jĕnt) A cleansing or purging agent, usually salts of long-chain aliphatic bases or acids that, through a surface action that depends on their possessing both hydrophilic and hydrophobic properties, exert cleansing (i.e., oil-dissolving) and antibacterial effects. [L. *de-tergeo,* pp. *-tersus,* to wipe off]

de•te•ri•o•ra•tion (dĕ-tēr′i-ŏr-ā′shŭn) The process or condition of becoming worse. [L. *deterior,* worse]

de•ter•mi•nant (dĕ-tĕr′mi-nănt) The factor that contributes to the generation of a trait. [L. *determinans,* determining, limiting]

de•ter•mi•na•tion (dĕ-tĕr′mi-nā′shŭn) **1.** A change, for the better or for the worse, in the course of a disease. **2.** A general move toward a given point. **3.** The measurement or estimation of any quantity or quality in scientific or laboratory investigation. **4.** Discernment of a state or category (e.g., in diagnosis). **5.** A process, both necessary and sufficient, whereby an effect is caused. **6.** Judicial decision resolving controversy. [L. *de-termino,* pp. *-atus,* to limit, determine, fr. *terminus,* a boundary]

de•ter•mi•nism (dē-tĕr′mi-nizm) The proposition that all behavior is caused exclusively by genetic and environmental influences with no random components, and independent of free will. [L. *determino,* to limit, fr. *terminus,* boundary + -ism]

de•tox•i•cate (dē-tok′si-kāt) SYN detoxify.

de•tox•i•ca•tion (dē-tok′si-kā′shŭn) SYN detoxification.

de•tox•i•fi•ca•tion (dē-tok′si-fi-kā′shŭn) **1.** Recovery from the toxic effects of a drug. **2.** Removal of the toxic properties from a poison. **3.** Metabolic conversion of pharmacologically active principles to pharmacologically less active principles. SYN detoxication.

de•tox•i•fy (dē-tok′si-fī) To diminish or remove the poisonous quality of any substance; to lessen the virulence of any pathogenic organism. SYN detoxicate. [L. *de*, from, + *toxicum*, poison]

de•train•ing (dē-trān′ing) SYN reversal.

de•tri•tion (dĕ-trish′ŭn) A wearing away by use or friction. [L. *de-tero*, pp. *-tritus*, to rub off]

de•tri•tus (dĕ-trī′tŭs) Any broken-down material, carious or gangrenous matter, or gravel. [L. (SEE detrition)]

de•tru•sor (dĕ-trū′sŏr) A muscle that has the action of expelling a substance. [L. *detrudo*, to drive away]

de•tru•sor•rha•phy (dē-trū-sōr′ă-fē) A procedure in which bladder muscle (detrusor) is reconstructed around the ureterovesical junction to form a competent one-way valve. SEE ALSO ureteroneocystostomy. SYN extravesical reimplantation. [detrusor + G. *rhaphē*, a seam]

de•tu•mes•cence (dē′tū-mes′ĕns) Subsidence of a swelling. [L. *de*, from, + *tumesco*, to swell up, fr. *tumeo*, to swell]

deu•ter•an•o•pi•a (dū′tĕr-ă-nō′pē-ă) A congenital abnormality of the retina in which there are two rather than three retinal cone pigments (dichromatism) and complete insensitivity to middle wavelengths (green). [G. *deuteros*, second, + anopia]

♲ **deuterio-** Prefix meaning "containing deuterium."

deu•te•ri•um (dū-tēr′ē-ŭm) SYN hydrogen 2. [G. *deuteros*, second]

♲ **deutero-**, **deut-**, **deuto-** Combining forms meaning two, or second (in a series); secondary. [G. *deuteros*, second]

deu•ter•o•my•ce•tes (dū′tĕr-ō-mī-sē′tēz) Members of the class Deuteromycetes or the phylum Deuteromycota; characterized by lack of sexual reproductive form and recognized by their asexual structures, called conidia.

deu•ter•o•path•ic (dū′tĕr-ō-path′ik) Relating to a deuteropathy.

deu•ter•op•a•thy (dū′tĕr-op′ă-thē) A secondary disease or symptom. [deutero- + G. *pathos*, suffering]

deu•ter•o•plasm (dū′tĕr-ō-plazm) SYN deutoplasm. [deutero- + G. *plasma*, thing formed]

deu•to•nymph (dū′tō-nimf) The third stage of a mite.

deu•to•plasm (dū′tō-plazm) The yolk of a meroblastic egg; the nonliving material in the cytoplasm, especially that stored in the oocyte as food for the developing embryo, the commonest types being lipoid droplets and yolk granules. SYN deuteroplasm. [deuto- + G. *plasma*, thing formed]

de•vas•cu•lar•i•za•tion (dē-vas′kyū-lăr-ī-zā′shŭn) Occlusion of all or most of the blood vessels to any part or organ. [L. *de*, away, + *vasculum*, small vessel, + G. *izo*, to cause]

de•vel•op•er (dĕ-vel′ŏp-ĕr) **1.** A person who or procedure that develops. **2.** SYN eluent. **3.** The chemicals used to develop film by reducing the light-activated silver halide molecules to atomic silver.

de•vel•op•ment (dĕ-vel′ŏp-mĕnt) **1.** The act or process of natural progression in physical and psychological maturation from a previous, lower, or embryonic stage to a later, more complex, or adult stage. **2.** The process of chromatography.

de•vel•op•men•tal age (DA) (dĕ-vel′ŏp-men′tăl āj) **1.** Age estimated by anatomic development since fertilization. **2.** Age of a person estimated from the degree of anatomic, physiologic, mental, and emotional maturation.

de•vel•op•men•tal a•nat•o•my (dĕ-vel′ŏp-men′tăl ă-nat′ŏ-mē) Anatomy of the structural changes of a person from fertilization to adulthood; includes embryology, fetology, and postnatal development.

de•vel•op•men•tal a•nom•a•ly (dĕ-vel′ŏp-men′tăl ă-nom′ă-lē) An anomaly established during intrauterine life.

de•vel•op•men•tal a•prax•i•a of speech (DAS) (dĕ-vel′ŏp-men′tăl ă-prak′sē-ă spēch) Severe articulatory disturbance in childhood characterized by multiple and inconsistent errors in production of voluntary sequences of phonemes, but not due to weakness or spasticity of speech musculature (i.e., not dysarthria). SYN childhood apraxia, developmental dyspraxia of speech.

de•vel•op•men•tal de•lay (dĕ-vel′ŏp-men′tăl dĕ-lā′) Lack of normal intellectual growth and development. SEE ALSO mental retardation.

de•vel•op•men•tal dis•a•bil•i•ty (DD) (dĕ-vel′ŏp-men′tăl dis′ă-bil′i-tē) Loss of function brought on by prenatal and postnatal events in which the predominant disturbance is in the acquisition of cognitive, language, motor, or social skills; e.g., mental retardation, autistic disorder, learning disorder, and attention deficit hyperactivity disorder.

de•vel•op•men•tal do•mains (dĕ-vel′ŏp-men′tăl dō-mānz′) The five areas of child development: language, motor, cognitive, social-emotional, and self-help skills.

de•vel•op•men•tal dys•prax•i•a of speech (dĕ-vel′ŏp-men′tăl dis-prak′sē-ă spēch) SYN developmental apraxia of speech.

de•vel•op•men•tal grooves (dĕ-vel′ŏp-men′tăl grūvz) Fine lines found in the enamel of a tooth that mark the junction of the lobes of the crown in its development. SYN developmental lines.

de•vel•op•men•tal hip dys•pla•si•a (dĕ-vel′ŏp-men′tăl hip dis-plā′zē-ă) SYN congenital hip dysplasia.

de•vel•op•men•tal lines (dĕ-vel′ŏp-men′tăl līnz) SYN developmental grooves.

de•vel•op•men•tal•ly de•layed (dĕ-vel′ŏp-men′tă-lē dĕ-lād) Denotes lack of normal intellectual growth. SEE ALSO mental retardation.

de•vel•op•men•tal mile•stones (dĕ-vel′ŏp-men′tăl mīl′stōnz) The stages in the neuromuscular, mental, or social maturation of an infant or young child, generally marked by the attainment of a capacity or skill, such as rolling over, sitting with good head control, smiling spontaneously, laughing, and following moving objects with the eyes; most of these occur by the age of 2–4 months in the normal infant. See this page.

de•vel•op•men•tal psy•chol•o•gy (dĕ-vel′ŏp-men′tăl sī-kol′ŏ-jē) The study of the psychological, physiologic, and behavioral changes in an organism that occur from birth to old age.

de•vel•op•men•tal scis•sors grasp (dĕ-vel′ŏp-men′tăl siz′ŏrz grasp) A grasp pattern seen in the infant emerging in the 8th–9th month characterized by the thumb's trapping an object against the radial side of a flexed index finger; the ulnar digits are usually loosely flexed, providing stability for the radial digits; in this grasp, the thumb is not opposed but adducted.

De•ven•ter pel•vis (dĕ-ven′tĕr pel′vis) A pelvis with shortened anteroposterior diameter.

de•vi•ance (dē′vē-ăns) SYN deviation (3).

de•vi•ant (dē′vē-ănt) **1.** Denoting or indicative of deviation. **2.** An individual exhibiting deviation, especially sexual.

de•vi•ant be•hav•ior (dē′vē-ănt bē-hāv′yŏr) Activity that is prescribed by custom, social mores, or laws intended to curb or discourage such activity.

de•vi•a•tion (dē′vē-ā′shŭn) **1.** A turning away or aside from the normal point or course. **2.** An abnormality. **3.** PSYCHIATRY, BEHAVIORAL SCIENCES a departure from an accepted norm, role, or rule. SYN deviance. **4.** STATISTICS a measurement representing the difference between an individual value in a set of values and the mean value in that set. [L. *devio,* to turn from the straight path, fr. *de,* from, + *via,* way]

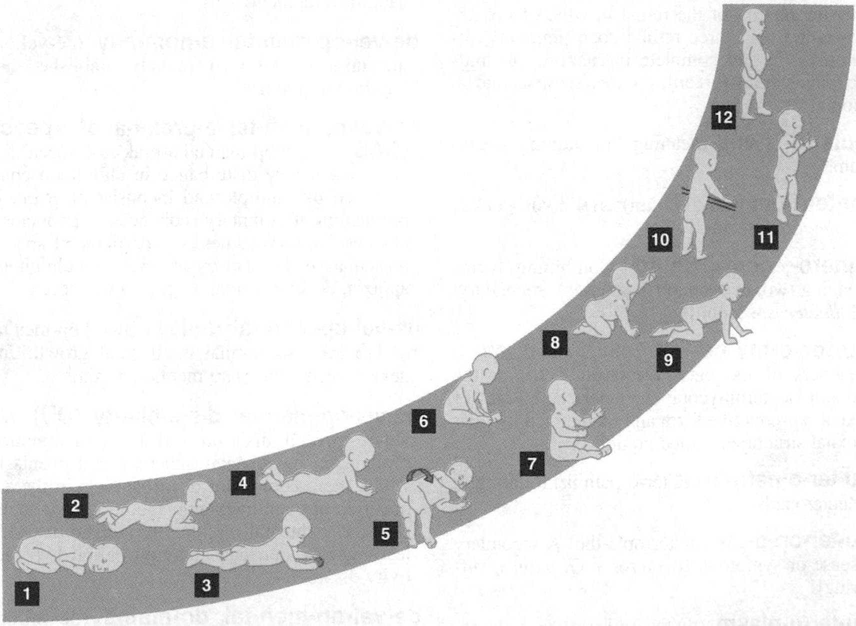

milestones in normal child development (shown by month): (1) moves largely by reflex; (2) holds head up when prone; (3) grasps objects; (4) raises chest and head when prone; (5) turns front to back; (6) sits, but only with some support; (7) sits securely without support; (8) reaches out in anticipation of being picked up; (9) creeps or crawls with abdomen lifted off the floor; (10) pulls self to standing position; (11) stands alone; (12) takes first steps

De•vic dis•ease (dĕ-vēk′ di-zēz′) SYN neuromyelitis optica.

de•vice (dĕ-vīs′) An appliance, usually mechanical, designed to perform a specific function (e.g., prosthesis or orthosis). [M.E., fr. O. Fr. *devis*, fr. L. *divisum*, divided]

dev•il's dung (dev′ilz dŭng) SYN asafoetida.

dev•il's grip (dev′ilz grip) SYN epidemic pleurodynia. SEE ALSO hand-foot-and-mouth disease.

de•vi•om•e•ter (dē′vē-om′ĕ-tĕr) A form of strabismometer.

de•vi•tal•ized (dē-vī′tăl-īzd) Devoid of life; dead.

de•vi•tal tooth (dē-vī′tăl tūth) A misnomer for a pulpless tooth.

de Weck•er scis•sors (dĕ wek-ĕr′ siz′ŏrz) Small scissors with sharp points for intraocular cutting of the iris and lens capsule.

DEXA Acronym for dual-energy x-ray absorptiometry.

dex•ter (deks′tĕr) Located on or relating to the right side. [L. fem. *dextra*, neut. *dextrum*]

dex•ter•i•ty (deks-ter′i-tē) SYN fine motor coordination. [L. *dexter*, right (hand)]

dex•trad (deks′trad) Toward the right side. [L. *dexter*, right, + *ad*, to]

dex•tral (deks′trăl) SYN right-handed.

dex•tral•i•ty (deks-tral′i-tē) Right-handedness; preference for the right hand in performing manual tasks.

dex•tran•ase (deks′tră-nās) An enzyme hydrolyzing 1,6-α-D-glucosidic linkages in dextran; used in the prevention of caries.

dex•trase (deks′trās) Nonspecific term for the complex of enzymes that converts dextrose (D-glucose) into lactic acid.

dex•tri•nase (deks′tri-nās) Any of the enzymes catalyzing the hydrolysis of dextrins; e.g., amylo-1,6-glucosidase, dextrin dextranase.

dex•trin dex•tran•ase (deks′trin deks′tră-nās) A glucosyltransferase transferring 1,4-α-D-glucosyl residues, thus catalyzing the synthesis of dextrans from dextrins by glucose transfer.

dex•tri•no•sis (deks′trin-ō′sis) SYN glycogenosis.

dex•tri•nu•ri•a (deks′tri-nyūr′ē-ă) The passage of dextrin in the urine.

♲ **dextro-, dextr-** Combining forms meaning right, toward, on the right side, or dextrorotatory. [L. *dexter*, on the right-hand side]

dex•tro•am•phet•a•mine sul•fate (deks′trō-am-fet′ă-mēn sul′fāt) Similar in action to racemic amphetamine sulfate, but more stimulating to the central nervous system; sympathomimetic and appetite depressant. SYN dextroamphetamine sulphate.

dextroamphetamine sulphate [Br.] SYN dextroamphetamine sulfate.

dex•tro•car•di•a (deks-trō-kahr′dē-ă) Displacement of the heart to the right, either as dextroposition, with simple displacement to the right, or as cardiac heterotaxia, with complete transposition of the right and left chambers, resulting in a heart that is the mirror image of a normal heart. [dextro- + G. *kardia*, heart]

dex•tro•car•di•a with si•tus in•ver•sus (deks-trō-kahr′dē-ă sī′tus in-vĕr′sŭs) Displacement of the heart to the right side of the thorax with mirror transposition of the cardiac chambers together with transposition of the abdominal viscera.

dex•tro•gas•tri•a (deks′trō-gas′trē-ă) Condition in which the stomach is displaced to the right; may represent either simple displacement or situs inversus. Usually associated with dextrocardia. [dextro- + G. *gastēr*, stomach]

dex•tro•gy•ra•tion (deks′trō-jī-rā′shŭn) A twisting to the right. [dextro- + L. *gyro*, pp. *-atus*, to turn in a circle, fr. *gyrus*, circle]

dex•trop•e•dal (deks-trop′ĕ-dăl) Denoting one who uses the right leg in preference to the left. SYN right-footed. [dextro- + L. *pes* (*ped-*), foot]

dex•tro•po•si•tion (deks′trō-pŏ-zish′ŭn) Abnormal right-sided location or origin of a normally left-sided structure, e.g., origin of the aorta from the right ventricle.

dex•tro•po•si•tion of the heart (deks′trō-pŏ-zish′ŭn hahrt) SEE dextrocardia.

dex•tro•ro•ta•to•ry (deks′trō-rō′tă-tōr-ē) Denoting dextrorotation, or certain crystals or solutions capable of such action; as a chemical prefix, usually abbreviated *d-*. Cf. levorotatory.

dex•trose (deks′trōs) SEE glucose.

dex•tro•si•nis•tral (deks′trō-sin′is-trăl) In a direction from right to left. [dextro- + L. *sinister*, left]

dex•tro•tor•sion (deks′trō-tōr′shŭn) **1.** A twisting to the right. **2.** OPHTHALMOLOGY a conjugate rotation of the upper pole of both corneas to the right. [dextro- + L. *torsio*, a twisting]

dex•tro•tro•pic (deks′trō-trō′pik) Turning to the right. [dextro- + G. *tropos*, a turn]

dex•tro•ver•sion (deks′trō-vĕr-zhŭn) **1.** Version toward the right. **2.** OPHTHALMOLOGY a conjugate rotation of both eyes to the right. [dextro- + L. *verto*, pp. *versus*, to turn]

df, DF Abbreviation for decayed and/or filled teeth.

DFE Abbreviation for dietary folate equivalent.

DGI Abbreviation for dynamic gait index.

dGMP Abbreviation for deoxyguanylic acid.

DHEA Abbreviation for dehydroepiandrosterone.

DHEA-S A steroid secreted by the cortex of suprarenal gland and the testis; a precursor of testosterone. Limited studies suggest that DHEA reduces the percentage of body fat, perhaps by blocking the storage of energy as fat. Commercial formulations of DHEA are marketed as dietary supplements, although it is neither a nutrient nor a component of the human food chain. It has been promoted for the prevention of degenerative diseases including atherosclerosis, Alzheimer dementia, and parkinsonism and other effects of aging, but none of the alleged benefits has been confirmed in large, randomized clinical trials. Long-term administration to postmenopausal women has been associated with insulin resistance, hypertension, and reduction of LDL cholesterol.

DHT Abbreviation for dihydrotestosterone.

DI Abbreviation for diabetes insipidus.

♻**di-** **1.** Prefix meaning two, twice. **2.** CHEMISTRY often used in place of bis- when not likely to be confusing; e.g., dichloro compounds. Cf. bi-, bis-. [G. *dis,* two]

♻**dia-** Prefix meaning through, throughout, completely. [G. *dia,* through]

di•a•be•tes (dī-ă-bē′tēz) Either diabetes insipidus or diabetes mellitus; term refers to a condition in which the pituitary gland increases urinary output (diabetes insipidus) or a disorder in which the pancreas produces defects in insulin production or action, thus inducing hyperglycemia (diabetes mellitus). Both diseases have in common the symptom polyuria; when used without qualification, refers to diabetes mellitus. [G. *diabētēs,* a compass, a siphon, diabetes]

di•a•be•tes in•sip•i•dus (DI) (dī-ă-bē′tēz in-sip′i-dŭs) Chronic excretion of very large amounts of pale urine of low specific gravity, causing dehydration and extreme thirst; ordinarily results from inadequate output of pituitary antidiuretic hormone. SEE ALSO nephrogenic diabetes insipidus.

di•a•be•tes in•ter•mit•tens (dī-ă-bē′tēz in-tĕr-mit′tenz) Diabetes mellitus in which there are periods of relatively normal carbohydrate metabolism followed by relapses to the previous diabetic state.

di•a•be•tes mel•li•tus (DM) (dī-ă-bē′tēz mel′i-tŭs) A metabolic disease in which carbohydrate use is reduced and that of lipid and protein enhanced; it is caused by an absolute or relative deficiency of insulin and is characterized, in more severe cases, by chronic hyperglycemia, glycosuria, water and electrolyte loss, ketoacidosis, and coma; long-term complications include neuropathy, retinopathy, nephropathy, generalized degenerative changes in large and small blood vessels, and increased susceptibility to infection. SEE ALSO Type 1 diabetes, Type 2 diabetes. [L. sweetened with honey]

di•a•bet•ic (dī-ă-bet′ik) Relating to or having diabetes.

di•a•bet•ic ac•i•do•sis (dī-ă-bet′ik as-i-dō′sis) Decreased pH and bicarbonate concentration in the body fluids caused by accumulation of ketone bodies in diabetes mellitus. SEE ALSO diabetic ketoacidosis.

di•a•bet•ic a•my•ot•ro•phy (dī-ă-bet′ik ă′mī-ot′rŏ-fē) A type of diabetic neuropathy that primarily affects elderly patients with diabetes mellitus; clinically characterized by unilateral or bilateral anterior thigh pain, weakness, and atrophy; one type of diabetic polyradiculopathy. Sometimes referred to, erroneously, as diabetic femoral neuropathy.

di•a•bet•ic co•ma (dī-ă-bet′ik kō′mă) State that develops in severe and inadequately treated diabetes mellitus and is commonly fatal, unless appropriate therapy is instituted promptly; results from reduced oxidative metabolism of the central nervous system that, in turn, stems from severe ketoacidosis and possibly also from the histotoxic action of the ketone bodies and disturbances in water and electrolyte balance.

di•a•bet•ic der•mop•a•thy (dī-ă-bet′ik dĕr-mop′ă-thē) Small macules and papules of the extensor surfaces of the extremities, most commonly the shins of diabetic patients, which become atrophic, hyperpigmented, and occasionally undergo ulceration with scarring; may be a manifestation of microangiopathy.

di•a•bet•ic di•et (dī-ă-bet′ik dī′ĕt) A dietary adjustment for patients with diabetes mellitus intended to decrease the need for insulin or oral diabetic agents and control weight by adjusting caloric and carbohydrate intake.

di•a•bet•ic foot in•fec•tion (dī-ă-bet′ik fut in-fek′shŭn) Disease of the foot and its digits usually due to diabetes mellitus or other neurologic disorder.

di•a•bet•ic glo•mer•u•lo•scle•ro•sis (dī-ă-bet′ik glo-mĕr′ū-lō-skler-ō′sis) Rounded hyaline or laminated nodules in the periphery of the glomeruli with capillary basement membrane thickening and increased mesangial matrix occurring in long-standing diabetes, proteinuria, and ultimately renal failure. SYN intercapillary glomerulosclerosis.

di•a•bet•ic ke•to•ac•i•do•sis (DKA) (dī-ă-bet′ik kē′tō-as′i-dō′sis) Buildup of ketones in blood due to breakdown of stored fats for energy; a complication of diabetes mellitus. Untreated, can lead to coma and death.

di•a•bet•ic neph•rop•a•thy (dī-ă-bet′ik nĕfrop′ă-thē) A syndrome occurring in people with diabetes mellitus; associated with damage to blood vessels that supply the glomerula at the kidney; characterized by albuminuria, hypertension, and progressive renal insufficiency.

di•a•bet•ic neu•rop•a•thy (dī-ă-bet′ik nūr-op′ă-thē) A generic term for any diabetes mellitus–related disorder of the peripheral nervous system, autonomic nervous system, and some cranial nerves. This most commonly occurring of the chronic complications of diabetes takes two forms, peripheral (with dulling of the sensations of pain, temperature, and pressure, especially in the lower legs and feet), and autonomic (with alternating bouts of diarrhea and constipation, impotence, and reduced cardiac function).

di•a•bet•ic ret•i•nop•a•thy (dī-ă-bet′ik ret′i-nop′ă-thē) Retinal changes occurring in diabetes of long duration, marked by hemorrhages, microaneurysms, and sharply defined waxy deposits, or by proliferative retinopathy.

di•a•be•to•gen•ic (dī-ă-bet′ō-jen′ik) Causing diabetes.

di•a•be•tog•en•ous (dī′ă-bē-toj′ĕn-ŭs) Caused by diabetes.

di•a•be•tol•o•gy (dī′ă-bē-tol′ŏ-jē) The field of medicine concerned with diabetes.

di•a•ce•tic ac•id (dī-ă-sē′tik as′id) SYN acetoacetic acid.

di•a•ce•tyl•mon•ox•ime (dī-as′ĕ-til-mon-ok′sēm) A 2-oxo-oxime that can reactivate phosphorylated acetylcholinesterase in vitro and in vivo; it penetrates the blood-brain barrier.

di•a•chron•ic (dī-ă-kron′ik) Systematically observed over time in the same subjects throughout as opposed to synchronic or cross-sectional. [dia- + G. *chronos,* time]

di•a•chron•ic stu•dy (dī-ă-kron′ik stŭd′ē) A study of the natural course of a life or disorder in which a cohort of subjects is serially observed over a period of time and no assumptions need be made about the stability of the system.

di•a•crit•ic, di•a•crit•i•cal (dī-ă-krit′ik, -i-kăl) Distinguishing; diagnostic; allowing of distinction. [G. *diakritikos,* able to distinguish]

di•ad (dī′ad) **1.** The transverse tubule and a cisterna in cardiac muscle fibers. **2.** SYN dyad (1).

di•ad•o•cho•ki•ne•si•a, di•ad•o•cho•ki•ne•sis (dī-ad′ŏ-kō-ki-nē′zē-ă, -ki-nē′sis) The normal power of alternately bringing a limb into opposite positions, as of flexion and extension or of pronation and supination. [G. *diadochos,* working in turn, + *kinēsis,* movement]

di•ad•o•cho•ki•net•ic (dī-ad′ŏ-kō-ki-net′ik) Relating to diadochokinesia.

diaeretic [Br.] SYN dieretic.

di•a•gen•e•sis (dī-ă-jen′ĕ-sĭs) The process of converting sediment to rock.

di•ag•nose (dī-ăg-nōs′) To make a diagnosis.

di•ag•no•sis (dī-ăg-nō′sis) The determination of the nature of a disease, injury, or congenital defect. SEE ALSO nursing diagnosis. [G. *diagnōsis,* a deciding]

di•ag•no•sis by ex•clu•sion (dī-ăg-nō′sis eks-klū′zhŭn) A determination made by excluding those diseases to which only some of the patient's symptoms might belong, leaving one disease as the most likely diagnosis, although no definitive tests or findings establish that diagnosis.

di•ag•no•sis code (dī′ăg-nō′sis kōd) A number assigned to a diagnosis using the International Classification of Diseases manual.

di•ag•no•sis-re•lat•ed group (DRG) (dī-ăg-nō′sis-rĕ-lāt′ĕd grūp) A classification of patients by diagnosis or surgical procedure (sometimes including age) into major diagnostic categories (each containing specific diseases, disorders, or procedures) for the purpose of determining payment of hospitalization charges, based on the premise that treatment of similar medical diagnoses generates similar costs.

di•ag•nos•o•gen•ic the•o•ry (dī-ăg-nos′ŏ-jen′ik thē′ŏr-ē) As applied to stuttering, a theory that attributes the disorder to misdiagnosis of normal disfluency in a young child; the resultant anxiety exacerbates the disfluency and establishes stuttering as a disorder.

di•ag•nos•tic (dī-ăg-nos′tik) **1.** Relating to or aiding in diagnosis. **2.** Establishing or confirming a diagnosis.

di•ag•nos•ti•cian (dī′ăg-nos-tish′ăn) One who is skilled in making diagnoses.

di•ag•nos•tic o•ver•kill (dī′ăg-nos′tik ō′vĕr-kil) The excessive use of tests for either medical or legal reasons in the determination of the nature of a disease, injury, or congenital defect.

di•ag•nos•tic ra•di•o•logy (dī-ăg-nos′tik rā′dē-ol′ŏ-jē) SYN radiology (2).

di•ag•nos•tic sen•si•tiv•i•ty (dī-ăg-nos′tik sen′si-tiv′i-tē) SYN clinical sensitivity.

di•ag•nos•tic spec•i•fic•i•ty (dī-ăg-nos′tik spes′i-fis′i-tē) **1.** The probability (P) that, given the absence of disease (D), a normal test result (T) excludes disease; i.e., P(T/D). **2.** Specificity (%) = number of patients without the disease who test negative × 100 ÷ total number tested without the disease.

***Di•ag•nos•tic and Sta•tis•ti•cal Man•u•al of Men•tal Dis•or•ders* (DSM)** (dī-ăg-nos′tik stă-tis′ti-kăl man′yū-ăl men′tăl dis-ōr′dĕrz) An American Psychiatric Association publication that classifies mental illnesses. Currently in its fourth edition (i.e., *DSM-IV*), the manual provides health care practitioners with a comprehensive system for diagnosing mental illnesses based on specific ideational and behavioral symptoms.

di·ag·nos·tic ul·tra·sound (dī-ăg-nos′tik ŭl′tră-sownd) The use of ultrasound to obtain images for medical diagnostic purposes.

di·ag·o·nal con·ju·gate (dī-ag′ŏ-năl kon′jŭ-găt) The anteroposterior dimension of the inlet; the clinical distance from the promontory of the sacrum to the lower margin of the symphysis pubica. SYN false conjugate (1).

di·a·gram (dī′ă-gram) A simple, graphic depiction of an idea or object.

di·a·ki·ne·sis (dī′ă-ki-nē′sis) Final stage of prophase in meiosis I, in which the chromosomes continue to shorten and the nucleolus and nuclear membrane disappear. [G. *dia,* through, + *kinēsis,* movement]

di·a·lect (dī′ă-lekt) The aggregate of generally local shifts in pronunciation, grammar, and vocabulary from a perceived less localized standard.

di·al·y·sance (dī-al′i-săns) The number of milliliters of blood completely cleared of any substance by an artificial kidney or by peritoneal dialysis in a unit of time; conventional clearance formulas are expressed as mm/min. [fr. dialysis]

di·al·y·sate (dī-al′i-sāt) That part of a mixture that passes through a dialyzing membrane. SYN diffusate.

di·al·y·sis (dī-al′i-sis) **1.** A form of filtration to separate crystalloid from colloid substances (or smaller molecules from larger ones) in a solution by interposing a semipermeable membrane between the solution and water; the crystalloid (smaller) substances pass through the membrane into the water on the other side, the colloids do not. SYN diffusion (2). **2.** The separation of substances across a semipermeable membrane on the basis of particle size and/or concentration gradients. **3.** A method of artificial kidney function. [G. a separation, fr. *dialyo,* to separate]

di·al·y·sis en·ceph·a·lop·a·thy syn·drome, di·al·y·sis de·men·ti·a (dī-al′i-sis en-sef′ă-lop′ă-thē sin′drōm, dī-al′i-sis dĕ-men′shē-ă) A progressive, often fatal, diffuse encephalopathy occurring in patients on chronic hemodialysis.

di·al·y·sis ret·i·nae (dī-al′i-sis ret′i-nē) Congenital or traumatic separation of the peripheral sensory retina from the retinal pigment epithelium at the ora serrata, often causing a retinal detachment.

di·a·lyz·er (dī′ă-lī-zĕr) The apparatus for performing dialysis; a membrane used in dialysis.

di·a·me·li·a (dī-ă-mē′lē-ă) Absence of two limbs. [di- + g. *a* priv. + *melos,* limb, + -ia]

di·am·e·ter (dī-am′ĕ-tĕr) **1.** A straight line connecting two opposite points on the surface of a more or less spheric or cylindric body, or at the boundary of an opening or foramen, passing through the center of such body or opening. **2.** The distance measured along such a line. [G. *diametros,* fr. *dia,* through, + *metron,* measure]

Di·a·mond-Black·fan syn·drome (dī′mŏnd blak′fan sin′drōm) SYN congenital hypoplastic anemia.

Di·a·mond TYM med·i·um (dī′mŏnd mē′dē-ŭm) Culture base of *t*rypticase, *y*east extract, *m*altose, and serum used to detect the presence of *Trichomonas vaginalis.*

Di·an·a com·plex (dī-an′ă kom′pleks) Ideas leading to the adoption of masculine traits and behavior in a female. [*Diana,* L. myth. char.]

di·a·pause (dī′ă-pawz) A period of biologic quiescence or dormancy with decreased metabolism; an interval in which development is arrested or greatly slowed. [dia- + G. *pausis,* pause]

di·a·pe·de·sis (dī′ă-pĕ-dē′sis) The passage of blood, or any of its formed elements, through the intact walls of blood vessels. SYN migration (2). [G. *dia,* through, + *pēdēsis,* a leaping]

di·a·per der·ma·ti·tis, di·a·per rash (dī′pĕr dĕr′mă-tī′tis, dī′pĕr rash) Colloquially referred to as diaper, ammonia, or napkin rash; dermatitis of thighs and buttocks resulting from exposure to urine and feces in infants' diapers. Formerly attributed to ammonia formation; moisture, bacterial growth, and alkalinity may all induce lesions.

di·aph·a·no·scope (dī-af′ă-nō-skōp) An instrument for illuminating the interior of a cavity to determine the translucency of its walls. [G. *diaphanēs,* transparent, + *skopeō,* to examine]

di·aph·a·nos·co·py (dī-af′ă-nos′kŏ-pē) Examination of a cavity with a diaphanoscope.

di·a·phe·met·ric (dī′ă-fē-met′rik) Relating to the determination of the degree of tactile sensibility. [G. *dia,* through, + *haphē,* touch, + *metron,* measure]

di·a·pho·re·sis (dī′ă-fŏr-ē′sis) SYN perspiration (1). [G. *diaphorēsis,* fr. *dia,* through, + *phoreō,* to carry]

di·a·pho·ret·ic (dī′ă-fŏr-et′ik) **1.** Relating to, or causing, perspiration. **2.** An agent that increases perspiration.

di·a·phragm (dī′ă-fram) **1.** The musculomembranous partition between the abdominal and thoracic cavities. SYN diaphragma (2) [TA], midriff. **2.** A thin disc pierced with an opening, used in a microscope, camera, or other optic instrument to shut out the marginal rays of light, thus giving a more direct illumination. **3.** A flexible ring covered with a dome-shaped sheet of elastic

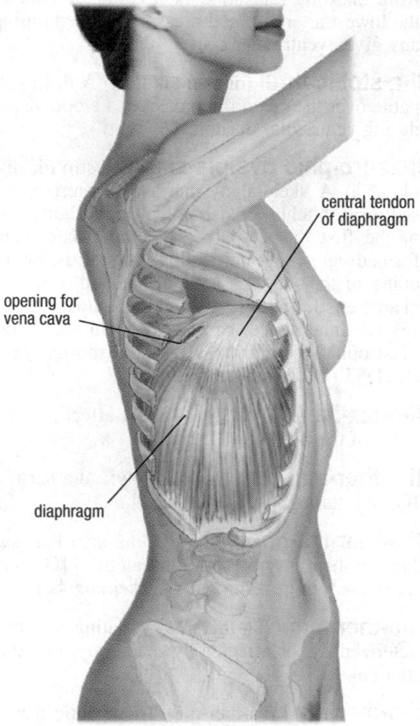

diaphragm

material placed in the vagina to prevent pregnancy. **4.** RADIOGRAPHY a grid (2). See this page. [G. *diaphragma*]

di•a•phrag•ma, pl. **di•a•phrag•ma•ta** (dī-ă-frag′mă, -mă-tă) [TA] **1.** A thin partition separating adjacent regions. **2.** [TA] SYN diaphragm (1). [G. *diaphragma,* a partition wall, midriff]

di•a•phrag•ma sel•lae (dī-ă-frag′mă sel′ē) [TA] A fold of dura mater extending transversely across the sella turcica and roofing over the hypophysial fossa; it is perforated in its center for the passage of the infundibulum. SYN diaphragm of sella turcica.

di•a•phrag•mat•ic (dī′ă-frag-mat′ik) Relating to a diaphragm. SYN phrenic (1).

di•a•phrag•mat•ic flut•ter (dī′ă-frag-mat′ik flŭt′ĕr) Rapid rhythmic contractions (average, 150 per minute) of the diaphragm, simulating atrial flutter clinically and sometimes electrocardiographically.

di•a•phrag•mat•ic her•ni•a (dī′ă-frag-mat′ik hĕr′nē-ă) Protrusion of abdominal contents into the chest through a weakness in the respiratory diaphragm; a common type is the hiatal hernia.

di•a•phrag•mat•ic lig•a•ment of the mes•o•neph•ros (dī′ă-frag-mat′ik lig′ă-mĕnt mez′ō-nef′rōs) The segment of the urogenital ridge that extends from the mesonephros to the diaphragm; becomes the suspensory ligament of the ovary.

di•a•phrag•mat•ic pleu•ri•sy (dī′ă-frag-mat′ik plūr′i-sē) SYN epidemic pleurodynia.

di•a•phragm of sel•la tur•ci•ca (dī′ă-fram sel′ă tŭr′si-kă) SYN diaphragma sellae.

di•a•phy•sec•to•my (dī′ă-fi-sek′tŏ-mē) Partial or complete removal of the shaft of a long bone. [diaphysis + G. *ektomē,* excision]

di•a•phys•i•al (dī-ă-fiz′ē-ăl) Relating to a diaphysis.

di•aph•y•sis, pl. **di•aph•y•ses** (dī-af′i-sis, -sēz) [TA] SYN shaft. [G. a growing between]

di•a•pi•re•sis (dī′ă-pī-rē′sis) Passage of colloidal or other small particles of suspended matter through the unruptured walls of the blood vessels. SEE ALSO diapedesis. [G. *diapeirō,* to drive through, fr. *peirō,* to pierce]

di•ar•rhe•a (dī′ă-rē′ă) An abnormally frequent discharge of semisolid or fluid fecal matter from the bowel. SYN diarrhoea. [G. *diarrhoia,* fr. *dia,* through, + *rhoia,* a flow, a flux]

di•ar•rhe•a•gen•ic (dī′ă-rē-ă-jen′ik) Pertains to diarrhea-causing microorganisms (e.g., *Escherichia coli*).

di•ar•rhe•al, **di•ar•rhe•ic** (dī′ă-rē′ăl, -ik) Relating to diarrhea. SYN diarrhetic, diarrhoeal.

di•ar•rhet•ic (dī′ă-rĕt′ik) SYN diarrheal.

diarrhoea [Br.] SYN diarrhea.

diarrhoeal [Br.] SYN diarrheal.

diarrhoeic [Br.] SYN diarrheic.

di•ar•thric (dī-ahr′thrik) Relating to two joints. SYN biarticular, diarticular. [G. *di-,* two, + *arthron,* joint]

di•ar•thro•di•al joint (dī′ahr-thrō′dē-ăl joynt) SYN synovial joint.

di•ar•thro•sis, pl. **di•ar•thro•ses** (dī′ahr-thrō′sis, dī′ahr-thrō′sēz) SYN synovial joint. [G. articulation]

di•ar•tic•u•lar (dī-ahr-tik′yū-lăr) SYN diarthric.

di•as•chi•sis (dī-as′ki-sis) A sudden inhibition of function produced by an acute focal disturbance in a portion of the brain at a distance from the original seat of injury, but anatomically connected with it through fiber tracts. [G. a splitting]

di•a•scope (dī′ă-skōp) A flat glass plate through which one can examine superficial skin lesions by means of pressure. [G. *dia,* through, + *skopeō,* to view]

di•as•co•py (dī-as′kŏ-pē) Examination of superficial skin lesions with a diascope. [G. *dia,* through, + *skopeō,* to see]

di•a•stal•sis (dī′ă-stal′sis) The type of peristalsis in which a region of inhibition precedes the wave of contraction, as seen in the intestinal tract. [G. an arrangement]

di•a•stal•tic (dī′ă-stal′tik) Pertaining to diastalsis.

di•as•ta•sis (dī-as′tă-sis) **1.** Any simple separation of normally joined parts. SYN divarication. **2.** The midportion of diastole when the blood enters the ventricle slowly or ceases to enter before atrial systole. Diastasis duration is in inverse proportion to heart rate and is absent at very high heart rates. [G. a separation]

di•as•tas•u•ri•a (dī′as-tās-yūr′ē-ă) SYN amylasuria.

di•a•stat•ic (dī′ă-stat′ik) Relating to a diastasis.

di•a•stat•ic frac•ture (dī′ă-stat′ik frak′shŭr) **1.** Separation of cranial bones at a suture. **2.** Fracture with marked separation of bone fragments.

di•a•ste•ma, pl. **di•a•ste•ma•ta** (dī′ă-stē′mă, -mă-tă) [TA] **1.** Fissure or abnormal opening in any part, especially if congenital. **2.** Space between two adjacent teeth in the same dental arch. **3.** A space between teeth not due to missing teeth. **4.** A space between the upper central incisors in humans, or a space between two adjacent teeth in the same dental arch, especially that between the upper lateral incisor and the adjacent canine, into which the lower canine closes in the Carnivora, such as dogs. SYN space (2). [G. *diastēma,* an interval]

di•a•ste•ma•to•cra•ni•a (dī′ă-stē′mă-tō-krā′nē-ă) Congenital sagittal fissure of the cranium. [G. *diastēma,* an interval, + *kranion,* skull]

di•a•ste•ma•to•my•e•li•a (dī′ă-stē′mă-tō-mī-ē′lē-ă) Complete or incomplete sagittal division of the spinal cord by an osseous or fibrocartilaginous septum. [G. *diastēma,* interval, + *myelon,* marrow]

di•as•to•le (dī-as′tŏ-lē) Normal postsystolic dilation of the heart cavities, during which they fill with blood; diastole of the atria precedes that of the ventricles; diastole of either chamber alternates rhythmically with systole or contraction of that chamber. [G. *diastolē,* dilation]

di•a•stol•ic (dī′ă-stol′ik) Relating to diastole.

di•a•stol•ic blood pres•sure (dī′ă-stol′ik blŭd presh′ŭr) Intracardiac pressure during or due to diastolic relaxation in a cardiac chamber.

di•a•stol•ic fil•ling (dī′ă-stol′ik fil′ing) Time between opening of the mitral valve and tricuspid valve; includes passive rapid ventricular filling and the atrial contribution.

di•a•stol•ic mur•mur (DM) (dī′ă-stol′ik mŭr′mŭr) A murmur heard during diastole.

di•a•stol•ic pres•sure (dī′ă-stol′ik presh′ŭr) The intracardiac pressure during or resulting from diastolic relaxation of a cardiac chamber; the lowest arterial blood pressure reached during any given ventricular cycle.

di•a•stol•ic thrill (dī′ă-stol′ik thril) A thrill palpable over the precordium or over a blood vessel during ventricular diastole.

di•as•tro•phic dys•pla•si•a (dī′ă-strō′fik dis-plā′zē-ă) A skeletal dysplasia characterized by scoliosis, hitchhiker's thumb due to shortening of the first metacarpal bone, cleft palate, malformed ear with calcification, chondritis, shortening of the Achilles tendon, clubbed foot, and characteristic radiologic findings; autosomal recessive inheritance, caused by mutation in the diastrophic dysplasia sulfate transporter gene (DTDST) on chromosome 5q.

di•a•tax•i•a (dī′ă-tak′sē-ă) Ataxia affecting both sides of the body.

di•a•ther•mal (dī′ă-thĕr′măl) SYN diathermic. [G. *dia,* through, + *thermē,* heat]

di•a•ther•ma•nous (dī′ă-thĕr′mă-nŭs) Permeable by heat rays. SYN transcalent. [G. *diathermaino,* to heat through, fr. *thermos,* hot]

di•a•ther•mic (dī′ă-thĕr′mik) Relating to, characterized by, or affected by diathermy. SYN diathermal.

di•a•ther•my (dī′ă-thĕr-mē) Therapeutic use of short or ultrashort waves of electromagnetic energy to heat muscular tissue. [G. *dia,* through, + *thermē,* heat]

di•ath•e•sis (dī-ath′ĕ-sis) The constitutional or inborn state disposing to a disease, group of diseases, or metabolic or structural anomaly. [G. arrangement, condition]

di•a•thet•ic (dī′ă-thet′ik) Relating to a diathesis.

di•a•to•ma•ceous earth (dī′ă-tŏ-mā′shē-ŭs ĕrth) A powder made of desiccated diatom material; used as a filtering agent, adsorbent, and abrasive in many chemical operations.

di•a•tom•ic (dī′ă-tom′ik) **1.** Denoting a compound with a molecule made up of two atoms. **2.** Denoting any ion or atomic grouping composed of two atoms only.

♻ **diazo-** Prefix denoting a compound containing the ≡C–N=N–X grouping, where X is not carbon (except for CN), or the grouping N_2 attached by one atom to carbon. Cf. azo-. [G. *di-,* two, + Fr. *azote,* nitrogen]

di•ba•sic (dī-bā′sik) Having two replaceable hydrogen atoms, denoting an acid with two ionizable hydrogen atoms.

di•benz*(b,f)*-1:4-ox•a•ze•pine (dī-benz oks-az′ĕ-pēn) A riot-control agent (NATO code CR) with higher potency and a greater safety margin than *o*-chlorobenzylidene malononitrile (CS).

di•bu•caine num•ber test (DN) (dī′byū-kān

nŭm′bĕr test) A procedure to differentiate one of several forms of atypical pseudocholinesterases that are unable to inactivate succinylcholine at normal rates; based on percentage of inhibition of the enzymes by dibucaine. SEE ALSO fluoride number.

DIC Abbreviation for disseminated intravascular coagulation.

di·car·box·yl·ic ac·id cy·cle (dī′kahr-bok-sil′ik as′id sī′kĕl) **1.** That portion of the tricarboxylic acid cycle involving the dicarboxylic acids (succinic, fumaric, malic, and oxaloacetic acids). **2.** A cyclic scheme in which certain steps of the tricarboxylic acid cycle are used with the glyoxylate cycle; important in the use of glyoxylic acid in microorganisms.

di·cen·tric (dī-sen′trik) Having two centromeres, an abnormal state.

di·chlor·o·di·phe·nyl-tri·chlor·o·eth·ane (DDT) (dī-klōr′ō-dī-fen′ăl trī-klōr′ō-eth′ān) A restricted-use insecticide.

di·chlor·o·for·mox·ime (dī-klōr′ō-fōr-moks′ēm) SYN phosgene oxime.

di·cho·ri·al di·cho·ri·on·ic (dī-kōr′ē-ăl, ē-on′ik) Showing evidence of two chorions. [G. *di-*, two, + chorion]

di·cho·ri·on·ic di·am·ni·on·ic pla·cen·ta (dī′kōr′ē-on′ik dī′am-nē-on′ik plă-sen′tă) SEE twin placenta.

di·chro·ic (dī-krō′ik) Relating to dichroism.

di·chro·ism (dī′krō-izm) The property of seeming to be differently colored when viewed from emitted light and from transmitted light. [G. *di-*, two, + *chrōa,* color]

di·chro·mate (dī-krō′māt) A compound containing the radical $Cr_2O_7^{=}$.

di·chro·mat·ic (dī′krō-mat′ik) **1.** Having or exhibiting two colors. **2.** Relating to dichromatism (2).

di·chro·ma·tism (dī-krō′mă-tizm) **1.** The state of being dichromatic (1). **2.** The abnormality of color vision in which only two of the three retinal cone pigments are present, as in protanopia, deuteranopia, and tritanopia. SYN dichromatopsia. [G. *di-*, two, + *chrōma,* color]

di·chro·ma·top·si·a (dī′krō-mă-top′sē-ă) SYN dichromatism (2). [G. *di-*, two, + *chrōma,* color, + *opsis,* vision]

Dick·ens shunt (dik′ĕnz shŭnt) SYN pentose phosphate pathway.

Dick test (dik test) An intracutaneous test of susceptibility to the erythrogenic toxin of *Streptococcus pyogenes* responsible for the rash and other manifestations of scarlet fever.

DICOM (dī′kom) Acronym for Digital Imaging and Communications in Medicine, a joint standard of the American College of Radiology and National Equipment Manufacturers Association; specifies entities (or objects) and functions (or services) to allow communication between various image sources and other computer devices, such as archives or workstations.

di·co·ri·a (dī-kōr′ē-ă) SYN diplocoria. [G. *di-*, two, + *korē,* pupil]

Di·cro·coe·li·um (dik′rō-sē′lē-ŭm) A genus of digenetic trematodes inhabiting the biliary tract of herbivores. The lancet fluke, *D. dentriticum,* is rarely found in humans but is an important parasite of sheep. [G. *dikroos,* forked, + *koilia,* belly]

di·crot·ic (dī-krot′ik) Relating to dicrotism. [G. *dikrotos,* double-beating]

di·crot·ic notch (dī-krot′ik noch) The acute drop in arterial pressure pulse curves following the systolic peak, corresponding to the incisura of the displacement pulse curve.

di·crot·ic pulse (dī-krot′ik pŭls) A pulse that is marked by a double beat, the second, due to a palpable dicrotic wave, being weaker than the first.

di·crot·ic wave (dī-krot′ik wāv) The second rise in the tracing of a dicrotic pulse.

di·cro·tism (dī′krŏ-tizm) That form of the pulse in which a double beat can be appreciated at any arterial pulse for each beat of the heart; due to accentuation of the dicrotic wave. [G. *di-,* two, + *krotos,* a beat]

dicta- Prefix meaning two hundred. [G.]

dic·ta·tion (dik-tā′shŭn) An oral record of a patient's care created by a health care professional that is used by a medical transcriptionist to create a printed record. [L. *dicto*, fr. *dico*, to say]

dic·ta·tor (dik′tā-tŏr) SYN author. [L.]

dic·ty·o·ma (dik′tē-ō′mă) A benign tumor of the ciliary epithelium with a netlike structure resembling embryonic retina. SYN embryonal medulloepithelioma. [G. *dikyton,* net (retina), + *-oma,* tumor]

di·dac·tic (dī-dak′tik) Instructive; denoting medical teaching by lectures or textbooks, as distinguished from clinical demonstrations with patients or laboratory exercises. [G. *didaktikos,* fr. *didaskō,* to teach]

di·dac·ty·lism (dī-dak′ti-lizm) Congenital condition of having two fingers on a hand or two toes on a foot. [G. *di-*, two, + *daktylos,* finger or toe]

di·del·phic (dī-del′fik) Having or relating to a double uterus. [G. *di-*, two, + *delphys,* womb]

DIDMOAD (did′mōd) Acronym for Wolfram syndrome, which comprises *d*iabetes *i*nsipidus, *d*iabetes *m*ellitus, *o*ptic *a*trophy, and *d*eafness.

didym-, didymo- Combining forms meaning the didymus, testis. [G. *didymos,* twin]

did·y·mus (did′i-mŭs) SYN testis. [G. *didymos,* a twin, pl. *didymoi,* testes]

-didymus Suffix meaning a conjoined twin, with the first element of the complete word designating fused parts. SEE ALSO -dymus, -pagus. [G. *didymos,* twin]

di·e·cious (dī-ē′shŭs) Denoting animals or plants that are sexually distinct, the individuals being of one or the other sex. [G. *di-*, two, + *oikia,* house]

di·en·ceph·a·lon, pl. **di·en·ceph·a·la** (dī′en-sef′ă-lon, -sef′ă-lă) That part of the prosencephalon composed of the epithalamus, dorsal thalamus, subthalamus, and hypothalamus. [G. *dia,* through, + *enkephalos,* brain]

Di·en·ta·moe·ba fra·gil·is (dī′ent-ă-mē′bă frā-jil′ŭs) A species of small amebalike flagellates related to *Trichomonas*, parasitic in the large intestine of humans and certain monkeys; usually nonpathogenic, but sometimes causing low-grade inflammation with mucous diarrhea.

di·ent·a·moe·bi·a·sis (dī-ent′ă-mē-bī′ă-sis) Infection with protozoa of the genus *Dientamoeba*.

di·er·e·sis (dī-ĕr′ĕ-sis) SYN solution of continuity. [G. *diairesis,* a division]

di·e·ret·ic (dī′ĕr-et′ik) 1. Relating to dieresis. 2. Dividing; ulcerating; corroding. SYN diaeretic.

di·es·trous (dī-es′trŭs) Pertaining to diestrus. SYN dioestrous.

di·es·trus (dī-es′trŭs) A period of sexual quiescence intervening between two periods of estrus. SYN dioestrus. [G. *dia,* between, + *oistros,* desire]

di·et (dī′ĕt) **1.** Food and drink in general. **2.** A prescribed course of eating and drinking in which the amount and kind of food, as well as the times at which it is to be taken, are regulated for therapeutic purposes. **3.** Reduction of caloric intake so as to lose weight. **4.** To follow any prescribed or specific diet. [G. *diaita,* a way of life; a diet]

di·e·tar·y (dī′ĕ-tār-ē) Relating to the diet.

di·e·ta·ry al·low·anc·es (dī′ă-tār-ē ă-low′ăns-ĕz) Nutrient intake judged proper and healthful in quantity and type.

di·e·tar·y a·men·or·rhe·a (dī′ĕ-tār-ē ā-men′ŏr-ē′ă) Loss of menstrual function due to severe weight loss or gain.

di·e·tar·y fi·ber (dī′ĕ-tār-ē fī′bĕr) The plant polysaccharides and lignin that are resistant to hydrolysis by the digestive enzymes in humans.

di·e·ta·ry fo·late e·quiv·a·lent (DFE) (dī′ĕ-tār′ē fō′lāt ē-kwiv′ă-lĕnt) The amount of folate available to the body based on differences in absorbability from different sources. 1 mg DFE = 1 mg food folate = 0.6 mg of folic acid from fortified food or supplement.

Di·e·tar·y Guide·lines for A·mer·i·cans (dī′ĕ-tār-ē gīd′līnz ă-mer′i-kănz) The recommendations of the U.S. Departments of Agriculture and Health and Human Services for dietary intakes to reduce chronic diseases related to food intake (e.g., heart disease, diabetes, obesity).

Di·e·ta·ry Re·fer·ence In·take (DRI) (dī′ĕ-tār-ē ref′ĕr-ĕns in′tāk) A set of values for the dietary nutrient intakes of healthy people in the U.S. and Canada, used for planning and assessing diets. Includes the Recommended Dietary Allowance (RDA), the Adequate Intake (AI), the Tolerable Upper Limit (TUL), and the Estimated Average Intake (EAI); has eventually replaced the U.S. Recommended Daily Allowance and the Canadian Recommended Nutrient Intake (RNI). See Appendix.

Die·ter·le stain (dē′tĕr-lē stān) Stain used to demonstrate spirochetes and Leishman-Donovan bodies; employs silver nitrate and uranium nitrate.

di·e·tet·ic (dī′ĕ-tet′ik) **1.** Relating to diet. **2.** Descriptive of food that, naturally or through processing, has a low caloric content.

di·e·tet·ics (dī′ĕ-tet′iks) The practical application of diet in the prophylaxis and treatment of disease.

di·eth·yl·stil·bes·trol (DES) (dī-eth′il-stil-bes′trol) A synthetic nonsteroidal estrogenic compound; sometimes previously used as a postcoital antipregnancy agent to prevent implantation of the fertilized oocyte. The first demonstrated transplacental carcinogen responsible for a delayed clear-cell vaginal carcinoma in girls born to mothers who took the drug during pregnancy when it was erroneously thought to prevent miscarriage. SYN stilboestrol.

di·e·ti·tian (dī′ĕ-tish′ŭn) An expert in dietetics.

Die·tl cri·sis (dē′tĕl krī′sis) Intermittent pain, sometimes with nausea and emesis, caused by intermittent proximal obstruction of ureter or disention of the renal pelvis.

di·et qua·li·ty in·dex (dī′ĕt kwahl′i-tē in′deks) A measure of the value of a dietary regimen using a composite of eight recommendations regarding the consumption of foods and nutrients from the U.S. National Academy of Sciences (NAS). Meeting the standard is assigned a value of 0, within 30% of goal a value of 1, differing by more than 30% a 2. The resulting index can be a figure between 0–16, the lower the better. The NAS recommendations include reducing total fat intake to 30% or less of total energy; reducing saturated fatty acid intake to less than 10% of energy; reducing cholesterol intake to less than 300 mg daily; eating five or more servings daily of vegetables and fruits; increasing intake of starches and other complex carbohydrates by eating six or more servings daily of bread, cereal, and legumes; maintaining protein intake at moderate levels (i.e., levels lower than twice the RDA); limiting total daily intake of sodium to 2400 mg or less; and maintaining adequate calcium intake (approximately the RDA).

Dieu·la·foy le·sion (dyū-lah-fwah′ lē′zhŭn) An abnormally large submucosal artery located in the proximal stomach, which may be the site of acute and recurrent episodes of massive hemorrhage.

dif- (L.) Prefix meaning separation, taking apart, in two, reversal, not, or un-.

dif·fer·ence (dif′ĕr-ĕns) Degree of variation found in the comparison of two similar items.

dif·fer·ence li·men (dif′ĕr-ĕns lī′men) A barely noticeable change in the intensity or frequency of a stimulus.

dif·fer·en·tial di·ag·no·sis (dif′ĕr-en′shăl dī-ăg-nō′sis) The determination of which of two or more diseases with similar symptoms is the one the patient has, by a systematic comparison and contrasting of the clinical findings. SYN differentiation (2).

dif·fe·ren·tial dis·play (dif′ĕr-en′shăl dis-plā′) Use of reverse transcriptase and polymerase chain reaction technologies to amplify mRNA from specific cells or tissues and then to compare them directly with amplified mRNA from another cell or tissue.

dif·fer·en·tial field di·ag·no·sis (dif′ĕr-en′shăl fēld dī′ăg nō′sis) Determination of possible causes of patient condition by EMS providers. SYN field diagnosis.

dif·fer·en·tial u·re·ter·al cath·e·ter·i·za·tion test (dif′ĕr-en′shăl yūr-ē′tĕr-ăl kath′ĕ-tĕr-ī-zā′shŭn test) A study performed to determine various functional parameters of one kidney compared with the other; ureteral catheters are inserted at cystoscopy into the ureter or renal pelvis bilaterally, and simultaneous measurements are made of urine flow rate, insulin, or *p*-aminohippuric acid (if infused), endogenous creatinine, or various urinary solutes.

dif·fer·en·ti·a·tion (dif′ĕr-en-shē-ā′shŭn) **1.** The acquisition or possession of one or more characteristics or functions different from that of the original type. SYN specialization (2). **2.** SYN differential diagnosis. **3.** Partial removal of a stain from a histologic section to accentuate the staining differences of tissue components.

dif·frac·tion (di-frak′shŭn) Deflection of the rays of light from a straight line in passing by the edge of an opaque body or in passing an obstacle of about the size of the wavelength of the light. [L. *dif- fringo,* pp. *-fractus,* to break in pieces]

dif·fu·sate (di-fyū′zāt) SYN dialysate. [L. *dif-fundo,* pp. *-fusus,* to pour in different directions]

dif·fuse **1.** (di-fyūz′) To disseminate; to spread about. **2.** (di-fyūs′) Disseminated; spread about; not restricted. [L. *dif-fundo,* pp. *-fusus,* to pour in different directions]

dif·fuse ab·scess (di-fyūs′ ab′ses) A collection of pus not circumscribed by a well-defined capsule.

dif·fuse ax·o·nal in·jur·y (di-fyūs′ ax′ŏn-ăl in′jŭr-ē) Axonal damage (e.g., tearing, sheaving of axon clusters, reactive swelling of surrounding tissue) resulting from acceleration or deceleration movements of the brain matter with accompanying fast rotational forces of the brain and the skull.

dif·fuse cu·ta·ne·ous leish·man·i·a·sis (di-fyūs′ kyū-tā′nē-ŭs lēsh′mă-nī′ă-sis) A disorder caused by several New and Old World species and strains of *Leishmania*. The condition is associated with a suppressed cell-mediated immune response.

dif·fuse cu·ta·ne·ous mas·to·cy·to·sis (di-fyūs′ kyū-tā′nē-ŭs mas′tō-sī-tō′sis) A benign process consisting of focal cutaneous infiltrates composed of mast cells; lesions are flat or slightly elevated, form wheals, and itch when stroked; bone lesions may occur.

dif·fuse hy·per·ker·a·to·sis of palms and soles (di-fyūs′ hī′pĕr-ker′a-tō′sis pahlmz sōlz) An autosomal dominant disorder with onset in early infancy; characterized by hyperkeratotic, scaling plaques and often hyperhidrosis on the palms and soles.

dif·fuse id·i·o·path·ic skel·e·tal hy·per·os·to·sis (di-fyūs′ id′ē-ō-path′ik skel′ĕ-tăl hī′pĕr-os-tō′sis) A generalized spinal and extraspinal articular disorder characterized by calcification and ossification of ligaments, particularly of the anterior longitudinal ligament; distinct from ankylosing spondylitis or degenerative joint disease. SYN Forestier disease.

dif·fuse in·ju·ries (di-fyūs′ in′jŭr-ēz) Extensive bodily damage usually resulting from encounters with low velocity-high mass forces.

dif·fuse la·mel·lar ker·a·ti·tis (DLK) (dif-yūs′ lă-mel′ăr ker′ă-tī′tis) Inflammation in the interface of a surgically induced lamellar cut in the cornea in LASIK surgery. SYN sands of Sahara.

dif·fuse Le·wy body dis·ease (di-fyūs′ lā′vē bod′ē di-zēz′) A degenerative cerebral disorder of old people, characterized initially by progressive dementia or psychosis, and subsequently by parkinsonian findings, usually with severe rigidity; other manifestations include involuntary movements, myoclonus, dysphagia, and orthostatic hypotension. Pathologically, Lewy bodies are present diffusely in the nuclei of the hypothalamus, basal forebrain, and brainstem. SYN Lewy body dementia.

dif·fuse ob·struc·tive em·phy·se·ma (di-fyūs′ ŏb-strŭk′tiv em′fi-sē′mă) The major component of chronic obstructive pulmonary disease.

dif·fuse un·i·la·ter·al sub·a·cute neu·ro·re·tin·i·tis (DUSN) (di-fyūs′ yū′ni-lat′ĕr-ăl sŭb′ă-kyūt′ nūr′ō-ret-i-nī′tis) Inflammation of the neurosensory retina caused by infiltration by a roundworm such as *Baylis ascaris* or *Ancylostoma* species.

dif·fuse wax·y spleen (di-fyūs′ waks′ē splēn) A condition of amyloid degeneration of the spleen, affecting chiefly the extrasinusoidal tissue spaces of the pulp.

dif·fus·i·ble (di-fyūz′i-bĕl) Capable of diffusing.

dif·fus·i·ble stim·u·lant (di-fyūz′i-bĕl stim′yū-lănt) A stimulant that produces a rapid but temporary effect.

dif·fus·ing ca·pac·i·ty (di-fyūz′ing kă-pas′i-tē) (symbol, D, followed by subscripts indicating location and chemical species) The amount of oxygen taken up by pulmonary capillary blood per minute per unit average oxygen pressure gradient between alveolar gas and pulmonary capillary blood; units are: mL/min/mmHg; also applied to other gases such as carbon monoxide.

dif·fu·sion (di-fyū′zhŭn) **1.** The random movement of molecules or ions or small particles in solution or suspension toward a uniform distribution throughout the available volume. **2.** SYN dialysis (1).

dif·fu·sion an·ox·i·a (di-fyū′zhŭn an-ok′sē-ă) Diffusion hypoxia severe enough to result in the absence of oxygen in alveolar gas.

dif·fu·sion co·ef·fi·cient (di-fyū′zhŭn kō′ĕ-fish′ĕnt) The mass of material diffusing across a unit area in unit time under a concentration gradient of unity.

dif·fu·sion hy·pox·i·a (di-fyū′zhŭn hī-pok′sē-ă) Decrease in alveolar oxygen tension when room air is inhaled at the conclusion of nitrous oxide anesthesia, because nitrous oxide diffusing out of the blood dilutes the alveolar oxygen.

dif·fu·sion res·pi·ra·tion (di-fyū′zhŭn res′pir-ā′shŭn) Maintenance of oxygenation during apnea by intratracheal insufflation of oxygen at high flow rates.

di·gas·tric (dī-gas′trik) **1.** Having two bellies; denoting especially a muscle with two fleshy parts separated by an intervening tendinous part. SYN biventral. SEE digastric muscle. **2.** Relating to the digastric muscle; denoting a fossa or groove with which it is in relation and a nerve supplying its posterior belly. [G. *di-*, two, + *gastēr*, belly]

di·gas·tric fos·sa (dī-gas′trik fos′ă) A hollow on the posterior surface of the base of the mandible, on either side of the median plane, giving attachment to the anterior belly of the digastric muscle.

di·gas·tric mus·cle (dī-gas′trik mŭs′ĕl) **1.** One of the suprahyoid group of muscles consisting of two bellies united by a central tendon that is connected to the body of the hyoid bone; *origin*, by posterior belly from the digastric groove medial to the mastoid process; *insertion*, by anterior belly into lower border of mandible near midline; *action*, elevates the hyoid when mandible is fixed; depresses the mandible when hyoid is fixed; *nerve supply*, posterior belly from facial, anterior belly by nerve to the mylohyoid from the mandibular division of trigeminal. **2.** A muscle with two fleshy bellies separated by a fibrous insertion; SYN musculus digastricus [TA].

di·gas·tric tri·an·gle (dī-gas′trik trī′ang-gĕl) SYN submandibular triangle.

di·gen·e·sis (dī-jen′ĕ-sis) Reproduction in distinctive patterns in alternate generations, as seen in the nonsexual (invertebrate) and the sexual (vertebrate) cycles of digenetic trematode parasites. [G. *di-*, two, + G. *genesis,* generation]

di·ge·net·ic (dī′jĕ-net′ik) **1.** Pertaining to or characterized by digenesis. SYN heteroxenous. **2.** Pertaining to the digenetic fluke.

Di·George syn·drome (di-jōrj′ sin′drōm) Congenital absence of the thymus gland. This results in a complete absence of functional T cells. Normal B-cell function is present.

di·gest (di-jest′) **1.** To soften by moisture and heat. **2.** To hydrolyze or break up into simpler chemical compounds by means of hydrolyzing enzymes or chemical action. **3.** The materials resulting from digestion or hydrolysis. [L. *digero,* pp. *-gestus,* to force apart, divide, dissolve]

di·ges·tant (di-jes′tănt) **1.** Aiding digestion. **2.** An agent that favors or assists the process of digestion. SYN digestive (2).

di·ges·tion (di-jes′chŭn) The mechanical, chemical, and enzymatic process whereby ingested food is converted into material suitable for assimilation for synthesis of tissues or liberation of energy. [L. *digestio.* See digest]

di·ges·tive (di-jes′tiv) **1.** Relating to digestion. **2.** SYN digestant (2).

di·ges·tive sys·tem (di-jes′tiv sis′tĕm) The digestive tract from the mouth to the anus with all its associated glands and organs. See page A26.

di·ges·tive tract (di-jes′tiv trakt) The passage leading from the mouth to the anus through the pharynx, esophagus, stomach, and intestine. SYN alimentary canal, alimentary tract.

di·ges·tive tract gas (dī-jes′tive trakt gas) SEE flatus.

dig•it (dij′it) A finger or toe. SYN digitus [TA], dactyl, dactylus. [L. *digitus*]

dig•i•tal (dij′i-tăl) **1.** Relating to or resembling a digit or digits or an impression made by them. **2.** Based on numeric methodology.

dig•i•tal col•lat•er•al ar•ter•y (dij′i-tăl kŏ-lat′ĕr-ăl ahr′tĕr-ē) SYN proper palmar digital artery.

dig•i•tal crease (dij′i-tăl krēs) One of the grooves on the palmar surface of a finger, at the level of an interphalangeal joint.

dig•i•tal dic•ta•tion (dij′i-tăl dik-tā′shŭn) System in which health care professionals' dictation is digitized.

dig•i•tal hear•ing aid (dij′i-tăl hēr′ing ād) Programmable hearing aid that can be customized to the extent of the user's hearing loss.

dig•i•tal in•tu•ba•tion (dij′i-tăl in′tū-bā′shŭn) Placement of an endotracheal tube guided by the fingers inserted into the patient's mouth. Fingers are used to locate glottis and guide tube into glottic opening. Used in the prehospital setting when direct visualization through laryngoscope not possible.

Di•gi•tal•is (dij′i-tā′lis) A perennial flowering plant that is the main source for some cardioactive steroid glycosides useful in therapy for CHF and other cardiac disease. SYN foxglove. [Mod.L., thimble, referring to shape of blossoms, fr. L. *digitus*, finger]

digitalisation [Br.] SYN digitalization.

dig•i•tal•i•za•tion (dij′i-tăl-ī-zā′shŭn) Administration of digitalis until sufficient amounts are present in the body to produce the desired therapeutic effects. SYN digitalisation.

dig•i•tal ra•di•og•ra•phy (dij′i-tăl rā′dē-og′ră-fē) Computed radiography or computer processing of a digitized image from a conventional image-intensifier and video camera. SEE ALSO digital subtraction angiography.

dig•i•tal rays of foot (dij′i-tăl rāz fut) SYN foot rays.

dig•i•tal rays of hand (dij′i-tăl rāz hand) SYN hand rays.

dig•i•tal re•flex (dij′i-tăl rē′fleks) SYN Hoffmann sign (2).

dig•i•tal sub•trac•tion an•gi•og•ra•phy (DSA) (dij′i-tăl sŭb-trak′shŭn an′jē-og′ră-fē) Computer-assisted radiographic angiography permitting visualization of vascular structures without superimposed bone and soft tissue density; images made before and after contrast injection allow subtraction (separation and removal) of opacities not enhanced by the contrast medium. Other image-processing can be performed. Contrast material may be injected intravenously or in lower-than-usual amount intraarterially. SEE digital radiography.

dig•i•tal ther•mom•e•ter (dij′i-tăl thĕr-mom′ĕ-tĕr) An instrument that measures the temperature of something or someone in an LCD readout; most common type used in health care in North America today, supplanting the mercury thermometer.

dig•i•tate (dij′i-tāt) Marked by a number of fingerlike processes or impressions. [L. *digitatus*, having fingers, fr. *digitus*, finger]

dig•i•ta•tion (dij′i-tā′shŭn) A process resembling a finger. [Mod. L. *digitatio*]

dig•i•tus, pl. **di•gi•ti** (dij′i-tŭs, -tī) [TA] SYN digit. [L.]

dig•i•tus man•us (dij′i-tŭs man′ŭs) [TA] SYN finger.

di•glos•si•a (dī-glos′ē-ă) A developmental defect that results in a longitudinal split in the tongue. SEE ALSO bifid tongue. [G. *di-*, two, + *glōssa*, tongue]

di•het•er•o•zy•gote (dī-het′ĕr-ō-zī′gōt) An individual heterozygous at two loci of interest, especially in genetic linkage analysis.

di•hy•drate (dī-hī′drāt) A compound with two molecules of water of crystallization.

di•hy•dric al•co•hol (dī-hī′drik al′kŏ-hol) Alcohol containing two OH groups in its molecule; e.g., ethylene glycol.

dihydro- Prefix indicating the addition of two hydrogen atoms. [G. *di*, two + *hydōr*, water]

7,8-di•hy•dro•fo•lic ac•id (dī-hī-drō-fō′lik as′id) Intermediate between folic acid and 5,6,7,8-tetrahydrofolic acid.

di•hy•dro•gen (dī-hī′drŏ-jĕn) SYN hydrogen (2).

di•hy•dro•lip•o•am•ide ace•tyl•trans•fer•ase (dī-hī′drō-lip-ō-am′īd ă-sē′til-trans′fĕr-ās) An enzyme transferring acetyl from S^6-acetyldihydrolipoamide to coenzyme A. A part of many enzyme complexes (e.g., pyruvate dehydrogenase complex). SYN lipoate acetyltransferase, thioltransacetylase A.

di•hy•dro•or•o•tate (dī-hī′drō-ōr′ŏ-tāt) L-5,6-dihydroorotate; an intermediate in the biosynthesis of pyrimidines.

di•hy•dro•pte•ro•ic ac•id (dī-hī′drop-ter-ō′ik as′id) An intermediate in the formation of folic acid; a compound of 6-hydroxymethylpterin and *p*-aminobenzoic acid, the combining of which is inhibited by sulfonamides.

di•hy•dro•ur•i•dine (dī-hī′drō-yūr′i-dēn) Uridine in which the 5,6-double bond has been saturated by addition of two hydrogen atoms; a rare constituent of transfer ribonucleic acids.

dihydroxy- Prefix denoting addition of two hydroxyl groups; as a suffix, becomes -diol.

di·hy·drox·y·ac·e·tone (dī′hī-drok′sē-as′e-tōn) The simplest ketose.

2,8-di·hy·drox·y·a·de·nine li·thi·a·sis (dī′hī-drok′sē-ad′ĕ-nēn li-thī′ă-sis) Formation of calculi of 2,8-dihydroxyadenine due to a deficiency or reduced activity of adenine phosphoribosyltransferase.

di·i·o·dide (dī-ī′ō-dīd) A compound containing two atoms of iodine per molecule.

♻ **diiodo-** Prefix indicating two atoms of iodine. [G. *di-,* two, + *ioeidēs,* violet flower color]

di·i·o·do·ty·ro·sine (DIT) (dī-ī′ŏ-dō-tī′rō-sēn) An intermediate in the biosynthesis of thyroid hormone.

di·ke·tone (dī-kē′tōn) A molecule containing two carbonyl groups; e.g., acetylacetone ($CH_3COCH_2COCH_3$).

di·ke·to·pi·per·a·zines (dī-kē′tō-pī-per′ă-zēnz) A class of organic compounds with a closed ring structure formed from two α-amino acids by the joining of the α-amino group of each to the carboxyl group of the other.

di·lac·er·a·tion (dī-las′ĕr-ā′shŭn) Displacement of some portion of a developing tooth, which is then further developed in its new relation, so that its root or crown is sharply angulated. [L. *di-lacero,* pp. *laceratus,* to tear in pieces, fr. *lacer,* mangled]

di·late (dī′lāt) To perform or undergo dilation.

di·la·ted car·di·o·my·op·a·thy (dī′lāt-ĕd kahr′dē-ō-mī-op′ă-thē) SYN Becker disease.

di·lat·ed pore (dī′lāt-ĕd pōr) An enlarged follicular opening of the skin, with a keratinous plug and occasional lanugo or mature hair.

di·la·tion, dil·a·ta·tion (dī-lā′shŭn, dil′ă-tā′shŭn) **1.** Physiologic or artificial enlargement of a hollow structure or opening. **2.** The act of stretching or enlarging an opening or the lumen of a hollow structure. [L. *dilato,* pp. *dilatatus,* to spread out, dilate]

di·la·tion and cu·ret·tage (D & C) (dī-lā′shŭn kūr′ĕ-tahzh′) Dilation of the cervix and curettement of the endometrium.

di·la·tion and e·vac·u·a·tion (D & E) (dī-lā′shŭn ĕ-vak′yū-ā′shŭn) Dilation of the cervix and removal of the products of conception.

di·la·tion and ex·trac·tion (dī-lā′shŭn ek-strak′shŭn) A form of abortion in which the cervix is dilated and the fetus extracted in pieces using surgical forceps; technique used to complete a second trimester spontaneous abortion or as a form of induced abortion.

di·la·tion and suc·tion (dī-lā′shŭn sŭk′shŭn) SYN suction curettage.

di·la·tor, dil·a·ta·tor (dī′lā-tŏr, dil′ă-tā-tŏr) **1.** An instrument designed for enlarging a hollow structure or opening. **2.** A muscle that pulls open an orifice. **3.** A substance that causes dilation or enlargement of an opening or the lumen of a hollow structure.

di·la·tor mus·cle (dī′lā-tŏr mŭs′ĕl) A muscle that opens an orifice or dilates the lumen of an organ; it is the dilating or opening component of a pylorus (the other component is the sphincter muscle).

di·la·tor pu·pil·lae mus·cle (dī′lā-tŏr pyū-pil′ē mŭs′ĕl) The radial muscular fibers extending from the sphincter pupillae to the ciliary margin; some anatomists regard them as elastic, not muscular, in humans. SYN musculus dilatator pupillae [TA].

di·la·tor tu·bae mus·cle (dī′lā-tōr tū′bē mŭs′ĕl) That portion of the musculus tensor veli palatini that attaches to the mucous membrane of the auditory tube; formerly described as a separate muscle. SYN musculus dilatator tubae [TA].

di·lep·tic sei·zure (dī-lep′tik sē′zhŭr) Attack characterized by impaired awareness of, interaction with, or memory of ongoing events.

dil·u·ent (dil′yū′ĕnt) **1.** Ingredient in a medicinal preparation that lacks pharmacologic activity but is pharmaceutically necessary or desirable. May be a liquid for the dissolution of drugs to be injected, ingested, or inhaled. **2.** Diluting; denoting that which dilutes. USAGE NOTE Often misspelled dilutent, or erroneously so pronounced.

di·lute (di-lūt′) **1.** To reduce the concentration, strength, quality, or purity of a solution or mixture. **2.** Diluted; denoting a solution or mixture so altered. [L. *di-luo,* to wash away, dilute]

di·lute Rus·sell vi·per ven·om test (DRVVT) (di-lūt′ rŭs′ĕl vī′pĕr ven′ŏm test) A test used to confirm the presence of a lupus anticoagulant.

di·lu·tion (di-lū′shŭn) **1.** The act of being diluted. **2.** A diluted solution or mixture. **3.** MICROBIOLOGY a method for counting the number of viable cells in a suspension; a sample is diluted to the point at which an aliquot, when plated, yields a countable number of separate colonies.

di·me·li·a (dī-mē′lē-ă) Congenital duplication of the whole or a part of a limb. [G. *di-,* two, + *melos,* limb]

di·men·sion (di-men′shŭn) Scope, size, magnitude; denoting, in the plural, linear measurements of length, width, and height.

di·mer (dī′mĕr) A compound or unit produced by the combination of two like molecules; in the strictest sense, without loss of atoms (thus nitrogen tetroxide, N_2O_4, is the dimer of nitrogen dioxide, NO_2), but usually by elimination of H_2O or a similar small molecule between the two (e.g., a disaccharide), or by simple noncovalent association (as of two identical protein molecules); higher orders of complexity are called trimers, tetramers, oligomers, and polymers. [G. *di-*, two, + *meros*]

di•mer•ic (dī-mĕr′ik) Having the characteristics of a dimer.

di•meth•yl sulf•ox•ide (DMSO) (dī-meth′il sŭl-foks′īd) A potent organic solvent with mild analgesic and antiinflammatory properties; used to enhance cutaneous absorption of topical agents and in the treatment of interstitial cystitis. SYN dimethyl sulphoxide.

dimethyl sulphoxide [Br.] SYN dimethyl sulfoxide.

di•mor•phic (dī-mōr′fik) **1.** MYCOLOGY growth and reproduction in two forms: mold and yeast. SYN dimorphous (2). **2.** SYN dimorphous (1).

di•mor•phism (dī-mōr′fizm) Existence in two shapes or forms; denoting a difference of crystalline form exhibited by the same substance, or a difference in form or outward appearance between individuals of the same species. [G. *di-*, two, + *morphē,* shape]

di•mor•phous (dī-mōr′fŭs) **1.** Having the property of dimorphism. SYN dimorphic (2). **2.** SYN dimorphic (1).

dim•ple (dim′pĕl) **1.** A natural indentation, usually circular and of small area, in the chin, cheek, or sacral region. **2.** A depression of similar appearance to a dimple, resulting from trauma or the contraction of scar tissue. **3.** To cause dimples.

dimp•ling (dim′pling) **1.** Causing dimples. **2.** A condition marked by the formation of dimples, natural or artificial.

di•ni•tro•phen•yl•hy•dra•zine test (dī′nī-trō-fē′nil-hī′dră-zēn test) A screening test for maple syrup urine disease; the addition of 2,4-dinitrophenylhydrazine in HCl to urine gives a chalky white precipitate in the presence of ketoacids.

din•ner pad (din′ĕr pad) A pad of moderate thickness placed over the pit of the stomach before the application of a plaster jacket; after the plaster has set, the pad is removed, leaving space for varying degrees of abdominal distention.

Di•no•fla•gel•li•da (dī′nō-flă-jel′i-dă) An order in the phylum Sarcomastigophora characterized by the presence of two flagella so placed as to cause the organism to have a whirling motility. Its outer surface is composed of cellulose-containing plates, the size and number of which vary with genus and species.

di•ode (dī′ōd) A bipolar device that permits a flow of electrons in only one direction. SYN silicone diode. [di- + *-ode* fr. *anode, cathode*]

dioestrous [Br.] SYN diestrous.

dioestrus [Br.] SYN diestrus.

♻ **-diol** **1.** Suffix form of the prefix dihydroxy. **2.** Suffix indicating a member of a class of compounds containing two hydroxyl groups.

di•op•ter (D, Δ, δ) (dī-op′tĕr) The unit of refracting power of lenses, denoting the reciprocal of the focal length expressed in meters. [G. *dioptra,* a leveling instrument]

di•op•tric ab•er•ra•tion (dī-op′trik ab′ĕr-ā′shŭn) SYN spheric aberration.

di•op•trics (dī-op′triks) The branch of optics concerned with the refraction of light.

di•o•tic (dī-ot′ik) Simultaneous presentation of the same sound to each ear. [di- + otic]

di•ov•u•lar (dī-ov′yū-lăr) Relating to two oocytes. SYN biovular. [di- + Mod. L. *ovulum,* dim. of L. *ovum,* egg]

di•ov•u•la•to•ry (dī-ōv′yŭ-lă-tōr-ē) Releasing two oocytes in one ovarian cycle.

di•ox•ide (dī-ok′sīd) A molecule containing two atoms of oxygen; e.g., carbon dioxide, CO_2.

di•ox•in (dī-ok′sin) **1.** A ring consisting of two oxygen atoms, four CH groups, and two double bonds; the positions of the oxygen atoms are specified by prefixes, as in 1,4-dioxin. **2.** A contaminant in the herbicide, 2,4,5-T; its potential toxicity, carcinogenicity, and teratogenicity are controversial.

di•ox•y•gen•ase (dī-oks′ē-jĕn-ās) An oxidoreductase that incorporates two atoms of oxygen (from one molecule of O_2) into the (reduced) substrate.

DIP Abbreviation for distal interphalangeal joint(s).

dip (dip) **1.** A downward inclination or slope. **2.** A preparation for coating a surface by submersion, as for the destruction of skin parasites. [M.E. *dippen*]

di•pep•ti•dase (dī-pep′ti-dās) [EC 3.4.13.11.] A hydrolase catalyzing the hydrolysis of a dipeptide to its constituent amino acids.

di•pep•tide (dī-pep′tīd) A combination of two amino acids by means of a peptide (–CO–NH–) link.

di•pep•ti•dyl pep•ti•dase (dī-pep′ti-dil pep′ti-dās) A hydrolase occurring in two forms: dipeptidyl peptidase I, dipeptidyl transferase, cleaving dipeptides from the amino end of polypeptides; dipeptidyl peptidase II, with properties similar to those of I, has a different specificity.

di•pep•ti•dyl trans•fer•ase (dī-pep′ti-dil trans′fĕr-ās) Cleaving dipeptides from the amino end of polypeptides. SEE dipeptidyl peptidase.

di•phal•lus (dī-fal′ŭs) Congenital duplication, partial or complete, of the penis. May also be associated with exstrophy of the urinary bladder. [G. *di-*, two, + *phallos,* penis]

di•pha•sic (dī-fā′zik) Occurring in or characterized by two phases or stages.

di•phen•yl (dī-fen′il) Colorless liquid that is used as a heat transfer agent, frequently as a polychlorinated biphenyl (PCB); used as fungistat for oranges and in organic syntheses. Produces convulsions and central nervous system depression. SYN biphenyl, phenylbenzene.

di•phen•yl•a•mine•ar•sine (dī-fen′il-am′ēn-ahr′sēn) SEE Adamsite.

2,5-di•phen•yl•ox•a•zole (PPO) (dī-fen′il-oks′ă-zōl) A scintillator used in radioactivity measurements by scintillation counting.

di•phos•pha•tase (dī-fos′fă-tās) SYN pyrophosphatase.

1,3-di•phos•pho•glyc•er•ate (dī-fos′fō-glis′ĕr-āt) An intermediate in glycolysis that enzymatically reacts with ADP to generate ATP and 3-phosphoglycerate.

2,3-di•phos•pho•glyc•er•ate (dī-fos′fō-glis′ĕr-āt) An intermediate in the Rapoport-Luebering shunt, formed between 1,3-P_2Gri and 3-phosphoglycerate; an important regulator of the affinity of hemoglobin for oxygen; an intermediate of phosphoglycerate mutase.

di•phos•pho•py•ri•dine nu•cle•o•tide (DPN) (dī-fos′fō-pir′i-dēn nū′klē-ō-tīd) SYN nicotinamide adenine dinucleotide.

diph•the•ri•a (dif-thēr′ē-ă) A specific infectious disease due to *Corynebacterium diphtheriae* and its highly potent toxin; marked by severe inflammation with formation of a thick membranous coating of the pharynx, the nose, and sometimes the tracheobronchial tree; the toxin produces degeneration in peripheral nerves, heart muscle, and other tissues. Symptoms include fever, fatigue, sore throat, difficulty in swallowing, and nausea. Adult morbidity ranges from 5 to 10%; in children younger than 5 years of age, mortality approaches 20%. [G. *diphthera,* leather]

diph•the•ri•al, **diph•the•rit•ic** (dif-thēr′ē-ăl, dif′thĕ-rit′ik) Relating to diphtheria, or the membranous exudate characteristic of this disease.

diph•the•ri•a tox•oid, tet•a•nus tox•oid, and per•tus•sis vac•cine (dif-thēr′ē-ă toks′oyd tet′ă-nŭs toks′oyd pĕr-tus′is vak-sēn′) A vaccine available in three forms: 1) diphtheria and tetanus toxoids plus pertussis vaccine (DTP); 2) tetanus and diphtheria toxoids, adult type (Td); and 3) tetanus toxoid (T). Used for active immunization against diphtheria, tetanus, and pertussis.

diph•the•rit•ic mem•brane (dif′thĕ-rit′ik mem′brān) The false membrane forming on the mucous surfaces in diphtheria.

diph•the•roid (dif′thĕ-royd) **1.** One of a group of local infections suggesting diphtheria, but caused by microorganisms other than *Corynebacterium diphtheriae.* SYN pseudodiphtheria. **2.** Any microorganism resembling *Corynebacterium diphtheriae.* [diphtheria + G. *eidos,* resemblance]

di•phyl•lo•both•ri•a•sis (dī-fil′ō-both-rī′ă-sis) Infection with the cestode *Diphyllobothrium latum;* human infection is caused by ingestion of raw or inadequately cooked fish infected with the plerocercoid larva. Leukocytosis and eosinophilia may occur; if the worm is high enough in the alimentary canal, it may preempt the supply of vitamin B_{12} or alter its absorption, leading to hyperchromic macrocytic anemia.

Di•phyl•lo•both•ri•um (dī-fil′lō-both′rē-ŭm) A large genus of tapeworms (order Pseudophyllidea) characterized by a spatulate scolex with dorsal and ventral sucking grooves, or bothria. Several species are found in humans, although only one, *Diphyllobothrium latum,* is of widespread importance. [G. *di-,* two, + *phyllon,* leaf, + *bothrion,* little ditch]

di•phy•o•dont (dī-fī′ō-dont) Developing two successive sets of teeth, as occurs in humans and most other mammals. [G. *di-,* two, + *phyō,* to produce, + *odous* (*odont-*), tooth]

dip•la•cu•sis (dip′lă-kū′sis) Abnormal perception of sound, either in time or in pitch, so that one sound is heard as two. SEE ALSO binaural diplacusis. [G. *diplous,* double, + *akousis,* a hearing]

di•ple•gi•a (dī-plē′jē-ă) Paralysis of corresponding parts on both sides of the body. [G. *di-,* two, + *plēgē,* a stroke]

♻ **diplo-** Combining form meaning double, twofold. SEE haplo-. [G. *diploos,* double]

dip•lo•ba•cil•lus (dip′lō-bă-sil′ŭs) Two rod-shaped bacterial cells linked end to end. [diplo- + bacillus]

dip•lo•bac•te•ri•a (dip′lō-bak-tēr′ē-ă) Bacterial cells linked together in pairs.

dip•lo•blas•tic (dip′lō-blas′tik) Formed of two germ layers. [diplo- + G. *blastos,* germ]

dip•lo•car•di•a (dip′lō-kahr′dē-ă) An anomaly in which the two lateral halves of the heart are separated to varying degrees by a central fissure. [diplo- + G. *kardia,* heart]

dip•lo•coc•cus, pl. **dip•lo•coc•ci** (dip′lō-kok′ŭs, dip′lō-kok′sī) Spheric or ovoid bacterial cells joined together in pairs. [diplo- + G. *kokkos,* berry]

dip•lo•co•ri•a (dip′lō-kōr′ē-ă) The occurrence of two pupils in the eye. SYN dicoria. [diplo- + G. *korē,* pupil]

dip•lo•gen•e•sis (dip′lō-jen′ĕ-sis) Production of a double fetus or of one with some parts doubled. [diplo- + G. *genesis,* production]

di•plo•ic vein (dip-lō′ik vān) One of the veins

in the diploë of the cranial bones, connected with the cerebral sinuses by emissary veins; the main diploic veins are the frontal, anterior temporal, posterior temporal, and occipital. SYN Dupuytren canal.

dip·loid (dip′loyd) Denoting the state of a cell containing two haploid sets derived from the father and from the mother respectively; the normal chromosome complement of somatic cells (in humans, 46 chromosomes). [diplo- + G. *eidos*, resemblance]

dip·loi·dy (dip′loy-dē) Denotes having two sets of homologous chromosomes.

dip·lo·my·e·li·a (dip′lō-mī-ē′lē-ă) Complete or incomplete doubling of the spinal cord; may be accompanied by a bony septum of the vertebral canal. [diplo- + G. *myelon*, marrow]

dip·lo·ne·ma (dip′lō-nē′mă) The doubled form of the chromosome strand visible at the diplotene stage of meiosis. [diplo- + G. *nēma*, thread]

dip·lop·a·gus (dip-lop′ă-gŭs) General term for conjoined twins, each with fairly complete bodies, although one or more internal organs may be shared in common. SEE conjoined twins. [diplo- + G. *pagos*, something fixed]

di·plo·pho·ni·a (dip′lō-fō′nē-ă) Vibration of both the ventricular folds and the vocal folds, producing two simultaneous voice tones. [diplo- + -phonia]

di·plo·pi·a (dip-lō′pē-ă) The condition in which a single object is perceived as two objects. SYN double vision. [diplo- + G. *ōps*, eye]

dip·lo·some (dip′lō-sōm) Paired allosomes; the pair of centrioles of mammalian cells. [diplo- + G. *sōma*, body]

dip·lo·so·mi·a (dip′lō-sō′mē-ă) Condition in which twins who seem functionally independent are joined at one or more points. SEE conjoined twins. [diplo- + G. *sōma*, body]

dip·lo·tene (dip′lō-tēn) The late stage of prophase in meiosis in which the paired homologous chromosomes begin to repel each other and move apart. [diplo- + G. *tainia*, band]

di·po·lar i·ons (dī-pō′lăr ī′onz) Ions possessing both a negative charge and a positive charge, each localized at a different point in the molecule, which thus has both positive and negative "poles." SYN zwitterions.

di·pole (dī′pōl) A pair of separated electrical charges, one or more positive and one or more negative; or a pair of separated partial charges. SYN doublet (2).

dip·se·sis (dip-sē′sis) An abnormal or excessive thirst, or a craving for unusual forms of drink. SYN dipsosis. [G. *dipseō*, to thirst]

♻**-dipsia**, **-dipsy** Combining form indicating thirst.

dip·so·ma·ni·a (dip′sō-mā′nē-ă) A recurring compulsion to drink alcoholic beverages to excess. SEE alcoholism. [G. *dipsa*, thirst, + *mania*, madness]

dip·so·sis (dip-sō′sis) SYN dipsesis. [G. *dipsa*, thirst, + *-osis*, condition]

dip·so·ther·a·py (dip′sō-thār′ă-pē) Treatment of certain diseases by abstention, as far as possible, from liquids.

dip·stick (dip′stik) A strip of plastic or paper bearing one or more dots or squares of reagent, used to perform qualitative or semiquantitative tests on urine; chemical reaction occurs in the presence of serum, plasma, or urine. Results of tests are read as color changes.

Dip·ter·a (dip′tĕr-ă) An important order of insects (the two-winged flies and gnats); it includes many significant disease vectors (e.g., mosquito, tsetse fly, sandfly, and biting midge). [G. *di-*, two, + *pteron*, wing]

dip·ter·an (dip′tĕr-an) Denoting insects of the order Diptera.

dip·ter·ous (dip′tĕr-ŭs) **1.** Having two wings. **2.** Relating to or characteristic of the order Diptera.

dip·y·li·di·a·sis (dip′i-li-dī′ă-sis) Infection of carnivores and humans with the cestode *Dipylidium caninum.*

Dip·y·lid·i·um ca·ni·num (dip-lid′ē-ŭm kā-nī′nŭm) The most common species of dog tapeworm, the double-pored tapeworm, the larvae of which are harbored by dog fleas or lice; the worm occasionally infects humans. [G. *dipylos*, with two entrances; L. ntr. of *caninus*, pertaining to *canis*, dog]

di·rect cal·o·rim·e·try (dĭr-ekt′ kal′ōr-im′ĕ-trē) Measurement of the heat produced by a reaction, as distinguished from measurement of something other than heat production.

di·rect cur·rent (DC) (dĭr-ekt′ kŭr′ĕnt) An electrical current that flows only in one direction; e.g., that derived from a battery; sometimes referred to as galvanic current.

di·rect flap (dĭr-ekt′ flap) A flap raised completely and transferred at the same stage. SYN immediate flap.

di·rect frac·ture (dĭr-ekt′ frak′shŭr) A fracture, especially of the skull, occurring at the point of injury.

di·rect im·mu·no·fluor·es·cence (dĭr-ekt′ im′yū-nō-flōr-es′ĕns) Fluorescence microscopy of tissue from lesions after application of labeled antibody. SEE ALSO fluorescent antibody technique.

di·rec·tion·al ath·e·rec·to·my (DCA) (dĭr-ek′shŭn-ăl ath′thĕr-ek′tŏ-mē) Excision of an atheroma with a motor-driven shaver mounted on an arterial catheter.

di·rec·tion·al pre·pon·der·ance (dĭr-ek′shŭn-ăl prē-pon′dĕr-ăns) A right or left predominance of nystagmus calculated from the responses to the binaural, bithermal caloric test.

di·rec·tion·al weak·ness (dĭr-ek′shŭn-ăl wēk′nĕs) A right or left decrement of nystagmus, calculated from the responses to the binaural, bithermal caloric test.

di·rect lar·yn·gos·co·py (dĭr-ekt′ lar′in-gos′kŏ-pē) Inspection of the larynx by means of either a rigid, hollow instrument or a fiberoptic cable.

di·rect med·i·cal con·trol (dĭr-ekt′ med′i-kăl kŏn-trōl′) Medical control provided directly to a prehospital provider by a physician or authorized health care provider; usually provided through the Emergency Medical Service radio system base station.

di·rect nu·cle·ar di·vi·sion (dĭr-ekt′ nū′klē-ăr di-vizh′ŭn) SYN amitosis.

di·rect oph·thal·mo·scope (dĭr-ekt′ of-thal′mŏ-skōp) An instrument designed to visualize the interior of the eye, with the instrument relatively close to the subject's eye and the observer viewing an upright magnified image.

di·rec·tor (di-rek′tŏr) **1.** A smoothly grooved instrument used with a knife to limit the incision of tissues. SYN staff (2). **2.** The head of a service or specialty division. [L. *dirigo,* pp. *-rectus,* to arrange, set in order]

di·rect re·act·ing bil·i·ru·bin (dĭr-ekt′ rē-akt′ing bil′i-rū′bin) The fraction of serum bilirubin that has been conjugated with glucuronic acid in the liver cell to form bilirubin diglucuronide; so called because it reacts directly with the Ehrlich diazo reagent; increased levels are found in hepatobiliary diseases, especially of the obstructive variety.

di·rect trans·fu·sion (dĭr-ekt′ trans-fyū′zhŭn) Transfusion of blood from the donor to the recipient, either through a tube connecting their blood or by suturing the vessels together. SYN immediate transfusion.

di·rect vi·sion (dĭr-ekt′ vizh′ŭn) SYN central vision.

di·rect wet mount ex·am·i·na·tion (dĭr-ekt′ wet mownt eg-zam′i-nā′shŭn) Microscopic review at low (100×) and high dry (400×) total magnifications of saline and fresh fecal specimen to detect parasites, including motile protozoan trophozoites.

dir. prop. Abbreviation for L. *directio propria,* with proper direction.

dirt-eat·ing (dĭrt ēt′ing) SYN geophagia.

dir·ty bomb (dĭr′tē bom) A mass-casualty weapon that combines some sort of radioactive material with conventional explosives; intended not only to cause panic and immediate harm to people nearby, but also to transmit radioactive material through the air.

♻ **dis-** Combining form denoting in two, apart; un-, not; very. Cf. dys-. [L. separation]

dis·a·bil·i·ty (dis′ă-bil′i-tē) **1.** Diminished capacity to perform within a prescribed range. **2.** An impairment or defect of one or more organs or members.

dis·a·bil·i·ty-ad·just·ed life years (DALYs) (dis′ă-bil′i-tē ă-jŭs′tĕd līf yērz) A measure of the burden of disease on a defined population, based on adjustment of life expectancy to allow for long-term disability as estimated from official statistics. SEE ALSO global burden of disease.

dis·a·bil·i·ty man·age·ment in·ter·ven·tion team (DMIT) (dis′ă-bil′i-tē man′ăj-mĕnt in′tĕr-ven′shŭn tēm) An interdisplinary group that derives, coordinates, and resolves individualized disability management programs for workers based on collective information established from occupational handicap assessments. Team members include a worker, union representative, direct supervisor, case coordinator, physician, and other health care professionals.

dis·a·ble·ment (dis-ā′bĕl-mĕnt) The process of becoming disabled; generally thought to include biological, functional, and social components. SEE ALSO disability.

di·sac·cha·ride (dī-sak′ă-rīd) A condensation product of two monosaccharides by elimination of water.

dis·ag·gre·ga·tion (dis-ag′rĕ-gā′shŭn) **1.** A breaking up into component parts. **2.** An inability to coordinate various sensations and failure to comprehend their mutual relations. [L. *dis-,* separating, + *ag- grego* (*adg-*), pp. *-gregatus,* to add to something]

dis·ar·tic·u·la·tion (dis′ahr-tik′yū-lā′shŭn) Amputation of a limb through a joint, without cutting of bone. SYN exarticulation. [L. *dis-,* apart, + *articulus,* joint]

dis·as·so·ci·a·tion (dis′ă-sō′sē-ā′shŭn) SYN dissociation (1).

DISASTER (di-zas′tĕr) An acronymic paradigm developed by the American Medical Association to assist in organizing the reaction to a mass-casualty incident. The components of the acronym are *D* for *disaster*, *I* for *incident command*, *S* for *scene security and safety*, *A* for *assess hazards*, *S* for *support*, *T* for *triage and treatment*, *E* for *evacuation*, and *R* for *recovery*.

dis·as·ter med·i·cine (diz-as′tĕr med′i-sin) SEE triage.

disc (disk) **1.** A round, flat plate; any approximately flat circular structure. **2.** DENTISTRY a circular piece of thin paper or other material, coated with an abrasive substance, used for cutting and polishing teeth and fillings. **3.** MICROBIOLOGY a plate coated with an antibiotic to measure susceptibility and resistance. **4.** The optic nerve head as viewed during ophthalmoscopy. [L. *discus;* G. *diskos,* a quoit, disc]

disc•ec•to•my (disk-ek′tŏ-mē) Excision, in part or whole, of an intervertebral disc. SYN discotomy. [disco- + G. *ektomē,* excision]

disc e•lec•tro•pho•re•sis (disk ĕ-lek′trō-fŏr-ē′sis) A modification of gel electrophoresis in which a discontinuity (pH, gel pore size) is introduced near the origin to produce a lamina (disc) of the materials being separated; the separating bands retain their discoid shape as they move through the gel.

dis•charge (DC) (dis′chahrj) **1.** That which is emitted or evacuated, as an excretion or a secretion. **2.** The activation or firing of a neuron.

dis•charge di•ag•no•sis (dis′chahrj dī′ăg-nō′sis) The final diagnosis given a patient before her release from the hospital after all testing, surgery, and workup are complete.

dis•charge plan•ning (dis′chahrj plan′ing) NURSING interdisplinary, collaborative process that involves evaluating patient's needs and developing and implementing a comprehensive plan for continuing, follow-up, or rehabilitation care.

disc her•ni•a•tion (disk hĕr′nē-ā′shŭn) Extension of disc material beyond the posterior anulus fibrosus and posterior longitudinal ligament and into the spinal canal.

dis•chro•na•tion (dis′krō-nā′shŭn) A disturbance in the consciousness of time. [L. *dis-*, apart, + G. *chronos,* time]

dis•ci (dis′ī) Plural of discus.

dis•ci•form (dis′i-fōrm) Disc-shaped. [disc + -form]

dis•ci•form de•gen•er•a•tion (dis′i-fōrm dĕ-jen′ĕr-ā′shŭn) Subretinal neovascularization with retinal separation and hemorrhage leading finally to a circular mass of fibrous tissue with marked loss of visual acuity. SYN disciform scar.

dis•ci•form ker•a•ti•tis (dis′i-fōrm ker′ă-tī′tis) Large disc-shaped infiltration of the central or paracentral corneal stroma. This lesion is deep and nonsuppurative and is seen in viral infections, particularly herpetic.

dis•ci•form scar (dis′i-fōrm skahr) SYN disciform degeneration.

dis•cis•sion (di-sizh′ŏn) **1.** Incision or cutting through a part. **2.** OPHTHALMOLOGY opening of the capsule and breaking up of the cortex of the lens with a needle knife or laser. [L. *discindo,* pp. *-scissus,* to tear asunder]

dis•ci•tis (dis-kī′tis) Nonbacterial inflammation of an intervertebral disc or disc space.

disc kid•ney (disk kid′nē) SYN pancake kidney.

dis•clos•ing a•gent (dis-klōz′ing ā′jĕnt) A selective dye in solution or tablet form used to visualize and identify soft debris, pellicle, and bacterial plaque on the surfaces of the teeth; in dental offices, a solution is most commonly used; chewable tablets are available for use in home dental care.

dis•clos•ing so•lu•tion (dis-klōz′ing sŏ-lū′shŭn) SEE disclosing agent.

dis•clos•ing tab•let (dis-klōz′ing tab′lĕt) SEE disclosing agent.

dis•clo•sure (dis-klō′zhŭr) Communicating confidential patient information to others in accordance with legal guidelines. SYN release of information.

disco- A disc; disc-shaped. [G. *diskos*]

dis•co•gen•ic (dis′kō-jen′ik) Denoting a disorder originating in or from an intervertebral disc. [disco- + G. *genesis,* origin]

dis•coid (dis′koyd) **1.** Resembling a disc. **2.** DENTISTRY an excavating or carving instrument having a circular blade with a cutting edge around the periphery. [disco- + G. *eidos,* appearance]

dis•coid lu•pus er•y•the•ma•to•sus (dis′koyd lū′pŭs er′ă-thē-mă-tō′sŭs) A form of lupus erythematosus in which cutaneous lesions appear on the face and elsewhere; these are atrophic plaques with erythema, hyperkeratosis, follicular plugging, and telangiectasia. See this page.

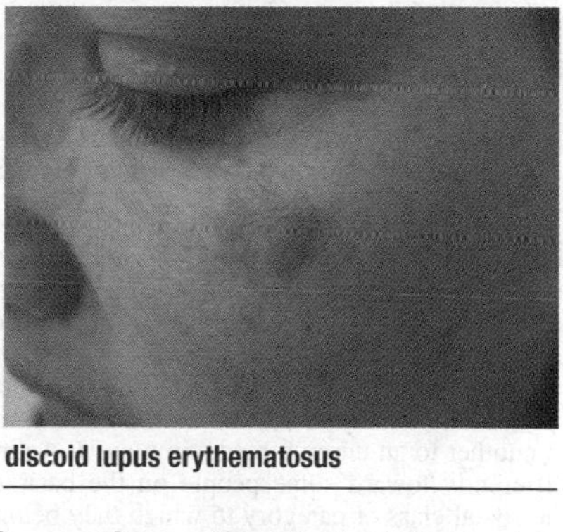

discoid lupus erythematosus

dis•con•tin•u•a•tion test (dis′kŏn-tin′yū-ā′shŭn test) A test to determine whether a certain drug is responsible for a reaction by observing a remission of symptoms following cessation of its use.

dis•cop•a•thy (dis-kop′ă-thē) Disease of a disc, particularly of an invertebral disc. [disco- + G. *pathos,* disease]

dis•co•pla•cen•ta (dis′kō-plă-sen′tă) A placenta of discoid shape.

dis•cor•dance (dis-kōr′dăns) Dissociation of

two characteristics in the members of a sample from a population; used as a measure of dependence. Cf. concordance.

dis·cor·dant al·ter·nans (dis-kōr′dănt awl-ter′nanz) Presence of right ventricular and pulmonary artery alternans with peripheral pulsus alternans, but with the strong beat of the right ventricle coinciding with the weak beat of the left and vice versa.

dis·cor·dant al·ter·na·tion (dis-kōr′dănt awl′tĕr-nā′shŭn) Alternation in cardiac activities of either the systemic or the pulmonary circulation, but not of both, or in both but oppositely directed in each.

dis·cor·dant chan·ges e·lec·tro·car·di·o·gram (dis-kōr′dănt chānj′ĕz ĕ-lek′trō-kahr′dē-ō-gram) The presence of more than one waveform change, each in a different direction (polarity).

dis·cot·o·my (dis-kot′ŏ-mē) SYN discectomy. [disco- + G. *tomē,* incision]

dis·crete (dis-krēt′) Separate; distinct; not joined to or incorporated with another; denoting especially certain lesions of the skin. [L. *discerno,* pp. *-cretus,* to separate]

dis·crete a·na·ly·zer (dis-krēt′ an′ă-līz-ĕr) An automated chemical analyzer in which the instrument performs tests on samples that are kept in discrete containers, in contrast to a continuous flow analyzer.

dis·crete skill (dis-krēt′ skil) A task or motor pattern that has a well-defined beginning and end (e.g., moving from sitting to standing, catching a ball).

dis·crim·i·nant stim·u·lus (dis-krim′i-nănt stim′yū-lŭs) A stimulus that can be differentiated from all other stimuli in the environment because it has been, and continues to serve as, an indicator of a potential reinforcer.

dis·crim·i·na·tion (dis-krim′i-nā′shŭn) **1.** The act of distinguishing between different things; ability to perceive different things as different, or to respond to them differently. **2.** PSYCHOLOGY responding differently, as when the subject responds in one way to a reinforced stimulus and in another to an unreinforced stimulus. **3.** Acting differently toward some people on the basis of the social class or category to which they belong rather than their individual qualities. [L. *discrimino,* pp. *-atus,* to separate]

dis·cri·mi·na·tion score (dis-krim′i-nā′shŭn skōr) The percentage of words that a subject can repeat correctly from a list of phonetically balanced words presented at 25–40 dB above the speech reception threshold.

disc syn·drome (disk sin′drōm) A constellation of symptoms and signs, including pain, paresthesia, sensory loss, weakness, and impaired reflexes, due to a compressive radiculopathy caused by intervertebral disc pressure.

dis·cus ner·vi op·ti·ci (dis′kŭs nĕr′vī op′ti-sī) [TA] SYN optic disc.

dis·ease (diz′ēz) **1.** An interruption, cessation, or disorder of body functions, systems, or organs. SYN illness, morbus, sickness. **2.** A morbid entity characterized usually by at least two of these criteria: recognized etiologic agent(s), identifiable group of signs and symptoms, or consistent anatomic alterations. SEE ALSO syndrome. [Eng. *dis-* priv. + ease]

dis·ease de·ter·mi·nants (di-zēz′ dĕ-tĕr′mi-nănts) Any variables that directly or indirectly influence the frequency of occurrence and/or the distribution of any given disease; they include specific disease agents, host characteristics, and environmental factors.

dis·ease-mod·i·fy·ing an·ti·rheu·mat·ic drugs (DMARD) (di-zēz′mod′i-fī-ing an′tē-rū-mat′ik drŭgz) Agents that apparently alter the course and progression of rheumatoid arthritis, as opposed to more rapidly acting substances that suppress inflammation and decrease pain, but do not prevent cartilage or bone erosion or progressive disability.

dis·en·fran·chise·ment (dis′ĕn-fran′chīz-mĕnt) Denial of a person's rights (e.g., the right to health care).

dis·en·gage·ment (dis-ĕn-gāj′mĕnt) **1.** The act of setting free or extricating; in childbirth, the emergence of the head from the vulva. **2.** Ascent of the presenting part from the pelvis after the inlet has been negotiated. [Fr.]

dis·e·qui·lib·ri·um (dis-ē-kwi-lib′rē-ŭm) A disturbance or absence of balance.

dis·flu·en·cy (dis-flū′ĕn-sē) SEE dysfluency.

dis·flu·ent (dis-flū′ĕnt) Relating to disfluency.

dis·im·pac·tion (dis-im-pak′shŭn) **1.** Separation of impaction in a fractured bone. **2.** Removal of impacted feces, usually manually.

dis·in·fect (dis-in-fekt′) To destroy pathogenic microorganisms in or on any substance or to inhibit their growth and vital activity.

dis·in·fec·tant (dis-in-fek′tănt) **1.** Capable of destroying pathogenic microorganisms or inhibiting their growth. **2.** An agent that possesses the capacity to disinfect.

dis·in·fec·tion (dis-in-fek′shŭn) Destruction of pathogenic microorganisms or their toxins or vectors by direct exposure to chemical or physical agents.

dis·in·te·gra·tion (dis-in′tĕ-grā′shŭn) **1.** Loss or separation of the component parts of a substance, as in catabolism or decay. **2.** Disorganization of psychic and behavioral processes. SYN decay (7). [dis- + L. *integer*, whole, intact]

dis·junc·tion (dis-jŭngk′shŭn) The normal separation of pairs of chromosomes at the anaphase stage of meiosis I or II. [dis- + L. *junctio*, a joining, fr. *jungo*, pp. *junctum*, to join]

disk (disk) SEE disc.

dis•lo•cate (dis′lō-kāt) To luxate; to put out of joint.

dis•lo•ca•tion frac•ture (dis-lō-kā′shŭn frak′shŭr) A fracture of a bone near an articulation with its concomitant dislocation from that joint.

dis•lo•ca•tions (dis-lō-kā′shŭnz) Displacements of an organ or any part; specifically disturbance or disarrangement of the normal relation of the bones entering into the formation of a joint. See this page. SYN luxation (1). [L. *dislocatio*, fr. *dis-*, apart, + *locatio*, a placing]

dis•mem•ber (dis-mem′bĕr) To amputate an arm or leg.

dis•mu•tase (dis-myū′tās) Generic name for enzymes catalyzing the reaction of two identical molecules to produce two molecules in differing states of oxidation or phosphorylation.

dis•or•der (dis-ōr′dĕr) A disturbance of function or structure, resulting from a genetic or embryologic failure in development or from exogenous factors such as poison, trauma, or disease.

dis•or•ga•nized schiz•o•phre•ni•a (dis-ōr′găn-īzd skits′ō-frē′nē-ă) A severe form of schizophrenia characterized by the predominance of incoherence; blunted, inappropriate, or silly affect; and the absence of systematized delusions.

dis•o•ri•en•ta•tion (dis-ōr′ē-ĕn-tā′shŭn) Loss of the sense of familiarity with one's surroundings (time, place, and person); loss of one's bearings.

dis•pen•sa•ry (dis-pen′săr-ē) **1.** A physician's office, especially the office of one who dispenses medicines. **2.** The office of a hospital pharmacist, where medicines are distributed on physicians' orders. **3.** An outpatient department of a hospital. [L. *dis-penso*, pp. *-atus*, to distribute by weight, fr. *penso*, to weigh]

Dis•pen•sa•to•ry (dis-pen′să-tōr-ē) A work originally intended as a commentary on the *Pharmacopeia*, but now more of a supplement to that work, which contains an account of the sources, mode of preparation, physiologic action, and therapeutic uses of most of the agents, official and nonofficial, used in the treatment of disease. [L. *dispensator*, a manager, steward; see dispensary]

dis•pense (dis-pens′) To prepare and give out medicine and other necessities to the sick; to fill a medical prescription.

dis•pense as writ•ten (DAW) (dis-pens′ rit′ĕn) Instruction by a physician to a pharmacist not to substitute a generic form of the drug. SEE triage.

di•sper•my, di•sper•mi•a (dī′spĕr-mē, -mē-ă) Entrance of two sperms into one oocyte. [di- + sperm]

dis•perse (dis-pĕrs′) To dissipate, to cause disappearance of, to scatter, to dilute.

dis•per•sion (dis-pĕr′zhŭn) **1.** The act of dispersing or of being dispersed. **2.** Incorporation of the particles of one substance into the mass of another, including solutions, suspensions, and colloidal dispersions (solutions). **3.** Specifically, what is usually called a colloidal solution. **4.** The extent or degree to which values of a statistical frequency distribution are scattered about a mean or median value. [L. *dispersio*]

dis•per•sion me•di•um (dis-pĕr′zhŭn mē′dē-ŭm) SYN external phase.

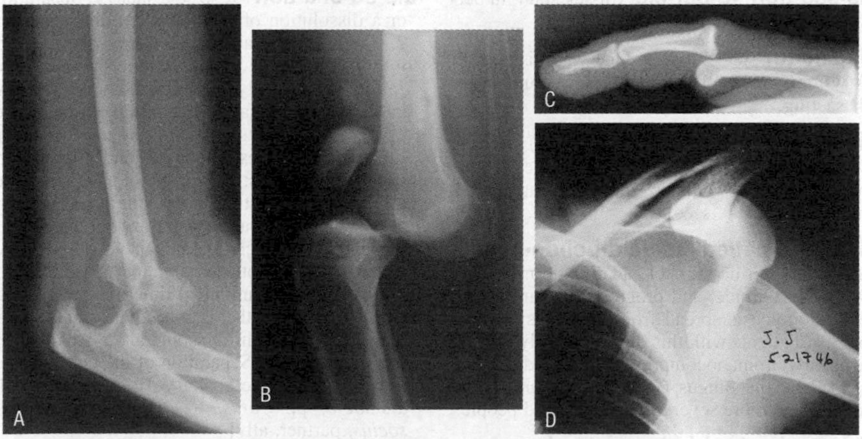

dislocations: (A) posterior dislocation of both radius and ulna at elbow joint; (B) anterior dislocation of the proximal tibia with an intact posterior cruciate ligament; (C) finger dislocation at the proximal interphalangeal joint with dorsal displacement of the distal segment; (D) subglenoid dislocation of the humeral head

di·spi·reme (dī-spī′rēm) The double chromatin skein in the telophase of mitosis. [G. *di-*, twice, + *speirēma*, coil, convolution]

dis·placed frac·ture (dis-plāst′ frak′shŭr) A fracture in which the fragments are separated and are not in alignment.

dis·place·ment (dis-plās′mĕnt) **1.** Removal from the normal location or position. **2.** The adding to a fluid (particularly a gas) in an open vessel one of greater density whereby the first is expelled. **3.** CHEMISTRY a change in which one element, radical, or molecule is replaced by another, or in which one element exchanges electric charges with another by reduction or oxidation. **4.** PSYCHIATRY the transfer of impulses from one expression to another, as from fighting to talking.

dis·po·si·tion (dis′pŏ-zish′ŭn) Follow-up list detailed in the health care record, after the initial episode of care, of services and treatments to be provided to the patient.

dis·pro·por·tion (dis′prŏ-pōr′shŭn) Lack of proportion or symmetry.

dis·sect (di-sekt′) **1.** To cut apart or separate the tissues of the body for study. **2.** SURGERY to separate structures along natural lines or planes of cleavage. [L. *dis-seco,* pp. *-sectus,* to cut asunder]

dis·sect·ing an·eu·rysm (di-sek′ting an′yūr-izm) Splitting or dissection of an arterial wall by blood entering through an intimal tear or by interstitial hemorrhage; more common in the aorta.

dis·sect·ing cel·lu·li·tis (di-sek′ting sel′yū-lī′tis) A chronic dissecting folliculitis of the scalp.

dis·sec·tion (di-sek′shŭn) The act of dissecting. SYN anatomy (3), necrotomy (1).

dis·sec·tion tu·ber·cle (di-sek′shŭn tū′bĕr-kĕl) SYN postmortem wart.

dis·sec·tor (di-sek′tŏr) **1.** One who dissects. **2.** A written guide for dissection. **3.** Instrument for dissecting.

dis·sem·i·nat·ed (di-sem′i-nā-tĕd) Widely scattered throughout an organ, tissue, or the body. [L. *dis-semino,* pp. *-atus,* to scatter seed, fr. *semen* (*-min-*), seed]

dis·sem·i·nat·ed coc·cid·i·oi·do·my·co·sis (di-sem′i-nā-tĕd kok-sid′ē-oy′dō-mī-kō′sis) A severe, chronic, and progressive form of coccidioidomycosis spread from the lungs to other organs. Patients with this disease usually are significantly immunocompromised. The disease is caused by the fungus *Coccidioides immitis* and tends to be more severe in dark-skinned people.

dis·sem·i·nat·ed in·tra·vas·cu·lar co·ag·u·la·tion (DIC) (di-sem′i-nā′tĕd in′tră-vas′kyū-lăr kō-ag′yū-lā′shŭn) A hemorrhagic syndrome that occurs following the uncontrolled activation of clotting factors and fibrinolytic enzymes throughout small blood vessels; fibrin is deposited, platelets and clotting factors are consumed, and fibrin degradation products inhibit fibrin polymerization, resulting in tissue necrosis and bleeding. SEE ALSO consumption coagulopathy.

dis·sem·i·nat·ed lu·pus er·y·the·ma·to·sus (di-sem′i-nā-tĕd lū′pŭs er′ă-thē-mă-tō′sŭs) SYN systemic lupus erythematosus.

dis·sem·i·nat·ed tu·ber·cu·lo·sis (di-sem′i-nā-tĕd tū-bĕr′kyū-lō′sis) SYN acute tuberculosis.

dis·sim·u·la·tion (di-sim′yū-lā′shŭn) Concealment of the truth about a situation, especially about a state of health or during a mental status examination, as by a malingerer or someone with a factitious disorder. [L. *dissimulatio*, fr. *dissimulo*, to feign, fr. *dis*, apart, + *simillis*, same]

dis·so·ci·at·ed an·es·the·si·a (dis-sō′sē-ā-tĕd an′es-thē′zē-ă) Loss of some types of sensation with persistence of others; most often used in context of nerve blocks, wherein a loss of sensation for pain and temperature occurs without loss of tactile sense.

dis·so·ci·at·ed hor·i·zon·tal de·vi·a·tion (dis-sō′sē-ā-tĕd hōr′i-zon′tăl dē-vē-ā′shŭn) A tendency, often associated with repaired congenital esotropia, in which an eye abducts when it is covered, in violation of Hering law.

dis·so·ci·at·ed nys·tag·mus (di-sō′sē-āt-ĕd nis-tag′mŭs) A nystagmus in which the movements of the two eyes are dissimilar in direction, amplitude, and periodicity.

dis·so·ci·at·ed ver·ti·cal de·vi·a·tion (di-sō′sē-āt-ĕd vĕr′ti-kăl dē-vē-ā′shŭn) A tendency, often associated with congenital esotropia, in which an eye elevates, abducts, and extorts when covered, in violation of Hering law.

dis·so·ci·a·tion (di-sō′sē-ā′shŭn) **1.** Separation, or a dissolution of relations. SYN disassociation. **2.** The change of a complex chemical compound into a simpler one by any lytic reaction, by ionization, by heterolysis, or by homolysis. **3.** An unconscious separation of a group of mental processes from the rest, resulting in an independent functioning of these processes and a loss of the usual associations; for example, a separation of affect from cognition. SEE multiple personality. **4.** A state used as an essential part of a technique for healing in psychology and psychotherapy, for instance in hypnotherapy or the neurolinguistic programming technique of time-line therapy. SEE ALSO Time-Line therapy. **5.** The translocation between a large chromosome and a small supernumerary one. **6.** Separation of the nuclear components of a heterokaryotic dikaryon. [L. *dis-socio,* pp. *-atus,* to disjoin, separate, fr. *socius,* partner, ally]

dis·so·ci·a·tion move·ment (di-sō′sē-ā′shŭn mūv′mĕnt) **1.** Physical movement that evidences the ability to differentiate among movements of different parts of the body; e.g., rolling segmentally, which entails leading with the head, followed by the shoulders and then the pelvis, instead of "logrolling", in which the body rolls as a single unit. **2.** Stabilization of one part of the body or movement of one part in the opposite direction of another (e.g., pelvic trunk as used in ambulation).

dis·so·ci·a·tion sen·si·bil·i·ty (di-sō′sē-ā′shŭn sens′i-bil′i-tē) The loss of the pain and the thermal senses with preservation of tactile sensibility or vice versa.

dis·so·ci·a·tion syn·drome (dis-ō′sē-ā′shŭn sin′drōm) Mental disease involving disturbances of identity, memory, and consciousness.

dis·so·ci·a·tive an·es·the·si·a (di-sō′sē-ă-tiv an′es-thē′zē-ă) A form of general anesthesia, but not necessarily complete unconsciousness, characterized by catalepsy, catatonia, and amnesia, especially that produced by phenylcyclohexylamine compounds, including ketamine.

dis·so·ci·a·tive iden·ti·ty dis·or·der (di-sō′sē-ă-tiv ī-den′ti-tē dis-ōr′dĕr) A disorder in which two or more distinct conscious personalities alternately prevail in the same person, sometimes without any one personality being aware of the other(s).

dis·so·ci·a·tive re·ac·tion (di-sō′sē-ă-tiv rē-ak′shŭn) Reaction characterized by such dissociative behavior as amnesia, fugues, sleepwalking, and dream states.

dis·solve (di-zolv′) To change or cause to change from a solid to a dispersed form by immersion in a fluid of suitable properties. [L. *dissolvo,* pp. *-solutus,* to loose asunder, to dissolve]

dis·so·nance (di′sō-năns) SOCIAL PSYCHOLOGY an aversive state that arises when a person is minimally aware of internal inconsistency or conflict. [L. *dissonus,* discordant, confused]

dis·tad (dis′tad) Toward the periphery; in a distal direction.

dis·tal (dis′tăl) **1.** Situated away from the center of the body, or from the point of origin; specifically applied to the extremity or distant part of a limb or organ. **2.** DENTISTRY away from the median sagittal plane of the face, following the curvature of the dental arch. SYN distalis. [L. *distalis*]

dis·tal an·gle (dis′tăl ang′gĕl) The angle formed by the meeting of the distal with the labial, buccal, or lingual surface of a tooth.

dis·tal end (dis′tăl end) The posterior extremity of a dental appliance. SYN heel (2).

dis·tal il·e·i·tis, re·gion·al il·e·i·tis (dis′tăl il′ē-ī′tis, rē′jŭn-ăl il′ē-ī′tis) SYN regional enteritis.

dis·tal in·ter·pha·lan·ge·al joints (DIP) (dis′tăl in′tĕr-fă-lan′jē-ăl joynts) The synovial joints between the middle and distal phalanges of the fingers and of the toes.

dis·tal in·tes·ti·nal ob·struc·tive syn·drome (dis′tăl in-tes′ti-năl ŏb-strŭk′tiv sin′drōm) A syndrome seen in cystic fibrosis secondary to impaction with feces and inspissated mucus.

dis·ta·lis (dis-tā′lis) SYN distal.

dis·tal oc·clu·sion (dis′tăl ŏ-klū′zhŭn) **1.** A tooth occluding in a position distal to normal. SYN retrusive occlusion (2). **2.** SYN distoclusion.

dis·tal ra·di·o·ul·nar joint (dis′tăl rā′dē-ō-ŭl′năr joynt) The pivot synovial joint between the head of the ulna and the ulnar notch on the radius; an articular disc passes across the distal part of the joint.

dis·tal sple·no·re·nal shunt (dis′tăl splē′nō-rē′năl shŭnt) Anastomosis of the splenic vein to the left renal vein, usually end-to-side, for control of portal hypertension.

dis·tal tongue bud (dis′tăl tŭng bŭd) SYN lateral lingual swelling.

dis·tance (dis′tăns) The amount of space between two objects, points, or places. [L. *distantia,* fr. *di-sto,* to stand apart, be distant]

dis·tance ed·u·ca·tion (dis′tăns ej′yū-kā′shŭn) Planned learning pursued in a place other than where the instruction is offered, using computer technology.

dis·tant flap (dis′tănt flap) A flap in which the donor site is distant from the recipient area.

dis·tem·per (dis-tem′pĕr) The colloquial usage for canine distemper caused by an RNA virus of the genus Morbillivirus, a member of the family Paramyxoviridae.

dis·ten·tion, dis·ten·sion (dis-ten′shŭn) The act or state of being distended or stretched. SEE ALSO dilation. [L. *dis-tendo,* to stretch apart]

dis·til·late (dis′ti-lāt) The product of distillation.

dis·til·la·tion (dis′ti-lā′shŭn) Volatilization of a liquid by heat and subsequent condensation of the vapor; in a liquid mixture, a means of separating the volatile from the nonvolatile, or the more volatile from the less volatile part. [L. *de-(di-)stillo,* pp. *-atus,* to drop down]

dis·to·buc·cal (dis′tō-bŭk′ăl) Relating to the distal and buccal surfaces of a tooth; denoting the angle formed by their junction.

dis·to·buc·co·oc·clu·sal (dis′tō-bŭk′ō-ŏ-klū′zăl) Relating to the distal, buccal, and occlusal surfaces of a premolar or molar tooth; denoting especially the angle formed by the junction of these surfaces.

dis·to·buc·co·pul·pal (dis′tō-bŭk′ō-pŭl′păl) Relating to the point (trihedral) angle formed by the junction of a distal, buccal, and pulpal walls of a cavity.

dis·to·cer·vi·cal (dis′tō-sĕr′vi-kăl) Relating to

the line angle formed by the junction of the distal and cervical (gingival) walls of a class V cavity.

dis·to·clu·sal (dis′tō-klū′zăl) **1.** Relating to or characterized by distoclusion. **2.** Denoting a compound cavity or restoration involving the distal and occlusal surfaces of a tooth. **3.** Denoting the line angle formed by the distal and occlusal walls of a class V cavity.

dis·to·clu·sion (dis′tō-klū′zhŭn) A malocclusion in which the mandibular arch articulates with the maxillary arch in a position distal to normal; in Angle classification, a class II malocclusion. SYN distal occlusion (2).

dis·to·gin·gi·val (dis′tō-jin′ji-văl) Relating to the junction of the distal and gingival walls of a tooth cavity.

dis·to·in·ci·sal (dis′tō-in-sī′zăl) Relating to the line (dihedral) angle formed by the junction of the distal and incisal walls of a class V cavity in an anterior tooth or formed by the distal and incisal surfaces of a tooth.

dis·to·la·bi·al (dis′tō-lā′bē-ăl) Relating to the distal and labial surfaces of a tooth; denoting the angle formed by their junction.

dis·to·la·bi·o·pul·pal (dis′tō-lā′bē-ō-pŭl′păl) Relating to the point (trihedral) angle formed by the junction of distal, labial, and pulpal walls of the incisal part of a class IV (mesioincisal) cavity.

dis·to·lin·gual (dis′tō-ling′gwăl) Relating to the distal and lingual surfaces of a tooth; denoting the angle formed by their junction.

dis·to·lin·guo·oc·clu·sal (dis′tō-ling′gwō-ŏ-klū′zăl) Relating to the distal, lingual, and occlusal surfaces of a bicuspid or molar tooth; denoting especially the angle formed by the junction of these surfaces.

dis·to·mo·lar (dis′tō-mō′lăr) A supernumerary tooth located in the region posterior to the third molar tooth.

dis·to·pul·pal (dis′tō-pŭl′păl) Relating to the line (dihedral) angle formed by the junction of the distal and pulpal walls of a cavity.

dis·tor·tion (dis-tōr′shŭn) **1.** PSYCHIATRY a defense mechanism that helps to repress or disguise unacceptable thoughts. **2.** DENTISTRY the permanent deformation of the impression material after the registration of an imprint. **3.** A twisting out of normal shape or form. **4.** OPHTHALMOLOGY unequal magnification over a field of view. [L. *distortio*, fr. *dis-torqueo*, to wrench apart]

dis·tor·tion ab·er·ra·tion (dis-tōr′shŭn ab-ĕr-ā′shŭn) The faulty formation of an image arising because the magnification of the peripheral part of an object is different from that of the central part when viewed through a lens.

dis·tor·tion-pro·duct o·to·a·cous·tic e·mis·sion (dis-tōr′shŭn prod′ŭkt ō′tō-ă-kū′stik ē-mish′ŭn) A form of evoked otoacoustic emission in which a third frequency is produced when two pure tones are used as the stimulus.

dis·to·ver·sion (dis′tō-vĕr-zhŭn) Malposition of a tooth distal to normal, in a posterior direction following the curvature of the dental arch.

dis·trac·ti·bil·i·ty (dis-trak′ti-bil′i-tē) Level at which competing sensory stimuli are capable of drawing attention away from a given task.

dis·trac·tion (dis-trak′shŭn) **1.** Difficulty or impossibility of concentration or fixation of the mind. **2.** Manipulation or traction of a limb to separate bony fragments or joint surfaces. [L. *dis-traho,* pp. *-tractus,* to pull in different directions]

dis·trac·tion os·te·o·gen·e·sis (dis-trak′shŭn os′tē-ō-jen′ĕ-sis) A technique of inducing new bone formation by dividing a bone and applying tension through an external fixation device to lengthen the bone.

dis·tress (dis-tres′) Mental or physical suffering or anguish. [L. *distringo,* to draw asunder]

dis·trib·ut·ed prac·tice (dis-trib′yū-tĕd prak′tis) Exercise activity in which more time is spent resting than practicing.

dis·tri·bu·tion (dis′tri-byū′shŭn) **1.** The passage of the branches of arteries or nerves to the tissues and organs. **2.** The area in which the branches of an artery or a nerve terminate, or the area supplied by such an artery or nerve. **3.** Passage of an agent through blood or lymph to body sites remote from the site(s) of contact and absorption; thus called systemic distribution. **4.** The relative numbers of people in each of various categories or populations, such as in different age, sex, or occupational samples. **5.** The pattern of occurrence of a substance within or between cells, tissues, organisms, or taxa. [L. *dis-tribuo,* pp. *-tributus,* to distribute, fr. *tribus,* a tribe]

dis·trix (dis′triks) Splitting of the hairs at their ends. [G. *dis,* twice, + *thrix,* hair]

dis·tro·pin (dis-trō′pin) SYN dystrophin.

dis·tur·bance (dis-tŭr′băns) A troubling or upsetting of a previous condition of order or tranquility. [L. *disturbo*, to agitate, confuse]

di·sul·fate (dī-sŭl′fāt) A molecule containing two sulfates. SYN disulphate.

di·sul·fide (dī-sŭl′fīd) **1.** A molecule containing two atoms of sulfur to one of the reference element, e.g., CS_2, carbon disulfide. **2.** A compound containing the –S–S– group, e.g., cystine. SYN disulphide.

di·sul·fide bond (dī-sŭl′fīd bond) A single bond between two sulfurs; specifically, the —S—S— link binding two peptide chains (or different parts of one peptide chain). SYN disulphide bond.

disulphate [Br.] SYN disulfate.

disulphide [Br.] SYN disulfide.

disulphide bond [Br.] SYN disulfide bond.

DIT Abbreviation for diiodotyrosine.

di•ter•penes (dī-tĕr′pēnz) Hydrocarbons or their derivatives containing four isoprene units, hence containing 20 carbon atoms and four branched methyl groups (e.g., vitamin A, retinene, aconitine).

Ditt•rich plug (dit′rik plŭg) A minute, dirty-grayish, foul-smelling mass of bacteria and fatty acid crystals in the sputum in pulmonary gangrene and fetid bronchitis.

di•u•re•sis (dī-yūr-ē′sis) Excretion of urine; commonly denotes production of unusually large volumes. [G. *dia,* throughout, completely, + *ourēsis,* urination]

di•u•ret•ic (dī-yūr-et′ik) **1.** Promoting excretion of urine. **2.** An agent that increases the amount of urine excreted.

di•ur•nal (dī-ŭr′năl) **1.** Pertaining to the daylight hours; opposite of nocturnal. **2.** Repeating once each 24 hours (e.g., a diurnal variation or a diurnal rhythm). Cf. circadian. [L. *diurnus,* of the day]

di•va•lence, **di•va•len•cy** (dī-vā′lĕns, -lĕn-sē) SYN bivalence.

di•va•lent (dī-vā′lĕnt) SYN bivalent (1).

di•var•i•ca•tion (dī′var-i-kā′shŭn) SYN diastasis (1). [L. *divaric.,* to spread asunder]

di•ver•gence (di-vĕr′jĕns) **1.** A moving or spreading apart or in different directions. **2.** The spreading of branches of the neuron to form synapses with several other neurons. [L. *di-,* apart, + *vergo,* to incline]

di•ver•gence in•suf•fi•cien•cy (di-vĕr′jĕns in′sŭ-fish′ĕn-sē) That condition in which an exophoria or exotropia is more marked for near vision than for far vision.

di•ver•gence pa•re•sis (di-vĕr′jĕns pă-rē′sis) An esodeviation of the eyes that is greater in the distance than near, which may be a sign of central nervous system disease or a mild bilateral sixth nerve palsy.

di•ver•gent (di-vĕr′jĕnt) Moving in different directions; radiating.

di•ver•gent stra•bis•mus (di-vĕr′jĕnt stră-biz′mŭs) SYN exotropia.

di•ver•sion (di-vĕr′zhŭn) The process of rerouting an ambulance to another facility other than the closest appropriate facility.

di•ver•tic•u•la (dī′vĕr-tik′yū-lă) Plural of diverticulum.

di•ver•tic•u•la of co•lon (dī′vĕr-tik′yū-lă kō′lŏn) Diverticula that are herniations of mucosa and submucosa between fibers of the major muscle layer (muscularis propria) of the colon; can cause bleeding and episodes of severe inflammation.

di•ver•tic•u•lar (dī′vĕr-tik′yū-lăr) Relating to a diverticulum.

di•ver•tic•u•lec•to•my (dī′vĕr-tik′yū-lek′tŏ-mē) Excision of a diverticulum.

di•ver•tic•u•li•tis (dī′vĕr-tik′yū-lī′tis) Inflammation of a diverticulum, especially of the small pockets in the wall of the colon that fill with stagnant fecal material and become inflamed; rarely, may cause obstruction, perforation, or bleeding.

di•ver•tic•u•lo•ma (dī′vĕr-tik′yū-lō′mă) Development of a granulomatous mass in the wall of the colon. [diverticulum + G. *-oma,* tumor]

di•ver•tic•u•lo•sis (dī′vĕr-tik′ū-lō′sis) Presence of a number of diverticula of the intestine, common in middle age; the lesions are acquired pulsion diverticula. See page B17.

di•ver•tic•u•lum, pl. **di•ver•tic•u•la** (dī′vĕr-tik′yū-lŭm, -lă) A pouch or sac opening from a tubular or saccular organ, such as the gut or bladder. [L. *deverticulum* (or *di-*), a by-road, fr. *de-verto,* to turn aside]

di•vid•ed dose (di-vīd′ĕd dōs) A definite fraction of a full dose; given at shorter intervals than a full dose.

div•ing goi•ter (dīv′ing goy′tĕr) A freely movable goiter that is sometimes above and sometimes below the sternal notch. SYN wandering goiter.

div•ing re•flex (dīv′ing rē′fleks) A reflex by which immersing the face or body in water, especially cold water, tends to cause bradycardia and peripheral vasoconstriction; relatively minor in most humans.

di•vi•si•o (di-viz′ē-ō) SYN division.

di•vi•si•o au•to•nom•i•ca sys•tem•a•tis ner•vo•si per•i•pher•i•ci (di-viz′ē-ō aw-tō-nō′mi-ka sis-tĕm′ă-tis ner-vō′sī per-i-fer′ĭ-sī) [TA] SYN autonomic division of nervous system.

di•vi•si•o la•ter•a•lis dex•tra he•pa•tis (di-viz′ē-ō lat-ĕr-ā′lis deks′tră hē-pā′tis) [TA] SYN right lateral division of liver.

di•vi•si•o la•ter•a•lis si•nis•tra he•pa•tis (di-viz′ē-ō lat-ĕr-ā′lis sin′is-tră hē-pā′tis) [TA] SYN left lateral division of liver.

di•vi•si•o me•di•a•lis dex•tra he•pa•tis (di-viz′ē-ō mē-dē-ā′lis deks′tră hē-pā′tis) [TA] SYN right medial division of liver.

di•vi•si•o me•di•a•lis si•nis•tra he•pa•tis (di-viz′ē-ō mē-dē-ā′lis sin′is-tră hē-pā′tis) [TA] SYN left medial division of liver.

di•vi•sion (di-vizh′ŭn) A separating into two or more parts. SYN divisio.

di•vi•sion•al block (di-vizh′ŭn-ăl blok) Arrest of the impulse in one of the assumed two main divisions of the left branch of the bundle of His; i.e., in either the anterior (superior) division or the posterior (inferior) division.

di•vul•sion (di-vŭl′shŭn) **1.** Removal of a part by tearing. **2.** Forcible dilation of the walls of a cavity or canal.

di•vul•sor (di-vŭl′sŏr) An instrument for forcible dilation of the urethra or other canal or cavity.

Dix-Hall•pike ma•neu•ver (diks-hawl′pīk mă-nū′vĕr) Test for eliciting paroxysmal vertigo and nystagmus in which the patient is brought from the sitting to the supine position with the head hanging over the examining table and turned to the right or left; vertigo and nystagmus are elicited when the head is rotated toward the affected ear.

di•zy•got•ic, **di•zy•gous** (dī-zī-got′ik, dī-zī′gŭs) Relating to twins derived from two zygotes but sharing a common intrauterine environment. [G. *di-*, two, + *zygotos,* yoked together]

di•zy•got•ic twins (dī-zī-got′ik twinz) Twins derived from two zygotes. SYN fraternal twins, heterologous twins.

diz•zi•ness (diz′ē-nĕs) Imprecise term commonly used by patients in an attempt to describe various symptoms such as faintness, vertigo, disequilibrium, or unsteadiness. SEE ALSO vertigo. [A. S. *dyzig,* foolish]

djen•kol poi•son•ing (jeng′kol poy′zŏn-ing) Any poisoning believed to result from eating excessive amounts of a bean, *Pitecolobium lobatum;* symptoms are renal pain, dysuria, and later anuria; the djenkol bean has a high vitamin B content and is used for food despite its toxic qualities. The beans are grown widely in tropic regions (e.g., Thailand, Myanmar). Clinically, associated acute renal failure is analogous to acute uric acid nephropathy.

DKA Abbreviation for diabetic ketoacidosis.

DL- Prefix (in small capital letters) denoting a substance consisting of equal quantities of the two enantiomorphs, D and L; replaces the older *dl-* (in lower case italics) as a more exact definition of structure.

DLEK Abbreviation for deep lamellar endothelial keratoplasty.

DLK Abbreviation for diffuse lamellar keratitis.

DM Abbreviation for diabetes mellitus; diastolic murmur; dopamine; NATO code for the vomiting agent Adamsite.

DMARD (dē′mahrd) Abbreviation (and acronym) for disease-modifying antirheumatic drugs.

DMD Abbreviation for Doctor of Dental Medicine.

DME Abbreviation for durable medical equipment.

DMERC Abbreviation for durable medical equipment regional carrier.

DMF car•ies in•dex (kār′ēz in′deks) An index of past caries experience that includes decayed, missing, and filled permanent teeth. The abbreviation DMFT is used when "complete" permanent teeth are referred to; DMFS is the abbreviation for the index that includes only the surfaces of permanent teeth.

DMIT Abbreviation for disability management intervention team.

DMSO Abbreviation for dimethyl sulfoxide.

DN Abbreviation for dibucaine number test.

DNA Abbreviation for deoxyribonucleic acid. See this page.

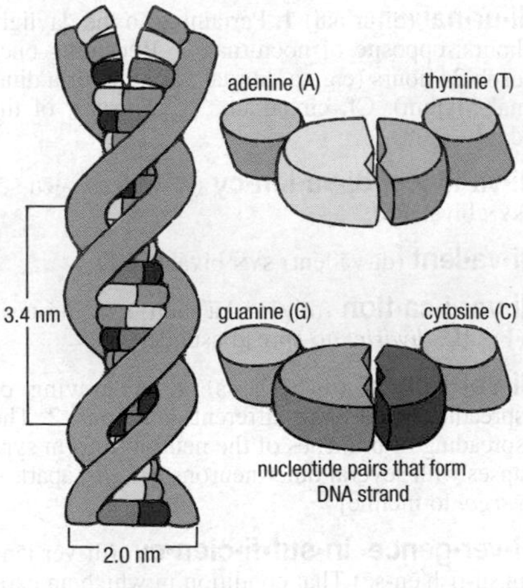

DNA (deoxyribonucleic acid)

DNA fin•ger•print•ing (fing′gĕr-print′ing) A technique used to compare people using molecular genotyping. DNA is isolated from a specific person, digested, and fractionated according to size. A Southern hybridization with a radiolabeled repetitive DNA probe provides an autoradiographic pattern unique to that person. DNA fingerprinting offers a statistical basis for evaluating the probability that samples of blood, hair, semen, or tissue have originated from a given individual.

DNA he•lix (hē′liks) SYN Watson-Crick helix.

DNA mar•kers (mahr′kĕrz) Segments of chromosomal DNA known to be linked with heritable traits or diseases. Although the markers themselves do not produce the conditions, they exist in concert with the genes responsible and are passed on with them. Certain markers, restriction fragment length polymorphisms, consist of segments of DNA that can be identified on autoradiographs (produced after digestion of the DNA by restriction enzymes and segregation of the resulting fragments through gel electrophoresis).

DNA mi•cro•ar•ray (mī′krō-ă-rā′) A technique used to identify the entire gene expression of bacterial cells. Microscopic spots of DNA are placed on a solid support in an array, and unknown samples fluorescently labeled are hybridized to the DNA on the array. A scanner is used to identify hybrids.

DNA pol•y•mor•phism (pol′ē-mōr′fizm) A condition in which one of two different but normal nucleotide sequences can exist at a particular site in DNA.

DNAR Abbreviation for do not attempt resuscitation.

DNA-RNA hy•brid (hī′brid) Double-stranded polynucleic acids in which one strand is DNA and the other strand is the complementary RNA; formed during transcription and during multiplication of oncogenic RNA viruses.

DNase Abbreviation for deoxyribonuclease.

DNA vi•rus (vī′rŭs) A major group of animal viruses in which the core consists of deoxyribonucleic acid (DNA); it includes parvoviruses, papovaviruses, adenoviruses, herpesviruses, poxviruses, and other unclassified DNA viruses. SYN deoxyribovirus.

DNR Abbreviation for do not resuscitate.

dns, DNS Abbreviation for dansyl.

DNSc Abbreviation for Doctor of Nursing Science.

DOA Abbreviation for dead on arrival.

DOB Abbreviation for date of birth.

Do•bra•va-Bel•grade vi•rus (dō′brā-vă bel′ grād vī′rŭs) A species of hantavirus in the Balkans causing hemorrhagic fever with renal syndrome. [after Dobrava, Slovenia (where first isolated from field mice) and Belgrade, the part of the former nation of Yugoslavia (where first isolated from humans)]

doc•tor (dok′tŏr) **1.** A title conferred by a university on one who has followed a prescribed course of study, or given as a title of distinction; as doctor of medicine, laws, philosophy, and other disciplines. **2.** A physician, especially one on whom has been conferred the degree of M.D. or D.O. degree. More generally, an independent practitioner in any health care profession (e.g., dentistry, optometry, podiatry). [L. a teacher, fr. *doceo,* pp. *doctus,* to teach]

Doc•tor of Na•tur•o•path•ic Med•i•cine (dok′tŏr nach′ŭr-ō-path′ik med′i-sin) Degree awarded after candidate completes a 4-year program similar in the scope of the basic sciences to the equivalent of a medical course. These students do not usually proceed to internship or residency. Focus of training is on complementary and alternative medicine, used in preference to clinical modalities.

Doc•tor of Pharm•a•cy (Phar.D.) (dok′tŏr fahr′mă-sē) The first-level professional degree or professional doctorate that prepares the graduate for pharmacy practice. The multidisciplinary curriculum may focus on pharmacy-biomedical sciences, pharmaceutical sciences, social and administrative sciences, clinical sciences and experiential training. Entrance into a Phar.D. (Pharm.D.) program generally does not require prior reception of a college degree, although most accepted applicants hold one. SEE pharmacist. SYN Pharm.D.

Doc•tor of Phys•i•cal Ther•a•py (D.P.T.) (dok′tŏr fiz′i-kăl thār′ă-pē) Highest degree conferred on students in the profession of physical therapy.

doc•tor shop•ping (dok′tŏr shop′ing) A practice in which patients go from one health care professional to one or more others so as to procure the diagnosis or therapy desired, rather than required, in the opinion of the first physician.

doc•u•men•ta•tion trail (dok′yū-mĕn-ta′shŭn trāl) A detailed sequential record of events pertaining to a particular matter; used as a risk management technique. SYN audit trail.

Dö•der•lein ba•cil•lus (dĕr′der-līn bă-sil′ŭs) A large, gram-positive bacterium occurring in normal vaginal secretions; thought by some to be identical with *Lactobacillus acidophilus.*

dol (dōl) A unit measure of pain. [L. *dolor,* pain]

♻ **dolicho-** Prefix meaning long. [G. *dolichos*]

dol•i•cho•ce•phal•ic, dol•i•cho•ceph•a•lous (dol′i-kō-sĕ-fal′ik, -sef′ă-lŭs) Having a disproportionately long head; denoting a cranium with a cephalic index less than 75. [dolicho- + G. *kephalē,* head]

dol•i•cho•fa•cial (dol′i-kō-fā′shăl) SYN dolichoprosopic.

dol•i•chol (dol′i-kol) Polyisoprenes in which the terminal member is saturated and oxidized to an alcohol, usually phosphorylated, and often glycosylated; found in endoplasmic reticulum, but not in mitochondrial or plasma membranes; urinary levels are elevated in disorders exhibiting abnormal skin, rectal, or brain profiles in electron microscopy of biopsies.

dol•i•cho•pel•lic, dol•i•cho•pel•vic (dol′i-kō-pel′ik, -pel′vik) Having a disproportionately long pelvis; denoting a pelvis with a pelvic index exceeding 95. [dolicho- + G. *pellis,* bowl (pelvis)]

dol·i·cho·pel·lic pel·vis (dol′i-kō-pel′ik pel′vis) A pelvis in which the anteroposterior diameter is longer than the transverse.

dol·i·cho·pro·sop·ic, dol·i·cho·pros·o·pous (dol′i-kō-pros-ō′pik, -kō-pros′ō-pŭs) Having a disproportionately long face. SYN dolichofacial. [dolicho- + G. *prosōpikos,* facial]

doll's eye sign (dolz ī sīn) Reflex movement of the eyes in the opposite direction to that in which the head is moved, e.g., the eyes being lowered as the head is raised, and the reverse (Cantelli sign); an indication of functional integrity of the brainstem tegmental pathways and cranial nerves involved in eye movement.

doll's head ma·neu·ver (dolz hed mă-nū′vĕr) A test to assess CNS damage in a patient with coma; failure of the eyes to deviate when the head is turned side to side indicates damage to brainstem.

do·lor (dō′lōr) Pain, as one of the four signs of inflammation (d., calor, rubor, tumor) enunciated by Celsus. [L.]

do·lo·rif·ic (dō-lōr-if′ik) Pain-producing.

do·lo·rim·e·try (dō-lōr-im′ĕ-trē) The measurement of pain. [L. *dolor,* pain, + G. *metron,* measure]

do·main (dō-mān′) **1.** Homologous unit of 110–120 amino acids, groups of which make up the light and heavy chains of the immunoglobulin molecule; each serves a specific function. The light chain has two domains, one in the variable region and one in the constant region of the chain; the heavy chain has four to five domains, depending on the class of immunoglobulin, one in the variable region and the remaining ones in the constant region. **2.** A region of a protein having some distinctive physical feature or role. **3.** An independently folded, globular structure composed of one section of a polypeptide chain. A domain may interact with another domain; it may be associated with a particular function. Domains can vary in size. [Fr. *domaine,* fr. L. *dominium,* property, dominion]

do·mes·tic vi·o·lence (dŏ-mĕs′tik vī′ŏ-lĕns) Intentionally inflicted injury perpetrated by and on family member(s); varieties include spouse abuse, child abuse, and sexual abuse, including incest. Various kinds of abuse (e.g., sexual abuse) also happen outside of the family unit.

dom·i·cil·i·at·ed (dom′i-sil′ē-āt-ĕd) A state of close association of an organism within human abodes or activities, such that partial domestication results, leading to the organism's dependence on continued association with the human environment; this frequently results in the domiciliated organism becoming a noxious pest, a vector, or an intermediate host of human disease. [L. *domicilium,* a dwelling]

dom·i·nance (dom′i-năns) The state of being dominant.

dom·i·nance of traits (dom′i-năns trāts) An expression of the apparent physiologic relationship existing between two or more genes that may occupy the same chromosomal locus (alleles). At a specific locus there are three possible combinations of two allelic genes, *A* and *a*: two homozygous (*AA* and *aa*) and one heterozygous (*Aa*). If a heterozygous individual presents only the hereditary characteristic determined by gene *A*, but not *a*, *A* is said to be dominant and *a* recessive; in this case, *AA* and *Aa*, although genotypically distinct, should be phenotypically indistinguishable. If *AA*, *Aa*, and *aa* are distinguishable, each from the others, *A* and *a* are codominant.

dom·i·nant (dom′i-nănt) **1.** Ruling or controlling. **2.** GENETICS denoting an allele possessed by one of the parents of a hybrid that is expressed in the latter to the exclusion of a contrasting allele (the recessive) from the other parent. [L. *dominans*, pres. p. of *dominor*, to rule, fr. *dominus*, lord, master, fr. *domus*, house]

dom·i·nant char·ac·ter (dom′i-nănt kar′ăk-tĕr) An inherited character expressed in either the homozygous or heterozygous state. SEE phenotype.

dom·i·nant eye (dom′i-nănt ī) The eye that is customarily used for monocular tasks.

dom·i·nant gene (dom′i-nănt jēn) SEE dominance of traits.

dom·i·nant hem·i·sphere (dom′i-nănt hem′is-fēr′) That cerebral hemisphere containing the representation of speech and controlling the arm and leg used preferentially in skilled movements; usually the left hemisphere.

dom·i·nant i·de·a (dom′i-nănt ī-dē′ă) An idea that governs all one's actions and thoughts.

dom·i·nant in·her·i·tance (dom′i-nănt in-her′i-tăns) SEE dominance of traits.

dom·i·nant op·tic at·ro·phy (dom′i-nănt op′tik at′rŏ-fē) An autosomal dominant bilateral optic neuropathy characterized by insidious preschool vision loss. SYN Kjer optic atrophy.

dom·i·nant trait (dom′i-nănt trāt) An outstanding mental or physical characteristic; SEE dominance of traits.

DOMS Abbreviation for delayed onset muscle soreness.

Do·nath-Land·stein·er an·ti·bod·y (dō′naht-lahnd′shtī-nĕr an′ti-bod-ē) An IgG antibody associated with paroxysmal cold hemoglobinuria. The antibody is biphasic, reacting with erythrocytes at temperatures lower than 15°C, which fixes complement to the cell membrane. On reaching body temperature, the antibody detaches, but the terminal complement components are activated on the cell membrane, causing hemolysis. SEE ALSO hemoglobinuria.

Do•nath-Land•stei•ner phe•nom•e•non (dō′naht lahnd′shtī-nĕr fē-nom′ĕ-non) The hemolysis that results in a sample of blood of a patient with paroxysmal hemoglobinuria when the sample is cooled to around 5°C and then rewarmed.

Don•ders law (don′dĕrz law) The rotation of the eyeball is determined by the distance of the object from the median plane and the line of the horizon.

dong quai (dōng kī) SYN angelica.

Don Juan (don-hwahn′, don jū′an) PSYCHIATRY a term used to denote men with compulsive sexual or romantic overactivity, usually with a succession of female partners. [legendary Spanish nobleman]

do•nor (dō′nŏr) **1.** A person from whom blood, tissue, or an organ is taken for transplantation. **2.** A compound that will transfer an atom or a radical to an acceptor. **3.** An atom that readily yields electrons to an acceptor. [L. *dono,* pp. *donatus,* to donate, to give]

do not at•tempt re•sus•ci•ta•tion (DNAR) (dū not ă-tempt′ rē-sus′i-tā′shŭn) Directive to health care workers from a patient who has expressed in writing a wish not to be resuscitated in the event of cardiac or respiratory arrest.

do not hos•pi•ta•lize (dū not hos′pi-tăl-īz) Written order indicating that a patient with a terminal illness is not to be admitted to the hospital.

Don•o•van bod•ies (don′ŏ-văn bod′ēz) Clusters of blue- or black-staining, bipolar chromatin condensations in large mononuclear cells in granulation tissue infected with *Calymmatobacterium granulomatis*.

don•o•va•no•sis (don′ō-vă-nō′sis) SYN granuloma inguinale.

do•pa, DOPA (dō′pă) An intermediate in the catabolism of L-phenylalanine and L-tyrosine, and in the biosynthesis of norepinephrine, epinephrine, and melanin; the L form, levodopa, is biologically active.

do•pa•mine (DM) (dō′pă-mēn) An intermediate in tyrosine metabolism and precursor of norepinephrine and epinephrine.

dop•ing (dōp′ing) The administration of foreign substances to a human or animal; often used in reference to athletes who try to enhance physiologic function and exercise performance. SEE ALSO blood doping.

Dop•pler (dop′lĕr) A diagnostic instrument that emits an ultrasonic beam into the body; the ultrasound reflected from moving structures changes its frequency (Doppler effect). Of diagnostic value in peripheral vascular and cardiac disease.

Dopp•ler co•lor flow (dop′lĕr kŏl′ŏr flō) A computer-generated color image produced by Doppler ultrasonography in which different directions of flow are represented by different hues. SEE Doppler ultrasonography.

Dopp•ler ech•o•car•di•og•ra•phy (dop′lĕr ek′ō-kahr-dē-og′ră-fē) Use of Doppler ultrasonography techniques to augment two-dimensional echocardiography by allowing velocities to be registered within the echocardiographic image. SEE ALSO duplex ultrasonography, Doppler ultrasonography.

Dopp•ler ef•fect (dop′lĕr e-fekt′) A change in frequency observed when the sound and observer are in relative motion away from or toward each other. SEE ALSO Doppler shift.

Dopp•ler shift (dop′lĕr shift) The magnitude of the frequency change in hertz when sound and observer are in relative motion away from or toward each other. SEE ALSO Doppler effect.

Dopp•ler ul•tra•so•nog•ra•phy (dop′lĕr ŭl′tra-sŏ-nog′ră-fē) Application of the Doppler effect in ultrasound to detect movement of scatterers (usually red blood cells) by the analysis of the change in frequency of the returning echoes. See this page.

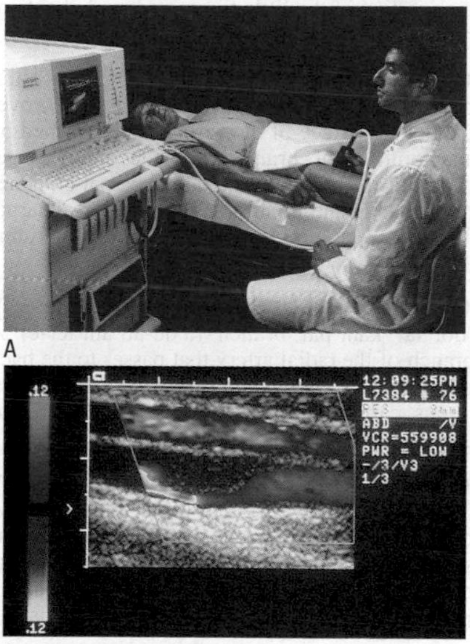

A

B

Doppler ultrasonography: (A) vascular imaging, (B) color flow Doppler showing femoral vein thrombus

Do•rel•lo ca•nal (dōr-el′lō kă-nal′) A bony canal sometimes found at the tip of the temporal bone enclosing the abducens nerve and inferior petrosal sinus as these two structures enter the cavernous sinus.

Do•ren•dorf sign (dōr′ĕn-dōrf sīn) Fullness of one supraclavicular groove in aneurysm of the aortic arch.

Dor fun•do•pli•ca•tion (dōr fŭn′dō-pli-kā′shŭn) A partial (180 degree) and anterior fundoplication, popular in Europe and South America and most often used along with a myotomy for the treatment of achalasia.

dor•sa (dōr′să) Plural of dorsum.

dor•sad (dōr′sad) Toward or in the direction of the back. [L. *dorsum,* back, + *ad,* to]

dor•sal (dōr′săl) **1.** Pertaining to the back or any dorsum. **2.** SYN posterior (2). See page B29. [Mediev. L. *dorsalis,* fr. *dorsum,* back]

dor•sal ar•ter•y of clit•o•ris (dōr′săl ahr′tĕr-ē klit′ŏr-is) One of the two terminal branches of the internal pudendal artery in the female, the other being the deep artery of the clitoris. SYN arteria dorsalis clitoridis [TA].

dor•sal ar•ter•y of pe•nis (dōr′săl ahr′tĕr-ē pē′nis) The dorsal terminal branch of the internal pudendal artery in the male. SYN arteria dorsalis penis [TA].

dor•sal branch of ul•nar nerve (dōr′săl branch ŭl′năr nĕrv) Branch arising from the ulnar nerve proximal to the wrist for distribution to the medial side of the dorsum of the hand and proximal portion of the little finger and medial side of ring finger. SYN ramus dorsalis nervi ulnaris.

dor•sal car•pal ar•ter•i•al arch (dōr′săl kahr′păl ahr-tēr′ē-ăl ahrch) A vascular network over the dorsal surface of the carpal joints, formed by anastomoses of branches of the anterior and posterior interosseous and dorsal carpal branches of the radial and ulnar arteries. SYN dorsal carpal network, rete carpale dorsale, rete carpi posterius.

dor•sal car•pal branch of ra•di•al ar•ter•y (dōr′săl kahr′păl branch rā′dē-ăl ahr′tĕr-ē) A branch of the radial artery that passes to the back of the wrist to join the dorsal carpal network. SYN ramus carpalis dorsalis arteriae radialis, ramus carpeus dorsalis arteriae radialis.

dor•sal car•pal branch of ul•nar ar•ter•y (dōr′săl kahr′păl branch ŭl′năr ahr′tĕr-ē) A branch of the ulnar artery that passes to the dorsal side of the carpus to enter the dorsal carpal network. SYN ramus carpalis dorsalis arteriae ulnaris, ramus carpeus dorsalis arteriae ulnaris.

dor•sal car•pal net•work (dōr′săl kahr′păl net′wŏrk) SYN dorsal carpal arterial arch.

dor•sal dig•i•tal ar•ter•y (dōr′săl dij′i-tăl ahr′tĕr-ē) One of the collateral digital branches of the dorsal metatarsal arteries in the foot, or of the dorsal metacarpal arteries in the hand.

dor•sal dig•i•tal nerves of foot (dōr′săl dij′i-tăl nĕrvz fut) Nerves supplying the skin of the dorsal aspect of the proximal and middle phalanges of the toes. SYN nervi digitales dorsales pedis [TA].

dor•sal dig•i•tal nerves of hand (dōr′săl dij′i-tăl nĕrvz hand) Terminal branches of the radial and ulnar nerves in the hand supplying the skin of the dorsal surface of the proximal and middle phalanges of the fingers. SYN nervi digitales dorsales manus [TA].

dor•sal flex•ure (dōr′săl flek′shŭr) A flexure in the middorsal region in the embryo.

dor•sal•gi•a (dōr-sal′jē-ă) Pain in the upper back. [L. *dorsum,* back, + G. *algos,* pain]

dor•sal hy•po•thal•a•mic ar•e•a (dōr′săl hī′pō-thal′ă-mik ār′ē-ă) A relatively small region of the hypothalamus located ventral to the hypothalamic sulcus; contains the following nuclei: portions of the dorsomedial nucleus (nucleus dorsomedialis [TA]), endopeduncular nucleus (nucleus endopeduncularis [TA]), and portions of the nucleus of the ansa lenticularis (nucleus ansae lenticularis [TA]).

dor•sal in•ter•os•se•i (in•ter•os•se•ous mus•cles) of foot (dōr′săl in′tĕr′os′ē-ī in′tĕr-os′sē-ŭs mŭs′ĕlz fut) Four intrinsic muscles of fourth layer of plantar muscles; *origin,* from sides of adjacent metatarsal bones; *insertion,* first into medial, second into lateral side of proximal phalanx of second toe, third and fourth into lateral side of proximal phalanx of third and fourth toes; *action,* abduct toes 2–4 from an axis through the second toe; *nerve supply,* lateral plantar. SYN musculi interossei dorsales pedis.

dor•sal in•ter•os•se•i (in•ter•os•se•ous mus•cles) of hand (dōr′săl in′tĕr-os′ē-ī in′tĕr-os′ē-ŭs mŭs′ĕlz hand) Four intrinsic muscles of hand; *origin,* sides of adjacent metacarpal bones; *insertion,* proximal phalanges and extensor expansion, first on radial side of index, second on radial side of middle finger; *action,* abduct fingers 2–4 from axis of middle finger; *nerve supply,* ulnar. SYN musculi interossei dorsales manus.

dor•sal in•ter•os•se•ous ar•ter•y (dōr′săl in′tĕr-os′ē-ŭs ahr′tĕr-ē) SYN posterior interosseous artery.

dor•sa•lis pe•dis ar•ter•y (dor-sā′lis ped′is ahr′tĕr-ē) Continuation of anterior tibial artery after crossing ankle; *branches,* lateral tarsal, arcuate, dorsal metatarsal; *anastomosis,* lateral plantar, forms the plantar arch.

dor•sa•lis pe•dis pulse (dōr-sā′lis ped′is pŭls) A palpable rhythmic expansion of the dorsalis pedis artery just distal to the ankle, an indication of adequate circulation to the foot.

dor•sal me•di•al cu•ta•ne•ous nerve (dōr′săl mē′dē-ăl kyū-tā′nē-ŭs nĕrv) SYN medial dorsal cutaneous nerve.

dor•sal me•ta•car•pal ar•ter•y (dōr′săl met′ă-kahr′păl ahr′tĕr-ē) One of four arteries taking origin from the dorsal carpal arch and running on the posterior aspect of the interosseous muscles of the hand. SYN arteria metacarpalis dorsalis.

dor·sal me·ta·tar·sal ar·ter·y (dōr′săl met′ă-tahr′săl ahr′tĕr-ē) One of four arteries arising from the dorsalis pedis (I) and arcuate (II–IV) arteries and running on the dorsa of the interosseous muscles of the foot. SYN arteria metatarsalis dorsalis.

dor·sal mid·brain syn·drome (dōr′săl mid′ brān sin′drōm) SYN Parinaud syndrome.

dor·sal na·sal ar·ter·y (dōr′săl nā′zăl ahr′tĕr-ē) *Origin*, ophthalmic; external artery of the nose; *distribution*, skin of side of root of nose; *anastomoses*, angular artery. SYN external nasal artery.

dor·sal nerve of clit·o·ris (dōr′săl nĕrv klit′ ŏr-is) The deep terminal branch of the pudendal, supplying especially the glans clitoridis after passing through the musculature of the urogenital diaphragm, to run along the dorsum of the clitoral shaft. SYN nervus dorsalis clitoridis [TA].

dor·sal nerve of pe·nis (dōr′săl nĕrv pē′nis) The deep terminal branch of the pudendal nerve that runs through the urogenital diaphragm giving branches, then runs along the dorsum of the penis, supplying the skin of the penis, the prepuce, the corpora cavernosa, and the glans. SYN nervus dorsalis penis [TA].

dor·sal nu·cle·us of thal·a·mus (dōr′săl nū′klē-ŭs thal′ă-mŭs) One of the major subdivisions of the thalamus; the composite dorsal nucleus includes the nucleus lateralis anterior or dorsalis, nucleus lateralis intermedius, nucleus lateralis posterior, and pulvinar; together, these cell groups form most of the free dorsal surface of the posterior half of the thalamus and project to a very large region of parietal, occipitoparietal, and temporal cortex; its afferent connections are largely obscure, but the nucleus lateralis posterior and the pulvinar receive a projection from the superior colliculus.

dor·sal nu·cle·us of va·gus nerve (dōr′săl nū′klē-ŭs vā′gŭs nĕrv) The visceral motor nucleus located in the vagal trigone (ala cinerea) of the floor of the fourth ventricle. It gives rise to the parasympathetic fibers of the vagus nerve innervating the heart muscle and the smooth musculature and glands of the respiratory and intestinal tracts.

dor·sal ra·di·o·car·pal lig·a·ment (dōr′săl rā′dē-ō-kahr′păl lig′ă-mĕnt) The ligament that extends from the distal end of the radius posteriorly to the proximal row of carpal bones.

i **dor·sal re·cum·bent po·si·tion** (dōr′săl rē-kŭm′bĕnt pŏ-zish′ŭn) SYN supine. See page B29.

dor·sal root (dōr′săl rūt) The sensory root of a spinal nerve, having a dorsal root ganglion containing the nerve cell bodies of the fibers conveyed by the root in its distal end.

dor·sal scap·u·lar ar·ter·y (dōr′săl skap′yū-lăr ahr′tĕr-ē) *Origin*, subclavian or as the deep branch of the transverse cervical; *distribution*, passes deep to the rhomboid muscles, supplying them and other muscles and skin along the vertebral border of the scapula; *anastomoses*, suprascapular and scapular circumflex.

dor·sal scap·u·lar nerve (dōr′săl skap′yū-lăr nĕrv) Arises from ventral primary rami of the fifth to seventh cervical nerves and passes downward to supply the levator scapulae and the rhomboideus major and minor muscles. SYN nervus dorsalis scapulae [TA].

dor·sal scap·u·lar vein (dōr′săl skap′yū-lăr vān) The vena comitans of the descending scapular artery; it is a tributary to the subclavian or the external jugular vein.

Dor·set cul·ture egg me·di·um (dōr′sĕt kŭl′chŭr eg mē′dē-ŭm) A medium for cultivating *Mycobacterium tuberculosis;* consists of fresh whole eggs and a solution of sodium chloride.

dor·si·flex·ion (dōr-si-flek′shŭn) Turning upward of the foot or toes or of the hand or fingers.

dor·si·spi·nal (dōr-si-spī′năl) Relating to the vertebral column, especially to its dorsal aspect.

dor·so·ceph·a·lad (dōr-sō-sef′ă-lad) Toward the occiput, or back of the head. [L. *dorsum,* back, + G. *kephalē,* head, + L. *ad,* to]

dor·so·lat·er·al (dōr-sō-lat′ĕr-ăl) Relating to the back and the side.

dor·so·lat·er·al fas·cic·u·lus (dōr-sō-lat′ĕr-ăl fă-sik′kyū-lŭs) A longitudinal bundle of thin, unmyelinated, and poorly myelinated fibers capping the apex of the posterior horn of the spinal gray matter, composed of posterior root fibers and short association fibers that interconnect neighboring segments of the posterior horn.

dor·so·lat·er·al sul·cus (dōr-sō-lat′ĕr-ăl sŭl′kŭs) SYN posterolateral sulcus.

dor·so·lum·bar (dōr-sō-lŭm′bahr) Referring to the back in the region of the lower thoracic and upper lumbar vertebrae.

dor·so·ven·trad (dōr-sō-ven′trad) In a direction from the dorsal to the ventral aspect.

dor·sum, gen. **dor·si**, pl. **dor·sa** (dōr′sŭm, -sī, -să) [TA] **1.** The back of the body. **2.** The upper or posterior surface, or the back, of any part. [L. back]

DOS Abbreviation for date of service.

dos·age (dō′săj) **1.** The giving of medicine or other therapeutic agent in prescribed amounts. **2.** The size, frequency, and number of doses of medicine to be given. USAGE NOTE sometimes incorrectly used for dose. Cf. dose.

dose (dōs) **1.** The quantity of a drug or other remedy to be taken or applied all at one time or in fractional amounts within a given period. USAGE NOTE Sometimes incorrectly used for dosage.

Cf. dosage (2). **2.** NUCLEAR MEDICINE amount of energy absorbed per unit mass of irradiated material (absorbed dose). SEE ALSO dosage. **3.** RADIATION THERAPY the energy absorbed per unit mass of irradiated material. [G. *dosis*, a giving]

dose e·quiv·a·lent (dōs ē-kwiv′ă-lĕnt) In radiation therapy, product of absorbed dose and the quality factor; the SI unit of dose equivalent is sievert (Sv).

dose e·qui·va·lent li·mits (dōs ĕ-kwiv′ă-lĕnt lim′its) Radiation exposure limits for radiation workers. Will replace earlier term "maximum permissible dose."

dose rate (dōs rāt) In radiation therapy, rate at which radiation is delivered.

dose-re·sponse re·la·tion·ship (dōs rē-spons′ rē-lā′shŭn-ship) Direct association between a stimulus and a desired outcome (e.g., quantity of physical activity and good health).

do·sim·e·ter (dō-sim′ĕ-tĕr) **1.** A device for measuring radiation, especially x-rays. **2.** In pulmonary function testing, a device that can be triggered automatically by a sensor near the subject's mouth or manually by a technician and that allows for the delivery of a reproducible dose from a nebulizer. [G. *dosis,* dose, + *metron*, measure]

do·sim·e·try (dō-sim′ĕ-trē) Measurement of radiation exposure, especially x-rays or gamma rays; calculation of radiation dose from internally administered radionuclides.

dot·age (dō′tăj) The deterioration of previously intact mental powers, common in old age.

DOT la·bel (lā′bĕl) The U.S. Department of Transportation (DOT) label shows the type of hazard, the U.N. hazard class number, and an identifying number.

dou·ble blind ex·per·i·ment (dŭb′ĕl blīnd eks-per′i-mĕnt) An investigation conducted with neither experimenter nor subjects knowing which experiment is the control; prevents bias in recording results. SEE ALSO double-masked experiment.

dou·ble bond (dŭb′ĕl bond) A covalent bond resulting from the sharing of two pairs of electrons; e.g., $H_2C{=}CH_2$ (ethylene).

dou·ble-chan·nel cath·e·ter (dŭb′ĕl-chan′ĕl kath′ĕ-tĕr) A catheter with two lumens, allowing irrigation and aspiration. SYN two-way catheter.

doub·le chin (dŭb′ĕl chin) SYN buccula.

dou·ble com·part·ment hy·dro·ceph·a·lus (dŭb′ĕl kŏm-pahrt′mĕnt hī′drō-sef′ă-lŭs) Independent supratentorial and infratentorial hydrocephalus usually due to a veil occlusion of the cerebral aqueduct.

dou·ble con·trast en·e·ma (dŭb′ĕl kon′trast en′ĕ-mă) SYN air contrast enema.

dou·ble crush syn·drome (dŭb′ĕl krŭsh sin′drōm) A situation in which a peripheral nerve is mechanically disrupted at more than one location.

dou·ble e·le·va·tor pal·sy (dŭb′ĕl el′ĕ-vā-tŏr pawl′zē) Limited elevation of an eye in abduction and adduction, implying paresis of the superior rectus and inferior oblique muscles, although many cases are due to restriction of the inferior rectus muscle.

dou·ble flap am·pu·ta·tion (dŭb′ĕl amp′yū-tā′shŭn) Surgical procedure in which a flap is cut from the soft parts on either side of the limb.

dou·ble he·lix (dŭb′ĕl hē′liks) SYN Watson-Crick helix.

dou·ble-masked ex·per·i·ment (dŭb′ĕl-māskt eks-per′i-mĕnt) A double-blind study conducted so that neither the subject nor the observer knows the identity of the control or variable.

dou·ble per·son·al·i·ty (dŭb′ĕl pĕr′sŏn-al′i-tē) SYN dual personality.

dou·ble pneu·mo·ni·a (dŭb′ĕl nū-mō′nē-ă) Lobar pneumonia involving both lungs.

dou·ble poin·ted nee·dle (dŭb′el poyn′tĕd nē′dĕl) A blood drawing needle used with an evacuated tube system to allow the user to collect more than one tube of blood without contaminating the tube or holder (also known as multisample needle).

dou·ble pro·duct (dŭb′ĕl prod′ŭkt) The product of systolic blood pressure multiplied by the heart frequency; a measure of heart work load. SEE ALSO Robinson index.

dou·ble re·frac·tion (dŭb′ĕl rĕ-frak′shŭn) The property of having more than one refractive index according to the direction of the transmitted light. SYN birefringence.

dou·ble ring sign (dŭb′ĕl ring sīn) Two concentric rings around the optic nerve characteristic of optic nerve hypoplasia.

dou·ble stain (dŭb′ĕl stān) A mixture of two dyes, each of which stains different portions of a tissue or cell.

dou·ble step gait (dŭb′ĕl step gāt) Dysfunctional mode of ambulation in which strides vary in length depending on which limb leads in the process.

dou·blet (dŭb′lĕt) **1.** A combination of two lenses designed to correct the chromatic and spheric aberration. **2.** SYN dipole. **3.** Any sequence of two nucleotides in a polynucleotide strand. **4.** A closely spaced pair of peaks or lines in a spectrum. **5.** Text repeated in a printed document.

dou·ble vi·sion (dŭb′ĕl vizh′ŭn) SYN diplopia.

dou·bling dose (dŭb′ling dōs) Amount of radiation that doubles the incidence of stochastic effects.

dou·bling time (dŭb′ling tīm) The time it takes for the number of cells in a neoplasm to double, with shorter doubling times implying more rapid growth.

doub·ly armed su·ture (dŭb′lē ahrmd sū′chŭr) A suture with a needle attached at both ends. SYN cobbler's suture.

doub·ly het·er·o·zy·gous (dŭb′lē het′ĕr-ō-zī′gŭs) Denoting that genotype in which a parent is heterozygous at both loci, the state that on average contains the maximum information about the linkage.

doub·ly la·beled wa·ter (dŭb′lē lā′bĕld waw′tĕr) Noncalorimetric technique for measuring energy expenditure in free-living subjects using an oral dose of water containing stable nonradioactive isotopes, ^{2}H and ^{18}O. Derived CO_2 production is used to calculate energy expenditure using indirect calorimetry formulas.

douche (dūsh) **1.** A current of water, gas, or vapor directed against a surface or projected into a cavity. **2.** An instrument for giving a douche. **3.** To apply a douche. [Fr. fr. *doucher,* to pour]

douche bath (dūsh bath) The local application of water in the form of a large jet or stream.

Doug·las bag (dŭg′lăs bag) A large bag in which expired gas is collected for several minutes to determine oxygen consumption in humans under conditions of actual work.

Doug·las pouch, **Doug·las space** (dug′lăs powch, spās) Rectouterine pouch lined with parietal peritoneum; mass in this area is palpable during rectal examination.

dou·la (dū′lă) A woman who assists at labor and birth and in postpartum care of mother and baby. Doulas are trained and certified according to various requirements of local jurisdictions. They are helpful in educating the new family and in helping build their confidence as new parents. [G. *doulē,* female slave]

dove·tail stress-bro·ken a·but·ment (dŭv′tāl stres′brō-kĕn ă-bŭt′mĕnt) An abutment connected to a fixed partial denture by a nonrigid connector that is trapezoidal in cross-section.

dow·a·ger hump (dow′ă-jĕr hŭmp) Postmenopausal cervical kyphosis of older women due to osteoporosis and compression fractures of vertebra.

dow·el graft (dow′ĕl graft) A circular bone graft harvested with special instruments, used in orthopedic surgery as a structural bone graft to obtain fusion between two adjacent vertebrae.

down code (down kōd) Assigning a code for a procedure or service lower than that actually performed.

Dow·ney cell (dow′nē sel) The atypical lymphocyte of infectious mononucleosis.

down·growth (down′grōth) Something that grows downward; the process of growing in a downward direction.

down·reg·u·la·tion (down-reg-yū-lā′shŭn) Development of a refractory or tolerant state consequent on repeated administration of a pharmacologically or physiologically active substance; often accompanied by an initial decrease in affinity of receptors for the agent and a subsequent diminution in the number of receptors.

Downs a·nal·y·sis (downz ă-nal′i-sis) A series of cephalometric criteria used as an aid in orthodontic diagnosis.

Down syn·drome (down sin′drōm) A chromosomal dysgenesis syndrome consisting of a variable constellation of abnormalities caused by triplication or translocation of chromosome 21. The abnormalities include mental retardation, retarded growth, flat hypoplastic face with short nose, prominent epicanthic skin folds, small, low-set ears with prominent antihelix, fissured and thickened tongue, laxness of joint ligaments, pelvic dysplasia, broad hands and feet, stubby fingers, and transverse palmar crease. Lenticular opacities and heart disease are common. The incidence of leukemia is increased and Alzheimer disease is almost inevitable by age 40. SYN trisomy 21 syndrome.

down·time (down′tīm) As used in EMS parlance, temporal duration from cardiac arrest until beginning of CPR or ACLS.

dox·a·cu·ri·um chlo·ride (doks-a-kyūr′ē-ŭm klōr′īd) A nondepolarizing neuromuscular blocking drug similar to pancuronium but without cardiovascular side effects.

Do·yère em·i·nence (dō-yer em′i-nĕns) A slight elevation on the surface of a striated muscle corresponds to the site of the motor endplate.

Doyle op·er·a·tion (doyl op-ĕr-ā′shŭn) Paracervical uterine denervation.

DPI Abbreviation for dry powder inhaler.

DPN Abbreviation for diphosphopyridine nucleotide.

DPN^{+} Abbreviation for oxidized diphosphopyridine nucleotide.

DPT Abbreviation for diphtheria-pertussis-tetanus (vaccine).

D.P.T. Abbreviation for Doctor of Physical Therapy.

DR Abbreviation for reaction of degeneration.

dr Abbreviation for dram.

dra·cun·cu·li·a·sis, **dra·cun·cu·lo·sis** (dră-kŭng-kyū-lī′ă-sis, -kyū-lō′sis) Infection with *Dracunculus medinensis.*

Dra•cun•cu•lus (dră-kŭng′kyū-lŭs) A genus of nematodes with some resemblance to true filarial worms; adults are larger and the intermediate host is a freshwater crustacean rather than an insect. [L. dim. of *draco,* serpent]

draft (draft) **1.** A current of air in a confined space. **2.** A quantity of liquid medicine ordered as a single dose.

drag•on•wort (drag′ŏn-wōrt) SYN bistort.

drag-to gait (drag-tū gāt) Dysfunctional mode of crutch-assisted ambulation in which the feet are not lifted correctly.

drain (drān) **1.** To remove fluid from a cavity (e.g., to drain an abscess). **2.** A device, usually in the shape of a tube or wick, for removing fluid as it collects in a cavity, especially a wound cavity. [A. S. *drehnian,* to draw off]

drain•age (drān′ăj) Continuous flow or withdrawal of fluids from a wound or other cavity.

drain•age tube (drān′ăj tūb) A tube introduced into a wound or cavity to facilitate removal of a fluid.

dram (dr) (dram) A unit of weight in apothecary measurement: 1/8 oz.; 60 gr. apothecaries' weight; 1/16 oz., avoirdupois weight. Cf. fluidram.

drape (drāp) **1.** To cover parts of the body other than those to be examined or operated on. **2.** The cloth or materials used for such cover. [M.E., fr. L.L. *drappus,* cloth]

Dra•per law (drā′pĕr law) A chemical change is produced in a photochemical substance only by those light rays that are absorbed by that substance.

draw (draw) **1.** To extract blood from a vein for various diagnostic purposes or in the process of blood donation and collection. **2.** To drag or pull by applying a steady force. [O.E. *dragan*]

draw•er sign (drōr sīn) In a knee examination, abnormal forward or backward sliding of the tibia with respect to the femur indicating laxity or tear of the anterior (forward slide) or posterior (backward slide) cruciate ligaments of the knee. SYN drawer test.

draw•er test (drōr test) SYN drawer sign.

dream (drēm) Mental activity during sleep in which events, thoughts, emotions, and images are experienced as real.

dream•y state (drē′mē stāt) The semiconscious state associated with an epileptic attack.

drep•a•no•cyte (drep′ă-nō-sīt) SYN sickle cell. [G. *drepanē,* sickle, + *kytos,* a hollow (cell)]

drep•a•no•cyt•ic (drep′ă-nō-sit′ik) Relating to or resembling a sickle cell.

drep•a•no•cyt•ic a•ne•mi•a (drep′ă-nō-sit′ik ă-nē′mē-ă) SYN sickle cell anemia.

dress•ing (dres′ing) The material applied, or the application itself of material, to a wound for protection, absorbance, and drainage.

dress•ing for•ceps (dres′ing fōr′seps) A forceps for general use in dressing wounds, removing fragments of necrotic tissue, small foreign bodies, and other functions.

Dress•ler beat (dres′lĕr bēt) Fusion beat interrupting a ventricular tachycardia and producing a normally narrow QRS complex as a result of the fusion of two impulses, one impulse from the ventricular tachycardia and the other from a supraventricular focus; Dressler beats strongly support the diagnosis of ventricular tachycardia by interruption of it.

Dress•ler syn•drome (dres′lĕr sin′drōm) Recurrent pericarditis following acute myocardial infarction, or inflammation of the pericardium resulting from previous injury to the heart muscles. Symptoms may develop weeks to months after myocardial infarction or open heart surgery.

DRG Abbreviation for diagnosis-related group.

DRI Abbreviation for Dietary Reference Intake.

drift (drift) **1.** A gradual movement, as from an original position. **2.** A gradual change in the value of a random variable over time as a result of various factors, some random and some systematic effects of trend or manipulation.

drill-out (dril-owt) A drilling away; scooping out.

Drin•ker res•pi•ra•tor (dringk′ĕr res′pir-ā′tŏr) A mechanical ventilator in which the body except the head is encased within a metal tank, which is sealed at the neck with an airtight gasket; artificial ventilation is induced by making the air pressure inside the tank alternately negative and positive. SYN iron lung.

drip (drip) **1.** To flow a drop at a time. **2.** A flowing in drops; often associated with intravenous infusion.

Dripps clas•si•fi•ca•tion (drips klas′i-fi-kā′shŭn) System used by anesthesiologists to describe physical status of patient. SYN ASA classification.

drive (drīv) **1.** A basic compelling urge. **2.** PSYCHOLOGY classified as either innate (e.g., hunger) or learned (e.g., hoarding) and appetitive (e.g., hunger, thirst, sex) or aversive (e.g., fear, pain, grief). SEE ALSO motive.

driv•ing (drīv′ing) The induction of a frequency in the electroencephalogram by sensory stimulation at this frequency.

drom•o•graph (drom′ō-graf) An instrument for recording the rapidity of the blood circulation. [G. *dromos,* a running, + *graphō,* to record]

drom•o•ma•ni•a (drom′ō-mā′nē-ă) An uncontrollable impulse to wander or travel. [G. *dromos,* a running, + *mania,* insanity]

dro•mo•tro•pic (drom′ō-trō′pik) Influencing the velocity of conduction of excitation, as in nerve or cardiac muscle fibers. [G. *dromos,* a running, + *tropē,* a turn]

drop (drop) **1.** To fall, or to be dispensed or poured in globules. **2.** A liquid globule. **3.** A volume of liquid regarded as a unit of dosage, equivalent in the case of water to about 1 minim (20 drops are equal to 1 mL. [A.S. *droppan*]

drop arm test (drop ahrm test) Maneuver used to determine integrity of the supraspinatus muscle and tendon. With the shoulder abducted 90 degrees, the patient is asked to lower the arm of the affected shoulder. A positive result shows the patient cannot lower the arm slowly and smoothly.

drop at•tack (drop ă-tak′) An episode of sudden falling that occurs during standing or walking, without warning and without loss of consciousness, vertigo, or postictal behavior. The patients are usually elderly and have normal findings on electroencephalograms; of unknown cause.

drop•foot, **drop foot** (drop′fut, drop fut) SEE footdrop.

drop hand (drop hand) SYN wrist-drop.

drop•let (drop′lĕt) A diminutive drop, such as a particle of moisture discharged from the mouth during coughing, sneezing, or speaking; these may transmit infections to others by their airborne passage. [drop + *-let,* dim. suffix]

drop•let in•fec•tion (drop′lĕt in-fek′shŭn) Infection acquired through the inhalation of droplets or aerosols of saliva or sputum containing virus or other microorganisms expelled by another person during sneezing, coughing, laughing, or talking.

drop•let pre•cau•tions (drop′lĕt prē-kaw′shŭnz) Procedures that reduce the risk of droplet-borne infections. Transmission through droplets occurs when the droplets contact the conjunctivae or the nasal or oral mucous membranes of a susceptible patient. Droplets do not usually travel more than 3 feet. Masks as well as standard precautions must be used when in the infected patient's room. SEE standard precautions, Universal Precautions.

drown•ing (drow′ning) Death from suffocation induced by immersion in water or other fluid, with filling of pulmonary air spaces and passages with fluid to the detriment of gas exchange. [M.E. *drounen*]

drows•i•ness (drow′zē-nĕs) A state of impaired awareness associated with a desire or inclination to sleep.

DRR Abbreviation for digitally reconstructed radiograph.

drug (drŭg) **1.** A therapeutic agent; any substance, other than food, used in the prevention, diagnosis, alleviation, treatment, or cure of disease. For types or classifications of drugs, see the specific name. SEE ALSO agent, medication. **2.** To administer or take a drug, usually implying that an excessive quantity or a narcotic is involved. **3.** General term for any substance, stimulating or depressing, that can be habituating or addictive, especially a narcotic. [M.E. *drogge*]

drug a•buse (drŭg ă-byūs′) Habitual use of drugs not needed for therapeutic purposes (e.g., such as solely to alter one's mood, affect, or state of consciousness) or to affect a body function unnecessarily (e.g., laxative abuse); nonmedical use of drugs.

drug-e•lut•ing cor•o•nar•y stent (drŭg′ē-lūt′ing kōr′ō-nar-ē stent) A widely used device with metal surfaces that are coated with a drug to prevent restenosis; used to maintain luminal patency; recent study results suggest that when the drug wears off and leaves the bare metal exposed, there is a possibility of acute heart attack and sudden death.

drug e•rup•tion (drŭg ĕr-ŭp′shŭn) Any eruption caused by the ingestion, injection, or inhalation of a drug, most often the result of allergic sensitization; reactions to drugs applied to the cutaneous surface are not generally designated as drug eruptions, but as contact-type dermatitis. SYN dermatitis medicamentosa, dermatosis medicamentosa, drug rash.

drug-fast (drŭg-fast) Pertaining to microorganisms that resist or become tolerant to an antibacterial agent.

drug hol•i•day (drŭg hol′i-dā) Intervals when a chronically medicated patient temporarily stops taking a prescribed medication; used to allow some recuperation of normal functions or to maintain sensitivity to the drug(s).

drug in•ter•ac•tions (drŭg in-tĕr-ak′shŭnz) The pharmacologic result, either desirable or undesirable, of drugs interacting with other drugs, with endogenous physiologic chemical agents (e.g., MAOIs with epinephrine), with components of the diet, and with chemicals used in diagnostic tests or the results of such tests.

drug o•ver•dose (OD) (drŭg ō′vĕr-dōs) The ingestion, accidentally or intentionally, of sufficient drug or drugs to cause injury or death.

drug psy•cho•sis (drŭg sī-kō′sis) Psychosis following or precipitated by ingestion of a drug.

drug rash (drŭg rash) SYN drug eruption.

drug re•sis•tance (drŭg rĕ-zis′tăns) The capacity of disease-causing pathogens to withstand drugs previously toxic to them; achieved by spontaneous mutation or through selective pressure after exposure to the drug in question.

drug-re·sis·tant hy·per·ten·sion (drŭg-rē-zis′tănt hī′pĕr-ten′shŭn) A disordered condition involving high blood pressure that is not relieved by multiple pharmacotherapy.

drug tet·a·nus (drŭg tet′ă-nŭs) Tonic spasms caused by strychnine or other tetanic agents. SYN toxic tetanus.

drug use e·val·u·a·tion (drŭg yūs ĕ-val′yū-ā′shŭn) SYN drug use review.

drug use re·view (drŭg yūs rĕ-vyū′) An authorized, structured, ongoing program that collects, analyzes, and interprets drug use patterns to improve the quality of drug use and patient outcomes. SYN clinical drug trial, drug use evaluation, drug utilization review.

drug u·ti·li·za·tion re·view (drŭg yū′til-ī-zā′shŭn rĕ-vyū′) SYN drug use review.

drum, drum·head (drŭm, drŭm′hed) SYN tympanic membrane.

drum mem·brane (drŭm mem′brān) SYN tympanic membrane.

Drum·mond sign (drŭm′ŏnd sīn) In certain cases of aortic aneurysm, a puffing sound, synchronous with cardiac systole, heard from the nostrils, when the mouth is closed.

drunk·en·ness (drung′kĕn-nĕs) Intoxication, usually alcoholic.

dru·sen (drū′sĕn) Small, bright structures seen in the retina and in the optic disc. See page B26. [Ger. pl. of *Druse,* stony nodule, geode]

DRVVT Abbreviation for dilute Russell viper venom test.

dry ab·scess (drī ab′ses) The remains of an abscess after the pus has been absorbed.

dry cough (drī kawf) A cough not accompanied by expectoration; a nonproductive cough.

dry eye syn·drome (drī ī sin′drōm) SYN keratoconjunctivitis sicca.

dry gan·grene (drī gang′grēn) A form of gangrene in which the involved part is dry and shriveled. See this page. SYN mummification (1).

dry joint (drī joynt) A joint affected with atrophic desiccating changes.

dry la·bor (drī lā′bŏr) Obsolete term for labor after spontaneous loss of the amniotic fluid.

***Dry·o·pi·the·cus* pat·tern** (drī-ō-pith′ĕ-kŭs pat′ĕrn) **1.** The ancestral pattern of cusps and grooves in humans. **2.** A Y-5 cusp-and-groove pattern. SEE ALSO cusp and groove pattern. [*Dryopithicus*, a genus of anthropoid apes of the Miocene epoch]

dry pleu·ri·sy (drī plūr′i-sē) Pleurisy with a

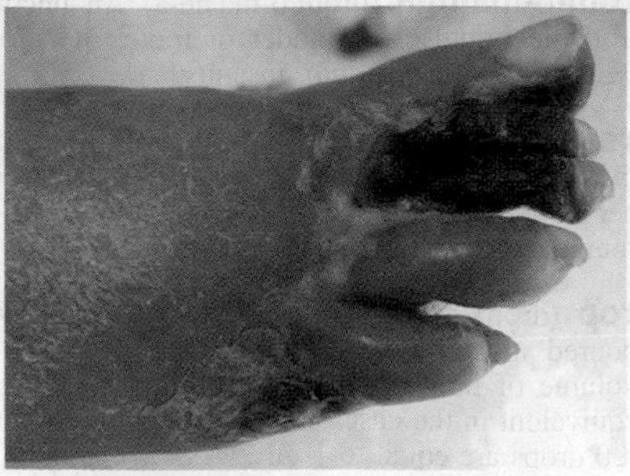

dry gangrene: toes

fibrinous exudation, without an effusion of serum, resulting in adhesion between the opposing surfaces of the pleura. SYN adhesive pleurisy, fibrinous pleurisy, plastic pleurisy.

dry rale (drī rahl) A harsh or musical breath sound produced by a constriction in a bronchial tube or the presence of a viscid secretion narrowing the lumen.

dry soc·ket (drī sok′ĕt) Localized inflammation of a tooth socket following extraction due to infection or loss of blood clot.

dry syn·o·vi·tis (drī sin′ō-vī′tis) Synovitis with little serous or purulent effusion. SYN synovitis sicca.

dry vom·it·ing (drī vom′it-ing) SYN retching.

DSA Abbreviation for digital subtraction angiography.

DSEK Abbreviation for Descemet stripping endothelial keratoplasty.

DSM Abbreviation for *Diagnostic and Statistical Manual of Mental Disorders* of the American Psychiatric Association.

DT Abbreviation for duration tetany.

dT Abbreviation for deoxythymidine.

DTaP Abbreviation for diphtheria, tetanus, and acellular pertussis vaccine.

dTDP Abbreviation for thymidine 5′-diphosphate.

dThd Abbreviation for thymidine.

dTMP Abbreviation for deoxythymidylic acid.

DTR Abbreviation for deep tendon reflex.

DTs Abbreviation for delirium tremens.

du·al-con·trolled ven·ti·la·tion (dū′ăl kŏn-trōld′ ven′ti-lā′shŭn) A mode of ventilation in which the ventilator uses both volume and pressure as feedback signals to control the size of the breath.

du·al-en·er·gy x-ray ab·sorp·ti·om·e·try

(DEXA) (dū′ăl en′ĕr-jē eks′rā ăb-sorp′shē-om′ĕ-trē) SEE dual x-ray absorptiometry.

du•al•ism (dū′ăl-izm) **1.** CHEMISTRY theory that every compound, no matter how many elements enter into it, is composed of two parts, one electrically negative, the other positive; applicable to polar compounds but not to nonpolar compounds. **2.** HEMATOLOGY the concept that blood cells have two origins, i.e., lymphogenous and myelogenous. **3.** The theory that the mind and body are two distinct systems, independent and different in nature. [L. *dualis,* relating to two, fr. *duo,* two]

du•al per•son•al•i•ty (dū′ăl pĕr′sŏn-al′i-tē) A form of mental disturbance in which someone assumes alternately two different identities; neither is conscious of the existence of the other. SYN double personality.

du•al x-ray ab•sorp•ti•om•e•try (DXA) (dū′ăl eks′rā ăb-sorp′shē-om′ĕ-trē) Use of low-dose x-radiation of two different energies to measure bone mineral content at different anatomic sites.

Du•bois ab•scess•es (dū′bwah ab′ses-ĕz) Small cysts of the thymus containing polymorphonuclear leukocytes but lined by squamous epithelium; reported in congenital syphilis but also found in the absence of syphilis.

Du•Bois for•mu•la (dū′bwah fōrm′yū-lă) A formula for predicting a human's surface area based on weight and height: $A = 71.84W^{0.425} H^{0.725}$, where A = surface area in cm^2, W = weight in kg, and H = height in cm, and a constant 0.007184.

Du•bo•witz score (dū′bŏ-wits skōr) A method of clinical assessment of gestational age in the newborn that includes neurologic criteria for the infant's maturity and other physical criteria to determine the gestational age of the infant; useful from birth to 5 days of life.

Du•chenne-A•ran dis•ease (dū-shen′ ah-rahn′ di-zēz′) SYN amyotrophic lateral sclerosis.

Du•chenne dys•tro•phy (dū-shen′ dis′trŏ-fē) The most common childhood muscular dystrophy, with onset usually before age 6 years. Characterized by symmetric weakness and wasting of first the pelvic and crural muscles and then the pectoral and proximal upper extremity muscles; pseudohypertrophy of some muscles, especially the calf; heart involvement; sometimes mild mental retardation; progressive course and early death, usually in adolescence. X-linked inheritance (affects males and transmitted by females).

Du•chenne-Erb pa•ral•y•sis (dū-shen′ ārb păr-al′i-sis) SYN Erb palsy.

Du•chenne sign (dū-shen′ sīn) Falling in of the epigastrium during inspiration in paralysis of the diaphragm.

duck wad•dle (dŭk wah′dĕl) A peculiar pattern of walking associated with congenital hip dysplasia.

duck walk (dŭk wawk) SYN metatarsus valgus.

Duck•worth phe•nom•e•non (duk′wŏrth fĕ-nom′ĕ-non) Respiratory arrest before cardiac arrest as a result of intracranial disease.

Duc•rey ba•cil•lus (dū-krā′ bă-sil′ŭs) SYN *Haemophilus ducreyi.*

duct (dŭkt) A tubular structure giving exit to the secretion of a gland, or conducting any fluid. SEE ALSO canal. SYN ductus [TA]. [L. *duco,* pp. *ductus,* to lead]

duc•tal (dŭk′tăl) Relating to a duct.

duc•tal an•eu•rysm (dŭk′tăl an′yūr-izm) Aneurysm of the patent ductus arteriosus, occurs either in infants or adults. SYN ductus diverticulum.

duct of His (dŭkt his) SYN His canal.

duc•tile (dŭk′tīl) Denoting the property of a material that allows it to be bent, drawn out (as a wire), or otherwise deformed without breaking. [L. *ductilis,* capable of being led or drawn]

duct•less (dŭkt′lĕs) Having no duct; denoting certain glands having only an internal secretion.

duct•less glands (dŭkt′lĕs glandz) SYN endocrine glands.

duc•tu•lar (dŭk′tū-lăr) Relating to a ductule.

duc•tule (dŭk′tūl) A minute duct. SYN ductulus [TA].

duc•tu•li bil•i•fe•ri (dukt′yū-lī bil-i-fer′ī) SYN biliary ductules.

duc•tu•li ef•fe•ren•tes tes•tis (dukt′yū-lī ĕf-ĕr′en-tēz tes′tis) [TA] SYN efferent ductules of testis.

duc•tu•li pros•ta•ti•ci (dukt′yū-lī pros-tat′i-sī) [TA] SYN prostatic ductules.

duc•tu•lus, pl. **duc•tu•li** (dŭk′tyū-lŭs, -lī) [TA] SYN ductule. [Mod. L. dim. of L. *ductus,* duct]

duc•tu•lus al•ve•o•la•ris, pl. **duc•tu•li al•ve•o•la•res** (dŭk′tyū-lŭs al-vē-ō-lā′ris, dŭk′tyū-lī al-vē-ō-lā-rēz) SYN alveolar duct.

duc•tus, gen. and pl. **duc•tus** (dŭk′tŭs, dŭk′tŭs) [TA] SYN duct. [L. a leading, fr. *duco,* pp. *ductus,* to lead]

duc•tus ar•te•ri•o•sus (dŭk′tŭs ahr-tē-rē-ō′sŭs) A fetal vessel connecting the left pulmonary artery with the descending aorta; in the first 2 months after birth, it normally changes into a fibrous cord, the ligamentum arteriosum; occasional postnatal failure to close causes a surgically correctable cardiovascular handicap. SYN arterial canal, arterial duct, Botallo duct.

duc•tus def•er•ens (dŭk′tŭs def′ĕr-enz) [TA]

The secretory duct of the testicle, running from the epididymis, of which it is the continuation, to the prostatic urethra where it terminates as the ejaculatory duct. SYN arteriola glomerularis efferens [TA], deferent duct, spermatic duct, spermiduct (1), vas deferens.

duc•tus di•ver•ti•cu•lum (dŭk′tŭs dī′vĕr-tik′yū-lŭm) SYN ductal aneurysm.

duc•tus pan•cre•at•i•cus ac•ces•so•ri•us (dŭk′tŭs pan-krē-at′i-kŭs ak-ses-ōr′ē-ŭs) [TA] SYN accessory pancreatic duct.

duc•tus ve•no•sus (dŭk′tŭs vē-nō′sŭs) In the fetus, continuation of the left umbilical vein through the liver to the inferior vena cava; after birth, its lumen is obliterated, forming the ligamentum venosum.

duct of Va•ter (dŭkt fah′tĕr) SYN His canal.

due dil•i•gence (dū dil′i-jĕns) In health care, making certain that rules and procedures are followed to avoid harming patients and staff.

Du•gas test (dū-gah′ test) In the case of an injured shoulder, if the elbow cannot be made to touch the chest while the hand rests on the opposite shoulder, the injury is a dislocation and not a fracture of the humerus.

Du•hot line (dū-ō′ līn) Hypothetic demarcation running from the sacral apex to the superior iliac spine.

Duh•ring dis•ease (dū′ring di-zēz′) SYN dermatitis herpetiformis.

Dührs•sen in•ci•sions (dēr′sen in-sizh′ŭnz) Three surgical incisions of an incompletely dilated cervix, corresponding roughly to positions at 2-, 6-, and 10-o'clock, used as a means of effecting immediate delivery of the fetus when there is an entrapped head during a breech delivery.

Duke ac•tiv•i•ty stat•us in•dex (dūk ak-tiv′i-tē stat′ŭs in′deks) A questionnaire used to estimate the subject's activity status and functional capacity in the absence of a stress test. [Duke Univeristy, U.S.]

Dukes clas•si•fi•ca•tion (dūks klas′i-fi-kā′shŭn) A classification of the extent of invasion of a resected adenocarcinoma of the colon or rectum commonly modified as follows: A (Dukes A), confined to the mucosa; B_1, into the muscularis mucosae; B_2, through the muscularis mucosae; C_1, limited to the bowel wall, with nodal metastases; C_2, through the bowel wall, with nodal metastases.

Dukes dis•ease (dūks di-zēz′) SYN exanthema subitum.

Duke test (dūk test) Procedure to measure bleeding time.

dull (dŭl) Not sharp or acute, in any sense; qualifying a surgical instrument, the action of the mind, pain, a sound (especially the percussion note), or other qualities. [M.E. *dul*]

Du•mont•pal•lier pes•sa•ry (dū-mōn[h]-pal-yā′ pes′ăr-ē) An elastic ring pessary. SYN Mayer pessary.

dump•ing syn•drome (dŭmp′ing sin′drōm) A syndrome that occurs after eating, most often seen in patients with shunts of the upper alimentary canal; characterized by flushing, sweating, dizziness, weakness, and vasomotor collapse, occasionally with pain and headache; results from rapid passage of large amounts of food into the small intestine, with an osmotic effect removing fluid from plasma and causing hypovolemia. SYN early dumping syndrome, postgastrectomy syndrome.

Dun•can dis•ease (dŭng′kăn di-zēz′) SYN X-linked lymphoproliferative syndrome.

Dun•can mech•a•nism (dŭng′kăn mek′ă-nizm) Passage of the placenta from the uterus with the rough side foremost.

Dun•can pla•cen•ta (dŭng′kăn plă-sen′tă) A separated placenta that appears at the vulva with the chorionic surface outward.

du•o•de•nal (dū′ō-dē′năl, dū-od′ĕ-năl) Relating to the duodenum.

du•o•de•nal am•pul•la (dū′ō-dē′năl am-pul′lă) The dilated portion of the superior part of the duodenum; SEE ALSO duodenal cap.

du•o•de•nal cap (dū′ō-dē′năl kap) The first portion of the duodenum, as seen in a roentgenogram or by fluoroscopy.

du•o•de•nal glands (dū′ō-dē′năl glandz) Small, branched, coiled tubular glands that occur mostly in the submucosa of the first third of the duodenum; they secrete an alkaline mucoid substance that serves to neutralize gastric juice. SYN Brunner glands.

du•o•de•nec•to•my (dū′ō-dĕ-nek′tŏ-mē) Excision of the duodenum. [duodenum + G. *ektomē,* excision]

du•o•de•ni•tis (dū-od′ĕ-nī′tis) Inflammation of the duodenum.

♻ **duodeno-** Combining form relating to the duodenum. [L. *duodenum (digitorum),* breadth of 12 fingers]

du•o•de•no•cho•lan•gi•tis (dū′ō-dē′nō-kō-lan-jī′tis) Inflammation of the duodenum and common bile duct. [duodeno- + G. *cholē,* bile, + *angeion,* vessel, + *-itis,* inflammation]

du•o•de•no•cho•le•cys•tos•to•my (dū′ō-dē′nō-kō′lē-sis-tos′tŏ-mē) SYN cholecystoduodenostomy. [duodeno- + G. *cholē,* bile, + *kystis,* bladder, + *stoma,* mouth]

du•o•de•no•cho•led•o•chot•o•my (dū′ō-dē′nō-kō′led-ō-kot′ŏ-mē) Incision into the common bile duct and the adjacent portion of the duodenum. [duodeno- + G. *choledochus,* bile duct, + *tomē,* incision]

du•o•de•no•cys•tos•to•my (dū'ō-dē'nō-sis-tos'tŏ-mē) **1.** SYN cholecystoduodenostomy. **2.** SYN cystoduodenostomy. **3.** SYN pancreatic cystoduodenostomy.

du•o•de•no•en•ter•os•to•my (dū'ō-dē'nō-en-tĕr-os'tŏ-mē) Establishment of communication between the duodenum and another part of the intestinal tract. [duodeno- + G. *enteron,* intestine, + *stoma,* mouth]

du•o•de•no•je•ju•nal flex•ure (dū'ō-dē'nō-jĕ-jū'năl flek'shŭr) An abrupt bend in the small intestine at the junction of the duodenum and jejunum. SYN flexura duodenojejunalis [TA].

du•o•de•no•je•ju•nos•to•my (dū'ō-dē'nō-jĕ-jū-nos'tŏ-mē) Operative formation of an artificial communication between the duodenum and the jejunum. [duodeno- + jejunum, + G. *stoma,* mouth]

du•o•de•nol•y•sis (dū'ō-dĕ-nol'i-sis) Incision of adhesions to the duodenum. [duodeno- + G. *lysis,* a freeing]

du•o•de•nor•rha•phy (dū'ō-dĕ-nōr'ă-fē) Suture of a tear or incision in the duodenum. [duodeno- + G. *rhaphē,* a seam]

du•o•de•nos•co•py (dū'ō-dĕ-nos'kŏ-pē) Inspection of the interior of the duodenum through an endoscope. [duodeno- + G. *skopeō,* to examine]

du•o•de•nos•to•my (dū'ō-dĕ-nos'tŏ-mē) Establishment of a fistula into the duodenum. [duodeno- + G. *stoma,* mouth]

du•o•de•not•o•my (dū'ō-dĕ-not'ŏ-mē) Incision of the duodenum. [duodeno- + G. *tomē,* incision]

du•o•de•num, gen. **du•o•de•ni**, pl. **du•o•de•na** (dū'ō-dē'nŭm, -nī, -nă) [TA] The first division of the small intestine, about 25 cm in length, extending from the pylorus to the junction with the jejunum at the level of the first or second lumbar vertebra on the left side. It is divided into the superior part, the first part of which is the duodenal cap, the descending part, into which the bile and pancreatic ducts open; the horizontal (inferior) part; and the ascending part, terminating at the duodenojejunal junction. [Mediev. L. fr. L. *duodeni,* twelve]

du•plex kid•ney (dū'pleks kid'nē) A kidney in which two pelviocalyceal systems are present.

du•plex ul•tra•so•nog•ra•phy (dū'pleks ŭl'tră-sŏ-nog'ră-fē) The combination of real-time and Doppler ultrasonography.

du•plex u•ter•us (dū'pleks yū'tĕr-ŭs) Any uterus with two lumina (uterus didelphys, uterus bicornis bicollis, or septate uterus).

du•pli•ca•tion (dū'pli-kā'shŭn) **1.** A doubling. SEE ALSO reduplication. **2.** GENETICS Inclusion of two copies of the same genetic material in a genome; an important step in diversification of genomes, as in the evolution of the (nonallelic) hemoglobin chains from a common ancestor. [L. *duplicatio*, a doubling, fr. *duplico*, to double]

du•pli•ca•tion of chro•mo•somes (dū'pli-kā'shŭn krō'mŏ-sōmz) A chromosome aberration resulting from unequal crossing over or exchange of segments between two homologous chromosomes; one chromosome of the pair loses a small segment, while the other gains this segment; the chromosome gaining the segment has undergone duplication whereas its homologue has undergone deletion.

Du•puy-Du•temps op•er•a•tion (dū-pwē' dū-tōn[h]' op-ĕr-ā'shŭn) A modified dacryocystorhinostomy for stenosis of the lacrimal duct.

Du•puy•tren am•pu•ta•tion (dū-pwē'trahn[h] amp'yū-tā'shŭn) Surgical removal of the arm at the shoulder joint.

Du•puy•tren ca•nal (dū-pwē'trahn[h] kă-nal') SYN diploic vein.

Du•puy•tren con•trac•ture (dū-pwē'trahn[h] kŏn-trak'shŭr) A disease of the palmar fascia resulting in thickening and shortening of fibrous bands on the palmar surface of the hand and fingers resulting in a characteristic flexion deformity of the fourth and fifth digits.

Du•puy•tren dis•ease of the foot (dū-pwē' trahn[h] di-zēz' fut) SYN plantar fibromatosis.

Du•puy•tren frac•ture (dū-pwē'trahn[h] frak' shŭr) A break at the lower part of the fibula, with dislocation of ankle.

Du•puy•tren hy•dro•cele (dū-pwē'trahn[h] hī'drō-sēl) Bilocular hydrocele in which the sac fills the scrotum and also extends into the abdominal cavity beneath the peritoneum.

Du•puy•tren sign (dū-pwē'trahn[h] sīn) **1.** In congenital dislocation, free up and down movement of the head of the femur occurs on intermittent traction. **2.** A crackling sensation on pressure over the bone in certain cases of sarcoma.

Du•puy•tren su•ture (dū-pwē'trahn[h] sū' chŭr) A continuous Lembert suture.

Du•puy•tren tour•ni•quet (dū-pwē'trahn[h] tŭr'ni-kĕt) An instrument for compression on the abdominal aorta.

du•ra (dū'ră) SYN dura mater. [L. fem. of *durus,* hard]

dur•a•ble med•i•cal e•quip•ment (DME) (dūr'ă-bĕl med'i-kăl ĕ-kwip'mĕnt) Rented or purchased medical equipment ordered by a health care provider for use in the home. These items must be reusable (e.g., hospital beds, wheelchairs, lifts).

dur•a•ble med•i•cal e•quip•ment re•gion•

al car•ri•er (DMERC) (dūr′ă-bĕl med′i-kăl ĕ-kwip′mĕnt rē′jŭn-ăl kar′ē-ĕr) A private company in the U.S. that contracts with Medicare to pay bills for durable medical equipment.

dur•a•ble pow•er of at•tor•ney (dūr′ă-bĕl pow′ĕr ă-tŏr′nē) **1.** SYN advance directive. **2.** SYN living will.

du•ral (dūr′ăl) Relating to the dura mater.

dur•al cav•er•nous si•nus fis•tu•la (dūr′ăl kav′ĕr-nŭs sī′nŭs fis′chū-lă) A vascular shunt between the meningeal branches of the internal or external carotid arteries and the cavernous sinus.

du•ral sheath (dūr′ăl shēth) An extension of the dura mater that ensheathes the roots of spinal nerves or, more particularly, the vagina externa nervi optici.

du•ral ve•nous si•nus•es (dūr′ăl vē′nŭs sī′nŭs-ĕz) Endothelium-lined venous channels in the dura mater. SYN venous sinuses.

du•ra mat•er (dūr′ă mā′tĕr) [TA] Pachymeninx (as distinguished from leptomeninx, the combined pia mater and arachnoid); a tough, fibrous membrane forming the outer covering of the central nervous system. SYN dura. [L. hard mother, mistransl. of Ar. *umm al-jāfīyah,* tough protector or covering]

du•ra•tion (dūr-ā′shŭn) A continuous period of time.

du•ra•tion of ac•tion (dŭr-ā′shŭn ak′shŭn) The amount of time that a measurable drug effect persists.

du•ra•tion tet•a•ny (dūr-ā′shŭn tet′ă-nē) A tonic spasm occurring in degenerated muscles on application of a strong galvanic current.

Dürck nodes (dĕrk nōdz) Perivascular chronic inflammatory infiltrates in the brain, occurring in human trypanosomiasis.

Du•ret hem•or•rhage (dū-rā′ hem′ŏr-ăj) Small brainstem hemorrhage resulting from brainstem distortion secondary to transtentorial herniation.

Du•ret le•sion (dū-rā′ lē′zhŭn) Small hemorrhage(s) in the floor of the fourth ventricle or beneath the aqueduct of Sylvius.

Dur•ham rule (dūr′ăm rūl) A U.S. test of criminal responsibility (1954): "an accused is not criminally responsible if his unlawful act was the product of mental disease or mental defect."

Dur•ham tube (dūr′ăm tūb) A jointed tracheotomy tube.

Du•ro•zi•ez dis•ease (dū-rō′zē-ā′ di-zēz′) Congenital stenosis of the mitral valve.

Du•ro•zi•ez mur•mur (dū-rō′zē-ā′ mŭr′mŭr) A two-phase murmur over peripheral arteries, especially the femoral artery, due to rapid ebb and flow of blood during aortic insufficiency. Murmur is audible when pressure is applied to the area just distal to the stethoscope.

DUSN Abbreviation for diffuse unilateral subacute neuroretinitis.

dust cell (dŭst sel) SYN alveolar macrophage.

Dut•ton dis•ease (dŭt′ŏn di-zēz′) African tick-borne relapsing fever caused by *Borrelia duttonii* and spread by a soft tick, *Ornithodoros moubata.*

du•ty cy•cle (t_i:t_{tot}) (dū′tē sī′kĕl) The ratio of inspiratory (t_i) time to total-breathing-cycle time (t_{tot}).

Du•ven•hage vi•rus (dū-ven-ahj′ vī′rŭs) A species of Lyssavirus causing a rabieslike disease in humans in Africa; transmitted by the bite of insectivorous bats. [named after its first victim, a man infected near Pretoria, South Africa.]

Du•ver•ney frac•ture (dū-ver-nā frak′shŭr) Break in the ilium below the anterior superior spine.

DV Abbreviation for daily value.

DVT Abbreviation for deep venous thrombosis.

dwarf (dwōrf) An abnormally undersized person with disproportion among the bodily parts. SEE dwarfism. [A.S. *dweorh*]

dwarf•ism (dwōrf′izm) A condition in which the standing height of the subject is below the third percentile. See page B30.

Dwy•er os•te•ot•o•my (dwī′er os′tē-ot′ŏ-mē) A surgical procedure to correct clubfoot.

DXA Abbreviation for dual x-ray absorptiometry.

Dy Abbreviation for dysprosium.

dy•ad (dī′ad) **1.** A pair. SYN diad (2). **2.** CHEMISTRY a bivalent element. **3.** Two people in an interactional situation, e.g., patient and therapist, husband and wife. **4.** The double chromosome resulting from the splitting of a tetrad during meiosis. [G. *dyas,* the number two, duality]

dye (dī) A stain or coloring matter; a compound consisting of chromophore and auxochrome groups attached to one or more benzene rings, its color being due to the chromophore and its dyeing affinities to the auxochrome. Dyes are used for intravital coloration of living cells, staining tissues and microorganisms, as antiseptics and germicides, and some as stimulants of epithelial growth. Commonly used for radiographic contrast medium. [A.S. *deah, deag*]

dye dis•ap•pear•ance test (dī dis-ă-pēr′ăns test) SYN fluorescein instillation test.

-dymus **1.** Suffix that is used with number roots; e.g., didymus, tridymus, tetradymus. **2.** Suffix occasionally used for -didymus. [G. *-dymos,* fold]

dy•nam•ic as•sess•ment (dī-nam′ik ă-ses′mĕnt) **1.** A process used in intervention that tests a hypothesis generated within the evaluation process facilitating evaluation of intervention efficacy. **2.** Assessing the interaction among the person, the environment, and the activity to understand more about the person's approach to a given activity; allows for adjustments in the intervention plan.

dy•nam•ic bal•ance (dī-nam′ik bal′ăns) The ability to anticipate and react to changes in balance as the body moves through space.

dy•nam•ic com•pli•ance (dī-nam′ik kŏm-plī′ăns) Compliance measured during cyclic variations in the volume of a distensible vessel; the ratio of the change in volume to the change in distending pressure when the pressure change is measured between points in time at which the rate of volume change is zero.

dy•nam•ic con•stant ex•ter•nal re•sis•tance train•ing (dī-nam′ik kon′stănt eks-tĕr′năl rĕ-zis′tăns trān′ing) Resistance training in which external resistance does not change; joint flexion and extension occur with each repetition. Formerly (but incorrectly) referred to as isotonic exercise.

dy•nam•ic e•qui•lib•ri•um (dī-nam′ik ē′kwi-lib′rē-ŭm) SYN equilibrium (2).

dy•nam•ic gait in•dex (DGI) (dī-nam′ik gāt in′deks) Assessment tool to measure a patient's ability to change gait with varying demands.

dy•nam•ic hy•per•in•fla•tion (dī-nam′ik hī′pĕr-in-flā′shŭn) The increase in lung volume that occurs during mechanical ventilation when insufficient exhalation time prevents the respiratory system from returning to its resting end-expiratory equilibrium volume between breath cycles.

dy•nam•ic il•e•us (dī-nam′ik il′ē-ŭs) Intestinal obstruction due to spastic contraction of a segment of the bowel. SYN spastic ileus.

dy•nam•ic pos•tur•og•ra•phy (dī-nam′ik pos′chŭr-og′ră-fē) A measurement of postural stability under varying visual and proprioceptive inputs. SYN posturography.

dy•nam•ic psy•chi•a•try (dī-nam′ik sī-kī′ă-trē) SYN psychoanalytic psychiatry.

dy•nam•ic psy•chol•o•gy (dī-nam′ik sī-kol′ŏ-jē) A psychological approach that concerns itself with the causes of behavior.

dy•nam•ic re•frac•tion (dī-nam′ik rĕ-frak′shŭn) Refraction of the eye during accommodation.

dy•nam•ics (dī-nam′iks) **1.** The science of motion in response to forces. **2.** PSYCHIATRY the determination of how emotional and mental disorders develop. **3.** BEHAVIORAL SCIENCES any of the numerous intrapersonal and interpersonal influences or phenomena associated with personality development and interpersonal processes. **4.** Factors that may contribute to a condition or situation. [G. *dynamis,* force]

dy•nam•ic splint (dī-nam′ik splint) A splint using springs or elastic bands that aids in movements initiated by the patient by controlling the plane and range of motion. SYN active splint, functional splint (1).

♻**dynamo-** Combining form meaning force, energy. [G. *dynamis,* power]

dy•na•mo•gen•e•sis (dī′nă-mō-jen′ĕ-sis) The production of force, especially of muscular or nervous energy. [dynamo- + G. *genesis,* production]

dy•na•mo•gen•ic (dī′nă-mō-jen′ik) Producing power or force, especially nervous or muscular power or activity.

dy•nam•o•graph (dī-nam′ŏ-graf) An instrument for recording the degree of muscular power. [dynamo- + G. *graphō,* to write]

dy•na•mom•e•ter (dī′nă-mom′ĕ-tĕr) An instrument for measuring the degree of muscular power. SYN ergometer (1). [dynamo- + G. *metron,* measure]

dyne (dīn) The unit of force in the CGS system, replaced in the SI by the newton (1 newton = 10^5 dynes), which gives a body of 1 g mass an acceleration of 1 cm/sec^2; expressed as F (dynes) = m (grams) × a (cm/sec^2). [G. *dynamis,* force]

dyn•ein (dīn′ēn) A protein associated with motile structures, exhibiting adenosine triphosphatase activity; it forms "arms" on the outer tubules of cilia and flagella. SEE ALSO tubulin. [dyne + protein]

♻**-dynia** Suffix denoting pain.

♻**dys-** Prefix meaning bad, difficult, un-, mis-; opposite of eu-. Cf. dis-. [G.]

dys•a•cu•sis, dys•a•cu•si•a, dys•a•cou•si•a (dis-ă-kyū′sis, -zē-ă, -zē-ă) **1.** Any impairment of hearing involving difficulty in processing details of sound as opposed to any loss of sensitivity to sound. **2.** Pain or discomfort in the ear from exposure to sound. [dys- + G. *akousis,* hearing]

dysaesthesia [Br.] SYN dysesthesia.

dys•a•phi•a (dis-ā′fē-ă) Impairment of the sense of touch. [dys- + G. *haphē,* touch]

dys•ar•te•ri•ot•o•ny (dis′ahr-tēr′ē-ot′ŏ-nē) Abnormal blood pressure, either too high or too low. [dys- + G. *artēria,* artery, + *tonos,* tension]

dys•ar•thri•a (dis-ahr′thrē-ă) A disturbance of speech due to paralysis, incoordination, or spasticity of the muscles used for speaking. SYN dysarthrosis (1). [dys- + G. *arthroō,* to articulate]

dys·ar·thri·a–clum·sy hand syn·drome (dis-ar′thrē-ă-klŭm′zē hand sin′drōm) A disorder characterized by dysarthria and a clumsiness of one hand, caused by a lacunar stroke in the basis pontis.

dys·ar·thric (dis-ahr′thrik) Relating to dysarthria.

dys·ar·thro·sis (dis′ahr-thrō′sis) **1.** SYN dysarthria. **2.** Malformation of a joint. **3.** A false joint. [dys- + G. *arthrōsis,* joint]

dys·au·to·no·mi·a (dis′aw-tō-nō′mē-ă) Abnormal functioning of the autonomic nervous system. [dys- + G. *autonomia,* self-government]

dys·ba·rism (dis′băr-izm) General term for the symptom complex resulting from exposure to decreased or changing barometric pressure, including all physiologic effects resulting from such changes with the exception of hypoxia, and including the effects of rapid decompression. [dys- + G. *baros,* weight]

dys·ba·si·a (dis-bā′zē-ă) **1.** Difficulty in walking. **2.** The difficult or distorted walking that occurs in people with certain mental disorders. [dys- + G. *basis,* a step]

dys·bu·li·a (dis-bū′lē-ă) Weakness and uncertainty of will. [dys- + G. *boulē,* will]

dys·bu·lic (dis-bū′lik) Relating to, or characterized by, dysbulia.

dys·cal·cu·li·a (dis′kal-kyū′lē-ă) Difficulty in performing simple mathematical problems; commonly seen in parietal lobe lesions. [dys- + L. *calculo*, to compute, fr. *calculus*, pebble, counter]

dys·ce·pha·li·a (dis′sĕ-fā′lē-ă) Malformation of the head and face. [dys- + G. *kephalē,* head]

dys·chei·ral, **dys·chi·ral** (dis-kī′răl, dis-kī′răl) Relating to dyscheiria.

dys·cheir·i·a, **dis·chi·ri·a, dys·chir·i·a** (dis-kī′rē-ă) A disorder of sensory processing in which the patient is unable to tell which side of the body has been touched (acheiria) or refers the stimulus to the wrong side (allocheiria) or to both sides (syncheiria). [dys- + G. *cheir*, hand, + -ia]

dys·che·zi·a (dis-kē′zē-ă) Difficulty in defecation. [dys- + G. *chezō,* to defecate]

dys·chon·dro·gen·e·sis (dis′kon-drō-jen′ĕ-sis) Abnormal development of cartilage. [dys- + G. *chondros,* cartilage, + *genesis,* production]

dys·chon·dro·pla·si·a (dis′kon-drō-plā′zē-ă) SYN enchondromatosis. [dys- + G. *chondros,* cartilage, + *plasis,* a forming]

dys·chro·ma·top·si·a (dis′krō-mă-top′sē-ă) A condition in which the ability to perceive colors is not fully normal. Cf. dichromatism, monochromatism, chromatopsia. [dys- + G. *chrōma,* color, + *opsis,* vision]

dys·chro·mi·a (dis-krō′mē-ă) Any abnormality in the color of the skin.

dys·co·ri·a (dis-kōr′ē-ă) Abnormality in the shape of the pupil. [dys- + G. *korē,* pupil of eye]

dys·cra·si·a (dis-krā′zē-ă) **1.** A morbid general state resulting from the presence of abnormal material in the blood, usually applied to diseases affecting blood cells or platelets. **2.** Old term indicating disease. [G. bad temperament, fr. dys- + *krasis,* a mixing]

dys·cra·sic, **dys·crat·ic** (dis-krā′sik, -krat′ik) Pertaining to or affected with dyscrasia.

dys·en·ter·ic (dis′en-ter′ik) Relating to or suffering from dysentery.

dys·en·ter·y (dis′ĕn-ter′ē) A disease marked by frequent watery stools, often with blood and mucus, and characterized clinically by pain, tenesmus, fever, and dehydration. [G. *dysenteria,* fr. *dys-*, bad, + *entera,* bowels]

dys·er·e·thism (dis-er′ĕ-thizm) A condition of slow response to stimuli. [dys- + G. *erethismos,* irritation]

dys·er·gi·a (dis-ĕr′jē-ă) Lack of harmonious action between the muscles concerned in executing any definite voluntary movement. [dys- + G. *ergon,* work]

dys·es·the·si·a (dis′es-thē′zē-ă) **1.** Impairment of sensation short of anesthesia. **2.** A condition in which a disagreeable sensation is produced by ordinary stimuli; caused by lesions of the sensory pathways, peripheral or central. **3.** Abnormal sensations experienced in the absence of stimulation. SYN dysaesthesia. [G. *dysaisthēsia,* fr. *dys-*, hard, difficult, + *aisthēsis,* sensation]

dysfibrinogenaemia [Br.] SYN dysfibrinogenemia.

dys·fi·brin·o·ge·ne·mi·a (dis′fī-brin′ō-jĕ-nē′mē-ă) An autosomal dominant disorder of qualitatively abnormal fibrinogens of various types, resulting in abnormalities of coagulation tests (bleeding time, clotting time, thrombin time); symptoms vary from none to abnormal bleeding and excessive clotting. SYN dysfibrinogenaemia.

dys·flu·en·cy (dis-flū′ĕn-sē) Speech interrupted in its forward flow by hesitations, repetitions, or prolongations of sounds; common manifestation of a stuttering disorder, and are also present in normal speech, particularly during speech development in young children. SEE stuttering. SYN nonfluency.

dys·func·tion (dis-fŭngk′shŭn) Difficult or abnormal function.

dys·func·tion·al la·bor (dis-fungk′shŭn-ăl lā′bŏr) Presentation in which impedance or delay causes difficulty.

dysgammaglobulinaemia [Br.] SYN dysgammaglobulinemia.

dys·gam·ma·glob·u·lin·e·mi·a (dis-gam′ă-glob′yū-li-nē′mē-ă) An immunoglobulin abnormality, especially a disturbance of the percentage distribution of γ-globulins. SYN dysgammaglobulinaemia.

dys·gen·e·sis (dis-jen′ĕ-sis) Defective development. [dys- + G. *genesis,* generation]

dys·gen·ic (dis-jen′ik) Applying to factors that have a detrimental effect on hereditary qualities, physical or mental.

dys·ger·mi·no·ma (dis′jĕr-mi-nō′mă) A rare malignant neoplasm of the ovary composed of undifferentiated gonadal germinal cells and occurring more frequently in patients younger than 20 years of age. The neoplasms contain foci of necrosis and hemorrhage and tend to be encapsulated; characteristically, they spread by way of lymphatic vessels, but widespread metastases also occur. [dys- + L. *germen,* a bud or sprout, + G. *-ōma,* tumor]

dys·geu·si·a (dis-gū′sē-ă) Impairment or perversion of the gustatory sense. [dys- + G. *geusis,* taste]

dys·gna·thi·a (dis-gnā′thē-ă) Any abnormality that extends beyond the teeth and includes the maxilla or mandible, or both. [dys- + G. *gnathos,* jaw]

dys·gnath·ic (dis-gnā′thik) Pertaining to or characterized by abnormality of the maxilla and mandible.

dys·gno·si·a (dis-gnō′zē-ă) Any cognitive disorder (i.e., any mental illness). [G. *dysgnōsia,* difficulty of knowing]

dyshaematopoiesis [Br.] SYN dyshematopoiesis.

dyshaematopoietic [Br.] SYN dyshematopoietic.

dyshaemopoiesis [Br.] SYN dyshemopoiesis.

dyshaemopoietic [Br.] SYN dyshemopoietic.

dys·har·mo·ni·ous re·tin·al cor·re·spon·dence (dis′hahr-mō′nē-ŭs ret′i-năl kōr′ĕ-spon′dĕns) A type of anomalous retinal correspondence in which the angle of the visual direction of the two retinas is different from the objective angle of the strabismus.

dys·hem·a·to·poi·e·sis, **dys·he·mo·poi·e·sis** (dis-hē′mă-tō-poy-ē′sis, -mō-poy-ē′sis) Defective formation of the blood. SYN dyshaematopoiesis. [dys- + G. *haima* (*haimat-*), blood, + *poiēsis,* making]

dys·hem·a·to·poi·et·ic, **dys·he·mo·poi·et·ic** (dis-hē′mă-tō-poy-et′ik, -mō-poy-et′ik) Pertaining to or characterized by dyshematopoiesis. SYN dyshaematopoietic.

dys·hi·dro·sis, **dys·hi·drot·ic ec·ze·ma** (dis′hi-drō′sis, dis′hi-drot′ik ek′zĕ-mă) A vesicular or vesicopustular eruption of multiple causes that occurs primarily on the volar surfaces of the hands and feet; the lesions spread peripherally but have a tendency to central clearing. SYN cheiropompholyx, chiropompholyx. [dys- + G. *hidrōs,* sweat]

dys·kar·y·o·sis (dis-kar′ē-ō′sis) Abnormal maturation seen in exfoliated cells that have normal cytoplasm but hyperchromatic nuclei, or irregular chromatin distribution; may be followed by the development of a malignant neoplasm. [dys- + G. *karyon,* nucleus, + *-ōsis,* condition]

dys·kar·y·ot·ic (dis′kar-ē-ot′ik) Pertaining to or characterized by dyskaryosis.

dys·ker·a·to·ma (dis-ker′ă-tō′mă) A skin tumor exhibiting dyskeratosis. [dys- + G. *keras,* horn, + *-oma,* tumor]

dys·ker·a·to·sis (dis-ker′ă-tō′sis) **1.** Premature keratinization in individual epithelial cells that have not reached the keratinizing surface layer; dyskeratotic cells generally become rounded, and they may break away from adjacent cells and fall off. **2.** Epidermalization of the conjunctival and corneal epithelium. **3.** A disorder of keratinization. [dys- + G. *keras,* horn, + *-osis,* condition]

dys·ker·a·tot·ic (dis-kar′ă-tot′ik) Relating to or characterized by dyskeratosis.

dys·ki·ne·si·a, **dys·ki·ne·sis** (dis′ki-nē′sē-ă, -nē′sis) Difficulty in performing voluntary movements. Term usually used in relation to various extrapyramidal disorders. [dys- + G. *kinēsis,* movement]

dys·ki·ne·si·a al·ge·ra (dis′ki-nē′sē-ă al-jē′ră) A hysteric condition in which active movement causes pain.

dys·ki·ne·si·a in·ter·mit·tens (dis′ki-nē′sē-ă in-tĕr-mit′tenz) Intermittent disability of the limbs due to impairment of circulation.

dys·ki·ne·si·a syn·drome (dis′ki-nē′sē-ă sin′drōm) A genetic disorder in which the clearance of mucus is sluggish and bronchiectasis is prevalent and intractable. Evidence suggests the defect lies in dynein, a protein in the cilia. The pattern of inheritance is apparently autosomal recessive.

dys·ki·net·ic (dis′ki-net′ik) Denoting or characteristic of dyskinesia.

dys·lex·i·a (dis-lek′sē-ă) Impaired reading ability with a competence level below that expected on the basis of the person's level of intelligence, and in the presence of normal vision, letter recognition, and normal recognition of the meaning of pictures and objects. [dys- + G. *lexis,* word, phrase]

dys·lex·ic (dis-lek′sik) Relating to, or characterized by, dyslexia.

dys·lip·i·de·mi·a (dis-lip′i-dē′mē-ă) Any biochemical disorder characterized by one or more abnormal levels of blood lipids.

dys•lo•gi•a (dis-lō′jē-ă) Impairment of speech and reasoning as the result of a mental disorder. [dys- + G. *logos,* speaking, reason]

dys•ma•ture (dis′mă-chŭr) **1.** Denoting faulty development or ripening; often connoting structural or functional abnormalities. **2.** OBSTETRICS denoting an infant whose birth weight is inappropriately low for its gestational age. **3.** Immature development of the placenta so that normal function does not occur.

dys•ma•tu•ri•ty (dis′mă-chŭr′i-tē) Syndrome of an infant born with relative absence of subcutaneous fat, wrinkling of the skin, prominent finger and toe nails, and meconium staining of skin and placental membranes; often associated with postmaturity or placental insufficiency.

dys•ma•tu•ri•ty syn•drome (dis′mă-chŭr′i-tē sin′drōm) SYN Ballantyne disease.

dys•me•li•a (dis-mē′lē-ă) Congenital abnormality characterized by missing or foreshortened limbs, sometimes with associated vertebral column abnormalities; caused by metabolic disturbance at the time of primordial limb development. SEE amelia, phocomelia. [dys- + G. *melos,* limb]

dys•men•or•rhe•a (dis-men′ōr-ē′ă) Difficult and painful menstruation. SYN dysmenorrhoea, menorrhalgia. [dys- + G. *mēn,* month, + *rhoia,* a flow]

dysmenorrhoea [Br.] SYN dysmenorrhea.

dys•me•tri•a (dis-mē′trē-ă) An aspect of ataxia, in which the ability to control the distance, power, and speed of an act is impaired; used to describe abnormalities of movement caused by cerebellar disorders. SEE ALSO hypermetria, hypometria. [dys- + G. *metron,* measure]

dys•mor•phism (dis-mōr′fizm) Abnormality of shape. [G. *dysmorphia,* badness of form]

dys•mor•pho•gen•e•sis (dis′mōr-fō-jen′ĕ-sis) The process of abnormal tissue formation. [dys- + G. *morphē,* form, + *genesis,* production]

dys•mor•phol•o•gy (dis′mōr-fol′ō-jē) The study of developmental structural defects. A branch of clinical genetics. [dys- + G. *morphē,* form, + *logos,* study]

dys•mor•pho•pho•bi•a (dis-mōr′fō-fō′bē-ă) SYN body dysmorphic disorder.

dys•my•o•to•ni•a (dis′mī-ō-tō′nē-ă) Abnormal muscular tonicity (either incresed or decreased). SEE dystonia. [dys- + G. *mys,* muscle, + *tonos,* tension, tone]

dys•nys•tax•is (dis′nis-tak′sis) A condition of half sleep. SYN light sleep. [dys- + G. *nystaxis,* drowsiness]

dys•o•don•ti•a•sis (dis′ō-don-tī′ă-sis) **1.** Difficulty or irregularity in the eruption of the teeth. **2.** An imperfect dentition. [dys- + G. *odous,* tooth, + *-iasis,* condition]

dys•on•to•gen•e•sis (dis′on-tō-jen′ĕ-sis) Defective embryonic development. [dys- + G. *ōn,* being, + *genesis,* origin]

dys•on•to•ge•net•ic (dis′on-tō-jĕ-net′ik) Characterized by dysontogenesis.

dys•o•rex•i•a (dis′ōr-ek′sē-ă) Diminished or perverted appetite, associated with emotional or psychological disorders. [dys-+ G. *orexis,* appetite]

dys•os•mi•a (dis-oz′mē-ă) Altered sense of smell. [dys- + G. *osmē,* smell]

dys•os•te•o•gen•e•sis (dis-os′tē-ō-jen′ĕ-sis) Defective bone formation. SYN dysostosis. [dys- + G. *osteon,* bone, + *genesis,* production]

dys•os•to•sis (dis′os-tō′sis) SYN dysosteogenesis. [dys- + G. *osteon,* bone, + -osis]

dys•pa•reu•ni•a (dis′păr-ū′nē-ă) Pain experienced during sexual intercourse. [dys- + G. *pareunos,* lying beside, fr. *para,* beside, + *eunē,* a bed]

dys•pep•si•a (dis-pep′sē-ă) Impaired gastric function or "upset stomach" due to some stomach disorder; characterized by epigastric pain, burning, nausea, and gaseous eructation. SYN gastric indigestion. [dys- + G. *pepsis,* digestion]

dys•pep•tic (dis-pep′tik) Relating to or having dyspepsia.

dys•pha•gi•a, dys•pha•gy (dis-fā′jē-ă, dis′fă-jē) Difficulty in swallowing. SYN aglutition. [dys- + G. *phagō,* to eat]

dys•pha•si•a (dis-fā′zē-ă) SYN aphasia. [dys- + G. *phasis,* speaking]

dys•pha•sic (dis-fā′zik) SYN aphasiac.

dys•phe•mi•a (dis-fē′mē-ă) Disordered phonation, articulation, or hearing due to emotional or mental deficits. [dys- + G. *phēmē,* speech]

dys•pho•ni•a (dis-fō′nē-ă) Any disorder of phonation affecting voice quality or ability to produce voice. SEE aphonia. [dys- + G. *phōnē,* voice]

dys•pho•ri•a (dis-fōr′ē-ă) A mood of general dissatisfaction, restlessness, depression, and anxiety; a feeling of unpleasantness or discomfort. [dys- + G. *phora,* a bearing]

dys•phra•si•a (dis-frā′zē-ă) SYN aphasia. [dys- + G. *phrasis,* speaking]

dys•pig•men•ta•tion (dis-pig′men-tā′shŭn) Any abnormality in the formation or distribution of pigment, especially in the skin; usually applied to an abnormal reduction in pigmentation (depigmentation).

dys·pla·si·a (dis-plā'zē-ă) Abnormal tissue development. SEE ALSO heteroplasia. [dys- + G. *plasis,* a molding]

dys·pla·si·a ep·i·phys·i·a·lis mul·ti·plex (dis-plā'zē-ă ep'i-fis-ē-ā'lis mŭl'ti-pleks) SYN multiple epiphysial dysplasia.

dys·plas·tic (dis-plas'tik) Pertaining to or marked by dysplasia.

dys·plas·tic mel·a·not·ic ne·vi (dis-plas'tik mĕl-ă-not'ik nē'vī) Cutaneous pigmented lesions with notched, irregular borders; considered premalignant and marker for increased risk of melanoma. Seen in 5% of white patients.

dys·plas·tic ne·vus syn·drome, dys·plas·tic ne·vus (dis-plas'tik nē'vŭs sin'drōm, dis-plas'tik nē'vŭs) Clinically atypical nevi having variable pigmentation and ill-defined borders, with an increased risk for development of cutaneous malignant melanoma; biopsies show melanocytic dysplasia.

dysp·ne·a (disp-nē'ă) Shortness of breath, a subjective difficulty or distress in breathing, usually associated with disease of the heart or lungs; occurs normally during intense physical exertion or at high altitude. [G. *dyspnoia,* fr. *dys-,* bad, + *pnoē,* breathing]

dysp·ne·a scale (disp-nē'ă skāl) Subjective four-step scale used to describe shortness of breath (+1 mild to +4 severe).

dysp·ne·ic (disp-nē'ik) Out of breath; relating to or suffering from dyspnea.

dys·prax·i·a (dis-prak'sē-ă) Difficulty in performing motor tasks. [dys- + G. *praxis,* a doing]

dys·prax·i·a of speech (dis-prak'sē-ă spēch) SYN apraxia of speech.

dys·pro·si·um (Dy) (dis-prō'sē-ŭm) A metallic element of the lanthanide (rare earth) series, atomic no. 66, atomic wt. 162.50. [G. *dysprositos,* hard to get at]

dys·pros·od·y, dys·pro·sod·i·a (dis-pros'ō-dē, dis'prō-sō'dē-ă) Impairment in ability to apply normal speech intonation patterns. SEE ALSO aprosody.

dysproteinaemia [Br.] SYN dysproteinemia.

dysproteinaemic [Br.] SYN dysproteinemic.

dys·pro·tein·e·mi·a (dis-prō'tēn-ē'mē-ă) An abnormality in plasma proteins, usually in immunoglobulins. SYN dysproteinaemia.

dys·pro·tein·e·mic (dis-prō'tēn-ē'mik) Relating to dysproteinemia. SYN dysproteinaemic.

dys·ra·phism, dys·raph·i·a (dis'ră-fizm, -raf'ē-ă) Defective fusion, especially of the neural folds, resulting in status dysraphicus or neural tube defect. [dys- + G. *rhaphē,* suture]

dys·re·flex·i·a (dis'rē-flek'sē-ă) A condition of disordered or inappropriate responses to stimuli. [dys- + reflex + -ia]

dys·rhyth·mi·a (dis-ridh'mē-ă) Defective rhythm. See also entries under rhythm. Cf. arrhythmia. [dys- + G. *rhythmos,* rhythm]

dys·rhyth·mo·gen·ic (dis-ridh'mō-jen'ik) SYN arrhythmogenic.

dys·se·ba·ci·a, dys·se·ba·ce·a (dis'sē-bā'shē-ă, dis'sē-bā'shē-ă) SYN seborrheic dermatitis. [dys- + L. *sebum,* grease]

dys·som·ni·a (dis-som'nē-ă) Disturbance of normal sleep or rhythm pattern.

dys·sta·si·a (dis-stā'sē-ă) Difficulty in standing. [dys- + G. *stasis,* standing]

dys·stat·ic (dis-tat'ik) Marked by difficulty in standing.

dys·syn·er·gi·a (dis'sin-ĕr'jē-ă) An aspect of ataxia, in which an act is not performed smoothly or accurately because of lack of harmonious association of its various components; usually used to describe abnormalities of movement caused by cerebellar disorders. [dys- + G. *syn,* with, + *ergon,* work]

dys·syn·er·gi·a cer·e·bel·lar·is my·o·clo·ni·ca (dis'sin-ĕr'jē-ă ser'ĕ-bel-ā'ris mī-ō'klō'ni-kă) A familial disorder beginning in late childhood, characterized by progressive cerebellar ataxia, action myoclonus, and preserved intellect. Probably due to multiple causes, among them, mitochondrial abnormalities.

dys·thy·mi·a (dis-thī'mē-ă) A chronic mood disorder manifested as depression for most of the day, more days than not, accompanied by some of the following symptoms: poor appetite or overeating, insomnia or hypersomnia, low energy or fatigue, low self-esteem, poor concentration, difficulty making decisions, and feelings of hopelessness. SEE endogenous depression, exogenous depression. [dys- + G. *thymos,* mind, emotion]

dys·thy·mic (dis-thī'mik) Relating to dysthymia.

dys·thy·mic dis·or·der (dis-thī'mik dis-ōr'dĕr) A chronic disturbance of mood characterized by mild depression or loss of interest in usual activities. SEE depression.

dys·thy·roid or·bit·o·pa·thy (dis-thī'royd ōr-bi-top'ă-thē) Immune-mediated inflammation of the orbit associated with thyroid disease. SYN Graves orbitopathy, thyroid ophthalmopathy.

dys·to·ci·a (dis-tō'sē-ă) Difficult childbirth. [G. *dystokia,* fr. *dys-,* difficult, + *tokos,* childbirth]

dys·to·ni·a (dis-tō'nē-ă) A state of abnormal (either hypo- or hyper-) tonicity in any tissue, particularly skeletal muscle. SYN torsion spasm. [dys- + G. *tonos,* tension]

dys·to·ni·a mus·cu·lo·rum de·for·mans (dis-tō′nē-ă mŭs-kyū-lō′rŭm de-form′anz) A genetic, environmental, or idiopathic disorder, usually beginning in childhood or adolescence, marked by muscular contractions that distort the spine, limbs, hips, and sometimes the cranial-innervated muscles. The abnormal movements are increased by excitement and, at least initially, abolished by sleep. The musculature is hypertonic when in action, hypotonic when at rest.

dys·ton·ic (dis-ton′ik) Pertaining to dystonia.

dys·ton·ic re·ac·tion (dis-ton′ik rē-ak′shŭn) A state of abnormal tension or muscle tone, similar to dystonia, produced as a side effect of certain antipsychotic medication; a severe form, where the eyes appear to roll up into the head, is called oculogyric crisis.

dys·to·pi·a (dis-tō′pē-ă) Faulty or abnormal position of a part or organ. SYN malposition. [dys- + G. *topos,* place]

dys·top·ic (dis-top′ik) Pertaining to, or characterized by, dystopia. SEE ALSO ectopic.

dys·tro·phi·a (dis-trō′fē-ă) SYN dystrophy. [L. fr. G. *dys-*, bad, + *trophē,* nourishment]

dys·tro·phi·a ad·i·po·so·ge·ni·ta·lis (dis-trō′fē-ă ad-i-pō′sō-jen-i-tā′lis) A disorder characterized primarily by obesity and hypogonadotrophic hypogonadism in adolescent boys; dwarfism is rare, and when present is thought to reflect hypothyroidism. Visual loss, behavioral abnormalities, and diabetes insipidus may occur. The most common causes are pituitary and hypothalamic neoplasms. SYN adiposogenital dystrophy, Fröhlich syndrome, hypophysial syndrome.

dys·tro·phi·a e·pi·the·li·al·is cor·ne·ae (dis-trō′fē-ă ep′i-thē-lē-ā′lis kōr′nē-ē) A corneal dystrophy causing stromal edema and epithelial bullae, erosions, and scarring. SYN Fuchs epithelial dystrophy.

i dys·tro·phi·a un·gui·um (dis-trō′fē-ă ŭn′gwin-ŭm) Dystrophy of the nails. See this page.

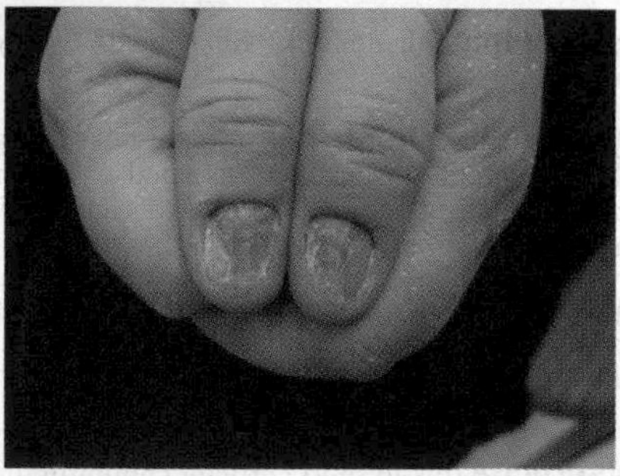

dystrophia unguium

dys·tro·phic (dis-trō′fik) Relating to dystrophy.

dys·tro·phic cal·ci·fi·ca·tion (dis-trō′fik kal′si-fi-kā′shŭn) Calcification occurring in degenerated or necrotic tissue, as in hyalinized scars, degenerated foci in leiomyomas, and caseous nodules.

dys·tro·phin (dis-trō′fin) A protein found in the sarcolemma of normal muscle; it is missing in individuals with pseudohypertrophic muscular dystrophy and in other forms of muscular dystrophy. SYN distropin, dystropin.

dys·tro·phy (dis′trŏ-fē) Abnormal development or growth of a tissue or organ, usually resulting from nutritional deficiency. SYN dystrophia. [dys- + G. *trophē,* nourishment]

dys·tro·pin (dis-trō′pin) SYN dystrophin.

dys·u·ri·a (dis-yūr′ē-ă) Difficulty or pain in urination. [dys- + G. *ouron,* urine]

dys·u·ric (dis-yūr′ik) Relating to or having dysuria.

dys·ver·sion (dis-vĕr′zhŭn) A turning in any direction, less than inversion; particularly dysversion of the optic nerve head (situs inversus of the optic disc). [dys- + L. *verto,* to turn]

D-zone test (zōn test) Assessment tool used to detect inducible clindamycin resistance in staphylococci and beta-hemolytic streptococci.

H, η The Greek letter eta.

ε **1.** The Greek letter epsilon. SEE epsilon. **2.** Molar absorption coefficient.

E 1. Abbreviation for exa-; extraction ratio; glutamic acid; energy; electromotive force; glutamyl; internal energy. **2.** As a subscript, refers to expired gas.

E Abbreviation for entgegen.

e Elementary charge; base of natural logarithms (2.71828...).

Ea·gle ba·sal me·di·um (ē′gĕl bā′săl mē′dē-ŭm) A solution of various salts containing 13 naturally occurring amino acids, several vitamins, two antibiotics, and phenol red; used as a tissue culture medium.

Ea·gle min·i·mum es·sen·tial me·di·um (ē′gĕl min′i-mŭm ĕ-sen′shăl mē′dē-ŭm) A tissue culture medium similar to Eagle basal medium but with different amounts and a few exclusions (e.g., antibiotics and phenol red).

Eales dis·ease (ēlz di-zēz′) Peripheral retinal periphlebitis causing recurrent retinal or intravitreous hemorrhages in young adults.

EAP Abbreviation for employee assistance program.

EAR Abbreviation for estimated average requirement. SEE ALSO Dietary Reference Intake.

ear (ēr) The organ of hearing: composed of the external ear, which includes the auricle and the external acoustic, or auditory, meatus; the middle ear, or the tympanic cavity with its ossicles; and the internal ear or inner ear, or labyrinth, which includes the semicircular canals, vestibule, and cochlea. SEE ALSO auricle. See this page, B28. SYN auris [TA]. [A.S. *eare*]

ear·ache (ēr′āk) Pain in the ear. SYN otalgia, otodynia.

ear bones (ēr bōnz) SYN auditory ossicles.

ear·drum (ēr′drŭm) SYN tympanic membrane.

Earle so·lu·tion (ĕrl sŏ-lū′shŭn) A tissue culture medium containing $CaCl_2$, $MgSO_4$, KCl, $NaHCO_3$, NaCl, $NaH_2PO_4{\cdot}H_2O$, and glucose.

ear lobe crease (ēr lōb krēs) A diagonal crease found on one or both earlobes with a possible connection to coronary heart disease in males.

ear·ly dis·charge (ĕr′lē dis′chahrj) Exit of a woman and her newborn from the hospital within 24 hours of a vaginal delivery.

ear·ly dump·ing syn·drome (ĕr′lē dump′ing sin′drōm) SYN dumping syndrome.

ear·ly in·ter·ven·tion (ĕr′lē in′tĕr-ven′shŭn) A multidisciplinary, coordinated, natural environment–based system (i.e., least restrictive environment) of service provision to eligible children birth to 3 or 5 years of age and their families (depending on governmental jurisdiction); provided under the U.S. Individuals with Disabilities Education Act, Part C. Services are designed to address identified developmental delays and at risk situations of the child and/or the family. SYN E.I. program.

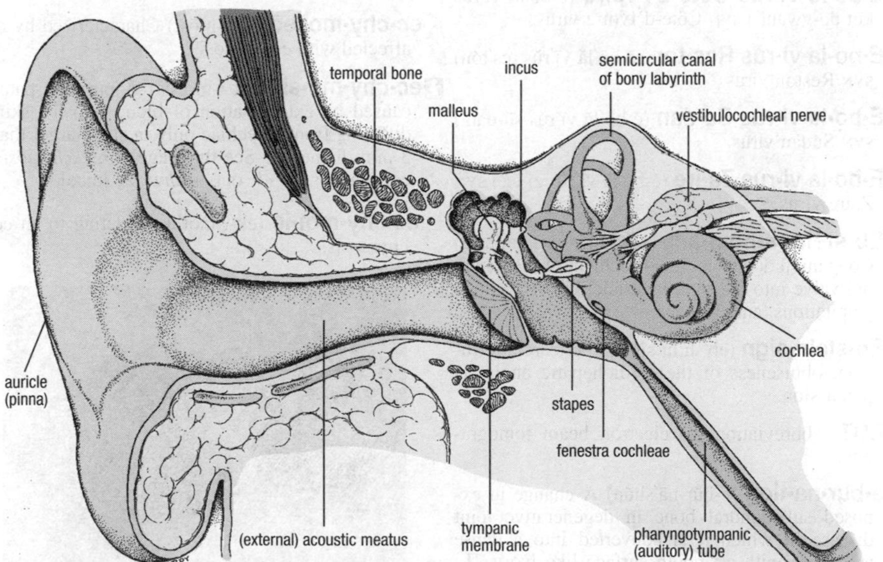

temporal (coronal) section of ear

ear•mold (ēr′mōld) Any of various types of fittings, usually made of plastic, designed to fit in the auricle of the ear and conduct amplified sound from a hearing aid to the ear canal.

ear•piece (ēr′pēs) A part of a device inserted into the external auditory canal to deliver sound to the ear.

ear•plug (ēr′plŭg) Generic term for occlusive devices for the external auditory canal for protection against noise-induced hearing loss or to prevent water from getting into the ear. SEE ALSO hearing protector.

earth (ĕrth) **1.** Soil; the soft material of the land, as opposed to rock and sand. **2.** An easily pulverized mineral. **3.** An insoluble oxide of aluminum or of certain other elements characterized by a high melting point. [A.S. *eorthe*]

eat•ing dis•or•ders (ēt′ing dis-ōr′dĕrz) A class of mental disorders including anorexia nervosa, bulimia nervosa, and pica.

eat•ing ep•i•lep•sy (ēt′ing ep′i-lep′sē) Epileptic seizures provoked by eating; a type of reflex epilepsy.

Ea•ton a•gent (ē′tŏn ā′jĕnt) SYN *Mycoplasma pneumoniae.*

E•berth lines (ā′bĕrt līnz) Lines appearing between the cells of the myocardium when stained with silver nitrate.

E•bo•la vi•rus (ē-bō′lă vī′rŭs) A virus morphologically similar to but antigenically distinct from Marburg virus, in the family Filoviridae, which causes viral hemorrhagic fever.

E•bo•la vi•rus Côte-d'I•voire (ē-bō′lă vī′rŭs kōt dē-vwahr′) SYN Côte-d'Ivoire virus.

E•bo•la vi•rus Res•ton (ē-bō′lă vī′rŭs res′tŏn) SYN Reston virus.

E•bo•la vi•rus Su•dan (ē-bō′lă vī′rŭs sū-dan′) SYN Sudan virus.

E•bo•la vi•rus Za•ire (ē-bō′lă vī′rŭs zī-ēr′) SYN Zaire virus.

Eb•stein a•nom•a•ly (eb′shtīn ă-nom′ă-lē) Congenital downward displacement of the tricuspid valve into the right ventricle; causes fatigue, palpitations, and dyspnea.

Eb•stein sign (eb′shtīn sīn) In pericardial effusion, obtuseness of the cardiohepatic angle on percussion.

EBT Abbreviation for electron beam tomography.

e•bur•na•tion (ē-bŭr-nā′shŭn) A change in exposed subchondral bone in degenerative joint disease in which it is converted into a dense substance with a smooth surface like ivory. [L. *eburneus,* of ivory]

e•bur•ni•tis (ē-bŭr-nī′tis) Increased density and hardness of the dentin, which may occur after the dentin is exposed. [L. *eburneus,* of ivory, + G. -itis, inflammation]

EBV Abbreviation for Epstein-Barr virus.

EC Abbreviation for enteric coated.

ec- Prefix meaning out of, away from. [G.]

ec•cen•tric (ek-sen′trik) **1.** Abnormal or peculiar in ideas or behavior. **2.** Situated away from a center or proceeding from a center. Cf. centrifugal (2). **3.** SYN peripheral. [G. *ek,* out, + *kentron,* center]

ec•cen•tric con•trac•tion (ek-sen′trik kŏn-trak′shŭn) A lengthening action in which a muscle's attachments are drawn away from one another by an external resistance, even though the muscle is activated. Often called negative work.

ec•cen•tric hy•per•tro•phy (ek-sen′trik hī-pĕr′trō-fē) Thickening of the wall of the heart or other cavity, with dilation.

ec•cen•tric oc•clu•sion (ek-sen′trik ŏ-klū′zhŭn) Any occlusion other than centric that results in premature contact of the teeth.

ec•chon•dro•ma, ec•chon•dro•sis (ek-kon-drō′mă, ek-kon-drō′sis) **1.** A neoplasm arising from cartilage as a mass protruding from the articular surface of a bone. **2.** An enchondroma that has burst through the shaft of a bone and become pedunculated. [G. *ek,* from, + *chondros,* cartilage, + *-oma,* tumor]

ec•chy•mo•ma (ek-i-mō′mă) A slight hematoma following a bruise. [G. *ek,* out, + *chymos,* juice, + *-oma,* tumor]

ec•chy•mosed (ek′i-mōst) Characterized by or affected with ecchymosis.

ec•chy•mo•sis (ek-i-mō′sis) A purplish patch caused by extravasation of blood into the skin, differing from petechiae only in size (larger than 3 mm diameter). See this page. [G. *ekchymōsis,* ecchymosis, fr. *ek,* out, + *chymos,* juice]

ec•chy•mot•ic (ek-i-mot′ik) Relating to an ecchymosis.

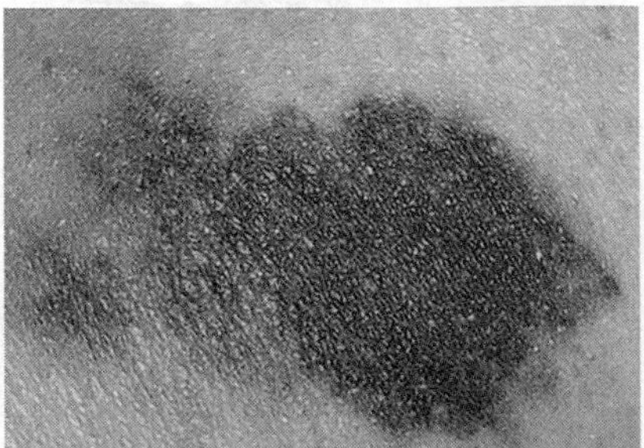

ecchymosis

ec•chy•mot•ic mask (ek-i-mot′ik mask) A dusky discoloration of the head and neck occurring when the trunk has been subjected to sudden and extreme compression, as in traumatic asphyxia.

ec•crine (ek′rin) **1.** SYN exocrine (1). **2.** Denoting the flow of sweat. [G. *ek-krino,* to secrete]

ec•crine gland (ek′rin gland) A type of coiled tubular sweat gland (other than apocrine glands) that occurs in the skin on almost all parts of the body.

ec•crine po•ro•ma (ek′rin pōr-ō′mă) A poroma or acrospiroma of the eccrine sweat glands, usually occurring on the sole of the foot.

ec•cri•sis (ek′ri-sis) **1.** The removal of waste products. **2.** Any waste product; excrement. [G. separation]

ec•cy•e•sis (ek-sī-ē′sis) SYN ectopic pregnancy. [G. *ek,* out, + *kyēsis,* pregnancy]

ec•dem•ic (ek-dem′ik) Denoting a disease brought into a region from without. [G. *ekdēmos,* foreign, from home, fr. *dēmos,* people]

ECF Abbreviation for extracellular fluid.

ECF-A Abbreviation for eosinophil chemotactic factor of anaphylaxis.

ECG Abbreviation for electrocardiogram.

ech•i•na•ce•a (ek′i-nā′shă) (*Echinacea angustifolia, E. pallida, E. purpurea*) A widely used herbal supplement claimed to act against infectious diseases; some clinical studies suggest value in preventing and treating the common cold; severe adverse reactions include anaphylaxis and angioedema. SYN comb flower, cornflower, Missouri (Kansas) snakeroot, snakeroot.

Ech•i•na•ce•a pur•pu•re•a (ek′i-nā′shă pūr-pūr′ē-ă) A species of plant in North America purported to heal infections and boost the body's immune system.

♻ **echino-, echin-** Combining forms meaning prickly, spiny. [G. *echinos,* hedgehog, sea urchin]

echi•no•coc•co•sis (ĕ-kī′nō-kok-kō′sis) Infection with *Echinococcus;* larval infection is called hydatid disease. Humans may serve as intermediate or dead-end hosts by harboring metacestode larvae.

Echi•no•coc•cus (ĕ-kī′nō-kok′ŭs) A genus of very small tapeworms; adults are found in various carnivores but not in humans; larvae, in the form of hydatid cysts, are found in the liver and other organs of ruminants, pigs, horses, rodents, and, under certain epidemiologic circumstances, humans (in whom disease is called hydatid disease). Worm has been studied in offensive biowarfare programs. [echino- + G. *kokkos,* a berry]

e•chi•no•coc•cus cyst (ĕ-kī′nō-kok′ŭs sist) SYN hydatid cyst.

ECHO (ek′ō) Acronym for enteric cytopathic human orphan [virus].

ech•o (ek′ō) **1.** A reverberating sound sometimes heard during auscultation of the chest. **2.** ULTRASONOGRAPHY the acoustic signal received from scattering or reflecting structures, or the corresponding pattern of light on a CRT or ultrasonogram. **3.** MAGNETIC RESONANCE IMAGING the signal detected following an inverting pulse. [G.]

ech•o•a•cou•si•a (ek′ō-ă-kū′sē-ă) A subjective disturbance of hearing in which a sound appears to be repeated. [echo + G. *akouō,* to hear]

ech•o•a•or•tog•ra•phy (ek′ō-ā-ōr-tog′ră-fē) Application of ultrasound techniques to the diagnosis and study of the aorta. [echo + aortography]

🅸 **ech•o•car•di•o•gram** (ek′ō-kahr′dē-ō-gram) The ultrasonic record obtained by echocardiography. SEE ultrasonography. See page B21.

ech•o•car•di•og•ra•phy (ek′ō-kahr-dē-og′ră-fē) The use of ultrasound in the investigation of the structure and motion of the heart and great vessels and diagnosis of cardiovascular lesions. SYN ultrasound cardiography. [echo + cardiography]

ech•o•en•ceph•a•log•ra•phy (ek′ō-en-sef-ă-log′ră-fē) The use of reflected ultrasound in the diagnosis of intracranial processes. [echo + encephalography]

ech•o•gen•ic (ek′ō-jen′ik) Pertaining to a structure or medium (e.g., tissue) that is capable of producing echoes. Contrast with the terms hypoechoic, hyperechoic, and anechoic, which refer to the paucity, abundance, and absence of echoes displayed on the image.

ech•o•gram (ek′ō-gram) A record obtained using high-frequency acoustic reflection techniques in any one of the various display modes, especially an echocardiogram. SEE ALSO ultrasonogram. [echo + G. *gramma,* a diagram]

ech•og•ra•phy (e-kog′ră-fē) SYN ultrasonography. [echo + G. *graphō,* to write]

ech•o•la•li•a (ek′ō-lā′lē-ă) Involuntary parrotlike repetition of a word or sentence just spoken by someone else; usually seen with schizophrenia. SYN echophrasia. [echo + G. *lalia,* a form of speech]

ech•o•mim•i•a (ek′ō-mim′ē-ă) SYN echopathy. [echo + G. *mimēsis,* imitation]

ech•o•mo•tism (ek′ō-mō′tizm) SYN echopraxia. [echo + L. *motio,* motion]

ech•op•a•thy (e-kop′ă-thē) A form of psychopathology, usually associated with schizophrenia, in which the words (echolalia) or actions (echopraxia) of another are imitated and repeated. SYN echomimia. [echo + G. *pathos,* suffering]

ech•o•phra•si•a (ek'ō-frā'zē-ă) SYN echolalia. [echo + *phrasis,* speech]

ech•o plan•ar (ek'ō plā'năr) A method of magnetic resonance imaging that allows quick image acquisition during free induction decay, using rapidly oscillating radiofrequency gradients.

echo•prax•i•a (ek'ō-prak'sē-ă) Involuntary imitation of movements made by another. SEE echopathy. SYN echomotism. [echo + G. *praxis,* action]

ech•o train (ĕk'ō trān) Series of 180-degree rephasing pulse and echoes in a fast-spin echo pulse sequence used in magnetic resonance imaging.

ECHO vi•rus, ech•o•vi•rus (ek'ō vī'rŭs, ek'ō-vī-rŭs) An enterovirus isolated from humans; although there are many inapparent infections, certain of the several serotypes are associated with fever and aseptic meningitis, and some appear to cause mild respiratory disease.

Eck fis•tu•la (ek fis'chū-lă) Transposition of the portal circulation to the systemic by making an anastomosis between the vena cava and portal vein, and then ligating the latter close to the liver.

ec•la•bi•um (ek-lā'bē-ŭm) Eversion of a lip. [G. *ek,* out, + L. *labium,* lip]

ec•lamp•si•a (ek-lamp'sē-ă) Occurrence of one or more convulsions, not attributable to other cerebral conditions such as epilepsy or cerebral hemorrhage, in a patient with preeclampsia. [G. *eklampsis,* a shining forth]

ec•lamp•tic (ek-lamp'tik) Relating to eclampsia.

ec•lamp•to•gen•ic, ec•lamp•tog•e•nous (ek'lamp'tō-jen'ik, ek'lamp-toj'ĕ-nŭs) Causing eclampsia.

e•clipse pe•ri•od (ē-klips' pēr'ē-ŏd) The time between infection by (or induction of) a bacteriophage, or other virus, and the appearance of mature virus within the cell; an interval of time during which infective viral material cannot be recovered.

ECMO Abbreviation for extracorporeal-membrane oxygenation.

♻ **eco-** Prefix meaning related to the environment. [G. *oikos,* house, household, habitation]

ec•o•log•ic chem•is•try (ek'ō-loj'ik kem'is-trē) **1.** Chemistry that concentrates on the effects of synthetic chemicals on the environment as well as the development of agents that are not harmful to the environment. **2.** The study of the molecular interactions between species and between species and the environment.

ec•o•log•ic stu•dy (ek'ō-loj'ik stŭd'ē) Epidemiologic study in which the units of analysis are populations or groups of people rather than individual people.

e•col•o•gy (ē-kol'ŏ-jē) The branch of biology concerned with interrelationships among living organisms, encompassing the relations of organisms to each other, to the environment, and to the energy balance within a given ecosystem. [eco- + G. *logos,* study]

e•col•o•gy of hu•man per•for•mance (ē-kol'ŏ-jē hyū'măn pĕr-fōr'măns) Framework for understanding human performance as a transactional process through which the person, the context, and performance of the task affect each other. Each transaction affects a person's future performance range and options.

e•co•sys•tem (ē'kō-sis-tĕm) **1.** The fundamental unit in ecology, comprising the living organisms and the nonliving elements that interact in a defined region. **2.** A biocenosis (biotic community) and its biotope.

e•co•tax•is (ē-kō-tak'sis) Migration of lymphocytes from the thymus and bone marrow into tissues possessing an appropriate microenvironment. [eco- + G. *taxis,* order, arrangement]

ec•o•tro•pic vi•rus (ek'ō-trō'pik vī'rŭs) An oncornavirus that does not produce disease in its natural host but does replicate in tissue culture cells derived from the host species.

ECP Abbreviation for eosinophil cationic protein.

ec•phy•ma (ek-fī'mă) A warty growth or protuberance. [G. a pimply eruption]

ECS Abbreviation for electrocerebral silence.

ec•sta•sy (ek'stă-sē) A drug of abuse used especially at clubs and raves; increases energy, heightens sexual urges, and induces euphoria. Even small recreational dosage *can* lead to hazardous reactions.

ECT Abbreviation for electroconvulsive therapy; electrochemotherapy; energy conservation techniques.

ECt_{50} SYN effective Ct_{50}.

ec•tad (ek'tad) Outward. [G. *ektos,* outside, + L. *ad,* to]

ec•tal (ek'tăl) Outer; external. [G. *ektos,* outside]

ec•ta•si•a, ec•ta•sis (ek-tā'zē-ă, ek'tă-sis) Dilation of a tubular structure. [G. *ektasis,* a stretching]

♻ **-ectasia, -ectasis** Combining forms meaning dilation, expansion. [G. *ektasis,* a stretching]

ec•ta•si•a cor•dis (ek-tā'zē-ă kōr'dis) Dilation of the heart. SYN cardiectasia.

ec•tat•ic (ek-tat'ik) Relating to, or marked by, ectasis.

ec·tat·ic em·phy·se·ma (ek-tat′ik em′fi-sē′mă) Obstructive airway disease with areas of dilatation of alveoli acini. Seen primarily in association with inherited deficiency of alpha-1-protease inhibitor. SEE panlobular emphysema.

ec·ten·tal (ek-ten′tăl) Relating to both ectoderm and endoderm; denoting the line where these two layers join. [G. *ektos,* outside, + *entos,* within]

ec·thy·ma (ek-thī′mă) A pyogenic infection of the skin initiated by β-hemolytic streptococci and characterized by adherent crusts beneath which ulceration occurs; the ulcers heal with scar formation. [G. a pustule]

ecto-, ect- Combining forms meaning outer, on the outside. SEE ALSO exo-. [G. *ektos,* outside]

ec·to·an·ti·gen (ek′tō-an′ti-jen) Any toxin or other excitor of antibody formation, separate or separable from its source. SYN exoantigen.

ec·to·blast (ek′tō-blast) **1.** SYN ectoderm. **2.** As used by some experimental embryologists, the original outer cell layer from which the primary germ layers are formed; in this sense, synonymous with protoderm. **3.** A cell wall. [ecto- + G. *blastos,* germ]

ec·to·car·di·a (ek′tō-kahr′dē-ă) Congenital displacement of the heart. SYN exocardia. [ecto- + G. *kardia,* heart]

ec·to·cer·vi·cal (ek′tō-sĕr′vi-kăl) Pertaining to the pars vaginalis of the cervix uteri that is lined with stratified squamous epithelium.

ec·to·derm (ek′tō-dĕrm) The outer layer of cells in the embryo, after establishment of the three primary germ layers (e.g., ectoderm, mesoderm, endoderm). SYN ectoblast (1). [ecto + G. *derma,* skin]

ec·to·der·mal (ek′tō-dĕr′măl) Relating to the ectoderm.

ec·to·en·tad (ek′tō-en′tad) From without inward.

ec·to·en·zyme (ek′tō-en′zīm) An enzyme that is excreted externally and that acts outside the organism.

ec·tog·e·nous (ek-toj′ĕ-nŭs) SYN exogenous. [ecto- + G. *-gen,* producing]

ec·to·glob·u·lar (ek′tō-glob′yū-lăr) Not within a globular body; specifically, not within a red blood cell.

ec·to·mere (ek′tō-mēr) One of the blastomeres involved in formation of ectoderm. [ecto- + G. *meros,* part]

ec·to·morph (ek′tō-mōrf) A constitutional body type or build (biotype or somatotype) in which tissues originating from the ectoderm predominate; from a morphologic standpoint, the limbs predominate over the trunk. [ecto- + G. *morphē,* form]

ec·to·mor·phic (ek′tō-mōrf′ik) Relating to, or having the characteristics of, an ectomorph.

-ectomy Suffix meaning removal of an anatomic structure. SEE ALSO -tomy. [G. *ektomē,* a cutting out]

ec·top·a·gus (ek-top′ă-gŭs) Conjoined twins whose bodies are joined laterally. SEE conjoined twins. [ecto- + G. *pagos,* something fixed]

ec·to·par·a·site (ek′tō-par′ă-sīt) A parasite that lives on the surface of the host body.

ec·to·pi·a (ek-tō′pē-ă) Congenital displacement or malposition of any organ or part of the body. SYN ectopy, heterotopia (1). [G. *ektopos,* out of place, fr. *ektos,* outside, + *topos,* place]

ec·to·pi·a cor·dis (ek-tō′pē-ă kōr′dis) Congenital condition in which the heart is exposed on the thoracic wall because of maldevelopment of the sternum and pericardium.

ec·to·pi·a len·tis (ek-tō′pē-ă len′tis) Displacement of the lens of the eye.

ec·to·pi·a len·tis et pu·pil·lae (ek-tō′pē-ă len′tis pyū-pil′ē) Disorder characterized by corectopia and a subluxed or dislocated lens.

ec·to·pi·a pu·pil·lae con·gen·i·ta (ek-tō′pē-ă pyū-pil′ē kon-jen′i-tă) Displacement of the pupil present at birth.

ec·to·pi·a tes·tis (ek-tō′pē-ă tes′tis) SYN parorchidium. SYN parorchidium.

ec·top·ic (ek-top′ik) **1.** Out of place; said of an organ not in its proper position, or of a pregnancy occurring elsewhere than in the cavity of the uterus. SYN aberrant (3), heterotopic (1), imperforate anus (2). **2.** CARDIOGRAPHY denoting a heartbeat that has its origin in some focus other than the sinuatrial node. [see ectopia]

ec·top·ic beat (ek-top′ik bēt) A cardiac beat originating elsewhere than at the sinuatrial node.

ec·top·ic bone (ek-top′ik bōn) Proliferation of bone in an abnormal place.

ec·top·ic fo·cus (ek-top′ik fō′kŭs) An irritable zone of myocardium capable of initiating ectopic beats or assuming the function of a pacemaker.

ec·top·ic preg·nan·cy (ek-top′ik preg′năn-sē) The development of an impregnated ovum outside the cavity of the uterus. See page 484. SYN eccyesis.

ec·top·ic schis·to·so·mi·a·sis (ek-top′ik shis′tō-sō-mī′ă-sis) A clinical form of schistosomiasis that occurs outside of the normal site of parasitism (mesenteric vein or hepatic portals).

ec·top·ic tach·y·car·di·a (ek-top′ik tak′i-kahr′dē-ă) A tachycardia originating in a focus other than the sinus node (e.g., atrial, A-V junctional, or ventricular tachycardia).

ec·top·ic tes·tis (ek-top′ik tes′tis) A variant of

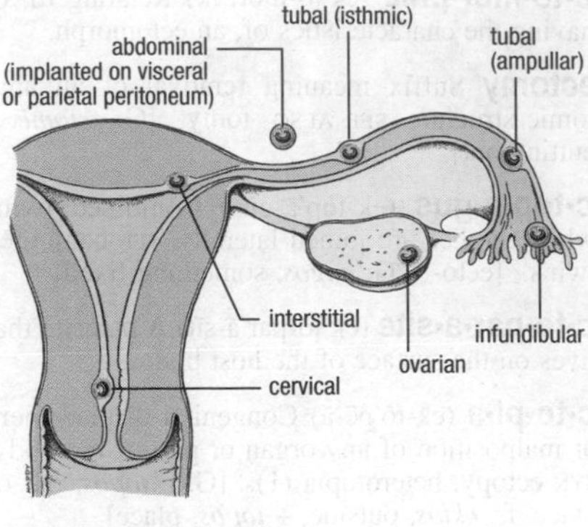

ectopic pregnancy: sites

undescended testis wherein testicular position is outside the usual pathway of descent. SEE ALSO ectopia testis.

ec·top·ic u·re·ter·o·cele (ek-top′ik yūr-ē′tĕr-ō-sēl) A ureterocele extending distal to the bladder neck.

ec·to·py (ek′tō-pē) SYN ectopia.

ec·tos·te·al (ek-tos′tē-ăl) Relating to the external surface of a bone. [ecto- + G. *osteon*, bone]

ec·tos·to·sis (ek′tos-tō′sis) Ossification in cartilage beneath the perichondrium, or formation of bone beneath the periosteum. [ecto- + G. *osteon*, bone, + *-osis*, condition]

ec·to·thrix (ek′tō-thriks) A sheath of spores (conidia) on the outside of a hair. [ecto- + G. *thrix*, hair]

♻ **ectro-** Prefix meaning congenital absence of a part. [G. *ektrōsis*, miscarriage]

ec·tro·dac·ty·ly, ec·tro·dac·tyl·i·a, ec·tro·dac·tyl·ism (ek′trō-dak′ti-lē, -dak-til′ē-ă, -dak′ti-lizm) Congenital absence of all or part of one or more fingers or toes. Known also as split-hand/foot deformity, lobster claw. There are several varieties and the pattern of inheritance is usually irregular. [ectro- + G. *daktylos*, finger]

ec·tro·dac·ty·ly–ec·to·der·mal dys·pla·si·a–cleft·ing syn·drome (ek′trō-dak′ti-lē-ek′tō-dĕr′măl dis-plā′zā-ă-kleft′ing sin′drōm) An autosomal recessive disorder resulting in defects of hands and feet; the ectodermal dysplasia causes anodontia and cleft palate.

ec·tro·gen·ic (ek′trō-jen′ik) Relating to ectrogeny.

ec·trog·e·ny (ek-troj′ĕ-nē) Congenital absence or defect of any body part. [ectro- + G. *-gen*, producing]

ec·tro·me·li·a (ek′trō-mē′lē-ă) **1.** Congenital hypoplasia or aplasia of one or more limbs. **2.** A disease of mice caused by the ectromelia virus; characterized by gangrenous loss of feet and necrotic areas in the internal organs; in laboratory mouse colonies, it usually results in high mortality rates. [ectro- + G. *melos*, limb]

ec·tro·mel·ic (ek′trō-mel′ik) Pertaining to, or characterized by, ectromelia.

ec·tro·pi·on, ec·tro·pi·um (ek-trō′pē-on, ek-trō′pē-ŭm) A rolling outward of the margin of a part, e.g., of an eyelid. [G. *ek*, out, + *tropē*, a turning]

ec·tro·pi·on u·ve·ae (ek-trō′pē-on ū′vē-ē) Eversion of the pigmented posterior epithelium of the iris at the pupillary margin.

ec·trop·o·dy (ek-trop′ŏ-dē) Total or partial absence of a foot. [ectro- + G. *pous*, foot]

ec·tro·syn·dac·ty·ly (ek′trō-sin-dak′ti-lē) Congenital anomaly marked by the absence of one or more fingers or toes and the fusion of others. [ectro- + G. *syn*, together, + *daktylos*, finger]

ECVT Abbreviation for electroconvulsive therapy.

ec·ze·ma (ek′sĕ-mă) Generic term for inflammatory conditions of the skin, particularly with vesiculation in the acute stage, typically erythematous, edematous, papular, and crusting; followed often by lichenification and scaling and occasionally by duskiness of the erythema and, infrequently, hyperpigmentation; often accompanied by sensations of itching and burning; the vesicles form by intraepidermal spongiosis. [G. fr. *ekzeō*, to boil over]

ec·ze·ma her·pe·ti·cum (ek′sĕ-mă her-pet′i-kŭm) A febrile condition caused by cutaneous dissemination of herpesvirus type 1, occurring most commonly in children, consisting of a widespread eruption of vesicles rapidly becoming umbilicated pustules.

ec·ze·ma mar·gi·na·tum (ek′sĕ-mă mar-ji-nā′tŭm) SYN tinea cruris.

ec·zem·a·toid (ek-sem′ă-toyd) Resembling eczema in appearance.

ec·zem·a·tous (ek-sem′ă-tŭs) Marked by or resembling eczema.

ED Abbreviation for effective dose, emergency department.

ED_{50} Abbreviation for median effective dose.

e·de·ma (ĕ-dē′mă) An accumulation of an excessive amount of watery fluid in cells, tissues, or serous cavities. SYN oedema. [G. *oidēma*, a swelling]

e·dem·a·tous (e-dem′ă-tŭs) Marked by edema. SYN oedematous.

e·den·tate (ē-den′tāt) SYN edentulous. [L. *edentatus*]

e·den·tu·lous (ē-den′chū-lŭs) Toothless, having lost the natural teeth. SYN edentate. [L. *edentulus,* toothless]

Ed•er-Pus•tow bou•gie (ed′ĕr pus′tof bū-zhē′) A metal olive-shaped bougie with a flexible metal dilating system (for esophageal stricture).

ed•e•tate (ed′ĕ-tāt) Contraction for ethylenediaminetetraacetate approved by the U.S. Adopted Names Council.

EDI Abbrevation for electronic data interchange.

Ed•i•son ef•fect (ed′i-sŏn e-fekt′) SYN thermionic emission.

ed•it•ing (ed′i-ting) Process in which a medical transcriptionist makes minor changes in a dictated report such as grammatical errors, inconsistencies, redundancies, or inappropriate remarks without altering the dictator's style. SEE ALSO verbatim transcription.

EDM Abbreviation for multiple epiphysial dysplasia.

EDS Abbreviation for excessive daytime sleepiness.

EDSS Abbreviation for expanded disability status scale.

EDTA Abbreviation for ethylenediaminetetraacetic acid.

ed•u•ca•tion (ej′ū-kā′shŭn) NURSING teaching patient, family, community member, staff, and others by planning and implementing learning activities to meet intended outcomes. SEE ALSO discharge.

EDV Abbreviation for end diastolic volume.

Ed•wards-Col•let clas•si•fi•ca•tion (ed′wărdz kol′ĕt klas′i-fi-kā′shŭn) System used to describe congenital heart malformations.

Ed•wards syn•drome (ed′wărdz sin′drōm) Trisomy in Group E chromosomes (16–18); second in incidence to trisomy 21 (i.e., Down syndrome) in frequency. Findings include mental retardation, congenital heart disease, spina bifida, and esophageal and biliary atresia. Affected patients generally die within 2 years of birth.

EEG Abbreviation for electroencephalogram; electroencephalography.

eel (ēl) A scaleless, snakelike fish. [M.E. *ele,* fr. O.E. *ael*]

EENT **1.** Abbreviation for eye, ear, nose, and throat. SEE ALSO ENT. **2.** Abbreviation for eyes, ears, nose, and throat (specialist).

EER Abbreviation for estimated energy requirement.

EF Abbreviation for ejection fraction.

EFA Abbreviation for essential fatty acid.

ef•face•ment (ē-fās′mĕnt) The thinning out of the cervix just before or during labor.

ef•fect (e-fekt′) The result or consequence of an action. [L. *efficio,* pp. *effectus,* to accomplish, fr. *facio,* to do]

ef•fec•tive con•ju•gate (e-fek′tive kon′jŭ-găt) The internal conjugate measured from the nearest lumbar vertebra to the symphysis, in spondylolisthesis. SYN false conjugate (2).

ef•fec•tive Ct_{50} (ECt_{50}) (e-fek′tiv) The Ct product required to produce a given effect on 50% of an exposed group. SYN ECt_{50}.

ef•fec•tive dose (ED) (e-fek′tiv dōs) **1.** The dose that produces the desired effect; when followed by a subscript (generally "ED_{50}"), it denotes the dose having such an effect on a certain percentage (e.g., 50%) of the test animals; ED_{50} is the median effective dose. **2.** In radiation protection, the sum of the equivalent doses in all tissues and organs of the body weighted for tissue effects of different types of radiation. The unit of effective dose is the sievert (Sv) or rem.

ef•fec•tive•ness (e-fek′tiv-nĕs) **1.** A measure of the accuracy or success of a diagnostic or therapeutic technique when carried out in an average clinical environment. **2.** The extent to which a treatment achieves its intended purpose.

ef•fec•tive os•mot•ic pres•sure (e-fek′tiv oz-mot′ik presh′ŭr) That part of the total osmotic pressure of a solution that governs the tendency of its solvent to pass across a boundary, usually a semipermeable membrane.

ef•fec•tive re•nal blood flow (ERBF) (e-fek′tiv rē′năl blŭd flō) The amount of blood flowing to the parts of the kidney that are involved with production of constituents of urine.

ef•fec•tive re•nal plas•ma flow (ERPF) (e-fek′tiv rē′năl plaz′mă flō) The amount of plasma flowing to the parts of the kidney that have a function in the production of constituents of urine; the clearance of substances such as iodopyracet and *p*-aminohippuric acid, assuming that the extraction ratio in the peritubular capillaries is 100%.

ef•fec•tive tem•per•a•ture (e-fek′tiv tem′pĕr-ă-chŭr) A comfort index or scale that takes into account the temperature of air, its moisture content, and movement.

ef•fec•tor (ĕ-fek′tŏr) **1.** A peripheral tissue that receives nerve impulses and reacts by contraction (muscle), secretion (gland), or a discharge of electricity (electric organ of certain bony fishes). **2.** A small metabolic molecule that, by combining with a repressor gene, depresses the activity of an operon. **3.** A small molecule that binds to a protein and, in so doing, alters the activity of that protein. **4.** A substance, technique, procedure, or individual that causes an effect. [L. producer]

ef•fem•i•na•tion (ĕ-fem′i-nā′shŭn) Acquisition

of appearance or manner described as feminine, either physiologically as part of female maturation, or pathologically by individuals of either sex. [L. *ef-femino,* pp. *-atus,* to make feminine, fr. *ex,* out, + *femina,* woman]

ef•fer•ent (ef′ĕr-ĕnt) Conducting outward from an organ or part; e.g., the efferent connections of a group of nerve cells, efferent blood vessels, or the excretory duct of an organ. [L. *efferens,* fr. *effero,* to bring out]

ef•fer•ent duc•tules of tes•tis (ef′ĕr-ĕnt dŭk′tyūlz tes′tis) The 12–14 small seminal ducts leading from the testis to the head of the epididymis. SYN ductuli efferentes testis [TA].

ef•fer•ent glo•mer•u•lar ar•te•ri•ole (ef′ĕr-ĕnt glō-mer′yū-lăr ahr-tēr′ē-ōl) The vessel that carries blood from the glomerular capillary network to the capillary bed of the proximal convoluted tubule. SYN vas efferens (2) [TA], efferent vessel.

ef•fer•ent nerve (ef′ĕr-ĕnt nĕrv) A nerve conveying impulses from the central nervous system to the periphery. SYN centrifugal nerve.

ef•fer•ent ves•sel (ef′ĕr-ĕnt ves′ĕl) SYN efferent glomerular arteriole.

ef•fer•ves•cent salts (ef′ĕr-ves′ĕnt sawlts) Preparations made by adding sodium bicarbonate and tartaric and citric acids to the active salt; when thrown into water, the acids break up the sodium bicarbonate, setting free carbonic acid gas.

ef•fi•ca•cy (ef′i-kă-sē) **1.** NURSING the success or effectiveness of a treatment. **2.** The power to produce a desired effect.

ef•fi•cien•cy (ĕ-fish′ĕn-sē) **1.** The production of the desired effects or results with minimum waste of time, effort, or skill. **2.** A measure of effectiveness; specifically, the useful work output divided by the energy input.

ef•fleur•age (ef-lūr-ahj′) A form of massage consisting of superficial or deep long, unbroken strokes in which the hand conforms to the surface and follows the fiber direction of underlying structures. SEE ALSO pétrissage. [Fr. *effleurer,* to touch lightly]

ef•flo•resce (ef′lōr-es′) To become powdery by losing the water of crystallization on exposure to a dry atmosphere. [L. *ef-floresco* (*exf-*), to blossom, fr. *flos* (*flor-*), flower]

ef•flu•vi•um, pl. **ef•flu•vi•a** (ĕ-flū′vē-ŭm, -ē-ă) Shedding of hair. SEE ALSO defluxion (1). [L. a flowing out, fr. *ef-fluo,* to flow out]

ef•fu•sion (ĕ-fyu′zhŭn) **1.** The escape of fluid from the blood vessels or lymphatics into the tissues or a cavity. **2.** A collection of the fluid effused. [L. *effusio,* a pouring out]

EFT Abbreviation for electronic funds transfer.

e.g. For example. [L. *exempli gratia*]

EGD Abbreviation for esophagogastroduodenoscopy.

e•ges•ta (ē-jes′tă) Unabsorbed food residues that are discharged from the digestive tract. [L. *e-gero,* pp. *-gestus,* to carry out, discharge]

EGFR Abbreviation for epidermal growth factor receptor .

egg (eg) The female sexual cell or gamete. (This term is *not* used in relation to humans.) SEE ALSO oocyte. [A.S. *aeg*]

egg al•bu•min (eg al-bū′min) SYN ovalbumin.

egg clus•ter (eg klŭs′tĕr) One of the clumps of cells resulting from the breaking up of the gonadal cords in the ovarian cortex; these clumps later develop into primary ovarian follicles.

egg mem•brane (eg mem′brān) A primary egg membrane is produced from ovarian cytoplasm (e.g., a vitelline membrane); a secondary egg membrane is the product of the ovarian follicle (e.g., the zona pellucida); a tertiary egg membrane is secreted by the lining of the oviduct (e.g., a shell).

egg•shell cal•ci•fi•ca•tion (eg′shel kal′si-fi-kā′shŭn) A thin layer of calcification around an intrathoracic lymph node, usually in silicosis, seen on a chest radiograph.

e•go (ē′gō) PSYCHOANALYSIS one of the three components of the psychic apparatus in the freudian structural framework, the other two being the id and superego. The ego occupies a position between the primal instincts (pleasure principle) and the demands of the outer world (reality principle), and therefore mediates between the person and external reality by performing the important functions of perceiving the needs of the self, both physical and psychologic, and the qualities and attitudes of the environment. It is also responsible for certain defensive functions to protect the person against the demands of the id and superego. [L. I]

e•go•bron•choph•o•ny (ē′gō-brong-kof′ŏ-nē) Egophony with bronchophony. [G. *aix* (*aig-*), goat, + *bronchos,* bronchus, + *phōnē,* voice]

e•go•cen•tric (ē′gō-sen′trik) Marked by extreme concentration of attention on oneself, i.e., self-centered. SYN egotropic. [ego + G. *kentron,* center]

e•go-dys•ton•ic (ē′gō-dis-ton′ik) Repugnant to or at variance with the aims of the ego and related psychologic needs of the individual (e.g., an obsessive thought or compulsive behavior); the opposite of ego-syntonic. [ego + G. *dys,* bad, + *tonos,* tension]

e•go-dys•ton•ic ho•mo•sex•u•al•i•ty (ē′gō-dis-ton′ik hō′mō-sek′shū-al′i-tē) A psychological or psychiatric disorder in which a person experiences persistent distress associated with same-sex preference and a strong need to change the behavior or, at least, to alleviate the distress associated with the homosexuality.

e•go ide•al (ē′gō ī-dēl′) The part of the personality that comprises the goals, aspirations, and aims of the self, usually growing out of the emulation of a significant person with whom one has identified.

e•go iden•ti•ty (ē′gō ī-den′ti-tē) The ego's sense of self.

e•go•ma•ni•a (ē′gō-mā′nē-ă) Extreme self-centeredness, self-appreciation, or self-content. [ego + G. *mania,* frenzy]

e•go•phon•ic (ē′gō-fon′ik) Relating to egophony.

e•goph•o•ny (ē-gof′ŏ-nē) A peculiar broken quality in voice sounds, like the bleating of a goat, heard about the upper level of the fluid in association with cases of pleurisy with effusion. [G. *aix* (*aig-*), goat, + *phōnē,* voice]

e•go-syn•ton•ic (ē′gō-sin-ton′ik) Acceptable to the aims of the ego and the related psychological needs of the individual (e.g., a delusion); the opposite of ego-dystonic. [ego + G. *syn,* together, + *tonos,* tension]

e•go•tro•pic (ē′gō-trō′pik) SYN egocentric. [ego + G. *tropē,* a turning]

EGTA Abbreviation for esophageal gastric tube airway.

E•gyp•tian oph•thal•mi•a (ē-jip′shŭn of-thal′mē-ă) SYN trachoma.

e-health (ē′helth) Health services and information on the Internet.

EHEC Abbreviation for enterohemorrhagic *Escherichia coli.*

Eh•lers-Dan•los syn•drome (ā′lerz dahn′lōs sin′drōm) An inherited disorder of connective tissue characterized by fragile hyperelastic skin and hypermobility of the joints. At least 14 variant forms have been identified and named.

EHR Abbreviation for electronic health record.

Eh•ret phe•nom•e•non (er′ā fē-nom′ĕ-non) A sudden throb felt by a finger on the brachial artery, as the pressure in the cuff falls during a blood pressure estimation; said to indicate fairly accurately the diastolic pressure.

Ehr•lich ac•id he•ma•tox•y•lin stain (er-lik as′id hē′mă-toks′i-lin stān) An alum type of hematoxylin stain used as a regressive staining method for nuclei, followed by differentiation to required staining intensity; the solution may be allowed to ripen naturally in sunlight or partially oxidized with sodium iodate.

Ehr•lich a•ne•mi•a (er-lik ă-nē′mē-ă) SYN aplastic anemia.

Ehr•lich an•i•line crys•tal vi•o•let stain (er-lik an′i-līn kris′tăl vī′ŏ-lĕt stān) A stain for gram-positive bacteria.

Ehr•lich benz•al•de•hyde re•ac•tion (er-lik benz-al′dĕ-hīd rē-ak′shŭn) A test for urobilinogen in the urine, by dissolving 2 g of dimethyl-*p*-aminobenzaldehyde in 100 mL of 5% hydrochloric acid and adding this reagent to urine; a red color in cold temperatures indicates the presence of an excessive amount of urobilinogen.

Ehr•li•chi•a (er-lik′ē-ă) A genus of small, often pleomorphic, coccoid to ellipsoidal, nonmotile, gram-negative bacteria (order Rickettsiales) that occur either singly or in compact inclusions in circulating mammalian leukocytes; species are the etiologic agents of ehrlichiosis and are transmitted by ticks. The type species is *Ehrlichia canis.*

Ehr•li•chi•a chaf•fe•en•sis (er-lik′ē-ă chaf′ē-en′sis) A bacterial species associated with human monocytic ehrlichiosis; carried by a tick vector, *Amblyomma americanum,* the Lone Star tick, and transmitted by various hard-bodied ticks.

Ehr•li•chi•a e•qui (er-lik′ē-ă ek′wī) A bacterial species that causes human granulocytic ehrlichiosis; occurs in the Mid-Atlantic, southern New England, and southern Midwest and is spread by ticks (*Ixodes*).

Ehr•li•chi•a pha•go•cy•to•phil•a (er-lik′ē-ă fā-gō-sī-tō-fil′a) SEE *Anaplasma phagocytophilum.*

Ehr•lich in•ner body (er-lik in′ĕr bod′ē) A round oxyphil body found in the red blood cell in hemolysis due to a specific blood poison. SYN Heinz-Ehrlich body.

ehr•lich•i•o•sis (er-lik′ē-ō′sis) A tick-borne infection of humans, dogs, and many other mammals caused by bacteria from the *Neorickettsia, Anaplasma,* and *Ehrlichia* groups; produces manifestations similar to those of Rocky Mountain spotted fever.

Ehr•lich phe•nom•e•non (er-lik fē-nom′ĕ-non) The difference between the amount of diphtheria toxin that will exactly neutralize one unit of antitoxin and that which, added to one unit of antitoxin, will leave one lethal dose free is greater than one lethal dose of toxin; i.e., it is necessary to add more than one lethal dose of toxin to a neutral mixture of toxin and antitoxin to make the mixture lethal (the basis of the L_+ dose).

Ehr•lich the•o•ry (er-lik thē′ŏr-ē) SEE side-chain theory.

Ehr•lich tri•ac•id stain (er-lik trī-as′id stān) A differential leukocytic stain comprised of saturated solutions of orange G, acid fuchsin, and methyl green.

Ehr•lich tri•ple stain (er-lik trip′ĕl stān) A mixture of indulin, eosin Y, and aurantia.

EIA Abbreviation for enzyme immunoassay; exercise-induced asthma.

Eich·horst cor·pus·cles (īk′hōrst kōr′pŭs-ĕlz) The globular forms sometimes occurring in the poikilocytosis of pernicious anemia.

Eich·horst neu·ri·tis (īk′hōrst nūr-ī′tis) SYN interstitial neuritis.

Eick·en meth·od (ī′kĕn meth′ŏd) Facilitation of hypopharyngoscopy by means of forward traction on the cricoid cartilage by a laryngeal probe.

ei·co·sa·noids (ī-kō′să-noydz) The physiologically active substances derived from arachidonic acid (e.g., the prostaglandins, leukotrienes, and thromboxanes); synthesized through a cascade pathway. [G. *eicosa-*, twenty, + *eidos,* form]

EIEC Abbreviation for enteroinvasive *Escherichia coli.*

eighth cra·ni·al nerve [CN VIII] (āth krā′nē-ăl nĕrv) SYN vestibulocochlear nerve [CN VIII].

Ei·ke·nel·la cor·ro·dens (ī-kĕ-nel′ă kō-rō′denz) A species of nonmotile, rod-shaped, gram-negative, facultatively anaerobic bacteria that is part of the normal flora of the adult human oral cavity but may be an opportunistic pathogen, especially in immunocompromised hosts; member of the HACEK group.

EIN Abbreviation for employer identification number.

Ei·nar·son gal·lo·cy·a·nin-chrome al·um stain (īn′ăr-sŏn gal′ō-sī′ă-nin-krōm al′ŭm stān) A method for staining both RNA and DNA a deep blue; with proper controls, nucleic acid content of stained cells and nuclei may be estimated by cytophotometry; also useful for Nissl substance.

ein·stein (īn′stīn) A unit of energy equal to 1 mol quantum, hence to 6.0221367×10^{23} quanta. The value of einstein, in kJ, is dependent upon the wavelength.

ein·stein·i·um (Es) (īn-stī′nē-ŭm) An artificially prepared transuranium element, atomic no. 99, atomic wt. 252.0; it has many isotopes, all of which are radioactive (^{252}Es has the longest known half-life, 1.29 years).

Ein·tho·ven law (īn′tō-vĕn law) ELECTROCARDIOGRAPHY the potential of any wave or complex in lead II is equal to the sum of its potentials in leads I and III.

Ein·tho·ven tri·an·gle (īn′tō-vĕn trī′ang-gĕl) An imaginary equilateral triangle with the heart at its center, its equal sides representing the three standard limb leads of the electrocardiogram.

E.I. pro·gram (prō′gram) SYN early intervention.

Ei·sen·men·ger com·plex (ī′zĕn-meng′ĕr kom′pleks) The combination of ventricular septal defect with pulmonary hypertension and consequent right-to-left shunt through the defect, with or without an associated overriding aorta.

Ei·sen·men·ger syn·drome (ī′zĕn-meng′ĕr sin′drōm) Cardiac failure with significant right-to-left shunt producing cyanosis due to higher pressure on the right side of the shunt. Usually due to the Eisenmenger complex, a ventricular septal defect with right ventricular hypertrophy and dilatation, severe pulmonary hypertension, and frequent straddling of the defect by a misplaced aortic root.

e·jac·u·late (ē-jak′yū-lāt) **1.** To expel suddenly; as of semen. **2.** (ē-jak′yu-lăt) Semen expelled in ejaculation. SEE ALSO ejaculation.

e·jac·u·la·ti·o (ē-jak′yū-lā′shē-ō) SYN ejaculation.

e·jac·u·la·tion (ē-jak′yū-lā′shŭn) The process that results in propulsion of semen from the genital ducts and urethra to the exterior; caused by the rhythmic contractions of the muscles surrounding the internal genital organs and the ischiocavernous and bulbocavernous muscles, resulting in an increase in pressure on the semen in the internal genital glands and the internal urethra. SYN ejaculatio. [L. *e-iaculo,* pp. *-atus,* to shoot out]

ejac·u·la·to·ry (ē-jak′yū-lă-tōr-ē) Relating to an ejaculation.

e·jac·u·la·to·ry duct (ē-jak′yū-lă-tōr-ē dŭkt) The duct formed by the union of the deferent duct and the excretory duct of the seminal vesicle, which opens into the prostatic urethra. SYN spermiduct (2).

e·jec·ta (ē-jek′tă) SYN ejection (2). [L. ntr. pl. of *ejectus,* pp. of *ejicio,* to throw out]

e·jec·tion (ē-jek′shŭn) **1.** The act of driving or throwing out by physical force from within. **2.** That which is ejected. SYN ejecta. [L. *ejectio,* from *ejicio,* to cast out]

e·jec·tion frac·tion (EF) (ē-jek′shŭn frak′shŭn) The fraction of blood contained in the ventricle at the end of diastole that is expelled during its contraction.

e·jec·tion mur·mur (ē-jek′shŭn mŭr′mŭr) A diamond-shaped systolic murmur produced by the ejection of blood into the aorta or pulmonary artery and ending by the time of the second heart sound component produced, respectively, by closing of the aortic or pulmonic valve.

e·jec·tion pe·ri·od (ē-jek′shŭn pēr′ē-ŏd) SYN sphygmic interval.

♻**eka-** Prefix used to denote an undiscovered or just discovered element in the periodic system before a proper and official name is assigned by authorities; e.g., eka-osmium, now plutonium. [Sanskrit *eka,* one]

EKG Abbreviation for electrocardiogram, more correctly given as ECG.

e•lab•o•ra•tion (ē-lab′ŏr-ā′shŭn) The process of working out in detail by labor and study. [L. *e-laborō,* pp. *-atus,* to labor, endeavor, fr. *labor,* toil, to work out]

elas•tance (ē-las′tăns) **1.** A measure of the stiffness of a chamber expressed as a change in pressure per unit change in volume; the reciprocal of compliance. **2.** INTERNAL MEDICINE, PHYSIOLOGY usually a measure of the tendency of a hollow viscus (e.g., lung, urinary bladder, gallbladder) to recoil toward its original dimensions on removal of a distending or compressing force.

e•las•tase (ĕ-las′tās) A serine proteinase hydrolyzing elastin.

e•las•tic (ĕ-las′tik) **1.** Having the property of returning to the original shape after being compressed, bent, or otherwise distorted. **2.** A rubber or plastic band used in orthodontics as either a primary or adjunctive source of force to move teeth. The term is generally modified by an adjective to describe the direction of the force or the location of the terminal connecting points. [G. *elastreō,* epic form of *elaunō,* drive, push]

e•las•tic ban•dage (ĕ-las′tik ban′dăj) A bandage containing stretchable material; used to exert local pressure.

e•las•tic car•ti•lage (ĕ-las′tik kahr′ti-lăj) Cartilage in which cells are surrounded by a territorial capsular matrix outside of which is an interterritorial matrix containing elastic fiber networks in addition to collagen fibers and ground substance. SYN yellow cartilage.

e•las•tic fi•bers (ĕ-las′tik fī′bĕrz) Fibers that are 0.2–2 mcm in diameter but may be larger in some ligaments; they branch and anastomose to form networks and fuse to form fenestrated membranes; the fibers and membranes consist of microfibrils about 10 nm wide and an amorphous substance containing elastin. SYN yellow fibers.

e•las•ti•cin (ĕ-las′ti-sin) SYN elastin.

e•las•tic•i•ty (ĕ-las-tis′i-tē) The quality or condition of being elastic.

e•las•tic la•mel•la (ĕ-las′tik lă-mel′ă) A thin sheet or membrane composed of elastic fibers.

e•las•tic lam•i•nae of ar•ter•ies (ĕ-las′tik lam′i-nē ahr′tĕr-ēz) External: the layer of elastic connective tissue lying immediately outside the smooth muscle of the tunica media. Internal: a fenestrated layer of elastic tissue of the tunica intima. SYN elastic layers of arteries.

e•las•tic lay•ers of ar•ter•ies (ĕ-las′tik lā′ĕrz ahr′tĕr-ēz) SYN elastic laminae of arteries.

e•las•tic mem•brane (ĕ-las′tik mem′brān) A membrane formed of elastic connective tissue, present as fenestrated lamellae in the coats of the arteries and elsewhere.

e•las•tic tis•sue (ĕ-las′tik tish′ū) A form of connective tissue in which the elastic fibers predominate; it constitutes the ligamenta flava of the vertebrae and the ligamentum nuchae, especially of quadrupeds; it occurs also in the walls of the arteries and of the bronchial tree, and connects the cartilages of the larynx.

e•las•tin (ĕ-las′tin) A yellow elastic fibrous mucoprotein that is the major connective tissue protein of elastic structures (large blood vessels, tendons, and ligaments). SYN elasticin.

e•las•to•fi•bro•ma (ĕ-las′tō-fī-brō′mă) A nonencapsulated slow-growing mass of poorly cellular, collagenous, fibrous and elastic tissue; occurs usually in subscapular adipose tissue of old people. [G. *elastos,* beaten, + L. *fibra, -oma* tumor]

e•las•toid de•gen•er•a•tion (ĕ-las′toyd dĕ-jen′ĕr-ā′shŭn) **1.** SYN elastosis (2). **2.** Hyaline degeneration of the elastic tissue of the arterial wall, seen during involution of the uterus.

e•las•to•ma (ĕ-las-tō′mă) A tumorlike deposit of elastic tissue.

e•las•to•sis (ĕ-las-tō′sis) **1.** Degenerative change in elastic tissue. **2.** Degeneration of collagen fibers, with altered staining properties resembling elastic tissue, or formation by fibroblast-activated ultraviolet or mast cell mediators of abnormal fibers. SYN elastoid degeneration (1), elastotic degeneration.

e•las•tot•ic de•gen•er•a•tion (ĕ-las-tot′ik dĕ-jen′ĕr-ā′shŭn) SYN elastosis (2).

e•laun•in (ē-law′nin) A component of elastic fibers formed from a deposition of elastin between oxytalan fibers; found in the connective tissue of the dermis, particularly in association with sweat glands. [G. *elaunō,* to drive]

el•bow (el′bō) **1.** The region of the upper limb between arm and forearm surrounding the elbow joint, especially posteriorly. **2.** The joint between the arm and the forearm. SYN cubitus (1) [TA]. **3.** An angular body resembling a flexed elbow. [A.S. *elnboga*]

el•bow bone (el′bō bōn) SYN olecranon.

el•bowed bou•gie (el′bōd bū-zhē′) A bougie with a sharply angulated bend near its tip.

el•bow joint (el′bō joynt) A compound hinge synovial joint between the humerus and the bones of the forearm; it consists of the articulatio humeroradialis and the articulatio humeroulnaris. See page 490. SYN cubital joint.

el•der a•buse (el′dĕr ă-byūs′) The physical or emotional abuse, including financial exploitation, of an elderly person, by one or more of the person's children, nursing facility caregivers, or any others.

el•der•ly pri•mi•gra•vi•da (el′dĕr-lē prī-mi-grav′i-dă) Dated term referring to a woman older than 35 years who is pregnant for the first time.

e-learn·ing (lĕrn′ing) Electronic learning; using computer technology for health care education.

e·lec·tive a·bor·tion (ĕ-lek′tiv ă-bōr′shŭn) An abortion without medical justification but done in a legal way, as in the U.S.

e·lec·tive mut·ism (ĕ-lek′tiv myū′tizm) Mutism due to psychogenic causes.

e·lec·tive sur·ger·y (ĕ-lek′tiv sŭr′jĕr-ē) Surgery a patient chooses to undergo although its need is neither vital nor urgent.

E·lec·tra com·plex (ĕ-lek′tră kom′pleks) Unresolved conflicts during childhood toward the father that subsequently influence a woman's relationships with men. [*Electra,* daughter of Agamemnon in Greek myth]

e·lec·tri·cal al·ter·nans (ĕ-lek′tri-kăl awl-ter′nanz) Alternation in the amplitude of P waves, QRS complexes, or T waves as observed by electrocardiography.

e·lec·tri·cal al·ter·na·tion of heart (ĕ-lek′tri-kăl awl-tĕr-nā′shŭn hahrt) A disorder in which the ventricular or atrial complexes or both are regular in time but of alternating pattern; detected by electrocardiography.

e·lec·tri·cal ax·is (ĕ-lek′tri-kăl ak′sis) The net direction of the electromotive forces developed in the heart during its activation, usually represented in the frontal plane.

e·lec·tri·cal burn (ĕ-lek′tri-kăl bŭrn) Tissue damage resulting from flow of an electrical current with temperatures as high as 5000°C. Entry and exit points occur but most burned tissue remains invisible at surface levels.

e·lec·tri·cal di·as·to·le (ĕ-lek′tri-kăl dī-as′tŏ-lē) Period from end of T wave to beginning of next Q wave.

e·lec·tri·cal fail·ure (ĕ-lek′tri-kăl fāl′yŭr) Failure in which the cardiac inadequacy is secondary to disturbance of the electrical impulse.

e·lec·tri·cal sys·to·le (ĕ-lek′tri-kăl sis′tŏ-lē) The duration of the QRS-T complex (i.e., from the earliest Q wave to the end of the latest T wave on the ECG).

e·lec·tric shock (ĕ-lek′trik shok) A traumatic state following the passage of an electrical current through the body.

electro- Combining form meaning electric, electricity. [G. *ēlektron,* amber (on which static electricity can be generated by friction)]

e·lec·tro·ac·u·punc·ture (ĕ-lek′trō-ak′yū-pungk-shŭr) Acupuncture in which needles are attached to a source of electric current.

electroanaesthesia [Br.] SYN electroanesthesia.

e·lec·tro·an·al·ge·si·a (ē-lek′trō-an-ăl-jē′zē-ă) Analgesia induced by the passage of an electric current.

e·lec·tro·an·es·the·si·a (ē-lek′trō-an-es-thē′zē-ă) Anesthesia produced by an electric current. SYN electroanaesthesia.

e·lec·tro·car·di·o·gram (ECG, EKG) (ĕ-lek′trō-kahr′dē-ō-gram) Graphic record of cardiac action currents obtained with the electrocardiograph. [electro- + G. *kardia,* heart, + *gramma,* a drawing]

e·lec·tro·car·di·o·graph (ĕ-lek′trō-kahr′dē-ō-graf) An instrument for recording the potential of the electrical currents that traverse the heart.

e·lec·tro·car·di·og·ra·phy (ĕ-lek′trō-kahr-dē-og′ră-fē) **1.** A method of recording the electrical activity of the heart: impulse formation, conduction, depolarization, and repolarization of atria and ventricles. **2.** The study and interpretation of electrocardiograms. See page 491.

e·lec·tro·cau·ter·i·za·tion (ĕ-lek′trō-kaw′tĕr-ī-zā′shŭn) Cauterization by passage of high fre-

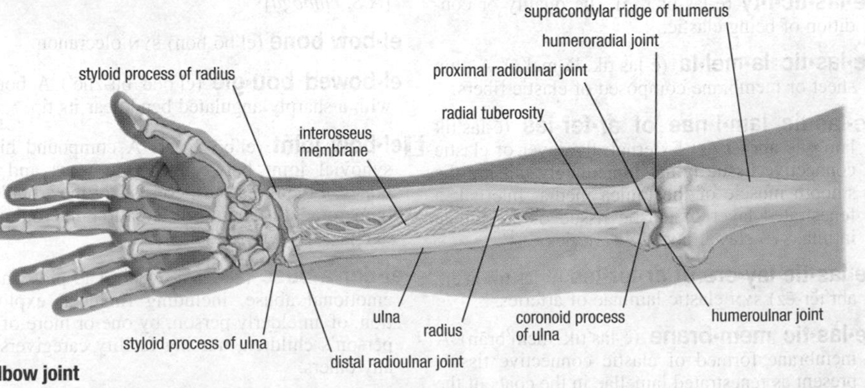

elbow joint

quency current through tissue or by metal that has been electrically heated.

e•lec•tro•cau•ter•y (ĕ-lek′trō-kaw′tĕr-ē) An instrument for directing a high frequency current through a local area of tissue.

e•lec•tro•ce•re•bral si•lence (ECS) (ĕ-lek′trō-ser′ĕ-brăl sī′lĕnts) Flat or isoelectric encephalogram; an electroencephalogram with absence of cerebral activity from symmetrically placed electrode pairs; if such a record is present for 30 minutes in a clinically brain-dead adult and if drug intoxication, hypothermia, and recent hypotension have been excluded, the diagnosis of cerebral death is supported. SYN flat electroencephalogram.

e•lec•tro•chem•i•cal (ĕ-lek′trō-kem′i-kăl) Denoting chemical reactions involving electricity, and the mechanisms involved.

e•lec•tro•che•mo•ther•a•py (ECT) (ĕ-lek′trō-kē′mō-thār′ă-pē) Anticancer therapy used in treatment of basal cell carcinoma of the skin; combination of bleomycin sulfate and chemotherapeutic agent injected directly into tumor followed by electrical impulses to the lesion through an electrode. This alternative therapy to surgical excision has demonstrated 98% effectiveness.

e•lec•tro•co•ag•u•la•tion (ĕ-lek′trō-kō-ag′yū-lā′shŭn) Coagulation produced by an electrocautery.

e•lec•tro•co•chle•o•gram (ĕ-lek′trō-kok′lē-ō-gram) The record obtained by electrocochleography.

e•lec•tro•co•chle•og•ra•phy (ĕ-lek′trō-kok-lē-og′ră-fē) A measurement of the electrical potentials generated in the inner ear as a result of sound stimulation. [electro- + L. *cochlea,* snail shell, + G. *graphō,* to write]

e•lec•tro•con•trac•til•i•ty (ĕ-lek′trō-kon-trak-til′i-tē) The power of contraction of muscular tissue in response to an electrical stimulus.

e•lec•tro•con•vul•sive (ĕ-lek′trō-kŏn-vŭl′siv) Denoting a convulsive response to an electrical stimulus. SEE electroshock therapy.

e•lec•tro•con•vul•sive ther•a•py (ECT, ECVT) (ĕ-lek′trō-kŏn-vŭl′siv thār′ă-pē) SYN electroshock therapy.

e•lec•tro•cor•ti•co•gram (ĕ-lek′trō-kōr′ti-kō-gram) A record of electrical activity derived directly from the cerebral cortex.

e•lec•tro•cor•ti•cog•ra•phy (ĕ-lek′trō-kor′ti-kog′ră-fē) The technique of recording the electri-

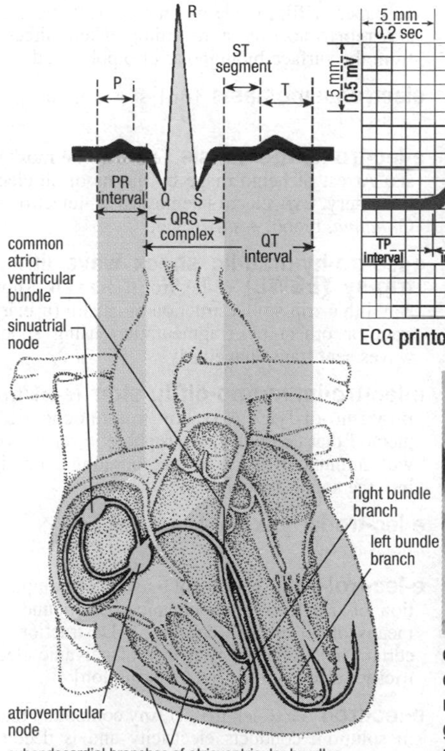

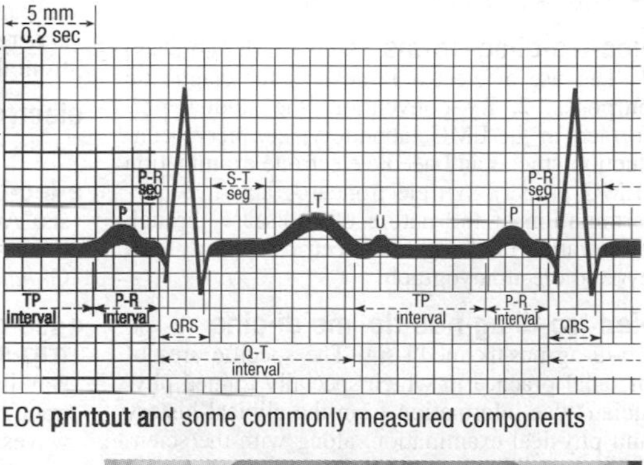

ECG printout and some commonly measured components

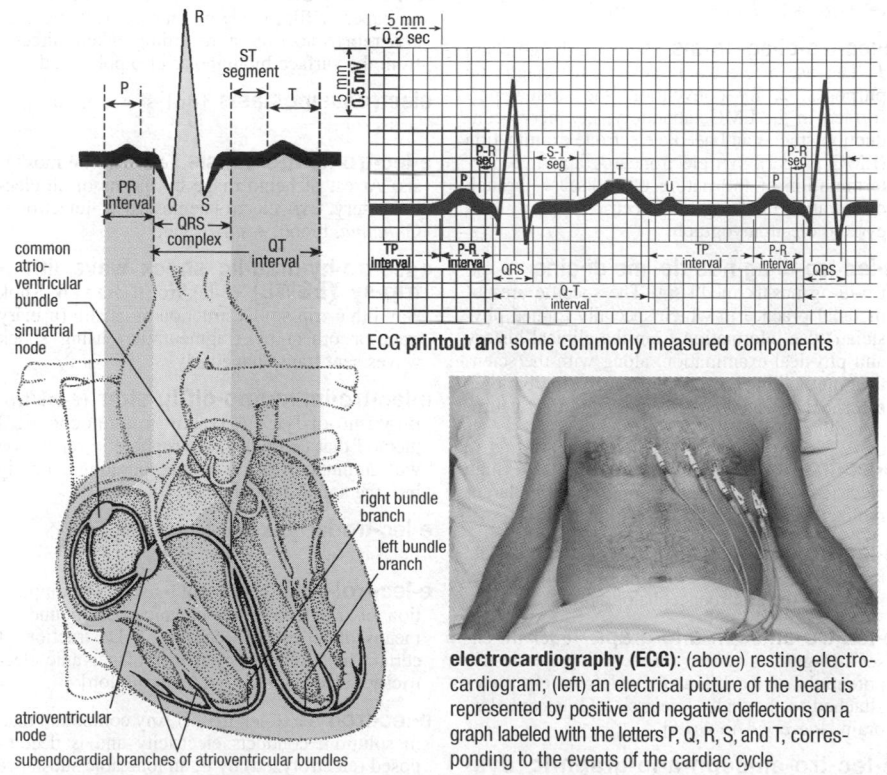

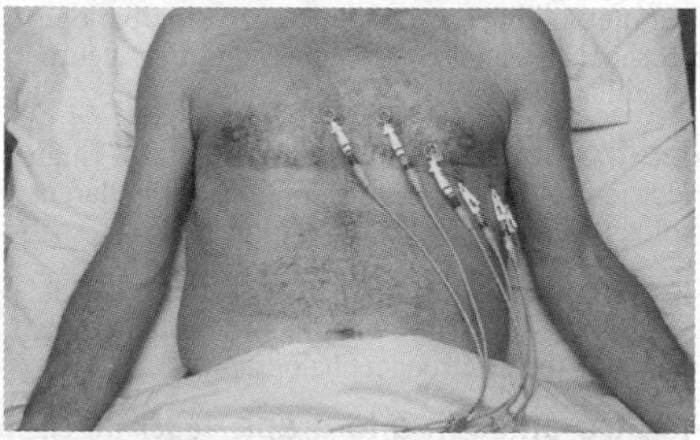

electrocardiography (ECG): (above) resting electrocardiogram; (left) an electrical picture of the heart is represented by positive and negative deflections on a graph labeled with the letters P, Q, R, S, and T, corresponding to the events of the cardiac cycle

cal activity of the cerebral cortex by means of electrodes placed directly on it.

e•lec•trode (ĕ-lek′trōd) **1.** Device to record one of the two extremities of an electric circuit; one of the two poles of an electric battery or of the end of the conductors connected thereto. **2.** An electrical terminal specialized for a particular electrochemical reaction. [electro- + G. *hodos,* way]

e•lec•trode cath•e•ter ab•la•tion (ĕ-lek′trōd kath′ĕ-tĕr ăb-lā′shŭn) A method of ablating the site of origin of arrhythmias whereby high energy electric shocks are delivered by intravascular catheters.

e•lec•tro•der•mal (ĕ-lek′trō-dĕr′măl) Pertaining to electric properties of the skin, usually referring to altered resistance. [electro- + G. *derma,* skin]

e•lec•tro•der•mal au•di•om•e•try (ĕ-lek′trō-dĕr′măl aw′dē-om′ĕ-trē) A form of electrophysiologic audiometry used to determine hearing thresholds by measuring changes in skin resistance as a conditioned response to noise stimuli.

e•lec•tro•des•ic•ca•tion (ĕ-lek′trō-des-i-kā′shŭn) Destruction of lesions or sealing off of blood vessels (usually of the skin, but also of available surfaces of mucous membrane) by monopolar high-frequency electric current. [electro- + L. *desicco,* to dry up]

e•lec•tro•di•ag•no•sis (ĕ-lek′trō-dī-ăg-nō′sis) **1.** The use of electronic devices for diagnostic purposes. **2.** By convention, the studies performed in the EMG laboratory, i.e., nerve conduction studies and needle electrode examination (EMG proper). SYN electroneurography. **3.** Determination of the nature of a disease through observation of changes in electrical activity. SYN evoked electromyography.

e•lec•tro•di•ag•nos•tic me•di•cine (ĕ-lek′trō-dī-ăg-nos′tik med′i-sin) The specific area of medical practice in which specially trained physicians use information from the clinical history and physical examination, along with the scientific method of recording and analyzing biologic electrical potentials, to diagnose and treat neuromuscular disorders.

e•lec•tro•di•al•y•sis (ĕ-lek′trō-dī-al′i-sis) In an electric field, the removal of ions from larger molecules and particles.

e•lec•tro•en•ceph•a•lo•gram (EEG) (ĕ-lek′trō-en-sef′ă-lō-gram) The record obtained by means of the electroencephalograph.

e•lec•tro•en•ceph•a•lo•graph (ĕ-lek′trō-en-sef′ă-lō-graf) A system for recording the electric potentials of the brain derived from electrodes attached to the scalp. [electro- + G. *encephalon,* brain, + *graphō,* to write]

e•lec•tro•en•ceph•a•lo•graph•ic dys•rhyth•mi•a (ĕ-lek′trō-en-sef′ă-lō-graf′ik dis-ridh′mē-ă) A diffusely irregular brain wave tracing.

e•lec•tro•en•ceph•a•log•ra•phy (EEG) (ĕ-lek′trō-en-sef′ă-log′ră-fē) Registration of the electrical potentials recorded by an electroencephalograph. See page 493.

e•lec•tro•en•dos•mo•sis (ĕ-lek′trō-en-dos-mō′sis) Endosmosis produced by means of an electric field.

e•lec•tro•gas•tro•gram (ĕ-lek′trō-gas′trō-gram) The record obtained using an electrogastrograph.

e•lec•tro•gas•tro•graph (ĕ-lek′trō-gas′trō-graf) An instrument used in electrogastrography. [electro- + G. *gastēr,* stomach, + *graphō,* to write]

e•lec•tro•gas•trog•ra•phy (ĕ-lek′trō-gas-trog′ră-fē) The recording of the electrical phenomena associated with gastric secretion and motility.

e•lec•tro•glot•to•graph (ĕ-lek′trō-glot′ō-graf) An instument that measures the impedance between two electrodes placed externally on either side of the larynx. The impedance is reduced whenever the vocal folds come in contact, thus creating a record of the cycles of glottal opening and closure.

e•lec•tro•gram (ĕ-lek′trō-gram) **1.** Any record on paper or film made by an electrical event. **2.** ELECTROPHYSIOLOGY a recording taken directly from the surface by unipolar or bipolar leads.

electrohaemostasis [Br.] SYN electrohemostasis.

e•lec•tro•he•mo•sta•sis (ĕ-lek′trō-hē-mos′tă-sis) Arrest of hemorrhage by means of an electrocautery. SYN electrohaemostasis. [electro- + G. *haima,* blood, + *stasis,* halt]

e•lec•tro•hy•drau•lic shock wave lith•o•trip•sy (ESWL) (ĕ-lek′trō-hī-drawl′ik shok wāv lith′ō-trip-sē) Destruction of calculi (urinary tract or other) by fragmentation using shock waves sent transcutaneously.

e•lec•tro•im•mu•no•dif•fu•sion (ĕ-lek′trō-im′yū-nō-di-fyū′zhŭn) An immunochemical method that combines electrophoretic separation with immunodiffusion by incorporating antibody into the support medium.

e•lec•tro•lar•ynx (ĕ-lek′trō-lar′ingks) SYN artificial larynx.

e•lec•trol•y•sis (ĕ-lek-trol′i-sis) **1.** Decomposition of a salt or other chemical compound by means of an electric current. **2.** Destruction of certain hair follicles by means of galvanic electricity. [electro- + G. *lysis,* dissolution]

e•lec•tro•lyte (ĕ-lek′trō-līt) Any compound that, in solution, conducts electricity and is decomposed (electrolyzed) by it; an ionizable substance in solution. [electro- + G. *lytos,* soluble]

e•lec•tro•lyt•ic (ĕ-lek′trō-lit′ik) Referring to or caused by electrolysis.

e•lec•tro•mag•ne•tic ra•di•a•tion, e•lec•tro•mag•ne•tic spec•trum (ĕ-lek′trō-mag-net′ik rā′dē-ā′shŭn, spek′trŭm) Wavelike energy propagated through matter or space; varies widely in wavelength, frequency, photon energy, and properties; may be natural or artificial and includes radiowaves, microwaves, heat waves, visible light, ultraviolet light, x-rays, gamma rays, and cosmic radiation.

e•lec•tro•me•chan•i•cal dis•so•ci•a•tion (ĕ-lek′trō-mĕ-kan′i-kăl di-sō′sē-ā′shŭn) Persistence of electrical activity in the heart without associated mechanical contraction; often a sign of cardiac rupture. SYN pulseless electrical activity.

e•lec•tro•mech•an•i•cal sys•tole (ĕ-lek′trō-mĕ-kan′i-kăl sis′tŏ-lē) The period from the beginning of the QRS complex to the first (aortic) vibration of the second heart sound. SYN QS_2 interval.

e•lec•trom•e•ter (ĕ-lek-trom′ĕ-ter) A device for measuring the electromotive force (voltage) of a source of electricity.

e•lec•tro•mo•til•i•ty (ĕ-lek′trō-mō-til′i-tē) The motility of the auditory outer hair cells in response to electrical stimulation.

e•lec•tro•mo•tive force (EMF) (ĕ-lek′trō-mō′tiv fōrs) The force (measured in volts) that causes the flow of electricity from one point to another.

e•lec•tro•my•o•gram (EMG) (ĕ-lek′trō-mī′ō-gram) A graphic representation of the electric currents associated with muscular action.

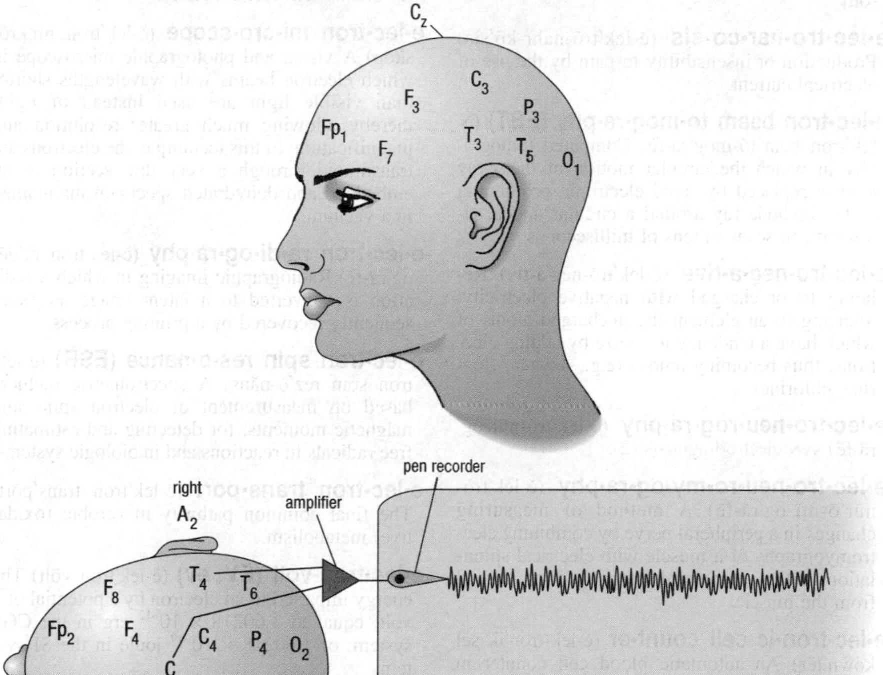

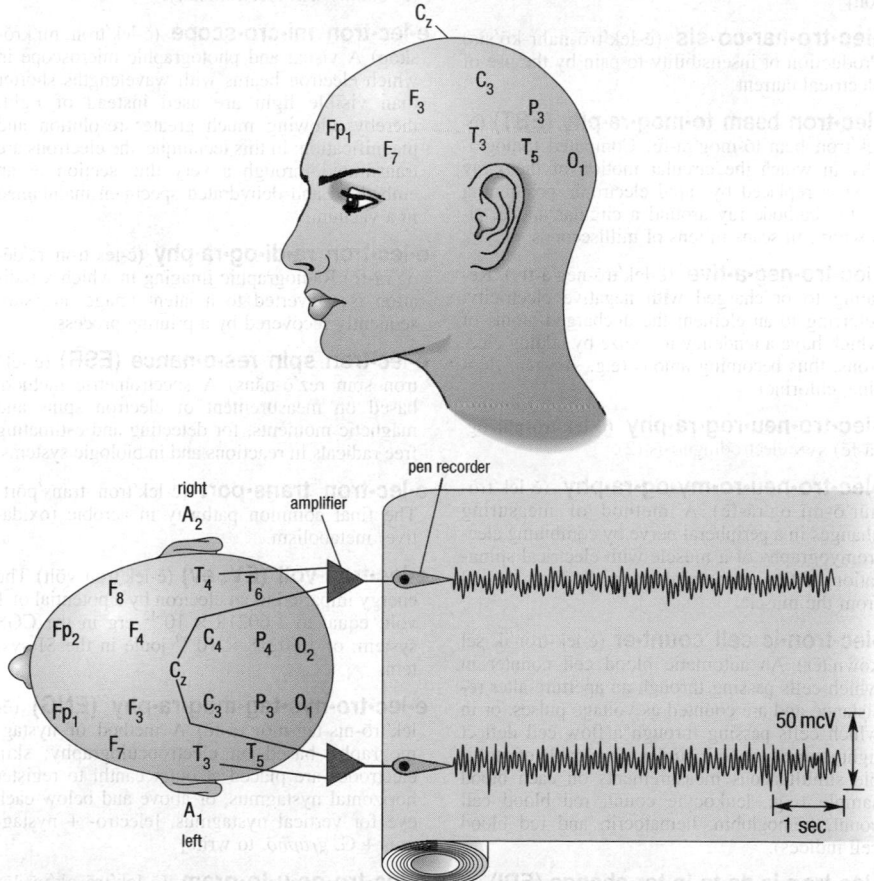

standard positions for the placement of EEG electrodes: A, auricle (or ear); C, central; Cz, vertex; F, frontal; Fp, frontal pole; O, occipital; P, parietal; T, temporal. Wires from pairs of electrodes are fed to amplifiers, and each recording measures voltage differences between two points on the scalp. The output of each amplifier drives a pen recorder or is stored in computer memory

e•lec•tro•my•o•graph (ĕ-lek′trō-mī′ō-graf) An instrument for recording electrical currents generated in an active muscle.

e•lec•tro•my•og•ra•phy (ĕ-lek′trō-mī-og′ră-fē) **1.** The recording of electrical activity generated in muscle for diagnostic purposes; both surface and needle recording electrodes can be used, although characteristically the latter are employed. **2.** Umbrella term for the entire electrodiagnostic study performed in the EMG laboratory, including not only the needle electrode examination, but also nerve conduction studies. [electro- + G. *mys,* muscle, + *graphō,* to write]

e•lec•tron (β–) (ĕ-lek′tron) One of the negatively charged subatomic particles that are distributed about the positive nucleus and with it constitute the atom; in mass they are estimated to be 1/1836.15 of a proton; when emitted from inside the nucleus of a radioactive substance, electrons are called beta particles. [electro- + -on]

e•lec•tro•nar•co•sis (ĕ-lek′trō-nahr-kō′sis) Production of insensibility to pain by the use of electrical current.

e•lec•tron beam to•mog•ra•phy (EBT) (ĕ-lek′tron bēm tō-mog′ră-fē) Computed tomography in which the circular motion of the x-ray tube is replaced by rapid electronic positioning of the cathode ray around a circular anode, allowing full scans in tens of milliseconds.

e•lec•tro•neg•a•tive (ĕ-lek′trō-neg′ă-tiv) Relating to or charged with negative electricity; referring to an element the uncharged atoms of which have a tendency to ionize by adding electrons, thus becoming anions (e.g., oxygen, fluorine, chlorine).

e•lec•tro•neu•rog•ra•phy (ĕ-lek′trō-nūr-og′ră-fē) SYN electrodiagnosis (2).

e•lec•tro•neu•ro•my•og•ra•phy (ĕ-lek′trō-nūr′ō-mī-og′ră-fē) A method of measuring changes in a peripheral nerve by combining electromyography of a muscle with electrical stimulation of the nerve trunk carrying fibers to and from the muscle.

e•lec•tron•ic cell count•er (ĕ-lek-tron′ik sel kown′tĕr) An automatic blood cell counter in which cells passing through an aperture alter resistance and are counted as voltage pulses, or in which cells passing through a flow cell deflect light; some types of counter are capable of multiple simultaneous measurements on each blood sample (e.g., leukocyte count, red blood cell count, hemoglobin, hematocrit, and red blood cell indices).

e•lec•tron•ic da•ta in•ter•change (EDI) (ĕ-lek-tron′ik dā′tă in′tĕr-chānj) In health care information services, provision of patients' data in a format useable to both sender and receiver.

e•lec•tron•ic funds trans•fer (EFT) (ĕ-lek-tron′ik fŭndz trans′fĕr) The automatic deposit of funds from one account to another account; often used in third-party reimbursement to health care providers. SYN automated deposit.

e•lec•tron•ic health re•cord (EHR) (ĕ-lek-tron′ik helth rek′ŏrd) SYN electronic medical record.

e•lec•tron•ic med•i•cal re•cord (EMR) (ĕ-lek-tron′ik med′i-kăl rek′ŏrd) A computerized (i.e., digitized) system for maintaining patient health information that generally includes patient complaints, history of prior illnesses, prior diagnostic testing, and prior medical treatments. Electronic records are used as a substitute for the traditional paper medical record; material is easy to access and update. SYN electronic health record.

e•lec•tron•ic re•mit•tance ad•vice (ERA) (ĕ-lek-tron′ik rē-mit′ăns ad-vīs′) Explanation of payments made by the health insurance company for claims sent electronically.

e•lec•tron mi•cro•scope (ĕ-lek′tron mī′krŏ-skōp) A visual and photographic microscope in which electron beams with wavelengths shorter than visible light are used instead of light, thereby allowing much greater resolution and magnification; in this technique, the electrons are transmitted through a very thin section of an embedded and dehydrated specimen maintained in a vacuum.

e•lec•tron ra•di•og•ra•phy (ĕ-lek′tron rā′dē-og′ră-fē) Radiographic imaging in which x-radiation is converted to a latent image and subsequently recovered by a printing process.

e•lec•tron spin res•o•nance (ESR) (ĕ-lek′tron spin rez′ŏ-năns) A spectrometric method, based on measurement of electron spins and magnetic moments, for detecting and estimating free radicals in reactions and in biologic systems.

e•lec•tron trans•port (ĕ-lek′tron trans′pōrt) The final common pathway in aerobic (oxidative) metabolism.

e•lec•tron-volt (EV, ev) (ĕ-lek′tron vōlt) The energy imparted to an electron by a potential of 1 volt; equal to 1.60218×10^{-12} erg in the CGS system, or 1.60218×10^{-19} joule in the SI system.

e•lec•tro•nys•tag•mog•ra•phy (ENG) (ĕ-lek′trō-nis-tag-mog′ră-fē) A method of nystagmography based on electrooculography; skin electrodes are placed at outer canthi to register horizontal nystagmus, or above and below each eye for vertical nystagmus. [electro- + nystagmus + G. *graphō,* to write]

e•lec•tro•oc•u•lo•gram (ĕ-lek′trō-ok′yū-lō-gram) A record of electric currents in electrooculography.

e•lec•tro•oc•u•log•ra•phy (EOG) (ĕ-lek′trō-ok′yū-log′ră-fē) Oculography in which electrodes placed on the skin adjacent to the eyes measure changes in standing potential between the front and back of the eyeball as the eyes move; a sensitive electrical test for detection of retinal pigment epithelium dysfunction.

e·lec·tro·ol·fac·to·gram (EOG) (ĕ-lek′trō-ōl-fak′tō-gram) An electronegative wave of potential occurring on the surface of the olfactory epithelium in response to stimulation by an odor.

e·lec·tro·pher·o·gram (ĕ-lek′trō-fer′ō-gram) The densitometric or colorimetric pattern obtained from filter paper or similar porous strips on which substances have been separated by electrophoresis; may also refer to the strips themselves. SYN electrophoretogram.

e·lec·tro·phil, **e·lec·tro·phile** (ĕ-lek′trō-fil, -fīl) **1.** The electron-attracting atom or agent in an organic reaction. Cf. nucleophil. **2.** Relating to an electrophil. SYN electrophilic. [electro- + G. *philos,* fond]

e·lec·tro·phil·ic (ĕ-lek′trō-fil′ik) SYN electrophil (2).

e·lec·tro·pho·re·sis (ĕ-lek′trō-fōr-ē′sis) The movement of particles in an electric field toward anode or cathode. SEE ALSO electropherogram. SYN ionophoresis, phoresis (1). [electro- + G. *phorēsis,* a carrying]

e·lec·tro·pho·ret·ic (ĕ-lek′trō-fōr-et′ik) Relating to electrophoresis, as an electrophoretic separation. SYN ionophoretic.

e·lec·tro·pho·ret·o·gram (ĕ-lek′trō-fōr-et′ō-gram) SYN electropherogram.

e·lec·tro·phren·ic res·pi·ra·tion (ĕ-lek′trō-fren′ik res′pir-ā′shŭn) The rhythmic electrical stimulation of the phrenic nerve by an electrode applied to the skin at the motor points of the phrenic nerve; it is used in paralysis of the respiratory center resulting from acute bulbar poliomyelitis.

e·lec·tro·por·a·tion ther·a·py (EPT) (ĕ-lek′trō-pōr-ā′shŭn thār′ă-pē) Investigational therapy involving use of electric fields to open pores in human cells; provides for easier and more efficient entry of genes or pharmaceutical products.

e·lec·tro·ret·i·no·gram (ERG) (ĕ-lek′trō-ret′i-nō-gram) A record of the retinal action currents produced in the retina by an adequate light stimulus. [electro- + retina + G. *gramma,* something written]

e·lec·tro·ret·i·nog·ra·phy (ĕ-lek′trō-ret′i-nog′ră-fē) The recording and study of the retinal action currents.

e·lec·tro·scis·sion (ĕ-lek′trō-sizh′ŭn) Division of tissues by means of an electrocautery knife. [electro- + L. *scissio,* a splitting, fr. *scindo,* to split]

e·lec·tro·shock (ĕ-lek′trō-shok′) SEE electroshock therapy.

e·lec·tro·shock ther·a·py (EST) (ĕ-lek′trō-shok′ thār′ă-pē) A form of treatment of mental disorders in which convulsions are produced by the passage of an electric current through the brain. SYN electroconvulsive therapy.

e·lec·tro·stat·ic bond (ĕ-lek′trō-stat′ik bond) Bond between atoms or groups carrying opposite charges (or, in some cases, partial charges).

e·lec·tro·sur·gery (ĕ-lek′trō-sŭr′jĕr-ē) Division of tissues by high frequency current applied locally with a metal instrument or needle. SEE ALSO electrocautery.

e·lec·tro·tax·is (ĕ-lek′trō-tak′sis) Reaction of plant or animal protoplasm to either an anode or a cathode. SEE ALSO tropism. SYN electrotropism. [electro- + G. *taxis,* orderly arrangement]

e·lec·tro·ther·a·peu·tics, **e·lec·tro·ther·a·py** (ĕ-lek′trō-thār′ă-pyū′tiks, ĕ-lek′trō-thār′ă-pē) Use of electricity in the treatment of disease.

e·lec·tro·ton·ic (ĕ-lek′trō-ton′ik) Relating to electrotonus.

e·lec·trot·o·nus (ĕ-lek-trot′ō-nŭs) Changes in excitability and conductivity in a nerve or muscle cell caused by the passage of a constant electric current. [electro- + G. *tonos,* tension]

e·lec·trot·ro·pism (ĕ-lek-trot′rō-pizm) SYN electrotaxis. [electro- + G. *tropē,* a turning]

e·lec·tro·vi·bra·to·ry mas·sage (ĕ-lek′trō-vī′bră-tōr-ē mă-sazh′) Use of an electronic vibrating device in massage.

e·le·i·din (ĕ-lē′i-din) A refractile and weakly staining keratin present in the cells of the stratum lucidum of the palmar and plantar epidermis.

el·e·ment (el′ĕ-mĕnt) **1.** A substance composed of atoms of only one kind, i.e., of identical atomic (proton) number, which therefore cannot be decomposed into two or more elements, and which can lose its chemical properties only by union with some other element or by a nuclear reaction changing the proton number. **2.** An indivisible structure or entity. **3.** A functional entity, frequently exogenous, within a bacterium, such as an extrachromosomal element. [L. *elementum,* a rudiment, beginning]

el·e·men·ta·ry gran·ule (el′ĕ-men′tăr-ē gran′yūl) A particle of blood dust, or hemoconia.

el·e·men·ta·ry par·ti·cle (el′ĕ-men′tăr-ē pahr′ti-kĕl) **1.** SYN platelet. **2.** One of the units occurring on the matrical surface of mitochondrial cristae; the particles may be concerned with the electron transport system.

♲ **eleo-** Prefix meaning oil. SEE ALSO oleo-. [G. *elaion,* olive oil]

el·e·phan·ti·ac, **el·e·phan·ti·as·ic** (el′ĕ-fan′tē-ak, el′ă-fan′tē-as′ik) Relating to elephantiasis.

el·e·phan·ti·a·sis (el′ĕ-fan-tī′ă-sis) Hypertrophy and fibrosis of the skin and subcutaneous tissue, especially of the lower extremities and genitalia, caused by long-standing obstruction of lymphatic vessels, most commonly after years of infection by the filarial worms *Wuchereria bancrofti* or *Brugia malayi*, coupled with secondary bacterial infection alone or combined with a fungal infection. See this page, B8. [G. fr. *elephas*, elephant]

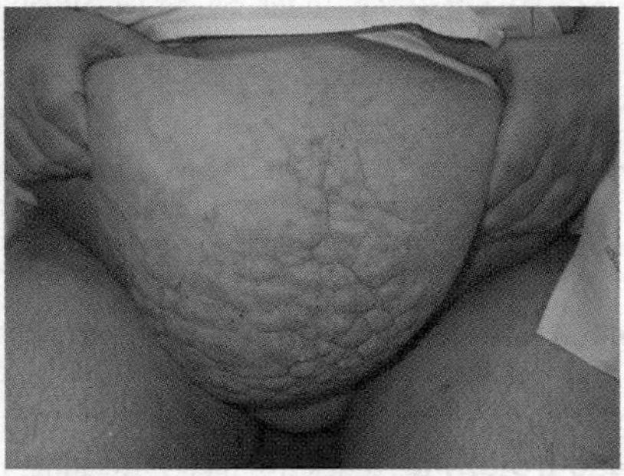

elephantiasis

el•e•phan•ti•a•sis scro•ti (el′ĕ-fan-tī′ă-sis skro′tī) Brawny swelling of the scrotum as a result of chronic lymphatic obstruction. SYN chyloderma.

el•e•phant man dis•ease (el′ĕ-fănt man di-zēz′) **1.** SYN Proteus syndrome. **2.** SYN neurofibromatosis.

el•e•phan•toid fe•ver (el′ĕ-fan′toyd fē′vĕr) Lymphangitis and fever marking the beginning of endemic elephantiasis (filariasis).

el•e•va•tion (el′ĕ-vā′shŭn) SYN torus (2).

el•e•va•tion res•o•lu•tion (el′e-vā′shŭn rez′ō-lū′shŭn) SYN azimuth resolution.

el•e•va•tor (el′ĕ-vā-tŏr) **1.** An instrument for prying up a sunken part, such as the depressed fragment of bone in fracture of the skull, or for elevating tissues. **2.** A surgical instrument used to luxate and remove teeth and roots that cannot be engaged by the beaks of a forceps, or to loosen teeth and roots prior to forceps application. [L. fr. *elevo*, pp. *-atus*, to lift up]

el•e•va•tor mus•cle of rib (el′ĕ-vā-tŏr mŭs′ĕl rib) SYN levator costarum muscles.

el•e•va•tor mus•cle of scap•u•la (el′ĕ-vā-tŏr mŭs′ĕl skap′yū-lă) SYN levator scapulae muscle.

el•e•va•tor mus•cle of soft pal•ate (el′ĕ-vā-tŏr mŭs′ĕl sawft pal′ăt) SYN levator veli palatini muscle.

el•e•va•tor mus•cle of up•per eye•lid (el′ĕ-vā-tŏr mŭs′ĕl ŭp′ĕr ī′lid) SYN levator palpebrae superioris muscle.

e•lev•enth cra•ni•al nerve [CN XI] (ĕ-lev′ĕnth krā′nē-ăl nĕrv) SYN accessory nerve [CN XI].

el•fin fa•cies syn•drome (el′fin fash′ē-ēz sin′drōm) SYN Williams syndrome.

e•lim•i•na•tion (ĕ-lim′i-nā′shŭn) Expulsion; removal of waste material from the body; the getting rid of anything. [L. *elimino*, pp. *-atus*, to turn out of doors, fr. *limen*, threshold]

e•lim•i•na•tion di•et (ĕ-lim′i-nā′shŭn dī′ĕt) A diet designed to detect which component of the diet causes allergic manifestations in the patient; food items to which the patient may be sensitive are withdrawn separately and successively from the diet until that which causes the symptoms is discovered.

ELISA (e-lē′să) Abbreviation for enzyme-linked immunosorbent assay.

elix. Abbreviation for elixir.

e•lix•ir (elix.) (ĕ-lik′sĭr) A clear, sweetened, hydroalcoholic liquid intended for oral use; elixirs contain flavoring substances and are used either as vehicles or for the therapeutic effect of the active medicinal agents. [Mediev. L., fr. Ar. *al-iksir*, the philosopher's stone]

El•li•ot op•er•a•tion (el′ē-ŏt op-ĕr-ā′shŭn) Trephining of the eyeball at the corneoscleral margin to relieve tension in glaucoma.

El•li•ot po•si•tion (el′ē-ŏt pŏ-zish′ŏn) A supine position on a double inclined plane or on a single inclined plane, with a cushion under the back at the level of the liver; used to facilitate abdominal section.

El•li•ott law (el′ē-ŏt law) Adrenaline acts on those structures innervated by sympathetic nerve fibers.

el•lip•soid joint (ē-lip′soyd joynt) A modified ball-and-socket synovial joint in which the joint surfaces are elongated or ellipsoid; it is a biaxial joint, i.e., having two axes of motion at right angles to each other. SYN condylar joint.

el•lip•tic am•pu•ta•tion (ē-lip′tik amp′yū-tā′shŭn) Circular amputation in which the sweep of the knife is not exactly vertical to the axis of the limb, the outline of the cut surface being therefore elliptic.

el•lip•to•cyte (ē-lip′tō-sīt) An elliptic red blood corpuscle found normally in the lower vertebrates with the exception of Cyclostomata; in mammals it normally occurs only in camels, hence cameloid cell. See page B3. SYN ovalocyte. [G. *elleipsis*, a leaving out, an ellipse, + *kytos*, cell]

el•lip•to•cy•to•sis (ē-lip′tō-sī-tō′sis) A hereditary abnormality of hemopoiesis in which 50–90% of the red blood cells consist of rod forms and elliptocytes, often with an associated hemolytic anemia. SYN ovalocytosis.

El•oes•ser flap (el-es′ĕr flap) A surgically created open skin-lined tract for chronic drainage of an empyema, often following pneumonectomy.

e•lon•ga•tion (ē-lon-gā′shŭn) RADIOLOGY radiographic distortion in which the image appears longer than it is; caused by insufficient vertical angulation.

e•lon•ga•tion fac•tor (ē-lon-gā′shŭn fak′tŏr) Proteins that catalyze the elongation of peptide chains during protein biosynthesis. SYN transfer factor (3).

Els•berg syn•drome (els′bĕrg sin′drōm) Acute urinary retention due to neurologic dysfunction in association with genital herpes.

El•schnig spots (elsh′nig spots) Isolated choroidal bright yellow or red spots with black pigment flecks at their borders, seen ophthalmoscopically in advanced hypertensive retinopathy.

el•u•ant (el′yū-ănt) The material that has been eluted.

el•u•ate (el′yū-āt) The solution emerging from a column or paper in chromatography. SEE ALSO elution.

el•u•ent (el′yū-ĕnt) The mobile phase in chromatography. SEE ALSO elution. SYN developer (2).

e•lute (ē-lūt′) To perform or accomplish an elution.

e•lu•tion (ē-lū′shŭn) **1.** The separation, by washing, of one solid from another. **2.** The removal, by means of a suitable solvent, of one material from another that is insoluble in that solvent, as in column chromatography. **3.** The removal of antibodies absorbed onto the erythrocyte surface. [L. *eluo,* pp. *lutus,* to wash out]

E•ly sign (ē′lī sīn) Indicator of femoral nerve irritation, lateral thigh contracture, or tightness of the rectus femoris muscle if the patient, when prone, flexes the calf onto the thigh and the gluteus muscles retract and the hip abducts.

♻ **elytro-** Prefix meaning the vagina. SEE ALSO colpo-, vagino-. [G. *elytron,* sheath (vagina)]

E/M Abbreviation for evaluation and management.

♻ **em-** SEE en-.

EMA Abbreviation for epithelial membrane antigen.

e•ma•ci•a•tion (ĕ-mā′shē-ā′shŭn) Abnormal thinness resulting from extreme loss of flesh. SYN wasting (1). [L. *emacio*, pp. *-atus,* to make thin]

em•a•na•tion (em′ă-nā′shŭn) **1.** Any substance that flows out or is emitted from a source or origin. **2.** The radiation from a radioactive element. [L. *e- mano,* pp. *-atus,* to flow out]

e•man•ci•pat•ed mi•nor (ē-man′si-pā-tĕd mī′nŏr) A young person who is legally entitled to be treated as an adult through a court order, marriage, military service, or being a parent.

e•mas•cu•la•tion (ē-mas′kyū-lā′shŭn) Castration of the male by removal of the testes and/or penis. [L. *emasculo,* pp. *-atus,* to castrate, fr. *e-* priv. + *masculus,* masculine]

EMB Abbreviation for eosin-methylene blue. SEE eosin-methylene blue agar.

em•balm (em-bahlm′) To treat a dead body with chemicals to preserve it from decay. [L. *in,* in, + *balsamum,* balsam]

Emb•den-Mey•er•hof path•way (em′dĕn mī′ĕr-hof path′wā) The anaerobic glycolytic pathway by which D-glucose (most notably in muscle) is converted to lactic acid. Cf. glycolysis.

em•bo•le (em′bō-lē) **1.** Reduction of a limb dislocation. **2.** Formation of the gastrula by invagination. SYN emboly. [G. *embolē,* insertion]

em•bo•lec•to•my (em′bō-lek′tŏ-mē) Removal of an embolus. [G. *embolos,* a plug (embolus), + *ektomē,* excision]

em•bo•li (em′bō-lī) Plural of embolus.

em•bol•ic (em-bol′ik) Relating to an embolus or to embolism.

em•bol•i•form nu•cle•us (em-bol′i-fōrm nū′klē-ŭs) A small wedge-shaped nucleus in the central white substance of the cerebellum just internal to the hilus of the dentate nucleus; receives axons of Purkinje cells of the intermediate area of the cerebellar cortex; axons of these cells exit the cerebellum through the superior cerebellar peduncle. SYN embolus (2).

embolisation [Br.] SYN embolization.

🛈 **em•bo•lism** (em′bŏ-lizm) Obstruction or occlusion of a vessel by an embolus. See page 498. [G. *embolisma,* a piece or patch; lit. something thrust in]

em•bo•li•za•tion (em′bol-ī-zā′shŭn) **1.** The formation and release of an embolus into the circulation. **2.** Therapeutic introduction of various substances into the circulation to occlude vessels, either to arrest or prevent hemorrhaging or to devitalize a structure or organ by occluding its blood supply. SYN embolisation.

em•bo•lo•la•li•a, em•bo•lo•phra•si•a (em′bō-lō-lā′lē-ă, em′bō-lō-frā′zē-ă) Interjection of meaningless words into a sentence when speaking. [G. *embolos,* something thrown in, fr. *emballo,* to throw in, + *lalia,* speaking]

em•bo•lo•ther•a•py (em′bō-lō-thār′ă-pē) Occlusion of arteries by insertion of blood clots, coils, or balloons using an angiographic catheter; used to control inoperable hemorrhage or to provide preoperative management of highly vascular neoplasms. [G. *embolos,* plug, + *therapeia,* medical treatment]

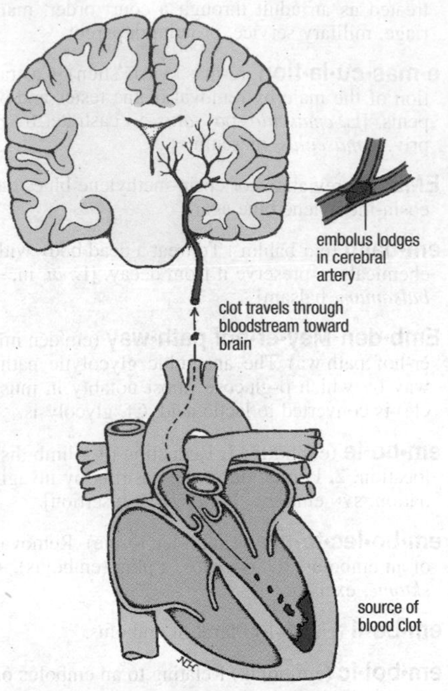

cerebral embolism (embolus arising from a mural thrombus of the left ventricle)

em•bo•lus, pl. **em•bo•li** (em′bō-lŭs, -lī) **1.** A plug, composed of a detached thrombus or vegetation, mass of bacteria, quantity of air or gas or foreign body, which occludes a vessel. **2.** SYN emboliform nucleus. [G. *embolos,* a plug, wedge or stopper]

em•bo•ly (em′bō-lē) SYN embole (2).

em•bra•sure (em-brā′shŭr) DENTISTRY an opening that widens outwardly or inwardly; specifically, that space adjacent to the interproximal contact area that spreads toward the facial, gingival, lingual, occlusal, or incisal aspect. [Fr. an opening in a wall for cannon]

em•bry•o (em′brē-ō) **1.** An organism in the early stages of development. **2.** In humans, the developing organism from conception until the end of the eighth week; developmental stages from this time to birth are commonly designated as fetal. **3.** A primordial plant within a seed. See page B1, B21. [G. *embryon,* fr. *en,* in, + *bryō,* to be full, swell]

embryo- Prefix denoting related to the embryo. [G. *embryon,* a young one]

em•bry•o•blast (em′brē-ō-blast) The cells at the embryonic pole of the blastocyst concerned with formation of the embryo *per se*. SYN inner cell mass. [embryo- + G. *blastos,* germ]

em•bry•o•car•di•a (em′brē-ō-kahr′dē-ă) A condition in which the cadence of the heart sounds resembles that of the fetus, the first and second sounds becoming alike and evenly spaced; a sign of serious myocardial disease. [embryo- + G. *kardia,* heart]

em•bry•o•gen•e•sis (em′brē-ō-jen′ĕ-sis) That phase of prenatal development involved in establishment of the characteristic configuration of the embryo; in humans, embryogenesis is usually regarded as extending from the end of the second week, when the embryonic disc is formed, to the end of the eighth week, after which the conceptus is usually called a fetus. [embryo- + G. *genesis,* origin]

em•bry•o•gen•ic, **em•bry•o•ge•net•ic** (em′brē-ō-jen′ik, -jĕ-net′ik) Producing an embryo; relating to the formation of an embryo.

em•bry•og•e•ny (em′brē-oj′ĕ-nē) The origin and growth of an embryo.

em•bry•ol•o•gist (em′brē-ol′ŏ-jist) One who specializes in embryology.

em•bry•ol•o•gy (em′brē-ol′ŏ-jē) Science of the origin and development of the organism from fertilization of the oocyte to the end of the eighth week and, by extension, all subsequent stages up to birth. See page B1. [embryo- + G. *logos,* study]

em•bry•o•ma (em′brē-ō′mă) SYN embryonal tumor.

em•bry•o•nal (em′brē-ōn′ăl) Relating to an embryo.

em•bry•o•nal ar•e•a, **em•bry•on•ic ar•e•a** (em′brē-ōn′ăl ār′ē-ă, em′brē-on′ik) The area of the blastoderm on either side of, and immediately cephalic to, the primitive streak where the component cell layers have become thickened.

em•bry•o•nal car•ci•no•ma (em′brē-ōn′ăl kahr′si-nō′mă) A malignant neoplasm of the testis, composed of large anaplastic cells with indistinct cellular borders; embryonal carcinomas may be malignant teratomas without differentiated elements.

em•bry•o•nal leu•ke•mi•a (em′brē-ōn′ăl lū-kē′mē-ă) SYN stem cell leukemia.

em•bry•o•nal me•dul•lo•ep•i•the•li•o•ma (em′brē-ōn′ăl mĕ-dŭl′ō-ep′i-thē-lē-ō′mă) SYN dictyoma.

em•bry•o•nal rhab•do•my•o•sar•co•mas (em′brē-ōn′ăl rab′dō-mī′ō-sahr-kō′măz) Malignant neoplasms occurring in children, consisting of loose, spindle-celled tissue with rare cross-striations, and arising in many parts of the body in addition to skeletal muscles.

em•bry•o•nal tu•mor, **em•bry•on•ic tu•mor** (em′brē-ōn′ăl tū′mŏr, em′brē-on′ik) A neoplasm, usually malignant, which arises during intrauterine or early postnatal development from an organ rudiment or immature tissue. It forms immature structures characteristic of the part from which it arises and may form other tissues as well. The term includes neuroblastoma and Wilms tumor and is also used to include certain neoplasms presenting in later life, this usage being based on the belief that such tumors arise from embryonic rests, which are fragments of embryonic tissue that are still present after the embryonic period. SEE ALSO teratoma. SYN embryoma.

em•bry•on•ic mem•brane (em′brē-on′ik mem′brān) SYN fetal membrane.

em•bry•on•ic pole (em′brē-on′ik pōl) The area of contact between the embryoblast and the overlying polar trophoblast of the blastocyst.

em•bry•on•ic shield (em′brē-on′ik shēld) A thickened area of the embryonic blastoderm from which the embryo develops.

em•bry•on•i•za•tion (em′brē-ŏn-ī-zā′shŭn) Reversion of a cell or tissue to an embryonic form.

em•bry•o•noid (em′brē-ō-noyd) Resembling an embryo or a fetus. [embryo- + G. *eidos,* appearance]

em•bry•o•ny (em′brē-ō-nē) The forming of an embryo.

em•bry•o•path•ic cat•a•ract (em′brē-ō-path′ ik kat′ăr-akt) Congenital cataract as a result of intrauterine infection, e.g., by the rubella virus.

em•bry•op•a•thy (em′brē-op′ă-thē) A morbid condition in the embryo or fetus. SYN fetopathy. [embryo- + G. *pathos,* disease]

em•bry•o•plas•tic (em′brē-ō-plas′tik) **1.** Producing an embryo. **2.** Relating to the formation of an embryo. [embryo- + G. *plassō,* to form]

em•bry•ot•o•my (em′brē-ot′ŏ-mē) Any mutilating operation on the fetus to make possible its removal when delivery is impossible by natural means. [embryo- + G. *tomē,* cutting]

em•bry•o•tox•ic•i•ty (em′brē-ō-tok-sis′i-tē) Injury to the embryo, which may result in death or abnormal development of a part, owing to substances that enter the placental circulation.

em•bry•o•tox•on (em′brē-ō-tok′son) Congenital opacity of the periphery of the cornea, caused by thickening and anterior displacement of the Schwalbe line. SYN Axenfeld anomaly. [embryo- + G. *toxon,* bow]

em•bry•o•troph (em′brē-ō-trōf) **1.** Nutritive material supplied to the embryo during development. Cf. hemotroph. **2.** In the implantation stages of deciduate placental mammals (e.g., humans), fluid adjacent to the blastocyst; a mixture of the secretion of the uterine glands, cellular debris resulting from the trophoblastic invasion of the endometrium, and exuded plasma.

em•bry•o•tro•phic (em′brē-ō-trō′fik) Relating to any process or agency involved in the nourishment of the embryo.

em•bry•ot•ro•phy (em′brē-ot′rŏ-fē) The nutrition of the embryo. [embryo- + G. *trophē,* nourishment]

E&M codes (kōdz) Abbreviation for Evaluation and Management codes.

e•med•ul•late (ē-med′yū-lāt) To extract any marrow. [L. *e-,* from, + *medulla,* marrow]

e•mei•o•cy•to•sis (ē′mē-ō-sī-tō′sis) SYN exocytosis (2). [L. *emitto,* to send forth, + G. *kytos,* cell, + *-osis,* condition]

e•mer•gence (ē-mĕr′jĕns) **1.** A stage in recovery from general anesthesia that includes a return to spontaneous breathing, voluntary swallowing, and normal consciousness. **2.** In microbiology, the appearance and identification of new microorganisms or strains of previously identified species. [L. *emergo,* arise, come forth]

e•mer•gen•cy con•tra•cep•tive (ē-mĕr′jĕn-sē kon′tră-sep′tiv) SYN morning after pill.

e•mer•gen•cy de•part•ment (ē-mĕr′jĕn′sē dĕ-pahrt′mĕnt) That section of a hospital or other health care facility that is designed, staffed, and equippped to treat injured people and those afflicted with sudden, severe illness. SYN emergency room.

e•mer•gen•cy doc•trine (ē-mĕr′jĕn-sē dok′ trin) In medical jurisprudence, an assumption that a disabled or nonresponsive patient will agree to life-saving measures. SYN implied consent (1).

e•mer•gen•cy hor•mo•nal con•tra•cep•tion (ē-mĕr′jĕn-sē hōr-mō′năl kon′tră sep′shŭn) SYN morning after pill.

e•mer•gen•cy med•i•cal ser•vices (EMS) (ē-mĕr′jĕn-sē med′i-kăl sĕr′vis-ĕz) An agency that provides prehospital care and transport to the sick and wounded. SYN ambulance service, emergency medical service system.

e•mer•gen•cy med•i•cal ser•vice sys•tem (EMSS) (ē-mĕr′jĕn-sē med′i-kăl sĕr′vis sis′tĕm) SYN emergency medical services.

e•mer•gen•cy med•i•cal tech•ni•cian (ē-mĕr′jĕn-sē med′i-kăl tek-nish′ăn) SYN prehospital provider.

e•mer•gen•cy med•i•cal tech•ni•cian–ba•sic (EMT-B) (ē-mĕr′jĕn-sē med′i-kăl tek-nish′ ăn-bā′sik) A certified prehospital provider who can perform basic life support (BLS); uses assessment-based approach to patient management. Minimum level of certification required to staff a BLS ambulance. SEE ALSO basic life support.

e•mer•gen•cy med•i•cal tech•ni•cian–in•ter•me•di•ate (EMT-I) (ē-mĕr′jĕn-sē med′i-kăl tek-nish′ăn-in′tĕr-mē′dē-ăt) A certified prehospital provider who can perform intermediate-level advanced life support (ALS); usually works under direct medical control. Minimum level of certification required to staff an ALS ambulance. SEE ALSO advanced cardiac life support. SYN cardiac care technician, cardiac rescue technician.

e•mer•gen•cy med•i•cal tech•ni•cian–par•a•med•ic (EMT-P) (ē-mĕr′jĕn-sē med′i-kăl tek-nish′ăn-par′ă-med′ik) A licensed prehospital provider who can perform all aspects of advanced life support; usually works according to standing orders or protocols and uses a diagnostic approach to patient management. SEE ALSO prehospital provider.

e•mer•gen•cy med•i•cine (ē-mĕr′jĕn-sē med′i-sin) That branch of health care involved with remediation or therapy of patients who are acutely ill or traumatized.

e•mer•gen•cy nurse prac•ti•tion•er (ENP) (ē-mĕr′jĕn-sē nŭrs prak-tish′ŏn-ĕr) Nurse practicing in an emergency department who is specifically trained to deal with minor injuries without the need for supervision by a physician.

e•mer•gen•cy room (ē-mĕr′jĕn-sē rūm) SYN emergency department.

e•mer•gen•cy sur•ger•y (ē-mĕr′jĕn-sē sŭr′jĕr-ē) Previously unanticipated surgery carried out in response to a sudden condition that may threaten a patient's well-being.

e•mer•gen•cy the•o•ry (ē-mĕr′jĕn-sē thē′ŏr-ē) A theory of the emotions, advanced by W.B. Cannon, that animal and human organisms respond to emergency situations by increased sympathetic nervous system activity including an increased catecholamine production with associated increases in blood pressure, heart and respiratory rates, and skeletal muscle blood flow.

e•mer•gent (ē-mĕr′jĕnt) **1.** Arising suddenly and unexpectedly, calling for quick judgment and prompt action. **2.** Coming out; leaving a cavity or other part.

em•e•sis (em′ĕ-sis) **1.** SYN vomiting. **2.** Combining form, used in the suffix position, for vomiting. [G. fr. *emeō,* to vomit]

♻ **-emesis** Suffix denoting vomiting, vomitus.

em•e•sis ba•sin (em′ĕ-sis bā′sin) A kidney-shaped container, usually plastic, intended to catch vomitus at the bedside.

em•e•sis grav•i•da•rum (em′ĕ-sis grav′i-dā′rŭm) Vomiting due to pregnancy.

e•met•ic (ĕ-met′ik) **1.** Relating to or causing vomiting. **2.** An agent that causes vomiting. [G. *emetikos,* producing vomiting, fr. *emeō,* to vomit]

em•e•to•ca•thar•tic (em′ĕ-tō-kă-thahr′tik) **1.** Both emetic and cathartic. **2.** An agent that causes both vomiting and purging.

EMF Abbreviation for electromotive force.

EMG Abbreviation for electromyogram.

EMG bi•o•feed•back (bī′ō-fēd′bak) A form of biofeedback that uses an electromyographic measure of muscle tension as the physical symptom to be deconditioned, such as tension in the frontalis muscle in the head that can cause headaches.

♻ **-emia** Suffix meaning blood. SYN -aemia. [G. *haima*]

em•i•gra•tion (em-i-grā′shŭn) The passage of white blood cells through the endothelium and wall of small blood vessels. [L. *emigro,* pp. *-atus,* to emigrate]

em•i•nence (em′i-nĕns) A circumscribed area raised above the general level of the surrounding surface, particularly on a bone surface. SYN eminentia [TA]. [L. *eminentia*]

em•i•nen•ti•a, pl. **em•i•nen•ti•ae** (em-i-nen′shē-ă, -shē-ē) [TA] SYN eminence. [L. prominence, fr. *emineo,* to stand out, project]

em•i•nen•ti•a py•ra•mi•da•lis (em-i-nen′shē-ă pi-ram-i-dā′lis) [TA] A conic projection posterior to the vestibular window in the middle ear; it is hollow and contains the stapedius muscle.

em•i•o•cy•to•sis (ē′mē-ō-sī-tō′sis) SYN exocytosis (2). [L. *emitto,* to send forth, + G. *kytos,* cell, + *-osis,* condition]

em•is•sar•y (em′i-sar-ē) **1.** Relating to, or providing, an outlet or drain. **2.** SYN emissary vein. [see emissarium]

em•is•sar•y vein (em′i-sar-ē vān) One of the channels of communication between the venous sinuses of the dura mater and the veins of the diploë and the scalp. SYN emissary (2).

e•mis•sion (ē-mish′ŭn) A discharge; referring usually to a discharge of the male internal genital organs into the internal urethra; the contents of the organs, including sperm cells, prostatic fluid, and seminal vesicle fluid, mix in the internal urethra with mucus from the bulbourethral glands to form semen. [L. *emissio,* fr. *e- mitto,* to send out]

EMIT (ē-mit′) Abbreviation for enzyme-multiplied immunoassay technique.

em•men•i•a (ĕ-men′ē-ă) SYN menses. [G. *emmēnos,* monthly]

em•men•ic (ĕ-men′ik) SYN menstrual.

em•men•i•op•a•thy (ĕ-men′ē-op′ă-thē) Any disorder of menstruation. [G. *emmēnos,* monthly, + *pathos,* suffering]

Em•met nee•dle (em′ĕt nē′dĕl) A strong needle with the eye in the point, having a wide curve, and set in a handle, used to pass a ligature around an undissected structure.

Em•met op•er•a•tion (em′ĕt op-ĕr-ā′shŭn) SYN trachelorrhaphy.

em•me•tro•pi•a (em′eĕ-trō′pē-ă) The state of refraction of the eye in which parallel rays, when the eye is at rest, are focused exactly on the retina. [G. *emmetros,* according to measure, + *ōps,* eye]

em•me•tro•pic (em′ĕ-trō′pik) Pertaining to or characterized by emmetropia.

Em•mon•si•a par•va* var. *cres•cens (em-on′sē-ă pahr′vă kres′enz) The main fungal species causing adiaspiromycosis in animals and the only agent of human adiaspiromycosis; infection is acquired by inhaling conidia from the fungus growing in soil. Also known as chrysosporium.

Em•mon•si•a par•va* var. *par•va (em-on′sē-ă pahr′vă pahr′vă) A fungal species causing adiaspiromycosis in animals.

e•mol•li•ent (ē-mol′ē-ent) **1.** Soothing to the skin or mucous membrane. **2.** An agent that softens the skin or soothes irritation in the skin or mucous membrane. [L. *emolliens,* pres. p. of *emollio,* to soften]

e•mol•li•ent en•e•ma (ē-mol′ē-ĕnt en′ĕ-mă) SYN oil retention enema.

e•mo•tion (ē-mō′shŭn) A strong feeling, aroused mental state, or intense state of drive or unrest directed toward a definite object and evidenced in both behavior and in psychologic changes, with accompanying autonomic nervous system manifestations. [L. *emoveo,* pp. *-motus,* to move out, agitate]

e•mo•tion•al (ē-mō′shŭn-ăl) Relating to or marked by an emotion.

e•mo•tion•al dep•ri•va•tion (ē-mō′shŭn-ăl dep′ri-vā′shŭn) Lack of adequate and appropriate interpersonal or environmental experiences, or both, usually in the early developmental years.

e•mo•tion•al dis•or•der (ē-mō′shŭn-ăl dis-ōr′dĕr) SEE mental illness, behavior disorder.

em•path•ic (em-path′ik) Relating to or marked by empathy.

em•pa•thize (em′pă-thīz) To feel empathy in relation to another person; to put oneself in another's place.

em•pa•thy (em′pă-thē) **1.** The ability to sense the emotions, feelings, and reactions intellectually and emotionally that another person is experiencing and to communicate that understanding to the person effectively. Cf. sympathy (3). **2.** The anthropomorphization or humanizing of objects and the feeling of oneself as being in and part of them. [G. *en* (*em*), in, + *pathos,* feeling]

i **em•phy•se•ma** (em′fi-sē′mă) **1.** Presence of air in the interstices of the connective tissue of a part. **2.** A condition of the lung characterized by increase beyond the normal in the size of air spaces distal to the terminal bronchiole (those parts containing alveoli), with destructive changes in their walls and reduction in their number. Clinical manifestation is breathlessness on exertion, due to the combined effect (in varying degrees) of reduction of alveolar surface for gas exchange and collapse of smaller airways with trapping of alveolar gas in expiration; this causes the chest to be held in the position of inspiration ("barrel chest"), with prolonged expiration and increased residual volume. Symptoms of chronic bronchitis often, but not necessarily, coexist. Two structural varieties are panlobular (panacinar) emphysema and centrilobular (centriacinar) emphysema; paracicatricial, paraseptal, and bullous emphysema are also common. SYN pulmonary emphysema. See page 502. [G. inflation of stomach, etc. fr. *en,* in, + *physēma,* a blowing, fr. *physa,* bellows]

em•phy•sem•a•tous (em′fi-sem′ă-tŭs) Relating to or affected with emphysema.

em•pir•ic (em-pir′ik) **1.** Founded on practical experience, rather than on reasoning alone, but not proved scientifically, in contrast to rational (1). **2.** Based on careful observational testing of a hypothesis; rational. [G. *empeirikos;* fr. *empeiria,* experience, fr. *en,* in, + *peira,* a trial]

em•pir•ic for•mu•la (em-pir′ik fōrm′yū-lă) CHEMISTRY a formula indicating the kind and number of atoms in the molecules of a substance, or its composition, but not the relation of the atoms to each other or the intimate structure of the molecule.

em•pir•ic hor•op•ter (em-pir′ik hōr-op′tĕr) An experimentally determined ellipse passing through the optic centers of two eyes by which points adjacent to the point of fixation, both lying on the ellipse, are perceived to be stimulating corresponding retinal points.

em•pir•ic risk (em-pir′ik risk) Risk that is based on empiric evidence alone, without any appeal to formal theory or surmise.

em•pir•ic treat•ment (em-pir′ik trēt′mĕnt) Therapy based on practical experience, rather than theoretic postulates.

em•ploy•ee as•sis•tance pro•gram (EAP) (em-ploy′ē ă-sis′tăns prō′gram) A means established to help workers overcome psychosocial or behavioral problems that impair work performance.

em•ploy•er i•den•ti•fi•ca•tion num•ber (EIN) (em-ploy′ĕr ī-dent′i-fi-kā′shŭn nŭm′bĕr) A numeric specifier obtained from the government for identification of business/employer tax information; often it is the patient's social security number.

em•por•i•at•rics (em-pōr′ē-at′riks) The specialty of travel medicine, dealing with diseases that travelers can acquire, especially in the trop-

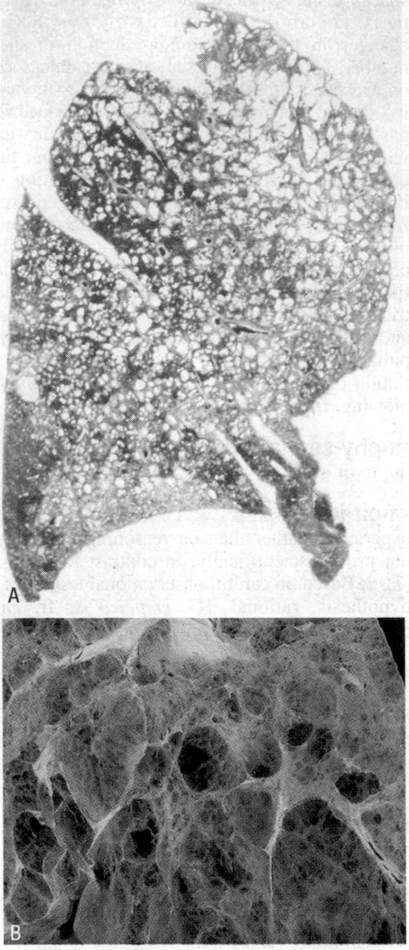

panlobular emphysema: (A) left lung from patient with severe emphysema reveals widespread destruction of pulmonary parenchyma; (B) lung from patient with α1-antitrypsin deficiency shows panacinar pattern of emphysema; loss of alveolar walls has resulted in markedly enlarged air spaces

ics. [G. *emporion,* market, fr. *emporos,* traveler, merchant, + *(technē) iatrikē,* medical art]

em•pros•thot•o•nos (em′pros-thot′ŏ-nŭs) A tetanic contraction of the flexor muscles, curving the back with concavity forward. [G. *emprosthen,* forward, + *tonos,* tension]

em•py•e•ma (em′pī-ē′mă) Pus in a body cavity; when used without qualification, refers specifically to pyothorax. [G. *empyēma,* suppuration, fr. *en,* in, + *pyon,* pus]

em•py•e•mic (em′pī-ē′mik) Relating to empyema.

em•py•e•sis (em′pī-ē′sis) A pustular eruption. [G. suppuration]

EMR Abbreviation for electronic medical record.

EMS Abbreviation for emergency medical services.

EMSS Abbreviation for emergency medical service system.

EMT-B Abbreviation for emergency medical technician–basic.

EMT-I Abbreviation for emergency medical technician–intermediate.

EMT-P Abbreviation for emergency medical technician–paramedic.

e•mul•si•fi•er (ē-mŭl′si-fī-ĕr) An agent (e.g., gum arabic or egg yolk), used to make an emulsion of a fixed oil. Soaps, detergents, steroids, and proteins can act as emulsifiers.

e•mul•si•fy (ē-mul′si-fī) To produce an emulsion by dispersing one fluid, in the form of small globules, in another fluid. SEE ALSO cardiomyopathy, ejection period, sphygmic interval, emulsion, emulsifier.

e•mul•sion (ē-mŭl′shŭn) A system containing two immiscible liquids in which one is dispersed, in the form of very small globules (internal phase), throughout the other (external phase). [Mod. L. fr. *e-mulgeo,* pp. *-mulsus,* to milk or drain out]

e•mul•soid (ē-mŭl′soyd) A colloidal dispersion in which the dispersed particles are more or less liquid and exert a certain attraction on and absorb a certain quantity of the fluid in which they are suspended.

♻**en-** Prefix meaning in; appears as em- before b, p, or m. [G.]

e•nam•el (ĕ-nam′ĕl) The hard, acellular, inert substance covering the tooth. In its mature form, it is composed of an inorganic portion made up of 90% hydroxyapatite and 6–8% calcium carbonate, calcium fluoride, and magnesium carbonate, the remainder consisting of an organic matrix of protein and glycoprotein; structurally, it is made up of oriented rods each of which consists of a stack of rodlets encased in an organic prism sheath. [M.E., fr. Fr. *enamailer,* to apply enamel, fr. *en,* on, + *amail,* enamel, fr. Germanic]

e•nam•el cap (ĕ-nam′ĕl kap) The enamel covering the crown of a tooth.

e•nam•el crypt (ĕ-nam′ĕl kript) The narrow, mesenchyme-filled space between the dental ledge and an enamel organ.

e•nam•el germ (ĕ-nam′ĕl jĕrm) The enamel organ of a developing tooth; one of a series of knoblike projections from the dental lamina, later becoming bell-shaped and receiving the dental papilla in its hollow.

e•nam•el hy•po•cal•ci•fi•ca•tion (ĕ-nam′ĕl hī′pō-kal′si-fi-kā′shŭn) A disturbance in the maturation of enamel due to improper calcification of the enamel matrix, resulting in the appearance of chalky, smooth surfaces on the crown. SEE ALSO enamel hypoplasia, fluorosis.

e•nam•el hy•po•pla•si•a (ĕ-nam′ĕl hī′pō-plā′zē-ă) A disturbance in the developing ameloblasts during enamel matrix formation resulting in a pitted surface of the crown. SEE ALSO enamel hypocalcification, fluorosis.

e•nam•el•ins (ĕ-nam′ĕl-inz) Proteins that form the organic matrix of mature tooth enamel. [enamel + -in]

e•nam•el lay•er (ĕ-nam′ĕl lā′ĕr) SYN ameloblastic layer.

e•nam•el mem•brane (ĕ-nam′ĕl mem′brān) The internal layer of the enamel organ formed by the enamel cells.

e•nam•el•o•gen•e•sis (ĕ-nam′ĕl-ō-jen′ĕ-sis) SYN amelogenesis.

e•nam•el•o•ma, **e•nam•el pearl** (ĕ-nam′ĕl-ō′mă, ĕ-nam′ĕl pĕrl) A developmental anomaly in which there is a small nodule of enamel below the cementoenamel junction, usually at the bifurcation of molar teeth.

e•nam•el or•gan (ĕ-nam′ĕl ōr′găn) A circumscribed mass of ectodermal cells budded off from the dental lamina; it develops the ameloblast layer of cells, which produces the enamel cap of a developing tooth. SYN dental organ.

en•an•them, **en•an•the•ma** (en-an′them, en′an-thē′mă) A mucous membrane eruption, especially one occurring in connection with one of the exanthemas. Cf. exanthema. [G. *en,* in, + *anthēma,* bloom, eruption, fr. *antheō,* to bloom]

en•an•them•a•tous (en′an-them′ă-tŭs) Relating to an enanthem.

en•an•the•sis (en′an-thē′sis) The skin eruption of a general disease, such as scarlatina or typhoid fever. [G. *en,* in, + *anthēsis,* full bloom]

en•ar•thro•di•al (en′ahr-thrō′dē-ăl) Relating to an enarthrosis.

en•ar•thro•di•al joint (en′ahr-thrō′dē-ăl joynt) SYN ball-and-socket joint.

en•ar•thro•sis (en′ahr-thrō′sis) SYN ball-and-socket joint. [G. *en-arthrōsis,* a jointing where the ball is deep set in the socket]

en bloc (on[h] blok) In a lump; as a whole; referring to a surgical or autopsy procedure in which organs or tissues are removed from the body in continuity, without prior dissection. [Fr., in a lump]

en•cap•su•la•tion (en-kap′sū-lā′shŭn) Enclosure in a capsule or sheath. [L. *in* + capsula, dim. of *capsa,* box]

en•ceph•a•lal•gi•a (en-sef′ă-lal′jē-ă) SYN headache. [encephalo- + G. *algos,* pain]

en•ceph•a•la•tro•phic (en-sef′ă-lă-trō′fik) Relating to encephalatrophy.

en•ceph•a•lat•ro•phy (en-sef′ă-lat′rŏ-fē) Atrophy of the brain. [encephalo- + G. *a-* priv. + *trophē,* nourishment]

en•ce•phal•ic (en′se-fal′ik) Relating to the brain, or to the structures within the cranium.

en•ceph•a•lit•ic (en-sef′ă-lit′ik) Relating to encephalitis.

en•ceph•a•li•tis, pl. **en•ceph•a•lit•i•des** (en-sef′ă-lī′tis, en-sef′ă-lit′i-dēz) Inflammation of the brain parenchyma. Cf. meningoencephalitis. SYN cephalitis. [G. *enkephalos,* brain, + *-itis,* inflammation]

en•ceph•a•li•tis per•i•ax•i•a•lis dif•fu•sa (en-sef′ă-lī′tis per′ē-aks-ā′lis di-fyū′să) SYN Schilder disease.

En•ceph•a•lit•o•zo•on (en-sef′ă-lit-ō-zō′on) A genus of protozoan parasites, formerly considered part of the family Toxoplasmatidae, class Sporozoea, but now recognized as a member of the protozoan phylum Microspora, family Nosematidae. *E. cuniculi* is considered the primary microsporan parasite of mammals, commonly found in the brain and kidney tubules of rodents and carnivores; causes nosematosis in rabbits. [encephalitis + G. *zōon,* animal]

En•ceph•a•lit•o•zo•on hel•lem (en-sef′ă-lit-ō-zō′on hel′ĕm) A species of *Encephalitozoon* described in human ophthalmic infections; causes punctate keratopathy and corneal ulceration in AIDS patients.

En•ceph•a•lit•o•zo•on in•tes•ti•nal•e (en-sef′ă-lit-ō-zō′on in-tes-ti-nā′lē) A diarrheogenic microsporidian described in HIV-infected patients; disease may be localized to the gastrointestinal tract or may disseminate intravascularly.

♻ **encephalo-**, **encephal-** Combining forms meaning the brain. Cf. cerebro-. [G. *enkephalos,* brain]

en•ceph•a•lo•cele (en-sef′ă-lō-sēl) A congenital gap in the cranium with herniation of brain substance. SYN craniocele. [encephalo- + G. *kēlē,* hernia]

en•ceph•a•lo•gram (en-sef′ă-lō-gram) The record obtained by encephalography. [encephalo- + G. *gramma,* a drawing]

en•ceph•a•log•ra•phy (en-sef′ă-log′ră-fē) Radiographic representation of the brain. [encephalo- + G. *graphō,* to write]

en•ceph•a•loid (en-sef′ă-loyd) Resembling brain substance; denoting a carcinoma of soft, brainlike consistency. [encephalo- + G. *eidos,* resemblance]

en·ceph·a·lo·lith (en-sef′ă-lō-lith) A concretion in the brain or one of its ventricles. [encephalo- + G. *lithos,* stone]

en·ceph·a·lo·ma (en-sef′ă-lō′mă) Herniation of brain substance. SYN cerebroma.

en·ceph·a·lo·ma·la·ci·a (en-sef′ă-lō-mă-lā′shē-ă) Abnormal softness of the cerebral parenchyma often due to ischemia or infarction. SYN cerebromalacia. [encephalo- + G. *malakia,* softness]

en·ceph·a·lo·men·in·gi·tis (en-sef′ă-lō-men-in-jī′tis) SYN meningoencephalitis. [encephalo- + G. *mēninx,* membrane, + *-itis,* inflammation]

en·ceph·a·lo·me·nin·go·cele (en-sef′ă-lō-me-ning′gō-sēl) SYN meningoencephalocele. [encephalo- + G. *mēninx,* membrane, + *kēlē,* hernia]

en·ceph·a·lo·men·in·gop·a·thy (en-sef′ă-lō-men′in-gop′ă-thē) SYN meningoencephalopathy.

en·ceph·a·lo·mere (en-sef′ă-lō-mēr) A neuromere. [encephalo- + G. *meros,* a part]

en·ceph·a·lom·e·ter (en-sef′ă-lom′ĕ-tĕr) An apparatus for indicating on the skull the location of the cortical centers. [encephalo- + G. *metron,* measure]

en·ceph·a·lo·my·e·li·tis (en-sef′a-lō-mī′ĕ-lī′tis) Inflammation of the brain and spinal cord. [encephalo- + G. *myelon,* marrow, + *-itis,* inflammation]

en·ceph·a·lo·my·e·lo·cele (en-sef′ă-lō-mī′ĕ-lō-sēl) Congenital cranial defect usually in the occipital region and cervical vertebrae, with herniation of the meninges and neural tissue. [G. *enkephalos,* brain, + *myelon,* marrow, + *kēlē,* hernia]

en·ceph·a·lo·my·e·lo·neu·rop·a·thy (en-sef′ă-lō-mī′ĕ-lō-nūr-op′ă-thē) A disease involving the brain, spinal cord, and peripheral nerves.

en·ceph·a·lo·my·e·lop·a·thy (en-sef′ă-lō-mī′ĕ-lop′ă-thē) **1.** Any disease of both brain and spinal cord. [G. *enkephalos,* brain, + *myelon,* marrow, + *pathos,* suffering]

en·ceph·a·lo·my·e·lo·ra·dic·u·li·tis (en-sef′ă-lō-mī′ĕ-lō-ră-dik′yū-lī′tis) SYN encephalomyeloradiculopathy.

en·ceph·a·lo·my·e·lo·ra·dic·u·lop·a·thy (en-sef′ă-lō-mī′ĕ-lō-ră-dik′yū-lop′ă-thē) A disease process involving the brain, spinal cord, and spinal roots. SYN encephalomyeloradiculitis.

en·ceph·a·lo·my·o·car·di·tis (en-sef′ă-lō-mī′ō-kahr-dī′tis) Associated encephalitis and myocarditis; often caused by a viral infection such as in poliomyelitis.

en·ceph·a·lo·my·o·car·di·tis vi·rus (en-sef′ă-lō-mī′ō-kahr-dī′tis vī′rŭs) A picornavirus, probably of rodents; occasionally causes febrile illness with central nervous system involvement in humans.

en·ceph·a·lon, pl. **en·ceph·a·la** (en-sef′ă-lon, -lă) [TA] That portion of the cerebrospinal axis contained within the cranium, composed of the prosencephalon, mesencephalon, and rhombencephalon. [G. *enkephalos,* brain, fr. *en,* in, + *kephalē,* head]

en·ceph·a·lop·a·thy (en-sef′a-lop′ă-thē) **1.** Any disorder of the brain. **2.** A disorder of the brain parenchyma, as distinct from a disorder of the meninges. SYN cephalopathy, cerebropathy, encephalosis. [encephalo- + G. *pathos,* suffering]

en·ceph·a·los·chi·sis (en-sef′ă-los′ki-sis) Developmental failure of closure of the rostral part of the neural tube. [encephalo- + G. *schisis,* fissure]

en·ceph·a·lo·scle·ro·sis (en-sef′ă-lō-skler-ō′sis) A sclerosis, or hardening, of the brain. SEE ALSO cerebrosclerosis. [encephalo- + G. *sklērōsis,* hardening]

en·ceph·a·lo·sis (en-sef′ă-lō′sis) SYN encephalopathy.

en·ceph·a·lot·o·my (en-sef′ă-lot′ŏ-mē) Dissection or incision of the brain. [encephalo- + G. *tomē,* incision]

en·chon·dro·ma (en′kon-drō′mă) A benign cartilaginous growth starting within the medullary cavity of a bone originally formed from cartilage; enchondromas may distend the cortex, especially of small bones, and may be solitary or multiple (endochondromatosis). [Mod. L. fr. G. *en,* in, + *chondros,* cartilage, + *-oma,* tumor]

en·chon·dro·ma·to·sis (en-kon′drō-mă-tō′sis) A rare familial, and probably hamartomatous, proliferation of cartilage in the metaphyses of several bones, most commonly of the hands and feet, causing distorted growth in length or pathologic fractures; chondrosarcoma frequently develops. When combined with hemangiomas in the cutaneous or visceral regions, it is called Maffucci syndrome. SYN dyschondroplasia.

en·chon·drom·a·tous (en′kon-drō′mă-tŭs) Relating to or having the elements of enchondroma.

en·clave (en′klāv) An enclosure; a detached mass of tissue enclosed in tissue of another kind; seen especially in the case of isolated masses of gland tissue detached from the main gland. [Fr. fr. L. *clavis,* key]

en·cod·ing (en-kōd′ing) The first stage in the memory process, followed by storage and retrieval, involving processes associated with receiving or briefly registering stimuli through one or more of the senses and modifying that information.

en·cop·re·sis (en′kō-prē′sis) The repeated, generally involuntary passage of feces into inappropriate places (e.g., clothing); considered a mental disorder if it occurs in a child over 4 years old. [G. *enkopros,* full of manure]

en·coun·ter (en-kown′tĕr) A health care contact between the patient and the provider who is responsible for diagnosing and treating the patient.

en·coun·ter form (en-kown′tĕr fōrm) A service form also called a superbill that lists health care procedure codes completed during a patient's office visit.

en·coun·ter group (en-kown′tĕr grūp) A form of psychological sensitivity training that emphasizes the experiencing of individual relationships within the group and minimizes intellectual and didactic input; the group focuses on the present rather than concerning itself with the past or outside problems of its members.

en·cryp·tion (en-krip′shŭn) The scrambling of electronic information being stored and sent so that if someone wrongly receives such information it will not be readable.

en·cyst·ed (en-sis′tĕd) Encapsulated by a membranous bag. [G. *kystis,* bladder]

en·cyst·ed cal·cu·lus (en-sis′tĕd kal′kyū-lŭs) A urinary calculus enclosed in a sac developed from the wall of the bladder. SYN pocketed calculus.

end·an·gi·i·tis, end·an·ge·i·tis (end-an′jē-ī′tis) Inflammation of the intima of a blood vessel. SYN endovasculitis. [endo + G. *angeion,* vessel, + *-itis,* inflammation]

end·a·or·ti·tis (end′ā-ōr-tī′tis) Inflammation of the intima of the aorta.

end·ar·ter·ec·to·my (end′ahr-tĕr-ek′tŏ-mē) Excision of diseased endothelial and media or most of the media of an artery, and also of occluding atheromatous deposits, so as to leave a smooth lining, mostly consisting of adventitia. [endo- + artery + G. *ektomē,* excision]

end·ar·te·ri·tis (end′ahr-tĕr-ī′tis) Inflammation of the intima of an artery. SYN endoarteritis.

end·ar·te·ri·tis ob·li·te·rans, ob·lit·er·at·ing end·ar·te·ri·tis (end′ahr-tĕr-ī′tis ob-lit′ĕr-anz, ob-lit-ĕr-ā′ting end′ahr-tĕr-ī′tis) An extreme degree of endarteritis proliferans closing the lumen of the artery. SYN arteritis obliterans, obliterating arteritis.

end·ar·te·ri·tis pro·li·fe·rans, pro·lif·er·at·ing end·ar·te·ri·tis (end′ahr-tĕr-ī′tis prō-lif′ĕr-anz, prō-lif′ĕr-āt′ing end′ahr-tĕr-ī′tis) Chronic endarteritis accompanied by a marked increase of fibrous tissue in the intima.

end ar·ter·y (end ahr′tĕr-ē) An artery with insufficient anastomoses to maintain viability of the tissue supplied if occlusion of the artery occurs. SYN terminal artery.

end·au·ral (end-awr′ăl) Within the ear. [endo- + L. *auris,* ear]

end·brain (end′brān) SYN telencephalon.

end bud (end bŭd) SYN caudal eminence.

end bulb (end bŭlb) One of the oval or rounded bodies in which the sensory nerve fibers terminate in mucous membrane.

end di·a·stol·ic vol·ume (EDV) (end dī′ă-stol′ik vol′yūm) The amount of blood in the ventricle immediately before a cardiac contraction begins; a measurement of cardiac filling between beats, related to diastolic function.

en·dec·to·cide (en-dek′tō-sīd) A drug effective against both endoparasites and ectoparasites (e.g., the macrolide antibiotic avermectin). [*en*doparasite + *ecto*parasite + -cide]

en·dem·ic (en-dem′ik) Present in a community or among a group of people; said of a disease prevailing continually in a region. Cf. epidemic, sporadic. [G. *endēmos,* native, fr. *en,* in, + *dēmos,* the people]

en·dem·ic dis·ease (en-dem′ik di-zēz′) Continued prevalence of a disease in a specific population or geographic area. SEE ALSO endemic.

en·dem·ic he·ma·tu·ri·a (en-dem′ik hē′mă-tyūr′ē-ă) SYN schistosomiasis haematobium.

en·dem·ic neu·ri·tis (en-dem′ik nūr-ī′tis) SYN beriberi.

en·dem·ic sta·bil·i·ty (en-dem′ik stă-bil′i-tē) A situation in which all factors influencing disease occurrence are relatively stable, resulting in little fluctuation in disease incidence over time; changes in one or more of these factors (e.g., reduction in proportion of people with immunity from exposure to infectious agent) can lead to an unstable situation in which major disease outbreaks occur. SYN enzootic stability.

en·dem·ic ty·phus (en-dem′ik tī′fŭs) SYN murine typhus.

en·dem·o·ep·i·dem·ic (en-dem′ō-ep-i-dem′ik) Denoting a temporary large increase in the number of cases of an endemic disease.

end·er·gon·ic (en′dĕr-gon′ik) Referring to a chemical reaction that takes place with absorption of energy from its surroundings (i.e., a positive change in Gibbs free energy). Cf. exergonic. [endo- + G. *ergon,* work]

end-feel (end′fēl) The texture of resistance felt when a joint reaches the end of its range of motion. Can be bony (bone-to-bone contact), springy (soft tissue approximation), abrupt (limited by protective muscle spasm), or empty (pain is felt well before the end of a normal range of motion, but no organic resistance is identified). Abnormal end-feel can indicate causes of joint dysfunction.

end-feet (end′fēt) SYN axon terminals.

end•ing (end′ing) **1.** A termination or conclusion. **2.** A nerve ending.

♻**endo-, end-** Prefixes indicating within, inner, absorbing, or containing. SEE ALSO ento-. [G. *endon,* within]

En•do a•gar (en′dō ā′gahr) A medium containing peptone, lactose, dipotassium phosphate, agar, sodium sulfite, basic fuchsin, and distilled water; originally developed for the isolation of *Salmonella typhi*, this medium is now most useful in the bacteriologic examination of water; coliform organisms ferment the lactose, and their colonies become red and color the surrounding medium; non-lactose-fermenting organisms produce clear, colorless colonies against the faint pink background of the medium. SYN Endo medium.

en•do•an•eu•rys•mo•plas•ty (en′dō-an-yūr-iz′mō-plas-tē) SYN aneurysmoplasty.

en•do•an•eu•rys•mor•rha•phy (en′dō-an-yūr-iz-mōr′ă-fē) SYN aneurysmoplasty. [endo- + G. *aneurysma,* aneurysm, + *rhaphē,* suture]

en•do•ar•te•ri•tis (en′dō-ahr-tĕr-ī′tis) SYN endarteritis.

en•do•ar•ter•i•tis ob•lit•e•rans (en′dō-ahr-tĕr-ī′tis ō-blit′ĕr-anz) SYN Buerger disease.

en•do•blast (en′dō-blast) Entoderm. [endo- + G. *blastos,* germ]

en•do•bron•chi•al tube (en′dō-brong′kē-ăl tūb) A single- or double-lumen tube with an inflatable cuff at the distal end that, after being passed through the larynx and trachea, is positioned so that ventilation is restricted to one lung; a single-lumen tube is placed in the mainstem bronchus of the lung; a double-lumen tube is positioned at the tracheal carina to permit ventilation of either or both lungs.

en•do•car•di•al heart tube (en′dō-kahr′dē-ăl hahrt tūb) The two endothelial tubes that meet in the midthoracic region of the embryo and fuse to form the primordial cardiac or heart tube, the primordium of the heart.

en•do•car•dit•ic (en′dō-kahr-dit′ik) Relating to endocarditis.

en•do•car•di•tis (en′dō-kahr-dī′tis) Inflammation of the endocardium.

en•do•car•di•um, pl. **en•do•car•di•a** (en′dō-kahr′dē-ŭm, -ē-ă) The innermost tunic of the heart, which includes endothelium and subendothelial connective tissue; in the atrial wall, smooth muscle and numerous elastic fibers also occur. [endo- + G. *kardia,* heart]

en•do•cer•vi•cal (en′dō-sĕr′vi-kăl) **1.** Within any cervix, specifically within the cervix uteri. SYN intracervical. **2.** Relating to the endocervix.

en•do•cer•vi•ci•tis (en′dō-sĕr-vi-sī′tis) Inflammation of the mucous membrane of the cervix uteri. SYN endotrachelitis.

en•do•cer•vix (en′dō-sĕr′viks) The mucous membrane of the cervical canal.

en•do•chon•dral bone (en′dō-kon′drăl bōn) A bone that develops in a cartilage environment after the latter is partially or entirely destroyed by calcification and subsequent resorption. SYN cartilage bone.

en•do•chon•dral os•si•fi•ca•tion (en′dō-kon′drăl os′i-fi-kā′shŭn) Formation of osseous tissue by the replacement of calcified cartilage; long bones grow in length by endochondral ossification at the epiphysial cartilage plate where osteoblasts form bone trabeculae on a framework of calcified cartilage. SYN intrachondral ossification.

en•do•co•ag•u•la•tion (en′dō-kō-ag′yū-lā′shŭn) SYN thermocoagulation.

en•do•coch•le•ar po•ten•tial (en′dō-kok′lē-ăr pō-ten′shăl) The standing direct current potential in the endolymph relative to the perilymph, measuring positive 80 mV.

en•do•co•li•tis (en′dō-kō-lī′tis) Simple catarrhal inflammation of the colon.

en•do•cra•ni•al (en′dō-krā′nē-ăl) **1.** Within the cranium. **2.** Relating to the endocranium.

en•do•cra•ni•um (en′dō-krā′nē-ŭm) The lining membrane of the cranium, or dura mater of the brain.

en•do•crine (en′dō-krin) **1.** Secreting internally, most commonly into the systemic circulation; of or pertaining to such secretion. Cf. paracrine. **2.** The internal or hormonal secretion of a ductless gland. **3.** Denoting a gland that furnishes an internal secretion. [endo- + G. *krinō,* to separate]

en•do•crine glands (en′dō-krin glandz) Glands that have no ducts, their secretions being absorbed directly into the blood. SYN ductless glands.

en•do•crine sys•tem (en′dō-krin sis′tĕm) Collective designation for those tissues capable of secreting hormones.

en•do•cri•nol•o•gist (en′dō-kri-nol′ŏ-jist) One who specializes in endocrinology.

en•do•cri•nol•o•gy (en′dō-kri-nol′ŏ-jē) The science and medical specialty concerned with the internal or hormonal secretions and their physiologic and pathologic relations. [endocrine + G. *logos,* study]

en•do•cri•no•ma (en′dō-kri-nō′mă) A tumor

with endocrine tissue that retains the function of the parent organ, usually to an excessive degree.

en·do·crin·o·path·ic (en′dō-krin′ō-path′ik) Relating to or having an endocrinopathy.

en·do·cri·nop·a·thy (en′dō-kri-nop′ă-thē) A disorder in the function of an endocrine gland and the consequences thereof. [endocrine + G. *pathos*, disease]

en·do·cys·ti·tis (en′dō-sis-tī′tis) Inflammation of the mucous membrane of the bladder. [endo- + G. *kystis,* bladder, + *-itis,* inflammation]

en·do·cy·to·sis (en′dō-sī-tō′sis) Internalization of substances from the extracellular environment through the formation of vesicles formed from the plasma membrane. SEE ALSO phagocytosis. Cf. exocytosis (2). [endo- + G. *kytos,* cell, + *-osis,* condition]

en·do·derm (en′dō-dĕrm) The innermost of the three primary germ layers of the embryo (ectoderm, mesoderm, endoderm); from it are derived the epithelial lining of the primodrial gut and the epithelial component of the glands and other structures (e.g., lower respiratory system) that develop as outgrowths from the gut tube. SYN entoderm, hypoblast. [endo- + G. *derma,* skin]

en·do·der·mal cells (en′dō-dĕr′măl selz) Embryonic cells forming the umbilical vesicle (yolk sac) and giving rise to the epithelium of the alimentary and respiratory tracts and to the parenchyma of associated glands. SYN entodermal cell.

en·do·der·mal cyst (en′dō-dĕr′măl sist) Cyst lined by columnar epithelium; presumed dermal in origin.

en·do·don·tics, en·do·don·ti·a, en·do·don·tol·o·gy (en′dō-don′tiks, -shē-ă, -don-tol′ō-jē) A field of dentistry concerned with the diseases and injuries of the dental pulp and periapical tissues, and with the prevention, diagnosis, and treatment of diseases and injuries in these tissues. [endo- + G. *odous,* tooth]

en·do·don·tist (en′dō-don′tist) One who specializes in the practice of endodontics.

en·do·en·ter·i·tis (en′dō-en-tĕr-ī′tis) Inflammation of the intestinal mucous membrane. [endo- + G. *enteron,* intestine, *-itis,* inflammation]

end-of-life care (end līf kār) Multidimensional and multidisciplinary physical, emotional, and spiritual care of the patient with terminal illness, including support of family and caregivers.

en·dog·a·my (en-dog′ă-mē) Reproduction by conjugation between sister cells, the descendants of one original cell. [endo- + G. *gamos,* marriage]

en·do·gen·ic tox·i·co·sis (en′dō-jen′ik tok-si-kō′sis) SYN autointoxication.

en·dog·e·nous (en-doj′ĕ-nŭs) Originating or produced within the organism or one of its parts. [endo- + G. *-gen,* production]

en·dog·e·nous de·pres·sion (en-doj′ĕ-nŭs dĕ-presh′ŭn) A descriptive syndrome for a cluster of symptoms and features occurring in the absence of external precipitants and believed to have a biologic origin (e.g., anhedonia, psychomotor agitation or retardation, diurnal mood variation with increased severity in the morning, early morning awakening and insomnia in the middle of the night, weight loss, self-reproach or guilt, and lack of reactivity to one's environment).

en·dog·e·nous hy·per·glyc·er·i·de·mi·a (en-doj′ĕ-nŭs hī′pĕr-glis′ĕr-i-dē′mē-ă) Type IV familial hyperlipoproteinemia or, more commonly, a nonfamilial sporadic variety.

en·dog·e·nous in·fec·tion (en-doj′ĕ-nŭs in-fek′shŭn) A disorder caused by an infectious agent already present in the body, the previous infection having been inapparent.

en·dog·e·nous py·ro·gen (EP) (en-doj′ĕ-nŭs pī′rō-jen) An endogenous protein that induces fever. Several (about 11) have been identified, including cytokines formed by components of the immune system, especially macrophages (e.g., interleukins 1 and 6, interferons, and tumor necrosis factors). Cf. bioregulator.

en·do·glin (en′dō-glin) A protein on the surface of endothelial cells that binds to transforming growth factor-β.

en·do·in·tox·i·ca·tion (en′dō-in-tok′si-kā′shŭn) Poisoning by an endogenous toxin.

en·do·lith (en′dō-lith) A calcified body found in the pulp chamber of a tooth; may be composed of irregular dentin (true denticle) or due to ectopic calcification of pulp tissue (false denticle). SYN denticle (1), pulp stone. [endo- + G. *lithos,* stone]

en·do·lymph (en′dō-limf) The fluid contained within the membranous labyrinth of the inner ear.

en·do·lym·phat·ic ap·pen·dage (en′dō-lim-fat′ik ă-pen′dăj) SYN endolymphatic diverticulum.

en·do·lym·phat·ic di·ver·tic·u·lum (en′dō-lim-fat′ik dī′vĕr-tik′yū-lŭm) An outgrowth from the otic vesicle that elongates to form the endolymphatic duct and sac. SYN endolymphatic appendage.

en·do·lym·phat·ic duct (en′dō-lim-fat′ik dŭkt) A small membranous canal, connecting with both saccule and utricle of the membranous labyrinth, passing through the aqueduct of the vestibule, and terminating in a dilated blind extremity, the endolymphatic sac, on the posterior surface of the petrous portion of the temporal bone beneath the dura mater.

en•do•lym•phat•ic hy•drops (en′dō-lim-fat′ik hī′drops) SYN Ménière disease.

en•do•lym•phat•ic sac (en′dō-lim-fat′ik sak) The dilated blind extremity of the endolymphatic duct. SYN saccus endolymphaticus [TA], Böttcher space.

en•do•lym•phat•ic sac sur•ger•y (en′dō-lim-fat′ik sak sŭr′jĕr-ē) A generic term for several operations performed on the endolymphatic sac for the treatment of Ménière disease.

en•do•lym•phat•ic shunt op•er•a•tion (en′dō-lim-fat′ik shŭnt op-ĕr-ā′shŭn) An operation to establish a communication between the endolymphatic sac and the cerebrospinal fluid space for the treatment of Ménière disease.

en•do•lym•phic (en′dō-lim′fik) Relating to the endolymph.

En•do me•di•um (en′dō mē′dē-ŭm) SYN Endo agar.

en•do•me•tri•a (en′dō-mē′trē-ă) Plural of endometrium.

en•do•me•tri•al (en′dō-mē′trē-ăl) Relating to or composed of endometrium.

en•do•met•ri•al ab•la•tion (en′dō-mē′trē-ăl ab-lā′shŭn) Therapeutic selective endometrial destruction.

en•do•met•ri•al hy•per•pla•si•a (en′dō-mē′trē-ăl hī′pĕr-plā′zē-ă) Increase in the number of endometrial glands, usually secondary to hyperestrinism; classified as simple hyperplasia, complex hyperplasia, or complex hyperplasia with atypia; the latter may progress to adenocarcinoma.

en•do•me•tri•al stro•mal sar•co•ma (en′dō-mē′trē-ăl strō′măl sahr-kō′mă) A term sometimes used for a relatively rare sarcoma believed to be a form of endometriosis in which the lesions form multiple foci in the myometrium and in vascular spaces in other sites, and which consist of histologic and cytologic elements that resemble those of the endometrial stroma.

en•do•me•tri•oid (en′dō-mē′trē-oyd) Microscopically resembling endometrial tissue.

en•do•me•tri•oid car•ci•no•ma (en′dō-mē′trē-oyd kahr′si-nō′mă) Adenocarcinoma of the ovary or prostate resembling endometrial adenocarcinoma, possibly arising from ovarian foci of endometriosis.

en•do•me•tri•oid tu•mor (en′dō-mē′trē-oyd tū′mŏr) A tumor of the ovary containing epithelial or stromal elements resembling tumors of the endometrium.

en•do•me•tri•o•ma (en′dō-mē-trē-ō′mă) Circumscribed mass of ectopic endometrial tissue in endometriosis. [endometrium + *-oma*, tumor]

en•do•me•tri•o•sis (en′dō-mē-trē-ō′sis) Ectopic occurrence of endometrial tissue, frequently forming cysts containing altered blood. See this page. [endometrium + *-osis*, condition]

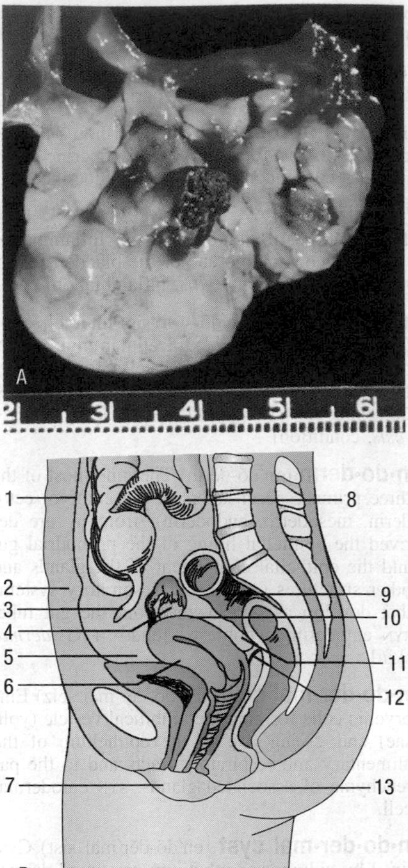

endometriosis: (A) implants of endometriosis on the ovary appear as red-blue nodules; (B) common sites of endometriosis formation–(1) umbilicus, (2) scar on abdominal wall, (3) appendix, (4) ovary, (5) anterior cul-de-sac and bladder, (6) uterine wall, (7) vulva, (8) ileum, (9) pelvic colon, (10) posterior surface of uterus and uterosacral ligaments, (11) posterior cul-de-sac, (12) rectovaginal septum, (13) perineum

en•do•me•tri•tis (en′dō-mē-trī′tis) Inflammation of the endometrium. [endometrium + *-itis*, inflammation]

en•do•me•tri•um, pl. **en•do•me•tri•a** (en′dō-mē′trē-ŭm, -ă) [TA] The mucous membrane forming the inner layer of the uterine wall; it consists of a simple columnar epithelium and a lamina propria that contains simple tubular uterine glands. The structure, thickness, and state of the endometrium undergo marked change with the menstrual cycle. [endo- + G. *mētra,* uterus]

en·do·mi·to·sis (en′dō-mī-tō′sis) SYN endopolyploidy.

en·do·morph (en′dō-mōrf) A constitutional body type or build (biotype or somatotype) in which tissues that originated in the endoderm prevail; from a morphologic standpoint, the trunk predominates over the limbs. [endo- + G. *morphē,* form]

en·do·mor·phic (en′dō-mōr′fik) Relating to, or having the characteristics of, an endomorph.

En·do·my·ce·ta·les (en′dō-mī-sē-tā′lēz) An order of Ascomycota that includes the yeasts.

en·do·my·o·car·di·al (en′dō-mī-ō-kahr′dē-ăl) Relating to the endocardium and the myocardium.

en·do·my·o·car·di·al fi·bro·sis (en′dō-mī-ō-kahr′dē-ăl fī-brō′sis) Thickening of the ventricular endocardium by fibrosis, involving the subendocardial myocardium, and sometimes the atrioventricular valves, with mural thrombosis, leading to progressive right and left ventricular failure with mitral and tricuspid insufficiency; occurs in adults and is endemic to parts of Africa.

en·do·my·o·car·di·tis (en′dō-mī′ō-kahr-dī′tis) Inflammation of both endocardium and myocardium.

en·do·my·o·me·tri·tis (en′dō-mī-ō-mē-trī′tis) Sepsis involving the tissues of the uterus. [endo- + G. *mys,* muscle, + *mētra,* uterus, + *-itis,* inflammation]

en·do·mys·i·um (en′dō-miz′ē-ŭm) The fine connective tissue sheath surrounding a muscle fiber. [endo- + G. *mys,* muscle]

en·do·neu·ri·um (en′dō-nūr′ē-ŭm) The innermost connective tissue supportive structure present in peripheral nerve trunks, found within the fascicles. With the perineurium and epineurium, the endoneurium comprises the peripheral nerve stroma. SYN Henle sheath. [endo- + G. *neuron,* nerve]

en·do·nu·cle·ase (en′dō-nū′klē-ās) A nuclease (phosphodiesterase) that cleaves polynucleotides (nucleic acids) at interior bonds, thus producing polynucleotide or oligonucleotide fragments of varying size. Cf. exonuclease.

en·do·par·a·site (en′dō-par′ă-sīt) A parasite living within the body of its host.

en·do·pep·ti·dase (en′dō-pep′ti-dās) An enzyme catalyzing the hydrolysis of a peptide chain at points well within the chain, not near termini (e.g., pepsin, trypsin). Cf. exopeptidase.

en·do·per·i·car·di·tis (en′dō-per′i-kahr-dī′tis) Simultaneous inflammation of the endocardium and pericardium. [endo- + G. *peri,* around, + *kardia,* heart, + *-itis,* inflammation]

en·do·per·i·my·o·car·di·tis (en′dō-per′i-mī-ō-kahr-dī′tis) Simultaneous inflammation of the heart muscle and of the endocardium and pericardium. [endo- + G. *peri,* around, + *mys,* muscle, + *kardia,* heart, + *-itis,* inflammation]

en·do·per·i·to·ni·tis (en′dō-per′i-tō-nī′tis) Superficial inflammation of the peritoneum.

en·do·phle·bi·tis (en′dō-flĕ-bī′tis) Inflammation of the intima of a vein. [endo- + G. *phleps (phleb-),* vein, + *-itis,* inflammation]

en·doph·thal·mi·tis (en′dof-thal-mī′tis) Inflammation of the tissues within the eyeball. See page B26. [endo- + G. *ophthalmos,* eye, + *-itis,* inflammation]

en·do·plasm (en′dō-plazm) The inner or medullary part of the cytoplasm, as opposed to the ectoplasm, containing the cell organelles.

en·do·plas·mic re·tic·u·lum (ER) (en′dō-plas′mik rĕ-tik′yū-lŭm) The network of cytoplasmic tubules or flattened sacs (cisternae) with (rough ER) or without (smooth ER) ribosomes on the surface of their membranes in eukaryotes.

en·do·pol·y·ploid (en′dō-pol′ē-ployd) Relating to endopolyploidy.

en·do·pol·y·ploi·dy (en′dō-pol′ē-ploy-dē) The process or state of duplication of the chromosomes without accompanying spindle formation or cytokinesis, resulting in a polyploid nucleus. SYN endomitosis. [endo- + polyploidy]

en·do·rec·tal pull-through pro·ce·dure (en′dō-rek′tăl pul′thrū prŏ-sē′jŭr) Removal of diseased rectal mucosa along with resection of the lower bowel, followed by anastomosis of the proximal stump to the anus, to spare rectal muscle function.

en·do·re·du·pli·ca·tion (en′dō-rē-dū-pli-kā′shŭn) A form of polyploidy or polysomy by redoubling of chromosomes, giving rise to four-stranded chromosomes at prophase and metaphase.

end or·gan (end ōr′găn) The special structure containing the terminal of a nerve fiber in peripheral tissue such as muscle, tissue, skin, mucous membrane, or glands.

en·dor·phin (ĕn-dōr′fin) A natural substance produced in the brain that binds to opioid receptors, thus dulling the perception of pain; postulated to trigger "exercise high," a state of euphoria and exhilaration during intense exercise.

en·dor·phin·er·gic (en-dōr′fin-ĕr′jik) Relating to nerve cells or fibers that employ an endorphin as their neurotransmitter. [endorphin + G. *ergon,* work]

en·do·sac (en′dō-sak) A sac or bag used in laparoscopic surgery in which tissue is placed to facilitate removal or morcellation.

en•do•sal•pin•gi•tis (en′dō-sal-pin-jī′tis) Inflammation of the lining membrane of the eustachian or the fallopian tube. [endo- + G. *salpinx* (*salping-*), tube, + *-itis,* inflammation]

en•do•scope (en′dō-skōp) An instrument for the examination of the interior of a tubular or hollow organ. [endo- + G. *skopeō,* to examine]

en•do•scop•ic bi•op•sy (en′dō-skop′ik bī′op-sē) Biopsy obtained by instruments passed through an endoscope or obtained by a needle introduced under endoscopic guidance.

en•do•scop•ic ret•ro•grade chol•an•gi•o•pan•cre•a•tog•ra•phy (ERCP) (en′dō-skop′ik ret′rō-grād kō-lan′jē-ō-pan′krē-ă-tog′ră-fē) A method of cholangiopancreatography using an endoscope to inspect and cannulate the ampulla of Vater, with injection of contrast medium for radiographic examination of the pancreatic, hepatic, and common bile ducts.

en•dos•co•pist (en-dos′kŏ-pist) A specialist trained in the use of an endoscope.

en•dos•co•py (en-dos′kŏ-pē) Examination of the interior of a canal or hollow viscus by means of a special instrument, such as an endoscope. SEE endoscope. See page B17.

en•do•skel•e•ton (en′dō-skel′ĕ-tŏn) The internal bony framework of the body; the skeleton in its usual context as distinguished from the exoskeleton.

en•do•so•nos•co•py (en′dō-son-os′kŏ-pē) A sonographic study carried out by transducers inserted into the body as miniature probes in the esophagus, urethra, bladder, vagina, or rectum.

en•do•spore (en′dō-spōr) **1.** A body formed within the vegetative cells of some bacteria, particularly those belonging to the genera *Bacillus* and *Clostridium.* **2.** A fungus spore borne within a cell or within the tubular end of a sporophore, as in the spherule of *Coccidioides immitis.* [endo- + G. *sporos,* seed]

en•dos•se•ous im•plant (en-dos′sē-ŭs im′plant) SYN endosteal implants.

en•dos•te•al (en-dos′tē-ăl) Relating to the endosteum.

en•dos•te•al im•plants (en-dos′tē-ăl im′plants) Those devices that are inserted into the alveolar and/or basal bone and protrude through the mucoperiosteum. See this page. SYN endosseous implant.

en•dos•te•i•tis, en•dos•ti•tis (en-dos′tē-ī′tis, en′dos-tī′tis) Inflammation of the endosteum or of the medullary cavity of a bone. SYN central osteitis (2), perimyelitis. [endo- + G. *osteon,* bone, + *-itis,* inflammation]

en•dos•te•o•ma (en-dos′tē-ō′mă) A benign neoplasm of bone tissue in the medullary cavity of a bone. SYN endostoma. [endo- + G. *osteon,* bone, + *-ōma,* tumor]

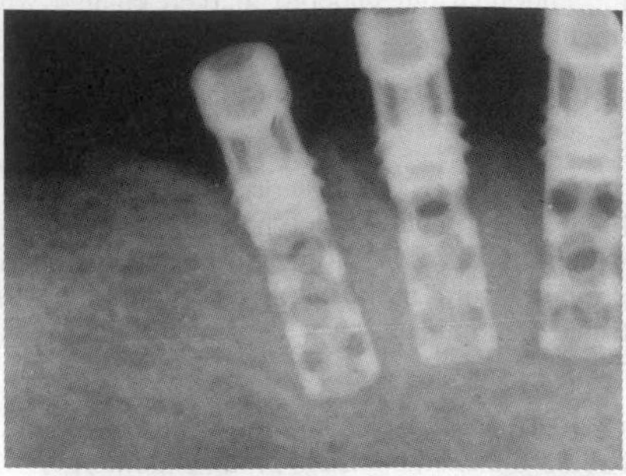

endosteal implants in alveolar bone: crowns not yet in place

en•dos•te•um (en-dos′tē-ŭm) [TA] A layer of cells lining the inner surface of bone in the central medullary cavity. SYN medullary membrane. [endo- + G. *osteon,* bone]

en•dos•to•ma (en′dō-stō′mă) SYN endosteoma.

en•do•ten•din•e•um (en′dō-ten-din′ē-ŭm) The fine connective tissue surrounding secondary fascicles of a tendon. [endo- + L. *tendon,* tendon, + *-eus,* adj.; the whole, in its neuter form, used substantively]

en•do•the•li•a (en′dō-thē′lē-ă) Plural of endothelium.

en•do•the•li•al (en′dō-thē′lē-ăl) Relating to the endothelium.

en•do•the•li•al cell (en′dō-thē′lē-ăl sel) One of the simple squamous cells forming the lining of blood and lymph vessels and the inner layer of the endocardium.

en•do•the•li•al dys•tro•phy of cor•ne•a (en′dō-thē′lē-ăl dis′trŏ-fē kōr′nē-ă) Spontaneous loss of corneal endothelium leading to edema of the corneal stroma and epithelium.

en•do•the•li•al leu•ko•cyte (en′dō-thē′lē-ăl lū′kō-sīt) Older term for a monocyte thought to be derived from reticuloendothelial tissue.

en•do•the•li•al my•e•lo•ma (en′dō-thē′lē-ăl mī-ĕ-lō′mă) SYN Ewing tumor.

en•do•the•li•oid (en′dō-thē′lē-oyd) Resembling endothelium.

en•do•the•li•o•ma (en′dō-thē-lē-ō′mă) Generic term for a group of neoplasms, particularly benign tumors, derived from the endothelial tissue of blood vessels or lymphatic channels; endotheliomas may be benign or malignant. [endothelium + *-oma,* tumor]

en•do•the•li•o•sis (en′dō-thē-lē-ō′sis) Proliferation of endothelium.

en·do·the·li·um, pl. **en·do·the·li·a** (en′dō-thē′lē-ŭm, en′dō-thē′lē-ă) A layer of flat cells that line the blood vessels, lymphatic vessels, and the heart. [endo- + G. *thēlē,* nipple]

en·do·ther·mic (en′dō-thĕr′mik) Denoting a chemical reaction during which heat is absorbed. Cf. exothermic (1). [endo- + G. *thermē,* heat]

en·do·tho·rac·ic fas·ci·a (en′dō-thōr-as′ik fash′ē-ă) The extrapleural fascia that lines the wall of the thorax; it extends over the cupula of the pleura as the suprapleural membrane and also forms a thin layer between the diaphragm and pleura (phrenicopleural fascia).

en·do·thrix (en′dō-thriks) Fungal spores (conidia) invading the interior of a hair shaft; there is no conspicuous external sheath of spores, as there is with ectothrix. [endo- + G. *thrix,* hair]

endotoxaemia [Br.] SYN endotoxemia.

en·do·tox·e·mi·a (en′dō-tok-sē′mē-ă) Presence in the blood of endotoxins, which, if derived from gram-negative, rod-shaped bacteria, may cause a generalized Shwartzman phenomenon with shock. SYN endotoxaemia.

en·do·tox·ic (en′dō-tok′sik) Denoting an endotoxin.

en·do·tox·i·co·sis (en′dō-tok-si-kō′sis) Poisoning by an endotoxin.

en·do·tox·in (en′dō-tok′sin) **1.** A bacterial toxin not freely liberated into the surrounding medium, in contrast to exotoxin. **2.** The complex phospholipid-polysaccharide macromolecules that form an integral part of the cell wall of strains of gram-negative bacteria. The toxins may cause a state of shock accompanied by severe diarrhea, and, in smaller doses, fever and leukopenia followed by leukocytosis. SYN intracellular toxin.

en·do·tra·che·al (en′dō-trā′kē-ăl) Within the trachea.

en·do·tra·che·al an·es·the·si·a (en′-dō-trā′kē-ăl an′es-thē′zē-ă) Inhalation anesthesia technique in which anesthetic and respiratory gases pass through a tube placed in the trachea through the mouth or nose.

en·do·tra·che·al in·tu·ba·tion (en′dō-trā′kē-ăl in-tū-bā′shŭn) Passage of a tube through the nose or mouth into the trachea for maintenance of the airway during anesthesia or for maintenance of an imperiled airway.

en·do·tra·che·al tube (ET) (en′dō-trā′kē-ăl tūb) SYN tracheal tube.

en·do·trac·he·li·tis (en′dō-trā′kĕ-lī′tis) SYN endocervicitis.

en·do·vas·cu·li·tis (en′dō-vas′kyū-lī′tis) SYN endangiitis.

end-piece (end′pēs) The terminal part of the tail of a spermatozoon consisting of the axoneme and the flagellar membrane.

end·plate, end-plate (end′plāt) The ending of a motor nerve fiber in relation to a skeletal muscle fiber.

end point (end poynt) Overused jargon for termination or conclusion.

end-po·si·tion·al nys·tag·mus (end′pŏ-zish′ŭn-ăl nis-tag′mŭs) A jerky physiologic form of the disorder that occurs in an otherwise normal patient, when attempts are made to focus on a visual point at the limits of the field of vision.

end·prod·uct (end′prod-ŭkt) In health care, the final state of a manufacturing, therapeutic, or statistical process.

end stage (end stāj) The late, fully developed phase of a disease.

end sys·tol·ic vol·ume (ESV) (end sis-tol′ik vol′yūm) The amount of blood held remaining in each ventricle of the heart after systole (contraction) and before filling; approximately 50–60 mL.

end-ti·dal (end-tī′dăl) At the end of a normal expiration.

end-to-end a·nas·to·mo·sis (end end ă-nas′tŏ-mō′sis) Anastomosis performed after cutting each structure to be joined in a plane perpendicular to the ultimate flow through the structures.

en·dur·ance (en-dūr′ăns) Ability of muscle (e.g., cardiac or skeletal) and the musculoskeletal system to sustain a force, or generate a force repeatedly over time.

en·dur·ance phase (en-dūr′ăns fāz) This phase is used to develop the cardiorespiratory fitness of the participant. It includes 20 to 60 minutes of continuous or intermittent aerobic exercise. SYN cardiorespiratory training, endurance training.

en·dur·ance train·ing (en-dūr′ăns trān′ing) SYN endurance phase.

♻ **-ene** Suffix applied to a chemical name indicating the presence of a carbon-carbon double bond; e.g., propene (unsaturated propane, CH_3—CH=CH_2). [G. *enos,* origin]

en·e·ma (en′ĕ-mă) A rectal injection to clear out the bowel or to administer drugs or food. [G.]

en·er·gy (E) (en′ĕr-jē) The exertion of power; the capacity to do work, taking the forms of kinetic energy, potential energy, chemical energy, electrical energy, and other types. [G. *energeia,* fr. *en,* in, + *ergon,* work]

en·er·gy bal·ance e·qua·tion (en′ĕr-jē bal′ăns ĕ-kwā′zhŭn) Statement stating that body mass remains constant when caloric intake equals caloric expenditure. Any chronic imbalance on either side of the equation causes body mass to change.

en•er•gy con•ser•va•tion tech•niques (ECT) (en-ĕr′jē kon-sĕr-vā′shŭn tek-nēks′) Applying various measures to encourage the concept of saving energy in a physical environment may include activity restriction, modification of tasks, time management, work simplification techniques, ergonomics, or the reorganization of work stations or platforms to emphasize efficiency.

en•er•gy ex•pen•di•ture (en′ĕr-jē eks-pen′di-chŭr) SEE kilocalorie, calorie.

en•er•gy sub•trac•tion (en′ĕr-jē sŭb-trak′shŭn) Digital radiography using higher- and lower-energy exposures, either by double exposure at 2-kV levels or by interposing a copper filter that absorbs the lower-energy photons between two phosphor plates, with computer calculation of high-Z and low-Z images (bone and soft tissues, respectively); makes use of the fact that lower-energy x-rays are absorbed by more high-Z substances, such as calcium and copper, because of the photoelectric effect.

en•er•va•tion (en′ĕr-vā′shŭn) Failure of nerve force; weakening. [L. *enervo,* pp. *-atus,* to enervate, fr. *e-* priv. + *nervus,* nerve]

ENG Abbreviation for electronystagmography.

en•gage•ment (en-gāj′mĕnt) OBSTETRICS the mechanism by which the biparietal diameter of the fetal head enters the plane of the inlet.

En•glish lock (ing′glish lok) Articulation of the blades of obstetric forceps consisting of a socket on the shank at the junction with the handle in a similar socket on the other shank; used in Simpson forceps.

en•gorged (en-gōrjd′) Absolutely filled; distended with fluid. SEE ALSO congested, hyperemic. [O. Fr. fr. Mediev. L. *gorgia,* throat, narrow passage, fr. L. *gurges,* a whirlpool]

en•gorge•ment (en-gorj′mĕnt) OBSTETRICS swelling of breasts and local congestion of lymph and blood vessels associated with lactation. Engorgement is relieved by nursing the infant. [O.Fr. *engorgier,* to devour greedily]

en•gram (en′gram) In the mnemonic hypothesis, a physical habit or memory trace made on the protoplasm of an organism by the repetition of stimuli. [G. *en,* in, + *gramma,* mark]

en•graph•i•a (en-graf′ē-ă) The formation of engrams.

en•hance•ment (en-hans′mĕnt) **1.** The act of augmenting. **2.** IMMUNOLOGY the prolongation of a process or event by suppressing an opposing process.

en•hanc•er (en-hans′ĕr) A genetic element that is important in the function of a specific promoter. [M.E. *enhauncen,* raise, increase, fr. O. Fr. *enhaucier,* fr. L.L. *inalto,* fr. *altus,* high, + *-er,* agent suffix]

en•keph•a•lin•er•gic (en-kef′ă-lin-ĕr′jik) Relating to nerve cells or fibers that employ an enkephalin as their neurotransmitter. [enkephalin + G. *ergon,* work]

en•large•ment (en-lahrj′mĕnt) **1.** An increase in size; an anatomic swelling, enlargement, or prominence. **2.** An intumescence or swelling. SYN intumescence (1), intumescentia.

en•large•ment of the ves•tib•u•lar a•que•duct (en-lahrj′mĕnt ves-tib′yū-lăr ahk′wă-dŭkt) Recessive hereditary hearing impairment associated with a large vestibular aqueduct.

♻ **-enoic** Suffix indicating an unsaturated acid. [-ene + -ic]

e•nol (ē′nol) A compound possessing a hydroxyl group (alcohol) attached to a doubly bonded (ethylenic) carbon atom (–CH=CH(OH)–). [-ene + -ol]

e•no•lase (ē′nō-lās) An enzyme catalyzing the reversible dehydration of 2-phospho-D-glycerate to phospho*enol*pyruvate and water; a step in both glycolysis and gluconeogenesis; several isozymes exist; requires magnesium ion and is inhibited by F^{-}.

e•nol•o•gy (ē-nol′ŏ-jē) The study of wine. SYN oenology. [G. *oinos,* wine + *logos,*study]

en•oph•thal•mos (en′of-thal′mos) Recession of the eyeball within the orbit. [G. *en,* in, + *ophthalmos,* eye]

en•os•to•sis (en′os-tō′sis) A mass of proliferating bone tissue within a bone. [G. *en,* in, + *osteon,* bone, + *-osis,* condition]

en•o•yl (ē′nō-il) The acyl radical of an unsaturated aliphatic acid. [-ene + -oyl]

ENP Abbreviation for emergency nurse practitioner.

en•rolled nurse (en-rōld′ nŭrs) A second-level nurse who provides patient care under the direction of a registered nurse; in Canada, this title is graduate nurse. SYN auxiliary nurse.

en•si•form (en′si-fōrm) SYN xiphoid. [L. *ensis,* sword, + *forma,* appearance]

en•si•form pro•cess (en′si-fōrm pros′es) SYN xiphoid process.

ENT Abbreviation for ears, nose, and throat. SEE otorhinolaryngology.

en•tad (en′tad) Toward the interior. [G. *entos,* within, + L. *ad,* to]

en•tal (en′tăl) Relating to the interior; inside. [G. *entos,* within]

ent•am•e•bi•a•sis (ent′ă-mē-bī′ă-sis) Infection

with *Entamoeba histolytica*. SEE amebiasis, amebic dysentery. SYN entamoebiasis.

En•ta•moe•ba (ent′ă-mē′bă) A genus of ameba parasitic in the oral cavity, cecum, and large bowel of humans and other primates and in many domestic and wild mammals and birds; with the exception of *E. histolytica*, members of the genus appear to be relatively harmless inhabitants of the host. USAGE NOTE often spelled incorrectly as *Entameba*. [G. *entos,* within + *amoibē,* change]

Ent•a•moe•ba co•li (ent′ă-mē′bă kō′lī) Nonpathogenic strain of the parasite that occurs in the human large intestine; often confused with *E. histolytica*. See page B7.

En•ta•moe•ba dis•par (ent′ă-mē′bă dis′pahr) Nonpathogenic species of ameba that occurs in the large intestine of humans; formerly classed with *E. histolytica*, *E. dispar* is now recognized as a separate species; it is nonpathogenic and is not associated with symptomatic amebiasis in humans. Morphologically it resembles *E. histolytica;* however, the trophozoites are never found to contain ingested red blood cells.

Ent•a•moe•ba gin•gi•va•lis (ent′ă-mē′bă jin-ji-vā′lis) Species of ameba found in the human oral cavity.

Ent•a•moe•ba his•to•lyt•i•ca (ent′ă-mē′bă his-tō-lit′i-kă) Species of ameba that is the only distinct pathogen in the species; causes amebic dysentery. See this page.

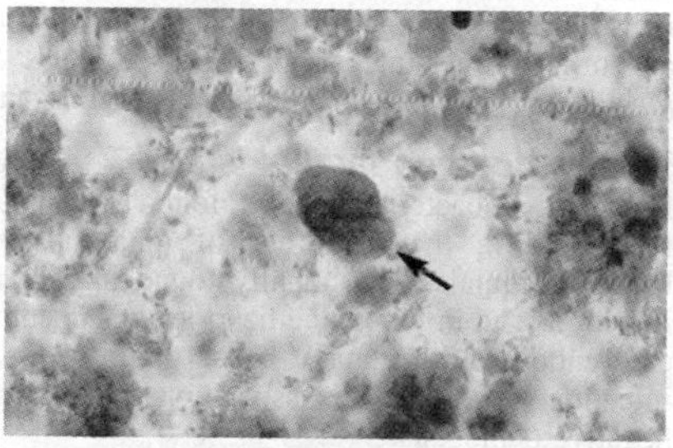

Entamoeba histolytica: stool smear shows a trophozoite of ***E. histolytica*** that has a pseudopodium (arrow), trichrome, ×3400

En•ta•moe•ba po•lec•ki (ent′ă-mē′bă pō′lek-ī) A species of ameba commonly found in the intestines of pigs; also parasitizes monkeys, cattle, goats, sheep, and dogs; also found in humans, where it does not produce symptoms; clinical importance lies in the possibility of confusing the organism with *E. histolytica*.

entamoebiasis [Br.] SYN entamebiasis.

en•ter•al (en′tĕr-ăl) Within, or by way of, the intestine or gastrointestinal tract, especially as distinguished from parenteral. A term used to describe tube feedings. [G. *enteron,* intestine]

en•ter•al feed•ing (en′tĕr-ăl fēd′ing) A form of tube alimentation.

en•ter•al•gi•a (en′tĕr-al′jē-ă) Enterdynia; severe abdominal pain accompanying spasm of the bowel. SYN enterodynia. [entero- + G. *algos,* pain]

en•ter•al hy•per•al•i•men•ta•tion (en′tĕr-ăl hī′pĕr-al-i-men-tā′shŭn) Hyperalimentation by the administration of elemental nutrients using a catheter placed within the intestinal tract; usually used in patients with at least a portion of functional small intestine.

en•ter•al nu•tri•tion (en′tĕr-ăl nū-trish′ŭn) Alimentation provided by means of a tube into the intestine or gastrointestinal tract.

en•ter•ec•ta•sis (en′tĕr-ek′tă-sis) Dilation of the bowel. [entero- + G. *ektasis,* a stretching]

en•ter•ec•to•my (en′tĕr-ek′tŏ-mē) Resection of a segment of the intestine. [entero- + G. *ektomē,* excision]

en•ter•el•co•sis (en′tĕr-el-kō′sis) Ulceration of the bowel. [entero- + G. *helkos,* ulcer]

en•ter•ic (en-ter′ik) Relating to the intestine. [G. *enterikos,* from *entera,* bowels]

ent•er•ic-coat•ed tab•let (en-ter′ik kōt′ĕd tab′lĕt) A tablet covered with a substance that delays release of the medication until the tablet has passed through the stomach and into the intestine.

en•ter•ic fe•ver (en-ter′ik fē′vĕr) **1.** SYN typhoid fever. **2.** The group of typhoid and paratyphoid fevers.

en•ter•ic i•so•la•tion (en-ter′ik ī′sō-lā′shŭn) Sequestration used for patients with infections of the intestinal tract.

en•ter•i•coid fe•ver (en-ter′i-koyd fē′vĕr) A fever, neither paratyphoid nor typhoid, resembling the latter.

en•ter•ic or•phan vi•rus•es (en-ter′ik ōr′făn vī′rŭs-ĕz) Enteroviruses isolated from humans and other animals, "orphan" implying lack of known association with disease when isolated; many viruses of the group are now known to be pathogenic; they include ECBO viruses, ECHO viruses, and ECSO viruses.

en•ter•ic tu•ber•cu•lo•sis (en-ter′ik tū-bĕr′kyū-lō′sis) A complication of cavitary pulmonary tuberculosis usually resulting from expectoration and swallowing of bacilli that then infect areas of the digestive tract. SEE ALSO tuberculous enteritis.

en•ter•ic vi•rus•es (en-ter′ik vī′rŭs-ĕz) Viruses of the genus enterovirus.

en•ter•i•tis (en′tĕr-ī′tis) Inflammation of the intestine, especially of the small intestine. [entero- + G. *-itis,* inflammation]

en·ter·i·tis ne·cro·ti·cans (en′tĕr-ī′tis ne-krot′i-kanz) Condition involving necrosis of the bowel wall caused by *Clostridium welchii.* SYN pigbel.

entero-, enter- Combining forms indicating the intestines. [G. *enteron,* intestine]

en·ter·o·ag·gre·ga·tive *Esch·e·rich·i·a co·li* (en′tĕr-ō-ag′rĕ-gā-tiv esh′ĕr-ik′ē-ă kō′lī) Pathogenic *E. coli* strains defined by their attachment to HEp-2 cells; cause persistent pediatric diarrhea.

en·ter·o·a·nas·to·mo·sis (en′tĕr-ō-ă-nas′tō-mō′sis) SYN enteroenterostomy.

En·ter·o·bac·ter (en′tĕr-ō-bak′tĕr) A genus of aerobic, facultatively anaerobic, non-spore-forming, motile bacteria (family Enterobacteriaceae) containing gram-negative rods. The cells are peritrichous, and some strains have encapsulated cells. Glucose is fermented with the production of acid and gas. The Voges-Proskauer test result is usually positive. These organisms occur in the feces of humans and other animals and in sewage, soil, water, and dairy products; recognized as an agent of common nosocomial infections of the urinary tract, lungs, or blood; somewhat resistant to antibiotics. This genus characteristically acquires resistance rapidly, in part because of the presence of inducible beta-lactamases. The type species is *E. cloacae.*

En·ter·o·bac·ter aer·o·ge·nes (en′tĕr-ō-bak′tĕr ār-oj′ĕ-nēz) A bacterial species often recovered from wounds, urine, blood, and spinal fluid of hospitalized patients.

En·ter·o·bac·ter sa·ka·za·ki·i (en′tĕr-ō-bak′tĕr sah-kah-zah′kē-ī) A bacterial species especially associated with nursery-acquired neonatal meningitis.

en·ter·o·bi·a·sis (en′tĕr-ō-bī′ă-sis) Infection with *Enterobius vermicularis,* the human pinworm.

En·te·ro·bi·us (en′tĕr-ō′bī-ŭs) A genus of nematode worms that includes the pinworms (*E. vermicularis*). See this page. [entero- + G. *bios,* life]

***En·te·ro·bi·us* gran·u·lo·ma** (en′tĕr-ō′bī-ŭs gran′yū-lō′mă) Lesions containing dead worms and eggs of the nematode are found in the vagina, cervix, fallopian tubes, omentum, peritoneum, liver, kidneys, and lungs.

en·ter·o·cele (en′tĕr-o-sēl) **1.** A hernial protrusion through a defect in the rectovaginal or vesicovaginal pouch. [entero- + G. *kēlē,* hernia] **2.** SYN abdominal cavity. [entero- + G. *koilia,* a hollow] **3.** An intestinal hernia. [see 1]

en·ter·o·cen·te·sis (en′tĕr-ō-sen-tē′sis) Puncture of the intestine with a hollow needle (trocar and cannula) to withdraw substances. [entero- + G. *kentēsis,* puncture]

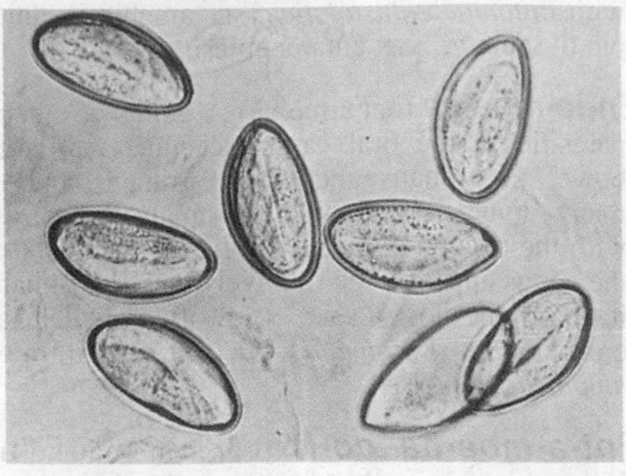

Enterobius vermicularis (pinworm ova): transparent tape preparation

en·ter·o·ci·dal (en′ter-ō-sī′dal) An agent that kills parasites residing in the gastrointestinal tract.

en·ter·o·clei·sis (en′tĕr-ō-klī′sis) Occlusion of the lumen of the alimentary canal. [entero- + G. *kleisis,* a closing]

en·ter·o·cly·sis (en′tĕr-ō-klī′sis) **1.** SYN high enema. **2.** In radiography of the small intestine, filling by introduction of contrast medium through a catheter advanced into the duodenum or jejunum from above. [entero- + G. *klysis,* a washing out]

En·ter·o·coc·cus (en′ter-ō-kok′ŭs) Genus of facultatively anaerobic, generally nonmotile, non-spore-forming, gram-positive bacteria. Found in the intestinal tract of humans and animals, enterococci cause intraabdominal, wound, and urinary tract infections. Type species is *E. faecalis. E. faecium* is also clinically significant.

En·ter·o·coc·cus fae·cal·is (en′tĕr-ō-kok-ŭs fā-kā′lis) A bacterial species found in human feces and in the intestines of many warm-blooded animals; occasionally found in urinary infections and in blood and heart lesions in subacute endocarditis; a major cause of nosocomial infection, especially in association with gram-negative pathogens.

En·ter·o·coc·cus fae·ci·um (en′tĕr-ō-kok-ŭs fē′shē-ŭm) Bacterial species of this genus recovered in human infection; this species has low-level resistance to ampicillin, and in the U.S. and other countries where vancomycin is used frequently, resistant strains have been rapidly appearing as causes of nosocomial infections; in cases of septicemia in immunocompromised patients, fatality rates in cases of septicemia are high in immunocompromised patients.

en·ter·o·co·li·tis (en′tĕr-ō-kō-lī′tis) Inflammation of the mucous membrane of both small and large intestines. SYN coloenteritis. [entero- + G. *kolon,* colon, + *-itis,* inflammation]

en·ter·o·co·los·to·my (en′tĕr-ō-kŏ-los′tŏ-mē) Establishment of an artificial opening between the small intestine and the colon. [entero- + G. *kōlon,* colon, + *stoma,* mouth]

en·ter·o·cyst, en·ter·o·cys·to·ma (en′tĕr-ō-sist, en′tĕr-ō-sis-tō′mă) A cyst of the wall of the intestine. [entero- + G. *kystis,* bladder]

en·ter·o·cys·to·cele (en′tĕr-ō-sis′tō-sēl) A hernia of both intestine and bladder wall. [entero- + G. *kystis,* bladder, + *kēlē,* hernia]

en·ter·o·dyn·i·a (en′tĕr-ō-din′ē-ă) SYN enteralgia. [entero- + G. *odynē,* pain]

en·ter·o·en·do·crine cells (en′tĕr-ō-en′dō-krin selz) A family of cells with argyrophilic granules occurring throughout the digestive tract and believed to produce at least 20 gastrointestinal hormones and neurotransmitters.

en·ter·o·en·ter·os·to·my (en′tĕr-ō-en-tĕr-os′tō-mē) Establishment of a new communication between two segments of intestine. SYN enteroanastomosis, intestinal anastomosis.

en·ter·o·gas·tric re·flex (en′tĕr-ō-gas′trik rē′fleks) Peristaltic contraction of the small intestine induced by the entrance of food into the stomach. SEE ALSO gastrocolic reflex.

en·ter·o·gas·tri·tis (en′tĕr-ō-gas-trī′tis) SYN gastroenteritis. [entero- + G. *gastēr,* belly, + *-itis,* inflammation]

en·ter·o·gas·trone (en′tĕr-ō-gas′trōn) A hormone obtained from the intestinal mucosa that inhibits gastric secretion and motility; secretion of enterogastrone is stimulated by exposure of duodenal mucosa to dietary lipids.

en·ter·og·e·nous (en′tĕr-oj′ĕ-nŭs) Of intestinal origin. [entero- + G. *-gen,* producing]

en·ter·og·e·nous cy·a·no·sis (en′tĕr-oj′ĕ-nŭs sī′ă-nō′sis) Apparent cyanosis caused by the absorption of nitrites or other toxic materials from the intestine with the formation of methemoglobin or sulfhemoglobin; the skin color change is due to the chocolate color of methemoglobin.

en·ter·og·e·nous cyst (en′tĕr-oj′ĕ-nŭs sist) Mediastinal cyst derived from cells sequestered from the primitive foregut; may be classified histologically as bronchogenic, esophageal, or gastric.

en·ter·o·hem·or·rhag·ic *Esch·e·rich·i·a co·li* (EHEC) (en′tĕr-ō-hem-ŏr-aj′ik esh-ĕ-rik′ē-ă kō′lī) Strain of *E. coli,* usually of the serotype 0157:H7; produces a toxin resembling that produced by *Shigella;* associated with damage to the epithelium, ischemia of the bowel, and necrosis of the colon. Apparently responsible for a hemorrhagic form of colitis without fever, which can be very severe and is spread primarily by contaminated beef. May also cause microangiopathic hemolytic anemia, renal failure, and the hemolytic uremic syndrome.

en·ter·o·he·pat·ic cir·cu·la·tion (en′tĕr-ō-hĕ-pat′ik sĭr′kyū-lā′shŭn) Absorption from the intestine of hepatic products, notably bile salts, by the portal system; secreted again in bile, these may be recycled several times.

en·ter·o·hep·a·ti·tis (en′tĕr-ō-hep-ă-tī′tis) Inflammation of both the intestine and the liver. [entero- + G. *hēpar* (*hēpat-*), liver, + *-itis,* inflammation]

en·ter·o·hep·a·to·cele (en′tĕr-ō-hep′ă-tō-sēl) Congenital umbilical hernia containing intestine and liver. SEE omphalocele. [entero- + G. *hēpar* (*hēpat-*), liver, + *kēlē,* hernia]

en·ter·o·in·va·sive *Esch·e·rich·i·a co·li* (EIEC) (en′tĕr-ō-in-vā′siv esh-ĕ-rik′ē-ă kō′lī) Strain of *E. coli* that penetrates gut mucosa and multiplies in colon epithelial cells, resulting in shigellosislike changes of the mucosa. This strain produces a severe diarrheal illness that can resemble shigellosis except for the absence of vomiting and a shorter duration of illness.

en·ter·o·ki·ne·sis (en′tĕr-ō-ki-nē′sis) Muscular contraction of the alimentary canal. SEE ALSO peristalsis. [entero- + G. *kinēsis,* movement]

en·ter·o·ki·net·ic (en′tĕr-ō-ki-net′ik) Relating to, or producing, enterokinesis.

en·ter·o·lith (en′tĕr-ō-lith) An intestinal calculus formed of layers of soaps and earthy phosphates surrounding a nucleus of some hard body, such as a swallowed fruit stone or other indigestible substance. [entero- + G. *lithos,* stone]

en·ter·o·li·thi·a·sis (en′tĕr-ō-li-thī′ă-sis) Presence of calculi in the intestine.

en·ter·ol·o·gy (en′tĕr-ol′ŏ-jē) The branch of medical science concerned especially with the intestinal tract. [entero- + G. *logos,* study]

en·ter·ol·y·sis (en′tĕr-ol′i-sis) Division of intestinal adhesions. [entero- + G. *lysis,* dissolution]

en·ter·o·meg·a·ly, en·ter·o·me·ga·li·a (en′tĕr-ō-meg′ă-lē, -ō-mĕ-gā′lē-ă) SYN megaloenteron. [entero- + G. *megas,* great]

en·ter·o·my·co·sis (en′tĕr-ō-mī-kō′sis) An intestinal disease of fungal origin. [entero- + G. *mykēs,* fungus, + *-osis,* condition]

en·ter·o·pa·re·sis (en′tĕr-ō-păr-ē′sis) Rarely used term for a state of diminished or absent peristalsis with flaccidity of the muscles of the intestinal walls. [entero- + G. *paresis,* slackening, relaxation]

en·ter·o·path·o·gen (en′tĕr-ō-path′ŏ-jen) An organism capable of producing disease in the intestinal tract.

en·ter·o·path·o·gen·ic (en′tĕr-ō-path′ŏ-jen′ik) Capable of producing disease in the intestinal tract.

en·ter·o·path·o·gen·ic *Esch·e·rich·i·a co·li* (EPEC) (en′tĕr-ō-path′ō-jen′ik esh-ĕ-rik′ē-ă kō′lī) Organisms that adhere to small bowel mucosa and produce characteristic changes in the microvilli. This strain produces symptomatic, sometimes serious, gastrointestinal illnesses, especially severe in neonates and young children; typically produces toxins.

en·ter·op·a·thy (en′tĕr-op′ă-thē) An intestinal disease. [entero- + G. *pathos,* suffering]

en·ter·o·pep·ti·dase (en′tĕr-ō-pep′ti-dās) An intestinal proteolytic glycoenzyme from the duodenal mucosa that converts trypsinogen into trypsin (removes a hexapeptide from trypsinogen).

en·ter·o·pex·y (en′tĕr-ō-pek-sē) Fixation of a segment of the intestine to the abdominal wall. [entero- + G. *pēxis,* fixation]

en·ter·op·to·sis, en·ter·op·to·si·a (en′tĕr-op-tō′sis, -tō′sē-ă) Abnormal descent of the intestines in the abdominal cavity, usually associated with falling of the other viscera. [entero- + G. *ptōsis,* a falling]

en·ter·op·tot·ic (en′tĕr-op-tot′ik) Relating to or suffering from enteroptosis.

en·ter·or·rha·gi·a (en′tĕr-ōr-ā′jē-ă) Bleeding within the intestinal tract. [entero- + G. *rhēgnymi,* to burst forth]

en·ter·or·rha·phy (en′tĕr-ōr′ă-fē) Suture of the intestine. [entero- + G. *rhaphē,* suture]

en·ter·o·sep·sis (en′tĕr-ō-sep′sis) Sepsis occurring in or derived from the alimentary canal. [entero- + G. *sēpsis,* putrefaction]

en·ter·o·spasm (en′tĕr-ō-spazm) Increased, irregular, and painful peristalsis. [entero- + G. *spasmos,* spasm]

en·ter·o·sta·sis (en′tĕr-ō-stā′sis) Intestinal stasis; a retardation or arrest of the passage of the intestinal contents; older term for ileus. [entero- + G. *stasis,* a standing]

en·ter·o·ste·no·sis (en′tĕr-ō-sten-ō′sis) Narrowing of the lumen of the intestine. [entero- + G. *stenōsis,* narrowing]

i **en·ter·os·to·my** (en′tĕr-os′tŏ-mē) An artificial anus or fistula into the intestine through the abdominal wall. See this page. [entero- + G. *stoma,* mouth]

en·ter·ot·o·my (en′tĕr-ot′ŏ-mē) Incision into the intestine.

enterotoxaemia [Br.] SYN enterotoxemia.

en·ter·o·tox·e·mi·a (en′tĕr-ō-tok-sē′mē-ă) The presence of an enterotoxin in the blood. SYN enterotoxaemia. [enterotoxin + G. *haima,* blood]

en·ter·o·tox·i·gen·ic (en′tĕr-ō-tok-si-jen′ik) Denoting an organism containing or producing a toxin specific for cells of the intestinal mucosa.

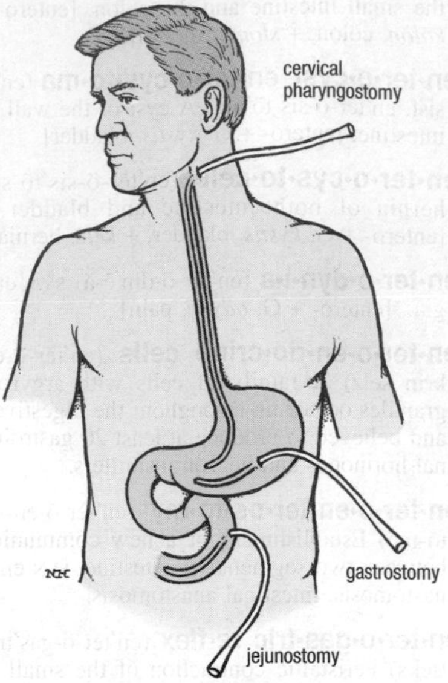

enterostomy tubes: flexible tubes passing through surgical openings into selected portions of the gastrointestinal tract, providing access for liquid food; a temporary alternative to enterostomy

en·ter·o·tox·i·gen·ic *Esch·e·rich·i·a co·li* (ETEC) (en′tĕr-ō-tok-si-jen′ik esh-ĕ-rik′ē-ă kō′lī) Strain that attaches to the duodenum or proximal small intestine mucosa, where it forms heat-stable and heat-labile toxins that activate adenylate cyclase, causing wasting diarrhea. Responsible for 40–70% of traveler's diarrhea; chiefly water borne in human feces.

en·ter·o·tox·in (en′tĕr-ō-tok′sin) A cytotoxin specific for the cells of the intestinal mucosa.

en·ter·o·tro·pic (en′tĕr-ō-trō′pik) Attracted by or affecting the intestine. [entero- + G. *tropikos,* turning]

En·te·ro·vi·rus (en′tĕr-ō-vī-rŭs) A large and diverse group of viruses that includes poliovirus types 1–3, coxsackievirus A and B, echoviruses, and those enteroviruses identified since 1969 that were assigned type numbers.

en·ter·o·zo·ic (en′tĕr-ō-zō′ik) Relating to an enterozoon.

en·ter·o·zo·on (en′tĕr-ō-zō′on) An animal parasite in the intestine. [entero- + G. *zōon,* animal]

ent·ge·gen (*E*) (ent′gā-gen) Term used when the two higher ranking groups, attached to different carbon atoms in a carbon-carbon double bond, are on opposite sides of the double bond (hence, analogous to trans-). [Ger. opposite]

en·thal·py (*H*) (en′thal-pē) Heat content, symbolized as *H;* a thermodynamic function, defined as $E + PV$, where E is the internal energy of a system, P the pressure, and V the volume; the heat of a reaction, measured at constant pressure, is ΔH. SYN heat (3). [G. *enthalpō*, to warm in]

en·the·si·tis (en′thĕ-sī′tis) Traumatic disease occurring at the insertion of muscles where recurring concentration of stress provokes inflammation with a strong tendency toward fibrosis and calcification. [G. *enthetos*, implanted, + *-itis*, inflammation]

en·the·so·path·ic (en′thĕ-sō-path′ik) Denoting or characteristic of enthesopathy.

en·the·sop·a·thy (en′thĕ-sop′ă-thē) A disease process occurring at the site of insertion of muscle tendons and ligaments into bones or joint capsules. [G. *en*, in, + *thesis*, a placing, + *pathos*, suffering]

ento-, ent- Combining forms meaning inner, or within. SEE ALSO endo-. [G. *entos*, within]

en·to·blast (en′tō-blast) **1.** Pertaining to entoderm. **2.** Cell nucleolus. [ento- + G. *blastos*, germ]

en·to·cele (en′tō-sēl) An internal hernia. [ento- + G. *kēlē*, hernia]

en·to·cho·roi·de·a (en′tō-kōr-oyd′ē-ă) SYN choriocapillary layer. [ento- + G. *chorioeidēs*, choroid]

en·to·co·nid (en′tō-kō′nid) **1.** The distolingual cusp of human lower molars. **2.** One of the three cusps that make up the talonid of the molars. SEE ALSO hypoconid, hypoconulid. [ento- + G. *kōnos*, cone]

en·to·derm (en′tō-dĕrm) SYN endoderm. [ento- + G. *derma*, skin]

en·to·der·mal cell (en′tō-dĕr′măl sel) SYN endodermal cells.

en·to·ec·tad (en′tō-ek′tad) From within outward. [G. *entos*, within, + *ektos*, without,+ L. *ad*, to]

En·to·lo·ma si·nu·a·tum (en-tō-lō′mă sī-nū-ā′tŭm) A species of mushroom capable of producing mycetismus gastrointestinalis.

en·to·mi·on (en-tō′mē-on) The tip of the mastoid angle of the parietal bone. [G. *entomē*, notch]

en·to·mol·o·gy (en′tŏ-mol′ŏ-jē) The science concerned with the study of insects. [G. *entomon*, insect, + *logos*, study]

En·to·moph·tho·ra (en-tō-mof′thō-ră) SEE *Conidiobolus.*

En·to·moph·tho·ra co·ro·na·ta (en-tō-mof′thō-ră kō-rō-nā′tă) SEE *Conidiobolus.*

En·to·moph·thor·a·les (en-tō-mof′thō-rā′lēz) An order of the fungal class Zygomycetes. The genera include *Conidiobolus*, which causes a chronic granulomatous inflammation of a nasal and paranasal sinus mucosa (conidiobolomycosis) and *Basidiobolus*, which causes a chronic subcutaneous granuloma (basidiobolomycosis). When conidiobolomycosis and basidiobolomycosis are considered together, they are called entomophthoramycosis.

en·to·moph·tho·ra·my·co·sis (en′tō-mof-thōr′ă-mī-kō′sis) A disease caused by fungi of the genera *Basidiobolus* or *Conididiobolus;* tissues are invaded by broad nonseptate hyphae that become surrounded by eosinophilic material. A form of zygomycosis. [Entomophthorales (order name) + G. *mykēs*, fungus + -osis, condition]

En·to·mo·pox·vi·rus (en′tō-mō-poks-vī′rŭs) The genus of viruses (family Poxviridae) that comprises the poxviruses of insects; they do not seem to multiply in vertebrates. [G. *entomon*, insect]

en·top·ic (en-top′ik) Placed within; occurring or situated in the normal place; opposed to ectopic. [G. *en*, within, + *topos*, place]

en·top·tic (en-top′tik) Within the eyeball. Often used to describe visual phenomena generated by mechanical or electrical stimulations of the retina. [ento- + G. *optikos*, relating to vision]

en·to·ret·i·na (en′tō-ret′i-nă) The layers of the retina from the outer plexiform to the nerve fiber layer inclusive.

en·to·zo·al (en′tō-zō′ăl) Relating to entozoa.

en·to·zo·on, pl. **en·to·zo·a** (en′tō-zō′on, -ă) An animal parasite with a habitat in any of the internal organs or tissues. [ento- + G. *zōon*, animal]

en·train·ment mask (en-trān′mĕnt mask) A face mask designed to entrain atmospheric air to provide a constant fractional dilution of a pressurized gas, most commonly oxygen.

en·trap·ment neu·rop·a·thy (en-trap′mĕnt nūr-op′ă-thē) A focal nerve lesion produced by constriction or mechanical distortion of the nerve, within a fibrous or fibroosseous tunnel, or by a fibrous band.

en·tro·pi·on, en·tro·pi·um (en-trō′pē-on, -pē-ŭm) **1.** Inversion or turning inward of a part. **2.** The infolding of the margin of an eyelid. [G. *en*, in, + *tropē*, a turning]

en·tro·py (*S*) (en′trŏ-pē) That fraction of heat (energy) content not available for the performance of work, usually because (in a chemical reaction) it has been used to increase the random motion of the atoms or molecules in the system; thus, entropy is a measure of randomness or disorder. [G. *entropia*, a turning towards]

en·ty·py (en′ti-pē) A type of gastrulation seen in some early mammalian embryos in which the endoderm covers the embryonic and amniotic ectoderm; part of the preplacental trophoblast may also be covered. [G. *entypē,* pattern]

e•nu•cle•ate (ē-nū′klē-āt) To remove entirely; to shell like a nut, as in the removal of an eye from its capsule or a tumor from its enveloping capsule.

e•nu•cle•a•tion (ē-nū′klē-ā′shŭn) **1.** Removal of an entire structure (e.g., an eyeball, tumor), without rupture, as one shells the kernel of a nut. **2.** Removal or destruction of the nucleus of a cell. [L. *enucleo,* to remove the kernel, fr. *e,* out, + *nucleus,* nut, kernel]

en•u•re•sis (en-yūr-ē′sis) Urinary incontinence; particularly nocturnal (i.e., bed wetting). [G. *en-oureō,* to urinate in]

en•ve•lope (en′vĕ-lōp) ANATOMY any structure that encloses or covers.

en•vel•ope of mo•tion (en′vĕ-lōp mō′shŭn) SEE border movement.

en•ven•om•a•tion (en-ven′ō-mā′shŭn) The act of injecting a poisonous material (venom) by sting, spine, bite, or other venom apparatus.

en•vi•ron•ment (en-vī′rŏn-mĕnt) The milieu; the aggregate of all of the external conditions and influences affecting the life and development of an organism. [Fr. *environ,* around]

en•vi•ron•men•tal med•i•cine (en-vī′rŏn-men′tăl med′i-sin) That branch of health care involved with therapy of patients who are afflicted by causes related to the environment (e.g., duststorms, heat, overcrowding); also studies role of diet and environmental allergens on health and illness, among many other considerations.

en•vi•ron•men•tal psy•chol•o•gy (en-vī′rŏn-men′tăl sī-kol′ŏ-jē) The study and application by behavioral scientists and architects of how changes in physical space and related physical stimuli produce an impact on the behavior of individuals. SEE ALSO personal space.

en•zo•ot•ic (en′zō-ot′ik) Denoting a temporal pattern of disease occurrence in an animal population in which the disease occurs with predictable regularity with only relatively minor fluctuations in its frequency over time. SEE epizootic, sporadic. Cf. epizootic, sporadic. [G. *en,* in, + *zōon,* animal]

en•zo•ot•ic sta•bil•i•ty (en′zō-ot′ik stă-bil′i-tē) SYN endemic stability.

en•zy•got•ic (en′zī-got′ik) Derived from a single fertilized oocyte; denoting twins so derived. [G. *eis (en),* one, + zygote]

en•zy•got•ic twins (en′zī-got′ik twinz) SYN monozygotic twins.

en•zy•mat•ic (en′zī-mat′ik) Relating to an enzyme.

en•zyme (en′zīm) A protein that acts as a catalyst to induce chemical changes in other substances, while remaining apparently unchanged itself by the process. Enzymes, with the exception of those discovered long ago (e.g., pepsin, emulsin), are generally named by adding -ase to the name of the substrate on which the enzyme acts (e.g., glucosidase), the substance activated (e.g., hydrogenase), or the type of reaction (e.g., oxidoreductase, transferase, hydrolase, lyase, isomerase, ligase or synthetase—these being the six main groups in the Enzyme Nomenclature Recommendations of the International Union of Biochemistry). [G. + L. *en,* in + *zymē,* leaven]

en•zyme im•mu•no•as•say (EIA) (en′zīm im′yū-nō-as′ā) Procedure measuring antibodies to detect the analyte of interest and an enzyme linked to the antigen-antibody complex. The enzyme reacts with a substrate to produce a product that is measured to quantitate the amount of antigen-antibody formed. SEE ALSO enzyme-linked immunosorbent assay, enzyme-multiplied immunoassay technique.

en•zyme-linked im•mu•no•sor•bent as•say (ELISA) (en′zīm-lingkt im′yū-nō-sōr′bĕnt as′ā) A sensitive method for serodiagnosis of specific infectious diseases; an in vitro competitive binding assay in which an enzyme and its substrate rather than a radioactive substance serve as the indicator system; in positive test results, the two yield a colored or other easily recognizable substance; the enzyme is linked to known immunoglobulin (or antigen) and in positive test results remains as part of the antigen-antibody complex available to react with its substrate when added.

en•zyme-mul•ti•plied im•mu•no•as•say tech•nique (EMIT) (en′zīm-mŭl′ti-plīd im′yū-nō-as′ā tek-nēk′) A type of test in which the ligand is labeled with an enzyme. SEE ALSO competitive binding assay, enzyme-linked immunosorbent assay.

en•zy•mol•o•gy (en′zi-mol′ŏ-jē) The branch of chemistry concerned with the properties and actions of enzymes. [enzyme + G. *logos,* study]

en•zy•mol•y•sis (en′zi-mol′i-sis) **1.** The splitting or cleavage of a substance into smaller parts by means of enzymatic action. **2.** Lysis by the action of an enzyme. [enzyme + G. *lysis,* dissolution]

en•zy•mop•a•thy (en′zi-mop′ă-thē) Any disturbance of enzyme function, including genetic deficiency or defect in specific enzymes. [enzyme + G. *pathos,* disease]

EOA Abbreviation for esophageal obturator airway.

EOB Abbreviation for explanation of benefits.

EOG Abbreviation for electrooculography; electroolfactogram.

e•o•sin (ē′ō-sin) A fluorescent acid dye used for

cytoplasmic stains and counterstains in histology and in Romanowsky-type blood stains. [G. *ēōs,* dawn]

e·o·sin B (ē′ō-sin) The disodium salt of 4′,5′-dibromo-2′,7′-dinitrofluorescein. SYN eosin I bluish. [CI 45400]

e·o·sin I blu·ish (ē′ō-sin blū′ish) SYN eosin B.

e·o·sin-meth·yl·ene blue a·gar (ē′ō-sin-meth′i-lēn blū ā′gahr) Agar composed of peptone, lactose, sucrose, eosin, and methylene blue; inhibits growth of most gram-positive bacteria; used thus to distinguish between lactose-fermenting and non-lactose-fermenting, gram-negative bacteria.

e·o·sin·o·pe·ni·a (ē′ō-sin-ō-pē′nē-ă) An abnormally small number of eosinophils in the peripheral bloodstream. [eosino(phil) + G. *penia,* poverty]

e·o·sin·o·phil, e·o·sin·o·phile (ē′ō-sin′ō-fil, ē′ō-sin′ō-fīl) SYN eosinophilic leukocyte. See page B2. [eosin + G. *philos,* fond]

e·o·sin·o·phil ad·e·no·ma (ē′ō-sin′ō-fil ad′ē-nō′mă) SYN acidophil adenoma.

e·o·sin·o·phil ca·ti·on·ic pro·tein (ECP) (ē′ō-sin′ō-fil kat′ī-on′ik prō′tēn) A protein the level of which in serum of clotted blood reflects the rate of activation of circulating eosinophils.

e·o·sin·o·phil che·mo·tac·tic fac·tor of an·a·phy·lax·is (ē′ō-sin′ō-fil kē′mō-tak′tik fak′tŏr an′ă-fi-lak′sis) A peptide that is chemotactic for eosinophilic leukocytes and is released from disrupted mast cells.

e·o·sin·o·phil·i·a (ē′ō-sin-ō-fil′ē-ă) SYN eosinophilic leukocytosis.

e·o·sin·o·phil·i·a-my·al·gi·a syn·drome (ē′ō-sin-ō-fil′ē-ă mī-al′jē-ă sin′drōm) A probable autoimmune disorder precipitated by ingestion of contaminated L-tryptophan tablets, and characterized by fatigue, low-grade fever, myalgias, muscle tenderness and cramps, weakness, paresthesias of the extremities, and skin indurations; marked eosinophilia is noted on peripheral blood studies; serum aldolase is increased and biopsies of peripheral nerve, muscle, skin, and fascia show microangiopathy and inflammation in connective tissue.

e·o·sin·o·phil·ic (ē′ō-sin-ō-fil′ik) Staining readily with eosin dyes; denoting such cell or tissue elements.

e·o·sin·o·phil·ic gran·u·lo·ma (ē′ō-sin-ō-fil′ik gran′yū-lō′mă) A lesion observed more frequently in children and adolescents, occasionally in young adults, which occurs chiefly as a solitary focus in one bone, although multiple involvement is sometimes observed and similar foci may develop in the lung; characterized by numerous Langerhans cells and eosinophils, and occasional foci of necrosis; may be related to Hand-Schüller-Christian disease, possibly representing a benign form.

e·o·sin·o·phil·ic leu·ke·mi·a, e·o·sin·o·phil·o·cyt·ic leu·ke·mi·a (ē′ō-sin-ō-fil′ik lū-kē′mē-ă, ē-ō-sin′ō-fil-ō-sit′ik) A form of granulocytic leukemia in which there are conspicuous numbers of eosinophilic granulocytes in the tissues and circulating blood, or in which such cells are predominant.

e·o·sin·o·phil·ic leu·ko·cyte (ē′ō-sin-ō-fil′ik lū′kō-sīt) A polymorphonuclear white blood cell characterized by prominent cytoplasmic granules that are bright yellow-red or orange when treated with Wright stain; the nuclei are usually larger than those of neutrophils and characteristically have two lobes; these leukocytes are motile phagocytes with distinctive antiparasitic functions. SYN eosinophil, eosinophile, oxyphil (2), oxyphile, oxyphilic leukocyte.

e·o·sin·o·phil·ic leu·ko·cy·to·sis (ē′ō-sin-ō-fil′ik lū′kō-sī-tō′sis) A form of relative leukocytosis in which the greatest proportionate increase is in the eosinophils. SYN eosinophilia.

e·o·sin·o·phil·ic leu·ko·pe·ni·a (ē′ō-sin-ō-fil′ik lū′kō-pē′nē-ă) A decrease in the number of eosinophilic granulocytes normally present in the circulating blood.

e·o·sin·o·phil·ic pneu·mo·ni·a (ē′ō-sin-ō-fil′ik nū-mō′nē-ă) **1.** An immunologic disorder characterized by radiologic evidence of infiltrates accompanied by either peripheral blood eosinophilia or histopathologic evidence of eosinophilic infiltrates in lung tissue. **2.** Eosinophilic infiltration of the lung secondary to infection or allergic reaction.

e·o·sin·o·phil·ic pus·tu·lar fol·lic·u·li·tis (ē′ō-sin-ō-fil′ik pŭs′chū-lăr fō-lik′yū-lī′tis) A dermatosis characterized by sterile pruritic papules and pustules that coalesce to form plaques with papulovesicular borders; spontaneous exacerbations and remissions may be accompanied by peripheral leukocytosis, eosinophilia, or both, and may result in eventual destruction of hair follicles and formation of eosinophilic abscesses. The disease has been reported in AIDS, and a possibly separate form of eosinophilic pustular folliculitis occurs in infants. SYN Ofuji disease.

e·o·sin·o·phil·u·ri·a (ē′ō-sin′ō-fil-yūr-ē′ă) Presence of eosinophils in the urine.

e·o·sin y, e·o·sin Ys, e·o·sin yel·low·ish (ē′ō-sin, ē′ō-sin yel′ō-ish) The disodium salt of 2′,4′,5′,7′-tetrabromofluorescein. [C.I. 45380]

EP Abbreviation for endogenous pyrogen.

ep·ax·i·al (ep-ak′sē-ăl) Above or behind any axis, such as the spinal axis or the axis of a limb. [G. *epi,* on, + L. *axis,* axis]

EPEC Abbreviation for enteropathogenic *Escherichia coli.*

ep·en·dy·ma (ĕ-pen′di-mă) [TA] The cellular membrane lining the central canal of the spinal cord and the brain ventricles. [G. *ependyma,* an upper garment]

ep·en·dy·mal (ĕ-pen′di-măl) Relating to the ependyma.

ep·en·dy·mal cell (ĕ-pen′di-măl sel) A cell lining the central canal of the spinal cord (those of pyramidal shape) or one of the brain ventricles (those of cuboidal shape).

ep·en·dy·mi·tis (ĕ-pen′di-mī′tis) Inflammation of the ependyma.

ep·en·dy·mo·blast (ĕ-pen′di-mō-blast) An embryonic ependymal cell. [ependyma + G. *blastos,* germ]

ep·en·dy·mo·cyte (ĕ-pen′di-mō-sīt) An ependymal cell. [ependyma + G. *kytos,* cell]

ep·en·dy·mo·ma (ĕ-pen′di-mō′mă) A glioma derived from relatively undifferentiated ependymal cells; ependymomas may originate from the lining of any of the ventricles or, more commonly, from the central canal of the spinal cord.

e·phapse (ē′faps) A place where two or more nerve cell processes (e.g., axons, dendrites) touch without forming a typical synaptic contact; some form of neural transmission may occur at such nonsynaptic contact sites. [G. *ephapsis,* contact]

e·phap·tic (ē-fap′tik) Relating to an ephapse.

e·phe·bic (ĕ-fē′bik) Rarely used term relating to the period of puberty or to a youth. [G. *ephēbikos,* relating to youth, fr. *hēbē,* youth]

e·phed·ra (e-fed′ră) (*Ephedra sinica* and other spp.) An herbal supplement now banned in the United States, where it was used as a weight-loss supplement. Severe toxicities and adverse effects reported (e.g., stroke, cardiac arrest, seizure, psychotic attacks); over 800 reports of related illness; the compounds also included substances banned for use by athletes. SYN ma-huang, Mormon tea, popotillo. [L., horsetail, fr. G. *ephedros,* sitting on]

e·phe·lis, pl. **e·phe·li·des** (ĕ-fē′lis, ĕ-fē′li-dēz) SYN freckles. [G.]

♻ **epi-** Prefix meaning on, following, or subsequent to. [G.]

ep·i·an·dros·ter·one (ep′i-an-dros′tĕr-ōn) Inactive isomer of androsterone; found in urine and in testicular and ovarian tissue.

ep·i·blast (ep′i-blast) The component of the bilaminar embryonic disc that gives rise to ectoderm and mesoderm. The mesoderm then displaces the hypoblast cells and forms the entodermal cell layer on its inner surface. [epi- + G. *blastos,* germ]

ep·i·blas·tic (ep′i-blas′tik) Relating to epiblast.

ep·i·bleph·a·ron (ep-i-blef′ă-ron) A congenital horizontal skin fold near the margin of the eyelid, caused by abnormal insertion of muscle fibers. In the upper lid, it simulates blepharochalasis; in the lower lid, it causes a turning inward of the lashes. [epi- + G. *blepharon,* eyelid]

e·pib·o·ly, e·pib·o·le (ē-pib′ŏ-lē, ē-pib′ŏ-lē) **1.** A process involved in gastrulation of telolecithal eggs in which, as a result of differential growth, some cells of the protoderm move over the surface toward the lips of the blastopore. **2.** Growth of epithelium in an organ culture to surround the underlying mesenchymal tissue. [G. *epibolē,* a throwing or laying on]

ep·i·bul·bar (ep′i-bŭl′bahr) On a bulb of any kind; specifically, on the eyeball.

ep·i·can·thal fold (ep′i-kan′thăl fōld) A fold of skin extending from the root of the nose to the medial termination of the eyebrow, overlapping the medial angle of the eye; its presence is normal in fetal life and in Asians.

ep·i·car·di·a (ep′i-kahr′dē-ă) The portion of the esophagus from where it passes through the diaphragm to the stomach. [epi- + G. *kardia,* heart]

ep·i·car·di·al (ep′i-kahr′dē-ăl) **1.** Relating to the epicardia. **2.** Relating to the epicardium.

ep·i·con·dy·lal·gi·a (ep′i-kon-di-lal′jē-ă) Pain in an epicondyle of the humerus or in the tendons or muscles originating therefrom. [epicondyle + G. *algos,* pain]

ep·i·con·dyle (ep′i-kon′dīl) A projection from a long bone near the articular extremity above or on the condyle. SYN epicondylus [TA]. [epi- + G. *kondylos,* a knuckle]

ep·i·con·dy·li·tis (ep′i-kon-di-lī′tis) Infection or inflammation of an epicondyle, or of associated tendons and other soft tissues, particularly the medial or lateral epicondyle of the humerus.

ep·i·con·dy·lus, pl. **ep·i·con·dy·li** (ep′i-kon′di-lŭs, -lī) [TA] SYN epicondyle. [L.]

ep·i·cra·ni·al ap·o·neu·ro·sis (ep′i-krā′nē-ăl ap′ō-nūr-ō′sis) The aponeurosis or intermediate tendon connecting the frontalis and occipitalis muscles to form the epicranius. SYN galea (2).

ep·i·cra·ni·um (ep′i-krā′nē-ŭm) The muscle, aponeurosis, and skin covering the cranium. [epi- + G. *kranion,* skull]

ep·i·cra·ni·us (ep′i-krā′nē-ŭs) SEE epicranius muscle.

ep·i·cra·ni·us mus·cle (ep′i-krā′nē-ŭs mŭs′ĕl) Composed of the epicranial aponeurosis and the muscles inserting into it, i.e., the occipitofrontalis musculus and temporoparietalis musculus. SYN musculus epicranius [TA].

ep·i·cri·sis (ep′i-krī-sis) A secondary crisis; a crisis terminating a recrudescence of morbid symptoms following a primary crisis.

ep·i·crit·ic, **ep·i·crit·ic sen·si·bil·i·ty** (ep′i-krit′ik, ep′i-krit′ik sens′i-bil′i-tē) The aspect of somatic sensation that permits the discrimination and the topographic localization of the finer degrees of touch and temperature stimuli. Cf. protopathic. [G. *epikritikos,* adjudicatory, fr. *epi,* on, + *krinō,* to separate, judge]

ep·i·cys·ti·tis (ep′i-sis-tī′tis) Inflammation of the cellular tissue around the bladder. [epi- + G. *kystis,* bladder, + *-itis,* inflammation]

ep·i·dem·ic (ep′i-dem′ik) The occurrence in a community or region of cases of an illness, specific health-related behavior, or other health-related events clearly in excess of normal expectancy. Cf. endemic, sporadic. [epi- + G. *dēmos,* the people]

ep·i·dem·ic dis·ease (ep′i-dem′ik di-zēz′) Marked increase in prevalence of a disease in a specific population or geographic area, usually with an environmental cause, such as an infectious or toxic agent.

ep·i·dem·ic gas·tro·en·ter·i·tis vi·rus (ep′i-dem′ik gas′trō-en-tĕr-ī′tis vī′rŭs) An RNA virus, about 27 nm in diameter, which has not been cultured in vitro; it is the cause of epidemic nonbacterial gastroenteritis; at least five antigenically distinct serotypes have been recognized, including the Norwalk agent. These viruses are classified with the Caliciviruses in the family Caliciviridae. SYN gastroenteritis virus type A.

ep·i·dem·ic he·mo·glo·bi·nu·ri·a (ep′i-dem′ik hē′mō-glō-bi-nyūr′ē-ă) The presence of hemoglobin in the urine of young infants, attended with cyanosis, jaundice, and other conditions; may be due to secondary methemoglobinemia. SYN Winckel disease.

ep·i·dem·ic hem·or·rhag·ic fe·ver (ep′i-dem′ik hem′ŏr-aj′ik fē′vĕr) Hantavirus infection, an acute febrile disease transmitted to human beings by exposure to feces of infected rodents; besides fever, myalgia, headache, and anorexia, it causes a petechial eruption and acute renal failure, manifested by oliguria, proteinuria, azotemia, and hypertension. SEE Hantavirus.

ep·i·de·mic·i·ty (ep′i-dĕ-mis′i-tē) The state of prevailing disease in epidemic form.

ep·i·dem·ic ker·a·to·con·junc·ti·vi·tis (ep′i-dem′ik ker′ă-tō-kŏn-jŭngk′ti-vī′tis) Follicular conjunctivitis followed by subepithelial corneal infiltrates; often caused by adenovirus type 8, less commonly by other types. SYN viral keratoconjunctivitis.

ep·i·dem·ic ker·a·to·con·junc·ti·vi·tis vi·rus (ep′i-dem′ik ker′ă-tō-kŏn-jŭngk-ti-vī′tis vī′rŭs) An adenovirus (type 8) causing epidemic keratoconjunctivitis, especially among shipyard workers, and also associated with outbreaks of swimming pool conjunctivitis. SYN shipyard eye.

ep·i·dem·ic my·al·gi·a (ep′i-dem′ik mī-al′jē-ă) SYN epidemic pleurodynia.

ep·i·dem·ic my·o·si·tis, **my·o·si·tis ep·i·dem·i·ca a·cu·ta** (ep′i-dem′ik mī-ō-sī′tis, mī′ō-sī-tis ep-i-dem′i-kă ă-kyūt′ă) SYN epidemic pleurodynia.

ep·i·dem·ic neu·ro·my·as·the·ni·a (ep′i-dem′ik nūr′ō-mī-ăs-thē′nē-ă) An epidemic disease characterized by stiffness of the neck and back, headache, diarrhea, fever, and localized muscular weakness; probably viral in origin. Cf. chronic fatigue syndrome. SYN benign myalgic encephalomyelitis, Iceland disease.

ep·i·dem·ic pa·rot·i·di·tis (ep′i-dem′ik pă-rot′i-dī′tis) An acute infectious and contagious disease caused by a paramyxovirus and characterized by fever, inflammation and swelling of the parotid gland, and sometimes of other salivary glands, and occasionally by inflammation of the testis, ovary, pancreas, or meninges. SYN mumps.

ep·i·dem·ic par·o·ti·tis vi·rus (ep′i-dem′ik pă-rot′i-tis vī′rŭs) SYN mumps virus.

ep·i·dem·ic pleu·ro·dyn·i·a (ep′i-dem′ik plūr′ō-din′ē-ă) An acute infectious disease usually occurring in epidemic form, characterized by paroxysms of pain, usually in the chest, and associated with strains of coxsackievirus type B. SYN Bornholm disease, Daae disease, devil's grip, diaphragmatic pleurisy, epidemic myalgia, epidemic myositis, myositis epidemica acuta, Sylvest disease.

ep·i·dem·ic pleu·ro·dyn·i·a vi·rus (ep′i-dem′ik plūr′ō-din′ē-ă vī′rŭs) A coxsackievirus, type B, which causes epidemic pleurodynia. SYN Bornholm disease virus.

ep·i·dem·ic pol·y·ar·thri·tis (ep′i-dem′ik pol′ē-ahr-thrī′tis) A mild febrile illness of humans in Australia characterized by polyarthralgia and rash, caused by the Ross River virus and transmitted by mosquitoes.

ep·i·dem·ic ro·se·o·la (ep′i-dem′ik rō′zē-ō′lă) SYN rubella.

ep·i·dem·ic ty·phus (ep′i-dem′ik tī′fŭs) Disease caused by *Rickettsia prowazekii* and spread by body lice; marked by high fever, mental and physical depression, and a macular and papular eruption; lasts about 2 weeks and occurs when large crowds are brought together and personal hygiene is poor; recrudescences can occur. SYN jail fever.

ep·i·de·mi·o·log·ic ge·net·ics (ep′i-dē′mē-ŏ-loj′ik jĕ-net′iks) The study of genetics as a phenomenon of defined populations by the criteria, methods, and objectives of epidemiology rather than of population genetics.

ep·i·de·mi·ol·o·gist (ep′i-dē′mē-ol′ŏ-jist) An investigator who studies the occurrence of disease or other health-related conditions, states, or events in specified populations; one who practices epidemiology; the control of disease usually is also considered a task of the epidemiologist.

ep·i·de·mi·ol·o·gy (ep′i-dē′mē-ol′ŏ-jē) The study of the distribution and determinants of health-related states or events in specified populations, and the application of this study to control of health problems. [G. *epidēmios,* epidemic, + *logos,* study]

ep·i·der·mal, ep·i·der·mat·ic (ep′i-dĕr′măl, ep′i-dĕr-mat′ik) Relating to the epidermis. SYN epidermic.

ep·i·der·mal cyst (ep′i-dĕr′măl sist) A cyst formed of a mass of epidermal cells that, as a result of trauma, has been pushed beneath the epidermis; the cyst is lined with stratified squamous epithelium and contains concentric layers of keratin.

ep·i·der·mal growth fac·tor re·cep·tor (EGFR) (ep′i-dĕr′măl grōth fak′tŏr rĕ-sep′tŏr) Receptor often upregulated in epithelial tumors.

ep·i·der·mal·i·za·tion (ep′i-dĕr′mal-ī-zā′shŭn) SYN squamous metaplasia.

e·pi·der·mal-mel·an·in u·nit (ep′i-dĕr′măl-mel′ă-nin yū′nit) An association of one melanocyte with several surrounding epidermal keratinocytes, presumably one that favors the transfer of melanin granules from the melanocyte to the keratinocytes.

ep·i·der·mal ridg·es (ep′i-dĕr′măl rij′ĕz) Ridges of the epidermis of the palms and soles, where the sweat pores open. SYN skin ridges.

ep·i·der·mic (ep′i-dĕr′mik) SYN epidermal.

ep·i·der·mis, pl. **ep·i·derm·i·des** (ep′i-dĕrm′is, -i-dēz) [TA] **1.** The superficial epithelial portion of the skin (cutis). The epidermis of the palms and soles has the following strata: stratum corneum (horny layer), stratum lucidum (clear layer), stratum granulosum (granular layer), stratum spinosum (prickle cell layer), and stratum basale (basal cell layer); in other parts of the body, the stratum lucidum may be absent. **2.** BOTANY the outermost layer of cells in leaves and the young parts of plants. SYN cuticle (3), cuticula (2). [G. *epidermis,* the outer skin, fr. *epi,* on, + *derma,* skin]

ep·i·der·mi·tis (ep′i-dĕr-mī′tis) Inflammation of the epidermis or superficial layers of the skin.

ep·i·der·mo·dys·pla·si·a (ep′i-dĕr′mō-dis-plā′zē-ă) Faulty growth or development of the epidermis. [epidermis + G. *dys-,* bad, + *plasis,* a molding]

ep·i·der·moid (ep′i-dĕr′moyd) **1.** Resembling epidermis. **2.** A cholesteatoma or other cystic tumor arising from aberrant epidermal cells. [epidermis + G. *eidos,* appearance]

ep·i·der·moid car·ci·no·ma (ep′i-dĕr′moyd kahr′si-nō′mă) Squamous cell carcinoma of the skin.

ep·i·der·moid cyst (ep′i-dĕr′moyd sist) A spheric, unilocular cyst of the dermis, composed of encysted keratin and sebum; the cyst is lined by a keratinizing epithelium resembling the epidermis derived from the follicular infundibulum.

ep·i·der·mol·y·sis (ep′i-dĕr-mol′i-sis) A condition in which the epidermis is loosely attached to the corium, readily exfoliating or forming blisters. [epidermis + G. *lysis,* loosening]

i ep·i·der·mol·y·sis bul·lo·sa (ep′i-dĕr-mol′i-sis bul-ō′să) A group of inherited chronic noninflammatory skin diseases in which large bullae and erosions result from slight mechanical trauma; a form limited to the hands and feet is also called Weber-Cockayne syndrome. See this page.

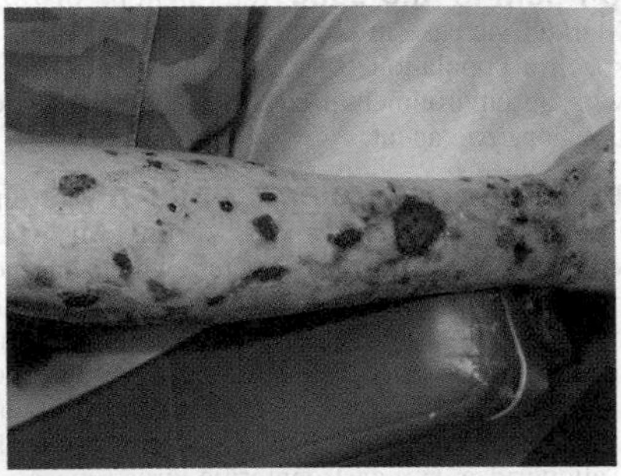

epidermolysis bullosa

Ep·i·der·mo·phy·ton (ep′i-dĕr-mof′i-ton, -dĕr-mō-fī′ton) A genus of fungi wih macroconidia that are clavate and smooth-walled. The only species, *E. floccosum*, is a common cause of tinea pedis and tinea cruris. [epidermis + G. *phyton,* plant]

ep·i·der·mot·ro·pism (ep′i-dĕr-mot′rō-pizm) Movement toward the epidermis, as in the migration of T lymphocytes into the epidermis in mycosis fungoides. [epidermis + G. *tropē,* a turning]

ep·i·did·y·mal (ep′i-did′i-măl) Relating to the epididymis.

ep·i·did·y·mec·to·my (ep′i-did-i-mek′tŏ-mē) Operative removal of the epididymis. [epididymis + G. *ektomē,* excision]

ep·i·did·y·mis, gen. **ep·i·did·y·mi·dis**, pl. **ep·i·did·y·mi·des** (ep-i-did′i-mis, ep-i-did-i-mī′dis, ep-i-did-i-mī′dēz) [TA] An elongated structure connected to the posterior surface of the testis, consisting of the head of the epididymis, body of epididymis, and tail of epididymis, which turns sharply on itself to become the ductus deferens; the main component is the very convoluted duct of the epididymis, within the tail and the beginning of the ductus deferens; stores and matures spermatozoa and transports them from testis to ductus deferens (vas deferens)

[Mod. L. fr. G. *epididymis,* fr. *epi,* on, + *didymos,* twin, in pl. testes]

ep•i•did•y•mi•tis (ep′i-did′i-mī′tis) Inflammation of the epididymis.

ep•i•did•y•mo-or•chi•tis (ep′i-did′i-mō-ōr-kī′tis) Simultaneous inflammation of both epididymis and testis. [epididymis + G. *orchis,* testis]

ep•i•did•y•mo•plas•ty (ep′i-did′i-mō-plas-tē) Surgical repair of the epididymis. [epididymis + G. *plastos,* formed]

ep•i•did•y•mot•o•my (ep′i-did′i-mot′ŏ-mē) Incision into the epididymis, as in preparation for epididymovasostomy or for drainage of purulent material. [epididymis + G. *tomē,* a cutting]

ep•i•did•y•mo•vas•ec•to•my (ep′i-did′i-mō-vă-sek′tŏ-mē) Surgical removal of the epididymis and vas deferens. [epididymis + vasectomy]

ep•i•did•y•mo•vas•os•to•my (ep-i-did′i-mō-va-sos′tŏ-mē) Surgical anastomosis of the vas deferens to the epididymis. [epididymis + vasostomy]

ep•i•du•ral (ep′i-dūr′ăl) On (or outside) the dura mater.

ep•i•du•ral an•es•the•si•a (ep′i-dūr′ăl an′es-thē′zē-ă) Regional anesthesia produced by injection of local anesthetic solution into the peridural space. See this page. SYN peridural anesthesia.

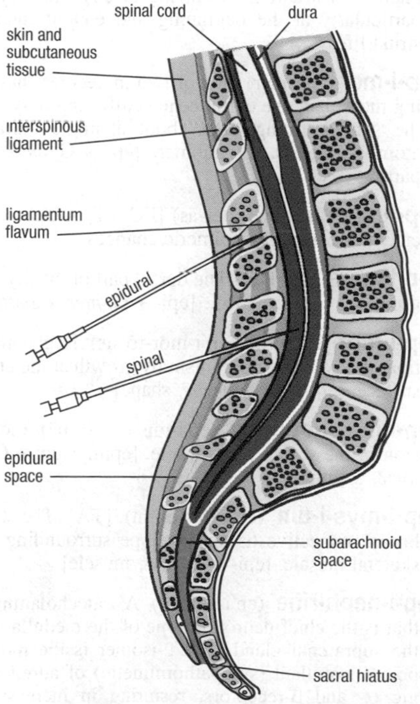

injection sites for spinal and epidural anesthesia

ep•i•du•ral block (ep′i-dūr′ăl blok) An obstruction in the epidural space; used inaccurately to refer to epidural anesthesia.

ep•i•du•ral cav•i•ty (ep′i-dūr′ăl kav′i-tē) The space between the walls of the vertebral canal and the dura mater of the spinal cord.

ep•i•du•ral he•ma•to•ma (ep′i-dūr′ăl hē′mă-tō′mă) SYN extradural hemorrhage.

ep•i•du•ral in•jec•tion (ep′i-dūr′ăl in-jek′shŭn) Subcutaneous or intramuscular injection of a pharmacotherapeutic or anesthetic agent into the epidural space.

ep•i•du•rog•ra•phy (ep′i-dūr-og′ră-fē) Radiographic visualization of the epidural space following the regional instillation of a radiopaque contrast medium.

ep•i•es•tri•ol (ep′ē-es′trē-ol) SEE estriol.

ep•i•gas•tral•gi•a (ep′i-gas-tral′jē-ă) Pain in the epigastric region. [epigastrium + G. *algos,* pain]

ep•i•gas•tric (ep′i-gas′trik) Relating to the epigastrium.

ep•i•gas•tric fos•sa (ep′i-gas′trik fos′ă) The slight depression in the midline just inferior to the xiphoid process of the sternum.

ep•i•gas•tric her•ni•a (ep′i-gas′trik hĕr′nē-ă) Hernia through the linea alba above the navel.

ep•i•gas•tric re•gion (ep′i-gas′trik rē′jŭn) The region of the abdomen located between the costal margins and the subcostal plane. SYN epigastrium.

ep•i•gas•tri•um (ep′i-gas′trē-ŭm) SYN epigastric region.

ep•i•gen•e•sis (ep′i-jen′ĕ-sis) **1.** Development of offspring from a zygote. **2.** Regulation of the expression of gene activity without alteration of genetic structure. [epi- + G. *genesis,* creation]

ep•i•ge•net•ic (ep′i-jĕ-net′ik) Relating to epigenesis.

ep•i•glot•tic, ep•i•glot•tid•e•an (ep′i-glot′ik, ep′i-glo-tid′ē-ăn) Relating to the epiglottis.

ep•i•glot•tic car•ti•lage (ep′i-glot′ik kahr′ti-lăj) A thin lamina of elastic cartilage forming the central portion of the epiglottis. SYN cartilago epiglottica [TA].

ep•i•glot•ti•dec•to•my (ep′i-glot-i-dek′tŏ-mē) Excision of the epiglottis. [epiglottis + G. *ektomē,* excision]

ep•i•glot•tis (ep′i-glot′is) [TA] A leaf-shaped plate of elastic cartilage, covered with mucous membrane, at the root of the tongue, which serves as a diverter valve over the superior aperture of the larynx during the act of swallowing; it stands erect when liquids are being swallowed but is passively bent over the aperture by solid foods that are being swallowed. [G. *epiglōttis,* fr. *epi,* on, + *glōttis,* the mouth of the windpipe]

ep·i·glot·ti·tis, **ep·i·glot·ti·di·tis** (ep′i-glot-ī′tis, ep′i-glot-i-dī′tis) Inflammation of the epiglottis, which may cause respiratory obstruction, especially in children; frequently due to infection by *Haemophilus influenzae* type b.

ep·i·ker·a·to·pha·ki·a (ep′i-ker′ă-tō-fā′kē-ă) Modification of refractive error by application of a donor cornea to the anterior surface of the patient's cornea from which epithelium has been removed. [epi- + G. *keras,* horn, + *phakos,* lens]

ep·i·late (ep′i-lāt) To extract a hair; to remove the hair from a part by forcible extraction, electrolysis, or loosening at the root by chemical means. Cf. depilate. [L. *e,* out, + *pilus,* a hair]

ep·i·la·tion (ep′i-lā′shŭn) The act or result of removing hair. SYN depilation.

e·pil·a·to·ry (e-pil′ă-tōr-ē) **1.** Pertaining to removal of hair by any method that also removes the entire hair shaft, as in plucking or the application of heated wax products that harden, allowing the patient to remove an entire mass of hair at the same time. **2.** An agent having this action. Cf. depilatory.

ep·i·lem·ma (ep′i-lem′ă) The connective tissue sheath of nerve fibers near their termination. [epi- *lemma,* husk]

ep·i·lep·sy (ep′i-lep′sē) A chronic disorder characterized by paroxysmal brain dysfunction due to excessive neuronal discharge, and usually associated with some alteration of consciousness. The clinical manifestations of the attack may vary from complex abnormalities of behavior including generalized or focal convulsions to momentary spells of impaired consciousness. These clinical states have been subjected to a variety of classifications, none universally accepted to date and, accordingly, the terminologies used to describe the different types of attacks remain purely descriptive and nonstandardized; they are variously based on the clinical manifestations of the seizure (motor, sensory, reflex, psychic, or vegetative); the pathologic substrate (hereditary, inflammatory, degenerative, neoplastic, traumatic, or cryptogenic); the location of the epileptogenic lesion (rolandic, temporal, diencephalic regions); and the time period during which the attacks occur (nocturnal, diurnal, menstrual). SYN fit (3), seizure disorder. [G. *epilēpsia,* seizure]

ep·i·lep·tic (ep′i-lep′tik) Relating to, characterized by, or suffering from epilepsy.

e·pi·lep·tic spasm (ep′i-lep′tik spazm) Spasm characterized by a sudden flexion-extension, or mixed extension-flexion, predominantly proximal (including truncal muscles), which is usually more sustained than a myoclonic movement but not as sustained as a tonic seizure. Occurs frequently in clusters, with the individual events ranging in duration from myoclonic to tonic seizure components.

ep·i·lep·ti·form (ep′i-lep′ti-fōrm) SYN epileptoid.

ep·i·lep·to·gen·ic, **ep·i·lep·tog·e·nous** (ep′i-lep-tō-jen′ik, ep′i-lep-toj′ĕ-nŭs) Causing epilepsy.

ep·i·lep·to·gen·ic zone (ep′i-lep-tō-jen′ik zōn) A cortical region that on stimulation reproduces the patient's spontaneous seizure or aura.

ep·i·lep·toid (ep′i-lep′toyd) Resembling epilepsy; denoting certain convulsions, especially of functional nature. SYN epileptiform. [G. *epilēpsia,* seizure, epilepsy, + *eidos,* resemblance]

ep·i·lu·min·es·cence mi·cros·co·py (ep′i-lū-mi-nes′ĕns mī-kros′kŏ-pē) Low-power microscopy (×50–100), commonly a television microscope, applied to a glass slide covering mineral oil on the surface of a skin lesion, e.g., to determine malignancy in pigmented lesions. SYN surface microscopy.

ep·i·man·dib·u·lar (ep′i-man-dib′yū-lăr) On the lower jaw. [epi- + L. *mandibulum,* mandible]

ep·i·men·or·rha·gi·a (ep′i-men-ōr-ā′jē-ă) Prolonged and profuse menstruation occurring at any time, but most frequently at the beginning and end of menstrual life.

ep·i·men·or·rhe·a (ep′i-men-ōr-ē′ă) Too frequent menstruation, occurring at any time, but particularly at the beginning and end of menstrual life.

ep·i·mer (ep′i-mĕr) One of two molecules (having more than one chiral center) differing only in the spatial arrangement about a single chiral atom. SEE sugars. Cf. anomer. [epi- + G. *meros,* part]

ep·i·mer·ase (ep′i-mĕr-ās) [EC 5.1] A class of enzymes catalyzing epimeric changes.

ep·i·mere (ep′i-mēr) The dorsal part of the myotome. SEE myotome (3). [epi- + G. *meros,* part]

ep·i·mor·pho·sis (ep′i-mōr-fō′sis) Regeneration of a part of an organism by growth at the cut surface. [epi- + G. *morphē,* shape]

ep·i·mys·i·ot·o·my (ep′i-mis-ē-ot′ŏ-mē) Incision of the sheath of a muscle. [epimysium + G. *tomē,* a cutting]

ep·i·mys·i·um (ep′i-mis′ē-ŭm) [TA] The fibrous connective tissue envelope surrounding a skeletal muscle. [epi- + G. *mys,* muscle]

ep·i·neph·rine (ep′i-nef′rin) A catecholamine that is the chief neurohormone of the medulla of the suprarenal gland. The L-isomer is the most potent stimulant (sympathomimetic) of adrenergic α- and β-receptors, resulting in increased heart rate and force of contraction, vasoconstriction or vasodilation, relaxation of bronchiolar and intestinal smooth muscle, glycogenolysis, lipolysis, and other metabolic effects; used in the treatment of bronchial asthma, acute allergic disorders, open-angle glaucoma, and heart block, and as a topical and local vasoconstrictor. SYN adrenaline. [epi- + G. *nephros*, kidney, + -ine]

ep•i•neph•ros (ep′i-nef′ros) SYN suprarenal gland. [epi- + G. *nephros*, kidney]

ep•i•neu•ral (ep′i-nūr′ăl) On a neural arch of a vertebra.

ep•i•neu•ri•al (ep′i-nūr′ē-ăl) Relating to the epineurium.

ep•i•neu•ri•um (ep′i-nūr′ē-ŭm) [TA] The outermost supporting structure of peripheral nerve trunks, consisting of a condensation of areolar connective tissue; subdivided into those layers that surround the whole nerve trunk (epifascicular epineurium), and those layers that extend between the nerve fascicles (interfascicular epineurium). With the endoneurium and perineurium, the epineurium comprises the peripheral nerve stroma. [epi- + G. *neuron*, nerve]

ep•i•ot•ic cen•ter (ep′ē-ot′ik sen′tĕr) The center of ossification of the petrous part of the temporal bone that appears posterior to the posterior semicircular canal.

ep•i•phar•ynx (ep′i-far′ingks) SYN nasopharynx. [G. *epi*, on, over, + pharynx]

ep•i•phe•nom•e•non (ep′i-fĕ-nom′ĕ-non) A symptom appearing during the course of a disease, not of usual occurrence, and not necessarily associated with the disease.

e•piph•o•ra (ē-pif′ōr-ă) An overflow of tears on the cheek, due to imperfect drainage by the tear-conducting passages or excess lacrimal production. SYN tearing. [G. a sudden flow, fr. *epi*, on, + *pherō*, to bear]

ep•i•phys•i•al ar•rest (ep′i-fiz′ē-ăl ă-rest′) Early and premature fusion between epiphysis and diaphysis.

ep•i•phys•i•al car•ti•lage (ep′i-fiz′ē-ăl kahr′ti-lăj) Particular type of new cartilage produced by the epiphysis of a growing long bone; located on the epiphysial (distal) side of the zone of growth cartilage, it is a zone of relatively quiescent chondrocytes (the resting zone) of the epiphysial (growth) plate that unites the epiphysis with the shaft. SEE ALSO epiphysial plate.

ep•i•phys•i•al frac•ture (ep′i-fiz′ē-ăl frak′shŭr) Injury to the growth plate of a long bone in children and adolescents.

ep•i•phys•i•al line (ep′i-fiz′ē-ăl līn) The line of junction of the epiphysis and diaphysis of a long bone where growth in length occurs. SYN linea epiphysialis [TA].

ep•i•phys•i•al plate (ep′i-fiz′ē-ăl plāt) The disc of cartilage between the metaphysis and the epiphysis of an immature long bone permitting growth in length. SYN cartilago epiphysialis [TA], growth plate.

ep•i•phys•i•ol•y•sis (ep′i-fiz-ē-ol′i-sis) **1.** Loosening or separation, either partial or complete, of an epiphysis from the shaft of a bone. **2.** Arrest of growth by ablation of the growth plate cartilage. [epiphysis + G. *lysis*, loosening]

e•piph•y•sis, pl. **e•piph•y•ses** (e-pif′i-sis, -sēz) [TA] A part of a long bone developed from a center of ossification distinct from that of the shaft and separated at first from the latter by a layer of cartilage. [G. an excrescence, fr. *epi*, upon, + *physis*, growth]

e•piph•y•si•tis (e-pif′i-sī′tis) Inflammation of an epiphysis.

ep•i•pi•al (ep′i-pī′ăl) On the pia mater.

epiplo- Combining form meaning omentum. SEE ALSO omento-. [G. *epiploon*]

ep•i•plo•ic (ep′i-plō′ik) SYN omental.

ep•i•plo•ic fo•ra•men (ep′i-plō′ik fōr-ā′mĕn) The passage, below and behind the porta hepatis, connecting the two sacs of the peritoneum; it is bounded anteriorly by the hepatoduodenal ligament and posteriorly by a peritoneal fold over the inferior vena cava.

ep•i•scle•ra (ep′i-skler′ă) The connective tissue between the sclera and the conjunctiva. [epi- + sclera]

ep•i•scle•ral (ep′i-skler′ăl) **1.** On the sclera. **2.** Relating to the episclera.

ep•i•scle•ral ar•ter•y (ep′i-skler′ăl ahr′tĕr-ē) One of many small branches of the anterior ciliary arteries that arise as they perforate the sclera near the corneoscleral junction, and course on the sclera. SYN arteria episcleralis [TA].

ep•i•scle•ral space (ep′i-skler′ăl spās) The area between the fascial sheath of the eyeball and the sclera.

ep•i•scle•ral veins (ep′i-skler′ăl vānz) A series of small venules in the sclera close to the corneal margin that empty into the anterior ciliary veins.

ep•i•scle•ri•tis (ep′i-skler-ī′tis) Inflammation of the episcleral connective tissue. SEE ALSO scleritis. See page B27.

episio- Prefix meaning the vulva. SEE ALSO vulvo-. [G. *episeion*, pubic region]

ep•i•si•o•per•i•ne•or•rha•phy (e-piz′ē-ō-per′i-nē-ōr′ă-fē) Repair of an incised or a ruptured perineum and lacerated vulva or repair of a surgical incision of the vulva and perineum. [episio- + G. *perinaion*, perineum, + *rhaphē*, a stitching]

ep•i•si•o•plas•ty (e-piz′ē-ō-plas-tē) Surgical repair of the vulva. [episio- + G. *plastos*, formed]

ep•i•si•or•rha•phy (e-piz′ē-ōr′ră-fē) Repair of

a lacerated vulva or an episiotomy. [episio- + G. *rhaphē,* a stitching]

ep•i•si•o•ste•no•sis (e-piz′ē-ō-stĕ-nō′sis) Narrowing of the vulvar orifice. [episio- + G. *stenōsis,* narrowing]

ep•i•si•ot•o•my (e-piz′ē-ot′ŏ-mē) Surgical incision of the vulva to prevent laceration at the time of delivery or to facilitate vaginal surgery. [episio- + G. *tomē,* incision]

ep•i•sode (ep′i-sōd) An important event or series of events taking place in the course of continuous events (e.g., an episode of depression).

ep•i•sode of care (ep′i-sōd kār) All services provided to a patient with a medical problem within a specific period of time across a continuum of care in an integrated health care system.

ep•i•so•dic hy•per•ten•sion (ep′i-sod′ik hī′pĕr-ten′shŭn) Hypertension manifested intermittently, triggered by anxiety or emotional factors. SYN paroxysmal hypertension.

ep•i•some (ep′i-sōm) An extrachromosomal element (plasmid) that may either integrate into the bacterial chromosome of the host or replicate and function stably when physically separated from the chromosome. [epi- + G. *sōma,* body (chromosome)]

ep•i•spa•di•as (ep′i-spā′dē-ăs) A malformation in which the urethra opens on the dorsum of the penis; frequently associated with exstrophy of the bladder. [epi- + G. *spaō,* to tear or gouge]

ep•i•sple•ni•tis (ep′i-splē-nī′tis) Inflammation of the capsule of the spleen.

e•pis•ta•sis (e-pis′tă-sis) **1.** The formation of a pellicle or scum on the surface of a liquid, especially on standing urine. **2.** Phenotypic interaction of nonallelic genes. **3.** A form of gene interaction whereby one gene masks or interferes with the phenotypic expression of one or more genes at other loci; the gene with the expressed phenotype is said to be epistatic, the phenotype altered or suppressed is then said to be hypostatic. [G. scum; epi- + G. *stasis,* a standing]

ep•i•stat•ic (ep′i-stat′ik) Relating to epistasis.

ep•i•stax•is (ep′i-stak′sis) Profuse bleeding from the nose. SYN nosebleed. [G. fr. *epistazō,* to bleed at the nose, fr. *epi,* on, + *stazō,* to fall in drops]

ep•i•sten•o•car•di•ac per•i•car•di•tis (ep′i-sten-ō-kahr′dē-ak per′i-kahr-dī′tis) Inflammation of the pericardium with transmural myocardial infarction and limited to the area over the infarct.

ep•i•ster•nal (ep′i-stĕr′năl) **1.** Over or on the sternum. **2.** Relating to the episternum.

ep•i•stro•phe•us (ep′i-strō′fē-ŭs) SYN axis (5). [G. the pivot]

ep•i•ten•din•e•um (ep′i-ten-din′ē-ŭm) The white fibrous sheath surrounding a tendon. [L.]

ep•i•thal•a•mus (ep′i-thal′ă-mŭs) [TA] A small dorsomedial area of the thalamus corresponding to the habenula and its associated structures, the medullary stria, pineal body, and habenular commissure. [epi- + thalamus]

ep•i•the•li•a (ep′i-thē′lē-ă) Plural of epithelium.

ep•i•the•li•al (ep′i-thē′lē-ăl) Relating to or consisting of epithelium.

ep•i•the•li•al down•growth (ep′i-thē′lē-ăl down′grōth) The invasion of surface epithelium into the interior of the eye as a consequence of a penetrating ocular wound.

ep•i•the•li•al dys•tro•phy (ep′i-thē′lē-ăl dis′trŏ-fē) Corneal dystrophy affecting primarily the epithelium and its basement membrane.

ep•i•the•li•al•i•za•tion (ep′i-thē′lē-ăl-ī-zā′shŭn) Formation of epithelium over a denuded surface. SYN epithelization.

ep•i•the•li•al lam•i•na (ep′i-thē′lē-ăl lam′i-nă) The layer of modified ependymal cells that forms the inner layer of the tela choroidea, facing the ventricle.

ep•i•the•li•al mem•brane an•ti•gen (EMA) (ep′i-thē′lē-ăl mem′brān an′ti-jen) A heavily glycosylated, 70-kD protein complex, first isolated in human milk fat globulin; this antigen is present in a variety of glandular epithelia, especially in breast carcinoma cells, but may also be seen in cultured fibroblasts, lymphoid cells, and some stromal cells. Immunohistochemical staining may be used as a diagnostic aid in tissue diagnosis.

ep•i•the•li•al pearl (ep′i-thē′lē-ăl pĕrl) SYN keratin pearl.

ep•i•the•li•al plug (ep′i-thē′lē-ăl plŭg) A mass of epithelial cells temporarily occluding an embryonic opening; the term is most commonly used with reference to the external nares.

ep•i•the•li•oid (ep′i-thē′lē-oyd) Resembling or having some of the characteristics of epithelium. [epithelium + G. *eidos,* resemblance]

ep•i•the•li•oid cell (ep′i-thē′lē-oyd sel) **1.** A nonepithelial cell having certain characteristics of epithelium. **2.** Large mononuclear histiocytes having certain epithelial characteristics, particularly in tubercles where they are polygonal and have eosinophilic cytoplasm.

ep•i•the•li•o•lyt•ic (ep′i-thē′lē-ō-lit′ik) Destructive to epithelium.

ep•i•the•li•o•ma (ep′i-thē′lē-ō′mă) **1.** An epithelial neoplasm or hamartoma of the skin, especially of skin appendage origin. **2.** A carcinoma of the skin derived from squamous, basal, or adnexal cells. [epithelium + G. *-ōma,* tumor]

ep·i·the·li·om·a·tous (ep′i-thē′lē-ō′mă-tŭs) Pertaining to epithelioma.

ep·i·the·li·op·a·thy (ep′i-thē′lē-op′ă-thē) Disease involving epithelium. [epithelium + G. *pathos,* suffering]

ep·i·the·li·um, pl. **ep·i·the·li·a** (ep′i-thē′lē-ŭm, -ă) [TA] The purely cellular avascular layer covering all the free surfaces, cutaneous, mucous, and serous, including the glands and other structures derived therefrom. See this page. [G. *epi,* upon, + *thēlē,* nipple, a term applied originally to the thin skin covering the nipples and the papillary layer of the border of the lips]

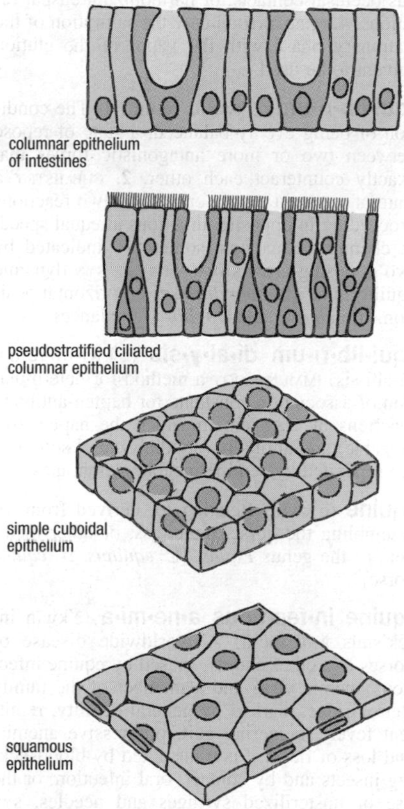

types of epithelium (simplified schematic)

ep·i·the·li·za·tion (ep′i-thē′li-zā′shŭn) SYN epithelialization.

ep·i·tope (ep′i-tōp) The simplest form of an antigenic determinant, on a complex antigenic molecule, that can combine with antibody or T-cell receptor. [epi- + -tope]

ep·i·trich·i·um (ep′i-trik′ē-ŭm) SYN periderm. [epi- + G. *trichion,* dim. of *thrix,* (*trich-*), hair]

ep·i·tym·pan·ic (ep′i-tim-pan′ik) Above, or in the upper part of, the tympanic cavity or membrane.

ep·i·tym·pan·ic re·cess (ep′i-tim-pan′ik rē′ses) The upper portion of the tympanic cavity above the tympanic membrane; it contains the head of the malleus and the body of the incus.

ep·i·zo·ic (ep′i-zō′ik) Living as a parasite on the skin surface.

ep·i·zo·ol·o·gy (ep′i-zō-ol′ŏ-jē) SYN epizootiology. [epi- + G. *zōon,* animal, + *logos,* study]

ep·i·zo·on, pl. **ep·i·zo·a** (ep′i-zō′on, -zō′ă) An animal parasite living on the body surface. [epi- + G. *zōon,* animal]

ep·i·zo·ot·ic (ep′i-zō-ot′ik) **1.** Disease occurrence in an animal population with a frequency clearly in excess of the expected. **2.** An outbreak (epidemic) of disease in an animal population; often with the implication that it may also affect human populations. [epi- + G. *zōon,* animal]

ep·i·zo·ot·i·ol·o·gy (ep′i-zō-ot′ē-ol′ŏ-jē) Epidemiology of disease in animal populations. SYN epizoology. [epi- + G. *zōon,* animal, + *logos,* study]

ep·i·zote (ep′i-zōt) (*Chenopodium ambrosioides*) An herb of the U.S. Southwest with some similarity to cilantro (coriander); used in the nineteenth century as a digestive; of possible value as an antiflatulent. Clinical studies are ongoing. The safety of this agent has not been confirmed. SYN American wormseed.

EPO Abbreviation for exclusive provider organization.

EPOC Abbreviation for excess postexercise oxygen consumption.

ep·o·nych·i·a (ep′ō-nik′ē-ă) Infection involving the proximal nail fold.

ep·o·nych·i·um (ep′ō-nik′ē-ŭm) [TA] **1.** The thin, condensed, eleidin-rich layer of epidermis that precedes and initially covers the nail plate in the embryo. It normally degenerates by the eighth month, except at the nail base, where it remains as the cuticle of the nail. **2.** The corneal layer of epidermis overlapping and in direct contact with the nail root proximally or the sides of the nail plate laterally, forming the undersurface of the nail wall or nail folds. SYN perionychium. **3.** The thin skin adherent to the nail at its proximal portion. [G. *epi,* upon, + *onyx* (*onych-*), nail]

ep·o·nym (ep′ŏ-nim) The name of a disease, structure, operation, or procedure, usually derived from the name of the person who first discovered or described it. SYN eponymic (2). [G. *epōnymos,* named after]

ep·o·nym·ic (ep′ŏ-nim′ik) **1.** Relating to an eponym. **2.** SYN eponym.

ep·ox·y (ē-pok′sē) Chemical term describing an oxygen atom bound to two linked carbon atoms .

Generally, any cyclic ether, but commonly applied to a three-membered ring; important chemical intermediates, and the basis of epoxy resins (polymers) formed from epoxy monomers.

ep•sil•on (ε) (ep′si-lon) **1.** Fifth letter of the Greek alphabet. **2.** Extinction coefficient. **3.** CHEMISTRY a position of a substituent located on the fifth atom from the carboxyl or other primary functional group.

ep•si•lon clos•tri•di•al tox•in (ep′si-lon klos-trid′ē-ăl toks′in) A toxin produced by *Clostridium perfringens* and considered by the U.S. Centers for Disease Control and Prevention to be a Category B agent.

ep•si•lon wave (ep′si-lon wāv) Late R wave (in lead V_1) of delayed right ventricular activation in arrhythmogenic RV dysplasia.

Ep•stein-Barr vi•rus (EBV) (ep′stīn bahr vī′rŭs) A herpesvirus that causes infectious mononucleosis and is also found in cell cultures of Burkitt lymphoma; associated with nasopharyngeal carcinoma. SYN human herpesvirus 4.

Ep•stein pearls (ep′stīn pĕrlz) Multiple small, white, epithelial inclusion cysts found in the midline of the palate in newborn infants.

Ep•stein sign (ep′stīn sīn) Lid retraction in an infant giving it a frightened expression and a "wild glance." SEE setting sun sign, Collier sign.

EPT Abbreviation for electroporation therapy.

ep•u•lis (ep-yū′lis) A nonspecific exophytic gingival mass. [G. *epoulis,* a gumboil]

ep•u•loid (ep′yū-loyd) A gingival mass that resembles an epulis.

e•qua•tion (ĕ-kwā′zhŭn) A statement expressing the equality of two things, usually by means of mathematical or chemical symbols. [L. *aequare,* to make equal]

e•qua•tion of mo•tion (ĕ-kwā′zhŭn mō′shŭn) **1.** An expression of Newton's second law that relates forces, displacements, and their derivatives for a mechanical system. **2.** For the respiratory system, an equation that relates the forces involved in breathing to the displacements they produce. Typically, pressure differences are used to represent generalized forces and volume changes are used to represent generalized displacements. The simplest equation of motion written for the lungs states that the change in transpulmonary pressure is equal to the sum of an elastic term plus a flow resistive term: transpulmonary pressure change = elastance × tidal volume + resistance × change in flow.

e•qua•to•ri•al plane (ek′wă-tōr′ē-ăl plān) In metaphase of mitosis, the plane that touches all the centromeres and their spindle attachments.

e•qua•to•ri•al plate (ek′wă-tōr′ē-ăl plāt) The assembly of chromosomes in mitosis.

e•qua•to•ri•al staph•y•lo•ma (ek′wă-tōr′ē-ăl staf′i-lō′mă) A staphyloma occurring in the area of exit of the vortex veins. SYN scleral staphyloma.

e•qui•ax•i•al (ē′kwi-ak′sē-ăl) Having axes of equal length.

e•quil•i•bra•tion (ē′kwi-li-brā′shŭn) **1.** The act of maintaining an equilibrium or balance. **2.** The act of exposing a liquid (e.g., blood or plasma) to a gas at a certain partial pressure until the partial pressures of the gas within and without the liquid are equal. **3.** DENTISTRY modification of occlusal forms of the teeth by grinding, with the intent of equalizing occlusal stress, producing simultaneous occlusal contacts, or harmonizing cuspal relations. **4.** CHROMATOGRAPHY the saturation of the stationary phase with the vapor of the elution solvent to be used.

e•qui•lib•ri•um (ē′kwi-lib′rē-ŭm) **1.** The condition of being evenly balanced; a state of repose between two or more antagonistic forces that exactly counteract each other. **2.** CHEMISTRY a state of apparent repose created by two reactions proceeding in opposite directions at equal speed; in chemical equations, sometimes indicated by two opposing arrows (↔) or (↔). SYN dynamic equilibrium. [L. *aequilibrium,* a horizontal position, fr. *aequus,* equal, + *libra,* a balance]

e•qui•lib•ri•um di•al•y•sis (ē′kwi-lib′rē-ŭm dī-al′i-sis) IMMUNOLOGY a method for determination of association constants for hapten-antibody reactions in a system in which the hapten (dialyzable) and antibody (nondialyzable) solutions are separated by semipermeable membranes.

e•quine (ē′kwīn) Relating to, derived from, or resembling the horse, mule, ass, or other members of the genus *Equus.* [L. *equinus,* fr. *equus,* horse]

e•quine in•fec•tious a•ne•mi•a (ē′kwīn in-fek′shŭs ă-nē′mē-ă) A worldwide disease of horses and other equids, caused by equine infectious anemia virus and a member of the family Retroviridae, marked by general debility, remittent fever, staggering gait, progressive anemia, and loss of flesh; it is transmitted by bloodsucking insects and by contact, oral infection, or the use of unsterilized syringes and needles. SYN swamp fever (1).

e•quine mor•bil•li•vi•rus (ē′kwīn mōr-bil′i-vī′rŭs) A species causing a fatal respiratory disease in horses and humans in Australia, with encephalitis also seen in some human cases. SYN Hendra virus.

e•qui•no•val•gus (ē′kwī-nō-val′gŭs, ek′wi-nō-) SYN talipes equinovalgus.

e•qui•no•var•us (ē′kwī-nō-vā′rŭs) SYN talipes equinovarus.

e•quip•ment (ĕ-kwip′mĕnt) Supplies, tools, or other materials required to perform a specific task or function. [O.Fr. *equiper*, to equip, fr. Germanic]

e·qui·tox·ic (ē′kwi-tok′sik) Of equivalent toxicity.

e·quiv·a·lence, **e·quiv·a·len·cy** (ē-kwiv′ă-lĕns, -lĕn-sē) The property of an element or radical of combining with or displacing, in definite and fixed proportion, another element or radical in a compound. [L. *aequus,* equal, + *valentia,* strength (valence)]

e·quiv·a·lent (ē-kwiv′ă-lĕnt) **1.** Equal in any respect. **2.** That which is equal in size, weight, force, or any other quality to something else. **3.** Having the capability to counterbalance or neutralize each other. **4.** Having equal valences. **5.** SYN gram equivalent. [see equivalence]

ER Abbreviation for endoplasmic reticulum; emergency room.

Er Symbol for erbium.

ERA Abbreviation for electronic remittance advice.

E·ran·ko fluo·res·cence stain (ĕ-ran′kō flōr-es′ĕns stān) Exposure of frozen sections to formaldehyde, which produces a strong yellow-green fluorescence from cells containing norepinephrine.

ERBF Abbreviation for effective renal blood flow.

er·bi·um (Er) (ĕr′bē-ŭm) A rare earth (lanthanide) element, atomic no. 68, atomic wt. 167.26. [from Ytterby, a village in Sweden]

Erb pal·sy, **Erb pa·ral·y·sis** (erb pawl′zē, păr-al′i-sis) A type of brachial palsy in which there is paralysis of the muscles of the upper arm and shoulder girdle (deltoid, biceps, brachialis, and brachioradialis muscles) due to a lesion of the upper trunk of the brachial plexus or of the roots of the fifth and sixth cervical roots. SYN Duchenne-Erb paralysis.

Erb point (erb poynt) A point posterior to the sternocleidomastoid muscle 2–3 cm above the clavicle, overlying the transverse process of the sixth cervical vertebra and the emergence of cutaneous branches of the cervicle plexus.

Erb-West·phal sign (erb vest′fahl sīn) Abolition of the patellar tendon reflex, in tabes and certain other diseases of the spinal cord, and occasionally also in brain disease. SYN Westphal sign.

ERCP Abbreviation for endoscopic retrograde cholangiopancreatography.

e·rec·tile (ĕ-rek′tīl) Capable of erection.

e·rec·tile dys·func·tion (ĕ-rek′tīl dis-fŭngk′shŭn) Any disorder of penile erection that prevents successful performance of coitus.

e·rec·tile tis·sue (ĕ-rek′tīl tish′ū) A tissue with numerous vascular spaces that may become engorged with blood.

e·rec·tion (ĕ-rek′shŭn) The condition of erectile tissue when filled with blood, which then becomes hard and unyielding; denoting especially this state of the penis. [L. *erectio,* fr. *erigo,* pp. *erectus,* to set up]

e·rec·tor (ĕ-rek′tŏr) **1.** One who or that which raises or makes erect. **2.** Denoting specifically certain muscles having such action. SYN arrector. [Mod. L.]

e·rec·tor mus·cles of hairs (ĕ-rek′tŏr mŭs′ĕlz hārz) SYN arrector muscle of hair.

e·rec·tor spi·nae mus·cles, **e·rec·tor mus·cle of spine** (ĕ-rek′tŏr spī′nē mŭs′ĕlz, ĕ-rek′tŏr mŭs′ĕl spīn) *Origin*, from sacrum, ilium, and spines of lumbar vertebrae; it divides into three columns, iliocostalis musculus, longissimus musculus, and spinalis musculus, which insert into ribs and vertebrae with additional muscle slips joining the columns at successively higher levels; *action*, extends vertebral column; *nerve supply*, dorsal primary rami of spinal nerves. See this page. SYN musculus erector spinae [TA].

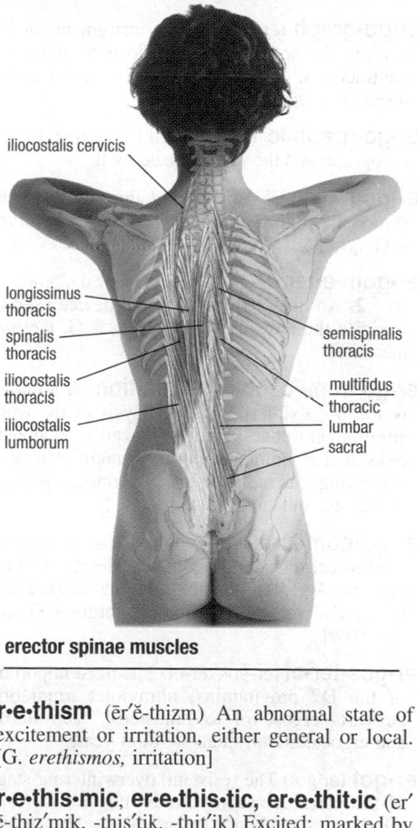

erector spinae muscles

er·e·thism (ĕr′ĕ-thizm) An abnormal state of excitement or irritation, either general or local. [G. *erethismos,* irritation]

er·e·this·mic, er·e·this·tic, er·e·thit·ic (er′ē-thiz′mik, -this′tik, -thit′ik) Excited; marked by or causing erethism; irritable.

ERG Abbreviation for electroretinogram.

erg (ĕrg) The unit of work in the CGS system; the amount of work done by 1 dyne acting through 1 cm, 1 g cm^2 s^{-2}; in the SI, 1 erg equals 10^{-7} joule. [G. *ergon,* work]

er•ga•si•a (ĕr-gā′zē-ă) **1.** Any form of activity, especially mental. **2.** The total of functions and reactions of an individual. [G. work]

er•gas•to•plasm (ĕr-gas′tō-plazm) SYN granular endoplasmic reticulum. [G. *ergastēr,* a workman, + *plasma,* something formed]

ergo- Combining form meaning work. [G. *ergon*]

er•go•cal•cif•er•ol (ĕr′gō-kal-sif′ĕr-ol) Activated ergosterol, the vitamin D of plant origin; it arises from ultraviolet irradiation of ergosterol; used in prophylaxis and treatment of vitamin D deficiency. SYN calciferol, vitamin D2.

er•go•gen•ic aid (ĕr′gō-jen′ik ād) Ergogenic aids have been classified as nutritional, pharmacologic, physiologic, or psychological; methods to enhance athletic performance range from use of accepted techniques such as carbohydrate loading to illegal and unsafe approaches such as use of anabolic-androgenic steroids.

er•go•graph (ĕr′gō-graf) An instrument for recording the amount of work done by muscular contractions, or the amplitude of contraction. [ergo- + G. *graphō,* to write]

er•go•graph•ic (ĕr′gō-graf′ik) Relating to the ergograph and the record made by it.

er•go•lyt•ic (ĕr′gō-lit′ik) Pertaining to any substance that impairs exercise performance. [ergo- + G. *lysis,* a loosening]

er•gom•e•ter (ĕr-gom′ĕ-tĕr) **1.** SYN dynamometer. **2.** An indoor rower or pedal device used to exercise the arms and legs. [ergo- + G. *metron,* measure]

er•go•nom•ic job e•val•u•a•tion (ĕr′gō-nom′ik job ĕ-val′yū-ā′shŭn) An analysis of the work environment that identifies hazards, evaluates risks, and recommends possible modifications in predicting interactions arising among people, processes, and environments.

er•go•nom•ics (ĕr′gō-nom′iks) The science of workplace, tools, and equipment designed to reduce worker discomfort, strain, and fatigue and to prevent work-related injuries. [ergo- + G. *nomos,* law]

er•gos•ter•ol (ĕr-gos′tĕr-ol) The most important of the D2 provitamins; ultraviolet irradiation converts ergosterol to lumisterol, tachysterol, and ergocalciferol; main sterol in yeast.

er•got (ĕr′got) The resistant, overwintering stage of the parasitic ascomycetous fungus *Claviceps purpurea,* a pathogen of cereal rye that transforms the seed of rye into a compact, spurlike mass of fungal pseudotissue (the sclerotium) containing five or more optically isomeric pairs of alkaloids. The levorotary isomers induce uterine contractions, control bleeding, and alleviate certain localized vascular disorders (migraine headaches). [O. Fr. *argot,* cock's spur]

er•got•ism (ĕr′got-izm) Poisoning by a toxic substance contained in the sclerotia of the fungus *Claviceps purpura,* growing on cereal rye; characterized by necrosis of the extremities (gangrene) due to contraction of the peripheral vascular bed. SYN ergot poisoning, Saint Anthony fire (1).

er•got poi•son•ing (ĕr′got poy′zŏn-ing) SYN ergotism.

Er•len•mey•er flask (er′len-mī-er flask) A glass container with a flat base and a funnel-shaped body, the top of which forms the pour spout, usually with a wide opening.

e•rode (ē-rōd′) **1.** To cause, or to be affected by, erosion. **2.** To remove by ulceration. [L. *erodo,* to gnaw away]

e•rog•e•nous (ĕ-roj′ĕ-nŭs) Capable of producing sexual excitement when stimulated. [G. *eros,* love, + *genos,* birth]

e•rog•e•nous zone, e•ro•to•gen•ic zone (ĕ-roj′ĕ-nŭs zōn, er′ō-tō-jen′ik) Areas of the body, such as genitals and nipples, which elicit sexual arousal when stimulated.

e•ros (ār′os) PSYCHOANALYSIS the life principle representing all instinctual tendencies toward procreation and life. [G. love]

E-ro•sette test (ē-rō-zet′ test) An assay to identify T lymphocytes by mixing purified blood lymphocytes with serum and sheep erythrocytes; rosettes of erythrocytes form around human T lymphocytes on incubation.

e•ro•sion (ē-rō′zhŭn) **1.** A wearing away or a state of being worn away, as by friction or pressure. **2.** A shallow ulcer; in the stomach and intestine, an ulcer limited to the mucosa, with no penetration of the muscularis mucosae. **3.** The wearing away of a tooth by nonbacterial chemical action; when the cause is unknown, it is referred to as idiopathic erosion. SYN odontolysis. See page B15. [L. *erosio,* fr. *erodo,* to gnaw away]

e•ro•sive (ē-rō′siv) **1.** Having the property of eroding or wearing away. **2.** An eroding agent.

e•rot•ic (ĕ-rot′ik) Lustful; relating to sexual passion; having the quality to produce sexual arousal. [G. *erōtikos,* relating to love, fr. *erōs,* love]

e•ro•to•gen•ic (ĕ-rot′ō-jen′ik) Capable of causing sexual excitement or arousal. [G. *erōs,* love, + *-gen,* production]

er•o•to•ma•ni•a (ĕ-rot′ō-mā′nē-ă) **1.** Excessive or morbid inclination to erotic thoughts and behavior. **2.** The delusional belief that one is involved in a relationship with another, generally of higher socioeconomic status. [G. *erōs,* love, + *mania,* frenzy]

er•o•to•man•ic dis•or•der (ĕ-rot′ō-man′ik dis-ōr′dĕr) The false belief that one is loved by another, such as a movie star or a casual acquaintance.

er•o•to•path•ic (ĕ-rot′ō-path′ik) Relating to erotopathy.

er•o•top•a•thy (er′ō-top′ă-thē) Any abnormality of the sexual impulse. [G. *erōs,* love, + *pathos,* suffering]

er•o•to•pho•bi•a (ĕ-rot′ō-fō′bē-ă) Morbid aversion to the thought of sexual love and to its physical expression. [G. *erōs,* love, + *phobos,* fear]

ERPF Abbreviation for effective renal plasma flow.

er•ror (er′ŏr) **1.** A defect in structure or function. **2.** BIOSTATISTICS a mistaken decision, as in hypothesis testing or classification by a discriminant function; or the difference between the true value and the observed value of a variate, ascribed to randomness or misreading by an observer. **3.** A false or mistaken belief; in biomedical and other sciences, there are many varieties of error, for example due to bias, inaccurate measurements, or faulty instruments.

er•ror of the first kind (er′ŏr fĭrst kīnd) In a Neyman-Pearson test of a statistical hypothesis, the possibility of rejecting the null hypothesis when it is true. SYN alpha (α) error.

er•ror-prone po•ly•mer•ase chain re•ac•tion (PCR) (er′ŏr-prōn pol′im-ĕr-ās chān rē-ak′shŭn) Use of PCR under conditions in which misincorporation of bases is favored, e.g., where random mutants are sought for a portion of amplified DNA.

er•ror of the sec•ond kind (er′ŏr sek′ŏnd kīnd) In a Neyman-Pearson test of a statistical hypothesis, the possibility of accepting the null hypothesis when it is false. SYN beta (β) error.

er•rors and o•mis•sions in•sur•ance (ĕr′ŏrz ō-mish′ŭnz in-shŭr′ăns) Professional liability insurance for medical transcriptionists.

ERT Abbreviation for estrogen replacement therapy.

e•ruc•ta•tion (ē-rŭk-tā′shŭn) The voiding of gas or of a small quantity of acid fluid from the stomach through the mouth. SYN belching. [L. *eructo,* pp. *-atus,* to belch]

e•rup•tion (ĕr-up′shŭn) **1.** A breaking out, especially the appearance of lesions on the skin. **2.** A rapidly developing dermatosis of the skin or mucous membranes, especially when appearing as a local manifestation of one of the exanthemata; an eruption is characterized, according to the nature of the lesion, as macular, papular, vesicular, pustular, bullous, nodular, erythematous, among other classifications. **3.** The passage of a tooth through the alveolar process and perforation of the gums until it reaches occlusion or contact with the opposing tooth. SEE ALSO emergence. [L. *erumpo,* pp. *-ruptus,* to break out]

e•rup•tive (ĕr-up′tiv) Characterized by eruption.

e•rup•tive xan•tho•ma (ĕr-up′tiv zan-thō′mă) The sudden appearance of groups of waxy, yellow or yellowish-brown papules with an erythematous halo, especially over extensors of the elbows and knees, and on the back and buttocks of patients with severe hyperlipemia, often familial or, more rarely, in severe diabetes.

ERV Abbreviation for expiratory reserve volume.

er•y•sip•e•las (er′i-sip′ĕ-lăs) A specific, acute, cutaneous inflammatory disease caused by β-hemolytic streptococci and characterized by hot, red, edematous, brawny, and sharply defined eruptions; usually accompanied by severe constitutional symptoms. See this page. [G., fr. *erythros,* red + *pella,* skin]

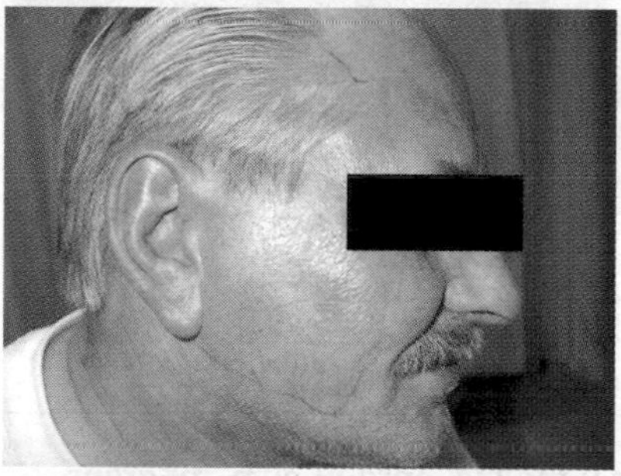

erysipelas: right side of face

er•y•si•pel•a•tous (er′i-si-pel′ă-tŭs) Relating to erysipelas.

er•y•sip•e•loid (er′i-sip′ĕ-loyd) A specific, usually self-limiting, cellulitis of the hand caused by *Erysipelothrix rhusiopathiae;* appears as a dusky erythema with diamondlike configuration of the skin at the site of a wound sustained in handling fish or meat and may become generalized, with plaques of erythema and bullae and, occasionally, severe toxemia. [G. *erysipelas* + *eidos,* resemblance]

Er•y•sip•e•lo•thrix (er′i-sip′ĕ-lō-thriks) A genus of bacteria containing nonmotile, gram-positive, rod-shaped organisms that have a tendency to form long filaments. Members of this genus are parasitic on mammals, birds, and fish. The type species is *E. rhusiopathiae*. [erysipelas + G. *thrix,* hair]

er•y•the•ma (er′i-thē′mă) Redness of the skin due to capillary dilatation. [G. *erythēma,* flush]

er•y•the•ma ab ig•ne (er′i-thē′mă ig′nē) SYN erythema caloricum.

er•y•the•ma an•u•la•re (er′i-thē′mē-ă an-yū-lā′rē) Rounded or ringed lesions.

er•y•the•ma an•u•lare cen•tri•fu•gum (er′i-thē′mă an-yū-lā′rē sen-trif′fyū-gŭm) A chronic, recurring erythematous eruption consisting of small and large anular lesions, with a scant marginal scale, usually of unknown cause.

er•y•the•ma ar•thri•ti•cum ep•i•de•mi•cum (er′i-thē′mă ahr′thrit′i-kŭm ep-i-dem′i-kŭm) SYN Haverhill fever. SEE ALSO rat-bite fever.

er•y•the•ma ca•lo•ri•cum (er′i-thē′mă ka-lōr′i-kŭm) A reticulated, pigmented, macular eruption that occurs, mostly on the shins, of bakers, stokers, and others exposed to radiant heat. See this page. SYN erythema ab igne.

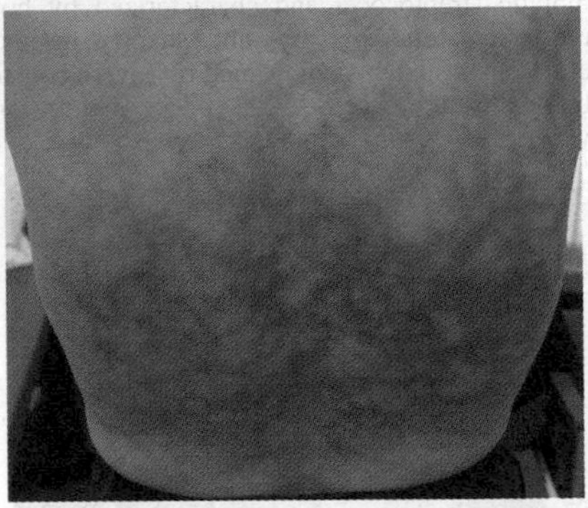

erythema caloricum: back

er•y•the•ma chro•ni•cum mi•grans (er′i-thē′mă krō′nē-kŭm mī′granz) A raised erythematous ring with advancing indurated borders and central clearing, radiating from the site of a tick bite such as that by *Ixodes scapularis;* the characteristic skin lesion of Lyme disease, due to the spirochete *Borrelia burgdorferi*.

er•y•the•ma dose (er′i-thē′mă dōs) The minimum dose of x-rays or other forms of radiation sufficient to produce erythema.

er•y•the•ma in•du•ra•tum (er′i-thē′mă in-dū-rā′tŭm) Recurrent hard subcutaneous nodules that frequently break down and form necrotic ulcers, usually on the calves and less frequently on the thighs or arms of middle-aged women; probably a form of nodular vasculitis. SYN Bazin disease.

er•y•the•ma in•fec•ti•o•sum (er′i-thē′mă in-fek-shē-ō′sŭm) A mild infectious exanthema of childhood characterized by an erythematous maculopapular eruption, resulting in a lacelike facial rash or "slapped cheek" appearance. Fever and arthritis may also accompany infection; caused by parvovirus B 19. SYN fifth disease.

er•y•the•ma i•ris (er′i-thē′mă ī′ris) Concentric rings of erythema varying in intensity, characteristic of erythema multiforme. SYN herpes iris (1).

er•y•the•ma mar•gi•na•tum (er′i-thē′mă mahr-ji-nā′tŭm) A variant of erythema multiforme seen in rheumatic fever.

er•y•the•ma mul•ti•for•me (er′i-thē′mă mŭl-ti-fōr′mē) An acute eruption of macules, papules, or subdermal vesicles presenting a multiform appearance, the characteristic lesion being the target or iris form of lesion over the dorsal aspect of the hands and forearms; its origin may be allergic, seasonal, or from drug sensitivity, and the eruption, although usually self limited, may be recurrent or may run a severe course, sometimes with fatal termination (Stevens-Johnson syndrome). SYN herpes iris (2).

er•y•the•ma no•do•sum (er′i-thē′mă nō-dō′sŭm) A panniculitis marked by the sudden formation of painful nodes on the extensor surfaces of the lower extremities, with lesions that are self limiting but tend to recur; associated with arthralgia and fever; may be the result of drug sensitivity or associated with sarcoidosis and various infections. Deep biopsies show a septal panniculitis (i.e., inflammation of fatty connective tissue), with infiltration by lymphocytes and scattered multinucleated giant cells. See this page.

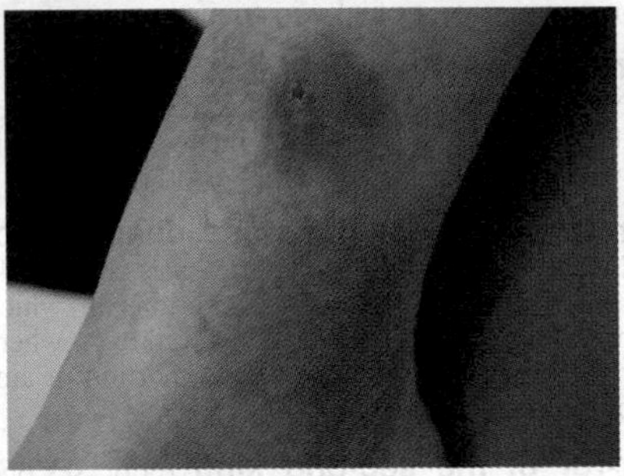

erythema nodosum: leg

er•y•the•ma nu•chae (er′i-thē′mă nū′kē) SYN Unna nevus.

er•y•the•ma per•ni•o (er′i-thē′mă per′nē-ō) SYN chilblain.

er•y•them•a•tous (er′i-them′ă-tŭs) Relating to or marked by erythema.

er•y•the•ma•to•ve•sic•u•lar (er′i-thē′mă-tō-vē-sik′y-ū-lăr) Denoting a condition characterized by erythema and vesiculation, as in allergic contact dermatitis.

er•y•the•ma tox•i•cum (er′i-thē′mă tok′si-kŭm) Flushing of the skin due to allergic reaction to some toxic substance.

er•y•the•ma tox•i•cum ne•o•na•to•rum (er′

i-thē′mă tok′si-kŭm nē-o-nā-tŏ′rum) A common transient idiopathic eruption of erythema, small papules, and occasionally pustules filled with eosinophilic leukocytes overlying hair follicles of the newborn.

erythraemia [Br.] SYN erythremia.

erythraemic myelosis [Br.] SYN erythremic myelosis.

er•y•thral•gi•a (er′i-thral′jē-ă) Painful redness of the skin. SEE ALSO erythromelalgia. [erythro- + G. *algos,* pain]

er•y•thras•ma (er′i-thraz′mă) An eruption of well-circumscribed reddish-brown patches, in the axillae and groins especially, due to the presence of *Corynebacterium minutissimum* in the stratum corneum. [G. *erythrainō,* to redden]

e•ryth•re•de•ma (ĕ-rith′rĕ-dē′mă) SYN acrodynia (2). [erythro- + G. *oidēma,* swelling]

er•y•thre•mi•a (er′i-thrē′mē-ă) SYN polycythemia vera. SYN erythraemia. [erythro- + G. *haima,* blood]

er•y•threm•ic my•e•lo•sis (er′i-thrē′mik mī-ĕ-lō′sis) A neoplastic process of erythropoietic tissue, characterized by anemia, irregular fever, splenomegaly, hepatomegaly, hemorrhagic disorders, and numerous erythroblasts in blood. Acute and chronic forms are recognized, but in the latter there is less prominence of the immature cells; the former is also called Di Guglielmo disease and acute erythremia. SYN erythraemic myelosis.

er•y•thrism (er′i-thrizm) Redness of the hair with a ruddy, freckled complexion. [G. *erythros,* red]

er•y•thris•tic (er′i-thris′tik) Relating to or marked by erythrism; having a ruddy complexion and reddish hair. SYN rufous.

♻**erythro-, erythr-** **1.** Combining forms denoting red or red blood cell; corresponds to L. *rub-*. **2.** Indicates the structure of erythrose in a larger sugar; used as such, it is italicized (e.g., 2-deoxy-D-*erythro*-pentose). [G. *erythros,* red]

e•ryth•ro•blast (ĕ-rith′rō-blast) The first generation of cells in the red blood cell series that can be distinguished from precursor endothelial cells. In normal maturation, four stages of development can be recognized: pronormoblast, basophilic normoblast, polychromatic normoblast, and orthochromatic normoblast. [erythro- + G. *blastos,* germ]

erythroblastaemia [Br.] SYN erythroblastemia.

e•ryth•ro•blas•te•mi•a (ĕ-rith′rō-blas-tē′mē-ă) The presence of nucleated red blood cells in peripheral blood. SYN erythroblastaemia. [erythroblast + G. *haima,* blood]

e•ryth•ro•blas•to•pe•ni•a (ĕ-rith′rō-blas-tō-pē′nē-ă) A primary deficiency of erythroblasts in bone marrow, seen in aplastic anemia. [erythroblast + G. *penia,* poverty]

e•ryth•ro•blas•to•sis (ĕ-rith′rō-blas-tō′sis) The presence of many erythroblasts in the blood. [erythroblast + *-osis,* condition]

e•ryth•ro•blas•to•sis fe•ta•lis (ĕ-rith′rō-blas-tō′sis fē-tā′lis) A grave hemolytic anemia that, in most instances, results from development in the mother of anti-Rh antibody in response to the Rh factor in the (Rh-positive) fetal blood; characterized by many erythroblasts in the circulation, and often generalized edema (hydrops fetalis) and enlargement of the liver and spleen; sometimes caused by antibodies for antigens other than Rh. SYN congenital anemia, hemolytic disease of newborn, neonatal anemia, Rh antigen incompatibility.

e•ryth•ro•blas•tot•ic (ĕ-rith′rō-blas-tot′ik) Pertaining to erythroblastosis, especially erythroblastosis fetalis.

er•y•throc•la•sis (er′i-throk′lă-sis) Fragmentation of the red blood cells. [erythro- + G. *klasis,* a breaking]

e•ryth•ro•clas•tic (ĕ-rith′rō-klas′tik) Pertaining to erythroclasis; destructive to red blood cells.

e•ryth•ro•cy•a•no•sis (ĕ-rith′rō-sī-ă-nō′sis) A condition seen in girls and young women in which exposure of the limbs to cold causes them to become swollen and dusky red; it results from direct exposure to cold, but not freezing, temperatures. [erythro- + G. *kyanos,* blue, + *-osis,* condition]

e•ryth•ro•cyte (ĕ-rith′rŏ-sīt) A mature red blood cell. See this page. SYN hemacyte, red blood cell, red cell, red corpuscle. [erythro- + G. *kytos,* cell]

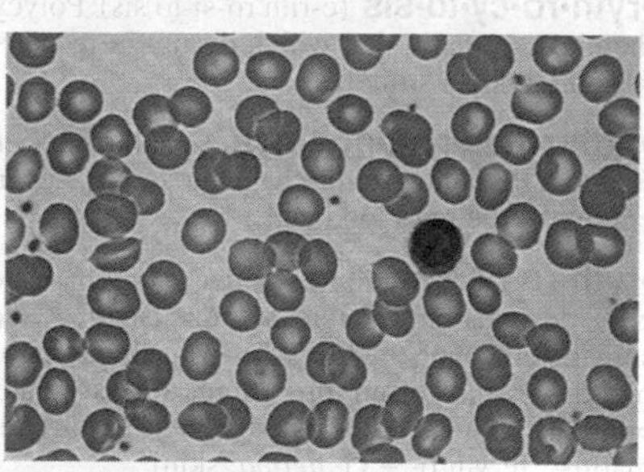

erythrocytes: in blood smear

e•ryth•ro•cyte count (ĕ-rith′rŏ-sīt kownt) SYN red blood cell count.

e•ryth•ro•cyte in•di•ces (ĕ-rith′rŏ-sīt in′di-sēz) Calculations for determining the average size, hemoglobin content, and concentration of hemoglobin in red blood cells, specifically mean cell volume, mean cell hemoglobin, and mean cell hemoglobin concentration.

e•ryth•ro•cyte sed•i•men•ta•tion rate (ESR) (ĕ-rith′rō-sīt sed′i-mĕn-tā′shŭn rāt) The rate of settling of red blood cells in anticoagulated blood; increased rates are often associated with anemia or inflammatory states.

erythrocythaemia [Br.] SYN erythrocythemia.

e•ryth•ro•cy•the•mi•a (ĕ-rith′rō-sī-thē′mē-ă) SYN polycythemia. SYN erythrocythaemia. [erythro- + G. *kytos,* cell, + *haima,* blood]

e•ryth•ro•cyt•ic (ĕ-rith′rō-sit′ik) Pertaining to an erythrocyte.

e•ryth•ro•cy•tic cycle (ĕ-rith′rō-sit′ik sī′kĕl) That pathogenic portion of the vertebrate phase of the life cycle of malarial organisms that takes place in the red blood cells.

e•ryth•ro•cyt•ic se•ries (ĕ-rith′rō-sit′ik sēr′ēz) The cells in the various stages of development in the red bone marrow leading to the formation of the erythrocyte, e.g., erythroblasts, normoblasts, erythrocytes.

e•ryth•ro•cy•tol•y•sin (ĕ-rith′rō-sī-tol′i-sin) SYN hemolysin (1).

e•ryth•ro•cy•tol•y•sis (ĕ-rith′rō-sī-tol′i-sis) SYN hemolysis. [erythrocyte + G. *lysis,* loosening]

e•ryth•ro•cy•tor•rhex•is (ĕ-rith′rō-sī-tŏr-ek′sis) A partial erythrocytolysis in which particles of protoplasm escape from the red blood cells, which then become crenated and deformed. SYN erythrorrhexis. [erythrocyte + G. *rhēxis,* rupture]

e•ryth•ro•cy•tos•chi•sis (ĕ-rith′rō-sī-tos′ki-sis) A breaking up of the red blood cells into small particles that morphologically resemble platelets. [erythrocyte + G. *schisis,* a splitting]

e•ryth•ro•cy•to•sis (ĕ-rith′rō-sī-tō′sis) Polycythemia, especially that which occurs in response to some known stimulus.

e•ryth•ro•de•gen•er•a•tive (ĕ-rith′rō-dē-jen′ĕr-ă-tiv) Pertaining to or characterized by degeneration of the red blood cells.

e•ryth•ro•der•ma (ĕ-rith′rō-dĕr′mă) A nonspecific designation for intense and usually widespread reddening of the skin from dilatation of blood vessels, often preceding, or associated with exfoliation. See this page. SYN erythrodermatitis. [erythro- + G. *derma,* skin]

e•ryth•ro•der•ma des•qua•ma•ti•vum (ĕ-rith′rō-dĕr′mă des-kwah′mă-tī′vŭm) Severe, extensive seborrheic dermatitis with exfoliative dermatitis, generalized lymphadenopathy, and diarrhea in the newborn; frequently occurs in undernourished, cachectic children. SYN Leiner disease.

e•ryth•ro•der•ma pso•ri•a•ti•cum (ĕ-rith′rō-dĕr′mă sōr-ē-at′i-kŭm) Extensive exfoliative dermatitis simulating psoriasis.

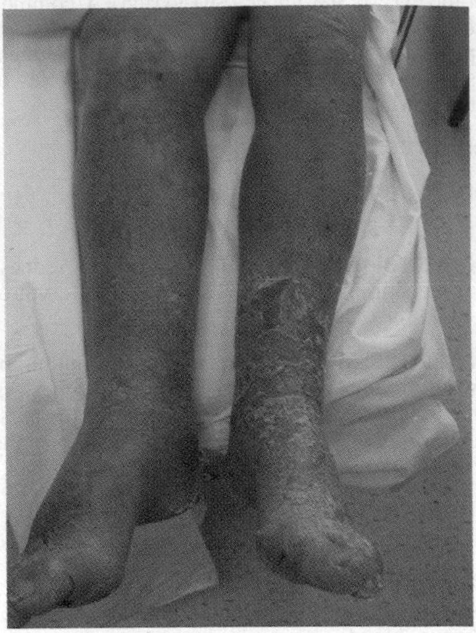

erythroderma: leg, eczematous form

e•ryth•ro•der•ma•ti•tis (ĕ-rith′rō-dĕr-mă-tī′tis) SYN erythroderma.

e•ryth•ro•don•ti•a (ĕ-rith′rō-don′shē-ă) Reddish discoloration of the teeth, as may occur in porphyria. [erythro- + G. *odous,* tooth]

erythroedema [Br.] SYN acrodynia (2).

e•ryth•ro•gen•ic (ĕ-rith′rō-jen′ik) **1.** Producing red, as causing an eruption or a red color sensation. **2.** Pertaining to the formation of red blood cells. [erythro- + *-gen,* producing]

e•ryth•ro•gen•ic tox•in (ĕ-rith′rō-jen′ik tok′sin) SYN streptococcus erythrogenic toxin.

er•y•throid (e-rith′royd) Of a reddish color.

e•ryth•ro•ker•a•to•der•mi•a (ĕ-rith′rō-ker-ă-tō-dĕr′mē-ă) A neurocutaneous syndrome characterized by papulosquamous erythematous plaques with onset shortly after birth; ataxia, nystagmus, dysarthria, and decreased tendon reflexes appear later in life; symmetric progressive erythrokeratodermia is inherited as an autosomal dominant disorder and does not involve the palms and soles. [erythro- + G. *keras,* horn, + *derma,* skin, + *-ia,* condition]

e•ryth•ro•ker•a•to•der•mi•a va•ri•a•bi•lis (ĕ-rith′rō-ker-ă-tō-dĕr′mē-ă vah-rē-ă-bil′is) A dermatosis characterized by hyperkeratotic plaques of bizarre, geographic configuration, associated with erythrodermic areas that may vary remarkably in size, shape, and position from day to day; hair, nails, and teeth are not affected; onset is usually in the first year of life; autosomal dominant or recessive inheritance, caused by mutation in the connexin gene encoding gap junction protein β-3 (GJB3) on 1p.

e·ryth·ro·ki·net·ics (ĕ-rith′rō-ki-net′iks) The kinetics of erythrocytes from their generation to destruction. [erythro- + G. *kinēsis,* movement]

erythroleukaemia [Br.] SYN erythroleukemia.

e·ryth·ro·leu·ke·mi·a (ĕ-rith′rō-lū-kē′mē-ă) Simultaneous neoplastic proliferation of erythroblastic and leukoblastic tissues. SYN erythroleukaemia.

e·ryth·ro·leu·ko·sis (ĕ-rith′rō-lū-kō′sis) A condition resembling leukemia in which the erythropoietic tissue is affected in addition to the leukopoietic tissue.

er·y·throl·y·sin (er′i-throl′i-sin) SYN hemolysin (1).

er·y·throl·y·sis (er′i-throl′i-sis) SYN hemolysis.

e·ryth·ro·mel·al·gi·a (ĕ-rith′rō-mel-al′jē-ă) **1.** Paroxysmal throbbing and burning pain in the skin often precipitated by exertion or heat, affecting the hands and feet, accompanied by a dusky mottled redness of the parts with increased skin temperature; may be associated with myeloproliferative disorders. **2.** A rare disorder of middle age, characterized by paroxysmal attacks of severe burning pain, reddening, hyperalgesia, and sweating, involving one or more extremities, usually both feet; the attacks can be triggered by warmth, and are usually relieved by cold and limb elevation. See this page. SYN Mitchell disease, red neuralgia. [erythro- + G. *melos,* limb, + *algos,* pain]

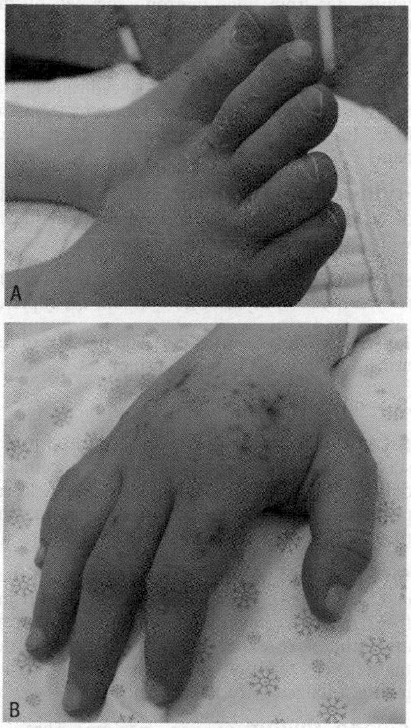

erythromelalgia: (A) foot; (B) hand

er·y·thron (er′i-thron) The total mass of circulating red blood cells, and that part of the hematopoietic tissue from which they are derived.

e·ryth·ro·ne·o·cy·to·sis (ĕ-rith′rō-nē-ō-sī-tō′sis) The presence in the peripheral circulation of regenerative forms of red blood cells. [erythrocyte + G. *neos,* new, + *kytos,* cell, + *-osis,* condition]

e·ryth·ro·pe·ni·a (ĕ-rith′rō-pē′nē-ă) Deficiency in the number of red blood cells. [erythrocyte + G. *penia,* poverty]

e·ryth·ro·pha·gi·a (ĕ-rith′rō-fā′jē-ă) Phagocytic destruction of red blood cells. [erythrocyte + G. *phagō,* to eat, + -ia]

e·ryth·ro·phag·o·cy·to·sis (ĕ-rith′rō-fag′ō-sī-tō′sis) Phagocytosis of erythrocytes.

e·ryth·ro·phil (ĕ-rith′rō-fil) **1.** Staining readily with red dyes. SYN erythrophilic. **2.** A cell or tissue element that stains red. [erythro- + G. *philos,* fond]

e·ryth·ro·phil·ic (ĕ-rith′rō-fil′ik) SYN erythrophil (1).

e·ryth·ro·pla·ki·a (ĕ-rith′rō-plā′kē-ă) A red, velvety, plaquelike lesion of mucous membrane that often represents malignant change. [erythro- + G. *plax,* plate]

e·ryth·ro·pla·si·a (ĕ-rith′rō-plā′zē-ă) Erythema and dysplasia of the epithelium. [erythro- + G. *plassō,* to form]

e·ryth·ro·pla·si·a of Quey·rat (ĕ-rith′rō-plā′zē-ă kā-rah′) Carcinoma in situ of the glans penis.

e·ryth·ro·poi·e·sis (ĕ-rith′rō-poy-ē′sis) The formation of red blood cells. [erythrocyte + G. *poiēsis,* a making]

e·ryth·ro·poi·et·ic (ĕ-rith′rō-poy-et′ik) Pertaining to or characterized by erythropoiesis.

e·ryth·ro·poi·et·ic por·phyr·i·a (ĕ-rith′rō-poy-et′ik pōr-fir′ē-ă) A classification of porphyria that includes congenital erythropoietic porphyria and erythropoietic protoporphyria.

e·ryth·ro·poi·et·ic pro·to·por·phyr·i·a (ĕ-rith′rō-poy-et′ik prō′tō-pōr-fir′ē-ă) A benign disorder of porphyrin metabolism due to a deficiency of ferrochelatase and characterized by enhanced fecal excretion of protoporphyrin and increased protoporphyrin IX in red blood cells, plasma, and feces; solar urticaria or eczema develops on exposure to sunlight.

e·ryth·ro·poi·e·tin (ĕ-rith′rō-poy′ĕ-tin) A protein that enhances erythropoiesis by stimulating formation of proerythroblasts and release of reticulocytes from bone marrow; secreted by the kidney and possibly by other tissues.

e•ryth•ro•pros•o•pal•gi•a (ĕ-rith′rō-pros-ō-pal′jē-ă) A disorder similar to erythromelalgia, but with the pain and redness occurring in the face. [erythro- + G. *prosōpon,* face, + *algos,* pain]

e•ryth•rop•si•a (er′ith-rop′sē-ă) An abnormality of vision in which all objects appear to be tinged with red. [erythro- + G. *ōps,* eye]

e•ryth•ror•rhex•is (ĕ-rith′rō-rek′sis) SYN erythrocytorrhexis. [erythrocyte + G. *rhēxis,* rupture]

er•y•thru•ri•a (er′i-thyūr′ē-ă) The passage of red urine. [erythro- + G. *ouron,* urine]

Es Symbol for einsteinium.

es•cape (es-kāp′) CARDIOLOGY term used to describe the situation when a higher pacemaker defaults or A-V conduction fails and a lower pacemaker assumes the function of pacemaking for one or more beats.

es•cape beat, **es•caped beat** (es-kāp′ bēt, es-kāpt′ bēt) An automatic beat, usually arising from the A-V junction or ventricle, occurring after the next expected normal beat has defaulted; it is therefore always a late beat, terminating a longer cycle than the normal.

es•cape rhythm (es-kāp′ ridh′ŭm) Three or more consecutive impulses at a rate not exceeding the upper limit of the inherent pacemaker.

es•char (es′kahr) A thick, coagulated crust or slough that develops following a thermal burn or chemical or physical cauterization of the skin. [G. *eschara,* a fireplace, a scab caused by burning]

es•cha•rot•ic (es′kă-rot′ik) Caustic or corrosive. [G. *escharōtikos*]

es•cha•rot•o•my (es′kă-rot′ŏ-mē) Surgical incision in an eschar to lessen constriction, as might be done following a burn. [eschar + G. *tomē,* incision]

i ***Esch•e•rich•i•a*** (esh-ĕ-rik′ē-ă) A genus of aerobic, facultatively anaerobic bacteria containing short, motile or nonmotile, gram-negative rods. Motile cells are peritrichous. Glucose and lactose are fermented with the production of acid and gas. These organisms are found in feces; some are pathogenic to humans, causing conditions such as enteritis, peritonitis, and cystitis. It is the type genus of the family Enterobacteriaceae. The type species is *E. coli*. See page B7.

Esch•e•rich•i•a co•li (esh-ĕ-rik′ē-ă kō′lī) A bacterial species that occurs normally in the intestines of humans and other vertebrates, is widely distributed in nature, and is a frequent cause of infections of the urogenital tract and of diarrhea in infants; enteropathogenic strains (serovars) of *E. coli* cause diarrhea due to enterotoxin, the production of which seems to be associated with a transferable episome. Serious outbreaks of disease, with fatalities, occurred in Walkerton, Ontario and N. Battleford, Saskatchewan.

E se•lec•tin (sĕ-lek′tin) Cell surface receptor produced by endothelium.

e•soph•a•ge•al (ĕ-sof′ă-jē′ăl) Relating to the esophagus. SYN oesophageal.

e•soph•a•ge•al a•cha•la•si•a (ĕ-sof′ă-jē′ăl ak′ă-lā′zē-ă) An obstruction to the passage of food that develops in the terminal esophagus; caused by an autonomic nervous system abnormality. SYN achalasia of the cardia, cardiospasm, oesophageal achalasia.

e•soph•a•ge•al ar•ter•ies (ĕ-sof′ă-jē′ăl ahr′tĕr-ēz) Esophageal branches of the inferior thyroid artery; left gastric artery; thoracic aorta.

e•soph•a•ge•al a•tre•si•a (ĕ-sof′ă-jē′ăl ă-trē′zē-ă) Neonatal condition in which the proximal end of the esophagus ends in a blind pouch. Food cannot enter the stomach through the esophagus.

e•soph•a•ge•al gas•tric tube air•way (EGTA) (ĕ-sof′ă-jē′ăl gas′trik tūb ār′wā) In emergency respiratory therapy, a device used in cardiopulmonary resuscitation consisting of a mask for delivery of oxygen under positive pressure and an inflatable occlusive tube placed in the esophagus to prevent gastric inflation and regurgitation during resuscitation; used in unconscious patients for resuscitation. SYN esophageal obturator airway, Gordon-Don Michael tube.

e•soph•a•ge•al hi•a•tus (ĕ-sof′ă-jē′ăl hī-ā′tŭs) The opening in the right crus of the diaphragm, between the central tendon and the hiatus aorticus, through which pass the esophagus and the two vagus nerves. SYN oesophageal hiatus.

e•soph•a•ge•al lead (ĕ-sof′ă-jē′ăl lēd) An electrocardiographic lead passed down the throat into the esophagus to record the electrocardiogram at various levels of the esophagus; especially useful for certain types of arrhythmias. Similarly, a transducer for echocardiography can be passed into the esophagus. SYN oesophageal lead.

e•soph•a•ge•al ner•vous plex•us (ĕ-sof′ă-jē′ăl nĕrv′ŭs plĕks′ŭs) One of two nervous plexuses, posterior and anterior, on the walls of the esophagus; the first is formed by branches from the right vagus and left recurrent, the second by the anastomosing trunks of the vagus after leaving the pulmonary plexuses; branches supply the mucous and muscular coats of the esophagus. SYN plexus gulae, plexus nervosus esophageus.

e•soph•a•ge•al ob•tu•ra•tor air•way (EOA) (ĕ-sof′ă-jē′ăl ob′tŭr-ā-tŏr ār′wā) SYN esophageal gastric tube airway.

e•soph•a•ge•al re•flux, **gas•tro•e•soph•a•ge•al re•flux** (ĕ-sof′ă-jē′ăl rē′flŭks, gas′trō-ĕ-sō-fā′jē-ăl rē′flŭks) SEE gastroesophageal reflux disease. SYN oesophageal reflux.

e·soph·a·ge·al speech (ĕ-sof′ă-jē′ăl spēch) A technique for speaking after total laryngectomy; phonation results from introducing air into the upper esophagus to allow vibration of the pharyngoesophageal (PE) segment. SYN oesophageal speech.

e·soph·a·ge·al tra·che·al air·way (ĕ-sof′ă-jē′ăl trā′kē-ăl ār′wā) SYN pharyngeal tracheal multiple balloon system.

e·soph·a·ge·al va·ri·ces (ĕ-sof′ă-jē′ăl var′i-sēz) Longitudinal venous varices at the lower end of the esophagus as a result of portal hypertension; they are superficial and liable to ulceration and massive bleeding. See page B16. SYN oesophageal varices.

e·soph·a·ge·al veins (ĕ-sof′ă-jē′ăl vānz) Series of veins draining the submucous venous plexus of the esophagus; proceeding inferiorly from the cervical portion of the esophagus, they drain to the inferior thyroid vein, the superior intercostal veins, the azygos, accessory hemiazygos, and hemiazygos veins, all of which are ultimately tributaries of the superior vena cava; the most inferior esophageal veins, from the cardiac portion of the esophagus, drain through the esophageal branches of the left gastric vein, a tributary of the portal vein. Thus, the submucosal veins of the inferior esophagus form a portocaval anastomosis, and are subject to the formation of varicosities in portal hypertension. SYN oesophageal veins.

e·soph·a·gec·ta·sis, e·soph·a·gec·ta·si·a (ĕ-sof-ă-jek′tă-sis, -jek-tā′zē-ă) Dilation of the esophagus SYN oesophagectasis. [esophagus + G. *ektasis,* a stretching]

e·soph·a·gec·to·my (ĕ-sof-ă-jek′tŏ-mē) Excision of any part of the esophagus. SYN oesophagectomy. [esophagus + G. *ektomē,* excision]

e·soph·a·gi (ĕ-sof′ă-jī) Plural of esophagus. SYN oesophagi.

e·soph·a·gism (ĕ-sof′ă-jizm) Esophageal spasm causing dysphagia. SYN oesophagism.

e·soph·a·gi·tis (ĕ-sof′ă-jī′tis) Inflammation of the esophagus. SYN oesophagitis.

e·soph·a·go·car·di·o·plas·ty (ē-sof′ă-gō-kahr′dē-ō-plas-tē) Surgical repair of the esophagus and cardiac end of the stomach. SYN oesophagocardioplasty.

e·soph·a·go·cele (ĕ-sof′ă-gō-sēl) Protrusion of the mucous membrane of the esophagus through a tear in the muscular coat. SYN oesophagocele. [esophagus + G. *kēlē,* hernia]

e·soph·a·go·du·o·den·os·to·my (ĕ-sof′ă-gō-dū′ō-dĕ-nos′tŏ-mē) Surgical formation of a direct communication between the esophagus and the duodenum, with or without removal of the stomach. SYN oesophagoduodenostomy.

e·soph·a·go·en·ter·os·to·my (ĕ-sof′ă-gō-en-tĕr-os′tŏ-mē) Surgical formation of a direct communication between the esophagus and intestine. SYN oesophagoenterostomy. [esophagus + G. *enteron,* intestine, + *stoma,* mouth]

e·soph·a·go·gas·trec·to·my (ĕ-sof′ă-gō-gas-trek′tŏ-mē) Removal of a portion of the lower esophagus and proximal stomach for treatment of neoplasms or strictures of those organs, especially those lesions located at or near the cardioesophageal junction. SYN oesophagogastrectomy.

e·soph·a·go·gas·tric junc·tion (ĕ-sof′ă-gō-gas′trik jŭngk′shŭn) Terminal end of esophagus and beginning of stomach at the cardiac orifice; site of the physiologic inferior esophageal sphincter. SYN oesophagogastric junction.

e·soph·a·go·gas·tro·a·nas·to·mo·sis (ĕ-sof′ă-gō-gas′trō-ă-nas-tŏ-mō′sis) SYN esophagogastrostomy. SYN oesophagogastroanastomosis.

esoph·a·go·gas·tro·du·o·de·nos·co·py (EGD) (ĕ-sof′ă-gō-gas′trō-dū′ō-den-os′kŏ-pē) Endoscopic examination of the esophagus, stomach, and duodenum, usually performed using a fiberoptic instrument. Motility evaluation, secretion, collection, and tissue sampling may be done. Patient is sedated before the procedure to assess the gag reflex postprocedure, which is necessary before intake of food and drink may be resumed. See page B16. SYN oesophagogastroduodenoscopy.

e·soph·a·go·gas·tro·plas·ty (ĕ-sof′ă-gō-gas′trō-plas-tē) SYN cardioplasty. SYN oesophagogastroplasty.

e·soph·a·go·gas·tros·to·my (ĕ-sof′ă-gō-gas-tros′tŏ-mē) Anastomosis of esophagus to stomach, usually following esophagogastrectomy. SYN esophagogastroanastomosis, gastroesophagostomy, oesophagogastrostomy. [esophagus + G. *gastēr,* stomach, + *stoma,* mouth]

e·soph·a·go·gram (ĕ-sof′ă-gō-gram) A radiograph of the esophagus. SYN oesophagogram.

e·soph·a·gog·ra·phy (ĕ-sof′ă-gog′ră-fē) Radiography of the esophagus using swallowed or injected radiopaque contrast media; the technique of obtaining an esophagogram. SYN oesophagography. [esophagus + G. *graphō,* to write]

e·soph·a·go·ma·la·ci·a (ĕ-sof′ă-gō-mă-lā′shē-ă) Softening of the walls of the esophagus. SYN oesophagomalacia. [esophagus + G. *malakia,* softness]

e·soph·a·go·my·ot·o·my (ĕ-sof′ă-gō-mī-ot′ō-mē) Treatment of esophageal achalasia by longitudinal division of the lowest part of the esophageal muscle down to the submucosal layer; some muscle fibers of the cardia may also be divided. SYN oesophagomyotomy. [esophagus + G. *mys,* muscle, + *tomē,* incision]

e·soph·a·go·plas·ty (ĕ-sof′ă-gō-plas-tē) Surgical repair of the wall of the esophagus. SYN oesophagoplasty. [esophagus + G. *plastos,* formed]

e·soph·a·go·pli·ca·tion (ĕ-sof′ă-gō-pli-kā′shŭn) Reduction in size of a dilated esophagus or of a pouch in it by making longitudinal folds or tucks in its wall. SYN oesophagoplication. [esophagus + L. *plico,* to fold]

e·soph·a·gop·to·sis, **e·soph·a·gop·to·si·a** (ĕ-sof′ă-gō-tō′sis, -tō′sē-ă) Relaxation and downward displacement of the walls of the esophagus. SYN oesophagoptosis. [esophagus + G. *ptōsis,* a falling]

e·soph·a·go·scope (ĕ-sof′ă-gō-skōp) An endoscope for inspecting the interior of the esophagus. SYN oesophagoscope. [esophagus + G. *skopeō,* to examine]

e·soph·a·gos·co·py (ĕ-sof′ă-gos′kŏ-pē) Inspection of the interior of the esophagus by means of an endoscope. SYN oesophagoscopy. [esophagus + G. *skopeō,* to examine]

e·soph·a·go·spasm (ĕ-sof′ă-gō-spazm) Spasm of the walls of the esophagus. SYN oesophagospasm.

e·soph·a·go·ste·no·sis (ĕ-sof′ă-gō-stĕ-nō′sis) Stricture or a general narrowing of the esophagus. SYN oesophagostenosis. [esophagus + G. *stenōsis,* a narrowing]

e·soph·a·go·sto·mi·a·sis (ĕ-sof′ă-gō-stō-mī′ă-sis) Intestinal parasitization by nematodes of the genus *Oesophagostomum.* SYN oesophagostomiasis.

e·soph·a·gos·to·my (ĕ-sof-ă-gos′tŏ-mē) Surgical formation of an opening directly into the esophagus from without. SYN oesophagostomy. [esophagus + G. *stoma,* mouth]

e·soph·a·got·o·my (ĕ-sof-ă-got′ŏ-mē) An incision through the wall of the esophagus. SYN oesophagotomy. [esophagus + G. *tomē,* an incision]

e·soph·a·gus, pl. **e·soph·a·gi** (ĕ-sof′ă-gŭs, -gī; -jī) The portion of the digestive canal between the pharynx and stomach. It is about 25 cm long and consists of three parts: the cervical, from the cricoid cartilage to the thoracic inlet; the thoracic, from the thoracic inlet to the diaphragm; and the abdominal, below the diaphragm to the cardiac opening of the stomach. SYN oesophagus. [G. *oisophagos,* gullet]

es·o·pho·ri·a (es′ō-fōr′ē-ă) A tendency for the eyes to turn inward, prevented by binocular vision. [G. *esō,* inward, + *phora,* a carrying]

es·o·phor·ic (es′ō-fōr′ik) Relating to or marked by esophoria.

es·o·tro·pi·a (es′ō-trō′pē-ă) The form of strabismus in which the visual axes converge; may be paralytic or concomitant, monocular or alternating, accommodative or nonaccommodative. SYN convergent strabismus. [G. *esō,* inward, + *tropē,* turn]

es·o·tro·pic (es′ō-trō′pik) Relating to or marked by esotropia.

ESP Abbreviation for extrasensory perception.

es·pun·di·a (es-pūn′dē-ă) A type of American leishmaniasis caused by *Leishmania braziliensis* that affects the mucous membranes, particularly in the nasal and oral region, resulting in grossly destructive changes; may develop metastatically from sores originally found elsewhere on the body. SYN Breda disease. [Sp., fr. L. *spongia,* sponge]

ESR Abbreviation for erythrocyte sedimentation rate; electron spin resonance.

es·sen·tial (ĕ-sen′shăl) **1.** Necessary, indispensable (e.g., essential amino acids, essential fatty acids). **2.** Characteristic of. **3.** Determining. **4.** Of unknown etiology. **5.** Relating to an essence (e.g., essential oil). **6.** SYN intrinsic.

es·sen·tial a·mi·no ac·ids (ĕ-sen′shăl ă-mē′nō as′idz) The α-amino acids nutritionally required by an organism that must be supplied in its diet (i.e., cannot be synthesized by the organism), either as free amino acid or in proteins.

es·sen·tial dys·men·or·rhe·a (ĕ-sen′shăl dis-men′ŏr-ē′ă) SYN primary dysmenorrhea.

es·sen·tial fat·ty ac·id (EFA) (ĕ-sen′chăl fat′ē as′id) The 18-carbon fatty acids that are nutritionally required by humans and must be consumed through dietary sources. The EFAs are linoleic acid or C18:2 (n-6) and alpha-linolenic acid or C18:2 (n-3).

es·sen·tial hy·per·ten·sion (e-sen′shăl hī′pĕr-ten′shŭn) Hypertension with no known cause; accounts for approximately between 90 and 95% of patients diagnosed with hypertension. SYN primary hypertension.

es·sen·tial nu·tri·ent (e-sen′shăl nū′trē-ĕnt) Dietary substances required for optimal health that must be consumed because they are not provided by the body.

es·sen·tial oil (ĕ-sen′shăl oyl) A plant product, usually somewhat volatile, giving the odors and tastes characteristic of the particular plant; usually, the steam distillates of plants or of oils obtained by pressing the rinds of plants. SEE ALSO volatile oil.

es·sen·tial pru·ri·tus (ĕ-sen′shăl prū-rī′tŭs) Itching that occurs independently of skin lesions.

es·sen·tial tel·an·gi·ec·ta·si·a (ĕ-sen′shăl tel-an′jē-ek-tā′zē-ă) **1.** Localized capillary dilation of undetermined origin. **2.** SYN angioma serpiginosum.

es•sen•tial throm•bo•cy•to•pe•ni•a (ĕ-sen′shăl throm′bō-sī-tō-pē′nē-ă) A primary form of this disorder (in contrast to secondary forms that are associated with metastatic neoplasms, tuberculosis, and leukemia involving the bone marrow, or with direct suppression of bone marrow by the use of chemical agents, or with other conditions).

es•sen•tial trem•or (ĕ-sen′shăl trem′ŏr) An action tremor of 4–8 Hz frequency that usually begins in early adult life and is limited to the upper limbs and head; called familial when it appears in several family members.

Es•ser graft (es′ĕr graft) SYN inlay graft.

EST Abbreviation for electroshock therapy.

es•tab•lished pa•tient (es-tab′lisht pā′shĕnt) Denotes someone who has been seen by a physician or member of a health care group within a 3-year period. SEE ALSO EIN.

es•ter (es′tĕr) An organic compound containing the grouping, –X(O)–O–R (X = carbon, sulfur, phosphorus; R = radical of an alcohol), formed by the elimination of H_2O between the –OH of an acid group and the –OH of an alcohol group.

es•ter•ase (es′tĕr-ās) A generic term for enzymes that catalyze the hydrolysis of esters.

es•ter•i•fi•ca•tion (es-ter′i-fi-kā′shŭn) The process of forming an ester, as in the reaction of ethanol and acetic acid to form ethyl acetate.

es•the•si•a (es-thē′zē-ă) SYN perception. SYN aesthesia. [G. *aisthēsis*, sensation]

esthesio- Prefix meaning sensation, perception. SYN aesthesio-. [G. *aesthēsis,* sense perception]

es•the•si•od•ic (es-thē′zē-od′ik) Conveying sensory impressions. SYN aesthesodic, esthesodic. [esthesio- + G. *hodos,* way]

es•the•si•o•gen•e•sis (es-thē′zē-ō-jen′ĕ-sis) The production of sensation, especially of nervous erethism. SYN aesthesiogenesis. [esthesio- + G. *genesis,* origin]

es•the•si•o•gen•ic (es-thē′zē-ō-jen′ik) Producing a sensation. SYN aesthesiogenic.

es•the•si•om•e•ter (es-thē′zē-om′ĕ-tĕr) An instrument for determining the state of tactile and other forms of sensibility. SYN aesthesiometer, tactometer. [esthesio- + G. *metron,* measure]

es•the•si•om•e•try (es-thē′zē-om′ĕ-trē) Measurement of the degree of tactile or other sensibility. SYN aesthesiometry.

es•the•si•o•neu•ro•sis (es-thē′zē-ō-nūr-ō′sis) Any sensory impairment (e.g., anesthesia, hyperesthesia, paraesthesia). SYN aesthesioneurosis.

es•the•si•o•phys•i•ol•o•gy (es-thē′zē-ō-fiz-ē-ol′ŏ-jē) The physiology of sensation and the sense organs. SYN aesthesiophysiology.

es•the•sod•ic (es′thĕ-zod′ik) SYN esthesiodic.

es•thet•ic (es-thet′ik) **1.** Pertaining to the sensations. **2.** Pertaining to esthetics (i.e., beauty). SYN aesthetic. [G. *aisthēsis,* sensation]

es•thet•ics (es-thet′iks) The branch of philosophy concerned with art and beauty, especially with the components thereof. SYN aesthetics.

es•ti•mate (es′ti-măt) **1.** A measurement or a statement about the value of some quantity that is known, believed, or suspected to incorporate some degree of error. **2.** The result of applying any estimator to a random sample of data. It is not a random variable but a realization of one, a fixed quantity, and it has no variance although commonly it also furnishes an estimate of what the variance of the estimator is. USAGE NOTE not to be confused with an estimator, which is a prescription for obtaining an estimate. [L. *aestimo*, pp. *aestimatum,* to appraise]

es•ti•mat•ed av•er•age re•quire•ment (EAR) (es′ti-mā′ted av′răj rĕ-kwīr′mĕnt) The daily intake of a specific nutrient estimated to meet the requirement in 50% of healthy people in an age- and gender-specific group. The EAR is used to calculate the recommended dietary allowance.

es•ti•ma•ted en•er•gy re•quire•ment (EER) (est′ti-mā-tĕd en′ĕr-jē rē-kwīr′mĕnt) Intake of a nutrient that meets the estimated needs of 50% of the population.

es•ti•val (es′ti-văl) Relating to or occurring in the summer. SYN aestival. [L. *aestivus,* summer (adj.)]

es•ti•va•tion (es′ti-vā′shŭn) Living through the summer in a quiescent, torpid state. SYN aestivation.

es•ti•vo•au•tum•nal (es′ti-vō-aw-tŭm′năl) Relating to or occurring in summer and autumn. SYN aestivoautumnal. [L. *aestivus,* summer (adj.), + *autumnalis,* autumnal]

Est•land•er op•er•a•tion (est′lahnd-ĕr op-ĕr-ā′shŭn) Use of an Estlander flap in plastic surgery of the lips.

es•tra•di•ol (es-tră-dī′ol) The most potent naturally occurring estrogen, formed by the ovary, placenta, testes, and possibly the cortex of the suprarenal gland. SYN oestradiol.

es•tri•ol (es′trē-ol) An estrogenic metabolite of estradiol, usually the predominant estrogenic metabolite found in urine (especially during pregnancy). SYN oestriol.

es•tro•gen (es′trŏ-jen) Generic term for any substance, natural or synthetic, which exerts biologic effects characteristic of estrogenic hormones; formed by the ovary, placenta, testes, and possibly the adrenal cortex, as well as by certain plants; stimulates secondary sexual characteristics and exert systemic effects, such as growth and maturation of long bones; until recently given after menopause or oophorectomy to prevent heart attack and prevent osteoporosis; also used to prevent or stop lactation, suppress ovulation, and palliate carcinoma of the breast and prostate. SYN oestrogen. [G. *oistrus,* estrus, + *-gen,* producing]

es•tro•gen•ic (es′trŏ-jen′ik) **1.** Causing estrus in animals. **2.** Having an action similar to that of an estrogen. SYN oestrogenic.

es•tro•gen re•cep•tor (es′trŏ-jen rĕ-sep′tŏr) Receptor for estrogens; its presence conveys a better prognosis for breast cancers. SYN oestrogen receptor.

es•tro•gen re•place•ment ther•a•py (ERT) (es′trŏ-jen rĕ-plās′mĕnt thār′ă-pē) Administration of sex hormones to women after menopause or oophorectomy. SYN hormone replacement therapy, oestrogen replacement therapy.

es•trone (es′trōn) A metabolite of 17β-estradiol, commonly found in urine, ovaries, and placenta, with considerably less biologic activity than the parent hormone. SYN oestrone.

es•trous (es′trŭs) Pertaining to estrus. SYN estrual.

es•trous cy•cle (es′trŭs sī′kĕl) The series of cyclic uterine, ovarian, and other changes that occur in higher animals. SYN oestrous cycle.

es•tru•al (es′trū-ăl) SYN estrous. SYN oestrual.

es•tru•a•tion (es′trū-ā′shŭn) SYN estrus. SYN oestruation.

es•trus (es′trŭs) That portion or phase of the sexual cycle of female animals characterized by willingness to permit coitus; readily detectable behavioral and other signs are exhibited by animals during this period. SYN estruation, heat (2), oestrus. [G. *oistros,* mad desire]

ESV Abbreviation for end systolic volume.

ESWL Abbreviation for electrohydraulic shock wave lithotripsy; extracorporeal shock wave lithotripsy.

ET Abbreviation for endotracheal tube.

Et Abbreviation for ethyl.

e•ta (H, η) (ā′tă) The seventh letter of the Greek alphabet. **1.** CHEMISTRY denotes the position seven atoms from the carboxyl group or other primary functional group. **2.** Viscosity.

et al. And others. [L. *et alii*]

etc. And so forth. [L. *et cetera*]

ETEC Abbreviation for enterotoxigenic *Escherichia coli.*

eth•ane•di•ni•trile (eth′ān-dī-nī′tril) A toxic chemical compound, N≡C—C≡N. SYN cyanogen (1).

eth•a•nol (eth′ăn-ol) SYN alcohol (2).

eth•a•nol test (eth′ă-nol test) Measurement of alcohol consumption in drivers who are determined to have acted in a manner suggesting impairment; may involve blood, urine, or breath testing.

eth•en•yl (eth′ĕ-nil) SYN vinyl.

e•ther (ē′thĕr) **1.** Any organic compound in which two carbon atoms are independently linked to a common oxygen atom, thus containing the group –C–O–C–. SEE ALSO epoxy. **2.** Loosely used to refer to diethyl ether. [G. *aithēr,* the pure upper air]

e•the•re•al (ē-thēr′ē-ăl) Relating to or containing ether. [G. *aitherios,* etherial, fr. *aithēr,* the upper air]

e•the•re•al oil (ē-thēr′ē-ăl oyl) SYN volatile oil.

eth•i•cal (eth′i-kăl) Relating to ethics; in conformity with the rules governing personal and professional conduct.

eth•ics (eth′iks) **1.** The branch of philosophy that deals with the distinction between right and wrong, with the moral consequences of human actions. **2.** NURSING philosophy or code about what is ideal in human character and conduct; principles of right or wrong accepted by individual or group; study of morals and moral choices. [G. *ethikos,* arising from custom, fr. *ethos,* custom]

♻ **ethmo-** Prefix meaning ethmoid; the ethmoid bone. [G. *ēthmos,* sieve]

eth•moid (eth′moyd) **1.** Resembling a sieve. **2.** Relating to the ethmoid bone. SYN ethmoidal. [G. *ēthmos,* sieve, + *eidos,* resemblance]

eth•moi•dal (eth-moy′dăl) SYN ethmoid.

eth•moid bone (eth′moyd bōn) An irregularly shaped bone lying between the orbital plates of the frontal and anterior to the sphenoid bone; it consists of two lateral masses of thin plates enclosing air cells, attached above to a perforated horizontal lamina, the cribriform plate, from which descends a median vertical or perpendicular plate in the interval between the two lateral masses; the bone articulates with the sphenoid, frontal, maxillary, lacrimal, and palatine bones, the inferior nasal concha, and the vomer; it enters into the formation of the anterior cranial fossa, the orbits, and the nasal cavity.

eth•moid crest (eth′moyd krest) Bony ridge that articulates with, or provides attachment for, any part of the ethmoid bone, especially the middle nasal concha.

eth•moi•dec•to•my (eth′moy-dek′tŏ-mē) Removal of all or part of the mucosal lining and bony partitions between the ethmoid sinuses. [ethmo- + G. *ektomē,* excision]

eth•moid fo•ra•men (eth′moyd fōr-ā′mĕn)

Either of two foramina formed by grooves on either edge of the ethmoidal notch of the frontal bone, and completed by similar grooves on the ethmoid bone: anterior ethmoid foramen, located in an anterior position; posterior ethmoid foramen located in a posterior position.

eth•moid in•fun•dib•u•lum (eth′moyd in′fŭn-dib′yū-lŭm) A passage from the middle meatus of the nose communicating with the anterior ethmoid cells and frontal sinus.

eth•moid•i•tis (eth′moy-dī′tis) Inflammation of the ethmoid sinuses.

eth•moid lab•y•rinth (eth′moyd lab′i-rinth) A mass of air cells with thin bony walls forming part of the lateral wall of the nasal cavity; the cells are arranged in three groups, anterior, middle, and posterior, and are closed laterally by the orbital plate, which forms part of the wall of the orbit.

eth•moid veins (eth′moyd vānz) Accompany the anterior and posterior ethmoid arteries and pass into the superior ophthalmic vein; they drain the ethmoid sinuses.

eth•mo•tur•bi•nals (eth′mō-tŭr′bi-nălz) The conchae of the ethmoid bone; the superior and middle conchae; occasionally a third, the supreme concha, exists.

eth•nic group (eth′nik grūp) A social group characterized by a distinctive social and cultural tradition maintained from generation to generation, a common history and origin, and a sense of identification with the group.

eth•no•cen•trism (eth′nō-sen′trizm) The tendency to evaluate other groups according to the values and standards of one's own ethnic group, especially with the conviction that one's own ethnic group is superior to other groups. [G. *ethnos,* race, tribe, + *kentron,* center of a circle]

eth•o•phar•ma•col•o•gy (eth′ō-fahr-mă-kol′ŏ-jē) The study of drug effects on behavior, relying on observation and description of species-specific elements (acts and postures during social encounters). [G. *ethos,* character, habit, + pharmacology]

e•thox•y (eth-ok′sē) The monovalent radical, CH_3CH_2O–.

eth•yl (Et) (eth′il) The hydrocarbon radical CH_3CH_2–.

eth•yl al•co•hol (eth′il al′kŏ-hol) SYN alcohol (2).

eth•yl•ate (eth′i-lāt) A compound in which the hydrogen of the hydroxyl group of ethanol is replaced by a metallic atom, usually sodium or potassium (e.g., C_2H_5ONa, sodium ethylate).

eth•yl•di•chlo•ro•ar•sine (eth′il-dī-klōr-ō-ahr′sēn) A blister agent used during World War I; irritating to the respiratory tract.

eth•yl•ene•di•a•mine•tet•ra•a•cet•ic ac•id (EDTA) (eth′i-lēn-dī′ă-mēn-tet′ră-ă-sē′tik as′id) A chelating agent and anticoagulant; added to blood specimens for hematologic and other tests.

eth•yl•i•dyne (eth-il′i-dīn) The radical $CH_3C\equiv$.

e•ti•o•la•tion (ē′tē-ō-lā′shŭn) **1.** Pallor resulting from absence of light, as in people confined because of illness or imprisonment, or in plants bleached by being deprived of light. **2.** The process of blanching, bleaching, or making pale by withholding light. [Fr. *étioler,* to blanch]

e•ti•o•log•ic, e•ti•o•log•ic•al (ē′tē-ŏ-loj′ik, -loj′ik-ăl) Relating to etiology. SYN aetiologic, aetiological.

e•ti•ol•o•gy (ē′tē-ol′ŏ-jē) **1.** The science and study of the causes of disease and their mode of operation. Cf. pathogenesis. **2.** The science of causes, causality; in common usage, cause. SYN aetiology. [G. *aitia,* cause, + *logos,* treatise, discourse]

Eu Symbol for europium.

eu- Combining form meaning good, well; opposite of dys-, caco-. [G.]

EUA Abbreviation for examination under anesthetic.

Eu•bac•te•ri•um (yū′bak-tēr′ē-ŭm) A genus of anaerobic, non-spore-forming, nonmotile bacteria containing straight or curved gram-positive rods that usually occur singly, in pairs, or in short chains. Usually these organisms attack carbohydrates. They are often associated with mixed infections involving the abdomen, pelvis, or genitourinary tract. The type species is *E. limosum.*

Eu•ces•to•da (yū′ses-tō′dă) The subclass of *Cestoda* that includes tapeworms. SEE ALSO Cestoda.

eu•chlor•hy•dri•a (yū′klōr-hī′drē-ă) A condition in which free hydrochloric acid exists in normal amounts in the gastric juice. [eu- + cholohydric (acid) + -ia]

eu•cho•li•a (yū-kō′lē-ă) A normal state of the bile as regards quantity and quality. [eu- + G. *cholē,* bile]

eu•chro•ma•tin (yū-krō′mă-tin) The parts of chromosomes that, during interphase, are uncoiled dispersed threads and not stained by ordinary dyes; metabolically active, in contrast to the inert heterochromatin.

Eu•co•le•us (yu-kō′lē-us) One of three trichurid nematode genera, commonly referred to as *Capillaria.*

eu•di•a•pho•re•sis (yū-dī′ă-fŏr-ē′sis) Normal free sweating. [eu- + G. *diaphorēsis,* perspiration]

eu•gen•ic (yū-jen′ik) Relating to eugenics.

eu·gen·ics (yū-jen′iks) **1.** Practices and policies, as of mate selection or of sterilization, which tend to better the innate qualities of progeny and human stock. **2.** Practices and genetic counseling directed to anticipating genetic disability and disease. [G. *eugeneia,* nobility of birth, fr. *eu,* well, + *genesis,* production]

eu·glob·u·lin (yū-glob′yū-lin) That fraction of the serum globulin less soluble in $(NH_4)_2SO_4$ solution than the pseudoglobulin fraction.

euglycaemia [Br.] SYN euglycemia.

euglycaemic [Br.] SYN euglycemic.

eu·gly·ce·mi·a (yū′glī-sē′mē-ă) A normal blood glucose concentration. SYN euglycaemia, normoglycemia. [eu- + G. *glykys,* sweet, + *haima,* blood]

eu·gly·ce·mic (yū′glī-sē′mik) Denoting, characteristic of, or promoting euglycemia. SYN euglycaemic, normoglycemic.

eu·gna·thi·a (yū-gnā′thē-ă) An abnormality that is limited to the teeth and their immediate alveolar supports. [eu- + G. *gnathos,* jaw]

eu·gon·ic (yū-gon′ik) A term used to indicate that the growth of a bacterial culture is rapid and relatively luxuriant; used especially in reference to the growth of cultures of the human tubercle bacillus (*Mycobacterium tuberculosis*). [G. *eugonos,* productive, fr. *eu,* well, + *gonos,* seed, offspring]

Eu·kar·y·o·tae, Eu·car·y·o·tae (yū-kar-ē-ō′tē) A superkingdom of organisms characterized by eukaryotic cells; acellular members (kingdom Protoctista) are characterized by a single eukaryotic unit; more complex (multicellular) members have been assigned to the kingdoms Fungi, Plantae, and Animalia.

eu·kar·y·ote (yū-kar′ē-ōt) **1.** A cell containing a membrane-bound nucleus with chromosomes of DNA, RNA, and proteins, with cell division involving a form of mitosis in which mitotic spindles (or some microtubule arrangement) are involved; mitochondria are present, and, in photosynthetic species, plastids are found. Possession of a eukaryote type of cell characterizes the four kingdoms above the Monera or prokaryote level of complexity: Protoctista, Fungi, Plantae, and Animalia, combined into the superkingdom Eukaryotae. **2.** Common name for members of the Eukaryotae. [eu- + G. *karyon,* kernel, nut]

eu·kar·y·ot·ic (yū′kar-ē-ot′ik) Pertaining to or characteristic of a eukaryote.

Eu·len·burg dis·ease (oy′lĕn-bĕrg di-zēz′) SYN congenital paramyotonia.

eu·me·tri·a (yū-mē′trē-ă) Graduation of the strength of nerve impulses to match the need. [G. moderation, goodness of meter]

eu·my·ce·to·ma (yū′mī-sē-tō′mă) Mycetoma caused by fungi. Cf. actinomycetoma.

eu·nuch (yū′nŭk) A male whose testes have been removed or have never developed. [G. *eunouchos,* chamberlain, fr. *eunē,* bed, + *echō,* to have]

eu·nuch·oid (yū′nŭ-koyd) Resembling, or having the general characteristics of, a eunuch; usually indicating the physical habitus of a male in whom hypogonadism occurred before puberty. [G. *eunouchos,* eunuch, + *eidos,* resembling]

eu·nuch·oid gi·gan·tism (yū′nŭ-koyd jī-gant′izm) Gigantism with deficient development of sexual organs; may be of pituitary or gonadal origin; gigantism accompanied by body proportions typical of hypogonadism during adolescence.

eu·nuch·oid·ism (yū′nŭ-koyd-izm) A state in which testes are present but fail to function normally; may be of gonadal or pituitary origin.

eu·pep·si·a (yū-pep′sē-ă) Good digestion. [G., fr. *eu,* well, + *pepsis,* digestion]

eu·pep·tic (yū-pep′tik) Digesting well; having a good digestion.

eu·pep·tide (yū-pep′tīd) A peptide containing normal peptide bonds (between α-carboxyl groups and α-amino groups). Cf. peptide. [G. *eu-*, normal, usual + peptide]

eu·pho·ret·ic (yū′fōr-et′ik) SYN euphoriant.

eu·pho·ri·a (yū-fōr′ē-ă) A feeling of well-being, commonly exaggerated and not necessarily well founded. [eu- + G. *pherō,* to bear]

eu·pho·ri·ant (yū-fōr′ē-ănt) **1.** Having the capability to produce a sense of well-being. **2.** An agent with such a capability. SYN euphoretic.

eu·plas·tic lymph (yū-plas′tik limf) Lymph that contains relatively few leukocytes but a comparatively high concentration of fibrinogen; such lymph clots fairly well and tends to become organized with fibrous tissue.

eu·ploid (yū′ployd) Relating to euploidy.

eu·ploid·y (yū-ploy′dē) The state of a cell containing whole haploid sets. [eu- + G. *-ploos,* -fold]

eup·ne·a (yūp-nē′ă) Easy, free respiration; the type observed in a normal individual under resting conditions. [G. *eupnoia,* fr. *eu,* well, + *pnoia,* breath]

eu·prax·i·a (yū-prak′sē-ă) Normal ability to perform coordinated movements. [eu- + G. *praxis,* a doing]

eu·rhyth·mi·a (yū-ridh′mē-ă) Harmonious body relationships of the separate organs. [eu- + G. *rhythmos,* rhythm]

Eu·ro·pe·an bat lys·sa·vi·rus (yūr′ŏ-pē-ăn bat lis′ă-vī′rŭs) Two species (1 and 2) causing rabieslike diseases in humans in Europe; transmitted by bite of insectivorous bats.

Eu•ro•pe•an blue•ber•ry (yŭr′ŏ-pē′ăn blū′ber-ē) SYN bilberry.

eu•ro•pi•um (Eu) (yū-rō′pē-ŭm) An element of the rare earth (lanthanide) group, atomic no. 63, atomic wt. 151.965. [L. *Europa,* Europe]

eury- Prefix meaning broad, wide; opposite of steno-. [G. *eurys,* wide]

eu•ry•bleph•a•ron (yūr′ē-blef′ă-ron) A congenital anomaly characterized by sagging of the lateral aspect of the lower eyelid away from the eye. [eury- + G. *blepharon,* eyelid]

eu•ry•ce•phal•ic, eu•ry•ceph•a•lous (yūr′ē-sĕ-fal′ik, -sef′ă-lŭs) Having an abnormally broad head; sometimes used in reference to a brachycephalic head. [eury- + G. *kephalē,* head]

eu•ryg•nath•ic (yūr′ig-nath′ik) Having a wide jaw. [G. *eurys* wide + *gnathos* jaw]

eu•ry•on (yūr′ē-on) The extremity, on either side, of the greatest transverse diameter of the head; a point used in craniometry. [G. *eurys,* broad]

eu•sta•chi•an (yū-stā′shăn) Described by or attributed to Bartolomeo Eustachio (1524–1574); usually referring to the pharyngotympanic (auditory) tube.

eu•sta•chi•an tube (yū-stā′shăn tūb) SYN pharyngotympanic (auditory) tube.

eu•stron•gyl•oi•des (yū-stron-jil-oy′dēz) A nematode found in fish, amphibians, and reptiles; human infections, manifested by gastrointestinal symptoms, are rare and related to consumption of raw fish; larvae are pinkish-red.

eu•sys•to•le (yū-sis′tŏ lē) A condition in which the cardiac systole is normal in force and time. [eu- + systole]

eu•sys•tol•ic (yū′sis-tol′ik) Relating to eusystole.

eu•tec•tic al•loy (yū-tek′tik al′oy) An alloy, generally brittle and subject to tarnish and corrosion, with a fusion temperature lower than that of any of its components; used in dentistry mainly in solders.

eu•tha•na•si•a (yū′thă-nā′zhē-ă) **1.** The intentional putting to death of a person with an incurable or painful disease, intended as an act of mercy. **2.** A quiet, painless death. SYN man-made death (1). [eu- + G. *thanatos,* death]

eu•then•ics (yū-then′iks) The science concerned with establishing optimal living conditions for plants, animals, or humans, especially through proper provisioning and environment. [G. *eutheneō,* to thrive]

eu•ther•mic (yū-thĕr′mik) At an optimal temperature. [eu- + G. *thermos,* warm]

eu•ton•ic (yū-ton′ik) SYN normotonic (1). [eu- + G. *tonos,* tone]

eu•tro•phi•a (yū-trō′fē-ă) A state of normal nourishment and growth. [G. fr. *eu,* well, + *trophē,* nourishment]

eu•tro•phic (yū-trō′fik) Relating to, characterized by, or promoting eutrophia.

EV, ev Abbreviation for electron-volt.

e•vac•u•ant (ē-vak′yū-ănt) **1.** Promoting an excretion, especially of the bowels. **2.** An agent that increases excretion, especially a cathartic.

e•vac•u•a•ted tube (ē-vak′yū-āt-ĕd tūb) A plastic or glass sealed vacuum tube used to collect a blood specimen obtained through venipuncture.

e•vac•u•a•tion (ē-vak′yū-ā′shŭn) **1.** Removal of material, especially wastes, from the bowels by defecation. **2.** SYN stool (2). **3.** Removal of air from a closed vessel; production of a vacuum. **4.** Orderly removal of people from danger.

e•vac•u•a•tor (ē-vak′yū-ā-tŏr) A mechanical evacuant; an instrument for the removal of fluid or small particles from a body cavity, or of impacted feces from the rectum.

e•vag•i•na•tion (ē-vaj′i-nā′shŭn) Protrusion of some part or organ from its normal position. [L. *e,* out, + *vagina,* sheath]

e•val•u•at•ing (ĕ-val′yū-ā′ting) A part of the nursing process in which the extent to which the established goals of care have been met is determined and recorded.

e•val•u•a•tion (ĕ-val′yū-ā′shŭn) **1.** NURSING determining whether expected outcomes were met; measuring effectiveness of nursing care, medical care, and forms of health care by other providers. **2.** Synthesis of examination findings into a defined cluster of diagnostic classifications. SYN assessment (1).

e•val•u•a•tion and man•age•ment (E/M) (ĕ-val′yū-ā′shŭn man′ăj-mĕnt) General term denoting procedures done to determine the course of the patient's therapy.

E•val•u•a•tion and Man•age•ment codes (E&M codes) (ĕ-val′yū-ā′shŭn man′ăj-mĕnt kōdz) CPT codes that describe patient encounters with health care professionals; used to evaluate and manage health.

ev•a•nes•cent (ev-ă-nes′ĕnt) Of short duration. [L. *e,* out, + *vanesco,* to vanish]

Ev•ans blue (ev′ănz blū) [CI 23860] A diazo dye used for the determination of the blood volume on the basis of the dilution of a standard solution of the dye in the plasma after its intravenous injection; binds to proteins; used as a vital stain for following diffusion through blood vessel walls.

Ev•ans syn•drome (ev′ănz sin′drōm) Acquired hemolytic anemia and thrombocytopenia.

e•vap•o•rate (ē-vap′ŏr-āt) To cause or undergo evaporation.

e•vap•o•ra•tion (ē-vap′ŏr-ā′shŭn) **1.** A change from liquid to vapor form. **2.** Loss of volume of a liquid by conversion into vapor. SYN volatilization. [L. *e,* out, + *vaporo,* to emit vapor]

e•ven ech•o re•pha•sing (ē′vĕn ek′ō rē-fāz′ing) Use of evenly spaced echoes to reduce artifact in magnetic resonance imaging.

event (ē-vent′) Specific occurrence, such as an episode of illness; often used in terminology of clinical trials. [L. *eventus,* outcome, fr. *e-,* out, + *venio,* to come]

e•ven•tra•tion (ē′ven-trā′shŭn) **1.** Protrusion of omentum and/or intestine through an opening in the abdominal wall. SYN evisceration (2). **2.** Removal of the contents of the abdominal cavity. [L. *e,* out, + *venter,* belly]

e•ven•tra•tion of the di•a•phragm (ē′ven-trā′shŭn dī′ă-fram) Extreme elevation of a half or part of the diaphragm, which is usually atrophic and abnormally thin.

e•ver•sion (ē-vĕr′zhŭn) A turning outward, as of the eyelid or foot. [L. *e-everto,* pp. *-versus,* to overturn]

e•vert (ē-vĕrt′) To turn outward. [L. *e-verto,* to overturn]

ev•i•dence-based med•i•cine (ev′i-dĕns-bāst med′i-sin) The process of applying relevant information derived from peer-reviewed medical literature to address a specific clinical problem; the application of simple rules of science and common sense to determine the validity of the information; and the application of the information to the clinical problem. SEE ALSO Cochrane collaboration, clinical practice guidelines.

ev•i•dence-based prac•tice (ev′i-dĕns-bāst prak′tis) The formulation of treatment decisions by using the best available research evidence and integrating this evidence with the practitioner's skill and experience.

e•vis•cer•a•tion (ē-vis′ĕr-ā′shŭn) **1.** Removal of the contents of the eyeball, leaving the sclera and sometimes the cornea. **2.** SYN eventration (1). [L. *eviscero,* to disembowel]

e•vo•ca•tion (ev′ō-kā′shŭn) Induction of a particular tissue produced by the action of an evocator during embryogenesis. [L. *evoco,* pp. *evocatus,* to call forth, evoke]

e•vo•ca•tor (ev′ō-kā-tŏr) A factor in the control of morphogenesis in the early embryo.

e•voked e•lec•tro•my•og•ra•phy (ē-vōkt′ ĕ-lek′trō-mī-og′ră-fē) SYN electrodiagnosis.

e•voked o•to•a•cous•tic e•mis•sion (ē-vōkt′ ō′tō-ă-kūs′tik ē-mish′ŭn) A form resulting from acoustic stimulation, as opposed to spontaneous otoacoustic emission.

e•voked re•sponse (ē-vōkt′ rĕ-spons′) An alteration in the electrical activity of a region of the nervous system through which an incoming sensory stimulus is passing.

ev•o•lu•tion (ev′ŏ-lū′shŭn) **1.** A continuing process of change from one state, condition, or form to another. **2.** A progressive distancing between the genotype and the phenotype in a line of descent. [L. *e-volvo,* pp. *-volutus,* to roll out]

ev•o•lu•tion•ar•y fit•ness (ev′ŏ-lū′shŭn-ar-ē fit′nĕs) The probability that the line of descent from an individual with a specific trait will not eventually die out.

e•vul•sion (ē-vŭl′shŭn) A forcible pulling out or extraction. Cf. avulsion. [L. *evulsio,* fr. *e-vello,* pp. *-vulsus,* to pluck out]

Ew•art pro•ce•dure (yu′ărt prŏ-sē′jŭr) Elevation of the larynx between the thumb and forefinger to elicit tracheal tugging.

Ew•art sign (yu′ărt sīn) In large pericardial effusions, an area of dullness with bronchial breathing and bronchophony below the angle of the left scapula. SYN Pins sign.

Ew•ing sar•co•ma (ū′ing sahr-kō′mă) SYN Ewing tumor.

Ew•ing sign (ū′ing sīn) Tenderness at the upper inner angle of the orbit at the point of attachment of the pulley of the superior oblique muscle, denoting closure of the outlet of the frontal sinus.

Ew•ing tu•mor (ū′ing tū′mŏr) A malignant neoplasm that occurs usually before the age of 20 years, about twice as frequently in males, and in about 75% of patients involves bones of the extremities, including the shoulder girdle, with a predilection for the metaphysis; histologically, there are conspicuous foci of necrosis in association with irregular masses of small, regular, rounded, or ovoid cells (2–3 times the diameter of erythrocytes), with very scanty cytoplasm. SYN endothelial myeloma, Ewing sarcoma.

♻ **ex-** Prefix meaning out of, from, away from. [L. and G. out of]

♻ **exa- (E)** Prefix used in the SI and metric system to signify one quintillion (10^{18}).

ex•ac•er•ba•tion (eg-zas′ĕr-bā′shŭn) An increase in the severity of a disease or any of its signs or symptoms. [L. *exacerbo,* pp. *-atus,* to exasperate, increase, fr. *acerbus,* sour]

exaemia [Br.] SYN exemia.

exaeresis [Br.] SYN exeresis.

ex•am•i•na•tion (eg-zam′i-nā′shŭn) Any investigation or inspection made for the purpose of diagnosis; usually qualified by the method used.

ex•an•them (eg-zan′thĕm) SYN exanthema.

ex•an•the•ma (ek′san-thē′mă) A skin eruption occurring as a symptom of an acute viral or coccal disease, as in scarlet fever or measles. Cf. enanthem, enanthema. SYN exanthem. [G. efflorescence, an eruption, fr. *anthos,* flower]

ex·an·the·ma sub·i·tum (ek′san-thē′mă sū′bē-tŭm) A disease due to human herpesvirus-6 of infants and young children, marked by sudden onset with fever lasting several days (sometimes with convulsions) and followed by a fine macular (sometimes maculopapular) rash that appears within a few hours to a day after the fever has subsided. SYN Dukes disease, roseola infantilis, roseola infantum, sixth disease.

ex·an·them·a·tous (ek′san-them′ă-tŭs) Relating to an exanthema.

ex·ar·tic·u·la·tion (eks′ahr-tik-yū-lā′shŭn) SYN disarticulation. [L. *ex,* out, + *articulus,* joint]

ex·cal·a·tion (eks′kă-lā′shŭn) Absence, suppression, or failure of development of one of a series of structures, as of a digit or vertebra. [G. *ex,* from, + *chalaō,* to abate, release]

ex·ca·va·ti·o (eks-kă-vā′shē-ō) [TA] SYN excavation (1). [L. fr. *ex-cavo,* pp. *-cavatus,* to hollow out, fr. *ex,* out, + *cavus,* hollow]

ex·ca·va·tion (eks′kă-vā′shŭn) **1.** A natural cavity, pouch, or recess. SYN excavatio [TA]. **2.** A cavity formed artificially or as the result of a pathologic process.

ex·ca·va·ti·o rec·to·u·te·ri·na (eks-kă-vā′shē-ō rek′tō-yū-tĕ-rī′nă) [TA] SYN rectouterine pouch.

ex·ca·va·ti·o rec·to·ve·si·ca·lis (eks-kă-vā′shē-ō rek′tō-ves-i-kā′lis) [TA] SYN rectovesical pouch.

ex·ca·va·tor (eks′kă-vā-tŏr) **1.** An instrument like a large sharp spoon or scoop, used to scrape out pathologic tissue. **2.** DENTISTRY an instrument, generally a small spoon or curette, used to clean out and shape a carious cavity before filling it.

ex·ce·men·to·sis (ek′sē-men-tō′sis) A nodular outgrowth of cementum on the root surface of a tooth.

ex·cen·tric (ek-sen′trik) Alternative spelling for eccentric (2, 3).

ex·cep·tion (ek-sep′shŭn) That which is omitted, excluded, or set apart. [L. *excipio,* to exclude]

ex·cess post·ex·er·cise ox·y·gen con·sump·tion (EPOC) (eks′es pōst-eks′ĕr-sīz ok′si-jĕn kŏn-sŭmp′shŭn) Elevated aerobic metabolism following exercise that restores the body to its preexercise condition; duration varies with intensity and duration of exercise performed. SYN recovery oxygen consumption.

ex·change (eks-chānj′) To substitute one thing for another, or the act of such substitution.

ex·change list (ĕks-chānj′ list) A system in which commonly consumed foods are sorted into categories roughly according to their proportions of carbohydrate, protein, and fat. Originally developed for people with diabetes, it is now commonly used for general diet planning.

ex·change trans·fu·sion (eks-chānj′ trans-fyū′zhŭn) Removal of most of a patient's blood followed by introduction of an equal amount from donors. SYN substitution transfusion, total transfusion.

ex·ci·mer la·ser (ek′si-mĕr lā′zĕr) Laser used particularly for refractive procedures, consisting of photons in the ultraviolet spectrum emitted by unstable dimers of argon and fluoride. [*exc*ited d*imer*]

ex·cip·i·ent (ek-sip′ē-ĕnt) A more or less inert substance added in a prescription as a diluent or vehicle or to give form or consistency when the remedy is given in pill form. [L. *excipiens;* pres. p. of *ex- cipio,* to take out]

ex·cise (ek′sīz) To cut out. SEE ALSO resect.

ex·ci·sion (ek-sizh′ŭn) **1.** The act of cutting out; the surgical removal of part or all of a structure or organ. SYN resection (3). SEE ALSO resection. **2.** MOLECULAR BIOLOGY a recombination event in which a genetic element is removed. SYN exeresis. [L. *excido,* to cut out]

ex·ci·sion bi·op·sy (ek-sizh′ŭn bī′op-sē) Excision of tissue for gross and microscopic examination in such a manner that the entire lesion is removed.

ex·cit·a·bil·i·ty (ek-sī′tă-bil′i-tē) Having the capability of being excited. The cellular property that enables it to react to irritation or stimulation.

ex·cit·a·ble (ek-sī′tă-bĕl) **1.** Capable of quick response to a stimulus; having potentiality for emotional arousal. Cf. irritable. **2.** NEUROPHYSIOLOGY referring to a tissue, cell, or membrane capable of undergoing excitation in response to an adequate stimulus.

ex·cit·a·ble ar·e·a (ek-sī′tă-bĕl ar′ē-ă) SYN motor cortex.

ex·ci·ta·tion (ek′sī-tā′shŭn) **1.** The act of increasing the rapidity or intensity of physical or mental processes. **2.** NEUROPHYSIOLOGY the complete all-or-none response of a nerve or muscle to an adequate stimulus, ordinarily including propagation of excitation along the membranes of the cell or cells involved. SEE ALSO stimulation. **3.** The process whereby radiation causes a bound electron to vibrate or oscillate within its orbit.

ex·ci·ta·tion wave (ek′sī-tā′shŭn wāv) A wave of altered electrical conditions that is propagated along a muscle fiber preparatory to its contraction.

ex·cit·a·to·ry post·syn·ap·tic po·ten·tial

(ek-sī′tă-tōr-ē pōst′si-nap′tik pŏ-ten′shăl) The change in potential that is produced in the membrane of the next neuron when an impulse that has an excitatory influence arrives at the synapse; it is a local change in the direction of depolarization; summation of these potentials can lead to discharge of an impulse by the neuron.

ex•cit•ed state (ek-sī′tĕd stāt) The condition of an atom or molecule after absorbing energy, which may be the result of exposure to light, electricity, elevated temperature, or a chemical reaction; such activation may be a necessary prelude to a chemical reaction or to the emission of light.

ex•cite•ment (ek-sīt′mĕnt) An emotional state sometimes characterized by its potential for impulsive or poorly controlled activity.

ex•cit•ing eye (ek-sī′ting ī) The injured eye in sympathetic ophthalmia.

ex•ci•to•mo•tor (ek-sī′tō-mō′tŏr) Causing or increasing the rapidity of motion. SYN centrokinetic (2).

ex•ci•to•re•flex nerve (ek-sī′tō-rē′fleks nĕrv) A visceral nerve the special function of which is to cause reflex action.

ex•ci•tor nerve (ek-sī′tŏr nĕrv) A nerve conducting impulses that stimulate to increase function.

ex•clave (eks-klāv′) An outlying, detached portion of a gland or other part, such as the thyroid or pancreas; an accessory gland. [L. *ex,* out, + *-clave* (in enclave)]

ex•clu•sion (eks-klū′zhŭn) A shutting out; disconnection from the main portion. [L. *ex- cludo,* pp. *-clusus,* to shut out]

ex•clu•sive pro•vi•der or•gan•i•za•tion (EPO) (eks-klū′siv prō-vī′dĕr ōr′găn-ī-zā′shŭn) A managed care plan in the U.S. in which enrollees must receive their care from affiliated providers; treatment provided outside the approved network must be paid for by the patients. SEE ALSO managed care.

ex•co•ri•ate (eks-kōr′ē-āt) To scratch or otherwise denude the skin by physical means.

ex•co•ri•a•tion (eks-kōr′ē-ā′shŭn) A scratch mark; a linear break in the skin surface, usually covered with blood or serous crusts. See page B11. [L. *excorio,* to skin, strip, fr. *corium,* skin, hide]

ex•cre•ment (eks′krĕ-mĕnt) Waste matter or any excretion cast out of the body; e.g., feces. [L. *ex- cerno,* pp. *-cretus,* to separate]

ex•cre•men•ti•tious (eks′krĕ-men-tish′ŭs) Relating to any excrement.

ex•cres•cence (eks-kres′ĕns) Any outgrowth from a surface. [L. *ex- cresco,* pp. *-cretus,* to grow forth]

ex•cre•ta (eks-krē′tă) SYN excretion (2). [L. neut. pl. of *excretus,* pp. of *ex-cerno,* to separate]

ex•crete (eks-krēt′) To separate from the blood and cast out; to perform excretion.

ex•cre•tion (eks-krē′shŭn) **1.** The process whereby the undigested residue of food and the waste products of metabolism are eliminated, material is removed to regulate the composition of body fluids and tissues, or substances are expelled to perform functions on an exterior surface. **2.** The product of a tissue or organ that is material to be passed out of the body. SYN excreta. SEE excrement. Cf. secretion.

ex•cre•to•ry (eks′krĕ-tōr-ē) Relating to excretion.

ex•cre•to•ry duct (eks′krĕ-tōr-ē dŭkt) A duct carrying the secretion from a gland or a fluid from any reservoir.

ex•cre•to•ry gland (eks′krĕ-tōr-ē gland) A gland separating excrementitious or waste material from the blood.

ex•cy•clo•pho•ri•a (ek-sī′klō-fōr′ē-ă) A cyclophoria in which the upper poles of each cornea tend to rotate laterally. [ex- + cyclo- + G. *phora,* a carrying]

ex•cys•ta•tion (ek′sis-tā′shŭn) The action of an encysted organism in escaping from its envelope.

ex•e•mi•a (eg-sē′mē-ă) A condition, as in shock, in which a considerable portion of the blood is removed from the main circulation but remains within blood vessels in certain areas where it is stagnant. SYN exaemia. [G. *ex,* out of, + *haima,* blood]

ex•en•ce•phal•ic (eks′en-sĕ-fal′ik) Relating to exencephaly.

ex•en•ceph•a•ly (eks′en-sef′ă-lē) Condition in which the neurocranium is defective with the brain exposed or extruding. [G. *ex,* out, + *enkephalos,* brain]

ex•en•ter•a•tion (ek-sen′tĕr-ā′shŭn) Removal of internal organs and tissues, usually radical removal of the contents of a body cavity. [G. *ex,* out, + *enteron,* bowel]

ex•en•ter•i•tis (ek-sen′tĕr-ī′tis) Inflammation of the peritoneal covering of the intestine. [G. *exō,* on the outside, + enteritis]

ex•er•cise (ek′sĕr-sīz) **1.** *Active:* Planned repetitive physical activity structured to improve and maintain physical fitness. **2.** *Passive:* motion of limbs without effort by the patient.

ex•er•cise ca•pac•i•ty (eks′ĕr-sīz kă-pas′i-tē) SEE maximal oxygen consumption.

ex•er•cise com•pli•ance (eks′ĕr-sīz kŏm-plī′

ăns) A person's conformity to a prescribed or self-prescribed fitness program.

ex•er•cise e•con•omy (eks′ĕr-sīz ĕ-kon′ŏ-mē) Energy required (usually measured as oxygen consumption) to maintain a constant velocity of movement. SYN movement economy.

ex•er•cise high (eks′ĕr-sīz hī) A state of euphoria and exhilaration as duration of moderate-to-intense exercise increases, triggered by release of endorphins.

ex•er•cise im•mu•nol•o•gy (eks′ĕr-sīz im′yū-nŏl′ŏ-jē) Field of study on the interactions of physical, environmental, and psychological factors on immune function.

ex•er•cise-in•duced an•a•phy•lax•is (eks′ĕr-sīz-in-dūst′ an′ă-fi-laks′is) Profound allergic reaction due to exercise.

ex•er•cise-in•duced a•ne•mi•a (eks′ĕr-sīz-in-dūst′ ă-nē′mē-ă) Reduction in hemoglobin concentration to levels approaching clinical anemia, believed due to intense exercise training; generally occurs in the early phase of training and parallels the disproportionately large expansion in plasma volume in relation to total hemoglobin with training. SEE ALSO anemia. SYN sports anemia.

ex•er•cise-in•duced asth•ma (EIA), ex•er•cise-in•duced bron•cho•spasm (eks′ĕr-sīz-in-dūst′ az′mă, brong′kō-spazm) Bronchial spasm, edema, and mucus secretion brought about by exercise, particularly in cool, dry environment. Recovery usually occurs spontaneously within 90 minutes. A 10–15% reduction in preexercise values for FEV_1/FVC confirms diagnosis. SEE ALSO asthma.

ex•er•cise-in•duced ur•ti•car•i•a (eks′ĕr-sīz-in-dūst′ ŭr′ti-kar′ē-ă) A variant of cholinergic urticaria with larger lesions, induced by physical activity.

ex•er•cise phys•i•ol•o•gy (eks′ĕr-sīz fiz′ē-ol′ŏ-jē) Body of knowledge concerning physiologic, metabolic, and structural responses to short-term and long-term physical activity.

ex•er•cise pre•scrip•tion (eks′ĕr-sīz prĕ-skrip′shŭn) Formulation of individualized exercise program based on exercise frequency, intensity, and duration with consideration for the specificity of the training response, specific to the prescribed exercise method. SEE ALSO prescription, specificity of training principle.

ex•er•cise pres•sor re•flex (eks′ĕr-sīz pres′ŏr rē′fleks) Reflex afferent neural input to cardiovascular center in medulla from proprioceptors (mechanoreceptors and metaboreceptors) in active muscles during exercise.

ex•er•cise ra•di•o•nu•clide an•gi•o•car•di•og•ra•phy (eks′ĕr-sīz rā′dē-ō-nū′klīd an′jē-ō-kahr-dē-og′ră-fē) Radionuclide angiocardiography while performing exercise, such as on a treadmill or bicycle.

ex•er•cise stress test (eks′ĕr-sīz stres test) SYN stress test.

ex•er•cise tol•er•ance (eks′ĕr-sīz tol′ĕr-ăns) The point at which a participant in a physical activity attains the limit of acceptable effort before succumbing to weariness.

ex•er•e•sis (ek-ser′ĕ-sis) SYN excision. SYN exaeresis. [G. *exairesis,* a taking out, fr. *haireō,* to take, grasp]

ex•er•gon•ic (ek′sĕr-gon′ik) Referring to a chemical reaction that takes place with release of Gibbs free energy to its surroundings. Cf. endergonic. [exo- + G. *ergon,* work]

ex•er•tion•al head•ache (eg-zĕr′shŭn-ăl hed′āk) The form of headache brought on by exercise.

ex•er•tion•al hy•po•ten•sion (eg-zĕr′shŭn-ăl hī′pō-ten′shŭn) Lowered systolic blood pressure in response to exercise. May occur in patients with coronary artery disease, cardiomyopathy, or serious arrhythmias.

ex•fo•li•a•tion (eks′fō-lē-ā′shŭn) **1.** Detachment and shedding of superficial cells from any tissue surface. **2.** Scaling or desquamation of the horny layer of epidermis. **3.** Loss of deciduous teeth following physiologic loss of root structure. [Mod. L. fr. L. *ex,* out, + *folium,* leaf]

ex•fo•li•a•tive (eks-fō′lē-ă-tiv) Marked by exfoliation, desquamation, or profuse scaling. [Mod. L. *exfoliativus*]

ex•fo•li•a•tive cy•tol•o•gy (eks-fō′lē-ă-tiv sī-tol′ŏ-jē) The examination, for diagnostic purposes, of cells denuded from a neoplasm or an epithelial surface, recovered from exudate, secretions, or washings from tissue (e.g., sputum, vaginal secretion, gastric washings, urine). SYN cytopathology (2).

ex•fo•li•a•tive der•ma•ti•tis (eks-fō′lē-ă-tiv dĕr′mă-tī′tis) Generalized exfoliation with scaling of the skin and usually with erythema (erythroderma); may be a drug reaction or associated with various benign dermatoses, lupus erythematosus, lymphomas, or of undetermined cause. See page 548. SYN pityriasis rubra, Wilson disease (2).

ex•fo•li•a•tive gas•tri•tis (eks-fō′lē-ă-tiv gas-trī′tis) Gastritis with excessive shedding of mucosal epithelial cells.

ex•fol•i•a•tive psor•i•a•sis (eks-fō′lē-ă-tiv sōr-ī′ă-sis) Exfoliative dermatitis developing from chronic psoriasis, sometimes resulting from overtreatment of psoriasis.

ex•ha•la•tion (eks′hă-lā′shŭn) **1.** Breathing out. SYN expiration (1). **2.** The giving forth of gas or vapor. **3.** Any exhaled or emitted gas or vapor. [L. *ex-halo,* pp. *-halatus,* to breathe out]

ex•hale (eks-hāl′) **1.** To breathe out. SYN expire (1). **2.** To emit a gas, vapor, or odor.

ex•haus•tion (eg-zaws′chŭn) **1.** Extreme fatigue; inability to respond to stimuli. **2.** Removal of contents; depletion of a supply of anything. **3.** Extraction of the active constituents of a drug by treating with water, alcohol, or other solvent. [L. *ex-haurio,* pp. *-haustus,* to draw out, empty]

ex•hi•bi•tion•ism (ek′si-bish′ŭn-izm) A morbid compulsion to expose a part of the body, especially the genitals, with the intent of provoking sexual interest in the viewer.

ex•hi•bi•tion•ist (ek′si-bish′ŭn-ist) One who engages in exhibitionism.

♻ **exo-** Prefix meaning exterior, external, or outward. SEE ALSO ecto-. [G. *exō,* outside]

ex•o•an•ti•gen (ek′sō-an′ti-jen) SYN ectoantigen.

ex•o•car•di•a (ek′sō-kahr′dē-ă) SYN ectocardia.

ex•o•ce•lom•ic mem•brane (eks′ō-sē-lom′ik mem′brān) A layer of cells delaminated from the inner surface of the blastocystic cytotrophoblast and from the envelope of the primary yolk sac during the second week of embryonic life.

ex•o•crine (ek′sō-krin) **1.** Denoting glandular secretion delivered to an apical or luminal surface. SYN eccrine (1). **2.** Denoting a gland that secretes outwardly through excretory ducts. [exo- + G. *krinō,* to separate]

ex•o•crine gland (ek′sō-krin gland) A gland from which secretions reach a free surface of the body by ducts.

ex•o•cy•to•sis (ek′sō-sī-to′sis) **1.** The appearance of migrating inflammatory cells in the epidermis. **2.** The process whereby secretory granules or droplets are released from a cell; the membrane around the granule fuses with the cell membrane, which ruptures, and the secretion is discharged. SYN emeiocytosis, emiocytosis. Cf. endocytosis. [exo- + G. *kytos,* cell, + *-osis,* condition]

ex•o•de•vi•a•tion (ek′sō-dē-vē-ā′shŭn) **1.** SYN exophoria. **2.** SYN exotropia.

ex•o•don•ti•a (ek′sō-don′shē-ă) The branch of dental practice concerned with the extraction of teeth. [exo- + G. *odous,* tooth]

ex•o•don•tist (ek′sō-don′tist) One who specializes in the extraction of teeth.

ex•o•en•zyme (ek′sō-en-zīm) SYN extracellular enzyme.

ex•o•e•ryth•ro•cyt•ic stage (eks′ō-ĕ-rith′rō-sit′ik stāj) Developmental stage of the malaria parasite (*Plasmodium*) in liver parenchyma cells of the vertebrate host before erythrocytes are invaded. The initial generation produces cryptozoites, the next generation metacryptozoites; reinfection of liver cells from blood cells apparently does not occur.

ex•og•a•my (eks-og′ă-mē) Sexual reproduction

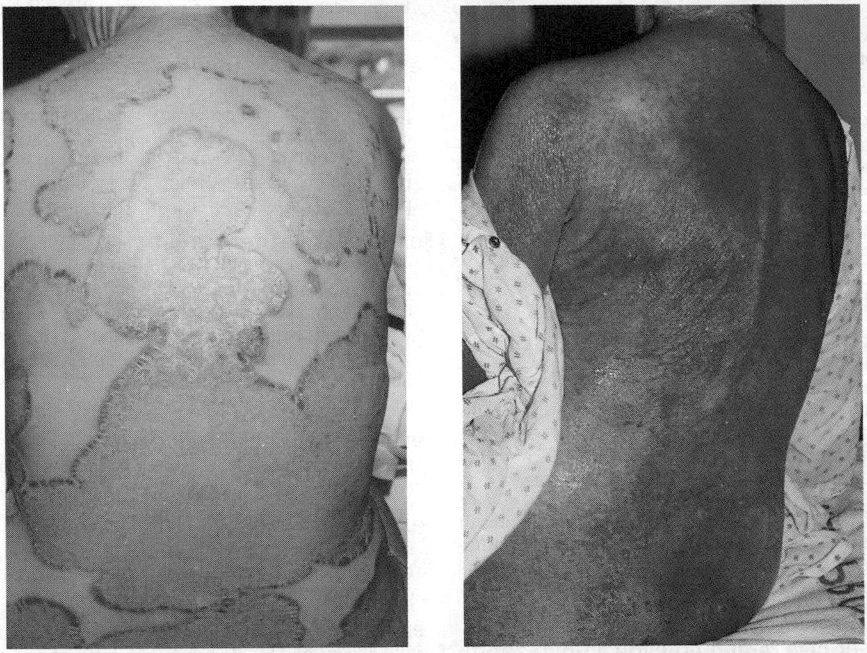

exfoliative dermatitis

by means of conjugation of two gametes of different ancestry, as in certain protozoan species. [exo- + G. *gamos,* marriage]

ex•o•gas•tru•la (eks′ō-gas′trū-lă) An abnormal embryo in which the primordial gut is everted.

ex•og•e•nous (eks-oj′ĕ-nŭs) Originating or produced outside of the organism. SYN ectogenous. [exo- + G. *-gen,* production]

ex•og•e•nous buf•fer (eks-oj′ĕ-nŭs bŭf′ĕr) Sodium bicarbonate or sodium citrate taken orally before competition by sprint-type athletes to raise extracellular pH; enhances performance in short-term, maximal exercise that generates high levels of muscle and blood lactate.

ex•og•e•nous de•pres•sion (eks-oj′ĕ-nŭs dĕ-presh′ŭn) Disorder with signs and symptoms similar to those of endogenous depression but the precipitating factors are social or environmental and outside the person.

ex•og•e•nous fi•bers (eks-oj′ĕ-nŭs fī′bĕrz) Nerve fibers by which a given region of the central nervous system is connected with other regions; the term applies to both afferent and efferent fiber connections.

ex•og•e•nous hy•per•glyc•er•i•de•mi•a (eks-oj′ĕ-nŭs hī′pĕr-glis′ĕr-i-dē′mē-ă) Persistent form of the disorder due to retarded rate of removal from plasma of chylomicrons of dietary origin.

ex•og•e•nous in•fec•tion (eks-oj′ĕ-nŭs in-fek′shŭn) A form of infection caused by a pathogen or agent not normally present in the body.

ex•og•e•nous o•be•si•ty (eks-oj′ĕ-nŭs ō-bē′si-tē) State of overweight caused by overeating rather than another cause.

ex•og•e•nous py•ro•gens (eks-oj′ĕ-nŭs pī′rō-jenz) Drugs or substances that are formed by microorganisms and induce fever. Among the latter are lipopolysaccharides and lipoteichoic acid.

ex•om•pha•los (eks-om′fă-lŏs) **1.** Protrusion of the umbilicus. SYN exumbilication (1). **2.** SYN umbilical hernia. **3.** SYN omphalocele. [G. *ex,* out, + *omphalos,* umbilicus]

ex•on (ek′son) A portion of a DNA that codes for a section of the mature messenger RNA from that DNA, and is therefore expressed ("translated" into protein) at the ribosome. [ex- + on]

ex•o•nu•cle•ase (eks′ō-nū′klē-ās) A nuclease that releases one nucleotide at a time, serially, beginning at one end of a polynucleotide (nucleic acid). Cf. endonuclease.

ex•o•pep•ti•dase (eks′ō-pep′ti-dās) An enzyme that catalyzes the hydrolysis of the terminal amino acid of a peptide chain (e.g., carboxypeptidase). Cf. endopeptidase.

Ex•o•phi•a•la (ek-sō-fī′ă-lă) A genus of pathogenic fungi having dematiaceous conidiophores. They cause mycetoma or phaeohyphomycosis; in cases of mycetoma, black granules develop in subcutaneous abscesses; in cases of phaeohyphomycosis, sclerotic bodies are found in tissues. [*exo* + G. *phialē,* a broad flat vessel]

Ex•o•phi•a•la (eks′ō-fī-ā′la) A fungal species that causes tinea nigra.

Ex•o•phi•a•la jean•sel•me•i (ek-sō-fī′ă-lă zhahn-sel′mē-ī′) A species found in cases of mycetoma or phaeohyphomycosis.

ex•o•pho•ri•a (eks′ō-fōr′ē-ă) Tendency of the eyes to deviate outward when fusion is suspended. SYN exodeviation (1). [exo- + G. *phora,* a carrying]

ex•o•phor•ic (eks′ō-fōr′ik) Relating to exophoria.

ex•oph•thal•mi•a (eks′of-thal′mē-ă) SEE exophthalmos.

ex•oph•thal•mic (eks′of-thal′mik) Relating to exophthalmos; a condition marked by prominence of the eyeball.

ex•oph•thal•mic goi•ter (eks′of-thal′mik goy′tĕr) Any of the various forms of hyperthyroidism in which the thyroid gland is enlarged and exophthalmos is present.

ex•oph•thal•mic oph•thal•mo•ple•gi•a (eks′of-thal′mik of′thal-mō-plē′jē-ă) Condition causing protrusion of the eyeballs due to increased water content of orbital tissues incidental to thyroid disorders, usually hyperthyroidism.

ex•oph•thal•mom•e•ter (eks′of-thal-mom′ĕ-tĕr) An instrument to measure the distance between the anterior pole of the eye and a fixed reference point, often the zygomatic bone. [exophthalmos + G. *metron,* measure]

ex•oph•thal•mos, **ex•oph•thal•mus** (eks′of-thal′mos, eks′of-thal′mŭs) Protrusion of one or both eyeballs; can be congenital and familial, or due to pathology, such as a retroorbital tumor (usually unilateral) or thyroid disease (usually bilateral). SYN proptosis. [G. *ex,* out, + *ophthalmos,* eye]

ex•o•phyte (eks′ō-fīt) An exterior or external plant parasite. [exo- + G. *phyton,* plant]

ex•o•phyt•ic (eks′ō-fit′ik) **1.** Pertaining to an exophyte. **2.** Denoting a neoplasm or lesion that grows outward from an epithelial surface.

ex•o•se•ro•sis (eks′ō-sĕ-rō′sis) Serous exudation from the skin surface, as in eczema or abrasions.

ex•o•skel•e•ton (eks′ō-skel′ĕ-tŏn) **1.** All hard parts (e.g., hair, teeth, nails, feathers, dermal plates, and scales), developed from the ectoderm or somatic mesoderm in vertebrates. **2.** Outer chitinous envelope of insects, some crustaceous, and other invertebrates.

ex•os•to•sis, **ex•os•to•ses**, pl. **ex•os•to•ses** (eks′os-tō′sis, -sēz, -sēz) A cartilage-capped bony projection arising from any bone that develops from cartilage. SEE ALSO osteochondroma. See this page, B28. SYN hyperostosis (2), poroma (2). [exo- + G. *osteon,* bone, + *-osis,* condition]

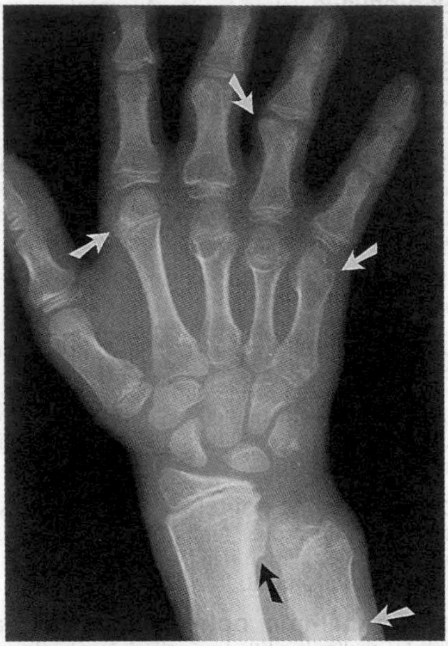

exostosis: several small osteochondromas (arrows)

ex•o•ter•ic (eks′ō-ter′ik) Of external origin; arising outside the organism. [G. *exōterikos,* outer]

ex•o•ther•mic (eks′ō-thĕr′mik) **1.** Denoting a chemical reaction during which heat (i.e., enthalpy) is emitted. Cf. endothermic. **2.** Relating to the external warmth of the body. [exo- + G. *thermē,* heat]

ex•o•tox•ic (eks′ō-tok′sik) **1.** Relating to an exotoxin. **2.** Relating to the introduction of an exogenous poison or toxin.

ex•o•tox•in (eks′ō-tok′sin) A specific, soluble, antigenic, usually heat labile, injurious substance elaborated by certain bacteria; it is formed within the cell but is released into the environment where it is rapidly active in extremely small amounts; most exotoxins are proteinaceous in nature. SYN extracellular toxin.

ex•o•tro•pi•a (ek′sō-trō′pē-ă) That type of strabismus in which the visual axes diverge; may be paralytic or concomitant, monocular or alternating, constant or intermittent. SYN divergent strabismus, exodeviation (2), wall-eye. [exo- + G. *tropē,* turn]

ex•pand•a•ble stent (eks-pan′di-bĕl stent) Stent placed within the lumen of a structure, often percutaneously, which then shortens in its longitudinal dimension and increases its diameter, thereby increasing the inside dimension of the structure.

ex•pan•ded dis•a•bil•i•ty sta•tus scale (EDSS) (eks-pand′ĕd dis′ă-bil′i-tē stat′us skāl) A commonly used rating system for evaluating the degree of neurologic impairment in multiple sclerosis, based on neurologic findings, and not symptoms; there are 10 grades in all, in steps and half-steps (e.g., 4, 4.5, 5), with "1" neurologically normal and "10" dead. SYN Kurtzke multiple sclerosis disability scale.

ex•pan•sion (eks-pan′shŭn) **1.** An increase in size as of chest or lungs. **2.** The spreading out of any structure, as a tendon. **3.** An expanse; a wide area. [L. *ex-pando,* pp. *-pansus,* to spread out]

ex•pec•to•rant (eks-pek′tŏr-ănt) **1.** Promoting secretion from the mucous membrane of the air passages or facilitating its expulsion. **2.** An agent (e.g., guaifenesin) that thins respiratory tract mucus and promotes its removal from the tracheobronchial passages. [L. *ex,* out, + *pectus,* chest]

ex•pec•to•rate (eks-pek′tŏr-āt) To cough up and spit out mucus from the lower respiratory tract.

ex•pec•to•ra•tion (eks-pek′tŏr-ā′shŭn) **1.** The act of coughing and spitting out mucus from the lower respiratory tract. **2.** Mucus or other material so expelled.

ex•pen•di•ture (eks-pen′di-chŭr) The act of expending; an amount expended or used up. [L. *expendo,* to weigh out, pay]

ex•pense (eks-pens′) That which is given in exchange for something else; cost. [L. *expendo,* to pay out]

ex•pe•ri•ence (ek-spēr′ē-ĕns) The feeling of emotions and sensations, as opposed to thinking; involvement in what is happening rather than abstract reflection on an event or interpersonal encounter. [L. *experientia,* fr. *experior,* to try]

ex•per•i•en•tial au•ra (eks-pēr′ē-en′shăl awr′ă) Epileptic aura characterized by altered perception of one's internal or external environment; may involve auditory, visual, olfactory, gustatory, somatosensory, or emotional altered perceptions. When one of the altered perceptions is clearly predominant, the specific aura classification should be used. SEE ALSO aura (1).

ex•per•i•ment (eks-per′i-mĕnt) **1.** A study in which the investigator intentionally alters one or more factors under controlled conditions to study the effects of doing so. **2.** MAGNETIC RESONANCE pulse sequence. [L. *experimentum,* fr. *experior,* to test, try]

ex•per•i•men•tal de•sign (eks-per′i-men′tăl dĕ-zīn′) RESEARCH a study design used to test cause and effect relationships between variables.

ex•per•i•men•tal er•ror (eks-per′i-men′tăl er′

ŏr) The total error of measurement ascribed to the conduct of an empiric observation. It is commonly expressed as the standard deviation of replicated experiments. There may be many components, including those in the sampling procedure, the measurements, injudicious choice of a model, observer bias, etc.

ex·per·i·men·tal group (eks-per′i-men′tăl grūp) The group of subjects exposed to the variable of an experiment, as opposed to the control group.

ex·per·i·men·tal med·i·cine (eks-per′i-men′tăl med′i-sin) The scientific investigation of medical problems by experimentation on animals or by clinical research.

ex·per·i·men·tal psy·chol·o·gy (eks-per′i-men′tăl sī-kol′ŏ-jē) **1.** A subdiscipline within the science of psychology that is concerned with the study of conditioning, learning, perception, motivation, emotion, language, and thinking. **2.** Also used in relation to subject-matter areas in which experimental, in contrast to correlational or socioexperiential, methods are emphasized.

ex·per·i·ment·er ef·fects (eks-pēr′i-men′tĕr e-fekts′) The influence of the experimenter's behavior, personality traits, or expectancies on the results of that person's own research.

ex·pert wit·ness (eks′pĕrt wit′nĕs) In health care, someone with special training who testifies for the defense or prosecution in a court case to clarify esoteric points for the jury or judge.

ex·pi·ra·tion (eks′pir-ā′shŭn) **1.** SYN exhalation (1). **2.** Death. [L. *expiro* or *ex-spiro,* pp. *-atus,* to breathe out]

ex·pi·ra·tion date (eks′pir-ā′shŭn dāt) The date or time at which a product is no longer potent or of therapeutic value, determined by manufacturer.

ex·pi·ra·to·ry (eks-pī′ră-tōr-ē) Relating to expiration.

ex·pi·ra·to·ry re·serve vol·ume (ERV) (eks-pī′ră-tōr-ē rē-zĕrv′ vol′yūm) The maximal volume of air (about 1000 mL) that can be expelled from the lungs after a normal expiration. SYN reserve air, supplemental air.

ex·pi·ra·to·ry stri·dor (eks-pī′ră-tōr-ē strī′dŏr) A singing sound due to the semiapproximated vocal folds offering resistance to the escape of air.

ex·pire (eks-pīr′) **1.** SYN exhale (1). **2.** To die. **3.** PHARM to pass the expiration date. SEE ALSO expiration date.

ex·pired gas (eks-pīrd′ gas) **1.** Any gas that has been expired from the lungs. **2.** Often used synonymously with mixed expired gas.

ex·plan·a·tion of be·ne·fits (EOB) (eks′plă-nā′shŭn ben′ĕ-fits) The report from an insurance carrier that explains benefits, deductibles, copayment responsibilities, and reasons for noncoverage of claims.

ex·plant (eks-plant′) Living tissue transferred from an organism to an artificial medium for culture.

ex·plo·ra·tion (eks′plŏr-ā′shŭn) An active examination, usually involving endoscopy or a surgical procedure, to ascertain conditions present as an aid in diagnosis. [L. *ex-ploro,* pp. *-ploratus,* to explore]

ex·plor·a·to·ry (eks-plōr′ă-tōr-ē) Relating to, or with a view to, exploration.

ex·plor·er (eks-plōr′ĕr) A sharp pointed dental instrument used to investigate natural or restored tooth surfaces to detect caries, other defects, or dental deposits (e.g., calculus).

ex·pos·ed dose (eks-pōzd′ dōs) The amount of a compound that contacts an epithelial barrier such as the skin, eyes, respiratory tract, or gastrointestinal tract before absorption occurs. SYN external dose.

ex·po·sure (eks-pō′zhŭr) Contact of a compound with an epithelial barrier such as the skin, eyes, respiratory tract, or gastrointestinal tract before absorption occurs. SEE ALSO exposed dose, external dose.

ex·po·sure dose (eks-pō′zhŭr dōs) The radiation dose, expressed in roentgens, delivered at a point in free air.

ex·po·sure ker·a·ti·tis (eks-pō′zhŭr ker′ă-tī′tis) Inflammation of the cornea resulting from irritation caused by inability to close the eyelids.

ex·press (eks-pres′) To press or squeeze out. [L. *ex-premo,* pp. *-pressus,* to press out]

ex·pressed skull frac·ture (eks-prest′ skŭl frak′shŭr) A fracture with outward displacement of a part of the cranium.

ex·pres·sion (eks-presh′ŭn) **1.** Squeezing out; expelling by pressure. **2.** Mobility of the features giving a particular emotional significance to the face. SYN facies (3) [TA]. **3.** Something that manifests something else.

ex·pres·sion vec·tor (eks-presh′ŭn vek′tŏr) An agent (plasmid, yeast, or animal virus genome) used experimentally to introduce foreign genetic material into a propagatable host cell to replicate and amplify the foreign DNA sequences as a recombinant molecule (recombinant DNA cloning of sequences).

ex·pres·sive a·pha·si·a (eks-pres′iv ă-fā′zē-ă) A type of aphasia in which the greatest deficit is in speech production or language output; usually accompanied by a deficit in communicating by writing, signs, or other means. The patient is aware of his impairment. The lesion typically includes the posterior frontal lobe. SYN Broca aphasia (2), motor aphasia, nonfluent aphasia.

ex•pres•sive lan•guage dis•or•der (eks-pres′iv lang′gwăj dis-ōr′dĕr) Any problem related to oral communication; may have physical or emotional causes.

ex•pul•sive (eks-pŭl′siv) Tending to force out or expel. [L. *ex-pello,* pp. *-pulsus,* to drive out]

ex•pul•sive pains (eks-pŭl′siv pānz) Effective labor pains, associated with contraction of the uterine muscle.

ex•qui•site (eks-kwiz′it) Extremely intense, keen, sharp; said of pain or tenderness. [L. *exquiro,* pp. *exquisitus,* to search out]

ex•san•gui•nate (ek-sang′gwi-nāt) **1.** To remove or withdraw the circulating blood; to make bloodless. **2.** SYN exsanguine. [L. *ex,* out, + *sanguis* (*-guin*), blood]

ex•san•gui•na•tion (ek-sang′gwi-nā′shŭn) Removal of blood; making exsanguine.

ex•san•guine (ek-sang′gwin) Deprived of blood. SYN exsanguinate (2).

Ex•se•ro•hi•lum (eks′ĕr-ō-hī′lŭm) A genus of fungi; a cause of human phaeohyphomycosis. Found in the environment, on grasses and, other plants.

ex•sic•cant (ek-sik′ănt) SYN desiccant.

ex•sic•cate (ek′si-kāt) SYN desiccate.

ex•sic•ca•tion (ek′si-kā′shŭn) **1.** SYN desiccation. **2.** The removal of water of crystallization. SYN dehydration (3). [L. *ex sicco,* pp. *siccatus,* to dry up]

ex•sorp•tion (ek-sōrp′shŭn) Movement of substances from the blood into the lumen of the gut. [L. *ex,* out, + *sorbeo,* to suck]

ex•stro•phy (eks′trŏ-fē) Congenital eversion of a hollow organ. [G. *ex,* out, + *strophē,* a turning]

ex•stro•phy of the blad•der (eks′trŏ-fē blad′ĕr) A congenital gap in the anterior wall of the bladder and the adjacent abdominal wall, the interior and posterior wall of the bladder being exposed.

ex•tem•po•ra•ne•ous com•pound•ing (eks-tem′pŏr-ā′nē-ŭs kom′pound-ing) A medication or product made specifically for an individual patient.

ex•tend (eks-tend′) To straighten a limb, to diminish or extinguish the angle formed by flexion; to place the distal segment of a limb in such a position that its axis is continuous with that of the proximal segment. [L. *ex- tendo,* pp. *-tensus,* to stretch out]

ex•ten•ded-care fa•cil•i•ty (eks-ten′dĕd-kār fă-sil′i-tē) Health care supplier of skilled care after hospitalization or severe illness or injury. SYN nursing home, residential care.

ex•ten•ded fam•i•ly (eks-ten′dĕd fam′i-lē) The traditional or nuclear family, including any relatives.

ex•ten•ded me•di•a•sti•nos•cop•y (eks-ten′dĕd mē′dē-as′ti-nos′kŏ-pē) Cervical mediastinoscopy in which, in addition to the standard pretracheal and paratracheal exploration, the mediastinoscope is passed anterior to the innominate artery and aortic arch to provide access to the subaortic (aortopulmonary window) and anterior mediastinal lymph nodes; an alternative to the Chamberlain procedure.

ex•tend•ed rad•i•cal mas•tec•to•my (eks-ten′dĕd rad′i-kăl mas-tek′tŏ-mē) Excision of the entire breast including the nipple, areola, and overlying skin, as well as the pectoral muscles and the lymphatic-bearing tissues of the axilla and chest wall and internal mammary chain of lymph nodes.

ex•ten•ded thy•mec•to•my (eks-ten′dĕd thī-mek′tŏ-mē) Thymectomy performed using combined sternotomy and a cervical incision to allow removal of all extraglandular thymic tissue. SYN maximal thymectomy.

ex•ten•der (eks-tend′ĕr) A person who or thing that spreads, stretches, or increases. [L. *extendo,* to stretch]

ex•ten•sion (eks-ten′shŭn) **1.** The act of bringing the distal portion of a joint in continuity with the long axis of the proximal portion. **2.** A pulling or dragging force exerted on a limb in a distal direction. **3.** To straighten a joint (i.e., the elbow is in extension when fully straightened). [L. *extensio,* a stretching out]

ex•ten•sor (eks-ten′sŏr) A muscle the contraction of which causes movement at a joint with the consequence that the limb or body assumes a straighter line, or so that the distance between the parts proximal and distal to the joint is increased or extended; the antagonist of a flexor. SEE muscle. [L. one who stretches, fr. *ex-tendo,* to stretch out]

ex•ten•sor car•pi ra•di•a•lis bre•vis mus•cle (eks-ten′sŏr kahr′pī rā-dē-ā′lis brev′is mŭs′ĕl) *Origin,* lateral epicondyle of humerus; *insertion,* base of third metacarpal bone; *action,* extends and abducts wrist radially; *nerve supply,* radial. SYN musculus extensor carpi radialis brevis [TA], short radial extensor muscle of wrist.

ex•ten•sor car•pi ra•di•a•lis lon•gus mus•cle (eks-ten′sŏr kahr′pī rā-dē ā′lis long′gus mŭs′ĕl) *Origin,* lateral supracondylar ridge of humerus; *insertion,* back of base of second metacarpal bone; *action,* extends and deviates wrist radialward; *nerve supply,* radial. SYN musculus extensor carpi radialis longus [TA], long radial extensor muscle of wrist.

ex•ten•sor car•pi ul•na•ris mus•cle (eks-ten′sŏr kahr′pī ŭl-nā′ris mŭs′ĕl) *Origin,* lateral epicondyle of humerus (humeral head) and oblique line and posterior border of ulna (ulnar head); *insertion*, base of fifth metacarpal bone; *action*, extends and abducts wrist ulnarward; *nerve supply*, radial (posterior interosseous). SYN musculus extensor carpi ulnaris [TA], ulnar extensor muscle of wrist.

ex·ten·sor di·gi·ti mi·ni·mi mus·cle (eks-ten′sŏr dij′ĭ-tī min′i-mī mŭs′ĕl) *Origin*, lateral epicondyle of humerus; *insertion*, dorsum of proximal, middle, and distal phalanges of little finger; *action*, extends fingers; *nerve supply*, radial (posterior interosseous). SYN musculus extensor digiti minimi [TA], extensor muscle of little finger.

ex·ten·sor di·gi·to·rum bre·vis mus·cle (eks-ten′sŏr dij-i-tō′rŭm brev′is mŭs′ĕl) *Origin*, dorsal surface of calcaneus; *insertion*, by four tendons fusing with those of the extensor digitorum longus, and by a slip attached independently to the base of the proximal phalanx of the great toe; *action*, extends toes; *nerve supply*, deep peroneal. See this page. SYN musculus extensor digitorum brevis [TA], short extensor muscle of toes.

ex·ten·sor di·gi·to·rum lon·gus mus·cle (eks-ten′sŏr dij-i-tō′rŭm long′gus mŭs′ĕl) *Origin*, lateral condyle of tibia, upper two thirds of anterior margin of fibula; *insertion*, by four tendons to the dorsal surfaces of the bases of the proximal, middle, and distal phalanges of the second to fifth toes; *action*, extends the four lateral toes; *nerve supply*, deep branch of peroneal. See this page. SYN musculus extensor digitorum longus [TA], long extensor muscle of toes.

extensor digitorum brevis muscle

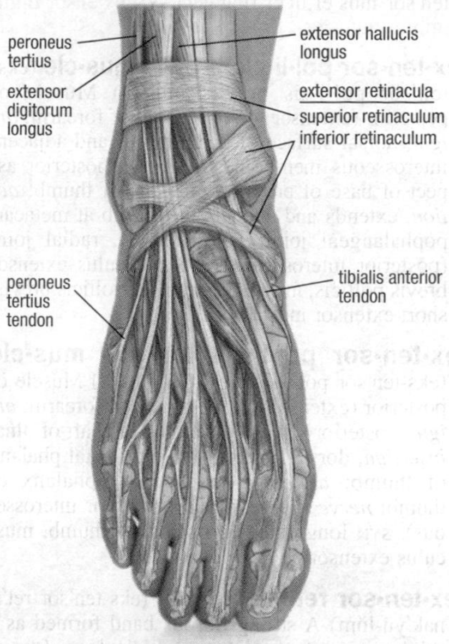

extensor digitorum longus muscle

ex·ten·sor di·gi·to·rum mus·cle (eks-ten′sŏr dij-i-tō′rŭm mŭs′ĕl) *Origin*, lateral epicondyle of humerus; *insertion*, by four tendons into the base of the proximal and middle and base of the distal phalanges; *action*, extends fingers; *nerve supply*, radial (posterior interosseous). See page 554. SYN musculus extensor digitorum [TA], extensor muscle of fingers, musculus extensor digitorum communis.

ex·ten·sor hal·lu·cis bre·vis mus·cle (eks-ten′sŏr hal′ū-sis brev′is mŭs′ĕl) The medial belly of extensor digitorum brevis, the tendon of which is inserted into the base of the proximal phalanx of the great toe. SYN musculus extensor hallucis brevis [TA], short extensor muscle of great toe.

ex·ten·sor hal·lu·cis lon·gus mus·cle (eks-ten′sŏr hal′ū-sis long′gus mŭs′ĕl) *Origin*, lateral surface of tibia and interosseous membrane; *insertion*, base of distal phalanx of great toe; *action*, extends the great toe; *nerve supply*, anterior tibial. SYN musculus extensor hallucis longus [TA].

ex·ten·sor in·di·cis mus·cle (eks-ten′sŏr in′di-sis mŭs′ĕl) *Origin*, dorsal surface of ulna; *insertion*, dorsal extensor aponeurosis of index finger; *action*, assists in extending the forefinger; *nerve supply*, radial. SYN musculus extensor indicis [TA], index extensor muscle.

ex·ten·sor mus·cle of fin·gers (eks-ten′sŏr mŭs′ĕl fing′gĕrz) SYN extensor digitorum muscle.

ex·ten·sor mus·cle of lit·tle fin·ger (eks-

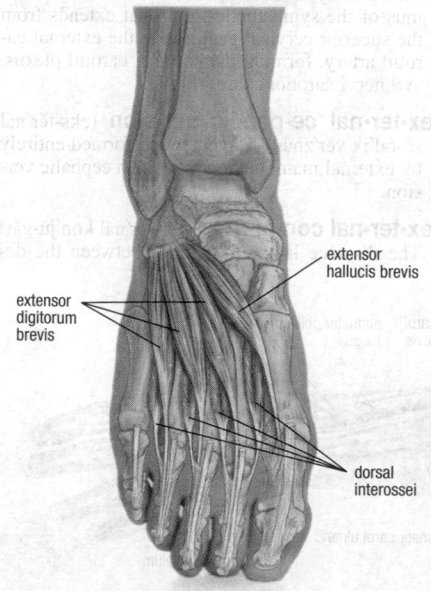

ten′sŏr mŭs′ĕl lit′ĕl fing′gĕr) SYN extensor digiti minimi muscle.

ex•ten•sor pol•li•cis brev•is mus•cle (eks-ten′sŏr pol′i-sis brev′is mŭs′ĕl) Muscle of posterior (extensor) compartment of forearm; *origin*, dorsal surface of distal radius and adjacent interosseous membrane; *insertion*, posterior aspect of base of proximal phalanx of thumb; *action*, extends and abducts the thumb at metacarpophalangeal joint; *nerve supply*, radial joint (posterior interosseous). SYN musculus extensor brevis pollicis, musculus extensor pollicis brevis, short extensor muscle of thumb.

ex•ten•sor pol•li•cis lon•gus mus•cle (eks-ten′sŏr pol′i-sis long′gus mŭs′ĕl) Muscle of posterior (extensor) compartment of forearm; *origin*, posterior surface of middle of shaft of ulna; *insertion*, dorsal aspect of base of distal phalanx of thumb; *action*, extends distal phalanx of thumb; *nerve supply*, radial (posterior interosseous). SYN long extensor muscle of thumb, musculus extensor pollicis longus.

ex•ten•sor ret•i•nac•u•lum (eks-ten′sŏr ret′i-nak′yū-lŭm) A strong fibrous band formed as a thickening of the antebrachial deep fascia, stretching obliquely across the back of the wrist, attaching deeply to ridges on the dorsal aspect of the radius, triquetral and pisiform bones, binding down the extensor tendons of the fingers and thumb. See page 555.

exteriorise [Br.] SYN exteriorize.

ex•te•ri•or•ize (eks-tēr′ē-ōr-īz) **1.** To direct interests, thoughts, or feelings into a channel leading outside the self, to some definite aim or object. **2.** To expose an organ temporarily for observation, or permanently for purposes of physiologic experiment. SYN exteriorise.

ex•tern (eks′tĕrn) An advanced student or recent graduate who assists in the medical or surgical care of hospital patients. [F. *externe,* outside, a day scholar]

ex•ter•nal (eks-tĕr′năl) On the outside or farther from the center. USAGE NOTE Often incorrectly used to mean lateral. [L. *externus*]

ex•ter•nal a•cous•tic me•a•tus (eks-tĕr′năl ă-kūs′tik mē-ā′tŭs) The passage leading inward through the tympanic portion of the temporal bone, from the auricle to the tympanic membrane; it consists of a bony (inner) portion and a fibrocartilaginous (outer) portion, the cartilaginous external acoustic meatus.

ex•ter•nal a•nal sphinc•ter mus•cle (eks-tĕr′năl ā′năl sfingk′tĕr mŭs′ĕl) Fusiform ring of striated muscular fibers surrounding anus, attached posteriorly to the coccyx and anteriorly to the central tendon of the perineum. SYN external sphincter muscle of anus, musculus sphincter ani externus.

ex•ter•nal au•dit (eks-tĕr′năl aw′dit) A verification of health care records by someone outside the organization to be sure that the health care facility is maintaining professional standards.

ex•ter•nal base of skull (eks-tĕr′năl bās skŭl) External aspect of the base of the cranium.

ex•ter•nal cap•sule (eks-tĕr′năl kap′sŭl) A thin lamina of white substance separating the claustrum from the putamen. It joins the internal capsule at either extremity of the putamen, forming a capsule of white matter external to the lenticular nucleus. SYN capsula externa [TA].

ex•ter•nal ca•rot•id ar•ter•y (eks-tĕr′năl kă-rot′id ahr′tĕr-ē) *Origin*, common carotid at C-4 vertebral level; *branches*, superior thyroid, lingual, facial, occipital, posterior auricular, ascending pharyngeal, and *terminal branches*, maxillary and superficial temporal at level of neck of mandible. SYN arteria carotis externa.

ex•ter•nal ca•rot•id nerves (eks-tĕr′năl kă-rot′id nĕrvz) A number of sympathetic nerve fibers conveyed through the cephalic arterial ramus of the sympathetic trunk that extends from the superior cervical ganglion to the external carotid artery, forming the external carotid plexus. SYN nervi carotici externi [TA].

ex•ter•nal ce•pha•lic ver•sion (eks-tĕr′năl sĕ-fal′ik vĕr′zhŭn) Movement performed entirely by external manipulation. SEE ALSO cephalic version.

ex•ter•nal con•ju•gate (eks-tĕr′năl kon′jŭ-găt) The distance in a straight line between the de-

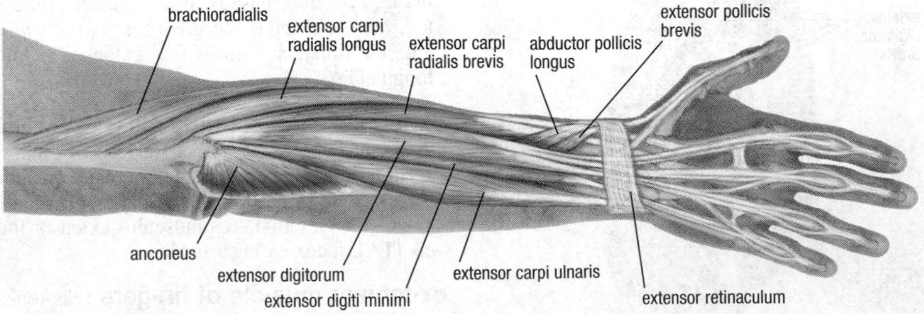

extensor digitorum muscle

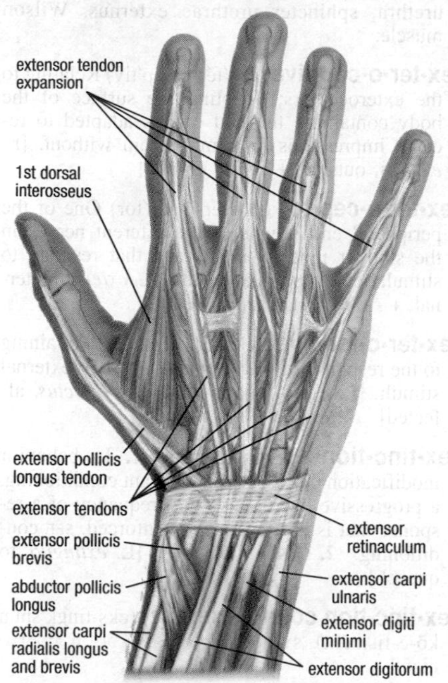

extensor retinaculum

pression under the last spinous process of the lumbar vertebrae and the upper edge of the pubic symphysis.

ex·ter·nal dose (eks-tĕr′năl dōs) SYN exposed dose.

ex·ter·nal ear (eks-tĕr′năl ēr) SEE ear. SEE ALSO auricle, pinna.

ex·ter·nal fis·tu·la (eks-tĕr′năl fis′chū-lă) A fistula between a hollow viscus and the skin.

ex·ter·nal fix·a·tion (eks-tĕr′năl fik-sā′shŭn) Fixation of fractured bones by splints, plastic dressings, or transfixion pins.

ex·ter·nal gen·i·ta·li·a (eks-tĕr′năl jen′i-tā′lē-ă) The vulva and clitoris in the female, and the penis and scrotum in the male.

ex·ter·nal in·ter·cos·tal mus·cle (eks-tĕr′nal in′tĕr-kos′tăl mŭs′ĕl) Flat muscle of thorax arising from lower border of one rib and passing obliquely downward and forward to be inserted into upper border of rib below; *action*, contracts during inspiration to elevate ribs; also to maintain tension in intercostal spaces to resist inward movement during inspiration; *nerve supply*, intercostal. SYN musculus intercostalis externus.

ex·ter·nal mam·ma·ry ar·ter·y (eks-tĕr′nal mam′ăr-ē ahr′tĕr-ē) SYN lateral thoracic artery.

ex·ter·nal na·sal ar·ter·y (eks-tĕr′năl nā′zăl ahr′tĕr-ē) SYN dorsal nasal artery.

ex·ter·nal na·sal branch·es of in·fra·or·bi·tal nerve (eks-tĕr′năl nā′zăl branch′ĕz in′fră-ōr′bi-tăl nĕrv) Branches to external aspect of nose, including those of infraorbital nerve, rami nasales externi nervi infraorbitalis [NA], and nasociliary nerve, rami nasales externi nervi ethmoidalis anterioris [NA]. SYN rami nasales externi nervi infraorbitalis.

ex·ter·nal na·sal veins (eks-tĕr′năl nā′zăl vānz) Several vessels that drain the external nose, emptying into the angular or facial vein.

ex·ter·nal nose (eks-tĕr′năl nōz) The visible portion of the nose that forms a prominent feature of the face; it consists of a root, dorsum, and apex from above downward and is perforated inferiorly by two nostrils separated by a septum. SYN nasus (1).

ex·ter·nal ob·lique mus·cle (eks-tĕr′năl ō-blēk′ mŭs′ĕl) *Origin*, fifth to twelfth ribs; *insertion*, anterior half of lateral lip of iliac crest, inguinal ligament, and anterior layer of the rectus sheath; *action*, diminishes capacity of abdomen, draws thorax downward; *nerve supply*, thoracoabdominal nerves. See this page. SYN musculus obliquus externus abdominis [TA].

ex·ter·nal ob·tu·ra·tor mus·cle (eks-tĕr′năl ob′tŭr-ā-tōr mŭs′ĕl) SYN obturator externus muscle.

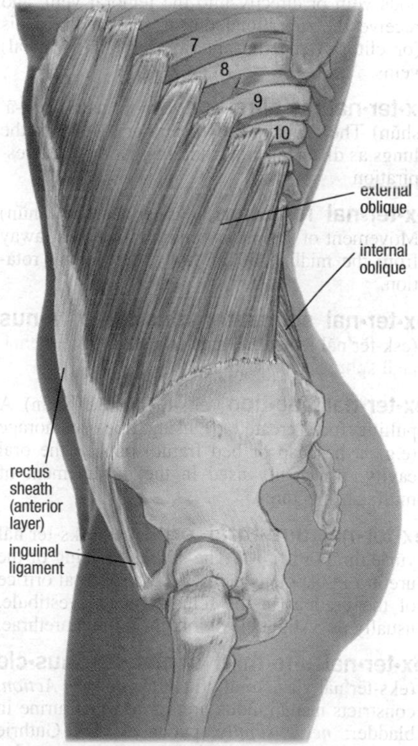

external oblique muscle

ex·ter·nal oc·cip·i·tal crest (eks-tĕr′năl ok-sip′i-tăl krest) A ridge extending from the external occipital protuberance to the border of the foramen magnum.

ex·ter·nal oph·thal·mop·a·thy (eks-tĕr′năl of′thăl-mop′ă-thē) Any disease of the conjunctiva, cornea, or adnexa of the eye.

ex·ter·nal oph·thal·mo·ple·gi·a (eks-tĕr′năl of′thăl-mō-plē′jē-ă) SYN ophthalmoplegia externa.

ex·ter·nal os of u·ter·us (eks-tĕr′năl os yū′tĕr-ŭs) The vaginal opening of the uterus.

ex·ter·nal phase (eks-tĕr′năl fāz) The medium or fluid in which a disperse is suspended. SYN dispersion medium.

ex·ter·nal pte·ry·goid mus·cle (eks-tĕr′năl ter′i-goyd mŭs′ĕl) SYN lateral pterygoid muscle.

ex·ter·nal pu·den·dal ar·ter·ies (eks-tĕr′năl pū-den′dăl ahr′tĕr-ēz) *Origin*, femoral; *distribution*, skin over pubes, skin over penis, and skin of scrotum or labium majus through anterior scrotal (labial) arteries; *anastomoses*, dorsal artery of penis or clitoris, posterior scrotal or labial arteries. SYN arteriae pudendae externae [TA].

ex·ter·nal pu·den·dal veins (eks-tĕr′năl pū-den′dăl vānz) These correspond to the arteries of the same name; they empty into the great saphenous vein or directly into the femoral vein, and receive the superficial dorsal vein of the penis (or clitoris) and the anterior scrotal (or labial) veins.

ex·ter·nal res·pi·ra·tion (eks-tĕr′năl res′pir-ā′shŭn) The exchange of respiratory gases in the lungs as distinguished from internal or tissue respiration.

ex·ter·nal ro·ta·tion (eks-tĕr′năl rō-tā′shŭn) Movement of a joint, around its long axis, away from the midline of the body. SYN lateral rotation.

ex·ter·nal sphinc·ter mus·cle of a·nus (esk-tĕr′năl sfingk′tĕr mŭs′ĕl ā′nŭs) SYN external anal sphincter muscle.

ex·ter·nal trac·tion (eks-tĕr′năl trak′shŭn) A pulling force created by using fixed anchorage (e.g., a headcap or bed frame) outside the oral cavity; principally used in the management of midfacial fractures.

ex·ter·nal u·re·thral or·i·fice (eks-tĕr′năl yūr-ē′thrăl ōr′i-fis) **1.** The slitlike opening of the urethra in the glans penis. **2.** The external orifice of the urethra (in the female) in the vestibule, usually on a slight elevation, the papilla urethrae.

ex·ter·nal u·re·thral sphinc·ter mus·cle (eks-tĕr′năl yūr-ē′thrăl sfingk′tĕr mŭs′ĕl) *Action*, constricts membranous urethra to retain urine in bladder; *nerve supply*, pudendal. SYN Guthrie muscle, musculus constrictor urethrae, musculus sphincter urethrae externus, sphincter muscle of urethra, sphincter urethrae externus, Wilson muscle.

ex·ter·o·cep·tive (eks′tĕr-ō-sep′tiv) Relating to the exteroceptors; denoting the surface of the body containing the end organs adapted to receive impressions or stimuli from without. [L. *exterus,* outside, + *capio,* to take]

ex·ter·o·cep·tor (eks′tĕr-ō-sep′tŏr) One of the peripheral end organs of the afferent nerves in the skin or mucous membrane that respond to stimulation by external agents. [L. *exterus,* external, + *receptor,* receiver]

ex·ter·o·fec·tive (eks′tĕr-ō-fek′tiv) Pertaining to the response of the nervous system to external stimuli. [L. *extero,* from outside, + *affectus,* affected]

ex·tinc·tion (eks-tingk′shŭn) **1.** In behavior modification or classical or operant conditioning, a progressive decrease in the frequency of a response that is not positively reinforced. SEE conditioning. **2.** SYN absorbance. [L. *extinguo,* to quench]

ex·tinc·tion co·ef·fi·cient (ε) (eks-tingk′shŭn kō-ĕ-fish′ĕnt) SYN specific absorption coefficient.

ex·tin·guish (eks-ting′gwish) **1.** To abolish; to quench, as a flame; to cause loss of identity; to destroy. **2.** PSYCHOLOGY to abolish a conditioned response. SEE conditioning. [L. *extinguo,* to quench]

ex·tir·pa·tion (eks′tĭr-pā′shŭn) Complete removal of an organ or diseased tissue. [L. *extirpo,* to root out, fr. *stirps,* a stalk, root]

ex·tor·sion (eks-tōr′shŭn) **1.** Outward rotation of a limb or of an organ. **2.** Conjugate rotation of the upper poles of each cornea outward. [L. *extorsio,* fr. *ex- torqueo,* to twist out]

extra- Prefix meaning without, outside of. [L.]

ex·tra·ax·i·al (eks′tră-aks′ē-ăl) Off the axis; applied to intracranial lesions that do not arise from the brain itself.

ex·tra·cap·su·lar an·ky·lo·sis (eks′tră-kap′sŭ-lăr ang′ki-lō′sis) Stiffness of a joint due to induration or heterotopic ossification of the surrounding tissues. SYN spurious ankylosis.

ex·tra·cap·su·lar lig·a·ments (eks′tră-kap′sŭ-lăr lig′ă-mĕnts) Ligaments associated with a synovial joint but separate from and external to its articular capsule.

ex·tra·cel·lu·lar (eks′tră-sel′yŭ-lăr) Outside the cells.

ex·tra·cel·lu·lar en·zyme (eks′tră-sel′yŭ-lăr en′zīm) An enzyme performing its functions outside a cell (e.g., the various digestive enzymes). SYN exoenzyme.

ex·tra·cel·lu·lar flu·id (ECF) (eks′tră-sel′yŭ-lăr flū′id) **1.** The interstitial fluid and the plasma, constituting about 20% of the weight of the body; **2.** Sometimes used to mean all fluid outside of cells, usually excluding transcellular fluid.

ex•tra•cel•lu•lar tox•in (eks′tră-sel′yū-lăr tok′sin) SYN exotoxin.

ex•tra•chro•mo•som•al el•e•ment, ex•tra•chro•mo•som•al ge•net•ic el•e•ment (eks′tră-krō-mō-sō′măl el′ĕ-mĕnt, jĕ-net′ik el′ĕ-mĕnt) SYN plasmid.

ex•tra•chro•mo•som•al in•her•i•tance (eks′tră-krō-mō-sŏ′măl in-her′i-tăns) Transmission of characters dependent on some factor not connected with the chromosomes.

ex•tra•cor•po•re•al (eks′tră-kōr-pōr′ē-ăl) Outside, or unrelated to, the body or any anatomic corpus.

ex•tra•cor•po•re•al cir•cu•la•tion (eks′tră-kōr-pōr′ē-ăl sĭr′kyū-lā′shŭn) The circulation of blood outside of the body through a machine that temporarily assumes an organ's functions (e.g., through a heart-lung machine or artificial kidney).

ex•tra•cor•po•re•al-mem•brane ox•y•gen•a•tion (ECMO) (eks′tră-kōr-pōr′ē-ăl- mem′brān oks′i-jĕn-ā′shŭn) A system to augment alveolar ventilation by gaseous diffusion across membranes outside the patient's body.

ex•tra•cor•po•re•al shock wave lith•o•trip•sy (ESWL) (eks′tră-kōr-pōr′ē-ăl shok wāv lith′ō-trip′sē) Breaking up of renal or ureteral calculi by focused ultrasound energy.

ex•tract (eks′trakt) **1.** (ek′strakt) A concentrated preparation of a drug obtained by removing the active constituents with suitable solvents, evaporating all or nearly all of the solvent, and adjusting the residual mass or powder to the prescribed standard. **2.** (ek-strakt′) To remove part of a mixture with a solvent. **3.** To perform extraction. [L. *ex-traho*, pp. *-tractus*, to draw out]

ex•tract•ing for•ceps (eks-trak′ting fōr′seps) SYN dental forceps.

ex•trac•tion (ek-strak′shŭn) **1.** Luxation and removal of a tooth from its alveolus. **2.** Partitioning of material (solute) into a solvent. **3.** The active portion of a drug; the making of an extract. **4.** Surgical removal by pulling out. **5.** Removal of the fetus from the uterus or vagina at or near the end of pregnancy, either manually or with instruments. **6.** Removal by suction of the products of conception before a menstrual period has been missed. [L. *ex-traho,* pp. *-tractus,* to draw out]

ex•trac•tion co•ef•fi•cient (ek-strak′shŭn kō-ĕ-fish′ĕnt) The percentage of a substance removed from the blood or plasma in a single passage through a tissue.

ex•trac•tion ra•ti•o (E) (ek-strak′shŭn rā′shē-ō) The fraction of a substance removed from the blood flowing through the kidney.

ex•trac•tives (ek-strak′tivz) Substances present in vegetable or animal tissue that can be separated by successive treatment with solvents and recovered by evaporation of the solution.

ex•trac•tor (ek-strak′tŏr) Instrument for use in drawing or pulling out any natural part, as a tooth, or a foreign body.

ex•tra•cys•tic (eks′tră-sis′tik) Outside of, or unrelated to, the gallbladder or urinary bladder or any cystic tumor.

extradural haemorrhage [Br.] SYN extradural hemorrhage.

ex•tra•du•ral hem•or•rhage (eks′tră-dūr′ăl hem′ŏr-ăj) An accumulation of blood between the skull and the dura mater. SYN epidural hematoma, extradural haemorrhage.

ex•tra•em•bry•on•ic (eks′tră-em′brē-on′ik) Outside the body of the embryo; referring, e.g., to membranes providing protection and nutrition but discarded at birth without being incorporated in the body.

ex•tra•em•bry•on•ic ce•lom (eks′tră-em′brē-on′ik sē′lŏm) SYN chorionic cavity.

ex•tra•he•pat•ic (eks-tră-he-pat′ik) Outside the liver.

ex•tra lean (eks′tră lēn) A product so labeled contains, by F.D.A. order, less than 5 g fat, 2 g saturated fat, and 95 mg cholesterol per serving.

ex•tra•mam•ma•ry Pa•get dis•ease (eks′tră-mam′ăr-ē pa′jĕt di-zēz′) An intraepidermal form of mucinous adenocarcinoma, most commonly in the anogenital region. SYN Paget disease (3).

ex•tra•no•dal mar•gin•al zone lymph•o•ma (eks′tră-nō′dăl mahr′ji-năl zōn lim-fō′mă) SYN MALToma.

ex•tra•oc•u•lar mus•cles (eks′tră-ok′yū-lăr mŭs′ĕlz) The muscles within the orbit including the four rectus muscles (superior, inferior, medial, and lateral), two oblique muscles (superior and inferior), and the levator of the superior eyelid (levator palpebrae superioris).

ex•tra•per•i•to•ne•al fas•ci•a (eks′tră-per′i-tŏ-nē′ăl fash′ē-ă) The thin layer of fascia and adipose tissue between the peritoneum and fascia transversalis. SYN fascia subperitonealis [TA].

ex•tra•phys•i•o•log•ic (eks′tră-fiz′ē-ō-loj′ik) Outside of the domain of physiology; more than physiologic, therefore pathologic.

ex•tra•py•ram•i•dal (eks′tră-pir-am′i-dăl) Outside or not involving the pyramidal tract.

ex•tra•py•ram•i•dal dis•ease (eks′tră-pir-am′i-dăl di-zēz′) A general term for a number of disorders caused by abnormalities of the basal ganglia or certain brain stem or thalamic nuclei; characterized by motor deficits, loss of postural reflexes, bradykinesia, tremor, rigidity, and various involuntary movements.

ex•tra•py•ram•i•dal dys•ki•ne•si•a (eks′tră-pir-am′i-dăl dis′ki-nē′zē-ă) Abnormal involuntary movement attributed to pathologic states of one or more parts of the striate body and characterized by insuppressible, stereotyped, automatic movements that cease only during sleep (e.g., Parkinson disease; chorea; athetosis; hemiballism).

ex•tra•py•ram•i•dal mo•tor sys•tem (eks′tră-pir-am′i-dăl mō′tŏr sis′tĕm) Literally: all those brain structures affecting bodily (somatic) movement, excluding the motor neurons, the motor cortex, and the pyramidal (corticobulbar and corticospinal) tract. Despite its very wide literal connotation, the term is commonly used to denote in particular the striate body (basal ganglia), its associated structures (substantia nigra; subthalamic nucleus), and its descending connections with the midbrain.

ex•tra•sac•cu•lar her•ni•a (eks′tră-sak′yŭ-lăr hĕr′nē-ă) SYN sliding hernia.

ex•tra•sen•so•ry (eks′tră-sen′sŏr-ē) Outside or beyond the ordinary senses; not limited to the senses, as in extrasensory perception.

ex•tra•sen•so•ry per•cep•tion (ESP) (eks′tră-sen′sŏr-ē pĕr-sep′shŭn) Arrival at understanding by means other than through the ordinary senses (e.g., telepathy, clairvoyance, precognition).

ex•tra•sys•to•le (eks′tră-sis′tŏ-lē) An ectopic beat from any source in the heart. SYN premature systole.

ex•tra•tho•rac•ic air•way ob•struc•tion (eks′tră-thōr-as′ik ār′wā ŏb-strŭk′shŭn) Form of airway obstruction in which the site of airway narrowing is above the thoracic inlet; can be variable (reduction in inspiratory but not expiratory flows) or fixed (reduction in both inspiratory and expiratory flows).

ex•trav•a•sate (eks-trav′ă-sāt) **1.** To exude from or pass out of a vessel into the tissues, said of blood, lymph, or urine. **2.** The substance thus exuded. SYN suffusion (4). [L. *extra,* out of, + *vas,* vessel]

ex•trav•a•sa•tion (eks-trav′ă-sā′shŭn) The act of extravasating. [extra- + L. *vas,* vessel]

ex•tra•vas•cu•lar flu•id (eks′tră-vas-kyŭ-lăr flū′id) All fluid outside the blood vessels, i.e., intracellular, interstitial, and transcellular fluids; it constitutes about 48–58% of the body weight.

ex•tra•ver•sion (eks′tră-vĕr′zhŭn) SYN extroversion.

ex•tra•ves•i•cal re•im•plan•ta•tion (eks′tră-ves′i-kăl rē′im-plan-tā′shŭn) SYN detrusorrhaphy.

ex•tre•mal quo•tient (eks-trē′măl kwō′shĕnt) The ratio of the rate in the jurisdiction with the highest rate of interventions, such as surgical procedures, to the rate in the jurisdiction with the lowest rate.

ex•trem•i•tas (eks-trem′i-tĕs) [TA] SYN extremity. SEE limb. [L. fr. *extremus,* last, outermost]

ex•trem•i•ty (eks-trem′i-tē) One of the ends of an elongated or pointed structure. Incorrectly used to mean limb. SYN extremitas [TA].

ex•trin•sic (eks-trin′zik) Originating outside of the part where found or on which it acts; denoting especially a muscle, such as extrinsic muscles of hand. [L. *extrinsecus,* from without]

ex•trin•sic al•ler•gic al•ve•o•li•tis (eks-trin′zik ă-lĕr′jik al-vē′ŏ-lī′tis) Pneumoconiosis resulting from hypersensitivity to organic dust, usually specified according to occupational exposure; in the acute form, respiratory symptoms and fever start several hours after exposure to the dust; in the chronic form, there is eventual diffuse pulmonary fibrosis after exposure over several years. SYN hypersensitivity pneumonitis.

ex•trin•sic co•a•gu•la•tion path•way (eks-trin′zik kō-ag′yŭ-lā′shŭn path′wā) A part of the coagulation pathway that is activated by contact of factor VII in the blood with tissue factor (TF), an integral membrane protein of extravascular plasma membranes. The integrity of this pathway can be tested by the prothrombin time (PT).

ex•trin•sic fac•tor (eks-trin′zik fak′tŏr) Dietary vitamin B12.

ex•trin•sic in•cu•ba•tion pe•ri•od (eks-trin′zik in′kyū-bā′shŭn pēr′ē-ŏd) Time required for the development of a disease agent in a vector, from the time of uptake of the agent to the time when the vector is infective.

ex•trin•sic PEEP (eks-trin′zik pēp) SYN auto-PEEP.

ex•trin•sic sphinc•ter (eks-trin′zik sfingk′tĕr) A sphincter provided by circular muscular fibers extraneous to the organ.

ex•tro•ver•sion (eks′trō-vĕr′zhŭn) **1.** A turning outward. **2.** A personality patterned on the presence of others. Cf. introversion. SYN extraversion. [incorrectly formed fr. L. *extra,* outside, + *verto,* pp. *versus,* to turn]

ex•tro•vert, ex•tra•vert (eks′trŏ-vĕrt, -tră-vĕrt) A gregarious person whose chief interests lie outside the self, and who is socially self-confident and involved in the affairs of others. Cf. introvert.

ex•trude (eks-trūd′) To thrust, force, or press out.

ex•tru•sion (eks-trū′zhŭn) **1.** A thrusting or

forcing out of a normal position. **2.** The overeruption or migration of a tooth beyond its normal occlusal position.

ex·tru·sion re·flex (eks-trū′zhŭn rē′fleks) When a spoon is put into an infant's mouth, the tongue automatically thrusts forward.

ex·tu·ba·tion (eks′tū-bā′shŭn) Removal of a tube from an organ, structure, or orifice. Often associated with removal of the endotracheal tube after ventilation or surgical procedure. [L. *ex,* out, + *tuba,* tube]

ex·u·ber·ant (eg-zū′bĕr-ănt) Denoting excessive proliferation or growth, as of granulation tissue. [L. *exubero,* to abound, be abundant]

ex·u·date (eks′yū-dāt) Any fluid that has exuded out of a tissue or its capillaries because of injury or inflammation. Cf. transudate. SYN exudation (2). [L. *ex,* out, + *sudo,* to sweat]

ex·u·da·tion (eks′yū-dā′shŭn) **1.** The act or process of exuding. **2.** SYN exudate.

ex·u·da·tion cyst (eks′yū-dā′shŭn sist) A cyst resulting from distention of a closed cavity, such as a bursa, by an excessive secretion of its normal fluid contents.

ex·ud·a·tive (eks′yū′dă-tiv) Relating to the process of exudation or to an exudate.

ex·u·da·tive dru·sen (eks-yū′dă-tiv drū′sĕn) Accumulations of an amorphous and granular material, cytoplasmic processes, and bent fibers between the basement membrane of the retinal pigment epithelium and the inner collagenous zone of the lamina basalis choroidae; types of exudative drusen include hard drusen and soft drusen. SYN typical drusen.

ex·ud·a·tive in·flam·ma·tion (eks-yū′dă-tiv in′flă-mā′shŭn) Any inflammatory process with formation of a conspicuous exudate that may be fibrinous, mucous, or cellular.

ex·ud·a·tive ret·i·ni·tis, ret·i·ni·tis ex·u·da·ti·va (eks-yū′dă-tiv ret′i-nī′tis, ret-i-nī′tis eks-yū-da-tī′vă) A chronic abnormality characterized by deposition of cholesterol and cholesterol esters in outer retinal layers and subretinal space. In adults, often preceded by uveitis; in children, often preceded by retinal vascular abnormalities.

ex·ude (eks-yūd′) In general, to ooze or pass gradually out of a body structure or tissue. [L. *ex,* out, + *sudo,* to sweat]

ex·um·bil·i·ca·tion (eks′ŭm-bil′i-kā′shŭn) **1.** SYN exomphalos (1). **2.** SYN umbilical hernia. **3.** SYN omphalocele. [L. *ex,* out, + *umbilicus,* navel]

ex vi·vo (ex vē′vō) Referring to the use or positioning of a tissue or cell after removal from an organism while the tissue or cells remain viable. [L. from the living]

eye (ī) **1.** The organ of vision that consists of the eyeball and the optic nerve. SYN oculus [TA]. **2.** The area of the eye, including lids and other accessory organs of the eye; the contents of the orbit (common). See this page, B26. [A.S. *eāge*]

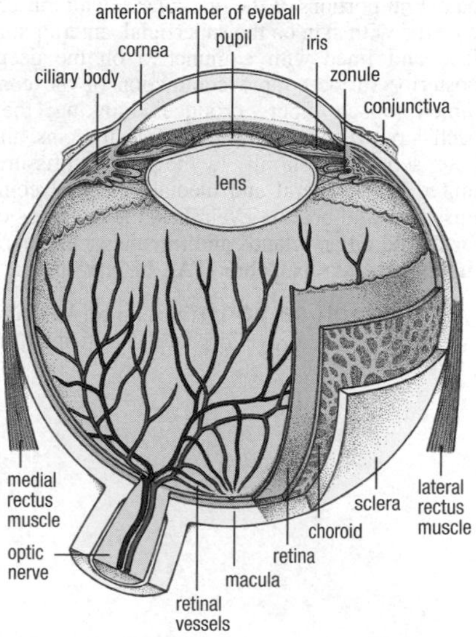

eye (cutaway superior view)

eye·ball (ī′bawl) The eye proper without the appendages. SYN bulbus oculi [TA], bulb of eye.

eye balm (ī bawlm) SYN goldenseal.

eye bank (ī bangk) A place where corneas of eyes removed after death are preserved for subsequent keratoplasty.

eye·brow (ī′brow) The crescentic line of hairs at the superior edge of the orbit. SYN supercilium (1) [TA].

eye-clo·sure pu·pil re·ac·tion (ī-klō′zhŭr pyū′pil rē-ak′shŭn) A constriction of both pupils when an effort is made to close eyelids forcibly held apart. A variant of the pupil response to near vision. SYN Galassi pupillary phenomenon, Gifford reflex, Westphal pupillary reflex.

eye cup (ī kŭp) A small oval receptacle used to apply a liquid to the external eye.

eye·glass·es (ī′glas-ĕz) SYN spectacles.

eye-hand co·or·di·na·tion (ī-hand kō-ōr′di-nā′shŭn) SYN visual-motor control.

eye·lash (ī′lash) One of the stiff hairs projecting from the margin of the eyelid. SYN cilium (1).

eye·lash sign (ī′lash sīn) In a case of apparent unconsciousness due to functional disease, such as conversion hysteria, stroking the eyelashes will occasion movement of the lids, but no such reflex will occur in case of severe organic brain lesion such as apoplexy, fracture of the skull, or other traumatism.

eye•lid (ī′lid) One of the two movable folds covering the front of the eyeball when closed; formed of a fibrous core (tarsal plate) and the palpebral portions of the orbicularis oculi muscle covered with skin on the superficial, anterior surface and lined with conjunctiva on the deep, posterior surface; rapid contraction of the contained muscle fibers produces blinking; they each have fixed (orbital) and free margins, the latter separated centrally by the palpebral fissure, united at the lateral and medial palpebral commissures, and bearing eyelashes, the openings of tarsal and ciliary glands and (medially) the lacrimal puncta. SYN palpebra [TA], blepharon, lid.

eye•lid im•bri•ca•tion (ī′lid im′bri-kā′shŭn) An abnormality of eyelid position by which the upper eyelid overrides the lower eyelid on closure, leading to chronic ocular irritation.

eye patch•ing (ī pach′ing) Covering the eye for the purposes of therapy after trauma or surgery, or by an obstructing spectacle lens in mild cases of amblyopia in children.

eye•piece (ī′pēs) The compound lens at the end of the microscope tube nearest the eye; it magnifies the image made by the objective.

eye spec•u•lum (ī spek′yū-lŭm) An instrument for keeping the eyelids apart during inspection of or operation on the eye. SYN blepharostat.

eye•strain (ī′stān) SYN asthenopia.

eye tooth (ī tūth) SYN canine tooth.

F

F Abbreviation for fractional concentration, followed by subscripts indicating location and chemical species; free energy; farad; faraday; Fahrenheit; visual field; fluorine; force; filial generation, followed by subscript numerals indicating indicating specified matings; phenylalanine; focus (1).

F0 Abbreviation for fundamental frequency.

F1.2 Abbreviation for prothrombin fragment 1.2.

F Abbreviation for faraday, Faraday constant, force; free energy.

f Abbreviation for femto-; respiratory frequency; fugacity; formyl.

FAAFP Abbreviation for Fellow of the American Academy of Family Physicians.

FAAMT Abbreviation for Fellow of the American Association for Medical Transcription.

FAB SEE French-American-British classification system.

Fab SEE Fab fragment.

FAB class•i•fi•ca•tion (klas'i-fi-kā'shŭn) SEE French-American-British classification system.

fa•bel•la (fă-bel'lă) A sesamoid bone in the tendon of the lateral head of the gastrocnemius muscle. [Mod. L. dim. of *faba,* bean]

Fab frag•ment (fab frag'mĕnt) The antigen-binding fragment of an immunoglobulin molecule, consisting of both a light chain and part of a heavy chain.

Fa•bry dis•ease (fah'brē di-zēz') A disorder resulting from deficient α-galactosidase and characterized by abnormal accumulations of neutral glycolipids (e.g., globotriaosylceramide) in endothelial cells in blood vessel walls; clinical findings include angiokeratomas on the thighs, buttocks, and genitalia; hypohidrosis; paresthesia in extremities; cornea verticillata; and spokelike posterior subcapsular cataracts. Death results from renal, cardiac, or cerebrovascular complications. An X-linked recessive inheritance that is caused by mutation of the α-galactosidase gene (GLA) on Xq. SYN Anderson-Fabry disease, Ruiter-Pompen disease, Sweeley-Klionsky disease.

FACCP Abbreviation for Fellow of the American College of Chest Physicians.

face (fās) **1.** The front portion of the head; the visage including the eyes, nose, mouth, forehead, cheeks, and chin, but not the ears. SYN facies (1) [TA]. **2.** SYN surface.

face-bow (fās'bō) A caliperlike device used to record the relationship of the jaws to the temporomandibular joints; the record may then be used to orient a cast or model of the maxilla to the opening and closing axis of the articulator.

face-lift (fās'lift) SEE rhytidectomy.

FACEP Abbreviation for Fellow of the American College of Emergency Physicians.

face pre•sen•ta•tion (fās prez'ĕn-tā'shŭn) SEE cephalic presentation.

fac•et, fa•cette (fas'ĕt, fă-set') **1.** A small, smooth area on a bone or other firm structure. **2.** A worn spot on a tooth, produced by chewing or grinding. [Fr. *facette*]

fac•e•tec•to•my (fas'ĕ-tek'tŏ-mē) Excision of a facet. [facet + G. *ektomē,* excision]

fac•et joint (fas'ĕt joynt) The synovial joint between the vertebral facets or between vertebrae and ribs. SYN zygapophysial joint.

fa•cial (fā'shăl) Relating to the face.

fa•cial ar•ter•y (fā'shăl ahr'tĕr-ē) *Origin,* external carotid; *branches,* ascending palatine, tonsillar and glandular branches, submental, inferior labial, superior labial, masseteric, buccal, lateral nasal branches, and angular. SYN arteria facialis [TA].

fa•cial ax•is (fā'shăl ak'sis) SYN basifacial axis.

fa•cial bones (fā'shăl bōnz) The bones surrounding the mouth and nose and contributing to the orbits; they are the paired maxillae, zygomatic, nasal, lacrimal, palatine, and inferior nasal conchae; and the unpaired ethmoid, vomer, mandible, and hyoid. See this page.

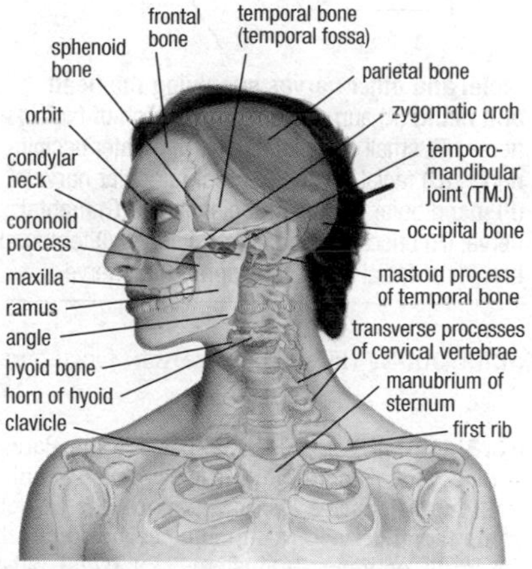

facial bones

fa•cial ca•nal (fā'shăl kă-nal') The bony passage in the temporal bone through which the facial nerve passes; the facial canal commences at the internal auditory meatus with the horizontal part which passes at first anteriorly (medial crus of facial canal) then turns posteriorly at the geniculum of the facial canal to pass medial to the tympanic cavity (lateral crus of facial canal);

finally, it turns downward (descending part of facial canal) to reach the stylomastoid foramen.

fa·cial hem·i·ple·gi·a (fā′shăl hem′ē-plē′jē-ă) Paralysis of one side of the face, the muscles of the extremities being unaffected.

fa·cial nerve [CN VII] (fā′shăl nĕrv) Nerve with origin in the tegmentum of the lower portion of the pons; it emerges from the brain at the posterior border of the pons; it leaves the cranial cavity through the internal acoustic meatus where it is joined by the intermediate nerve, traverses the facial canal in the petrous portion of the temporal bone, and makes its exit through the stylomastoid foramen; after supplying the stapedius, occipitalis, auricular, stylohyoid, and posterior belly of the digastric muscles; its main trunk ramifies within the parotid gland forming the intraparotid plexus, the various branches of which pass to the muscles of facial expression. See this page. SYN nervus facialis [CN VII] [TA], seventh cranial nerve [CN VII].

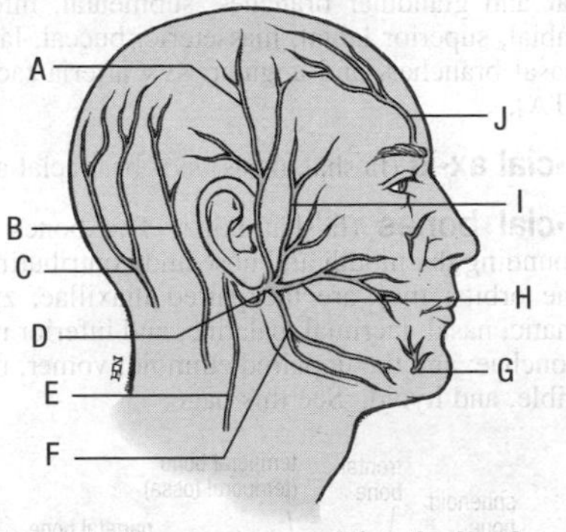

facial and other nerves supplying the head and neck: (A) auriculotemporal branch of facial nerve; (B) small occipital nerve; (C) greater occipital nerve; (D) facial nerve; (E) great auricular nerve; (F) mandibular branch of facial nerve; (G) mental nerve; (H) buccal branch of facial nerve; (I) temporal branch of facial nerve; (J) supraorbital nerve

fa·cial pal·sy (fā′shăl pawl′zē) SYN facial paralysis.

fa·cial pa·ral·y·sis (fā′shăl păr-al′i-sis) Paresis or paralysis of the facial muscles, usually unilateral, due to either a lesion involving the nucleus or the facial nerve or a supranuclear lesion in the cerebrum or upper brainstem. SYN facial palsy, facioplegia, prosopoplegia.

fa·cial re·cess ap·proach (fā′shăl rē′ses ă-prōch′) A surgical approach to the middle ear from the mastoid through the recess lateral to the facial nerve canal.

fa·cial spasm (fā′shăl spazm) SYN facial tic.

fa·cial tic (fā′shăl tik) Involuntary twitching of the facial muscles, sometimes unilateral. SYN Bell spasm, facial spasm, palmus (1), prosopospasm.

fa·cial vein (fā′shăl vān) A continuation of the angular vein at the medial angle of the eye; it passes diagonally downward and outward, uniting with the retromandibular vein below the border of the lower jaw before emptying into the internal jugular vein.

-facient Generally, a combining form meaning causing; one who or that which brings something about. [L. *facio,* to make]

fa·ci·es, pl. **fa·ci·es** (fash′ē-ēz, fash′ē-ēz) [TA] **1.** SYN face (1). **2.** SYN surface. **3.** SYN expression (2). [L.]

fa·cil·i·ta·ted com·mu·ni·ca·tion (fă-sil′i-tā-tĕd kŏ-myū′ni-kā′shŭn) Method in which people who are unable to communicate effectively are aided by a facilitator who physically assists them to use augmentative communication systems (e.g., communication board or typewriter). SEE augmentative and alternative communication. SEE ALSO communication board.

fa·cil·i·ta·tion (fă-sil′i-tā′shŭn) Enhancement or reinforcement of a reflex or other nervous activity by the arrival at the reflex center of other excitatory impulses. [L. *facilitas,* fr. *facilis,* easy]

fac·ing (fās′ing) A tooth-colored material (usually plastic or porcelain) used to hide the buccal or labial surface of a metal crown to give the outward appearance of a natural tooth.

facio- Combining form meaning the face. SEE ALSO prosopo-. [L. *facies*]

fa·ci·o·plas·ty (fā′shē-ō-plas-tē) Surgical repair involving the face. [facio- + G. *plastos,* formed]

fa·ci·o·ple·gi·a (fā′shē-ō-plē′jē-ă) SYN facial paralysis. [facio- + G. *plēgē,* a stroke]

FACNM Abbreviation for Fellow of the American College of Nurse-Midwives.

FACR Abbreviation for Fellow of the American College of Radiology; Fellow of the American College of Rheumatology.

FACS Abbreviation for fluorescence-activated cell sorter.

FACT (fakt) An acronym for Foundation for the Accreditation of Cellular Therapy.

F-ac·tin (ak′tin) The association of G-actin subunits into a fibrous (F) protein.

fac·ti·tious (fak-tish′ŭs) Artificial; self-induced; not naturally occurring. [L. *factitius,* made by art, fr. *facio,* to make]

fac·ti·tious dis·or·der (fak-tish′ŭs dis-ōr′dĕr) A mental condition in which the patient intentionally induces symptoms of illness for psychological reasons.

fac·tor (fak′tŏr) **1.** A contributing cause in any

action. **2.** One of the components that, by multiplication, make up a number or expression. **3.** SYN gene. **4.** A vitamin or other essential element. **5.** An event, characteristic, or other definable entity that brings about a change in a health condition. **6.** A categoric independent variable used to identify, by means of numeric codes, membership in a qualitatively identifiable group (e.g., "overcrowding is a factor in disease transmission."). [L. maker, causer, fr. *facio,* to make]

fac•tor I (fak′tŏr) In the clotting of blood, a factor that is converted to fibrin through the action of thrombin. SEE ALSO fibrinogen.

fac•tor II (fak′tŏr) A glycoprotein converted in the clotting of blood to thrombin by factor Xa, platelets, calcium ions, and factor V. SEE ALSO prothrombin.

fac•tor IIa (fak′tŏr) SYN thrombin.

fac•tor III (fak′tŏr) In the clotting of blood, tissue factor, or thromboplastin, initiates the extrinsic pathway by reacting with factor VII and calcium to form factor VIIa. SEE ALSO thromboplastin.

fac•tor IV (fak′tŏr) In the clotting of blood, calcium ions.

fac•tor V (fak′tŏr) A plasma factor in blood coagulation; does not have enzymatic action but participates in the common pathway of coagulation by binding factor Xa to platelet surfaces; deficiency of this factor leads to a rare hemorrhagic tendency known as parahemophilia or hypoproaccelerinemia. SYN accelerator factor, plasma accelerator globulin, proaccelerin, prothrombin accelerator.

fac•tor VII (fak′tŏr) A plasma factor in blood coagulation, forms a complex with tissue thromboplastin and calcium to activate factor X; accelerates the conversion of prothrombin to thrombin, in the presence of tissue thromboplastin, calcium, and factor V. SYN cothromboplastin, proconvertin, serum accelerator, serum prothrombin conversion accelerator.

fac•tor VIII (fak′tŏr) A plasma factor in blood coagulation; participates in the clotting of the blood by forming a complex with factor IXa, platelets, and calcium and enzymatically catalyzing the activation of factor X; deficiency is associated with classic hemophilia A. **Factor VIII:C** is the coagulant component of factor VIII, which circulates in the plasma complexed with **factor VIIIR** (von Willebrand factor), a glycoprotein that is synthesized by endothelial cells and megakaryocytes, and binds to arteries that have lost their endothelial cell linings, creating a surface to which platelets adhere. Disorders involving factor VIIIR form a heterogenous group of abnormalities called von Willebrand disease. SYN antihemophilic factor A, antihemophilic globulin A, proserum prothrombin conversion accelerator.

fac•tor IX (fak′tŏr) In the clotting of blood, required for the formation of intrinsic blood thromboplastin; deficiency causes hemophilia B. SYN antihemophilic globulin B, Christmas factor, plasma thromboplastin component.

fac•tor IX com•plex (fak′tŏr kom′plĕks) A hemostatic containing factors II, VII, IX, and X.

fac•tor X (fak′tŏr) A plasma coagulation factor that assists in the conversion of prothrombin to thrombin. Deficiency impairs blood coagulation. SYN prothrombinase, Stuart factor, Stuart-Prower factor.

fac•tor Xa (fak′tŏr) The active form of factor X; it is formed from factor X by limited proteolysis via factor VIIa and tissue factor (extrinsic pathway) or factor IXa, VIIIa (intrinsic pathway). Factor Xa forms a complex with factor Va, phospholipid, and calcium to convert prothrombin to thrombin.

fac•tor XI (fak′tŏr) A plasma coagulation factor; a component of the contact system that is absorbed from plasma and serum by glass and similar surfaces. Deficiency of factor XI results in a hemorrhagic tendency. SYN plasma thromboplastin antecedent.

fac•tor XII (fak′tŏr) A plasma coagulation factor. When activated by glass or other substance to its active form, factor XIIa (EC 3.4.21.38), a serine proteinase, it activates factors VII and XI and converts factor XI to its active form, factor XIa. Deficiency of this factor greatly prolongs clotting time of venous blood, but only rarely in a hemorrhagic tendency. SYN Hageman factor.

fac•tor XIII (fak′tŏr) A plasma coagulation factor catalyzed by thrombin into its active form, factor XIIIa, which cross-links subunits of the fibrin clot to form insoluble fibrin. SYN Laki-Lorand factor.

fac•to•ri•al ex•per•i•ments (fak-tōr′ē-ăl eks-per′i-mĕnts) An experimental design in which two or more series of treatments are tried in all combinations.

fac•ul•ta•tive (fak′ŭl-ta′tiv) Able to live under more than one specific set of environmental conditions; possessing an alternative pathway.

fac•ul•ta•tive an•aer•obe (fak′ŭl-tā′tiv an′ăr-ōb) An anaerobe that grows in the presence of air or under conditions of reduced oxygen tension.

fac•ul•ta•tive hy•per•o•pi•a (fak′ŭl-tā′tiv hī′pĕr-ō′pē-ă) SYN manifest hyperopia.

fac•ul•ta•tive par•a•site (fak′ŭl-tā′tiv par′ă-sīt) An organism that may either lead an independent existence or live as a parasite, in contrast to an obligate parasite.

fac•ul•ty (fak′ŭl-tē) A natural or specialized power of a living organism.

FAD Abbreviation for flavin adenine dinucleotide.

fad di•et (fad dī′ĕt) A nutritional regimen, generally of an extreme nature, intended to produce results more quickly than a traditional diet-exercise combination; often of a dubious nature.

Fa•den su•ture (fā′dĕn sū′chŭr) A suture anchoring an ocular rectus muscle to the posterior sclera to limit excessive action of the eyeball. [Ger. *Faden,* thread, twine]

FAE Abbreviation for fetal alcohol effects.

faecal [Br.] SYN fecal.

faecal abscess [Br.] SYN fecal abscess.

faecal concentration [Br.] SYN fecal concentration.

faecal examination [Br.] SYN fecal examination.

faecal fistula [Br.] SYN fecal fistula.

faecalith [Br.] SYN fecalith.

faecaloid [Br.] SYN fecaloid.

faecaloma [Br.] SYN fecaloma.

faecaluria [Br.] SYN fecaluria.

faecal vomiting [Br.] SYN fecal vomiting.

faeces [Br.] SYN feces.

fag•ot cell (fag′ŏt sel) A neoplastic promyelocyte with bundles of Auer rods, found in hypergranular promyelocytic leukemia (M3).

Fahr dis•ease (fahr di-zēz′) Progressive calcific deposition in the walls of blood vessels of the basal ganglia, in young to middle-aged people; occasionally associated with mental retardation and extrapyramidal symptoms.

Fahr•en•heit scale (far′ĕn-hīt skāl) A thermometer scale in which the freezing point of water is 32°F and the boiling point of water 212°F; 0°F indicates the lowest temperature Fahrenheit could obtain by a mixture of ice and salt in 1724; °C = (5/9)(°F − 32).

fail•ure (fāl′yŭr) The state of insufficiency or nonperformance.

fail•ure to thrive (fāl′yŭr thrīv) A condition in which an infant's weight gain and growth are far below usual levels for age.

faint (fānt) **1.** Extremely weak; threatened with syncope. **2.** An episode of syncope. SEE ALSO syncope. [M.E., fr. O. Fr. *feindre,* to feign]

faith heal•ing (fāth hēl′ing) Therapy involving prayer and manual interventions.

fal•cate (fal′kāt) SYN falciform.

fal•ces (fal′sēz) Plural of falx.

fal•ci•form (fal′si-fōrm) Having a crescentic or sickle shape. SYN falcate. [L. *falx,* sickle, + *forma,* form]

fal•ci•form lig•a•ment (fal′si-fōrm lig′ă-mĕnt) SYN falciform process.

fal•ci•form lig•a•ment of liv•er (fal′si-fōrm lig′ă-mĕnt liv′ĕr) A crescentic fold of peritoneum extending to the surface of the liver from the diaphragm and anterior abdominal wall; the round ligament lies in its free inferior border; remnant of embryonic ventral mesogastrium. SYN ligamentum falciforme hepatis [TA].

fal•ci•form pro•cess (fal′si-fōrm pros′es) A continuation of the inner border of the sacrotuberous ligament upward and forward on the inner aspect of the ramus of the ischium. SYN processus falciformis [TA], falciform ligament.

fal•cip•a•rum ma•lar•i•a (fal-sip′ă-rŭm mă-lar′ē-ă) Disease caused by *Plasmodium falciparum* and characterized by intense malarial paroxysms that after synchronization occur every 48 hours with acute cerebral, renal, or gastrointestinal manifestations in severe cases, chiefly caused by the large number of red blood cells affected and the tendency for infected red blood cells to become sticky and then clump, thus blocking capillaries. SYN malignant tertian malaria.

fal•cu•la (fal′kyū-lă) SYN falx cerebelli. [L. dim. of *falx*]

fal•cu•lar (fal′kyū-lăr) **1.** Resembling a sickle or falx. **2.** Relating to the falx cerebelli or cerebri.

fal•lo•pi•an (fă-lō′pē-ăn) Described by or attributed to Gabriele Fallopio (1523–1562); usually referring to the uterine tube.

fal•lo•pi•an tube (fă-lō′pē-ăn tūb) SYN uterine tube.

Fal•lot tet•rad (fă-lō′ tet′rad) SYN tetralogy of Fallot.

Fal•lot tri•ad (fă-lō′ trī′ad) SYN trilogy of Fallot.

false a•ne•mi•a (fawls ă-nē′mē-ă) SYN pseudoanemia.

false an•eu•rysm (fawls an′yūr-izm) **1.** Pulsating, encapsulated hematoma in communication with the lumen of a ruptured vessel; **2.** Ventricular pseudoaneurysm, a cardiac rupture contained and loculated by pericardium, which forms its external wall. **3.** An aneurysm with walls that consist of adventitia, periarterial fibrous tissue, and hematoma.

false an•ky•lo•sis (fawls ang′ki-lō′sis) SYN fibrous ankylosis.

false bleph•a•rop•to•sis (fawls blef′ă-rop-tō′sis) SYN pseudoptosis.

false cast (fawls kast) An elongated, ribbonlike mucous thread with poorly defined edges and pointed or split ends, often confused with a true urinary cast. SYN pseudocast.

false chor•dae ten•din•e•ae (fawls kōr′dē ten-din′ē-ē) Tendinous cords that, unlike the true chordae tendineae, do not attach to the leaflets of the atrioventricular valves. Instead they connect papillary muscles to each other or to the ventricular wall (including the interventricular septum), or merely pass between two points on the ventricular wall (including the septum). SYN chordae tendineae falsae [TA], chordae tendineae spuriae.

False Claims Act (FCA) (fawls klāmz akt) U.S. federal legislation that prohibits anyone from knowingly presenting a false or fraudulent claim to the U.S. government for payment. The act defines "knowingly" as either having actual knowledge that information is false or acting with reckless disregard of the truth or falsity of information.

false con•ju•gate (fawls kon′jŭ-găt) **1.** SYN diagonal conjugate. **2.** SYN effective conjugate.

false di•ver•tic•u•lum (fawls dī′vĕr-tik′yū-lŭm) A diverticulum of the intestine that passes through a defect in the muscular wall of the gut and thus does not include a layer of muscle in its wall.

false he•ma•tu•ri•a (fawls hē′mă-tyūr′ē-ă) SYN pseudohematuria.

false her•maph•ro•dit•ism (fawls hĕr-maf′rō-dīt-izm) SYN pseudohermaphroditism.

false im•age (fawls im′ăj) The image in the deviating eye in strabismus.

false joint (fawls joynt) SYN pseudarthrosis.

false la•bor (fawls lā′bŏr) Braxton Hicks contraction that causes the patient physical discomfort.

false lu•men (fawls lū′mĕn) In a dissecting aneurysm, the abnormal channel within the wall of the involved artery.

false mem•brane (fawls mem′brān) A thick, tough fibrinous exudate on the surface of a mucous membrane or the skin, as seen in diphtheria. SYN croupous membrane, neomembrane, plica (2), pseudomembrane.

false mem•o•ry syn•drome (fawls mem′ŏr-ē sin′drōm) An apparent memory of an imagined event, usually traumatic and remote in time; generally used pejoratively to imply that the memory was engendered by the therapist facilitating its recovery; a controversial concept.

false neg•a•tive (fawls neg′ă-tiv) **1.** A test result that erroneously excludes a person from a specific diagnostic or reference group. **2.** A person excluded by erroneous test results from a particular diagnostic group. **3.** A false-negative test result.

false-neg•a•tive rate (fawls-neg′ă-tiv rāt) Percentage of incorrect results that are, in fact, positive.

false-neg•a•tive re•ac•tion (fawls-neg′ă-tiv rē-ak′shŭn) An erroneous or mistakenly negative response.

false neu•ro•ma (fawls nūr-ō′mă) SYN traumatic neuroma.

false pel•vis (fawls pel′vis) SYN greater pelvis.

false pos•i•tive (fawls poz′i-tiv) **1.** A test result that erroneously assigns a person to a specific diagnostic or reference group. **2.** A person included by erroneous test results in a particular diagnostic group. **3.** A false-positive test result.

false-pos•i•tive rate (fawls-poz′i-tiv rāt) Percentage of incorrect results that are, in fact, negative.

false-pos•i•tive re•ac•tion (fawls-poz′i-tiv rē-ak′shŭn) An erroneous or mistakenly positive response.

false preg•nan•cy (fawls preg′năn-sē) A condition in which some signs and symptoms suggest pregnancy, although the woman is not pregnant. SYN pseudocyesis, pseudopregnancy (1).

false ribs (fawls ribz) Five lower ribs on either side that do not articulate with the sternum directly. SYN costae spuriae [TA].

false su•ture (fawls sū′chŭr) A suture with opposing margins that are smooth or present only a few ill-defined projections.

fal•set•to (fawl-set′tō) High-pitched voice produced by vibration of the anterior third of the vocal folds while the posterior folds are tightly adducted. SEE ALSO voice. [Ital., unnatural voice, fr. *falso,* false, + *-etto,* dim. suff.]

false vo•cal cord (fawls vō′kăl kōrd) SYN vestibular fold.

false wa•ters (fawls waw′tĕrs) A leakage of fluid before or in beginning labor, before the rupture of the amnion.

fal•si•fi•ca•tion (fawl′si-fi-kā′shŭn) The deliberate act of misrepresentation so as to deceive. [L. *falsus,* false, + *facio,* to make]

falx, pl. **fal•ces** (fawlks, fal′sēz) [TA] A sickle-shaped structure. [L. sickle]

falx ce•re•bel•li (fawlks ser-ĕ-bel′ī) [TA] A short process of dura mater projecting forward from the internal occipital crest below the tentorium; it occupies the posterior cerebellar notch and the vallecula, and bifurcates below into two diverging limbs passing to either side of the foramen magnum. SYN falcula.

falx ce•re•bri (fawlks se-rē′brī) [TA] The sickle-shaped fold of dura mater in the longitudinal fissure between the two cerebral hemispheres; it is attached anteriorly to the crista galli of the ethmoid bone and caudally to the upper surface of the tentorium.

falx in•gui•na•lis (fawlks ing-gwi-nā′lis) [TA] SYN inguinal falx.

fa·mil·i·al (fă-mil′ē-ăl) Affecting more members of the same family than can be accounted for by chance, usually within a single sibship; commonly but incorrectly used to mean genetic. [L. *familia,* family]

fa·mil·i·al ad·e·no·mat·ous pol·y·po·sis (FAP) (fă-mil′ē-ăl ad′ĕ-nō′mă-tŭs pol′i-pō′sis) Polyposis of the colon that usually begins in childhood; polyps increase in number, causing symptoms of chronic colitis; pigmented retinal lesions are frequently found; carcinoma of the colon almost invariably develops in untreated cases; autosomal dominant inheritance, caused by mutation in the adenomatous polyposis coli gene (APC) on 5q. In Gardner syndrome, which is allelic to FAP, there are extracolonic changes (desmoid tumors, osteomas, jaw cysts). SYN adenomatous polyposis coli, familial polyposis coli.

fa·mil·i·al ag·gre·ga·tion (fă-mil′ē-ăl ag′rĕ-gā′shŭn) Occurrence of a trait in more members of a family than can be readily accounted for by chance; presumptive but not cogent evidence of the operation of genetic factors.

fa·mil·i·al a·min·o·gly·co·side o·to·tox·i·ci·ty (fă-mil′ē-ăl ă-mē′nō-glī′kō-sīd ō′tō-tok-sis′i-tē) Inherited susceptibility to sensory hearing loss on administration of aminoglycoside antibiotics due to a mutation in the mitochondrial genome.

fa·mil·i·al am·y·loid neu·rop·a·thy (fă-mil′ē-ăl am′i-loyd nūr-op′ă-thē) A disorder in which various peripheral nerves are infiltrated with amyloid and their functions disturbed, an abnormal prealbumin is also formed and is present in the blood; characteristically, it begins during midlife and is found largely in people of Portuguese descent; autosomal dominant inheritance. Other rare clinical types occur.

fa·mil·i·al dys·au·to·no·mi·a (fă-mil′ē-ăl dis′aw-tō-nō′mē-ă) A congenital syndrome with aberrations in autonomic nervous system function such as indifference to pain, diminished lacrimation, poor vasomotor homeostasis, motor incoordination, labile cardiovascular reactions, hyporeflexia, frequent attacks of bronchial pneumonia, hypersalivation with aspiration and difficulty in swallowing, hyperemesis, emotional instability, and an intolerance for anesthetics.

fa·mil·i·al e·ryth·ro·pha·go·cy·tic lym·pho·his·ti·o·cy·to·sis (FEL) (fă-mil′ē-ăl ă-rith′rō-făg′ō-sit′ik lim′fō-his′tē-ō-sī-tō′sis) SYN familial hemophagocytic lymphohistiocytosis.

fa·mil·i·al fat-in·duced hy·per·li·pe·mi·a (fă-mil′ē-ăl fat′in-dūst′ hī′pĕr-li-pē′mē-ă) SYN type I familial hyperlipoproteinemia.

fa·mil·i·al goi·ter (fă-mil′ē-ăl goy′tĕr) A group of heritable thyroid disorders in which goiter is commonly apparent first during childhood; often associated with skeletal or mental retardation, and with other signs of hypothyroidism that may develop with age.

fa·mil·i·al he·mo·pha·go·cy·tic lymph·o·his·ti·o·cy·to·sis (FMLH) (fă-mil′ē-ăl hē′mō-făg′ō-sit′ik lim′fō-his′tē-ō-sī-tō′sis) An extremely rare, usually fatal disease of childhood characterized by multiorgan infiltration with activated macrophages and lymphocytes. The disease is often familial and appears to be inherited as an autosomal recessive trait. SYN familial erythrophagocytic lymphohistiocytosis.

fa·mil·i·al hy·per·cho·les·ter·ol·e·mi·a (fă-mil′ē-ăl, hī′pĕr-kŏ-les′tĕr-ol-ē′mē-ă) SYN type II familial hyperlipoproteinemia.

fa·mil·i·al hy·per·cho·les·ter·ol·e·mi·a with hy·per·li·pe·mi·a (fă-mil′ē-ăl hī′pĕr-kŏ-les′tĕr-ol-ē′mē-ă hī′pĕr-li-pē′mē-ă) SYN type III familial hyperlipoproteinemia.

fa·mil·i·al hy·per·chy·lo·mi·cro·ne·mi·a (fă-mil′ē-ăl hī′pĕr-kī′lō-mī′krō-nē′mē-ă) SYN type I familial hyperlipoproteinemia.

fa·mi·li·al hy·per·lip·o·pro·tein·e·mi·a (fă-mil′ē-ăl, hī′pĕr-lip′ō-prō-tēn-ē′mē-ă) A group of diseases characterized by changes in concentration of β-lipoproteins and pre-β-lipoproteins and the lipids associated with them.

fa·mil·i·al hy·per·tri·glyc·er·i·de·mi·a (fă-mil′ē-ăl hī′pĕr-trī-glis′ĕr-i-dē′mē-ă) **1.** SYN type I familial hyperlipoproteinemia. **2.** SYN type IV familial hyperlipoproteinemia.

fa·mil·i·al hy·per·tro·phic car·di·o·my·op·a·thy (fă-mil′ē-ăl hī′pĕr-trō′fik kahr′dē-ō-mī-op′ă-thē) Familial form of hypertrophic cardiomyopathy.

fa·mil·i·al jaun·dice (fă-mil′ē-ăl jawn′dis) SYN hereditary spherocytosis.

fa·mil·i·al non·he·mo·lyt·ic jaun·dice (fă-mil′ē-ăl non′hē-mō-lit′ik jawn′dis) Mild form of the hepatic disorder due to increased amounts of unconjugated bilirubin in the plasma without evidence of liver damage, biliary obstruction, or hemolysis; thought to be due to an inborn error of metabolism in which the excretion of bilirubin by the liver is defective. SYN Gilbert disease.

fa·mil·i·al par·ox·ys·mal pol·y·ser·o·si·tis (fă-mil′ē-ăl păr-ok-siz′măl pol′ē-sēr′ō-sī′tis) Transient recurring attacks of abdominal pain, fever, pleurisy, arthritis, and rash; the condition is asymptomatic between attacks.

fa·mil·i·al par·tial lip·o·dys·tro·phy (fă-mil′ē-ăl pahr′shăl lip′ō-dis′trŏ-fē) Characterized by symmetric lipoatrophy of the trunk and limbs but the face is spared; with full rounded face, xanthomata, acanthosis nigricans, and insulin-resistant hyperglycemia; fat accumulates around the neck, shoulders, and genitalia. SYN Kobberling-Dunnigan syndrome.

fa·mil·i·al pe·ri·od·ic pa·ral·y·sis (fă-mil′ē-ăl pĕr′ē-od′ik păr-al′i-sis) Inherited muscle disorder manifested as recurrent episodes of marked generalized weakness. SEE hyperkalemic periodic paralysis, hypokalemic periodic paralysis, normokalemic periodic paralysis.

fa·mil·i·al pol·yp·o·sis co·li (fă-mil′ē-ăl pol′i-pō′sis kō′lī) SYN familial adenomatous polyposis.

fa·mil·i·al pseu·do·in·flam·ma·to·ry mac·u·lar de·gen·er·a·tion (fă-mil′ē-ăl sū′dō-in-flam′ă-tōr-ē mak′yŭ-lăr dĕ-jen′ĕr-ā′shŭn) Macular degeneration that occurs during the fifth decade of life, with sudden development of a central scotoma in one eye followed rapidly by a similar lesion in the opposite eye. SYN Sorsby macular degeneration.

fa·mil·i·al screen·ing (fă-mil′ē-ăl skrēn′ing) Examination directed at close relatives of probands with diseases that may lie latent, as in age-dependent dominant traits, or that may involve risk to progeny, as in X-linked traits.

fam·i·ly (fam′i-lē) **1.** A group of two or more people linked by blood, adoptive, or marital ties, or the common-law equivalent. **2.** In biologic classification, a taxonomic grouping at the level intermediate between the order and the tribe or genus. **3.** A group of substances closely related structurally. **4.** A group of proteins with characteristic sequence, pharmacologic, and/or signaling profiles. [L. *familia*]

fam·i·ly-cen·tered care (fam′i-lē-sen′tĕrd kār) The application of services, therapies, and interventions that are based on the concerns and priorities of the family and not primarily on establishing diagnosis.

fam·i·ly his·to·ry (fam′i-lē his′tŏr-ē) A written documentation made after questioning the patient about the presence or absence of diseases or conditions that might have an effect on the health of the patient (e.g., coronary disease, alcoholism, diabetes mellitus). Use generally involves a form filled out by a new patient (or surrogate) during intake.

fam·i·ly med·i·cine (fam′i-lē med′ĭ-sin) The medical specialty concerned with providing continuous comprehensive care to all age groups, from first patient contact to terminal care, with special emphasis on care of the family as a unit.

fam·i·ly nurs·ing (fam′i-lē nŭrs′ing) A nursing specialty concerned with understanding people's experiences of health and illness within the context of their family. (The term family is defined by the patient.) Nurses collaborate with families to create situations that reduce and alleviate emotional, physical, and spiritual suffering from illness.

fam·i·ly prac·tice (fam′i-lē prak′tis) A specialty of medicine in which the physician takes responsibility for the health and medical care of all members of a family group, regardless of age or gender, but usually does limited amounts of obstetrics and surgery.

fam·i·ly prac·tice phy·si·cian (fam′i-lē prak′tis fi-zish′ŭn) The trained health care professional who attends most of the needs of her patients through diagnosis to pharmacotherapy. Previously, the first caregiver seen by patients.

fam·i·ly ther·a·py (fam′i-lē thār′ă-pē) A type of group psychotherapy in which a family in conflict meets as a group with the therapist to explore its relationships and processes; focus is on the resolution of current issues between members rather than on individual members.

Fan·co·ni a·ne·mi·a (fahn-kō′nē ă-nē′mē-ă) A type of idiopathic refractory anemia characterized by pancytopenia, hypoplasia of the bone marrow, and congenital anomalies, occurring in members of the same family (an autosomal recessive trait in at least five nonallelic types); the anemia is normocytic or slightly macrocytic, macrocytes and target cells may be found in the circulating blood, and the leukopenia usually is due to neutropenia. Congenital anomalies include short stature; microcephaly; hypogenitalism; strabismus; anomalies of the thumbs, radii, kidneys, and urinary tract; mental retardation; and microphthalmia. SYN Fanconi syndrome (1).

Fan·co·ni syn·drome (fahn-kō′nē sin′drōm) **1.** SYN Fanconi anemia. **2.** A group of conditions with characteristic disorders of renal tubular function, which may be classified as: cystinosis, an autosomal recessive disease of early childhood; adult Fanconi syndrome, a rare hereditary form, probably due to a recessive gene different from that found in cystinosis, characterized by the tubular malfunction seen in cystinosis and by osteomalacia, but without cystine deposit in tissues; acquired Fanconi syndrome, which may be associated with multiple myeloma or may result from chemical poisoning, injury, or persisting damage of proximal tubular epithelium due to various causes, leading to multiple defects of tubular function.

fan·ta·sy (fan′tă-sē) Imagery that is more or less coherent, as in dreams and daydreams, yet unrestricted by reality. SYN phantasia. [G. *phantasia*, idea, image]

FAP Abbreviation for familial adenomatous polyposis.

F.A.P.E. Abbreviation for free appropriate public education. SEE ALSO IDEA.

Fa·ra·beuf am·pu·ta·tion (fahr′ă-buf amp′yū-tā′shŭn) **1.** Surgical removal of the leg, the flap being large and on the outer side; **2.** Surgical removal of the foot; disarticulation of the foot through the subtalar joint and the talonavicular joint.

Fa·ra·beuf tri·an·gle (fahr′ă-buf trī′ang-gĕl) The area formed by the internal jugular and facial veins and the hypoglossal nerve.

far·ad (F) (fahr′ăd) A practical unit of electrical capacity; the capacity of a condenser having a charge of 1 coulomb under an electromotive force of 1 volt. [M. *Faraday*]

far·a·day (F, *F*) (far′ă-dā) 96,485.309 coulombs per mole, the amount of electricity required to reduce one equivalent of a monovalent ion. [M. *Faraday*]

Far·a·day con·stant (*F*) (far′ă-dā kon′stănt) SEE faraday.

Far·a·day ef·fect (far′ă-dā e-fekt′) Result of planar rotation of polarized light seen when solutions are placed in a magnetic field.

Far·a·day laws (far′ă-dā lawz) **1.** The amount of an electrolyte decomposed by an electric current is proportional to the amount of the current; **2.** When the same current is passed through several electrolytes, the amounts of the different substances decomposed are proportional to their chemical equivalents.

far-and-near su·ture (fahr′-and-nēr sū′chŭr) A suture consisting of alternate near and far stitches, used to approximate fascial edges.

far·del (fahr′del) The total measurable penalty that is incurred as a result of the occurrence of a genetic disease in one individual; one of two major quantitative considerations in the prognostic aspects of genetic counseling, the other being risk of occurrence. [M.E., fr. O. Fr., fr. Ar. *fardah*, bundle]

far in·fra·red (fahr in′fră-red) Portion of light spectrum between 1500 and 12,500 nm.

farm·er's lung (far′mĕrz lŭng) A hypersensitivity pneumonitis characterized by fever and dyspnea, caused by inhalation of organic dust from moldy hay containing spores of actinomycetes and certain true fungi, which may thrive in the elevated temperatures of hay lofts and silos.

far point (fahr poynt) That point in conjugate focus with the retina when the eye is not accommodating.

Far·rant mount·ing flu·id (far′ănt mownt′ing flū′id) An aqueous solution containing gum arabic, arsenic trioxide, glycerol, and water, used in mounting histologic sections directly from water; some modifications involve addition of potassium acetate to bring the pH up to neutrality and substitution of other preservatives like cresol or thymol for arsenic trioxide.

Farr laws (fahr lawz) A set of mathematical formulas, axioms, and laws first enunciated in the annual reports submitted by William Farr to the Registrar General of England and Wales from 1839–1883. The laws deal with the relationship of incidence to prevalence, the natural history of epidemics, and mathematic features of common types of epidemic.

Farr test (fahr test) Measures capacity of radiolabeled antigen to bind with antibody (which is precipitated using ammonium sulfate); can be used for all classes of immunoglobulin.

far·sight·ed·ness (fahr′sīt′ĕd-nĕs) SYN hyperopia.

fart·lek train·ing (fahrt′lek trān′ing) Relatively unstructured interval-type training for aerobic fitness; consists of alternating intervals of fast- and slow-paced training over natural terrain (usually hilly countryside). SYN speed play. [Swed. *fart*, speed, + *lek*, play]

far ul·tra·vi·o·let (fahr ul′tră-vī′ŏ-lĕt) Portion of light spectrum between 180–290 nm.

FAS Abbreviation for fetal alcohol syndrome.

Fas (fas) A receptor present in cells that binds with Fas ligand to induce apoptosis. SEE ALSO Fas ligand.

i fas·ci·a, pl. **fas·ci·ae** (fash′ē-ă, fash′ē-ē) [TA] A sheet of fibrous tissue that envelops the body beneath the skin; it also encloses muscles and groups of muscles, and separates their several layers or groups. See this page. [L. a band or fillet]

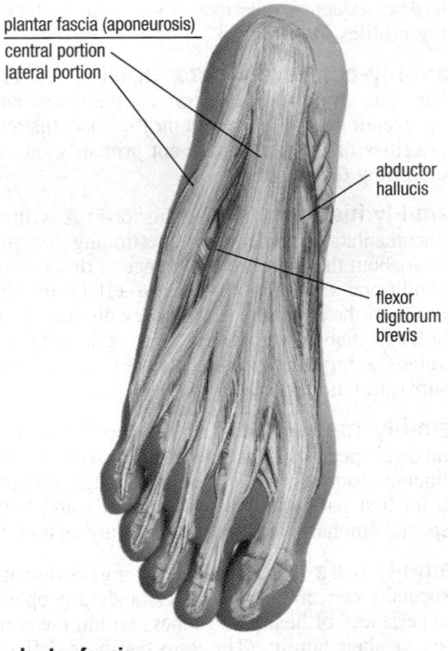

plantar fascia

fas·ci·a ad·he·rens (fash′ē-ă ad-hē′renz) A broad intercellular junction in the intercalated disc of cardiac muscle that anchors actin filaments.

fas·ci·a graft (fash′ē-ă graft) A graft of fibrous tissue, usually the fascia lata.

fas·ci·al (fash′ē-ăl) Relating to any fascia.

fas·ci·al sheath of eye·ball (fash′ē-ăl shēth

ī′bawl) A condensation of connective tissue on the outer aspect of the sclera from which it is separated by a narrow cleftlike episcleral space; the sheath is attached to the sclera near the sclerocorneal junction and blends with the fascia of the extraocular muscles. SYN Tenon capsule.

fas•ci•a mus•cu•li quad•ra•ti lum•bor•um (fash′ē-ă mŭs′kyū-lī kwah-drā′tī lŭm-bō′rŭm) SYN anterior layer of thoracolumbar fascia.

fas•ci•a pe•ri•ne•i su•per•fi•ci•a•lis (fash′ē-ă per-in′ē-ī sū-pĕr-fish-ē-ā′lis) [TA] SYN superficial fascia of perineum.

fas•ci•a sub•per•i•to•ne•a•lis (fash′ē-ă sŭb-per-i-tō-nē-ā′lis) [TA] SYN extraperitoneal fascia.

fas•ci•cle (fas′i-kĕl) A band or bundle of fibers, usually of muscle or nerve fibers; a nerve fiber tract. SYN fasciculus (1) [TA].

fas•cic•u•lar (fă-sik′yū-lăr) Relating to a fasciculus; arranged in the form of a bundle or collection of rods.

fas•cic•u•lar de•gen•er•a•tion (fă-sik′yū-lăr dĕ-jen′ĕr-ā′shŭn) Muscular degeneration due to loss of motor neurons in the spinal cord or brainstem.

fas•cic•u•lar graft (fă-sik′yū-lăr graft) A nerve graft in which each bundle of fibers is approximated and sutured separately.

fas•cic•u•la•tion (fă-sik′yū-lā′shŭn) **1.** An arrangement in the form of fasciculi. **2.** Involuntary contractions, or twitchings, of groups (fasciculi) of muscle fibers, a coarser form of muscular contraction than fibrillation.

fas•cic•u•li (fa-sik′yū-lī) Plural of fasciculus.

fas•cic•u•li pro•pri•i (fă-sik′yū-lī prō′prē-ī) [TA] Flechsig fasciculi or ground bundles (fasciculus anterior proprius and fasciculus lateralis proprius or lateral ground bundle); intersegmental fasciculi; ascending and descending association fiber systems of the spinal cord that lie deep in the anterior, lateral, and posterior funiculi adjacent to the gray matter. SYN ground bundles.

fas•cic•u•lus, gen. and pl. **fas•cic•u•li** (fă-sik′kyū-lŭs, -yū-lī) [TA] **1.** SYN fascicle. **2.** SYN cord (1). **3.** [TA] SYN bundle. [L. dim. of *fascis,* bundle]

fas•cic•u•lus lon•gi•tu•di•na•lis in•fe•ri•or (fă-sik′yū-lus lon-ji-tū-di-nā′lis in-fēr′ē-ŏr) [TA] SYN inferior longitudinal fasciculus.

fas•cic•u•lus lon•gi•tu•di•na•lis su•pe•ri•or (fă-sik′yū-lus lon-ji-tū-di-nā′lis sŭ-pēr′ē-ŏr) [TA] SYN superior longitudinal fasciculus.

fas•ci•ec•to•my (fash-ē-ek′tŏ-mē) Excision of strips of fascia. [fascia + G. *ektomē,* excision]

fas•ci•i•tis (fash-ē-ī′tis) **1.** Inflammation in fascia. **2.** Reactive proliferation of fibroblasts in fascia.

♻**fascio-** Prefix indicating a fascia. [L. *fascia,* a band or fillet]

fas•ci•od•e•sis (fash-ē-od′ĕ-sis) Surgical attachment of a fascia to another fascia or a tendon. [fascio- + G. *desis,* a binding together]

fas•ci•o•la, pl. **fas•ci•o•lae** (fă′shē-ō′lă, fă′shē-ō′lē) A small band or group of fibers. [L. dim. of *fascia,* band, fillet]

fas•ci•o•lar (fă-sī′ō-lăr) Relating to the gyrus fasciolaris.

fas•ci•o•plas•ty (fash′ē-ō-plas-tē) Plastic surgery of a fascia. [fascia + G. *plastos,* formed]

fas•ci•or•rha•phy (fash′ē-ōr′ă-fē) Suture of a fascia or aponeurosis. SYN aponeurorrhaphy. [fascio- + G. *rhaphē,* suture]

fas•ci•ot•o•my (fash′ē-ot′ŏ-mē) Incision through a fascia; used in the treatment of certain vascular disorders and injuries when marked swelling is anticipated, which could compromise blood flow; fasciotomy may be combined with embolectomy in the treatment of acute arterial embolism. [fascio- + G. *tomē,* incision]

Fas li•gand (fas lī′gand) A molecule on the surface of cytotoxic T cells that binds to its receptor, Fas, on the surface of other cells, initiating apoptosis in the target cell. SEE ALSO Fas.

Fas re•cep•tor (fas rĕ-sep′tŏr) SEE Fas.

fast (fast) **1.** Durable; resistant to change; applied to stained microorganisms that cannot be decolorized. SEE ALSO acid-fast. **2.** Abstinence from ingesting food. [A.S. *foest,* firm, fixed]

fast com•po•nent of ny•stag•mus (fast kŏm-pō′nĕnt nis-tag′mŭs) Compensatory movement of the eyes in the vestibuloocular reflex.

fast gly•co•lyt•ic (FG) fi•bers (fast glī′kō-lit′ik fī′bĕrz) SYN fast-twitch fibers.

fas•tid•i•ous (fas-tid′ē-ŭs) BACTERIOLOGY having complex nutritional requirements.

fas•tig•i•al nu•cle•us (fas-tij′ē-ăl nū′klē-ŭs) The most medial of the cerebellar nuclei, lying medial to the interpositus nucleus, near the midline, in the white matter underneath the vermis of the cerebellar cortex. It receives the axons of Purkinje cells from all parts of the vermis. Its major projection is to the vestibular nuclei and medullary reticular formation.

fas•tig•i•um (fas-tij′ē-ŭm) **1.** [TA] Apex of the roof of the fourth ventricle of the brain, an angle formed by the anterior and posterior medullary vela extending into the substance of the vermis. **2.** The acme or period of full development of a disease. [L. top, as of a gable; a pointed extremity]

fast•ing blood sug•ar (fast′ing blŭd shug′ăr) SYN fasting plasma glucose.

fast•ing plas•ma glu•cose (FPG) (fast′ing

plaz′mă glū′kōs) Blood levels of the substance measured after patient has not eaten for a given duration; generally assessed by phlebotomy first thing in the morning. SYN fasting blood sugar.

fast-neu·tron ra·di·a·tion ther·a·py (fast-nū′tron rā′dē-ā′shŭn thār′ă-pē) Radiation therapy using high-energy neutrons from cyclotrons or proton accelerators.

fast-ox·i·da·tive-gly·co·lyt·ic (FOG) fi·bers (fast-oks′i-dā-tive-glī′kō-lit′ik fī′bĕrz) SYN fast-twitch fibers.

fast smear (fast smēr) A cytologic smear containing material from the vaginal pool and pancervical scrapings, mixed and prepared on one microscopic slide, smeared, and fixed immediately; used principally for routine screening of ovaries, endometrium, cervix, vagina, and hormonal states.

fast-twitch fi·bers (fast-twich fī′bĕrz) Histologically distinct skeletal muscle fibers that generate energy rapidly and are active in quick, powerful actions; subclassified as types IIa and IIb. SYN fast glycolytic (FG) fibers, fast-oxidative-glycolytic (FOG) fibers, Type II fibers.

fat (fat) **1.** SYN adipose tissue. **2.** Common colloquial term for obese. **3.** A greasy, soft-solid material, found in animal tissues and many plants, composed of a mixture of glycerol esters; together with oils they make up the homolipids. **4.** A triacylglycerol or a mixture of triacylglycerols. [A.S. *faet*]

fa·tal (fā′tăl) Pertaining to or causing death; denoting especially inevitability or inescapability of death. [L. *fatalis*, of or belonging to fate]

fa·tal·i·ty rate (fă-tal′i-tē rāt) The death rate observed in a designated series of people affected by a simultaneous event such as a disaster.

fat cell (fat sel) A connective tissue cell distended with one or more fat globules, the cytoplasm usually being compressed into a thin envelope, with the nucleus at one point in the periphery. SYN adipocyte, adipose cell.

fat cell the·o·ry (fat sel thē′ŏr-ē) Proposal that the number and size of the fat cells determines the quantity of fat stored.

fat em·bo·lism (fat em′bŏ-lizm) The occurrence of fat globules in the circulation following fractures of a long bone, in burns, in parturition, and in association with fatty degeneration of the liver; the emboli most commonly block pulmonary or cerebral vessels when symptoms referable to either or both of these regions appear.

fat-free (fat-frē′) A product so labeled contains, by F.D.A. order, less than 0.5 g fat per serving.

fat-free bod·y mass (FFM) (fat′frē bod′ē mas) Body mass devoid of storage fat; a theoretic entity that contains the small percentage of non-sex-specific essential fat equivalent to approximately 3% of body mass (located chiefly within the central nervous system, bone marrow, and internal organs). SYN lean body mass.

fat·i·ga·bil·i·ty (fat′i-gă-bil′i-tē) A condition in which fatigue is easily induced.

fa·tigue (fă-tēg′) **1.** That state, following a period of mental or bodily activity, characterized by a lessened capacity for work and reduced efficiency of accomplishment, usually accompanied by a feeling of weariness, sleepiness, or irritability; may also supervene when, from any cause, energy expenditure outstrips restorative processes and may be confined to a single organ. **2.** Sensation of boredom and lassitude due to absence of stimulation, monotony, or lack of interest in one's surroundings. [Fr., fr. L. *fatigo*, to tire]

fa·tigue fe·ver (fă-tēg′ fē′vĕr) A benign fever and muscle pain caused by accumulation of metabolites following overexertion.

fa·tigue frac·ture (fă-tēg′ frak′shŭr) Breakage that occurs in bone subjected to repetitive stress; most often transverse in configuration. See page B25. SYN stress fracture.

fa·tigue state (fă-tēg′ stāt) Exhaustion or loss of strength and/or endurance following a strenuous activity.

fat mass (fat mas) That portion of the human body that is composed strictly of fat (as opposed to fat-free mass).

fat ne·cro·sis (fat nĕ-krō′sis) The death of adipose tissue, characterized by the formation of small (1–4 mm), dull, chalky, gray or white foci. SYN steatonecrosis.

fat-pad, fat pad (fat-pad, fat pad) An accumulation of somewhat encapsulated adipose tissue.

fat-sol·u·ble vi·ta·mins (fat-sol′yū-bĕl vī-tă′minz) Those vitamins, soluble in fat solvents (nonpolar solvents) and relatively insoluble in water, marked in chemical structure by the presence of large hydrocarbon moieties in the molecule (e.g., vitamins A, D, E, K).

fat-stor·ing cell (fat-stōr′ing sel) A multilocular fat-filled cell present in the perisinusoidal space in the liver. SYN lipocyte.

fat sub·sti·tutes (fat sŭb′sti-tūts) Substances that have some of the same properties as fat but are not recognized by the body as such and are thereby not absorbed.

fat tide (fat tīd) An increase in the fat content of blood and lymph following a meal.

fat·ty (fat′ē) Oily or greasy; relating in any sense to fat.

fat·ty ac·id (fat′ē as′id) Any acid derived from fats by hydrolysis (e.g., oleic, palmitic, or stearic acids); any long-chain monobasic organic acid;

they accumulate in disorders associated with the peroxisomes.

fat·ty ac·id–bind·ing pro·tein (fat′ē as′id-bīnd′ing prō′tēn) SYN Z-protein.

fat·ty ac·id ox·i·da·tion cy·cle (fat′ē as′id oks′i-dā′shŭn sī′kĕl) A series of reactions involving acyl-coenzyme A compounds; the major pathway of fatty acid catabolism in living tissue. SEE ALSO beta (β)-oxidation.

fat·ty cir·rho·sis (fat′ē sir-ō′sis) Early nutritional cirrhosis, especially in people with alcoholism, in which the liver is enlarged by fatty change, with mild fibrosis.

fat·ty de·gen·er·a·tion (fat′ē dĕ-jen′ĕr-ā′shŭn) Abnormal formation of microscopically visible droplets of fat in the cytoplasm of cells, as a result of injury. SYN adipose degeneration, steatosis (2).

fat·ty heart (fat′ē hahrt) **1.** Fatty degeneration of the myocardium. **2.** Accumulation of adipose tissue on the external surface of the heart with occasional infiltration of fat between the muscle bundles of the heart wall. SYN adiposis cardiaca, cor adiposum.

fat·ty her·ni·a (fat′ē hĕr′nē-ă) SYN pannicular hernia.

fat·ty in·fil·tra·tion (fat′ē in′fil-trā′shŭn) Abnormal accumulation of fat droplets in the cytoplasm of cells, particularly of fat derived from outside the cells. SEE ALSO fatty degeneration.

fat·ty kid·ney (fat′ē kid′nē) A kidney in which there is fatty metamorphosis of the parenchymal cells, especially fatty degeneration.

fat·ty liv·er (fat′ē liv′ĕr) Yellow discoloration of the liver due to fatty degeneration of liver parenchymal cells.

fat·ty met·a·mor·pho·sis (fat′ē met′ă-mōr′fō-sis) The appearance of microscopically visible droplets of fat in the cytoplasm of cells. SEE ALSO fatty degeneration.

fat·ty oil (fat′ē oyl) An oil derived from both animals and plants; chemically, a glyceride of a fatty acid that is converted into a soap by substitution of the glycerine with an alkaline base; a fatty oil, in contrast to a volatile oil, is permanent and not capable of distillation.

fau·ces, gen. **fau·ci·um** (faw′sēz, -sē-ŭm) [TA] The space between the cavity of the mouth and the pharynx, bounded by the soft palate and the base of the tongue. [L. the throat]

fau·cial (faw′shăl) Relating to the fauces.

fau·cial ton·sil (faw′shăl ton′sil) SYN palatine tonsil.

faul·ty un·ion (fawl′tē yūn′yŭn) SYN fibrous union. SEE ALSO vicious union.

fau·na (faw′nă) The animal forms of a continent, district, locality, or habitat. [Mod. L. application of *Fauna,* sister of *Faunus,* a rural deity]

fa·ve·o·late (fă-vē′ō-lāt) Pitted.

fa·ve·o·lus, pl. **fa·ve·o·li** (fă-vē-ō′lus, -lī) A small pit or depression. [Mod. L. dim. of *favus,* honeycomb]

fa·vid (fā′vid) An allergic reaction in the skin observed in patients who have favus, which is a type of tinea capitis.

fa·vism (fā′vizm) An acute condition seen following the ingestion of certain species of beans, e.g., *Vicia faba,* or inhalation of the pollen of its flower, in patients with genetic erythrocytic deficiency of glucose 6-phosphate dehydrogenase; characterized by fever, headache, abdominal pain, severe anemia, prostration, and coma. [Ital. *favismo,* from *fava,* bean]

Fav·re dys·tro·phy (fahv′rĕ dis′trŏ-fē) SYN vitreotapetoretinal dystrophy.

Fav·re-Ra·cou·chot dis·ease (fahv′rĕ-rah-kū-shō′ di-zēz′) Comedones developing on sun-damaged skin due to obstruction of pilosebaceous follicles by solar elastosis. SYN solar comedo.

fa·vus (fā′vŭs) A severe type of chronic ringworm of the scalp and nails; it occurs more frequently in Mediterranean countries, southeastern Europe, southern Asia, and northern Africa. Differences in severity are related to hygiene. [L. honeycomb]

Fa·zi·o-Londe dis·ease (fahz′ē-ō-lōnd′ di-zēz′) A progressive bulbar palsy affecting the brainstem; due to motor neuron degeneration; a variant of spinal muscular atrophy.

FBS Abbreviation for fasting blood sugar.

FCA Abbreviation for U.S. False Claims Act.

FCE Abbreviation for functional capacity evaluation.

Fc frag·ment, **Fc** (frag′mĕnt) The crystallizable fragment of an immunoglobulin molecule composed of part of the heavy chains and responsible for binding to antibody receptors on cells and the Clq component of complement.

F.D.A., **FDA** Abbreviation for U.S. Food and Drug Administration of the U.S. Department of Health and Human Services.

F.D.A. clas·si·fi·ca·tion of med·i·cal de·vi·ces (klas′i-fi-kā′shŭn med′i-kăl dĕ-vīs′ĕz) An assessment instrument of health care implants and procedures based on use of legal and ethical controlled experiments formulated by the U.S. Food and Drug Administration.

F.D.I. den·tal no·men·cla·ture (den′tăl nō′mĕn-klā-chŭr) A system of identifying teeth; used worldwide, which identifies each dental quadrant (1–4 for the permanent teeth and 5–8 for the deciduous teeth) and each tooth with a number indicating its location from the midline; e.g., 36 is the lower left first permanent molar and 62 is the upper left deciduous lateral incisor; devised by the Fédération Dentaire Internationale (International Dental Federation). SEE ALSO Palmer dental nomenclature, universal dental nomenclature.

Fe Symbol for iron. [L. *ferrum,* iron]

fear (fēr) Apprehension; dread; alarm; by having an identifiable stimulus, fear is differentiated from anxiety, which has no easily identifiable stimulus. [A.S. *faer*]

feath•er edge (fedh′ĕr ej) The thinnest area of a blood smear, where the differential count is performed.

feb•ri•fuge (feb′ri-fyūzh) A substance that reduces fever.

feb•rile (feb′ril) Denoting or relating to fever. SYN feverish (1), pyretic.

feb•rile con•vul•sion (feb′ril kŏn-vŭl′shŭn) A brief seizure, lasting less than 15 minutes, seen in a neurologically normal infant or young child, associated with fever.

feb•rile de•lir•i•um (feb′ril dĕ-lir′ē-ŭm) An acute reversible state of confusion as a result of a high body temperature.

fe•cal (fē′kăl) Relating to feces. SYN faecal.

fe•cal ab•scess (fē′kăl ab′ses) SYN stercoral abscess. SYN faecal abscess.

fe•cal con•cen•tra•tion (fē′kăl kon′sĕn-trā′shŭn) Preparation using centrifugation and either flotation or sedimentation methods to separate parasitic elements from fecal debris. SYN faecal concentration.

fe•cal ex•am•i•na•tion (fē′kăl eg-zam′i-nā′shŭn) Microscopic review of direct wet mounts, concentration methods, and permanent stained smears to recover and identify parasites from stool specimens. SYN faecal examination.

fe•cal fat test (fē′kăl fat test) Laboratory-based measurement of lipid matter in stool to determine disorders.

fe•cal fis•tu•la (fē′kăl fis′chū-lă) SYN intestinal fistula. SYN faecal fistula.

fe•ca•lith (fē′kă-lith) SYN coprolith. SYN faecalith. [L. *faeces,* feces, + G. *lithos,* stone]

fe•cal•oid (fē′kă-loyd) Resembling feces. SYN faecaloid. [L. *faeces,* feces, + G. *eidos,* resemblance]

fe•ca•lo•ma (fē′kă-lō′mă) SYN coproma. SYN faecaloma.

fe•ca•lu•ri•a (fē′kăl-yūr′ē-ă) The commingling of feces with urine passed from the urethra in people with a fistula connecting the intestinal tract and bladder. SYN faecaluria. [L. *faeces,* feces, + G. *ouron,* urine]

fe•cal vom•it•ing (fē′kăl vom′it-ing) Vomitus with appearance or odor of feces suggestive of long-standing distal small-bowel or colonic obstruction. SYN copremesis, faecal vomiting, stercoraceous vomiting.

fe•ces (fē′sēz) The matter discharged from the bowel during defecation, consisting of the undigested residue of food, epithelium, intestinal mucus, bacteria, and waste material from the food. SYN faeces, stercus. [L., pl. of *faex* (*faec-*), dregs]

Fech•ner-Web•er law (fek′ner vā′ber law) SYN Weber-Fechner law.

fec•u•lent (fek′yū-lĕnt) Foul. [L. *faeculentus,* full of excrement, fr. *faeces,* dregs, feces]

fe•cund (fē′kŭnd) SYN fertile (1). [L. *fecundus,* fruitful]

fec•un•da•tion (fē′kŭn-dā′shŭn) The act of rendering fertile. SEE ALSO fertilization.

fe•cun•di•ty (fē′kŭn′di-tē) The ability to produce live offspring.

feed•back (fēd′bak) **1.** In a given system, the return, as input, of some of the output, as a regulatory mechanism (e.g., regulation of a furnace by a thermostat). **2.** An explanation for the learning of motor skills: sensory stimuli set up by muscle contractions modulate the activity of the motor system. **3.** The feeling evoked by another person's reaction to oneself. SEE biofeedback.

feed•back in•hi•bi•tion (fēd′bak in′hi-bish′ŭn) Inhibition of activity by an end product of the pathway of which that activity is a part. SYN feedback mechanism.

feed•back mech•an•ism (fēd′bak mek′ă-nizm) SYN feedback inhibition.

feed•ing (fēd′ing) Giving food or nourishment.

feed•ing tube (fēd′ing tūb) A flexible tube passed through the oral pharynx and into the esophagus and stomach, through which liquid food is fed.

fee-for-ser•vice (fē-fōr-sĕr′vis) Payment made at the time of health care service; the amount varies according to the provider's estimate of the costs involved.

fee-for-ser•vice in•sur•ance (fē-fōr-sĕr′vis in-shŭr′ăns) Coverage in the U.S. that reimburses participants and providers following submission of a claim. Participants have few, if any, restrictions on which hospitals or doctors to use.

Feer dis•ease (făr di-zēz′) SYN acrodynia (2).

FEES (fēz) Acronym and abbreviation for fiberoptic endoscopic examination of swallowing.

fee sched•ule (fē skej′ūl) A listing of the fees normally charged by a given health care provider for specific therapies and procedures provided.

FEF Abbreviation for forced expiratory flow.

Fein•gold di•et (fīn′gōld dī′ĕt) A dietary regimen postulated to reduce hyperkinetic behavior in attention deficit hyperactivity disorder; eliminates patient's ingestion of salicylates, preservatives, and artificial colors and flavors.

Fein•gold the•o•ry (fīn′gōld thē′ŏr-ē) Food additives and colors may cause hyperactivity in children; some studies have suggested that these substances may play a role in 5% of patients with attention deficit hyperactivity disorder.

Feiss line (fīs līn) A line from the medial malleolus to the plantar aspect of the first metatarsophalangeal joint, used to measure pronation of the foot during weight bearing.

FEL (fel) Abbreviation and acronym for familial erythrophagocytic lymphohistiocytosis.

Fel•den•krais meth•od (fel′den-krīs meth′ŏd) Series of gentle low-impact exercises to retard loss of muscle mass and movement; intended for older patients or those recovering from surgical procedures or hospitalization.

fe•line in•fec•tious a•ne•mi•a (FIA) (fē′līn in-fek′shŭs ă-nē′mē-ă) An acute or chronic anemia of domestic cats caused by the rickettsia *Haemobartonella felis*.

fel•la•ti•o (fĕ-lā′shē-ō) Oral stimulation of the penis. [L.]

fel•on (fel′ŏn) A purulent infection or abscess involving the bulbous distal end of a finger. SYN whitlow. [M.E. *feloun*, malignant]

fel•on herb (fel′ŏn ĕrb) SYN carline thistle.

fel•on•wort (fel′ŏn-wōrt) SYN celandine.

felt•work (felt′wŏrk) **1.** A fibrous network. **2.** A close plexus of nerve fibrils. SEE neuropil.

fe•male (fē′māl) ZOOLOGY denoting the gender that produces oocytes (or ova) and thus bears the young.

fe•male ath•lete tri•ad (fē′māl ath′lēt trī′ad) A combination of disordered eating, amenorrhea, and osteoporosis, commonly seen in adolescent and young adult female athletes. SYN female triad.

fe•male cath•e•ter (fē′māl kath′ĕ-tĕr) A short, nearly straight catheter for passage into the female bladder.

fe•male cir•cum•ci•sion (fē′māl sĭr′kŭm-si′zhŭn) A broad term referring to many forms of female genital cutting, ranging from removal of the clitoral prepuce to the removal of the clitoris, labia minora, and parts of the labia majora, and of infibulation; done for cultural, not medical, reasons.

fe•male con•dom (fē′māl kon′dŏm) An intravaginal bag, usually latex, which lines the vulva and vagina and is intended to prevent contraception during coitus.

fe•male gen•i•tal mu•ti•la•tion (fē′māl jen′i-tăl myū′ti-lā′shŭn) SEE female circumcision.

fe•male gen•i•tal sys•tem (fē′māl jen′i-tăl sis′tĕm) The female reproductive system consisting of the ovaries, uterine ducts, uterus, vagina, and external genitalia. See page A14.

fe•male pat•tern al•o•pe•ci•a (fē′māl pat′ĕrn al′ō-pē′shē-ă) Diffuse partial hair loss in the centroparietal area of the scalp, with preservation of the frontal and temporal hair lines; the most frequent type of androgenic alopecia in women.

fe•male pseu•do•her•ma•phro•di•tism (fē′māl sū′dō-hĕr-maf′rŏ-di-tizm) Pseudohermaphroditism with skeletal and genital anomalies (ambiguous external genitalia, e.g., clitoral enlargement) but with female gonads (ovaries). SYN androgyny (1).

fe•male tri•ad (fē′māl trī′ad) SYN female athlete triad.

fem•i•nin•i•ty com•plex (fem′i-nin′i-tē kom′pleks) PSYCHOANALYSIS the unconscious fear, in boys and men, of castration at the hands of the mother with resultant identification with the aggressor and envious desire for breasts and vagina.

fem•i•nist (fem′i-nist) Theories, beliefs, and practices that seek to understand the views and the effects of views about women's abilities and realities. Hierarchical structures and power inequities have been found to significantly influence the experience of patients and nurses.

fem•i•ni•za•tion (fem′i-nī-zā′shŭn) Development of what are superficially external female characteristics by a male.

fem•o•ral (fem′ŏr-ăl) Relating to the femur or thigh.

fem•o•ral an•te•ver•sion (fem′ŏr-ăl an′tē-vĕr-zhŭn) A condition of abnormal medial rotation of the thigh at the hip joint.

fem•o•ral ar•ter•y (fem′ŏr-ăl ahr′tĕr-ē) *Origin*, continuation of external iliac, beginning at inguinal ligament; *branches*, external pudendal, superficial epigastric, superficial circumflex iliac, profunda femoris, descending genicular, terminating as the popliteal artery as it passes through the adductor hiatus to enter the popliteal space. SYN arteria femoralis [TA].

fem•o•ral ca•nal (fem′ŏr-ăl kă-nal′) The medial compartment of the femoral sheath. SYN canalis femoralis [TA].

fem•o•ral her•ni•a (fem′ŏr-ăl hĕr′nē-ă) Hernia through the femoral ring. SYN crural hernia, femorocele.

fem•o•ral nerve (fem′ŏr-ăl nĕrv) Arises from the second, third, and fourth lumbar nerves in the substance of the psoas muscle and enters the thigh through the muscular lacuna beneath the inguinal ligament, lateral to the femoral vessels; it arborizes within the femoral triangle into muscle branches to the sartorius, pectineus, and quadriceps muscles and anterior femoral cutaneous nerves to the skin of the anterior and medial region of the thigh; its terminal branch is the saphenous nerve by which it supplies the skin of the medial leg and foot. SYN nervus femoralis [TA].

fem•o•ral nut•ri•ent ar•ter•y (fem′ŏr-ăl nū′trē-ĕnt ahr′tĕr-ē) One of two arteries, superior and inferior, arising from the first and third perforating arteries, respectively (sometimes second and fourth).

fem•o•ral pulse (fem′ŏr-ăl pŭls) A palpable rhythmic expansion of the femoral artery in the groin.

fem•o•ral sheath (fem′ŏr-ăl shēth) The fascia enclosing the femoral vessels, formed by the transversalis fascia anteriorly and the iliac fascia posteriorly; two septa divide the sheath into three compartments, the lateral of which contains the femoral artery and the femoral branch of the genitofemoral nerve, the middle the femoral vein, and the medial is the femoral canal. SYN crural sheath.

fem•o•ral tri•an•gle (fem′ŏr-ăl trī′ang-gĕl) A triangular space at the upper part of the thigh, bounded by the sartorius and adductor longus muscles and the inguinal ligament, with a floor formed laterally by the iliopsoas muscle and medially by the pectineus muscle; the branches of the femoral nerve are distributed within the femoral triangle; it is bisected by the femoral vessels, which enter the adductor canal at its apex. SYN trigonum femorale [TA], Scarpa triangle.

fem•o•ral vein (fem′ŏr-ăl vān) A continuation of the popliteal vein; it accompanies the femoral artery through the adductor canal and into the femoral triangle where it lies within the femoral sheath; it becomes the external iliac vein as it passes deep to inguinal ligament. SYN vena femoralis [TA].

fem•o•ro•cele (fem′ŏr-ō-sēl) SYN femoral hernia. [L. *femur,* thigh, + G. *kēlē,* hernia]

fem•o•ro•tib•i•al (fem′ŏr-ō-tib′ē-ăl) Relating to the femur and the tibia.

femto- (f) Prefix indicating unit of measure in the SI and metric system signifying one quadrillionth (10^{-15}). [Danish and Norwegian *femten,* fifteen]

fe•mur, gen. **fe•mo•ris**, pl. **fem•o•ra** (fē′mŭr, fem′ŏr-is, -ă) [TA] **1.** The thigh. **2.** The long bone of the thigh, articulating with the hip bone proximally and the tibia and patella distally. See this page. SYN thigh bone. [L. thigh]

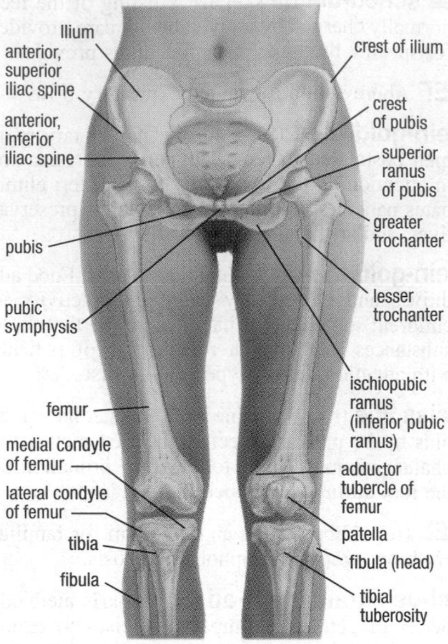

femur

fe•nes•tra, pl. **fe•nes•trae** (fĕ-nes′tră, -trē) [TA] **1.** An anatomic aperture, often closed by a membrane. **2.** An opening left in a cast or other form of fixed dressing to permit access to a wound or inspection of the part. **3.** The opening in one of the blades of an obstetric forceps. **4.** A lateral opening in the sheath of an endoscopic instrument that allows lateral viewing or operative maneuvering through the sheath. **5.** Openings in the wall of a tube, catheter, or trocar designed to promote better flow of air or fluids. SYN window. [L. window]

fe•nes•tra co•chle•ae (fĕ-nes′tră kōk′lē-ē) [TA] An opening on the medial wall of the middle ear leading into the cochlea, closed in life by the secondary tympanic membrane. SYN round window.

fen•es•trat•ed (fen′ĕs-trāt-ĕd) Having fenestrae or windowlike openings.

fen•es•trat•ed cap•il•lar•y (fen′ĕs-trāt-ĕd kap′i-lar-ē) A capillary, found in renal glomeruli, intestinal villi, and some glands, in which ultramicroscopic pores of variable size occur.

fen•es•trat•ed mem•brane (fen′ĕs-trāt-ĕd mem′brān) An elastic membrane, as in elastic laminae of arteries.

fen•es•tra•tion (fen′ĕs-trā′shŭn) **1.** The presence of openings or fenestrae in a part. **2.** Making openings in a dressing to allow inspection of the parts. **3.** DENTISTRY a surgical perforation of the mucoperiosteum and alveolar process to expose the root tip of a tooth to permit drainage of tissue exudate. **4.** SURGERY an opening created to gain access to the cavity within an organ or a bone.

fe·nes·tra ves·tib·u·li (fĕ-nes′tră ves-tib′yū-lī) [TA] An oval opening on the medial wall of the tympanic cavity leading into the vestibule, closed by the foot of the stapes. SYN oval window.

feng shui (fŭng shwā) An ancient Chinese belief system used to configure one's living or work environment to promote health, happiness, and prosperity, by enhancement of energy flow (chi); includes use of space, color, and order as factors in satisfaction.

fen·u·greek (fen′yū-grēk) (*Trigonella foenum-graecum*) Purported therapeutic use in GI disorders; also used topically; may cause bleeding disorders and hypoglycemia. SYN Greek hay. [L. *faenum graecum* Greek hay]

Fer·gu·son ref·lex (fĕr′gŭ-sŏn rē′fleks) Enhancement of uterine activity due to mechanical stretching of the lower uterine segment and cervix.

Fer·gus·son in·ci·sion (fĕr′gŭ-sŏn in-sizh′ŭn) An incision used in maxillectomy, along the junction of the nose and cheek, and bisecting the upper lip.

fer·ment (fĕr-ment′) To cause or to undergo fermentation. [L. *fermentum,* leaven]

fer·men·ta·tion (fĕr′mĕn-tā′shŭn) **1.** A chemical change induced in a complex organic compound by the action of an enzyme, whereby the substance is split into simpler compounds. **2.** BACTERIOLOGY the anaerobic dissimilation of substrates with the production of energy and reduced compounds; the mechanism of fermentation does not involve a respiratory chain or cytochrome, hence oxygen is not the final electron acceptor as it is in oxidation. [L. *fermento,* pp. *-atus,* to ferment, from L. *fermentum,* yeast]

fer·ment·a·tive (fĕr-ment′ă-tiv) Causing or having the ability to cause fermentation.

fer·mi·um (Fm) (fĕr′mē-ŭm) Radioactive element, artificially prepared in 1955; atomic no. 100, atomic wt. 257.095; ^{257}Fm has the longest known half-life (100.5 days).

fern·ing (fĕrn′ing) Pattern of arborization produced by a thin film of cervical mucus, secreted at midcycle, on drying, which somewhat resembles a fern or a palm leaf.

fern test (fĕrn test) **1.** A measurement of estrogenic activity; cervical mucus smears form a fern pattern at those times when estrogen secretion is elevated, as at the time of ovulation. **2.** A test to detect ruptured amniotic membranes.

Fer·ra·ta cell (fer-rah′tah sel) SYN hemohistioblast.

fer·re·dox·ins (fer′ĕ-dok′sinz) Proteins containing iron and (labile) sulfur in equal amounts, displaying electron-carrier activity but no classical enzyme function. Ferredoxins are found in green plants, algae, and anaerobic bacteria, and are involved in several oxidation-reduction reactions in living organisms (e.g., nitrogen fixation).

Fer·rein pyr·a·mid (fer-ān[h]′ pir′ă-mid) SYN medullary ray.

Fer·rein va·sa a·ber·ran·ti·a (fer-ān[h]′ vā′să ā-ber-an′shē-ă) Biliary canaliculi that are not connected with hepatic lobules.

♻ **ferri-** Prefix designating the presence of a ferric ion in a compound. [L. *ferrum,* iron]

fer·ric (fer′ik) **1.** Relating to iron in its valence state of 3+ (Fe^{3+}). **2.** A compound in which iron exists in its valence state of Fe^{3+}.

fer·ri·heme (fer′i-hēm) SYN hematin.

fer·ri·tin (fer′i-tin) An iron protein complex, containing up to 23% iron, formed by the union of ferric iron with apoferritin; it is found in the intestinal mucosa, spleen, bone marrow, reticulocytes, and liver, and regulates iron storage and transport from the intestinal lumen to plasma.

♻ **ferro-** Combining form designating the presence of metallic iron or of the divalent ion Fe^{2+}. [L. *ferrum,* iron]

fer·ro·ki·net·ics (fer′ō-ki-net′iks) The study of iron metabolism using radioactive iron. [L. *ferrum,* iron, + G. *kinēsis,* movement]

fer·ro·pro·teins (fer′ō-prō′tēnz) Proteins containing iron in a prosthetic group (e.g., heme, cytochrome).

fer·rous (fer′ŭs) **1.** Relating to iron in its valence state, Fe^{2+}. **2.** A compound in which iron exists in its valence state of $^{2+}$. [L. *ferreus,* made of iron]

fer·ru·gi·na·tion (fĕ-rū′ji-nā′shŭn) Deposition of mineral including iron in the walls of small blood vessels and at the site of a dead neuron. [L. *ferrugo,* iron-rust]

fer·ru·gi·nous (fĕ-rū′ji-nŭs) **1.** Iron bearing; associated with or containing iron. **2.** Of the color of iron rust. [L. *ferrugineus,* iron rust, rust-colored]

Fer·ry line (fer′ē līn) An iron line occurring in the corneal epithelium anterior to a filtering bleb.

fer·tile (fĕr′til) **1.** Fruitful; capable of conceiving and bearing young. SYN fecund. **2.** Impregnated; fertilized. [L. *fertilis,* fr. *fero,* to bear]

fer·tile pe·ri·od (fĕr′til pēr′ē-ŏd) The period in a regularly menstruating woman's cycle, during which conception is most likely.

fer·til·i·ty (fĕr-til′i-tē) The capacity to conceive and bear offspring; refers to production of live offspring and hence does not include stillbirths.

fer·til·i·za·tion (fĕr′til-ī-zā′shŭn) The process

beginning with penetration of the secondary oocyte by the sperm and completed by fusion of the male and female pronuclei.

fer•ti•li•za•tion age (fĕr′til-ī-zā′shŭn āj) The age of an embryo or fetus defined by the time elapsed since the estimated date of fertilization of the oocyte. SYN conceptual age.

FES Abbreviation for functional electrical stimulation.

FESS Abbreviation for functional endoscopic sinus surgery.

fes•ter (fes′tĕr) **1.** To form pus or putrefy. **2.** To make inflamed. [L. *fistula*]

fes•ti•nant (fes′ti-nănt) Rapid; hastening; accelerating. [L. *festino,* to hasten]

fes•ti•nat•ing gait, **fes•ti•na•tion** (fes′ti-nā′ting gāt, fes′ti-nā′shŭn) Locomotion in which the trunk is flexed, legs are flexed at the knees and hips, but stiff, whereas the steps are short and progressively more rapid; characteristically seen with parkinsonism (1) and other neurologic diseases.

fes•toon (fes-tūn′) **1.** A carving in the base material of a denture that simulates the contours of the natural tissue that is being replaced by the denture. **2.** A distinguishing characteristic of certain hard tick species, consisting of small rectangular areas separated by grooves along the posterior margin of the dorsum of both males and females. [thr. Fr. fr. L. *festum,* festival, hence festive decorations]

fes•toon•ing (fes-tūn′ing) Undulating, like the pattern of dermal papillae beneath a subepidermal blister.

FET Abbreviation for forced expiratory time.

fe•tal (fē′tăl) **1.** Relating to a fetus; **2.** Development in utero after the eighth week. SYN foetal.

fe•tal al•co•hol ef•fects (FAE) (fē′tăl al′kō-hol ē′feks) Alterations in growth and mental development resulting in behavioral and learning difficulties; observed in mothers with a history of moderate alcohol consumption throughout pregnancy.

fe•tal al•co•hol syn•drome (FAS) (fē′tăl al′kŏ-hol sin′drōm) Malformation or alteration present in varying degrees that includes growth deficiency, hyperactivity, craniofacial anomalies, and limb defects, found among offspring of mothers with long-term alcoholism during pregnancy; mental retardation is often demonstrated later.

fe•tal as•pir•a•tion syn•drome (fē′tăl as′pir-ā′shŭn sin′drōm) A manifestation resulting from aspiration of amniotic fluid and meconium by the fetus, usually caused by hypoxia and often leading to aspiration pneumonia. SYN meconium aspiration syndrome.

fe•tal death (fē′tăl deth) Demise before the complete expulsion or extraction from the mother of a product of conception, irrespective of the duration of pregnancy. Fetal death is considered early if it occurs in the first 20 weeks of gestation; middle (intermediate) if it occurs from 21–28 weeks, and late if it occurs after 28 weeks.

fe•tal dys•to•ci•a (fē′tăl dis-tō′sē-ă) Dystocia due to an abnormality of the fetus.

fe•tal growth re•stric•tion (fē′tăl grōth rĕ-strik′shŭn) Fetal weight in the fifth percentile or lower for gestational age.

fe•tal heart rate (FHR) (fē′tăl hahrt rāt) In the fetus, the number of heartbeats per minute, normally 120–160.

fe•tal hy•drops, **hy•drops fe•ta•lis** (fē′tăl hī′drops, hī′drops fē-tā′lis) Abnormal accumulation of serous fluid in the fetal tissues, as in erythroblastosis fetalis.

fe•tal med•i•cine (fē′tăl med′i-sin) Study of the growth, development, care, and treatment of the fetus, and of environmental factors harmful to the fetus. SYN fetology.

fe•tal mem•brane (fē′tăl mem′brān) A structure (e.g., chorion) or tissue that develops from the zygote but does not form part of the embryo proper. SYN embryonic membrane.

fe•tal part of pla•cen•ta, **pla•cen•ta fe•ta•lis** (fē′tăl pahrt plă-sen′tă, plă-sen′tă fē-tā′lis) The chorionic portion of the placenta, containing the fetal blood vessels, from which the umbilical cord develops; specifically, in humans, it develops from the chorion frondosum or villous chorion.

fe•tal pre•sen•ta•tion (fē′ăl prez′ĕn-tā′shŭn) SEE presentation.

fe•tal scalp stim•u•la•tion (fē′tăl skalp stim′yŭ-lā′shŭn) Intrapartum test for fetal well-being; acceleration of the fetal heart rate in response to digital or forceps stimulation of scalp is associated with a normal scalp blood pH.

fe•tal souf•fle (fē′tăl sū′fĕl) A blowing murmur, synchronous with the fetal heart beat, sometimes only systolic and sometimes continuous, heard on auscultation over the pregnant uterus.

fe•tal was•tage (fē′tăl wā′stăj) Loss of an embryo or fetus through spontaneous abortion or stillbirth; usually expressed as a rate per 1000 pregnancies with respect to a particular cause, such as maternal infection or drug addiction.

fe•ti•cide (fē′ti-sīd) Destruction of the embryo or fetus in the uterus. [L. *fetus* + *caedo,* to kill]

fet•id (fet′id) Foul-smelling. [L. *foetidus*]

fet•ish (fet′ish) An inanimate object or nonsexual body part that is regarded as endowed with magic or erotic qualities. [Fr. *fétiche,* fr. L. *factitius,* made by art, artificial]

fet·ish·ism (fet′ish-izm) The act of worshipping or using for sexual arousal and gratification that which is regarded as a fetish.

fe·to·glob·u·lins (fē′tō-glob′yū-linz) One of several types of proteins found in fetal blood, of unknown function; occur in normal amounts in adults and in larger amounts in the fetus and pregnant mother, especially in the second trimester; elevated levels are also detected in adult patients with liver disease and neoplasms.

fe·tol·o·gy (fē-tol′ŏ-jē) SYN fetal medicine. [L. *fetus* + G. *logos,* study]

fe·tom·e·try (fē-tom′ĕ-trē) Estimation of the size of the fetus, especially of its head, before delivery. [L. *fetus* + G. *metron,* measure]

fe·top·a·thy (fē-top′ă-thē) SYN embryopathy. [L. *fetus* + G. *pathos,* suffering, disease]

fe·to·pla·cen·tal (fē′tō-plă-sen′tăl) Relating to the fetus and its placenta. SYN foetoplacental.

fe·to·pro·tein, **al·pha (α)-fe·to·pro·tein (AFP), gam·ma (γ)-fe·to·pro·tein, be·ta (β)-fe·to·pro·tein** (fē′tō-prō′tēn, al′fă, gam′ă) Fetal proteins found in small amounts in adults in the following forms: 1) AFP increases in maternal blood during pregnancy; when detected by amniocentesis, is an important indicator of neural tube defects (e.g., spina bifida); used as a tumor marker in adults with hepatocellular carcinoma; 2) beta (β)-fetoprotein, although a fetal liver protein, has been detected in adult patients with liver disease; and 3) gamma (γ)-fetoprotein occurs in association with various neoplasms. SEE ALSO fetoglobulins.

fe·tor (fē′tōr) A very offensive odor. [L. an offensive smell, fr. *feteo,* to stink]

fe·tor he·pat·i·cus (fē′tōr hē-pat′i-kŭs) A peculiar odor to the breath in people with severe liver disease; caused by volatile aromatic substances that accumulate in the blood and urine due to defective hepatic metabolism.

fe·to·scope (fē′tō-skōp) **1.** A fiberoptic endoscope used in fetology. **2.** A stethoscope designed for listening to fetal heart sounds.

fe·tos·co·py (fē-tos′kŏ-pē) Use of a fiberoptic endoscope to view the fetus and the fetal surface of the placenta transabdominally, and also for collection of fetal blood from the umbilical vein for prenatal diagnosis of fetal disorders.

fe·to·tox·ic (fē′tō-tok′sik) A substance that is poisonous to a fetus. SYN foetotoxic.

fe·tu·in (fē-tū′in) A low molecular-weight globulin that constitutes nearly the total globulin in fetal blood. [fetus + -in]

fe·tus, pl. **fe·tus·es** (fē′tŭs, -ĕz) **1.** The unborn young of a viviparous animal after it has taken form in the uterus. **2.** In humans, the product of conception from the end of the eighth week to the moment of birth. See this page, B1, B21. SYN foetus. [L. offspring]

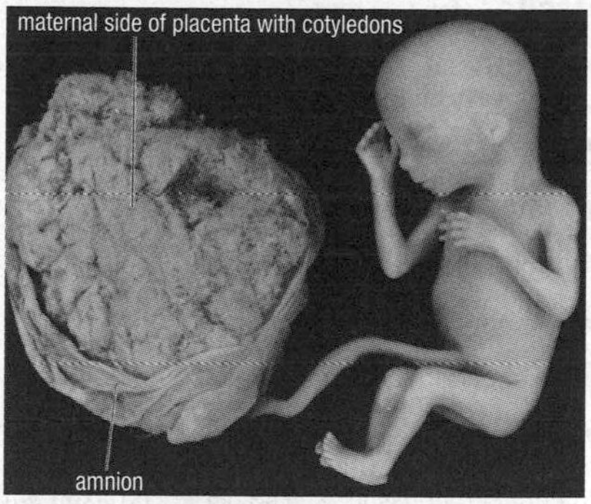

fetus: an 18-week-old example connected to the placenta by its umbilical cord; the skin of the fetus is thin because of lack of subcutaneous fat (note the placenta with its cotyledons and the amnion)

fe·tus pap·y·ra·ce·us (fē′tŭs pap-i-rā′shē-ŭs) One of twin fetuses that has died and been pressed flat against the uterine wall by the growth of the living fetus.

Feul·gen cy·to·met·ry (foyl′gen sī-tom′ĕ-trē) A form of cytometry using Feulgen-stained nuclei to characterize the chromatin pattern and nuclear distribution of DNA of cells.

FEV Abbreviation for forced expiratory volume, with subscript indicating time interval in seconds.

fe·ver (fē′vĕr) A complex physiologic response to disease mediated by pyrogenic cytokines and characterized by a rise in core temperature, generation of acute phase reactants, and activation of immunologic systems. SYN pyrexia. [A.S. *fefer*]

fe·ver blis·ter (fē′vĕr blis′tĕr) Colloquialism for herpes simplex of the lips.

fe·ver·few (fē′vĕr-fyū) (*Chrysanthemum multiflorum*) Herbal agent used in migraine headache and fever. Associated with ulceration of oral cavity, labial edema, and hypersensitivity reactions. SYN bachelor's button, Santa Maria. [L. *febrifuga,* febrifuge]

fe·ver·ish (fē′vĕr-ish) **1.** SYN febrile. **2.** Having a fever.

fe·ver of un·known or·i·gin (FUO) (fē′vĕr ŭn′nōn ōr′i-jin) A sustained elevation of temperature, lasting 2 weeks or longer, for which no explanation can be found despite vigorous diagnostic evaluation. SYN pyrexia of unknown origin.

fe·ver·wort (fē′vĕr-wōrt) SYN boneset.

FF Abbreviation for filtration fraction.

F fac·tor (fak′tŏr) SYN F plasmid.

F-fac·tor (fak′tŏr) Abbreviation for roentgen to rad conversion factor.

FFD Abbreviation for focal-film distance.

FFM Abbreviation for fat-free body mass.

FG Abbreviation for frozen gait.

FHR Abbreviation for fetal heart rate.

FIA Abbreviation for feline infectious anemia.

fi·ber (fī′bĕr) **1.** A strand or filament; especially the extracellular filamentous structures peculiar to connective tissue. **2.** The nerve cell axon with its glial envelope. SYN fibra [TA]. **3.** Elongated, hence threadlike, cells such as muscle cells and the epithelial cells composing the major part of the eye lens. **4.** Nutrients in the diet that are not digested by gastrointestinal enzymes. SYN fibre. [L. *fibra*]

fi·ber·op·tic (fī′bĕr-op′tik) Pertaining to fiberoptics. SYN fibre-optic.

fi·ber·op·tic en·dos·cop·ic ex·am·i·na·tion of swal·low·ing (FEES) (fī′bĕr-op′tik en′dŏ-skop′ik eg-zam′i-nā′shŭn swah′lō-ing) A diagnostic technique for evaluation of deviant swallowing patterns, using a transnasal fiberoptic endoscope to visualize the larynx and pharynx. SEE ALSO fiberoptics, endoscope.

fi·ber·op·tics (fī′bĕr-op′tiks) An optic system in which flexible glass or plastic fibers are used to transmit light around curves and corners; of particular use in endoscopy. SYN fibre-optics.

fi·ber·scope (fī′bĕr-skōp) An optic instrument that transmits light and carries images back to the observer through a flexible bundle of small glass or plastic fibers. It is used to inspect interior portions of the body. SEE ALSO fiberoptics.

fi·bra (fī′bră) [TA] SYN fiber (2). [L.]

fi·brae me·rid·i·o·na·les mus·cu·lar·is cil·i·ar·is (fī′brē me-rid-ē-ō-nā′lēzmŭs-kū-lā′ris sil-ē-ā′ris) [TA] SYN meridional fibers of ciliary muscle.

fibre [Br.] SYN fiber.

fibre-optic [Br.] SYN fiberoptic.

fibre-optics [Br.] SYN fiberoptics.

fi·bril (fī′bril) A minute fiber or component of a fiber. SYN fibrilla. [Mod. L. *fibrilla*]

fi·bril·la, pl. **fi·bril·lae** (fī-bril′ă, -ē) SYN fibril. [Mod. L. dim. of L. *fibra,* a fiber]

fi·bril·lar, **fi·bril·lar·y** (fī′bri-lăr, fī′bri-lar-ē) **1.** Relating to a fibril. **2.** Denoting the fine rapid contractions or twitchings of fibers or of small groups of fibers in skeletal or cardiac muscle. SYN filar (1).

fi·bril·lar·y as·tro·cyte, **fi·brous as·tro·cyte** (fī′bri-lar-ē as′trō-sīt, fī′brŭs as′trō-sīt) A stellate astrocytic cell with long processes found mainly in the white matter of the brain and spinal cord and characterized by having bundles of glial filaments in its cytoplasm; origin of most astrocytomas.

fi·bril·lar·y con·trac·tions (fī′bri-lar-ē kŏn-trak′shŭnz) Contractions occurring spontaneously in individual muscle fibers.

fi·bril·late (fī′bri-lāt) **1.** To make or to become fibrillar. **2.** SYN fibrillated. **3.** To be in a state of fibrillation (3).

fi·bril·lat·ed (fī′bri-lā-tĕd) Composed of fibrils. SYN fibrillate (2).

fi·bril·la·tion (fib′ri-lā′shŭn) **1.** The condition of being fibrillated. **2.** The formation of fibrils. **3.** Exceedingly rapid contractions or twitching of muscular fibrils, but not of the muscle as a whole. **4.** Vermicular twitching, usually slow, of individual muscular fibers; commonly occurs in atria or ventricles of the heart as well as in recently denervated skeletal muscle fibers.

fi·bril·lo·gen·e·sis (fī′bril-ō-jen′ĕ-sis) The development of fine fibrils (as seen with the electron microscope) normally present in collagenous fibers of connective tissue.

fi·brin (fī′brin) An elastic filamentous protein derived from fibrinogen by the action of thrombin, which releases fibrinopeptides A and B from fibrinogen in coagulation of the blood; a component of thrombi, vegetations, and acute inflammatory exudates such as in diphtheria and lobar pneumonia. [L. *fibra,* fiber]

fi·brin·ase (fī′brin-ās) **1.** Former term for factor XIII. **2.** SYN plasmin.

fi·brin cal·cu·lus (fī′brin kal′kyū-lŭs) A urinary calculus formed largely from fibrinogen in blood.

fi·brin/fi·brin·o·gen deg·ra·da·tion pro·ducts (fī′brin-fī-brin′ō-jen deg′ră-dā′shŭn prod′ŭkts) Several poorly characterized small peptides that result from the action of plasmin on fibrinogen and fibrin in the fibrinolytic process.

♻**fibrino-** Combining form meaning fibrin. [L. *fibra,* fiber]

fi·bri·no·cel·lu·lar (fī′bri-nō-sel′yū-lăr) Composed of fibrin and cells, as in certain types of exudates resulting from acute inflammation.

fi·brin·o·gen (fī-brin′ō-jen) A globulin of the blood plasma that is converted into fibrin by the action of thrombin in the presence of ionized calcium to produce coagulation of the blood; the only coagulable protein in the blood plasma of vertebrates; absent in afibrinogenemia and defective in dysfibrinogenemia.

fi·brin·o·ge·ne·mi·a (fī′brin-ō-jĕ-nē′mē-ă) SYN hyperfibrinogenemia. SYN fibrogenaemia.

fi•bri•no•gen•e•sis (fī′bri-nō-jen′ĕ-sis) Formation or production of fibrin.

fi•bri•no•gen•ic, fi•bri•nog•e•nous (fī′brin-ō-jen′ik, fī′bri-noj′ĕ-nŭs) **1.** Pertaining to fibrinogen. **2.** Producing fibrin.

fi•brin•o•gen•ol•y•sis (fī-brin′ō-jĕ-nol′i-sis) The inactivation or dissolution of fibrinogen in the blood. [fibrinogen + G. *lysis,* dissolution]

fi•brin•o•gen•o•pe•ni•a (fī-brin′ō-jen′ō-pē′nē-ă) A subnormal concentration of fibrinogen in the blood. [fibrinogen + G. *penia,* poverty]

fi•brin•oid (fī′bri-noyd) **1.** Resembling fibrin. **2.** A deeply or brilliantly acidophilic, homogeneous, refractile, proteinaceous material that: 1) is frequently formed in the walls of blood vessels and in connective tissue of patients with such diseases as disseminated lupus erythematosus, polyarteritis nodosa, scleroderma, dermatomyositis, and rheumatic fever; and 2) is sometimes observed in healing wounds, chronic peptic ulcers, the placenta, necrotic arterioles of malignant hypertension, and other unrelated conditions. [fibrin + G. *eidos,* resemblance]

fi•brin•oid de•gen•er•a•tion, fi•brin•ous de•gen•er•a•tion (fī′bri-noyd dĕ-jen′ĕr-ā′shŭn, fī′brin-ŭs) A process resulting in acidophilic refractile deposits with staining reactions that resemble fibrin, occurring in connective tissue, blood vessel walls, and other sites.

fi•bri•nol•y•sin (fī′brin-ol′ī-sin) SYN plasmin.

fi•bri•nol•y•sis (fī′bri-nol′i-sis) Hydrolysis of fibrin. [fibrino- + G. *lysis,* dissolution]

fi•bri•no•lyt•ic (fī′brin-ō-lit′ik) Denoting, characterized by, or causing fibrinolysis.

fi•bri•no•lyt•ic pur•pu•ra (fī′brin-ō-lit′ik pŭr′pyŭr-ă) A disorder in which bleeding is associated with rapid fibrinolysis of the clot.

fi•brin•o•pep•tide (fī′brin-ō-pep′tīd) One of two pairs of peptides (A and B) released from the amino-terminal ends of 2α- and 2β-chains of fibrinogen by the action of thrombin to form fibrin; has a vasoconstrictive effect.

fi•bri•no•pu•ru•lent (fī′brin-ō-pyūr′yū-lĕnt) Pertaining to pus or suppurative exudate that contains a relatively large amount of fibrin.

fi•brin•ous (fī′brin-ŭs) Pertaining to or composed of fibrin.

fi•brin•ous bron•chi•tis (fī′brin-ŭs brong-kī′tis) Inflammation of the bronchial mucous membrane, accompanied by a fibrinous exudation, with obstruction of air flow. SYN pseudomembranous bronchitis.

fi•brin•ous in•flam•ma•tion (fī′brin-ŭs in′flă-mā′shŭn) An exudative inflammation in which there is a disproportionately large amount of fibrin.

fi•brin•ous per•i•car•di•tis (fī′brin-ŭs per′i-kahr-dī′tis) Acute pericarditis with fibrinous exudate.

fi•brin•ous pleu•ri•sy (fī′brin-ŭs plūr′i-sē) SYN dry pleurisy.

fi•brin•ous pol•yp (fī′brin-ŭs pol′ip) A misnomer for a mass of fibrin retained within the uterine cavity after childbirth.

fi•bri•nu•ri•a (fī-brin-yūr′ē-ă) The passage of urine that contains fibrin. [fibrin + G. *ouron,* urine]

fibro-, fibr- Combining forms meaning fiber. [L. *fibra*]

fi•bro•ad•e•no•ma (fī′brō-ad-ĕ-nō′mă) A benign neoplasm derived from glandular epithelium, in which there is a conspicuous stroma of proliferating fibroblasts and connective tissue elements; commonly occurs in breast tissue. See page B19. SYN fibroid adenoma, adenoma fibrosum.

fi•bro•ad•i•pose (fī′brō-ad′i-pōs) Relating to or containing both fibrous and fatty structures.

fi•bro•a•re•o•lar (fī′brō-ă-rē′ō-lăr) Denoting connective tissue that is both fibrous and areolar in character.

fi•bro•blast (fī′brō-blast) A stellate or spindle-shaped cell with cytoplasmic processes present in connective tissue, capable of forming collagen fibers; an inactive fibroblast is sometimes called a fibrocyte.

fi•bro•blas•tic (fī′brō-blas′tik) Relating to fibroblasts.

fi•bro•car•ci•no•ma (fī′brō-kahr-si-nō′mă) SYN scirrhous carcinoma.

fi•bro•car•ti•lage (fī′brō-kahr′ti-lăj) A variety of cartilage that contains visible type I collagen fibers; appears as a transition between tendons or ligaments or bones. SYN fibrocartilago.

fi•bro•car•ti•lag•i•nous (fī′brō-kahr-ti-laj′i-nŭs) Relating to or composed of fibrocartilage.

fi•bro•car•ti•la•go (fī′brō-kahr-ti-lā′gō) [TA] SYN fibrocartilage.

fi•bro•cel•lu•lar (fī′brō-sel′yū-lăr) Both fibrous and cellular.

fi•bro•chon•dri•tis (fī′brō-kon-drī′tis) Inflammation of a fibrocartilage.

fi•bro•chon•dro•ma (fī′brō-kon-drō′mă) A benign neoplasm of cartilaginous tissue, in which there is a relatively large amount of fibrous stroma.

fi•bro•cyst (fī′brō-sist) Any cystic lesion circumscribed by or situated within a conspicuous amount of fibrous connective tissue.

fi·bro·cys·tic (fī-brō-sis′tik) Pertaining to or characterized by the presence of fibrocysts.

fi·bro·cys·tic breast dis·ease (fī-brō-sis′tik brest di-zēz′) Common benign female breast disorder of unknown etiology. It can be manifest by multiple dense breast masses and multiple tiny lumps. Masses enlarge and shrink with menstrual cycle.

fi·bro·cys·to·ma (fī′brō-sis-tō′mă) A benign neoplasm, usually derived from glandular epithelium, characterized by cysts within a conspicuous fibrous stroma.

fi·bro·e·las·tic (fī′brō-ĕ-las′tik) Composed of collagen and elastic fibers.

fibrogenaemia [Br.] SYN fibrinogenemia.

fi·broid (fī′broyd) **1.** Resembling or composed of fibers or fibrous tissue. **2.** Old term for certain types of leiomyoma, especially those occurring in the uterus. **3.** SYN fibroleiomyoma. [fibro- + G. *eidos*, resemblance]

fi·broid ad·e·no·ma, **ad·e·no·ma fi·bro·sum** (fī′broyd ad′ĕ-nō′mă, ad′ĕ-nō′mă fī-brō′sŭm) SYN fibroadenoma.

fi·broid cat·a·ract, **fi·brin·ous cat·a·ract** (fī′broyd kat′ăr-akt, fī′brin-ŭs kat′ăr-akt) A sclerotic hardening of the capsule of the lens, following exudative iridocyclitis.

fi·broid·ec·to·my (fī′broyd-ek′tō-mē) Removal of a fibroid tumor. [fibroid + G. *ektomē*, excision]

fi·bro·la·mel·lar liv·er cell car·ci·no·ma (fī′brō-lă-mel′ăr liv′ĕr sel kahr′si-nō′mă) Primary hepatic carcinoma in which malignant hepatocytes are intersected by fibrous lamellated bands. SYN oncocytic hepatocellular tumor.

fi·bro·lei·o·my·o·ma (fī′brō-lī′ō-mī-ō′mă) A leiomyoma containing nonneoplastic collagenous fibrous tissue, which may make the tumor hard; fibroleiomyoma usually arises in the myometrium, and the proportion of fibrous tissue increases with age. SYN fibroid (3), leiomyofibroma.

fi·bro·li·po·ma (fī′brō-li-pō′mă) A lipoma with an abundant stroma of fibrous tissue.

fi·bro·ma (fī-brō′mă) A benign neoplasm derived from fibrous connective tissue. [fibro- + G. *-oma*, tumor]

fi·bro·ma·toid (fī-brō′mă-toyd) A nodule or mass of proliferating fibroblasts that resembles a fibroma but is not regarded as neoplastic.

fi·bro·ma·to·sis (fī′brō-mă-tō′sis) **1.** A condition characterized by the occurrence of many fibromas, with a relatively large distribution. **2.** Abnormal hyperplasia of fibrous tissue.

fi·bro·ma·tous (fī-brō′mă-tŭs) Pertaining to, or of the nature of, a fibroma.

fi·bro·mus·cu·lar (fī′brō-mŭs′kyū-lăr) Both fibrous and muscular; relating to both fibrous and muscular tissues.

fi·bro·my·al·gi·a, **fi·bro·my·al·gi·a syn·drome** (fī′brō-mī-al′jē-ă, fī′brō-mī-al′jē-ă sin′drōm) A condition involving lack of stage IV sleep and chronic diffuse widespread aching and stiffness of muscles and soft tissues; diagnosis requires 11 of 18 specific tender points including the occiput, neck, shoulders, chest, elbows, gluteus, greater trochanter, and knees; 4/Kg touch pressure elicits painful response; tender points are found on both sides of the body and above and below the waist. SEE ALSO tender point.

fi·bro·my·ec·to·my (fī′brō-mī-ek′tŏ-mē) Excision of a fibromyoma.

fi·bro·my·o·ma (fī′brō-mī-ō′mă) A leiomyoma that contains a relatively abundant amount of fibrous tissue.

fi·bro·my·o·si·tis (fī′brō-mī′ō-sī′tis) Chronic inflammation of a muscle with an overgrowth, or hyperplasia, of connective tissue. [fibro- + G. *mys*, muscle, + *-itis*, inflammation]

fi·bro·myx·o·ma (fī′brō-mik-sō′mă) A myxoma that contains a relatively abundant amount of mature fibroblasts and connective tissue. [fibro- + G. *myxa*, mucus, + *-ōma*, tumor]

fi·bro·nec·tin (fī′brō-nek′tin) Any of various glycoproteins found on cell membranes and in blood and other body fluids; thought to function as adhesive ligandlike molecules. Possible roles in other processes include transformation to malignancy. Deficiency of fibronectin is associated with Ehlers-Danlos syndrome. [L. *fibra*, fiber, + *nexus*, interconnection]

fi·bro·neu·ro·ma (fī′brō-nūr-ō′mă) SYN neurofibroma.

fi·bro·pap·il·lo·ma (fī′brō-pap-i-lō′mă) A papilloma characterized by a conspicuous amount of fibrous connective tissue at the base and forming the cores on which the neoplastic epithelial cells are massed.

fi·bro·pla·si·a (fī′brō-plā′zē-ă) Production of fibrous tissue, usually implying an abnormal increase of nonneoplastic fibrous tissue. [fibro- + G. *plasis*, a molding]

fi·bro·plas·tic (fī′brō-plas′tik) Producing fibrous tissue. [fibro- + G. *plastos*, formed]

fi·bro·re·tic·u·late (fī′brō-re-tik′yū-lāt) Relating to or consisting of a network of fibrous tissue.

fi·bro·sar·co·ma (fī′brō-sahr-kō′mă) A malignant neoplasm derived from deep fibrous tissue, characterized by bundles of immature proliferating fibroblasts arranged in a distinctive herringbone pattern with variable collagen formation, which tends to invade locally and metastasize by the bloodstream.

fi·bro·se·rous (fī′brō-sēr′ŭs) Composed of fibrous tissue with a serous surface; denoting any serous membrane.

fi·bros·ing co·lon·op·a·thy (fī-brōs′ing kō′lŏn-op′ă-thē) Colonic fibrosis seen in cystic fibrosis patients, thought to be due to pancreatins.

fi·bro·sis (fī-brō′sis) Formation of fibrous tissue as a reparative or reactive process, as opposed to formation of fibrous tissue as a normal constituent of an organ or tissue.

fi·bro·sit·ic head·ache (fī′brō-sit′ik hed′āk) Headache centered in the occipital region due to fibrositis of the occipital muscles; tender areas are present and, commonly, tender nodules are found in the scalp in the lower occipital region.

fi·bro·si·tis (fī′brō-sī′tis) **1.** Inflammation of fibrous tissue. **2.** Obsolete term for fibromyalgia. [fibro- + G. *-itis,* inflammation]

fi·brot·ic (fī-brot′ik) Pertaining to or characterized by fibrosis.

fi·brous (fī′brŭs) Composed of or containing fibroblasts, and also the fibrils and fibers of connective tissue formed by such cells.

fi·brous an·ky·lo·sis (fī′brŭs ang′ki-lō′sis) Stiffening of a joint due to the presence of fibrous bands between and about the bones forming the joint. SYN false ankylosis, pseudankylosis.

fi·brous ar·tic·u·lar cap·sule (fī′brŭs ahr-tik′yū-lăr kap′sŭl) The outer fibrous part of the capsule of a synovial joint, which may in places be thickened to form capsular ligaments.

fi·brous cap·sule (fī′brŭs kap′sŭl) Any fibrous envelope of a part; the fibrous capsule of an organ.

fi·brous cap·sule of kid·ney (fī′brŭs kap′sŭl kid′nē) A fibrous membrane ensheathing the kidney.

fi·brous cap·sule of liv·er (fī′brŭs kap′sŭl liv′ĕr) A layer of connective tissue enshcathing the hepatic artery, portal vein, and bile ducts as these ramify within the liver. SYN capsula fibrosa perivascularis hepatis [TA], Glisson capsule.

fi·brous cor·ti·cal de·fect (fī′brŭs kōr′ti-kăl dē-fekt′) A common 1–3 cm defect in the cortex of a bone, most commonly the lower femoral shaft of a child, filled with fibrous tissue. Nonosteogenic or nonossifying fibroma by convention refers to lesions larger than 3 cm in diameter. SYN nonosteogenic fibroma.

fi·brous de·gen·er·a·tion (fī′brŭs dĕ-jen′ĕr-ā′shŭn) Not a decline in itself, but rather a reparative process; cells and foci of tissue previously affected with degenerative processes and necrosis are replaced by cellular fibrous tissue.

fi·brous dys·pla·si·a of bone (fī′brŭs dis-plā′zē-ă bōn) A disturbance in which bone undergoing physiologic lysis is replaced by abnormal fibrous tissue, resulting in asymmetric distortion and expansion of bone; may be confined to a single bone (monostotic fibrous dysplasia) or involve multiple bones (polyostotic fibrous dysplasia).

fi·brous goi·ter (fī′brŭs goy′tĕr) A firm hyperplasia of the thyroid and its capsule.

fi·brous joint (fī′brŭs joynt) A union of two bones by fibrous tissue such that there is no joint cavity and almost no motion possible; the types of fibrous joints are sutures, syndesmoses, and gomphoses. SYN immovable joint, synarthrodia, synarthrodial joint (1).

fi·brous tis·sue (fī′brŭs tish′ū) A tissue composed of bundles of collagenous white fibers between which are rows of connective tissue cells; the tendons, ligaments, aponeuroses, and some membranes, such as the dura mater.

fi·brous tu·ber·cle (fī′brŭs tū′bĕr-kĕl) A tubercle in which fibroblasts proliferate about the periphery (and into the cellular zones), eventually resulting in a rim or wall of cellular fibrous tissue or collagenous material around the tubercle.

fi·brous un·ion (fī′brŭs yūn′yŭn) Union of fracture by fibrous tissue. SEE nonunion, vicious union. SYN faulty union.

fib·u·la (fib′yū-lă) The lateral and smaller of the two bones of the leg; it does not bear weight and articulates with the tibia above and the tibia and talus below. SYN calf bone. [L. *fibula* (contr. fr. *figibula*), that which fastens, a clasp, buckle, fr. *figo,* to fix, fasten]

fib·u·lar (fib′yū-lăr) Relating to the fibula. [L. *fibularis*]

fib·u·lar ar·ter·y (fib′yū-lăr ahr′tĕr-ē) SYN peroneal artery.

fib·u·la·ris lon·gus mus·cle (fib-yū-lā′ris long′gŭs mŭs′ĕl) *Origin*, upper two thirds of outer surface of fibula and lateral condyle of tibia; *insertion*, by tendon passing bchind lateral malleolus and across sole of foot to medial cuneiform and base of first metatarsal; *action*, plantarflexion and eversion of foot; *nerve supply*, superficial peroneal. SYN long fibular muscle, long peroneal muscle, musculus fibularis longus, musculus peroneus longus, peroneus longus muscle.

fib·u·lar·is ter·ti·us mus·cle (fib-yū-lā′ris tĕr′shē-ŭs mŭs′ĕl) *Origin*, in common with musculus extensor digitorum longus; *insertion*, dorsum of base of fifth metatarsal bone; *nerve supply*, deep branch of peroneal; *action*, assists in dorsiflexion and eversion of foot. SYN musculus fibularis tertius, musculus peroneus tertius, peroneus tertius muscle, third peroneal muscle.

fib·u·lar nut·ri·ent ar·ter·y (fib′yū-lăr nū′trē-ĕnt ahr′tĕr-ē) *Origin*, fibular (peroneal); *distribution*, fibula.

fib•u•lar tar•sal ten•din•ous sheaths (fib′yū-lăr tahr′săl ten′di-nŭs shēths) Synovial tendon sheaths of flexor tendons enabling movement of tendons posterior to the lateral malleolus and across tarsal bones, passing deep to the fibular retinacula; includes (1) the common tendinous sheath of fibulares (peronei) muscles (vagina communis tendinum musculorum fibularium (peroneorum) [TA]); and (2) the plantar tendinous sheath of fibularis (peroneus) (vagina plantaris tendinis musculi fibularis (peronei) longi [TA]).

fib•u•lar veins (fib′yū-lăr vānz) SYN peroneal veins.

fib•u•lo•cal•ca•ne•al (fib′yū-lō-kal-kā′nē-ăl) Relating to the fibula and the calcaneus.

Fick laws of dif•fu•sion (fik lawz di-fyū′zhŭn) **1.** The direction of movement of solutes by diffusion is always from a higher to a lower concentration and the diffusive flux J_A of solute A across a plane at x is proportional to the concentration gradient of A at x; i.e., $J_A = -D(C_A/x)$; **2.** The increase of concentration of solute A with time, C_A/t, is directly proportional to the change in the concentration gradient, i.e., $C_A/t = D(fl^2/x^2)$.

Fick meth•od (fik meth′ŏd) A method of calculating cardiac output or organ blood flow from measurements of oxygen consumption and of the difference in oxygen concentration between arterial and venous.

Fi•coll-Hy•paque tech•nique (fī′kol-hī′păk tek-nēk′) A density-gradient centrifugation technique for separating lymphocytes from other formed elements in the blood; the sample is layered onto a Ficoll-sodium metrizoate gradient of specific density; following centrifugation, lymphocytes are collected from the plasma-Ficoll interface.

FID Abbreviation for free induction decay.

Fied•ler my•o•car•di•tis (fēd′ler mī′ō-kahr-dī′tis) SYN acute isolated myocarditis.

field (fēld) A definite area of plane surface, considered in relation to some specific object. [A.S. *feld*]

field balm (fēld bawlm) SYN catnip.

field block (fēld blok) Regional anesthesia produced by infiltration of local anesthetic solution into tissues surrounding an operative field.

field di•ag•no•sis (fēld dī′ăg-nō′sis) SYN differential field diagnosis.

Field rap•id stain (fēld rap′id stān) A stain to permit rapid positive diagnosis of malaria in endemic areas by using thick films; it employs methylene blue and azure B in a phosphate buffer, with the preparation counterstained by eosin in a phosphate buffer.

field size (fēld sīz) The projection that, on a plane perpendicular to the beam axis of the light field, corresponds to the area being treated by radiation. SYN portal (3).

field test (fēld test) An evaluation of physical fitness performed outside the laboratory environment that can be easily administered to large numbers of subjects with little or no equipment (e.g., 6-minute walk test, 1.5 mile run test, step test).

field of view (FOV) (fēld vyū) Area of anatomy included in an image.

fifth cra•ni•al nerve [CN V] (fifth krā′nē-ăl nĕrv) SYN trigeminal nerve [CN V].

fifth dis•ease (fifth di-zēz′) SYN erythema infectiosum. [after scarlatina, morbilli, rubella, and fourth d.]

fight bite (fīt bīt) A laceration of the digits of the hand resulting from a punch or blow that connects with the teeth of the victim.

FIGLU (fig′lū) Acronym for formiminoglutamic acid.

fig•ure (fig′yŭr) **1.** A form or shape. **2.** A person representing the essential aspects of a particular role. **3.** A form, shape, outline, or representation of an object or person. [L. *figura*, fr *fingo*, to shape, fashion]

fig•ure and ground (fig′yŭr grownd) That aspect of perception wherein the perceived is separated into at least two parts, each with different attributes but influencing one another. Figure is the most distinct; ground the least formed; e.g., a bird or tree (figure) seen against the sky (ground).

fig•ure-of-8 ban•dage (fig′yŭr-āt′ ban′dăj) A bandage applied alternately to two parts, usually two segments of a limb above and below the joint, in such a way that the turns describe the figure 8; used primarily for the treatment of fractures of the clavicle.

fi•la (fī′lă) Plural of filum. [L.]

fi•la•ceous (fī-lā′shŭs) SYN filamentous. [L. *filum,* a thread]

fil•a•ment (fil′ă-mĕnt) **1.** SYN filamentum. **2.** BACTERIOLOGY a fine threadlike form, unsegmented or segmented without constrictions. [L. *filamentum,* fr. *filum,* a thread]

fil•a•men•tous (fil′ă-men′tŭs) **1.** Threadlike in structure. SYN filiform (1). **2.** Composed of filaments or threadlike structures. SYN filaceous, filar (2).

fil•a•men•tum, pl. **fil•a•men•ta** (fil-ă-men′tŭm, -tă) A fibril, fine fiber, or threadlike structure. SYN filament (1). [L.]

fi•lar (fī′lăr) **1.** SYN fibrillar. **2.** SYN filamentous. [L. *filum,* a thread]

Fi•lar•i•a (fi-lar′ē-ă) Nematodes classified in several genera of the family Onchocercidae; e.g., *Wuchereria bancrofti*, *Brugia malayi*, *Onchocerca volvulus*, *Mansonella perstans*, *M. streptocerca*, *M. ozzardi*, *Loa loa*, and *Dirofilaria*. SEE ALSO filaria.

fi•lar•i•a, pl. **fi•lar•i•ae** (fi-lar′ē-ă, -ē-ē) Common name for nematodes of the family Onchocercidae and the superfamily Filarioidea, which live as adults in the blood, tissue fluids, tissues, or body cavities of many vertebrates. The females lay partially embryonated eggs; the embryos uncoil and circulate in blood or tissue fluids as microfilariae; if the embryos are ingested by an appropriate bloodsucking arthropod, larval stages develop; later, infective larvae may be injected into another vertebrate host's skin when the arthropod seeks another blood meal. [L. *filum,* a thread]

fi•lar•i•al (fi-lar′ē-ăl) Pertaining to a filaria (or filariae), including the microfilaria stage.

fil•a•ri•a•sis (fil′ă-rī′ă-sis) Presence of filariae in the tissues of the body or in blood (microfilaremia) or tissue fluids (microfilariasis), occurring in tropical and subtropical regions; living adult worms cause minimal tissue reaction, which may be asymptomatic, but death of the adult worms may cause granulomatous inflammation and permanent fibrosis. Certain species of filarial worms can damage lymphatic channels, thus permitting onset of obstruction of the lymphatic channels from dense hyalinized scars in the subcutaneous tissues; the most serious consequence is elephantiasis or pachyderma.

fi•lar•i•ci•dal (fi-lar′i-sī′dăl) Fatal to filariae.

fi•lar•i•cide (fi-lar′i-sīd) An agent that kills filariae. [filaria + L. *caedo,* to kill]

fi•lar•i•form (fi-lar′i-fōrm) **1.** Resembling filariae or other types of small nematode worms. **2.** Thin or hairlike.

Fi•la•tov flap (fē′lah-tof flap) SYN tubed flap.

Fi•la•tov-Gil•lies flap (fē′lah-tof gil′ēz flap) SYN tubed flap.

fil•i•al (fil′ē-ăl) Denoting the relationship of offspring to parents. SEE filial generation. [L. *filialis,* fr. *filius,* son, *filia,* daughter]

fil•i•al gen•er•a•tion (F) (fil′ē-ăl jen′ĕr-ā′shŭn) The offspring of a genetically specified mating: first filial generation (symbol F_1), the offspring of parents of contrasting genotypes; second filial generation (F_2), the offspring of two F_1 individuals; third filial generation (F_3), fourth filial generation (F_4), and so on; the offspring in succeeding generations of continued inbreeding of F_1 descendents.

fi•li•form (fil′i-fōrm) **1.** SYN filamentous (1). **2.** BACTERIOLOGY denoting an even growth along the line of inoculation, either stroke or stab. [L. *filum,* thread]

fi•li•form bou•gie (fil′i-fōrm bū-zhē′) A very slender bougie most often used for gentle exploration of strictures or sinus tracts of small diameter where false passages can be encountered or created; the trailing end usually consists of a threaded cylinder into which the screw tip of a following bougie can be inserted.

fi•li•form pa•pil•lae (fil′i-fōrm pă-pil′ē) Numerous elongated conic keratinized projections on the dorsum of the tongue.

fil•let (fil′et) **1.** SYN lemniscus. **2.** A skein, loop of cord, or tape used for making traction on a part of the fetus. [Fr. *filet,* a band]

fill•ing (fil′ing) Colloquial term for a dental restoration.

fill•ing de•fect (fil′ing dē-fekt′) Displacement of contrast medium by a space-occupying lesion in a radiographic study of a contrast-filled hollow viscus, such as a polyp on a barium enema; also applied to defects in the otherwise uniform distribution of radionuclide in an organ, such as a metastasis in the liver on a ^{99m}Tc-sulfur colloid scan.

film (film) **1.** A thin sheet of flexible material coated with a light-sensitive or x-ray-sensitive substance used in taking photographs or radiographs. **2.** A thin layer or coating. **3.** Colloquially, a radiograph.

film badge (film baj) Small packet of x-ray film and filters worn by radiation workers to monitor exposure to radiation on a monthly basis. SEE ALSO pocket dosimeter, thermoluminescent dosimeter.

film•less ra•di•o•gra•phy (film′lĕs rā′dē-og′ră-fē) Electronic acquisition and distribution of radiographic images, eliminating the handling and storage of film. SEE ALSO PACS.

fi•lo•pres•sure (fī′lō-presh′ŭr) Temporary pressure on a blood vessel by a ligature, which is removed when the flow of blood has ceased. [L. *filum,* thread]

fil•ter (fil′tĕr) **1.** A porous substance through which a liquid or gas is passed to separate it from contained particulate matter or impurities. SYN filtrum. **2.** To use or to subject to the action of a filter. **3.** RADIOLOGY a device, used in both diagnostic and therapeutic radiology, which permits passage of useful x-rays and absorbs those with a lower and less desirable energy. **4.** A device used in spectrophotometric analysis to isolate a segment of the spectrum. **5.** A mathematic algorithm applied to image data for the purpose of enhancing image quality, usually by suppression of high spatial frequency noise. **6.** A passive electronic circuit or device that selectively permits the passage of certain electrical signals. **7.** A device placed in the inferior vena cava to prevent pulmonary embolism from low extremity clot. **8.** RADIATION PHYSICS material placed in an x-ray beam that is used to improve the beam's quality by removing low-energy beams. [Mediev. L. *filtro,* pp. *-atus,* to strain through felt, fr. *filtrum,* felt]

fil·ter·ing bleb (fil′tĕr-ing bleb) A blister of conjunctiva resulting from glaucoma surgery by which a flap of sclera is created in the eye wall, allowing aqueous humor to percolate out of the eye and underneath the conjunctiva, thus lowering intraocular pressure.

fil·ter·ing op·er·a·tion (fil′tĕr-ing op-ĕr-ā′shŭn) A surgical procedure for creation of a fistula between the anterior chamber of the eye and the subconjunctival space in treatment of glaucoma.

fil·tra·ble, fil·ter·a·ble (fil′tră-bĕl, fil′tĕr-ă-bĕl) Capable of passing through a filter; frequently applied to smaller viruses and some bacteria.

fil·trate (fil′trāt) That which has passed through a filter.

fil·tra·tion (fil-trā′shŭn) **1.** The process of passing a liquid or gas through a filter. **2.** RADIOLOGY the process of attenuating and hardening a beam of x-rays or gamma rays by interposing a filter (3) between the radiation source and the object being irradiated; inherent filtration is that which is caused by the apparatus itself, such as the glass of an x-ray tube, without addition of a filter. SYN percolation (1).

fil·tra·tion an·gle (fil-trā′shŭn ang′gĕl) SYN iridocorneal angle.

fil·tra·tion co·ef·fi·cient (fil-trā′shŭn kō-ĕ-fish′ĕnt) A measure of a membrane's permeability to water; specifically, the volume of fluid filtered in unit time through a unit area of membrane per unit pressure difference, taking into account both hydraulic and osmotic pressures.

fil·tra·tion frac·tion (FF) (fil-trā′shŭn frak′shŭn) The portion of the plasma entering the kidney that filters into the lumen of the renal tubules, determined by dividing the glomerular filtration rate by the renal plasma flow; normally, it is around 0.17.

fil·trum (fil′trŭm) SYN filter (1). [Mediev. L.]

fi·lum, pl. **fi·la** (fī′lum, -lă) A structure of filamentous or threadlike appearance. [L. thread]

fi·lum of spi·nal du·ra mat·er (fī′lum spī′năl dūr′ă mā′tĕr) The threadlike termination of the spinal dura mater, surrounding and fused to the filum terminale of the cord, and attached to the deep dorsal sacrococcygeal ligament; extends from S_{2-3} to Co_2 vertebral levels.

fi·lum ter·mi·na·le (fī′lum ter-mē-nā′lē) The slender threadlike termination of the spinal cord. See this page.

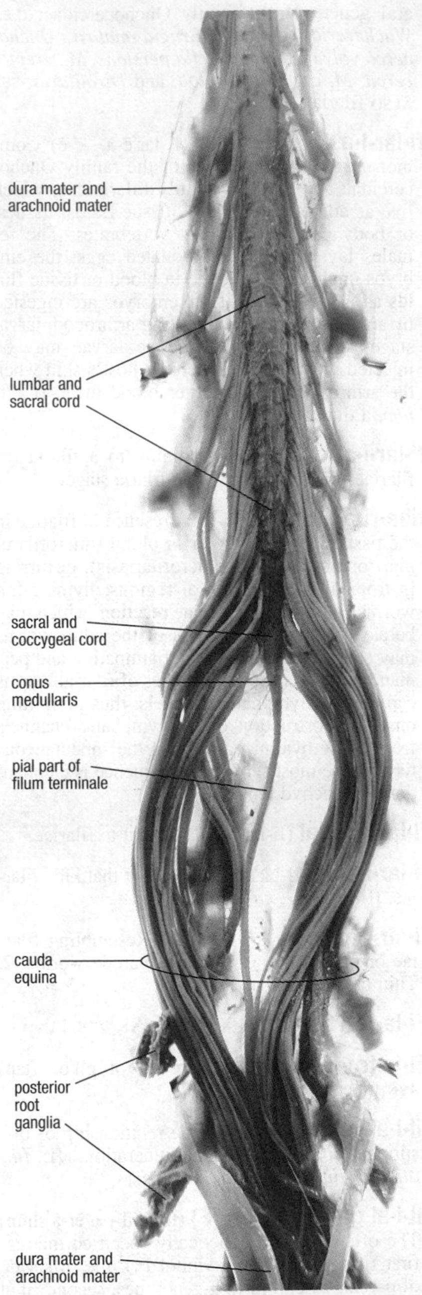

filum terminale with distal spinal cord and cauda equina

FIM Abbreviation for functional independence measure.

fim·bri·a, pl. **fim·bri·ae** (fim′brē-ă, -brē-ē) **1.** Any fringelike structure. **2.** SYN pilus (2). [L. fringe]

fim·bri·ae ova·ri·cae (fim-brē′ē ō-vā-rī′sē) [TA] SYN fimbriae of uterine tube.

fim•bri•ae of u•ter•ine tube (fim′brē-ē yū′tĕr-in tūb) The irregularly branched or fringed processes surrounding the ampulla at the abdominal opening of the uterine tube; most of the lining epithelial cells have cilia that beat toward the uterus. SYN fimbriae ovaricae [TA].

fim•bri•a hip•po•cam•pi (fim′brē-ă hip-ō-kam′pī) [TA] A narrow sharp-edged crest of white fiber matter, continuous with the alveus hippocampi, attached to the medial border of the hippocampus; composed of efferent fibers of the hippocampus that form the fornix, fibers of the hippocampal commissure, and septohippocampal fibers. SYN corpus fimbriatum (1).

fim•bri•ate, fim•bri•at•ed (fim′brē-āt, -ā-ted) Having fimbriae.

fim•bri•o•cele (fim′brē-ō-sēl) Hernia of the corpus fimbriatum of the oviduct. [L. *fimbria*, fringe, + G. *kēlē*, hernia]

fine co•or•di•na•tion (fīn kō-ōr′di-nā′shŭn) SYN fine motor coordination.

fine mo•tor con•trol (fīn mō′tŏr kŏn-trōl′) SYN fine motor coordination.

fine mo•tor co•or•di•na•tion (FMC) (fīn mō′tŏr kō-ōr′di-nā′shŭn) Ability to perform delicate manipulations with the hand requiring steadiness, muscle control, and simultaneous discrete finger movements. SYN dexterity, fine coordination, fine motor control.

fine nee•dle bi•op•sy (fīn nē′dĕl bī′op-sē) Removal of tissue or suspensions of cells through a small needle.

fin•ger (fing′gĕr) One of the digits of the hand. See this page. SYN digitus manus. [A.S.]

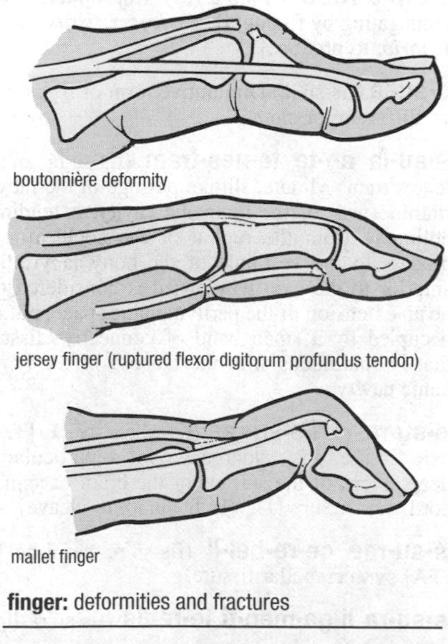

finger: deformities and fractures

fin•ger ag•no•si•a (fing′gĕr ag-nō′zē-ă) Inability to name or recognize individual fingers, of one's own or those of other people; most often caused by lesion of or near the angular gyrus of the dominant hemisphere.

fin•ger-nose test (fing′gĕr-nōz test) A test of voluntary eye-motor coordination of the upper limb(s); the subject is asked to slowly touch the tip of the nose with the extended index finger; assesses cerebellar function.

fin•ger•print (fing′gĕr-print′) **1.** An impression of the inked bulb of the distal phalanx of a finger, showing the configuration of the surface ridges, used as a means of identification. SEE ALSO dermatoglyphics, Galton system of classification of fingerprints. **2.** Term, sometimes used informally, referring to any analytic method capable of making fine distinctions between similar compounds or gel patterns (e.g., the pattern of an infrared absorption curve or of a two-dimensional paper chromatograph). **3.** GENETICS analysis of DNA fragments to determine the identity of a person or the paternity of a child.

fin•ger•spel•ling (fing′gĕr-spel′ing) Method of communication using specific finger and hand movements, representing letters of the alphabet, to spell words. SEE ALSO American Manual Alphabet.

fin•ger-thumb re•flex (fing′gĕr-thŭmb rē′fleks) SYN basal joint reflex.

fin•ger-to-fin•ger test (fing′gĕr fing′gĕr test) A test for coordination and position sense of the upper limbs; the subject is asked to approximate the ends of the index fingers; assesses cerebellar function.

Fin•kel•stein test (fing′kĕl-shtīn test) Assay to detect de Quervain tenosynovitis in which the thumb is flexed into the palm and is covered by the remaining four digits; the wrist is then bent toward the ulna; positive result of test produces pain and crepitus along the path of the involved tendon.

Finn Cham•ber test (fin chām′bĕr tĕst) Device to test skin sensitivity; patch with small aluminum cups that hold material or agents to be tested for allergic reaction; taped against the patient's skin.

Fin•ney op•er•a•tion (fin′ē op-ĕr-ā′shŭn) Gastroduodenostomy that creates, by the technique of closure, a large opening to ensure free emptying from the stomach.

fire ant (fīr ant) Any of several species in the genus *Solenopsis* the bite of which causes a fiery burning sensation and sometimes severe allergic reactions.

fire•wall (fīr′wawl) **1.** A special building material that is placed in walls between buildings or rooms to prevent the spread of fire. **2.** A software program designed to prevent unauthorized persons from getting into a computer system.

first aid (fĭrst ād) Immediate assistance administered in the case of injury or sudden illness by a bystander or other lay person, before the arrival of trained medical personnel.

first aid plant (fĭrst ād plant) SYN *Aloe vera.*

first cra·ni·al nerve [CN I] (fĭrst krā′nē-ăl nĕrv) SYN olfactory nerve [CN I].

first-de·gree AV block (fĭrst-dĕ-grē′ blok) SEE atrioventricular block.

first-de·gree burn (fĭrst-dĕ-grē′ bŭrn) SYN superficial burn.

first-de·gree pro·lapse (fĭrst dĕ-grē′ prō′laps) Form of cervical prolapse where the cervix of the prolapsed uterus is well within the vaginal orifice.

first heart sound (S_1) (fĭrst hahrt sownd) Occurs with ventricular systole and is mainly produced by closure of the atrioventricular valves.

first in·ten·tion (fĭrst in-ten′shŭn) Healing by fibrous adhesion, without suppuration or granulation tissue formation. SEE ALSO second intention, third intention.

first mo·lar, first per·ma·nent mo·lar (fĭrst mō′lăr, pĕr′mă-nĕnt mō′lăr) Sixth permanent tooth or fourth deciduous tooth in the maxilla and mandible on either side of the midsagittal plane of the head following the arch form.

first-pass me·tab·o·lism, first-pass ef·fect (fĭrst-pas mĕ-tab′ŏ-lizm, e-fekt′) The intestinal and hepatic degradation or alteration of a drug or substance taken by mouth, after absorption, removing some of the active substance from the blood before it enters the general circulation.

first phar·yng·e·al arch car·ti·lage (fĭrst făr-in′jē-ăl ahrch kahr′ti-lăj) SYN mandibular cartilage.

first re·spon·der (fĭrst rĕ-spon′dĕr) **1.** The first person to arrive at the emergency scene (medical incident or trauma) to assist the patient or render immediate life-sustaining aid. **2.** The basic level of training and certification for prehospital medical responders (i.e., fire fighters and law enforcement personnel).

first and sec·ond pos·ter·i·or in·ter·cos·tal ar·ter·ies (fĭrst sek′ŏnd pos-tēr′ē-ŏr in-tĕr-kos′tăl ahr′tĕr-ēz) Terminal branches of the superior intercostal artery (from costocervical trunk) supplying upper two intercostal spaces. SYN arteriae intercostales posteriores I et II, posterior intercostal arteries 1–2.

fis·cal in·ter·me·di·ar·y (fis′kăl in′tĕr-mē′dē-ar-ē) An outside contractor that processes claims for U.S. government programs such as Medicare and Medicaid.

Fi·scher sign, Fi·scher symp·tom (fish′ĕr sīn, simp′tŏm) An obsolete sign: in tuberculosis of the mediastinal or peribronchial glands, after the patient's head is bent back as far back as possible, auscultation over the manubrium sterni will sometimes reveal a continuous loud murmur caused by the pressure of the enlarged glands on the large mediastinal vessels.

FISH (fish) Acronym for fluorescent in situ hybridization.

Fish·berg con·cen·tra·tion test (fish′bĕrg kon′sĕn-trā′shŭn test) A test of renal water conservation; after overnight fluid deprivation, morning urine samples are collected and specific gravity is measured.

Fish·er ex·act test (fish′ĕr eg-zakt′ test) Measurement for association in a two-by-two table that is based on the exact distribution of the frequencies within the table.

Fish·er syn·drome (fish′ĕr sin′drōm) A syndrome characterized by ophthalmoplegia, ataxia, and areflexia; a form of polyneuroradiculitis.

fish·mouth (fish′mowth) **1.** Rubefaction of the orifice of the urethra due to infection with *Neisseria gonorrhoeae*. **2.** An incision so shaped to allow drainage of infection or putrefaction.

fis·sion (fish′ŭn) **1.** The act of splitting, e.g., amitotic division of a cell or its nucleus. **2.** Splitting of the nucleus of an atom. [L. *fissio,* a cleaving, fr. *findo,* pp. *fissus,* to cleave]

fis·sion pro·duct (fish′ŭn prod′ŭkt) An atomic species produced in the course of the fission of a larger atom such as ^{235}U.

fis·si·par·i·ty (fis′i-par′i-tē) SYN schizogenesis. [L. *fissio,* cleaving, fr. *findo,* to cleave, + *pario,* to bring forth]

fis·sip·a·rous (fi-sip′ă-rŭs) Reproducing or propagating by fission. [L. *findo,* pp. *fissus,* split, + *pario,* to produce]

fis·su·la (fis-sū′lă) Diminutive form of fissure; a small fissure or cleft.

fis·su·la an·te fe·nes·tram (fis-sū′lă an′tē fen-es′tram) Minute, slitlike passage in the labyrinthine wall of the tympanic cavity, extending obliquely from the region of the cochleaform process to the vestibule of the bony labyrinth, anterior to the oval window; it is considered to be an extension of the perilymphatic space, but is occupied by a small band of connective tissue that is continuous with the mucosa of the tympanic cavity.

fis·su·ra, pl. **fis·su·rae** (fis-sū′ră, -rē) **1.** [TA] SYN fissure. **2.** NEUROANATOMY a particularly deep sulcus of the surface of the brain or spinal cord. SYN fissure (1). [L. fr. *findo,* to cleave]

fis·su·rae ce·re·bel·li (fis-sū′rē ser-ĕ-bel′ī) [TA] SYN cerebellar fissure.

fis·su·ra li·ga·men·ti te·re·tis (fis-sū′ră lig-ă-men′tī ter′i-tis) [TA] SYN fissure of round ligament of liver.

fis•su•ra li•ga•men•ti ve•no•si (fis-sū′ră lig-ă-men′tī vē-nō′sī) [TA] SYN fissure of ligamentum venosum.

fis•sure (fish′ŭr) **1.** A deep furrow, cleft, or slit. SYN fissura (2). SEE ALSO sulcus. **2.** DENTISTRY a developmental break or fault in the tooth enamel. See page B11. SYN fissura (1). [L. *fissura*]

fis•sured frac•ture (fish′ŭrd frak′chŭr) SYN linear fracture.

fis•sured ton•gue (fish′ŭrd tŭng) A painless condition of the tongue characterized by numerous grooves or furrows on the dorsal surface.

fis•sure of lig•a•men•tum ve•no•sum (fish′ŭr lig-ă-men′tŭm vē-nō′sŭm) A deep cleft extending from the porta hepatis and the inferior vena cava between the left lobe and the caudate lobe; it lodges the ligamentum venosum and is thus a vestige of the fossa of the ductus venosus. SYN fissura ligamenti venosi [TA].

fis•sure of round lig•a•ment of li•ver (fish′ŭr rownd lig′ă-mĕnt liv′ĕr) A cleft on the inferior surface of the liver, running from the inferior border to the left extremity of the porta hepatis; it lodges the round ligament of the liver. SYN fissura ligamenti teretis [TA].

fis•tu•la, pl. **fis•tu•lae**, **fis•tu•las** (fis′chū-lă, -lē, -lăz) An abnormal passage from one epithelialized surface to another, either congenital, caused by disease or injury, or created surgically. [L. a pipe, a tube]

fis•tu•la•tion, **fis•tu•li•za•tion** (fis′chū-lā′shŭn, -lī-zā′shŭn) Formation of a fistula in a part; becoming fistulous.

fis•tu•lec•to•my (fis′chū-lek′tŏ-mē) Excision of a fistula. SYN syringectomy. [fistula + G. *ektomē,* excision]

fis•tu•lot•o•my (fis′chū-lot′ŏ-mē) Incision or surgical enlargement of a fistula. SYN syringot omy. [fistula + G. *tomē,* incision]

fis•tu•lous (fis′chū-lŭs) Relating to or containing a fistula.

fit (fit) **1.** An attack of an acute disease or the sudden appearance of some symptom, such as coughing. **2.** A convulsion. **3.** SYN epilepsy. **4.** DENTISTRY the adaptation of any dental restoration, e.g., of an inlay to the cavity preparation in a tooth, or of a denture to its basal seat. [A.S. *fitt*]

FITC Abbreviation for fluorescein isothiocyanate.

fit•ness (fit′nĕs) **1.** Well-being. **2.** Suitability. **3.** POPULATION GENETICS a measure of the relative survival and reproductive success of a given individual or phenotype, or of a population subgroup. **4.** A set of attributes, primarily respiratory and cardiovascular, relating to the ability to perform tasks requiring expenditures of energy.

fit test•ing (fit tes′ting) A process in which all people who are required to wear negative-pressure respirators are examined and interviewed to determine which mask best conforms to their facial features; a rigorous protocol in which the tester challenges the face-to-facepiece seal with a chemical agent.

five-el•e•ment the•o•ry (fīv-el′ĕ-mĕnt thē′ŏr-ē) A traditional medical system for interpreting a person's mental, emotional, and physical states as manifested in five distinct types of energy: wood, air, fire, water and earth (Asian) or ether, air, fire, water, and earth (Ayurvedic). SEE ALSO polarity therapy, acupressure, shiatsu, chi, shakra.

five-year sur•viv•al rate (fīv′yēr sŭr-vī′văl rāt) The proportion of patients still alive 5 years after a diagnosis or form of treatment is completed. Usually applied to statistics of survival of cancer patients, because, after 5 years, recurrences are less likely.

fix•a•tion (fik-sā′shŭn) **1.** The condition of being firmly attached or set. **2.** HISTOLOGY the rapid killing of tissue elements and their preservation and hardening to retain as nearly as possible the same relations they had in the living body. SYN fixing. **3.** CHEMISTRY the conversion of a gas into solid or liquid form by chemical reactions, with or without the help of living tissue. **4.** PSYCHOANALYSIS the quality of being firmly attached to a particular person or object or period in one's development. **5.** PHYSIOLOGIC OPTICS the coordinated positioning and accommodation of both eyes that results in bringing or maintaining a sharp image of a stationary or moving object on the fovea of each eye. [L. *figo,* pp. *fixus,* to fix, fasten]

fix•a•tion nys•tag•mus (fik-sā′shŭn nis-tag′mŭs) Nystagmus aggravated or induced by ocular fixation, arising as optokinetic nystagmus, or resulting from midbrain lesions.

fix•a•tion sup•pres•sion (fik-sā′shŭn sŭ-presh′ŭn) The reduction in induced or spontaneous nystagmus that occurs with visual fixation.

fix•a•tive (fik′să-tiv) **1.** Serving to fix, bind, or make firm or stable. **2.** A substance used for the preservation of gross and histologic specimens of tissue, or individual cells, usually by denaturing and precipitating or cross-linking the protein constituents. SEE ALSO fluid, solution.

fix•a•tor (fik-sā′tŏr) **1.** A device providing rigid immobilization through external skeletal fixation by means of rods (fixators) attached to pins that are placed in or through the bone. **2.** A muscle or muscle group that works to stabilize a joint or body region while other muscles initiate movement.

fix•a•tor mus•cle (fik-sā′tŏr mŭs′ĕl) A muscle

that acts as a stabilizer of one part of the body during movement of another part.

fixed drug e·rup·tion (fikst drŭg ĕr-up′shŭn) A type of drug eruption that recurs at a fixed site (or sites) after administration of a particular drug.

fixed end (fikst end) For a given movement, the end of a bone that is held stationary (as a consequence of attachment or muscular fixation) while the other end of the bone (the mobile end) moves in response to muscle activity or gravity. SYN punctum fixum.

fixed i·de·a (fikst ī-dē′ă) **1.** An exaggerated notion, belief, or delusion that persists, despite evidence to the contrary, and controls the mind. **2.** The obstinate conviction of a psychotic person regarding the correctness of a delusion.

fixed mac·ro·phage (fikst mak′rō-fāj) A relatively immotile macrophage found in connective tissue, lymph nodes, spleen, and bone marrow.

fixed par·tial den·ture (fikst pahr′shăl den′chŭr) A restoration of one or more missing teeth that cannot be readily removed by the patient or dentist; it is permanently attached to natural teeth or roots, which furnish the primary support to the appliance. SYN bridge (3).

fixed pu·pil (fikst pyū′pil) A stationary pupil unresponsive to all stimuli.

fixed-rate pace·mak·er (fikst-rāt pās′mā-kĕr) An artificial pacemaker that emits electrical stimuli at a constant frequency.

fixed vi·rus (fikst vī′rŭs) Rabies virus with virulence for rabbits that has been stabilized by numerous passages through this experimental host. SEE ALSO street virus.

fix·er (fiks′ĕr) In photography and radiography, a solution that removes both the unexposed and undeveloped silver halide crystals from the film emulsion and hardens the gelatin.

fix·ing (fik′sing) SYN fixation (2).

flac·cid (flak′sid) Relaxed, flabby, or without tone. [L. *flaccidus*]

flac·cid dys·arth·ri·a (flak′sid dis-ahr′thrē-ă) Dysarthria associated with peripheral muscle weakness usually due to lower motor neuron disorders, causing hypernasality, imprecise consonants, breathy voice, and monotony of pitch. SEE hypernasality.

flac·cid·i·ty (flak-sid′i-tē) The condition or state of being flaccid.

flag (flag) MEDICAL TRANSCRIPTION warning or caution by the transcriptionist to the author of a report, pointing out problems (e.g., missing date, dictation errors, equipment problems, or potentially inflammatory remarks). Flags contribute to risk management.

fla·gel·la (flă-jel′ă) Plural of flagellum.

fla·gel·lar (flă-jel′ăr) Relating to a flagellum or to the extremity of a protozoan.

fla·gel·lar an·ti·gen (flă-jel′ăr an′ti-jen) The heat-labile antigens associated with bacterial flagella, in contrast to somatic antigen. SEE ALSO H antigen.

flag·el·late (flaj′ĕ-lāt) **1.** Possessing one or more flagella. **2.** A member of the class Mastigophora.

flag·el·lat·ed (flaj′ĕ-lā-tĕd) Possessing one or more flagella.

flag·el·la·tion (flaj′ĕ-lā′shŭn) **1.** Whipping either oneself or another as a means of arousing or heightening sexual feeling. **2.** The pattern of formation of flagella. [L. *flagellatus,* fr. *flagello,* to whip or scourge]

fla·gel·li·form (flă-jel′i-fōrm) Whiplike in structure.

flag·el·lo·sis (flaj′ĕ-lō′sis) Infection with flagellated protozoa in the intestinal or genital tract (e.g., trichomoniasis).

fla·gel·lum, pl. **fla·gel·la** (flă-jel′ŭm, -ă) A whiplike locomotory organelle of constant structural arrangement consisting of nine double peripheral microtubules and two single central microtubules; it arises from a deeply staining basal granule, often connected to the nucleus by a fiber, the rhizoplast. [L. dim. of *flagrum,* a whip]

flag·ging re·ports (flag′ing rĕ-pōrts′) Process in which a medical transcriptionist calls a dictator's attention to an area in the dictation that needs clarification due to the dictation's unintelligibility or inconsistentcy.

flail chest (flāl chest) Flapping chest wall; condition in which three or more consecutive ribs on the same side of the chest have been fractured in at least two places, with resulting instability of the chest wall, paradoxic respiratory movements of the injured segment, and loss of respiratory efficiency.

flail joint (flāl joynt) A joint with loss of function caused by loss of ability to stabilize the joint in any plane within its normal range of motion.

flame cell (flām sel) Primitive, ciliated excretory cell in trematodes; the movement of the cilia on this cell within the miracidium larva within a schistosome egg indicates egg viability.

flange (flanj) That part of the denture base that extends from the cervical ends of the teeth to the border of the denture.

flank (flangk) SYN latus.

flank in·ci·sion (flangk in-sizh′ŭn) An incision usually made near and parallel to the 12th rib or between the iliac crest and the rib.

flank po·si·tion (flangk pŏ-zish′ŏn) A lateral recumbent position, but with the lower leg flexed, the upper leg extended, and convex extension of the upper side of the body; used for nephrectomy.

flap (flap) **1.** Mass of partially detached tissue. SEE ALSO pedicle flap, local flap, distant flap. **2.** An uncontrolled movement, as of the hands. SEE asterixis. [M.E. *flappe*]

flap am•pu•ta•tion (flap amp′yū-tā′shŭn) An amputation in which flaps of the muscular and cutaneous tissues are shaped to cover the end of the bone. SYN flap operation (1).

flap•less am•pu•ta•tion (flap′lĕs amp′yū-tā′shŭn) An amputation without any tissue to cover the stump.

flap op•er•a•tion (flap op-ĕr-ā′shŭn) **1.** SYN flap amputation. **2.** DENTAL SURGERY an operation in which a portion of the mucoperiosteal tissues is surgically detached from the underlying bone or impacted tooth for better access and visibility in exploring the area covered by the tissue. SEE ALSO flap.

flap•ping trem•or (flap′ing trem′ŏr) SYN asterixis.

flare (flār) **1.** A gradual tapering or spreading outward. **2.** A diffuse redness of the skin extending beyond the local reaction to the application of an irritant; it is due to dilation of the arterioles and capillaries; depends on an axon reflex set up by the liberation of a histaminelike substance in skin when injured. SEE ALSO triple response. **3.** Protein in aqueous fluid.

flash (flash) **1.** A sudden and brief burst of light or heat. **2.** Excess material extruded between the sections of a flask in the process of molding denture bases or other dental restorations.

flash•back (flash′bak) An involuntary recurrence of some aspect of a hallucinatory experience or perceptual distortion occurring some time after ingestion of the hallucinogen that produced the original effect and without subsequent ingestion of the substance.

flash blind•ness (flash blīnd′nĕs) A temporary loss of vision produced when retinal light-sensitive pigments are bleached by light more intense than that to which the retina is physiologically adapted at that moment.

flash-lag ef•fect (flash-lag e-fekt′) The apparent lagging behind a moving object of a portion of it that flashes briefly.

flash meth•od (flash meth′ŏd) Sterilization of milk by raising it rapidly to a temperature of 161°F, holding it there for a short time, and reducing it rapidly to 40°F.

flask (flask) A small receptacle, usually glass, used for holding liquids, powder, or gases. [M.E. keg, fr. Fr. *flasque*, fr. Germanic]

flat af•fect (flat a′fekt) Absence of or diminution in the amount of emotional tone or outward emotional reaction (e.g., facial expression, posture) typically shown by oneself or others under similar circumstances; may include lack of vocal expression; often a symptom of mental disorders; a milder form is termed blunted affect.

Fla•tau law (flah′tow law) A law concerning the excentric position of the long spinal tracts; the greater the distance the nerve fibers run lengthwise in the cord, the more they tend to be situated toward its periphery.

flat bone (flat bōn) A type of bone characterized by its thin, flattened shape, such as the scapula or certain of the cranial bones.

flat chest (flat chest) A thorax in which the anteroposterior diameter is shorter than the average.

flat con•dy•lo•ma (flat kon-di-lō′mă) **1.** SYN condyloma latum. **2.** A condyloma of the uterine cervix or other site caused by human papillomavirus infection and characterized histologically by koilocytosis without papillomatosis.

flat e•lec•tro•en•ceph•a•lo•gram (flat ĕ-lek′trō-en-sef′ă-lō-gram) SYN electrocerebral silence.

flat flap (flat flap) A flap in which during transfer the pedicle is left flat or open, i.e., untubed. SYN open flap.

flat•foot (flat′fut) SYN talipes planus.

flat pel•vis (flat pel′vis) A pelvis in which the anteroposterior diameter is uniformly contracted, the sacrum being dislocated forward between the iliac bones.

flat•u•lence (flat′yū-lĕns) Presence of an excessive amount of gas in the stomach and intestines. [Mod. L. *flatulentus*, fr. L. *flatus*, a blowing, fr. *flo*, pp. *flatus*, to blow]

flat•u•lent (flat′yū-lĕnt) Relating to or suffering from flatulence.

fla•tus (flā′tŭs) Gas or air in the gastrointestinal tract that may be expelled through the anus. [L. a blowing]

fla•tus vag•i•na•lis (flā′tŭs vaj′i-nā′lis) Expulsion of gas from the vagina, typically by means of a rectovaginal fistula.

flat wart (flat wōrt) SYN verruca plana.

flat•worm (flat′wŏrm) A member of the phylum Platyhelminthes, including the parasitic tapeworms and flukes.

fla•vin, fla•vine (flā′vin, flā′vēn) SYN riboflavin. [L. *flavus*, yellow]

fla•vin ad•e•nine di•nu•cle•o•tide (FAD) (flā′vin ad′ĕ-nēn dī-nū′klē-ō-tīd) A condensation product of riboflavin and adenosine 5′-diphosphate; the coenzyme of various aerobic dehydrogenases, e.g., D-amino-acid oxidase and aldehyde dehydrogenase; strictly speaking, FAD is not a dinucleotide because it contains a sugar alcohol.

fla•vin mon•o•nu•cle•o•tide (FMN) (flā′vin mon′ō-nū′klē-ō-tīd) Riboflavin 5′-phosphate; the coenzyme of a number of oxidation-reduction enzymes; e.g., NADH dehydrogenase and L-amino acid oxidase. Strictly speaking, FMN is not a nucleotide because it contains a sugar alcohol instead of a sugar.

fla•vi•vi•rus (flā′vi-vī-rŭs) A genus in the family Flaviviridae that includes yellow fever, dengue, and St. Louis encephalitis viruses. [L. *flavus,* yellow, + virus]

Fla•vo•bac•te•ri•um (flā′vō-bak-tēr′ē-ŭm) A genus of aerobic to facultatively anaerobic, nonspore-forming, motile and nonmotile bacteria containing gram-negative rods. These organisms characteristically produce yellow, orange, red, or yellow-brown pigments. They are found in soil and fresh and salt water. Some species are pathogenic. [L. *flavus,* yellow]

fla•vo•en•zyme (flā′vō-en′zīm) Any enzyme that possesses a flavin nucleotide as coenzyme; e.g., xanthine oxidase, succinate dehydrogenase.

fla•vo•pro•tein (flā′vō-prō′tēn) A compound protein possessing a flavin as prosthetic group. Cf. flavoenzyme.

flea (flē) An insect of the order Siphonaptera, distinguished by lateral compression, sucking mouthparts, extraordinary jumping powers, and ectoparasitic adult life in the hair and feathers of warm-blooded animals.

fleece•flow•er (flēs′flow-ĕr) SYN flo-ti.

Flei•scher ring (flīsh′er ring) An iron line in the corneal epithelium often present at the base of the keratoconus cone; caused by deposition of hemosiderin.

Fleisch•ner lines (flīsh′nĕr līnz) Coarse linear shadows on a chest radiograph, indicating bands of subsegmental atelectasis.

Flem•ming fix•a•tive (flem′ing fiks′a-tiv) A mixture of chromic acid, osmic acid, and acetic acid that makes an excellent cytoplasmic and chromosomal fixative, especially when acetic acid is omitted; disadvantages are that it penetrates poorly, requires lengthy washing, and deterioriates rapidly.

Flem•ming tri•ple stain (flem′ing trip′ĕl stān) A stain composed of safranin, methyl violet, and orange G.

flesh (flesh) **1.** Living tissue, especially soft tissues as contrasted with bone. **2.** SYN muscular tissue. **3.** The meat of animals used for food. [A.S. *flaesc*]

flesh fly (flesh flī) Genera of dipteran flies including *Wohlfahrtia*, *Sarcophaga*, and *Parasarcophaga*, which feed on feces and decaying meat or fish; can cause human disease.

Flet•cher fac•tor (flech′ĕr fak′tōr) SYN prekallikrein.

fleur-de-lis (flūr-dĕ-lē) SYN blue flag. [Fr., lily flower]

flex (fleks) To bend; to move a joint in such a direction as to approximate the two parts which it connects. [L. *flecto,* pp. *flexus,* to bend]

flex•i•bil•i•tas ce•re•a (flek-si-bil′i-tahs sē′rē-ă) The rigidity of catalepsy that may be overcome by slight external force, but which returns at once, holding the limb firmly in the new position. [L. waxy flexibility]

flex•i•bil•i•ty (fleks′i-bil′i-tē) Range of motion about a joint dependent on the condition of surrounding structures. SEE range of motion.

flex•i•ble en•do•scope (fleks′i-bĕl en′dō-skōp) An optic instrument that transmits light and carries images back to the observer through a flexible bundle of small (about 10 mcm) transparent fibers. It is used to inspect interior portions of the body. These instruments are generally equipped with mechanisms for steering and may have additional ports for allowing sampling or operative instruments along their axis to the internal site. SEE ALSO fiberoptics.

flex•i•ble hy•ster•o•scope (fleks′i-bĕl his′tĕr-ō-skōp) Steerable flexible hysteroscope of small diameter for operative or diagnostic procedures that does not require an outer sheath, has fiberoptics for visualization, and must be used with a distending gas.

flex•ion (flek′shŭn) **1.** The act of flexing or bending, e.g., bending of a joint so as to approximate the parts it connects; bending of the spine so that the concavity of the curve looks forward. **2.** The condition of being flexed or bent. SYN open-packed position (2). [L. *flecto,* pp. *flexus,* to bend]

flex•ion-ex•ten•sion in•ju•ry (flek′shŭn-eks-ten′shŭn in′jŭr-ē) Forceful application of a forward and backward movement of the unsupported head that may produce an injury to the cervical spine or the brain.

flex•ion-tear•drop frac•ture (flek′shŭn-tēr′ drop frak′shŭr) Breaking of the spinal cord due to massive flexure in the structure.

Flex•ner ba•cil•lus (fleks′nĕr bă-sil′ŭs) SYN *Shigella flexneri.*

flex•o•me•ter (fleks-om′ĕ-tĕr) SYN goniometer (3).

flex•or (fleks′ŏr) A muscle the action of which is to flex a joint.

flex•or car•pi ra•di•a•lis mus•cle (fleks′ŏr kahr′pī rā-dē-ā′lis mŭs′ĕl) *Origin*, common flexor origin of the medial condyle of humerus; *insertion*, anterior surface of the base of the second and most often sending a slip to that of the third metacarpal bone; *action*, flexes and abducts wrist radialward; *nerve supply*, median; its tendon travels in its own canal roofed by a layer of the transverse carpal ligament. SYN musculus flexor carpi radialis [TA], radial flexor muscle of wrist.

flex•or car•pi ul•na•ris mus•cle (fleks′ŏr kahr′pī ŭl-nā′ris mŭs′ĕl) *Origin*, humeral head from medial condyle of humerus, ulnar head from olecranon and upper three fifths of posterior border of ulna; *insertion*, pisiform bone, but is continued to the fifth metacarpal bone through the pisometacarpal ligament; *action*, flexes and abducts wrist ulnarward; *nerve supply*, ulnar. SYN musculus flexor carpi ulnaris [TA], ulnar flexor muscle of wrist.

flex•or di•gi•ti mi•ni•mi brev•is mus•cle of foot (fleks′ŏr dij′i-tī mi′ni-mī brev′is mŭs′ĕl fut) *Origin*, base of metatarsal bone of the little toe and sheath of musculus peroneus longus; *insertion*, lateral surface of base of proximal phalanx of little toe; *action*, flexes the proximal phalanx of the little toe; *nerve supply*, lateral plantar. SYN musculus flexor digiti minimi brevis pedis [TA], short flexor muscle of little toe.

flex•or di•gi•ti mi•ni•mi brev•is mus•cle of hand (fleks′ŏr dij′i-tī min′i-mī brev′is mŭs′ĕl hand) *Origin*, hamulus of hamate bone; *insertion*, medial side of proximal phalanx of little finger; *action*, flexes proximal phalanx of little finger; *nerve supply*, ulnar. See this page. SYN musculus flexor digiti minimi brevis manus [TA], short flexor muscle of little finger.

flex•or di•gi•to•rum brev•is mus•cle (fleks′ŏr dij-i-tō′rŭm brev′is mŭs′ĕl) *Origin*, medial tubercle of calcaneus and central portion of plantar fascia; *insertion*, middle phalanges of four lateral toes by tendons perforated by those of the flexor longus; *action*, flexes lateral four toes; *nerve supply*, medial plantar. See this page. SYN musculus flexor digitorum brevis [TA], short flexor muscle of toes.

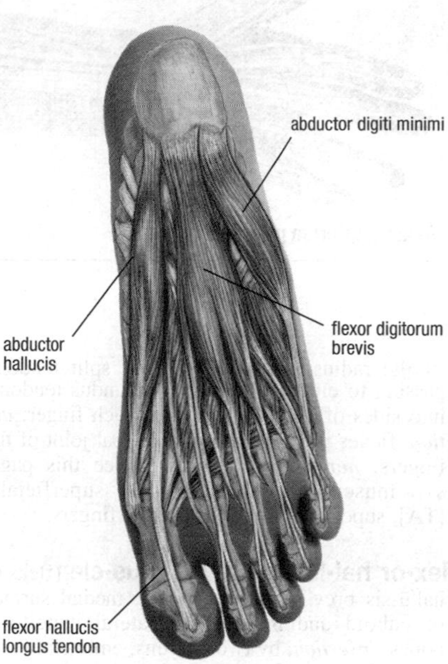

flexor digitorum brevis muscle

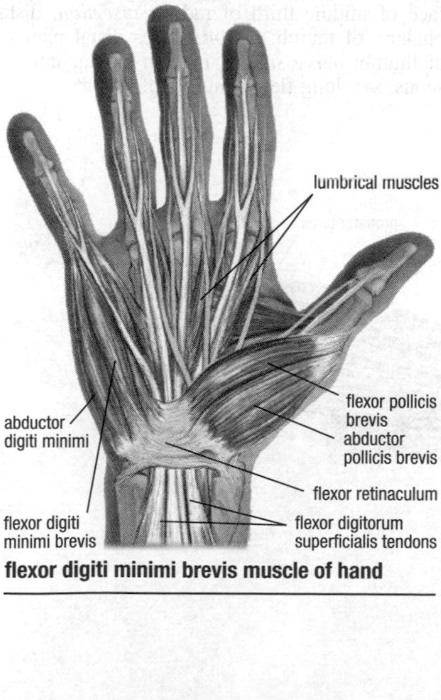

flexor digiti minimi brevis muscle of hand

flex•or di•gi•to•rum lon•gus mus•cle (fleks′ŏr dij-i-tō′rŭm long′gŭs mŭs′ĕl) *Origin*, middle third of posterior surface of tibia; *insertion*, by four tendons, perforating those of the flexor brevis, into bases of distal phalanges of four lateral toes; *action*, flexes second to fifth toes; *nerve supply*, tibial nerve. SYN musculus flexor digitorum longus [TA], long flexor muscle of toes.

flex•or di•gi•to•rum pro•fun•dus mus•cle (fleks′ŏr dij-i-tō′rŭm prō-fŭn′dŭs mŭs′ĕl) *Origin*, anterior surface of upper third of ulna; *insertion*, by four tendons, piercing those of the superficialis, into base of distal phalanx of each finger; *action*, flexes distal interphalangeal joint of fingers; *nerve supply*, ulnar and median (anterior interosseous muscle). See page 592. SYN musculus flexor digitorum profundus [TA].

flex•or di•gi•to•rum su•per•fi•ci•a•lis mus•cle (fleks′ŏr dij-i-tō′rŭm sū′pĕr-fish-ē-ā′lis mŭs′ĕl) *Origin*, humeroulnar head from the medial epicondyle of the humerus, the medial border of the coronoid process, and a tendinous arch between these points, radial head from the oblique line and middle third of the lateral border

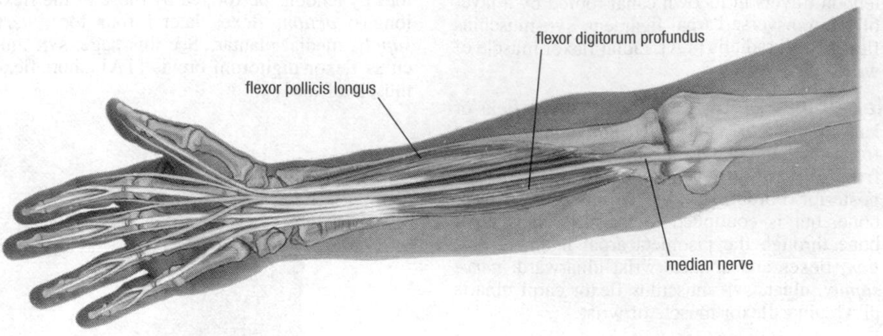

flexor digitorum profundus muscle

of the radius; *insertion*, by four split tendons, passing to either side of the profundus tendons, into sides of middle phalanx of each finger; *action*, flexes proximal interphalangeal joint of the fingers; *nerve supply*, median. See this page. SYN musculus flexor digitorum superficialis [TA], superficial flexor muscle of fingers.

flex•or hal•lu•cis brev•is mus•cle (fleks′ŏr hal′ū-sis brev′is mŭs′ĕl) *Origin*, medial surface of cuboid and middle and lateral cuneiform bones; *insertion*, by two tendons, embracing that of the flexor longus hallucis, into the sides of the base of the proximal phalanx of the great toe; *action*, flexes great toe; *nerve supply*, medial and lateral plantar. SYN short flexor muscle of great toe.

flex•or hal•lu•cis lon•gus mus•cle (fleks′ŏr hal′ū-sis long′gŭs mŭs′ĕl) *Origin*, lower two thirds of posterior surface of fibula; *insertion*, base of distal phalanx of great toe; *action*, flexes great toe; *nerve supply*, medial plantar. SYN long flexor muscle of great toe.

flex•or pol•li•cis brev•is mus•cle (fleks′ŏr pol′li-sis brev′is mŭs′ĕl) *Origin*, superficial portion from flexor retinaculum of wrist, deep portion from ulnar side of first metacarpal bone; *insertion*, base of proximal phalanx of thumb; *action*, flexes proximal phalanx of thumb; *nerve supply*, median (superficial head) and deep branch of ulnar (deep head). Some authors consider the deep head to be the first in a series of four palmar interossei muscles of the hand. SYN short flexor muscle of thumb.

flex•or pol•li•cis lon•gus mus•cle (fleks′ŏr pol′li-sis long′gŭs mŭs′ĕl) *Origin*, anterior surface of middle third of radius; *insertion*, distal phalanx of thumb; *action*, flexes distal phalanx of thumb; *nerve supply*, median palmar interosseous. SYN long flexor muscle of thumb.

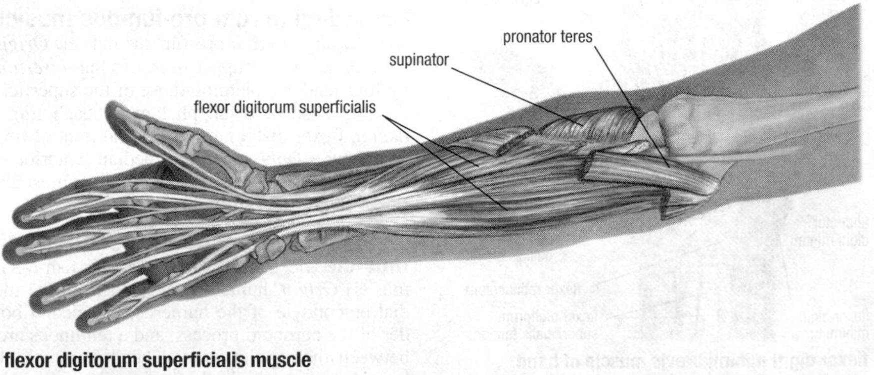

flexor digitorum superficialis muscle

flex•or re•flex (fleks′ŏr rē′fleks) Flexion of ankle, knee, and hip when the foot is painfully stimulated; the crossed extension reflex occurs in association with it.

flex•or ret•i•nac•u•lum of low•er limb (fleks′ŏr ret′i-nak′yū-lŭm lō′ĕr lim) A wide band passing from the medial malleolus to the medial and upper border of the calcaneus and to the plantar surface as far as the navicular bone; it holds in place the tendons of the tibialis posterior, flexor digitorum longus, and flexor hallucis longus.

flex•u•ra, pl. **flex•u•rae** (flek-shūr′ă, -ē) [TA] SYN flexure. [L. a bending]

flex•u•ra co•li dex•tra (flek-shūr′ă kō′lī deks′ tră) [TA] SYN right colic flexure.

flex•u•ra co•li si•nis•tra (flek-shūr′ă kō′lī sin′ is-tră) [TA] SYN left colic flexure.

flex•u•ra du•o•de•no•je•ju•na•lis (flek-shūr′ ă dū-ō-dē-nō-jē-jū-nā′lis) [TA] SYN duodenojejunal flexure.

flex•ur•al (flek′shŭr-ăl) Relating to a flexure.

flex•ur•al psor•i•a•sis (flek′shŭr-ăl sōr-ī′ă-sis) Psoriasis involving intertriginous folds (e.g., axillary and inguinal skin); may resemble seborrheic dermatitis.

flex•ure (flek′shŭr) A bend, as in an organ or structure. SYN flexura [TA]. [L. *flexura*]

Flie•rin•ga ring (flēr-ing′gă ring) A stainless steel ring sutured to the sclera to prevent collapse of the globe in difficult intraocular operations.

flight (flīt) **1.** The motion of an object through air. **2.** Escape. [O.E. *flyht*]

flight of i•de•as (flīt ī′dē-ăz) An uncontrollable symptom of the manic phase of a bipolar depressive disorder in which streams of unrelated words and ideas occur to the patient at a rate that is impossible to vocalize despite a marked increase in the person's overall output of words. SEE ALSO mania.

flight in•to dis•ease (flīt di-zēz′) Benefit through falling ill or assuming the sick role. SEE primary gain, secondary gain.

flight in•to health (flīt helth) DYNAMIC PSYCHOTHERAPY the early but often only temporary disappearance of the symptoms that ostensibly brought the patient into therapy; a defense against the anxiety engendered by the prospect of further psychoanalytic exploration of the patient's conflicts.

flight-or-fight re•sponse (flīt fīt rĕ-spons′) SEE emergency theory.

Flin•ders Is•land spot•ted fe•ver (flin′dĕrz ī′lănd spot′ĕd fē′vĕr) A febrile disease caused by the bacterium *Rickettsia honei* in southeastern Australia and characterized by headache, myalgia, and maculopapular rash. [named after Flinders Island in Tasmania, Australia, where the first cases of the disease were identified]

Flint ar•cade (flint ahr-kād′) A series of vascular arches at the bases of the pyramids of the kidney.

Flint mur•mur (flint mŭr′mŭr) A diastolic murmur, similar to that of mitral stenosis, heard best at the cardiac apex. SYN bicuspid murmur.

flip an•gle (flip ang′gĕl) In a magnetic resonance imaging sequence, the rotation of the average axis of the protons induced by radiofrequency signals; low angles are used in rapid-imaging sequences and to show a signal from flowing blood.

flit•ter (flit′ĕr) SYN impure flutter.

float•er (flōt′ĕr) **1.** Colloquial term for a cadaver removed from a body of water. **2.** An object in the field of vision that originates in the vitreous body.

float•ing (flōt′ing) **1.** Free or unattached. **2.** Unduly movable; out of the normal position; denoting an occasional abnormal condition of certain organs (e.g., kidneys, liver, spleen).

float•ing car•ti•lage (flōt′ing kahr′ti-lăj) A loose piece of cartilage within a joint cavity, detached from the articular cartilage or from a meniscus.

float•ing kid•ney (flōt′ing kid′nē) The abnormally mobile kidney in nephroptosis. SYN wandering kidney.

float•ing pa•tel•la (flōt′ing pă-tel′ă) SYN ballottable patella.

float•ing ribs [XI–XII] (flōt′ing ribz) The two lower ribs on either side that are not attached anteriorly. SYN costae fluctuantes [XI–XII] [TA], vertebral ribs.

float•ing spleen (flōt′ing splēn) A spleen that is palpable because of excessive mobility from a relaxed or lengthened pedicle rather than because of enlargement. SYN lien mobilis, movable spleen.

floc•cil•la•tion (flok′si-lā′shŭn) An aimless plucking at the bedclothes, as if one were picking off threads or tufts of cotton. [Mod. L. *flocculus*]

floc•cose (flok′ōs) BACTERIOLOGY describes a growth of short, curving filaments or chains closely but irregularly disposed. [L. *floccus,* a flock of wool]

floc•cu•lar (flok′yū-lăr) Relating to a flocculus of any sort; specifically to the flocculus of the cerebellum.

floc•cu•late (flok′yū-lāt) To become flocculent.

floc•cu•la•tion (flok′yū-lā′shŭn) Precipitation

from solution in the form of fleecy masses; the process of becoming flocculent.

floc·cu·lent (flok′yū-lĕnt) **1.** Resembling tufts of cotton or wool; denoting a fluid, such as urine, containing numerous shreds or fluffy particles of gray-white or white mucus or other material. **2.** BACTERIOLOGY denoting a fluid culture in which numerous colonies are either floating in the fluid medium or are loosely deposited at the bottom.

floc·cu·lus, pl. **floc·cu·li** (flok′yū-lŭs, -lī) **1.** A tuft or shred of cotton or wool or anything resembling it. **2.** [TA] A small lobe of the cerebellum at the posterior border of the middle cerebellar peduncle anterior to the biventer lobule; it is associated with the nodulus of the vermis; together, these two structures compose the vestibular part of the cerebellum. [Mod. L. dim. of L. *floccus,* a tuft of wool]

flood (flŭd) **1.** To bleed profusely from the uterus, as after childbirth or in cases of menorrhagia. **2.** Colloquialism for a profuse menstrual discharge. [A.S. *flōd*]

flood·ing (flŭd′ing) **1.** Bleeding profusely from the uterus, especially after childbirth or in severe cases of menorrhagia. **2.** A type of behavior therapy; a therapeutic strategy at the beginning of therapy, in which the patients imagine the most anxiety-producing scene and fully immerse (flood) themselves in it.

floor plate (flōr plāt) Ventral midline thinning of the developing neural tube, a continuity between the basal plates of either side; opposite of roof plate. SYN ventral plate.

flop·py in·fant (flop′ē in′fănt) A young child afflicted with neuromuscular or muscular disorders such that the limbs cannot move independently.

flop·py in·fant syn·drome, flop·py ba·by syn·drome (flop′ē in′fănt sin′drōm, flop′ē bā′bē sin′drōm) Colloquial usage to describe pediatric patients with low muscle tone.

flo·ra (flō′ră) **1.** Plant life, usually of a certain locality or district. **2.** The population of microorganisms inhabiting the internal and external surfaces of healthy conventional animals. [L. *Flora,* goddess of flowers, fr. *flos* (*flor-*), a flower]

flor·id (flōr′id) **1.** Of a bright red color; denoting certain cutaneous lesions. **2.** Fully developed. [L. *floridus,* flowery]

flo·ta·tion (flō-tā′shŭn) A process for separating solids by their tendency to float upon or sink into a liquid.

flo·ta·tion con·stant (S_f) (flō-tā′shŭn kon′stănt) Characteristic sedimentation behavior of a lipoprotein fraction of plasma in a centrifugal field in a medium of appropriate density, achieved by adding a salt or D_2O to the plasma. SYN Svedberg of flotation.

flo·ta·tion meth·od (flō-tā′shŭn meth′ŏd) Flotation of helminth eggs on the surface of a liquid of high specific gravity when eggs are difficult to find in direct examination.

flo-ti (flō-tē) (*Polygonum multiflorum*) Agent purported to lower blood pressure, induce fertility, and provide purgation; potentially hepatotoxic. SYN fleeceflower.

flow (flō) **1.** To bleed from the uterus less profusely than in flooding. **2.** The menstrual discharge. **3.** Movement of a liquid or gas; specifically, the volume of liquid or gas passing a given point per unit of time. **4.** RHEOLOGY A permanent deformation of a body that proceeds with time. [A.S. *flōwan*]

flow-con·trolled ven·ti·la·tor (flō′kŏn-trōld′ ven′til-ā-tŏr) A device designed to deliver mandatory breaths with a preset flow waveform.

flow cy·tom·e·try (flō sī-tom′ĕ-trē) A method of measuring fluorescence from stained cells that are in suspension and flowing through a narrow orifice, usually with one or two lasers to activate the dyes; used to measure cell size, number, viability, and nucleic acid content.

flow di·a·gram (flō dī′ă-gram) A diagram composed of blocks connected by arrows representing steps in a process such as decision analysis.

flow·ers (flow′ĕrz) A mineral substance in a powdery state after sublimation.

flow·me·ter (flō′mē-tĕr) **1.** A device for measuring the flow of liquid or gas. SEE ALSO pneumotachometer. **2.** A device for controlling the flow of medical gases, as in the delivery of air or oxygen to a nebulizer.

flow-vol·ume loop stud·ies (flō-vol′yūm lūp stŭd′ēz) Diagnostic methods in which inspiratory and expiratory flow-volume curves are used to determine the location of an obstruction in the tracheobronchial tree.

flu (flū) SYN influenza.

fluc·tu·ate (flŭk′shū-āt) **1.** To move in waves. **2.** To vary, to change from time to time, as in referring to any quantity or quality (blood pressure, concentration of substance in urine or blood, secretory activity). [L. *fluctuo,* pp. *-atus,* to flow in waves]

flu·ence (flū′ĕns) A measure of the quantity of x-radiation in a beam in diagnostic radiology, either particle fluence, the number of photons entering a sphere of unit cross-sectional area, or energy fluence, the sum of the energies of the photons passing through a unit area. Cf. flux. [L. *fluentia,* a flowing, fr. *fluo,* to flow]

flu·en·cy (flū′ĕn-sē) The smooth flow of speech sounds in connected discourse, without interruptions or repetitions. [L. *fluentia,*a flowing, fr. *fluo,* to flow]

flu·ent a·pha·si·a (flū'ĕnt ă-fā'zē-ă) SYN receptive aphasia.

flu·id (flū'id) **1.** A nonsolid substance, such as a liquid or gas, which tends to flow or conform to the shape of the container. **2.** Consisting of particles or distinct entities that can readily change their relative positions; tending to move or capable of flowing. [L. *fluidus,* fr. *fluo,* to flow]

flu·id bal·ance chart (flū'id bal'ăns chahrt) Record used to monitor input and output of fluids. Input includes oral fluids and infused intravenous fluids and blood products. Output includes fluid loss as urine, emesis, and wound drainage. SYN input and output record.

flu·id ex·tract (flū'id-eks'trakt) Pharmacopeial liquid preparation of a vegetable drug, made by percolation, containing alcohol as a solvent or as a preservative, or both, and so made that each milliliter contains the therapeutic constituents of 1 g of the standard drug that it represents.

flu·id·ounce (flū'id-owns') A measure of capacity: 8 fluidrams. The imperial fluid ounce is a measure that contains 1 avoirdupois ounce, 437.5 grains, of distilled water at 15.6°C, and equals 28.4 mL; the U.S. fluidounce is 1/128 gallon, contains 454.6 grains of distilled water at 25°C, and equals 29.57 mL.

flu·i·dram (flū'i-dram') A measure of capacity: 1/8 of a fluid ounce; a teaspoonful. The imperial fluidram contains 54.8 grains of distilled water, and equals 3.55 mL; the U.S. fluidram contains 57.1 grains of distilled water and equals 3.70 mL. Cf. dram.

fluke (flūk) Common name for members of the class Trematoda. All flukes of mammals (subclass Digenea) are internal parasites in the adult stage and are characterized by complex digenetic life cycles involving a snail initial host, in which larval multiplication occurs, and the release of swimming larvae (cercariae) that directly penetrate the skin of the final host (as in schistosomes), encyst on vegetation (as in *Fasciola*), or encyst in or on another intermediate host (as in *Clonorchis* and other fish-borne flukes). Blood flukes live in the mesenteric-portal bloodstream and associated vesical and pelvic venous plexuses; they include *Schistosoma haematobium* (the vesical blood fluke), *S. mansoni* (Manson intestinal blood fluke), and *S. japonicum* (the Oriental blood fluke). Other important flukes are *Paragonimus westermani* (bronchial or lung fluke), *Opisthorchis felineus* (cat liver fluke), *C. sinensis* (Chinese liver or Oriental fluke), *Heterophyes heterophyes* (Egyptian or small intestinal fluke), *Fasciolopsis buski* (large intestinal fluke), *Dicrocoelium dendriticum* (lancet fluke), *Fasciola hepatica* (liver or sheep liver fluke), and *Paramphistomum* (rumen fluke). Members of the genus *Paragonimus* are potential biothreat agents. [A.S. *flōc,* flatfish]

flu·men, pl. **flu·mi·na** (flū'mĕn, -mi-nă) A flowing, or stream. [L.]

♻**fluor-**, **fluoro-** Combining forms meaning fluorine.

fluo·ra·pa·tite (flōr-ap'ă-tīt) A form of hydroxyapatite in which fluoride ions have replaced some of the hydroxyl ions; as a component of teeth, fluorapatite resists acids from plaque-forming bacteria and high carbohydrate intake. SEE ALSO apatite, hydroxyapatite.

fluo·res·ce·in (flōr-es'ē-in) [C.I. 45350] An orange-red crystalline powder that yields a bright green fluorescence in solution, and is reduced to fluorescin; a nontoxic, water-soluble indicator used diagnostically to trace water flow and to visualize corneal abrasions or ulcers.

fluo·res·ce·in in·stil·la·tion test (flōr-es'sē-in in'sti-lā'shŭn test) A test for patency of the lacrimal system; fluorescein instilled in the conjunctival sac can be recovered from the inferior nasal meatus. SYN dye disappearance test, Jones test.

fluo·res·ce·in i·so·thi·o·cy·a·nate (FITC) (flōr-es'sē-in ī'sō-thī-ō-sī'ă-nāt) A fluorochrome dye frequently coupled to antibodies that are used to locate and identify specific antigens.

fluo·res·cence (flōr-es'ĕns) Emission of a longer wavelength radiation by a substance as a consequence of absorption of energy from a shorter wavelength radiation, continuing only as long as the stimulus is present; distinguished from phosphorescence in that, in the latter, emission persists for a perceptible period of time after the stimulus has been removed. [*fluor*spar + *-escence*, inchoative suffix]

fluo·res·cence-ac·ti·vat·ed cell sort·er (FACS) (flōr-es'ĕns ak'ti-vāt-ĕd sel sōr'tĕr) A machine that can separate and analyze cells, such as lymphocytes, which are labeled with fluorochrome-conjugated antibody, by their fluorescence and light scattering patterns.

fluo·res·cence mi·cros·co·py (flōr-es'ĕns mī-kros'kŏ-pē) A procedure based on the fact that fluorescent materials emit visible light when they are irradiated with ultraviolet or violet-blue visible rays; some materials manifest this property naturally, whereas others may be treated with fluorescent solutions (somewhat analogous to staining).

fluo·res·cent (flōr-es'ĕnt) Possessing the quality of fluorescence.

fluo·res·cent an·ti·bod·y tech·nique (flōr-es'ĕnt an'ti-bod-ē tek-nēk') A procedure to test for antigen with a fluorescent antibody by one of two methods: direct, in which immunoglobulin (antibody) conjugated with a fluorescent dye is added to tissue and combines with specific antigen (microbe, or other), the resulting antigen-antibody complex being located by fluorescence microscopy; or indirect, in which unlabeled immunoglobulin (antibody) is added to tissue and combines with specific antigen, after which the antigen-antibody complex may be labeled with fluorescein-conjugated anti-immunoglobulin antibody, the resulting triple complex then being located by fluorescence microscopy.

fluo•res•cent screen (flōr-es′ĕnt skrēn) A screen coated with fluorescent crystals such as the calcium tungstate used in the fluoroscope.

fluo•res•cent in si•tu hy•brid•i•za•tion (FISH), fluo•res•cence in si•tu hy•brid•i•za•tion (flōr-es′ĕnt in sī′tū hī′brid-ī-zā′shŭn, flōr-es′ĕns in sī′tū hī′brid-ī-zā′shŭn) A method used to determine the chromosomal location or expression pattern of genomic DNA or cDNA fragments. The piece of DNA to be mapped (the "probe") is labeled with a fluorescent dye and hybridized to a chromosome preparation or to a tissue section. The probe anneals to complementary DNA or RNA sequences. Examination of the chromosomes or tissue section under a fluorescence microscope reveals the number, size, and location of the target sequences.

fluo•res•cent stain (flōr-es′ĕnt stān) A staining procedure that uses a fluorescent dye or substance that combines selectively with certain tissue components and then fluoresces on irradiation with ultraviolet or violet-blue light.

fluo•res•cent trep•o•ne•mal an•ti•bod•y-ab•sorp•tion test (flōr-es′ĕnt trep-ō-nē′măl an′ti-bod-ē-ab-sōrp′shŭn test) A sensitive and specific serologic assay for syphilis using a suspension of the Nichols strain of *Treponema pallidum* as antigen; the presence or absence of antibody in the patient's serum is indicated by an indirect fluorescent antibody technique.

fluo•ri•dat•ed tooth (flōr′i-dā-tĕd tūth) A tooth exposed to fluorine salts during odontogenesis.

fluo•ri•da•tion (flōr′i-dā′shŭn) Addition of fluorides to a community water supply, usually 1 ppm or less, to reduce incidence of dental decay.

fluo•ride (flōr′īd) A compound of fluorine with a metal, a nonmetal, or an organic radical; the anion of fluorine; inhibits enolase; found in bone and tooth apatite; fluoride has a cariostatic effect; high levels are toxic.

fluo•ride num•ber (flōr′īd nŭm′bĕr) The percentage inhibition of pseudocholinesterase produced by fluorides; used to differentiate normal from atypical pseudocholinesterases. SEE ALSO dibucaine number test.

fluo•ri•di•za•tion (flōr′i-dī-zā′shŭn) Therapeutic use of fluorides to reduce the incidence of dental decay; sometimes used to refer to the topical application of fluoride agents to the teeth.

fluo•rine (F) (flōr-ēn′) A gaseous chemical element; atomic no. 9, atomic weight 18.9984032; ^{18}F (half-life of 1.83 hours) is used as a diagnostic aid in various tissue scans. [L. *fluere*, flow]

fluo•ro•chrome (flōr′ō-krōm) Any fluorescent dye used to label or stain.

fluo•rog•ra•phy (flōr-og′ră-fē) SYN photofluorography.

fluo•ro•im•mu•no•as•say (flōr′ō-im′yū-nō-as′ā) An immunoassay that has antigen or antibody labeled with a fluorophore.

fluo•rom•e•ter (flōr-om′ĕ-tĕr) A device employing an ultraviolet source, monochromators for selection of wavelength, and a detector of visible light; used in fluorometry.

fluo•rom•e•try (flōr-om′ĕ-trē) An analytic method for detecting fluorescent compounds, using a beam of ultraviolet light that excites the compounds and causes them to emit visible light. [fluoro- + G. *metron*, measure]

fluo•ro•pho•tom•e•try (flōr′ō-fŏ-tom′ĕ-trē) Photomultiplier tube measurement of fluorescence emitted from the interior of the eye after intravenous administration of fluorescein; used to measure the rate of formation of aqueous humor or integrity of the retinal vasculature.

fluo•ro•scope (flōr′ō-skōp) An apparatus for rendering visible the patterns of x-rays that have passed through a body under examination, by interposing a glass plate coated with fluorescent materials, such as calcium tungstate; to examine a patient by fluoroscopy. [fluorescence + G. *skopeō*, to examine]

fluo•ro•scop•ic (flōr-ō-skop′ik) Relating to or effected by means of fluoroscopy.

fluo•ros•co•py (flōr-os′kŏ-pē) Examination of the tissues and deep structures of the body by x-ray, using a fluoroscope.

fluo•ro•sis (flōr-ō′sis) A condition caused by an excessive intake of fluorides, characterized mainly by mottling, staining, or hypoplasia of the enamel of the teeth.

flush (flŭsh) **1.** To wash out with a full stream of fluid. **2.** A transient erythema due to heat, exertion, stress, or disease. **3.** Flat, or even with another surface, as a flush stoma.

flut•ter (flŭt′ĕr) Agitation; tremulousness. [A.S. *floterian*, to float about]

flut•ter de•vice (flŭt′ĕr dĕ-vīs′) Forced expiratory breathing implement that vibrates to facilitate coughing.

flut•ter-fi•bril•la•tion (flut′ĕr-fib′ri-lā′shŭn) SYN impure flutter.

flux (flŭks) **1.** The discharge of a fluid material in large amount from a cavity or surface of the body. SEE ALSO diarrhea. **2.** Material discharged from the bowels. **3.** A material used to remove oxides from the surface of molten metal and to protect it during casting; serves a similar purpose in soldering operations. Also, an ingredient in dental porcelain that by its lower melting temperature helps to bond the silica particles. **4.** (*J*) The moles of a substance crossing through a unit area of a boundary layer or membrane per unit of time. **5.** Bidirectional movement of a substance at a membrane or surface. **6.** DIAGNOSTIC RADIOLOGY photon fluence per unit time. [L. *fluxus,* a flow]

flux·ion·ar·y hy·per·e·mi·a (flŭk′shŭn-ar-ē hī′pĕr-ē′mē-ă) SYN active hyperemia.

fly (flī) A two-winged insect in the order Diptera. Important members include *Simulium* (black fly), *Calliphora* (bluebottle fly), *Piophila casei* (cheese fly), *Chrysops* (deer fly), *Siphona irritans* (horn fly), *Fannia scolaris* (latrine fly), *Oestrus ovis* and *Gasterophilus hemorrhoidalis* (nose fly), *Cochliomyia hominivorax* (primary screw-worm fly) and *C. macellaria* (secondary screw-worm fly), *Stomoxys calcitrans* (stable fly), *Glossina* (tsetse fly). Members of the insect order Trichoptera are also commonly called flies. [A.S. *fleóge*]

Fm Symbol for fermium.

FMC Abbreviation for fine motor coordination.

FMLH Abbreviation for familial hemophagocytic lymphohistiocytosis.

FMN Abbreviation for flavin mononucleotide.

FMR1 SYN fragile X syndrome.

FNA Abbreviation for fine needle aspiration biopsy.

foam cells (fōm selz) Cells with abundant, pale-staining, finely vacuolated cytoplasm, usually histiocytes that have ingested or accumulated material that dissolves during tissue preparation, especially lipids. SEE ALSO lipophage.

foam·y vi·rus·es (fō′mē vī′rŭs-ĕz) Retroviruses found in primates and other mammals; so named because of lacelike changes produced in monkey kidney cells; syncytia are also produced.

fo·cal (fō′kăl) **1.** Denoting a focus. **2.** Relating to a localized area.

fo·cal am·y·loi·do·sis (fō′kăl am′i-loy-dō′sis) SYN nodular amyloidosis.

fo·cal depth, depth of fo·cus (fō′kăl depth, depth fō′kŭs) The greatest distance through which an object point can be moved while remaining in focus.

fo·cal dis·tance (fō′kăl dis′tăns) The distance from the center of a lens to its focus.

fo·cal ep·i·lep·sy (fō′kăl ep′i-lep′sē) Epilepsy of various etiologies characterized by focal seizures or secondarily generalized tonic-clonic seizures. Ictal symptoms are often related to the brain region where the seizure begins focally. SYN localization-related epilepsy (2).

fo·cal-film dis·tance (FFD) (fō′kăl-film dis′tăns) The distance from the source of radiation (the focal spot of the x-ray tube) to the film or other image-receptor. SYN source-to-image distance.

fo·cal glo·mer·u·lo·ne·phri·tis (fō′kăl glō-mer′yū-lō-nĕ-frī′tis) Glomerulonephritis affecting a small proportion of renal glomeruli that commonly presents with hematuria and may be associated with acute upper respiratory infection in young males, not usually due to streptococci; associated with IgA deposits in the glomerular mesangium and may also be associated with systemic disease, as in Henoch-Schönlein purpura. SYN Berger disease, Berger focal glomerulonephritis.

fo·cal in·fec·tion (fō′kăl in-fek′shŭn) Local infection that can serve as a source of disseminated or metastatic infection

fo·cal in·ju·ry (fō′kăl in′jŭr-ē) Injury to a small, concentrated area, usually caused by high velocity–low mass forces.

fo·cal ne·cro·sis (fō′kăl nĕ-krō′sis) Occurrence of numerous small, well-circumscribed zones of tissue that manifest coagulative, caseous, or gummatous necrosis.

fo·cal point (fō′kăl poynt) SEE anterior focal point, posterior focal point.

fo·cal re·ac·tion (fō′kăl rē-ak′shŭn) A reaction that occurs at the point of entrance of an infecting organism or of an injection, as in the Arthus phenomenon. SYN local reaction.

fo·cal seg·men·tal glo·mer·u·lo·scle·ro·sis (fō′kăl seg-men′tăl glo-mer′yū-lō-skler-ō′sis) Segmental collapse of glomerular capillaries with thickened basement membranes and increased mesangial matrix; seen in some glomeruli of patients with nephrotic syndrome or mesangial proliferative glomerulonephritis.

fo·cal spot (fō′kăl spot) The area made of tungsten on the anode of a diagnostic x ray tube. The electrons interact with it to produce x-rays.

fo·cus, pl. **fo·ci** (fō′kŭs, -sī) **1.** (F) The point at which the light rays meet after passing through a convex lens. **2.** The center, or the starting point, of a disease process. [L. a hearth]

fo·cused his·to·ry and phy·si·cal ex·am·i·na·tion (fō′kŭst his′tŏr-ē fiz′i-kăl eg-zam′i-nā′shŭn) The second stage of patient assessment conducted by prehospital providers after the initial assessment of the stable responsive patient designed to identify additional injuries or conditions requiring emergency intervention.

fo·cused me·di·cal as·sess·ment (fō′kŭst med′i-kăl ă-ses′mĕnt) Physical examination of a prehospital patient that focuses on body areas and systems as indicated by the patient's chief complaint and initial assessment.

fo·cused trau·ma as·sess·ment (fō′kŭst traw′mă ă-ses′mĕnt) Physical examination, focusing on a specific injury or suspected area of injury, of a prehospital patient before transport.

fo·cus group (fō′kŭs grūp) Small group of people gathered together for purpose of identifying and discussing points of view about topic; discussion led by facilitator from outside the group.

foetal [Br.] SYN fetal.

foetoplacental [Br.] SYN fetoplacental.

foetotoxic [Br.] SYN fetotoxic.

foetus [Br.] SYN fetus.

fog (fawg) Droplets dispersed in the atmosphere or a respiratory device.

Fo•gar•ty cath•e•ter, **Fo•gar•ty em•bo•lec•to•my cath•e•ter** (fō′găr-tē kath′ĕ-tĕr, fō′găr-tē em′bō-lek′tŏ′mē kath′ĕ-tĕr) A catheter with an inflatable balloon at its tip; commonly used to remove arterial emboli and thrombi from major veins or to remove stones from the biliary ducts. SYN balloon-tip catheter (3).

fog•ging (fawg′ing) A method of refraction in which accommodation is relaxed by overcorrection with a convex spherical lens.

fog•ging ef•fect (fawg′ing ĕ-fekt′) In computed tomography and magnetic resonance imaging, inability to determine or visualize results of a cerebral stroke several days after the insult's occurrence.

fo•late (fō′lāt) A salt or ester of folic acid.

fold (fōld) **1.** A ridge or margin apparently formed by the doubling back of a lamina. SEE ALSO plica. **2.** In the embryo, a transient elevation or reduplication of tissue in the form of a lamina.

fold•a•ble in•tra•oc•u•lar lens (fōld′ă-bĕl in-tră-ok′yū-lăr lenz) A lens usually made of silicone or an acrylic polymer that may be doubled over for implantation into the eye following cataract removal.

fold•ed-lung syn•drome (fōld′ĕd-lŭng sin′drōm) Collapse of part of the lung caught between shrinking fibrous pleural scars, sometimes resulting from pleural asbestosis.

Fo•ley cath•e•ter (fō′lē kath′ĕ-tĕr) A urethral catheter with a retaining balloon; used to drain the bladder. See this page.

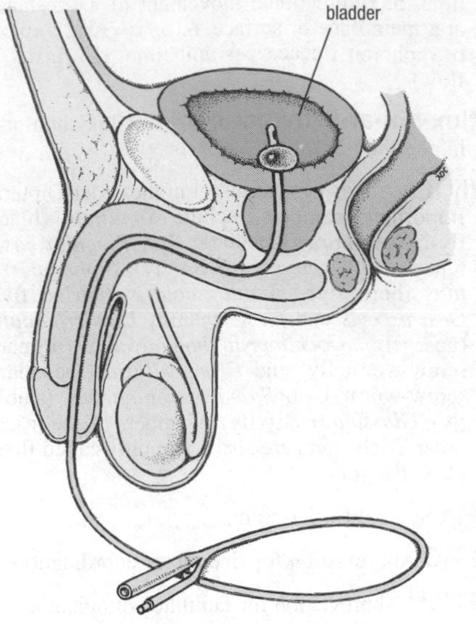

Foley catheter

fo•li•a (fō′lē-ă) Plural of folium.

fo•li•ate pa•pil•lae (fō′lē-āt pă-pil′ē) Numerous projections arranged in several transverse folds on the lateral margins of the tongue just in front of the palatoglossus muscle.

fo•lic ac•id (fō′lik as′id) **1.** Collective term for pteroylglutamic acids and their oligoglutamic acid conjugates. **2.** Pteroylmonoglutamic acid, a member of the vitamin B complex necessary for the production of red blood cells; present in liver, green vegetables, and yeast; used to treat folate deficiency and megaloblastic anemia.

fo•lic ac•id an•ta•go•nist (fō′lik as′id an-tag′ŏ-nist) Modified pterins, such as aminopterin and amethopterin, which interfere with the action of folic acid and thus produce the symptoms of folic acid deficiency; have been used in cancer chemotherapy.

fo•lie (fō-lē′) Old term for madness or insanity. [Fr. madness]

fo•lie du doute (fō-lē′ dū dūt) An excessive doubting about all the affairs of life and a morbid scrupulousness concerning minutiae. [Fr. from doubt]

fo•li•nate (fō′li-nāt) A salt or ester of folinic acid.

fo•lin•ic ac•id (fō-lin′ik as′id) The active form of folic acid, which acts as a formyl group carrier in transformylation reactions; the calcium salt, leucovorin calcium, has therapeutic use. SYN citrovorum factor.

Fo•lin re•ac•tion (fō′lin rē-ak′shŭn) The reaction of amino acids in alkaline solution with 1,2-naphthoquinone-4-sulfonate (Folin reagent) to yield a red color; useful for quantitative assay.

fo•li•um, pl. **fo•li•a** (fō′lē-ŭm, -ă) A broad, thin, leaflike structure. [L. a leaf]

folk med•i•cine (fōk med′i-sin) Treatment of ailments with remedies and simple measures based on experience and knowledge handed on from generation to generation.

fol•lib•er•in (fol-lib′ĕr-in) A decapeptide of hypothalamic origin capable of accelerating pituitary secretion of follitropin. SYN follicle-stimulating hormone-releasing factor, follicle-stimulating hormone-releasing hormone. [follicle-stimulating hormone + L. *libero*, to free, + -in]

fol·li·cle (fol′i-kĕl) **1.** A more or less spheric mass of cells usually containing a cavity. **2.** A crypt or minute cul-de-sac or lacuna, such as the depression in the skin from which the hair emerges. SYN folliculus [TA]. [L. *folliculus*, a small sac, dim. of *follis*, a pair of bellows]

fol·li·cle-stim·u·lat·ing hor·mone (fol′i-kĕl-stim′yū-lā-ting hōr′mōn) SYN follitropin.

fol·li·cle-stim·u·lat·ing hor·mone-re·leas·ing fac·tor, fol·li·cle-stim·u·lat·ing hor·mone-re·leas·ing hor·mone (fol′i-kĕl-stim′yū-lā-ting hōr′mōn-rē-lēs′ing fak′tŏr, hōr′mōn) SYN folliberin.

fol·lic·u·lar (fŏ-lik′yū-lăr) Relating to a follicle or follicles.

fol·lic·u·lar car·ci·no·ma (fŏ-lik′yū-lăr kahr′si-nō′mă) Carcinoma of the thyroid composed of well or poorly differentiated epithelial follicles without papillary formation, which is difficult to distinguish from adenoma; the criteria include blood vessel invasion and the finding of metastases of follicular thyroid tissue in other structures such as cervical lymph nodes and bone; follicular carcinoma may take up radioactive iodine.

fol·lic·u·lar cell (fŏ-lik′yū-lăr sel) An epithelial cell lining a follicle, such as that of the thyroid or ovary.

fol·lic·u·lar cyst (fŏ-lik′yū-lăr sist) **1.** An odontogenic cyst that arises from the epithelium of a tooth bud and dental lamina. **2.** SYN dentigerous cyst.

fol·lic·u·lar cys·ti·tis (fŏ-lik′yū-lăr sis-tī′tis) Chronic cystitis characterized by small mucosal nodules due to lymphocytic infiltration.

fol·lic·u·lar goi·ter (fŏ-lik′yū-lăr goy′tĕr) SYN parenchymatous goiter.

fol·lic·u·lar lym·pho·ma (fŏ-lik′yū-lăr lim-fo′mă) SYN nodular lymphoma.

fol·lic·u·lar stig·ma (fŏ-lik′yū-lăr stig′mă) The point where the graafian follicle is about to rupture on the surface of the ovary. SYN stigma (2).

fol·lic·u·li (fō-lik′yū-lī) Plural of folliculus.

fol·lic·u·li glan·du·lae thy·roi·de·ae (fō-lik′yū-lī glan′dyū-lē thī-roy′dē-ē) [TA] SYN thyroid follicles.

fol·lic·u·li lin·gua·les (fō-lik′yū-lī ling′gwā′lēz) [TA] SYN lingual follicles.

fol·lic·u·li lym·pha·ti·ci li·e·na·les (fō-lik′yū-lī lim-fat′i-shē lī-ĕ-nā′lēz) SYN splenic lymph follicles.

fol·lic·u·li·tis (fŏ-lik′yū-lī′tis) An inflammatory reaction in hair follicles; the lesions may be papules or pustules. See page B4.

fol·lic·u·li·tis bar·bae (fō-lik′yū-lī-tis bahr′bē) SYN tinea barbae.

fol·lic·u·li·tis de·cal·vans (fō-lik′yū-lī′tis dē-kal′vanz) A papular or pustular inflammation of the hair follicles of the scalp seen mostly in men, resulting in scarring and loss of hair in the affected area.

fol·lic·u·li·tis ke·loi·da·lis (fō-lik′yū-lī′tis kē-loy-dā′lis) SYN acne keloid.

fol·lic·u·li·tis u·ler·y·the·ma·to·sa re·ti·cu·la·ta (fō-lik′yū-lī′tis yū′lĕr-i-thē-mā-tō′să rē-tik-yū-lā′tă) Erythematous "ice-pick" or pitted scars on the cheeks; a scarring type of folliculitis, associated with keratosis pilaris.

fol·lic·u·lo·ma (fŏ-lik′yū-lō′mă) **1.** SYN granulosa cell tumor. **2.** Cystic enlargement of a graafian follicle.

fol·lic·u·lose (fŏ-lik′yū-lōs) Denotes anything composed of follicles.

fol·lic·u·lo·sis (fŏ-lik′yū-lō′sis) Presence of lymph follicles in abnormally great numbers.

fol·lic·u·lus, pl. **fol·lic·u·li** (fŏ-lik′yū-lŭs, -lī) [TA] SYN follicle. [L. a small sac, dim. of *follis*, bellows]

fol·lic·u·lus lym·phat·i·cus (fŏ-lik′yū-lŭs lim-fat′i-kŭs) SYN lymph follicle.

fol·lic·u·lus pi·li (fŏ-lik′yū-lŭs pil′ī) [TA] SYN hair follicle.

Fol·ling dis·ease (fahl′ing di-zēz′) SYN phenylketonuria.

fol·li·stat·in (fol′i-stat′in) A peptide synthesized by granulosa cells in response to FSH, which suppresses FSH activity, probably by binding activins. [*follic*le + -stat + -in]

fol·li·tro·pin (fol′i-trō′pin) An acidic glycoprotein hormone of the anterior pituitary that stimulates the ovarian follicles and promotes follicular maturation and the secretion of estradiol; in the male, it stimulates the epithelium of the seminiferous tubules and is partially responsible for inducing spermatogenesis. SYN follicle-stimulating hormone. [follicle + G. *tropē*, a turning, + -in]

fol·li·tro·pin-re·leas·ing hor·mone (FRH) (fol′i-trō′pin rĕ-lēs′ing hōr′mōn) A hypothalamic hormone that stimulates release of follitropin and luteotropin by the adenohypophysis.

fol·low·ing bou·gie (fol′ō-ing bū-zhē′) A flexible tapered bougie with a screw tip that is attached to the trailing end of a filiform bougie, to allow progressive dilation without danger of creating false passages.

fol·low up (fol′ō-ŭp) Phrasal verb meaning to provide continuing or further attention to something. SEE ALSO follow-up.

fol·low-up, fol·low·up (fol′ō-ŭp) Noun or adjective meaning the act of providing continuing or further attention to something. SEE ALSO follow up.

fo•mes, pl. **fom•i•tes** (fō′mēz, -mī-tēz) Objects such as clothing, towels, and utensils that may harbor a disease agent and are capable of transmitting it; usually used in the plural. [L. tinder, fr. *foveo,* to keep warm]

Fo•ni•o so•lu•tion (fō′nē-ō sŏ-lū′shŭn) A diluent with magnesium sulfate, used for stained smears of blood platelets.

Fon•se•ca•ea pe•dro•so•i (fon-sē′sē-ă pedrō′sō-ī) A slow-growing dematiaceous fungal species that produces skin and subcutaneous tissue infections (i.e., chromoblastomycosis). Infections usually result from traumatic inoculation. Conidial arrangement helps in the identification.

fon•ta•nelle, **fon•ta•nel** (fon′tă-nel′) One of several membranous intervals at the margins of the cranial bones in the infant. SYN fonticulus [TA]. [Fr. dim. of *fontaine,* fountain, spring]

fon•tic•u•lus, pl. **fon•tic•u•li** (fon-tik′yū-lŭs, -lī) [TA] SYN fontanelle. [L. dim. of *fons* (*font-*), fountain, spring]

food (fūd) That which is eaten to supply necessary nutritive elements. [A.S. *fōda*]

food a•dul•ter•ant (fūd ă-dŭlt′ĕr-ănt) Any substance added to a foodstuff or beverage that makes it unfit for human consumption.

food ball (fūd bawl) SYN phytobezoar.

Food and Drug Ad•min•i•stra•tion (F.D.A., FDA) (fūd drŭg ad-min′i-strā′shŭn) The U.S. federal agency charged with oversight of all issues related to the safety of pharmaceuticals and alimentation.

food ex•change list (fūd eks-chānj′list) A table of foodstuffs with listings of their caloric and carbohydrate content intended to ease the maintenance of correct diet in patients with diabetes mellitus and hypoglycemia; frequently misunderstood by patients.

Food Guide Py•ra•mid (fūd gīd pir′ă-mid) U.S. Department of Agriculture guidelines for sound nutrition that emphasize grains, vegetables, and fruits and downplay food sources high in animal protein, lipids, and dairy products. Recommendation for regular physical activity (at least 30 minutes) is included in guidelines. SYN My Pyramid.

Food Guide Pyr•a•mid for the El•der•ly (fūd gīd pir′ă-mid el′dĕr-lē) The Food Guide Pyramid adapted to the dietary needs and constraints of old people.

food hy•per•sen•si•tiv•i•ty re•ac•tion (fūd hī′pĕr-sen-si-tiv′i-tē rē-ak′shŭn) A disorder or disease process resulting from ingestion of a foodstuff that the patient is more or less unable to tolerate (e.g., suffocation, urticaria, nausea and vomiting).

food in•tol•er•ance (fūd in-tol′ĕr-ăns) A condition similar to a food allergy, but generally with less severe findings (e.g., flatus, dyspepsia).

food la•bel (fūd lā′bĕl) In the United States, the wrapper on a foodstuff that must contain nutritional information for the use of the consumer according to a specified format and size.

food poi•son•ing (fūd poy′zŏn-ing) Illness related to the ingestion of a foodstuff tainted by pathogens of any type.

food ren•der•ing (fūd ren′dĕr-ing) Conversion of waste and scrap matter from industrial slaughterhouses into animal feed; has been associated with spread of Creutzfeldt-Jakob disease (q.v.).

food re•quire•ments (fūd rē-kwīr′mĕnts) The generalized need for nutrients across a broad spectrum of people or animals, subject to amendment in individuals.

food se•cur•i•ty (fūd sĕ-kyūr′i-tē) A state in which a person, or all people in a collective (e.g., family, community, nation) have consistent physical and economic access to a nutritionally adequate and culturally acceptable diet, through nonemergency sources.

FOOSH (fūsh) Acronym for fall onto outstretched hand.

i **foot** (fut) **1.** The distal part of the leg. SYN pes (1) [TA]. **2.** A unit to measure length, containing 12 inches, equal to 30.48 cm. See page A16. [A.S. *fōt*]

foot•can•dle (fut′kan-dĕl) Illumination or brightness equivalent to 1 lumen per square foot; replaced in the SI nomenclature by the candela.

foot•drop (fut′drop) Partial or total inability to dorsiflex the foot, as a consequence of which the toes drag on the ground during walking unless a steppage gait is used; most often ultimately due to weakness of the dorsiflexor muscles of the foot (especially the tibialis anterior), but has many causes, including disorders of the central nervous system, motor unit, tendons, and bones.

foot of hip•po•cam•pus (fut hip′ō-kam′pŭs) The anterior thickened extremity of the hippocampus.

foot•ling (fut′ling) A fetal foot, particularly one that descends into the birth canal in an incomplete breech presentation. [foot, fr. A. S. *fot,* + *-ling,* dim. suffix]

foot•ling pre•sen•ta•tion, **foot pre•sen•ta•tion** (fut′ling prez′ĕn-tā′shŭn, fut prez′ĕn-tā′shŭn) SEE breech presentation.

foot•plate, **foot-plate** (fut′plāt, fut′plāt) **1.** SYN base of stapes. **2.** SYN pedicel.

foot-pound (fut′pownd) Energy expended, or

work done, in raising a mass of 1 pound a height of 1 foot vertically against gravitational force.

foot-pound·al (fut′pownd′ăl) Energy exerted, or work done, when a force of 1 poundal displaces a body 1 foot in the direction of the force; equal to about 0.01 calorie.

foot-pound-sec·ond sys·tem (FPS, fps) (fut′pownd-sek′ŏnd sis′tĕm) A system of absolute units based on the foot, pound, and second.

foot-pound-sec·ond u·nit, FPS u·nit, fps unit (fut′pownd-sek′ŏnd yū′nit, yū′nit, yū′nit) An absolute unit of the foot-pound-second system.

foot pro·cess (fut pros′es) SYN pedicel.

foot rays (fut rāz) The four radial grooves that separate five slightly thicker areas of the foot plates; they indicate formation of the metatarsals and phalanges of the hand. SYN digital rays of foot.

Foot re·tic·u·lin im·preg·na·tion stain (fut rĕ-tik′yū-lin im-preg-nā′shŭn stān) A silver stain in which reticulin stains black and collagen stains golden brown; sections are floated on the surface of solutions to avoid contamination with silver debris.

fo·ra·men, pl. **fo·ram·i·na** (fōr-ā′mĕn, fō-ra′mē-nă) [TA] An aperture or perforation through a bone or a membranous structure. [L. an aperture, fr. *foro,* to pierce]

fo·ra·men ce·cum me·dul·lae ob·lon·ga·tae (fōr-ā′mĕn sē′kŭm me-dŭl′ē ob-long-gā′tē) [TA] A small triangular depression at the lower boundary of the pons that marks the upper limit of the median fissure of the medulla oblongata.

fo·ra·men mag·num (fōr-ā′mĕn mag′nŭm) [TA] The large opening in the basal part of the occipital bone through which the spinal cord becomes continuous with the medulla oblongata. SYN great foramen.

fo·ra·men man·di·bu·lae (fōr-ā′mĕn man-dib′yū-le) [TA] SYN mandibular foramen.

fo·ra·men ob·tu·ra·tum (fōr-ā′mĕn ob-tū-rā′tŭm) [TA] SYN obturator foramen.

fo·ra·men o·va·le, **o·val fo·ra·men** (fōr-ā′mĕn ō-vā′lē, ō′văl fōr-ā′mĕn) **1.** The oval opening in the septum secundum in the embryonic and fetal heart; the persistent part of the septum primum acts as a valve for this interatrial communication during fetal life and normally postnatally becomes fused to the septum secundum to close it. **2.** foramen ovale [TA] a large oval opening in the base of the greater wing of the sphenoid bone, transmitting the mandibular nerve and a small meningeal artery; SYN Botallo foramen.

fo·ra·men ro·tun·dum (fōr-ā′mĕn rō-tŭn′dŭm) [TA] An opening in the base of the greater wing of the sphenoid bone, transmitting the maxillary nerve.

fo·ra·men sphe·no·pa·la·ti·num (fōr-ā′mĕn sfē′nō-pal-ă-tī′nŭm) [TA] SYN sphenopalatine foramen.

fo·ra·men spi·no·sum (fōr-ā′mĕn spī-nō′sŭm) [TA] An opening in the base of the greater wing of the sphenoid bone, anterior to the spine of the sphenoid, transmitting the middle meningeal artery.

fo·ra·men su·pra·or·bi·ta·le (fōr-ā′mĕn sū′pră-ōr-bi-tā′lē) [TA] SYN supraorbital foramen.

fo·ra·men zy·go·ma·ti·co·fa·ci·a·le (fōr-ā′mĕn zī-gō-mat′i-kō-fā-shē-ā′lē) [TA] SYN zygomaticofacial foramen.

fo·ra·men zy·go·ma·ti·co·or·bi·ta·le (fōr-ā′mĕn zī-gō-mat′i-kō-ōr-bi-tā′lē) [TA] SYN zygomaticoorbital foramen.

fo·ra·men zy·go·ma·ti·co·tem·po·ra·le (fōr-ā′mĕn zī-gō-mat′i-kō-tem-pō-rā′lē) [TA] SYN zygomaticotemporal foramen.

fo·ram·i·na (fō-ram′ē-nă) Plural of foramen.

fo·ram·i·na pa·la·ti·na mi·no·ra (fō-ra′mē-nă pal-ă-tī′nă mi-nō′ră) [TA] SYN lesser palatine foramina.

Forbes dis·ease (fōrbz di-zēz′) SYN glycogenosis type 3.

force (F, *F*) (fōrs) **1.** That which tends to produce motion in a body. **2.** Application of energy to initiate motion. [L. *fortis,* strong]

forced beat (fōrst bēt) **1.** An extrasystole supposedly precipitated in some way by the preceding normal beat to which it is coupled; **2.** An extrasystole caused by artificial stimulation of the heart.

forced ex·pi·ra·to·ry flow (FEF) (fōrst eks-pī′ră-tōr-ē flō) Expiratory flow during measurement of forced vital capacity; subscripts specify the exact parameter measured.

forced ex·pi·ra·to·ry time (FET) (fōrst eks-pī′ră-tōr-ē tīm) The time taken to expire a given volume or a given fraction of vital capacity during measurement of forced vital capacity; subscripts specify the exact parameters measured.

forced ex·pi·ra·to·ry vol·ume (FEV) (fōrst eks-pī′ră-tōr-ē vol′yūm) The maximal volume that can be expired in a specific time interval when starting from maximal inspiration.

forced feed·ing, **forc·i·ble feed·ing** (fōrst fēd′ing, fōr′si-bĕl) **1.** Giving liquid food through a nasal tube that passes into the stomach. **2.** Forcing a person to eat more food than desired.

forced vi·tal ca·pac·i·ty (FVC) (fōrst vī′tăl kă-pas′i-tē) Vital capacity measured with the subject exhaling as rapidly as possible.

force of mas•ti•ca•tion (fōrs mas-ti-kā′shŭn) The force created by the action of the muscles during mastication. SYN masticatory force.

for•ceps (fōr′seps) **1.** An instrument for seizing a structure and making compression or traction. Cf. clamp. **2.** [TA] Bands of white fibers in the brain, major forceps and minor forceps. [L. a pair of tongs]

for•ceps de•liv•er•y (fōr′seps dĕ-liv′ĕr-ē) Assisted birth of the child by an instrument designed to grasp the fetal head.

for•ci•pres•sure (fōr′si-presh-ŭr) A method of arresting hemorrhage by compressing a blood vessel with forceps.

For•dyce an•gi•o•ker•a•to•ma (fōr′dīs an′jē-ō-ker-ă-tō′mă) An asymptomatic vascular papule appearing on the scrotum in adults.

For•dyce spots, For•dyce gran•ules, For•dyce dis•ease (fōr′dīs spotz, gran′yūlz, di-zēz′) A condition marked by the presence of numerous small, yellowish-white bodies or granules on the inner surface and vermilion border of the lips; histologically the lesions are ectopic sebaceous glands.

fore•arm (fōr′ahrm) The segment of the upper limb between the elbow and the wrist. See this page. SYN antebrachium [TA].

fore•brain (fōr′brān) SYN prosencephalon.

fore•con•scious (fōr′kon-shŭs) Denoting memories, not at present in the consciousness, which can be evoked from time to time, or an unconscious mental process that becomes conscious only on the fulfillment of certain conditions. Cf. preconscious.

fore•foot (fōr′fut) The part of the foot containing the metatarsal bones and phalanges; the front part of the foot.

fore•gut (fōr′gŭt) The cephalic endodermal portion of the primordial digestive tube in the embryo. From it arises the epithelial lining of the pharynx, trachea, lungs, esophagus, and stomach, the first part and cranial half of the second part of the duodenum, and the parenchyma of the liver, gallbladder, and pancreas.

fore•head (fōr′hed) The part of the face between the eyebrows and the hairy scalp. SYN brow (2), frons.

for•eign bod•y (fōr′ĕn bod′ē) Anything in the tissues or cavities of the body that has been introduced there, not present under normal circumstances, and is not rapidly absorbable. See page B27.

for•eign bod•y gran•u•lo•ma (fōr′ĕn bod′ē gran′yū-lō′mă) A granuloma caused by the presence of foreign particulate material in tissue, characterized by a histiocytic reaction with foreign body giant cells.

Fo•rel de•cus•sa•tion (fō-rel′ dē-kŭs-ā′shŭn) SEE tegmental decussations (2).

fore•milk (fōr′milk) SYN colostrum.

fo•ren•sic (fŏr-en′sik) Pertaining or applicable to personal injury, murder, and other legal proceedings. [L. *forensis*, of a forum]

fo•ren•sic den•tis•try (fŏr-en′sik den′tis-trē) **1.** The relation and application of dental facts to legal problems, as in using the teeth of a corpse to help establish identity. **2.** The law in its bearing on the practice of dentistry.

fo•ren•sic med•i•cine (fŏr-en′sik med′i-sin) **1.** The relation and application of medical facts to legal matters. **2.** The law in its bearing on the practice of medicine. SYN legal medicine.

for•en•sic o•don•tol•o•gist (fŏr-en′sik ō-don-tol′ŏ-jist) Dental clinician who practices in the field of forensic dentistry.

fo•ren•sic psy•chi•a•try, le•gal psy•chi•a•try (fŏr-en′sik sī-kī′ă-trē, lē′găl) The application of psychiatry in courts of law, e.g., in determinations for commitment, competency, fitness to stand trial, responsibility for crime.

fo•ren•sic psy•chol•o•gy (fŏr-en′sik sī-kol′ŏ-jē) The application of psychology to legal matters in a court of law.

fore•play (fōr′plā) Stimulative sexual activity preceding sexual intercourse.

fore•quar•ter am•pu•ta•tion (fōr′kwōr-tĕr amp′yū-tā′shŭn) Amputation of the arm with re-

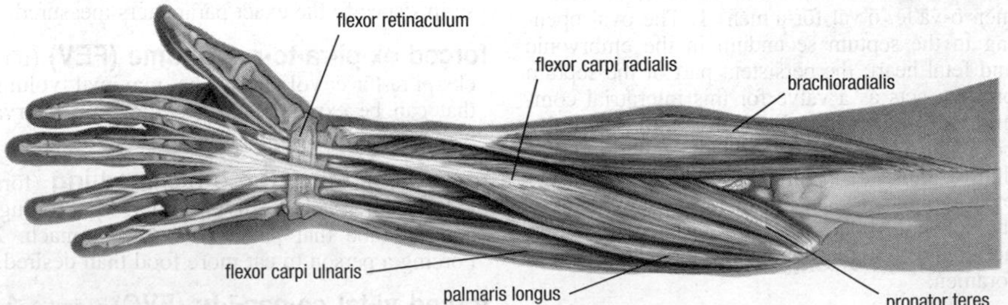

muscles of the anterior forearm

moval of the scapula and a portion of the clavicle.

fore·shor·ten·ing (fōr′shōrt-ĕn-ing) RADIOLOGY radiographic distortion occurring where the image appears shorter than the actual image. Caused by excessive vertical angulation.

fore·skin (fōr′skin) SYN prepuce.

For·es·ti·er dis·ease (fō-res-tē-ā′ di-zēz′) SYN diffuse idiopathic skeletal hyperostosis.

fore·wa·ters (fōr′waw′tĕrz) Colloquialism for the bulging fluid-filled amniotic membrane presenting in front of the fetal head.

fork (fōrk) A pronged instrument used for holding or lifting.

form (fōrm) Shape; mold. [L. *forma*]

-form Suffix meaning in the form, shape of; equivalent to -oid. SEE morpho-. [L. *-formis*]

For·mad kid·ney (fōr′mad kid′nē) An enlarged and deformed kidney sometimes seen in chronic alcoholism.

for·ma·lin-e·ther se·di·men·ta·tion con·cen·tra·tion (fōr′mă-lin-ē′thĕr sed′i-mĕn-tā′shŭn kon-sĕn-trā′shŭn) A sedimentation method to separate parasitic elements from fecal debris through centrifugation and the use of ether to trap debris in a separate layer from the parasites.

for·ma·lin-eth·yl a·ce·tate se·di·men·ta·tion con·cen·tra·tion (fōr′mă-lin-eth′il as′ĕ-tāt sed′i-mĕn-tā′shŭn kon-sĕn-trā′shŭn) A sedimentation method to separate parasitic elements from fecal debris through centrifugation and the use of ethyl acetate (a substitute for ether) to trap debris in a separate layer from the parasites.

for·ma·lin pig·ment (fōr′mă-lin pig′mĕnt) A pigment formed when acid aqueous solutions of formaldehyde act on blood-rich tissues.

for·mam·i·dase (fōr-mam′i-dās) An enzyme catalyzing the hydrolysis of N-formyl-L-kynurenine to L-kynurenine and formate, a reaction of significance in L-tryptophan catabolism. SYN formylase.

for·mant (fōr′mănt) Tones and their overtones resulting from the production of vowel phonemes.

for·mate (fōr′māt) A salt or ester of formic acid; i.e., the monovalent radical HCOO– or the anion $HCOO^-$.

for·ma·ti·o, pl. **for·ma·ti·o·nes** (fōr-mā′shē-ō, -ō′nēz) [TA] **1.** SYN formation. **2.** A structure of definite shape or cellular arrangement. [L. fr. *formo,* pp. *-atus,* to form]

for·ma·tion (fōr-mā′shŭn) **1.** Shape, configuration, arrangement; the way in which anything is formed. **2.** That which is formed. **3.** The act of giving form and shape. SYN formatio (1) [TA].

for·ma·ti·o re·tic·u·la·ris (fōr-mā′shē-ō re-tik-yū-lā′ris) [TA] SYN reticular formation.

form con·stan·cy (fōrm kon′stăns-ē) Recognition of forms and objects as the same although they appear in various environments, positions, and sizes.

forme fruste, pl. **formes frustes** (fōrm frūst) A partial, arrested, or inapparent form of disease. [Fr. unfinished form]

for·mic ac·id (fōr′mik as′id) The smallest carboxylic acid; a strong caustic, used as an astringent and counterirritant.

for·mi·ca·tion (fōr-mi-kā′shŭn) A form of paresthesia or tactile hallucination; a sensation as if small insects were creeping under the skin. [L. *formica,* ant]

for·mim·i·no·glu·tam·ic ac·id (FIGLU) (fōr-mim′i-nō-glū-tam′ik as′id) An intermediate metabolite in L-histidine catabolism in the conversion of L-histidine to L-glutamic acid, with the formimino group being transferred to tetrahydrofolic acid; it may appear in the urine of patients with folic acid or vitamin B_{12} deficiency or with liver disease.

for·min (fōr′min) A family of proteins that participates in cell polarization, cytokinesis, and vertebrate limb formation. [L. *forma,* form, + -in]

for·mol-gel test (fōr′mol-jel′ test) A test to detect the greatly increased serum proteins in visceral leishmaniasis; one drop of full-strength formalin is added to 1 mL of serum, with rapid and complete coagulation indicating the positive reaction.

for·mu·la, pl. **for·mu·las**, **for·mu·lae** (fōrm′yū-lă, -lăz, -lē) **1.** A recipe or prescription containing directions for the compounding of a medicinal preparation. **2.** CHEMISTRY a symbol or collection of symbols expressing the number of atoms of the element or elements forming one molecule of a substance, together with, on occasion, information such as the arrangement of the atoms within the molecule, their electronic structure, their charge, and the nature of the bonds within the molecule. **3.** An expression by symbols and numbers of the normal order or arrangement of parts or structures. [L. dim. of *forma,* form]

for·mu·la·ry (fōrm′yū-lār-ē) **1.** A collection of formulas for the compounding of medicinal preparations. SEE National Formulary, Pharmacopeia. **2.** An official list of drugs approved for prescription or administration to patients of a hospital or health maintenance organization (HMO) or to beneficiaries of a health insurance program, or to residents of Canadian provinces that use such an instrument.

for·myl (f) (fōr′mil) The radical, HCO–.

for·my·lase (fōr′mi-lās) SYN formamidase.

***N*-for•myl•me•thi•o•nine** (en-fōr′mil-me-thī′ō-nēn) Methionine acylated on the NH_2 group by a formyl (–CHO) group. This is the starting amino acid residue for virtually all bacterial polypeptides. It is also observed in mitochondria and chloroplasts of eukaryotes. SEE ALSO initiating codon.

for•ni•cate (fōr′ni-kāt) **1.** Vaulted or arched; resembling a fornix. [L. *fornicatus,* arched, fr. *fornix,* vault, arch] **2.** To have sexual intercourse with anyone to whom one is not then married. SEE fornication.

for•ni•cate gy•rus (fōr′ni-kāt jī′rŭs) The horseshoe-shaped cortical convolution bordering the hilus of the cerebral hemisphere; its upper limb is formed by the cingulate gyrus, its lower by the parahippocampal gyrus; SYN gyrus fornicatus (1).

for•ni•ca•tion (fōr-ni-kā′shŭn) Sexual intercourse between partners then unmarried to each other. [L. *fornicatio,* an arched or vaulted basement (brothel)]

for•nix, gen. **for•ni•cis**, pl. **for•ni•ces** (fōr′niks, -ni-sis, -ni-sēz) **1.** [TA] In general, an arch-shaped structure; often the arch-shaped roof (or roof portion) of an anatomic space. **2.** The compact, white fiber bundle by which the hippocampus of each cerebral hemisphere projects to the contralateral hippocampus and to the septum, anterior nucleus of the thalamus, and mammillary body. Arising from pyramidal cells of the Ammon's horn, the fibers of the fornix form the alveus hippocampi and the fimbria hippocampi, and in their further course compose, sequentially, the commissure of the fornix, also called the hippocampal commissure (commissura hippocampi [TA]), the crus of fornix (crus fornicis [TA]), the body of fornix (corpus fornicis [TA]), and the column of fornix (columna fornicis [TA]), which divides into a smaller portion of precommissural fibers that pass anterior to the anterior commissure to the septal area and a larger portion of postcommissural fibers that pass posterior to the anterior commissure to end mainly in the mammillary nuclei and to a lesser extent in the anterior thalamic nucleus. [L. arch, vault]

for•nix of stom•ach (fōr′niks stŏm′ăk) The domed or pocketlike portion of the stomach that lies superior to and to the left of the cardial orifice, in which, in the upright position, gas is often contained; formerly considered synonymous with fundus of stomach; in *Terminologia Anatomica,* the fundus is the uppermost portion of the body of the stomach, with mucosa that includes the greatest density of fundic cells.

For•si•us-Er•iks•son al•bin•ism (fōr′sē-ŭs-er′ik-sŏn al′bi-nizm′) SYN ocular albinism 2.

forsk•o•lin (fōr′skŏ-lin) A phorbol ester that binds to and activates protein kinase C, thus mimicking the actions of diacylglycerol. [fr. *Coleus forskohlii,* taxonomic name of botanical source]

För•ster u•ve•i•tis (fĕr′ster yū-vē-ī′tis) Syphilitic inflammation, with diffuse nodules involving the choroid and retinal vasculitis.

Fort Bragg fe•ver (fōrt brag fē′vĕr) SYN pretibial fever.

for•ti•fi•ca•tion spec•trum (fōr-ti-fi-kā′shŭn spek′trŭm) The zigzag banding of light, resembling the walls of fortified medieval towns, which marks the margin of the scintillating scotoma of migraine.

for•ward heart fail•ure (fōr′wărd hahrt fāl′yŭr) A concept that maintains that the phenomena of congestive heart failure result from the inadequate cardiac output, and especially from the consequent inadequacy of renal blood flow with resulting retention of sodium and water. Cf. backward heart failure.

fos•sa, gen. and pl. **fos•sae** (fos′ă, -ē) [TA] A depression usually more or less longitudinal in shape below the level of the surface of a part. [L. a trench or ditch]

fos•sa a•ce•ta•bu•li (fōs′ă ā-sē-tab′yū-lī) [TA] SYN acetabular fossa.

fos•sa for gall•blad•der (fos′ă gawl′blad-ĕr) A depression on the visceral surface of the liver anteriorly, between the quadrate and the right lobes, lodging the gallbladder.

fos•sa o•va•lis (fos′ă ō-vā′lis) **1.** [TA] An oval depression on the lower part of the septum of the right atrium; it is a vestige of the foramen ovale, and its floor corresponds to the septum primum of the fetal heart. **2.** SYN saphenous opening.

fos•sa of ves•ti•bule of va•gi•na (fos′ă ves′ti-byūl vă-jī′nă) The portion of the vestibule of the vagina between the frenulum of the labia minora and the posterior labial commissure of the vulva. SYN fossa vestibuli vaginae [TA].

fos•sa ves•tib•u•li va•gi•nae (fos′ă ves-tib′yū-lī vaj′i-nē) [TA] SYN fossa of vestibule of vagina.

fos•sette (fo-set′) **1.** SYN fossula. **2.** A seldom-used term for corneal ulcer of small diameter. [Fr. dim. of *fosse,* a ditch]

fos•su•la, pl. **fos•su•lae** (fos′yū-lă, -lē) [TA] **1.** A small fossa. **2.** A minor fissure or slight depression on the surface of the cerebrum. SYN fossette (1). [L. dim. of *fossa,* ditch]

fos•su•la post fe•nes•tram (fos′yū-lă pōst fĕ-nes′trăm) The small passage filled with connective tissue posterior to the oval window of the cochlea; a site of predilection for otosclerosis.

Fos•ter frame (faws′tĕr frām) A reversible bed similar to a Stryker frame.

Fos•ter Ken•ne•dy syn•drome (faws′tĕr ken′ĕ-dē sin′drōm) SYN Kennedy syndrome.

Foth•er•gill dis•ease (foth′ĕr-gil di-zēz′) **1.**

SYN trigeminal neuralgia. **2.** SYN anginose scarlatina.

Foth•er•gill neu•ral•gi•a (foth′ĕr-gil nūr-al′jē-ă) SYN trigeminal neuralgia.

Foth•er•gill op•er•a•tion (foth′ĕr-gil op-ĕr-ā′shŭn) SYN Manchester operation.

Foth•er•gill sign (foth′ĕr-gil sīn) In rectus sheath hematoma, the hematoma produces a mass that does not cross the midline and remains palpable when the rectus muscle is tense.

Fou•chet stain (fū-shā′ stān) Reagent employed to demonstrate bile pigments; paraffin sections are used for conjugated bile pigments, frozen sections for unconjugated ones.

fou•lage (fū-lahz[h]′) Kneading and pressure of the muscles, constituting a form of massage. [Fr. impression]

foun•da•tion (fown-dā′shŭn) A base; a supporting structure. [L. *fundo*, to found, establish, fr. *fundus*, bottom]

Foun•da•tion for the Ac•cred•i•ta•tion of Cel•lu•lar Ther•a•py (FACT) (fown-dā′shŭn ă-kred′i-tā′shŭn sel′yū-lăr thār′ă-ē) An accrediatation program that encompasses all phases of hematopoietic collection, processing, and transplantation.

found•er prin•ci•ple (fown′dĕr prin′si-pĕl) The conditional probabilities of the frequencies of a set of genes at any future date depend on the initial composition of the founders of the population and have in general no tendency to revert to the composition of the population from which the founders were themselves derived.

foun•tain de•cus•sa•tion (fown′tăn dē-kŭs-ā′shŭn) SEE tegmental decussations (1).

foun•tain sy•ringe (fown′tăn sĭr-inj′) An apparatus consisting of a reservoir for holding fluid, to the bottom of which is attached a tube with a suitable nozzle; used for vaginal or rectal injections, irrigating wounds, and other purposes, the force of the flow being regulated by the height of the reservoir above the point of discharge.

four•chette (fur′shet) The tense band of mucous membrane connection formed by the dorsal ends of the labia minora. It is often damaged in childbirth. [Fr. little fork]

Four Cor•ners vi•rus (fōr kōr′nĕrz vī′rŭs) SYN Sin Nombre virus. [from the point in the western U.S. where New Mexico, Colorado, Utah, and Arizona meet, site of a major outbreak of this disease]

Fou•ri•er a•nal•y•sis (fūr-ē-ā′ ă-nal′i-sis) A mathematical approximation of a function as the sum of periodic functions (sine waves) of different frequencies; used in reconstruction of magnetic resonance images and computed tomographs and analysis of any kind of signal for its frequency content.

Fou•ri•er trans•form (fūr-ē-ā′ trans′fōrm) A mathematical technique of dividing a time-varying function or signal into components at different frequencies, giving the phase and amplitude of each; used in computed tomography and magnetic resonance image reconstruction transformation.

four-point gait (fōr-poynt gāt) In physical therapy, crutch-assisted ambulation with which the crutch moves in tandem with the opposite limb.

fourth cra•ni•al nerve [CN IV] (fōrth krā′nē-ăl nĕrv) SYN trochlear nerve [CN IV].

fourth heart sound (S_4) (fōrth hahrt sownd) The sound produced in late diastole in association with ventricular filling due to atrial systole and related to reduced ventricular compliance. It may be normal at older ages but is nearly always abnormal at younger ages. It is common in ventricular hypertrophy, particularly with hypertension, and is almost invariable during acute myocardial infarction. Fourth heart sounds may arise from the right or left ventricle or both.

fourth lum•bar nerve [L4] (fōrth lŭm′bahr nĕrv) The ventral branch of the nerve is forked to enter into the formation of both lumbar and sacral plexuses.

fourth toe [IV] (fōrth tō) Fourth digit of foot.

fourth ven•tri•cle (fōrth ven′tri-kĕl) A cavity of irregular shape extending from the obex rostrad to its communication with the sylvian aqueduct, enclosed between the cerebellum dorsally and the rhombencephalic tegmentum ventrally, having a rhomboid-shaped floor (rhomboid fossa) and a tentlike roof that in its caudal part is formed by the tela choroidea and the posterior medullary velum, in its middle part by the white matter of the cerebellum, and in its narrowing rostral part (recessus superior) by the anterior medullary velum. The fourth ventricle reaches its greatest width at the pontomedullary transition, where it expands laterally behind the cerebellar peduncles into the spoutlike lateral recess, and its greatest height at the fastigial recess, which reaches up into the cerebellar white matter. Direct communication between the ventricular system and the subarachnoid space is established at the level of the fourth ventricle by a median opening in the tela choroidea, the medial aperture of the foramen of Magendie, which opens into the cerebellomedullary cistern, and on both sides by the lateral aperture or foramen of Luschka, which connects the lateral recess with the interpeduncular cistern.

FOV Abbreviation of field of view.

fo•ve•a, pl. **fo•ve•ae** (fō′vē-ă, -ē) [TA] Any natural depression on the surface of the body, such as the axilla, or on the surface of a bone. Cf. dimple. [L. a pit]

fo•ve•a cen•tra•lis mac•u•lae lu•te•ae (fō′

vē-ă sen-trā′lis mak′yū-lē lū′tē-ē) [TA] SYN central retinal fovea.

fo•ve•ate, fo•ve•at•ed (fō′vē-āt, -ā-ted) Pitted; having foveae or depressions on the surface.

fo•ve•a•tion (fō-vē-ā′shŭn) Pitted scar formation, as in chickenpox. [L. *fovea,* a pit]

fo•ve•o•la, pl. **fo•ve•o•lae** (fō-vē′ō-lă, -lē) [TA] A minute fovea or pit. [Mod. L. dim. of L. *fovea,* pit]

fo•ve•o•lar (fō-vē′ō-lăr) Pertaining to a foveola.

fo•ve•o•late (fō′vē-ō-lāt) Having minute pits (foveolae) or small depressions on the surface.

Fo•ville syn•drome (fō-vēl′ sin′drōm) A form of alternating hemiplegia characterized by abducens paralysis on one side, paralysis of the extremities on the other.

Fow•ler po•si•tion (fowl′ĕr pŏ-zish′ŭn) SYN semirecumbent. See page B29.

Fow•ler test (fowl′ĕr tĕst) Measurement of anterior shoulder instability; the supine patient's shoulder is abducted and externally rotated while posterior force is applied to the humerus. If movement is detected, the test is positive and instability is presumed to be present.

fox•ber•ry (foks′ber-ē) SYN bearberry.

fox•glove (foks′glŏv) SYN *Digitalis.*

fox•tail grass (foks′tāl gras) SYN barley.

FPG Abbreviation for fasting plasma glucose.

F plas•mid (plaz′mid) The prototype conjugative plasmid associated with conjugation in the K-12 strain of *Escherichia coli.* SYN F factor.

FPS, fps Abbreviation for foot-pound-second. SEE foot-pound-second system.

Fr 1. Symbol for francium. **2.** Abbreviation for French scale.

frac•tals (frak′tălz) Mathematical patterns developed by Benoit Mandelbrot in 1977, in which small parts have the same shape as the whole. Blood vessels and the bronchial tree behave as fractals; some infections and neoplasms also behave as fractals. [Fr., fr. L. *fractus,* broken, pp. of *frango,* to break, + -al]

frac•tion (frak′shŭn) **1.** The quotient of two quantities. **2.** An aliquot portion or any portion.

frac•tion•al in•jec•tion (frak′shŭn-ăl in-jek′shŭn) The instillation of a pharmacotherapeutic or anesthetic agent in small amounts to improve toleration or benefit.

frac•tion•a•tion (frak-shŭn-ā′shŭn) **1.** Separation of the components of a mixture into its basic constituents. **2.** The administration of a course of therapeutic radiation of a neoplasm in a planned series of fractions of the total dose, most often once a day for several weeks, to minimize radiation damage of contiguous normal tissues.

frac•ture (frak′shŭr) **1.** To break. **2.** A break, especially the breaking of a bone or cartilage. **3.** A break in the continuity of the bone and damage to surrounding tissues. See this page. [L. *fractura,* a break]

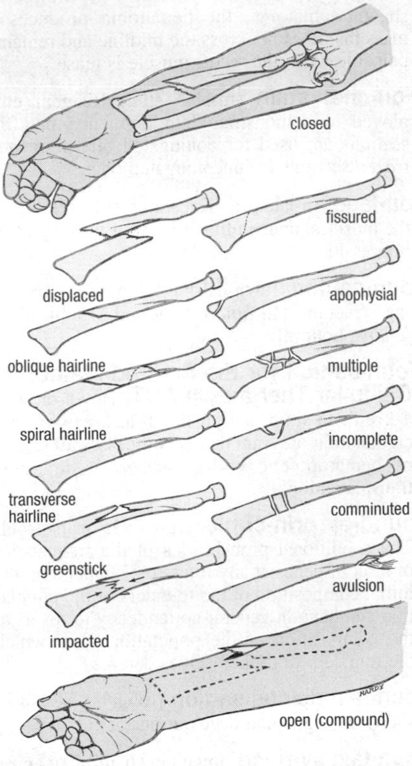

types of fractures

frac•ture blis•ter (frak′shŭr blis′tĕr) Superficial epidermolysis that occurs in association, most commonly, with fractures of the leg and ankle and forearm and wrist; etiology represents a combination of excessive swelling and torsional injury to the overlying soft tissues.

frac•ture by con•tre•coup (frak′shŭr kōn′trĕ-kū′) Skull fracture at a point distant from the site of impact.

frac•ture dis•lo•ca•tion (frak′shŭr dis′lō-kā′shŭn) Dislocation associated with or accompanied by a fracture of one of the bones forming the articulation.

frac•ture of fifth me•ta•car•pal (frak′shŭr fifth met-ă-kar′păl) SYN boxer's fracture.

frag•ile site (fraj′il sīt) A nonstaining gap at a specific point on a chromosome, usually involving both chromatids, always at the same point on chromosomes of different cells from an individual or kindred.

frag•ile X chro•mo•some (fraj′il krō′mō-sōm) An X chromosome with a weak (i.e., fragile) site near the end of the long arm, resulting in the appearance of an almost detached fragment; frequently associated with X-linked mental retardation.

frag•ile X syn•drome (FMR1) (fraj′il sin′drōm) The disorder has a sex-linked recessive character. Patients have a mutation in the FMR1 gene in the manufacture of the protein fMRP; most common cause of inherited mental impairment (findings include mild-to-severe learning disabilities and autism). SYN FMR1, marker X syndrome, Martin-Bell syndrome.

fra•gil•i•ty (fră-jil′i-tē) Brittleness; liability to break, burst, or disintegrate. [L. *fragilitas*]

fra•gil•i•ty of the blood (fră-jil′i-tē blŭd) SYN osmotic fragility.

fra•gil•i•ty test (fră-jil′i-tē test) A measurement of the resistance of erythrocytes to hemolysis in hypotonic saline solutions; erythrocytes to be tested are added to varying concentrations of saline and beginning and complete hemolysis are measured; in hereditary spherocytosis, the fragility of the erythrocytes is markedly increased, whereas in thalassemia and sickle cell anemia, the fragility of the erythrocytes is usually reduced.

frag•ment (frag′mĕnt) A small part broken from a larger entity.

frag•men•ta•tion (frag-men-tā′shŭn) The breaking of an entity into smaller parts. SYN spallation (1).

frail el•der (frāl el′dĕr) Colloquial usage (considered offensive by some patients) for a very old person who may experience difficulties with activities of daily living due to disease or overall decrepitude.

fram•be•si•a (fram-bē′zē-ă) SYN yaws. SYN framboesia. [Fr. *framboise,* raspberry]

fram•be•si•o•ma (fram-bē′zē-ō′mă) SYN mother yaw. [frambesia + *-oma,* tumor]

framboesia [Br.] SYN frambesia.

frame (frām) A supporting or integrating structure made of parts fitted together.

frame•work (frām′wŏrk) A structure that supports or encloses something.

frame•work re•gion (frām′wŏrk rē′jŭn) IMMUNOLOGY a conserved sequence of amino acids on either side of the hypervariable regions in the variable domains of an immunoglobulin chain.

Fran•ci•sel•la (fran-si-sel′lă) A genus of nonmotile, non-spore-forming, aerobic bacteria that contain small, gram-negative cocci and rods. Capsules are rarely produced, and the cells may show bipolar staining. These organisms are highly pleomorphic; they do not grow on plain agar or in liquid media without special enrichment; they are pathogenic and cause tularemia in humans. The type species is *Francisella tularensis.*

Fran•ci•sel•la tu•la•ren•sis (fran-si-sel′lă tū-lă-ren′sis) A bacterial species that causes tularemia in humans, transmitted to them from wild animals by bloodsucking insects or by contact with infected animals such as rabbits and ticks; it can penetrate unbroken skin to cause infection. It is the type species of the genus *Francisella.*

fran•ci•um (Fr) (fran′sē-ŭm) Radioactive element of the alkali metal series; atomic no. 87; half-life of most stable known isotope, ^{223}Fr, is 21.8 minutes. [*France,* native country of Marguerite Perey, the discoverer]

Franc•ke nee•dle (frahng′kĕ nē′dĕl) A small lancet-shaped, spring-activated needle, used to evacuate a small effusion of blood.

frank (frangk) Unmistakable; manifest; clinically evident.

frank breech pre•sen•ta•tion (frangk brēch prez′ĕn-tā′shŭn) SEE breech presentation.

frank•en•food (frangk′ĕn-fūd) SYN genetically modified food. [*Frankenstein* + food]

Frank•fort hor•i•zon•tal plane (frahngk′fōrt hōr′i-zon′tăl plān) **1.** A cephalometric plane that passes through the inferior borders of the bony orbits and the upper margins of the auditory meatus. **2.** A reference plane in orthodontic diagnosis and treatment planning. [Frankfurt-am-Main Agreement, Germany, site of 1884 anatomy convention]

frank•in•cense (frangk′in-sens) SYN olibanum.

Frank-Star•ling curve (frangk stahr′ling kŭrv) SYN Starling curve.

Fränt•zel mur•mur (frent′sel mŭr′mŭr) Murmur of mitral stenosis when louder at its beginning and end than in its midportion.

Fra•ser syn•drome (frā′zer sin′drōm) An association of cryptophthalmus with multiple anomalies, including middle and outer ear malformations, cleft palate, laryngeal deformity, displacement of umbilicus and nipples, digital malformations, separation of symphysis pubis, maldevelopment of kidneys, and masculinization of genitalia in females; autosomal recessive inheritance.

fra•ter•nal twins (fră-tĕr′năl twinz) SYN dizygotic twins.

fraud (frawd) An act of deliberate deception performed to acquire an unlawful benefit, such as the improper coding of health services in a claim for payment. [L. *fraus*]

Fraun•ho•fer line (frown′hōf-ĕr līn) Any one of the more prominent absorption lines of the solar spectrum.

Fra•zier nee•dle (frā′zhĕr nē′dĕl) A needle for draining lateral ventricles of brain.

Fra•zier-Spil•ler op•er•a•tion (frā′zhĕr spil′ĕr op-ĕr-ā′shŭn) SEE trigeminal rhizotomy.

FRC Abbreviation for functional residual capacity.

freck•les (frek′ĕlz) Yellowish or brownish macules developing on the exposed parts of the skin, especially in people with light complexion; the lesions increase in number on exposure to the sun; the epidermis is microscopically normal except for increased melanin. SEE ALSO lentigo. SYN ephelis. [O. E. *freken*]

Fre•det-Ram•stedt op•er•a•tion (fre-dā′ rahm′shtet op-ĕr-ā′shŭn) SYN pyloromyotomy.

Fred•rick•son clas•si•fi•ca•tion (fred′rik-sŏn klas′i-fi-kā′shŭn) A classification system of hyperlipoproteinemia that uses plasma appearance, triglyceride values, and total cholesterol values. There are five types: I, II, III, IV, and V. SEE ALSO hyperlipoproteinemia.

free ap•pro•pri•ate pub•lic ed•u•ca•tion (frē ă-prō′prē-ăt pŭb′lik ej′yū-kā′shŭn) An aspect of the Handicapped Children Act of 1975 (currently I.D.E.A.) that mandated free appropriate public education for all children with disabilities.

free as•so•ci•a•tion (frē ă-sō′sē-ā′shŭn) An investigative psychoanalytic technique in which the patient verbalizes, without reservation or censorship, the passing contents of his or her mind; the conflicts verbalized are the basis of the psychoanalyst's interpretations.

free en•er•gy (F, *F*) (frē en′ĕr-jē) A thermodynamic function symbolized as *F*, or *G* (Gibbs free energy), $=H - TS$, where *H* is the enthalpy of a system, *T* the absolute temperature, and *S* the entropy; chemical reactions proceed spontaneously in the direction that involves a net decrease in the free energy of the system (i.e., $\Delta G < 0$).

free flap (frē flap) Island flap in which the donor vessels are severed proximally, the flap is transported as a free object to the recipient area, and the flap is revascularized by anastomosing its supplying vessels to vessels there.

free gin•gi•va (frē jin′ji-vă) That portion of the gingiva that surrounds the tooth but is not directly attached to the tooth surface; the outer wall of the gingival sulcus.

free graft (frē graft) A graft transplanted without its normal attachments, or a pedicle, from one site to another.

free in•duc•tion de•cay (FID) (frē in-dŭk′shŭn dĕ-kā′) MAGNETIC RESONANCE IMAGING the decay curve that is detected by the radiofrequency coil after the application of an excitation pulse, without additional pulses (free).

free mac•ro•phage (frē mak′rō-fāj) An actively motile macrophage typically found in sites of inflammation.

free nerve end•ings (frē nĕrv end′ingz) A form of peripheral ending of sensory nerve fibers in which the terminal filaments end freely in the tissue.

free rad•i•cal (frē rad′i-kăl) A radical in its (usually transient) uncombined state; an atom or atom group carrying an unpaired electron and no charge. Free radicals may be involved as short-lived, highly active intermediates in various reactions in living tissue, notably in photosynthesis. The free radical nitric oxide, NO·, plays an important role in vasodilation. SYN radical (4).

free•way space (frē′wā spās) The space between the occluding surfaces of the maxillary and mandibular teeth when the mandible is in physiologic resting position. SYN interocclusal distance (2).

freeze-dry•ing (frēz′drī-ing) SYN lyophilization.

freeze frac•ture (frēz frak′shŭr) A procedure for preparing cells or other biologic samples for electron microscopy during which the sample is frozen quickly and then broken with a sharp blow. SYN cryofracture.

freez•ing (frēz′ing) Congealing, stiffening, or hardening by exposure to cold.

freez•ing point de•pres•sion (frēz′ing poynt dĕ-prĕs′shŭn) A method used to determine osmotic concentration by comparing freezing point of a solution with values of a pure solvent. The lower the freezing point, the higher the osmotic pressure.

Frei•berg dis•ease (frī′bĕrg di-zēz′) Osteonecrosis of second metatarsal head.

Frej•ka pil•low splint (frāj′kah pil′ō splint) A pillow splint used for abduction and flexion of the femurs in treatment of congenital hip dysplasia or dislocation in infants.

frem•i•tus (frem′i-tŭs) A vibration imparted to the hand resting on the chest or other part of the body. SEE ALSO thrill. [L. a dull roaring sound, fr. *fremo,* pp. *-itus,* to roar, resound]

frem•i•tus pec•to•ral•is (frem′i-tŭs pek-tō-rā′lis) Vibration on the chest wall produced by phonation.

fre•na (frē′nă) Plural of frenum.

fre•nal (frē′năl) Relating to any frenum.

French-A•mer•i•can-Bri•tish clas•si•fi•ca•tion sys•tem (FAB) (french′ă-mer′i-kăn-brit′ish klas′i-fi-kā′shŭn sis′tĕm) A classification and nomenclature system for acute leukemias based

HUMAN ANATOMY

CONTENTS

INDEX

A

B

C

D

E

F

G

H

I

J

K

L

M

N

O

P

Q

R

S

T

U

V

W

X

Z

PLATE 1: ANTERIOR AND POSTERIOR VIEW OF THE SKULL

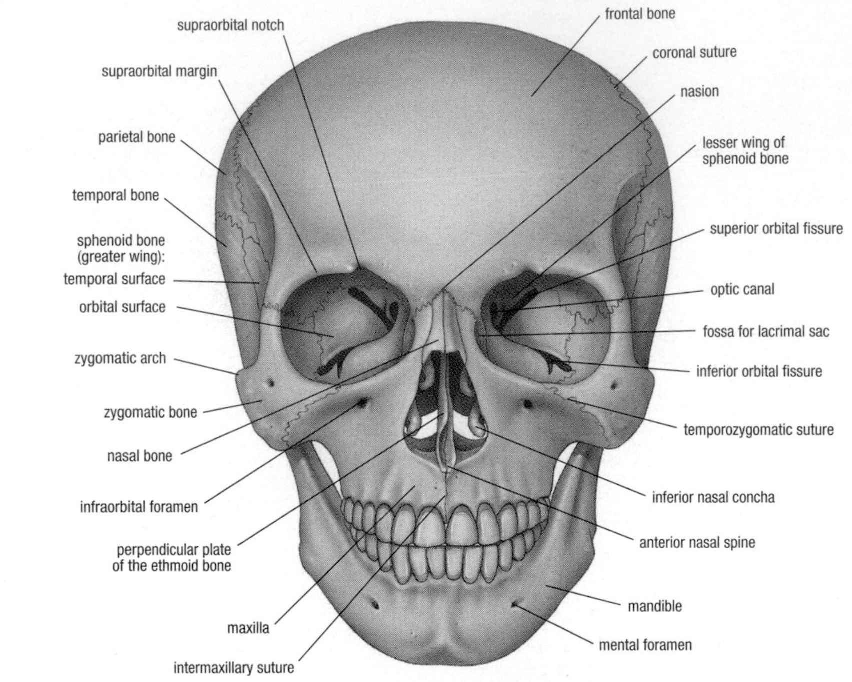
frontal bone
supraorbital notch
coronal suture
supraorbital margin
nasion
parietal bone
lesser wing of
sphenoid bone
temporal bone
superior orbital fissure
sphenoid bone
(greater wing):
temporal surface
optic canal
orbital surface
fossa for lacrimal sac
zygomatic arch
inferior orbital fissure
zygomatic bone
temporozygomatic suture
nasal bone
inferior nasal concha
infraorbital foramen
anterior nasal spine
perpendicular plate
of the ethmoid bone
mandible
maxilla
mental foramen
intermaxillary suture

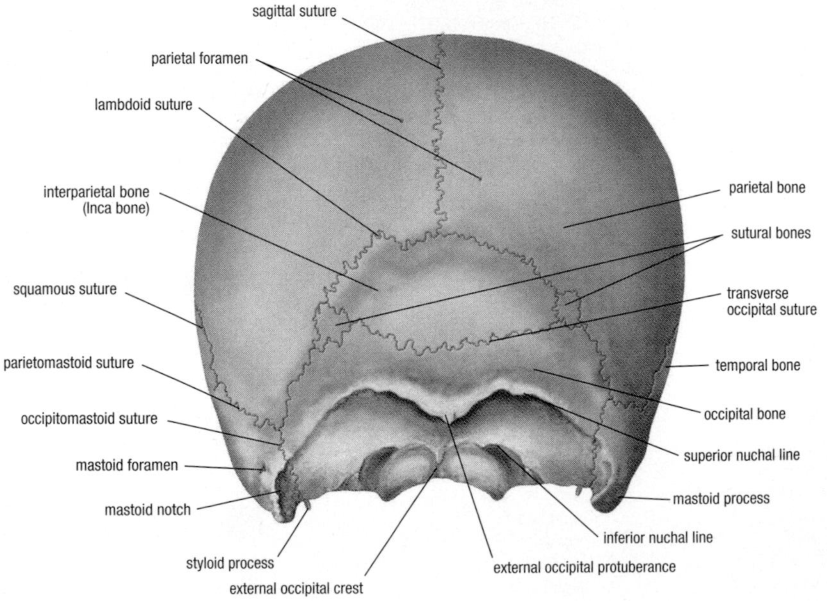
sagittal suture
parietal foramen
lambdoid suture
interparietal bone
(Inca bone)
parietal bone
sutural bones
squamous suture
transverse
occipital suture
parietomastoid suture
temporal bone
occipital bone
occipitomastoid suture
superior nuchal line
mastoid foramen
mastoid process
mastoid notch
inferior nuchal line
styloid process
external occipital protuberance
external occipital crest

PLATE 2: LATERAL VIEW OF THE SKULL

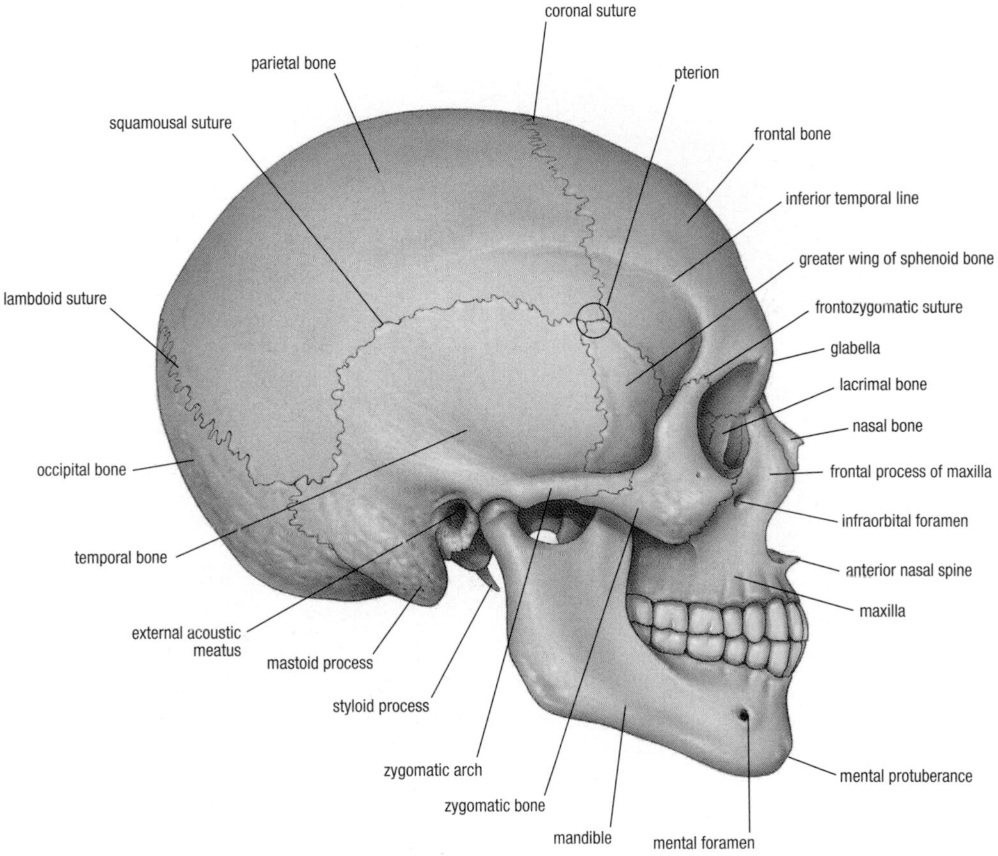

coronal suture
parietal bone
pterion
squamousal suture
frontal bone
inferior temporal line
greater wing of sphenoid bone
lambdoid suture
frontozygomatic suture
glabella
lacrimal bone
nasal bone
occipital bone
frontal process of maxilla
infraorbital foramen
temporal bone
anterior nasal spine
maxilla
external acoustic meatus
mastoid process
styloid process
zygomatic arch
mental protuberance
zygomatic bone
mandible
mental foramen

PLATE 3: SAGITTAL SECTION OF THE SKULL

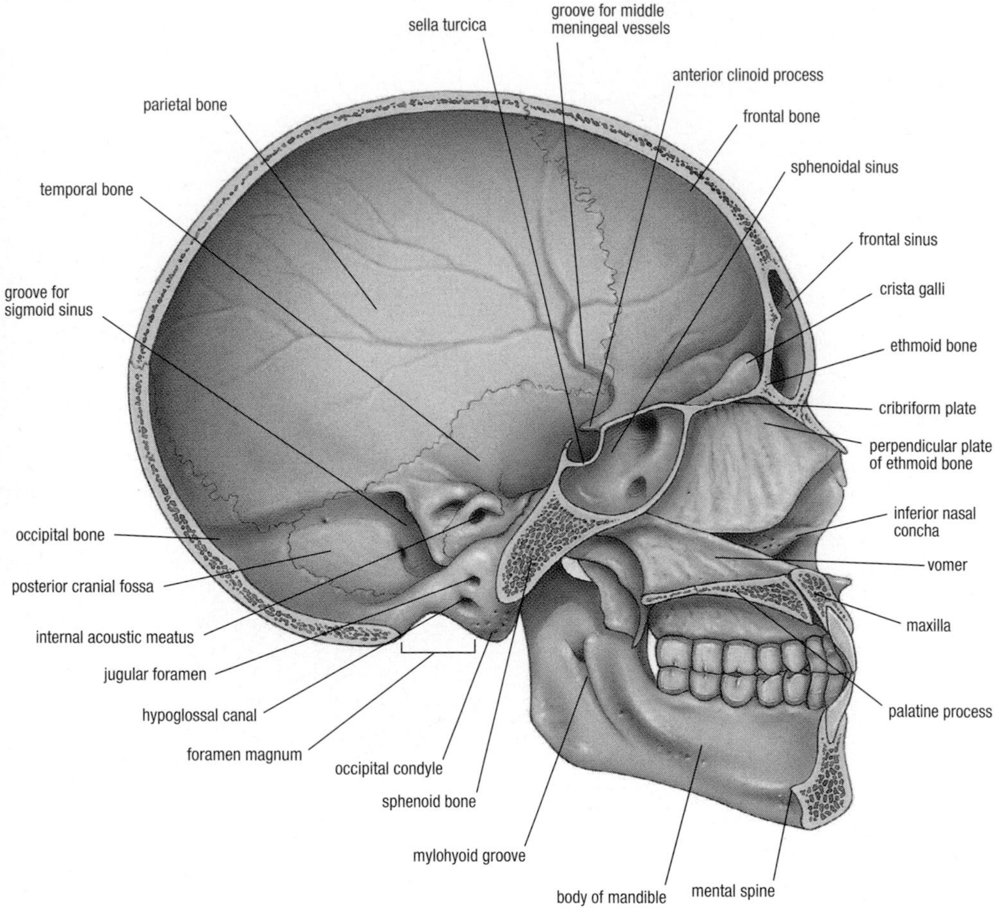

sella turcica
groove for middle meningeal vessels
anterior clinoid process
parietal bone
frontal bone
sphenoidal sinus
temporal bone
frontal sinus
groove for sigmoid sinus
crista galli
ethmoid bone
cribriform plate
perpendicular plate of ethmoid bone
inferior nasal concha
occipital bone
vomer
posterior cranial fossa
maxilla
internal acoustic meatus
jugular foramen
palatine process
hypoglossal canal
foramen magnum
occipital condyle
sphenoid bone
mylohyoid groove
body of mandible
mental spine

PLATE 4: MUSCULAR ANATOMY OF HEAD AND NECK

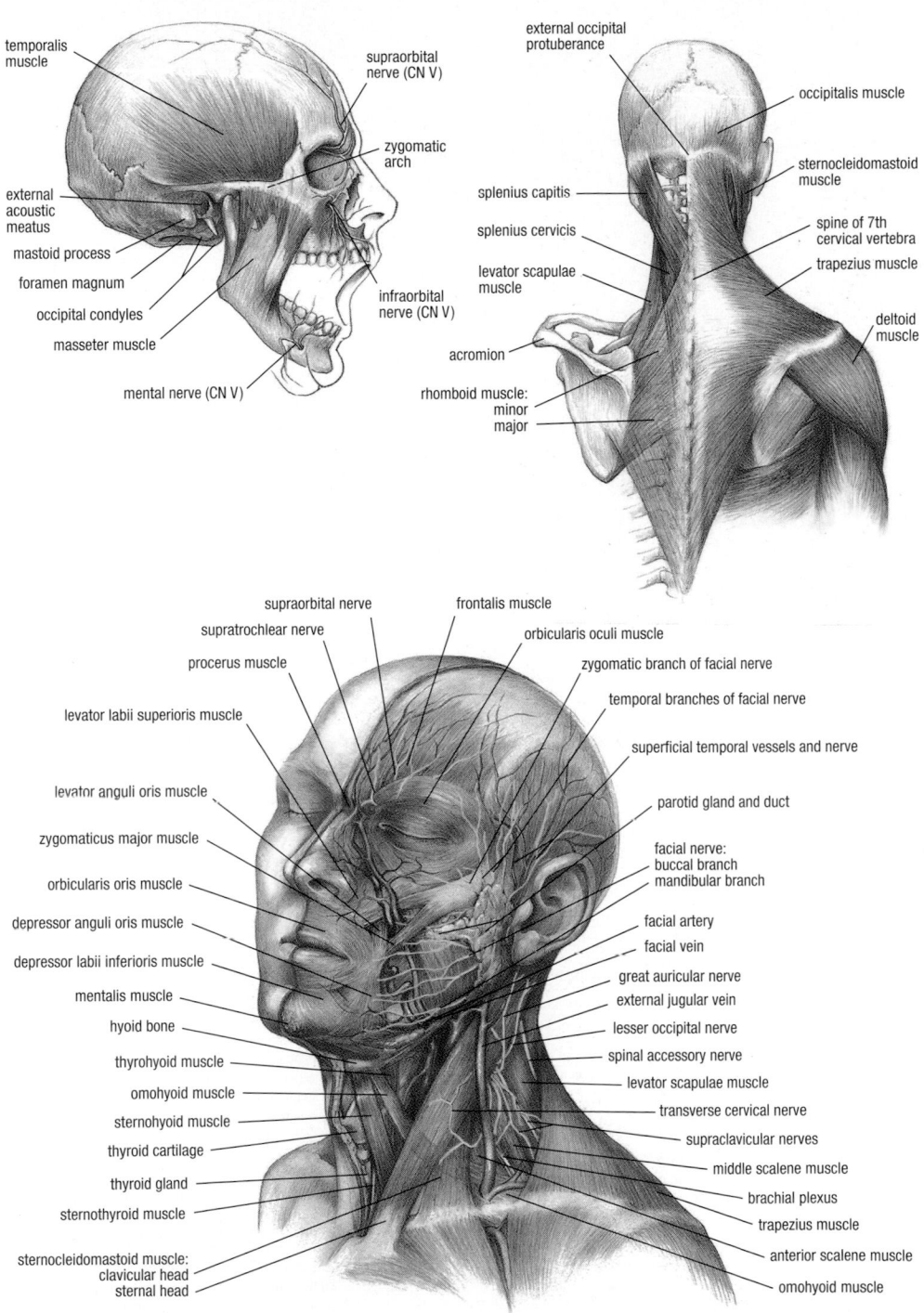

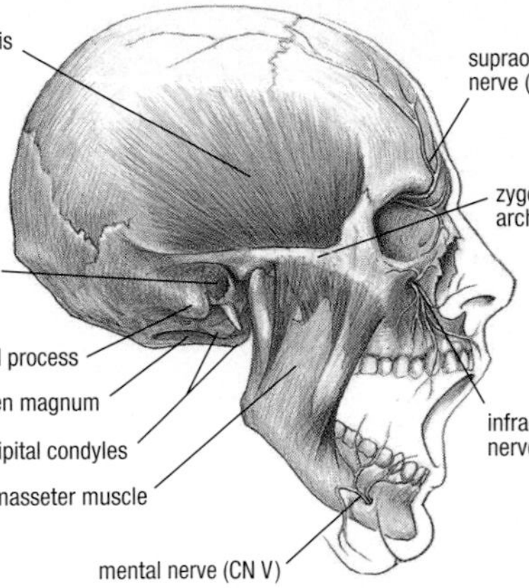
temporalis muscle
supraorbital nerve (CN V)
zygomatic arch
external acoustic meatus
mastoid process
foramen magnum
occipital condyles
masseter muscle
infraorbital nerve (CN V)
mental nerve (CN V)

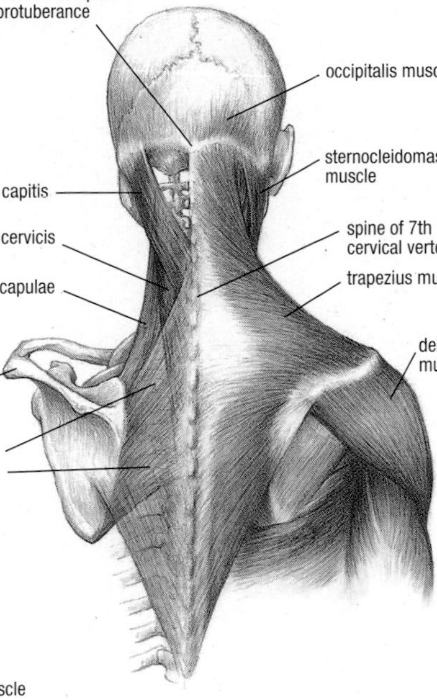
external occipital protuberance
occipitalis muscle
sternocleidomastoid muscle
splenius capitis
splenius cervicis
spine of 7th cervical vertebra
trapezius muscle
levator scapulae muscle
deltoid muscle
acromion
rhomboid muscle:
minor
major

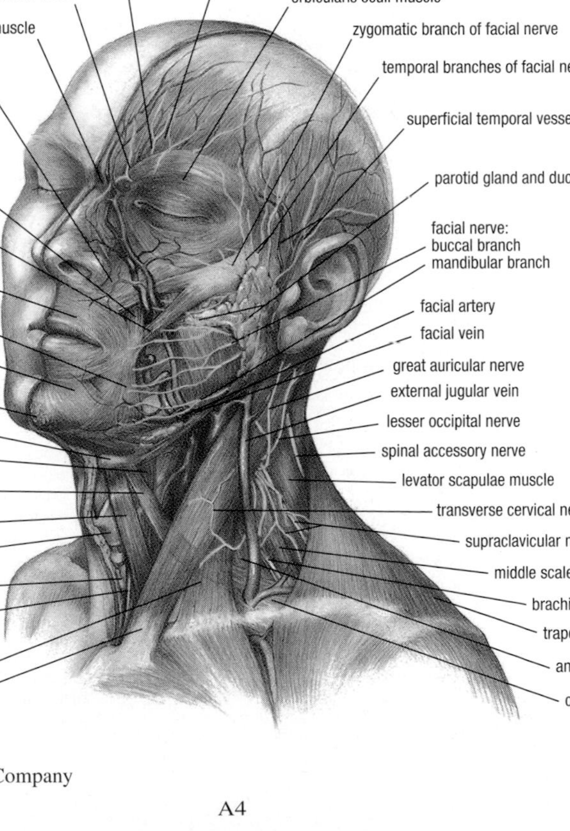
supraorbital nerve
frontalis muscle
supratrochlear nerve
orbicularis oculi muscle
procerus muscle
zygomatic branch of facial nerve
temporal branches of facial nerve
levator labii superioris muscle
superficial temporal vessels and nerve
levator anguli oris muscle
parotid gland and duct
zygomaticus major muscle
facial nerve:
buccal branch
mandibular branch
orbicularis oris muscle
depressor anguli oris muscle
facial artery
facial vein
depressor labii inferioris muscle
great auricular nerve
mentalis muscle
external jugular vein
hyoid bone
lesser occipital nerve
thyrohyoid muscle
spinal accessory nerve
levator scapulae muscle
omohyoid muscle
transverse cervical nerve
sternohyoid muscle
supraclavicular nerves
thyroid cartilage
middle scalene muscle
thyroid gland
brachial plexus
sternothyroid muscle
trapezius muscle
anterior scalene muscle
sternocleidomastoid muscle:
clavicular head
sternal head
omohyoid muscle

PLATE 5: CEREBRAL HEMISPHERES

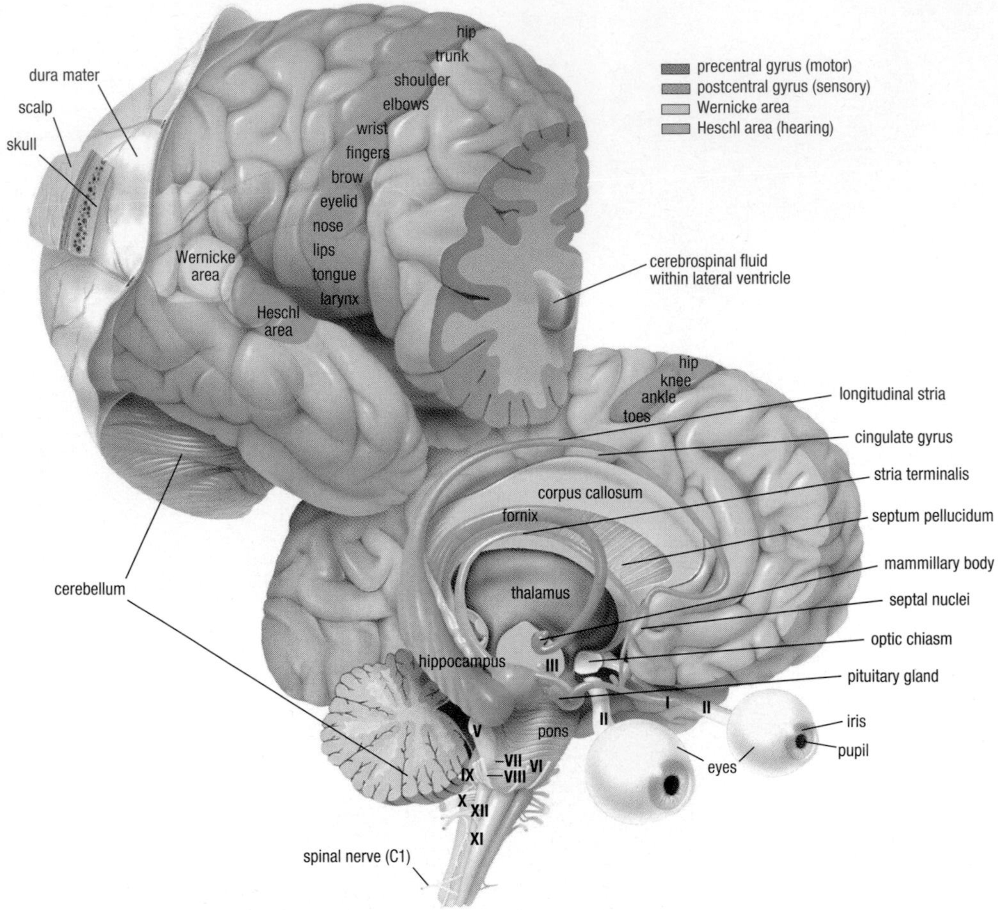

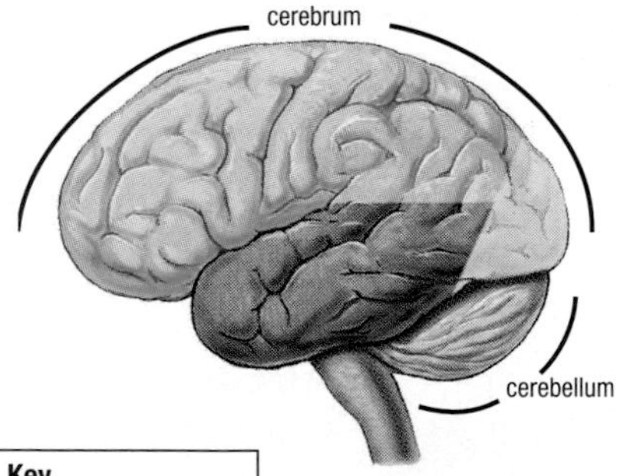

Key

- frontal lobe
- parietal lobe
- temporal lobe
- occipital lobe

Key

Cranial nerves

I olfactory nerve — smell
II optic nerve — sight
III oculomotor nerve — eye movement
IV trochlear nerve — eye movement (not illustrated)
V trigeminal nerve — face (sensory)
VI abducens nerve — eye movement
VII facial nerve — face (motor), taste
VIII vestibulocochlear nerve — hearing and balance
IX glossopharyngeal nerve — swallowing, taste, sensation
X vagus nerve — gastrointestinal tract, swallowing, heart rate, peristalsis
XI accessory nerve — shoulder muscles
XII hypoglossal nerve — tongue

PLATE 6: VERTEBRAL AND INTERVERTEBRAL DISC ANATOMY

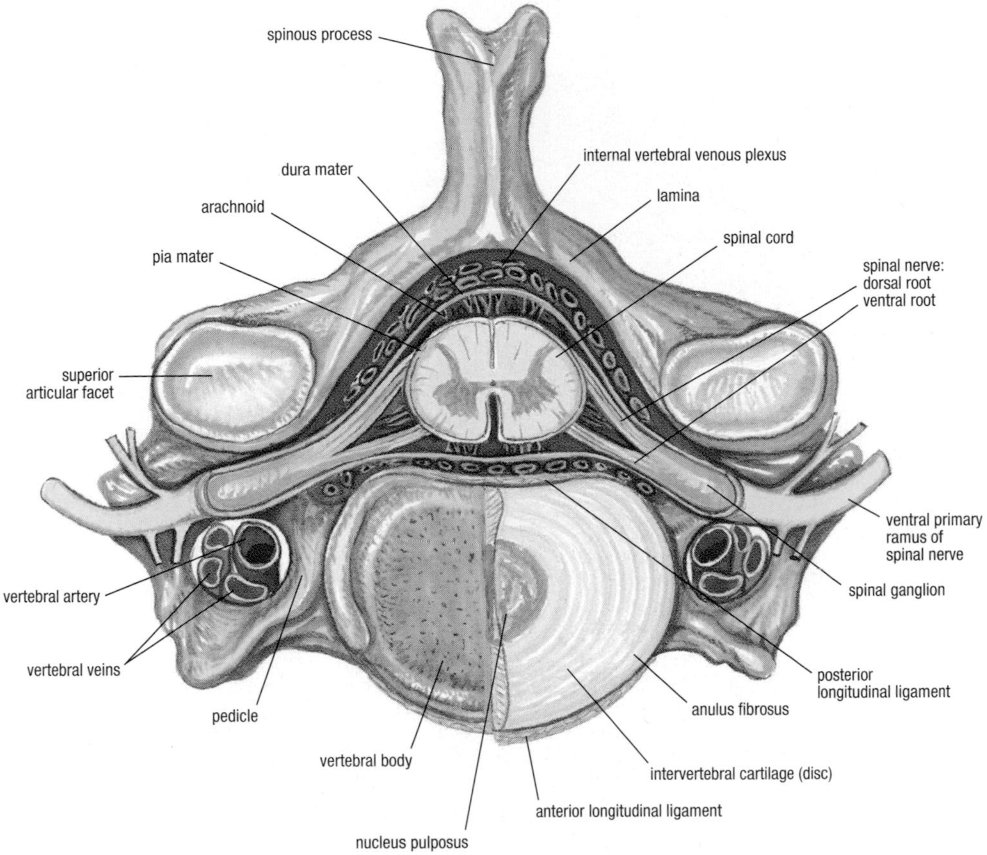

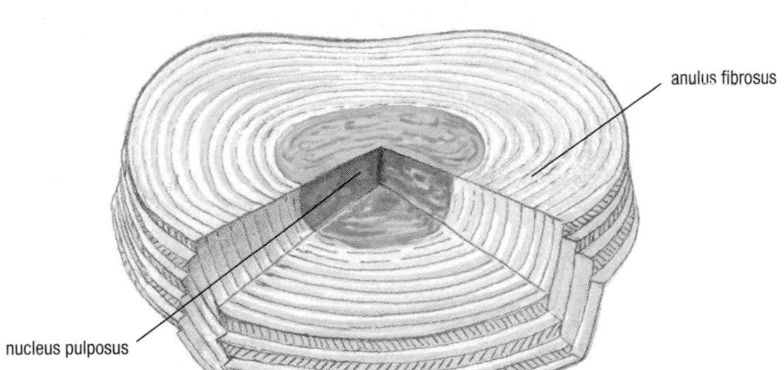

PLATE 7: NERVOUS SYSTEM OF THORAX AND UPPER LIMB, ANTERIOR VIEW

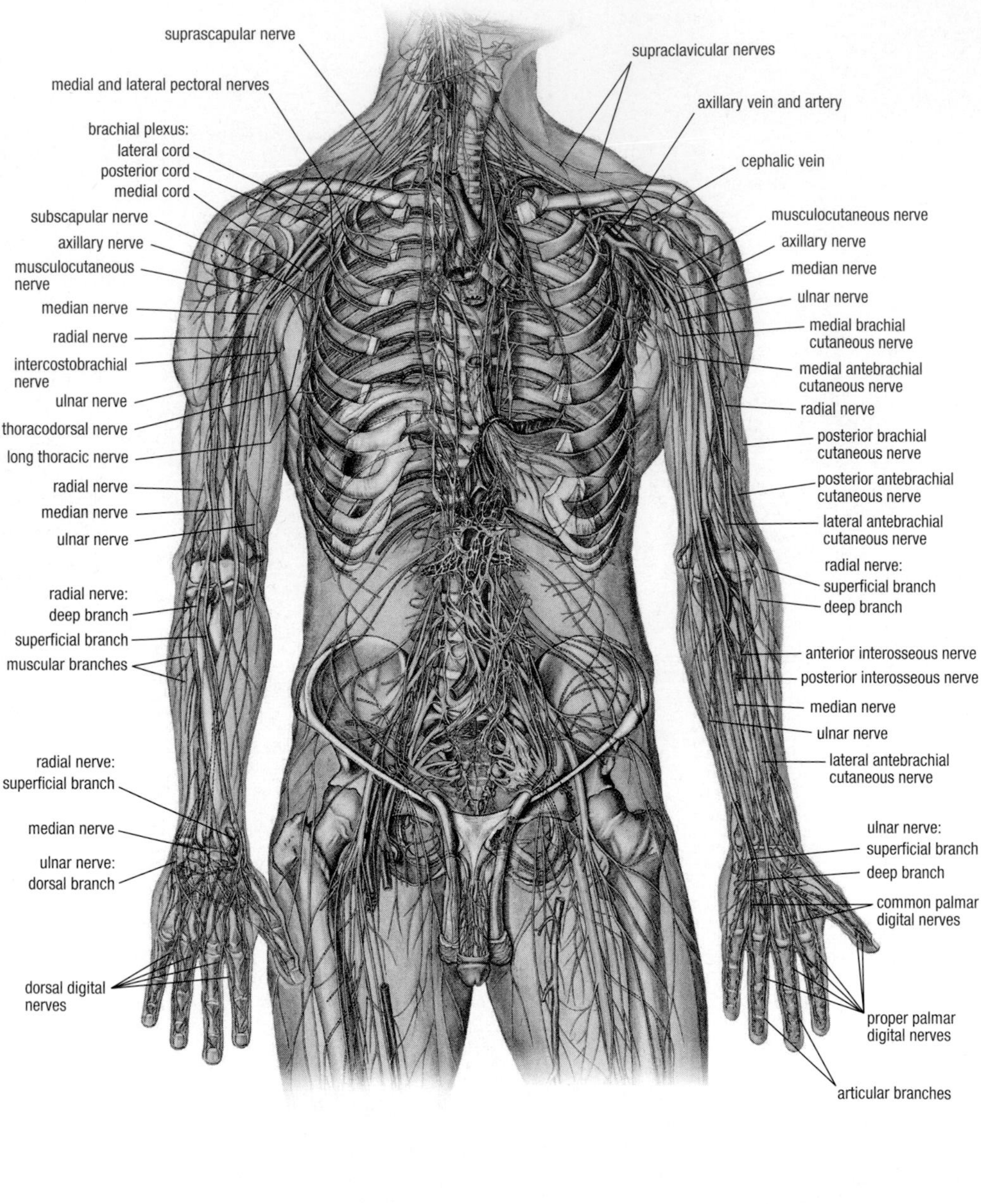

PLATE 8: MUSCULAR AND SKELETAL ANATOMY OF WRIST AND HAND, PALMAR VIEW

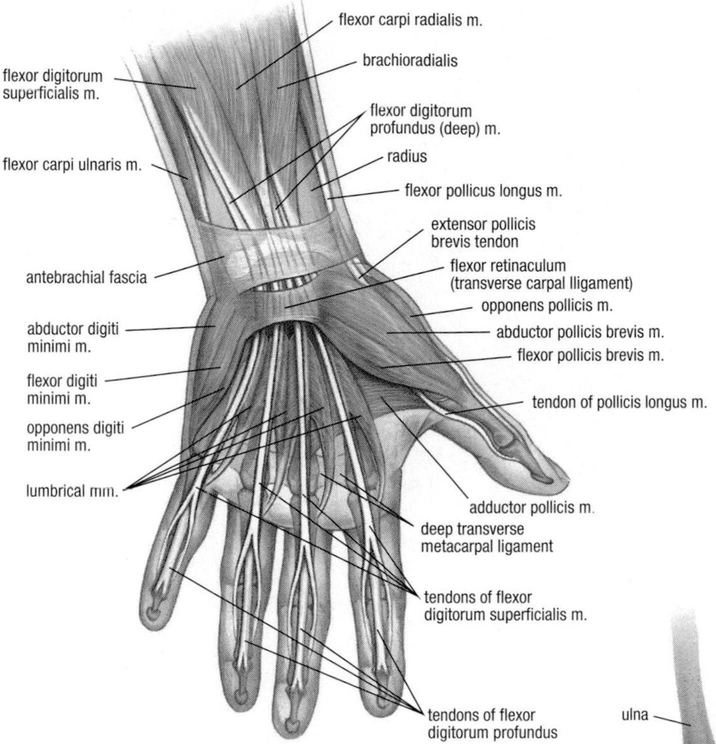

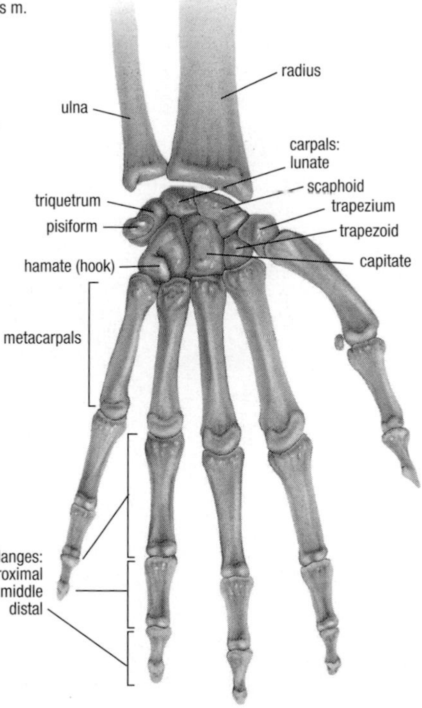

Imagery © Anatomical Chart Company

PLATE 9: VISCERA OF THORAX, ANTERIOR VIEW

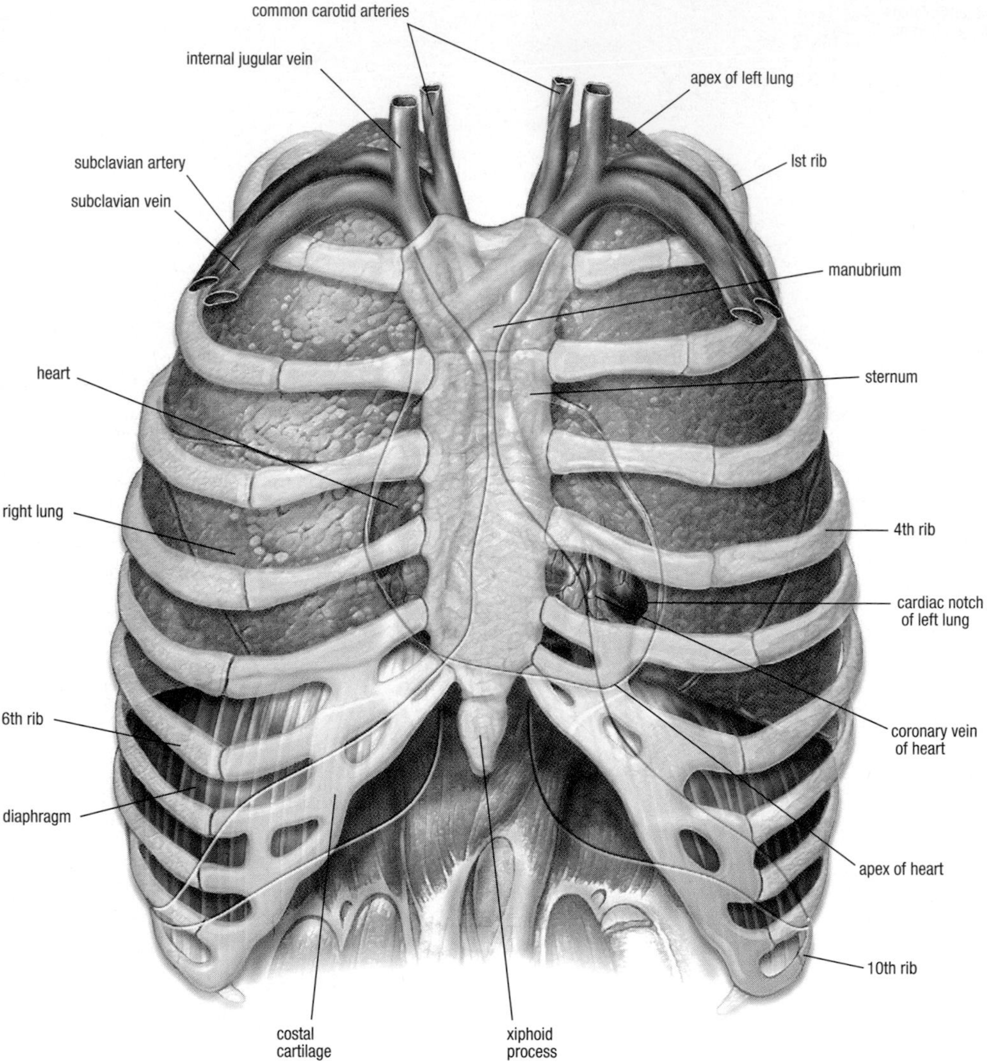

PLATE 10: ANATOMY OF HEART, ANTERIOR VIEW

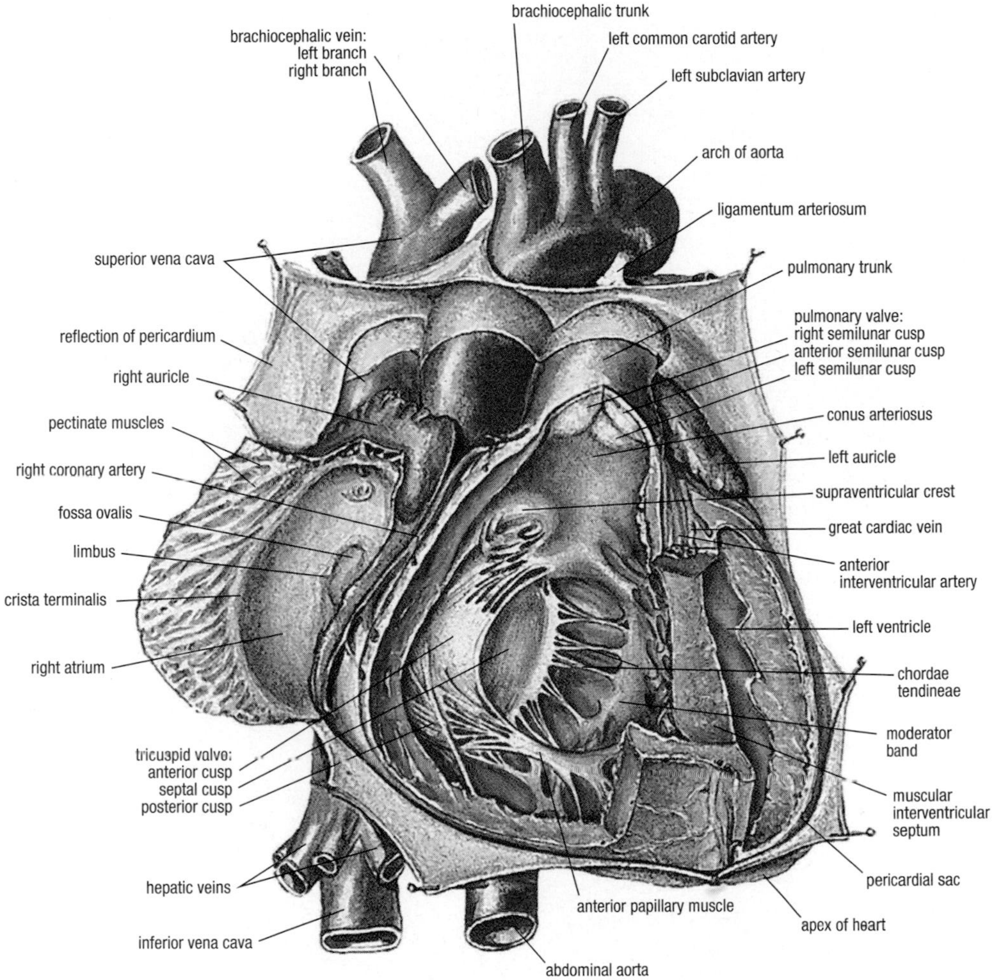
brachiocephalic trunk
brachiocephalic vein:
left branch
right branch
left common carotid artery
left subclavian artery
arch of aorta
ligamentum arteriosum
superior vena cava
pulmonary trunk
reflection of pericardium
pulmonary valve:
right semilunar cusp
anterior semilunar cusp
left semilunar cusp
right auricle
pectinate muscles
conus arteriosus
right coronary artery
left auricle
supraventricular crest
fossa ovalis
great cardiac vein
limbus
anterior
interventricular artery
crista terminalis
left ventricle
right atrium
chordae
tendineae
moderator
band
tricuspid valve:
anterior cusp
septal cusp
posterior cusp
muscular
interventricular
septum
hepatic veins
pericardial sac
anterior papillary muscle
apex of heart
inferior vena cava
abdominal aorta

PLATE 11: ABDOMINAL VISCERA, ANTERIOR VIEW

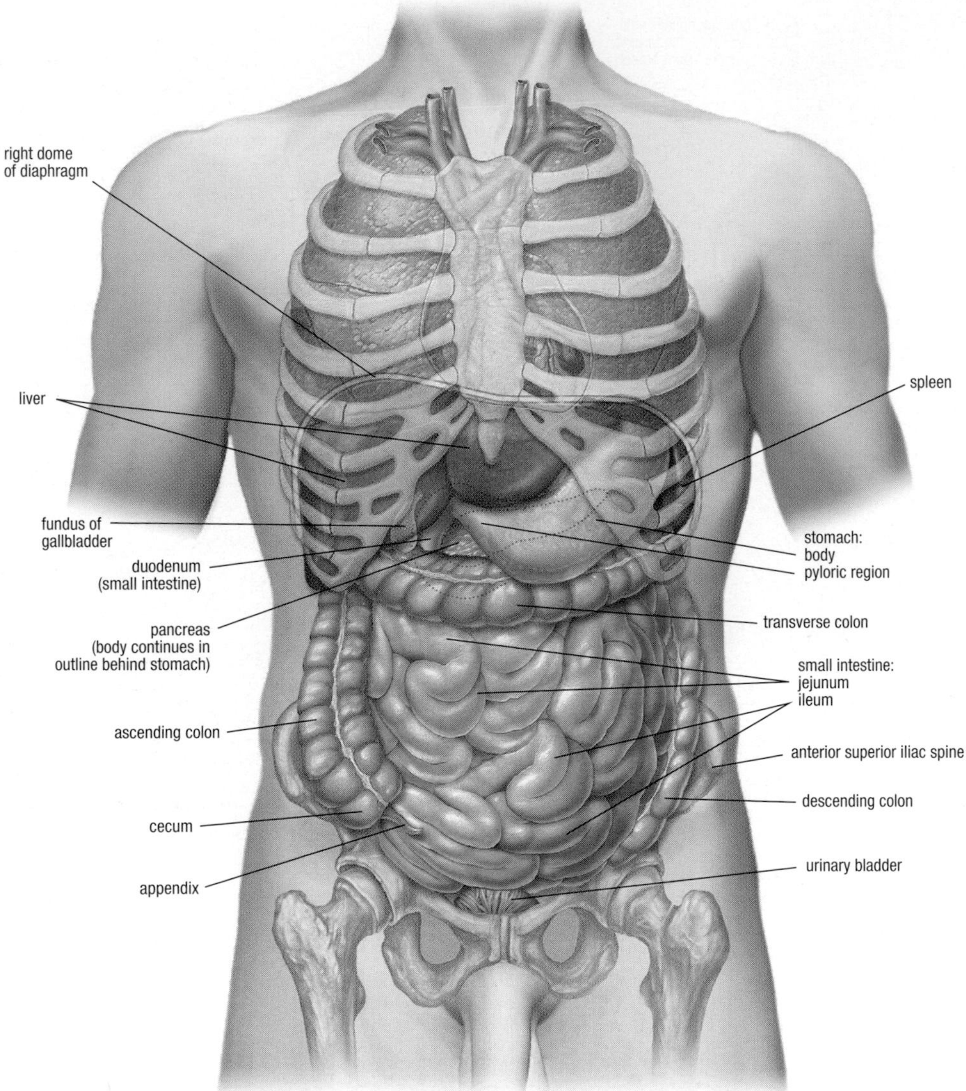

PLATE 12: ABDOMINAL VISCERA, POSTERIOR VIEW

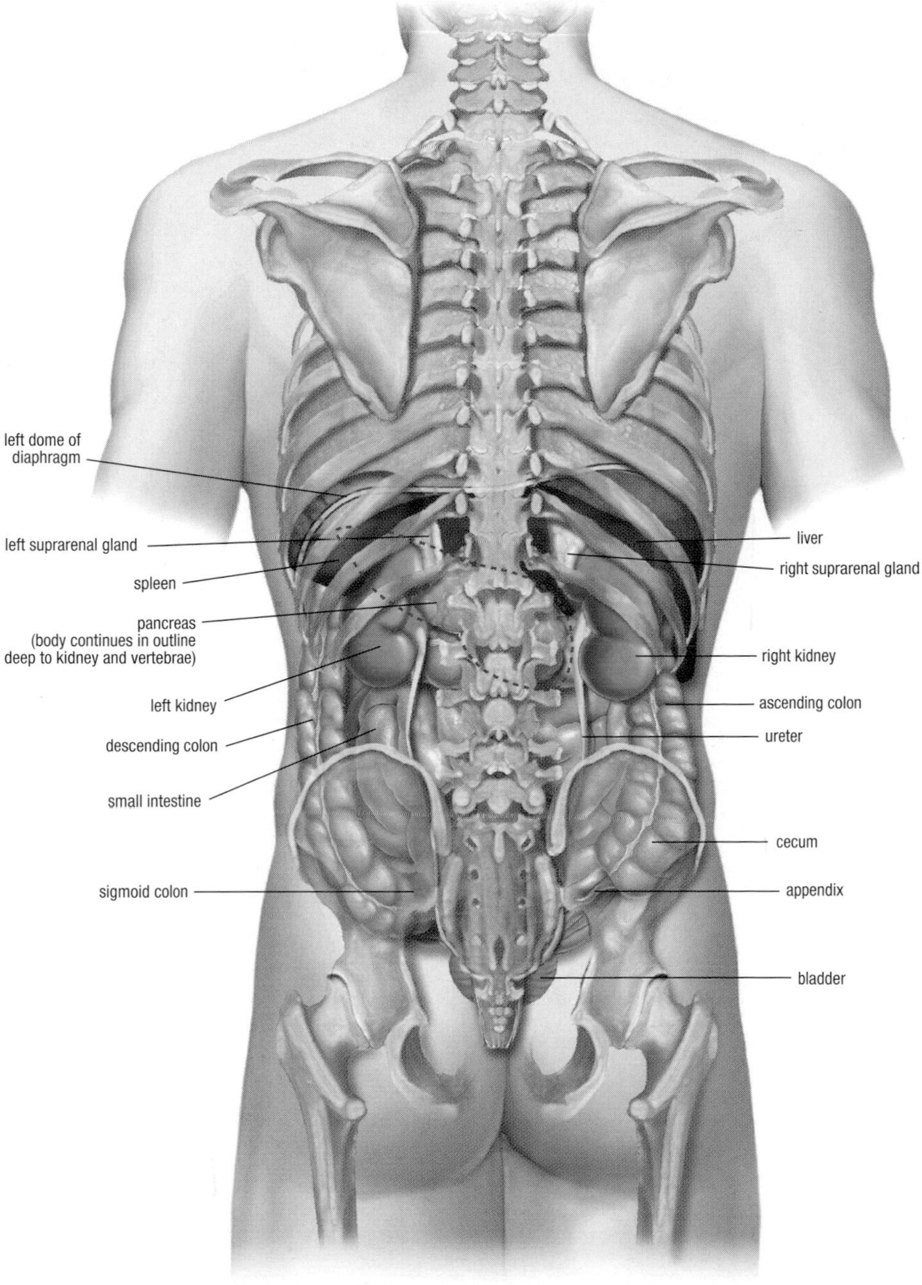

PLATE 13: MALE UROGENITAL SYSTEM, MIDSAGITTAL VIEW

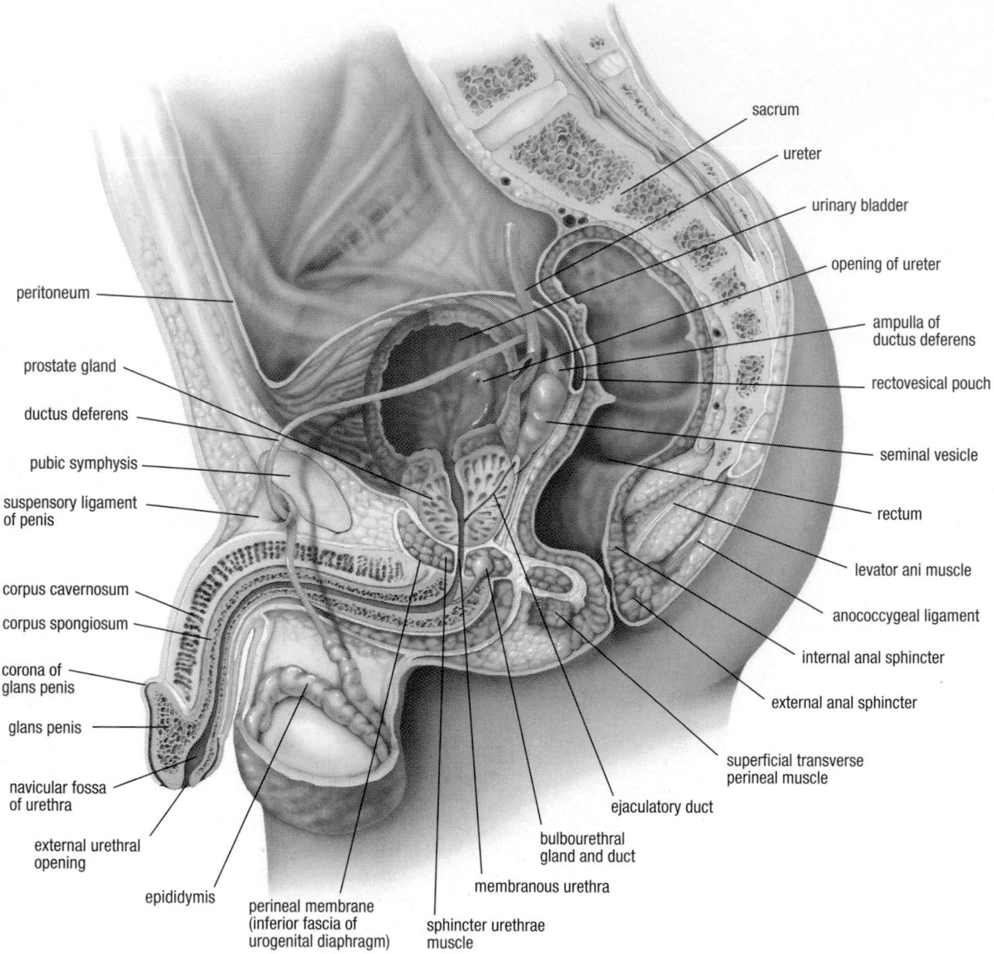

sacrum
ureter
urinary bladder
opening of ureter
peritoneum
ampulla of ductus deferens
prostate gland
rectovesical pouch
ductus deferens
seminal vesicle
pubic symphysis
suspensory ligament of penis
rectum
levator ani muscle
corpus cavernosum
anococcygeal ligament
corpus spongiosum
internal anal sphincter
corona of glans penis
external anal sphincter
glans penis
superficial transverse perineal muscle
navicular fossa of urethra
ejaculatory duct
external urethral opening
bulbourethral gland and duct
membranous urethra
epididymis
perineal membrane (inferior fascia of urogenital diaphragm)
sphincter urethrae muscle

PLATE 14: FEMALE UROGENITAL SYSTEM, MIDSAGITTAL VIEW

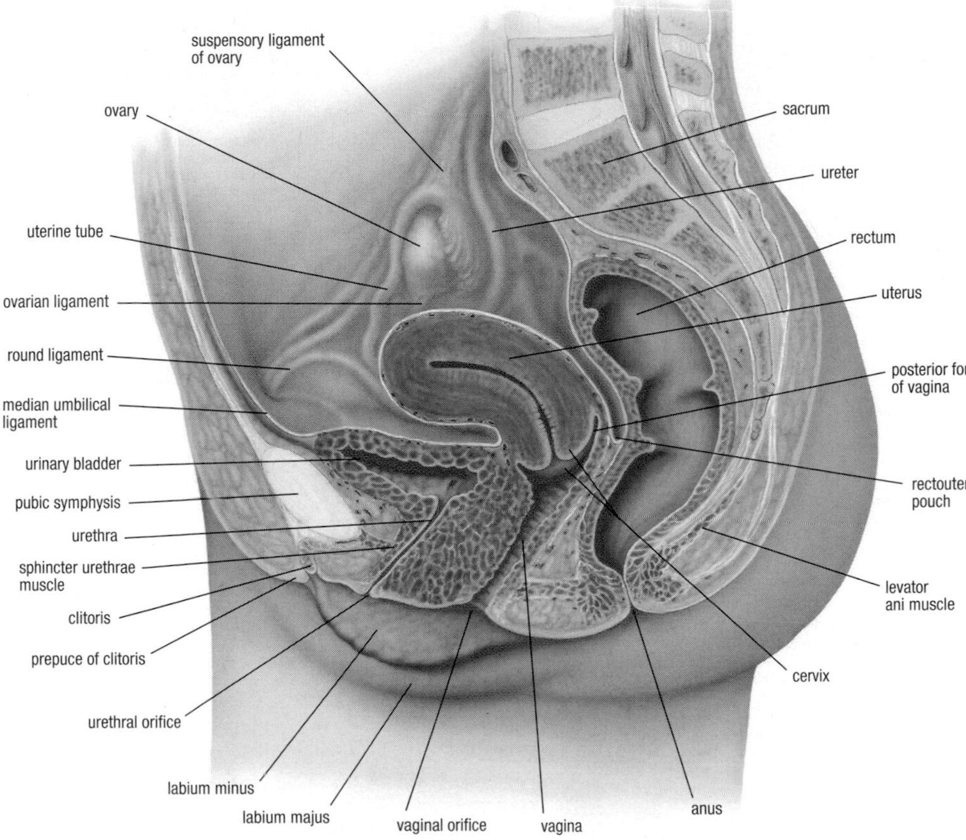

Imagery © Anatomical Chart Company

PLATE 15: NERVOUS SYSTEM OF PELVIS AND LOWER LIMB, ANTERIOR VIEW

Key

Nerves of lower limb

Abdomen
- **1** hepatic plexus
- **2** L1 nerve
- **3** L2 nerve
- **4** iliohypogastric nerve
- **5** ilioinguinal nerve
- **6** sympathetic trunk

Pelvis and perineum
- **7** L5 nerve
- **8** obturator nerve
- **9** lumbosacral trunk
- **10** S1 nerve
- **11** S3 nerve
- **12** sympathetic trunk
- **13** sciatic nerve
- **14** posterior femoral cutaneous nerve
- **15** inferior gluteal nerves
- **16** S5 nerve

Lower limb
- **17** femoral nerve
- **18** muscular branch (femoral nerve)
- **19** femoral artery and vein
- **20** anterior branch (obturator nerve)
- **21** posterior branch (obturator nerve)
- **22** inferior cluneal nerves

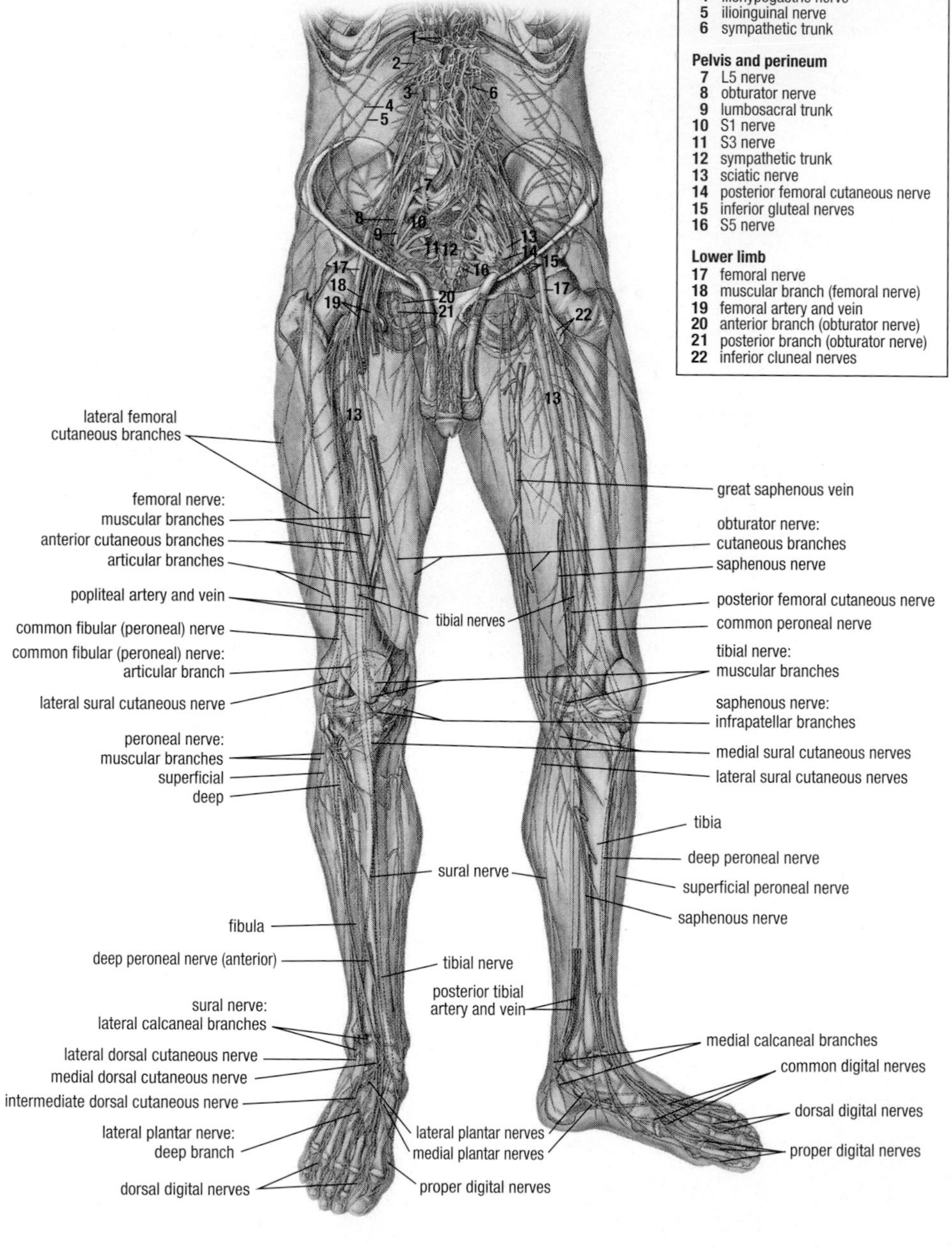

PLATE 16: MUSCULAR AND SKELETAL ANATOMY OF ANKLE AND FOOT, ANTERIOR VIEW

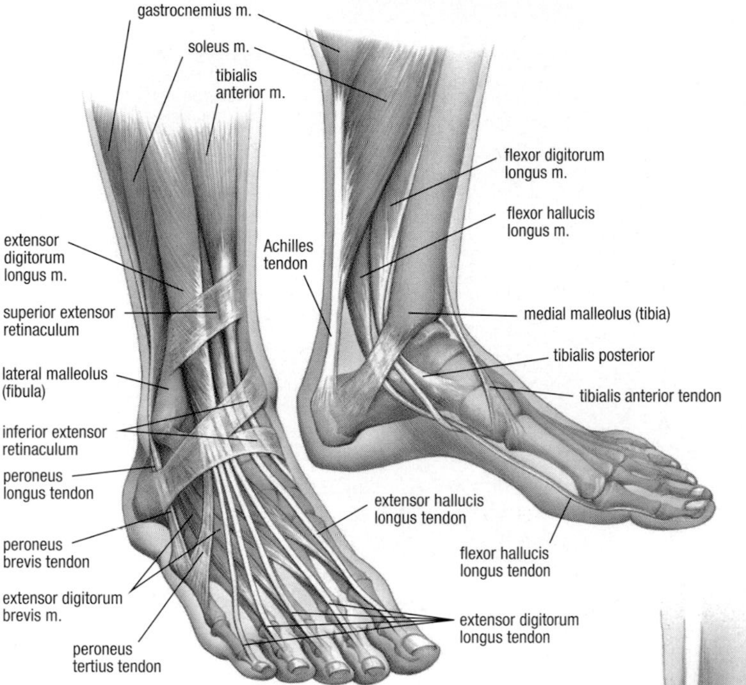
gastrocnemius m.
soleus m.
tibialis anterior m.
flexor digitorum longus m.
flexor hallucis longus m.
extensor digitorum longus m.
Achilles tendon
superior extensor retinaculum
medial malleolus (tibia)
tibialis posterior
lateral malleolus (fibula)
tibialis anterior tendon
inferior extensor retinaculum
peroneus longus tendon
extensor hallucis longus tendon
peroneus brevis tendon
flexor hallucis longus tendon
extensor digitorum brevis m.
extensor digitorum longus tendon
peroneus tertius tendon

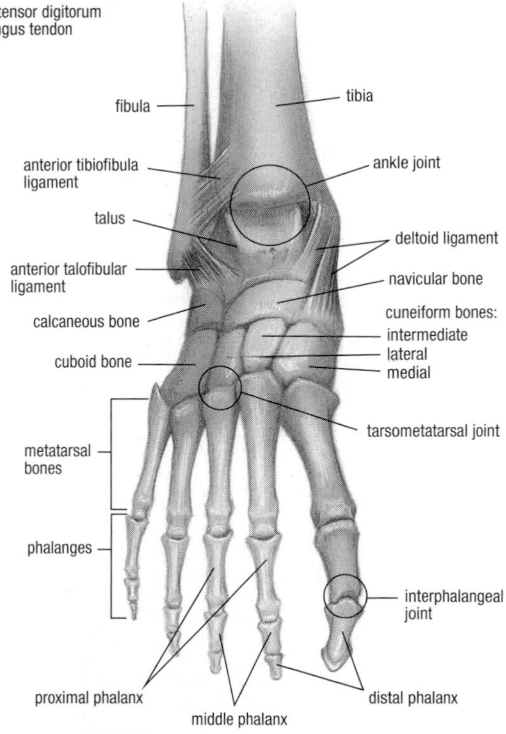
fibula
tibia
anterior tibiofibula ligament
ankle joint
talus
deltoid ligament
anterior talofibular ligament
navicular bone
calcaneous bone
cuneiform bones:
intermediate
lateral
medial
cuboid bone
tarsometatarsal joint
metatarsal bones
phalanges
interphalangeal joint
proximal phalanx
middle phalanx
distal phalanx

PLATE 17: SKELETAL ANATOMY, ANTERIOR VIEW

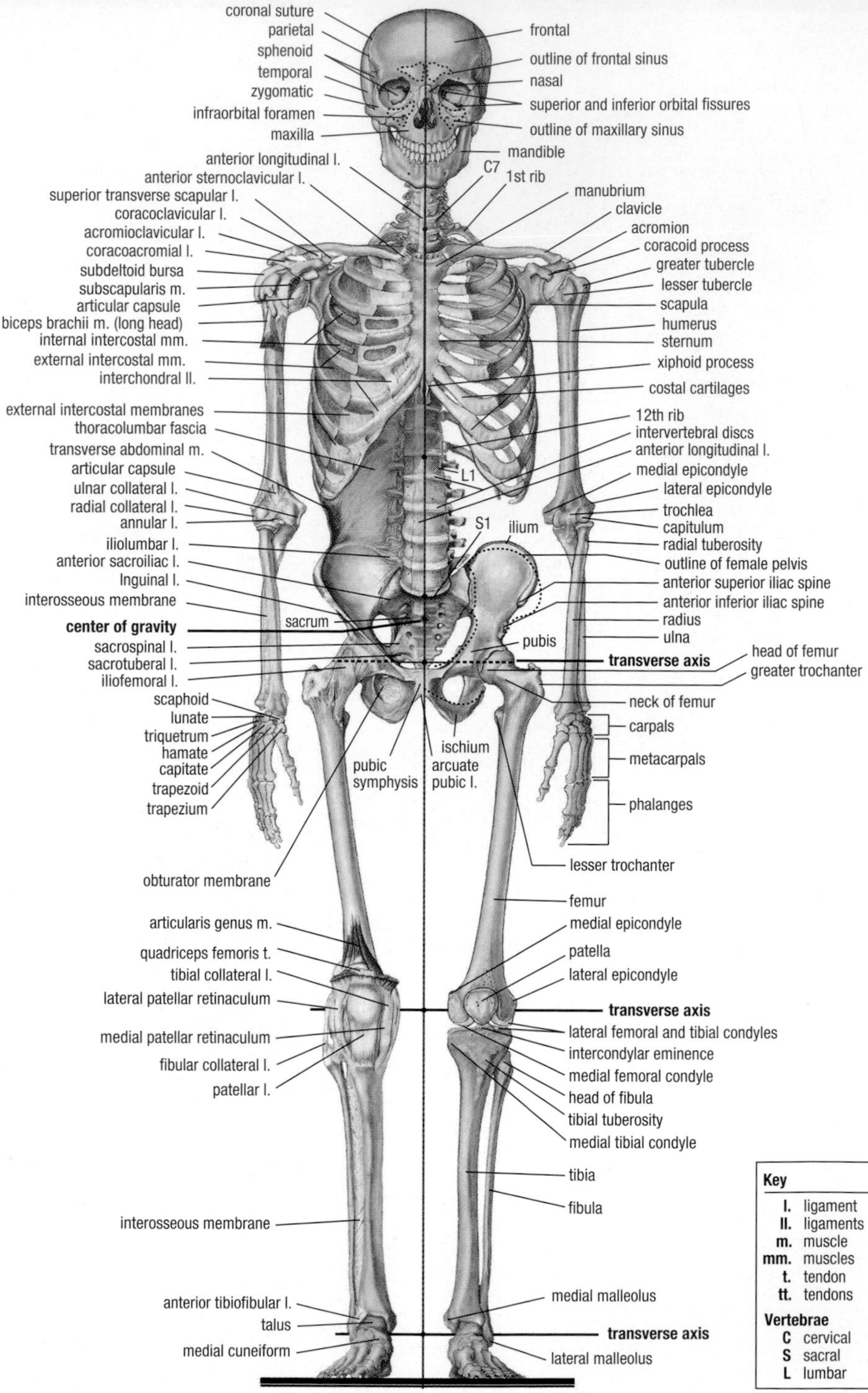

coronal suture
parietal
sphenoid
temporal
zygomatic
infraorbital foramen
maxilla
anterior longitudinal l.
anterior sternoclavicular l.
superior transverse scapular l.
coracoclavicular l.
acromioclavicular l.
coracoacromial l.
subdeltoid bursa
subscapularis m.
articular capsule
biceps brachii m. (long head)
internal intercostal mm.
external intercostal mm.
interchondral ll.
external intercostal membranes
thoracolumbar fascia
transverse abdominal m.
articular capsule
ulnar collateral l.
radial collateral l.
annular l.
iliolumbar l.
anterior sacroiliac l.
Inguinal l.
interosseous membrane
center of gravity
sacrum
sacrospinal l.
sacrotuberal l.
iliofemoral l.
scaphoid
lunate
triquetrum
hamate
capitate
trapezoid
trapezium
pubic symphysis
ischium
arcuate pubic l.
obturator membrane
articularis genus m.
quadriceps femoris t.
tibial collateral l.
lateral patellar retinaculum
medial patellar retinaculum
fibular collateral l.
patellar l.
interosseous membrane
anterior tibiofibular l.
talus
medial cuneiform
frontal
outline of frontal sinus
nasal
superior and inferior orbital fissures
outline of maxillary sinus
mandible
C7
1st rib
manubrium
clavicle
acromion
coracoid process
greater tubercle
lesser tubercle
scapula
humerus
sternum
xiphoid process
costal cartilages
12th rib
intervertebral discs
anterior longitudinal l.
medial epicondyle
L1
lateral epicondyle
trochlea
capitulum
S1
ilium
radial tuberosity
outline of female pelvis
anterior superior iliac spine
anterior inferior iliac spine
radius
ulna
pubis
transverse axis
head of femur
greater trochanter
neck of femur
carpals
metacarpals
phalanges
lesser trochanter
femur
medial epicondyle
patella
lateral epicondyle
transverse axis
lateral femoral and tibial condyles
intercondylar eminence
medial femoral condyle
head of fibula
tibial tuberosity
medial tibial condyle
tibia
fibula
medial malleolus
transverse axis
lateral malleolus

Key

l.	ligament
ll.	ligaments
m.	muscle
mm.	muscles
t.	tendon
tt.	tendons

Vertebrae

C	cervical
S	sacral
L	lumbar

PLATE 18: SKELETAL ANATOMY, POSTERIOR VIEW

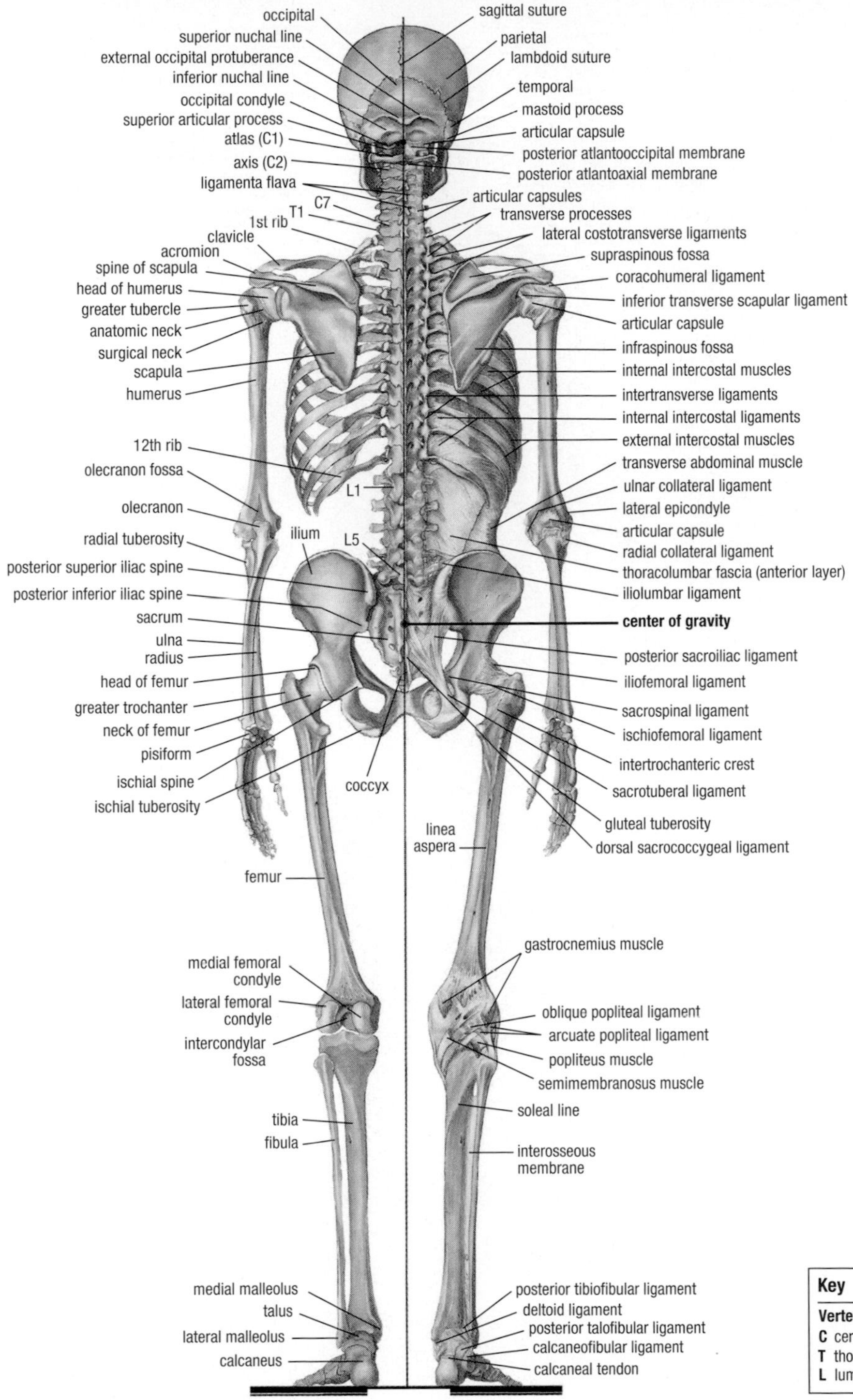

occipital
superior nuchal line
external occipital protuberance
inferior nuchal line
occipital condyle
superior articular process
atlas (C1)
axis (C2)
ligamenta flava
C7
T1
1st rib
clavicle
acromion
spine of scapula
head of humerus
greater tubercle
anatomic neck
surgical neck
scapula
humerus
12th rib
olecranon fossa
olecranon
radial tuberosity
posterior superior iliac spine
posterior inferior iliac spine
sacrum
ulna
radius
head of femur
greater trochanter
neck of femur
pisiform
ischial spine
ischial tuberosity
L1
ilium
L5
coccyx
femur
linea aspera
medial femoral condyle
lateral femoral condyle
intercondylar fossa
tibia
fibula
medial malleolus
talus
lateral malleolus
calcaneus
sagittal suture
parietal
lambdoid suture
temporal
mastoid process
articular capsule
posterior atlantooccipital membrane
posterior atlantoaxial membrane
articular capsules
transverse processes
lateral costotransverse ligaments
supraspinous fossa
coracohumeral ligament
inferior transverse scapular ligament
articular capsule
infraspinous fossa
internal intercostal muscles
intertransverse ligaments
internal intercostal ligaments
external intercostal muscles
transverse abdominal muscle
ulnar collateral ligament
lateral epicondyle
articular capsule
radial collateral ligament
thoracolumbar fascia (anterior layer)
iliolumbar ligament
center of gravity
posterior sacroiliac ligament
iliofemoral ligament
sacrospinal ligament
ischiofemoral ligament
intertrochanteric crest
sacrotuberal ligament
gluteal tuberosity
dorsal sacrococcygeal ligament
gastrocnemius muscle
oblique popliteal ligament
arcuate popliteal ligament
popliteus muscle
semimembranosus muscle
soleal line
interosseous membrane
posterior tibiofibular ligament
deltoid ligament
posterior talofibular ligament
calcaneofibular ligament
calcaneal tendon

Key

Vertebrae
C cervical
T thoracic
L lumbar

PLATE 19: MUSCULAR SYSTEM, ANTERIOR VIEW

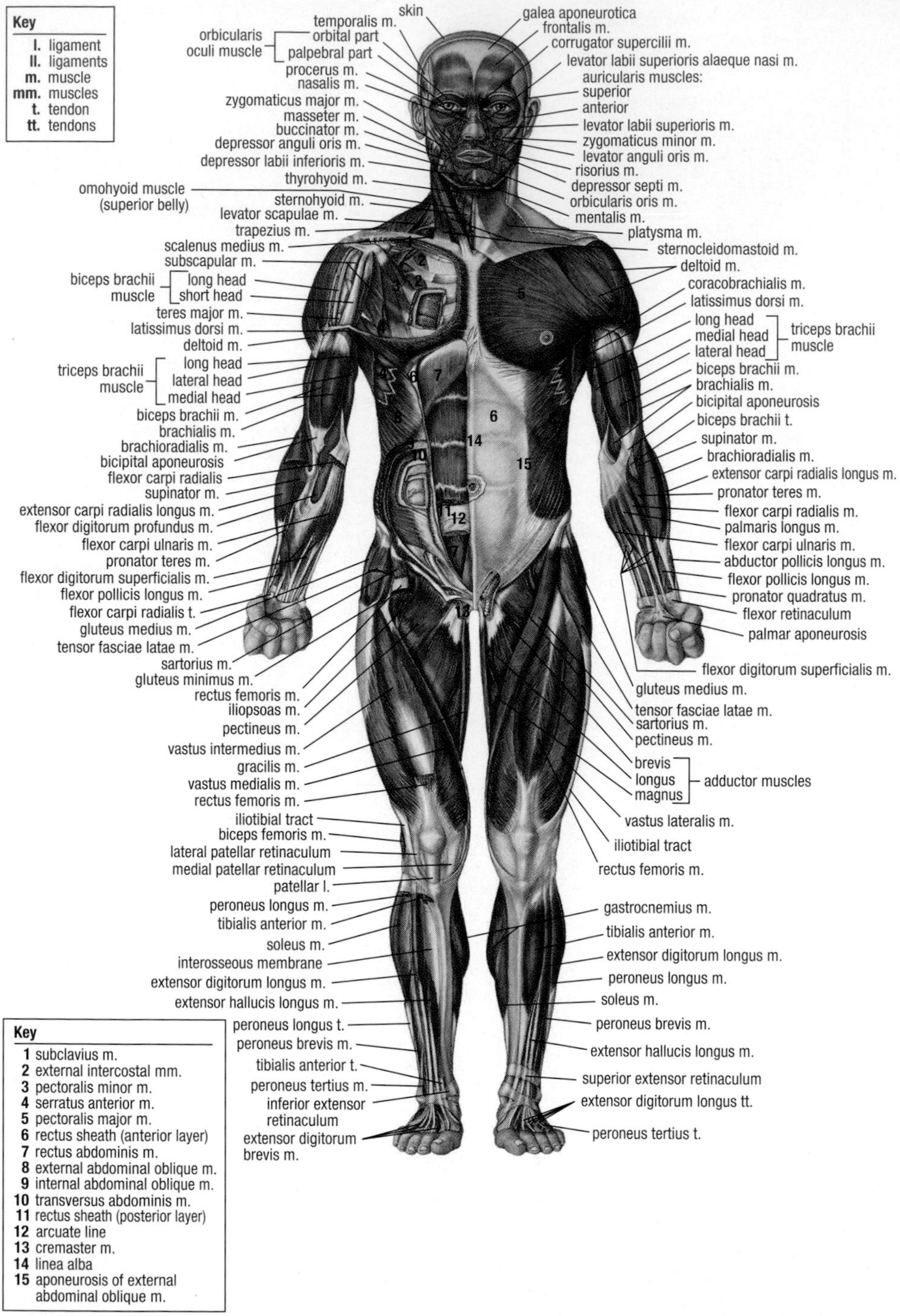
Key
I. ligament
II. ligaments
m. muscle
mm. muscles
t. tendon
tt. tendons
skin
temporalis m.
orbicularis oculi muscle
orbital part
palpebral part
procerus m.
nasalis m.
zygomaticus major m.
masseter m.
buccinator m.
depressor anguli oris m.
depressor labii inferioris m.
thyrohyoid m.
omohyoid muscle (superior belly)
sternohyoid m.
levator scapulae m.
trapezius m.
scalenus medius m.
subscapular m.
biceps brachii muscle
long head
short head
teres major m.
latissimus dorsi m.
deltoid m.
triceps brachii muscle
long head
lateral head
medial head
biceps brachii m.
brachialis m.
brachioradialis m.
bicipital aponeurosis
flexor carpi radialis
supinator m.
extensor carpi radialis longus m.
flexor digitorum profundus m.
flexor carpi ulnaris m.
pronator teres m.
flexor digitorum superficialis m.
flexor pollicis longus m.
flexor carpi radialis t.
gluteus medius m.
tensor fasciae latae m.
sartorius m.
gluteus minimus m.
rectus femoris m.
iliopsoas m.
pectineus m.
vastus intermedius m.
gracilis m.
vastus medialis m.
rectus femoris m.
iliotibial tract
biceps femoris m.
lateral patellar retinaculum
medial patellar retinaculum
patellar l.
peroneus longus m.
tibialis anterior m.
soleus m.
interosseous membrane
extensor digitorum longus m.
extensor hallucis longus m.
peroneus longus t.
peroneus brevis m.
tibialis anterior t.
peroneus tertius m.
inferior extensor retinaculum
extensor digitorum brevis m.
galea aponeurotica
frontalis m.
corrugator supercilii m.
levator labii superioris alaeque nasi m.
auricularis muscles:
superior
anterior
levator labii superioris m.
zygomaticus minor m.
levator anguli oris m.
risorius m.
depressor septi m.
orbicularis oris m.
mentalis m.
platysma m.
sternocleidomastoid m.
deltoid m.
coracobrachialis m.
latissimus dorsi m.
long head
medial head
lateral head
triceps brachii muscle
biceps brachii m.
brachialis m.
bicipital aponeurosis
biceps brachii t.
supinator m.
brachioradialis m.
extensor carpi radialis longus m.
pronator teres m.
flexor carpi radialis m.
palmaris longus m.
flexor carpi ulnaris m.
abductor pollicis longus m.
flexor pollicis longus m.
pronator quadratus m.
flexor retinaculum
palmar aponeurosis
flexor digitorum superficialis m.
gluteus medius m.
tensor fasciae latae m.
sartorius m.
pectineus m.
brevis
longus
magnus
adductor muscles
vastus lateralis m.
iliotibial tract
rectus femoris m.
gastrocnemius m.
tibialis anterior m.
extensor digitorum longus m.
peroneus longus m.
soleus m.
peroneus brevis m.
extensor hallucis longus m.
superior extensor retinaculum
extensor digitorum longus tt.
peroneus tertius t.
Key
1 subclavius m.
2 external intercostal mm.
3 pectoralis minor m.
4 serratus anterior m.
5 pectoralis major m.
6 rectus sheath (anterior layer)
7 rectus abdominis m.
8 external abdominal oblique m.
9 internal abdominal oblique m.
10 transversus abdominis m.
11 rectus sheath (posterior layer)
12 arcuate line
13 cremaster m.
14 linea alba
15 aponeurosis of external abdominal oblique m.

PLATE 20: MUSCULAR SYSTEM, POSTERIOR VIEW

Key

l. ligament
ll. ligaments
m. muscle
mm. muscles
t. tendon
tt. tendons

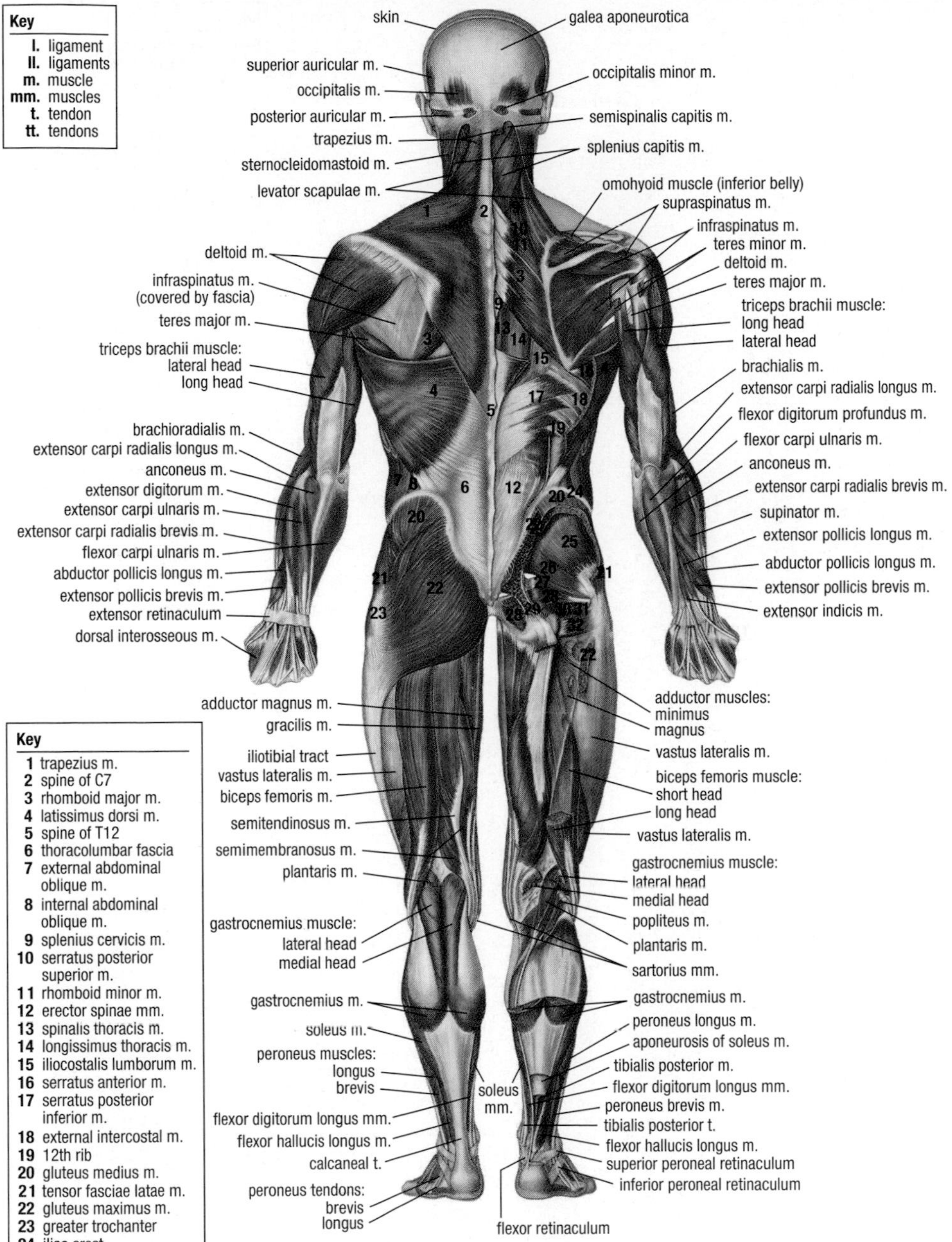

Key

1 trapezius m.
2 spine of C7
3 rhomboid major m.
4 latissimus dorsi m.
5 spine of T12
6 thoracolumbar fascia
7 external abdominal oblique m.
8 internal abdominal oblique m.
9 splenius cervicis m.
10 serratus posterior superior m.
11 rhomboid minor m.
12 erector spinae mm.
13 spinalis thoracis m.
14 longissimus thoracis m.
15 iliocostalis lumborum m.
16 serratus anterior m.
17 serratus posterior inferior m.
18 external intercostal m.
19 12th rib
20 gluteus medius m.
21 tensor fasciae latae m.
22 gluteus maximus m.
23 greater trochanter
24 iliac crest
25 gluteus minimus m.
26 piriformis m.
27 superior gemellus m.
28 obturator internus m.
29 sacrotuberal l.
30 inferior gemellus m.
31 obturator externus m.
32 quadratus femoris m.

PLATE 21: SPINAL AND CRANIAL NERVES

Key

Peripheral nerve origins

C5, C6	axillary nerve
L4, L5, S1, S2	common fibular (peroneal) nerve
L2, L3, L4	femoral nerve
L1, L2	genitofemoral nerve
L1	iliohypogastric nerve
L1	ilioinguinal nerve
L5, S1, L2	inferior gluteal nerve
C5, C6, C7	lateral cord
L2, L3	lateral femoral cutaneous nerve
C5, C6, C7	long thoracic nerve
C8, T1	medial cord
C6, C7, C8, T1	median nerve
C5, C6, C7	musculocutaneous nerve
L2, L3, L4	obturator nerve
C5, C6, C7, C8, T1	posterior cord
S1, S2, S3	posterior femoral cutaneous nerve
S2, S3, S4	pudendal nerve
C5, C6, C7, C8	radial nerve
L4, L5, S1, S2, S3	sciatic nerve
C6, C7, C8	superficial branch of radial nerve
L4, L5, S1	superior gluteal nerve
L4, L5, S1, S2, S3	tibial nerve
C8, T1	ulnar nerve

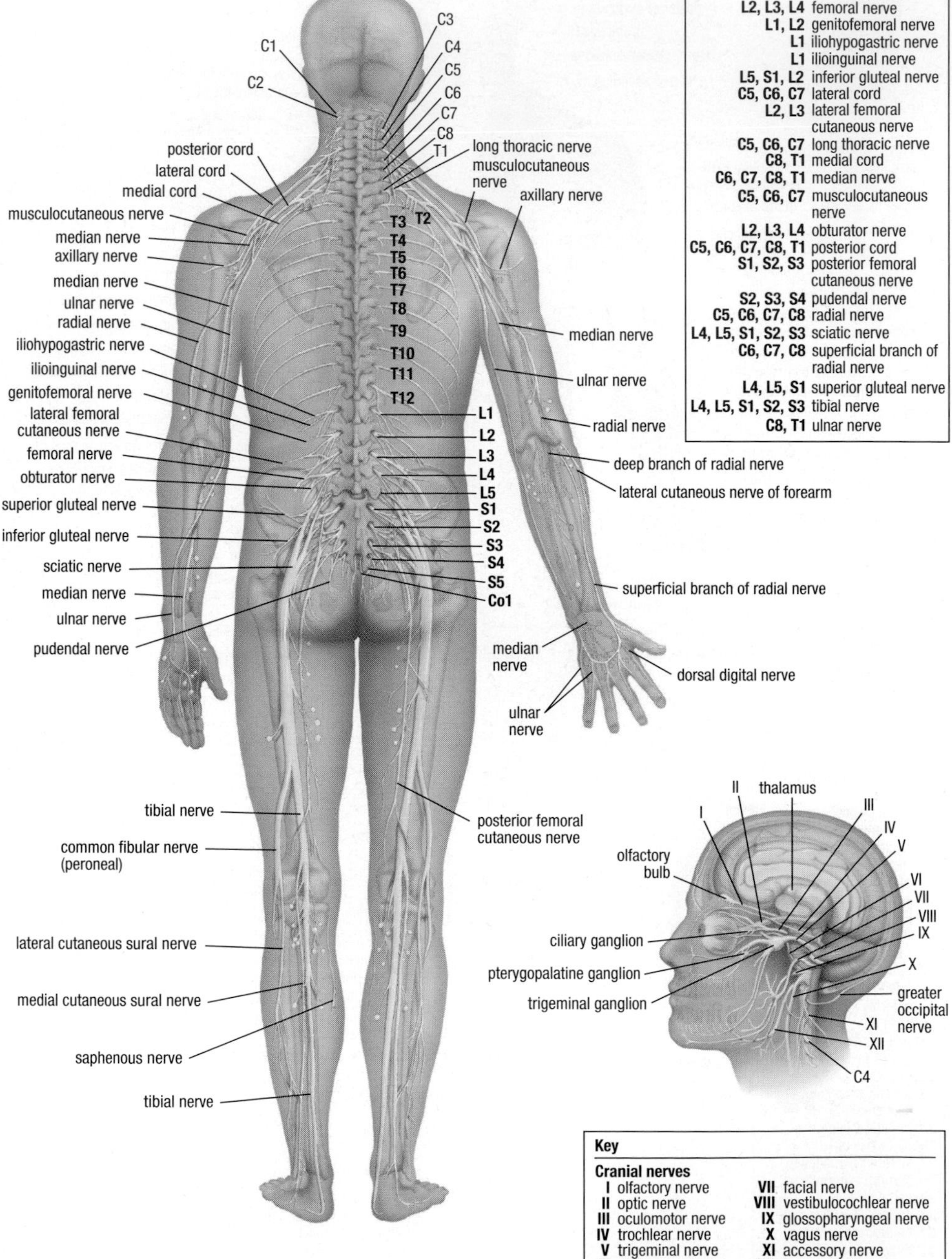

Key

Cranial nerves

I	olfactory nerve	**VII**	facial nerve
II	optic nerve	**VIII**	vestibulocochlear nerve
III	oculomotor nerve	**IX**	glossopharyngeal nerve
IV	trochlear nerve	**X**	vagus nerve
V	trigeminal nerve	**XI**	accessory nerve
VI	abducens nerve	**XII**	hypoglossal nerve

PLATE 22: ARTERIAL SYSTEM, ANTERIOR VIEW

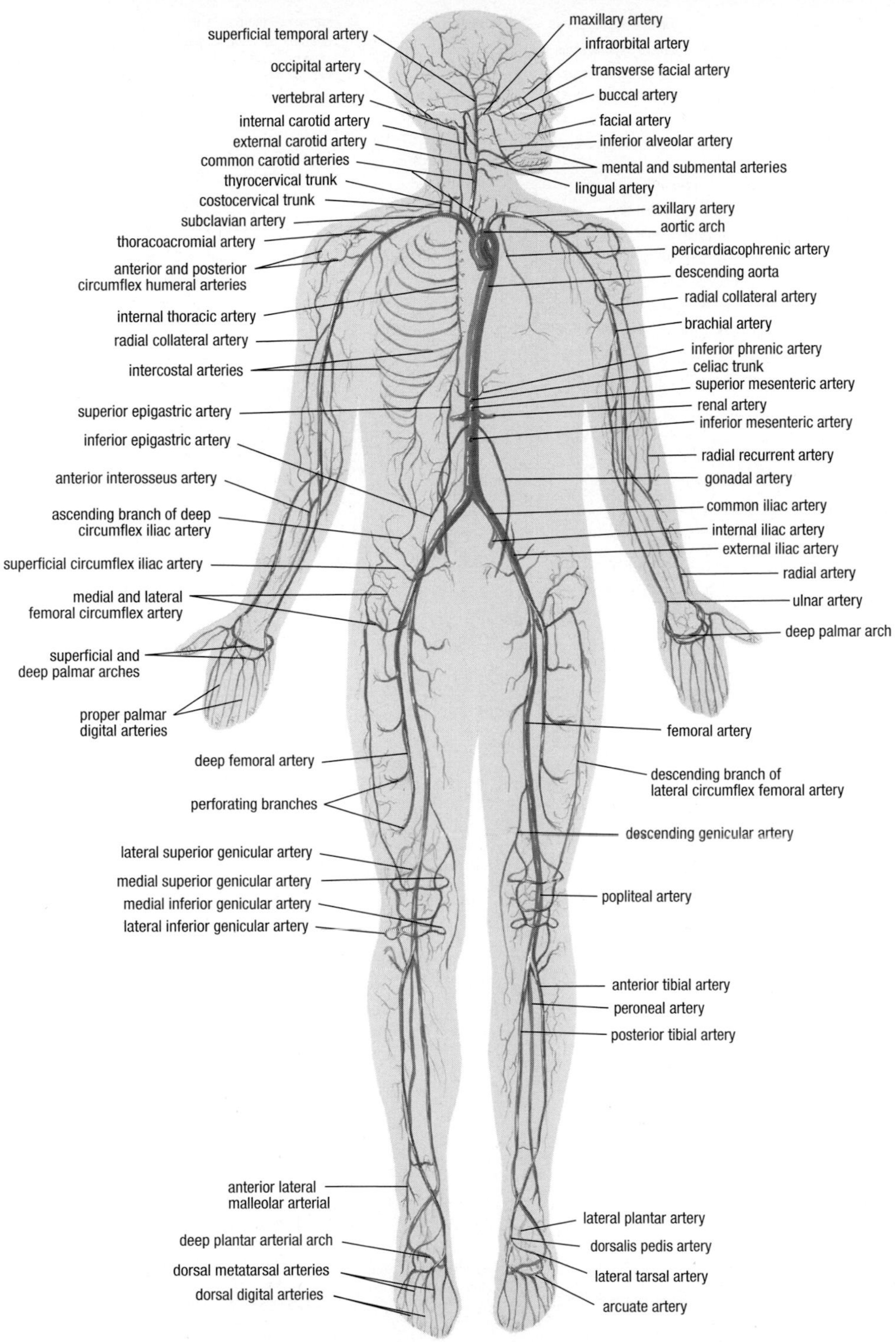

superficial temporal artery
occipital artery
vertebral artery
internal carotid artery
external carotid artery
common carotid arteries
thyrocervical trunk
costocervical trunk
subclavian artery
thoracoacromial artery
anterior and posterior circumflex humeral arteries
internal thoracic artery
radial collateral artery
intercostal arteries
superior epigastric artery
inferior epigastric artery
anterior interosseus artery
ascending branch of deep circumflex iliac artery
superficial circumflex iliac artery
medial and lateral femoral circumflex artery
superficial and deep palmar arches
proper palmar digital arteries
deep femoral artery
perforating branches
lateral superior genicular artery
medial superior genicular artery
medial inferior genicular artery
lateral inferior genicular artery
anterior lateral malleolar arterial
deep plantar arterial arch
dorsal metatarsal arteries
dorsal digital arteries
maxillary artery
infraorbital artery
transverse facial artery
buccal artery
facial artery
inferior alveolar artery
mental and submental arteries
lingual artery
axillary artery
aortic arch
pericardiacophrenic artery
descending aorta
radial collateral artery
brachial artery
inferior phrenic artery
celiac trunk
superior mesenteric artery
renal artery
inferior mesenteric artery
radial recurrent artery
gonadal artery
common iliac artery
internal iliac artery
external iliac artery
radial artery
ulnar artery
deep palmar arch
femoral artery
descending branch of lateral circumflex femoral artery
descending genicular artery
popliteal artery
anterior tibial artery
peroneal artery
posterior tibial artery
lateral plantar artery
dorsalis pedis artery
lateral tarsal artery
arcuate artery

PLATE 23: VENOUS SYSTEM, ANTERIOR VIEW

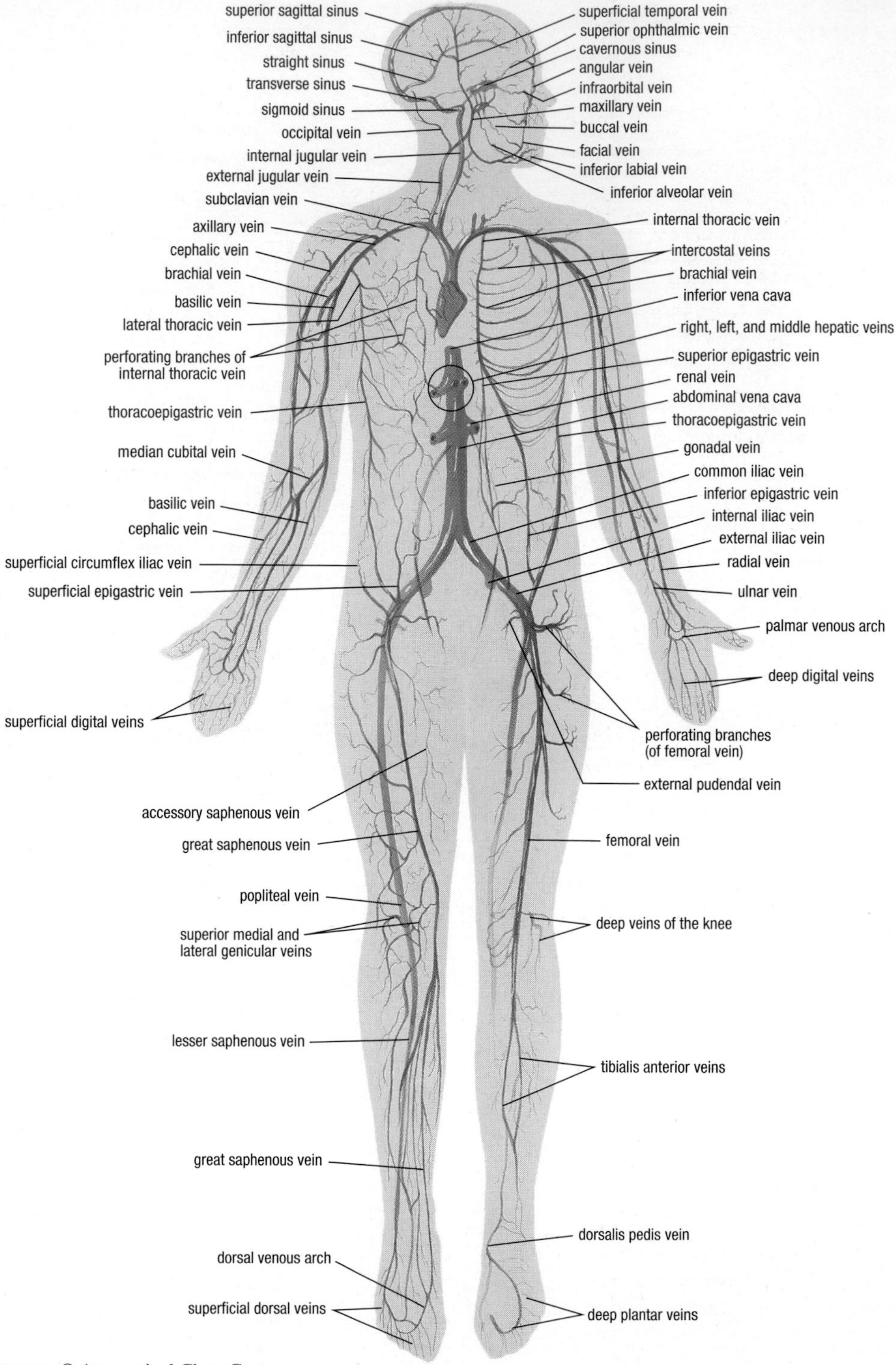

superior sagittal sinus
inferior sagittal sinus
straight sinus
transverse sinus
sigmoid sinus
occipital vein
internal jugular vein
external jugular vein
subclavian vein
axillary vein
cephalic vein
brachial vein
basilic vein
lateral thoracic vein
perforating branches of internal thoracic vein
thoracoepigastric vein
median cubital vein
basilic vein
cephalic vein
superficial circumflex iliac vein
superficial epigastric vein
superficial digital veins
accessory saphenous vein
great saphenous vein
popliteal vein
superior medial and lateral genicular veins
lesser saphenous vein
great saphenous vein
dorsal venous arch
superficial dorsal veins
superficial temporal vein
superior ophthalmic vein
cavernous sinus
angular vein
infraorbital vein
maxillary vein
buccal vein
facial vein
inferior labial vein
inferior alveolar vein
internal thoracic vein
intercostal veins
brachial vein
inferior vena cava
right, left, and middle hepatic veins
superior epigastric vein
renal vein
abdominal vena cava
thoracoepigastric vein
gonadal vein
common iliac vein
inferior epigastric vein
internal iliac vein
external iliac vein
radial vein
ulnar vein
palmar venous arch
deep digital veins
perforating branches (of femoral vein)
external pudendal vein
femoral vein
deep veins of the knee
tibialis anterior veins
dorsalis pedis vein
deep plantar veins

PLATE 24: LYMPHATIC SYSTEM, ANTERIOR VIEW

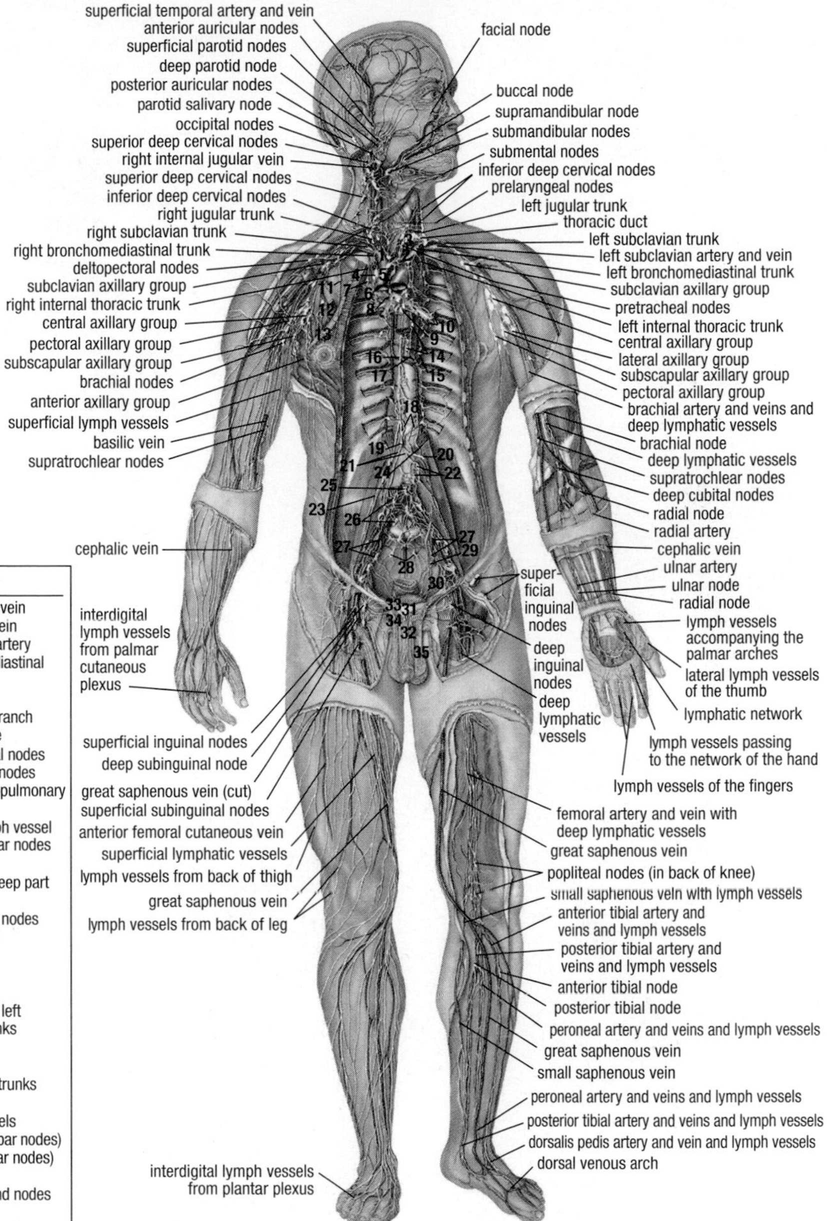

Key

1 right brachiocephalic vein
2 left brachiocephalic vein
3 left common carotid artery
4 anterior superior mediastinal nodes
5 superior vena cava
6 right cardiac lymph branch
7 internal thoracic node
8 right tracheobronchial nodes
9 left tracheobronchial nodes
10 right and left bronchopulmonary nodes
11 internal thoracic lymph vessel ending in subclavicular nodes
12 interpectoral nodes
13 lymph vessels from deep part of breast
14 posterior mediastinal nodes
15 intercostal nodes and lymph vessels
16 thoracic duct
17 thoracic aorta
18 descending right and left intercostal lymph trunks
19 cisterna chyli
20 intestinal trunk
21 right and left lumbar trunks
22 lumbar nodes
23 testicular lymph vessels
24 retroaortic node (lumbar nodes)
25 preaortic node (lumbar nodes)
26 common iliac nodes
27 internal iliac artery and nodes
28 sacral nodes
29 lymph vessels to internal iliac nodes
30 obturator vessels and nerve
31 presymphysial node
32 collecting lymph vessels from glans penis
33 superficial lymph vessels from the penis
34 lymph vessels from the scrotum
35 lymph vessels of testis and epididymus

PLATE 25: RESPIRATORY SYSTEM, ANTERIOR VIEW

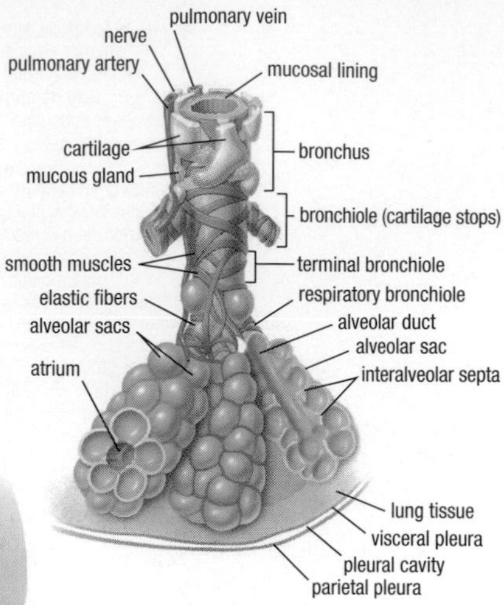

pulmonary vein
nerve
pulmonary artery
mucosal lining
cartilage
mucous gland
bronchus
bronchiole (cartilage stops)
smooth muscles
terminal bronchiole
elastic fibers
respiratory bronchiole
alveolar sacs
alveolar duct
alveolar sac
atrium
interalveolar septa
lung tissue
visceral pleura
pleural cavity
parietal pleura

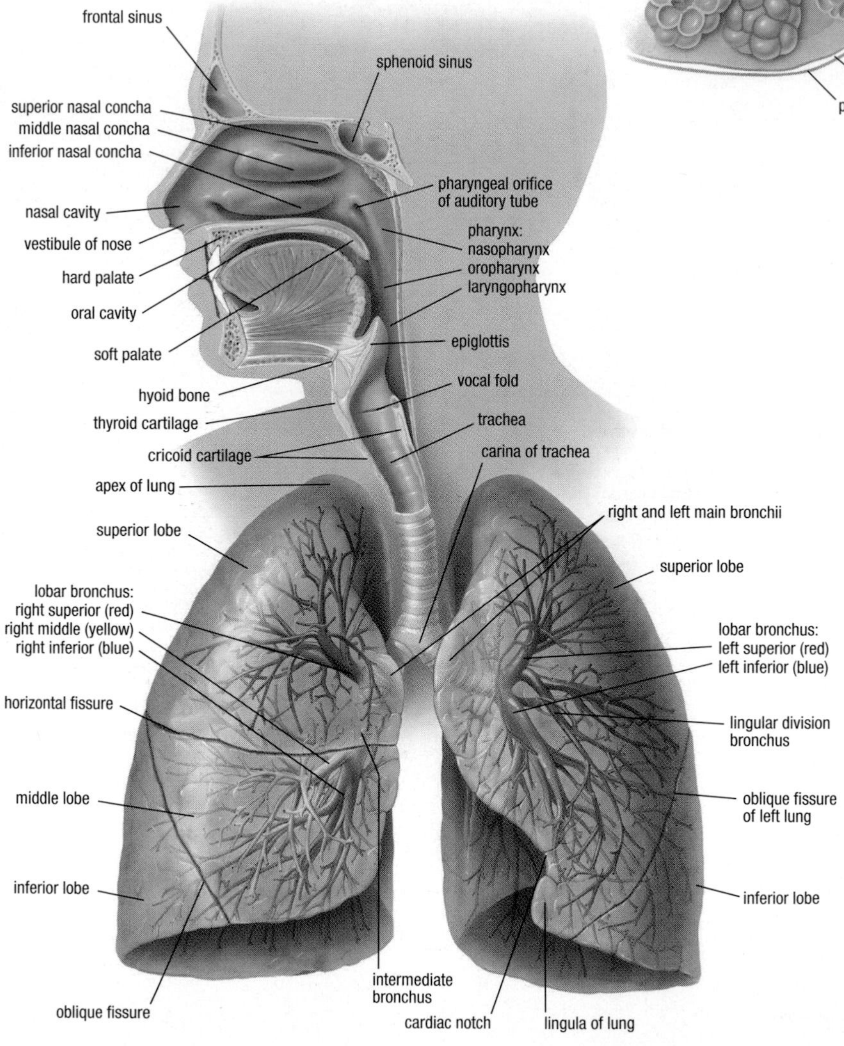

frontal sinus
sphenoid sinus
superior nasal concha
middle nasal concha
inferior nasal concha
pharyngeal orifice of auditory tube
nasal cavity
vestibule of nose
pharynx:
nasopharynx
oropharynx
laryngopharynx
hard palate
oral cavity
epiglottis
soft palate
hyoid bone
vocal fold
thyroid cartilage
trachea
cricoid cartilage
carina of trachea
apex of lung
right and left main bronchii
superior lobe
superior lobe
lobar bronchus:
right superior (red)
right middle (yellow)
right inferior (blue)
lobar bronchus:
left superior (red)
left inferior (blue)
horizontal fissure
lingular division bronchus
middle lobe
oblique fissure of left lung
inferior lobe
inferior lobe
intermediate bronchus
oblique fissure
cardiac notch
lingula of lung

PLATE 26: DIGESTIVE SYSTEM, ANTERIOR VIEW

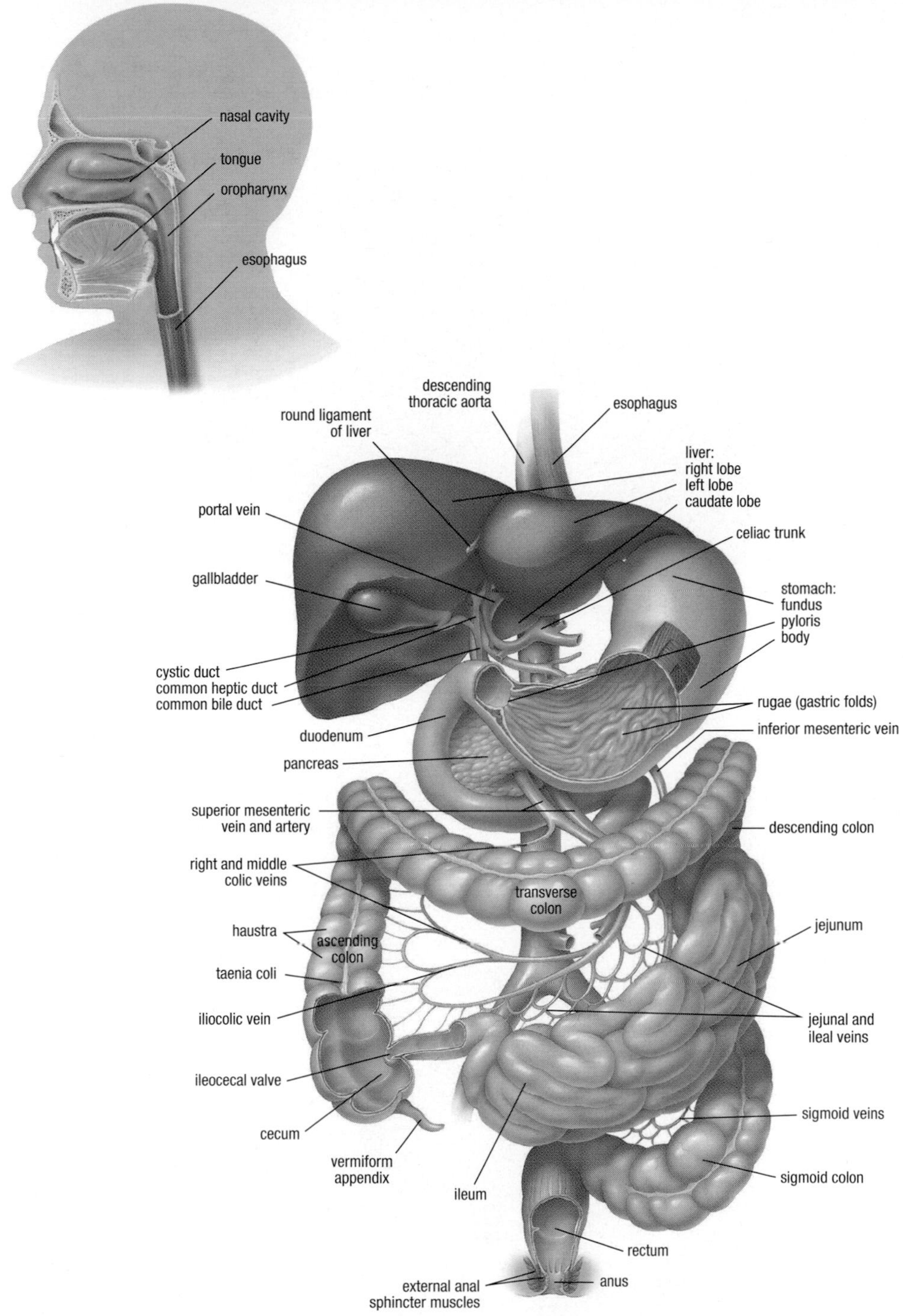

PLATE 27: URINARY SYSTEM, ANTERIOR VIEW

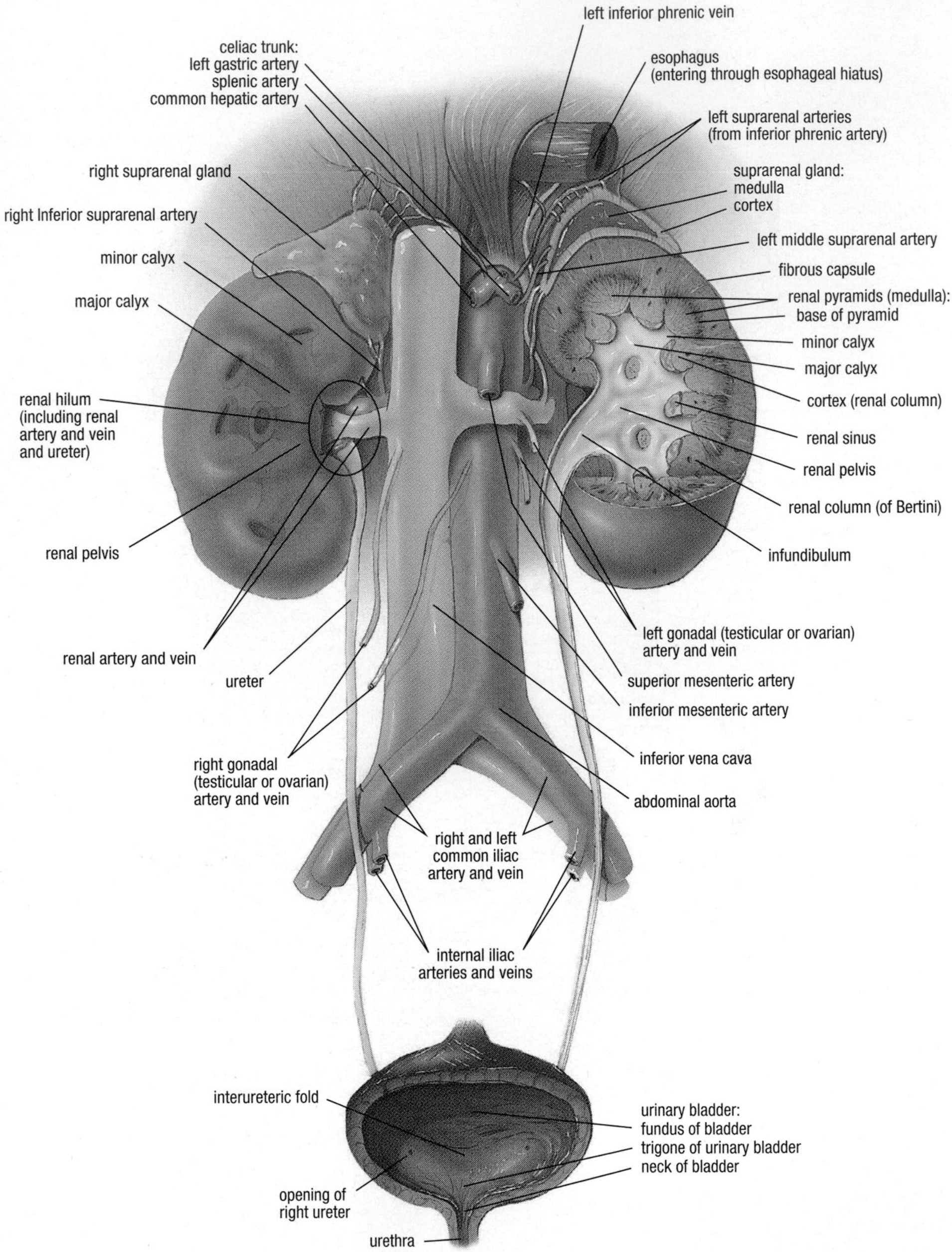

left inferior phrenic vein
celiac trunk:
left gastric artery
splenic artery
common hepatic artery
esophagus
(entering through esophageal hiatus)
left suprarenal arteries
(from inferior phrenic artery)
right suprarenal gland
suprarenal gland:
medulla
cortex
right Inferior suprarenal artery
left middle suprarenal artery
minor calyx
fibrous capsule
major calyx
renal pyramids (medulla):
base of pyramid
minor calyx
major calyx
renal hilum
(including renal
artery and vein
and ureter)
cortex (renal column)
renal sinus
renal pelvis
renal column (of Bertini)
renal pelvis
infundibulum
left gonadal (testicular or ovarian)
artery and vein
renal artery and vein
ureter
superior mesenteric artery
inferior mesenteric artery
right gonadal
(testicular or ovarian)
artery and vein
inferior vena cava
abdominal aorta
right and left
common iliac
artery and vein
internal iliac
arteries and veins
interureteric fold
urinary bladder:
fundus of bladder
trigone of urinary bladder
neck of bladder
opening of
right ureter
urethra

on morphologic characteristics and cytochemical stain reactions. The acute myeloid leukemias are subdivided into eight FAB groups: M0, M1, M2, M3, M4, M5, M6, and M7. The acute lymphoid leukemias are subdivided into three groups: L1, L2, and L3. The myelodysplastic syndromes have also been subdivided by the FAB group into five subgroups: RA, RARS, RAEB, RAEB-T, and CMML. SEE ALSO myelodysplastic syndrome.

French scale (Fr) (french skāl) Assessment tool for grading sizes of sounds, tubules, and catheters as based on a measurement of 1/3 mm and equaling 1 Fr on the scale (e.g., 3 Fr = 1 mm).

fre•nec•to•my (frē-nek′tŏ-mē) Removal of any frenum. [frenum + G. *ektomē,* excision]

fre•net•ic (frĕ-net′ik) **1.** Frenzied; maniacal. **2.** A person exhibiting such behavior. [G. *phrenitikos,* frenzied]

fre•not•o•my (frē-not′ŏ-mē) Division of any frenum or frenulum, especially that of the tongue. [frenum + G. *tomē,* a cutting]

fren•u•lo•plas•ty (fren′yū-lō-plas-tē) Correction of an abnormally attached frenum by surgically repositioning it. [frenum + G. *plastos,* formed]

fren•u•lum, pl. **fren•u•la** (fren′yū-lŭm, -lă) A small frenum or bridle. SYN habenula (1) [TA], frenum (3). [Mod. L. dim. of L. *frenum,* bridle]

fren•u•lum at•tach•ment (fren′yū-lŭm ă-tach′mĕnt) SEE ankyloglossia.

fren•u•lum cli•to•ri•dis (fren′yū-lūm kli-tōr′i-dis) [TA] SYN frenulum of clitoris.

fren•u•lum of clit•o•ris (fren′yū-lŭm klit′ŏr-is) The line of union of the labia minora on the undersurface of the glans clitoridis. SYN frenulum clitoridis [TA].

fren•u•lum of il•e•al or•i•fice (fren′yū-lŭm il′ē-ăl ōr′i-fis) A fold, more evident in cadavers, running from the junction of the two commissures of the ileocecal valve on either side along the inner wall of the cecocolic junction. SYN Morgagni retinaculum.

fren•u•lum of the la•bi•a mi•no•ra (fren′yū-lŭm lā′bē-ă mi-nō′ră) The fold connecting the two labia minora posteriorly. SYN frenulum labiorum pudendi [TA].

fren•u•lum la•bi•i in•fe•ri•or•is (fren′yū-lŭm lā′bē-ī in-fēr′ē-ō′ris) [TA] SYN frenulum of lower lip.

fren•u•lum la•bi•o•rum pu•den•di (fren′yū-lŭm lā-bē-ō′rŭm pū-den′dī) [TA] SYN frenulum of the labia minora.

fren•u•lum of low•er lip (fren′yū-lŭm lō′ĕr lip) The folds of mucous membrane extending from the gingiva to the midline of the lower (frenulum of the lower lip) and upper lips (frenulum of the upper lips), respectively. SYN frenulum labii inferioris [TA].

fren•u•lum of pre•puce (fren′yū-lŭm prē′pyūs) A fold of mucous membrane passing from the undersurface of the glans penis to the deep surface of the prepuce. SYN frenulum preputii [TA].

fren•u•lum pre•pu•ti•i (fren′yū-lŭm prē-pyū′tē-ī) [TA] SYN frenulum of prepuce.

fren•u•lum of tongue (fren′yū-lŭm tŭng) Fold of mucous membrance extending from floor of mouth to midline of the undersurface of tongue. SYN lingual frenulum.

fre•num, pl. **fre•na**, **fre•nums** (frē′nŭm, -nă, -nŭmz) **1.** A narrow reflection or fold of mucous membrane passing from a more fixed to a movable part, serving to check undue movement of the part. **2.** An anatomic structure resembling such a fold. **3.** SYN frenulum. [L. a bridle, curb]

fre•quen•cy (ν) (frē′kwĕn-sē) **1.** The number of regular recurrences in a given time, e.g., heartbeats, sound vibrations. **2.** ACOUSTICS the number of cycles of compression and rarefaction of a sound wave that occur in 1 second, expressed in hertz (Hz). **3.** The rate of vocal fold vibration (i.e., the number of times the glottis opens and closes in 1 second) during phonation; perceived as voice pitch. [L. *frequens,* repeated, often, constant]

fre•quen•cy en•cod•ing (frē′kwĕn-sē en-kōd′ing) Locating a signal according to its frequency.

fresh•en•ing (fresh′ĕn-ing) Preparation of an open, partially healed wound for secondary closure by removal of fibrin, granulations, and early scar tissue.

Fres•nel prism (fre′nel prizm) A membranous prismatic lens that can be attached temporarily to the spectacle lens of the nondominant eye in diplopia.

fret•ting (fret′ing) Abrasive polishing and wear of two metallic surfaces at their interface due to repetitive motion. [M.E., fr. O.E. *fretan,* to devour]

freud•i•an (froyd′ē-ăn) Relating to or described by the Viennese psychiatrist Sigmund Freud (1856–1939).

freud•i•an psy•cho•a•nal•y•sis (froyd′ē-ăn sī′kō-ă-nal′i-sis) The theory and practice of psychoanalysis and psychotherapy as developed by Sigmund Freud, based on: 1) his theory of personality, which postulates that psychic life is made up of instinctual and socially acquired forces, or the id, the ego, and a superego; 2) his discovery that the free-associated technique of verbalizing for the analyst all thoughts reveals the areas in conflict within a patient's personality; 3) that the vehicle for gaining this insight and readjusting one's personality is the learning a patient does, first developing a stormy emotional bond with the analyst (transference relationship) and next successfully learning to break this bond.

freud·i·an slip (froyd′ē-ăn slip) A mistake in speech or deed that presumably suggests some underlying motive, often sexual or aggressive.

Freud the·o·ry (froyd thē′ŏr-ē) A comprehensive theory of how personality is formed and develops in normal and emotionally disturbed individuals; e.g., that an attack of conversion hysteria is due to a psychic trauma that has not adequately reacted to at the time it was received, and persists as an affect memory. SEE ALSO psychoanalysis.

Freund ad·ju·vant (froynd ad′jū-vănt) SEE adjuvant.

Freund a·nom·a·ly (froynd ă-nom′ă′lē) A narrowing of the upper aperture of the thorax by shortening of the first rib and its cartilage; formerly believed to predispose to tuberculosis because of defective expansion of the lung apex.

Freund com·plete ad·ju·vant (froynd kŏm-plēt′ ad′jū-vănt) Water-in-oil emulsion of antigen, to which killed mycobacteria or tuberculosis bacteria are added.

Freund in·com·plete ad·ju·vant (froynd in′kŏm-plēt′ ad′jū-vănt) Water-in-oil emulsion of antigen, without mycobacteria.

Freund op·er·a·tion (froynd op-ĕr-ā′shŭn) **1.** Total abdominal hysterectomy for uterine cancer. **2.** Chondrotomy to relieve Freund anomaly.

Frey hairs (frī hārz) Short hairs of varying degrees of stiffness, set at right angles into the end of a light wooden handle; used for assessing sensation.

FRH Abbreviation for follitropin-releasing hormone.

fri·a·ble (frī′ă-bĕl) **1.** Said of tissue that readily tears, fragments, or bleeds when gently palpated or manipulated. **2.** Easily reduced to powder. **3.** BACTERIOLOGY denoting a dry and brittle culture falling into powder when touched or shaken. [L. *friabilis,* fr. *frio,* to crumble]

fric·a·tive (frik′ă-tiv) Speech sound made by forcing the air stream through a narrow orifice, created by apposition of the teeth, tongue, or lips in producing consonantal phonemes such as f, v, s, and z.

fric·tion (frik′shŭn) **1.** The act of rubbing the surface of an object against that of another; especially rubbing the limbs of the body to aid the circulation. **2.** The force required for relative motion of two bodies that are in contact. **3.** A group of movements in massage intended to move superficial layers over deeper structures, to reach deeper tissues, or to create heat. Includes static, cross-fiber, with-fiber, and circular frictions. [L. *frictio*, fr. *frico*, to rub]

fric·tion rub (frik′shŭn rŭb) SYN friction sound.

fric·tion sound (frik′shŭn sownd) The sound, heard on auscultation, made by the rubbing of two opposed serous surfaces roughened by an inflammatory exudate, or, if chronic, by nonadhesive fibrosis. SYN friction rub.

Fried·länd·er ba·cil·lus (frēd′lān-der bă-sil′ŭs) SYN *Klebsiella pneumoniae.*

Fried·länd·er pneu·mo·ni·a (frēd′lān-der nū-mō′nē-ă) A form of pneumonia caused by infection with *Klebsiella pneumoniae* (Friedländer bacillus), characteristically severe and lobar in distribution.

Fried·man curve (frēd′măn kŭrv) SYN partogram.

Fried·reich a·tax·i·a (frēd′rīk ă-tak′sē-ă) A neurologic disorder characterized by ataxia, dysarthria, scoliosis, high-arched foot or pes cavus, and paralysis of the muscles, especially of the lower extremities; onset usually in childhood or youth with sclerosis of the posterior and lateral columns of the spinal cord; autosomal recessive inheritance, caused by mutation involving trinucleotide repeat expansion in Friedreich ataxia gene (FRDA) on chromosome 9q.

Fried·reich sign (frēd′rīk sīn) In adherent pericardium, sudden collapse of the previously distended veins of the neck at each diastole of the heart.

frig·id (frij′id) **1.** SYN cold. **2.** Temperamentally, especially sexually, unresponsive. [L. *frigidus,* cold]

fri·gid·i·ty (fri-jid′i-tē) **1.** Inability in the female to achieve orgasm or any other satisfactory level of sexual response. **2.** The state of being frigid (2).

fringe (frinj) Colloquial adjectival usage for unproven or incompletely accepted health care modalities; often perceived as pejorative by practitioners of these alternative methods.

frit (frit) A substance used in making dental porcelain powders. It is produced by plunging hot, partially or fully fused porcelain into water; as the material cracks and fractures, the procelain is reduced to powder. [Fr. *frit*, fried]

frog leg po·si·tion (frawg leg pŏ-zish′ŏn) Supine with soles of feet together and knees apart to expose the perineum.

Fröh·lich dwarf·ism (froy′lik dwōrf′izm) Dwarfism with Fröhlich syndrome.

Fröh·lich syn·drome (froy′lik sin′drōm) SYN dystrophia adiposogenitalis.

Fro·in syn·drome (frwahn[h] sin′drōm) An alteration in the cerebrospinal fluid, which is yellowish and coagulates spontaneously in a few seconds after withdrawal, owing to its greatly increased protein (albumin and globulin) content; noted in loculated portions of the subarachnoid space isolated from spinal fluid circulation by an inflammatory or neoplastic obstruction.

Fro•ment sign (frō-mōn[h] sīn) A maneuver used to determine ulnar nerve damage, whereby the person examined grasps a piece of paper between thumb and forefinger. The clinician attempts to pull the paper away. The test result is positive if the distal phalanx of the thumb flexes to hold the paper.

fron•do•sum (fron-dō′sŭm) Bearing villi or other leaflike structures. [L. full of leaves]

frons, gen. **fron•tis** (fronz, fron′tis) SYN forehead. [L.]

front•ad (frŏn′tad) Toward the front.

fron•tal (frŏn′tăl) **1.** In front; relating to the anterior part of a body. **2.** Referring to the frontal (coronal) plane or to the frontal bone or forehead. SYN frontalis.

fron•tal ar•e•a (frŏn′tăl ār′ē-ă) SYN frontal cortex.

fron•tal ar•ter•y (frŏn′tăl ahr′tĕr-ē) SYN supratrochlear artery.

fron•tal bel•ly of oc•cip•i•to•fron•tal•is mus•cle (frŏn′tăl bel′ē ok-sip′i-tō-frŏn-tā′lis mŭs′ĕl) The anterior belly of the occipitofrontalis muscle.

fron•tal bone (frŏn′tăl bōn) The large single bone forming the forehead and the upper margin and roof of the orbit on either side; it articulates with the parietal, nasal, ethmoid, maxillary, and zygomatic bones, and with the lesser wings of the sphenoid.

fron•tal cor•tex (frŏn′tăl kōr′teks) Cortex of the frontal lobe of the cerebral hemisphere. SYN frontal area.

fron•tal crest (frŏn′tăl krest) A ridge arising at the termination of the sagittal sulcus on the cerebral surface of the frontal bone and ending at the foramen cecum.

fron•tal gait (frŭnt′ăl gāt) Ambulation disorder caused by stroke, neoplasm, or cerebral insult.

fron•ta•lis (frŏn-tā′lis) SYN frontal. [L.]

fron•tal lobe of cer•e•brum (frŏn′tăl lōb ser′ĕ-brŭm) The portion of each cerebral hemisphere anterior to the central sulcus.

fron•tal lobe ep•i•lep•sy (frŏn′tăl lōb ep′i-lep-sē) A disorder with seizures originating in the frontal lobe. Frontal lobe epilepsies have been divided into several specific syndromes including the syndrome of supplementary motor seizures, cingulate seizures, anterior frontal polar region seizures, orbital frontal seizures, dorsolateral seizures, opercular seizures, and seizures of the motor cortex.

fron•tal nerve (frŏn′tăl nĕrv) A branch of the ophthalmic nerve that divides within the orbit into the supratrochlear and the supraorbital nerves. SYN nervus frontalis [TA].

fron•tal plane (frŏn′tăl plān) SYN coronal plane.

fron•tal pole of cer•e•brum (frŏn′tăl pōl ser′ĕ-brŭm) The most anterior promontory of each cerebral hemisphere.

fron•tal si•nus (frŏn′tăl sī′nŭs) A hollow paranasal sinus formed on either side in the lower part of the squama of the frontal bone; it communicates by the ethmoidal infundibulum with the middle meatus of the nasal cavity of the same side.

fron•tal su•ture (frŏn′tăl sū′chŭr) The suture between the two halves of the frontal bone, usually obliterated by about the sixth year; if persistent it is called a metopic suture.

fron•tier med•i•cine (frŭn-tēr′ med′i-sin) SEE fringe.

fron•to•an•te•ri•or po•si•tion (frŏn′tō-an-tēr′ē-ŏr pŏ-zish′ŏn) A cephalic presentation of the fetus with its forehead directed toward the right (right frontoanterior, RFA) or to the left (left frontoanterior, LFA) of the acetabulum of the mother.

fron•to•ma•lar (frŏn′tō-mā′lăr) SYN frontozygomatic.

fron•to•max•il•lar•y (frŏn′tō-mak′si-la-rē) Relating to the frontal and the maxillary bones.

fron•to•na•sal (frŏn′tō-nā′zăl) Relating to the frontal and the nasal bones.

fron•to•oc•cip•i•tal (frŏn′tō-ok-sip′i-tăl) Relating to the frontal and the occipital bones, or to the forehead and the occiput.

fron•to•pa•ri•e•tal (frŏn′tō-păr-ī′ĕ-tăl) Relating to the frontal and the parietal bones.

fron•to•pos•te•ri•or po•si•tion (frŏn′tō-pos-tēr′ē-ŏr pŏ-zish′ŏn) A cephalic presentation of the fetus with its forehead directed toward the right (right frontoposterior, RFP) or to the left (left frontoposterior, LFP) sacroiliac articulation of the mother.

fron•to•tem•po•ral (frŏn′tō-tem′pŏr-ăl) Relating to the frontal and the temporal bones.

fron•to•trans•verse po•si•tion (frŏn′tō-tranz-vĕrs′ pŏ-zish′ŏn) A cephalic presentation of the fetus with its forehead directed toward the right (right frontotransverse, RFT) or to the left (left frontotransverse, LFT) iliac fossa of the mother.

fron•to•zy•go•mat•ic (frŏn′tō-zī-gō-mat′ik) Relating to the frontal and zygomatic bones. SYN frontomalar.

frost (frawst) A deposit resembling that of frozen vapor or dew.

frost•bite (frawst′bīt) Local tissue destruction resulting from exposure to extreme or prolonged cold. In mild cases, it results in superficial, reversible freezing followed by erythema and slight pain; in severe cases, it can be painless or paresthetic and result in blistering, persistent edema, and gangrene.

fros•ted branch an•gi•i•tis (frawst′ĕd branch an′jē-ī′tis) Angiitis characterized by inflammation of blood vessels with sheathing giving the appearance of branches on a tree.

frost•ed liv•er (frawst′ĕd liv′ĕr) Hyaloserositis of the liver.

Frost su•ture (frawst sū′chŭr) Intermarginal suture between the eyelids to protect the cornea.

frot•tage (frō-tahzh′) **1.** The rubbing movement in massage. **2.** SYN frotteurism. [Fr., a rubbing]

frot•teur•ism (fraw′tur-izm) Sexual gratification derived from rubbing a bodily area against another person, often a stranger, in an inappropriate way. SYN frottage (2). [Fr. *frotteur,* one who rubs, fr. *frotter,* to rub, + -ism]

fro•zen gait (FG) (frō′zĕn gāt) SEE parkinsonism.

fro•zen pel•vis (frō′zĕn pel′vis) A condition in which the true pelvis is indurated throughout, especially by carcinoma.

fro•zen sec•tion (frō′zĕn sek′shŭn) A thin slice of tissue cut from a frozen specimen, often used for rapid microscopic diagnosis.

fro•zen watch•ful•ness (frō′zĕn wahch′fulnĕs) A condition seen in abused infants involving hopelessness and profoundly guarded affect.

FRT Abbreviation for functional reach test.

♻ **fructo-** Chemical prefix denoting the fructose configuration. [L. *fructus,* fruit]

fruc•to•fu•ra•nose (fruk′tō-fūr′ă-nōs) Fructose in furanose form.

fruc•to•ki•nase (fruk′tō-kī′nās) A liver enzyme that catalyzes the reaction of ATP and D-fructose to form fructose 6-phosphate and ADP; deficient in patients with essential fructosuria (hepatic fructokinase deficiency).

fructosaemia [Br.] SYN fructosemia.

fruc•tose (fruk′tōs) A ketohexase; the D-isomer (also called fruit sugar, levulose, and D-*arabino*-2-hexulose) found in fruits and honey and is a product of sucrose hydrolysis. It can be metabolized or converted to glucose. [L. *fructus*, fruit, + -ose]

fruc•to•se•mi•a (fruk′tō-sē′mē-ă) Presence of fructose in the circulating blood. SYN fructosaemia.

fruc•to•side (fruk′tō-sīd) Fructose in –C–O– linkage where the –C–O– group is the original 2 group of the fructose.

fruc•to•su•ri•a (fruk′tō-syūr′ē-ă) Excretion of fructose in the urine. [fructose + G. *ouron,* urine]

♻ **fructosyl-** Chemical prefix indicating fructose in -C-R- (not -C-O-R-) linkage through its carbon-2 (R usually C).

fruit sug•ar (frūt shug′ăr) D-fructose. SEE fructose.

frus•tra•tion (frŭs-trā′shŭn) The thwarting of or inability to gratify a desire or to satisfy an urge or need. [L. *frustro,* pp. *-atus,* to deceive, disappoint, fr. *frustra* (adv.), in vain]

FTA-ABS Abbreviation for fluorescent treponemal antibody absorption. SEE fluorescent treponemal antibody-absorption test.

FTD Abbreviation for fixing to die.

Fuchs ad•e•no•ma (fūks ad′ĕ-nō′mă) A benign epithelial tumor of the nonpigmented epithelium of the ciliary body, rarely exceeding 1 mm in diameter.

Fuchs black spot (fūks blak spot) An area of pigment proliferation in the macular region in degenerative myopia.

Fuchs col•o•bo•ma (fūks kol-ō-bō′mă) A congenital inferior crescent on the choroid at the edge of the optic disc; not associated with myopia.

Fuchs en•do•the•li•al dys•tro•phy (fūks en′dō-thē′lē-ăl dis′trŏ-fē) Common corneal dystrophy with autosomal dominant inheritance, characterized by keratopathia guttata with loss of endothelium and progressive corneal edema.

Fuchs e•pi•the•li•al dys•tro•phy (fūks ep′i-thē′lē-ăl dis′trŏ-fē) SYN dystrophia epithelialis corneae.

Fuchs het•er•o•chro•mic cy•cli•tis (fūks het′ĕr-ō-krō′mik sik-lī′tis) SYN Fuchs syndrome.

fuch•sin (fūk′sin) A nonspecific term referring to any of several red rosanilin dyes used as stains in histology and bacteriology.

fuch•sin•o•phil (fuk-sin′ō-fil) **1.** Staining readily with fuchsin dyes. SYN fuchsinophilic. **2.** A cell or histologic element that stains readily with fuchsin. [fuchsin + G. *philos,* fond]

fuch•sin•o•phil gran•ule (fuk-sin′ō-fil gran′yūl) A granule that has an affinity for fuchsin.

fuch•sin•o•phil•ic (fuk-sin′ō-fil′ik) SYN fuchsinophil (1).

Fuchs spur (fūks spŭr) Epithelial outgrowth of the dilator muscle of the pupil about midway in the breadth of the sphincter; part of the insertion of the dilator muscle onto the iris sphincter.

Fuchs syn•drome (fūks sin′drōm) A syndrome characterized by corneal degeneration, heterochromia of the iris, iridocyclitis, keratic precipitates, and cataract; probably autosomal dominant inheritance. SYN Fuchs heterochromic cyclitis.

Fuchs u•ve•i•tis (fūks yū-vē-ī′tis) SYN heterochromic uveitis.

fu•cose (fū′kōs) 6-Deoxygalactose; a methylpentose, the L-configuration of which occurs in the mucopolysaccharides of the blood group substances, in human milk (as a polysaccharide), and elsewhere in nature. The D-configuration has been found in certain antibiotics.

fu•gac•i•ty (f) (fyū-gas′i-tē) The tendency of the molecules in a fluid, as a result of all forces acting on them, to leave a given site in the body; the escaping tendency of a fluid, as in diffusion, evaporation, and the like. [L. *fuga,* flight]

-fugal Suffix meaning movement away from the part indicated by the main portion of the word. [L. *fugio,* to flee]

-fuge Suffix meaning flight, denoting the place from which flight takes place or that which is put to flight. [L. *fuga* a running away]

fugue (fyūg) A condition in which a person suddenly abandons a present activity or lifestyle and starts a new and different one, often in a different city; afterward, alleges amnesia for events occurring during the fugue period, although earlier events are remembered and habits and skills are usually unaffected. [Fr. fr. L. *fuga,* flight]

ful•crum, pl. **ful•cra**, **ful•crums** (ful′krŭm, -kră, -krŭmz) A support or the point thereon on which a lever turns. [L. a bedpost, fr. *fulcio,* to prop up]

ful•gu•rant (ful′gŭr-ănt) Sharp and piercing. Cf. fulminant. SYN fulgurating (1). [L. *fulgur,* flashing lightning]

ful•gu•rat•ing (ful′gŭr-āt-ing) **1.** SYN fulgurant. **2.** Relating to fulguration.

ful•gu•ra•tion (ful′gŭr-ā′shŭn) Destruction of tissue by means of a high-frequency electric current: **direct fulguration** uses an insulated electrode with a metal point, which is connected to the uniterminal of the high-frequency apparatus, from which a spark of electricity is allowed to impinge on the area to be treated; **indirect fulguration** involves directly connecting the patient by a metal contact to the uniterminal and utilizing an active electrode to complete an arc from the patient. [L. *fulgur,* lightning stroke]

full den•ture (ful den′chŭr) SYN complete denture.

ful•ler's earth (ful′ĕrz ĕrth) **1.** An amorphous variety of kaolin of varying composition, containing an aluminum magnesium silicate. **2.** A refined clay sometimes used as a dusting powder or applied moistened with water as a poultice. Used as decolorizer for oils and other liquids, filtering medium, filler for rubber, and in agricultural formulations. [fr. *fulling,* an old process of cleaning wool with earth or clay]

full thick•ness burn (ful thik′nĕs bŭrn) A burn involving destruction of the entire skin; deep thick burns extend into subcutaneous fat, muscle, or bone and often cause much scarring. SYN third-degree burn.

full-thick•ness graft (ful-thik′nĕs graft) A graft of the full thickness of mucosa and submucosa or of skin and subcutaneous tissue.

ful•mi•nant (ful′mi-nănt) Occurring suddenly, with lightninglike rapidity, and with great intensity or severity. Cf. fulgurant. [L. *fulmino,* pp. *-atus,* to hurl lightning, fr. *fulmen,* lightning]

ful•mi•nat•ing (ful′mi-nāt-ing) Running a speedy course, with rapid worsening.

fu•ma•rate hy•dra•tase (fū′măr-āt hī′dră-tās) An enzyme catalyzing the reversible interconversion of fumaric acid and water to malic acid, a reaction of importance in the tricarboxylic acid cycle. Deficiency leads to mental retardation.

fu•mar•ic ac•id (fyū-mar′ik as′id) A trans-Butanedioic acid; an unsaturated dicarboxylic acid occurring as an intermediate in the tricarboxylic acid cycle.

fu•mi•gant (fyū′mi-gănt) A substance used in fumigation.

fu•mi•gate (fyū′mi-gāt) To expose to the action of smoke or fumes as a means of disinfection or eradication. [L. *fumigo* pp. *-atus,* to fumigate, fr. *fumus,* smoke, + *ago,* to drive]

fu•mi•ga•tion (fyū′mi-gā′shŭn) The act of fumigating; the use of a fumigant.

fum•ing (fyūm′ing) Giving forth a visible vapor, a property of concentrated nitric, sulfuric, and hydrochloric acids, and of certain other substances. [L. *fumus,* smoke]

func•ti•o lae•sa (fŭnk′shē-ō lē′să) Impaired function; a fifth sign of inflammation added by Galen to those enunciated by Celsus (rubor, tumor, calor, and dolor). [L.]

func•tion (fŭngk′shŭn) **1.** The special action or physiologic property of an organ or other part of the body. **2.** To perform its special work or office, said of an organ or other part of the body. **3.** The general properties of any substance, depending on its chemical character and relation to other substances, according to which it may be grouped among acids, bases, alcohols, esters, or other groups. **4.** A particular reactive grouping in a molecule; e.g., a functional group, such as the –OH group of an alcohol. **5.** A quality, trait, or fact that is so related to another as to be dependent on and to vary with this other. [L. *functio,* fr. *fungor,* pp. *functus,* to perform]

func•tion•al (fŭngk′shŭn-ăl) **1.** Relating to a function. **2.** Not organic in origin; denoting a disorder with no known or detectable organic basis to explain the symptoms. SEE neurosis.

func•tion•al ac•ti•vi•ty (fŭngk′shŭn-ăl ak-tiv′i-tē) **1.** A task or act that allows one to meet the demands of the environment and daily life. **2.** An activity that is essential to support the physical, social, and psychological well-being of a person and allows that person to function in society. SEE ALSO functional test.

func•tion•al a•nat•o•my (fŭngk′shŭn-ăl ă-nat′ŏ-mē) The study of bodily structure as it relates to function.

func•tion•al blind•ness (fŭngk′shŭn-ăl blīnd′nĕs) Apparent loss of vision without discernible physical cause.

func•tion•al ca•pac•i•ty (fungk′shŭn-ăl kă-pas′i-tē) The extent to which a person can increase exercise intensity and maintain increased levels, dependent largely on cardiovascular fitness.

func•tion•al ca•pac•i•ty e•val•u•a•tion (FCE) (fungk′shŭn-ăl kă-pas′i-tē ē-val′yū-ā′shŭn) A comprehensive evaluation to determine a person's physical functional limitations and capabilities. SYN Work-Capacity Evaluation.

func•tion•al cas•tra•tion (fŭngk′shŭn-ăl kas-trā′shŭn) Gonadal atrophy produced by prolonged treatment with sex hormones or gonadotropin-releasing hormone superagonists or antagonists. SYN medical castration.

func•tion•al con•ges•tion (fŭngk′shŭn-ăl kŏn-jes′chŭn) Hyperemia occurring during functional activity of an organ. SYN physiologic congestion.

func•tion•al deaf•ness (fŭngk′shŭn-ăl def′nĕs) SYN psychogenic deafness.

func•tion•al dis•or•der, func•tion•al dis•ease (fŭngk′shŭn-ăl dis-ōr′dĕr, di-zēz′) A physical disorder with no known or detectable organic basis to explain the symptoms. SEE behavior disorder, neurosis.

func•tion•al dys•men•or•rhe•a (fŭngk′shŭn-ăl dis-men′ōr-ē′ă) SYN primary dysmenorrhea.

func•tion•al ef•fi•cien•cy (fungk′shŭn-ăl ē-fish′ĕn-sē) The ability of the neuromuscular system to monitor and manipulate movement during a functional activity so as to expend the least possible amount of energy.

func•tion•al e•lec•tric stim•u•la•tion (FES) (fŭngk′shŭn-ăl ĕ-lek′trik stim′yŭ-lā′shŭn) A multiple-channel electrotherapeutic modality that uses pulsatile waveforms to activate a muscle or group of muscles in a functional activity (e.g., walking, reaching up).

func•tion•al en•do•scop•ic si•nus sur•ger•y (FESS) (fŭngk′shŭn-ăl en′dō-skop′ik sī′nŭs sŭr′jĕr-ē) A group of operations performed on the paranasal sinuses, with illumination and magnification through an endoscope.

func•tion•al fi•ber (fungk′shŭn-ăl fī′bĕr) Indigestible food that offers health benefits for the gastrointestinal tract.

func•tion•al food (fŭngk′shŭn-ăl fūd) Foodstuff demonstrated to confer physiologic benefits, reduce the risk of chronic disease, or act as a nutrient. Cf. nutraceutical.

func•tion•al ge•no•mics (fŭngk′shŭn-ăl jē-nō′miks) The study of expressed genes in organisms, including the identity of the genes and the factors that control differential expression.

func•tion•al hand po•si•tion (fŭngk′shŭn-ăl hand pŏ-zish′ŏn) A position for a nonfunctional hand to prevent contractures and deformity. Position includes 20–30 degrees of wrist extension, 45 degrees of metacarpal joint flexion, 30 degrees of proximal interphalangeal (PIP) joint flexion, and 20 degrees of distal interphalangeal joint (DIP) flexion.

func•tion•al im•po•tence (fŭngk′shŭn-ăl im′pŏ-tĕns) An intermittent erectile dysfunction that is more psychogenic than physiologic in source; varies in degree depending on circumstance and sexual partner.

func•tion•al in•de•pen•dence mea•sure (FIM) (fungk′shŭn-ăl in′dĕ-pend′ĕns mezh′ŭr) An instrument used to measure the extent of disability based on the responses to 18 items covering self-care, sphincter control, mobility, locomotion, communication, and social cognition.

func•tion•al mur•mur (fŭngk′shŭn-ăl mŭr′mŭr) A cardiac murmur not associated with a significant heart lesion (e.g., such a sound related to anemia rather than an organic heart disorder). SYN innocent murmur.

func•tion•al neck dis•sec•tion (fŭngk′shŭn-ăl nek di-sek′shŭn) Operation to remove metastases to the lymph nodes of the neck; differs from a radical neck dissection by preserving any of the following structures: the sternocleidomastoid muscle, the spinal accessory nerve, and the internal jugular vein. SYN limited neck dissection.

func•tion•al neu•ro•sur•ger•y (fŭngk′shŭn-ăl nūr′ō-sŭr′jĕr-ē) Destruction or chronic excitation of a part of the brain to treat disordered behavior or function.

func•tion•al oc•clu•sion (fŭngk′shŭn-ăl ŏ-klū′zhŭn) **1.** Any tooth contacts made within the functional range of the opposing teeth surfaces. **2.** Occlusion that occurs during function.

func•tion•al reach (fungk′shŭn-ăl rēch) The distance a person can reach forward or to the side beyond arm's length while keeping a fixed base of support in a standing position.

func•tion•al reach test (FRT) (fŭngk′shŭn-ăl rēch test) An assessment of balance in which the patient stands erect and stretches out her or his arms; a reach measuring 6 inches or less suggests a predisposition to falling.

func•tion•al re•sid•u•al air (fŭngk′shŭn-ăl rĕ-zid′yū-ăl ār) SYN functional residual capacity.

func•tion•al re•sid•u•al ca•pac•i•ty (FRC) (fŭngk′shŭn-ăl rĕ-zid′yū-ăl kă-pas′i-tē) The volume of gas remaining in the lungs at the end of a normal expiration; it is the sum of expiratory reserve volume and residual volume. SYN functional residual air.

func•tion•al splint (fŭngk′shŭn-ăl splint) **1.** SYN dynamic splint. **2.** The joining of two or more teeth into a rigid unit by means of fixed restorations that cover all or part of the abutment teeth.

func•tion•al test (fŭngk′shŭn-ăl test) The measurement or qualification of activities identified by someone as essential to personal ADLs. SEE ALSO functional activity.

fun•dal mas•sage (fŭnd′ăl mă-sahzh′) In obstetrics, manipulation of the postpartum uterus through the abdominal wall to avert the risk of postpartum hemorrhage due to uterine atony.

fun•da•men•tal fre•quen•cy (F0) (fŭn′dă-men′tăl frē′kwĕn-sē) **1.** ACOUSTICS the basic frequency of a vibrating object or sound as opposed to its harmonics, or the principal component of a complex sound wave. **2.** The frequency of vocal fold vibration at the glottis, unaffected by resonance. SEE ALSO optimal pitch.

fun•dec•to•my (fŭn-dek′tŏ-mē) SYN fundusectomy. [fundus + G. *ektomē,* excision]

fun•dic (fŭn′dik) Relating to a fundus.

fun•di•form (fŭn′di-fōrm) Looped; sling-shaped. [L. *funda,* a sling, + *forma,* shape]

fun•do•pli•ca•tion (fŭn′dō-pli-kā′shŭn) Suture of the fundus of the stomach around the esophagus to prevent reflux in repair of hiatal hernia. [fundus + L. *plico,* to fold]

fun•dus, pl. **fun•di** (fŭn′dŭs, -dī) The bottom or lowest part of a sac or hollow organ; that part farthest removed from the opening or exit; occasionally a broad cul-de-sac. See page B26. [L. bottom]

fun•du•scope (fŭn′dŭ-skōp) SYN ophthalmoscope.

fun•du•sec•to•my (fŭn′dŭ-sek′tŏ-mē) Excision of the fundus of an organ. SYN fundectomy. [L. *fundus,* + G. *ektomē,* excision]

fun•dus of eye (fŭn′dŭs ī) The portion of the interior of the eyeball around the posterior pole, visible through the ophthalmoscope. SYN fundus oculi.

fun•dus of gall•blad•der (fŭn′dŭs gawl′blad-ĕr) The wide closed end of the gallbladder situated at the inferior border of the liver.

fun•dus oc•u•li (fŭn′dŭs ok′yū-lī) SYN fundus of eye.

fun•dus of stom•ach (fŭn′dŭs stŏm′ăk) The portion of the stomach that lies above the cardiac notch. SYN fundus ventriculi.

fun•dus of ur•i•nar•y blad•der (fŭn′dŭs yūr′i-nar-ē blad′ĕr) The fundus is formed by the posterior wall, which is somewhat convex. SYN fundus vesicae urinariae.

fun•dus of u•ter•us (fŭn′dŭs yū′tĕr-ŭs) The upper rounded extremity of the uterus above the openings of the uterine (fallopian) tubes.

fun•dus ven•tric•u•li (fŭn′dŭs ven-trik′yū-lī) SYN fundus of stomach.

fun•dus ve•si•cae u•ri•na•ri•ae (fŭn′dŭs ves′i-kē yūr-i-nā′rē-ē) SYN fundus of urinary bladder.

fungaemia [Br.] SYN fungemia.

fun•gal (fŭng′găl) Relating to a fungus. SYN fungous.

fun•gal in•fec•tion (fŭng′găl in-fek′shŭn) Any invasion of the body by a pathogenic fungus.

fun•gate (fŭng′gāt) To grow exuberantly, like a fungus.

fun•ge•mi•a (fŭn-jē′mē-ă) Fungal infection disseminated by way of the bloodstream. SYN fungaemia.

Fun•gi (fŭng′gī) A division of eukaryotic organisms that grow in irregular masses, without roots, stems, or leaves, and are devoid of chlorophyll or other pigments capable of photosynthesis. Each organism (thallus) is unicellular to filamentous and possesses branched somatic structures (hyphae) surrounded by cell walls containing cellulose or chitin or both, and containing true nuclei. They reproduce sexually or asexually (spore formation), and may obtain nutrition from other living organisms as parasites or from dead organic matter as saprobes (saprophytes). [L. *fungus,* a mushroom]

fun•gi (fŭng′gī) Plural of fungus.

fun•gi•ci•dal (fŭn-ji-sī′dăl) Having a killing action on fungi. [fungus + L. *caedo,* to kill]

fun•gi•cide (fŭn′ji-sīd) Any substance that has a killing action on fungi.

fun•gi•form (fŭn′ji-fōrm) Shaped like a fungus or mushroom; applied to any structure with a broad, often branched, free portion and a narrower base.

fun•gi•form pa•pil•lae (fŭn′ji-fōrm pă-pil′ē) Numerous minute elevations on the dorsum of the tongue, of a fancied mushroom shape, the tip being broader than the base; the epithelium of many of these papillae has taste buds.

Fun·gi Im·per·fec·ti (fŭng′gī im-pĕr-fek′tī) A phylum of fungi in which sexual reproduction is not known or in which one of the mating types has not yet been discovered. Cf. imperfect fungus.

fun·gi·stat·ic (fŭn′ji-stat′ik) Having an inhibiting action on the growth of fungi. [fungus + G. *statos,* standing]

fun·gi·tox·ic (fŭn′ji-tok′sik) Poisonous or in any way deleterious to the growth of fungi.

fun·goid (fŭng′goyd) Resembling a fungus; denoting an exuberant morbid growth on the surface of the body.

fun·gos·i·ty (fŭng-gos′i-tē) A fungoid growth.

fun·gous (fŭng′gŭs) SYN fungal.

fun·gus, pl. **fun·gi** (fŭng′gŭs, -gī) A general term used to encompass the diverse morphologic forms of yeasts and molds. Originally classified as primitive plants without chlorophyll, the fungi are placed in the kingdom Fungi and some in the kingdom Protista, along with algae, protozoa, and slime molds. Fungi share with bacteria an ability to break down complex organic substances and are essential to the recycling of carbon and other elements. Fungi are important as foods and to the fermentation process in the development of substances of industrial and medical importance, including alcohol, the antibiotics, other drugs, and antitoxins. Relatively few fungi are pathogenic for humans, whereas most plant diseases are caused by fungi. [L. *fungus,* a mushroom]

fun·gus ball (fŭng′gŭs bawl) A compact mass of fungal mycelium and cellular debris, 1–5 cm in diameter, residing within a lung cavity; usually produced by *Aspergillus fumigatus*. SEE ALSO aspergilloma (2).

fu·nic (fyū′nik) Relating to the funis, or umbilical cord. SYN funicular (2).

fu·ni·cle (fyū′ni-kĕl) SYN cord (1).

fu·nic·u·lar (fyū-nik′yū-lăr) **1.** Relating to a funiculus. **2.** SYN funic.

fu·nic·u·lar graft (fyū-nik′yū-lăr graft) A nerve graft in which each funiculus (composed of two or more fasciculi) is approximated and sutured separately.

fu·nic·u·lar pro·cess (fū-nik′yū-lăr pros′es) The tunica vaginalis surrounding the spermatic cord.

fu·nic·u·li·tis (fyū-nik′yū-lī′tis) **1.** Inflammation of a funiculus, especially of the spermatic cord. **2.** Inflammation of the umbilical cord usually associated with chorioamnionitis. [funiculus + G. *-itis,* inflammation]

fu·nic·u·lo·pexy (fyū-nik′yū-lō-pek-sē) Suturing of the spermatic cord to the surrounding tissue in the correction of an undescended testicle. [funiculus + G. *pēxis,* a fixing]

fu·nic·u·lus, pl. **fu·nic·u·li** (fyū-nik′yū-lŭs, -lī) [TA] SYN cord (1). [L. dim. of *funis,* cord]

fu·nic·u·lus sper·ma·ti·cus (fyū-nik′yū-lŭs spĕr-mat′i-kŭs) [TA] SYN spermatic cord.

fu·nic·u·lus um·bi·li·ca·lis (fyū-nik′yū-lŭs ŭm-bil-i-kā′lis) [TA] SYN umbilical cord.

fu·ni·form (fyū′ni-fōrm) Ropelike. [L. *funis,* cord, + *forma,* shape]

fu·ni·punc·ture (fyū′ni-pŭngk-chŭr) SYN cordocentesis. [L. *funis,* cord, + puncture]

fu·nis (fyū′nis) **1.** SYN umbilical cord. **2.** A cordlike structure. [L. a rope, cord]

fu·ni·si·tis (fyū′ni-sī′tis) Inflammation of the umbilical cord. [funis + -itis]

fun·nel (fŭn′ĕl) **1.** A hollow conic vessel with a tube of variable length proceeding from its apex, used in pouring fluids from one container to another, in filtering, and other tasks. **2.** ANATOMY an infundibulum.

fun·nel breast, **fun·nel chest** (fŭn′ĕl brest, chest) SYN pectus excavatum.

fun·nel chest (fun′ĕl chest) An abnormality of the thoracic cage that gives a concave appearance to the anterior chest.

fun·nel plot (fŭn′ĕl plot) A graphic method of detecting publication bias. The estimate of risk derived from a set of epidemiologic studies used in a metaanalysis is plotted against sample size. If there is no publication bias, the plot is funnel shaped; if studies giving significant results are more likely to be published than negative studies, the plot is asymmetric. SEE ALSO metaanalysis.

fun·nel-shaped pel·vis (fŭn′ĕl-shāpt pel′vis) A pelvis in which the pelvic inlet dimensions are normal, but the outlet is contracted in the transverse or in both transverse and anteroposterior diameters.

fun·ny bone (fŭn′ē bōn) Colloquial usage for the tip of the olecranon.

FUO Abbreviation for fever of unknown origin.

fu·ra-2 (fūr′ă) A fluorescent indicator that binds calcium; it is more excited at longer wavelengths when free of calcium than when calcium is bound; the ratio of fluorescence intensity at two excitation wavelengths provides a measure of free calcium ion concentration; may be injected into cells to monitor moment-to-moment changes in intracellular free calcium ion concentration. SEE ALSO aequorin.

fu·ra·nose (fyūr′ă-nōs) A saccharide unit or

molecule containing the furan grouping. [furan + -ose(1)]

fur·cal (fŭr′kăl) Forked.

fur·ca·tion (fŭr-kā′shŭn) **1.** A forking, or a fork-like part or branch. **2.** DENTISTRY the region of a multirooted tooth where the roots divide. [L. *furca,* fork]

fur·ca·tion probe (fŭr-kā′shŭn prōb) SYN Naber probe.

fur·fu·ra·ceous (fŭr′fŭr-ā′shŭs) Branny, or composed of small scales; denoting a form of desquamation. SYN pityroid. [L. *furfuraceus,* fr. *furfur,* bran]

fu·ror ep·i·lep·ti·cus (fyūr′ōr ep-i-lep′ti-kŭs) Attacks of anger to which people with epilepsy are occasionally subject, occurring without apparent provocation and without disturbance of consciousness.

fur·row (fŭr′rō) A groove or sulcus. [A.S. *furh*]

fu·run·cle (fŭr-ŭng′kĕl) A localized pyogenic infection, most frequently by *Staphylococcus aureus,* originating deep in a hair follicle. See page B10. SYN boil, furunculus. [L. *furunculus,* a petty thief]

fu·run·cu·lar (fū-rŭng′kyū-lăr) Relating to a furuncle. SYN furunculous.

fu·run·cu·loid (fŭr-ŭng′kyū-loyd) Resembling a furuncle. [furunculus + G. *eidos,* resemblance]

fu·run·cu·lo·sis (fŭr-ŭng′kyū-lō′sis) A condition marked by the presence of furuncles, often chronic and recurrent.

fu·run·cu·lous (fŭr-ŭng′kyū-lŭs) SYN furuncular.

fu·run·cu·lus, pl. **fu·run·cu·li** (fŭr-ŭng′kyū-lŭs, -lī) SYN furuncle. [L. a petty thief, a boil, dim. of *fur,* a thief]

Fu·sar·i·um (fyū-sā′rē-ŭm) A genus of rapidly growing fungi producing characteristic sickle-shaped, multiseptate macroconidia that can be mistaken for those produced by some dermatophytes. A few species can produce corneal ulcers; some are common colonizers of burned skin, and some may cause disseminated hyalohyphomycosis. See page B5. [L. *fusus,* spindle]

fused kid·ney (fyūzd kid′nē) A single, anomalous organ resulting from fusion of the two primordia of the kidneys.

fused teeth (fyūzd tēth) Teeth joined by dentin as a result of embryologic fusion or juxtaposition of two adjacent tooth germs.

fu·si·form (fyū′si-fōrm) Spindle-shaped; tapering at both ends. [L. *fusus,* a spindle, + *forma,* form]

fu·si·form an·eu·rysm (fyū′si-fōrm an′yūr-izm) An elongated spindle-shaped dilation of an artery.

fu·si·form gy·rus (fyū′si-fōrm jī′rŭs) An extremely long convolution extending lengthwise over the inferior aspect of the temporal and occipital lobes, demarcated medially by the collateral sulcus from the lingual gyrus and the anterior part of the parahippocampal gyrus, laterally by the inferior temporal sulcus from the inferior temporal gyrus.

fu·si·mo·tor (fyū′si-mō′tŏr) Pertaining to the efferent innervation of intrafusal muscle fibers by gamma motor neurons. SEE ALSO neuromuscular spindle. [L. *fusus,* spindle, + *moveo,* to move]

fu·sin (fyū′zin) A G protein–linked receptor present on certain human cells that is thought to be required for HIV fusion with a target cell. [fuse, fr. L. *fundo,* pp. *fusum,* to melt, + -in]

fu·sion (fyū′zhŭn) **1.** Liquefaction, as by melting by heat. **2.** Union, as by joining together. **3.** The blending of slightly different images from each eye into a single perception. **4.** The joining of two or more adjacent teeth during their development by a dentinal union. SEE ALSO concrescence. **5.** Joining of two genes, often neighboring genes. **6.** The joining of two bones into a single unit, thereby obliterating motion between the two. [L. *fusio,* a pouring, fr. *fundo,* pp. *fusus,* to pour]

fu·sion beat (fyū′zhŭn bēt) A beat triggered by more than a single electrical impulse, when the wave fronts coincide to act together on a single final pathway of activity; in the electrocardiogram, the atrial or ventricular complex when either atria or ventricles are activated jointly by two simultaneous or nearly simultaneous invading impulses.

fu·sion pro·tein (fyū′zhŭn prō′tēn) Biotechnologic product targeting malignant cells and some normal lymphocytes containing interleukin-2 (IL-2) receptors; used for treatment of patients with advanced and recurrent cutaneous T-cell lymphoma.

Fu·so·bac·ter·i·um (fū′zō-bak-tēr′ē-ŭm) A genus of bacteria containing gram-negative, nonspore-forming, obligately anaerobic rods that produce butyric acid as a major metabolic product. These organisms are found in cavities of humans and other animals; some species are pathogenic. [L. *fusus,* a spindle, + bacterium]

Fu·so·bac·te·ri·um nu·cle·a·tum (fū′zō-bak-tēr′ē-ŭm nū-klē-ā′tŭm) A species that is found indigenously in gingival crevices; involved in infections of the upper respiratory tract and pleural cavity. SYN Vincent bacillus.

fu·so·cel·lu·lar (fyū′zō-sel′yū-lăr) Spindle-celled.

fusospirochaetal [Br.] SYN fusospirochetal.

fu·so·spi·ro·chet·al (fyū′zō-spī-rō-kē′tăl) Referring to the associated fusiform and spirochetal organisms found in the lesions of Vincent angina. SYN fusospirochaetal.

fu·so·spi·ro·chet·al gin·gi·vi·tis (fyū′zō-spī-rō-kē′tăl jin′ji-vī′tis) SYN necrotizing ulcerative gingivitis.

Fut·cher line (fuch′ĕr līn) A dorsoventral line of pigmentation occurring symmetrically and bilaterally for about 10 cm along the lateral edge of the biceps muscle.

fu tzu (fū tsū) SYN aconite. [Mandarin]

FVC Abbreviation for forced vital capacity.

f wave, **ff waves** (wāv, wāvz) Atrial fibrillation wave.

F waves (wāvz) The waves of atrial flutter usually best seen in ECG leads 2, 3, and AVF. (A lowercase f indicates atrial fibrillation).

G

γ **1.** Gamma (q.v.). **2.** Abbreviation for activity coefficient; surface tension.

G Abbreviation for newtonian constant of gravitation, gap (3); gauss; giga-; D-glucose, as in UDPG; guanosine, as in GDP; glycine; guanine.

G G_{act} or $G^{\ddagger}$. Unit of acceleration based on the acceleration produced by the earth's gravitational attraction, where 1 g = 980.621 cm/sec^2 (about 32.1725 ft/sec^2) at sea level and 45° latitude. At 30° latitude, g equals 969.329 cm/sec^2.

g Abbreviation for gram.

g Abbreviation for unit of acceleration based on the acceleration produced by the earth's gravitational attraction, where 1 g = 980.621 cm/sec^2 (about 32.1725 ft/sec^2) at sea level and 45° latitude. At 30° latitude, g equals 979.329 cm/sec^2.

GA NATO code for tabun.

Ga Symbol for gallium.

GABA Acronym for gamma (γ)-aminobutyric acid.

G-ac•tin (akt′in) The globular (G) subunits of the actin molecule, having a molecular weight of 57,000 and containing one molecule of ATP.

gad•o•lin•i•um (Gd) (gad′ō-lin′ē-ŭm) An element of the lanthanide group; atomic no. 64, atomic wt. 157.25. The magnetic properties of this element are used in contrast media for magnetic resonance imaging. [mineral, gadolinite, from Johan *Gadolin,* Finnish chemist, 1760–1852]

Gaens•len sign (genz′len sīn) Pain on hyperextension of the hip with pelvis fixed by flexion of opposite hip; causes a torsion stress at the sacroiliac and lumbosacral joints.

gag (gag) **1.** To retch; to cause to retch or heave. **2.** To prevent from talking. **3.** An instrument adjusted between the teeth to keep the mouth from closing during operations in the mouth or throat.

G a•gents (ā′jĕnts) Abbreviation for G-series nerve agents.

gag re•flex (gag rē′fleks) Contact of a foreign body with the mucous membrane of the fauces causing retching or gagging.

gag rule (gag rūl) As generally used in the health care setting, a U.S. legal directive that obligates physicians not to discuss modes of termination of pregnancy.

gain (gān) **1.** Profit; advantage. **2.** The ratio of output to input of an amplifying system, generally expressed in decibels. [M.E. *gayne,* booty, fr. O.Fr., fr. Germanic]

Gaird•ner dis•ease (gārd′ner di-zēz′) Attacks of cardiac distress accompanied by apprehension.

Gais•böck syn•drome (gīs′bĕrk sin′drōm) SYN polycythemia hypertonica.

gait (gāt) Manner of walking, characterized by rhythm, cadence, step length, stride length, and velocity.

Gal Abbreviation for galactose.

ga•lac•ta•cra•si•a (gă-lak′tă-krā′zē-ă) Abnormal composition of mother's milk. [galact- + G. *akrasia,* bad mixture, fr. *a-* priv. + *krasis,* a mixing]

ga•lac•ta•gogue (gă-lak′tă-gog) An agent that promotes the secretion and flow of milk. [galact- + G. *agōgos,* leading]

ga•lac•tic (gă-lak′tik) Pertaining to milk; promoting the flow of milk.

galacto-, galact- Combining forms denoting milk. Cf. lact-. [G. *gala*]

ga•lac•to•cele (gă-lak′tō-sēl) Retention cyst caused by occlusion of a lactiferous duct. SYN lactocele. [galacto- + G. *kēlē,* tumor]

ga•lac•to•ki•nase (gă-lak′tō-kī′nās) An enzyme (phosphotransferase) that, in the presence of ATP, catalyzes the phosphorylation of D-galactose to D-galactose 1-phosphate, the first step in the metabolism of D-galactose; galactokinase is deficient in one form of galactosemia.

ga•lac•to•phore (gă-lak′tō-fōr) SYN lactiferous ducts. [galacto- + G. *phoros,* bearing]

ga•lac•to•pho•ri•tis (gă-lak′tō-fŏr-ī′tis) Inflammation of the milk ducts. [galacto- + G. *phoros,* carrying, + -itis, inflammation]

ga•lac•toph•o•rous (gal′ak-tof′ŏr-ŭs) Conveying milk.

ga•lac•to•poi•e•sis (gă-lak′tō-poy-ē′sis) Milk production. [galacto- + G. *poiēsis,* forming]

ga•lac•to•poi•et•ic (gă-lak′tō-poy-et′ik) Pertaining to galactopoiesis.

ga•lac•tor•rhe•a (gă-lak′tŏr-ē′ă) **1.** A flow of milk from the breasts other than normal lactation. **2.** Any white discharge from a nipple. SYN galactorrhoea, lactorrhea. [galacto- + G. *rhoia,* a flow]

galactorrhoea [Br.] SYN galactorrhea.

galactosaemia [Br.] SYN galactosemia.

ga•lac•tos•a•mine (gă-lak-tō′să-mēn) The 2-amino-2-deoxy derivative of galactose, in which the NH_2 replaces the 2-OH group; the D-isomer occurs in various mucopolysaccharides, notably of chondroitin sulfuric acid and of B blood group substance; usually found as the *N*-acetyl derivative.

ga•lac•tos•am•i•no•gly•can (gă-lak′tōs-ă-mē′nō-glī′kan) SEE mucopolysaccharide.

ga•lac•tose (Gal) (gă-lak′tōs) An aldohexose found (in D form) as a constituent of lactose, cerebrosides, gangliosides, mucoproteins, in galactoside or galactosyl combination; an epimer of D-glucose.

ga•lac•tose cat•a•ract (gă-lak′tōs kat′ăr-akt) A neonatal cataract associated with intralenticular accumulation of galactose alcohol. SEE galactosemia.

ga•lac•to•se•mi•a (gă-lak′tō-sē′mē-ă) An inborn error of galactose metabolism due to congenital deficiency of the enzyme galactosyl-1-phosphate uridyltransferase, resulting in tissue accumulation of galactose 1-phosphate; manifested by nutritional failure, hepatosplenomegaly with cirrhosis, cataracts, mental retardation, galactosuria, aminoaciduria, and albuminuria, which regress or disappear if galactose is removed from the diet. SYN galactosaemia. [galactose + G. *haima,* blood]

ga•lac•tose-1-phos•phate (gă-lak′tōs-fos′fāt) A phosphorylated derivative of galactose that is key in galactose metabolism; accumulates in certain types of galactosemia.

ga•lac•to•side (gă-lak′tō-sīd) A compound in which the H of the OH group on carbon-1 of galactose is replaced by an organic radical.

ga•lac•to•sis (gă-lak-tō′sis) Formation of milk by the lacteal glands. [galacto- + G. *-osis,* condition]

ga•lac•tos•u•ri•a (gă-lak′tō-syūr′ē-ă) The excretion of galactose in the urine. [galactose + G. *ouron,* urine]

ga•lac•to•syl (gă-lak′tō-sil) A compound in which the –OH attached to carbon-1 of galactose is replaced by an organic radical.

ga•lac•to•ther•a•py (gă-lak′tō-thār′ă-pē) Treatment of disease by means of an exclusive or nearly exclusive milk diet. SYN lactotherapy.

Ga•lant re•flex (gă-lahnt′ rē-fleks) A deep abdominal reflex in which there is a contraction of the abdominal muscles on tapping the anterior superior iliac spine.

Ga•las•si pu•pil•lar•y phe•nom•e•non (gah-lah′sē pyū′pi-lar-ē fĕ-nom′ĕ-non) SYN eye-closure pupil reaction.

ga•le•a (gā′lē-ă) **1.** A body structure shaped like a helmet. **2.** SYN epicranial aponeurosis. **3.** A form of bandage covering the head. **4.** SYN caul (1). [L. a helmet]

Ga•le•az•zi frac•ture (gah-lā-ahts′sē frak′shŭr) Fracture of the shaft of the radius with dislocation of the distal radioulnar joint. See page B25.

ga•len•i•cals (gā-len′i-kălz) **1.** Herbs and other vegetable drugs, as distinguished from the mineral or chemical remedies. **2.** Crude drugs and the tinctures, decoctions, and other preparations made from them, as distinguished from the alkaloids and other active principles. **3.** Remedies prepared according to an official formula.

Gal•la•var•din phe•nom•e•non (gah-lah-vahr′din fĕ-nom′ĕ-non) Dissociation between the noisy and musical elements of the ejection murmur of aortic stenosis, the musical element being better heard at the left sternal border and at the cardiac apex whereas the noisy element is better heard at the aortic area; projection of the aortic stenotic murmur to the low left sternal edge.

gall•blad•der (gawl′blad-ĕr) A pear-shaped receptacle on the inferior surface of the liver, in a hollow between the right lobe and the quadrate lobe; it serves as a storage reservoir for bile. See page B21. SYN vesica biliaris [TA], cholecyst, cholecystis.

Gal•le•go dif•fer•en•ti•at•ing so•lu•tion (gah-yā′gō sŏ-lū′shŭn) A dilute solution of formaldehyde and acetic acid used in a modified Gram stain to differentiate and enhance the basic fuchsin binding to gram-negative microorganisms.

Gal•lie trans•plant (gal′ē trans′plant) Narrow strips of the femoral fascia lata used for suture material.

gal•li•um (Ga) (gal′ē-ŭm) A rare metal; atomic no. 31, atomic wt. 69.723. [L. *Gallia,* France]

gal•li•um 67 (gal′ē-ŭm) A cyclotron-produced radionuclide with a half-life of 3.260 days and major gamma ray emissions; as a tumor- and inflammation-localizing radiotracer.

gal•li•um 68 (gal′ē-ŭm) A positron emitter with a radioactive half-life of 1.130 hours.

gal•lon (gal′ŏn) A measure of U.S. liquid capacity containing 4 quarts, 231 cubic inches, or 8.3293 pounds of distilled water at 20°C; it is the equivalent of 3.785412 liters. The British imperial gallon contains 277.4194 cubic inches. [O.Fr. *galon*]

gal•lop, **gal•lop rhythm** (gal′ŏp, gal′ŏp ridh′ŭm) A triple cadence to the heart sounds due to an abnormal third or fourth heart sound being heard in addition to the first and second sounds; sometimes indicative of serious disease. SYN cantering rhythm, Traube bruit.

gall•stone (gawl′stōn) A concretion in the gallbladder or a bile duct, composed chiefly of a mixture of cholesterol, calcium bilirubinate, and calcium carbonate, occasionally as a pure stone composed of just one of these substances. SYN cholelith.

gal•lus ad•e•no•like vi•rus (gal′ŭs ad′ĕ-nō-līk vī′rŭs) SYN GAL virus.

Gal•ton law (gawl′tŏn law) In a population mating at random, the progeny of a parent with an extreme value for a measurable phenotype will tend on average to have values nearer the population mean than in the extreme parent.

Gal•ton sys•tem of clas•si•fi•ca•tion of fin•ger•prints (gawl′tŏn sis′tĕm klas′i-fi-kā′shŭn fing′gĕr-prints) A classification scheme based on the variations in the patterns of the ridges, which are grouped into arches, loops, and whorls. SEE ALSO dermatoglyphics.

Gal•ton whis•tle (gawl′tŏn wis′ĕl) A cylindric whistle, attached to a compressible bulb, with a screw attachment that changes the frequency; used to test hearing.

gal•van•ic cur•rent (gal-van′ik kŭr′rĕnt) Low-voltage direct current.

gal•van•ic skin re•sponse (GSR) (gal-van′ik skin rĕ-spons′) A measure of changes in emotional arousal recorded by attaching electrodes to any part of the skin and recording changes in moment-to-moment perspiration and related autonomic nervous system activity.

gal•va•nom•e•ter (gal′vă-nom′ĕ-ter) An instrument for measuring the strength of an electric current.

GAL vi•rus (gal vī′rŭs) Fowl adenovirus not known to be pathogenic for humans. SYN gallus adenolike virus.

Gam•bi•an try•pan•o•so•mi•a•sis (gam′bē-ăn trī-pan′ō-sō-mī′ă-sis) A chronic disease of humans caused by *Trypanosoma brucei gambiense* in Africa; characterized by splenomegaly, drowsiness, an uncontrollable urge to sleep, and the development of psychotic changes; basal ganglia and cerebellar involvement commonly lead to chorea and athetosis; the terminal phase of the disease is characterized by wasting, anorexia, and emaciation that gradually leads to coma and death, usually from intercurrent infection. SYN chronic trypanosomiasis.

game•keep•er's thumb (gām′kēp-ĕrz thŭmb) Rupture of the volar ligament at the first metacarpophalangeal joint due to forceful abduction of the thumb while extended.

ga•mete (gam′ēt) **1.** One of two haploid cells undergoing karyogamy. **2.** Any germ cell, whether oocyte or sperm. [G. *gametēs,* husband; *gametē,* wife]

ga•mete in•tra•fal•lo•pi•an trans•fer (GIFT) (gam′ēt in′tră-fă-lō′pē-ăn trans′fĕr) Placement of the oocyte and sperm into the ampulla of the fallopian tube; a form of assisted reproduction.

gameto- Combining form meaning a gamete. [G. *gametēs*, husband, *gametē*, wife, fr. *gameō*, to marry]

ga•me•to•cide (gă-mē′tō-sīd) An agent destructive of gametes, specifically the malarial gametocytes. [gameto- + L. *caedo,* to kill]

ga•me•to•cyte (gă-mē′tō-sīt) A cell capable of dividing to produce gametes, e.g., a spermatocyte or oocyte. [gameto- + G. *kytos,* cell]

ga•me•to•gen•e•sis (gam′ĕ-tō-jen′ĕ-sis) The process of formation and development of gametes. [gameto- + G. *genesis,* production]

gam•ma (γ) (gam′ă) **1.** Third letter in the Greek alphabet. **2.** CHEMISTRY the third in a series, the fourth carbon in an aliphatic acid, or position 2 removed from the α position in the benzene ring. **3.** Symbol for 10^{-4} gauss. **4.** For terms with the prefix γ, see the specific term.

gamma (γ)-a•mi•no•bu•tyr•ic ac•id (GABA) (gam′ă ă-mē′nō-byū-tēr′ik as′id) 4-aminobutyric acid; The principal inhibitory neurotransmitter, used in the treatment of epilepsy.

gam•ma an•gle (gam′ă ang′gĕl) The angle formed between a line joining the fixation point to the center of the eye and the optic axis.

gam•ma (γ)-be•ta (β)-D-ri•bo•fur•a•no•syl•ad•e•nine (gam′ă bā′tă rī-bō-fyūr′ă-nō-sil-ad′ĕ-nēn) SYN adenosine (2).

gam•ma-bu•ty•ro•lac•tone (GBL) (gam′ă-byū′tir-ō-lak′tōn) An industrial and household solvent that is readily metabolized after oral ingestion to gamma-hydroxybutyrate (GHB). Like GHB, it is marketed illicitly as a euphoriant, appetite suppressant, antidepressant, and sleep aid. It is more potent than GHB and has both a more rapid onset and a longer duration of action, but its pharmacologic and toxic properties are essentially the same: nausea, bradycardia, and CNS depression ranging from drowsiness and confusion to seizures, coma, and death. Dependency and severe withdrawal symptoms have been reported.

gam•ma cam•er•a (gam′ă kam′ĕr-ă) Any one of several scintigraphic cameras that record simultaneously counts from the entire operative field of view. See page B23. SYN scintillation camera.

gam•ma fi•bers (gam′ă fī′bĕrz) Nerve fibers that have a conduction rate of about 20 m/sec.

Gam•ma•her•pes•vir•i•nae (gam′ă-her′pēz-vir′i-nē) A subfamily of Herpesviridae containing Epstein-Barr virus and others that cause lymphoproliferation.

gam•ma (γ)-hy•drox•y•bu•ty•rate (GHB) (gam′a hī-drok′sē-byū′tir-āt) A naturally occurring short-chain fatty acid, a metabolite of γ-aminobutyric acid (GABA) found in all body tissues, with the highest concentration in the brain; it affects levels of GABA, dopamine, 5-hydroxytryptamine, and acetylcholine, and may itself be a neurotransmitter. Accumulation of GHB in people with an inherited disorder in the metabolism of GABA causes ataxia and mental retardation. Synthetic GHB, formerly used in anesthesia and in the treatment of narcolepsy and alcohol withdrawal, has been banned by the U.S. Food and Drug Administration because of severe neurologic, cardiovascular, respiratory, and gastrointestinal side effects. SYN 4-hydroxybutyrate.

gam•ma knife (gam′ă nīf) A minimally invasive radiosurgical system used in the treatment of benign and malignant intracranial neoplasms and arteriovenous malformations.

gam•ma low•er mo•tor neu•ron (gam′ă lō′ ĕr mō′tŏr nūr′on) SYN gamma motor neuron.

gam•ma mo•tor neu•ron (gam′ă mō′tŏr nūr′ on) Motor neuron that terminates in skeletal muscle, and synapses with sensory neuromuscular spindles. Gamma motor neurons work with neuromuscular spindles to regulate skeletal muscle tone below levels of conscious control. Cf. alpha (α) motor neuron. SYN gamma lower motor neuron.

gam•ma ra•di•a•tion (gam′ă rā′dē-ā′shŭn) Ionizing electromagnetic radiation resulting from nuclear processes, such as radioactive decay or fission.

gam•ma ray (gam′ă rā) Electromagnetic radiation emitted from radioactive substances; they are high-energy x-rays but originate from the nucleus rather than the orbital shell and are not deflected by a magnet.

gam•mop•a•thy (gă-mop′ă-thē) A primary disturbance in immunoglobulin synthesis.

Gam•na dis•ease (gahm′nă di-zēz′) A form of chronic splenomegaly characterized by conspicuous thickening of the capsule and the presence of multiple, small, rustlike, brown foci (Gamna-Gandy bodies), which contain iron; this condition may be observed in fibrocongestive splenomegaly, sickle cell disease, and some examples of hemochromatosis.

gam•o•gen•e•sis (gam′ō-jen′ĕ-sis) SYN sexual reproduction. [G. *gamos,* marriage, + *genesis,* production]

gan•gli•a (gang′glē-ă) Plural of ganglion.

gan•gli•a of au•to•nom•ic plex•us•es (gang′glē-ă aw′tō-nom′ik plek′sŭs-ĕz) Autonomic ganglia lying in plexuses of autonomic fibers (e.g., the celiac and inferior mesenteric ganglia of the sympathetic, and the small parasympathetic ganglia of the myenteric plexus). SYN ganglia plexuum autonomicorum.

gan•gli•al (gang′glē-ăl) SYN ganglionic.

gan•gli•a plex•u•um au•to•no•mi•co•rum (gang′glē-ă pleks′yū-ŭm aw-tō-nō-mī-kō′rŭm) SYN ganglia of autonomic plexuses.

gan•gli•a of sym•pa•thet•ic trunk (gang′ glē-ă sim′pă-thet′ik trŭngk) The clusters of postganglionic neurons located at intervals along the sympathetic trunks, including the superior cervical, middle cervical, and cervicothoracic (stellate) ganglion, the thoracic, lumbar, and sacral ganglia, and the ganglion impar. SYN ganglia trunci sympathici, paravertebral ganglia.

gan•gli•ate, gan•gli•at•ed (gang′glē-āt, gang′ glē-ā-tĕd) Having ganglia. SYN ganglionated.

gan•gli•at•ed nerve (gang′glē-ā-tĕd nĕrv) A sympathetic nerve.

gan•gli•a trun•ci sym•pa•thi•ci (gang′glē-ă trŭn′sī sim-path′i-sī) SYN ganglia of sympathetic trunk.

gan•gli•ec•to•my (gang′glē-ek′tŏ-mē) SYN ganglionectomy.

gan•gli•form (gang′gli-fōrm) Having the form or appearance of a ganglion. SYN ganglioform.

gan•gli•i•tis (gang′glē-ī′tis) SYN ganglionitis.

gan•gli•o•blast (gang′glē-ō-blast) An embryonic cell from which ganglion cells develop. [ganglion + G. *blastos,* germ]

gan•gli•o•cyte (gang′glē-ō-sīt) SYN ganglion cell.

gan•gli•o•cy•to•ma (gang′glē-ō-sī-tō′mă) A rare lesion that contains neuronal (ganglion) cells in a sparse glial stoma. SYN central ganglioneuroma. [ganglion + G. *kytos*, cell, + *-oma*, tumor]

gan•gli•o•form (gang′glē-ō-fōrm) SYN gangliform.

gan•gli•o•gli•o•ma (gang′glē-ō-glē-ō′mă) A rare tumor consisting of a glioma component and an atypical neuronal (ganglion) cell component; in younger patients often associated with seizures.

gan•gli•ol•y•sis (gang′glē-ol′i-sis) The dissolution or breaking up of a ganglion.

gan•gli•o•ma (gang′glē-ō′mă) SYN ganglioneuroma.

gan•gli•on, pl. **gan•gli•a, gan•gli•ons** (gang′glē-ŏn, -ă, -onz) **1.** [TA] An aggregation of nerve cell bodies located in the peripheral nervous system. SYN neuroganglion. **2.** A cyst containing mucopolysaccharide-rich fluid within a fibrous capsule; usually attached to a tendon sheath in the hand, wrist, or foot, or connected with the underlying joint. SYN myxoid cyst, synovial cyst. See page 623. [G. a swelling or knot]

gan•gli•on•at•ed (gang′glē-ō-nā-tĕd) SYN gangliate.

gan•gli•on cell (gang′glē-ŏn sel) A neuron the cell body of which is located outside the limits of the brain and spinal cord, hence forming part of the peripheral nervous system; ganglion cells are either 1) the pseudounipolar cells of the sensory spinal and cranial nerves (sensory ganglia), or 2) the peripheral multipolar motor neurons innervating the viscera (visceral or autonomic ganglia). SYN gangliocyte.

gan•gli•on cer•vi•co•thor•a•ci•cum (gang′ glē-ŏn sĕr′vi-kō-thō-ras′i-kŭm) [TA] SYN cervicothoracic ganglion.

gan•gli•on cyst (gang′glē-ŏn sist) Collection of

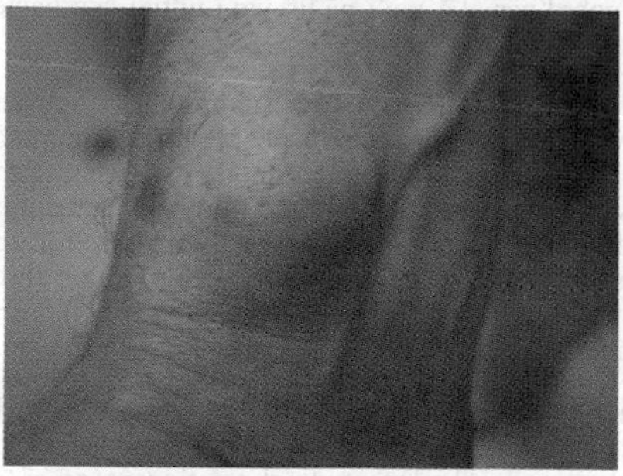

ganglion: wrist

fluid or benign tumor mass within tendons of the wrist or ankle, most commonly on the dorsal aspect of the wrist.

gan•gli•on•ec•to•my (gang′glē-ō-nek′tŏ-mē) Excision of a ganglion. SYN gangliectomy. [ganglion + G. *ektomē,* excision]

gan•gli•o•neu•ro•blas•to•ma (gang′lē-ō-nūr′ō-blas-tō′ma) A tumor of mixed cellular type, with elements of neuroblastoma and ganglioneuroma.

gan•gli•o•neu•ro•ma (gang′glē-ō-nūr-ō′mă) A benign neoplasm composed of mature ganglionic neurons, in varying numbers, scattered singly or in clumps within a relatively abundant and dense stroma of neurofibrils and collagenous fibers; usually found in the posterior mediastinum and retroperitoneum, sometimes in relation to the suprarenal glands. SYN ganglioma. [ganglion + G. *neuron,* nerve, + *-oma,* tumor]

gan•gli•on•ic (gang′glē-on′ik) Relating to a ganglion. SYN ganglial.

gan•gli•on•ic block•ade (gang′glē-on′ik blok-ād′) Inhibition of nerve impulse transmission at autonomic ganglionic synapses by drugs such as nicotine or hexamethonium.

gan•gli•on•ic block•ing a•gent (gang′glē-on′ik blok′ing ā′jĕnt) An agent that impairs the passage of impulses in autonomic ganglia.

gan•gli•on•ic branch•es of max•il•lar•y nerve (gang′glē-on′ik branch′ĕz mak′si-lar-ē nĕrv) The ganglionic branches, two short sensory branches of the maxillary nerve in the pterygopalatine fossa, the fibers of which pass through the pterygopalatine ganglion without synapse. SYN nervi pterygopalatini [TA].

gan•gli•on•ic branch of in•ter•nal ca•rot•id ar•ter•y (gang′glē-on′ik branch in-tĕr′năl kă-rot′id ahr′tĕr-ē) Branch to trigeminal ganglion; a small branch of the cavernous part of the internal carotid artery to the trigeminal ganglion.

gan•gli•on im•par (gang′glē-ŏn im′pahr) The most inferior, unpaired ganglion of the sympathetic trunk; inconstant. SYN coccygeal ganglion, Walther ganglion.

gan•gli•on in•fe•ri•us ner•vi va•gi (gang′glē-ŏn in-fē′rē-ŭs nĕr′vī vā′jī) [TA] SYN inferior ganglion of vagus nerve.

gan•gli•on•i•tis (gang′glē-ŏn-ī′tis) **1.** Inflammation of a lymphatic ganglion. **2.** Inflammation of a nerve ganglion. SYN gangliitis.

gan•gli•o•nos•to•my (gang′glē-ŏn-os′tŏ-mē) Making a surgical opening into a ganglion (2). [ganglion + G. *stoma,* mouth]

gan•gli•o•ple•gic (gang′glē-ō-plē′jik) A pharmacologic compound that paralyzes an autonomic ganglion, usually for a relatively short time. [ganglion + G. *plēgē,* stroke, shock]

gan•gli•o•side (gang′glē-ō-sīd) A glycosphingolipid chemically similar to cerebrosides but containing one or more sialic acid residues; found principally in nerve tissue, spleen, and thymus; G_{M1} accumulates in generalized gangliosidosis; G_{M2} accumulates in Tay-Sachs disease.

gan•gli•o•si•do•sis (gang′glē-ō-si-dō′sis) Any disease characterized, in part, by the abnormal accumulation within the nervous system of specific gangliosides (e.g., G_{M2} gangliosidosis, Tay-Sachs disease), caused by hexosaminidase A enzyme deficiency with accumulation of G_{M2} ganglioside.

gang rape (gang rāp) Forcible sexual congress involving intrusive contact perpetrated by a group (nearly always male) on a nonconsenting victim.

gan•grene (gang-grēn′) **1.** Necrosis due to obstruction, loss, or diminution of blood supply; it may be localized to a small area or involve an entire extremity or organ (e.g., bowel), and may be wet or dry. SYN mortification. **2.** Extensive necrosis from any cause, e.g., gas gangrene. See this page. [G. *gangraina,* an eating sore, fr. *graō,* to gnaw]

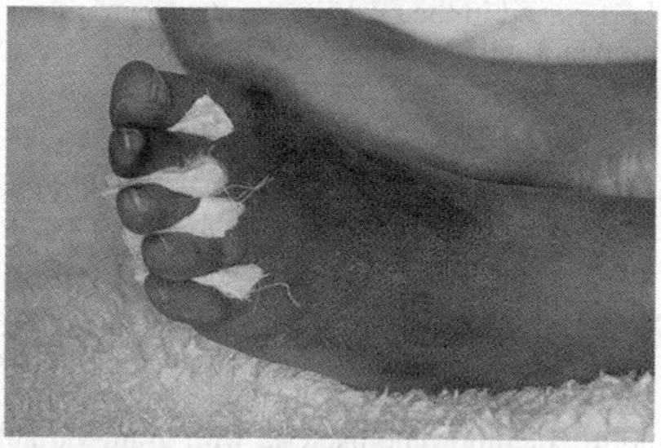

gangrene of the toes: result of severe ischemia

gan•gre•nous (gang′grĕ-nŭs) Relating to or affected with gangrene. SYN mortified.

gan•gre•nous sto•ma•ti•tis (gang′grĕ-nŭs

stō′mă-tī′tis) Condition characterized by necrosis of oral tissue. SEE noma.

Gan•ser syn•drome (gahn′ser sin′drōm) A psychotic-like condition, without the symptoms and signs of a traditional psychosis, occurring typically in prisoners who feign insanity; e.g., such a person, when asked to multiply 6 by 4, may give 23 as the answer, or will call a key a lock.

Gant clamp (gant klamp) A right-angled clamp used in hemorrhoidectomy.

gan•try (gan′trē) A frame housing the x-ray tube, collimators, and detectors in a CT machine, with a large opening into which the patient is inserted; a mechanical support for mounting a device to be moved in a circular path. [M.E., fr. O. Fr., fr. L. *cantherius,* wooden frame, fr. G. *kanthēlia,* pack saddle, fr. *kanthos,* pack ass]

gap (gap) **1.** A hiatus or opening in a structure. **2.** An interval or discontinuity in any series or sequence. **3.** (G) A period in the cell cycle.

gap 1 (gap) In the somatic cell cycle, the pause that follows mitosis and is followed by synthesis in preparation for the next cycle.

gap 2 (gap) In the somatic cell cycle, a pause between completion of synthesis and the onset of cell division.

gap junc•tion (gap jŭngk′shŭn) **1.** An intercellular junction having a 2-nm gap between apposed cell membranes; the gap contains subunits in the form of polygonal lattices; it occurs in epithelia, between certain nerve cells, and in smooth and cardiac muscle. SEE ALSO synapse. **2.** Areas of increased electrochemical communication between myometrial cells that aid in the propagation of the contractions of labor. SYN nexus.

gap pe•ri•od (gap pēr′ē-ŏd) Phase of a cell no longer in the cell cycle and thus at least temporarily incapable of division.

gap phe•nom•e•non (gap fĕ-nom′ĕ-non) A short period in the cycle of the atrioventricular or intraventricular conduction allowing passage of an impulse that at other times would be blocked in transit.

Gard•ner-Di•a•mond syn•drome (gahrd′nĕr dī′mŏnd sin′drōm) SYN autoerythrocyte sensitization syndrome.

Gard•ner•el•la (gahrd-nĕr-el′ă) A genus of facultatively anaerobic, oxidase- and catalase-negative, non-spore-forming, nonencapsulated, nonmotile, pleomorphic bacteria with gram-variable rods.

Gard•ner•el•la vag•i•na•lis (gahrd-nĕr-el′ă vaj-i-nā′lis) A species that is the etiologic agent of bacterial vaginosis.

***Gard•ner•el•la vag•i•na•lis* vag•i•ni•tis** (gahrd′nĕr-el′ă vaj′i-nā′lis vaj′i-nī′tis) SEE bacterial vaginosis.

Gard•ner syn•drome (gahrd′nĕr sin′drōm) Multiple polyposis predisposing to carcinoma of the colon; also multiple tumors, osteomas of the skull, epidermoid cysts, and fibromas; autosomal dominant inheritance, caused by mutation in the adenomatous polyposis coli gene (APC) on chromosome 5q. This disorder is allelic to familial adenomatous polyposis.

Gard•ner-Wells tongs (gahrd′nĕr-welz tawngz) A metal fixation device attached to the skull to apply longitudinal traction in cases of cervical fracture. See this page.

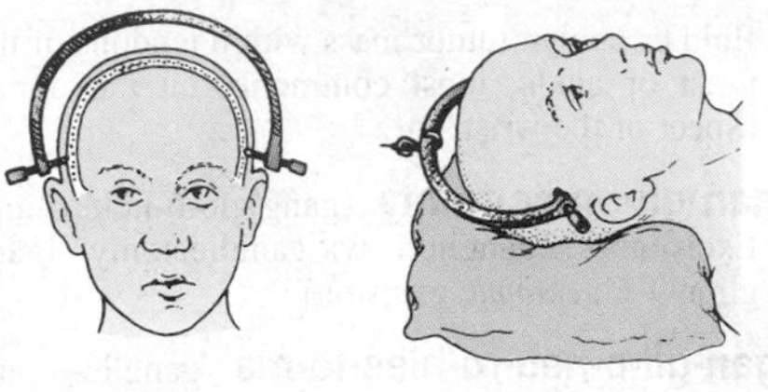

Gardner-Wells traction tongs: used for cervical traction

gar•gle (gahr′gĕl) **1.** To rinse the fauces with fluid through which expired breath is forced to produce a bubbling effect while the head is held far back. **2.** A medicated fluid used for gargling; a throat wash. [O. Fr., fr. L. *gurgulio,* gullet, windpipe]

gar•goyl•ism (gahr′goyl-izm) A grossly offensive term describing appearance of patients suffering the constellation of symptoms and findings associated with Hurler syndrome (q.v.).

Ga•ri•el pes•sa•ry (gahr-ē-el′ pes′ă-rē) An hollow inflatable rubber pessary made in the form of a ring or a pear.

Gar•land tri•an•gle (gahr′lănd trī′ang-gĕl) A triangular area of relative resonance in the lower back near the spine, found on the same side as a pleural effusion.

gar•lic (gahr′lik) A herbal product promoted for treatment of vascular disease, dyslipidemias, and hypertension.

Gar•ré dis•ease (gah-rā′ di-zēz′) SYN sclerosing osteitis.

Gar•ré os•te•o•my•e•li•tis (gah-rā′ os′tē-ō-mī-ĕ-lī′tis) Chronic osteomyelitis with proliferative periostitis. A focal gross thickening of the periosteum with peripheral reactive bone formation resulting from mild infection.

Gart•ner cyst (gahrt′nĕr sist) A lesion of the principal duct in the vestigial structures of the paroophoron in the cervix or anterolateral vaginal wall, corresponding to the sexual portion of mesonephros in the male. SYN Gartner duct cyst.

Gart•ner duct cyst (gahrt′nĕr dŭkt sist) SYN Gartner cyst.

Gärt•ner meth•od (gārt′ner meth′ŏd) A method of measuring venous pressure, based on Gärtner vein phenomenon; with the patient sitting erect, a vein is selected on the back of the hand, which is held dependent, well below the level of the right atrium, and then is raised slowly; when the vein is observed to collapse, the distance between its level and that of the atrium is measured with a millimeter rule; this distance gives the venous pressure in millimeters of blood; thus the vein itself is used as a manometer communicating with the right atrium; highly inaccurate, especially in elderly patients.

Gärt•ner to•nom•e•ter (gārt′ner tō-nom′ĕ-ter) An apparatus for estimating the blood pressure by noting the force, expressed by the height of a column of mercury, needed to arrest pulsation in a finger encircled by a compressing ring.

gas (gas) **1.** Fluid, like air, capable of indefinite expansion but convertible by compression and cold into a liquid and, eventually, a solid. **2.** In clinical practice, a substance entirely in its vapor phase at 1 atmosphere of pressure because ambient temperature is above its boiling point.

gas ab•scess (gas ab′ses) An abscess containing gas caused by *Enterobacter aerogenes*, *Escherichia coli*, or other microorganisms.

gas ba•cil•lus (gas bă-sil′ŭs) SYN *Clostridium perfringens.*

gas chro•ma•tog•ra•phy (gas krō′mă-tog′ră-fē) A chromatographic procedure in which the mobile phase is a mixture of gases or vapors, which are separated by their differential adsorption on a stationary phase.

gas em•bo•lism (gas em′bŏ-lizm) Occlusion of one or more small blood vessels, especially in muscles, tendons, and joints, caused by expanding gas bubbles.

gas•e•ous (gas′ē-ŭs) Of the nature of gas.

gas ex•change in•dex (gas eks-chānj′ in′deks) Assessment tool to gauge respiration.

gas gan•grene (gas gang-grēn′) Gangrene occurring in a wound that is infected with various anaerobic spore-forming bacteria, especially *Clostridium perfringens* and *C. novyi*, which cause crepitation of the surrounding tissues, due to gas liberated by bacterial fermentation, and constitutional septic symptoms.

Gas•kell clamp (gas′kĕl klamp) An instrument for crushing the atrioventricular bundle in experimental animals and thus producing heart block.

gas-liq•uid chro•ma•tog•ra•phy (GLC) (gas-lik′wid krō′mă-tog′ră-fē) A chromatographic technique in which the mobile phase is an inert gas and the stationary phase is liquid rather than solid.

gas mask (gas mask) A device worn over the nose and mouth as protection against airborne toxic gases.

gas•o•met•ric (gas′ō-met′rik) Relating to gasometry.

gas•om•e•try (gas-om′ĕ-trē) Measurement of gases; determination of the relative proportion of gases in a mixture.

gas per•i•to•ni•tis (gas per′i-tŏ-nī′tis) Inflammation of the peritoneum accompanied by an intraperitoneal accumulation of gas.

gas•sing (gas′ing) Poisoning by irrespirable or otherwise noxious gases.

gas•ter (gas′tĕr) [TA] SYN stomach. [G. *gastēr,* belly]

gas•trad•e•ni•tis (gas′trad-ĕ-nī′tis) Inflammation of the glands of the stomach. [gastr- + G. *adēn,* gland, + *-itis,* inflammation]

gas•trec•ta•sis, **gas•trec•ta•si•a** (gas-trek′tă-sis, gas-trek-tā′zē-ă) Dilation of the stomach. [gastr- + G. *ektasis,* extension]

gas•trec•to•my (gas-trek′tŏ-mē) Excision of a part or all of the stomach. [gastr- + G. *ektomē,* excision]

gas•tric (gas′trik) Relating to the stomach.

gas•tric a•nal•y•sis (gas′trik ă-nal′i-sis) Measurement of pH and acid output of stomach contents; basal acid output can be determined by collecting the overnight gastric secretion or by a 1-hour collection; maximal acid output is determined following injection of histamine; output is measured by titration with a strong base.

gas•tric ar•ter•ies (gas′trik ahr′tĕr-ēz) Arteries supplying the stomach along the lesser curvature.

gas•tric by•pass (gas′trik bī′pas) High division of the stomach, anastomosis of the small upper pouch of the stomach to the jejunum, and closure of the distal part of the stomach that is retained; used for treatment of morbid obesity. See page 626.

gas•tric di•ges•tion (gas′trik di-jes′chŭn) That part of digestion, chiefly of the proteins, carried on in the stomach by the enzymes of the gastric juice. SYN peptic digestion.

gas•tric feed•ing (gas′trik fēd′ing) Giving of nutriment directly into the stomach by means of a tube inserted through the nasopharynx and esophagus or directly through the abdominal wall.

gas•tric fis•tu•la (gas′trik fis′chū-lă) A fistulous tract from the stomach to the abdominal wall.

gas•tric fol•li•cle (gas′trik fol′i-kĕl) SYN gastric glands.

gas•tric glands (gas′trik glandz) Branched tu-

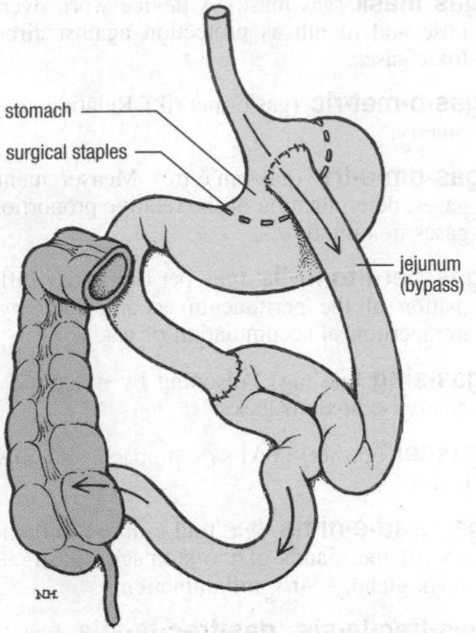

gastric bypass: in the gastrojejunostomy procedure, a small stomach pouch is created to limit food intake and the jejunum is attached to the pouch, allowing food to bypass the lower stomach, thus reducing the amount of nutrients and calories absorbed

bular glands lying in the mucosa of the fundus and body of the stomach; such glands contain parietal cells that secrete hydrochloric acid, zymogen cells that produce pepsin, and mucous cells. SYN gastric follicle.

gas•tric in•di•ges•tion (gas′trik in′di-jes′chŭn) SYN dyspepsia.

gas•tric in•hib•i•to•ry pol•y•pep•tide (GIP), gas•tric in•hib•i•to•ry pep•tide (GIP) (gas′trik in-hib′i-tōr-ē pol′ē-pep′tīd, pep′tīd) A peptide hormone, secreted by the stomach, which stimulates intestinal secretions and insulin release as part of the digestive process; GIP inhibits the secretion of acids and of pepsin.

gas•tric la•vage (gas′trik lă-vahzh′) Washing out the stomach with water or saline solution. Performed to remove ingested poisons and also to empty the stomach before general anesthesia. SEE ALSO lavage.

gas•tric sta•pling (gas′trik stāp′ling) Partitioning of the stomach by rows of staples; used to treat morbid obesity.

gas•tric tet•a•ny (gas′trik tet′ă-nē) Tetany associated with a gastric disorder, especially with loss of HCl by vomiting.

gas•tric ul•cer (gas′trik ŭl′sĕr) An ulcer of the stomach. See this page. SYN Cruveilhier ulcer.

gas•tric ver•ti•go (gas′trik vĕr′ti-gō) Sensation of imbalance symptomatic of disease of the stomach.

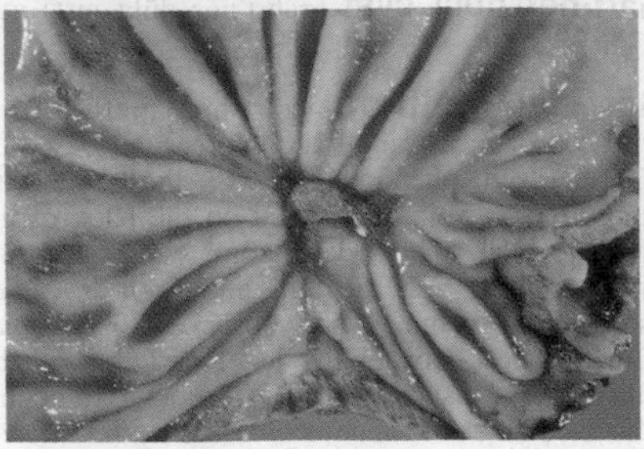

gastric ulcer: base of ulcer is gray owing to fibrin deposition

gas•tri•no•ma (gas′tri-nō′mă) A gastrin-secreting tumor associated with the Zollinger-Ellison syndrome.

gas•trins (gas′trinz) Hormones secreted in the pyloric-antral mucosa of the mammalian stomach that stimulate secretion of HCl by the parietal cells of the gastric glands; a competitive inhibitor of gastrins is cholecystokinin. [G. *gastēr*, stomach, + -in]

gas•tri•tis (gas-trī′tis) Inflammation, especially mucosal, of the stomach. [gastr- + G. *-itis*, inflammation]

gastro-, gastr- Combining forms meaning the stomach, abdomen. [G. *gastēr*, the belly]

gas•tro•a•nas•to•mo•sis (gas′trō-an-as-tō-mō′sis) Anastomosis of the cardiac and antral segments of the stomach, for relief from marked hour-glass contraction of the stomach. SYN gastrogastrostomy.

gas•tro•car•di•ac (gas′trō-kahr′dē-ak) Relating to both the stomach and the heart.

gas•tro•cele (gas′trō-sēl) Hernia of part of the stomach. [gastro- + G. *kēlē*, hernia]

gas•troc•ne•mi•us (gas′trok-nē′mē-ŭs) SYN gastrocnemius muscle. [G. *gastroknēmia*, calf of the leg, fr. *gaster* (*gastr-*), belly, + *knēmē*, leg]

gas•troc•ne•mi•us mus•cle (gas′trok-nē′mē-ŭs mŭs′ĕl) *Origin*, by two heads (lateral and medial) from the lateral and medial condyles of the femur; *insertion*, with soleus by tendo calcaneus into lower half of posterior surface of calcaneus; *action*, plantar flexion of foot; *nerve supply*, tibial. SYN musculus gastrocnemius [TA], gastrocnemius.

gas•tro•co•lic (gas′trō-kol′ik) Relating to the stomach and the colon.

gas•tro•co•lic re•flex (gas′trō-kol′ik rē′fleks) A mass movement of the contents of the colon, frequently preceded by a similar movement in the small intestine, which sometimes occurs immediately following the entrance of food into the stomach.

gas·tro·co·li·tis (gas′trō-kō-lī′tis) Inflammation of both stomach and colon.

gas·tro·co·los·to·my (gas′trō-kŏ-los′tŏ-mē) Establishment of a communication between stomach and colon. [gastro- + G. *kōlon,* colon, + *stoma,* mouth]

gas·tro·du·o·de·nal (gas′trō-dū-ō-dē′năl) Relating to the stomach and duodenum.

gas·tro·du·o·de·nal ar·ter·y (gas′trō-dū-ō-dē′năl ahr′tĕr-ē) *Origin*, hepatic; terminal *branches,* right gastroepiploic, superior pancreaticoduodenal. SYN arteria gastroduodenalis [TA].

gas·tro·du·o·de·ni·tis (gas′trō-dū-ō-dĕ-nī′tis) Inflammation of both stomach and duodenum.

gas·tro·du·o·de·nos·co·py (gas′trō-dū-ō-dĕ-nos′kŏ-pē) Visualization of the interior of the stomach and duodenum by a gastroscope. [gastro- + duodenum, + G. *skopeō,* to view]

gas·tro·du·o·de·nos·to·my (gas′trō-dū-ō-dĕ-nos′tŏ-mē) Establishment of a communication between the stomach and the duodenum. [gastro- + duodenum + G. *stoma,* mouth]

gas·tro·en·ter·ic (gas′trō-en-ter′ik) SYN gastrointestinal.

gas·tro·en·ter·i·tis (gas′trō-en-tĕr-ī′tis) Inflammation of the mucous membrane of both stomach and intestine. SYN enterogastritis. [gastro- + G. *enteron,* intestine, + *-itis,* inflammation]

gas·tro·en·ter·i·tis vi·rus type A (gas′trō-en-tĕr-ī′tis vī′rŭs tīp) SYN epidemic gastroenteritis virus.

gas·tro·en·ter·i·tis vi·rus type B (gas′trō-en-tĕr-ī′tis vī′rŭs tīp) SYN Rotavirus.

gas·tro·en·ter·o·co·li·tis (gas′trō-en′tĕr-ō-kō-lī′tis) Inflammatory disease involving the stomach and intestines. [gastro- + G. *enteron,* intestine, + *kōlon,* colon, + *-itis,* inflammation]

gas·tro·en·ter·ol·o·gist (gas′trō-en-tĕr-ol′ŏ-jist) A specialist in gastroenterology.

gas·tro·en·ter·ol·o·gy (gas′trō-en-tĕr-ol′ŏ-jē) The medical specialty concerned with the function and disorders of the gastrointestinal tract, including stomach, intestines, and associated organs. [gastro- + G. *enteron,* intestine, + *logos,* study]

gas·tro·en·ter·op·a·thy (gas′trō-en-tĕr-op′ă-thē) Any disorder of the alimentary canal. [gastro- + G. *enteron,* intestine, + *pathos,* suffering]

gas·tro·en·ter·o·plas·ty (gas′trō-en′tĕr-ō-plas-tē) Operative repair of defects in the stomach and intestine. [gastro- + G. *enteron,* intestine, + *plassō,* to form]

gas·tro·en·ter·op·to·sis (gas′trō-en-tĕr-op-tō′sis) Downward displacement of the stomach and a portion of the intestine. [gastro- + G. *enteron,* intestine, + *ptōsis,* a falling]

gas·tro·en·ter·os·to·my (gas′trō-en-tĕr-os′tŏ-mē) Establishment of a new opening between the stomach and the intestine, either anterior or posterior to the transverse colon. [gastro- + G. *enteron,* intestine, + *stoma,* mouth]

gas·tro·en·ter·ot·o·my (gas′trō-en-tĕr-ot′ŏ-mē) Section into both stomach and intestine. [gastro- + G. *enteron,* intestine, + *tomē,* incision]

gas·tro·ep·i·plo·ic (gas′trō-ep-i-plō′ik) Relating to the stomach and the greater omentum (epiploon).

gas·tro·ep·i·plo·ic ar·ter·ies (gas′trō-ep-i-plō′ik ahr′tĕr-ēz) SYN gastroomental arteries.

gas·tro·e·soph·a·ge·al (gas′trō-ĕ-sŏ-fă′jē-ăl) Relating to both stomach and esophagus. SYN gastro-oesophageal. [gastro- + G. *oisophagos,* gullet (esophagus)]

gas·tro·e·soph·a·ge·al her·ni·a (gas′trō-ĕ-sŏ-fă′jē-ăl hĕr′nē-ă) A hiatal hernia into the thorax. SYN gastro-oesophageal hernia.

gas·tro·e·soph·a·ge·al re·flux dis·ease (GERD) (gas′trō-ĕ-sŏ-fă′jē-ăl rē′flŭks di-zēz′) A syndrome of chronic or recurrent epigastric or retrosternal pain, accompanied by varying degrees of belching, nausea, cough, or hoarseness, due to reflux of acid gastric juice into the lower esophagus; results from malfunction of the lower esophageal sphincter (LES) and disordered gastric motility; may lead to peptic esophagitis, ulceration, stricture, or Barrett esophagus. SYN gastro-oesophageal reflux disease.

gas·tro·e·soph·a·gi·tis (gas′trō-ĕ-sof-ă-jī′tis) Inflammation of the stomach and esophagus. SYN gastro-oesophagitis.

gas·tro·e·soph·a·gos·to·my (gas′trō-ĕ-sof-ă-gos′tŏ-mē) SYN esophagogastrostomy. SYN gastro-oesophagostomy. [gastro- + G. *oisophagos,* gullet (esophagus), + *stoma,* mouth]

gas·tro·gas·tros·to·my (gas′trō-gas-tros′tŏ-mē) SYN gastroanastomosis.

gas·tro·ga·vage (gas′trō-gă-vahzh′) SYN gavage (1).

gas·tro·gen·ic (gas′trō-jen′ik) Deriving from or caused by the stomach.

gas·tro·he·pat·ic (gas′trō-he-pat′ik) Relating to the stomach and the liver. [gastro- + G. *hēpar* (*hēpat-*), liver]

gas·tro·il·e·ac re·flex (gas′trō-il′ē-ak rē′fleks) Opening of the ileocolic valve induced by entrance of food into the stomach.

gas·tro·il·e·i·tis (gas′trō-il-ē-ī′tis) Inflammation of the alimentary canal in which the stomach and ileum are primarily involved.

gas·tro·il·e·os·to·my (gas′trō-il-ē-os′tŏ-mē)

A surgical joining of stomach to ileum; a technical error in which the ileum instead of jejunum is selected for the site of a gastrojejunostomy.

gas·tro·in·tes·ti·nal (GI) (gas′trō-in-tes′ti-năl) Relating to the digestive tract from mouth to anus. SYN gastroenteric.

gas·tro·in·tes·ti·nal au·to·nom·ic nerve tu·mor (gas′trō-in-tes′ti-năl aw′tō-nom′ik nĕrv tū′mŏr) Benign or malignant tumor of stomach and small intestine histogenetically related to myenteric plexus; may be familial and related to gastrointestinal neuronal dysplasia.

gas·tro·in·tes·ti·nal (GI) tract (gas′trō-in-tes′ti-năl trakt) The stomach, small intestine, and large intestine; often used as a synonym of digestive tract.

gas·tro·in·tes·ti·nal stro·mal tu·mor (gas′trō-in-tes′ti-năl strō′măl tū′mŏr) Benign or malignant tumor composed of unclassifiable spindle cells; immunohistochemically distinct from smooth muscle and Schwann cell tumors.

gas·tro·je·ju·no·co·lic (gas′trō-jĕ-jū′nō-kol′ik) Referring to the stomach, jejunum, and colon.

gas·tro·je·ju·nos·to·my (gas′trō-jĕ-jū-nos′tŏ-mē) Establishment of a direct communication between the stomach and the jejunum. [gastro- + jejunum G. *stoma,* mouth]

gas·tro·li·e·nal (gas′trō-lī′ē-năl) SYN gastrosplenic. [gastro- + L. *lien,* spleen]

gas·tro·lith (gas′trō-lith) A concretion in the stomach. [gastro- + G. *lithos,* stone]

gas·tro·li·thi·a·sis (gas′trō-li-thī′ă-sis) Presence of one or more calculi in the stomach. [gastro- + G. *lithos,* stone + *-iasis,* condition]

gas·trol·y·sis (gas-trol′i-sis) Division of perigastric adhesions. [gastro- + G. *lysis,* loosening]

gas·tro·ma·la·ci·a (gas′trō-mă-lā′shē-ă) Softening of the walls of the stomach. [gastro- + G. *malakia,* softness]

gas·tro·meg·a·ly (gas′trō-meg′ă-lē) **1.** Enlargement of the stomach. **2.** Enlargement of the abdomen. [gastro- + G. *megas* (*megal-*), large]

gas·tro·myx·or·rhe·a (gas′trō-mik-sō-rē′ă) Excessive secretion of mucus in the stomach. SYN gastromyxorrhoea. [gastro- + G. *myxa,* mucus, + *rhoia,* a flow]

gastromyxorrhoea [Br.] SYN gastromyxorrhea.

gastro-oesophageal [Br.] SYN gastroesophageal.

gastro-oesophageal hernia [Br.] SYN gastroesophageal hernia.

gastro-oesophageal reflux [Br.] SYN gastroesophageal reflux.

gastro-oesophageal reflux disease [Br.] SYN gastroesophageal reflux disease.

gastro-oesophagitis [Br.] SYN gastroesophagitis.

gastro-oesophagostomy [Br.] SYN gastroesophagostomy.

gas·tro·o·men·tal ar·ter·ies (gas-trō′ō-men′tăl ahr′tĕr-ēz) Arteries that supply the stomach and greater omentum as they course along the greater curvature of the stomach. SYN gastroepiploic arteries.

gas·tro·pa·ral·y·sis (gas′trō-păr-al′i-sis) Paralysis of the muscular coat of the stomach.

gas·tro·pa·re·sis (gas′trō-păr-ē′sis) A slight degree of gastroparalysis. [gastro- + G. *paresis,* a letting go, paralysis]

gas·tro·path·ic (gas′trō-path′ik) Denoting gastropathy.

gas·trop·a·thy (gas-trop′ă-thē) Any disease of the stomach. [gastro- + G. *pathos,* disease]

gas·tro·pex·y (gas′trō-pek-sē) Attachment of the stomach to the abdominal wall or diaphragm. [gastro- + G. *pēxis,* fixation]

gas·tro·phren·ic (gas′trō-fren′ik) Relating to the stomach and the diaphragm. [gastro- + G. *phrēn,* diaphragm]

gas·tro·plas·ty (gas′trō-plas-tē) **1.** Surgical treatment of a defect in the stomach or lower esophagus that uses the stomach wall for the reconstruction. **2.** The production of a staple line across the upper portion of the stomach to limit uptake, used in cases of severe obesity. [gastro- + G. *plastos,* formed]

gas·tro·pli·ca·tion (gas′trō-pli-kā′shŭn) An operation to reduce the size of the stomach by suturing a longitudinal fold with the peritoneal surfaces in apposition. SYN gastrorrhaphy (2). [gastro- + L. *plico,* to fold]

gas·trop·to·sis, gas·trop·to·si·a (gas′trop-tō′sis, -tō′zē-ă) Downward displacement of the stomach. [gastro- + G. *ptosis,* a falling]

gas·tro·pul·mo·nar·y (gas′trō-pul′mŏ-nar-ē) SYN pneumogastric.

gas·tro·py·lor·ec·to·my (gas′trō-pī-lōr-ek′tŏ-mē) SYN pylorectomy.

gas·tro·py·lor·ic (gas′trō-pī-lōr′ik) Relating to the stomach as a whole and to the pylorus.

gas·tror·rha·gi·a (gas′trō-rā′jē-ă) Hemorrhage from the stomach. [gastro- + G. *rhēgnymi,* to burst forth]

gas·tror·rha·phy (gas-trōr′ă-fē) **1.** Suture of a perforation of the stomach. **2.** SYN gastroplication. [gastro- + G. *rhaphē,* a stitching]

gas·tror·rhe·a (gas′trōr-ē′ă) Excessive secretion of gastric juice or of mucus (gastromyxorrhea) by the stomach. SYN gastrorrhoea. [gastro- + G. *rhoia,* a flow]

gastrorrhoea [Br.] SYN gastrorrhea.

gas•tros•chi•sis (gas-tros′ki-sis) A defect in the anterior abdominal wall; usually accompanied by protrusion of viscera. [gastro- + G. *schisis,* a fissure]

gas•tro•scope (gas′trō-skōp) An endoscope for inspecting the inner surface of the stomach. [gastro- + G. *skopeō,* to examine]

gas•tro•scop•ic (gas′trō-skop′ik) Relating to gastroscopy.

gas•tros•co•py (gas-tros′kŏ-pē) Inspection of the inner surface of the stomach through an endoscope.

gas•tro•spasm (gas′trō-spazm) Spasmodic contraction of the walls of the stomach.

gas•tro•splen•ic (gas′trō-splen′ik) Relating to the stomach and the spleen. SYN gastrolienal.

gas•tro•stax•is (gas′trō-stak′sis) Oozing of blood from the mucous membrane of the stomach. [gastro- + G. *staxis,* trickling]

gas•tro•ste•no•sis (gas′trō-stĕ-nō′sis) Diminution in size of the cavity of the stomach. [gastro- + G. *stenōsis,* narrowing]

gas•tros•to•la•vage (gas-tros′tō-lă-vahzh′) Lavage of the stomach through a gastric fistula.

gas•tros•to•my (gas-tros′tŏ-mē) Establishment of a new opening into the stomach. [gastro- + G. *stoma,* mouth]

gas•tros•to•my tube (gas-tros′tŏ-mē tūb) SYN percutaneous endoscopic gastrostomy tube.

gas•trot•o•my (gas-trot′ŏ-mē) Incision into the stomach. [gastro- + G. *tomē,* incision]

gas•tro•to•nom•e•try (gas′trō-tō-nom′ĕ-trē) The measurement of intragastric pressure. [gastro- + G. *tonos,* tension, + *metron,* measure]

gas•tro•tro•pic (gas′trō-trō′pik) Affecting the stomach. [gastro- + G. *tropikos,* turning]

gas•tru•la (gas′trū-lă) The embryo in the stage of development following the blastula or blastocyst formation; in the human embryo, the absence of yolk allows for a rapid, direct "putting in place" of the germ layers (ectoderm and endoderm), which are derived from the pluripotential embryonic disc. [Mod. L. dim. of G. *gastēr,* belly]

gas•tru•la•tion (gas′trū-lā′shŭn) Transformation of the blastula or blastocyst into the gastrula; the development and invagination of the embryonic germ layers.

gate-con•trol the•o•ry (gāt′kŏn-trōl′ thē′ŏr-ē) A theory to explain the mechanism of pain; small-fiber afferent stimuli, particularly pain, entering the substantia gelatinosa can be modulated by large-fiber afferent stimuli and descending spinal pathways so that their transmission to ascending spinal pathways is blocked (gated).

gat•ed ra•di•o•nu•clide an•gi•o•car•di•og•ra•phy (gāt′ĕd rā′dē-ō-nū′klīd an′jē-ō-kahr-dē-og′ră-fē) Radionuclide angiocardiography using cardiac gating to combine images from several cardiac cycles to improve the quality of the images of separate phases (e.g., systole and diastole).

gate•keep•er (gāt′kēp-ĕr) A health care professional, typically a physician or nurse, who has the first encounter with a patient and who thus controls the patient's entry into the health care system.

gat•ing (gāt′ing) **1.** In a biologic membrane, the opening and closing of a channel, believed to be associated with changes in integral membrane proteins. **2.** A process in which electrical signals are selected by a gate, which passes such signals only when the gate pulse is present to act as a control signal, or passes only the signals that have certain characteristics.

gat•ing mech•a•nism (gāt′ing mek′ă-nizm) **1.** Occurrence of the maximum refractory period among cardiac conducting cells approximately 2 mm proximal to the terminal Purkinje fibers in the ventricular muscle; gating mechanism may be a cause of ventricular aberration, bidirectional tachycardia, and concealed extrasystoles. **2.** A mechanism by which painful impulses may be blocked from entering the spinal cord. Cf. gate-control theory.

Gauch•er cells (gō-shā′ selz) Large, finely, and uniformly vacuolated cells derived from the reticuloendothelial system and found especially in the spleen, lymph nodes, liver, and bone marrow of patients with Gaucher disease; Gaucher cells contain kerasin (a cerebroside), which accumulates as a result of a genetically determined absence of the enzyme glucosylceramidase.

Gauch•er dis•ease (gō-shā′ di-zēz′) A lysosomal storage disease resulting from glycocerebroside accumulation due to a genetic deficiency of glucocerebrosidase; may occur in adults but occurs most severely in infants; marked by hepatosplenomegaly, regression of neurologic maturation, and characteristic histiocytes (Gaucher cells) in the viscera.

gau•cho tea (gowch′ō tē) SYN yerba maté.

gauge (gāj) A measuring device.

gaunt•let ban•dage (gawnt′lĕt ban′dăj) A figure-of-8 bandage covering the hand and fingers.

gauss (G) (gows) A unit of magnetic field intensity, equal to 10^{-4} tesla. [J.K.F. *Gauss*]

gaus•si•an (gows′ē-ăn) Relating to or described by Johann K. F. Gauss.

gaus•si•an dis•tri•bu•tion (gow′sē-ăn dis′tri-byū′shŭn) The statistical distribution of members of a population around the population mean. In a gaussian distribution, 68.2% of values fall within ± 1 standard deviation (SD); 95.4% fall within ± 2 SD of the mean; and 99.7% fall within ± 3 SD of the mean. SYN bell-shaped curve, normal distribution.

Gauss sign (gows sīn) Marked mobility of the uterus in the early weeks of pregnancy.

gauze (gawz) A bleached cotton cloth of plain weave, used for dressings, bandages, and absorbent sponges; petrolatum gauze is saturated with petrolatum. [Fr. *gaze,* fr. Ar. *gazz,* raw silk]

ga•vage (gă-vahzh′) **1.** Forced feeding by stomach tube. SYN gastrogavage. **2.** Therapeutic use of a high-potency diet administered by stomach tube. [Fr. *gaver,* to gorge fowls]

gay (gā) **1.** A homosexual, especially male. **2.** Denoting a homosexual individual or the male homosexual lifestyle. SEE ALSO lesbian.

gay bow•el syn•drome (gā bow′ĕl sin′drōm) Gastrointestinal discomfort experienced by homosexual males that includes abdominal pain, cramps, bloating, flatulence, nausea, vomiting, or diarrhea caused by enteric bacteria, viruses, fungi, zooparasites, or trauma.

Gay-Lus•sac e•qua•tion (gā-lū-sahk ĕ-kwā′zhŭn) The overall chemical equation for alcoholic fermentation; $C_6H_{12}O_6 = 2CO_2 + 2CH_3CH_2OH$.

Gay-Lus•sac law (gā-lū-sahk law) SYN Charles law.

gaze (gāz) The act of looking steadily at an object.

GB NATO code for sarin.

G-band•ing stain (band′ing stān) A chromosome-staining technique used in human cytogenetics to identify individual chromosomes, which produces characteristic bands; it uses acetic acid, proteolytic enzymes, salts, heat, detergents, or urea, and finally Giemsa stain; chromosome bands appear similar to those fluorochromed by Q-banding stain.

GBL Abbreviation for gamma-butyrolactone.

GB vi•rus•es (vī-rŭs′ĕz) Members of the family Flaviviridae; GBV-A and GBV-B have been isolated from tamarins infected with human viral agents; GBV-C is a human pathogen related to hepatitis G virus.

G cells (selz) Enteroendocrine cells that secrete gastrin, found primarily in the mucosa of the pyloric antrum of the stomach.

GCP Abbreviation for Good Clinical Practices.

G-CSF Abbreviation for granulocyte colony-stimulating factor.

GD NATO code for soman.

Gd Symbol for gadolinium.

GDM Abbreviation for gestational diabetes mellitus.

GDS Abbreviation for Geriatric Depression Scale.

Ge Symbol for germanium.

ge•gen•halt•en (gā′gen-hahlt-en) German (with a capital G, as with all German nouns) for counterpressure, the term is nonetheless used in English to describe a certain type of neurologic or muscular opposition to resistance associated with various catatonic states.

Gei•gel re•flex (gī′gel rē′fleks) In the female, a contraction of the muscular fibers at the upper edge of the Poupart ligament on gently stroking the inner thigh; analogue of the cremasteric reflex in males.

Gei•ger-Muel•ler Coun•ter (gī′ger-mil′er kown′tĕr) An instrument used to detect and monitor radiation. Typically used to locate radioactive sources. (Mueller is a variant spelling for Müller.)

gel (jel) **1.** A jelly, or the solid or semisolid phase of a colloidal solution. **2.** To form a gel or jelly; to convert a solution into a gel. [Mod. L. *gelatum*]

gel•a•tin (jel′ă-tin) A derived protein formed from the collagen of tissues by boiling in water; it swells up when put in cold water, but dissolves only in hot water; used as a hemostat, plasma substitute, and protein food adjunct in the treatment of malnutrition. It is also used in the manufacture of capsules. [L. *gelo,* pp. *gelatus,* to freeze, congeal]

ge•lat•i•nize (jĕ-lat′i-nīz) **1.** To convert into gelatin. **2.** To become gelatinous.

ge•lat•i•nous (jĕ-lat′i-nŭs) **1.** Pertaining to or characteristic of gelatin. **2.** Jellylike or resembling gelatin.

gel•a•tin•ous drop•like cor•ne•al dys•tro•phy (jĕ-lat′i-nŭs drop′līk kōr′nē-ăl dis′trŏ-fē) A bilateral, autosomal recessive condition characterized by mulberrylike elevated amyloid deposits involving the epithelium and anterior corneal stroma.

ge•lat•i•nous sub•stance (jĕ-lat′i-nŭs sub′stăns) The apical part of the posterior horn (dorsal horn; posterior gray column) of the gray matter of the spinal cord, composed largely of very small nerve cells; its gelatinous appearance is due to its very low content of myelinated nerve fibers.

ge•la•tion (jĕ-lā′shŭn) COLLOIDAL CHEMISTRY the transformation of a solution into a gel.

gel dif•fu•sion pre•cip•i•tin tests (jel di-fyū'zhŭn prē-sip'i-tin tests) Precipitin tests in which the immune precipitate forms in a gel medium (usually agar) into which one or both reactants have diffused; generally classified in two types, in one dimension, and in two dimensions.

Gé·li·neau syn·drome (zhā-lē-nō' sin'drōm) SYN narcolepsy.

Gé·ly su·ture (zhā-lē' sū'chŭr) A cobbler's suture used in closing intestinal wounds.

Ge·mel·la (jĕ-mel'ă) A genus of motile, aerobic, facultatively anaerobic, coccoid bacteria (family Streptococcaceae) that occur singly or in pairs, with flattened adjacent sides. They are gram indeterminate but have a cell wall like that of gram-positive bacteria, and are parasitic on mammals. The type species is *G. haemolysans*, which is found in bronchial secretions and in mucus from the respiratory tract. [L. dim. of *geminus,* twin]

Ge·mel·la mor·bil·lor·um (jĕ-mel'ă mōr-bi-lō'rŭm) A microaerophilic bacterium, formerly called *Streptococcus morbillorum*, which fails to produce β-hemolysis of blood agar and lacks distinguishing serogroup antigens; causes serious infections in some patients similar to those seen with viridans streptococci.

ge·mel·lus (jĕ-mel'ŭs) SYN inferior gemellus muscle.

gem·i·nate (jem'i-nāt) Occurring in pairs. [L. *gemino,* pp. *-atus,* to double, fr. *geminus,* twin]

gem·i·na·tion (jem'i-nā'shŭn) Embryologic partial division of a primordium. For example, gemination of a single tooth germ results in two partially or completely separated crowns on a single root. [L. *geminatio,* a doubling]

gem·ma·tion (jem-ā'shŭn) A form of fission in which the parent cell does not divide but puts out a small budlike process (daughter cell) with its proportionate amount of chromatin; the daughter cell then separates to begin independent existence. SYN budding. [L. *gemma,* a bud]

gem·mule (jem'yūl) **1.** A small bud that projects from the parent cell, and finally becomes detached, forming a cell of a new generation. **2.** SYN dendritic spines. [L. *gemmula,* dim. of *gemma,* bud]

♻ **gen-** Prefix denoting being born, producing, coming to be. [G. *genos,* birth]

♻ **-gen** Suffix denoting "precursor of." SEE ALSO pro- (2).

ge·na (jē'nă) SYN cheek. [L.]

ge·nal (jē'năl) Relating to the gena, or cheek.

ge·nal glands (jē'năl glandz) SYN buccal glands.

gen·der (jen'dĕr) Category to which a person is assigned by self or others, on the basis of sex. Cf. sex, gender role.

gen·der i·den·ti·ty (jen'dĕr i-den'ti-tē) The sex role adopted by a person; the degree to which a person acts out a stereotypical masculine or feminine role in everyday behavior. Cf. gender role, sex role.

gen·der role (jen'dĕr rōl) The sex of a child assigned by a parent; when opposite to the child's anatomic sex (e.g., due to genital ambiguity at birth or to the parents' strong wish for a child of the opposite sex), the basis is set for postpubertal dysfunctions. SEE sex role, sex reversal.

gen·der-spe·cif·ic med·i·cine (jen'dĕr-spĕ-sif'ik med'i-sin) That branch of therapy that limits itself to care of one gender or the other, usually in the care of gender-related illness or genetics.

gene (jēn) A functional unit of heredity that occupies a specific place (locus) on a chromosome, is capable of reproducing itself exactly at each cell division, and directs the formation of an enzyme or other protein. The gene as a functional unit consists of a discrete segment of a giant DNA molecule containing the purine (adenine and guanine) and pyrimidine (cytosine and thymine) bases in the correct sequence to code the sequence of amino acids of a specific peptide. Protein synthesis is mediated by molecules of messenger-RNA formed on the chromosome with the gene acting as a template. The RNA then passes into the cytoplasm and becomes oriented on the ribosomes where it in turn acts as a template to organize a chain of amino acids to form a peptide. In organisms reproducing sexually, genes normally occur in pairs in all cells except gametes, as a consequence of the fact that all chromosomes are paired except the sex chromosomes (X and Y) of the male. SYN factor (3). [G. *genos,* birth]

ge·ne·al·o·gy (jē'nē-ol'ŏ-jē) **1.** Heredity. **2.** The explicit assembly of the descent of a person or family; it may be of any length. [G. *genea,* descent, + *logos,* study]

gene dos·age com·pen·sa·tion (jēn dō'săj kom'pĕn-sā'shŭn) The putative mechanism that adjusts the X-linked phenotypes of males and females to compensate for the haploid state in males and the diploid state in females. It is now largely ascribed to lyonization, which compensates the mean of the dose but not its variance, which is greater in females.

gene ex·pres·sion (jēn eks-presh'ŭn) **1.** The detectable effect of a gene. **2.** Appearance of an inherited trait; for many reasons, a gene may not be expressed at all.

gene fam·i·ly (jēn fam'i-lē) Group of genes related by sequence similarity.

gen·er·a (jen'ĕ-ră) Plural of genus.

gen•er•al ad•ap•ta•tion re•ac•tion (jen′ĕr-ăl ad′ap-tā′shŭn rē-ak′shŭn) SEE general adaptation syndrome.

gen•er•al ad•ap•ta•tion syn•drome (jen′ĕr-ăl ad′ap-tā′shŭn sin′drōm) A term introduced by Hans Selye to describe marked physiologic changes in various organ systems of the body, especially the pituitary-endocrine system, as a result of exposure to prolonged physical or psychological stress.

gen•er•al a•nat•o•my (jen′ĕr-ăl ă-nat′ŏ-mē) The study of gross and microscopic structures as well as of the composition of the body, its tissues, and fluids.

gen•er•al an•es•the•si•a (jen′ĕr-ăl an′es-thē′zē-ă) Loss of ability to perceive pain associated with loss of consciousness produced by intravenous or inhalation anesthetic agents.

gen•er•al an•es•thet•ic (jen′ĕr-ăl an′es-thet′ik) A compound that produces loss of sensation associated with loss of consciousness.

gen•er•al du•ty nurse (jen′ĕr-ăl dū′tē nŭrs) Nurse prepared to work as a generalist, as distinguished from a nurse prepared to function within a specialty practice.

gen•er•al im•mu•ni•ty (jen′ĕr-ăl i-myū′ni-tē) Immunity associated with widely diffused mechanisms that tend to protect the body as a whole, as compared with local immunity.

generalisation [Br.] SYN generalization.

generalised [Br.] SYN generalized.

gen•er•al•ist (jen′ĕr-ăl-ist) A general physician or family physician; a physician trained to take care of the majority of nonsurgical diseases, sometimes including obstetrics.

gen•er•al•i•za•tion (jen′ĕr-ăl-ī-zā′shŭn) **1.** Rendering or becoming general, diffuse, or widespread, as when a primarily local disease becomes systemic. **2.** The reasoning by which a basic conclusion is reached, which applies to different items, each having some common factor. **3.** Categorization that obscures differences between people or situations (e.g., age categories). SYN generalisation.

gen•er•al•ized (jen′ĕr-ă-līzd) Involving the whole of an organ, as opposed to a focal or regional process. SYN generalised.

gen•er•al•ized an•a•phy•lax•is (jen′ĕr-al-īzd an′ă-fi-lak′sis) The immediate response, involving smooth muscles and capillaries throughout the body, that follows injection of antigen (allergen). SEE ALSO anaphylactic shock. SYN systemic anaphylaxis.

gen•er•al•ized anx•i•e•ty dis•or•der (jen′ĕr-ă-līzd ang-zī′ĕ-tē dis-ōr′dĕr) Chronic, repeated episodes of anxiety or dread accompanied by autonomic changes. SEE ALSO anxiety.

gen•er•al•ized len•tig•i•no•sis (jen′ĕr-ă-līzd len-tij′i-nō′sis) Lentigines occurring singly or in groups from infancy onward.

gen•er•al•ized plane xan•tho•ma•to•sis (jen′ĕr-ă-līzd plān zan′thō-mă-tō′sis) Widespread xanthomatosis associated with multiple myeloma, familial hyperlipoproteinemia, or less commonly with primary biliary cirrhosis, or with no underlying disease.

gen•er•al•ized Shwartz•man phe•nom•e•non (jen′ĕr-ă-līzd shvahrts′mahn fĕ-nom′ĕ-non) When both the primary injection of endotoxin-containing filtrate and the secondary injection are given intravenously 24 hours apart, the animal usually dies within 24 hours after the second inoculation. This reaction has no immunologic basis.

gen•er•al•ized ton•ic-clo•nic sei•zure, gen•er•al•ized ton•ic-clo•nic ep•i•lep•sy (jen′ĕr-ăl-īzd ton′ik-klon′ik sē′zhŭr, ep′i-lep′sē) A generalized seizure characterized by the sudden onset of tonic contraction of the muscles often associated with a cry or moan, and frequently resulting in a fall to the ground. The tonic phase of the seizure gradually gives way to clonic convulsive movements occurring bilaterally and synchronously before slowing and eventually stopping, followed by a variable period of unconsciousness and gradual recovery. SYN grand mal.

gen•er•al•ized tu•ber•cu•lo•sis (jen′ĕr-ă-līzd tū-bĕr′kyū-lō′sis) SYN miliary tuberculosis.

gen•er•al mas•sage (jen′ĕr-ăl mă-sahzh′) Manual stimulation of the body often used in connection with warm baths to improve muscular and circulatory disorders.

gen•er•al prac•tice (jen′ĕr-ăl prak′tis) SEE family practice.

gen•er•al prac•ti•tion•er (GP) (jen′ĕr-ăl prak-tish′ŭn-ĕr) SEE family practice physician.

gen•er•al re•lax•a•tion (jen′ĕr-ăl rē′laks-ā′shŭn) Lessened muscular stress affecting the body as a whole.

gen•er•al stim•u•lant (jen′ĕr-ăl stim′yū-lănt) A stimulant that affects the entire body.

gen•er•al symp•tom (jen′ĕr-ăl simp′tŏm) A finding related to the entirety of the organism, rather than only a constituent part.

gen•er•a•tion (jen-ĕr-ā′shŭn) **1.** SYN reproduction (2). **2.** A discrete stage in succession of descent; e.g., father, son, and grandson are three generations. [L. *generatio,* fr. *genero,* pp. *-atus,* to beget]

gen•er•a•tive (jen′ĕr-ă-tiv) Pertaining to the process of generating.

gen•er•a•tor (jen′ĕr-ă-tŏr) An apparatus for conversion of chemical, mechanical, atomic, or other forms of energy into electricity. [*generator*, a begetter, producer]

ge•ner•ic (jĕ-ner′ik) **1.** Relating to or denoting a genus. **2.** General. **3.** Characteristic or distinctive. [L. *genus* (*gener-*), birth]

ge•ner•ic drug (gĕ-ner′ik drŭg) A medicine distributed under its generic (nonproprietary) name.

ge•ner•ic e•quiv•a•lent (jĕ-ner′ik ē-kwiv′ă-lĕnt) SEE generic substitution.

ge•ner•ic name (jĕ-ner′ik nām) **1.** CHEMISTRY a noun that indicates the class or type of a single compound (e.g., salt, saccharide (sugar), hexose, alcohol, aldehyde, lactone, acid, amine, alkane, steroid, vitamin). "Class" is more appropriate and more often used than is "generic." **2.** In the pharmaceutical and commercial fields, a misnomer for nonproprietary name. **3.** BIOLOGIC SCIENCES the first part of the scientific name (Latin binary combination or binomial) of an organism; written with an initial capital letter and in italics. **4.** BACTERIOLOGY the species name consists of two parts (comprising one name): the generic name and the specific epithet; in other biologic disciplines, the species name is regarded as being composed of two names: the generic name and the specific name.

ge•ner•ic sub•sti•tu•tion (jĕ-ner′ik sŭb′sti-tū′shŭn) The dispensing of a chemically equivalent, less expensive drug in place of a brand-name or proprietary product.

gen•e•sis (jen′ĕ-sis) An origin or beginning process; also used as combining form in suffix position. [G.]

gene splic•ing (jēn splīs′ing) SYN splicing (1).

gene ther•a•py (jēn thār′ă-pē) The process of inserting a gene into an organism to replace or repair gene function to treat a disease or genetic defect.

ge•net•ic (jĕ-net′ik) Pertaining to genetics; genetical.

ge•net•i•cal•ly mod•i•fied food (jĕ-net′ik-ă-lē mod′i-fīd fūd) Scientifically altered foodstuffs intended to limit exposure of the plants or animals to disease or spoilage. Concerns about safety and efficacy have been raised worldwide. SYN frankenfood.

ge•net•ic am•pli•fi•ca•tion (jĕ-net′ik amp′li-fi-kā′shŭn) A process for producing an increase in pertinent genetic material, particularly for increasing the proportion of plasmid DNA to that of bacterial DNA. Includes the production of extrachromosomal copies of the genes for RNA.

ge•net•ic as•so•ci•a•tion (jĕ-net′ik ă-sō′sē-ā′shŭn) The occurrence together in a population, more often than can be readily explained by chance, of two or more traits of which at least one is known to be genetic.

ge•net•ic code (jĕ-net′ik kōd) The genetic information carried by the specific DNA molecules of the chromosomes; specifically, the system whereby particular combinations of three consecutive nucleotides in a DNA molecule control the insertion of one particular amino acid in equivalent places in a protein molecule.

ge•net•ic coun•sel•ing (jĕ-net′ik kown′sĕl-ing) The process whereby an expert in genetic disorders provides information about risk and clinical burden of a disorder or disorders to patients or relatives in families with genetic disorders as an aid to making informed and responsible decisions about marriage, children, early diagnossi, and prognosis.

ge•net•ic coun•sel•or (jĕ-net′ik kown′sĕ-lŏr) A physician or scientist who specializes in diseases or conditions closely linked to inheritance.

ge•net•ic de•ter•mi•nant (jĕ-net′ik dĕ-tĕr′mi-nănt) Any antigenic determinant or identifying characteristic, particularly those of allotypes.

ge•net•ic dis•or•der (jĕ-net′ik dis-ōr′dĕr) A widely used by nonetheless imprecise term that denotes a condition or illness related to biologic inheritance.

gen•et•ic ep•i•de•mi•o•lo•gy (jĕ-net′ik ep′i-dē-mē-ol′ŏ-jē) The branch of epidemiology that studies the role of genetic factors and their interactions with environmental factors in the occurrence of disease in various populations.

ge•net•ic fe•male (jĕ-net′ik fē′māl) **1.** A person with a normal female karyotype, including two X chromosomes. **2.** A person whose cell nuclei contain Barr sex chromatin bodies, which are normally absent in males.

ge•net•ic fit•ness (jĕ-net′ik fit′nĕs) In a phenotype, the mean number of surviving offspring that it generates in its lifetime, usually expressed as a fraction or percentage of the average genetic fitness of the population.

ge•net•i•cist (jĕ-net′i-sist) A specialist in genetics.

ge•net•ic le•thal (jĕ-net′ik lē′thăl) A disorder that prevents effective reproduction by those affected.

ge•net•ic load (jĕ-net′ik lōd) The aggregate of more or less harmful genes that are carried, mostly hidden, in the genome and may be transmitted to descendants and cause disease.

ge•net•ic map (jĕ-net′ik map) An abstract representation of the ordered array of genetic loci such that the interval between entries has algebraic signs and magnitude proportional to the expected number of crossings over between them and distances are algebraically additive; e.g., on a genetic map the combined distance between locus A and locus C is the algebraic sum of the two distances between loci A and B, and B and C.

ge•net•ic mark•er (jĕ-net′ik mahr′kĕr) SEE genetic determinant.

ge•net•ic psy•chol•o•gy (jĕ-net′ik sī-kol′ŏ-jē) A science dealing with the evolution of behavior and the relation to each other of the different types of mental activity.

ge•net•ics (jĕ-net′iks) **1.** The branch of science concerned with the means and consequences of transmission and generation of the components of biologic inheritance. **2.** The genetic features and constitution of any single organism or set of organisms. [G. *genesis,* origin or production]

ge•net•ic screen•ing (jĕ-net′ik skrēn′ing) SEE familial screening.

ge•net•o•tro•phic (jĕ-net′ō-trō′fik) Relating to inherited individual distinctions in nutritional requirements. [G. *genesis,* origin, + *trophē,* nourishment]

ge•ni•al, **ge•ni•an** (jĕ-nī′ăl, -nī′an) SYN mental (2). [G. *geneion,* chin]

ge•ni•al tu•ber•cle (jĕ-nī′ăl tū′bĕr-kĕl) SYN mental spine.

-genic Suffix meaning producing, forming; produced, formed by. [G. *genos,* birth]

ge•nic•u•la (jĕ-nik′yū-lă) Plural of geniculum.

ge•nic•u•lar (jĕ-nik′yū-lăr) Commonly used to mean genual.

ge•nic•u•lar ar•ter•ies (jĕ-nik′yū-lăr ahr′tĕr-ēz) Arteries contributing to the articular network of the knee.

ge•nic•u•late (jĕ-nik′yū-lāt) **1.** Bent like a knee. **2.** Referring to the geniculum of the facial nerve, denoting the ganglion there present. **3.** Denoting the lateral or medial geniculate body. [L. *geniculo,* pp. *-atus,* to bend the knee, fr. *genu,* knee]

ge•nic•u•late bod•y (jĕ-nik′yū-lāt bod′ē) SEE lateral geniculate body, medial geniculate body.

ge•nic•u•late gan•gli•on (jĕ-nik′yū-lāt gang′glē-on) A ganglion of the nervus intermedius fibers conveyed by the facial nerve, located within the facial canal at the genu of the canal and containing the sensory neurons innervating the taste buds on the anterior two thirds of the tongue and a small area on the external ear.

ge•nic•u•late neu•ral•gi•a (jĕ-nik′yū-lāt nūr-al′jē-ă) A severe paroxysmal lancinating pain deep in the ear, on the anterior wall of the external meatus, and on a small area just in front of the pinna. SYN Hunt neuralgia, neuralgia facialis vera.

ge•nic•u•lum, pl. **ge•nic•u•la** (jĕ-nik′yū-lŭm, -lă) **1.** A small genu or angular kneelike structure. **2.** A knotlike structure. [L. dim. of *genu,* knee]

ge•ni•o•glos•sus (jĕ′nē-ō-glos′ŭs) SYN genioglossus muscle.

ge•ni•o•glos•sus mus•cle (jē′nē-ō-glos′ŭs mŭs′ĕl) One of the paired lingual muscles; *origin,* mental spine of the mandible; *insertion,* lingual fascia beneath the mucous membrane and epiglottis; *action,* depresses and protrudes the tongue; *nerve supply,* hypoglossal. SYN musculus genioglossus [TA], genioglossus, musculus geniohyoglossus.

ge•ni•o•hy•oid mus•cle (jē′nē-ō-hī′oyd mŭs′ĕl) *Origin,* mental spine of mandible; *insertion,* body of hyoid bone; *action,* draws hyoid forward, or depresses jaw when hyoid is fixed; *nerve supply,* fibers from ventral primary rami of first and second cervical spinal nerves accompanying hypoglossal. SYN musculus geniohyoideus [TA].

ge•ni•on (jĕ′nē-on) The tip of the mental spine, a point in craniometry. [G. *geneion,* chin]

ge•ni•o•plas•ty (jĕ′nē-ō-plas-tē) SYN mentoplasty. [G. *geneion,* chin, cheek, + *plastos,* formed]

gen•i•tal (jen′i-tăl) **1.** Relating to reproduction or generation. **2.** Relating to the primary female or male sex organs or genitals. **3.** Relating to or characterized by genitality. [L. *genitalis,* pertaining to reproduction, fr. *gigno,* to bring forth]

gen•i•tal am•bi•gu•i•ty (jen′i-tăl am′bi-gyū′i-tē) Incomplete development of fetal genitalia as a result of excessive androgen action on a female fetus or inadequate amounts of androgen in a male fetus.

gen•i•tal cord (jen′i-tăl kōrd) One of a pair of mesenchymal ridges bulging into the caudal part of the celom of a young embryo and containing the mesonephric and paramesonephric ducts.

gen•i•tal cor•pus•cles (jen′i-tăl kor′pŭs-ĕlz) Special encapsulated nerve endings found in the skin of the genitalia and nipples. SYN corpuscula genitalia [TA].

gen•i•tal fur•row (jen′i-tăl fur′ō) SYN urethral groove.

gen•i•tal groove (jen′i-tăl grūv) SYN urethral groove.

gen•i•tal her•pes (jen′i-tăl hĕr′pēz) Herpetic lesions on the penis of the male or on the cervix, perineum, vagina, or vulva of the female, caused by herpes simplex virus type 2. SYN herpes genitalis.

gen•i•ta•li•a (jen′i-tā′lē-ă) The organs of reproduction or generation, external and internal. SYN genitals. [L. neut. pl. of *genitalis,* genital]

gen•i•tal•i•ty (jen′i-tal′i-tē) PSYCHOANALYSIS a term referring to the genital components of sexuality (i.e., the penis and vagina), as opposed, for example, to orality and anality.

gen•i•tal phase (jen′i-tăl fāz) In psychoanalytic personality theory, the final stage of psychosexual development, occurring during puberty, in which the person's psychosexual development is so organized that sexual gratification can be achieved from genital-to-genital contact and the capacity exists for a mature affectionate relationship with another person. SEE ALSO phallic phase.

gen•i•tals (jen′i-tălz) SYN genitalia.

gen•i•tal self-ex•am•i•na•tion (jen′i-tăl self′ eg-zam′i-nā′shŭn) Scrutiny of the external genitals by the patient using manual manipulation and visual inspection to look for abnormalities (e.g., lumps, lesions).

gen•i•tal tract (jen′i-tăl trakt) The genital passages of the urogenital apparatus.

gen•i•tal wart (jen′i-tăl wōrt) SYN condyloma acuminatum.

gen•i•to•fem•o•ral (jen′i-tō-fem′ŏr-ăl) Relating to the genitalia and the thigh; denoting the genitofemoral nerve.

gen•i•to•fem•o•ral nerve (jen′i-tō-fem′ŏr-ăl nĕrv) Arises from the first and second lumbar nerves, passes distad along the anterior surface of psoas major muscle and divides into genital and femoral branches. SYN nervus genitofemoralis [TA].

gen•i•to•ur•i•nar•y (GU) (jen′i-tō-yūr′i-nar-ē) Relating to the organs of reproduction and urination. SYN urogenital.

gen•i•to•ur•i•nar•y surgeon (jen′i-tō-yūr′i-nar-ē sŭr′jŏn) SYN urologist.

gen•o•cop•y (jen′ō-kop-ē) A genotype at one locus that produces a phenotype that at some levels of resolution is indistinguishable from that produced by another genotype; e.g., two types of elliptocytosis that are genocopies of each other, but are distinguished by the fact that one is linked to the Rh blood group locus and the other is not.

ge•no•der•ma•to•sis (jen′ō-dĕr-mă-tō′sis) A skin condition of genetic origin.

ge•nome (jē′nōm) **1.** A complete set of chromosomes derived from one parent, the haploid number of a gamete. **2.** The total gene complement of a set of chromosomes found in higher life forms (the haploid set in a eukaryotic cell), or the functionally similar but simpler linear arrangements found in bacteria and viruses. SEE ALSO Human Genome Project. [gene + chromosome]

ge•nome map (jē′nōm map) A representation, usually in graphic form, or the entire composition of the DNA of a given genus and species.

ge•nom•ic (jē-nom′ik) Relating to a genome.

ge•nom•ic clone (jē-nom′ik klōn) A cell with a vector containing a fragment of DNA from a different organism.

ge•nom•ic im•print•ing (jē-nom′ik im′print-ing) Epigenetic process that leads to inactivation of paternal or maternal allele of certain genes susceptible to epigenetic regulation; accounts, among others, for the Angelman and Prader-Willi syndromes.

gen•om•ics (jē-nō′miks) Study of the structure of the genome of particular organisms, including mapping and sequencing.

ge•no•spe•cies (jē′nō-spē-shēz) A group of organisms in which interbreeding is possible, as evidenced by genetic transfer and recombination.

ge•note (jē′nōt) MICROBIAL GENETICS an element of recombination in which one of the pair is not a complete chromosome; commonly used as a suffix (e.g., endogenote, exogenote, F genote). [gene + G. *-ōtēs,* toponymic suffix]

ge•no•tox•ic (jē′nō-toks′ik) Denoting a substance that by damaging DNA may cause mutation or cancer. [gene + toxic]

gen•o•type (jē′nō-tīp) **1.** The genetic constitution of an individual. **2.** Gene combination at one specific locus or any specified combination of loci. [G. *genos,* birth, descent, + *typos,* type]

gen•o•typ•i•cal (jē′nō-tip′i-kăl) Relating to the genotype.

gen•tian•o•phil, gen•tian•o•phile (jen′shŭn-ō-fil, jen′shŭn-ō-fīl) Staining readily with gentian violet. [gentian + G. *philos,* fond]

gen•tian•o•pho•bic (jen′shŭn-ō-fō′bik) Not taking a gentian violet stain, or taking it poorly. [gentian + G. *phobos,* fear]

gen•tian vi•o•let (jen′shŭn vī′ŏ-lĕt) An unstandardized dye mixture of violet rosanilins.

gen•ti•o•bi•ose (jen′shē-ō-bī′ōs) A disaccharide containing two D-glucopyranose molecules linked β-1,6; a structural moiety in many compounds (amygdalin). SYN amygdalose.

gen•u, pl. **gen•u•a** (jē′nyū, -yū-ă) [TA] **1.** The joint between the thigh and the leg. SYN knee (1) [TA]. SEE ALSO knee joint, geniculum. **2.** Any structure of angular shape resembling a flexed knee. [L.]

gen•u•al (jen′yū-ăl) Relating to the knee. [L. *genu,* knee]

gen•u•cu•bi•tal po•si•tion (jen′yū-kyū′bi-tăl pŏ-zish′ŏn) SYN knee-elbow position.

gen•u•pec•to•ral po•si•tion (jen′yū-pek′tōr-ăl pŏ-zish′ŏn) SYN knee-chest position.

gen•u re•cur•va•tum (jē′nyū rē-kŭr-vā′tŭm) Hyperextension of the knee, the lower limb having a forward curvature.

ge•nus, pl. **gen•er•a** (jē′nŭs, jen′ĕr-ă) In natural history classification, the taxonomic level of division between the family, or tribe, and the species; a group of species alike in the broad features of their organization but different in detail, and incapable of fertile mating. [L. birth, descent]

gen·u val·gum (jē′nyū val′gŭm) A deformity marked by lateral angulation of the leg in relation to the thigh. SYN knock-knee, tibia valga.

gen·u va·rum (jē′nyū vā′rŭm) A deformity marked by medial angulation of the leg in relation to the thigh; an outward bowing of the lower limbs. SYN bowleg, bow-leg, tibia vara.

geo- Prefix indicating the earth, soil. [G. *gē,* earth]

ge·ode (jē′ōd) A cystlike space (or spaces) with or without an epithelial lining, observed radiologically in subarticular bone, usually in arthritic disorders. [Fr., fr. L. *geodes,* precious stone, fr. G. *gē,* earth, + *-ōdēs,* appearance]

ge·o·graph·ic in·for·ma·tion sys·tem (jē′ō-graf′ik in′fōr-mā′shŭn sis′tĕm) A computer-based system that combines cartographic capabilities with electronic data processing to rapidly produce customized maps for use in epidemiologic studies.

ge·o·graph·ic ker·a·ti·tis (jē′ō-graf′ik ker′ă-tī′tis) keratitis with coalescence of superficial lesions in herpes keratitis.

ge·o·graph·ic re·tin·al a·tro·phy (jē′ō-graf′ik ret′i-năl at′rŏ-fē) A pattern of well-demarcated retinal pigment epithelial atrophy associated with choriocapillary layer and photoreceptor atrophy leading to vision loss.

ge·o·graph·ic tongue (jē′ō-graf′ik tŭng) Idiopathic, asymptomatic erythematous circinate macules, often bounded peripherally by a white band, as a result of atrophy of the filiform papillae; with time the lesions resolve, coalesce, and change in distribution; frequently associated with fissured tongues. See page B15. SYN glossitis areata exfoliativa, lingua geographica, pityriasis linguae.

ge·o·met·ric i·som·er·ism (jē′ō-met′trik ī-som′ĕr-izm) A form of isomerism displayed by unsaturated or ring compounds where free rotation about a bond (usually a carbon-carbon bond) is restricted. Cf. cis-, trans-.

ge·o·met·ric mean (jē′ō-met′rik mēn) The mean calculated as the antilogarithm of the arithmetic mean of the logarithms of the individual values; it can also be calculated as the *n*th root of the product of *n* values.

ge·o·met·ric sense (jē′ō-met′rik sens) One or other of two directions along a curve in which something is moving (e.g., clockwise or counterclockwise).

ge·o·met·ric un·sharp·ness (jē′ō-met′rik ŭn-shahrp′nĕs) SYN penumbra.

ge·o·pha·gi·a, ge·oph·a·gism, ge·oph·a·gy (jē′ō-fā′jē-ă, jē-of′ă-jizm, -of′ă-jē) The practice of eating dirt or clay. SYN dirt-eating. [geo- + G. *phagō,* to eat]

ge·o·phil·ic (jē′ō-fil′ik) Soil-loving; refers to microorganisms indigenous to soil.

ge·o·tri·cho·sis (jē′ō-tri-kō′sis) An opportunistic systemic hyalohyphomycosis caused by *Geotrichum candidum;* ascribed symptoms are diverse and suggestive of secondary or mixed infections. [geo- + G. *thrix,* hair, + *-osis,* condition]

Ge·o·tri·chum can·di·dum (jē′o′trī-kŭm kan′dī-dŭm) A fungal species occasionally associated with wound infections. Colonies of *Geotrichum* may first appear as white, creamy, and yeastlike; white, powdery mold is also produced. Barrel-shaped arthroconidia that do not alternate are produced.

ge·phy·rin (je-fir′in fon′tă-nel′) A protein in the ataxia telangiectasia mutation-related family, essential for glycine receptor clustering on neuronal membranes.

GERD (gĕrd) Acronym for gastroesophageal reflux disease.

Ger·dy fon·ta·nelle (zher-dē′ fon′tă-nel′) SYN sagittal fontanelle.

ger·i·at·ric (jer-ē-at′rik) Relating to old age.

Ger·i·at·ric De·pres·sion Scale (GDS) (jer′ē-at′rik dĕ-presh′ŭn skāl) A self-administered tool of assessment, with 30 questions, used to determine the presence of long-term depression in old people; higher scores indicate greater levels of disability.

ger·i·at·rics (jer′ē-at′riks) The branch of medicine concerned with the medical problems and care of old people. [G. *gēras,* old age, + *iatrikos,* healing]

Ger·li·er dis·ease (zher-lē-ā′ di-zēz′) SYN vestibular neuronitis.

germ (jĕrm) **1.** A microbe; a microorganism. **2.** A primordium; the earliest trace of a structure within an embryo. [L. *germen,* sprout, bud, germ]

ger·ma·ni·um (Ge) (jĕr-mā′nē-ŭm) A metallic element; atomic no. 32, atomic wt. 72.61. [L. *Germania,* Germany]

Ger·man mea·sles (jĕr′măn mē′zĕlz) SYN rubella.

Ger·man mea·sles vi·rus (jĕr′mĕn mē′zĕlz vī′rŭs) SYN rubella virus.

germ cell (jĕrm sel) SYN sex cell.

ger·mi·ci·dal (jĕr′mi-sī′dăl) SYN germicide (1).

ger·mi·cide (jĕr′mi-sīd) **1.** Destructive to germs or microbes. SYN germicidal. **2.** An agent with this action. [germ + L. *caedo,* to kill]

ger·mi·nal (jĕr′mi-năl) Relating to a germ or, in botany, to germination.

ger·mi·nal ar·e·a, ar·e·a ger·mi·na·ti·va (jĕr′mi-năl ār′ē-ă, ār′ē-ă jĕr-mi-nā-tī′vă) The place in the blastoderm where the embryo begins to be formed.

ger·mi·nal cell (jĕr′mi-năl sel) A cell from which other cells proliferate.

ger·mi·nal cords (jĕr′mi-năl kōrdz) SYN primordial sex cords.

ger·mi·nal disc, germ disc (jĕr′mi-năl disk, jĕrm disk) The point in a telolecithal oocyte where the embryo begins to form.

ger·mi·nal ep·i·the·li·um (jĕr′mi-năl ep′i-thē′lē-ŭm) A cuboidal layer of peritoneal epithelium covering the gonads, formerly thought to be the source of germ cells.

ger·mi·nal lo·cal·i·za·tion (jĕr′mi-năl lō′kăl-ī-zā′shŭn) Determination in very young embryos of the presumptive areas for specific organs or structures.

ger·mi·nal pole (jĕr′mi-năl pōl) SYN animal pole.

ger·mi·no·ma (jĕr′mi-nō′mă) A neoplasm of the germinal tissue of gonads, mediastinum, or pineal region, such as seminoma. [L. *germen*, bud, + *-oma*, tumor]

germ line (jĕrm līn) A collection of haploid cells derived from the specialized cells of the primitive gonad.

germ mem·brane, ger·mi·nal mem·brane (jĕrm mem′brān, jĕr′mi-năl mem′brān) SYN blastoderm.

♲**gero-, geront-, geronto-** Combining forms meaning old age. SEE ALSO presby-. [G. *gerōn*, old man]

ger·o·der·ma (jer′ō-dĕr′mă) **1.** The atrophic skin of the aged. **2.** Any condition in which the skin is thinned and wrinkled, resembling the integument of old age. [gero- + G. *derma*, skin]

ger·o·don·tics, ger·o·don·tol·o·gy (jer′ō-don′tiks, -don-tol′ŏ-jē) SYN dental geriatrics. [gero- + G. *odous*, tooth]

ge·ron·tal (jer-on′tăl) Relating to old age.

ger·on·tol·o·gist (jer′ŏn-tol′ŏ-jist) One who specializes in gerontology.

ger·on·tol·o·gy (jer′ŏn-tol′ŏ-jē) The scientific study of the process and problems of aging. [geronto- + G. *logos*, study]

ger·on·tox·on (jer′on-tok′son) SYN arcus senilis. [geronto- + G. *toxon*, bow]

Ge·ro·ta cap·sule (gā-rō′tah kap′sŭl) SYN renal fascia.

Ge·ro·ta fas·ci·a (gā-rō′tah fash′ē-ă) SYN renal fascia.

Ge·ro·ta meth·od (gā-rō′tah meth′ŏd) Injection of the lymphatics with a dye that is soluble in chloroform or ether but not in water; alkannin, red sulfide of mercury, and Prussian blue are said to be suitable for this purpose.

Ge·sell Pre·school Test (gĕ-zel′ prē′skūl test) A norm-referenced test for children 30 months to 6 years of age that assesses personal, social, and communication skills and gross and fine motor coordination.

ges·ta·gen (jes′tă-jen) Any of several gestagenic substances, which are usually steroid hormones.

ge·stalt, ge·stalt phe·nom·e·non (ge-stahlt′, ge-stahlt′ fĕ-nom′ĕ-non) A perceived entity so integrated as to constitute a functional unit with properties not derivable from its parts. SEE ALSO gestaltism. [Ger. shape]

ge·stalt·ism, ge·stalt psy·chol·o·gy (ge-stahlt′izm, ges-tahlt′ sī-kol′ŏ-jē) The theory in psychology that the objects of mind come as complete forms or configurations that cannot be split into parts; e.g., a square is perceived as such rather than as four discrete lines. [see gestalt]

ge·stalt ther·a·py (ge-stahlt′ thār′ă-pē) A type of psychotherapy, used with individual people or groups, which emphasizes treatment of the person as a whole: the person's biologic component parts and her or his organic functioning, perceptual configuration, and interrelationships with the external world.

ges·ta·tion (jes-tā′shŭn) SYN pregnancy. [L. *gestatio*, from *gesto*, pp. *gestatus*, to bear]

ges·ta·tion·al age (jes-tā′shŭn-ăl āj) The age of a fetus expressed in elapsed time since the first day of the last normal menstrual period.

ges·ta·tion·al di·a·be·tes mel·li·tus (GDM) (jes-tā′shŭn-ăl dī-ă-bē′tēz mel′i-tŭs) Carbohydrate intolerance during pregnancy usually resolving after delivery.

ges·ta·tion·al e·de·ma (jes-tā′shŭn-ăl ĕ-dē′mă) A generalized and excessive accumulation of fluid in the tissues of greater than 1+ pitting after 12 hours' bed rest, or of a weight gain of 5 pounds or more in 1 week due to the influence of pregnancy.

ges·ta·tion·al hy·per·ten·sion (jes-tā′shŭn-ăl hī′pĕr-ten′shŭn) Hypertension during pregnancy in a previously normotensive woman or aggravation of hypertension during pregnancy in a hypertensive woman. SYN pregnancy-induced hypertension.

ges·ta·tion·al pro·tein·u·ri·a (jes-tā′shŭn-ăl prō′tē-nūr′ē-ă) The presence of protein in urine during or under the influence of pregnancy in the absence of hypertension, edema, renal infection, or known intrinsic renovascular disease.

ges·ta·tion·al ring (jes-tā′shŭn-ăl ring) The white ring identified by pulse echosonography that signals an early stage of pregnancy.

ges·ta·tion·al sac (jes-tā′shŭn-ăl sak) Cystic structure of early pregnancy that represents the amnionic sac, fluid, and placenta; in humans, the fused amnion and chorion.

ges·to·sis, pl. **ges·to·ses** (jes-tō′sis, -sēz) Any disorder of pregnancy. [L. *gesto,* to carry, to bear, + G. *-osis,* condition]

Gey so·lu·tion (gā sŏ-lū′shŭn) A salt solution usually used in combination with naturally occurring body substances (e.g., blood serum, tissue extracts) or more complex chemically defined, nutritive solutions for culturing animal cells.

GF NATO coe for cyclosarin.

GFR Abbreviation for glomerular filtration rate.

G_{M1} gan·gli·o·si·do·sis (gang′glē-ō-si-dō′sis) A disease characterized by accumulation of a specific monosialoganglioside, G_{M1}. Three forms exist: infantile or generalized, juvenile, and adult. Attributable to a deficiency of G_{M1}-β-galactosidase.

G_{M2} gan·gli·o·si·do·sis (gang′glē-ō-si-dō′sis) One of the hereditary metabolic disorders; several forms exist, including Tay-Sachs disease, Sandhoff disease, AV variant and adult onset; characterized by accumulation of a specific metabolite, G_{M2} ganglioside, due to deficiency of hexosaminidase A or B, or G_{M2} activator factor.

GH Abbreviation for growth hormone.

GHB Abbreviation for gamma (γ)-hydroxybutyrate.

Ghon tu·ber·cle (gon tū′bĕr-kĕl) Calcification seen in pulmonary parenchyma (usually midlung) resulting from earlier, usually childhood, infection with tuberculosis; sometimes confused with a combination of parenchymal lesion and calcified lymph node, which is properly termed a Ranke complex.

ghost cell (gōst sel) **1.** A dead cell in which the outline remains visible, but without other cytoplasmic structures or stainable nucleus. **2.** An erythrocyte after loss of its hemoglobin.

ghost cor·pus·cle (gōst kōr′pŭs-ĕl) SYN achromocyte.

ghre·lin (grel′in) A peptide hormone secreted by endocrine cells in the gastrointestinal tract. Acts as a growth hormone secretagogue and as an orexigenic agent mediated by the hypothalamic hormones neuropeptide Y (NPY) and agouti growth-related peptide (AGRP). [groth *h*ormone *rel*ease + -in]

GHRF, **GH-RF** Abbreviation for growth hormone–releasing factor.

GHRH, **GH-RH** Abbreviation for growth hormone–releasing hormone.

GHz Abbreviation for gigahertz, equal to one billion (10^9) hertz; used in ultrasound.

GI Abbreviation for gastrointestinal; Gingival Index.

gi·ant ax·o·nal neu·rop·a·thy (jī′ănt ak′sŏ-năl nūr-op′ă-thē) A rare disorder beginning at or after the third year of life, and presenting clinically with kinky hair, progressive clumsiness, muscle weakness and atrophy, sensory loss, and areflexia.

gi·ant cell (jī′ănt sel) A cell of large size, often with many nuclei.

gi·ant cell ar·te·ri·tis (jī′ănt sel ahr′tĕr-ī′tis) SYN temporal arteritis.

gi·ant cell car·ci·no·ma (jī′ănt sel kahr′si-nō′mă) A malignant epithelial neoplasm characterized by unusually large anaplastic cells.

gi·ant cell fi·bro·ma (jī′ănt sel fī-brō′mă) A tumor of the oral mucosa composed of fibrous connective tissue with large stellate and multinucleate fibroblasts. Cf. giant cell granuloma.

gi·ant cell gli·o·blas·to·ma mul·ti·for·me (jī′ănt sel glī′ō-blas-tō′mă mŭl-ti-fōr′mē) A histologic form of glioblastoma with large, often multinucleated, bizarre tumor cells.

gi·ant cell gran·u·lo·ma (jī′ănt sel gran′yū-lō′mă) A nonneoplastic lesion characterized by a proliferation of granulation tissue containing numerous multinucleated giant cells; it occurs on the gingiva and alveolar mucosa (occasionally on other soft tissues) where it presents as a soft red-blue hemorrhagic nodular swelling; it also occurs within the mandible or maxilla as a unilocular or multilocular radiolucency. Identical bony lesions may be seen in hyperparathyroidism and cherubism. SEE ALSO giant cell tumor of bone. Cf. giant cell fibroma.

gi·ant cell my·e·lo·ma (jī′ănt sel mī-ĕ-lō′mă) SYN giant cell tumor of bone.

gi·ant cell pneu·mo·ni·a (jī′ănt sel nū-mō′nē-ă) A rare complication of measles, with a postmortem finding of multinucleated giant cells lining alveoli. SYN interstitial pneumonia.

gi·ant cell tu·mor of bone (jī′ănt sel tū′mŏr bōn) A soft, reddish-brown, sometimes malignant, osteolytic tumor composed of multinucleated giant cells and ovoid or spindle-shaped cells, occurring most frequently in an end of a long tubular bone of young adults. SYN giant cell myeloma, osteoclastoma.

gi·ant cell tu·mor of ten·don sheath (jī′ănt sel tū′mŏr ten′dŏn shēth) A nodule arising commonly from the flexor sheath of the fingers and thumb; composed of fibrous tissue, lipid- and hemosiderin-containing macrophages, and multinucleated giant cells. SYN localized nodular tenosynovitis.

gi•ant con•dy•lo•ma (jī′ănt kon′di-lō′mă) A large type of condyloma acuminatum found in the anus, vulva, or preputial sac of the penis of middle-aged, uncircumcised men; it tends to extend deeply and recur.

gi•ant•ism (jī′ăn-tizm) SYN gigantism.

gi•ant pap•il•lar•y con•junc•ti•vi•tis (jī′ănt pap′i-lar-ē kŏn-jŭngk′ti-vī′tis) Conjunctival inflammation characterized by large papillae and associated with sensitization to antigenic material present on the surface of a contact lens.

gi•ant ur•ti•car•i•a (jī′ănt ŭr′ti-kar′ē-ă) SYN angioedema.

Gi•ar•di•a (jē-ahr′dē-ă) A genus of flagellates that parasitize the small intestine of human beings, domestic and wild mammals, and birds. See page B7.

gi•ar•di•a•sis (jē′ahr-dī′ă-sis) Infection with the protozoan parasite *Giardia lamblia*, sometimes asymptomatic but often manifested by diarrhea, dyspepsia, and malabsorption. SYN lambliasis.

gib•bous (gib′ŭs) Humped; humpbacked; denoting a sharp angle in the flexion of the spine. [L. *gibbosus*]

Gibbs the•o•rem (gibz thē′ŏr-ĕm) Substances that lower the surface tension of the pure dispersion medium tend to collect in its surface, whereas substances that raise the surface tension tend to remain out of the surface film.

gib•bus (gib′ŭs) Extreme kyphosis, hump, or hunch; a deformity of spine in which there is a sharply angulated segment, the apex of the angle being posterior. [L. a hump]

Gib•ney boot (gib′nē būt) Adhesive tape treatment of a sprained ankle or similar condition, applied in a basket-weave fashion under the sole of the foot and around the back of the lower leg.

Gib•ney fix•a•tion ban•dage (gib′nē fix-ā′shŭn ban′dăj) Herring-bone strapping of the foot and leg for sprain of the ankle.

Gib•son ban•dage (gib′sŏn ban′dăj) A bandage, resembling a Barton bandage, for stabilizing fracture of the mandible.

Gib•son mur•mur (gib′sŏn mŭr′mŭr) SYN machinery murmur.

Giem•sa stain (gēm′să stān) Compound of methylene blue–eosin and methylene blue used for demonstrating Negri bodies, *Tunga* species, spirochetes and protozoans, and differential staining of blood smears; also used for chromosomes, sometimes after hydrolyzing the cytologic preparation in hot hydrochloric acid, and for showing chromosome G bands.

Gier•ke dis•ease (gēr′kē di-zēz′) SYN glycogenosis type 1.

Gif•ford re•flex (gif′ŏrd rē′fleks) SYN eye-closure pupil reaction.

GIFT (gift) Acronym for gamete intrafallopian transfer.

giga- (G) Prefix used in the SI and metric system to signify one billion (10^9). [G. *gigas,* giant]

gi•gan•tism (jī-gant′izm) A condition of abnormal size or overgrowth of the entire body or of any of its parts. SYN giantism. [G. *gigas,* giant]

giganto- Prefix meaning huge, gigantic. [G. *gigas,* one of the race of giants]

gi•gan•to•mas•ti•a (jī-gan′tō-mas′tē-ă) Massive hypertrophy of the breast. [giganto- + G. *mastos,* breast]

Gig•li saw (jē′lyē saw) A hand-held wire saw for use in craniotomy.

GIH Abbreviation for growth hormone–inhibiting hormone.

Gil•bert dis•ease (zhēl′bār di-zēz′) SYN familial nonhemolytic jaundice.

Gil•christ dis•ease (gil′krist di-zēz′) SYN blastomycosis.

Gilles de la Tou•rette syn•drome (zhēl dĕ lah tūr-et′ sin′drōm) SYN Tourette syndrome.

Gil•les•pie syn•drome (gi-les′pē sin′drōm) Congenital absence of the iris, mental retardation, and cerebellar ataxia; possibly due to a heritable mutation.

Gil•li•am op•er•a•tion (gil′ē-ăm op-ĕr-ā′shŭn) An operation for retroversion of the uterus by suturing round ligaments to abdominal wall fascia.

Gil•lies op•er•a•tion (gil′ēz op-ĕr-ā′shŭn) A technique for reducing fractures of the zygoma and the zygomatic arch through an incision in the temporal region above the hairline.

gin•gi•va, gen. and pl. **gin•gi•vae** (jin′ji-vă, -vē) [TA] The dense fibrous tissue, covered by mucous membrane, that envelops the alveolar processes of the upper and lower jaws and surrounds the necks of the teeth. SYN gum (2). [L.]

gin•gi•val (jin′ji-văl) Relating to the gums.

gin•gi•val ab•scess (jin′ji-văl ab′ses) An abscess confined to the gingival soft tissue. SYN gumboil, parulis.

Gin•gi•val In•dex (GI) (jin′ji-văl in′deks) Measurement of periodontal disease based on the severity and location of the lesion.

gin•gi•val line (jin′ji-văl līn) The position of the margin of the gingiva in relation to the teeth in the dental arch. SYN gum line.

gin·gi·val mar·gin (jin′ji-văl mahr′jin) **1.** The most coronal portion of the gingiva surrounding the tooth. **2.** The edge of the free gingiva.

gin·gi·val mas·sage (jin′ji-văl mă-sahzh′) Mechanical stimulation of the gingiva by rubbing or pressure to improve tissue tone and blood circulation.

Gin·gi·val-Per·i·o·don·tal In·dex (GPI) (jin′ji-văl per′ē-ō-don′tăl in′deks) An index of gingivitis, gingival irritation, and advanced periodontal disease.

gin·gi·val sul·cus (jin′ji-văl sŭl′kŭs) SYN sulcus (4).

gin·gi·vec·to·my (jin′ji-vek′tŏ-mē) Surgical resection of unsupported gingival tissue; performed to arrest development of periodontal disease. SYN gum resection. [gingiva + G. *ektomē,* excision]

gin·gi·vi·tis (jin′ji-vī′tis) Inflammation of the gingiva with no apical migration of the junctional epithelium beyond the cementoenamel junction. [gingiva + G. *-itis,* inflammation]

♻**gingivo-** Combining form meaning the gingivae, the gums of the mouth. [L. *gingiva*]

gin·gi·vo·glos·si·tis (jin′ji-vō-glos-ī′tis) Inflammation of both the tongue and gingival tissues. SEE ALSO stomatitis.

gin·gi·vo·lin·guo·ax·i·al (jin′ji-vō-ling′gwō-ak′sē-ăl) Referring to the point angle formed by the gingival, lingual, and axial walls of a cavity.

gin·gi·vo·os·se·ous (jin′ji-vō-os′ē-ŭs) Referring to the gingiva and its underlying bone.

gin·gi·vo·plas·ty (jin′ji-vō-plas-tē) A surgical procedure that reshapes and recontours the gingival tissue to attain esthetic, physiologic, and functional form.

gin·gi·vo·sis (jin′ji-vō′sis) SYN chronic desquamative gingivitis.

gin·gi·vo·sto·ma·ti·tis (jin′ji-vō-stō′mă-tī′tis) Inflammation of the gingiva and other oral mucous membranes. [gingivo- + G. *stoma,* mouth, + *-itis,* inflammation]

gin·gly·form (jing′gli-fōrm) SYN ginglymoid. [G. *ginglymos,* a hinge joint, + L. *forma,* form]

gin·glym·o·ar·thro·di·al (jing′gli-mō-ahr-thrō′dē-ăl) Denoting a joint having the form of both ginglymus and arthrodia, or hinge joint and sliding joint.

gin·gly·moid (jing′gli-moyd) Relating to or resembling a hinge joint. SYN ginglyform. [G. *ginglymos,* a hinge joint, + *eidos,* resembling]

gin·gly·moid joint (jing′gli-moyd joynt) SYN hinge joint.

gin·gly·mus (jing′gli-mŭs) SYN hinge joint. [G. *ginglymos*]

Gink·go bi·lo·ba (ging′kō bi-lō′bă) Extremely widely used herbal native to China but extinct in the wild, surviving only in cultivation that is claimed to improve vascular insufficiency; and palliate symptoms of Alzheimer disease; adverse effects include subdural hematoma and bleeding disorders. Prescribed as a drug in some countries of the European Union.

gin·seng (jin′seng) (*Panax quinquefolius*) Herbal with dozens of purported therapeutic properties (e.g., antidepressant, aphrodisiac, sleep aid, systemic panacea); used worldwide by enormous numbers of people.

GIP Abbreviation for gastric inhibitory polypeptide; gastric inhibitory peptide.

Gi·rard re·a·gent (ji-rahr′ rē-ā′jĕnt) The hydrazine of betaine chloride, used to extract ketonic steroids by forming water-soluble hydrazones with them.

gir·dle (gĭr′dĕl) A belt; a zone. A structure that has the form of a belt or girdle. SYN cingulum (1) [TA]. [A.S. *gyrdel*]

gir·dle an·es·the·si·a (gĭr′dĕl an′es-thē′zē-ă) Anesthesia distributed as a band encircling the trunk.

gir·dle sen·sa·tion (gĭr′dĕl sen-sā′shŭn) SYN zonesthesia.

gla·bel·la (glă-bel′ă) **1.** A smooth prominence, most marked in the male, on the frontal bone above the root of the nose. **2.** The most forward projecting point of the forehead in the midline at the level of the supraorbital ridges. SYN intercilium, mesophryon. SEE ALSO antinion. [L. *glabellus,* hairless, smooth, dim. of *glaber*]

gla·brous, gla·brate (glā′brŭs, -brāt) Smooth or hairless; denoting areas of the body where hair does not normally grow, i.e., palms or soles. [L. *glaber,* smooth]

gland (gland) An organized aggregation of cells functioning as a secretory or excretory organ. SYN glandula (1). [L. *glans,* acorn]

glan·des (glan′dēz) Plural of glans.

glan·di·lem·ma (glan′di-lem′ă) The capsule of a gland. [L. *glandula,* gland, + G. *lemma,* sheath]

glands of the fe·male u·re·thra (glandz fē′māl yūr-ē′thră) Numerous mucous glands in the wall of the female urethra.

glands of the male u·re·thra (glandz māl yūr-ē′thră) Numerous mucous glands in the wall of the penile urethra.

glan·du·la, pl. **glan·du·lae** (glan′dyū-lă, -lē) **1.** SYN gland. **2.** SYN glandule. [L. gland, dim. of *glans,* acorn]

glan·du·lae ce·ru·mi·no·sae (glan′dyū-lē sĕ-rū-mi-nō′sē) [TA] **1.** SYN ceruminous glands. **2.** Tubuloalveolar glands of the external auditory meatus believed to be modified apocrine sweat glands; they secrete cerumen.

glan•du•lar (glan′dyū-lăr) Relating to a gland. SYN glandulous.

glan•du•lar ep•i•the•li•um (glan′dyū-lăr ep′i-thē′lē-ŭm) Epithelium composed of secretory cells.

glan•dule (glan′dyūl) A small gland. SYN glandula (2). [L. *glandula*]

glan•du•lous (glan′dyū-lŭs) SYN glandular.

glans, pl. **glan•des** (glanz, glan′dēz) A conic acorn-shaped structure. [L. acorn]

glans cli•to•ri•dis (glanz kli-tō′ri-dis) [TA] SYN glans of clitoris.

glans of clit•o•ris (glanz klit′ŏr-is) A small mass of highly sensitized erectile tissue capping the body of the clitoris. SYN glans clitoridis [TA].

glans pe•nis (glanz pē′nis) [TA] The conic expansion of the corpus spongiosum which forms the head of the penis.

glan•u•lar (glan′yū-lăr) Pertaining to the glans penis. [irreg. fr. *glans*, by analogy with *glandular*]

Glanz•mann throm•bas•the•ni•a (glahnts′mahn throm′bas-thē′nē-ă) A hemorrhagic diathesis characterized by normal or prolonged bleeding time, normal coagulation time, defective clot retraction, and normal platelet count but morphologic or functional abnormality of platelets; several kinds of platelet abnormalities have been described; caused by defect in platelet membrane glycoprotein IIb-IIIa complex; autosomal recessive inheritance, caused by mutation in the platelet-membrane glycoprotein IIb-IIIa complex gene (ITGA2B) on chromosome 17.

gla•se•ri•an fis•sure (glā-sēr′ē-ăn fish′ŭr) SYN petrotympanic fissure.

Glas•gow Co•ma Scale (glas′gō kō′mă skāl) A measure used to assess level of consciousness and reaction to stimuli in a neurologically impaired patient based on performance in three categories: eye opening, verbal response-performance, and motor responsiveness. The three scores are added. Lower scores predict poorer outcomes. The scale was originally worked out in Glasgow in Scotland. SYN outcome score. [Glasgow, Scotland]

Glas•gow sign (glas′gō sīn) A systolic murmur heard over the brachial artery in aneurysm of the aorta.

glass (glas) A transparent substance composed of silica and oxides of various bases. [A.S. *glaes*]

glass•es (glas′ĕz) SYN spectacles.

glass i•o•no•mer ce•ment (glas ī-on′ō-mĕr sĕ-ment′) A fluoride-releasing restorative cement produced by mixing calcium aluminosilicate glass with an aqueous solution of polyacrylic acid. [ion + -mer (1)]

glas•sy mem•brane (glas′ē mem′brān) **1.** The basement membrane present between the stratum granulosum and the theca interna of a vesicular ovarian follicle; it becomes very prominent in large atretic follicles. **2.** The basement membrane and associated connective tissue of the hair follicle. SYN hyaline membrane (2).

glau•co•ma (glaw-kō′mă) A disease of the eye associated with increased intraocular pressure and excavation and atrophy of the optic nerve; produces defects in the visual field and may result in blindness; may be primary or secondary, acute or chronic, open or closed. See this page. [G. *glaukōma*, opacity of the crystalline lens, fr. *glaukos*, bluish green]

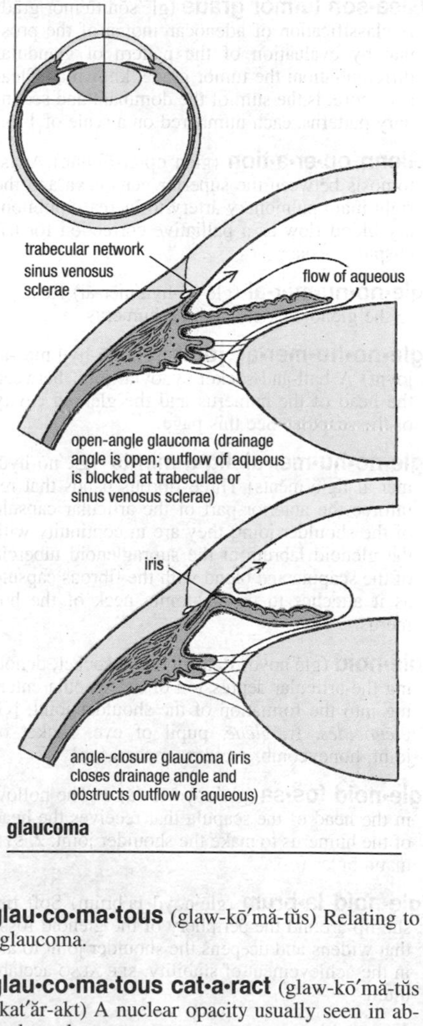

glaucoma

glau•co•ma•tous (glaw-kō′mă-tŭs) Relating to glaucoma.

glau•co•ma•tous cat•a•ract (glaw-kō′mă-tŭs kat′ăr-akt) A nuclear opacity usually seen in absolute glaucoma.

glau•co•ma•tous cup (glaw-kō′mă-tŭs kŭp) A deep depression of the optic disc combined with optic atrophy; caused by glaucoma. See page B26. SYN glaucomatous excavation.

glau•co•ma•tous ex•ca•va•tion (glaw-kō′mă-tŭs eks′kă-vā′shŭn) SYN glaucomatous cup.

glau•co•ma•tous ha•lo (glaw-kō′mă-tŭs hā′lō) **1.** A yellowish white ring surrounding the optic disc, indicating atrophy of the choroid in glaucoma. **2.** A halo surrounding lights, caused by corneal edema in closed-angle granule closure glaucoma.

GLC Abbreviation for gas-liquid chromatography.

Glc, GlcA, GlcN, GlcNAc, GlcUA Symbols for the radicals of D-glucose, gluconic and glucuronic acid, glucosamine, *N*-acetylglucosamine, and glucuronic acid, respectively.

Glea•son tu•mor grade (glē′sŏn tū′mŏr grād) A classification of adenocarcinoma of the prostate by evaluation of the pattern of glandular differentiation; the tumor grade, known as Gleason score, is the sum of the dominant and secondary patterns, each numbered on a scale of 1–5.

Glenn op•er•a•tion (glen op-ĕr-ā′shŭn) Anastomosis between the superior vena cava and the right main pulmonary artery to increase pulmonary blood flow as a palliative correction for tricuspid atresia.

gle•no•hu•mer•al (glē′nō-hyū′mĕr-ăl) Relating to the glenoid cavity and the humerus.

gle•no•hu•mer•al joint (glē′nō-hyū′mĕr-ăl joynt) A ball-and-socket synovial joint between the head of the humerus and the glenoid cavity of the scapula. See this page.

gle•no•hu•mer•al lig•a•ments (glē′nō-hyū′mĕr-ăl lig′ă-mĕnts) Three fibrous bands that reinforce the anterior part of the articular capsule of the shoulder joint; they are in continuity with the glenoid labrum at the supraglenoid tubercle of the scapula and blend with the fibrous capsule as it attaches to the anatomic neck of the humerus.

gle•noid (glē′noyd) Resembling a socket; denoting the articular depression of the scapula entering into the formation of the shoulder joint. [G. *glēnoeidēs,* fr. *glēnē,* pupil of eye, socket of joint, honeycomb, + *eidos,* appearance]

gle•noid fos•sa (glē′noyd fos′ă) **1.** The hollow in the head of the scapula that receives the head of the humerus to make the shoulder joint. **2.** SYN mandibular fossa.

gle•noid la•brum (glē′noyd lā′brŭm) Soft tissue lip around the periphery of the glenoid fossa that widens and deepens the shoulder joint to aid in the achievement of stability. SEE ALSO acetabulum.

gli•a (glī′ă) SYN neuroglia. [G. glue]

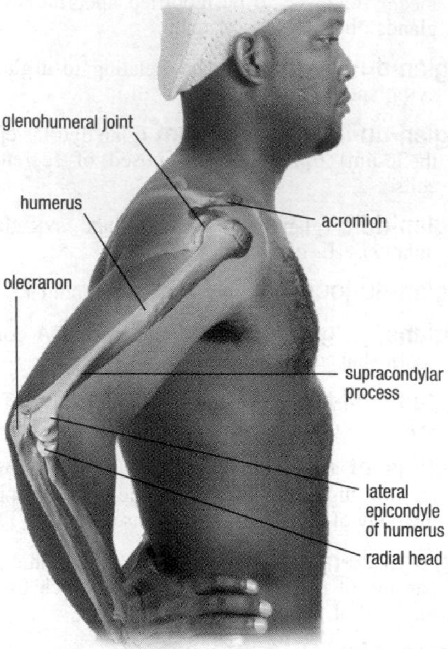

glenohumeral joint

gli•a cells (glī′ă selz) SEE neuroglia.

gli•a•cyte (glī′ă-sīt) A neuroglia cell. SEE neuroglia. [G. *glia,* glue, + *kytos,* cell]

gli•a•din (glī′ă-din) A class of protein, separable from wheat and rye glutens, that contains up to 40% L-glutamine; a member of the prolamins, which are insoluble in water, absolute alcohol, and neutral solvents, but soluble in 50–90% alcohol.

gli•al (glī′ăl) Pertaining to glia or neuroglia.

gli•al fib•ril•lar•y a•cid•ic pro•tein (glī′ăl fib′ri-lar-ē a-sid′ik prō′tēn) A cytoskeletal protein of 51 kD found in fibrous astrocytes; stains for this protein are frequently used to assist in the differential diagnosis of neurologic lesions.

glide•wire (glīd′wīr) A hydrophilic or lubricated guidewire, generally used in the urinary tract. SEE ALSO guidewire.

glid•ing joint (glīd′ing joynt) SYN plane joint.

glio- Prefix meaning glue, gluelike (relating specifically to the neuroglia). [G. *glia,* glue]

gli•o•blast (glī′ō-blast) An early neural cell developing from the early ependymal cell of the neural tube; gives rise to neuroglial and ependymal cells, astrocytes, and oligodendrocytes. SEE ALSO spongioblast. [glio- + G. *blastos,* germ]

gli•o•blas•to•ma mul•ti•for•me (glī′ō-blas-tō′mă mŭl′ti-fōr′mē) A glioma consisting chiefly of undifferentiated anaplastic cells of glial origin that show marked nuclear pleomorphism, necrosis, and vascular endothelial proliferation; frequently, tumor cells are arranged radially about an irregular focus of necrosis; these neoplasms grow rapidly, invade extensively, and occur most frequently in the cerebrum of adults. SYN grade IV astrocytoma. [G. *glia,* glue, + *blastos,* germ, + *-oma,* tumor]

gli•o•ma (glī-ō′mă) Any neoplasm derived from one of the various types of cells that form the interstitial tissue of the brain, spinal cord, pineal gland, posterior pituitary gland, and retina. [G. *glia,* glue, + *-oma,* tumor]

gli•o•ma•to•sis (glī′ō-mă-tō′sis) Neoplastic growth of neuroglial cells in the brain or spinal cord; the term is used especially with reference to a relatively large neoplasm or to multiple foci. SYN neurogliomatosis.

gli•o•ma•tous (glī-ō′mă-tŭs) Pertaining to or characterized by a glioma.

gli•o•neu•ro•ma (glī′ō-nūr-ō′mă) A ganglioneuroma derived from neurons, with numerous glial cells and fibers in the matrix.

gli•o•sar•co•ma (glī′ō-sahr-kō′mă) A glioblastoma multiforme with an associated malignant mesenchymal component. Sometimes used as a term for a malignant neoplasm derived from connective tissue (e.g., that associated with blood vessels in the brain) in which there are proliferating glial cells.

gli•o•sis (glī-ō′sis) Overgrowth of the astrocytes in an area of damage in the brain or spinal cord.

GLIP (glip) Acronym for glucagonlike insulinotropic peptide.

Glis•son cap•sule (glis′ĕn kap′sŭl) SYN fibrous capsule of liver.

Glis•son cir•rho•sis (glis′ĕn sir-ō′sis) Chronic perihepatitis with thickening and subsequent contraction, resulting in atrophy and deformity of the liver.

Gln Abbreviation for glutamine or its acyl radical, glutaminyl.

glob•al (glō′băl) Complete, generalized, overall, or total.

glob•al a•pha•si•a (glō′băl ă-fā′zē-ă) Disorder in which all aspects of speech and communication are severely impaired. At best, patients can understand or speak only a few words or phrases; they can neither read nor write. SYN mixed aphasia, total aphasia.

glob•al bur•den of dis•ease (glō′băl bŭr′dĕn di-zēz′) Mathematical measure of loss of healthy life years due to disabling diseases in a country's population. SEE ALSO disability-adjusted life years.

glob•al warm•ing (glō′băl wōrm′ing) A nonspecific colloquialism for the phenomena related to changes in weather pattern caused by generalized elevation of ocean temperature. Although still in slight dispute in some quarters, recognized as a dangerous and potentially overwhelming ecologic crisis; some scientists believe it may be possible to reverse the trend through limitation of greenhouse gas emissions, which are thought responsible for the rise in global temperatures.

glo•bi (glō′bī) **1.** Plural of globus. **2.** Brown bodies sometimes found in the granulomatous lesions of leprosy.

glo•bin (glō′bin) The protein of hemoglobin; α-globin and β-globin represent the two types of chains found in adult hemoglobin. SYN hematohiston.

glo•bo•side (glō′bō-sīd) A glycosphingolipid isolated from kidney and erythrocytes; accumulates in patients with Sandhoff disease.

glo•bo•tri•a•o•syl•cer•a•mide (glō′bō-trī-ă′ō-sil-ser′ă-mīd) A sphingolipid containing three sugar moieties that accumulates in patients with Fabry disease.

glob•ule (glob′yūl) **1.** A small spheric body of any kind. **2.** A fat droplet in milk. [L. *globulus,* dim. of *globus,* a ball]

glob•u•lin (glob′yū-lin) A family of proteins precipitated from plasma by ammonium sulfate. Globulins may be further fractionated by solubility, electrophoresis, ultracentrifugation, and other separation methods into many subgroups, the main groups being α-, β-, and γ-globulin; including immunoglobulins, lipoproteins, gluco- or mucoproteins, and metal-binding and metal-transporting proteins. [L. *globulus,* globule]

glob•u•li•nu•ri•a (glob′yū-li-nyūr′ē-ă) The excretion of globulin in the urine, usually, if not always, in association with serum albumin.

glo•bus, pl. **glo•bi** (glō′bŭs, -bī) **1.** A round body; ball. **2.** SEE globi. [L.]

glo•bus hys•ter•i•cus (glō′bŭs his-ter′i-kŭs) Difficulty in swallowing; a sensation as if a ball was in the throat or as if the throat compressed; a symptom of conversion disorder.

glo•bus pal•li•dus (glō′bŭs pal′i-dŭs) [TA] The inner and lighter gray portion of the lentiform nucleus. SEE ALSO paleostriatum. SYN pallidum.

glo•mal (glō′măl) Relating to or involving a glomus.

glo•man•gi•o•ma (glō-man′jē-ō′mă) A variant of glomus tumor, characterized by multiple tumors resembling cavernous hemangioma.

glo•man•gi•o•sis (glō-man′jē-ō′sis) The occurrence of multiple complexes of small vascular channels, each resembling a glomus.

glo•mec•to•my (glō-mek′tŏ-mē) Excision of a

glomus tumor. [L. *glomus* + G. *ektomē,* cutting out]

glom·er·a (glom′ĕr-ă) Plural of glomus.

glo·mer·u·lar (glō-mer′yū-lăr) Relating to or affecting a glomerulus or the glomeruli.

glo·mer·u·lar cap·sule (glō-mer′yū-lăr kap′ sŭl) The expanded beginning of a nephron composed of an inner and outer layer: the visceral layer consists of podocytes which surround a tuft of capillaries (glomerulus); the parietal layer is simple squamous epithelium which becomes cuboidal at the tubular pole.

glo·mer·u·lar cyst (glō-mer′yū-lăr sist) cyst formed by dilation of Bowman capsule, found in rare cases of congenital polycystic kidneys.

glo·mer·u·lar fil·tra·tion rate (GFR) (glō-mer′yū-lăr fil-trā′shŭn rāt) The volume of water filtered out of the plasma through glomerular capillary walls into Bowman capsules per unit time; it is considered to be equivalent to inulin clearance.

glo·mer·u·lar ne·phri·tis (glō-mer′yū-lăr nĕ-frī′tis) SYN glomerulonephritis.

glom·er·ule (glom′ĕr-yūl) SYN glomerulus.

glo·mer·u·li·tis (glō-mer′yū-lī′tis) Inflammation of a glomerulus, specifically of the renal glomeruli, as in glomerulonephritis.

glo·mer·u·lo·ne·phri·tis (glō-mer′yū-lō-nĕ-frī′tis) Renal disease characterized by inflammatory changes in glomeruli that are not the result of infection of the kidneys. SYN glomerular nephritis. [glomerulus + G. *nephros,* kidney, + *-itis,* inflammation]

glo·mer·u·lop·a·thy (glō-mer′yū-lop′ă-thē) Glomerular disease of any type. [glomerulus + G. *pathos,* suffering]

glo·mer·u·lo·sa cell (glō-mer′yū-lō′să sel) A cell of the zona glomerulosa of the cortex of the suprarenal gland that is the source of aldosterone; the cells are arranged in spheric or oval groups.

glo·mer·u·lo·scle·ro·sis (glō-mer′yū-lō-skler-ō′sis) Hyaline deposits or scarring within the renal glomeruli, a degenerative process occurring in association with renal arteriosclerosis or diabetes mellitus. [glomerulus + G. *sklērōsis,* hardness]

glo·mer·u·lus, pl. **glo·mer·u·li** (glō-mer′yū-lŭs, -ū-lī) **1.** A plexus of capillaries. **2.** A tuft formed of capillary loops at the beginning of each nephric tubule in the kidney; this tuft with its capsule constitutes the renal corpusculum (malpighian body). **3.** The twisted secretory portion of a sweat gland. **4.** A cluster of dendritic ramifications and axon terminals forming a complex synaptic relationship and surrounded by a glial sheath. SYN Bowman capsule, glomerule. [Mod. L. dim. of L. *glomus,* a ball of yarn]

glo·mus, pl. **glom·er·a** (glō′mŭs, glom′ĕr-ă) **1.** A small globular body. **2.** A highly organized arteriolovenular anastomosis forming a tiny nodular focus in the nailbed, pads of the fingers and toes, ears, hands, and feet and many other organs of the body. The anastomosis is convoluted and richly innervated and drains into a periglomic vein and then into one of the veins of the skin. The glomus functions as a shunt or bypass regulating mechanism in the flow of blood, temperature, and conservation of heat in the part as well as in the indirect control of the blood pressure and other functions of the circulatory system. [L. *glomus,* a ball]

glo·mus ju·gu·la·re tu·mor (glō′mŭs jŭg-yū-lā′rē tū′mŏr) SYN chemodectoma.

glo·mus tu·mor (glō′mŭs tū′mŏr) An unusual vascular neoplasm composed of specialized pericytes, usually in nodular masses, which occurs almost exclusively in the skin; it is exquisitely tender and may be so painful that patients voluntarily immobilize an extremity. SEE ALSO glomangioma.

glo·mus tym·pan·i·cum tu·mor (glō′mŭs tim-pan′i-kŭm tū′mŏr) A glomus tumor arising on the medial wall of the middle ear.

glos·sa (glos′ă) SYN tongue (1). [G.]

glos·sal (glos′ăl) SYN lingual (1).

glos·sal·gi·a (glos-al′jē-ă) SYN glossodynia. [gloss- + G. *algos,* pain]

glos·sec·to·my (glos-ek′tŏ-mē) Resection or amputation of the tongue. SYN lingulectomy (1). [gloss- + G. *ektomē,* excision]

Glos·si·na (glos-ī′nă) A genus of bloodsucking Diptera (tsetse flies) confined to Africa; they serve as vectors of the trypanosomes that cause African sleeping sickness. [G. *glōssa,* tongue]

glos·si·tis (glos-ī′tis) Inflammation of the tongue. [gloss- + G. *-itis,* inflammation]

glos·si·tis ar·e·a·ta ex·fo·li·a·ti·va (glos-ī′tis ar-ē-ā′tă eks-fō-lē-ă-tī′vă) SYN geographic tongue.

♻**glosso-**, **gloss-** Combining forms indicating language; corresponds to L. *linguo-*. Cf. linguo-. [G. *glōssa,* tongue]

glos·so·cele (glos′ō-sēl) A swelling and protrusion of the tongue from the mouth, owing to its excessive size. SEE ALSO macroglossia. [glosso- + G. *kēlē,* tumor, hernia]

glos·so·dyn·i·a (glos′ō-din′ē-ă) A condition characterized by burning or painful tongue. SYN burning tongue, glossalgia. [glosso- + G. *odynē,* pain]

glos·so·ep·i·glot·tic, **glos·so·ep·i·glot·tid·e·an** (glos′ō-ep-i-glot′ik, glos′ō-ep-i-glō-tid′ē-ăn) Relating to the tongue and the epiglottis.

glos•so•hy•al (glos′ō-hī′ăl) SYN hyoglossal.

glos•so•la•li•a (glos′ō-lā′lē-ă) Rarely used term for unintelligible jargon or babbling. [glosso- + G. *lalia,* talk, chat]

glos•sop•a•thy (glos-op′ă-thē) A disease of the tongue. [glosso- + G. *pathos,* suffering]

glos•so•pha•ryn•ge•al (glos′ō-făr-in′jē-ăl) Relating to the tongue and the pharynx.

glos•so•pha•ryn•ge•al breath•ing (glos′ō-făr-in′jē-ăl brēdh′ing) Respiration unaided by the usual primary muscles of respiration; the air is forced into the lungs by use of the tongue and muscles of the pharynx.

glos•so•pha•ryn•ge•al nerve [CN IX] (glos′ō-făr-in′jē-ăl nĕrv) Cranial nerve that emerges from the rostral end of the medulla and passes through the jugular foramen to supply sensation, including taste, to the pharynx and posterior third of the tongue; it also carries somatic motor fibers to the stylopharyngeus muscle and secretomotor presynaptic parasympathetic fibers to the otic ganglion for innervation of the parotid gland. SYN nervus glossopharyngeus [CN IX] [TA], ninth cranial nerve [CN IX].

glos•so•plas•ty (glos′ō-plas-tē) Surgical repair of the tongue. [glosso- + G. *plastos,* formed]

glos•sor•rha•phy (glos-ōr′ă-fē) Suture of a wound of the tongue. [glosso- + G. *rhaphē,* suture]

glos•so•spasm (glos′ō-spazm) Spasmodic contraction of the tongue.

glos•sot•o•my (glos-ot′ŏ-mē) Any cutting operation on the tongue, usually to obtain access to further reaches of the pharynx. [glosso- + G. *tomē,* incision]

glos•so•trich•i•a (glos′ō-trik′ē-ă) SYN hairy tongue. [glosso- + G. *thrix,* hair]

glot•tal (glot′ăl) Relating to the glottis.

glot•tal at•tack (glot′ăl ă-tak′) Excessive glottal closure before phonation resulting in loud and sudden voice onset.

glot•tal fry (glot′ăl frī) Vocal fold vibration in the lowest part of the pitch range, characterized by a creaky, pulsed type of phonation. SYN gravel voice.

glot•tal•iz•a•tion (glot′al-ī-zā′shŭn) SYN vocal fry.

glot•tic (glot′ik) Relating to (1) the tongue or (2) the glottis.

glot•tis, pl. **glot•ti•des** (glot′is, -i-dēz) [TA] The vocal apparatus of the larynx, consisting of the vocal folds of mucous membrane investing the vocal ligament and vocal muscle on each side, the free edges of which are the vocal cords, and of a median fissure, the rima glottidis. [G. *glōttis,* aperture of the larynx]

glot•ti•tis (glo-tī′tis) Inflammation of the glottic portion of the larynx.

glove an•es•the•si•a (glŏv an′es-thē′zē-ă) Loss of sensation in the distal upper limb, i.e., the hand and fingers.

glov•er's su•ture (glŏv′ĕrz sū′chŭr) A continuous suture in which each stitch is passed through the loop of the preceding one.

GLP-1 Abbreviation for glucagonlike peptide.

Glu Abbreviation for glutamic acid or its acyl radical, glutamyl.

glu•ca•gon (glū′kă-gon) A hormone produced by pancreatic alpha cells. Parenteral administration of 0.5–1 mg results in prompt mobilization of hepatic glycogen, thus elevating blood glucose concentration. It is used in the treatment of glycogen storage disease (von Gierke) and hypoglycemia, particularly hypoglycemic coma due to exogenously administered insulin. [glucose + G. *agō,* to lead]

glu•ca•gon•like in•su•lin•o•trop•ic pep•tide (GLIP) (glū′kă-gon-līk in′sū-lin-ō-trō′pik pep′tīd) An insulinotropic substance originating in the gastrointestinal tract and released into the circulation following ingestion of a meal containing glucose.

glu•ca•gon•like pep•tide (GLP-1) (glū′kă-gon-līk pep′tīd) A gut hormone that slows gastric emptying and stimulates insulin secretion. It may become useful in the future in the treatment of Type 2 diabetes, perhaps administered by patch, inhaler, or buccal pellet formulation.

glu•ca•gon•o•ma (glū′kă-gon-ō′mă) A glucagon-secreting tumor, usually derived from pancreatic islet cells.

glu•can (glū′kan) A polyglucose; e.g., callose, cellulose, starch amylose, glycogen amylose.

1,4-α-D-glu•can-branch•ing en•zyme (glū-kan-branch′ing en′zīm) amylo-(1,4→1,6)-transglucosylase; or transglucosidase; an enzyme in muscle and in plants (Q enzyme) that cleaves α-1,4 linkages in glycogen or starch, transferring the fragments into α-1,6 linkages, creating branches in the polysaccharide molecules; in plants, it converts amylose to amylopectin; this enzyme is deficient in individuals with glycogen storage disease type IV.

1,4-α-D-glu•can 6-α-D-glu•co•syl•trans•fer•ase, α-glu•can-branch•ing gly•co•syl•trans•fer•ase (glū′kan glū-kō′sil-tranz′fĕr-ās, glū′kan-branch′ing glī-kō′sil-trans′fĕr-ās) A glucosyltransferase that transfers an α-glucosyl residue in a 1,4-α-glucan to the primary hydroxyl group of glucose in a 1,4-α-glucan.

4-α-D-β-glu•can•o•trans•fer•ase (glū-′kă-nō-trans′fĕr-ās) A 4-glycosyltransferase that converts maltodextrins into amylose and glucose by transferring parts of 1,4-glucan chains to new 4-positions on glucose or other 1,4-glucans.

♲**gluco-** Combining form meaning glucose. SEE ALSO glyco-. [G. *gleukos*, sweet new wine, sweetness]

glu·co·cer·e·bro·side (glū′kō-ser′ĕ-brō-sīd) SYN glucosylceramide.

glu·co·cor·ti·coid (glū′kō-kōr′ti-koyd) **1.** Any steroidlike compound capable of significantly promoting hepatic glycogen deposition, influencing intermediate metabolism, and exerting a clinically useful antiinflammatory effect. Cortisol is the most potent of the naturally occurring glucocortocoids; most semisynthetic glucocortocoids are cortisol derivatives. **2.** Denoting this type of biologic activity. SYN glycocorticoid.

glu·co·fu·ra·nose (glū′kō-fyūr′ă-nōs) Glucose in furanose form.

glu·co·gen·e·sis (glū′kō-jen′ĕ-sis) Formation of glucose. [gluco- + G. *genesis*, production]

glu·co·gen·ic (glū′kō-jen′ik) Giving rise to or producing glucose.

glu·co·ki·nase (glū′kō-kī′nās) Phosphotransferase that catalyzes the conversion of D-glucose and ATP D-glucose 6-phosphate and ADP; the liver enzyme has a higher K_m value for D-glucose than does hexokinase.

glu·co·ki·net·ic (glū′kō-ki-net′ik) Tending to mobilize glucose; usually evidenced by a reduction of the glycogen stores in the tissues to produce an increase in the concentration of glucose circulating in the blood.

glu·co·lip·ids (glū′kō-lip′idz) Glycosphingolipids that contain D-glucose.

glu·com·e·ter (glū′kō-mē′tĕr) A device used to measure sugar levels in blood.

glu·co·ne·o·gen·e·sis (glū′kō-nē′ō-jen′ĕ-sis) The formation of glucose from noncarbohydrates, such as protein or fat. Cf. glyconeogenesis.

glu·con·ic ac·id (glū-kon′ik as′id) The hexonic (aldonic) acid derived from glucose by oxidation of the –CHO group to –COOH.

glu·co·pro·tein (glū′kō-prō′tēn) A glycoprotein in which the sugar is glucose.

glu·co·pyr·a·nose (glū′kō-pir′ă-nōs) Glucose in its pyranose form.

glu·co·san (glū′kō-san) A polysaccharide yielding glucose on hydrolysis (e.g., callose, cellulose, glycogen, starch, dextrins).

glu·cose (glū′kōs) A dextrorotatory monosaccharide found in a free form in fruits and other parts of plants, and in combination in glucosides, glycogen, disaccharides, and polysaccharides (starch cellulose); the chief source of energy in human metabolism, the final product of carbohydrate digestion, and the principal sugar of the blood; insulin is required for the use of glucose by cells; in diabetes mellitus, the level of glucose in the blood is excessive, and it also appears in the urine. SYN D-glucose.

D-glu·cose (G, Glc) (glū′kōs) SYN glucose.

glu·cose-de·pen·dent in·su·lin·o·tro·pic po·ly·pep·tide (glū′kōs-dĕ-pen′dĕnt in′sŭ-lin-ō-trō′pik pol′ē-pep′tīd) An insulinotropic substance originating in the gastrointestinal tract and released into the circulation following ingestion of a meal containing glucose.

glu·cose ox·i·dase meth·od (glū′kōs ok′si-dās meth′ŏd) A highly specific method for measurement of glucose in serum or plasma by reaction with glucose oxidase, in which gluconic acid and hydrogen peroxide are formed.

glu·cose 6-phos·phate (glū′kōs fos′fāt) An ester of glucose with phosphoric acid; made in the course of glucose metabolism by mammalian and other cells; a normal constituent of resting muscle.

glu·cose-6-phos·phate de·hy·dro·gen·ase (G6PD) de·fi·cien·cy (glū′kōs fos′fāt dē-hī-droj′ĕ-nās dĕ-fish′ĕn-sē) Congenital deficiency of glucose-6-phosphate dehydrogenase, an enzyme important for maintaining cellular concentrations of reduced nucleotides; can cause a variety of anemias, including favism, primaquine sensitivity and other drug-sensitivity anemias, anemia of the newborn, and chronic nonspherocytic hemolytic anemia.

glu·cose tol·er·ance test (GTT) (glū′kōs tol′ĕr-ăns test) A test for diabetes, or for hypoglycemic states such as may be seen rarely in patients with insulinomas. Following ingestion of 75 g of glucose while the patient is fasting, the blood sugar promptly rises and then falls to normal within 2 hours; in diabetic patients, the increase is greater and the return to normal unusually prolonged; in hypoglycemic patients, depressed glucose levels may be observed in 3-, 4-, or 5-hour measurements.

glu·cose trans·port max·i·mum (glū′kōs trans′pōrt mak′si-mŭm) The maximal rate of reabsorption of glucose from the glomerular filtrate; it amounts to approximately 320 mg/minute in humans.

α-glu·co·si·dase in·hib·i·tor (glū-kō′si-dās in-hib′i-tŏr) An oral agent that aids in the control of diabetes mellitus by delaying the absorption of glucose from the digestive system.

glu·co·si·dase in·hib·i·tors (glū-kō′sid′ās in-hib′i-tŏrz) Agents such as acarbose that reduce gastrointestinal absorption of carbohydrates. This group of drugs, known popularly as "starch blockers," lowers plasma glucose levels and tend to cause weight loss. Flatulence is a limiting side effect.

glu·co·si·das·es (glū-kō′sid-ās-ĕz) Enzymes that hydrolyze glucosides.

glu·co·side (glū′kō-sīd) A compound of glucose with an alcohol or other R–OH compound involving loss of the H atom of the 1-OH (hemiacetal) group of the glucose, yielding a –C–O–R link from the C-1 of the glucose; a glycoside of glucose.

glu·co·sin·o·lates (glū′kō-sin′ō-lāts) A group of secondary plant metabolites occurring in cruciferous plants, especially *Brassica* vegetables (e.g., cabbage); hydrolyzed into wide range of biologically active compounds, including isothiocyanates, which show anticarcinogenic activity.

glu·cos·u·ri·a (glū′kō-syūr′ē-ă) The urinary excretion of glucose, usually in enhanced quantities. SYN glycosuria (1), glycuresis (1). [glucose + G. *ouron,* urine]

glu·co·syl·cer·a·mide (glū′kō-sil-ser′ă-mīd) A neutral glycolipid containing equimolar amounts of fatty acid, glucose, and sphingosine (or a derivative thereof); accumulates in people with Gaucher disease. SYN glucocerebroside.

glu·co·syl·trans·fer·ase (glū′kō-sil-trans′fĕr-ās) Any enzyme transferring glucosyl groups from one compound to another.

glu·cu·ro·nate (glū-kyūr′ō-nāt) A salt or ester of glucuronic acid.

glu·cu·ron·ic ac·id (glū′kyūr-on′ik as′id) The uronic acid of glucose in which C-6 is oxidized to a carboxyl group; the D-isomer detoxicates or inactivates various substances (e.g., benzoic acid, phenol, camphor, and the female sex hormones), the glucuronides so formed being excreted in the urine.

glu·cu·ro·nide, **glu·cu·ro·no·side** (glū-kyūr′ō-nīd, glū′kyūr-on′ō-sīd) A glycoside of glucuronic acid; many foreign chemicals, as well as catabolic products of normal body constituents (e.g., steroid hormones), are commonly excreted in the urine as D-glucuronides, the conjugation taking place in the liver.

glue-foot·ed gait (glū-fūt-ĕd gāt) SYN Bruns ataxia.

glue-sniff·ing (glū′snif-ing) Inhalation of fumes from plastic cements; the solvents, which include toluene, xylene, and benzene, induce central nervous system stimulation followed by depression.

glu·ta·mate (glū′tă-māt) A salt or ester of glutamic acid.

glu·tam·ic ac·id (E, Glu) (glū-tam′ik as′id) An amino acid that occurs in proteins; the sodium salt is monosodium glutamate. Cf. glutamate.

glu·tam·ic-ox·a·lo·a·ce·tic trans·am·i·nase (GOT) (glū-tam′ik-oks′ă-lō-ă-sē′tik trans-am′i-nās) SYN aspartate aminotransferase.

glu·tam·ic-py·ru·vic trans·am·i·nase (GPT) (glū-tam′ik-pī-rū′vik trans-am′i-nās) SYN alanine aminotransferase.

glu·ta·min·ase (glū-tam′in-ās) An enzyme in kidney and other tissues that catalyzes the hydrolysis of L-glutamine to ammonia and L-glutamic acid; an important enzyme for urinary ammonia formation.

glu·ta·mine (Gln, Q) (glū′tă-mēn) The δ-amide of glutamic acid, derived by oxidation from proline in the liver or by the combination of glutamic acid with ammonia; the L-isomer is present in proteins and in blood and other tissues, and is an important source of urinary ammonia.

glu·tam·i·nyl (Glx, Gln, Q) (glū-tam′i-nil) The acyl radical of glutamine.

glu·tam·o·yl (glū-tam′ō-il) The radical of glutamic acid from which both α- and δ-hydroxyl groups have been removed.

glu·tam·yl (Glx, E, Glu) (glū′tă-mil) The radical of glutamic acid from which either the α- or the δ-hydroxyl group has been removed.

glu·tar·al·de·hyde (glū′tăr-al′dĕ-hīd) High-level disinfectant; registred as a sterilant/disinfectant chemical with the U.S. Environmental Protection Agency.

glu·tar·ic ac·id (glū-tar′ik as′id) An intermediate in tryptophan catabolism; accumulates in glutaric acidemia.

glu·ta·thi·one (GSH) (glū′tă-thī′ōn) **1.** The principal low molecular weight thiol compound of living plant cells; used in the course of intermediary metabolism as a donor of thiol (SH) groups; essential for detoxification of acetaminophen. **2.** Compound has a wide variety of roles in a cell. A deficiency can cause hemolysis with oxidative stress.

glu·te·al (glū′tē-ăl) Relating to the buttocks. [G. *gloutos,* buttock]

glu·te·al fold, **glu·te·al fur·row** (glū′tē-ăl fōld, fŭr′ō) A prominent fold that marks the upper limit of the thigh and the lower limit of the buttock; it coincides with the lower border of the gluteus maximus muscle.

glu·te·al tu·ber·os·i·ty (glū′tē-ăl tū′bĕr-os′i-tē) The roughened area of insertion on the upper portion of the shaft of the femur of the deep, lesser part of the gluteus maximus muscle; when markedly developed, this tuberosity is called the third trochanter.

glu·ten (glū′tĕn) The insoluble protein (prolamines) constituent of wheat and other grains; a mixture of gliadin, glutenin, and other proteins; believed to be an agent in celiac disease. [L. *gluten,* glue]

glu·ten a·tax·i·a (glū′tĕn ă-tak′sē-ă) Ataxia resulting from immunologic damage to cerebellulm, posterior spinal columns, and peripheral nerves in gluten-senstive people.

glu•ten en•ter•op•a•thy (glū′tĕn en′tĕr-op′ă-thē) SYN celiac disease.

glu•ten-free di•et (glūt′ten-frē dī′ĕt) Elimination of all wheat, rye, barley, and oat gluten from the diet; treatment for gluten-sensitive enteropathy. SEE celiac disease.

glu•te•o•fem•o•ral (glū′tē-ō-fem′ŏr-ăl) Relating to the buttocks and thighs.

glu•te•us max•i•mus gait (glū-tē′ŭs maks′i-mŭs gāt) Compensatory backward propulsion of trunk to maintain center of gravity over the supporting lower extremity.

glu•te•us max•i•mus mus•cle (glū′tē-ŭs maks′i-mŭs mŭs′ĕl) *Origin*, ilium behind posterior gluteal line, posterior surface of sacrum and coccyx, and sacrotuberous ligament; *insertion*, iliotibial band of fascia lata (superficial three quarters) and gluteal ridge (deep inferior one quarter) of femur; *action*, extends thigh, especially from the flexed position, as in climbing stairs or rising from a sitting position; *nerve supply*, inferior gluteal. See this page. SYN musculus gluteus maximus [TA].

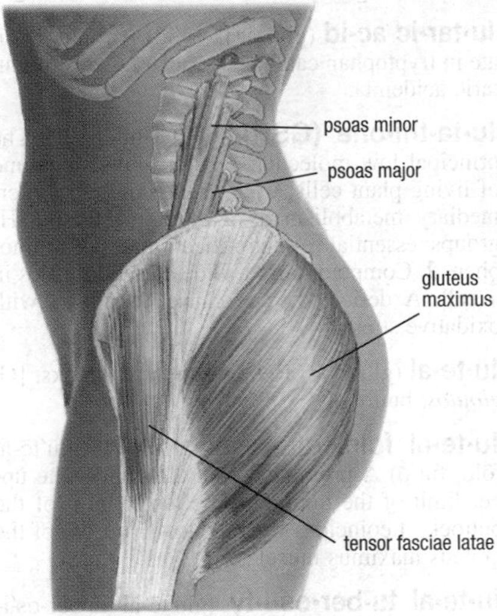

gluteus maximus muscle

glu•te•us me•di•us gait (glū-tē′ŭs mē′dē-ŭs gāt) Compensatory action during the stance phase of gait list of body (or throw of trunk) to the weak gluteal side, to place the center of gravity over the supporting lower extremity.

glu•te•us me•di•us mus•cle (glū′tē-ŭs mē′dē-ŭs mŭs′ĕl) *Origin*, ilium between anterior and posterior gluteal lines; *insertion*, lateral surface of greater trochanter; *action*, abducts and rotates

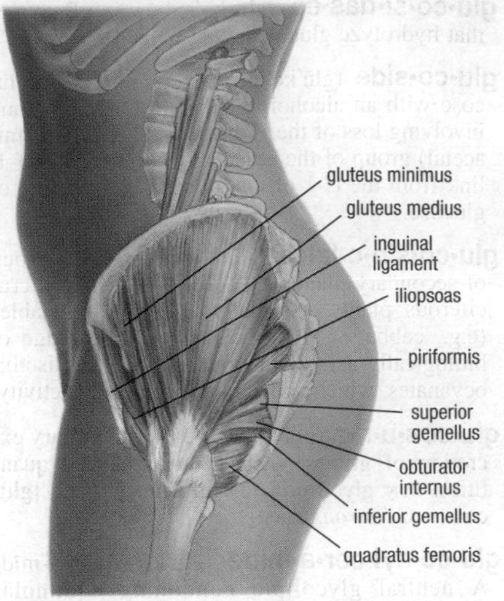

gluteus medius muscle

thigh; *nerve supply*, superior gluteal. See this page. SYN musculus gluteus medius [TA].

glu•te•us mi•ni•mus mus•cle (glū′tē-ŭs min′i-mŭs mŭs′ĕl) *Origin*, ilium between anterior and inferior gluteal lines; *insertion*, greater trochanter of femur; *action*, abducts thigh; *nerve supply*, superior gluteal. SYN musculus gluteus minimus [TA].

glu•ti•nous (glū′tin-ŭs) Sticky.

glu•ti•tis (glū-tī′tis) Inflammation of the muscles of the buttock. [G. *gloutos*, buttock, + *-itis*, inflammation]

Glx Abbreviation for glutaminyl; glutamyl.

Gly Abbreviaton for glycine or its acyl radical, glycyl.

glycaemia [Br.] SYN glycemia.

gly•can (glī′kan) SYN polysaccharide.

gly•ca•ted he•mo•glo•bin (glī′kāt-ĕd hē′mō-glō-bin) Any one of four hemoglobin A fractions to which glucose and related monosaccharides bind; concentrations are increased in the erythrocytes of patients with diabetes mellitus. The glycated hemoglobin levels change slowly and can be used as a retrospective index of glucose control over the previous 8–10 weeks in such patients. SYN glycohemoglobin.

gly•ce•mi•a (glī-sē′mē-ă) The presence of glucose in the blood. SYN glycaemia. [G. *glykys*, sweet, + *haima*, blood]

gly•ce•mic in•dex (glī-sē′mik in′deks) A relative measurement of the rise in blood glucose levels 2 hours after ingestion of any food containing 50 g. of a carbohydrate.

glyc·er·al·de·hyde (glis′ĕr-al′dĕ-hīd) A triose and the simplest optically active aldose; the dextrorotatory isomer is taken as the structural reference point for all D compounds, the levorotatory isomer for all L compounds.

gly·cer·ic ac·id (glī-ser′ik as′id) The fatty acid analog of glycerol; occurs particularly in the form of phosphorylated derivatives, as an intermediate in glycolysis.

L-gly·cer·ic ac·i·du·ri·a (glī-ser′ik as′i-dyūr′ē-ă) Excretion of L-glyceric acid in the urine; a primary metabolic error due to deficiency of D-glyceric dehydrogenase, resulting in excretion of L-glyceric and oxalic acids and leading to the clinical syndrome of oxalosis with frequent formation of oxalate renal calculi.

glyc·er·i·das·es (glis′ĕr-i-dās-ĕz) General term for enzymes catalyzing the hydrolysis of glycerol esters (glycerides); e.g., triacylglycerol lipase.

glyc·er·ide (glis′ĕr-īd) An ester of glycerol.

glyc·er·ol, glyc·er·in (glis′ĕr-ol, -in) A sweet oily fluid obtained by the saponification of fats and fixed oils; used as a solvent, as a skin emollient, by injection or in suppository form for constipation, orally to reduce ocular tension, and as a vehicle and sweetening agent.

glyc·er·ol de·hy·dra·tion test (glis′ĕr-ol dē′hī-drā′shŭn test) Transient hearing improvement in some patients with Ménière disease after an oral glycerol dose resulting in an osmotic diuresis.

glyc·er·yl (glis′ĕr-il) The trivalent radical, $C_3H_5^{\equiv}$, of glycerol; often used in error for glycero- or glycerol.

gly·cine (G, Gly) (glī′sēn) The simplest amino acid; a major component of gelatin and silk fibroin; used as a nutrient and dietary supplement, and in solution for irrigation.

gly·cine am·i·di·no·trans·fer·ase (glī′sēn am′i-dē′nō-trans′fĕr-ās) An enzyme catalyzing the transfer of an amidine group from L-arginine to glycine, forming guanidinoacetate and L-ornithine; an important reaction in creatine synthesis; it can also act on canavanine.

gly·ci·nu·ri·a (glī′si-nyūr′ē-ă) The excretion of glycine in the urine. [glycine + G. *ouron,* urine]

♲ **glyco-** Combining form denoting relationship to sugars (e.g., glycogen), or to glycine (e.g., glycocholate). SEE ALSO gluco-. [G. *glykys,* sweet]

gly·co·ca·lyx (glī′kō-kā′liks) A filamentous coating on the apical surface of certain epithelial cells, composed of carbohydrate moieties of proteins that protrude from the free surface of the plasma membrane; gives positive test result to periodic acid-Schiff procedure. [glyco- + G. *kalyx,* husk, shell]

gly·co·cho·late (glīprime;kō-kō′lāt) A salt or ester of glycocholic acid.

gly·co·cho·lic ac·id (glī′kō-kō′lik as′id) *N*-cholylglycine; one of the major bile acid conjugates, formed by condensation of the —COOH group of cholic acid and the amino group of glycine; water-soluble and a powerful detergent.

gly·co·con·ju·gates (glī′kō-kon′jŭ-găts) A general class of sugar-containing macromolecules of the body including glycolipids, glycoproteins, and proteoglycans.

gly·co·cor·ti·coid (glī′kō-kōr′ti-koyd) SYN glucocorticoid.

gly·co·gen (glī′kō-jen) A glucosan of high molecular weight, resembling amylopectin in structure [with α(1,4) linkages] but with even more highly branched [α(1,6) linkages, as well as a small number of α(1,3) linkages], found in most of the tissues of the body, especially those of the liver and muscle; as the principal carbohydrate reserve, it is readily converted into glucose. SYN animal starch.

gly·co·gen·e·sis (glī′kō-jen′ĕ-sis) Formation of glycogen from D-glucose by means of glycogen synthase and dextrin dextranase; the first enzyme catalyzes formation of a polyglucose with α-1,4 links from UDP glucose, the second cleaves fragments from one chain and transfers them to an α-1,6 linkage in another. [glyco- + G. *genesis,* production]

gly·co·ge·net·ic (glī′kō-jĕ-net′ik) Glycogenic (2); relating to glycogenesis.

gly·co·gen gran·ule (glī′kō-jen gran′yūl) Glycogen occurring in cells as beta granules that average about 300 Å in diameter, or as alpha granules that are aggregates measuring 900 Å of smaller particles.

gly·co·gen load·ing (glī′kō-jen lōd′ing) SYN carbohydrate loading.

gly·co·gen·ol·y·sis (glī′kō-jĕ-nol′i-sis) The hydrolysis of glycogen to glucose.

gly·co·ge·no·sis (glī′kō-jĕ-nō′sis) Any glycogen deposition disease characterized by accumulation of glycogen of normal or abnormal chemical structure in tissue; there may be enlargement of the liver, heart, or striated muscle, including the tongue, with progressive muscular weakness. SYN dextrinosis.

gly·co·ge·no·sis type 1 (glī′kō-jĕ-nō′sis tīp) Disorder due to glucose 6-phosphatase deficiency, resulting in accumulation of excessive glycogen of normal chemical structure, particularly in liver and kidney. SYN Gierke disease, von Gierke disease.

gly·co·ge·no·sis type 2 (glī′kō-jĕ-nō′sis tīp) Disorder due to lysosomal α-1,4-glucosidase deficiency, resulting in accumulation of excessive glycogen of normal chemical structure in heart, muscle, liver, and nervous system. SYN Pompe disease.

gly·co·ge·no·sis type 3 (glī′kō-jĕ-nō′sis tīp) Disorder due to amylo-1,6-glucosidase deficiency, resulting in accumulation of abnormal glycogen with short outer chains in liver and muscle. SYN Cori disease, Forbes disease.

gly·co·ge·no·sis type 4 (glī′kō-jĕ-nō′sis tīp) Familial cirrhosis with storage of abnormal glycogen; glycogenosis due to deficiency of 1,4-α-glucan branching enzyme, resulting in accumulation of abnormal glycogen with long inner and outer chains in liver, kidney, muscle, and other tissues. SYN Andersen disease.

gly·co·ge·no·sis type 5 (glī′kō-jĕ-nō′sis tīp) Disorder due to muscle glycogen phosphorylase deficiency, resulting in accumulation of glycogen of normal chemical structure in muscle tissue. SYN McArdle disease, McArdle-Schmid-Pearson disease.

gly·co·ge·no·sis type 6 (glī′kō-jĕ-nō′sis tīp) Disorder due to hepatic glycogen phosphorylase deficiency, resulting in accumulation of glycogen of normal chemical structure in liver tissue and leukocytes. SYN Hers disease.

gly·co·gen su·per·com·pen·sa·tion (glī′kō-jen sū′pĕr-kom′pĕn-sa′shŭn) SYN carbohydrate loading.

glycohaemoglobin [Br.] SYN glycohemoglobin.

gly·co·he·mo·glo·bin (glī′kō-hē′mō-glō′bin) SYN glycated hemoglobin. SYN glycohaemoglobin.

gly·col·al·de·hyde (glī′kol-al′dĕ-hīd) The simplest two-carbon sugar; the aerobic deamination product of ethanolamine.

gly·col·ic ac·id (glī-kol′ik as′id) An intermediate in the interconversion of glycine and ethanolamine.

gly·col·ic ac·i·du·ri·a (glī-kol′ik as′i-dyūr′ē-ă) Excessive excretion of glycolic acid in the urine; a primary metabolic defect due to deficiency of 2-hydroxy-3-oxoadipate carboxylase, resulting in excretion of glycolic and oxalic acids, leading to the clinical syndrome of oxalosis.

gly·co·lip·id (glī′kō-lip′id) A lipid with one or more covalently attached sugars.

gly·co·lyl (glī′kō-lil) The acyl radical of glycolic acid, replacing acetyl in some sialic acids; the products are called *N*-glycolylneuraminic acids.

gly·col·y·sis (glī-kol′i-sis) The energy-yielding conversion of D-glucose to lactic acid (instead of pyruvate oxidation products) in various tissues, notably muscle, when sufficient oxygen is not available; given that molecular oxygen is not consumed in the process, this is frequently referred to as "anaerobic glycolysis" [glyco- + G. *lysis,* a loosening]

gly·co·lyt·ic (glī′kō-lit′ik) Relating to glycolysis.

gly·co·ne·o·gen·e·sis (glī′kō-nē′ō-jen′ĕ-sis) Formation of glycogen from noncarbohydrates, such as protein or fat, by conversion of the latter to D-glucose. SEE ALSO glycogenesis. Cf. gluconeogenesis. [glyco- + G. *neos,* new, + *genesis,* production]

gly·co·pe·ni·a (glī′kō-pē′nē-ă) A deficiency of any or all sugars in an organ or tissue. [glyco- + G. *penia,* poverty]

gly·co·pep·tide (glī′kō-pep′tīd) A compound containing sugar(s) linked to amino acids (or peptides), with the latter preponderant, as in bacterial cell walls. Cf. peptidoglycan.

gly·co·phil·i·a (glī′kō-fil′ē-ă) A condition in which there is a distinct tendency to develop hyperglycemia, even after the ingestion of a relatively small quantity of glucose. [glyko- + G. *phileō,* to love]

gly·co·pro·tein (glī′kō-prō′tēn) **1.** One of a group of protein-carbohydrate compounds (conjugated proteins), among which the most important are the mucins, mucoid, and amyloid. **2.** Sometimes restricted to proteins containing small amounts of carbohydrate, in contrast to mucoids or mucoproteins. SEE ALSO mucoprotein.

gly·co·pty·a·lism (glī′kō-tī′ă-lizm) SYN glycosialia. [glyco- + G. *ptyalon,* saliva]

gly·cor·rha·chi·a (glī′kō-rā′kē-ă) Presence of sugar in the cerebrospinal fluid. [glyco- + G. *rhachis,* spine]

gly·cor·rhe·a (glī′kōr-ē′ă) Discharge of sugar from the body, as in glucosuria, especially in unusually large quantities. SYN glycorrhoea. [glyco- + G. *rhoia,* a flow]

glycorrhoea [Br.] SYN glycorrhea.

gly·co·se·cre·to·ry (glī′kō-sĕ-krē′tŏr-ē) Causing or involved in the secretion of glycogen.

gly·co·si·a·li·a (glī′kō-sī-ā′lē-ă) Presence of sugar in the saliva. SYN glycoptyalism. [glyco- + G. *sialon,* saliva]

gly·co·si·a·lor·rhe·a (glī′kō-sī′ă-lōr′ē′ă) An excessive secretion of saliva that contains sugar. SYN glycosialorrhoea. [glyco- + G. *sialon,* saliva, + *rhoia,* a flow]

glycosialorrhoea [Br.] SYN glycosialorrhea.

gly·co·side (glī′kō-sīd) Condensation product of a sugar with any other radical involving the loss of the H of the hemiacetal or hemiketal OH of the sugar, leaving the O of this OH as the link.

gly·co·sphing·o·lip·id (glī′kō-sfing′gō-lip-id) A ceramide linked to one or more sugars through the terminal OH group; included as glycosphingolipids are cerebrosides, gangliosides, and ceramide oligosaccharides (oligoglycosylceramides). The prefix glyc- may be replaced by gluc-, galact-, lact-.

gly•co•stat•ic (glī′kō-stat′ik) Indicating the property of certain extracts of the anterior hypophysis that permits the body to maintain its glycogen stores in muscle, liver, and other tissues.

gly•cos•ur•i•a (glī′kō-syūr′ē-ă) **1.** SYN glucosuria. **2.** Urinary excretion of glucose. SYN glycuresis (2). [glyco- + G. *ouron,* urine]

gly•co•syl (glī′kō-sil) The radical resulting from detachment of the OH of the hemiacetal or hemiketal of a saccharide. Cf. glycoside.

gly•co•syl•at•ed he•mo•glo•bin (glī-kō′si-lāt-ĕd hē′mō-glō-bin) Any one of four hemoglobin A fractions (A_{Ia1}, A_{Ia2}, A_{Ib}, or A_{Ic}) to which D-glucose and related monosaccharides bind; concentrations are increased in the erythrocytes of patients with diabetes mellitus and can be used as a retrospective index of glucose control over time in such patients.

gly•co•sy•la•tion (glī′kō-si-lā′shŭn) Formation of linkages with glycosyl groups, as between D-glucose and the hemoglobin chain to form the fraction hemoglobin A_{Ic}, the level of which rises in association with the raised blood D-glucose concentration in poorly controlled or uncontrolled diabetes mellitus. SEE ALSO glycosylated hemoglobin.

gly•co•syl•trans•fer•ase (glī-kō′sil-trans′fĕr-ās) Any enzyme (EC subclass 2.4) that transfers glycosyl groups from one compound to another.

gly•co•tro•pic fac•tor (glī′kō-trō′pik fak′tŏr) A principle in extracts of the anterior lobe of the hypophysis that raises the blood sugar and antagonizes the action of insulin; purified pituitary growth hormone produces an identical effect. Cf. bioregulator. SYN insulin-antagonizing factor.

gly•cu•re•sis (glī′kyūr-ē′sis) **1.** SYN glucosuria. **2.** SYN glycosuria (2). [glyco- + G. *ourēsis,* urination]

gly•cu•ron•ate (glī′kyūr′ŏn-āt) A salt or ester of a glycuronic acid.

gly•cyl (Gly) (glī′sil) The acyl radical of glycine.

GM-CSF Abbreviation for granulocyte-macrophage colony-stimulating factor.

GMP Abbreviation for guanylic acid.

GN Abbreviation for graduate nurse.

gnat (nat) A midge; general term applied to several species of minute insects, including species of *Simulium* (buffalo gnat) and *Hippelates* (eye gnat). [A.S. *gnaet*]

gnath•ic (nath′ik) Relating to the jaw or alveolar process. [G. *gnathos,* jaw]

gnath•ic in•dex (nath′ik in′deks) Relation between the basialveolar (basion to alveolar point) and basinasal (basion to nasion) lengths: (basialveolar length × 100)/basinasal length; the result indicates the degree of projection of the maxilla or upper jaw.

gnath•i•on (nath′ē-on) The most inferior point of the mandible in the midline. In cephalometrics, it is the midpoint between the most anterior and inferior point on the bony chin, measured at the intersection of the mandibular baseline and the nasion-pogonion line. [G. *gnathos,* jaw]

♻ **gnatho-, gnath-** Combining forms denoting the jaw. [G. *gnathos*]

gnath•o•dy•nam•ics (nath′ō-dī-nam′iks) The study of the relationship of the magnitude and direction of the forces developed by and on the components of the masticatory system during function. [gnatho- + G. *dynamis,* power]

gnath•o•dy•na•mom•e•ter (nath′ō-dī′nă-mom′ĕ-tĕr) A device for measuring biting pressure. [gnatho- + dynamometer]

gnath•o•log•ic (nath′ō-loj′ik) Pertaining to gnathodynamics.

gnath•o•plas•ty (nath′ō-plas-tē) Plastic and reconstructive surgery of the jaw. [gnatho- + G. *plastos,* formed]

Gna•thos•to•ma (nath-os′tō-mă) A genus of spiruroid nematode worms (family Gnathostomatidae) characterized by several rows of cuticular spines about the head and by multiple-host aquatic life cycles; it includes pathogenic parasites of cats, cattle, and swine. [gnatho- + G. *stoma,* mouth]

♻ **-gnomonic, -gnomonical** Combining form denoting acknowledgment of elements of a disorder.

♻ **-gnomy** Combining form denoting elements taken collectively.

gno•si•a (nō′sē-ă) The perceptive faculty enabling one to recognize the form and the nature of people and things; the faculty of perceiving and recognizing. [G. *gnōsis,* knowledge]

♻ **-gnosia** Combining form denoting perception of something.

♻ **-gnosis** Combining form denoting knowledge about something.

gno•to•bi•ol•o•gy (nō′tō-bī-ol′ŏ-jē) The study of animals in the absence of contaminating microorganisms; i.e., of "germ-free" animals. [G. *gnotos,* known, + *bios,* life, + *logos,* study]

gno•to•bi•o•ta (nō′tō-bī-ō′tă) Living colonies or species assembled from pure isolates. [G. *gnotos,* known, + Mod. L. *biota,* fr. G. *bios,* life]

gno·to·bi·ot·ic (nō′tō-bī-ot′ik) Denoting germ-free or formerly germ-free organisms in which the composition of any associated microbial flora, if present, is fully defined. [see gnotobiota]

GnRH Abbreviation for gonadotropin-releasing hormone.

goal-or·i·ent·ed move·ments (gōl-ōr′ē-en-tĕd mūv′mĕnts) In physical and rehabilitation therapy, a term describing those motions intended to result in an outcome, as distinguished from those enacted in reaction to a stimulus or need.

goat thorn (gōt thōrn) SYN *Astragalus.*

gob·let cell (gob′lĕt sel) An epithelial cell that becomes distended with a large accumulation of mucous secretory granules at its apical end, giving it the appearance of a goblet. SYN beaker cell.

Gog·gi·a sign (gōj′ē-ă sīn) The fibrillation of the biceps muscle, when pinched and tapped, is confined to a limited area in cases of debilitating disease, whereas in health it is general.

goi·ter (goy′tĕr) A chronic enlargement of the thyroid gland, not due to a neoplasm, occurring endemically in certain localities, especially regions where glaciation occurred and the soil is low in iodine, and sporadically elsewhere. SYN goitre, struma. [Fr. from L. *guttur,* throat]

goitre [Br.] SYN goiter.

goi·tro·gen·ic (goy′trō-jen′ik) Causing goiter.

goi·trous (goy′trŭs) Denoting or characteristic of a goiter.

gold (Au) (gōld) A yellow metallic element, atomic no. 79, atomic wt. 196.96654; ^{198}Au (half-life of 2.694 days) is used in the treatment of certain tumors and in imaging. SYN aurum.

Gold·blatt hy·per·ten·sion (gōld′blat hī′pĕr-ten′shŭn) Increased blood pressure following obstruction of blood flow to one kidney.

Gold·blatt kid·ney (gōld′blat kid′nē) A kidney with an arterial blood supply that has been compromised, as a consequence of which arterial (renovascular) hypertension develops.

Gol·den·har syn·drome (gōl′dĕn-hahr sin′drōm) A congenital syndrome characterized by ear, eye, and oral anomalies. Ear anomalies include auricular appendices, unilateral posteriorly placed ear, unilateral microtia, atresia of external auditory meatus, and blind fistulae. See this page. [Maurice Goldenhar, 1924–2001, Swiss physician]

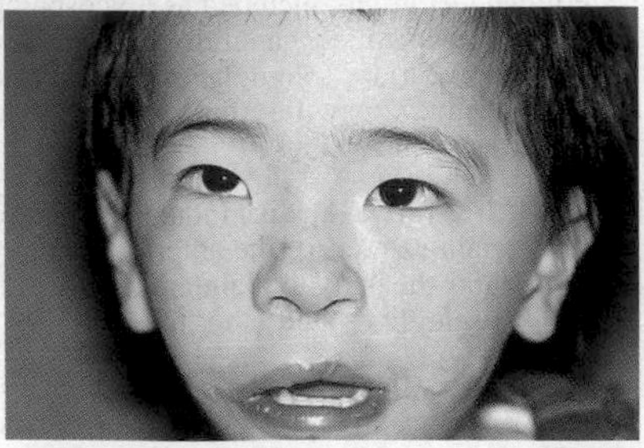

Goldenhar syndrome: note hypoplasia of left side of face, telecanthus, flat malar regions, low-set ears, and micrognathia

gol·den hour (gol′dĕn owr) Phrase used to describe the maximum amount of time from injury to definitive care for a trauma victim.

gold·en·seal (gōld′ĕn sēl) (*Hydrastis canadensis*) Herbal remedy that claims unsubstantiated benefit in treatment of anorexia nervosa, cancer, GI disease, pruritus, and other conditions. Widely reported adverse effects (e.g., seizures, cardiac problems, respiratory depression). Death has been reported after overdose. Among the most commonly used of all herbal preparations. SYN eye balm, yellow paint, yellow puccoon.

Gold·flam dis·ease (gōld′flahm di-zēz′) SYN myasthenia gravis.

Gold·mann ap·pla·na·tion to·nom·e·ter (gōld′mahn ap′lă-nā′shŭn tō-nom′ĕ-tĕr) An applanation tonometer that flattens only 3 sq. mm of cornea, used with a slitlamp; used to measure intraocular pressure.

Gold·mann-Fa·vre syn·drome (gōld′mahn fahv′rĕ sin′drōm) An autosomal recessive, progressive vitreotapetoretinal degeneration.

Gold·mann to·nom·e·ter (gōld′man tō-nom′ĕ-tĕr) Device fixed to a slit-lamp microscope that is used to measure intraocular pressure. SEE Goldmann applanation tonometer. [Hans Goldmann, 1899–1991, Swiss ophthalmologist]

Gold·schei·der test (gōlt′shī-der test) Determination of the temperature sense by touching the skin with a sharp-pointed metallic rod heated to varying degrees.

gold stan·dard (gōld stan′dărd) Jargonistic term meaning ideal or basic measurement; usage best avoided.

Gold·stein toe sign (gōld′stīn tō sīn) Increased space between the great toe and its neighbor, seen in Down syndrome, occasionally in cretinism, and as a normal variant.

gold-top tube (gōld-top tūb) A container color indicating the presence of a clot activator and serum gel separator—used for various chemical, serologic, and immunologic tests.

Gol·gi ap·pa·ra·tus (gol′jē ap′ă-rat′ŭs) A membranous system of cisternae and vesicles located between the nucleus and the secretory pole or surface of a cell; concerned with the investment and intracellular transport of membrane-bounded secretory proteins.

Gol•gi cells (gōl′jē selz) SEE Golgi type I neuron, Golgi type II neuron.

Gol•gi-Maz•zo•ni cor•pus•cle (gol′jē mahts-tsō′nē kŏr′pŭs-ĕl) An encapsulated sensory nerve ending similar to a pacinian corpuscle but simpler in structure.

Gol•gi os•mi•o•bi•chro•mate fix•a•tive (gōl′jē oz′mē-ō-bī-crō′māt fiks′ă-tiv) An osmicbichromate mixture used to demonstrate nerve cells and their processes.

Gol•gi stain (gōl′jē stān) Any of several methods for staining nerve cells, nerve fibers, and neuroglia using fixation and hardening in formalin-osmic-dichromate combinations for various times, followed by impregnation in silver nitrate.

Gol•gi ten•don or•gan (GTO) (gol′jē ten′dŏn ōr′găn) A proprioceptive sensory nerve ending embedded among the fibers of a tendon, often near the musculotendinous junction; it is activated by any increase of tension in the tendon, caused either by active contraction or passive stretch of the corresponding muscle. See this page. SYN neurotendinous spindle.

Gol•gi ten•don or•gan re•flex (gol′jē ten′dŏn ōr′găn rē′fleks) The relaxation or inhibitory response in muscles to protect them from excessive force or speed: elicited by Golgi tendon organs. Cf. myotactic reflex.

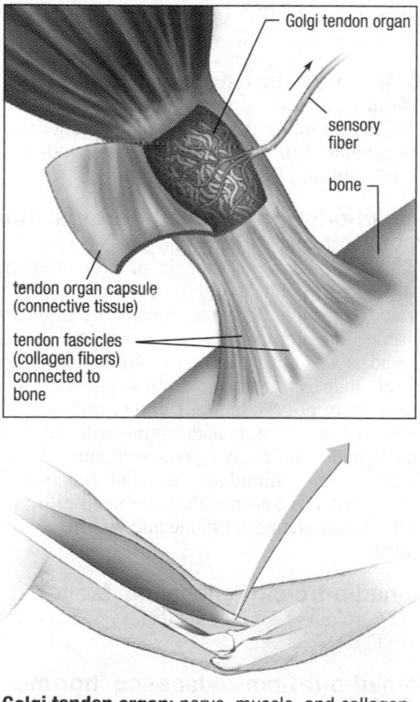

Golgi tendon organ: nerve, muscle, and collagen fibers entwined in a spindle-shaped capsule; may play a role in central inhibition of excessive muscle contraction

Gol•gi type I neu•ron (gōl′jē nūr′on) Nerve cells with long axons that leave the gray matter of which they form a part.

Gol•gi type II neu•ron (gōl′jē nūr′on) Nerve cells with short axons that ramify in the gray matter.

gom•i•to•li (gō-mit′ō-lī) Intricately coiled and looped capillary vessels present largely in the upper infundibular stem of the stalk of the pituitary gland; they make up a portion of the pituitary portal circulation. [It. *gomitolo,* coil]

Go•mo•ri al•de•hyde fuch•sin stain (gō-mōr′ē al′dĕ-hīd fūk′sin stān) A stain used to demonstrate beta cells of the pancreas, storage form of thyrotrophic hormone in beta cells of the anterior pituitary, hypophysial neurosecretory substance, mast cells, granules, elastic fibers, sulfated mucins, and gastric chief cells.

Go•mo•ri chrome al•um he•ma•tox•y•lin-phlox•ine stain (gō-mōr′ē krōm al′ŭm hē′mă-toks′i-lin stān) A technique used to demonstrate cytoplasmic granules, after Bouin or formalin-Zenker fixatives, using oxidized hematoxylin plus phloxine; in the pancreas, beta cells are blue, alpha and delta cells are red, and zymogen granules are red to unstained; in the pituitary, alpha cells are pink, beta cells and chromophobes are gray-blue, and nuclei are purple to blue.

Go•mo•ri meth•en•a•mine-sil•ver stain (gō-mōr′ē meth-en′ă-mēn sil′vĕr stān) Techniques for 1) *argentaffin cells:* a method using a methenamine-silver solution in combination with gold chloride, sodium thiosulfate, and safranin O; argentaffin granules appear brown-black against a green background; 2) *urates:* warm sections are treated directly with a hot methenamine-silver solution to produce a blackening of urates; 3) *fungi:* SEE Grocott-Gomori methenamine-silver stain; 4) *melanin,* which reduces silver nitrate.

Go•mo•ri non•spe•cif•ic ac•id phos•pha•tase stain (gō-mōr′ē non′spĕ-sif′ik as′id fos′fă-tās stān) A method in which formalin-fixed frozen sections are incubated in a substrate containing sodium β-glycerophosphate and lead nitrate at pH 5.0; the insoluble lead phosphate produced is treated with ammonium sulfide to give a black lead sulfide.

Go•mo•ri non•spe•cif•ic al•ka•line phos•pha•tase stain (gō-mōr′ē non′spĕ-sif′ik al′kă-lin fos′fă-tās stān) A calcium-cobalt sulfide method using frozen sections or cold acetone- or formalin-fixed paraffin sections, plus sodium β-glycerophosphate as a substrate at pH 9.0–9.5 with Mg^{2+} as activator; calcium ions precipitate the liberated phosphate, cobalt salt replaces the calcium phosphate, and ammonium sulfide converts the product to a black cobalt sulfide.

Go•mo•ri one-step tri•chrome stain (gō-mōr′ē wŭn-step trī′krōm stān) A connective tissue stain that uses hematoxylin and a dye mixture containing chromotrope 2R and light green or aniline blue; muscle fibers appear red, collagen is green (or blue if aniline blue is used), and nuclei are blue to black.

Go•mo•ri sil•ver im•preg•na•tion stain (gō-mōr′ē sil′vĕr im′preg-nā′shŭn stān) A reliable method for reticulin, as an aid in the diagnosis of neoplasm and early cirrhosis of the liver; the staining solution employs silver nitrate, potassium hydroxide, and ammonia water carefully prepared to avoid having silver precipitate.

Gom•pertz law (gom′pĕrts law) The proportional relationship of mortality to age; after age 35–40, the increase in mortality with age tends to be logarithmic.

gom•pho•sis (gom-fō′sis) [TA] A form of fibrous joint in which a peglike process fits into a hole, as the root of a tooth into the socket in the alveolus. [G. *gomphos,* bolt, nail, + *-osis,* condition]

go•nad (gō′nad) An organ that produces sex cells; a testis or an ovary. [Mod. L. fr. G. *gonē,* seed]

go•nad•al (gō-nad′ăl) Relating to a gonad.

go•nad•al cords (gō-nad′ăl kōrdz) Primordial sex cords formed by columns of germinal and follicle cells penetrating centripetally into the embryonic ovarian or testicular cortex.

go•nad•al dys•gen•e•sis (gō-nad′ăl dis-jen′ĕ-sis) Defective gonadal development; types include gonadal aplasia or agenesis, rudimentary gonads, congenitally defective gonads, and true hermaphroditism.

go•nad•al ridge (gō-nad′ăl rij) An elevation of thickened mesothelium and underlying mesenchyme on the ventromedial border of the embryonic mesonephros; the primordial germ cells become embedded in it, establishing it as the primordium of the testis or ovary.

go•nad•ec•to•my (gon′ă-dek′tŏ-mē) Excision of ovary or testis. [gonado- + G. *ektomē,* excision]

♻ **gonado-, gonad-** Combining forms indicating the gonads. [G. *gonē,* seed]

go•nad•o•blas•to•ma (gō-nad′ō-blas-tō′mă) Rare, benign neoplasm composed of germ cells, sex cord derivatives, and stromal cells; appears in cases of mixed or pure gonadal dysgenesis; usually small (1–3 cm) and partially calcified but may give rise to malignant germ-cell tumors, most often seminoma and dysgerminoma or embryonal; usually bilateral; found in patients with gonadal dysgenesis.

go•nad•o•crins (gō-nad′ō-krinz) Peptides that stimulate release of both follicle-stimulating hormone and luteinizing hormone from the pituitary; found in ovarian follicular fluid in rats. Cf. bioregulator. [gonad + G. *krinō,* to secrete]

go•nad•o•lib•er•in (gō-nad′ō-lib′ĕr-in) **1.** A hypothalamic substance causing the release of gonadotropin. SYN gonadotropin-releasing factor, gonadotropin-releasing hormone. **2.** A decapeptide from pig hypothalami that induces release of both lutropin and follitropin in constant proportions and thus acts as both luliberin and folliberin. SYN luteinizing hormone/follicle-stimulating hormone-releasing factor. Cf. bioregulator. [gonad + L. *libero,* to free, + -in]

gon•a•dop•athy (gon′ă-dop′ă-thē) Disease affecting the gonads. [gonado- + G. *pathos,* suffering]

go•nad•o•rel•in hy•dro•chlo•ride (gō-nad′ō-rel′in hī′drō-klōr′īde) A gonadotropin-releasing hormone obtained from sheep, pigs, or other animals and used to evaluate the functional capacity of the gonadotrophs of the anterior pituitary. [*gonado*tropin-*rel*easing + -in]

go•nad•o•troph (gō-nad′ō-trōf) An endocrine cell of the adenohypophysis that affects certain cells of the ovary or testis.

go•nad•o•tro•phic (gō-nad′o-trō′fik) SYN gonadotropic. [gonado- + G. *trophē,* nourishment]

go•nad•o•tro•phin (gō-nad′ō-trō′fin) SYN gonadotropin (1).

go•nad•o•tro•pic (gō-nad′ō-trō′pik) **1.** Descriptive of or relating to the actions of a gonadotropin. **2.** Promoting the growth and/or function of the gonads. SYN gonadotrophic. [gonado- + G. *tropē,* a turning]

go•nad•o•tro•pin, go•nad•o•tro•pic hor•mone (gō-nad′ō-trō′pin, gō-nad′ō-trō′pik hōr′mōn) **1.** A hormone capable of promoting gonadal growth and function; such effects, as exerted by a single hormone, usually are limited to discrete functions or histologic components of a gonad, such as stimulation of follicular growth or of androgen formation; most gonadotropins exert their effects in both sexes, although the effect of a given gonadotropin will differ in males and females. SYN gonadotrophin. **2.** Any hormone that stimulates gonadal function. **3.** Any substance that has the combined effects of follicle-stimulating hormone and luteinizing hormone.

go•nad•o•tro•pin-re•leas•ing fac•tor (gō-nad′ō-trō′pin-rĕ-lēs′ing fak′tŏr) SYN gonadoliberin (1).

go•nad•o•tro•pin-re•leas•ing hor•mone (GnRH) (gō-nad′ō-trō′pin-rĕ-lēs′ing hōr′mōn) SYN gonadoliberin (1).

gon•a•duct (gon′ă-dŭkt) **1.** SYN seminal duct. **2.** SYN uterine tube. [gonado- + duct]

go•nal•gi•a (gō-nal′jē-ă) Pain in the knee. [G. *gony,* knee, + *algos,* pain]

gon•an•gi•ec•to•my (gon′an-jē-ek′tŏ-mē) SYN vasectomy. [G. *gonē,* seed. + *angeion,* vessel, + *ektome,* excision, + -y]

gon•ar•thri•tis (gon′ahr-thrī′tis) Inflammation of the knee joint. [G. *gony,* knee, + *arthron,* joint, + *-itis,* inflammation]

gon•ar•throt•o•my (gon′ahr-throt′ŏ-mē) Incision into the knee joint. [G. *gony,* knee, + *arthron,* joint, + *tomē,* incision]

gon•e•cyst, **gon•e•cys•tis** (gon′ĕ-sist, -sis′tis) SYN seminal vesicle. [G. *gonē,* seed, + *kystis,* bladder]

go•ni•a (gō′nē-ă) Plural of gonion.

gonio- Combining form denoting an angle. [G. *gōnia*]

go•ni•om•e•ter (gō′nē-om′ĕ-tĕr) **1.** An instrument for measuring joint angles. **2.** An appliance used in the static test of labyrinthine disease. It consists of a plank, one end of which may be raised to any desired height; as one end of the plank is gradually raised, the point at which a patient loses balance is noted. **3.** A calibrated device used to measure the arc or range of motion of a joint. SYN arthrometer, flexometer. [G. *gōnia,* angle, + *metron,* measure]

go•ni•on, pl. **go•ni•a** (gō′nē-on, -ă) [TA] The lowest posterior and most outward point of the angle of the mandible. In cephalometrics, it is measured by bisecting the angle formed by the tangents to the lower and the posterior borders of the mandible; when the angles of both sides of the mandible appear on the lateral radiograph, a point midway between the right and left side is used. [G. *gōnia,* angle]

go•ni•o•punc•ture (gō′nē-ō-pŭngk-chŭr) An operation for congenital glaucoma in which a puncture is made in the filtration angle of the anterior chamber.

go•ni•o•scope (gō′nē-ō-skōp) A lens designed to study the angle of the anterior chamber of the eye. [G. *gōnia,* angle, + *skopeō,* to examine]

go•ni•os•co•py (gō′nē-os′kŏ-pē) Examination of the angle of the anterior chamber of the eye with a gonioscope or with a contact prism lens.

go•ni•o•syn•ech•i•a (gō′nē-ō-si-nek′ē-ă) Adhesion of the iris to the posterior surface of the cornea in the angle of the anterior chamber; associated with angle-closure glaucoma. [G. *gōnia,* angle, + *synechis,* holding together]

go•ni•ot•o•my (gō′nē-ot′ŏ-mē) Surgical opening of the trabecular meshwork in congenital glaucoma. [G. *gōnia,* angle, + *tomē,* incision]

gon•o•cele (gon′ō-sēl) A cystic lesion of the epididymis or rete testis, resulting from obstruction and containing secretions from the testis. [G. *gonē,* seed, + *kēlē,* tumor]

gonococcaemia [Br.] SYN gonococcemia.

gon•o•coc•cal (gon′ō-kok′ăl) Relating to the gonococcus. SYN gonococcic.

gon•o•coc•cal ar•thri•tis (gon′ō-kok′ăl ahr-thrī′tis) Joint space infection in humans caused by disseminated *Neisseria gonorrhoeae;* characteristically monarticular, but may be polyarticular.

gon•o•coc•cal con•junc•ti•vi•tis (gon′ō-kok′ăl kŏn-jŭngk′ti-vī′tis) A type of hyperacute, purulent conjunctivitis.

gon•o•coc•ce•mi•a (gon′ō-kok-sē′mē-ă) The presence of gonococci in the circulating blood. See page B4. SYN gonococcaemia. [gonococcus + G. *haima,* blood]

gon•o•coc•cic (gon′ō-kok′sik) SYN gonococcal.

gon•o•coc•cus, pl. **gon•o•coc•ci** (gon′ō-kok′ŭs, -sī) SYN *Neisseria gonorrhoeae.* [G. *gonē,* seed, + *kokkos,* berry]

gon•o•phore, **gon•oph•o•rus** (gon′ŏ-fōr, gō-nof′ŏr-ŭs) Any structure serving to store up or conduct the sex cells; oviduct, spermatic duct, uterus, or seminal vesicle; an accessory generative organ. [G. *gonē,* seed, + *phoros,* bearing]

gon•or•rhe•a (gon′ŏr-ē′ă) A contagious catarrhal inflammation of the genital mucous membrane, acquired through sexual contact and due to *Neisseria gonorrhoeae;* may involve the lower or upper genital tract, especially the urethra, endocervix, and uterine tubes, or may spread to the peritoneum and rarely to the heart, joints, or other structures by way of the bloodstream. See page B4. SYN gonorrhoea. [G. *gonorrhoia,* fr. *gonē,* seed, + *rhoia,* a flow]

gon•or•rhe•al (gon′ŏr-ē′ăl) Relating to gonorrhea. SYN gonorrhoeal.

gon•or•rhe•al oph•thal•mi•a (gon′ŏr-ē′ăl of-thal′mē-ă) Acute purulent conjunctivitis due to *Neisseria gonorrhoeae.* SYN gonorrhoeal ophthalmia.

gonorrhoea [Br.] SYN gonorrhea.

gonorrhoeal [Br.] SYN gonorrheal.

gonorrhoeal ophthalmia [Br.] SYN gonorrheal ophthalmia.

go•ny•camp•sis (gon′i-kamp′sis) Ankylosis or any abnormal curvature of the knee. [G. *gony,* knee, + *kampsis,* a bending or curving]

good cho•les•ter•ol (gud kŏ-les′tĕr-ol) Colloquial usage for HDL cholesterol (q.v.).

Good Clin•i•cal Prac•tic•es (GCP) (gud klin′i-kăl prak′tis-ĕz) A standard of quality for use in assessment of clinical trials in humans;

intended to standardize concepts and data management of health care statistics worldwide.

good death (gud deth) Colloquial usage for treatment of a patient in accord with the patient's stated (usually written) wishes and in maintenance of appropriate palliation of pain.

Good•ell sign (gud′el sīn) Softening of the cervix and vagina as being usually indicative of pregnancy.

Good•e•nough draw-a-man test (gud′ĕ-nō draw-ă-man test) A brief test for assessing a person's level of intelligence based on how accurately drawn and how many elements are included when a child or adult is given a pencil and sheet of white paper and asked to draw a human. Also called the Goodenough draw-a-person test and, in its current form, the Goodenough-Harris drawing test.

Good•e•nough-Har•ris draw•ing test (gud′ĕ-nō-har′is draw′ing test) Refinement of Goodenough draw-a-person test that evaluates inclusion of body details and clothing. SEE Goodenough draw-a-man test.

Good Man•u•fac•tur•ing Prac•tice (gud man-yū-fak′shŭr-ing prak′tis) Regulations related to the production, storage, and distribution of drugs and medical equipment.

Good•pas•ture stain (gud′pas-chŭr stān) A stain for gram-negative bacteria, using aniline fuchsin.

Good•pas•ture syn•drome (gud′pas-chŭr sin′drōm) Glomerulonephritis of the anti-basement membrane type associated with or preceded by hemoptysis; the nephritis usually progresses rapidly to produce death from renal failure, and the lungs at autopsy show extensive hemosiderosis or recent hemorrhage.

Good Sa•mar•i•tan leg•is•la•tion (gud să-mar′i-tăn lej′is-lā′shŭn) State laws passed to protect suppliers of emergency medical assistance from litigation except in cases of gross malfeasance.

Good Source of... (gud sōrs) This phrase, when used in food labeling, means that, according to F.D.A. regulations, the food so labeled contains at least 10% of the MDR of a given nutrient.

goose•flesh (gūs′flesh) SYN cutis anserina.

Gop•a•lan syn•drome (gō′pah-lahn sin′drōm) Severe discomfort of the feet associated with elevated skin temperature and excessive sweating.

Gor•don-Don Mi•chael tube (gōr′don-dŏn mī′kăl tūb) SYN esophageal gastric tube airway.

gor•get (gōr′jet) A director or guide with wide groove for use in lithotomy.

gork (gōrk) A jargonistic and abusive notation on a dying or dead patient's chart indicating that no proper diagnosis was reached. Used as a verb and noun.

Gor•lin sign (gōr′lin sīn) Unusual ease in touching the tip of the nose with the tongue; seen in Ehlers-Danlos syndrome.

Gor•lin syn•drome (gōr′lin sin′drōm) SYN basal cell nevus syndrome.

gos•er•e•lin (gō′sĕr-el′in) A synthetic decapeptide agonist analogue of the luteinizing hormone–releasing hormone (GnRH); it inhibits pituitary gonadotropin secretion and is used in the treatment of prostate cancer, breast cancer, endometriosis, and for thinning the endometrium before endometrial ablation or resection.

Gos•se•lin frac•ture (gō-slen[h]′ frak′shŭr) V-shaped fracture of distal end of tibia.

gos•sy•pol (gos′i-pol) (*Gossypium hirsutum*) This plant's parts are thought to be of value as a male contraceptive (clinical studies done); other uses are as an antineoplastic and vaginal spermicide. Adverse effects reported include heart failure, hepatotoxicity, nephrotoxicity, and, with oral ingestion of seeds, death by poisoning. SYN cotton. [*gossypium,* + *-ol*]

GOT (got) Abbreviation for glutamic-oxaloacetic transaminase.

gouge (gowj) A strong, curved chisel used in operations on bone.

Gould su•ture (gūld sū′chŭr) An intestinal mattress suture in which each loop is invaginated in such a way that the tissue at the loop is bulged out, becoming convex instead of concave.

Gou•ley cath•e•ter (gū′lē kath′ĕ-tĕr) A solid curved steel instrument grooved on its inferior surface so that it can be passed over a guide through a urethral stricture.

i gout (gowt) A disorder of purine metabolism, occurring especially in men, characterized by a raised but variable blood uric acid level and severe recurrent acute arthritis of sudden onset resulting from deposition of crystals of sodium urate in connective tissues and articular cartilage; usually inherited, resulting from a variety of abnormalities of purine metabolism. See page B24. [L. *gutta,* drop]

gou•ty (gow′tē) Relating to or characteristic of gout.

gou•ty ar•thri•tis (gow′tē ahr-thrī′tis) Inflammation of the joints in gout.

i gou•ty to•phus (gow′tē tō′fŭs) A deposit of uric acid and urates in periarticular fibrous tissue, cartilage of the external ear, or kidney, in gout. See page 657.

gov•ern•ance (gŏv′ĕr-năns) The act or power of exercising authority or control. [fr. L. *guberno,* fr. G. *kubernō,* to steer a ship, + - ance]

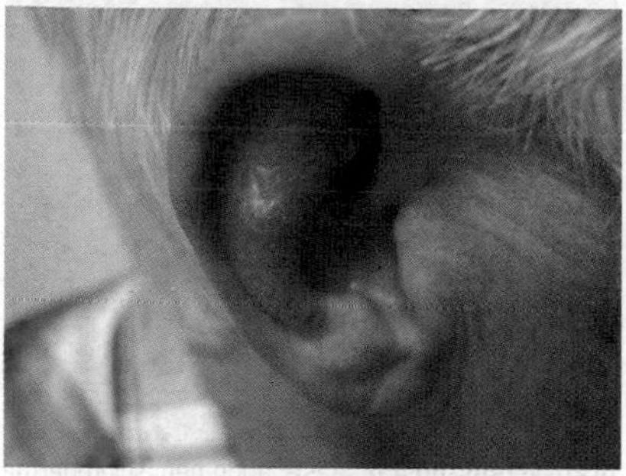

gouty tophus: right ear

Gow•ers syn•drome (gow′ĕrz sin′drōm) Syndrome consisting of palpitation, chest pain, respiratory difficulties, and disturbances in gastric motility; formerly attributed to vagal stimulation, now considered psychogenic (anxiety neurosis).

Gow•ers tract (gow′ĕrz trakt) SYN anterior spinocerebellar tract.

GP Abbreviation for general practitioner.

GPI Abbreviation for Gingival-Periodontal Index.

GPN Abbreviation for graduate professional nurse.

G pro•tein dis•eas•es (prō′tēn di-zēz′ĕz) A widely variant group of diseases resulting from mutations in G proteins; these include endocine adenomas, cholera, and night blindness.

GPT Abbreviation for glutamic-pyruvic transaminase.

GPWW Abbreviation for group practice without walls.

gr Abbreviation for grain (3).

graaf•i•an fol•li•cle (grah′fē-ăn fol′i-kĕl) SYN vesicular ovarian follicle.

Gra•cey cu•rettes (grā′sē kyūr-ets′) SYN area-specific curettes.

grac•ile fas•cic•u•lus (gras′il fă-sik′kyū-lŭs) The smaller medial subdivision of the posterior funiculus.

gra•cile lob•ule (gras′il lob′yūl) The anterior portion of the posteroinferior lobule of the cerebellum, the posterior portion being the semilunar lobule inferior; the two are continuous with the tuber of the vermis. SYN lobulus paramedianus [TA].

grac•ile nu•cle•us (gras′il nū′klē-ŭs) The medial one of the three nuclei of the dorsal column, the other two being the cuneate nucleus and the accessory cuneate nucleus, which corresponds to the clava. It receives dorsal-root fibers conveying sensory innervation of the leg and lower trunk and projects, by way of the medial lemniscus, to the ventral nucleus posterior nucleus of the thalamus.

grac•i•lis mus•cle (gras′i-lis mŭs′ĕl) *Origin*, ramus of pubis near symphysis; *insertion*, shaft of tibia below medial tuberosity (SEE pes anserinus); *action*, adducts thigh, flexes knee, rotates leg medially; *nerve supply*, obturator. SYN musculus gracilis [TA].

grade (grād) **1.** A rank, division, or level on the scale of a value system. **2.** In cancer pathology, a classification of the degree of malignancy or differentiation of tumor tissue; e.g., well, moderately well, or poorly differentiated, and undifferentiated or anaplastic. **3.** EXERCISE TESTING measurement of a vertical rise or fall as a percentage of horizontal distance traveled. [L. *gradus,* step]

grad•ed ac•tiv•i•ty (grād′ĕd ak-tiv′i-tē) A task that has been modified in one or more ways to provide an appropriate therapeutic demand or challenge for a client.

gra•ded ex•er•cise test (GXT) (grād′ĕd eks′ĕr-sīz test) Multistage exercise testing (usually on treadmill or bicycle ergometer) in which exercise intensity is progressively increased (graded) through levels that bring the test subject to a self-imposed fatigue level. SEE stress test, Astrand-Ryhming Cycle Ergometer Test.

grade I as•tro•cy•to•ma (grād as′trō-sī-tō′mă) Solid or cystic astrocytoma of high differentiation or low grade.

grade II as•tro•cy•to•ma (grād as′trō-sī-tō′mă) astrocytoma of low to intermediate grade.

grade III as•tro•cy•to•ma (grād as′trō-sī-tō′mă) astrocytoma of intermediate grade. SEE ALSO glioblastoma multiforme.

grade IV as•tro•cy•to•ma (grād as′trō-sī-tō′mă) SYN glioblastoma multiforme.

Gra•de•ni•go syn•drome (grah-dā-nē′gō sin′drōm) A syndrome consisting of otorrhea, headache, diplopia, and retroorbital pain in petrositis due to an epidural abscess at the apex of the anterior surface of the petrous pyramid causing compression of the abducens nerve in Dorello canal and irritation of the trigeminal ganglion.

gra•di•ent (grā′dē-ĕnt) Rate of change of temperature, pressure, or other variable, as a function of factors of distance or time.

gra•di•ent am•pli•fi•er (grā′dē-ĕnt amp′li-fī-ĕr) A device that supplies power to the gradient coils during magnetic resonance imaging.

gra•di•ent ech•o (grā-dē′ĕnt ek′ō) Echo produced as a result of gradient rephasing.

gra•di•ent ech•o pulse se•quence (grā′dē-ĕnt ek′ō pŭls sē′kwĕns) MAGNETIC RESONANCE IMAGING modality that uses a gradient to regenerate an echo.

gra•di•ent-re•called ac•qui•si•tion in the stead•y state (GRASS) (grā′dē-ĕnt-rē-kawld′ ak′wi-zish′ŭn sted′ē stāt) A type of gradient echo sequence with free induction decay sampling in magnetic resonance imaging; also called "fast imaging with steady-state precession." This family of sequences is faster than spin echo techniques, and is used for magnetic resonance angiography and cardiac imaging.

grad•u•at•ed (graj′ū-āt′ĕd) **1.** Marked by lines or in other ways to denote capacity, degrees, percentages, or other discrete instruments. **2.** Divided or arranged in levels, grades, or successive steps.

grad•u•at•ed te•not•o•my (graj′ū-āt′ĕd te-not′ŏ-mē) Partial incisions of the tendon of an eye muscle for correction of strabismus.

grad•u•ate nurse (GN) (graj′ū-ăt nŭrs) A nurse who has been granted a degree by a state-certified nursing program but has not yet passed a licensing examination; may be diploma, associate degree, baccalaureate, or master's level.

grad•u•ate pro•fes•sion•al nurse (GPN) (graj′ū-ăt prŏ-fesh′ŭn-ăl nŭrs) A nurse who has been granted a degree by a state-certified nursing program but has not yet passed a licensing examination. Generally speaking, a baccalaureate-prepared nurse

Grae•fe knife (grā′fĕ nīf) A narrow-bladed knife used in making a section of the cornea.

Grae•fe op•er•a•tion (grā′fĕ op-ĕr-ā′shŭn) **1.** Removal of cataract by a limbal incision with capsulotomy and iridectomy. Both operations were landmarks in the field of ophthalmic surgery. **2.** Iridectomy for glaucoma.

Grae•fe sign (grā′fĕ sīn) In Graves disease, lag of the upper eyelid as it follows the rotation of the eyeball downward. SYN von Graefe sign.

Graf•fi vi•rus (grah′fē vī′rŭs) A type C mouse myeloleukemia virus from filtrates of transplantable tumors; possibly related to Gross virus.

graft (graft) **1.** Any free (unattached) tissue or organ for transplantation. **2.** To transplant such structures. SEE ALSO flap, implant, transplant. [A.S. *graef*]

graft•ing (graft′ing) Surgical transplantation of living tissue. [O.Fr. *graffe*]

graft-ver•sus-host dis•ease (GVHD) (graft vĕr′sŭs hōst di-zēz′) An incompatibility reaction (which may be fatal) in a subject (host) of low immunologic competence (deficient lymphoid tissue) who has been the recipient of immunologically competent lymphoid tissue from a donor who lacks at least one antigen possessed by the recipient host; the reaction, or disease, is the result of action of the transplanted cells against those host tissues that possess the antigen not possessed by the donor. See this page.

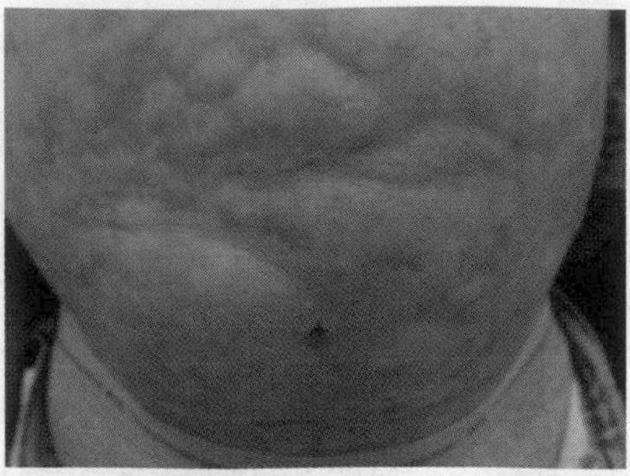

graft-versus-host disease: abdomen, scleroderma like changes

graft-ver•sus-host re•ac•tion (GVHR) (graft vĕr′sŭs hōst rē-ak′shŭn) Clinical and histologic changes of graft-versus-host disease occurring in a specific organ.

Gra•ham law (grā′ăm law) The relative rapidity of diffusion of two gases varies inversely as the square root of their densities, i.e., their molecular weights.

Gra•ham Steell mur•mur (grā′ăm stēl mŭr′mŭr) An early diastolic murmur of pulmonic insufficiency secondary to pulmonary hypertension, as in mitral stenosis and various congenital defects associated with pulmonary hypertension. SYN Steell murmur.

grain (grān) **1.** Cereal plants (e.g., corn, wheat, or rye), or a seed of one of them. **2.** A minute, hard particle of any substance, as of sand. **3. (gr)** A unit of weight, 1/60 dram (apoth. or troy), 1/437.5 avoirdupois ounce, 1/480 troy ounce, 1/5760 troy pound, 1/7000 avoirdupois pound; the equivalent of 0.064799 gram. [L. *granum*]

grains of par•a•dise (grānz par′ă-dīs) SYN amomum.

gram (g) (gram) A unit of weight in the metric or centesimal system, the equivalent of 15.432358 grains or 0.03527 avoirdupois ounce.

-gram Suffix meaning a recording, usually by an instrument. Cf. -graph. [G. *gramma,* character, mark]

gram cal•o•rie (gram kal′ŏr-ē) SYN small calorie.

gram-cen•ti•me•ter (gram-sen′ti-mē-tĕr) The energy exerted, or work done, when a mass of 1 g is raised a height of 1 cm; equal to 9.807×10^{-5} joules or newton-meters.

Gram-chro•mo•trope stain (gram-krō′mō-trōp stān) A modified trichrome stain for microsporidian spores that combines Gram-stain reagents in the procedure.

gram e•qui•va•lent (gram ĕ-kwiv′ă-lĕnt) **1.** The weight in grams of an element that combines with or replaces 1 gram of hydrogen. **2.** The atomic or molecular weight in grams of an atom or group of atoms involved in a chemical reaction divided by the number of electrons donated, taken up, or shared by the atom or group of atoms in the course of that reaction. **3.** The weight of a substance contained in 1 liter of normal solution; a variant of (1). SYN equivalent (5).

Gram i•o•dine (gram ī′ō-dīn) A solution containing iodine and potassium iodide, used in a Gram stain.

gram-i•on (gram-ī′on) The weight in grams of an ion that is equal to the sum of the atomic weights of the atoms making up the ion.

gram-me•ter (gram-mē′tĕr) A unit of energy equal to 100 gram-centimeters.

gram-mol•e•cule (gram-mol′i-kyūl) The amount of a substance with a mass in grams equal to its molecular weight; e.g., a gram-molecule of hydrogen weighs 2.016 g, that of water 18.015 g.

gram-neg•a•tive (gram-neg′ă-tiv) Refers to the inability of a bacterium to resist decolorization with alcohol after being treated with Gram crystal violet. However, following decolorization, these bacteria can be readily counterstained with safranin, imparting a pink or red color to the bacterium when viewed by light microscopy. SEE Gram stain.

gram-pos•i•tive (gram-poz′i-tiv) Refers to the ability of a bacterium to resist decolorization with alcohol after being treated with Gram crystal violet stain, imparting a violet color to the bacterium when viewed by light microscopy. SEE Gram stain.

Gram stain (gram stān) A method for differential staining of bacteria; smears are fixed by flaming, stained in a solution of crystal violet, treated with iodine solution, rinsed, decolorized, and then counterstained with safranin O; gram-positive organisms stain purple-black, and gram-negative organisms stain pink. Useful in bacterial taxonomy and identification and for indicating fundamental differences in cell wall structure.

grand•daugh•ter cyst (grand′daw-tĕr sist) A tertiary cyst sometimes developed within a daughter cyst, as in the hydatid cyst of *Echinococcus*.

grand mal (grōn[h] mal) SYN generalized tonic-clonic seizure.

grand rounds (grand rowndz) A regularly scheduled didactic presentation at a teaching hospital in which one or more actual cases are used to illustrate a selected medical topic to health care professionals, particularly those in training.

Gran•ger line (grān′jĕr līn) On lateral skull radiographs, the line produced by the groove of the optic chiasm or sulcus prechiasmaticus.

gran•ny knot (gran′ē not) A double knot in which the free ends of the second loop are asymmetric and not in the same plane as the free ends of the first loop.

gran•u•lar (gran′yū-lăr) **1.** Composed of or resembling granules or granulations. **2.** Particles with strong affinity for nuclear stains, seen in many bacterial species.

gran•u•lar cell tu•mor (gran′yū-lăr sel tū′mŏr) A microscopically specific, generally benign tumor, often involving peripheral nerves in skin, mucosa, or connective tissue, derived from Schwann cells; the abundant cytoplasm contains lysosomal granules, the cells infiltrate between adjacent tissues although growth is slow, and adjacent surface epithelium may show hyperplasia.

gran•u•lar con•junc•ti•vi•tis (gran′yū-lăr kŏn-jŭngk′ti-vī′tis) SYN trachomatous conjunctivitis.

gran•u•lar cor•ne•al dys•tro•phy (gran′yū-lăr kōr′nē-ăl dis′trŏ-fē) An autosomal dominant disorder characterized by hyaline deposits in the corneal stroma.

gran•u•lar cor•tex (gran′yū-lăr kōr′teks) SEE cerebral cortex.

gran•u•lar en•do•plas•mic re•tic•u•lum (gran′yū-lăr en′dō-plaz′mik rĕ-tik′yū-lŭm) Endoplasmic reticulum in which ribosomal granules are applied to the cytoplasmic surface of the cisternae; involved in the synthesis and secretion of protein through membrane-bound vesicles to the extracellular space. SYN ergastoplasm.

gran•u•lar leu•ko•cyte (gran′yū-lăr lū′kō-sīt) Any one of the polymorphonuclear leukocytes, especially a neutrophilic leukocyte. SEE ALSO granulocyte, basophilic leukocyte, eosinophilic leukocyte.

gran•u•lar oph•thal•mi•a (gran′yū-lăr of-thal′mē-ă) SYN trachoma.

gran•u•lar pits (gran′yū-lăr pits) Pits on the inner surface of the skull, along the course of the superior sagittal sinus, in which are lodged the arachnoidal granulations.

gra•nu•la•ti•o, pl. **gran•u•la•ti•o•nes** (gran′yū-lā′shē-ō, gran′yū-lā-shē-ō′nēz) SYN granulation. [L.]

gran•u•la•tion (gran′yū-lā′shŭn) **1.** Formation into grains or granules; the state of being granular. **2.** A granular mass in or on the surface of any organ or membrane or one of the individual granules forming the mass. **3.** The formation of minute, rounded, fleshy connective tissue projections on the surface of a wound, ulcer, or inflamed tissue surface during healing; one of the fleshy granules composing this surface. SEE ALSO granulation tissue. **4.** PHARMACOLOGY the formation of crystals by constant agitation of a supersaturated solution of a salt. SYN granulatio. [L. *granulatio*]

gran·u·la·ti·o·nes ar·ach·noi·de·a·les (gran′yū-lā-shē-ō′nēz ă-rak′noy-dē-ā′lēz) [TA] SYN arachnoid granulations. SEE ALSO arachnoid villi.

gran·u·la·tion tis·sue (gran′yū-lā′shŭn tish′ū) Vascular connective tissue forming granular projections on the surface of a healing wound, ulcer, or inflamed surface. SEE ALSO granulation.

gran·ule (gran′yūl) **1.** A grainlike particle; a granulation; a minute discrete mass. **2.** A very small pill, usually gelatin- or sugar-coated, containing a drug to be given in a small dose. **3.** A colony of the bacterium or fungus causing a disease or simply colonizing the tissues of the patient. **4.** A small particle that can be seen by electron microscopy; contains stored material. [L. *granulum,* dim. of *granum,* grain]

gran·ule cells (gran′yūl selz) **1.** Small nerve cell bodies in the external and internal granular layers of the cerebral cortex. **2.** Small nerve cell bodies in the granular layer of the cerebellar cortex.

granulo- Prefix meaning granular, granules. [L. *granulum,* a small grain.]

gran·u·lo·cyte (gran′yū-lō-sīt) A mature granular leukocyte, including neutrophilic, acidophilic, and basophilic types of polymorphonuclear leukocytes, i.e., respectively, neutrophils, eosinophils, and basophils. [granulo- + G. *kytos,* cell]

gran·u·lo·cyte col·o·ny-stim·u·lat·ing fac·tor (G-CSF) (gran′yū-lō-sīt kol′ŏ-nē stim′yū-lā-ting fak′tŏr) Glycoproteins that are synthesized by a variety of cells and are involved in growth and differentiation of hematopoietic stem cells. SEE ALSO colony-stimulating factors.

gran·u·lo·cyte-mac·ro·phage col·o·ny-stim·u·lat·ing fac·tor (GM-CSF) (gran′yū-lō-sīt-mak′rō-fāzh kol′ŏ-nē-stim′yū-lā-ting fak′tŏr) A glycoprotein secreted by macrophages or bone stromal cells that functions as a growth factor for myeloid progenitor cells, such as granulocytes, macrophages, and eosinophils. SEE ALSO colony-stimulating factors.

gran·u·lo·cyt·ic leu·ke·mi·a (gran′yū-lō-sit′ik lū-kē′mē-ă) A form of the hematologic disorder characterized by an uncontrolled proliferation of myelopoietic cells in the bone marrow and in extramedullary sites, and the presence of large numbers of immature and mature granulocytic forms in various tissues (and organs) and in the circulating blood. The predominant cell is usually of the neutrophilic series, but in a few instances eosinophilic or basophilic granulocytes, or even megakaryocytes, may represent the chief form. SYN myelocytic leukemia, myelogenic leukemia, myelogenous leukemia, myeloid leukemia.

gran·u·lo·cyt·ic sar·co·ma (gran′yū-lō-sit′ik sahr-kō′mă) A malignant tumor of immature myeloid cells, frequently subperiosteal, associated with or preceding granulocytic leukemia. SEE ALSO chloroma. SYN myeloid sarcoma.

gran·u·lo·cyt·ic se·ries (gran′yū-lō-sit′ik sēr′ēz) The cells in the several stages of development in the bone marrow leading to the mature granulocyte of the circulation, e.g., myeloblasts, different stages of the myelocyte, granulocytes.

gran·u·lo·cy·to·pe·ni·a (gran′yū-lō-sī′tō-pē′nē-ă) Less than the normal number of granular leukocytes in the blood. SYN granulopenia. [granulocyte + G. *penia,* poverty]

gran·u·lo·cy·to·poi·e·sis (gran′yū-lō-sī′tō-poy-ē′sis) SYN granulopoiesis.

gran·u·lo·cy·to·poi·et·ic (gran′yū-lō-sī′tō-poy-et′ik) SYN granulopoietic. [granulocyte + G. *poieō,* to make]

gran·u·lo·cy·to·sis (gran′yū-lō-sī-tō′sis) A condition characterized by more than the normal number of granulocytes in the circulating blood or in the tissues.

gran·u·lo·ma (gran′yū-lō′mă) A nodular inflammatory lesion, firm and persistent and usually either small or granular, which includes epithelial cells and may also contain other compactly grouped modified phagocytes such as giant cells and other macrophages; often bordered by lymphocytes. SEE ALSO granulomatosis. See page B14. [granulo- + G. *-oma,* tumor]

gran·u·lo·ma in·gui·na·le (gran′yū-lō′mă ing-gwī-nā′lē) A specific granuloma, classified as a sexually transmitted disease and caused by *Calymmatobacterium granulomatis* observed in macrophages as Donovan bodies; the ulcerating granulomatous lesions occur in the inguinal regions and on the genitalia. SYN donovanosis, granuloma venereum, ulcerating granuloma of pudenda.

gran·u·lo·ma mul·ti·for·me (gran′yū-lō′mă mŭl-ti-fōr′mē) A chronic granulomatous anular eruption of the skin on the upper body in older adults in central Africa; of unknown cause.

gran·u·lo·ma·to·sis (gran′yū-lō′mă-tō′sis) Any condition characterized by the presence of granulomas.

gran·u·lo·ma·tous (gran′yū-lom′ă-tŭs) Having the characteristics of a granuloma.

gran·u·lo·ma·tous co·li·tis (gran′yū-lom′ă-tŭs kō-lī′tis) Changes, identical to those of regional enteritis, involving the colon.

gran·u·lo·ma·tous en·ceph·a·lo·my·e·li·tis (gran′yū-lom′ă-tŭs en-sef′a-lō-mī′ĕ-lī′tis) An encephalomyelitis in which granulomas occur.

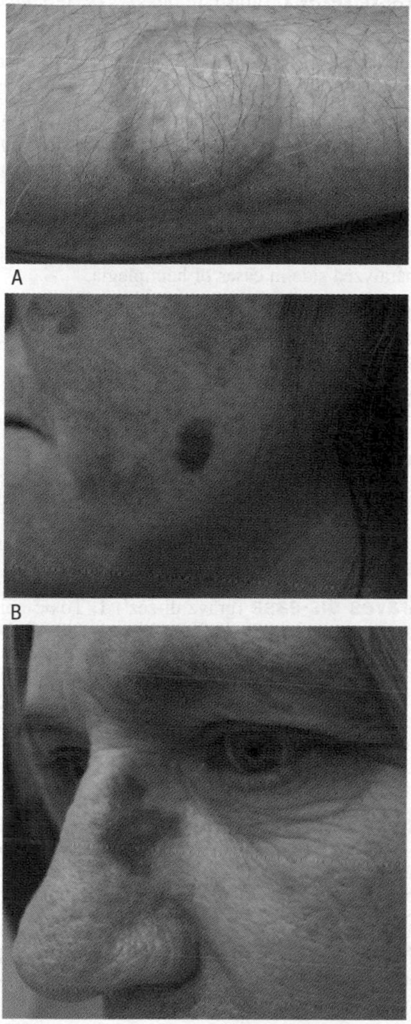

granuloma: (A) arm; (B) cheek; (C) nose

gran•u•lo•ma•tous en•ter•i•tis (gran′yū-lom′ă-tŭs en′tĕr-ī′tis) SYN regional enteritis.

gran•u•lo•ma•tous in•flam•ma•tion (gran′yū-lom′ă-tŭs in′flă-mā′shŭn) A form of proliferative inflammation SEE ALSO granuloma.

gran•u•lo•ma trop•i•cum (gran′yū-lō′mă trop′i-kŭm) SYN yaws.

gran•u•lo•ma ve•ne•re•um (gran′yū-lō′mă vĕ-nē′rē-ŭm) SYN granuloma inguinale.

gran•u•lo•mere (gran′yū-lō-mēr) The central part of a blood platelet. SYN chromomere (2). [granulo- + G. *meros,* a part]

gran•u•lo•pe•ni•a (gran′yū-lō-pē′nē-ă) SYN granulocytopenia.

gran•u•lo•plas•tic (gran′yū-lō-plas′tik) Forming granules.

gran•u•lo•poi•e•sis (gran′yū-lō-poy-ē′sis) Production of granulocytes. In adults, granulocytes are produced chiefly in the red bone marrow of flat bones. SYN granulocytopoiesis. [granulo(cyte) + G. *poiēsis,* a making]

gran•u•lo•poi•et•ic (gran′yū-lō-poy-et′ik) Pertaining to granulopoiesis. SYN granulocytopoietic.

gran•u•lo•sa cell (gran′yū-lō′să sel) A cell of the membrana granulosa lining the vesicular ovarian follicle that becomes a luteal cell of the corpus luteum after ovulation.

gran•u•lo•sa cell tu•mor (gran′yū-lō′să sel tū′mŏr) A benign or malignant tumor of the ovary arising from the membrana granulosa of the ovarian (graafian) follicle and frequently secreting estrogen. SYN folliculoma (1).

gran•u•lo•sis (gran′yū-lō′sis) A mass of minute granules of any character.

-graph **1.** Suffix indicating something written, as in monograph, radiograph. **2.** Suffix indicating the instrument for making a recording, as in kymograph. Cf. -gram. [G. *graphō,* to write]

graphanaesthesia [Br.] SYN graphanesthesia.

graph•an•es•the•si•a (graf′an-es-thē′zē-ă) Tactual inability to recognize figures or letters written on the skin; may be due to spinal cord or brain disease. SYN graphanaesthesia. [G. *graphē,* writing + *anaisthēsia,* fr. *an-* priv. + *aisthēsis,* perception]

-graphia Suffix denoting relationship to writing.

graph•or•rhe•a (graf-ŏ-rē′ă) Rarely used term for the writing of long lists of meaningless words, associated with a schizophrenic disorder. SYN graphorrhoea. [grapho- + G. *rhoia,* flow]

graphorrhoea [Br.] SYN graphorrhea.

-graphy Suffix indicating a writing, a description. [G. *graphō,* to write]

grasp (grasp) To seize or clasp, especially with the hand. [M.E. *graspen*]

grasp•ing re•flex (grasp′ing rē′fleks) An involuntary flexion of the fingers to tactile or tendon stimulation on the palm of the hand, producing an uncontrollable grasp; physiologic in the newborn, otherwise usually associated with frontal lobe lesions. Cf. darwinian reflex.

grasp pat•tern (grasp pat′ĕrn) A program of coordinated movements used to pick up and hold an object in the hand; during the first year of life, it develops steadily in complexity and in the degree of motor control required. SEE ALSO reflexive squeeze grasp. See page 662.

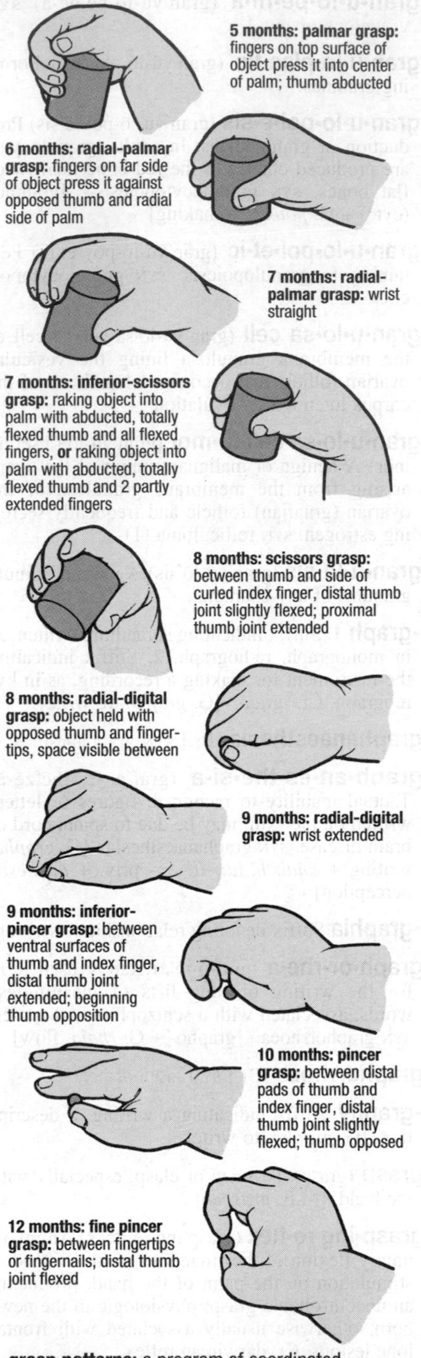
5 months: palmar grasp: fingers on top surface of object press it into center of palm; thumb abducted
6 months: radial-palmar grasp: fingers on far side of object press it against opposed thumb and radial side of palm
7 months: radial-palmar grasp: wrist straight
7 months: inferior-scissors grasp: raking object into palm with abducted, totally flexed thumb and all flexed fingers, **or** raking object into palm with abducted, totally flexed thumb and 2 partly extended fingers
8 months: scissors grasp: between thumb and side of curled index finger, distal thumb joint slightly flexed; proximal thumb joint extended
8 months: radial-digital grasp: object held with opposed thumb and finger-tips, space visible between
9 months: radial-digital grasp: wrist extended
9 months: inferior-pincer grasp: between ventral surfaces of thumb and index finger, distal thumb joint extended; beginning thumb opposition
10 months: pincer grasp: between distal pads of thumb and index finger, distal thumb joint slightly flexed; thumb opposed
12 months: fine pincer grasp: between fingertips or fingernails; distal thumb joint flexed

grasp patterns: a program of coordinated movements used in picking up and holding an object in the hand; during the first year of life the grasp pattern steadily develops in complexity and in the degree of motor control required

grasp re·flex (grasp rē′fleks) SYN reflexive squeeze grasp.

GRASS (gras) Acronym for gradient-recalled acquisition in the steady state.

Gras·set phe·nom·e·non (grah-sā′ fĕ-nom′ĕ-non) In organic paralysis of the lower extremity, the supine patient can raise either limb separately, but not both together.

Gras·set sign (grah-sā′ sīn) Normal contraction of the sternocleidomastoid muscle on the paralyzed side in cases of hemiplegia.

grat·tage (gră-tazh′) Scraping or brushing an ulcer or surface with sluggish granulations to stimulate the healing process. [Fr. scraping]

grave (grāv) Denoting symptoms of a serious or dangerous character. [L. *gravis,* heavy, grave]

grav·el (grav′ĕl) Small concretions, usually of uric acid, calcium oxalate, or phosphates, formed in the kidney and passed through the ureter, bladder, and urethra. [M.E., fr. O.Fr.]

gra·vel voice (grav′ĕl voys) SYN glottal fry.

Graves dis·ease (grāvz di-zēz′) **1.** Toxic goiter characterized by diffuse hyperplasia of the thyroid gland, a form of hyperthyroidism; exophthalmos is a common, but not invariable, concomitant. **2.** Thyroid dysfunction and all or any of its clinical associations. **3.** An organ-specific autoimmune disease of the thyroid gland. SEE thyrotoxicosis, Hashimoto disease, goiter, myxedema. SYN Parry disease.

Graves oph·thal·mop·a·thy (grāvz of-thal-mop′ă-thē) Exophthalmos caused by increased water content of retroocular orbital tissues; associated with thyroid disease, usually hyperthyroidism.

Graves op·tic neu·rop·a·thy (grāvz op′tik nūr-op′ă-thē) Visual dysfunction due to optic nerve compression in Graves ophthalmopathy.

Graves or·bi·top·a·thy (grāvz ōr′bi-top′ă-thē) SYN dysthyroid orbitopathy.

grav·id (grav′id) SYN pregnant.

grav·i·da (grav′i-dă) A pregnant woman. Gravida followed by a roman numeral or preceded by a Latin prefix (primi-, secundi-, and so on) designates the number of pregnancies; e.g., **gravida I**, primigravida: a woman in her first pregnancy; **gravida II**, secundigravida: a woman in her second pregnancy. Also, gravida (or G) 1, 2, etc. Cf. para. [L. *gravidus* {adj.}, fem. *gravida,* fr. *gravis,* heavy]

grav·i·dar·um (grā-vē-dā′rum) Of pregnant women. [L.]

gra·vid·ic (gră-vid′ik) Relating to pregnancy or a pregnant woman.

gra·vid·i·ty (gră-vid′i-tē) The number of pregnancies (complete or incomplete) experienced by a woman. [L. *graviditas,* pregnancy]

grav·id u·ter·us (grav′id yū′tĕr-ŭs) The condition of the uterus in pregnancy.

grav·i·met·ric (grav′i-met′rik) Relating to or determined by weight.

grav·i·re·cep·tor (grav′i-rĕ-sep′tŏr) A highly specialized receptor organ and nerve ending in the inner ear, joints, tendons, and muscles that give the brain information about body position, equilibrium, direction of gravitational forces, and the sensation of "down" or "up." [L. *gravis,* heavy, + receptor]

grav·i·ta·tion·al in·se·cu·ri·ty (grav′i-tā′shŭn-ăl in′sĕ-kyūr′i-tē) Excessive reaction to or fear of ordinary movement or change in head position; avoidance or pronounced emotional response to situations normally requiring adjustment of sense of balance. SYN postural insecurity.

grav·i·ta·tion·al ul·cer (grav′i-tā′shŭn-ăl ŭl′sĕr) A chronic ulcer of the leg with impaired healing because of the incompetence of the valves of varicose veins; the venous return stagnates and creates hypoxemia. SEE ALSO varicose ulcer.

grav·i·ty (grav′i-tē) The attraction toward the Earth that makes any mass exert downward force or have weight. [L. *gravitas*]

grav·i·ty con·cen·tra·tion (grav′i-tē kon′sĕn-trā′shŭn) A method of separating parasites from debris through gravity sedimentation of fecal suspensions.

gray (Gy) (grā) The SI unit of absorbed dose of ionizing radiation, equivalent to 1 J/kg of tissue; 1 Gy = 100 rad. [Louis H. *Gray,* British radiologist, 1905–1965]

gray cat·a·ract (grā kat′ăr-akt) A cataract of gray color, usually seen in senile, mature, or cortical cataract.

gray col·umns (grā kol′ŭmz) The three somewhat ridge-shaped masses of gray matter (anterior, posterior, and lateral columns) that extend longitudinally through the center of each lateral half of the spinal cord; in transverse sections these columns appear as gray horns and are therefore commonly called ventral or anterior, dorsal or posterior, and lateral horn, respectively. SYN columnae griseae [TA].

gray de·gen·er·a·tion (grā dĕ-jen′ĕr-ā′shŭn) degeneration of the white substance of the spinal cord, the fibers of which lose their myelin sheaths and become darker in color.

gray fi·bers (grā fī′bĕrz) SYN unmyelinated fibers.

gray hep·a·ti·za·tion (grā hep′ă-tī-zā′shŭn) The second stage of hepatization in pneumonia, when the exudate is beginning to degenerate before breaking down; the color is a yellowish gray or mottled.

gray in·du·ra·tion (grā in-dūr-ā′shŭn) A condition occurring in lungs during and after pneumonic processes in which there is failure of resolution; there is an increase in fibrous tissue but usually not a prominent degree of pigmentation, unless chronic passive congestion is also present.

gray lit·er·a·ture (grā lit′ĕr-ă-chŭr) Reports and other documents that are unpublished or have limited distribution, such as local health department reports, conference proceedings, and academic theses and dissertations; limited indexing, inaccessibility, and questionable authenticity all diminish the usefulness of such materials.

gray mat·ter (grā mat′ĕr) Those regions of the brain and spinal cord that are made up primarily of the cell bodies and dendrites of nerve cells rather than myelinated axons. SYN substantia grisea [TA], gray substance.

gray-scale ul·tra·so·nog·ra·phy (grā-skāl ŭl′tră-sŏ-nog′ră-fē) The display of the ultrasound echo amplitude or signal intensity as different shades of gray, improving image quality compared with the obsolete black-and-white presentation.

gray sub·stance (grā sub′stăns) SYN gray matter.

gray syn·drome, gray ba·by syn·drome (grā sin′drōm, grā bā′bē sin′drōm) Ashen appearance of an infant at birth and during the neonatal period that can be caused by transplacental toxic effects of the drug chloramphenicol taken by the mother during late pregnancy; the syndrome may be fatal.

gray-top tube (grā-top tūb) A container with potassium oxalate used as an anticoagulant and sodium fluoride as a preservative; used to maintain glucose in whole blood and for some special chemistry tests.

great ad·duc·tor mus·cle (grāt ă-dŭk′tŏr mŭs′ĕl) SYN adductor magnus muscle.

great a·nas·to·mot·ic ar·ter·y (grāt ă-nas′tŏ-mot′ik ahr′tĕr-ē) SYN inferior ulnar collateral artery.

great au·ric·u·lar nerve (grāt awr-ik′yū-lăr nĕrv) Arises from the ventral primary rami of the second and third cervical spinal nerves, supplies the skin of part of the auricle, adjacent portion of the scalp, and that overlying the angle of the jaw; it also innervates the parotid sheath, conveying from it the pain fibers stimulated by stretching of the sheath during parotitis (mumps). SYN nervus auricularis magnus [TA].

great car·di·ac vein (grāt kahr′dē-ak vān) Begins at the apex of the heart (anastomose with the middle cardiac vein), runs first with the anterior interventricular artery as it ascends the anterior interventricular groove, then turns to the left as it approaches or reaches the coronary groove to run with the circumflex branch of the left coronary artery; it merges with the oblique vein of the left atrium to form the coronary sinus.

great ce•re•bral vein of Ga•len (grāt ser′ĕ-brăl vān gā′len) A large, unpaired vein formed by the junction of the two internal cerebral veins in the caudal part of the tela choroidea of the third ventricle; it passes caudally between the splenium of the corpus callosum and the pineal gland, curving dorsally to merge with the inferior sagittal sinus to form the straight sinus.

great•er a•lar car•ti•lage (grā′tĕr ā′lăr kahr′ti-lăj) One of a pair of cartilages that form the tip of the nose. It consists of a medial crus that extends into the nasal septum with its fellow of the opposite side, and a lateral crus that forms the anterior part of the wing of the nose.

great•er cur•va•ture of stom•ach (grā′tĕr kŭr′vă-chŭr stŏm′ăk) The border of the stomach to which the greater omentum is attached.

great•er mult•ang•u•lar bone (grā′tĕr mŭl-tang′gyū-lăr bōn) SYN trapezium.

great•er oc•cip•i•tal nerve (grā′tĕr ok-sip′i-tăl nĕrv) Medial branch of the dorsal primary ramus of the second cervical nerve; sends branches to the semispinalis capitis and multifidus cervicis, but is mainly sensory, supplying the back part of the scalp, meningeal branches to the posterior cranial fossa, and pain and proprioceptive branches to the first cervical nerve for the suboccipital muscles.

great•er o•men•tum (grā′tĕr ō-men′tŭm) A peritoneal fold passing from the greater curvature of the stomach to the transverse colon, hanging like an apron in front of the intestines. SYN caul (2), cowl, velum (3).

great•er pal•a•tine ca•nal (grā′tĕr pal′ă-tīn kă-nal′) The canalis formed between the maxilla and palatine bones; it transmits the descending palatine artery and the greater palatine nerve. SYN pterygopalatine canal.

great•er pal•a•tine fo•ra•men (grā′tĕr pal′ă-tīn fōr-ā′mĕn) An opening in the posterolateral corner of the hard palate opposite the last molar tooth, marking the lower end of the pterygopalatine canal.

great•er pal•a•tine nerve (grā′tĕr pal′ă-tīn nĕrv) A branch of the pterygopalatine ganglion that passes downward through the greater palatine canal to supply the mucosa and glands of the hard palate, and the anterior part of the soft palate. SYN nervus palatinus major [TA].

great•er pan•cre•at•ic ar•ter•y (grā′tĕr pan-krē-ăt′ik ahr′tĕr-ē) *Origin*, splenic; *distribution*, tail of pancreas; *anastomoses*, inferior pancreatic artery and arteries of pancreatic tail. SYN arteria pancreatica magna.

great•er pec•tor•al mus•cle (grāt′ĕr pek′tŏr-ăl mŭs′ĕl) SYN pectoralis major muscle.

great•er pel•vis (grā′tĕr pel′vis) The expanded portion of the pelvis above the brim. SYN false pelvis.

great•er pe•tro•sal nerve (grā′tĕr pĕ-trō′săl nĕrv) A branch from the genu of the facial nerve exiting by way of the hiatus of the facial canal and running in a groove on the anterior surface of the petrous part of the temporal bone beside the foramen lacerum to join the deep petrosal nerve, thus forming the nerve of the pterygoid canal, which passes through the pterygoid canal to reach the pterygopalatine ganglion. SYN greater superficial petrosal nerve, nervus petrosus major, parasympathetic root of pterygopalatine ganglion.

great•er pos•te•ri•or rec•tus mus•cle of head (grā′tĕr pos-tēr′ē-ŏr rek′tŭs mŭs′ĕl hed) SYN rectus capitis posterior major muscle.

great•er pso•as mus•cle (grā′tĕr sō′ăs mŭs′ĕl) SYN psoas major muscle.

great•er rhom•boid mus•cle (grā′tĕr rom′boyd mŭs′ĕl) SYN rhomboid major muscle.

great•er splanch•nic nerve (grā′tĕr splangk′nik nĕrv) Uppermost of the abdominopelvic splanchnics, which arises from the fifth or sixth to the ninth or tenth thoracic sympathetic ganglia in the thorax and passes downward along the bodies of the thoracic vertebrae, penetrating the diaphragm to join the celiac plexus; conveys presynaptic sympathetic fibers to the celiac ganglia, and visceral afferent fibers from the celiac plexus. SYN nervus splanchnicus major [TA].

great•er su•per•fi•cial pe•tro•sal nerve (grā′tĕr sū′pĕr-fish′ăl pĕ-trō′săl nĕrv) SYN greater petrosal nerve.

great•er su•pra•cla•vi•cu•lar fos•sa (grā′tĕr sū′pră-klă-vik′yū-lăr fos′ă) A depressed area above the middle of the clavicle, lateral to the sternocleidomastoid muscle, overlying the omoclavicular triangle, a subdivision of the posterior triangle of the neck.

great•er tro•chan•ter (grā′tĕr trō-kan′tĕr) A strong process at the proximal and lateral part of the shaft of the femur, overhanging the root of the neck; it gives attachment to the gluteus medius and minimus, piriformis, obturator internus and externus, and gemelli muscles. SYN trochanter major [TA].

great•er tu•ber•cle of the hu•mer•us (grā′tĕr tū′bĕr-kăl hyū′mĕr-ŭs) The larger and more lateral prominence of the two tubercles at the proximal end of the humerus.

great•er ves•tib•u•lar gland (grā′tĕr ves-tib′yū-lăr gland) One of two mucoid-secreting tubuloalveolar glands on either side of the lower part of the vagina, the equivalent of the bulbourethral glands in the male; ensheathed with vestibular bulbs by ischiocavernosus muscles; contraction of which causes secretion into vestibule of vagina. SYN Bartholin gland.

great·er wing of sphe·noid bone (grā′tĕr wing sfē′noyd bōn) Strong squamous processes extending in a broad superolateral curve from the body of the sphenoid bone. The greater wing presents these surfaces (facies): 1) cerebral surface forms anterior third of the floor of the lateral portion of the middle cranial fossa; 2) temporal surface forms the deepest portion of the temporal fossa; 3) infratemporal surface forms the "roof" of the infratemporal fossa; 4) orbital surface forms posterolateral wall of orbit. The greater wing forms the inferior border of the supraorbital fissure and is perforated at its root by the foramina rotundum, ovale, and spinosum and the pterygoid canal.

great·er zy·go·mat·ic mus·cle (grā′tĕr zī′gō-mat′ik mŭs′ĕl) SYN zygomaticus major muscle.

great fo·ra·men (grāt fōr-ā′mĕn) SYN foramen magnum.

great seg·men·tal med·ul·lar·y ar·ter·y (grāt seg-men′tăl med′ŭ-lar′ē ahr′tĕr-ē) Largest of the medullary arteries that supply the spinal cord by anastomosing with the anterior (longitudinal) spinal artery. It arises from a lower intercostal or upper lumbar artery (on the left side about 65% of the time) supplying most of the blood to the lower two-thirds of the anterior spinal artery. SEE medullary arteries of brain.

great toe (grāt tō) The first digit of the foot.

Greek hay (grēk hā) SYN fenugreek.

Green·field fil·ter (grēn′fēld fil′tĕr) A multistrutted spring-styled filter usually placed in the inferior vena cava to prevent venous emboli from reaching the pulmonary circulation from the lower extremity.

green·stick frac·ture (grēn′stik frak′shŭr) A fracture in which the bone is partially broken and partially bent; a type of incomplete fracture that occurs primarily in children. See this page.

green-top tube (grēn-top tūb) A container with a lining of lithium heparin, ammonium heparin, or sodium heparin used as anticoagulants.

Greig ce·pha·lo·po·ly·syn·dac·ty·ly syn·drome (greg sef′ă-lō-pol′ē-sin-dak′ti-lē sin′drōm) An autosomal dominant disorder characterized by polysyndactyly of the hands and feet, macrocephaly, frontal bossing, hypertelorism, and flat nasal bridge, caused by mutation in the GLI3 gene on chromosome 7p13.

Greig syn·drome (greg sin′drōm) SYN ocular hypertelorism.

grenz ray (grenz rā) Very soft x-rays, closely allied to the ultraviolet rays in their wavelength (i.e., long) and in their biologic action on tissues; they are produced by a specially built vacuum tube with a hot cathode operating from a transformer delivering not more than 8 kw. [Ger. *Grenze*, borderline, boundary]

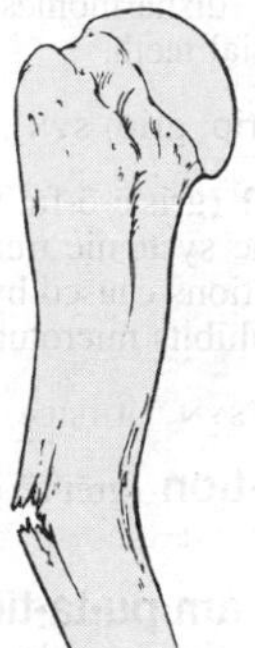

greenstick fracture

Grey Tur·ner sign (grā tŭr′nĕr sīn) Local areas of discoloration about the umbilicus and in the region of the loins, in acute hemorrhagic pancreatitis and other causes of retroperitoneal hemorrhage.

grid (grid) **1.** A chart with horizontal and perpendicular lines for plotting curves. **2.** X-RAY IMAGING a device formed of lead strips for preventing scattered radiation from reaching the x-ray film. [M.E. *gridel*, fr. L. *craticula*, lattice]

Grid·ley stain (grid′lē stān) A silver staining method for reticulum.

Grid·ley stain for fun·gi (grid′lē stān fŭng′gī) A method for fixed tissue sections based on Bauer chromic acid leucofuchsin stain with the addition of Gomori aldehyde fuchsin stain and metanil yellow as counterstains; against a yellow background, hyphae, conidia, yeast capsules, elastin, and mucin appear in different shades of blue to purple.

grief (grēf) A normal emotional response to an external loss; distinguished from a depressive disorder because it usually subsides after a reasonable time.

Grie·sing·er dis·ease (grē′zing-ger di-zēz′) Bilious typhoid of Griesinger, a severe form of louse-borne relapsing fever caused by *Borrelia recurrentis;* findings include high fever, epistaxis, dyspnea, intense jaundice, purpura, and splenomegaly.

Grie·sing·er sign (grē′zing-ger sīn) Erythema and edema over the posterior part of the mastoid process due to septic thrombosis of the mastoid emissary vein and indicating thrombophlebitis of the sigmoid sinus.

grind·ing (grīnd′ing) SYN abrasion (3).

grind·ing-in (grīnd′ing-in′) The act of correcting occlusal disharmonies by grinding the natural or artificial teeth.

grip, grippe (grip, grip) SYN influenza.

gris•e•o•ful•vin (gris′ē-ō-ful′vin) A fungistatic agent used in the systemic treatment of superficial fungal infections caused by certain dermatophytes, which inhibits microtubule assembly.

gris•tle (gris′ĕl) SYN cartilage. [A.S.]

Grit•ti op•er•a•tion (grēt′tē op-ĕr-ā′shŭn) SYN Gritti-Stokes amputation.

Grit•ti-Stokes am•pu•ta•tion (grēt′tē stōks amp′yū-tā′shŭn) Supracondylar amputation of the femur, the patella being preserved and applied to the end of the bone, its articular cartilage being removed so as to obtain union. SYN Gritti operation.

Groc•co sign (grok′kō sīn) **1.** Acute dilation of the heart following a muscular effort, described in Graves disease; also occurring in various forms of myocardiopathy. **2.** Extension of liver dullness several centimeters to the left of the midspinal line in cases of enlargement of that organ.

Groc•co tri•an•gle (grok′kō trī′ang-gĕl) A triangular patch of dullness at the base of the chest alongside the spinal column, on the side opposite a pleural effusion.

gro•cer's itch (grō′sĕrz ich) SYN baker's itch.

Groe•nouw cor•ne•al dys•tro•phy (grer′nō kor′nē-ăl dis′trŏ-fē) **1.** A granular type of corneal dystrophy, with autosomal dominant inheritance, caused by mutation in the transforming growth factor, beta-induced, gene (TGFβ1) encoding keratoepithelin on chromosome 5q. **2.** A progressive macular type of corneal dystrophy, characterized by punctate opacities and episodes of photophobia, corneal erosion, and foreign body sensation; autosomal recessive inheritance.

groin (groyn) **1.** SYN inguinal region. **2.** Sometimes used to indicate just the crease in the junction of the thigh with the trunk.

groove (grūv) A narrow elongated depression or furrow on any surface. SEE ALSO sulcus.

groove of nail ma•trix (grūv nāl mā′triks) SYN sulcus matricis unguis.

gross (grōs) Coarse or large; large enough to be visible to the naked eye.

gross a•nat•o•my (grōs ă-nat′ŏ-mē) General anatomy, so far as it can be studied without the use of the microscope; commonly used to denote the study of anatomy by dissection of a cadaver. SYN macroscopic anatomy.

gross mo•tor skills (grōs mō′tŏr skilz) Those abilities related to activity controlled by the large muscle groups.

Gross vi•rus (grōs vī′rŭs) The first strain of mouse leukemia virus that was isolated clinically.

gross vis•u•al skills (grōs vizh′ū-ăl skilz) Those abilities related to ocular acuity free from interference by nerves or muscles.

ground bun•dles (grownd bŭn′dĕlz) SYN fasciculi proprii.

ground glass (grownd glas) Opacity in radiologic imaging that may indicate various disease states.

ground-glass pat•tern (grownd-glas pat′ĕrn) Radiographic or CT appearance of hazy opacity that does not obscure underlying anatomic detail.

ground la•mel•la (grownd lă-mel′ă) SYN interstitial lamella.

ground state (grownd stāt) The normal, inactivated state of an atom from which, on activation, the singlet, triplet, and other excited states are derived.

ground sub•stance (grownd sub′stăns) The amorphous material in which structural elements occur; in connective tissue, it is composed of proteoglycans, plasma constituents, metabolites, water, and ions present between cells and fibers.

group (grūp) **1.** A number of similar or related objects. **2.** CHEMISTRY a radical.

group ag•glu•ti•na•tion (grūp ă-glū′ti-nā′shŭn) Agglutination by antibodies specific for minor (group) antigens common to several microorganisms, each of which possesses its own major specific antigen.

group ag•glu•ti•nin (grūp ă-glū′ti-nin) An immune agglutinin specific for a group antigen. SYN cross-reacting agglutinin.

group an•ti•gens (grūp an′ti-jenz) Antigens that are shared by related genera of microorganisms.

group A strep•to•coc•cal (GAS) nec•ro•tiz•ing fas•ci•i•tis (grūp strep′tō-kok′ăl gas nek′rō-tīz-ing fash′ē-ī′tis) A complication of infection with GAS in which the bacteria attack and destroy muscle tissue.

group home (as a residential facility) (grūp hōm) SYN ICF.

group med•i•cine (grūp med′i-sin) Therapy in which health care is provided by individual physicians who have allied themselves as a collective, usually with practitioners of various disciplines located within a building or complex.

group mod•el HMO (grūp mod′ĕl) An HMO that contracts with a single medical practice to be the sole source of care for its subscribers; two types of practice exist under this model: the "captive" group, which is formed by an HMO to serve its subscribers, and the "independent" group, a previously independent practice that contracts with the HMO.

group prac·tice (grūp prak′tis) The cooperative practice of medicine by a group of physicians, each of whom as a rule specializes in some particular field; such a group often shares a common suite of consulting rooms, laboratories, staff, equipment, and like facilities. Cf. group practice without walls.

group prac·tice with·out walls (GPWW) (grūp prak′tis with-owt′ wawlz) A physicians' consortium, in which several practices merge with the intention of providing consulting to each other and to share expenses, but not within the same premises. Cf. group practice.

group ther·a·py (grūp thār′ă-pē) A meeting in which several patients with the same condition meet with a single counselor to discuss a condition or problem shared by all patients; generally thought helpful because patients may share perceptions and understandings.

Gro·ver dis·ease (grō′vĕr di-zēz′) SYN transient acantholytic dermatosis.

grow·ing pains (grō′ing pānz) Aching pains, frequently felt at night, in the limbs of growing children; attributed variously to growth, rheumatic state, faulty posture, fatigue, or ill-defined psychic causes.

growth (grōth) The increase in size of a living being or any of its parts occurring in the process of development; as measured in increments of weight, volume, or linear dimensions. Cf. bioregulator.

growth hor·mone (GH) (grōth hōr′mōn) SYN somatotropin.

growth hor·mone–in·hib·it·ing hor·mone (GIH) (grōth-hōr′mōn-in-hib′i-ting hōr′mōn) SYN somatostatin.

growth hor·mone–pro·duc·ing ad·e·no·ma (grōth hōr′mōn-prŏ-dus′ing ad′ĕ-nō′mă) An adenoma that produces the clinical picture of gigantism or acromegaly, although a third of the cells have no granules or are a mixture of acidophils and chromophobes; some tumors may secrete both growth hormone and prolactin; often an acidophil or eosinophil adenoma.

growth hor·mone–re·leas·ing fac·tor (GHRF, GH-RF) (grōth hōr′mōn-rĕ-lēs′ing fak′tōr) SYN somatoliberin.

growth hor·mone–re·leas·ing hor·mone (GHRH, GH-RH) (grōth hōr′mōn-rĕ-lēs′ing hōr′mōn) SYN somatoliberin.

growth-on·set di·a·be·tes (grōth-on′set dī-ă-bē′tēz) SYN Type 1 diabetes.

growth plate (grōth plāt) SYN epiphysial plate.

growth rate (grōth rāt) Absolute or relative growth increase, expressed per unit of time.

Gru·ber meth·od (grū′ber meth′ŏd) A modification of the Politzer method in which the patient does not swallow, but says "hoc" at the instant of compression of the bag.

gru·mous (grū′mŭs) Thick and lumpy, as clotting blood. [L. *grumus,* a little heap]

Gru·nert spur (grū′nĕrt spŭr) Epithelial outgrowth of the dilator muscle of the pupil at the junction of the iris and the ciliary body; part of the origin of the iris dilator muscle.

grunt (grŭnt) During labored breathing, a characteristic sound created by rhythmic closure of the glottis; usually observed in newborns with RDS.

Gryn·feltt tri·an·gle (grin′felt trī′ang-gĕl) A triangular space bounded above by the end of the last rib and the serratus posterior inferior muscle, anteriorly by the internal oblique, and posteriorly by the quadratus lumborum; lumbar hernia occurs in this space. SYN Lesshaft triangle.

gry·po·sis (grip-ō′sis) An abnormal curvature. [G. *grypos,* hooked, + *-osis,* condition]

G-se·ries nerve a·gents (sēr′ēz nĕrv ā′jĕnts) Nonpersistent nerve agents developed by Germany before and during World War II and subsequently assigned NATO codes beginning with G. They include tabun (GA), sarin (GB), soman (GD), and cyclosarin (GF). These agents were not used on the battlefield during World War II, but several have been used subsequently, notably during the Iran-Iraq war in the 1980s.

GSH Abbreviation for glutathione.

GSR Abbreviation for galvanic skin response.

GSSG Abbreviation for glutathione disulfide.

GSW Abbreviation for gunshot wound.

gt Abbreviation for gutta, drop (q.v.).

GTO Abbreviation for Golgi tendon organ.

GTP Abbreviation for guanosine 5′-triphosphate.

GTT Abbreviation for glucose tolerance test.

G-tube (tūb) SYN percutaneous endoscopic gastrostomy tube.

GU Abbreviation for genitourinary.

guai·ac test (gwī′ak test) A screening procedure for occult blood in stool.

Guan·a·ri·to vi·rus (gwahn-ah-rē′tō vī′rŭs) A species of arenavirus causing Venezuelan hemorrhagic fever. [After municipality in Venezuela where all initial cases of Venezuelan hemorrhagic fever were confirmed]

gua·nase (gwahn′ās) SYN guanine deaminase.

gua·ni·di·no·ac·e·tate *N*-meth·yl·trans·fer·ase (gwahn′i-dē′nō-as′ĕ-tāt meth′il-trans′fĕr-ās) The enzyme catalyzing the transfer of a methyl group from *S*-adenosyl-L-methionine ("active methionine") to guanidinoacetate (glycocyamine), forming creatine and *S*-adenosyl-L-homocysteine.

gua•nine (G) (gwah′nēn) One of the two major purines (the other being adenine) occurring in all nucleic acids.

gua•nine de•am•i•nase (gwah′nēn dē-am′i-nās) A deaminase of the liver that catalyzes the hydrolysis of guanine into xanthine and ammonia; the first step in purine degradation. SYN guanase.

gua•nine de•ox•y•ri•bo•nu•cle•o•tide (gwah′nēn dē-oks′ē-rī′bō-nū′klē-ō-tīd) SYN deoxyguanylic acid.

gua•nine ri•bo•nu•cle•o•tide (gwah′nēn rī′bō-nū′klē-ō-tīd) SYN guanylic acid.

gua•no•sine (G, Guo) (gwah′nō-sēn) A major constituent of RNA and of guanine nucleotides.

gua•no•sine 5′-tri•phos•phate (GTP) (gwah′nō-sēn trī-fos′fāt) An immediate precursor of guanine nucleotides in RNA; similar to ATP; has a crucial role in microtubule formation.

gua•nyl•ic ac•id (GMP) (gwă-nil′ik as′id) A major component of ribonucleic acids. SYN guanine ribonucleotide.

guar•an•tor (gar′ăn-tōr) The patient, caregiver, or entity responsible for payment of the health care bill.

guard (gahrd) **1.** To watch over so as to protect or maintain control. **2.** A person or thing performing such a function.

guard•i•an (gahr′dē-ăn) An adult considered legally responsible for the care and custody of a minor or another adult determined unable to provide self-care.

guard•ing (gahrd′ing) A spasm of muscles to minimize motion or agitation of sites affected by injury or disease.

gu•ber•nac•u•lum (gū′bĕr-nak′yū-lŭm) **1.** A fibrous cord connecting two structures. **2.** A mesenchymal column of tissue that connects the fetal testis to the developing scrotum; it appears to play a role in guiding testicular descent. The gubernaculum in female embryos attaches to the ovaries and uterus. SYN gubernaculum testis [TA]. [L. a helm]

gu•ber•nac•u•lum den•tis (gū′bĕr-nak′yū-lŭm den′tis) A connective tissue band uniting the tooth sac with the gum.

gu•ber•nac•u•lum tes•tis (gū′bĕr-nak′yū-lŭm tes′tis) [TA] SYN gubernaculum (2).

Gub•ler syn•drome (goo-blā′ sin′drōm) A form of alternating hemiplegia characterized by contralateral hemiplegia and ipsilateral facial paralysis.

Gué•neau de Mus•sey point (gā-nō′ dĕ mū-sē′ poynt) A point, painful under pressure, at the junction of a line prolonging the left border of the sternum and a horizontal line at the level of end of the bony portion of the tenth rib; it is present in cases of diaphragmatic pleurisy.

Gué•rin frac•ture (gā-rin[h]′ frak′shŭr) SYN horizontal maxillary fracture.

guide (gīd) **1.** To lead in a set course. **2.** Any device or instrument by which another is led into its proper course, e.g., a grooved director, a catheter guide. [M.E., fr. O.Fr. *guier,* to show the way, fr. Germanic]

guid•ed im•ag•e•ry (gī′dĕd im′ăj-rē) Theoretic therapy that posits the power of the mind to affect physiology directly; used in a variety of medical settings to reduce stress, calm the mind, decrease pain, stimulate the immune system, and slow the heart rate.

gui•ded tis•sue re•gen•er•a•tion (gīd′ĕd tish′ū rē-jen′ĕr-ā′shŭn) Regeneration of tissue directed by the physical presence or chemical activities of a biomaterial; often involves placement of barriers to exclude one or more cell types during healing or regeneration of tissue.

guide•line (gīd′līn) **1.** A marking in the form of a line that serves as a guide or reference. **2.** A rule or directive outlining a policy or procedure. SEE ALSO clinical practice guidelines.

guide•wire (gīd′wīr) A long and flexible fine spring used to introduce and position an intravascular angiographic catheter (see Seldinger technique).

Guil•lain-Bar•ré syn•drome (gē-ahn[h]′ bah-rā′ sin′drōm) A self-limiting demyelinating syndrome related to autoimmune dysfunction, surgical complication, some vaccines, Hodgkin disease, and some types of drug reactions. Motor and/or sensory dysfunction begins in the extremities and moves proximally, sometimes leading to respiratory failure, before function is restored within weeks or months. SYN Landry paralysis, Landry syndrome, polyradiculoneuritis.

guil•lo•tine (gil′ō-tēn, gē′ō-tēn) An instrument in the shape of a metal ring through which runs a sliding knifeblade, used in cutting off an enlarged tonsil. [Fr. an instrument for execution by decapitation]

Gulf War syn•drome (gŭlf wōr sin′drōm) A constellation of findings (e.g., dermatologic disorders, mental problems) comprising a condition experienced by those who fought in the first Gulf War in 1990; still subject to diagnostic dispute by some clinicians.

gul•let (gŭl′ĕt) SYN throat (1). [L. *gula,* throat]

Gull•strand slit•lamp (gūl′strahnd slit-lamp) SYN slitlamp.

gum (gŭm) **1.** The dried exuded sap from a variety of trees and shrubs, forming an amorphous brittle mass; usually forms a mucilaginous solution in water. [L. *gummi*] **2.** SYN gingiva. [A.S. *goma,* jaw]

gum ar•a•bic (gŭm ār′ă-bik) SYN *Acacia.*

gum•boil (gŭm′boyl) SYN gingival abscess.

gum cam•phor (gŭm kam′fŏr) A ketone distilled from *Cinnamomum camphora* used in the oral cavity to treat infection.

gum line (gŭm līn) SYN gingival line.

gum•ma, pl. **gum•ma•ta, gum•mas** (gŭm′ă, ă-tă, -ĕz) An infectious granuloma that is characteristic of tertiary syphilis. Gummata are characterized by an irregular central portion that is firm, sometimes partially hyalinized, and consisting of coagulative necrosis in which "ghosts" of structures may be recognized; a poorly defined middle zone of epithelioid cells, with occasional multinucleated giant cells; and a peripheral zone of fibroblasts and numerous capillaries, with infiltrated lymphocytes and plasma cells. SYN syphiloma. [L. *gummi,* gum, fr. G. *kommi*]

gum•ma•tous (gŭm′ă-tŭs) Pertaining to or characterized by the features of a gumma.

gum re•sec•tion (gŭm rē-sek′shŭn) SYN gingivectomy.

Gunn cross•ing sign (gŭn kraws′ing sīn) Retinal arteriovenous crossing with venous compression in hypertensive disease.

Gunn dots (gŭn dots) Minute, highly glistening, white or yellowish specks usually seen in the posterior part of the fundus; nonpathologic.

Gunn sign (gŭn sīn) **1.** Compression of the underlying vein at arteriovenous crossings seen ophthalmoscopically in arteriolar sclerosis. **2.** On alternate stimulation with light, the pupil of an eye with optic nerve transmission defect constricts poorly or even dilates when stimulated (a relative afferent pupillary defect). SYN Marcus Gunn sign.

Gunn syn•drome (gŭn sin′drōm) SYN jaw-winking syndrome.

gun•shot wound (GSW) (gŭn′shot wūnd) Injury caused by a bullet or other projectile from a firearm that hits a human or animal.

gun•stock de•for•mi•ty (gŭn′stok dĕ-fōrm′i-tē) A form of cubitus varus resulting from condylar fracture at the elbow in which the axis of the extended forearm is not continuous with that of the arm but is displaced toward midline.

Guo Abbreviation for guanosine.

gur•gling rale (gŭr′gling rahl) Coarse sound heard over large cavities or over trachea nearly filled with secretions.

gur•ney (gŭr′nē) A stretcher or cot with wheels used to transport hospital patients. [Scottish *gurn,* to grimace in pain]

gush•er (gŭsh′er) An abundant flow of fluid.

Gus•sen•bau•er su•ture (gŭs′en-bow′er sū′chŭr) A figure-of-8 suture for the intestine, resembling the Czerny-Lembert suture but not including the mucous membrane.

gus•ta•tion (gŭs-tā′shŭn) **1.** The act of tasting. **2.** The sense of taste. See this page. [L. *gustatio,* fr. *gusto,* pp. *-atus,* to taste]

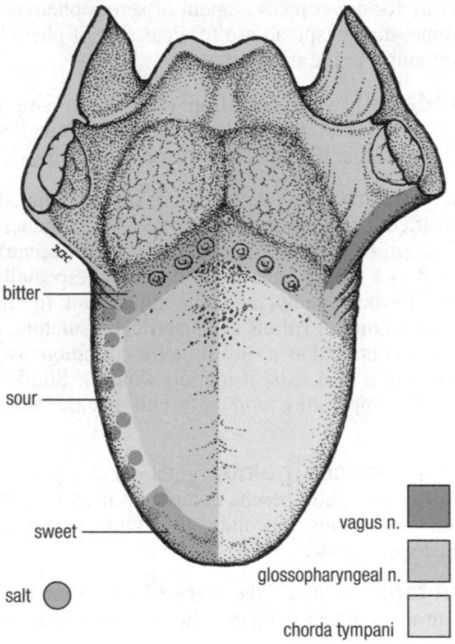

gustation: regions of taste perception and their gustatory nerves

gus•ta•to•ry (gŭs′tă-tōr-ē) Relating to gustation, or taste.

gus•ta•to•ry ag•no•si•a (gŭs′tă-tōr-ē ag-nō′zē-ă) Inability to classify or identify a tastant, even though the ability to distinguish between or recognize tastants may be normal; may be general, partial, or specific.

gus•ta•tory au•ra (gŭs′tă-tōr-ē awr′ă) Epileptic aura characterized by illusions or hallucinations of taste. SEE ALSO aura (1).

gus•ta•to•ry cells (gŭs′tă-tōr-ē selz) SYN taste cells.

gus•ta•to•ry hy•per•hi•dro•sis (gŭs′tă-tōr-ē hī′pĕr-hī-drō′sis) Excessive sweating of the lips, nose, and forehead after eating certain foods.

gus•ta•to•ry rhi•nor•rhe•a (gŭs′tă-tōr-ē rī′nōr-ē′ă) Watery nasal discharge associated with stimulation of the sense of taste.

gut (gŭt) **1.** SYN intestine. **2.** Embryonic digestive tube. **3.** Abbreviated term for catgut. SEE ALSO suture.

gut·as·so·ci·a·ted lym·phoid tis·sue (gŭt′ ă-sō′sē-ā-tĕd lim′foyd tish′ū) Lymphoid tissue of the gastrointestinal mucosa that contains both B cells and T cells. This tissue is responsible for localized immunity to pathogens such as bacteria, viruses, and parasites.

Guth·rie mus·cle (gŭth′rē mŭs′ĕl) SYN external urethral sphincter muscle.

Guth·rie test (gŭth′rē test) Bacterial inhibition assay for direct measurement of serum phenylalanine; in widespread use for detection of phenylketonuria in the newborn.

gut·ta (gt) (gŭt′ă) **1.** A drop. (abbrev. gt, [sing.], gtt. [pl.]. **2.** A rubberlike polyterpene found in gutta-percha. Cf. chicle, gutta-percha. [L.]

gut·ta-per·cha (gut′ă-pĕr′chă) The coagulated, purified, dried, milky juice of trees of the genera *Palaguium* and *Payena* (family Sapotaceae); used as a filling material in dentistry, especially to fill root canals in endodontics, and in the manufacture of splints and electrical insulators; a solution is used as a substitute for collodion, as a protective, and to seal incised wounds. Solid at room temperature and soft and plastic when heated.

gut·ta-per·cha points (gut′ă-pĕr′chă poynts) Cones of a gutta-percha compound used for filling root canals in conjunction with a cement, paste, or plastic.

gut·tate (gŭt′āt) Of the shape of, or resembling, a drop, characterizing certain cutaneous lesions.

gut·ter dys·tro·phy of cor·ne·a (gŭt′ĕr dis′ trŏ-fē kōr′nē-ă) A marginal furrow usually inferiorly about 1 mm from the limbus; sometimes bilateral. SYN keratoleptynsis (1).

gut·ter frac·ture (gŭt′ĕr frak′shŭr) A long, narrow, depressed fracture of the skull.

gut·ter wound (gŭt′ĕr wūnd) A tangential wound that makes a furrow without perforating the skin.

Gutt·man scale (gūt′mahn skāl) A measurement scale that ranks categories of responses to a question, with each unit representing an increasingly strong expression of an attribute such as pain or disability.

gut·tur·al (gŭt′ŭr-ăl) Relating to the throat.

Guy·on am·pu·ta·tion (gē-yōn[h]′ amp′yū-tā′ shŭn) Surgical removal of the foot and ankle joint, carried out just above the malleoli, a modification of Syme amputation.

Guy·on ca·nal (gē-yōn[h]′ kă-nal′) The superficial canal between the flexor retinaculum of the hand and flexor carpi ulnaris through which pass the ulnar nerve and vasculature between forearm and hand.

Guy·on sign (gē-yōn[h]′ sīn) **1.** Ballottement of the kidney in cases of nephroptosis, especially when there is also a renal tumor. **2.** The hypoglossal nerve lies directly on the external carotid artery, whereby this vessel may be distinguished from the internal carotid when ligation is necessary.

Guy·on tun·nel syn·drome (gē-yōn[h]′ tŭn′ el sin′drōm) Entrapment or compression of the ulnar nerve within Guyon canal as the ulnar nerve passes into the wrist.

GVHD Abbreviation for graft-versus-host disease.

GVHR Abbreviation for graft-versus-host reaction.

GXT Abbreviation for graded exercise test.

Gy Abbreviation for Gray (unit of absorbed radiation).

Gym·no·din·i·um (jim-nō-dī′nē-um) Genus of marine dinoflagellates that includes the unicellular organism that causes red tide.

Gym·no·din·i·um brev·e (jim-nō-dī′nē-um brev′ē) A species of microscopic algae that causes red tide; it produces a toxin that affects the central nervous system of fish, paralyzing and killing them.

Gym·no·phal·loi·des (jim-nō-fă-loy′dēz) Small trematode (family Gymnophallidae) normally found in birds; often reported in human intestine in Korea; the intermediate host is presumed to be a marine oyster or clam.

Gym·no·phal·loi·des se·o·i (jim-nō-fă-loy′ dēz sē′ō-ī) Trematode found in inhabitants of an island southwest of the Korean peninsula; infection produces vague intestinal symptoms; it is a human parasite under natural conditions. Migrating birds are natural definitive hosts.

GYN Abbreviation for gynecology.

♻**gyn-, gyne-, gy·ne·co-, gyno-** Combining forms meaning female. [G. *gynē*, woman]

gynae- [Br.] SYN gyne-.

gynaecic [Br.] SYN gynecic.

gynaeco- [Br.] SYN gyneco-.

gynaecoid [Br.] SYN gynecoid.

gynaecoid obesity [Br.] SYN gynecoid obesity.

gynaecoid pelvis [Br.] SYN gynecoid pelvis.

gynaecologic [Br.] SYN gynecologic.

gynaecologist [Br.] SYN gynecologist.

gynaecology [Br.] SYN gynecology.

gynaecomastia [Br.] SYN gynecomastia.

gynaecomasty [Br.] SYN gynecomasty.

gynaephobia [Br.] SYN gynephobia.

gy•nan•drism (gī-nan′drizm) A developmental abnormality characterized by hypertrophy of the clitoris and union of the labia majora, simulating in appearance the penis and scrotum. SEE hermaphroditism, pseudohermaphroditism. [gyn- + G. *anēr* {*andr-*}, man]

gy•nan•dro•blas•to•ma (gī-nan′drō-blas-tō′mă) **1.** SYN arrhenoblastoma. **2.** A rare variety of arrhenoblastoma of the ovary, containing granulosa or theca cell elements and producing simultaneous androgenic and estrogenic effects.

gy•nan•droid (gī-nan′droyd) Someone exhibiting gynandrism. [gyn- + G. *anēr* {*andr-*}, man, + *eidos,* resemblance]

gy•nan•dro•mor•phism (gī-nan′drō mōr′fizm) **1.** An abnormal combination of male and female characteristics. **2.** The presence of male and female sex chromosome complements in different tissues; sex chromosome mosaicism. [gyn- + G. *anēr* {*andr-*}, a male human, + *morphē,* form]

gy•nan•dro•mor•phous (gī-nan′drō-mōr′fŭs) Having both male and female characteristics.

gy•ne•cic (gī-nē′sik) Pertaining to or associated with women. SYN gynaecic.

gy•ne•coid (gī′nĕ-koyd) **1.** Resembling a woman in form and structure. **2.** OBSTETRICS referring to the shape of the normal female pelvis. SYN gynaecoid. [gyneco- + G. *eidos,* resemblance]

gy•ne•coid o•be•si•ty (gī′nĕ-koyd ō-bē′si-tē) Obesity with fat excess mainly in the femoral-gluteal region (pear shape). SYN gynaecoid obesity.

gy•ne•coid pel•vis (gī′nĕ-koyd pel′vis) The normal female pelvis. SYN gynaecoid pelvis.

gy•ne•co•log•ic (gī′nĕ-kŏ-loj′ik) Relating to gynecology. SYN gynaecologic.

gy•ne•co•log•ic ex•am•i•na•tion (gī′nĕ-kŏ-loj′ik eg-zam′i-nā′shŭn) Investigation and assessment of the female urogenital system for the purposes of diagnosis and to rule out the presence of disease or injury.

gy•ne•col•o•gist (gī′nĕ-kol′ŏ-jist) A physician specializing in gynecology. SYN gynaecologist.

gy•ne•col•o•gy (GYN) (gī′nĕ-kol′ŏ-jē) The medical specialty concerned with diseases of the female genital tract, as well as endocrinology and reproductive physiology of the female. SYN gynaecology. [gyneco- + G. *logos,* study]

gy•ne•co•ma•sti•a, gy•ne•co•mas•ty (gī′nĕ-kō-mas′tē-ă, -mas′tē) Excessive development of the male mammary glands, due mainly to ductal proliferation with periductal edema; frequently secondary to increased estrogen levels, but mild gynecomastia may occur in normal adolescents. SYN gynaecomastia. [gyneco- + G. *mastos,* breast]

gy•ne•pho•bi•a (gī′nĕ-fō′bē-ă) Morbid fear of women or of the female sex. SYN gynaephobia. [gyne- + G. *phobos,* fear]

gy•no•gen•e•sis (gī′nō-jen′ĕ-sis) Oocyte development activated by a sperm, but to which the male gamete contributes no genetic material. [gyno- + G. *genesis,* production]

gy•no•plas•tics (gī′nō-plas-tiks) SEE gynoplasty.

gy•no•plas•ty (gī′nō-plas-tē) Reparative or plastic surgery of the female genital organs. [gyno- + G. *plassō,* to form]

gyp•sy weed (jip′sē wēd) SYN bugleweed.

gy•rate (jī′rāt) **1.** Of a convoluted or ring shape. **2.** To revolve. [L. *gyro,* pp. *gyratus,* to turn round in a circle, *gyrus*]

gy•rec•to•my (jī-rek′tŏ-mē) Excision of a cerebral gyrus. [G. *gyros,* ring, + *ektomē,* excision]

gy•ri (jī′rī) Plural of gyrus. [L.]

gy•ro•mag•net•ic ra•ti•o (jī′rō-mag-net′ik rā′shē-ō) The precessional frequency of an element at 1.0 tesla.

Gy•ro•mi•tra es•cu•len•ta (jī-rō-mī′tră es-kyū-len′tă) A species of mushroom that may produce a monomethylhydrazine toxin that causes nausea, diarrhea, and other symptoms; in severe cases death may ensue.

gy•rose (jī′rōs) Marked by irregular curved lines like the surface of a cerebral hemisphere. [G. *gyros,* circle]

gy•ro•spasm (jī′rō-spazm) Spasmodic rotary movements of the head. [G. *gyros,* circle, + *spasmos,* spasm]

gy•rus, gen. and pl. **gy•ri** (jī′rŭs, -rī) One of the prominent rounded elevations or convolutions that form the cerebral hemispheres, each consisting of an exposed superficial portion and a portion hidden from view in the wall and floor of the sulcus. [L. fr. G. *gyros,* circle]

gy•rus for•ni•ca•tus (jī′rŭs fōr-nī-kā′tus) **1.** SYN fornicate gyrus. **2.** Used previously to refer to the entire limbic system.

H

H Abbreviation for hyperopia or hyperopic; horizontal; Hauch; henry, unit of electrical inductance; hydrogen; the Fraunhofer line at λ 3968 due to calcium; histidine; magnetic field strength; heroin; NATO code for sulfur mustard (q.v.), especially the unpure type produced by the Löwenstein process.

H^+ Abbreviation for hydrogen ion, the proton.

^1H Abbreviation for hydrogen-1.

^2H Abbreviation for hydrogen-2.

^3H Abbreviation for hydrogen-3.

H Abbreviation for enthalpy; heat content, in the equation for free energy.

h Abbreviation for hecto-; height; hour; haustus.

h Abbreviation for Planck constant; $h = h/2\pi$.

HA Abbreviation for headache.

haar·schei·be tu·mor (hahr′shī-bĕ tū′mŏr) SYN trichodiscoma. [Ger. *Haar,* hair, + *Scheibe,* disc]

HAART (hahrt) Acronym and abbreviation for highly active antiretroviral therapy.

Haa·se rule (hah′sĕ rūl) The length of the fetus in centimeters, divided by 5, is the duration of pregnancy in months, i.e., the age of the fetus.

ha·be·na, pl. **ha·be·nae** (hă-bē′nă, -bē′nē) **1.** A frenum or restricting fibrous band. **2.** A restraining bandage. **3.** SYN habenula (2). [L. strap]

hab·e·nal, ha·be·nar (hă-bē′năl, -năr) Relating to a habena.

ha·ben·u·la, pl. **ha·ben·u·lae** (hă-ben′yū-lă, -lē) [TA] **1.** SYN frenulum. **2.** NEUROANATOMY the term originally denoted the stalk of the pineal gland (pineal habenula; pedunculus of pineal body), but gradually came to refer to a neighboring group of nerve cells with which the pineal gland was believed to be associated, the habenular nucleus. Currently, the term, as defined by TA, refers exclusively to this circumscript cell mass in the caudal and dorsal aspect of the dorsal thalamus, embedded in the posterior end of the medullary stria from which it receives most of its afferent fibers. By way of the retroflex fasciculus (habenulointerpeduncular tract) it projects to the interpeduncular nucleus and other paramedian cell groups of the midbrain tegmentum. Despite its proximity to the pineal stalk, no habenulopineal fiber connection is known to exist. It is a part of the epithalamus. SYN habena (3). [L.]

ha·ben·u·lar (hă-ben′yū-lăr) Relating to a habenula, especially the stalk of the pineal body.

Ha·ber syn·drome (hah′ber sin′drōm) A permanent flushing and telangiectasia of the cheeks, nose, forehead, and chin, with prominent follicular openings, small papules with scaling, and minute pitted areas; occasionally accompanied by scaly and keratotic lesions of the trunk.

hab·it (hab′it) **1.** An act, behavioral response, practice, or custom established in one's repertoire by frequent repetition of the same act. SEE ALSO addiction. **2.** A basic variable in the study of conditioning and learning used to designate a new response learned either by association or by being followed by a reward or reinforced event. SEE conditioning, learning. **3.** An autonomic behavior integrated into a more complex pattern to function on a daily basis. [L. *habeo,* pp. *habitus,* to have]

hab·it cough (hab′it kawf) A persistent cough due to a tic or to psychological causes.

hab·it spasm (hab′it spazm) SYN tic.

ha·bit·u·al a·bor·tion (hă-bich′ū-ăl ă-bōr′shŭn) A condition in which a woman has had three or more consecutive, spontaneous abortions.

ha·bit·u·al cen·tric (hă-bich′ū-ăl sen′trik) SYN centric occlusion.

ha·bit·u·al pitch (hă-bich′ū-ăl pich) Central tendency of pitch, or fundamental frequency, most often used by a person. Voice strain or vocal pathology may result when the habitual pitch is significantly different from the optimal pitch. SEE optimal pitch. SYN modal frequency, modal pitch.

ha·bit·u·a·tion (hă-bich′ū-ā′shŭn) **1.** The process of forming a habit, referring generally to psychological dependence on the continued use of a drug to maintain a sense of well-being, which can result in drug addiction. **2.** The method by which the nervous system reduces or inhibits responsiveness during repeated stimulation.

hab·i·tus (hab′i-tŭs) The physical characteristics of a person. [L. habit]

HACCP Abbreviation fro Hazard Analysis Critical Control Point.

HACE Abbreviation for high altitude cerebral edema.

HACEK group (has′ek grūp) A group of gram-negative bacteria that includes *Haemophilus aphrophilus*, *Actinobacillus actinomycetemcomitans*, *Cardiobacterium hominis*, *Eikenella corrodens*, and *Kingella kingae*. Bacteria in this group have in common a culture requirement of an enhanced carbon dioxide atmosphere and ability to infect human heart valves.

Ha·der·up den·tal no·men·cla·ture (hah′der-ŭp den′tăl nō′mĕn-klā-chūr) **1.** European system of identifying teeth by use of a number for each permanent tooth and a + or − sign to indicate the position of each tooth, e.g., 6 + is the upper right first permanent molar. **2.** A system for deciduous teeth analogous to that for the permanent teeth in which a 0 is added before the tooth number, e.g., 03+ is the upper right deciduous canine.

Haeck•el law (hek′ĕl law) SYN recapitulation theory.

haem [Br.] SYN heme.

haem [Br.] SYN heme.

haem- [Br.] SYN hem-.

haema- [Br.] SYN hema-.

haemachrome [Br.] SYN hemachrome.

haemacyte [Br.] SYN hemacyte.

haemacytometer [Br.] SYN hemacytometer.

haemadsorption [Br.] SYN hemadsorption.

haemadsorption virus type 1 [Br.] SYN hemadsorption virus type 1.

haemadsorption virus type 2 [Br.] SYN hemadsorption virus type 2.

haemagglutination [Br.] SYN hemagglutination.

haemagglutinin [Br.] SYN hemagglutinin.

haemagglutinin-protease [Br.] SYN hemagglutinin-protease.

haemagogic [Br.] SYN hemagogic.

haemal [Br.] SYN hemal.

haemalum [Br.] SYN hemalum.

haemanalysis [Br.] SYN hemanalysis.

haemangiectasia [Br.] SYN hemangiectasia.

haemangiectasis [Br.] SYN hemangiectasis.

haemangio- [Br.] SYN hemangio-.

haemangioblast [Br.] SYN hemangioblast.

haemangioblastoma [Br.] SYN hemangioblastoma.

haemangioendothelioblastoma [Br.] SYN hemangioendothelioblastoma.

haemangioendothelioma [Br.] SYN hemangioendothelioma.

haemangiofibroma [Br.] SYN hemangiofibroma.

haemangioma [Br.] SYN hemangioma.

haemangiomatosis [Br.] SYN hemangiomatosis.

haemangiopericytoma [Br.] SYN hemangiopericytoma.

haemangiosarcoma [Br.] SYN hemangiosarcoma.

haemapophysis [Br.] SYN hemapophysis.

haemarthrosis [Br.] SYN hemarthrosis.

haemastatic [Br.] SYN hemostatic.

haemat- [Br.] SYN hemat-.

haematein [Br.] SYN hematein.

haematemesis [Br.] SYN hematemesis.

haematencephalon [Br.] SYN hematencephalon.

haematic [Br.] SYN hematic.

haematidrosis [Br.] SYN hematidrosis.

haematin [Br.] SYN hematin.

haematinaemia [Br.] SYN hematinemia.

haematin chloride [Br.] SYN hematin chloride.

haematinic [Br.] SYN hematinic.

haemato- [Br.] SYN hemato-.

haematoblast [Br.] SYN hematoblast.

haematocele [Br.] SYN hematocele.

haematocephaly [Br.] SYN hematocephaly.

haematochezia [Br.] SYN hematochezia.

haematochyluria [Br.] SYN hematochyluria.

haematocolpometra [Br.] SYN hematocolpometra.

haematocolpos [Br.] SYN hematocolpos.

haematocrit [Br.] SYN hematocrit.

hae•ma•toc•ry•a Cold-blooded vertebrates. [hemato- + G. *kryos,* cold]

haematocystis [Br.] SYN hematocystis.

haematogenesis [Br.] SYN hematogenesis.

haematogenic [Br.] SYN hematogenic.

haematogenous [Br.] SYN hematogenous.

haematogenous jaundice [Br.] SYN hematogenous jaundice.

haematogenous metastasis [Br.] SYN hematogenous metastasis.

haematohiston [Br.] SYN hematohiston.

haematoid [Br.] SYN hematoid.

haematoidin [Br.] SYN hematoidin.

haematologist [Br.] SYN hematologist.

haematology [Br.] SYN hematology.

haematolymphangioma [Br.] SYN hematolymphangioma.

haematolysis [Br.] SYN hematolysis.

haematolytic [Br.] SYN hematolytic.

haematoma [Br.] SYN hematoma.

haematometra [Br.] SYN hematometra.

haematomphalocele [Br.] SYN hematomphalocele.

haematomyelia [Br.] SYN hematomyelia.

haematomyelopore [Br.] SYN hematomyelopore.

haematopathology [Br.] SYN hematopathology.

hae•ma•to•phi•li•na A division of Cheiroptera that includes bloodsucking (vampire) bats. [hemato- + G. *philos,* fond]

haematoplast [Br.] SYN hematoplast.

haematoplastic [Br.] SYN hematoplastic.

haematopoiesis [Br.] SYN hematopoiesis.

haematopoietic [Br.] SYN hematopoietic.

haematopoietic gland [Br.] SYN hematopoietic gland.

haematopoietic growth factor [Br.] SYN hematopoietic growth factor.

haematopoietic system [Br.] SYN hematopoietic system.

haematoporphyrin [Br.] SYN hematoporphyrin.

haematopsia [Br.] SYN hematopsia.

haematorrhachis [Br.] SYN hematorrhachis.

haematorrhachis externa [Br.] SYN hematorrhachis externa.

haematorrhachis interna [Br.] SYN hematorrhachis interna.

haematosalpinx [Br.] SYN hematosalpinx.

haematosin [Br.] SYN hematosin.

haematosis [Br.] SYN hematosis.

haematospermatocele [Br.] SYN hematospermatocele.

haematostatic [Br.] SYN hematostatic.

haematostaxis [Br.] SYN hematostaxis.

haematosteon [Br.] SYN hematosteon.

haematotherma [Br.] SYN hematotherma.

haematothermal [Br.] SYN hematothermal.

haematothorax [Br.] SYN hemothorax.

haematotoxic [Br.] SYN hematotoxic.

haematotoxin [Br.] SYN hematotoxin.

haematotropic [Br.] SYN hematotropic.

haematoxic [Br.] SYN hematoxic.

haematoxylin [Br.] SYN hematoxylin.

haematoxylin and eosin stain [Br.] SYN hematoxylin and eosin stain.

haematozoon [Br.] SYN hematozoon.

haematuria [Br.] SYN hematuria.

haemerythrin [Br.] SYN hemerythrin.

haemic [Br.] SYN hemic.

haemic murmur [Br.] SYN hemic murmur.

haemin [Br.] SYN hemin.

haemo- [Br.] SYN hemo-.

haemobilia [Br.] SYN hemobilia.

haemoblast [Br.] SYN hemoblast.

haemoblastosis [Br.] SYN hemoblastosis.

haemocatheresis [Br.] SYN hemocatheresis.

haemocatheretic [Br.] SYN hemocatheretic.

Haemoccult test [Br.] SYN Hemoccult test.

haemochorial placenta [Br.] SYN hemochorial placenta.

haemochromatosis [Br.] SYN hemochromatosis.

haemochrome [Br.] SYN hemochrome.

haemochromogen [Br.] SYN hemochromogen.

haemochromometer [Br.] SYN hemochromometer.

haemoclasia [Br.] SYN hemoclasia.

haemoclasis [Br.] SYN hemoclasis.

haemoclastic [Br.] SYN hemoclastic.

haemocoel [Br.] SYN hemocele.

haemocoele [Br.] SYN hemocele.

haemoconcentration [Br.] SYN hemoconcentration.

haemoconia [Br.] SYN hemoconia.

haemoconiosis [Br.] SYN hemoconiosis.

haemocyanin [Br.] SYN hemocyanin.

haemocyte [Br.] SYN hemocyte.

haemocytoblast [Br.] SYN hemocytoblast.

haemocytocatheresis [Br.] SYN hemocytocatheresis.

haemocytolysis [Br.] SYN hemocytolysis.

haemocytoma [Br.] SYN hemocytoma.

haemocytometer [Br.] SYN hemocytometer.

haemocytometry [Br.] SYN hemocytometry.

haemocytotrypsis [Br.] SYN hemocytotripsis.

haemodiafiltration [Br.] SYN hemodiafiltration.

haemodiagnosis [Br.] SYN hemodiagnosis.

haemodialyser [Br.] SYN hemodialyzer.

haemodialysis [Br.] SYN hemodialysis.

haemodilution [Br.] SYN hemodilution.

haemodynamics [Br.] SYN hemodynamics.

haemoendothelial placenta [Br.] SYN hemoendothelial placenta.

haemofiltration [Br.] SYN hemofiltration.

haemoflagellate [Br.] SYN hemoflagellate.

haemofuscin [Br.] SYN hemofuscin.

haemogenesis [Br.] SYN hemogenesis.

haemogenic [Br.] SYN hemogenic.

haemoglobin [Br.] SYN hemoglobin.

haemoglobin A [Br.] SYN hemoglobin A.

haemoglobinaemia [Br.] SYN hemoglobinemia.

haemoglobin Bart [Br.] SYN hemoglobin Bart.

haemoglobin C [Br.] SYN hemoglobin C.

haemoglobin F [Br.] SYN hemoglobin F.

haemoglobinolysis [Br.] SYN hemoglobinolysis.

haemoglobinometry [Br.] SYN hemoglobinometry.

haemoglobinopathy [Br.] SYN hemoglobinopathy.

haemoglobinophilic [Br.] SYN hemoglobinophilic.

haemoglobin S [Br.] SYN hemoglobin S.

haemoglobins [Br.] SYN hemoglobin.

haemoglobinuria [Br.] SYN hemoglobinuria.

haemoglobinuric [Br.] SYN hemoglobinuric.

haemoglobinuric nephrosis [Br.] SYN hemoglobinuric nephrosis.

haemogram [Br.] SYN hemogram.

haemohistioblast [Br.] SYN hemohistioblast.

haemolith [Br.] SYN hemolith.

haemolutein [Br.] SYN hemolutein.

haemolymph [Br.] SYN hemolymph.

haemolysate [Br.] SYN hemolysate.

haemolysin [Br.] SYN hemolysin.

haemolysinogen [Br.] SYN hemolysinogen.

haemolysin unit [Br.] SYN hemolysin unit.

haemolysis [Br.] SYN hemolysis.

haemolytic [Br.] SYN hemolytic.

haemolytic anaemia [Br.] SYN hemolytic anemia.

haemolytic disease of newborn [Br.] SYN hemolytic disease of newborn.

haemolytic jaundice [Br.] SYN hemolytic jaundice.

haemolytic plaque assay [Br.] SYN hemolytic plaque assay.

haemolytic splenomegaly [Br.] SYN hemolytic splenomegaly.

haemolytic unit [Br.] SYN hemolytic unit.

haemolytic uremic syndrome [Br.] SYN hemolytic uremic syndrome.

haemomediastinum [Br.] SYN hemomediastinum.

haemometra [Br.] SYN hemometra.

haemonchiasis [Br.] SYN hemonchiasis.

Hae•mon•chus (hē-mong′kŭs) An economically important genus of nematodes (family Nematostrongylidae); parasitizes the abomasum of cattle, sheep, goats, and other ruminants, causing anemia; human infection occasionally occurs.

haemonectin [Br.] SYN hemonectin.

haemoparasite [Br.] SYN hemoparasite.

haemopathology [Br.] SYN hemopathology.

haemopathy [Br.] SYN hemopathy.

haemoperfusion [Br.] SYN hemoperfusion.

haemopericardium [Br.] SYN hemopericardium.

haemoperitoneum [Br.] SYN hemoperitoneum.

haemopexin [Br.] SYN hemopexin.

haemophagocyte [Br.] SYN hemophagocyte.

haemophil [Br.] SYN hemophil.

haemophile [Br.] SYN hemophile.

haemophilia [Br.] SYN hemophilia.

haemophilia A [Br.] SYN hemophilia A.

haemophilia B [Br.] SYN hemophilia B.

haemophiliac [Br.] SYN hemophiliac.

haemophilic [Br.] SYN hemophilic.

haemophilioid [Br.] SYN hemophilioid.

Hae•moph•i•lus (hē-mof′i-lŭs) A genus of aerobic to facultatively anaerobic, nonmotile bacteria (family Brucellaceae) containing minute, gram-negative, rod-shaped cells that sometimes form threads and are pleomorphic. These organisms are strictly parasitic, growing best, or only, on media containing blood. They may or may not be pathogenic. They occur in various lesions and secretions, as well as in normal respiratory tracts, of vertebrates. The type species is *H. influenzae*. [G. *haima,* blood, + *philos,* fond]

Hae•moph•i•lus ac•tin•o•my•ce•tem•com•i•tans (hē-mof′i-lŭs ak′tin-ō-mī′sē-tem′-ko-m′i-tanz) A bacterial species of oral flora in humans; frequently associated with human periodontal disease as well as subacute and chronic endocarditis; occurs with actinomycetes in actinomycotic lesions. A member of the HACEK group of organisms (*Haemophilus* sp., *Actinobacillus actinomycetemcomitans, Cardiobacterium hominis, Eikenella corrodens*, and *Kingella* species).

Hae•moph•i•lus ae•gyp•ti•us (hē-mof′i-lŭs ē-jip′ti-kŭs) A biotype of *H. influenzae* that causes acute or subacute infectious conjunctivitis in warm climates. SYN Koch-Weeks bacillus.

Hae•moph•i•lus du•cre•yi (hē-mof′i-lŭs dū-krā′ī) A bacterial species that causes soft chancre (chancroid). SYN Ducrey bacillus.

Hae•moph•i•lus in•flu•en•zae (hē-mof′i-lŭs in-flū-en′zē) A bacterial species found in the respiratory tract that causes acute respiratory infections including pneumonia, acute conjunctivitis, bacterial meningitis, and purulent meningitis in children, rarely in adults; originally considered to be the cause of influenza, it is the type species of the genus *Haemophilus*. See page B4. SYN Pfeiffer bacillus, Weeks bacillus.

***Hae•moph•i•lus in•flu•en•zae* type B** (hē-mof′i-lŭs in-flū-en′zē) The most virulent serotype (there are six, A–F, based on antigenic typing of the polysaccharide capsule); bacterial species responsible for meningitis and respiratory infections in young children.

***Hae•moph•i•lus in•flu•en•zae* type B vac•cine** (hē-mof′i-lŭs in-flū-en′zē tīp vak-sēn′) A conjugate of oligosaccharides of the capsular antigen of *H. influenzae* type B and diphtheria CRM protein.

Hae•moph•i•lus pa•ra•trop•i•ca•lis (hē-mof′i-lŭs par-ă-trop-i-kā′lis) A relatively nonpathogenic bacterial species that has been associated with human infection, including cases of endocarditis.

Hae•moph•i•lus seg•nis (hē-mof′i-lŭs seg′nis) A usually saprophytic bacterial species that occasionally causes endocarditis, meningitis, and other infections in humans.

haemophoresis [Br.] SYN hemophoresis.

haemophthalmia [Br.] SYN hemophthalmia.

haemophthalmus [Br.] SYN hemophthalmus.

haemoplastic [Br.] SYN hemoplastic.

haemopneumopericardium [Br.] SYN hemopneumopericardium.

haemopneumothorax [Br.] SYN hemopneumothorax.

haemopoiesis [Br.] SYN hemopoiesis.

haemopoietic [Br.] SYN hemopoietic.

haemoporphyrin [Br.] SYN hemoporphyrin.

haemoprecipitin [Br.] SYN hemoprecipitin.

haemoprotein [Br.] SYN hemoprotein.

haemoptysis [Br.] SYN hemoptysis.

haemorheology [Br.] SYN hemorheology.

haemorrhachis [Br.] SYN hemorrhachis.

haemorrhage [Br.] SYN hemorrhage.

haemorrhagic [Br.] SYN hemorrhagic.

haemorrhagic ascites [Br.] SYN hemorrhagic ascites.

haemorrhagic colitis [Br.] SYN hemorrhagic colitis.

haemorrhagic cyst [Br.] SYN hemorrhagic cyst.

haemorrhagic cystitis [Br.] SYN hemorrhagic cystitis.

haemorrhagic disease of the newborn [Br.] SYN hemorrhagic disease of the newborn.

haemorrhagic endovasculitis [Br.] SYN hemorrhagic endovasculitis.

haemorrhagic fever [Br.] SYN hemorrhagic fever.

haemorrhagic fever with renal syndrome [Br.] SYN hemorrhagic fever with renal syndrome.

haemorrhagic infarct [Br.] SYN hemorrhagic infarct.

haemorrhagic measles [Br.] SYN hemorrhagic measles.

haemorrhagic plague [Br.] SYN hemorrhagic plague.

haemorrhagic shock [Br.] SYN hemorrhagic shock.

haemorrhagins [Br.] SYN hemorrhagins.

haemorrhoidal [Br.] SYN hemorrhoidal.

haemorrhoidectomy [Br.] SYN hemorrhoidectomy.

haemosiderin [Br.] SYN hemosiderin.

haemosiderosis [Br.] SYN hemosiderosis.

haemospermia [Br.] SYN hemospermia.

Hae•mo•spo•ri•na (hē′mō-spō-rī′nă) A suborder of Coccidia (class Sporozoea); heteroxenous, with sporogony in bloodsucking insects and merogony in vertebrates including humans; includes the genus *Plasmodium*.

haemostasis [Br.] SYN hemostasis.

haemostat [Br.] SYN hemostat.

haemostatic [Br.] SYN hemostatic.

haemostatic forceps [Br.] SYN hemostatic forceps.

haemotherapeutics [Br.] SYN hemotherapeutics.

haemotherapy [Br.] SYN hemotherapy.

haemothorax [Br.] SYN hemothorax.

haemotoxic [Br.] SYN hemotoxic.

haemotoxin [Br.] SYN hemotoxin.

haemotroph [Br.] SYN hemotroph.

haemotrophe [Br.] SYN hemotrophe.

haemotropic [Br.] SYN hemotropic.

haemotympanum [Br.] SYN hemotympanum.

haemoximeter [Br.] SYN hemoximeter.

haemoximetry [Br.] SYN hemoximetry.

haemozoon [Br.] SYN hemozoon.

haem protein [Br.] SYN heme protein.

haemprotein [Br.] SYN heme protein.

Haff•kine vac•cine (hahf′kīn vak-sēn′) **1.** A killed culture of *Vibrio cholerae* in two strengths, a weaker one for the initial inoculation and a stronger for the second inoculation 7–10 days later. **2.** A killed plague bacillus (*Yersinia pestis*) vaccine.

haf•ni•um (Hf) (haf′nē-ŭm) A rare chemical element, atomic no. 72, atomic wt. 178.49. [L. *Hafnia*, Copenhagen]

Hage•man fac•tor (hāg′măn fak′tŏr) SYN factor XII.

H ag•glu•ti•nin (ă-glū′ti-nin) An agglutinin that is formed as the result of stimulation by, and that reacts with, the thermolabile antigen(s) in the flagella of motile strains of microorganisms.

Hag•lund dis•ease (hahg′lŭnd di-zēz′) An abnormal prominence of the posterior superior lateral aspect of the os calcis.

hahn•i•um (hahn′ē-ŭm) Name proposed for the artificially made element 105.

Hai•din•ger brush•es (hī′ding-er brŭsh′ĕz) The perception of two dark yellowish brushes or sheaves radiating about 5 degrees from the point of fixation when an evenly illuminated surface, such as the blue sky, is viewed through a polarizing lens.

Hai•ley and Hai•ley dis•ease (hā′lē hā′lē di-zēz′) SYN keratosis follicularis.

hair (hār) **1.** One of the fine, keratinized filamentous epidermal growths arising from the skin of the body of mammals except the palms, soles, and flexor surfaces of the joints; the full length and texture of hair varies markedly in different body sites. **2.** One of the fine, hairlike processes of the auditory cells of the labyrinth, and of other sensory cells, called auditory hair, sensory hair, and other types. SYN thrix. [A.S. *haer*]

HAIR-AN syn•drome (hār′an sin′drōm) Acronymic disorder comprising hyperandrogenism, insulin resistance, and acanthosis nigricans; virilization in pubertal girls associated with markedly elevated insulin levels and normal levels of luteinizing hormone and follicle-stimulating hormone. [hyperandrogenism, insulin resistance, acanthosis nigricans]

hair ball (hār bawl) SYN trichobezoar.

hair cell (hār sel) Sensory epithelial cells present in the spiral organ (organ of Corti), in the maculae and cristae of the membranous labyrinth of the ear, and in taste buds; they are characterized by having long stereocilia or kinocilia (or both) that, with the light microscope, appear as fine hairs. SEE ALSO taste cells.

hair fol•li•cle (hār fol′i-kĕl) A tubelike invagination of the epidermis from which the hair shaft develops and into which the sebaceous glands open; the follicle is lined by cellular inner and outer root sheaths of epidermal origin and is invested with a fibrous sheath derived from the dermis. SYN folliculus pili [TA].

hair•line frac•ture (hār′līn frak′shŭr) A fracture without separation of the fragments, the line of break being hairlike, as seen sometimes in the skull. SYN capillary fracture.

hair pa•pil•la (hār pă-pil′ă) SYN papilla pili.

hair•pin ves•sels (hār′pin ves′ĕlz) Atypical blood vessels that double back on themselves, seen on colposcopy of the cervix; their presence indicates early invasive cervical cancer. SYN corkscrew vessels.

hair root (hār rūt) The part of a hair that is embedded in the hair follicle, its lower succulent extremity capping the dermal papilla pili in the deep bulbous portion of the follicle.

hair-trans•plant (hār′trans-plant) Dermatologic and reconstructive surgery performed to correct scalp hair deficiencies.

hair whorls (hār wōrlz) A spiral arrangement of the hairs, as at the crown of the head.

hair•y (hār′ē) **1.** Of or resembling hair. **2.** Covered with hair. SEE ALSO hirsutism. SYN pilar, pilary, pileous, pilose.

hair·y cell (hār′ē sel) Medium-sized leukocytes that have features of reticuloendothelial cells and multiple cytoplasmic projections (hairs) on the cell surface, but may be a variety of B lymphocyte; found in hairy cell leukemia.

hair·y cell leu·ke·mi·a (hār′ē sel lū-kē′mē-ă) A rare, usually chronic disorder characterized by proliferation of hairy cells in reticuloendothelial organs and blood.

hair·y leu·ko·pla·ki·a (hār′ē lū′kō-plā′kē-ă) A white lesion appearing on the tongue or buccal mucosa of immunocompromised patients; the lesion appears raised, with a corrugated or "hairy" surface. Seen in patients with HIV/AIDS, it has been associated with Epstein-Barr virus. Condition is usually benign and subsides with therapy.

hair·y mole (hār′ē mōl) SYN nevus pilosus.

hair·y pol·yp (hār′ē pol′ip) A tissue mass arising from a more slender stalk with a piliated appearance; usually found in the oral cavity.

i **hair·y tongue** (hār′ē tŭng) A tongue with abnormal elongation of the filiform papillae, resulting in a thickened furry appearance; may be a benign side effect of some antibiotic therapy. See page B15. SYN glossotrichia, trichoglossia.

ha·lal, ha·lāl, ha·laal (hah-lahl) Denotes food that was prepared in accord with the dietary laws required in observant Muslims; it forbids consumption of some foods and drink (e.g., ethanol) altogether and dictates how Muslim butchers prepare meats and poultry.

ha·la·tion (hă-lā′shŭn) Blurring of the visual image by glare.

Hal·dane ef·fect (hawl′dān e-fect′) The promotion of carbon dioxide dissociation by oxygenation of hemoglobin.

Hale col·loi·dal i·ron stain (hāl kŏ-loyd′ăl ī′ŏrn stān) A stain used to distinguish acid mucopolysaccharides (e.g., hyaluronic acid); may be combined with PAS to visualize carbohydrate-containing proteins and glycoproteins.

half-and-half nail (haf haf nāl) Division of the nail by a transverse line into a proximal dull white part and a distal pink or brown part; seen in uremia.

half-life (haf′līf) **1.** The period in which the radioactivity or number of atoms of a radioactive substance decreases by half; similarly applied to any substance whose quantity decreases exponentially with time. Cf. half-time. **2.** Time required for the serum concentration of a drug to decline by 50%.

half-time (haf′tīm) The time, in a first-order chemical (or enzymic) reaction, for half of the substance (substrate) to be converted or to disappear. Cf. half-life.

half-val·ue la·yer (HVL) (haf-val′yū lā′ĕr) The thickness of a specific absorber (e.g., aluminum) that will reduce the intensity of a beam of radiation to one-half its initial value. SEE ALSO filter.

half·way house (haf′wā hows) A facility for patients who no longer require the complete facilities of a hospital or institution but are not yet prepared to return to independent living.

hal·ide (hal′īd) A salt of a halogen.

hal·i·to·sis (hal-i-tō′sis) A foul odor of the breath. [L. *halitus,* breath, + G. *-osis,* condition]

hal·i·tus (hal′i-tŭs) Any exhalation, as of a breath or vapor. [L., fr. *halo,* to breathe]

Hal·lé point (ah-lā′ poynt) A point at the intersection of a horizontal line touching the anterior superior spine of the ilium and a perpendicular line drawn from the spine of the pubis; here, the ureter can be most readily palpated.

Hal·ler arch·es (hahl′er ahrch′ĕz) SEE lateral arcuate ligaments, medial arcuate ligaments.

Hal·ler cir·cle (hahl′er sĭr′kĕl) **1.** SYN vascular circle of optic nerve. **2.** SYN areolar venous plexus.

Hal·ler·vor·den-Spatz syn·drome (hah′lĕr-fōr′den-shpahts sin′drōm) A disorder characterized by dystonia with other extrapyramidal dysfunctions appearing in the first two decades of life; associated with large amounts of iron in the globus pallidus and substantia nigra.

Hall·gren syn·drome (hahl′gren sin′drōm) Vestibulocerebellar ataxia, pigmentary retinal dystrophy, congenital deafness, and cataract.

Hall·pike ma·neu·ver (hawl′pīk mă-nū′vĕr) Test for vertigo; positive result if rising from a sitting to a standing posture with head tilted to one side causes dizziness and nystagmus.

hal·lu·cal (hal′ŭ-kăl) Relating to the hallux.

hal·lu·ci·na·tion (hă-lū′si-nā′shŭn) The subjective perception of an object or event when no such stimulus or situation is present; may be visual, auditory, olfactory, gustatory, or tactile. [L. *alucinor,* to wander in mind]

hal·lu·ci·no·gen (hă-lū′si-nō-jen) A mind-altering chemical, drug, or agent that elicits optic or auditory hallucinations, depersonalization, perceptual disturbances, and disturbances of thought processes. [L. *alucinor,* to wander in mind, + G. *-gen,* producing]

hal·lu·ci·no·gen·ic (hă-lū′si-nō-jen′ik) SYN psychedelic.

hal·lu·ci·no·sis (hă-lū′si-nō′sis) A syndrome, usually of organic origin (e.g., alcoholic hallucinosis characterized by more or less persistent hallucinations), in which the patient perceives as real things that do not, in fact, exist.

hal•lux, pl. **hal•lu•ces** (hal′ŭks, -ŭ-sēz) [TA] The great toe; the first digit of the foot. [a Mod. L. form for L. *hallex* (*hallic-*), great toe]

hal•lux do•lo•ro•sus (hal′ŭks dō-lō-rō′sŭs) A condition, usually associated with flatfoot, in which walking causes severe pain in the metatarsophalangeal joint of the great toe.

hal•lux flex•us (hal′ŭks flek′sŭs) Hammer toe involving the first toe.

hal•lux rig•id•us (hal′ŭks rij′i-dŭs) A condition in which there is stiffness in the first metatarsophalangeal joint; the joint may be the site of osteoarthritis.

hal•lux val•gus (hal′ŭks val′gŭs) A deviation of the tip of the great toe, or main axis of the toe, toward the outer or lateral side of the foot.

hal•lux var•us (hal′ŭks var′ŭs) Deviation of the main axis of the great toe to the inner side of the foot away from its neighbor.

ha•lo (hā′lō) **1.** A reddish yellow ring surrounding the optic disc, due to a widening of the scleral ring making the deeper structures visible. **2.** An anular flare of light surrounding a luminous body or a depigmented ring around a mole. SEE halo nevus. **3.** SYN areola (4). **4.** A circular metal band used in a halo cast or halo brace, attached to the skull with pins. [G. *halōs,* threshing floor on which oxen trod a circle; the halo round the sun or moon]

ha•lo ef•fect (hā′lō e-fekt′) **1.** The usually beneficial effect that the manner, attention, and caring of a provider have on a patient during a medical encounter, regardless of which medical procedure or services the encounter involves. **2.** The influence on an observation of the observer's perception of the characteristics of the person observed (other than the characteristics under study) or the influence of the observer's recollection or knowledge of findings on a previous occasion.

hal•o•gen (hal′ō-jen) One of the chlorine group (fluorine, chlorine, bromine, iodine, astatine) of elements; halogens form monobasic acids with hydrogen, and their hydroxides (fluorine forms none) are also monobasic acids. [G. *hals,* salt, + *-gen,* producing]

hal•o•gen•o•der•ma (hal′ō-jen′ō-dĕr′mă) Dermatosis caused by ingestion or injection of halogens, most notably bromides and iodides. [halogen + G. *derma,* skin]

ha•lom•e•ter (hal-om′ĕ-tĕr) An instrument used to measure the diffraction halo of a red blood cell; based on the premise that the halo of the large erythrocyte of pernicious anemia is smaller than that of the normal cell; the hazy, colorless halo of normal size is characteristic of secondary anemia.

ha•lo ne•vus (hā′lō nē′vŭs) A benign, sometimes multiple, melanocytic nevus in which involution occurs with a central brown mole surrounded by a uniformly depigmented zone or halo. SYN Sutton nevus.

hal•o•phil, hal•o•phile (hal′ō-fil, -fīl) A microorganism with growth that is enhanced by or dependent on a high salt concentration. [G. *hals,* salt, + *philos,* fond]

hal•o•phil•ic (hal′ō-fil′ik) Requiring a high concentration of salt for growth.

ha•lo sign (hā′lō sīn) Elevation of the subcutaneous fat layer over the fetal skull in a dead or dying fetus; said to be the most common radiologic sign of fetal death.

ha•lo vest (hā-lō′ vest) An orthopedic device used to help immobilize the neck and head.

Hal•sted law (hawl′sted law) Transplanted tissue will grow only if there is an anatomic or physiologic deficiency of such tissue in the host.

Hal•sted op•er•a•tion (hawl′sted op-ĕr-ā′shŭn) **1.** An operation for the radical correction of inguinal hernia. **2.** SYN radical mastectomy.

Hal•sted su•ture (hawl′sted sū′chŭr) A suture placed through the subcuticular fascia; used for exact skin approximation.

ha•mar•ti•a (ham-ahr′shē-ă) A localized developmental disturbance characterized by abnormal arrangement and/or combinations of the tissues normally present in the area. [G. *hamartion,* a bodily defect]

ham•ar•to•blas•to•ma (ham-ahr′tō-blas-tō′mă) A malignant neoplasm of undifferentiated anaplastic cells thought to be derived from a hamartoma. [hamartoma + blastoma]

ham•ar•to•ma (ham′ahr-tō′mă) A focal malformation that resembles a neoplasm, grossly and even microscopically, but that results from faulty development, with a disproportion or abnormal mixture of tissue elements normally present at the site; develops and grows at virtually the same rate as normal tissue and is not likely to compress or invade adjacent structures (in contrast to a neoplasm). [G. *hamartia,* a bodily defect, + *-oma,* tumor]

ham•ar•tom•a•tous (ham′ahr-tō′mă-tŭs) Relating to hamartoma.

ha•mate (ham′āt) SEE hamate bone.

ha•mate bone (ham′āt bōn) The bone on the medial (ulnar) side of the distal row of the carpals; it articulates with the fourth and fifth metacarpal, triquetral, lunate, and capitate. SYN os hamatum [TA], unciform bone.

Ham•bur•ger law (hahm′bŭr-gĕr law) Albumins and phosphates pass from red corpuscles to serum and chlorides pass from serum to cells when blood is acid; the reverse occurs when blood is alkaline.

Ham·bur·ger phe·nom·e·non (hahm′bŭr-gĕr fĕ-nom′ĕ-non) SYN chloride shift.

Ham·il·ton an·xi·e·ty rat·ing scale (ham′il-ton ang-zī′ĕ-tē rāt′ing scāl) A list of specific symptoms used as a measure of severity of anxiety.

Ham·il·ton de·pres·sion rat·ing scale (ham′il-ton dĕ-presh′ŭn rāt′ing scāl) A list of specific symptoms used as a measure of severity of depression.

Ham·man mur·mur (ham′ăn mŭr′mŭr) A crunching precordial sound synchronous with the heartbeat; heard in mediastinal emphysema; also known as Hamman crunch.

Ham·man-Rich syn·drome (ham′ăn-rich′ sin′drōm) SYN idiopathic pulmonary fibrosis.

Ham·man sign (ham′ăn sīn) A crunching, rasping sound, synchronous with heart beat, heard over the precordium and sometimes at a distance from the chest in mediastinal emphysema.

Ham·man syn·drome (ham′ăn sin′drōm) Spontaneous mediastinal emphysema, resulting from rupture of alveoli.

ham·mer (ham′ĕr) SYN malleus.

Ham·mer·schlag meth·od (hah′mer-shlahg meth′ŏd) A hydrometric method of determining the specific gravity of the blood by allowing a drop of blood to fall into each of a series of tubes containing mixtures of chloroform and benzene of known graded specific gravities; the specific gravity of that mixture in which the drop remains exactly suspended, neither rising nor falling, corresponds to the specific gravity of the blood sample.

ham·mer toe (ham′ĕr tō) Permanent flexion at the midphalangeal joint of one or more of the toes.

Ham·mond dis·ease (ham′ŏnd di-zēz′) SYN athetosis.

Hamp·ton hump (hamp′tŏn hŭmp) A juxtapleural pulmonary soft tissue density on a chest radiograph, convex toward the hilum, usually at the costophrenic angle; described as a manifestation of pulmonary infarction, due to pulmonary embolism.

i **ham·string** (ham′string) One of the tendons bounding the popliteal space on either side; the **medial hamstring** comprises the tendons of the semimembranosus, semitendinosus, gracilis, and sartorius muscles; the **lateral hamstring** is the tendon of the biceps femoris muscle. Hamstring muscles (a) have origin from the ischial tuberosity, (b) act across (at) both the hip and knee joints (producing extension and flexion, respectively), and (c) are innervated by the tibial portion of the sciatic nerve. The medial hamstring contributes to medial rotation of the leg at the flexed knee joint, whereas the lateral hamstring contributes to lateral rotation. See this page.

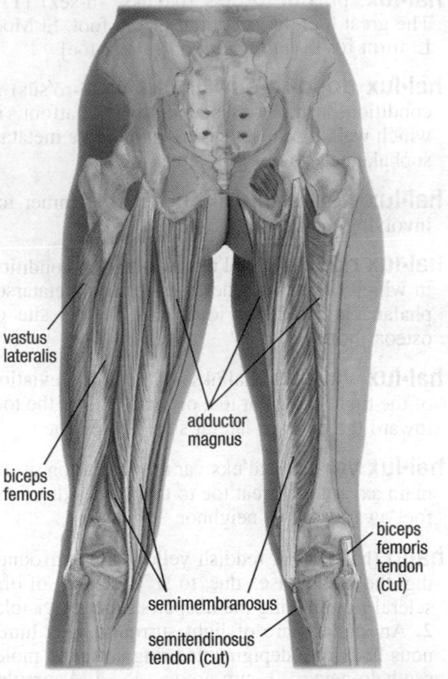

hamstring

ham·string ten·don (ham′string ten′dŏn) SEE hamstring.

Ham test (ham test) SYN acidified serum test.

ham·u·lar (ham′yū-lăr) Hook-shaped; unciform. [L. *hamulus, q.v.*]

ham·u·lus, gen. and pl. **ham·u·li** (ham′yū-lŭs, -lī) Any hooklike structure. SYN hook (2). [L. dim. of *hamus,* hook]

Han·cock am·pu·ta·tion (han′kok amp′yū-tā′shŭn) Surgical removal of the foot through the astragalus (talus).

i **hand** (hand) The portion of the upper limb distal to the radiocarpal joint, comprising the wrist, palm, and fingers. See page A8. SYN manus [TA]. [A.S.]

hand·ed·ness (hand′ĕd-nĕs) Preference for the use of one hand, most commonly the right, associated with dominance of the opposite cerebral hemisphere; may also be the result of training or habit.

hand-foot-and-mouth dis·ease (hand-fut-mowth di-zēz′) An exanthematous eruption of small, pearl-gray vesicles of the fingers, toes, palms, and soles, accompanied by painful vesicles and ulceration of the buccal mucous membrane and the tongue and by slight fever; the disease lasts 4–7 days, and is usually caused by

Coxsackie virus type A-16, but other types have been identified. This disease is highly contagious and affects many children.

hand•i•cap (hand′ē-kap) **1.** A physical, mental, or emotional condition that interferes with normal functioning. **2.** Reduction in the capacity to fulfill a social role as a consequence of an impairment, inadequate training for the role, or other circumstances. SEE ALSO disability. [fr. *hand in cap* (game)]

hand•ling (hand′ling) Application of hands in a trained manner to parts of a patient's body to decrease the frequency of abnormal patterns of movement, improve muscle tone, and increase the occurrence of automatic normal movement.

hand-o•ver-mouth ex•er•cise (H.O.M.E.) (hand ō′vĕr mowth eks′ĕr-sīz) A patient-management technique for pedodontic dental patients where the dentist gently places his or her hand over the child's mouth and tells the child that his hand will be removed as soon as the child is quiet and can listen without being loud and disruptive. **This method can only be employed by the dentist, not the dental auxiliaries, and must never include obstructing the nasal airway, which is illegal.**

hand rays (hand rāz) The four radial grooves that separate five slightly thicker areas of the hand plates; they indicate the formation of the metacarpals and phalanges of the hand. SYN digital rays of hand.

Hand-Schül•ler-Chris•tian dis•ease (hahnt shēl′er kris′chĕn di-zēz′) The chronic disseminated form of Langerhans cell histiocytosis. The classic triad of signs consists of diabetes insipidus, exophthalmos, and bony lesions composed of histiocytes. SYN Christian disease (1), Christian syndrome, Schüller syndrome.

hand•shapes (hand′shāps) Manual symbols of speech sounds used in cued speech.

hang•man's frac•ture (hang′mănz frak′shŭr) A break in the cervical spine through the pedicles of C-2; may be associated with an anterior dislocation of the C-2 vertebral body with respect to C-3. See page B25.

hang•nail (hang′nāl) A loose triangular tag of skin attached at the proximal portion in the medial or lateral nail fold.

Hanks so•lu•tion (hangks sŏ-lū′shŭn) A salt solution usually used in combination with naturally occurring body substances (e.g., blood serum, tissue extracts) or more complex chemically defined nutritive solutions for culturing animal cells; two variations contain $CaCl_2$, $MgSO_4{\cdot}7H_2O$, KCl, KH_2PO_4, $NaHCO_3$, NaCl, $Na_2HPO_4{\cdot}2H_2O$, and D-glucose.

Han•no•ver ca•nal (hahn′ō-ver kă-nal′) The potential space between the ciliary zonule and the vitreous body.

Han•sen ba•cil•lus (hahn′sen bă-sil′ŭs) SYN *Mycobacterium leprae.*

Han•sen dis•ease (hahn′sen di-zēz′) SYN leprosy.

Han•ta•vi•rus (hahn′tă-vī′rŭs) A genus of Bunyaviridae responsible for pneumonia and hemorrhagic fevers. Four members of the genus are recognized thus far: Hantaan, Puumala, Seoul, and Prospect Hill; the first three are known human pathogens, and Hantaan virus causes Korean hemorrhagic fever. Various rodent species are the asymptomatic carriers of these viruses, which are shed in saliva, urine, and feces. Human infection is direct, or by the respiratory route from contaminated specimens; person-to-person spread has not been demonstrated. Affected people may have a mild to fatal course. The most seriously ill have hemorrhagic fevers accompanied by renal failure and sometimes respiratory collapse. This virus was isolated from patients in Arizona and New Mexico in 1992.

Han•ta•vi•rus pul•mo•na•ry syn•drome (hahn′tă-vī′rŭs pul′mŏ-nar-ē sin′drōm) A febrile disease caused by several species of hantavirus (Andes, Bayou, Black Creek Canal, New York, and Sin Nombre viruses) in North and South America and characterized by thrombocytopenia, leukocytosis, and capillary leakage in the lungs, with death due to shock and cardiac complications.

H an•ti•gen (an′ti-jen) **1.** The antigen in the flagella of motile bacteria; SEE ALSO O antigen. **2.** The chemical precursor of antigens of the ABO blood group locus.

HA-P Abbreviation for hemagglutinin-protease.

HAP Abbreviation for hospital-acquired pneumonia.

HAPE Abbreviation for high altitude pulmonary edema.

haph•al•ge•si•a (haf′al-jē′zē-ă) Pain or an extremely disagreeable sensation caused by the merest touch. SYN Pitres sign (1). [G. *haphē,* touch, + *algēsis,* sense of pain]

haplo- Combining form meaning simple, single. [G. *haplous*]

hap•loid (hap′loyd) Denoting the number of chromosomes in sperm or ova, which is half the number in somatic (diploid) cells; the haploid number in normal human beings is 23. [G. *haplos*, simple, + *eidos*, appearance]

hap•lo•pro•tein (hap′lō-prō′tēn) The functional complex between an apoprotein and the prosthetic group that together are responsible for biological activity.

hap•lo•scope (hap′lō-skōp) An instrument for presenting separate views to each eye so that they may be seen as one.

hap·lo·scop·ic (hap′lō-skop′ik) Relating to a haploscope.

hap·lo·type (hap′lō-tīp) **1.** The genetic constitution of an individual with respect to one member of a pair of allelic genes; individuals are of the same haplotype (but of different genotypes) if alike with respect to one allele of a pair but different with respect to the other allele of a pair. **2.** IMMUNOGENETICS that portion of the phenotype determined by a set of closely linked genes inherited from one parent (i.e., genes located on one of the pair of chromosomes). The human major histocompatability complex comprises 4 recognized loci (A, B, C, and D) for which there are more than 50 alleles. Similarly, the allotypic markers (antigens) of the immunoglobulin subclasses IgG1, IgG2, IgG3, and IgA2 occur in combinations and are inherited as units almost always unchanged in transmission; the alleles that control these various haploptypes are not linked to those controlling the antigens of the κ type L chains. [haplo- + G. *typos,* impression, model]

HapMap (hap′map) A catalogue of human genetic variables being gathered worldwide to help increase understanding of genetic diseases and disorders.

hap·ten (hap′tĕn) A molecule that is incapable, alone, of causing the production of antibodies but can, however, combine with a larger antigenic molecule called a carrier. SYN incomplete antigen, partial antigen. [G. *haptō,* to fasten, bind]

hap·tics (hap′tiks) The science concerned with the tactile sense. [G. *haptō,* to grasp, touch]

hap·to·glo·bin (hap′tō-glō′bin) A group of α_2-globulins in human serum, so called because of their ability to combine with hemoglobin; variant types form a polymorphic system, with α- and β-polypeptide chains controlled by separate genetic loci. [G. *haptō,* to grasp, + hemoglobin]

Ha·ra·da-i·to pro·ce·dure (hah-rah′dah-ē′tō prŏ-sē′jŭr) A procedure designed to correct ocular extorsion due to fourth nerve palsy by selectively tightening the anterior fibers of the superior oblique tendon.

Ha·ra·da-Mo·ri fil·ter pa·per strip cul·ture (hah-rah′dah-mōr′ē fil′tĕr pā′pĕr strip kŭl′chŭr) A combination of filter paper, fecal specimen, and tap water placed in a centrifuge tube; provides an environment for nematode eggs to hatch and larvae to develop.

Ha·ra·da syn·drome, Ha·ra·da dis·ease (hah-rah′dah sin′drōm, hah-rah′dah di-zēz′) Bilateral retinal edema, uveitis, choroiditis, and retinal detachment, with temporary or permanent deafness, graying of the hair (poliosis), and alopecia; related to the Vogt-Koyanagi syndrome and sympathetic ophthalmia.

hard chan·cre (hahrd shang′kĕr) SYN chancre.

hard corn (hahrd kōrn) The usual form of clavus over a toe joint. SYN heloma durum.

hard dru·sen (hahrd drū′sĕn) Type of exudative or typical drusen that appears ophthalmoscopically as discrete, yellow nodules characterized histopathologically by well-defined accumulations of hyaline material in the inner and outer collagenous zones of the Bruch membrane.

hard·en·ing (hahrd′ĕn-ing) **1.** A condition of lessened reactions to allergens from repeated or prolonged nontherapeutic exposure, similar to hyposensitization. **2.** Any procedure in tissue preparation for examinations, such as sectioning for microscopy, which renders the tissue firmer.

hard pal·ate (hahrd pal′ăt) **1.** The anterior part of the palate, consisting of the bony palate covered above by the mucous membrane of the floor of the nasal cavity and below by the mucoperiosteum of the roof of the mouth that contains the palatine vessels, nerves, and mucous glands. **2.** CEPHALOMETRICS a line connecting the anterior and posterior nasal spines to represent the position of the bony palate.

hard pulse (hahrd pŭls) A pulse that strikes forcibly against the tip of the finger and is with difficulty compressed, suggesting hypertension.

hard tu·ber·cle (hahrd tū′bĕr-kĕl) A tubercle lacking necrosis.

hard ul·cer (hahrd ŭl′sĕr) SYN chancre.

Har·dy-Rand-Rit·ter test (hahr′dē rand rit′ĕr test) Assessment of color vision deficiency using pseudoisochromatic cards. These excellent cards have not been reprinted by the American Optical Company because the plates were accidentally destroyed in 1965.

Har·dy-Wein·berg law (hahr′dē wīn′bĕrg law) If mating occurs at random with respect to any one autosomal locus in a population in which the gene frequencies are equal in the two sexes, and the factors tending to change gene frequencies (mutation, differential selection, migration) are either absent or negligible, then in one generation the probabilities of all possible genotypes will on average equal the same proportions as if the genes were assembled at random. The law does not apply to two or more loci jointly, nor to X-linked traits where the initial gene frequencies differ in the two sexes.

hare·lip (hār′lip) SYN cleft lip.

har·le·quin fe·tus (hahr′lĕ-kwin fē′tŭs) Severe form of collodion in a newborn, usually premature; a form of ichthyosiform erythroderma characterized by encasement of the body in grayish brown, often fissured plaques resembling plates of armor, and by grotesque deformity of the face, hands, and feet; usually fatal within a few days.

har·mon·ic mean (hahr-mon′ik mēn) The mean calculated as the number of values being averaged, divided by the sum of their reciprocals.

har•mon•ic su•ture (hahr-mon′ik sū′chŭr) SYN plane suture.

har•mo•ni•ous ret•i•nal cor•re•spon•dence (hahr-mō′nē-ŭs ret′i-năl kōr′ĕ-spon′dĕns) A type of anomalous retinal correspondence in which the angle of the visual direction of the two retinas is equal to the objective angle of strabismus.

Har•ring•ton rods (har′ring-tŏn rodz) Metal stabilizing rods used in surgery to lessen scoliosis.

Har•ris-Ben•e•dict e•qua•tion (har′is-ben′ĕ-dikt ē-kwā′zhŭn) An equation based on a person's height, age, and weight that is used for estimating caloric needs.

Har•ris he•ma•tox•y•lin (har′is hē′mă-toks′i-lin) An alum type of hematoxylin similar to Delafield hematoxylin, but which uses chemical ripening to produce oxidation of hematoxylin for immediate use.

Har•ri•son groove (har′i-sŏn grūv) A deformity of the ribs that results from the pull of the diaphragm on ribs weakened by rickets or other softening of the bone.

Hart•mann cu•rette (hahrt′măn kyūr-et′) A blade-edged implement for the removal of adenoids.

Hart•mann op•er•a•tion (hahrt′măn op-ĕr-ā′shŭn) Resection of the sigmoid colon beginning at or just above the peritoneal reflexion and extending proximally, with closure of the rectal stump and end-colostomy.

Hart•mann pouch (hahrt′măn powch) Infundibulum of gallbladder; sometimes described as abnormal pouching at the gallbladder neck.

Hart•mann so•lu•tion (hahrt′măn sŏ-lū′shŭn) **1.** SYN lactated Ringer solution. **2.** A solution used to desensitize dentin in dental operations; contains thymol, ethyl alcohol, and diethyl ether.

Hart•nup dis•ease, **Hart•nup syn•drome** (hahrt′nŭp di-zēz′, sin′drōm) A congenital metabolic disorder consisting of aminoaciduria due to a defect in renal tubular absorption of neutral α-amino acids and urinary excretion of tryptophan derivatives, which occurs because defective intestinal absorption leads to bacterial degradation of unabsorbed tryptophan in the gut; characterized by a pellagralike, light-sensitive skin rash with temporary cerebellar ataxia.

har•vest (hahr′vĕst) To obtain cells, tissues, or organs for grafting or transplantation, from either a donor or the patient.

Ha•shi•mo•to di•sease (hahsh-ē-mō′tō di-zēz′) Chronic autoimmune disease of thyroid resulting from antibodies to thyroglobulin and microsomes; most common cause of hypothyroidism in the U.S. Also called Hashimoto struma and thyroiditis.

hash•ish (hah-shēsh′) A form of cannabis that consists largely of resin from the flowering tops and sprouts of cultivated female hemp plants of the species *Cannabis sativa;* contains the highest concentration of cannabinols among preparations derived from cannabis. [Ar. hay]

Has•sall bod•ies, **Has•sall con•cen•tric cor•pus•cle** (has′ăl bod′ēz, kŏn-sen′trik kōr′pŭs-ĕl) SYN thymic corpuscle.

Has•son can•nu•la (has′ŏn kan′yū-lă) A laparoscopic instrument for open (rather than blind needle insufflation) placement of the initial port. The Hasson has a blunt-tipped obturator instead of a sharp trocar and a balloon on the distal portion of the sheath to hold it in place.

hatch•ing flask (hach′ing flask) A flask painted a dark color, so that only a small area of dechlorinated water at the top is exposed to light in simulation of pond water conditions, which stimulates hatching of any live schistosome eggs in fresh stool and urine sediment added to the flask; the released miracidium larvae will be searching for appropriate snail intermediate hosts.

Hauch (H) (howk[h]) A term used to designate the flagellar antigen of bacteria. SEE ALSO H antigen. [Ger. breath]

haus•tral (haws′trăl) Relating to a haustrum.

haus•tra•tion (haws′trā′shŭn) **1.** The process of formation of a haustrum. **2.** An increase in prominence of the haustra.

haus•trum, pl. **haus•tra** (haws′trŭm, -tră) [TA] One of a series of saccules or pouches, so called because of a fancied resemblance to the buckets on a water wheel. [L. a machine for drawing water, fr. *haurio,* pp. *haustus,* to draw up, drink up]

haus•tus (h) (haw′stŭs) A potion; medicinal beverage. [L., a drink, draft]

HAV Abbreviation for hepatitis A virus.

Ha•ver•hill fe•ver (hav′ĕr-hil fē′ver) An infection by *Streptobacillus moniliformis,* usually due to a rat bite, marked by initial chills and high fever (gradually subsiding), by arthritis usually in the larger joints and spine, and by a rash occurring chiefly over the joints and on the extensor surfaces of the extremities. SYN erythema arthriticum epidemicum. [*Haverhill,* MA, where an epidemic occurred in 1926]

ha•ver•sian (hă-vĕr′zē-ăn) Relating to Clopton Havers and the various osseous structures described by him.

ha•ver•sian ca•nals (hă-vĕr′zē-ăn kă-nalz′) Vascular canals that run longitudinally in the center of haversian systems of compact osseous tissue.

ha•ver•sian la•mel•la (hă-vĕr′zē-ăn lă-mel′ă) SYN concentric lamella.

ha•ver•sian spac•es (hă-vĕr′zē-ăn spās′ĕz) Spaces in bone formed by the enlargement of haversian canals.

ha•ver•sian sys•tem (hă-vĕr′zē-ăn sis′tĕm) SYN osteon.

HA1 vi•rus (vī′rŭs) Abbreviaton for hemadsorption virus type 1. SEE parainfluenza viruses.

HA2 vi•rus (vī′rŭs) Abbreviation for hemadsorption virus type 2. SEE parainfluenza viruses.

Haw•kins im•pinge•ment sign (haw′kinz im-pinj′mĕnt sīn) Pain produced by forced internal rotation of the humerus in 90 degrees of abduction.

Ha•yem so•lu•tion (āh-yem sŏ-lū′shŭn) A blood diluent used before red blood cells are counted.

hay fe•ver (hā fē′vĕr) A form of atopy characterized by an acute irritative inflammation of the mucous membranes of the eyes and upper respiratory passages accompanied by itching and profuse watery secretion, followed occasionally by bronchitis and asthma; the episode recurs annually at the same or nearly the same time of the year, in spring, summer, or late summer and autumn, caused by an allergic reaction to the pollen of trees, grasses, weeds, and flowers.

Hay•flick lim•it (hā′flik lim′it) The limit of human cell division in subcultures; such cells typically divide only about 50 times before dying out.

Hay•garth nodes (hā′gahrth nōdz) Exostoses from the margins of the articular surfaces and from the periosteum and bone in the neighborhood of the joints of the fingers, leading to ankylosis and associated with lateral deflection of the fingers toward the ulnar side, which occur in rheumatoid arthritis.

Hay test (hā test) Sulfur is added to urine; test result is positive for bile salts if sulfur sinks to the bottom of sample.

Haz•ard A•nal•y•sis Crit•i•cal Con•trol Point (HACCP) (haz′ărd ă-nal′ă-sis krit′i-kăl kon′trōl poynt) A food safety system that identifies points in food production where risk of bacterial contamination is high.

Hb Abbreviation for hemoglobin.

Hb A Abbreviation for hemoglobin A.

HB_cAb Abbreviation for antibody to the hepatitis B core antigen.

HB_cAg Abbreviation for hepatitis B core antigen.

HB_sAg Abbreviation for hepatitis B surface antigen.

H band (band) The paler area in the center of the A band of a striated muscle fiber, comprising the central portion of thick (myosin) filaments that are not overlapped by thin (actin) filaments.

Hb C Abbreviation for hemoglobin C.

HBE Abbreviation for His bundle electrogram.

HBe, HB_eAg Abbreviation for hepatitis B e antigen.

Hb F Abbreviation for hemoglobin F.

HBIG Abbreviation for hepatitis B immune globulin.

Hb S Abbreviation for hemoglobin S; sickle cell hemoglobin.

HBV Abbreviation for hepatitis B virus.

HCFA Abbreviation for Health Care Financing Administration.

HCFA-1450 SYN CMS-1450.

HCFA-1500 SYN CMS-1500.

hCG Abbreviation for human chorionic gonadotropin.

HCl Chemical formula for hydrochloric acid.

HCN Chemical formula for hydrogen cyanide.

HCPCS Abbreviation for Healthcare Common Procedure Coding System.

HCS Abbreviation for human chorionic somatomammotropic hormone.

HC smoke (smōk) NATO designation for a military obscurant smoke consisting of zinc oxide and hexachloroethane mixed with a small quantity of grained aluminum. Combustion of the compound results in a toxic smoke containing zinc chloride and various other harmful chemical compounds. HC smoke can cause pulmonary edema and late-onset cryptogenic organizing pneumonia and bronchiolitis obliterans with organizing pneumonia.

HCT Abbreviation for Hearing Conservation Program.

Hct Abbreviation for hematocrit.

HCV Abbreviation for hepatitis C virus.

HD NATO code for pure (distilled, neat) sulfur mustard.

HDI Abbreviation for high-definition imaging.

HDL Abreviation for high density lipoprotein. SEE lipoprotein.

HDL-C Abbreviation for high density lipoprotein-cholesterol.

HDN Abbreviation for ABO hemolytic disease of the newborn.

HDV Abbreviation for hepatitis D virus.

He Symbol for helium.

head (hed) **1.** The upper or anterior extremity of the animal body, containing the brain and the organs of sight, hearing, taste, and smell. **2.** The upper, anterior, or larger extremity, expanded or rounded, of any body, organ, or other anatomic structure. **3.** The rounded extremity of a bone. **4.** That end of a muscle that is attached to the less movable part of the skeleton. [A.S. *heāfod*]

head•ache (HA) (hed′āk) Pain in various parts of the head, not confined to the area of distribution of any nerve. SEE ALSO cephalodynia. SYN cephalalgia, encephalalgia.

Head ar•e•as (hed ār′ē-ăz) Areas of skin exhibiting reflex hyperesthesia and hyperalgesia due to visceral disease.

head cap (hed kap) A device fitted closely to the skull; used for fixed anchorage in external traction.

head cold (hed kōld) An upper respiratory viral infection characterized by rhinitis, headache, and cough.

head-drop•ping test (hĕd drop′ing test) A test used in the diagnosis of disease of the extrapyramidal or striatal system (e.g., parkinsonism, Wilson disease); with the patient supine and relaxed, the examiner briskly lifts the head with the right hand and then allows it to drop on the palm of the left hand; the head of a normal person drops suddenly like a dead weight, whereas in striatal disease, the head falls slowly, gently, and almost hesitantly.

head of fib•u•la (hed fib′yū-lă) The superior extremity of the fibula, which articulates by a facet with the undersurface of the lateral condyle of the tibia.

Head lines, Head zones (hed līnz, hed zōnz) Bands of cutaneous hyperesthesia associated with acute or chronic inflammation of the viscera.

head-tilt/chin-lift ma•neu•ver (hĕd′tilt-chin′ lift mă-nū′vĕr) Basic procedure used in CPR to open the patient's airway. Rescuers one hand tilts head back while other hand is placed under the chin to lift the mandible and displace the tongue. SYN manual airway maneuver, rescue breathing.

heal (hēl) **1.** To restore to health, especially to cause an ulcer or wound to cicatrize or unite. **2.** To become well, to be cured; to cicatrize or close, said of an ulcer or wound. [A.S. *healan*]

heal•ing (hēl′ing) **1.** Restoring to health; promoting the closure of wounds and ulcers. **2.** The process of a return to health. **3.** Closing of a wound. SEE ALSO union.

heal•ing by first in•ten•tion (hēl′ing fĭrst inten′shŭn) Healing by fibrous adhesion, without suppuration or granulation tissue formation. SYN primary adhesion, primary union.

heal•ing by sec•ond in•ten•tion (hēl′ing sek′ŏnd in-ten′shŭn) Delayed closure of two granulating surfaces. SYN secondary adhesion, secondary union.

heal•ing by third in•ten•tion (hēl′ing thĭrd in-ten′shŭn) The slow filling of a wound cavity or ulcer by granulations, with subsequent cicatrization.

health (helth) **1.** The state of an organism when it functions optimally without evidence of disease or abnormality. **2.** A state characterized by anatomic, physiologic, and psychological integrity; ability to perform personally valued family, work, and community roles; ability to deal with physical, biologic, psychological, and social stress; a feeling of well-being; and freedom from the risk of disease and untimely death. **3.** Complete physical, mental, and social well-being, not just the absence of disease, as defined by the World Health Organization. [A.S. *haelth*]

Health Ca•na•da (helth kan′ă-dă) Canadian federal ministry that develops national health policy, enforces national health regulations, and promotes disease prevention.

Health Care Fi•nanc•ing Ad•mi•ni•stra•tion (HCFA) (helth kār fī′nan-sing ad-min′i-strā′shŭn) SEE Centers for Medicare and Medicaid Services.

Health•care Com•mon Pro•ce•dure Cod•ing Sys•tem (HCPCS) (helth′kār kom′ŏn prŏ-sē′jŭr kōd′ing sis′tĕm) The alphanumeric coding system for reporting outpatient health care services for Medicare beneficiaries.

health care pro•vi•der (helth kār prŏ-vīd′ĕr) General term for any institution or member of the health care team providing health care. SEE ALSO doctor, physician, nurse, nurse practitioner, physical therapist, hospital, occupational therapist, home health care.

health care prox•y (helth kār proks′ē) Printed form used legally to allow another person to make health care decisions for a patient when the patient is unable or no longer able to make such decisions personally.

health care ra•tion•ing (helth kār rash′ŭning) NURSING planning for and implementing an equitable allocation or distribution of available health care resources.

health care sys•tem (helth kār sis′tĕm) Organized system of providers and services for health care; may include hospitals, clinics, home care, long-term care facilities, assisted living, physicians, health plans, and other services.

health dis•par•i•ties (helth dis-par′i-tēz) Differences in measures of health and availability of health care across populations.

health ed•u•ca•tion (helth e′jū-kā′shŭn) NURSING education to gain knowledge, skills, values, and attitudes for maintaining and improving health in patients.

health in•for•mat•ics (helth in′fōr-mat′iks) The practice and technology of collecting, storing, and analyzing health care data electronically and transferring data between computer systems.

health in•for•ma•tion ma•nage•ment (HIM) (helth in′fōr-mā′shŭn man′ăj-mĕnt) Collection and analysis of health care data to provide information for health care decisions involving patient care, institutional management, health care policies and planning, and research; formerly known as medical records management. SEE ALSO record.

health in•for•ma•tion sys•tem (helth in′fōr-mā′shŭn sis′tĕm) Combination of vital and health statistical data from multiple sources, used to derive information about the health needs, health resources, use of health services, and outcomes of use by the people in a defined region or jurisdiction.

health in•sur•ance (helth in-shŭr′ăns) A commercial product designed to protect consumers from the financial risks of illness and injury. SYN medical insurance.

Health In•sur•ance Claim Form (helth in-shŭr′ăns klām fōrm) SYN CMS-1500.

Health In•sur•ance Por•ta•bil•i•ty and Ac•count•a•bil•i•ty Act (HIPAA) (helth in-shŭr′ăns pōr-tă-bil′i-tē ă-kownt′ă-bil′i-tē akt) U.S. federal legislation designed to preserve health insurance coverage for workers and their families when they change or lose their jobs. Includes security and privacy standards to protect personal health information and avoid misuse or inappropriate disclosure. It was established in 1996 and is administered by the U.S. Department of Health and Human Services.

health lit•er•a•cy (helth lit′ĕr-ă-sē) NURSING ability of members of the public to read, understand, and interpret health care information.

health main•te•nance or•ga•ni•za•tion (HMO) (helth mān′tĕn-ăns ōr′găn-ī-zā′shŭn) A comprehensive prepaid system of managed health care with emphasis on the prevention and early detection of disease, and continuity of care. HMOs may be nonprofit or profit-making ventures; along with preferred provider organizations (PPOs) and other managed care plans, they have begun to dominate the health care market. HMOs generally offer a package of services; however, the choice of physician is frequently limited to those participating in the HMO. SEE ALSO managed care, preferred provider organization.

Health On the Net Foun•da•tion (helth net fown-dā′shŭn) Not-for-profit portal to medical information on the Internet; developed HONcode of ethical guidelines for health care Web site developers.

Health Plan Em•ploy•er Da•ta and In•for•ma•tion Set (HEDIS) (helth plan em-ploy′ĕr dā′tă in′fōr-mā′shŭn set) A set of standardized measures for comparing health plans; developed and maintained by the National Committee for Quality Assurance (NCQA).

health pro•mo•tion (helth prŏ-mō′shŭn) Providing clients with information to enhance health and prevent disease. Lifestyles that influence good health are encouraged. SEE ALSO primary preventive nursing.

health re•cord (helth rek′ōrd) A comprehensive compilation of information traditionally placed in the medical record but also covering aspects of the patient's physical, mental, and social health that do not necessarily relate directly to the condition under treatment. SEE ALSO record (1).

health-re•la•ted phy•si•cal fit•ness (helth-rĕ-lā′tĕd fiz′i-kăl fit′nĕs) Components of physical fitness (most commonly, aerobic fitness, body composition, muscular strength and endurance, and lower back and hamstring muscular flexibility) that are associated with some aspect of overall good health or disease prevention.

health-re•lat•ed qual•i•ty of life (H.R.Q.O.L.) (helth-rē-lā′tĕd kwah′li-tē līf) An assessment of a person's well-being with regard to her or his physical health.

Health Re•sour•ces and Ser•vi•ces Ad•mi•ni•stra•tion (HRSA) (helth rĕ-sors′ĕz sĕr′vi-sĕz ad-min′i-strā′shŭn) A U.S. federal agency responsible for managing national data banks, such as the National Practitioner Data Bank, as well as other health care programs.

health risk ap•prais•al (helth risk ă-prā′zăl) A method of describing a person's chance of falling ill or dying of a specified condition, based on actuarial calculations that allow for known exposure to risk; expressed as the expected age at which death or disease will occur, and intended as a way of drawing the person's attention to the probable consequences of risk behavior.

health sta•tus (helth stat′ŭs) Level of health of an individual person, a group, or a population as assessed by that individual or by objective measures.

health•y (hel′thē) **1.** The amorphous term is understood by the F.D.A. to signify the product so labeled is low in fats, cholesterol, and sodium and that it contains 10% of the required daily amounts of Vitamins A and C, as well as calcium, iron, protein, and fiber. **2.** Well; in a state of normal functioning; free from disease.

Health•y Peo•ple 2010 (helth′ē pē′pĕl) Comprehensive, nationwide health promotion and disease prevention agenda by U.S. Department of Health and Human Services; contains 467 objectives for improving health of all people in U.S. during first decade of 21st century.

Hea•ney op•er•a•tion (hē′nē op-ĕr-ā′shŭn) Technique for vaginal hysterectomy.

hear•ing (hēr′ing) The ability to perceive sound; the sensation of sound as opposed to vibration. SYN -acousis (2), -acusis, audition.

hear•ing aid (hēr′ing ād) An electronic amplifying device designed to bring sound more effectively into the ear; it consists of a microphone, amplifier, and receiver. See this page. SYN hearing instrument.

Hear•ing Con•ser•va•tion Pro•gram (hēr′ing kon′sĕr-vā′shŭn prō′gram) A formal program of protection of personal hearing, and engineered control of noise, required by U.S. federal law.

Hear•ing Han•di•cap In•ven•tory for the El•der•ly (HHIE-S) (hēr′ing hand′ē-kap in′vĕn-tōr-ē el′dĕr-lē) Screening test that uses a communication scale to determine whether older adults have difficulty hearing and understanding speech.

hear•ing im•pair•ment, hear•ing loss (hēr′ing im-pār′mĕnt, laws) A reduction in the ability to perceive sound; may range from slight inability to complete deafness. SEE ALSO deafness.

hear•ing in•stru•ment (hēr′ing in′strŭ-mĕnt) SYN hearing aid.

hear•ing pro•tec•tor (hēr′ing prŏ-tek′tŏr) Occlusive devices for the external auditory canal made of pliable material or fluid (usually glycerin)-filled ear muffs for protection against noise-induced hearing loss.

heart (hahrt) A hollow muscular organ that receives the blood from the veins and propels it into the arteries. It is divided by a musculomembranous septum into two halves (right or venous and left or arterial) each of which consists of a receiving chamber (atrium) and an ejecting chamber (ventricle). See page 688, A10. SYN cor, [TA], coeur. [A.S. *heorte*]

heart at•tack (hahrt ă-tak′) SYN myocardial infarction.

heart•beat (hahrt′bēt) A single complete cycle of contraction and dilation of heart muscle.

heart•burn (hahrt′bŭrn) SYN pyrosis.

heart cham•ber re•mo•del•ing (hahrt chām′bĕr rē-mod′ĕl-ing) An architectural change in any cardiac chamber (usually one or both ventricles) due to a pathologic or normal (neonatal) stimulus.

heart fail•ure (hahrt fāl′yŭr) **1.** Inadequacy of the heart so that as a pump it fails to maintain the circulation of blood, with the result that congestion and edema develop in the tissues. SYN cardiac insufficiency, congestive heart failure, myocardial insufficiency. SEE ALSO forward heart failure, backward heart failure, right ventricular failure, left ventricular failure. **2.** Resulting clinical syndromes including shortness of breath, pit-

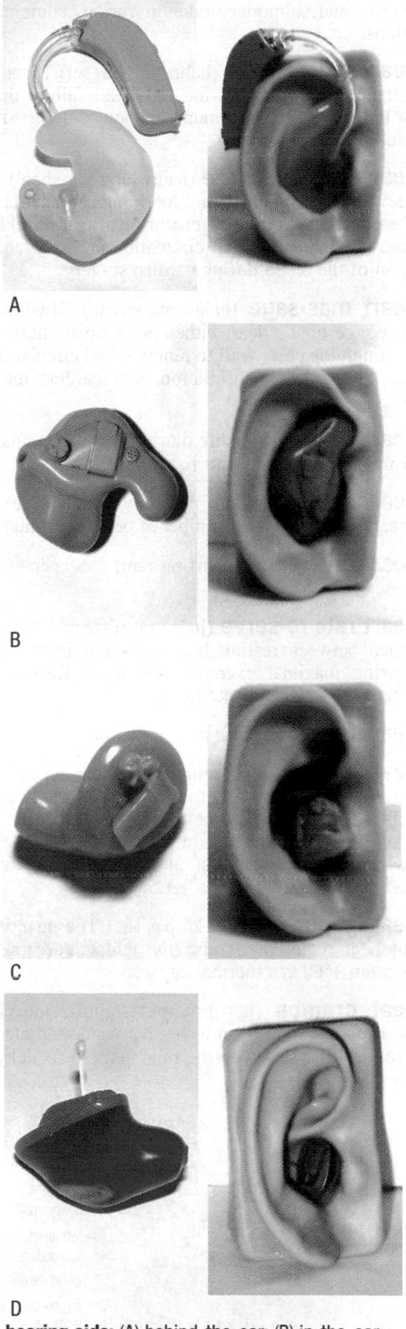

hearing aids: (A) behind-the-ear; (B) in-the-ear; (C) in-the-canal; (D) completely in the canal

ting edema, enlarged tender liver, engorged neck veins, and pulmonary rales in various combinations.

heart fail·ure cell (hahrt fāl′yŭr sel) Macrophage in the lung during left heart failure that often carries large amounts of hemosiderin. SEE ALSO siderophore.

heart-lung ma·chine (hahrt-lŭng mă-shēn′) A device incorporating a blood pump (artificial heart) and a blood oxygenator (artificial lung) to provide extracorporeal circulation and oxygenation of the blood during cardiac surgery.

heart mas·sage (hahrt mă-sahzh′) Rhythmic massage of the heart either in an open chest or through the chest wall to renew failed circulation during cardiac resuscitation. SYN cardiac massage.

heart mur·mur (hahrt mŭr′mŭr) A colloquialism for cardiac murmur (q.v.).

heart rate (hahrt rāt) Velocity of the heart's beat, recorded as the number of beats per minute.

heart rate range (hahrt rāt rānj) SYN heart rate reserve.

heart rate re·serve (hahrt rāt rē-zĕrv′) Difference between resting heart rate and heart rate during maximal exercise. SEE ALSO Karvonen method. SYN heart rate range.

heart sac (hahrt sak) SYN pericardium.

heat (hēt) **1.** A high temperature; the sensation produced by proximity to fire or an incandescent object, as opposed to cold. The basis of heat is the kinetic energy of atoms and molecules, which becomes zero at absolute zero. **2.** SYN estrus. **3.** SYN enthalpy. [A.S. *haete*]

heat ca·pac·i·ty (hēt kă-pas′i-tē) The quantity of heat required to raise the temperature of a system 1°C. SYN thermal capacity.

heat cramps (hēt kramps) Painful muscle spasms resulting from excessive water and electrolyte loss. SEE hyperthermia. SEE ALSO dehydration.

heat of e·vap·o·ra·tion (hēt ē-vap′ŏr-ā′shŭn) Heat absorbed in the evaporation of water, sweat, or other liquid; for water it amounts to 540 cal/g at 100°C. SYN heat of vaporization.

heat ex·haus·tion (hēt eg-zaws′chŭn) A form of reaction to heat marked by prostration, weakness, and collapse, resulting from severe dehydration.

heat-la·bile (hēt′lā′bīl) Destroyed or altered by heat.

heat lamp (hēt lamp) A lamp that emits infrared light and produces heat; used to apply topical heat to the skin.

heat of va·por·i·za·tion (hēt vā′pŏr-ī-zā′shŭn) SYN heat of evaporation.

heat rash (hēt rash) SYN miliaria rubra.

heat stress in·dex (hēt stres in′deks) Measure of environment's potential to cause heat injury; based on ambient air temperature and relative humidity.

heat·stroke, heat stroke (hēt′strōk, hēt strōk) A severe and often fatal illness produced by exposure to excessively high temperatures, especially when accompanied by marked exertion; characterized by headache, vertigo, confusion, hot dry skin, and a slight rise in body temperature; in severe cases, very high fever, vascular collapse, and coma develop.

heat ur·ti·car·i·a (hēt ŭr′ti-kar′ē-ă) SYN cholinergic urticaria.

heav·y chain (hev′ē chān) A polypeptide chain of high molecular weight determining the class and subclass of an immunoglobulin.

heav·y chain dis·ease (hev′ē chān di-zēz′) A term used for a group of diseases, the paraproteinemias, characterized by production of homogeneous immunoglobulins or fragments, and associated with malignant disorders of the plasmacytic and lymphoid cell series.

heav·y work (hev′ē wŏrk) A physical demand level, described as the exertion of up to 100

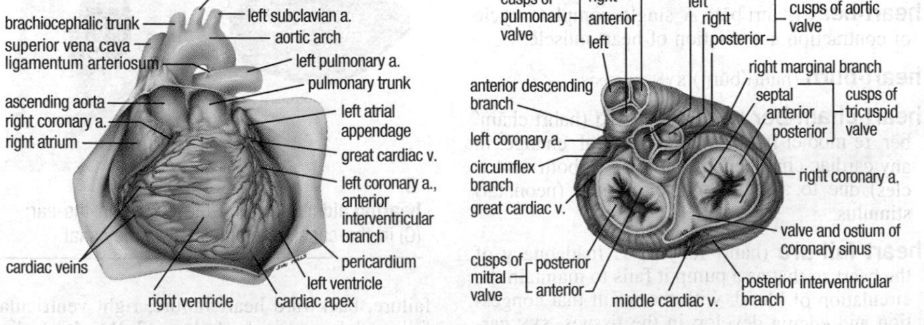

human heart: (left) ventral view with pericardium opened; (right) transverse section at the level of the valves

pounds of force occasionally, or up to 50 pounds of force frequently, or 20 pounds of force constantly to move objects. SEE ALSO very heavy work.

he•be•phre•ni•a (hē′bĕ-frē′nē-ă) A syndrome characterized by shallow and inappropriate affect, giggling, and silly, regressive behavior and mannerisms; a subtype of schizophrenia now renamed disorganized schizophrenia (q.v.). [G. *hēbē,* puberty, + *phrēn,* the mind]

he•be•phren•ic (hē′bĕ-fren′ik) Relating to or characterized by hebephrenia.

Heb•er•den nodes (hē′bĕr-dĕn nōdz) Exostoses no larger than a pea found on the terminal phalanges of the fingers in osteoarthritis, which are enlargements of the tubercles at the articular extremities of the distal phalanges. SYN tuberculum arthriticum (1).

he•bet•ic (hē-bet′ik) Pertaining to youth. [G. *hēbētikos,* youthful, fr. *hēbē,* youth]

he•bi•at•rics (hē′bē-at′riks) SYN adolescent medicine. [G. *hēbē,* youth, + *iatrikos,* relating to medicine]

He•bra pru•ri•go (hā′brah prūr-ī′gō) A severe form of chronic dermatitis with secondary infection in which there are constantly recurring, intensely itchy papules and nodules, often associated with atopy.

hec•a•ter•o•mer•ic (hek′ă-ter′ō-mer′ik) Denoting a spinal neuron the axon of which divides and gives off processes to both sides of the cord; usually the same as a heteromeric neuron. [G. *hekateros,* each of two, + *meros,* part]

hecto- (h) Prefix used in the SI and metric system to signify one hundred (10^2). [G. *hekaton,* one hundred]

hec•to•me•ter (hek′tō-mē-tĕr) 100 meters. SYN hectometre.

hectometre [Br.] SYN hectometer. SEE hectometer.

HEDIS (hed′is) Acronym for Health Plan Employer Data and Information Set.

hed•ro•cele (hed′rō-sēl) Prolapse of the intestine through the anus. [G. *hedra,* a seat, the fundament, + *kēlē,* hernia]

heel (hēl) **1.** SYN calx (2). **2.** SYN distal end. [A.S. *hēla*]

heel bone (hēl bōn) SYN calcaneus (1).

heel pad (hēl pad) An encapsulated body of fat beneath the plantar surface of the calcaneus, which cushions during weight bearing and walking.

heel spur (hēl spŭr) An abnormal bony growth on the calcaneus. SEE ALSO bone spur. SYN calcaneal spur.

heel ten•don (hēl ten′dŏn) SYN tendo calcaneus.

Heer•fordt dis•ease (hār′fōrt di-zēz′) SYN uveoparotid fever.

He•gar di•la•tors (hā′gahr dī′lā-tŏrz) A series of cylindric bougies of graduated sizes used to dilate the cervical canal.

He•gar sign (hā′gahr sīn) Softening and compressibility of the lower segment of the uterus in early pregnancy (about the seventh week) that, on bimanual examination, is felt by the finger in the vagina as though the neck and body of the uterus were separated, or connected by only a thin band of tissue. See this page.

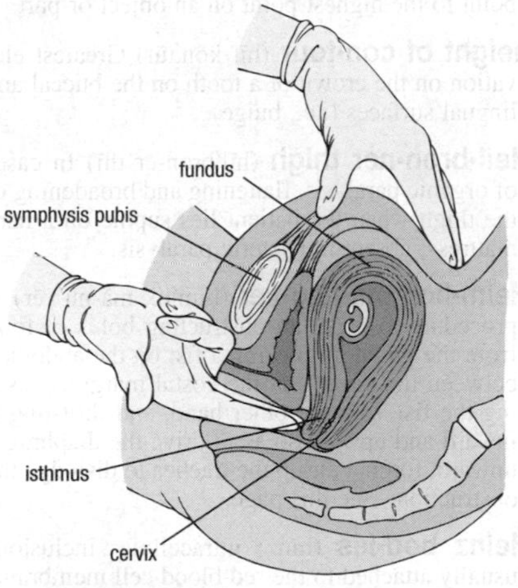

positive Hegar sign

Hegg•lin a•nom•a•ly (heg′lin ă-nom′ă-lē) A disorder in which neutrophils and eosinophils contain basophilic structures known as Döhle or Amato bodies and in which there is faulty maturation of platelets, with thrombocytopenia; autosomal dominant inheritance.

Hegg•lin syn•drome (heg′lin sin′drōm) ELECTROCARDIOGRAPHY dissociation between electromechanical systole (QS_2 interval) and electrical systole (QT interval) so that the second heart tone (SII) is recorded before the end of the T wave; described by Hegglin as an energy-dynamic cardiac insufficiency during diabetic coma and other metabolic disorders.

Hei•den•hain Az•an stain (hī′den-hīn ā′zan stān) A technique using azocarmine B or G followed by aniline blue to stain nuclei and erythrocytes red, muscle orange, glia fibrils reddish, mucin blue, and collagen and reticulum dark blue. [*az*ocarmine + *an*iline blue]

Hei•den•hain i•ron he•ma•tox•y•lin stain (hī′den-hīn ī′ŏrn hē′mă-toks′i-lin stān) An iron alum hematoxylin stain used for staining muscle striations and mitotic structures blue-black.

Hei•den•hain law (hī′den-hīn law) Glandular secretion is always accompanied by an alteration in the structure of the gland.

Hei•den•hain mod•i•fi•ca•tion of Mal•lo•ry-Az•an stain (hī′den-hīn mod′i-fi-kā′shŭn mal′ŏr-ē ā′zan stān) Procedure to visualize tissues of the upper esophagus that uses azocarmine, aniline blue, and orange G stains.

Hei•den•hain pouch (hī′den-hīn powch) Surgical separation of small stomach pouch from rest of stomach, which drains to exterior, used in studies of stomach physiology.

height (h) (hīt) The distance from the lowest point to the highest point on an object or part.

height of con•tour (hīt kon′tūr) Greatest elevation on the crown of a tooth on the buccal and lingual surfaces (i.e., bulge).

Heil•bron•ner thigh (hīl′bron-er thī) In cases of organic paralysis, flattening and broadening of the thigh when the patient lies supine on a hard mattress; absent in hysteric paralysis.

Heim•lich ma•neu•ver (hīm′lik mă-nū′vĕr) A procedure to expel an obstructing bolus of food from the throat by placing a fist on the abdomen between the navel and the costal margin, grasping the fist with the other hand, and thrusting it inward and upward so as to drive the diaphragm upward, forcing air up the trachea to dislodge the obstruction. See this page.

Heinz bod•ies (hīnz) intracellular inclusions usually attached to the red blood cell membrane, composed of dentured hemoglobin; they occur in thalassemia, enzymopathies, hemoglobinopathies, and after splenectomy. Visualization of these usually requires examination of red blood cells using supravital stains or by phase microscopy. See page B3.

Heinz-Ehr•lich bod•y (hīnts-er′lik bod′ē) SYN Ehrlich inner body.

HeLa (hē′lă) Referring to cells of the first continuously cultured (human cervical) carcinoma strain.

hel•i•cal (hel′i-kăl) **1.** Relating to a helix. SYN helicine (2). **2.** SYN helicoid. [G. *helix,* a coil]

hel•i•ces (hel′i-sēz) Plural of helix.

hel•i•cine (hel′i-sēn) **1.** Coiled. **2.** SYN helical (1). [G. *helix,* a coil]

Hel•i•co•bac•ter (hel′i-kō-bak′tĕr) A genus of gram-negative helical, curved, or straight microaerophilic bacteria with rounded ends and numerous sheathed flagella (unipolar or bipolar and lateral) with terminal bulbs. Form nonpigmented, translucent colonies, 1–2 mm in diameter. Catalase and oxidase positive. Found in gastric mucosa of ferrets and primates, including human

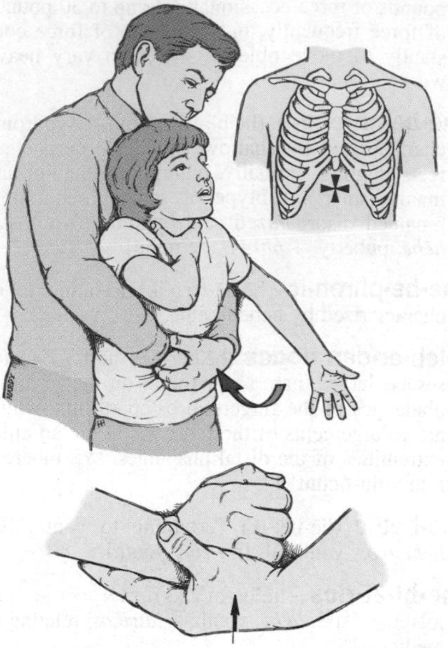

Heimlich maneuver: bottom image shows view from above

beings. Some species are associated with gastric and peptic ulcers and predispose to gastric carcinoma. The type species is *H. pylori.*

Hel•i•co•bac•ter ci•nae•di (hel′i-kō-bak′tĕr sī-nē′dī) A bacterial species associated with cases of proctitis and colitis in homosexual men.

Hel•i•co•bac•ter fen•nel•li•ae (hel′i-kō-bak′tĕr fen-ĕl-lī′ē) A bacterial species associated with proctitis and colitis in homosexual men.

Hel•i•co•bac•ter heil•man•ni•i (hel′i-kō-bak′tĕr hī′mahn′nē-ī) A bacterial species observed in gastric mucosa. This agent has a low prevalence (less than 1% of patients), has not been cultured in vitro, and is of unknown pathogenic significance.

Hel•i•co•bac•ter py•lor•i (hel′i-kō-bak′ter pī-lō′rī) A bacterial species that produces urease and is associated with several gastroduodenal diseases, including gastritis and peptic ulcer. The type species of the genus *Helicobacter.*

hel•i•coid (hel′i-koyd) Resembling a helix. SYN helical (2). [G. *helix,* a coil, + *eidos,* resemblance]

hel•i•co•pod gait (hel′i-kō-pod gāt) A gait, seen in some conversion reactions or hysteric disorders, in which the feet move in half circles. SYN helicopodia.

hel•i•co•po•di•a (hel′i-kō-pō′dē-ă) SYN helicopod gait. [G. *helix,* a coil, + *pous,* foot]

hel•i•co•tre•ma (hel′i-kō-trē′mă) A semilunar

opening at the apex of the cochlea through which the scala vestibuli and the scala tympani of the cochlea communicate with one another. [G. *helix,* a spiral, + *trēma,* a hole]

he•li•en•ceph•a•li•tis (hē′lē-en-sef′ă-lī′tis) Inflammation of the brain following sunstroke. [G. *helios,* sun, + *enkephalos,* brain, + *-itis,* inflammation]

he•li•o•ther•a•py (hē′lē-ō-thār′ă-pē) Use of sunlight (and more generally) light from any source to provide palliation of disease; usually for dermatologic disorders, but sometimes used in seasonal affective disorder (q.v.). SYN solar therapy.

he•li•ox (hē′lē-oks) Mixture of helium and oxygen.

he•li•um (He) (hē′lē-ŭm) A gaseous element present in minute amounts in the atmosphere (0.000524% of dry volume); atomic no. 2, atomic wt. 4.002602; used as a diluent of medicinal gases, particularly oxygen [G. *hēlios,* sun]

he•li•um di•lu•tion meth•od (hē′lē-ŭm di-lū′shŭn meth′ŏd) A procedure for indirect determination of residual lung volume.

he•li•um ther•a•py (hē′lē-ŭm thār′ă-pē) The use of a helium-gas mixture (usually helium and oxygen) in the management of obstruction of the airways; the density of helium is much lower than that of either air or oxygen; as a result, the gaseous mixture will move past an airway obstruction more easily.

he•lix, pl. **hel•i•ces** (hē′liks, hel′i-sēz) **1.** [TA] The margin of the auricle; a folded rim of cartilage forming the upper part of the anterior, the superior, and the greater part of the posterior edges of the auricle. **2.** A line in the shape of a coil (or a spring, or the threads on a bolt), each point being equidistant from a straight line that is the axis of the cylinder in which each point of the helix lies. USAGE NOTE: Often mistakenly applied to a spiral. [L. fr. G. *helix,* a coil]

Hel•ler•work (hel′ĕr-wŏrk) A modality of therapy that establishes connections among movement, body alignment, and personal awareness with the belief that the body, mind, and spirit are inseparable. SEE ALSO holistic medicine.

Hel•lin law (hel′in law) Twins occur once in 89 births, triplets once in 89^2, and quadruplets once in 89^3. If the frequency of twins in a population is p, the frequency of triplets is p^2, and the frequency of quadruplets is p^3.

Hel•ly fix•a•tive (hel′ē fiks′ă-tiv) A combination of potassium dichromate, mercuric chloride, formaldehyde, and distilled water, used as a microanatomic fixative for cytoplasmic granules and nuclear staining; has the same disadvantages as Zenker fixative.

Helm•holtz en•er•gy (A) (helm′hōlts en′ĕr-jē) Energy equivalent to the internal energy minus the entropy contribution (TS).

hel•minth (hel′minth) Any intestinal vermiform parasite, primarily nematodes, cestodes, trematodes, and acanthocephalans. [G. *helmins,* worm]

hel•min•tha•gogue (hel-minth′ă-gog) SYN anthelmintic (1). [G. *helmins,* worm, + *agōgos,* leading]

hel•min•them•e•sis (hel′min-them′ĕ-sis) The vomiting or expelling of intestinal worms through the mouth. [G. *helmins,* worm, + *emesis,* vomiting]

hel•min•thi•a•sis (hel′min-thī′ă-sis) The condition of having vermiform parasites anywhere inside the body.

hel•min•tho•ma (hel′min-thō′mă) A discrete nodule of granulomatous inflammation (including the healed stage) caused by a helminth or its products. [G. *helmins,* worm, + *-oma,* tumor]

Hel•min•tho•spo•ri•um (hel-min-thō-spōr′ē-ŭm) A saprobic fungus, often isolated in clinical laboratories.

he•lo•ma (hē-lō′mă) SYN clavus. [G. *hēlos,* nail, + *-oma,* tumor]

he•lo•ma du•rum (hē-lō′mă dū′rŭm) SYN hard corn.

he•lo•ma mol•le (hē-lō′mă mol′ē) SYN soft corn.

he•lot•o•my (hē-lot′ŏ-mē) Surgical treatment of corns. [heloma + G. *tomē,* cutting]

help•er cells (hel′pĕr selz) SYN T-helper cells.

help•er vi•rus (hel′pĕr vī′rŭs) A virus with replication that renders it possible for a defective virus or a virusoid (also present in the host cell) to develop into a fully infectious agent.

HELPP syn•drome (help sin′drōm) Condition of pregnancy characterized by raised liver enzymes, hemolysis, and low platelet count with preeclampsia.

♻ **hem-, hema-** Combining forms meaning blood. SEE ALSO hemat-, hemato-, hemo-. SYN haem-. [G. *haima*]

he•ma•chrome (hē′mă-krōm) The coloring matter of the blood, hemoglobin, or hematin. SYN haemachrome. [hema- + G. *chrōma,* color]

he•ma•cyte (hē′mă-sīt) SYN erythrocyte. SYN haemacyte.

he•ma•cy•tom•e•ter (hē′mă-sī-tom′ĕ-tĕr) SYN hemocytometer. SYN haemacytometer.

he•mad•sorp•tion (hēm′ad-sŏrp′shŭn) A phenomenon manifested by an agent or substance adhering to or being adsorbed on the surface of a red blood cell. SYN haemadsorption.

he•mad•sorp•tion vi•rus type 1 (HA1 vi•rus) (hēm′ad-sōrp′shŭn vī′rŭs tīp) Parainfluenza virus type 3. SEE parainfluenza viruses. SYN haemadsorption virus type 1.

he•mad•sorp•tion vi•rus type 2 (HA2 vi•rus) (hēm′ad-sōrp′shŭn vī′rŭs tīp) Parainfluenza virus type 1. SEE parainfluenza viruses. SYN haemadsorption virus type 2.

he•mag•glu•ti•na•tion (hē′mă-glū-ti-nā′shŭn) The agglutination of red blood cells; may be immune (as a result of specific antibody to red blood cell antigens or other antigens that coat the red blood cells), or nonimmune (as in hemagglutination caused by viruses or other microbes). SYN haemagglutination.

he•mag•glu•ti•nin (hē′mă-glū′ti-nin) a substance, antibody or other, which causes hemagglutination. SYN haemagglutinin.

he•mag•glu•tin•in-pro•te•ase (HA-P) (hē′mă-glū′ti-nin-prō′tē-ās) A cytotoxic enzyme produced by *Vibrio cholerae* that alters epithelial structure and barrier function. SYN haemagglutinin-protease.

he•ma•gog•ic (hī′mă-goj′ik) Promoting a flow of blood. SYN haemagogic.

he•mal (hē′măl) **1.** Relating to the blood or blood vessels. **2.** Referring to the ventral side of the vertebral bodies or their precursors, where the heart and great vessels are located, as opposed to neural (2). SYN haemal. [G. *haima,* blood]

he•mal•um (hī′mă-lŭm) A solution of hematoxylin and alum used as a nuclear stain in histology, especially with eosin as a counterstain. SYN haemalum.

he•ma•nal•y•sis (hē′mă-nal′i-sis) Analysis of the blood; an examination of blood, especially with reference to chemical methods. SYN haemanalysis. [G. *haima,* blood, + analysis]

♻ **hemangi-** Combining form meaning blood vessel. [G. *haima*, blood, + *angeion*, vessel]

he•man•gi•ec•ta•sis, he•man•gi•ec•ta•si•a (hē-man′jē-ek′tă-sis, hē-man′jē-ek-tā′zē-ă) Dilation of blood vessels. SYN haemangiectasis. [G. *haima,* blood, + *angeion,* vessel, + *ektasis,* a stretching]

♻ **hemangio-** Combining form meaning the blood vessels. SYN haemangio-. [G. *haima,* blood, + *angeion,* vessel]

he•man•gi•o•blast (hē-man′jē-ō-blast) A primordial embryonic cell of mesodermal origin producing cells from which are derived vascular endothelium, reticuloendothelial elements, and blood-forming cells of all types. SYN haemangioblast. [hemangio- + G. *blastos,* germ]

he•man•gi•o•blas•to•ma (hē-man′jē-ō-blas-tō′mă) A benign cerebellar neoplasm composed of capillary vessel-forming endothelial cells and stromal cells; a slowly growing tumor that affects, primarily, middle-aged individuals; increased incidence in von Hippel-Lindau disease. SYN angioblastoma, haemangioblastoma, Lindau tumor.

he•man•gi•o•en•do•the•li•o•blas•to•ma (hē-man′jē-ō-en′dō-thē′lē-ō-blas-tō′mă) Hemangioendothelioma in which the endothelial cells seem to be especially immature forms. SYN haemangioendothelioblastoma. [hemangio- + endothelium + G. *blastos,* germ, + *-oma,* tumor]

he•man•gi•o•en•do•the•li•o•ma (hē-man′jē-ō-en′dō-thē′lē-ō′mă) A neoplasm derived from blood vessels, characterized by numerous prominent endothelial cells that occur singly, in aggregates, and as the lining of congeries of vascular tubes or channels; in the elderly, may be malignant (angiosarcoma or hemangiosarcoma), but in children are benign and probably represent a growing stage of capillary hemangioma. SYN haemangioendothelioma. [hemangio- + endothelium + G. *-oma,* tumor]

he•man•gi•o•fi•bro•ma (hē-man′jē-ō-fī-brō′mă) A hemangioma with an abundant fibrous tissue framework. SYN haemangiofibroma.

he•man•gi•o•ma (hē-man′jē-ō′mă) A congenital anomaly, in which proliferation of blood vessels leads to a mass that resembles a neoplasm; it can occur anywhere in the body but is most frequently observed in the skin and subcutaneous tissues. SEE ALSO nevus. SYN haemangioma. [hemangio- + G. *-oma,* tumor]

he•man•gi•o•ma•to•sis (hē-man′jē-ō-mă-tō′sis) A condition in which there are numerous hemangiomas. SYN haemangiomatosis.

he•man•gi•o•per•i•cy•to•ma (hē-man′jē-ō-per′i-sī-tō′mă) An uncommon vascular, usually benign, neoplasm composed of round and spindle cells that are derived from the pericytes and surround endothelium-lined vessels. SYN haemangiopericytoma. [hemangio- + pericyte + G. *-oma,* tumor]

he•man•gi•o•sar•co•ma (hē-man′jē-ō-sahr-kō′mă) A rare malignant neoplasm characterized by rapidly proliferating, extensively infiltrating, anaplastic cells derived from blood vessels and lining irregular blood-filled or lumpy spaces. SYN haemangiosarcoma.

he•ma•poph•y•sis (hēm′ă-pof′i-sis) The sternal extremity of a rib with its cartilage, representing the second element in each half of a hemal arch. SYN haemapophysis. [hem- + apophysis]

he•mar•thro•sis (hēm′ahr-thrō′sis) Blood in a joint. SYN haemarthrosis. [G. *haima,* blood, + *arthron,* joint]

♻ **hemat-** Combining form meaning blood. SEE ALSO hem-, hemato-, hemo-. SYN haemat-. [G. *haima* (*haimat-*)]

he•ma•te•in (hē′mă-tē′in) An oxidation product of hematoxylin. SYN haematein.

he•ma•tem•e•sis (hē′mă-tem′ĕ-sis) Vomiting blood. SYN haematemesis. [hemat- + G. *emesis,* vomiting]

he•mat•en•ceph•a•lon (hē′mat-en-sef′ă-lon, hem′at-) SYN cerebral hemorrhage. SYN haematencephalon. [hemat- + G. *enkephalos,* brain]

he•mat•ic (hē-mat′ik) **1.** Relating to blood. SYN hemic. **2.** SYN hematinic (2). SYN haematic.

he•ma•ti•dro•sis (hē′mă-tid-rō′sis) Excretion of blood or blood pigment in the sweat; an extremely rare disorder. SYN haematidrosis, hemidrosis (1). [hemat- + G. *hidrōs,* sweat]

hem•a•tin (hē′mă-tin) Heme in which the iron is Fe(III) (Fe^{3+}); the prosthetic group of methemoglobin. SYN ferriheme, haematin, hematosin, oxyheme, oxyhemochromogen.

hem•a•tin chlo•ride (hē′mă-tin klōr′īd) SYN hemin. SYN haematin chloride.

he•ma•ti•ne•mi•a (hē′mă-ti-nē′mē-ă, hem′ă-) The presence of heme in the circulating blood. SYN haematinaemia. [hematin + G. *haima,* blood]

hem•a•tin•ic (hē′mă-tin′ik) **1.** Improving the condition of the blood. **2.** An agent that increases the number of erythrocytes or the hemoglobin concentration of the blood. SYN hematic (2). SYN haematinic.

he•ma•tin•o•me•ter (hē′mă-tin-om′ĕ-tĕr) SYN hemoglobinometry.

♻**hemato-** Combining form denoting blood. SEE ALSO hem-, hemat-, hemo-. SYN haemato-. [G. *haima* (*haimat-*)]

he•ma•to•blast (hē′mă-tō-blast) A primordial, undifferentiated form of blood cell from which erythroblasts, lymphoblasts, myeloblasts, and other immature blood cells are derived; in normal bone marrow, present only in small numbers and difficult to identify in smears, because hematoblasts are fragile and easily disintegrated. SYN haematoblast, hematocytoblast. [hemato- + G. *blastos,* germ]

he•ma•to•cele (hē′mă-tō-sēl) **1.** SYN hemorrhagic cyst. **2.** Effusion of blood into a canal or a cavity of the body. **3.** Swelling due to effusion of blood into the tunica vaginalis testis. SYN haematocele. [hemato- + G. *kēlē,* tumor]

hem•a•to•ceph•a•ly (hē′mă-tō-sef′ă-lē) Intracranial effusion of blood, commonly in a fetus. SYN haematocephaly. [hemato- + G. *kephalē,* head]

he•ma•to•che•zi•a (hē′mă-tō-kē′zē-ă) Passage of bloody stools, in contradistinction to melena, or tarry stools. SYN haematochezia. [hemato- + G. *chezō,* to go to stool]

he•ma•to•chy•lu•ri•a (hē′mă-tō-kīl-yūr′ē-ă) Presence of blood and chyle in the urine. SYN haematochyluria. [hemato- + G. *chylos,* juice, + *ouron,* urine]

he•ma•to•col•po•me•tra (hē′mă-tō-kol′pō-mē′tră) Accumulation of blood in the uterus and vagina resulting from an imperforate hymen or other lower vaginal obstruction. SYN haematocolpometra. [hemato- + G. *kolpos,* vagina, + *mētra,* womb]

he•ma•to•col•pos (hē′mă-tō-kol′pŏs) An accumulation of menstrual blood in the vagina in consequence of imperforate hymen or other obstruction. SYN haematocolpos, retained menstruation. [hemato- + G. *kolpos,* vagina]

he•mat•o•crit (Hct) (hē-mat′ō-krit) Percentage of the volume of a blood sample occupied by cells. Cf. plasmacrit. SYN haematocrit. [hemato- + G. *krinō,* to separate]

he•ma•to•cry•al (hē′mă-tok′rē-ăl) SYN poikilothermic.

he•ma•to•cyst (hē′mă-tō-sist) SYN hemorrhagic cyst.

he•ma•to•cys•tis (hē′mă-tō-sis′tis) An effusion of blood into the bladder. SYN haematocystis. [hemato- + G. *kystis,* bladder]

he•ma•to•cy•to•blast (hē′mă-tō-sī′tō-blast) SYN hematoblast.

he•ma•to•gen•e•sis (hē′mă-tō-jen′ĕ-sis) SYN hemopoiesis. SYN haematogenesis. [hemato- + G. *genesis,* production]

he•ma•to•gen•ic, he•ma•tog•e•nous (hē′mă-tō-jen′ik, hem′ă-; -toj′ĕ-nŭs) **1.** SYN hemopoietic. **2.** Pertaining to anything produced from, derived from, or transported by the blood. SYN haematogenic.

he•ma•tog•e•nous jaun•dice (hē′mă-toj′ĕ-nŭs jawn′dis) SYN hemolytic jaundice. SYN haematogenous jaundice.

he•ma•tog•e•nous me•tas•ta•sis (hē′mă-toj′ĕ-nŭs mĕ-tas′tă-sis) SYN haematogenous metastasis. SEE metastasis.

he•ma•to•his•ton (hē′mă-tō-his′tŏn) SYN globin. SYN haematohiston.

he•ma•toid (hē′mă-toyd) Resembling blood. SYN haematoid. [hemato- + G. *eidos,* resemblance]

he•ma•toi•din (hē-mă-toy′din) A pigment derived from hemoglobin that contains no iron but is closely related to or similar to bilirubin. Hematoidin is formed intracellularly, presumably within reticuloendothelial cells, but is often found extracellularly after 5–7 days in foci of previous hemorrhage. SYN haematoidin, hemolutein. [hemato- + G. *eidos,* resemblance, + -in]

he•ma•tol•o•gist (hē′mă-tol′ŏ-jist) A physician

trained and experienced in hematology, i.e., skilled in performing diagnostic examinations of blood and bone marrow, or in treatment of such diseases, or both. SYN haematologist.

he•ma•tol•o•gy (hē′mă-tol′ŏ-jē) The medical specialty that pertains to the anatomy, physiology, pathology, symptomatology, and therapeutics related to the blood and blood-forming tissues. SYN haematology. [hemato- + G. *logos,* study]

he•ma•to•lymph•an•gi•o•ma (hē′mă-tō-limf′an-jē-ō′-mă) A congenital anomaly consisting of numerous, closely packed, variably sized lymphatic vessels and larger channels, in association with a moderate number of blood vessels of a similar type. SYN haematolymphangioma.

he•ma•tol•y•sis (hē′mă-tol′i-sis) SYN hemolysis. SYN haematolysis.

he•ma•to•lyt•ic (hē′mă-tō-lit′ik) SYN hemolytic. SYN haematolytic.

he•ma•to•ma (hē′mă-tō′mă) A localized mass of extravasated blood that is relatively or completely confined within an organ or tissue, a space, or a potential space; the blood is usually clotted, and, depending on how long it has been there, may manifest various degrees of organization and decolorization. See this page. SYN haematoma. [hemato- + G. *-oma,* tumor]

he•ma•to•me•tra (hē′mă-tō-mē′tră) A collection or retention of blood in the uterine cavity. SYN haematometra, hemometra. [hemato- + G. *mētra,* uterus]

he•ma•tom•e•try (hē′mă-tom′ĕ-trē) Examination of the blood to determine any or all of the following: 1) the total number, types, and relative proportions of various blood cells; 2) the number or proportion of other formed elements; 3) the percentage of hemoglobin. In some instances, hematometry is used to include a determination of blood pressure. [hemato- + G. *metron,* measure]

he•mat•om•pha•lo•cele (hē′mat-om-fal′ō-sēl) Umbilical hernia into which an effusion of blood has taken place. SYN haematomphalocele. [hemato- + G. *omphalos,* umbilicus, + *kēlē,* hernia]

he•ma•to•my•e•li•a (hē′mă-tō-mī-ē′lē-ă) Hemorrhage into the substance of the spinal cord; it is usually a posttraumatic lesion but may also be encountered in instances of spinal cord capillary telangiectases. SYN haematomyelia, hematorrhachis interna, myelapoplexy, myelorrhagia. [hemato- + G. *myelos,* marrow]

he•ma•to•my•e•lo•pore (hē′mă-tō-mī′ĕ-lō-pōr) Formation of porosities in the spinal cord as a result of hemorrhages. SYN haematomyelopore. [hemato- + G. *myelos,* marrow, + *poros,* a pore]

he•ma•to•pa•thol•o•gy (hē′mă-tō-path-ol′ŏ-jē) The division of pathology concerned with diseases of the blood and of hemopoietic and lymphoid tissues. SYN haematopathology, hemopathology. [hemato- + G. *pathos,* suffering, + *logos,* study]

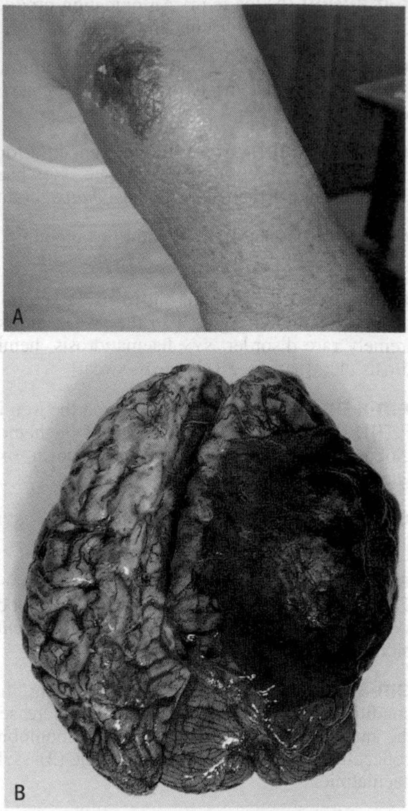

hematoma: (A) subcutanteous hematoma (arm with cellulitis); (B) subdural hematoma

he•ma•to•plast (hē′mă-tō-plast) SYN hemocytoblast. SYN haematoplast.

he•ma•to•plas•tic (hē′mă-tō-plas′tik) SYN hemopoietic. SYN haematoplastic. [hemato- + G. *plassō,* to form]

he•ma•to•poi•e•sis (hē′mă-tō-poy-ē′sis) SYN hemopoiesis. SYN haematopoiesis.

he•ma•to•poi•et•ic (hē′mă-tō-poy-et′ik) SYN hemopoietic. SYN haematopoietic.

he•ma•to•poi•et•ic gland (hē′mă-tō-poy-et′ik gland) A blood-forming organ (e.g., spleen). SYN haematopoietic gland.

he•ma•to•poi•et•ic growth fac•tor (HGF) (hē′mă-tō-poy-et′ik grōth fak′tŏr) Any of several glycoproteins that regulate the survival, self-renewal, proliferation, and differentiation of hematopoietic progenitor cells. There are two nomenclature groups: interleukins (IL) and colony-stimulating factors (CSF). SYN haematopoietic growth factor.

he·ma·to·poi·et·ic sys·tem (hē′mă-tō-poy-et′ik sis′tĕm) The blood-making organs; in the embryo at different ages these are the yolk sac, liver, thymus, spleen, lymph nodes, and bone marrow; after birth they are principally the bone marrow, spleen, thymus, and lymph nodes. SYN haematopoietic system.

he·ma·to·por·phy·rin (hē′mă-tō-pōr′fir-in) A porphyrin resulting from the decomposition of hemoglobin; chemical composition is that of heme with the iron removed and the two vinyl groups hydrated to hydroxyethyl. SYN haematoporphyrin, hemoporphyrin.

he·ma·top·si·a (hē′mă-top′sē-ă) SYN hemophthalmia. SYN haematopsia. [hemato- + G. *opsis,* vision]

he·ma·tor·rha·chis (hē′mă-tōr′ă-kis) A spinal hemorrhage. SYN haematorrhachis, hemorrhachis. [hemato- + G. *rhachis,* spine]

he·ma·tor·rha·chis ex·ter·na (hē′mă-tōr′ă-kis eks-ter′nă) Hemorrhage into the spinal canal external to the cord, either within or outside the dura. SYN haematorrhachis externa.

he·ma·tor·rha·chis in·ter·na (hē′mă-tōr′ă-kis in-ter′nă) SYN hematomyelia. SYN haematorrhachis interna.

he·ma·to·sal·pinx (hē′mă-tō-sal′pingks) Collection of blood in a tube, often associated with a tubal pregnancy. SYN haematosalpinx, hemosalpinx. [hemato- + G. *salpinx,* a trumpet]

hem·a·to·sin (hē′mă tō′sin) SYN hematin. SYN haematosin.

hem·a·to·sis (hē′mă-tō′sis) Oxygenation of venous blood in the lungs. Cf. hemopoiesis. SYN haematosis.

he·ma·to·sper·mat·o·cele (hē′mă-tō-spĕr-mat′ō-sēl) A spermatocele that contains blood. SYN haematospermatocele.

he·ma·to·sper·mi·a (hē′mă-tō-spĕr′mē-ă) The presence of blood in seminal ejaculate.

he·ma·to·stat·ic (hē′mă-tō-stat′ik) **1.** Variant of hemostatic. **2.** Due to stagnation or arrest of blood flow. SYN haematostatic.

he·ma·to·stax·is (hē′mă-tō-stak′sis) Spontaneous bleeding due to a disease of the blood. SYN haematostaxis. [hemato- + G. *staxis,* a dripping]

he·ma·tos·te·on (hē′mă-tos′tē-on) Bleeding in the medullary cavity of a bone. SYN haematosteon. [hemato- + G. *osteon,* bone]

hem·a·to·ther·ma (hē′mă-tō-thĕr′mă) The warm-blooded vertebrates (birds and mammals). SYN haematotherma. [hemato- + G. *thermos,* warm]

he·ma·to·therm·al (hē′mă-tō-thĕr′măl) SYN homeothermic. SYN haematothermal.

he·ma·to·tox·in (hē′mă-tō-toks′in) SYN hemotoxin. SYN haematotoxin.

he·ma·to·tro·pic (hē′mă-tō-trō′pik) SYN hemotropic. SYN haematotropic.

he·ma·tox·y·lin (hē′mă-toks′i-lin) [CI 75290] A crystalline compound containing the coloring matter of *Haematoxylon campechianum* (logwood), from which it is obtained by extraction with ether. It is used as a dye in histology, especially for cell nuclei and chromosomes, muscle cross-striations, and enterochromaffin cells, and as an indicator (red to yellow at pH 0.0–1.0, yellow to violet at pH 5.0–6.0). SYN haematoxylin.

he·ma·tox·y·lin and e·o·sin stain (hē′mă-toks′i-lin ē′ō-sin stān) The most generally useful staining method for tissues; nuclei are stained a deep blue-black with hematoxylin, and cytoplasm is stained pink after counterstaining with eosin, usually in water. SYN haematoxylin and eosin stain.

hem·a·to·zo·on (hē′mă-tō-zō′on) SYN hemozoon. SYN haematozoon.

he·ma·tu·ri·a (hē′mă-tyūr′-ē-ă) Any condition in which urine contains blood or red blood cells. SYN haematuria. [hemato- + G. *ouron,* urine]

heme (hēm) **1.** The porphyrin chelate of iron in which the iron is Fe(II) (Fe^{2+}); the oxygen-carrying, color-furnishing, prosthetic group of hemoglobin. **2.** Iron complexed with nonporphyrins but related tetrapyrrole structures (e.g., biliverdin heme). SYN haem, haem, reduced hematin. [G. *haima,* blood]

heme pro·tein (hēm prō′tēn) Any protein containing an iron-porphyrin (heme) prosthetic group resembling that of hemoglobin. SYN haem protein, haemprotein.

hem·er·a·lo·pia (hem′ĕr-ă-lō′pē-ă) Inability to see as distinctly in a bright light as in reduced illumination; seen in patients with impaired cone function. SYN day blindness. [G. *hēmera,* day, + *alaos,* obscure, + *ōps,* eye]

hem·e·ryth·rin (hēm′ĕ-rith′rin) Any of several iron-containing, oxygen-binding circulatory proteins in certain invertebrates, with molecular weights similar to that of hemoglobin but lacking porphyrin groups. SYN haemerythrin. [hem- + G. *erythros,* red, + in]

♻ **hemi-** Combining form meaning one half. Cf. semi-. [G.]

hem·i·ac·e·tal (hem′ē-as′ĕ-tăl) A product of the addition of an alcohol to an aldehyde (an acetal is formed by the addition of an alcohol to a hemiacetal). In the aldose sugars, the hemiacetal formation is internal and labile, brought about by the 4-OH or 5-OH attack on the carbonyl O, yielding the furanose or pyranose structures; the hemiacetal forms of the sugars are involved in all polysaccharides, as glycosyls or glycosides. SEE ALSO hemiketal, acetal.

hem•i•a•geu•si•a (hem′ē-ă-gū′sē-ă) Loss of sense of taste from one side of the tongue. [hemi- + G. *a-* priv. + *geusis,* taste]

hemianaesthesia [Br.] SYN hemianesthesia.

hem•i•an•al•ge•si•a (hem′ē-an-ăl-jē′zē-ă) Analgesia affecting one side of the body.

hem•i•an•en•ceph•a•ly (hem′ē-an-en-sef′ă-lē) Meroencephaly on one side only, or involving one side much more extensively than the other.

hem•i•an•es•the•si•a (hem′ē-an-es-thē′zē-ă) Anesthesia on one side of the body. SYN hemianaesthesia, unilateral anesthesia.

hem•i•a•no•pi•a (hem′ē-ă-nō′pē-ă) Loss of vision for one half of the visual field of one or both eyes.

hem•i•an•os•mi•a (hem′ē-an-oz′mē-ă) Loss of the sense of smell on one side. [hemi- + G. *an-* priv. + *osmē,* smell]

hem•i•a•prax•i•a (hem′ē-ă-prak′sē-ă) Apraxia affecting one side of the body.

hem•i•a•tax•i•a (hem′ē-ă-tak′sē-ă) Ataxia affecting one side of the body.

hem•i•ath•e•to•sis (hem′ē-ath-ĕ-tō′sis) Athetosis affecting one hand, or one hand and foot, only.

hem•i•at•ro•phy (hem′ē-at′rŏ-fē) Atrophy of one lateral half of a part or of an organ, as the face or tongue.

hem•i•a•zy•gos vein (hem′ē-az′i-gŏs vān) Formed by the merger of the left ascending lumbar vein with the left subcostal vein or a communication from the inferior vena cava, it pierces the left crus of the diaphragm, ascends along the left side of the bodies of the lower thoracic vertebrae, opposite the eighth vertebra, crosses the midline behind the aorta, thoracic duct, and esophagus, and empties into the azygos vein, sometimes in common with the accessory hemiazygos vein.

hem•i•bal•lis•mus (hem′ē-bal-iz′mŭs) Ballism involving one side of the body. [hemi- + G. *ballismos,* jumping about]

hem•i•block (hem′ē-blok) Arrest of the impulse in one of the two main divisions of the left branch of the bundle of His; i.e., in either the anterior (superior) division or the posterior (inferior) division.

he•mic (hē′mik) SYN hematic (1). SYN haemic.

hem•i•car•di•a (hem′ē-kahr′dē-ă) **1.** Either lateral half, including atrium and ventricle, of the heart. **2.** A congenital malformation of the heart in which only two of the usual four chambers are formed. [hemi- + G. *kardia,* heart]

hem•i•cel•lu•lose (hem′ē-sel′yū-lōs) An indigestible carbohydrate similar to cellulose, found in a plant's water-absorbing outer layer.

hem•i•cel•lu•los•es (hem′ē-sel′yū-lōs-ēz) Polysaccharides in foods that are fermented more easily than cellulose.

hem•i•cen•trum (hem′ē-sen′trŭm) One of the two lateral halves of the body of the vertebra. [hemi- + G. *kentron,* center]

hem•i•ceph•a•lal•gi•a (hem′ē-sef-ă-lal′jē-ă) The unilateral headache characteristic of migraine. SYN hemicrania (2). [hemi- + G. *kephalē,* head, + *algos,* pain]

hem•i•ce•pha•li•a (hem′ē-sĕ-fā′lē-ă) Congenital failure of the cerebrum to develop normally; usually the cerebellum and basal ganglia are represented at least in rudimentary form. [hemi- + G. *kephalē,* head]

hem•i•cho•re•a (hem′ē-kōr-ē′ă) Chorea involving the muscles on one side only.

he•mic mur•mur (hē′mik mŭr′mŭr) SYN anemic murmur. SYN haemic murmur.

hem•i•col•ec•to•my (hem′ē-kō-lek′tō-mē) Removal of the right or left side of the colon. [hemi- + G. *kolon,* colon, + *ektomē,* excision]

hem•i•cor•po•rec•to•my (hem′ē-kōr-pō-rek′tŏ-mē) Surgical removal of the lower half of the body, including the lower extremities, bony pelvis, genitalia, and various of the pelvic contents including the lower part of the rectum to the anus. [hemi- + L. *corpus,* body, + G. *ektomē,* excision]

hem•i•cra•ni•a (hem′ē-krā′nē-ă) **1.** SYN migraine. **2.** SYN hemicephalalgia. [hemi- + G. *kranion,* skull]

hem•i•cra•ni•o•sis (hem′ē-krā-nē-ō′sis) Enlargement of one side of the cranium.

hem•i•des•mo•somes (hem′ē-des′mō-sōmz) Half desmosomes that occur on the basal surface of the stratum basale of stratified squamous epithelium.

hem•i•di•a•pho•re•sis (hem′ē-dī-ă-fŏr-ē′sis) Diaphoresis, or sweating, on one side of the body. SYN hemidrosis (2), hemihidrosis.

hem•i•dro•sis (hem′i-drō′sis) **1.** SYN hematidrosis. **2.** SYN hemidiaphoresis.

hemidysaesthesia [Br.] SYN hemidysesthesia.

hem•i•dys•es•the•si•a (hem′ē-dis-es-thē′zē-ă) Dysesthesia affecting one side of the body. SYN hemidysaesthesia.

hem•i•dys•tro•phy (hem′ē-dis′trŏ-fē) Underdevelopment of one lateral half of the body.

[hemi- + G. *dys-*, ill, + *trophē*, nourishment, growth]

hem·i·ec·tro·me·li·a (hem′ē-ek-trō-mē′lē-ă) Defective development of the limbs on one side of the body. [hemi- + ectromelia]

hem·i·fa·cial (hem′ē-fā′shăl) Pertaining to one side of the face.

he·mi·fa·cial spasm (hem′ē-fā′shăl spazm) A facial nerve disorder, with onset in late adult life, characterized by episodes of irregular, sometimes painful, myoclonic contractions of various facial muscles; triggered by voluntary or reflex movements of the face, spasm typically begins in the orbicularis oculi muscle and then spreads; occasionally a sequela of Bell palsy, but more often the result of proximal compression of the facial nerve by an aberrant blood vessel or neoplasm.

hem·i·gas·trec·to·my (hem′ē-gas-trek′tŏ-mē) Excision of the distal half of the stomach.

he·mi·glo·bin (hem′ē-glō-bin) SYN methemoglobin. [variant of *hemoglobin* to reflect shift from ferr*ous* to ferr*ic* state]

he·mi·glo·bi·ne·mi·a (hem′ē-glō-bi-nē′mē-ă) SYN methemoglobinemia.

he·mi·glo·bi·nu·ri·a (hem′ē-glō-bi-nyūr′ē-ă) SYN methemoglobinuria.

hem·i·glos·sec·to·my (hem′ē-glos-ek′tŏ-mē) Surgical removal of half of the tongue. [hemi- + G. *glōssa,* tongue, + *ektomē,* excision]

hem·i·glos·si·tis (hem′ē-glos-ī′tis) A vesicular eruption on one side of the tongue and the corresponding inner surface of the cheek, probably herpetic. [hemi- + G. *glōssa,* tongue, + *-itis,* inflammation]

hem·i·gna·thi·a (hem′ē-gnā′thē-ă) Incomplete development of one side of the mandible. [hemi- + G. *gnathos,* jaw]

hem·i·hi·dro·sis (hem′ē-hī-drō′sis) SYN hemidiaphoresis.

hemihypaesthesia [Br.] SYN hemihypesthesia.

hem·i·hyp·al·ge·si·a (hem′ē-hīp′al-je′zē-ă) Hypalgesia affecting one side of the body.

hemihyperaesthesia [Br.] SYN hemihyperesthesia.

hem·i·hy·per·es·the·si·a (hem′ē-hī′pĕr-es-thē′zē-ă) Hyperesthesia, or increased tactile and painful sensibility, affecting one side of the body. SYN hemihyperaesthesia.

hem·i·hy·per·to·ni·a (hem′ē-hī′pĕr-tō′nē-ă) Exaggerated muscular tonicity on one side of the body. [hemi- + G. *hyper,* over, + *tonos,* tone]

hem·i·hy·per·tro·phy (hem′ē-hī-pĕr′trō-fē) Muscular or osseous hypertrophy of one side of the face or body.

hem·i·hyp·es·the·si·a (hem′ē-hīp′es-thē′zē-ă) Diminished sensibility in one side of the body. SYN hemihypaesthesia. [hemi- + G. *hypo,* under, + *aesthēses,* sensation]

hem·i·hy·po·to·ni·a (hem′ē-hī-pō-tō′nē-ă) Partial loss of muscular tonicity on one side of the body. [hemi- + G. *hypo,* under, + *tonos,* tone]

hem·i·ke·tal (hem′ē-kē′tăl) A product of the addition of an alcohol to a ketone. In the ketose sugars, the hemiketal formation is from an attack by an internal OH on the ketone carbonyl leading to intramolecular cyclization (furanose or pyranose); the hemiketal forms of the sugars are involved in polysaccharide formation, as glycosyls or glycosides. SEE ALSO hemiacetal, ketal.

hem·i·lam·i·nec·to·my (hem′ē-lam-i-nek′tŏ-mē) Removal of a portion of a vertebral lamina, usually performed for exploration of, access to, or decompression of the intraspinal contents. [hemi- + L. *lamina,* layer, + G. *ektomē,* excision]

hem·i·lar·yn·gec·to·my (hem′ē-lar-in-jek′tŏ-mē) Excision of one lateral half of the larynx. [hemi- + G. *larnyx* (*laryng-*), larynx, + *ektomē,* excision]

hem·i·lat·er·al (hem′ē-lat′ĕr-ăl) Relating to one lateral half.

hem·i·mor·phic (hem′ē-mōr′fik) Asymmetric. [hemi- + G. *morphē,* form, shape, + -ic]

he·min (hēm′in) Chloride of heme in which Fe^{2+} has become Fe^{3+}. Hemin crystals are called Teichmann crystals. SYN haemin, hematin chloride.

hem·i·pa·re·sis (hem′ē-pă-rē′sis) Weakness affecting one side of the body.

hem·i·pel·vec·to·my (hem′ē-pel-vek′tŏ-mē) Amputation of an entire leg together with the os coxae. SYN interpelviabdominal amputation, Jaboulay amputation. [hemi- + L. *pelvis,* basin (pelvis), + G. *ektomē,* excision]

hem·i·ple·gi·a (hem′ē-plē′jē-ă) Paralysis of one side of the body. [hemi- + G. *plēgē,* a stroke]

hem·i·ple·gic (hem′ē-plē′jik) Relating to hemiplegia.

hem·i·ple·gic gait (hem′ē-plē′jik gāt) Gait in which the leg is stiff, without flexion at knee and ankle, and with each step is rotated away from the body, then toward it, forming a semicircle. SYN spastic gait.

hem·i·sen·so·ry (hem′ē-sen′sŏr-ē) Loss of sensation on one side of the body. Cf. hemianesthesia.

hem·i·spasm (hem′ē-spazm) A spasm affecting one or more muscles of one side of the face or body.

hem•i•sphere (hem′is-fēr′) Half of a spheric structure. SYN cerebral hemisphere (1). SYN hemisphericum. [hemi- + G. *sphaira,* ball, globe]

hem•i•sphere of cer•e•bel•lum HII–HX (hem′is-fēr′ ser′ă-bel′ŭm) The large part of the cerebellum lateral to the vermis cerebelli. SYN hemispherium (2).

hem•i•spher•i•cum (hem′is-fēr′i-kŭm) SYN hemisphere.

hem•i•sphe•ri•um (hem′is-fēr′ē-ŭm) **1.** SYN cerebral hemisphere. **2.** SYN hemisphere of cerebellum HII–HX. [G. *hemisphairion*]

hem•i•sys•to•le (hem′ē-sis′tŏ-lē) Contraction of the left ventricle following every second atrial contraction only, so that there is one pulse beat to every two heartbeats.

hem•i•tho•rax (hem′ē-thōr′aks) One side of the thorax.

hem•i•trun•cus (hem′ē-trŭngk′ŭs) A variant truncus arteriosus in which only one pulmonary artery originates from the truncal artery.

hem•i•ver•te•bra (hem′ē-vĕr′tĕ-bră) A congenital defect of a vertebra in which one side of a vertebra fails to develop completely.

hem•i•zy•gos•i•ty (hem′ē-zī-gos′i-tē) The state of being hemizygous.

hem•i•zy•gote (hem′ē-zī′gōt) An individual hemizygous with respect to one or more specified loci; e.g., a normal male is a hemizygote with respect to the gene for all X-linked or Y-linked genes in his genome. [hemi- + G. *zygōtos,* yoked]

hem•i•zy•got•ic (hem′ē-zī-got′ik) SYN hemizygous.

hem•i•zy•gous (hem′ē-zī′gŭs) Having unpaired genes in an otherwise diploid cell; males are normally hemizygous for genes on both sex chromosomes. SYN hemizygotic.

Hem•lock So•ci•e•ty (hem′lok sŏ-sī′ĕ-tē) An organization devoted to the theories and procedures of suicide and euthanasia, whether by the patient's acting alone or with the assistance of the physician. Now restructured and renamed Compassion and Choices.

♻ **hemo-** Combining form denoting blood. SEE ALSO hem-, hemat-, hemato-. SYN haemo-. [G. *haima*]

he•mo•bil•i•a (hē′mō-bil′ē-ă) The presence of blood in the bile. SYN haemobilia.

he•mo•blast (hē′mō-blast) SYN hemocytoblast. SYN haemoblast.

he•mo•blas•to•sis (hē′mō-blas-tō′sis) A proliferative condition of the hematopoietic tissues in general. SYN haemoblastosis.

he•mo•ca•ther•e•sis (hē′mō-kă-ther′ĕ-sis) Destruction of the blood cells, especially of erythrocytes (hemocytocatheresis). SYN haemocatheresis. [hemo- + G. *kathairesis,* destruction]

he•mo•cath•e•ret•ic (hē′mō-kath-ĕ-ret′ik) Pertaining to or characterized by hemocatheresis. SYN haemocatheretic.

Hem•oc•cult test (hēm′ŏ-kŭlt′ test) A qualitative assay for occult blood in stool based on detecting the peroxidase activity of hemoglobin; a test kit can be used at home and the specimen produced mailed to a laboratory for evaluation. SYN Haemoccult test.

hem•o•cele (hē′mō-sēl) The system of interconnected spaces within the bodies of arthropods containing blood or hemolymph. SYN haemocoel, haemocoele. [hemo- + G. *koilōma,* cavity]

he•mo•cho•ri•al pla•cen•ta (hē′mō-kōr′ē-ăl plă-sen′tă) The type of placenta, as in humans and some rodents, in which maternal blood is in direct contact with the chorionic villi. SYN haemochorial placenta.

he•mo•chro•ma•to•sis (hē′mō-krō-mă-tō′sis) A disorder of iron metabolism characterized by excessive absorption of ingested iron, saturation of iron-binding protein, and deposition of hemosiderin in tissue, particularly in the liver, pancreas, and skin; cirrhosis of the liver, diabetes mellitus (bronze diabetes), bronze pigmentation of the skin, and, eventually heart failure may occur; also can result from administration of large amounts of iron orally, by injection, or in forms of blood transfusion therapy. SYN haemochromatosis. [hemo- + G. *chrōma,* color, + *-osis,* condition]

he•mo•chrome (hē′mō-krōm) SYN hemochromogen. SYN haemochrome.

he•mo•chro•mo•gen (hē′mō-krō′mō-jen) Any compound in which 1 mol of ferro- or ferriporphyrin is combined with 2 mol of a nitrogenous base or protein. SYN haemochromogen, hemochrome. [hemo- + G. *chrōma,* color, + *-gen,* producing]

he•mo•chro•mom•e•ter (hē′mō-krō-mom′ĕ-tĕr) SYN hemoglobinometry. SYN haemochromometer.

he•moc•la•sis, he•mo•cla•si•a (hē-mok′lă-sis, hē′mō-klā′zē-ă) Rupture, dissolution (hemolysis), or other type of destruction of red blood cells. SYN haemoclasis. [hemo- + G. *klasis,* a breaking]

he•mo•clas•tic (hē′mō-klas′tik) Pertaining to hemoclasis. SYN haemoclastic.

he•mo•con•cen•tra•tion (hē′mō-kon′sĕn-trā′shŭn) Decrease in the volume of plasma in relation to the number of red blood cells; increase in the concentration of red blood cells in the circulating blood. SYN haemoconcentration.

he•mo•co•ni•a (hē′mō-kō′nē-ă) Small, refractive particles in the circulating blood, probably lipid material associated with fragmented stroma from red blood cells. SYN haemoconia. [hemo- + G. *konis,* dust]

he•mo•co•ni•o•sis (hē′mō-kō′nē-ō′sis) A condition in which there is an abnormal concentration of hemoconia in the blood. SYN haemoconiosis.

he•mo•cy•a•nin (hē′mō-sī′ă-nin) An oxygen-carrying pigment in some mollusks, crustacea, and arthropods; contains copper rather than heme; used as an experimental antigen. SYN haemocyanin. [hemo- + G. *kyanos,* blue material, + -in]

he•mo•cyte (hē′mō-sīt) Any cell or formed element of the blood. SYN haemocyte. [hemo- + G. *kytos,* a hollow (cell)]

he•mo•cy•to•blast (hē′mō-sī′tō-blast) A blood cell derived from embryonic mesenchyme, characterized by basophilic cytoplasm and a relatively large nucleus with a spongy, loose network of chromatin and several nucleoli; mitochondria are extremely fine and delicate. Hemocytoblasts represent the primordial stem cells of the monophyletic theory of the origin of blood and can develop into erythroblasts, young forms of the granulocytic series; and megakaryocytes. SYN haemocytoblast, hematoplast, hemoblast. [hemo- + G. *kytos,* cell, + *blastos,* germ]

he•mo•cy•to•ca•ther•e•sis (hē′mō-sī′tō-kă-ther′ĕ-sis) Hemolysis or other type of destruction of red blood cells. SYN haemocytocatheresis. [hemo- + G. *kytos,* a hollow (cell), + *kathairesis,* destruction]

he•mo•cy•tol•y•sis (hē′mō-sī-tol′i-sis) The dissolution of blood cells, including hemolysis. SYN haemocytolysis. [hemo- + G. *kytos,* cell, + *lysis,* dissolution]

he•mo•cy•to•ma (hē′mō-sī-tō′mă) A tumor made up of undifferentiated blood cells. SYN haemocytoma. [hemo- + G. *kytos,* cell, + -oma]

he•mo•cy•tom•e•ter (hē′mō-sī-tom′ĕ-tĕr) An apparatus for estimating the number of blood cells in a quantitatively measured volume of blood; consists of a glass pipette with an ampulla for collecting and diluting the blood, and a counting chamber marked in squares. SYN haemocytometer, hemacytometer. [hemo- + G. *kytos,* cell, + *metron,* measure]

he•mo•cy•tom•e•try (hē′mō-sī-tom′ĕ-trē) The counting of red blood cells. SYN haemocytometry.

he•mo•cy•to•trip•sis (hē′mō-sī′tō-trip′sis) Fragmentation or disintegration of blood cells by means of mechanical trauma, e.g., compression between hard surfaces. SYN haemocytotrypsis. [hemo- + G. *kytos,* cell, + *tripsis,* a grinding]

he•mo•di•a•fil•tra•tion (hē′mō-dī′ă-fil-trā′shŭn) A combination of hemodialysis for diffusion of smaller molecular weight solutes with hemofiltration for convective transport of those of larger molecular weight. SYN haemodiafiltration.

he•mo•di•ag•no•sis (hē′mō-dī′ăg-nō′sis) Diagnosis made by means of examination of the blood. SYN haemodiagnosis.

he•mo•di•al•y•sis (hē′mō-dī-al′i-sis) Dialysis of soluble substances and water from the blood by diffusion through a semipermeable membrane; separation of cellular elements and colloids from soluble substances is achieved by pore size in the membrane and rates of diffusion. SYN haemodialysis.

he•mo•di•a•lyz•er (hē′mō-dī′ă-līz-ĕr) A machine for hemodialysis in acute or chronic renal failure; toxic substances in the blood are removed by exposure to dialyzing fluid across a semipermeable membrane. SYN artificial kidney, haemodialyser.

he•mo•di•lu•tion (hē′mō-di-lū′shŭn) Increase in the volume of plasma in relation to red blood cells; reduced concentration of red blood cells in the circulation. SYN haemodilution.

he•mo•dy•nam•ic (hē′mō-dī-nam′ik) Relating to the physical aspects of blood circulation.

he•mo•dy•nam•ics (hē′mō-dī-nam′iks) The study of the dynamics of blood circulation. SYN haemodynamics. [hemo- + G. *dynamis,* power]

he•mo•en•do•the•li•al pla•cen•ta (hē′mō-en′dō-thē′lē-ăl plă-sen′tă) The type of placenta, as in rabbits, in which the trophoblast becomes so attenuated that, by light microscopy, maternal blood appears to be separated from fetal blood only by the endothelium of the chorionic capillaries. SYN haemoendothelial placenta.

he•mo•fil•tra•tion (hē′mō-fil-trā′shŭn) A process, similar to hemodialysis, by which blood is dialyzed using ultrafiltration and simultaneous reinfusion of physiologic saline solution. SYN haemofiltration.

he•mo•flag•el•late (hē′mō-flaj′ĕ-lāt) Protozoan flagellates that are parasitic in the blood; they include the genera *Leishmania* and *Trypanosoma*, several species of which are important pathogens. SYN haemoflagellate. [hemo- + L. *flagellum,* dim. of *flagrum,* a whip]

he•mo•fus•cin (hē′mō-fŭs′in) A brown pigment derived from hemoglobin that occurs in urine occasionally along with hemosiderin, usually indicative of increased red blood cell destruction; occurs also in the liver with hemosiderin in cases of hemochromatosis. SYN haemofuscin.

he•mo•gen•e•sis (hē′mō-jen′ĕ-sis) SYN hemopoiesis. SYN haemogenesis.

he•mo•gen•ic (hē′mō-jen′ik) SYN hemopoietic. SYN haemogenic.

he•mo•glo•bin (Hgb, Hb) (hē′mō-glō′bin) The red respiratory protein of erythrocytes, consisting of approximately 3.8% heme and 96.2% globin, with a molecular weight of 64,450, which as oxyhemoglobin (HbO_2) transports oxygen from the lungs to the tissues where the oxygen is readily released and HbO_2 becomes Hb. When Hb is exposed to certain chemicals, its normal respiratory function is blocked; thus, oxygen in HbO_2 is easily displaced by carbon monoxide, a process that results in the formation of fairly stable carboxyhemoglobin (HbCO), as in asphyxiation resulting from inhalation of exhaust fumes from gasoline engines. When the iron in Hb is oxidized from the ferrous to ferric state, as in poisoning with nitrates and certain other chemicals, a nonrespiratory compound, methemoglobin (MetHb), is formed. Further oxidation produces sulfmethemoglobin. SYN haemoglobin, haemoglobins.

he•mo•glo•bin A (Hb A) (hē′mō-glō′bin) Normal adult hemoglobin, consisting of two variants, designated Hb A (by far the more prevalent) and Hb A_2. SYN haemoglobin A.

he•mo•glo•bin Bart (hē′mō-glō′bin bahrt) An Hb homotetramer (all four polypeptides identical) of formula γ_4, found in the early embryo and in α-thalassemia 2; not effective in oxygen transport; does not display a Bohr effect. SYN haemoglobin Bart.

he•mo•glo•bin C (Hb C) (hē′mō-glō′bin) An abnormal hemoglobin that affects the physical properties of erythrocytes, causing hemolytic anemia; often found in patients also having sickle cell disease or thalassemia. SYN haemoglobin C.

he•mo•glo•bi•ne•mi•a (hē′mō-glō′bi-nē′mē-ă) The presence of free hemoglobin in the blood plasma, as when intravascular hemolysis occurs. SYN haemoglobinaemia.

he•mo•glo•bin F (Hb F) (hē′mō-glō′bin) Normal fetal hemoglobin; production is greatly reduced after infancy except in certain congenital or acquired hematologic disorders. SYN haemoglobin F.

he•mo•glo•bi•nol•y•sis (hē′mō-glō′bi-nol′i-sis) Destruction or chemical splitting of hemoglobin. SYN haemoglobinolysis. [hemoglobin + G. *lysis,* dissolution]

he•mo•glob•i•nom•e•try (hē′mō-glō′bi-nom′ĕ-trē) Measurement of the hemoglobin concentration of the blood. SYN haemoglobinometry, hematinometer, hemochromometer.

he•mo•glo•bi•nop•a•thy (hē′mō-glō′bi-nop′ă-thē) A disorder or disease caused by or associated with the presence of hemoglobins in the blood. SYN haemoglobinopathy. [hemoglobin + G. *pathos,* disease]

he•mo•glo•bi•no•phil•ic (hē′mō-glō′bi-nō-fil′ik) Denoting certain microorganisms that cannot be cultured except in the presence of hemoglobin. SYN haemoglobinophilic. [hemoglobin + G. *phileō,* to love]

he•mo•glo•bin S (Hb S) (hē′mō-glō′bin) An abnormal hemoglobin that renders erythrocytes subject to sickling and hemolysis at reduced oxygen tension; makes up 70–100% of hemoglobin in people with sickle cell anemia. SYN haemoglobin S, sickle cell hemoglobin.

he•mo•glo•bi•nu•ri•a (hē′mō-glō′bi-nyūr′ē-ă) The presence of hemoglobin in the urine, including certain closely related pigments formed from slight alteration of the hemoglobin molecule; indicative of intravascular hemolysis or of bleeding into the urinary tract, with hemolysis there. The urine may be reddish-yellow to dark red. SYN haemoglobinuria. [hemoglobin + G. *ouron,* urine]

he•mo•glo•bi•nu•ric (hē′mō-glō′bi-nyūr′ik) Relating to or marked by hemoglobinuria. SYN haemoglobinuric.

he•mo•glo•bi•nu•ric ne•phro•sis (hē′mō-glō′bi-nyūr′ik nĕ-frō′sis) Acute oliguric renal failure associated with hemoglobinuria, due to massive intravascular hemolysis. SYN haemoglobinuric nephrosis.

he•mo•gram (hē′mō-gram) A complete detailed record of the findings in a thorough examination of the blood, especially with reference to the numbers, proportions, and morphologic features of the formed elements. SYN haemogram. [hemo- + G. *gramma,* a drawing]

he•mo•his•ti•o•blast (hē′mō-his′tē-ō-blast) A primordial type of mesenchymal cell believed to be capable of developing into all types of blood cells, including monocytes, and into histiocytes. SYN Ferrata cell, haemohistioblast. [hemo- + G. *histion,* web, + *blastos,* germ]

he•mo•lith (hē′mō-lith) A concretion in the wall of a blood vessel. SYN haemolith. [hemo- + G. *lithos,* stone]

he•mo•lu•te•in (hē′mō-lū′tē-in) SYN hematoidin. SYN haemolutein. [hemo- + L. *luteus,* yellow, + -in]

he•mo•lymph (hē′mō-limf) **1.** Blood and lymph, considered together. **2.** The nutrient fluid of certain invertebrates. SYN haemolymph.

he•mol•y•sate (hē-mol′i-sāt) Preparation resulting from the lysis of erythrocytes. SYN haemolysate.

he•mol•y•sin (hē-mol′i-sin) **1.** Any substance elaborated by a living agent and capable of lysing red blood cells and liberating their hemoglobin. SYN erythrocytolysin, erythrolysin. **2.** A sensitizing (complement-fixing) antibody that combines with red blood cells of the antigenic type that stimulated formation of the hemolysin, so that complement fixes with the antibody-cell union and causes dissolution of the cells. SYN haemolysin.

he•mo•ly•sin•o•gen (hē′mol-i-sin′ŏ-jen) The antigenic material in red blood cells that stimulates the formation of hemolysin. SYN haemolysinogen.

he•mo•ly•sin u•nit, he•mo•lyt•ic u•nit (hē-mol′i-sin yū′nit, hē′mō-lit′ik) The smallest quantity (highest dilution) of inactivated immune serum (hemolysin) that will sensitize the standard suspension of erythrocytes so that the standard complement will cause complete hemolysis. SYN haemolysin unit.

he•mol•y•sis (hē-mol′i-sis) Alteration, dissolution, or destruction of red blood cells in such a manner that hemoglobin is liberated into the medium in which the cells are suspended. SYN erythrocytolysis, erythrolysis, haemolysis, hematolysis. [hemo- + G. *lysis,* destruction]

he•mo•lyt•ic (hē′mō-lit′ik) Destructive to blood cells, resulting in liberation of hemoglobin. SYN haemolytic, hematolytic, hemotoxic (2), hematotoxic, hematoxic.

he•mo•lyt•ic a•ne•mi•a (hē′mō-lit′ik ă-nē′mē-ă) Any anemia resulting from an increased rate of erythrocyte destruction. See this page. SYN haemolytic anaemia.

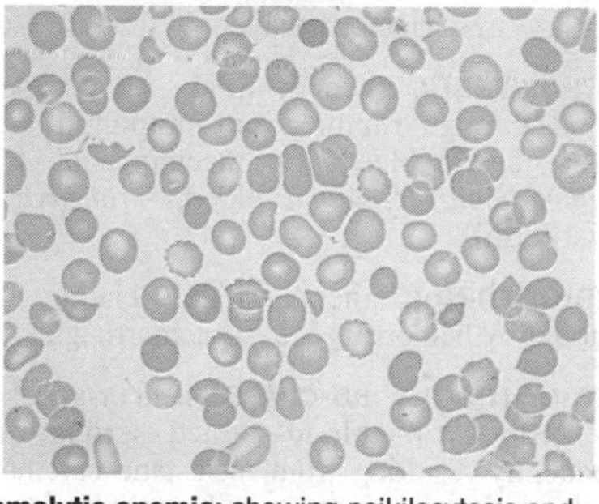

hemolytic anemia: showing poikilocytosis and absence of platelets, but no signs of hemolysis

he•mo•lyt•ic dis•ease of new•born (hē′mō-lit′ik di-zēz′ nū′bōrn) SYN erythroblastosis fetalis. SYN haemolytic disease of newborn.

he•mo•lyt•ic jaun•dice (hē′mō-lit′ik jawn′dis) Hepatic disorder that results from increased production of bilirubin from hemoglobin as a result of any process (e.g., toxic, genetic, or immune) causing increased destruction of erythrocytes. SYN haemolytic jaundice, hematogenous jaundice.

he•mo•ly•tic plaque as•say (hē′mō-lit′ik plak as′ā) SYN Jerne plaque assay. SYN haemolytic plaque assay.

he•mo•lyt•ic sple•no•meg•a•ly (hē′mō-lit′ik splē′nō-meg′ă-lē) Enlargement of the spleen associated with congenital hemolytic jaundice. SYN haemolytic splenomegaly.

he•mo•lyt•ic u•re•mic syn•drome (hē′mō-lit′ik yūr-ē′mik sin′drōm) Combination of hemolytic anemia and thrombocytopenia that occurs with acute renal failure. In children, characterized by sudden onset of gastrointestinal bleeding, hematuria, oliguria, and microangiopathic hemolytic anemia in association with intestinal infection by *Shigella*, *Salmonella*, or *Escherichia coli* strain O157:H7; in adults, associated with complications of pregnancy following normal delivery, with oral contraceptive use, or with infection. SYN haemolytic uremic syndrome.

he•mo•lyze (hē′mō-līz) To produce hemolysis or liberation of the hemoglobin from red blood cells.

he•mo•lyzed (hē′mō-līzd) Condition of a specimen of plasma or serum that has broken blood cells dissolved in it.

he•mo•me•di•as•ti•num (hē′mō-mē′dē-ă-stī′nŭm) Blood in the mediastinum. SYN haemomediastinum.

he•mo•me•tra (hē′mō-mē′tră) SYN hematometra. SYN haemometra.

he•mon•chi•a•sis (hē′mong-kī′a-sĭs) Infestation with nematodes of the genus *Haemonchus*. SYN haemonchiasis.

he•mo•nec•tin (hē′mō-nek′tin) An extracellular protein found in bone marrow matrix that promotes adhesion and differentiation of cells in the granulocyte line. SYN haemonectin. [hemo- + L. *necto,* to fasten, + -in]

he•mo•pa•ra•site (hē′mō-par′ă-sīt) A parasite that inhabits the bloodstream of the host. SYN haemoparasite.

he•mo•pa•thol•o•gy (hē′mō-pă-thol′ŏ-jē) SYN hematopathology. SYN haemopathology.

he•mop•a•thy (hē-mop′ă-thē) Any abnormal condition or disease of the blood or hemopoietic tissues. SYN haemopathy. [hemo- + G. *pathos,* suffering]

he•mo•per•fu•sion (hē′mō-pĕr-fyū′zhŭn) Passage of blood through columns of adsorptive material, such as activated charcoal, to remove toxic substances. SYN haemoperfusion. [hemo- + L. *perfusio,* to pass through]

he•mo•per•i•car•di•um (hē′mō-per′ē-kahr′dē-ŭm) Blood in the pericardial sac. SYN haemopericardium.

he•mo•per•i•to•ne•um (hē′mō-per′i-tō-nē′ŭm) Blood in the peritoneal cavity. SYN haemoperitoneum.

he•mo•pex•in (hē′mō-peks′in) A serum protein related to β-globulins, important in binding heme and porphyrins, preventing excretion, and perhaps regulating heme in drug metabolism. SYN haemopexin. [hemo- + G. *pēxis,* fixation, + -in]

he•mo•phag•o•cyte (hē′mō-fag′ō-sīt) A cell that engulfs and destroys blood cells, especially erythrocytes. SYN haemophagocyte.

he•mo•phil, **he•mo•phile** (hē′mō-fil, -fīl) A microorganism growing preferably in media containing blood. SYN haemophil. [hemo- + G. *philos,* fond]

he•mo•phil•i•a (hē′mō-fil′ē-ă) An inherited disorder of blood coagulation characterized by a permanent tendency to hemorrhages, spontaneous or traumatic, due to a defect in the blood coagulating mechanism. SYN haemophilia. [hemo- + G. *philos,* fond]

he•mo•phil•i•a A (hē′mō-fil′ē-ă) The inherited blood disorder resulting from a deficiency of factor VIII, occurring almost exclusively in males, and characterized by prolonged clotting time, decreased formation of thromboplastin, and diminished conversion of prothrombin. SYN classic hemophilia, haemophilia A.

he•mo•phil•i•a B (hē′mō-fil′ē-ă) A clotting disorder resembling hemophilia A, caused by hereditary deficiency of factor IX. SYN Christmas disease, haemophilia B.

he•mo•phil•i•ac (hē′mō-fil′ē-ak) A person suffering from hemophilia. SYN haemophiliac.

he•mo•phil•ic (hē′mō-fil′ik) Relating to hemophilia. SYN haemophilic.

he•mo•phi•li•oid (hē′mō-fil′ē-ōyd) Any disorder that resembles but does not result from any deficiency of factor VIII. SYN haemophilioid.

he•mo•pho•re•sis (hē′mō-fŏr-ē′sis) Blood convection or irrigation of tissues. SYN haemophoresis. [hemo- + G. *phoreō,* to bear]

he•moph•thal•mi•a, **he•moph•thal•mus** (hē′mof-thal′mē-ă, -mof-thal′mŭs) A blood-filled eye. SYN haemophthalmia, hematopsia. [hemo- + G. *ophthalmos,* eye]

he•mo•plas•tic (hē′mō-plas′tik) SYN hemopoietic. SYN haemoplastic.

he•mo•pneu•mo•per•i•car•di•um (hē′mō-nū′mō-per-i-kahr′dē-ŭm) The occurrence of blood and air in the pericardium. SYN haemopneumopericardium, pneumohemopericardium. [hemo- + G. *pneuma,* air, + pericardium]

he•mo•pneu•mo•tho•rax (hē′mō-nū′mō-thō′raks) Accumulation of air and blood in the pleural cavity. SYN haemopneumothorax, pneumohemothorax. [hemo- + G. *pneuma,* air, + thorax]

he•mo•poi•e•sis (hē′mō-poy-ē′sis) The process of formation and development of the various types of blood cells and other formed elements. SYN haemopoiesis, hematogenesis, hematopoiesis, hemogenesis, sanguification. [hemo- + G. *poiēsis,* a making]

he•mo•poi•et•ic (hē′mō-poy-et′ik) Pertaining to or related to the formation of blood cells. SYN haemopoietic, hematogenic (1), hematogenous, hematoplastic, hematopoietic, hemogenic, hemoplastic, sanguifacient.

he•mo•por•phy•rin (hē′mō-pōr′fir-in) SYN hematoporphyrin. SYN haemoporphyrin.

he•mo•pre•cip•i•tin (hē′mō-prē-sip′i-tin) An antibody that combines with and precipitates soluble antigenic material from erythrocytes. SYN haemoprecipitin.

he•mo•pro•tein (hē′mō-prō′tēn) Protein linked to a metal-porphyrin compound (e.g., cytochromes, myoglobin, catalase). SYN haemoprotein.

he•mop•ty•sis (hē-mop′ti-sis) The spitting of blood derived from the lungs or bronchial tubes as a result of pulmonary or bronchial hemorrhage. SYN haemoptysis. [hemo- + G. *ptysis,* a spitting]

he•mo•rhe•o•lo•gy (hē′mō-rē-ol′ŏ-jē) The science of the flow of blood in relation to the pressures, flow, volumes, and resistances in blood vessels, especially with respect to blood viscosity and red blood cell deformation in the microcirculation. SYN haemorheology. [hemo- + G. *rheos,* flow, + *logos,* study]

he•mor•rha•chis (hē-mōr′ă-kis) SYN hematorrhachis. SYN haemorrhachis.

hem•or•rhage (hem′ŏr-ăj) **1.** An escape of blood through ruptured or unruptured vessel walls. **2.** To bleed. SYN haemorrhage. [G. *haimorrhagia,* fr. *haima,* blood, + *rhēgnymi,* to burst forth]

hem•or•rhag•ic (hem′ŏr-aj′ik) Relating to or marked by hemorrhage. SYN haemorrhagic.

hem•or•rhag•ic as•ci•tes (hem′ŏr-aj′ik ă-sī′tēz) Bloody or blood-stained serous fluid, frequently resulting from metastatic carcinoma, in the peritoneal cavity. SYN haemorrhagic ascites.

hem•or•rhag•ic co•li•tis (hem′ŏr-aj′ik kō-lī′tis) Abdominal cramps and bloody diarrhea, without fever, attributed to a self-limited infection by a strain of *Escherichia coli.* SYN haemorrhagic colitis.

hem•or•rhag•ic cyst (hem′ŏr-aj′ik sist) A cyst containing blood or resulting from the encapsulation of a hematoma. SYN blood cyst, haemorrhagic cyst, hematocele (1), hematocyst.

hem•or•rhag•ic cys•ti•tis (hem′ŏr-aj′ik sis-tī′tis) Bladder inflammation with macroscopic hematuria. Generally the result of a chemical or other traumatic insult to the bladder (chemother-

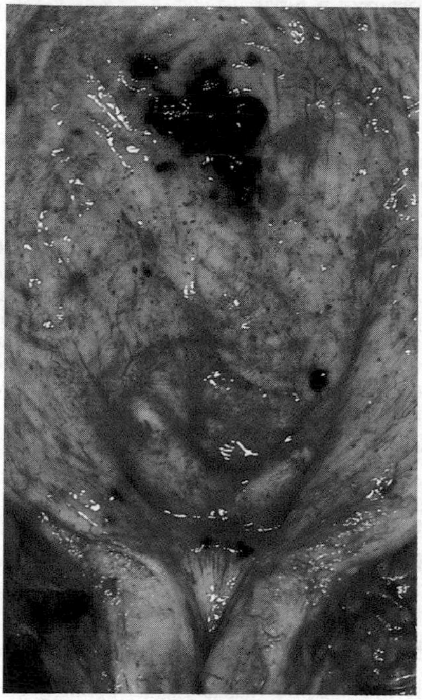

acute hemorrhagic cystitis: patient died 2 days after surgery, cystitis caused by indwelling catheter

apy, radiation therapy). See this page. SYN haemorrhagic cystitis.

hem•or•rhag•ic dis•ease of the new•born (hem′ŏr-aj′ik di-zēz′ nū′bōrn) A syndrome characterized by spontaneous internal or external bleeding accompanied by hypoprothrombinemia, slightly decreased platelet counts, and markedly elevated bleeding and clotting times, usually occurring between the third and sixth days of life and effectively treated with vitamin K. SYN haemorrhagic disease of the newborn.

hem•or•rhag•ic en•do•vas•cu•li•tis (hem′ŏr-aj′ik en′dō-vas′kyū-lī′tis) Endothelial and medial hyperplasia of placental blood vessels with thrombosis, fragmentation, and diapedesis of red blood cells resulting in stillbirth or fetal developmental disorders. SYN haemorrhagic endovasculitis.

hem•or•rhag•ic fe•ver (hem′ŏr-aj′ik fē′vĕr) An infectious syndrome caused by several different viruses. Some types of hemorrhagic fever are tick borne, others mosquito borne, and some airborne; others are zoonoses; clinical manifestations are high fever, scattered petechiae, bleeding in gastrointestinal tract and other organs, hypotension, and shock; kidney damage may be severe, especially in Korean hemorrhagic fever, and neurologic signs may appear, especially in the Argentine-Bolivian types. Four types of hemorrhagic fever are transmissible person-to-person: Lassa fever, Ebola fever, Marburg virus disease, and Crimean-Congo hemorrhagic fever. SEE ALSO epidemic hemorrhagic fever. SYN haemorrhagic fever.

hem•or•rhag•ic fe•ver with re•nal syn•drome (hem′ŏr-aj′ik fē′vĕr rē′năl sin′drōm) A condition caused by a Hantavirus, which is transmitted to humans by contact with or inhalation of contaminated rodent body fluids. Cf. epidemic hemorrhagic fever. SYN haemorrhagic fever with renal syndrome.

hem•or•rhag•ic in•farct (hem′ŏr-aj′ik in′fahrkt) An infarct that turns red due to infiltration of blood from collateral vessels into the necrotic area. SYN haemorrhagic infarct.

hem•or•rhag•ic mea•sles (hem′ŏr-aj′ik mē′zĕlz) A severe form in which the eruption is dark because of the effusion of blood into affected areas of the skin. SYN haemorrhagic measles.

hem•or•rhag•ic plague (hem′ŏr-aj′ik plāg) The hemorrhagic form of bubonic plague. SEE ALSO plague. SYN haemorrhagic plague.

hem•or•rhag•ic shock (hem′ŏr-aj′ik shok) Hypovolemic shock resulting from acute hemorrhage, characterized by hypotension; tachycardia; pale, cold, and clammy skin; and oliguria. SYN haemorrhagic shock.

hem•or•rhag•ins (hem′ŏr-aj′inz) Toxins found in certain venoms and poisonous material from some plants, e.g., rattlesnake venom and ricin; cause degeneration and lysis of endothelial cells in capillaries and small vessels, thereby resulting in numerous small hemorrhages in the tissues. SYN haemorrhagins. [hemorrhage + -in]

hem•or•rhoi•dal (hem′ŏr-oy′dăl) Relating to hemorrhoids. SYN haemorrhoidal.

hem•or•rhoid•ec•to•my (hem′ŏr-oy-dek′tŏ-mē) Surgical removal of hemorrhoids; usually accomplished by excision of hemorrhoidal tissues by sharp dissection, or by application of elastic ligature at the base of the hemorrhoidal bundles to produce ischemic necrosis and ultimate ablation of the hemorrhoidectomy. SYN haemorrhoidectomy. [hemorrhoids + G. *ektomē*, excision]

hem•or•rhoids (hem′ŏr-oydz) A varicose condition of the external or internal rectal veins causing painful swellings at the anus. SYN piles. [G. *haimorrhois*, pl. *haimorrhoides*, veins likely to bleed, fr. *haima*, blood, + *rhoia*, a flow]

he•mo•sal•pinx (hē′mō-sal′pingks) SYN hematosalpinx.

he•mo•sid•er•in (hē′mō-sid′ĕr-in) A yellow or brown protein produced by phagocytic digestion of hematin; found in most tissues, but especially in the liver; at higher levels, it stains blue with Perl Prussian blue stain. SYN haemosiderin. [hemo- + G. *sidēros*, iron, + -in]

he•mo•sid•er•o•sis (hē′mō-sid-ĕr-ō′sis) Accumulation of hemosiderin in tissue, particularly in liver and spleen. SEE hemochromatosis. SYN haemosiderosis. [hemosiderin + *-osis*, condition]

he•mo•sper•mi•a (hē′mō-spĕr′mē-ă) The presence of blood in the seminal fluid. SYN haemospermia. [hemo- + G. *sperma,* seed]

he•mo•sta•sis (hē′mō-stā′sis) **1.** The arrest of bleeding. **2.** The arrest of circulation in a part. **3.** Stagnation of blood. SYN haemostasis. [hemo- + G. *stasis,* a standing]

he•mo•stat (hē′mō-stat) **1.** Any agent that arrests, chemically or mechanically, the flow of blood from an open vessel. **2.** An instrument for arresting hemorrhage by compression of the bleeding vessel. SYN haemostat.

he•mo•stat•ic (hē′mō-stat′ik) **1.** Arresting the flow of blood within the vessels. **2.** SYN antihemorrhagic. SYN haemastatic, haemostatic.

he•mo•stat•ic for•ceps (hē′mō-stat′ik fōr′seps) A forceps with a catch for locking the blades, used for seizing the end of a blood vessel to control hemorrhage. SYN artery forceps, haemostatic forceps.

he•mo•ther•a•py, he•mo•ther•a•peu•tics (hē′mō-thār′ă-pē, -thār-ă-pyū′tiks) Treatment of disease by the use of blood or blood derivatives, as in transfusion. SYN haemotherapy.

he•mo•tho•rax (hē′mō-thōr′aks) Blood in the pleural cavity. SYN haematothorax, haemothorax.

he•mo•tox•ic, he•ma•to•tox•ic, he•ma•tox•ic (hē′mō-tok′sik, hē′mă-tō-toks′ik, hē′mă-toks′ik) **1.** Causing blood poisoning. **2.** SYN hemolytic. SYN haemotoxic.

he•mo•tox•in (hē′mō-tok′sin) Any substance that destroys red blood cells, including various hemolysins; usually used with reference to substances of biologic origin, in contrast to chemicals. SYN haemotoxin, hematotoxin.

he•mo•troph, he•mo•trophe (hē′mō-trōf) The nutritive materials supplied to the embryos of placental mammals through the maternal bloodstream. Cf. embryotroph. SYN haemotroph. [hemo- + G. *trophē,* food]

he•mo•trop•ic (hē′mō-trō′pik) Pertaining to the mechanism by which a substance in or on blood cells, especially the erythrocytes, attracts phagocytic cells; the latter change direction and migrate toward the hemotropic cells. SYN haemotropic, hematotropic. [hemo- + G. *tropos,* direction (or *tropē,* a turning)]

he•mo•tym•pa•num (hē′mō-tim′pă-nŭm) The presence of blood in the middle ear. SYN haemotympanum.

hem•ox•im•e•ter (hēm′oks-im′ĕ-ter′) SYN oximeter. SYN haemoximeter.

hem•ox•im•e•try (hēm′oks-im′ĕ-trē) Spectrophotometric analysis of blood for determination of the saturation of oxyhemoglobin and of dyshemoglobins (e.g., carboxyhemoglobin, methemoglobin). SYN haemoximetry.

he•mo•zo•on (hē′mō-zō′on) A parasitic animal that resides in the blood of the host. SYN haemozoon, hematozoon. [hemo- + G. *zōon,* animal]

Hen•der•son-Has•sel•balch e•qua•tion (hen′dĕr-sŏn hahs′ĕl-bawlk ĕ-kwā′zhŭn) A formula relating the pH value of a solution to the pK_a value of the acid in the solution and the ratio of the acid and the conjugate base concentrations: $pH = pK_a + \log([A^-]/[HA])$ where $[A^-]$ is the concentration of the conjugate base and [HA] is the concentration of the protonated acid.

Hen•der•son•u•la tor•u•loi•de•a (hen-dĕr-sŏn′yū-lă tōr-yū-loy′dē-ă) A species of black yeast capable of producing chronic infections of the nails as well as of the skin of the feet.

Hend•ra vi•rus (hen′dră vī′rŭs) SYN equine morbillivirus. [from Hendra, the suburb of Brisbane, Australia, where it was first isolated]

Hen•le an•sa (hen′lē an′să) SYN nephron loop.

Hen•le glands (hen′lē glandz) Formerly considered accessory lacrimal glands, these epithelial invaginations are located near the fornices in the medial part of the palpebral conjunctiva; they open on the conjunctiva surface along with the Krause gland, and secrete into the basal aqueous tear layer.

Hen•le lay•er (hen′lē lā′ĕr) The outer layer cells of the inner root sheath of the hair follicle.

Hen•le lig•a•ment (hen′lē lig′ă-mĕnt) SYN inguinal falx.

Henle loop (hen′lē lūp) SYN nephron loop.

Hen•le re•ac•tion (hen′lē rē-ak′shŭn) Dark brown staining of the medullary cells of the adrenal bodies when treated with the salts of chromium, the cortical cells remaining unstained.

Hen•le sheath (hen′lē) SYN endoneurium.

Hen•ne•bert sign (en′ĕ-bār sīn) Nystagmus produced by pressure applied to a sealed external auditory canal; may be seen in labyrinthine fistula or with intact tympanic membrane in syphilitic involvement of the otic capsule. SEE ALSO Tullio phenomenon.

He•noch pur•pu•ra (hen′awk pŭr′pyŭr-ă) SYN Henoch-Schönlein purpura.

He•noch-Schön•lein pur•pu•ra (hen′awk shĕrn′līn pŭr′pyŭr-ă) An eruption of nonthrombocytopenic purpuric lesions due to dermal leukocytoclastic vasculitis with IgA in vessel walls associated with joint pain and swelling, colic, and passage of bloody stools, and occurring characteristically in young children; glomerulonephritis may occur during an initial episode or develop later. SYN anaphylactoid purpura (2), Henoch purpura, Schönlein purpura.

hen•ry (H) (hen′rē) The unit of electrical inductance, when 1 volt is induced by a change in current of 1 ampere/second. [Joseph *Henry*]

Hen•ry law (hen′rē law) At equilibrium, at a given temperature, the amount of gas dissolved in a given volume of liquid is directly proportional to the partial pressure of that gas in the gas phase (this only holds for gases that do not react chemically with the solvent).

Hen•sen cell (hen′sĕn sel) One of the supporting cells in the organ of Corti, immediately to the outer side of the cells of Deiters.

Hen•sen node (hen′sen nōd) SYN primitive node.

HEPA (hep′ă) Acronym for high-efficiency particulate air-filters.

He•pad•na•vi•ri•dae (hē-pad-nă-vir′ă-dē) A family of DNA-containing viruses. The principal genus Hepadnavirus is associated with hepatitis B. [*hepa*titis + DNA + virus]

he•par, gen. **hep•a•tis** (hē′par, hē-pā′tis) [TA] SYN liver. [L. borrowed fr. G. *hēpar,* gen. *hēpatos,* the liver]

hep•a•rin (hep′ăr-in) An anticoagulant that is a component of various tissues (especially liver and lung) and mast cells. Its principal active constituent is a glycosaminoglycan composed of D-glucuronic acid and D-glucosamine. In conjunction with a serum protein cofactor (the so-called heparin cofactor), heparin acts as an antithrombin and an antiprothrombin by preventing platelet agglutination and consequent thrombus formation.

hep•a•rin•ize (hep′ăr-in-īz) To perform therapeutic administration of heparin.

hep•a•rin lock (hep′ăr-in lok) An indwelling venous catheter used when intravenous infusions or withdrawal of venous blood for testing must be performed repeatedly over an extended period; between uses it is filled with the anticoagulant heparin.

hepat-, hepatico-, hepato- Combining forms meaning the liver. [G. *hēpar* (*hēpat-*)]

hep•a•ta•tro•phi•a, hep•a•tat•ro•phy (hepat′ă-trō′fē-ă, hep′ă-tat′rŏ-fē) Atrophy of the liver.

hep•a•tec•to•my (hep′ă-tek′tŏ-mē) Removal of the liver, whole or in part. [hepat- + G. *ektomē,* excision]

he•pat•ic (hĕ-pat′ik) Relating to the liver. [G. *hēpatikos*]

he•pat•ic ad•e•no•ma (hĕ-pat′ik ad′ĕ-nō′mă) A benign tumor of the liver, usually occurring in women in association with lengthy oral contraceptive use.

he•pat•ic ar•ter•y prop•er (hĕ-pat′ik ahr′tĕr-ē prop′ĕr) *Origin,* common hepatic; *branches,* right and left hepatic. SYN arteria hepatica propria.

he•pat•ic branch•es of an•te•ri•or va•gal trunk (hĕ-pat′ik branch′ĕz an-tēr′ē-ŏr vā′găl trŭngk) Branches of the anterior and posterior vagal trunks distributed to the liver.

he•pat•ic co•ma (hĕ-pat′ik kō′mă) State that occurs with advanced hepatic insufficiency and portal-systemic shunts, caused by elevated blood ammonia levels; characteristic findings include asterixis in the precoma stage and paroxysms of bilaterally synchronous triphasic waves on EEG examination.

he•pat•ic di•ver•tic•u•lum (he-pat′ik dī′vĕr-tik′yū-lŭm) An outgrowth of endodermal epithelium from the caudal part of the embryonic foregut (future site of duodenum); it gives rise to the liver, gallbladder, cystic duct, and bile ducts. See page 706. SYN liver bud.

he•pat•ic duct (hĕ-pat′ik dŭkt) SEE common hepatic duct.

he•pat•ic en•ceph•a•lop•a•thy (hĕ-pat′ik en-sef′a-lop′ă-thē) **1.** SYN portal-systemic encephalopathy. **2.** SYN Reye syndrome.

he•pat•ic flex•ure (hĕ-pat′ik flek′shŭr) SYN right colic flexure.

he•pat•ic lob•ule (hĕ-pat′ik lob′yūl) SYN lobules of liver.

he•pat•i•co•do•chot•o•my (he-pat′i-kō-dō-kot′ŏ-mē) Combined hepaticotomy and choledochotomy.

he•pat•i•co•du•o•de•nos•to•my (he-pat′i-kō-dū′ō-dē-nos′tŏ-mē) Establishment of a communication between the hepatic ducts and the duodenum. [hepatico- + duodenostomy]

he•pat•i•co•en•ter•os•to•my (he-pat′i-kō-en-tĕr-os′tŏ-mē) Establishment of a communication between the hepatic ducts and the intestine. [hepatico- + enterostomy]

he•pat•i•co•gas•tros•to•my (he-pat′i-kō-gas-tros′tŏ-mē) Establishment of a communication between the hepatic duct and the stomach. [hepatico- + gastrostomy]

he•pat•i•co•li•thot•o•my (he-pat′i-kō-li-thot′ŏ-mē) Removal of a stone from a hepatic duct. [hepatico- + G. *lithos,* stone, + *tomē,* a cutting]

he•pat•i•co•lith•o•trip•sy (he-pat′i-kō-lith′ō-trip-sē) The crushing or fragmentation of a biliary calculus in the hepatic duct. [hepatico- + G. *lithos,* stone, + *tripsis,* a rubbing]

he•pat•i•cos•to•my (he-pat′i-kos′tŏ-mē) Estab-

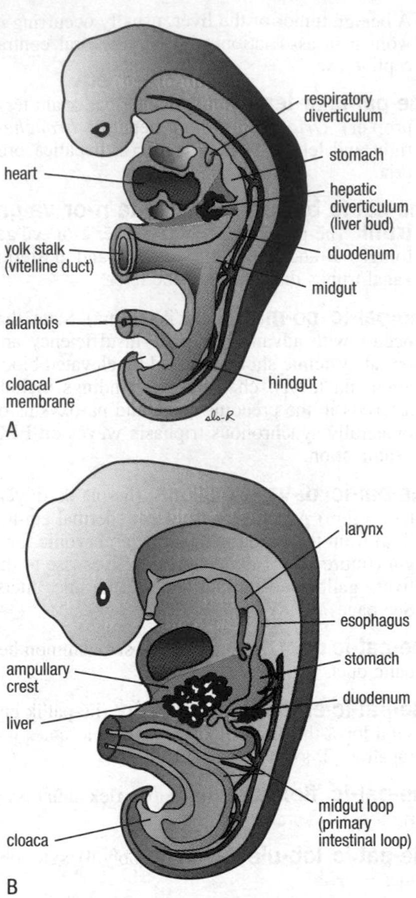

liver development in the embryo: (A) an embryo (approximately 25 days) showing the primordial gastrointestinal tract and formation of the liver (the hepatic diverticulum is formed from endoderm lining the foregut); (B) an embryo (approximately 32 days) showing epithelial liver cords penetrating the mesenchyme of the septum transversum

lishment of an opening into the hepatic duct. [hepatico- + G. *stoma,* mouth]

he•pat•i•cot•o•my (he-pat′i-kot′ŏ-mē) Incision into the hepatic duct. [hepatico- + G. *tomē,* incision]

he•pat•ic por•phyr•i•a (hĕ-pat′ik pōr-fir′ē-ă) A category of porphyria that includes porphyria cutanea tarda, variegate porphyria, and coproporphyria.

he•pat•ic por•tal vein (hĕ-pat′ik pōr′tăl vān) SYN portal vein.

he•pat•ic veins (hĕ-pat′ik vānz) Having drained the liver, these collect blood from the central veins and terminate in three large veins opening into the inferior vena cava below the diaphragm and several small inconstant veins entering the vena cava at more inferior levels.

hep•a•tit•ic (hep′ă-tit′ik) Relating to hepatitis.

hep•a•ti•tis (hep′ă-tī′tis) Inflammation of the liver; usually from a viral infection, a drug, and sometimes from toxic agents. [hepat- + G. *-itis,* inflammation]

hep•a•ti•tis A (hep′ă-tī′tis) SYN viral hepatitis type A.

hep•a•ti•tis A vi•rus (HAV) (hep′ă-tī′tis vī′rŭs) An RNA virus, the causative agent of viral hepatitis type A. See page B6. SYN infectious hepatitis virus.

hep•a•ti•tis B (hep′ă-tī′tis) SYN viral hepatitis type B.

hep•a•ti•tis B core an•ti•gen (HB$_c$Ab, HB$_c$Ag) (hep′ă-tī′tis kōr an′ti-jen) The antigen found in the core of the Dane particle (which is the complete virus) and also in hepatocyte nuclei in hepatitis B infections.

hep•a•ti•tis B e an•ti•gen (HBe, HB$_e$Ag) (hep′ă-tī′tis an′ti-jen) An antigen, or group of antigens, associated with hepatitis B infection and distinct from the surface antigen (HB$_s$Ag) and the core antigen (HB$_c$Ag). Its presence indicates that the virus is replicating and the person is potentially infectious.

hep•a•ti•tis B im•mune glob•u•lin (HBIG) (hep′ă-tī′tis i-myūn′ glob′yū-lin) A high-titer passive immune globulin directed against type B hepatitis virus (HBV). Passive immunity to type B hepatitis can be conferred by administration of this immune serum globulin. It is recommended for those exposed to fluids from people infected with HBV.

hep•a•ti•tis B sur•face an•ti•gen (HB$_s$Ag) (hep′ă-tī′tis sŭr′făs an′ti-jen) Antigen of the small (20 nm) spheric and filamentous forms of hepatitis B antigen, and a surface antigen of the larger (42 nm) Dane particle (complete infectious hepatitis B virus). SEE ALSO hepatitis B e antigen.

hep•a•ti•tis B vi•rus (HBV) (hep′ă-tī′tis vī′rŭs) A DNA virus, the causative agent of viral hepatitis type B. See page B6. SYN serum hepatitis virus.

hep•a•ti•tis C (hep′ă-tī′tis) A viral hepatitis, usually mild but often progressing to a chronic stage; the most prevalent type of posttransfusion hepatitis.

hep•a•ti•tis C vi•rus (HCV) (hep′ă-tī′tis vī′rŭs) A non-A, non-B RNA virus that causes posttransfusion hepatitis.

hep•a•ti•tis D vi•rus, hep•a•ti•tis del•ta vi•rus (HDV) (hep′ă-tī-tis vī′rŭs, del′tă vī′rŭs) A small "defective" RNA virus that requires the presence of hepatitis B virus for replication. The clinical course is variable but is usually more severe than other hepatitides. SYN delta agent.

hep·a·ti·tis E (hep′ă-tī′tis) A viral hepatitis occurring chiefly in the tropics; transmitted by the fecal-oral route, it does not become chronic or lead to a carrier state, but has a higher mortality than hepatitis A, particularly in pregnancy.

hep·a·ti·tis E vi·rus (HEV) (hep′ă-tī′tis vī′rŭs) An RNA virus that is the principal cause of enterically transmitted, waterborne, or epidemic non-A, non-B hepatitis occurring primarily in Asia and Africa.

hep·a·ti·tis F (hep′ă-tī′tis) A disease caused by a still poorly characterized DNA virus.

hep·a·ti·tis G (hep′ă-tī′tis) A disease caused by an RNA virus similar to hepatitis virus.

hep·a·ti·tis G vi·rus (HGV) (hep′ă-tī′tis vī′rŭs) An RNA virus related to the hepatitis C virus, and which may cause coinfection with that agent.

hep·a·ti·za·tion (hep′ă-tī-zā′shŭn) Conversion of a loose tissue into a firm mass like the substance of the liver macroscopically, denoting especially such a change in the lungs in the consolidation of pneumonia.

hep·a·to·bil·i·ar·y hep·a·ti·tis (hē-pat′ō-bil′ē-ar-ē hep′ă-tī′tis) Interruption of the normal bile flow with resulting inflammation of liver tissue. Caused by cholelithasis or cholestasis. Often linked to the use of oral contraceptives and allopurinols.

hep·a·to·blas·to·ma (hep′ă-tō-blas-tō′mă) A malignant neoplasm occurring in young children, primarily in the liver, composed of tissue resembling embryonal or fetal hepatic epithelium, or mixed epithelial and mesenchymal tissues.

hep·a·to·car·ci·no·ma (hep′ă-tō-kahr-si-nō′mă) SYN malignant hepatoma.

hep·a·to·cele (hĕ-pat′ō-sēl) Protrusion of part of the liver through the abdominal wall or the diaphragm. [hepato- + G. *kēlē,* hernia]

hep·a·to·cel·lu·lar car·ci·no·ma (hep′ă-tō-sel′yū-lăr kahr′si-nō′mă) SYN malignant hepatoma.

hep·a·to·cel·lu·lar jaun·dice (hep′ă-tō-sel′yū-lăr jawn′dis) Liver disorder resulting from diffuse injury or inflammation or failure of function of the hepatic cells, usually referring to viral or toxic hepatitis.

hep·a·to·chol·an·gi·o·je·ju·nos·to·my (hep′ă-tō-kō-lan′jē-ō-jĕ-jū-nos′tŏ-mē) Union of the hepatic duct to the jejunum. [hepato- + G. *cholē,* bile, + *angeion,* vessel, + jejunostomy]

hep·a·to·chol·an·gi·os·to·my (hep′ă-tō-kō-lan′jē-os′tŏ-mē) Creation of an opening into the common bile duct to establish drainage.

hep·a·to·chol·an·gi·tis (hep′ă-tō-kō-lan-jī′tis) Inflammation of the liver and biliary tree.

hep·a·to·cys·tic (hep′ă-tō-sis′tik) Relating to the gallbladder, or to both liver and gallbladder. [hepato- + G. *kystis,* bladder]

hep·a·to·cyte (hep′ă-tō-sīt) A parenchymal liver cell.

hep·a·to·en·ter·ic (hep′ă-tō-en-ter′ik) Relating to the liver and the intestine. [hepato- + G. *enteron,* intestine]

hep·a·to·fu·gal (hep′ă-tō-fyū′găl) Away from the liver, usually referring to portal blood flow.

hep·a·to·gas·tric (hep′ă-tō-gas′trik) Relating to the liver and the stomach.

hep·a·to·gen·ic, hep·a·tog·e·nous (hep′ă-tō-jen′ik, -toj′ĕn-ŭs) Of hepatic origin; formed in the liver.

hep·a·tog·e·nous jaun·dice (hep-ă-toj′ĕn-ŭs jawn′dis) Condition resulting from disease of the liver, as distinguished from that due to blood changes.

hep·a·tog·raphy (hep′ă-tog′ră-fē) Radiography of the liver. [hepato- + G. *graphē,* a writing]

hep·a·toid (hep′ă-toyd) Resembling or like the liver. [hepato- + G. *eidos,* resemblance]

hep·a·to·jug·u·lar re·flux (hep′ă-tō-jŭg′yū-lăr rē′flŭks) An elevation of venous pressure visible in the jugular veins and measurable in the veins of the arm, produced in active or impending congestive heart failure by firm pressure with the flat hand over the liver for 30–60 seconds.

hep·a·to·len·tic·u·lar de·gen·er·a·tion (hep′ă-tō-len-tik′yū-lăr dĕ-jen′ĕr-ā′shŭn) **1.** A familial disorder characterized by copper deposition in the liver, causing chronic hepatitis and eventually cirrhosis; degeneration of the lenticular (pallidal and putaminal) nuclei, and marked hyperplasia of astrocytes in the cerebral cortex, cerebellum, basal ganglia, and brainstem nuclei; plasma levels of ceruloplasmins and copper are decreased, urinary excretion of copper is increased, and the amounts of copper in the liver, brain, and kidneys is high; clinical features include deposition of golden brown pigment in the cornea (Kayser-Fleischer rings), dysphasia and dysarthria, rigidity, and a coarse resting tremor, which increases when the limbs are outstretched ("wing-beating" tremor). **2.** SYN Wilson disease (1).

hep·a·to·lith (hep′ă-tō-lith) A concretion or calculus in the liver. [hepato- + G. *lithos,* stone]

hep·a·to·li·thec·to·my (hep′ă-tō-li-thek′tŏ-mē) Removal of a calculus from the liver. [hepato- + G. *lithos,* stone, + *ektomē,* excision]

hep·a·to·li·thi·a·sis (hep′ă-tō-li-thī′ă-sis) Presence of calculi in the liver. [hepato- + G. *lithiasis,* presence of a calculus]

hep·a·tol·o·gy (hep′ă-tol′ŏ-jē) The branch of medicine concerned with diseases of the liver. [hepato- + G. *logos,* study]

hep·a·tol·y·sin (hep′ă-tol′i-sin) A cytolysin that destroys parenchymal cells of the liver.

hep·a·to·ma (hep′ă-tō′mă) SEE malignant hepatoma. [hepato- + G. *-oma,* tumor]

hep·a·to·meg·a·ly, **hep·a·to·me·ga·li·a** (hep′ă-tō-meg′ă-lē, -mĕ-gā′lē-ă) Enlargement of the liver. SYN megalohepatia. [hepato- + G. *megas,* large]

hep·a·to·mel·a·no·sis (hep′ă-tō-mel-ă-nō′sis) Heavy pigmentation of the liver. [hepato- + G. *melas,* black, + *-osis,* condition]

hep·a·tom·pha·lo·cele (hep′ă-tom′fă-lō-sēl) Umbilical hernia with involvement of the liver. [hepato- + omphalocele]

hep·a·to·neph·ric (hep′ă-tō-nef′rik) SYN hepatorenal.

hep·a·to·pan·cre·at·ic am·pul·la (hep′ă-tō-pan′krē-at′ik am-pul′lă) The dilation within the major duodenal papilla that normally receives both the common bile duct and the main pancreatic duct.

hep·a·to·path·ic (hep′ă-tō-path′ik) Damaging the liver.

hep·a·top·a·thy (hep′ă-top′ă-thē) Disease of the liver. [hepato- + G. *pathos,* suffering]

hep·a·to·pet·al (hep′ă-top′ĕ-tăl) Toward the liver, usually referring to the normal direction of portal blood flow.

hep·a·to·pex·y (hep′ă-tō-pek′sē) Anchoring of the liver to the abdominal wall. [hepato- + G. *pēxis,* fixation]

hep·a·to·pneu·mon·ic (hep′ă-tō-nū-mon′ik) Relating to the liver and the lungs. SYN hepatopulmonary. [hepato- + G. *pneumonikos,* pulmonary]

hep·a·to·por·tal (hep′ă-tō-pōr′tăl) Relating to the portal system of the liver.

hep·a·to·pul·mo·nary (hep′ă-tō-pul′mŏ-nar′ē) SYN hepatopneumonic.

hep·a·to·re·nal (hep′ă-tō-rē′năl) Relating to the liver and the kidney. SYN hepatonephric. [hepato- + L. *renalis,* renal, fr. *renes,* kidneys]

hep·a·to·re·nal syn·drome, **hep·a·to·ne·pho·ric syn·drome** (hep′ă-tō-rē′năl sin′drōm, hep′ă-tō-nĕ-fōr′ik sin′drōm) The occurrence of acute renal failure in patients with disease of the liver or biliary tract.

hep·a·tor·rha·phy (hep′ă-tōr′ă-fē) Suture of a wound of the liver. [hepato- + G. *rhaphē,* a suture]

hep·a·tor·rhex·is (hep′ă-tōr-ek′sis) Rupture of the liver. [hepato- + G. *rhēxis,* rupture]

hep·a·tos·co·py (hep′ă-tos′kŏ-pē) Examination of the liver. [hepato- + G. *skopeō,* to examine]

hep·a·to·sple·ni·tis (hep′ă-tō-splē-nī′tis) Inflammation of the liver and spleen.

hep·a·to·sple·nog·ra·phy (hep′ă-tō-splē-nog′ră-fē) The use of a contrast medium to outline or depict the liver and spleen radiographically.

hep·a·to·splen·o·meg·a·ly (hep′ă-tō-splē-nō-meg′ă-lē) Enlargement of the liver and spleen. [hepato- + G. *splēn,* spleen, + *megas,* large]

hep·a·to·sple·nop·a·thy (hep′ă-tō-splē-nop′ă-thē) Disease of the liver and spleen.

hep·a·tot·o·my (hep′ă-tot′ŏ-mē) Incision into the liver. [hepato- + G. *tomē,* incision]

hepatotoxaemia [Br.] SYN hepatotoxemia.

hep·a·to·tox·e·mi·a (hep′ă-tō-tok-sē′mē-ă) Autointoxication assumed to be due to improper functioning of the liver. SYN hepatotoxaemia. [hepato- + G. *toxikon,* poison, + *haima,* blood]

hep·a·to·tox·ic (hep′ă-tō-tok′sik) Relating to an agent that damages the liver, or pertaining to any such action.

hep·a·to·tox·in (hep′ă-tō-tok′sin) A toxin that is destructive to parenchymal cells of the liver.

♻ **hepta-, hept-** Combining forms denoting seven. Cf. septi-, sept-. [G. *hepta*]

hep·tose (hep′tōs) A sugar with seven carbon atoms in its molecule; e.g., sedoheptulose.

herb (ĕrb) **1.** A plant that lasts for a single season, or more, generally lying close to the ground; no wooden structures within the plant exist; some herbs are used as flavoring agent in the preparation of foodstuffs and in the manufacture of herbals (q.v.). SEE ALSO naturopathic medicine. **2.** Somewhat antiquated slang for marijuana (q.v.).

her·ba de la pas·to·ra (er′bă dā lah pahs-tōr′ă) SYN damiana.

herb·al (ĕr′băl) An imprecise but common usage for any agent in any form intended to improve or affect health; sold over the counter, without prescription and without F.D.A. oversight about potency, appropriateness, or purity. SEE ALSO naturopathic medicine.

herb·al·ist (ĕr′băl-ist) A sometimes trained, but uncertified, healer who provides nonprescription therapies often derived from the classic treatments of Europe, Asia, Africa, and in Native American traditions. SEE ALSO naturopathic medicine.

herb·al med·i·cine (ĕr′băl, hĕr′băl med′i-sin) SEE naturopathic medicine, herbal.

herb·al ther·a·py (ĕr′băl thār′ă-pē) The use of herbs and other plants for their medicinal qualities. SYN phytomedicine, phytotherapy.

herb bath (ĕrb, hĕrb bath) Immersion in a tub of water that is used as an infusion to cure dermatologic or other complaints.

her·bi·cide (ĕr-bi′sīd) Any chemical compound designed to kill plants. Herbicides have been used in military operations for deforestation, but the U.S. military excludes herbicides from being classified as chemical-warfare agents.

herb·i·cide poi·son·ing (ĕr′bi-sīd poy′zŏn-ing) Intoxication or poisoning caused by chemical agents intended to kill insects and other sources of damage to plants; especially common among agricultural workers.

her·biv·o·rous (hĕr-biv′ŏr-ŭs) Feeding exclusively on vegetable foods. Cf. carnivorous.

herb tea (ĕrb tē) An infusion of herbal material in boiling water intended to ameliorate or palliate various disorders.

herd (hĕrd) A group of people or animals in a given area. [O.E. *heord*]

herd im·mu·ni·ty (hĕrd i-myū′ni-tē) The resistance to invasion and spread of an infectious agent in a group or community, based on the resistance to infection of a high proportion of individual members of the group.

herd in·stinct (hĕrd in′stingkt) Tendency or inclination to band together with and share the customs of others of a group, and to conform to the opinions and adopt the views of the group.

he·red·i·tar·y (hĕr-ed′i-tar-ē) Transmissible from parent to offspring by information encoded in the parental germ cell. [L. *hereditarius;* fr. *heres* (*hered-*), an heir]

he·red·i·tar·y be·nign te·lan·gi·ec·ta·si·a (hĕr-ed′i-tar-ē bĕ-nīn′ tel-an′jē-ek-tā′zē-ă) An autosomal dominant disorder in which the face, upper trunk, and arms develop telangiectases.

he·red·i·tar·y cer·e·bel·lar a·tax·i·a (hĕr-ed′i-tar-ē ser′ĕ-bel′ăr ă-tak′sē-ă) **1.** A disease of later childhood and early adult life, marked by ataxic gait, hesitating and explosive speech, nystagmus, and sometimes optic neuritis. **2.** Collective term for a number of hereditary disorders in which cerebellar signs are the most prominent finding.

he·red·i·tar·y cho·re·a (hĕr-ed′i-tar-ē kōr-ē′ă) SYN Huntington chorea.

he·red·i·tar·y club·bing (hĕr-ed′i-tar-ē klŭb′ing) Clubbing of the digits without associated pulmonary or other progressive disease.

he·red·i·tar·y deaf·ness (hĕr-ed′i-tar-ē def′nĕs) SEE hereditary hearing impairment.

he·red·i·tar·y hear·ing im·pair·ment (hĕr-ed′i-tar-ē hēr′ing im-pār′mĕnt) Hearing impairment occurring in syndromic forms (in which there are other anomalies in addition to the hearing impairment) and nonsyndromic forms (in which hearing impairment is the only unusual finding) with autosomal dominant and recessive, X-linked, and mitochondrial modes of transmission; may be congenital, of early onset in childhood, or late onset in mid-life and advanced age.

he·red·i·tar·y non·pol·y·po·sis co·lo·rec·tal can·cer (hĕr-ed′i-tar-ē non′pol-i-pō′sis kō′lŏr-ek′tăl kan′sĕr) An autosomal dominant predisposition to cancer of the colon and rectum.

he·red·i·tar·y pro·gres·sive ar·thro·oph·thal·mop·a·thy (hĕr-ed′i-tar-ē prŏ-gres′iv ahr′thrō-of-thal-mop′ă-thē) A skeletal dysplasia associated with multiple dysplasia of the epiphyses, overtubulation of long bones with metaphysial widening, flattened vertebral bodies, pelvic bone abnormalities, hypermobility of joints, cleft palate, progressive myopia, retinal detachment, and deafness. Autosomal dominant inheritance caused by mutation in either the COL2A1 gene on 12q, COL11A1 gene on 1p, or COL11A2 gene on 6p. SYN Stickler syndrome.

he·red·i·tar·y sphe·ro·cy·to·sis (hĕr-ed′i-tār-ē sfēr′ō-sī-tō′sis) A congenital defect of spectrin, the main component of the erythrocyte cell membrane, which becomes abnormally permeable to sodium, resulting in thickened and almost spheric erythrocytes that are fragile and susceptible to spontaneous hemolysis, with decreased survival in the circulation; results in chronic anemia with reticulocytosis, episodes of mild jaundice due to hemolysis, and acute crises with gallstones, fever, and abdominal pain. SYN familial jaundice, spherocytic anemia.

he·red·i·tar·y spi·nal a·tax·i·a (hĕr-ed′i-tar-ē spī′năl ă-tak′sē-ă) Sclerosis of the posterior and lateral columns of the spinal cord, occurring in children and marked by ataxia in the lower extremities, extending to the upper, followed by paralysis and contractures. SEE ALSO spinocerebellar ataxia.

he·red·i·ty (hĕ-red′i-tē) **1.** The transmission of characteristics from parent to offspring by information encoded in the parental germ cells. **2.** Genealogy. [L. *hereditas,* inheritance, fr. *heres* (*hered-*), heir]

♻**heredo-** Prefix meaning heredity. [L. *heres,* heir]

Her·ing-Breu·er re·flex (her′ing broy′er rē′fleks) The effects of afferent impulses from the pulmonary vagi in the control of respiration, e.g., inflation of the lungs arrests inspiration, with expiration then ensuing, whereas deflation of the lungs brings on inspiration.

Her•ing law (her′ing law) States that paired agonist muscles from each eye operating in the same field of gaze receive equal innervation while paired antagonist muscles receive equal inhibition.

Her•ing nerve (her′ing něrv) Branch of glossopharyngeal nerve running to the carotid sinus; supplies visceral afferent fibers mediating physiologic status to pressure receptors and chemoreceptors.

Her•ing test (her′ing test) A test of binocular vision; the subject looks through an apparatus having at its far end a thread near which a small sphere is dropped; with binocular vision the observer recognizes the location of the sphere in front of or behind the thread; with monocular vision this is not possible.

Her•ing the•o•ry of col•or vi•sion (her′ing thē′ŏr-ē kŏl′ŏr vizh′ŭn) That there are three opponent visual processes: blue-yellow, red-green, and white-black.

her•i•ta•bil•i•ty (her′i-tă-bil′i-tē) **1.** PSYCHOMETRICS a statistical term used to denote the extent of variance of a subject's total score or response that is attributable to a presumed genetic component, in contrast to an acquired component. **2.** GENETICS a statistical term used to denote the proportion of phenotypic variance due to variance in genotypes that is genetically determined, denoted by the traditional symbol h^2. [see heredity]

Her•mann fix•a•tive (her′mahn fiks′ă-tiv) A hardening fixative of glacial acetic acid, osmic acid, and platinum chloride.

her•maph•ro•dite (hĕr-maf′rō-dīt) An individual (e.g., human or animal) with hermaphroditism. [G. *Hermaphroditos,* the son of *Hermēs,* Mercury, + *Aphroditē,* Venus]

her•maph•ro•dit•ism (hĕr-maf′rō-dīt-izm) The presence in one individual of both ovarian and testicular tissue; i.e., true hermaphroditism.

her•met•ic (hĕr-met′ik) Airtight; denoting a vessel closed or sealed in such a way that air can neither enter it nor issue from it.

her•ni•a (hĕr′nē-ă) Protrusion of a part or structure through the tissues normally containing it. SYN rupture (1). [L. rupture]

her•ni•a knife (hĕr′nē-ă nīf) A knife with a slender blade that has a short cutting edge, for dividing the constricting tissues at the mouth of the hernial sac. SYN herniotome.

her•ni•al (hĕr′nē-ăl) Relating to hernia.

her•ni•al sac (hĕr′nē-ăl sak) The peritoneal envelope of a hernia.

her•ni•at•ed (hĕr′nē-ā-tĕd) Denoting any structure protruded through a hernial opening.

i **her•ni•at•ed disc** (hĕr′nē-ā-tĕd disk) Protrusion of a degenerated or fragmented intervertebral disc into the intervertebral foramen with potential compression of a nerve root or into the spinal canal with potential compression of the cauda equina in the lumbar region or the spinal cord at higher levels. See page 711. SYN protruded disc, ruptured disc.

her•ni•a•tion (hĕr′nē-ā′shŭn) Protrusion of an anatomic structure (e.g., intervertebral disc) from its normal anatomic position.

♻ **hernio-** Prefix meaning a hernia. [L. *hernia,* rupture]

her•ni•oid (hĕr′nē-oyd) Resembling hernia. [hernio- + G. *eidos,* resemblance]

her•ni•o•plas•ty (hĕr′nē-ō-plas-tē) SYN herniorrhaphy. [hernio- + G. *plastos,* formed]

her•ni•or•rha•phy (hĕr′nē-ōr′ă-fē) Surgical repair of a hernia. SYN hernioplasty. [hernio- + G. *rhaphē,* a seam]

her•ni•o•tome (her′nē-ō-tōm) SYN hernia knife.

her•ni•ot•o•my (hĕr-nē-ot′ŏ-mē) Surgical division of the constriction or strangulation of a hernia, often followed by herniorrhaphy. [hernio- + G. *tomē,* a cutting]

he•ro•ic (hē-rō′ik) Denoting an aggressive, daring procedure in a dangerously ill patient that may endanger the patient but that also has a possibility of being successful, whereas lesser action would result in failure. [G. *hērōikos,* pertaining to a hero]

her•o•in (H) (her′ō-in) An alkaloid prepared from morphine by acetylation; formerly used for the relief of cough. Except for research, its use in the United States is prohibited by federal law because of its potential for abuse. Epidemic levels of addiction have been reported in the Vancouver, British Columbia, Downtown East-Side district, but rates of addiction are also high in Montréal.

her•pan•gi•na (hĕr-pan′ji-nă) A disease caused by types of coxsackievirus and marked by vesiculopapular lesions around the fauces that break down to form grayish yellow ulcers. [G. *herpēs,* vesicular eruption, + L. *angina,* quinsy, fr. *ango,* to strangle]

her•pes (her′pēz) A papular, vesicular, or ulcerative eruption of skin or mucous membranes caused by local infection with herpesvirus 1 or 2 (herpes simplex) or by reactivation of the varicella-zoster virus. SYN serpigo (2). [G. *herpēs,* a spreading skin eruption, shingles, fr. *herpō,* to creep]

her•pes cor•ne•ae (hĕr′pēz kōr′nē-ē) SYN herpetic keratitis.

her•pes fa•ci•a•lis (hĕr′pēz fā-sē-ā′lis) SYN herpes simplex.

her·pes feb·ri·lis (hĕr′pēz feb-rī′lis) SYN herpes simplex.

her·pes gen·i·tal·is (hĕr′pēz jen-i-tā′lis) SYN genital herpes.

her·pes ges·ta·ti·o·nis (hĕr′pēz jes-tā′shē-ō′nis) A polymorphous, bullous eruption beginning in the second or third trimester of pregnancy, flaring about the time of delivery, and subsequently resolving.

her·pes i·ris (her′pēz ī′ris) **1.** SYN erythema iris. **2.** SYN erythema multiforme.

her·pes la·bi·a·lis (hĕr′pēz lā-bē-ā′lis) SYN herpes simplex.

her·pes men·stru·a·lis (hĕr′pēz men′strū-ā′lis) Recurrence of herpes simplex during menses.

her·pes sim·plex (her′pēz sim′pleks) A variety of infections caused by herpesvirus types 1 and 2; type 1 infections are marked most commonly by the eruption of one or more groups of vesicles on the vermilion border of the lips or at the external nares, type 2 by such lesions on the genitalia; both types often are recrudescent and reappear during other febrile illnesses or even physiologic states such as menstruation. See page 712. SYN herpes facialis, herpes febrilis, herpes labialis, Simplexvirus.

her·pes sim·plex en·ceph·a·li·tis (hĕr′pēz sim′pleks en-sef′ă-lī′tis) The most common acute encephalitis, caused by HSV-1; affects people of any age; preferentially involves the inferomedial portions of the temporal lobe and the orbital portions of the frontal lobes; pathologically, severe hemorrhagic necrosis is present along with, in the acute stages, intranuclear eosinophilic inclusion bodies in the neurons and glial cells.

her·pes sim·plex test (hĕr′pēz sim′pleks test) Clinical or laboratory hematologic or microscopic assessment of the presence of herpes simplex virus.

her·pes sim·plex vi·rus (HSV) (hĕr′pēz sim′pleks vī′rŭs) SEE herpes simplex.

her·pes·vi·rus, her·pes vi·rus (hĕr′pēz-vī′

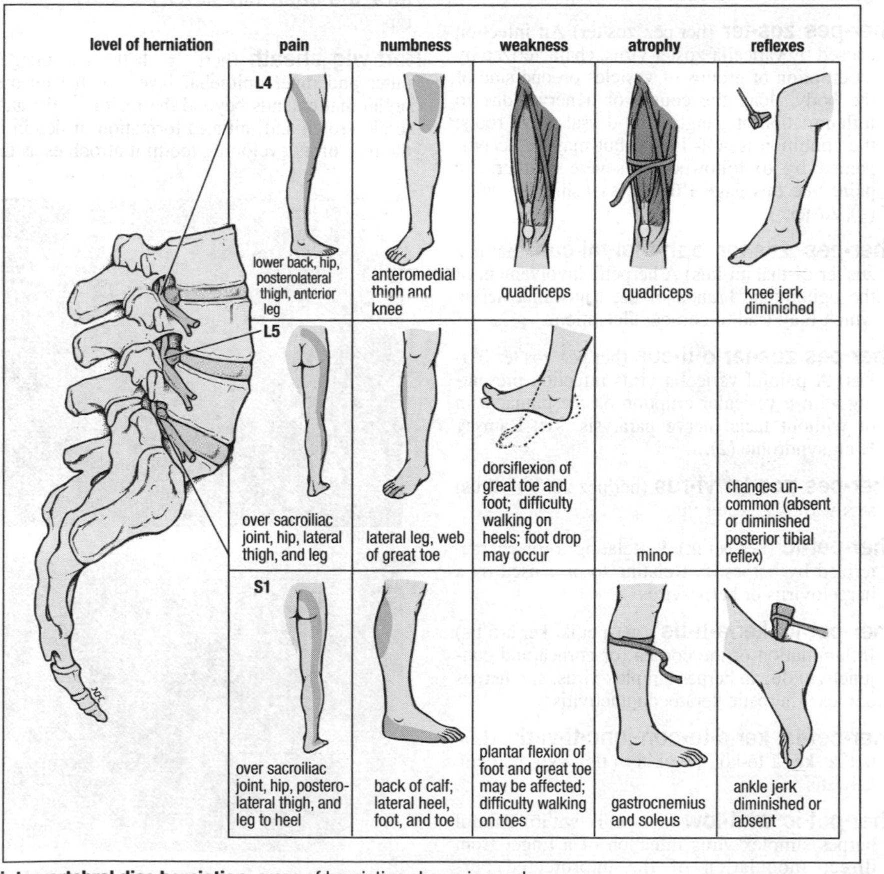

level of herniation
pain
numbness
weakness
atrophy
reflexes
L4
lower back, hip, posterolateral thigh, anterior leg
anteromedial thigh and knee
quadriceps
quadriceps
knee jerk diminished
L5
over sacroiliac joint, hip, lateral thigh, and leg
lateral leg, web of great toe
dorsiflexion of great toe and foot; difficulty walking on heels; foot drop may occur
minor
changes uncommon (absent or diminished posterior tibial reflex)
S1
over sacroiliac joint, hip, posterolateral thigh, and leg to heel
back of calf; lateral heel, foot, and toe
plantar flexion of foot and great toe may be affected; difficulty walking on toes
gastrocnemius and soleus
ankle jerk diminished or absent

intervertebral disc herniation: areas of herniation shown in purple

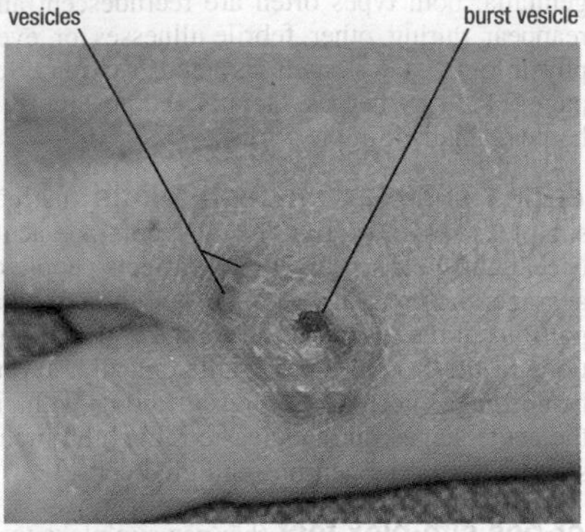

herpes simplex infection: hand involvement

rŭs, herʹpēz vīʹrŭs) Any virus belonging to the family Herpesviridae.

her•pes•vi•rus sai•mi•ri (hĕrʹpēz-vīʹrŭs sī-mirʹē) The cause of an ubiquitous infection of squirrel monkeys, which is highly oncogenic when injected into other monkey species.

her•pes zos•ter (hĕrʹpēz zosʹtĕr) An infection caused by varicella-zoster virus, characterized by an eruption of groups of vesicles on one side of the body along the course of a nerve, due to inflammation of ganglia and dorsal nerve roots; the condition is self-limited but may be accompanied by or followed by severe postherpetic pain. See this page B6, B9. SYN shingles, zona (2), zoster.

her•pes zos•ter oph•thal•mi•cus (hĕrʹpēz zosʹtĕr of-thalʹmi-kŭs) A herpetic involvement of the ophthalmic branch of the trigeminal nerve, which may lead to corneal ulceration.

her•pes zos•ter o•ti•cus (hĕrʹpēz zosʹtĕr ōʹti-kŭs) A painful varicella virus infection presenting with a vesicular eruption on the pinna, with or without facial nerve paralysis. SYN Ramsay Hunt syndrome (2).

her•pes zos•ter vi•rus (hĕrʹpēz zosʹtĕr vīʹrŭs) SYN varicella-zoster virus.

her•pet•ic (hĕr-petʹik) **1.** Relating to or characterized by herpes. **2.** Relating to or caused by a herpetovirus or herpesvirus.

her•pet•ic ker•a•ti•tis (hĕr-petʹik kerʹă-tīʹtis) Inflammation of the cornea (or cornea and conjunctiva) due to herpes simplex virus. SYN herpes corneae, herpetic keratoconjunctivitis.

her•pet•ic ker•a•to•con•junc•ti•vi•tis (hĕr-petʹik kerʹă-tō-kŏn-jŭngkʹti-vīʹtis) SYN herpetic keratitis.

her•pet•ic whit•low (hĕr-petʹik witʹlō) Painful herpes simplex virus infection of a finger from direct inoculation of the unprotected perionychial fold, often accompanied by lymphangitis and regional adenopathy, lasting up to several weeks; most common in physicians, dentists, and nurses as a result of exposure to the virus in a patient's mouth. Some older sources term this condition felon. See page 713.

her•pet•i•form (hĕr-petʹi-fōrm) Resembling herpes.

her•pet•i•form aph•thae (hĕr-petʹi-fōrm afʹthē) A variant of oral aphthae, of unknown etiology, characterized by up to several dozen ulcers, 2–3 mm in diameter, organized in a clustered herpetiform distribution.

Herr•mann syn•drome (hĕrʹmăn sinʹdrōm) A multisystem disorder beginning in late childhood or early adolescence, with photomyoclonus and hearing loss followed by diabetes mellitus, progressive dementia, pyelonephritis, and glomerulonephritis; progressive sensorineural hearing loss is of later onset; probably autosomal dominant inheritance with incomplete penetrance.

her•sage (ār-sahzhʹ) Separating the individual fibers of a nerve trunk. [Fr. (from L. *hirpex*, a large rake), a harrowing]

Hers dis•ease (ārz di-zēzʹ) SYN glycogenosis type 6.

Hert•wig sheath (hertʹvig shēth) The merged outer and inner epithelial layers of the enamel organ that extends beyond the region of the anatomic crown and initiates formation of dentin in the root of a developing tooth; it atrophies as the

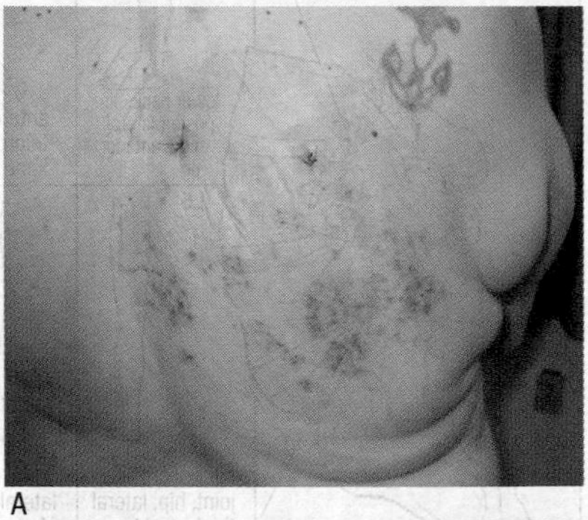
A

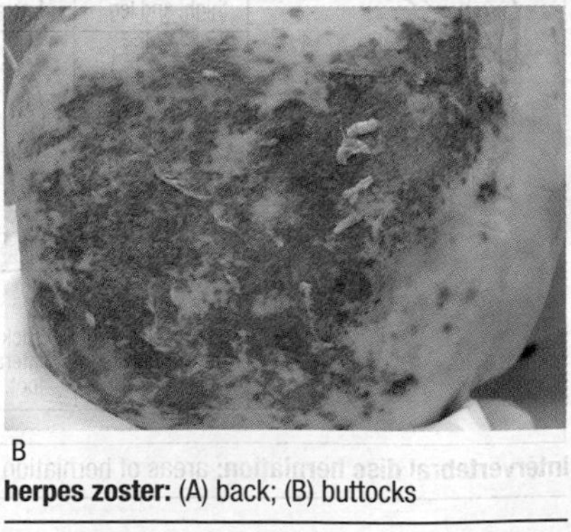
B

herpes zoster: (A) back; (B) buttocks

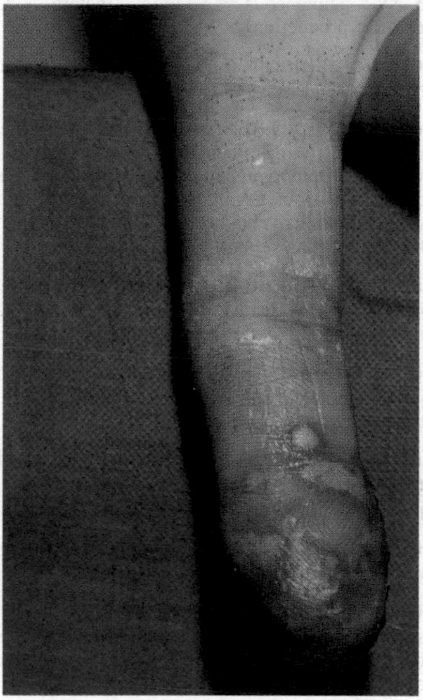

herpetic whitlow (felon): index finger

root is formed, and any of the cells that persist are called Malassez epithelial rests.

hertz (Hz) (hĕrts) A unit of sound or alternating current frequency, 1 Hz is equivalent to 1 cycle per second. [H.R. *Hertz*]

Herx•hei•mer re•ac•tion (herks′hīm-er rē-ak′shŭn) A systemic inflammatory reaction affecting the skin, mucous membranes, nervous system, or viscera occurring after antimicrobial treatment of treponemal disease (e.g., syphilis, Lyme disease); believed to be due to a rapid release of treponemal antigen with an associated allergic reaction in the patient. SYN Jarisch-Herxheimer reaction.

hes•i•tan•cy (hez′i-tăns-ē) An involuntary delay or inability in starting the urinary stream.

hes•i•tant (hez′i-tănt) Term used to descibe the state of RNA polymerase when it is susceptible to pause, arrest, or termination signals. SEE ALSO overdrive, antitermination.

Hes•sel•bach her•ni•a (hes′ĕl-bahk hĕr′nē-ă) Hernia with diverticula through the cribriform fascia, presenting a lobular outline.

Hes•sel•bach tri•an•gle (hes′ĕl-bahk trī′ang-gĕl) SYN inguinal triangle.

Hess law (hes law) The amount of heat generated by a reaction is the same whether the reaction takes place in one step or several steps; i.e., ΔH values (and thus ΔG values) are additive.

heteraesthesia [Br.] SYN heteresthesia.

het•er•ax•i•al (het′ĕr-ak′sē-ăl) Having mutually perpendicular axes of unequal length.

het•er•e•cious (het′ĕr-ē′shŭs) Having more than one host; said of a parasite passing different stages of its life cycle in different animals. [heter- + G. *oikion,* home]

het•er•e•cism (het′ĕr-ē-sizm) The occurrence, in a parasite, of two cycles of development passed in two different hosts. [heter- + G. *oikion,* home]

het•er•es•the•si•a (het′ĕr-es-thē′zē-ă) A change occurring in the degree (either plus or minus) of the sensory response to a cutaneous stimulus as the latter crosses a certain line on the surface. SYN heteraesthesia. [heter- + G. *aisthēsis,* sensation]

♻ hetero-, heter- Combining forms meaning the other, different; opposite of homo-. [G. *heteros,* other]

het•er•o•ag•glu•ti•nin (het′ĕr-ō-ă-glū′ti-nin) A form of hemagglutinin, which agglutinates the red blood cells of species other than that in which the heteroagglutinin occurs. SEE ALSO hemagglutinin.

het•er•o•an•ti•bod•y (het′ĕr-ō-an′ti-bod-ē) Antibody that is heterologous with respect to antigen, in contradistinction to isoantibody.

het•er•o•an•ti•se•rum (het′ĕr-ō-an′tē-sēr′ŭm) Antiserum developed in one animal species against antigens or cells of another species.

het•er•o•blas•tic (het′er-ō-blas′tik) Developing from more than a single type of tissue. [hetero- + G. *blastos,* germ]

het•er•o•cel•lu•lar (het′ĕr-ō-sel′yū-lăr) Formed of cells of different kinds.

het•er•o•chro•ma•tin (het′ĕr-ō-krō′mă-tin) The part of the chromonema that remains tightly coiled and condensed during interphase and thus stains readily.

het•er•o•chro•mi•a (het′ĕr-ō-krō′mē-ă) A difference in coloration in two structures that are normally alike in color. [hetero- + G. *chrōma,* color]

het•er•o•chro•mic u•ve•i•tis (het′ĕr-ō-krō′mik yū′vē-ī′tis) Anterior uveitis and depigmentation of the iris. SYN Fuchs uveitis.

het•er•o•chro•mo•some (het′ĕr-ō-krō′mō-sōm) SYN allosome.

het•er•o•chro•mous (het′ĕr-ō-krō′mŭs) Having an abnormal difference in coloration.

het•er•o•chro•ni•a (het′ĕr-ō-krō′nē-ă) Origin or development of tissues or organs at an unusual time or out of the regular sequence. Cf. synchronia. [hetero- + G. *chronos,* time]

het•er•o•chron•ic (het′er-ō-kron′ik) SYN heterochronous.

het•er•och•ro•nous (het′ĕr-ok′rŏ-nŭs) Relating to heterochronia. SYN heterochronic.

het•er•o•crine (het′ĕr-ō-krin) Denoting the secretion of two or more kinds of material. Cf. bioregulator. [hetero- + G. *krinō,* to separate]

het•er•o•cy•to•tro•pic (het′ĕr-ō-sī′tō-trō′pik) Having an affinity for cells of a different species. [hetero- + G. *kytos,* cell, + *tropē,* a turning toward]

het•er•o•cy•to•tro•pic an•ti•bod•y (het′ĕr-ō-sī′tō-trō′pik an′ti-bod-ē) A cytotropic antibody (chiefly of the IgG class) similar in activity to homocytotropic antibody, but having an affinity for cells of a different species rather than for cells of the same or a closely related species.

het•er•o•dont (het′ĕr-ō-dont) Having teeth that are morphologically different, as in humans. [hetero- + G. *odous,* tooth]

het•er•od•ro•mous (het′ĕr-od′rŏ-mŭs) Moving in the opposite direction. [hetero- + G. *dromos,* running]

het•er•o•e•rot•ic (het′ĕr-ō-ĕr-ot′ik) SYN alloerotic.

het•er•o•er•o•tism (het′ĕr-ō-er′ŏ-tizm) SYN alloerotism.

het•er•o•ga•met•ic (het′ĕr-ō-gă-met′ik) Having sex gametes of contrasting types; human males are heterogametic. [hetero- + G. *gametikos,* connubial]

het•er•og•a•mous (het′ĕr-og′ă-mŭs) Relating to heterogamy.

het•er•og•a•my (het′ĕr-og′ă-mē) **1.** Conjugation of unlike gametes. **2.** Bearing different types of flowers. **3.** Reproduction by indirect methods of pollination. [hetero- + G. *gamos,* marriage]

het•er•o•ge•ne•i•ty (het′ĕr-ō-jĕ-nē′i-tē) Heterogeneous state or quality.

het•er•o•ge•ne•ous (het′ĕr-ō-jē′nē-ŭs) Comprising elements with various and dissimilar properties.

het•er•o•ge•ne•ous ra•di•a•tion (het′ĕr-ō-jē′nē-ŭs rā′dē-ā′shŭn) Radiation consisting of different frequencies, various energies, or a variety of particles.

het•er•o•ge•ne•ous sys•tem (het′ĕr-ō-jē′nē-ŭs sis′tĕm) CHEMISTRY a system that contains various distinct and mechanically separable parts or phases; e.g., a suspension or an emulsion.

het•er•o•gen•e•sis (het′ĕr-ō-jen′ĕ-sis) **1.** Alternation of generations. **2.** SYN asexual generation. **3.** SYN spontaneous generation. [hetero- + G. *genesis,* production]

het•er•o•ge•net•ic (het′ĕr-ō-jĕ-net′ik) Relating to heterogenesis.

het•er•o•ge•net•ic an•ti•gen (het′ĕr-ō-jĕ-net′ik an′ti-jen) An antigen that is possessed by a variety of phylogenetically unrelated species; e.g., the various organ- or tissue-specific antigens, the alpha- and beta-crystalline protein of the lens of the eye, and Forssman antigen.

het•er•o•ge•net•ic par•a•site (het′ĕr-ō-jĕ-net′ik par′ă-sīt) A parasite with a life cycle that involves an alternation of generations.

het•er•o•gen•ic, het•er•o•ge•ne•ic (het′ĕr-ō-jen′ik, -jĕ-nē′ik) Having different gene constitutions, especially in diverse species.

het•er•o•gen•ic en•ter•o•bac•te•ri•al an•ti•gen (het′ĕr-ō-jen′ik en′tĕr-ō-bak-tēr′ē-ăl an′ti-jen) SYN common antigen.

het•er•og•e•nous (het′ĕr-oj′ĕ-nŭs) Of foreign origin. Commonly confused with heterogeneous.

het•er•o•gon•ic life cy•cle (het′ĕr-ō-gon′ik līf sī′kĕl) Free-living stage of the life cycle of an organism (e.g., *Strongyloides stercoralis*) that also has a parasitic stage.

het•er•o•graft (het′ĕr-ō-graft) SYN xenograft.

het•er•o•ki•ne•sis (het′ĕr-ō-ki-nē′sis) Differential distribution of X and Y chromosomes during meiotic cell division. [hetero- + G. *kinēsis,* movement]

het•er•o•la•li•a (het′ĕr-ō-lā′lē-ă) The habitual substitution of meaningless or inappropriate words for those intended; a form of aphasia. SYN heterophemia, heterophemy. [hetero- + G. *lalia,* speech]

het•er•o•lat•er•al (het′ĕr-ō-lat′ĕr-ăl) SYN contralateral. [hetero- + L. *latus,* side]

het•er•ol•o•gous (het′ĕr-ol′ŏ-gŭs) **1.** Pertaining to cytologic or histologic elements occurring where they are not normally found. SEE ALSO xenogeneic. **2.** Derived from an animal of a different species; thus the serum of a horse is heterologous for a rabbit. [hetero- + G. *logos,* ratio, relation]

het•er•ol•o•gous graft (het′ĕr-ol′ŏ-gŭs graft) SYN xenograft.

het•er•ol•o•gous stim•u•lus (het′ĕr-ol′ŏ-gŭs stim′yū-lŭs) A stimulus that acts on any part of the sensory apparatus or nerve tract.

het•er•ol•o•gous tu•mor (het′ĕr-ol′ŏ-gŭs tū′mŏr) A tumor composed of a tissue unlike that from which it springs.

het•er•ol•o•gous twins (het′ĕr-ol′ŏ-gŭs twinz) SYN dizygotic twins.

het•er•ol•y•sis (het′ĕr-ol′i-sis) Dissolution or

digestion of cells or protein components from one species by a lytic agent from a different species. [hetero- + G. *lysis,* a loosening]

het•er•o•lyt•ic (het′ĕr-ō-lit′ik) Pertaining to heterolysis or to the effect of a heterolysin.

het•er•o•mer•ic (het′ĕr-ō-mer′ik) **1.** Having a different chemical composition. **2.** Denoting spinal neurons that have processes passing over to the opposite side of the cord. [hetero- + G. *meros,* part]

het•er•o•met•a•pla•si•a (het′ĕr-ō-met-ă-plā′zē-ă) Tissue transformation resulting in production of a tissue foreign to the part where produced.

het•er•o•met•ric au•to•reg•u•la•tion (het′ĕr-ō-met′rik aw′tō-reg-yŭ-lā′shŭn) Intrinsic regulation of the strength of cardiac contraction as a function of diastolic fiber length (volume), independent of afterload, autonomic nerves, and other extrinsic influences. Heterometric autoregulation is also known as the length-tension relationship, the relationship of end diastolic volume to end diastolic pressure, Starling law of the heart, and the Frank-Starling mechanism.

het•er•o•me•tro•pi•a (het′ĕr-ō-mĕ-trō′pē-ă) A condition in which the refraction is different in the two eyes. SYN anisometropia. [hetero- + G. *metron,* measure, + *ōps,* eye]

het•er•o•mor•pho•sis (het′ĕr-ō-mōr-fō′sis) **1.** Development of one tissue from tissue of another kind or type. **2.** Embryonic development of tissue or an organ inappropriate to its site. [hetero- + G. *morphōsis,* a molding]

het•er•o•mor•phous (het′ĕr-ō-mōr′fŭs) Differing from the normal form.

het•er•on•o•mous (het′ĕr-on′ŏ-mŭs) **1.** Different from the type; abnormal. **2.** Subject to the direction or control of another; not self-governing. [hetero- + G. *nomos,* law]

het•er•on•o•my (het′ĕr-on′ŏ-mē) The condition or state of being heteronomous. [hetero- + G. *nomos,* law]

het•er•op•a•thy (het′ĕr-op′ă-thē) **1.** Abnormal sensitivity to stimuli. **2.** SYN allopathy. [hetero- + G. *pathos,* suffering]

het•er•oph•a•gy (het′ĕr-of′ă-jē) Digestion within a cell of a substance phagocytized from without. [hetero- + G. *phagō,* to eat]

het•er•o•phe•mi•a, **het•er•oph•e•my** (het′ĕr-ō-fē′mē-ă, -of′ĕ-mē) SYN heterolalia. [hetero- + G. *phēmē,* a speech]

het•er•o•phil, **het•er•o•phile** (het′ĕr-ō-fil, -fīl) **1.** The neutrophilic leukocyte. **2.** Pertaining to heterogenetic antigens occurring in different species or to antibodies directed against such antigens. [hetero- + G. *philos,* fond]

het•er•o•pho•ni•a (het′ĕr-ō-fō′nē-ă) **1.** The change of voice at puberty. **2.** Any abnormality in the voice sounds. [hetero- + G. *phōnē,* voice]

het•er•o•pho•ri•a (het′ĕr-ō-fōr′ē-ă) A tendency for deviation of the eyes from parallelism, prevented by binocular vision. [hetero- + G. *phora,* movement]

het•er•oph•thal•mus (het′ĕr-of-thal′mŭs) A seldom-used term for a difference in the appearance of the two eyes, usually due to heterochromia iridis. [hetero- + G. *ophthalmos,* eye]

het•er•o•phy•i•a•sis (het′ĕr-ō-fī-ī′ă-sis) Infection with a heterophyid trematode, particularly *Heterophyes heterophyes.*

het•er•o•pla•si•a (het′ĕr-ō-plā′zē-ă) **1.** Development of cytologic and histologic elements that are not normal for the organ or part in question (e.g., the growth of bone in a site where there is normally fibrous connective tissue). **2.** Malposition of tissue or a part that is otherwise normal (e.g., a ureter that develops at the lower pole of a kidney). [hetero- + G. *plasis,* a forming]

het•er•o•plas•tic (het′ĕr-ō-plas′tik) **1.** Pertaining to or manifesting heteroplasia. **2.** Relating to heteroplasty.

het•er•o•ploid (het′ĕr-ō-ployd) Relating to heteroploidy.

het•er•o•ploi•dy (het′ĕr-ō-ploy-dē) The state of a cell possessing some number of complete haploid sets other than the normal. [hetero- + G. *ploides,* in form]

het•er•o•pyk•no•sis (het′ĕr-ō-pik-nō′sis) Any state of variable density or condensation, usually in different chromosomes or between different regions of the same chromosome; a region may be attentuated (negative heteropyknosis) or accentuated (positive heterpyknosis). [hetero- + G. *pyknos,* dense]

het•er•o•pyk•not•ic (het′ĕr-ō-pik-not′ik) Relating to or characterized by heteropyknosis.

het•er•o•re•cep•tor (het′ĕr-ō-rĕ-sep′tōr) A site on a neuron that binds a modulatory neuroregulator other than that released by the neuron. [hetero- + receptor]

het•er•o•sex•ism (het′ĕr-ō-sek′sizm) A belief that heterosexuality is the only normal and acceptable sexual orientation and is superior to other orientations. Heterosexism discriminates against and excludes people on the basis of sexual orientation.

het•er•o•sex•u•al (het′ĕr-ō-sek′shū-ăl) **1.** A person whose sexual orientation is toward people of the opposite sex. **2.** Relating to or characteristic of heterosexuality. **3.** One whose interests and behavior are characteristic of heterosexuality.

het•er•o•sex•u•al•i•ty (het′ĕr-ō-sek′shū-al′i-tē) Erotic attraction, predisposition, or activity, including sexual congress, between persons of the opposite sex.

het•er•o•sug•ges•tion (het′ĕr-ō-sŭg-jes′chŭn) Hypnotic suggestion received from another person; opposed to autosuggestion.

het•er•o•tax•i•a (het′ĕr-ō-taks′ē-ă) Abnormal arrangement of organs or parts of the body in relation to each other. [hetero- + G. *taxis,* arrangement]

het•er•o•tax•ic (het′ĕr-ō-taks′ik) Abnormally placed or arranged.

het•er•o•to•ni•a (het′ĕr-ō-tō′nē-ă) Abnormality or variation in tension or tonus. [hetero- + G. *tonos,* tension]

het•er•o•to•pi•a (het′ĕr-ō-tō′pē-ă) **1.** SYN ectopia. **2.** NEUROPATHOLOGY displacement of gray matter, typically into the deep cerebral white matter. [hetero- + G. *topos,* place]

het•er•o•top•ic (het′ĕr-ō-top′ik) **1.** SYN ectopic (1). **2.** Relating to heterotopia (2). [hetero- + *topos*, place, + suffix *-ic*, pertaining to]

het•er•o•top•ic os•si•fi•ca•tion (het′ĕr-ō-top′ik os′i-fi-kā′shŭn) Growth of calcium deposits within soft tissue, usually at the site of a hematoma due to blunt trauma or in tissue atrophied due to central nervous system injury. SYN myositis ossificans.

het•er•ot•o•pous (het′ĕr-ot′ŏ-pŭs) Heterotopic, especially in reference to teratomas composed of tissues that are out of place in the region where found.

het•er•o•trans•plan•ta•tion (het′ĕr-ō-trans-plan-tā′shŭn) Transfer of a heterograft (xenograft).

het•er•o•tri•cho•sis (het′ĕr-ō-tri-kō′sis) A condition characterized by hair growth of variegated color. [hetero- + G. *trichōsis,* growth of hair]

het•er•o•troph (het′ĕr-ō-trōf) A microorganism that obtains its carbon, as well as its energy, from organic compounds. SEE ALSO autotroph. [hetero- + G. *trophē,* nourishment]

het•er•o•tro•phic (het′ĕr-ō-trō′fik) **1.** Relating to or exhibiting the properties of heterotrophy. **2.** Relating to a heterotroph.

het•er•o•tro•pi•a, **het•er•ot•ro•py** (het′ĕr-ō-trō′pē-ă, -ot′rō-pē) SYN strabismus. [hetero- + G. *tropē,* a turning]

het•er•o•trop•ic preg•nan•cies (het′ĕr-ō-trō′pik preg′năn-sēz) Pregnancies occurring simultaneously in different sites, e.g., intrauterine and ampullary.

het•er•o•typ•ic (het′ĕr-ō-tip′ik) Of a different or unusual type or form.

het•er•o•typ•i•cal chro•mo•some (het′ĕr-ō-tip′i-kăl krō′mŏ-sōm) SYN allosome.

het•er•o•typ•ic cor•tex (het′ĕr-ō-tip′ik kōr′teks) SYN allocortex.

het•er•o•xan•thine (het′ĕr-ō-zan′thēn) 7-Methylxanthine; one of the alloxuric bases in urine, representing end products of purine metabolism.

het•er•ox•e•nous (het′ĕr-oks′ĕ-nŭs) SYN digenetic (1). [hetero- + G. *xenos,* stranger]

het•er•ox•e•nous par•a•site (het′ĕr-oks′ĕ-nŭs par′ă-sīt) A parasite that has more than one obligatory host in its life cycle.

het•er•o•zy•gos•i•ty, **het•er•o•zy•go•sis** (het′ĕr-ō-zī-gos′i-tē, -zī-gō′sis) The state of being heterozygous. [hetero- + G. *zygon,* a yoke]

het•er•o•zy•gote (het′ĕr-ō-zī′gōt) A heterozygous individual. [hetero- + G. *zygotos,* yoked]

het•er•o•zy•gous (het′ĕr-ō-zī′gŭs) Having different allelic genes at one locus or (by extension) many loci; heterotic.

Heub•ner ar•te•ri•tis (hoyb′ner ahr′tĕr-ī′tis) Inflammation of arteries within the circle of Willis secondary to chronic basal meningitis from tubercle bacillus or a fungus such as *Cryptococcus*, *Histoplasma*, or *Coccidiodes*.

HEV Abbreviation for hepatitis E virus.

♻**hexa-**, **hex-** Combining forms meaning six. [G. *hex*]

hex•ad (heks′ad) A sexivalent element or radical.

hex•a•dac•ty•ly, **hex•a•dac•tyl•ism** (hek′să-dak′ti-lē, -lizm) The presence of six fingers or six toes on one or both hands or feet. [hexa- + G. *daktylos,* finger]

hex•ad•no•vi•rus (heks-ad′nō-vī′rŭs) A genus in the family Hepadnaviridae, which is the cause of hepatitis B.

hex•a•mer (heks′ă-mĕr) **1.** SEE virion. **2.** A complex or compound containing six subunits or moieties. [hexa- + G. *meros,* part]

hex•ane (heks′ān) A saturated hydrocarbon, C_6H_{14}, of the paraffin series.

hex•a•ploi•dy (heks′ă-ploy-dē) SEE polyploidy.

hex•i•tol (heks′i-tol) The polyol (sugar alcohol) obtained on the reduction of a hexose (e.g., D-sorbitol).

hex•o•ki•nase (heks′ō-kī′nās) A phosphotransferase present in yeast, muscle, brain, and other tissues that catalyzes the phosphorylation of D-glucose and other hexoses to form D-glucose 6-phosphate (or other hexose 6-phosphate) (phosphate is transferred from ATP, which is converted to ADP); the first step in glycolysis; a deficiency of hexokinase can result in hemolytic anemia and impaired glycolysis.

hex•o•ki•nase meth•od (heks′ō-kī′nās meth′ŏd) The most specific method for measuring glucose in serum or plasma, involving hexokinase,

ATP, glucose 6-phosphate NADP, and glucose 6-phosphate dehydrogenase.

hex•one ba•ses, his•tone ba•ses (heks′ōn bās′ēz, his′tōn) The α-amino acids arginine, histidine, and lysine, which are basic by virtue of the presence in the side chains of a guanidine, imidazole, and amine group, respectively.

hex•os•a•mine (heks-;ōs′ă-mēn) The amine derivative (NH_2 replacing OH) of a hexose (e.g., glucosamine).

hex•os•a•min•i•dase (heks-ōs′ă-min′i-dās) General term for enzymes cleaving *N*-acetylhexose residues from gangliosidelike oligosaccharides.

hex•o•sans (hek′sō-sanz) Polysaccharides with the general formula $(C_6H_{10}O_5)_x$ that, on hydrolysis, yield hexoses; included are glucosans (glucans), mannans, galactans, and fructosans (fructans).

hex•ose (heks′ōs) A monosaccharide containing six carbon atoms in the molecule ($C_6H_{12}O_6$); D-glucose is the principal hexose in nature.

hex•ose phos•pha•tase (heks′ōs fos′fă-tās) An enzyme catalyzing the hydrolysis of a hexose phosphate to a hexose (e.g., glucose-6-phosphatase).

hex•u•lose (heks′yū-lōs) SYN ketohexose.

hex•yl (heks′il) The radical of hexane, $CH_3(CH_2)_4CH_2$-.

Hey am•pu•ta•tion (hā amp′yū-tā′shŭn) Amputation of the foot in front of the tarsometatarsal joint.

Heyde syn•drome (hād sin′drōm) A gastrointestinal disorder involving hemorrhage and anemia secondary to aortic valve stenosis. These symptoms resolve after repair or replacement of the damaged aortic valve.

Hey•er-Pu•denz valve (hī′ĕr-pū′denz valv) A valve used in the shunting procedure for hydrocephaly; consisting of a catheter-valve system in which the ventricular catheter leads the cerebrospinal fluid into a one-way pump through which the cerebrospinal fluid passes down the distal catheter into the right atrium of the heart.

Hey her•ni•a (hā hĕr′nē-ă) SYN Cooper hernia.

Hf Symbol for hafnium.

HFO Abbreviation for high frequency oscillation.

HFPPV Abbreviation for high frequency positive pressure ventilation.

HFPV Abbreviation for high frequency percussive ventilation.

HFV Abbreviation for high-frequency ventilation.

Hg Symbol for mercury (hydrargyrum).

Hgb Abbreviation for hemoglobin.

HGE Abbreviation for human granulocytic ehrlichiosis.

HGF Abbreviation for hematopoietic growth factor; human growth factor; hyperglycemic-glycogenolytic factor.

HGSIL Abbreviation for high-grade squamous intraepithelial lesion.

HGV Abbreviation for hepatitis G virus.

H&H Abbreviation for hemoglobin and hematocrit.

HHIE-S Hearing Handicap Inventory for the Elderly screening form.

HHS Abbreviation for U.S. Department of Health and Human Services.

hi•a•tal (hī-ā′tăl) Relating to a hiatus.

hi•a•tal her•ni•a, hi•a•tus her•ni•a (hī-ā′tăl hĕr′nē-ă, hī-ā′tŭs hĕr′nē-ă) Protrusion of a part of the stomach through the esophageal hiatus of the diaphragm. See this page.

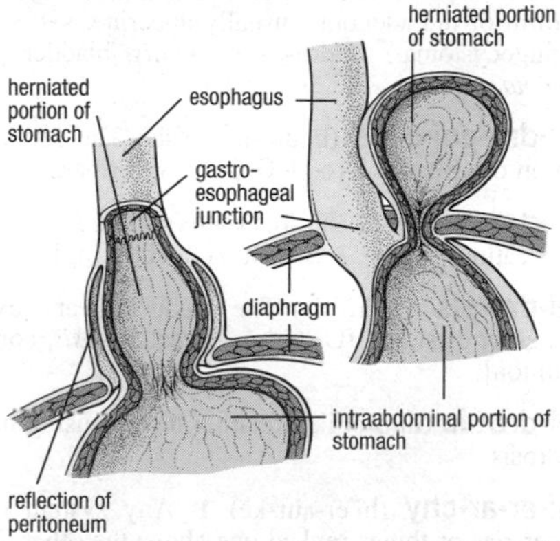

sliding esophageal and paraesophageal hernias: in sliding esophageal hernias (left), the upper stomach and cardioesophageal junction slide in and out of the thorax; in paraesophageal hernias (right), all or part of the stomach pushes through the diaphragm next to the gastroesophageal junction

hi•a•tus, pl. **hi•a•tus** (hī-ā′tŭs) An aperture, opening, or foramen. [L. an aperture, fr. *hio*, pp. *hiatus,* to yawn]

hi•a•tus of ca•nal of les•ser pe•tro•sal nerve (hī-ā′tŭs kă-nal′ les′ĕr pĕ-trō′săl nĕrv) The small opening in the petrous bone lateral to the hiatus of facial canal that gives passage to the lesser petrosal nerve.

Hib Vaccine given to children against *Haemophilus influenzae* serotype B meningitis.

hi•ber•na•ting gland (hī′bĕr-nāt-ing gland) SYN brown fat.

hi•ber•no•ma (hī′bĕr-nō′mă) A rare benign neoplasm consisting of brown fat that resembles the fat in certain hibernating animals. [L. *hibernus,* pertaining to winter, + G. *-ōma,* tumor]

hic•cup, hic•cough (hik′ŭp, hik′ŭp) A diaphragmatic spasm causing a sudden inhalation that is interrupted by a spasmodic closure of the glottis, producing a noise.

hi•drad•e•ni•tis (hī′drad-ĕ-nī′tis) Inflammation of the sweat glands. [G. *hidrōs,* sweat, + *adēn,* gland, + *-itis,* inflammation]

hi•drad•e•ni•tis sup•pu•ra•ti•va (hī′drad-ĕ-nī′tis sŭp′ū-rā-tī′vă) Chronic suppurative folliculitis of apocrine sweat-gland–bearing skin producing abscesses or sinuses with scarring.

hi•drad•e•no•ma (hī-drad′ĕ-nō′mă) A benign neoplasm derived from epithelial cells of sweat glands. [G. *hidrōs,* sweat, + *adēn,* gland, + *-oma,* tumor]

♻ **hidro-, hidr-** Combining forms meaning sweat, sweat glands. Cf. sudor-. [G. *hidrōs*]

hi•dro•cys•to•ma (hī′drō-sis-tō′mă) A cystic form of hidradenoma, usually apocrine. SYN syringocystoma. [hidro- + G. *kystis,* bladder, + *-ōma,* tumor]

hi•dro•poi•e•sis (hī′drō-poy-ē′sis) The formation of sweat. [hidro- + G. *poiēsis,* formation]

hi•dros•che•sis (hī-dros′kĕ-sis) Suppression of sweating. [hidro- + G. *schesis,* a checking]

hi•dro•sis (hī-drō′sis) The production and excretion of sweat. [G. *hidrōs,* sweat, + *-osis,* condition]

hi•drot•ic (hī-drot′ik) Relating to or causing hidrosis.

hi•er•ar•chy (hī′ĕr-ahr-kē) **1.** Any system of persons or things ranked one above the other. **2.** PSYCHOLOGY/PSYCHIATRY an organization of habits or concepts in which simpler components are combined to form increasingly complex integrations. [G. *hierarchia,* rule or power of the high priest]

high (hī) Elevated, lofty; above some basis or point of comparison. [O.E. *hēah*]

high al•ti•tude ce•re•bral e•de•ma (hī al′ti-tūd ser′ĕ-brăl ĕ-dē′mă) Brain swelling related to a fast ascent. Signs and symptoms may include fatigue, nausea, vomiting, ataxia, and altered mentation.

high al•ti•tude pul•mo•nar•y e•de•ma (hī al′ti-tūd pul′mŏ-nar-ē ĕ-dē′mă) A severe form of acute mountain sickness with subtle onset of symptoms.

high-def•i•ni•tion im•ag•ing (HDI) (hī′def-i-nish′ŭn im′ăj-ing) Ultrasound assessment of mammary tissue to determine presence of possibly cancerous lesions.

high den•si•ty lip•o•pro•tein-cho•les•ter•ol (HDL-C) (hī den′si-tē lip′ō-prō′tēn-kŏ-les′tĕr-ol) The so-called good cholesterol, which, because of its high protein:lipid ratio, is thought to be cardioprotective.

high-dose-rate brach•y•ther•a•py (hī-dōs-rāt brak′ē-thār′ă-pē) Brachytherapy consisting of brief exposure, usually on an outpatient basis, to a high-dose radiation source.

high en•do•the•li•al post•cap•il•lar•y ven•ules (hī en′dō-thē′lē-ăl pōst′kap′i-lar′ē ven′yūlz) Venules in the lymph nodes, tonsils, and Peyer patches that have a high-walled endothelium through which blood lymphocytes migrate into the lymphatic parenchyma.

high en•e•ma (hī en′ĕ-mă) An enema instilled far up into the colon. SYN enteroclysis (1).

high-en•er•gy com•pounds (hī-en′ĕr-jē kom′powndz) Classically, a group of phosphoric esters the hydrolysis of which takes place with a standard free energy change of –5 to –15 kcal/mol (or –20 to –63 kJ/mol) (in contrast to –1 to –4 kcal/mol, or –4 to –17 kJ/mol) for simple phosphoric esters like glucose 6-phosphate or α-glycerophosphates, thus being capable of driving energy-consuming reactions in living cells or reconstituted cell-free systems; adenosine 5′-triphosphate, with respect to the β- and γ-phosphates, is the best known and is regarded as the immediate energy source for most metabolic syntheses. Other examples include acid anhydrides, phosphoric esters of enols, phosphamic acid ($R–NH–PO_3H_2$) derivatives, acyl thioesters (e.g., of coenzyme A), sulfonium compounds ($R_3–S^+$), and aminoacyl esters of ribosyl moieties. SEE ALSO high-energy phosphates.

high-en•er•gy phos•phate bond (hī-en′ĕr-jē fos′fāt bond) SEE high-energy phosphates.

high-en•er•gy phos•phates (hī-en′ĕr-jē fos′fāts) Those phosphate esters and phosphoanhydrides that, on hydrolysis, yield an unusually large amount of energy; e.g., nucleotide polyphosphates such as ATP, enol phosphates such as phospho*enol*pyruvate. SEE ALSO high-energy compounds.

high•er or•der preg•nan•cy (hī′ĕr ōr′dĕr preg′năn-sē) A pregnancy that has three fetuses (triplets) or more.

high•est in•ter•cos•tal ar•ter•y (hī′ĕst in′tĕr-kos′tăl ahr′tĕr-ē) SYN supreme intercostal artery.

high•est in•ter•cos•tal vein (hī′ĕst in′tĕr-kos′tăl vān) Drains the first intercostal space into either the vertebral or the brachiocephalic vein.

high•est thor•a•cic ar•ter•y (hī′ĕst thōr-as′ik ahr′tĕr-ē) SYN superior thoracic artery.

high-fi•ber (hī-fī′bĕr) A product so labeled contains, by F.D.A. order, more than 5 g of dietary fiber per serving.

high-fi•ber di•et (hī-fī′bĕr dī′ĕt) A diet high in the nondigestible part of plants, i.e., fiber. Fiber is found in fruits, vegetables, whole grains, and legumes. Insoluble fiber increases stool bulk, decreases transit time of food in the bowel, and decreases constipation and the risk of colon cancer. Soluble fiber delays absorption of glucose, which helps to control blood sugar in diabetes mellitus, and delays absorption of lipids, which helps to control hyperlipidemia. Recommended in treatment of diverticular disease of the colon.

high Fow•ler po•si•tion (hī fowl′ĕr pŏ-zish′ŏn) Patient position in which the head of the bed is raised to a 90 degree angle. See page B29.

high-fre•quen•cy cur•rent (hī-frē′kwĕn-sē kŭr′ĕnt) An alternating electric current having a frequency of 10,000 or more cycles per second; it produces no muscular contractions and does not affect the sensory nerves.

high-fre•quen•cy hear•ing im•pair•ment (hī-frē′kwĕn-sē hēr′ing im-pār′mĕnt) Selective loss of hearing for high frequencies, usually associated with sensory damage; common in acoustic trauma and noise-induced hearing loss.

high fre•quen•cy os•cil•la•tion (HFO) (hī frē′kwĕn-sē os′i-lā′shŭn) A type of mechanical ventilation.

high fre•quen•cy per•cus•sive ven•ti•la•tion (HFPV) (hī frē′kwĕn-sē pĕr-kus′iv ven′ti-lā′shŭn) A type of mechanical ventilation.

high fre•quen•cy pos•i•tive pres•sure ven•ti•la•tion (HFPPV) (hī frē′kwĕn-sē poz′i-tiv presh′ŭr ven′ti-lā′shŭn) A type of mechanical ventilation.

high-fre•quen•cy trans•duc•tion (hī-frē′kwĕn-sē trans-dŭk′shŭn) Specialized transduction in which the donor bacterium contains not only the transducing, defective probacteriophage but also the nondefective prophage that serves as "helper" virus, enabling most of the defective prophage particles to develop sufficiently to function as transducing agents.

high-fre•quen•cy ven•ti•la•tion (HFV) (hī-frē′kwĕn-sē ven′ti-lā′shŭn) Technique of positive-pressure ventilation in which breathing frequency is above normal and tidal volume is below normal. The ventilatory pattern is similar to that of an animal panting.

high-grade ex•plo•sive (hī-grād eks-plō′siv) A device that generates both a supersonic pressure front (blast wave, q.v.) and also a subsonic pressure front (blast wind, q.v.) when it explodes.

high-grade squa•mous in•tra•e•pi•the•li•al le•sion (HSIL, HGSIL) (hī-grād skwā′mŭs in′tră-ep-i-thē′lē-ăl lē′zhŭn) Term used in the Bethesda system for reporting cervical-vaginal cytologic diagnosis to describe a spectrum of noninvasive cervical epithelial abnormalities, including moderate and severe dysplasia, carcinoma in situ, and cervical intraepithelial neoplasia grades 2 and 3. SEE ALSO Bethesda system, ASCUS, atypical glandular cells of undetermined significance, low-grade squamous intraepithelial lesion.

high•ly ac•tive an•ti•ret•ro•vi•ral ther•a•py (HAART) (hī′lē ak′tiv an′ti-ret′rō-vī′răl thār′ă-pē) A combination of anti-AIDS medications usually consisting of two NRTIs with one or two protease inhibitors, or two NRTIs with an NNRTI.

high•ly arched pal•ate (hī′lē ahrcht pal′ăt) SEE secondary palate.

high mo•lec•u•lar weight ki•nin•o•gen (HMWK) (hī mŏ-lek′yū-lăr wāt ki-nin′ō-jen) A plasma protein of 110,000 molecular weight that normally exists in plasma in a 1:1 complex with prekallikrein. The complex is a cofactor in the activation of coagulation factor XII. The product of this reaction, XIIa, in turn activates prekallikrein to kallikrein.

High•more bod•y (hī′mōr bod′ē) SYN mediastinum testis.

high mus•cle tone (hī mŭs′ĕl tōn) SYN hypertonicity.

high-per•for•mance liq•uid chro•ma•tog•ra•phy (HPLC) (hī pĕr-fōr′măns lik′wid krō′mă-tog′ră-fē) A chromatographic technology used to separate and quantitate mixtures of substances in solution. The technique is used to measure organic compounds, including steroid hormones, pesticides and poisons, toxic and carcinogenic compounds, and drugs. SYN high-pressure liquid chromatography.

high-pres•sure liq•uid chro•ma•to•gra•phy (HPLC) (hī-presh′ŭr lik′wid krō′mă-tog′ră-fē) SYN high-performance liquid chromatography.

high-pro•tein di•et (hī-prō′tēn dī′ĕt) A controversial regimen that provides large amounts of protein, either to resolve states of depletion or to allow intake of greater levels of protein than normal for athletic reasons. Reports suggest possible kidney disease as a result of this diet.

high-res•o•lu•tion com•put•ed to•mog•ra•phy (HRCT) (hī-rez′ō-lū′shŭn kŏm-pyū′tĕd tŏ-mog′ră-fē) Computed tomography with narrow collimation to reduce volume-averaging and an edge-enhancing reconstruction algorithm to sharpen the image, sometimes with a restricted field of view to minimize the size of pixels in the region imaged; used particularly for lung imaging.

high, rich in, or ex•cel•lent source of (hī rich, ek′sĕ-lĕnt sōrs) These terms, when used in food labeling, mean that, according to F.D.A. regulations, the food so labeled contains at least 25% more of a given nutrient or ingredient than a similar product.

high-risk in•fant (hī-risk in′fănt) A newborn considered to be in greater danger of health problems than the norm in the first month of life. Premature infants are more likely to be so categorized than infants carried to term.

high-risk re•gis•ter (HRR) (hī risk rej′is-tĕr) AUDIOLOGY checklist of conditions known to exhibit a higher-than-normal prevalence of hearing loss. Conditions include familial history of hearing loss, congenital infections, craniofacial anomalies, low birth weight, hyperbilirubinemia, ototoxic medications, bacterial meningitis, and severe CNS depression at birth. SEE screening.

high-step•page gait (hī′-step′ăj gāt) A gait in which the foot is raised high to avoid catching a drooping foot and brought down suddenly in a flapping manner; often seen in peroneal nerve palsy (i.e., foot-drop) and tabes.

high-tech med•i•cine (hī-tek med′i-sin) Colloquial and imprecise term for therapy related to use of advanced modalities.

high TENS (hī tenz) A transcutaneous electrical nerve stimulator applied at the sensory level characterized by high-frequency and short-duration pulses.

high ve•loc•i•ty sig•nal loss (hī vĕ-los′i-tē sig′năl laws) Increase in time of flight due to an increase in the velocity of flow in magnetic resonance imaging.

high ve•ron•i•ca (hī vĕr-on′i-kă) SYN black root.

high volt e•lec•tri•cal stim•u•la•tion (HVES) (hī vōlt ĕ-lek′trik-ăl stim′yū-lā′shŭn) An electrotherapeutic modality that delivers a twin peak monophasic pulsed current at either a negative or a positive polarity to facilitate the reduction of pain or edema or to promote healing.

hi•la (hī′lă) Plural of hilum.

hi•lar (hī′lăr) Pertaining to a hilum.

hi•li•tis (hī-lī′tis) Inflammation of the lining membrane of any hilus.

Hill cri•ter•i•a of e•vi•dence (hil krī-tēr′ē-ă ev′i-dĕns) A calculation of epidemiologic criteria that helps to indicate whether a statistically significant relationship obtained in epidemiologic and other studies is a causal relationship. A. B. Hill's criteria (in descending order of importance) are strength, consistency, specificity, temporality, biologic gradient (i.e., dose-response relationship), biologic plausibility, coherence, experimental evidence from animal studies, and analysis. Temporality is the only absolute criterion: the putative cause must precede the effect in time.

Hill e•qua•tion (hil ĕ-kwā′zhŭn) The equation $y(1 - y) = [S]^n/K_d$, where y is the fractional degree of saturation, [S] is the binding ligand concentration, n is the Hill coefficient, and K_d is the dissociation constant for the ligand. The Hill coefficient is a measure of the cooperativity of the protein; the larger the value, the higher the cooperativity. This coefficient cannot be higher than the number of binding sites. For the oxygen binding curve of hemoglobin, an association constant, K_a, is used and the equation becomes $y/(1 - y) = K_a[S]^n$. For human hemoglobin, $n = 2.5$.

hil•lock (hil′lok) ANATOMY any small elevation or prominence.

Hill op•er•a•tion (hil op-ĕr-ā′shŭn) Repair of hiatus hernia; narrowing the esophagogastric junction and attaching it to the right medial arcuate ligament.

Hill-Sachs le•sion (hil saks lē′zhŭn) An articular cartilage defect on the posterior aspect of the humeral head, often caused by injury to the humeral head by the rim of the glenoid fossa after anterior glenohumeral dislocation.

Hill sign (hil sīn) In aortic insufficiency, greater systolic blood pressure in the legs than in the arms; normal arterial systolic pressure in the leg is 10–20 mm of Hg above that in the arm, whereas in aortic insufficiency the difference may be 60–100 mm of Hg.

Hil•ton law (hil′tŏn law) The nerve supplying a joint that also supplies the muscles that move the joint and the skin covering the articular insertion of those muscles.

Hil•ton meth•od (hil′tŏn meth′ŏd) Division of the nerves supplying a part, for the relief of pain in ulcers.

hi•lum, pl. **hi•la** (hī′lŭm, -lă) [TA] **1.** The part of an organ where the nerves and vessels enter and leave. SYN porta (1). **2.** A depression or slit resembling the hilum in the olivary nucleus of the brain. [L. a small bit or trifle]

hi•lus (hī′lŭs) Hilum. [a British variant of L. *hilum*]

hi•lus cells (hī′lŭs selz) Cells in the hilus of the ovary that produce androgens; they are thought to be the ovarian counterpart of the interstitial cells of the testis.

HIM (him) Acronym for health information management.

hind•brain (hīnd′brān) SYN rhombencephalon.

hind•foot (hīnd′fut) The rear part of the foot consisting of the calcaneus and talus.

hind•foot val•gus (hīnd′fut val′gŭs) Eversion of the calcaneus relative to the tibia. SYN rearfoot pronation.

hind•foot va•rus (hīnd′fut var′ŭs) Inversion of the calcaneus relative to the tibia. SYN rearfoot supination.

hind•gut (hīnd′gŭt) **1.** The caudal or terminal part of the embryonic gut. **2.** The left part of transverse colon, descending and sigmoid colon, rectum, and superior part of anal canal.

hind•wa•ter (hīnd′waw′tĕr) Colloquialism for amniotic fluid in utero behind the presenting part of the fetus.

hinged flap (hinjd flap) A turnover flap transferred by lifting it over on its pedicle as if the pedicle were a hinge.

hinge joint (hinj joynt) A uniaxial joint in which a broad, transversely cylindric convexity on one bone fits into a corresponding concavity on the other, allowing of motion in one plane only. SYN ginglymoid joint, ginglymus.

hinge re•gion (hinj rē′jŭn) **1.** That part of a tRNA structure that is deformed, bending a "cloverleaf" (two-dimensional) model to form an "L" model (crystal form, as seen by electron microscopy). **2.** In an immunoglobulin, a short sequence of amino acids that lies between two longer sequences and allows the latter to bend about the former.

hip (hip) **1.** The lateral prominence of the pelvis from the waist to the thigh. **2.** The joint between femur and pelvis. **3.** Colloquially, the head, neck, and greater trochanter of femur, as in the phrases "hip fracture" and "hip replacement." [A.S. *hype*]

HIPAA Abbreviation for Health Insurance Portability and Accountability Act.

hip bath (hip bath) SYN sitz bath.

hip bone (hip bōn) A large flat bone formed by the fusion of the ilium, ischium, and pubis (in the adult), constituting the lateral half of the pelvis; it articulates with its fellow anteriorly, with the sacrum posteriorly, and with the femur laterally. SYN coxa (1), innominate bone, os coxa.

hip frac•ture (hip frak′shŭr) Vernacular term for fracture of the femoral neck, typically resulting from a fall in an old person with osteoporosis; more common in women; requires surgical repair with internal fixation and can lead to prolonged or permanent loss of mobility and shortened life span.

hip joint (hip joynt) The ball-and-socket synovial joint between the head of the femur and the acetabulum. SYN coxa (2).

hip•po•cam•pal (hip′ō-kam′păl) Relating to the hippocampus.

hip•po•cam•pal sul•cus (hip′ō-kam′păl sŭl′kŭs) A shallow groove between the dentate gyrus and the parahippocampal gyrus; the remains of a fissure extending deep into the hippocampus between Ammon horn and the dentate gyrus that becomes obliterated during fetal development.

hip•po•cam•pus (hip′ō-kam′pŭs) [TA] The complex, internally convoluted structure that forms the medial margin of the cerebral hemisphere, bordering the choroid fissure of the lateral ventricle, and composed of two gyri (Ammon horn and the dentate gyrus), together with their white matter, the alveus, and fimbria hippocampi. In humans the hippocampus is confined to the temporal lobe by the massive development of the corpus callosum. The hippocampus forms part of the limbic system. Its major afferent connections are with the entorhinal area of the parahippocampal gyrus, and transparent septum; by way of the fornix it projects to the septum, anterior nucleus of the thalamus, and mammillary body. [G. *hippocampos,* seahorse]

hip•po•crat•ic (hip′ō-krat′ik) Relating to, described by, or attributed to Hippocrates.

hip•po•crat•ic face (hip′ō-krat′ik fās) SYN hippocratic facies.

hip•po•crat•ic fa•ci•es (hip′ō-krat′ik fash′ē-ēz) A pinched expression of the face, with sunken eyes, concavity of cheeks and temples, relaxed lips, and leaden complexion; observed in one close to death after severe and prolonged illness. SYN hippocratic face.

hip•po•crat•ic fin•gers (hip′ō-krat′ik fing′gĕrz) SEE clubbing.

hip•po•crat•ic nails (hip′ō-krat′ik nālz) The coarse curved nails capping clubbed digits (hippocratic fingers).

Hip•po•crat•ic Oath (hip′ō-krat′ik ōth) An oath taken by physicians about to enter the practice of their profession, which, although usually attributed to Hippocrates of Cos, is probably an ancient oath of the Asclepiads.

hip•po•crat•ic suc•cus•sion sound (hip′ō-krat′ik sŭ-kŭsh′ŭn sownd) A splashing sound elicited by shaking a patient with hydro- or pyopneumothorax, the physician's ear is applied to the chest.

hip poin•ter (hip poynt′ĕr) Contusion of the iliac crest.

hip•pus (hip′ŭs) Intermittent pupillary dilation and constriction, independent of illumination, convergence, or psychic stimuli. [G. *hippos,* horse, from a fancied suggestion of galloping movements]

hir•cus, gen. and pl. **hir•ci** (hir′kŭs, -sī) **1.** The odor of the axillae. **2.** One of the hairs growing in the axillae. **3.** SYN tragus (1). [L. he-goat]

Hirsch•berg meth•od (hĕrsh′berg meth′ŏd) A method of estimating the amount of deviation of a strabismic eye, by observing the reflection of a light fixated by the straight eye on the cornea of the deviating eye.

Hirsch•berg test (hĕrsh′berg test) A test of binocular motor alignment by which a penlight is shone at the eyes and the position of the light reflex on the cornea observed, allowing an estimate of the amount of deviation, if present.

Hirsch·feld ca·nals (hĕrsh′feld kă-nalz′) SYN interdental canals.

Hirsch·sprung dis·ease (hĕrsh′sprŭng di-zēz′) SYN congenital megacolon.

hir·sute (hir-sūt′) Relating to or characterized by hirsutism. [L. *hirsutus,* shaggy]

hir·su·tism (hir′sū-tizm) Presence of excessive bodily and facial terminal hair, in a male pattern, especially in women; may be present in normal adults as an expression of an ethnic characteristic or may develop in children or adults as the result of androgen excess due to tumors or drugs (e.g., nonandrogenetic drugs). See page B12. [L. *hirsutus,* shaggy]

hir·u·di·cide (hir-ū′di-sīd) An agent that kills leeches. [L. *hirudo,* leech, + *caedo,* to kill]

hir·u·din (hir-ū′din) An antithrombin substance extracted from the salivary glands of the leech that has the property of preventing coagulation of the blood. [L. *hirudo,* leech]

Hir·u·din·e·a (hir′ū-din′ē-ă) The leeches, a class of worms in the phylum Annelida with flat, segmented bodies, a sucker at the posterior end, and often a smaller sucker at the anterior end; they are predatory on invertebrate tissues, or feed on blood and tissue exudates of vertebrates. The class includes parasitic forms. [L. *hirudo,* leech]

Hir·u·do (hi-rū′dō) A genus of leeches; used in traditional medicine for blood letting or as an antithrombin. [L. leech]

His Abbreviation for histidine.

–His Combining form for histidino.

His- Histidyl.

His bun·dle (hiz bŭn′dĕl) SYN atrioventricular bundle.

His bun·dle e·lec·tro·gram (HBE) (hiz bŭn′dĕl ĕ-lek′trō-gram) An electrogram recorded from the His bundle, either in the experimental animal or in humans during cardiac catheterization.

His ca·nal (hiz kă-nal′) Structural opening in a fetus between the posterior tongue and the developing thyroid. Distal part may form a thyroidal pyramidal lobe and the proximal part is usually obliterated. SYN Bochdalek duct, duct of His, duct of Vater, thyroglossal duct.

His line (hiz līn) A line extending from the tip of the anterior nasal spine (acanthion) to the hindmost point on the posterior margin of the foramen magnum (opisthion), dividing the face into an upper and a lower, or dental, part.

Hiss stain (his stān) A stain for demonstrating the capsules of microorganisms, using gentian violet or basic fuchsin followed by a copper sulfate wash.

His·ta·log test (his′tă-lawg test) A test for measurement of maximal production of gastric acidity or anacidity; it is similar to the histamine test, but uses Histalog (betazole hydrochloride), an analogue of histamine.

histaminaemia [Br.] SEE histaminemia.

his·ta·mine (his′tă-mēn) A depressor amine derived from histidine and present in ergot and in animal tissues. It is a powerful stimulant of gastric secretion, a constrictor of bronchial smooth muscle and a vasodilator (capillaries and arterioles) that causes a fall in blood pressure. Histamine is liberated in the skin as a result of injury; when injected intradermally in high dilution, it causes the triple response.

his·ta·mine-fast (his′tă-mēn-fast) Indicating the absence of the normal response to histamine, especially in speaking of true gastric anacidity.

his·ta·mi·ne·mi·a (his′tă-min-ē′mē-ă) The presence of histamine in the circulating blood. [histamine + G. *haima,* blood]

his·ta·mine-re·leas·ing fac·tor (his′tă-mēn-rĕ-lēs′ing fak′tŏr) A lymphokine produced from antigen-stimulated lymphocytes that induces the release of histamine from basophils.

his·ta·mine test (his′tă-mēn test) A test for maximal production of gastric acidity or anacidity; after preliminary administration of an antihistamine, histamine acid phosphate is injected subcutaneously, followed by analysis of gastric contents. SEE ALSO Histalog test.

his·ta·min·ic head·ache (his′tă-min′ik hed′āk) SYN cluster headache.

his·ta·mi·nu·ri·a (his′tă-mi-nyūr′ē-ă) The excretion of histamine in the urine. [histidine + G. *ouron,* urine]

his·ti·dase (his′ti-dās) SYN histidine ammonia-lyase.

his·ti·dine (His, H) (his′ti-dēn) The L-isomer is a basic amino acid found in most proteins.

his·ti·dine am·mo·ni·a-ly·ase (his′ti-dēn ă-mō′nē-ă-lī′ās) An enzyme catalyzing deamination of L-histidine; this enzyme is absent or deficient in people with histidinemia. SYN histidase.

his·ti·dine de·car·box·yl·ase (his′ti-dēn dē′kahr-bok′sil-ās) An enzyme catalyzing the decarboxylation of L-histidine to histamine and CO_2; it plays a role in constriction of bronchial smooth muscle.

his·ti·din·o (–His) (his′ti-din-ō) The radical of histidine produced by removal of a hydrogen from a nitrogen atom.

his·ti·di·nu·ri·a (his′ti-di-nyūr′ē-ă) Excretion of considerable amounts of histidine in the urine;

frequently observed in later months of pregnancy, and in histidinemia.

his•ti•dyl (His-) (his′ti-dil) The acyl radical of histidine.

♻ **histio-** Combining form indicating tissue, especially connective tissue. [G. *histion,* web]

his•ti•o•blast (his′tē-ō-blast) A tissue-forming cell. SYN histoblast. [histio- + G. *blastos,* germ]

his•ti•o•cyte (his′tē-ō-sīt) A macrophage present in connective tissue. SYN histocyte. [histio- + G. *kytos,* cell]

his•ti•o•cy•to•ma (his′tē-ō-sī-tō′mă) A tumor composed of histiocytes. [histio- + G. *kytos,* cell, + *-ōma,* tumor]

his•ti•o•cy•to•sis (his′tē-ō-sī-tō′sis) A generalized multiplication of histiocytes. SYN histocytosis.

his•ti•o•cy•to•sis X (his′tē-ō-sī-tō′sis) Proliferation of Langerhans cells of undetermined clinical type, possibly Hand-Schüller-Christian disease, Letterer-Siwe disease, and eosinophilic granuloma.

his•ti•o•gen•ic (his′tē-ō-jen′ik) SYN histogenous.

♻ **histo-** Combining form meaning tissue. [G. *histos,* web (tissue)]

his•to•blast (his′tō-blast) SYN histioblast.

his•to•chem•is•try (his′tō-kem′is-trē) SYN cytochemistry.

his•to•com•pat•i•bil•i•ty (his′tō-kŏm-pat′i-bil′i-tē) A state of immunologic similarity (or identity) that permits successful homograft transplantation.

his•to•com•pa•ti•bil•i•ty com•plex (his′tō-kŏm-pat′i-bil′i-tē kom′pleks) A family of 50 or more genes on the sixth human chromosome that code for cell surface proteins and play a role in the immune response. Histocompatibility genes control the production of proteins on the outer membranes of tissue and blood cells, especially lymphocytes, and are vital elements in cell-cell recognition. The proteins also determine the level and type of immune response, and may serve other biochemical or immunologic functions. In the case of allografts, it is necessary to determine whether donor and recipient possess compatible sets of proteins (histocompatibility antigens), to minimize the likelihood of rejection. Histocompatibility testing (human leukocyte antigen tissue typing) provides this information.

his•to•com•pat•i•bil•i•ty test•ing (his′tō-kŏm-pat′i-bil′i-tē test′ing) A testing system for human leukocyte antigens, of major importance in transplantation.

his•to•cyte (his′tō-sīt) SYN histiocyte.

his•to•cy•to•sis (his′tō-sī-tō′sis) SYN histiocytosis.

his•to•dif•fer•en•ti•a•tion (his′tō-dif′ĕr-en-shē-ā′shŭn) The morphologic appearance of tissue characteristics during development.

his•to•gen•e•sis (his′tō-jen′ĕ-sis) The origin of a tissue; the formation and development of the tissues of the body. [histo- + G. *genesis,* origin]

his•to•ge•net•ic (his′tō-jĕ-net′ik) Relating to histogenesis.

his•tog•e•nous (his-toj′ĕ-nŭs) Formed by the tissues (e.g., the histogenous cells in an exudate arising from proliferation of the fixed tissue cells). SYN histiogenic. [histo- + G. *-gen,* producing]

his•to•gram (his′tō-gram) A bar chart representing a frequency distribution; heights of the bars indicate degree of frequency. [*histo*ry + -gram]

his•toid (his′toyd) **1.** Resembling in structure one of the tissues of the body. **2.** The histologic structure of a neoplasm derived from and consisting of a single, relatively simple type of neoplastic tissue that closely resembles the normal. [histo- + G. *eidos,* resemblance]

his•toid lep•ro•sy (his′toyd lep′rŏ-sē) A form of lepromatous leprosy with lesions microscopically resembling dermatofibromas or other spindle-celled tumors.

his•to•in•com•pat•i•bil•i•ty (his′tō-in′kŏm-pat′i-bil′i-tē) A state of immunologic dissimilarity of tissues sufficient to cause rejection of a homograft when tissue is transplanted from one person to another; implies a difference in histocompatibility genes in donor and recipient.

his•to•log•ic, his•to•log•i•cal (his′tō-loj′ik, i-kăl) Pertaining to histology.

his•to•log•ic ac•com•mo•da•tion (his′tō loj′ik ă-kom′ŏ-dā′shŭn) Change in shape of cells to meet altered physical conditions, as the flattening of cuboidal cells in cysts as a result of pressure.

his•tol•o•gist (his-tol′ŏ-jist) One who specializes in the science of histology. SYN microanatomist.

his•tol•o•gy (his-tol′ŏ-jē) The science concerned with the minute structure of cells, tissues, and organs in relation to their function. SEE ALSO microscopic anatomy. SYN microanatomy. [histo- + G. *logos,* study]

his•tol•y•sis (his-tol′i-sis) Disintegration of tissue. [histo- + G. *lysis,* dissolution]

his•to•ma (his-tō′mă) A benign neoplasm in which the cytologic and histologic elements are closely similar to those of normal tissue from which the neoplastic cells are derived. [histo- + G. *-oma,* tumor]

his·to·met·a·plas·tic (his′tō-met-ă-plas′tik) Exciting tissue metaplasia.

his·to·mo·ni·a·sis (his′tō-mō-nī′ă-sis) A disease chiefly affecting turkeys, caused by *Histomonas meleagridis* and characterized by ulcerative and necrotic lesions of the liver and cecum, acute onset, and a high mortality rate. It is transmitted inside the eggs of the nematode *Heterakis gallinae*, which is primarily responsible for maintaining and spreading the infection. SYN blackhead (2).

his·tone (his′tōn) One of a number of simple proteins (often found in the cell nucleus) that contains a high proportion of basic amino acids, are soluble in water, dilute acids, and alkalies, and are not coagulable by heat.

his·to·nu·ri·a (his′tō-nyūr′ē-ă) The excretion of histone in the urine, as observed in certain instances of leukemia, febrile illnesses, and wasting diseases. [histone + G. *ouron,* urine]

his·to·path·o·gen·e·sis (his′tō-path-ō-jen′ĕ-sis) Abnormal embryonic development or growth of tissue. [histogenesis + pathogenesis]

his·to·pa·thol·o·gy (his′tō-pă-thol′ŏ-jē) The science or study dealing with the cytologic and histologic structure of abnormal or diseased tissue.

his·to·phys·i·ol·o·gy (his′tō-fiz-ē-ol′ŏ-jē) The microscopic study of tissues in relation to their functions.

His·to·plas·ma cap·su·la·tum (his-tō-plaz′mă kap-sū-lā′tŭm) A dimorphic fungus species that causes histoplasmosis; its ascomycetous state is *Ajellomyces capsulatum.* The organism's natural habitat is soil fertilized with bird and bat droppings, where it grows as a mold, fragments of which, following inhalation, produce the primary pulmonary infection; within the mammalian host, inhaled mycelial fragments grow as uninuclear yeasts that reproduce by budding. *H. capsulatum* is encountered primarily in Africa. [histo- + G. *plasma,* something formed]

his·to·plas·min (his′tō-plaz′min) An antigenic extract of *Histoplasma capsulatum*, used in immunologic tests for the diagnosis of histoplasmosis; also used in skin test surveys of populations to determine the geographic distribution of the fungus and to predict those that are endemic for histoplasmosis.

his·to·plas·mo·ma (his′tō-plaz-mō′mă) An infectious granuloma caused by *Histoplasma capsulatum.*

his·to·plas·mo·sis (his′tō-plaz-mō′sis) A widely distributed infectious disease caused by *Histoplasma capsulatum* and occurring frequently in epidemics; usually acquired by inhalation of spores of the fungus in soil dust and manifested by a primary benign pneumonitis; occasionally, the primary disease progresses to produce localized lesions in the lung, such as pulmonary cavitation, or the typical disseminated disease of the reticuloendothelial system that is manifested by fever, emaciation, splenomegaly, and leukopenia. Often spreads to the eye where it causes retinal lesions.

his·tor·rhex·is (his′tō-rek′sis) Breakdown of tissue by some agency other than infection. [histo- + G. *rhēxis,* rupture]

his·to·ry (his′tŏr-ē) In health care, record of a patient's symptoms, illness, and treatment thereof, as well as other life details related to health.

his·to·ry of pres·ent ill·ness (HPI) (his′tŏr′ē prez′ĕnt il′nĕs) A detailed formal statement of available historical data about a patient's presenting complaint.

his·to·tome (his′tō-tōm) SYN microtome. [histo- + G. *tomē,* cut]

his·tot·o·my (his-tot′ŏ-mē) SYN microtomy.

his·to·tope (his′tō-tōp) That part of the Class II major histocompatibility molecule that interacts with the T-cell receptor. [histo- + -tope]

his·to·tox·ic (his′tō-tok′sik) Relating to poisoning of the respiratory enzyme system of the tissues.

his·to·tox·ic an·ox·i·a (his′tō-tok′sik ă-nok′sē-ă) Poisoning of the respiratory enzyme systems of the tissues, as in the inhibition of cytochrome oxidase by cyanides; owing to the inability of tissue cells to use oxygen, its tension in arterial and capillary blood is usually greater than normal.

his·to·tro·phic (his′tō-trō′fik) Providing nourishment for or favoring the formation of tissue. [histo- + G. *trophē,* nourishment]

his·to·tro·pic (his′tō-trō′pik) Attracted toward the tissues; denoting certain parasites, stains, and chemical compounds. [histo- + G. *tropikos,* turning]

hitch·hik·er thumb (hich′hī′kĕr thŭm) Malposition of the thumb, which, as a result of shortness of the first metacarpal, stands at right angles to the radial border of the hand and in the same plane with it; a characteristic sign of diastrophic dwarfism.

hit·ting the wall (hit′ing wawl) A term athletes use to describe an abrupt decline in the ability to maintain the desired intensity of endurance exercise performance; associated with accumulation of blood lactate and depletion of liver and muscle glycogen reserves.

HIV Abbreviation for human immunodeficiency virus.

HIV-1 Abbreviation for human immunodeficiency virus-1.

HIV-2 Abbreviation for human immunodeficiency virus 2.

hives (hīvz) **1.** SYN urticaria. **2.** SYN wheal.

HIV ex•cep•tion•al•ism (ek-sep′shŭn-ăl-izm) A concept whereby the privacy concerns of those infected with HIV are considered to be more important than public health concerns.

HIV 1 ma•jor (Group M) and HIV 1 out•li•er (Group O) Mutated forms of HIV-1.

HIV was•ting syn•drome (wāst′ing sin′drōm) SYN wasting syndrome.

hK3 Abbreviation for human glandular kallikrein 3.

HL-7 Health Level 7, a medical informatics standard that facilitates communication among different digital systems.

HLA com•plex (kom′pleks) The major histocompatibility complex in humans.

HLA typ•ing (tīp′ing) Tests done to determine whether a patient has antibodies against a potential donor's HLAs. The presence of antibodies means that a graft will be rejected.

HMB-45 An antibody to a premelanosome glycoprotein found to be present in melanomas and other tumors derived from melanocytes.

HMD Abbreviation for hyaline membrane disease.

HME Abbreviation for human monocytic ehrlichiosis.

HMG CoA-re•duc•tase in•hib•i•tors (rĕ-dŭk′tās in-hib′i-tŏrz) Drugs that interfere with the biosynthesis of cholesterol; used to treat hyperlipidemia.

HMO Abbreviation meaning health maintenance organization; hospital medical officer; hypothetic mean organism.

HMWK Abbreviation for high molecular weight kininogen.

HN NATO code for nitrogen mustards.

H_2O Symbol for water.

Ho Symbol for holmium.

Hoag•land sign (hōg′lănd sīn) Eyelid edema in infectious mononucleosis.

hoarse (hōrs) Having a rough, harsh voice. [A.S. *hās*]

hob•nail cell (hob′nāl sel) A cell characteristic of a clear cell adenocarcinoma; a round expansion of clear cytoplasm projects into the lumen of neoplastic tubules, but the basal part of the cell containing the nucleus is narrow.

hob•nail liv•er (hob′nāl liv′ĕr) In Laënnec cirrhosis, the contraction of scar tissue and hepatic cellular regeneration that causes a nodular appearance of the liver's surface.

Ho•bo•ken nod•ules (hō′bō-kĕn nod′yūlz) Gross dilations on the outer surface of the umbilical arteries. SEE ALSO Hoboken valves.

Ho•bo•ken valves (hō′bō-kĕn valvz) The flangelike protrusions into the lumen of the umbilical arteries where they are twisted or kinked in their course through the umbilical cord.

Hodge pes•sa•ry (hoj pes′ŏr-ē) A double-curve oblong pessary employed for the correction of retrodeviations of the uterus.

Hodg•kin dis•ease (hoj′kin di-zēz′) A disease marked by chronic enlargement of the lymph nodes, often local at the onset and later generalized, together with enlargement of the spleen and often of the liver, no pronounced leukocytosis, and commonly anemia and continuous or remittent (Pel-Ebstein) fever; considered to be a malignant neoplasm of lymphoid cells of uncertain origin (Reed-Sternberg cells), associated with inflammatory infiltration of lymphocytes and eosinophilic leukocytes and fibrosis; can be classified into lymphocytic predominant, nodular sclerosing, mixed cellularity, and lymphocytic depletion type; a similar disease occurs in domestic cats. See page B31.

Hodg•kin sar•co•ma (hoj′kin sahr-kō′mă) Lymphocyte depletion form of Hodgkin disease.

Hodg•son dis•ease (hoj′sŏn di-zēz′) An aneurysmal dilation of the arch of the aorta associated with insufficiency of the aortic valve.

ho•do•scope (hō′dō-skōp) An instrument designed to follow charged particles in a magnetic field.

Hof•fa op•er•a•tion (hawf′ă op-ĕr-ā′shŭn) In congenital dislocation of the hip, a rarely used operation consisting of hollowing out the acetabulum and reduction of the head of the femur after severing the muscles inserted into the upper portion of the bone.

Hoff•mann mus•cu•lar at•ro•phy (hawf′mahn mŭs′kyū-lăr at′rŏ-fē) SYN spinal muscular atrophy, type I.

Hoff•mann phe•nom•e•non (hawf′mahn fĕ-nom′e-non) Excessive irritability of the sensory nerves due to electrical or mechanical stimuli in tetany.

Hoff•mann sign, Hoff•mann re•flex (hawf′mahn sīn, rē′fleks) **1.** In latent tetany, mild mechanical stimulation of the trigeminal nerve causes severe pain. **2.** Flexion of the terminal phalanx of the thumb and of the second and third phalanges of one or more of the fingers when the volar surface of the terminal phalanx of the fingers is flicked. SYN digital reflex.

Hof•mei•ster op•er•a•tion (hawf′mī-stĕr op-ĕr-ā′shŭn) Partial gastrectomy with closure of a portion of the lesser curvature and retrocolic anastomosis of the remainder to the jejunum.

Hog·ben num·ber (hog′bĕn nŭm′bĕr) Unique personal identifying number constructed by using a sequence of digits for birth date, sex, birthplace, and other identifiers. They are the basis for identification numbers in many primary care facilities and are used in many record linkage systems.

hog·weed (hawg′wēd) SYN broom.

hol·an·dric (hol-an′drik) Related to genes located on the Y chromosome. [G. *holos,* entire, + *aner,* human male]

hol·an·dric gene (hol-an′drik jēn) SYN Y-linked gene.

ho·lism (hō′lizm) **1.** Principle that an organism, or one of its actions, is not equal to merely the sum of its parts but must be perceived or studied as a whole. **2.** The approach to the study of a psychological phenomenon through the analysis of a phenomenon as a complete entity in itself. [G. *holos,* entire]

ho·lis·tic (hō-lis′tik) Pertaining to the characteristics of holism or holistic psychologies.

ho·lis·tic care (hō-lis′tik kār) Care that incorporates the whole of a person, that is, physical, psychological, emotional, and spiritual dimensions. SYN holistic medicine.

ho·lis·tic med·i·cine (hō-lis′tik med′i-sin) SYN holistic care.

Hol·len·horst plaques (hol′ĕn-hōrst plaks) Glittering, orange-yellow, atheromatous emboli in the retinal arterioles that contain cholesterin crystals and originate in the carotid artery or great vessels.

hol·low (hol′ō) A concavity or depression.

hol·low bone (hol′ō bōn) SYN pneumatic bone.

hol·low-cath·ode lamp (hol′ō-kath′ōd lamp) A lamp consisting of a metal cathode and an inert gas that can emit a line spectrum of specific wavelength; used in atomic absorption spectrophotometry.

hol·ly·hock (hol′ē-hok) SYN althea.

Holmes-A·die pu·pil (hōlmz ā′dē pyū′pil) SYN Adie syndrome.

Holmes-A·die syn·drome (hōlmz ā′dē sin′drōm) SYN Adie syndrome.

Holmes stain (hōlmz stān) A silver nitrate staining method for nerve fibers.

Holm·gren wool test (hōlm′gren wul test) A test for color blindness, in which the subject matches variously colored skeins of wool.

hol·mi·um (Ho) (hol′mē-ŭm) An element of the lanthanide group, atomic no. 67, atomic wt. 164.93032. [L. *Holmia,* for Stockholm]

♻**holo-** Prefix meaning whole, entire, complete. [G. *holos*]

hol·o·blas·tic (hol′ō-blas′tik) Denoting the involvement of the entire oocyte in cleavage. [holo- + G. *blastos,* germ]

hol·o·cord (hol′ō-kōrd) Relating to the entire spinal cord, extending from the cervicomedullary junction to the conus medullaris.

hol·o·crine (hol′ō-krin) SEE holocrine gland. [holo- + G. *krinō,* to separate]

hol·o·crine gland (hol′ō-krin gland) A gland with secretion that consists of disintegrated cells of the gland itself, e.g., a sebaceous gland, in contrast to a merocrine gland.

hol·o·di·a·stol·ic (hol′ō-dī-ă-stol′ik) Relating to or occupying the entire diastolic period. SYN pandiastolic.

hol·o·en·dem·ic (hol′ō-en-dem′ik) Endemic in the entire population.

hol·o·en·zyme (hol′ō-en′zīm) A complete enzyme, i.e., apoenzyme plus coenzyme, cofactor, metal ion, and/or prosthetic group.

hol·o·gram (hōl′ō-gram) A three-dimensional image produced by wavefront reconstruction and recorded on a photographic plate. [holo- + G. *gramma,* something written]

hol·o·gyn·ic (hol′ō-jin′ik) Related to characters manifest only in females. [holo- + G. *gynē,* woman]

hol·o·pros·en·ceph·a·ly (hol′ō-pros-en-sef′ă-lē) Failure of the forebrain or prosencephalon to divide into hemispheres or lobes; cyclopia occurs in the severest form. It is often accompanied by a deficit in midline facial development. [holo- + G. *prosō,* forward, + *enkephalos,* brain]

hol·o·ra·chis·chi·sis (hol′ō-ră-kis′ki-sis) Spina bifida of the entire spinal column. [holo- + G. *rhachis,* spine, + *schisis,* fissure]

hol·o·sys·tol·ic (hol′ō-sis-tol′ik) SYN pansystolic.

Hol·ter mon·i·tor (hōl′tĕr mon′i-tŏr) A technique for long-term, continuous recording of electrocardiographic signals on magnetic tape for scanning and selection of significant but fleeting changes that might otherwise escape notice. The device is used as the patient conducts normal ADLs.

Holt·house her·ni·a (hōlt′hows hĕr′nē-ă) Inguinal hernia with extension of the loop of intestine along the Poupart ligament.

holy this·tle (hō′lē this′ĕl) SYN blessed thistle.

Ho·mans sign (hō′mĕnz sīn) Pain in the calf when the ankle is slowly and gently dorsiflexed (with the knee bent), indicative of incipient or established thrombosis in the veins of the leg.

hom·ax·i·al (hōm-ak′sē-ăl) Having all the axes alike, as a sphere. [G. *homos,* the same, + axis]

H.O.M.E. (hōm) Acronym for hand-over-mouth exercise.

home-based med·i·cal trans·crip·tion (hōm′ bāst med′i-kăl tran-skrip′shŭn) System in which medical transcriptionists transcribe at home rather than in a facility; such transcriptionists may be either employees or independent contractors.

home health care (hōm helth cār) Care of patients delivered within their residence rather than a clinical setting; usually provided by nurses, home health aides, and other professionals on a regularly scheduled visit.

home·less per·son (hōm′lĕs pĕr′sŏn) A colloquial term describing a person of no fixed residence; such people generally have little access to health care and are often beset with multiple psychological, physical, and addictive disorders. Their lack of mailing address generally makes follow-up difficult, so those with chronic illnesses remain sick, get sicker, and in the case of those with infectious diseases (e.g., TB) represent a continuing threat to others.

home main·te·nance as·sist·ance (hōm man′tĕ-năns ă-sis′tăns) Provision of services to a patient or client within the patient's residence; usually related to problems with IADLs and disease course.

♲ **homeo-** Combining form meaning the same, alike. SEE ALSO homo- (1). [G. *homoios,* similar]

ho·me·o·met·ric au·to·reg·u·la·tion (hō′mē-ō-met′rik aw′tō-reg-yŭ-lā′shŭn) Intrinsic regulation of strength of cardiac contraction in response to influences that do not depend on change in fiber length, i.e., the Frank-Starling mechanism, (e.g., the Anrep effect in which strength increases in response to increased afterload, and the Bowditch staircase effect [treppe] in which strength increases in response to increased heart rate) and do not depend on extrinsic regulation (e.g., in which strength increases in response to sympathetic nerve stimulation or norepinephrine).

ho·me·o·mor·phous (hō′mē-ō-mōr′fŭs) Of similar shape, but not necessarily of the same composition. [homeo- + G. *morphē,* shape]

ho·me·o·path (hō′mē-ō-path) SYN homeopathist.

ho·me·o·path·ic (hō′mē-ō-path′ik) **1.** Relating to homeopathy. SYN homeotherapeutic (1). **2.** Denoting an extremely small dose of a pharmacologic agent, such as might be used in homeopathy; more generally, a dose believed to be too small to produce the effect usually expected from that agent. Cf. pharmacologic (2), physiologic (4). [homeo- + G. *pathos,* disease]

ho·me·op·a·thist (hō′mē-op′ă-thist) A medical practitioner of homeopathy. SYN homeopath.

ho·me·op·a·thy (hō′mē-op′ă-thē) A system of therapy developed by Samuel Hahnemann based on the "law of infinitesimal doses" in *similia similibus curantur* (likes are cured by likes), which holds that a medicinal substance that can evoke certain symptoms in healthy people may be effective in the treatment of illnesses having symptoms closely resembling those produced by the substance. [homeo- + G. *pathos,* suffering]

ho·me·o·pla·si·a (hō′mē-ō-plā′zē-ă) The formation of new tissue of the same character as that already existing in the part. [homeo- + G. *plasis,* a molding]

ho·me·o·plas·tic (hō′mē-ō-plas′tik) Relating to or characterized by homeoplasia.

ho·me·o·sta·sis (hō′mē-ō-stā′sis) **1.** The state of equilibrium (balance between opposing pressures) in the body with respect to various functions and to the chemical compositions of the fluids and tissues. **2.** The processes through which such bodily equilibrium is maintained. [homeo- + G. *stasis,* a standing]

ho·me·o·stat·ic (hō′mē-ō-stat′ik) Relating to homeostasis.

ho·me·o·ther·a·peu·tic (hō′mē-ō-thār-ă-pyū′tik) **1.** SYN homeopathic (1). **2.** Relating to homeotherapy.

ho·me·o·ther·a·py, **ho·me·o·ther·a·peu·tics** (hō′mē-ō-thār′ă-pē, -thār-ă-pyū′tiks) Treatment or prevention of a disease using the principles of homeopathy.

ho·me·o·ther·mic (hō′mē-ō-thĕr′mik) Pertaining to, or having the essential characteristic of homeotherms. SYN hematothermal.

♲ **homo-** **1.** Combining form meaning the same, alike; opposite of hetero-. SEE ALSO homeo-. **2.** CHEMISTRY prefix used to indicate insertion of one more carbon atom in a chain. [G. *homos,* the same]

ho·mo·bi·o·tin (hō′mō-bī′ō-tin) A compound resembling biotin except for the substitution of an oxygen atom for the sulfur and the presence of an additional CH_2 group in the side chain; an active biotin antagonist.

ho·mo·blas·tic (hō′mō-blas′tik) Developing from a single type of tissue. [homo- + G. *blastos,* germ]

ho·mo·car·no·sine (hō′mō-kahr′nō-sēn) A constituent of the brain formed from L-histidine and γ-aminobutyric acid.

ho·mo·car·no·sin·o·sis (hō′mō-kahr′nō-sēn-ō′sis) An inborn error in metabolism in which homocarnosine levels are elevated, particularly in the cerebrospinal fluid.

ho•mo•cit•rul•li•nu•ri•a (hō′mō-sit′rū-li-nyūr′ē-ă) An inherited disorder associated with elevated urinary levels of homocitrulline.

ho•mo•cys•te•ine (hō′mō-sis′tē-ēn) A homologue of cysteine, produced by the demethylation of methionine, and an intermediate in the biosynthesis of L-cysteine from L-methionine via L-cystathionine. Elevation in serum levels increase risk of atherosclerosis.

homocystinaemia [Br.] SYN homocystinemia.

ho•mo•cys•tine (hō′mō-sis′tēn) The disulfide resulting from the mild oxidation of homocysteine; an analogue of cystine.

ho•mo•cys•ti•ne•mi•a (hō′mō-sis-ti-nē′mē-ă) Presence of an excess of homocystine in the plasma, as in homocystinuria. SYN homocystinaemia.

ho•mo•cy•to•tro•pic (hō′mō-sī-tō-trō′pik) Having an affinity for cells of the same or a closely related species. [homo- + G. *kytos,* cell, + *tropē,* a turning toward]

ho•mo•cy•to•tro•pic an•ti•bod•y (hō′mō-sī-tō-trō′pik an′ti-bod-ē) Antibody of the IgE class that has an affinity for tissues (notably mast cells) of the same or a closely related species and that, on combining with specific antigen, triggers the release of pharmacologic mediators of anaphylaxis from the cells to which it is attached. SYN reaginic antibody.

ho•mo•dont (hō′mō-dont) Having teeth that are morphologically of the same type, as in the alligator. [homo- + G. *odous,* tooth]

ho•mo•ga•met•ic (hō′mō-gă-met′ik) Producing only one type of gamete with respect to sex chromosomes; in humans and most animals, the female is homogametic. SYN monogametic. [homo- + G. *gametikos,* connubial]

ho•mog•a•my (hō-mog′ă-mē) Similarity of husband and wife in a specific trait. [homo- + G. *gamos,* marriage]

ho•mo•ge•ne•ous (hō′mō-jē′nē-ŭs) Of uniform structure or composition throughout. [homo- + G. *genos,* race]

ho•mo•ge•ne•ous ra•di•a•tion (hō′mō-jē′nē-ŭs rā′dē-ā′shŭn) Radiation consisting of a narrow band of frequencies, the same energy, or a single type of particle.

ho•mo•ge•ne•ous sys•tem (hō′mō-jē′nē-ŭs sis′tĕm) CHEMISTRY a system with parts that cannot be mechanically separated, and is therefore uniform throughout and possesses in every part identically physical properties; e.g., a solution of sodium chloride in water.

ho•mo•gen•e•sis (hō′mō-jen′ĕ-sis) Production of offspring similar to the parents, in contrast to heterogenesis. [homo- + G. *genesis,* production]

ho•mog•e•nous (hō-moj′ĕ-nŭs) Having a structural similarity because of descent from a common ancestor. Commonly confused with homogeneous. [homo- + G. *genos,* family, kind]

ho•mo•gen•tis•ic ac•id (hō′mō-jen-tis′ik as′id) An intermediate in L-phenylalanine and L-tyrosine catabolism; if made alkaline, it oxidizes rapidly in air to a quinone that polymerizes to a melaninlike material; elevated levels are observed in individuals having alcaptonuria. SYN alcapton, alkapton.

ho•mo•gon•ic life cy•cle (hō′mō-gon′ik līf sī′kĕl) Parasitic stage of life cycle of an organism (e.g., *Strongyloides stercoralis*) that also has a free-living stage.

ho•mo•graft (hō′mō-graft) Type of skin graft from another person or a cadaver used in the treatment of burns.

ho•mo•lat•er•al (hō′mō-lat′ĕr-ăl) SYN ipsilateral. [homo- + L. *latus,* side]

ho•mol•o•gous (hŏ-mol′ō-gŭs) **1.** BIOLOGY denoting organs or parts corresponding in evolutionary origin and similar to some extent in structure, but not necessarily similar in function. **2.** CHEMISTRY denoting a single chemical series, differing by fixed increments. **3.** GENETICS denoting chromosomes or chromosome parts identical with respect to their construction and genetic content. **4.** IMMUNOLOGY denoting serum or tissue derived from members of a single species, or an antibody with respect to the antigen that produced it.

ho•mol•o•gous chro•mo•somes (hŏ-mol′ō-gŭs krō′mŏ-sōmz) Members of a single pair of chromosomes.

ho•mol•o•gous graft (hŏ-mol′ō-gŭs graft) SYN allograft.

ho•mol•o•gous re•com•bi•na•tion (hŏ-mol′ō-gŭs rē-kom′bi-nā′shŭn) The exchange of corresponding stretches of DNA between two sister chromosomes.

ho•mol•o•gous stim•u•lus (hŏ-mol′ō-gŭs stim′yū-lŭs) A stimulus that acts only on the nerve terminations in a special sense organ.

ho•mol•o•gous tu•mor (hŏ-mol′ō-gŭs tū′mŏr) A tumor composed of tissue of the same sort as that from which it springs.

ho•mol•y•sin (hō-mol′i-sin) A sensitizing hemolytic antibody (hemolysin) formed as the result of stimulation by an antigen derived from an animal of the same species. [homo- + hemolysin]

ho•mol•y•sis (hō-mol′i-sis) Lysis of red blood cells by a homolysin and complement.

ho•mo•mor•phic (hō′mō-mōr′fik) Denoting

two or more structures of similar size and shape. [homo- + G. *morphē,* shape, appearance]

ho•mon•o•mous (hō-mon′ŏ-mŭs) Denoting parts, having similar form and structure, arranged in a series, as the fingers or toes. [G. *homonomos,* under the same laws, fr. *homos,* same, + *nomos,* law]

ho•mon•y•mous (hō-mon′i-mŭs) Having the same name or expressed in the same terms, e.g., the corresponding halves (right or left, superior or inferior) of the retinas. [G. *homōnymos,* of the same name, fr. *onyma,* name]

hom•on•y•mous dip•lo•pi•a (hō-mon′ŏ-mŭs di-plō′pē-ă) Visual defect in which the image observed by the right eye appears shifted to the right of the image observed by the left eye.

hom•on•y•mous hem•i•an•op•i•a (hō-mon′ŏ-mŭs hem′ē-ă-nō′pē-ă) Visual deficit affecting the same side (right or left) of each visual field. SYN homonymous hemianopsia.

hom•on•y•mous hem•i•an•op•si•a (hō-mon′ŏ-mŭs hem′ē-an-op′sē-ă) SYN homonymous hemianopia.

ho•mon•y•mous im•ag•es (hō-mon′i-mŭs im′ăj-ĕz) Double images produced by stimuli arising from points proximal to the horopter.

ho•mo•phil (hō′mō-fil) Denoting an antibody that reacts only with the specific antigen that induced its formation. [homo- + G. *philos,* fond]

ho•mo•pho•bi•a (hō′mō-fō′bē-ă) Irrational fear of homosexual feelings, thoughts, behaviors, or people.

ho•mo•plas•tic (hō′mō-plas′tik) Similar in form and structure, but not in origin. [homo- + G. *plastos,* formed]

ho•mo•plas•tic graft (hō′mō-plas′tik graft) SYN allograft.

ho•mo•plas•ty (hō′mō-plas-tē) Repair of a defect by a homograft.

ho•mo•pol•y•mer (hō′mō-pol′i-mĕr) A polymer composed of a series of identical radicals; e.g., polylysine, poly(adenylic acid), polyglucose.

hom•or•gan•ic (hom′ōr-gan′ik) Produced by the same organs, or by homologous organs.

Ho•mo sa•pi•ens (hō′mō sā′pē-ĕnz) The genus and species of humankind.

ho•mo•ser•ine (hō′mō-ser′ēn) A hydroxyamino acid differing from serine in the possession of an additional CH_2 group; formed in the conversion of L-methionine to L-cysteine.

ho•mo•sex•u•al (hō′mō-sek′shū-ăl) **1.** Relating to or characteristic of homosexuality. **2.** One whose interests and behavior are characteristic of homosexuality. SEE gay, lesbian.

ho•mo•sex•u•al in•ter•course (hō′mō-sek′shū-ăl in′tĕr-kōrs) Oral, manual, and anal sexual stimulation between members of the same sex.

ho•mo•sex•u•al•i•ty (hō′mō-sek′shū-al′i-tē) Erotic attraction, predisposition, or activity, including sexual congress, between people of the same sex, especially past puberty.

ho•mo•sex•u•al pan•ic (hō′mō-sek′shū-ăl pan′ik) An acute, severe attack of anxiety based on unconscious conflicts regarding homosexuality.

ho•mo•ton•ic (hō′mō-ton′ik) Of uniform tension or tonus.

ho•mo•top•ic (hō′mō-top′ik) Pertaining to or occurring at the same place or part of the body. [homo- + G. *topos,* place]

ho•mo•type (hō′mō-tīp) Any part or organ of the same structure or function as another, especially as one on the opposite side of the body. [homo- + G. *typos,* type]

ho•mo•typ•ic, **ho•mo•typ•i•cal** (hō′mō-tip′ik, i-kăl) Of the same type or form; corresponding to the other one of two paired organs or parts.

ho•mo•va•nil•lic ac•id (HVA) (hō′mō-vă-nil′ik as′id) A phenol found in human urine; produced through the methylation of homoprotocatechuic acid on the *meta*-OH group.

ho•mo•zy•gos•i•ty, **ho•mo•zy•go•sis** (hō′mō-zī-gos′i-tē, -zī-gō′sis) The state of being homozygous. [homo- + G. *zygon,* yoke]

ho•mo•zy•gote (hō′mō-zī′gōt) A homozygous individual. [homo- + G. *zygōtos,* yoke]

ho•mo•zy•gous (hō′mō-zī′gŭs) Having identical genes at one or more loci.

ho•mo•zy•gous by de•scent (hō′mō-zī′gŭs dĕ-sent′) Possessing two genes at a given locus that are descended from a single source, as may occur in consanguineous mating.

ho•mun•cu•lus (hō-mŭngk′yū-lŭs) The figure of a human sometimes superimposed on pictures of the surface of the brain to represent the motor or sensory regions of the body represented there. [L. dim. of *homo,* man]

hon•ey•comb lung (hŏn′ē-kōm lŭng) The radiologic and gross appearance of the lungs resulting from interstitial fibrosis and cystic dilation of bronchioles and distal air spaces; a sequel of any of several diseases, including eosinophilic granuloma and sarcoidosis.

hon•ey•comb pat•tern (hŏn′ē-kōm pat′ĕrn) Dense, slightly irregular circular shadows, most common next to the pleura at the lung base, on chest radiographs or CT; caused by chronic interstitial fibrosis of diverse causes.

Hong Kong in•flu•en•za (hawng-kawng in-flū-en′ză) Influenza caused by a serotype of influenza virus type A that was first identified in Hong Kong.

hood (hud) SYN laminar flow hood. SEE ALSO horizontal laminar flow hood, vertical laminar flow hood.

hook (huk) **1.** An instrument curved or bent near its tip, used for fixation of a part or traction. **2.** SYN hamulus. [A.S. *hōk*]

Hooke law (huk law) The stress applied to stretch or compress a body is proportional to the strain, or change in length thus produced, so long as the limit of elasticity of the body is not exceeded.

hook•worm (huk′wŏrm) Common name for bloodsucking nematodes, chiefly members of the genera *Ancylostoma* (Old World hookworm), *Necator*, and *Uncinaria*, and including the species *A. caninum* (dog hookworm) and *N. americanus* (New World hookworm). See page B7.

hook•worm dis•ease (huk′wŏrm di-zēz′) SEE ancylostomiasis, necatoriasis.

Hoo•ver signs (hū′vĕr sīnz) **1.** A subject lying supine, when asked to raise one leg, involuntarily creates counterpressure with the heel of the other leg; if this leg is paralyzed, whatever muscular power is preserved in it will be exerted in this way; or if the patient attempts to lift a paralyzed leg, counterpressure will be made with the other heel, whether any movement occurs in the paralyzed limb or not; not present in hysteria or malingering. **2.** A modification in the movement of the costal margins during respiration, caused by a flattening of the diaphragm; suggestive of empyema or other intrathoracic condition causing a change in the contour of the diaphragm.

Hop•kins rod-lens tel•e•scope (hop′kinz rod′lenz tel′ĕ-skōp) An endoscopic telescope in which the air-containing spaces between the conventional series of lenses are replaced with glass rods with polished ends separated by small "air-lenses." This system transmits more light, yields greater magnification and provides greater depth and breadth of field than conventional lens systems.

Hop•mann pap•il•lo•ma (hop′mahn pap-i-lō′mă) A papillomatous overgrowth of the nasal mucous membrane.

hor•de•o•lum (hōr′dē′ō-lŭm) A suppurative inflammation of a gland or hair follicle of the eyelid. SYN sty, stye. [Mod. L., *hordeolus,* a sty in the eye, dim. of *hordeum,* barley]

hor•de•o•lum ex•ter•num (hōr′dē′ō-lŭm ekstĕr′nŭm) Inflammation of the sebaceous gland of an eyelash.

hor•i•zon•tal fis•sure of cer•e•bel•lum (hōr′i-zon′tăl fish′ŭr ser′ĕ-bel′ŭm) Horizontal fissure that divides the ansiform lobule into its major parts, crus I (superior semilunar lobule) and crus II (inferior semilunar lobule).

hor•i•zon•tal heart (hōr′i-zon′tăl hahrt) Description of the heart's electrical position; recognized in the electrocardiogram when the electrical axis lies between −30 and +30 degrees.

hor•i•zon•tal lam•i•nar flow hood (hōr′i-zon′tăl lam′i-năr′ flō hud) A laminar flow hood in which the air is pushed through a filter horizontally toward the user to maintain a sterile environment.

hor•i•zon•tal la•ryn•gec•tomy (hōr′i-zon′tăl lar′in-jek′tŏ-mē) SYN partial laryngectomy.

hor•i•zon•tal max•il•lar•y frac•ture (hōr′i-zon′tăl mak′si-lar-ē frak′shŭr) A horizontal fracture at the base of the maxillae above the apices of the teeth. SYN Guérin fracture, Le Fort I fracture.

hor•i•zon•tal o•ver•lap (hōr′i-zon′tăl ō′vĕr-lap) The projection of the upper anterior or posterior teeth beyond their antagonists in a horizontal direction. SYN overjet, overjut.

hor•i•zon•tal plane (hōr′i-zon′tăl plān) Plane parallel and relative to the horizon; in the anatomic position, horizontal planes are transverse planes; in the supine or prone positions, horizontal planes are frontal (coronal planes).

hor•i•zon•tal tear (hōr′i-zon′tăl tār) A tear of articular cartilage roughly perpendicular to the long axis of the bone.

hor•i•zon•tal trans•mis•sion (hōr′i-zon′tăl trans-mish′ŭn) Transmission of infectious agents from an infected individual to a susceptible contemporary, in contradistinction to vertical transmission.

hor•mo•nal (hōr-mōn′ăl) Pertaining to hormones. Cf. bioregulator.

hor•mo•nal gin•gi•vi•tis (hōr-mōn′ăl jin′ji-vī′tis) Gingivitis in which the host response to bacterial plaque is presumably exacerbated by hormonal alterations occurring during puberty, pregnancy, oral contraceptive use, or menopause. SYN pregnancy gingivitis.

hor•mone (hōr′mōn) A chemical substance formed in a tissue or organ and carried in the blood; stimulates or inhibits the growth or function of one or more other tissues or organs. [G. *hormōn,* pres. part. of *hormaō,* to rouse or set in motion]

hor•mone re•place•ment ther•a•py (HRT) (hōr′mōn rĕ-plās′mĕnt thār′ă-pē) SYN estrogen replacement therapy.

hor•mo•no•gen•e•sis (hōr′mō-nō-jen′ĕ-sis) The formation of hormones. SYN hormonopoiesis.

hor•mo•no•gen•ic (hōr′mō-nō-jen′ik) Pertaining to the formation of a hormone. SYN hormonopoietic.

hor•mo•no•poi•e•sis (hōr′mō-nō-poy-ē′sis) SYN hormonogenesis. [hormone + G. *poiēsis,* production]

hor•mo•no•poi•et•ic (hōr′mō-nō-poy-et′ik) SYN hormonogenic.

horn (hōrn) **1.** A hard projection; consisting largely of compact keratin, tapering to a point, usually paired, on the head of certain mammals. **2.** Any structure resembling a horn in shape. SYN cornu (1). [A.S.]

Hor•ner pu•pil (hōr′nĕr pyū′pil) Constricted pupil due to impairment of sympathetic nerve innervation of the dilator muscle of the pupil. SEE ALSO Horner syndrome.

Hor•ner syn•drome (hōr′nĕr sin′drōm) Ptosis, miosis, and anhidrosis on the side of a sympathetic palsy. Enophthalmos is more apparent than real. The affected pupil is visibly slow to dilate in dim light; due to a lesion of the cervical sympathetic chain or its central pathways.

Hor•ner teeth (hōr′nĕr tēth) Incisor teeth having a horizontal, hypoplastic groove.

Hor•ner-Tran•tas dots (hōr′nĕr-trahn′tăs dotz) Evanescent white cellular infiltrates occurring in vernal keratoconjunctivitis.

horn•y (hōrn′ē) Of the nature or structure of horn. SYN corneous, keratic, keratinous (2), keratoid (1), keroid.

horn•y la•yer (hōr′nē lā′ĕr) SYN stratum corneum epidermidis.

hor•rip•i•la•tion (ho′rip-i-lā′shŭn) Erection of the fine hairs on contraction of the arrectores pilorum. [L. *horreo,* to bristle, + *pilus,* hair]

horse chest•nut (hōrs chest′nŭt) (*Aesculus hippocastanum*) The nuts from this tree, after preparation, are made into a liquid used for its purported value as a tonic and narcotic.

horse•rad•ish per•ox•i•das•es (hōrs′rad-ish pĕr-ok′si-dās-ĕz) An enzyme used in immunohistochemistry to label the antigen-antibody complex.

horse•shoe fis•tu•la (hōrs′shū fis′chū-lă) An anal fistula partially encircling the anus and opening at both extremities on the cutaneous surface.

horse•shoe kid•ney (hōrs′shū kid′nē) Poles of the two kidneys, usually the inferior ones; occasionally, the poles of the kidneys are joined by a band that extends across the midline.

horse•tail (hōrs′tāl) (*Equisetum arvense*) An herbal remedy purported to have value in wound healing and other internal uses; serious adverse reactions have been reported after its use.

Hor•te•ga cells (ōr-tā′gă selz) SYN microglia.

Hor•te•ga neu•rog•li•a stain (ōr-tā′gă nūr-og′lē-ă stān) One of several silver carbonate methods to demonstrate astrocytes, oligodendroglia, and microglia.

Hor•ton ar•te•ri•tis (hōr′tŏn ahr′tĕr-ī′tis) SYN temporal arteritis.

Hor•ton head•ache (hōr′tŏn hed′āk) SYN cluster headache.

hose (hōz) Thin, form-fitting leg covering; in medicine, used in the treatment of circulatory problems, to promote venous return. SEE ALSO TED hose.

hos•pice (hos′pis) An institution that provides a centralized program of palliative and supportive services to dying patients and their families, in the form of physical, psychological, social, and spiritual care; such services are provided by an interdisciplinary team of professionals and volunteers who are available to provide assistance at home and in specialized inpatient settings. [L. *hospitium*, hospitality, lodging, fr. *hospes*, guest]

hos•pi•tal (hos′pi-tăl) A health care facility or institution equipped for medical diagnosis, treatment, and care for both inpatients and outpatients and for clinical training of physicians, nurses, and allied care personnel. [L. *hospitalis,* for a guest, fr. *hospes* (*hospit-*), a host, a guest]

hos•pi•tal-ac•quired in•fec•tion (hos′pi-tăl-ă-kwīd′ in-fek′shŭn) SEE nosocomial (2).

hos•pi•tal-based phy•si•cian (hos′pi-tăl-bāst fī-zish′ŭn) SYN hospitalist (1).

hos•pi•tal bed syn•drome (hos′pi-tăl bed sin′drōm) An event whereby a disabled, usually aged, patient, manages to get out of a hospital bed even though the sides are elevated, either out of agitation, altered mentation, or suicidal ideation.

hos•pi•tal in•for•ma•tion syst•em (hos′pi-tăl in′fōr-mā′shŭn sis′tĕm) Integrated computer system to store, manipulate, and retrieve clinical, nonclinical, and administrative information in health care organization.

hospitalisation [Br.] SYN hospitalization.

hos•pi•tal•ist (hos′pit-ăl-ist) **1.** A physician whose professional activities are performed chiefly within a hospital (e.g., anesthesiologist, emergency department physician, intensivist (intensive care specialist), pathologist, and radiologist). SYN hospital-based physician. **2.** A primary care physician (not a house officer) who assumes responsibility for the observation and treatment of hospitalized patients and returns them to the care of their private physicians when they are discharged from the hospital. [hospital + -ist]

hos•pi•tal•i•za•tion (hos′pi-tăl-ī-zā′shŭn) Placing a patient in a hospital for diagnostic study and treatment. SYN hospitalisation.

hos·pi·ta·lize (hos'pi-tăl-īz) To place in a hospital.

hos·pi·tal rec·ord (hos'pi-tăl rek'ŏrd) The medical record generated during hospitalization, containing a history and physical examination report, physicians' progress notes and treatment orders, notes of nurses' observations and treatments administered, reports of laboratory tests, x-ray and other diagnostic studies, surgical procedures, consultants' opinions, and a discharge summary or autopsy record.

host (hōst) The organism in or on which a parasite lives, thus deriving its body substance or energy. [L. *hospes,* a host]

host cell (hōst sel) A cell (e.g., a bacterium) in which a vector can be propagated.

hot com·press (hot kom'pres) A pad of flannel or gauze wrung out of hot water or physiologic saline and firmly applied to a body surface to promote local pain relief, muscular relaxation, or pointing of an abscess.

hot flash, hot flush (hot flash, hot flŭsh) Colloquialism for one of the vasomotor symptoms of the climacteric that may involve the whole body as a flash of heat.

hot line (hot līn) In health care, a direct telephone link for emergency services.

hot nod·ule (hot nod'yūl) A thyroid nodule with a much higher uptake of radioactive iodine than the surrounding parenchyma; usually benign but sometimes causing hyperthyroidism.

hot pep·per (hot pep'ĕr) SYN capsicum.

hot spot (hot spot) A region in a gene in which there is a putatively high rate of mutation.

hot tub dis·ease (hot tŭb di-zēz') Dermatologic and respiratory illness related to pathogens present in the water of a hot tub.

hot tub fol·lic·u·li·tis (hot tŭb fŏ-lik'yū-lī'tis) Pruritic papules and pustules in body areas covered by a bathing suit after prolonged immersion in a hot tub; caused by *Pseudomonas aeruginosa.* See page B4.

hot-wire flow-mea·sur·ing de·vice (hot' wīr flō'mezh'ĕr-ing dĕ-vīs') A device used to measure flow; it relies on the effect of convective cooling as a stream of air passes over a small heated filament (thermistor).

hour·glass con·trac·tion (owr'glas kŏn-trak' shŭn) Constriction of the middle portion of a hollow organ, such as the stomach or the gravid uterus.

hour·glass mur·mur (owr'glas mŭr'mŭr) One in which there are two areas of maximum loudness decreasing to a point midway between the two.

hour·glass stom·ach (owr'glas stŏm'ăk) A condition in which there is a central constriction of the wall of the stomach dividing it into two cavities, cardiac and pyloric.

house·keep·ing de·part·ment (hows'kēp-ing dĕ-pahrt'mĕnt) In health care, the agency in a hospital or long-term nursing facility responsible for care of the facility, rather than the patient.

house·maid's knee (hows'mādz nē) An adventitious occupational bursitis occurring over the tibial tuberosity, the area of contact when kneeling; not to be confused with infrapatellar bursitis.

house of·fi·cer (hows awf'i-sĕr) An intern or resident employed by a hospital to provide service to patients while receiving training in a medical specialty.

house or·gan (hows ōr'găn) A colloquial term used to describe a publication offering news of a business or institution (e.g., hospital); now largely supplanted by online services and Web sites.

house phy·si·cian (hows fi-zish'ŭn) A doctor responsible for patient care within an institution under the guidance of an attending physician.

house staff (hows staf) Physicians and surgeons in specialty training at a hospital who care for the patients under the direction and responsibility of the attending staff.

house·wives' ec·ze·ma (hows'wīvz eks'ĕ-mă) Colloquial usage describing rashes related to the use of cleaning fluids (e.g., harsh soaps or astringents) involved in cleaning the home.

Hous·ton-Har·ris syn·drome (hyū'stŏn-har' is sin'drōm) SYN achondrogenesis type IA.

How·ell-Jol·ly bod·ies (how'ĕl zhō-lē' bod' ēz) Spheric or ovoid eccentrically located granules, approximately 1 mcm in diameter, occasionally observed in the stroma of circulating erythrocytes after splenectomy or in megaloblastic or severe hemolytic anemia.

How·ship la·cu·nae (how'ship lă-kū'nē) Tiny depressions, pits, or irregular grooves in bone that is being resorbed by osteoclasts. SYN resorption lacunae.

H&P Abbreviation for history and physical.

HPA ax·is Abbreviation for hypothalamic-pituitary-adrenal axis.

HPI Abbreviation for history of present illness.

HPLC Abbreviation for high-pressure liquid chromatography; high-performance liquid chromatography.

HPV Abbreviation for human papillomavirus.

HR con·duc·tion time (kŏn-dŭk'shŭn tīm) SEE intraventricular conduction.

HRCT Abbreviation for high-resolution computed tomography.

H.R.Q.O.L. Abbreviation for health-related quality of life. SEE ALSO Q.O.L.

HRR Abbreviation for high-risk register.

HRSA Abbreviation for Health Resources and Services Administration.

HRT Abbreviation for hormone replacement therapy.

Hru•by lens (rū′bē lenz) A non-contact lens mounted on a slitlamp used for evaluating the retina.

HSCT Abbreviation for hematopoietic stem cell transplantation.

hsiang-dan (shahng-dahn) SYN *Aloe vera.*

HSIL Abbreviation for high-grade squamous intraepithelial lesion.

HSV Abbreviation for herpes simplex virus.

5-HT Abbreviation for 5-hydroxytryptamine.

Ht Abbreviation for total hyperopia.

HTLV Abbreviation for human T-cell lymphoma/leukemia virus.

HTLV-I Abbreviation for human T-cell lymphotrophic virus type I; human lymphotropic virus, type 1.

HTLV-II Abbreviation for human T-cell lymphotrophic virus type II; human lymphotropic virus, type 2.

HTLV-III Abbreviation for human T-cell lymphotropic virus type III. SEE human immunodeficiency virus.

HTN Abbreviation for hypertension.

huang chi (hwahng chē) SYN *Astragalus.*

hub (hŭb) The expanded portion of a hollow needle that serves as a handle for manipulation and as a site of attachment for a syringe, infusion tube, or some other appliance.

Hüc•kel rule (hē′kĕl rūl) The number of depolarized electrons in an aromatic ring is equal to $4n + 2$ where n is 0 or any positive integer; L-tyrosine, L-phenylalanine, L-tryptophan, and L-histidine (when the imidazole ring is deprotonated) obey this rule.

huck•le•ber•ry (hŭk′ĕl-ber-ē) SYN bilberry.

Hue•ter ma•neu•ver (hē′tĕr mă-nū′vĕr) Pressing the patient's tongue downward and forward with the left forefinger in passing a stomach tube.

huff cough•ing (hŭf kawf′ing) A type of deep breathing and coughing exercise taught to postoperative patients. Patients inhale deeply while leaning forward and exhale sharply while making a "huff" sound. This mobilizes secretions and helps to keep airway open and clear.

Hüf•ner e•qua•tion (hēf′ner ĕ-kwā′zhŭn) An equation expressing the relationship between myoglobin dissociation and oxygen partial pressure: $([MBO_2]/[Mb]) = (K \times pO_2)$.

HUGO (hyū′gō) Abbreviation for Human Genome Organization.

Hull tri•ad (hŭl trī′ad) The association of diastolic gallop, anasarca, and small pulse pressure.

hum (hŭm) A low continuous murmur. [echoic]

hu•man an•ti•he•mo•phil•ic fac•tor (hyū′măn an′tē-hē-mō-fil′ik fak′tŏr) A lyophilized concentrate of factor VIII, obtained from fresh normal human plasma; used as a hemostatic agent in hemophilia.

hu•man bite (hyū′măn bīt) A wound caused by human teeth; because the human oral cavity harbors multiple pathogens, such wounds must be thoroughly cleaned to prevent serious infection.

hu•man ca•lor•i•me•ter (hyū′măn kal′ŏr-im′ĕ-tĕr) A device to measure the heat output of the human body during various levels of physical exertion. It consists of a chamber with closed air circulation and a means of comparing the temperature of water entering a coil completely surrounding the subject with the temperature of water leaving the coil.

hu•man cho•ri•on•ic go•nad•o•tro•pin (hCG) (hyū′măn kōr′ē-on′ik gō-nad′ō-trō′pin) SEE chorionic gonadotropin.

hu•man cho•ri•on•ic so•ma•to•mam•mo•tro•pic hor•mone (HCS) (hyū′măn kōr′ē-on′ik sō′mă-tō-mam′ō-trō′pik hōr′mōn) SYN human placental lactogen.

hu•man com•mu•ni•ca•tion (hyū′măn kŏ-myū′ni-kā′shŭn) The production and reception of oral, written, signed, or gestured information among human beings; involves the use of symbols known as language received through the auditory, tactile, proprioceptive, and visual systems and generated through voice and speech, writing, manual signs, and gestures; communication among humans may at times involve the vestibular, olfactory, and gustatory senses.

hu•man dip•loid cell vac•cine (hyū′măn dip′loyd sel vak-sēn′) An iodinated virus vaccine used for protection against rabies vaccine usually prepared in the human diploid cell WI-38.

hu•man e•col•o•gy (hyū′măm ē-kol′ŏ-jē) The study and science of the natural world as related to *Homo sapiens* and the place of the species within the world.

hu•man e•o•sin•o•phil•ic en•ter•i•tis (hyū′măn ē′ō-sin-ō-fil′ik en′tĕr-ī′tis) Segmental eosinophilic inflammation of the gastrointestinal tract in humans; suspect etiologic agent is *Ancylos-*

toma caninum; laboratory indicators are eosinophilia and increased IgE.

hu•man gam•ma glob•u•lin (hyū′măn gam′ă glob′yū-lin) A preparation of the proteins of liquid human plasma, containing the antibodies of normal adults; it is obtained from pooled liquid human plasma from a number of donors.

hu•man ge•net•ics (hyū′măn jĕ-net′iks) The study of the genetic aspects of humans as a species. Cf. medical genetics.

Hu•man Ge•nome Or•ga•ni•za•tion (HUGO) (hyū′măn jē′nōm ōr′găn-ī-zā′shŭn) An international association of geneticists and specialists in the related sciences founded in 1989 and dedicated to the exploration of all ramifications of genetic studies.

Hu•man Ge•nome Pro•ject (hyū′măn jē′nōm proj′ekt) A comprehensive effort by molecular biologists worldwide to map the human genome, which consists of about 100,000 genes, or 3 billion DNA base pairs. The wholesale sequencing of the genome would not be possible without the automated method of gene sequencing, invented by Leroy Hood.

hu•man glan•du•lar kal•li•kre•in 3 (hK3) (hyū′măn glan′dyū-lăr kal′i-krē′in) SYN prostate-specific antigen.

hu•man gran•u•lo•cyt•ic ehr•lich•i•o•sis (HGE) (hū′măn gran′yū-lō-sit′ik er-lik′ē-ō′sis) A febrile disease causing headache and myalgia and sometimes involving the respiratory, digestive, and central nervous systems; caused by *Anaplasma phagocytophaga*, which is transmitted by ixodid ticks; laboratory findings include leukopenia, thrombocytopenia, and inclusion bodies (morulae) in neutrophils.

hu•man her•pes•vi•rus 1 (hyū′măn hĕr′pēz-vī′rŭs) Herpes simplex virus, type 1. SEE herpes simplex.

hu•man her•pes•vi•rus 2 (hyū′măn hĕr′pēz-vī′rŭs) Herpes simplex virus, type 2. SEE herpes simplex.

hu•man her•pes•vi•rus 3 (hyū′măn hĕr′pēz-vī′rŭs) SYN varicella-zoster virus.

hu•man her•pes•vi•rus 4 (hyū′măn hĕr′pēz-vī′rŭs) SYN Epstein-Barr virus.

hu•man her•pes•vi•rus 5 (hyū′măn hĕr′pēz-vī′rŭs) SYN cytomegalovirus.

hu•man her•pes•vi•rus 6 (hyū′măn hĕr′pēz-vī′rŭs) A herpesvirus found in certain lymphoproliferative disorders, and associated with roseola (exanthema subitum).

human her•pes•vi•rus 7 (hyū′măn hĕr′pēz-vī′rŭs) Virus found in association with human T lymphocytes and is shed in the saliva of most adults; however, a causal relationship to any known disease has not been determined.

hu•man her•pes•vi•rus 8 (hyū′măn hĕr′pēz-vī′rŭs) A linear double-stranded DNA virus that induces Kaposi sarcoma (KS) in immunodeficient people. DNA sequences unique to this virus are regularly found in KS specimens from HIV-negative people as well. The virus is also associated with several uncommon lymphoproliferative syndromes in AIDS patients, including multicentric Castleman disease and primary effusion lymphoma (body cavity-based lymphoma).

hu•man im•mu•no•de•fi•cien•cy vi•rus 2 (HIV-2) (hyū′măn im′yū-nō-dĕ-fish′ĕn-sē vī′rŭs) A virus, found primarily in West Africa, which causes a less virulent form of AIDS and is more closely related to simian virus strains. SEE ALSO AIDS.

hu•man im•mu•no•de•fi•cien•cy vi•rus (HIV) (hyū′măn im′yū-nō-dĕ-fish′ĕn-sē vī′rŭs) Human T-cell lymphotropic virus type III; a cytopathic retrovirus that is the etiologic agent of acquired immunodeficiency syndrome (AIDS) (q.v.). See this page, B6 . SYN lymphadenopathy-associated virus.

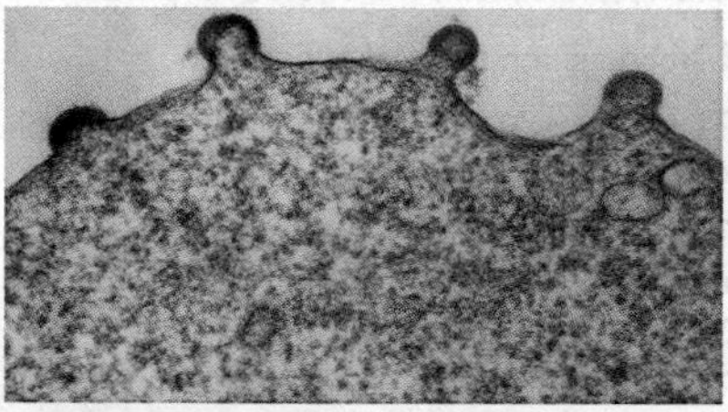

budding of virions from the plasma membrane of an HIV-infected cell

hu•man in•su•lin (hyū′măn in′sŭ-lin) A protein that has the normal structure of insulin produced by the human pancreas, prepared by recombinant DNA techniques and by semisynthetic processes.

hu•man leu•ko•cyte an•ti•gen (hyū′măn lū′kō-sīt an′ti-jen) Any of several members of a system consisting of the gene products of at least four linked loci (A, B, C, and D) and a number of subloci on the sixth human chromosome that have been shown to have a strong influence on human allotransplantation, transfusions in refractory patients, and certain disease associations; more than 50 alleles are recognized, most of which are at loci HLA-A and HLA-B; autosomal dominant inheritance.

hu•man men•o•pau•sal go•nad•o•tro•pin (hyū′măn men′ō-paw′zăl gō-nad′ō-trō′pin) A pituitary hormone originally obtained from the urine of postmenopausal women but now produced synthetically; used to induce ovulation. SEE ALSO menotropins. Cf. bioregulator.

hu•man mo•no•cy•tic ehr•lich•i•o•sis (HME) (hyū′măn mon-ō-sit′ik er-lik-ē-ō′sis) A febrile disease caused by *Ehrlichia chaffeensis* and transmitted by the Lone Star tick (*Ambly-*

omma americanum); similar to human granulocytic ehrlichiosis, except that inclusions are found in monocytes.

hu·man pap·il·lo·ma·vi·rus (HPV) (hyū′măn pap-i-lō′mă-vī′rŭs) DNA virus of the genus papillomavirus; certain types cause cutaneous and genital warts in humans, including verruca vulgaris and condyloma acuminatum; other types are associated with severe cervical intraepithelial neoplasia and anogenital and laryngeal carcinomas. Over 70 types have been characterized on the basis of DNA relatedness. SYN infectious papillomavirus.

hu·man pla·cen·tal lac·to·gen (hyū′măn plă-sen′tăl lak′tō-jen) Any agent to stimulate human milk production that has been isolated from human placentas; its biologic activity mimics that of somatotropin and prolactin; secreted into maternal circulation; deficiency during pregnancy leads to abnormal intrauterine and postnatal growth. Cf. bioregulator. SYN chorionic growth hormone-prolactin, human chorionic somatomammotropic hormone, placental growth hormone.

hu·man plas·ma pro·tein frac·tion (hyū′măn plaz′mă prō′tēn frak′shŭn) A solution of selected proteins derived from the plasma of human donors, containing 4.5–5.5 g of protein per 100 mL, of which 83–90% is albumin and the remainder is α- and β-globulins; used as a blood volume supporter.

hu·man T-cell lym·pho·ma/leu·ke·mi·a vi·rus (HTLV) (hyū′măn sel lim-fō′mă-lū-kē′mē-ă vī′rŭs) A group of viruses (subfamily Oncovirinae, family Retroviridae) that are lymphotropic with a selective affinity for the helper/inducer cell subset of T lymphocytes and are associated with adult T-cell leukemia and lymphoma.

hu·mec·tant (hyū-mek′tănt) An agent that promotes retention of moisture; a substance added to a powder, e.g., a dentifrice, to prevent hardening on exposure to air. [L. *humectus,* moist, fr. *humor,* moisture]

hu·mer·al (hyū′mĕr-ăl) Relating to the humerus.

hu·mer·al joint (hyū′mĕr-ăl joynt) SYN shoulder joint.

hu·mer·o·ra·di·al (hyū′mĕr-ō-rā′dē-ăl) Relating to both humerus and radius; denoting especially the ratio of length of one to the other.

hu·mer·o·ra·di·al joint (hyū′mĕr-ō-rā′dē-ăl joynt) The portion of the elbow joint between the capitulum of the humerus and the head of the radius.

hu·mer·o·scap·u·lar (hyū′mĕr-ō-skap′yū-lăr) Relating to both humerus and scapula.

hu·mer·o·ul·nar (hyū′mĕr-ō-ŭl′năr) Relating to both humerus and ulna; denoting especially the ratio of length of one to the other.

hu·mer·o·ul·nar joint (hyū′mĕr-ō-ŭl′năr joynt) The portion of the elbow joint between the trochlea of the humerus and the trochlear notch of the ulna.

i **hu·mer·us**, gen. and pl. **hu·mer·i** (hyū′mĕr-ŭs, -ī) [TA] The bone of the arm, articulating with the scapula above and the radius and ulna below. See this page. [L. shoulder]

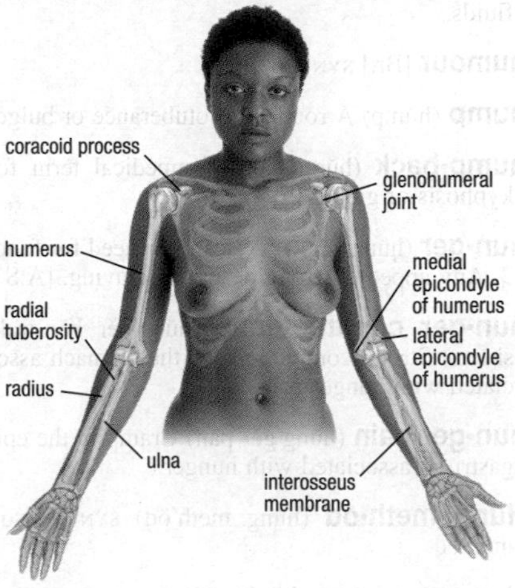

humerus

hu·mid·i·fi·er (hyū-mid′i-fī-ĕr) A device for increasing the water vapor content of a gas or of ambient air.

hu·mid·i·ty (hyū-mid′i-tē) Moisture or dampness, as of the air. [L. *humiditas,* dampness]

Hum·mels·heim op·er·a·tion (hŭm′elz-hīm op-ĕr-ā′shŭn) Transplantation of a normal ocular rectus muscle, to substitute for a paralyzed muscle.

Hum·mels·heim pro·ce·dure (hŭm′elz-hīm prŏ-sē′jŭr) Surgical procedure to correct an ocular deviation due to a sixth nerve palsy by which the superior and inferior rectus tendons are split and transferred laterally.

hu·mor, gen. **hu·mor·is** (hyū′mŏr, hyū-mōr′is) **1.** Any clear fluid or semifluid hyaline anatomic substance. **2.** One of the elemental body fluids that were the basis of the physiologic and pathologic teachings of the hippocratic school: blood, yellow bile, black bile, and phlegm. SYN humour. [L. correctly, *umor,* liquid]

hu·mor·al (hyū′mŏr-ăl) Relating to a humor in any sense.

humoral hypercalcaemia of benignancy [Br.] SYN humoral hypercalcemia of benignancy.

hu·mor·al hy·per·cal·ce·mi·a of be·nig·nan·cy (hyū′mŏr-ăl hī′pĕr-kal-sē′mē-ă bĕ-nig′năn-sē) An excess of calcium induced by parathyroid hormonelike protein of benign tumor. SYN humoral hypercalcaemia of benignancy.

hu•mor•al im•mu•ni•ty (hyū′mŏr-ăl i-myū′ni-tē) Immunity associated with circulating antibodies, in contradistinction to cellular immunity.

hu•mor•al reg•u•la•tor (hyū′mŏr-ăl reg′yū-lā′tŏr) A substance that acts as a result of contact with targets for activity through blood or body fluids.

humour [Br.] SYN humor.

hump (hŭmp) A rounded protuberance or bulge.

hump•back (hŭmp′bak) Nonmedical term for kyphosis or gibbus.

hun•ger (hŭng′gĕr) **1.** A desire or need for food. **2.** Any appetite, strong desire, or craving. [A.S.]

hun•ger con•trac•tions (hŭng′gĕr kŏn-trak′shŭnz) Strong contractions of the stomach associated with hunger pains.

hun•ger pain (hŭng′gĕr pān) Cramp in the epigastrium associated with hunger.

Hung meth•od (hŭng meth′ŏd) SYN Wilson method.

Hun•ner ul•cer (hŭn′ĕr ŭl′sĕr) A focal and often multiple lesion involving all layers of the bladder wall in chronic interstitial cystitis; the surface epithelium is destroyed by inflammation and the initially pale lesion cracks and bleeds with distention of the bladder.

Hun•ter ca•nal (hŭn′tĕr kă-nal′) SYN adductor canal.

Hun•ter op•er•a•tion (hŭn′tĕr op-ĕr-ā′shŭn) Ligation of an artery proximal and distal to an aneurysm.

Hun•ter syn•drome (hŭn′tĕr sin′drōm) An error of mucopolysaccharide metabolism characterized by deficiency of iduronate sulfatase, with excretion of dermatan sulfate and heparan sulfate in the urine; clinically similar to Hurler syndrome but distinguished by less severe skeletal changes, an absence of corneal clouding, and X-linked recessive inheritance; caused by mutation in the iduronate sulfatase gene (IDS) on chromosome Xq.

Hun•ter-Thomp•son dwarf•ism (hŭn′tĕr-tom′sŏn dwōrf′izm) A severe form of acromesomelic dwarfism, characterized by shortening of the distal segments of the limbs; the lower limbs are more severely affected than the upper limbs; often associated with dislocations of elbows, knees, and hips. Autosomal recessive inheritance, caused by mutations in the cartilage-derived morphogenetic protein 1 (CDMP1) gene on chromosome 20q.

hun•ting re•sponse (hŭnt′ing rĕ-spons′) Alternating vasodilatation and vasoconstriction in one or more extremities during application of ice or generalized hypothermia.

Hun•ting•ton cho•re•a (hŭn′ting-tŏn kŏ-rē′ă) A neurodegenerative disorder, with onset usually in the third or fourth decade, characterized by chorea and dementia; pathologically, there is bilateral marked atrophy of the putamen and the head of the caudate nucleus. Autosomal dominant inheritance with complete penetrance, caused by mutation associated with trinucleotide repeat expansion in the Huntington gene (HD) on chromosome 4p. SYN hereditary chorea.

Hunt neu•ral•gi•a (hŭnt nūr-al′gē′ă) SYN geniculate neuralgia.

Hunt par•a•dox•ic phe•nom•e•non (hŭnt par-ă-doks′ik fĕ-nom′ĕ-non) In dystonia musculorum deformans, if an attempt is made at plantar flexion of the foot when the foot is in dorsal spasm the only response is an increase of the extensor, or dorsal, spasm; if, however, the patient is told to extend the foot that is already in a state of strong dorsal flexion, there will be a sudden movement of plantar flexion; the same phenomenon, *mutatis mutandis*, is observed when there is a condition of strong plantar flexion.

Hunt syn•drome (hŭnt sin′drōm) **1.** An intention tremor beginning in one extremity, gradually increasing in intensity, and subsequently involving other parts of the body. **2.** Facial paralysis, otalgia, and herpes zoster resulting from viral infection of the seventh cranial nerve and geniculate ganglion. **3.** A form of juvenile paralysis agitans associated with primary atrophy of the pallidal system. SYN Ramsay Hunt syndrome (1).

Hur•ler syn•drome (hĕr′lĕr sin′drōm) Mucopolysaccharidosis with a deficiency of α-L-iduronidase, an accumulation of an abnormal intracellular material, and excretion of dermatan sulfate and heparan sulfate in the urine; also characterized by severe abnormality in development of skeletal cartilage and bone, with dwarfism, kyphosis, deformed limbs, limitation of joint motion, spadelike hand, corneal clouding, hepatosplenomegaly, mental retardation, and gargoyle-like facies.

Hurst dis•ease (hŭrst di-zēz′) SYN acute necrotizing hemorrhagic encephalomyelitis.

Hürth•le cell ad•e•no•ma (hĕrt′lĕ sel ad′ĕ-nō′mă) An uncommon type of thyroid tumor characterized by abundant eosinophilic cytoplasm containing numerous mitochondria. Often malignant with widespread metastases; rarely takes up radioiodine. SYN oncocytic adenoma.

Hürth•le cell car•ci•no•ma (hĕrt′lĕ sel kahr′si-nō′mă) SYN Hürthle cell tumor. SYN oncocytic carcinoma, oxyphilic carcinoma.

Hürth•le cell tu•mor (hĕrt′lĕ sel tū′mŏr) A neoplasm of the thyroid gland composed of polyhedral acidophilic cells, thought by some to be oncocytes; it may be benign or malignant, the behavior of the latter depending on the general microscopic pattern, whether follicular, papillary, or undifferentiated. SEE ALSO Hürthle cell adenoma. SYN Hürthle cell carcinoma.

Hutch•in•son cres•cen•tic notch (hŭch′in-sŏn krĕ-sent′ik noch) The semilunar notch on the incisal edge of Hutchinson teeth, encountered in congenital syphilis.

Hutch•in•son fa•ci•es (hŭch′in-sŏn fash′ē-ēz) The peculiar facial expression produced by the drooping eyelids and motionless eyes in external ophthalmoplegia.

Hutch•in•son frac•ture (hŭch′in-sŏn frak′shŭr) Radial styloid fracture. SYN chauffeur's fracture.

Hutch•in•son freck•le (hŭch′in-sŏn frek′ĕl) SYN lentigo maligna.

Hutch•in•son-Gil•ford dis•ease (hŭch′in-sŏn gil′fŏrd di-zēz′) SYN progeria.

Hutch•in•son in•ci•sors (hŭch′in-sŏn in-sī′zŏrz) SYN Hutchinson teeth.

Hutch•in•son pu•pil (hŭch′in-sŏn pyū′pil) Dilation of the pupil on the side of the lesion as part of a third nerve palsy; often due to herniation of the uncus of the temporal lobe through the tentorial notch.

Hutch•in•son teeth (hŭch′in-sŏn tēth) The incisors of congenital syphilis in which the incisal edge is notched and narrower than the cervical area giving a screwdriver appearance. SEE ALSO Hutchinson crescentic notch. SYN Hutchinson incisors.

Hutch•in•son tri•ad (hŭch′in-sŏn trī′ad) Parenchymatous keratitis, labyrinthine disease, and Hutchinson teeth, significant of congenital syphilis.

Hux•ley lay•er (hŭks′lē lā′ĕr) A layer of cells interposed between Henle layer and the cuticle of the inner root sheath of the hair follicle.

Huy•gens prin•ci•ple (hoy′genz prin′si-pĕl) Used in ultrasound technology; the principle that any wave phenomenon can be analyzed as the sum of many simple sources properly chosen with regard to phase and amplitude.

HVA Abbreviation for homovanillic acid.

HV con•duc•tion time (kŏn-dŭk′shŭn tīm) SEE intraventricular conduction.

HVES Abbreviation for high volt electrical stimulation.

HV in•ter•val (in′tĕr-văl) The time from the initial deflection of the His bundle (H) potential and the onset of ventricular activity (normally 35–45 msec).

HVL Abbreviation for half-value layer.

hy•a•lin (hī′ă-lin) A clear, eosinophilic, homogeneous substance occurring in degeneration (e.g., in arteriolar walls in arteriolar sclerosis and in glomerular tufts in diabetic glomerulosclerosis). [G. *hyalos,* glass]

hy•a•line (hī′ă-lēn) Transparent or colorless. SYN hyaloid. [G. *hyalos,* glass]

hy•a•line bod•ies (hī′ă-lēn bod′ēz) Homogeneous eosinophilic inclusions in the cytoplasm of epithelial cells; in renal tubules, hyaline bodies represent droplets of protein reabsorbed from the lumen. SEE ALSO Mallory bodies, drusen.

hy•a•line car•ti•lage (hī′ă-lēn kahr′ti-lăj) Cartilage with a frosted-glass appearance, with interstitial substance containing fine collagen fibers.

hy•a•line de•gen•er•a•tion (hī′ă-lēn dĕ-jen′ĕr-ā′shŭn) A group of degenerative processes that affect various cells and tissues, resulting in rounded masses ("droplets") or broad bands of substances that are homogeneous, translucent, refractile, and acidophilic; may occur in the collagen of old fibrous tissue, smooth muscle of arterioles or the uterus, and as droplets in parenchymal cells.

hy•a•line mem•brane (hī′ă-lēn mem′brān) **1.** The thin, clear basement membrane beneath certain epithelia. **2.** SYN glassy membrane (2).

hy•a•line mem•brane disease (HMD) (hī′ă-lēn mem′brān di-zēz′) SYN respiratory distress syndrome of the newborn.

hy•a•line tu•ber•cle (hī′ă-lēn tū′bĕr-kĕl) A form of fibrous tubercle in which the cellular fibrous tissue and collagenous fibers become altered and merged into a fairly homogeneous, acellular, deeply acidophilic, firm mass.

hy•a•lin•i•za•tion (hī′ă-lin-ī-zā′shŭn) The formation of hyalin.

hy•a•li•no•sis (hī′ă-li-nō′sis) Hyaline degeneration, especially that of relatively extensive degree.

hy•a•lin•ur•i•a (hī′ă-lin-yūr′ē-ă) The excretion of hyalin or casts of hyaline material in the urine. [hyalin + G. *ouron,* urine]

hy•a•li•tis (hī′ă-lī′tis) SYN vitreitis.

♻ **hyalo-, hyal-** Combining forms meaning glassy, hyalin; vitreous. Cf. vitreo-. [G. *hyalos,* glass]

hy•al•o•gens (hī-al′ō-jenz) Substances similar to mucoids that are found in many animal structures (e.g., cartilage, vitreous humor, hydatid cysts) and yield sugars on hydrolysis.

hy•a•lo•hy•pho•my•co•sis (hī′ă-lō-hī′fō-mī-kō′sis) An infection caused by a fungus with hyaline (colorless) mycelia in tissue, usually with a decrease in body resistance due to surgery, indwelling catheters, steroid therapy, or immunosuppressive drugs or cytotoxins. [hyalo-

+ G. *hyphē*, web, + *mykēs*, fungus, + *-osis*, condition]

hy·a·loid (hī′ă-loyd) SYN hyaline. [hyalo- + G. *eidos*, resemblance]

hy·a·loid ar·ter·y (hī′ă-loyd ahr′tĕr-ē) Artery in the embryo, which forms an extensive ramification in the primary vitreous and a vascular tunic around the lens; by 8-1/2 months, these vessels have atrophied almost completely, but a few persistent remnants are evident entoptically as muscae volitantes. SYN arteria hyaloidea [TA].

hy·a·loid bod·y (hī′ă-loyd bod′ē) SYN vitreous body.

hy·a·loid fos·sa (hī′ă-loyd fos′ă) A depression on the anterior surface of the vitreous body in which lies the lens.

hy·al·o·mere (hī′ă-lō-mēr) The clear periphery of a blood platelet. [hyalo- + G. *meros*, part]

hy·a·lo·pha·gi·a, **hy·a·loph·a·gy** (hī′ă-lō-fā′jē-ă, -lof′ă-jē) The eating or chewing of glass. [hyalo- + G. *phagō*, to eat]

hy·a·lo·plasm, **hy·a·lo·plas·ma** (hī′ă-lō-plazm, -plaz′mă) The protoplasmic fluid substance of a cell. [hyalo- + G. *plasma*, thing formed]

hy·a·lo·sis (hī′ă-lō′sis) Degenerative changes in the vitreous body. [hyalo- + G. *-osis*, condition]

hy·al·o·some (hī-al′ō-sōm) An oval or round structure within a cell nucleus that stains faintly but otherwise resembles a nucleolus. [hyalo- + G. *sōma*, body]

hy·al·u·ro·nate (hī′ă-lūr′ō-nāt) A salt or ester of hyaluronic acid.

hy·al·u·ron·ic ac·id (hī′ă-lūr-on′ik as′id) A mucopolysaccharide forming a gelatinous material in the tissue spaces and acting as a lubricant and shock absorbant; hydrolyzed by hyaluronidase.

H-Y an·ti·gen (an′ti-jen) An antigen factor, dependent on the Y chromosome, responsible for the differentiation of the human embryo into the male phenotype by inducing the initially bipotential embryonic gonad to develop into a testis; in the absence of this antigen, the indifferent gonad develops into an ovary.

hy·brid (hī′brid) **1.** An individual (plant or animal) with parents that are different varieties of the same species or that belong to different but closely allied species. **2.** Fused tissue culture cells, as in a hybridoma. [L. *hybrida*, offspring of a tame sow and a wild boar, fr. G. *hybris*, violation, wantonness]

hy·brid cap·ture (hī′brid kap′shŭr) A signal amplification method. An RNA probe is annealed to target DNA; then a captured antibody binds the DNARNA hybrid to a solid surface.

hybridisation [Br.] SYN hybridization.

hy·brid·i·za·tion (hī′brid-ī-zā′shŭn) **1.** The process of breeding a hybrid. **2.** Crossing over between related but nonallelic genes. **3.** The specific association of complementary strands of polynucleic acids, e.g., the formation of a DNA-RNA hybrid. SYN hybridisation.

hy·brid·o·ma (hī′brid-ō′mă) A tumor of hybrid cells used in the production in vitro of specific monoclonal antibodies; produced by fusion of an established tissue culture line of lymphocyte tumor cells and specific antibody-producing cells. [G. *hybris*, violation, wantonness, + *-ōma*, tumor]

hy·dan·to·in (hī-dan′tō-in) A crystalline heterocyclic compound derived from urea or from allantoin; the NH–CH_2–CO group is prototypical of α-amino acids.

hy·da·tid (hī′dă-tid) **1.** SYN hydatid cyst. **2.** A vesicular structure resembling an *Echinococcus* cyst. [G. *hydatis*, a drop of water, a hyatid]

hy·da·tid cyst (hī′dă-tid sist) A cyst formed in the liver, brain, and many other body sites by the larval metacestode stage of *Echinococcus*, chiefly in herbivores and humans; two morphologic forms caused by metacestodes of *E. granulosus* are found in humans; the unilocular hydatid cyst and the osseous hydatid cyst; two other forms in humans include the alveolar hydatid cyst, caused by the metacestode of *E. multilocularis* and the polycystic hydatid, caused by *E. vogeli* and *E. oligarthus*. SYN echinococcus cyst, hydatid (1).

hy·da·tid dis·ease (hī′dă-tid di-zēz′) Infection with the metacestode larvae of tapeworms of the genus *Echinococcus*.

hy·da·tid frem·i·tus (hī′dă-tid frem′i-tŭs) SYN hydatid thrill.

hy·da·tid·i·form (hī′dă-tid′i-fōrm) Having the form or appearance of a hydatid.

hy·da·tid·i·form mole, **hy·da·tid mole** (hī′dă-tid′i-fōrm mōl, hī′dă-tid) A vesicular or polycystic mass resulting from the proliferation of the trophoblast, with hydropic degeneration and avascularity of the chorionic villi.

hy·da·tid·o·cele (hī′dă-tid′ō-sēl) A cystic mass composed of one or more hydatids formed in the scrotum. [hydatid + G. *kēlē*, tumor]

hy·da·ti·do·ma (hī′dă-tid-ō′mă) A benign neoplasm in which there is prominent formation of hydatids. [hydatid + G. *-oma*, tumor]

hy·da·tid·o·sis (hī′dă-tid-ō′sis) The morbid state caused by the presence of hydatid cysts.

hy·da·ti·dos·to·my (hī′dă-ti-dos′tŏ-mē) Surgical evacuation of a hydatid cyst. [hydatid + G. *stoma*, mouth]

hy·da·tid thrill (hī′dă-tid thril) The peculiar

trembling or vibratory sensation felt on palpation of a hydatid cyst. SYN Blatin syndrome, hydatid fremitus.

hydraemia [Br.] SYN hydremia.

hy•dram•ni•os, hy•dram•ni•on (hī-dram′nē-os, -on) Presence of an excessive amount of amniotic fluid, usually over 2,000 mL. [G. *hydōr,* water, + amnion]

hy•dran•en•ceph•a•ly (hī′dran-en-sef′ă-lē) Complete or nearly complete absence of cerebral hemispheres, which have been replaced by fluid-filled sacs lined by leptomeninges. The cranium and its fossae are normal. [hydr- + G. *an-* priv. + *enkephalos,* brain]

hy•drar•gyr•i•a, hy•drar•gyr•ism (hī-drahr-jir′ē-ă, hī-drahr′jir-izm) SYN mercury poisoning. [L. *hydrargyrum,* mercury]

hy•drar•thro•di•al (hī′drahr-thrō′dē-ăl) Relating to hydrarthrosis.

hy•drar•thro•sis (hī′drahr-thrō′sis) Effusion of a serous fluid into a joint cavity. [hydr- + G. *arthron,* joint]

hy•drase (hī′drās) Former name for hydratase.

hy•dra•tase (hī′dră-tās) Certain hydrolyases (EC class 4.2.1) catalyzing hydration-dehydration.

hy•drate (hī′drāt) An aqueous solvate (in older terminology, a hydroxide); a compound crystallizing with one or more molecules of water.

hy•dra•tion (hī-drā′shŭn) **1.** Chemically, the addition of water; differentiated from hydrolysis, where the union with water is accompanied by a splitting of the original molecule and the water molecule. **2.** Clinically, the taking in of water; used commonly in the sense of reduced hydration or dehydration.

hy•dre•mi•a (hī-drē′mē-ă) A condition in which the blood volume is increased as a result of an increase in the water content of plasma. SYN hydraemia. [hydr- + G. *haima,* blood]

hy•dren•ceph•a•lo•cele (hī′dren-sef′ă-lō-sēl) Protrusion, through a defect in the cranium, of brain substance expanded into a sac containing fluid. SYN hydrocephalocele, hydroencephalocele. [hydr- + G. *enkephalos,* brain, + *kēlē,* tumor]

hy•dren•ceph•a•lo•me•nin•go•cele (hī′dren-sef′ă-lō-mĕ-ning′gō-sēl) Protrusion, through a defect in the cranium, of a sac containing meninges, brain substance, and cerebrospinal fluid.

hy•dric (hī′drik) Relating to hydrogen in chemical combination.

hy•dride (hī′drīd) A negatively charged hydrogen (i.e., $H:^-$) or a compound of hydrogen in which it assumes a formal negative charge.

♻ **hydro-, hydr-** **1.** Combining forms meaning water, watery. **2.** Containing or combined with hydrogen. **3.** A hydatid. [G. *hydōr,* water]

hy•dro•a (hī-drō′ă) Any bullous eruption. [hydro- + G. *ōon,* egg]

hy•dro•a vac•ci•ni•for•me (hī-drō′ă vak-sin-i-fōr′mē) A recurrent eruption of erythema evolving to umbilicated bullae, occurring on exposure to the sun and affecting chiefly male children with resolution before adult life.

hy•dro•cal•y•co•sis (hī′drō-kal-i-kō′sis) A usually symptomless anomaly of the renal calyx that is dilated from obstruction of the infundibulum; usually discovered incidentally at pyelography or autopsy; may become infected. [hydro- + G. *kalyx,* cup of a flower]

hy•dro•car•bon (hī′drō-kahr′bŏn) A compound containing only hydrogen and carbon.

hy•dro•cele (hī′drō-sēl) A collection of serous fluid in a sacculated cavity; specifically, such a collection in the space of the tunica vaginalis testis, or in a separate pocket along the spermatic cord. [hydro- + G. *kēlē,* hernia]

hy•dro•ce•lec•to•my (hī′drō-sē-lek′tŏ-mē) Excision of a hydrocele. [hydrocele + G. *ektomē,* excision]

hy•dro•ce•phal•ic (hī′drō-sĕ-fal′ik) Relating to or suffering from hydrocephalus.

hy•dro•ceph•a•lo•cele (hī′drō-sef′ă-lō-sēl) SYN hydrencephalocele.

hy•dro•ceph•a•loid (hī′drō-sef′ă-loyd) **1.** Resembling hydrocephalus. **2.** A condition in infants suffering from diarrhea or other debilitating disease, with dehydration and general symptoms resembling those of hydrocephalus without, however, any abnormal accumulation of cerebrospinal fluid.

hy•dro•ceph•a•lus (hī′drō-sef′ă-lŭs) A condition marked by an excessive accumulation of cerebrospinal fluid resulting in dilation of the cerebral ventricles and raised intracranial pressure; may also result in enlargement of the cranium and atrophy of the brain. SYN hydrocephaly. [hydro- + G. *kephalē,* head]

hy•dro•ceph•a•lus ex vac•u•o (hī′drō-sef′ă-lŭs eks vak′yū-ō) Hydrocephalus due to loss or atrophy of brain tissue; less commonly associated with raised intracranial pressure.

hy•dro•ceph•a•ly (hī′drō-sef′ă-lē) SYN hydrocephalus.

hy•dro•chlo•ric ac•id (HCl) (hī′drō-klōr′ik as′id) The acid of gastric juice. The gas and the concentrated solution are strong irritants.

hy•dro•chlo•ride (hī′drō-klōr′īd) A compound formed by the addition of a hydrochloric acid molecule to an amine or related substance.

hy·dro·cho·le·re·sis (hī′drō-kō-lĕr-ē′sis) Increased output of a watery bile of low specific gravity, viscosity, and solid content. [hydro- + G. *cholē,* bile, + *hairesis,* a taking]

hy·dro·cho·le·ret·ic (hī′drō-kō′lĕr-et′ik) Pertaining to hydrocholeresis.

hy·dro·col·loid (hī′drō-kol′oyd) A gelatinous colloid in unstable equilibrium with its contained water, useful in dentistry for impressions because of its dimensional stability under controlled conditions.

hy·dro·col·po·cele, hy·dro·col·pos (hī′drō-kol′pō-sēl, -kol′pos) Accumulation of mucus or other nonsanguineous fluid in the vagina. [hydro- + G. *kolpos,* bosom (vagina)]

hy·dro·cor·ti·sone (hī′drō-kōr′ti-sōn) A steroid hormone secreted by the cortex of suprarenal gland and the most potent of the naturally occurring glucocorticoids in humans. SYN cortisol.

hy·dro·cyst (hī′drō-sist) A cyst with clear, watery contents. [hydro- + G. *kystis,* bladder]

hy·dro·den·si·tom·e·try (hī′drō-dens′i-tom′ĕ-trē) SYN underwater weighing.

hy·dro·dy·nam·ic the·o·ry (hī′drō-dī-nam′ik thē′ŏr-ē) Widely accepted theory that explains pain impulse conduction to dental pulp resulting from fluid movement within the dentinal tubules, stimulating the nerve endings, which cause pain and hypersensitivity.

hy·dro·en·ceph·a·lo·cele (hī′drō-en-sef′ă-lō-sēl) SYN hydrencephalocele.

hy·dro·gel (hī′drō-jel) A colloid in which the particles are in the external or dispersion phase and water in the internal or dispersed phase.

hy·dro·gen (H) (hī′drō-jen) **1.** A gaseous element, atomic no. 1, atomic wt. 1.00794. **2.** The molecular form of the element, H_2. SYN dihydrogen. [hydro- + G. *-gen,* producing]

hy·dro·gen 1 (^1H) (hī′drō-jen) The common hydrogen-1 isotope, making up 99.985% of the hydrogen-1 atoms occurring in nature.

hy·dro·gen 2 (^2H) (hī′drō-jen) The isotope of hydrogen 2 of atomic weight 2; the less common stable isotope of hydrogen-2 making up 0.015% of the hydrogen-2 atoms occurring in nature. SYN deuterium.

hy·dro·gen 3 (^3H) (hī′drō-jen) A hydrogen isotope of atomic weight 3; weakly radioactive, emitting beta particles to become the stable helium-3; half-life, 12.32 years. SYN tritium.

hy·dro·gen·ase (hī-droj′ĕn-ās) Any enzyme that removes a hydride ion (or $H:^-$) from NADH (or NADPH) or adds hydrogen to ferricytochrome or to ferredoxin.

hy·dro·gen·a·tion (hī-droj′ĕ-nā′shŭn) Addition of hydrogen to a compound, especially to an unsaturated fat or fatty acid; thus, soft fats or oils are solidified or "hardened."

hy·dro·gen bond (hī′drō-jen bond) A bond arising from the sharing of a hydrogen atom, covalently bound to an electronegative element (e.g., N or O), with another electronegative element (e.g., N, O, or a halogen).

hy·dro·gen chlo·ride (hī′drō-jen klōr′īd) A highly soluble gas that, in solution, forms hydrochloric acid.

hy·dro·gen cy·a·nide (HCN) (hī′drō-jen sī′ăn-īd) A highly toxic cellular asphyxiant, HCN, used as a fumigant and also as a chemical-warfare agent. Its NATO code is AC.

hy·dro·gen do·nor (hī′drō-jen dō′nŏr) A metabolite from which hydrogen is removed (by a dehydrogenase system) and transferred by a hydrogen carrier to another metabolite, which is thus reduced.

hy·dro·gen ex·po·nent (hī′drō-jen eks-pō′nĕnt) The logarithm of the hydrogen ion concentration in blood or other fluid; its negative is the pH of that fluid.

hy·dro·gen ion (H^+) (hī′drō-jen ī′on) A hydrogen atom minus its electron and therefore carrying a unit positive charge (i.e., a proton); in water, it combines with a water molecule to form hydronium ion, H_3O^+.

hy·dro·gen pump (hī′drō-jen pŭmp) Molecular mechanism for acid secretion from gastric parietal cells based on the activity of a H^+-K^+-ATPase.

hy·dro·gen trans·port (hī′drō-jen trans′pōrt) The transfer of hydrogen from one metabolite (hydrogen donor) to another (hydrogen acceptor) through the action of an enzyme system; the donor is thus oxidized and the acceptor reduced.

hy·dro·ki·net·ic (hī′drō-ki-net′ik) Pertaining to the motion of fluids and the forces giving rise to such motion.

hy·dro·las·es (hī′drō-lās-ĕz) Enzymes (EC class 3) cleaving substrates with addition of H_2O at the point of cleavage.

hy·dro·ly·as·es (hī′drō-lī′ās-ĕz) A class of lyases (EC class 4.2.1) comprising enzymes removing H and OH as water, leading to formation of new double bonds within the affected molecule.

hy·drol·y·sate (hī-drol′i-sāt) A solution containing the products of hydrolysis.

hy·drol·y·sis (hī-drol′i-sis) A chemical process whereby a compound is cleaved into two or more simpler compounds with the uptake of the H and OH parts of a water molecule on either side of the chemical bond cleaved; hydrolysis is effected by the action of acids, alkalies, or enzymes. Cf. hydration. [hydro- + G. *lysis,* dissolution]

hy·dro·lyt·ic (hī′drō-lit′ik) Referring to or causing hydrolysis.

hy·dro·ma (hī-drō′mă) SYN hygroma.

hy·dro·me·nin·go·cele (hī′drō-mĕ-ning′gō-sēl) Protrusion of the meninges of brain or spinal cord through a defect in the cranium or vertebral column, the sac so formed containing cerebrospinal fluid. [hydro- + G. *mēninx,* membrane, + *kēlē,* hernia]

hy·drom·e·ter (hī-drom′ĕ-tĕr) An instrument for determining the specific gravity of a liquid. [hydro- + G. *mĕron,* measure]

hy·dro·me·tra (hī′drō-mē′tră) Accumulation of thin mucus or other watery fluid in the cavity of the uterus. [hydro- + G. *mētra,* uterus]

hy·dro·met·ric (hī′drō-met′rik) Relating to hydrometry or the hydrometer.

hy·dro·me·tro·col·pos (hī′drō-me′trō-kol′pos) Distention of uterus and vagina by fluid other than blood or pus. [hydro- + G. *mētra,* uterus, + *kolpos,* bosom (vagina)]

hy·drom·e·try (hī-drom′ĕ-trē) Determination of the specific gravity of a fluid by means of a hydrometer.

hy·dro·mi·cro·ceph·a·ly (hī′drō-mī′krō-sef′ă-lē) Microcephaly associated with an increased amount of cerebrospinal fluid.

hy·dro·my·e·li·a (hī′drō-mī-ē′lē-ă) An increase of fluid in the dilated central canal of the spinal cord, or in congenital cavities elsewhere in the cord substance. [hydro- + G. *myelos,* marrow]

hy·dro·my·e·lo·cele (hī′drō-mī′ĕ-lō-sēl) Protrusion of a portion of the spinal cord, thinned out into a sac distended with cerebrospinal fluid, through a vertebral column, spina bifida. [hydro- + G. *myelos,* marrow, + *kēlē,* tumor, hernia]

hy·dro·my·o·ma (hī′drō-mī-ō′mă) A leiomyoma that contains cystlike foci of proteinaceous fluid; hydromyomas occur more frequently in leiomyomas of the uterus, as a result of degenerative changes. [hydro- + G. *mys,* muscle, + *-oma,* tumor]

hy·dro·ne·phro·sis (hī′drō-nĕ-frō′sis) Dilation of the pelvis and calyces of one or both kidneys resulting from obstruction to the flow of urine. See this page. SYN pelvocaliectasis, uronephrosis. [hydro- + G. *nephros,* kidney, + *-osis,* condition]

hy·dro·ne·phrot·ic (hī′drō-nĕ-frot′ik) Relating to hydronephrosis.

hy·dro·per·i·car·di·tis (hī′drō-per′i-kahr-dī′tis) Pericarditis with a large serous effusion.

hy·dro·per·i·car·di·um (hī′drō-per′i-kahr′dē-ŭm) A noninflammatory accumulation of fluid in the pericardial sac.

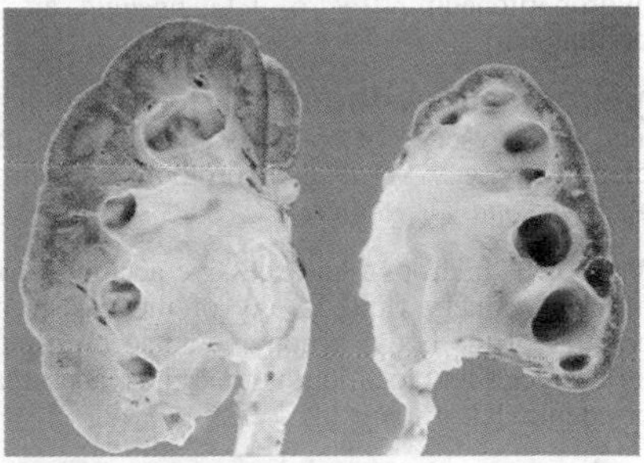

hydronephrosis: kidney on right shows severe parenchymal atrophy

hy·dro·per·i·to·ne·um, hy·dro·per·i·to·ni·a (hī′drō-per′i-tō-nē′ŭm, -tō′nē-ă) SYN ascites. [hydro- + peritoneum]

hy·dro·phil·i·a (hī′drō-fil′ē-ă) **1.** Associating freely with water. **2.** A tendency of the blood and tissues to absorb fluid. [hydro- + G. *philos,* fond]

hy·dro·phil·ic (hī′drō-fil′ik) Denoting the property of attracting or associating with water molecules, possessed by polar radicals or ions, as opposed to hydrophobic (2).

hy·dro·pho·bi·a (hī′drō-fō′bē-ă) SYN rabies. [hydro- + G. *phobos,* fear]

hy·dro·pho·bic (hī′drō-fō′bik) **1.** Relating to or suffering from hydrophobia. **2.** Lacking an affinity for water molecules, as opposed to hydrophilic.

hy·droph·thal·mos (hī′drof-thal′mŏs) SEE buphthalmia.

hy·drop·ic (hī-drop′ik) Containing water or a watery fluid.

hy·drop·ic de·gen·er·a·tion (hī-drop′ik dĕ-jen′ĕr-ā′shŭn) SYN cloudy swelling.

hy·dro·pneu·ma·to·sis (hī′drō-nū′mă-tō′sis) Combined emphysema and edema; the presence of liquid and gas in tissues. [hydro- + G. *pneuma,* breath, spirit]

hy·dro·pneu·mo·go·ny (hī′drō-nū-mō′gŏ-nē) Injection of air into a joint to determine the amount of effusion. [hydro- + G. *pneuma,* air, + *gony,* knee]

hy·dro·pneu·mo·per·i·car·di·um (hī′drō-nū′mō-per′i-kahr′dē-ŭm) The presence of a serous effusion and of gas in the pericardial sac. SYN pneumohydropericardium. [hydro- + G. *pneuma,* air, + pericardium]

hy·dro·pneu·mo·per·i·to·ne·um (hī′drō-nū′mō-per′i-tō-nē′ŭm) The presence of gas and serous fluid in the peritoneal cavity. SYN pneumohydroperitoneum. [hydro- + G. *pneuma,* air, + peritoneum]

hy•dro•pneu•mo•tho•rax (hī′drō-nū′mō-thōr′aks) The presence of both gas and fluids in the pleural cavity. SYN pneumohydrothorax. [hydro- + G. *pneuma,* air, + thorax]

hy•drops (hī′drops) An excessive accumulation of clear, watery fluid in any of the tissues or cavities of the body; synonymous, according to its character and location, with ascites, anasarca, or edema. [G. *hydrōps*]

hy•dro•py•o•ne•phro•sis (hī′drō-pī′ō-nĕ-frō′sis) Presence of purulent urine in the pelvis and calyces of the kidney following obstruction of the ureter. [hydro- + G. *pyon,* pus, + nephrosis]

hy•dror•rhe•a (hī′drō-rē′ă) A profuse discharge of watery fluid from any part of the body. SYN hydrorrhoea. [hydro- + G. *rhoia,* flow]

hydrorrhoea [Br.] SYN hydrorrhea.

hy•dro•sal•pinx (hī′drō-sal′pingks) Accumulation of serous fluid in the uterine tube, often an end result of pyosalpinx. [hydro- + G. *salpinx,* trumpet]

hy•dro•sar•co•cele (hī′drō-sahr′kō-sēl) A chronic swelling of the testis complicated with hydrocele. [hydro- + G. *sarx,* flesh, + *kēlē,* tumor]

hy•dro•stat•ic (hī′drō-stat′ik) Relating to the pressure of fluids or to their properties when in equilibrium.

hy•dro•stat•ic weigh•ing (hī′drō-stat′ik wā′ing) SYN underwater weighing.

hy•dro•sy•rin•go•my•e•li•a (hī′drō-sir-ing′gō-mī-ē′lē-ă) SYN syringomyelia. [hydro- + G. *hydōr,* water, + *syrinx,* a tube, + *myelos,* marrow]

hy•dro•tax•is (hī′drō-tak′sis) The movement of cells or organisms in relation to water. [hydro- + G. *taxis,* arrangement]

hy•dro•ther•a•py (hī′drō-thār′ă-pē) The external application of water as a liquid, solid, or vapor for therapeutic purposes. [hydro- + G. *therapeia,* therapy]

hydrothionaemia [Br.] SYN hydrothionemia.

hy•dro•thi•o•ne•mi•a (hī′drō-thī′ō-nē′mē-ă) The presence of hydrogen sulfide in the circulating blood. SYN hydrothionaemia. [hydro- + G. *theion,* sulfur, + *haima,* blood]

hy•dro•thi•o•nur•i•a (hī′drō-thī′ō-nyūr′ē-ă) The excretion of hydrogen sulfide in the urine. [hydro- + G. *theion,* sulfur, + *ouron,* urine]

hy•dro•tho•rax (hī′drō-thōr′aks) Presence of fluid in one or both pleural cavities, usually resulting from cardiac failure.

hy•drot•ro•pism (hī′drot′rŏ-pizm) The property in growing organisms of turning toward a moist surface (positive hydrotropism) or away from a moist surface (negative hydrotropism). [hydro- + G. *tropos,* a turning]

hy•dro•tu•ba•tion (hī′drō-tū-bā′shŭn) Injection of a liquid medication or saline solution through the cervix into the uterine cavity and uterine tubes for dilation or treatment of the tubes.

hy•dro•u•re•ter (hī′drō-yūr′ē-tĕr) Distention of the ureter with urine, due to blockage from any cause.

hy•dro•va•ri•um (hī′drō-var′ē-ŭm) A collection of fluid in the ovary.

hy•drox•ide (hī-drok′sīd) A compound containing a potentially ionizable hydroxyl group; particularly a compound that liberates OH^- on dissolving in water.

hy•drox•o•co•bal•a•min (hī-drok′sō-kō-bal′ă-min) SYN hydroxycobalamin.

♻ **hydroxy-** Prefix indicating addition or substitution of the –OH group to or in the compound named after it. SEE ALSO oxa-, oxo-, oxy-.

hy•drox•y•ap•a•tite (hī-drok′sē-ap′ă-tīt) A natural mineral structure resembling the crystal lattice of bones and teeth; used in chromatography of nucleic acids; also found in pathologic calcifications. SEE ALSO apatite.

4-hy•drox•y•bu•ty•rate (hī-drok′sē-byū′tir-āt) SYN gamma (γ)-hydroxybutyrate.

hy•drox•y•co•bal•a•min (hī-drok′sē-kō-bal′ă-min) A chemical compound, also called vitamin B12a, which is the immediate precursor to cyanocobalamin (vitamin B12) in the body and that has also been investigated as an antidote in cyanide poisoning, although it is not currently approved for such use in the U.S. SEE ALSO amyl nitrite, sodium nitrite, sodium thiosulfate. SYN hydroxocobalamin.

17-hy•drox•y•cor•ti•co•ste•roid test (hī-droks′ē-kōr-ti-kō′ster′oyd) A test (dependent on the Porter-Silber reaction) that is used as a measure of adrenocortical function and is performed on urine. Low values are seen in Addison disease and hypopituitarism; high values are seen in Cushing syndrome and extreme stress.

hy•drox•yl (hī-drok′sil) The radical, –OH.

11-hy•drox•y•lase de•fi•cien•cy (hī-drok′si-lās dĕ-fish′ĕn-sē) A type of congenital adrenal hyperplasia, with various manifestations, including hypertensive types and salt-wasting varieties.

21-hy•drox•y•lase de•fi•ci•en•cy (hī-drok′si-lās dĕ-fish′ĕn-sē) One form of congenital adrenal hyperplasia, with variable presentations, including simple virilizing, salt-wasting, and nonclassic types.

hy•drox•y•las•es (hī-drok′si-lā-sĕz) Enzymes catalyzing formation of hydroxyl groups by addition of an oxygen atom, hence oxidizing the substrate.

hy•drox•y•phen•yl•u•ri•a (hī-drok′sē-fen′il-yūr′ē-ă) Urinary excretion of tyrosine and phenylalanine, as a result of ascorbic acid deficiency; occurs notably in those premature infants who lack this vitamin.

21-hy•drox•y•pro•ges•ter•one (hī-drok′sē-prō-jest′tĕr-ōn) SYN deoxycorticosterone.

5-hy•drox•y•tryp•ta•mine (5-HT) (hī-drok-sē-trip′tă-mēn) SYN serotonin.

hy•giene (hī′jēn) **1.** The science of health and its maintenance. **2.** Cleanliness that promotes health and well-being, especially of a personal nature. [G. *hygieinos,* healthful, fr. *hygiēs,* healthy]

hy•giene hy•poth•e•sis (hī′jēn hī-poth′ĕ-sis) The tenet that improved cleanliness and modern medical care may be lowering the ability of people to deal with otherwise nonlethal pathogens and disease.

hy•gien•ic (hī-jen′ik) Healthful; relating to hygiene; tending to maintain health.

hy•gien•ist (hī-jē′nist) One who is skilled in the science of health and its maintenance.

♻ **hygro-, hygr-** Combining forms meaning moisture, humidity; opposite of xero-. [G. *hygros,* moist]

hy•gro•ma (hī-grō′mă) A cystic swelling containing a serous fluid. SYN hydroma. [hygro- + G. *-oma,* tumor]

hy•grom•e•try (hī-grom′ĕ-trē) SYN psychrometry.

hy•gro•scop•ic (hī′grō-skop′ik) Denoting a substance capable of readily absorbing and retaining moisture; e.g., NaOH, $CaCl_2$.

hy•gro•scop•ic con•den•ser hu•mid•i•fi•er (hī′grō-skop′ik kŏn-den′sĕr hyū-mid′i-fī-ĕr) A passive humidification device that works by collecting heat and moisture on exhalation and returning it to inhaled gas SYN artificial nose.

hy•men (hī′mĕn) [TA] A thin membranous fold, highly variable in appearance, which partly occludes the ostium of the vagina before its rupture, which may occur for a variety of reasons. It is frequently absent, even in virgins, although remnants are commonly present as hymenal tags (caruncula). [G. *hymēn,* membrane]

hy•men•al (hī′mĕn-ăl) Relating to the hymen. USAGE NOTE often misspelled hymeneal, or so mispronounced.

hy•men•ec•to•my (hī′mĕ-nek′tŏ-mē) Excision of the hymen. [G. *hymēn,* membrane, + *ektomē,* excision]

hy•me•ni•tis (hī′mĕ-nī′tis) Inflammation of the hymen.

hy•men•ol•o•gy (hī′mĕ-nol′ŏ-jē) The branch of anatomy and physiology concerned with the membranes of the body. [G. *hymēn,* membrane, + *logos,* study]

hy•men•ot•o•my (hī′mĕ-not′ŏ-mē) Surgical division of a hymen. [G. *hymēn,* membrane, + *tomē,* incision]

hy•o•ep•i•glot•tic (hī′ō-ep-i-glot′ik) Relating to the hyoid bone and the epiglottis; denoting the elastic hyoepiglottic ligament connecting the two structures.

hy•o•glos•sal (hī′ō-glos′ăl) Relating to the hyoid bone and the tongue. SYN glossohyal.

hy•o•glos•sal mem•brane (hī′ō-glos′ăl mem′brān) Posterior widening of the lingual septum connecting the root of the tongue to the hyoid bone; the inferior fibers of the genioglossus are attached to it and by this means to the upper anterior body of the hyoid bone near the midline.

hy•o•glos•sal mus•cle (hī′ō-glos′ăl mŭs′ĕl) SYN hyoglossus muscle.

hy•o•glos•sus (hī′ō-glos′ŭs) SYN hyoglossus muscle.

hy•o•glos•sus mus•cle (hī′ō-glos′ŭs mŭs′ĕl) *Origin*, body and greater horn of hyoid bone; *insertion*, side of the tongue; *action*, retracts and pulls down side of tongue; *nerve supply*, motor by hypoglossal, sensory by lingual. SYN musculus hyoglossus [TA], hyoglossal muscle, hyoglossus.

hy•oid (hī′oyd) U-shaped or V-shaped; denoting the os hyoideum and the apparatus hyoideus. [G. *hyoeidēs,* shaped like the letter upsilon, υ]

hy•oid arch (hī′oyd ahrch) The second visceral, or pharyngeal (branchial in fish), arch; the second postoral arch in the pharyngeal arch series.

hy•oid bone (hī′oyd bōn) A U-shaped bone lying between the mandible and the larynx, suspended from the styloid processes by slender stylohyoid ligaments.

♻ **hyp-** Variation of the prefix hypo-, often used before a vowel. Cf. sub-.

hy•pa•cu•sis (hī′pă-kū′sis) Hearing impairment of a conductive or neurosensory nature. SYN hypoacusis. [hypo- + G. *akousis,* hearing]

hypaesthesia [Br.] SYN hypesthesia.

hypalbuminaemia [Br.] SYN hypalbuminemia.

hyp•al•bu•mi•ne•mi•a (hīp′al-bū′mi-nē′mē-ă) SYN hypoalbuminemia. SYN hypalbuminaemia. [G. *hypo,* under, + albuminemia]

hyp•al•ge•si•a (hīp′al-jē′zē-ă) Decreased sensibility to pain. SYN hypoalgesia. [G. *hypo,* under, + *algēsis,* sense of pain]

hyp•al•ge•sic, hyp•al•get•ic (hīp′al-jē′sik,

-jet′ik) Relating to hypalgesia; having diminished sensitiveness to pain.

♻ **hyper-** Prefix meaning excessive, above normal; opposite of hypo-. [G. *hyper,* above, over]

hy·per·ab·duc·tion syn·drome (hī′pĕr-ab-dŭk′shŭn sin′drōm) SYN thoracic outlet syndrome.

hy·per·a·cid·i·ty (hī′pĕr-ă-sid′i-tē) An abnormally high degree of acidity, as of the gastric juice.

hy·per·ac·tiv·i·ty (hī′pĕr-ak-tiv′i-tē) **1.** SYN superactivity. **2.** General restlessness or excessive movement such as that characterizing children with attention deficit disorder or hyperkinesis.

hy·per·a·cu·sis, **hy·per·a·cu·si·a** (hi′pĕr-ă-kū′sis, -kū′sē-ă) Heightened auditory acuity, sometimes accompanied by painful sensitivity to ordinary environmental sounds. USAGE NOTE The term is not synonymous with recruitment or hypersensitivity. [hyper- + G. *akousis,* hearing]

hy·per·ad·e·no·sis (hī′pĕr-ad′ĕ-nō′sis) Glandular enlargement, especially of the lymphatic glands. [hyper- + G. *adēn,* gland, + *-ōsis,* condition]

hy·per·ad·i·po·sis, **hy·per·ad·i·pos·i·ty** (hī′pĕr-ad′i-pō′sis, -pos′i-tē) An extreme degree of adiposis or fatness.

hyperaemic [Br.] SYN hyperemic.

hyperaesthesia [Br.] SYN hyperesthesia.

hyperaesthetic [Br.] SYN hyperesthetic.

hy·per·al·do·ste·ron·ism (hī′pĕr-al-dos′tĕr-ōn-izm) SYN aldosteronism.

hy·per·al·ge·si·a (hī′pĕr-al-jē′zē-ă) Extreme sensitivity to painful stimuli. [hyper- + G. *algos,* pain]

hy·per·al·ge·sic, **hy·per·al·get·ic** (hī′pĕr-al-jē′sik, -jet′ik) Relating to hyperalgesia.

hy·per·al·i·men·ta·tion (hī′pĕr-al′i-men-tā′shŭn) Administration or consumption of nutrients beyond minimum normal requirements, in an attempt to replace nutritional deficiencies.

hyperamylasaemia [Br.] SYN hyperamylasemia.

hy·per·am·y·la·se·mi·a (hī′pĕr-am′i-lā-sē′mē-ă) Elevated serum amylase, usually seen as one of the manifestations of acute pancreatitis. SYN hyperamylasaemia. [hyper- + amylase, + G. *haima,* blood]

hy·per·an·a·ki·ne·si·a, **hy·per·an·a·ki·ne·sis** (hī′pĕr-an′ă-ki-nē′zē-ă, -ki-nē′sis) Excessive to-and-fro movement, e.g., of the stomach or intestine. [hyper- + G. *anakinēsis,* to-and-fro movement]

hy·per·a·phi·a (hī′pĕr-ā′fē-ă) Extreme sensitivity to touch. [hyper- + G. *haphē,* touch]

hy·per·aph·ic (hī′pĕr-af′ik) Marked by hyperaphia.

hy·per·bar·ic (hī′pĕr-bar′ik) **1.** Pertaining to pressure of ambient gases exceeding 1 atmosphere. **2.** Concerning solutions, more dense than the diluent or medium; e.g., in spinal anesthesia, a hyperbaric solution has a density greater than that of spinal fluid. [hyper- + G. *baros,* weight]

hy·per·bar·ic cham·ber (hī′pĕr-bar′ik chām′bĕr) A chamber providing pressures greater than atmospheric, commonly used to treat decompression sickness and to provide hyperbaric oxygenation.

hy·per·bar·ic ox·y·gen, **high pres·sure ox·y·gen** (hī′pĕr-bar′ik ok′si-jĕn, hī presh′ŭr) Oxygen at a pressure greater than 1 atmosphere.

hy·per·bar·ic ox·y·gen ther·a·py (hī′pĕr-bar′ik ok′si-jĕn thār′ă-pē) Treatment in which oxygen is provided in a sealed chamber at an ambient pressure greater than 1 atmosphere.

hy·per·bar·ism (hī′pĕr-bar′izm) Disturbances in the body resulting from the pressure of ambient gases at greater than 1 atmosphere (e.g., nitrogen narcosis, oxygen toxicity, bends). [hyper- + G. *baros,* weight]

hyperbilirubinaemia [Br.] SYN hyperbilirubinemia.

hy·per·bil·i·ru·bi·ne·mi·a (hī′pĕr-bil′i-rū-bi-nē′mē-ă) An abnormally large amount of bilirubin in the circulating blood, resulting in clinically apparent icterus or jaundice when the concentration is sufficient. SYN hyperbilirubinaemia.

hypercalcaemia [Br.] SYN hypercalcemia.

hy·per·cal·ce·mi·a (hī′pĕr-kal-sē′mē-ă) An abnormally high concentration of calcium compounds in the circulating blood; commonly used to indicate an elevated concentration of calcium ions in the blood. SYN calcemia, hypercalcaemia.

hy·per·cal·ci·u·ri·a (hī′pĕr-kal′sē-yū′rē-ă) Excretion of abnormally large amounts of calcium in the urine.

hy·per·cap·ni·a (hī′pĕr-kap′nē-ă) Abnormally increased arterial carbon dioxide tension. SYN hypercarbia. [hyper- + G. *kapnos,* smoke, vapor]

hy·per·cap·nic a·cid·o·sis (hī′pĕr-kap′nik as′i-dō′sis) SYN respiratory acidosis.

hy·per·car·bi·a (hī′pĕr-kahr′bē-ă) SYN hypercapnia.

hy·per·ca·tab·o·lism (hī′pĕr-kă-tab′ŏ-lizm) An increase in basal metabolic rate and in breakdown of muscle and adipose tissue as a result of injury, metabolic stress, or sepsis. SEE ALSO catabolism.

hy·per·ce·men·to·sis (hī′pĕr-sē′mĕn-tō′sis)

Excessive deposition of secondary cementum on the root of a tooth, which may be caused by localized trauma or inflammation, excessive tooth eruption, or osteitis deformans, or may occur idiopathically. [hyper- + L. *caementum,* a rough quarry stone, + *-osis,* condition]

hyperchloraemia [Br.] SYN hyperchloremia.

hy•per•chlor•e•mi•a (hī′pĕr-klōr-ē′mē-ă) An abnormally large concentration of chloride ions in the circulating blood. SYN hyperchloraemia.

hy•per•chlor•hy•dri•a (hī′pĕr-klōr-hī′drē-ă) Presence of an excessive amount of hydrochloric acid in the stomach. SYN chlorhydria. [hyper- + chlorhydric (acid)]

hypercholesteraemia [Br.] SYN hypercholesteremia.

hy•per•cho•les•ter•e•mi•a (hī′pĕr-kŏ-les′tĕr-ē′mē-ă) SYN hypercholesterolemia. SYN hypercholesteraemia.

hypercholesterolaemia [Br.] SYN hypercholesterolemia.

hy•per•cho•les•ter•ol•e•mi•a (hī′pĕr-kŏ-les′tĕr-ol-ē′mē-ă) The presence of an abnormally large amount of cholesterol in the blood. SYN hypercholesteremia, hypercholesterolaemia.

hy•per•cho•li•a (hī′pĕr-kō′lē-ă) A condition in which an abnormally large amount of bile is formed in the liver. [hyper- + G. *cholē,* bile]

hy•per•chro•ma•si•a (hī′pĕr-krō-mā′zē-ă) SYN hyperchromatism.

hy•per•chro•mat•ic (hī′pĕr-krō-mat′ik) **1.** Abnormally highly colored, excessively stained, or overpigmented. SYN hyperchromic (1). **2.** Showing increased chromatin. [hyper- + G. *chrōma,* color]

hy•per•chro•ma•tism (hī′pĕr-krō′mă-tizm) **1.** Excessive pigmentation. **2.** Increased staining capacity, especially of cell nuclei for hematoxylin. **3.** An increase in chromatin in cell nuclei. SYN hyperchromasia, hyperchromia. [hyper- + G. *chrōma,* color]

hy•per•chro•mi•a (hī′pĕr-krō′mē-ă) SYN hyperchromatism.

hy•per•chro•mic (hī′pĕr-krōm′ik) **1.** SYN hyperchromatic (1). **2.** Denoting increased light absorption.

hy•per•chro•mic a•ne•mi•a, hy•per•chro•mat•ic a•ne•mi•a (hī′pĕr-krō′mik ă-nē′mē-ă, hī′pĕr-krō-mat′ik) Hematologic disorder characterized by a decrease in the ratio of the weight of hemoglobin to the volume of the erythrocyte, i.e., the mean corpuscular hemoglobin concentration is less than normal.

hy•per•chy•li•a (hī′pĕr-kī′lē-ă) Excessive secretion of gastric juice. [hyper- + G. *chylos,* juice]

hyperchylomicronaemia [Br.] SYN hyperchylomicronemia.

hy•per•chy•lo•mi•cro•ne•mi•a (hī′pĕr-kī′lō-mī′krō-nē′mē-ă) Increased plasma concentrations of chylomicrons. SYN hyperchylomicronaemia.

hy•per•cor•ti•coid•ism (hī′pĕr-kōr′ti-koyd-izm) **1.** Excessive secretion of one or more steroid hormones of the cortex of suprarenal gland. **2.** The state produced by therapeutic administration of large quantities of steroids having glucocorticoid activity (e.g., hydrocortisone). SEE ALSO Cushing syndrome.

hy•per•cor•ti•so•nism (hī′pĕr-kōr′ti-sōn-izm) A condition that appears as a result of intensive steroid therapy. Signs are moon face, hirsutism, obesity, and fat pads on belly and back (buffalo hump). SEE ALSO hypercorticoidism.

hypercryaesthesia [Br.] SYN hypercryesthesia.

hy•per•cry•al•ge•si•a (hī′pĕr-krī′al-jē′zē-ă) SYN hypercryesthesia. [hyper- + G. *kryos,* cold, + *algēsis,* the sense of pain]

hy•per•cry•es•the•si•a (hī′pĕr-krī′es-thē′zē-ă) Extreme sensibility to cold. SYN hypercryaesthesia, hypercryalgesia. [hyper- + G. *kryos,* cold, + *aisthēsis,* sensation]

hypercupraemia [Br.] SYN hypercupremia.

hy•per•cu•pre•mi•a (hī′pĕr-kyū-prē′mē-ă) An abnormally high level of plasma copper. SYN hypercupraemia. [hyper- + L. *cuprum,* copper, + G. *haima,* blood]

hy•per•cy•a•not•ic (hī′pĕr-sī′ă-not′ik) Marked by extreme cyanosis.

hypercythaemia [Br.] SYN hypercythemia.

hy•per•cy•the•mi•a (hī′pĕr-sī-thē′mē-ă) The presence of an abnormally high number of red blood cells in the circulating blood. SYN hypercythaemia, hypererythrocythemia. [hyper- + G. *kytos,* cell, + *haima,* blood]

hy•per•cy•to•sis (hī′pĕr-sī-tō′sis) Any condition in which there is an abnormal increase in the number of cells in the circulating blood or the tissues; frequently used synonymously with leukocytosis.

hy•per•di•crot•ic (hī′pĕr-dī-krot′ik) Markedly dicrotic.

hy•per•ech•o•ic (hī′pĕr-ĕ-kō′ik) **1.** Denoting a region in an ultrasound image in which the echoes are stronger than normal or than surrounding structures. **2.** ULTRASONOGRAPHY pertaining to material that produces echoes of higher amplitude or density than the surrounding medium.

hy•per•ek•plex•i•a (hī′pĕr-ek-pleks′ē-ă) A hereditary disorder in which there are pathologic startle responses, i.e., protective reactions to unanticipated, potentially threatening, stimuli of any type, particularly auditory; the stimuli induce often widespread and violent sudden contractions of the head, neck, spinal, and sometimes limb musculature, resulting in involuntary shouting, jerking, jumping, and falling; autosomal dominant and recessive inheritance forms, with the responsible gene localized to chromosome 5q; probably the result of lack of inhibitory neurotransmitters, glycine, or GABA. SYN kok disease, startle disease. [hyper- + G. *ekplēxia,* sudden shock, fr. *ekplēssō,* to startle]

hy·per·em·e·sis (hī′pĕr-em′ĕ-sis) Excessive vomiting. [hyper- + G. *emesis,* vomiting]

hy·per·em·e·sis grav·i·da·rum (hī′pĕr′ē-mē′sis grā-vē′dā-rum) Nausea and vomiting during pregnancy severe enough to result in dehydration, acidosis, and weight loss. May require hospitalization; if untreated, can be fatal.

hy·per·e·met·ic (hī′pĕr-ĕ-met′ik) Marked by excessive vomiting.

hy·per·e·mi·a (hī′pĕr-ē′mē-ă) The presence of an increased amount of blood in a part or organ. SEE ALSO congestion. [hyper- + G. *haima,* blood]

hy·per·e·mic (hī′pĕr-ē′mik) Denoting hyperemia. SYN hyperaemic.

hy·per·en·ceph·a·ly (hī′pĕr-en-sef′ă-lē) A fetal developmental deficiency of the neurocranium, exposing the poorly formed brain. [hyper- + G. *enkephalos,* brain]

hy·per·en·dem·ic dis·ease (hī′pĕr-en-dem′ik di-zēz′) A disease that is constantly present at a high incidence and/or prevalence rate and affects all age groups equally.

hy·per·e·o·sin·o·phil·i·a (hī′pĕr-ē′ō-sin-ō-fil′ē-ă) A greater degree of increase in the number of eosinophilic granulocytes in the circulating blood or the tissues than would be expected in the disease or condition causing the increase.

hy·per·e·o·sin·o·phil·ic syn·drome (hī′pĕr-ē′ō-sin-ō-fil′ik sin′drōm) Persistent peripheral eosinophilia with later infiltration into bone marrow, heart, and other organ systems; accompanied by nocturnal sweating, coughing, anorexia and weight loss, itching, various skin lesions, and symptoms of Löffler endocarditis.

hy·per·er·ga·si·a (hī′pĕr-ĕr-gā′zē-ă) Increased or excessive functional activity. [hyper- + G. *ergasia,* work]

hy·per·er·gi·a (hī′pĕr-ĕr′jē-ă) An allergic hypersensitivity. SYN hypergia.

hy·per·er·gic (hī′pĕr-ĕr′jik) Relating to hyperergia. SYN hypergic.

hypererythrocythaemia [Br.] SYN hypererythrocythemia.

hy·per·e·ryth·ro·cy·the·mi·a (hī′pĕr-ĕ-rith′rō-sī-thē′mē-ă) SYN hypercythemia. SYN hypererythrocythaemia.

hy·per·es·o·pho·ri·a (hī′pĕr-es′ō-fōr′ē-ă) A tendency of one eye to deviate upward and inward, prevented by binocular vision. [hyper- + G. *esō,* inward, + *phora,* movement]

hy·per·es·the·si·a (hī′pĕr-es-thē′zē-ă) Abnormal acuteness of sensitivity to touch, pain, or other sensory stimuli. SYN hyperaesthesia, oxyesthesia. [hyper- + G. *aisthēsis,* sensation]

hy·per·es·thet·ic (hī′pĕr-es-thet′ik) Marked by hyperesthesia. SYN hyperaesthetic.

hy·per·ex·o·pho·ri·a (hī′pĕr-ek′sō-fōr′ē-ă) A tendency of one eye to deviate upward and outward, prevented by binocular vision. [hyper- + G. *exō,* outward, + *phora,* movement]

hy·per·ex·ten·sion (hī′pĕr-eks-ten′shŭn) Extension of a limb or part beyond the normal limit.

hy·per·ex·ten·sion-hy·per·flex·ion in·jur·y (hī′pĕr-eks-ten′shŭn-hī′pĕr-flek′shŭn in′jŭr-ē) Violence to the body causing the unsupported head to move rapidly backward and forward resulting in hyperextension and hyperflexion of the neck; does not imply any specific resultant trauma or pathology.

hyperferraemia [Br.] SYN hyperferremia.

hy·per·fer·re·mi·a (hī′pĕr-fĕr-ē′mē-ă) High serum iron level; found in hemochromatosis. SYN hyperferraemia.

hyperfibrinogenaemia [Br.] SYN hyperfibrinogenemia.

hy·per·fi·brin·o·ge·ne·mi·a (hī′pĕr-fī-brin′ō-jĕ-nē′mē-ă) An increased level of fibrinogen in the blood. SYN fibrinogenemia, hyperfibrinogenaemia.

hy·per·fi·bri·nol·y·sis (hī′pĕr-fī-brin-ol′i-sis) Markedly increased fibrinolysis, as in subdural hematomas.

hy·per·flex·ion (hī′pĕr-flek′shŭn) Flexion of a limb or part beyond the normal limit.

hy·per·frac·tion·at·ed ra·di·a·tion (hī′pĕr-frak′shŭn-ā-tĕd rā′dē-ā′shŭn) Smaller fractions of a dose of radiation given more frequently than daily.

hy·per·func·tion·al oc·clu·sion (hī′pĕr-fŭngk′shŭn-ăl ŏ-klū′zhŭn) Occlusal stress of a tooth or teeth that exceeds normal physiologic demands.

hy·per·gal·ac·to·sis (hī′pĕr-gă-lak-tō′sis) Excessive secretion of milk. [hyper- + G. *gala,* milk, + *-ōsis,* condition]

hypergammaglobulinaemia [Br.] SYN hypergammaglobulinemia.

hy·per·gam·ma·glob·u·lin·e·mi·a (hī′pĕr-gam′ă-glob′yū-lin-ē′mē-ă) An increased concentration of gammaglobulins in the plasma. SYN hypergammaglobulinaemia.

hy•per•gen•e•sis (hī′pĕr-jen′ĕ-sis) Excessive development or redundant production of parts or organs of the body. [hyper- + G. *genesis,* production]

hy•per•ge•net•ic (hī′pĕr-jĕ-net′ik) Relating to hypergenesis.

hy•per•gen•i•tal•ism (hī′pĕr-jen′i-tăl-izm) Abnormal overdevelopment of genitalia.

hy•per•geu•si•a (hī′pĕr-gū′sē-ă) Abnormal acuteness of the sense of taste. SYN oxygeusia. [hyper- + G. *geusis,* taste]

hy•per•gi•a (hī-pĕr′jē-ă) SYN hyperergia.

hy•per•gic (hī-pĕr′jik) SYN hyperergic.

hy•per•glan•du•lar (hī′pĕr-glan′dyū-lăr) Characterized by overactivity or increased size of a gland.

hy•per•glob•u•lin•e•mi•a (hī′pĕr-glob′yū-lin-ē′mē-ă) An abnormally high concentration of globulins in the circulating blood plasma.

hyperglycaemia [Br.] SYN hyperglycemia.

hy•per•gly•ce•mi•a (hī′pĕr-glī-sē′mē-ă) An abnormally high concentration of glucose in the blood, a feature of diabetes mellitus. SYN hyperglycaemia. [hyper- + G. *glykys,* sweet, + *haima,* blood]

hyperglyceridaemia [Br.] SYN hyperglyceridemia.

hy•per•glyc•er•i•de•mi•a (hī′pĕr-glis′ĕr-i-dē′mē-ă) Elevated plasma concentration of glycerides; normal if transiently present after absorption of a meal containing lipids, abnormal if a persistent state. SYN hyperglyceridaemia.

hyperglycinaemia [Br.] SYN hyperglycinemia.

hy•per•gly•ci•ne•mi•a (hī′pĕr-glī′si-nē′mē-ă) Elevated plasma glycine concentration. SYN hyperglycinaemia.

hy•per•gly•ci•nu•ri•a (hī′pĕr-glī′si-nyūr′ē-ă) Enhanced urinary excretion of glycine.

hy•per•gly•co•gen•ol•y•sis (hī′pĕr-glī′kō-jĕ-nol′i-sis) Excessive glycogenolysis. [hyper- + glycogen + G. *lysis,* loosening]

hy•per•gly•cor•rha•chi•a (hī′pĕr-glī′kō-rā′kē-ă) Excessive sugar in the cerebrospinal fluid. [hyper- + G. *glykys,* sweet, + *rhachis,* spine]

hy•per•gly•co•su•ri•a (hī′pĕr-glī′kō-syūr′ē-ă) Persistent excretion of unusually large amounts of glucose in the urine.

hy•per•go•nad•ism (hī′pĕr-gō′nad-izm) A clinical state resulting from enhanced secretion of gonadal hormones.

hy•per•go•nad•o•tro•pic (hī′pĕr-gō-nad′ō-trō′pik) Indicating an increased production or excretion of gonadotropic hormones.

hy•per•go•nad•o•tro•pic eu•nuch•oid•ism (hī′pĕr-gō-nad′ō-trō′pik yū′nŭ-koyd-izm) Eunuchoidism of gonadal origin, commonly accompanied by enhanced levels of pituitary gonadotropins in the blood and urine, as in Klinefelter syndrome.

hyperhaemoglobinaemia [Br.] SYN hyperhemoglobinemia.

hy•per•he•mo•glo•bi•ne•mi•a (hī′pĕr-hē′mō-glō-bin-ē′mē-ă) An unusually large amount of hemoglobin in the circulating blood plasma. SYN hyperhaemoglobinaemia.

hy•per•hi•dro•sis (hī′pĕr-hī-drō′sis) Excessive or profuse sweating. SYN hyperidrosis, polyhidrosis, polyidrosis. [hyper- + hidrosis]

hy•per•hy•dra•tion (hī′pĕr-hī-drā′shŭn) Excess water content of the body.

hy•per•i•dro•sis (hī′pĕr-ī-drō′sis) SYN hyperhidrosis.

hy•per-IgM syn•drome (hī′pĕr sin′drōm) An X-linked immunodeficiency disorder with very low serum concentrations of IgG and IgA with a normal or a markedly elevated concentration of polyclonal IgM; affected boys develop recurrent bacterial infections in the first or second year of life.

hy•per•im•mu•no•glob•u•lin E syn•drome (hī′pĕr-im′yū-nō-glob′yū-lin sin′drōm) An immunodeficiency disorder characterized by high levels of plasma IgE concentrations, a leukocyte chemotactic defect, and recurrent staphylococcal infections of the skin, upper respiratory tract, and other sites.

hy•per•in•fec•tion (hī′pĕr-in-fek′shŭn) Infection by very large numbers of organisms as a result of immunologic deficiency.

hy•per•in•fla•tion (hī′pĕr-in-flā′shŭn) Overdistention of pulmonary alveoli with air as a result of local or general airway obstruction.

hyperinsulinaemia [Br.] SYN hyperinsulinemia.

hy•per•in•su•li•ne•mi•a (hī′pĕr-in′sŭ-lin-ē′mē-ă) Increased levels of insulin in the plasma due to increased secretion of insulin by the beta cells of the pancreatic islets. SYN hyperinsulinaemia, hyperinsulinism.

hy•per•in•su•lin•ism (hī′pĕr-in′sŭ-lin-izm) SYN hyperinsulinemia.

hy•per•in•vo•lu•tion (hī′pĕr-in-vō-lū′shŭn) SYN superinvolution.

hy•per•i•so•ton•ic (hī′pĕr-ī′sō-ton′ik) SYN hypertonic.

hyperkalaemia [Br.] SYN hyperkalemia.

hyperkalaemic periodic paralysis [Br.] SYN hyperkalemic periodic paralysis.

hy•per•ka•le•mi•a (hī′pĕr-kă-lē′mē-ă) A greater than normal concentration of potassium ions in the circulating blood. SYN hyperkalaemia, hyperpotassemia. [hyper- + Mod. L. *kalium,* potash, + G. *haima,* blood]

hy•per•ka•le•mic pe•ri•od•ic pa•ral•y•sis (hī′pĕr-kă-lē′mik pēr′ē-od′ik păr-al′i-sis) A form of periodic paralysis in which the serum potassium level is elevated during attacks; onset occurs in infancy, attacks are frequent but relatively mild, and myotonia is often present. SYN hyperkalaemic periodic paralysis.

hy•per•ker•a•tin•i•za•tion (hī′pĕr-ker′a-tin-ī-zā′shŭn) SYN hyperkeratosis.

hy•per•ker•a•to•sis (hī′pĕr-ker′ă-tō′sis) Thickening of the horny layer of the epidermis or mucous membrane. SEE ALSO keratoderma, keratosis. SYN hyperkeratinization.

hyperketonaemia [Br.] SYN hyperketonemia.

hy•per•ke•to•ne•mi•a (hī′pĕr-kē′tō-nē′mē-ă) Elevated concentrations of ketone bodies in the blood. SYN hyperketonaemia.

hy•per•ke•ton•u•ri•a (hī′pĕr-kē′tō-nyūr′ē-ă) Increased urinary excretion of ketonic compounds.

hyperkinaemia [Br.] SYN hyperkinemia.

hy•per•ki•ne•mi•a (hī′pĕr-ki-nē′mē-ă) Increased circulation rate; increased volume flow through the circulation; supernormal cardiac output. SYN hyperkinaemia. [hyper- + G. *kineō,* to move, + *haima,* blood]

hy•per•ki•ne•sis, **hy•per•ki•ne•si•a** (hī′pĕr-ki-nē′sis, -nē′zē-ă) **1.** Excessive motility. **2.** Excessive muscular activity. SYN supermotility. [hyper- + G. *kinēsis,* motion]

hy•per•ki•net•ic (hī′pĕr-ki-net′ik) Pertaining to or characterized by hyperkinesia.

hy•per•ki•ne•tic dys•arth•ri•a (hī′pĕr-ki-net′ik dis-ahr′thrē-ă) Dysarthria associated with disorders of the extrapyramidal motor system resulting in involuntary movements of the articulatory and respiratory systems that cause variations in voice loudness and rate and in interruptions in ongoing speech. SEE ALSO extrapyramidal motor system, myoclonus, athetosis, Tourette syndrome.

hy•per•ki•net•ic syn•drome (hī′pĕr-ki-net′ik sin′drōm) A condition marked by pathologically excessive energy seen sometimes in young children with brain injury, mental illness, and attention deficit disorder, and in epileptics; the chief characteristics are hypermotility and emotional instability; distractibility, inattention, and lack of shyness and fear are common accompaniments.

hy•per•ky•pho•sis (hī′pĕr-kī-fō′sis) An abnormal exaggeration of the normal forward (flexion) curvature of the thoracic spine.

hy•per•ky•phot•ic (hī′pĕr-kī-fot′ik) Having a pathologically exaggerated kyphotic curve of the thoracic spine. This is most often a complication of Sheuermann disease or osteoporosis. SEE ALSO Scheuermann disease, osteoporosis.

hy•per•leu•ko•cy•to•sis (hī′pĕr-lū′kō-sī-tō′sis) An increase in the number and proportion of leukocytes in the circulating blood or the tissues greater than that ordinarily observed in most instances of leukocytosis.

hyperlipaemia [Br.] SYN hyperlipemia.

hy•per•li•pe•mi•a (hī′pĕr-li-pē′mē-ă) An elevated level of lipids in the blood. SEE ALSO lipemia. SYN hyperlipaemia. [hyper- + G. *lipos,* fat, + *haima,* blood]

hyperlipidaemia [Br.] SYN hyperlipidemia.

hy•per•lip•id•e•mi•a (hī′pĕr-lip′i-dē′mē-ă) SYN lipemia. SYN hyperlipidaemia.

hyperlipoidaemia [Br.] SYN hyperlipoidemia.

hy•per•lip•oi•de•mi•a (hī′pĕr-lip′oy-dē′mē-ă) SYN lipemia. SYN hyperlipoidaemia.

hyperlipoproteinaemia [Br.] SYN hyperlipoproteinemia.

hy•per•lip•o•pro•tein•e•mi•a (hī′pĕr-lip′ō-prō-tēn-ē′mē-ă) An increase in the lipoprotein concentration of the blood. SYN hyperlipoproteinaemia.

hy•per•lith•ur•i•a (hī′pĕr-li-thyūr′ē-ă) An excessive excretion of uric (lithic) acid in the urine.

hy•per•lor•do•sis (hī′pĕr-dō′sis) An abnormal anteriorly convex curvature of the spine, usually lumbar.

hy•per•lor•dot•ic (hī′lōr-dot′ik) Having a pathologically exaggerated lordotic curve of the lumbar spine; colloquial term is "swayback."

hy•per•lu•cent (hī′pĕr-lū′sĕnt) A region on a chest radiograph showing greater than normal film blackening resulting from increased transmission of x-rays. [hyper- + L. *lucens,* shining, fr. *luceo,* to shine]

hy•per•lu•cent lung (hī′pĕr-lū′sĕnt lŭng) The radiographic finding that a lung or portion thereof is less dense than normal, e.g., from air trapping by a bronchial foreign body, asymmetric emphysema, or decreasing blood flow.

hyperlysinaemia [Br.] SYN hyperlysinemia.

hy•per•ly•si•ne•mi•a (hī′pĕr-lī-si-nē′mē-ă) A metabolic disorder characterized by mental retardation, convulsions, anemia, and asthenia; associated with an abnormal increase of the amino acid lysine in the circulating blood due to a deficiency of lysine-ketoglutarate reductase. One variant is associated with a deficiency of α-aminoadipic semialdehyde synthase, resulting in hyperlysinemia and saccharopinemia. SYN hyperlysinaemia, lysinemia.

hy·per·ly·sin·ur·i·a (hī′pĕr-lī-si-nyūr′ē-ă) The presence of abnormally high concentrations of lysine in the urine; a form of aminoaciduria that occurs in cystinuria, hepatolenticular degeneration, and Fanconi syndrome.

hypermagnesaemia [Br.] SYN hypermagnesemia.

hy·per·mag·ne·se·mi·a (hī′pĕr-mag′nĕ-sē′mē-ă) Excessive magnesium in blood; may be a result of chronic renal insufficiency, overuse of magnesium-containing laxatives or antacids, or severe dehydration. Signs include weakness, paralysis, drowsiness, confusion, bradycardia, hypotension, nausea, and vomiting. SYN hypermagnesaemia.

hy·per·mas·ti·a (hī′pĕr-mas′tē-ă) **1.** SYN polymastia. **2.** Excessively large breasts. [hyper- + G. *mastos,* breast]

hy·per·ma·ture cat·a·ract (hī′pĕr-mă-chūr′ kat′ăr-akt) A cataract in which the lens cortex becomes liquid, with the nucleus gravitating within the capsule (Morgagni cataract).

hy·per·men·or·rhe·a (hī′pĕr-men-ŏr-ē′ă) Excessively prolonged or profuse menses. SYN hypermenorrhoea, menorrhagia, menostaxis. [hyper- + G. *mēn,* month, + *rhoia,* flow]

hypermenorrhoea [Br.] SYN hypermenorrhea.

hy·per·me·tab·o·lism (hī′pĕr-mĕ-tab′ŏ-lizm) Heat production by the body above normal, as in thyrotoxicosis.

hy·per·me·tri·a (hī′pĕr-mē′trē-ă) Unusual range of motion characterized by overreaching a desired object or goal; usually seen with cerebellar disorders. Cf. hypometria. [hyper- + G. *metron,* mcasurc]

hy·per·me·tro·pi·a (hī′pĕr-mē-trō′pē-ă) SYN hyperopia. [hyper- + G. *metron,* measure, + *ōps,* eye]

hy·per·mo·bile pa·tel·la (hī′pĕr-mō′bil pă-tel′ă) A range of patellar movement equal to three or more quadrants of the patella.

hy·per·mo·tor sei·zure (hī′pĕr-mō′tŏr sē′zhŭr) Attack characterized by automatisms involving predominantly proximal limb muscles and producing marked limb displacement.

hy·per·my·o·to·ni·a (hī′pĕr-mī′ō-tō′nē-ă) Extreme muscular tonus. [hyper- + G. *mys,* muscle, + *tonos,* tension]

hy·per·my·ot·ro·phy (hī′pĕr-mī-ot′rŏ-fē) Muscular hypertrophy. [hyper- + G. *mys,* muscle, + *trophē,* nourishment]

hy·per·na·sal·i·ty (hī′pĕr-nā-zal′i-tē) Speech produced with excessive resonance in the nasal cavity, often due to dysfunction of the soft palate. SYN hyperrhinophonia.

hypernatraemia [Br.] SYN hypernatremia.

hypernatraemic encephalopathy [Br.] SYN hypernatremic encephalopathy.

hy·per·na·tre·mi·a (hī′pĕr-nă-trē′mē-ă) An abnormally high plasma concentration of sodium ions. SYN hypernatraemia. [hyper- + natrium, + G. *haima,* blood]

hy·per·na·tre·mic en·ceph·a·lop·a·thy (hī′pĕr-nă-trē′mik en-sef′a-lop′ă-thē) Subarachnoid and subdural effusions in infants with hypernatremic dehydration. SYN hypernatraemic encephalopathy.

hy·per·ne·o·cy·to·sis (hī′pĕr-nē′ō-sī-tō′sis) Hyperleukocytosis in which there are considerable numbers of immature and young cells (especially in the granulocytic series). [hyper- + G. *neos,* new, + *kytos,* cell, + *-osis,* condition]

hypernoea [Br.] SYN hypernoia.

hy·per·noi·a (hī′pĕr-noy′ă) Great rapidity of thought; excessive mental activity or imagination, as seen in the manic phase of bipolar disorder. SYN hypernoea. [hyper- + G. *noeō,* to think]

hy·per·on·cot·ic (hī′pĕr-on-kot′ik) Indicating an oncotic pressure higher than normal, e.g., of blood plasma.

hy·per·o·nych·i·a (hī′pĕr-ō-nik′ē-ă) Hypertrophy of the nails. [hyper- + G. *onyx,* (*onych-*), nail]

hy·per·o·pi·a (H) (hī′pĕr-ō′pē-ă) An ocular condition in which only convergent rays can be brought to focus on the retina. See page 750. SYN farsightedness, hypermetropia. [hyper- + G. *ōps,* eye]

hy·per·o·pic (H) (hī′pĕr-ō′pik) Pertaining to hyperopia.

hy·per·o·pic a·stig·ma·tism (hī′pĕr-ō′pik ă-stig′mă-tizm) Astigmatism in which one meridian is hyperopic and the one at a right angle to it is without a refractive error.

hy·per·or·chi·dism (hī′pĕr-ōr′ki-dizm) Increased size or functioning of the testes. [hyper- + G. *orchis,* testis]

hy·per·or·tho·cy·to·sis (hī′pĕr-ōr′thō-sī-tō′sis) Hyperleukocytosis in which the relative percentages of the various types of white blood cells are within the normal range. [hyper- + G. *orthos,* correct, + *kytos,* cell, + *-osis,* condition]

hy·per·os·mi·a (hī′pĕr-oz′mē-ă) An exaggerated or abnormally acute sense of smell. [hyper- + G. *osmē,* sense of smell]

hy·per·os·mo·lal·i·ty (hī′pĕr-oz′mō-lal′i-tē) Increased concentration of a solution expressed as osmoles of solute per kilogram of serum water.

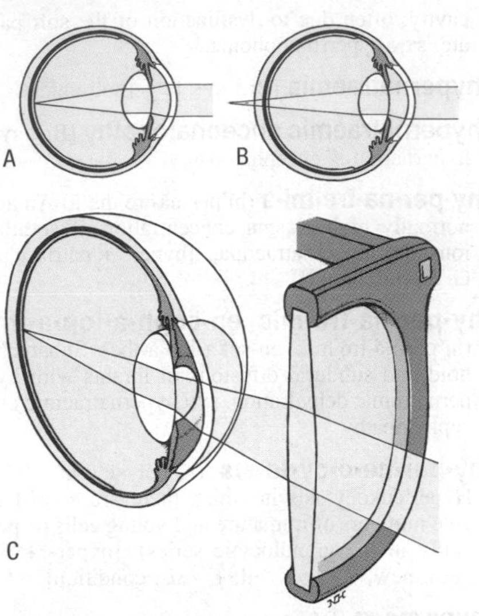

hyperopia: (A) normal (20/20) vision, light rays focus sharply on retina; (B) hyperopic (farsighted) vision, light rays from close objects come to sharp focus behind the retina; (C) hyperopia corrected by eyeglasses with convex lenses

hy·per·os·mo·lar (hy·per·gly·cem·ic) non·ke·tot·ic co·ma (hī′pĕr-oz-mō′lăr hī′per-glī-sē′mik non′kē-tot′ik kō′mă) A complication seen in diabetes mellitus in which marked hyperglycemia occurs (e.g., levels exceeding 800 mg/dL), causing osmotic shifts in water in brain cells and resulting in coma; can be fatal or lead to permanent neurologic damage; ketoacidosis does not occur.

hy·per·os·mo·lar·i·ty (hī′pĕr-oz′mō-lar′i-tē) An increase in the osmotic concentration of a solution expressed as osmoles of solute per liter of solution.

hy·per·os·mot·ic (hī′pĕr-oz-mot′ik) **1.** Having an osmolality greater than that of another fluid, ordinarily assumed to be plasma or extracellular fluid. **2.** Relating to increased osmosis.

hy·per·os·te·oi·do·sis (hī′pĕr-os′tē-oyd-ō′sis) Excessive formation of osteoid, as seen in rickets and osteomalacia.

hy·per·os·to·sis (hī′pĕr-os-tō′sis) **1.** Hypertrophy of bone. **2.** SYN exostosis. [hyper- + G. *osteon,* bone, + *-ōsis,* condition]

hy·per·o·var·i·an·ism (hī′pĕr-ō-var′ē-ăn-izm) Sexual precocity in young girls due to premature development of ovaries and secretion of ovarian hormones. SYN true precocious puberty.

hy·per·ox·al·u·ri·a (hī′pĕr-ok-să-lyūr′ē-ă) Presence of an unusually large amount of oxalic acid or oxalates in the urine. SYN oxaluria.

hy·per·ox·i·a (hī′pĕr-ok′sē-ă) **1.** An increased amount of oxygen in tissues and organs. **2.** A greater oxygen tension than normal.

hyperoxygenised [Br.] SYN hyperoxygenized.

hy·per·o·xy·gen·ized (hī′pĕr-oks′i-jĕn-īzd) Combined with a large amount of oxygen. SYN hyperoxygenised.

hy·per·par·a·sit·ism (hī′pĕr-par′ă-sīt-izm) A condition in which a secondary parasite develops within a previously existing parasite.

hy·per·par·a·thy·roid·ism (hī′pĕr-par′ă-thī′royd-izm) A condition due to an increase in the secretion of the parathyroids, causing elevated serum calcium, decreased serum phosphorus, and increased excretion of both calcium and phosphorus, calcium stones, and sometimes generalized osteitis fibrosa cystica.

hy·per·pep·sin·i·a (hī′pĕr-pep-sin′ē-ă) An excess of pepsin in the gastric juice.

hy·per·per·i·stal·sis (hī′pĕr-per′i-stal′sis) Excessive rapidity of the passage of food through the stomach and intestine.

hyperphenylalaninaemia [Br.] SYN hyperphenylalaninemia.

hy·per·phen·yl·al·a·ni·ne·mi·a (hī′pĕr-fen′il-al′ă-ni-nē′mē-ă) The presence of abnormally high blood levels of phenylalanine in newborn infants associated with phenylketonuria, maternal phenylketonuria, or transient deficiency of phenylalanine hydroxylase or *p*-hydroxyphenylpyruvic acid oxidase. SYN hyperphenylalaninaemia.

hy·per·pho·ne·sis (hī′pĕr-fō-nē′sis) An increase in the percussion sound or of the voice sound in auscultation. [hyper- + G. *phōnēsis,* a sounding]

hy·per·pho·ri·a (hī′pĕr-fōr′ē-ă) A tendency of the visual axis of one eye to deviate upward, prevented by binocular vision. [hyper- + G. *phora,* motion]

hyperphosphataemia [Br.] SYN hyperphosphatemia.

hy·per·phos·pha·te·mi·a (hī′pĕr-fos′fă-tē′mē-ă) Elevation of phosphorus concentration in blood; may be due to consumption of large amounts of phosphorus-rich foods and drinks or to renal insufficiency. It may also be caused by hypocalcemia, hyperparathyroidism, or overuse of phosphate-containing laxatives or antacids. With concurrent hypocalcemia, tetany and seizures may occur. SYN hyperphosphataemia.

hy·per·phos·pha·tu·ri·a (hī′pĕr-fos′fă-tyūr′ē-ă) An increased excretion of phosphates in the urine.

i hy·per·pig·men·ta·tion (hī′pĕr-pig-men-tā′shŭn) An excess of pigment in a tissue or part. See page 751.

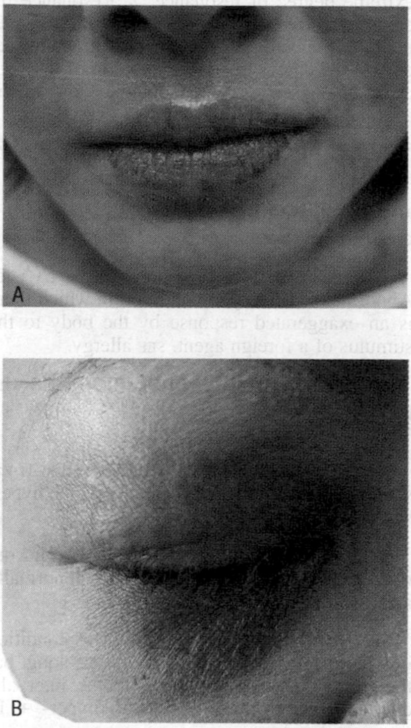

hyperpigmentation: (A) drug-induced, lips; (B) postinflammatory, periorbital

hy·per·pi·tu·i·ta·rism (hī′pĕr-pi-tū′i-tă-rizm) Excessive production of anterior pituitary hormones, especially growth hormone; may result in gigantism or acromegaly.

hy·per·pla·si·a (hī′pĕr-plā′zē-ă) An increase in the number of cells in a tissue or organ, excluding tumor formation, whereby the bulk of the part or organ may be increased. SEE ALSO hypertrophy. Cf. hypoplasia. See this page. [hyper- + G. *plasis,* a molding]

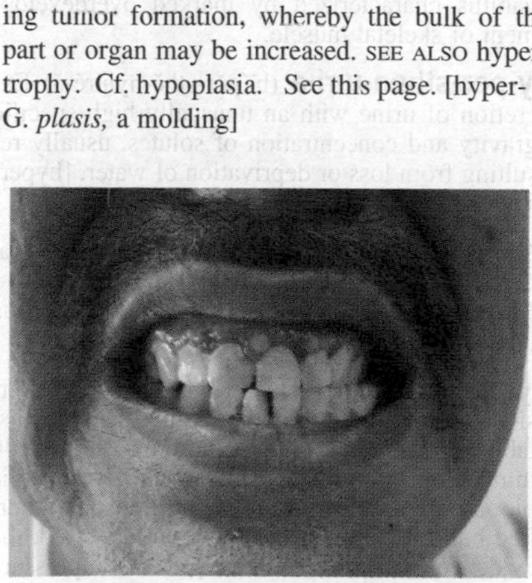

drug-induced gingival hyperplasia: caused by phenytoin

hy·per·plas·tic (hī′pĕr-plas′tik) Relating to hyperplasia.

hy·per·plas·tic gin·gi·vi·tis (hī′pĕr-plas′tik jin′ji-vī′tis) Gingivitis of long-standing duration in which the gingivae become enlarged and firm due to proliferation of fibrous connective tissue.

hy·per·plas·tic in·flam·ma·tion (hī′pĕr-plas′tik in′flă-mā′shŭn) SYN proliferative inflammation.

hy·per·plas·tic pol·yp (hī′pĕr-plas′tik pol′ip) A benign small sessile polyp of the large bowel showing lengthening and cystic dilation of mucosal glands; also applied to nonneoplastic gastric mucosal polyps. See this page. SYN metaplastic polyp.

hy·per·plas·tic pulp·i·tis (hī′pĕr-plas′tik pŭl-pī′tis) Hyperplastic granulation tissue growing out of the exposed pulp chamber of a grossly decayed tooth.

hy·per·pne·a (hī′pĕrp-nē′ă) Breathing that is deeper and more rapid than is normal at rest. SYN hyperpnoea. [hyper- + G. *pnoē,* breathing]

hyperpnoea [Br.] SYN hyperpnea.

hy·per·po·lar·i·za·tion (hī′pĕr-pō′lăr-ī-zā′shŭn) An increase in polarization of membranes of nerves or muscle cells; the reverse change from that associated with excitatory action.

hy·per·po·ne·sis (hī′pĕr-pō-nē′sis) Exaggerated activity within the motor portion of the nervous system. [hyper- + G. *ponos,* toil]

hyperpotassaemia [Br.] SYN hyperpotassemia

hy·per·po·tas·se·mi·a (hī′pĕr-pō′tă-sē′mē-ă) SYN hyperkalemia. SYN hyperpotassaemia.

hyperprebetalipoproteinaemia [Br.] SYN hyperprebetalipoproteinemia.

hy·per·pre·be·ta·lip·o·pro·tein·e·mi·a (hī′pĕr-prē′bā′tă-lip′ō-prō′tēn-ē′mē-ă) Increased concentrations of pre-β-lipoproteins in the blood. SYN hyperprebetalipoproteinaemia.

hyperproinsulinaemia [Br.] SYN hyperproinsulinemia.

hy·per·pro·in·su·li·ne·mi·a (hī′pĕr-prō-in′sŭl-i-nē′mē-ă) Elevated plasma levels of proinsulin or proinsulinlike material. SYN hyperproinsulinaemia.

hyperprolactinaemia [Br.] SYN hyperprolactinemia.

hy·per·pro·lac·ti·ne·mi·a (hī′pĕr-prō-lak′ti-nē′mē-ă) Elevated levels of prolactin in the blood; a normal physiologic reaction during lactation, but pathologic otherwise; often due to physical or emotional stress or rapid weight loss, sometimes to pituitary adenoma; amenorrhea is usually present. SYN hyperprolactinaemia.

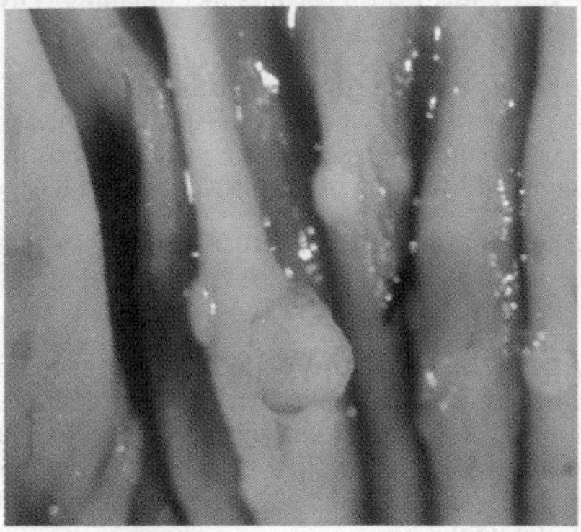

hyperplastic polyp

hyperprolinaemia [Br.] SYN hyperprolinemia.

hy•per•pro•li•ne•mi•a (hī′pĕr-prō′li-nē′mē-ă) A metabolic disorder characterized by enhanced plasma proline concentrations and urinary excretion of proline, hydroxyproline, and glycine; autosomal recessive inheritance. Type I hyperprolinemia is associated with a deficiency of proline oxidase and renal disease; Type II hyperprolinemia is associated with a deficiency of Δ-pyrroline-5-carboxylate dehydrogenase, mental retardation, and convulsions and is caused by mutation in the δ-pyrroline 5 carboxylate gene (P5CD) on 1p. SYN hyperprolinaemia.

hyperproteinaemia [Br.] SYN hyperproteinemia.

hy•per•pro•tein•e•mi•a (hī′pĕr-prō′tēn-ē′mē-ă) An abnormally large concentration of protein in plasma. SYN hyperproteinaemia.

hy•per•pro•te•o•sis (hī′pĕr-prō′tē-ō′sis) A condition resulting from an excessive amount of protein in the diet.

hy•per•py•ret•ic (hī′pĕr-pī-ret′ik) Relating to hyperpyrexia. SYN hyperpyrexial.

hy•per•py•rex•i•a (hī′pĕr-pī-rek′sē-ă) Extremely high fever. [hyper- + G. *pyrexis,* feverishness]

hy•per•py•rex•i•al (hī′pĕr-pī-rek′sē-ăl) SYN hyperpyretic.

hy•per•re•ac•tive ma•lar•i•ous sple•no•meg•a•ly (hī′pĕr-ak′tiv mă-lar′ē-ŭs splē′nō-meg′ă-lē) A syndrome characterized by persistent splenomegaly, exceptionally high serum IgM and malaria antibody levels, and hepatic sinusoidal lymphocytosis. SYN tropical splenomegaly syndrome.

hy•per•re•flex•i•a (hī′pĕr-rē-flek′sē-ă) A condition in which the deep tendon reflexes are exaggerated.

hy•per•res•o•nance (hī′pĕr-rez′ŏ-năns) **1.** An extreme degree of resonance. **2.** Resonance increased above the normal, and often of lower pitch, on percussion of an area of the body; occurs in the chest due to overinflation of the lung as in emphysema or pneumothorax and in the abdomen over a distended bowel.

hy•per•rhi•no•pho•ni•a (hī′pĕr-rī′nō-fō′nē-ă) SYN hypernasality.

hy•per•sal•i•va•tion (hī′pĕr-sal′i-vā′shŭn) Increased salivation.

hy•per•sen•si•tiv•i•ty (hī′per-sen′si-tiv′i-tē) Abnormal sensitivity, a condition in which there is an exaggerated response by the body to the stimulus of a foreign agent. SEE allergy.

hy•per•sen•si•tiv•i•ty pneu•mo•ni•tis (hī′pĕr-sen′si-tiv′i-tē nū′mō-nī′tis) SYN extrinsic allergic alveolitis.

hy•per•sen•si•ti•za•tion (hī′pĕr-sen′si-tī-zā′shŭn) The immunologic process by which hypersensitivity is induced.

hy•per•sex•u•al (hī′pĕr-sek′shū-ăl) PSYCHIATRY referring to a person who exhibits abnormally increasd sexual activity.

hy•per•som•ni•a (hī′pĕr-som′nē-ă) A condition in which sleep periods are excessively long, but the person responds normally in the intervals; distinguished from somnolence. [hyper- + L. *somnus,* sleep]

hy•per•splen•ism (hī′pĕr-splēn′izm) Any condition in which the cellular components of the blood or platelets are removed at an abnormally high rate by the spleen.

hy•per•sthe•ni•a (hī′pĕr-sthē′nē-ă) Excessive tension or strength. [hyper- + G. *sthenos,* strength]

hy•per•sthen•ic (hī′pĕr-sthen′ik) **1.** Pertaining to or marked by hypersthenia. **2.** Pertaining to a habitus characterized by marked overdevelopment of skeletal muscle.

hy•per•sthen•u•ri•a (hī′pĕr-sthĕ-nyū′rē-ă) Excretion of urine with an unusually high specific gravity and concentration of solutes, usually resulting from loss or deprivation of water. [hyper- + G. *sthenos,* strength, + *ouron,* urine]

hy•per•tel•or•ism (hī′pĕr-tel′ŏr-izm) Abnormal distance between two paired organs. [hyper- + G. *tēle,* far off, + *horizō,* to separate, fr. *horos,* a boundary]

hy•per•ten•sion (HTN) (hī′pĕr-ten′shŭn) Persisting high arterial blood pressure; generally established guidelines are values exceeding 140 mmHg systolic or exceeding 90 mmHg diastolic blood pressure. Despite many discrete and inherited but rare forms that have been identified, the evidence is that for the most part blood pressure is a multifactorial, perhaps galtonian, trait. Hypertension is considered a risk factor for developing heart disease, stroke, and kidney disease.

Its signs and symptoms include dizziness and headache. [hyper- + L. *tensio,* tension]

hy·per·ten·sive (hī′pĕr-ten′siv) **1.** Marked by an increased blood pressure. **2.** Denoting a person suffering from high blood pressure.

hy·per·ten·sive ar·te·ri·op·a·thy (hī′pĕr-ten′siv ahr-tēr′ē-op′ă-thē) Arterial degeneration resulting from hypertension.

hy·per·ten·sive ar·te·ri·o·scle·ro·sis (hī′pĕr-ten′siv ahr-tēr′ē-ō-skler-ō′sis) Progressive increase in muscle and elastic tissue of arterial walls, resulting from hypertension; in long-standing hypertension, elastic tissue forms numerous concentric layers in the intima and there is replacement of muscle by collagen fibers and hyaline thickening of the intima of arterioles; such changes can develop with increasing age in the absence of hypertension and may then be referred to as senile arteriosclerosis.

hy·per·ten·sive ret·i·nop·a·thy (hī′pĕr-ten′siv ret′i-nop′ă-thē) A retinal condition occurring in accelerated vascular hypertension, marked by arteriolar constriction, flame-shaped hemorrhages, cotton-wool patches, star-figure edema at the macula, and papilledema.

hy·per·ten·sive up·per e·so·pha·ge·al sphinc·ter (hī′pĕr-ten′siv ŭp′ĕr ĕ-sof′ă-jē′ăl sf-ingk′tĕr) SYN cricopharyngeal achalasia.

hy·per·ten·sor (hī′pĕr-ten′sŏr) SYN pressor.

hy·per·the·co·sis (hī′pĕr-thē-kō′sis) Diffuse hyperplasia of the thecal cells of the graafian follicles.

hy·per·thel·i·a (hī′pĕr-thē′lē-ă) SYN polythelia. [hyper- + G. *thēlē,* nipple]

hy·per·ther·mal·ge·si·a (hī′pĕr-thĕrm′al-jē′zē-ă) Extreme sensitivity to heat. [hyper- + G. *thermē,* heat, + *algēsis,* pain]

hy·per·ther·mi·a (hī′pĕr-thĕr′mē-ă) Hyperpyrexia, often (but not necessarily) induced therapeutically . [hyper- + G. *thermē,* heat]

hyperthrombinaemia [Br.] SYN hyperthrombinemia.

hy·per·throm·bi·ne·mi·a (hī′pĕr-throm′bi-nē′mē-ă) An abnormal increase of thrombin in the blood, frequently resulting in a tendency to intravascular coagulation. SYN hyperthrombinaemia.

hy·per·thy·mic (hī′pĕr-thī′mik) **1.** Pertaining to hyperthymia. **2.** Pertaining to hyperthymism.

hy·per·thy·roid·ism (hī′pĕr-thī′royd-izm) An abnormality of the thyroid gland in which secretion of thyroid hormone is usually increased and is no longer under regulatory control of hypothalamic-pituitary centers; characterized by a hypermetabolic state, usually with weight loss, tremulousness, elevated plasma levels of thyroxin and/or triiodothyronine; often associated with exophthalmos (Graves disease).

hyperthyroxinaemia [Br.] SYN hyperthyroxinemia.

hy·per·thy·rox·i·ne·mi·a (hī′pĕr-thī-rok′si-nē′mē-ă) An elevated thyroxine concentration in the blood. SYN hyperthyroxinaemia.

hy·per·to·ni·a (hī′pĕr-tō′nē-ă) Extreme tension of the muscles or arteries. [hyper- + G. *tonos,* tension]

hy·per·ton·ic (hī′pĕr-tŏn′ik) **1.** Having a greater degree of tension. SYN spastic (1). **2.** Having a greater osmotic pressure than a reference solution, which is ordinarily assumed to be blood plasma or interstitial fluid; more specifically, refers to a fluid in which cells shrink. SYN hyperisotonic.

hy·per·to·ni·cit·y (hī′pĕr-tō-nis′i-tē) Abnormally increased muscle tone or strength. The condition is sometimes associated with genetic or CNS disorders (e.g., trisomy 18) and may be mainfest in arm or leg deformities. SEE ALSO spasticity. SYN high muscle tone.

hy·per·ton·ic la·bor (hī′pĕr-ton′ik lā′bŏr) Labor in which the uterus does not relax between contractions and general myometrial spasm prevents expulsion of the fetus.

hy·per·ton·ic sa·line (hī′pĕr-ton′ik sā′lēn) Solution containing 1 to 15% w/v sodium choloride.

hy·per·tri·cho·sis (hī′pĕr-tri-kō′sis) Growth of hair in excess of the normal. SEE ALSO hirsutism. [hyper- + G. *trichōsis,* being hairy]

hypertriglyceridaemia [Br.] SYN hypertriglyceridemia.

hy·per·tri·glyc·er·i·de·mi·a (hī′pĕr-trī-glis′ĕr-i-dē′mē-ă) Elevated triglyceride concentration in the blood. SYN hypertriglyceridaemia.

hy·per·tro·phic (hī′pĕr-trō′fik) Relating to or characterized by hypertrophy.

hy·per·tro·phic ar·thri·tis (hī′pĕr-trō′fik ahr-thrī′tis) SYN osteoarthritis.

hy·per·tro·phic car·di·o·my·op·a·thy (hī′pĕr-trō′fik kahr′dē-ō-mī-op′ă-thē) Cardiac hypertrophy of unknown cause, possibly genetic, with impairment of left ventricular filling, emptying, or both. Signs and symptoms include fatigue and syncope when an increased demand for cardiac output cannot be met. SEE ALSO sudden death.

hy·per·tro·phic pul·mo·nar·y os·te·o·ar·throp·a·thy (hī′pĕr-trō′fik pul′mŏ-nar-ē os′tē-ō-ahr-throp′ă-thē) Expansion of the distal ends, or the entire shafts, of the long bones, sometimes with erosions of the articular cartilages and thickening and villous proliferation of the synovial membranes, and frequent clubbing of fingers; the disorder occurs in chronic pulmonary disease, in heart disease, and occasionally in other acute and chronic disorders. SYN Bamberger-Marie disease.

hy·per·tro·phic py·lor·ic ste·no·sis (hī′pĕr-trō′fik pī-lōr′ik stĕ-nō′sis) Muscular hypertrophy of the pyloric sphincter, associated with projectile vomiting beginning in the second or third week of life, usually in males. SYN congenital pyloric stenosis.

hy·per·tro·phic rhi·ni·tis (hī′pĕr-trō′fik rī-nī′tis) Chronic rhinitis with permanent thickening of the mucous membrane.

hy·per·tro·phy (hī-pĕr′trō-fē) General increase in bulk of a part or organ, due to increase in size, but not in number, of the individual tissue elements. SEE ALSO hyperplasia. See this page. [hyper- + G. *trophē*, nourishment]

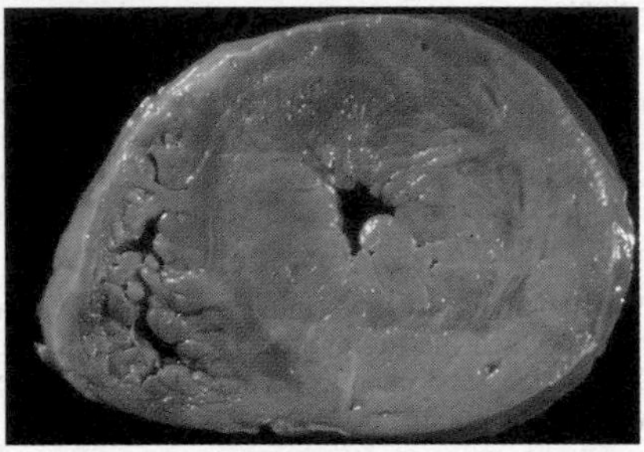

myocardial hypertrophy

hy·per·tro·pi·a (hī′pĕr-trō′pē-ă) An ocular deviation with one eye higher than the other. [hyper- + G. *tropē*, a turn]

hyperuricaemia [Br.] SYN hyperuricemia.

hyperuricaemic [Br.] SYN hyperuricemic.

hy·per·u·ri·ce·mi·a (hī′pĕr-yūr′i-sē′mē-ă) Enhanced blood concentrations of uric acid. SYN hyperuricaemia.

hy·per·u·ri·ce·mic (hī′pĕr-yūr′i-sē′mik) Relating to or characterized by hyperuricemia. SYN hyperuricaemic.

hypervalinaemia [Br.] SYN hypervalinemia.

hy·per·val·i·ne·mi·a (hī′pĕr-val′i-nē′mē-ă) Abnormally high plasma concentrations of valine, a common finding in maple syrup urine disease. SYN hypervalinaemia.

hy·per·vas·cu·lar (hī′pĕr-vas′kyū-lăr) Abnormally vascular; containing an excessive number of blood vessels. [hyper- + L. *vas*, a vessel]

hy·per·ven·ti·la·tion (hī′pĕr-ven′ti-lā′shŭn) Increased alveolar ventilation relative to metabolic carbon dioxide production, so that alveolar carbon dioxide pressure decreases to below normal.

hy·per·ven·ti·la·tion tet·a·ny (hī′pĕr-ven′ti-lā′shŭn tet′ă-nē) A neurologic disorder caused by forced overbreathing, due to reduced levels of CO_2 in the blood.

hy·per·vi·ta·min·o·sis (hī′pĕr-vī′tă-mi-nō′sis) A condition resulting from the ingestion of an excessive amount of a vitamin preparation, with symptoms varying according to the particular vitamin.

hypervolaemia [Br.] SYN hypervolemia.

hypervolaemic [Br.] SYN hypervolemic.

hy·per·vo·le·mi·a (hī′pĕr-vō-lē′mē-ă) Abnormally increased volume of blood. SYN circulatory overload, hypervolaemia, plethora (1), repletion (1). [hyper- + L. *volumen*, volume, + G. *haima*, blood]

hy·per·vo·le·mic (hī′pĕr-vō-lē′mik) Pertaining to or characterized by hypervolemia. SYN hypervolaemic.

hyp·es·the·si·a (hīp′es-thē′zē-ă) Diminished sensitivity to stimulation. SYN hypaesthesia, hypoesthesia. [G. *hypo*, under, + *aisthēsis*, feeling]

hy·pha, pl. **hy·phae** (hī′fă, -fē) A branching tubular cell characteristic of the filamentous fungi (molds). Intercommunicating hyphae constitute a mycelium, the visible colony on natural substrates or artificial laboratory media. [G. *hyphē*, a web]

hyphaema [Br.] SYN hyphema.

hyphaemia [Br.] SYN hyphemia.

hyp·he·do·nia (hīp′hē-dō′nē-ă) A habitually lessened or attenuated degree of pleasure from that which should normally give great pleasure. [G. *hypo*, under, + *hēdonē*, pleasure]

hy·phe·ma (hī-fē′mă) Blood in the anterior chamber of the eye. See page 755. SYN hyphaema. [G. *hyphaimos*, suffused with blood]

hy·phe·mi·a (hī-fē′mē-ă) SYN hypovolemia. SYN hyphaemia. [hypo- + G. *haima*, blood]

hyp·na·gog·ic (hip′nă-goj′ik) Denoting a transitional state, related to the hypnoidal, preceding sleep; applied also to various hallucinations that may manifest themselves at that time. SEE ALSO hypnoidal. [hypno- + G. *agōgos*, leading]

hyp·na·gog·ic hal·lu·cin·a·tion (hip′nă-goj′ik hă-lū′si-nā′shŭn) A common symptom in narcolepsy characterized by vivid, dreamlike perceptions occurring with sleep onset. Often these perceptions involve fearful situations that are described as realistic and include visual, tactile, and auditory hallucinations.

hyp·na·gog·ic star·tle (hip′nă-goj′ik stahr′tĕl) A twitch or myoclonus that occurs when the sleeper awakes suddenly, often accompanied by a sensation of falling through space.

hyp·na·gogue (hip′nă-gog) An agent that induces sleep. [hypno- + G. *agōgos*, leading]

hyp·nap·a·gog·ic (hip-nap′ă-goj′ik) Denoting a state similar to the hypnagogic, through which the mind passes in coming out of sleep; denoting

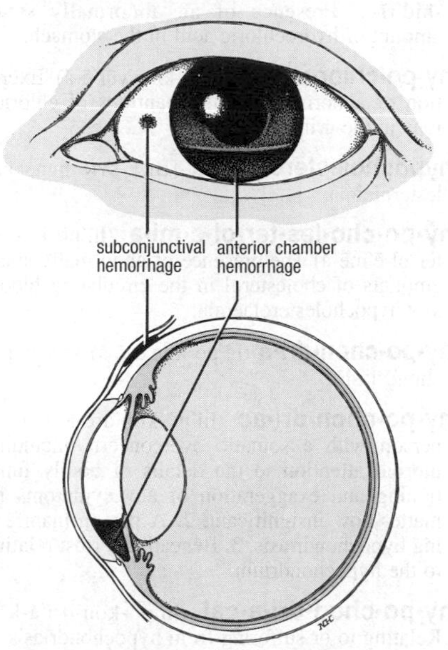

hyphema (anterior chamber hemorrhage) and subconjunctival hemorrhage

also hallucinations experienced at such time. [hypno- + G. *apo,* from, + *agōgos,* leading]

hypno-, hypn- Combining forms meaning sleep, hypnosis. [G. *hypnos,* sleep]

hyp•no•a•nal•y•sis (hip′nō-ă-nal′i-sis) Psychoanalysis or other psychotherapy that employs hypnosis as an adjunctive technique.

hyp•no•gen•e•sis (hip′nō-jen′ĕ-sis) The induction of sleep or of the hypnotic state. [hypno- + G. *genesis,* production]

hyp•no•gen•ic, hyp•nog•e•nous (hip′nō-jen′ik, -noj′ĕ-nŭs) **1.** Relating to hypnogenesis. **2.** An agent capable of inducing a hypnotic state. SEE hypnosis.

hyp•no•gen•ic spot (hip′nō-jen′ik spot) A pressure-sensitive point on the body of certain susceptible people, which, when pressed, causes the induction of sleep.

hyp•noi•dal (hip-noy′dăl) Resembling hypnosis; denoting the subwaking state, a mental condition intermediate between sleeping and waking. SEE ALSO hypnagogic. [hypno- + G. *eidos,* resemblance]

hyp•no•pom•pic hal•lu•ci•na•tion (hip′nō-pom′pik hă-lū′si-nā′shŭn) Vivid hallucinations that occur when wakening from sleep; occurs with narcolepsy, but grouped with hypnagogic hallucination.

hyp•no•sis (hip-nō′sis) An artificially induced trancelike state, resembling somnambulism, in which the subject is highly susceptible to suggestion and responds readily to the commands of the hypnotist. SEE ALSO mesmerism. [G. *hypnos,* sleep, + *-osis,* condition]

hyp•no•ther•a•py (hip′nō-thār′ă-pē) **1.** Psychotherapeutic treatment by means of hypnotism. **2.** Treatment of disease by inducing a trancelike sleep.

hyp•not•ic (hip-not′ik) **1.** Causing sleep. **2.** An agent that promotes sleep. **3.** Relating to hypnotism. [G. *hypnōtikos,* causing one to sleep]

hyp•not•ic sug•ges•tion (hip-not′ik sŭg-jes′chŭn) A direction given to a hypnotized subject for an activity that occurs during the trance or after; subject is not aware of such order and is purported to follow such direction regardless (e.g., smoking cessation). SYN posthypnotic suggestion.

hyp•not•ic trance (hip-not′ik trans) That state of somnolence or dissociation experienced by someone subjected to hypnosis.

hyp•no•tism (hip′nō-tizm) **1.** The process or act of inducing hypnosis. **2.** The practice or study of hypnosis. SEE mesmerism. [G. *hypnos,* sleep]

hyp•no•tist (hip′nō-tist) One who practices hypnotism.

hyp•no•tize (hip′nō-tīz) To induct someone into hypnosis.

hyp•no•zo•ite (hip′nō-zō′īt) Exoerythrocytic schizozoite of *Plasmodium vivax* or *P. ovale* in the human liver, characterized by delayed primary development; thought to be responsible for malarial relapse.

hypo- **1.** Prefix meaning deficient, below normal. SEE ALSO hyp-. Cf. sub-. **2.** CHEMISTRY denoting the lowest, or least rich in oxygen, of a series of chemical compounds. [G. *hypo,* under]

hy•po•a•cid•i•ty (hī′pō-a-sid′i-tē) A subnormal degree of acidity as in gastric juice.

hy•po•ac•tiv•i•ty (hī′pō-ak-tiv′i-tē) A state in which there is less movement than expected.

hy•po•a•cu•sis (hī′pō-ă-kyū′sis) SYN hypacusis.

hy•po•a•dre•nal•ism (hī′pō-ă-drē′năl-izm) **1.** Reduced function of both the cortices and medullae of the suprarenal gland. **2.** Reduced adrenal cortical function, hypocorticoidism.

hypoaesthesia [Br.] SYN hypoesthesia.

hypoalbuminaemia [Br.] SYN hypoalbuminemia.

hy•po•al•bu•mi•ne•mi•a (hī′pō-al-bū′mi-nē′mē-ă) An abnormally low concentration of albumin in the blood. SYN hypalbuminemia, hypoalbuminaemia.

hy•po•al•do•ster•on•u•ri•a (hī′pō-al-dos′tĕr-on-yūr′ē-ă) Abnormally low levels of aldosterone in the urine.

hy·po·al·ge·si·a (hī′pō-al-jē′zē-ă) SYN hypalgesia. [hypo- + G. *algēsis,* a sense of pain]

hy·po·az·ot·u·ri·a (hī′pō-az′ō-tyūr′ē-ă) Excretion of abnormally small quantities of nonprotein nitrogenous material (especially urea) in the urine. [hypo- + Fr. *azote,* nitrogen, + G. *ouron,* urine]

hy·po·bar·ic (hī′pō-bar′ik) **1.** Pertaining to pressure of ambient gases less than 1 atmosphere. **2.** With respect to solutions, less dense than the diluent or medium; e.g., in spinal anesthesia, a hypobaric solution has a density lower than that of spinal fluid. [hypo- + G. *baros,* weight]

hy·po·bar·ism (hī′pō-bar′izm) Dysbarism resulting from decreasing barometric pressure on the body without hypoxia; gas in body cavities tends to expand, and gases dissolved in body fluids tend to come out of solution as bubbles. Cf. decompression sickness, bends.

hy·po·ba·rop·a·thy (hī′pō-bar-op′ă-thē) Sickness produced by reduced barometric pressure. [hypo- + G. *baros,* weight, + *pathos,* suffering]

hypobetalipoproteinaemia [Br.] SYN hypobetalipoproteinemia.

hy·po·be·ta·lip·o·pro·tein·e·mi·a (hī′pō-bā′tă-lip′ō-prō-tēn-ē′mē-ă) Abnormally low levels of β-lipoproteins in the plasma, occasionally with acanthocytosis and neurologic signs. SEE ALSO abetalipoproteinemia. SYN hypobetalipoproteinaemia.

hy·po·blast (hī′pō-blast) SYN endoderm. [hypo- + G. *blastos,* germ]

hy·po·blas·tic (hī′pō-blas′tik) Relating to or derived from the hypoblast.

hypocalcaemia [Br.] SYN hypocalcemia.

hy·po·cal·ce·mi·a (hī′pō-kal-sē′mē-ă) Abnormally low levels of calcium in the circulating blood; commonly denotes subnormal concentrations of calcium ions. SYN hypocalcaemia.

hy·po·cal·ci·fi·ca·tion (hī′pō-kal′si-fi-kā′shŭn) Deficient calcification of bone or teeth.

hy·po·cap·ni·a (hī′pō-kap′nē-ă) Abnormally decreased arterial carbon dioxide tension. SYN hypocarbia. [hypo- + G. *kapnos,* smoke, vapor]

hy·po·car·bi·a (hī′pō-kahr′bē-ă) SYN hypocapnia.

hypochloraemia [Br.] SYN hypochloremia.

hy·po·chlor·e·mi·a (hī′pō-klōr-ē′mē-ă) An abnormally low level of chloride ions in the circulating blood. SYN hypochloraemia.

hy·po·chlor·hy·dri·a (hī′pō-klōr-hī′drē-ă, -hid′rī-ă) Presence of an abnormally small amount of hydrochloric acid in the stomach.

hy·po·chlor·u·ri·a (hī′pō-klōr-yūr′ē-ă) Excretion of abnormally small quantities of chloride ions in the urine.

hypocholesterolaemia [Br.] SYN hypocholesterolemia.

hy·po·cho·les·ter·ol·e·mi·a (hī′pō-kŏ-les′tĕr-ol-ē′mē-ă) The presence of abnormally small amounts of cholesterol in the circulating blood. SYN hypocholesterolaemia.

hy·po·chon·dri·a (hī′pō-kon′drē-ă) SYN hypochondriasis.

hy·po·chon·dri·ac (hī′pō-kon′drē-ak) **1.** A person with a somatic overconcern, including morbid attention to the details of bodily functioning and exaggeration of any symptoms no matter how insignificant. **2.** A person manifesting hypochondriasis. **3.** Beneath the ribs; relating to the hypochondrium.

hy·po·chon·dri·a·cal (hī′pō-kon-drī′ă-kăl) Relating to or suffering from hypochondriasis.

hy·po·chon·dri·a·cal mel·an·cho·li·a (hī′pō-kon-drī′ă-kăl mel′ăn-kō′lē-ă) Melancholia with many associated physical complaints, often with no identifiable physical cause.

hy·po·chon·dri·ac re·gion (hī′pō-kon′drē-ak rē′jŭn) The region on each side of the abdomen covered by the costal cartilages; it is lateral to the epigastric region.

hy·po·chon·dri·a·sis (hī′pō-kon-drī′ă-sis) A morbid concern about one's own health and exaggerated attention to any unusual bodily or mental sensations; a delusion that one is suffering from some disease for which no physical basis is evident. SYN hypochondria. [fr. hypochondrium, regarded as the site of hypochondria, + G. *-iasis,* condition]

hy·po·chon·dro·pla·si·a (hī′pō-kon′drō-plā′zē-ă) Dwarfism similar to achondroplasia, not evident until midchildhood; the cranium and facies are normal. [hypo- + G. *chondros,* cartilage, + *plasis,* a molding]

hy·po·chro·ma·si·a (hī′pō-krō-mā′zē-ă) SYN hypochromia.

hy·po·chro·mat·ic (hī′pō-krō-mat′ik) Containing a small amount of pigment, or less than the normal amount for the individual tissue. SYN hypochromic (1). [hypo- + G. *chrōma,* color]

hy·po·chro·ma·tism (hī′pō-krō′mă-tizm) **1.** The condition of being hypochromatic. **2.** SYN hypochromia.

hy·po·chro·mi·a (hī′pō-krō′mē-ă) An anemic condition in which the percentage of hemoglobin in the red blood cells is less than the normal range. SYN hypochromasia, hypochromatism (2). [hypo- + G. *chrōma,* color]

hy·po·chro·mic (hī′pō-krō′mik) **1.** SYN hypochromatic. **2.** Denoting decrease in light absorption with a shift in λ inferior to a lower wavelength.

hy·po·chro·mic a·ne·mi·a (hī′pō-krō′mik ă-nē′mē-ă) A disorder characterized by a decrease in the ratio of the weight of hemoglobin to the volume of the erythrocyte, i.e., the mean corpuscular hemoglobin concentration is subnormal. See page B3.

hy·po·cone (hī′pō-kōn) **1.** The distolingual cusp of human upper molars. **2.** A cusp appearing late in the evolution of the molars. SYN talon. [hypo- + G. *kōnos*, pine cone]

hy·po·con·id (hī′pō-kon′id) **1.** The distobuccal cusp of human lower molars. **2.** One of the cusps that comprises the talonid of the molars. [hypocone + id (2)]

hy·po·con·u·lid (hī′pō-kon′yū-lid) 1. The distal cusp of the lower molars. 2. One of the cusps of the talonid. [hypo- + Mod. L. dim. of L. *conus*, cone]

hy·po·cor·ti·coid·ism (hī′pō-kōr′ti-koyd-izm) SYN adrenocortical insufficiency.

hypocupraemia [Br.] SYN hypocupremia.

hy·po·cu·pre·mi·a (hī′pō-kyū-prē′mē-ă) Reduced copper content of the blood; found in Wilson disease because the level of ceruloplasmin is depressed, even though the level of copper attached to serum albumin is increased. SYN hypocupraemia. [hypo- + L. *cuprum*, copper, + G. *haima*, blood]

hy·po·cy·cloi·dal (hī′pō-sī-kloy′dăl) A tricyclic motion used by mechanical tomography units to optimize blurring and reduce artifacts. [hypo- + G. *kuklos*, circle, + *-oeidēs*, appearance]

hypocythaemia [Br.] SYN hypocythemia.

hy·po·cy·the·mi·a (hī′pō-sī-thē′mē-ă) Hypocytosis of the circulating blood, such as that observed in aplastic anemia. SYN hypocythaemia. [hypo- + G. *kytos*, cell, + *haima*, blood]

hy·po·dac·ty·ly, hy·po·dac·tyl·ia, hy·po·dac·tyl·ism (hī′pō-dak′ti-lē, -dak-til′ē-ă, -dak′til-izm) A condition of having fewer than the normal complement of fingers or toes. SYN oligodactyly, oligodactylia. [hypo- + G. *daktylos*, finger]

hy·po·der·mic (hī′pō-dĕr′mik) SYN subcutaneous.

hy·po·der·mic im·plan·ta·tion (hī′pō-dĕr′mik im′plan-tā′shŭn) Instillation of a device, usually metallic or plastic, which delivers dosage of a medication over a long duration.

hy·po·der·mic in·jec·tion (hī′pō-dĕr′mik in-jek′shŭn) The administration of a remedy in liquid form by injection into the subcutaneous tissues.

hy·po·der·mic sy·ringe (hī′pō-dĕr′mik sir-inj′) A small syringe with a barrel (which may be calibrated), perfectly matched plunger, and tip; used with a hollow needle for subcutaneous injections and for aspiration.

hy·po·der·mic tab·let (hī′pō-dĕr′mik tab′lĕt) A compressed or molded tablet that dissolves completely in water to form an injectable solution.

hy·po·der·mis (hī′pō-dĕr′mis) SYN superficial fascia.

hy·po·der·moc·ly·sis (hī′pō-dĕr-mok′li-sis) Subcutaneous injection of a saline or other solution. [hypo- + G. *derma*, skin, + *klysis*, a washing out]

hy·po·dip·si·a (hī′pō-dip′sē-ă) A reduced sense of thirst; a physiologic condition, perhaps caused by hypertonicity of body fluids; loosely, oligodipsia. [hypo- + G. *dipsa*, thirst]

hy·po·don·ti·a (hī′pō-don′shē-ă) A condition of having fewer than the normal complement of teeth, either congenital or acquired. SYN oligodontia. [hypo- + G. *odous*, tooth]

hy·po·dy·nam·ic (hī′pō-dī-nam′ik) Possessing or exhibiting subnormal power or force.

hy·po·ec·cri·sis (hī′pō-ek′ri-sis) Reduced excretion of waste matter. [hypo- + G. *eccrisis*, separation]

hy·po·ec·crit·ic (hī′pō-ĕ-krit′ik) Characterized by hypoeccrisis.

hy·po·ech·o·ic (hī′pō-ĕ-kō′ik) Pertaining to a region in an ultrasound image in which the echoes are weaker or fewer than normal or in the surrounding regions. [hypo- + echo + -ic]

hy·po·es·o·pho·ri·a (hī′pō-es′ō-fōr′ē-ă) A tendency of the visual axis of one eye to deviate downward and inward, prevented by binocular vision. [hypo- + G. *esō*, within, + *phoros*, bearing]

hy·po·es·the·si·a (hī′pō-es-thē′zē-ă) SYN hypesthesia. SYN hypoaesthesia.

hy·po·ex·o·pho·ri·a (hī′pō-eks′ō-fōr′ē-ă) A tendency of the visual axis of one eye to deviate downward and outward, prevented by binocular vision. [hypo- + G. *exō*, without, + *phoros*, bearing]

hypoferraemia [Br.] SYN hypoferremia.

hy·po·fer·re·mi·a (hī′pō-fĕr-ē′mē-ă) A deficiency of iron in the circulating blood. SYN hypoferraemia.

hypofibrinogenaemia [Br.] SYN hypofibrinogenemia.

hy·po·fi·brin·o·ge·ne·mi·a (hī′pō-fī-brin′ō-jĕ-nē′mē-ă) Abnormally low concentration of fibrinogen in the circulating blood plasma. SYN hypofibrinogenaemia.

hy·po·frac·tion·at·ed ra·di·a·tion (hī′pō-frak′shŭn-ā-tĕd rā′dē-ā′shŭn) Larger fractions of a dose of radiation given less frequently than daily.

hy·po·fron·tal·i·ty (hī′pō-frŭn-tal′i-tē) A decrease in the neuronal activity of various areas of the frontal lobes, arising from various causes and associated with a number of clinical symptoms or disorders.

hy·po·func·tion (hī′pō-fŭngk′shŭn) Reduced, low, or inadequate function.

hy·po·ga·lac·ti·a (hī′pō-gă-lak′shē-ă) Less than normal milk secretion. [hypo- + G. *gala,* milk]

hy·po·ga·lac·tous (hī′pō-gă-lak′tŭs) Producing or secreting a less than normal amount of milk.

hypogammaglobulinaemia [Br.] SYN hypogammaglobulinemia.

hy·po·gam·ma·glob·u·lin·e·mi·a (hī′pō-gam′ă-glob′yū-li-nē′mē-ă) Decreased gamma fraction of serum globulin; associated with increased susceptibility to pyogenic infections. SYN hypogammaglobulinaemia.

hy·po·gan·gli·o·no·sis (hī′pō-gang′glē-ŏ-nō′sis) A reduction in the number of ganglionic nerve cells.

hy·po·gas·tric (hī′pō-gas′trik) Relating to the hypogastrium.

hy·po·gas·tric ar·ter·y (hī′pō-gas′trik ahr′tĕr-ē) SYN internal iliac artery.

hy·po·gas·tric nerve (hī′pō-gas′trik nĕrv) One of the two nerve trunks (right and left) that lead from the superior hypogastric plexus into the pelvis to join the inferior hypogastric plexuses. SYN nervus hypogastricus [TA].

hy·po·gas·tros·chi·sis (hī′pō-gas-tros′ki-sis) Congenital fissure of the anterior abdominal wall in the hypogastric region. [hypogastrium + G. *schisis,* cleaving]

hy·po·gen·e·sis (hī′pō-jen′ĕ-sis) Congenital defect of growth with underdevelopment of parts or organs of the body. [hypo- + G. *genesis,* origin]

hy·po·ge·net·ic (hī′pō-jĕ-net′ik) Relating to hypogenesis.

hy·po·gen·i·tal·ism (hī′pō-jen′i-tăl-izm) Partial or complete failure of maturation of the genitalia; commonly, a consequence of hypogonadism.

hy·po·geu·si·a (hī′pō-gū′sē-ă) Blunting of the sense of taste. [hypo- + G. *geusis,* taste]

hy·po·glos·sal (hī′pō-glos′ăl) **1.** Below the tongue. **2.** Relating to the twelfth cranial nerve, nervus hypoglossus. [L. *hypoglossus* fr. hypo- + *glossus,* tongue]

hy·po·glos·sal ca·nal (hī′pō-glos′ăl kă-nal′) The canal through which the hypoglossal nerve emerges from the skull. SYN canalis hypoglossalis [TA], anterior condyloid foramen.

hy·po·glos·sal nerve [CN XII] (hī′pō-glos′ăl nĕrv) Arises from an oblong nucleus in the medulla and emerges by several root filaments between the pyramid and the olive through the preolivary groove; it passes through the hypoglossal canal, then courses downward and forward to supply the intrinsic and four of five extrinsic muscles of the tongue. SYN nervus hypoglossus [CN XII] [TA], twelfth cranial nerve [CN XII].

hy·po·glos·sal nu·cle·us (hī′pō-glos′ăl nū′klē-ŭs) The motor nucleus innervating the intrinsic and four of the five extrinsic muscles of the tongue; it is located in the medulla oblongata near the midline, immediately beneath the floor of the inferior recess of the rhomboid fossa.

hy·po·glot·tis (hī′pō-glot′is) The undersurface of the tongue. [G. *hypoglōssis,* or *-glōttis,* undersurface of tongue, fr. *hypo,* under, + *glōssa,* tongue]

hypoglycaemia [Br.] SYN hypoglycemia.

hypoglycaemic [Br.] SYN hypoglycemic.

hypoglycaemic coma [Br.] SYN hypoglycemic coma.

hy·po·gly·ce·mi·a (hī′pō-glī-sē′mē-ă) An abnormally low concentration of glucose in the circulating blood. SYN hypoglycaemia.

hy·po·gly·ce·mic (hī′pō-glī-sē′mik) Pertaining to or characterized by hypoglycemia. SYN hypoglycaemic.

hy·po·gly·ce·mic a·gent (hī′pō-glī-sē′mik ā′jĕnt) Oral medications used in the management of Type 2 diabetes mellitus, but ineffective in Type 1 diabetes.

hy·po·gly·ce·mic co·ma (hī′pō-glī-sē′mik kō′mă) A metabolic encephalopathy caused by hypoglycemia; usually seen in diabetic patients, and due to exogenous insulin excess. SYN hypoglycaemic coma.

hy·po·gly·cor·rhach·i·a (hī′pō-glī-kō-rā′kē-ă) Depressed concentration of glucose in the cerebrospinal fluid; a characteristic of bacterial, fungal, and tuberculous meningitis. [hypo- + G. *glykys,* sweet, + *rhachis,* spine]

hy·pog·na·thous (hī-pog′na-thŭs) Having an abnormally small mandible. [hypo- + G. *gnathos,* jaw]

hy·po·go·nad·ism (hī′pō-gō′nad-izm) Inadequate gonadal function, as manifested by deficiencies in gametogenesis or the secretion of gonadal hormones.

hy·po·go·nad·o·tro·pic (hī′pō-gon′ă-dō-trō′

pik) Indicating inadequate secretion of gonadotropins and its consequences.

hy•po•hi•dro•sis (hī′pō-hī-drō′sis) Diminished perspiration.

hy•po•hi•drot•ic (hī′pō-hi-drot′ik) Characterized by diminished sweating. See page B12.

hy•po•hy•dra•tion (hī′pō-hī-drā′shŭn) Decrease in body water content. New steady-state condition of decreased water content.

hypokalaemia [Br.] SYN hypokalemia.

hy•po•ka•le•mi•a (hī′pō-kă-lē′mē-ă) The presence of an abnormally small concentration of potassium ions in the circulating blood; occurs in familial periodic paralysis and in potassium depletion due to excessive loss from the gastrointestinal tract or kidneys. The changes of hypokalemia may include vacuolation of renal tubular epithelial cytoplasm with impairment of urinary concentrating power and acidification, flattening of the T wave of the electrocardiogram, and muscle weakness. SYN hypokalaemia, hypopotassemia. [hypo- + Mod. L. *kalium,* potassium, + G. *haima,* blood]

hy•po•ka•le•mic pe•ri•od•ic pa•ral•y•sis (hī′pō-kă-lē′mik pēr′ē-od′ik păr-al′i-sis) Periodic paralysis in which the serum potassium level is low during attacks; attacks may be precipitated by cold, high carbohydrate meals, or alcohol, may last hours to days, and may cause respiratory paralysis. SYN hypolakaemic periodic paralysis.

hy•po•ki•ne•sis, hy•po•ki•ne•si•a (hī′pō-ki-nē′sis, -nē′zē-ă) Diminished or slow movement. SYN hypomotility. [hypo- + G. *kinēsis,* movement]

hy•po•ki•net•ic (hī′pō-ki-net′ik) Relating to or characterized by hypokinesis.

hy•po•ki•ne•tic dys•arth•ri•a (hī′pō-ki-net′ik dis-ahr′thrē-ă) Dysarthria associated with disorders of the extrapyramidal motor system resulting in reduction and rigidity of movement, causing monotony of pitch and loudness, reduced stress, and imprecise enunciation of consonants. SEE ALSO extrapyramidal motor system, parkinsonian dysarthria.

hypolakaemic periodic paralysis [Br.] SYN hypokalemic periodic paralysis.

hy•po•ley•dig•ism (hī′pō-lī′dig-izm) Subnormal secretion of androgens by the interstitial (Leydig) cells of the testes.

hypolipoproteinaemia [Br.] SYN hypolipoproteinemia.

hy•po•lip•o•pro•tein•e•mi•a (hī′pō-lip′ō-prō-tēn-ē-mē′ă) An abnormally low level of lipoprotein in plasma. SYN hypolipoproteinaemia.

hypomagnesaemia [Br.] SYN hypomagnesemia.

hy•po•mag•ne•se•mi•a (hī′pō-mag′nĕ-sē′mē-ă) Deficiency of magnesium in blood; may be caused by chronic alcoholism, dehydration, diabetic acidosis, and chronic diarrhea, malabsorption syndrome, postoperative complication of bowel surgery, prolonged nasogastric suction, prolonged diuretic therapy, or starvation. Signs include arrhythmias, neuromuscular irritability, leg cramps, mood changes, confusion, hallucinations, or seizures. SYN hypomagnesaemia.

hy•po•mas•ti•a (hī′pō-mas′tē-ă) Atrophy or congenital smallness of the breasts. [hypo- + G. *mastos,* breast]

hy•po•me•li•a (hī′pō-mē′lē-ă) General term for hypoplasia of some or all parts of one or more limbs. [hypo- + G. *melos,* limb]

hy•po•men•or•rhe•a (hī′pō-men-ōr-ē′ă) Diminution of the flow or a shortening of the duration of menstruation. SYN hypomenorrhoea. [hypo- + G. *mēn,* month, + *rhoia,* flow]

hypomenorrhoea [Br.] SYN hypomenorrhea.

hy•po•mere (hī′pō-mēr) **1.** The portion of the myotome that extends ventrolaterally to form body-wall and limb muscle, innervated by the primary anterior ramus of a spinal nerve. **2.** Somatic and splanchnic layers of the lateral mesoderm that give rise to the lining of the celom. [hypo- + G. *meros,* part]

hy•po•me•tab•o•lism (hī′pō-mĕ-tab′ō-lizm) Reduced metabolism.

hy•po•me•tri•a (hī′pō-mē′trē-ă) Ataxia characterized by underreaching an object or goal; seen with cerebellar disease. Cf. hypermetria. [hypo- + G. *metron,* measure]

hy•pom•ne•si•a (hī′pom-nē′zē-ă) Impaired memory. [hypo- + G. *mnēmē,* memory]

hy•po•mo•bile pa•tel•la (hī′pō-mō′bil pă-tel′ă) A range of patellar movement equal to one quadrant patella or less.

hy•po•morph (hī′pō-mōrf) **1.** A person whose standing height is short in proportion to sitting height, owing to shortness of the lower limbs. Cf. endomorph. **2.** A mutant gene that causes a partial decrease in the activity controlled by the gene. [hypo- + G. *morphē,* form]

hy•po•mo•til•i•ty (hī′pō-mō-til′i-tē) SYN hypokinesis.

hy•po•mo•tor sei•zure (hī′pō-mō′tŏr sē′zhŭr) Seizure characterized by complete or partial arrest of ongoing motor activity in a patient whose level of consciousness cannot be determined accurately (e.g., newborns, infants, mentally retarded patients).

hy•po•my•e•li•na•tion, hy•po•my•e•lin•o•gen•e•sis (hī′pō-mī′ĕ-lin-ā′shun, -ō-jen′ĕ-sis) Defective formation of myelin in the spinal cord and brain; the basis for a number of demyelinating diseases.

hy·po·my·o·to·ni·a (hī′pō-mī′ō-tō′nē-ă) A condition of diminished muscular tonus. [hypo- + G. *mys* (*myo-*) muscle, + *tonos,* tension]

hy·po·myx·i·a (hī′pō-mik′sē-ă) A condition in which the secretion of mucus is diminished. [hypo- + G. *myxa,* mucus]

hy·po·na·sal·i·ty (hī′pō-nā-zal′i-tē) Insufficient nasal resonance during speech, usually due to obstruction of the nasal tract. SYN hyporhinophonia.

hyponatraemia [Br.] SYN hyponatremia.

hy·po·na·tre·mi·a (hī′pō-nă-trē′mē-ă) Abnormally low concentrations of sodium ions in the circulating blood. SYN hyponatraemia. [hypo- + natrium, + G. *haima,* blood]

hy·po·ne·o·cy·to·sis (hī′pō-nē′ō-sī-tō′sis) Leukopenia associated with the presence of immature and young leukocytes (especially in the granulocytic series). [hypo- + G. *neos,* new, + *kytos,* cell, + *-osis,* condition]

hy·po·nych·i·al (hī′pō-nik′ē-ăl) **1.** SYN subungual. **2.** Relating to the hyponychium.

hy·po·nych·i·um (hī′pō-nik′ē-ŭm) The epithelium of the nail bed, particularly its proximal part in the region of the nail root and lunula, forming the nail matrix. [hypo- + G. *onyx,* nail]

hy·pon·y·chon (hī-pon′i-kon) An ecchymosis beneath a fingernail or toenail. [hypo- + G. *onyx,* nail]

hy·po·or·tho·cy·to·sis (hī′pō-ōr′thō-sī-tō′sis) Leukopenia in which the relative numbers of the various types of white blood cells are within normal ranges. [hypo- + G. *orthos,* correct, + *kytos,* cell, + *-osis,* condition]

hy·po·pan·cre·a·tism (hī′pō-pan′krē-ă-tizm) A condition of diminished activity of digestive enzyme secretion by the pancreas.

hy·po·par·a·thy·roid·ism (hī′pō-par′ă-thī′royd-izm) A condition due to diminution or absence of the secretion of the parathyroid hormones, with low serum calcium, tetany, and sometimes increased bone density. SEE ALSO pseudohypoparathyroidism.

hy·po·pha·lan·gism (hī′pō-fă-lan′jizm) Congenital absence of one or more of the phalanges of a finger or toe.

hy·po·pha·ryn·ge·al di·ver·tic·u·lum (hī′pō-făr-in′jē-ăl dī′vĕr-tik′yū-lŭm) SYN pharyngoesophageal diverticulum.

hy·po·phar·ynx (hī′pō-far′ingks) SYN laryngopharynx.

hy·po·pho·ne·sis (hī′pō-fō-nē′sis) In percussion or auscultation, a sound that is diminished or fainter than usual. [hypo- + G. *phōnēsis,* a sounding]

hy·po·pho·ri·a (hī′pō-fōr′ē-ă) A tendency of the visual axis of one eye to deviate downward, prevented by binocular vision. [hypo- + G. *phora,* motion]

hypophosphataemia [Br.] SYN hypophosphatemia.

hy·po·phos·pha·ta·si·a (hī′pō-fos′fă-tā′zē-ă) An abnormally low content of alkaline phosphatase in the circulating blood.

hy·po·phos·pha·te·mi·a (hī′pō-fos-fă-tē′mē-ă) Deficiency of phosphorus in blood; may be due to chronic diarrhea, deficiency of vitamin D, hyperparathyroidism with hypercalcemia, hypomagnesemia, malnutrition, chronic alcoholism, or malabsorption syndrome. Signs include anorexia, muscle wasting, paresthesia, and tremors. SYN hypophosphataemia.

hy·po·phos·pha·tu·ri·a (hī′pō-fos′fă-tyūr′ē-ă) Reduced urinary excretion of phosphates.

hy·poph·y·sec·to·my (hī-pof′i-sek′tŏ-mē) Surgical removal of the hypophysis or pituitary gland.

hy·po·phys·e·o·priv·ic (hī′pō-fiz′ē-ō-priv′ik) SYN hypophysioprivic.

hy·po·phys·e·o·tro·pic (hī′pō-fiz′ē-ō-trō′pik) SYN hypophysiotropic.

hy·po·phy·si·al (hī′pō-fiz′ē-ăl) Relating to a hypophysis.

hy·po·phy·si·al ca·chex·i·a (hī′pō-fiz′ē-ăl kă-kek′sē-ă) SYN Simmonds disease, panhypopituitarism.

hy·po·phy·si·al di·ver·tic·u·lum (hī′pō-fiz′ē-ăl dī′vĕr-tik′yū-lŭm) An upgrowth from the ectodermal roof of the stomodeum of the embryo that is adjacent to the floor of the diencephalon; it forms the adenohypophysis (glandular segment of the pituitary gland). SYN adenohypophysial pouch, pituitary diverticulum, Rathke pocket, Rathke pouch.

hy·po·phy·si·al fos·sa (hī′pō-fiz′ē-ăl fos′ă) Fossa of the sphenoid bone housing the pituitary gland. SEE ALSO sella turcica.

hy·po·phy·si·al syn·drome (hī′pō-fiz′ē-ăl sin′drōm) SYN dystrophia adiposogenitalis.

hy·po·phys·i·o·priv·ic (hī′pō-fiz′ē-ō-priv′ik) Pertaining to absence or depressed function of the pituitary gland. SYN hypophyseoprivic. [hypophysis + L. *privus,* deprived of]

hy·po·phys·i·o·sphe·noi·dal syn·drome (hī′pō-fiz′ē-ō-sfē-noy′dăl sin′drōm) Neoplastic invasion of the base of the skull in the region of the sphenoidal sinus, often with destruction of the dorsum sellae.

hy·po·phys·i·o·tro·pic (hī′pō-fiz′ē-ō-trō′pik) Denoting a stimulatory hormone that acts on the pituitary gland (hypophysis). SYN hypophyseotropic.

hy·poph·y·sis (hī-pof′i-sis) [TA] An unpaired compound gland suspended from the base of the hypothalamus by a short extension of the infundibulum, the infundibular or pituitary stalk. The hypophysis consists of two major subdivisions: 1) the neurohypophysis, comprising the infundibulum and its bulbous termination, the neural part or infundibular process (posterior lobe), which is composed of neuroglia-like pituicytes, blood vessels, and unmyelinated nerve fibers of the hypothalamohypophyseal tract with cell bodies that reside in the supraoptic and paraventricular nuclei of the hypothalamus, and convey to the lobe for storage and release the neurosecretory hormones oxytocin and antidiuretic hormone; 2) the adenohypophysis, comprising the larger distal part, a sleevelike extension of this lobe (infundibular part), which invests the infundibular stalk, and a thin intermediate part (poorly developed in humans) between the anterior and posterior lobes; the anterior lobe consists of cords of cells of several different types interspersed with capillaries of the hypothalamohypophysial portal system; secretion of somatotropins, prolactin, thyroid-stimulating hormone, gonadotropins, adrenal corticotropin, and other related peptides in the adenohypophysis is regulated by releasing and inhibiting factors elaborated by neurons in the hypothalamus that are taken up by a primary plexus of capillaries in the median eminence and transported through portal vessels in the infundibular part and infundibular stem to a secondary plexus of capillaries in the distal part. SEE ALSO hypothalamus. SYN pituitary gland. [G. an undergrowth]

hy·poph·y·si·tis (hī-pof′i-sī′tis) Inflammation of the hypophysis.

hy·po·pl·e·sis (hī′pō-pī-ē′sis) SYN hypotension (1). [hypo- + G. *piesis,* pressure]

hy·po·pig·men·ta·tion (hī′pō-pig′mĕn-tā′shŭn) Deficiency of cutaneous melanin relative to surrounding skin. SEE albinism. See this page. [hypo- + pigmentation]

hy·po·pi·tu·i·ta·rism (hī′pō-pi-tū′i-tăr-izm) A condition due to diminished activity of the anterior lobe of the hypophysis, with inadequate secretion of one or more anterior pituitary hormones.

hy·po·pla·si·a (hī′pō-plā′zē-ă) **1.** Underdevelopment of a tissue or organ, usually due to a decrease in the number of cells. **2.** Atrophy due to destruction of some of the elements of a tissue or organ, and not merely to their general reduction in size. Cf. hyperplasia. [hypo- + G. *plasis,* a molding]

hy·po·plas·tic (hī′pō-plas′tik) Pertaining to or characterized by hypoplasia.

hy·po·plas·tic a·ne·mi·a (hī′pō-plas′tik ă-nē′mē-ă) Progressive nonregenerative anemia resulting from greatly depressed, inadequately functioning bone marrow; as the process persists, aplastic anemia may occur.

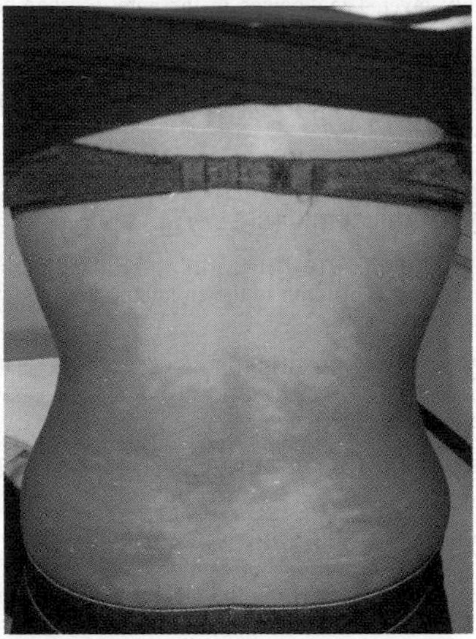

hypopigmentation: postinflammatory, following tinea infection

hy·pop·ne·a (hī-pop′nē-ă) Breathing that is shallower, or slower, than normal. SYN hypopnoea, oligopnea. [hypo- + G. *pnoē,* breathing]

hypopnoea [Br.] SYN hypopnea.

hy·po·po·si·a (hī′pō-pō′sē-ă) Hypodipsia, with emphasis on a reduced tendency to drink rather than on the reduced sensation of thirst. [hypo- + G. *posis,* drinking]

hypopotassaemia [Br.] SYN hypopotassemia.

hy·po·po·tas·se·mi·a (hī′pō-pō-tă-sē′mē-ă) SYN hypokalemia. SYN hypopotassaemia.

hy·po·prax·i·a (hī′pō-prak′sē-ă) Deficient activity. [hypo- + G. *praxis,* action, + *-ia,* condition]

hypoproteinaemia [Br.] SYN hypoproteinemia.

hy·po·pro·tein·e·mi·a (hī′pō-prō′tēn-ē′mē-ă) Abnormally small amounts of total protein in the blood. SYN hypoproteinaemia.

hypoprothrombinaemia [Br.] SYN hypoprothrombinemia.

hy·po·pro·throm·bin·e·mi·a (hī′pō-prō-throm′bin-ē′mē-ă) Abnormally small amounts of prothrombin in the circulating blood. SYN hypoprothrombinaemia.

hy·pop·ty·a·lism (hī′pop-tī′ă-lizm) SYN hyposalivation. [hypo- + G. *ptyalon,* saliva]

hy·po·py·on (hī-pō′pē-on) The presence of visibly layered leukocytes in the anterior chamber of the eye. [hypo- + G. *pyon,* pus]

hy·po·re·flex·i·a (hī′pō-rē-flek′sē-ă) A condition in which the deep tendon reflexes are weakened.

hyporeninaemia [Br.] SYN hyporeninemia.

hyporeninaemic [Br.] SYN hyporeninemic.

hy·po·ren·i·ne·mi·a (hī′pō-rē′ni-nē′mē-ă) Low levels of renin in the circulating blood. SYN hyporeninaemia.

hy·po·ren·i·ne·mic (hī′pō-rē′ni-nē′mik) Denoting or characterized by hyporeninemia. SYN hyporeninaemic.

hy·po·rhi·no·pho·ni·a (hī′pō-rī′nō-fō′nē-ă) SYN hyponasality.

hy·po·ri·bo·fla·vin·o·sis (hī′pō-rī′bō-flā-vi-nō′sis) NUTRITION a condition produced by a deficiency of riboflavin in the diet, characterized by cheilosis and magenta tongue and usually associated with other manifestations of B vitamin deficiency. A more correct term than the more commonly used ariboflavinosis.

hy·po·sal·i·va·tion (hī′pō-sal′i-vā′shŭn) Reduced salivation. SYN hypoptyalism.

hy·po·scle·ral (hī′pō-skler′ăl) Beneath the sclerotic coat of the eyeball.

hy·po·sen·si·tiv·i·ty (hī′pō-sen′si-tiv′i-tē) A condition of subnormal sensitivity, in which the response to a stimulus is unusually delayed or lessened in degree.

hy·pos·mi·a (hī-poz′mē-ă) Diminished sense of smell. [hypo- + G. *osmē,* smell]

hy·po·so·ma·to·tro·pism (hī′pō-sō-mat′ō-trō′pizm) A state characterized by deficient secretion of pituitary growth hormone (somatotropin).

hy·po·spa·di·ac (hī′pō-spā′dē-ak) Relating to hypospadias.

hy·po·spa·di·as (hī′pō-spā′dē-ăs) A developmental anomaly characterized by a defect on the ventral surface of the penis so that the urethral meatus (urethral opening) is more proximal than normal; may be associated with chordee; also, a similar defect in the female in which the urethra opens into the vagina. Cf. epispadias. SYN urogenital sinus anomaly. [hypo- + G. *spaō,* to tear or gouge]

hy·po·sphyg·mi·a (hī′pō-sfig′mē-ă) Abnormally low blood pressure with sluggishness of the circulation. [hypo- + G. *sphyxis,* pulse]

hy·po·splen·ism (hī′pō-splēn′izm) Absent or reduced splenic function, usually due to surgical removal, congenital aplasia, tumor replacement, or splenic vascular accident.

hy·pos·ta·sis (hi-pos′tă-sis) **1.** Formation of a sediment at the bottom of a liquid. **2.** SYN hypostatic congestion. **3.** The phenomenon whereby the phenotype that would ordinarily be manifested at one locus is obscured by the genotype at another epistatic locus. [G. *hypo-stasis,* a standing under, sediment]

hy·po·stat·ic (hī′pō-stat′ik) **1.** Sedimentary; resulting from a dependent position. **2.** Relating to hypostasis.

hy·po·stat·ic con·ges·tion (hī′pō-stat′ik kŏn-jes′chŭn) Congestion due to pooling of venous blood in a dependent part. SYN hypostasis (2).

hy·po·stat·ic ec·ta·si·a (hī′pō-stat′ik ek-tā′zē-ă) Dilation of a blood vessel, usually a vein, in a dependent portion of the body, as in varicose veins of the leg.

hy·po·stat·ic pneu·mo·ni·a (hī′pō-stat′ik nū-mō′nē-ă) Pneumonia resulting from infection developing in the dependent portions of the lungs due to decreased ventilation of those areas, with resulting failure to drain bronchial secretions; occurs primarily in old people or those debilitated by disease who lie in the same position for long periods.

hy·pos·the·ni·a (hī′pos-thē′nē-ă) Weakness. SEE asthenia. [hypo- + G. *sthenos,* strength]

hy·pos·then·ic (hī′pos-then′ik) **1.** Weak. **2.** Pertaining to a slender habitus, with underdevelopment of skeletal muscle.

hy·pos·the·nu·ri·a (hī′pos-thĕ-nyūr′ē-ă) The excretion of urine of low specific gravity, due to inability of the renal tubules to produce concentrated urine; also occurs following excessive water ingestion in association with diabetes insipidus. [hypo- + G. *sthenos,* strength, + *ouron,* urine]

hy·po·sto·mi·a (hī′pō-stō′mē-ă) A form of microstomia in which the oral opening is a small vertical slit. [hypo- + G. *stoma,* mouth]

hy·po·tel·or·ism (hī′pō-tel′ŏr-izm) Abnormal closeness of eyes. [hypo- + G. *tēle,* far off, + *horizō,* to separate, fr. *horos,* boundary]

hy·po·ten·sion (hī′pō-ten′shŭn) **1.** Subnormal arterial blood pressure. SYN hypopiesis. **2.** Reduced pressure or tension of any kind. [hypo- + L. *tensio,* a stretching]

hy·po·ten·sive (hī′pō-ten′siv) Characterized by low blood pressure or causing reduction in blood pressure.

hy·po·tha·lam·ic in·fun·dib·u·lum (hī′pō-thă-lam′ik in′fŭn-dib′yū-lŭm) The apical portion of the tuber cinereum extending into the stalk of the hypophysis.

hy·po·thal·a·mic-pi·tu·i·ta·ry-a·dre·nal ax·is (HPA ax·is) (hī′pō-thă-lam′ik-pi-tū′i-tar-ē ă-dre′năl ak′sis) A major component of the stress response system, consisting of the hypothalamus, anterior pituitary, cortex, and the cortex of the suprarenal gland. The HPA axis regulates secretion of cortisol from the adrenal gland in response to stress.

hy•po•thal•a•mo•hy•po•phy•si•al por•tal sys•tem (hī′pō-thal′ă-mō-hī′pō-fiz′ē-ăl pōr′tăl sis′tĕm) SYN portal hypophysial circulation.

hy•po•thal•a•mus (hī′pō-thal′ă-mŭs) [TA] The ventral and medial region of the diencephalon forming the walls of the ventral half of the third ventricle; delineated from the thalamus by the hypothalamic sulcus, lying medial to the internal capsule and subthalamus, continuous with the precommissural septum anteriorly and with the mesencephalic tegmentum and central gray substance posteriorly. Its ventral surface is marked by, from before backward, the optic chiasma, the unpaired infundibulum, which extends by way of the infundibular stalk into the posterior lobe of the hypophysis, and the paired mammillary bodies. The nerve cells of the hypothalamus are grouped into the supraoptic paraventricular, lateral preoptic, lateral hypothalamic, tuberal, anterior hypothalamic, ventromedial, dorsomedial, arcuate, posterior hypothalamic, and premammillary nuclei and into the mammillary body. It has afferent fiber connections with the mesencephalon, limbic system, cerebellum, and efferent fiber connections with the same structures and with the posterior lobe of the hypophysis; its functional connection with the anterior lobe of the hypophysis is established by the hypothalamohypophysial portal system. The hypothalamus is prominently involved in the functions of the autonomic nervous system and, through its vascular link with the anterior lobe of the hypophysis, in endocrine mechanisms; it also appears to play a role in neural mechanisms underlying moods and motivational states. SEE ALSO hypophysis. [hypo- + thalamus]

hy•po•the•nar (hī′pō-thē′năr) **1.** [TA] SYN hypothenar eminence. **2.** Denoting any structure in relation with the hypothenar eminence or its underlying collective components. [hypo- + G. *thenar,* the palm]

hy•po•the•nar em•i•nence (hī′pō-thē′năr em′i-nĕns) The fleshy mass at the medial side of the palm. See this page. SYN hypothenar (1).

hy•po•ther•mal (hī′pō-thĕr′măl) Denoting hypothermia.

hy•po•ther•mi•a (hī′pō-thĕr′mē-ă) A core body temperature significantly lower than 98.6°F (37°C). [hypo- + G. *thermē,* heat]

hy•poth•e•sis (hī-poth′ĕ-sis) A conjecture cast in a form that is amenable to confirmation or refutation by experiment and the assembly of data; not to be confused with assumption, postulation, or unfocused speculation. SEE ALSO postulate, theory. [G. foundation, assumption, fr. *hypotithēmi,* to lay down]

hy•po•thet•ic mean or•ga•nism (HMO) (hī′pō-thet′ik mēn ōr′gă-nizm) A hypothetical organism with characters that are the means of the positive characters of the organisms that belong to the same taxon as the HMO, as opposed to the calculated mean organism.

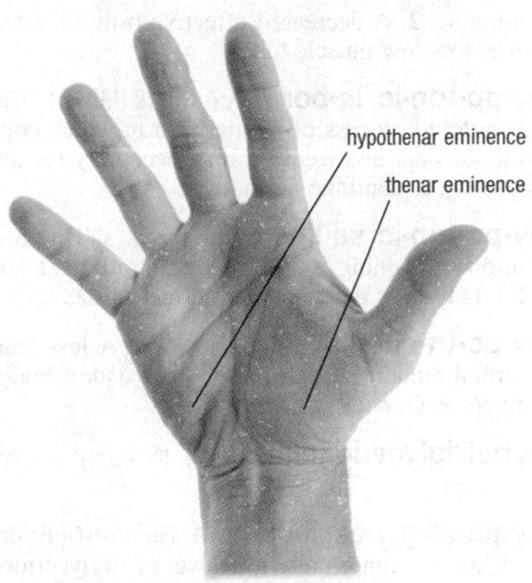

hypothenar eminence

hypothrombinaemia [Br.] SYN hypothrombinemia.

hy•po•throm•bi•ne•mi•a (hī′pō-throm′bin-ē′mē-ă) Abnormally small amounts of thrombin in the circulating blood. SYN hypothrombinaemia.

hy•po•thy•mi•a (hī′pō-thī′mē-ă) Depression of spirits; the "blues." [hypo- + G. *thymos,* mind, soul]

hy•po•thy•mic (hī′pō-thī′mik) Denoting or characteristic of hypothymia.

hy•po•thy•roid (hī′pō-thī′royd) Marked by reduced thyroid function.

hy•po•thy•roid•ism (hī′pō-thī′royd-izm) Diminished production of thyroid hormone, leading to clinical manifestations of thyroid insufficiency, including somnolence, slow mentation, dryness and loss of hair, subnormal temperature, hoarseness, muscle weakness, delayed relaxation of tendon reflexes, and sometimes myxedema. [hypo- + G. *thyreoeidēs,* thyroid]

hy•po•to•ni•a (hī′pō-tō′nē-ă) **1.** Reduced tension in any part, as in the eyeball. **2.** Relaxation of the arteries. **3.** A condition in which there is a diminution or loss of muscular tonicity, in consequence of which the muscles may be stretched beyond their normal limits. SYN hypotonicity (1). [hypo- + G. *tonos,* tone]

hy•po•ton•ic (hī′pō-ton′ik) **1.** Having a lesser degree of tension. **2.** Having a lesser osmotic pressure than a reference solution, ordinarily plasma or interstitial fluid.

hy•po•to•nic•i•ty (hī′pō-tō-nis′i-tē) **1.** SYN hypotonia. **2.** A decreased effective osmotic pressure. SYN low muscle tone.

hy·po·ton·ic la·bor (hī′pō-ton′ik lā′bŏr) The disordered process of giving birth in which contractions are less frequent than necessary for the delivery to continue normally.

hy·po·ton·ic sa·line (hī′pō-ton′ik sā′lēn) Solution containing a lower concentration of sodium chloride than isotonic normal saline.

hy·po·tri·cho·sis (hī′pō-tri-kō′sis) A less than normal amount of hair on the head and/or body. [hypo- + G. *trichōsis,* hairiness]

hypotriglyceridaemia [Br.] SYN hypotriglyceridemia.

hy·po·tri·gly·cer·i·de·mi·a (hī′pō-trī-glis′ĕr-i-dē′mē-ă) Abnormally low level of triglycerides in plasma. SYN hypotriglyceridaemia.

hy·po·tro·pi·a (hī′pō-trō′pē-ă) An ocular deviation with one eye lower than the other. [hypo- + G. *tropē,* turn]

hy·po·tym·pa·not·o·my (hī′pō-tim-pă-not′ŏ-mē) Surgical extirpation, without sacrifice of hearing, of small tumors confined to the lower tympanic cavity. [hypo- + G. *tympanon,* tympanum, + *tomē,* incision]

hy·po·tym·pa·num (hī′pō-tim′pă-nŭm) The lower part of the tympanic cavity.

hypouricaemia [Br.] SYN hypouricemia.

hy·po·u·ri·ce·mi·a (hī′pō-yūr′i-sē′mē-ă) Reduced blood concentration of uric acid. SYN hypouricaemia.

hy·po·u·ri·cu·ri·a (hī′pō-yūr′i-kyū′rē-ă) Reduced excretion of uric acid in the urine.

hy·po·ven·ti·la·tion (hī′pō-ven-ti-lā′shŭn) Reduced alveolar ventilation relative to metabolic carbon dioxide production, so that alveolar carbon dioxide pressure increases above normal.

hy·po·vi·ta·min·o·sis (hī′pō-vī′tă-min-ō′sis) Insufficiency of one or more vitamins in the diet; manifested first by depletion of tissue levels, then by functional changes, and finally by appearance of morphologic lesions. Cf. avitaminosis.

hypovolaemia [Br.] SYN hypovolemia.

hypovolaemic [Br.] SYN hypovolemic.

hypovolaemic shock [Br.] SYN hypovolemic shock.

hy·po·vo·le·mi·a (hī′pō-vō-lē′mē-ă) A decreased amount of blood volume in the body. SYN hyphemia, hypovolaemia. [hypo- + L. *volumen,* volume, + G. *haima,* blood]

hy·po·vo·le·mic (hī′pō-vō-lē′mik) Pertaining to or characterized by hypovolemia. SYN hypovolaemic.

hy·po·vo·le·mic shock (hī′pō-vō-lē′mik shok) Shock caused by a reduction in volume of blood, as from hemorrhage or dehydration. SYN hypovolaemic shock.

hy·po·vo·li·a (hī′pō-vō′lē-ă) Diminished water content or volume of a given compartment; e.g., extracellular hypovolia. [hypo- + L. *volumen,* volume]

hypoxaemia [Br.] SYN hypoxemia.

hy·po·xan·thine (hī′pō-zan′thēn) A purine present in the muscles and other tissues, formed during purine catabolism by deamination of adenine; elevated in molybdenum-cofactor deficiency.

hy·pox·e·mi·a (hī′pok-sē′mē-ă) Subnormal oxygenation of arterial blood, short of anoxia. SYN hypoxaemia. [hypo- + oxygen, + G. *haima,* blood]

hy·pox·i·a (hī-pok′sē-ă) Lower than normal levels of oxygen in inspired gases, arterial blood, or tissue, short of anoxia. [hypo- + oxygen]

hy·pox·ic (hī-pok′sik) Denoting or characterized by hypoxia.

hy·pox·ic hy·pox·i·a (hī-pok′sik hī-pok′sē-ă) Condition resulting from a defective mechanism of oxygenation in the lungs.

hy·pox·ic ne·phro·sis (hī-pok′sik nĕ-frō′sis) Acute oliguric renal failure following hemorrhage, burns, shock, or other causes of hypovolemia and reduced renal blood flow.

hyp·sa·rhyth·mi·a (hip′să-ridh′mē-ă) The abnormal and characteristically chaotic electroencephalogram in patients with infantile spasms. [G. *hypsi,* high, + *a-* priv. + *rhythmos,* rhythm]

hyp·so·dont (hip′sō-dont) Having long teeth; in some animals both the crown and body of the tooth are elongated, whereas in others there is a marked elongation of the cusps. [hypso- + G. *odous,* tooth]

Hyr·tl loop (hēr′tĕl lūp) A communicating loop between the right and left hypoglossal nerves, lying between the geniohyoid and genioglossus muscles or in the substance of the geniohyoid; it is found in about 1 in 10 people.

hys·ter·al·gi·a (his′tĕr-al′jē-ă) Pain in the uterus. SYN hysterodynia, metrodynia. [hystero- + G. *algos,* pain]

hys·ter·a·tre·si·a (his′tĕr-ă-trē′zē-ă) Atresia of the uterine cavity, usually resulting from inflammatory endocervical adhesions.

hys·ter·ec·to·my (his′tĕr-ek′tŏ-mē) Removal of the uterus; unless otherwise specified, usually denotes complete removal of the uterus (corpus and cervix). [hystero- + G. *ektomē,* excision]

hys·ter·e·sis (his′tĕr-ē′sis) **1.** Failure of either one of two related phenomena to keep pace with the other; or any situation in which the value of one depends on whether the other has been increasing or decreasing. **2.** The lag of a magnetic effect behind its cause. **3.** The temperature differential that exists when a substance melts at one temperature and solidifies at another. **4.** A type of cooperativity in enzyme-catalyzed reactions in which the degree of cooperativity is associated with a slow conformational change of the enzyme. Cf. allosterism. [G. *hysterēsis,* a coming later]

hys•ter•eu•ry•sis (his′tĕr-yūr-ē′sis) Dilation of the lower segment and cervical canal of the uterus. [hystero- + G. *eurynō,* to dilate, fr. *eurys,* wide]

hys•te•ri•a (his-tĕr′ē-ă) A somatoform disorder in which there is an alteration or loss of physical functioning that suggests a physical disorder such as paralysis of an arm or disturbance of vision, but that is instead apparently an expression of a psychological conflict or need. [G. *hystera,* womb, from the original notion of womb-related disturbances in women]

hys•ter•ic a•pho•ni•a (his-ter′ik ā-fō′nē-ă) SEE conversion disorder.

hys•ter•ic a•tax•i•a (his-ter′ik ă-taks′ē-ă) SEE conversion disorder.

hys•ter•ic blind•ness (his-tĕr′ik blīnd′nĕs) Loss of vision or blurring of vision following a highly traumatic event.

hys•ter•ic cho•re•a (his-ter′ik kŏr-ē′ă) SEE conversion chorea.

hys•ter•ic con•vul•sion (his-ter′ik kŏn-vŭl′shŭn) Convulsions resulting from conversion disorder (for which hysteria is an older form).

hys•ter•ic joint (his-tĕr′ik joynt) A simulation of joint disease, with symptoms of pain, possible swelling, and impairment of motion.

hys•ter•ic psy•cho•sis (his-tĕr′ik sī-kō′sis) **1.** A psychotic disturbance with predominantly hysteric symptoms. **2.** A mental disorder resembling conversion hysteria but of psychotic severity. **3.** A brief reactive psychosis, often culture bound.

hys•ter•ics (his-tĕr′iks) An expression of emotion accompanied often by crying, laughing, and screaming.

♻**hystero-**, **hyster-** **1.** Combining forms meaning the uterus. SEE ALSO metr-, utero-. [G. *hystera,* womb (uterus)] **2.** Hysteria. [G. *hystera,* womb (uterus)] **3.** Later, following. [G. *hysteros,* later]

hys•ter•o•cat•a•lep•sy (his′tĕr-ō-kat′ă-lep-sē) Hysteria with cataleptic manifestations, including rigid body posture and a generalized trance-like state.

hys•ter•o•cele (his′tĕr-ō-sēl) **1.** An abdominal or perineal hernia containing part or all of the uterus. **2.** Protrusion of uterine contents into a weakened, bulging area of uterine wall. [hystero- + G. *kēlē,* hernia]

hys•ter•o•clei•sis (his′tĕr-ō-klī′sis) Operative occlusion of the uterus. [hystero- + G. *kleisis,* closure]

hys•ter•o•dyn•i•a (his′tĕr-ō-din′ē-ă) SYN hysteralgia. [hystero- + G. *odynē,* pain]

hys•ter•o•ep•i•lep•sy (his′tĕr-ō-ep′i-lep-sē) Hysteric convulsions.

hys•ter•o•gen•ic, **hys•ter•og•en•ous** (his′tĕr-ō-jen′ik, -oj′ĕ-nŭs) Causing hysteric symptoms or reactions. [hysteria + G. *-gen,* producing]

hys•ter•o•gram (his′tĕr-ō-gram) **1.** Radiologic examination of the uterus, usually using a contrast medium. **2.** A recording of the strength of uterine contractions.

hys•ter•o•graph (his′tĕr-ō-graf) Apparatus for recording the strength of uterine contractions.

hys•ter•og•ra•phy (his′tĕr-og′ră-fē) **1.** Radiographic examination of the uterine cavity filled with a contrast medium. **2.** Graphic procedure used to record uterine contractions. [hystero- + G. *graphō,* to write]

hys•ter•oid (his′tĕr-oyd) Resembling or simulating hysteria. [hystero- + G. *eidos,* resemblance]

hys•ter•ol•y•sis (his′tĕr-ol′i-sis) Breaking up of adhesions between the uterus and neighboring parts. [hystero- + G. *lysis,* dissolution]

hys•ter•om•e•ter (his′tĕr-om′ĕ-tĕr) A graduated sound for measuring the depth of the uterine cavity. SYN uterometer. [hystero- + G. *metron,* measure]

hys•ter•o•my•o•ma (his′tĕr-ō-mī-ō′mă) A myoma of the uterus. [hystero- + G. *mys,* muscle, + *-oma,* tumor]

hys•ter•o•my•o•mec•to•my (his′tĕr-ō-mī′ō-mek′tŏ-mē) Operative removal of a uterine myoma. [hysteromyoma + G. *ektomē,* excision]

hys•ter•o•my•ot•o•my (his′tĕr-ō-mī-ot′ŏ-mē) Incision into the muscles of the uterus. [hystero- + G. *mys,* muscle, + *tomē,* incision]

hys•ter•o•o•oph•o•rec•to•my (his′tĕr-ō-ō-of′ŏr-ek′tŏ-mē) Surgical removal of the uterus and ovaries. [hystero- + G. *ōon,* egg, + *phoros,* bearing, + *ektomē,* excision]

hys•ter•op•a•thy (his′tĕr-op′ă-thē) Any disease of the uterus. [hystero- + G. *pathos,* suffering]

hys•ter•o•pex•y (his′tĕr-ō-pek-sē) Fixation of a displaced or abnormally movable uterus. SYN uterofixation, uteropexy. [hystero- + G. *pēxis,* fixation]

hys•ter•o•plas•ty (his′tĕr-ō-plas-tē) SYN uteroplasty.

hys•ter•or•rha•phy (his′tĕr-ōr′ă-fē) Sutural repair of a lacerated uterus. [hystero- + G. *rhaphē,* suture]

hys•ter•or•rhex•is (his′tĕr-ō-rek′sis) Rupture of the uterus. [hystero- + G. *rhēxis,* rupture]

hys•ter•o•sal•pin•gec•to•my (his′tĕr-ō-sal-pin-jek′tŏ-mē) Operation for the removal of the uterus and one or both uterine tubes. [hystero- + G. *salpinx,* a trumpet, + *ektomē,* excision]

hys•ter•o•sal•pin•gog•ra•phy (his′tĕr-ō-sal-ping-gog′ră-fē) Radiography of the uterus and uterine tubes after the injection of radiopaque material. SYN hysterotubography, metrosalpingography, uterosalpingography, uterotubography. [hystero- + G. *salpinx,* a trumpet, + *graphō,* to write]

hys•ter•o•sal•pin•go•o•oph•o•rec•to•my (his′tĕr-ō-sal-ping′gō-ō-of′ŏr-ek′tŏ-mē) Excision of the uterus, oviducts, and ovaries. [hystero- + G. *salpinx,* trumpet, + *ōon,* egg, + *phoros,* bearing, + *ektomē,* excision]

hys•ter•o•sal•pin•gos•to•my (his′tĕr-ō-sal-ping-gos′tŏ-mē) Operation to restore patency of a uterine tube. [hystero- + G. *salpinx,* trumpet, + *stoma,* mouth]

hys•ter•o•scope (his′tĕr-ō-skōp) An endoscope used in direct visual examination of the uterine cavity. SYN metroscope, uteroscope. [hystero- + G. *skopeō,* to view]

hys•ter•os•co•py (his′tĕr-os′kŏ-pē) Visual instrumental inspection of the uterine cavity. SYN uteroscopy.

hys•ter•o•spasm (his′tĕr-ō-spazm) Spasm of the uterus.

hys•ter•ot•o•my (his′tĕr-ot′ŏ-mē) Incision of the uterus. SYN uterotomy. [hystero- + G. *tomē,* incision]

hys•ter•o•tra•chel•ec•to•my (his′tĕr-ō-trā′kĕ-lek′tŏ-mē) Removal of the cervix of uterus. [hystero- + G. *trachēlos,* neck, + *ektomē,* excision]

hys•ter•o•tra•chel•o•plas•ty (his′tĕr-ō-tra′kĕ-lō-plas-tē) Surgical repair of the cervix of uterus. [hystero- + G. *trachēlos,* neck, + *plastos,* formed, shaped]

hys•ter•o•tra•che•lor•rha•phy (his′tĕr-ō-trā′kĕ-lōr′ă-fē) Sutural repair of a lacerated cervix of uterus. [hystero- + G. *trachēlos,* neck, + *rhaphē,* a seam]

hys•ter•o•tra•chel•ot•o•my (his′tĕr-ō-trā′kĕ-lot′ŏ-mē) Incision of the cervix of uterus. [hystero- + G. *trachēlos,* neck, + *tomē,* incision]

hys•ter•o•tu•bog•ra•phy (his′tĕr-ō-tū-bog′ră-fē) SYN hysterosalpingography.

Hz Abbreviation for hertz.

ι (ī-ō′ta) Iota (q.v.).

I **1.** Symbol or abbreviation for iodine; luminous intensity or radiant intensity; ionic strength (in mol/L); isoleucine; inosine; intensity of electrical current, expressed in amperes. **2.** As a subscript, symbol for inspired gas. **3.** Designation for I blood group.

IA Abbreviation for intraarterial.

-ia Combining form meaning condition, used in formation of names of many diseases. Cf. -ism. [G. *-ia,* an ancient noun-forming suffix]

IADL Abbreviation for instrumental activities of daily living. SEE ALSO ADL, BADL.

I and O Abbreviation for (fluid) intake and output.

IAP Abbreviation for intermittent acute porphyria.

-iasis Combining form meaning a condition or state, especially an unhealthy one. [G. suffix forming nouns from verbs]

i•at•ric (ī-at′rik) Pertaining to medicine or to a physician or healer. [G. *iatros,* physician]

-iatrist, **-iatrician** Combining forms denoting a specialist in a given field of medicine.

iatro- Combining form meaning physicians, medicine, treatment. Cf. medico-. [G. *iatros,* physician]

i•at•ro•gen•ic (ī-at′rō-jen′ik) Denoting response to medical or surgical treatment, as induced by the treatment itself; usually used for unfavorable responses. [iatro- + G. *-gen,* producing]

i•at•ro•gen•ic di•a•be•tes mel•li•tus (ī-at′rō-jen′ik dī′ă-bē-tēs mel′i-tŭs) The disease as found after surgical or hospital interventions.

i•at•ro•gen•ic pneu•mo•thor•ax (ī-at′rō-jen′ik nū′mō-thōr′aks) Pneumothorax caused by a medical procedure, most often central venous catheter insertion, thoracentesis, or transbronchial and transthoracic lung biopsy.

i•at•ro•gen•ic trans•mis•sion (ī-at′rō-jen′ik trans-mish′ŭn) Transmission of infectious agents due to medical interference (e.g., transmission by contaminated needles).

I band (band) A light band on each side of the Z line of striated muscle fibers, comprising a region of the sarcomere where thin (actin) filaments are not overlapped by thick (myosin) filaments.

IBD Abbreviation for inflammatory bowel disease.

IBS Abbreviation for irritable bowel syndrome.

-ic **1.** Suffix denoting of, pertaining to. **2.** Chemical suffix denoting an element in a compound in one of its highest valencies. Cf. -ous (1). **3.** Suffix indicating an acid. [L. *-icus,* fr. G. *-ikos*]

ICAO stan•dard at•mos•phere (stan′dărd at′mŏs-fēr) The standard atmosphere adopted by the International Civil Aviation Organization, used for calibrating altimeters and for expressing hypobaric chamber pressures in terms of equivalent altitude.

ic•co•somes (ī′kō-sōmz) Beaded cytoplasmic structures on follicular dendrite cells; thought to be a repository for antigens. [*i*mmune *c*omplex *c*oated + -some]

ICD Abbreviation for International Classification of Diseases; implantable cardioverter defibrillator; intravenous contraceptive device.

ICDA *International Classification of Diseases, Adapted for Use in the United States.*

Ice•land dis•ease (īs′lănd di-zēz′) SYN epidemic neuromyasthenia.

I cell (sel) A cultured skin fibroblast containing membrane-bound inclusions; characteristic of mucolipidosis II. SEE ALSO immunocyte. SYN inclusion cell.

ice pick head•ache (īs pik hed′āk) SYN idiopathic stabbing headache.

ICF Abbreviation for intracellular fluid; intermediate care facility; International Classification of Functioning, Disability, and Health. SYN group home (as a residential facility).

ICH Abbreviation for intracranial hypertension, intracerebral hemorrhage, International Conference on Harmonization.

i•chor (ī′kōr) Rarely used term for a thin watery discharge from an ulcer or unhealthy wound. [G. *ichōr,* serum]

ichorhaemia [Br.] SYN ichorrhemia.

i•cho•roid (ī′kō-royd) Denoting a thin purulent discharge. [G. *ichōr,* serum, + *eidos,* resemblance]

i•chor•ous (ī′kōr-ŭs) Relating to or resembling ichor.

i•chor•rhe•a (ī′kō-rē′ă) A profuse ichorous discharge. SYN ichorrhoea. [G. *ichōr,* serum, + *rhoia,* a flow]

i•chor•rhe•mi•a (ī′kō-rē′mē-ă) Sepsis resulting from infection accompanied by an ichorous discharge. SYN ichorhaemia.

ichorrhoea [Br.] SYN ichorrhea.

ich•thy•ism (ik′thē-izm) Poisoning caused by eating stale or otherwise unfit fish. [G. *ichthys,* fish]

ichthyo- Combining form denoting fish. [G. *ichthys*]

ich•thy•oid (ik′thē-oyd) Fish-shaped. [ichthyo- + G. *eidos,* resemblance]

ich•thy•o•si•form e•ryth•ro•der•ma (ik′thē-ō′si-fōrm ĕ-rith′rō-dĕr′mă) SYN congenital ichthyosiform erythroderma.

ich•thy•o•sis (ik′thē-ō′sis) Congenital disorders of keratinization characterized by noninflammatory dryness and scaling of the skin, often associated with other defects and with abnormalities of lipid metabolism; distinguishable genetically, clinically, and microscopically and by epidermal cell kinetics. See this page. [ichthyo- + G. *-osis,* condition]

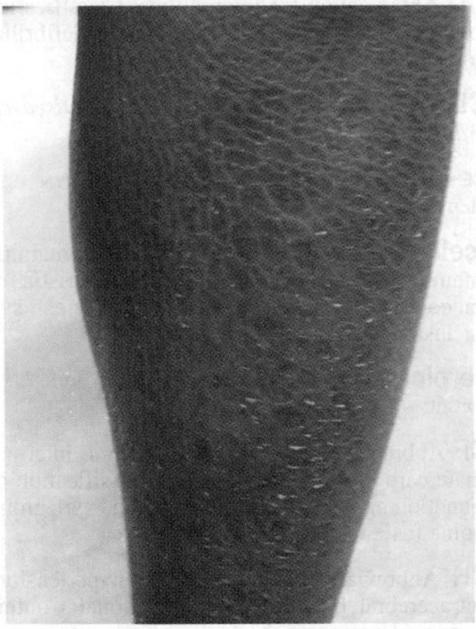

ichthyosis vulgaris: leg

ich•thy•ot•ic (ik′thē-ot′ik) Relating to ichthyosis.

ich•thy•o•tox•ism (ik′thē-ō-tok′sizm) Poisoning caused by fish. [ichthyo- + G. *toxikon,* poison]

ICM Abbreviation for International Confederation of Midwives.

ICN Abbreviation for International Council of Nurses.

icon (ī′kon) Any visual image used as a marker.

ICP Abbreviation for intracranial pressure.

ICS Abbreviation for incident command system.

-ics Suffix meaning organized knowledge, practice, treatment. [-ic + -s]

ICSD Abbreviation for International Classification of Sleep Disorders.

ICSH Abbreviation for interstitial cell-stimulating hormone.

ICt_{50} Abbreviation for incapacitating Ct_{50}.

ic•tal (ik′tăl) Relating to or caused by a stroke or seizure. [L. *ictus,* a stroke]

ic•ter•ic (ik-ter′ik) Relating to or marked by jaundice. [G. *ikterikos,* jaundiced]

ictero- Combining form related to jaundice. [G. *ikteros,* jaundice]

ic•ter•o•gen•ic (ik′tĕr-ō-jen′ik) Causing jaundice. [ictero- + G. *-gen,* producing]

icterohaemorrhagic fever [Br.] SYN icterohemorrhagic fever.

ic•ter•o•hem•or•rhag•ic fe•ver (ik′tĕr-ō-hem′ŏr-aj′ik fē′vĕr) **1.** Any pyrexia accompanied by icterus and evidence of hemorrhage (e.g., Rift Valley fever may be present as icterohemorrhagic fever). **2.** Infection with the variety of *Leptospira interrogans* serotype known as icterohemorrhagiae, characterized by fever, jaundice, hemorrhagic lesions, azotemia, and central nervous system manifestations. SYN icterohaemorrhagic fever.

ic•ter•o•hep•a•ti•tis (ik′tĕr-ō-hep′ă-tī′tis) Inflammation of the liver with jaundice as a prominent symptom. [ictero- + G. *hēpar,* liver, + *-itis,* inflammation]

ic•ter•oid (ik′tĕr-oyd) Yellow hued, or seemingly jaundiced. [ictero- + G. *eidos,* resemblance]

ic•ter•us (ik′tĕr-us) SYN jaundice. [G. *ikteros*]

ic•ter•us gra•vis (ik′tĕr-us grav′is) Jaundice associated with high fever and delirium; seen in severe hepatitis and other diseases of the liver with severe functional failure. SYN malignant jaundice.

ic•ter•us ne•o•na•to•rum (ik′tĕr-ŭs nē-ō′nā-tō′rŭm) Icterus in the newborn; sometimes normal but can be induced or accentuated by excessive hemolysis, sepsis, neonatal hepatitis, or congenital atresia of the biliary system. SYN jaundice of the newborn, physiologic icterus, physiologic jaundice.

ic•tus (ik′tŭs) **1.** A stroke or attack. **2.** A beat. [L.]

ic•tus cor•dis (ik′tŭs kōr′dis) SYN apex beat.

ICU Abbreviation for intensive care unit.

ICU psy•cho•sis (sī-kō′sis) Psychotic episode(s) occurring within 24 hours after entering the ICU in people with no previous history of psychosis; related to sleep deprivation, overstimulation, and time spent on life support systems.

ID Abbreviation for intradermal.

id (id) **1.** PSYCHOANALYSIS one of three components of the psychic apparatus in the freudian structural framework, the other two being the ego and superego. It is completely in the unconscious realm, is unorganized, is the reservoir of psychic energy or libido, and is under the influence of the primary processes. **2.** The total of all psychic energy available from the innate biologic hungers, appetites, bodily needs, drives, and impulses in a newborn infant. [L. *id,* that]

-id 1. Suffix denoting a state of sensitivity of the skin in which a part remote from the primary lesion reacts ("-id reaction") to the pathogen, giving rise to a secondary inflammatory lesion; the lesion manifesting the reaction is designated by the use of -id as a suffix. [G. *-eidēs,* resembling, through Fr. *-ide*] **2.** Small, young specimen. [G. *-idion,* a diminutive ending]

IDC Abbreviation for indwelling catheter.

IDD Abbreviation for iodine deficiency disorder.

-ide 1. Combining form denoting the more electronegative element in a binary chemical compound. **2.** Combining form (in a sugar name) indicating substitution for the H of the hemiacetal OH; e.g., glycoside.

IDEA (ī-dē′ă) Acronym for U.S. Individuals with Disabilities Education Act.

i•de•a (ī-dē′ă) Any mental image or concept. [G. semblance]

i•deal (ī-dēl′) A standard of perfection.

i•de•a of ref•er•ence (ī-dē′ă ref′rĕns) The misinterpretation that other people's statements or acts or neutral objects in the environment are directed toward one's self when, in fact, they are not.

i•de•a•tion (ī′dē-ā′shŭn) The formation of ideas or thoughts.

i•de•a•tion•al (ī′dē-ā′shŭn-ăl) Relating to ideation.

i•dée fixe (ē-dā′ fēks) French for fixed idea (q.v.).

i•den•ti•cal twins (ī-dent′ti-k′ăl twinz) SYN monozygotic twins.

i•den•ti•fi•ca•tion (ī-den′ti-fi-kā′shŭn) **1.** Act or process of determining classification or nature of. **2.** A sense of oneness, or psychic continuity with another person or group; one of the freudian defense mechanisms common to everyone whereby anxiety regarding one's personal identity or worth is dissipated through the mechanism of perceiving oneself as having characteristics in common with a person in the public eye, or in childhood identifying with a more powerful person such as a parent. [Mediev. L. *identicus,* fr. L. *idem,* the same, + *facio,* to make]

i•den•ti•fi•er (ī-den′ti-fī-ĕr) A person or thing that establishes or marks the identity or specific nature of anything. [L. Lat. *identitas*, identity, fr. L. *iem*, the same]

i•den•ti•ty (ī-den′ti-tē) **1.** The sum of characteristics by which a person is recognized (by self and others). **2.** A composite definition of the self that includes an interpersonal aspect (e.g., roles, relationships); an aspect of possibility or potential (i.e., who one might become) and a values-oriented aspect that provides a basis for choices and decisions, including self-esteem and self-concept, both in reflecting and being influenced by the society in which one functions.

i•den•ti•ty cri•sis (ī-den′ti-tē krī′sis) A disorientation concerning one's sense of self, values, and role in society, often of acute onset and related to a particular and significant event in one's life.

i•den•ti•ty dis•or•der (ī-den′ti-tē dis-ōr′dĕr) A mental disorder of childhood or adolescence in which one suffers severe distress regarding one's ability to reconcile aspects of the self into a coherent acceptable sense of self.

ideo- Prefix meaning ideas; ideation Cf. idio-. [G. *idea,* form, notion]

i•de•o•ki•net•ic a•prax•i•a, id•e•o•mo•tor a•prax•i•a (id′ē-ō-ki-net′ik ă-prak′sē-ă, id′ē-ō-mō′tŏr) A motor disorder in which simple acts are incapable of being performed, presumably because the connections between the cortical centers that control volition and the motor cortex are interrupted.

i•de•ol•o•gy (ī′dē-ol′ŏ-jē) The powerful and authoritative messages communicated through language or culture that tell us who we are and how we are to behave. [idea + -logy]

idio- Prefix meaning private, distinctive, peculiar to. Cf. ideo-. [G. *idios,* one's own]

id•i•o•glos•si•a (id′ē-ō-glos′ē-ă) 1. A unique spoken language invented by a person, differing markedly from normal speech and for the most part unintelligible to listeners, so that it is not a useful form of communication; usually a sign of psychosis or mental retardation. 2. A type of spoken communication developed by and used between twins. SYN idiolalia. [idio- + G. glōssa, tongue, + -ia]

id•i•o•gram (id′ē-ō-gram) **1.** SYN karyotype. **2.** Diagrammatic representation of chromosome morphology characteristic of a species or population. [idio- + G. *gramma,* something written]

id•i•o•het•er•o•ag•glu•ti•nin (id′ē-ō-het′ĕr-ō-ă-glū′tin-in) An idioagglutinin occurring in the blood of one animal, but capable of combining with the antigenic material from another species. [idio- + G. *heteros,* another, + agglutinin]

id•i•o•het•er•ol•y•sin (id′ē-ō-het-ĕr-ol′i-sin) An idiolysin occurring in the blood of one species, but capable of hemolyzing red blood cells of another species.

id•i•o•i•so•ag•glu•ti•nin (id′ē-ō-ī′sō-ă-glū′tin-in) An idioagglutinin occurring in the blood of a certain species, capable of agglutinating cells from animals of the same species. [idio- + G. *isos,* equal, + agglutinin]

id·i·o·i·sol·y·sin (id′ē-ō-ī-sol′i-sin) An idiolysin occurring in the blood of an animal of a certain species, capable of hemolyzing red blood cells from animals of the same species.

id·i·o·la·li·a (id′ē-ō-lā′lē-ă) SYN idioglossia.

id·i·ol·y·sin (id′ē-ol′i-sin) A lysin that occurs naturally in the blood of a person or an animal, without the injection of a stimulating antigen or the passive transfer of antibody.

id·i·o·mus·cu·lar con·trac·tion (id′ē-ō-mŭs′kyū-lăr kŏn-trak′shŭn) SYN myoedema.

id·i·o·path·ic (id′ē-ō-path′ik) Denoting a disease of unknown cause. SYN agnogenic. [idio- + G. *pathos,* suffering]

id·i·o·path·ic al·do·ste·ron·ism (id′ē-ō-path′ik al-dos′tĕr-ōn-izm) SYN primary aldosteronism.

id·i·o·path·ic en·vi·ron·men·tal in·tol·er·ance (IEI) (id′ē-ō′path-ik en-vī′rŏn-men′tăl in-tol′ĕr-ăns) A puzzling condition in which nonspecific symptoms involving many organ systems arise by unknown mechanisms after putative environmental exposures to very low levels of diverse chemicals. SYN multiple chemical sensitivity.

id·i·o·path·ic hy·per·cal·ce·mi·a of in·fants (id′ē-ō-path′ik hī′pĕr-kal-sē′mē-ă in′fănts) Persistent hypercalcemia of unknown cause in very young children, associated with osteosclerosis, renal insufficiency, and sometimes hypertension.

id·i·o·path·ic hy·per·tro·phic sub·a·or·tic ste·no·sis (id′ē-ō-path′ik hī′pĕr-trō′fik sŭb′ā-ōr′tik stĕ-nō′sis) Left ventricular outflow obstruction due to hypertrophy, usually congenital, of the ventricular septum.

id·i·o·path·ic neu·ral·gi·a (id′ē-ō-path′ik nūr-al′jē-ă) Nerve pain not due to any apparent cause.

id·i·o·path·ic pul·mo·nar·y fi·bro·sis (IPF) (id′ē-ō-path′ik pul′mŏ-nar-ē fī-brō′sis) Subacute form also called Hamman-Rich syndrome; an acute to chronic inflammatory process of the lungs, the healing stage of diffuse alveolar damage or acute interstitial pneumonia, either idiopathic or associated with collagen-vascular diseases. SYN cryptogenic fibrosing alveolitis, Hamman-Rich syndrome.

id·i·o·path·ic stab·bing head·ache (id′ē-ō-path′ik stab′ing hed′āk) Brief repetitive sharp pains in the temporal-parietal area of the head. SYN ice pick headache.

id·i·o·path·ic sub·glot·tic ste·no·sis (id′ē-ō-path′ik sŭb-glot′ik stĕ-nō′sis) Narrowing of the infraglottic lumen, of unknown cause; apparently occurring only in women.

id·i·o·path·ic throm·bo·cy·to·pe·nic pur·pu·ra (ITP) (id′ē-ō-path′ik throm′bō-sī-tō-pē′nik pŭr′pyŭr-ă) A systemic illness characterized by extensive ecchymoses and hemorrhages from mucous membranes and very low platelet counts; resulting from destruction in the spleen of platelets to which an autoimmune globulin is bound; childhood cases, which often follow viral infection, are mild and transitory; in adults, bleeding may be recurrent and severe. SYN immune thrombocytopenic purpura, purpura hemorrhagica, thrombopenic purpura.

id·i·op·a·thy (id′ē-op′ă-thē) An idiopathic disease. [idio- + G. *pathos,* suffering]

id·i·o·phren·ic (id′ē-ō-fren′ik) Relating to, or originating in, the mind or brain alone, not reflex or secondary. [idio- + G. *phrēn,* mind]

id·i·o·syn·cra·sy (id′ē-ō-singk′ră-sē) **1.** A person's mental, behavioral, or physical characteristic or peculiarity. **2.** PHARMACOLOGY an abnormal reaction to a drug, sometimes specified as genetically determined. [G. *idiosynkrasia,* fr. *idios,* one's own, + *synkrasis,* a mixing together]

id·i·o·syn·crat·ic (id′ē-ō-sin-krat′ik) Relating to or marked by an idiosyncrasy.

id·i·ot-sa·vant (ē′dē-ō′sah-vawn[h]′) A person of low general intelligence who possesses an unusual facility in performing certain mental tasks that most normal people cannot do. [Fr.]

id·i·o·type (id′ē-ō-tīp) A determinant that confers on an immunoglobulin molecule an antigenic "individuality" and is frequently a unique attribute of a given antibody in a given animal. [idio- + G. *typos,* model]

id·i·o·typ·ic an·ti·bod·y (id′ē-ō-tip′ik an′ti-bod-ē) An antibody that binds to an idiotope of another antibody.

id·i·o·ven·tric·u·lar (id′ē-ō-ven-trik′yū-lăr) Pertaining to or associated with the cardiac ventricles alone.

id·i·o·ven·tric·u·lar rhythm (id′ē-ō-ven-trik′yū-lăr ridh′ŭm) A slow independent ventricular rhythm under control of an ectopic ventricular center; occurs in heart block and sinus arrest. SYN ventricular rhythm.

IDLH Abbreviation for Immediate Danger to Life and Health level.

id re·ac·tion (id rē-ak′shŭn) An allergic manifestation of candidiasis, the dermatophytoses, and other mycoses characterized by itching, vesicular lesions that appear in response to superficial infections that are distant from the id reaction itself. SEE ALSO dermatophytid, -id (1).

IDU Abbreviation for injection drug user.

i.e. That is. [L. *id est*]

IEI Abbreviation for idiopathic environmental intolerance.

IEP Abbreviation for U.S. Individualized Education Program.

IF Abbreviation for initiation factor; intrinsic factor.

IFC Abbreviation for interferential current.

IFN Abbreviation for interferon.

IFSP Abbreviation for individualized family service plan.

Ig Abbreviation for immunoglobulin.

IgA Abbreviation for immunoglobulin A.

IgD Abbreviation for immunoglobulin D.

IgE Abbreviation for immunoglobulin E.

IGF Abbreviation for insulinlike growth factors.

IgG Abbreviation for immunoglobulin G.

IgM Abbreviation for immunoglobulin M.

ig•ni•punc•ture (ig′ni-pŭngk-shŭr) The original procedure of closing a retinal separation by transfixation with cautery. [L. *ignis,* fire, + puncture]

IGRT Abbreviation for intensity guided radiation therapy.

I.H.P. Abbreviation for individual habilitation plan.

IL Abbrevation for interleukin.

ILA Abbreviation for insulinlike activity.

il•e•ac (il′ē-ak) **1.** Relating to ileus. **2.** Relating to the ileum.

il•e•al (il′ē-ăl) Of or pertaining to the ileum.

il•e•al ar•ter•ies (il′ē-ăl ahr′tĕr-ēz) *Origin*, superior mesenteric; *distribution*, ileum; *anastomoses*, other branches of superior mesenteric. SYN arteriae ileales [TA].

il•e•al di•ver•tic•u•lum (il′ē-ăl dī′vĕr-tik′yū-lŭm) SYN Meckel diverticulum.

il•e•al or•i•fice (il′ē-ăl ōr′i-fis) The opening of the terminal ileum into the large intestine at the transition between the cecum and the ascending colon. SYN ileocecal valve, ileocolic valve, ileocolic vein, ostium ileale.

il•e•al u•re•ter (il′ē-ăl yŭr′ē-tĕr) SYN ureteroileoneocystostomy.

il•e•al veins (il′ē-ăl vānz) SEE jejunal and ileal veins.

il•e•ec•to•my (il′ē-ek′tŏ-mē) Removal of the ileum. [ileum + G. *ektomē,* excision]

il•e•i•tis (il′ē-ī′tis) Inflammation of the ileum.

♻ **ileo-** Combining form denoting the ileum; bottom of the small intestine. [New L. *ileum,* groin]

il•e•o•a•nal (il′ē-ō-ā′năl) Denoting a relationship to the ileum and the anus.

ileocaecal [Br.] SYN ileocecal.

ileocaecostomy [Br.] SYN ileocecostomy.

il•e•o•ce•cal (il′ē-ō-sē′kăl) Relating to both ileum and cecum. SYN ileocaecal.

il•e•o•ce•cal or•i•fice (il′ē-ō-sē′kăl ōr′i-fis) SEE ileal orifice.

il•e•o•ce•cal valve (il′ē-ō-sē′kăl valv) SYN ileal orifice.

il•e•o•ce•cos•to•my (il′ē-ō-sē-kos′tŏ-mē) Anastomosis of the ileum to the cecum. SYN cecoileostomy, ileocaecostomy.

il•e•o•co•lic (il′ē-ō-kol′ik) Relating to the ileum and the colon.

il•e•o•co•lic ar•ter•y (il′ē-ō-kol′ik ahr′tĕr-ē) *Origin,* superior mesenteric, often by a common trunk with the right colic; *distribution*, terminal part of ileum, cecum, vermiform appendix, and ascending colon; *anastomoses,* right colic and ileal. SYN arteria ileocolica [TA].

il•e•o•co•lic valve (il′ē-ō-kol′ik valv) SYN ileal orifice.

il•e•o•co•lic vein (il′ē-ō-kol′ik vān) SYN ileal orifice.

il•e•o•co•li•tis (il′ē-ō-kō-lī′tis) Inflammation of both ileum and colon.

il•e•o•co•los•to•my (il′ē-ō-kō-los′tŏ-mē) Establishment of a new communication between the ileum and the colon. [ileo- + colostomy]

il•e•o•cys•to•plas•ty (il′ē-ō-sis′tō-plas-tē) Surgical reconstruction of the bladder involving the use of an isolated intestinal segment to augment bladder capacity. [ileo- + G. *kystis,* bladder, + *plastos,* formed]

il•e•o•il•e•os•to•my (il′ē-ō-il-ē-os′tŏ-mē) **1.** Establishment of a communication between two segments of the ileum. **2.** The opening so established. [ileum + ileum + G. *stoma,* mouth]

il•e•o•je•ju•ni•tis (il′ē-ō-jĕ′jū-nī′tis) A chronic inflammatory condition involving the jejunum and of the ileum.

il•e•o•pex•y (il′ē-ō-pek-sē) Surgical fixation of ileum. [ileo- + G. *pēxis,* fixation]

il•e•o•proc•tos•to•my (il′ē-ō-prok-tos′tŏ-mē) Establishment of a communication between the ileum and the rectum. [ileo- + G. *prōktos,* anus (rectum), + *stoma,* mouth]

il•e•or•rha•phy (il′ē-ōr′ă-fē) Suturing the ileum. [ileo- + G. *rhaphē,* suture]

il•e•o•sig•moid•os•to•my (il′ē-ō-sig′moyd-os′

tŏ-mē) Establishment of a communication between the ileum and the sigmoid colon. [ileo- + sigmoid, + G. *stoma,* mouth]

il·e·os·to·my (il′ē-os′tŏ-mē) **1.** Establishment of a fistula through which the ileum discharges the bowel's contents directly to the outside of the body. **2.** A type of fecal diversion. See this page. [ileo- + G. *stoma,* mouth]

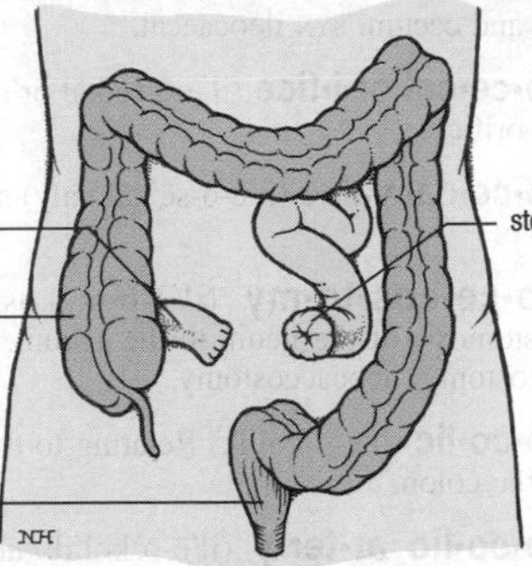

ileostomy: stoma opens on anterior abdominal wall

il·e·ot·o·my (il′ē-ot′ŏ-mē) Incision into the ileum. [ileo- + G. *tomē,* incision]

il·e·um (il′ē-ŭm) [TA] The third portion of the small intestine, about 3.6 m (12 ft) in length, extending from the jejunum to the ileocecal opening. [L. fr. G. *eileō,* to roll up, twist]

il·e·us (il′ē-ŭs) Mechanical, dynamic, or adynamic obstruction of the intestines; may be accompanied by severe colicky pain, abdominal distention, vomiting, absence of passage of stool, and often fever and dehydration. [G. *eileos,* intestinal colic, fr. *eilō,* to roll up tight]

il·e·us sub·par·ta (il′ē-ŭs sŭb-pahr′tā) Obstruction of the large bowel by pressure of the pregnant uterus.

il·i·ac (il′ē-ak) Relating to the ilium.

il·i·ac bone (il′ē-ak bōn) SYN ilium.

il·i·ac co·lon (il′ē-ak kō′lŏn) That portion of the descending colon that occupies the left iliac fossa, between the crest of the left ilium and the pelvic brim.

il·i·ac crest (il′ē-ak krest) The long, curved upper border of the wing of the ilium. See this page.

il·i·ac mus·cle (il′ē-ak mŭs′ĕl) SYN iliacus muscle.

il·i·a·cus mus·cle (il-ē-ā′kŭs mŭs′ĕl) *Origin,* iliac fossa; *insertion,* tendon of psoas, anterior surface of lesser trochanter, and capsule of hip joint; *action,* flexes thigh and rotates it medially;

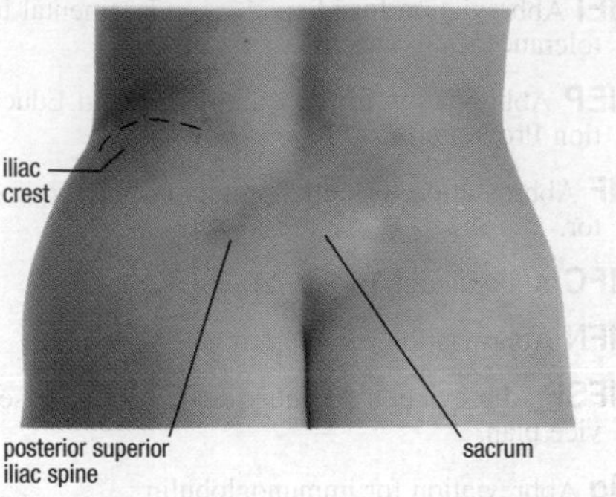

iliac crest

nerve supply, lumbar plexus. SYN musculus iliacus [TA], iliac muscle.

ilio- Combining form meaning the ilium; top of hip bone. [L. *ilium*]

il·i·o·coc·cyg·e·al (il′ē-ō-kok-sij′ē-ăl) Relating to the ilium and the coccyx.

il·i·o·coc·cyg·e·al mus·cle (il′ē-ō-kok-sij′ē-ăl mŭs′ĕl) SYN iliococcygeus muscle.

il·i·o·coc·cyg·e·us mus·cle (il′ē-ō-kok-sij′ē-ŭs mŭs′ĕl) The posterior part of the levator ani arising from the tendinous arch of the levator ani muscle and inserting on the anococcygeal ligament and coccyx. SYN musculus iliococcygeus [TA], iliococcygeal muscle.

il·i·o·cos·ta·lis cer·vi·cis mus·cle (il′ē-ō-kos-tā′lis sĕr′vis-is mŭs′ĕl) *Origin,* angles of upper six ribs; *insertion,* transverse processes of middle cervical vertebrae; *action,* extends, abducts, and rotates cervical vertebrae; *nerve supply,* dorsal branches of upper thoracic nerves.

il·i·o·cos·ta·lis lum·bo·rum mus·cle (il′ē-ō-kos-tā′lis lum-bō′rŭm mŭs′ĕl) *Origin,* with erector spinae; *insertion,* the angles of lower six ribs; *action,* extends, abducts, and rotates lumbar vertebrae; *nerve supply,* dorsal branches of thoracic and lumbar nerves. SYN lumbar iliocostal muscle.

il·i·o·cos·ta·lis mus·cle (il′ē-ō-kos-tā′lis mŭs′ĕl) The lateral division of the erector spinae, having three subdivisions: iliocostalis lumborum musculus, iliocostalis thoracis musculus, and iliocostalis cervicis musculus. SYN musculus iliocostalis [TA], iliocostal muscle.

il·i·o·cos·tal mus·cle (il′ē-ō-kos′tăl mŭs′ĕl) SYN iliocostalis muscle.

il·i·o·fem·o·ral (il′ē-ō-fem′ŏr-ăl) Relating to the ilium and the femur.

il·i·o·fem·o·ral lig·a·ment (il′ē-ō-fem′ŏr-ăl lig′ă-mĕnt) A triangular ligament attached by its apex to the anterior inferior spine of the ilium and rim of the acetabulum, and by its base to the anterior intertrochanteric line of the femur; the strong medial band is attached to the lower part of the intertrochanteric line; the strong lateral part is fixed to the tubercle at the upper part of this line; the bands diverge, forming a Y-like figure with a weak area between; among the strongest of ligaments, it limits extension at the hip joint. SYN ligamentum iliofemorale [TA], Y-shaped ligament.

il·i·o·fem·o·ral tri·an·gle (il′ē-ō-fem′ŏr-ăl trī′ang-gĕl) SYN Bryant triangle.

il·i·o·hy·po·gas·tric nerve (il′ē-ō-hī-pō-gas′trik nĕrv) Arises from the first lumbar nerve; it supplies the abdominal muscles and the skin of the lower part of the anterior abdominal wall. SYN nervus iliohypogastricus [TA].

il·i·o·in·gui·nal (il′ē-ō-ing′gwi-năl) Relating to the iliac region and the groin.

il·i·o·in·gui·nal nerve (il′ē-ō-ing′gwi-năl nĕrv) Arises from the first lumbar nerve, passes through the inguinal canal and superficial inguinal ring to supply the skin of the upper medial thigh, mons pubis, and scrotum or labium majus. SYN nervus ilioinguinalis [TA].

il·i·o·lum·bar (il′ē-ō-lŭm′bahr) Relating to the iliac and the lumbar regions.

il·i·o·lum·bar ar·ter·y (il′ē-ō-lŭm′bahr ahr′tĕr-ē) *Origin*, internal iliac; *distribution*, pelvic muscles and bones; *anastomoses*, deep circumflex iliac, lumbar. SYN arteria iliolumbalis [TA].

il·i·o·lum·bar vein (il′ē-ō-lŭm′bahr vān) Accompanying the artery of the same name, anastomosing with the lumbar and deep circumflex iliac veins, and emptying into the internal iliac vein. SYN vena iliolumbalis [TA].

il·i·o·pec·tin·e·al (il′ē-ō-pek-tin′ē-ăl) Relating to the ilium and the pubis.

il·i·o·pec·tin·e·al arch (il′ē-ō-pek-tin′ē-ăl ahrch) A thickened band of fused iliac and psoas fascia passing posteriorly from the posterior aspect of the inguinal ligament across the anterior aspect of the femoral nerve to attach to the iliopectineal eminence of the hip bone. The iliopectinal arch thus forms a septum that subdivides the space deep to the inguinal ligament into a lateral muscular lacunae and a medial vascular lacunae. When a psoas minor muscle is present, its tendon of insertion blends with the iliopectineal arch.

il·i·o·pec·tin·e·al line (il′ē-ō-pek-tin′ē-ăl līn) SYN linea terminalis.

il·i·op·so·as mus·cle (il′ē-op-sō′ăs mŭs′ĕl) A compound muscle, consisting of the iliacus musculus and psoas major musculus. SYN musculus iliopsoas [TA].

il·i·o·pu·bic tract (il′ē-ō-pyū′bik trakt) Thickened inferior margin of the transversalis fascia seen as a fibrous band running parallel and posterior (deep) to the inguinal ligament, contributing to the posterior wall of the inguinal canal as it bridges the external iliac-femoral vessels from the iliopectineal arch to the superior pubic ramus. It marks the inferior edge of the deep inguinal ring and the medial margin of the femoral canal. Seen only when the inguinal region is viewed from its internal aspect, it is a useful landmark in laparoscopy of this region, as for repair of inguinal herniae. SYN tractus iliopubicus [TA].

il·i·o·tib·i·al band fric·tion syn·drome (il′ē-ō-tib′ē-ăl band frik′shŭn sin′drōm) A painful condition affecting the hip, thigh, or knee; produced by irritation of the iliotibial tract as it glides over the greater trochanter, anterior superior iliac spine, Gerdy tubercle, or the lateral femoral condyle; sometimes associated with a snapping or grating sensation.

il·i·o·tib·i·al band syn·drome (il′ē-ō-tib′ē-ăl band sin′drōm) A syndrome of knee pain that may result from inflammation due to mechanical friction of the iliotibial band and the lateral femoral epicondyle.

il·i·o·tib·i·al tract (il′ē-ō-tib′ē-ăl trakt) A fibrous reinforcement of the fascia lata on the lateral surface of the thigh, extending from the crest of the ilium to the lateral condyle of the tibia. See this page.

il·i·o·tro·chan·ter·ic (il′ē-ō-trō′kan-ter′ik) Re-

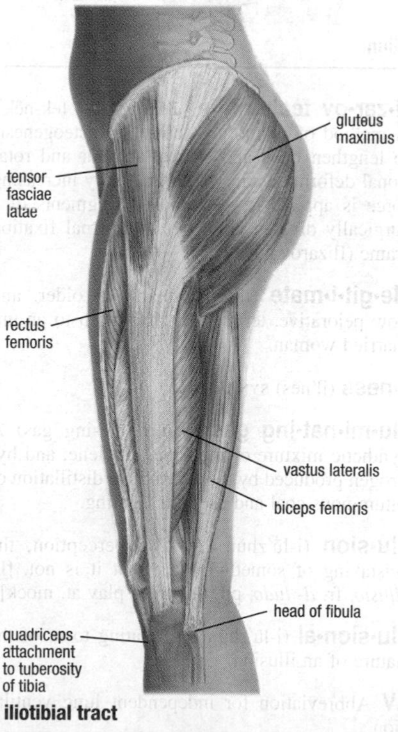

iliotibial tract

lating to the ilium and the great trochanter of the femur.

il•i•o•tro•chan•ter•ic lig•a•ment (il′ē-ō-trō′kan-ter′ik lig′ă-mĕnt) The lateral strong band of the Y-shaped iliofemoral ligament; it is attached below to the tubercle at the upper part of the intertrochanteric line.

il•i•um, pl. **il•i•a** (il′ē-ŭm, -ă) [TA] The broad, flaring portion of the hip bone, distinct at birth but later becoming fused with the ischium and pubis; it consists of a body, which joins the pubis and ischium to form the acetabulum and a broad thin portion, called the ala or wing. See this page. SYN iliac bone. [L. groin, flank]

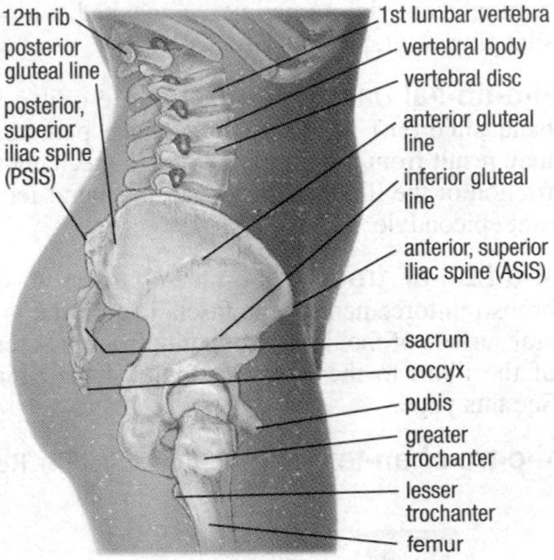

ilium

Il•i•zar•ov tech•nique (ē′lē-zawr′av tek-nēk′) A method of promoting controlled osteogenesis to lengthen bone and correct angular and rotational deformities, in which gradually increasing force is applied to the apposed fragments of a surgically divided bone by an external fixation frame (Ilizarov device).

il•le•git•i•mate (il′lĕ-jit′i-măt) An older, and now pejorative, term for a child born to an unmarried woman.

ill•ness (il′nes) SYN disease (1).

il•lu•mi•nat•ing gas (i-lū′mi-nāt-ing gas) A synthetic mixture of methane, ethylene, and hydrogen produced by the destructive distillation of bituminous coal and used for lighting.

il•lu•sion (i-lū′zhŭn) A false perception; the mistaking of something for what it is not. [L. *illusio,* fr. *il- ludo,* pp. *-lusus,* to play at, mock]

il•lu•sion•al (i-lū′zhŭn-ăl) Relating to or of the nature of an illusion.

ILV Abbreviation for independent lung ventilation.

IM Abbreviation for internal medicine; intramuscular(ly).

im•age (im′ăj) **1.** Representation of an object made by the rays of light emanating or reflected from it. **2.** Representation produced by x-rays, ultrasound, tomography, thermography, radioisotopes, or other modalities. **3.** To produce such a representation. [L. *imago,* likeness]

im•age am•pli•fi•er (im′ăj am′pli-fī′ĕr) A device for converting a low light level fluoroscopic image to one that can be seen by the eye in a lighted environment; usually consists of an electronic light amplifier chained to a television tube.

im•ag•e•ry (im′ăj-rē) A technique in behavior therapy in which the client or patient is conditioned to substitute pleasant fantasies to counter the unpleasant feelings associated with anxiety.

i•mag•ing (im′ăj-ing) Production of a clinical image using x-rays, ultrasound, computed tomography, magnetic resonance, radionuclide scanning, or thermography; especially, cross-sectional imaging (e.g., ultrasonography, CT, MRI). SEE image.

i•ma•go, pl. **i•mag•i•nes** (i-mā′gō, -maj′i-nēz) **1.** The last stage of an insect after it has completed all its metamorphoses through the egg, larva, and pupa; the adult insect form. **2.** SYN archetype (2). [L. image]

im•bal•ance (im-bal′ăns) **1.** Lack of equality between opposing forces. **2.** Lack of equality in some aspect of binocular vision, such as muscle balance or image size. [L. *in-* neg. + *bi-lanx* (*-lanc-*), having two scales, fr. *bis,* twice, + *lanx,* dish, scale of a balance]

im•bi•bi•tion (im′bi-bish′ŭn) **1.** Absorption of fluid by a solid body without resultant chemical change in either. **2.** Taking up of water by a gel. [L. *im-bibo,* to drink in (*in* + *bibo*)]

im•bri•cate, **im•bri•cat•ed** (im′bri-kāt, im′bri-kāt′ĕd) Overlapping, like shingles. [L. *imbricatus,* covered with tiles]

im•bri•ca•tion (im′bri-kā′shŭn) The operative overlapping of layers of tissue in the closure of wounds or the repair of defects. [L. *imbrex,* roofing tile, fr. *imber,* rain]

IME Abbreviation for independent medical evaluation.

IMF Abbreviation for inframammary fold.

IMI Abbreviation for intramuscular injection.

im•id•a•zole (i-mid′i-zōl) A five-membered heterocyclic compound occurring in L-histidine and other biologically important compounds.

im•ide (im′īd) The radical or group, =NH, attached to two –CO– groups.

♻ **imido-** Prefix denoting the radical of an imide, formed by the loss of the H of the =NH group.

im•i•dole (im′i-dōl) SYN pyrrole.

♻ **-imine** Suffix denoting the group =NH.

♻ **imino-** Prefix denoting the group =NH.

i•mi•no ac•ids (i′mĕ-nō as′idz) Compounds with molecules containing both an acid group and an imino group.

Im•lach fat-pad (im′lăk fat′pad) Fat surrounding the round ligament of the uterus in the inguinal canal.

im•ma•ture cat•a•ract (i′mă-chŭr kat′ăr-akt) A stage of partial lens opacification.

im•me•di•ate al•ler•gy (i-mē′dē-ăt al′ĕr-jē) A type I allergic reaction; so called because in a sensitized subject the reaction becomes evident usually within minutes after contact with the allergen (antigen), reaches its peak within an hour or so, then rapidly recedes. SEE ALSO immediate reaction, anaphylaxis. Cf. delayed allergy.

im•me•di•ate aus•cul•ta•tion, di•rect aus•cul•ta•tion (i-mē′dē-ăt aws′kŭl-tā′shŭn, dĭr-ekt′) Listening to body sounds by application of the ear or a stethoscope to the surface of the body.

Im•me•di•ate Dan•ger to Life and Health lev•el (IDLH) (i-mē′dē-ăt dān′jĕr līf helth lev′ĕl) Exposure levels to toxic agents set by NIOSH at which serious illness or death may occur.

im•me•di•ate den•ture (i-mē′dē-ăt den′chŭr) A removable complete or partial denture constructed for insertion immediately following the removal of natural teeth to maintain a normal appearance and the ability to chew food.

im•me•di•ate en•er•gy sys•tem (i-mē′dē-ăt en′ĕr-jē sis′tĕm) Intramuscular nonaerobic energy system composed of high-energy phosphates ATP–PCr; powers all-out physical effort for up to 6–8 seconds.

im•me•di•ate flap (i-mē′dē-ăt flap) SYN direct flap.

im•me•di•ate per•cus•sion (i-mē′dē-ăt pĕr-kŭsh′ŭn) The striking of the part under examination directly with the finger or a plessor, without the intervention of another finger or plessimeter.

im•me•di•ate re•ac•tion (i-mē′dē-ăt rē-ak′shŭn) Local or generalized immune response that begins within a few minutes to about an hour after exposure to an antigen to which the individual has been sensitized. SEE ALSO skin test, wheal-and-erythema reaction.

im•me•di•ate trans•fu•sion (i-mē′dē-ăt trans-fyū′zhŭn) SYN direct transfusion.

im•mer•sion (i-mĕr′zhŭn) **1.** The placing of a body under water or other liquid. **2.** MICROSCOPY filling the space between the objective lens and the top of the cover glass with a fluid, such as water or oil, to reduce spheric aberration and increase effective numeric aperture. [L. *immergo,* pp. *-mersus,* to dip in (*in* + *mergo*)]

im•mer•sion foot (i-mĕr′zhŭn fut) A condition resulting from prolonged exposure to damp and cold; the extremity is initially cold and anesthetic, but on rewarming becomes hyperemic, paresthetic, and hyperhidrotic; recovery is often slow. SYN immersion injury (2), trenchfoot.

im•mer•sion in•ju•ry (i-mĕr′zhŭn in′jŭr-ē) **1.** Trauma related to near drowning. **2.** SYN immersion foot.

im•mer•sion ob•jec•tive (i-mĕr′zhŭn ŏb-jek′tiv) A high power objective used with a drop of oil between the lens and the specimen on the slide, allowing a greater numeric aperture; similar lenses are available for use with water as the immersing liquid.

im•mis•ci•ble (i-mis′i-bĕl) Incapable of mutual solution; e.g., oil and water. [L. *immisceo,* to mix in (*in* + *misceo*)]

im•mis•sion (i-mish′ŭn) Environmental concentration of a pollutant, resulting from a combination of emissions and dispersals; often synonymous with exposure. [L. *immissio,* introduction, fr. *im- mitto,* to introduce]

im•mit•tance (i-mit′ăns) AUDIOLOGY a general term describing measurements of tympanic membrane impedance, compliance, or admittance. SYN admittance. [L. *immitto,* to send in]

immobilisation [Br.] SYN immobilization.

im•mo•bil•i•ty (i′mō-bil′i-tē) The absence of movement, or inability to move.

im•mo•bil•i•za•tion (i-mō′bi-lī-zā′shŭn) The act or process of fixing or rendering immobile. SYN immobilisation.

im•mo•bi•lize (i-mō′bi-līz) To render fixed or incapable of moving. [L. *in-*, neg., + *mobilis,* movable]

immortalisation [Br.] SYN immortalization.

im•mor•tal•i•za•tion (i-mōr′tăl-ī-zā′shŭn) Conferring on normal cells cultured in vitro the property of an infinite lifespan, as from spontaneous mutation, by exposure to chemical carcinogens, or by viral infection. SYN immortalisation.

im•mov•a•ble joint (i-mū′vă-bĕl joynt) SYN fibrous joint.

im•mune (i-myūn′) **1.** Free from the possibility of acquiring a given infectious disease; resistant to an infectious disease. **2.** Pertaining to cell-mediated or humoral immunity, whereby an organism is so altered by previous contact with an antigen that it responds quickly and upon specifically subsequent contact; also to reactions in vitro with antibody-containing serum from such sensitized organisms. [L. *immunis,* free from service, fr. *in,* neg., + *munus* (*muner-*), service]

im•mune ad•her•ence (i-myūn′ ad-hēr′ĕns) The binding of antigen-antibody complexes or cells coated with antibodies or complement to cells bearing the appropriate complement or Fc receptors.

im•mune ad•sorp•tion (i-myūn′ ad-sōrp′shŭn) **1.** Removal of antibody from antiserum by use of specific antigen. **2.** Removal of antigen by specific antiserum.

im•mune com•plex (i-myūn′ kom′pleks) Antigen combined with specific antibody, to which complement may also be fixed and may precipitate or remain in solution. Frequently associated with autoimmune disease.

im•mune com•plex dis•ease (i-myūn′ kom′pleks di-zēz′) Immunologic category of diseases evoked by the deposition of antigen-antibody or antigen-antibody-complement complexes on cell surfaces, with subsequent development of vasculitis; nephritis is common. Most of the connective tissue diseases may belong in this immunologic category; immune complex diseases can also occur during a variety of diseases of known etiology, such as subacute bacterial endocarditis. SEE ALSO autoimmune disease.

im•mune e•lec•tron mi•cros•co•py (i-myūn′ ĕ-lek′tron mī-kros′kŏ-pē) Electron microscopy of biologic specimens to which specific antibody has been bound.

im•mune pa•ral•y•sis (i-myūn′ păr-al′i-sis) The induction of tolerance due to injection of large amounts of antigen. The antigen is poorly metabolized and the paralysis remains only during the persistence of the above.

im•mune re•ac•tion (i-myūn′ rē-ak′shŭn) Antigen-antibody reaction indicating a certain degree of resistance.

im•mune re•sponse (i-myūn′ rĕ-spons′) **1.** Any response of the immune system to an antigen including antibody production or cell-mediated immunity. **2.** The response of the immune system to an antigen (immunogen) that leads to the condition of induced sensitivity; the immune response to the initial antigenic exposure (primary immune response) is detectable, as a rule, only after a lag period of from several days to 2 weeks; the immune response to a subsequent stimulus (secondary immune response) by the same antigen is more rapid than in the case of the primary immune response.

im•mune re•sponse genes (i-myūn′ rĕ-spons′ jēnz) Genes in the HLA-D region of the histocompatibility complex of human chromosome-6 that control the immune response to specific antigens.

im•mune se•rum (i-myūn′ sēr′ŭm) SYN antiserum.

im•mune sur•veil•lance (i-myūn′ sŭr-vā′lăns) A theory that the immune system destroys tumor cells, which are constantly arising during the life of the individual. SYN immunologic surveillance.

im•mune sys•tem (i-myūn′ sis′tĕm) An intricate complex of interrelated cellular, molecular, and genetic components, which provides a defense (immune response) against foreign organisms or substances and aberrant native cells.

im•mune throm•bo•cy•to•pe•nic pur•pu•ra (i-myūn′ throm′bō-sī-tō-pē′nik pŭr′pyŭr-ă) SYN idiopathic thrombocytopenic purpura.

im•mu•ni•fa•cient (im′yū-ni-fā′shĕnt) Making immune after a specific disease. [L. *immunis,* exempt, + *faciens,* making, pr. part. of *facio*]

im•mu•ni•ty (i-myū′ni-tē) The status or quality of being immune (1). SYN insusceptibility. [L. *immunitas* (see immune)]

im•mu•ni•za•tion (im′myū-nī-zā′shŭn) Protection of susceptible individuals from communicable diseases by administration of a living modified agent, a suspension of killed organisms, or an inactivated toxin. SEE ALSO vaccination.

im•mu•nize (im′yū-nīz) To render immune.

♻**immuno-** Combining form meaning immune, immunity. [L. *immunis,* immune]

im•mu•no•ad•ju•vant (im′yū-nō-ad′jū-vănt) SEE adjuvant (2).

im•mu•no•as•say (im′yū-nō-as′ā) Detection and assay of substances by serologic (immunologic) methods. SEE ALSO radioimmunoassay, radioimmunoelectrophoresis, immunologic pregnancy test. SYN immunochemical assay.

im•mu•no•blast (im′yū-nō-blast) An antigenically stimulated lymphocyte; a large cell with well-defined basophilic cytoplasm, a large nucleus with prominent nuclear membrane, distinct nucleoli, and clumped chromatin. [immuno- + G. *blastos,* germ]

im•mu•no•blot, im•mu•no•blot•ting (im′yū-nō-blot′, -blot′ing) Process by which antigens can be separated by electrophoresis and blotted to nitrocellulose sheets, where they bind and are subsequently identified by staining with labeled antibodies. SEE ALSO Western blot analysis.

im•mu•no•chem•i•cal as•say (im′yū-nō-kem′i-kăl as′ā) SYN immunoassay.

im•mu•no•com•pe•tence (im′yū-nō-kom′pĕ-tĕns) The ability to produce a normal immune response.

im•mu•no•com•pe•tent (im′yū-nō-kom′pĕ-tĕnt) Possessing the ability to mount a normal immune response.

im•mu•no•com•pro•mised (im′yū-nō-kom′prŏ-mīzd) Denoting an individual with deficient immunologic mechanisms either because of an immunodeficiency disorder or because the system has been rendered so by immunosuppressive agents.

im•mu•no•com•pro•mised host (im′yū-nō-kom′prŏ-mīzd hōst) A person whose immune system's defenses have been weakened by exposure to disease, drugs, or radiotherapy.

im•mu•no•con•glu•ti•nin (im′yū-nō-kŏn-glū′ti-nin) An autoantibodylike immunoglobulin (IgM) formed by an organism against its own complement, following injection of complement-containing complexes or sensitized bacteria.

im•mu•no•cyte (im′yū-nō-sīt) An immunologically competent leukocyte capable of producing antibodies or reacting in cell-mediated immunity reactions. SEE ALSO I cell. [immuno- + G. *kytos*, cell]

im•mu•no•cy•to•ad•her•ence (im′yū-nō-sī′tō-ad-hēr′ĕns) A method for determining cell surface properties, in which immunoglobulin or receptors on the surface of one cell population cause cells with corresponding molecular configurations on their surface to adhere in rosettes around the cells.

im•mu•no•cy•to•chem•is•try (im′yū-nō-sī′tō-kem′is-trē) The study of cell constituents by immunologic methods, such as the use of fluorescent antibodies.

im•mu•no•de•fi•cien•cy (im′yū-nō-dĕ-fish′ĕn-sē) A condition resulting from a defective immune mechanism; may be primary (due to a defect in the immune mechanism itself) or secondary (dependent on another disease process). SYN immunologic deficiency.

im•mu•no•de•fi•cien•cy dis•ease (im′yū-nō-dĕ-fish′ĕn-sē di-zēz′) A disorder or condition related to a defective or suppressed immune response.

im•mu•no•de•fi•cient (im′yū-nō-dĕ-fish′ĕnt) Lacking in some essential function of the immune system.

im•mu•no•dif•fu•sion (im′yū-nō-di-fyū′zhŭn, im-ū′nō-) A technique of studying antigen-antibody reactions by observing precipitates formed by combination of specific antigen and antibodies that have diffused in a gel in which they have been separately placed.

im•mu•no•e•lec•tro•pho•re•sis (im′yū-nō-ē-lek′trō-fŏr-ē′sis) A kind of precipitin test in which the components of one group of immunologic reactants are first separated on the basis of electrophoretic mobility, the separated components then being identified on the basis of precipitates formed by reaction with components of the other group of reactants.

im•mu•no•en•hance•ment (im′yū-nō-en-hans′mĕnt) IMMUNOLOGY the potentiating effect of specific antibody in establishing and in delaying rejection of a tumor allograft. SYN immunologic enhancement.

im•mu•no•en•hanc•er (im′yū-nō-en-hans′ĕr) Any specific or nonspecific substance that increases the degree of the immune response.

im•mu•no•flu•o•res•cence (im′yū-nō-flŏr-es′ĕns) An immunohistochemical technique using labeling of antibodies by fluorescent dyes to identify bacterial, viral, or other antigenic material specific for the labeled antibody; the binding of antibody can be determined microscopically by the application of ultraviolet rays to the preparation. SEE ALSO fluorescent antibody technique.

im•mu•no•flu•o•res•cent stain (im′yū-nō-flŏr-es′sĕnt stān) Stain resulting from combination of fluorescent antibody with antigen specific for the antibody portion of the fluorochrome conjugate.

im•mu•no•gen (i-myū′nō-jen) SYN antigen.

im•mu•no•ge•net•ics (im′yū-nō-jĕ-net′iks) The study of the genetics of transplantation and tissue rejection, histochemical loci, immunologic response, immunoglobulin structure, and immunosuppression.

im•mu•no•gen•ic (im′yū-nō-jen′ik) SYN antigenic.

im•mu•no•ge•nic•i•ty (im′yū-nō-jĕ-nis′i-tē) SYN antigenicity.

im•mu•no•glob•u•lin (Ig) (im′yū-nō-glob′yū-lin) One of a class of structurally related proteins, each consisting of two pairs of polypeptide chains, one pair of light (L) [low molecular weight] chains (κ or λ), and one pair of heavy (H) chains (γ, α, δ, and ε), all four linked together by disulfide bonds. On the basis of the structural and antigenic properties of the H chains, Igs are classified (in order of relative amounts present in normal human serum) as IgG (7 S in size, 80%), IgA (10–15%), IgM (19 S, a pentamer of the basic unit, 5–10%), IgD (less than 0.1%), and IgE (less than 0.01%). These classes are all homogeneous and susceptible to amino acid sequence analysis. Each class of H chain can associate with either κ or λ L chains. Subclasses of Igs, based on differences in the H chains, are referred to as IgG1, and so on.

When split by papain, IgG yields three pieces: the Fc piece, consisting of the C-terminal portion of the H chains, with no antibody activity but capable of fixing complement, and crystallizable; and two identical Fab pieces, carrying the antigen-binding sites and each consisting of an L chain bound to the remainder of an H chain.

Antibodies are Igs, and all Igs probably function as antibodies. However, Ig refers not only to the usual antibodies, but also to a great number of pathologic proteins classified as myeloma proteins, which appear in multiple myeloma along with Bence Jones proteins, myeloma globulins, and Ig fragments.

From the amino acid sequences of Bence Jones proteins, it is known that all L chains are divided into a region of variable sequence (V_L) and one of constant sequence (C_L), each comprising about half the length of the L chain. The constant regions of all human L chains of the same type (κ or λ) are identical except for a single amino acid substitution, under genetic controls. H chains are similarly divided, although the V_H region, although similar in length to the V_L region, is only one third or one fourth the length of the C_H region. Binding sites are a combination of V_L and V_H protein regions. The large number of possible combinations of L and H chains make up the "libraries" of antibodies of each individual.

im•mu•no•glob•u•lin do•mains (im′yū-nō-glob′yū-lin dō-mānz′) Structural units of immunoglobulin heavy or light chains that are composed of approximately 110 amino acids. Light chains of an immunoglobulin are composed of one constant domain and one variable domain. Heavy chains are composed of either three or four constant domains and one variable domain.

im•mu•no•his•to•chem•is•try (im′yū-nō-his′tō-kem′is-trē) Demonstration of specific antigens in tissues by the use of markers that are either fluorescent dyes or enzymes.

im•mu•no•log•ic com•pe•tence (im′yū-nō-loj′ik kom′pĕ-tĕns) Capability of mounting an immunologic response.

im•mu•no•log•i•c de•fi•cien•cy (im′yū-nō-loj′ik dĕ-fish′ĕn-sē) SYN immunodeficiency.

im•mu•no•log•ic en•hance•ment (im′yū-nō-loj′ik en-hans′mĕnt) SYN immunoenhancement.

im•mu•no•log•ic mech•a•nism (im′yū-nō-loj′ik mek′ă-nizm) The groups of cells (chiefly lymphocytes and cells of the reticuloendothelial system) that function in establishing active acquired immunity (induced sensitivity, allergy).

im•mu•no•log•ic pa•ral•y•sis (im′yū-nō-loj′ik păr-al′i-sis) Lack of specific antibody production after exposure to large doses of an antigen; immunologic paralysis disappears when the antigen is eliminated.

im•mu•no•log•ic preg•nan•cy test (im′yū-nō-loj′ik preg′năn-sē test) A general term for assays to detect increased human chorionic gonadotropin in serum or urine by immunologic techniques including latex particle agglutination, hemagglutination inhibition, radioimmunoassay, and radioreceptor assays.

im•mu•no•log•ic sur•veil•lance (im′yū-nō-loj′ik sŭr-vā′lăns) SYN immune surveillance.

im•mu•no•log•ic tol•er•ance (im′yū-nō-loj′ik tol′ĕr-ăns) Lack of immune response to antigen. Theories of tolerance induction include clonal deletion and clonal anergy. In clonal deletion, the actual clone of cells is eliminated whereas in clonal anergy the cells are present but nonfunctional.

im•mu•nol•o•gist (im′yū-nol′ŏ-jist) A specialist in the science of immunology.

im•mu•nol•o•gy (im′yū-nol′ŏ-jē) **1.** The science concerned with the various phenomena of immunity, induced sensitivity, and allergy. **2.** Study of the structure and function of the immune system. [immuno- + G. *logos,* study]

im•mu•no•mod•u•la•to•ry (im′yū-nō-mod′yū-lă-tōr-ē) **1.** Capable of modifying or regulating one or more immune functions. **2.** An immunological adjustment, regulation, or potentiation.

im•mu•no•per•ox•i•dase tech•nique (im′yū-nō-pĕr-oks′i-dās tek-nēk′) An immunologic test that uses antibodies chemically conjugated to the enzyme peroxidase.

im•mu•no•phil•in (im′yū-nō-fil′in) Any of several high-affinity receptor proteins in the cytoplasm that combine with immunosuppressant drugs leading to rotamase inhibition and, in T cells, thus to interruption of cell activation. [*immune* + G. *philos,* fond, + in]

im•mu•no•po•ten•ti•a•tion (im′yū-nō-pō-ten′shē-ā′shŭn) Enhancement of the immune response by increasing its rate or prolonging its duration.

im•mu•no•po•ten•ti•a•tor (im′yū-nō-pō-ten′shē-ā-tŏr) Any substance that on inoculation enhances or augments an immune response.

im•mu•no•pro•lif•er•a•tive dis•or•ders (im′myū-nō-prō-lif′ĕr-ă-tiv dis-ōr′dĕrz) Disorders in which there is a continuing proliferation of cells of the immunocyte complex associated with autoallergic disturbances and immunoglobulin abnormalities, such as in chronic lymphocytic leukemia, the so-called macroglobulinemias, and multiple myeloma.

im•mu•no•ra•di•o•met•ric as•say (im′yū-nō-rā′dē-ō-met′rik as′ā) A procedure in which an unknown antigen binds to an excess of antibody that has a radioactive label. The unbound antibody is removed in a subsequent step. The amount of antigen present is directly proportional to the amount of measured radioactivity.

im•mu•no•re•ac•tive (im′yū-nō-rē-ak′tiv) Denoting or exhibiting immunoreaction.

im•mu•no•sor•bent (im′yū-nō-sōr′bĕnt) An antibody (or antigen) used to remove specific antigen (or antibody) from solution or suspension.

im•mu•no•sup•pres•sant (im′yū-nō-sŭ-pres′ănt) An agent that induces immunosuppression. SYN immunosuppressive (2).

im•mu•no•sup•pres•sion (im′yū-nō-sŭ-presh′ŭn) Prevention or interference with the development of immunologic response; may reflect natural immunologic unresponsiveness (tolerance), may be artificially induced by chemical, biologic, or physical agents, or may be caused by disease.

im·mu·no·sup·pres·sive (im′yū-nō-sŭ-pres′iv) **1.** Denoting or inducing immunosuppression. **2.** SYN immunosuppressant.

im·mu·no·sup·pres·sive ther·a·py (im′yū-nō-sŭ-pres′iv thār′ă-pē) Medication given to patients to curb response by their immune systems (e.g., patients who have undergone organ or tissue transplantation).

im·mu·no·sur·veil·lance (im′yū-nō-sŭr-vā′lăns) Theory that holds that the immune system eliminates tumor cells that arise spontaneously.

im·mu·no·ther·a·py (im′yū-nō-thār′ă-pē) Originally, therapeutic administration of serum or immune globulin containing preformed antibodies produced by another person; currently, immunotherapy includes nonspecific systemic stimulation, adjuvants, active specific immunotherapy, and adoptive immunotherapy. New forms of immunotherapy include the use of monoclonal antibodies. This method has been widely adopted in oncology, particularly in cases that fail to respond to other treatment. Immunotherapy seeks to boost immune system function, as with the administration of interferons and interleukin-2, or to attack cancerous cells directly, as with the injection of monoclonal antibodies. Various immunotherapeutic techniques have also been used in the treatment of AIDS. In addition, a number of alternative medical practices are claimed to enhance immune function, and various over-the-counter substances have gained popularity for this supposed property. SYN biologic immunotherapy.

im·mu·no·trans·fu·sion (im′yū-nō-trans-fyū′zhŭn) An indirect transfusion in which the donor is first immunized by injections of antigen from microorganisms isolated from the recipient; later, the donor's blood is collected, defibrinated, and then administered to the patient; the latter is thus passively immunized by antibody formed in the donor.

IMP Abbevation for inosine 5′-monophosphate.

im·pact·ed (im-pak′tĕd) Wedged or pressed closely so as to be immovable.

im·pact·ed fe·tus (im-pak′tĕd fē′tŭs) A fetus that, because of its large size or narrowing of the pelvic canal, has become wedged and incapable of spontaneous advance or recession.

im·pact·ed frac·ture (im-pak′tĕd frak′shŭr) A fracture in which one of the fragments is driven into the cancellous tissue of the other fragment.

im·pact·ed tooth (im-pak′tĕd tūth) **1.** A tooth the normal eruption of which is prevented by adjacent teeth or bone. **2.** A tooth that has been driven into the alveolar process or surrounding tissue as a result of trauma.

im·pact fac·tor (im′pakt fak′tŏr) Mathematic expression of frequency with which a particular medical journal's original articles are cited in other medical journals.

im·paired cog·ni·tion syn·drome (im-pārd′kog-nish′ŭn sin′drōm) First of three identified types of Gulf War syndrome (q.v.).

im·pair·ment (im-pār′mĕnt) Any loss or abnormality of psychological, physiologic, or anatomic structure or function.

im·par (im′pahr) Unpaired, azygous. [L. *im*, not + *par*, equal, a pair]

im·ped·ance (im-pē′dăns) **1.** Opposition to flow of gases, liquids, or electrical current. **2.** Resistance of an acoustic system to being set in motion.

im·ped·ance match·ing (im-pē′dăns mach′ing) The force delivered through the mechanical advantages of the tympanic ossicles and the area ratio of the tympanic membrane to the oval window to overcome the acoustic impedance between the ambient air and the fluid in the inner ear.

im·per·fect fun·gus (im-pĕr′fĕkt fŭng′gŭs) A fungus in which the means of sexual reproduction is not yet recognized; these fungi generally reproduce by means of asexual structures called conidia. Cf. Fungi Imperfecti.

im·per·fect stage (im-pĕr′fĕkt stāj) A mycologic term used to describe the asexual life cycle phase of a fungus.

im·per·fo·rate (im-pĕr′fŏr-āt) SYN atretic.

im·per·fo·rate a·nus (im-pĕr′fŏr-āt ā′nŭs) **1.** SYN anal atresia. **2.** SYN ectopic (1).

im·per·fo·ra·tion (im′pĕr-fŏr-ā′shŭn) Condition of being atretic, occluded, or closed. [L. *im*- neg. + *per-foro*, pp. *-atus*, to bore through]

im·per·me·a·ble (im-pĕr′mē-ă-bĕl) Not permitting the passage of liquids, gases, or heat through a membrane or other structure. [L. *impermeabilis*, not to be passed through]

im·pe·tig·i·nous (im′pe-tij′i-nŭs) Relating to impetigo.

im·pe·ti·go (im-pĕ-tī′gō) A contagious superficial pyoderma, caused by *Staphylococcus aureus* or group A streptococci that begins with a superficial flaccid vesicle that ruptures to form a thick yellowish crust, most commonly occurring on the faces of children. See page 780, B4, B11. SYN impetigo contagiosa, impetigo vulgaris. [L. a scabby eruption, fr. *im-peto* (*inp-*), to rush upon, attack]

im·pe·ti·go con·ta·gi·o·sa (im-pĕ-tī′gō kon-tā-jē-ō′să) SYN impetigo.

im·pe·ti·go her·pet·i·for·mis (im-pĕ-tī′gō hĕr-pet-i-fōr′mis) A rare pyoderma, occurring most commonly in the third trimester of preg-

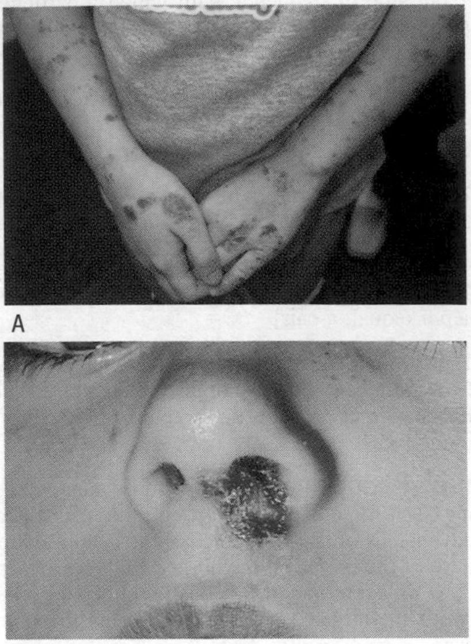

A

B

impetigo: (A) forearms and hands; (B) nostril

nancy as an eruption of small closely aggregated pustules accompanied by severe constitutional symptoms and fetal death.

im·pe·ti·go ne·o·na·to·rum (im-pĕ-tī′gō nē-ō′nā-tō′rum) **1.** SYN dermatitis exfoliativa infantum. **2.** SYN bullous impetigo of newborn.

im·pe·ti·go vul·ga·ris (im-pĕ-tī′gō vul′gā′ris) SYN impetigo.

im·pinge·ment sign (im-pinj′mĕnt sīn) Pain in patients with rotator cuff tendinitis or tears within the subacromial space elicited by provocative physical examination maneuvers.

im·pingement syn·drome (im-pinj′mĕnt sin′drōm) Chronic shoulder pain and disability due to trauma to the rotator cuff (particularly the supraspinatus tendon) by surrounding bony processes and ligaments, such as occurs during overhead work.

im·pinge·ment test (im-pinj′mĕnt test) Diagnostic test in which local anesthetic is injected into the subacromial space of a patient with impingement signs; relief of pain following the injection during provocative maneuvers is helpful in confirming the subacromial space as the source of the symptoms.

im·plant **1.** (im-plant′) To graft or insert. **2.** (im′plant) Material inserted or grafted into tissues. SEE ALSO graft, transplant. **3.** DENTISTRY a graft or insert set in or onto the alveolar recess prepared for its insertion. SEE ALSO implant denture. **4.** ORTHOPAEDICS a metallic or plastic device employed in joint reconstruction. [L. *im-*, in, + *planto,* pp. *-atus,* to plant, fr. *planta,* a sprout, shoot]

im·plan·ta·tion (im′plan-tā′shŭn) **1.** Attachment of the blastocyst to the endometrium, and its subsequent embedding in the compact layer, occurring 6–7 days after fertilization of the oocyte in humans. **2.** The process of placing a device or substance within the body, e.g., placement of a saline-filled device beneath the breast mound. **3.** Insertion of a natural tooth into an artificially constructed alveolus. **4.** Tissue grafting. SEE ALSO transplantation.

im·plant den·ture (im′plant den′chŭr) A denture that receives its stability and retention from a substructure that is partially or wholly implanted under the soft tissues of the denture basal seat.

im·plant·ed su·ture (im-plant′ĕd sū′chŭr) Passage of a pin through each lip of the wound parallel to the line of incision, the pins then being looped together with sutures.

im·ple·men·ta·tion (im′plĕ-mĕn-tā′shŭn) A step of the nursing process. It follows assessment, nursing diagnosis, and planning. In this stage, the nursing actions are carried out. SYN intervention (3).

im·pli·cit learn·ing (im-pli′sit lĕrn-ing) Observable improvements in a person's motor performance but of which the person has no awareness.

im·plied con·sent (im′plīd kon′sent) **1.** SYN emergency doctrine. **2.** Granting of permission for health care without formal agreement, when a patient makes an appointment with a physician.

im·plo·sion (im-plō′zhŭn) **1.** A sudden collapse, as of an evacuated vessel, in which there is a bursting inward rather than outward as in explosion. **2.** A type of behavior therapy, similar to flooding, during which the patient is given massive exposure to extreme anxiety-arousing stimuli.

im·po·tence, im·po·ten·cy (im′pŏ-tĕns, -tĕn-sē) **1.** Weakness; lack of power. **2.** Inability of the male to achieve and/or maintain penile erection and thus engage in copulation; a manifestation of neurologic, vascular, or psychological dysfunction. [L. *impotentia,* inability, fr. *in-*, neg., + *potentia,* power]

im·preg·nate (im-preg′nāt) **1.** To fertilize or fecundate; to cause to conceive. **2.** To permeate or saturate with another substance. SEE ALSO saturate. [L. *im-*, in, + *praegnans,* with child]

im·pres·si·o, pl. **im·pres·si·o·nes** (im-pres′ē-ō, -ō′nēz) [TA] SYN impression. [L.]

im·pres·sion (im-presh′ŭn) **1.** A mark seemingly made by the pressure of one structure or organ on another, seen especially in cadaveric dissections. See also *groove* for the various impressions of the lungs, e.g., descending aorta, subclavian artery, and vena cavae. **2.** An effect produced on the mind by some external object acting through the organs of sense. **3.** An imprint or negative likeness; especially, the negative form of the teeth and/or other tissues of the oral cavity, made in a plastic material that becomes relatively hard or set while in contact with these tissues, made to reproduce a positive form or cast of the recorded tissues; classified, according to the materials of which they are made, as reversible and irreversible hydrocolloid impression, modeling elastic gel impression, plaster impression, and wax impression. SYN impressio [TA]. [L. *impressio,* fr. *im- primo,* pp. *-pressus,* to press on]

im•pres•sion tray (im-presh′ŭn trā) A U-shaped receptacle that holds the material used for making a dental impression; can be metal or plastic, and prefabricated or custom made in the dental laboratory.

im•print•ing (im′print-ing) A particular kind of learning characterized by its occurrence in the first few hours of life, which determines species-recognition behavior.

im•prop•er dose quan•ti•ty (im-prop′ĕr dōs kwahn′ti-tē) Drug error in which the health care provider gives the wrong dose or quantity.

im•prove•ment (ĭm-prūv′mĕnt) The act or process of making better.

im•pulse (im′pŭls) **1.** A sudden pushing or driving force. **2.** A sudden, often unreasoning, determination to perform some act. **3.** The action potential of a nerve fiber. [L. *im-pello,* pp. *-pulsus,* to push against, impel (*inp-*)]

im•pulse con•trol dis•or•der (im′pŭls kŏn-trōl′ dis-ōr′dĕr) A class of mental disorders characterized by failure to resist an impulse to perform some act harmful to oneself or to others; includes pathologic gambling, pedophilia, kleptomania, pyromania, trichotillomania, and intermittent or isolated explosive disorders.

im•pul•sion (im-pŭl′shŭn) An abnormal urge to perform a certain activity.

im•pul•sive (im-pŭl′siv) Relating to or actuated by an impulse, rather than controlled by reason or careful deliberation.

im•pul•sive ob•ses•sion (im-pŭl′siv ŏb-sesh′ ŭn) An obsession accompanied by action, sometimes becoming a mania.

im•pure flut•ter (im-pyūr′ flŭt′ĕr) Mixture of atrial flutter (FF) waves and fibrillation (ff) waves in the electrocardiogram. SYN flitter, flutter-fibrillation.

IMRT Abbreviation for intensity modulated radiation therapy.

IMV Abbreviation for intermittent mandatory ventilation. SEE ALSO mode of ventilation.

In **1.** Symbol for indium. **2.** Abbreviation for inulin.

♻**in-** Prefix meaning (1) Not, akin to G. *a-*, *an-* or Eng. *un-;* (2) In, within, inside; (3) Very; appears as im- before b, p, or m. [L.]

in•ac•ti•vate (in-ak′ti-vāt) To destroy the biologic activity or the effects of an agent or substance.

in•ac•ti•vat•ed po•li•o•vi•rus vac•cine (in-ak′ti-vā-tĕd pō′lē-ō-vī′rŭs vak-sēn′) SEE poliovirus vaccine (1).

in•ac•tive re•pres•sor (in-ak′tiv rĕ-pres′ŏr) A repressor that cannot combine with an operator gene until it has combined with a corepressor (usually a product of a protein pathway); after activation, the repressor arrests production of the proteins controlled by the operator gene; a homeostatic mechanism for regulation of repressible enzyme systems. SYN aporepressor.

in•ad•e•quate per•son•al•i•ty (in-ad′ĕ-kwăt pĕr′sŏn-al′i-tē) A personality disorder, characterized by personal and social ineptness plus emotional and physical instability, which renders the person unable to cope with the normal vicissitudes of life.

in•ad•e•quate stim•u•lus (in-ad′ĕ-kwăt stim′ yū-lŭs) A stimulus too weak to evoke a response.

in•an•i•mate (in-an′i-măt) Not alive. [L. *in-* neg. + *anima,* breath, soul]

in•a•ni•tion (in′ă-nish′ŭn) Severe weakness and wasting as results from lack of food, defect in assimilation, or neoplastic disease. [L. *inanis,* empty]

in•ap•pe•tence (in-ap′ĕ-tĕns) Lack of desire or of craving. [L. *in-* neg. + *ap-peto,* pp. *-petitus,* to strive after, long for (*adp-*)]

in•ar•tic•u•late (in′ahr-tik′yū-lăt) **1.** Not fluent in the form of intelligible speech. **2.** Unable to satisfactorily express oneself in words.

in•as•sim•i•la•ble (in′ă-sim′il-ă-bĕl) Not easily incorporated; not capable of undergoing assimilation. SEE assimilation.

in•born (in′bōrn) Implanted during development in utero. In the specific context of inborn error of metabolism, it connotes a genetic disruption of an enzyme. SEE inborn errors of metabolism. SYN innate.

in•born er•rors of me•tab•o•lism (ĭn′bōrn er′ŏrz mĕ-tab′ŏ-lizm) A group of disorders, each of which involves a disorder of a single unique enzyme, genetic in origin and operating from birth; effects are ascribable to accumulation of the substrate on which the enzyme normally acts (e.g., phenylketonuria), to deficiency of the product of the enzyme (e.g., albinism), or to forced metabolism through an auxiliary pathway (e.g., oxaluria).

in•bred (in′bred) Denoting populations (e.g., groups, genetic lines) descended over several generations almost exclusively from a small set of ancestors, and hence having a high degree of consanguinity.

in•breed•ing (in′brēd-ing) **1.** Mating between organisms that are genetically more closely related than organisms selected at random from the population. **2.** A practice of mating animals that are closely related.

in•ca•pac•i•tat•ing chem•i•cal a•gent (in′kă-pas′i-tā-ting kem′i-kăl ā′jĕnt) **1.** In U.S. military parlance, a chemical agent designed for use on the battlefield to cause temporary impairment of a soldier's performance. The U.S. military usage specifically excludes riot-control agents and refers solely to anticholinergic compounds designed to cause lethargy and confusion. The only official U.S. military incapacitating agent is 3-quinuclidinyl benzilate, or QNB (NATO code BZ). **2.** In a more extended sense, any chemical compound designed to cause temporary impairment rather than serious illness or death. Examples include riot-control agents and opioids. Because in certain circumstances (e.g., high doses) these compounds can cause death, they should not be called *nonlethal agents.*

in•ca•pac•i•ta•ting Ct_{50} (ICt_{50}) (in′kă-pas′i-tā-ting) The Ct product required to produce incapacitation (temporary decrement in performance) in 50% of an exposed group.

in•ca•pac•i•ta•ting dose (in′kă-pas′i-tā-ting dōs) The dose of a chemical or biologic preparation (e.g., a bacterial exotoxin or a suspension of bacteria) that is likely to cause incapacitation; it varies in relation to the type of animal and the route of administration; when followed by a subscript (generally "ID_{50}" or median incapacitating dose), it denotes the dose likely to cause incapacitation in a certain percentage (e.g., 50%) of the test animals; median incapacitating dose is ID_{50}, absolute incapacitating dose is ID_{100} and minimal lethal dose is ID_{05}.

in•car•cer•at•ed (in-kahr′sĕr-ā-tĕd) Confined; imprisoned; trapped. [L. *in,* in, + *carcero,* pp. *-atus,* to imprison, fr. *carcer,* prison]

in•car•cer•at•ed her•ni•a (in-kahr′sĕr-ā-tĕd hĕr′nē-ă) SYN irreducible hernia.

in•cen•tive pay sys•tem (in-sen′tiv pā sis′tĕm) System whereby medical transcriptionists are paid based on how much they produce in addition to meeting quality requirements.

in•cen•tive spi•rom•e•ter (in-sen′tiv spī-rom′ĕ-tĕr) A device used in bronchial hygiene therapy that provides the patient with visual or other feedback during efforts to achieve a predetermined respiratory flow or volume; useful in increasing inspiratory volume, improving inspiratory muscle performance, maintaining airway patency, and preventing or reversing atelectasis. See this page.

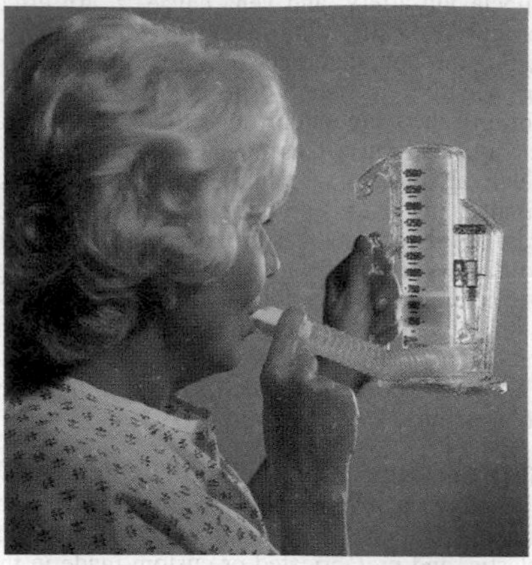

incentive spirometer: hand-held device helps postoperative patients, those with chest injuries, and others at risk of atelectasis to gauge lung expansion and air flow rates achieved during deep-breathing exercises

in•cest (in′sest) **1.** Sexual relations between people closely related by blood, especially between parents and their children, and between sibs. **2.** The crime of sexual relations between people related by blood, where such cohabitation is prohibited by law. [L. *incestus,* unchaste, fr. *in-,* not, + *castus,* chaste]

in•ces•tu•ous (in-ses′chū-ŭs) **1.** Pertaining to incest. **2.** Guilty of incest.

in•ci•dence (in′si-dĕns) **1.** The number of specified new events, e.g., people falling ill with a specified disease, during a specified period in a specified population. **2.** OPTICS intersection of a ray of light with a surface. [L. *incido,* to fall into or on, to happen]

in•ci•dent (in′si-dĕnt) **1.** Going toward; impinging on, as incident rays. **2.** (n.) An occurrence or event, generally an untoward, or unwelcome occurrence, e.g. a complication of an existing disease, a mishap affecting a patient in hospital. [L. *incido,* pp. *-casus,* to fall into, to meet with]

in•ci•dent•a•lo•ma (in′si-den′tă-lō′mă) Mass lesion, noted fortuitously during computed tomographic examinations performed for other reasons. [incidental + *-oma,* tumor]

in•ci•den•tal par•a•site (in′si-den′tăl par′ă-sīt) A parasite that normally lives on a host other than its present host. SYN accidental parasite.

in•ci•dent com•mand sys•tem (ICS) (in′si-dĕnt kŏ-mand′ sis′tĕm) A standardized but flexible disaster-management structure, mandated in the National Incident Management System (NIMS) (q.v.), for responding to mass-casualty incidents. It includes command, planning, operations, logistics, and finance/administration sections as well as other cells that are filled as needed.

in•ci•dent man•age•ment sys•tem (in′si-dĕnt man′ăj-mĕnt sis′tĕm) A nationally recognized system of unified command and control for dealing with mass casualties or disasters.

in•ci•dent point (in′si-dĕnt poynt) The point at which a light ray enters an optic system.

in•ci•dent re•port (in′si-dĕnt rē-pōrt′) Formal written description of an unusual occurrence, particularly an error or accident that has or may have adverse consequences.

in•ci•dent to (in′si-dĕnt tū) Term denoting when health care services are provided to a covered patient by allied health professionals (e.g., nurses, technicians, and other types of therapists) under the direct supervision of a physician.

in•ci•sal (in-sī′zăl) Cutting; relating to the cutting edges of the incisor and canine teeth. [L. *incido,* pp. *-cisus,* to cut into]

in•ci•sal guide an•gle (in-sī′zăl gīd ang′gĕl) The angle formed with the horizontal plane by drawing a line in the sagittal plane between incisal edges of the maxillary and mandibular central incisors when the teeth are in centric occlusion.

in•cise (in-sīz′) To cut with a knife.

in•cised wound (in-sīzd′ wūnd) A clean cut, as by a sharp instrument.

i **in•ci•sion** (in-sizh′ŭn) A cut; a surgical wound; a division of the soft parts made with a knife. See this page. [L. *incisio*]

in•ci•sion•al her•ni•a (in-si′zhŭn-ăl hĕr′nē-ă) Hernia occurring through a surgical incision or scar.

in•ci•sion bi•op•sy (in-sizh′ŭn bī′op-sē) Removal of only a part of a lesion by incising into it.

in•ci•sive (in-sī′siv) **1.** Cutting; having the power to cut. **2.** Relating to the incisor teeth.

in•ci•sive bone (in-sī′siv bōn) SYN os incisivum.

in•ci•sive ca•nal, in•ci•sor ca•nal (in-sī′siv kă-nal′, in-sī′zŏr) One of several bony canals leading from the floor of the nasal cavity into the incisive fossa on the palatal surface of the maxilla; they convey the nasopalatine nerves and branches of the greater palatine arteries that anastomose with the septal branch of the sphenopalatine artery. SYN canalis incisivus [TA].

in•ci•sive ca•nal cyst (in-sī′siv kă-nal′ sist) A cyst in or near the incisive canal, arising from proliferation of epithelial remnants of the nasopalatine duct; the most common maxillary developmental cyst.

in•ci•sive fo•ra•men (in-sī′siv fōr-ā′mĕn) One of several (usually four) openings of the incisive canals into the incisive fossa.

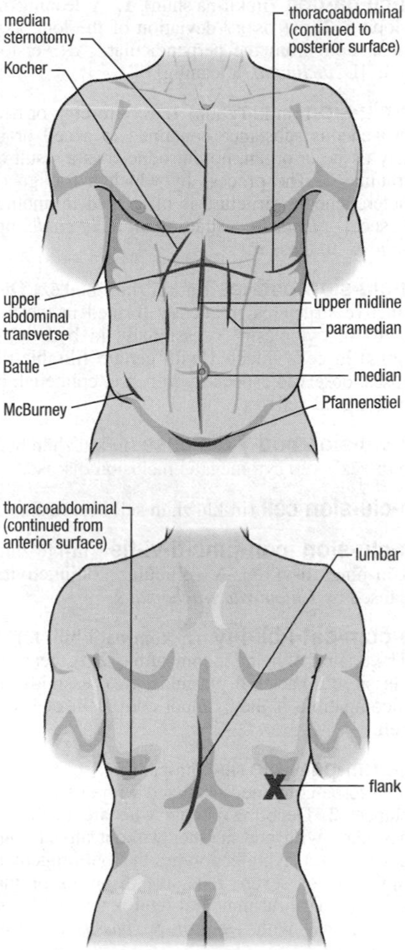

surgical incisions

in•ci•sive pa•pil•la (in-sī′siv pă-pil′ă) A slight elevation of the mucosa at the anterior extremity of the raphe of the palate; lying directly anterior to the underlying incisive fossa.

in•ci•sor (in-sī′zŏr) SYN incisor tooth. [L. *incido,* to cut into]

in•ci•sor tooth (in-sī′zŏr tūth) A tooth with a chisel-shaped crown and a single conic tapering root; there are four of these teeth in the anterior part of each jaw, in both the deciduous and the permanent dentitions (e.g., central and lateral teeth). SYN dens incisivus [TA], incisor.

in•ci•su•ra, pl. **in•ci•su•rae** (in′sis-ū′ră, -rē) [TA] SYN notch. [L. a cutting into]

in•ci•sure (in-sī′zhūr) SYN notch. [L. *incisura*]

in·cli·na·tion (in′kli-nā′shŭn) **1.** A leaning or sloping. **2.** DENTISTRY deviation of the long axis of a tooth from the perpendicular. SYN version (3). [L. *inclinatio,* a leaning]

in·clu·sion (in-klū′zhŭn) **1.** Any foreign or heterogeneous substance contained in a cell or in any tissue or organ, not introduced as a result of trauma. **2.** The process by which a foreign or heterogeneous structure is misplaced in another tissue. [L. *inclusio,* a shutting in, fr. *in-cludo,* pp. *-clusus,* to close in]

in·clu·sion bod·ies (in-klū′zhŭn bod′ēz) Distinctive structures frequently formed in the nucleus or cytoplasm (occasionally in both locations) in cells infected with certain filtrable viruses, observed especially in nerve, epithelial, or endothelial cells.

in·clu·sion bod·y dis·ease (in-klū′zhŭn bod′ē di-zēz′) SYN cytomegalic inclusion disease.

in·clu·sion cell (in-klū′zhŭn sel) SYN I cell.

in·clu·sion con·junc·ti·vi·tis (in-klū′zhŭn kŏn-jŭngk′ti-vī′tis) A follicular conjunctivitis caused by *Chlamydia trachomatis.*

in·com·pat·i·bil·i·ty (in′kŏm-pat′i-bil′i-tē) **1.** The quality of being incompatible. **2.** A means of classifying bacterial plasmids; two plasmids are incompatible if they cannot coexist in one host cell.

in·com·pat·i·ble (in-kŏm-pat′i-bĕl) **1.** Not suitable to be combined or mixed with another substance. **2.** Denoting people who are unable to associate with one another without anxiety and conflict. **3.** Having genotypes that put progeny at high risk of severe recessive disorders or that promote harmful maternal-fetal reaction. [L. *in-* neg., + *con-,* with, + *patior,* pp. *passus,* to suffer, tolerate]

in·com·pe·tence, in·com·pe·ten·cy (in-kom′pĕ-tĕns, -tĕn-sē) **1.** The quality of being incompetent or incapable of performing the allotted function, especially failure of cardiac or venous valves to close completely. SYN insufficiency (2). **2.** FORENSIC PSYCHIATRY the inability to distinguish right from wrong or to manage one's affairs. **3.** Inability of the cervix to remain closed and thereby continue pregnancy to term. [L. *in-,* neg. + *com-peto,* strive after together]

in·com·pe·tent cer·vi·cal os (in-kom′pĕ-tĕnt sĕr′vi-kăl os) A defect in the strength of the internal os allowing premature dilation of the cervix.

in·com·plete a·bor·tion (in′kŏm-plēt′ ă-bōr′shŭn) Abortion in which parts of the products of conception have been passed but some others (usually the placenta) remain in the uterus.

in·com·plete an·ti·bod·y (in′kŏm-plēt′ an′ti-bod-ē) **1.** SYN univalent antibody. **2.** SYN serum agglutinin.

in·com·plete an·ti·gen (in′kŏm-plēt′ an′ti-jen) SYN hapten.

in·com·plete fis·tu·la (in′kŏm-plēt′ fis′chū-lă) SYN blind fistula.

in·com·plete foot pre·sen·ta·tion (in′kŏm-plēt′ fut prez′ĕn-tā′shŭn) SEE breech presentation.

in·com·plete frac·ture (in′kŏm-plēt frak′shŭr) A fracture in which the bone is not completely divided.

in·com·plete pro·tein (in′kŏm-plēt′ prō′tēn) A protein food that lacks all essential amino acids.

in·con·stant (in-kon′stănt) **1.** Irregular. **2.** ANATOMY denoting a structure, such as an artery, or nerve, that may or may not be present.

in·con·ti·nence (in-kon′ti-nĕns) **1.** Inability to prevent the discharge of urine or feces. **2.** Lack of restraint of the appetites, especially sexual. SYN incontinentia. [L. *in-continentia,* fr. *in-,* neg., + *con-tineo,* to hold together, fr. *teneo,* to hold]

in·con·ti·nent (in-kon′ti-nĕnt) Denoting incontinence.

in·con·ti·nen·ti·a (in-kon′ti-nen′shē-ă) SYN incontinence. [L.]

in·co·or·di·na·tion (in′kō-ōr′di-nā′shŭn) SYN ataxia. [L. *in-,* neg., + coordination]

in·crease (in′krēs) Any growth in quantity.

in·cre·ment (in′krĕ-mĕnt) A change in the value of a variable; usually an increase, with "decrement" applied to a decrease, although "increment" can also correctly be applied to both. [L. *incrementum,* increase]

in·cre·tin (in-krē′tin) Generic term for all insulinotropic substances originating in the gastrointestinal tract that are released into the circulation by meals containing glucose. One is glucose-dependent insulinotropic polypeptide, which is released into the circulation from crypt cells in the proximal duodenum and jejunum after meals containing glucose or long-chain fatty acids. Another is proglucagon-derived polypeptide, cleavage product of glucagon, which is further processed into glucagonlike peptide-1 and then to glucagonlike insulinotropic peptide. Cf. bioregulator.

in·cre·tion (in-krē′shŭn) The functional activity of an endocrine gland. [in- + secretion]

in·crus·ta·tion (in′krŭs-tā′shŭn) **1.** Formation of a crust or a scab. **2.** A coating of some adventitious material or an exudate; a scab. [L. *incrusto,* pp. *-atus,* to incrust, fr. *crusta,* crust]

in·cu·ba·tion (in′kyū-bā′shŭn) **1.** Maintaining controlled environmental conditions to favor growth or development of microbial or tissue cultures. **2.** Maintaining artificial environment for an infant, usually one who is premature or hypoxic, by providing proper temperature, humidity, and, usually, oxygen. **3.** Developing, without sign or symptom, an infection from the time the infectious agent gains entry until the appearance of the first signs or symptoms. [L. *incubo,* to lie on]

in·cu·ba·tion pe·ri·od (in′kyū-bā′shŭn pēr′ē-ŏd) **1.** The interval between invasion of the body by an infecting organism and the appearance of the first sign or symptom it causes. SYN incubative stage, latent period (3), latent stage, prodromal stage. **2.** In a disease vector, the period between entry of the disease organism and the time at which the vector is capable of transmitting the disease to another human host.

in·cu·ba·tive stage (in′kyū-bā′tiv stāj) SYN incubation period (1).

in·cu·ba·tor (in′kyū-bā-tŏr) **1.** A container in which controlled environmental conditions can be maintained (e.g., for culturing microorganisms). **2.** An apparatus for maintaining an infant (usually premature) in an environment of proper oxygenation, humidity, and temperature.

in·cu·bus (in′kyū-bŭs) **1.** Originally, an evil spirit that lay on and oppressed sleeping people, especially, a male spirit that copulated with sleeping women. Cf. succubus. **2.** SYN nightmare. [L. fr. *incubo,* to lie on]

in·cu·dal (in′kū-dăl) Relating to the incus.

in·cu·dec·to·my (in′kū-dek′tŏ-mē) Removal of the incus of the tympanum. [incus + G. *ektomē,* excision]

in·cu·des (in-kū′dēz) Plural of incus. [L.]

in·cu·do·sta·pe·di·al (in-kū′dō-stā-pē′dē-ăl) Relating to the incus and the stapes; denoting the articulation between the incus and the stapes in the middle ear.

in·cur·va·tion (in′kŭr-vā′shŭn) An inward curvature; a bending inward.

in·cus, gen. **in·cu·dis**, pl. **in·cu·des** (ing′kŭs, in-kū′dis, -dēz) [TA] The middle of the three ossicles in the middle ear; it has a body and two limbs or processes (long crus and short crus); at the tip of the long crus is a small knob, the lenticular process that articulates with the head of the stapes. SYN anvil. [L. anvil]

in·cy·clo·duc·tion (in-sī′klō-dŭk′shŭn) A cycloduction in which the upper pole of the cornea is rotated inward (medially). [in- + cyclo- + L. *duco*, pp. *ductus*, to lead]

in·cy·clo·pho·ri·a (in-sī′klō-fōr′ē-ă) A cyclophoria in which the 12-o'clock position in the iris tends to twist medially. [L. in- + cyclo- + G. *phora,* a carrying]

in·cy·clo·tro·pi·a (in-sī′klō-trō′pē-ă) A cyclotropia in which the upper poles of the corneas are rotated inward (medially) to each other. [in- + cyclo- + G. *tropē*, a turning]

IND Abbreviation for investigational new drug.

in·dem·ni·ty (in-dem′ni-tē) The agreement between an insurance company or other financial entity to underwrite the expenses incurred by a policyholder for covered services.

in·de·pen·dent liv·ing (in′dĕ-pen′dĕnt liv′ing) A philosophy for self-determination and equal opportunity for people with disabilities that includes the right to live with the same opportunities and choices as someone who does not have a disablility.

in·de·pen·dent liv·ing mod·el (in-dĕ-pen′dĕnt liv′ing mod′ĕl) Service delivery model that identifies the consumer as the decision maker regarding health care and other daily living needs on presentation of choices by health care providers.

in·de·pen·dent lung ven·ti·la·tion (ILV) (in′dĕ-pen′dĕnt lŭng ven′ti-lā′shŭn) A mode of mechanical ventilation.

in·de·pen·dent med·i·cal e·val·u·a·tion (IME) (in′dĕ-pen′dĕnt mĕd′i-kăl ĕ-val′yū-ā-shŭn) Used by insurers to determine a patient's diagnosis, need for continued treatment, degree and permanency of disability, or ability to return to work.

in·de·pen·dent nurs·ing ac·tions (in′dĕ-pen′dĕnt nŭrs′ing ak′shŭnz) Nurse-initiated interventions; actions prescribed independently by nurses for patient care; initiated without supervision.

in·de·pen·dent prac·tice as·so·ci·a·tion (in′dĕ-pen′dĕnt prak′tis ă-sō′sē-ā′shŭn) An association of independent physicians or small groups of physicians formed for the purpose of contracting with one or more managed health care organizations. Member physicians provide medical services for patients enrolled in those organizations in their own offices and are allowed to maintain private practices. SEE ALSO managed care, health maintenance organization.

in·de·pen·dent prac·tice as·so·ci·a·tion HMO (in′dĕ-pen′dĕnt prak′tis ă-sō′sē-ā′shŭn) An arrangement by which physician providers are paid by the HMO on a fee-for-service basis for each patient seen, under terms negotiated with the HMO.

in·de·pen·dent var·i·a·ble (in′dĕ-pen′dĕnt var′ē-ă-bĕl) STATISTICS a variable that is manipulated by the researcher and measured by the effect it has on the dependent variable or variables.

in·dex, gen. **in·di·cis**, pl. **in·di·ces**, **in·dex·es** (in′deks, -di-sis, -di-sēz, -dek-sĕz) **1.** [TA] SYN index finger. **2.** A guide, standard, indicator, symbol, or number denoting the relation in respect to size, capacity, or function, of one part or thing to another. SEE ALSO quotient, ratio. **3.**

A core or mold used to record or maintain the relative position of a tooth or teeth to one another or to a cast. **4.** A guide, usually made of plaster, used to reposition teeth, casts, or parts. **5.** EPIDEMIOLOGY a rating scale. [L. one that points out, an informer, the forefinger, an index, fr. *in-dico,* pp. *-atus,* to declare]

in·dex case (in′deks kās) The first case in the investigation of the outbreak of a potentially epidemic disease.

in·dex ex·ten·sor mus·cle (in′deks eks-ten′sŏr mŭs′ĕl) SYN extensor indicis muscle.

in·dex fin·ger (in′deks fing′gĕr) The second finger (the thumb being counted as the first). SYN index (1).

in·dex my·o·pi·a (in′deks mī-ō′pē-ă) A form of shortsightedness related to the refractive index in the ocular media.

In·di·an gin·seng (in′dē-ăn jin′seng) SYN ashwagandha.

In·di·an paint (in′dē-ăn pānt) SYN blood root.

in·di·can·i·dro·sis (in′di-kan′i-drō′sis) Excretion of indican in the sweat. [indican + G. *hidrōs,* sweat]

in·di·can·u·ri·a (in′di-kan-yūr′ē-ă) An increased urinary excretion of indican, a derivative of indol formed chiefly in the intestine when protein is putrefied; indol is also formed during the putrefaction of protein in other sites.

in·di·ca·tion (in′di-kā′shŭn) The basis or rationale for using a particular treatment or diagnostic test; may be furnished by a knowledge of the cause (causal indication), by the symptoms present (symptomatic indication), or by the nature of the disease (specific indication). [L., fr. *in-dico,* pp. *-atus,* to point out, fr. *dico,* to proclaim]

in·di·ca·tor (in′di-kā-tŏr) **1.** CHEMICAL ANALYSIS a substance that changes color within a certain definite range of pH or oxidation potential, or in any way renders visible the completion of a chemical reaction (e.g., litmus, phenolsulfonphthalein). **2.** An isotope that is used as a tracer. **3.** The labeled substance the distribution of which between reactants of a system is used to determine the amount of analyte present. [L. one that points out]

in·di·ces (in′di-sēz) Alternative plural of index.

in·dif·fer·ent go·nad (in-dif′ĕr-ĕnt gō′nad) The primordial organ in an embryo before its differentiation into testis or ovary.

in·dif·fer·ent tis·sue (in-dif′ĕr-ĕnt tish′ū) Undifferentiated, nonspecialized, embryonic tissue.

in·di·gent (in′dij-ĕnt) Having insufficient income to pay for medical care or other living necessities.

in·di·ges·tion (in′di-jes′chŭn) Nonspecific term for various symptoms resulting from a failure of proper digestion and absorption of food in the alimentary tract.

in·di·rect cal·o·rim·e·try (in′di-rekt′ kal′ŏr-im′ĕ-trē) Determination of heat production of an oxidation reaction by measuring uptake of oxygen or liberation of carbon dioxide and nitrogen excretion.

in·di·rect Coombs test (in′di-rekt′ kūmz test) SYN Coombs indirect test.

in·di·rect frac·ture (in′di-rekt′ frak′shŭr) A fracture, especially of the skull, which occurs at a point not at the site of impact.

in·di·rect he·mag·glu·ti·na·tion test (in′di-rekt′ hē′mă-glū′ti-nā′shŭn test) SYN passive hemagglutination.

in·di·rect im·mu·no·flu·o·res·cence (in′di-rekt′ im′yū-nō-flōr-es′ĕns) Fluorescence microscopy of normal tissue after application of the patient's serum, to detect antibodies to normal tissue components (autoantibodies). SEE ALSO fluorescent antibody technique.

in·di·rect lar·yn·gos·co·py (in′di-rekt′ lar′in-gos′kŏ-pē) Inspection of the larynx by means of a reflected image on a mirror.

in·di·rect nu·cle·ar di·vi·sion (in′di-rekt′ nū′klē-ĕr di-vizh′ŭn) SYN mitosis.

in·di·rect oph·thal·mo·scope (in′di-rekt′ of-thal′mŏ-skōp) An instrument designed to visualize the interior of the eye, with the instrument at arm's length from the subject's eye and the observer viewing an inverted image through a convex lens located between the instrument and the subject's eye.

in·di·rect re·act·ing bil·i·ru·bin (in′di-rekt′ rē-ak′ting bil′i-rū′bin) The fraction of serum bilirubin that has not been conjugated with glucuronic acid in the liver cell; so called because it reacts with the Ehrlich diazo reagent only when alcohol is added; increased levels are found in hepatic disease and hemolytic conditions.

in·di·rect trans·fu·sion (in′di-rekt′ trans-fyū′zhŭn) Transfusion into a patient of blood previously obtained from a donor and stored in a suitable container.

in·di·rect vi·sion (in′di-rekt′ vizh′ŭn) SYN peripheral vision.

in·di·um (In) (in′dē-ŭm) A metallic element, atomic no. 49, atomic wt. 114.82. [*indigo,* because of its blue line in the spectrum]

in·di·vid·u·al ha·bil·i·ta·tion plan (I.H.P.) (in′di-vij′yū-ăl hab-il′i-tā′shŭn plan) A document that outlines the provision of services provided to people with disabilities who reside in a group living arrangement to promote engagement in activities of daily living and functional independence.

In·di·vid·u·al·ized Ed·u·ca·tion Pro·gram (IEP) (in′di-vij′yū-ăl-īzd ej′ū-kā′shŭn prō′gram) In the U.S., an education program tailored to a particular student with a disability, the provision of which is mandated by law. Mandated by IDEA, an IEP has two parts; the plan itself and the written document supporting it. SEE ALSO Individuals with Disabilities Education Act.

in·di·vid·u·a·lized fam·i·ly ser·vice plan (IFSP) (in′di-vij′yū-ăl-īzd fam′i-lē sĕr′vis plan) The written contract that identifies the early intervention services designed for individual children and their families who are eligible for these services under the IDEA.

in·di·vid·u·al li·cen·sure (in′di-vij′ū-ăl lī′sĕn-shŭr) In health care regulation, granting a licence to a health care practitioner upon completion of her or his training and subsequent investigation by authorizing bodies.

in·di·vid·u·al prac·tice as·so·ci·a·tion (IPA) (in′di-vij′ū-ăl prak′tis ă-sō′sē-ā′shŭn) Form of HMO in which the patient does not need a referral or permission to see any physician in the plan.

in·di·vid·u·al psy·chol·o·gy (in′di-vij′yū-al sī-kol′ŏ-jē) SYN adlerian psychology.

In·di·vid·u·als with Dis·a·bil·i·ties Ed·u·ca·tion Act (IDEA) (in′di-vij′yū-ălz dis-ă-bil′i-tēz ej′ū-kā′shŭn akt) U.S. federal law (Public Law 94-142, enacted in 1975 and subsequently amended) guaranteeing all students with disabilities, ages 3–21 years, the right to a free and appropriate public education designed to meet their individual needs. SEE ALSO Individualized Education Program.

in·di·vid·u·a·tion (in′di-vij′yū-ā′shŭn) **1.** Development of the individual from the specific. **2.** JUNGIAN PSYCHOLOGY the process by which one's personality is differentiated, developed, and expressed. **3.** Regional activity in an embryo as a response to an organizer.

in·di·vid·u·a·tion field (in′di-vij′yū-ā′shŭn fēld) The field within which an organizer can bring about the rearrangement of primordial tissues in such a manner that a complete embryo is formed.

in·do·cy·a·nine green (in′dō-sī′ă-nēn grēn) A tricarbocyanine dye that binds to serum albumin and is used in blood volume determinations and in liver function tests.

in·do·cy·an·ine green an·gi·og·ra·phy (in′dō-sī′ă-nēn grēn an′jē-og′ră-fē) A test for studying choroidal vasculature by which indocyanine green dye, which absorbs infrared light at 805 nm and emits at 835 nm, is injected intravenously and photographed as it flows through the retinal and choroidal vessels.

in·dol·ac·e·tu·ri·a (in′dōl-as′ĕ-tyūr′ē-ă) Excretion of an appreciable amount of indoleacetic acid in the urine; a manifestation of Hartnup disease.

in·dol·a·mine (in-dol′ă-mēn) An indole or indole derivative containing a primary, secondary, or tertiary amine group.

in·dole (in′dōl) **1.** 2,3-benzopyrrole; basis of many biologically active substances (e.g., serotonin, tryptophan); formed in degradation of tryptophan. SYN ketole. **2.** Any of many alkaloids containing the indole (1) structure.

in·do·lent (in′dō-lĕnt) Inactive; sluggish; painless or nearly so, said of a morbid process. [L. *in-*, neg., + *doleo,* pr. p. *dolens* (*-ent-*), to feel pain]

in·do·lent bu·bo (in′dō-lĕnt bū′bō) A painless, chronic enlargement of an inguinal node.

in·do·lic ac·ids (in-dō′lik as′idz) Metabolites of L-tryptophan formed within the body or by intestinal microorganisms.

in·dox·yl (in-dok′sil) The radical of 3-hydroxyindole; a product of intestinal bacterial degradation of indoleacetic acid; increased amounts are excreted in the urine in phenylketonuria.

in·dox·yl·u·ri·a (in-dok′sil-yūr′ē-ă) The excretion of indoxyl, especially indoxyl sulfate, in the urine; indoxyluria may be associated with indicanuria, inasmuch as hydrolysis of indican results in formation of indoxyl.

in·duced a·bor·tion (in-dūst′ ă-bōr′shŭn) Abortion brought on deliberately by drugs or mechanical means.

in·duced en·zyme, **in·duc·i·ble en·zyme** (in′dūst en′zīm, in-dū′si-bĕl) An enzyme that can be detected in a growing culture of a microorganism, after the addition of a particular substance (inducer) to the culture medium, but not before the addition.

in·duced e·ryth·ro·cy·the·mi·a (in-dūst′ ĕ-rith′rō-sī-thē′mē-ă) SYN blood doping.

in·duced hy·po·ten·sion, **con·trolled hy·po·ten·sion** (in-dūst′ hī′pō-ten′shŭn, kŏn-trōld′) Deliberate acute reduction of arterial blood pressure to reduce operative blood loss by pharmacologic means during anesthesia and surgery.

in·duc·er (in-dūs′ĕr) A molecule, usually a substrate of a specific enzyme pathway, that combines with and deactivates an active repressor (produced by a regulator gene); this allows an operator gene previously repressed to activate the structural genes controlled by it to resume enzyme production.

in·duc·tance (in-dŭk′tăns) The coefficient of electromagnetic induction; the unit of inductance is the henry. SEE induction.

in·duc·tion (in-dŭk′shŭn) **1.** Production or causation. **2.** Production of an electric current or magnetic state in a body by electricity or magnetism in another body close to the first body. **3.** The period from the start of anesthesia to the establishment of a depth of anesthesia adequate for a surgical procedure. **4.** EMBRYOLOGY the influence exerted by an organizer or evocator on the differentiation of adjacent cells or on the development of an embryonic structure. **5.** A modification imposed on the offspring by the action of environment on the germ cells of one or both parents. **6.** MICROBIOLOGY a change from probacteriophage to vegetative phage, which may occur spontaneously or after stimulation by certain physical and chemical agents. **7.** ENZYMOLOGY the process of increasing the amount or the activity of a protein. SEE ALSO inducer. **8.** A stage in the process of hypnosis. **9.** Causal analysis; a method of reasoning in which an inference is made from one or more specific observations to a more general statement. Cf. deduction. [L. *inductio,* a leading in]

in•duc•tion of fol•lic•u•lo•gen•e•sis (in-duk′shŭn fŏ-lik′yū-lō-gen′ĕ-sis) Production of follicles by use of pharmacotherapeutic agents or hormones.

in•duc•tion of la•bor (in-duk′shŭn lā′bŏr) Medical attempt to improve the process of giving birth through drugs or surgical interventions and manipulation.

in•duc•tion pe•ri•od (in-dŭk′shŭn pēr′ē-ŏd) **1.** The period required for a specific agent to produce a disease. **2.** The interval from the causal action of a factor to initiation of disease. **3.** The interval between an initial injection of antigen and the appearance of demonstrable antibodies in the blood.

in•duc•tor (in-dŭk′tŏr) **1.** That which brings about induction. **2.** EMBRYOLOGY an evocator or an organizer.

in•du•rat•ed (in′dūr-ā-tĕd) Hardened, usually used with reference to soft tissues becoming extremely firm but not as hard as bone. [L. *in-duro,* pp. *-duratus,* to harden, fr. *durus,* hard]

in•du•ra•tion (in′dūr-ā′shŭn) **1.** The process of becoming extremely firm or hard, or having such physical features. SEE indurated. **2.** A focus or region of indurated tissue. SYN sclerosis (1). [L. *induratio*]

in•du•ra•tive (in-dūr′ă-tiv) Pertaining to, causing, or characterized by induration.

in•du•si•um, pl. **in•du•si•a** (in-dū′zē-ŭm, -zē-ă) **1.** A membranous layer or covering. **2.** The amnion. [L. a woman's undergarment, fr. *induo,* to put on]

in•du•si•um gris•e•um (in-dū′zē-ŭm gris′ē-ŭm) [TA] A thin layer of gray matter on the dorsal surface of the corpus callosum in which the medial and lateral longitudinal striae lie embedded. The indusium griseum is a rudimentary component of the hippocampus, continuous caudally around the splenium of the corpus callosum with the fasciolar gyrus, a slender convolution in turn continuous with the dentate gyrus of the hippocampus; rostrally the indusium griseum curves around the genu and rostrum of the corpus callosum and extends ventralward to the olfactory trigone as the tenia tecta or rudimentum hippocampi, hidden in the depth of the posterior parolfactory sulcus that marks the anterior border of the subcallosal gyrus or precommissural septum.

in•dus•tri•al dis•ease (in-dŭs′trē-ăl di-zēz′) A morbid condition resulting from exposure to an agent discharged by a commercial enterprise into the environment. Cf. occupational disease.

in•dus•tri•al hear•ing loss (in-dŭs′trē-ăl hēr′ ing loss) SYN noise-induced hearing loss.

in•dus•tri•al hy•giene (in-dŭs′trē-ăl hī′jēn) Practices adopted by an industrial concern to minimize occupation-related disease and injury.

in•dwell•ing cath•e•ter (IDC) (in′dwel-ing kath′ĕ-tĕr) A catheter left in place in the bladder, usually a balloon catheter.

in•e•bri•ant (in-ē′brē-ănt) **1.** Making drunk; intoxicating. **2.** An intoxicant, such as alcohol. SEE inebriation.

in•e•bri•a•tion (in-ē′brē-ā′shŭn) Intoxication, especially by alcohol. SEE inebriant. [L. *in-*, intensive + *ebrietas,* drunkenness]

In•er•mi•cap•si•fer (in-er-mī-kap′si-fer) Genus of tapeworm (order Cyclophyllidae) first recognized in humans in 1935; an arthropod is thought to be involved in disease transmission (rodent to human, human to human).

In•er•mi•cap•si•fer ma•da•gas•car•i•en•sis (in-er-mī-kap′si-fer mad′ă-gas-kar-ē-en′sis) An uncommon tapeworm infection in humans in Cuba, Madagascar, and in Africa. It is mainly found in children 1–3 years old, causing vague intestinal symptoms; suspected arthropod vector; proglottids, eggs, and egg capsules resemble those of *Raillietina* spp.

in•ert (in-ĕrt′) **1.** Slow in action; sluggish; inactive. **2.** Devoid of active chemical properties, as the inert gases. **3.** Denoting a drug or agent having no pharmacologic or therapeutic action. [L. *iners,* unskillful, sluggish, fr. *in,* neg. + *ars,* art]

in•ert gas•es (in-ĕrt′ gas′ĕz) SYN noble gases.

in•er•ti•a (in-ĕr′shē-ă) **1.** The tendency of a physical body to oppose any force tending to move it from a position of rest or to change its uniform motion. **2.** Denoting inactivity or lack of force, lack of mental or physical vigor, or sluggishness of thought or action. [L. want of skill, laziness]

in•er•ti•a time (in-ĕr′shē-ă tīm) The interval elapsing between the reception of the stimulus from a nerve and the contraction of the muscle.

in·ev·i·ta·ble a·bor·tion (in-ev′i-tă-bĕl ă-bōr′shŭn) Rupture of fetal membranes, onset of labor, or both before the fetus is viable.

in·ex·suf·fla·tor (in′eks′sŭf-lā-tŏr) Device that provides alternating positive and negative pressures to facilitate coughing.

in ex·tre·mis (in eks-trē′mis) At the point of death. [L. *extremus,* last]

in·fan·cy (in′făn-sē) Babyhood; the earliest period of extrauterine life; roughly, the first year of life.

in·fant (in′fănt) A child younger than 1 year of age; more specifically, a newborn baby. [L. *infans,* not speaking]

in·fant grasp re·flex (in′fănt′ grasp rē′fleks) SYN palmar reflex.

in·fan·ti·cide (in-fan′ti-sīd) **1.** The killing of an infant. **2.** One who murders an infant. [infant + L. *caedo,* to kill]

in·fan·tile (in′făn-tīl) **1.** Relating to, or characteristic of, infants or infancy. **2.** Denoting childish behavior.

in·fan·tile ac·ro·pus·tu·lo·sis (in′făn-tīl ak′rō-pŭs′tyū-lō′sis) A recurrent papulopustular and crusting pruritic eruption, usually in black children.

in·fan·tile au·tism (in′făn-tīl aw′tizm) A severe emotional disturbance of childhood characterized by qualitative impairment in reciprocal social interaction and in communication, language, and social development. SYN Kanner syndrome.

in·fan·tile ec·ze·ma (in′făn-tīl ek′sĕ-mă) Eczema in infants; the clinical appearance varies according to the dominant causative mechanism, e.g., contact-type hypersensitivity, candidiasis, atopy, seborrhea, or a combination including intertrigo and diaper dermatitis.

in·fan·tile hy·po·thy·roid·ism (in′făn-tīl hī′pō-thī′royd-izm) Disorder that may result from endemic congenital goiter; nonendemic cases are usually due to defective thyroidal embryogenesis, defective hypothalamic-pituitary function, congenital defects in thyroid hormone synthesis or action, or intrauterine exposure to goitrogenic agents.

in·fan·tile neu·ro·ax·o·nal dys·tro·phy (in-făn-tīl nūr′ō-ak-sŏ′năl dis′trŏ-fē) A rare, familial disorder of early childhood manifested as progressive psychomotor deterioration, increased reflexes, Babinski sign, hypotonia, and progressive blindness.

in·fan·tile os·te·o·ma·la·ci·a, ju·ve·nile os·te·o·ma·la·ci·a (in′făn-tīl os′tē-ō-mă-lā′shē-ă, jū′vĕ-nil) SYN rickets.

in·fan·tile pu·ru·lent con·junc·ti·vi·tis (in′făn-tīl pyūr′u-lĕnt kŏn-jŭngk′ti-vī′tis) SYN ophthalmia neonatorum.

in·fan·tile scur·vy (in′făn-tīl skŭr′vē) A cachectic condition in infants, resulting from malnutrition and marked by pallor, fetid breath, coated tongue, diarrhea, and subperiosteal hemorrhages; probably a combination of scurvy and rickets due to combined deficiency of vitamins C and D. SYN Barlow disease, osteopathia hemorrhagica infantum.

in·fan·tile sex·u·al·i·ty (in′făn-tīl sek′shū-al′i-tē) PSYCHOANALYSIS the body of theories concerning psychosexual development in infants and children; encompasses the overlapping oral, anal, and phallic phases during the first 5 years of life.

in·fan·tile spi·nal mus·cu·lar at·ro·phy (in′făn-til spī′năl mŭs′kyū-lăr at′rŏ-fē) Transmitted as autosomal recessive on chromosome 5q. Progressive dysfunction of the anterior horn cells in the spinal cord and brainstem cranial nerves with profound weakness and bulbar dysfunction occurring in the first 2 years of life. Three groups, based on age of clinical onset, are recognized.

in·fan·ti·lism (in-fan′ti-lizm) **1.** A state marked by slow development of mind and body. **2.** Childishness, as characterized by a temper tantrum of an adolescent or adult. **3.** Underdevelopment of the sexual organs.

in·fant mor·tal·i·ty rate (in′fănt mōr-tal′i-tē rāt) A measure of the rate of deaths of liveborn infants before their first birthday; the numerator is the number of infants less than 1 year of age born alive in a defined region during a calendar year who die before they are 1 year old; the denominator is the total number of live births.

in·farct (in′fahrkt) An area of necrosis resulting from a sudden insufficiency of arterial or venous blood supply. SYN infarction (2). [L. *in-farcio,* pp. *-fartus* (*-ctus,* an incorrect form), to stuff into]

in·farc·tion (in-fahrk′shŭn) **1.** Sudden insufficiency of arterial or venous blood supply due to emboli, thrombi, vascular torsion, or pressure that produces a macroscopic area of necrosis; the heart, brain, spleen, kidney, intestine, lung, and testes are likely to be affected, as are tumors, especially of the ovary or uterus. **2.** SYN infarct.

in·farc·tus my·o·car·di·i (in-fahrk′tŭs mī-ō-kahr′dē-ī) SYN myocardial infarction.

in·fect (in-fekt′) **1.** To enter, invade, or inhabit another organism, causing infection or contamination. **2.** To dwell internally, endoparasitically, as opposed to externally (infest). [L. *in-ficio,* pp. *-fectus,* to dip into, dye, corrupt, infect, fr. *in* + *facio,* to make]

in·fect·ed a·bor·tion (in-fek′tĕd ă-bōr′shŭn) A septic complication of an abortion.

in·fec·tion (in-fek′shŭn) Invasion of the body

by organisms that have the potential to cause disease.

in·fec·tion-ex·haus·tion psy·cho·sis (in-fek′shŭn-eg-zaws′chŭn sī-kō′sis) A mental disorder following an acute infection, shock, or chronic intoxication; begins as delirium followed by pronounced mental confusion with hallucinations and unsystematized delusions, and sometimes stupor.

in·fec·tion im·mu·ni·ty (in-fek′shŭn i-myū′ni-tē) The paradoxic immune status in which resistance to reinfection coincides with the persistence of the original infection.

in·fec·tion trans·mis·sion pa·ram·e·ter (in-fek′shŭn trans-mish′ŭn păr-am′ĕ-tĕr) The proportion of total possible contacts between infectious cases and susceptibles that lead to new infections. SEE ALSO serial interval, mass action principle.

in·fec·tious (in-fek′shŭs) **1.** Capable of being transmitted by infection, with or without actual contact. **2.** Caused by infection of the body by pathogenic organisms; *not* a synonym for *contagious*. SYN contagion, contagious. SYN infective.

in·fec·tious bo·vine ker·a·to·con·junc·ti·vi·tis (in-fek′shŭs bō′vīn ker′ă-tō-kŏn-jŭngk′ti-vī′tis) A disease of cattle caused by the bacterium *Moraxella bovis* and characterized by blepharospasm, conjunctivitis, lacrimation, and corneal opacity and ulceration. SYN pinkeye (2).

in·fec·tious crys·tal·line ker·a·top·a·thy (in-fek′shŭs kris′tă-lēn ker′ă-top′ă-thē) Fernlike, needle-shaped deposits that may be seen in bacterial keratitis, particularly that due to α-hemolytic streptococci.

in·fec·tious dis·ease, in·fec·tive dis·ease (in-fek′shŭs di-zēz′, in-fek′tiv) A disease resulting from the presence and activity of a microbial agent.

in·fec·tious ec·zem·a·toid der·ma·ti·tis (in-fek′shŭs ek-zem′ă-toyd dĕr′mă-tī′tis) An inflammatory reaction of skin adjacent to the site of a pyogenic infection; thought to be due to a local sensitization to the resident organisms.

in·fec·tious en·do·car·di·tis, in·fec·tive en·do·car·di·tis (in-fek′shŭs en′dō-kahr-dī′tis, in-fek′tiv) Endocarditis due to infection by microorganisms.

in·fec·tious hep·a·ti·tis vi·rus (in-fek′shŭs hep′ă-tī′tis vī′rŭs) SYN hepatitis A virus.

in·fec·tious mon·o·nu·cle·o·sis (in-fek′shŭs mon′ō-nū-klē-ō′sis) An acute febrile illness caused by the Epstein-Barr virus; frequently spread by saliva transfer; characterized by fever, sore throat, enlargement of lymph nodes and spleen, lymphocytosis with abnormal lymphocytes similar to monocytes, and heterophil antibody in serum.

in·fec·tious·ness (in-fek′shŭs-nĕs) The state or quality of being infectious.

in·fec·tious pap·il·lo·ma·vi·rus (in-fek′shŭs pap′i-lō′mă-vī′rŭs) SYN human papillomavirus.

in·fec·tive (in-fek′tiv) SYN infectious.

in·fec·tive dose (in-fek′tiv dōs) The number of organisms necessary to produce either an infection or an immunologic response in a host. Cf. minimal infecting dose.

in·fec·tive em·bo·lism (in-fek′tiv em′bō-lizm) SYN pyemic embolism.

in·fec·tiv·i·ty (in′fek-tiv′i-tē) **1.** The characteristic of a disease agent that embodies its capability to enter, survive in, and multiply in a susceptible host. **2.** The proportion of exposures in defined circumstances that result in infection.

in·fe·ri·or (in-fēr′ē-ŏr) **1.** Situated below or directed downward. **2.** ANATOMY situated nearer the soles of the feet in relation to a specific reference point; opposite of superior. **3.** Less useful or of poorer quality. [L. lower]

in·fe·ri·or al·ve·o·lar ar·ter·y (in-fēr′ē-ŏr al-vē′ŏ-lăr ahr′tĕr-ē) *Origin*, first part of maxillary artery; *distribution*, through mandibular foramen and canal to lower teeth and chin; *branches*, artery to mylohyoid, mental artery, dental arteries.

in·fe·ri·or al·ve·o·lar nerve (in-fēr′ē-ŏr al-vē′ŏ-lăr nĕrv) One of the terminal branches of the mandibular, it enters the mandibular canal to be distributed to the lower teeth, periosteum, and gingiva of the mandible; a branch, the mental nerve, passes through the mental foramen to supply the skin and mucosa of the lower lip and chin. SYN nervus alveolaris inferior [TA].

in·fe·ri·or a·nal nerves (in-fēr′ē-ŏr ā′năl nĕrvz) Several branches of the pudendal nerve that pass to the external anal sphincter and skin of the anal region. SYN nervi rectales inferiores [TA], inferior hemorrhoidal nerves, inferior rectal nerves, nervi anales inferiores.

in·fe·ri·or ba·sal vein (in-fēr′ē-ŏr bā′săl vān) Tributary to the common basal vein draining the medial and posterior part of the inferior lobe in each lung.

in·fe·ri·or bor·der (in-fēr′ē-ŏr bōr′dĕr) The caudal or lowermost margin of a structure.

in·fe·ri·or cer·e·bel·lar pe·dun·cle (in-fēr′ē-ŏr ser′ĕ-bel′ăr pĕ-dŭngk′ĕl) Large paired bundles of nerve fibers that develop on the dorsolateral surfaces of the upper medulla, extend under the lateral recesses of the rhomboid fossa and curve dorsally into the cerebellum medial to the middle cerebellar peduncle; composed of a larger (lateral) bundle, the restiform body, and a small (medial) bundle, the juxtarestiform body. Fibers forming this composite bundle originate from spinal neurons and medullary relay nuclei.

The largest constituent (restiform body) is crossed fibers from the inferior olive; it also contains the dorsal spinocerebellar tract and cerebellar projections from the lateral reticular nucleus, the accessory cuneate nucleus, the paramedian reticular nuclei, and the perihypoglossal nuclei. Vestibulocerebellar fibers are placed medially in the inferior cerebellar peduncle and are usually separately identified as the juxtarestiform body.

in•fe•ri•or ce•re•bral veins (in-fēr′ē-ŏr ser′ē-brăl vānz) Numerous cerebral veins that drain the undersurface of the cerebral hemispheres and empty into the cavernous and transverse sinuses.

in•fe•ri•or cer•vi•cal car•di•ac nerve (in-fēr′ē-ŏr sĕr′vi-kăl kahr′dē-ak nĕrv) A nerve passing from the stellate ganglion to the cardiac plexus.

in•fe•ri•or clu•ne•al nerves (in-fēr′ē-ŏr klū′nē-ăl nĕrvz) Branches of the posterior femoral cutaneous nerve that emerge from under the inferior border of the gluteus maximus to supply the skin of the lower half of the gluteal region. SYN nervi clunium inferiores.

in•fe•ri•or con•stric•tor mus•cle of phar•ynx (in-fēr′ē-ŏr kŏn-strik′tŏr mŭs′ĕl far′ingks) *Origin*, outer surfaces of thyroid (thyropharyngeal part) and cricoid (cricopharyngeal part, musculus cricopharyngeus; superior or upper esophageal sphincter muscle) cartilages; *insertion*, pharyngeal raphe in the posterior portion of wall of pharynx; *action*, narrows lower part of pharynx in swallowing, the cricopharyngeal part has a sphincteric function for the esophagus, allowing some voluntary control of eructation and reflux; *nerve supply*, pharyngeal plexus. SYN laryngopharyngeus, musculus constrictor pharyngis inferior, musculus laryngopharyngeus, superior esophageal sphincter.

in•fe•ri•or ep•i•gas•tric vein (in-fēr′ē-ŏr ep′i-gas′trik vān) Corresponds to the artery of the same name and empties into the external iliac vein just proximal to the inguinal ligament.

in•fe•ri•or ex•ten•sor ret•i•nac•u•lum (in-fēr′ē-ŏr eks-ten′sŏr ret′i-nak′yū-lŭm) A Y-shaped ligament restraining the extensor tendons of the foot distal to the ankle joint.

in•fe•ri•or fib•u•lar ret•i•nac•u•lum (in-fēr′ē-ŏr fib′yū-lăr ret′i-nak′yū-lŭm) Broad thickened band of deep fascia overlying fibularis longus and brevis tendons as they pass along the lateral margin of the foot, anchoring the tendons and their associated bursae in place; it is a lateral continuation of the stem of the Y-shaped inferior extensor retinaculum that attaches to the fibular trochlea of the calcaneus (which intervenes between the two tendons) and then continues to attach to the inferolateral aspect of the calcaneous. SYN inferior peroneal retinaculum.

in•fe•ri•or gan•gli•on of glos•so•pha•ryn•ge•al nerve (in-fēr′ē-ŏr gang′glē-ŏn glos′ō-făr-in′jē-ăl nĕrv) The lower of two sensory ganglions on the glossopharyngeal nerve as it traverses the jugular foramen.

in•fe•ri•or gan•gli•on of va•gus nerve (in-fēr′ē-ŏr gang′glē-ŏn vā′gŭs nĕrv) A large sensory ganglion of the vagus, anterior to the internal jugular vein. SYN ganglion inferius nervi vagi [TA].

in•fe•ri•or ge•mel•lus mus•cle (in-fēr′ē-ŏr jĕ-mel′ŭs mŭs′ĕl) *Origin*, tuberosity of ischium; *insertion*, tendon of musculus obturator internus; *action*, rotates thigh laterally; *nerve supply*, sacral plexus. SYN gemellus, musculus gemellus inferior.

in•fe•ri•or glu•te•al ar•ter•y (in-fēr′ē-ŏr glū′tē-ăl ahr′tĕr-ē) *Origin*, internal iliac; *distribution*, hip joint and gluteal region; *anastomoses*, branches of internal pudendal, lateral sacral, superior gluteal, obturator, medial, and lateral circumflex femoral. SYN arteria glutea inferior, arteria ischiadica.

in•fe•ri•or glu•te•al nerve (in-fēr′ē-ŏr glū′tē-ăl nĕrv) Arises as a branch of the sacral plexus, conveying fibers from the fifth lumbar and first and second sacral nerves, and supplies the gluteus maximus muscle. It is subject to injury by compression and ischemia in sedentary people, resulting in difficulty in rising from a sitting position and difficulty climbing stairs. SYN nervus gluteus inferior.

in•fe•ri•or hem•or•rhoid•al ar•ter•y (in-fēr′ē-ŏr hem′ŏr-oyd′ăl ahr′tĕr-ē) SYN inferior rectal artery.

in•fe•ri•or hem•or•rhoid•al nerves (in-fēr′ē-ŏr hem′ŏr-oyd′ăl nĕrvz) SYN inferior anal nerves.

in•fe•ri•or hy•po•gas•tric (nerve) plex•us (in-fēr′ē-ŏr hī′pō-gas′trik nĕrv pleks′ŭs) One of the bilateral mixed (sympathetic, parasympathetic) autonomic plexus in the pelvis distributed to the pelvic viscera; it receives the hypogastric nerves and the pelvic splanchnic nerves and conveys visceral afferent fibers.

in•fe•ri•or•i•ty (in-fēr′ē-ōr′i-tē) The condition or state of being or feeling inadequate or inferior, especially relative to one's peers or to others similarly situated.

in•fe•ri•or•i•ty com•plex (in-fēr′ē-ōr′i-tē kom′pleks) A sense of inadequacy that is expressed in extreme shyness, diffidence, or timidity, or as a compensatory reaction in exhibitionism or aggressiveness.

in•fe•ri•or la•bi•al ar•ter•y (in-fēr′ē-ŏr lā′bē-ăl ahr′tĕr-ē) SYN inferior labial branch of facial artery.

in•fe•ri•or la•bi•al branch of fa•cial ar•ter•y (in-fēr′ē-ŏr lā′bē-ăl branch fā′shăl ahr′tĕr-ē) *Origin*, facial; *distribution*, structures of lower lip; *anastomoses*, the artery from the opposite side, mental and sublabial. SYN arteria labialis inferior, inferior labial artery, ramus labialis inferior arteriae facialis.

in·fe·ri·or la·bi·al vein (in-fēr′ē-ŏr lā′bē-ăl vān) A tributary of the facial vein draining the lower lip.

in·fe·ri·or lin·gual mus·cle (in-fēr′ē-ŏr ling′gwăl mŭs′ĕl) SYN inferior longitudinal muscle of tongue.

in·fe·ri·or lin·gu·lar ar·ter·y (in-fēr′ē-ŏr ling′gyū-lăr ahr′tĕr-ē) Branch (of the lingular branch) of the left pulmonary artery serving the inferior lingular segment of the superior lobe of the left lung. SYN arteria lingularis inferior, inferior lingular branch (of lingular branch) of left pulmonary artery, ramus lingularis inferior.

in·fe·ri·or lin·gu·lar branch (of lin·gu·lar branch) of left pul·mon·ar·y ar·ter·y (in-fēr′ē-ŏr ling′gyū-lăr branch ling′gyū-lăr branch left pul′mŏ-nar-ē ahr′tĕr-ē) SYN inferior lingular artery.

in·fe·ri·or lin·gu·lar (bron·cho·pul·mon·ar·y) seg·ment (in-fēr′ē-ŏr ling′gyū-lăr brong′kō-pul′mŏ-nar-ē seg′mĕnt) Of the four bronchopulmonary segments that typically comprise the superior lobe of the left lung, the most inferior, supplied by the inferior lingular bronchus and inferior lingular segmental (pulmonary) artery; corresponds approximately in position to the medial segment of the middle lobe of the right lung; the lingula is a feature of this part of the left lung.

in·fe·ri·or lon·gi·tu·di·nal fas·cic·u·lus (in-fēr′ē-ŏr lon′ji-tū′di-năl fă-sik′kyū-lŭs) A well-marked bundle of long association fibers running the whole length of the occipital and temporal lobes of the cerebrum, in part parallel with the inferior horn of the lateral ventricle. SYN fasciculus longitudinalis inferior [TA].

in·fe·ri·or lon·gi·tu·di·nal mus·cle of tongue (in-fēr′ē-ŏr lon′ji-tū′di-năl mŭs′ĕl tŭng) A cylindric, intrinsic muscle of tongue, occupying underpart on either side; *action*, shortens lower part of tongue; *nerve supply*, motor by hypoglossal, sensory by lingual. SYN inferior lingual muscle, musculus longitudinalis inferior linguae.

in·fe·ri·or lum·bar tri·an·gle (in-fēr′ē-ŏr lŭm′bahr trī′ang-gĕl) Area of the back (posterior abdominal wall) bounded by edges of the latissimus dorsi and external oblique muscles and iliac crest; herniations occasionally occur here. SYN Petit lumbar triangle.

in·fe·ri·or mac·u·lar ar·te·ri·ole (in-fēr′ē-ŏr mak′yū-lăr ahr-tēr′ē-ōl) *Origin*, central artery of retina; *distribution*, inferior part of macula. SYN arteriola macularis inferior [TA].

in·fe·ri·or med·ul·lar·y ve·lum (in-fēr′ē-ŏr med′ŭ-lar′ē vē′lŭm) A thin sheet of white matter, hidden by the cerebellar tonsil, attached along the peduncle of the flocculus and, at or near the midline, to the nodulus of the vermis; it is continuous caudally with the epithelial lamina and choroid plexus of the fourth ventricle.

in·fe·ri·or me·sen·ter·ic ar·ter·y (in-fēr′ē-ŏr mez′en-ter′ik ahr′tĕr-ē) *Origin*, abdominal aorta; *branches*, left colic, sigmoid, superior rectal; *anastomoses*, middle colic and middle rectal. SYN arteria mesenterica inferior.

in·fe·ri·or mes·en·ter·ic (nerve) plex·us (in-fēr′ē-ŏr mez′en-tĕr′ik nĕrv pleks′ŭs) An autonomic plexus, derived from the abdominal aortic plexus, surrounding the inferior mesenteric artery and sending branches to the descending colon, sigmoid, and rectum.

in·fe·ri·or nas·al con·cha (in-fēr′ē-ŏr nā′zăl kong′kă) **1.** A thin, spongy, bony plate with curved margins, on the lateral wall of the nasal cavity, separating the middle from the inferior meatus; it articulates with the ethmoid, lacrimal, maxilla, and palate bones. **2.** The above bony plate and its thick mucoperiosteum containing an extensive cavernous vascular bed for heat exchange.

in·fe·ri·or o·blique mus·cle (in-fēr′ē-ŏr ō-blēk′ mŭs′ĕl) *Origin*, orbital plate of maxilla lateral to the lacrimal groove; *insertion*, sclera between the superior and lateral recti; *action*, primary, extorsion; secondary, elevation and abduction; *nerve supply*, oculomotor (inferior branch). SYN musculus obliquus inferior [TA].

in·fe·ri·or o·blique mus·cle of head (in-fēr′ē-ŏr ō-blēk′ mŭs′ĕl hed) SYN obliquus capitis inferior muscle.

in·fe·ri·or ol·i·var·y nu·cle·us (in-fēr′ē-ŏr ol′i-var-ē nū′klē-ŭs) A large aggregate of small densely packed nerve cells arranged in folded laminae shaped like a purse with the opening (hilum) directed medially. It corresponds in position to the oliva, projects to all parts of the contralateral half of the cerebellar cortex by way of the olivocerebellar tract, and is the only source of cerebellar climbing fibers. Its afferent connections include fibers from the spinal cord, the dentate nucleus and motor cortex, but its major input appears to be the central tegmental tract originating from multiple nuclei at midbrain levels.

in·fe·ri·or or·bi·tal fis·sure (in-fēr′ē-ŏr ōr′bi-tăl fish′ŭr) A gap or cleft between the greater wing of the sphenoid and the orbital plate of the maxilla, through which pass the maxillary nerve and the inferior ophthalmic vein or its communicating branches to the pterygoid venous plexus in the infratemporal fossa.

in·fe·ri·or pal·pe·bral (ar·te·ri·al) arch (in-fēr′ē-ŏr pal′pĕ-brăl ahr-tēr′ē-ăl ahrch) Formed by the medial palpebral artery, which communicates with a branch of the lacrimal artery along the tarsal margin.

in·fe·ri·or pan·cre·at·i·co·du·o·de·nal ar·

ter•y (in-fēr′ē-ŏr, pan′krē-at′ik-ō-dū′ō-dē′năl ahr′tĕr-ē) *Origin*, superior mesenteric; one of two arteries, anterior and posterior; *distribution*, head of pancreas, duodenum; *anastomoses*, superior pancreaticoduodenal. SYN arteria pancreaticoduodenalis inferior.

in•fe•ri•or pel•vic ap•er•ture (in-fēr′ē-ŏr pel′vik ap′ĕr-chŭr) The lower opening of the true pelvis, bounded anteriorly by the pubic arch, laterally by the rami of the ischium and the sacrotuberous ligament on either side, and posteriorly by these ligaments and the tip of the coccyx.

in•fe•ri•or per•o•ne•al re•ti•nac•u•lum (in-fēr′ē-ŏr pĕr′ō-nē′ăl ret′i-nak′yū-lŭm) SYN inferior fibular retinaculum.

in•fe•ri•or phren•ic ar•ter•y (in-fēr′ē-ŏr fren′ik ahr′tĕr-ē) *Origin*, the first paired branch from the abdominal aorta inferior to the diaphragm; *distribution*, diaphragm; *anastomoses*, superior phrenic, internal thoracic, and musculophrenic. SYN arteria phrenica inferior.

in•fe•ri•or pos•te•ri•or ser•ra•tus mus•cle (in-fēr′ē-ŏr pos-tēr′ē-ŏr ser′ă-tŭs mŭs′ĕl) SYN serratus posterior inferior muscle.

in•fe•ri•or pu•bic lig•a•ment (in-fēr′ē-ŏr pyū′bik lig′ă-mĕnt) The ligament that arches across the inferior aspect of the pubic symphysis.

in•fe•ri•or pu•bic ra•mus (in-fēr′ē-ŏr pyū′bik rā′mŭs) Inferior extension from body of pubic bone that meets with the ramus of the ischium to form the ischiopubic ramus.

in•fe•ri•or rec•tal ar•ter•y (in-fēr′ē-ŏr rek′tăl ahr′tĕr ē) *Origin*, internal pudendal; *distribution*, anal canal, muscles and skin of the anal region, and skin of the buttock; *anastomoses*, middle rectal, perineal, and gluteal. SYN arteria rectalis inferior, inferior hemorrhoidal artery.

in•fe•ri•or rec•tal nerves (in-fēr′ē-ŏr rek′tăl nĕrvz) SYN inferior anal nerves.

in•fe•ri•or rec•tus mus•cle (in-fēr′ē-ŏr rek′tŭs mŭs′ĕl) *Origin*, inferior part of the common tendinous ring; *insertion*, inferior part of sclera of the eye; *action*, primary, depression; secondary, adduction and extorsion; *nerve supply*, oculomotor (inferior branch). SYN musculus rectus inferior [TA].

in•fe•ri•or re•nal seg•ment (in-fēr′ē-ŏr rē′năl seg′mĕnt) Portion of the kidney exclusively supplied by the inferior segmental (renal) artery.

in•fe•ri•or seg•ment (in-fēr′ē-ŏr seg′mĕnt) A delimited part or section of an organ or other structure that lies at the lowest level (nearest the feet) compared with the other similar parts or sections.

in•fe•ri•or su•pra•re•nal ar•ter•y (in-fēr′ē-ŏr sū′pră-rē′năl ahr′tĕr-ē) *Origin*, renal; *distribution*, suprarenal gland. SYN arteria suprarenalis inferior.

in•fe•ri•or tem•po•ral line (in-fēr′ē-ŏr tem′pŏr-ăl līn) The lower of two curved lines on the parietal bone; it marks the outer limit of attachment of the temporalis muscle.

in•fe•ri•or tem•po•ral re•ti•nal ar•te•ri•ole (in-fēr′ē-ŏr tem′pŏr-ăl ret′i-năl ahr-tēr′ē-ōl) The branch of the central artery of the retina that passes laterally below the macula to supply the lower lateral or temporal part of the retina.

in•fe•ri•or tem•po•ral sul•cus (in-fēr′ē-ŏr tem′pŏr-ăl sŭl′kŭs) The sulcus on the basal aspect of the temporal lobe that separates the fusiform gyrus from the inferior temporal gyrus on its lateral side.

in•fe•ri•or tha•lam•ic pe•dun•cle (in-fēr′ē-ŏr thă-lam′ik pĕ-dŭngk′ĕl) A large fiber bundle emerging from the anterior part of the thalamus in the ventral direction, in part joining the medial fibers of the internal capsule, in other part curving laterally around the medial margin of the capsule into the innominate substance. Many of its fibers establish a reciprocal connection of the mediodorsal nucleus of the thalamus with the orbital gyri of the frontal lobe, but numerous other fibers constitute a conduction system from the amygdala and olfactory cortex to the mediodorsal nucleus. SEE ALSO ansa peduncularis.

in•fe•ri•or thal•a•mo•stri•ate veins (in-fēr′ē-ŏr thal′ă-mō-strī′āt vānz) Veins draining the thalamus and striate body exiting the anterior perforated substance; tributary to the basal vein. SYN striate veins.

in•fe•ri•or thy•roid ar•ter•y (in-fēr′ē-ŏr thy′royd ahr′tĕr-ē) *Origin*, terminal branch of thyrocervical trunk (with ascending cervical artery); *branches*, inferior laryngeal, muscular, esophageal, and tracheal. SYN arteria thyroidea inferior.

in•fe•ri•or ul•nar col•lat•e•ral ar•ter•y (in-fēr′ē-ŏr ŭl′năr kŏ-lat′ĕr-al ahr′tĕr-ē) *Origin*, brachial; *distribution*, arm muscles at back of elbow; *anastomoses*, anterior and posterior ulnar recurrent, superior ulnar collateral, profunda brachii, and recurrent interosseous, as part of the articular network of the elbow. SYN arteria anastomotica magna, arteria collateralis ulnaris inferior, great anastomotic artery.

in•fe•ri•or ve•na ca•va (IVC) (in-fēr′ē-ŏr vē′nă kā′vă) Receives the blood from the lower limbs and the greater part of the pelvic and abdominal organs; it begins at the level of the fifth lumbar vertebra on the right side by the merger of the right and left common iliac veins, pierces the diaphragm at the level of the eighth thoracic vertebra, and empties into the posteroinferior aspect of the right atrium of the heart. SYN postcava.

in•fe•ri•or ves•i•cal ar•ter•y (in-fēr′ē-ŏr ves′i-kăl ahr′tĕr-ē) *Origin*, internal iliac; *distribution*, base of bladder, ureter, and (in the male) seminal vesicles, ductus deferens, and prostate; *anasto-*

moses, middle rectal, and other vesical branches. SYN arteria vesicalis inferior.

in•fer•til•i•ty (in′fĕr-til′i-tē) Diminished or absent ability to produce offspring; does not imply sterility. [L. *in-*, neg., + *fertilis,* fruitful]

in•fest (in-fest′) To dwell on or in a host as a parasite. [L. *infesto,* pp. *-atus,* to attack]

in•fes•ta•tion (in′fes-tā′shŭn) Parasitization of a host; usually refers to multicellular parasites (worms, arthropods).

in•fib•u•la•tion (in-fib′yū-la′shŭn) Closure of the vaginal vestibule by creating a fusion of the labia majora; typically done after excision of the labia minora and clitoris and incision of the labia majora to create raw surfaces that can be surgically joined by pinning so that they will eventually grow together; done for cultural, not medical, reasons. SEE ALSO female circumcision. [L. *infibulo,* to pin or clasp together, to join surgically (Celsus), fr. *in-* + *fibula,* pin, clasp]

in•fil•trate (in′fil-trāt) **1.** To perform or undergo infiltration. **2.** SYN infiltration (2). **3.** Infiltration (1) in the lung as inferred from appearance of a localized, ill-defined opacity on a chest radiograph. [L. *in* + Mediev. L. *filtro,* pp. *-atus,* to strain through felt, fr. *filtrum,* felt]

in•fil•tra•tion (in′fil-trā′shŭn) **1.** The act of permeating or penetrating into a substance, cell, or tissue; said of gases, fluids, or matter held in solution. **2.** The gas, fluid, or dissolved matter that has entered any substance, cell, or tissue. SYN infiltrate (2). **3.** Injection of solution into tissues, as in infiltration anesthesia. **4.** Extravasation of solutions intended for intravascular injection.

in•fil•tra•tion an•es•the•si•a (in′fil-trā′shŭn an′es-thē′zē-ă) Anesthesia produced by injection of local anesthetic solution directly into an area that is painful or about to be operated on.

in•fi•nite dis•tance (in′fi-nit dis′tăns) The limit of distant vision, the rays entering the eyes from an object at that point being practically parallel.

in•firm (in-fĭrm′) Weak or feeble because of old age or disease. [L. *in-firmus,* fr. *in-* neg., + *firmus,* strong]

in•fir•ma•ry (in-fĭr′măr-ē) A clinic or small hospital, especially in a school or college. SEE ALSO infirm. [L. *infirmarium*]

in•fir•mi•ty (in-fĭr′mi-tē) A weakness; an abnormal, more or less disabling, condition of mind or body. SEE ALSO infirm.

in•flam•ma•tion (in′flă-mā′shŭn) A fundamental, stereotyped complex of cytologic and chemical reactions that occur in affected blood vessels and adjacent tissues in response to an injury or abnormal stimulation caused by a physical, chemical, or biologic agent. [L. *inflammo,* pp. *-atus,* fr. *in,* in, + *flamma,* flame]

in•flam•ma•to•ry (in-flam′ă-tōr-ē) Pertaining to, characterized by, causing, resulting from, or becoming affected by inflammation.

in•flam•ma•to•ry bow•el dis•ease (IBD) (in-flam′ă-tōr-ē bow′ĕl di-zēz′) General term for Crohn disease and ulcerative colitis, chronic disorders of the small and large intestine, of unknown cause, with conspicuous inflammatory features and distinctive but overlapping signs and symptoms.

in•flam•ma•to•ry car•ci•no•ma (in-flam′ă-tōr-ē kahr′si-nō′mă) Carcinoma of the breast presenting with edema, hyperemia, tenderness, and rapid enlargment of the breast; microscopically, there is extensive invasion of dermal lymphatics by the carcinoma.

in•flam•ma•tor•y lin•e•ar ver•ru•cous ep•i•der•mal ne•vus (in-flam′ă-tōr-ē lin′ē-ăr ver-ū′kŭs ep′i-dĕr′măl nē′vŭs) Rare pruritic confluent scaly erythematous papules in linear array, usually appearing in early childhood on a limb and resolving before adulthood.

in•flam•ma•to•ry lymph (in-flam′ă-tōr-ē limf) A faintly yellow, usually coagulable fluid (i.e., euplastic lymph) that collects on the surface of an acutely inflamed membrane or cutaneous wound.

in•flam•ma•to•ry pap•il•lar•y hy•per•pla•si•a (in-flam′ă-tōr-ē pap′i-lar-ē hī′pĕr-plā′zē-ă) Closely arranged papules of the palatal mucosa underlying an ill-fitting denture.

in•flam•ma•to•ry pseu•do•tu•mor (in-flam′ă-tōr-ē sū′dō-tū′mŏr) A tumorlike mass in the lungs or other sites, composed of fibrous or granulation tissue infiltrated by inflammatory cells.

in•flam•ma•to•ry rheu•ma•tism (in-flam′ă-tōr-ē rū′mă-tizm) Rheumatoid arthritis or other cause of joint inflammation.

in•flare (in′flār) A dysfunction of the pelvic girdle characterized by medial rotation of the iliosacral joint.

in•fla•tion (in-flā′shŭn) Distention by a fluid or gas. SYN vesiculation (2). [L. *inflatio,* fr. *in-flo,* pp. *-flatus,* to blow into, inflate]

in•flec•tion, in•flex•ion (in-flek′shŭn, in-flek′shŭn) An inward bending. [L. *in-flecto,* pp. *-flexus,* to bend]

in•flu•en•za (in-flū-en′ză) An acute infectious respiratory disease, caused by influenza viruses; attacks the respiratory epithelial cells and produces a catarrhal inflammation; characterized by sudden onset, chills, fever of short duration, severe prostration, headache, muscle aches, and a cough that usually is dry until secondary infection occurs. The disease commonly occurs in epidemics, sometimes in pandemics; strain-specific immunity develops, but mutations in the virus are frequent, and the immunity usually does not protect against antigenically different strains. SYN flu, grip, grippe. [It. influence (of planets or stars), fr. L. *influentia,* fr. *in-fluo,* to flow in]

in•flu•en•zal (in′flū-en′zăl) Relating to, marked by, or resulting from influenza.

in•flu•en•zal pneu•mo•ni•a (in′flū-en′zăl nū-mō′nē-ă) **1.** A pulmonary disorder complicating influenza. **2.** Any such disorder due to *Haemophilus influenzae.*

In•flu•en•za•vi•rus (in′flū-en′ză-vī-rŭs) The family of Orthomyxoviridae contains three genera: Influenzavirus A, B; Influenzavirus C; and "Thogoto-like viruses." Each type of virus has a stable nucleoprotein group antigen common to all strains of the type, but distinct from that of the other types; the genome is negative-sense single-stranded RNA in 6–8 segments; each also has a mosaic of surface antigens (hemagglutinin and neuraminidase) that characterize the strains and are subject to variations of two kinds: 1) a rather continual drift that occurs independently within the hemagglutinin and neuraminidase antigens; 2) after a period of years, a sudden shift (notably in type A virus of human origin) to a different hemagglutinin or neuraminidase antigen. The sudden major shifts are the basis of subdivisions of type A virus of human origin, which occur following infection of the animal host with two different strains at the same time, resulting in a hybrid virus. Strain notations indicate type, geographic origin, year of isolation, and, in the case of type A strains, the characterizing subtypes of hemagglutinin and neuraminidase antigens (e.g., A/Hong Kong/1/68 (H_3 N_2); B/Hong Kong/5/72).

in•for•mal ad•mis•sion (in-fōr′măl ad-mish′ŭn) Entry of a patient into a psychiatric care facility voluntarily; such patients are free to leave without staff permission.

in•for•ma•tics (in′fōr-mat′iks) **1.** The study of information and ways to process and handle it, especially by means of information technology, i.e., computers and other electronic devices for rapid transfer, processing, and analysis of large amounts of data. **2.** The science of arranging and organizing the results of genomic and functional genomic studies. SEE ALSO bioinformatics. [*information* + -ics]

in•for•ma•tion (in′fōr-mā′shun) Knowledge; a collection of facts or data. [L. *informo,* to shape or fashion]

in•for•ma•tion the•o•ry (in′fōr-mā′shŭn thē′ŏr-ē) BEHAVIORAL SCIENCES a system for studying the communication process through the detailed analysis, often mathematical, of all aspects of the process including the encoding, transmission, and decoding of signals; not concerned in any direct sense with the meaning of a message.

in•formed con•sent (in-fōrmd′ kŏn-sent′) Voluntary agreement given by a person or a responsible proxy (e.g., a parent) for participation in a study, immunization program, or treatment regimen, after being informed of the purpose, methods, procedures, benefits, and risks. The essential criteria of informed consent are that the subject has both knowledge and comprehension, that consent is freely given without duress or undue influence, and that the right of withdrawal at any time is clearly communciated to the subject.

in•for•mo•fers (in-fōrm′ō-fĕrz) Name suggested for the protein particles that appear when RNA is removed from nucleoprotein particles. [*information* + -fer]

in•for•mo•somes (in-fōrm′ō-sōmz) Name suggested for the bodies composed of messenger (informational) RNA and protein that are found in the cytoplasm of animal cells. [*information* + G. *sōma,* body]

♻ **infra-** Prefix denoting a position below the part denoted by the word to which it is joined. [L. below]

in•fra•bulge (in′fră-bŭlj) **1.** That portion of the crown of a tooth gingival to the height of contour. **2.** That area of a tooth where the retentive portion of a clasp of a removable partial denture is placed.

in•fra•cla•vic•u•lar fos•sa (in′fră-klă-vik′yū-lăr fos′ă) A triangular depression bounded by the clavicle and the adjacent borders of the deltoid and pectoralis major muscles.

in•fra•clu•sion (in′fră-klū′zhŭn) The state wherein a tooth has failed to erupt to the maxillomandibular plane of interdigitation. SYN infra-occlusion, infraversion (3).

in•frac•tion (in-frak′shŭn) A fracture; especially one without displacement. [L. *infractio,* a breaking, fr. *infringere,* to break]

in•fra•di•an (in-frā′dē-ăn) Relating to biologic variations or rhythms occurring in cycles less frequent than every 24 hours. Cf. circadian, ultradian. [infra- + L. *dies,* day]

in•fra•di•an rhythm (in-frā′dē-ăn ridh′ĕm) A biorhythm whose cycles last less than 1 day or 24 hours.

in•fra•glot•tic (in′fră-glot′ik) Inferior to the glottis.

in•fra•hy•oid (in′fră-hī′oyd) Inferior to the hyoid bone.

in•fra•mam•il•lar•y (in′fră-mam′i-lar-ē) Relating to that which is situated below a nipple.

in•fra•mam•ma•ry fold (IMF) (in′fră-mam′ăr-ē fōld) A crescentic zone on the chest wall below the female breast consisting of regular arrays of collagen in the dermis and an underlying condensation of superficial fascia, imparting shape to the breast and binding it to the pectoralis fascia.

in·fra·man·dib·u·lar (in′fră-man-dib′yū-lăr) SYN submandibular.

in·fra·mar·gin·al (in′fră-mahr′ji-năl) Below any margin or edge.

in·fra·max·il·lar·y (in′fră-mak′si-lar-ē) SYN mandibular.

in·fra·nod·al ex·tra·sys·to·le (in′fră-nō′dăl eks′tră-sis′tŏ-lē) SYN ventricular extrasystole.

in·fra·oc·clu·sion (in′fră-ŏ-klū′zhŭn) SYN infraclusion.

in·fra·or·bit·al ar·ter·y (in′fră-ōr′bi-tăl ahr′tĕr-ē) *Origin*, third part of maxillary; *distribution*, upper canine and incisor teeth, inferior rectus and inferior oblique muscles, lower eyelid, lacrimal sac, maxillary sinus, and upper lip; *anastomoses*, branches of ophthalmic, facial, superior labial, transverse facial, and buccal. SYN arteria infraorbitalis [TA].

in·fra·or·bit·al ca·nal (in′fră-ōr′bi-tăl kă-nal′) A canal running beneath the orbital margin of the maxilla from the infraorbital groove, in the floor of the orbit, to the infraorbital foramen; it transmits the infraorbital artery and nerve. SYN canalis infraorbitalis [TA].

in·fra·or·bit·al fo·ra·men (in′fră-ōr′bi-tăl fōr-ā′mĕn) The external opening of the infraorbital canal, on the anterior surface of the body of the maxilla.

in·fra·or·bit·al nerve (in′fră-ōr′bi-tăl nĕrv) The continuation of the maxillary nerve after it has entered the orbit, through the infraorbital fissure, traversing the infraorbital canal to reach the face; it supplies the mucosa of the maxillary sinus, the upper incisors, canine and premolars, the upper gums, the inferior eyelid and conjunctiva, part of the nose and the superior lip. SYN nervus infraorbitalis [TA].

in·fra·or·bit·o·me·a·tal line (in′fră-ōr′bi-tō-mē-ā′tăl līn) Line drawn between the infraorbital margin and the external acoustic meatus, used to adjust the position of the cranium during imaging procedures.

in·fra·pa·tel·lar fat pad (in′fră-pă-tel′ăr fat pad) The fatty mass that occupies the area between the patellar ligament and the infrapatellar synovial fold of the knee joint.

in·fra·psy·chic (in′fră-sī′kik) Denoting ideas or actions originating below the level of consciousness.

in·fra·red (in′fră-red) That portion of the electromagnetic spectrum with wavelengths between 770–1000 nm.

in·fra·red mi·cro·scope (in′fră-red mī′krŏ-skōp) A microscope that is equipped with infrared transmitting optics and that measures the infrared absorption of minute samples with the aid of photoelectric cells; images may be observed with image converters or television.

in·fra·son·ic (in′fră-son′ik) Denoting those frequencies that lie below the range of human hearing. [infra- + L. *sonus*, sound]

in·fra·spi·na·tus bur·sa (in′fră-spī-nā′tus bŭr′să) The bursa located between the tendon of the infraspinatus and the capsule of the shoulder joint.

in·fra·spi·na·tus mus·cle (in′fră-spī-nā′tus mŭs′ĕl) *Origin*, infraspinous fossa of scapula; *insertion*, middle facet of greater tubercle of humerus; *action*, extends arm and rotates it laterally; *nerve supply*, suprascapular (from fifth to sixth cervical spinal nerves). See this page. SYN musculus infraspinatus [TA].

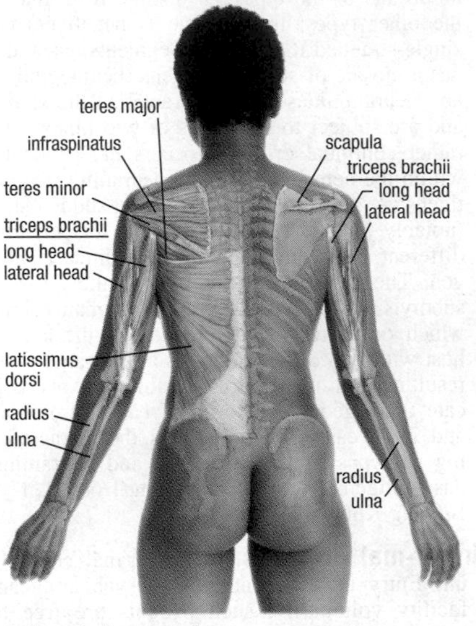

infraspinatus muscle

in·fra·spi·nous fos·sa (in′fră-spī′nŭs fos′ă) The concavity on the dorsal aspect of the scapula below its spine.

in·fra·tem·po·ral ap·proach (in′fră-tem′pŏr-ăl ă-prōch′) Surgical approach to the base of the skull and its contents from inferior to the temporal bone.

in·fra·tem·po·ral crest (in′fră-temp′ŏr-ăl krest) A rough ridge marking the angle of union of the temporal and infratemporal surfaces of the greater wing of the sphenoid bone.

in·fra·tem·po·ral fos·sa (in′fră-tem′pŏr-ăl fos′ă) The cavity on the side of the skull bounded laterally by the zygomatic arch and ramus of the mandible, medially by the lateral pterygoid plate, anteriorly by the zygomatic process of the maxilla, posteriorly by the articular tubercle of the temporal bone and the posterior border of the lateral pterygoid plate, and above by the squama of the temporal bone and the infratemporal crest on the greater wing of the sphenoid bone.

in·fra·troch·le·ar nerve (in′fră-trok′lē-ăr nĕrv) A terminal branch of the nasociliary nerve running beneath the pulley of the superior oblique muscle to the front of the orbit, and supplying the skin of the eyelids and root of the nose. SYN nervus infratrochlearis [TA].

in·fra·ver·sion (in′fră-vĕr′zhŭn) **1.** A turning (version) downward. **2.** PHYSIOLOGIC OPTICS rotation of both eyes downward. **3.** SYN infraclusion.

in·fun·dib·u·la (in′fŭn-dib′yū-lă) Plural of infundibulum.

in·fun·dib·u·lar (in′fŭn-dib′yū-lăr) Relating to an infundibulum.

in·fun·dib·u·lar stalk (in′fŭn-dib′yū-lăr stawk) SYN infundibular stem.

in·fun·dib·u·lar stem (in′fŭn-dib′yū-lăr stem) The neural component of the pituitary stalk that contains nerve tracts passing from the hypothalamus to the pars nervosa. SYN infundibular stalk.

in·fun·dib·u·lec·to·my (in′fŭn-dib′yū-lek′tŏ-mē) Excision of an infundibulum, especially of hypertrophied ventricular septal myocardium encroaching on the ventricular outflow tract. [infundibulum + G. *ektomē,* excision]

in·fun·dib·u·lo·fol·lic·u·li·tis (in′fŭn-dib′yū-lō-fŏ-lik′yū-lī′tis) Inflammation of the follicular infundibulum, the superficial part of the hair follicle above the opening of the sebaceous gland.

in·fun·dib·u·lo·ma (in′fŭn-dib′yū-lō′mă) A pilocytic astrocytoma arising in the neurohypophysis of the pituitary. [infundibulum + G. *-oma,* tumor]

in·fun·dib·u·lum, pl. **in·fun·dib·u·la** (in′fŭn-dib′yū-lŭm, -lă) **1.** [TA] A funnel or funnel-shaped structure or passage. **2.** SYN infundibulum of uterine tube. **3.** The expanding portion of a calyx as it opens into the pelvis of the kidney. **4.** SYN arterial cone. **5.** Termination of a bronchiole in the alveolus. **6.** Termination of the cochlear canal beneath the cupola. **7.** The funnel-shaped, unpaired prominence of the base of the hypothalamus behind the optic chiasm, enclosing the infundibular recess of the third ventricle and continuous below with the stalk of the hypophysis. **8.** The contact surface indentation in the incisor and cheek teeth of a horse. SYN mark (2). [L. a funnel]

in·fun·dib·u·lum of di·en·ceph·a·lon (in′fŭn-dib′yū-lŭm dī′en-sef′ă-lon) SYN neurohypophysial diverticulum.

in·fun·dib·u·lum tu·bae u·te·ri·nae (in′fŭn-dib′yū-lŭm tū′bē yū-tĕ-rī′nē) [TA] SYN infundibulum of uterine tube.

in·fun·dib·u·lum of u·ter·ine tube (in′fŭn-dib′yū-lŭm yū′tĕr-in tūb) The funnellike expansion of the abdominal extremity of the uterine (fallopian) tube. SYN infundibulum tubae uterinae [TA], infundibulum (2).

in·fu·sion (in-fyū′zhŭn) **1.** The process of steeping a substance in water, either cold or hot (below the boiling point), to extract its soluble principles. **2.** A medicinal preparation obtained by steeping the crude drug in water. **3.** The introduction of fluid other than blood, e.g., saline solution, into a vein. [L. *infusio,* fr. *in-fundo,* pp. *-fusus,* to pour in]

in·fu·sion-as·pi·ra·tion drain·age (in-fyū′zhŭn-as′pir-ā′shŭn drān′ăj) A type of drainage in which antibiotics are continuously infused into a cavity at the same time fluid is being drained (aspirated) from the cavity.

In·gel·fin·ger rule (ing′gĕl-fing′gĕr rūl) A principle developed by Franz Ingelfinger for use in the editorial offices of the *New England Journal of Medicine*, stating that original articles submitted for publication will be reviewed on the understanding that the same information will not be submitted for publication elsewhere during the period of review; has been adopted by many other peer-reviewed medical journals.

in·ges·ta (in-jes′tă) Solid or liquid nutrients taken into the body. [pl. of L. *ingestum,* ntr. pp. of *in-gero, -gestus,* to carry in]

in·ges·tion (in-jes′chŭn) **1.** Introduction of food and drink into the stomach. **2.** Incorporation of particles into the cytoplasm of a phagocytic cell by invagination of a portion of the cell membrane as a vacuole. [L. *in-gero,* to carry in]

in·ges·tive (in-jes′tiv) Relating to ingestion.

in·gra·ves·cent (in′gră-ves′ĕnt) Increasing in severity. [L. *ingravesco,* to grow heavier, fr. *gravis,* heavy]

in·grown hair (in′grōn hār) Hair that grows at more acute angles than is normal, and in all directions; it incompletely clears the follicle, turns back in, and causes pseudofolliculitis.

in·grown nail (in′grōn nāl) A toenail, one edge of which is overgrown by the nailfold, producing a pyogenic granuloma; due to faulty trimming of the toenails or pressure from a tight shoe.

in·gui·nal (ing′gwi-năl) Relating to the groin.

in·gui·nal ca·nal (ing′gwi-năl kă-nal′) The obliquely directed passage through the layers of the lower abdominal wall that transmits the spermatic cord in the male and the round ligament in the female. SYN canalis inguinalis [TA].

in·gui·nal falx (ing′gwi-năl fawlks) Common tendon of insertion of the transversus and internal oblique muscles into the crest and tubercle of the pubis and iliopectineal line; it is frequently largely muscular rather than aponeurotic and may be poorly developed; forms posterior wall of medial inguinal canal. SYN falx inguinalis [TA], Henle ligament.

in·gui·nal her·ni·a (ing′gwi-năl hĕr′nē-ă) A hernia at the inguinal region: direct inguinal hernia involves the abdominal wall between the deep epigastric artery and the edge of the rectus muscle; indirect inguinal hernia involves the internal inguinal ring and passes into the inguinal canal. See this page.

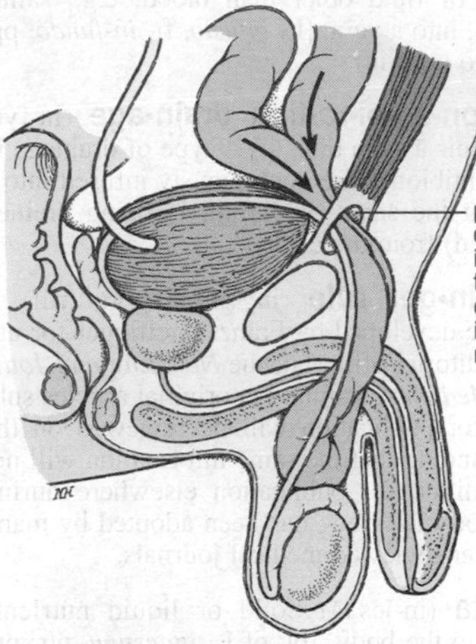

indirect inguinal hernia

in·gui·nal lig·a·ment (ing′gwi-năl lig′ă-mĕnt) A fibrous band formed by the thickened inferior border of the aponeurosis of the external oblique muscle that extends from the anterior superior spine of the ilium to the pubic tubercle, bridging muscular and vascular lacunae; forms the floor of the inguinal canal; gives origin to the lowermost fibers of internal oblique and transversus abdominis muscles. See this page. SYN ligamentum inguinale [TA].

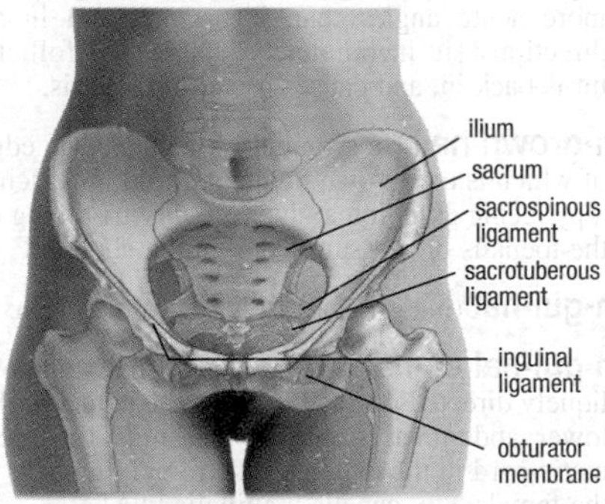

inguinal ligament

in·gui·nal re·gion (ing′gwi-năl rē′jŭn) The topographic area of the inferior abdomen related to the inguinal canal, lateral to the pubic region. See this page. SYN groin (1).

in·gui·nal tri·an·gle (ing′gwi-năl trī′ang-gĕl)

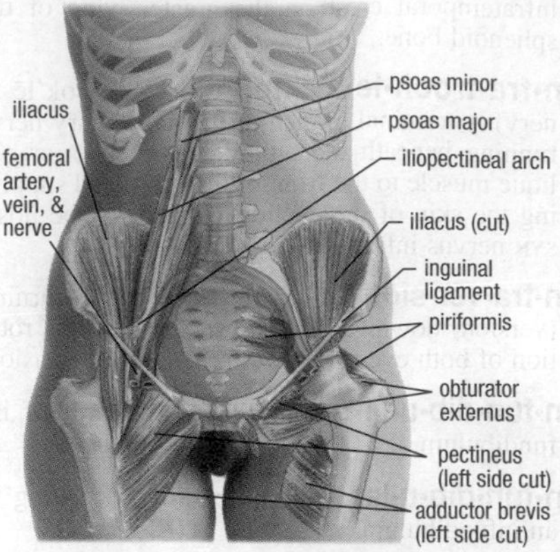

inguinal region

The triangular area in the lower abdominal wall bounded by the inguinal ligament below, the border of the rectus abdominis medially, and the inferior epigastric vessels (lateral umbilical fold) laterally. It is the site of direct inguinal hernia. SYN trigonum inguinale [TA], Hesselbach triangle, inguinal trigone.

in·gui·nal tri·gone (ing′gwi-năl trī′gōn) SYN inguinal triangle.

in·gui·no·cru·ral (ing′gwi-nō-krūr′ăl) Relating to the groin and the thigh.

in·gui·no·dyn·i·a (ing′gwi-nō-din′ē-ă) Rarely used term for pain in the groin. [L. *inguen* (*inguin-*), groin, + G. *odynē*, pain]

in·gui·no·la·bi·al (ing′gwi-nō-lā′bē-ăl) Relating to the groin and the labium.

in·gui·no·per·i·to·ne·al (ing′gwi-nō-per′i-tō-nē′ăl) Relating to the groin and the peritoneum.

in·gui·no·scro·tal (ing′gwi-nō-skrō′tăl) Relating to the groin and the scrotum.

INH Abbreviation for isonicotinic acid hydrazide.

in·hal·ant (in-hāl′ănt) **1.** That which is inhaled; a remedy given by inhalation. **2.** A drug (or combination of drugs) with high vapor pressure, carried by an air current into the nasal passage, where it produces its effect. **3.** Group of products consisting of finely powdered or liquid drugs that are carried to the respiratory passages by the use of special devices such as low-pressure aerosol containers. SYN insufflation (2). SEE ALSO inhalation, aerosol.

in·ha·la·tion (in′hă-lā′shŭn) **1.** The act of drawing in the breath. SYN inspiration. **2.** Drawing a medicated vapor in with the breath. **3.** A solution of a drug or combination of drugs for administration as a nebulized mist intended to reach the respiratory tree. [L. *in-halo,* pp. *-halatus,* to breathe at or in]

in·ha·la·tion an·es·the·si·a (in′hă-lā′shŭn

an′es-thē′zē-ă) General anesthesia resulting from breathing of anesthetic gases or vapors.

in·ha·la·tion an·es·thet·ic (in′hă-lā′shŭn an′es-thet′ik) A gas or a liquid with sufficient vapor pressure to produce general anesthesia when inhaled.

in·ha·la·tion in·ju·ry (in′hă-lā′shŭn in′jŭr-ē) Trauma to the throat, lungs, and associated areas caused by fire, exposure to toxins, or lethal gases.

in·ha·la·tion ther·a·py (in′hă-lā′shŭn thār′ă-pē) Treatment with a substance that is introduced into the patient's respiratory tract through breathing in, spontaneously or with the aid of a mechanical device.

in·hale (in-hāl′) To draw in the breath. SYN inspire.

in·hal·er (in-hāl′ĕr) An apparatus for administering medicines by inhalation. SYN metered-dose inhaler.

in·her·ent (in-her′ĕnt) Occurring as a natural part or consequence; intrinsic. [L. *inhaerens,* sticking to, adhering]

in·her·i·tance (in-her′i-tăns) **1.** Characters or qualities that are transmitted from parent to offspring by coded cytologic data; that which is inherited. **2.** Cultural or legal endowment. **3.** The act of inheriting. [L. *heredito,* inherit, fr. *heres* (*hered-*), an heir]

in·her·it·ed (in-her′it-ĕd) Derived from a preformed genetic code present in the parents. Contrast with acquired.

in·her·it·ed char·ac·ter (in-her′it-ĕd kar′ăk-tĕr) A single attribute of an animal or plant that is transmitted at one locus from generation to generation in accordance with mendelian laws. SEE gene.

in·her·i·ted dis·or·der (in-hār′i-tĕd dis-ōr′dĕr) An illness or disease that is derived from genetic aberration.

in·her·i·ted trait (in-hār′i-tĕd trāt) Any characteristic that is passed from one generation to the next.

in·hib·it (in-hib′it) To curb or restrain.

in·hi·bi·tion (in′hi-bish′ŭn) **1.** Depression or arrest of a function. SEE ALSO inhibitor. **2.** PSYCHOANALYSIS the restraining of instinctual or unconscious drives or tendencies, especially if they conflict with one's conscience or with societal demands. **3.** PSYCHOLOGY the gradual attenuation, masking, and extinction of a previously conditioned response. [L. *in-hibeo,* pp. *-hibitus,* to keep back, fr. *habeo,* to have]

in·hib·i·tor (in-hib′i-tŏr) **1.** An agent that restrains or retards physiologic, chemical, or enzymatic action. **2.** A nerve, stimulation of which represses activity. SEE ALSO inhibition.

in·hib·i·to·ry (in-hib′i-tōr-ē) Restraining; tending to inhibit.

in·hib·i·to·ry fi·bers (in-hib′i-tōr-ē fī′bĕrz) Nerve fibers that inhibit the activity of the nerve cells with which they have synaptic connections, or of the effector tissue (smooth muscle, heart muscle, glands) in which they terminate.

in·hib·i·to·ry nerve (in-hib′i-tōr-ē nĕrv) A nerve conveying impulses that diminish functional activity in a part.

in·hib·i·to·ry ob·ses·sion (in-hib′i-tōr-ē ŏb-sesh′ŭn) An obsession involving an impediment to action, usually representing a phobia.

in·hib·i·to·ry post·syn·ap·tic po·ten·tial (in-hib′i-tōr-ē pōst′si-nap′tik pŏ-ten′shăl) The change in potential produced in the membrane of the next neuron when an impulse that has an inhibitory influence arrives at the synapse; it is a local change in the direction of hyperpolarization; frequency of discharge of a given neuron is determined by the extent to which impulses that lead to excitatory postsynaptic potentials predominate over those that cause inhibitory postsynaptic potentials.

in-house med·i·cal tran·scrip·tion (in′hows med′i-kăl tran-skrip′shŭn) System in which medical transcriptionists work on the premises of a health care facility.

in·i·on (in′ē-on) A point located on the external occipital protuberance at the intersection of the midline with a line drawn tangent to the uppermost convexity of the right and left superior nuchal lines. [G. nape of the neck]

i·ni·tial as·sess·ment (i-nish′ăl ă-ses′mĕnt) First evaluation of a patient by EMS personnel to identify immediate threats to life. SYN primary survey.

i·ni·tial heat (i-nish′ăl hēt) The first burst of heat produced after the beginning of a muscle twitch, described by A.V. Hill.

in·i·tial·ism (i-ni′shăl-izm) Abbreviation formed from the initial letter of each word or selected words in a phrase (e.g., CPK).

in·i·ti·at·ing a·gent (i-nish′ē-ā-ting ā′jĕnt) SEE initiation.

in·i·ti·at·ing co·don (i-nish′ē-ā-ting kō′don) The trinucleotide AUG (or sometimes GUG) that codes for the first amino acid in protein sequences, formylmethionine; the latter is often removed posttranscriptionally.

in·i·ti·a·tion (i-nish′ē-ā′shŭn) **1.** The first stage of tumor induction by a carcinogen; subtle alteration of cells by exposure to a carcinogenic agent so that they are likely to form a tumor on subsequent exposure to a promoting agent (promotion). **2.** Starting point of replication or translation in macromolecule biosynthesis. **3.** Start of chemical or enzymatic reaction.

in·i·ti·a·tion co·don (i-nish′ē-ā′shŭn kō′don) A specific mRNA sequence (usually AUG, but sometimes GUG) that is the signal for the addition of fMet-tRNA and the beginning of translation.

in·i·ti·a·tion fac·tor (IF) (i-nish′ē-ā′shŭn fak′tŏr) One of several soluble proteins involved in the initiation of protein or RNA synthesis.

in·i·tis (in-ī′tis) **1.** Inflammation of fibrous tissue. **2.** SYN myositis. [G. *is* (*in-*), fiber, + *-itis,* inflammation]

in·ject (in-jekt′) To introduce into the body; denoting a fluid forced beneath the skin or into a blood vessel. [L. *injicio,* to throw in]

in·ject·ed (in-jek′tĕd) **1.** Denoting a fluid introduced into the body by injection. **2.** Denoting a surface with blood vessels that are visibly dilated.

in·jec·tion (in-jek′shŭn) **1.** Introduction of a medicinal substance or nutrient material into the subcutaneous tissue (subcutaneous or hypodermic injection), the muscular tissue (intramuscular injection), a vein (intravenous injection), an artery (intraarterial injection), the rectum (rectal injection or enema), the vagina (vaginal injection or douche), the urethra, or other canals or cavities of the body. **2.** An injectable pharmaceutical preparation. **3.** Congestion or hyperemia. See this page. [L. *injectio,* a throwing in, fr. *in-jicio,* to throw in]

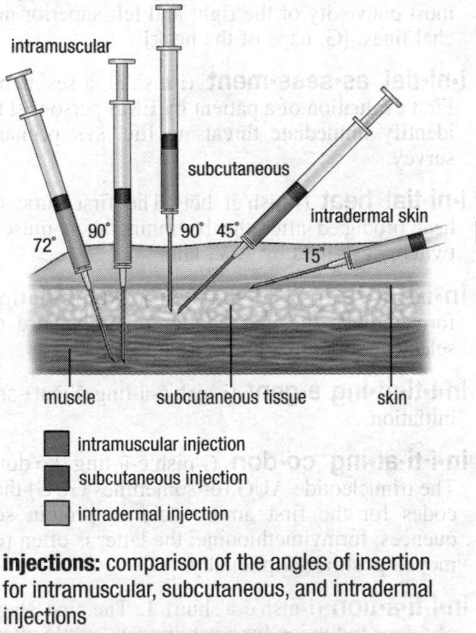

injections: comparison of the angles of insertion for intramuscular, subcutaneous, and intradermal injections

in·jec·tion drug us·er (IDU) (in-jek′shŭn drŭg yū′zĕr) A person who uses a hypodermic to administer drugs, usually illegally (e.g., heroin, methamphetamines); often leads to dermatologic and hematologic disorders resulting from unclean site or equipment; widely associated with transmission of HIV; also called injecting drug user. SYN intravenous drug user.

in·ju·ry (in′jŭr-ē) Damage, harm, or loss, to a person particularly as the result of external force. [L. *injuria,* fr. *in-* neg. + *jus (jur-),* right]

ink·blot test (ingk′blot test) SYN Rorschach test.

in·lay (in′lā) **1.** DENTISTRY a prefabricated restoration sealed into the prepared cavity with cement. **2.** A graft of bone into a bone cavity. **3.** A graft of skin into a wound cavity for epithelialization. **4.** ORTHOPAEDICS an orthomechanical device inserted into a shoe; commonly called an "arch support."

in·lay graft (in′lā graft) A skin graft wrapped (raw side out) around a bolus of dental compound and inserted into a prepared surgical pocket. SYN Esser graft.

in·let (in′lĕt) A passage leading into a cavity. SYN aditus [TA].

in·nate (i-nāt′) SYN inborn. [L. *in-nascor,* pp. *-natus,* to be born in, pp. as adj. inborn, innate]

in·nate im·mu·ni·ty (i-nāt′ i-myū′ni-tē) Resistance manifested by an organism that has not been sensitized by previous infection or vaccination; innate immunity is nonspecific and is not stimulated by specific antigens. SEE ALSO self. SYN natural immunity, nonspecific immunity.

in·ner cell mass (in′ĕr sel mas) SYN embryoblast.

in·ner·most in·ter·cos·tal mus·cle (in′ĕr-mōst in′tĕr-kos′tăl mŭs′ĕl) flat muscle of thorax that occurs as a layer parallel to and is essentially part of internal intercostal muscle but separated from it by intercostal vessels and nerves. SYN musculus intercostalis intimus.

in·ner·va·tion (in′ĕr-vā′shŭn) The supply of motor and sensory nerve fibers functionally connected with an organ or region. See page 801. [L. *in,* in, + *nervus,* nerve]

in·nid·i·a·tion (i-nid′ē-ā′shŭn) The growth and multiplication of abnormal cells in a location to which they have been transported by means of lymph or the blood stream, or both. SEE ALSO metastasis. [L. *in,* in, + *nidus,* nest]

in·no·cent (in′ō-sĕnt) **1.** Not apparently harmful. **2.** Free from moral wrong. [L. *innocens* (*-ent-*), fr. *in,* neg., + *noceo,* to injure]

in·no·cent mur·mur (in′ō-sĕnt mŭr′mŭr) SYN functional murmur.

in·noc·u·ous (i-nok′yū-ŭs) Harmless. [L. *innocuus*]

in·nom·i·nate (i-nom′i-nāt) SYN anonyma. [L. *innominatus,* fr. *in-* neg. + *nomen* (*nomin-*), name]

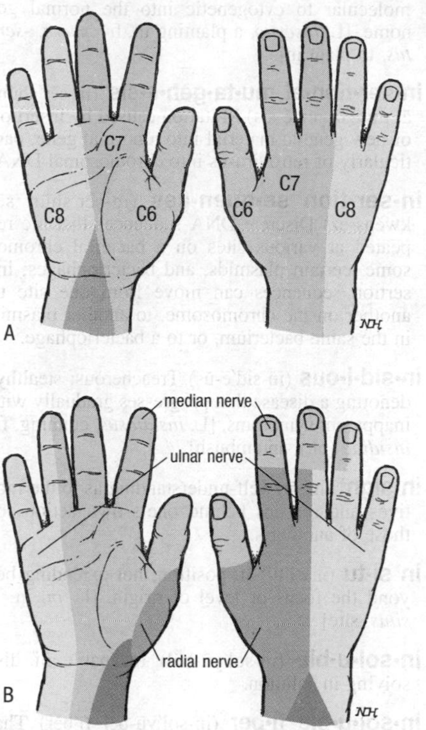

innervation of the hand and wrist: (A) segmental dermatomes, (B) cutaneous nerve distribution

in•nom•i•nate ar•ter•y (i-nom′i-nāt ahr′tĕr-ē) Obsolete term for brachiocephalic trunk.

in•nom•i•nate bone (i-nom′i-nāt bōn) SYN hip bone. [L. *innominatus,* unnamed]

in•nom•i•nate veins (i-nom′i-nāt vānz) SYN brachiocephalic veins.

INO Abbreviation for internuclear ophthalmoplegia; inhaled nitric oxide.

Ino Abbreviation for inosine.

in•oc•u•la•bil•i•ty (i-nok′yū-lă-bil′i-tē) The quality of being inoculable.

in•oc•u•la•ble (i-nok′yū-lă-bĕl) **1.** Transmissible by inoculation. **2.** Susceptible to a disease transmissible by inoculation.

in•oc•u•late (i-nok′yū-lāt) **1.** To introduce the agent of a disease or other antigenic material into the subcutaneous tissue or a blood vessel, or through an abraded or absorbing surface for preventive, curative, or experimental purposes. **2.** To implant microorganisms or infectious material into or on culture media. **3.** To communicate a disease by transferring its virus. [L. *inoculo,* pp. *-atus,* to ingraft]

in•oc•u•la•tion (i-nok′yū-lā′shŭn) Introduction into the body of the causative organism of a disease.

in•oc•u•lum (i-nok′yū-lŭm) The microorganism or other material introduced by inoculation.

in•op•er•a•ble (in-op′ĕr-ă-bĕl) Denoting that which cannot be operated on, or cannot be corrected or removed by an operation.

in•or•gan•ic (in′ōr-gan′ik) **1.** Not organic; not formed by living organisms. **2.** SEE inorganic compound. **3.** Not containing carbon.

in•or•gan•ic ac•id (in′ōr-gan′ik as′id) An acid made up of molecules not containing organic radicals; e.g., HCl, H_2SO_4, H_3PO_4.

in•or•gan•ic chem•is•try (in′ōr-gan′ik kem′is-trē) The science concerned with compounds not involving carbon-containing molecules.

in•or•gan•ic com•pound (in′ōr-gan′ik kom′pownd) A compound in which the atoms or radicals consist of elements other than carbon and are typically held together by electrostatic forces rather than by covalent bonds; often are capable of dissociation into ions in polar solvents (e.g., H_2O). Cf. organic compound.

in•or•gan•ic or•tho•phos•phate (P_i, P_1) (in′ōr-gan′ik ōr′thō-fos′fāt) Any ion or salt form of phosphoric acid.

inosaemia [Br.] SYN inosemia.

in•os•a•mine (in-ōs′ă-mēn) An inositol in which an –OH group is replaced by an $-NH_2$ group.

in•os•co•py (in-os′kŏ-pē) Microscopic examination of biologic materials (e.g., tissue, sputum, clotted blood) after dissection or chemical digestion of the fibrillary elements and strands of fibrin. [ino- + G. *skopeō,* to look at]

in•o•se•mi•a (in′ō-sē′mē-ă) The presence of inositol in the circulating blood. SYN inosaemia. [inose + G. *haima,* blood]

in•o•sine (I, Ino) (in′ō-sēn) A nucleoside formed by the deamination of adenosine.

in•o•sine 5′-mon•o•phos•phate (IMP) (in′ō-sēn mon′ō-fos′fāt) SYN inosinic acid.

in•o•sine 5′-tri•phos•phate (ITP) (in′ō-sēn trī-fos′-fāt) Inosine with triphosphoric acid esterified at its 5′ position; participates in a number of enzyme-catalyzed reactions.

in•o•sin•ic ac•id (in′ō-sin′ik as′id) A mononucleotide found in muscle and other tissues; a key intermediate in purine biosynthesis; also produced in relatively high levels in muscle. SYN inosine 5′-monophosphate.

in•o•si•tol (in-ō′si-tol) A member of the vitamin B complex.

in·o·si·tu·ri·a (in′ō-si-tyūr′ē-ă) The excretion of inositol in the urine. [inositol + G. *ouron,* urine]

in·o·tro·pic (in′ō-trō′pik) Influencing the contractility of muscular tissue. [ino- + G. *tropos,* a turning]

in·pa·tient (in′pā-shĕnt) Patient who is admitted to and is assigned a bed in a health care facility while undergoing diagnosis and receiving treatment and care.

in·put and out·put rec·ord (in′put owt′put rek′ŏrd) SYN fluid balance chart.

in·quest (in′kwest) A legal inquiry into the cause of sudden, violent, or mysterious death. [L. *in,* in, + *quaero,* pp. *quaesitus,* to seek]

INR Abbreviation for international normalized ratio.

in·sane (in-sān′) **1.** Of unsound mind; severely mentally impaired; deranged; crazy. **2.** Relating to insanity. [L. *in-* neg. + *sanus,* sound, sane]

in·san·i·tary (in-san′i-tar-ē) Injurious to health, usually in reference to an unclean or contaminated environment. SYN unsanitary. [L. *in-* neg. + *sanus,* sound]

in·san·i·ty (in-san′i-tē) **1.** A nonmedical term referring to severe mental illness or psychosis. **2.** LAW that degree of mental illness that negates the person's legal responsibility or capacity. [L. *in-* neg. + *sanus,* sound]

in·scrip·tion (in-skrip′shŭn) **1.** The main part of a prescription; that which indicates the drugs and the quantity of each to be used in the mixture. **2.** A mark, band, or line. [L. *inscriptio*]

in·sec·ti·cide (in-sek′ti-sīd) An agent that kills insects. [insect + L. *caedō,* to kill]

in·se·cu·ri·ty (in′sĕ-kyūr′i-tē) A feeling of vulnerability and helplessness.

in·sem·i·na·tion (in-sem′i-nā′shŭn) Deposit of seminal fluid within the vagina, normally during coitus. SYN semination. [L. *in-semino,* pp. *-atus,* to sow or plant in, fr. *semen,* seed]

in·se·nes·cence (in′sĕ-nes′ĕns) The process of growing old. [L. *insenesco,* to begin to grow old]

in·sen·si·ble (in-sen′si-bĕl) **1.** SYN unconscious. **2.** Not appreciable by the senses. [L. *in-sensibilis,* fr. *in,* neg. + *sentio,* pp. *sensus,* to feel]

in·sen·si·ble pers·pi·ra·tion (in-sen′si-bĕl pĕrs′pir-ā′shŭn) perspiration that evaporates before it is perceived as moisture on the skin; the term sometimes includes evaporation from the lungs.

in·ser·tion (in-sĕr′shŭn) **1.** A putting in. **2.** The attachment of a muscle to the more movable part of the skeleton, as distinguished from origin. **3.** DENTISTRY the intraoral placing of a dental prosthesis. **4.** Intrusion of fragments of any size from molecular to cytogenetic into the normal genome. [L. *insertio,* a planting in, fr. *insero, -sertus,* to plant in]

in·ser·tion·al mu·ta·gen·e·sis (in-sĕr′shŭn-ăl myū′tă-jen′ĕ-sis) Mutation caused by insertion of new genetic material into a normal gene, particularly of retroviruses into chromosomal DNA.

in·ser·tion se·quen·ces (in-sĕr′shŭn sē′kwĕns-ĕz) Discrete DNA sequences that are repeated at various sites on a bacterial chromosome, certain plasmids, and bacteriophages; insertion sequences can move from one site to another on the chromosome, to another plasmid in the same bacterium, or to a bacteriophage.

in·sid·i·ous (in-sid′ē-ŭs) Treacherous; stealthy; denoting a disease that progresses gradually with inapparent symptoms. [L. *insidiosus,* cunning, fr. *insidiae* (pl.), an ambush]

in·sight (in′sīt) Self-understanding as to the motives and reasons behind one's own actions or those of another's.

in si·tu (in sī′tū) In position; not extending beyond the focus or level of origin. [L. *in,* in, + *situs,* site]

in·sol·u·ble (in-sol′yū-bĕl) Incapable of dissolving in solution.

in·sol·u·ble fi·ber (in-sol′yū-bĕl fī′bĕr) That portion of a foodstuff (e.g., bran) that cannot be digested and is passed through the alimentary system without change.

in·som·ni·a (in-som′nē-ă) Inability to sleep, in the absence of external impediments (e.g., noise, a bright light) during the period when sleep should normally occur; may vary in degree from restlessness or disturbed slumber to a curtailment of the normal length of sleep or to absolute wakefulness. [L. fr. *in-* priv. + *somnus,* sleep]

in·som·ni·ac (in-som′nē-ak) **1.** A sufferer from insomnia. **2.** Exhibiting, tending toward, or producing insomnia.

in·sorp·tion (in-sōrp′shŭn) Movement of substances from the lumen of the gut into the blood. [L. *in,* in, + *sorbeo,* to suck]

in·sper·sion (in-spĕr′zhŭn) Sprinkling with a fluid or a powder. [L. *inspersio,* fr. *in-spergo,* pp. *-spersus,* to scatter on, fr. *spargo,* to scatter]

in·spi·ra·tion (in′spir-ā′shŭn) SYN inhalation (1). [L. *inspiratio,* fr. *in-spiro,* pp. *-atus,* to breathe in]

in·spi·ra·to·ry (in′spir-ă-tōr-ē) Relating to or timed during inhalation.

in·spi·ra·to·ry ca·pac·i·ty (in′spir-ă-tōr-ē kă-pas′i-tē) The volume of air that can be inspired after a normal expiration; it is the sum of the tidal volume and the inspiratory reserve volume. SYN complementary air.

in·spi·ra·to·ry re·serve vol·ume (IRV) (in′spir-ă′tōr-ē rē-zĕrv′ vol′yūm) The maximal volume of air that can be inspired after a normal inspiration; the inspiratory capacity less the tidal volume. SYN complemental air.

in·spi·ra·to·ry stri·dor (in′spir-ă-tōr-ē strī′dŏr) A crowing sound during the inspiratory phase of respiration due to pathology involving the epiglottis or larynx.

in·spire (in-spīr′) SYN inhale.

in·spired gas (I) (in-spīrd′ gas) **1.** as symbol for gas, subscrip I [e.g., X_I]; Any gas that is being inhaled; **2.** Specifically, that gas after it has been humidified at body temperature.

in·spis·sate (in-spis′āt) To perform or undergo inspissation.

in·spis·sa·tion (in′spi-sā′shŭn) **1.** The act of thickening or condensing, as by evaporation or absorption of fluid. **2.** An increased thickening or diminished fluidity. [L. *in,* intensive, + *spisso,* pp. *-atus,* to thicken]

in·sta·bil·i·ty (in′stă-bil′i-tē) **1.** The state of being unstable, or lacking stability. **2.** The abnormal tendency of a joint to subluxate or dislocate with normal activities and stresses. SEE ALSO laxity.

in·star (in′stahr) Any of the successive nymphal or larval stages in the metamorphosis of insects. [L. form]

in·step (in′step) The arch, or highest part of the dorsum of the foot. SEE ALSO tarsus.

in·stil·la·tion (in′sti-lā′shŭn) Dropping liquid on or into a part. [L. *instillatio,* fr. *in-stillo,* pp. *-atus,* to pour in by drops, fr. *stilla,* a drop]

in·stinct (in′stingkt) **1.** An enduring disposition or tendency to act in an organized and biologically adaptive manner. **2.** The unreasoning impulse to perform some purposive action without an immediate consciousness of the end to which that action may lead. **3.** PSYCHOANALYTIC THEORY the forces assumed to exist behind the tension caused by the needs of the id. [L. *instinctus,* impulse]

in·stinc·tive, in·stinc·tu·al (in-stingk′tiv, -stingk′shū-ăl) Relating to instinct.

In·sti·tute of Med·i·cine (IOM) (in′sti-tūt med′i-sin) The IOM was chartered in 1970 as a component of the U.S. National Academy of Sciences. The Institute provides a vital service by working outside the framework of government to ensure scientifically informed analysis and independent guidance. The IOM's mission is to serve as adviser to the U.S. to improve health. The IOM provides unbiased, evidence based, and authoritative information and advice concerning health and science policy to policy-makers, professionals, leaders in every sector of society, and the general public.

in·sti·tu·tion·al li·cen·sure (in′sti-tū′shŭn-ăl lī′sĕn-shŭr) Credentials granted to a unitary institution, rather than to its individual practitioners, which allows such institution the right to provide health care services as specified and permitted by the operative authority.

In·sti·tu·tion·al Re·view Board (IRB) (in′sti-tū′shŭn-ăl rĕ-vyū′ bōrd) The standing committee in a hospital or other facility that is charged with responsibility for ensuring the safety and well-being of human subjects involved in research.

in·stru·ment (in′strŭ-mĕnt) A tool or implement. [L. *instrumentum*]

in·stru·men·tal ac·tiv·i·ties of dail·y liv·ing (IADL) (in′strŭ-men′tăl ak-tiv′i-tēz dā′lē liv′ing) Activities oriented to interactions with the environment, more complex than activities of daily living (ADL); usually optional or can be delegated (e.g., care of pets, financial management, meal preparation, clean up and shopping). SYN personal activities of daily living.

in·stru·men·tal la·bor (in′strŭ-men′tăl lā′bŏr) Delivery that is completed or improved by use of mechanical devices.

in·stru·men·tar·i·um (in′strŭ-mĕn-tār′ē-ŭm) A collection of instruments and other equipment for an operation or for a medical or dental procedure.

in·stru·men·ta·tion (in′strŭ-men-tā′shŭn) **1.** In dentistry, application of an armamentarium in a restorative procedure. **2.** The use of dental instruments.

in·su·date (in′sū-dāt) Fluid swelling within an arterial wall (ordinarily serous), differing from an exudate in that it does not come to lie extramurally. [L. *in,* in, + *sudo,* pp. *-atus,* to sweat]

in·suf·fi·cien·cy (in′sŭ-fish′ĕn-sē) **1.** Lack of completeness of function or power. **2.** SYN incompetence (1). [L. *in-,* neg. + *sufficientia,* fr. *sufficio* to suffice]

in·suf·fi·cient sleep syn·drome (in′sŭ-fish′ĕnt slēp sin′drōm) A condition in which patients typically get less sleep than they need, due to stress, chemical agents (e.g., caffeine), or neurologic disorder.

in·suf·flate (in′sŭ-flāt) To blow air, gas, or fine powder into a cavity. [L. *in-sufflo,* to blow on or into]

in·suf·fla·tion (in′sŭ-flā′shŭn) **1.** The act or process of insufflating. **2.** SYN inhalant (3).

in·suf·fla·tion an·es·the·si·a (in′sŭ-flā′shŭn an′es-thē′zē-ă) Maintenance of inhalation anesthesia by delivery of anesthetic gases or vapors directly to the airway of a spontaneously breathing patient.

in·suf·fla·tor (in′sŭf-lā′tŏr) An instrument used in insufflation.

in•su•la, gen. and pl. **in•su•lae** (in′sū-lă, -lē) **1.** An oval region of the cerebral cortex overlying the extreme capsule, lateral to the lenticular nucleus, buried in the depth of the fissura lateralis cerebri (sylvian fissure). SYN island of Reil. **2.** SYN island. **3.** Any circumscribed body or patch on the skin. [L. island]

in•su•lar (in′sŭ-lăr) Relating to any insula, especially the island of Reil.

in•su•lar gy•ri (in′sŭ-lăr jī′rī) The short gyri of insula and long gyrus of insula.

in•su•lin (in′sŭ-lin) A polypeptide hormone, secreted by beta cells in the islets of Langerhans, that promotes glucose use, protein synthesis, and the formation and storage of neutral lipids; available in a variety of preparations including genetically engineered human insulin, which is presently favored, insulin is used parenterally in the treatment of diabetes mellitus. Cf. bioregulator. [L. *insula*, island, + -in]

insulinaemia [Br.] SYN insulinemia.

in•su•lin-an•tag•o•niz•ing fac•tor (in′sŭ-lin-an-tag′ō-nīz-ing fak′tŏr) SYN glycotropic factor.

in•su•lin-de•pen•dent di•a•be•tes mel•li•tus (in′sŭ-lin-dĕ-pen′dĕnt dī′ă-bē′tēz mel′i-tŭs) Former designation for Type 1 diabetes (q.v.); term declared obsolete by the American Diabetes Association.

in•su•lin•e•mi•a (in′sŭ-li-nē′mē-ă) Literally, insulin in the circulating blood; usually connotes an abnormally large concentration of insulin. SYN insulinaemia.

in•su•lin•like ac•tiv•i•ty (ILA) (in′sŭ-lin-līk ak-tiv′i-tē) A measure of substances, usually in plasma, that exert biologic effects similar to those of insulin in various bioassays; sometimes used as a measure of plasma insulin concentrations; always gives higher values than immunochemical techniques for the measurement of insulin.

in•su•lin•like growth fac•tors (IGF) (in′sŭ-lin-līk grōth fak′tŏrs) Peptides with formation that is stimulated by growth hormone. These peptides bring about peripheral tissue effects of that hormone and have high (about 70%) homology to human insulin.

in•su•lin•o•gen•e•sis (in′sŭ-lin-ō-jen′ĕ-sis) Production of insulin. [insulin + G. *genesis*, production]

in•su•lin•o•gen•ic, in•su•lo•gen•ic (in′sŭ-lin-ō-jen′ik, -lō-jen′ik) Relating to insulinogenesis.

in•su•li•no•ma (in′sŭ-li-nō′mă) An islet cell adenoma that secretes insulin. SYN insuloma.

in•su•lin pump (in′sŭ-lin pŭmp) Device used to deliver insulin subcutaneously by continuous basal infusion and intermittent bolus injections. See this page.

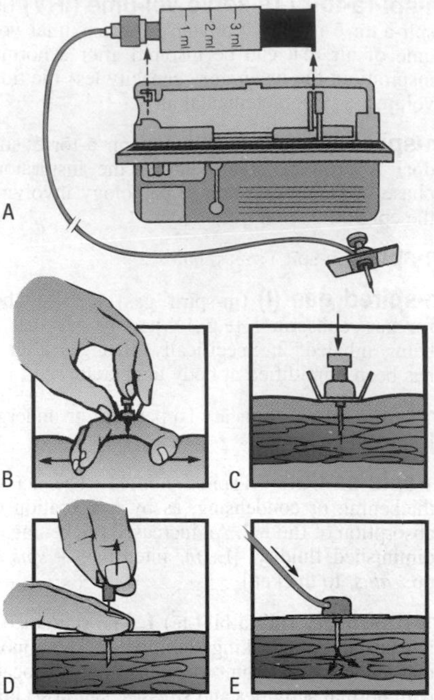

insulin pump: (A) diagram showing syringe in place inside pump and connection of pump via tubing to needle site; (B-E) insertion site before, during, and after needle and catheter have been inserted

in•su•lin re•cep•tor sub•strate-1 (IRS-1) (in′sŭ-lin rĕ-sep′tŏr sŭb′strāt) A cytoplasmic protein that is a direct substrate of the activated insulin receptor kinase. Insulin exposure results in its rapid phosphorylation at multiple tyrosine residues. Its phosphorylated sites associate with high affinity to certain cellular proteins. IRS-1 thus acts as an adaptor molecule that links the receptor kinase to various cellular activities regulated by insulin. IRS-1 is also phosphorylated after stimulation by insulinlike growth factor-1 and several interleukins.

in•su•lin re•sis•tance (in′sŭ-lin rĕ-zis′tăns) Diminished effectiveness of insulin in lowering blood sugar levels; arbitrarily defined as requiring 200 U or more of insulin per day to prevent hyperglycemia or ketosis; usually due to insulin binding by antibodies, but abnormalities in insulin receptors on cell surfaces also occur; associated with obesity, ketoacidosis, infection, and certain rare conditions.

in•su•lin-re•sis•tance syn•drome (in′sū-lin rĕ-zis′tĕns sin′drōm) SYN metabolic syndrome.

in•su•lin shock (in′sŭ-lin shok) Severe hypoglycemia produced by administration of insulin, manifested by sweating, tremor, anxiety, vertigo, and diplopia, followed by delirium, convulsions, and collapse.

in·su·li·tis (in′sŭ-lī′tis) Inflammation of the islands of Langerhans, with lymphocytic infiltration that may result from viral infection and be the initial lesion of Type 1 diabetes mellitus. [L. *insula,* island, + *-itis,* inflammation]

in·su·lo·ma (in′sŭ-lō′mă) SYN insulinoma. [L. *insula,* island, + *-oma,* tumor]

in·sult (in′sŭlt) An injury, attack, or trauma. [L. *insultus,* fr L. *insulto,* to spring on]

in·sur·ance (in-shŭr′ăns) A contractual arrangement whereby one party agrees to indemnify the other against financial or other specified loss during a stated period in the future. [O.Fr. *enseurer,* fr. L. *securus,* without worry]

in·sured (in-shŭrd′) SYN beneficiary.

in·sus·cep·ti·bil·i·ty (in′sŭ-sep′ti-bil′i-tē) SYN immunity. [L. *suscipio,* pp. *-ceptus,* to take upon one, fr. *sub,* under, + *capio,* to take]

in·take (in′tāk) **1.** The act of consuming or absorbing anything. **2.** That which is taken n. Cf. output. [in + take]

in·te·gra·tion (in′tĕ-grā′shŭn) **1.** The state of being combined, or the process of combining, into a complete and harmonious whole. SEE ALSO sensory integration. **2.** PHYSIOLOGY the process of building up (e.g., as by accretion, anabolism). **3.** MATHEMATICS the process of ascertaining a function from its differential. **4.** MOLECULAR BIOLOGY a recombination event in which a genetic element is inserted. [L. *integro,* pp. *-atus,* to make whole, fr. *integer,* whole]

in·te·gra·tive med·i·cine (in′tĕ-grā-tiv med′i-sin) Combines mainstream medical therapies with complementary and alternative medical therapies for which there is some reliable scientific evidence of safety and effectiveness.

in·teg·ri·ty (in-teg′ri-tē) Soundness or completeness of structure; a sound or unimpaired condition.

in·teg·u·ment (in-teg′yū-mĕnt) **1.** The enveloping membrane of the body; includes, in addition to the epidermis and dermis, all of the derivatives of the epidermis, e.g., hairs, nails, sudoriferous and sebaceous glands, and mammary glands. **2.** The rind, capsule, or covering of any body or part. SYN integumentum commune [TA], tegument. [L. *integumentum,* a covering, fr. *in-tego,* to cover]

in·teg·u·men·ta·ry (in-teg′yū-men′tăr-ē) Relating to the integument. SEE ALSO cutaneous, dermal.

in·teg·u·men·tum com·mu·ne (in-teg-yū-men′tŭm kō-myū′nē) [TA] SYN integument.

in·tel·lec·tu·al·i·za·tion (in′tĕ-lek′shū-ăl-ī-zā′shŭn) An unconscious defense mechanism in which reasoning, logic, or focusing on and verbalizing intellectual minutiae is used in an attempt to avoid confrontation with an objectionable impulse, affect, or interpersonal situation. [L. *intellectus,* perception, discernment]

in·tel·li·gence (in-tel′i-jĕns) **1.** A person's aggregate capacity to act purposefully, think rationally, and deal effectively with the environment, especially in meeting challenges and solving problems. **2.** PSYCHOLOGY A person's relative standing on two quantitative indices, those that measured intelligence and the effectiveness of adaptive behavior; a quantitative score or similar index on both indices constitutes the operational definition of intelligence. [L. *intelligentia*]

in·tel·li·gence quo·tient (IQ) (in-tel′i-jĕns kwō′shĕnt) The psychologist's index of intelligence as one part of a two-part determination, the other part being an index of adaptive behavior. IQ is ordinarily expressed as a ratio between the person's score on a given test and the score that the average individual of comparable age attained on the same test.

in·ten·si·ty (in-ten′si-tē) Marked tension; great activity; often used simply to denote a measure of the degree or amount of some quality. [L. *intendo,* pp. *-tensus,* to stretch out]

in·ten·si·ty mod·u·lat·ed ra·di·a·tion ther·a·py (IMRT) (in-ten′si-tē moj′yū-lā-tĕd rā′dē-ā′shŭn thār′ă-pē) In radiation therapy, technique in which the intensity of the beam is regulated to allow an increased dose to the tumor volume while reducing the dose to normal tissue; uses inverse treatment planning.

in·ten·sive care u·nit (ICU) (in-ten′siv kār yū′nit) A hospital facility for provision of intensive nursing and medical care of critically ill patients, characterized by high quality and quantity of continuous nursing and medical supervision and by use of sophisticated monitoring and resuscitative equipment; may be organized for the care of specific patient groups, e.g., neonatal or newborn ICU, neurological ICU, pulmonary ICU. SYN critical care unit.

in·ten·tion (in-ten′shŭn) **1.** An objective. **2.** SURGERY a process or operation. [L. *intentio,* a stretching out; intention]

in·ten·tion spasm (in-ten′shŭn spazm) A spasmodic contraction of the muscles occurring when a voluntary movement is attempted.

in·ten·tion-to-treat an·al·y·sis (in-ten′shŭn-trēt ă-nal′i-sis) Method of assessing results of a randomized controlled trial that includes in the analysis all the cases that should have received a treatment regimen but for some reason did not. All cases allocated to each arm of the trial are analyzed together as representing that treatment arm, regardless of whether they received or completed the prescribed regimen.

in·ten·tion trem·or (in-ten′shŭn trem′ŏr) A

tremor that occurs during the performance of precise voluntary movements, caused by disorders of the cerebellum or its connections. SYN volitional tremor (2).

♻**inter-** Combining form meaning among, between. [L. *inter,* between]

in·ter·ac·tion (in′tĕr-ak′shŭn) **1.** The reciprocal action between two entities in a common environment, as in chemical, ecologic, and social interaction. **2.** The effects when two entities concur that would not be observed with either in isolation. **3.** STATISTICS, PHARMACOLOGY, QUANTITATIVE GENETICS the phenomenon that the combined effects of two causes differ from the sum of the effects separately (as in synergism and antagonism). **4.** Independent operation of two or more causes to produce or prevent an effect. **5.** STATISTICS the necessity for a product term in a linear model.

in·ter·al·ve·o·lar sep·tum (in′tĕr-al-vē′ō-lăr sep′tŭm) **1.** The tissue intervening between two adjacent pulmonary alveoli; it consists of a close-meshed capillary network covered on both surfaces by very thin alveolar epithelial cells. **2.** One of the bony partitions between the tooth sockets.

in·ter·arch dis·tance (in′tĕr-ahrch dis′tăns) **1.** The vertical distance between the maxillary and mandibular arches under conditions of vertical dimensions that must be specified. **2.** The vertical distance between maxillary and mandibular ridges.

in·ter·ar·y·te·noid fold (in′tĕr-ar-i-tē′noyd fōld) The soft tissue between the arytenoid cartilages.

in·ter·a·tri·al block (in′tĕr-ā′trē-ăl blok) SYN intraatrial block.

in·ter·a·tri·al con·duc·tion time (in′tĕr-ā′trē-ăl kŏn-dŭk′shŭn tīm) SYN intraatrial conduction time (2).

in·ter·a·tri·al sep·tum (in′tĕr-ā′trē-ăl sep′tŭm) The wall between the atria of the heart. SYN septum interatriale [TA].

in·ter·au·ral (in′tĕr-awr′ăl) Referring to differences between ears, particularly temporal events occurring in or emanating from the ears.

in·ter·au·ral at·ten·u·a·tion (in′tĕr-awr′ăl ă-ten′yū-ā′shŭn) The reduction in intensity the head provides sound presented to one ear canal before it gets to the other ear; for air conduction, the reduction approximates 35 dB, but for bone conduction, it is only about 10 dB.

in·ter·bod·y (in′tĕr-bod′ē) Between the bodies of two adjacent vertebrae.

in·ter·ca·dence (in′tĕr-kā′dĕns) The occurrence of an extra beat between two regular pulse beats. [inter- + L. *cado,* pr. p. *cadens* (*-ent-*), to fall]

in·ter·ca·dent (in′tĕr-kā′dĕnt) Irregular in rhythm; characterized by intercadence.

in·ter·ca·lar·y (in-tĕr′kă-lar′ē) **1.** Occurring between two others; as in a pulse tracing, an upstroke interposed between two normal pulse beats. **2.** In fungi, located in a hypha or between hyphal segments, not at a hyphal terminus. [L. *intercalarius,* concerning an insertion]

in·ter·ca·lat·ed (in-tĕr′kă-lā-tĕd) Interposed; inserted between two others. [L. *intercalatus*]

in·ter·ca·lat·ed disc (in-tĕr′kă-lā-tĕd disk) A histologic feature of cardiac muscle, occurring at the junction of two myocardial cells; site of intercellular passage of ions and electrical impulses.

in·ter·ca·lat·ed ducts (in-tĕr′kă-lā-tĕd dŭkts) The minute ducts of glands, such as the salivary and the pancreas, that lead from the acini; they are lined by low cuboidal cells.

in·ter·cap·il·lar·y glo·mer·u·lo·scle·ro·sis (in′tĕr-kap′i-lar-ē glo-mer′yū-lō-skler-ō′sis) SYN diabetic glomerulosclerosis.

in·ter·ca·pit·u·lar veins (in′tĕr-kă-pich′yū-lăr vānz) Connect the dorsal and palmar veins in the hand, or the dorsal and plantar veins in the foot.

in·ter·ca·rot·id bod·y (in′tĕr-kă-rot′id bod′ē) SYN carotid body.

in·ter·car·pal joints (in′tĕr-kahr′păl joynts) The synovial joints between the carpal bones. SYN carpal joints (1).

in·ter·car·pal lig·a·ments (in′tĕr-kahr′păl lig′ă-mĕnts) Three sets of short fibrous bands that bind together the two rows of carpal bones; according to their location they are named dorsal intercarpal ligaments (ligamenta intercarpalia dorsalia), interosseous intercarpal ligaments (ligamenta intercarpalia interossea), and palmar intercarpal ligaments (ligamenta intercarpalia palmaria).

in·ter·cav·er·nous si·nus·es (in′tĕr-kav′ĕr-nŭs sī′nŭs-ĕz) The anterior and posterior anastomoses between the cavernous sinuses, passing anterior and posterior to the hypophysis and forming, with the cavernous sinuses, the circular sinus (1).

in·ter·cel·lu·lar bridg·es (in′tĕr-sel′yū-lăr brij′ĕz) Slender cytoplasmic strands connecting adjacent cells; in histologic sections the bridges are shrinkage artifacts; true bridges with cytoplasmic confluence exist between incompletely divided germ cells. SYN cell bridges, cytoplasmic bridges.

in·ter·cel·lu·lar can·a·lic·u·lus (in′tĕr-sel′yū-lăr kan′ă-lik′yŭ-lŭs) One of the fine channels between adjoining secretory cells, such as those between serous cells in salivary glands.

in·ter·cil·i·um (in′tĕr-sil′ē-ŭm) SYN glabella (2). [inter- + L. *cilium,* eyelid]

in·ter·cos·tal mem·branes (in′tĕr-kos′tăl mem′brānz) The membranous layers between ribs.

in·ter·cos·tal nerves (in′tĕr-kos′tăl nĕrvz) Ventral primary rami of the thoracic nerves. SYN nervi intercostales [TA].

in·ter·cos·tal space (in′tĕr-kos′tăl spās) An interval between the ribs, occupied by intercostal muscles, veins, arteries, and nerves.

in·ter·cos·to·brach·i·al nerves (in′tĕr-kos′tō-bra′kē-ăl nĕrz) Lateral cutaneous branches of the second and third intercostal nerves that pass to the skin of the medial side of the arm. SYN nervi intercostobrachiales [TA].

in·ter·course (in′tĕr-kōrs) Communication or dealings between or among people. SEE ALSO coitus. [L. *intercursus,* a running between]

in·ter·cri·co·thy·rot·o·my (in′tĕr-krī′kō-thī-rot′ŏ-mē) SYN cricothyrotomy.

in·ter·crines (in′tĕr-krīnz) SYN chemokines. [inter- + G. *krinō,* to separate, secrete]

in·ter·cross (in′tĕr-kraws) A mating between two individuals both heterozygous at a specified locus or loci.

in·ter·cur·rent (in′tĕr-kŭr′ĕnt) Intervening; said of a disease attacking a person who already has another disease. [inter- + L. *curro,* pr. p. *currens* (*-ent-*), to run]

in·ter·cus·pal po·si·tion (in′tĕr-kŭs′păl pŏ-zish′ŏn) SYN centric occlusion.

in·ter·cus·pa·tion (in′tĕr-kŭs-pā′shŭn) **1.** The cusp-to-fossa relation of the maxillary and mandibular posterior teeth to each other. **2.** The interlocking or fitting together of the cusps of opposing teeth. SYN interdigitation (4).

in·ter·den·tal (in′tĕr-den′tăl) **1.** Between the teeth. **2.** Denoting the relationship between the proximal surfaces of the teeth of the same arch. [inter- + L. *dens,* tooth]

in·ter·den·tal ca·nals (in′tĕr-den′tăl kă-nalz′) Canals that extend vertically through alveolar bone between roots of mandibular and maxillary incisor and maxillary bicuspid teeth. SYN Hirschfeld canals.

in·ter·den·tal pa·pil·la (in′tĕr-den′tăl pă-pil′ă) The gingiva that fills the interproximal space between two adjacent teeth.

in·ter·den·tal sep·tum (in′tĕr-den′tăl sep′tŭm) The bony interval separating two adjacent teeth in a dental arch.

in·ter·den·tal splint (in′tĕr-den′tăl splint) A splint for a fractured jaw, consisting of two metal or acrylic resin bands wired to the teeth of the upper and lower jaws, respectively, then fastened together to keep the jaws immovable.

in·ter·den·ti·um (in′tĕr-den′shē-ŭm) The interval between any two contiguous teeth.

in·ter·dig·it (in′tĕr-dij′it) That part of the hand or foot lying between any two adjacent fingers or toes.

in·ter·di·gi·tat·ing re·tic·u·lum cell (in′tĕr-dij′i-tāt-ing rĕ-tik′yū-lŭm sel) An antigen-presenting cell in the paracortex of lymph nodes, interacting with T lymphocytes.

in·ter·dig·i·ta·tion (in′tĕr-dij′i-tā′shŭn) **1.** The mutual interlocking of toothed or fingerlike processes. **2.** The processes thus interlocked. **3.** Infoldings or plicae of adjacent cell or plasma membranes. **4.** SYN intercuspation (2). [inter- + L. *digitus,* finger]

in·ter·dis·ci·pli·nar·y (in′tĕr-dis′i-pli-nār-ē) Denoting the overlapping interests of different fields of medicine and science. [inter- + L. *disciplina,* instruction, teaching]

in·ter·face (in′tĕr-fās) **1.** A surface that forms a common boundary of two bodies. **2.** The boundary between regions of different radiopacity, acoustic, or magnetic resonance properties; the projection of the interface between tissues of different such properties on an image. **3.** The connection between discrete parts of a computer system.

in·ter·fa·cial ca·nals (in′tĕr-fā-shăl kă-nalz′) Intercellular spaces occurring in relation to intercellular attachments by desmosomes in stratified squamous epithelium, generally resulting from shrinkage of an artifact of fixation.

in·ter·fer·ence (in′tĕr-fēr′ĕns) **1.** The coming together of waves in various media in such a way that the crests of one series correspond to the hollows of the other, the two thus neutralizing each other; or so that the crests of the two series correspond, thus increasing the excursions of the waves. **2.** Collision within the myocardium of two waves of excitation at the junction of territories controlled by each, as is seen in A-V dissociation. **3.** Also, in A-V dissociation, the disturbance of the regular rhythm of the ventricles by a conducted impulse from the atria, e.g., by a ventricular capture (interference beat). **4.** The condition in which infection of a cell by one virus prevents superinfection by another virus, or in which superinfection prevents effects that would result from infection by either virus alone, even though both viruses persist. **5.** Effect of a component on the accuracy of measurement of the desired analyte. [inter- + L. *ferio,* to strike]

in·ter·fe·ren·tial cur·rent (IFC) (in′tĕr-fĕr-en′shăl kŭr′rĕnt) An electrotherapeutic modality that employs the interference of two polyphasic sine waves to decrease the perception of pain.

in·ter·fer·on (IFN) (in′tĕr-fēr′on) A class of small protein and glycoprotein cytokines (15–28 kD) produced by T cells, fibroblasts, and other cells in response to viral infection and other biologic and synthetic stimuli. Interferons bind to specific receptors on cell membranes; their effects include inducing enzymes, suppressing cell proliferation, inhibiting viral proliferation, enhancing the phagocytic activity of macrophages, and augmenting the cytotoxic activity of T lymphocytes. Interferons are divided into five major classes (alpha, beta, gamma, tau, and omega) and several subclasses (indicated by Arabic numerals and letters) on the basis of physicochemical properties, cells of origin, mode of induction, and antibody reactions. [interfere + -on]

in·ter·fer·on-al·pha (α) (in′tĕr-fēr′on-al′fă) The major interferon made by virus-induced leukocytes; several different subtypes exist that are elaborated by leukocytes in response to viral infection or to stimulation with double-stranded RNA.

in·ter·fer·on al·pha (α) 2b (in′tĕr-fēr′on al′fă) A water-soluble protein (MW 19,271) secreted by cells infected by virus; used to treat hairy cell leukemia, malignant melanoma, condylomata acuminata, AIDS-associated Kaposi sarcoma, and chronic infection of hepatitis C virus.

in·ter·fer·on be·ta (β) 1b (in′tĕr-fēr′on bā′tă) A purified protein containing 165 amino acids (MW approximately 18,500) with antiviral and immunomodulatory effects; used in the treatment of relapsing-remitting multiple sclerosis to reduce the frequency of clinical exacerbations.

in·ter·fer·on o·me·ga (ω) (in′tĕr-fēr′on ō-mā′gă) A form of interferon known as interferon-alpha-2.

in·ter·fer·on tau (τ) (in′tĕr-fēr′on tow) An interferon secreted by bovine conceptus, with potent antiretroviral activity; in experimental use. SYN trophoblast interferon, trophoblastin.

in·ter·fer·on type I (in′tĕr-fēr′on tīp) Antiviral interferons, including interferon-α, and interferon-β.

in·ter·fer·on type II (in′tĕr-fēr′on tīp) Immune interferon, interferon-gamma.

in·ter·gan·gli·on·ic branches of sym·pa·thet·ic trunk (in′tĕr-gan′glē-on′ik branch′ĕz sim′pă-thet′ik trŭngk) The nerve strands interconnecting the ganglia of the sympathetic trunk; they consist of presynaptic sympathetic and visceral afferent fibers passing to higher or lower levels of the trunk.

in·ter·glo·bu·lar den·tin (in′tĕr-glob′yū-lăr den′tin) Imperfectly calcified matrix of dentin situated between the calcified globules near the dentinal periphery.

in·ter·ic·tal (in′tĕr-ik′tăl) The period between convulsions. [inter- + L. *ictus,* stroke]

in·ter·im den·ture (in′tĕr-im den′chŭr) A dental prosthesis to be used for a short time for reasons of esthetics, mastication, occlusal support, or convenience, or to condition the patient to accept an artificial substitute for missing natural teeth until more definite prosthetic dental treatment can be provided. SYN temporary denture.

in·ter·ki·ne·sis (in′tĕr-ki-nē′sis) Period between the first and second divisions of meiosis; comparable with interphase of mitosis. [inter- + G. *kinēsis,* movement]

in·ter·lam·i·nar jel·ly (in′tĕr-lam′i-năr jel′ē) The gelatinous material between ectoderm and endoderm that serves as the substrate on which mesenchymal cells migrate.

in·ter·leu·kin (IL) (in′tĕr-lū′kin) The name given to a group of multifunctional cytokines after their amino acid structure is known. They are synthesized by lymphocytes, monocytes, macrophages, and certain other cells. SEE ALSO lymphokine, cytokine. [inter- + *leuk*ocyte + -in]

in·ter·leu·kin-1 (in′tĕr-lū′kin) A cytokine, derived primarily from mononuclear phagocytes, which enhances the proliferation of T-helper cells and growth and differentiation of B cells.

in·ter·leu·kin-2 (in′tĕr-lū′kin) A cytokine derived from T-helper lymphocytes that causes proliferation of T lymphocytes and activated B lymphocytes.

in·ter·leu·kin-3 (in′tĕr-lū′kin) A cytokine derived from monocytes, fibroblasts, and endothelial cells that increases production of monocytes. SYN multicolony-stimulating factor.

in·ter·leu·kin-4 (in′tĕr-lū′kin) A cytokine derived from T4 lymphocytes that causes differentiation of B lymphocytes. SYN B-cell differentiating factor.

in·ter·leu·kin-5 (in′tĕr-lū′kin) A cytokine derived from T lymphocytes that causes activation of B lymphocytes and differentiation of eosinophils.

in·ter·leu·kin-6 (in′tĕr-lū′kin) A cytokine derived from fibroblasts, macrophages, and tumor cells that increases synthesis and secretion of immunoglobulins by B lymphocytes. SYN B-cell stimulatory factor 2.

in·ter·leu·kin-7 (in′tĕr-lū′kin) A cytokine derived from bone marrow cells that causes proliferation of B and T lymphocytes.

in·ter·leu·kin-8 (in′tĕr-lū′kin) A cytokine derived from endothelial cells, fibroblasts, keratinocytes, macrophages, and monocytes which causes chemotaxis of neutrophils and T-cell lymphocytes. SYN anionic neutrophil-activating peptide, monocyte-derived neutrophil chemotactic factor, neutrophil-activating factor.

in·ter·leu·kin-9 (in′tĕr-lū′kin) A cytokine derived from T cells that causes growth and proliferation of T cells.

in·ter·leu·kin-10 (in′tĕr-lū′kin) A cytokine derived from helper T-cell lymphocytes, B-cell lymphocytes, and monocytes that inhibits gamma-interferon (IFNγ) secretion by T-cell lymphocytes and it inhibits mononuclear cell inflammation.

in•ter•leu•kin-11 (in′tĕr-lū′kin) A cytokine derived from bone marrow stromal cells (endothelial cells, macrophages, and preadipocytes) that stimulates increased plasma concentrations of acute phase proteins.

in•ter•leu•kin-12 (in′tĕr-lū′kin) A cytokine derived from B lymphocytes, T lymphocytes, and macrophages that induces interferon-γ gene expression in T lymphocytes and NK cells.

in•ter•leu•kin-13 (in′tĕr-lū′kin) A cytokine derived from helper T-cell lymphocytes that inhibits mononuclear cell inflammation.

in•ter•leu•kin-14 (in′tĕr-lū′kin) A cytokine derived from T cells that stimulates B cell proliferation and inhibits Ig secretion.

in•ter•leu•kin-15 (in′tĕr-lū′kin) A cytokine derived from T cells that stimulates T-cell proliferation and NK cell activation.

in•ter•leu•kin-16 (in′tĕr-lū′kin) A cytokine made by T cells that is a potent chemotactant for $CD4^+$ T cells.

in•ter•leu•kin-17 (in′tĕr-lū′kin) A proinflammatory cytokine made by T cells.

in•ter•leu•kin-18 (in′tĕr-lū′kin) A cytokine made by macrophages; a potent inducer of interferon-γ by T cells and natural killer cells.

in•ter•lo•bar duct (in′tĕr-lō′bahr dŭkt) A duct draining the secretion of the lobe of a gland and formed by the junction of a number of interlobular ducts.

in•ter•lo•bar veins of kid•ney (in′tĕr-lō′bahr vānz kid′nē) Those that parallel the interlobar arteries, receive blood from arcuate veins, and terminate in the renal vein.

in•ter•lo•bi•tis (in′tĕr-lō-bī′tis) Inflammation of the pleura separating two pulmonary lobes.

in•ter•lob•u•lar ar•ter•ies (in′tĕr-lob′yū-lăr ahr′tĕr-ēz) Arteries that pass between lobules of an organ. SYN arteriae interlobulares [TA].

in•ter•lob•u•lar duct (in′tĕr-lob′yū-lăr dŭkt) Any duct leading from a lobule of a gland and formed by the junction of the fine ducts draining the acini.

in•ter•lob•u•lar em•phy•se•ma (in′tĕr-lob′yū-lăr em′fi-sē′mă) Interstitial emphysema in the connective tissue septa between the pulmonary lobules.

in•ter•lob•u•lar pleu•ri•sy (in′tĕr-lob′yū-lăr plūr′i-sē) Inflammation limited to the pleura in the sulci between the pulmonary lobes.

in•ter•lob•u•lar veins of kid•ney (in′tĕr-lob′yū-lăr vānz kid′nē) Running parallel to the interlobular arteries, they drain the peritubular capillary plexus, emptying into the arcuate veins.

in•ter•lob•u•lar veins of liv•er (in′tĕr-lob′yū-lăr vānz liv′ĕr) Terminal branches of the portal vein that course in the portal canals between the conceptual liver lobules and empty into the liver sinusoids.

in•ter•max•il•lar•y bone (in′tĕr-mak′si-lar-ē bōn) SYN os incisivum.

in•ter•max•il•lar•y su•ture (in′tĕr-mak′si-lar-ē sū′chŭr) The line of union of the two maxillae.

in•ter•me•di•ar•y nerve (in′tĕr-mē′dē-ār-ē nĕrv) A root of the facial nerve containing sensory fibers for taste from the anterior two thirds of tongue with cell bodies that are located in the geniculate ganglion and presynaptic parasympathetic autonomic fibers with cell bodies that are located in the superior salivatory nucleus, i.e., the fibers eventually conveyed through the chorda tympani branch of the facial nerve to the lingual nerve. SYN nervus intermedius [TA], intermediate nerve.

in•ter•me•di•ate (in′tĕr-mē′dē-ăt) **1.** Between two extremes; interposed; intervening. **2.** A substance formed in the course of chemical reactions that then proceeds to participate rapidly in further reactions, so that at any given moment it is present in minute concentrations only; such substances, when appearing in the course of the reactions involved in metabolism, are metabolic intermediates. **3.** DENTISTRY a cement base. **4.** An element or organ between right and left (or lateral and medial) structures. SYN intermedius.

in•ter•me•di•ate ba•sil•ic vein (in′tĕr-mē′dē-ăt bă-sil′ik vān) Medial branch of the median antebrachial vein that joins the basilic vein.

in•ter•me•di•ate care fa•cil•i•ty (ICF) (in′tĕr-mē′dē-ăt kār fă-sil′i-tē) A residential option for patients who cannot live alone and also need more supervision than in-home services offer but who do not need the level of care found in skilled nursing facilities. SEE nursing facility.

in•ter•me•di•ate ce•phal•ic vein (in′tĕr-mē′dē-ăt sĕ-fal′ik vān) Lateral branch of the median antebrachial vein that joins the cephalic vein near the elbow.

in•ter•me•di•ate cu•ne•i•form bone (in′tĕr-mē′dē-ăt kyū-nē′i-fōrm bōn) A bone of the distal row of the tarsus; it articulates with the medial and lateral cuneiform, navicular, and second metatarsal bones. SYN wedge bone.

in•ter•me•di•ate heart (in′tĕr-mē′dē-ăt hahrt) Description of the heart's electrical axis when this is directed at approximately between +30°–+60°.

in•ter•me•di•ate host, in•ter•me•di•ar•y host (in′tĕr-mē′dē-ăt hōst, in′tĕr-mē′dē-ār-ē) **1.** One in which larval or developmental stages occur. **2.** A host through which a microorganism can pass or contains an asexual stage of a parasite.

in·ter·me·di·ate nerve (in′tĕr-mē′dē-ăt nĕrv) SYN intermediary nerve.

in·ter·me·di·ate sa·cral crest (in′tĕr-mē′dē-ăt sā′krăl krest) Crests formed by the fusion of articular processes of all the sacral vertebrae. SYN articular crest.

in·ter·me·di·ate su·pra·cla·vic·u·lar nerve (in′tĕr-mē′dē-ăt sū′pră-klă-vik′yū-lăr nĕrv) One of several nerves arising from C3-C4 part of cervical plexus that run across top of shoulder and pass down across shaft of clavicle to supply skin of top of shoulder and in infraclavicular region. SYN middle supraclavicular nerve, nervus supraclavicularis intermedius.

in·ter·me·di·ate trait (in′tĕr-mē′dē-ăt trāt) A measurable trait in which there is some evidence of the operation of a simple major cause, but in which the variation within the putative categories is such as to cause overlap and hence ambiguity in classification of any particular reading.

in·ter·me·di·ate vas·tus mus·cle (in′tĕr-mē′dē-ăt vas′tŭs mŭs′ĕl) SYN vastus intermedius muscle.

in·ter·me·di·o·lat·er·al nu·cle·us (in′tĕr-mē′dē-ō-lat′ĕr-ăl nū′klē-ŭs) The cell column that forms the lateral horn of the spinal gray matter. Extending from the first thoracic through the second lumbar segment, the column contains the autonomic motor neurons that give rise to the preganglionic fibers of the sympathetic system.

in·ter·me·di·o·me·di·al fron·tal branch of cal·lo·so·mar·gin·al ar·ter·y (in′tĕr-mē′dē-ō-mē′dē-ăl frŏn′tăl branch kă-lō′sō-mahr′ji-năl ahr′tĕr-ē) Branch of middle portion of callosomarginal artery to anterosuperior portion of medial aspect of frontal lobe of cerebrum.

in·ter·me·di·o·me·di·al nu·cle·us (in′tĕr-mē′dē-ō-mē′dē-ăl nū′klē-ŭs) A small group of scattered visceral motor neurons immediately ventral to the thoracic nucleus in the thoracic and upper two lumbar segments of the spinal cord; considered to receive visceral afferent fibers at all spinal levels.

in·ter·me·di·us (in′tĕr-mē′dē-ŭs) SYN intermediate. [L.]

in·ter·men·stru·al pain (in′tĕr-men′strū-ăl pān) **1.** Pelvic discomfort occurring approximately at the time of ovulation, usually at the midpoint of the menstrual cycle. **2.** SYN mittelschmerz.

in·ter·met·a·car·pal joint (in′tĕr-met′ă-kahr′păl joynt) The synovial joints between the bases of the second, third, fourth, and fifth metacarpal bones.

in·ter·met·a·tar·sal joint (in′tĕr-met′ă-tahr′săl joynt) The synovial joints between the bases of the five metatarsal bones.

in·ter·mit·tent (in′tĕr-mit′ĕnt) Marked by intervals of complete quietude between two periods of activity.

in·ter·mit·tent a·cute por·phyr·ia (IAP) (in′tĕr-mit′ĕnt ă-kyūt′ pōr-fir′ē-ă) Disorder caused by the hepatic overproduction of δ-aminolevulinic acid, with a great increase in urinary excretion of it and of porphobilinogen, due to a deficiency of porphobilinogen deaminase; characterized by intermittent acute attacks of hypertension, abdominal colic, psychosis, and polyneuropathy, but with no photosensitivity; exacerbated by ingestion of certain drugs (e.g., barbiturates). SYN acute intermittent porphyria, acute porphyria.

in·ter·mit·tent clau·di·ca·tion (in′tĕr-mit′ĕnt klaw′di-kā′shŭn) A condition caused by ischemia of the muscles; characterized by attacks of lameness and pain, brought on by walking, chiefly in the calf muscles; however, the condition may occur in other muscle groups. SYN Charcot syndrome, myasthenia angiosclerotica.

in·ter·mit·tent com·pres·sion (in′tĕr-mit′ĕnt kŏm-presh′ŭn) **1.** A treatment procedure that employs intermittent external pressure to reduce edema in an extremity. **2.** A neurodevelopmental treatment technique to facilitate contraction by applying pressure directly to the muscles surrounding a joint requiring better stabilization. SYN pressure tapping.

in·ter·mit·tent cramp (in′tĕr-mit′ĕnt kramp) **1.** SYN tetany. **2.** SYN benign tetanus.

in·ter·mit·tent ex·plo·sive dis·or·der (in′tĕr-mit′ĕnt eks-plō′siv dis-ōr′dĕr) An uncommon disorder that begins in early childhood, characterized by repeated acts of violent, aggressive behavior in otherwise normal people that is markedly out of proportion to the event that provokes it.

in·ter·mit·tent man·da·to·ry ven·ti·la·tion (IMV) (in′tĕr-mit′ĕnt man′dă-tōr-ē ven′ti-lā′shŭn) A mode of mechanical ventilation in which the patient can trigger spontaneous breaths between or during preset mandatory breaths.

in·ter·mit·tent per·cus·sive ven·ti·la·tion (IPV) (in′tĕr-mit′ĕnt pĕr-kus′iv ven′ti-lā′shŭn) A ventilatory technique that delivers short high velocity bursts of respiratory gas through a full face mask at a rapid rate (80–650 cycles/min) in addition to a steady flow of gas at a physiologic level. The percussive effect dilates airways and enhances clearance of bronchial secretions.

in·ter·mit·tent pos·i·tive pres·sure breath·ing (IPPB) (in′tĕr-mit′ĕnt poz′i-tiv presh′ŭr brēdh′ing) SYN controlled mechanical ventilation.

in·ter·mit·tent tet·a·nus (in′tĕr-mit′ĕnt tet′ă-nŭs) SYN tetany.

in·ter·mus·cu·lar sep·tum (in′tĕr-mŭs′kyū-lăr sep′tŭm) A term applied to aponeurotic sheets separating various muscles of the limbs; these are anterior and posterior crural, lateral and medial femoral, lateral and medial humeral.

in·tern (in′tĕrn) An advanced student or recent graduate undertaking further education by assisting in the medical or surgical care of hospital patients, with supervision and instruction; formerly, one who resided within the institution. [F. *interne,* inside]

in·ter·nal (in-tĕr′năl) Away from the surface. USAGE NOTE: Often incorrectly used to mean medial. [L. *internus*]

in·ter·nal ad·he·sive per·i·car·di·tis (in-tĕr′năl ad-hē′siv per′i-kahr-dī′tis) SYN concretio cordis.

in·ter·nal au·dit (in-tĕr′năl aw′dit) An assessment of records and data in a business or professional organization by an employee of that organization to verify that documentation and operations are accurate and legal.

in·ter·nal au·di·to·ry veins (in-tĕr′năl aw′di-tōr-ē vānz) SYN labyrinthine veins.

in·ter·nal base of skull (in-tĕr′năl bās skŭl) The interior aspect of the skull base on which the brain rests; the floor of the cranial cavity. SEE ALSO base of skull.

in·ter·nal branch of trunk of ac·ces·so·ry nerve (in-tĕr′năl branch trŭngk ak-ses′ŏr-ē nĕrv) Branch of the accessory nerve trunk that carries fibers from the cranial root and that unites with the vagus nerve in the jugular foramen. SEE ALSO accessory nerve [CN XI].

in·ter·nal cap·sule (in-tĕr′năl kap′sŭl) A massive layer (8–10 mm thick) of white matter separating the caudate nucleus and thalamus (medial) from the more laterally situated lentiform nucleus (globus pallidus and putamen). It consists of 1) fibers ascending from the thalamus to the cerebral cortex that compose, among others, the visual, auditory, and somatic sensory radiations, and 2) fibers descending from the cerebral cortex to the thalamus, subthalamic region, midbrain, hindbrain, and spinal cord. The internal capsule is the major route by which the cerebral cortex is connected with the brainstem and spinal cord. Laterally and superiorly it is continuous with the corona radiata which forms a major part of the white matter of the cerebral hemisphere; caudally and medially it continues, much reduced in size, as the crus cerebri that contains, among others, the pyramidal tract. On horizontal section it appears in the form of a V opening out laterally; the V's obtuse angle is called genu (knee); its anterior and posterior limbs, respectively, the crus anterior and crus posterior. SYN capsula interna [TA].

in·ter·nal ca·rot·id ar·ter·y (in-tĕr′năl kă-rot′id ahr′tĕr-ē) arises from the common carotid opposite upper border of thyroid cartilage (C4 vertebral level) and terminates in the middle cranial fossa by dividing into the anterior and middle cerebral arteries. SYN arteria carotis interna.

in·ter·nal ca·rot·id nerve (in-tĕr′năl kă-rot′id nĕrv) The cephalic arterial ramus conveying postsynaptic sympathetic fibers from the superior cervical ganglion to the internal carotid artery to form the internal carotid plexus. SYN nervus caroticus internus [TA].

in·ter·nal ce·phal·ic ver·sion (in-tĕr′năl sĕ-fal′ik vĕr′zhŭn) Version performed by means of one hand within the vagina. SEE ALSO cephalic version.

in·ter·nal ce·re·bral veins (in-tĕr′năl ser′ĕ-brăl vānz) Paired veins passing caudally near the midline in the tela choroidea of the third ventricle, formed by the union of the choroid vein, thalamostriate (terminal) vein, and vein of septum pellucidum, and uniting caudally so as to form the great cerebral vein. SYN venae internae cerebri [TA].

in·ter·nal dose (in-tĕr′năl dōs) The amount of a compound that is absorbed by the body by penetrating an epithelial barrier such as the skin, eyes, respiratory tract, or gastrointestinal tract.

in·ter·nal ear (in-tĕr′năl ēr) SEE ear. SEE ALSO labyrinth.

in·ter·nal en·er·gy (U, *U*) (in-tĕr′năl en′ĕr-jē) Energy of a system measured by the heat absorbed from the system's surroundings and the amount of work done on the system by its surroundings.

in·ter·nal fis·tu·la (in-tĕr′năl fis′chū-lă) A fistula between hollow viscera.

in·ter·nal fix·a·tion (in-tĕr′năl fik-sā′shŭn) Stabilization of fractured bony parts by direct fixation to one another with surgical wires, screws, pins, rods, plates, or methylmethacrylate.

in·ter·nal hem·or·rhage (in-tĕr′năl hem′ŏr-ăj) Bleeding into organs or cavities of the body. SYN concealed hemorrhage.

in·ter·nal il·i·ac ar·ter·y (in-tĕr′nal il′ē-ak ahr′tĕr-ē) *Origin*, common iliac; *branches*, from anterior division obturator, inferior gluteal, umbilical, superior vesical, inferior vesical, middle rectal, and internal pudendal; from posterior division: iliolumbar, lateral sacral, superior gluteal. SYN arteria hypogastrica, arteria iliaca interna, hypogastric artery.

in·ter·nal il·i·ac vein (in-tĕr′năl il′ē-ak vān) Runs from the upper border of the greater sciatic notch to the brim of the pelvis where it joins the external iliac vein to form the common iliac vein; it drains most of the territory supplied by the internal iliac artery.

in·ter·nal in·ju·ry (in-tĕr′năl in′jŭr-ē) Any trauma that involves organs or cavities of the body.

in·ter·nal in·ter·cos·tal mus·cle (in-tĕr′năl in′tĕr-kos′tăl mŭs′ĕl) Each arises from lower border of rib and passes obliquely downward and backward to be inserted into upper border of rib below; *action*, contract during expiration, also maintain tension in the intercostal spaces to resist mediolateral movement; *nerve supply*, intercostal.

in·ter·nal·i·za·tion (in-tĕr′năl-ī-zā′shŭn) Adopting as one's own the standards and values of another person or society.

in·ter·nal·ized ho·mo·pho·bi·a (in-tĕr′năl-izd hō′mō-fō′bē-ă) A psychological trait occurring in a homosexual, often associated with self-loathing, self-censure, and self-censorship.

in·ter·nal jug·u·lar vein (in-tĕr′năl jŭg′yū-lăr vān) Main venous structure of the neck, formed as a continuation of the sigmoid sinus of the dura mater, contained within the carotid sheath as it descends the neck uniting, behind the sternoclavicular joint, with the subclavian vein to form the brachiocephalic vein.

in·ter·nal med·i·cine (IM) (in-tĕr′năl med′i-sin) The branch of medicine concerned with nonsurgical diseases in adults, but not including diseases limited to the skin or to the nervous system.

in·ter·nal o·blique mus·cle (in-tĕr′năl ō-blēk′ mŭs′ĕl) *Origin*, iliac fascia deep to lateral part of inguinal ligament, anterior half of crest of ilium, and lumbar fascia; *insertion*, tenth to twelfth ribs and sheath of rectus; some of the fibers from inguinal ligament terminate in the conjoint tendon; *action*, diminishes capacity of abdomen, flexes lumbar vertebral column (bends thorax forward); *nerve supply*, lower thoracic. See this page. SYN musculus obliquus internus abdominis [TA].

in·ter·nal ob·tu·ra·tor mus·cle (in-tĕr′năl ob′tŭr-ā-tŏr mŭs′ĕl) SYN obturator internus muscle.

in·ter·nal oc·cip·i·tal crest (in-tĕr′ăl ok-sip′i-tăl krest) A ridge running from the internal occipital protuberance to the posterior margin of the foramen magnum, giving attachment to the falx cerebelli.

in·ter·nal oph·thal·mop·a·thy (in-tĕr′năl of′thăl-mop′ă-thē) Any disease of the internal structures of the eyeball.

in·ter·nal oph·thal·mo·ple·gi·a (in-tĕr′năl of-thal′mō-plē′jē-ă) SYN ophthalmoplegia interna.

in·ter·nal phase (in-tĕr′năl fāz) The particles contained in a colloid solution.

in·ter·nal po·dal·ic ver·sion (in-tĕr′năl pō-dal′ik vĕr′zhŭn) Maneuver to deliver the fetus by inserting a hand into the uterine cavity, grasping one or both feet, and drawing them through the cervix; rarely indicated today except for the delivery of a second twin.

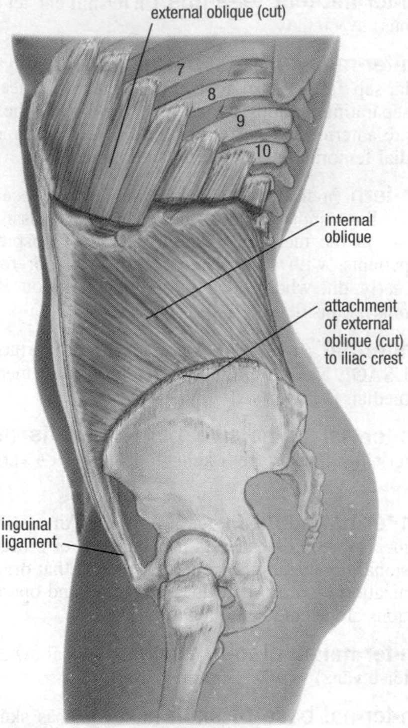

internal oblique muscle

in·ter·nal pter·y·goid mus·cle (in-tĕr′năl ter′i-goyd mŭs′ĕl) SYN medial pterygoid muscle.

in·ter·nal pu·den·dal ar·ter·y (in-tĕr′năl pyū-den′dăl ahr′tĕr-ē) *Origin*, internal iliac; *branches*, inferior rectal, perineal, posterior scrotal (or labial), urethral, artery of bulb of penis (or of vestibule), deep artery of penis (or clitoris), dorsal artery of penis (or clitoris).

in·ter·nal pu·den·dal vein (in-tĕr′năl pyū-den′dăl vān) A tributary of the internal iliac vein that accompanies the internal pudendal artery as a single or double vessel. It drains the perineum.

in·ter·nal rep·re·sen·ta·tion (in-tĕr′năl rep′rĕ-zen-tā′shŭn) Term used by neurolinguistic programming to denote the way people use mental imagery (visual, auditory, or kinesthetic) to encode experience, the composite of which comprises their internal and external reality.

in·ter·nal res·pi·ra·tion (in-tĕr′năl res′pir-ā′shŭn) SYN tissue respiration.

in·ter·nal ro·ta·tion (in-tĕr′năl rō-tā′shŭn) Movement of a joint, around its long axis, toward the midline of the body. SYN medial rotation.

in·ter·nal trac·tion (in-tĕr′năl trak′shŭn) A pulling force created by using one of the cranial bones, above the point of fracture, for anchorage.

in·ter·nal u·re·thral or·i·fice (in-tĕr′năl yūr-ē′thrăl ōr′i-fis) The internal opening or orifice of the urethra, at thc anterior and inferior angle of the trigone.

in·ter·na·sal su·ture (in′tĕr-nā′zăl sū′chŭr) Line of union between the two nasal bones.

In·ter·na·tion·al Clas·si·fi·ca·tion of Dis·eas·es (ICD) (in′tĕr-nash′ŭn-ăl klas′i-fi-kā′shŭn di-zēz′ĕz) The enumeration of specific conditions and groups of conditions determined by an internationally representative expert committee that advises the World Health Organization, which publishes the complete list in a periodically revised book, the *Manual of the International Statistical Classification of Diseases, Injuries and Causes of Death*. The tenth revision (ICD-10) came into use in 1992; it has 20 chapters, each with a hierarchical arrangement of subdivisions (rubrics) some chapters are etiologic; others relate to body systems, classes of conditions, or procedures.

In·ter·na·tion·al Clas·si·fi·ca·tion of Func·tion·ing, Dis·a·bil·i·ty, and Health (in′tĕr-nash′ŭn-ăl klas′i-fi-kā′shŭn fungk′shŭn-ing dis′ă-bil′i-tē helth) The World Health Organization's health classification mode.

In·ter·na·tion·al Clas·si·fi·ca·tion of Health Prob·lems in Pri·ma·ry Care (in′tĕr-nash′ŭn-ăl klas′i-fi-kā′shŭn helth prob′lĕmz prī′mar-ē kār) A classification of diseases, conditions, and problems arranged for use in primary care where diagnostic precision is seldom possible.

In·ter·na·tion·al Clas·si·fi·ca·tion of Im·pair·ments, Dis·a·bil·i·ties and Hand·i·caps (in′tĕr-nash′ŭn-ăl klas′i-fi-ka′shŭn im-pār′mĕnts dis′ă-bil′i-tēz han′dē-kaps) A WHO-sponsored numeric taxonomy of the impairments, disabilities, and handicaps consequent on injury and disease.

In·ter·na·tion·al Clas·si·fi·ca·tion of Sleep Dis·or·ders (ICSD) (in′tĕr-nash′ŭn-ăl klas′i-fi-kā′shŭn slēp dis-ōr′dĕrz) Coded listing, last revised in 2005, published by the American Academy of Sleep Medicine; used for diagnosis of disorders and disease states related to or active during periods of sleep.

In·ter·na·tion·al Con·fed·e·ra·tion of Mid·wives (ICM) (in′tĕr-nash′ŭn-ăl kŏn-fed′ĕr-ā′shŭn mid′wīvz) A professional organization that seeks to improve the lives of women and infants through strengthening the position and training of the midwife as a valued health care practitioner.

In·ter·na·tion·al Con·fer·ence on Har·mo·ni·za·tion (ICH) (in′tĕr-nash′ŭn-ăl kon′fĕr-ĕns hahr′mŏ-nī-zā′shŭn) A worldwide regulatory and investigatory authority that intends to investigate and combine the research and development of new drugs according to a single standard.

In·ter·na·tion·al Coun·cil of Nurs·es (ICN) (in-tĕr-nash′ŭn-ăl kown′sil nŭr′sĕz) A professional nursing organization; its focus is more on education than on everyday labor issues.

in·ter·na·tion·al nor·mal·ized ra·ti·o (INR) (in′tĕr-nash′ŭn-ăl nōr′măl-īzd rā′shē-ō) The prothrombin time ratio that would have been obtained if a standard reagent had been used in a prothrombin time determination; the prothrombin time ratio is expressed as the patient's prothrombin time divided by the mean of the prothrombin time reference interval; the prothrombin time ratio is obtained for a working reagent in the laboratory through use of a parameter designated the international sensitivity index. SEE ALSO international sensitivity index.

In·ter·na·tion·al Pho·net·ic Al·pha·bet (IPA) (in′tĕr-nash′ŭn-ăl fō-net′ik al′fă-bet) System of orthographic symbols devised for representing speech sounds; can be used for any language or to represent the sounds of disordered speech.

In·ter·na·tion·al Red Cross So·ci·e·ty (in′tĕr-nash′ŭn-ăl red kraws sŏ-sī′ĕ-tē) A benevolent organization, based in Geneva with aims similar to those of the American Red Cross. It provides humanitarian aid to refugees, prisoners of war, and victims of natural disaster.

in·ter·na·tion·al sen·si·ti·vi·ty in·dex (ISI) (in′tĕr-nash′ŭn-ăl sen′si tiv′i-tē in′deks) The slope of the line of best fit relating the log prothrombin time obtained with a standard reagent to the log prothrombin time obtained with the working reagent for both normal people and patients who receive stable oral anticoagulant therapy; the standard reagents used for this value assignment are reference preparations calibrated against the World Health Organization standard reagent. SEE ALSO international normalized ratio.

In·ter·na·tion·al Sys·tem of U·nits (SI) (in′tĕr-nash′ŭn-ăl sis′tĕm yū′nits) A system of measurements, based on the metric system, adopted at the 11th General Conference on Weights and Measures of the International Organization for Standardization (1960) to cover both the coherent units (basic, supplementary, and derived units) and the decimal multiples and submultiples of these units formed by use of prefixes proposed for general international scientific and technologic use. SI proposes seven basic units: meter (m), kilogram (kg), second (s), ampere (A), Kelvin (K), candela (cd), and mole (mol) for the basic quantities of length, mass, time, electric current, temperature, luminous intensity, and amount of substance; supplementary units proposed include the radian (rad) for plane angle and steradian (sr) for solid angle; derived units (e.g., force, power, frequency) are stated in terms of the basic units (e.g., velocity is in meters per second, m/sec^{-1}). Multiples (prefixes) in descending order are: exa- (E, 10^{18}), peta- (P, 10^{15}), tera- (T, 10^{12}), giga- (G, 10^{9}), mega- (M, 10^{6}), kilo- (k, 10^{3}), hecto- (h, 10^{2}), deca- (da, 10^{1}), deci- (d, 10^{-1}), centi- (c, 10^{-2}), milli- (m, 10^{-3}), micro- (μ, 10^{-6}), nano- (n, 10^{-9}), pico- (p, 10^{-12}), femto- (f, 10^{-15}), atto- (a, 10^{-18}). The prefix zepto (z) has been proposed for 10^{-21}. [Fr. *Système International d'Unités*]

in·ter·na·tion·al u·nit (in′tĕr-nash′ŭn-ăl yū′nit) The amount of a substance (e.g., drug, hormone, vitamin, enzyme) that produces a specific effect as defined by an international body and accepted internationally. SYN unit (4).

interneurones [Br.] SYN interneurons.

in·ter·neu·rons (in′tĕr-nūr′onz) Combinations or groups of neurons between sensory and motor neurons that govern coordinated activity. SYN interneurones.

in·tern·ist (in-tĕr′nist) A physician trained in internal medicine.

in·ter·nod·al seg·ment (in′tĕr-nō′dăl seg′mĕnt) The portion of a myelinated nerve fiber between two successive nodes. SYN internode.

in·ter·node (in′tĕr-nōd) SYN internodal segment.

in·ter·nu·cle·ar (in′tĕr-nū′klē-ăr) Between nerve cell groups in the brain or retina.

in·ter·nu·cle·ar oph·thal·mo·ple·gi·a (INO) (in′tĕr-nū′klē-ăr of-thal′mō-plē′jē-ă) Ophthalmoplegia in lesions of the medial longitudinal fasciculus, with failure of adduction in horizontal gaze but with retention of convergence.

in·ter·nun·ci·al (in′tĕr-nun′sē-ăl) **1.** Indicating a neuron functionally interposed between two or more other neurons. **2.** Acting as a medium of communication between two organs. [L. *internuntius* (or *-nuncius*), a messenger between two parties, fr. *inter,* between, + *nuncius,* a messenger]

in·ter·nun·ci·al neu·ron (in′tĕr-nun′sē-ăl nūr′on) A neuron interposed between and connecting two other neurons.

in·ter·ob·serv·er er·ror (in′tĕr-ŏb-zĕr′vĕr er′ŏr) The differences in interpretation by two or more people making observations of the same phenomenon.

in·ter·oc·clu·sal dis·tance (in′tĕr-ŏ-klū′zăl dis′tăns) **1.** The vertical distance between the opposing occlusal surfaces, assuming rest relation unless otherwise designated. **2.** SYN freeway space.

in·ter·o·cep·tive (in′tĕr-ō-sep′tiv) Relating to the sensory nerve cells innervating the viscera (thoracic, abdominal and pelvic organs, and the cardiovascular system), their sensory end organs, or the information they convey to the spinal cord and the brain. [inter- + L. *capio,* to take]

in·ter·o·cep·tor (in′tĕr-ō-sep′tŏr) One of the various forms of small sensory end organs (receptors) situated within the walls of the respiratory and gastrointestinal tracts or in other viscera. [inter- + L. *capio,* to take]

in·ter·os·se·ous car·ti·lage (in′tĕr-os′ē-ŭs kahr′ti-lăj) SYN connecting cartilage.

in·ter·os·se·ous mem·brane of fore·arm (in′tĕr-os′ē-ŭs mem′brān fōr′ahrm) The dense membrane that connects the interosseous margins of the radius and ulna, forming the radioulnar syndesmosis, and with those bones separating the flexor and extensor compartments of the forearm.

in·ter·os·se·ous mus·cles (in′tĕr-os′ē-ŭs mŭs′ĕlz) Muscles that arise from and run between long (metacarpal and metatarsal) bones of the hand and foot, extending to and moving digits. SEE ALSO dorsal interossei (interosseous muscles) of foot, dorsal interossei (interosseous muscles) of hand, palmar interosseous muscle, plantar interosseous muscle. SYN musculi interossei.

in·ter·pa·ri·e·tal su·ture (in′tĕr-păr-ī′ĕ-tăl sū′chŭr) SYN sagittal suture.

in·ter·par·ox·ys·mal (in′tĕr-par′ok-siz′măl) Occurring between successive paroxysms of a disease.

in·ter·pe·dun·cu·lar fos·sa (in′tĕr-pĕ-dungk′yū-lăr fos′ă) Deep depression on the inferior surface of the mesencephalon, between the crura cerebri, the floor of which is formed by the posterior perforated substance.

in·ter·pe·dun·cu·lar nu·cle·us (in′tĕr-pĕ-dungk′yū-lăr nū′klē-ŭs) A median, unpaired, ovoid cell group at the base of the midbrain tegmentum between the cerebral peduncles; it receives the retroflex fasciculus from the habenula, and projects to the raphe region (raphe nuclei) and periaqueductal gray substance of the midbrain.

in·ter·pel·vi·ab·dom·i·nal am·pu·ta·tion (in′tĕr-pel′vē-ab-dom′i-năl amp′yū-tā′shŭn) SYN hemipelvectomy.

in·ter·pha·lan·ge·al (in′tĕr-fă-lan′jē-ăl) Between two phalanges; denoting the finger or toe joints.

in·ter·pha·lan·ge·al joints of hand (in′tĕr-fă-lan′jē-ăl joynts hand) The hinge synovial joints between the phalanges of the fingers.

in·ter·phase (in′tĕr-fāz) The stage between two successive divisions of a cell nucleus in which the biochemical and physiologic functions of the cell are performed and replication of chromatin occurs.

in·ter·phy·let·ic (in′tĕr-fī-let′ik) Denoting the

transitional forms between two kinds of cells during the course of metaplasia. [inter- + G. *phylē,* tribe]

in·ter·pleu·ral space (in′tĕr-plūr′ăl spās) SYN mediastinum (2).

in·ter·po·lat·ed ex·tra·sys·to·le (in-tĕr′pō-lā′tĕd eks′tră-sis′tŏ-lē) A ventricular extrasystole that, instead of being followed by a compensatory pause, is sandwiched between two consecutive sinus cycles.

in·ter·pre·ta·tion (in-tĕr′prĕ-tā′shŭn) **1.** PSYCHOANALYSIS the characteristic therapeutic intervention of the analyst. **2.** CLINICAL PSYCHOLOGY drawing inferences and formulating the meaning in terms of the psychological dynamics inherent in a person's responses to psychological tests or during psychotherapy.

in·ter·prox·i·mal (in′tĕr-prok′si-măl) Between adjoining surfaces.

in·ter·prox·i·mal space (in′tĕr-prok′si-măl spās) The space between adjacent teeth in a dental arch; it is divided into the embrasure occlusal to the contact area, and the septal space gingival to the contact area.

in·ter·pu·bic disc (in′tĕr-pyū′bik disk) The disc of fibrocartilage that unites the pubic bones at the pubic symphysis.

in·ter·ra·dic·u·lar space (in′tĕr-ră-dik′yū-lăr spās) The space between the roots of multirooted teeth.

in·ter·rupt·ed su·ture (in′tĕr-ŭp′tĕd sū′chŭr) A single stitch fixed by tying ends together.

in·ter·scap·u·lar gland (in′tĕr skap′yū-lăr gland) SYN brown fat.

in·ter·scap·u·lar hi·ber·no·ma (in′tĕr-skap′yū-lăr hī′bĕr-nō′mă) SYN brown fat.

in·ter·sec·ti·o, pl. **in·ter·sec·ti·o·nes** (in′tĕr-sek′shē-ō, -ō′nēz) SYN intersection. [L.]

in·ter·sec·tion (in′tĕr-sek′shŭn) The site of crossing of two structures. SYN intersectio.

in·ter·seg·men·tal vein (in′tĕr-seg-men′tăl vān) A vein receiving blood from adjacent bronchopulmonary segments; it emerges from the inferior margin of a segment to become a tributary of a branch of a pulmonary vein.

in·ter·space (in′tĕr-spās) Any space between two similar objects, such as a costal interspace or interval between two ribs.

in·ter·spi·na·les mus·cles (in′tĕr-spī-nā′lēz mŭs′ĕlz) The paired muscles between spinous processes of adjacent vertebrae; subdivided into cervical, thoracic, and lumbar muscles. SYN musculi interspinales [TA], interspinal muscles.

in·ter·spi·nal mus·cles (in′tĕr-spī′năl mŭs′ĕlz) SYN interspinales muscles.

in·ter·spi·nal plane (in′tĕr-spī′năl plān) A horizontal plane passing through the anterior superior iliac spines; it marks the boundary between the lateral and umbilical regions superiorly and the inguinal and pubic regions inferiorly.

in·ter·stice, pl. **in·ter·stic·es** (in-tĕr′stis, -sti-sēz) SYN interstitium. [L. *interstitium,* fr. *sisto,* to stand]

in·ter·sti·tial (in′tĕr-stish′ăl) **1.** Relating to spaces or interstices in any structure. **2.** Relating to spaces within a tissue or organ, but excluding such spaces as body cavities or potential space. Cf. intracavitary. See page B18.

in·ter·sti·tial cells (in′tĕr-stish′ăl selz) **1.** Cells between the seminiferous tubules of the testis that secrete testosterone. SYN Leydig cells. **2.** cells derived from the theca interna of atretic follicles of the ovary; they resemble luteal cells and are an important source of estrogens. **3.** Pineal cells similar to glial cells with long processes.

in·ter·sti·tial cell-stim·u·lat·ing hor·mone (ICSH) (in′tĕr-stish′ăl sel′stim′yū-lā-ting hōr′mōn) SYN lutropin.

in·ter·sti·tial cys·ti·tis (in′tĕr-stish′ăl sis-tī′tis) A chronic inflammatory condition of unknown etiology involving the mucosa and muscularis of the bladder, resulting in reduced bladder capacity, pain relieved by voiding, and severe bladder irritative symptoms. SEE ALSO Hunner ulcer. See page 816.

in·ter·sti·tial dis·ease (in′tĕr-stish′ăl di-zēz′) A disease occurring chiefly in the connective-tissue framework of an organ, the parenchyma suffering secondarily.

in·ter·sti·tial em·phy·se·ma (in′tĕr-stish′ăl em′fi-sē′mă) **1.** Presence of air in the pulmonary tissues consequent upon rupture of the air cells. **2.** Presence of air or gas in the connective tissue.

in·ter·sti·tial flu·id (in′tĕr-stish′ăl flū′id) The fluid in spaces between the tissue cells, constituting about 16% of the weight of the human body; closely similar in composition to lymph.

in·ter·sti·tial gas·tri·tis (in′tĕr-stish′ăl gas-trī′tis) Inflammation of the stomach involving the submucosa and muscle coats.

in·ter·sti·tial ges·ta·tion (in′tĕr-stish′ăl jes-tā′shŭn) SYN intramural pregnancy.

in·ter·sti·tial growth (in′tĕr-stish′ăl grōth) Growth from a number of different centers within an area; in contrast with appositional growth, it can occur only when the materials involved are nonrigid.

in·ter·sti·tial her·ni·a (in′tĕr-stish′ăl hĕr′nē-ă) A hernia in which the protrusion is between any two of the layers of the abdominal wall.

in·ter·sti·tial im·plant (in′tĕr-stish′ăl im′plant)

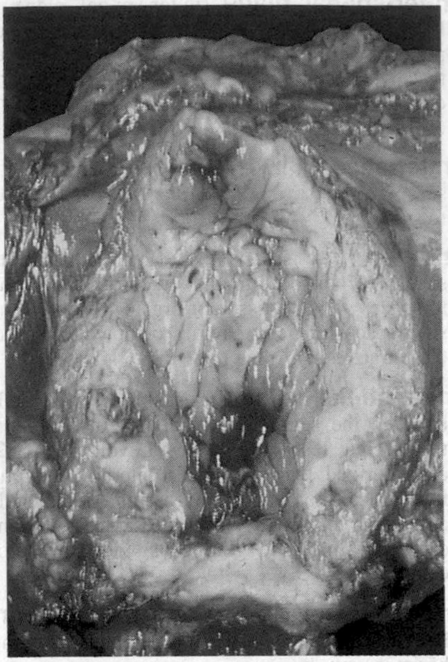

interstitial cystitis

Introduction of a radioactive mechanical device into a tumor directly so as to lessen the likelihood of spread of radiation into unaffected tissue.

in·ter·sti·tial in·flam·ma·tion (in′tĕr-stish′ăl in′flă-mā′shŭn) Inflammation in which the inflammatory reaction occurs chiefly in the supportive fibrous connective tissue or stroma of an organ.

in·ter·sti·tial ker·a·ti·tis (in′tĕr-stish′ăl ker′ă-tī′tis) An inflammation of the corneal stroma, often with neovascularization.

in·ter·sti·tial la·mel·la (in′tĕr-stish′ăl lă-mel′ă) One of the lamellae of partially resorbed osteons occurring between newer, complete osteons. SYN ground lamella.

in·ter·sti·tial ne·phri·tis (in′tĕr-stish′ăl nĕ-frī′tis) A form of nephritis in which the interstitial connective tissue is chiefly affected.

in·ter·sti·tial neu·ri·tis (in′tĕr-stish′ăl nūr-ī′tis) Inflammation of the connective tissue framework of a nerve. SYN Eichhorst neuritis.

in·ter·sti·tial nu·cle·us (in′tĕr-stish′ăl nū′klē-ŭs) SYN Cajal nucleus.

in·ter·sti·tial plas·ma cell pneu·mo·ni·a (in′tĕr-stish′ăl plaz′mă sel nū-mō′nē-ă) SYN *Pneumocystis jiroveci* pneumonia.

in·ter·sti·tial pneu·mo·ni·a (in′tĕr-stish′ăl nū-mō′nē-ă) SYN giant cell pneumonia.

in·ter·sti·tial preg·nan·cy (in′tĕr-stish′ăl preg′năn-sē) SYN intramural pregnancy.

in·ter·sti·tial ra·di·a·tion ther·a·py (in′tĕr-stish′ăl rā′dē-ā′shŭn) Use of sealed radioactive sources in the form of needles, wires, or seeds inserted directly into malignant tissue; may be temporary or permanent.

in·ter·sti·tial ther·a·py (in′tĕr-stish′ăl thār′ă-pē) Radiation therapy by means of radioactive seeds or needles implanted directly into the tissues to be irradiated.

in·ter·sti·tial tis·sue (in′tĕr-stish′ăl tish′ū) SYN connective tissue.

in·ter·stit·i·um (in′tĕr-stish′ē-ŭm) A small area, space, or gap in the substance of an organ or tissue. SEE ALSO connective tissue. SYN interstice. [L.]

in·ter·tar·sal (in′tĕr-tahr′săl) Denoting the articulations of the tarsal bones with each other.

in·ter·tar·sal joints (in′tĕr-tahr′săl joynts) The synovial joints that unite the tarsal bones. SYN tarsal joints.

in·ter·trans·ver·sar·i·i mus·cles (in′tĕr-trans-vĕr-sā′rē-ī mŭs′ĕlz) The paired muscles between transverse processes of adjacent vertebrae; there are anterior and posterior muscles in the cervical region; lateral and medial muscles in the lumbar region; and single muscles in the thoracic region. SYN musculi intertransversarii [TA], intertransverse muscles.

in·ter·trans·verse lig·a·ment (in′tĕr-trans-vĕrs′ lig′ă-mĕnt) One of the ligaments that connect the transverse processes of adjacent vertebrae.

in·ter·trans·verse mus·cles (in′tĕr-trans-vĕrs′ mŭs′ĕlz) SYN intertransversarii muscles.

in·ter·tri·go (in′tĕr-trī′gō) Irritant dermatitis occurring between folds or juxtaposed surfaces of the skin, such as between the scrotum and the thigh, caused by friction, sweat retention, moisture, warmth, and concomitant overgrowth of resident microorganisms. [L. a galling of the skin, fr. *inter,* between, + *tero,* to rub]

in·ter·tro·chan·ter·ic crest (in′tĕr-trō′kan-ter′ik krest) The rounded ridge that connects the greater and lesser trochanters of the femur posteriorly and marks the junction of the neck and shaft of the bone.

in·ter·tro·chan·ter·ic frac·ture (in′tĕr-trō′kan-ter′ik frak′shŭr) Fracture of the proximal femur located in the metaphyseal bone in the region between the greater and lesser trochanters.

in·ter·tro·chan·ter·ic line (in′tĕr-trō′kan-ter′ik līn) A rough line that separates the neck and shaft of the femur anteriorly; it passes downward and medially from the greater trochanter to the lesser trochanter and continues into the medial lip of the linea aspera. SYN linea intertrochanterica [TA].

in·ter·tu·ber·cu·lar groove (in′tĕr-tū-bĕr′kyū-lăr grūv) The furrow running longitudinally down the humerus between the lesser and greater tubercles; this is the location of the tendon of the long head of the biceps brachii muscle.

in·ter·tu·ber·cu·lar sheath (in′tĕr-tū-bĕr′kyū-lăr shēth) The extension of the synovial membrane of the shoulder joint downward in the intertubercular groove to surround the tendon of the long head of the biceps.

in·ter·u·re·ter·ic fold (in′tĕr-yūr′ĕ-ter′ik fōld) A fold of mucous membrane extending from the orifice of the ureter of one side to that of the other side. SYN plica interureterica [TA].

in·ter·val (in′tĕr-văl) A time or space between two periods or objects; a break in continuity. [L. *inter-vallum,* space between breastworks in a camp, an interval, fr. *vallum,* a rampart, wall]

in·ter·val train·ing (in′tĕr-văl trān′ing) Application of highly structured exercise with rest intervals using "supermaximum" effort to overload the specific systems of energy transfer; allows performance of inordinately high exercise intensities with relatively minimal fatigue.

in·ter·ve·nous tu·ber·cle (in′tĕr-vē′nŭs tū′bĕr-kĕl) The slight projection on the wall of the right atrium between the orifices of the venae cavae.

in·ter·ven·tion (in′tĕr-ven′shŭn) **1.** An action or ministration that produces an effect or that is intended to alter the course of a pathologic process. **2.** BIOWARFARE Any action, ministration, or device intended to prevent or alter the course of deliberate release of a mass-casualty agent. SYN countermeasure. SEE ALSO absorption. **3.** SYN implementation. [L. *inter-ventio*, a coming between, fr *inter-venio*, to come between]

in·ter·ven·tion·al (in′tĕr-ven′shŭn-ăl) Pertaining to an overt act or process intended to alter or prevent some event or outcome. [L. *intervenio*, to come between]

in·ter·ven·tion ap·proach (in′tĕr-ven′shŭn ă-prōch′) Using selected strategies to direct the process of intervention based on desired outcomes, evaluation data, and evidence that can serve to promote health, establish or restore skill and function, maintain existing status, teach compensation or adapted methods, or prevent further disability or related problems.

in·ter·ven·tion im·ple·men·ta·tion (in′tĕr-ven′shŭn im′plĕ-mĕn-tā′shŭn) The skilled process of effecting change in a person's performance leading to engagement in occupations or activities to support participation within a context (e.g., physical, spiritual, social or cultural).

in·ter·ven·tion re·view (in′tĕr-ven′shŭn rĕ-vyū′) An ongoing process of reevaluating and reviewing an intervention plan, its efficacy, and progress made toward targeted outcomes.

in·ter·ven·tric·u·lar fo·ra·men (in′tĕr-ven-trik′yū-lăr fōr-ā′mĕn) The short, often slitlike passage that, on both the left and right sides, connects the third brain ventricle (of the diencephalon) with the lateral ventricles (of the cerebral hemispheres); the passage is bounded anteriomedially by the column of fornix and posterolaterally by the anterior pole of the thalamus. SYN Monro foramen, porta (2).

in·ter·ven·tri·cu·lar sep·tal branch·es of left-right cor·o·nar·y ar·ter·y (in′tĕr-ven-trik′yū-lăr sep′tăl branch′ĕz left-rīt kōr′ŏ-nar-ē ahr′tĕr-ē) The interventricular septal branches; branches of the anterior and posterior interventricular arteries distributed to the muscle of the interventricular septum.

in·ter·ven·tric·u·lar sep·tum (in′tĕr-ven-trik′yū-lăr sep′tŭm) The wall between the ventricles of the heart.

in·ter·ver·te·bral disc (in′tĕr-vĕr′tĕ-brăl disk) A disc interposed between the bodies of adjacent vertebrae. It is composed of an outer fibrous part (anulus fibrosus) that surrounds a central gelatinous mass (nucleus pulposus).

in·ter·ver·te·bral for·a·men (in′tĕr-vĕr′tĕ-brăl fōr-ā′mĕn) The lateral opening to the vertebral canal that allows for the emergence of spinal nerve roots. The intervertebral foramen is composed of inferior and superior vertebral pedicles.

in·ter·ver·te·bral vein (in′tĕr-vĕr′tĕ-brăl vān) One of numerous veins accompanying the spinal nerves through the intervertebral foramina, draining spinal cord and vertebral venous plexuses, and emptying in the neck into the vertebral vein, in the thorax into the intercostal veins, in the lumbar and sacral regions into the lumbar and sacral veins.

in·ter·vil·lous la·cu·na (in′tĕr-vil′ŭs lă-kū′nă) One of the blood spaces in the placenta into which the chorionic villi project.

in·ter·vil·lous spac·es (in′tĕr-vil′ŭs spās′ĕz) The spaces containing maternal blood, located between chorionic villi; they are lined with syncytiotrophoblast.

in·tes·ti·nal (in-tes′ti-năl) Relating to the intestine.

in·tes·ti·nal a·nas·to·mo·sis (in-tes′ti-năl ă-nas′tŏ-mō′sis) SYN enteroenterostomy.

in·tes·ti·nal an·gi·na (in-tes′ti-năl an′ji-nă) SYN abdominal angina.

in·tes·ti·nal ar·ter·ies (in-tes′ti-năl ahr′tĕr-ēz) SEE ileal arteries, jejunal arteries.

in·tes·ti·nal a·tre·si·a (in-tes′ti-năl ă-trē′zē-ă) An obliteration of the lumen of the small intestine, with the ileum involved in 50% of cases and the jejunum and duodenum next in frequency; most frequent cause of intestinal obstruction in the newborn; etiology may be related to a failure of recanalization during early development or to some impairment of blood supply during intrauterine life.

in•tes•ti•nal col•ic (in-tes′i-năl kol′ik) Intermittent sharp abdominal pain due to intestinal spasm.

in•tes•ti•nal di•ges•tion (in-tes′ti-năl di-jes′chŭn) That part of digestion carried on in the intestine; it affects all cellular nutrients: starches, fats, and proteins.

in•tes•ti•nal dys•pep•si•a (in-tes′ti-năl dis-pep′sē-ă) Indigestion that originates in the intestines rather than in the stomach.

in•tes•ti•nal em•phy•se•ma (in-tes′ti-năl em′fi-sē′mă) SYN pneumatosis cystoides intestinalis.

in•tes•ti•nal fis•tu•la (in-tes′ti-năl fis′chū-lă) A tract leading from the lumen of the small intestine to the exterior. SYN fecal fistula.

in•tes•ti•nal flo•ra (in-tes′ti-năl flōr′ă) Collective term for those bacteria that normally reside within the intestines and assist in digestion and evacuation.

in•tes•ti•nal flu (in-tes′ti-năl flū) A colloquial expression for acute viral gastroenteritis.

in•tes•ti•nal fluke (in-tes′ti-năl flūk) Any of various trematodes parasitizing the human small intestine; severe infection may cause ulceration, malabsorption, and obstruction.

in•tes•ti•nal fol•li•cles (in-tes′ti-năl fol′i-kĕlz) SYN intestinal glands.

in•tes•ti•nal gas (in-tes′ti-năl gas) Gas resident in the intestines caused by pathogens or certain foodstuffs. Cf. flatus

in•tes•ti•nal glands (in-tes′ti-năl glandz) The tubular glands in the mucous membrane of the small and large intestines. SYN intestinal follicles, Lieberkühn glands.

in•tes•ti•nal vil•li (in-tes′ti-năl vil′ī) Projections (0.5–1.5 mm in length) of the mucous membrane of the intestine; they are leaf-shaped in the duodenum and become shorter, more finger-shaped, and sparser in the ileum.

in•tes•tine (in-tes′tin) **1.** The digestive tube passing from the stomach to the anus. It is divided primarily into the intestinum tenue (small intestine) and the intestinum crassum (large intestine). **2.** Inward; inner. See this page. SYN intestinum [TA], bowel, gut (1). [L. *intestinum*]

in•tes•ti•num, pl. **in•tes•ti•na** (in-tes-tī′num, -nă) [TA] SYN intestine. [L. *intestinus,* internal, neuter, as noun, the entrails, fr. *intus,* within]

in-the-ca•nal hear•ing aid (kă-nal′ hēr′ing ād) A device to improve hearing that is placed in the external auditory canal but is still visible.

in-the-ear hear•ing aid (ēr hēr′ing ād) A device to improve hearing that fits into the shell of the ear.

in•ti•ma (in′ti-mă) Innermost. SEE tunica intima. [L. fem. of *intimus,* inmost]

in•ti•mal (in′ti-măl) Relating to the intima or inner coat of a vessel.

in•ti•mate part•ner vi•o•lence (in′ti-măt pahrt′nĕr-vī′ŏ-lĕns) SEE domestic violence.

in•ti•mi•tis (in′ti-mī′tis) Inflammation of an intima, as in endangiitis. [intima + G. *-itis,* inflammation]

in•toe (in′tō) Medial deviation of the axis of the foot. SYN metatarsus varus.

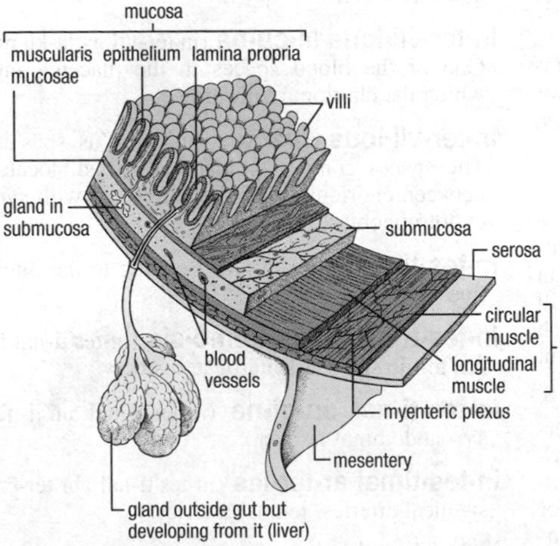

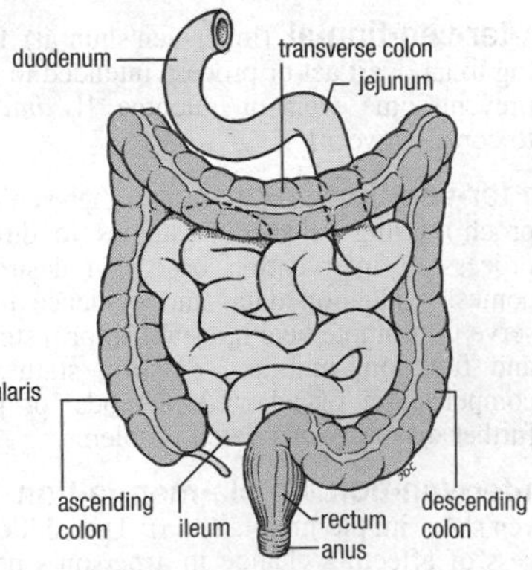

intestines: (left) diagram of four main layers of the wall of the digestive tube: mucosa, submucosa, muscularis, and serosa (below the diaphragm); (right) anterior view of the abdominal intestines

in·tol·er·ance (in-tol′ĕr-ăns) Abnormal metabolism, excretion, or other disposition of a given substance; term often used to indicate impaired use or disposal of dietary constituents.

in·to·na·tion (in′tō-nā′shŭn) During speech, a pattern of change in voice used to convey linguistic information such as syllabic accent stress or pitch variations to signal interrogation, declaration, or exclamation; used to convey emotion by patterns of change in pitch, loudness, and speech rate.

in·tor·sion (in-tōr′shŭn) Conjugate rotation of the upper poles of each cornea inward. [L. *intorqueo,* pp. *tortus,* to twist]

in·tor·tor (in-tōr′tŏr) A muscle that turns a part medialward. SEE ALSO invertor.

in·tox·i·cant (in-tok′si-kănt) **1.** Having the power to intoxicate. **2.** An intoxicating agent, such as alcohol. SYN toxicant.

in·tox·i·ca·tion (in-tok′si-kā′shŭn) **1.** SYN poisoning. **2.** Temporary acute alcoholism. [L. *in,* in, + G. *toxikon,* poison]

♻ **intra-** Prefix meaning inside, within; opposite of extra-. SEE ALSO endo-, ento-. [L. within]

in·tra·ab·dom·i·nal pres·sure (in′tră-ab-dom′i-năl presh′ŭr) Pain or discomfort located in the abdominal cavity.

in·tra·al·ve·o·lar in·jec·tion (in′tră-al-vē′ō-lăr in-jek′shŭn) In dentistry, introduction of an anesthetic agent into soft tissue near the tooth to be worked on.

in·tra·a·or·tic bal·loon (in′tră-ā-or′tik bă-lūn′) SEE intraaortic balloon pump.

in·tra·a·or·tic bal·loon pump (in′tră-ā-ōr′tik bă-lūn′ pŭmp) An externally actuated and intermittently inflatable balloon placed into the descending aorta and that, on activation during diastole, augments blood pressure and organ perfusion by its pulsatile thrust; then, on deflation, decreases the cardiac work with each systole—the so-called counterpulsation principle—by reducing cardiac afterload.

in·tra·ar·ter·i·al (IA) (in′tră-ahr-tēr′ē-ăl) Route by which medications are administered directly into an artery.

in·tra·ar·tic·u·lar frac·ture (in′tră-ahr-tik′yū-lăr frak′shŭr) Fracture occurring through the articular surface into the joint.

in·tra·a·tri·al block (in′tră-ā′trē-ăl blok) Impaired conduction through the atria, manifested by widened and often notched P waves in the electrocardiogram. SYN interatrial block.

in·tra·a·tri·al con·duc·tion (in′tră-ā′trē-ăl kŏn-dŭk′shŭn) Conduction of the cardiac impulse through the atrial myocardium, represented by the P wave in the electrocardiogram.

in·tra·a·tri·al con·duc·tion time (in′tră-ā′trē-ăl kŏn-dŭk′shŭn tīm) **1.** The total duration of electrical activity of the atria in one cardiac cycle. **2.** The time between right atrial and left atrial activation. SYN interatrial conduction time.

in·tra·au·ric·u·lar (in′tră-awr-ik′yū-lăr) Within an auricle (e.g., of the ear).

in·tra·cap·su·lar frac·ture (in′tră-kap′sŭ-lăr frak′shŭr) A fracture near a joint and within the line of insertion of the joint capsule.

in·tra·cap·su·lar lig·a·ments (in′tră-kap′sŭ-lăr lig′ă-mĕnts) Ligaments located within and separate from the articular capsule of a synovial joint. SYN ligamenta intracapsularia [TA].

in·tra·car·di·ac cath·e·ter (in′tră-kahr′dē-ak kath′ĕ-tĕr) A catheter that can be passed into the heart through a vein or artery, to withdraw samples of blood, measure pressures within the heart's chambers or great vessels, and inject contrast media; used mainly in the diagnosis and evaluation of congenital, rheumatic, and coronary artery lesions and to evaluate systolic and diastolic cardiac function. SYN cardiac catheter.

in·tra·car·di·al in·jec·tion (in′tră-kahr′dē-ăl in-jek′shŭn) Introduction of an agent via tube or needle directly into the heart.

in·tra·cath·e·ter (in′tră-kath′ĕ-tĕr) A plastic tube, usually attached to the puncturing needle, inserted into a blood vessel for infusion, injection, or pressure monitoring.

in·tra·cav·i·tar·y (in′tră-kav′i-tar-ē) Within an organ or body cavity.

in·tra·cav·i·tar·y ra·di·a·tion ther·a·py (in′tră-kav′i-tar-ē rā′dē-ā′shŭn thār′ă-pē) Use of sealed radioactive sources placed within a body cavity adjacent to a malignant tumor.

in·tra·cel·lu·lar (in′tră-sel′yū-lăr) Within a cell or cells.

in·tra·cel·lu·lar can·a·lic·u·lus (in′tră-sel′yū-lăr kan′ă-lik′yŭ-lŭs) A fine canal formed by invagination of the cell membrane into the cytoplasm of a cell, such as those of the parietal cells of the stomach.

in·tra·cel·lu·lar flu·id (ICF) (in′tră-sel′yū-lăr flū′id) The fluid within the tissue cells, constituting about 30–40% of the body weight. SYN intracellular water.

in·tra·cel·lu·lar tox·in (in′tră-sel′yū-lăr tok′sin) SYN endotoxin.

in·tra·cel·lu·lar wa·ter (in′tră-sel′yū-lăr waw′tĕr) SYN intracellular fluid.

in·tra·ce·re·bral (in′tră-ser′ă-brăl) Within the cerebrum.

in·tra·ce·re·bral he·ma·to·ma (in′tră-ser′ă-brăl hē′mă-tō′mă) An accumulation of blood within the substance of the brain, usually due to blunt trauma.

in·tra·cer·vi·cal (in′tră-sĕr′vi-kăl) SYN endocervical (1).

in·tra·chon·dral os·si·fi·ca·tion (in′tră-kon′drăl os′i-fi-kā′shŭn) SYN endochondral ossification.

in·tra·cor·ne·al im·plants (in′tră-kōr′nē-ăl im′plants) Inserts placed within corneal pockets to alter the refractive power of the eye.

in·tra·cor·o·nar·y stent·ing (in′tră-kōr′ŏ-nar-ē stent′ing) SYN percutaneous coronary intervention.

in·tra·cor·po·re·al (in′tră-kōr-pōr′ē-ăl) **1.** Within the body. **2.** Within any structure anatomically styled a corpus. [intra- + L. *corpus,* body]

in·tra·cra·ni·al an·eur·ysm (in-tră-krā′nē-ăl an′yūr-izm) Any aneurysm located within the cranium.

in·tra·cra·ni·al cav·i·ty (in′tră-krā′nē-ăl kav′i-tē) SYN cranial cavity.

in·tra·cra·ni·al hem·or·rhage (in′tră-krā′nē-ăl hem′ŏr-ăj) Escape of blood within the cranium due to loss of integrity of vascular channels, frequently forming a hematoma.

in·tra·cra·ni·al hy·per·ten·sion (ICH) (in′tră-krā′nē-ăl hī′pĕr-ten′shŭn) Increased pressure within the skull due to tumor, disease, or trauma.

in·tra·cra·ni·al pres·sure (ICP) (in′tră-krā′nē-ăl presh′ŭr) Pressure within the cranial cavity, particularly the pressure of the cerebrospinal fluid as measured by cisternal or lumbar pressure. See this page.

in·tra·crine (in′tră-krin) Denoting self-stimulation through cellular production of a factor that acts within the cell. [intra- + G. *krinō,* to separate, secrete]

in·trac·ta·ble (in-trak′tă-bĕl) **1.** SYN refractory (1). **2.** SYN obstinate (1). [L. *in-tractabilis,* fr. *in-* neg. + *tracto,* to draw, haul]

in·tra·cu·ta·ne·ous re·ac·tion, in·tra·der·mal re·ac·tion (in′tră-kyū-tā′nē-ŭs rē-ak′shŭn, in′tră-dĕr′măl) A reaction following the injection of antigen into the skin of a sensitive subject, such as in the case of the tuberculin test.

in·tra·cy·to·plas·mic sperm in·jec·tion (in′tră-sī-tō-plaz′mik spĕrm in-jek′shŭn) A procedure in which a single sperm cell is injected into the oocyte during in vitro fertilization.

in·trad (in′trad) Toward the inner part.

in·tra·der·mal in·jec·tion (in′tră-dĕr′măl in-jek′shŭn) An injection into the corium, or substance of the skin.

in·tra·der·mal ne·vus (in′tră-dĕr′măl nē′vŭs) A nevus in which nests of melanocytes are found in the dermis, but not at the epidermal-dermal junction; benign pigmented nevi in adults are most commonly intradermal.

in·tra·der·mal test (in′tră-dĕr′măl test) SYN skin test.

in·tra·em·bry·on·ic (in′tră-em′brē-on′ik) Within the embryonic body; referring to the portion of the umbilical vein within the embryo. Cf. extraembryonic.

in·tra·em·bry·on·ic ce·lom (in′tră-em′brē-on′ik sē′lŏm) The part of the celom in the embryo between the somatopleuric and splanchnopleuric mesoderm; the principal body cavities of the trunk (e.g., thoracic, abdominal, and pelvic) arise from this embryonic part of the celom.

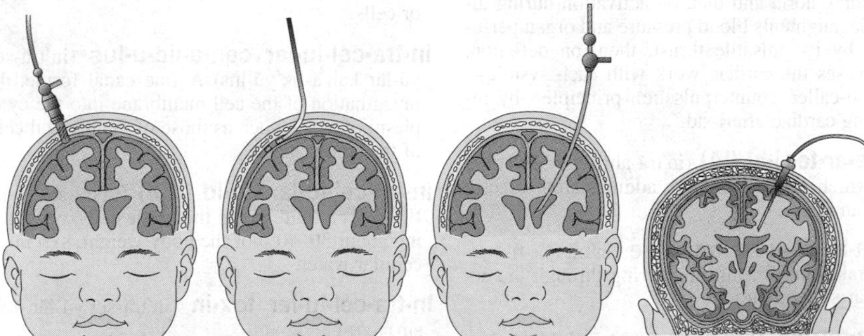

intracranial pressure monitoring: (A) anterior view of head of infant, a subarachnoid screw passes through a bur hole in the skull ending in the epidural space; (B) fiberoptic sensor is implanted into the epidural space; (C) an intraventricular catheter has been inserted through the anterior fontanelle and threaded into the lateral ventricle; (D) posterior view of head of infant, a fiber-optic transducer-tipped catheter has been inserted through a subarachnoid bolt into the white matter of the brain

in·tra·fi·lar (in′tră-fī′lăr) Lying within the meshes of a network. [intra- + L. *filum*, thread]

in·tra·fu·sal (in′tră-fyū′zăl) Applied to structures within the muscle spindle.

in·tra·fu·sal fi·bers (in′tră-fyū′zăl fī′bĕrz) Muscle fibers present within a neuromuscular spindle.

in·tra·he·pat·ic cho·le·sta·sis of preg·nan·cy (in′tră-hĕ-pat′ik kō′lē-stā′sis preg′năn-sē) Intrahepatic cholestasis with centrilobular bile staining without inflammatory cells or proliferation of mesenchymal cells; clinically characterized by pruritus and/or icterus; of unknown cause but associated with high estrogen levels. SYN cholestasis of pregnancy, recurrent jaundice of pregnancy.

in·tra·lig·a·men·ta·ry preg·nan·cy (in′tră-lig′ă-men′tăr-ē preg′năn-sē) Pregnancy within the broad ligament.

in·tra·lin·gual in·jec·tion (in′tră-ling′gwăl in-jek′shŭn) Introduction of medication into the tongue with a needle or syringe.

in·tra·lob·u·lar duct (in′tră-lob′yū-lăr dŭkt) A duct that lies within a lobule of a gland.

in·tra·med·ul·lar·y trans·fu·sion (in′tră-med′ŭ-lar-ē tranz-fyū′zhŭn) Transfusion, most commonly in infants, into the medullary cavity of a long bone, usually the femur or tibia.

in·tra·mu·ral he·ma·to·ma (in′tră-myūr′ăl hē′mă-tō′mă) A hematoma in the wall of a structure, such as the bowel or bladder, usually resulting from trauma.

in·tra·mu·ral preg·nan·cy (in′tră-myūr′ăl preg′năn-sē) Development of the fertilized ovum in the uterine portion of the uterine tube. SYN interstitial gestation, interstitial pregnancy.

in·tra·mus·cu·lar (IM) (in′tră-mŭs′kyū-lăr) Within the substance of a muscle.

in·tra·mus·cu·lar in·jec·tion (IMI) (in′tră-mŭsk′yū-lar in-jek′shŭn) Injection of fluid into deep muscle. Usual sites for intramuscular injections include ventrogluteal, vastus lateralis, and deltoid muscles. Absorption is faster than subcutaneous and up to 3 mL can be given by this method.

in·tra·na·sal an·es·the·si·a (in′tră-nā′zăl an′es-thē′zē-ă) **1.** Insufflation anesthesia in which an inhalation anesthetic is added to inhaled air passing through the nose or nasopharynx. **2.** Anesthesia of nasal passages by infiltration and topical application of local anesthetic solution to nasal mucosa.

in·tra·ob·serv·er er·ror (in′tră-ŏb-zĕr′vĕr er′ŏr) The differences in interpretation by a person making observations of the same phenomenon at different times.

in·tra·oc·u·lar (in′tră-ok′yū-lăr) Within the eyeball.

in·tra·oc·u·lar lens (IOL) (in′tră-ok′yū-lăr lenz) A mechanical transplant used in ophthalmology to replace the natural lens that has ceased to function due to disease (e.g., cataract) or otherwise functionally disrupted.

in·tra·oc·u·lar pres·sure (IOP) (in′tră-ok′yū-lăr presh′ŭr) The pressure of the intraocular fluid, usually measured in millimeters of mercury.

in·tra·op·er·a·tive (in′tră-op′ĕr-ă-tiv) Denotes that which occurs during an operation.

in·tra·op·er·a·tive hy·per·ther·mi·a (in′tră-op′ĕr-ă-tiv hī′pĕr-thĕr′mē-ă) Intentional elevation of the temperature of a body part or surgical area to aid in healing.

in·tra·op·er·a·tive ra·di·a·tion ther·a·py (IORT) (in′tră-op′ĕr-ă-tiv rā′dē-ā′shŭn thār′ă-pē) Radiation treatment delivered directly to the tumor or tumor bed after the area has been surgically exposed; allows normal healthy tissue to be displaced from the treatment field.

in·tra·o·ral (in′tră-ōr′ăl) Inside the mouth.

in·tra·o·ral an·es·the·si·a (in′tră-ōr′ăl an′es-thē′zē-ă) **1.** Insufflation anesthesia in which an inhalation anesthetic is added to inhaled air passing through the mouth. **2.** Regional anesthesia of the mouth and associated structures when local anesthetic solutions are used by topical application to oral mucosa, by local infiltration, or as nerve blocks.

in·tra·o·ral cam·er·a (in′tră-ōr′ăl kam′ĕr-ă) A camera that uses a small wand to take digital pictures (still or video) in the oral cavity for immediate viewing by the dental staff and patient. This method allows for viewing small areas that would be difficult to see without the camera's use.

in·tra·os·se·ous (in′tră-os′ē-ŭs) Route for delivery of fluid, blood, or medication through a needle inserted directly into the marrow of long bones.

in·tra·os·se·ous an·es·the·si·a (in′tră-os′ē-ŭs an′es-thē′zē-ă) Injection of anesthetic into bone as a supplemental or primary technique in routine dental procedures.

in·tra·os·se·ous in·jec·tion (in′tră-os′ē-ŭs in-jek′shŭn) Injection of anesthetic into the intraradicular bone around a tooth. It is usually performed by penetrating the cortical bone with a dental bur, followed by injection of the anesthetic solution into the cancellous bone.

in·tra·pa·ri·e·tal sul·cus (in′tră-păr-ī′ĕ-tăl sŭl′kŭs) A horizontal sulcus extending back from the postcentral sulcus over some distance, then dividing perpendicularly into two branches so as to form, with the postcentral sulcus, a figure H.

It divides the parietal lobe into superior and inferior parietal lobules.

in·tra·pa·rot·id plex·us of fa·cial nerve (in′tră-păr-ot′id plek′sŭs fā′shăl nĕrv) The diverging branches of the facial nerve passing through the substance of the parotid gland, connected by numerous looped anastomoses. SYN pes anserinus (1).

in·tra·par·tum (in′tră-pahr′tŭm) During labor and delivery or childbirth. Cf. antepartum, postpartum. [intra- + L. *partus,* childbirth]

in·tra·par·tum hem·or·rhage (in′tră-pahr′tŭm hem′ŏr-ăj) Hemorrhage occurring in the course of normal labor and delivery.

in·tra·per·i·to·ne·al (in′tră-per-i-tō-nē′ăl) Route by which medication is administered directly into the peritoneal cavity.

in·tra·per·i·to·ne·al in·jec·tion (in′tră-per′i-tō-nē′ăl in-jek′shŭn) Injection of an agent into the peritoneal cavity.

in·tra·psy·chic (in′tră-sī′kik) Denoting the psychological dynamics that occur inside the mind without reference to the person's exchanges with other persons or events.

in·tra·seg·men·tal bron·chi (in′tră-seg-ment′ăl brong′kī) Branches of segmental bronchi to the bronchopulmonary segments of the lungs. SYN bronchi intrasegmentales.

in·tra·the·cal (IT) (in′tră-thē′kăl) **1.** Within a sheath. **2.** Within the subarachnoid or subdural space.

in·tra·tho·ra·cic air·way ob·struc·tion (in′tră-thōr-as′ik ār′wā ŏb-strŭk′shŭn) Form of airway obstruction in which the site of airway narrowing is below the thoracic inlet; can be variable (reduction in expiratory but not inspiratory flows) or fixed (reduction in both inspiratory and expiratory flows).

in·tra·tra·che·al (in′tră-trā′kē-ăl) Method of giving medications through the trachea.

in·tra·u·ter·ine am·pu·ta·tion (in′tră-yū′tĕr-in amp′yū-tā′shŭn) SYN congenital amputation.

in·tra·u·ter·ine de·vice (IUD), in·tra·u·ter·ine con·tra·cep·tive de·vice (IUCD) (in′tră-yū′tĕr-in dĕ-vīs′, kon′tră-sep′tiv dĕ-vīs′) Pieces of plastic or metal of various shapes (e.g., coil, loop, bow) inserted into the uterus to exert a contraceptive effect.

in·tra·u·ter·ine frac·ture (in′tră-yū′tĕr-in frak′shŭr) A fracture of one or more bones of a fetus occurring before birth.

in·tra·u·ter·ine growth re·tar·da·tion (IUGR) (in′tră-yū′tĕr-in grōth rē′tahr-dā′shŭn) Inhibition of fetal intrauterine growth. May be caused by maternal, placental, and fetal factors.

in·tra·u·ter·ine in·sem·i·na·tion (IUI) (in′tră-yū′tĕr-in in-sem′i-nā′shŭn) Placement of sperm that have been washed of seminal fluid directly into the uterus to bypass the cervix.

in·tra·vas·cu·lar flu·id (in′tră-vas′kyū-lăr flū′id) The totality of the bodily fluids present in the cardiovascular system and within the lymphatic vessels.

in·tra·vas·cu·lar lig·a·ture (in′tră-vas′kyū-lăr lig′ă-chŭr) Balloon occlusion of the feeding vessels of a cerebral arteriovenous malformation.

in·tra·ve·nous (IV) (in′tră-vē′nŭs) Through the veins. See this page.

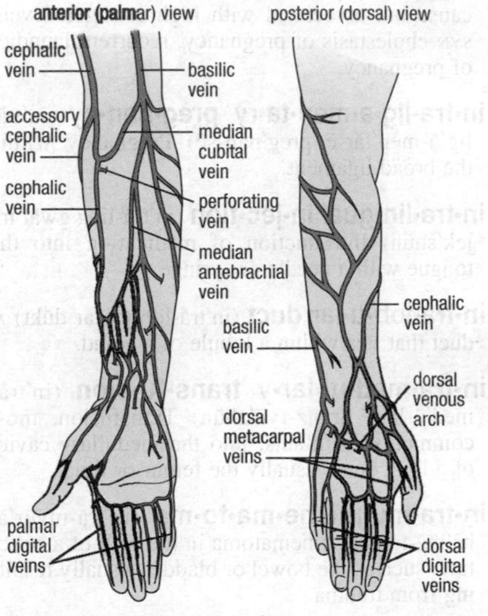

intravenous cannulation sites

in·tra·ve·nous al·i·men·ta·tion (in′tră-vē′nŭs al′i-mĕn-tā′shŭn) SYN parenteral nutrition.

in·tra·ve·nous an·es·the·si·a (in′tră-vē′nŭs an′es-thē′zē-ă) General anesthesia produced by injection of central nervous system depressants into the venous circulation.

in·tra·ve·nous bo·lus (in′tră-vē′nŭs bō′lŭs) **1.** A relatively large volume of fluid or dose of a drug or test substance given intravenously and rapidly to hasten or magnify a response. **2.** RADIOLOGY rapid injection of a large dose of contrast medium to increase opacification of blood vessels.

in·tra·ve·nous cath·e·ter (in′tră-vē′nŭs kath′ĕ-tĕr) A catheter that is surgically introduced into a vein to supply pharmacotherapeutic agents.

in·tra·ve·nous chol·an·gi·og·ra·phy (in′tră-vē′nŭs kō-lan′jē-og′ră-fē) Investigation of bile ducts opacified by hepatic secretion of an intravenously injected contrast medium.

in·tra·ve·nous drip (in′tră-vē′nŭs drip) The

slow but continuous introduction of solutions intravenously, one drop at a time.

in•tra•ven•ous drug user (IVDU) (in′tră-vē′nŭs drŭg yū′zĕr) SYN injection drug user.

in•tra•ve•nous in•jec•tion (IVI) (in′tră-vē′nŭs in-jek′shŭn) Injection of fluid directly into a vein. Allows larger amounts of fluid to be administered and provides means for rapid absorption of medication.

in•tra•ve•nous push (IVP) (in′tră-vē′nŭs push) A method of quickly injecting medications into a vein.

in•tra•ve•nous py•el•o•gram/py•el•og•ra•phy (IVP) (in′tră-vē′nŭs pī′ĕ-lō-gram-pī′ĕ-log′ră-fē) SEE intravenous urography.

in•tra•ve•nous re•gion•al an•es•the•si•a (in′tră-vē′nŭs rē′jŭn-ăl an′es-thē′zē-ă) Regional anesthesia by intravenous injection of local anesthetic solution distal to an occlusive tourniquet in an extremity previously exsanguinated by pressure or gravity. SYN Bier method (1).

in•tra•ve•nous ur•og•ra•phy, ex•cre•to•ry ur•og•ra•phy (in′tră-vē′nŭs yūr-og′ră-fē, eks′krĕ-tōr-ē) Radiography of kidneys, ureters, and bladder following injection of contrast medium into a peripheral vein.

in•tra•ven•tric•u•lar block, IV block (in′tră-ven-trik′yū-lăr blok, blok) Delayed conduction within the ventricular conducting system or myocardium, including bundle-branch block, periinfarction blocks, the fascicular blocks, excitation, and the Wolff-Parkinson-White (preexcitation) syndrome; widens QRS duration in ECG.

in•tra•ven•tric•u•lar con•duc•tion (in′tră-ven-trik′yū-lăr kŏn-dŭk′shŭn) Transference of the cardiac impulse through the ventricular myocardium, represented by the QRS complex in the electrocardiogram. SYN ventricular conduction.

in•tra•ven•tric•u•lar hem•or•rhage (IVH) (in′tră-ven-trik′yū-lăr hem′ŏr-ăj) Type of intracranial hemorrhage primarily affecting premature babies.

in•tra•vi•tal stain (in′tră-vī′tăl stān) A stain that is taken up by living cells after parenteral administration, e.g., intravenously or subcutaneously.

in•tra vi•tam (in′tră vī′tăm) During life. [L. *vita,* life]

in•tra•vox•el de•phas•ing (in′tră-voks′ĕl dē-fāz′ing) Phase difference between flow and stationary nuclei in a voxel.

in•trin•sic (in-trin′zik) **1.** Belonging entirely to a part. **2.** ANATOMY denoting those muscles the origin and insertion of which are both within the structure under consideration, distinguished from the extrinsic muscles, which have their origin outside of the structure under consideration; applied especially to the limbs but also to the ciliary muscle as distinguished from the recti and other orbital muscles which are outside the eyeball. SYN essential (6). [L. *intrinsecus,* on the inside]

in•trin•sic asth•ma (in-trin′zik az′mă) A nonallergic, nonseasonal form of asthma that first occurs later in life, tending to become chronic and persistent rather than episodic; triggered by inhalation of irritants, exposure to cold, physical exercise, or anxiety.

in•trin•sic co•ag•u•la•tion path•way (in-trin′zik kō-ag′yū-lā′shŭn path′wā) A part of the coagulation pathway that is activated by contact of coagulation proteins with negatively charged surfaces. All components are within the bloodstream and include factors XII, XI, IX, VII, HMWK, and prekallikrein. The activated partial thromboplastin time tests for abnormalities in this pathway.

in•trin•sic dys•men•or•rhe•a (in-trin′zik dis-men′ŏr-ē′ă) SYN primary dysmenorrhea.

in•trin•sic fac•tor (IF) (in-trin′zik fak′tŏr) A relatively small mucoprotein secreted by the neck cell of the gastric glands and required for adequate absorption of vitamin B12; deficiency results in pernicious anemia.

in•trin•sic PEEP (in-trin′zik pēp) SYN auto-positive-end-expiratory-pressure.

in•trin•sic re•flex (in-trin′zik rē′fleks) A reflex muscular contraction elicited by the application of a stimulus, usually stretching, to the muscle itself as opposed to a muscular contraction caused by an extrinsic stimulus, e.g., skin, as in the abdominal skin reflexes.

in•trin•sic sphinc•ter (in-trin′zik sfingk′tĕr) A thickening of the circular fibers of the muscular coat of an organ.

in•trin•sic sphinc•ter de•fi•cien•cy (ISD) (in-trin′zik sfingk′tĕr dĕ-fish′ĕn-sē) Refers to grade 3 of the stress urinary incontinence scale, which is the inability of the urethral walls to remain compressed with an increase in abdominal pressure as in straining at stool.

♲ **intro-** Prefix meaning inwardly, into; opposite of extra-. Cf. intra-. [L. *intro,* into]

in•tro•duc•er (in′trō-dūs′ĕr) An instrument, such as a catheter, needle, or endotracheal tube, for introduction of a flexible device. [L. *intro-duco,* to lead into, introduce]

in•tro•duc•to•ry mas•sage (in′trŏ-duk′tŏr-ē mă-sahzh′) In massage therapy, stroking around, rather than on, a painful area when direct touch would be contraindicated.

in•tro•flec•tion, in•tro•flex•ion (in′trō-flek′shŭn, in′trō-flek′shŭn) A bending inward. [intro- + L. *flecto,* pp. *flectus,* to bend]

in•tro•i•tus (in-trō′i-tŭs) The entrance into a canal or hollow organ, as the vagina. [L. entrance, fr. *intro-eo,* to go into]

in•tro•ject (in′trō-jekt′) The dynamically endowed, enduring internal representation of an object.

in•tro•jec•tion (in′trō-jek′shŭn) A psychological defense mechanism involving appropriation of an external happening and its assimilation by the personality, making it a part of the self. [intro- + L. *jacto,* to throw]

in•tro•mis•sion (in′trō-mish′ŭn) The insertion or introduction of one part into another. [intro- + L. *mitto,* to send]

in•tro•mit•tent (in′trō-mit′ĕnt) Conveying or sending into a body or cavity.

in•tron (in′tron) A portion of DNA that lies between two exons, is transcribed into RNA, but does not appear in that RNA after maturation, and so is not expressed (as protein) in protein synthesis. [inter- + -on]

in•tro•spec•tion (in′trō-spek′shŭn) Looking inward; self-scrutinizing; contemplating one's own mental processes. [intro- + L. *specto,* to look at, inspect]

in•tro•spec•tive (in′trō-spek′tiv) Relating to introspection.

in•tro•sus•cep•tion (in′trō-sŭs-sep′shŭn) SYN intussusception.

in•tro•ver•sion (in′trō-vĕr′zhŭn) **1.** The turning of a structure into itself. SEE ALSO intussusception, invagination. **2.** A trait of preoccupation with oneself, as practiced by an introvert. Cf. extraversion. [intro- + L. *verto,* pp. *versus,* to turn]

in•tro•vert 1. (in′trō-vert) One who tends to be unusually shy, introspective, self-centered, and avoids becoming concerned with or involved in the affairs of others. Cf. extrovert. **2.** (in-trō-vert′) To turn a structure into itself.

in•tu•bate (in′tū-bāt) To perform intubation.

in•tu•ba•tion (in′tū-bā′shŭn) Insertion of a tubular device into a canal, hollow organ, or cavity; specifically, passage of an orotracheal or nasotracheal tube for anesthesia or for control of pulmonary ventilation. [L. *in,* in, + *tuba,* tube]

in•tu•i•tive stage (in-tū′i-tiv stāj) PSYCHOLOGY a stage of development, usually occurring between 4–7 years of age, in which the most prominent aspects of the stimuli to which a child is exposed, rather than any form of logical thought, determine the child's thought processes.

in•tu•mesce (in′tū-mes′) To swell up; to enlarge. [L. *in-tumesco,* to swell up, fr. *tumeo,* to swell]

in•tu•mes•cence (in′tū-mes′ĕns) **1.** SYN enlargement. **2.** The process of enlarging or swelling; used to describe the spinal enlargements.

in•tu•mes•cent (in′tū-mes′ĕnt) Enlarging; becoming enlarged or swollen.

in•tu•mes•cen•ti•a (in′tū-mes-sen′shē-ă) SYN enlargement. [Mod. L.]

in•tus•sus•cep•tion (in′tŭ-sŭ-sep′shŭn) **1.** The taking up or receiving of one part within another, especially the enfolding of one segment of the intestine within another. SEE ALSO introversion, invagination. **2.** The incorporation of new material in the growth of the cell wall. SYN introsusception. [L. *intus,* within, + *sus-cipio,* to take up, fr. *sub* + *capio,* to take]

in•tus•sus•cep•tive (in′tŭ-sŭ-sep′tiv) Relating to or characterized by intussusception.

in•tus•sus•cep•tum (in′tŭ-sŭ-sep′tŭm) The inner segment in an intussusception; the part of the bowel that is received within the other part.

in•tus•sus•cip•i•ens (in′tŭ-sŭ-sip′ē-ĕnz) The portion of the bowel, in intussusception, which receives the other portion. [L. *intus,* within, + *suscipiens,* pr. p. of *suscipio,* to take up]

in•u•lin (In) (in′yū-lin) A fructose polysaccharide from the rhizome of *Inula* and other plants; used by intravenous injection to determine the rate of glomerular filtration. Cf. inulin clearance.

in•u•lin clear•ance (in′yū-lin klēr′ăns) An accurate measure of the rate of filtration through the renal glomeruli, because inulin filters freely with water and is neither excreted nor reabsorbed through tubule walls. Inulin is not a normal constituent of plasma and must be infused continously to maintain a steady plasma concentration and a steady rate of urinary excretion during the measurement.

in•unc•tion (in-ŭngk′shŭn) Administration of a drug in ointment form by rubbing to cause absorption of the active ingredient. [L. *inunctio,* an anointing, fr. *inunguo,* pp. *-unctus,* to smear on]

in u•ter•o (in yū′tĕr-ō) Within the womb; not yet born. [L.]

in•vag•i•nate (in-vaj′i-nāt) To ensheathe, infold, or insert a structure within itself or another. [L. *in,* in, + *vagina,* a sheath]

in•vag•i•na•tion (in-vaj′i-nā′shŭn) **1.** The ensheathing, enfolding, or insertion of a structure within itself or another. **2.** The state of being invaginated. SEE ALSO introversion, intussusception.

in•va•lid (in′vă-lid) **1.** Weak; sick. **2.** A person partially or completely disabled. [L. *in-* neg. + *validus,* strong]

in•va•sion (in-vā′zhŭn) **1.** The beginning or incursion of a disease. **2.** Local spread of a malignant neoplasm by infiltration or destruction of adjacent tissue; for epithelial neoplasms, invasion signifies infiltration beneath the epithelial basement membrane. **3.** Entrance of foreign cells into a tissue, such as polymorphonuclear leukocytes in inflammation. [L. *invasio,* fr. *in-vado,* pp. *-vasus,* to go into, attack]

in•va•sion of pri•va•cy (in-vā′zhŭn prī′vă-sē) In health care, illicit (i.e., unauthorized) use of documentary materials related to treatment or condition.

in•va•sive (in-vā′siv) **1.** Denoting or characterized by invasion. **2.** Denoting a procedure requiring insertion of an instrument or device into the body through the skin or a body orifice for diagnosis or treatment.

in•va•sive car•ci•no•ma (in-vā′siv kahr′si-nō′mă) Carcinoma that has spread from its site of origin to adjacent tissues by direct extension.

in•va•sive mole (in-vā′siv mōl) SYN chorioadenoma destruens.

in•va•sive pro•ce•dure (in-vā′siv prō-sē′jŭr) Any surgical or exploratory activity in which the body is pierced by a device or instrument or by manual digitation.

in•ven•to•ry (in′vĕn-tōr-ē) A detailed, often descriptive, list of items.

in•verse ra•ti•o ven•ti•la•tion (IRV) (in-vĕrs′ rā′shē-ō ven′ti-lā′shŭn) A mode of mechanical ventilation.

in•verse square law (in′vĕrs skwār law) In radiation therapy, proposition that intensity of a radiation beam is inversely proportional to the square of the distance from the source of radiation.

in•ver•sion (in-vĕr′zhŭn) **1.** A turning inward, upside down, or in any direction contrary to the existing one. **2.** Conversion of a disaccharide or polysaccharide by hydrolysis into a monosaccharide; specifically, the hydrolysis of sucrose to D-glucose and D-fructose; so called because of the change in optical rotation. **3.** Alteration of a DNA molecule made by removing a fragment, reversing its orientation, and putting it back into place. **4.** Heat-induced transition of silica, in which the quartz tridymite or cristobalite changes its physical properties as to thermal expansion. [L. *inverto,* pp. *-versus,* to turn upside down, to turn about]

in•ver•sion of the u•ter•us (in-vĕr′zhŭn yū′tĕr-ŭs) A turning of the uterus inside out, usually following childbirth.

in•ver•te•brate (in-vĕr′tĕ-brăt) **1.** Not possessed of a spinal or vertebral column. **2.** Any animal that has no spinal column.

in•ver•tor (in-vĕr′tŏr) A muscle that inverts or causes inversion or turns a part, such as the foot, inward. SEE inversion.

in•vert sug•ar (in′vĕrt shug′ăr) A mixture of equal parts of D-glucose and D-fructose produced by hydrolysis of sucrose (inversion).

in•ves•ti•ga•tion•al new drug (IND) (in-ves′ti-gā′shŭn-ăl nū drŭg) A pharmacotherapeutic agent that has not been approved for general use by the U.S. Food and Drug Administration, but is in the course of being tested on humans.

in•vet•er•ate (in-vet′ĕr-ăt) Long seated; firmly established; said of a disease or of confirmed habits. [L. *in-vetero,* pp. *-atus,* to render old, fr. *vetus,* old]

in•vis•ca•tion (in′vis-kā′shŭn) **1.** Smearing with mucilaginous matter. **2.** The mixing of the food, during mastication, with the buccal secretions. [L. *in,* in, on, + *viscum,* birdlime]

in vi•tro (in vē′trō) In an artificial environment, referring to a process or reaction occurring therein, as in a test tube or culture media. Cf. in vivo. [L. in glass]

in vi•tro fer•ti•li•za•tion (IVF) (in vē′trō fĕr′til-ī-zā′shŭn) A process whereby (usually multiple) ova are placed in a medicum to which sperm are added for fertilization. The zygote thus produced is then introduced into the uterus and allowed to develop to term.

in vi•vo (in vē′vō) In the living body, referring to a process or reaction occurring therein. Cf. in vitro. [L. in the living being]

in vi•vo fer•til•i•za•tion (IVF) (in vē′vō fĕr′til-ī-zā′shŭn) **1.** Aspiration of mature oocytes from ovarian follicles during laparoscopy; the oocytes are placed in a Petri dish containing a special culture medium and sperms; cleaving zygotes are transferred to the uterus by introducing a catheter through the vagina and cervical canal. **2.** Fertilization of a mature oocyte within the distal uterine tube of a fertile donor female (rather than in an artificial medium), for subsequent nonsurgical transfer to an infertile recipient.

in•vo•lu•crum, pl. **in•vo•lu•cra** (in′vō-lū′krŭm, -lū′kră) **1.** An enveloping membrane, e.g., a sheath or sac. **2.** The sheath of new bone that forms around a sequestrum. [L. a wrapper, fr. *involvo,* to roll up]

in•vol•un•tar•y (in-vol′ŭn-tār-ē) **1.** Independent of the will; not volitional. **2.** Contrary to the will. [L. *in-* neg. + *voluntarius,* willing, fr. *volo,* to wish]

in•vol•un•tar•y mus•cles (in-vol′ŭn-tār-ē mŭs′ĕlz) Those muscles not ordinarily under control of the will; except in the case of the heart, they are smooth (nonstriated) muscles, innervated by the autonomic nervous system.

in•vol•un•tar•y pa•tient (in-vol′ŭn-tār-ē pā′shĕnt) In psychiatry, a patient confined to a facility without the patient's consent.

in•vo•lu•tion (in′vō-lū′shŭn) **1.** Return of an enlarged organ to normal size. **2.** Turning inward of the edges of a part. **3.** PSYCHIATRY mental decline associated with advanced age. SYN catagenesis. [L. *in-volvo,* pp. *-volutus,* to roll up]

in•vo•lu•tion•al (in′vō-lū′shŭn-ăl) Relating to involution.

in•vo•lu•tion•al de•pres•sion (in′vō-lū′shŭn-ăl dĕ-presh′ŭn) Depression or psychosis first occurring in the involutional years (40–55 for women, 50–65 for men).

in•vo•lu•tion•al mel•an•cho•li•a (in′vō-lū′shŭn-ăl mel′ăn-kō′lē-ă) A depressive disorder of middle life, commonly associated with the climacteric.

in•vo•lu•tion•al pto•sis (in-vō-lū′shŭn-al tō′sis) SYN aponeurotic ptosis.

in•volved field (in-volvd′ fēld) In radiation treatment, the area of the tumor itself.

i•o•dide (ī′ō-dīd) Negative ion of iodine, I^-.

i•o•dide ac•ne (ī′ō-dīd ak′nē) A follicular eruption on the face, trunk, and extremities, due to injection or ingestion of iodide in a hypersensitive person. SEE ALSO iododerma.

i•o•di•nate (ī-ō′di-nāt) To treat or combine with iodine.

i•o•di•nat•ed ^{131}I hu•man se•rum al•bu•min (ī-ō′di-nāt′ĕd hyū′măn sēr′ŭm al-bū′min) A sterile, buffered, isotonic solution prepared to contain not less than 10 mg of radioiodinated normal human serum albumin per mL, and adjusted to provide not more than 1 mCi of radioactivity per mL; used as a diagnostic aid in the measurement of blood volume and cardiac output.

i•o•di•nat•ed ^{125}I se•rum al•bu•min (ī-ō′di-nāt′ĕd sēr′ŭm al-bū′min) A sterile, buffered, isotonic solution prepared to contain not less than 10 mg of radioiodinated normal human serum albumin per mL, and adjusted to provide not more than 1 mCi of radioactivity per mL; used as a diagnostic aid in determining blood volume and cardiac output.

i•o•dine (I) (ī′ō-dīn, ī′ō-dēn) A nonmetallic chemical element, atomic no. 53, atomic wt. 126.90447; used as a catalyst, reagent, tracer, constituent of radiographic contrast media, therapy in thyroid disease, antidote for alkaloidal poisons, and component of certain stains and solutions. [G. *iōdēs,* violet-like, fr. *ion,* a violet, + *eidos,* form]

i•o•dine de•fi•cien•cy dis•or•der (ī′ō-dīn dĕ-fish′ĕn-sē dis-ōr′dĕr) A lack of iodine that causes growth and development disorders.

i•o•dine-fast (ī′ō-dīn-fast) Denoting hyperthyroidism unresponsive to iodine therapy, which develops frequently in most patients so treated.

i•o•dine stain (ī′ō-dīn stān) A stain to detect amyloid, cellulose, chitin, starch, carotenes, and glycogen, and to stain amebae by virtue of their glycogen; feces and other wet preparations are stained directly with Lugol iodine solution; smears are treated with Schaudinn fixative and then stained with alcoholic iodine, followed by Heidenhain iron hematoxylin.

i•o•din•o•phil, **i•o•din•o•phile** (ī′ō-din′ō-fil, -fīl) **1.** Staining readily with iodine. SYN iodinophilous. **2.** Any histologic element that stains readily with iodine. [iodine + G. *philos,* fond]

i•o•din•oph•i•lous (ī′ō-din-of′i-lŭs) SYN iodinophil (1).

i•o•dism (ī′ō-dizm) A condition marked by acute rhinitis, an acneform eruption, weakness, salivation, and foul breath, caused by the continuous administration of iodine or one of the iodides.

i•o•dize (ī′ō-dīz) To treat or impregnate with iodine.

i•o•dized salt (ī′ō-dīzd sawlt) Dietary sodium chloride that has been treated with iodine to prevent goiter. Most commonly available table salt in the United States has been so altered.

i•o•do•der•ma (ī-ō′dō-dĕr′mă) An eruption of follicular papules and pustules, or a granulomatous lesion, caused by iodine toxicity or sensitivity. SEE ALSO iodide acne.

i•o•do•form gauze (ī-ō′dō-fōrm gawz) Sterile strips of gauze impregnated with iodoform; used to pack abscesses, acting as a wick to promote drainage.

i•o•do•met•ric (ī′ō′dō-met′rik) Relating to iodometry.

i•o•dom•e•try (ī′ō-dom′ĕ-trē) Analytic techniques involving titrations in which iodine is either formed or consumed, the sudden appearance or disappearance of iodine marking the end point. [iodine + G. *metron,* measure]

i•o•do•phil•i•a (ī-ō′dō-fil′ē-ă) An affinity for iodine, as manifested by some leukocytes in certain conditions. [iodine + G. *phileō,* to love]

i•o•do•phor (ī-ō′dō-fōr) Any compound in which iodine is combined with an organic carrier; an intermediate-level disinfectant registered with the U.S. Environmental Protection Agency as hospital disinfectant with tuberculocidal action. Available in topical antiseptics and hard-surface disinfectant form. [io- + G. *phoros,* carrying]

i•o•dop•sin (ī′ō-dop′sin) A visual pigment, composed of 11-*cis*-retinal bound to an opsin, found in the cones of the retina. SYN visual violet. [G. *ion,* violet, + *ōps,* eye, + -in]

i•o•do•ther•a•py (ī-ō′dō-thār′ă-pē) Treatment with iodine.

i•o•du•ri•a (ī′ō-dyūr′ē-ă) Urinary excretion of iodine.

IOL Abbreviation for intraocular lens.

IOM Abbreviation for Institute of Medicine.

i•on (ī′on) An atom or group of atoms carrying an electric charge by virtue of having gained or lost one or more electrons. Ions charged with negative electricity (anions) travel toward a positive pole (anode); those charged with positive electricity (cations) travel toward a negative pole (cathode). Ions may exist in solid, liquid, or gaseous environments, although those in liquid (electrolytes) are more common and familiar. [G. *iōn,* going]

i•on chan•nel dis•or•ders (ī′on chan′ĕl dis-ōr′dĕrz) A number of diseases, mostly inherited and episodic in nature, caused by dysfunction of the calcium, chloride, potassium, or sodium channels of nerve or muscle; the inherited myotonias and periodic paralyses are included in this category; there is usually dominant inheritance, with the primary defect due to mutations of gene encoding on locus 7q32, 17q, or 1q31-32. SYN channelopathies.

i•on ex•change (ī′on eks-chānj′) SEE anion exchange, cation exchange, ion-exchange chromatography.

i•on-ex•change chro•ma•tog•ra•phy (ī′on-eks-chānj′ krō′mă-tog′ră-fē) Chemical investigation in which cations or anions in the mobile phase are separated by electrostatic interactions with the stationary phase. SEE ALSO anion exchange, cation exchange.

i•on-ex•change res•in (ī′on-eks-chānj′ rez′in) SEE anion exchange, cation exchange, ion-exchange chromatography.

i•on•ic (ī-on′ik) Relating to an ion.

i•on•ic strength (I) (ī-on′ik strengkth) Symbolized as Γ/2 or I and set equal to $0.5\Sigma m_i z_i^2$, where m_i equals the molar concentration and z_i the charge of each ion present in solution; if molar concentrations (c_i) are used instead of molality (and the solution is dilute), then $I = 0.5(1/\rho_o)\Sigma c_i z_i^2$ where ρ_o is the density of the solvent; a number of biochemically important events (e.g., protein solubility and rates of enzyme action) vary with the ionic strength of a solution.

i•on•i•za•tion (ī′on-ī-zā′shŭn) **1.** Dissociation into ions, occurring when an electrolyte is dissolved in water or certain liquids or when molecules are subjected to electrical discharge or ionizing radiation. **2.** Production of ions as a result of interaction of radiation with matter; process by which a neutral force becomes either positive or negative. **3.** SYN iontophoresis.

i•on•i•za•tion cham•ber (ī′on-ī-zā′shŭn chām′bĕr) A chamber for detecting ionization of the enclosed gas; used for determining intensity of ionizing radiation.

i•on•ize (ī′on-īz) To separate into ions; to dissociate atoms or molecules into electrically charged atoms or radicals.

i•on•iz•ing ra•di•a•tion (ī′on-īz′ing rā′dē-ā′shŭn) Corpuscular (e.g., neutrons, electrons) or electromagnetic (e.g., x-ray, gamma) radiation of sufficient energy to ionize the irradiated material.

i•o•none (ī′ō-nōn) One of two cyclic terpene ketones with an odor of violets or cedar wood.

i•on•o•phore (ī-on′ō-fōr) A compound or substance that forms a complex with an ion and transports it across a membrane. [ion + G. *phore,* a bearer]

i•on•o•pho•re•sis (ī-on′ō-fŏr-ē′sis) SYN electrophoresis. [ion + G. *phorēsis,* a carrying]

i•on•o•pho•ret•ic (ī-on′ō-fŏr-et′ik) SYN electrophoretic.

i•on•to•pho•re•sis (ī-on′tō-fŏr-ē′sis) The introduction, by means of electric current, of ions of soluble substances into tissue for therapeutic purposes. SYN ionization (3). [ion + G. *phorēsis,* a carrying]

i•on•to•pho•ret•ic (ī-on′tō-fŏr-et′ik) Relating to iontophoresis.

IOP Abbreviation for intraocular pressure.

i•o•pro•mide (ī′ō-prō′mīd) A monomeric, nonionic, water-soluble, low osmolar radiographic contrast medium for intravenous urography or angiography.

IORT Abbreviation for intraoperative radiation therapy.

i•o•ta (ι) (ī-ō′tă) **1.** The ninth letter in the Greek alphabet. **2.** CHEMISTRY denotes the ninth in a series, or the ninth atom from a carboxyl group or other functional group. **3.** A tiny or minute amount.

IPA Abbreviation for International Phonetic Alphabet; isopropyl alcohol; individual practice association.

ip•e•cac•u•a•nha (ip′ĕ-kak-wahn′ă) The dried root of *Uragoga (Cephaelis) ipecacuanha* (family Rubiaceae), a shrub found in Brazil and other parts of South America; contains emetine, cephaeline, emetamine, ipecacuanhic acid, psychotrine, and methylpsychotrine; has expectorant, emetic, and antidysenteric properties. [native Brazilian word]

IPF Abbreviation for idiopathic pulmonary fibrosis.

i•po•date (ī′pō-dāt) A radiographic contrast medium, given orally as the sodium or, more often, the calcium salt, for opacification of the gallbladder and central biliary tree.

I•po•mo•e•a (ī′pō-mē′ă) A plant genus of the family *Convolvulaceae.*

IPPB Abbreviation for intermittent positive pressure breathing.

ip·si·lat·er·al (ip′si-lat′ĕr-ăl) On the same side, with reference to a given point, e.g., a dilated pupil on the same side as an extradural hematoma. SYN homolateral. [L. *ipse,* same, + *latus* (*later-*), side]

IPV Abbreviation for intermittent percussive ventilation.

IQ Abbreviation for intelligence quotient.

IR Abbreviation for infrared.

Ir Symbol for iridium.

IRB Abbreviation for Institutional Review Board.

ir·i·dal (ir′i-dăl) Relating to the iris. SYN iridial, iridian, iridic.

ir·i·dec·to·my (ir′i-dek′tŏ-mē) **1.** Excision of a portion of the iris. **2.** The hole in the iris produced by a surgical iridectomy. [irido- + G. *ektomē,* excision]

ir·i·den·clei·sis (ir′i-den-klī′sis) The incarceration of a portion of the iris by corneoscleral incision in glaucoma to effect filtration between the anterior chamber and subconjunctival space. [irido- + G. *enkleiō,* to shut in]

irideraemia [Br.] SYN irideremia.

ir·i·de·re·mi·a (ir′i-dĕr-ē′mē-ă) Condition wherein the iris is so rudimentary as to appear to be absent. Cf. aniridia. SYN irideraemia. [irido- + G. *erēmia,* absence]

ir·i·des (ir′i-dēz) Plural of iris. [G.]

ir·id·e·sis (ī-rid′ĕ-sis) Ligature of a portion of the iris brought out through an incision in the cornea. [irido- + G. *desis,* a binding together]

ir·id·i·al, i·rid·i·an, ir·id·ic (ī-rid′ē-ăl, -ē-ăn, -rid′ik) SYN iridal.

ir·id·i·um (Ir) (ī-rid′ē-ŭm) A white, silvery metallic element, atomic no. 77, atomic wt. 192.22; ^{192}Ir is a radioisotope that has been used in the interstitial treatment of certain tumors. [L. *iris,* rainbow]

♻ **irido-, irid-** Combining forms meaning the iris. [G. *iris* (*irid-*), rainbow]

ir·i·do·a·vul·sion (ir′i-dō-ă-vŭl′shŭn) Avulsion, or tearing away, of the iris.

ir·i·do·cele (ī-rid′ō-sēl) Herniation of a portion of the iris through a corneal defect. [irido- + G. *kēlē,* hernia]

ir·i·do·cho·roid·i·tis (ir′i-dō-kōr′oyd-ī′tis) Inflammation of both iris and choroid.

ir·i·do·col·o·bo·ma (ir′i-dō-kol′ō-bō′mă) A coloboma or congenital defect of the iris. [irido- + G. *kolobōma,* coloboma]

ir·i·do·cor·ne·al an·gle (ir′i-dō-kōr′nē-ăl ang′gĕl) The acute area between the iris and the cornea at the periphery of the anterior chamber of the eye. SYN angulus iridocornealis [TA], angle of iris, filtration angle.

ir·i·do·cor·ne·al en·do·the·li·al syn·drome (ir′i-dō-kōr′nē-ăl en′dō-thē′lē-ăl sin′drōm) A congenital disorder comprising glaucoma, iris atrophy, decreased corneal endothelium, anterior peripheral synechia, and multiple iris nodules. SYN Cogan-Reese syndrome, iris-nevus syndrome.

ir·i·do·cy·clec·to·my (ir′i-dō-sī-klek′tŏ-mē) Removal of the iris and ciliary body for excision of a tumor. [irido- + G. *kyklos,* circle (ciliary body), + *ektomē,* excision]

ir·i·do·cy·cli·tis (ir′i-dō-sī-klī′tis) Inflammation of both iris and ciliary body. SEE ALSO iritis, uveitis. [irido- + G. *kyklos,* circle (ciliary body), + *-itis,* inflammation]

ir·i·do·cy·clo·cho·roid·i·tis (ir′i-dō-sī′klō-kōr′oyd-ī′tis) Inflammation of the iris, involving the ciliary body and the choroid. SYN panuveitis.

ir·i·do·cys·tec·to·my (ir′i-dō-sis-tek′tŏ-mē) An operation for making an artificial pupil when posterior synechiae follow extracapsular extraction of cataract. [irido- + G. *kystis,* bladder (capsule), + *ektomē,* excision]

ir·i·do·di·al·y·sis (ir′i-dō-dī-al′i-sis) Separation of the iris root from the scleral; often results from trauma. [irido- + G. *dialysis,* loosening]

ir·i·do·di·la·tor (ir′i-dō-dī′lāt-ŏr) Causing dilation of the pupil; applied to the musculus dilator pupillae.

ir·i·do·do·ne·sis (ir′i-dō-dō-nē′sis) Agitated motion of the iris. [irido- + G. *doneō,* to shake to and fro]

ir·i·do·ki·net·ic (ir′i-dō-ki-net′ik) Relating to the movements of the iris. SYN iridomotor.

ir·i·do·ma·la·ci·a (ir′i-dō-mă-lā′shē-ă) Degenerative softening of the iris. [irido- + G. *malakia,* softness]

ir·i·do·me·so·di·al·y·sis (ir′i-dō-me′sō-dī-al′i-sis) Separation of adhesions around the inner margin of the iris. [irido- + G. *mesos,* middle, + *dialysis,* loosening]

ir·i·do·mo·tor (ir′i-dō-mō′tŏr) SYN iridokinetic.

ir·i·do·pa·ral·y·sis (ir′i-dō-păr-al′i-sis) SYN iridoplegia.

ir·i·dop·a·thy (ir′i-dop′ă-thē) Pathologic lesions in the iris.

ir·i·do·ple·gi·a (ir′i-dō-plē′jē-ă) Paralysis of the musculus sphincter iridis. SYN iridoparalysis. [irido- + G. *plēgē,* stroke]

ir·i·dop·to·sis (ir′i-dop-tō′sis) Prolapse of the iris. [irido- + G. *ptōsis,* a falling]

ir•i•dor•rhex•is (ir′i-dō-rek′sis) Deliberate, surgical tearing of the iris from the scleral spur to increase the breadth of a coloboma. [irido- + G. *rhēxis,* rupture]

ir•i•dos•chi•sis (ir′i-dos′ki-sis) Separation of the anterior layer of the iris from the posterior layer; ruptured anterior fibers float in the aqueous humor. [irido- + G. *schisma,* cleft]

ir•i•do•scle•rot•o•my (ir′i-dō-skler-ot′ŏ-mē) An incision involving both sclera and iris. [irido- + sclera, + G. *tomē,* incision]

ir•i•dot•o•my (ir′i-dot′ŏ-mē) **1.** Transverse division of some of the fibers of the iris, forming an artificial pupil. **2.** Creating a hole in the iris to prevent or treat angle closure glaucoma. [irido- + G. *tomē,* incision]

IRI:G ra•ti•o (rā′shē-ō) The relationship of immunoreactive insulin to serum or plasma glucose.

i•ris, pl. **ir•i•des** (ī′ris, ir′i-dēz) [TA] The anterior division of the vascular tunic of the eye, a diaphragm, perforated in the center (the pupil), attached peripherally to the scleral spur; it is composed of stroma and a double layer of pigmented retinal epithelium from which are derived the sphincter and dilator muscles of the pupil. [G. rainbow, the iris of the eye]

I•rish tops (īr′ish tops) SYN broom.

iris-naevus syndrome [Br.] SYN iris-nevus syndrome.

i•ris-ne•vus syn•drome (ī′ris-nē′vŭs sin′drōm) SYN iridocorneal endothelial syndrome. SYN iris-naevus syndrome.

i•ris pit (ī′ris pit) Coloboma affecting the stroma of the iris with pigment epithelium intact.

i•ris spat•u•la (ī′ris spach′ŭ-lă) A flat surgical instrument used for repositioning an iris that has prolapsed through a wound.

i•rit•ic (ī-rit′ik) Relating to iritis.

i•ri•tis (ī-rī′tis) Inflammation of the iris. SEE ALSO iridocyclitis, uveitis.

IRMA (ĕrma) Acronym for immunoradiometric assay.

i•ron (Fe) (ī′ŏrn) A metallic element, atomic no. 26, atomic wt. 55.847, that occurs in the heme of hemoglobin, myoglobin, transferrin, ferritin, and iron-containing porphyrins, and is an essential component of enzymes such as catalase, peroxidase, and the various cytochromes; its salts are used medicinally. [A.S. *iren*]

i•ron 59 (ī′ŏrn) An iron isotope; a gamma and beta emitter with a half-life of 44.51 days; used as tracer in study of iron metabolism, determination of blood volume, and in blood transfusion studies.

i•ron bind•ing ca•pac•i•ty (ī′ŏrn bīnd′ing kă-pas′i-tē) Ability of iron-binding protein in serum (transferrin) to bind serum iron.

i•ron de•fi•cien•cy a•ne•mi•a (ī′ŏrn dĕ-fish′ĕn-sē ă-nē′mē-ă) Hypochromic microcytic anemia characterized by low serum iron, increased serum iron-binding capacity, decreased serum ferritin, and decreased marrow iron stores.

i•ron fil•ings (ī′ŏrn fil′ingz) Small packets of *Paragonimus* spp. eggs that can be seen in the sputum; the egg clumps tend to be yellow-brown.

i•ron line (ī′ŏrn līn) Deposition of iron in the corneal epithelium.

i•ron lung (ī′ŏrn lŭng) SYN Drinker respirator.

i•ron me•tab•o•lism (ī′ŏrn mĕ-tab′ŏ-lizm) The sum of the chemical and physical processes whereby iron is introduced into or evacuated from the body.

i•ron o•ver•load (ī′ŏrn ō′vĕr-lōd) A variable level of toxicity caused by nonphysiologic or intolerable levels of iron within the body.

i•ron poi•son•ing (ī′ŏrn poy′zŏn-ing) Measurable toxicity related to the presence of nonphysiologic levels of iron in the body.

i•ron-stor•age dis•ease (ī′ŏrn-stōr′ăj di-zēz′) The storage of excess iron in the parenchyma of many organs, as in idiopathic hemochromatosis or transfusion hemosiderosis.

ir•ra•di•ate (ir-rā′dē-āt) To apply radiation from a source to a structure or organism. SEE irradiation.

ir•ra•di•a•tion (ir-rā′dē-ā′shŭn) **1.** The subjective enlargement of a bright object seen against a dark background. **2.** Exposure to the action of electromagnetic radiation (e.g., heat, light, x-rays). **3.** The spreading of nervous impulses from one area in the brain or cord, or from a tract, to another tract. SEE ALSO radiation. **4.** A process of preparation in which food is exposed to low doses of radiation to decrease bacteria and improve shelf life. [L. *ir-radio,* (*in-r*), pp. *-radiatus,* to beam forth]

ir•ra•tion•al (ir-rash′ŭn-ăl) Not rational; unreasonable (contrary to reason) or unreasoning (not exercising reason). [L. *irrationalis,* without reason]

ir•re•duc•i•ble (ir′rĕ-dū′si-bĕl) **1.** Not reducible; incapable of being made smaller. **2.** CHEMISTRY incapable of being made simpler, or of being replaced, hydrogenated, or reduced in positive charge.

ir•re•duc•i•ble her•ni•a (ir′rĕ-dū′si-bĕl hĕr′nē-ă) A hernia that cannot be reduced without operation. SYN incarcerated hernia.

ir•reg•u•lar a•stig•ma•tism (ir-reg′yū-lăr ă-stig′mă-tizm) Astigmatism in which different parts of the same meridian have different degrees of curvature.

ir·reg·u·lar bone (ir-reg′yū-lăr bōn) One of a group of bones having peculiar or complex forms, e.g., vertebrae, many of the skull bones.

ir·reg·u·lar den·tin, ir·ri·ta·tion den·tin (ir-reg′yū-lăr den′tin, ir′i-tā′shŭn) SYN tertiary dentin.

ir·reg·u·lar pulse (i-reg′yū-lăr pŭls) An imprecise, but common, term involving variation in rate of impulses in an artery due to cardiac arrhythmia.

ir·re·sus·ci·ta·ble (ir′rĕ-sŭs′i-tă-bĕl) Incapable of being revived.

ir·re·ver·si·ble co·ma (ir′ĕ-vĕr′si-bĕl kō′mă) A state of profound unconsciousness that cannot be reversed. Cf. brain death

ir·re·vers·i·ble pulp·i·tis (ir′rĕ-vĕr′si-bĕl pŭl-pī′tis) Inflammation of the dental pulp from which the pulp is unable to recover; clinically, may be asymptomatic or characterized by pain that persists after thermal stimulation.

ir·ri·gate (ir′i-gāt) To perform irrigation. [L. *ir-rigo,* pp. *-atus,* to irrigate, fr. *in,* on, + *rigo,* to water]

ir·ri·ga·tion (ir′i-gā′shŭn) In surgery, washing out a body cavity, space, or wound with a fluid.

ir·ri·ta·bil·i·ty (ir′i-tă-bil′i-tē) The property inherent in protoplasm of reacting to a stimulus. [L. *irritabilitas,* fr. *irrito,* pp. *-atus,* to excite]

ir·ri·ta·ble (ir′i-tă-bĕl) **1.** Capable of reacting to a stimulus. **2.** Tending to react immoderately to a stimulus. Cf. excitable.

ir·ri·ta·ble bow·el syn·drome (IBS), ir·ri·ta·ble co·lon (ir′i-tă-bĕl bow′ĕl sin′drōm, kō′lŏn) A condition characterized by gastrointestinal signs and symptoms including constipation, diarrhea, gas and bloating, all in the absence of organic pathology. Associated with uncoordinated and inefficient contractions of the large intestine. SYN spastic colon.

ir·ri·tant (ir′i-tănt) **1.** Irritating; causing irritation. **2.** Any agent with this action.

ir·ri·tant con·tact der·ma·ti·tis (ir′i-tănt kon′takt dĕr′mă-tī′tis) Skin reactions ranging from erythema and scaling to necrotic burns resulting from nonimmunologic damage by chemicals in contact with the skin immediately or repeatedly.

ir·ri·ta·tion (ir′i-tā′shŭn) **1.** Inflammatory reaction of the tissues to an injury. **2.** The normal response of nerve or muscle to a stimulus. **3.** The evocation of a normal or exaggerated reaction in the tissues by the application of a stimulus. [L. *irritatio*]

ir·ri·ta·tion fi·bro·ma (ir′i-tā′shŭn fī-brō′mă) A slow-growing nodule on the oral mucosa, composed of fibrous tissue covered by epithelium; results from mechanical irritation caused by dentures, fillings, or from other sources, such as cheek biting.

ir·ri·ta·tive (ir′i-tā′tiv) Causing irritation.

ir·rup·tion (i-rŭp′shŭn) Act or process of breaking through to a surface. [L. *irruptio,* fr. *irrumpo,* to break in]

IRS-1 Abbreviation for insulin receptor substrate-1.

IRV Abbreviation for inspiratory reserve volume; inverse ratio ventilation.

Ir·vine-Gass syn·drome (ir′vīn gahs sin′drōm) Macular edema, associated with aphakia, and vitreous humor adherent to incision after cataract extraction.

I·saacs syn·drome, I·saacs-Mer·tons syn·drome (ī′zăks sin′drŏm, ī′zăks măr′tŏns sin′drōm) A rare disorder resulting from abnormal, spontaneous muscle activity of neural origin, manifested as continuous muscle stiffness and delayed relaxation after exercise, often accompanied by pain, cramps, fasciculations, hyperhydrosis, and muscle hypertrophy (on EMG, manifests as myokymia). Isaac syndrome usually begins in the lower extremities but can affect abdominal, upper extremity, vocal, and respiratory muscles; it is most often sporadic, although autosomal dominant inheritance has been reported. Probably it is an autoimmune disease, with antibodies against the potassium channels of peripheral nerves.

is·aux·e·sis (is′awk-sē′sis) Growth of parts at the same rate as growth of the whole. [G. *isos,* even, + *auxēsis,* increase]

ischaemia [Br.] SYN ischemia.

ischaemic [Br.] SYN ischemic.

ischaemic heart disease [Br.] SYN ischemic heart disease.

ischaemic hypoxia [Br.] SYN ischemic hypoxia.

ischaemic necrosis [Br.] SYN ischemic necrosis.

is·che·mi·a (is-kē′mē-ă) Local anemia due to mechanical obstruction (mainly arterial narrowing) of the blood supply; often marked by pain and by organ dysfunction. SYN ischaemia. [G. *ischō,* to keep back, + *haima,* blood]

is·che·mic (is-kē′mik) Relating to or affected by ischemia. SYN ischaemic.

is·che·mic con·trac·ture of the left ven·tri·cle (is-kē′mik kŏn-trak′shŭr left ven′tri-kĕl) Irreversible contraction of the left ventricle of the heart as a complication seen in the early period of cardiopulmonary bypass and now avoided by appropriate cardioplegic solutions. SYN stone heart.

is•che•mic heart dis•ease (is-kē′mik hahrt di-zēz′) A general term for diseases of the heart caused by insufficient blood supply to myocardium, e.g., atherosclerotic coronary artery disease, angina pectoris, unstable angina, and myocardial infarction. SYN ischaemic heart disease.

is•che•mic hy•pox•i•a (is-kē′mik hī-pok′sē-ă) Tissue hypoxia characterized by tissue oligemia and caused by arterial or arteriolar obstruction or vasoconstriction. SYN ischaemic hypoxia.

is•che•mic ne•cro•sis (is-kē′mik nĕ-krō′sis) Cell death caused by hypoxia resulting from local deprivation of blood supply, as by infarction. SYN ischaemic necrosis.

is•che•mic pain (is-kē′mik pān) SYN rest pain.

is•chi•a (is′kē-ă) Plural of ischium.

is•chi•ad•ic (is′kē-ad′ik) SYN sciatic (1).

is•chi•al (is′kē-ăl) SYN sciatic (1).

is•chi•al bone (is′kē-ăl bōn) SYN ischium.

is•chi•al bur•sa (is′kē-ăl bŭr′să) The bursa between the gluteus maximus muscle and the tuberosity of the ischium.

is•chi•al bur•si•tis (is′kē-ăl bŭr-sī′tis) Inflammation of the bursa overlying the ischial tuberosity of the pelvis.

is•chi•al•gi•a (is′kē-al′jē-ă) **1.** Pain in the hip; specifically, the ischium. SYN ischiodynia. **2.** Rarely used term for sciatica. [G. *ischion,* hip, + *algos,* pain]

is•chi•al spine (is′kē-ăl spīn) A pointed process from the posterior border of the ischium on a level with the lower border of the acetabulum; gives attachment to the sacrospinous ligament; the pudendal nerve passes dorsal to the ischial spine, which is palpable per vaginam or per rectum, and thus is used as a target for the needletip in administering a pudendal nerve block.

is•chi•al tu•ber•os•i•ty (is′kē-ăl tū′bĕr-os′i-tē) Landmark at the inferior aspect of the ischium: origin of the hamstring muscles.

is•chi•at•ic (is′kē-at′ik) SYN sciatic (1).

is•chi•at•ic her•ni•a (is′kē-at′ik hĕr′nē-ă) A hernia through the sacrosciatic foramen.

ischio- Combining form denoting ischium. [G. *ischion,* a hip-joint, haunch (ischium)]

is•chi•o•cap•su•lar (is′kē-ō-kap′sŭ-lăr) Relating to the ischium and the capsule of the hip joint; denoting the part of the capsule that is attached to the ischium.

is•chi•o•cav•ern•ous mus•cle (is′kē-ō-kav′ĕr-nŭs mŭs′ĕl) *Origin,* ramus of ischium; *insertion,* corpus cavernosum penis (or clitoridis); *action,* compresses the crus of the penis (or clitoris) forcing blood in its sinuses into the distal part of the corpus cavernosum; *nerve supply,* perineal. SYN musculus ischiocavernosus [TA].

is•chi•o•cele (is′kē-ō-sēl) SYN sciatic hernia. [ischio- + G. *kēlē,* hernia]

is•chi•o•coc•cyg•e•al (is′kē-ō-kok-sij′ē-ăl) Relating to the ischium and the coccyx.

is•chi•o•coc•cyg•e•us (is′kē-ō-kok-sij′ē-ŭs) SYN coccygeus muscle.

is•chi•o•dyn•i•a (is′kē-ō-din′ē-ă) SYN ischialgia (1). [ischio- + G. *odynē,* pain]

is•chi•o•fem•o•ral (is′kē-ō-fem′ŏr-ăl) Relating to the ischium, or hip bone, and the femur, or thigh bone.

is•chi•o•fib•u•lar (is′kē-ō-fib′yū-lăr) Relating to or connecting the ischium and the fibula.

is•chi•o•ni•tis (is′kē-ō-nī′tis) Inflammation of the ischium.

is•chi•o•tib•i•al (is′kē-ō-tib′ē-ăl) Relating to or connecting the ischium and the tibia.

is•chi•o•ver•te•bral (is′kē-ō-vĕr′tĕ-brăl) Relating to the ischium and the vertebral column.

is•chi•um, gen. **is•chi•i**, pl. **is•chi•a** (is′kē-ŭm, -ī, -ă) [TA] The lower and posterior part of the hip bone, distinct at birth but later becoming fused with the ilium and pubis; it consists of a body, where it joins the ilium and superior ramus of the pubis to form the acetabulum, and a ramus joining the inferior ramus of the pubis. SYN ischial bone. [Mod. L. fr. G. *ischion,* hip]

is•chu•ri•a (is-kyūr′ē-ă) Reduction in the flow of urine from any cause, including dehydration, inappropriate secretion of ADH, renal disease, atony of the bladder, and urinary tract obstruction. [G. *ischō,* to keep back, + *ouron,* urine]

ISD Abbreviation for intrinsic sphincter deficiency.

Ish•i•ha•ra test (ē′shē-hah′rah test) Assessment for color vision deficiency that uses a series of pseudoisochromatic plates on which numbers or letters are printed in dots of primary colors surrounded by dots of other colors; the figures are discernible by observers with normal color vision.

ISI Abbreviation for international sensitivity index.

is•land (ī′lănd) ANATOMY any isolated part, separated from the surrounding tissues by a groove, or marked by a difference in structure. SYN insula (2). [A.S. *īgland*]

is•land flap (ī′lănd flap) A flap in which the pedicle consists solely of the supplying artery and vein(s), sometimes including a nerve.

is·land of Reil (ī′lănd rīl) SYN insula (1).

is·let (ī′lĕt) A small island.

is·let cell (ī′lĕt sel) One of the cells of the pancreatic islets.

is·let cell tu·mor (ī′lĕt sel tū′mŏr) An endocrine tumor composed of cells equivalent or related to those in the normal islet of Langerhans; may be benign or malignant; usually hormonally active; comprises insulinomas, glucagonomas, vipomas, somatostatinomas, gastrinomas, pancreatic polypeptide-secreting tumors, and multihormonal or hormonally inactive pancreatic islet cell tumors.

is·lets of Lan·ger·hans (ī′lĕts lahng′er-hahnz) Cellular masses varying from a few to hundreds of cells lying in the interstitial tissue of the pancreas; they are the source of insulin and glucagon. See this page.

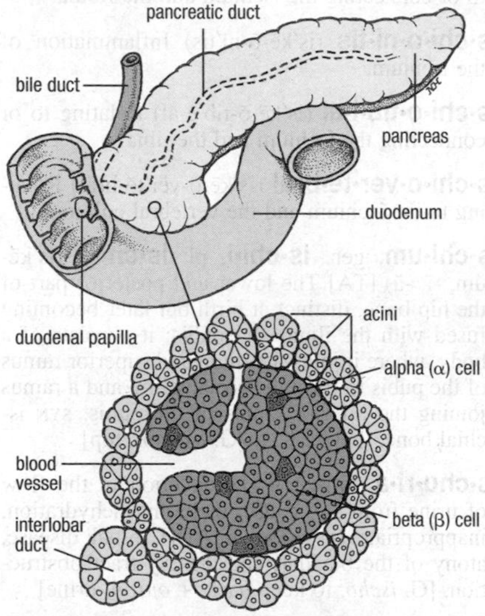

pancreas: an islet of Langerhans (endocrine function) surrounded by structures that secrete and transport pancreatic juice (exocrine function)

-ism Suffix meaning (1) A medical condition or a disease resulting from or involving some specified thing; (2) A practice, doctrine. Cf. -ia, -ismus. [G. *-isma, -ismos,* noun-forming suffix]

-ismus Suffix from L. for -ism; customarily used to imply spasm, contraction. [L. fr. G. *-ismos,* suffix forming nouns of action]

iso- **1.** Prefix meaning equal, like. **2.** CHEMISTRY prefix indicating "isomer of" (isomerism); e.g., isocyanate vs. cyanate. **3.** IMMUNOLOGY prefix designating similarity with respect to species; in recent years, the meaning has shifted to similarity with respect to genetic constitution of individual people. [G. *isos,* equal]

i·so·ag·glu·ti·na·tion (ī′sō-ă-glū′ti-nā′shŭn) Agglutination of red blood cells as a result of the reaction between an isoagglutinin and specific antigen in or on the cells. SYN isohemagglutination. [iso- + L. *ad,* to, + *gluten,* glue]

i·so·ag·glu·ti·nin (ī′sō-ă-glū′ti-nin) An isoantibody that causes agglutination of cells of genetically different members of the same species. SYN isohemagglutinin.

i·so·ag·glu·tin·o·gen (ī′sō-ă-glū-tin′ō-jen) An isoantigen that induces agglutination of the cells to which it is attached on exposure to its specific isoantibody.

i·so·am·y·lase (ī′sō-am′il-ās) A hydrolase that cleaves 1,6-α-D-glucosidic branch linkages in glycogen, amylopectin, and their β-limit dextrins; part of the complex known as debranching enzyme.

i·so·an·ti·bod·y (ī′sō-an′ti-bod-ē) **1.** An antibody that occurs only in some individuals of a species and reacts specifically with a particular foreign isoantigen. **2.** Sometimes used as a synonym of alloantibody. [G. *isos,* equal]

i·so·an·ti·gen (ī′sō-an′ti-jen) **1.** An antigenic substance that occurs only in some individuals of a species, such as the blood group antigens of humans. **2.** Sometimes used as a synonym of alloantigen.

i·so·bar (ī′sō-bahr) **1.** One of two or more nuclides having the same total number of protons plus neutrons, but with different distribution. **2.** The line on a map connecting points of equal barometric pressure. [iso- + G. *baros,* weight]

i·so·bar·ic (ī′sō-bar′ik) **1.** Having equal weights or pressures. **2.** With respect to solutions, having the same density as the diluent or medium.

i·so·cap·ni·a (ī′sō-kap′nē-ă) A state in which the arterial carbon dioxide pressure remains constant or unchanged. [iso- + G. *kapnos,* vapor]

i·so·cel·lu·lar (ī′sō-sel′yū-lăr) Composed of cells of equal size or of similar character. [iso- + L. *cellula,* dim. of *cella,* a storeroom]

i·so·cen·ter (ī′sō-sen′tĕr) The convergence of the three axes of rotation in radiation therapy; the intersecting point of the axis of rotation of the gantry, the collimator, and the treatment couch.

i·so·chro·mat·ic (ī′sō-krō-mat′ik) **1.** Of uniform color. **2.** Denoting two objects of the same color. [iso- + G. *chrōma,* color]

i·so·chro·mat·o·phil, i·so·chro·mat·o·phile (ī′sō-krō-mat′ō-fil, fīl) Having an equal affinity for the same dye; said of cells or tissues. [iso- + G. *chrōma,* color, + *philos,* fond]

i·so·chro·mo·some (ī′sō-krō′mŏ-sōm) A chromosomal aberration that arises as a result of transverse rather than longitudinal division of the centromere during meiosis; two daughter chromosomes are formed, each lacking one chromosome arm but with the other doubled.

i•so•chro•ni•a (ī′sō-krō′nē-ă) **1.** The state of having the same chronaxie. **2.** Agreement, with respect to time, rate, or frequency, between processes. [iso- + G. *chronos,* time]

i•soch•ro•nous (ī-sok′rō-nŭs) Occurring during the same time.

i•so•ci•trate (ī′sō-sit′rāt) A salt or ester of isocitric acid.

i•so•ci•trate de•hy•dro•gen•ase (ī′sō-sit′rāt dē′hī-droj′ĕn-ās) One of two enzymes that catalyze the conversion of *threo*-D_s-isocitrate to α-ketoglutarate (2-oxoglutarate) and CO_2.

i•so•cit•ric ac•id (ī′sō-sit′rik as′id) An intermediate in the tricarboxylic acid cycle.

i•so•co•ri•a (ī′sō-kōr′ē-ă) Equality in the size of the two pupils. [iso- + G. *korē,* pupil]

i•so•cor•tex (ī′sō-kōr′teks) The larger part of the mammalian cerebral cortex, distinguished from the allocortex by being composed of a larger number of nerve cells arranged in six layers. SEE ALSO cerebral cortex.

i•so•cy•tol•y•sin (ī′sō-sī-tol′i-sin) A cytolysin that reacts with the cells of certain other animals of the same species, but not with the cells of the individual that formed the isocytolysin.

i•so•dem•o•graph•ic map (ī′sō-dem′ō-graf′ik map) Diagrammatic method of displaying countries or administrative jurisdictions within a country in two-dimensional maps with each area directly proportional to the population density of the country or jurisdiction. [iso- + G. *dēmos,* people, + *graphō,* to write + -ic]

i•so•dense (ī′sō-dĕns) Denoting a tissue having a radiopacity (radiodensity) similar to that of another or adjacent tissue.

i•so•dose (ī′sō-dōs) Area of equivalent radiation dose. [iso- + dose]

i•so•dy•nam•ic (ī′sō-dī-nam′ik) **1.** Of equal force or strength. **2.** Relating to foods or other materials that liberate the same amount of energy on combustion. [iso- + G. *dynamis,* force]

i•so•e•lec•tric line (ī′sō-ĕ-lek′trik līn) The baseline of the electrocardiogram.

i•so•e•lec•tric pe•ri•od (ī′sō-ĕ-lek′trik pēr′ē-ŏd) The period occurring in the electrocardiogram between the end of the S wave and the beginning of the T wave during which electrical forces neutralize each other so that no difference exists in potential under the two electrodes. SYN abnormal ST segment.

i•so•e•lec•tric point (pI) (ī′sō-ĕ-lek′trik poynt) The pH at which an amphoteric substance, such as protein or an amino acid, is electrically neutral.

i•so•en•er•get•ic (ī′sō-en′ĕr-jet′ik) Exerting equal force; equally active.

i•so•en•zyme (ī′sō-en′zīm) One of a group of enzymes that catalyze the same reaction but may be differentiated by variations in physical properties, such as isoelectric point, electrophoretic mobility, kinetic parameters, or modes of regulation. SYN isozyme.

i•so•e•ryth•rol•y•sis (ī′sō-ĕ-rith-rol′i-sis) Destruction of erythrocytes by isoantibodies. [iso- + erythrocyte, + G. *lysis,* dissolution]

i•so•fla•vones (ī′sō-flā′vōnz) Plant chemicals that may help prevent cancer and heart disease.

i•so•ga•mete (ī′sō-gam′ēt) **1.** One of two or more similar cells that conjugate or fuse and subsequently divide, resulting in reproduction. **2.** A gamete of the same size as the gamete with which it unites. [iso- + G. *gametēs* or *gametē,* husband or wife]

i•sog•a•my (ī-sog′ă-mē) Conjugation between two equal gametes or two individual cells alike in all respects. [iso- + G. *gamos,* marriage]

i•so•ge•ne•ic, i•so•gen•ic (ī′sō-jĕ-nē′ik, -jen′ik) SYN syngeneic.

i•so•ge•ne•ic graft (ī′sō-jĕ-nē′ik graft) SYN syngraft.

i•sog•e•nous (ī-soj′ĕ-nŭs) Of the same origin, as in development from the same tissue or cell. [iso- + G. *genos,* family, kind]

i•so•graft (ī′sō-graft) SYN syngraft.

isohaemagglutinin [Br.] SYN isohemagglutinin.

isohaemolysin [Br.] SYN isohemolysin.

isohaemolysis [Br.] SYN isohemolysis.

i•so•he•mag•glu•ti•na•tion (ī′sō-hē′mă-glū′ti-nā′shŭn) SYN isoagglutination. [iso- + G. *haima,* blood, + L. *ad,* to, + *gluten,* glue]

i•so•he•mag•glu•ti•nin (ī′sō-hē′mă-glū′ti-nin) SYN isoagglutinin. SYN isohaemagglutinin.

i•so•he•mo•ly•sin (ī′sō-hē-mol′i-sin) An isolysin that reacts with red blood cells. SYN isohaemolysin.

i•so•he•mo•ly•sis (ī′sō-hē-mol′i-sis) Dissolution of red blood cells as a result of the reaction between an isolysin (isohemolysin) and specific antigen in or on the cells. SYN isohaemolysis. [iso- + G. *haima,* blood, + *lysis,* dissolution]

i•so•im•mu•ni•za•tion (ī′sō-im′yū-nī-zā′shŭn) Development of a significant titer of specific antibody as a result of antigenic stimulation with material contained on or in the red blood cells of another individual of the same species.

i•so•ki•net•ic ex•er•cise (ī′sō-ki-net′ik eks′ĕr-sīz) Exercises in which the muscle contracts at a consistent speed and tension throughout the entire range of movement.

i•so•late (ī′sŏ-lāt) **1.** To separate, to set apart from others; that which is so treated. **2.** To free of chemical contaminants. **3.** PSYCHOANALYSIS to separate experiences or memories from the affects pertaining to them. **4.** GROUP PSYCHOTHERAPY a person to whom others in the group do not respond. **5.** Viable organisms separated on a single occasion from a field sample in experimental hosts, culture systems, or stabilates. **6.** A population that for geographic, linguistic, cultural, social, religious, or other reasons is subject to little or no genetic flow. [It. *isolare;* Mediev. L. *insulo,* pp. *-atus,* to insulate, fr. L. *insula,* island]

i•so•lat•ed ex•plo•sive dis•or•der (ī′sŏ-lā-tĕd eks-plō′siv dis-ōr′dĕr) A disorder of impulse control characterized by a single episode of failure to resist a violent, externally directed act that has a harmful impact on others.

i•so•lat•ed pro•tein•ur•i•a (ī′sŏ-lā-tĕd prō′tē-nyūr′ē-ă) Protein-related disorder in the urine of a patient who is asymptomatic, has normal renal function and urinary sediment, and has no manifestation of systemic disease on initial examination.

i•so•la•tion (ī′sŏ-lā′shŭn) **1.** MICROBIOLOGY separation of an organism from others, usually by making serial cultures. **2.** Separation for the period of communicability of infected people or animals from others to prevent or limit the direct or indirect transmission of the infectious agent from those who are infected to those who are susceptible. Cf. quarantine.

i•so•lec•i•thal (ī′sō-les′i-thăl) Denoting an oocyte with a moderate amount of uniformly distributed yolk.

i•so•lette (ī′sŏ-let′) Individual clear basket used in nurseries for newborns.

i•so•leu•cine (I) (ī′sō-lū′sēn) An L-amino acid found in almost all proteins; an isomer of leucine and, like it, a dietary essential amino acid.

i•sol•o•gous (ī-sol′ŏ-gŭs) SYN syngeneic. [iso- + G. *logos,* ratio]

i•sol•o•gous graft (ī-sol′ŏ-gŭs graft) SYN syngraft.

i•sol•y•sin (ī-sol′i-sin) An antibody that combines with, sensitizes, and results in complement-fixation and dissolution of cells that contain the specific isoantigen; isolysins occur in the blood of some members of a species and they react with the cells of that species, but not with the cells of the individual (or the same type) in which the isolysins are naturally formed.

i•sol•y•sis (ī-sol′i-sis) Lysis or dissolution of cells as a result of the reaction between an isolysin and specific antigen in or on the cells. SEE ALSO isohemolysis. [iso- + G. *lysis,* dissolution]

i•so•lyt•ic (ī′sō-lit′ik) Pertaining to, characterized by, or causing isolysis.

i•so•malt•ose (ī′sō-mawl′tōs) A disaccharide in which two glucose molecules are attached by an α1,6 link, rather than an α1,4 link as in maltose.

i•so•mer (ī′sō-mĕr) **1.** One of two or more substances displaying isomerism. Cf. stereoisomer. **2.** One of two or more nuclides having the same atomic and mass numbers but differing in energy states for a finite period of time. [iso- + G. *meros,* part]

i•som•er•ase (ī-som′ĕr-ās) A class of enzymes (EC class 5) catalyzing the conversion of a substance to an isomeric form.

i•so•mer•ic (ī′sō-mer′ik) Relating to or characterized by isomerism.

i•som•er•ism (ī-som′ĕr-izm) The existence of a chemical compound in two or more forms that are identical with respect to percentage composition but differ as to the positions of one or more atoms within the molecules, and also in physical and chemical properties.

i•som•er•i•za•tion (ī-som′ĕr-ī-zā′shŭn) A process in which one isomer is formed from another, as in the action of isomerases.

i•so•met•ric (ī′sō-met′rik) **1.** Of equal dimensions. **2.** PHYSIOLOGY denoting the condition when the ends of a contracting muscle are held fixed so that contraction produces increased tension at a constant overall length. Cf. auxotonic, isotonic (3), isovolumic. [iso- + G. *metron,* measure]

i•so•met•ric con•trac•tion (ī′sō-met′rik kŏn-trak′shŭn) Force development at constant length. Cf. isotonic contraction.

i•so•met•ric ex•er•cise (ī′sō-met′rik ek′sĕr-sīz) Exercise consisting of muscular contractions without movement of the involved parts of the body.

i•so•met•ric pe•ri•od of car•di•ac cy•cle (ī′sō-met′rik pēr′ē-ŏd kahr′dē-ak sī′kĕl) That period in which the muscle fibers do not shorten although the cardiac muscle is excited and the pressure in the ventricles rises, extending from the closure of the atrioventricular valves to the opening of the semilunar valves (isovolumic constriction) or the reverse (isovolumic relaxation). SYN isovolumic period.

i•so•me•tro•pi•a (ī′sō-mĕ-trō′pē-ă) Equality in refraction in the two eyes. [iso- + G. *metron,* measure, + *ōps* (*ōp*-), eye]

i•so•mor•phic (ī′sō-mōr′fik) SYN isomorphous.

i•so•mor•phism (ī′sō-mōr′fizm) Similarity of form between two or more organisms or between parts of the body. [iso- + G. *morphē,* shape]

i•so•mor•phous (ī′sō-mōr′fŭs) Having the

same form or shape, or being morphologically equal. SYN isomorphic.

i•sop•a•thy (ī-sop′ă-thē) **1.** Treatment of disease by means of the causal agent or a product of the same disease. **2.** Treatment of a diseased organ by an extract of a similar organ from a healthy animal. SEE ALSO homeopathy. [iso- + G. *pathos,* suffering]

i•so•per•i•stal•tic a•nas•to•mo•sis (ī′sō-per′i-stawl′tik ă-nas′tō-mō′sis) An anastomosis allowing flow of contents in the same and normal direction.

i•soph•a•gy (ī-sof′ă-jē) SYN autolysis. [iso- + G. *phagō,* to eat]

i•so•phane in•su•lin (ī′sō-fān in′sŭ-lin) SYN NPH insulin.

i•so•plas•tic (ī′sō-plas′tik) SYN syngeneic. [iso- + G. *plassō,* to form]

i•so•plas•tic graft (ī′sō-plas′tik graft) SYN syngraft.

i•so•pre•cip•i•tin (ī′sō-prē-sip′i-tin) An antibody that combines with and precipitates soluble antigenic material in the plasma or serum, or in an extract of the cells, from another member, but not all members, of the same species. [iso- + precipitin]

i•so•prene (ī′sō-prēn) An unsaturated five-carbon hydrocarbon with a branched chain, the basis for the formation of isoprenoids (terpenes, carotenoids, and rubber). Fat-soluble vitamins either are isoprenoid or have isoprenoid side chains; steroids are synthesized through isoprenoid intermediates.

i•so•pre•noids (ī′sō-prēn′oydz) Polymers with carbon skeletons that consist in whole or in large part of isoprene units joined end to end.

i•sop•ter (ī-sop′tĕr) A line of equal retinal sensitivity in the visual field. [iso- + G. *optēr,* observer]

i•sor•rhe•a (ī′sō-rē′ă) Equality of intake and output of water; maintenance of water equilibrium. SYN isorrhoea. [iso- + G. *rhoia,* a flow]

isorrhoea [Br.] SYN isorrhea.

i•sos•best•ic point (ī′sos-bes′tik poynt) APPLIED SPECTROSCOPY a wavelength at which absorbance of two substances, one of which can be converted into the other, is the same.

i•so•sex•u•al (ī′sō-sek′shū-ăl) **1.** Relating to the existence of characteristics or feelings of both sexes in one person. **2.** Descriptive of an individual's somatic characteristics, or of internal processes, which are consonant with the sex of that individual.

i•sos•mot•ic (ī′sos-mot′ik) Having the same total osmotic pressure or osmolality as another fluid (ordinarily intracellular fluid); such a fluid is not isosmotic if it includes solutes that freely permeate cell membranes.

i ***I•sos•po•ra*** (ī-sos′pŏr-ă) A genus of coccidia chiefly parasitizing mammals. See page B7. [iso- + G. *sporos,* seed]

i•sos•po•ri•a•sis (ī-sos′pŏ-rī′ă-sis) Disease caused by infection with a species of *Isospora,* such as *I. belli* in humans; such disease usually is mild except in cases of immunosuppression, as in AIDS, where it may cause an intractable diarrhea.

i•sos•the•nu•ri•a (ī-sos′thĕ-nyūr′ē-ă) A state in chronic renal disease in which the kidney cannot form urine with a higher or a lower specific gravity than that of protein-free plasma; specific gravity of the urine becomes fixed around 1.010, irrespective of the fluid intake. [iso- + G. *sthenos,* strength, + *ouron,* urine]

i•so•ther•mal (ī′sō-thĕr′măl) Having the same temperature. [iso- + G. *thermē,* heat]

i•so•tone (ī′sō-tōn) One of several nuclides having the same number of neutrons in their nuclei. [iso- + G. *tonos,* stretching, tension]

i•so•to•ni•a (ī′sō-tō′nē-ă) A condition of tonic equality in which tension or osmotic pressure in two substances or solutions is the same. [iso- + G. *tonos,* tension]

i•so•ton•ic (ī′sō-ton′ik) **1.** Relating to isotonicity or isotonia. **2.** Having equal tension; denoting solutions possessing the same osmotic pressure; more specifically, limited to solutions in which cells neither swell nor shrink. Thus, a solution that is isosmotic with intracellular fluid will not be isotonic if it includes solute, such as urea, that freely permeates cell membranes. **3.** PHYSIOLOGY denoting the condition when a contracting muscle shortens against a constant load, as when lifting a weight. Cf. auxotonic, isometric (2).

i•so•ton•ic con•trac•tion (ī′sō-ton′ik kŏn-trak′shŭn) Shortening at constant force development. Cf. isometric contraction.

i•so•ton•ic ex•er•cise (ī′sō-ton′ik eks′ĕr-sīz) Exercise in which the muscle contracts against a fixed resistance, without movement.

i•so•to•nic•i•ty (ī′sō-tō-nis′i-tē) **1.** The quality of possessing and maintaining a uniform tone or tension. **2.** The property of a solution in being isotonic.

i•so•tope (ī′sŏ-tōp) One of two or more nuclides that are chemically identical, having the same number of protons, yet differ in mass number, because their nuclei contain different numbers of neutrons; individual isotopes are named with the inclusion of their mass number in the superior position (^{12}C) and the atomic number (nuclear protons) in the inferior position ($_{6}C$). [iso- + G. *topos,* part, place]

i•so•to•pic (ī′sō-top′ik) Of identical chemical

composition but differing in some physical property, such as atomic weight.

i•so•tro•pic, **i•sot•ro•pous** (ī′sō-trō′pik, ī-sot′rō-pŭs) Having properties which are the same in all directions. [iso- + G. *tropē,* a turn]

i•so•type (ī′sō-tīp) An antigenic determinant (marker) that occurs in all members of a subclass of an immunoglobulin class. [iso- + G. *typos,* model]

i•so•typ•ic (ī′sō-tip′ik) Pertaining to an isotype.

i•so•vol•u•mic (ī′sō-vol-yū′mik) Occurring without an associated alteration in volume, as when, in early ventricular systole, the muscle fibers initially increase their tension without shortening so that ventricular volume remains unaltered. SEE ALSO isometric.

i•so•vol•u•mic per•i•od (ī′sō-vol-yū′mik pēr′ē-ŏd) SYN isometric period of cardiac cycle.

i•so•zyme (ī′sō-zīm) SYN isoenzyme.

isth•mec•to•my (is-mek′tŏ-mē) Excision of the midportion of the thyroid. [G. *isthmos,* isthmus, + *ektomē,* excision]

isth•mic, **isth•mi•an** (is′mik, -mē-ăn) Denoting an anatomic isthmus.

isth•mo•pa•ral•y•sis (is′mō-păr-al′i-sis) Paralysis of the velum pendulum palati and the muscles forming the anterior pillars of the fauces. SYN isthmoplegia. [G. *isthmos,* isthmus, + paralysis]

isth•mo•ple•gi•a (is′mō-plē′jē-ă) SYN isthmoparalysis. [G. *isthmos,* isthmus, + *plēgē,* stroke]

isth•mus, pl. **isth•mi**, **isth•mus•es** (is′mŭs, -mī, -mŭs-ĕz) [TA] **1.** A constriction connecting two larger parts of an organ or other anatomic structure. **2.** A narrow passage connecting two larger cavities. **3.** The narrowest portion of the brainstem at the junction between midbrain and hindbrain. [G. *isthmos*]

isth•mus of au•di•to•ry tube (is′mŭs aw′di-tōr-ē tūb) The narrowest portion of the auditory tube at the junction of the cartilaginous and bony portions. SYN isthmus tubae auditivae [TA].

isth•mus tu•bae au•di•ti•vae (is′mŭs tū′bē aw-di-tī′vē) [TA] SYN isthmus of auditory tube.

IT Abbreviation for intrathecal.

itch (ich) **1.** A peculiar irritating sensation in the skin that arouses the desire to scratch. SYN pruritus (2). **2.** Common name for scabies. [A.S. *gikkan*]

itch•ing (ich′ing) An uncomfortable sensation of irritation of the skin or mucous membranes that causes scratching or rubbing of the affected parts. SYN pruritus (1).

-ite **1.** Suffix meaning of the nature of, resembling. **2.** A salt of an acid that has the termination -ous. **3.** COMPARATIVE ANATOMY a suffix denoting an essential portion of the part to the name of which it is attached. SEE ALSO -ites. [G. *-itēs,* fem. *-itis*]

i•ter (ī′tĕr) A passage leading from one anatomic part to another. SEE ALSO canaliculus. [L. *iter* (*itiner-*), a way, journey]

i•ter•al (ī′tĕr-ăl) Relating to an iter.

-ites Adjectival suffix to nouns, corresponding to L. *-alis, -ale,* or *-inus, -inum,* or Eng. *-y* or *-like,* or the hyphenated nouns; the adjective so formed is used without the qualified noun. SEE ALSO -ite. [G. *itēs,* m., or *-ites,* n.]

-itic Combining form denoting disorder of.

-itides Plural of -itis.

-itis SEE -ites. [G. fem. of *-ites*]

I•to ne•vus (ē′tō nē′vŭs) Pigmentation of skin innervated by lateral branches of the supraclavicular nerve and the lateral cutaneous nerve of the arm, due to scattered, heavily pigmented, dendritic melanocytes in the dermis.

ITP Abbreviation for idiopathic thrombocytopenic purpura; inosine 5′-triphosphate.

IUCD Abbreviation for intrauterine contraceptive device.

IUD Abbreviation for intrauterine device.

IUGR Abbreviation for intrauterine growth retardation.

IUI Abbreviation for intrauterine insemination.

-ium Combining form usually denoting a natural element (e.g., polonium).

^{131}I up•take test (ŭp′tāk test) A test of thyroid function in which ^{131}I-iodide is given orally; after 24 hours, the amount present in the thyroid gland is measured and compared with normal values.

IV Abbreviation for intravenous(ly).

IVC Abbreviation for inferior vena cava.

IVDU Abbreviation for intravenous drug user.

I•ve•mark syn•drome (ē′vĕ-mahrk sin′drōm) SYN polysplenia.

Ives disease (īvz di-zēz′) Increased skin hypersensitivity (“leopard spots”), swelling, and redness seen in old men. Treatment includes avoidance of exposure to sun, systemic adrenocortical steroid, and some other pharmaceuticals.

IVF Abbreviation for in vivo fertilization; in vitro fertilization.

IVH Abbreviation for intraventricular hemorrhage.

IVI Abbreviation for intravenous injection.

I•vor Lew•is e•soph•a•gec•to•my (ī′vōr-lū′ is ĕ-sof′ă-jek′tō-mē) Commonly used approach for esophagectomy using laparotomy and right thoracotomy, with intrathoracic anastomosis.

IVP Abbreviation for intravenous pyelogram/pyelography; intravenous push.

IV tub•ing (tū′bing) Modality used to connect the bag of medication to the patient; either gravity driven or forced by a pump calibrated to give the fluids over a longer period.

IVU Abbreviation for intravenous urogram.

Ix•o•des (ik-sō′dēz) A genus of hard ticks (family Ixodidae), many species of which are parasitic on humans and animals; they are characterized by an anal groove surrounding the anus anteriorly, absence of eyes and festoons, and marked sexual dimorphism; about 40 species have been described from North America. [G. *ixōdēs,* sticky, like bird-lime, fr. *ixos,* mistletoe, + *eidos,* form]

Ix•o•des red•i•kor•ze•vi (ik-sō′dēz red-i-kōr′ zē-vī) A Eurasian tick species that has caused human toxicosis in Israel.

Ix•o•des scap•u•lar•is (ik-sō′dēz skap-yū-lā′ ris) The black-legged or shoulder tick, a species found in the southern and eastern U.S.; the primary vector of Lyme disease and human granulocytic ehrlichiosis in the U.S.

ix•o•di•a•sis (ik′sō-dī′ă-sis) Skin lesions caused by the bites of certain ixodid ticks.

ix•od•ic (ik-sod′ik) Relating to or caused by ticks.

ix•o•did (ik′sō-did) Common name for members of the family Ixodidae.

Ix•od•i•dae (ik-sod′i-dē) A family of ticks, the so-called hard ticks, genera of which transmit many important human and animal diseases and cause tick paralysis.

J Abbreviation for joule; electric current density.

J Abbreviation for flux (4).

Ja•bou•lay am•pu•ta•tion (zhah′bū-lā′ amp′yū-tā′shŭn) SYN hemipelvectomy.

jack•et (jak′ĕt) **1.** A fixed bandage applied around the body to immobilize the spine. **2.** DENTISTRY an artificial crown composed of fired porcelain or acrylic resin. [M.E., fr. O.Fr. *jaquet*, dim. of *jaque*, tunic, fr. *Jacques*, nickname of Fr. peasants]

jack•pot syn•drome (jak′pot sin′drōm) Clinical and legal jargon phrase denoting action of a patient who seeks excessive remuneration for what the physician regards as a minor matter.

jack•so•ni•an sei•zure, **jack•so•ni•an ep•i•lep•sy** (jak-sō′nē-ăn sē′zhūr, ep′ĭ-lep-sē) A seizure originating in or near the rolandic neocortex, which clinically involves one part of the body; seizure spread is accompanied by progressive spread to other parts of the body on the same side; may become generalized.

Jack•son law (jak′sŏn law) Loss of mental functions due to disease retraces in reverse order its evolutionary development.

Jack•son mem•brane (jak′sŏn mem′brān) A thin vascular membrane or veillike adhesion, covering the anterior surface of the ascending colon from the cecum to the right flexure; it may cause obstruction by kinking of the bowel.

Jack•son rule (jak′sŏn rūl) After an epileptic attack, simple and quasiautomatic functions are less affected and more rapidly recovered than the more complex ones.

Jack•son sign (jak′sŏn sīn) During quiet respiration the movement of the paralyzed side of the chest may be greater than that of the opposite side, whereas in forced respiration the paralyzed side moves less than the other.

Ja•cob•son re•flex (jā′kŏb-sŏn rē′fleks) Flexion of the fingers elicited by tapping the flexor tendons over the wrist joint or the lower end of the radius.

jac•ti•ta•tion (jak′ti-tā′shŭn) Extreme restlessness or tossing about from side to side. [L. *jactatio,* a tossing, fr. *jacto,* pp. *-atus,* to throw]

JADA (jă′dă) Acronym for *Journal of the American Dental Association.*

Jae•ger test types (yā′gĕr test tīps) Type of different sizes used for testing the acuity of near vision.

Jahn•ke syn•drome (yahn′kĕ sin′drōm) Sturge-Weber syndrome without glaucoma.

jail fe•ver (jāl fē′vĕr) SYN epidemic typhus.

JAMA (jam′ă) The official name for the journal published by the American Medical Association.

Ja•mai•ca pep•per (jă-mā′kă pep′ĕr) SYN allspice.

ja•mais vu (zhah-mā vū) A lack of memory and sensation of disorientation in a patient, even though confirmation of an earlier act or circumstance can be found. SEE ALSO déjà vu. [Fr., never seen]

Ja•net test (zhah-nā′ test) A test for functional or organic anesthesia; the patient (with eyes closed) is told to say "yes" or "no" on feeling (or not) the touch of the examiner's finger; in the case of functional anesthesia the patient may say "no" when an anesthetic area is touched, but will say nothing, being unaware of being touched, in cases of organic anesthesia.

Jane•way gas•tros•to•my (jān′wā gas-tros′tŏ-mē) Surgical procedure and device used to gain permanent access to stomach. Full-thickness stomach flap is taken from the greater curvature and then closed around the catheter and brought out to skin surface. Mucocutaneous tissue is formed into a nipple at skin edge.

Jane•way le•sion (jān′wā lē′zhŭn) One of the stigmata of infectious endocarditis: irregular, erythematous, flat, painless macules on the palms, soles, thenar, and hypothenar eminences of the hands, tips of the fingers, and plantar surfaces of the toes.

jan•i•ceps (jan′i-seps) Conjoined twins having their two heads fused together, with the faces looking in opposite directions. SEE conjoined twins. [L. *Janus,* a Roman deity having two faces, + *caput,* head]

Jan•sen op•er•a•tion (yahn′sen op-ĕr-ā′shŭn) An operation for frontal sinus disease; the lower wall and lower portion of the anterior wall are removed and the mucous membrane is curetted away.

Ja•nus green B (jan′ŭs grēn) [CI 11050] diethylsafraninazodimethylaniline chloride; A basic dye used in histology and to stain mitochondria supravitally.

Jap•a•nese B en•ceph•a•li•tis (jap′ă-nēz en-sef′ă-lī′tis) An epidemic encephalitis or encephalomyelitis of Japan, Siberian Russia, and other parts of Asia; due to the Japanese B encephalitis virus (genus Flavivirus) and transmitted by mosquitoes; can occur as a symptomless, subclinical infection but may cause an acute meningoencephalomyelitis.

Jap•a•nese B en•ceph•a•li•tis vi•rus (jap′ă-nēz en-sef′ă-lī′tis vī′rŭs) A virus of the genus Flavivirus (group B arbovirus) normally present in humans, especially in children, as an inapparent infection, but may cause febrile response and sometimes encephalitis.

Jap•a•nese spot•ted fev•er (jap′ă-nēz′ spot′ĕd fē′vĕr) A febrile disease caused by the bacterium *Rickettsia japonica* and characterized by headache and exanthema; found in Japan.

jar·gon (jahr′gŏn) **1.** Language or terminology peculiar to a specific field, profession, or group. **2.** Nonsensical speech due to insult or trauma to the brain. [Fr. gibberish]

jar·gon a·pha·si·a (jahr′gŏn ă-fā′zē-ă) SYN paragrammatism.

Ja·risch-Herx·hei·mer re·ac·tion (yah′rish herks′hīm-er rē-ak′shŭn) SYN Herxheimer reaction.

Jar·man score (jahr′man skōr) Index of social and medical deprivation, used mainly by family practice doctors, especially in the U.K.

Jar·vik ar·ti·fi·cial heart (jahr′vik ahr′ti-fish′ ăl hahrt) A pneumatic artificial heart.

jaun·dice (jawn′dis) **1.** A yellowish staining of the integument, sclerae, and deeper tissues and of the excretions with bile pigments, which are increased in plasma. **2.** Symptom of various disorders, including liver disease. See this page. SYN icterus. [Fr. *jaune,* yellow]

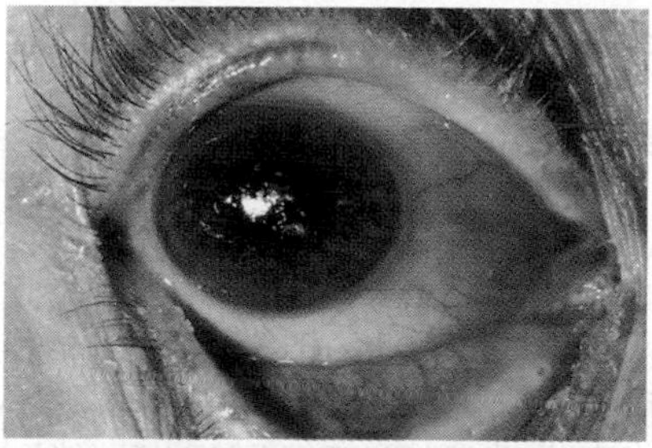

jaundice: patient in hepatic failure displays yellow sclera

jaun·dice ber·ry (jawn′dis ber′ē) SYN barberry.

jaun·dice of the new·born (jawn′dis nū′ bōrn) SYN icterus neonatorum.

jaw (jaw) **1.** One of the two bony structures, in which the teeth are set, forming the framework of the mouth. **2.** Common name for either the maxilla or the mandible. [A.S. *ceōwan,* to chew]

jaw bone (jaw bōn) SYN mandible.

jaw gra·da·tion (jaw grā-dā′shŭn) Controlled vertical mandibular movement during vocalization as a function of length, depth, and amount of muscular contraction.

Ja·wor·ski bod·ies (yĕ-vōr′skē bod′ēz) Mucous shreds in the gastric contents in hyperchlorhydria.

jaw re·flex (jaw rē′fleks) A spasmodic contraction of the temporal muscles following a downward tap on the loosely hanging mandible.

jaw re·trac·tion (jaw rĕ-trak′shŭn) An atypical oral pattern that includes excessive pulling back of the lower jaw, making it difficult to open the mouth fully for eating or verbal communication.

jaw thrust (jaw thrŭst) An atypical pattern seen when there is a strong, sudden downward extension of the lower jaw elicited when the bottle, breast, cup, or spoon is presented or when communication is attempted. It can be accompanied by an overall increase in extensor muscle tone throughout the body. This response can result in food loss from within the oral cavity and can also dislocate the temporomandibular joint.

jaw wink·ing (jaw wingk′ing) A paradoxic movement of eyelids associated with movements of the jaw.

jaw-wink·ing syn·drome (jaw′wingk′ing sin′ drōm) An increase in the width of the palpebral fissures during chewing, sometimes with a rhythmic elevation of the upper lid when the mouth is open and ptosis when the mouth is closed. SYN Gunn syndrome, Marcus Gunn phenomenon, Marcus Gunn syndrome.

JCAHO Abbreviation for Joint Commission on Accreditation of Healthcare Organizations.

J chain (chān) A glycopeptide disulfide that is bonded to polymeric IgA and IgM; its function is to ensure correct polymerization of the subunits of IgA and IgM. [*j*oining]

Jef·fer·son frac·ture (jef′ĕr-sŏn frak′shŭr) Fracture of the atlas, usually due to compressive trauma.

je·ju·nal (jĕ-jū′năl) Relating to the jejunum.

je·ju·nal ar·ter·ies (jĕ-jū′năl ahr′tĕr-ēz) *Origin,* superior mesenteric; *distribution,* jejunum; *anastomoses,* by a series of arches with each other and with ileal arteries. SYN arteriae jejunales [TA].

je·ju·nal and il·e·al veins (jĕ-jū′năl il′ē-ăl vānz) Structures that drain the jejunum and ileum; they terminate in the superior mesenteric vein.

je·ju·nec·to·my (jĕ′jū-nek′tŏ-mē) Excision of all or a part of the jejunum. [jejunum + G. *ektomē,* excision]

je·ju·ni·tis (jĕ′jū-nī′tis) Inflammation of the jejunum.

jejuno-, jejun- Combining forms meaning the jejunum, jejunal. [L. *jejunus,* empty]

je·ju·no·co·los·to·my (jĕ-jū′nō-kō-los′tŏ-mē) Establishment of a communication between the jejunum and the colon. [jejuno- + colon + G. *stoma,* mouth]

je·ju·no·il·e·al (jĕ-jū′nō-il′ē-ăl) Relating to the jejunum and the ileum.

je·ju·no·il·e·al by·pass, je·ju·no·il·e·al

shunt (jĕ-jū′nō-il′ē-ăl bī′pas, shŭnt) Anastomosis of the upper jejunum to the terminal ileum for treatment of morbid obesity. SYN bowel bypass.

je•ju•no•il•e•i•tis (jĕ-jū′nō-il′ē-ī′tis) Inflammation of the jejunum and ileum.

je•ju•no•il•e•os•to•my (jĕ-jū′nō-il′ē-os′tŏ-mē) Establishment of a new communication between the jejunum and the ileum. [jejuno- + ileum + G. *stoma,* mouth]

je•ju•no•je•ju•nos•to•my (jĕ-jū′nō-jĕ′jū-nos′tŏ-mē) An anastomosis between two portions of jejunum. [jejuno- + jejuno- + G. *stoma,* mouth]

je•ju•no•plas•ty (jĕ-jū′nō-plas-tē) A corrective surgical procedure on the jejunum. [jejuno- + G. *plastos,* molded]

je•ju•nos•to•my (jĕ′jū-nos′tŏ-mē) Operative establishment of an opening from the abdominal wall into the jejunum, usually with creation of a stoma on the abdominal wall. [jejuno- + G. *stoma,* mouth]

je•ju•not•o•my (jĕ′jū-not′ŏ-mē) Incision into the jejunum. [jejuno- + G. *tomē,* incision]

je•ju•num (je-jū′nŭm) [TA] The portion of small intestine, about 8 feet in length, between the duodenum and the ileum. The jejunum is distinct from the ileum in being more proximal, of larger diameter with a thicker wall, having larger, more highly developed plicae circulares, and being more vascular (redder in appearance), with the jejunal arteries forming fewer tiers of arterial arcades and longer vasa recta. [L. *jejunus,* empty]

jel•ly (jel′ē) A semisolid tremulous compound usually containing some form of gelatin in aqueous solution. [L. *gelo,* to freeze]

jel•ly•fish (jel′ē-fish) Marine coelenterates, including some poisonous species; toxin is injected into the skin by nematocysts on the tentacles, causing linear wheals. See page B8.

Jen•dras•sik ma•neu•ver (yen-drah′sik mă-nū′vĕr) A method of emphasizing the patellar reflex: the subject hooks the hands together by the flexed fingers and pulls against them with all possible strength.

Jen•ner stain (jen′ĕr stān) A methylene blue eosinate similar to Wright stain but differing in not using polychromed methylene blue; used for staining of blood smears.

Jen•sen dis•ease (yen′sĕn di-zēz′) SYN retinochoroiditis juxtapapillaris.

jerk (jĕrk) **1.** A sudden pull. **2.** SYN deep reflex.

jerk nys•tag•mus (jĕrk nis-tag′mŭs) Nystagmus in which there is a slow drift of the eyes in one direction, followed by a rapid recovery movement, always described in the direction of the recovery movement; it usually arises from labyrinthine or neurologic lesions or stimuli.

Jer•ne plaque as•say (yer′nĕ plak as′ā) An assay that enumerates individual antibody-forming cells. SYN hemolytic plaque assay.

jer•sey fin•ger (jĕr′zē fing′gĕr) Avulsion of the flexor digitorum profundus tendon from the distal phalanx due to abrupt passive extension of the actively flexed finger.

jet (jet) A region of high blood velocity immediately downstream of a vessel stenosis.

jet lag (jet lag) An imbalance of the normal circadian rhythm resulting from subsonic or supersonic travel through several time zones; leads to fatigue, irritability, and functional disturbances.

jet neb•u•liz•er (jet neb′yū-lī-zĕr) An atomizer that uses an air or gas stream to change a liquid into small particles.

Jeune syn•drome (zhūn sin′drōm) SYN asphyxiating thoracic dystrophy.

jew•el•er's for•ceps (jew′ĕl-ĕrz fōr′seps) A small thumb forceps with very fine pointed blades, used to grasp tissues in microsurgical procedures.

Jew•ett nail (jū′ĕt nāl) An intramedullary hip screw used in trochanteric fractures.

Jew•ett and Strong stag•ing (jew′ĕt strawng stāj′ing) Staging of bladder carcinoma: O, noninvasive; A, with submucosal invasion; B, with muscle invasion; C, with invasion of perivascular fat; D, with lymph node metastasis.

jew's harp plant (jūz hahrp plant) SYN trillium.

JH vi•rus (vī′rŭs) Human rhinovirus strain 1A. [*J*ohns *H*opkins University, where first isolated]

jig•ger (jig′ĕr) Common name for *Tunga penetrans.* SEE ALSO chigoe.

Jo•bert de Lam•balle su•ture (zhō-bār′ dĕ-lahm-bahl′ sū′chŭr) An interrupted intestinal suture, used for invaginating the margins of the intestines in circular enterorrhaphy.

Jo•cas•ta com•plex (jō-kas′tă kom′pleks) A mother's libidinous fixation on a son. [*Jocasta,* mother and wife of Oedipus in Greek mythology]

jock itch (jok ich) SYN tinea cruris.

Jod-Ba•se•dow phe•nom•e•non (yod-bah′zĕ-dō fĕ-nom′ĕ-non) Induction of thyrotoxicosis in a previously euthyroid person as a result of exposure to large quantities of iodine; occurs most often in areas of endemic iodine-deficient goiter and in patients with multinodular goiter; also can develop following use of iodine-containing agents for diagnostic studies.

Jof•froy re•flex (zhof-rwah′ rē′fleks) Twitching of the glutei muscles when firm pressure is made on the buttocks, in cases of spastic paralysis.

Jof•froy sign (zhof-rwah′ sīn) **1.** Disorder of the arithmetic faculty (the person being unable to do simple sums in addition or multiplication) in the early stages of organic brain disease. **2.** Absence of facial muscle contraction in exophthalmic goiter when patient directs her or his gaze upward.

John•son meth•od (jon′son meth′ŏd) SYN chloropercha method.

joint (joynt) ANATOMY the place of union, usually more or less movable, between two or more bones. Joints between skeletal elements exhibit a great variety of form and function, and are classified into three general morphologic types: fibrous joints; cartilaginous joints; and synovial joints. See this page. SYN arthrosis (1), articulation (1), junctura (1). [L. *junctura;* fr. *jungo,* pp. *junctus,* to join]

joint cap•sule (joynt kap′sŭl) SYN articular capsule.

Joint Com•mis•sion on Ac•cre•di•ta•tion of Health•care Or•ga•ni•za•tions (JCAHO) (joynt kŏ-mish′ŏn ă-kred-i-tā′shŭn helth′kār ōr-găn-i-zā′shŭns) An independent nonprofit organization that evaluates and accredits health care organizations and programs in the United States.

joint ef•fu•sion (joynt ĕ-fyu′zhŭn) Increased fluid in synovial cavity of a joint.

joint ex•ten•sion (joynt eks-ten′shŭn) SYN close-packed position.

joints of foot (joynts fut) Collective term comprising the talocrural, intertarsal, tarsometatarsal, intermetatarsal, metatarsophalangeal, and interphalangeal joints.

joints of hand (joynts hand) Collective term comprising the radiocarpal or wrist joint; intercarpal, carpometacarpal, intermetacarpal, metacarpophalangeal, and interphalangeal joints.

joint sta•bil•i•ty (joynt stă-bil′i-tē) Ability of the kinetic chain (i.e., nervous, skeletal, and muscular systems) to stabilize a joint during movement.

jo•jo•ba (hō-hō′bă) Herbal oil remedy pressed from *Simmondsia chinensis* and *S. californica;* alleged to grow hair and cure dermatologic disorders. [Mexican Sp.]

Jones I test (jōnz test) SYN primary dye test.

Jones II test (jōnz test) SYN secondary dye test.

Jones cri•ter•i•a (jōnz krī-tēr′ē-ă) Characteristics and findings (proposed by T.D. Jones in 1944 and modified in 1965) that are used to confirm the diagnosis of rheumatic fever. There are five major criteria: carditis, polyarthritis, chorea, erythema marginatum, and subcutaneous nodules; minor criteria include fever, arthralgia, elevated erythrocyte sedimentation rate or C reactive protein, and prolonged PR interval on ECG. Diagnosis requires evidence of recent group A β-hemolytic streptococcal infection, plus two major and one minor criteria, or one major and two minor criteria; revised Jones criteria allow the diagnosis when indolent carditis or chorea exists with no other cause, or in patients with a previous history of rheumatic fever who have one major or two minor criteria in association with a recent streptococcal infection.

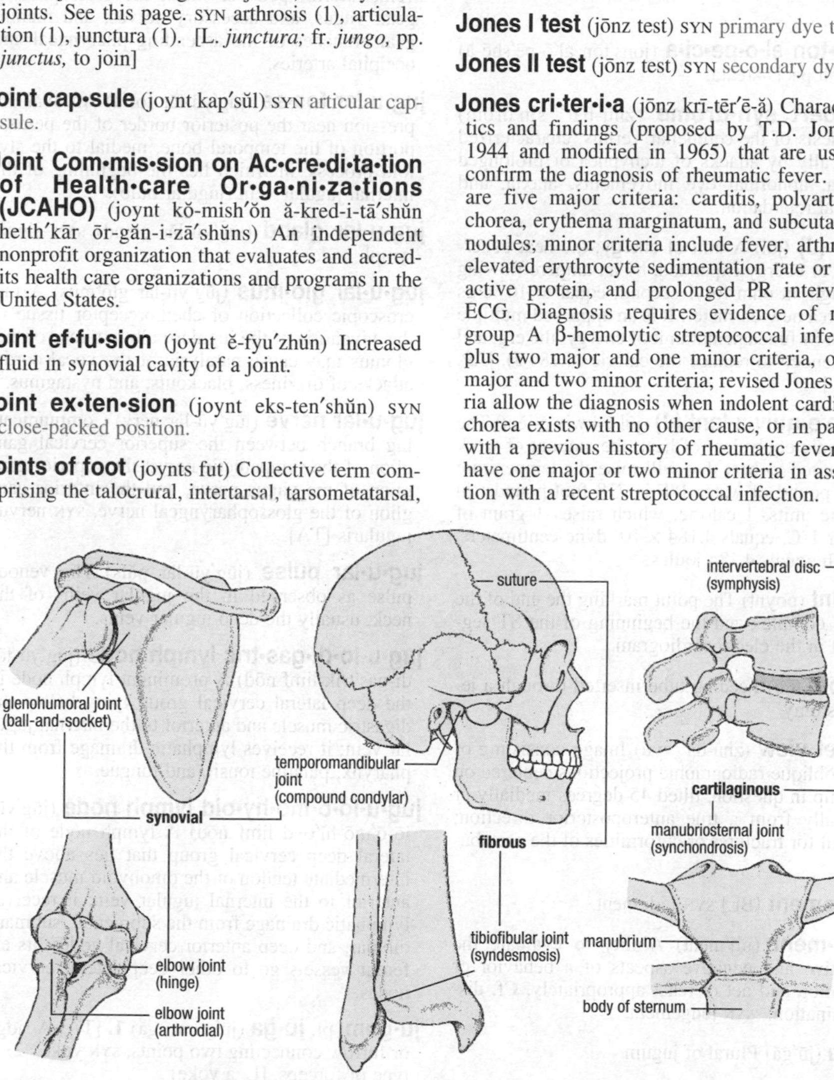

joints

Jones frac•ture (jōnz frak′shŭr) Transverse stress fracture of the proximal shaft of the fifth metatarsal.

Jo•ne•si•a den•i•trif•i•cans (jōnz′ē-ă den-i-trif′i-kanz) A species of motile, gram-positive bacteria formerly classified as *Listeria denitrificans;* the only member of the genus *Jonesia.*

Jones test (jōnz test) SYN fluorescein instillation test.

Jones trans•fer (jōnz trans′fĕr) Surgical procedure to treat claw deformities of the great toe in which the extensor hallucis longus tendon is transferred to the neck of the metatarsal; can also be used to correct claw deformities of the lesser toes.

Jons•ton al•o•pe•ci•a (jons′tŏn al′ō-pē′shē-ă) SYN alopecia areata.

Jou•bert syn•drome (zhū-bār′ sin′drōm) Agenesis of the cerebellar vermis, characterized clinically by attacks of tachypnea or prolonged apnea, abnormal eye movements, ataxia, and mental retardation.

joule (J) (jūl) A unit of energy; the heat generated, or energy expended, by an ampere flowing through an ohm for 1 second; equal to 10^7 ergs and to a newton-meter. It is an approved multiple of the SI fundamental unit of energy, the erg, and is intended to replace the calorie (4.184 J). [J.P. *Joule*]

Joule e•quiv•a•lent (J) (jūl ē-kwiv′ă-lĕnt) The dynamic equivalent of heat; the amount of work converted to heat that will raise the temperature of 1 pound of water 1°F is 778 foot-pounds; in metric units, 1 calorie, which raises 1 gram of water 1°C, equals 4.184×10^7 dyne-centimeters, which equals 4.184 joules.

J point (poynt) The point marking the end of the QRS complex and the beginning of the ST segment in the electrocardiogram.

J-tube (tūb) Feeding tube inserted through a jejunostomy.

Ju•det view (zhū-dā′ vyū) Image consisting of two oblique radiographic projections centered on the hip in question, tilted 45 degrees medially or laterally from a true anteroposterior direction; useful for fractures or deformities of the acetabulum.

judgement [Br.] SYN judgment.

judg•ment (jŭj′mĕnt) Ability to evaluate the positive and negative aspects of a behavior or situation and act or react appropriately. Cf. discrimination. SYN judgement.

ju•ga (jū′gă) Plural of jugum.

ju•gal (jū′găl) **1.** Connecting; yoked. **2.** Relating to the zygomatic bone. [L. *jugalis,* yoked together, fr. *jugum,* a yoke]

ju•gal bone (jū′găl bōn) SYN zygomatic bone.

ju•ga•le (jū-gā′lē) A craniometric point at the union of the temporal and frontal processes of the zygomatic bone. SYN jugal point.

ju•gal point (jū′găl poynt) SYN jugale.

jug•u•lar (jŭg′yū-lăr) **1.** Relating to the throat or neck. **2.** Relating to the jugular veins. **3.** A jugular vein. [L. *jugulum,* throat]

jug•u•lar fo•ra•men (jŭg′yū-lăr fōr-ā′mĕn) A passage between the petrous portion of the temporal bone and the jugular process of the occipital, sometimes divided into two by the intrajugular processes; it contains the internal jugular vein, inferior petrosal sinus, the glossopharyngeal, vagus, and accessory nerves, and meningeal branches of the ascending pharyngeal and occipital arteries.

jug•u•lar fos•sa (jŭg′yū-lăr fos′ă) An oval depression near the posterior border of the petrous portion of the temporal bone, medial to the styloid process, in which lies the beginning of the internal jugular vein (jugular bulb).

jug•u•lar gland (jŭg′yū-lăr gland) SYN signal lymph node.

jug•u•lar glo•mus (jŭg′yū-lăr glō′mŭs) A microscopic collection of chemoreceptor tissue in the adventitia of the jugular bulb; a tumor of this glomus may cause paralysis of the vocal cords, attacks of dizziness, blackouts, and nystagmus.

jug•u•lar nerve (jŭg′yū-lăr nĕrv) Communicating branch between the superior cervical ganglion of the sympathetic nerve, the superior ganglion of the vagus nerve, and the inferior ganglion of the glossopharyngeal nerve. SYN nervus jugularis [TA].

jug•u•lar pulse (jŭg′yū-lăr pŭls) The venous pulse as observed in the jugular veins of the neck, usually the deep jugular veins.

jug•u•lo•di•gas•tric lymph node (jŭg′yū-lō-dī-gas′trik limf nōd) A prominent lymph node in the deep lateral cervical group lying below the digastric muscle and anterior to the internal jugular vein; it receives lymphatic drainage from the pharynx, palatine tonsil, and tongue.

jug•u•lo•o•mo•hy•oid lymph node (jŭg′yū-lō-ō′mō-hī′oyd limf nōd) A lymph node of the lateral deep cervical group that lies above the intermediate tendon of the omohyoid muscle and anterior to the internal jugular vein; it receives lymphatic drainage from the submental, submandibular, and deep anterior cervical nodes; its efferent vessels go to other deep lateral cervical nodes.

ju•gum, pl. **ju•ga** (jū′gŭm, -gă) **1.** [TA] A ridge or furrow connecting two points. SYN yoke. **2.** A type of forceps. [L. a yoke]

juice (jūs) **1.** The interstitial fluid of a plant or animal. **2.** A digestive secretion. [L. *jus,* broth]

juice ther•a•py (jūs thār′ă-pē) The dietary and therapeutic administration of vegetables and fruits that have been mechanically converted to liquids.

jump flap (jŭmp flap) A distant flap transferred in stages through an intermediate carrier; e.g., an abdominal flap is attached to the wrist, then at a later stage the wrist is brought to the face.

jump•ing dis•ease, **jump•er dis•ease** (jŭmp′ing di-zēz′, jŭm′pĕr) One of the pathologic startle syndromes found in isolated parts of the world, characterized by greatly exaggerated responses, such as jumping, flinging the arms, and yelling, to minimal stimuli. SYN jumping Frenchmen of Maine syndrome.

jump•ing French•men of Maine syn•drome (jŭmp′ing french′mĕn mān sin′drōm) SYN jumping disease.

junc•ti•o (jŭngk′shē-ō) SYN junction.

junc•tion (jŭngk′shŭn) The point, line, or surface of union of two parts, mainly bones or cartilages. SYN junctio.

junc•tion•al ep•i•the•li•um (jŭngk′shŭn-ăl ep′i-thē′lē-ŭm) Surface located at the base of the gingival sulcus. It is a cufflike nonkeratinized band of squamous epithelium encircling and affixing itself to the dental surface.

junc•tion•al rhythm (jŭngk′shŭn-ăl ridh′ŭm) Rhythms originating anywhere within the A-V junction. Formerly termed "A-V nodal" or simply "nodal" rhythms.

junc•tion•al tach•y•car•di•a (jŭngk′shŭn-ăl tak′i-kahr′dē-ă) Cardiac activation arising from the atrioventricular junction with a ventricular response rate over 100 beats per minute.

junc•tion ne•vus (jŭngk′shŭn nē′vŭs) A nevus consisting of nests of melanocytes in the basal cell zone, at the junction of the epidermis and dermis, appearing as a slightly raised, small, flat, nonhairy pigmented (brown or black) tumor.

junc•tu•ra, pl. **junc•tu•rae** (jŭngk-tyūr′ă, -rē) **1.** [TA] SYN joint. **2.** The point, line, or surface of union of two parts, mainly bones or cartilages. SYN juncture. [L. a joining]

junc•ture (jŭngk′shūr) SYN junctura (2).

jung•i•an (yung′ē-ăn) The psychological system or the psychoanalytic form of treatment deriving from it developed by Carl Gustav Jung.

jung•i•an psy•cho•a•nal•y•sis (yung′ē-ăn sī′kō-ă-nal′i-sis) The theory of psychopathology and the practice of psychotherapy, according to the principles of C. G. Jung, which emphasized human beings' symbolic nature, and differs from freudian psychoanalysis especially in placing less significance upon instinctual (sexual) urges. SYN analytic psychology.

junk DNA (jŭngk) The portion of DNA that is not transcribed and expressed, comprising about 90% of the 3 billion base pairs of the human genome; its function is not known. SYN selfish DNA.

junk food (jŭngk fūd) A colloquial term for highly flavored but unwholesome food that is high in fat, salt, or sugar but deficient in protein, fiber, and vitamins.

Jur•kat cells (yūr′kăt selz) A line of T cells often employed in immunologic research, originally derived from a Burkitt lymphoma.

jus•tice (jŭs′tis) **1.** An ethical principle of fairness or equity, according equal rights to all and basing rewards on merit and punishments on guilt. **2.** NURSING ethical principle that individual people and groups with similar circumstances and conditions should be treated alike; fairness with equal distribution of goods and services. SEE ALSO Nursing Interventions Classification.

ju•ve•nile ar•thri•tis, **ju•ve•nile rheu•ma•toid ar•thri•tis** (jū′vĕ-nil ahr-thrī′tis, rū′mă-toyd ahr-thrī′tis) Chronic arthritis beginning in childhood, most cases of which are pauciarticular, i.e., affecting few joints. Several patterns of illness have been identified: in one subset, primarily affecting girls, iritis is common and antinuclear antibody is usually present; another subset, primarily affecting boys, frequently includes spinal arthritis resembling ankylosing spondylitis; some cases are true rheumatoid arthritis beginning in childhood and characterized by the presence of rheumatoid factor and destructive deforming joint changes, often undergoing remission at puberty. SEE ALSO Still disease.

ju•ve•nile cat•a•ract (jū′vĕ-nil kat′ăr-akt) A cataract occurring in a child or young adult.

ju•ve•nile cell (jū′vĕ-nil sel) SYN metamyelocyte.

ju•ve•nile de•lin•quen•cy (jū′vĕ-nil dĕ-lingk′wĕn-sē) An older term used to describe the behavior of teenagers acting in a manner inconsistent with societal expectations. Cf. sociopath, antisocial personality disorder

ju•ve•nile di•a•be•tes (jū′vĕ-nil dī′ă-bē′tēz) Term disallowed by the American Diabetes Association. See Type 1 diabetes.

ju•ve•nile ky•pho•sis (jū′vĕ-nil kī-fō′sis) SYN Scheuermann disease.

ju•ve•nile my•o•clon•ic ep•i•lep•sy (jū′vĕ-nil mī′ō-klon′ik ep′i-lep′sē) An inherited epilepsy syndrome typically beginning in early adolescence, and characterized by early morning myoclonic jerks that may progress into a generalized tonic-clonic seizure.

ju•ve•nile of•fend•er (jū′vĕ-nil ŏ-fend′ĕr) In law, a person who has yet to reach legal majority but who has broken an existing law.

ju·ve·nile-on·set di·a·be·tes (jū′vĕ-nil-on′ set dī-ă-bē′tēz) SYN Type 1 diabetes.

ju·ve·nile pel·vis (jū′vĕ-nil pel′vis) A pelvis justo minor in which the bones are slender.

ju·ve·nile per·i·o·don·ti·tis (jū′vĕ-nil per′ē-ō-don-tī′tis) A degenerative periodontal disease of adolescents in which the periodontal destruction is out of proportion to the local irritating factors present on the adjacent teeth; inflammatory changes become superimposed, and bone loss, migration, and extrusion are observed. Two forms are recognized: 1) localized, in which the destruction is limited to the incisors and first molars; 2) generalized, involving all of the teeth. SYN periodontosis.

ju·ve·nile plan·tar der·ma·to·sis (jū′vĕ-nil plan′tahr dĕr-mă-tō′sis) A painful dermatitis, occurring primarily in children, which causes the plantar skin to appear glazed and fissured; may be associated with hyperhidrosis.

ju·ve·nile spi·nal mus·cu·lar a·tro·phy (jū′vĕ-nil spī′năl mŭs′kyū-lăr at′rŏ-fē) Slowly progressive proximal muscular weakness and wasting, beginning in childhood, caused by degeneration of motor neurons in the anterior horns of the spinal cord; onset usually between 2 and 17 years of age; usually autosomal recessive inheritance.

jux·ta·col·ic ar·ter·y (jŭks′tă-col′ik ahr′tĕr-ē) SYN marginal artery of colon.

jux·ta·crine (jŭks′tă-krin) A mode of hormone action that requires the cell producing the effector to be in direct contact with the cell containing the appropriate receptor. [L. *juxta,* close to, + G. *krinō,* to separate]

jux·ta·ep·i·phys·i·al (jŭks′tă-ep-i-fiz′ē-ăl) Close to or adjoining an epiphysis.

jux·ta·e·soph·a·ge·al pul·mo·nar·y lymph nodes, jux·ta·e·soph·a·ge·al lymph nodes (jŭks′tă-ē-sof-ă′jē-ăl pul′mŏ-năr-ē limf nōdz, limf nōdz) Several nodes of the posterior mediastinal group located along either side of the esophagus; they receive lymph from both the esophagus and the lungs. SYN juxta-oesophageal pulmonary lymph nodes.

jux·ta·glo·mer·u·lar (jŭks′tă-glŏ-mĕr′yū-lăr) Close to or adjoining a renal glomerulus.

jux·ta·glo·mer·u·lar cells (jŭks′tă-glŏ-mĕr′ yū-lăr selz) Cells located at the vascular pole of the renal corpuscle that secrete renin and form a component of the juxtaglomerular complex; they are modified smooth muscle cells primarily of the afferent arteriole of the renal glomerulus.

jux·ta·glo·mer·u·lar cell tu·mor (jŭks′tă-glŏ-mĕr′yū-lăr sel tū′mŏr) A tumor of juxtaglomerular cell origin usually presenting with symptoms of secondary aldosteronism, including severe diastolic hypertension, which appears to be due to tumor-produced renin. The histologic appearance resembles that of a hemangiopericytoma.

jux·ta·glo·mer·u·lar gran·ules (jŭks′tă-glŏ-mĕr′yū-lăr gran′yūlz) Osmophilic secretory granules present in the juxtaglomerular cells, thought to contain renin.

jux·tal·lo·cor·tex (jŭks′tă-lō-kōr′teks) Collective term for regions of the cerebral cortex between the isocortex and the allocortex.

juxta-oesophageal lymph nodes [Br.] SYN juxtaesophageal lymph nodes.

juxta-oesophageal pulmonary lymph nodes [Br.] SYN juxtaesophageal pulmonary lymph nodes.

jux·ta·po·si·tion (jŭks′tă-pŏ-zish′ŭn) A position side by side. SEE ALSO apposition, contiguity. [L. *juxta,* near to, + *positio,* a placing, fr. *pono,* pp. *positus,* to place]

K

κ Kappa (q.v.).

k **1.** Abbreviation for kelvin; lysine; kilo-. **2.** OPTICS the coefficient of scleral rigidity. **3.** In contact lens fitting, the radius of curvature of the flattest meridian of the apical cornea.

K Abbreviation for potassium.

k Abbreviation for rate constants.

Kai·ser·ling fix·a·tive (kī′zĕr-ling fiks′ă-tiv) A method of preserving histologic and pathologic specimens without altering the color, by immersing them in an aqueous solution of potassium nitrate, potassium acetate, and formalin.

kak-, kako- SEE caco-.

kal-, kali- Combining forms indicating potassium; sometimes improperly written as *kalio-*. [L. *kalium,* potassium]

ka·la a·zar (kah′lah ah-zahr′) SYN visceral leishmaniasis. [Hind. *kala,* black, + *azar,* poison]

kalaemia [Br.] SYN kalemia.

ka·le·mi·a (kă-lē′mē-ă) The presence of potassium in the blood. SYN kalaemia.

ka·li·o·pe·ni·a (kā′lē-ō-pē′nē-ă) Insufficiency of potassium in the body. [Mod. L. *kalium,* potassium, + G. *penia,* poverty]

ka·li·o·pe·nic (kā′lē-ō-pē′nik) Relating to kaliopenia.

ka·li·um (k) (kā′lē-ŭm) SYN potassium. [Mod. L. fr. Ar. *qali,* potash]

ka·li·u·re·sis (kā′le-yūr-ē′sis) SYN kaluresis.

ka·li·u·ret·ic (kā′lē-yūr-et′ik) SYN kaluretic.

kal·lak (kal′ak) A pustular dermatitis observed among the Inuit. [Innu, skin disease]

kal·li·kre·in (kal′i-krē′in) A group of enzymes (e.g., plasma, tissue, pancreatic, urinary, submandibular kallikrein) that can convert kininogen by proteolysis to bradykinin or kallidin; trypsin and plasmin can also effect the conversion; plasma kallikrein activates the Hageman factor and acts on kininogen. Tissue kallikrein is a serine endopeptidase that can generate kallidin from kininogen. SYN kininogenase, kininogenin.

kal·u·re·sis (kal′yūr-ē′sis) Increased urinary excretion of potassium. SYN kaliuresis. [Mod. L. *kalium,* potassium, + G. *ourēsis,* urination]

kal·u·ret·ic (kal′yūr-et′ik) Relating to, causing, or characterized by kaluresis. SYN kaliuretic.

Ka·na·ga·wa phe·nom·e·non (kah-nah-gow′ă fĕ-nom′ĕ-non) Production of beta-hemolysis on a special high-salt mannitol medium (Wagatsuma agar) by most strains of *Vibrio parahaemolyticus,* which produces a heat-stable hemolysin. [Kanagawa, Japanese prefecture where first discovered]

Kan·ner syn·drome (ka′nĕr sin′drōm) SYN infantile autism.

ka·od·ze·ra (kah′od-zer′ā) A disease prevalent in Zimbabwe, similar to sleeping sickness, caused by *Trypanosoma rhodesiense.* SEE ALSO Rhodesian trypanosomiasis.

ka·o·lin clot·ting time (KCT) (kā′ō-lin klot′ ing tīm) A sensitive test of platelet-poor plasma for detecting lupus anticoagulants in mixtures of plasmas taken from patients and from control groups; kaolin initiates clotting through the contact factors and subsequently involves the other factors in the intrinsic pathway of coagulation.

ka·o·lin·o·sis (kā′ō-lin-ō′sis) Pneumonoconiosis caused by the inhalation of clay dust.

Kap·lan-Mei·er a·nal·y·sis (kap′lăn-mī′ĕr ă-nal′i-sis) A method of calculating survival of a patient population in which the increments are the actual survival times of the patients.

Kap·lan-Mei·er es·ti·mate (kap′lăn-mī′ĕr es′ ti-măt) Nonparametric method of compiling life tables or survival tables that combines calculated probabilities of survival with estimates to allow for censored (missing) observations; used mainly in survival studies of cancer and similar long-term diseases.

Kap·o·si sar·co·ma (kap′ŏ-zē sahr-kō′mă) A multifocal malignant neoplasm of primitive vasoformative tissue, occurring in the skin and sometimes in lymph nodes or viscera, consisting of spindle cells and irregular small vascular spaces frequently infiltrated by hemosiderin-pigmented macrophages and extravasated red blood cells; clinically manifested by cutaneous lesions consisting of reddish-purple to dark-blue macules, plaques, or nodules; seen most commonly in men older than 60 years of age and, in AIDS patients, as an opportunistic disease associated with human herpes virus 8 infection. See this page, B14.

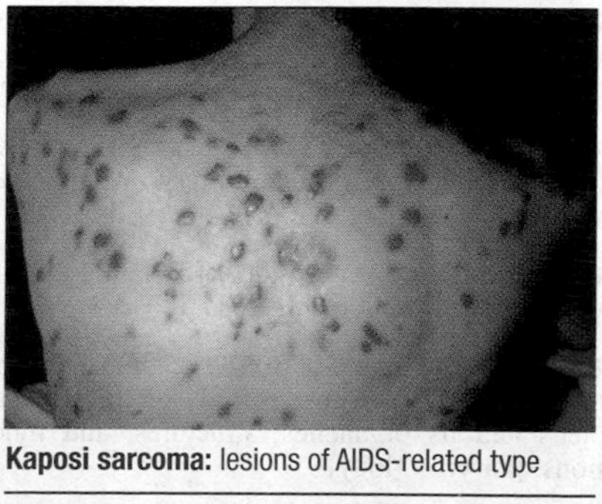

Kaposi sarcoma: lesions of AIDS-related type

Kap·o·si var·i·cel·li·form e·rup·tion (kap′ ŏ-zē var′i-sel′i-fōrm ĕr-up′shŭn) A rare complication of either herpes simplex or vaccinia superimposed on atopic dermatitis, with generalized vesicles and vesicopapules and high fever.

kap•pa (κ) (kap′ă) **1.** The 10th letter in the Greek alphabet. **2.** CHEMISTRY denotes the position of a substituent located on the 10th atom from the carboxyl or other functional group. **3.** A measure of the degree of nonrandom agreement between observers or measurements of the same categoric variable.

kap•pa an•gle (kap′ă ang′gĕl) The angle between the pupillary axis and the visual axis; it is positive when the pupillary axis is nasal to the visual axis, and negative when the pupillary axis is temporal to the visual axis.

Kar•nof•sky scale (kahr-nof′skē skāl) A performance scale for rating a person's usual activities; used to evaluate a patient's progress after a therapeutic procedure.

Kar•tag•e•ner syn•drome (kahr-tăg′ĕ-nĕr sin′drōm) Complete situs inversus associated with bronchiectasis and chronic sinusitis associated with ciliary dysmotility and impaired ciliary mucus transport in the respiratory epithelium; autosomal recessive inheritance with variable penetrance. The mechanism of the reversal of laterality remains an enigma, but it appears to be strictly an abolition (indifference) of laterality rather than a true reversal.

Kar•von•en meth•od (kahr-vahn′ĕn meth′ŏd) Method of determining the training heart rate by adding to the resting heart rate a given percentage (60–85%) of the heart rate reserve (the difference between resting heart rate and maximal heart rate).

♻**karyo-** Combining form meaning nucleus. Cf. nucleo-. [G. *karyon,* nucleus]

kar•y•o•cyte (kar′ē-ō-sīt) A young, immature normoblast. SYN rubricyte. [karyo- + G. *kytos,* cell]

kar•y•o•gam•ic (kar′ē-ō-gam′ik) Relating to or marked by karyogamy.

kar•y•og•a•my (kar′ē-og′ă-mē) Fusion of the nuclei of two cells, as occurs in fertilization or true conjugation. [karyo- + G. *gamos,* marriage]

kar•y•o•gen•e•sis (kar′ē-ō-jen′ĕ-sis) Formation of the nucleus of a cell. [karyo- + G. *genesis,* production]

kar•y•o•gen•ic (kar′ē-ō-jen′ik) Relating to karyogenesis; forming the nucleus.

kar•y•ol•o•gy (kar′ē-ol′ŏ-jē) The branch of cytology that deals with the study of the cell nucleus and its organelles, structures, and functions. [karyo + -logy]

kar•y•ol•y•sis (kar′ē-ol′i-sis) Destruction of the nucleus of a cell by swelling, with the loss of affinity of its chromatin for basic dyes. [karyo- + G. *lysis,* dissolution]

kar•y•o•lyt•ic (kar′ē-ō-lit′ik) Relating to karyolysis.

kar•y•o•mor•phism (kar′ē-ō-mōr′fizm) **1.** Development of the nucleus of a cell. **2.** Denoting the nuclear shapes of cells, especially leukocytes. [karyo- + G. *morphē,* form]

kar•y•on (kar′ē-on) SYN nucleus (1). [G. *karyon,* a nut, kernel]

kar•y•o•phage (kar′ē-ō-fāj) An intracellular parasite that feeds on the host nucleus. [karyo- + G. *phagō,* to devour]

kar•y•o•plast (kar′ē-ō-plast) A cell nucleus surrounded by a narrow band of cytoplasm and a plasma membrane. [karyo- + G. *plastos,* formed]

kar•y•o•pyk•no•sis (kar′ē-ō-pik-nō′sis) Cytologic characteristics of the superficial or cornified cells of stratified squamous epithelium in which there is shrinkage of the nuclei and condensation of the chromatin into structureless masses. [karyo- + G. *pyknos,* thick, crowded, + *-osis,* condition]

kar•y•or•rhex•is (kar′ē-ō-rek′sis) Fragmentation of the nucleus whereby its chromatin is distributed irregularly throughout the cytoplasm; a stage of necrosis usually followed by karyolysis. [karyo- + G. *rhexis,* rupture]

kar•y•o•some (kar′ē-ō-sōm) A mass of chromatin often found in the interphase cell nucleus representing a more condensed zone of chromatin filaments. [karyo- + G. *sōma,* body]

kar•y•o•type (kar′ē-ō-tīp) The chromosome characteristics of an individual cell or of a cell line, usually presented as a systematized array of metaphase chromosomes from a photomicrograph of a single cell nucleus arranged in pairs in descending order of size and according to the position of the centromere. SYN idiogram (1). [karyo- + G. *typos,* model]

Kas•a•bach-Mer•ritt syn•drome (kahs′ă-bok-mer′it sin′drōm) Large, bluish, progressive vascular malformations in extremities. Stagnation of blood in lesions can cause disseminated intravascular coagulation, platelet consumption, and bleeding. Condition usually affects infants; sudden growth of lesion causes depletion of platelets. Mortality rate is around 30%.

Ka•sai op•er•a•tion (kă-sī′ op-ĕr-ā′shŭn) SYN portoenterostomy.

Ka•so•ker•o vi•rus (kah′sō-ker′ō vī′rŭs) A virus of the family Bunyaviridae causing a febrile disease in humans characterized by headache, abdominal pain, diarrhea, severe myalgia, and arthralgia. [after the Kasokero Cave in Uganda where the virus was first isolated from bats]

Kas•ten fluo•res•cent Feul•gen stain (kahs′ten flōr-es′ĕnt foyl′gen stān) A fluorescent modification of the Feulgen stain, using any one of a variety of fluorescent basic dyes to which SO_2 is added; the brilliant fluorescence makes this method unusually sensitive and adaptable to cytofluorometric quantification of DNA.

Kas·ten fluo·res·cent per·i·od·ic a·cid–Schiff stain (kahs′ten flōr-es′ĕnt pĕr′ē-od′ik as′id shif stān) A fluorescent modification of the periodic acid–Schiff stain for polysaccharides, which uses a Kasten fluorescent Schiff reagent.

Kas·ten fluo·res·cent Schiff re·a·gents (kahs′ten flōr-es′ĕnt shif re-ā′jĕnts) Fluorescent analogues of Schiff reagent that are fluorescent basic dyes lacking acidic side groups and containing one or more primary amine groups; used in cytochemical detection of DNA in Kasten fluorescent Feulgen stain, polysaccharides in Kasten fluorescent PAS stain, and proteins in the ninhydrin-Schiff stain; such analogs include acriflavine, auramine O, and flavophosphine N.

Kast syn·drome (kăst sin′drōm) SYN Maffucci syndrome.

kat Abbreviation for katal.

kata- Alternative spelling for prefix cata-, meaning down. [G. *kata,* down]

kat·al (kat) (kat′ăl) Unit of catalytic activity equal to one mole of product formed (or substrate consumed) per second, as of the amount of enzyme that catalyzes transformation of one mole of substrate per second.

ka·thex·is (kath-eks′is) A rare disorder characterized by bone marrow retention of myeloid elements leading to severe peripheral neutropenia; neutrophils have a distinctly abnormal appearance; GM-CSF levels are undetectable and administration of this substance is therapeutically effective. SYN myelokathexis.

Katz in·dex (kats in′deks) Assessment of activities of daily living; correlates with recovery from hip fracture, placement in an assisted-living facility, and mortality rates.

ka·va, ka·va-ka·va (kah′vă, kah′vă-kah′vă) Agent derived from *Piper methysticum;* purported antiseizure properties; used to treat anxiety disorders, as a sleep aid, and for its suggested value in therapy for muscle spasms and sexually transmitted diseases. Adverse effects reported include hepatitis, cirrhosis, and parkinsonian syndrome. Some studies of this potentially dangerous product suggest that it may have clinical value as an anticarcinogenic. Reports have also been made of skin discoloration with long-term use. [Tongan, bitter]

Ka·wa·sa·ki dis·ease, Ka·wa·sa·ki syn·drome (kah-wă-sah′kē di-zēz′, sin′drōm) A systemic vasculitis of unknown origin that occurs primarily in children younger than 8 years of age. Symptoms include a fever lasting more than 5 days; polymorphic rash; erythematous, dry, cracking lips; conjunctival injection; swelling of the hands and feet; irritability; adenopathy; and a perineal desquamative rash. Approximately 20% of untreated patients may develop coronary artery aneurysms. Treatment includes oral aspirin at high dosage, immune globulin administered intravenously, and supportive care. As the child recovers from the illness, thrombocytosis and peeling of the fingertips occur. SYN mucocutaneous lymph node syndrome.

Kay·ser-Flei·scher ring (kā′sĕr flī′shĕr ring) A greenish yellow pigmented ring encircling the cornea just within the corneoscleral margin, seen in hepatolenticular degeneration, due to copper deposited in Descemet membrane.

Ka·zan·ji·an op·er·a·tion (kah-zan′jē-ăn op-ĕr-ā′shŭn) Surgical extension of the vestibular sulcus of edentulous ridges to increase their height and to improve denture retention.

kc Abbreviation for kilocycle.

kcal Abbreviation for kilogram calorie; kilocalorie.

K cells (selz) SYN killer cells.

KCT Abbreviation for kaolin clotting time.

Kearns-Sayre syn·drome (kernz sār sin′drōm) A form of chronic progressive external ophthalmoplegia with associated cardiac conduction defects, short stature, and hearing loss; a sporadically occurring mitochondrial myopathy presenting in childhood.

Keat·ing-Hart meth·od (kēt′ing-hahrt meth′ŏd) Fulguration in the treatment of external cancer or of the field of operation after the removal of a malignant growth.

Keen op·er·a·tion (kēn op-ĕr-a′shŭn) Removal of sections of the posterior branches of the spinal nerves to the affected muscles, and of the spinal accessory nerve, as a cure for torticollis.

Keg·el ex·er·cis·es (keg′ĕl eks′ĕr-sīz-ĕz) Alternate contraction and relaxation of perineal muscles for treatment of urinary stress incontinence.

Kehr sign (kār sīn) Pain referred to the left shoulder, due to splenic rupture.

Kel·ly op·er·a·tion (kel′ē op-ĕr-ā′shŭn) **1.** Correction of retroversion of the uterus by plication of uterosacral ligaments. **2.** Correction of urinary stress incontinence by vaginally placing sutures beneath the bladder neck.

Kel·ly rec·tal spec·u·lum (kel′ē rek′tăl spek′yŭ-lŭm) A tubular speculum with obturator for rectal examination.

ke·loid (kē′loyd) A nodular, firm, often linear mass of hyperplastic thickish scar tissue, consisting of irregularly distributed bands of collagen; occurs in the dermis, usually after trauma, surgery, a burn, or severe cutaneous disease. See page B11. [G. *kēlē*, a tumor (or *kēlis*, a spot), + *eidos*, appearance]

ke·loid ac·ne (kē′loyd ak′nē) A form of dermatologic disease most common in African Americans involving inflammation and pyogenesis about follicular structures, particularly on the back of the neck.

ke·loi·do·sis (kē′loy-dō′sis) Multiple keloids.

ke·lo·plas·ty (kē′lō-plas-tē) Surgical removal of a scar or keloid. [keloid + G. *plastos*, formed]

kel·vin (K) (kel′vin) A unit of thermodynamic temperature equal to 1/273.16 of the thermodynamic temperature of the triple point of water. SEE ALSO Kelvin scale. [Lord *Kelvin*]

Kel·vin scale (kel′vin skāl) Temperature scale in which the triple point of water is assigned the value of 273.16 K; °C = K − 273.15. SYN absolute scale.

Kemp ech·o (kemp ek′ō) Phenomenon noted by David Kemp in 1978, i.e., that otoacoustic emissions are generated in the normal cochlea either spontaneously or in response to acoustic stimulation. SEE ALSO otoacoustic emission.

Ken·dall (ken′dăl) SEE Abell-Kendall method.

Ken·ne·dy dis·ease (ken′ĕ-dē di-zēz′) An X-linked recessive disorder characterized by progressive spinal and bulbar muscular atrophy; associated features include distal degeneration of sensory axons, and signs of endocrine dysfunction, including diabetes mellitus, gynecomastia, and testicular atrophy. SYN X-linked recessive bulbospinal neuronopathy.

Ken·ne·dy syn·drome (ken′ĕ-dē sin′drōm) Ipsilateral optic atrophy with central scotoma and contralateral choked disc or papilledema, caused by a meningioma of the ipsilateral optic nerve. SYN Foster Kennedy syndrome.

Ken·ny-Caf·fey syn·drome (ken′ē-kaf′ē sin′drōm) A disorder characterized by intermittent hypocalcemia (associated with abnormalities in parathyroid hormone secretion) and bone and eye abnormalities; autosomal dominant and autosomal recessive forms exist.

Kent bun·dle (kent bŭn′dĕl) **1.** SYN atrioventricular bundle. **2.** A muscle fiber bundle occurring occasionally as an accessory conducting pathway between the atria and the ventricles, associated with Wolff-Parkinson-White syndrome.

Ker·an·del sign (ker′an-del′ sīn) Delayed sensation to pain indicative of African trypanosomiasis.

ker·a·tan sul·fate (ker′ă-tan sŭl′fāt) A type of sulfated mucopolysaccharide found in cartilage, bone, connective tissue, the cornea, aorta, and in the intervertebral discs; accumulates in Morquio syndrome. SYN keratosulfate.

ker·a·tec·to·my (ker′ă-tek′tŏ-mē) An operation to remove corneal tissue. [kerato- + G. *ektomē*, excision]

ke·rat·ic (ker-at′ik) SYN horny. [G. *keras* (*kerat-*), horn]

ke·rat·ic pre·cip·i·tates (ker-at′ik prĕ-sip′i-tāts) Inflammatory cells on the corneal endothelium.

ker·a·tin (ker′ă-tin) A scleroprotein or albuminoid present in hair and nails; it contains a relatively large amount of sulfur, is insoluble in gastric juice, and is sometimes used for coating tablets that are intended to be dissolved only in the intestine. SYN cytokeratin. [G. *keras (kerat-)*, horn, + -in]

ker·a·tin·as·es (ker′ă-tin-ās-ĕz) Hydrolases catalyzing the hydrolysis of keratin.

ker·a·tin·i·za·tion (ker′ă-tin-ī-zā′shŭn) Keratin formation or development of a horny layer; may also apply to premature formation of keratin. SYN cornification.

ke·rat·i·no·cyte (ke-rat′i-nō-sīt) A cell of the living epidermis and certain oral epithelium that produces keratin in the process of differentiating into the dead and fully keratinized cells of the stratum corneum.

ke·rat·i·no·some (ke-rat′i-nō-sōm) A granule located in the upper layers of the stratum spinosum of certain stratified squamous epithelia. SYN membrane-coating granule.

ke·rat·i·nous (ke-rat′i-nŭs) **1.** Relating to keratin. **2.** SYN horny.

ke·rat·i·nous cyst (ke-rat′i-nŭs sist) An epithelial cyst containing keratin.

ker·a·tin pearl (ker′ă-tin pĕrl) A focus of central keratinization within concentric layers of abnormal squamous cells; seen in squamous cell carcinoma. SYN epithelial pearl.

ker·a·ti·tis (ker′ă-tī′tis) Inflammation of the cornea. SEE ALSO keratopathy. [kerato- + G. *-itis*, inflammation]

♻ **kerato-, kerat-** Combining forms indicating the cornea; horny tissue or cells. SEE ALSO cerat-, cerato-. [G. *keras*, horn]

🅘 **ker·a·to·ac·an·tho·ma** (ker′ă-tō-ak′an-thō′mă) A rapidly growing, umbilicated tumor, usually occurring on exposed areas of the skin, which invades the dermis but remains localized and usually resolves spontaneously. See page B14. [kerato- + G. *akantha*, thorn, + *-oma*, tumor]

ker·a·to·cele (ker′ă-tō-sēl) Hernia of the Descemet membrane through a defect in the outer layers of the cornea. [kerato- + G. *kēlē*, hernia]

ker·a·to·con·junc·ti·vi·tis (ker′ă-tō-kŏn-jŭngk′ti-vī′tis) Inflammation of the conjunctiva and of the cornea.

ker•a•to•con•junc•ti•vi•tis sic•ca (ker′ă-tō-kŏn-jŭngk′ti-vī′tis sik′ă) A chronic mucopurulent conjunctivitis, sometimes leading to corneal ulceration and scarring, due to deficit of the aqueous component of tears. SYN dry eye syndrome.

ker•a•to•co•nus (ker′ă-tō-kō′nŭs) A conic protrusion of the cornea caused by thinning of the stroma; usually bilateral. SEE ALSO Fleischer ring, Munson sign. SYN conic cornea. [kerato- + G. *kōnos,* cone]

ker•a•to•cyst (ker′ă-tō-sist) Odontogenic cyst derived from remnants of the dental lamina and appearing as a unilocular or multilocular radiolucency that may produce jaw expansion; associated with the bifid rib basal cell nevus syndrome.

ker•a•to•cyte (ker′ă-tō-sīt) **1.** The fibroblastic stromal cell of the cornea. **2.** A variety of poikilocyte that owes its abnormal shape to fragmentation occurring as the cell flows through damaged small vessels. SYN schistocyte. See this page.

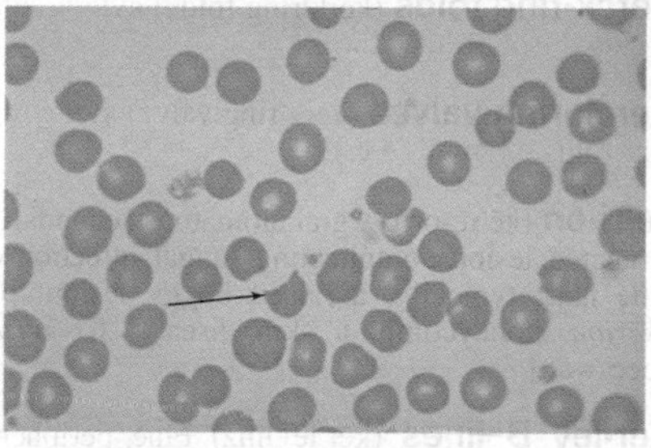

keratocyte

ker•a•to•der•ma (ker′ă-tō-dĕr′mă) **1.** Any horny superficial growth. **2.** A generalized thickening of the horny layer of the epidermis. [kerato- + G. *derma,* skin]

ker•a•to•der•ma blen•nor•rhag•i•cum (ker′ă-tō-dĕr′mă blen′ō-raj′i-kŭm) Scattered, thickened, hyperkeratotic skin lesions (e.g., pustules, crusts) seen in Reiter syndrome.

ker•a•to•der•ma plan•ta•re sul•ca•tum (ker′ă-tō-dĕr′mă plan-tā′rē sŭl-kā′tŭm) Hyperkeratosis and fissure formation on the soles. SYN cracked heel.

ker•a•to•der•ma•ti•tis (ker′ă-tō-dĕr′mă-tī′tis) Inflammation with proliferation of the horny layer of the skin.

ker•a•to•ec•ta•si•a (ker′ă-tō-ek-tā′zē-ă) A bulging forward of the cornea.

ker•a•to•ep•i•the•li•o•plas•ty (ker′ă-tō-ep-i-thē′lē-ō-plas-tē) A surgical procedure for the repair of persistent corneal epithelial defects. Corneal epithelium is removed and small pieces of donor cornea, with epithelium attached, are placed at the corneoscleral limbus. [kerato- + epithelio- + G. *plastos,* formed]

ker•a•tog•e•nous (ker′ă-toj′ĕ-nŭs) Causing a growth of cells that produce keratin and result in the formation of horny tissue (e.g., fingernails, scales, and feathers).

ker•a•tog•e•nous mem•brane (ker-ă-toj′ĕ-nŭs mem′brān) **1.** SYN nail matrix. **2.** SYN nail bed.

ker•a•to•hy•a•lin, ker•a•to•hy•a•lin gran•ules (ker′ă-tō-hī′ă-lin, ker′ă-tō-hī′ă-lin gran′yūlz) The substance in the large basophilic granules of the stratum granulosum of the epidermis. [kerato- + hyalin]

ker•a•toid (ker′ă-toyd) **1.** SYN horny. **2.** Resembling corneal tissue. [kerato- + G. *eidos,* resemblance]

ker•a•toid ex•an•the•ma (ker′ă-toyd ek-san-thē′mă) A symptom occurring in the secondary stage of yaws: patches of fine, light colored, furfuraceous desquamation, scattered irregularly over limbs and trunk.

ker•a•to•lep•tyn•sis (ker′ă-tō-lep-tin′sis) **1.** SYN gutter dystrophy of cornea. **2.** An operation for removing the surface of the cornea and replacement by bulbar conjunctiva for cosmetic reasons. [kerato- + G. *leptynsis,* a making thin]

ker•a•to•leu•ko•ma (ker′ă-tō-lū-kō′mă) A white corneal opacity. [kerato- + G. *leukos,* white, + *-ōma,* growth]

ker•a•tol•y•sis (ker′ă-tol′i-sis) **1.** Separation or loosening of the horny layer of the epidermis. **2.** A disease characterized by a shedding of the epidermis recurring at more or less regular intervals. [kerato- + G. *lysis,* loosening]

ker•a•to•lyt•ic (ker′ă-tō-lit′ik) Relating to keratolysis.

ker•a•to•ma (ker′ă-tō′mă) **1.** SYN callosity. **2.** A horny tumor. [kerato- + G. *-oma,* tumor]

ker•a•to•ma•la•ci•a (ker′ă-tō-mă-lā′shē-ă) Dryness with ulceration and perforation of the cornea occurring in cachectic children; results from severe vitamin A deficiency. [kerato- + G. *malakia,* softness]

ker•a•tome (ker′ă-tōm) A knife used for incising the cornea. SYN keratotome.

ker•a•tom•e•ter (ker′ă-tom′ĕ-tĕr) An instrument for measuring the curvature of the anterior corneal surface. SYN ophthalmometer. [kerato- + G. *metron,* measure]

ker•a•tom•e•try (ker′ă-tom′ĕ-trē) Measurement of the radii of anterior corneal curvature.

ker•a•to•mi•leu•sis (ker′ă-tō-mī-lū′sis) Surgical alteration of refractive error by changing the shape of a deep layer of the cornea. [fr. G. *keras* (*kerat-*), horn, cornea, + *smileusis,* carving]

ker•a•to•path•i•a (ker′ă-tō-path′ē-ă) SYN keratopathy.

ker•a•to•path•i•a gut•ta•ta (ker′ă-tō-path′ē-ă gut′ă-tă) Wartlike endothelial excrescence on the posterior surface of the cornea.

ker•a•top•a•thy (ker′ă-top′ă-thē) Any corneal disease, damage, dysfunction, or abnormality. SYN keratopathia. [kerato- + G. *pathos,* suffering, disease]

ker•a•to•pha•ki•a (ker′ă-tō-fā′kē-ă) Implantation of a donor cornea or plastic lens within the corneal stroma to modify refractive error. [kerato- + G. *phakos,* lens]

ker•a•to•plas•ty (ker′ă-tō-plas-tē) Removal of a portion of the cornea and the insertion in its place of a piece of cornea of the same size and shape removed from elsewhere. SYN corneal graft. [kerato- + G. *plassō,* to form]

ker•a•to•pros•the•sis (ker′ă-tō-pros-thē′sis) Replacement of the central area of an opacified cornea by an artificial lens. [kerato- + G. *prosthesis,* addition]

ker•a•to•rhex•is, ker•a•tor•rhex•is (ker′ă-tō-rek′sis, kĕr′ă-tō-rek′sis) Rupture of the cornea, due to trauma or perforating ulcer. [kerato- + G. *rhēxis,* a bursting]

ker•a•to•scle•ri•tis (ker′ă-tō-skler-ī′tis) Inflammation of both cornea and sclera.

ker•a•to•scope (ker′ă-tō-skōp) An instrument marked with lines or circles by means of which the corneal reflex can be observed. SYN Placido da Costa disc. [kerato- + G. *skopeō,* to examine]

ker•a•tos•co•py (ker′ă-tos′kŏ-pē) **1.** Examination of the reflections from the anterior surface of the cornea to determine the character and amount of corneal astigmatism. **2.** A term first applied by Cuignet to his method of retinoscopy. [kerato- + G. *skopeō,* to examine]

ker•a•tose (ker′ă-tōs) Keratotic, relating to or marked by keratosis.

ker•a•to•sis, pl. **ker•a•to•ses** (ker′ă-tō′sis, -sēz) Any lesion on the epidermis marked by the presence of circumscribed overgrowths of the horny layer. See page B14. [kerato- + G. *-osis,* condition]

ker•a•to•sis fol•lic•u•la•ris (ker′ă-tō′sis fol-ik-yū-lār′is) A familial eruption, beginning usually in childhood, in which keratotic papules originating from both follicles and interfollicular epidermis of the trunk, face, scalp, and axillae become crusted and verrucous; often intensely pruritic. See this page. SYN Darier disease, Hailey and Hailey disease.

ker•a•to•sul•fate (ker′ă-tō-sŭl′fāt) SYN keratan sulfate. SYN keratosulphate.

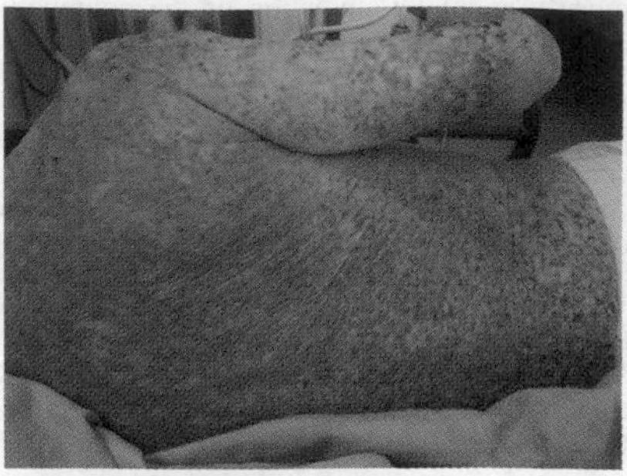

keratosis follicularis

keratosulphate [Br.] SYN keratosulfate.

ker•a•to•tome (ker-ăt′ō-tōm) SYN keratome.

ker•a•tot•o•my (ker′ă-tot′ŏ-mē) **1.** Any incision through the cornea. **2.** An operation making a partial thickness incision into the cornea to flatten it and reduce its refractive power in that meridian. [kerato- + G. *tomē,* incision]

Kerck•ring folds (kerk′ring fōldz) SYN circular folds of small intestine.

Kerck•ring valves (kerk′ring valvz) SYN circular folds of small intestine.

ke•ri•on (kē′rē-on) A granulomatous secondarily infected lesion complicating fungal infection of the hair; typically, a raised boggy lesion. [G. *kērion,* honeycomb; a skin disease, fr. *kēros,* beeswax]

Ker•ley B lines (kĕr′lē līnz) Fine peripheral septal lines.

KERMA (kĕr′mă) Acronym for kinetic energy released in a material.

ker•nic•ter•us (kĕr-nik′tĕr-ŭs) Yellow staining and degenerative lesions in basal ganglia associated with high levels of unconjugated bilirubin in infants; may occur with hemolytic disorder such as Rh or ABO erythroblastosis or G6PD deficiency as well as with neonatal sepsis or Crigler-Najjar syndrome; characterized by opisthotonos, high-pitched cry, lethargy, and poor sucking, as well as abnormal or absent Moro reflex, and loss of upward gaze; later consequences include deafness, cerebral palsy, other sensorineural deficits, and mental retardation. SYN bilirubin encephalopathy, nuclear jaundice. [Ger. *Kern,* kernel (nucleus), + *Ikterus,* jaundice]

Ker•nig sign (ker′nig sīn) When a subject is supine and the thigh is flexed to a right angle with the axis of the trunk, complete extension of the leg on the thigh is impossible; present in various forms of meningitis.

Ker•no•han notch (kĕr′nĕ-han noch) A notch in the cerebral peduncle caused by displacement of the brainstem against the incisura of the tentorium by a transtentorial herniation.

ker•oid (ker′oyd) SYN horny. [G. *keroeidēs,* hornlike]

Ke•shan dis•ease (kē′shăn di-zēz′) Cardiomyopathy due to the deficiency of selenium found in women and children in Keshan, China.

Kes•ten•baum num•ber (kes′ten-bowm nŭm′bĕr) The difference between the two pupil diameters when each eye is measured in bright light with the other eye tightly covered; an indicator of the relative afferent pupillary defect in patients with two normally innervated irises.

Kes•ten•baum pro•ce•dure (kes′ten-bowm prō-sē′jŭr) Surgical procedure on the extraocular muscles indicated for patients with torticollis associated with nystagmus.

Kes•ten•baum sign (kes′ten-bowm sīn) A decrease in the number of arterioles crossing optic disc margins as a sign of optic neuritis.

ke•tal (kē′tăl) A hydrated ketone in which both hydroxyl groups are esterified with alcohols.

♻**keto-** Combining form denoting a compound containing a ketone group; replaced by oxo- in systematic nomenclature. [Ger.]

ke•to ac•id (kē′tō as′id) An acid containing a ketone group (–CO–) in addition to the acid group(s).

ke•to•ac•i•do•sis (kē′tō-as-i-dō′sis) Acidosis, as in diabetes or starvation, caused by the enhanced production of ketone bodies.

ke•to•ac•i•du•ri•a (kē′tō-as-i-dyūr′ē-ă) Excretion of urine having an elevated content of ketonic acids.

ke•to•gen•e•sis (kē′tō-jen′ĕ-sis) Metabolic production of ketones or ketone bodies.

ke•to•gen•ic (kē′tō-jen′ik) Giving rise to ketone bodies in metabolism.

ke•to•gen•ic di•et (kē′tō-jen′ik dī′ĕt) A high-fat, low-carbohydrate, and normal protein diet causing ketosis.

ke•to•hep•tose (kē′tō-hep′tōs) A seven-carbon sugar possessing a ketone group.

ke•to•hex•ose (kē′tō-heks′ōs) A six-carbon sugar possessing a ketone group, e.g., fructose. SYN hexulose.

ke•tol (kē′tol) A ketone that has an OH group near the CO group.

ke•tole (kē′tōl) SYN indole (1).

ke•tole group (kē′tōl grūp) Carbons 1 and 2 of a 2-ketose ($HOCH_2CO$–).

ke•to•lyt•ic (kē′tō-lit′ik) Causing the dissolution of ketone or acetone substances, referring usually to oxidation products of glucose and allied substances.

ketonaemia [Br.] SYN ketonemia.

ke•tone (kē′tōn) A substance with the carbonyl group linking two carbon atoms; the most important in medicine and the simplest in chemistry is dimethyl ketone (acetone).

ke•tone bo•dy (kē′tōn bod′ē) One of a group of ketones that includes acetoacetic acid, β-hydroxybutyric acid, and acetone; high levels are found in tissues and body fluids in ketosis. SYN acetone body.

ke•to•ne•mi•a (kē′tō-nē′mē-ă) The presence of recognizable concentrations of ketone bodies in the plasma. SYN ketonaemia. [ketone + G. *haima,* blood]

ke•ton•u•ri•a (kē′tō-nyūr′ē-ă) Enhanced urinary excretion of ketone bodies.

ke•tose (kē′tōs) A carbohydrate containing the characteristic carbonyl group of the ketones.

ke•to•sis (kē-tō′sis) Enhanced production of ketone bodies, as in diabetes mellitus or starvation. [ketone + *-osis,* condition]

17-ke•to•ste•roids (kē′tō-ster′oydz) Any steroids with a ketone group on C-17; commonly used to designate urinary metabolites of androgenic and adrenocortical hormones that possess this structural feature. Cf. bioregulator. SYN 17-oxosteroids.

ke•to•tic (kē-tot′ik) Pertaining to ketone bodies; presence of acidosis due to excess ketone body production such as occurs in uncontrolled insulin-dependent diabetes.

key-in-lock ma•neu•ver (kē′-in-lok′ mă-nū′vĕr) A method by which obstetric forceps are used to rotate the fetal head.

kg Abbreviation for kilogram.

ki (kī) SYN chi.

kid•ney (kid′nē) One of the two organs that excrete urine. The kidneys are bean-shaped organs (about 11 cm long, 5 cm wide, and 3 cm thick) lying on either side of the vertebral column, posterior to the peritoneum, opposite the 12th thoracic and first three lumbar vertebrae. See page 852. SYN ren [TA]. [A.S. *cwith,* womb, belly, + *neere,* kidney (L. *ren*, G. *nephros*)]

kid•ney fail•ure (kid′nē fāl′yŭr) SYN renal failure.

kid•ney ma•chine (kid′nē mă-shēn′) Colloquialism for dialyzer.

kid•ney stone (kid′nē stōn) SYN renal calculus.

Kiel clas•si•fi•ca•tion (kēl klas′i-fi-kā′shŭn) Classification of non-Hodgkin lymphoma into low-grade malignancy (lymphocytic, lymphoplasmacytoid, centrocytic, and cen-

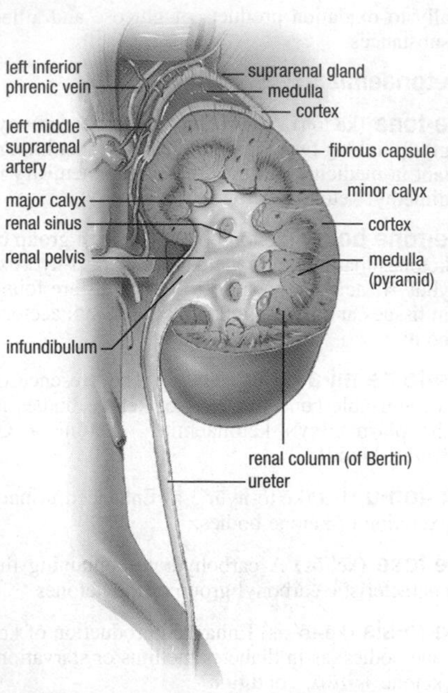

left kidney and adrenal gland: cross-section

troblastic-centrocytic types) and high-grade malignancy (centroblastic, lymphoblastic of Burkitt or convoluted cell, and immunoblastic types).

Kien•böck dis•ease (kēn′bek di-zēz′) Osteonecrosis of the lunate bone resulting from unknown etiolgy, although can occur after trauma.

Kien•böck dis•lo•ca•tion (kēn′bek dis′lō-kā′shŭn) Dislocation of the lunate bone.

Kier•nan space (kēr′năn spās) Interlobular space in the liver.

Kies•sel•bach ar•e•a (kē′sĕl-bahk ār′ē-ă) An area on the anterior portion of the nasal septum rich in capillaries (Kiesselbach plexus) and often the seat of epistaxis. SYN Little area.

Ki•ku•chi dis•ease (kē-kū′chē di-zēz′) Necrotizing lymphadenitis of unknown etiology, most often encountered in young women in Japan but also in other parts of the world; lymph node enlargement, associated with fever, subsides spontaneously.

kill•er cells (kil′lĕr selz) Cytotoxic cells involved in antibody-dependent, cell-mediated immune responses. SYN K cells, null cells (1), T-cytotoxic cells.

Kil•li•an bun•dle (kil′ē-ăn bŭn′dĕl) SEE inferior constrictor muscle of pharynx.

Kil•li•an op•er•a•tion (kil′ē-ăn op-ĕr-ā′shŭn) An operation for frontal sinus disease in which the entire anterior wall is removed and the mucous membrane is curetted away; the ethmoid cells are removed through an opening in the nasal process of the maxillary bone, and the upper portion of the medial wall of the orbit is removed as well.

Kil•li•an tri•an•gle (kil′ē-ăn trī′ang-gĕl) The triangular area of the cervical esophagus, bordered by the oblique fibers of the inferior constrictor muscle of the pharynx and the transverse fibers of the cricopharyngeus muscle, through which Zenker diverticulum occurs.

♻ **kilo- (k)** Prefix used in the SI and metric system to signify one thousand (10^3). [Fr. fr. G. *chilioi,* one thousand]

kil•o•cal•o•rie (kcal) (kil′ō-kal′ŏr-ē) The quantity of energy required to raise the temperature of 1 kg of water from 14.5–15.5°C; it is 1000 times the value of the small calorie. SYN kilogram calorie, large calorie.

kil•o•cy•cle (kc) (kil′ŏ-sī-kĕl) One thousand cycles per second.

kil•o•gram (kg) (kil′ŏ-gram) The SI unit of mass, 1000 g; equivalent to 15,432.358 gr, 2.2046226 lb. avoirdupois, or 2.6792289 lb. troy.

kil•o•gram cal•o•rie (kcal) (kil′ŏ-gram kal′ŏr-ē) SYN kilocalorie.

kil•o•gram-me•ter (kil′ŏ-gram-mē′tĕr) The energy exerted, or work done, when a mass of 1 kg is raised a height of 1 m; equal to 9.80665 J in the SI system. SYN kilogram-metre.

kilogram-metre [Br.] SYN kilogram-meter.

ki•lo•joule (kil′ŏ-jūl) 1000 joules.

kil•o•volt (kv) (kil′ŏ-vōlt) A unit of electrical potential, potential difference, or electromotive force, equal to 10^3 volts. [kilo + volt]

kil•o•volt peak (kVp) (kil′ŏ-vōlt pēk) The highest voltage applied across an x-ray tube; it influences the penetrating power of the x-ray beam.

Kim•mel•stiel-Wil•son syn•drome, Kim•mel•stiel-Wil•son dis•ease (kim′ĕl-stēl wil′sŏn sin′drōm, kim′ĕl-stēl wil′sŏn di-zēz′) Nephrotic syndrome and hypertension in diabetic people, associated with diabetic glomerulosclerosis.

kinaesthesia [Br.] SYN kinesthesia.

kinaesthesiometer [Br.] SYN kinesthesiometer.

kinaesthesis [Br.] SYN kinesthesis.

kinaesthetic [Br.] SYN kinesthetic.

kinaesthetic awareness [Br.] SYN kinesthetic awareness.

kinaesthetic sense [Br.] SYN kinesthetic sense.

kinanaesthesia [Br.] SYN kinanesthesia.

kin•an•es•the•si•a (kin′an-es-thē′zē-ă) A disturbance of deep sensibility in which there is inability to perceive either direction or extent of movement, the result being ataxia. SYN kinanaesthesia. [G. *kinēsis,* motion, + *an-* priv. + *aisthēsis,* sensation]

ki•nase (kī′nās) **1.** An enzyme catalyzing the conversion of a proenzyme to an active enzyme. **2.** An enzyme catalyzing the transfer of phosphate groups to form triphosphates (e.g., ATP).

kin•dred (kin′drĕd) An aggregate of genetically related people; distinguished from pedigree, which is a stylized representation of a kindred. [O.E. *kynrēde*, fr. *cyn*, kin, + *rēde*, condition]

kin•e•mat•ic chain (kin′ĕ-mat′ik chān) A combination of several joints linking several limb segments together during a specific movement or posture.

kin•e•mat•ics (kin′ĕ-mat′iks) PHYSIOLOGY the science concerned with movements of the parts of the body. [G. *kinēmatica,* things that move]

kin•e•mat•ic vis•cos•i•ty (ν, υ) (kin′ĕ-mat′ik vis-kos′i-tē) A measure used in studies of fluid flow; the dynamic viscosity, mc, in poises divided by the density of the material; units: stokes.

kin•e•plas•tics (kin′ĕ-plas′tiks) SYN cineplastic amputation.

kin•e•sal•gi•a, ki•ne•si•al•gi•a (kin′ĕ-sal′jē-ă, ki-nē′sē-al′jē-ă) Pain caused by muscular movement. [G. *kinēsis,* motion, + *algos,* pain]

♻**kinesi-, kinesio-, kineso-** Combining forms indicating motion. [G. *kinēsis*]

ki•ne•si•a (ki-nē′sē-ă) SYN motion sickness. [G. *kinēsis,* movement]

ki•ne•si•at•rics (ki-nē′sē-at′riks) SYN kinesitherapy. [G. *kinēsis,* movement, + *iatrikos,* relating to medicine]

ki•ne•sics (ki-nē′siks) The study of nonverbal, bodily motion in communication.

kin•e•sim•e•ter (kin′ĕ-sim′ĕ-tĕr) An instrument for measuring the extent of a movement. SYN kinesiometer. [G. *kinēsis,* movement, + *metron,* measure]

ki•ne•si•ol•o•gy (ki-nē′sē-ol′ŏ-jē) The science or the study of movement, and the active and passive structures involved. [G. *kinēsis,* movement, + *-logos,* study]

ki•ne•si•om•e•ter (ki-nē′sē-om′ĕ-tĕr) SYN kinesimeter.

ki•ne•sis (ki-nē′sis) Motion; as a termination, used to denote movement or activation, particularly the kind induced by a stimulus. [G.]

ki•ne•si•ther•a•py (ki-nē′si-thār′ă-pē) Physical therapy involving motion and range of motion exercises. SEE movement. SYN kinesiatrics.

kin•es•the•si•a, kin•es•the•sis (kin′es-thē′zē-ă, -sis) **1.** The sense perception of movement; the muscular sense. **2.** An illusion of moving in space. SYN kinaesthesia. [G. *kinēsis,* motion, + *aisthēsis,* sensation]

kin•es•the•si•om•e•ter (kin′es-thē′sē-om′ĕ-tĕr) An instrument for determining the degree of muscular sensation. SYN kinaesthesiometer. [kinesthesia, + G. *metron,* measure]

kin•es•thet•ic (kin′es-thet′ik) Relating to kinesthesia. SYN kinaesthetic.

kin•es•thet•ic a•ware•ness (kin′es-thet′ik ă-wār′nĕs) SYN body scheme. SYN kinaesthetic awareness.

kin•es•thet•ic sense (kin′es-thet′ik sens) SYN myesthesia. SYN kinaesthetic sense.

ki•net•ic (ki-net′ik) Relating to motion or movement. [G. *kinētikos,* of motion, fr. *kinētos,* moving]

ki•net•ic chain ex•er•cise (ki-net′ik chān eks′ĕr-sīz) Exercise in which musculoskeletal and nervous systems combine to produce movement.

ki•net•ic en•er•gy (ki-net′ik en′ĕr-jē) The energy of motion.

ki•net•ics (ki-net′iks) The study of motion, acceleration, or rate of change.

♻**kineto-** Combining form indicating motion. [G. *kinētos,* moving, movable]

ki•ne•to•car•di•o•gram (ki-nē′tō-kahr′dē-ō-gram) One type of graphic recording of the vibrations of the chest wall produced by cardiac activity.

ki•ne•to•car•di•o•graph (ki-nē′tō-kahr′dē-ō-graf) A device for recording precordial impulses due to cardiac movement; the absolute displacement of a point on the chest wall is recorded relative to a fixed reference point above the recumbent patient.

ki•ne•to•chore (ki-nē′tō-kōr) The structural portion of the chromosome to which microtubules attach. Cf. centromere. [kineto- + G. *chōra,* space]

ki•ne•to•gen•ic (ki-nē′tō-jen′ik) Causing or producing motion.

ki•ne•to•plast (ki-nē′tō-plast) An intensely staining extranuclear DNA structure found in parasitic flagellates near the base of the flagellum. Electron micrographs show it to be part of a single giant mitochondrion filling most of the cytoplasm of amastigote flagellates. SEE ALSO parabasal body. [kineto- + G. *plastos,* formed]

Kin•gel•la (king-gel′ă) Member of the family Neisseriaceae; a gram-negative coccus with a requirement of enhanced carbon dioxide for recovery in culture.

Kin•gel•la in•do•log•e•nes (king-gel′ă in-dō-loj′ĕ-nēz) SYN *Suttonella indologenes.*

Kin•gel•la kin•gae (king-gel′ă king′ē) A bacterial species that causes endocarditis, especially in immunocomprised people; associated with bone and joint infections in children. SEE ALSO HACEK group.

ki•nin (kī′nin) One of a number of substances having pronounced physiologic effects. Some are polypeptides, formed in blood in various pathologic processes, which stimulate visceral smooth muscle but relax vascular smooth muscle, thus producing vasodilation. [G. *kineō*, to move, + -in]

ki•nin•o•gen (ki-nin′ō-jen) The globulin precursor of a (plasma) kinin.

ki•nin•o•ge•nase (ki-nin′ō-jĕ-nās) SYN kallikrein.

ki•nin•o•gen•in (ki-nin′ō-jen′in) SYN kallikrein.

kink (kingk) An angulation, bend, or twist.

kin•ky-hair dis•ease (kingk′ē-hār′ di-zēz′) An inborn error of copper metabolism with onset within a few weeks of birth; manifested by short, sparse, poorly pigmented kinky hair; failure to thrive; development of seizures; spasticity; and progressive mental deterioration leading to death. X-linked recessive inheritance due to a defect of copper transport, caused by mutation in the Menkes gene (MNK), which encodes a copper-transporting ATPase on Xq. SYN Menkes syndrome.

♻ **kino-** Combining form indicating movement. [G. *kineō*, to move]

ki•no•cil•i•um (kin′ō-sil′ē-ŭm) A cilium, usually motile, having nine peripheral double microtubules and two single central ones. [kino- + cilium]

kin•ship (kin′ship) The state of being genetically related.

Kirk am•pu•ta•tion (kĭrk amp′yū-tā′shŭn) Amputation at the lower end of the femur, using the tendon of the quadriceps extensor to cover the end of the bone.

Kirsch•ner wire (kĭrsh′nĕr wīr) An apparatus for skeletal traction in long bone fracture or for fracture fixation.

Kisch re•flex (kish rē′fleks) Closure of the eye in response to stimulation of the skin at the depth of the external auditory meatus.

kis•sing punc•ta (kis′sing pŭngk′tă) A condition in which the upper punctum is apposed to the lower punctum when the eyes are open.

Ki•ta•sa•to ba•cil•lus (ki-tă-sah′tō bă-sil′ŭs) SYN *Yersinia pestis.*

Kjel•land for•ceps (kyel′ĕnd fōr′seps) An obstetric forceps with a sliding lock and little pelvic curve.

Kjer op•tic at•ro•phy (kyer op′tik at′rŏ-fē) SYN dominant optic atrophy.

Kleb•si•el•la (kleb-sē-el′ă) A genus of aerobic, facultatively anaerobic, nonmotile, non-spore-forming bacteria (family Enterobacteriaceae) containing gram-negative, encapsulated rods that occur singly, in pairs, or in short chains. These organisms produce acetylmethylcarbinol and lysine decarboxylase or ornithine decarboxylase; they do not usually liquefy gelatin. Citrate and glucose are ordinarily used as sole carbon sources. These organisms may or may not be pathogenic. They occur in the respiratory, intestinal, and urogenital tracts of humans as well as in soil, water, and grain. The type species is *K. pneumoniae*. [E. *Klebs*]

Kleb•si•el•la ox•y•to•ca (kleb-sē-el′ă ok-sē-tō′kă) A bacterial species characterized by its ability to produce indole. Clinically, it resembles *K. pneumoniae;* however, nosocomial strains exhibit a greater propensity to develop antibiotic resistance.

Kleb•si•el•la pneu•mo•ni•ae (kleb-sē-el′ă nū-mō′nē-ē) A bacterial species found in soil and water, on grain, and in the intestinal tract of humans and other animals; it also occurs in association with several pathologic conditions, urinary tract infections, sputum, feces, and metritis in mares; capsular types 1, 2, and 3 of this organism may be causative agents in pneumonia; commonly associated with lobar pneumonia among hospitalized patients. SYN Friedländer bacillus.

Klei•ger test (klē′gĕr test) Maneuver used to determine stability of the deltoid ligament. The examiner stabilizes the leg just above the ankle with one hand and everts the foot with the other. Pain or instability suggests injury to the deltoid ligament.

Klei•hau•er-Bet•ke tech•nique (klī′how-ĕr-bet′kĕ tek-nēk′) Procedure used to determine the concentration of fetal cells in maternal circulation.

Klei•hau•er stain (klī′how-ĕr stān) A combination of aniline blue and Biebrich scarlet red used for detection of fetal cells in the maternal blood.

klep•to•ma•ni•a (klep′tō-mā′nē-ă) A disorder of impulse control characterized by a morbid tendency to steal. [G. *kleptō*, to steal, + *mania*, insanity]

klep•to•ma•ni•ac (klep′tō-mā′nē-ak) A person exhibiting kleptomania.

Kline•fel•ter syn•drome (klīn′fel-tĕr sin′drōm) Anomaly in males with chromosome count 47, XXY sex chromosome constitution; usually have seminiferous tubule dysgenesis, elevated urinary gonadotropins, gynecomastia, and eunuchoid habitus. SYN XXY syndrome.

Klip•pel-Feil syn•drome (kli-pĕl′fīl′ sin′ drōm) A congenital abnormality of the spine characterized by a reduction in the number of cervical vertebrae and their fusion. See this page.

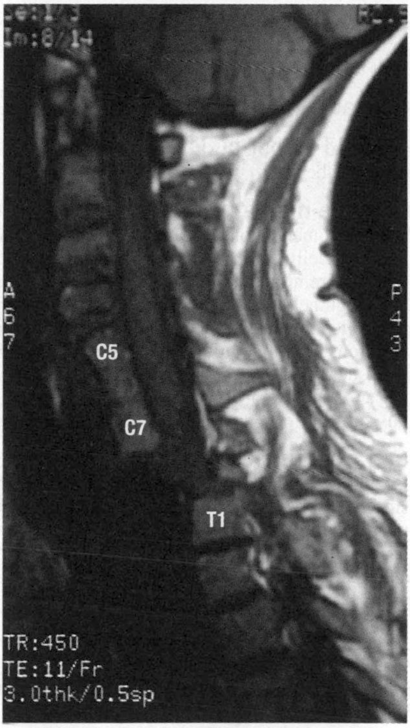

Klippel-Feil deformity: sagittal magnetic resonance imaging scan revealing the finding located at the C-5 to C-7 levels (also note the stage II distraction extension injury at the C-7, T-1 level)

Klump•ke-De•jer•ine pal•sy (klump′kĕ dā-jĕr-ēn pawl′zē) SYN Klumpke palsy.

Klump•ke pal•sy, Klump•ke pa•ral•y•sis (klump′kĕ pawl′zē, păr-al′i-sis) A type of brachial birth palsy in which there is paralysis of the muscles of the distal forearm and hand (all ulnar innervated muscles, plus more distal radial and median-innervated muscles), due to a lesion of the lower trunk of the brachial plexus, or of the C8 and T1 cervical roots. SYN Klumpke-Dejerine palsy.

kly•stron (klī′stron) Device within a linear accelerator that serves as a microwave amplifier. SEE ALSO magnetron. [G. *klyzō,* to dash against, + *-tron* fr. *electron*]

Knapp streaks (nap strēkz) SYN angioid streaks.

Knapp stri•ae (nap strī′ē) SYN angioid streaks.

knee (nē) [TA] **1.** SYN genu (1). **2.** Any structure of angular shape resembling a flexed knee. [A.S. *cneōw*]

knee-ank•le-foot orth•o•sis (nē-ang′kĕl-fut ōr-thō′sis) An orthosis extending from the upper portion of the thigh, crossing the knee and ankle, and terminating at the toes; designed to control knee and ankle motion.

knee•cap (nē′kap) SYN patella.

knee-chest po•si•tion (nē-chest pŏ-zish′ŏn) A prone posture resting on the knees and upper part of the chest, assumed for gynecologic or rectal examination. See page B29. SYN genupectoral position.

knee com•plex (nē kom′pleks) The tibiofemoral joint, the patellofemoral joint, and related musculature and connective tissue. SEE ALSO patellofemoral joint.

knee dis•ar•tic•u•la•tion am•pu•ta•tion (nē dis′ahr-tik′yū-lā′shŭn amp′yū-tā′shŭn) SYN Callander amputation.

knee-el•bow po•si•tion (nē-el′bō pŏ-zish′ŏn) A prone position resting on the knees and elbows, assumed for gynecologic or rectal examination or operation. SYN genucubital position.

knee-jerk re•flex (nē′-jĕrk rē′fleks) SYN patellar reflex.

knee joint (nē joynt) A compound condylar synovial joint consisting of the joint between the condyles of the femur and the condyles of the tibia, articular menisci (semilunar cartilages) being interposed, and the articulation between femur and patella. See this page.

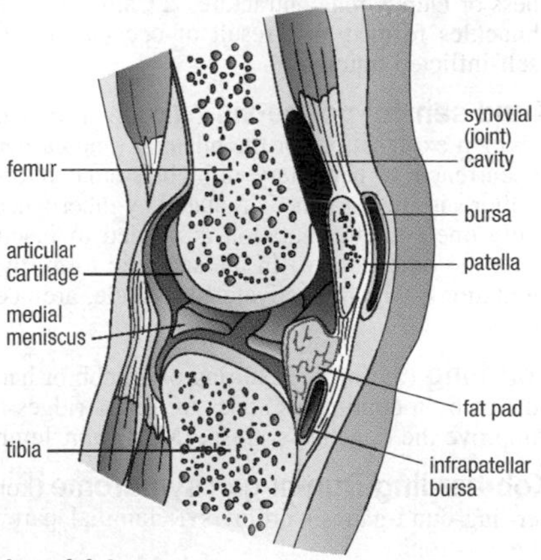

knee joint

knee pre•sen•ta•tion (nē prez′ĕn-tā′shŭn) SEE breech presentation.

knee re•flex (nē rē′fleks) SYN patellar reflex.

knife, pl. **knives** (nīf, nīvz) A cutting instrument used in surgery and dissection. [M.E. *knif,* fr. A.S. *cnif,* fr. O. Norse *knīfr*]

knit•ting (nit′ing) Nonmedical term denoting the process of union of the fragments of a broken bone or of the edges of a wound. [M.E., *knitten,* to knot, fr. A.S. *cnyttan*]

knob (nob) A protuberance; a mass; a nodule.

knock-knee (nok′nē) SYN genu valgum.

knock•out (nok′owt) A genetically engineered organism in which the genome has been altered by site-directed recombination so that a gene is deleted.

knock•out mouse (nok′owt mows) A mouse from whose genome a single gene has been artificially deleted.

knot (not) **1.** A compact intertwining of two or more cords or cordlike structures in such a way that they cannot spontaneously become separated; or a similar twining or infolding of a single cord on itself. **2.** ANATOMY, PATHOLOGY a node, ganglion, or circumscribed swelling suggestive of a knot. [A.S. *cnotta*]

Knott tech•nique (not tek-nēk′) Concentration procedure using blood and dilute formalin; designed to detect microfilariae.

knuck•le (nŭk′ĕl) **1.** A joint of a finger when the fist is closed, especially a metacarpophalangeal joint. **2.** A kink or loop of intestine, as in a hernia. [M.E. *knokel*]

knuck•le pads (nŭk′ĕl padz) **1.** An autosomal dominant trait, in which thick pads of skin appear over the proximal phalangeal joints; occasionally associated with leukonychia and deafness or Dupuytren contracture. **2.** Calluses of the knuckles formed as a result of occupational or self-inflicted trauma.

Knud•sen hy•po•the•sis (nūd′sĕn hī-poth′ĕ-sis) An explanation for the bilateral (and earlier) occurrence of hereditary retinoblastoma; if one tumor suppressor gene is mutated by inheritance, only one somatic mutation is needed to inactivate the other allele. In the sporadic form, two mutations, which inactivate each allele, are necessary.

knurl•ing (nŭr′ling) Texturing of a knob or handle as by a continuous series of milled ridges to improve the clinician's grasp. [M.E. *knor,* lump]

Kob•ber•ling-Dun•ni•gan syn•drome (kob′ĕr-ling-dun′i-găn sin′drōm) SYN familial partial lipodystrophy.

Ko•belt tu•bules (kō′bĕlt tū′byūlz) Remnants of the mesonephric tubules in the female, contained within the epoophoron.

Ko•ber re•ac•tion (kō′bĕr rē-ak′shŭn) In colorimetric analysis, detects estrogen in blood or urine; sulfuric or phenolsulfonic acid hydrolysis of sample turns pink if reaction is positive.

Koch ba•cil•lus (kōk bă-sil′ŭs) SYN *Mycobacterium tuberculosis.*

Ko•cher in•ci•sion (kōk′ĕr in-sizh′ŭn) An abdominal incision below and parallel to the costal margin.

Ko•cher sign (kō′kĕr sīn) In Graves disease, on upward gaze, the globe lags behind the movement of the upper eyelid.

Koch law (kōk law) SYN Koch postulate.

Koch old tu•ber•cu•lin (kōk ōld tū-bĕr′kyū-lin) SEE tuberculin.

Koch phe•nom•e•non (kōk fĕ-nom′ĕ-non) **1.** The phenomenon of infection immunity; living tubercle bacilli (*Mycobacterium tuberculosis*) do not cause reinfection when inoculated into tuberculous guinea pigs (i.e., the animals are "immune" to reinfection) even though the original infections continue to develop and eventually cause death of the animals. **2.** Rise of temperature and increase of the local lesion, in a tuberculous subject, following an injection of tuberculin.

Koch pos•tu•late (kōk pos′chū-lăt) To establish the specificity of a pathogenic microorganism, it must be present in all cases of the disease, inoculations of its pure cultures must produce disease in animals, and from these it must be again obtained and be propagated in pure cultures. SYN Koch law.

Koch tri•an•gle (kōk trī′ang-gĕl) A triangular area of the wall of the right atrium of the heart, which marks the approximate situation of the atrioventricular node.

Koch-Weeks ba•cil•lus (kōk-wēks bă-sil′ŭs) SYN *Haemophilus aegyptius.*

Kock pouch (kok powch) A continent ileostomy with a reservoir and valved opening fashioned from doubled loops of ileum.

Koeb•ner phe•nom•en•on (keb′nĕr fĕ-nom′ĕ-non) Heightened susceptibility to the effects of trauma and chemical exposure in those with psoriasis, lichen planus, and other chronic dermatoses.

KOH Formula of potassium hydroxide.

Köh•ler dis•ease (kā′ler di-zēz′) Osteonecrosis of the tarsal navicular bone or of the patella.

koi•lo•cyte (koy′lō-sīt) A squamous cell, often binucleated, showing a perinuclear halo; characteristic of condyloma acuminatum. [G. *koilos,* hollow, + *kytos,* cell]

koi•lo•cy•to•sis (koy′lō-sī-tō′sis) Perinuclear vacuolation. SEE ALSO koilocyte. [G. *koilos,* hollow, + *kytos,* cell, + *-osis,* condition]

koi•lo•nych•i•a (koy′lō-nik′ē-ă) A malformation of the nails in which the outer surface is concave; often associated with iron deficiency or softening by occupational contact with oils. SYN spoon nail. [G. *koilos,* hollow, + *onyx* (*onych-*), nail]

kok dis•ease (kōk di-zēz′) SYN hyperekplexia.

Ko•kos•kin stain (kō-kos′kin stān) A modified trichrome stain for microsporidian spores in which heat is used to shorten the staining times.

Koll•mann di•la•tor (kol′mahn dī′lā-tōr) A metallic expandable instrument used to dilate urethral strictures.

kolp- SEE colpo-.

ko•lyt•ic (kō-lit′ik) Denoting an inhibitory action. [G. *kolyō,* to hinder]

Kom•mer•ell di•ver•tic•u•lum (kom′ĕr-ĕl dī′vĕr-tik′yū-lŭm) Not a true diverticulum, but a bulblike swelling at the origin of the left subclavian artery due to a remnant of the left fourth aortic arch; associated vascular ring compression syndromes involve persistent right aortic arch; the left subclavian artery may pass behind the esophagus; the diverticulum may be large enough to compress the trachea and esophagus even after the vascular ring has been divided and may need to be resected or affixed to the chest wall or vertebral fascia.

Kon•do•le•on op•er•a•tion (kon-dō′lē-ŏn op-ĕr-ā′shŭn) Excision of strips of subcutaneous connective tissue for the relief of elephantiasis.

ko•ni•o•cor•tex (kō′nē-ō-kōr′teks) Regions of the cerebal cortex characterized by a particularly well developed inner granular layer (layer 4); this type of cerebral cortex is represented by the primary sensory area 17 of the visual cortex, areas 1–3 of the somatic sensory cortex, and area 41 of the auditory cortex. SEE ALSO cerebral cortex. [G. *konis,* dust, + L. *cortex,* bark]

kon•zo (kon′zō) A cyanide-caused upper motor neuron disease manifested principally as spastic paraplegia, seen in Africa; results from the consumption of improperly prepared cassava roots, which contain high concentrations of cyanogenetic glucosides. [Yaka, tired legs]

Kop•lik spots (kop′lik spotz) Small red spots on the buccal mucous membrane, in the center of each of which may be seen, in a strong light, a minute bluish white speck; they occur early in measles (morbilli), before the skin eruption, and are regarded as a pathognomonic sign of the disease.

kopro- SEE copro-.

Ko•re•an hand ac•u•punc•ture (kōr-ē′ăn hand ak′yū-pŭngk-shŭr) A form of the Asian therapy in which the hand is the focus of intervention, in the belief that its structures control those of the whole body.

Ko•re•an hem•or•rhag•ic fe•ver, Ko•re•an hem•or•rhag•ic fe•ver vi•rus (kōr-ē′ăn hem′ŏr-aj′ik fē′vĕr, vī′rŭs) An epidemic form of the disease caused by a Hantaan virus. Cf. hemorrhagic fever with renal syndrome, epidemic hemorrhagic fever.

Ko•re•an mint (kōr-ē′ăn mint) SYN agastache.

Ko•rot•koff sounds (kō-rot′kof sowndz) Aural findings heard during blood pressure determination using a stethoscope and sphygmomanometer. Sounds originating within the blood passing through the vessel or produced by a vibrating motion of the arterial wall.

Ko•rot•koff test (kō-rot′kof test) A test of collateral circulation; while the artery proximal to an aneurysm is compressed, the blood pressure in the distal circulation is estimated; if it is fairly high, the collateral circulation is good.

Kor•sa•koff syn•drome (kor′sĕ-kawf sin′drōm) An alcohol amnestic syndrome characterized by confusion and severe impairment of memory, especially for recent events, for which the patient compensates by confabulation; typically encountered in those with chronic alcoholism; delirium tremens may precede the syndrome, and Wernicke syndrome often coexists; the precise pathogenesis is uncertain, but direct toxic effects of alcohol are probably less important than severe nutritional deficiencies often associated with chronic alcoholism. SYN amnestic syndrome (1), polyneuritic psychosis.

ko•sher (kō′shĕr) Denotes a diet that follows the dietary laws required in observant Jews; it interdicts consumption of some food altogether and requires that dairy and meat items be consumed at different times and on different dishes. Kosher butchers prepare meats and poultry according to hygiene precepts stronger than those at use in nonkosher butchers.

Kr Symbol for krypton.

Kras•ke op•er•a•tion (kras′kĕ op-ĕr-ā′shŭn) Removal of the coccyx and excision of the left wing of the sacrum to afford approach for resection of the rectum for cancer or stenosis.

krau•ro•sis vul•vae (kraw-rō′sis vŭl′vē) Atrophy and shrinkage of the epithelium of the vagina and vulva, often accompanied by a chronic inflammatory reaction in the deeper tissues, as in lichen sclerosus. [G. *krauros,* dry, brittle]

Krau•se end bulb (krow′zĕ end bŭlb) Nerve terminals in skin, mouth, conjunctiva, and other parts, consisting of a laminated capsule of connective tissue enclosing the terminal, branched, convoluted ending of an afferent nerve fiber; generally believed to be sensitive to cold.

Krebs cy•cle (krebz sī′kĕl) SYN tricarboxylic acid cycle.

Krebs-Hen•se•leit cy•cle, Krebs or•ni•thine cy•cle, Krebs u•re•a cy•cle (krebz hen′sĕ-līt sī′kĕl, krebz ŏr′ni-thēn sī′kĕl, krĕbs yūr-ē′ă) SYN urea cycle.

krig•ing (krī′jing) A method first used in the

earth sciences to smooth data from spatially scattered point measurements, used in geographic epidemiology.

Krim•sky test (krim′skē test) A measurement of strabismus by which a penlight is shone at the eyes and the position of the light reflex centered with a prism, thus indicating the amount of deviation.

krin•gle (kring′gĕl) A structural motif or domain seen in certain proteins in which a fold of large loops is stabilized by disulfide bonds; an important structural feature in blood coagulation factors. [Ger. *Kringel*, curl]

Kro•nec•ker stain (krō′nek-ĕr stān) A 5% sodium chloride stain rendered faintly alkaline with sodium carbonate, used in the examination of fresh tissues under the microscope.

Krö•nig a•re•a (krār′nig ār′ē-ă) The narrow straplike portion of the resonant field that extends over the shoulder, connecting the larger areas of resonance over the pulmonary apex in front and behind.

Krö•nig steps (krār′nig steps) Extension of the lower part of the right border of absolute cardiac dullness in hypertrophy of the right heart.

Kru•ken•berg am•pu•ta•tion (krū′kĕn-berg amp′yū-tā′shŭn) A cineplastic amputation at the carpus with the distal end of the forearm used to create a forklike stump; especially valuable in the blind because the stump has proprioception.

Kru•ken•berg spin•dle (krū′kĕn-berg spin′dĕl) A vertical fusiform area of melanin pigmentation on the posterior surface of the central cornea.

Kru•ken•berg tu•mor (krū′kĕn-berg tū′mŏr) A metastatic carcinoma of the ovary, usually bilateral and secondary to a mucous carcinoma of the stomach, which contains signet-ring cells filled with mucus.

Kru•ken•berg veins (krū′kĕn-berg vānz) SYN central veins of liver.

Kru•se brush (krū′sĕ brŭsh) A bunch of fine platinum wires attached to a holder; used in bacteriologic work to spread material over the surface of a culture medium.

Krus•kal-Wal•lis sta•tis•ti•cal test (krūs′kăl-wahl′is stă-tis′tik-ăl test) Nonparametric equivalent of analysis of variants for more than three groups.

♻ **krymo-, kryo-** SEE crymo-, cryo-.

kryp•ton (Kr) (krip′ton) One of the inert gases, present in small amounts in the atmosphere (1.14 ppm by dry volume); atomic no. 36, atomic wt. 83.80; ^{85}Kr has been used in studies of cardiac abnormalities. [G. *kryptos*, concealed]

kryp•ton la•ser (krip′ton lā′zĕr) Device used for ophthalmic procedures, particularly retinal photocoagulation in the presence of vitreous hemorrhage, consisting of photons in the red (647 nm) spectrum.

KTP la•ser (lā′zĕr) Device in the blue-green to green (532 nm) spectrum, used for hemostasis; produced by doubling the frequency of an Nd:YAG laser by passing the beam through a KTP crystal. [K (potassium) Titanyl Phosphate]

KUB 1. Abbreviation for kidneys, ureters, and bladder. **2.** X-ray view of the abdomen to visualize these structures.

Küh•ne fi•ber (kē′nĕ fī′bĕr) Artificial muscle made by filling the intestine of an insect with a growth of myxomycetes; used to demonstrate the contractility of protoplasm.

Küh•ne meth•yl•ene blue (kē′nĕ meth′il-ēn blū) Methylene blue in absolute alcohol and phenol solution.

Küh•ne phe•nom•e•non (kē′nĕ fĕ-nom′ĕ-non) When a constant current is passed through a muscle, an undulation is seen to pass from the positive to the negative pole.

Küh•ne plate (kē′nĕ plāt) The endplate of a motor nerve fiber in a muscle spindle.

Kuhnt spac•es (kūnt spās′ĕz) Shallow diverticula or recesses between the ciliary body and ciliary zonule that open into the posterior chamber of the eye.

ku•ma•ri (kū-mah′rē) SYN *Aloe vera.*

küm•mel (kim′el) SYN caraway. [Ger., caraway seed]

Kupf•fer cells (kup′fĕr selz) Phagocytic cells of the mononuclear phagocyte series found on the luminal surface of the hepatic sinusoids.

Kür•stei•ner ca•nals (kēr-shtīn′ĕr kă-nalz′) A fetal complex of vesicular, canalicular, and glandlike structures derived from parathyroid or thymus; normally remain rudimentary but may persist postnatally as cystic structures.

Kurtz•ke mul•ti•ple scle•ro•sis dis•a•bil•i•ty scale (kurtz′kĕ mŭl′ti-pĕl skler-ō′sis dis′ă-bil′i-tē skāl) SYN expanded disability status scale.

ku•ru (kū′rū) A progressive, fatal form of spongiform encephalopathy, endemic in New Guinea and caused by prions. Transmission is believed to occur through ritual cannibalism. SEE prion. [native dialect, to shiver from fear or cold]

Kuss•maul res•pi•ra•tion (kūs′mowl res′pir-ā′shŭn) Deep, rapid respiration characteristic of diabetic or other types of acidosis.

Kuss•maul sign (kūs′mowl sīn) In constrictive pericarditis, a paradoxic increase in venous distention and pressure or failure to collapse during inspiration; seen occasionally in effusive-constrictive pericarditis when tamponading pericardial fluid overlies a constricting epicarditis.

kv Abbreviation for kilovolt.

Kveim an·ti·gen (kvīm an′ti-jen) A saline suspension of human sarcoid tissue prepared from the spleen of a person with active sarcoidosis; used in the Kveim test.

Kveim test (kvīm test) An intradermal test for the detection of sarcoidosis, done by injecting Kveim antigen (obtained from spleens of patients with sarcoidosis) and examining skin biopsies after 3 and 6 weeks; a positive test result is indicated by typical nodules showing evidence of sarcoid tissue.

KVO Abbreviation for keep vein open.

kVp Kilovolt peak, the highest instantaneous energy across an x-ray tube, corresponding to the highest energy x-rays emitted.

kwa·shi·or·kor (kwah-shē-ōr′kōr) A disease seen in African children 1–3 years old, due to dietary deficiency, particularly of protein; characterized by marked hypoalbuminemia, anemia, edema, pot belly, depigmentation of the skin, loss of hair or change in hair color to red, and bulky stools containing undigested food. [Ghanian Niger-Congo language, red boy or displaced child]

ky·ma·tism (kī′mă-tizm) SYN myokymia. [G. *kyma,* wave]

ky·mo·gram (kī′mō-gram) The graphic curve made by a kymograph.

ky·mo·graph (kī′mō-graf) An instrument for recording wavelike motions or modulation of body organs (e.g., heart, great blood vessels); it consists of a drum revolved by clockwork and covered with smoked paper on which the curve is inscribed by a writing point. [G. *kyma,* wave, + *graphō,* to record]

ky·mog·ra·phy (kī-mog′ră-fē) Use of the kymograph.

kyn·u·ren·ic ac·id (kin-yūr-ē′nik as′id) A product of the metabolism of L-tryptophan; appears in urine in pyridoxine deficiency.

kyn·u·ren·ine (kin-yūr′ĕ-nēn) A product of the metabolism of L-tryptophan, excreted in the urine.

ky·phos (kī′fos) A hump, the convex prominence in kyphosis. [G.]

ky·pho·sco·li·o·sis (kī′fō-skō-lē-ō′sis) Kyphosis combined with scoliosis; congestive heart failure is a late complication.

ky·pho·sis (kī-fō′sis) *Note: Although this term denotes both normal and pathologic states, the latter use is becoming less common.* **1.** An anteriorly concave curvature of the vertebral column, such as normally occurs in the thoracic and sacrococcygeal regions. **2.** Hyperkyphosis; excessive anteriorly concave curvature of a part of the spine, usually thoracic. Cf. hyperkyphotic. [G. *kyphōsis,* hump-back, fr. *kyphos,* bent, humpbacked]

ky·phot·ic (kī-fot′ik) Relating to or suffering from kyphosis.

ky·phot·ic pel·vis (kī-fot′ik pel′vis) Backward curvature of the lumbar spine causing contraction of pelvic measurements.

kyte (kīt) Stomach; belly (Scots dialect).

♻ **kyto-** SEE cyto-.

Λ, λ Greek character, the letter lambda.

L Abbreviation for liter; NATO code for Lewisite.

L Abbreviation for linking number.

♻**L- 1.** Abbreviation for levorotatory. Cf. *d*-. **2.** Prefix indicating a chemical compound to be structurally (sterically) related to L-glyceraldehyde. [L. *laevus,* on the left-hand side]

La Symbol for lanthanum.

La•band syn•drome (lă-band′ sin′drōm) Fibromatosis of the gingivae associated with hypoplasia of the distal phalanges, nail dysplasia, joint hypermotility, and sometimes hepatosplenomegaly; autosomal dominant inheritance.

la•bel (lā′bĕl) **1.** To incorporate into a compound a substance that is readily detected, such as a radionuclide, whereby its metabolism can be followed or its physical distribution detected. **2.** The substance so incorporated.

la belle in•dif•fer•ence (lah bel in′dēf-ār-ahns) A naive, inappropriate lack of emotion or concern for the perceptions by others of one's disability, typically seen in persons with conversion hysteria. [Fr.]

la•bi•a (lā′bē-ă) Plural of labium.

la•bi•al (lā′bē-ăl) **1.** Relating to the lips or any labia. **2.** Toward a lip. [L. *labium,* lip]

la•bi•al branch•es of men•tal nerve (lā′bē-ăl branch′ĕz men′tăl nĕrv) Branches of mental nerve to lower lip.

la•bi•al her•ni•a (lā′bē-ăl hĕr′nē-ă) Hernia through the canal of Nuck.

la•bi•al splint (lā′bē-ăl splint) An appliance made of plastic, metal, or in a combination of the two, made to conform to the outer aspect of the dental arch and used in the management of jaw and facial injuries.

la•bi•al ves•ti•bule (lā′bē-ăl ves′ti-byūl) That part of the oral vestibule related to the lips.

la•bi•a ma•jo•ra (lā′bē-ă mă-jōr′ă) Plural of labium majus.

la•bi•a mi•no•ra (lā′bē-ă mi-nō′ră) Plural of labium minus.

la•bile (lā′bīl) Unstable; unsteady, not fixed; denoting: (1) an adaptability to alteration or modification, i.e., relatively easily changed or rearranged; (2) constituents of serum affected by increases in heat; (3) an electrode that is kept moving over the surface during the passage of an electric current; (4) PSYCHOLOGY free and uncontrolled mood or behavioral expression of the emotions; (5) easily removable (e.g., a labile hydrogen atom). [L. *labilis,* liable to slip, fr. *labor,* pp. *lapsus,* to slip]

la•bil•i•ty (lă-bil′i-tē) The state of being labile.

♻**labio-** Prefix meaning relating to lips. SEE ALSO cheilo-. [L. *labium,* lip]

la•bi•o•cer•vi•cal (lā′bē-ō-sĕr′vi-kăl) Relating to a lip and a neck; specifically, to the labial or buccal surface of the neck of a tooth. [labio- + L. *cervix,* neck]

la•bi•o•cho•re•a (lā′bē-ō-kōr-ē′ă) A chronic spasm of the lips, interfering with speech. [labio- + G. *choreia,* dance]

la•bi•o•cli•na•tion (lā′bē-ō-kli-nā′shŭn) Inclination of position more toward the lips than is normal; said of a tooth.

la•bi•o•den•tal (lā′bē-ō-den′tăl) Relating to the lips and the teeth; denoting certain letters the sound of which is formed by both lips and teeth. [labio- + L. *dens,* tooth]

la•bi•o•gin•gi•val (lā′bē-ō-jin′ji-văl) Relating to the point of junction of the labial border and the gingival line on the distal or mesial surface of an incisor tooth.

la•bi•o•graph (lā′bē-ō-graf) An instrument for recording the movements of the lips in speaking. [labio- + G. *graphō,* to record]

la•bi•o•men•tal (lā′bē-ō-men′tăl) Relating to the lower lip and the chin. [labio- + L. *mentum,* chin]

la•bi•o•na•sal (lā′bē-ō-nā′zăl) **1.** Relating to the upper lip and the nose, or to both lips and the nose. **2.** Denoting a letter that is both labial and nasal in the production of its sound.

la•bi•o•pal•a•tine (lā′bē-ō-pal′ă-tīn) Relating to the lips and the palate.

la•bi•o•place•ment (lā′bē-ō-plās′mĕnt) Positioning (e.g., of a tooth) more toward the lips than normal.

la•bi•o•plas•ty (lā′bē-ō-plas-tē) Surgical repair of a lip. [labio- + G. *plastos,* formed]

la•bi•o•ver•sion (lā′bē-ō-vĕr′zhŭn) Malposition of an anterior tooth from the normal line of occlusion toward the lips.

la•bi•um, gen. **la•bi•i**, pl. **la•bi•a** (lā′bē-ŭm, -ī, -ă) [TA] **1.** SYN lip. **2.** Any lip-shaped structure. [L.]

la•bi•um ma•jus (lā′bē-ŭm mā′jŭs) One of two rounded folds of integument forming the lateral boundaries of the pudendal cleft. The labia majora are the female homologue of the scrotum.

la•bi•um mi•nus (lā′bē-ŭm mī′nŭs) One of two narrow longitudinal folds of mucous membrane enclosed in the pudendal cleft within the labia majora; posteriorly, they gradually merge into the labia majora and join to form the frenulum labiorum pudendi (fourchette); anteriorly, each labium divides into two portions that unite with those of the opposite side in front of the glans clitoridis to form the prepuce.

la•bor (lā′bŏr) The process of expulsion of the fetus and the placenta from the uterus. The stages of labor are: **first stage**, beginning with the onset of uterine contractions through the period of dilation of the os uteri; **second stage**, the period of expulsive effort, beginning with complete dilation of the cervix and ending with expulsion of the infant; **third stage**, or **placental stage**, the period beginning at the expulsion of the infant and ending with the completed expulsion of the placenta and membranes. SYN labour. [L. toil, suffering]

lab•o•ra•to•ri•an (lab′ŏr-ă-tōr′ē-ăn) One who works in a laboratory; in the medical and allied health professions; one who examines or performs tests (or supervises such procedures) with various types of chemical and biologic materials, chiefly as an aid in the diagnosis, treatment, and control of disease, or as a basis for health and sanitation practices.

lab•o•ra•tor•y (lab′ŏ-ră-tōr-ē, la-bōr′a-tōr′ē) A place equipped for the performance of tests, experiments, and investigative procedures and for the preparation of reagents and therapeutic and chemical materials. [Mediev. L. *laboratorium*, a workplace, fr. L. *laboro*, pp. *-atus*, to labor]

lab•o•ra•tor•y di•ag•no•sis (lab′ŏ-ră-tōr-ē dī-ăg-nō′sis) A diagnosis made by a chemical, microscopic, microbiologic, immunologic, or pathologic study of secretions, discharges, blood, or tissue.

lab•o•ra•tor•y in•for•ma•tion sys•tem (lab′ŏ-ră-tōr-ē in′fōr-ma′shŭn sis′tĕm) A complete software program for clinical laboratory collection, reporting, and quality assurance of specimens.

la•bor coach (lā′bŏr kōch) A layperson who assists a mother in giving birth, generally a friend or relative who has attended classes with the gravid patient to learn methods of breathing and body positioning.

la•bor curve (lā′bŏr kŭrv) SYN partogram. SYN labour curve.

la•bor pains (lā′bŏr pānz) Rhythmic uterine contractions that under normal conditions increase in intensity, frequency, and duration, culminating in vaginal delivery of the infant. SYN labour pains.

labour [Br.] SYN labor.

labour curve [Br.] SYN labor curve.

labour pains [Br.] SYN labor pains.

la•brum, pl. **la•bra** (lā′brŭm, -bră) [TA] **1.** A lip. **2.** A lip-shaped structure. [L.]

lab•y•rinth (lab′ĭ-rinth) **1.** The internal or inner ear, composed of the semicircular ducts, vestibule, and cochlea. **2.** Any group of communicating cavities, as in each lateral mass of the ethmoid bone. **3.** A group of communicating culture tubes used for separating motile from nonmotile microorganisms.

lab•y•rin•thec•to•my (lab′ĭ-rin-thek′tŏ-mē) Excision of the labyrinth; a destructive operation to destroy labyrinthine function. [labyrinth + G. *ektomē*, excision]

lab•y•rin•thine (lab′ĭ-rin′thēn) Relating to any labyrinth.

lab•y•rin•thine an•es•the•si•a test (lab-ĭ-rin′thēn an-es-thē′zē-ă test) Local anesthetic is instilled into the tympanic cavity of the affected ear and allowed to absorb through the round window into the inner ear. If temporary resolution or amelioration of vertigo or postural instability occurs, the test ear can be assumed to be the major source of the problems. This test can also identify residual labyrinthine function not detectable by caloric testing.

lab•y•rin•thine ar•ter•y (lab′ĭ-rin′thēn ahr′tĕr-ē) Internal acoustic meatal branch, a branch of the basilar artery that enters the labyrinth through the internal acoustic meatus.

lab•y•rin•thine dys•func•tion (lab-ĭ-rin′thēn dis-fŭngk′shŭn) Abnormal or decreased function of a portion of the labyrinthine sensors. The CNS's effectiveness in compensating for the abnormality is typically lower in proportion to the degree of labyrinthine instability and irregularity.

lab•y•rin•thine fis•tu•la (lab′ĭ-rin′thēn fis′chū-lă) A fistula between a fluid-filled compartment of the inner ear and another fluid-filled compartment in the inner ear (internal) or a space external to the inner ear as the middle ear or mastoid air cells or subarachnoid space (external); it may result in auditory and vestibular disturbances, depending on its location.

lab•y•rin•thine nys•tag•mus (lab′ĭ-rin′thēn nis-tag′mŭs) SYN vestibular nystagmus.

lab•y•rin•thine re•flex (lab′i-rin′thīn rē′fleks) Reflex initiated through stimulation of receptors in the utricle or semicircular canals.

lab•y•rin•thine right•ing re•flex•es (lab′ē-rin′thēn rīt′ing rē′fleks-ez) Postural movement whereby stimulation of the proprioceptors of the labyrinth cause change in the tone of the neck muscles, bringing the head into its natural position in space.

lab•y•rin•thine veins (lab′ĭ-rin′thēn vānz) One or more veins accompanying the labyrinthine artery; they drain the internal ear, pass out through the internal acoustic meatus, and empty into the transverse sinus or the inferior petrosal sinus. SYN internal auditory veins.

lab•y•rin•thine ver•ti•go (lab′ĭ-rin′thēn vĕr′ti-gō) SYN Ménière disease.

lab·y·rin·thi·tis (lab′ĭ-rin-thī′tis) Inflammation of the labyrinth (the internal ear), sometimes accompanied by vertigo and deafness. SYN otitis interna.

lab·y·rin·thot·o·my (lab′ĭ-rin-thot′ŏ-mē) Incision into the labyrinth. [labyrinth + G. *tomē,* incision]

lac·er·at·ed (las′ĕr-ā-tĕd) Torn; rent; having a ragged edge. [L. *lacero,* pp. *-atus,* to tear to pieces]

lac·er·a·tion (las′ĕr-ā′shŭn) **1.** A torn or jagged wound caused by blunt trauma; incorrectly applied to a cut. **2.** The process or act of tearing the tissues. [L. *lacero,* pp. *-atus,* to tear to pieces]

la·cer·tus (lă-sĕr′tŭs) **1.** The muscular part of the upper limb from shoulder to elbow. **2.** A fibrous band, bundle, or slip related to a muscle. [L.]

Lach·man test (lak′măn test) A maneuver to detect deficiency of the anterior cruciate ligament; with the knee flexed 20–30 degrees, the tibia is displaced anteriorly relative to the femur; a soft endpoint of greater than 4 mm displacement is positive (abnormal).

lac·ri·mal (lak′ri-măl) Relating to the tears, their secretion, the secretory glands, and the drainage apparatus. [L. *lacrima,* a tear]

lac·ri·mal ap·pa·ra·tus (lak′ri-măl ap′ă-rat′ŭs) Consisting of the lacrimal gland, the lacrimal lake, the lacrimal canaliculi, the lacrimal sac, and the nasolacrimal duct.

lac·ri·mal ar·ter·y (lak′ri-măl ahr′tĕr-ē) *Origin,* ophthalmic; *distribution,* lacrimal gland, lateral and superior rectus muscles, superior eyelid, forehead, and temporal fossa. SYN arteria lacrimalis [TA].

lac·ri·mal bone (lak′ri-măl bōn) An irregularly rectangular thin plate, forming part of the medial wall of the orbit behind the frontal process of the maxilla; it articulates with the inferior nasal concha, ethmoid, frontal, and maxillary bones.

lac·ri·mal can·a·lic·u·lus (lak′ri-măl kan′ă-lik′yū-lŭs) A curved canal beginning at the lacrimal punctum in the margin of each eyelid near the medial commissure and running transversely medially to empty with its fellow into the lacrimal sac.

lac·ri·mal ca·run·cle (lak′ri-măl kar′ŭng-kĕl) A small reddish body at the medial angle of the eye, containing modified sebaceous and sweat glands.

lac·ri·mal fold (lak′ri-măl fōld) A fold of mucous membrane guarding the lower opening of the nasolacrimal duct. SYN plica lacrimalis [TA].

lac·ri·mal fos·sa (lak′ri-măl fos′ă) A hollow in the orbital plate of the frontal bone, formed by the overhanging margin and zygomatic process, lodging the lacrimal gland.

lac·ri·mal gland (lak′ri-măl gland) The gland that secretes tears; it consists of 6–12 separate compound tubuloalveolar serous glands, located in the upper lateral part of the orbit, and is partially divided into a smaller palpebral part and a larger orbital part by the aponeurosis of the levator palpebrae muscle.

lac·ri·mal lake (lak′ri-măl lāk) The small cisternlike area of the conjunctiva at the medial angle of the eye, in which the tears collect after bathing the anterior surface of the eyeball and the conjunctival sac. SYN lacus lacrimalis [TA].

lac·ri·mal nerve (lak′ri-măl nĕrv) A branch of the ophthalmic nerve supplying sensory fibers to the lateral part of the upper eyelid, conjunctiva, and lacrimal gland. The secretomotor fibers of the latter were conveyed to the lacrimal nerve by the communicating branch of the zygomatic nerve (a branch of the maxillary nerve). SYN nervus lacrimalis [TA].

lac·ri·mal pa·pil·la (lak′ri-măl pă-pil′ă) A slight projection from the margin of each eyelid near the medial commissure, in the center of which is the lacrimal punctum (opening of the lacrimal duct).

lac·ri·mal punc·tum (lak′ri-măl pŭngk′tŭm) The minute circular opening of the lacrimal canaliculus, on the margin of each eyelid near the medial commissure.

lac·ri·mal sac (lak′ri-măl sak) The upper portion of the nasolacrimal duct into which empty the two lacrimal canaliculi. SYN saccus lacrimalis [TA], dacryocyst, tear sac.

lac·ri·mal vein (lak′ri-măl vān) Drains the lacrimal gland, passing posteriorly through the orbit with the lacrimal artery to empty into the superior ophthalmic vein.

lac·ri·ma·tion (lak′ri-mā′shŭn) The secretion of tears, especially in excess. [L. *lacrimatio*]

lac·ri·ma·tor (lak′ri-mā-tŏr) An agent that irritates the eyes and produces tears. [L. *lacrima,* tear]

lac·ri·ma·to·ry (lak′ri-mă-tōr-ē) Causing lacrimation.

lac·ri·mo·gus·ta·to·ry re·flex (lak′ri-mō-gŭs′tă-tōr-ē rē′fleks) Chewing of food causing secretion of tears. SEE ALSO crocodile tears syndrome.

lac·ri·mot·o·my (lak′ri-mot′ŏ-mē) The operation of incising the lacrimal duct or sac. [L. *lacrima,* tear, + G. *tomē,* incision]

♻**lact-, lacti-, lacto-** Combining forms for milk. SEE ALSO galacto-. [L. *lac, lactis*]

lac·tac·i·do·sis (lakt-as′i-dō′sis) Acidosis due to increased lactic acid.

lac·tam, lac·tim (lak′tam, lak′tim) Contractions of "lactoneamine" and "lactoneimine," applied to the tautomeric forms –NH–CO– and –N=C(OH)–, respectively, observed in many purines, pyrimidines, and other substances.

lac•tase (lak′tās) SYN beta (β)-D-galactosidase.

lac•tate (lak′tāt) **1.** A salt or ester of lactic acid. **2.** To produce milk in the mammary glands.

lac•tate de•hy•dro•gen•ase (LDH) (lak′tāt dē′hī-droj′ĕn-ās) Name for four enzymes. The first two transfer H to ferricytochrome *c;* the last two transfer it to NAD^+, in catalyzing the oxidation of lactate to pyruvate; the isozyme distribution of heart and muscle lactate dehydrogenase is of diagnostic use in myocardial infarction.

lac•tate de•hy•dro•gen•ase vi•rus (lak′tāt dē′hī-droj′ĕn-ās vī′rŭs) An arterivirus present perhaps as a "passenger" in various transplantable mouse tumors; the virus may cause a lifelong infection and be recognized by elevated plasma lactate dehydrogenose.

lac•tat•ed Ring•er so•lu•tion (lak′tāt-ĕd ring′ĕr sŏ-lū′shŭn) A solution containing NaCl, sodium lactate, $CaCl_2$(dihydrate), and KCl in distilled water; used for the same purposes as Ringer solution. SYN Hartmann solution (1).

lac•tate par•a•dox (lak′tāt par′ă-doks) Reduced capacity for lactate production by skeletal muscle during exercise at altitude despite reduction in arterial PO_2; related to an altitude-induced reduction in the glucose-mobilizing hormone epinephrine during exercise.

lac•tate thresh•old (lak′tāt thresh′ōld) A point, during exercise of increasing intensity, when a measurable increase in venous blood lactate levels occurs in conjunction with an exponential increase in respiratory frequency. SEE ALSO ventilatory threshold, anaerobic threshold. SYN onset of blood lactate accumulation.

lac•ta•tion (lak-tā′shŭn) **1.** Production of milk. **2.** Period following birth during which milk is secreted in the breasts. [L. *lactatio,* suckle]

lac•ta•tion a•men•or•rhe•a (lak-tā′shŭn ā-men-ŏr-ē′ă) Physiologic suppression of menses while nursing.

lac•te•al (lak′tē-ăl) **1.** Relating to or resembling milk; milky. **2.** A lymphatic vessel that conveys chyle from the intestine. SYN chyle vessel, lacteal vessel.

lac•te•al ves•sel (lak′tē-ăl ves′ĕl) SYN lacteal (2).

lac•tic ac•id (lak′tik as′id) A normal intermediate in the fermentation (oxidation, metabolism) of sugar.

lac•tic ac•i•de•mi•a (lak′tik as′i-dē′mē-ă) The presence of dextrorotatory lactic acid in the circulating blood. [lactic acid + G. *haima,* blood]

lac•tif•er•ous (lak-tif′ĕr-ŭs) Yielding milk. SYN lactigerous. [lacti- + L. *fero,* to bear]

lac•tif•er•ous ducts (lak-tif′ĕr-ŭs dŭkts) Ducts numbering 15–20, which drain the lobes of the mammary gland; they open at the nipple. SYN galactophore, mammillary ducts, milk ducts.

lac•tif•er•ous glands (lak-tif′ĕr-ŭs glandz) SYN mammary gland.

lac•tif•er•ous si•nus (lak-tif′ĕr-ŭs sī′nŭs) A circumscribed spindle-shaped dilation of the lactiferous duct just before it enters the nipple. In nursing mothers this dilation stores a droplet of milk that is expressed by compression as the infant begins to suckle; this is thought to encourage continual suckling while the let-down reflex ensues.

lac•tig•e•nous (lak-tij′ĕ-nŭs) Producing milk. [lacti- + *-gen,* producing]

lac•tig•er•ous (lak-tij′ĕr-ŭs) SYN lactiferous. [lacti- + L. *gero,* to carry]

Lac•to•ba•cil•lus (lak′tō-bă-sil′ŭs) A genus of microaerophilic or anaerobic, non-spore-forming, ordinarily nonmotile bacteria containing gram-positive rods which vary from long and slender cells to short coccobacilli; chains are commonly produced. These organisms are found in dairy products, the effluents of grain and meat products, water, sewage, beer, wine, fruits and fruit juices, pickled vegetables, and in sourdough and mash, and are part of the normal flora of the mouth, intestinal tract, and vagina of many warm-blooded animals, including humans; rarely are they pathogenic. The type species is *L. delbrueckii.* [lacto- + bacillus]

lac•to•ba•cil•lus (lak′tō-bă-sil′ŭs) A vernacular term used to refer to any member of the genus *Lactobacillus.*

Lac•to•ba•cil•lus ac•i•doph•i•lus (lak′tō-bă-sil′ŭs as′i-dof′i-lŭs) A bacterial species found in the feces of milk-fed infants and also in the feces of older persons on a high milk-, lactose-, or dextrin containing diet.

Lac•to•ba•cil•lus bul•gar•i•cus (lak′tō-bă-sil′ŭs bŭl-gā′ri-kŭs) A bacterial species used in the production of yogurt.

lac•to•cele (lak′tō-sēl) SYN galactocele. [lacto- + G. *kēlē,* tumor]

lac•to•fer•rin (lak′tō-fer′in) A transferrin found in the milk of several mammalian species and thought to be involved in the transport of iron to erythrocytes.

lac•to•gen (lak′tō-jen) An agent that stimulates milk production or secretion. [lacto- + G. *-gen,* producing]

lac•to•gen•e•sis (lak′tō-jen′ĕ-sis) Milk production. [lacto- + G. *genesis,* production]

lac•to•gen•ic (lak′tō-jen′ik) Pertaining to lactogenesis.

lac•to•gen•ic hor•mone (lak′tō-jen′ik hōr′mōn) SYN prolactin.

lac•to•glob•u•lin (lak′tō-glob′yŭ-lin) The globulin present in milk; it makes up 50–60% of bovine whey protein.

lac•tone (lak′tōn) An intramolecular organic anhydride formed from a hydroxyacid by the loss of water between an –OH and a –COOH group; a cyclic ester.

lac•to-o•vo•veg•e•ta•ri•an (lak′tō-ō′vō-vej′i-tār′ē-ăn) A vegetarian who consumes dairy products and eggs but does not eat animal flesh.

lac•to•phe•nol cot•ton blue stain (lak′tō-fē′nol kot′ŏn blū stān) A solution consisting of phenol crystals, glycerol, lactic acid, and distilled water to which cotton blue or crystal violet is added; used as a stain in mycology.

lac•tor•rhe•a (lak′tō-rē′ă) SYN galactorrhea. SYN lactorrhoea. [lacto- + G. *rhoia,* a flow]

lactorrhoea [Br.] SYN lactorrhea.

lac•tose (lak′tōs) A disaccharide present in cow's milk and used in food for infants and convalescents and in pharmaceutical preparations; large doses act as an osmotic diuretic and as a laxative. SYN milk sugar.

lac•tose in•tol•e•rance (lak′tōs in-tol′ĕr-ăns) SYN adult lactase deficiency.

lac•tos•u•ri•a (lak′tō-syūr′ē-ă) Excretion of lactose (milk sugar) in the urine; a common finding during pregnancy and lactation, and in newborn, especially premature, babies. [lactose + G. *ouron,* urine, + -ia]

lac•to•ther•a•py (lak′tō-thār′ă-pē) SYN galactotherapy.

lac•to•ve•ge•tar•i•an (lak′tō-vej-ĕ-tār′ē-ăn) One whose diet contains only vegetables and dairy products. SEE ALSO vegetarian, vegan.

la•cu•na, pl. **la•cu•nae** (lă-kū′nă, -kū′nē) **1.** [TA] A small space, cavity, or depression. **2.** A gap or defect. **3.** An abnormal space between strata or between the cellular elements of the epidermis. **4.** SYN corneal space. [L. a pit, dim. of *lacus,* a hollow, a lake]

la•cu•na mag•na (lă-kū′nă mag′nă) A recess on the roof of the fossa navicularis of the penis, formed by a fold of mucous membrane, the valve of the navicular fossa.

la•cu•nar (lă-kū′năr) Relating to a lacuna.

la•cu•nar am•ne•si•a, **lo•cal•ized am•ne•si•a** (lă-kū′năr am-nē′zē-ă, lō′kăl-īzd am-nē′zē-ă) Memory loss about isolated events.

la•cu•nar lig•a•ment (lă-kū′năr lig′ă-mĕnt) A curved fibrous band that passes horizontally backward from the medial end of the inguinal ligament to the pectineal line; it forms the medial boundary of the femoral ring. SYN ligamentum lacunare [TA].

la•cu•nule (lă-kū′nyūl) A very small lacuna. [Mod. L. *lacunula,* dim. of L. *lacuna*]

la•cus, pl. **la•cus** (lā′kŭs) SYN lake (1). [L. lake]

la•cus la•cri•ma•lis (lā′kŭs lak′ri-mā′lis) [TA] SYN lacrimal lake.

la•cus se•mi•na•lis (lā′kŭs sem-i-nā′lis) The vault of the vagina after insemination. SYN seminal lake.

LAD Abbreviation for leukocyte adhesion deficiency.

Ladd band (lad band) A peritoneal attachment of an incompletely rotated cecum, found in malrotation of the intestine; may cause obstruction of the duodenum.

lad•der splint (lad′ĕr splint) A flexible splint consisting of two stout parallel wires with finer cross wires.

Ladd op•er•a•tion (lad op-ĕr-ā′shŭn) Division of Ladd band to relieve duodenal obstruction in malrotation of the intestine.

La•dy Win•der•mere syn•drome (lā′dē win′dĕr-mēr sin′drōm) Nontuberculous mycobacterial pulmonary disease in frail women, usually elderly, often with pectus excavatum or scoliosis. Features include pulmonary infiltrates, involvement of the lingual or middle lobe, and absence of predisposing disease. It is caused primarily by the *Mycobacterium avium* complex and is most commonly seen after age 50 years in white women and women of Asian ancestry. [fr. the main character in Oscar Wilde's play, *Lady Windermere's Fan*]

La•ën•nec cir•rho•sis (lah-ĕ-nek′ sir-ō′sis) Hepatic disorder in which normal liver lobules are replaced by small regeneration nodules, sometimes containing fat, separated by a fairly regular framework of fine fibrous tissue strands (hobnail liver); usually due to chronic alcoholism. Can cause severe impairment of liver function, portal hypertension with ascites and esophageal varices, and life-threatening complications.

la•e•trile (lā′ĕ-tril) An allegedly antineoplastic drug consisting chiefly of amygdalin derived from apricot pits; no beneficial effect has been proven.

♻ **laev-** SYN levo-.

laevo- [Br.] SYN levo-.

laevocardia [Br.] SYN levocardia.

laevodopa [Br.] SYN levodopa.

laevorotation [Br.] SYN levorotation.

laevorotatory [Br.] SYN levorotatory.

La•fo•ra bod•y (lah-fō′rah bod′ē) An intraneural intracytoplasmic inclusion body composed of acid mucopolysaccharides, seen in familial myoclonus epilepsy.

la•ge•na, pl. **la•ge•nae** (lă-jē′nă, -jē-nē) **1.** SYN cupular cecum of the cochlear duct. **2.** One of the three parts of the membranous labyrinth of the internal ear of lower vertebrates; in mammals, the lagena becomes the cochlea. [L. flask]

lag•ging (lag′ing) Retarded or diminished ventilatory movement of the affected side of the chest due to pleural disease with muscle splinting or collapse of a lung.

♻ **-lagnia, -lagny** Combining forms denoting an improper sexual predilection.

lake (lāk) **1.** [TA] A small collection of fluid. SYN lacus. **2.** To cause blood plasma to become red as a result of the release of hemoglobin from erythrocytes. SEE ALSO lacuna. SEE ALSO lacuna. [A.S. *lacu,* fr. L. *lacus,* lake]

La•ki-Lor•and fac•tor (lā′kē lōr′and fak′tŏr) SYN factor XIII.

la•ky (lā′kē) Pertaining to the transparent bright red appearance of blood serum or plasma that develops as a result of hemoglobins released from destroyed red blood cells.

La Le•che League In•ter•na•tion•al (LLLI) (lă lā′chā lēg in′tĕr-nash′ŏ-năl) An organization that vigorously promotes the advantages of breast-feeding over other methods of nutrition and alimentation in the infant.

♻ **-lalia** Combining form denoting a speech disorder.

♻ **lal-, lalio-, lalo-** Combining forms pertaining to speech or speech organs.

lal•ling (lal′ing) A form of stammering in which the speech is almost unintelligible. [G. *laleō,* to chatter]

lal•o•che•zi•a (lal′ŏ-kē′zē-ă) Emotional discharge gained by uttering indecent or filthy words. [G. *lalia,* speech, + *chezō,* to relieve oneself]

la•lo•ple•gi•a (lal′ŏ-plē′jē-ă) Paralysis of the muscles concerned in the mechanism of speech. [G. *lalia,* speech, + *plēgē,* a stroke]

La•maze meth•od (lĕ-mahz′ meth′ŏd) A technique of psychoprophylactic preparation for childbirth, designed to minimize the pain of labor.

lamb•da (Λ, λ) (lam′dă) **1.** The 11th letter of the Greek alphabet. **2.** Symbol (λ) for Avogadro number; wavelength; radioactive constant; Ostwald solubility coefficient; molar conductivity of an electrolyte (Λ). **3.** CHEMISTRY the position of a substituent located on the 11th atom from the carboxyl or other functional group (λ). **4.** The craniometric point at the junction of the sagittal and lambdoid sutures.

lamb•doid (lam′doyd) Resembling the Greek letter lambda, as does the lambdoid suture. [lambda + G. *eidos,* resemblance]

lamb•doid su•ture (lam′doyd sū′chŭr) Line of union between the occipital and the parietal bones.

Lam•bert law (lam′bĕrt law) **1.** Each layer of equal thickness absorbs an equal fraction of the light that traverses it. **2.** The illumination of a surface on which the light falls normally from a point source is inversely proportional to the square of the distance from the source.

Lam•bl ex•cres•cence (lam′bĕl eks-kres′ĕns) A small pointed projection from the edge of an aortic cusp, of unknown significance.

Lam•bli•a in•tes•ti•na•lis (lam′blē-ă in-tes-ti-nā′lis) Old term for *Giardia lamblia,* still frequently used, especially by protozoologists in Russia and other countries in Eastern Europe and Central Asia.

lam•bli•a•sis (lam-blī′ă-sis) SYN giardiasis.

Lam•bri•nu•di op•er•a•tion (lam-bri-nū′dē op-ĕr-ā′shŭn) A form of triple arthrodesis done in such a manner as to prevent foot-drop such as occurs in poliomyelitis.

la•mel•la, pl. **la•mel•lae** (lă-mel′ă, -mel′ē) **1.** A thin sheet or layer, such as occurs in compact bone. **2.** A preparation in the form of a medicated gelatin disc, used as a means of making local applications to the conjunctiva in place of solutions. [L. dim. of *lamina,* plate, leaf]

la•mel•lar (lă-mel′ăr) **1.** Arranged in thin plates or scales. **2.** Relating to lamellae.

la•mel•lar bone (lă-mel′ăr bōn) The normal type of adult mammalian bone, whether cancellous or compact, composed of parallel lamellae in the former and concentric lamellae in the latter.

la•mel•lar cat•a•ract (lă-mel′ăr kat′ăr-akt) A cataract in which the opacity is limited to the cortex. SYN zonular cataract.

lam•el•lat•ed cor•pus•cles (lam′ĕ-lāt′ĕd kōr′pŭs-ĕlz) Small oval bodies in the skin of the fingers, in the mesentery, tendons, and elsewhere, formed of concentric layers of connective tissue with a soft core in which the axon of a nerve fiber runs, splitting up into a number of fibrils that terminate in bulbous enlargements; they are sensitive to pressure. SYN corpuscula lamellosa [TA], pacinian corpuscles.

la•mel•li•po•di•um, pl. **la•mel•li•po•di•a** (lă-mel′i-pō′dē-ŭm, -ă) A cytoplasmic veil produced on all sides of migrating polymorphonuclear leukocytes.

lam•i•na, pl. **lam•i•nae** (lam′i-nă, -nē) Thin plate or flat layer. SEE ALSO layer, stratum. [L]

lam•i•na ar•cus ver•te•brae (lam′i-nă ahr′ kŭs vĕr′tĕ-brē) [TA] SYN lamina of vertebral arch.

lam•i•na ba•sa•lis cho•roi•de•ae (lam′i-nă bā-sā′lis kō-roy′dē-ē) [TA] The transparent, nearly structureless inner layer of the choroid in contact with the pigmented layer of the retina. SYN basal layer of choroid, Bruch membrane, vitreous lamella, vitreous membrane (3).

lam•i•na cho•roid•o•ca•pil•la•ris (lam′i-nă kō-roy′dō-kap-i-lā′ris) [TA] SYN choriocapillary layer.

lam•i•na cri•bro•sa os•sis eth•moi•da•lis (lam′i-nă kri-brō′să ŏs′is eth-moy-dā′lis) [TA] SYN cribriform plate of ethmoid bone.

lam•i•na cri•bro•sa scler•ae (lam′i-nă krib-rō′să sklĕr′ē) The portion of the sclera through which pass the fibers of the optic nerve.

lam•i•na fus•ca of scle•ra (lam′i-nă fŭs′kă skler′ă) An exceedingly delicate layer of loose, pigmented connective tissue on the inner surface of the sclera, connecting it with the choroid.

lam•i•na•gram (lam′i-nă-gram) An image made by laminagraphy.

lam•i•na•graph (lam′i-nă-graf) A device for laminagraphy; a laminagram.

lam•i•na of lens (lam′i-nă lenz) One of a series of concentric layers composed of the lens fibers that make up the substance of the lens.

lam•i•na lim•i•tans an•te•ri•or cor•ne•ae (lam′i-nă lim′i-tanz an-tēr′ē-ŏr kōr′nē-ē) SYN anterior elastic lamina of cornea.

lam•i•na lim•i•tans pos•ter•i•or cor•ne•ae (lam′i-nă lim′i-tanz pos-tēr′ē-ŏr kōr′nē-ē) SYN posterior elastic lamina of cornea.

lam•i•na me•dul•la•ris me•di•a•lis (lam′i-nă med-yū-lā′ris mē-dē-ā′lis) [TA] SEE medullary laminae of thalamus.

lam•i•na me•dul•la•ris me•di•a•lis nu•cle•i len•ti•for•mis (lam′i-nă med-yū-lā′ris mē-dē-ā′ lis nū′klē-ī len-ti-fōr′mis) [TA] SYN medial medullary lamina of lentiform nucleus.

lam•i•na of mes•en•ce•phal•ic tec•tum (lam′i-nă mes-en-se-fal′ik tek′tŭm) The roofplate of the mesencephalon formed by the quadrigeminal bodies. SYN tectum of midbrain.

lam•i•na mul•ti•for•mis (lam′i-nă mŭl-ti-fōr′ mis) [TA] SYN multiform layer of cerebral cortex.

lam•i•na pro•pri•a (lam′i-nă prō′prē-ă) The layer of connective tissue underlying the epithelium of a mucous membrane.

lam•i•nar (lam′i-năr) **1.** Arranged in plates or laminae. **2.** Relating to any lamina.

lam•i•nar flow (lam′i-năr flō) The relative motion of elements of a fluid along smooth parallel paths, which occurs at lower values of Reynolds number.

lam•i•nar flow hood (lam′i-năr flō hud) An enclosure in which air flow is directed so as to prevent contamination of sterile materials by airborne organisms. SYN hood.

lam•i•nat•ed clot (lam′i-nā-tĕd klot) A clot formed in a succession of layers such as occurs in an aneurysm.

lam•i•nat•ed ep•i•the•li•um (lam′i-nā-tĕd ep′ i-thē′lē-ŭm) SYN stratified epithelium.

lam•i•na of ver•te•bral arch (lam′i-nă vĕr′tĕ-brăl ahrch) The flattened posterior portion of the vertebral arch extending between the pedicles and the midline, forming the dorsal wall of the vertebral foramen; the spinous process extends from the midline junction of right and left laminae. SYN lamina arcus vertebrae [TA], neurapophysis.

lam•i•na vis•ce•ra•lis (lam′i-nă vis-ĕr-ā′lis) [TA] SYN visceral layer.

lam•i•nec•to•my (lam′i-nek′tŏ-mē) Excision of a vertebral lamina; commonly used to denote removal of the posterior arch. [L. *lamina*, layer, + G. *ektomē*, excision]

lam•i•ni•tis (lam′i-nī′tis) Inflammation of any lamina.

lam•i•nog•ra•phy, lam•i•nag•ra•phy (lam′i-nog′ră-fē, lam′i-nag′ră-fē) Radiographic technique in which the images of tissues above and below the plane of interest are blurred out by movement of the x-ray tube and film holder, to show a specific area more clearly. SEE ALSO tomography. [lamina + G. *graphē*, a writing]

lam•i•not•o•my (lam-i-not′ŏ-mē) An operation on one or more vertebral laminae. SYN rachiotomy. [L. *lamina*, layer, + G. *tomē*, incision]

lamp (lamp) Illuminating device; source of light. SEE ALSO light.

Lan•cas•ter red-green test (lan′kas-tĕr red-green′ test) A determination to measure ocular deviations in various fields of gaze in adult patients with acquired strabismus and diplopia by placing a red filter over the right eye and a green filter over the left eye followed by alignment by the patient of a red or green light with light of opposite color projected by the examiner.

lance (lans) **1.** To incise a part, as an abscess or boil. **2.** A lancet. [L. *lancea*, a slender spear]

Lance•field clas•si•fi•ca•tion (lans′fēld klas′ i-fi-kā′shŭn) A serologic classification dividing hemolytic streptococci into groups (A–O) based on precipitation test results for group-specific carbohydrate substances.

lan•cet (lan′set) A surgical knife with a short, wide, sharp-pointed, two-edged blade. [Fr. *lancette*]

lan•ci•nat•ing (lan′si-nāt-ing) Denoting a sharp cutting or tearing pain. [L. *lancino,* pp. *-atus,* to tear]

Lan•ci•si sign (lan-chē′sē sīn) A large systolic jugular venous wave caused by tricuspid regurgitation replacing the normal negative systolic trough ("x" descent).

Lan•dau-Kleff•ner syn•drome (lan′dow-klef′nĕr sin′drōm) Childhood disorder characterized by generalized and psychomotor seizures associated with acquired aphasia; multifocal spikes and spike and wave discharges in the electroencephalogram. SYN acquired epileptic aphasia.

Lan•dau re•flex (lan′dow rē′fleks) Seen in infants aged 3 months–2 years. An extensor response of the neck, spine, and limbs, elicited by lifting the thorax of the prone subject. Extensor muscle tone ceases when the head is flexed passively.

Lan•dol•fi sign (lan-dol′fē sīn) In aortic insufficiency, systolic contraction and diastolic dilation of the pupil.

Lan•dry pa•ral•y•sis, Lan•dry syn•drome (lan′drē păr-al′i-sis, sin′drōm) SYN Guillain-Barré syndrome.

land•scape e•col•o•gy (land′skāp ē-kol′ŏ-jē) The study of the reciprocal effects of spatial pattern on ecologic processes.

Lane band (lān band) A congenital band on the distal ileum that may extend into the right iliac fossa causing stasis. SYN Lane kink.

Lane kink (lān kingk) SYN Lane band.

Lan•gen•beck tri•an•gle (lahng′ĕn-bek trī′ang-gĕl) The area formed by lines drawn from the anterior superior iliac spine to the surface of the greater trochanter and to the surgical neck of the femur; a penetrating wound in this area probably involves the hip joint.

Lan•gen•dorff meth•od (lahng′ĕn-dōrf meth′ŏd) Perfusion of the isolated mammalian heart by carrying fluid under pressure into the sectioned aorta, and thus into the coronary system.

Lan•ger•hans cell his•ti•o•cy•to•sis (lahng′er-hahnz sel his′tē-ō-sī-tō′sis) A set of closely related disorders unified by a common proliferating element, the Langerhans cell. Three overlapping clinical syndromes are recognized: a single site disease (eosinophilic granuloma), a multifocal unisystem process (Hand-Schüller-Christian syndrome), and a multifocal, multisystem histiocytosis (Letterer-Siwe syndrome.) Formerly this process was known as histiocytosis X. See this page.

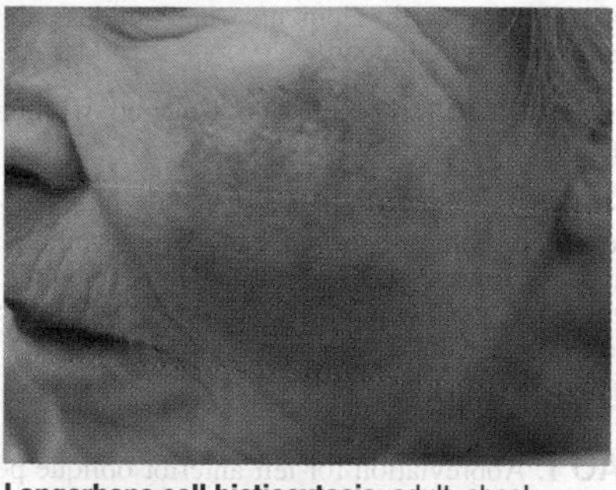

Langerhans cell histiocytosis: adult, cheek

Lan•ger•hans cells (lahng′er-hahnz selz) **1.** Dendritic clear cells in the epidermis containing distinctive granules but lacking tonofilaments, melanosomes, and desmosomes; they carry surface receptors for immunoglobulin (Fc) and complement (C3), and are believed to be antigen-fixing and processing cells of monocytic origin; active participants in cutaneous delayed hypersensitivity. **2.** Cells seen in eosinophilic granuloma and lymphoma of the lungs.

Lan•ger-Sal•di•no syn•drome (lang′ĕr-sal-dē′nō sin′drōm) SYN achondrogenesis type II.

Lang•hans cells (lahng′hahnz selz) **1.** Multinucleated giant cells seen in tuberculosis and other granulomatous diseases; the nuclei are arranged in an arciform manner at the periphery of the cells. SYN Langhans-type giant cells. **2.** SYN cytotrophoblastic cells.

Lang•hans-type gi•ant cells (lahng′hahnz-tīp gī′ănt selz) SYN Langhans cells (1).

lan•guage (lang′gwăj) The use of spoken, manual, written, and other symbols to express, represent, or receive communication. [L. *lingua*]

lan•guage board (lang′gwăj bōrd) SYN communication board.

lan•guage de•lay (lang′gwăj dĕ-lā′) In pediatrics and SLP, denotes a condition in which a child has not developed language skills at an age-appropriate level.

lano- Combining form meaning wool.

lan•o•lin (lan′ŏ-lin) SYN adeps lanae. [L. *lana,* wool, + *oleum,* oil]

lan•tha•nides (lan′thă-nīdz) Those elements with atomic numbers 57–71 that closely resemble one another chemically and were formerly difficult to differentiate. [*lanthanum,* first element of the series]

lan•tha•num (La) (lan′thă-nŭm) A metallic element, atomic no. 57, atomic wt. 138.9055; first of the rare earth elements (lanthanides). [G. *lanthanō,* to lie hidden]

la•nu•gi•nous (lă-nū′ji-nŭs) Covered with lanugo.

la•nu•go (lă-nū′gō) Fine, soft, lightly pigmented fetal hair with minute shafts and large papillae; it appears toward the end of the third month of gestation. SYN lanugo hair. [L. down, wooliness, from *lana,* wool]

la•nu•go hair (lă-nū′gō hār) SYN lanugo.

LAO 1. Abbreviation for left anterior oblique position. **2.** RADIOGRAPHY abbreviation used in assessment of the size of the left atrium and ventricle. **3.** Radiographic position in which the left anterior side of the body part being examined is closest to the film surface.

laparo- Prefix meaning the loins (less properly, the abdomen in general). [G. *lapara,* flank, loins]

lap•a•ro•cele (lap′ă-rō-sēl) SYN abdominal hernia. [laparo- + G. *kēlē,* hernia]

lap•a•ro•en•do•scop•ic (lap′ă-rō-en′dō-skop′ik) Having to do with the introduction of a laparoscope into the abdominal cavity for a variety of intracavitary procedures.

lap•a•ror•rha•phy (lap′ă-rōr′ă-fē) SYN celiorrhaphy.

lap•a•ro•scope (lap′ă-rŏ-skōp) An endoscope for examining the peritoneal cavity. SYN peritoneoscope. [laparo- + G. *skopeō,* to view]

lap•a•ro•scop•ic-as•sis•ted vag•i•nal hys•ter•ec•to•my (lap′ă-rō-skop′ik-ă-sist′ĕd vaj′i-năl his′tĕr-ek′tŏ-mē) Procedure in which the ovarian pedicle, broad ligament, and uterosacral ligaments are surgically severed using laparoscopic instruments and the procedure completed through a colpotomy done in the typical fashion.

lap•a•ro•scop•ic cho•le•cys•tot•o•my (lap′ă-rō-skop′ik kō′lĕ-sis-tot′ŏ-mē) Minimally invasive surgical technique for removal of the gallbladder that uses a laparoscope for visualization of the gallbladder and placement of instruments into the abdominal cavity through trocars. See this page.

lap•a•ro•scop•ic knot (lap′ă-rō-skop′ik not) Although placed intracorporally through a laparoscopic instrument, such a knot may be tied extracorporally and passed into the body through a cannula, or the knot may be both placed and tied intracorporally.

lap•a•ro•scop•ic ne•phrec•to•my (lap′ă-rō-skop′ik nef-rek′tŏ-mē) Removal of a kidney by percutaneous endoscopic technique.

lap•a•ro•scop•ic u•ter•o•sa•cral nerve ab•la•tion (lap′ă-rō-skop′ik yū′tĕr-ō-sā′krăl nĕrv ab-lā′shŭn) Laparoscopic transection using a laser (usually KTP or argon) of the uterosacral nerves for the treatment of primary dysmenorrhea.

lap•a•ros•co•py (lap′ă-ros′kŏ-pē) Examination of the contents of the peritoneum with a laparoscope. The abdomen is first inflated with carbon dioxide, and the laparoscope passed through a small incision in the abdominal wall. The device is frequently used to view the female reproductive organs, in particular where endometriosis or pelvic inflammatory disease is suspected. Fitted with grasping and cutting tools, the laparoscope

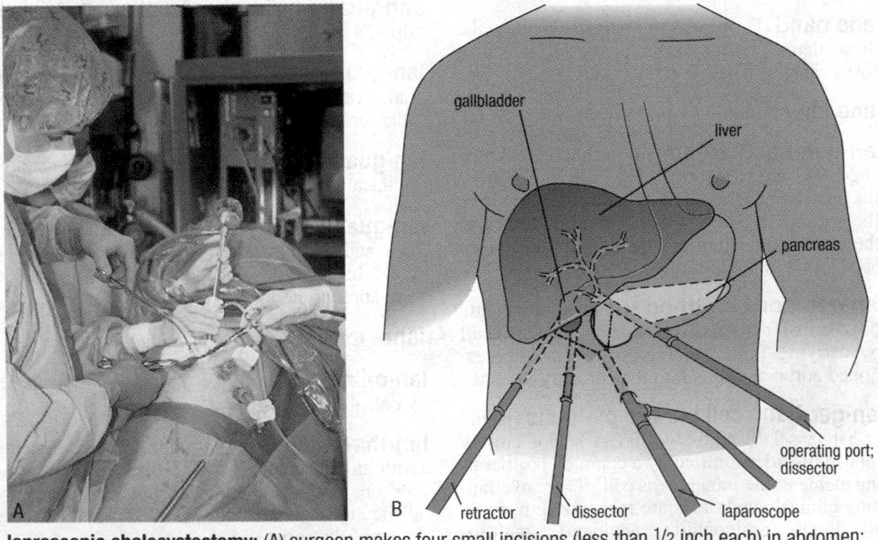

laproscopic cholecystectomy: (A) surgeon makes four small incisions (less than 1/2 inch each) in abdomen; (B) and inserts laparoscope with a miniature camera through umbilical incision can perform minor surgery and take tissue samples for biopsy. SEE ALSO peritoneoscopy.

lap•a•rot•o•my (lap'ă-rot'ŏ-mē) **1.** Incision into the loin. **2.** SYN celiotomy. [laparo- + G. *tomē,* incision]

lap•a•rot•o•my pad (lap'ă-rot'ŏ-mē pad) A compress made from several layers of gauze folded into a rectangular shape; used as a sponge or packing material in surgery. SYN abdominal pad.

La•picque law (la-pēk' law) The chronaxie is inversely proportional to the diameter of an axon.

lap•i•ni•za•tion (lap'i-nī-zā'shŭn) Serial passage of a virus or vaccine in rabbits. [Fr. *lapin,* rabbit]

lap•i•nized (lap'i-nīzd) Denoting viruses that have been adapted to develop in rabbits by serial transfers in this species. [Fr. *lapin,* rabbit]

La•place for•ceps (lah-plahs' fōr'seps) A forceps for approximating intestines during surgical anastomosis.

La•place law (lah-plahs' law) The equilibrium relationship between transmural pressure difference (ΔP), wall tension (T), and radius of curvature (R) in a concave surface; for a sphere: $\Delta P = 2T/R$; for a cylinder: $\Delta P = T/R$.

la•quer stain for al•co•hol•ic hy•a•lin (lak'ĕr stān al'kŏ-hol'ik hī'ă-lin) A combination of Altmann aniline-acid fuchsin stain with a Masson trichrome stain, which, on a gray-brown background, stains alcoholic hyalin red, collagen green, and nuclei brown.

large cal•o•rie (C) (lahrj kal'ŏr-ē) SYN kilocalorie.

large cell car•ci•no•ma (lahrj sel kahr'si-nō'mă) An anaplastic carcinoma, particularly bronchogenic, composed of cells that are much larger than those in oat cell carcinoma of the lung.

large cell lym•pho•ma (lahrj sel lim-fō'mă) Any such neoplasm composed of large mononuclear cells of undetermined type.

large for ges•ta•tion•al age (LGA) (lahrj jes'tā-shŭn-ăl āj) Infant whose birth weight falls above the ninetieth percentile. Can be due to a range of factors including heredity and maternal hyperglycemia.

large in•tes•tine (lahrj in-tes'tin) The portion of the digestive tube extending from the ileocecal valve to the anus; it comprises the cecum, colon, rectum, and anal canal.

La•ron-type dwarf•ism (lah-ron'-tīp dwōrf'izm) A disorder associated with deficiency of somatomedin C (insulinlike growth factor I) or abnormalities in receptor activity.

La•ro•yenne op•er•a•tion (lah-rō-yen' op-ĕr-ā'shŭn) Puncture of Douglas pouch to evacuate the pus and to secure drainage in cases of pelvic suppuration.

Lar•rey am•pu•ta•tion (lah-rā' amp'yū-tā'shŭn) Amputation at the shoulder joint.

Lar•son-Jo•hans•son dis•ease (lahr'sŏn-yō-hahn'sŏn di-zēz') Inflammation or partial avulsion of the lower pole of the patella due to traction forces. SEE ALSO Osgood-Schlatter disease.

lar•va, pl. **lar•vae** (lahr'vă, -vē) **1.** Developmental stage or stages of an insect or helminth. **2.** The second stage in the life cycle of a tick; the stage in which it hatches from the egg and, following engorgement, molts into the nymph. **3.** The young of fishes or amphibians that often differ in appearance from the adult. [L. a mask]

lar•va cur•rens (lahr'vă kŭr'enz) Cutaneous larva migrans caused by rapidly moving larvae of *Strongyloides stercoralis* (up to 10 cm/hour), typically extending from the anal area down the upper thighs and observed as a rapidly progressing linear urticarial trail. [L. *larva,* mask + *currens,* racing]

lar•val (lahr'văl) **1.** Relating to larvae. **2.** SYN larvate.

lar•va mi•grans (lahr'vă mī'granz) A larval animal, typically a nematode, which wanders for a time in the host tissues but does not develop to the adult stage; this usually occurs in abnormal hosts that inhibit normal development of the parasite. [L. *larva,* mask, + *migro,* to transfer, migrate]

lar•vate (lahr'vāt) Masked or concealed; applied to a disease with undeveloped, absent, or atypical symptoms. SYN larval (2). [L. *larva,* mask]

lar•vi•cid•al (lahr'vi-sī'dăl) Destructive to larvae.

lar•vi•cide (lahr'vi-sīd) An agent that kills larvae. [larva + L. *caedo,* to kill]

la•ryn•ge•al (lă-rin'jē-ăl) Relating in any way to the larynx.

i **la•ryn•ge•al mask** (lă-rin'jē-ăl mask) Oral airway with an inflatable cuff at its lower end that forms a seal above the laryngeal inlet rather than within the larynx. Used in prehospital care as an airway adjunct instead of an endotracheal tube. See page 870. SYN laryngeal mask airway.

la•ryn•ge•al mask air•way (LMA) (lă-rin'jē-ăl mask ār'wā) SYN laryngeal mask.

la•ryn•ge•al pap•il•lo•ma•to•sis (lă-rin'jē-ăl pap'i-lō'mă-tō'sis) Multiple squamous papillomas of the larynx in young children, usually due to infection by the human papillomavirus, which may be transmitted at birth from maternal condylomata.

la•ryn•ge•al prom•i•nence (lă-rin'jē-ăl prom'

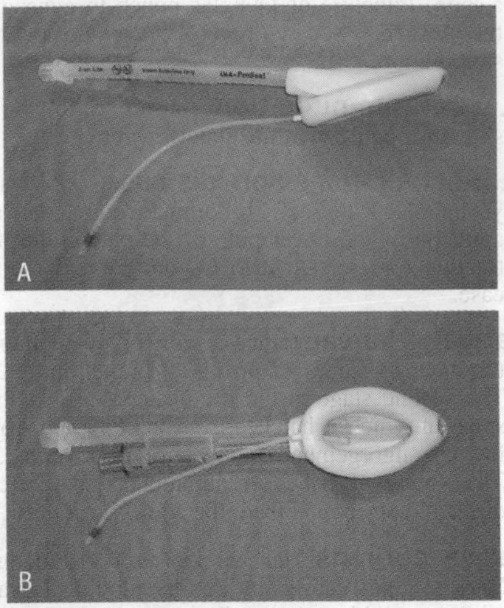

laryngeal mask: deflated. (A) side view; (B) front view

i-nĕns) The projection on the anterior portion of the neck formed by the thyroid cartilage of the larynx; serves as an external indication of the level of the fifth cervical vertebra.

la·ryn·ge·al ste·no·sis (lă-rin′jē-ăl stĕ-nō′sis) Narrowing or stricture of any or all areas of the larynx; may be congenital or acquired.

la·ryn·ge·al syn·co·pe (lă-rin′jē-ăl sing′kŏ-pē) A paroxysmal neurosis characterized by attacks of coughing, with unusual sensations, as of tickling, in the throat, followed by a brief period of unconsciousness.

lar·yn·ge·al ven·tri·cle (lă-rin′jē-ăl ven′tri-kĕl) The recess in each lateral wall of the larynx between the vestibular and vocal folds and into which the laryngeal sacculus opens. SYN Morgagni sinus (3).

la·ryn·ge·al web (lă-rin′jē-ăl web) Congenital anomaly consisting of mucous membrane–covered connective tissue between the vocal cords located ventrally and extending dorsally for varying distances; it causes airway obstruction and hoarse cry in the newborn.

la·ryn·gec·to·my (lar′in-jek′tŏ-mē) Excision of the larynx. [laryngo- + G. *ektomē,* excision]

la·ryn·ges (lă-rin′jēz) Plural of larynx. [L.]

lar·yn·gis·mus (lar′in-jiz′mŭs) A spasmodic narrowing or closure of the rima glottidis. [L. fr. G. *larynx,* + *-ismos,* -ism]

lar·yn·gis·mus stri·du·lus (lar′in-jiz′mŭs strid′yū-lŭs) A spasmodic closure of the glottis, lasting a few seconds, followed by a noisy inspiration. Cf. laryngitis stridulosa. SYN pseudocroup.

lar·yn·git·ic (lar′in-jit′ik) Relating to or caused by laryngitis.

lar·yn·gi·tis (lar′in-jī′tis) Inflammation of the mucous membrane of the larynx; accompanied by edema of the vocal cords, which produces hoarseness. [laryngo- + G. *-itis,* inflammation]

lar·yn·gi·tis sic·ca (lar′in-jī′tis sik′ă) Laryngitis characterized by dryness and crusting of the mucous membrane of the larynx.

lar·yn·gi·tis stri·du·lo·sa (lar′in-jī′tis stri-dyū-lō′să) Catarrhal inflammation of the larynx in children, accompanied by night attacks of spasmodic closure of the glottis, causing inspiratory stridor.

♻**laryngo-, laryng-** Combining forms denoting the larynx. [G. *larynx*]

la·ryn·go·cele (lă-ring′gō-sēl) An air sac communicating with the larynx through the ventricle, often bulging outward into the tissue of the neck, especially during coughing. [laryngo- + G. *kēlē,* hernia]

la·ryn·go·fis·sure (lă-ring′gō-fish′ŭr) Operative opening into the larynx, generally through the midline, commonly done for the excision of early carcinoma or the correction of laryngostenosis. SYN thyrotomy (2).

lar·yn·gol·o·gy (lar′ing-gol′ŏ-jē) The branch of medical science concerned with the larynx; the specialty of diseases of the larynx. [laryngo- + G. *logos,* study]

la·ryn·go·ma·la·ci·a (lă-ring′gō-mă-lā′shē-ă) The presence of soft laryngeal cartilage, especially of the epiglottis, in infants, resulting in inspiratory stridor. [laryngo- + G. *malakia,* a softness]

la·ryn·go·pa·ral·y·sis (lă-ring′gō-păr-al′i-sis) Paralysis of the laryngeal muscles. SYN laryngoplegia.

la·ryn·go·pha·ryn·ge·al (lă-ring′gō-fă-rin′jē-ăl) Relating to both larynx and pharynx or to the laryngopharynx.

la·ryn·go·phar·yn·gec·to·my (lă-ring′gō-far′in-jek′tŏ-mē) Resection or excision of both larynx and pharynx.

la·ryn·go·phar·yn·ge·us (lă-ring′gō-făr-in′jē-ŭs) SYN inferior constrictor muscle of pharynx.

la·ryn·go·phar·yn·gi·tis (lă-ring′gō-far-in-jī′tis) Inflammation of the larynx and pharynx.

la·ryn·go·phar·ynx (lă-ring′gō-far′ingks) The part of the pharynx lying below the aperture of the larynx and behind the larynx; it extends from the vestibule of the larynx to the esophagus at the level of the inferior border of the cricoid cartilage. SYN hypopharynx.

la·ryn·go·plas·ty (lă-ring′gō-plas-tē) Reparative or plastic surgery of the larynx. [laryngo- + G. *plassō,* to form]

la·ryn·go·ple·gi·a (lă-ring′gō-plē′jē-ă) SYN laryngoparalysis. [laryngo- + G. *plēgē,* stroke]

la·ryn·gop·to·sis (lă-ring′gop-tō′sis) An abnormally low position of the larynx; may occur as a normal variant at birth or with aging. [laryngo- + G. *ptōsis,* a falling]

la·ryn·go·scope (lă-ring′gō-skōp) Any of several types of hollow tubes, equipped with electric lighting, used in examining or operating on the interior of the larynx through the mouth. [laryngo- + G. *skopeō,* to inspect]

la·ryn·go·scop·ic (lă-ring′gō-skop′ik) Relating to laryngoscopy.

lar·yn·gos·co·py (lar′in-gos′kŏ-pē) Inspection of the larynx by means of the laryngoscope.

la·ryn·go·spasm (lă-ring′gō-spazm) Spasmodic closure of the glottic aperture.

la·ryn·go·ste·no·sis (lă-ring′gō-stĕ-nō′sis) Stricture or narrowing of the lumen of the larynx. [laryngo- + G. *stenōsis,* a narrowing]

lar·yn·gos·to·my (lar′in-gos′tŏ-mē) The establishment of a permanent opening from the neck into the larynx. [laryngo- + G. *stoma,* mouth]

lar·yn·got·o·my (lar′in-got′ŏ-mē) A surgical incision of the larynx. [laryngo- + G. *tomē,* incision]

la·ryn·go·tra·che·al (lă-ring′gō-trā′kē-ăl) Relating to both larynx and trachea.

la·ryn·go·tra·che·al di·ver·tic·u·lum (lă-ring′gō-trā′kē-ăl dī′vĕr-tik′yū-lŭm) The outgrowth from the caudal end of the floor of the pharynx that gives rise to the larynx, laryngotracheal tube, and the esophagus.

la·ryn·go·tra·che·al tube (lă-ring′gō-trā-kē-ăl tūb) The endodermal tube that forms when the laryngotracheal diverticulum is divided by the tracheoesophageal fold; its upper end forms the larynx and its middle, the trachea.

la·ryn·go·tra·che·i·tis (lă-ring′gō-trā′kē-ī′tis) Inflammation of both larynx and trachea.

la·ryn·go·tra·che·o·bron·chi·tis (lă-ring′gō-trā′kē-ō-brong-kī′tis) An acute respiratory infection involving the larynx, trachea, and bronchi. SEE croup.

la·ryn·go·trach·e·o·e·so·pha·ge·al cleft (lar-ing′gō-trā′kē-ō-ē′sō-fā′jē-ăl kleft) Absence of fusion of the musculature or cricoid cartilaginous laminae of varying severity: **type 1**, submucous cleft of the interarytenoid muscles (known also as occult posterior laryngeal cleft or submucous laryngeal cleft); **type 2**, partial cricoid cleft (known also as partial posterior laryngeal cleft); **type 3**, total cricoid cleft (known also as laryngotracheoesophageal cleft or total cricoid cleft); and **type 4**, extension of the cleft into the esophagus. SYN laryngotracheo-oesophageal cleft.

laryngotracheo-oesophageal cleft [Br.] SYN laryngotracheoesophageal cleft.

lar·yn·go·tra·che·o·plas·ty (lă-ring′gō-trā′kē-ō-plas′tē) Operation to repair subglottic stenosis.

lar·ynx, pl. **la·ryn·ges** (lar′ingks, lă-rin′jēz) [TA] The organ of voice production, which also serves a protective function for the airway; the part of the respiratory tract between the pharynx and the trachea: it consists of a framework of cartilages and elastic membranes housing the vocal folds and the muscles that control the position and tension of these elements. See this page. [Mod. L. fr. G.]

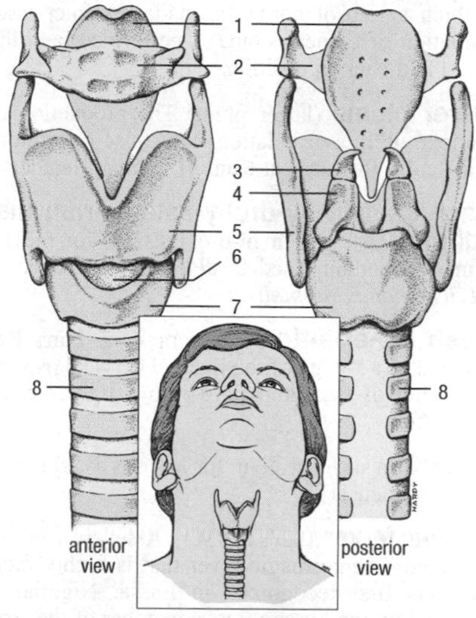

laryngeal cartilages: (1) epiglottis, (2) hyoid bone, (3) corniculate cartilage, (4) arytenoid cartilage, (5) thyroid cartilage, (6) cricothyroid ligament, (7) cricoid cartilage, (8) trachea

lase (lāz) To cut, divide, or dissolve a substance, or to treat an anatomic structure, with a laser beam. [Backformation from laser (q.v.)]

La·sègue sign (lah-seg′ sīn) When a subject is supine with hip flexed and knee extended, dorsiflexion of the ankle causing pain or muscle spasm in the posterior thigh indicates lumbar root or sciatic nerve irritation.

La·sègue syn·drome (lah-seg′ sin′drōm) In conversion hysteria, inability to move an anesthetic limb when the eyes are closed (i.e., without visualization).

LASEK (lā′sek) Acronym for laser-assisted epithelial keratoplasty.

la•ser (lā′zĕr) **1.** (noun) Device that concentrates high energies into an intense narrow beam of nondivergent monochromatic electromagnetic radiation; used in microsurgery, cauterization, and for a variety of diagnostic purposes. **2.** (verb) To treat a structure with a laser beam. [acronym coined from *l*ight *a*mplification by *s*timulated *e*mission of *r*adiation]

la•ser-as•sis•ted ep•i•the•li•al ker•a•to•plas•ty (lā′sĕr ă-sis′tĕd ep′i-thē′lē-ăl ker′ă-tō-plas-tē) Refractive surgery in which the epithelial layer of the cornea is removed, the excimer laser carves the corneal tissue into the desired refraction, after which the epithelial layer is replaced.

la•ser-as•sis•ted in si•tu ker•a•to•mi•leu•sis (LASIK) (lā′zĕr-ă-sis′tĕd in sī′tū ker′ă-tō-mī-lū′sis) A refractive procedure to correct myopia or hyperopia, with or without astigmatism in which a flap of cornea is made, excimer laser ablation of corneal stoma is performed, and the flap laid back in position.

la•ser plume (lā′zĕr plūm) The production of smoke with laser ablation; can cause respiratory difficulty for surgical team. [L. *pluma,* feather]

Lash ca•sein hy•drol•y•sate-se•rum me•di•um (lash kā′sēn hī-drol′i-sāt-sēr′ŭm mē′dē-ŭm) A medium used to detect the presence of *Trichomonas vaginalis.*

Lash op•er•a•tion (lash op-ĕr-ā′shŭn) Removal of a wedge of the internal cervical os with suturing of the internal os into a tighter canal structure.

LASIK (lā′sik) Acronym for laser-assisted in situ keratomileusis.

Las•sa fe•ver (lah′să fē′vĕr) A severe form of epidemic hemorrhagic fever that is highly fatal. It was first recognized in Lassa, Nigeria; is caused by the Lassa virus, a member of the Arenaviridae family, and characterized by high fever, sore throat, severe muscle aches, rash with hemorrhages, headache, abdominal pain, vomiting, and diarrhea. The multimammate rat *Mastomys natalensis* serves as a reservoir, but person-to-person transmission is also common.

Las•sa vi•rus (lah′să vī′rŭs) An arenavirus that causes Lassa fever, an acute febrile disease with a high mortality.

las•si•tude (las′i-tūd) A sense of weariness. [L. *lassitudo,* fr. *lassus,* weary]

la•tah (lah′tah) One of the pathologic startle syndromes. A culture-bound disorder characterized by an exaggerated physical response to being startled or to unexpected suggestion, those afflicted involuntarily uttering cries or executing movements in response to command or in imitation of what they hear or see in others. SEE ALSO jumping disease. [Malay, ticklish]

late au•di•to•ry-e•voked re•sponse (lāt aw′di-tōr-ē-ē-vōkt′ rĕ-spons′) Reaction of the auditory cortex to acoustic stimulation.

late dump•ing syn•drome (lāt dŭmp′ing sin′drōm) Disorder seen in patients who have had ablation of the pyloric sphincter mechanism; associated with flushing, sweating, dizziness, weakness, and vasomotor collapse 2–3 hours after a meal; caused by hypoglycemia resulting from the rapid absorption of a large carbohydrate load, which then stimulates insulin release. SEE ALSO dumping syndrome.

late ef•fect (lāt e-fekt′) Physical finding that occurs after onset of an acute illness or injury; generally considered as secondary to the disorder, rather than unrelated.

late lu•te•al phase dys•phor•i•a (lāt lū′tē-ăl fāz dis-fōr′ē-ă) SYN premenstrual syndrome.

la•ten•cy (lā′tĕn-sē) **1.** The state of being latent. **2.** In conditioning, or other behavioral experiments, the period of apparent inactivity between the time the stimulus is presented and the moment a response occurs. **3.** PSYCHOANALYSIS the period of time from approximately age five to puberty.

la•ten•cy phase, la•ten•cy pe•ri•od (lā′tĕn-sē fāz, pēr′ē-ŏd) **1.** PSYCHIATRY according to psychoanalytic personality theory, the period of psychosexual development in children, extending from about age 5 to the beginning of adolescence around age 12, during which the apparent cessation of sexual preoccupation stems from a strong, aggressive blockade of libidinal and sexual impulses in an effort to avoid oedipal relationships; during this phase, boys and girls are inclined to choose friends and join groups of their own sex. **2.** BIOWARFARE interval during which an organism lies dormant.

la•tent (lā′tĕnt) Not manifest; dormant, but potentially discernible. [L. *lateo,* pres. p. *latens* (*-ent-*), to lie hidden]

la•tent al•ler•gy (lā′tĕnt al′ĕr-jē) Allergy that causes no signs or symptoms but can be revealed by means of certain immunologic tests with specific allergens.

la•tent car•ri•er (lā′tĕnt kar′ē-ĕr) A person, typically a prospective parent, bearing the appropriate genotype of a trait (homozygous for recessive, homozygous or heterozygous for dominant, hemizygous or homozygous for X-linked) that manifests the trait only under certain conditions (e.g., age, an environmental insult).

la•tent con•tent (lā′tĕnt kon′tent) The hidden, unconscious meaning of thoughts or actions, especially in dreams or fantasies.

la•tent gout (lā′tĕnt gowt) Hyperuricemia without symptoms of gout; often used synonymously with interval gout.

la•tent hy•per•o•pi•a (lā′tĕnt hī′pĕr-ō′pē-ă) The component of total hyperopia that can be corrected by a physiologic response of the ciliary muscle; can be measured only after administration of a cycloplegic agent.

la•tent im•age (lā′tĕnt im′ăj) The undeveloped image on an exposed x-ray film; it becomes visible after chemical processing.

la•tent learn•ing (lā′tĕnt lĕrn′ing) Learning that is not evident to the observer at the time it occurs, but is inferred from later performance in which learning is more rapid than would be expected without the earlier experience.

la•tent mem•brane pro•tein (lā′tĕnt mem′brān prō′tēn) Gene product of Epstein-Barr virus.

la•tent nys•tag•mus (lā′tĕnt nis-tag′mŭs) Jerk nystagmus that is brought out by covering one eye. The fast phase is always away from the covered eye.

la•tent pe•ri•od (lā′tĕnt pēr′ē-ŏd) **1.** The duration elapsing between the application of a stimulus and the response, e.g., contraction of a muscle. **2.** BIOTERRORISM interval between exposure to a chemical, toxic, or radiologic agent and the first signs or symptoms. **3.** SYN incubation period (1).

la•tent re•flex (lā′tĕnt rē′fleks) A reflex that must be considered normal but usually appears only under some pathologic circumstance that lowers its threshold.

la•tent schiz•o•phre•ni•a (lā′tĕnt skits′ō-frē′nē-ă) A preexisting susceptibility for developing overt schizophrenia under strong emotional stress.

la•tent stage (lā′tĕnt stāj) SYN incubation period (1).

lat•er•ad (lat′ĕr-ad) Toward the side. [L. *latus,* side, + *ad,* to]

i **lat•er•al** (lat′ĕr-ăl) **1.** On the side. **2.** Farther from the median or midsagittal plane. **3.** DENTISTRY a position either right or left of the midsagittal plane. **4.** A radiograph made with the film in the sagittal plane; especially, the second view of a chest series. See page B29. [L. *lateralis,* lateral, fr. *latus,* side]

lat•er•al ab•er•ra•tion (lat′ĕr-ăl ab′ĕr-ā′shŭn) In spheric aberration, the distance between paraxial focus of central rays on the optic axis.

lat•er•al an•te•brach•i•al cu•ta•ne•ous nerve (lat′ĕr-ăl an′tē-brā′kē-al kyū-tā′nē-ŭs nĕrv) SYN lateral cutaneous nerve of forearm.

lat•er•al an•te•ri•or tho•rac•ic nerve (lat′ĕr-ăl an-tēr′ē-ŏr thōr-as′ik nĕrv) SYN lateral pectoral nerve.

lat•er•al ap•er•ture of fourth ven•tri•cle (lat′ĕr-ăl ap′ĕr-chŭr fōrth ven′tri-kĕl) One of the two lateral openings of the fourth ventricle into the subarachnoid space (the lateral cerebellomedullary cistern) at the cerebellopontine angle. SYN apertura lateralis ventriculi quarti [TA].

lat•er•al ar•cu•ate lig•a•ments (lat′ĕr-ăl ahrk′yū-āt lig′ă-mĕnts) A thickening of the fascia of the quadratus lumborum muscle between the transverse process of the first lumbar vertebra and the twelfth rib on either side that gives attachment to a portion of the diaphragm (one of the Haller arches).

lat•er•al ba•sal (bron•cho•pul•mon•ar•y) seg•ment [S IX] (lat′ĕr-ăl bā′săl brong′kō-pul′mŏ-nar-ē seg′mĕnt) Of the four bronchopulmonary segments of the inferior lobes of the right or left lung that contact the diaphragm, the one lying farthest to the right in the right lung, and farthest to the left in the left lung, supplied by the lateral basal segmental bronchi and lateral basal segmental (pulmonary) artery.

lat•er•al bor•der (lat′ĕr-ăl bōr′dĕr) The margin or edge of a structure that is farthest from the midline.

lat•er•al branch•es of ar•ter•y of tu•ber cin•er•e•um (lat′ĕr-ăl branch′ĕz ahr′tĕr-ē tū′bĕr si-nēr′ē-ŭm) Branches arising from the lateral aspect of the artery of tuber cinereum.

lat•er•al branch•es of pon•tine ar•ter•ies (lat′ĕr-ăl branch′ĕz pon′tēn ahr′tĕr-ēz) Longer branches of the basilar artery extending across the inferior surface of the pons to reach the lateral aspects.

lat•er•al car•ti•lage of nose (lat′ĕr-ăl kahr′ti-lăj nōz) The cartilage located in the lateral wall of the nose above the alar cartilage. SYN cartilago nasi lateralis [TA].

lat•er•al ce•re•bral sul•cus (lat′ĕr-ăl ser′ĕ-brăl sŭl′kŭs) The deepest and most prominent of the cortical fissures, extending from the anterior perforated substance first laterally at the deep incisure between the frontal and temporal lobes, then back and slightly upward over the lateral aspect of the cerebral hemisphere, with the superior temporal gyrus as its lower bank, the insula forming its greatly expanded floor. Two short side branches, the ramus anterior and ramus ascendens, divide the inferior frontal gyrus into an orbital part, triangular part, and opercular part.

lat•er•al cir•cum•flex ar•ter•y of thigh (lat′ĕr-ăl sĕr′kŭm-fleks ahr′tĕr-ē thī) SYN lateral circumflex femoral artery.

lat•er•al cir•cum•flex fem•o•ral ar•ter•y (lat′ĕr-ăl sĕr′kŭm-fleks fem′ŏr-ăl ahr′tĕr-ē) *Origin*, profunda femoris; *distribution*, hip joint, thigh muscles; *anastomoses*, medial circumflex femoral, inferior gluteal, superior gluteal. SYN arteria circumflexa femoris lateralis, lateral circumflex artery of thigh, lateral femoral circumflex artery.

lat•er•al col•umn (lat′ĕr-ăl kol′ŭm) A slight protrusion of the gray matter of the spinal cord into the lateral funiculus of either side, especially marked in the thoracic region where it encloses preganglionic motor neurons of the sympathetic division of the autonomic nervous system; it corresponds to the lateral horn appearing in transverse sections of the spinal cord. SEE ALSO gray columns.

lat·er·al con·dyle of fe·mur (lat'ĕr-ăl kon'dīl fē'mŭr) One of the two large rounded articular masses of the distal end of the femur, united anteriorly with its contralabial partner by the patellar surface but separated from it posteriorly and inferiorly by the intercondylar fossa; the lateral condyle is longer than the medial condyle.

lat·er·al cord of brach·i·al plex·us (lat'ĕr-ăl kōrd brā'kē-ăl plek'sŭs) In the brachial plexus, the bundle of nerve fibers formed by the anterior divisions of the superior and middle trunks that lies lateral to the axillary artery. This cord gives off the lateral pectoral nerve and terminates by dividing into the musculocutaneous nerve and the lateral root of the median nerve.

lat·er·al cor·ti·co·spi·nal tract (LCST) (lat'ĕr-ăl kōr'ti-kō-spī'năl trăkt) Contralateral descending motor tract. Upper motor neurons influence the lower either directly or indirectly.

lat·er·al cri·co·ar·y·te·noid mus·cle (lat'ĕr-ăl krī'kō-ar'i-te'noyd mŭs'ĕl) Intrinsic muscle of larynx; *origin*, upper margin of arch of cricoid cartilage; *insertion*, muscular process of arytenoid; *action*, adducts vocal folds (narrows rima glottidis); *nerve supply*, recurrent laryngeal. SYN musculus cricoarytenoideus lateralis.

lat·er·al cu·ne·i·form bone (lat'ĕr-ăl kyū-nē'i-fōrm bōn) A bone of the distal row of the tarsus; it articulates with the intermediate cuneiform, cuboid, navicular, and second, third, and fourth metatarsal bones. SYN wedge bone.

lat·er·al cu·ta·ne·ous nerve of fore·arm (lat'ĕr-ăl kyū-tā'nē-ŭs nĕrv fōr'ahrm) The terminal cutaneous branch of the musculocutaneous nerve, which emerges between biceps brachii and brachialis muscles to supply the skin of the radial side of the forearm. SYN lateral antebrachial cutaneous nerve, nervus cutaneus antebrachii lateralis.

lat·er·al cu·ta·ne·ous nerve of thigh (lat'ĕr-ăl kyū-tā'nē-ŭs nĕrv thī) Arises from the lumbar plexus, conveying fibers from the second and third lumbar nerves, supplies the skin of the anterolateral and lateral surfaces of the thigh. SYN lateral femoral cutaneous nerve, nervus cutaneus femoris lateralis.

lat·er·al ep·i·con·dyle of hu·mer·us (lat'ĕr-ăl ep'i-kon'dīl hyū'mĕr-ŭs) The epicondylus situated at the lateral side of the distal end of the bone.

lat·er·al ep·i·con·dy·li·tis (lat'ĕr-ăl ep'i-kon'di-lī'tis) Tension stress injury to the lateral epicondyle caused by repeated or forceful contraction of the wrist extensors; often seen in those involved in sports that use racquets. SYN lateral humeral epicondylitis, tennis elbow.

lat·er·al fem·o·ral cir·cum·flex ar·ter·y (lat'ĕr-ăl fem'ŏr-ăl sĭr'kŭm-fleks ahr'tĕr-ē) SYN lateral circumflex femoral artery.

lat·er·al fem·o·ral cu·ta·ne·ous nerve (lat'ĕr-ăl fem'ŏr-ăl kyū-tā'nē-us nĕrv) SYN lateral cutaneous nerve of thigh.

lat·er·al folds (lat'ĕr-ăl fōldz) Ventral foldings of the lateral margins of the embryonic disc, the development of which establishes the embryonic body form.

lat·er·al fu·nic·u·lus (lat'ĕr-ăl fyū-nik'yū-lŭs) The lateral white column of the spinal cord between the lines of exit and entrance of the anterior and posterior nerve roots.

lat·er·al ge·nic·u·late bo·dy (lat'ĕr-ăl jĕ-nik'yū-lăt bod'ē) The more lateral of a pair of small oval masses that protrude slightly from the posteroinferior aspects of the thalamus; its main (dorsal) subdivision serves as a processing station in the major pathway from the retina to the cerebral cortex, receiving fibers from the optic tract and giving rise to the geniculocalcarine radiation to the visual cortex in the occipital lobe. SYN corpus geniculatum laterale [TA].

lat·er·al her·maph·ro·dit·ism (lat'ĕr-ăl hĕr-maf'rō-dit-izm) A form in which a testis is present on one side and an ovary on the other.

lat·er·al hu·mer·al ep·i·con·dy·li·tis (lat'ĕr-ăl hyū'mĕr-ăl ep'i-kon'di-lī'tis) SYN lateral epicondylitis.

lat·er·al·i·ty (lat'ĕr-al'i-tē) Referring to a side of the body or of a structure; specifically, the dominance of one side of the brain or the body.

lat·er·al lin·gual bud (lat'ĕr-ăl ling'gwăl bŭd) SYN lateral lingual swelling.

lat·er·al lin·gual swel·ling (lat'ĕr-ăl lin'gwăl swel'ing) Either of two oval swellings in the floor of the primordial mouth, one on each side of the median lingual swelling; they converge to form the anterior two thirds of the tongue. SYN distal tongue bud, lateral lingual bud.

lat·er·al lon·gi·tu·di·nal stri·a (lat'ĕr-ăl lawn'ji-tū'di-năl strī'ă) A thin longitudinal band of nerve fibers accompanied by gray matter, near each outer edge of the upper surface of the corpus callosum under cover of the cingulate gyrus.

lat·er·al mal·le·o·lus (lat'ĕr-ăl ma-lē'ŏ-lŭs) The process at the lateral side of the lower end of the fibula, forming the projection of the lateral part of the ankle; the lateral malleolus extends farther inferiorly than the medial malleolus.

lat·er·al med·ul·lar·y branch·es of (in·tra·cra·ni·al part of) ver·te·bral ar·ter·y (lat'ĕr-ăl med'ŭ-lar'ē branch'ĕz in'tră-krā'nē-ăl pahrt vĕr'tĕ-brăl ahr'tĕr-ē) Minute branches of the vertebral artery (or its larger branches) that course laterally along the ventral aspect of the medulla oblongata.

lat•er•al me•nis•cus (lat′ĕr-ăl mĕ-nis′kŭs) Crescentic intraarticular cartilage of the knee joint attached to the lateral border of the upper articular surface of the tibia, occupying the space surrounding the contacting surfaces of the femur and tibia.

lat•er•al na•sal branch of fa•cial ar•te•ry (lat′ĕr-ăl nā′zăl branch fā′shăl ahr′tĕr-ē) Branch of facial artery to the side of the nose (ala and dorsum); anastomoses with its contralateral partner, as well as the septal and alar branches of the superior labial, the dorsal nasal branch of the ophthalmic, and the infraorbital branch of the maxillary artery.

lat•er•al oc•cip•i•tal ar•ter•y (lat′ĕr-ăl ok-sip′i-tăl ahr′tĕr-ē) One of the terminal branches of the posterior cerebral artery; it supplies, by several named branches, the lateral portions of the temporal lobe.

lat•er•al pec•to•ral nerve (lat′ĕr-ăl pek′tŏr-ăl nĕrv) A nerve that arises from the lateral cord of the brachial plexus usually passing medial to pectoralis minor to supply the sternoclavicular head of pectoralis major. SYN lateral anterior thoracic nerve, nervus pectoralis lateralis.

lat•er•al pinch (lat′ĕr-ăl pinch) A grasp pattern in which the object is held between the thumb pads and the radial side of the index finger. (Also referred to as a key grasp).

lat•er•al plan•tar ar•ter•y (lat′ĕr-ăl plan′tahr ahr′tĕr-ē) Larger of the two terminal branches of the posterior tibial artery; *distribution*, forms the plantar arch and through it supplies the sole of the foot and plantar surfaces of the toes; *anastomoses*, medial plantar, dorsalis pedis. SYN arteria plantaris lateralis.

lat•er•al plan•tar nerve (lat′ĕr-ăl plan′tahr nĕrv) One of two terminal branches of the tibial nerve; it courses along the lateral side of the sole, dividing into superficial and deep branches; it supplies the skin of the lateral aspect of the sole and the lateral 1-1/2 toes; it innervates the intrinsic muscles of the plantar part of the foot with the exception of the abductor hallucis and the flexor digitorum brevis; its distribution in the foot is similar to that of the ulnar nerve in the hand. SYN nervus plantaris lateralis.

lat•er•al plate (lat′ĕr-ăl plāt) A nonsegmented mass of mesoderm on the lateral periphery of the embryonic disc.

lat•er•al po•si•tion (lat′ĕr-ăl pŏ-zish′ŭn) The side-lying position.

lat•er•al pter•y•goid mus•cle (lat′ĕr-ăl ter′i-goyd mŭs′ĕl) Masticatory muscle of infratemporal fossa; *origin*, inferior head from lateral lamina of pterygoid process; superior head from infratemporal crest and adjacent greater wing of the sphenoid; *insertion*, into pterygoid fovea of mandible and articular disc and capsule of temporomandibular joint; *action*, protrudes lower jaw to enable opening of mouth; unilateral contraction deviates chin laterally, enabling grinding motion for chewing; *nerve supply*, nerve to lateral pterygoid from mandibular division of trigeminal. SYN external pterygoid muscle, musculus pterygoideus externus, musculus pterygoideus lateralis.

lat•er•al rec•tus mus•cle (lat′ĕr-ăl rek′tŭs mŭs′ĕl) *Origin*, lateral part of the common tendinous ring that bridges superior orbital fissure; *insertion*, lateral part of sclera of eye; *action*, abduction; *nerve supply*, abducens. SYN musculus rectus lateralis [TA], abducens oculi.

lat•er•al rec•tus mus•cle of the head (lat′ĕr-ăl rek′tŭs mŭs′ĕl hed) SYN rectus capitis lateralis muscle.

lat•er•al re•cum•bent po•si•tion (lat′ĕr-ăl rĕ-kŭm′bĕnt pŏ-zish′ŏn) SYN Sims position.

lat•er•al ro•ta•tion (lat′ĕr-ăl rō-tā′shŭn) SYN external rotation.

lat•er•al sa•cral ar•ter•ies (lat′ĕr-ăl sā′krăl ahr′tĕr-ēz) Usually one of two arteries that arise from the internal iliac artery or its branches; they supply muscles and skin in the neighborhood and send branches into the sacral canal, supply radicular and spinal arteries, and continue on to the skin and subcutaneous tissues overlying the sacrum. SYN arteriae sacrales laterales.

lat•er•al sa•cral veins (lat′ĕr-ăl sā′krăl vānz) Several veins that receive the drainage of the sacral venous plexus and sacral intervertebral veins, then accompany the corresponding artery and empty into the internal iliac vein on each side.

lat•er•al su•pra•cla•vic•u•lar nerve (lat′ĕr-ăl sū′pra-klă-vik′yŭ lăr nĕrv) One of several branches of C3–C4 portion of cervical plexus that descend to skin over acromion and deltoid region. SYN nervus supraclavicularis lateralis, posterior supraclavicular nerve.

lat•er•al tar•sal strip pro•ce•dure (lat′ĕr-ăl tahr′săl strip prŏ-sē′jŭr) A procedure designed to correct lower eyelid malposition due to horizontal lid laxity by shortening it at the lateral canthal end.

lat•er•al tho•rac•ic ar•ter•y (lat′ĕr-ăl thōr-as′ik ahr′tĕr-ē) *Origin*, third part of axillary; *distribution*, passes around lateral border of pectoral muscles, supplying them and other muscles of chest and mammary gland. SYN arteria thoracica lateralis, external mammary artery, long thoracic artery.

lat•er•al vas•tus mus•cle (lat′ĕr-ăl vas′tŭs mŭs′ĕl) SYN vastus lateralis muscle.

lat•er•al ven•tri•cle (lat′ĕr-ăl ven′tri-kĕl) A cavity shaped somewhat like a horseshoe in conformity with the general shape of the hemisphere; each lateral ventricle communicates with the third ventricle through the interventricular foramen of Monro, and expands from there forward into the frontal lobe as the anterior horn as well as caudally over the thalamus as the central part or cella media which, behind the thalamus, curves ventrally and laterally, then forward into the temporal lobe as the inferior horn; from the apex of the curve a variably sized posterior horn extends back into the white matter of the occipital lobe. The large choroid plexus of the lateral ventricle invades the cella media and the inferior horn (but not the anterior and posterior horn) from the medial side.

late rick•ets (lāt rik′ĕts) SYN osteomalacia.

latero- Combining form meaning lateral, to one side. [L. *lateralis,* lateral, fr. *latus,* side]

lat•er•o•de•vi•a•tion (lat′ĕr-ō-dē′vē-ā′shŭn) A bending or a displacement to one side. [latero- + L. *devio,* to turn aside, fr. *via,* a way]

lat•er•o•duc•tion (lat′ĕr-ō-dŭk′shŭn) A drawing to one side; denoting a movement of a limb or turning of the eyeball away from the midline. [latero- + L. *duco,* pp. *ductus,* to lead]

lat•er•o•flex•ion, lat•er•o•flec•tion (lat′ĕr-ō-fleks′shŭn, -shŭn) A bending or curvature to one side. [latero- + L. *flecto,* pp. *flexus,* to bend]

lat•er•o•tor•sion (lat′ĕr-ō-tōr′shŭn) A twisting to one side; denoting rotation of the eyeball around its anteroposterior axis, so that the top part of the cornea turns away from the sagittal plane. [latero- + L. *torsio,* a twisting]

lat•er•o•tru•sion (lat′ĕr-ō-trū′zhŭn) The outward thrust given by the muscles of mastication to the rotating mandibular condyle during movement of the mandible. [latero- + L. *trudo,* pp. *trusus,* to thrust]

lat•er•o•ver•sion (lat′ĕr-ō-vĕr′zhŭn) Version to one side or the other, denoting especially a malposition of the uterus. [latero- + L. *verto,* pp. *versus,* to turn]

late sys•to•le (lāt sis′tŏ-lē) SYN prediastole.

la•tex (lā′teks) **1.** An emulsion or suspension produced by some seed plants; contains suspended microscopic globules of natural rubber. **2.** Similar synthetic materials such as polystyrene and polyvinyl chloride. [L. liquid]

la•tex al•ler•gy (lā′teks al′ĕr-jē) Cutaneous hypersensitivity to natural rubber, used in the manufacture of rubber gloves, condoms, and other articles.

la•tex sen•si•tiv•i•ty (lā′teks sen′si-tiv′i-tē) Hypersensitivity to a specific protein found in processed natural rubber products causing contact dermatitis or anaphylaxis.

lath•y•rism (lath′i-rizm) A disease that occurs in Ethiopia, Algeria, and India, characterized by various nervous manifestations, tremors, spastic paraplegia, and paresthesias; prevalent in districts where vetches, khasari (*Lathyrus sativus*), and allied species are the main food. [L. *lathyrus,* vetch]

la•tis•si•mus dor•si mus•cle (lă-tis′i-mŭs dōr′sī mŭs′ĕl) *Origin,* spinous processes of the lower five or six thoracic and the lumbar vertebrae, median ridge of sacrum, and outer lip of iliac crest; *insertion,* with teres major into posterior lip of bicipital groove of humerus; *action,* adducts arm, rotates it medially, and extends it; *nerve supply,* thoracodorsal. See this page. SYN musculus latissimus dorsi [TA].

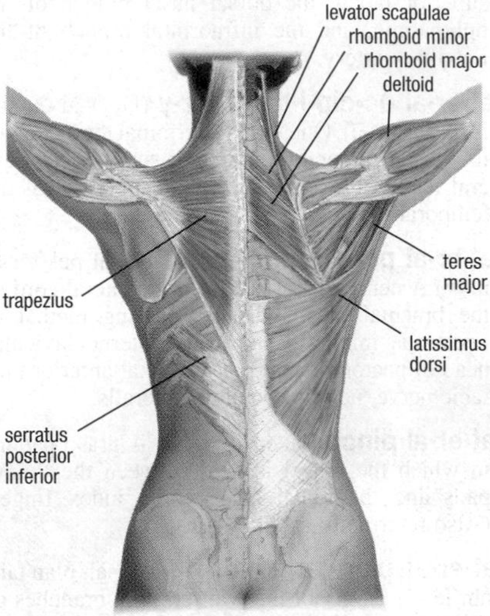

latissimus dorsi muscle

lat•i•tude (lat′i-tūd) The range of light or x-ray exposure acceptable with a given photographic emulsion. [L. *latitudo,* width, fr. *latus,* wide]

La•tro•dec•tus (lat-rō-dek′tŭs) A genus of relatively small spiders, the widow spiders, capable of inflicting highly poisonous, neurotoxic, painful bites. [L. *latro,* servant, robber, + G. *dēktēs,* a biter]

LATS (lats) Acronym for long-acting thyroid stimulator.

lat•us, gen. **lat•e•ris,** pl. **lat•e•ra** (lat′us, -ĕr-is, -ĕr-ă) [TA] The side of the body between the pelvis and the ribs. SYN flank. [L. broad]

Latz•ko ce•sar•e•an sec•tion (lahts′kō sē-zar′ē-ăn sek′shŭn) A cesarean section in which the uterus is entered by paravesical blunt dissection without entering the peritoneal cavity.

lau•da•num (law′dă-nŭm) An older medicinal syrup or tincture that contains opium.

laugh•ing gas (laf′ing gas) SYN nitrous oxide.

Lau•gi•er her•ni•a (lō-zhē-ā′ hĕr′nē-ă) A hernia passing through an opening in the lacunar ligament.

Lau•rence-Moon syn•drome (lawr′ĕns-mūn sin′drōm) Disorder characterized by mental retardation, pigmentary retinopathy, hypogenitalism, and spastic paraplegia; autosomal recessive inheritance. This syndrome is to be distinguished from Bardet-Biedl; in the past, the two syndromes have been lumped together under the designation of Laurence-Moon-Bardet-Biedl syndrome.

Lau•rer ca•nal (lowr′er kă-nal′) A tube originating on the surface of the ootype of trematodes, directed dorsally to or near the surface; it may have originally served as a vagina or possibly as a reservoir of excess shell material.

Lauth ca•nal (lōt kă-nal′) SYN scleral venous sinus.

Lauth vi•o•let (lōt vī′ō-lĕt) SYN thionine.

LAV Abbreviation for lymphadenopathy-associated virus.

la•vage (lă-vahzh′) The washing out of a hollow cavity or organ by copious injections and rejections of fluid. SEE ALSO gastric lavage. [Fr. from L. *lavo,* to wash]

la•va•tion (lă-vā′shŭn) To wash. [L. *lavatio*, fr. *lavo*, to wash]

lav•en•der-top tube (lav′ĕn-dĕr-top tūb) This type of tube contains EDTA as an anticoagulant; used for most hematologic procedures.

law (law) **1.** A principle or rule. **2.** A statement of a sequence or relation of phenomena that is invariable under the given conditions. SEE ALSO principle, rule, theorem. [A.S. *lagu*]

law of Bergonié and Tribondeau (law bār-gō-nyā′ trē-bon-dō′) Concept in radiobiology used to relate ionizing radiation effectiveness on cells that are actively mitotic and undifferentiated and have a long mitotic cycle.

law of con•ti•gu•i•ty (law kon′ti-gyū′i-tē) When two ideas or psychologically perceived events have once occurred in close association they are likely to so occur again, the subsequent occurrence of one tending to elicit the other; this law figures prominently in modern theories of conditioning and learning.

law of ex•ci•ta•tion (law ek′sī-tā′shŭn) A motor nerve responds, not to the absolute value, but to the alteration of value from moment to moment, of the electric current (i.e., rate of change of intensity of the current is a factor in determining its effectiveness).

law of the heart (law hahrt) The energy liberated by the heart when it contracts is a function of the length of its muscle fibers at the end of diastole.

law of in•de•pen•dent as•sort•ment (law in′dē-pen′dĕnt ă-sōrt′mĕnt) Different hereditary factors assort independently when the gametes are formed; traits at linked loci are an exception. SYN Mendel second law.

law of par•tial pres•sures (law pahr′shăl presh′shŭrz) SYN Dalton law.

law of re•ferred pain (law rĕ-fĕrd′ pān) Pain arises only from irritation of nerves that are sensitive to those stimuli that produce pain when applied to the surface of the body.

law of re•frac•tion (law rĕ-frak′shŭn) For two given media, the sine of the angle of incidence bears a constant relation to the sine of the angle of refraction. SYN Descartes law, Snell law.

law•ren•ci•um (Lr) (lawr-en′sē-ŭm) An artificial transplutonium element; atomic no. 103; atomic wt. 262.11.

law of seg•re•ga•tion (law seg′rĕ-gā′shŭn) Factors that affect development retain their individuality from generation to generation, do not become contaminated when mixed in a hybrid, and become sorted out from one another when the next generation of gametes is formed. SYN Mendel first law.

law of sim•i•lars (law sim′i-lărz) SEE similia similibus curantur.

lax•a•tive (lak′să-tiv) Any oral agent that promotes the expulsion of feces, including harsh stimulant laxatives (e.g., senna, bisacodyl), saline laxatives (e.g., magnesium citrate), stool softeners (e.g., docusate sodium), bulking laxatives (e.g., psyllium, methylcellulose), and lubricants (e.g., mineral oil). SYN aperient. [L. *laxativus,* fr. *laxo,* pp. *-atus,* to slacken, relax]

lax•i•ty (laks′i-tē) Looseness or freedom of movement in a joint, normal or excessive. SEE ALSO instability. [L. *laxitas,* looseness]

lay•er (lā′ĕr) A sheet of one substance lying on another and distinguished from it by a difference in texture or color or by not being continuous with it. SEE ALSO stratum, lamina.

la•zy eye (lā′zē ī) Central suppression of visual impulses from an eye with a severe refractive error or in strabismus. SYN amblyopia.

lb Abbreviation for pound (unit of weight).

LBW Abbreviation for low birth weight.

LCAT de•fi•cien•cy (dĕ-fish′ĕn-sē) A rare condition characterized by corneal opacities, hemolytic anemia, proteinuria, renal insufficiency, and premature atherosclerosis, and very low levels of lecithin cholesterol acyltransferase (LCAT) activity; results in accumulation of unesterfied cholesterol in plasma and tissues.

LCD Abbreviation for local coverage determination.

LCST Abbreviation for lateral corticospinal tract.

LCt_{50} Abbreviation for lethal Ct_{50}.

LD Abbreviation for lethal dose.

LDH Abbreviation for lactate dehydrogenase.

LDL Abbreviation for malondialdehyde-modified low-density lipoprotein.

LDL-C Abbreviation for low density lipoprotein-cholesterol.

L-do·pa (dō′pă) Abbreviation for levodopa.

L dos·es (dōs′ĕz) A group of terms that indicate the relative activity or potency of diphtheria toxin; the L doses are different from the minimal lethal dose and minimal reacting dose, inasmuch as the latter two represent the direct effects of toxin, whereas the L doses pertain to the combining power of toxin with specific antitoxin. ["L" for L. *limes*, limit, boundary]

LE, L.E. Abbreviation for left eye; lupus erythematosus.

leach·ing (lēch′ing) Removal of the soluble constituents of a substance by running water through it. [A.S. *leccan,* to wet]

lead (lēd) **1.** An electrical conductor carrying current or intermittent signals between an organ or tissue and an electrical or electronic device. **2.** The tracing obtained from a particular combination of electrode positions.

lead (Pb) (led) A metallic element, atomic no. 82, atomic wt. 207.2; occurs in nature as an oxide or one of the salts, but chiefly as the sulfide, or galena; ^{210}Pb (half-life equal to 22.6 years) has been used in the treatment of certain eye conditions. SYN plumbum.

lead en·ceph·a·lop·a·thy, lead en·ceph·a·li·tis (led en-sef′a-lop′ă-thē, en-sef′ă-lī′tis) A metabolic encephalopathy, caused by the ingestion of lead compounds and seen particularly in early childhood; it is characterized pathologically by extensive cerebral edema, status spongiosus, neurocytolysis, and some reactive inflammation; clinical manifestations include convulsions, delirium, and hallucinations. SEE ALSO lead poisoning.

lead poi·son·ing (led poy′zŏn-ing) Acute or chronic intoxication by lead or any of its salts; symptoms of **acute lead poisoning** usually are those of acute gastroenteritis in adults or encephalopathy in children; **chronic lead poisoning** is manifested chiefly by anemia, constipation, colicky abdominal pain, neuropathy with paralysis (especially wrist-drop involving the extensor muscles of the forearm) bluish lead line of the gums, and interstitial nephritis; saturnine gout, convulsions, and coma may occur. SYN plumbism.

lean (lēn) A product so labeled contains, by F.D.A. order, less than 10 g fat, 4.5 g saturated fat, and 95 mg cholesterol per serving.

lean bod·y mass (lēn bod′ē mas) SYN fat-free body mass.

Lear com·plex (lēr kom′pleks) A father's libidinous fixation on a daughter. [fr. King *Lear,* Shakespearean character]

learn (lĕrn) To gain knowledge, understanding, or skill through study or practice. [O.E. *leornian*]

learned drive (lĕrnd drīv) SYN motive (1).

learned help·less·ness (lĕrnd help′lĕs-nĕs) A laboratory model of depression involving both classical (respondent) and instrumental (operant) conditioning techniques; application of unavoidable shock is followed by failure to cope in situations where coping might otherwise be possible.

learn·ing (lĕrn′ing) **1.** Generic term for the relatively permanent change in behavior that occurs as a result of practice. SEE ALSO conditioning, memory. **2.** NURSING change in behavior (e.g., knowledge, skill, value/attitude) as result of experience.

learn·ing dis·a·bil·i·ty (lĕrn′ing dis′ă-bil′ĭ-tē) A disorder in one or more of the basic cognitive and psychological processes involved in understanding or using written or spoken language; may be manifested in age-related impairment in the ability to read, write, spell, speak, or perform mathematical calculations.

least con·fu·sion cir·cle (lēst kŏn-fyū′zhŭn sĭr′kĕl) In the configuration of rays emerging from a spherocylindric lens system, the place where diverging rays of the lens first forming a line image are balanced by converging rays of the second lens.

leath·er-bot·tle stom·ach (ledh′ĕr-bot′ĕl stŏm′ăk) Marked thickening and rigidity of the stomach wall, with reduced capacity of the lumen, although often without obstruction; nearly always due to scirrhous carcinoma, as in linitis plastica.

Le·ber con·gen·i·tal am·au·ro·sis (lā′bĕr kŏn-jen′i-tăl am′awr-ō′sis) Retinitis pigmentosa characterized by severe visual impairment, nystagmus, and a 'flat' electroretinogram.

Le·ber he·red·i·tar·y op·tic at·ro·phy (lā′bĕr hĕr-ed′i-tar-ē op′tik at′rŏ-fē) Degeneration of the optic nerve and papillomacular bundle with resulting loss of central vision and blindness, which is progressive for several weeks, then usually becomes stationary with permanent central scotoma; the age of onset is variable, most often in the third decade; more males than females are affected. Mitochondrial or cytoplasmic inheritance through the maternal lineage, caused by mutation in the mitochondrial gene(s) acting autonomously or in association with each other.

Le·ber id·i·o·path·ic stel·late ret·i·nop·a·thy (lā′bĕr id′ē-ō-path′ik stel′āt ret′in-op′ă-thē) SEE neuroretinitis.

LE cell (sel) A polymorphonuclear leukocyte containing an amorphous round body; formed in vitro in the blood of patients with systemic lupus erythematosus, or by the action of the patient's serum on normal leukocytes. SYN lupus erythematosus cell.

LE cell test (sel test) The in vitro incubation of the blood or bone marrow of patients with systemic lupus erythematosus, or action of their serum on normal leukocytes, causes formation of characteristic LE cells. SYN lupus erythematosus cell test.

Le Cha•te•lier law (lĕ-shah-tel-yā′ law) If external factors such as temperature and pressure disturb a system in equilibrium, adjustment occurs in such a way that the effect of the disturbing factors is reduced to a minimum.

lec•i•thal (les′i-thăl) Having a yolk or pertaining to the yolk of any egg; used especially as a suffix. [G. *lekithos,* egg yolk]

lec•i•thin (les′i-thin) Traditional term for phospholipids that on hydrolysis yield two fatty acid molecules and a molecule each of glycerophosphoric acid and choline. Lecithins are found in nervous tissue, especially in the myelin sheaths, in egg yolk, and as essential constituents of animal and vegetable cells. [G. *lekithos,* egg yolk]

lec•i•thi•nase (les′i-thi-nās) SYN phospholipase.

lec•i•thin:sphin•go•my•e•lin ra•ti•o (les′i-thin-sfing′gō-mī′ĕ-lin rā′shē-ō) A ratio used to determine fetal pulmonary maturity, found by testing the amniotic fluid; when the lungs are mature, lecithin exceeds sphingomyelin by 2:1.

lec•i•tho•blast (les′i-thō-blast) One of the cells proliferating to form the yolk-sac endoderm. [G. *lekithos,* egg yolk, + *blastos,* germ]

Le•cler•ci•a (le-kler′shē-ă) A genus in the family Enterobacteriaceae that resembles the genus *Escherichia*, but is separable by metabolic and genetic classification. Isolated from the feces of humans and animals, it has been recovered clinically from blood, sputum, urine, and wounds; its degree of pathogenicity is unclear.

lec•tin (lek′tin) A protein of primarily plant (usually seed) origin that binds to glycoproteins on the surface of cells causing agglutination, precipitation, or other phenomena resembling the action of specific antibody; lectins include plant agglutinins (phytoagglutinins, phytohemagglutinins), plant precipitins, and perhaps certain animal proteins; some have mitogenic properties. [L. *lego,* pp. *lectum,* to select, + -in]

lec•tin gly•co•his•to•chem•is•try (lek′tin glī′kō-his′tō-kem′is-trē) Technique for measuring the endogenous ligands for specific sugar moieties, such as peanut agglutinin, wheat germ agglutinin, and gorse seed agglutinin, in characterization of surface epithelium.

lec•tin path•way mol•e•cule (lek′tin path′wā mol′ĕ-kyūl) The binding of mannose-binding protein to bacterial carbohydrates resulting in activation of the complement pathway.

ledge (lej) In anatomy, a structure resembling a ledge. SEE ALSO lamina.

leech (lēch) **1.** Any bloodsucking aquatic annelid worm, including those of the class Hirudinea, sometimes used in medicine and plastic surgery for local withdrawal of blood. **2.** To treat medically by applying leeches. [A.S. *laece,* a physician; a leech, because of its therapeutic use]

LEEP (lēp) Acronym for loop electrocautery excision procedure.

Le Fort am•pu•ta•tion (lĕ-fōrt′ amp′yū-tā′shŭn) A modification of Pirogoff amputation; the calcaneus is sawed through horizontally instead of vertically so that the patient steps on the same part of the heel as before.

Le Fort I frac•ture (lĕ fōrt′ frak′shŭr) SYN horizontal maxillary fracture. See this page.

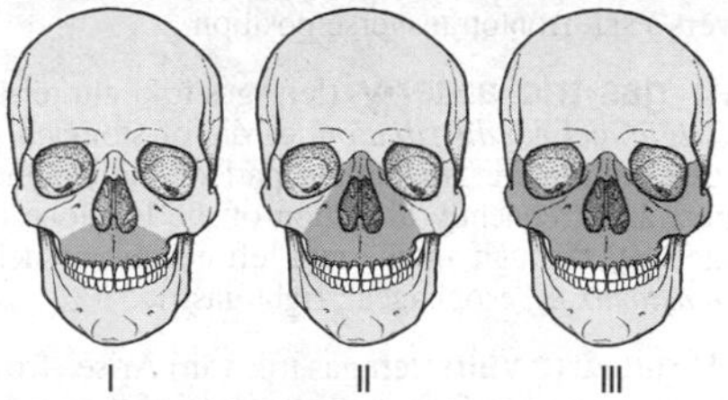

Le Fort classification of facial fractures: (I) horizontal maxillary (Guérin); (II) pyramidal; (III) craniofacial dysjunction

Le Fort II frac•ture (lĕ fōrt′ frak′shŭr) SYN pyramidal fracture. See this page.

Le Fort III frac•ture (lĕ fōrt′ frak′shŭr) SYN craniofacial dysjunction fracture. See this page.

left an•te•ri•or de•scend•ing ar•ter•y (left an-tēr′ē-ŏr dĕ-send′ing ahr′tĕr-ē) SYN anterior interventricular branch of left coronary artery.

left a•tri•um of heart (left ā′trē-ŭm hahrt) The upper chamber of the left side of the heart which receives the blood from the pulmonary veins. SYN atrium cordis sinistrum [TA], atrium pulmonale, atrium sinistrum cordis.

left bun•dle of a•tri•o•ven•tric•u•lar bun•dle (left bŭn′dĕl ā′trē-ō-ven-trik′yŭ-lăr bŭn′dĕl) The left limb or branch of the atrioventricular bundle that separates from the atrioventricular bundle just below the membranous portion of the interventricular septum to descend the septal wall of the left ventricle and begin to ramify subendocardially.

left col•ic ar•ter•y (left kol′ik ahr′tĕr-ē) *Origin,* inferior mesenteric; *distribution,* descending colon and splenic flexure; *anastomoses*, middle colic, sigmoid. SYN arteria colica sinistra.

left col·ic flex·ure (left kol′ik flek′shŭr) The bend at the junction of the transverse and descending colon. SYN flexura coli sinistra [TA], splenic flexure.

left cor·o·nar·y ar·ter·y (left kōr′ŏ-nar-ē ahr′tĕr-ē) *Origin*, left aortic sinus; *distribution*, it divides into two major branches, an anterior interventricular, which descends in the anterior interventricular sulcus, and a circumflex branch, which passes to the diaphragmatic surface of the left ventricle; gives atrial, ventricular, and atrioventricular branches. SYN arteria coronaria sinistra.

left-foot·ed (left-fut′ĕd) SYN sinistropedal.

left fron·to·an·te·ri·or (left frŭn′tō-an-tēr′ē-ŏr) SEE frontoanterior position.

left fron·to·pos·te·ri·or (left frŭn′tō-pos-tēr′ē-ŏr) SEE frontoposterior position.

left fron·to·trans·verse (left frŭn′tō-trans-vĕrs′) SEE frontotransverse position.

left gas·tric ar·ter·y (left gas′trik ahr′tĕr-ē) *Origin*, celiac; *distribution*, cardia of stomach at lesser curvature, abdominal part of the esophagus, and frequently a portion of the left lobe of the liver through an aberrant left hepatic branch; *anastomoses*, esophageal, right gastric.

left gas·tric vein (left gas′trik vān) Arises from a union of veins from both surfaces of the cardia of the stomach and an esophageal tributary from the cardiac portion of the esophagus; it runs in the lesser omentum and empties into the portal vein. SEE ALSO esophageal veins.

left gas·tro·ep·i·plo·ic ar·ter·y (left gas′trō-ep′i-plō′ik ahr′tĕr-ē) SYN left gastroomental artery.

left gas·tro·o·men·tal ar·ter·y (left gas′trō-ō-men′tăl ahr′tĕr-ē) *Origin*, splenic; *distribution*, greater curvature of stomach and greater omentum; *anastomoses*, right gastroepiploic and short gastric arteries. SYN arteria gastroepiploica sinistra, arteria gastroomentalis sinistra, left gastroepiploic artery.

left-hand·ed (left-hand′ĕd) Denoting the habitual or more skillful use of the left hand for writing and for most manual functions. SYN sinistromanual.

left heart (left hahrt) The left atrium and left ventricle.

left heart by·pass (left hahrt bī′pas) Any procedure that shunts blood returning from the pulmonary circulation to the systemic circulation without passing through the left heart. This is used during cardiac surgery and in severe left heart failure or cardiogenic shock.

left he·pat·ic duct (left hĕ-pat′ik dŭkt) The duct that drains bile from the left half of the liver, including the quadrate lobe and the left part of the caudate lobe.

left lat·er·al di·vi·sion of liv·er (left lat′ĕr-ăl di-vizh′ŭn liv′ĕr) The portion of the liver that lies to the left of the approximately vertical plane of the left hepatic vein and includes the left posterior and anterior lateral segments (hepatic segments II and III); it corresponds to the left anatomic lobe of the liver, and so is demarcated externally by the falciform ligament on the diaphragmatic surface and by the fissures for the ligamentum venosum and ligamentum teres on the viscera surface. SYN divisio lateralis sinistra hepatis [TA].

left liv·er (left liv′ĕr) Portion of the liver receiving blood from the left branches of the hepatic artery and portal vein, and from which bile is drained through the left hepatic duct; the plane of the middle hepatic vein separates left from right liver.

left lobe of liv·er (left lōb liv′ĕr) It is separated from the right lobe above and in front by the falciform ligament, and from the quadrate and caudate lobes by the fissure for the ligamentum teres and the fissure for the ligamentum venosum; the distribution of the portal vein, hepatic artery, and bile ducts does not correspond to the gross lobar divisions of the liver. It contains two segments, superior and inferior. SYN lobus hepatis sinister [TA].

left mar·gin·al ar·ter·y (left mahr′ji-năl ahr′tĕr-ē) A large ventricular branch of the circumflex branch of the left coronary artery that courses along the center of the left pulmonary surface (obtuse margin) of the heart, usually to the apex. SYN ramus marginalis sinister arteriae coronariae sinistrae.

left me·di·al di·vi·sion of liv·er (left mē′dē-ăl di-vizh′ŭn liv′ĕr) The portion of the liver that lies between the approximately vertical planes of the left and middle hepatic veins and includes the left medial segment (hepatic segment IV); on the diaphragmatic surface, it is approximately the left third of the anatomic right lobe of the liver; on the visceral surface, its inferior portion corresponds to the quadrate lobe. SYN divisio medialis sinistra hepatis [TA].

left pul·mo·na·ry ar·te·ry (left pul′mŏ-nar-ē ahr′tĕr-ē) The shorter of the two terminal branches of the pulmonary trunk, it pierces the pericardium to enter the hilum of the left lung. Its branches accompany the segmental and subsegmental bronchi. Branches to the superior lobe (rami lobi superioris [TA]) are apical (ramus apicalis [TA]), anterior ascending (ramus anterior ascendens [TA]), anterior descending (ramus anterior descendens [TA]), posterior (ramus posterior [TA]), and lingular (ramus lingularis [TA]), the last having inferior and superior branches (rami lingulares inferior et superior [TA]). Branches to the inferior lobe (rami lobi inferioris [TA]) are the superior branch of the inferior lobe (ramus superior lobi inferioris [TA]) and the medial (medialis), anterior, lateral (lateralis), and posterior basal branches (rami basales [TA]).

left-to-right shunt (left-rīt shŭnt) A diversion of blood from the left side of the heart to right (as through a septal defect), or from the systemic circulation to the pulmonary (as through a patent ductus arteriosus).

left um•bil•i•cal vein (left ŭm-bil′i-kăl vān) Returns the blood from the placenta to the embryo; traversing the umbilical cord, it enters the embryo body at the umbilicus and then passes into the liver, where it is joined by the portal vein; its blood then flows by way of the ductus venosus and the inferior vena cava to the right atrium; the right umbilical vein disappears during the seventh week. SYN vena umbilicalis [TA], umbilical vein.

left ven•tri•cle (left ven′tri-kĕl) The lower chamber on the left side of the heart that receives the arterial blood from the left atrium and drives it by the contraction of its walls into the aorta.

left-ven•tric•u•lar as•sist de•vice (left-ven-trik′yŭ-lăr ă-sist′ dĕ-vīs′) Mechanical pump inserted at some point in the circulation to parallel the activity of the left ventricle and thereby reduce its load.

left ven•tric•u•lar e•jec•tion time (LVET) (left ven-trik′yŭ-lăr ē-jek′shŭn tīm) The time measured clinically from onset to incisural notch of the carotid or other pulse; properly, the time of ejection of blood from the left ventricle, beginning with aortic valve opening and ending with aortic valve closing.

left ven•tric•u•lar fail•ure (left ven-trik′yŭ-lăr fāl′yŭr) Congestive heart failure manifested by signs of pulmonary congestion and edema.

left ven•tri•cu•lar vol•ume re•duc•tion sur•ger•y (left ven-trik′yŭ-lăr vol′yūm rĕ-dŭk′shŭn sŭr′jĕr-ē) Operation in which the volume of a dilated, nonaneurysmal left ventricle is reduced by myocardial resection in order to improve ventricular geometry and mechanical function and thereby treat end-stage congestive heart failure. SYN Battista operation, Battista procedure, partial left ventriculectomy, reduction left ventriculoplasty, ventricular reduction surgery.

leg (leg) **1.** The segment of the inferior limb between the knee and the ankle; commonly used to mean the entire inferior limb. **2.** A structure resembling a leg. SYN crus (1) [TA].

le•gal blind•ness (lē′găl blīnd′nĕs) Generally, visual acuity of less than 6/60 or 20/200 using Snellen test types, or visual field restriction to 20 degrees or less in the better eye; the criteria used to define legal blindness vary.

le•gal med•i•cine (lē′găl med′i-sin) SYN forensic medicine.

Le•gen•dre sign (lĕ-zhahn′drĕ sīn) In facial hemiplegia of central origin, when the examiner raises the lids of the actively closed eyes the resistance is less on the affected side.

Legg-Cal•vé-Per•thes dis•ease, Legg dis•ease, Legg-Per•thes dis•ease (leg′kal-vā′per′tĕz di-zēz′, leg di-zēz′, leg-per′tĕz di-zēz′) Self-limiting pediatric disease of the femoral head caused by poor circulation. The degeneration of the femoral head is followed by regeneration and absorption of bone. The process may take 4 years. Usually found in children aged 4–8 years. See this page. SYN coxa plana.

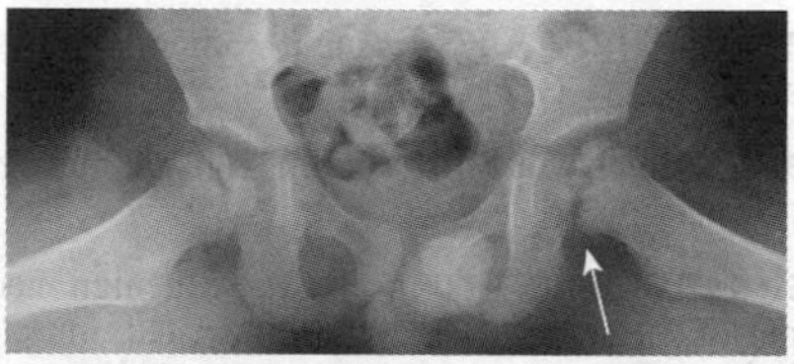

Legg-Calvé-Perthes disease: irregular and sclerotic femoral head of 3-year-old boy

-legia Suffix meaning reading, as distinguished from the G. derivatives, *-lexis* and *-lexy*, which signify speech, from G. *legō*, to say. [L. *lego*, to read]

Le•gion•el•la (lē-jŭ-nel′lă) A genus of aerobic, motile, non-acid-fast, nonencapsulated, gram-negative bacilli; they dwell in water and are borne by air; pathogenic for humans. The type species is *L. pneumophila.*

Le•gion•el•la boze•man•i•i (lē-jŭ-nel′lă bōz-man′ē-ī) A species that causes human pneumonia.

Le•gion•el•la mic•da•de•i (lē-jŭ-nel′lă mik-dā′dē-ī) A species that causes Pittsburgh pneumonia, a variant of Legionnaire disease. Accounts for approximately 60% of *Legionella* pneumonias other than those caused by *L. pneumophila*. SYN Pittsburgh pneumonia agent.

Le•gion•naires′ dis•ease (lē′jŭ-nārz′ di-zēz′) An acute infectious disease, caused by various species of *Legionella pneumophila*, with prodromal influenzalike symptoms and a rapidly rising high fever, followed by severe pneumonia and production of usually nonpurulent sputum, and sometimes mental confusion, hepatic fatty changes, and renal tubular degeneration. It has a high case-fatality rate; acquired from contaminated water, usually by aerosolization rather than transmission from person to person. [American *Legion* convention, in Philadelphia in 1976, at which many delegates were so affected]

Leigh dis•ease (lē di-zēz′) Subacute encephalomyelopathy affecting infants, causing seizures, spasticity, optic atrophy, and dementia; the genetic causation is heterogeneous; may be associated with deficiency of cytochrome *c* oxidase or

NADH-ubiquinone oxidoreductase or other enzymes involved in energy metabolism. Autosomal recessive, X-linked recessive and mitochondrial inheritance have been described; mutations have been identified in the surfeit-1 gene (SURF) on chromosome 9, in a mtDNA-encoded subunit of ATP synthase, in the X-linked E1-alpha subunit of pyruvate dehydrogenase, and in several subunits of mitochondrial complex I.

Lei•ner dis•ease (lī′nĕr di-zēz′) SYN erythroderma desquamativum.

♻**leio-** Combining form meaning smooth. [G. *leios*]

lei•o•der•mi•a (lī′ō-dĕr′mē-ă) Smooth, glossy skin. [leio- + G. *derma,* skin]

lei•o•my•o•fi•bro•ma (lī′ō-mī-ō-fī-brō′mă) SYN fibroleiomyoma.

lei•o•my•o•ma (lī′ō-mī-ō′mă) A benign neoplasm derived from smooth (nonstriated) muscle. [leio- + G. *mys,* muscle, + *-oma,* tumor]

lei•o•my•o•ma cu•tis (lī′ō-mī-ō′mă kyū′tis) Cutaneous eruption of multiple small painful nodules composed of smooth muscle fibers; derived from arrector muscles of hair. SYN dermatomyoma.

lei•o•my•o•ma•to•sis (lī′ō-mī′ō-mă-tō′sis) The state of having multiple leiomyomas throughout the body.

lei•o•my•o•ma•to•sis per•i•to•ne•a•lis dis•sem•i•na•ta (lī′ō-mī′ō-mă-tō′sis per′i-tō-nē-ā′lis di-sem-i-nā′tă) A benign condition characterized by multiple small nodules on abdominal and pelvic peritoneum, grossly mimicking disseminated ovarian cancer but with histologic characteristics of benign myoma; often associated with recent pregnancy.

lei•o•my•o•sar•co•ma (lī′ō-mī′ō-sahr-kō′mă) A malignant neoplasm derived from smooth (nonstriated) muscle. [leio- + myosarcoma]

Leish•man-Don•o•van bod•y (lēsh′măn don′ō-văn bod′ē) The intracytoplasmic, nonflagellated leishmanial form of certain intracellular parasites, such as species of *Leishmania* or the intracellular form of *Trypanosoma cruzi.* SYN amastigote.

Leish•man•i•a (lēsh-man′ē-ă) A genus of digenetic, asexual, protozoan flagellates that occur as amastigotes in the macrophages of vertebrate hosts, and as promastigotes in invertebrate hosts and in cultures.

leish•man•i•a, pl. **leish•man•i•ae** (lēsh-man′ē-ă, -ē) A member of the genus *Leishmania.*

leish•man•i•a•sis (lēsh′mă-nī′ă-sis) Infection with a species of *Leishmania* resulting in a group of diseases traditionally divided into four major types: 1) visceral leishmaniasis (kala azar); 2) Old World cutaneous leishmaniasis; 3) New World cutaneous leishmaniasis; and 4) mucocutaneous leishmaniasis. SEE ALSO tropical diseases.

Leish•man stain (lēsh′măn stān) A polychromed eosin–methylene blue stain used in the examination of blood films.

Lem•bert su•ture (lem-bār′ sū′chŭr) The second row of the Czerny-Lembert intestinal suture; an inverting suture for intestinal surgery, used either as a continuous suture or interrupted suture, producing serosal apposition and including the collagenous submucosal layer but not entering the lumen of the intestine.

Le•min•or•el•la (lem′in-ō-rel′ă) A genus in the family Enterobacteriaceae containing two species, *L. grimontii* and *L. richardii,* which have been isolated from clinical material, primarily from fecal samples. Its clinical importance remains unclear.

lem•mo•blast (lem′ō-blast) In an embryo, a cell of neural crest origin capable of forming a cell of the neurilemma sheath. [G. *lemma,* husk, + *blastos,* germ]

lem•mo•cyte (lem′ō-sīt) One of the cells of the neurolemma. [G. *lemma,* husk, + *kytos,* cell]

lem•nis•cus, pl. **lem•nis•ci** (lem-nis′kŭs, -nis′ī) A bundle of nerve fibers ascending from sensory relay nuclei to the thalamus. SYN fillet (1). [L. from G. *lēmniskos,* ribbon or fillet]

lem•on sign (lĕm′ŏn sīn) The ultrasound finding of frontal bone scalloping associated with Arnold-Chiari malformation.

Len•drum phlox•ine-tar•tra•zine stain (len′drŭm flox′ēn tahr′tră-zēn stān) A stain for demonstrating acidophilic inclusion bodies, which appear red on a yellow background; nuclei stain blue, but Negri bodies do not stain.

Le•nègre syn•drome (lĕ-neg′ sin′drōm) Isolated damage of the cardiac conduction system as a result of a sclerodegenerative lesion; characterized ordinarily as idiopathic fibrosis of the atrioventricular nodal, His bundle, or bundle branches with corresponding conduction block(s).

length (length) Linear distance between two points.

length-breadth in•dex (length-bredth in′deks) SYN cephalic index.

Len•nert lym•pho•ma (len′ert lim-fō′mă) Malignant lymphoma with a high proportion of diffusely scattered epithelioid cells, tonsillar involvement, and an unpredictable course.

Len•nox-Gas•taut syn•drome, **Len•nox syn•drome** (len′ŏks gahs-tō′ sin′drōm, len′ŏks sin′drōm) A generalized myoclonic astatic epilepsy in children, with mental retardation, resulting from various cerebral afflictions such as perinatal hypoxia, cerebral hemorrhage, encephalitides, maldevelopment or metabolic disorders of the brain; characterized by multiple seizure types (generalized tonic, atonic, myoclonic, tonic-clonic, and atypical absence) and background slowing and slow spike and wave pattern on EEG; patients are usually mentally retarded or developmentally delayed.

lens (lenz) **1.** A transparent material with one or both surfaces having a concave or convex curve; acts on electromagnetic energy to cause convergence or divergence of light rays. **2.** [TA] The transparent biconvex cellular refractive structure lying between the iris and the vitreous humor, consisting of a soft outer part (cortex) with a denser part (nucleus), and surrounded by a basement membrane (capsule); the anterior surface has a cuboidal epithelium, and at the equator the cells elongate to become lens fibers. [L. a lentil]

lens cap•sule (lenz kap′sŭl) The capsule enclosing the lens of the eye.

lens•ec•to•my (lenz-ek′tŏ-mē) Removal of the lens of the eye. [lens + G. *ektomē,* excision]

lens pits (lenz pitz) The paired depressions formed in the surface ectoderm of the embryonic head as the lens placodes sink in toward the optic cup; the external openings of the pits are closed as the lens vesicles form.

lens stars (lenz stahrz) **1.** SYN radii of lens. **2.** Congenital cataracts with opacities along the suture lines of the lens; may be anterior or posterior, or both.

lens ves•i•cle (lenz ves′i-kĕl) In the embryo, the ectodermal invagination that forms opposite the optic cup; it is the primordium of the lens of the eye.

len•ti•co•nus (len′ti-kō′nŭs) Conic projection of the anterior or posterior surface of the lens of the eye, occurring as a developmental anomaly. [lens + L. *conus,* cone]

len•tic•u•lar (len-tik′yŭ′lăr) Relating to or resembling a lens of any kind. [L. *lenticula,* a lentil]

len•tic•u•lar a•stig•ma•tism (len-tik′yŭ′lăr ă-stig′mă-tizm) Astigmatism due to defect in the curvature, position, or index of refraction of the lens.

len•tic•u•lar loop (len-tik′yŭ′lăr lūp) The pallidal efferent fibers curving around the medial border of the internal capsule.

len•tic•u•lar nu•cle•us (len-tik′yŭ′lăr nū′klē-ŭs) The large conic mass of gray matter forming the central core of the cerebral hemisphere. The convex base of the cone, oriented laterally and rostrally, is formed by the putamen which together with the caudate nucleus composes the striatum; the apical part, oriented medially and caudally, consists of the two segments of the globus pallidus. The nucleus is ventral and lateral to the thalamus and caudate nucleus, from which it is separated by the internal capsule, and together with the caudate nucleus composes the striate body.

len•tic•u•lar pro•cess of in•cus (len-tik′yŭ-lăr pros′es ing′kŭs) A knob at the tip of the long limb of the incus of the middle ear, which articulates with the stapes. SYN orbiculare.

len•tic•u•lo•pap•u•lar (len-tik′yŭ-lō-pap′yŭ-lăr) Indicating an eruption with dome-shaped or lens-shaped papules.

len•ti•form (len′ti-fōrm) Lens-shaped.

len•tig•i•no•sis (len-tij′i-nō′sis) Presence of lentigines in very large numbers or in a distinctive configuration.

len•ti•glo•bus (len′ti-glō′bŭs) Rare congenital anomaly with a spheroid elevation on the posterior surface of the lens of the eye. [lens + L. *globus,* sphere]

len•ti•go, pl. **len•tig•i•nes** (len-tī′gō, len-tij′i-nēz) A brown macule resembling a freckle except that the border is usually regular, and microscopic proliferation of rete ridges is present; scattered melanocytes are seen in the basal cell layer. It is usually caused by sun exposure in someone of middle age or older. SEE ALSO junction nevus. SYN lentigo simplex. [L. fr. *lens* (*lent-*), a lentil]

i **len•ti•go ma•lig•na** (len-tī′gō mă-lig′nă) A brown or black mottled, irregularly outlined, slowly enlarging lesion resembling a lentigo in which there are increased numbers of scattered atypical melanocytes in the epidermis, usually occurring on the face of older persons; after many years the dermis may be invaded and the lesion is then termed lentigo maligna melanoma. See page B14. SYN Hutchinson freckle.

len•ti•go sim•plex (len-tī′gō sim′pleks) SYN lentigo.

le•o•nine fa•ci•es (lē′ō-nīn fash′ē-ēz) SYN leontiasis.

le•on•ti•a•sis (lē′on-tī′ă-sis) A leonine appearance due to ridges and furrows on the forehead and cheeks of people with advanced lepromatous leprosy. SYN leonine facies. [G. *leōn* (*leont-*), lion]

leop•ard bane (lep′ărd bān) SYN arnica.

LEOPARD syn•drome (lep′ărd sin′drōm) A hereditary syndrome consisting of *l*entigines (multiple), *e*lectrocardiographic abnormalities, *o*cular hypertelorism, *p*ulmonary stenosis, *a*bnormalities of genitalia, *r*etardation of growth, and *d*eafness (sensorineural).

Le•o•pold ma•neu•vers (lā′ă-pōld mă-nū′vĕrz) Four maneuvers employed to determine fetal position: 1) determination of what is in the fundus; 2) evaluation of the fetal back and extremities; 3) palpation of the presenting part above the symphysis; and 4) determination of the direction and degree of flexion of the head.

lep•er (lep′ĕr) A person who has leprosy. [G. *lepra*]

le•pid•ic (lĕ-pid′ik) Relating to scales or a scaly covering layer. [G. *lepis* (*lepid-*), scale, rind]

lep•o•thrix (lep′ō-thriks) SYN trichomycosis axillaris. [G. *lepos,* rind, husk, + *thrix,* hair]

lep•re•chaun•ism (lep′rĕ-kawn-izm) Congenital dwarfism characterized by extreme growth retardation, endocrine disorders, and emaciation, with elfin facies and large, low-set ears. [Irish *leprechaun,* elf]

lep•rid (lep′rid) Early cutaneous lesion of leprosy. [G. *lepra,* leprosy, + *-id* (1)]

le•pro•ma (lĕ-prō′mă) A discrete focus of granulomatous inflammation, caused by *Mycobacterium leprae*. [G. *lepros,* scaly, + *-oma,* tumor]

lep•ro•ma•tous (lep-rō′mă-tŭs) Pertaining to, or characterized by, the features of a leproma.

lep•ro•ma•tous lep•ro•sy (lep-rō′mă-tŭs lep′rŏ-sē) A form of leprosy in which nodular cutaneous lesions are infiltrated, have ill-defined borders, and are bacteriologically positive.

lep•ro•min (lep′rō-min) An extract of tissue infected with *Mycobacterium leprae* used in skin tests to classify the stage of leprosy. SEE ALSO test.

lep•ro•min test (lep′rō-min test) An assay in which an intradermal injection of a lepromin is used to classify the stage of leprosy. It differentiates tuberculoid leprosy, in which there is a positive delayed reaction at the injection site, from lepromatous leprosy, in which there is no reaction.

lep•ro•sar•i•um (lep′rō-sar′ē-ŭm) An older term for a hospital specializing in the care of patients with leprosy.

lep•ro•stat•ic (lep′rō-stat′ik) **1.** Inhibiting to the growth of *Mycobacterium leprae*. **2.** An agent having this action.

lep•ro•sy (lep′rŏ-sē) **1.** A chronic granulomatous infection caused by *Mycobacterium leprae* affecting the cooler body parts, especially the skin, peripheral nerves, and testes. Leprosy is a spectrum of diseases ranging in type from lepromatous to tuberculoid; these two types representing extremes of immunologic response. **2.** A name used in the Bible to describe various cutaneous diseases, especially those of a chronic or contagious nature, which probably included psoriasis and leukoderma. SYN Hansen disease. [G. *lepra,* from *lepros,* scaly]

♻ **-lepsis, -lepsy** Combining forms indicating a seizure. [G. *lēpsis*]

lep•tin (lep′tin) A helical protein secreted by adipose tissue and acting on a receptor site in the ventromedial nucleus of the hypothalamus to curb appetite and increase energy expenditure as body fat stores increase. Leptin levels are 40% higher in women, and show a further 50% rise just before menarche, later returning to baseline levels; levels are lowered by fasting and increased by inflammation. [G. *leptos,* thin, + -in]

♻ **lepto-** A combining form meaning light, thin, frail. [G. *leptos,* slender, delicate, weak]

lep•to•ceph•a•lous (lep′tō-sef′ă-lŭs) Having an abnormally tall, narrow cranium. [lepto- + G. *kephalē,* head]

lep•to•ceph•a•ly (lep′tō-sef′ă-lē) A malformation characterized by an abnormally tall, narrow cranium. [lepto- + G. *kephalē,* head]

lep•to•cyte (lep′tō-sīt) SYN target cell. [lepto- + G. *kytos,* cell]

lep•to•cy•to•sis (lep′tō-sī-tō′sis) The presence of leptocytes in the circulating blood, as seen in thalassemia and after splenectomy.

lep•to•dac•ty•lous (lep′tō-dak′ti-lŭs) Having slender fingers. [lepto- + G. *daktylos,* finger]

lep•to•me•nin•ge•al (lep′tō-mĕ-nin′jē-ăl) Pertaining to the leptomeninges.

lep•to•me•nin•ges, sing. **lep•to•men•inx** (lep′tō-mĕ-nin′jēz, lep′tō-men′ingks) The two delicate layers of the meninges, the arachnoid mater and pia mater considered together. SEE ALSO arachnoid, pia mater. SYN pia-arachnoid, piarachnoid. [lepto- + G. *mēninx,* pl. *mēninges,* membrane]

lep•to•men•in•gi•tis (lep′tō-men′in-jī′tis) Inflammation of leptomeninges. SEE ALSO arachnoiditis. SYN pia-arachnitis.

lep•to•so•mat•ic, lep•to•som•ic (lep′tō-sō-mat′ik, -tō-sō′mik) Having a slender, light, or thin body. [lepto- + G. *sōma,* body]

Lep•to•spi•ra (lep′tō-spī′ră) A genus of aerobic bacteria containing thin, tightly coiled organisms 6–20 mcm in length. Associated with icterohemorrhagic fever. [lepto- + G. *speira,* a coil]

lep•to•spi•ral jaun•dice (lep′tō-spī′răl jawn′dis) Jaundice associated with infection by various species of *Leptospira*.

lep•to•spi•ro•sis (lep′tō-spī-rō′sis) An acute infectious disease caused by a spirochete, *Leptospira interrogans;* infection is zoonotic and distributed worldwide.

lep•to•spi•ru•ri•a (lep′tō-spīr-yūr′ē-ă) The presence of species of the genus *Leptospira* in the urine as a result of leptospirosis in the renal tubules.

lep•to•tene (lep′tō-tēn) Early stage of prophase in meiosis in which the chromosomes contract and become visible as long filaments well separated from each other. [lepto- + G. *tainia,* band, tape]

Lep•to•trich•i•a (lep′tō-trik′ē-ă) A genus of anaerobic, nonmotile bacteria containing gram-negative, straight or slightly curved rods, with one or both ends rounded or pointed. These organisms occur in the human oral cavity. The type species is *Leptotrichia buccalis*. [lepto- + G. *thrix,* hair]

Lep•to•trom•bid•i•um (lep′tō-trom-bid′ē-ŭm) An important genus of trombiculid mites, which includes all of the vectors of scrub typhus (tsutsugamushi disease).

Lep•to•trom•bid•i•um a•ka•mu•shi (lep′tō-trom-bid′ē-ŭm ah-kah-mū′shē) One of two species of trombiculid mites, the other being *L. deliensis* (*Trombicula deliensis*), implicated in the transmission of *Orientia tsutsugamushi*, agent of tsutsugamushi disease in Asia.

Le•riche op•er•a•tion (lĕ-rēsh′ op-ĕr-ā′shŭn) SYN periarterial sympathectomy.

Le•riche syn•drome (lĕ-rēsh′ sin′drōm) Aortoiliac occlusive disease producing distal ischemic symptoms and signs.

Le•ri sign (lĕ-rē′ sīn) Voluntary flexion of the elbow is impossible in a case of hemiplegia when the wrist on that side is passively flexed.

Ler•moy•ez syn•drome (ler-mwah-yā′ sin′drōm) Increasing hearing loss and tinnitus preceding an attack of vertigo, after which the hearing improves. Variant of Ménière disease.

LES Abbreviation for lower esophageal sphincter.

les•bi•an (lez′bē-ăn) **1.** A female homosexual or a female homosexual lifestyle. **2.** One who practices lesbianism. SEE ALSO gay.

les•bi•an•ism (lez′bē-ăn-izm) Homosexuality involving women. SYN sapphism. [G. *lesbios,* relating to the island of Lesbos]

Lesch-Ny•han syn•drome (lĕsh nī′ăn sin′drōm) Complete inborn deficiency of enzyme hypoxanthine phosphoribosyltransferase in purine metabolism pathway; causes mental retardation, self-mutilation, choreoathetosis, and hyperuricemia. Invariably fatal in childhood.

le•sion (lē′zhŭn) **1.** A wound or injury. **2.** A pathologic change in the tissues. **3.** One of the individual points or patches of a multifocal disease. See page 886. [L. *laedo,* pp. *laesus,* to injure]

les•ser a•lar car•ti•lag•es (les′ĕr ā′lăr kahr′ti-lăj-ĕz) The two to four cartilaginous plates of the wing of the nose posterior to the greater alar cartilage.

les•ser cur•va•ture of stom•ach (les′ĕr kŭr′vă-chŭr stŏm′ăk) The right border of the stomach to which the lesser omentum is attached.

les•ser in•ter•nal cu•ta•ne•ous nerve (lĕs′ĕr in-tĕr′năl kyū-tā′nē-ŭs nĕrv) SYN medial cutaneous nerve of forearm.

les•ser oc•ci•pi•tal nerve (les′ĕr ok-sip′i-tăl nĕrv) Arises from cervical plexus, conveying fibers from ventral primary rami of second and third cervical nerves; supplies skin of posterior surface of auricle and adjacent portion of the scalp posterior to auricle. SYN nervus occipitalis minor.

les•ser o•men•tum (les′ĕr ō-men′tŭm) A peritoneal fold passing from the margins of the porta hepatis and the bottom of the fissure of the ductus venosus to the lesser curvature of the stomach and to the upper border of the duodenum for a distance of about 2 cm beyond the gastroduodenal pylorus.

les•ser pal•a•tine ar•ter•y (les′ĕr pal′ă-tīn′ ahr′tĕr-ē) One of several posterior branches of the descending palatine in the greater palatine canal, distributed to the soft palate and tonsil. SYN arteria palatina minor.

les•ser pa•la•tine ca•nals (les′ĕr pal′ă-tīn kă-nalz′) Canals located in the posterior part of the palatine bone.

les•ser pal•a•tine fo•ram•i•na (les′ĕr pal′ă-tīn fŏr-am′i-nă) Openings on the hard palate of palatine canals that pass vertically through the tuberosity of the palatine bone and transmit the smaller palatine nerves and vessels. SYN foramina palatina minora [TA].

les•ser pal•a•tine nerves (les′ĕr pal′ă-tīn nĕrvz) Usually two, these emerge through the lesser palatine foramina and supply the mucosa and glands of the soft palate and uvula; they are branches of the pterygopalatine ganglion and contain postsynaptic parasympathetic and sensory fibers of the maxillary nerve. SYN nervi palatini minores [TA].

les•ser pel•vis (les′ĕr pel′vis) The cavity of the pelvis below the brim or superior aperture.

les•ser pe•tro•sal nerve (les′ĕr pĕ-trō′săl nĕrv) The parasympathetic root of the otic ganglion, derived from the tympanic plexus; it leaves the tympanic cavity through the canal for the lesser petrosal nerve and passes within the cranium to the sphenopetrosal fissure, or to the foramen ovale, or to the petrosal foramen, through which it descends to reach the otic ganglion; conveys presynaptic parasympathetic fibers from the glossopharyngeal nerve concerned with secretomotor innervation of the parotid gland. SYN lesser superficial petrosal nerve, nervus petrosus minor, parasympathetic root of otic ganglion, radix parasympathica ganglii otici.

les•ser rhom•boid mus•cle (les′ĕr rom′boyd mŭs′ĕl) SYN rhomboid minor muscle.

les•ser splanch•nic nerve (les′ĕr splangk′nik nĕrv) One of the abdominopelvic splanchnic nerves arising in the thorax from the last two thoracic sympathetic ganglia and passing through the diaphragm to the aorticorenal ganglion; conveys presynaptic sympathetic fibers and visceral afferent fibers. SYN nervus splanchnicus minor [TA].

les·ser su·per·fi·ci·al pe·tro·sal nerve (les′ĕr sū′pĕr-fish′ăl pĕ-trō′săl nĕrv) SYN lesser petrosal nerve.

Les·ser tri·an·gle (les′ĕr trī′ang-gĕl) The space between the bellies of the digastric muscle and the hypoglossal nerve.

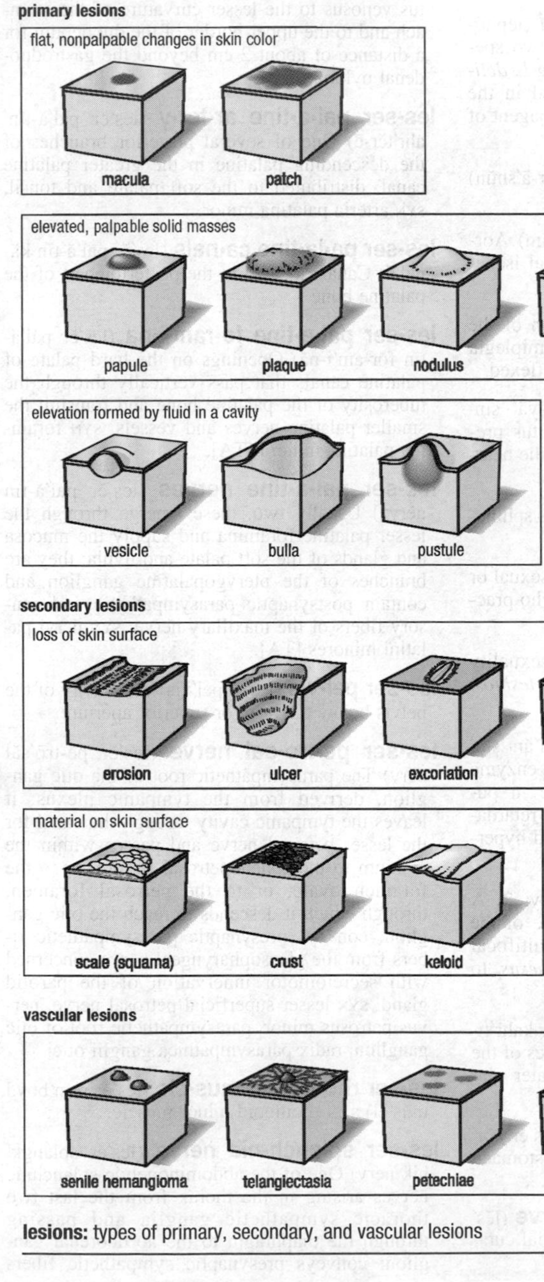

lesions: types of primary, secondary, and vascular lesions

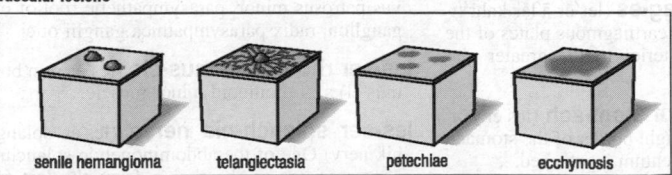

les·ser tro·chan·ter (les′ĕr trō-kan′tĕr) A pyramidal process projecting from the medial and proximal part of the shaft of the femur at the line of junction of the shaft and the neck; it receives the insertion of the psoas major and iliacus (iliopsoas) muscles.

less·er tu·ber·cle of the hu·mer·us (les′ĕr tū′bĕr-kăl hyū′mĕr-ŭs) The smaller and more

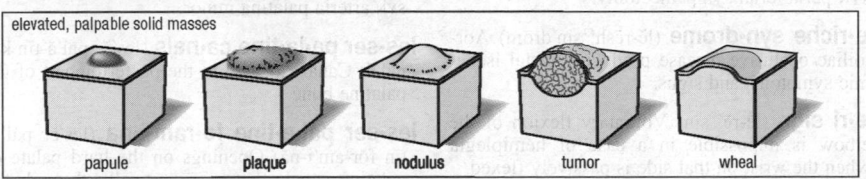

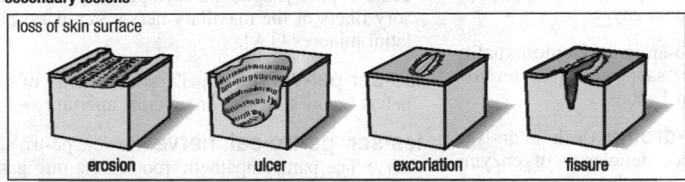

medial prominence of the two tubercles of the proximal end of the humerus.

les•ser ves•tib•u•lar glands (les'ĕr ves-tib'yŭ-lăr glandz) A number of minute mucous glands opening on the surface of the vestibule between the orifices of the vagina and urethra.

les•ser wing of sphe•noid bone (les'ĕr wing sfē'noyd bōn) One of a bilateral pair of triangular, pointed plates extending laterally from the anterolateral body of the sphenoid bone. Forming the posteriormost portion of the floor of the anterior cranial fossa, their sharp posterior edge forms the sphenoidal ridge separating anterior and middle cranial fossae. The medial end of the lesser wing attaches to the body by means of two pedicles, thus forming the optic canal. The wing itself forms the superior margin of the supraorbital fissure. SYN ala minor ossis sphenoidalis [TA].

les•ser zy•go•ma•tic mus•cle (les'ĕr zī'gō-mat'ik mŭs'ĕl) SYN zygomaticus minor muscle.

less fat (les fat) A product so labeled contains, by F.D.A. order, 25% or less fat than the comparison food.

less, few•er, or re•duced (les, fyū'ĕr, rē-dūst') These terms, when used in food labeling, mean that, according to F.D.A. regulations, the food so labeled contains at least 25% less of a given nutrient or ingredient than a similar product.

Less•haft tri•an•gle (les'hahft trī'ang-gĕl) SYN Grynfeltt triangle.

LET Abbreviation for linear energy transfer; leukocyte esterase test.

le•thal (lē'thăl) **1.** Pertaining to or causing death; denoting especially the causal agent. **2.** BIOWARFARE an agent that causes death in 10% or more of healthy adults. [L. *letalis,* fr. *letum,* death]

le•thal Ct$_{50}$ (LCt$_{50}$) (lē'thăl) The Ct product required to kill 50% of an exposed group.

le•thal dose (LD) (lē'thăl dōs) The dose of a chemical or biologic preparation (e.g., a bacterial exotoxin or a suspension of bacteria) that is likely to cause death; it varies in relation to the type of animal and the route of administration; when followed by a subscript (generally LD_{50}), it denotes the median LD likely to cause death in a certain percentage (e.g., 50%) of the test animals; median LD is LD_{50}, absolute lethal LD is LD_{100}, and minimal LD is LD_{05}.

le•thal fac•tor (lē'thăl fak'tŏr) SEE genetic lethal.

le•thal gene (lē'thăl jēn) A gene that produces a genotype that leads to death of the organism before reproduction is possible or that precludes reproduction; for a recessive gene the homozygous or hemizygous state is lethal.

le•thal mu•ta•tion (lē'thăl myū-tā'shŭn) A mutant trait that leads to a phenotype incompatible with effective reproduction.

leth•ar•gy (leth'ăr-jē) A state of deep and prolonged unconsciousness, resembling profound slumber, from which one can be aroused but into which one immediately relapses. [G. *lēthargis,* drowsiness]

LETS (letz) Acronym for large, external transformation-sensitive fibronectin.

Let•ter•er-Si•we dis•ease (let'er-er-sē'vē di-zēz') The acute disseminated form of Langerhans cell histiocytosis. SYN nonlipid histiocytosis.

♻ **leuc-, leuco-** Combining forms meaning white; white blood cell. SEE ALSO leuko-, leuk-. [G. *leukos,* white]

leucaemia [Br.] SYN leukemia.

leucapheresis [Br.] SYN leukapheresis.

leu•cine (lū'sēn) The L-isomer is one of the amino acids of proteins; a nutritionally essential amino acid.

leu•cin•u•ri•a (lū'si-nyūr'ē-ă) The excretion of leucine in the urine.

leucocidin [Br.] SYN leukocidin.

leucocyte [Br.] SYN leukocyte.

leucocytic [Br.] SYN leukocytic.

leucocytolysis [Br.] SYN leukocytolysis.

leucocytoma [Br.] SYN leukocytoma.

leucocytopenia [Br.] SYN leukopenia.

leucocytosis [Br.] SYN leukocytosis.

leucoderma [Br.] SYN leukoderma.

leucodystrophy [Br.] SYN leukodystrophy.

leucoencephalitis [Br.] SYN leukoencephalitis.

leucoencephalopathy [Br.] SYN leukoencephalopathy.

leucoerythroblastosis [Br.] SYN leukoerythroblastosis.

leucokininase [Br.] SYN leukokininase.

leucoma [Br.] SYN leukoma.

leuconychia [Br.] SYN leukonychia.

leucopenia [Br.] SYN leukopenia.

leucoplakia [Br.] SYN leukoplakia.

leucopoiesis [Br.] SYN leukopoiesis.

leucorrhoea [Br.] SYN leukorrhea.

leucosis [Br.] SYN leukosis.

leucotomy [Br.] SYN leukotomy.

leucotriene [Br.] SYN leukotrienes.

Leu•det tin•ni•tus (lū-dā′ tin′i-tŭs) A dry spasmodic click, also audible through the otoscope, heard in catarrhal inflammation of the pharyngotympanic (auditory) tube; caused by reflex spasm of the tensor palati muscle.

leukaemia [Br.] SYN leukemia.

leukaemia cutis [Br.] SYN leukemia cutis.

leukaemia inhibitory factor [Br.] SYN leukemia inhibitory factor.

leukaemic [Br.] SYN leukemic.

leukaemic retinopathy [Br.] SYN leukemic retinopathy.

leukaemid [Br.] SYN leukemid.

leukaemogen [Br.] SYN leukemogen.

leukaemogenesis [Br.] SYN leukemogenesis.

leukaemogenic [Br.] SYN leukemogenic.

leukaemoid [Br.] SYN leukemoid.

leukaemoid reaction [Br.] SYN leukemoid reaction.

leuk•a•phe•re•sis (lū′kă-fĕr-ē′sis) A procedure, analogous to plasmapheresis, in which leukocytes are removed from the withdrawn blood and the remainder of the blood is retransfused into the donor. SYN leucapheresis. [leuko- + G. *aphairesis,* a withdrawal]

leu•ke•mi•a (lū-kē′mē-ă) Progressive proliferation of abnormal leukocytes found in hemopoietic tissues, other organs, and usually in the blood in increased numbers. Leukemia is classified by the dominant cell type, and by duration from onset to death, which occurs in acute leukemia within a few months in most cases, and is associated with acute symptoms including severe anemia, hemorrhages, and slight enlargement of lymph nodes or the spleen. The duration of chronic leukemia exceeds 1 year, with a gradual onset of symptoms of anemia or marked enlargement of spleen, liver, or lymph nodes. SYN leucaemia, leukaemia. [leuko- + G. *haima,* blood]

leu•ke•mi•a cu•tis (lū-kē′mē-ă kyū′tis) Yellow-brown, red, blue-red, or purple, sometimes nodular lesions associated with diffuse infiltration of leukemic cells in the skin. SYN leukaemia cutis.

leu•ke•mi•a in•hib•i•to•ry fac•tor (lū-kē′mē-ă in-hib′i-tōr-ē fak′tōr) A lymphokine that inhibits the migration of neutrophils. SYN leukaemia inihibitory factor.

leu•ke•mic (lū-kē′mik) Pertaining to, or having the characteristics of, any form of leukemia. SYN leukaemic.

leu•ke•mic ret•i•nop•a•thy (lū-kē′mik ret′i-nop′ă-thē) Appearance of the retina in all types of leukemia, characterized by engorgement and tortuosity of veins, scattered hemorrhages, and edema of the retina and disc. SYN leukaemic retinopathy.

leu•ke•mid (lū-kē′mid) Any nonspecific type of cutaneous lesion that is associated with leukemia but is not a localized accumulation of leukemic cells (e.g., petechiae, vesicles, wheals, bullae, hematomas, and the lesions of exfoliative dermatitis and herpes zoster). SYN leukaemid. [leuko- + G. *haima,* blood, + *id* (1)]

leu•ke•mo•gen (lū-kē′mō-jen) Any substance or entity considered to be a causal factor in the occurrence of leukemia. SYN leukaemogen.

leu•ke•mo•gen•e•sis (lū-kē′mō-jen′ĕ-sis) The causation (or induction), development, and progression of a leukemic disease. SYN leukaemogenesis. [leukemia + G. *genesis,* production]

leu•ke•mo•gen•ic (lū-kē′mō-jen′ik) Pertaining to the causation, induction, and development of leukemia; manifesting the ability to cause leukemia. SYN leukaemogenic.

leu•ke•moid (lū-kē′moyd) Resembling leukemia in various signs and symptoms, especially with reference to changes in the circulating blood. SEE ALSO leukemoid reaction. SYN leukaemoid. [leukemia + G. *eidos,* resemblance]

leu•ke•moid re•ac•tion (lū-kē′moyd rē-ak′shŭn) Leukocytosis similar to that occurring in leukemia, but not the result of leukemic disease. Leukemoid reactions are sometimes observed as a feature of infectious disease (tuberculosis, diphtheria), intoxication (eclampsia, mustard gas poisoning), malignant neoplasms, and acute hemorrhage or hemolysis. SYN leukaemoid reaction.

♻ **leuko-, leuk-** Combining forms meaning white; white blood cells. For some words beginning this way, see leuc- and leuco-. [G. *leukos,* white]

leu•ko•ag•glu•ti•nin (lū′kō-ă-glū′ti-nin) An antibody that agglutinates white blood cells.

leu•ko•blast (lū′kō-blast) An immature white blood cell that is transitional between the lymphoidocyte and the promyelocyte; the cytoplasm is polychromatophilic, the nuclear chromatin is thicker, and the nucleoli less distinct. [leuko- + G. *blastos,* germ]

leu•ko•blas•to•sis (lū′kō-blas-tō′sis) A general term for the abnormal proliferation of leukocytes, especially as occurs in myelocytic and lymphocytic leukemia.

leu•ko•ci•din (lū′kō-sī′din) A heat-labile substance that is elaborated by many strains of *Staphylococcus aureus, Streptococcus pyogenes,* and pneumococci; manifests a destructive action on leukocytes, with or without lysis of the cells. SYN leucocidin. [leukocyte + L. *caedo,* to kill]

leu•ko•co•ri•a, **leu•ko•ko•ri•a** (lū′kō-kōr′ē-ă, lū′kō-kōr′ē-ă) Reflection from a white mass within the eye giving the appearance of a white pupil. [*leuko-* white, + G. *korē,* pupil]

leu•ko•cyte (lū′kō-sīt) A type of cell formed in the myelopoietic, lymphoid, and reticular portions of the reticuloendothelial system in various parts of the body, and normally present in those sites and in the circulating blood. Under various abnormal conditions, the total number of leukocytes may be increased or decreased or their relative proportions altered, and they may appear in other tissues and organs. Leukocytes represent three lines of development from primitive elements: myeloid, lymphoid, and monocytic series. On the basis of features observed with various methods of staining with polychromatic dyes, cells of the myeloid series are frequently termed granular leukocytes, or granulocytes; because the cytoplasmic granules of lymphocytes and monocytes are smaller and frequently not clearly visualized with routine methods, these cells are sometimes termed nongranular or agranular leukocytes. Granulocytes are commonly known as polymorphonuclear leukocytes (also polynuclear or multinuclear leukocytes), because in a mature cell the nucleus is divided into two to five rounded or ovoid lobes that are connected with thin strands or small bands of chromatin; they consist of three distinct types: neutrophils, eosinophils, and basophils, named on the basis of the staining reactions of the cytoplasmic granules. Cells of the lymphocytic series are smaller than other leukocytes and have relatively large, darkly staining, eccentrically placed nuclei. Cells of the monocytic series are usually larger than the other leukocytes and are characterized by a relatively abundant, slightly opaque, pale blue or blue-gray cytoplasm that contains many fine reddish-blue granules. Monocytes are usually indented, reniform, or shaped similarly to a horseshoe, but are sometimes rounded or ovoid; their nuclei are usually large and centrally placed and, even when eccentrically located, are completely surrounded by at least a small band of cytoplasm. SYN leucocyte, white blood cell. [leuko- + G. *kytos,* cell]

leu•ko•cyte ad•he•sion de•fi•cien•cy (LAD) (lū′kō-sīt ad-hē′zhŭn dĕ-fish′ĕn-sē) An inherited disorder in which there is a defective CD18 adherence complex that disturbs leukocyte chemotaxis. It is characterized by recurrent bacterial infections and impaired wound healing.

leu•ko•cyte es•ter•ase test (LET) (lū′kō-sīt es′tĕr-ās test) A chemical assay to determine the presence of lysed or intact white blood cells in urine, performed with a dipstick as part of routine urinalysis; serves as an adjunct to microscopic examination of urinary sediment, and used to screen asymptomatic people for urinary tract infection, especially chlamydial urethritis.

leu•ko•cyt•ic (lū′kō-sit′ik) Pertaining to or characterized by leukocytes. SYN leucocytic.

leu•ko•cy•to•blast (lū-kō-sī′tō-blast) A nonspecific term for any immature cell from which a leukocyte develops, including lymphoblasts and myeloblasts. [leukocyte + G. *blastos,* germ]

leu•ko•cy•toc•la•sis (lū′kō-sī-tok′lă-sis) Karyorrhexis of leukocytes. [leuko- + G. *kytos,* cell, + *klasia,* a breaking]

leu•ko•cy•to•clas•tic vas•cu•li•tis (lū′kō-sī-tō-klas′tik vas′kyū-lī′tis) Cutaneous acute vasculitis characterized clinically by palpable purpura, especially of the legs, and histologically by exudation of the neutrophils and sometimes fibrin around dermal venules, with nuclear dust and extravasation of red blood cells; may be limited to the skin or involve other tissues as in Henoch-Schönlein purpura. SEE ALSO cutaneous vasculitis. [G. *leukos,* white, + *kytos,* cell, + *klastos,* broken, fr. *klao,* to break]

leu•ko•cy•to•gen•e•sis (lū′kō-sī′tō-jen′ĕ-sis) The formation and development of leukocytes. [leukocyte + G. *genesis,* production]

leu•ko•cy•tol•y•sin (lū′kō-sī-tol′i-sin) Any substance (including lytic antibody) that causes dissolution of leukocytes. SYN leukolysin.

leu•ko•cy•tol•y•sis (lū′kō-sī-tol′i-sis) Dissolution or lysis of leukocytes. SYN leucocytolysis. [leukocyte + G. *lysis,* dissolution]

leu•ko•cy•to•lyt•ic (lū′kō-sī′tō-lit′ik) Pertaining to, causing, or manifesting leukocytolysis.

leu•ko•cy•to•ma (lū′kō-sī-tō′mă) A fairly well circumscribed, nodular, dense accumulation of leukocytes. SYN leucocytoma. [leukocyte + G. *-oma,* tumor]

leu•ko•cy•to•pe•ni•a (lū′kō-sī′tō-pē′nē-ă) SYN leukopenia.

leu•ko•cy•to•pla•ni•a (lū′kō-sī′tō-plā′nē-ă) Movement of leukocytes from the lumens of blood vessels through serous membranes, or in the tissues. [leukocyte + G. *planē,* a wandering]

leu•ko•cy•to•poi•e•sis (lū′kō-sī′tō-poy-ē′sis) SYN leukopoiesis. [leukocyte + G. *poiēsis,* a making]

leu•ko•cy•to•sis (lū′kō-sī-tō′sis) An actual increase in the total number of leukocytes in the blood, as distinguished from a relative increase (e.g., in dehydration). SYN leucocytosis.

leu•ko•cy•to•tac•tic (lū′kō-sī′tō-tak′tik) Pertaining to, characterized by, or causing leukocytotaxia. SYN leukotactic.

leu•ko•cy•to•tax•i•a (lū-kō-sī′tō-tak′sē-ă) **1.** The active ameboid movement of leukocytes, especially the neutrophilic granulocytes, either toward (positive leukocytotaxia) or away from (negative leukocytotaxia) certain microorganisms as well as various substances formed in inflamed tissue. **2.** The property of attracting or repelling leukocytes. SYN leukotaxia, leukotaxis. [leukocyte + G. *taxis,* arrangement]

leu•ko•cy•to•tox•in (lū′kō-sī′tō-tok′sin) Any substance that causes degeneration and necrosis of leukocytes, including leukolysin and leukocidin. SYN leukotoxin. [leukocyte + G. *toxikon,* poison]

leu•ko•cy•tu•ri•a (lū′kō-sī-tyūr′ē-ă) The presence of leukocytes in urine that is recently voided or collected by means of a catheter. [leukocyte + G. *ouron,* urine]

leu•ko•der•ma (lū′kō-dĕr′mă) An absence of pigment, partial or total, in the skin. SYN leucoderma, leukopathia, leukopathy. [leuko- + G. *derma,* skin]

leu•ko•dys•tro•phy (lū′kō-dis′trŏ-fē) A group of white matter diseases, some familial, characterized by progressive cerebral deterioration in early life and primary absence or degeneration of the myelin of the central and peripheral nervous systems; probably related to a defect in lipid metabolism; the adult type of Pelizaeus-Merzbacher disease is inherited as an autosomal dominant trait. SYN leucodystrophy. [leuko- + G. *dys,* bad, + *trophē,* nourishment]

leu•ko•e•de•ma (lū′kō-ĕ-dē′mă) A bluish-white opalescence of the buccal mucosa that becomes the normal mucosal color on stretching the tissue; may be considered a normal anatomic variation. SYN leuko-oedema.

leu•ko•en•ceph•a•li•tis (lū′kō-en-sef′ă-lī′tis) Encephalitis restricted to the white matter. SYN leucoencephalitis.

leu•ko•en•ceph•a•lop•a•thy (lū′kō-en-sef′ă-lop′ă-thē) White matter changes first described in children with leukemia, associated with radiation and chemotherapy injury, often associated with methotrexate; pathologically characterized by diffuse reactive astrocytosis with multiple areas of necrotic foci without inflammation. SYN leucoencephalopathy. [leuko- + G. *enkephalos,* brain, + *pathos,* suffering]

leu•ko•e•ryth•ro•blas•to•sis (lū′kō-ĕ-rith′rō-blas-tō′sis) Any anemic condition resulting from space-occupying lesions in the bone marrow; the blood contains immature cells of the granulocytic series and nucleated red blood cells. SYN leucoerythroblastosis, myelophthisic anemia, myelopathic anemia.

leu•ko•ki•ni•nase (lū′kō-kī′ni-nās) An enzyme that cleaves tuftsin to release leukokinin. SYN leucokininase.

leu•kol•y•sin (lū-kol′i-sin) SYN leukocytolysin.

leu•ko•ma (lū-kō′mă) A dense white opacity of the cornea. SYN leucoma. [G. whiteness, a white spot in the eye, fr. *leukos,* white]

leu•ko•ma•tous (lū-kō′mă-tŭs) Denoting leukoma.

leu•ko•my•e•lop•a•thy (lū′kō-mī′ĕ-lop′ă-thē) Any disease involving the white matter or the conducting tracts of the spinal cord. [leuko- + G. *myelos,* marrow, + *pathos,* suffering]

leu•ko•nych•i•a (lū′kō-nik′ē-ă) The occurrence of white spots, streaks, or patches under the nails, due to the presence of air bubbles between the nail and its bed. SYN leuconychia. [leuko- + G. *onyx* (*onych-*), nail]

leuko-oedema [Br.] SYN leukoedema.

leu•ko•path•i•a, **leu•kop•a•thy** (lū′kō-path′ē-ă, lū-kop′ă-thē) SYN leukoderma. [leuko- + G. *pathos,* disease]

leu•ko•pe•de•sis (lū′kō-pĕ-dē′sis) The movement of white blood cells (especially polymorphonuclear leukocytes) through the walls of capillaries and into the tissues. [leuko- + G. *pēdēsis,* a leaping]

leu•ko•pe•ni•a (lū′kō-pē′nē-ă) Any condition in which the number of leukocytes in the circulating blood is lower than normal, the lower limit of which is generally regarded as 4000–5000/mm^3 SYN leucocytopenia, leucopenia, leukocytopenia. [leuko(cyte) + G. *penia,* poverty]

leu•ko•pe•nic (lū′kō-pē′nik) Pertaining to leukopenia.

leu•ko•pe•nic in•dex (lū′kō-pē′nik in′deks) A significant decrease in the white blood cell count after ingestion of food to which a patient is hypersensitive, a count made during the normal fasting state being used as the basis for evaluation of the postprandial count.

leu•ko•pe•nic leu•ke•mi•a (lū′kō-pē′nik lū-kē′mē-ă) A form of lymphocytic, granulocytic, or monocytic leukemia in which the number of white blood cells is in the normal range or slightly depressed.

leu•ko•pla•ki•a (lū′kō-plā′kē-ă) A white patch of oral mucous membrane that cannot be wiped off and cannot be diagnosed clinically; the spots are smooth, irregular in size and shape, hard, and occasionally fissured. Often associated with pipe smoking. Biopsy may show malignant or premalignant changes. See this page. SYN leucoplakia. [leuko- + G. *plax,* plate]

leu•ko•pla•ki•a vul•vae (lū′kō-plā′kē-ă vŭl′vē)

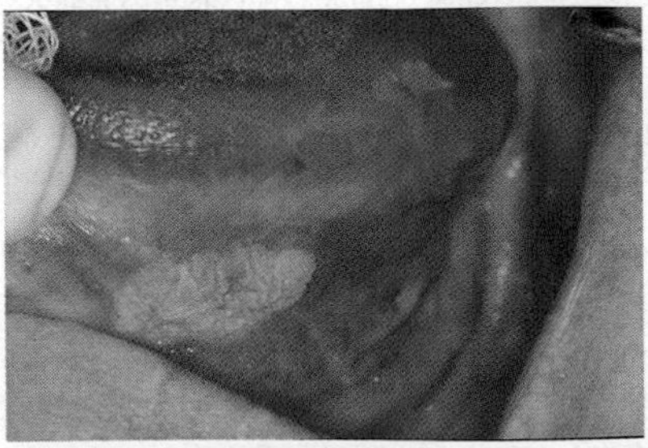

leukoplakia: with mild epithelial dysplasia

A clinical term for hyperkeratotic white patches of the vulvar epithelium; biopsy is necessary for specific diagnosis.

leu•ko•poi•e•sis (lū′kō-poy-ē′sis) Formation and development of the various types of white blood cells. SYN leucopoiesis, leukocytopoiesis. [leuko- + G. *poiēsis,* a making]

leu•ko•poi•et•ic (lū′kō-poy-et′ik) Pertaining to or characterized by leukopoiesis, as manifested by portions of the bone marrow and reticuloendothelial and lymphoid tissues, which form (respectively) the granulocytes, monocytes, and lymphocytes.

leu•kor•rha•gi•a (lū′kō-rā′jē-ă) SYN leukorrhea. [leuko- + G. *rhēgnymi,* to burst forth]

leu•kor•rhe•a (lū′kōr-ē′ă) Discharge from the vagina of a white or yellowish viscid fluid. SYN leucorrhoea, leukorrhagia, leukorrhoea. [leuko- + G. *rhoia,* flow]

leukorrhoea [Br.] SYN leukorrhea.

leu•ko•sis (lū-kō′sis) Abnormal proliferation of one or more of the leukopoietic tissues; the term includes myelosis, certain forms of reticuloendotheliosis, and lymphadenosis. SYN leucosis.

leu•ko•tac•tic (lū′kō-tak′tik) SYN leukocytotactic.

leu•ko•tax•i•a (lū′kō-tak′sē-ă) SYN leukocytotaxia.

leu•ko•tax•ine (lū′kō-tak′sēn) A cell-free nitrogenous material prepared from injured, acutely degenerating tissue and from inflammatory exudates.

leu•ko•tax•is (lū′kō-tak′sis) SYN leukocytotaxia.

leu•kot•ic (lū-kot′ik) Pertaining to, characterized by, or manifesting leukosis.

leu•kot•o•my (lū-kot′ŏ-mē) Incision into the white matter of the frontal lobe of the brain. SYN leucotomy. [leuko- + G. *tomē,* a cutting]

leu•ko•tox•in (lū′kō-tok′sin) SYN leukocytotoxin.

leu•ko•trich•i•a (lū′kō-trik′ē-ă) Whiteness of the hair. [leuko- + G. *thrix,* hair]

leu•ko•tri•enes (LT) (lū′kō-trī′ēnz) Products of eicosanoid metabolism with physiologic roles in inflammation and allergic reactions. SYN leucotriene.

LEU M1 The epitope for a monoclonal antibody generated to the human histiocytic cell line that localizes to neutrophils, adherent monocytes, and a subgroup of activated T cells.

le•va•tor (le-vā′tŏr) **1.** A surgical instrument for prying up the depressed part in a cranial fracture. **2.** One of several muscles the action of which is to raise the part into which it is inserted. [L. a lifter, fr. *levo,* pp. *-atus,* to lift, fr. *levis,* light]

le•va•tor an•gu•li o•ris mus•cle (le-vā′tŏr an′gyū-lī ō′ris mŭs′ĕl) *Origin,* canine fossa of maxilla; *insertion,* orbicularis oris and skin at angle of mouth; *action,* raises angle of mouth; *nerve supply,* facial. SYN musculus levator anguli oris [TA].

le•va•tor a•ni mus•cle (le-vā′tŏr ā′nī mŭs′ĕl) Formed by pubococcygeus and iliococcygeus muscles; *origin,* posterior body of pubis, tendinous arch of the levator ani, and spine of ischium; *insertion,* anococcygeal ligament, sides of the lower part of the sacrum and of coccyx; *action,* resists prolapsing forces and draws the anus upward following defecation; supports the pelvic viscera; *nerve supply,* nerve to levator ani (fourth sacral spinal nerve). SYN musculus levator ani [TA].

le•va•tor cos•ta•rum mus•cles (le-vā′tŏr kos-tā′rūm mŭs′ĕlz) Muscle of thorax; *origin,* tips of transverse processes of C7 and T1–T11 vertebrae; *insertion,* ribs, between tubercle and angle; *action,* elevate ribs for deep inspiration; *nerve,* dorsal rami of C8–T11 spinal nerves. SYN elevator muscle of rib, musculi levatores costarum.

le•va•tor la•bi•i su•pe•ri•o•ris a•lae•que na•si mus•cle (le-vā′tŏr lā′bē-ī sū-pēr-ē-ō′ris ă-lē′kwē nā′sī mŭs′ĕl) *Origin,* root of nasal process of maxilla; *insertion,* wing of nose and orbicularis oris muscle of upper lip; *action,* elevates upper lip and wing of nose; *nerve supply,* facial. SYN musculus levator labii superioris alaeque nasi [TA].

le•va•tor la•bi•i su•pe•ri•o•ris mus•cle (le-vā′tŏr lā′bē-ī sū-pēr-ē-ō′ris mŭs′ĕl) *Origin,* maxilla below infraorbital foramen; *insertion,* orbicularis oris of upper lip; *action,* elevates upper lip; *nerve supply,* facial. SYN musculus levator labii superioris [TA].

le•va•tor mus•cle of thy•roid gland (le-vā′tŏr mŭs′ĕl thī′royd gland) A fasciculus occasionally passing from the thyrohyoid muscle to the isthmus of the thyroid gland. SYN musculus levator glandulae thyroideae [TA].

le•va•tor pal•pe•brae su•pe•ri•o•ris mus•cle (le-vā′tŏr pal-pē′brē sū-pēr-ē-ō′ris mŭs′ĕl) *Origin,* orbital surface of the lesser wing of the sphenoid, above and anterior to the optic canal; *insertion,* skin of eyelid, tarsal plate, and orbital walls, by medial and lateral expansions of the aponeurosis of insertion; *action,* raises the upper eyelid; *nerve supply,* oculomotor. SYN musculus levator palpebrae superioris [TA], elevator muscle of upper eyelid.

le•va•tor pros•ta•tae mus•cle (le-vā′tŏr pros′tā-tē mŭs′ĕl) In the male, the most medial fibers of the levator ani (pubococcygeus) muscle that extend from the pubis into the fascia of the prostate. SYN musculus levator prostatae [TA].

le•va•tor scap•u•lae mus•cle (le-vā′tŏr skap′yū-lē mŭs′ĕl) *Origin,* from posterior tubercles of transverse processes of four upper cervical vertebrae; *insertion*, into superior angle of scapula; *action*, raises the scapula; *nerve supply*, dorsal scapular nerve. SYN musculus levator scapulae [TA], elevator muscle of scapula.

le•va•tor ve•li pa•la•ti•ni mus•cle (le-vā′tŏr vē′lī pal-ă-tē′nī mŭs′ĕl) *Origin*, apex of petrous portion of temporal bone and lower part of cartilaginous auditory (eustachian) tube; *insertion*, aponeurosis of soft palate; *action*, raises soft palate; through the expansion of its fleshy belly during contraction, it helps to "push" open the auditory tube; *nerve supply*, pharyngeal plexus (cranial root of accessory nerve). SYN musculus levator veli palatini [TA], elevator muscle of soft palate.

lev•el (lev′ĕl) Any rank, position, or status in a graded scale of values.

lev•el of con•scious•ness (lev′ĕl kon′shŭs-nĕs) The degree of a patient's alertness and awareness of self and environment, varying from wakefulness to coma. Decreases often measured with the Glasgow Coma Scale, a tool for standardizing uniformity in assessment by more than one observer as a way of standardizing subjective assessment data. SEE ALSO Glasgow Coma Scale.

lev•el-de•pen•dent fre•quen•cy re•sponse (lev′ĕl-dĕ-pen′dĕnt frē′kwĕn-sē rĕ-spons′) One of several strategies used in hearing aids to alter the balance in amplification between high- and low-frequency sounds.

Le•vey-Jen•nings chart (lē′vē-jen′ingz chahrt) SYN quality control chart.

lev•i•ga•tion (lev′i-gā′shŭn) Process of moistening a powdered chemical before mixing it into a cream or ointment to lessen the graininess of the drug. [L. *levigatio*, fr. *levis*, smooth]

Lev•in•stein pro•cess (lev′in-stīn pros′es) SEE Löwenstein process.

Le•vin tube (lĕ-vin′ tūb) A tube introduced through the nose into the upper alimentary canal, to facilitate intestinal decompression.

♻ **levo-** Combining form meaning left, toward or on the left side. SYN laev-, laevo-. [L. *laevus*]

le•vo•car•di•a (lē′vō-kahr′dē-ă) Situs inversus of the other viscera but with the heart normally situated on the left; congenital cardiac lesions are commonly associated. SYN laevocardia. [levo- + G. *kardia,* heart]

le•vo•do•pa (L-do•pa) (lē′vō-dō′pă) The biologically active form of dopa; an antiparkinsonian agent that is converted to dopamine. SYN laevodopa.

le•vo•duc•tion (lē′vō-dŭk′shŭn) Turning of one eye to the left. [levo- + L. *duco,* pp. *ductus,* to lead]

le•vo•ro•ta•tion (lē′vō-rō-tā′shŭn) **1.** A turning or twisting to the left; in particular, the counterclockwise twist given the plane of plane-polarized light by solutions of certain optically active substances. **2.** SYN sinistrotorsion. SYN laevorotation. [levo- + L. *roto,* to turn]

le•vo•ro•ta•to•ry (lē′vō-rō′tă-tōr-ē) Denoting levorotation, or crystals or solutions capable of causing it; as a chemical prefix, usually abbreviated *l-* or (−). Cf. dextrorotatory. SYN laevorotatory.

le•vo•tor•sion (lē′vō-tōr′shŭn) **1.** SYN sinistrotorsion. **2.** Rotation of the upper pole of the cornea of one or both eyes to the left. [levo- + L. *torsio,* a twisting]

le•vo•ver•sion (lē′vō-vĕr′zhŭn) **1.** Version toward the left. **2.** Conjugate turning of both eyes to the left. [levo- + L. *verto,* pp. *versus,* to turn]

Lev•ret for•ceps (lĕv-rā′ fōr′seps) A modification of the Chamberlen forceps, curved to correspond to the curve of the birth canal.

Lev syn•drome (lev sin′drōm) Bundle branch block in a patient with normal myocardium and normal coronary arteries resulting from fibrosis or calcification including the conducting system; affects the membranous septum, the apex of the muscular septum, and often the mitral and aortic valve rings.

Lew•is ac•id (lū′is as′id) An acid that is an electron pair acceptor.

Lew•is base (lū′is bās) A base that is an electron-pair donor.

Lew•i•site (L) (lū′is-īt) A chemical warfare vesicant (NATO Code L) that contains arsenic; developed near the end of World War I but produced mostly in Russia; differs from sulfur mustard in having a latency period of only seconds to a few minutes, in having a greater likelihood to cause pulmonary edema, and in having an antidote, dimercaprol (British anti-Lewisite).

Le•wy bod•y de•men•ti•a (lā′vē bod′ē dĕ-men′shē-ă) SYN diffuse Lewy body disease.

lex•i•cal (leks′i-kăl) Denoting the vocabulary related to or describing speech or language.

♻ **-lexis, -lexy** Combining forms that properly relate to speech, although often confused with -legia (Latin *-lego,* to read) and thus erroneously employed to relate to reading. [G. *lexis*, word, speech, from *legō*, to say]

Ley•den neu•ri•tis (lī′dĕn nūr-ī′tis) Fatty degeneration of the fibers of the affected nerve.

Ley•dig cells (lī′dig selz) SYN interstitial cells (1).

Ley•dig cell tu•mor (lī′dig sel tū′mŏr) A testicular and, less commonly, ovarian neoplasm composed of Leydig cells, usually benign but may be malignant; may secrete androgens or estrogens. Causes gynecomastia in adults and precocious sexual development in prepubescents.

LF Abbreviation for low frequency.

LFT Abbreviation for left frontotransverse position; liver function test.

LGA Abbreviation for large for gestational age.

LGSIL Abbreviation for low-grade squamous intraepithelial lesion.

LH Abbreviation for luteinizing hormone.

Lher•mitte sign (lār-mēt′ sīn) Sudden electriclike shocks extending down the spine on flexing the head.

Li Symbol for lithium.

li•a•ble (lī′ă-bĕl) In health care, denotes legal responsibility (e.g., proper therapy, billing).

lib•er•ins (lib′ĕr-inz) SYN releasing factors. [L. *libero,* to free, + -in]

li•bid•i•nous (li-bid′i-nŭs) Lascivious; invested with or arousing sexual desire or energy. [L. *libidinosus,* fr. *libido* (*libidin-*), pleasure, desire]

li•bi•do (li-bē′dō) **1.** Conscious or unconscious sexual desire. **2.** Any passionate interest or form of life force. **3.** In jungian psychology, synonymous with psychic energy. [L. lust]

Lib•man-Sacks en•do•car•di•tis, Lib•man-Sacks syn•drome (lib′măn saks en′dō-kahr-dī′tis, sin′drōm) Verrucous endocarditis sometimes associated with disseminated lupus erythematosus. SYN atypical verrucous endocarditis, nonbacterial verrucous endocarditis.

lice (līs) Plural of louse.

li•censed prac•ti•cal nurse (LPN) (lī′sĕnst prak′ti-kăl nŭrs) A nurse who has graduated from an accredited school of practical (vocational) nursing, and has been licensed by public authority after passing a qualifying examination.

li•censed vo•ca•tion•al nurse (LVN) (lī′sĕnst vō-kā′shŭn-ăl nŭrs) SYN practical nurse.

li•chen (lī′ken) A discrete flat papule or an aggregate of papules giving a patterned configuration resembling lichens growing on rocks. [G. *leichēn,* lichen; a lichenlike eruption]

li•chen•i•fi•ca•tion (lī′ken-i-fi-kā′shŭn) Leathery induration and thickening of the skin with hyperkeratosis, caused by scratching in atopic or chronic contact dermatitis. See page B11. [lichen + L. *facio,* to make]

li•chen myx•e•de•ma•to•sus (lī′ken miks′ĕ-dē′mă-tō′sŭs) A lichenoid eruption of papules or plaques of mucinous edema due to deposit of glycosaminoglycans in the skin and fibroblast proliferation, in the absence of endocrine disease. SYN papular mucinosis.

li•chen•oid (lī′kĕ-noyd) **1.** Resembling lichen. **2.** Accentuation of normal skin markings observed in cases of chronic eczema. **3.** Microscopically resembling lichen planus.

li•chen•oid der•ma•to•sis (lī′kĕ-noyd dĕr′mă-tō′sis) Any chronic skin eruption, characterized by induration and thickening of the skin with accentuation of skin markings.

li•chen•oid ker•a•to•sis (lī′kĕ-noyd ker′ă-tō′sis) A solitary benign papule or plaque, with microscopic features resembling lichen planus, occurring on sun-exposed or unexposed skin.

li•chen pla•nus, li•chen ru•ber pla•nus (lī′ken plā′nŭs, rū′bĕr plā′nŭs) Eruption of flat-topped, shiny, violaceous papules on flexor surfaces, male genitalia, and buccal mucosa of unknown cause; may form linear groups. Spontaneous resolution is common after months to years. See page 894.

li•chen scle•ro•sus et a•tro•phi•cus (lī′ken skler-ō′sŭs ă-trō′fi-kŭs) A chronic eruption, seen chiefly in the anogenital region, consisting of white atrophic papules which may be discrete or confluent and may contain a central depression or a black keratotic plug.

li•chen scrof•u•lo•so•rum (lī′ken skrō-fyū-lō-sō′rŭm) Small asymptomatic lichen papules on the trunk of children with tuberculosis. SYN papular tuberculid.

li•chen stri•a•tus (lī′ken strī-ā′tŭs) A self-limited papular eruption occurring primarily in children (more commonly in girls); the lesions are arranged in linear groups and usually occur on one extremity.

li•chen ur•ti•ca•tus (lī′ken ŭr-ti-kā′tŭs) SYN papular urticaria.

lid (lid) SYN eyelid.

lie (lī) Relationship of the long axis of the fetus to that of the mother.

Lie•ber•kühn glands (lē′ber-kēn glandz) SYN intestinal glands.

Lie•ber•mei•ster rule (lē′bĕr-mīs′tĕr rūl) In adult febrile tachycardia, about eight pulse beats correspond to an increase of 1°C.

Lie•big the•o•ry (lē′big thē′ŏr-ē) Theory that the hydrocarbons that oxidize readily and burn are aliments that produce the greatest quantity of animal heat.

lie de•tec•tor (lī dĕ-tek′tŏr) SYN polygraph (2).

li•en (lī′en) [TA] SYN spleen. [L.]

lien-, lieno- Combining forms related to the spleen. SEE spleno-. [L. *lien*]

li•en ac•ces•so•ri•us (lī′en ak-ses-sōr′ē-ŭs) SYN accessory spleen.

li•e•nal (lī-ē′năl) SYN splenic.

li·e·nal ar·ter·y (lī-ē′năl ahr′tĕr-ē) SYN splenic artery.

li·en mo·bi·lis (lī′en mō′bi-lis) SYN floating spleen.

li·en·ter·ic (lī′en-ter′ik) Relating to, or marked by, lientery.

li·en·ter·ic di·ar·rhe·a (lī′en-ter′ik dī′ă-rē′ă) Condition in which undigested food appears in the stools.

li·en·ter·y (lī′en-ter-ē) Passage of undigested food in the stools. [G. *leienteria,* fr. *leios,* smooth, + *enteron,* intestine]

life (līf) **1.** The quality or condition proper to living beings; the state of existence characterized by such functions as metabolism, growth, reproduction, adaptation, and response to stimuli. **2.** Living organisms such as animals and plants. [A.S. *life*]

life e·vents (līf ĕ-vents′) Occurrences in one's daily life, some of which act as stressors.

life in·stinct (līf in′stingkt) The instinct of self-preservation and sexual procreation; the basic urge toward preservation of the species.

life-span de·vel·op·ment (līf-span dĕ-vel′ŏp-mĕnt) Development and mastery (or loss) of differing biologic, intellectual, behavioral, and social skills in different stages of the life-span from the prenatal through the gerontologic periods of growth.

life stress (līf stres) Events or experiences that produce severe strain, e.g., failure on the job, marital separation, loss of a love object.

life·style (līf′stīl) Habits and customs influenced by the lifelong process of socialization, including social use of alcohol and tobacco, dietary habits, and exercise, all of which have important implications for health.

life ta·ble (līf tā′bĕl) A representation of the probable years of survivorship of a defined population of subjects.

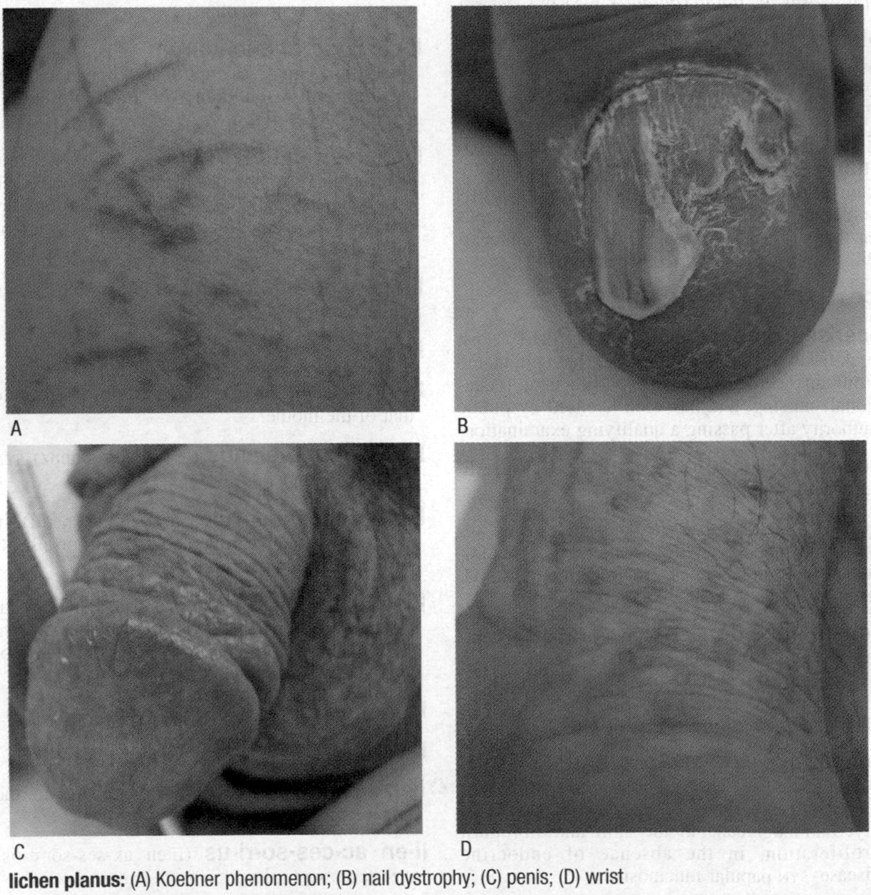

lichen planus: (A) Koebner phenomenon; (B) nail dystrophy; (C) penis; (D) wrist

lift (lift) **1.** To raise or elevate. **2.** The act of lifting. **3.** A device for lifting. [O.E., *lypta*]

lig•a•ment (lig′ă-mĕnt) **1.** A band or sheet of fibrous tissue connecting two or more bones, cartilages, or other structures, or serving as support for fascias or muscles. **2.** A fold of peritoneum supporting any of the abdominal viscera. **3.** Any structure resembling a ligament though not performing the function of such. **4.** [TA] The cordlike remains of a fetal vessel or other structure that has lost its original lumen. See this page. SYN ligamentum [TA]. [L. *ligamentum,* a band, bandage]

lig•a•men•ta in•tra•cap•su•la•ri•a (lig-ă-men′tă in′tră-kap-sū-lā′rē-ă) [TA] SYN intracapsular ligaments.

lig•a•men•ta sus•pen•so•ri•a mam•mae (lig-ă-men′tă sŭs-pen-sōr′ē-ă mam′ē) [TA] SYN suspensory ligaments of breast.

lig•a•ment of head of fe•mur (lig′ă-mĕnt hed fē′mŭr) A flattened ligament that passes from the fovea in the head of the femur to the borders of the acetabular notch (transverse acetabular ligament); the ligament does not contribute to the integrity of the joint or control movements there. SYN ligamentum capitis femoris [TA], round ligament of femur.

lig•a•men•to•pex•is, lig•a•men•to•pex•y (lig′ă-men′tō-pek′sis, -pek′sē) Shortening of any ligament of the uterus. [ligament + G. *pēxis,* fixation]

lig•a•men•tous (lig′ă-men′tŭs) Relating to or of the form or structure of a ligament.

lig•a•men•tum, pl. **lig•a•men•ta** (lig-ă-men′tŭm, -tă) [TA] SYN ligament. [L. a band, tie, fr. *ligo,* to bind]

lig•a•men•tum ca•pi•tis fem•o•ris (lig-ă-men′tŭm kap′i-tis fem′ŏ-ris) [TA] SYN ligament of head of femur.

lig•a•men•tum cor•a•co•ac•ro•mi•a•le (lig-ă-men′tŭm kōr′ă-kō-ă-krō-mē-ā′lē) [TA] SYN coracoacromial ligament.

lig•a•men•tum cor•a•co•cla•vi•cu•la•re (lig-ă-men′tŭm kōr′ă-kō-kla-vik-yū-lā′rē) [TA] SYN coracoclavicular ligament.

lig•a•men•tum cos•to•cla•vi•cu•la•re (lig-ă-men′tŭm kos′tō-kla-vik-yū-lā′rē) [TA] SYN costoclavicular ligament.

lig•a•men•tum cos•to•trans•ver•sa•ri•um (lig-ă-men′tŭm kos′tō-trans-vĕr-sā′rē-ŭm) [TA] SYN costotransverse ligament.

lig•a•men•tum cru•ci•a•tum an•te•ri•us (lig-ă-men′tŭm krū-shē-ā′tŭm an-tē′rē-ŭs) [TA] SYN anterior cruciate ligament.

lig•a•men•tum cru•ci•a•tum pos•te•ri•us (lig-ă-men′tŭm krū-shē-sē-ā′tŭm pos-tēr′ē-ŭs) [TA] SYN posterior cruciate ligament.

lig•a•men•tum del•toi•de•um (lig-ă-men′tŭm del-toy′dē-ŭm) SYN deltoid ligament.

lig•a•men•tum fal•ci•for•me hep•a•tis (lig-ă-men′tŭm fal-si-fōr′mē hē-pā′tis) [TA] SYN falciform ligament of liver.

lig•a•men•tum il•i•o•fem•o•ra•le (lig-ă-men′tŭm il′ē-ō-fem-ō-rā′lē) [TA] SYN iliofemoral ligament.

lig•a•men•tum in•gui•na•le (lig-ă-men′tŭm ing-gwi-nā′lē) [TA] SYN inguinal ligament.

lig•a•men•tum la•cu•na•re (lig-ă-ment′ŭm lak-yū-nā′rē) [TA] SYN lacunar ligament.

lig•a•men•tum la•tum u•ter•i (lig-ă-men′tŭm lā′tŭm yū′tĕr-ī) [TA] SYN broad ligament of the uterus.

lig•a•men•tum lon•gi•tu•di•na•le (lig-ă-men′tŭm lon′ji-tū-di-nā′lē) [TA] SYN longitudinal ligament.

lig•a•men•tum lum•bo•cos•ta•le (lig-ă-men′tŭm lŭm-bō-kos-tā′lē) [TA] SYN lumbocostal ligament.

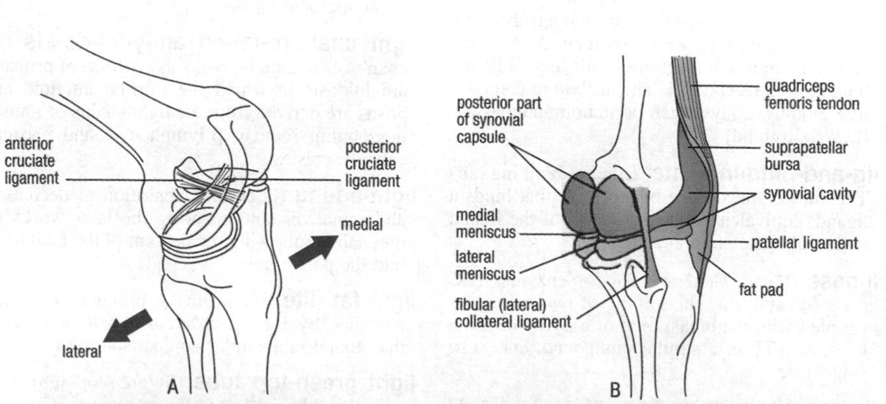

knee ligaments, tendons, and menisci: (A) anterolateral view; (B) posterolateral view

lig·a·men·tum nu·chae (lig-ă-men′tŭm nū′kē) [TA] A sagittal ligamentous band at the back of the neck, formed of thickened supraspinous ligaments; it extends from the external occipital protuberance to the posterior border of the foramen magnum cranially, and to the seventh cervical spinous process caudally. SYN nuchal ligament.

lig·a·men·tum pa·tel·lae (lig-ă-men′tŭm pă-tel′ē) [TA] SYN patellar ligament.

lig·a·men·tum pec·ti·ne·a·le (lig-ă-men′tŭm pek′tin-ē-ā′lē) [TA] SYN pectineal ligament.

lig·a·men·tum phre·ni·co·co·li·cum (lig-ă-men′tŭm fren′i-kō-kol′i-kŭm) [TA] SYN phrenicocolic ligament.

lig·a·men·tum pul·mo·na·le (lig-ă-men′tŭm pul-mō-nā′lē) [TA] SYN pulmonary ligament.

lig·a·men·tum splen·o·re·na·le (lig-ă-men′tŭm splē′nō-rē-nā′lē) [TA] SYN splenorenal ligament.

lig·a·men·tum sus·pen·so·ri·um o·va·ri·i (lig-ă-men′tŭm sŭs-pen-sōr′ē-ŭm ō-vā′rē-ī) [TA] SYN suspensory ligament of ovary.

lig·a·men·tum te·res hep·a·tis (lig-ă-men′tŭm ter′ēz hē-pā′tis) [TA] SYN round ligament of liver.

lig·a·men·tum te·res u·ter·i (lig-ă-men′tŭm ter′ēz yū′tĕr-ī) [TA] SYN round ligament of uterus.

lig·a·men·tum trans·ver·sum ge·nus (lig-ă-men′tŭm trans-vĕr′sŭm jē′nŭs) [TA] SYN transverse ligament of knee.

lig·a·men·tum trap·e·zoi·de·um (lig-ă-men′tŭm trap-ĕ-zoy′dē-ŭm) [TA] SYN trapezoid ligament.

lig·a·men·tum vo·ca·le (lig-ă-men′tŭm vō-kā′lē) [TA] SYN vocal ligament.

lig·and (lī′gand) **1.** An organic molecule attached to a central metal ion by multiple coordinate bonds. **2.** An organic molecule attached to a tracer element, e.g., a radioisotope. **3.** A molecule that binds to a macromolecule, e.g., a ligand binding to a receptor. **4.** The analyte in competitive binding assays, such as radioimmunoassay. [L. *ligo,* to bind]

lig·and-bind·ing site (lī′gand-bīnd′ing sīt) The site on the surface of a protein that binds a ligand; equivalent to the active site if the ligand is the substrate of an enzyme.

li·gase (lī′gās) Generic term for enzymes (EC class 6) catalyzing the joining of two molecules coupled with the breakdown of a pyrophosphate bond in ATP or a similar compound. SEE ALSO synthetase.

li·gase chain re·ac·tion (lī′gās chān rē-ak′shŭn) A technique for target amplification of DNA in which DNA ligase is used to join two complementary oligonucleotide probes that have bound to a target sequence in vitro. The ligation product is used as a template for ligation of complementary oligonucleotides that, through repeated enzymatic processing, allow for logarithmic accumulation of products that can be used to determine the presence of the target of interest.

li·gate (lī′gāt) To apply a ligature. [L. *ligo,* pp. *-atus,* to bind]

li·ga·tion (lī-gā′shŭn) **1.** Application of a ligature. **2.** The act of binding or annealing. [L. *ligatio,* fr. *ligo,* to bind]

lig·a·ture (lig′ă-chŭr) **1.** A thread, wire, fillet, or the like, tied tightly around a blood vessel, the pedicle of a tumor, or other structure to constrict it. **2.** ORTHODONTICS a wire or other material used to secure an orthodontic attachment or tooth to an archwire. [L. *ligatura,* a band or tie, fr. *ligo,* to tie]

light (līt) That portion of electromagnetic radiation to which the retina is sensitive. SEE ALSO lamp. [A.S. *leōht*]

light ad·ap·ta·tion (līt ad′ap-tā′shŭn) The visual adjustment occurring under increased illumination in which the retinal sensitivity to light is reduced. SEE ALSO light-adapted eye. SYN photopic adaptation.

light-a·dapt·ed eye (līt-ă-dap′tĕd ī) An eye that has been exposed to light, with bleaching of rhodopsin (visual purple) and insensitivity to low illumination. SYN photopic eye.

light blue-top tube (līt blū-top tūb) This color of tube indicates the container is treated with sodium citrate as an anticoagulant; used for collection of citrated plasma for coagulation studies.

light (cal·o·ries) (līt kal′ŏr-ēz) A product so labeled contains, by F.D.A. order, one-third fewer calories than a similar comparison food.

light chain (līt chān) A polypeptide chain with low molecular weight, as the κ or λ chains in immunoglobulin.

light chain-re·lat·ed am·y·loi·do·sis (līt chān′rĕ-lā′tĕd am′i-loy-dō′sis) A form of primary amyloidosis in which the fibrillar amyloid deposits are derived from the light chains of immunoglobulin; seen in β-lymphocyte and plasma-cells dyscrasias.

light·en·ing (līt′ĕn-ing) Sensation of decreased abdominal distention during the later weeks of pregnancy following the descent of the fetal head into the pelvic inlet.

light fat (lite) (līt fat līt) A product so labeled contains, by F.D.A. order, one half or less fat than found in a similar comparison food.

light green-top tube (līt grēn-top tūb) This color of tube indicates the container is treated with lithium heparin and gel separator; used for the collection of heparinized plasma for routine chemistry tests.

light re•flex (līt rē′fleks) **1.** SYN pupillary reflex. **2.** A red glow reflected from the fundus of the eye when a light is cast on the retina, as in retinoscopy. **3.** SYN Politzer luminous cone, Wilde triangle. SYN red reflex.

light sleep (līt slēp) SYN dysnystaxis.

light ther•a•py (līt thār′ă-pē) The therapeutic use of ultraviolet, colored, and laser lights to reestablish diurnal rhythms and alleviate pain and depression.

light treat•ment (līt trēt′mĕnt) SYN phototherapy.

light work (līt wŏrk) A physical demand level described as the exertion of up to 20 pounds of force occasionally, or up to 10 pounds of force frequently, or a negligible amount of force constantly to move objects. SEE ALSO sedentary work, medium work, medium-heavy work, very heavy work.

lig•nin (lig′nin) A water-insoluble fiber found in wheat bran, whole grains, and vegetables. [L. *lignum*, wood, + -in]

like•li•hood ra•ti•o (līk′lē-hud rā′shē-ō) The ratio of the probability of a test result among patients with a certain disease or disorder to the probability of that same test result among patients who do not have the targeted disease or disorder.

Li•kert scale (lī′kĕrt scāl) Ordinal scale of responses to a question or statement, ordered in hierarchic sequence from strongly negative to strongly positive. Used mainly in behavioral sciences and psychiatry.

Lil•lie al•lo•chrome con•nec•tive tis•sue stain (lil′ē al′ō-krōm kŏ-nek′tiv tish′ū stān) A procedure using PAS, hematoxylin, picric acid, and methyl blue; used for distinction between basement membrane and reticulin, and for demonstration of arteriosclerotic lesions.

Lil•lie az•ure-e•o•sin stain (lil′ē azh′ŭr-ē′ō-sin stān) A stain in which an azure eosinate solution is used to stain bacteria and rickettsiae in tissues.

Lil•lie fer•rous i•ron stain (lil′ē fer′ŭs ī′ŏrn stān) A method using potassium ferrocyanide in acetic acid that demonstrates melanins as a deep green color; lipofuscins and heme pigments are unreactive.

Lil•lie sul•fu•ric ac•id Nile blue stain (lil′ē sŭl-fyūr′ik as′id nīl blū stān) A technique for showing fatty acids when present in high concentrations.

limb (lim) **1.** An extremity; a member; an arm or leg. SYN member. **2.** A segment of any jointed structure. SEE ALSO leg. [A.S. *lim*]

limb bud (lim bŭd) An ectodermally covered mesenchymal outgrowth from the embryonic trunk giving rise to either the upper limb or lower limb.

limb-gir•dle mus•cu•lar dys•tro•phy (lim′ gĭr′dĕl mŭs′kyū-lăr dis′trŏ-fē) One of the less well-defined types of this disorder, it is characterized by weakness and wasting, usually symmetric, of the pelvic girdle muscles, the shoulder girdle muscles, or both, but not the facial muscles. Muscle pseudohypertrophy, heart involvement, and mental retardation are absent. Variable inheritance.

lim•bic (lim′bik) **1.** Relating to a limbus. **2.** Relating to the limbic system.

lim•bic sys•tem (lim′bik sis′tĕm) Collective term denoting a heterogeneous array of brain structures at or near the edge (limbus) of the medial wall of the cerebral hemisphere, in particular the hippocampus, amygdala, and fornicate gyrus; the term is often used so as to include also the interconnections of these structures, as well as their connections with the septal area, the hypothalamus, and a medial zone of mesencephalic tegmentum. By way of the latter connections, the limbic system exerts an important influence on the endocrine and autonomic motor systems; its functions also appear to affect motivational and mood states.

limb lead (lim lēd) One of the three standard leads (leads I, II, III) or one of the unipolar limb leads (aVR, aVL, aVF).

lim•bus, pl. **lim•bi** (lim′bŭs, -bī) [TA] The edge, border, or fringe of a part. [L. a border]

lim•bus of cor•ne•a (lim′bŭs kōr′nē-ă) The margin of the cornea overlapped by the sclera.

lime (līm) **1.** An alkaline earth oxide occurring in grayish-white masses (quicklime); on exposure to the atmosphere it becomes converted into calcium hydrate and calcium carbonate (air-slaked lime); direct addition of water to calcium oxide produces calcium hydrate (slaked lime). SYN calx (1). **2.** Fruit of the lime tree, *Citrus medica*, which is a source of ascorbic acid and acts as an antiscorbutic agent. [O.E. *līm*, birdlime]

li•men, pl. **lim•i•na** (lī′men, lim′i-nă) [TA] Entrance; the external opening of a canal or space, such as limen insulae. SYN threshold (4). [L.]

li•men in•su•lae (lī′men in′sū-lē) [TA] The band of transition between the anterior portion of the gray matter of the insula and the anterior perforated substance; it is formed by a narrow strip of olfactory cortex along the lateral side of the lateral olfactory stria.

li•men na•si (lī′men nā′sī) [TA] A ridge marking the boundary between the nasal cavity proper and the vestibule.

li•mes (lī′mēz) A boundary, limit, or threshold. SEE ALSO L doses. [L.]

lim·i·nal (lim′i-năl) **1.** Pertaining to a threshold. **2.** Pertaining to a stimulus just strong enough to excite a tissue, e.g., nerve or muscle. [L. *limen* (*limin-*), a threshold]

lim·it (lim′it) A boundary or end. [L. *limes,* boundary]

lim·it·ed neck dis·sec·tion (lim′i-tĕd nek di-sek′shŭn) SYN functional neck dissection.

lim·it·ed ra·di·og·ra·pher (lim′i-tĕd rā′dē-og′ră-fĕr) A medical professional who is licensed to perform specific x-ray procedures for diagnostic purposes. The specific duties of a limited radiographer vary according to state laws, but may include patient positioning, operation of x-ray equipment, and processing x-ray films.

lim·it·ing de·cis·ion (lim′i-ting dĕ-sizh′ŭn) An understanding of self achieved as a result of response to a significant or traumatic event. SEE ALSO Time-Line therapy.

limp (limp) A lame walk with a yielding step; asymmetric gait. SEE ALSO claudication.

Lin·dau tu·mor (lin′dow tū′mŏr) SYN hemangioblastoma.

Lind·ner bod·ies (lind′ner bod′ēz) Initial bodies resembling inclusion bodies found in scrapings of epithelial cells infected with trachoma.

line (līn) **1.** A long, narrow mark or a strand of material. **2.** ANATOMY any linear mark or streak distinguished from adjacent tissues by color, texture, or elevation. **3.** A strain of cells or organisms derived from a single ancestor or precursor. **4.** A section of tubing supplying fluid or conducting impulses for monitoring equipment (e.g., intravenous line, arterial line). SYN linea [TA]. [L. *linea,* a linen thread, a string, line, fr. *linum,* flax]

lin·e·a, gen. and pl. **lin·e·ae** (lin′ē-ă, -ē-ē) [TA] SYN line. [L.]

lin·e·a al·ba (lin′ē-ă al′bă) [TA] A fibrous band running vertically the entire length of the center of the anterior abdominal wall, receiving the attachments of the oblique and transverse abdominal muscles. SYN white line (1).

lin·e·a a·no·cu·ta·ne·a (lin′ē-ă ā′nō-kyū-tā′nē-ă) [TA] SYN pectinate line.

lin·e·a as·pe·ra (lin′ē-ă as′pĕr-ă) The rough ridge with two pronounced lips running the length of the posterior femur. [L., rough line]

lin·e·ae a·tro·phi·cae (lin′ē-ē ă-trof′ĭ-kē) SYN striae cutis distensae.

lin·e·a ep·i·phys·i·a·lis (lin′ē-ă ep′i-fi-sē-ā′lis) [TA] SYN epiphysial line.

lin·e·a in·ter·tro·chan·te·ri·ca (lin′ē-ă in′tĕr-trō-kan-ter′i-kă) [TA] SYN intertrochanteric line.

line an·gle (līn ang′gĕl) That area formed by the junction of two surfaces of a tooth or two surfaces of a cavity preparation.

lin·e·a ni·gra (lin′ē-ă nī′gră) The linea alba in pregnancy, which then becomes pigmented. See page B9.

lin·e·ar (lin′ē-ăr) Pertaining to or resembling a line.

lin·e·ar ac·cel·er·a·tor (lin′ē-ăr ak-sel′ĕr-ā-tŏr) A device imparting high velocity and energy to atomic and subatomic particles; an important device for radiation therapy.

lin·e·ar am·pli·fi·ca·tion (lin′ē-ăr am′pli-fi-kā′shŭn) A hearing aid circuit in which all frequencies receive equivalent amplification.

lin·e·ar at·ro·phy (lin′ē-ăr at′rŏ-fē) SYN striae cutis distensae.

li·ne·ar en·er·gy trans·fer (LET) (lin′ē-ăr en′ĕr-jē trans′fĕr) Rate at which a charged particle deposits energy as it travels through matter.

lin·e·ar frac·ture (lin′ē-ăr frak′shŭr) A fracture running parallel with the long axis of the bone. SYN fissured fracture.

lin·e·ar·i·ty (lin′ē-ar′i-tē) A relationship between two quantities whereby a change in one causes a directly proportional change in the other. [L. *linearis,* linear, fr. *linea,* line]

lin·e·ar scle·ro·der·ma (lin′ē-ăr skler′ō-dĕr′mă) Localized scleroderma with bandlike lesions of skin with induration, atrophy, hyper- or hypopigmentation, which may be disfiguring with extension into underlying tissues and joint contractures. Involvement of the forehead and scalp has been called coup de Sabre.

lin·e·a sem·i·lu·na·ris (lin′ē-ă sem-ē-lū-nā′ris) [TA] The slight groove in the external abdominal wall parallel to the lateral edge of the rectus sheath. SYN semilunar line, Spigelius line.

lin·e·a ster·na·lis (lin′ē-ă stĕr-nā′lis) [TA] SYN sternal line.

lin·e·a ter·mi·na·lis (lin′ē-ă tĕr-mi-nā′lis) [TA] An oblique ridge on the inner surface of the ilium and continued on the pubis, which forms the lower boundary of the iliac fossa; it separates the true from the false pelvis. SYN iliopectineal line, terminal line.

line of de·mar·ca·tion (līn dē′mahr-kā′shŭn) A zone of inflammatory reaction separating a gangrenous area from healthy tissue.

line of fix·a·tion (līn fik-sā′shŭn) A line joining the object (or point of fixation) with the fovea.

line of pull (līn pul) A description of the direction of force exerted by a muscle, depending on the orientation of its fibers, its skeletal attachments, the disposition of its tendons, and the axis of movement of any joints affected.

lines of Blasch·ko (līnz blash′kō) A pattern of distribution of skin lesions or pigmentary anomalies; linear on the extremities, S-shaped curves on the abdomen, and V-shaped on the back, thought to result from genetic mosaicism and the interplay of transverse clonal proliferation and longitudinal growth and flexion of the embryo.

line spec·trum (līn spek′trŭm) An emission spectrum of elements in which the emitted light bands cover a very narrow range of energies.

Lin·gels·hei·mi·a (ling′gels-hī′mē-ă) SYN *Acinetobacter.*

lin·gua, gen. and pl. **lin·guae** (ling′gwă, -gwē) [TA] **1.** SYN tongue (1). **2.** SYN tongue (2). [L. tongue]

lin·gua ge·o·gra·phi·ca (ling′gwă jē-ō-graf′i-kă) SYN geographic tongue.

lin·gual (ling′gwăl) **1.** Relating to the tongue or any tonguelike part. SYN glossal. **2.** Next to or toward the tongue.

lin·gual ar·ter·y (ling′gwăl ahr′tĕr-ē) *Origin*, external carotid; *distribution*, runs along under surface of tongue, terminates as deep lingual artery; *branches*, suprahyoid and dorsal lingual branches and sublingual artery.

lin·gual bar (ling′gwăl bahr) Major connector located lingually to dental arch joining two or more bilateral parts of a mandibular removable partial denture.

lin·gual crib (ling′gwăl crib) Wire orthodontic appliance placed in a position lingual to the maxillary incisors to help a child overcome the habits of thumb sucking and tongue thrusting.

lin·gual flange (ling′gwăl flanj) Portion of flange of a mandibular denture that occupies space adjacent to tongue.

lin·gual fol·li·cles (ling′gwăl fol′i-kĕlz) Collections of lymphoid tissue in the mucosa of the pharyngeal part of the tongue posterior to the terminal sulcus collectively forming the lingual tonsil. SYN folliculi linguales [TA].

lin·gual fren·u·lum SYN frenulum of tongue.

lin·gual gin·gi·va (ling′gwăl jin′ji-vă) Portion of gingiva that covers lingual surfaces of teeth and alveolar process.

lin·gual goi·ter (ling′gwăl goy′tĕr) A tumor of thyroid tissue involving the embryonic rudiment at the base of the tongue.

lin·gual gy·rus (ling′gwăl jī′rŭs) A relatively short horizontal convolution on the inferomedial aspect of the occipital and temporal lobes, demarcated from the lateral occipitotemporal or fusiform gyrus by the deep collateral sulcus, from the cuneus by the calcarine sulcus; its anterior extreme abuts the isthmus of the parahippocampal gyrus; the medial or upper strip of the gyrus forming the lower bank of the calcarine sulcus corresponds to the inferior half of the striate area or primary visual cortex and represents the contralateral upper quadrant of the binocular field of vision.

lin·gual nerve (ling′gwăl nĕrv) One of the branches of the mandibular nerve, passing medially to the lateral pterygoid muscle, between the medial pterygoid and the mandible, and beneath the mucous membrane of the floor of the mouth to the side of the tongue over the anterior two-thirds of which it is distributed; it also supplies the mucous membrane of the floor of the mouth. It passes close to the lingual side of the roots of the second and third lower molar teeth and is endangered during tooth extractions. SYN nervus lingualis [TA].

lin·gual pa·pil·la (ling′gwăl pă-pil′ă) **1.** One of numerous variously shaped projections of the mucous membrane of the dorsum of the tongue. **2.** The lingual portion of the gingiva filling the interproximal space between adjacent teeth; in molar and premolar areas, there may be separate lingual and buccal interdental papillae. SEE ALSO interdental papilla.

lin·gual rest (ling′gwăl rest) Metallic extension onto lingual surface of a tooth to provide support or indirect retention for a removable partial denture.

lin·gual ton·sil (ling′gwăl ton′sil) A collection of lymphoid follicles on the posterior or pharyngeal portion of the dorsum of the tongue. SYN tonsilla lingualis [TA].

lin·gual vein (ling′gwăl vān) It receives blood from the tongue, sublingual and submandibular glands, and muscles of the floor of the mouth; empties into the internal jugular or the facial vein.

lin·gua ni·gra (ling′gwă nī′gră) SYN black tongue.

lin·gui·form (ling′gwi-fōrm) Tongue-shaped.

lin·gu·la, pl. **lin·gu·lae** (ling′gyū-lă, -lē) [TA] **1.** A term applied to several tongue-shaped processes, particularly that of the cerebellum and of the upper lobe of the left lung. **2.** When not qualified, the lingula of the cerebellum. [L. dim. of *lingua*, tongue]

lin·gu·lar (ling′gyū-lăr) Pertaining to any lingula.

lin·gu·lec·to·my (ling′gyū-lek′tŏ-mē) **1.** SYN glossectomy. **2.** Excision of the lingular portion of the upper lobe of the left lung.

♻**linguo-** Combining form denoting the tongue. [L. *lingua*]

lin·guo·clu·sion (ling′gwō-klū′zhŭn) Displacement of a tooth toward the interior of the dental arch, or toward the tongue.

lin·guo·pap·il·li·tis (ling′gwō-pap′i-lī′tis)

Small, painful ulcers involving the papillae on the tongue margins.

lin•guo•ver•sion (ling′gwō-vĕr′zhŭn) Malposition of a tooth toward the tongue.

lin•i•ment (lin′i-mĕnt) A liquid preparation for external use, frequently applied by friction to the skin. [L., fr. *lino,* to smear]

li•ni•tis (li-nī′tis) Inflammation of cellular tissue, specifically of the perivascular tissue of the stomach. [G. *linon,* flax, linen cloth, + *-itis,* inflammation]

li•ni•tis plas•ti•ca (li-nī′tis plas′ti-kă) Infiltrating scirrhous carcinoma, causing extensive thickening of the wall of the stomach; often called leather-bottle stomach.

link•age (lingk′ăj) **1.** A chemical covalent bond. **2.** The relationship between syntenic loci sufficiently close that the respective alleles are not inherited independently by the offspring; a characteristic of loci, not genes.

link•age dis•e•qui•lib•ri•um (lingk′ăj dis-ē′kwi-lib′rē-ŭm) A state involving two loci in which the probability of a joint gamete is not equal to the product of the probabilities of the constituent genes. The difference between these quantities is the increase of the disequilibrium; there are many causes of the disequilibrium.

link•age mark•er (lingk′ăj mahr′kĕr) A locus at which there is a high probability of heterozygotes (indispensible state for linkage analysis), but in itself perhaps of no clinical interest.

linked (lingkt) Said of two genetic loci that exhibit genetic linkage.

link•er (lingk′ĕr) A fragment of synthetic DNA containing a restriction site that may be used for splicing genes.

link•ing num•ber (*L*) (lingk′ing nŭm′bĕr) A property of a long biopolymer (such as duplex DNA) equal to the number of twists (related to the frequency of turns around the central axis of the helix) plus the writhing number.

lip (lip) **1.** One of the two muscular folds that encircle the mouth anteriorly; each has an outer mucosa with a stratified squamous epithelial surface layer. **2.** Any liplike structure bounding a cavity or groove. SYN labium (1) [TA]. [A.S. *lippa*]

lipaemia [Br.] SYN lipemia.

lipaemia retinalis [Br.] SYN lipemia retinalis.

lipaemic [Br.] SYN lipemic.

li•pase (lip′ās) Any fat-splitting or lipolytic enzyme; a carboxylesterase.

lip•ec•to•my (lip-ek′tŏ-mē) Surgical removal of fatty tissue, as in cases of adiposity. [lipo- + G. *ektomē,* excision]

lip•e•de•ma (lip′ĕ-dē′mă) Chronic swelling, usually of the lower extremities, particularly in middle-aged women, caused by the widespread, even distribution of subcutaneous fat and fluid. [lipo- + G. *oidēma,* swelling]

li•pe•de•ma•tous al•o•pe•ci•a (lip′ĕ-dē′mă-tŭs al′ō-pē′shē-ă) Condition with itching, soreness, or tenderness of the scalp in black women; the scalp is thickened and soft, subcutaneous fat is increased, and the hair is sparse and short.

li•pe•mi•a (li-pē′mē-ă) The presence of an abnormally high concentration of lipids in the circulating blood. SYN hyperlipidemia, hyperlipoidemia, lipaemia, lipidemia, lipoidemia. [lipid + G. *haima,* blood]

li•pe•mi•a re•ti•na•lis (li-pē′mē-ă ret-i-nā′lis) A creamy appearance of the retinal blood vessels that occurs when the lipids of the blood exceed 5%. SYN lipaemia retinalis.

li•pe•mic (li-pē′mik) Relating to lipemia; describes milky appearance in serum and plasma. SYN lipaemic.

lip•id (lip′id) “Fat-soluble,” an operational term describing a solubility characteristic, not a chemical substance, i.e., denoting substances extracted from animal or vegetable cells by nonpolar solvents; included in the heterogeneous collection of materials thus extractable are fatty acids, glycerides, glyceryl ethers, phospholipids, sphingolipids, long-chain alcohols, waxes, terpenes, steroids, and “fat-soluble” vitamins such as A, D, and E. [G. *lipos,* fat]

lip•id A (lip′id) The glycolipid component of lipopolysaccharide responsible for its endotoxic activity.

lipidaemia [Br.] SYN lipidemia.

lip•i•de•mi•a (lip′i-dē′mē-ă) SYN lipemia. SYN lipidaemia.

lip•id gran•u•lo•ma•to•sis, lip•oid gran•u•lo•ma•to•sis (lip′id gran′yū-lō′mă-tō′sis, lip′oyd) SYN xanthomatosis.

lip•i•do•sis, pl. **lip•i•do•ses** (lip′i-dō′sis, -sēz) Hereditary abnormality of lipid metabolism that results in abnormal amounts of lipid deposition; classification is based on the responsible enzymatic deficiency and type of lipid involved. Such enzymatic activity takes place in the lysosomes, and the abnormal products appear as lysosomal storage diseases. Sphingolipidoses make up the largest portion of recognized lipidoses, including abnormal metabolism of gangliosides, ceramides, and cerebrosides. [lipid + G. *-ōsis,* condition]

lip•id pneu•mo•ni•a, lip•oid pneu•mo•ni•a (lip′id nū-mō′nē-ă, lip′oyd) Pulmonary condition marked by inflammatory and fibrotic changes in the lungs due to the inhalation of various oily or fatty substances, particularly liquid petrolatum, or resulting from accumulation in the lungs of endogenous lipid material, either cholesterol from obstructive pneumonitis or following fracture of a bone; phagocytes containing lipid are usually present.

♻ **lipo-, lip-** (lip) Combining forms meaning fatty, lipid. [G. *lipos,* fat]

lip•o•ar•thri•tis (lip′ō-ahr-thrī′tis) Inflammation of the periarticular fatty tissues of the knee. [lipo- + arthritis]

lip•o•ate (lip′ō-āt) A salt or ester of lipoic acid.

lip•o•ate a•ce•tyl•trans•fer•ase (lip′ō-āt ă-sē′til-trans′fĕr-ās) SYN dihydrolipoamide acetyltransferase.

lip•o•at•ro•phy (lip′ō-at′rŏ-fē) Loss of subcutaneous fat, which may be total, congenital, and associated with hepatomegaly, excessive bone growth, and insulin-resistant diabetes. [G. *lipos,* fat, + *a-,* priv. + *trophē,* nourishment]

lip•o•blast (lip′ō-blast) An embryonic fat cell. [lipo- + G. *blastos,* germ]

lip•o•blas•to•ma (lip′ō-blas-tō′mă) **1.** SYN liposarcoma. **2.** A benign subcutaneous tumor composed of embryonal fat cells separated into distinct lobules, occurring usually in infants.

lip•o•blas•to•ma•to•sis (lip′ō-blas-tō′mă-tō′sis) A diffuse form of lipoblastoma that infiltrates locally but does not metastasize.

lip•o•cer•a•tous (lip′ō-ser′ă-tŭs) SYN adipoceratous.

lip•o•cere (lip′ō-sēr) SYN adipocere. [lipo- + L. *cera,* wax]

lip•o•chrome (lip′ō-krōm) **1.** A pigmented lipid, e.g., lutein, carotene. **2.** More specifically, yellow pigments that seem identical to carotene and xanthophyll and are frequently found in the serum, skin, cortex of suprarenal gland, corpus luteum, and arteriosclerotic plaques, as well as in the liver, spleen, and adipose tissue. **3.** The pigment produced by certain bacteria. [lipo- + G. *chroma,* color]

lip•o•crit (lip′ō-krit) An apparatus and procedure for separating and volumetrically analyzing the amount of lipid in blood or other body fluids. [lipo- + G. *krinō,* to separate]

lip•o•cyte (lip′ō-sīt) SYN fat-storing cell. [lipo- + G. *kytos,* cell]

lip•o•der•moid (lip′ō-dĕr′moyd) Congenital, yellowish-white, fatty, benign tumor located subconjunctivally. [lipo- + dermoid]

lip•o•dys•tro•phy (lip′ō-dis′trŏ-fē) Defective metabolism of fat. [lipo- + G. *dys-,* bad, difficult, + *trophē,* nourishment]

lip•o•e•de•ma (lip′ō-ĕ-dē′mă) Edema of subcutaneous fat, causing painful swellings, especially of the legs in women. SYN cellulite (2), lipooedema.

lip•o•fi•bro•ma (lip′ō-fī-brō′mă) A benign neoplasm of fibrous connective tissue, with conspicuous numbers of adipose cells.

lip•o•fus•cin (lip′ō-fyūs′in) Brown pigment granules representing lipid-containing residues of lysosomal digestion and considered one of the aging or "wear and tear" pigments; found in liver, kidney, heart muscle, and ganglion cells.

lip•o•fus•ci•no•sis (lip′ō-fyūs′i-nō′sis) Abnormal storage of any one of a group of fatty pigments.

lip•o•gen•e•sis (lip′ō-jen′ĕ-sis) The production of fat, either fatty degeneration or fatty infiltration; also applied to the normal deposition of fat or to the conversion of carbohydrate or protein to fat. SYN adipogenesis. [lipo- + G. *genesis,* production]

lip•o•gen•ic (lip′ō-jen′ik) Relating to lipogenesis. SYN adipogenic, adipogenous, lipogenous.

li•pog•e•nous (li-poj′ĕ-nŭs) SYN lipogenic.

lip•o•gran•u•lo•ma (lip′ō-gran′yŭ-lō′mă) A nodule or focus of granulomatous inflammation (usually of the foreign-body type) in association with lipid material deposited in tissues, e.g., after the injection of certain oils. SEE ALSO paraffinoma.

lip•o•gran•u•lo•ma•to•sis (lip′ō-gran′yŭ-lō′mă-tō′sis) **1.** Presence of lipogranulomas. **2.** Local inflammatory reaction to necrosis of adipose tissue.

lip•oid (lip′oyd) **1.** Resembling fat. **2.** Former term for lipid. SYN adipoid. [lipo- + G. *eidos,* appearance]

lipoidaemia [Br.] SYN lipoidemia.

lip•oi•de•mi•a (lip′oy-dē′mē-ă) SYN lipemia. SYN lipoidaemia.

lip•oid gran•u•lo•ma (lip′oyd gran′yŭ-lō′mă) A lesion characterized by aggregates or accumulations of fairly large mononuclear phagocytes that contain lipid.

lip•oid ne•phro•sis (lip′oyd nĕ-frō′sis) Idiopathic nephrotic syndrome occurring most commonly in children, in which glomeruli show minimal changes with no thickening of the basement membranes, fat vacuoles in the tubular epithelium, and fusion of glomerular foot processes.

lip•oi•do•sis (lip′oy-dō′sis) Presence of anisotropic lipoids in the cells.

lip•oid the•o•ry of nar•co•sis (lip′oyd thē′ŏr-ē nahr-kō′sis) That narcotic efficiency parallels the coefficient of partition between oil and water, and that lipoids in the cell and on the cell membrane absorb the drug because of this affinity.

lip•o•in•jec•tion (lip′ō-in-jek′shŭn) Augmentation of tissue with fat cells after atrophy, as in vocal cord paralysis or scarring.

li•pol•y•sis (li-pol′i-sis) The splitting up (hydrolysis), or chemical decomposition, of fat. [lipo- + G. *lysis,* dissolution]

lip•o•lyt•ic (lip′ō-lit′ik) Relating to or causing lipolysis.

li•po•ma (li-pō′mă) A benign neoplasm of adipose tissue, composed of mature fat cells. [lipo- + G. *-oma,* tumor]

li•po•ma•toid (li-pō′mă-toyd) Resembling a lipoma, frequently said of accumulations of adipose tissue that are not thought to be neoplastic.

lip•o•ma•to•sis (lip′ō-mă-tō′sis) SYN adiposis.

li•po•ma•tous (li-pō′mă-tŭs) Pertaining to or manifesting the features of a lipoma, or characterized by the presence of a lipoma (or lipomas).

li•po•ma•tous in•fil•tra•tion (li-pō′mă-tŭs in′fil-trā′shŭn) Nonencapsulated adipose tissue forming a lipomalike mass, usually in the cardiac interatrial septum where it may cause arrhythmia and sudden death.

lip•o•me•nin•go•cele (lip′ō-mĕ-ning′gō-sēl) A lipoma of the cauda equina associated with a spina bifida. [lipo- + G. *mēninx,* membrane, + *kēlē,* tumor]

lipo-oedema [Br.] SYN lipoedema.

lip•o•pe•nia (lip′ō-pē′nē-ă) An abnormally small amount, or a deficiency, of lipids in the body. [lipo- + G. *penia,* poverty]

lip•o•phage (lip′ō-fāj) A cell that ingests fat. [G. *lipos,* fat, + *phagō,* to eat]

lip•o•pha•gic (lip′ō-fă′jik) Relating to lipophagy.

lip•oph•a•gy (lip-of′ă-jē) Ingestion of fat by a lipophage. [lipo- + G. *phagō,* to eat]

lip•o•phil (lip′ō-fil) A substance with lipophilic (i.e., hydrophobic) properties. [lipo- + G. *philos,* fond of]

lip•o•phil•ic (lip′ō-fil′ik) Capable of dissolving, of being dissolved in, or of absorbing lipids.

lip•o•pol•y•sac•cha•ride (lip′ō-pol′ē-sak′ă-rīd) A compound or complex of lipid and carbohydrate; the lipopolysaccharide (endotoxin) that is released from the cell walls of gram-negative organisms that produces septic shock.

lip•o•pro•tein (lip′ō-prō′tēn) Complexes or compounds containing lipid and protein. Almost all the lipids in plasma are present as lipoproteins and are therefore transported as such. Plasma lipoproteins are characterized by their flotation constants as chylomicra, very low density (VLDL), intermediate density (IDL), low density (LDL), high density (HDL), and very high density (VHDL). They range in molecular weight from 175,000 to 1×10^9. Gauging lipoprotein levels is important in assessing the risk of cardiovascular disease.

lip•o•pro•tein (alpha) [α] (lip′ō-prō′tēn) A lipoprotein consisting of an LDL particle to which a large glycoprotein, apolipoprotein (α), is covalently bonded. Elevation of the concentration in serum has been identified as a risk factor for coronary artery disease.

lip•o•pro•tein li•pase (lip′ō-prō′tēn lip′ās) An enzyme that hydrolyzes one fatty acid from a triacylglycerol; its activity is enhanced by heparin and inactivated by heparinase. SEE ALSO clearing factors.

lip•o•sar•co•ma (lip′ō-sahr-kō′mă) A malignant neoplasm of adults that occurs especially in the retroperitoneal tissues and the thigh; planes composed of well-differentiated fat cells, or may be dedifferentiated, either myxoid, round celled, or pleomorphic; recurrences are common, and dedifferentiated liposarcomas metastasize to the lungs or serosal surfaces. SYN lipoblastoma (1). [lipo- + *sarx,* flesh, + *-oma,* tumor]

li•po•sis (li-pō′sis) **1.** SYN adiposis. **2.** Fatty infiltration, neutral fats being present in the cells. [lipo- + G. *-osis,* condition]

lip•o•sol•u•ble (lip′ō-sol′yŭ-bĕl) Fat-soluble.

lip•o•suc•tion (lip′ō-sŭk′shŭn) Method of removing unwanted subcutaneous fat using percutaneously placed suction tubes.

lip•o•suc•tion•ing (lip′ō-sŭk′shŭn-ing) Removal of fat by high vacuum pressure; used in body contouring.

lip•o•tro•phic (lip′ō-trōf′ik) Relating to lipotrophy.

li•pot•ro•phy (li-pot′rŏ-fē) An increase of fat in the body. [lipo- + G. *trophē,* nourishment]

lip•o•tro•pic (lip′ō-trō′pik) **1.** Pertaining to substances preventing or correcting excessive fat deposits in liver such as occurs in choline deficiency. **2.** Relating to lipotropy.

lip•o•tro•pic hor•mone, lip•o•tro•pic pi•tu•i•tar•y hor•mone (lip′ō-trō′pik hōr′mōn, pi-tū′i-tār-ē) SYN lipotropin.

lip•o•tro•pin (lip′ō-trō′pin) A pituitary hormone mobilizing fat from adipose tissue. Cf. bioregulator. SYN lipotropic hormone, lipotropic pituitary hormone.

li•pot•ro•py (li-pot′rŏ-pē) **1.** Affinity of basic dyes for fatty tissue. **2.** Prevention of accumulation of fat in the liver. **3.** Affinity of nonpolar substances for each other. [lipo- + G. *tropē,* turning]

lip•o•vac•cine (lip′ō-vak-sēn′) A vaccine that has a vegetable oil as a solvent.

li•pox•i•dase (li-poks′i-dās) SYN lipoxygenase.

li•pox•y•ge•nase (li-poks'ē-jĕ-nās) An enzyme that catalyzes the oxidation of unsaturated fatty acids with O_2 to yield hydroperoxides of the fatty acids. SYN lipoxidase.

lip•ping (lip'ing) The formation of a liplike structure, as at the articular end of a bone in osteoarthritis.

Lipp•man-Cobb meth•od (lip-man'kob meth'ŏd) A procedure used to measure the degree of scoliotic angle.

lip read•ing (lip rēd'ing) SYN speech reading.

lip re•flex (lip rē'fleks) A pouting movement of the lips provoked in young infants by tapping near the angle of the mouth.

lip re•trac•tion (lip rĕ-trak'shŭn) An atypical oral pattern that occurs when the lips are drawn back to form a tight horizontal line over the mouth, making it difficult to assist with sucking liquids, removing food from a spoon or cup, and retaining food in the mouth.

li•pu•ri•a (li-pyūr'ē-ă) Presence of lipids in the urine. SYN adiposuria. [lipo- + G. *ouron,* urine]

li•pur•ic (li-pyūr'ik) Pertaining to lipuria.

liq•ue•fa•cient (lik'wĕ-fā'shĕnt) **1.** Making liquid; causing a solid to become liquid. **2.** Denoting a resolvent supposed to cause the resolution of a solid tumor by liquefying its contents. [L. *lique-facio,* pres. p. *-faciens,* to make fluid, fr. *liqueo,* to be liquid]

liq•ue•fac•tion (lik'wĕ-fak'shŭn) The act of becoming liquid; change from a solid to a liquid form. SEE liquefacient.

liq•ue•fac•tive ne•cro•sis (lik'wĕ-fak'tiv nĕ-krō'sis) A type of necrosis characterized by dull, opaque, partly or completely fluid remains of tissue. It is observed in abscesses and frequently in infarcts of the brain.

li•ques•cent (li-kwes'ĕnt) Becoming or tending to become liquid. [L. *liquesco,* to become liquid]

liq•uid (lik'wid) **1.** An inelastic substance, like water, that is neither solid nor gaseous and in which the molecules are relatively free to move with respect to each other yet still are restricted by intermolecular forces. **2.** Flowing like water. [L. *liquidus*]

liq•uid-liq•uid chro•ma•tog•ra•phy (lik'wid-lik'wid krō'mă-tog'ră-fē) Process in which both the moving phase and the stationary (or reverse-moving) phase are liquids, as in countercurrent distribution.

liq•uid pro•tein di•et (lik'wid prō'tēn dī'ĕt) Liquid nourishment or meal replacement that a person may consume to lose weight and/or gain muscle mass depending on the amount of protein and the frequency of consumption.

liq•uid scin•til•la•tor (lik'wid sin'ti-lā-tŏr) A liquid with the properties of a scintillator, in which the substance whose radioactivity is to be measured can be dissolved, to be placed in a well counter.

li•quor, gen. **li•quor•is**, pl. **li•quo•res** (lik'ŏr, lī'kwōr; lī-kwōr'is; -kwōr'ēz) **1.** Any liquid or fluid. **2.** A term for certain body fluids. **3.** The pharmacopeial term for any aqueous solution (not a decoction or infusion) of a nonvolatile substance and for aqueous solutions of gases. SEE ALSO solution. [L.]

li•quor am•ni•i (lī'kwōr ahm'nē-ī) SYN amnionic fluid.

LIS Abbreviation for laboratory information system; low-intensity stimulator.

Lisch nod•ule (lish nod'yūl) Iris hamartomas typically seen in association with type 1 neurofibromatosis.

Lis•franc am•pu•ta•tion (lis-frahngk' amp'yū-tā'shŭn) Removal of the foot at the tarsometatarsal joint, the sole being preserved to make the flap.

Lis•franc in•ju•ry (lis-frahngk' in'jŭr-ē) Disruption of the tarsometatarsal joint, with or without an associated fracture.

lisp•ing (lis'ping) Mispronunciation of the sibilants *s* and *z*.

lis•pro in•su•lin (lis'prō in'sŭ-lin) A modified version of natural human insulin, synthesized by a genetically programmed strain of nonpathogenic *Escherichia coli,* in which the amino acids lysine (Lys) and proline (Pro) near the end of the B chain are transposed. This chemical alteration yields an insulin with a much faster onset of action, which reaches its peak effect earlier than regular insulin. Unlike other insulins, it is available only by prescription. [Lys + Pro]

lis•sen•ce•pha•li•a (lis'en-sĕ-fā'lē-ă) SYN agyria. [G. *lissos,* smooth, + *enkephalos,* brain]

lis•sen•ce•phal•ic (lis'en-sĕ-fal'ik) Pertaining to, or characterized by, lissencephalia.

lis•sive (lis'iv) Having the property of relieving muscle spasm without causing flaccidity. [G. *lissos,* smooth]

lis•so•sphinc•ter (lis'ō-sfingk'tĕr) A sphincter of smooth musculature. [G. *lissos,* smooth, + sphincter]

list (list) A series of words collected or organized on a specific principle. [It. *lista,* fr. Germanic]

Lis•te•ri•a (lis-tēr'ē-ă) A genus of aerobic to microaerophilic, motile, bacteria (family Corynebacteriaceae) containing small, coccoid, gram-positive rods; found in the feces of humans and other animals, on vegetation, and in silage, and parasitic on poikilothermic and warm-blooded animals, including humans. The type species is *L. monocytogenes*. [Joseph *Lister*]

lis·te·ri·o·sis (lis-tēr′ē-ō′sis) A sporadic disease of animals and humans, particularly those who are immunocompromised or pregnant, caused by a bacterium, *Listeria monocytogenes*. [fr. organism *Listeria*]

lis·ter·ism (lis′tĕr-izm) SYN Lister method.

Lis·ter meth·od (lis′tĕr meth′ŏd) Antiseptic surgery, as first advocated by Lister in 1867; the operation was performed under a cloud of diluted carbolic acid spray, the instruments were dipped in a carbolic solution before use, and the wound was dressed with a thick layer of carbolized gauze; from this was developed the present practice of aseptic surgery. SYN listerism.

List·ing law (lis′ting law) When the eye leaves one object and fixes on another, it revolves about an axis perpendicular to a plane cutting both the former and the present lines of vision.

List·ing re·duced eye (lis′ting rĕ-dūst′ ī) A representation that simplifies calculations of retinal imagery: radius of anterior refracting surface, 5.1 mm; total length, 20 mm; distance of nodal point to retina, 15 mm.

li·ter (L) (lē′tĕr) A measure of capacity of 1000 cubic centimeters or 1 cubic decimeter; equivalent to 1.056688 quarts (U.S., liquid). SYN litre. [Fr., fr. G. *litra,* a pound]

lit·er·a·cy (lit′ĕr-ă-sē) Ability of a person to read, write, and speak in English, and solve problems sufficiently well to function in a job and in society. [L. *littera,* letter]

lit·er·a·ture (lit′ĕr-ă-chŭr) A body of written material. [L. *litteratura,* fr. *littera,* letter]

lith·a·gogue (lith′ă-gog) Causing the dislodgment or expulsion of calculi, especially urinary calculi. [litho- + G. *agōgos,* drawing forth]

li·thec·to·my (li-thek′tŏ-mē) SYN lithotomy. [litho- + G. *ektomē,* excision]

li·thi·a·sis (li-thī′ă-sis) Formation of calculi of any kind, especially of biliary or urinary calculi. [lith- + G. *-iasis,* condition]

lith·i·um (Li) (lith′ē-ŭm) An element of the alkali metal group, atomic no. 3, atomic wt. 6.941. Many salts have clinical applications. [Mod. L. fr. G. *lithos,* a stone]

♻ **litho-, lith-** Combining forms meaning a stone, calculus, calcification. [G. *lithos*]

lith·o·clast (lith′ō-klast) SYN lithotrite. [litho- + G. *klastos,* broken]

lith·o·gen·e·sis, li·thog·e·ny (lith′ō-jen′ĕ-sis, lith-oj′ĕ-nē) Formation of calculi. [litho- + G. *genesis,* production]

lith·o·gen·ic (lith′ō-jen′ik) Promoting the formation of calculi.

lith·og·e·nous (lith-oj′ĕ-nŭs) Calculus-forming.

li·thol·a·pax·y (li-thol′ă-pak-sē) The operation of crushing a stone in the bladder and washing out the fragments through a catheter. [litho- + G. *lapaxis,* an emptying out]

li·thol·y·sis (li-thol′i-sis) The dissolution of urinary calculi. [litho- + G. *lysis,* dissolution]

lith·o·lyt·ic (lith′ō-lit′ik) **1.** Tending to dissolve calculi. **2.** An agent having such properties. [litho- + G. *lysis,* dissolution]

lith·o·ne·phri·tis (lith′ō-nĕ-frī′tis) Interstitial nephritis associated with calculus formation.

lithopaedion [Br.] SYN lithopedion.

lithopaedium [Br.] SYN lithopedium.

lith·o·pe·di·on, lith·o·pe·di·um (lith′ō-pē′dē-on, -ŭm) A retained fetus, usually extrauterine in the abdominal cavity, that has become calcified. SYN lithopaedion. [litho- + G. *paidion,* small child]

li·thot·o·my (li-thot′ŏ-mē) Cutting for stone; a cutting operation for the removal of a calculus, especially a vesical calculus. SYN lithectomy. [litho- + G. *tomē,* incision]

i **li·thot·o·my po·si·tion** (li-thot′ŏ-mē pŏ-zish′ŏn) A supine position with buttocks at the end of the operating table, the hips and knees being fully flexed with feet strapped in position. See page B29.

lith·o·trip·sy (lith′ō-trip-sē) The crushing of a stone in the renal pelvis, ureter, or bladder, by mechanical force or sound waves. SYN lithotrity. [litho- + G. *tripsis,* a rubbing]

lith·o·trip·tic (lith′ō-trip′tik) **1.** Relating to lithotripsy. **2.** An agent that effects the dissolution of a calculus.

lith·o·trip·tos·co·py (lith′ō-trip-tos′kŏ-pē) Crushing of a stone in the bladder under direct vision by use of a lithotriptoscope. [litho- + G. *tribō,* to rub, crush, + *skopeō,* to view]

lith·o·trite (lith′ō-trīt) A mechanical instrument used to crush a urinary calculus in lithotripsy. SYN lithoclast. [litho- + L. *tero,* pp. *tritus,* to rub]

li·thot·ri·ty (li-thot′ri-tē) SYN lithotripsy.

lit·mus (lit′mŭs) A blue coloring material obtained from *Roccella tinctorial* and other lichens, the principal component of which is azolitmin; used as an indicator (reddened by acids and turned blue again by alkalies). [Dutch *lakmoes*]

litre [Br.] SYN liter.

lit·ter (lit′ĕr) **1.** A stretcher or portable couch for moving the sick or injured. **2.** A group of animals of the same parents, born at the same time. [Fr. *litière;* fr. *lit,* bed]

lit•tle a•dre•no•cor•ti•co•tro•pic hor•mone (ACTH) (lit′ĕl ă-drē′nō-kōr′ti-kō-trō′pik hōr′mōn) The conventional ACTH molecule when contrasted with big ACTH.

Lit•tle ar•ea (lit′ĕl ār′ē-ă) SYN Kiesselbach area.

Lit•tle League el•bow (lit′ĕl lēg el′bō) SYN medial epicondylitis.

Lit•tle League shoul•der (lit′ĕl lēg shōl′dĕr) Fracture of the growth plate of the humeral head in the adolescent, resulting from repetitive rotational stresses during the act of pitching a baseball.

lit•tle toe [V] (lit′ĕl tō) Fifth digit of the foot.

lit•to•ral cell (sel) The cells lining the lymphatic sinuses of lymph nodes and the blood sinuses of bone marrow. [L. *littoralis,* the seashore]

Lit•tré glands (lē-trā′ glandz) SYN Morgagni glands.

Lit•tré her•ni•a (lē-trā′ hĕr′nē-ă) **1.** SYN parietal hernia. **2.** Hernia of Meckel diverticulum.

Litz•mann ob•liq•ui•ty (litz′măn ō-blik′wi-tē) Inclination of the fetal head so that the biparietal diameter is oblique in relation to the plane of the pelvic brim, the posterior parietal bone presenting to the parturient canal. SYN posterior asynclitism.

live•born in•fant (līv′bōrn in′fănt) The product of a live birth; an infant who shows evidence of life after birth.

li•ve•do (li-vē′dō) A bluish discoloration of the skin, either in limited patches or generalized. [L. lividness, fr. *liveo,* to be black and blue]

liv•e•doid (liv′ĕ-doyd) Pertaining to or resembling livedo.

liv•e•doid der•ma•ti•tis (liv′ĕ-doyd dĕr′mă-tī′tis) A reddish blue mottled condition of the skin due to affection of the cutaneous vascular apparatus.

li•ve•do re•tic•u•la•ris (li-vē′dō re-tik-yū-lār′is) A persistent purplish network-patterned discoloration of the skin caused by dilation of capillaries and venules due to stasis or changes in underlying blood vessels including hyalinization. See this page.

liv•er (liv′ĕr) The largest gland of the body, lying beneath the diaphragm in the right hypochondrium and upper part of the epigastrium; it is of irregular shape and weighs from 1–2 kg, or about 1/40 the weight of the body. It secretes bile and is also of great importance in both carbohydrate and protein metabolism. SYN hepar [TA]. [A.S. *lifer*]

liv•er ac•i•nus (liv′ĕr as′i-nŭs) The smallest functional unit of the liver, comprising all of the liver parenchyma supplied by a terminal branch of the portal vein and hepatic artery.

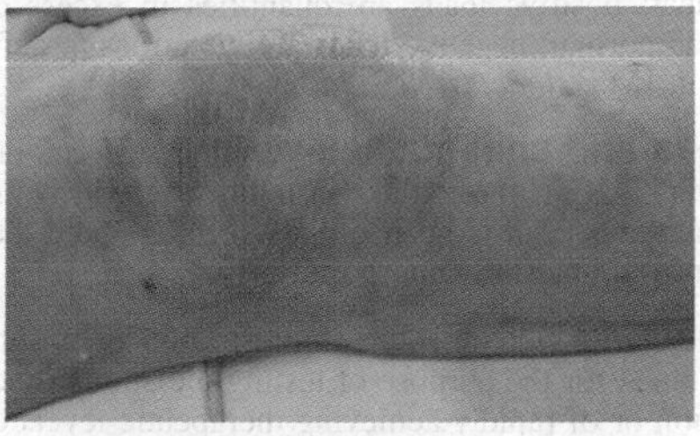

livedo reticularis: leg, adult

liv•er bud (liv′ĕr bŭd) SYN hepatic diverticulum.

liv•er lil•y (liv′ĕr lil′ē) SYN blue flag.

liv•er spot (liv′ĕr spot) SYN senile lentigo.

live vac•cine (līv vak-sēn′) Vaccine prepared from living, attenuated organisms.

liv•id (liv′id) Having a black and blue or a leaden or ashy gray color, as in discoloration from a contusion, congestion, or cyanosis. [L. *lividus,* being black and blue]

li•vid•i•ty (li-vid′i-tē) The state of being livid.

liv•ing and well (liv′ing wel) SYN alive and well.

liv•ing will (liv′ing wil) Legal document used to indicate one's preference to die rather than be sustained artificially if sick or injured beyond the prospect of recovery. SEE advance directive. SYN durable power of attorney (2).

li•vor (lī′vōr) The livid discoloration of the skin on the dependent parts of a corpse. [L. a black and blue spot]

LLLI Abbreviation for La Leche League International.

LM Abbreviation for licentiate in midwifery.

lm Abbreviation for lumen (2).

LMA Abbreviation for left mentoanterior position; laryngeal mask airway.

LMP Abbreviation for left mentoposterior position.

LMRP Abbreviation for Local Medical Review Policy.

LMT Abbreviation for left mentotransverse position.

LMWH Abbreviation for low molecular weight heparin.

LNPF Abbreviation for lymph node permeability factor.

load (lōd) **1.** The quantity of a measurable entity borne by an object or organism. **2.** A departure from normal body content, as of water, salt, or heat; positive loads are quantities in excess of the normal; negative loads are quantities in deficit. [M.E. *lode,* fr. A.S. *lād,*]

load-and-shift ma•neu•ver (lōd-shift mă-nū′vĕr) A test of shoulder instability in which the humeral head is pushed against the glenoid and moved anteriorly and posteriorly.

load•ing (lōd′ing) **1.** Administration of a substance for the purpose of testing metabolic function or of rapidly achieving therapeutic levels of a drug. **2.** Application of weight or resistance to a muscle or through a joint. SEE ALSO axial loading.

load•ing dose (lōd-ing′ dōs) The first dose of a medicine, which is much larger than the following doses, to reach a therapeutic level more rapidly.

Lo•a lo•a (lō′ă lō′ă) The African eye worm, a species of the family Onchocercidae that is the causal agent of loiasis. Humans are the only known definitive host, and parasites are transmitted by *Chrysops* flies; infective larvae from the latter require at least 3 years to mature in humans, and the adult forms may persist in humans for as long as 17 years. SEE ALSO loiasis.

lo•bar (lō′bahr) Relating to any lobe.

lo•bar pneu•mo•ni•a (lō′bahr nū-mō′nē-ă) Pulmonary disease affecting one or more lobes, or part of a lobe, of the lung in which the consolidation is virtually homogeneous; commonly due to infection by *Streptococcus pneumoniae;* sputum is scanty and usually of a rusty tint from altered blood.

lo•bate (lō′bāt) **1.** Divided into lobes. **2.** Lobe-shaped; denoting a bacterial colony with a deeply undulate margin.

lobe (lōb) **1.** One of the subdivisions of an organ or other part, bounded by fissures, connective tissue, septa, or other structural demarcations. SYN lobus [TA]. **2.** A rounded projecting part, as the lobe of the ear. SEE ALSO lobule. **3.** One of the larger divisions of the crown of a tooth, formed from a distinct point of calcification. SYN lobus [TA]. [G. *lobos,* lobe]

lo•bec•to•my (lō-bek′tŏ-mē) Excision of a lobe of any organ or gland. [G. *lobos,* lobe, + *ektomē,* excision]

lo•bi (lō′bī) Plural of lobus. [L.]

lo•bi•tis (lō-bī′tis) Inflammation of a lobe.

lo•bot•o•my (lō-bot′ŏ-mē) **1.** Incision into a lobe. **2.** Division of one or more nerve tracts in a lobe of the cerebrum. [G. *lobos,* lobe, + *tomē,* a cutting]

lob•u•lar (lob′yū-lăr) Relating to a lobule.

lob•u•lar cap•il•la•ry he•man•gi•o•ma (lob′yū-lăr kap′i-lar-ē hē-man′jē-ō′mă) SYN pyogenic granuloma.

lob•u•lar glo•mer•u•lo•ne•phri•tis (lob′yū-lăr glō-mer′yū-lō-nĕ-frī′tis) SYN membranoproliferative glomerulonephritis.

lob•u•late, lob•u•lat•ed (lob′yū-lāt, -ĕd) Divided into lobules.

lob•ule (lob′yūl) A small lobe or subdivision of a lobe. SYN lobulus [TA].

lob•ules of ep•i•did•y•mis (lob′yūlz ep′i-did′i-mis) The coiled portion of the efferent ductules that constitute the head of the epididymis; these join the ductus epididymidis. SYN lobuli epididymidis.

lob•ules of liv•er (lob′yūlz liv′ĕr) The conceptual polygonal histologic unit of the liver, consisting of masses of liver cells arranged around a central vein, a terminal branch of one of the hepatic veins; at the periphery are located preterminal and terminal branches of the portal vein, hepatic artery, and bile duct; in the human liver, hepatic lobules are distinguishable only when fibrous septa are present as a result of disease. SYN lobulus hepatis [TA], hepatic lobule.

lob•u•li ep•i•did•y•mi•dis (lob′yū-lī ep′i-did′i-mī′dis) SYN lobules of epididymis.

lob•u•lus, gen. and pl. **lob•u•li** (lob′yū-lŭs, yū-lī) [TA] SYN lobule. [Mod. L. dim. of *lobus,* lobe]

lob•u•lus hep•a•tis (lob′yū-lŭs hē-pă′tis) [TA] SYN lobules of liver.

lob•u•lus pa•ra•me•di•a•nus (lob′yū-lŭs par′ă-mē-dē-ā′nŭs) [TA] SYN gracile lobule.

lo•bus, gen. and pl. **lo•bi** (lō′bŭs, -bī) [TA] SYN lobe (1), lobe (3). [LL. fr. G. *lobos*]

lo•bus an•te•ri•or hy•po•phys•e•os (lō′bŭs an-tēr′ē-ŏr hī-po-fiz′ē-os) [TA] SYN adenohypophysis.

lo•bus cau•da•tus (lō′bŭs kaw-dā′tŭs) SYN posterior hepatic segment I. SYN caudate lobe.

lo•bus hep•a•tis dex•ter (lō′bŭs hē-pă′tis deks′tĕr) [TA] SYN right lobe of liver.

lo•bus hep•a•tis sin•is•ter (lō′bŭs hē-pă′tis si-nis′tĕr) [TA] SYN left lobe of liver.

lo•bus pos•te•ri•or hy•po•phys•e•os (lō′bŭs pos-tēr′ē-ŏr hī-pō-fiz′ē-os) [TA] SYN neurohypophysis. SEE ALSO hypophysis.

lo•bus tem•po•ra•lis (lō′bŭs tem-pō-rā′lis) [TA] SYN temporal lobe.

lo•cal (lō′kăl) Having reference or confined to a limited part; not general or systemic. [L. *localis,* fr. *locus,* place]

lo•cal an•a•phy•lax•is (lō′kăl an′ă-fi-lak′sis) The immediate, transient kind of response that follows the injection of antigen (allergen) into the skin of a sensitized individual and is limited to the area surrounding the site of inoculation. SEE ALSO skin test.

lo·cal an·es·the·si·a (lō′kăl an′es-thē′zē-ă) A general term referring to topical, infiltration, field block, or nerve block anesthesia but not usually to spinal or epidural anesthesia.

lo·cal as·phyx·i·a (lō′kăl as-fik′sē-ă) Stagnation of circulation, sometimes resulting in local gangrene, especially of the fingers; one of the symptoms usually associated with Raynaud syndrome.

lo·cal cov·er·age de·ter·mi·na·tion (LCD) (lō′kăl kŭv′ĕr-ăj dĕ-tĕr′mi-nā′shŭn) Advisories with detailed and updated information about coding and medical necessity of a specific service; used to ensure the accuracy of health care billing.

lo·cal death (lō′kăl deth) Death of a part of the body or of a tissue by necrosis.

lo·cal flap (lō′kăl flap) A flap transferred to an adjacent area.

lo·cal im·mu·ni·ty (lō′kăl i-myū′ni-tē) A natural or acquired immunity to certain infectious agents, as manifested by an organ or a tissue, as a whole or in part.

lo·cal·i·za·tion (lō′kăl-ī-zā′shŭn) **1.** Limitation to a definite area. **2.** The reference of a sensation to its point of origin. **3.** The determination of the location of a morbid process.

lo·cal·i·za·tion-re·lat·ed ep·i·lep·sy (lō′kăl-ī-zā′shŭn-rĕ-lā′tĕd ep′i-lep′sē) **1.** SYN myoclonus epilepsy. **2.** SYN focal epilepsy.

lo·cal·ized (lō′kăl-īzd) Restricted or limited to a definite part.

lo·cal·ized mu·ci·no·sis (lō′kăl-īzd myū′si-nō′sis) SEE mucinosis.

lo·cal·ized nod·u·lar ten·o·syn·o·vi·tis (lō′kăl-īzed nod′yŭ-lăr ten′ō-sin′ō-vī′tis) SYN giant cell tumor of tendon sheath.

lo·cal·ized scle·ro·der·ma (lō′kăl-īzd skler′ō-dĕr′mă) SYN morphea.

lo·cal·iz·ing symp·tom (lō-kal′ī-zing simp′tŏm) A symptom indicating clearly the seat of the morbid process.

Lo·cal Med·i·cal Re·view Pol·i·cy (LMRP) (lō′kăl med′i-kăl rĕ-vyū′ pol′i-sē) A guideline in the U.S. for making local medical coverage decisions in the absence of a specific Medicare statute, regulation, or national coverage policy, or as an adjunct to an existing national coverage policy; devised by coverage contractors in consultation with the local medical community.

lo·cal re·ac·tion (lō′kăl rē-ak′shŭn) SYN focal reaction.

lo·cal stim·u·lant (lō′kăl stim′yŭ-lănt) A stimulant with an action confined to the part to which it is applied.

lo·ca·tor (lō′kā-tŏr) An instrument or apparatus for finding the position of a foreign object in tissue.

lo·chi·a (lō′kē-ă) Discharge from the vagina of mucus, blood, and tissue debris, following childbirth. [G. neut. pl. of *lochios,* relating to childbirth, fr. *lochos,* childbirth]

lo·chi·al (lō′kē-ăl) Relating to the lochia.

lo·chi·o·me·tra (lō′kē-ō-mē′tră) Distention of the uterus with retained lochia. [G. *mētra,* womb]

lo·chi·or·rhe·a, **lo·chi·or·rha·gi·a** (lō′kē-ōr-ē′ă, -ā′jē-ă) Profuse flow of the lochia. SYN lochiorrhoea. [lochia + G. *rhoia,* a flow]

lochiorrhoea [Br.] SYN lochiorrhea.

lo·ci (lō′sī) Plural of locus.

lock (lok) **1.** An enclosing, fastening, or securing device. **2.** A mechanism that, when moved, permits or obstructs passage.

locked-in syn·drome (lokt-in sin′drōm) Basis pontis infarct resulting in tetraplegia, horizontal ophthalmoplegia, dysphagia, and facial diplegia with preserved consciousness; caused by basilar artery occlusion.

locked knee (lokt nē) A condition in which the knee lacks full extension and flexion because of internal derangement, usually the result of a torn medial meniscus.

locked twins (lokt twinz) A form of malpresentation in which a breech twin and a vertex twin become locked at the chin during labor and attempted delivery.

Locke so·lu·tion (lok sŏ-lū′shŭn) A solution containing NaCl, $CaCl_2$, KCl, $NaHCO_3$, and D-glucose; used in laboratory experiments to irrigate mammalian heart and other tissues; also used in combination with naturally occurring body substances (e.g., blood serum, tissue extracts) or more complex chemically defined nutritive solutions for culturing animal cells.

lock·ing su·ture (lok′ing sū′chŭr) A running suture in which the suture material is made to pass through the loop made from the previous stitch. SYN lock stitch.

lock·jaw (lok′jaw) SYN trismus.

lock stitch (lok stich) SYN locking suture.

lo·co·mo·tor (lō′kō-mō′tŏr) Relating to locomotion, or movement from one place to another. [L. *locus,* place, + L. *moveo,* pp. *motus,* to move]

loc·u·lar (lok′yū-lăr) Relating to a loculus.

loc·u·late (lok′yū-lāt) Containing numerous loculi.

loc•u•lat•ed pleu•ral ef•fu•sion (lok′yū-lāt-ĕd plūr′ăl ĕ-fyū′zhŭn) Pleural effusion that is confined to one or more fixed pockets in the pleural space.

loc•u•la•tion (lok′yū-lā′shŭn) **1.** A loculate region in an organ or tissue, or a loculate structure formed between surfaces of organs or mucous or serous membranes. **2.** The process that results in the formation of a loculus or loculi.

loc•u•lus, pl. **loc•u•li** (lok′yū-lŭs, -lī) A small cavity or chamber. [L. dim. of *locus,* place]

lo•cus, pl. **lo•ci** (lō′kŭs, -sī) **1.** A place; usually, a specific site. **2.** The position that a gene occupies on a chromosome. **3.** The position of a point, as defined by the coordinates on a graph. [L.]

lo•cus of con•trol (lō′kŭs kŏn-trōl′) **1.** A theoretic construct designed to assess a person's perceived control over personal behavior; classified as internal if the person feels in control of events, external if others are perceived to have that control. **2.** BIOWARFARE a place from which a terrorist event is evaluated and managed.

lod score (lod skōr) A number used in genetic linkage studies; logarithm (base 10) of the odds in favor of genetic linkage. [*l*ogarithm + *od*ds]

Loeb de•cid•u•o•ma (lōb dĕ-sid′yū-ō′mă) Mass of decidual tissue produced in the uterus, in the absence of a fertilized ovum, by means of mechanical or hormonal stimulation.

Loe•wen•stein Oc•cu•pa•tion•al Ther•a•py Cog•ni•tive As•sess•ment (LOTCA) (lō′ĕn-stīn ok′yū-pā′shŭn-ăl thār-ă′pē kog′nă-tiv′ ă-ses′mĕnt) Battery of cognitive tests for both primary assessment and ongoing evaluation of patients with traumatic brain injury.

Loe•wen•thal re•ac•tion (lĕr′vĕn-tahl rē-ak′shŭn) The agglutinative reaction in relapsing fever.

Löf•fler ba•cil•lus (lĕrf′lĕr bă-sil′ŭs) SYN *Corynebacterium diphtheriae.*

Löf•fler caus•tic stain (lĕrf′lĕr kaw′stik stān) A stain for flagella, using an aqueous solution of tannin and ferrous sulfate with the addition of an alcoholic fuchsin stain.

Löf•fler cul•ture me•di•um (lĕrf′lĕr kŭl′chŭr mē′dē-ŭm) A culture medium consisting of beef blood serum, sheep blood serum, and beef bouillon containing peptone, glucose, and sodium chloride; used for the isolation of *Corynebacterium diphtheriae.*

Löf•fler en•do•car•di•tis (lĕrf′lĕr en′dō-kahr-dī′tis) Fibroplastic constrictive parietal endocarditis with eosinophilia, an endocarditis of obscure cause characterized by progressive congestive heart failure, multiple systemic emboli, and eosinophilia.

Löf•fler pa•ri•e•tal fi•bro•plas•tic en•do•car•di•tis (lĕrf′lĕr pa-rī′e-tăl fī′brō-plas′tik en′dō-kahr-dī′tis) Sclerosis of the endocardium in the presence of a high eosinophil count.

Löf•fler stain (lĕrf′lĕr stān) A stain for flagella; the specimen is treated with a mixture of ferrous sulfate, tannic acid, and alcoholic fuchsin, then stained with aniline-water fuchsin or gentian violet made alkaline with sodium hydroxide solution.

Löf•fler syn•drome (lĕrf′lĕr sin′drōm) SYN pulmonary eosinophilia.

log•ag•no•si•a (lawg′ag-nō′zē-ă) SYN aphasia. [logo- + G. *agnosia,* ignorance]

log•a•graph•i•a (lawg′ă-graf′ē-ă) SYN agraphia. [logo- + G. *a-* priv. + *graphō,* to write]

log•am•ne•si•a (lawg′am-nē′zē-ă) SYN aphasia. [logo- + G. *amnēsia,* forgetfulness]

Lo•gan bow (lō′găn bō) Heavy stainless steel wire bent in an arc and taped to both cheeks to protect a freshly repaired cleft lip.

log•a•pha•si•a (lawg′ă-fā′zē-ă) Aphasia of articulation. [logo- + G. *aphasia,* speechlessness]

log•as•the•ni•a (lawg′as-thē′nē-ă) SYN aphasia. [logo- + G. *astheneia,* weakness]

♻ **-logia** Suffix meaning **1.** The study of the subject noted in the body of the word, or a treatise on the same; the English equivalent is -logy, or, with a connecting vowel, -ology [G. *logos,* discourse, treatise]. **2.** Collecting or picking. [G. *legō,* to collect]

Lo•gis•tic Or•gan Dys•func•tion Score (lŏ-jis′tik ōr′găn dis-fŭngk′shŭn skōr) An evaluation method used in intensive care that rates the level of dysfunction of each organ system and among organ systems; includes evaluation of degree of dysfunction of cardiovascular, hepatic, hematologic, pulmonary, renal, and nervous systems.

♻ **logo-, log-** Combining forms meaning speech, words. [G. *logos,* word, discourse]

log•o•ple•gi•a (lawg′ō-plē′jē-ă) Paralysis of the organs of speech. [logo- + G. *plēgē,* stroke]

log•or•rhe•a (lawg′ōr-ē′ă) Uncommon term for abnormal or pathologic talkativeness or garrulousness. SYN logorrhoea. [logo- + G. *rhoia,* a flow]

logorrhoea [Br.] SYN logorrhea.

♻ **-logy** SEE -logia. [G. *logos,* treatise, discourse]

lo•i•a•sis (lō-ī′ă-sis) A chronic disease caused by the filarial nematode *Loa loa;* symptoms first occur 3–4 years after a bite by an infected tabanid fly. When the larvae mature, the adult worms move about through connective tissue, frequently becoming visible beneath the skin and mucous membranes or while passing through the conjunctiva. The worms provoke hyperemia and exudation of fluid; the patient is annoyed by the perception of "creeping" in the tissues and intense itching, as well as occasional pain, especially when the swelling is in the region of tendons and joints.

loin (loyn) The part of the side and back between the ribs and the pelvis. SYN lumbus. [Fr. *longe;* E. *lumbus*]

Lom•bard re•flex (lom′bahrd rē′fleks) The increase in vocal intensity when talking in a background of noise. It is the speaker's unconscious effort to be heard over the noise.

lo•mi•lo•mi (lō′mē-lō′mē) A traditional Hawaiian system of massage that emphasizes the use of two-handled techniques, elbows, and forearms to apply strokes over a broad area. SEE ALSO Swedish massage. [Hawaiian]

lo•mus•tine (lō-mŭs′tēn) 1-(2-chloroethyl)-3-cyclohexyl-1-nitrosourea; an antineoplastic agent.

Lone Star tick (lōn stahr tik) *Amblyomma americanum;* primary insect vector of Rocky Mountain spotted fever. Tick is found in southern U.S. Hosts include dogs and farm animals. [fr. Lone Star State, nickname of Texas]

long ab•duc•tor mus•cle of thumb (lawng ab-dŭk′tŏr mŭs′ĕl thŭm) SYN abductor pollicis longus muscle.

long-act•ing thy•roid stim•u•la•tor (LATS) (lawng′ak′ting thī′royd stim′yū-lā-tŏr) A substance, found in the blood of some hyperthyroid patients, that exerts a prolonged stimulatory effect on the thyroid gland; associated in plasma with the IgG (7S γ-globulin) fraction and seems to be an antibody or, perhaps, an immune complex. Cf. bioregulator.

long ad•duc•tor mus•cle (lawng ă-dŭk′tŏr mŭs′ĕl) SYN adductor longus muscle.

long bone (lawng bōn) One of the elongated bones of the extremities, consisting of a tubular shaft (diaphysis) and two extremities (epiphyses) usually wider than the shaft; the shaft is composed of compact bone surrounding a central medullary cavity. Cf. short bone.

long cil•i•ar•y nerve (lawng sil′ē-ār-ē nĕrv) One of two or three branches of the nasociliary nerve that bypass the ciliary ganglion, supplying postsynaptic sympathetic fibers for the dilatator pupillae muscle and sensory fibers for the ciliary muscles, iris, and cornea. SYN nervus ciliaris longus.

lon•gev•i•ty (lawn-jev′i-tē) Duration of a particular life beyond the norm for the species.

long ex•ten•sor mus•cle of thumb (lawng eks-ten′sŏr mŭs′ĕl thŭm) SYN extensor pollicis longus muscle.

long ex•ten•sor mus•cle of toes (lawng eks-ten′sŏr mŭs′ĕl tōz) SYN extensor digitorum longus muscle.

long fib•u•lar mus•cle (lawng fib′yū-lăr mŭs′ĕl) SYN fibularis longus muscle.

long flex•or mus•cle of great toe (lawng fleks′ŏr mŭs′ĕl grāt tō) SYN flexor hallucis longus muscle.

long flex•or mus•cle of thumb (lawng fleks′ŏr mŭs′ĕl thŭm) SYN flexor pollicis longus muscle.

long flex•or mus•cle of toes (lawng fleks′ŏr mŭs′ĕl tōz) SYN flexor digitorum longus muscle.

long gy•rus of in•su•la (lawng jī′rŭs in′sū-lă) The most posterior and longest of the slender straight gyri that compose the insula.

lon•gis•si•mus ca•pi•tis mus•cle (lon-jis′i-mŭs kap′i-tŭs mŭs′ĕl) *Origin*, from transverse processes of upper thoracic and transverse and articular processes of lower and middle cervical vertebrae; *insertion*, into mastoid process; *action*, keeps head erect, draws it backward or to one side; *nerve supply*, dorsal primary rami of cervical spinal nerves. SYN musculus longissimus capitis [TA].

lon•gis•si•mus cer•vi•cis mus•cle (lon-jis′i-mŭs sĕr′vi-sis mŭs′ĕl) *Origin*, transverse processes of upper thoracic vertebrae; *insertion*, transverse processes of middle and upper cervical vertebrae; *action*, extends cervical vertebrae; *nerve supply*, dorsal primary rami of lower cervical and upper thoracic spinal nerves. SYN musculus longissimus cervicis [TA].

lon•gis•si•mus tho•ra•cis mus•cle (lon-jis′i-mŭs thō-rā′sis mŭs′ĕl) *Origin*, with iliocostalis and from transverse processes of lower thoracic vertebrae; *insertion*, by lateral slips into most or all of the ribs between angles and tubercles and into tips of transverse processes of upper lumbar vertebrae, and by medial slips into accessory processes of upper lumbar and transverse processes of thoracic vertebrae; *action*, extends vertebral column; *nerve supply*, dorsal primary rami of thoracic and lumbar spinal nerves. SYN musculus longissimus thoracis [TA], thoracic longissimus muscle.

lon•gi•tu•di•nal (lon′ji-tū′di-năl) **1.** Running lengthwise; in the direction of the long axis of the body or any of its parts. **2.** Studied over a period of time, diachronic; contrast with cross-sectional or synchronic, which give equivalent results only under certain strict conditions of stability and equilibrium. [L. *longitudo,* length]

lon•gi•tu•di•nal ab•er•ra•tion (lon′ji-tū′di-năl ab-ĕr-ā′shŭn) In spheric aberration, the distance separating the focus of paraxial and peripheral rays on the optic axis.

lon•gi•tu•di•nal dis•so•ci•a•tion (lon′ji-tū′di-năl di-sō′sē-ā′shŭn) Dissociation between parallel chambers of the heart, as between one atrium and the other or between one ventricle and the other, in contrast to dissociation between atria and ventricles.

lon·gi·tu·di·nal frac·ture (lon′ji-tū′di-năl frak′shŭr) A fracture involving the bone in the line of its axis.

lon·gi·tu·di·nal lie (lon′ji-tū′di-năl lī) That relationship in which the long axis of the fetus is longitudinal and roughly parallel to the long axis of the mother; the presenting part may be either the head or the breech.

lon·gi·tu·di·nal lig·a·ment (lon′ji-tū′di-năl lig′ă-mĕnt) One of two extensive fibrous bands running the length of the vertebral column: the anterior longitudinal ligament and the posterior longitudinal ligament. SYN ligamentum longitudinale [TA].

lon·gi·tu·di·nal pon·tine fas·cic·u·li (lon′ji-tū′di-năl pon′tēn fa-sik′yū-lī) The massive bundles of corticofugal fibers passing longitudinally through the ventral part of pons; they are composed of corticopontine, corticobulbar, and corticospinal fibers.

lon·gi·tu·di·nal pon·tine fi·bers (lon′ji-tū-di-năl pon′tēn fī′bĕrz) SEE longitudinal pontine fasciculi.

lon·gi·tu·di·nal re·lax·a·tion (long′ji-tū′di-năl rē′lak-sā′shŭn) MAGNETIC RESONANCE IMAGING the return of the magnetic dipoles of the hydrogen nuclei (magnetization vector) to equilibrium parallel to the magnetic field, after they have been flipped 90°; varies in rate in different tissues, taking up to 15 seconds for water. SEE TI.

lon·gi·tu·di·nal sec·tion (long′ji-tū′di-năl sek′shŭn) A cross-section attained by slicing in any plane parallel to the long or vertical axis, actually or through imaging techniques, the body or any part of the body or anatomic structure. Longitudinal sections include, but are not limited to, median, sagittal, and coronal sections.

lon·gi·tu·di·nal tear (lon′ji-tū′di-năl tār) A tear of articular cartilage roughly parallel to the long axis of the bone.

long le·va·to·res cos·ta·rum mus·cles (lawng lev-ă-tō′rēz kos-tā′rŭm mŭs′ĕlz) *Insertion*, the second rib below their origin; *action*, raise ribs; *nerve supply*, intercostal.

Long·mire op·er·a·tion (lawng′mīr op-ĕr-ā′shŭn) Intrahepatic cholangiojejunostomy with partial hepatectomy for biliary obstruction.

long mus·cle of head (lawng mŭs′ĕl hed) SYN longus capitis muscle.

long mus·cle of neck (lawng mŭs′ĕl nek) SYN longus colli muscle.

long pal·mar mus·cle (lawng pahl′mĕr mŭs′ĕl) SYN palmaris longus muscle.

long per·o·ne·al mus·cle (lawng pĕr′ō-nē′ăl mŭs′ĕl) SYN fibularis longus muscle.

long pos·te·ri·or cil·i·ar·y ar·ter·ies (lawng pos-tēr′ē-ŏr sil′ē-ār-ē ahr′tĕr-ēz) One of two branches of the ophthalmic running forward between the sclerotic and choroid coats to the iris, at the outer and inner margins of which they form two circles by anastomosis. SYN arteriae ciliares posteriores longae.

long QT syn·dromes (lawng sin′drōmz) Any of several congenital and acquired diseases in which the electrocardiographic QT interval is longer than established measurements for age and sex; the presence of long QT intervals presages arrhythmias and sudden death. SEE ALSO QT interval.

long ra·di·al ex·ten·sor mus·cle of wrist (lawng rā′dē-ăl eks-ten′sŏr mŭs′ĕl rist) SYN extensor carpi radialis longus muscle.

long slow dis·tance train·ing (lawng slō dis′tăns trān′ing) SYN continuous training.

long-term care fa·ci·li·ty (lawng′tĕrm kār fă-sil′i-tē) SYN nursing facility.

long-term mem·o·ry (LTM) (lawng′tĕrm mem′ŏ-rē) That phase of the memory process considered the permanent storehouse of information that has been registered, encoded, passed into the short-term memory, coded, rehearsed, and finally transferred and stored for future retrieval; material and information retained in LTM underlies cognitive abilities.

long tho·ra·cic ar·ter·y (lawng thōr-as′ik ahr′tĕr-ē) SYN lateral thoracic artery.

long tho·rac·ic nerve (lawng thōr-as′ik nĕrv) Arises from the fifth, sixth, and seventh cervical nerves (roots of brachial plexus), descends the neck behind the brachial plexus, and is distributed to the serratus anterior muscle; it is somewhat unusual in that it courses on the superficial aspect of the muscle it supplies; its paralysis results in "winged scapula." SYN nervus thoracicus longus [TA].

lon·gus ca·pi·tis mus·cle (long′gus kap′i-tis mŭs′ĕl) *Origin*, anterior tubercles of transverse processes of third to sixth cervical vertebrae; *insertion*, basilar process of occipital bone; *action*, twists or flexes neck anteriorly; *nerve supply*, cervical plexus. SYN musculus longus capitis [TA], long muscle of head.

lon·gus col·li mus·cle (long′gus kol′ī mŭs′ĕl) Medial part: *origin*, the bodies of the third thoracic to the fifth cervical vertebrae; *insertion*, the bodies of the second to fourth cervical vertebrae; superolateral part: *origin*, the anterior tubercles of the transverse processes of the third to fifth cervical vertebrae; *insertion*, the anterior tubercle of the atlas; inferolateral part: *origin*, the bodies of the first to third thoracic vertebrae; *insertion*, the anterior tubercles of the transverse processes of the fifth and sixth cervical vertebrae; *action*, for all three parts, twist neck and flex neck anteriorly; *nerve supply*, for all three parts, ventral primary rami of cervical spinal nerves (cervical plexus). SYN musculus longus colli [TA], long muscle of neck.

loop (lūp) **1.** A sharp curve or complete bend in a vessel, cord, or other elongate body, forming an oval or circular ring. SEE ALSO ansa. **2.** A wire (usually of platinum or nichrome) fixed into a handle at one end and bent into a circle at the other, rendered sterile by flaming, and used to transfer microorganisms. [M.E. *loupe*]

loop di•u•ret•ic (lūp dī′yūr-et′ik) A class of agents promoting evacuation of urine (e.g., furosemide, ethacrynic acid) that act by inhibiting reabsorption of sodium and chloride, not only in the proximal and distal tubules but also in the Henle loop.

loop e•lec•tro•cau•ter•y ex•ci•sion pro•ce•dure (LEEP) (lūp ĕ-lek′trō-kaw′tĕr-ē ek-sizh′ŭn prŏ-sē′jŭr) Electrocautery excisional biopsy of abnormal cervical tissue.

loop elec•tro•sur•gi•cal ex•ci•sion pro•ce•dure (lūp ĕ-lek′trō-sĭr′jik-ăl ek-sizh′ŭn prŏ-sē′jŭr) SYN loop excision.

loop ex•ci•sion (lūp ek-sizh′ŭn) A diagnostic and therapeutic gynecologic surgical technique for removing dysplastic cells from the cervix with a small wire loop. SYN loop electrosurgical excision procedure.

loops of spi•nal nerves (lūps spī′năl nĕrvz) Loops of the spinal nerves, connecting ventral primary rami of the spinal nerves. SYN ansae nervorum spinalium.

loose as•so•ci•a•tions (lūs as-sō′sē-ā′shŭnz) A manifestation of a thought disorder whereby the patient's responses do not relate to the interviewer's questions or one paragraph, sentence, or phrase is not logically connected to those that occur before or after.

loose bod•ies (lūs bod′ēz) Fragments of cartilage or bone within a joint cavity. They usually result from previous trauma not always symptomatic.

loos•en•ing of as•so•ci•a•tions (lūs′sĕn-ing ă-sō′sē-ā′shŭnz) A manifestation of a severe thought disorder characterized by the lack of an obvious connection between one thought or phrase and the next, or with the response to a question.

loose-packed po•si•tion (lūs′pakt pŏ-zish′ŏn) A position of a joint in which the joint surfaces are not congruent and the joint capsule is lax. SEE ALSO open-packed position.

loph•o•dont (lof′ŏ-dont) Having the crowns of the molar teeth formed in transverse or longitudinal crests or ridges, as in the herbivores. [G. *lophos*, ridge, + *odous*, tooth]

lor•do•sco•li•o•sis (lōr′dō-skō′lē-ō′sis) Combined backward and lateral curvature of the spine. [G. *lordos*, bent back, + *skoliōsis*, crookedness, fr. *skolios*, bent, aslant]

lor•do•sis (lōr-dō′sis) *Note: Although term correctly denotes normal and pathologic states, the latter usage is less common.* **1.** [TA] A normal anteriorly convex curvature of the vertebral column. **2.** Hyperlordosis; an abnormal anteriorly convex curvature of the spine, usually lumbar. Cf. hyperlordosis, hyperlordotic. [G. *lordōsis*, a bending backward]

lor•do•sis cer•vi•cis (lōr-dō′sis ser′vi-sis) [TA] SYN cervical lordosis.

lor•do•sis col•li (lōr-dō′sis kol′ī) SYN cervical lordosis.

lor•do•sis lum•ba•lis (lōr-dō′sis lŭm-bā′lis) [TA] SYN lumbar lordosis.

lor•dot•ic (lōr-dot′ik) Pertaining to or marked by lordosis.

lor•dot•ic po•si•tion (lōr-dot′ik pŏ-zish′ŏn) A radiographic position with exaggerated lumbar lordotic curve, allowing x-ray examination of the lung apices without the clavicles being superimposed.

Lo•schmidt num•ber (lō′shmit nŭm′bĕr) The number of molecules in 1 cm^3 of ideal gas at 0°C and 1 atm of pressure; Avogadro number divided by 22,414 (i.e., 2.6868×10^{19} cm^{-3}).

loss (laws) Deprivation, bereavement; failure to retain possession or control of something. [O.E. *los*]

LOT (lot) Acronym for left occipitotransverse position.

LOTCA Abbreviation for Loewenstein Occupational Therapy Cognitive Assessment.

lo•tion (lō′shŭn) A class of liquid suspensions or dispersions intended for external application. [L. *lotio*, a washing, fr. *lavo*, to wash]

loud•ness dis•com•fort lev•el (lowd′nĕs dis-kŏm′fŏrt lev′ĕl) The intensity at which sound, particularly speech, causes discomfort.

Lou Geh•rig dis•ease (lū ger′ig di-zēz′) SYN amyotrophic lateral sclerosis.

Lou•is an•gle, Lud•wig an•gle (lū-ē′ ang′gĕl, lud′vig) SYN sternal angle.

loupe (lūp) A magnifying lens. [Fr.]

louse, pl. **lice** (lows, līs) Common name for members of the ectoparasitic insect orders Anoplura (sucking lice) and Mallophaga (biting lice). See page B8. [A.S. *lūs*]

love-lies-bleed•ing (lŭv-līz-blēd′ing) SYN amaranth.

Lo•vi•bond an•gle (lō′vi-bond ang′gĕl) The

angle made at the meeting of the proximal nail fold and the nail plate when viewed from the radial aspect; normally, less than 180° but exceeding this in clubbing of the fingers.

low birth weight (LBW) (lō bĭrth wāt) Birth weight less than 2500 g. Can be due to a range of factors, including interference with intrauterine growth or premature birth.

low cal·o·rie (lō kal′ŏr-ē) A product so labeled contains, by F.D.A. order, fewer than 40 calories per serving.

low cho·les·ter·ol (lō kŏ-les′tĕr-ol) A product so labeled contains, by F.D.A. order, less than 20 mg cholesterol per serving and less than 2 g saturated fat per serving.

low den·si·ty li·po·pro·tein-cho·les·ter·ol (LDL-C) (lō den′si-tē lī′pō-prō′tēn kŏ-les′tĕr-ol) The so-called bad cholesterol; contains mostly lipids and few proteinaceous elements; its levels ought to be kept to a minimum to improve health.

Lö·wen·berg for·ceps (lĕr′vĕn-berg fōr′seps) Forceps with short curved blades ending in rounded grasping extremities devised for the removal of adenoid growths in the nasopharynx.

Löw·en·stein pro·cess (ler′ven-shtīn pros′ĕs) A technique from the time of World War I (1914–1918) to manufacture the chemical warfare agent sulfur mustard by bubbling dry ethylene through sulfur monochloride; also spelled Levinstein.

low·er air·way (lō′ĕr ār′wā) The portion of the respiratory tract that extends from the subglottis to and including the terminal bronchioles.

low·er e·soph·a·ge·al sphinc·ter (LES) (lō′ĕr ĕ-sof′ă-jē′ăl sfingk′tĕr) Musculature of the gastroesophageal junction that is tonically active except during swallowing.

low·er ex·trem·i·ty (lō′ĕr eks-trem′i-tē) SYN lower limb.

low·er limb (lō′ĕr lim) The hip, thigh, leg, ankle, and foot. SYN lower extremity.

low·er mo·tor neu·ron (lō′ĕr mō′tŏr nūr′on) The final motor neurons that innervate skeletal muscles; distinguished from upper motor neurons of the motor cortex that contribute to the pyramidal or corticospinal tract. SEE ALSO motor neuron.

low·est splanch·nic nerve (lō′est splangk′nik nĕrv) One of the abdominopelvic splanchnic nerves arising in the thorax and penetrating the diaphragm to supply presynaptic sympathetic fibers for the renal plexus; often combined with the lesser splanchnic nerve, but occasionally existing as an independent nerve. SYN nervus splanchnicus imus [TA].

low·est thy·roid ar·ter·y (lō′est thī′royd ahr′tĕr-ē) SYN thyroid ima artery.

low fat (lō fat) A product so labeled contains, by F.D.A. order, less than 3 g of fat per serving.

low-fre·quen·cy trans·duc·tion (lō-frē′kwĕn-sē trans-dŭk′shŭn) Specialized transduction in which only a small portion of the prophage particles, because of their defectiveness, are able to develop sufficiently to serve as effective transducing agents.

low-grade ex·plo·sive (lō-grād eks-plō′siv) A device that generates a subsonic pressure front (blast wind) but not a supersonic pressure front (blast wave) when it explodes.

low-grade squa·mous in·tra·ep·i·the·li·al le·sion (LGSIL, LSIL) (lō-grād skwā′mŭs in-tră-ep′i-thē′lē-ăl lē′zhŭn) Term used in the Bethesda system for reporting cervical/vaginal cytologic diagnosis to describe a spectrum of noninvasive cervical epithelial abnormalities; these lesions include the cellular changes associated with human papillomavirus cytopathologic effect and mild dysplasia (cervical intraepithelial neoplasia grade 1). SEE ALSO Bethesda system, reactive changes, ASCUS, atypical glandular cells of undetermined significance.

low-in·ten·si·ty stim·u·la·tor (LIS) (lō-in-ten′si-tē stim′yū-lā-tŏr) SYN microcurrent.

low, lit·tle, few, or low source of... (lō, lit′ĕl, fyū, lō sōrs) These terms, when used in food labeling, mean that, according to F.D.A. regulations, the food so labeled will allow someone frequent consumption of the product without exceeding the nutrient's daily values.

low mo·lec·u·lar weight hep·ar·in (LMWH) (lō mŏ-lek′yŭ-lăr wāt hep′ăr-in) A form of heparin with a longer half life and fewer adverse effects (e.g., thrombocytopenia).

low mo·lec·u·lar weight pro·tein (lō mŏ-lek′yŭ-lăr wāt prō′tēn) A gene product that is a component of a proteosome.

low mus·cle tone (lō mŭs′ĕl tōn) SYN hypotonicity.

low os·mo·lar con·trast a·gent (lō oz-mō′lăr kon′trast ā′jĕnt) Nonionic water-soluble radiographic contrast material. SYN low osmolar contrast medium, nonionic contrast agent.

low os·mo·lar con·trast me·di·um (lō oz-mō′lăr kon′trast mē′dē-ŭm) SYN low osmolar contrast agent.

low-pu·rine di·et (lō-pyūr′ēn dī′ĕt) A diet low in precursors of purines (such as tissues rich in cells with abundant nuclei, as in liver and glandular meats) to minimize formation of uric acid. Useful in treatment of patients with gout or urate-containing renal calculi.

low-salt di·et (lō-sawlt dī′ĕt) A diet with restricted amounts of sodium chloride, and other sodium salts, necessary in the treatment of some cases of hypertension, heart failure, and other syndromes characterized by fluid retention or edema formation.

low so·di·um (lō sō′dē-ŭm) A product so labeled contains, by F.D.A. order, no more than 140 mg of sodium per serving.

low TENS (lō tenz) A transcutaneous electrical nerve stimulator applied at the motor level characterized by low-frequency and long duration of pulses.

low-ten·sion glau·co·ma (lōw-ten′shŭn glaw-kō′mă) Optic nerve atrophy and excavation with typical field defects of glaucoma but without abnormal increase in intraocular pressure. SYN normal-tension glaucoma.

low-tone hear·ing loss (lō-tōn hēr′ing laws) Inability to hear low notes or frequencies.

lox·os·ce·lism (lok-sos′ĕ-lizm) Illness produced by the brown recluse spider, *Loxosceles reclusus;* characterized by gangrenous slough at the site of the bite, nausea, malaise, fever, hemolysis, and thrombocytopenia.

loz. Abbreviation for lozenge.

loz·enge (loz.) (loz′ĕnj) SYN troche. [Fr. *losange,* fr. *lozangé,* rhombic]

LPN Abbreviation for licensed practical nurse.

LPO Abbreviation for left posterior oblique. That radiographic position in which the left posterior side of the body part being examined is closest to the film.

Lr Symbol for lawrencium.

Lr dose, **L_r dose** (dōs, dōs) The limes reacting dose of diphtheria toxin, i.e., the smallest amount of toxin that, when mixed with one unit of antitoxin and injected intracutaneously in the shaved skin of a susceptible guinea pig, yields a minimal, positive reaction and inflammation localized to the region of the injection; the L_rd. closely approximates the L_0d., as would be expected, inasmuch as a slight excess of unneutralized toxin results in a reaction.

LSA Abbreviation for left sacroanterior position.

L se·lec·tin (sĕ-lek′tin) Cell surface receptor produced by leukocytes.

L shell (shell) The next lowest energy level of electrons in the atom, after the K shell.

LSIL Abbreviation for low-grade squamous intraepithelial lesion.

LSP Abbreviation for left sacroposterior position.

LST Abbreviation for left sacrotransverse position.

LT Abbreviation for leukotrienes, usually followed by another letter with a subscript number (e.g., LTA_4, LTC_4).

LTM Abbreviation for long-term memory.

LTOT Abbreviation for long-term oxygen therapy.

Lu Symbol for lutetium.

Lu·barsch crys·tals (lū′bahrsh kris′tălz) Intracellular crystals in the testis resembling sperm crystals.

lu·bri·cat·ing en·e·ma (lū′bri-kāt-ing en′ĕ-mă) SYN oil retention enema.

lu·cerne (lū-sĕrn′) SYN alfalfa. [Fr., fr. L. *lucerna,* lamp]

lu·cid (lū′sid) Clear, not obscured or confused, as in a lucid moment or lucid spoken expression. [L. *lucidus,* clear]

lu·cid·i·ty (lū-sid′i-tē) The quality or state of being lucid.

lu·cif·u·gal (lū-sif′yū-găl) Avoiding light. [L. *lux,* light, + *fugio,* to flee from]

Lu·cio lep·ro·sy (lū′syō lep′rŏ-sē) An acute form of pure diffuse lepromatous leprosy; during the reactive phase, can produce irregularly shaped, intensely erythematous, tender plaques, especially of the legs, with a tendency to ulceration and scarring.

lu·cip·e·tal (lū-sip′i-tăl) Seeking light. [L. *lux,* light, + *peto,* to seek]

Luc·ké vi·rus (luk′ā vī′rŭs) A herpesvirus associated with Lucké carcinoma.

Luc op·er·a·tion (lūk op-ĕr-ā′shŭn) SYN Caldwell-Luc operation.

Lud·wig an·gi·na (lud′vig an′ji-nă) Cellulitis, usually of odontogenic origin, bilaterally involving the submaxillary, sublingual, and submental spaces, resulting in painful swelling of the floor of the mouth, elevation of the tongue, dysphasia, dysphonia, and (at times) compromise of the airway. [W.F. Ludwig]

Lud·wig gan·gli·on (lud′vig gang′glē-ŏn) A small collection of parasympathetic nerve cells in the interatrial septum.

Lu·er a·dap·ter (lū′er ă-dap′tĕr) A device that connects the syringe to the needle tightly.

Lu·er sy·ringe (lū′ĕr sir-inj′) A glass syringe with a metal tip and locking device to secure the needle; used for hypodermic and intravenous injections and phlebotomy.

lu·es (lū′ēz) A plague or pestilence; specifically, syphilis. [L. pestilence]

lu·et·ic (lū-et′ik) SYN syphilitic.

lu·et·ic mask (lū-et′ik mask) A dirty brownish yellow pigmentation, blotchy in character, resembling that of chloasma, occurring on the forehead, temples, and sometimes the cheeks in patients with tertiary syphilis.

Luft dis·ease (luft di-zēz′) A metabolic disease

due to relative uncoupling of phosphorylation in skeletal muscle causing myopathy and general hypermetabolism; a mitochondial myopathy.

Luft po·tas·si·um per·man·ga·nate fix·a·tive (luft pŏ-tas′ē-ŭm pĕr-man′gă-nāt fiks′ă-tiv) A fixative useful in electron microscopy for cytologic preservation of lipoprotein complexes in membranes and myelin, because of its oxidative properties.

Lu·gol i·o·dine so·lu·tion (lū-gol′ ī′ō-dīn sŏ-lū′shŭn) An iodine-potassium iodide solution used as an oxidizing agent, for removal of mercurial fixation artifacts, and also in histochemistry to stain amebas.

lu-hui (lū-hwē) SYN *Aloe vera.*

lu·lib·er·in (lū-lib′ĕr-in) A decapeptide hormone from the hypothalamus that stimulates the anterior pituitary to release both follicle-stimulating hormone and luteinizing hormone. Cf. bioregulator. SYN luteinizing hormone-releasing hormone. [luteinizing hormone + L. *libero*, to free, + -in]

lum·ba·go (lŭm-bā′gō) Pain in mid and lower back; a descriptive term not specifying cause. SYN lumbar rheumatism. [L. fr. *lumbus,* loin]

lum·bar (lŭm′bahr) Relating to the loins, or the part of the back and sides between the ribs and the pelvis. [L. *lumbus,* a loin]

lum·bar ar·ter·y (lŭm′bahr ahr′tĕr-ē) *Origin,* abdominal aorta; one of four or five pairs; *distribution,* lumbar vertebrae, muscles of back, abdominal wall; *anastomoses,* intercostal, subcostal, superior and inferior epigastric, deep circumflex iliac, and iliolumbar. SYN arteriae lumbales [TA].

lum·bar flex·ure (lŭm′bahr flek′shŭr) The normal ventral curve of the vertebral column in the lumbar region.

lum·bar gan·gli·a (lŭm′bahr gang′glē-ă) Four or more paravertebral sympathetic ganglia on the medial border of the psoas major muscle on either side; they form, with the sacral and coccygeal ganglia and their interganglionic branches, the abdominopelvic part of the sympathetic trunk.

lum·bar her·ni·a (lŭm′bahr hĕr′nē-ă) A protrusion between the last rib and the iliac crest where the aponeurosis of the transversus muscle is covered only by the latissimus dorsi.

lum·bar il·i·o·cos·tal mus·cle (lŭm′bahr il′ē-ō-kos′tăl mŭs′ĕl) SYN iliocostalis lumborum muscle.

lum·bar·i·za·tion (lŭm′bahr-ī-zā′shŭn) A congenital anomaly of the lumbosacral junction characterized by development of the first sacral vertebra as a lumbar vertebra resulting in six lumbar vertebrae instead of five.

lum·bar lor·do·sis (lŭm′bahr lōr-dō′sis) The normal, anteriorly convex curvature of the lumbar segment of the vertebral column; a secondary curvature, acquired postnatally as the upright posture is assumed when one learns to walk. SYN lordosis lumbalis [TA].

lum·bar nerves [L1–L5] (lŭm′bahr nĕrvz) Five bilaterally paired spinal nerves emerging from the lumbar portion of the spinal cord; the first four nerves enter into the formation of the lumbar plexus, the fourth and fifth into that of the sacral plexus. SYN nervi lumbales [TA].

lum·bar plex·us (lŭm′bahr plek′sŭs) **1.** A nervous plexus, formed by the ventral rami of the first four lumbar nerves; it lies in the substance of the psoas muscle. **2.** A lymphatic plexus formed of about twenty lymph nodes and connecting vessels situated along the lower portion of the aorta and the common iliac vessels.

i **lum·bar punc·ture** (lŭm′bahr pungk′shŭr) A puncture into the subarachnoid space of the lumbar region to obtain spinal fluid for diagnostic or therapeutic purposes. See this page. SYN rachicentesis, rachiocentesis, spinal tap.

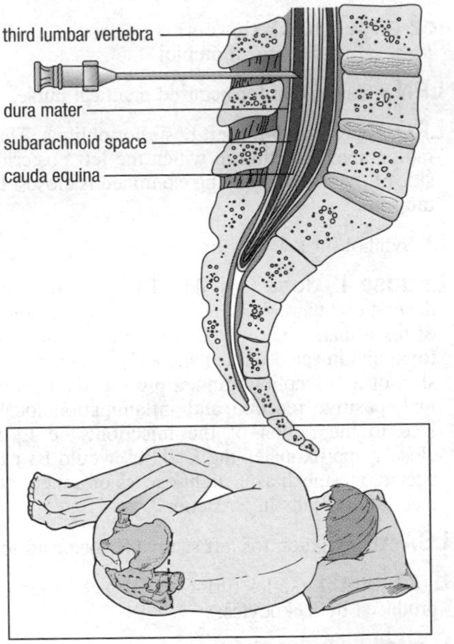

lumbar puncture: for a lumbar puncture, patient lies on side with back slightly rounded and knees flexed toward abdomen

lum·bar rheu·ma·tism (lŭm′bahr rū′mă-tizm) SYN lumbago.

lum·bar rib (lŭm′bahr rib) An occasional rib articulating with the transverse process of the first lumbar vertebra.

lum·bar splanch·nic nerves (lŭm′bahr splangk′nik nĕrvz) Branches from the lumbar sympathetic trunks that pass anteriorly to convey presynaptic sympathetic fibers to, and visceral afferents from, the celiac, intermesenteric, aortic, and superior hypogastric plexuses. SYN nervi splanchnici lumbales [TA].

lum•bar tri•an•gle (lŭm′bahr trī′ang-gĕl) An area in the posterior abdominal wall bounded by the edges of the latissimus dorsi and external oblique muscles and the iliac crest; herniations occasionally occur here. SYN trigonum lumbale.

lum•bar vein (lŭm′bahr vān) Veins accompanying the lumbar arteries, which drain the posterior body wall and the lumbar vertebral venous plexuses, and terminate anteriorly as follows: the first and second in the ascending lumbar vein, the third and fourth in the inferior vena cava, and the fifth in the iliolumbar vein; all communicate via the ascending lumbar veins.

lum•bar ver•te•brae [L1–L5] (lŭm′bahr vĕr′tĕ-brā) The vertebrae, usually five in number, located in the lumbar region of the back. SYN vertebrae lumbales [L1–L5].

lum•bi (lŭm′bī) Plural of lumbus. [L.]

lum•bo•cos•tal (lŭm′bō-kos′tăl) **1.** Relating to the lumbar and the hypochondriac regions. **2.** Relating to the lumbar vertebrae and the ribs; denoting a ligament connecting the first lumbar vertebra with the neck of the twelfth rib. [L. *lumbus,* loin, + *costa,* rib]

lum•bo•cos•tal lig•a•ment (lŭm′bō-kos′tăl lig′ă-mĕnt) A strong band that unites the twelfth rib with the tips of the transverse processes of the first and second lumbar vertebrae. SYN ligamentum lumbocostale [TA].

lum•bo•cos•to•ab•dom•i•nal tri•an•gle (lŭm′bō-kŏs′tō-ab-dom′i-năl tri′ang-gĕl) An irregular area bounded by the serratus posterior inferior, obliquus externus, obliquus internus, and erector spinae muscles.

lum•bo•in•gui•nal (lŭm′bō-ing′gwi-năl) Relating to the lumbar and the inguinal regions. [L. *lumbus,* loin, + *inguen* (*inguin-*), groin]

lum•bo•sa•cral (lŭm′bō-sā′krăl) Relating to the lumbar vertebrae and the sacrum. SYN sacrolumbar.

lum•bri•cal mus•cles of foot (lŭm′bri-kăl mŭs′ĕlz fut) Four intrinsic muscles of the foot; *origin*, first: from tibial side of tendon to second toe of flexor digitorum longus; second, third, and fourth: from adjacent sides of all four tendons of this musculus; *insertion*, tibial side of extensor tendon on dorsum of each of the four lateral toes; *action*, flex the proximal and extend the middle and distal phalanges; *nerve supply*, lateral (second to fourth lumbricals) and medial (first lumbrical) plantar. SYN musculus lumbricalis pedis [TA].

lum•bri•cal mus•cles of hand (lŭm′bri-kăl mŭs′ĕlz hand) Four intrinsic muscles of the hand; *origin*, the two lateral: from the radial side of the tendons of the flexor digitorum profundus going to the index and middle fingers; the two medial: from the adjacent sides of the second and third, and third and fourth tendons; *insertion*, radial side of extensor tendon on dorsum of each of the four fingers; *action*, flexes metacarpophalangeal joint and extends the proximal and distal interphalangeal joint; *nerve supply*, the two radial muscles by the median, the two ulnar muscles by the ulnar. See this page. SYN musculus lumbricalis manus [TA].

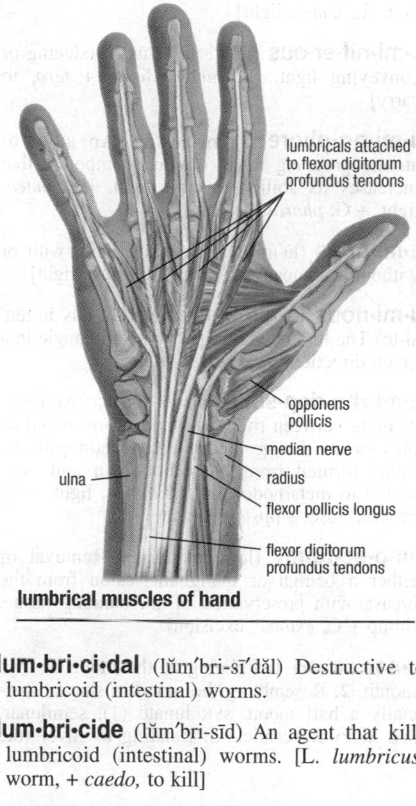

lumbrical muscles of hand

lum•bri•ci•dal (lŭm′bri-sī′dăl) Destructive to lumbricoid (intestinal) worms.

lum•bri•cide (lŭm′bri-sīd) An agent that kills lumbricoid (intestinal) worms. [L. *lumbricus,* worm, + *caedo,* to kill]

lum•bri•coid (lŭm′bri-koyd) Denoting or resembling a roundworm, especially *Ascaris lumbricoides*. SEE ALSO vermiform. [L. *lumbricus,* earthworm, + G. *eidos,* resemblance]

lum•bri•co•sis (lŭm′bri-kō′sis) Infection with round intestinal worms.

lum•bus, gen. and pl. **lum•bi** (lŭm′bŭs, -bī) SYN loin. [L.]

lu•men, pl. **lu•mi•na, lu•mens** (lū′mĕn, -mi-nă, -mĕnz) **1.** The space in the interior of a tubular structure, such as an artery or the intestine. **2.** **(lm)** The unit of luminous flux; the luminous flux emitted in a unit solid angle of 1 steradian by a uniform point source of light having a luminous intensity of 1 candela. [L. light, window]

lu·mi·nal (lū′mi-năl) Relating to the lumen of a blood vessel or other tubular structure. SYN luminalis.

lu·mi·na·lis (lū′mi-nā′lis) SYN luminal.

lu·mi·nance (lū′mi-năns) The brightness of an object, expressed as the luminous flux per unit solid angle per unit projected area, measured in lamberts or in candelas per square meter. [L. *lumino*, to light up, fr. *lumen*, light]

lu·mi·nes·cence (lū′mi-nes′ens) Emission of light from a body as a result of a chemical reaction. [L. *lumen*, light]

lu·mi·nif·er·ous (lū′mi-nif′ĕr-ŭs) Producing or conveying light. [L. *lumen*, light, + *fero*, to carry]

lu·mi·no·phore (lū′mi-nō-fōr) An atom or atomic grouping in an organic compound that increases its ability to emit light. [L. *lumen*, light, + G. *phoros*, bearing]

lu·mi·nous (lū′mi-nŭs) Emitting light, with or without accompanying heat. [L. *lumen*, light]

lu·mi·nous in·ten·si·ty (I) (lū′mi-nŭs in-ten′si-tē) The luminous flux per unit solid angle in a given direction. SYN radiant intensity.

lu·mi·rho·dop·sin (lū′mi-rō-dop′sin) An intermediate between rhodopsin and all-*trans*-retinal plus opsin during bleaching of rhodopsin by light; formed from bathorhodopsin and converted to metarhodopsin. [L. *lumen*, light, + G. *rhodon*, rose, + *opsis*, vision]

lump·ec·to·my (lŭmp-ek′tŏ-mē) Removal of either a benign or malignant lesion from the breast, with preservation of surrounding tissue. [lump + G. *ektomē*, excision]

lu·nar (lū′năr) **1.** Relating to the moon or to a month. **2.** Resembling the moon in shape, especially a half moon. SYN lunate (1), semilunar. SEE ALSO crescentic. **3.** Relating to silver (the moon was the symbol of silver in alchemy). [L. *luna*, moon]

lu·nate (lū′nāt) **1.** SYN lunar (2). **2.** Relating to the lunate bone.

lu·nate bone (lū′nāt bōn) One of the proximal row in the carpus between the scaphoid and triquetral; it articulates with the radius, scaphoid, triquetral, hamate, and capitate.

Lund-Brow·der chart (lund-brow′dĕr chahrt) A tabular scale used to determine the scope of burns in children. See this page.

lung (lŭng) One of a pair of viscera occupying the pulmonary cavities of the thorax, the organs of respiration in which aeration of the blood takes place. As a rule, the right lung is slightly larger than the left and is divided into three lobes (an upper, a middle, and a lower or basal), whereas the left has but two lobes (an upper and a lower or basal). Each lung is irregularly conic, presenting a blunt upper extremity (the apex), a concave base following the curve of the diaphragm, an outer convex surface (costal surface), an inner or mediastinal surface, a thin and sharp anterior border, and a thick and rounded posterior border. See page 917. SYN pulmo [TA]. [A.S. *lungen*]

lung bud (lŭng bŭd) SYN respiratory diverticulum.

lung com·pli·ance (lŭng kŏm-plī′ăns) The change in lung volume per unit change in transpulmonary pressure; may be static or dynamic.

lung vol·ume re·duc·tion sur·gery (lŭng vol′yūm rĕ-dŭk′shŭn sŭr′jĕr-ē) Procedure whereby nonfunctional lung tissue in emphysema patients is removed, allowing more room in the thoracic cavity for relatively healthy tissue and thus theoretically improving lung function. SEE ALSO emphysema.

lung·worms (lŭng′wŏrmz) Any of various species of nematode parasites that infest the lungs

relative percentages of areas affected by growth

	at birth	0 to 1 yr	1 to 4 yr	5 to 9 yr	10 to 15 yr	adult
A: half of head	9½%	8½%	6½%	5½%	4½%	3½%
B: half of thigh	2½%	3½%	4%	4½%	4½%	4½%
C: half of leg	2½%	2½%	2½%	3%	3½%	3½%

To determine the extent of an infant's or child's burns, use the diagrams shown here.

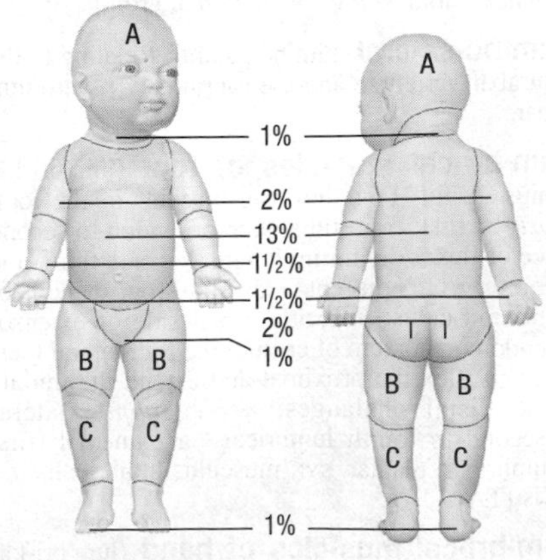

Lund-Browder chart

and air passage of sheep, cattle, and (rarely) human beings.

lu•nu•la, pl. **lu•nu•lae** (lūn′yū-lă, -lē) **1.** The pale arched area at the proximal portion of the nail plate. **2.** A small semilunar structure. [L. dim. of *luna,* moon]

lu•nule (lūn′yūl) **1.** SYN lunule of nail. **2.** A small semilunar structure.

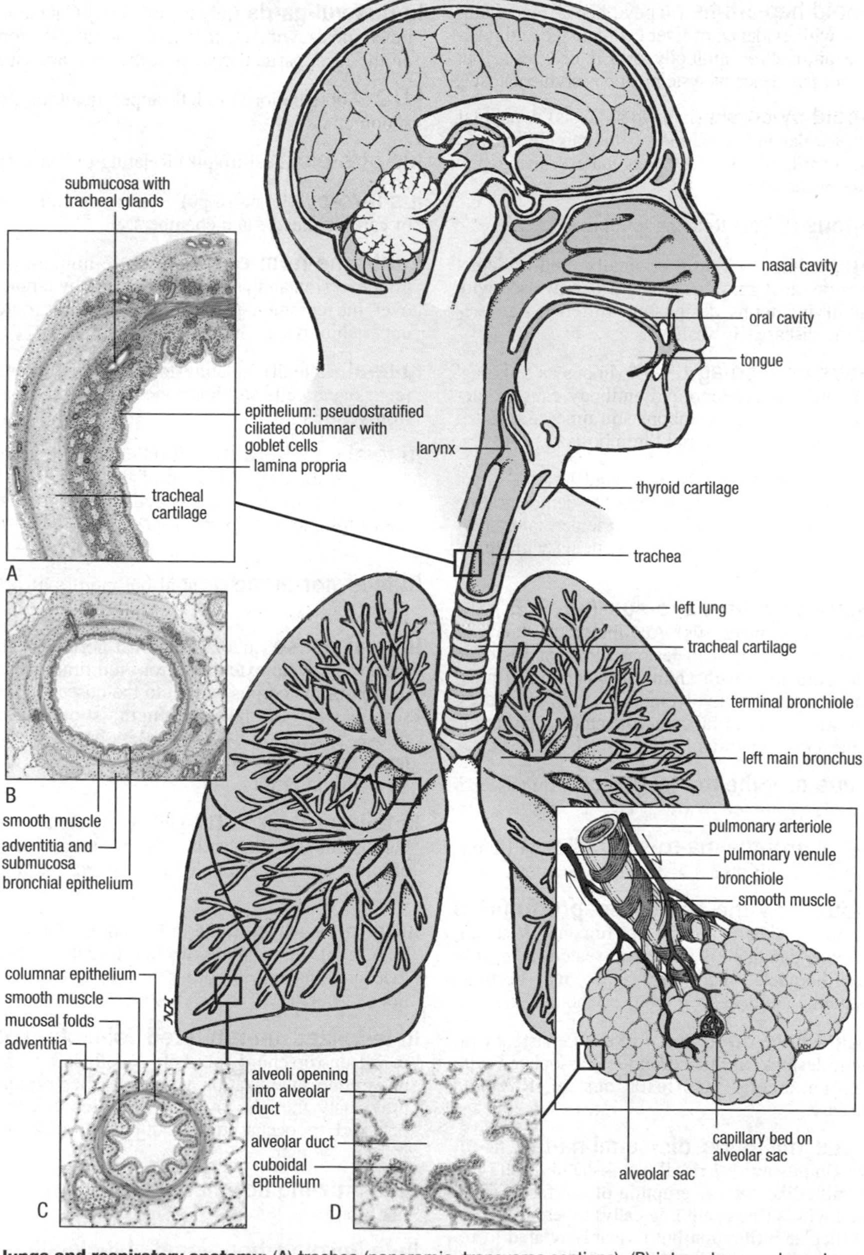

lungs and respiratory anatomy: (A) trachea (panoramic, transverse sections); (B) intrapulmonary bronchus; (C) terminal bronchiole; (D) respiratory bronchiole with alveoli

lu•nule of nail (lūn′yūl nāl) The pale arched area at the proximal portion of the nail plate. SYN lunule (1).

lu•pi•form (lū′pi-fōrm) SYN lupoid.

lu•poid (lū′poyd) Resembling lupus. SYN lupiform. [L. *lupus* + G. *eidos,* resemblance]

lu•poid hep•a•ti•tis (lū′poyd hep′ă-tī′tis) Jaundice with evidence of liver cell damage and positive antinuclear antibody or LE cell tests, but without evidence of systemic lupus erythematosus.

lu•poid sy•co•sis (lū′poyd sī-kō′sis) A papular or pustular inflammation of the hair follicles of the beard, followed by punctuate scarring and loss of the hair.

lu•pous (lū′pŭs) Relating to lupus.

lu•pus (lū′pŭs) A term originally used to depict erosion (as if gnawed) of the skin, now used with modifying terms designating different varieties of the disease. [L. wolf]

lu•pus an•ti•co•ag•u•lant (lū′pŭs an′tē-kō-ag′yŭ-lănt) Antiphospholipid antibody causing elevation in partial thromboplastin time; associated with venous and arterial thrombosis.

lu•pus band test (lū′pŭs band test) A direct immunofluorescent technique for demonstrating a band of immunoglobulins at the dermal-epidermal junction of the skin of patients with lupus erythematosus.

lu•pus er•y•the•ma•to•sus (LE, L.E.) (lū′pŭs ĕr-i′thĕ-mă-tō′sŭs) An illness that may be characterized by skin lesions alone or systemic (disseminated) with antinuclear antibodies present and usually involvement of vital structures. SEE ALSO discoid lupus erythematosus, systemic lupus erythematosus.

lu•pus er•y•the•ma•to•sus cell (lū′pŭs ĕr-i′thĕ-mă-tō′sŭs sel) SYN LE cell.

lu•pus er•y•the•ma•to•sus cell test (lū′pŭs ĕr-i′thĕ-mĕ-tō′sŭs sel test) SYN LE cell test.

lu•pus er•y•the•ma•to•sus pro•fun•dus (lū′pŭs ĕr-i′thĕ-mă-tō′sŭs prō-fun′dŭs) A subcutaneous panniculitis with deep-seated, firm, rubbery nodules, usually of the face; may occur in systemic and localized lupus erythematosus.

lu•pus li•ve•do (lū′pŭs li-vē′dō) Persistent cyanotic lesions on the extremities, associated with the cutaneous manifestations of Raynaud disease.

lu•pus mil•i•a•ris dis•se•mi•na•tus fa•ci•e•i (lū′pŭs mil-li-ā′ris dis′sem-i-nā′tŭs fash′ī-ā-ī) A milletlike papular eruption of the face associated with a (histopathologically) tuberculoid perifollicular infiltration but probably related to rosacea rather than tuberculous infection.

lu•pus ne•phri•tis (lū′pŭs nĕ-frī′tis) Glomerulonephritis occurring in some patients with systemic lupus erythematosus, characterized by hematuria and a progressive course culminating in renal failure.

lu•pus per•ni•o (lū′pŭs pĕr′nē-ō) Sarcoid lesions, clinically resembling frostbite and microscopically resembling lupus vulgaris, involving ears, cheeks, nose, hands, and fingers.

lu•pus vul•ga•ris (lū′pŭs vul′gā′ris) Cutaneous tuberculosis with characteristic nodular lesions on the face, particularly about the nose and ears.

LUQ Abbreviation for left upper quadrant (of abdomen).

lus•i•tro•pic (lū′si-trō′pik) Relating to lusitropy.

lus•it•ro•py (lū-sit′trŏ-pē) Relaxation functions of cardiac muscle and chambers.

Lust phe•nom•e•non (lūst fĕ-nom′ĕ-non) Foot eversion and dorsiflexion caused by tapping over the common peroneal nerve on the outer upper shin; occurs in tetany.

lu•te•al (lū′tē-ăl) Relating to the corpus luteum (e.g., luteal cells and hormones). [L. *luteus,* saffron-yellow]

lu•te•al cell, lu•te•in cell (lū′tē-ăl sel, lū′tē-in) A cell of the corpus luteum of the ovary that is derived from the granulosa cells of the preovulatory follicle; it secretes progesterone and estrogen.

lu•te•al hor•mone (lū′tē-ăl hōr′mōn) SYN progesterone.

lu•te•al phase (lū′tē-ăl fāz) That portion of the menstrual cycle extending from the time of formation of the corpus luteum to the onset of menses, usually 14 days in length; **short luteal phase**, a period of 10 days or less between ovulation and the onset of menses, frequently associated with infertility.

lu•te•in (lū′tē-in) **1.** The yellow pigment in the corpus luteum, the yolk of eggs, or any lipochrome. **2.** SYN xanthophyll. [L. *luteus,* saffron-yellow]

lu•te•in•i•za•tion (lū′tē-in-ī-zā′shŭn) Transformation of the mature ovarian follicle and its theca interna into a corpus luteum after ovulation.

lu•te•in•ized un•rup•tured fol•li•cle (lū′tē-in-īzd un-rŭp′chŭrd fol′i-kĕl) A follicle that has undergone luteinization without earlier rupture; previously thought to cause infertility but now believed to occur equally often in fertile and infertile women.

lu•te•i•niz•ing hor•mone (LH) (lū′tē-in-ī′zing hōr′mōn) SYN lutropin.

lu•te•i•niz•ing hor•mone/fol•li•cle-stim•u•lat•ing hor•mone-re•leas•ing fac•tor (lū′tē-in-ī′zing hōr′mōn-fol′i-kĕl-stim′yŭ-lā′ting hōr′mōn-rĕ-lē′sing fak′tŏr) SYN gonadoliberin (2).

lu·te·i·niz·ing hor·mone-re·leas·ing fac·tor (lū′tē-in-ī′zing hōr′mōn-rĕ-lē′sing fak′tŏr) Former name for luteinizing hormone-releasing hormone. Cf. bioregulator.

lu·te·i·niz·ing hor·mone-re·leas·ing hor·mone (lū′tē-in-ī′zing hōr′mōn-rĕ-lē′sing hōr′mōn) SYN luliberin.

Lu·tem·ba·cher syn·drome (lū′tem-bahk′er sin′drōm) A congenital cardiac abnormality consisting of a defect of the interatrial septum, mitral stenosis, and enlarged right atrium.

lu·te·o·hor·mone (lū′tē-ō-hōr′mōn) SYN progesterone.

lu·te·ol·y·sis (lū′tē-ol′i-sis) Degeneration or destruction of ovarian luteinized tissue.

lu·te·o·lyt·ic (lū′tē-ō-lit′ik) Promoting or characteristic of luteolysis.

lu·te·o·ma (lū′tē-ō′mă) An ovarian tumor of granulosa or theca-lutein cell origin, producing progesterone effects on the uterine mucosa.

lu·te·o·pla·cen·tal shift (lū′tē-ō-plă-sen′tăl shift) The change in site of production of the estrogen and progesterone essential for human pregnancy from the corpus luteum to the placenta; after the sixth week of pregnancy, a human placenta can produce enough of these hormones to prevent abortion despite ovariectomy.

lu·te·o·tro·pic, lu·te·o·tro·phic (lū′tē-ō-trō′pik, -trōf′ik) Having a stimulating action on the development and function of the corpus luteum.

lu·te·o·tro·pic hor·mone (lū′tē-ō-trō′pik hōr′mōn) SYN luteotropin.

lu·te·o·tro·pin (lū′tē-ō-trō′pin) An anterior pituitary hormone that acts to maintain the function of the corpus luteum. Cf. bioregulator. SYN luteotropic hormone.

lu·te·ti·um (Lu) (lū-tē′shē-ŭm) A rare earth element; atomic no. 71, atomic wt. 174.967. [L. *Lutetia,* Paris]

lu·tro·pin (lū-trō′pin) A glycoprotein hormone that stimulates the final ripening of an ovarian follicle, its secretion of progesterone, its rupture to release the egg, and the conversion of the ruptured follicle into the corpus luteum. Cf. bioregulator. SYN interstitial cell-stimulating hormone, luteinizing hormone.

Lutz-Splen·do·re-Al·mei·da dis·ease (lūts splen-dō′rē ahl-mā′dah di-zēz′) SYN paracoccidioidomycosis.

lux (lŭks) A unit of light or illumination; the reception of a luminous flux of 1 lumen per square meter of surface. SYN candle-meter, meter-candle. [L. light]

lux·a·tion (lŭk-sā′shŭn) **1.** SYN dislocations. **2.** DENTISTRY the dislocation or displacement of the condyle in the temporomandibular fossa, or of a tooth from the alveolus. [L. *luxatio*]

Lux·ol fast blue (lŭk′sol fast blū) Name for a group of closely related copper phthalocyanine dyes used as stains (with PAS, PTAH, hematoxylin, silver nitrate) for myelin in nerve fibers.

LVET Abbreviation for left ventricular ejection time.

LVN Abbreviation for licensed vocational nurse.

L&W Abbreviation for living and well.

ly·ase (lī′ās) Class name for enzymes removing groups nonhydrolytically (EC class 4); prefixes such as "hydro-," "ammonia-," etc., are used to indicate the type of reaction. Trivial names for lyases include synthases, decarboxylases, aldolases, dehydratases. Cf. synthase, synthetase.

ly·can·thro·py (lī-kan′thrŏ-pē) The morbid delusion that one is a wolf. [G. *lykos,* wolf, + *anthrōpos,* man]

lycopenaemia [Br.] SYN lycopenemia.

ly·co·pene (lī′kō-pēn) The red pigment of the tomato; the parent substance from which all natural carotenoid pigments are derived.

ly·co·pe·ne·mi·a (lī′kō-pĕ-nē′mē-ă) A condition in which there is a high concentration of lycopene in the blood, producing carotenoidlike yellowish pigmentation of the skin; found in people who consume excessive amounts of tomatoes or tomato juice, or other fruits and berries that contain lycopene. SYN lycopenaemia. [lycopene + G. *haima,* blood]

ly·co·per·do·no·sis (lī′kō-per′dō-nō′sis) A persisting pneumonitis following inhalation of fungal spores of the puffballs *Lycoperdon pyriforme* and *L. bovista*.

Ly·ell syn·drome (lī′ĕl sin′drōm) SYN toxic epidermal necrolysis.

Lyme ar·thri·tis (līm ahr-thrī′tis) The arthritic manifestation of Lyme disease.

Lyme dis·ease (līm di-zēz′) An inflammatory disorder typically contracted during the summer and caused by *Borrelia burgdorferi*, a spirochete transmitted by *Ixodes scapularis* in the eastern U.S. and *I. pacificus* in the western U.S., and by various *Ixodes* species in Europe. (*B. valaisiana* is another spirochete associated with Lyme disease). The characteristic skin lesion, erythema chronicum migrans, usually is preceded or accompanied by fever, malaise, fatigue, headache, and stiff neck; neurologic or cardiac manifestations, or arthritis (i.e., Lyme arthritis), may occur weeks to months later. Dogs, horses, and cattle are also affected. See page B4. [Lyme, CT, where first observed]

lymph (limf) A clear, sometimes faintly yellow and slightly opalescent fluid that is collected from the tissues throughout the body, flows in the lymphatic vessels, and through the lymph nodes, and is eventually added to the venous blood circulation. Lymph consists of a clear liquid portion, varying numbers of white blood cells (chiefly lymphocytes), and a few red blood cells. [L. *lympha,* clear spring water]

lym·phad·e·nec·to·my (lim-fad′ĕ-nek′tŏ-mē) Excision of lymph nodes. [lymphadeno- + G. *ektomē,* excision]

lym·phad·e·ni·tis (lim-fad′ĕ-nī′tis) Inflammation of a lymph node or lymph nodes. [lymphadeno- + G. *-itis,* inflammation]

♻**lymphadeno-, lymphaden-** Combining forms meaning the lymph nodes. [L. *lympha,* spring water, + G. *adēn,* gland]

lym·phad·e·nog·ra·phy (lim-fad′ĕ-nog′ră-fē) Radiographic visualization of lymph nodes after injection of a contrast medium; lymphography. [lymphadeno- + G. *graphō,* to write]

lym·phad·e·noid (lim-fad′ĕ-noyd) Relating to, or resembling, or derived from a lymph node. [lymphadeno- + G. *eidos,* resemblance]

lym·phad·e·nop·a·thy (lim-fad′ĕ-nop′ă-thē) Any disease process affecting a lymph node or lymph nodes. [lymphadeno- + G. *pathos,* suffering]

lymph·ad·e·nop·a·thy-as·so·ci·at·ed virus (LAV) (lim-fad′ĕ-nop′ă-thē-ă-sō′sē-āt-ĕd vī′rŭs) SYN human immunodeficiency virus.

lym·phad·e·no·sis (lim-fad′ĕ-nō′sis) The basic underlying proliferative process that results in enlargement of lymph nodes, as in lymphocytic leukemia and certain inflammations. [lymphadeno- + G. *-osis,* condition]

lymphaemia [Br.] SYN lymphemia.

lym·phan·gi·al (lim-fan′jē-ăl) Relating to a lymphatic vessel.

lym·phan·gi·ec·ta·sis, lym·phan·gi·ec·ta·si·a (lim-fan′jē-ek′tă-sis, -ek-tā′zē-a) Dilation of the lymphatic vessels, the basic process that may result in the formation of a lymphangioma. SYN lymphectasia. [lymphangio- + G. *ektasis,* a stretching]

lym·phan·gi·ec·tat·ic (lim-fan′jē-ek-tat′ik) Relating to or characterized by lymphangiectasis.

lym·phan·gi·ec·to·my (lim-fan′jē-ek′tŏ-mē) Excision of a lymph channel. [lymphangio- + G. *ektomē,* excision]

lym·phan·gi·i·tis (lim-fan′jē-ī′tis) SYN lymphangitis.

♻**lymphangio-, lymphangi-** Combining forms meaning the lymphatic vessels. [L. *lympha,* spring water, + G. *angeion,* vessel]

lym·phan·gi·o·en·do·the·li·o·ma (lim-fan′jē-ō-en′dō-thē′lē-ō′mă) A neoplasm consisting of irregular groups of endothelial cells, and intubate structures that are thought to be derived from lymphatic vessels. [lymphangio- + endothelium + *-oma,* tumor]

lym·phan·gi·og·ra·phy (lim-fan′jē-og′ră-fē) Radiographic demonstration of lymphatics and lymph nodes following the injection of a contrast medium; lymphography. [lymphangio- + G. *graphō,* to write]

lym·phan·gi·ol·o·gy (lim-fan′jē-ol′ŏ-jē) The branch of medical science concerned with the lymphatic vessels. SYN lymphology. [lymphangio- + G. *logos,* study]

lym·phan·gi·o·ma (lim-fan′jē-ō′mă) A well-circumscribed nodule of lymphatic vessels that are usually greatly dilated and lined with normal endothelial cells; lymphoid tissue is usually present in the peripheral portions of the lesions, which are present at birth or shortly therafter, and probably represent anomalous development of lymphatic vessels (rather than true neoplasms); they occur most frequently in the neck and axilla. [lymphangio- + G. *-oma,* tumor]

lym·phan·gi·o·phle·bi·tis (lim-fan′jē-ō-flĕ-bī′tis) Inflammation of the lymphatic vessels and veins.

lym·phan·gi·o·plas·ty (lim-fan′jē-ō-plas-tē) Surgical alteration of lymphatic vessels. [lymphangio- + G. *plastos,* formed]

lym·phan·gi·o·sar·co·ma (lim-fan′jē-ō-sahr-kō′mă) A malignant neoplasm derived from the endothelial cells of lymphatic vessels, usually developing in the arm several years after radical mastectomy.

lym·phan·gi·ot·o·my (lim-fan′jē-ot′ŏ-mē) Incision of lymphatic vessels. [lymphangio- + G. *tomē,* incision]

lym·phan·gi·tis (lim′fan-jī′tis) Inflammation of the lymphatic vessels. SYN lymphangiitis. [lymphangio- + G. *-itis,* inflammation]

lym·pha·phe·re·sis (lim′fă-fĕ-rē′sis) SYN lymphocytapheresis.

lym·phat·ic (lim-fat′ik) **1.** Pertaining to lymph. **2.** A vascular channel that transports lymph. **3.** Sometimes used to pertain to a sluggish or phlegmatic temperament. [L. *lymphaticus,* frenzied; Mod. L. use, of or for lymph]

lym·phat·ic duct (lim-fat′ik dŭkt) One of the two large lymph channels, right lymphatic duct or thoracic duct.

lym·phat·ic fil·a·ri·a·sis gran·u·lo·ma (lim-fat′ik fil′ă-rī′ă-sis gran′yū-lō′mă) Granulomatous lesion often found surrounding dead microfilariae.

lym·phat·ic leu·ke·mi·a (lim-fat′ik lū-kē′mē-ă) SYN lymphocytic leukemia.

lym•phat•ic node (lim-fat′ik nōd) SEE lymph node.

lym•phat•i•cos•to•my (lim-fat′i-kos′tŏ-mē) Making an opening into a lymphatic duct. [lymphatic + G. *stoma,* mouth]

lym•phat•ic plex•us (lim-fat′ik pleks′ŭs) A plexus of lymphatic capillaries, usually without valves, that opens into one or more larger lymphatic vessels.

lym•phat•ic si•nus (lim-fat′ik sī′nŭs) The channels in a lymph node crossed by a reticulum of cells and fibers and bounded by littoral cells; there are subcapsular, trabecular, and medullary sinuses.

lym•phat•ic tis•sue, lym•phoid tis•sue (lim-fat′ik tish′ū, lim′foyd) A three-dimensional network of reticular fibers and cells the meshes of which are occupied in varying degrees of density with lymphocytes; there is nodular, diffuse, and loose lymphatic tissue. SYN adenoid tissue.

lym•pha•ti•tis (lim′fă-tī′tis) Inflammation of the lymphatic vessels or lymph nodes. [lymphatic + G. *-itis,* inflammation]

lym•pha•tol•y•sis (lim′fă-tol′i-sis) Destruction of the lymphatic vessels or lymphoid tissue, or both. [lymphatic + G. *lysis,* dissolution]

lym•pha•to•lyt•ic (lim-fat′ō-lit′ik) Pertaining to or characterized by lymphatolysis.

lymph cap•il•lar•y (limf kap′i-lar-ē) The beginning of the lymphatic system of vessels; it is lined with a highly attenuated endothelium with poorly developed basement membrane and a lumen of variable caliber. SEE lacteal (2).

lymph cor•pus•cle, lym•phat•ic cor•pus•cle, lym•phoid cor•pus•cle (limf kōr′pŭs-ĕl, lim-fat′ik, lim′foyd) A mononuclear type of leukocyte formed in lymph nodes and other lymphoid tissue, and also in the blood.

lymph drain•age (limf drān′ăj) SYN manual lymph drainage.

lym•phec•ta•si•a (lim′fek-tā′zē-ă) SYN lymphangiectasis. [lymph + G. *ektasis,* a stretching]

lymph•e•de•ma (lim′fē-dē′mă) Swelling (especially in subcutaneous tissues) as a result of obstruction of lymphatic vessels or lymph nodes and the accumulation of large amounts of lymph in the affected region. SYN lymphoedema. [lymph + G. *oidēma,* a swelling]

lym•phe•mi•a (lim-fē′mē-ă) The presence of unusually large numbers of lymphocytes or their precursors, or both, in the circulating blood. SYN lymphaemia. [lymph(ocyte) + G. *haima,* blood]

lymph fol•li•cle, lym•phat•ic fol•li•cle (limf fol′i-kĕl, lim-fat′ik fol′i-kĕl) One of the spheric masses of lymphoid cells, frequently having a more lightly staining center. SYN folliculus lymphaticus, lymph nodule, nodulus lymphaticus.

lymph gland (limf gland) SYN lymph node.

lymph node (limf nōd) One of numerous round, oval, or bean-shaped bodies located along the course of lymphatic vessels, varying greatly in size (1–25 mm in diameter) and usually presenting a depressed area, the hilum, on one side through which afferent lymphatic vessels enter and efferent lymphatic vessels emerge. The structure consists of a fibrous capsule and internal trabeculae supporting lymphoid tissue and lymph sinuses; lymphoid tissue is arranged in nodules in the cortex and cords in the medulla of a node, with afferent vessels entering at many points of the periphery. See this page. SYN nodus lymphaticus [TA], nodus lymphoideus [TA], lymph gland, lymphoglandula, lymphonodus.

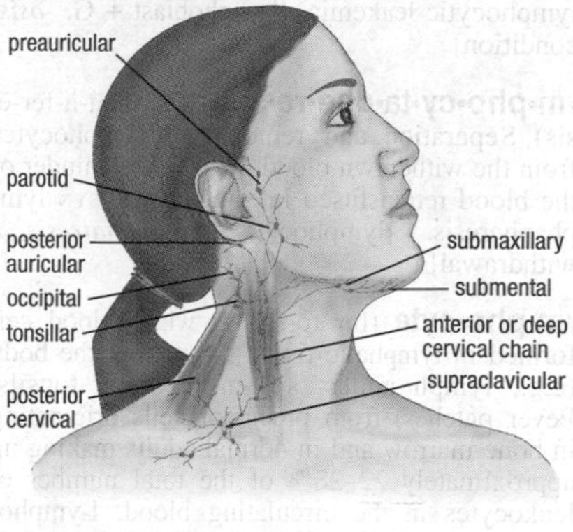

location of lymph nodes of the neck

lymph node per•me•a•bil•i•ty fac•tor (LNPF) (limpf nōd pĕr′mē-ă-bil′i-tē fak′tŏr) A substance, released by lymphocytes when stimulated or damaged, which increases capillary permeability and the accumulation of mononuclear cells.

lymph nod•ule (limf nod′yūl) SYN lymph follicle.

lympho-, lymph- Combining forms meaning lymph. [L. *lympha,* spring water]

lym•pho•blast (lim′fō-blast) An immature cell that matures into a lymphocyte and is characterized by more abundant cytoplasm than in a lymphocyte, a nucleus in which the chromatin is finer than in a lymphocyte (but coarser than in a myeloblast), and one or two prominent nucleoli. SYN lymphocytoblast. [lympho- + G. *blastos,* germ]

lym•pho•blas•tic (lim′fō-blas′tik) Pertaining to the production of lymphocytes.

lym•pho•blas•tic leu•ke•mi•a (lim′fō-blas′tik lū-kē′mē-ă) Acute lymphocytic leukemia in which the abnormal cells are chiefly (or almost totally) blast forms of the lymphocytic series, or in which unusually large numbers of the immature forms occur in association with adult lymphocytes.

lym•pho•blas•tic lym•pho•ma (lim′fō-blas′tik lim-fō′mă) A diffuse lymphoma in children, with supradiaphragmatic distribution and T lymphocytes having convoluted nuclei; many affected patients develop acute lymphoblastic leukemia.

lym•pho•blas•to•ma (lim′fō-blas-tō′mă) A form of malignant lymphoma in which the chief cells are lymphoblasts. [lymphoblast + G. *-oma,* tumor]

lym•pho•blas•to•sis (lim′fō-blas-tō′sis) The presence of lymphoblasts in the peripheral blood; sometimes used as a synonym for acute lymphocytic leukemia. [lymphoblast + G. *-osis,* condition]

lym•pho•cy•ta•phe•re•sis (lim′fō-sīt-ă-fĕr-ē′sis) Separation and removal of lymphocytes from the withdrawn blood, with the remainder of the blood retransfused into the donor. SYN lymphapheresis. [lymphocyte + G. *aphairesis,* a withdrawal]

lym•pho•cyte (lim′fō-sīt) A white blood cell formed in lymphatic tissue throughout the body (e.g., lymph nodes, spleen, thymus, tonsils, Peyer patches) from precursor cells originating in bone marrow and in normal adults making up approximately 22–28% of the total number of leukocytes in the circulating blood. Lymphocytes are generally small (7–8 mcm), but larger forms are common (10–20 mcm); with Wright (or a similar) stain, the nucleus is deeply colored (purple-blue), and is composed of dense aggregates of chromatin within a sharply defined nuclear membrane; the nucleus is usually round, but may be slightly indented, and is eccentrically situated within a relatively small amount of light blue cytoplasm that ordinarily contains no granules; especially in larger forms, the cytoplasm may be fairly abundant and may include several fine, bright red-violet granules; in contrast to granules of the myeloid series of cells, those in lymphocytes do not yield a positive oxidase or peroxidase reaction. Lymphocytes are divided into two principal groups, T cells and B cells, based on their surface molecules as well as their function. Natural killer cells, which are large granular lymphocytes, represent a small percentage of the lymphocyte population. See page B2. [lympho- + G. *kytos,* call]

lymphocythaemia [Br.] SYN lymphocythemia.

lym•pho•cy•the•mi•a (lim′fō-sī-thē′mē-ă) SYN lymphocytosis. SYN lymphocythaemia.

lym•pho•cyt•ic (lim′fō-sit′ik) Pertaining to or characterized by lymphocytes.

lym•pho•cyt•ic ad•e•no•hy•poph•y•si•tis (lim′fō-sit′ik ad′ĕ-nō-hī-pof′i-sī′tis) A diffuse lymphocytic infiltration of the adenohypophysis, often related to pregnancy; probably a disturbance in the immune system.

lym•pho•cyt•ic cho•ri•o•men•in•gi•tis (lim′fō-sit′ik kōr′ē-ō-men′in-jī′tis) Meningitis that usually occurs in young adults during the fall and winter months. Caused by a virus carried by the common house mouse. SEE ALSO lymphocytic choriomeningitis virus.

lym•pho•cyt•ic cho•ri•o•men•in•gi•tis vi•rus (lim′fō-sit′ik kōr′ē-ō-men′in-jī′tis vī′rŭs) An RNA virus that causes lymphocytic choriomeningitis; infection may be inapparent, but sometimes the virus causes influenzalike disease, meningitis, or, rarely, meningoencephalomyelitis.

lym•pho•cy•tic hy•po•phy•si•tis (lim′fō-sit′ik hī-pof′i-sī′tis) An acute anterior pituitary lymphocytic reaction characterized clinically by signs and symptoms of anterior pituitary insufficiency; probably an autoimmune disorder because antipituitary antibodies are present in the serum.

lym•pho•cyt•ic leu•ke•mi•a (lim′fō-sit′ik lū-kē′mē-ă) A variety of the hematologic disorder characterized by an uncontrolled proliferation and conspicuous enlargement of lymphoid tissue in various sites (e.g., lymph nodes, spleen, bone marrow, lungs) and the occurrence of increased numbers of cells of the lymphocytic series in the blood. See page B31. SYN lymphatic leukemia.

lym•pho•cyt•ic se•ries, lym•phoid se•ries (lim′fō-sit′ik sēr′ēz, lim′foyd) The cells at various states in the development in lymphoid tissue of the mature lymphocytes, e.g., lymphoblasts, young lymphocytes, mature lymphocytes.

lym•pho•cy•to•blast (lim′fō-sī′tō-blast) SYN lymphoblast. [lymphocyte + G. *blastos,* germ]

lym•pho•cy•to•ma (lim′fō-sī-tō′mă) A circumscribed nodule or mass of mature lymphocytes, grossly resembling a neoplasm. [lymphocyte + G. *-oma,* tumor]

lym•pho•cy•to•pe•ni•a (lim′fō-sī′tō-pē′nē-ă) SYN lymphopenia.

lym•pho•cy•to•poi•e•sis (lim′fō-sī′tō-poy-ē′sis) The formation of lymphocytes. [lymphocyte + G. *poiēsis,* a making]

lym•pho•cy•to•sis (lim′fō-sī-tō′sis) A form of leukocytosis in which there is an actual or relative increase in the number of lymphocytes. SYN lymphocythemia.

lym•pho•duct (lim′fō-dŭkt) A lymphatic vessel. [lympho- + L. *ductus,* a leading]

lymphoedema [Br.] SYN lymphedema.

lym•pho•ep•i•the•li•o•ma (lim′fō-ep′i-thē′lē-ō′mă) A poorly differentiated radiosensitive squamous cell carcinoma involving lymphoid tissue in the region of the tonsils and nasopharynx; metastasizes early to cervical lymph nodes. [lympho- + epithelium + *-oma*, tumor]

lym•pho•gen•ic (lim′fō-jen′ik) SYN lymphogenous (1).

lym•phog•e•nous (lim-foj′ĕ-nŭs) **1.** Originating from lymph or the lymphatic system. SYN lymphogenic. **2.** Producing lymph.

lym•phog•e•nous me•tas•ta•sis (lim-foj′ĕ-nŭs mĕ-tas′tă-sis) SEE metastasis.

lym•pho•glan•du•la (lim′fō-glan′dyū-lă) SYN lymph node.

lym•pho•gran•u•lo•ma (lim′fō-gran-yū-lō′mă) Old and nonspecific term used with reference to a few basically dissimilar diseases in which the pathologic processes result in granulomas or granulomalike lesions, especially in various groups of lymph nodes (which then become conspicuously enlarged).

lym•pho•gran•u•lo•ma ve•ne•re•um, ve•ne•re•al lymph•o•gran•u•lo•ma (lim′fō-gran-yū-lō′mă ve-nē′rē-ŭm, vĕ-nēr′ē-ăl lim′fō-gran′yū-lō′mă) A sexually transmitted infection usually caused by *Chlamydia trachomatis,* and characterized by a transient genital ulcer and inguinal adenopathy in the male; in the female, perirectal lymph nodes are involved and rectal stricture is a common occurrence. SYN tropical bubo.

lym•phog•ra•phy (lim-fog′ră-fē) Visualization of lymphatics (lymphangiography), lymph nodes (lymphadenography), or both by radiography following the intralymphatic injection of a contrast medium, usually an iodized oil. [lympho- + *graphō,* to write]

lym•pho•his•ti•o•cy•to•sis (lim′fō-his′tē-ō-sī-tō′sis) Proliferation or infiltration of lymphocytes and histiocytes.

lym•phoid (lim′foyd) **1.** Resembling lymph or lymphatic tissue, or pertaining to the lymphatic system. **2.** SYN adenoid (1). [lympho- + G. *eidos,* appearance]

lym•phoi•dec•to•my (lim′foy-dek′tŏ-mē) Excision of lymphoid tissue. [lymphoid + G. *ektomē,* excision]

lym•pho•kine (lim′fō-kīn) Hormonelike peptide, released by activated lymphocytes, that mediates immune response; a cytokine obtained from lymphocytes. [*lympho*cyte + G. *kineō,* to set in motion]

lym•pho•ki•ne•sis (lim′fō-ki-nē′sis) **1.** Circulation of lymph in the lymphatic vessels and through the lymph nodes. **2.** Movement of endolymph in the semicircular canals of the inner ear. [lympho- + G. *kinēsis,* movement]

lym•phol•o•gy (lim-fol′ŏ-jē) SYN lymphangiology. [lympho- + G. *logos,* study]

i **lym•pho•ma** (lim-fō′mă) Any neoplasm of lymphoid tissue; in general use, synonymous with malignant lymphoma. See page B14. [lympho- + G. *-oma,* tumor]

lym•pho•ma•toid (lim-fō′mă-toyd) Resembling a lymphoma.

lym•pho•ma•toid pol•y•po•sis (lim-fō′mă-toyd pol′i-pō′sis) Multifocal mantle cell lymphoma, producing numerous lymphoid polyps in the intestines.

lym•pho•ma•to•sis (lim′fō-mă-tō′sis) Any condition characterized by the occurrence of multiple, widely distributed sites of involvement with lymphoma.

lym•pho•ma•tous (lim-fō′mă-tŭs) Pertaining to or characterized by lymphoma.

lym•pho•myx•o•ma (lim′fō-mik-sō′mă) A soft nonmalignant neoplasm that contains lymphoid tissue in a matrix of loose, areolar connective tissue. [lympho- + G. *myxa,* mucus, + *-oma,* tumor]

lym•pho•no•dus (lim′fō-nō′dŭs) SYN lymph node.

lym•phop•a•thy (lim-fop′ă-thē) Any disease of the lymphatic vessels or lymph nodes. [lympho- + G. *pathos,* suffering]

lym•pho•pe•ni•a (lim′fō-pē′nē-ă) A reduction, relative or absolute, in the number of lymphocytes in the circulating blood. SYN lymphocytopenia. [lympho- + G. *penia,* poverty]

lym•pho•plas•ma•cel•lu•lar dis•or•ders (lim′fō-plaz-mă-sel′yū-lăr dis-ōr′dĕrz) Term used to refer to a group of disorders including plasmacytoma, multiple myeloma, lymphoplasmacytic lymphoma, MALT lymphoma, and amyloidosis.

lym•pho•plas•ma•phe•re•sis (lim′fō-plaz′mă-fĕr-ē′sis) Separation and removal of lymphocytes and plasma from the withdrawn blood, with the remainder of the blood retransfused into the donor. [lymphocyte + plasma + G. *aphairesis,* a withdrawal]

lym•pho•poi•e•sis (lim′fō-poy-ē′sis) The formation of lymphatic tissue. [lympho- + G. *poiēsis,* a making]

lym•pho•poi•et•ic (lim′fō-poy-et′ik) Pertaining to or characterized by lymphopoiesis.

lym•pho•re•tic•u•lo•sis (lim′fō-rĕ-tik′yū-lō′sis) Proliferation of the reticuloendothelial cells (macrophages) of the lymph glands.

lym•phor•rhe•a, lym•phor•rha•gi•a (lim′fō-rē′ă, -rā′jē-ă) An escape of lymph on the surface from ruptured, torn, or cut lymphatic vessels. SYN lymphorrhoea. [lympho- + G. *rhoia,* a flow]

lymphorrhoea [Br.] SYN lymphorrhea.

lym•phor•rhoid (lim′fŏ-royd) A dilation of a lymph channel, resembling a hemorrhoid.

[lymph + *-rrhoid*, tending to leak, on the analogy of *hemorrhoid*]

lym•phos•ta•sis (lim-fos′tă-sis) Obstruction of the normal flow of lymph. [lympho- + G. *stasis*, a standing still]

lym•pho•tax•is (lim′fō-tak′sis) The exertion of an effect that attracts or repels lymphocytes. [lympho- + G. *taxis*, orderly arrangement]

lym•pho•tox•ic•i•ty (lim′fō-tok-sis′i-tē) Toxicity to lymphocytes.

lym•pho•tox•in (lim-fō-tok′sin) A lymphokine that lyses or damages many cell types.

lymph ves•sels (limf ves′ĕlz) The vessels that convey the lymph; they anastomose freely with each other. SYN vasa lymphatica.

Lynch syn•drome (linch sin′drōm) **Type I**, familial colorectal cancer, generally occurring at an early age; **type II**, familial colorectal cancer occurring at an early age in conjunction with female genital cancer or cancers at other sites proximal to the bowel.

♻ **lyo-** Combining form denoting dissolution. SEE ALSO lyso-. [G. *lyō*, to loosen, dissolve]

Ly•on hy•poth•e•sis (lī′on hī-poth′ĕ-sis) SYN lyonization.

ly•on•i•za•tion (lī′on-ī-zā′shŭn) The normal phenomenon whereby wherever there are two or more haploid sets of X-linked genes in each cell, all but one of the genes are inactivated apparently at random and have no phenotypic expression. Its randomness explains the more variable expressivity of X-linked traits in women than in men. SEE ALSO gene dosage compensation. SYN Lyon hypothesis, X-inactivation.

Ly•on rat (lē-ōn[h]′ rat) Laboratory animal derived from the Sprague Dawley rat; used as a model to study sensitivity of blood pressure to oral calcium. [Lyons, France]

ly•o•phil, **ly•o•phile** (lī′ō-fil, -fīl) A substance that is lyophilic.

ly•o•phil•ic (lī′ō-fil′ik) COLLOID CHEMISTRY denoting a dispersed phase having a pronounced affinity for the dispersion medium; when the dispersed phase is lyophilic, the colloid is usually a reversible one. SYN lyotropic. [lyo- + G. *phileō*, to love]

ly•oph•i•li•za•tion (lī-of′i-lī-zā′shŭn) The process of isolating a solid substance from solution by freezing the solution and evaporating the ice under vacuum. SYN freeze-drying.

ly•o•phobe (lī′ō-fōb) A substance that is lyophobic.

ly•o•pho•bic (lī′ō-fō′bik) COLLOID CHEMISTRY denoting a dispersed phase having but slight affinity for the dispersion medium; when the dispersed phase is lyophobic, the colloid is usually an irreversible one. [lyo- + G. *phobos*, fear]

ly•o•tro•pic (lī′ō-trō′pik) SYN lyophilic. [lyo- + G. *tropē*, a turning]

Lys Abbreviation for lysine, or its radicals in peptides.

lysaemia [Br.] SYN lysemia.

ly•sate (lī′sāt) Material produced by the destructive process of lysis.

lyse (līs) To break up, to disintegrate, to effect lysis. SYN lyze.

ly•se•mi•a (lī-sē′mē-ă) Disintegration or dissolution of red blood cells and the occurrence of hemoglobin in the circulating plasma and in the urine. SYN lysaemia. [lyso- + G. *haima*, blood]

ly•sin (lī′sin) **1.** A complement-fixing antibody that acts destructively on cells and tissues; the various types are designated in accordance with the form of antigen that stimulates the production of the lysin, e.g., hemolysin, bacteriolysin. **2.** Any substance that causes lysis.

lysinaemia [Br.] SYN lysinemia.

ly•sine (k, Lys) (lī′sēn) A nutritionally essential α-amino acid found in many proteins; distinguished by an ε-amino group.

ly•sin•e•mi•a (lī′si-nē′mē-ă) SYN hyperlysinemia. SYN lysinaemia.

ly•sin•o•gen (lī-sin′ō-jen) An antigen that stimulates the formation of a specific lysin.

ly•sin•o•gen•ic (lī′si-nō-jen′ik) Having the property of a lysinogen.

ly•sin•u•ri•a (lī′si-nyūr′ē-ă) The presence of lysine in the urine.

ly•sis (lī′sis) **1.** Destruction of red blood cells, bacteria, and other structures by a specific lysin, usually referred to by the structure destroyed (e.g., hemolysis, bacteriolysis, nephrolysis); may be due to a direct toxin or an immune mechanism, such as antibody reacting with antigen on the surface of a target cell, usually by binding and activation of a series of proteins in the blood with enzymatic activity (complement system). **2.** Gradual subsidence of the symptoms of an acute disease; a form of the recovery process, as distinguished from crisis. [G. dissolution or loosening]

ly•sis of ad•he•sions (lī′sis ad-hē′zhŭnz) Surgical division of postinflammatory or postoperative adhesions, particularly abdominal (peritoneal) adhesions.

♻ **lyso-**, **lys-** Combining forms meaning lysis, dissolution. SEE ALSO lyo-. [G. *lysis*, a loosening]

ly•so•gen (lī′sō-jen) **1.** That which is capable of inducing lysis. **2.** A bacterium in the state of lysogeny. [lysin + G. *-gen*, producing]

ly·so·gen·e·sis (lī′sō-jen′ĕ-sis) The production of lysins.

ly·so·gen·ic (lī′sō-jen′ik) **1.** Causing or having the power to cause lysis, as the action of certain antibodies and chemical substances. **2.** Pertaining to bacteria in the state of lysogeny.

ly·so·gen·ic bac·te·ri·um (lī′sō-jen′ik bak-tēr′ē-ŭm) **1.** A bacterium in the symbiotic condition in which its genome includes the genome (probacteriophage) of a temperate bacteriophage; in occasional instances the probacteriophage dissociates from the bacterial genome, develops into vegetative bacteriophage, and then matures, causing lysis of the respective host bacterium and release into the culture medium of infective temperate bacteriophage. **2.** Formerly, a pseudolysogenic bacterial strain, i.e., a "carrier" strain of bacteriophage of low infectivity.

ly·so·ge·nic·i·ty (lī′sō-jĕ-nis′i-tē) The property of being lysogenic.

ly·sog·e·ny (lī-soj′ĕ-nē) The phenomenon by which a bacterium is infected by a temperate bacteriophage with DNA that is integrated into the bacterial genome and replicates along with the bacterial DNA but remains latent or unexpressed; triggering of the lytic cycle may occur spontaneously or by certain agents and will result in the production of bacteriophage and lysis of the bacterial cell.

ly·so·ki·nase (lī′sō-kī′nās) Term proposed for activator agents (e.g., streptokinase, urokinase, staphylokinase) that produce plasmin by indirect or multiple-stage action on plasminogen.

ly·so·so·mal dis·ease (lī′sō-sō′măl di-zēz′) A disease due to inadequate functioning of a lysosomal enzyme; most such diseases are associated with a storage disease.

ly·so·some (lī′sō-sōm) A cytoplasmic membrane-bound vesicle measuring 5–8 nm (primary lysosome) and containing a wide variety of glycoprotein hydrolytic enzymes active at an acid pH; serves to digest exogenous material, such as bacteria, as well as effete organelles of the cells. [lyso- + G. *soma,* body]

ly·so·type (li′sō-tīp) A type within a bacterial species determined by its reaction to specific phages. [lyso + type]

ly·so·zyme (lī′sō-zīm) An enzyme destructive to cell walls of certain bacteria; present in tears, egg white, and some plant tissues; used in the prevention of caries and in the treatment of infant formulas. SYN muramidase.

lys·sa (lis′ă) **1.** A cartilage in the tongue of the dog. **2.** Old term for rabies. [G. *madness*]

Lys·sa·vi·rus (lis′ă-vī′rŭs) A genus of viruses (family Rhabdoviridae) that includes the rabies virus group.

Lyth·o·glyph·op·sis (lith′ō-glif-op′sis) A genus of amphibious freshwater operculate snails of the family Hydrobiidae (subfamily Hydrobiinae; subclass Prosobranchiata). In the Mekong River delta in Vietnam, *L. aperta* serves as an intermediate host of the blood fluke, *Schistosoma mekongi.*

lyt·ic (lit′ik) Pertaining to lysis; used colloquially as an abbreviation for osteolytic.

lyze (līz) SYN lyse.

M

μ The Greek letter mu. USAGE NOTE The JCAHO directs that units including the prefix *micro-* be written in full (*microgram, microliter*) instead of abbreviated (as μ*g* and μ*L*) because the Greek letter is often misread as *m*.

***M*$_r$** Abbreviation for molecular weight ratio or relative molecular mass.

mM Abbreviation for millimolar (10^{-3} M).

M Abbreviation for moles per liter (also written M or *M*); molarity.

♻ ***m-*** SYN meta- (3).

MA Abbreviation for mental age; mentoanterior position.

ma, mA Abbreviation for milliampere.

MAC Abbreviation for *Mycobacterium avium* complex.

Mac•chi•a•vel•lo stain (mah′kē-ă-vel′ō stān) A basic fuchsin-citric acid-methylene blue sequence in smears that produces red staining of rickettsiae and inclusion bodies, with nuclei staining blue.

Mac•Con•key a•gar (mă-kongk′ē ā′gahr) Medium containing peptone, lactose, bile salts, neutral red, and crystal violet, used to recover gram-negative bacilli and characterize them according to their ferment lactose. Fermenters appear as red colonies, whereas nonfermenters are colorless.

mac•er•ate (mas′ĕr-āt) To soften by steeping or soaking. SEE ALSO maceration.

mac•er•a•tion (mas′ĕr-ā′shŭn) **1.** Softening by the action of a liquid. **2.** Softening of tissues after death by nonputrefactive (sterile) autolysis; seen especially in the stillborn, with bullous separation of the epidermis. [L. *macero,* pp. *-atus,* to soften by soaking]

Mac•ew•en sign (mĕ-kyū′ĕn sīn) Percussion of the skull gives a cracked-pot sound in cases of hydrocephalus.

Mac•ew•en tri•an•gle (mĕ-kyū′ĕn trī′ang-gĕl) SYN suprameatal triangle.

Ma•cha•do-Jo•seph dis•ease (mă-shah′dū-jō′sef di-zēz′) A rare form of hereditary ataxia, characterized by onset in early adult life of progressive spinocerebellar and extrapyramidal disease with external ophthalmoplegia, rigidity, dystonia, and often peripheral amyotrophy; found predominantly in people of Azorean ancestry; autosomal dominant inheritance, caused by a trinucleotide repeat expansion mutation in the Machado-Joseph gene (MJD1) on 14q. [Surnames of two families studied in major descriptions of the disease]

Mach band (mahk band) A relatively bright or dark band perceived in a zone where the luminance increases or decreases rapidly.

Mach ef•fect (mahk e-fekt′) The appearance of a light or dark line on a radiograph where there is a concave or convex interface in the subject, a physiologic optic form of edge enhancement.

ma•chine (mă-shēn′) Any mechanical apparatus or device. [L. *machina,* contrivance]

ma•chin•er•y mur•mur (mă-shēn′ĕr-ē mŭr′mŭr) The long "continuous" rumbling murmur of patent ductus arteriosus. SYN Gibson murmur.

Mac•ken•zie am•pu•ta•tion (mă-ken′zē amp′yū-tā′shŭn) A modification of the Syme amputation at the ankle joint, the flap being taken from the inner side.

Mac•leod syn•drome (mă-klowd′ sin′drōm) SYN unilateral lobar emphysema.

Mac•Neal tet•ra•chrome blood stain (măk-nēl′ tet′ră-krōm blŭd stān) A stain for blood smears composed of a mixture of methylene blue, azure A, methylene violet, and eosin Y.

mac•ren•ceph•a•ly, mac•ren•ce•pha•li•a (mak′ren-sef′ă-lē, mak′ren-sĕ-fā′lē-ă) Hypertrophy of the brain; the condition of having a large brain. [macro- + G. *enkephalos,* brain]

♻ **macro-, macr-** Combining forms meaning large, long. SEE ALSO mega-, megalo-. [G. *makros*]

mac•ro•ad•e•no•ma (mak′rō-ad′ĕ-nō′mă) A pituitary adenoma larger than 10 mm in diameter.

macroamylasaemia [Br.] SYN macroamylasemia.

mac•ro•am•y•lase (mak′rō-am′i-lās) A form of serum amylase in which the enzyme is joined to a globulin.

mac•ro•am•y•la•se•mi•a (mak′rō-am′i-lā-sē′mē-ă) A form of hyperamylasemia, in which a portion of serum amylase exists as macroamylase. SYN macroamylasaemia. [macroamylase + G. *haima,* blood]

mac•ro•bi•ot•ic (mak′rō-bī-ot′ik) **1.** Long-lived. **2.** Tending to prolong life. SEE ALSO macrobiotic diet.

mac•ro•bi•ot•ic di•et (mak′rō-bī-ot′ik dī′ĕt) A diet claimed to increase longevity, often by promoting an emphasis on whole-grain natural foods and restrictions on noncereal foods (especially animal products), as well as liquids.

mac•ro•blast (mak′rō-blast) A large erythroblast. [macro- + G. *blastos,* germ]

mac•ro•car•di•a (mak-rō-kahr′dē-ă) SYN cardiomegaly.

mac•ro•ce•phal•ic, mac•ro•ceph•a•lous (mak′rō-sĕ-fal′ik, mak′rō-sef′ă-lŭs) SYN megacephalic. [macro- + G. *kephalē,* head]

mac•ro•ceph•a•ly, mac•ro•ce•pha•li•a (mak′rō-sef′ă-lē, mak′rō-sĕ-fā′lē-ă) SYN megacephaly. [macro- + G. *kephalē,* head]

mac•ro•chei•li•a, mac•ro•chi•li•a (mak′rō-kī′lē-ă) **1.** Abnormally enlarged lips. **2.** Cavernous lymphangioma of the lip, a condition of permanent swelling resulting from the presence of greatly distended lymphatic spaces. [macro- + G. *cheilos,* lip]

mac•ro•chei•ri•a, mac•ro•chi•ri•a (mak′rō-kī′rē-ă) A condition characterized by abnormally large hands. SYN megalocheiria, megalochiria. [macro- + G. *cheir,* hand]

mac•ro•co•lon (mak′rō-kō′lŏn) A sigmoid colon of unusual length; a variety of megacolon.

mac•ro•cor•ne•a (mak′rō-kōr′nē-ă) An abnormally large cornea.

mac•ro•cra•ni•um (mak′rō-krā′nē-ŭm) An enlarged cranium, especially the bones containing the brain, as seen in hydrocephalus; the face appears relatively small in comparison.

mac•ro•cry•o•glob•u•li•ne•mi•a (mak′rō-krī′ō-glob′yū-lin-ē′mē-ă) The presence of cold-precipitating macroglobulins in the peripheral blood; such macrocryoglobulins are often called cold hemagglutinins.

mac•ro•cyte (mak′rō-sīt) A large erythrocyte, such as those observed in pernicious anemia; indicated by an elevated mean corpuscle volume. [macro- + G. *kytos,* a hollow (cell)]

macrocythaemia [Br.] SYN macrocythemia.

mac•ro•cy•the•mi•a (mak′rō-sī-thē′mē-ă) The occurrence of unusually large numbers of macrocytes in the circulating blood. SYN macrocythaemia, macrocytosis. [macrocyte + G. *haima,* blood]

mac•ro•cyt•ic a•ne•mi•a (mak′rō-sit′ik ă-nē′mē-ă) Any anemia in which the average size of circulating erythrocytes is larger than normal, i.e., the mean corpuscular volume is 94 mcm^3 or more (normal range, 82–92 mcm^3), including such syndromes as pernicious anemia, sprue, celiac disease, macrocytic anemia of pregnancy, anemia of diphyllobothriasis, and others.

mac•ro•cy•to•sis (mak′rō-sī-tō′sis) SYN macrocythemia. See page B3. [macrocyte + G. *-osis,* condition]

mac•ro•don•ti•a, mac•ro•don•tism (mak′rō-don′shē-ă, mak′rō-don′tizm) A condition in which a single tooth, pairs of teeth, or the entire dentition is disproportionately large. SYN megadontism, megalodontia.

mac•ro•el•e•ments (mak′rō-el′ĕ-mĕnts) Inorganic nutrients needed in relatively high daily amounts (i.e., more than 100 mg per day) (e.g., calcium, phosphorus, sodium).

mac•ro•ga•mete (mak′rō-gam′ēt) The female element in anisogamy; it is the larger of the two sex cells, with more reserve material, and usually nonmotile. [macro- + G. *gametē,* wife]

mac•ro•ga•me•to•cyte (mak′rō-gă-mē′tō-sīt) The female gametocyte or mother cell producing the female or macrogamete among fungi or protozoa that undergo anisogamy.

mac•ro•gen•i•to•so•mi•a (mak′rō-jen′i-tō-sō′mē-ă) Excessive bodily and genital development. [macro- + L. *genitalis,* genital, + G. *sōma,* body]

mac•rog•li•a (mak-rog′lē-ă) SYN astrocyte. [macro- + G. *glia,* glue]

macroglobulinaemia [Br.] SYN macroglobulinemia.

mac•ro•glob•u•lin•e•mi•a (mak′rō-glob′yū-li-nē′mē-ă) Increased levels of macroglobulins in the blood. SYN macroglobulinaemia.

mac•ro•glos•si•a (mak′rō-glos′ē-ă) Enlargement of the tongue, either developmental or due to a neoplasm or vascular hamartoma. SYN megaloglossia. [macro- + G. *glōssa,* tongue]

mac•ro•gna•thi•a (mak′rog-nā′thē-ă) Enlargement or elongation of the jaw. [macro- + G. *gnathos,* jaw]

mac•ro•lide (mak′rō-līd) A natural lactone, with a large ring, usually of 14–20 atoms; several antibiotics, including erythromycin, are macrolides. They inhibit protein biosynthesis.

mac•ro•mas•ti•a, mac•ro•ma•zi•a (mak′rō-mas′tē-ă, mak′rō-mā′zē-ă) Abnormally large breasts. SEE ALSO hypermastia (2). [macro- + G. *mastos,* breast]

mac•ro•me•li•a (mak′rō-mē′lē-ă) Abnormal size of one or more of the limbs. SYN megalomelia. [macro- + G. *melos,* limb]

mac•ro•mol•e•cule (mak′rō-mol′ĕ-kyūl) A molecule of colloidal size (e.g., proteins, polynucleic acids, polysaccharides).

mac•ro•mon•o•cyte (mak′rō-mon′ō-sīt) An unusually large monocyte.

mac•ro•my•e•lo•blast (mak′rō-mī′ĕ-lō-blast) An abnormally large myeloblast.

mac•ro•nor•mo•blast (mak′rō-nōr′mō-blast) **1.** A large normoblast. **2.** A large, incompletely hemoglobiniferous, nucleated red blood cell with a "cartwheel" nucleus.

mac•ro•nu•cle•us (mak′rō-nū′klē-ŭs) **1.** A nucleus that occupies a relatively large portion of the cell, or the larger nucleus where two or more are present in a cell. **2.** The larger of the two nuclei in ciliates, which governs vegetative metabolic functions and not reproduction. SEE ALSO micronucleus (2).

mac•ro•nu•tri•ent (mak′rō-nū′trē-ĕnt) Nutrients required in the greatest amount; e.g., carbohydrates, protein, fats.

mac•ro•nych•i•a (mak′rō-nik′ē-ă) Abnormally large fingernails or toenails. [macro- + G. *onyx*, nail]

mac•ro•pe•nis (mak′rō-pē′nis) An abnormally large penis.

mac•ro•phage (mak′rō-fāj) Any mononuclear, actively phagocytic cell arising from monocytic stem cells in bone marrow; these cells are widely distributed and vary in morphology and motility; most are large, long-lived cells with nearly round nuclei and abundant endocytic vacuoles, lysosomes, and phagolysosomes. Phagocytic activity is typically mediated by serum recognition factors, including certain immunoglobulins and components of the complement system, but also may be nonspecific for some inert materials and bacteria, as in the case of alveolar macrophages; macrophages also are involved in both the production of antibodies and in cell-mediated immune responses, participate in presenting antigens to lymphocytes, and secrete a variety of immunoregulatory molecules. [macro- + G. *phagō*, to eat]

mac•ro•phage col•o•ny-stim•u•lat•ing fac•tor (M-CSF) (mak′rō-fāj kol′o-nē-stim′yū-lā′ting fak′tōr) A glycoprotein growth factor that causes the committed cell line to proliferate and mature into macrophages. SEE ALSO colony-stimulating factors.

mac•ro•po•di•a (mak′rō-pō′dē-ă) Abnormally large feet. SYN megalopodia. [macro- + G. *pous*, foot]

mac•ro•pol•y•cyte (mak′rō-pol′ē-sīt) An unusually large polymorphonuclear neutrophilic leukocyte that contains a multisegmented nucleus (e.g., 8, 10, or more lobes); frequently observed in pernicious anemia and certain other forms of anemia. [macro- + G. *polys*, many, + *kytos*, cell]

mac•ro•pro•so•pi•a (mak′rō-prō-sō′pē-ă) A condition in which the face is too large in proportion to the size of the neurocranium or cranial vault. [macro- + G. *prosōpon*, face]

mac•ro•rhin•i•a (mak′rō-rīn′ē-ă) Excessive size of the nose, either congenital or pathologic. [macro- + G. *rhis* (*rhin-*), nose]

mac•ro•scop•ic (mak′rō-skop′ik) **1.** Of a size visible with the naked eye or without the use of a microscope. **2.** Relating to macroscopy.

mac•ro•scop•ic a•nat•o•my (mak′rō-skop′ik ă-nat′ŏ-mē) SYN gross anatomy.

ma•cros•co•py (mă-kros′kŏ-pē) Examination of objects with the naked eye. [macro- + G. *skopeō*, to view]

mac•ro•sig•moid (mak′rō-sig′moyd) Enlargement or dilation of the sigmoid colon.

mac•ro•so•mi•a (mak′rō-sō′mē-ă) Abnormally large size of the body. [macro- + G. *sōma*, body]

mac•ro•sto•mi•a (mak′rō-stō′mē-ă) Abnormally large mouth resulting from failure of fusion between the maxillary and mandibular prominences of the embryonic face. [macro- + G. *stoma*, mouth]

mac•ro•ti•a (mak-rō′shē-ă) Congenital enlargement of the auricle of the external ear, particularly the pinna. [macro- + G. *ous*, ear]

mac•ro•trau•ma (mak′rō-traw′mă) Tissue damage resulting from a single injury.

mac•u•la, pl. **mac•u•lae** (mak′yū-lă, -lē) **1.** A small spot, perceptibly different in color from the surrounding tissue. **2.** A small, discolored patch or spot on the skin, neither elevated above nor depressed below the skin's surface. **3.** In ocular anatomy, indicates that portion of the retina located within the major vascular arcades, temporal to the optic nerve. See page B10, B26. SYN macule, spot (1). [L. a spot]

mac•u•la ad•he•rens (mak′yū-lă ad-hē′rens) SYN desmosome.

mac•u•la a•tro•phi•ca (mak′yū-lă ā-trō′fi-kă) An atrophic glistening white spot on the skin.

mac•u•la ce•ru•le•a (mak′yū-lă sĕ-rū′lē-ă) A bluish stain on the skin caused by the bites of fleas or lice, seen especially in pediculosis pubis. SYN blue spot (1).

mac•u•la cor•ne•ae (mak′yū-lă kōr′nē-ē) A moderately dense opacity of the cornea.

mac•u•la cri•bro•sa, pl. **mac•u•lae cri•bro•sae** (mak′yū-lă kri-brō′să, mak-yū-lē kri-brō′sē) [TA] One of three areas on the wall of the vestibule of the labyrinth, marked by numerous foramina giving passage to nerve filaments supplying portions of the membranous labyrinth; **macula cribrosa inferior**, located in the posterior bony ampulla for passage of posterior ampullary nerve fibers; **macula cribrosa media**, area near the base of the cochlea through which the saccular nerve fibers pass; **macula cribrosa superior**, perforated area above the elliptic recess for passage of the utriculoampullary nerve fibers; **macula cribrosa quarta**, a name sometimes applied to the opening for the cochlear nerve.

mac•u•la den•sa (mak′yū-lă den′să) A closely packed group of densely staining cells in the distal tubular epithelium of a nephron, in direct apposition to the juxtaglomerular cells; they may function as either chemoreceptors or as baroreceptors feeding information to the juxtaglomerular cells.

mac•u•lae a•cus•ti•cae (mak-yū-lē ă-kū′sti-sē) SEE macula of saccule, macula of utricle.

mac•u•la fla•va (mak′yū-lă flā′vă) A yellowish spot at the anterior extremity of the rima glottidis where the two vocal folds join.

mac•u•lar, **mac•u•late** (mak′yū-lăr, -lāt) **1.**

Relating to or marked by macules. **2.** Denoting the central retina, especially the macula retinae.

mac•u•lar am•y•loi•do•sis (mak′yū-lahr am′i-loy-dō′sis) A localized form of amyloidosis cutis characterized by pruritic symmetric brown reticulated macules, especially on the upper back; microscopically, amyloid is deposited as small subepidermal globules.

mac•u•lar ar•ter•ies (mak′yū-lahr ahr′tĕr-ēz) SEE inferior macular arteriole, superior macular arteriole.

ma•cu•lar cor•ne•al dys•tro•phy (mak′yū-lahr kōr′nē-ăl dis′trŏ-fē) An autosomal recessive disorder characterized by glycosaminoglycan deposits in the corneal stroma.

mac•u•lar de•gen•er•a•tion (mak′yū-lahr dĕ-jen′ĕr-ā′shŭn) A progressive deterioration of the macula lutea resulting in the loss of central vision. SYN age-related macular degeneration.

mac•u•lar dys•tro•phy (mak′yū-lahr dis′trŏ-fē) SYN macular retinal dystrophy.

ma•cu•la of ret•i•na (mal′yū-lă ret′i-nă) An oval area of the sensory retina, 3–5 mm, temporal to the optic disc corresponding to the posterior pole of the eye; at its center is the central fovea, which contains only retinal cones. SYN macula retinae [TA].

mac•u•la ret•i•nae (mak′yū-lă rĕt-i-nē) [TA] SYN macula of retina.

mac•u•lar lep•ro•sy (mak′yū-lahr lep′rŏ-sē) A form of tuberculoid leprosy in which the lesions are small, hairless, and dry, erythematous in light skin and hypopigmented or copper colored in dark skin.

mac•u•lar ret•i•nal dys•tro•phy (mak′yū-lahr ret′i-năl dis′trŏ-fē) A group of disorders predominantly involving the posterior portion of the ocular fundus, due to degeneration in the sensory layer of the retina, retinal pigment epithelium, Bruch membrane, choroid, or a combination of these tissues. SEE Stargardt disease, Best disease. SYN macular dystrophy.

mac•u•la of sac•cule (mak′yū-lă sak′yūl) The oval neuroepithelial sensory receptor in the anterior wall of the saccule; hair cells of the neuroepithelium support the statoconial membrane and have terminal arborizations of vestibular nerve fibers around their bodies.

mac•u•la of u•tri•cle (mak′yū-lă yū′tri-kĕl) The neuroepithelial sensory receptor in the inferolateral wall of the utricle; hair cells of the neuroepithelium support the statoconial membrane and have terminal arborizations of vestibular nerve fibers around their bodies; sensitive to linear acceleration in the longitudinal axis of the body and to gravitational influences.

mac•ule (mak′yūl) SYN macula. See page B10. [L. *macula,* spot]

mac•u•lo•ce•re•bral (mak′ū-lō-ser′ĕ-brăl) Relating to the macula lutea and the brain; denoting a type of nervous disease marked by degenerative lesions in both the retina and the brain.

mac•u•lo•er•y•the•ma•tous (mak′yū-lō-ĕr-i-thē′mă-tŭs) Denoting lesions that are erythematous and macular, covering wide areas.

mac•u•lo•pap•ule (mak′yū-lō-pap′yūl) A lesion with a flat base surrounding a papule in the center.

mac•u•lop•a•thy (mak′yū-lop′ă-thē) Any pathologic condition of the macula lutea.

mad•a•ro•sis (mad′ă-rō′sis) SYN alopecia adnata.

mad-dog weed (mad-dawg wēd) SYN alisma.

Mad•dox rod (mad′ŏks rod) A glass rod (or a series of parallel glass rods) that converts the image of a light source into a streak of light perpendicular to the axis of the rod. The position of this streak in relation to the image of the light source seen by the fellow eye indicates the presence and amount of heterophoria.

Ma•de•lung de•for•mi•ty (mah′dĕ-lūng dĕ-fōrm′i-tē) A distal radioulnar subluxation due to a relative deficiency of axial growth of the medial side of the distal radius, which, as a consequence, is abnormally inclined proximally and ulnarwards.

Ma•de•lung neck (mah′dĕ-lūng nek) Multiple symmetric lipomatoses (Madelung disease) confined to the neck.

Mad Hat•ter syn•drome (mad hat′ĕr sin′drōm) **1.** Gastrointestinal and central nervous system manifestations of chronic mercury poisoning, including stomatitis, diarrhea, ataxia, tremor, hyperreflexia, sensorineural impairment, and emotional instability; previously seen in workers in lead manufacturing who put material that contains mercury in their mouths to make the material more pliable. **2.** The characteristic perceptual disturbances (including concrete, describable, visual hallucinations that decrease over time) caused by glycolate anticholinergic compounds that block the action of the neurotransmitter acetylcholine at muscarinic cholinergic receptors. The best-known of these compounds are 3-quinuclidinyl benzilate (QNB), NATO code name BZ, and a related compound, Agent-15, which was part of the chemical warfare arsenal of Iraq during the regime of Saddam Hussein (1979–2003). SEE ALSO anticholinergic toxidrome. [fr. character in *Alice in Wonderland*]

Mad•u•ra boil (mă-dū′rah boyl) SYN mycetoma (1).

Mad•u•rel•la (mad′yū-rel′ă) A genus of fungi including a number of species that cause mycetoma. [*Madura,* India]

ma•du•ro•my•co•sis (ma-dū′rō-mī-kō′sis) SYN mycetoma (1). [*Madura,* India, + mycosis]

M.A.Ed. Abbreviation for Master of Arts in Education.

Maf•fuc•ci syn•drome (mĕ-fū′chē sin′drōm) Enchondromas of the limbs in association with venous and lymphaticovenous malformation; propensity to develop other benign or malignant tumors. SYN Kast syndrome.

Ma•gen•die law (mah-zhahn-dē′ law) SYN Bell law.

mag•got (mag′ŏt) A fly larva or grub.

Ma•gill for•ceps (mă-gil′ fōr′seps) A bent blunt instrument used to facilitate nasotracheal intubation.

mag•ma (mag′mă) **1.** A soft mass left after extraction of the active principles. **2.** A salve or thick paste. [G. a soft mass or salve, fr. *massō,* to knead]

Mag•nan sign (mah-nyahn′ sīn) Paresthesia in the psychosis of cocaine addicts, who imagine they have a foreign body in the shape of a powder or fine sand under the skin, and that it is constantly changing its position. SYN coke bugs.

Mag•nan trom•bone move•ment (mah-ny-ahn′ trom-bōn′ mūv′mĕnt) An involuntary forward and back movement of the tongue when it is drawn out of the mouth; may be seen in several basal ganglia disorders.

mag•ne•si•um (Mg) (mag-nē′zē-ŭm) An alkaline earth element, atomic no. 12, atomic wt. 24.3050, that oxidizes to magnesia; a bioelement; many salts have clinical applications. [Mod. L. fr. G. *Magnēsia,* a region in Thessaly]

mag•net (mag′nĕt) **1.** A body that has the property of attracting particles of iron, cobalt, nickel, or any of various metallic alloys and that when freely suspended tends to assume a definite direction between the magnetic poles of the earth (magnetic polarity). **2.** A bar or horseshoe-shaped piece of iron or steel that has been made magnetic by contact with another magnet or, as in an electromagnet, by passage of electric current around a metallic (iron) core. **3.** An electromagnet built in a cylindric configuration to accommodate a patient in its core, for magnetic resonance imaging. [G. *magnēs*]

mag•net hos•pi•tal (mag′nĕt hos-pi′tal) A facility where nursing care standards are administered as established by the American Nurses Credentialing Center, a division of the American Nurses Association. Magnet status is awarded to a health care organization that has demonstrated excellence and provides the best nursing and patient care through its support of international nursing professional standards.

mag•net•ic gait (mag-net′ik gāt) **1.** SYN Bruns ataxia. **2.** SYN Bruns ataxia.

mag•net•ic re•son•ance an•gi•og•ra•phy (MRA) (mag-net′ik rez′ŏ-năns an′jē-og′ră-fē) Method of visualizing vessels that contain flowing nuclei by producing a contrast between them and the stationary nuclei. See page B22.

mag•net•ic res•o•nance im•ag•ing (MRI) (mag-net′ik rez′ŏ-năns im′ăj-ing) A diagnostic modality in which the magnetic nuclei (especially protons) of a patient are aligned in a strong, uniform magnetic field, absorb energy from tuned radiofrequency pulses, and emit radiofrequency signals as their excitation decays. These signals, which vary in intensity according to nuclear abundance and molecular chemical environment, are converted into sets of tomographic images by using field gradients in the magnetic field, which permits three-dimensional localization of the point sources of the signals. Unlike conventional radiography or computed tomography, MRI does not expose patients to ionizing radiation. See page B22.

mag•net•o•stric•tive ul•tra•son•ic de•vice (mag-nē′tō-strik′tiv ŭl′tră-son′ik dĕ-vīs′) An electronically powered tool that uses rapid energy vibrations of a powered instrument tip to fracture calculus from a tooth surface and clean the environment of a periodontal pocket. The magnetostrictive ultrasonic device consists of a portable unit that contains an electronic generator, a handpiece, and interchangeable instrument inserts. The instrument tip vibrates at 18,000–42,000 cycles per second.

mag•ne•tron (mag′nĕ-tron) Device within a linear accelerator that serves as a microwave amplifier and oscillator. SEE ALSO klystron. [*magnet* + *-tron* fr. *electron*]

mag•ni•fi•ca•tion (mag′ni-fi-kā′shŭn) **1.** The seeming increase in size of an object viewed under the microscope; when written, this increased size is expressed by a figure preceded by ×, indicating the number of times its diameter is enlarged. **2.** The increased amplitude of a tracing, as of a muscular contraction, caused by the use of a lever with a long writing arm. [L. *magnifico,* pp. *-atus,* to magnify]

mag•ni•fi•ca•tion ra•di•og•ra•phy (mag′ni-fi-kā′shŭn rā′dē-og′ră-fē) Radiography using a microfocal x-ray tube and increased subject-film distance to provide magnification of the subject without loss of sharpness or increase in radiation exposure.

mag•ni•tude im•age (mag′ni-tūd im′ăj) MAGNETIC RESONANCE IMAGING an image formed from the amplitude of the signal, distinct from the phase information. SEE ALSO magnetic resonance imaging.

mag•no•cel•lu•lar (mag′nō-sel′yū-lăr) Composed of cells of large size. [L. *magnus,* large, + cellular]

ma-huang (mah-hwahng) SYN ephedra.

MAI Abbreviation for *Mycobacterium avium-intracellulare*. SEE ALSO *Mycobacterium avium-intracellulare* complex.

mAi Abbreviation for milliampere-impulse.

MAIC Abbreviation for *Mycobacterium avium-intracellulare* complex.

main•stream aer•o•sol (mān′strēm ār′ō-sol) A system for administering an aerosol that directs the mainstream of inspired airflow through the aerosol generator.

main•stream•ing (mān′strēm-ing) Providing the least restrictive environment (socially, physically, and educationally) for people with chronic disabilities by introducing them into the natural environment rather than segregating them into homogeneous groups living in sheltered environments under constant supervision.

main•tain•er (mān-tān′ĕr) A device used to hold or keep teeth in a given position.

main•te•nance (mān′ten-ăns) **1.** A therapeutic regimen intended to preserve benefit. Cf. compliance (2), adherence (2). **2.** The extent to which the patient continues good heath practices without supervision, incorporating them into a general lifestyle. Cf. compliance. [M.E., fr. O.Fr., fr. Mediev. L. *manuteneo*, to hold in the hand]

main•te•nance of wake•ful•ness test (MWT) (mān′tĕ-năns wāk′ful-nĕs test) Assessment that lasts up to 8 hours in which a patient is studied during naps and wakefulness in a sleep-inducing environment.

Mai•son•neuve frac•ture (mā-zō-nūv′ frak′shŭr) Spiral fracture of the neck of the fibula, resulting from violent external rotation of the ankle.

ma•jor ag•glu•ti•nin (mā′jŏr ă-glū′ti-nin) Immune agglutinin present in greatest quantity in an antiserum and evoked by the most dominant of a mosaic of antigens. SYN chief agglutinin.

ma•jor his•to•com•pat•i•bil•i•ty com•plex (MHC) (mā′jŏr his′tō-kŏm-pat′i-bil′i-tē kom′pleks) A group of linked loci, collectively termed H-2 complex in the mouse and HLA complex in humans, that codes for cell-surface histocompatibility antigens and is the principal determinant of tissue type and transplant compatibility.

ma•jor min•er•als (mā′jŏr min′ĕr-ălz) Minerals required by adults in amounts greater than 100 mg/day.

ma•jor sal•i•var•y glands (mā′jor sal′i-var-ē glandz) A category of salivary glands that includes the three largest glands of the oral cavity, which also secrete most of the saliva: the parotid, submandibular, and sublingual glands.

ma•jor sub•lin•gual duct (mā′jŏr sŭb-ling′gwăl dŭkt) The duct that drains the anterior portion of the sublingual gland; it opens at the sublingual papilla.

mal (mahl) A disease or disorder. [Fr., Sp. fr. L. *malum*, an evil]

♻**mal-** Prefix meaning ill, bad; opposite of eu-. Cf. dys-, caco-. [L. *malus*, bad]

ma•la (mā′lă) **1.** SYN cheek. **2.** SYN zygomatic bone. [L. cheek bone]

Mal•a•bar car•da•mom (mal′ă-bahr kahr′dă-mŏm) SYN cardamom.

mal•ab•sorp•tion (mal′ab-sōrp′shŭn) Imperfect, inadequate, or otherwise disordered gastrointestinal absorption.

mal•ab•sorp•tion syn•drome (mal′ab-sōrp′shŭn sin′drōm) A state characterized by diverse features (e.g., diarrhea, weakness, edema, lassitude, weight loss, poor appetite, protuberant abdomen, pallor, bleeding tendencies, paresthesias, and muscle cramps), caused by any of several conditions in which there is ineffective absorption of nutrients (e.g., sprue, gluten-induced enteropathy, gastroileostomy, tuberculosis, and certain fistulae).

ma•la•ci•a (mă-lā′shē-ă) A softening or loss of consistency and contiguity in any of the organs or tissues. Also used as a combining form in the suffix position. SYN mollities (2). SYN malacosis. [G. *malakia*, a softness]

mal•a•co•pla•ki•a, mal•a•ko•pla•ki•a (mal′ă-kō-plā′kē-ă) Rare lesion most commonly seen in the mucosa of the urinary bladder, characterized by mottled yellow and gray soft nodules that consist of macrophages and calcospherites (Michaelis-Guttmann bodies). [malaco- + G. *plax*, plate, plaque]

mal•a•co•sis (mal′ă-kō′sis) SYN malacia.

mal•a•cot•ic (mal′ă-kot′ik) Pertaining to or characterized by malacia.

mal•ad•just•ment (mal′ad-jŭst′mĕnt) PSYCHOLOGY/PSYCHIATRY an inability to cope with the problems and challenges of everyday living. [mal- + *adjust*, fr. O.Fr. *adjuster*, fr. L.L. *adjuxto*, to put close to, + -ment]

mal•a•dy (mal′ă-dē) A disease or illness. [Fr. *maladie*, illness]

mal•aise (mă-lāz′) A feeling of general discomfort or uneasiness, an "out of sorts" feeling, often the first indication of an infection or other disease. [Fr. discomfort]

mal•a•lign•ment (mal′ă-līn′mĕnt) **1.** Improper alignment of structures. **2.** Displacement of a tooth or teeth from a normal position in the dental arch.

ma•lar (mā′lăr) Relating to the mala, the cheek or cheek bones.

ma•lar bone (mā′lăr bōn) SYN zygomatic bone.

ma•lar•i•a (mă-lar′ē-ă) A disease caused by the presence of the sporozoan *Plasmodium* in the erythrocyte phase, usually transmitted by the bite of an infected female mosquito of the genus *Anopheles*. Human infection begins with the exoerythrocytic cycle in liver parenchyma cells, followed by a series of erythrocytic schizogenous cycles repeated at regular intervals; production of gametocytes in other red blood cells provides future gametes for another mosquito infection; characterized by episodic severe chills and high fever, prostration, and occasionally death or immunologically mediated sequelae. SEE ALSO *Plasmodium,* tropical diseases. SYN swamp fever *(2).* [It. *mala,* bad, + *aria,* air, referring to the old theory of the miasmatic origin of the disease]

ma•lar•i•ae ma•lar•i•a (mă-lar′ē-ē mă-lar′ē-ă) A malarial fever with paroxysms that recur every 72 hours or every fourth day, reckoning the day of the paroxysm as the first; due to the schizogony and release of merozoites from infected cells, with invasion of new red blood corpuscles by *Plasmodium malariae*. SYN quartan malaria.

ma•lar•i•al (mă-lar′ē-ăl) Pertaining to or affected with malaria.

ma•lar•i•al cres•cent (mă-lar′ē-ăl kres′ĕnt) The male or female gametocyte(s) of *Plasmodium falciparum,* the presence of which in human red blood cells is diagnostic of falciparum malaria. SYN crescent (3).

ma•lar•i•o•ther•a•py (mă-lar′ē-ō-thār′a-pē) SYN therapeutic malaria.

Ma•las•sez ep•i•the•li•al rests (mal′ah-sā ep′i-thē′lē-ăl rests) Epithelial remains of Hertwig root sheath in the periodontal ligament.

Mal•as•se•zi•a (mal-ă-sē′zē-ă) A genus of fungi (family Cryptococcaceae) of low pathogenicity that lack the ability to synthesize medium-chain and long-chain fatty acids and require for growth an exogenous supply of these lipids as can be found in the skin. [L. C. *Malassez*]

Mal•as•se•zi•a fur•fur (mal-ă-sē′zē-ă fŭr′fŭr) A common cause of tinea versicolor, a superficial skin infection. This fungus has been associated with fungemia among neonates in intensive care units and in anorectic patients consuming a high-lipid diet.

mal•as•sim•i•la•tion (mal′ă-sim′i-lā′shŭn) Rarely used term for incomplete or faulty assimilation; malabsorption.

ma•late (mal′āt) A salt or ester of malic acid.

ma•late de•hy•dro•gen•ase (mal′āt dē-hī′drō-jĕ-nās) Any enzyme that catalyzes the dehydrogenation of malate to oxaloacetate. At least six are known; one is an enzyme in the tricarboxylic acid cycle.

mal•ax•a•tion (mal′ak-sā′shŭn) Formation of ingredients into a mass for pills and plasters. [L. *malaxo,* pp. *-atus,* to soften]

mal del pin•to (mal del pēn′tō) SYN pinta.

mal de mer (mahl dĕ mā;r) SYN seasickness.

mal de mo•ra•do (mal dā mō-rā′dō) Reddish purple skin discoloration seen in acute attacks of onchodermatitis caused by *Onchocerca volvulus* in Central America. [Sp. *mal,* disease, + *morado,* purple]

male (māl) **1.** ZOOLOGY denoting the sex to which those belong that produce spermatozoa; an individual of that sex. **2.** SYN masculine. [L. *masculus,* fr. *mas,* male]

male gen•i•tal sys•tem (māl jen′i-tăl sis′tĕm) The male reproductive system, consisting of the testes, genital ducts and glands, and external genitalia. See page A13.

male pat•tern al•o•pe•ci•a (māl pat′ĕrn al′ō-pē′shē-ă) The most common form of androgenic alopecia, seen in men as receding frontal and bilateral triangular temple hair lines, and a balding patch on the vertex, which may progress to complete alopecia.

mal•e•rup•tion (mal′ē-rŭp′shŭn) Faulty eruption of teeth.

mal•for•ma•tion (mal′fōr-mā′shŭn) Failure of proper or normal development; more specifically, a primary structural defect that results from a localized error of morphogenesis; e.g., cleft lip. Cf. deformation.

mal•func•tion (mal-fŭngk′shŭn) Disordered, inadequate, or abnormal function.

Mal•gaigne her•ni•a (mahl-gen′ hĕr′nē-ă) Infantile inguinal hernia before descent of the testis.

Mal•gaigne lux•a•tion (mahl-gen′ luk-sā′shŭn) SYN nursemaid's elbow.

Mal•her•be cal•ci•fy•ing ep•i•the•li•o•ma (mahl-ārb′ kal′si-fī-ing ep′i-thē′lē-ō′mă) SYN pilomatrixoma.

mal•ic ac•id (mal′ik as′id, mā′lik) Hydroxysuccinic acid; found in apples and various other tart fruits; an intermediate in the tricarboxylic acid cycle, the glyoxylate cycle, and in a shuttle system.

ma•lig•nan•cy (mă-lig′năn-sē) The property or condition of being malignant.

ma•lig•nant (mă-lig′nănt) **1.** Resistant to treatment; occurring in severe form and frequently fatal; tending to become worse. **2.** In reference to a neoplasm, having the properties of locally invasive and destructive growth and metastasis. [L. *maligno,* pres. p. *-ans* (*ant-*), to do anything maliciously]

ma•lig•nant a•ne•mi•a (mă-lig′nănt ă-nē′mē-ă) SYN pernicious anemia.

ma•lig•nant bu•bo (mă-lig′nănt bū′bō) The enlarged lymph node associated with bubonic plague.

ma•lig•nant cil•i•ar•y ep•i•the•li•o•ma (mă-lig′nănt sil′ē-ar-ē ep′i-thē′lē-ō′mă) Malignant hyperplasia of ciliary epithelium with frequent involvement of the pigmented layer.

ma•lig•nant dys•ker•a•to•sis (mă-lig′nănt dis′ker-ă-tō′sis) Dyskeratosis that may occur in precancerous or malignant lesions.

ma•lig•nant ex•ter•nal o•ti•tis (mă-lig′nănt eks-tĕr′năl ō-tī′tis) A life-threatening *Pseudomonas* osteomyelitis of the temporal bone in elderly people with diabetes that begins with ear pain and swelling of and discharge from the external auditory canal. SYN *Pseudomonas* osteomyelitis.

ma•lig•nant fi•brous his•ti•o•cy•to•ma (mă-lig′nănt fī′brŭs his′tē-ō-sī-tō′mă) A deeply situated tumor, especially on the extremities of adults, frequently recurring after surgery and metastasizing to the lungs; shows partial fibroblastic and histiocytic differentiation with a variable storiform pattern, myxoid areas, and giant cells.

ma•lig•nant gran•u•lo•ma (mă-lig′nănt gran′yū-lō′mă) SYN midline lethal granuloma.

ma•lig•nant hep•a•to•ma (mă-lig′nănt hep′ă-tō′mă) A carcinoma derived from parenchymal cells of the liver. SYN hepatocarcinoma, hepatocellular carcinoma.

ma•lig•nant his•ti•o•cy•to•sis (mă-lig′nănt his′tē-ō-sī-tō′sis) A rapidly fatal form of lymphoma, characterized by fever, jaundice, pancytopenia, and enlargement of the liver, spleen, and lymph nodes; the affected organs show focal necrosis and hemorrhage, with proliferation of histiocytes and phagocytosis of red blood cells.

ma•lig•nant hy•per•ten•sion (mă-lig′nănt hī′pĕr-ten′shŭn) Severe hypertension that runs a rapid course, causing necrosis of arteriolar walls in kidney and retina, hemorrhages, and death most frequently due to uremia or rupture of a cerebral vessel.

ma•lig•nant hy•per•ther•mi•a (mă-lig′nănt hī′pĕr-thĕr′mē-ă) Rapid onset of extremely high fever with muscle rigidity, precipitated by exogenous agents in genetically susceptible people, especially by halothane or succinylcholine.

ma•lig•nant jaun•dice (mă-lig′nănt jawn′dis) SYN icterus gravis.

ma•lig•nant lym•pho•ma (mă-lig′nănt lim-fō′mă) General term for malignant neoplasms of lymphoid and reticuloendothelial tissues that present as solid tumors composed of cells that appear primitive or resemble lymphocytes, plasma cells, or histiocytes. Lymphomas appear most frequently in lymph nodes, spleen, or other normal sites of lymphoreticular cells. Lymphomas are classified by cell type, degrees of differentiation, and nodular or diffuse pattern; Hodgkin disease and Burkitt lymphoma are special forms.

ma•lig•nant neph•ro•scle•ro•sis (mă-lig′nănt nef′rō-skler-ō′sis) The renal changes in malignant hypertension; subcapsular petechiae, necrosis in the walls of scattered afferent glomerular arterioles, and red blood cells and casts in the urine, with uremia as a common termination.

ma•lig•nant ter•tian ma•lar•i•a (mă-lig′nănt tĕr′shăn mă-lar′ē-ă) SYN falciparum malaria.

ma•lig•nant tu•mor (mă-lig′nănt tū′mŏr) A tumor that invades surrounding tissues, is usually capable of producing metastases, may recur after attempted removal, and is likely to cause death of the host unless adequately treated. SEE ALSO cancer.

ma•ling•er (mă-ling′gĕr) To pretend to be ill or disabled, or to feign slow recuperation from an illness or other disabling condition, to arouse sympathy, avoid work or other responsibilities, or continue to receive medical care, medical benefits, or other forms of attention or compensation. [Fr. *malingre*, fr. *mal-*, bad, + Old. Fr. *haingre, heingre*, thin, haggard]

ma•ling•er•er (mă-ling′gĕr-ĕr) One who engages in malingering.

ma•ling•er•ing (mă-ling′gĕr-ing) Feigning illness or inability to work resulting from an ulterior motive, such as to collect insurance benefits. [Fr. *malingre*, sickly]

mal•in•ter•dig•i•ta•tion (mal′in-tĕr-dij′i-tā′shŭn) Intercuspal relation of the upper and lower teeth.

mal•le•a•ble (mal′ē-ă-bĕl) Capable of being shaped by being beaten or by pressure; a property of certain metals such as gold and silver. [L. *malleus,* a hammer]

mal•le•ar folds (mal′ē-ăr fōldz) Two ligamentous bands, anterior and posterior, making folds on the tympanic side of the tympanic membrane extending from each extremity of the tympanic notch to the malleolar prominence; they mark the boundary between the tense and the flaccid portions of the tympanic membrane.

mal•le•o•in•cu•dal (mal′ē-ō-ing′kyū-dăl) Relating to the malleus and the incus in the tympanum.

mal•le•o•lar (mă-lē′ō-lăr) Relating to one or both malleoli.

mal•le•o•lar stri•a (mă-lē′ō-lăr strī′ă) A bright line seen through the membrana tympani, produced by the attachment of the manubrium of the malleus.

mal•le•o•lus, pl. **mal•le•o•li** (ma-lē′ō-lŭs, -lī) [TA] A rounded bony prominence such as those on either side of the ankle joint. [L. dim. of *malleus,* hammer]

mal·le·ot·o·my (mal′ē-ot′ō-mē) **1.** Division of the malleus. [malleus + G. *tomē*, incision] **2.** Division of the ligaments holding the malleoli in apposition to permit their separation in certain cases of clubfoot. [malleolus + G. *tomē*, incision]

mal·let fin·ger (mal′ĕt fing′gĕr) **1.** Flexion deformity of a distal phalanx due to avulsion of the extensor tendon by forceful passive flexion of the phalanx. **2.** SYN baseball finger.

mal·let toe (mal′et tō) A toe in neutral position at the metatarsophalangeal and proximal interphalangeal joints, but flexed at the distal interphalangeal joint.

mal·le·us, gen. and pl. **mal·le·i** (mal′ē-ŭs, -ī) The largest of the three auditory ossicles, resembling a club rather than a hammer; it is regarded as having a head, below which is the neck, and from this diverge the handle or manubrium, and the slender, anterior process; from the base of the manubrium the short lateral process arises. The manubrium and lateral process are firmly attached to the tympanic membrane, and the head articulates with a saddle-shaped surface on the body of the incus. SYN hammer. [L. a hammer]

Mall for·mu·la (mawl fōrm′yū-lă) A formula for determining the age (in days) of a human embryo, calculated as the square root of its length (measured from vertex to breech) in millimeters multiplied by 100.

Mal·lo·ry an·i·line blue stain (mal′ŏr-ē an′i-lĭn blū stān) SYN Mallory trichrome stain.

Mal·lo·ry bod·ies (mal′ŏr-ē bod′ēz) Large, poorly defined accumulations of eosinophilic material in the cytoplasm of damaged hepatic cells in certain forms of cirrhosis and marked fatty change especially due to alcoholism.

Mal·lo·ry col·la·gen stain (mal′ŏr-ē kol′a-jen stān) One of a number of staining methods using phosphomolybdic or phosphotungstic acid with an acid stain, such as aniline blue, or with hematoxylin for connective tissue staining.

Mal·lo·ry i·o·dine stain (mal′ŏr-ē ī′ō-dīn stān) Amyloid appears reddish brown after Gram iodine stain, then violet and blue after flooding with diluted sulfuric acid.

Mal·lo·ry phlox·ine stain (mal′ŏr-ē floks′ēn stān) A technique based on retention of phloxine by hyaline after overstaining and then decolorizing with lithium carbonate, used in combination with alum hematoxylin to give nuclear staining; hyaline appears red, older hyaline is pink to colorless, amyloid is pale pink, and nuclei are blue-black.

Mal·lo·ry phos·pho·tung·stic ac·id he·ma·tox·y·lin stain (mal′ŏr-ē fos′fō-tŭng′stik as′id hē′mă-toks′i-lin stān) SYN phosphotungstic acid hematoxylin.

Mal·lo·ry stain for ac·ti·no·my·ces (mal′ŏr-ē ak-tin′ō-mī′sēz stān) A stain using alum hematoxylin, followed by eosin; immersion in Ehrlich aniline crystal violet stain, and Weigert iodine solution; mycelia stain blue and clubs stain red.

Mal·lo·ry stain for he·mo·fuch·sin (mal′ŏr-ē stān hē′mō-fyūk′sin) Sections are stained sequentially in alum hematoxylin and basic fuchsin; the lipofuchsin-like pigment and ceroid stain bright red, nuclei stain blue, whereas melanin and hemosiderin appear unstained in their natural browns.

Mal·lo·ry tri·chrome stain (mal′ŏr-ē trī′krōm stān) A method especially suitable for studying connective tissue; sections are stained in acid fuchsin, aniline blue-orange G solution, and phosphotungstic acid; fibrils of collagen are blue; fibroglia, neuroglia, and muscle fibers are red; and fibrils of elastin are pink or yellow. SYN Mallory aniline blue stain, Mallory triple stain.

Mal·lo·ry tri·ple stain (mal′ŏr-ē tri′pĕl stān) SYN Mallory trichrome stain.

Mal·lo·ry-Weiss le·sion (mal′ŏr-ē wīs lē′zhŭn) Laceration of the gastric cardia, as seen in the Mallory-Weiss syndrome. SYN Mallory-Weiss tear.

Mal·lo·ry-Weiss syn·drome (mal′ŏr-ē wīs sin′drōm) Laceration of the lower end of the esophagus associated with bleeding or penetration into the mediastinum, with subsequent mediastinitis; usually caused by severe retching and vomiting.

Mal·lo·ry-Weiss tear (mal′ŏr-ē wīs tār) SYN Mallory-Weiss lesion.

mal·nu·tri·tion (mal′nū-trish′ŭn) Faulty nutrition resulting from malabsorption, poor diet, or overeating.

mal·oc·clu·sion (mal′ō-klū′zhŭn) **1.** Any deviation from a physiologically acceptable contact of opposing dentitions. **2.** Any deviation from an ideal occlusion.

ma·lon·di·al·de·hyde-mod·i·fied low-den·si·ty lip·o·pro·tein (LDL) (mal′on-dī-al′de-hīd-mod′i-fīd lō-den′si-tē lip′ō-prō′tēn) LDL molecule with aldehyde-substituted lysine residue(s) in the apoprotein moiety, resulting from oxidative reaction accompanying prostaglandin synthesis and platelet aggregation.

ma·lon·ic ac·id (mă-lon′ik as′id) A dicarboxylic acid of importance in intermediary metabolism; an inhibitor of succinate dehydrogenase.

mal·o·nyl-CoA (mal′ō-nil) The condensation product of malonic acid and coenzyme A, an intermediate in fatty acid biosynthesis.

mal·pi·ghi·an (mal-pig′ē-ăn) Described by or attributed to Marcello Malpighi.

mal·pi·ghi·an bod·ies (mal-pig′ē-ăn bod′ēz) SYN splenic lymph follicles.

mal•pi•ghi•an cap•sule (mal-pig′ē-ăn kap′sŭl) A thin fibrous membrane enveloping the spleen and continued over the vessels entering at the hilus.

mal•pi•ghi•an pyr•a•mid (mal-pig′ē-ăn pir′ă-mid) SYN renal pyramid.

mal•pi•ghi•an stig•mas (mal-pig′ē-ăn stig′măz) The points of entrance of the smaller veins into the larger veins of the spleen.

mal•pi•ghi•an stra•tum (mal-pig′ē-ăn strā′tŭm) The living layer of the epidermis comprising the stratum basale, stratum spinosum, and stratum granulosum.

mal•po•si•tion (mal′pō-zish′ŭn) SYN dystopia.

mal•prac•tice (mal-prak′tis) Mistreatment of a patient through ignorance, carelessness, neglect, or criminal intent.

mal•pre•sen•ta•tion (mal′prez-ĕn-tā′shŭn) Faulty presentation of the fetus; presentation of any part other than the occiput.

mal•ro•ta•tion (mal′rō-tā′shŭn) Failure during embryonic development of normal rotation of all or part of an organ or system such as the midgut or kidney.

mal•ro•ta•tion of the kid•ney (mal′rō-tā′shŭn kid′nē) Failure of a kidney to rotate during its ascent from the pelvis; usually its hilum faces anteriorly rather than anteriomedially.

MALT (mawlt) Acronym for mucosa-associated lymphoid tissue.

Mal•tese cross (mawl′tez kraws) A tetrad formation of the early ringlike parasites within the red blood cell seen in babesiosis.

MALToma (mawl′tō-mă) B-cell lymphoma of mucosa-associated lymphoid tissue. SYN extranodal marginal zone lymphoma.

mal•tose (mawl′tōs) A disaccharide formed in the hydrolysis of starch and consisting of two D-glucose residues.

ma•lum (mā′lŭm) A disease. [L. an evil]

mam•ma, gen. and pl. **mam•mae** (mam′ă, -ē) [TA] SYN breast. SEE ALSO mammary gland. [L.]

mam•mal•gi•a (mă-mal′jē-ă) SYN mastodynia. [L. *mamma,* breast, + G. *algos,* pain]

mam•ma•plas•ty (mam′ă-plas-tē) Surgical procedure of the breast to alter its shape, size, or position, or all of these. SYN mammoplasty, mastoplasty. [L. *mamma,* breast, + G. *plastos,* formed]

mam•ma•ry (măm′ă-rē) Relating to the breasts.

mam•ma•ry crest (măm′ă-rē krest) Bandlike thickening of ectoderm in the embryo extending on either side from just below the axilla to the inguinal region; in human embryos, the mammary glands arise from primordia in the thoracic part of the ridge. SYN mammary fold, milk line, milk ridge.

mam•ma•ry duct ec•ta•si•a (măm′ă-rē dŭkt ek-tā′zē-ă) Dilation of mammary ducts by lipid and cellular debris in older women; rupture of ducts may result in granulomatous inflammation and infiltration by plasma cells. SEE ALSO plasma cell mastitis.

mam•ma•ry fold (măm′ă-rē fōld) SYN mammary crest.

mam•ma•ry gland (măm′ă-rē gland) The compound alveolar apocrine secretory gland that forms the breast. It consists of 15–24 lobes, each consisting of many lobules, separated by adipose tissue and fibrous septa; the parenchyma of the resting gland consists of ducts; the alveoli develop only during pregnancy. SYN lactiferous glands.

mam•mec•to•my (mă-mek′tŏ-mē) SYN mastectomy. [L. *mamma,* breast, + *ektomē,* excision]

mam•mi•form (mam′i-fōrm) Resembling a breast; breast-shaped. SYN mammose (1). [L. *mamma,* breast, + *forma,* form]

♻ **mammil-, mammilli-** Combining forms indicating the mammillae. Cf. thelo-. [L. *mamilla,* nipple]

mam•mil•la, pl. **mam•mil•lae** (mă-mil′ă, -ē) **1.** A small rounded elevation resembling the female breast. **2.** SYN nipple. [L. nipple]

mam•mil•la•plas•ty (mă-mil′ă-plas-tē) Plastic surgery of the nipple and areola. SYN theleplasty. [L. *mammilla,* nipple, + G. *plastos,* formed]

mam•mil•la•re (mam′i-lar-ē) SYN mammillary. [L.]

mamm•il•lar•i•a (mam′i-lar′ē-ă) SEE mammillary body.

mam•mil•la•ry (mam′i-lar-ē) Relating to or shaped like a nipple. SYN mammillare.

mam•mil•la•ry bod•y (mam′i-lar-ē bod′ē) A small, round, paired cell group that protrudes into the interpeduncular fossa from the inferior aspect of the hypothalamus. It receives hippocampal fibers through the fornix and projects fibers to the anterior thalamic nuclei and into the brainstem tegmentum. SYN corpus mammillare [TA].

mam•mil•la•ry ducts (mam′i-lar-ē dŭkts) SYN lactiferous ducts.

mam•mil•la•ry line (mam′i-lar-ē līn) A vertical line that passes through the nipple on either side. SYN nipple line.

mam•mil•late, mam•mil•lat•ed (mam′i-lāt, -ĕd) Studded with nipplelike projections.

mam•mil•la•tion (mam′i-lā′shŭn) **1.** A nipplelike projection. **2.** The condition of being mammillated.

mam·mil·li·form (mă-mil′i-fōrm) Nipple-shaped. [L. *mamilla,* nipple, + *forma,* form]

mam·mil·li·tis (mam′i-lī′tis) Inflammation of the nipple. [L., *mamilla,* nipple, + G. *-itis,* inflammation]

mammo- Combining form indicating the breasts. Cf. masto-. [L. *mamma,* breast]

mam·mo·gram (mam′ō-gram) The record produced by mammography.

mam·mog·ra·phy (mă-mog′ră-fē) Imaging examination of the breast by means of x-rays; used for screening and diagnosis of breast disease. See page B19. [mammo- + G. *graphō,* to write]

Mam·mo·mon·o·ga·mus (mam′ō-mon-og′ă-mus) Genus of syngamid trematodes (family Syngamidae) found in the respiratory system of ruminants and occasionally reported in humans; worms usually joined together in a Y-shaped formation.

Mam·mo·mon·o·ga·mus la·ryn·ge·us (mam′ō-mon-og′ă-mus la-rin′jē-ŭs) Nematode found in the upper respiratory tract of some mammals; approximately 100 human cases have been reported, most from Caribbean islands; worm is red to reddish-brown; copulating male and female present in a Y shape; life cycle of pathogen not known.

mam·mo·plas·ty (mam′ō-plas-tē) SYN mammaplasty. [mammo- + G. *plastos,* formed]

mam·mose (mam′ōs) **1.** SYN mammiform. **2.** Having large breasts.

mam·mo·so·ma·to·troph cell ade·no·ma (mam′ō-sō-mat′ō-trōph sel ad′ĕ-nō′mă) A rare prolactin-producing and growth hormone-producing pituitary adenoma comprising ultrastructurally monomorphic cells with both somatotrophic and lactotrophic differentiation.

mam·mot·o·my (ma-mot′ō-mē) SYN mastotomy. [mammo- + G. *tomē,* incision]

mam·mo·tro·pic, mam·mo·tro·phic (mam′ō-trō′pik, -trō′fik) Having a stimulating effect on the development, growth, or function of the mammary glands. [mammo- + G. *tropos,* a turning]

man·aged care (man′ăjd kār) An arrangement in the U.S. whereby a third-party payer (e.g., insurance company, government, or corporation) mediates between physicians and patients, negotiating fees for service and overseeing the types of treatment given. The third-party payer may mandate second opinions, precertification review for patients requiring hospital admission, negotiate wholesale prices with physicians, and implement cost-containment measures (e.g., hospital audits and claims reviews). SEE health maintenance organization. SEE ALSO capitation.

man·age·ment (man′ăj-mĕnt) The process of supervising or controlling the affairs or activities of a group. [It. *maneggiare,* to control, fr. L. *manus,* hand]

Man·ches·ter op·er·a·tion (man′ches-tĕr op-ĕr-ā′shŭn) A vaginal operation for prolapse of the uterus, consisting of cervical amputation and parametrial fixation (cardinal ligaments) anterior to the uterus. SYN Fothergill operation. [*Manchester,* England]

man·dat·ed re·por·ter (man′dā-tĕd rē-pōr′tĕr) A professional person required by law to report evidence or suspicion that a child or elderly adult has been abused or neglected. Mandated reporters include, but are not limited to, physicians, surgeons, medical examiners, registered nurses, licensed practical nurses, social workers, residents, interns, and other hospital personnel involved in admission, care, examination, or treatment of patients.

man·da·to·ry breath (man′dă-tōr-ē breth) A breath for which either the timing or size is controlled by a ventilator; the machine initiates (i.e., triggers) or terminates (i.e., cycles) the breath.

man·di·ble (man′di-bĕl) A U-shaped bone, forming the lower jaw, articulating by its upturned extremities with the temporal bone on either side. SYN jaw bone, mandibula, submaxilla.

man·dib·u·la, pl. **man·dib·u·lae** (man-dib′yū-lă, -lē) SYN mandible. [L. a jaw, fr. *mando,* pp. *mansus,* to chew]

man·dib·u·lar (man-dib′yū-lăr) Relating to the lower jaw. SYN inframaxillary, submaxillary (1).

man·dib·u·lar arch (man-dib′yū-lăr ahrch) The first pharyngeal or postoral arch in the pharyngeal (branchial in fish) arch series. SYN mandibular process.

man·dib·u·lar car·ti·lage (man-dib′yū-lăr kahr′ti-lăj) A cartilage bar in the first pharyngeal arch (mandibular arch) that forms a temporary supporting structure in the embryonic mandible; the cartilaginous primordia of the malleus and incus develop from its proximal end, and it also gives rise to the sphenomandibular and anterior malleolar ligaments. SYN first pharyngeal arch cartilage, Meckel cartilage.

man·di·bu·lar for·a·men (man-dib′yū-lăr fōr-ā′mĕn) An opening on the medial surface of the ramus of the mandible through which the inferior alveolar artery, vein, and nerve pass to supply the lower teeth. SYN foramen mandibulae [TA].

man·dib·u·lar fos·sa (man-dib′yū-lăr fos′ă) A deep hollow in the squamous portion of the temporal bone at the root of the zygoma, in which rests the condyle of the mandible. SYN glenoid fossa (2).

man·dib·u·lar joint (man-dib′yū-lăr joynt) SYN temporomandibular joint.

man·dib·u·lar lymph node (man-dib′yū-lăr limf nōd) One of the facial lymph nodes located by the facial artery near the point where it crosses the mandible.

man·dib·u·lar nerve [CN V3] (man-dib′yū-lăr nĕrv) The third division of the trigeminal nerve formed by the union of sensory fibers from the trigeminal ganglion and the motor root of the trigeminal nerve in the foramen ovale, through which the nerve emerges; its branches are: meningeal, masseteric, deep temporal, lateral and medial pterygoid, buccal, auriculotemporal, lingual, and inferior alveolar; its sensory fibers are distributed to the auricle, external acoustic meatus, tympanic membrane, temporal region, cheek, skin overlying the mandible (except its angle), anterior two thirds of tongue, floor of mouth, lower teeth, and gingiva; its motor fibers innervate all the muscles of mastication plus the mylohyoid, anterior belly of the digastive, and the tensores veli palati and tympani. SYN nervus mandibularis [CN V3] [TA].

man·dib·u·lar pro·cess (man-dib′yū-lăr pros′es) SYN mandibular arch.

man·dib·u·lar sym·phy·sis (man-dib′yū-lăr sim′fi-sis) [TA] The fibrocartilaginous union of the halves of the mandible in the fetus; it becomes an osseus union during the first year. SYN mental symphysis.

man·dib·u·lo·ac·ral dys·pla·si·a (man-dib′yū-lō-ak′răl dis-plā′zē-ă) An autosomal recessive disorder characterized by dental crowding, acroosteolysis, stiff joints, and atrophy of the skin of the hands and feet; clavicles are hypoplastic, cranial sutures are wide, and multiple wormian bones are present.

man·dib·u·lo·fa·cial (man-dib′yū-lō-fā′shăl) Relating to the mandible and the face.

man·dib·u·lo·fa·cial dys·os·to·sis (man-dib′yū-lō-fā′shăl dis′os-tō′sis) SYN Treacher Collins syndrome.

man·dib·u·lo·oc·u·lo·fa·cial (man-dib′yū-lō-ok′yū-lō-fā′shăl) Relating to the mandible and the orbital part of the face.

man·drel, man·dril (man′drĕl, man′dril) **1.** The shaft or spindle to which a tool is attached and by means of which it is rotated. **2.** SYN mandrin. **3.** DENTISTRY an instrument used in a handpiece to hold a disc, stone, or cup used for grinding, smoothing, or finishing. [G. *mandra,* a stable; the bed in which a ring's stone is set]

man·drin (man′drin) A stiff wire or stylet inserted in the lumen of a soft catheter to give it shape and firmness while passing through a hollow tubular structure. SYN mandrel (2), mandril. [Fr. *mandrin,* mandrel]

ma·ne (mah′nā) In the morning. [L.]

ma·neu·ver (mă-nū′vĕr) A planned movement or procedure. SYN manoeuvre. [Fr. *manoeuvre,* fr. L. *manu operari,* to work by hand]

man·ga·nese (Mn) (mang′gă-nēz) A metallic element resembling and often associated, in ores, with iron; atomic no. 25, atomic wt. 54.94; manganous salts are sometimes used in medicine. [Mod. L. *manganesium, manganum,* an altered form of *magnesium*]

mange (mānj) A cutaneous disease of domestic and wild animals caused by any one of several genera of skin-burrowing mites; in humans, mite infestations are usually referred to as scabies. [Fr. *manger,* to eat]

ma·ni·a (mā′nē-ă) An emotional disorder characterized by euphoria or irritability, increased psychomotor activity, rapid speech, flight of ideas, decreased need for sleep, distractibility, grandiosity, and poor judgment; usually occurs in bipolar disorder. SEE manic-depressive. [G. frenzy]

-mania Suffix indicating an abnormal love for, or morbid impulse toward, some specific object, place, or action. [G. frenzy]

ma·ni·a·cal (mă-nī′ă-kăl) Relating to or characterized by mania. SYN manic.

man·ic (man′ik) SYN maniacal.

man·ic-de·pres·sive (man′ik dĕ-pres′siv) Pertaining to a manic-depressive psychosis (bipolar disorder). SEE ALSO mania, bipolar disorder.

man·ic-de·pres·sive psy·cho·sis (man′ik dĕ-pres′siv sī-kō′sis) SYN bipolar disorder.

man·ic ep·i·sode (man′ik ep′i-sōd) Manifestation of a major mood disorder in which there is a distinct period during which the predominant mood of the person is either elevated, expansive, or irritable, and there are associated symptoms of the excited or manic phase of the bipolar disorder. SEE affective disorder, endogenous depression.

man·i·fes·ta·tion (man′i-fes-tā′shŭn) The display or disclosure of characteristic signs or symptoms of an illness. [L. *manifestus,* caught in the act]

man·i·fest con·tent (man′i-fest kon′tent) Those elements of fantasy and dreams that are consciously available and reportable.

man·i·fest hy·per·o·pi·a (man′i-fest hī′pĕr-ō′pē-ă) The component of total hyperopia that cannot be corrected by a physiologic response of the ciliary muscle; measured without mydriasis. SYN facultative hyperopia.

man·i·fest·ing het·er·o·zy·gote (man′i-fest′ing het′ĕr-ō-zī′gōt) An organism heterozygous for what is ordinarily a recessive condition, which, as a result of special mechanisms (e.g., lyonization, allelic exclusion, or a deletion in the homologous chromosome), has phenotypic manifestations.

ma•nip•u•la•tion (mă-nip′yū-lā′shŭn) **1.** Skillful manual exploration of an object or person. SEE ALSO manual therapy, mobilization. **2.** A passive therapeutic intervention associated with small-amplitude high-velocity movement at the end of a subject's available range of motion in a joint.

man-made death (man-mād deth) **1.** SYN euthanasia. **2.** SYN slow code.

man•ner (măn′ĕr) The way in which something is done; style, method. [O.Fr. *maniere*, fr. L. *manus*, hand]

man•ner•ism (man′ĕr-izm) A peculiar or unusual characteristic mode of movement, action, or speech.

Mann•kopf sign (mahn′kopf sīn) Acceleration of the pulse when a painful point is pressed on.

Mann meth•yl blue-e•o•sin stain (man meth′il blū ē′ō-sin stān) A stain useful for anterior pituitary and viral inclusion bodies; a mixture of the two dyes stains alpha cell granules red, beta cell granules dark blue, chromophobes gray to pink, colloid red, erythrocytes orange-red, and collagen fibers blue; this method is also useful for enterochromaffin, goblet, Paneth, and pancreatic islet cells; Negri bodies appear red while their nuclei and central granules are blue.

man•nose (man′ōs) An aldohexose obtained from various plant sources (i.e., from mannans).

man•nose-bind•ing pro•tein (man′ōs bīnd′ ing prō′tēn) A protein involved in innate immunity that can bind mannosylated microorganisms and activate the complement pathway.

manoeuvre [Br.] SYN maneuver.

ma•nom•e•ter (mă-nom′ĕ-tĕr) An instrument for measuring the pressure of gases or liquids. [G. *manos,* thin, scanty, + *metron,* measure]

man•o•met•ric (man′ō-met′rik) Relating to a manometer.

ma•nom•e•try (mă-nom′ĕ-trē) Measurement of the pressure of gases by means of a manometer. SEE manometer.

Man•so•ni schis•to•so•mi•a•sis (man-sō′nī shis′tō-sō-mī′ă-sis) SYN schistosomiasis mansoni.

man•tle (man′tĕl) **1.** A covering layer. **2.** SYN pallium.

man•tle cell lym•pho•ma (man′tĕl sel lim-fō′ mă) A clinically and biologically distinct B-cell neoplasm with a recurring acquired genetic abnormality, the t(11;14) translocation, and a heterogeneous histologic appearance that may lead to confusion with reactive or other neoplastic lymphoproliferative disorders.

man•tle ra•di•o•ther•a•py (man′tĕl rā′dē-ō-thār′ă-pē) Radiotherapy with protection of uninvolved radiosensitive structures or organs.

Man•toux test (mahn-tū′ test) SEE tuberculin test.

man•u•al air•way man•eu•ver (man′yū-ăl ār′ wā mă-nū′vĕr) SYN head-tilt/chin-lift maneuver.

man•u•al Eng•lish (man′yū-ăl ing′lish) A means of communicating in English with a person with profound hearing impairment by a combination of signs, finger spelling, and gestures. Cf. American Sign Language.

man•u•al lymph drain•age (MLD, mld) (man′yū-ăl limf drān′ăj) A massage technique intended to promote the absorption of interstitial fluid by stimulating flow in lymphatic channels. SYN lymph drainage.

man•u•al mus•cle test•ing (MMT) (man′yū-ăl mŭs′ĕl test′ing) Assessment modality for the strength of a muscle through manual evaluation. Rating is done by moving the involved part through its full-range of motion against gravity and then against gravity with resistance.

man•u•al ther•ap•y (man′yū-ăl thār′ă-pē) The use of skilled hand movements to manipulate tissues of the body to restore movement, alleviate pain, promote general health, or induce relaxation.

man•u•al ven•ti•la•tion (man′yū-ăl ven′ti-lā′ shŭn) Intermittent compression of a gas-filled reservoir bag to force gases into a patient's lungs and thus maintain oxygenation and carbon dioxide elimination during apnea or hypoventilation.

man•u•al vis•u•al meth•od (man′yū-ăl vizh′ ū-ăl meth′ŏd) A method for the education of deaf children that emphasizes the role of vision in communication and the early and consistent use of ASL or other national sign languages. SEE ALSO oral auditory method, combined methods, total communication.

ma•nu•bri•o•ster•nal joint (mă-nū′brē-ō-stĕr′ năl joynt) The early union, by hyaline cartilage, of the manubrium and the body of the sternum, which later becomes a symphysial type of joint.

ma•nu•bri•um, pl. **ma•nu•bri•a** (mă-nū′brē-ŭm, -ă) [TA] The portion of the sternum or of the malleus that represents the handle. [L. handle]

ma•nu•bri•um of mal•le•us (mă-nū′brē-ŭm mal′ē-ŭs) The handle of the malleus; the portion that extends downward, inward, and backward from the neck of the malleus; it is embedded throughout its length in the tympanic membrane.

ma•nu•bri•um of ster•num (mă-nū′brē-ŭm stĕr′nŭm) The upper segment of the sternum, a flattened, roughly triangular bone, occasionally fused with the body of the sternum, forming with it a slight angle, the sternal angle.

ma•nus, gen. and pl. **ma•nus** (mā′nŭs) [TA] SYN hand. [L.]

MAOI Abbreviation for monoamine oxidase inhibitor.

map (map) A representation of a region or structure; e.g., of a stretch of DNA.

map·ping func·tion (map′ping fŭngk′shŭn) LINKAGE ANALYSIS a formula that converts the recombination fraction (which is on the probability scale) into map distance (in morgans).

Ma·ra·ñón sign (mahr-ahn-yōn′ sīn) In Graves disease, a vasomotor reaction following stimulation of the skin over the throat.

ma·ran·tic (mă-ran′tik) SYN marasmic. [G. *marantikos,* wasting]

ma·ras·mic (mă-raz′mik) Relating to or suffering from marasmus. SYN marantic.

ma·ras·mus (mă-raz′mŭs) Cachexia, especially in young children, primarily due to prolonged dietary deficiency of protein and calories. SYN Parrot disease (2). [G. *marasmos,* withering]

Mar·burg dis·ease (mahr′būrg di-zēz′) Infection caused by a virus of the order Mononegavirales and the family Filoviridae and of the genus *Marburg.* The virus is "pantropic" and affects most organ systems. The disease is characterized by a prominent rash and hemorrhages in many organs and often fatal. It was first seen in Marburg, Germany in 1967, among laboratory workers exposed to African green monkeys. Some person-to-person spread has been observed. Attempts to isolate the virus should be done only in high-security laboratories. SEE ALSO Marburg virus. SYN Marburg virus disease.

Mar·burg vi·rus (mahr′būrg vī′rŭs) An RNA-containing virus, genus *Filovirus,* first recognized at Marburg University (Germany), where it was the cause of a highly fatal hemorrhagic fever among laboratory workers and handlers of green monkeys. SEE ALSO Marburg disease.

Mar·burg vi·rus dis·ease (mahr′būrg vī′rŭs di-zēz′) SYN Marburg disease.

Mar·chand a·dre·nal (mahr-shahn′ ă-drē′năl) A small collection of accessory adrenal tissue in the broad ligament of the uterus or in the testis.

Mar·chand wan·der·ing cell (mahr-shahn′ wahn′dĕr-ing sel) A cell of the mononuclear phagocyte system.

march frac·ture (mahrch frak′shŭr) A stress fracture in the shaft of a metatarsal bone, most often at the first metatarsal due to prolonged running or walking in military recruits unaccustomed to such activity.

march he·mo·glo·bi·nu·ri·a (mahrch hē′mō-glō′bi-nyūr′ē-ă) A form occurring after marathon races, protracted marching, or heavy physical exercise.

Mar·chi·a·fa·va-Big·na·mi dis·ease (mahr-kē-ă-fah′vah-bēn-yah′mē di-zēz′) A disorder characterized by demyelination of the corpus callosum and cortical laminar necrosis involving the frontal and temporal lobes. Occurs predominantly in chronic alcoholics, particularly wine drinkers.

Mar·chi fix·a·tive (mahr′kē fiks′ă-tiv) A mixture of Müller fixative with osmium tetroxide, with potassium chlorate substituted for the potassium dichromate of the Müller fixative for better results; used to demonstrate degenerating myelin. SEE ALSO Marchi stain.

Mar·chi re·ac·tion (mahr′kē rē-ak′shŭn) Failure of the myelin sheath of a nerve to blacken when submitted to the action of osmic acid.

Mar·chi stain (mahr′kē stān) A staining method in which the specimen is hardened for 8–10 days in a modified Müller fixative, followed by immersion for 1–3 weeks in the same with the addition of osmic acid; fat and degenerating nerve fibers stain black.

Mar·cus Gunn phe·nom·e·non, Mar·cus Gunn syn·drome (mahr′kŭs gŭn fē-nom′ĕ-non, sin′drōm) SYN jaw-winking syndrome.

Mar·cus Gunn sign (mahr′kŭs-gŭn sīn) SYN Gunn sign.

Ma·rek dis·ease vi·rus (mahr′ek di-zēz′ vī′rŭs) SYN avian neurolymphomatosis virus.

ma·re·no·strin (mar′ē-nos′trin) SYN pyrin.

Ma·rey law (mah-rā′ law) The pulse rate varies inversely with the blood pressure; i.e., the pulse is slow when the pressure is high; an expression of baroreceptor reflex influences on heart rate.

mar·fa·noid (mahr′fahn-oyd) A term used of those whose phenotype bears a superficial resemblance to that of Marfan syndrome.

Mar·fan syn·drome (mahr-fahn′ sin′drōm) A connective tissue multisystemic disorder characterized by skeletal changes (arachnodactyly, long limbs, joint laxity, pectus excavatum), cardiovascular defects (aortic aneurysm which may dissect, mitral valve prolapse), and ectopia lentis; autosomal dominant inheritance, caused by mutation in the fibrillin-1 gene (FBN1) on chromosome 15q. See page 940.

mar·gin (mahr′jin) A boundary, edge, or border, as of a surface or structure. SEE ALSO border. SYN margo [TA]. [L. *margo,* border, edge]

mar·gi·nal (mahr′ji-năl) Relating to a margin.

mar·gi·nal ar·cade (mahr′ji-năl ahr-kād′) SYN marginal artery of colon.

mar·gi·nal ar·ter·y of col·on (mahr′ji-năl ahr′tĕr-ē kō′lŏn) Artery formed by anastomoses between the right and left colic arteries; it passes downward from the left colic flexure to the aboral end of the pelvic colon. SYN arcus marginalis coli, arteria juxtacolica, arteria marginalis coli, artery of Drummond, juxtacolic artery, marginal arcade, Riolan arch.

mar·gi·nal ridge (mahr′ji-năl rij) **1.** An eleva-

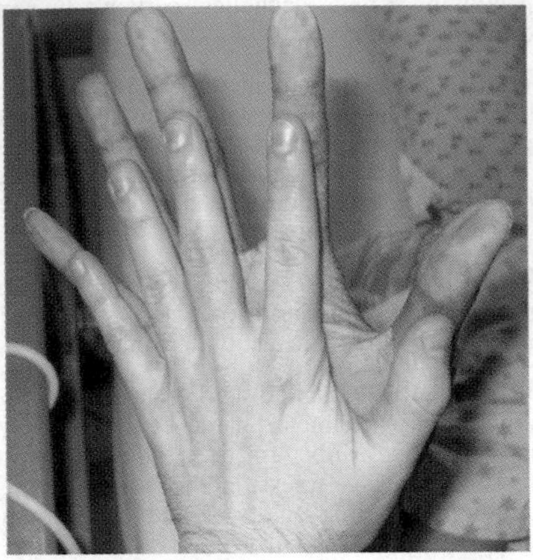

Marfan syndrome: hand

tion of enamel that forms the proximal boundaries of the occlusal surface of premolars and molars. **2.** An elevation on the mesial and distal portions of the lingual surface and, occasionally, the labial surface of incisors.

mar•gi•nal ten•to•ri•al branch of in•ter•nal ca•rot•id ar•ter•y (mahr′ji-năl ten-tōr′ē-ăl branch in-tĕr′năl kă-rot′id ahr′tĕr-ē) A small branch from the cavernous part of the internal carotid artery to the free margin of the tentorium.

mar•gi•nal zone (mahr′ji-năl zōn) A zone between the red and white pulp of the spleen containing numerous macrophages and a rich plexus of sinusoids supplied by white pulp arterioles carrying blood-borne antigens.

mar•gi•nal zone lym•pho•ma (mahr′ji-năl zōn lim-fō′mă) A heterogeneous group of neoplasms originating from the B-cell–rich zones of the lymph nodes, spleen, or extranodal lymphoid tissue. Those tumors originating from mucosa-associated lymphoid tissue (MALT), most often in the stomach, intestines, salivary glands, and lungs, are called MALTomas.

mar•gin•a•tion (mahr′ji-nā′shŭn) A phenomenon that occurs during the relatively early phases of inflammation; as a result of dilation of capillaries and slowing of the bloodstream, leukocytes tend to occupy the periphery of the cross-sectional lumen and adhere to the endothelial cells that line the vessels.

mar•gi•no•plas•ty (mahr′ji-nō-plas-tē) Plastic surgery of the tarsal border of an eyelid.

mar•gin of safe•ty (mahr′jin sāf′tē) The area between the minimal therapeutic dose and the minimal toxic dose of a drug. SYN safety margin.

mar•go, gen. **mar•gi•nis**, pl. **mar•gi•nes** (mahr′gō, -ji-nis, -nēz) [TA] SYN margin, border. [L.]

mar•go or•bi•ta•lis (mahr′gō ōr′bi-tā′lis) [TA] SYN orbital margin.

mar•i•jua•na (mar′i-hwahn′ă) Popular name for the dried flowering leaves of *Cannabis sativa*, which are smoked as cigarettes, "joints," or "reefers." In the U.S., marijuana includes any part of, or any extracts from, the female plant. Alternative spellings are mariguana, marihuana. SEE ALSO cannabis. [fr. Sp. *Maria Juana,* Mary Jane]

Mar•ine-Len•hart syn•drome (mah′rēn-len′hahrt sin′drōm) Toxic multinodular goiter.

Ma•ri•nes•co suc•cu•lent hand (mah-rē-nes′kō sŭk′yŭ-lĕnt hand) Edema of the hand with coldness and lividity of the skin, observed in syringomyelia.

Mar•i•on dis•ease (mar-ē-ōn′ di-zēz′) A congenital obstruction of the posterior urethra.

Mar•i•otte ex•per•i•ment (mar-ē-ot′ ek-sper′i-mĕnt) An experiment in which one looks fixedly with one eye (the other being closed) at a black dot on a card, on which is also marked a black cross; as the card is moved to or from the eye, at a certain distance the cross becomes invisible but appears again as the card is moved further; this proves the absence of photoreceptors where the optic nerve enters the eye.

Mar•i•otte law (mar-ē-ot′ law) SYN Boyle law.

Mar•jo•lin ul•cer (mahr′zhō-lan[h] ul-sĕr′) Well-differentiated but aggressive squamous cell carcinoma occurring in cicatricial tissue at the epidermal edge of a sinus draining underlying osteomyelitis.

mark (mahrk) **1.** Any spot, line, or other figure on the cutaneous or mucocutaneous surface, visible through difference in color, elevation, or other peculiarity. **2.** SYN infundibulum (8). [A.S. *mearc*]

mark•er (mahrk′ĕr) **1.** A device used to make a mark or to indicate measurement. **2.** A characteristic or factor by which a cell or molecule can be recognized or identified. **3.** A locus containing two or more alleles that, being harmless, are common and therefore yield high frequencies of heterozygotes that facilitate linkage analysis.

mark•er trait (mahr′kĕr trāt) A trait that may be of little importance in itself but which by association, linkage, or other means facilitates the detection, anticipation, or understanding of a disease or (for genetic diseases) the localization of the causative gene on the karyotype.

mark•er X syn•drome (mahr′kĕr sin′drōm) SYN fragile X syndrome.

Mark 1 kit (mahrk kit) Nerve agent antidote autoinjector kit consisting of atropine autoinjector and 2PAM C1 Autoinjector.

mar•mo•rat•ed (mahr′mō-rā-tĕd) Denoting a condition in which the appearance of the skin is streaked like marble. SEE ALSO cutis marmorata. [L. *marmoratus,* marbled]

Mar•quis re•a•gent (mahr-kē′ rē-ā′jent) A solution of formaldehyde in sulfuric acid used in color tests for formaldehyde.

mar•row (ma′rō) **1.** A highly cellular hematopoietic connective tissue filling the medullary cavities and spongy epiphyses of bones that becomes predominantly fatty with age, particularly in the long bones of the limbs. **2.** Any soft gelatinous or fatty material resembling the marrow of bone. SEE ALSO medulla. [A.S. *mearh*]

mar•row-mes•en•chyme con•nec•tions (mar′ō-mez-ĕn′kīm kon′nek-shŭns) Uninterrupted continuations between bone marrow and mesenchyme of fetal and newborn middle ears.

Mar•shall ob•lique vein (mahr′shăl ō-blēk′ vān) SYN oblique vein of left atrium.

marsh drain (mahrsh drān) SYN alisma.

marsh•mal•low root (mahrsh′mal-ō rūt) SYN althea.

marsh tre•foil (mahrsh tre′foyl) SYN bog bean.

mar•su•pi•al•i•za•tion (mahr-sū′pē-ăl-ī-zā′shŭn) Exteriorization of a cyst or other such enclosed cavity by resecting the anterior wall and suturing the cut edges of the remaining wall to adjacent edges of the skin, thereby creating a pouch. [L. *marsupium,* pouch]

Mar•te•gi•a•ni ar•e•a (mahr′te-je-ah′nē ār′ē-ă) SYN Martegiani funnel.

Mar•te•gi•a•ni fun•nel (mahr′te-jē-ah′nē fŭn′ĕl) The funnel-shaped dilation on the optic disc that indicates the beginning of the hyaloid canal. SYN Martegiani area.

Mar•tin ban•dage (mahr′tin ban′dăj) A roller bandage of soft rubber used to provide compression to a limb in the treatment of varicose veins or ulcers.

Mar•tin-Bell syn•drome (mahr′tin-bel sin′drōm) SYN fragile X syndrome.

Mar•ti•not•ti cell (mahr-ti-nawt′tē sel) A small multipolar nerve cell with short branching dendrites scattered through various layers of the cerebral cortex; its axon ascends toward the surface of the cortex.

Mar•tin tube (mahr′tin tūb) A drainage tube with a cross piece near the extremity to keep it from slipping out of a cavity.

Mar•to•rell syn•drome (mahr-tō-rel′ sin′drōm) SYN Takayasu arteritis.

Mar•y•land co•ma scale (mar′i-lănd kō′mă skāl) SEE coma scale.

mA-s Abbreviation for milliampere-second.

mas•cu•line (mas′kyū-lin) Relating to or marked by the characteristics of the male sex or gender. SYN male (2). [L. *masculus,* male, fr. *mas,* male]

mas•cu•line pel•vis (mas′kyū-lin pel′vis) **1.** A pelvis justo minor in which the bones are large and heavy. **2.** A slight degree of funnel-shaped pelvis in the woman, in which the shape approximates that of the male pelvis.

mas•cu•line u•ter•us (mas′kyū-lin yū′tĕr-ŭs) SYN prostatic utricle.

mas•cu•lin•i•ty (mas′kyū-lin′i-tē) The qualities and characteristics of a male.

mas•cu•lin•i•za•tion (mas′kyū-lin-ī-zā′shŭn) The condition marked by the attainment of male characteristics, such as facial hair, either physiologically as part of male maturation, or pathologically by individuals of either sex. [L. *masculus,* male]

mas•cu•li•nize (mas′kyū-li-nīz) To confer the qualities or characteristics peculiar to the male.

mask (mask) **1.** Any of a variety of disease states producing alteration or discoloration of the skin of the face. **2.** The expressionless appearance seen in certain diseases (e.g., Parkinson facies). **3.** A facial bandage. **4.** A shield designed to cover the mouth and nose for maintenance of aseptic conditions. **5.** A device designed to cover the mouth and nose for administration of inhalation anesthetics, oxygen, or other gases. SEE ALSO mission-oriented protective posture, gas mask.

masked vi•rus (maskt vī′rŭs) A virus ordinarily occurring in the host in a noninfective state, but that may be activated and demonstrated by special procedures such as blind passage in experimental animals.

mask•ing (mask′ing) **1.** The use of noise of any kind to interfere with the audibility of another sound. For any given intensity, low-pitched tones have a greater masking effect than those of a high pitch. **2.** AUDIOLOGY application of a noise applied to one ear while testing the hearing acuity of the other ear. **3.** The hiding of smaller rhythms in the brain wave record by larger and slower ones the wave form of which they distort. **4.** DENTISTRY an opaque covering used to camouflage the metal parts of a prosthesis. **5.** RADIOGRAPHY superimposition of an altered positive image on the original negative to produce an enhanced copy photographically.

mask•ing di•lem•ma (mask′ing di-lĕm′mă) A problem encountered in establishing the bone conduction thresholds in severe bilateral conductive hearing loss, in which the amount of masking of the nontest ear exceeds the interaural attenuation so that enough masking is too much masking.

mask•ing lev•el dif•fer•ence (mask′ing lev′ĕl dif′ĕr-ĕns) A technique of comparing threshold responses with masking noise presented in phase and out of phase with the test signal; release from masking is normal and indicates an intact brainstem auditory pathway.

mask·like face (mask′līk fās) SYN Parkinson facies.

mask of preg·nan·cy (mask preg′năn-sē) SYN melasma.

Mas·low hi·er·ar·chy (maz′lō hī′ĕr-ahr-kē) A ranking of needs that humans presumably fill successively in the order of lowest to highest: physiologic needs, love and belonging, self-esteem, and self-actualization.

mas·o·chism (mas′ō-kizm) **1.** Passive algolagnia; a form of perversion, often sexual in nature, in which a person experiences pleasure in being abused, humiliated, or maltreated. Cf. sadism. **2.** A general orientation in life that personal suffering relieves guilt and leads to a reward.

mas·o·chist (mas′ō-kist) The passive party in the practice of masochism.

mas·o·chis·tic per·son·al·i·ty (mas′ō-kis′tik pĕr′sŏn-al′i-tē) A personality disorder in which the person accepts exploitation and sacrifices self-interest while at the same time feeling morally superior or feigning moral superiority, attempting to elicit sympathy, and inducing guilt in others.

ma·son's lung (mā′sŏnz lŭng) Silicosis occurring in stone masons.

MASS (măs) **1.** An acronym proposed by the American Medical Association, to assist in triage in mass-casualty incidents. The components of the acronym are *M* for *move*, *A* for *assess*, *S* for *sort*, and *S* for *send*. **2.** Acronym for syndrome manifesting *m*itral valve prolapse, *a*ortic anomalies, *s*keletal changes, and *s*kin changes.

mass (mas) **1.** A lump or aggregation of coherent material. **2.** PHARMACY a soft but solid preparation containing an active medicinal agent, of such consistency that it can be divided into small pieces and rolled into pills. **3.** One of the seven fundamental quantities in the SI system; its unit is the kilogram (kg), defined as the mass of the international prototype of the kilogram, which is made of platinum-iridium and kept at the International Bureau of Weights and Measures. SYN massa. [L. *massa,* a dough-like mass]

mas·sa, gen. and pl. **mas·sae** (mas′să, -sē) SYN mass. [L.]

mass ac·tion prin·ci·ple (mas ak′shŭn prin′si-pĕl) The fundamental principle in epidemic theory: the incidence of an infectious disease is determined by the product of the current prevalence and the number of susceptibles in the population. SEE ALSO serial interval, infection transmission parameter.

mas·sage (mă-sahzh′) A method of manipulation of the body by rubbing, pinching, kneading, or tapping. [Fr. from G. *massō,* to knead]

mas·sage the·ra·py (mă-sahzh′ thār′ă-pē) A collection of modalities intended to improve health through manipulation of the body through human touch and the manipulation of soft tissues using rubbing, pinching, kneading, or tapping to increase circulation, improve muscle tone, and ameliorate the relaxation of the patient or client. SEE ALSO Swedish massage, deep tissue massage, sports massage, seated massage, reflexology, manual lymph drainage, craniosacral therapy, polarity therapy, shiatsu, acupressure, proprioceptive neuromuscular facilitation, Reiki, bodywork. SYN massotherapy, myotherapy.

mass-cas·u·al·ty in·ci·dent (mas-kazh′ū-ăl-tē in′si-dĕnt) Any event that overwhelms the abilities of on-site hospitals or receiving hospitals to treat casualties.

mass-ca·su·al·ty weap·ons (MCW) (mas-kazh′ū-ăl-tē wep′ŏnz) Weapons (e.g., chemical, biologic, and radiologic agents) intended to cause death or serious injury to large numbers of humans (or animals). Note that MCWs may cause widespread loss of life without destroying infrastructure, as weapons of mass destruction do.

massed prac·tice (mast prak′tis) A practice schedule in which rest periods are shorter in duration than practice times.

mas·se·ter·ic ar·ter·y (mas′ĕ-ter′ik ahr′tĕr-ē) *Origin*, maxillary; *distribution*, deep surface of masseter muscle; *anastomoses*, branches of transverse facial and masseteric branches of facial. SYN arteria masseterica [TA].

mas·se·ter·ic nerve (mas′ĕ-ter′ik nĕrv) A muscular branch of the mandibular nerve passing through the mandibular notch to the medial surface of the masseter muscle; which it supplies, and the temporomandibular joint. SYN nervus massetericus [TA].

mas·se·ter mus·cle (mă-sē′tĕr mŭs′ĕl) *Origin*, superficial part: inferior border of the anterior two thirds of the zygomatic arch; deep part: inferior border and medial surface of the zygomatic arch; *insertion*, lateral surface of ramus and coronoid process of the mandible; *action*, elevates mandible (closes jaw); *nerve supply*, masseteric branch of mandibular division of trigeminal. SYN musculus masseter [TA].

mass hys·te·ri·a (mas his-ter′ē-ă) **1.** Simultaneous identical physical or emotional symptoms among a group of people. **2.** A socially contagious frenzy of irrational behavior in a group of people as a reaction to an event. SYN mass sociogenic illness.

mass me·di·an aer·o·dy·nam·ic di·am·e·ter (MMAD) (mas mē′dē-ăn ār′ō-dī-nam′ik dī-am′ĕ-tĕr) The geometric mean of the aerodynamic diameters of a given sample of inhaled particles.

Mas•son ar•gen•taf•fin stain (mas-ōn′ ahr-jen′tă-fin stān) A stain used to stain enterochromaffin granules brown-black.

Mas•son-Fon•tan•a am•mo•ni•a•c sil•ver stain (mas-ōn′ fon-tan′ă a-mōn′ē-ak sil′vĕr stān) A stain used to demonstrate melanin and argentaffin granules.

Mas•son tri•chrome stain (mas-ōn′ trī′krōm stān) Original composition for multicolored tissue preparations including ponceau de xylidine, acid fuchsin, iron alum hematoxylin, and either aniline blue or fast green FCF; chromatin stains black, cytoplasm is in shades of red, granules of eosinophils and mast cells are deep red, erythrocytes are black, elastic fibers are red, and collagen fibers and mucus are dark blue (aniline blue) or green (fast green FCF); modifications substitute other dyes, such as Biebrich scarlet red and wool green stain.

mas•so•the•ra•py (mas′ō-thār′ă-pē) SYN massage therapy.

mass per•i•stal•sis (mas per′i-stal′sis) Forcible peristaltic movements of short duration, occurring only three or four times a day, which move the contents of the large intestine from one division to the next, as from the ascending to the transverse colon.

mass so•ci•o•gen•ic ill•ness (mas sō′sē-ō′jen′ik il′nĕs) SYN mass hysteria.

mass spec•trum (mas spek′trŭm) A distribution of charged particles arranged in the order of mass.

MAST (mast) Acronym for military antishock trousers.

mast•ad•e•ni•tis (mast′ad-ĕ-nī′tis) SYN mastitis. [masto- + G. *adēn,* gland, + *-itis,* inflammation]

mast•ad•e•no•ma (mast′ad-ĕ-nō′mă) An adenoma of the breast. [masto- + G. *adēn,* gland, + *-ōma,* tumor]

Mast•ad•e•no•vi•rus (mast-ad′ĕ-nō-vī′rŭs) A genus of adenoviruses with over 40 antigenic types (species) being infective for humans. They cause respiratory infections in children, epidemic acute respiratory disease in military recruits, acute follicular conjunctivitis in adults, and epidemic keratoconjunctivitis; many infections are inapparent. [G. *mastos,* breast, hence mammal, + adenovirus]

mas•tal•gi•a (mas-tal′jē-ă) SYN mastodynia. [masto- + G. *algos,* pain]

mas•tat•ro•phy, mas•ta•tro•phi•a (mas-tat′rŏ-fē, mast-ă-trō′fē-ă) Atrophy or wasting of the breasts. [masto- + atrophy]

mast cell (mast sel) A connective tissue cell that contains coarse, basophilic, metachromatic granules; secretes heparin and histamine. SYN mastocyte.

mast cell leu•ke•mi•a (mast sel lū-kē′mē-ă) SYN basophilic leukemia.

mas•tec•to•my (mas-tek′tŏ-mē) Excision of the breast. SYN mammectomy. [masto- + G. *ektomē,* excision]

mas•ter pa•tient in•dex (MPI) (mas′tĕr pā′shĕnt in′deks) Database of all patients ever treated at a given health care facility.

Mas•ter of Sci•ence in Nurs•ing (MSN) (mas′tĕr sī′ĕns nŭrs′ing) A degree granted after a prescribed graduate program of nursing education.

mas•ti•cate (mas′ti-kāt) To chew; to perform mastication.

mas•ti•ca•tion (mas′ti-kā′shŭn) The process of chewing food in preparation for deglutition and digestion; the act of grinding or comminuting with the teeth. See this page. [L. *mastico,* pp. *-atus,* to chew]

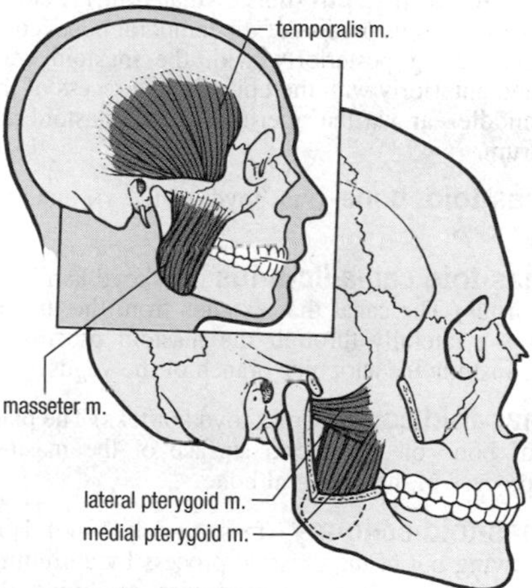

muscles of mastication

mas•ti•ca•to•ry (mas′ti-kă-tōr-ē) Relating to mastication.

mas•ti•ca•to•ry force (mas′ti-kă-tōr-ē fōrs) SYN force of mastication.

mas•ti•gote (mas′ti-gōt) An individual flagellate. [G. *mastix,* a whip]

mas•ti•tis (mas-tī′tis) Inflammation of the breast. SYN mastadenitis. [masto- + G. *-itis,* inflammation]

mast leu•ko•cyte (mast lū′kō-sīt) SYN basophilic leukocyte.

masto-, mast- Combining forms meaning the

breast; the mastoid. Cf. mammo-, mazo-. [G. *mastos*]

mas·to·cyte (mas′tō-sīt) SYN mast cell.

mas·to·cy·to·ma (mas′tō-sī-tō′mă) A fairly well-circumscribed accumulation or nodular focus of mast cells, grossly resembling a neoplasm. [mastocyte + G. *-oma,* tumor]

mas·to·cy·to·sis (mas′tō-sī-tō′sis) Abnormal proliferation of mast cells in a variety of tissues; may be systemic, involving various organs, or cutaneous (urticaria pigmentosa). [mastocyte + G. *-osis,* condition]

mas·to·dyn·i·a (mas′tō-din′ē-ă) Pain in the breast. SYN mammalgia, mastalgia. [masto- + G. *odynē,* pain]

mas·toid (mas′toyd) **1.** Resembling a breast; breast-shaped. **2.** Relating to the mastoid process, antrum, cells, and the like. [masto- + G. *eidos,* resemblance]

mas·toid air cells (mas′toyd ār selz) Numerous small intercommunicating cavities in the mastoid process of the temporal bone that empty into the mastoid or tympanic antrum.

mas·toid an·trum (mas′toyd an′trŭm) A cavity in the petrous portion of the temporal bone, communicating posteriorly with the mastoid cells and anteriorly with the epitympanic recess of the middle ear via the aperture of the mastoid antrum.

mas·toid bone (mas′toyd bōn) SYN mastoid process.

mas·toid can·a·lic·u·lus (mas′toyd kan′ă-lik′yŭ-lŭs) The canal that extends from the jugular fossa laterally through the mastoid process. It transmits the auricular branch of the vagus.

mas·toid cor·tex (mas′toyd kōr′teks) The plate of bone on the lateral surface of the mastoid process of the temporal bone.

mas·toid·ec·to·my (mas′toy-dek′tŏ-mē) Hollowing out of the mastoid process by curretting, gouging, drilling, or otherwise removing the bony partitions forming the mastoid cells. [mastoid (process) + G. *ektomē,* excision]

mas·toid fo·ra·men (mas′toyd fōr-ā′mĕn) An opening at the posterior portion of the mastoid process, transmitting the mastoid branch of the occipital artery to the dura and an emissary vein to the sigmoid sinus.

mas·toid·i·tis (mas′toy-dī′tis) Inflammation of any part of the mastoid process. See this page.

mas·toid pro·cess (mas′toyd pros′es) The nipplelike projection of the petrous part of the temporal bone. SYN mastoid bone.

mas·ton·cus (mas-tongk′ŭs) A tumor or swelling of the breasts. [masto- + G. *onkos,* mass]

mas·to-oc·cip·i·tal (mas′tō-ok-sip′i-tăl) Relating to the mastoid portion of the temporal bone and to the occipital bone, denoting the suture uniting them.

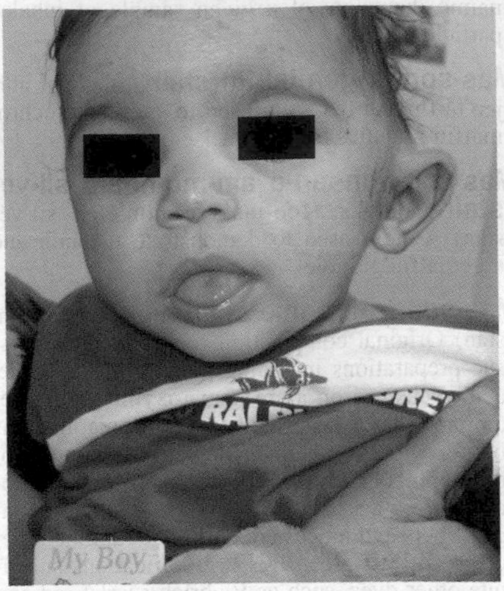

mastoiditis: frontal view

mas·to·pa·ri·e·tal (mas′tō-pă-rī′ĕ-tăl) Relating to the mastoid portion of the temporal bone and to the parietal bone, denoting the suture uniting them.

mas·top·a·thy (mas-top′ă-thē) Any disease of the breasts. [masto- + G. *pathos,* suffering]

mas·to·pexy (mas′tō-pek-sē) Surgical procedure to affix sagging breasts in a more elevated and normal position, often with some improvement in shape. [masto- + G. *pēxis,* fixation]

mas·to·pla·si·a (mas′tō-plā′zē-ă) Enlargement of the breast. [masto- + G. *plasis,* a molding]

mas·to·plas·ty (mas′tō-plas-tē) SYN mammaplasty. [masto- + G. *plastos,* formed]

mas·top·to·sis (mas′top-tō′sis) Ptosis or sagging of the breast. [masto- + G. *ptōsis,* a falling]

mas·tor·rha·gi·a (mas′tō-rā′jē-ă) Hemorrhage from a breast. [masto- + G. *rhēgnymi,* to burst forth]

mas·to·squa·mous (mas′tō-skwā′mŭs) Relating to the mastoid and the squamous portion of the temporal bone.

mas·tot·o·my (mas-tot′ŏ-mē) Incision of the breast. SYN mammotomy. [masto- + G. *tomē,* incision]

mas·tur·bate (mas′tŭr-bāt) To practice masturbation. [L. *masturbari,* pp. *masturbatus*]

mas·tur·ba·tion (mas′tŭr-bā′shŭn) Self-stimulation of the genitals for erotic pleasure, often resulting in orgasm.

MAT (mat) Acronym for multifocal atrial tachycardia.

matched groups (macht grūps) A method of experimental control in which subjects in one group are matched on a one-to-one basis with subjects in other groups concerning all organism variables (e.g., age, sex, height, weight) that the experimenter believes could influence the variable being investigated.

match•ing (mach′ing) The process of making a study group and a comparison group in an epidemiologic study comparable with respect to extraneous or confounding factors such as age, sex, and weight.

ma•ter (mā′ter) The "sheltering" coverings of the central nervous system. SEE arachnoid mater, dura mater, pia mater. [L. mother]

ma•te•ri•a al•ba (mă-tē′rē-ă al′bă) Accumulation or aggregation of microorganisms, desquamated epithelial cells, blood cells, and food debris loosely adherent to surfaces of plaques, teeth, gingiva, or dental appliances. [L. white matter]

ma•te•ri•al (mă-tēr′ē-ăl) That of which something is made or composed; the constituent element of a substance. [L. *materialis,* fr. *materia,* substance]

Ma•te•ri•al Safe•ty Da•ta Sheet (MSDS) (mă-tēr′ē-ăl sāf′tē dā′tă shēt) **1.** The document provided by chemical or industrial manufacturers that contains information on hazardous chemicals. MSDS includes: nature of the chemical, precautions to take in using the chemical, conditions of safe use, clean-up procedure during a spillage accident, and recommended disposal procedures. **2.** Information sheets generally prepared by manufacturers listing ingredients by generic name, toxic properties, recommendations for safe use and other important information.

ma•te•ri•a med•i•ca (mă-tē′rē-ă med′i-kă) **1.** That aspect of medical science concerned with the origin and preparation of drugs, their doses, and their mode of administration. **2.** Any agent used therapeutically. SEE ALSO pharmacognosy, pharmacology. [L. medical matter]

ma•ter•nal (mă-tĕr′năl) Relating to or derived from the mother. [L. *maternus,* fr. *mater,* mother]

ma•ter•nal death rate (mă-tĕr′năl deth rāt) The number of maternal deaths occurring as the direct result of the reproductive process per 100,000 live births. SYN maternal mortality ratio.

ma•ter•nal dys•to•ci•a (mă-tĕr′năl dis-tō′sē-ă) Dystocia caused by an abnormality or physical problem in the mother.

ma•ter•nal-fe•tal med•i•cine (mă-tĕr′năl-fē′tăl med′i-sin) A subspecialty of obstetrics/gynecology devoted to the study of the obstetric, medical, and surgical complications of pregnancy.

ma•ter•nal mor•bid•i•ty (mă-tĕr′năl mōr-bid′i-tē) Medical complications in a woman caused by pregnancy, labor, or delivery.

ma•ter•nal mor•tal•i•ty ra•ti•o (mă-tĕr′năl mōr-tal′i-tē rā′shē-ō) SYN maternal death rate.

ma•ter•nal part of pla•cen•ta (mă-tĕr′năl pahrt plă-sen′tă) The part of the placenta derived from the basal layer or decidua basalis of the endometrium. SYN pars uterina placentae [TA].

mat•er•nic•i•ty (mat′ĕr-nis′i-tē) The important emotional boding that happens between mother and newborn.

ma•ter•ni•ty (mă-tĕr′ni-tē) Motherhood. SEE maternal.

mat•ing (māt′ing) The pairing of male and female for the purpose of reproduction.

mat•ri•cal (mat′ri-kăl) Relating to any matrix.

ma•tri•ces (mā′tri-sēz) Plural of matrix. [L.]

mat•ri•cide (mat′ri-sīd) **1.** The killing of one's mother. **2.** One who commits such an act. [L. *mater,* mother, + *caedo,* to kill]

mat•ri•lin•e•al (mat′ri-lin′ē-ăl) Denoting descent through the female line. [L. *mater,* mother, + *linea,* line]

ma•trix, pl. **ma•tri•ces** (mā′triks; -tri-sēz, mat′ri-sēz) **1.** The formative portion of a tooth or a nail. **2.** The intercellular substance of a tissue. **3.** A surrounding substance within which something is contained or embedded. **4.** A mold in which anything is cast or swaged; a counterdie; a specially shaped instrument, plastic material, or metal strip used for holding and shaping the material used in filling a tooth cavity. **5.** A rectangular array of numbers or symbol quantities that simplify the execution of linear operations of tedious complexity; the theory of matrices is widely used in solving simultaneous equations and in population genetics. [L. womb; female breeding animal]

ma•trix band (mā′triks band) A metal or plastic band secured around the crown of a tooth to confine restorative material to be adapted into a prepared cavity.

ma•trix cal•cu•lus (mā′triks kal′kyū-lŭs) A yellowish-white to light tan urinary calculus containing calcium salts in an organic matrix and usually associated with chronic infection.

ma•trix me•tal•lo•pro•tein•ase (mā′triks mĕ-tal′ō-prō′tēn-ās) A subfamily of endopeptidases that hydrolyze extracellular proteins, especially collagens and elastin. By regulating the integrity and composition of the extracellular matrix, these enzymes play a pivotal role in the control of signals elicited by matrix molecules that regulate cell proliferation, differentiation, and death.

ma•trix un•guis (mā′triks ŭng′gwis) SYN nail bed.

mat•ter (mat′ĕr) SYN substance. [L. *materies,* substance]

mat•tress su•ture (mat-trĕs′ sū′chŭr) A suture using a double stitch that forms a loop about the tissue on both sides of a wound, producing eversion of the edges when tied.

mat•u•ra•tion (mach′ūr-ā′shŭn) **1.** Achievement of full development or growth. **2.** Developmental changes that lead to maturity. **3.** Processing of a macromolecule; e.g., posttranscriptional modification of RNA or posttranslational modification of proteins. [L. *maturatio,* a ripening, fr. *maturus,* ripe]

mat•u•ra•tion ar•rest (mach′ūr-ā′shŭn ă-rest′) Cessation of complete differentiation of cells at an immature stage; in spermatogenic maturation arrest, the seminiferous tubules contain spermatocytes, but no sperms develop.

mat•u•ra•tion in•dex (mach′ūr-ā′shŭn in′deks) An index indicating the degree of maturation attained by the vaginal epithelium as adjudged by the cell types being exfoliated; serves as an objective means of evaluating hormonal secretion or response; represents the percentage of parabasal cells/intermediate cells/superficialis, in that order; "shift to the left" indicates more immature cells on the surface (atrophy), whereas "shift to the right" indicates more mature epithelium.

ma•ture (mă-chūr′) **1.** Ripe; fully developed. **2.** To ripen; to become fully developed. [L. *maturus,* ripe]

ma•ture bac•te•ri•o•phage (mă-chūr′ bak-tēr′ē-ō-fāj) The complete, infective form of bacteriophage.

ma•ture cat•a•ract (mă-chūr′ kat′ăr-akt) A cataract in which both the nucleus and cortex are opaque.

ma•ture mi•nor (mă-chūr′ mī′nŏr) Person younger than 18 years of age, who nonetheless possesses an understanding of the nature and consequences of proposed treatment.

ma•ture on•set di•a•bet•es of youth (MODY) (mă-chūr′ on′set dī′ă-bē′tēz yūth) SEE Type 2 diabetes.

ma•tu•ri•ty (mă-chūr′i-tē) A state of full development or completed growth.

ma•tu•ri•ty-on•set di•a•be•tes (mă-chūr′ĭ-tē-on′set dī′ă-bē′tēz) SYN Type 2 diabetes.

Mau•rer dots (mow′rer dotz) Finely granular precipitates or irregular cytoplasmic particles that usually occur diffusely in red blood cells infected with the trophozoites of *Plasmodium falciparum*, occasionally those of *P. malariae;* rarely observed in blood smears of *P. falciparum* because its trophozoites are seldom seen in peripheral blood.

Mau•ri•ac syn•drome (mō′rē-ahk′ sin′drōm) Dwarfism with obesity and hepatosplenomegaly in children with poorly controlled diabetes mellitus.

Mau•ri•ceau ma•neu•ver (mō-rē-sō′ mă-nū′ vĕr) A method of assisted breech delivery in which the infant's body is astraddle the obstetrician's right forearm, and the middle finger of the right hand is in the fetal mouth to maintain flexion while traction is made on the shoulders by the other hand.

Mauth•ner sheath (mowt′ner shēth) SYN axolemma.

max•il•la, gen. and pl. **max•il•lae** (mak-sil′ă, -ē) [TA] An irregularly shaped bone, supporting the superior teeth and taking part in the formation of the orbit, hard palate, and nasal cavity. See this page. [L. jawbone]

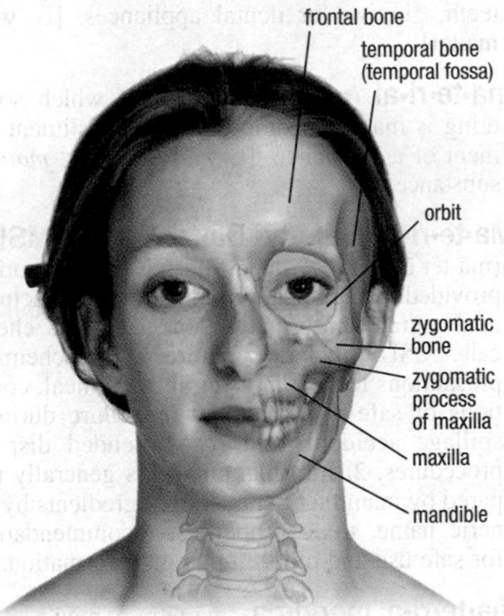

maxilla

max•il•lar•y (mak′si-lar-ē) Relating to the maxilla, or upper jaw.

max•il•lar•y ar•ter•y (mak′si-lar-ē ahr′tĕr-ē) *Origin,* external carotid; *branches,* deep auricular, anterior tympanic, middle meningeal, inferior alveolar, masseteric, deep temporal, buccal, posterior superior alveolar, infraorbital, descending palatine, artery of pterygoid canal, sphenopalatine. SYN arteria maxillaris [TA].

max•il•lar•y gland (mak′si-lar-ē gland) SYN submandibular gland.

max•il•lar•y nerve [CN V2] (mak′si-lar-ē nĕrv) The second division of the trigeminal nerve, passing from the trigeminal ganglion in the middle cranial fossa through the foramen rotundum into the pterygopalatine fossa, where it gives off ganglionic branches to the pterygopalatine ganglion and continues forward to give off the zygomatic nerve and enter the orbit, where it continues as the infraorbital nerve. Its sensory fibers are distributed to the skin and conjunctiva of the lower eyelid; the skin and mucosa of the upper lip and cheek; the palate, upper teeth and gingiva; the maxillary sinus; wings of the nose; and posterior/interior nasal cavity. SYN nervus maxillaris [CN V2] [TA].

max•il•lar•y pro•cess (mak′si-lar-ē pros′es) A thin plate of irregular form projecting from the middle of the upper border of the inferior concha, articulating with the maxilla bone and partly closing the orifice of the maxillary sinus.

max•il•lar•y si•nus (mak′si-lar-ē sī′nŭs) The largest of the paranasal sinuses, occupying the body of the maxilla and communicating with the middle meatus of the nose. SYN antrum of Highmore.

max•il•lar•y vein (mak′si-lar-ē vān) The posterior continuation of the pterygoid plexus; it joins the superficial temporal vein to form the retromandibular vein.

max•il•lo•den•tal (mak-sil′ō-den′tăl) Relating to the upper jaw and its associated teeth.

max•il•lo•fa•cial (mak-sil′ō-fā′shăl) Pertaining to the jaws and face, particularly with reference to specialized surgery of this region.

max•il•lo•man•dib•u•lar (mak-sil′ō-man-dib′yū-lăr) Relating to the upper and lower jaws.

max•il•lot•o•my (mak′si-lot′ŏ-mē) Surgical sectioning of the maxilla to allow movement of all or a part of the maxilla into the desired position. [maxilla + G. *tomē,* incision]

max•i•mal as•sis•tance (mak′si-măl ă-sis′tăns) Application at three or more points of contact by one or more persons to assist a patient to perform a desired activity safely, with contribution of 75% or more effort by caregivers and 25% or less by the patient.

max•i•mal dose (mak′si-măl dōs) The largest amount of a drug or physical procedure that an adult can take with safety.

max•i•mal ox•y•gen con•sump•tion (mak′si-măl ok′si-jĕn kŏn-sŭmp′shŭn) Highest amount of oxygen a person can consume during maximal exercise of several minutes' duration. It is demonstrated by a leveling off or decline in oxygen consumption with increasing intensity. SYN aerobic capacity, aerobic power, maximal oxygen uptake, VO_{2max}.

max•i•mal ox•y•gen up•take (mak′si-măl ok′si-jĕn ŭp′tāk) SYN maximal oxygen consumption.

max•i•mal thy•mec•tomy (mak′si-măl thī-mek′tŏ-mē) SYN extended thymectomy.

Max•i•mow stain for bone mar•row (mak′sē-mŏv stān bōn mar′ō) An alum-hematoxylin and azure II-eosin stain used to distinguish granulated leukocytes, mast cells, and cartilage.

max•i•mum (mak′si-mŭm) The greatest amount, value, or degree attained or attainable. [L. neuter of *maximus,* greatest]

max•i•mum breath•ing ca•pac•i•ty (MBC) (mak′si-mŭm brēdh′ing kă-pas′i-tē) SYN maximum voluntary ventilation.

max•i•mum ex•pi•ra•tory pres•sure (MEP) (mak′si-mŭm eks-pīr′ă-tōr-ē presh′ŭr) The maximum pressure within the alveoli that occurs during a forceful expiration; the measurement is made when the lungs are full of air.

max•i•mum in•spi•ra•tory pres•sure (MIP) (mak′si-mŭm in-spīr′ă-tōr-ē presh′ŭr) The maximum pressure within the alveoli that occurs during inspiration; the measurement of MIP provides a global assessment of inspiratory muscle function.

max•i•mum in•ten•si•ty pro•jec•tion (MIP) (mak′si-mŭm in-ten′si-tē prŏ-jek′shŭn) Computerized image display method used in magnetic resonance angiography and helical computed tomography; a series of slices are combined with display of the brightest pixel on any slice at each location, and suppression of the background; simulates a projection angiogram.

max•i•mum med•i•cal im•prove•ment (MMI) (maks′i-mŭm med′i-kăl im-prūv′mĕnt) The point during recovery as designated by a physician, at which recovery is maximal.

max•i•mum per•mis•si•ble dose (MPD) (mak′si-mŭm pĕr-mis′i-bĕl dōs) Defined by the International Commission on Radiological Protection as the greatest dose of radiation that, in the light of present knowledge, is not expected to cause detectable bodily injury to a person at any time during his or her lifetime. This dose has been reduced with each Commission report. The MPD is given in terms of acute or chronic exposure of the whole body or of organs, systems, or regions of the body, and differs for persons who are occupationally exposed versus the public at large.

max•i•mum pow•er out•put (mak′si-mŭm pow′ĕr owt′put) The greatest sound resulting from amplification that the instrument can produce; an indication of hearing aid performance.

max•i•mum ve•loc•i•ty (V_{max}) (mak′si-mŭm vĕ-los′i-tē) **1.** The maximum rate of an enzyme-catalyzed reaction that can be achieved by progressively increasing the substrate concentration at a given enzyme concentration; in cases of substrate inhibition. V_{max} is an extrapolated value in the absence of such inhibition. **2.** The maximum initial rate of shortening of a myocardial fiber that can be obtained under zero load; used to evaluate the contractility of the fiber.

max•i•mum vol•un•tar•y con•trac•tion (MVC) (mak′si-mum vol′ŭn-tar-ē kŏn-trak′shŭn)

The greatest amount of tension a muscle can generate and hold, however briefly, as in muscle testing.

max·i·mum vol·un·tar·y ven·ti·la·tion (MVV) (mak′si-mŭm vol′ŭn-tar-ē ven′ti-lā′shŭn) The volume of air breathed when an individual breathes as deeply and as quickly as possible for a given time. SYN maximum breathing capacity.

May·er he·mal·um stain (mī′ĕr hē′mă-lŭm stān) A progressive nuclear stain also used as a counterstain.

May·er mu·ci·car·mine stain (mī′ĕr myū′si-kar′mīn stān) SEE mucicarmine.

May·er mu·ci·he·ma·te·in stain (mī′ĕr myū-si-hē′mă-tē′in stān) SEE mucihematein.

May·er pes·sa·ry (mī′ĕr pes′a-rē) SYN Dumontpallier pessary.

May·er re·flex (mī′ĕr rē′fleks) SYN basal joint reflex.

Mayne·ord fac·tor (mā′nōrd fak′tŏr) An application of the inverse square law in radiation therapy; an inverse square correction of the percentage of depth of dose related to distance.

May·o op·er·a·tion (mā′ō op-ĕr-ā′shŭn) An operation for the radical cure of umbilical hernia; the neck of the sac is exposed by two elliptic incisions, the gut is returned to the abdomen, the sac and adherent omentum are cut away, and the fascial edges of the opening are overlapped with mattress sutures.

May·o-Rob·son point (mā′ō-rob′sŏn poynt) A point just above and to the right of the umbilicus, where tenderness on pressure exists in disease of the pancreas.

May·o-Rob·son po·si·tion (mā′ō-rob′sŏn pŏ-zish′ŏn) A supine position with a thick pad under the loins, causing a marked lordosis in this region; used in operations on the gallbladder.

May·o stand (mā′ō stand) A removable instrument tray set on a movable stand that is positioned over or adjacent to a surgical site; it provides a place for sterile instruments and supplies used during surgery.

May-White syn·drome (mā-wīt sin′drōm) Progressive myoclonus epilepsy with lipomas, deafness, and ataxia; probably a familial form of mitochondrial encephalomyopathy.

♻ **mazo-** Combining form indicating the breast. SEE ALSO masto-. [G. *mazos*]

Mb Abbreviation for myoglobin.

M band (band) SYN M line.

MBC Abbreviation for maximum breathing capacity.

MbCO Abbreviation for myoglobin in combination with CO.

MbO_2 Abbreviation for oxymyoglobin.

mc Abbreviation for millicurie.

mcΩ Abbreviation for microhm.

Mc·Ar·dle dis·ease (mik-ahr′dĕl di-zēz′) SYN glycogenosis type 5.

Mc·Ar·dle-Schmid-Pear·son dis·ease (mik-ahr′dĕl shmit pēr′sŏn di-zēz′) SYN glycogenosis type 5.

Mc·Bur·ney in·ci·sion (mik-ber′nē in-si′zhŭn) An incision parallel with the course of the external oblique muscle, 1–2 inches cephalad to the anterior superior spine of the ilium.

Mc·Bur·ney point (mik-ber′nē poynt) A site one third the distance from the anterior superior iliac spine to the umbilicus that with deep palpation produces rebound tenderness indicating appendicitis. SEE ALSO appendicitis.

Mc·Bur·ney sign (mik-ber′nē sīn) Tenderness at site two-thirds of the distance between the umbilicus and the anterior-superior iliac spine; seen in appendicitis.

Mc·Call cul·do·plas·ty pro·ce·dure (mik-kawl′ kŭl′dō-plast-tē prŏ-sē′jŭr) Method of supporting the vaginal cuff during a vaginal hysterectomy by attaching the uterosacral and cardinal ligaments to the peritoneal surface with suture material that, when tied, draws toward the midline, helping to close off the cul-de-sac.

Mc·Car·ey-Kauf·mann me·di·a (mik-kar′ē-kawf-măn mē′dē-ă) A culture solution used for storage of enucleated eyes or corneal tissue for corneal transplantation.

Mc·Car·thy re·flex·es (mi-kahr′thē rē′fleks-ez) SYN spinoadductor reflex.

mcCi Abbreviation for microcurie.

Mc·Cune-Al·bright syn·drome (mik-kyūn′-awl′brīt sin′drōm) Polyostotic fibrous dysplasia with irregular brown patches of cutaneous pigmentation and endocrine dysfunction, especially precocious puberty in girls. SEE ALSO pseudohypoparathyroidism. SYN Albright disease, Albright syndrome (1).

Mc·Don·ald ma·neu·ver (mik-don′ăld mă-nū′vĕr) Measurement of uterus from the upper border of the symphysis to a line tangential to the fundus over the abdomen with a tape to determine the height of the uterus; each centimeter approximately corresponds to the gestational age in weeks from 20–34 weeks' gestation.

mcg Abbreviation for microgram.

Mc·Goon tech·nique (mik-gūn′ tek-nēk′) Plastic reconstruction of an incompetent mitral valve, when the incompetence is due to rupture of chordae to the posterior leaflet, by plication of the redundant leaflet.

MCH Abbreviation for mean corpuscular hemoglobin.

MCHC Abbreviation for mean corpuscular hemoglobin concentration.

mCi Abbreviation for millicurie.

McKu·sick met·a·phys·i·al dys·pla·si·a (mik-kyū′sik met′ă-fiz′ē-ăl dis-plā′zē-ă) SYN cartilage-hair hypoplasia.

mcL, mcl Abbreviation for microliter.

mcM Abbreviation for micromolar.

mcm Abbreviation for micrometer.

McMas·ters cy·cle test (mik-mas′tĕrz sī′kĕl test) SYN submaximal exercise testing.

mcmc Abbreviation for micromicro-; micromicron.

mcmol Abbreviation for micromole.

mcmol/L Abbreviation for micromolar.

Mc·Mur·ray test (mik-mŭr′ē test) Rotation of the tibia on the femur to determine injury to meniscal structures.

Mc·Ne·mar test (mik′nĕ-mahr test) A form of Chi-square test for matched paired data.

MCP Abbreviation for metacarpophalangeal.

Mc·Ro·berts ma·neu·ver (mik-rob′ĕrts mă-nū′vĕr) Maneuver to reduce a fetal shoulder dystocia by flexion of the maternal hips.

MCS Abbreviation for multiple chemical sensitivity.

M-CSF Abbreviation for macrophage colony-stimulating factor.

MCUS Abbreviation for midstream urine specimen.

MCV Abbreviation for mean corpuscular volume.

mcV Abbreviation for microvolt.

Mc·Vay op·er·a·tion (mik-vā′ op-ĕr-ā′shŭn) Repair of inguinal and femoral hernias by suture of the transversus abdominis muscle and its associated fasciae (transversus layer) to the pectineal ligament.

MCW Abbreviation for mass-casualty weapons. SEE ALSO CBR, CBRNE, NBC, weapons of mass destruction.

MD Abbreviation for methyldichloroarsine.

M.D. Abbreviation for medical doctor.

Md Symbol for mendelevium.

M.D. An·der·son sys·tem (an′dĕr-sŏn sis′tĕm) Classification of melanoma: (1) lesion limited to dermatologic involvement, (2) regional lymph node involvement, (3) distant metastases.

MDF Abbreviation for myocardial depressant factor.

MDI Abbreviation for metered-dose inhaler.

MDS Abbreviation for minimum data set.

ME Abbreviation for myalgic encephalomyelitis; medical examiner.

mead·ow der·ma·ti·tis, mead·ow grass der·ma·ti·tis (mĕd′ō dĕr′mă-tī′tis, gras dĕr′mă-tī′tis) A photoallergic skin reaction to contact with a plant containing furocoumarin; often occurs after sunbathing. SYN phytophlyctodermatitis.

Mead·ows syn·drome (me′dōz sin′drōm) Cardiomyopathy developing during pregnancy or the puerperium.

meal (mēl) **1.** The food consumed at regular intervals or at a specified time. **2.** Ground flour from a grain.

mean (mēn) A statistical measurement of central tendency or average of a set of values, usually assumed to be the arithmetic mean unless otherwise specified. [M.E., *mene* fr. O.Fr., fr. L. *medianus*, in the middle]

mean cal·o·rie (mēn kal′ŏr-ē) One hundredth of the energy required to raise the temperature of 1 g of water from 0°C–100°C.

mean cor·pus·cu·lar he·mo·glo·bin (MCH) (mēn kōr-pŭs′kyū-lăr hē′mō-glō-bin) The hemoglobin content of the average red blood cell (RBC), calculated from the hemoglobin(Hgb) therein and the RBC count, in RBC indices. The calculation is: MCH = Hbg (g) × 10 ÷ RBC.

mean cor·pus·cu·lar he·mo·glo·bin con·cen·tra·tion (MCHC) (mēn kōr-pŭs′kyū-lăr hē′mō-glō-bin kon′sĕn-trā′shŭn) The average hemoglobin concentration in a given volume of packed red blood cells (RBC), calculated from the hemoglobin therein and the hematocrit (Hct), in RBC indices. The calculation is: MCHC = Hbg (g) × 100 ÷ Hct.

mean cor·pus·cu·lar vol·ume (MCV) (mēn kōr-pŭs′kū-lăr vol′yūm) The average volume of red blood cells (RBC), calculated from the hematocrit (Hct) and the RBC count, in RBC indices. The calculation is: MCV = Hct × 10 ÷ RBC.

mean life (mēn līf) The average lifetime of decay of a radioactive atom. SYN average life.

mean QRS ax·is (mēn ak′sis) The average direction of all the QRS complexes recorded in a standard 12-lead ECG.

mea·sles (mē′zĕlz) **1.** An acute exanthematous disease, caused by measles virus and marked by fever and other constitutional disturbances, a catarrhal inflammation of the respiratory mucous membranes, and a generalized maculopapular eruption of a dusky red color; the eruption occurs early on the buccal mucous membrane in the form of Koplik spots; incubation period is 10–12 days. SYN morbilli, rubeola. **2.** A disease of swine caused by the presence of *Cysticercus cellulosae*, the measle or larva of *Taenia solium*, the pork tapeworm. **3.** A disease of cattle caused by the presence of *Cysticercus bovis*, the measle or larva of *T. saginata*, the beef tapeworm. See page B30. [D. *maselen*]

mea•sles vi•rus (mē′zĕlz vī′rŭs) An RNA virus of the genus Morbillivirus that causes measles and is transmitted through the respiratory tract; possesses hemagglutinating, hemadsorbing, and hemolyzing properties. SYN rubeola virus.

mea•sure•ment (mezh′ŭr-mĕnt) Determination of a dimension or quantity.

me•a•tal (mē-ā′tăl) Relating to a meatus.

♻ **meato-** Combining form indicating meatus. [L. *meatus*, passage]

me•a•to•plas•ty (mē-at′ō-plas-tē) Surgical repair of a meatus or canal, e.g., the external auditory meatus or the urethral meatus.

me•a•tor•rha•phy (mē′ă-tōr′ă-fē) Closing by suture of the wound made by performing a meatotomy. [meato- + G. *rhaphē*, suture]

me•a•tos•co•py (mē-ă-tos′kŏ-pē) Inspection, usually instrumental, of any meatus, especially of the meatus of the urethra. [meato- + G. *skopeō*, to view]

me•a•tot•o•my (mē′ă-tot′ŏ-mē) An incision made to enlarge a meatus, e.g., of the urethra or ureter. [meato- + G. *tomē*, incision]

me•a•tus, pl. **me•a•tus** (mē-ā′tŭs) [TA] A passage or channel, especially the external opening of a canal. [L. a going, a passage, fr. *meo*, pp. *meatus*, to go, pass]

me•a•tus a•cus•ti•cus (mē-ā′tŭs ă-kū′sti-kŭs) SYN acoustic meatus.

me•a•tus na•si (mē-ā′tūs nā′sī) SYN nasal meatus.

me•chan•i•cal (mĕ-kan′i-kăl) **1.** Performed by means of some apparatus, not manually. **2.** Explaining phenomena in terms of mechanics. **3.** Automatic. [G. *mechanikos*, relating to a machine, fr. *mēchanē*, a contrivance, machine]

me•chan•i•cal an•ti•dote (mĕ-kan′i-kăl an′ti-dōt) A substance that prevents the absorption of a poison.

me•chan•i•cal dys•men•or•rhe•a (mĕ-kan′i-kăl dis-men′ōr-ē′ă) Disorder of menses resulting from obstruction of discharge of menstrual blood, as in cervical stenosis. SYN obstructive dysmenorrhea.

me•chan•i•cal ef•fi•ci•en•cy (mĕ-kan′i-kăl ē-fish′ĕn-sē) The ratio of work output to work input, expressed as a percentage.

me•chan•i•cal il•e•us (mĕ-kan′i-kăl il′ē-ŭs) Obstruction of the bowel due to some mechanical cause, e.g., volvulus, gallstone, adhesions.

me•chan•i•cal jaun•dice (mĕ-kan′i-kăl jawn′dis) SYN obstructive jaundice.

me•chan•i•cal vec•tor (mĕ-kan′i-kăl vek′tŏr) A vector that conveys pathogens to a susceptible individual without essential biologic development of the pathogens in the vector, as in the transfer of septic organisms on the feet or mouth parts of the housefly.

me•chan•i•cal ven•ti•la•tion (mĕ-kan′i-kăl ven′ti-lā′shŭn) The use of an automatic mechanical device to perform all or part of the work of breathing. SEE ALSO ventilator.

me•chan•ics (mĕ-kan′iks) The science of the action of forces in promoting motion or equilibrium. SEE mechanical.

mech•a•nism (mek′ă-nizm) **1.** An arrangement or grouping of the parts of anything that has a definite action. **2.** The means by which an effect is obtained. **3.** The chain of events in a particular process. **4.** The detailed description of a reaction pathway. **5.** BIOWARFARE a device or part of one intended to release a biologic or chemical agent. [G. *mēchanē*, a contrivance]

mech•a•nisms of la•bor (mĕk′ă-nizmz lā′bŏr) The passive fetal position adjustments made as the baby accommodates to the space in the birth canal. These movements in a vertex presentation are descent, flexion, engagement, internal rotation, extension, external rotation, and expulsion.

me•chan•o•e•lec•tric trans•duc•tion (mek′ă-nō-ē-lek′trik trans-dŭk′shŭn) The conversion of mechanical energy to electric energy by sensory cells such as auditory and vestibular hair cells.

mech•a•no•re•cep•tor (mek′ă-nō-rē-sep′tŏr) A receptor that responds to mechanical pressure or distortion; e.g., receptors in the carotid sinuses, touch receptors in the skin.

me•chlor•eth•a•mine (mek′lōr-eth′ă-mēn) SEE nitrogen mustards.

Mec•kel car•ti•lage (mek′el kahr′ti-lăj) SYN mandibular cartilage.

🅸 **Mec•kel di•ver•tic•u•lum** (mek′el dī′vĕr-tik′yū-lŭm) The remains of the yolk stalk of the embryo, which, when persisting abnormally as a blind sac or pouch in the adult, is located on the ileum a short distance above the cecum; it may be attached to the umbilicus and, if the lining includes gastric mucosa, peptic ulceration and bleeding can occur. See page 951. SYN ileal diverticulum.

Mec•kel scan (mek′el skan) Use of technetium-99m pertechnetate in a scan of the gastric mucosa to detect ectopic gastric mucosa in Meckel

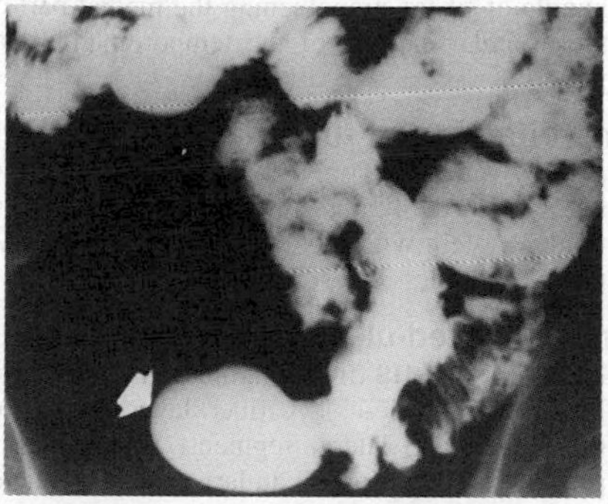

Meckel diverticulum: contrast radiograph of small intestine shows barium-filled diverticulum of the ileum

diverticulum; the pertechnetate anion is secreted by epithelial cells in the gastric mucosa.

me·co·ni·um (mē-kō′nē-ŭm) The greenish first intestinal discharges of the newborn infant, consisting of epithelial cells, mucus, and bile. [L., fr. G. *mēkōnion,* dim. of *mēkōn,* poppy]

me·co·ni·um as·pi·ra·tion (mē-kō′nē-ŭm as′pir-ā′shŭn) Intrauterine aspiration by the fetus of amniotic fluid contaminated by meconium resulting from fetal hypoxic distress.

me·co·ni·um as·pi·ra·tion syn·drome (mē-kō′nē-ŭm as′pir-ā′shŭn sin′drōm) SYN fetal aspiration syndrome.

me·co·ni·um il·e·us (mē-kō′nē-ŭm il′ē-ŭs) Intestinal obstruction in the fetus and newborn following inspissation of meconium; caused by lack of trypsin; associated with cystic fibrosis.

me·co·ni·um per·i·to·ni·tis (mē-kō′nē-ŭm per′i-tō-nī′tis) Peritonitis caused by intestinal perforation in the fetus or newborn; associated with congenital obstruction or fibrocystic disease of the pancreas.

me·co·ni·um plug (mē-kō′nē-ŭm plŭg) A plug of thick, inspissated meconium that may cause intestinal obstruction.

me·di·a (mē′dē-ă) **1.** SYN tunica media. **2.** Plural of medium. [L. fem. of *medius,* middle]

me·di·al (mē′dē-ăl) Relating to the middle or center; nearer to the median or midsagittal plane. [L. *medialis,* middle]

me·di·al an·te·bra·chi·al cu·ta·ne·ous nerve (mē′dē-ăl an′ti-brā′kē-ăl kyū-tā′nē-ŭs nĕrv) SYN medial cutaneous nerve of forearm.

me·di·al an·te·ri·or tho·rac·ic nerve (mē′dē-ăl an-tēr′ē-ŏr thōr-as′ik nĕrv) SYN medial pectoral nerve.

me·di·al ar·cu·ate lig·a·ments (mē′dē-ăl ahrk′yū-ăt lig′ă-mĕnts) One of the Haller arches; a tendinous thickening of the psoas fascia that extends from the body of the first lumbar vertebra to its transverse process on either side. A portion of the diaphragm arises from it.

me·di·al bra·chi·al cu·ta·ne·ous nerve (mē′dē-ăl brā′kē-ăl kyū-tā′nē-ŭs nĕrv) SYN medial cutaneous nerve of forearm.

me·di·al cir·cum·flex ar·ter·y of thigh (mē′dē-ăl sĭr′kŭm-fleks ahr′tĕr-ē thī) SYN medial circumflex femoral artery.

me·di·al cir·cum·flex fem·or·al ar·ter·y (mē′dē-ăl sĭr′kŭm-fleks fem′ŏr-ăl ahr′tĕr-ē) *Origin,* profunda femoris; *distribution,* hip joint, muscles of thigh; *anastomoses,* inferior gluteal, superior gluteal, lateral circumflex femoral. SYN arteria circumflexa femoris medialis, medial circumflex artery of thigh, medial femoral circumflex artery.

me·di·al clu·ne·al nerves (mē′dē-ăl klū′nē-ăl nĕrvz) Terminal branches of the dorsal primary rami of the sacral nerves, supplying the skin of the midgluteal region. SYN middle cluneal nerves, nervi clunium medii.

me·di·al col·lat·er·al ar·ter·y (me′dē-ăl kŏ-lat′ĕr-ăl ahr′tĕr-ē) SYN middle collateral artery.

me·di·al col·lat·er·al lig·a·ment (mē′dē-ăl kŏ-lat′ĕr-ăl lig′ă-mĕnt) A broad, flat band attached superiorly to the medial condyle of the femur and inferiorly to the medial condyle of the tibia; stabilizes the knee joint medially, resisting valgus stress. SYN tibial collateral ligament.

me·di·al con·dyle of fe·mur (mē′dē-ăl kon′dīl fē′mŭr) One of the two large rounded articular masses of the distal end of the femur, united anteriorly with its contralateral partner by the patellar surface but separated from it posteriorly and inferiorly by the intercondylar fossa; the medial condyle is the shorter condyle closest to the midline of the two femoral condyles.

me·di·al cru·ral cu·ta·ne·ous branch·es of sa·phe·nous nerve (mē′dē-al krūr′ăl kyū-tā′nē-ŭs branch′ĕz să-fē′nŭs nĕrv) SYN medial cutaneous nerve of leg.

me·di·al cru·ral cu·ta·ne·ous nerve (mē′dē-al krūr′ăl kyū-tā′nē-ŭs nĕrv) SYN medial cutaneous nerve of leg.

me·di·al cu·ne·i·form bone (mē′dē-ăl kyū-nē′i-fōrm bōn) The largest of the three cuneiform bones, the medial bone of the distal row of the tarsus, articulating with the intermediate cuneiform, navicular, and first and second metatarsal bones. SYN wedge bone.

me·di·al cu·ta·ne·ous nerve of arm (mē′dē-ăl kyū-tā′nē-ŭs nĕrv ahrm) Arises from the medial cord of the brachial plexus, unites in the axilla with the lateral cutaneous branch of the second intercostal nerve, and supplies the skin of the medial side of the arm.

me•di•al cu•ta•ne•ous nerve of fore•arm (mē′dē-ăl kyū-tā′nē-ŭs nĕrv fōr′ahrm) Arises from the medial cord of the brachial plexus, passes downward in company with the brachial artery and then the basilic vein, and supplies the skin of the anterior and ulnar surfaces of the forearm. SYN lesser internal cutaneous nerve, medial antebrachial cutaneous nerve, medial brachial cutaneous nerve, nervus cutaneus antebrachii medialis, nervus cutaneus brachii medialis, Wrisberg nerve.

me•di•al cu•ta•ne•ous nerve of leg (mē′dē-ăl kyū-tā′nē-ŭs nĕrv leg) Branches of saphenous nerve distributed to the skin of the medial side of the leg. SYN medial crural cutaneous branches of saphenous nerve, medial crural cutaneous nerve, rami cutanei cruris mediales nervi sapheni.

me•di•al dor•sal cu•ta•ne•ous nerve (mē′dē-al dōr′săl kyū-tā′nē-ŭs nĕrv) Medial terminal branch of the superficial fibular (peroneal) nerve, supplying the dorsum of the foot and dorsal nerves to toes (except adjacent sides of great and second toes). SYN dorsal medial cutaneous nerve, nervus cutaneus dorsalis medialis.

me•di•al ep•i•con•dyle of hu•mer•us (mē′dē-ăl ep′i-kon′dīl hyū′mĕr-ŭs) The epicondylus situated proximal and medial to the condyle.

me•di•al epi•con•dy•li•tis (mē′dē-ăl ep′i-kon′di-lī′tis) Inflammation of the medial epicondyle of the humurus due to overuse of the wrist flexors or to cumulative trauma, as in some athletes. SYN Little League elbow.

me•di•al fem•or•al cir•cum•flex ar•ter•y (mē′dē-ăl fem′ŏr-ăl sĭr′kŭm-fleks ahr′tĕr-ē) SYN medial circumflex femoral artery.

me•di•al fore•brain bun•dle (mē′dē-ăl fōr′brān bŭn′dĕl) A fiber system coursing longitudinally through the lateral zone of the hypothalamus, connecting the latter reciprocally with the midbrain tegmentum and with various components of the limbic system; it also carries fibers from norepinephrine-containing and serotonin-containing cell groups in the brainstem to the hypothalamus and cerebral cortex, as well as dopamine-carrying fibers from the substantia nigra to the caudate nucleus and putamen.

me•di•al ge•nic•u•late bod•y (mē′dē-ăl je-nik′yū-lāt bod′ē) The medial one of a pair of prominent cell groups in the posteroinferior parts of the thalamus; it functions as the last of a series of processing stations along the auditory conduction pathway to the cerebral cortex, receiving the brachium of the inferior colliculus and giving rise to the auditory radiation to the auditory cortex in the superior temporal gyrus.

med•i•al•i•za•tion (mē′dē-ăl-ī-zā′shŭn) An operation to move a part toward the midline, such as the arytenoid cartilage or vocal cord, in vocal cord paralysis.

me•di•al lig•a•ment (mē′dē-ăl lig′ă-mĕnt) The bundle of fibers strengthening the medial part of the articular capsule of the temporomandibular joint.

me•di•al lon•gi•tud•in•al fas•cic•u•lus (MLF) (mē′dē-ăl lon′ji-tū′di-nal fă-sik′kyū-lŭs) Pathway in the brainstem that connects the vestibular system with the cranial nerves that serve the eye muscles (e.g., CNs III, IV, VI).

me•di•al med•ul•lar•y la•mi•na of len•ti•form nu•cle•us (mē′dē-ăl med′ŭ-lar′ē lam′i-nă len′ti-fōrm nū′klē-ŭs) A fiber layer separating the medial and lateral segments of the globus pallidus. SYN lamina medullaris medialis nuclei lentiformis [TA].

me•di•al me•nis•cus (mē′dē-ăl mĕ-nis′kŭs) Attached to the medial border of the upper articular surface of the tibia. See this page.

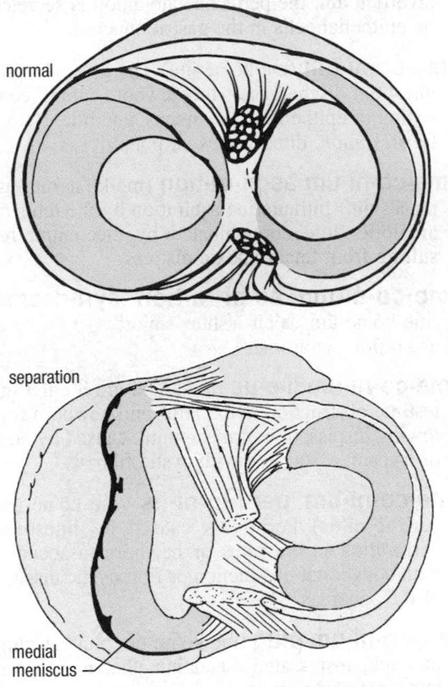

marginal separation of medial meniscus: right knee (normal menisci shown for comparison)

me•di•al oc•cip•i•tal ar•ter•y (mēd′dē-ăl ok-sip′i-tăl ahr′tĕr-ē) One of the terminal branches of the posterior cerebral artery; it is distributed, by several named branches, to the posterior corpus callosum and the medial and superolateral portions of the occipital lobe including the visual cortex.

me•di•al pec•tor•al nerve (mē′dē-al pek′tŏr-ăl nĕrv) Arises from medial cord of brachial plexus to supply pectoral muscles; usually pierces pectoralis minor, then continues to supply mainly the sternocostal portion of pectoralis major. SYN medial anterior thoracic nerve, nervus pectoralis medialis.

me•di•al plan•tar ar•ter•y (mē′dē-ăl plan′tahr ahr′tĕr-ē) One of the terminal branches of the posterior tibial; *distribution*, medial side of the sole of the foot; *anastomoses*, dorsalis pedis, lateral plantar. SYN arteria plantaris medialis.

me•di•al plan•tar nerve (mē′dē-ăl plan′tahr nĕrv) One of two terminal branches of the tibial nerve; courses along medial aspect of sole to supply abductor hallucis and flexor digitorum brevis and, by way of common and proper digital branches, to innervate skin of medial part of foot and medial 3-1/2 toes. SYN nervus plantaris medialis.

me•di•al pter•y•goid mus•cle (mē′dē-ăl ter′i-goyd mŭs′ĕl) Masticatory muscle of infratemporal fossa; *origin*, pterygoid fossa of sphenoid and tuberosity of maxilla; *insertion*, medial surface of mandible between angle and mylohyoid groove; *action*, elevates mandible closing jaw; *nerve supply*, nerve to medial pterygoid from mandibular division of trigeminal. SYN internal pterygoid muscle, musculus pterygoideus internus, musculus pterygoideus medialis.

me•di•al rec•tus mus•cle (mē′dē-ăl rek′tŭs mŭs′ĕl) *Origin*, medial part of the anulus tendineus communis; *insertion*, medial part of sclera of the eye; *action*, adduction; *nerve supply*, oculomotor. SYN musculus rectus medialis [TA].

me•di•al ro•ta•tion (mē′dē-ăl rō-tā′shŭn) SYN internal rotation.

me•di•al su•pra•cla•vic•u•lar nerve (me′dē-ăl sū′pra-klă-vĭk′yū-lar nĕrv) One of several nerves arising from C3–C4 loop of cervical plexus that supply skin over medial end of clavicle and upper medial part of thorax. SYN anterior supraclavicular nerve, nervus supraclavicularis medialis.

me•di•al vas•tus mus•cle (mē′dē-ăl vas′tŭs mŭs′ĕl) SYN vastus medialis muscle.

me•di•an (mē′dē-ăn) **1.** Central; middle; lying in the midline. **2.** The middle value in a set of measurements; like the mean, a measure of central tendency. [L. *medianus*, middle]

me•di•an an•te•brach•i•al vein (mē′dē-ăn an′ti-brā′kē-ăl vān) It begins at the base of the dorsum of the thumb, curves around the radial side, ascends the middle of the forearm, and just below the bend of the elbow divides into the intermediate basilic and intermediate cephalic veins; sometimes it divides lower down, one branch going to the basilic vein, the other to the intermediate vein of the elbow.

me•di•an ap•er•ture of fourth ven•tri•cle (mē-dē′ăn ap′ĕr-chŭr fōrth ven′tri-kĕl) The large midline opening in the posterior inferior part of the roof of the fourth ventricle, connecting the ventricle with the posterior cerebellomedullary cistern. SYN apertura mediana ventriculi quarti [TA].

me•di•an ar•ter•y (mē′dē-ăn ahr′tĕr-ē) *Origin*, anterior interosseous; *distribution*, accompanies median nerve to palm; *anastomoses*, branches of superficial palmar arch. SYN arteria mediana, comitant artery of median nerve.

me•di•an ax•il•lar•y line (mē′dē-ăn ak′si-lar-ē līn) [TA] SYN midaxillary line.

me•di•an cu•bi•tal vein (mē′dē-ăn kyū′bi-tăl vān) Passes across the anterior aspect of the elbow from the cephalic vein to the basilic vein; commonly this vein is replaced by intermediate basilic and intermediate cephalic veins. The median cubital vein is often used for venipuncture.

me•di•an ef•fec•tive dose (ED_{50}) (mē′dē-ăn e-fekt′iv dōs) SEE effective dose.

me•di•an e•pi•si•ot•o•my (mē′dē-ăn ĕ-piz′ē-ot′ŏ-mē) SYN midline episiotomy.

me•di•an groove of tongue (mē-dē′ăn grūv tŭng) Median groove or median longitudinal raphe of tongue; raphe linguae; a slight longitudinal depression running forward on the dorsal surface of the tongue from the foramen cecum.

me•di•an ling•ual swell•ing (mē′dē-ăn ling′gwăl swel′ling) A smooth swelling in the midline of the floor of the primordial mouth between the first and second pharyngeal arches; it is incorporated into the tongue but forms no recognizable part of it. SYN median tongue bud, tuberculum impar.

i **me•di•an nerve** (mē′dē-ăn nĕrv) Formed by the union of medial and lateral roots from the medial and lateral cords of the brachial plexus, respectively; it supplies all the muscles in the anterior compartment of the forearm with the exception of the flexor carpi ulnaris and ulnar half of the flexor digitorum profundus; it passes through the carpal tunnel to supply the thenar muscles (except adductor pollicis and the deep head of flexor pollicis brevis) via its recurrent thenar branch; its sensory fibers are distributed to the skin of the palmar and distal dorsal aspects of the radial three-and-a-half digits and adjacent palm. The median nerve is most commonly injured through compression in carpal tunnel syndrome, resulting in a loss of ability to oppose the thumb (thus creating "ape hand") and loss of sensation over the radial portion of the hand. See page 954.

me•di•an plane (mē′dē-ăn plān) A vertical plane through the midline of the body that divides the body into right and left halves. SYN midsagittal plane.

me•di•an rhi•nos•co•py (mē′dē-ăn rī-nos′kŏ-pē) Inspection of the roof of the nasal cavity and openings of the posterior ethmoid cells and sphenoidal sinus by means of a long-bladed nasal speculum or nasopharyngoscope.

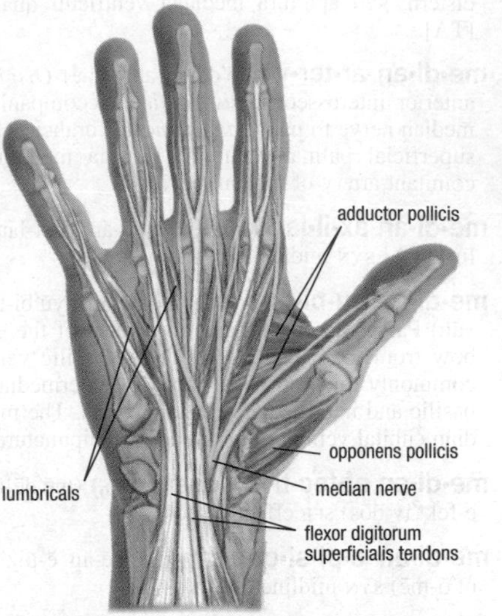

median nerve

me·di·an rhom·boid glos·si·tis (mē′dē-ăn rom′boyd glŏs-ī′tis) An asymptomatic, ovoid or rhomboid, macular or mamillated, erythematous lesion with papillary atrophy on the dorsum of the tongue just anterior to the circumvallate papillae; usually results from infection by *Candida albicans*.

me·di·an sa·cral crest (mē-dē′ăn sā′krăl krest) An unpaired crest formed by the fused spinous processes of the upper four sacral vertebrae.

me·di·an sa·cral vein (mē′dē-ăn sā′krăl vān) An unpaired vein accompanying the middle sacral artery receiving blood from the sacral venous plexus and emptying into the left common iliac vein.

me·di·an sec·tion (mē′dē-ăn sek′shŭn) A cross-section obtained by slicing in the median plane, actually or through imaging techniques, the body or any part of the body that occupies or crosses the median plane or by slicing any generally symmetric anatomic structure, such as a finger or a cell, in its midline. Because actual sectioning the median plane results in a right and a left half, an anatomical median section may be a two-dimensional view of the cut surface on the medial aspect of either half.

me·di·ant (mē′dē-ănt) In the middle of a range or process.

me·di·an tongue bud (mē′dē-ăn tŭng bŭd) SYN median lingual swelling.

me·di·as·ti·nal (mē′dē-as-tī′năl) Relating to the mediastinum.

me·di·as·ti·nal em·phy·se·ma (mē′dē-ă-stin′ăl em′fi-sē′mă) Deflection of air, usually from a ruptured emphysematous bleb in the lung, into the mediastinal tissue.

me·di·as·ti·nal fi·bro·sis (mē′dē-ă-stin′ăl fī-brō′sis) Fibrosis that may obstruct the superior vena cava, pulmonary arteries, veins, or bronchi; most common cause is histoplasmosis; less commonly tuberculosis or unknown.

me·di·as·ti·nal space (mē′dē-ă-stin′ăl spās) SYN mediastinum (2).

me·di·as·ti·nal veins (mē′dē-ă-stin′ăl vānz) Several small veins from the mediastinum emptying into the brachiocephalic veins or the superior vena cava.

me·di·as·ti·ni·tis (mē′dē-as-ti-nī′tis) Inflammation of the cellular tissue of the mediastinum.

me·di·as·ti·nog·ra·phy (mē′dē-as-ti-nog′ră-fē) Radiography of the mediastinum. [mediastinum + G. *graphō,* to write]

me·di·as·ti·no·per·i·car·di·tis (mē′dē-ă-stinō-per′i-kar-dī′tis) Inflammation of the pericardium and of the surrounding mediastinal cellular tissue.

me·di·as·tin·o·scope (mē′dē-as′tī-nō-skōp) An endoscope for inspection of mediastinum through a suprasternal incision.

me·di·as·ti·nos·co·py (mē′dē-as′ti-nos′kō-pē) Exploration of the mediastinum through a suprasternal incision, for biopsy of paratracheal lymph nodes. [mediastinum + G. *skopeō,* to view]

me·di·as·ti·not·o·my (mē′dē-as′ti-not′ŏ-mē) Incision into the mediastinum. [mediastinum + G. *tomē,* incision]

me·di·as·ti·num (me′dē-ă-stī′nŭm) [TA] **1.** A septum between two parts of an organ or a cavity. **2.** The median partition of the thoracic cavity, covered by the mediastinal part of the parietal pleura and containing all the thoracic viscera and structures except the lungs. It is divided arbitrarily into two major divisions: a superior mediastinum (mediastinum superius [TA]), which lies directly superior to a horizontal plane intersecting the sternal angle and approximately the T4–5 intervertebral disc, and an inferior mediastinum (mediastinum inferius [TA]) inferior to that plane; the latter is, in turn, subdivided in 3 parts: a middle mediastinum (mediastinum medium [TA]), which is coterminous with the pericardial sac containing the heart, a nearly potential anterior mediastinum (mediastinum anterius [TA]) lying in front, and a posterior mediastinum (mediastinum posterius [TA]) behind, containing the esophagus, descending aorta, and thoracic duct. SYN interpleural space, mediastinal space. [Mod. L. a middle septum, fr. Mediev. L. *mediastinus,* medial, fr. L. *mediastinus,* a lower servant, fr. *medius,* middle]

me·di·as·ti·num tes·tis (me′dē-ă-stī′nŭm tes′

tis) [TA] A mass of fibrous tissue continuous with the tunica albuginea, projecting into the testis from its posterior border. SYN Highmore body.

me•di•ate **1.** (mē′dē-it) Situated between; intermediate. **2.** (mē′dē-āt) To effect something by means of an intermediary substance, as in complement-mediated phagocytosis. [L. *mediatus,* fr. *medio,* pp. *-atus,* to divide in the middle]

me•di•ate aus•cul•ta•tion (mē′dē-at aws′kŭl-tā′shŭn) Listening to body sounds with a stethoscope.

me•di•at•ed trans•port (mē′dē-ā-tĕd trans′pōrt) Movement of a solution across a membrane with the aid of a transport agent (e.g., protein).

me•di•ate per•cus•sion (mē′dē-at pĕr-kŭsh′ŭn) Percussion effected by the intervention of a finger or a plessimeter between the striking finger or plessor and the part percussed.

me•di•a•tor com•plex (mē′dē-ā-tōr kom′pleks) Coactivation proteins involved in RNA polymerase transcription of DNA segments.

med•i•ca•ble (med′i-kă-bĕl) Treatable, with hope of a cure.

Med•i•caid (medi′i-kād) A nationwide health insurance program in the U.S. that provides coverage to certain low-income citizens and qualified legal residents; funded jointly by the state and federal governments, the program has federal guidelines that give the individual states wide discretion to determine eligibility and to set benefits; established in 1965 by an amendment to the Social Security Act. Cf. Medicare (1).

med•i•cal (med′i-kăl) **1.** Relating to medicine or the practice of medicine. SYN medicinal (2). **2.** SYN medicinal (1). [L. *medicalis,* fr *medicus,* physician]

med•i•cal as•sis•tant (med′i-kăl ă-sis′tănt) A person who supports a physician or other health care provider by performing administrative and clinical tasks.

med•i•cal cas•tra•tion (med′kăl kas-trā′shŭn) SYN functional castration.

med•i•cal di•a•ther•my (med′i-kăl dī′ă-thĕr-mē) Diathermy of mild degree causing no destruction of tissue.

med•i•cal di•rec•tor (med′i-kăl di-rek′tŏr) **1.** A physician designated by an emergency medical service (EMS) system or service to provide medical oversight. Advanced level prehospital providers usually function under the medical license of the medical director. **2.** A physician designated by an educational program or institution to provide medical oversight of an EMS education program or course.

med•i•cal er•ror (med′kăl er′ŏr) In nursing usage, any failure to implement a planned action as intended or the implementation of the wrong nursing plan.

med•i•cal eth•ics (med′i-kăl eth′iks) The moral conduct and principles that govern members of the medical profession.

med•i•cal ex•am•in•er (ME) (med′i-kăl eg-zam′in-ĕr) **1.** A physician who examines a person and reports on that person's physical condition to the company or individual at whose request the examination was made. **2.** In states or municipalities where the office of coroner has been abolished, a physician appointed to investigate all cases of sudden, violent, or suspicious death.

med•i•cal ge•net•ics (med′i-kăl jĕ-net′iks) The study of the etiology, pathogenesis, and natural history of human diseases that are at least partially genetic in origin. Cf. clinical genetics, human genetics.

med•i•cal in•sur•ance (med′i-kăl in-shūr′ăns) SYN health insurance.

med•i•cal in•ten•sive care u•nit (MICU) (med′i-kăl in-ten′siv kār yū′nit) Hospital unit designated for care of critically ill patients with nonsurgical conditions.

med•i•cal•i•za•tion (med′i-kăl-ī-zā′shŭn) Process by which life problems become articulated as health or mental health conditions.

med•i•cal lan•guage spe•cial•ist (MLS) (med′i-kăl lang′gwăj spesh′i-list) One who interprets dictation by physicians and other health care providers and converts it into printed format to provide a permanent record of patient care.

med•i•cal•ly nec•es•sar•y (med′i-kăl-ē nes′ĕ-sar-ē) Services or supplies needed for diagnosis, treatment, or care.

med•i•cal mod•el (med′i-kăl mod′ĕl) The traditional approach to the diagnosis and treatment of illness as practiced by physicians in the Western world; focuses on the defect or dysfunction.

med•i•cal psy•chol•o•gy (med′i-kăl sī-kol′ŏ-jē) The branch of psychology concerned with the application of psychological principles to the practice of medicine; the application of clinical psychology or clinical health psychology, usually in a hospital setting.

med•i•cal rec•ord (med′i-kăl rek′ŏrd) SEE record (1).

med•i•cal re•view of•fi•cer (MRO) (med′i-kal rĕ-vyū′ awf′i-sĕr) A physician trained and certified to review and analyze substance abuse testing results.

Med•i•cal Sub•ject Head•ings (MeSH) (med′i-kăl sŭb′jekt hed′ings) A huge controlled vocabulary (or metadata system) for the purpose of indexing journal articles and books in the life sciences. Created and updated by the United States National Library of Medicine (NLM), it is used by the MEDLINE article database and by NLM's catalog of book holdings. MeSH can be browsed and downloaded free of charge on the Internet; a printed version is published once a year.

med•i•cal tran•scrip•tion•ist (med′i-kăl tran-skrip′shŭn′ist) A person who performs machine transcription of physician-dictated medical records; a certified medical transcriptionist (CMT) has satisfied the requirements for certification by the American Association for Medical Transcription (AAMT).

med•i•cal tran•scrip•tion ser•vice (med′i-kăl tran-skrip′shŭn sĕr′vis) A business that contracts with physicians or health care facilities to transcribe dictated health care records.

Med•i•care (med′i-kār) **1.** A national health insurance plan managed by the U.S. government that covers Social Security and Railroad Retirement beneficiaries age 65 years and older, people who have been entitled for at least 24 months to receive Social Security or Railroad Retirement disability benefits, and certain people with end-stage renal disease; established in 1965 by an amendment to the Social Security Act. Cf. Medicaid. **2.** The universal public health insurance system of Canada, administered by the provincial governments under guidelines set by the Canadian federal government; initiated under the Canada Health Act in 1984. **3.** A national public health insurance system in Australia; provides for free care in public hospitals, and free or subsidized care in clinical settings for certain conditions; established in 1984.

Med•i•care Part A (mĕd′i-kār pahrt) The portion of the U.S. Medicare Program that covers inpatient hospital stays, skilled nursing facility care, hospice care, and some home health care.

Med•i•care Part B (med′i-kār pahrt) The portion of the U.S. Medicare Program that helps pay for physician services, outpatient hospital care, durable medical equipment, and some services not covered by Medicare Part A.

med•i•cate (med′i-kāt) **1.** To treat disease by the giving of drugs. **2.** To impregnate with a medicinal substance. [L. *medico,* pp. *-atus,* to heal]

med•i•ca•tion (med′i-kā′shŭn) **1.** The act of medicating. **2.** A medicinal substance or medicament.

med•i•ca•tion er•ror (med′i-kā′shŭn er′ŏr) Incorrect administration of a medication. May be due to incorrect dosage, drug, patient, time or route of administration, or interaction between incompatible medications.

med•i•ca•tion rec•on•cil•i•a•tion (med′i-kā′shŭn rek′ŏn-sil′ē-ā′shŭn) The process of comparing medications that the patient is taking with medications that the health care facility is about to provide so as to avoid harmful interactions.

me•dic•i•nal (mĕ-dis′i-năl) **1.** Relating to medicine having curative properties. SYN medical (2). **2.** SYN medical (1).

med•i•cine (med′i-sin) **1.** A drug. **2.** The art of preventing, diagnosing, and treating disease; the science concerned with disease in all its aspects. **3.** The study and treatment of general diseases or those affecting the internal parts of the body, especially those not usually requiring surgical intervention. [L. *medicina,* fr. *medicus,* physician]

♻ **medico-** Combining form meaning medical. Cf. iatro-. [L. *medicus,* physician]

med•i•co•chi•rur•gi•cal (med′i-kō-kī-rŭr′ji-kăl) Relating to both medicine and surgery, or to both physicians and surgeons. [medico- G. *cheirourgia,* surgery]

med•i•co•le•gal (med′i-kō-lē′găl) Relating to both medicine and the law. SEE ALSO forensic medicine. [medico- + L. *legalis,* legal]

Med•i•gap in•sur•ance (med′i-gap in-shŭr′ăns) A supplemental insurance policy designed to fill the "gap," that is, any care or services not covered under the Medicare program. SYN supplemental insurance.

♻ **medio-, medi-** Combining forms meaning middle, median. [L. *medius*]

me•di•o•car•pal (mē′dē-ō-kahr′păl) SYN midcarpal.

me•di•o•dor•sal (mē′dē-ō-dōr′săl) Relating to the median plane and the dorsal plane.

me•di•o•lat•er•al (mē′dē-ō-lat′ĕr-ăl) Relating to the median plane and a side.

me•di•o•ne•cro•sis (mē′dē-ō-nĕ-krō′sis) Necrosis of a tunica media.

me•di•o•tar•sal am•pu•ta•tion (mē′dē-ō-tahr′săl amp′yū-tā′shŭn) SYN Chopart amputation.

med•i•ta•tion (med′i-tā′shŭn) Any mental activity intended to keep the practitioner's attention in the present; has been used for several thousand years to balance physical, emotional, and mental states; sometimes employed as part of overall therapy for diverse medical conditions (e.g., providing pain relief, lowering blood pressure).

Med•i•ter•ra•ne•an di•et (med′i-tĕr-ā′nē-ăn dī′ĕt) A diet rich in grains, fruits, vegetables, and olive oil with small amounts of meat and poultry.

Med•i•ter•ra•ne•an er•y•the•ma•tous fe•ver (med′i-tĕ-rā′nē-ăn er′i-them′ă-tŭs fē′vĕr) A malignant form of Mediterranean spotted fever that causes skin redness; its course and other symptoms may be similar to those of Mediterranean exanthematous fever. SEE *Rickettsia conorii.*

Med•i•ter•ra•ne•an ex•an•them•a•tous fe•ver (med′i-tĕ-rā′nē-ăn ek′san-them′ă-tŭs fē′vĕr)

An affliction occurring sporadically in the Mediterranean littoral marked by a severe chill with abrupt rise of temperature, pain in the joints, tonsillitis, diarrhea, vomiting, and, on the 3rd–5th day, a rash of elevated nonconfluent macules beginning on the thighs and spreading to the entire body; lasts from 10 days–2 weeks and then disappears by rapid lysis without desquamation; probably caused by *Rickettsia conorii*, like Boutonneuse fever.

Med•i•ter•ra•ne•an spot•ted fe•ver (med′i-tĕ-rā′nē-ăn spot′ĕd fē′vĕr) Tick-borne infection with *Rickettsia conorii* seen in Africa, Europe, the Middle East, and India and known by different names in different areas, (e.g., Marseilles fever, Crimean fever, Indian tick typhus, and Kenya fever). Two forms are Mediterranean exanthematous fever, which manifests as skin eruptions, and Mediterranean erythematous fever, which manifests as skin redness. SEE ALSO *Rickettsia conorii.*

me•di•um, pl. **me•di•a** (mē′dē-ŭm, -ă) **1.** A means; that through which an action is performed. **2.** A substance through which impulses or impressions are transmitted. **3.** SYN culture medium. **4.** The liquid holding a substance in solution or suspension. [L. neuter of *medius,* middle]

me•di•um-heav•y work (mē′dē-ŭm-hev′ē wŏrk) A physical demand level described as the exertion of up to 75 pounds of force occasionally, or up to 35 pounds of force frequently, or 15 pounds of force constantly to move objects. SEE ALSO very heavy work.

me•di•um work (mē′dē-ŭm wŏrk) A physical demand level described as the exertion of up to 50 pounds of force occasionally, or up to 20 pounds of force frequently, or 10 pounds of force constantly to move objects. SEE ALSO sedentary work, light work, medium-heavy work, very heavy work.

MEDLARS (med′lahrz) Medical Literature Analysis and Retrieval System, a computerized system of databases and databanks maintained by the U.S. National Library of Medicine.

MEDLINE (med′līn) An early Internet database devoted to global coverage of biomedical literature; accessible through MEDSCAPE. [fr. MEDLARS online]

MEDLINEplus (med′līn-plŭs) Website with extensive and authoritative health information from National Library of Medicine and National Institutes of Health; links to Web resources with health care information.

me•dul•la, pl. **me•dul•lae** (mĕ-dŭl′ă, -ē) Any soft marrowlike structure, especially in the center of a part. SEE ALSO medulla oblongata. SYN substantia medullaris (1). [L. marrow, fr. *medius,* middle]

me•dul•la of hair shaft (mĕ-dŭl′ă hār shaft) The central axis of some hairs, containing a column of large vacuolated and keratinized cells; the medullary portion is surrounded by the cortex.

me•dul•la of lymph node (mĕ-dŭl′ă limf nōd) The central portion of a node consisting of cordlike masses of lymphocytes, plasma cells, and macrophages in a stroma of reticular fibers separated by lymph sinuses; it reaches the surface of the node at the hilum.

me•dul•la ob•lon•ga•ta (mĕ-dŭl′ă ob-long-gah′tă) [TA] The most caudal subdivision of the brainstem, continuous with the spinal cord, extending from the lower border of the decussation of the pyramid to the pons; its ventral surface resembles that of the spinal cord except for the bilateral prominence of the inferior olive; the dorsal surface of its upper half forms part of the floor of the fourth ventricle. Motor nuclei of the medulla oblongata include the hypoglossal nucleus, the dorsal motor nucleus, inferior salivatory nucleus, and the nucleus ambiguus; sensory nuclei include the nuclei of the posterior column (gracile and cuneate), the cochlear and vestibular nuclei, the mid and caudal portions of the spinal trigeminal nucleus, and the nucleus of the solitary tract. SEE ALSO medulla. SYN myelencephalon, oblongata.

me•dul•lar (me-dŭl′ăr) SYN medullary.

med•ul•lar•y (med′ŭ-lar′ē) Relating to the medulla or marrow. SYN medullar.

med•ul•lar•y ar•ter•ies of brain (med′ŭ-lar′ē ahr′tĕrēz brān) Branches of the cortical arteries that penetrate to and supply the white matter of the cerebrum.

med•ul•lar•y car•ci•no•ma (med′ŭ-lar′ē kahr′si-nō′mă) A malignant neoplasm, comparatively soft and brainlike in consistency, which consists chiefly of neoplastic epithelial cells, with only a scant amount of fibrous stroma.

med•ul•lar•y car•ci•no•ma of breast (med′ŭ-lar′ē kahr′si-nō′mă brest) A subtype of breast carcinoma composed of sheets of large epithelial cells surrounded by scant fibrous stroma; it is soft and well circumscribed and has a better prognosis than invasive ductal carcinoma.

med•ul•lar•y car•ci•no•ma of thy•roid (med′ŭ-lar′ē kahr′si-nō′mă thī′royd) A malignant thyroid neoplasm composed of calcitonin producing C-cells and amyloid rich stroma; it may be sporadic or familial; the familial form may be part of the multiple endocrine neoplasia syndrome, types 2A and 2B.

med•ul•lar•y cav•i•ty (med′ŭ-lar′ē kav′i-tē) The marrow cavity in the shaft of a long bone.

med•ul•lar•y cone (med′ŭ-lar′ē kōn) The tapering lower extremity of the spinal cord. SYN conus medullaris [TA].

med•ul•lar•y la•mi•nae of thal•am•us

(med′ŭ-lar′ē lam′i-nē thal′ă-mŭs) Layers of myelinated fibers that appear on transverse sections of the thalamus; the lamina medullaris lateralis [TA] (external medullary lamina) marks the ventral and lateral borders of the thalamus and delimits it from the subthalamus and reticular nucleus of thalamus; the lamina medullaris medialis [TA] (internal medullary lamina) is interposed between the mediodorsal and ventral nuclei of the thalamus and encloses the intralaminar nuclei (centromedian, paracentral, and central lateral nuclei).

med•ul•lar•y mem•brane (med′ŭ-lar′ē mem′brān) SYN endosteum.

med•ul•lar•y plate (med′ŭ-lar′ē plāt) SYN neural plate.

med•ul•lar•y pyr•a•mid (med′ŭ-lar′ē pir′ă-mid) SYN renal pyramid.

med•ul•lar•y ray (med′ŭ-lar′ē rā) The center of the renal lobule, which has the shape of a small, steep pyramid, consisting of straight tubular parts; these may be either ascending or descending limbs of the nephronic loop or collecting tubules. SYN Ferrein pyramid.

med•ul•lar•y space (med′ŭ-lar′ē spās) The central cavity and the cellular intervals between the trabeculae of bone, filled with marrow.

med•ul•lar•y spi•nal ar•ter•ies (med′ŭ-lar′ē spī′năl ahr′tĕr-ēz) SYN segmental medullary arteries.

med•ul•lar•y sponge kid•ney (med′ŭ-lar′-ē spŏnj kid′nē) Cystic disease of the renal pyramids associated with calculus formation and hematuria; differs from cystic disease of the renal medulla in that renal failure does not usually develop.

med•ul•lar•y stri•ae of fourth ven•tri•cle (med′ŭ-lar′ē strī′ē fōrth ven′tri-kĕl) Slender fascicles of fibers extending transversely below the ependymal floor of the ventricle from the median sulcus to enter the inferior cerebellar peduncle. They arise from the arcuate nuclei on the ventral surface of the medullary pyramid.

med•ul•lar•y stri•a of thal•a•mus (med′ŭ-lar′ē strīă thal′ă-mŭs) A narrow, compact fiber bundle that extends along the line of attachment of the roof of the third ventricle to the thalamus on each side and terminates posteriorly in the habenular nucleus. It is composed of fibers originating in the septal area, the anterior perforated substance, the lateral preoptic nucleus, and the medial segment of the globus pallidus.

med•ul•lar•y sub•stance (med′ŭ-lar′ē sŭb′stăns) **1.** The lipid material present in the myelin sheath of nerve fibers. **2.** Medulla of bones and other organs. SYN substantia medullaris (2).

me•dul•la spi•na•lis (mĕ-dŭl′ă spī-nā′lis) SYN spinal cord.

med•ul•lat•ed (med′ŭ-lā-tĕd) **1.** Having a medulla or medullary substance. **2.** SYN myelinated.

med•ul•lec•to•my (med′yū-lek′tŏ-mē) Excision of any medullary substance. [medulla + G. *ektomē,* excision]

med•ul•li•za•tion (med′ŭ-lī-zā′shŭn) Enlargement of the medullary spaces in rarefying osteitis.

♻ **medullo-** Combining form indicating the medulla. Cf. myel-. [L. *medulla*]

me•dul•lo•ar•thri•tis (mĕ-dŭl′ō-ar-thrī′tis) Inflammation of the cancellous articular extremity of a long bone.

me•dul•lo•blas•to•ma (mĕ-dŭl′ō-blas-tō′mă) A tumor consisting of neoplastic cells that resemble the undifferentiated cells of the primitive medullary tube; medulloblastomas are usually located in the vermis of the cerebellum, comprise approximately 3% of all intracranial neoplasms, and occur most frequently in children.

me•dul•lo•ep•i•the•li•o•ma (mĕ-dŭl′ō-ep′i-thē′lē-ō-′mă) A rare, primitive, rapidly growing intracranial neoplasm thought to originate from the cells of the embryonic medullary canal. [medullo- + epithelium + *-oma,* tumor]

Me•du•sa's head (mĕ-dū′săz hed) SYN caput medusae.

Mees line (māz līn) A horizontal white band of the nails seen in chronic arsenical poisoning, and occasionally in leprosy.

♻ **mega-** **1.** Combining form meaning large, oversize; opposite of micro-. SEE ALSO macro-, megalo-. **2.** Prefix used in the SI and metric systems to signify one million (10^6). [G. *megas,* big]

meg•a•bac•te•ri•um (meg′ă-bak-tēr′ē-ŭm) A bacterium of unusually large size.

me•ga•blad•der (meg′ă-blad-ĕr) SYN megacystis.

meg•a•ce•phal•ic (meg′ă-se-fal′ik) Relating to or characterized by megacephaly. SYN macrocephalic, macrocephalous, megacephalous.

meg•a•ceph•a•lous (meg′ă-sef′ă-lŭs) SYN megacephalic.

meg•a•ceph•a•ly (meg′ă-sef′ă-lē) A condition, either congenital or acquired, in which the head is abnormally large; usually applied to an adult cranium with a capacity of over 1450 mL. SYN macrocephaly, macrocephalia, megalocephaly, megalocephalia. [mega- + G. *kephalē,* head]

meg•a•co•lon (meg′ă-kō-lŏn) A condition of extreme dilation and hypertrophy of the colon.

meg•a•cy•cle (meg′ă-sī-kĕl) One million cycles per second.

meg•a•cys•tic syn•drome (meg′ă-sis′tik sin′

drōm) A combination of a large smooth thin-walled bladder, vesicoureteral regurgitation, and dilated ureters.

meg·a·cys·tis (meg′ă-sis′tis) Pathologically large bladder in children. SYN megabladder, megalocystis. [mega- + *kystis,* bladder]

meg·a·dac·ty·ly, **meg·a·dac·tyl·i·a, meg·a·dac·tyl·ism** (meg′ă-dak′ti-lē, -dak-til′ē-ă, -dak′ti-lizm) Condition characterized by enlargement of one or more digits (fingers or toes). SYN dactylomegaly. [mega- + G. *daktylos,* digit]

meg·a·don·tism (meg′ă-don′tizm) SYN macrodontia.

meg·a·dose (meg′ă-dōs) A very large or maximum dose beyond the known therapeutic range.

meg·a·e·soph·a·gus (meg′ă-e-sof′ă-gŭs) Great enlargement of the lower portion of the esophagus, as seen in patients with achalasia and Chagas disease. SYN mega-oesophagus.

meg·a·hertz (MHz) (meg′ă-hĕrts) One million hertz (Hz).

meg·a·kar·y·o·blast (meg-ă-kar′ē-ō-blast) The precursor of a megakaryocyte.

meg·a·kar·y·o·cyte (meg-ă-kar′ē-ō-sīt) A large cell with a multilobed nucleus; normally present in bone marrow, not in the circulating blood; gives rise to blood platelets (thrombocytes). SYN megalokaryocyte. [mega- + G. *karyon,* nut (nucleus), + *kytos,* hollow vessel (cell)]

meg·a·kar·y·o·cyte growth and de·vel·op·ment fac·tor (meg-ă-kar′ē-ō-sīt grōth dĕ-vel′ŏp-mĕnt fak′tŏr) SYN thrombopoietin.

meg·a·kar·y·o·cyt·ic leu·ke·mi·a (meg′ă-kar′ē-ō-sit′ik lū-kē′mē-ă) An unusual form of myelopoietic disease that is characterized by uncontrolled proliferation of megakaryocytes in the bone marrow, and sometimes by the presence of megakaryocytes in the blood.

meg·al·gi·a (meg-al′jē-ă) Very severe pain. [mega- + G. *algos,* pain]

♻ **megalo-**, **megal-** Combining forms meaning large; opposite of micro-. SEE ALSO macro-, mega-. [G. *megas* (*megal-*)]

meg·a·lo·blast (meg′ă-lō-blast) A large, nucleated, embryonic type of cell that is a precursor of erythrocytes in an abnormal erythropoietic process observed in pernicious anemia; a megaloblast's four stages of development are: 1) promegaloblast, 2) basophilic megaloblast, 3) polychromatic megaloblast, and 4) orthochromatic megaloblast. SEE ALSO erythroblast. [megalo- + G. *blastos,* + germ, sprout]

meg·a·lo·blas·tic a·ne·mi·a (meg′ă-lō-blast′ik ă-nē′mē-ă) Any anemia in which there is a predominant number of megaloblastic erythroblasts, and relatively few normoblasts, among the hyperplastic erythroid cells in the bone marrow (as in pernicious anemia).

meg·a·lo·car·di·a (meg′ă-lō-kahr′dē-ă) SYN cardiomegaly. [megalo- + G. *kardia,* heart]

meg·a·lo·ceph·a·ly, **meg·a·lo·ce·pha·li·a** (meg′ă-lō-sef′ă-lē, -sĕ-fā′lē-ă) SYN megacephaly.

meg·a·lo·chei·ri·a, **meg·a·lo·chi·ri·a** (meg′ă-lō-kī′rē-ă) SYN macrocheiria. [megalo- + G. *cheir,* hand]

meg·a·lo·cys·tis (meg′ă-lō-sis′tis) SYN megacystis. [megalo- + G. *kystis,* bladder]

meg·a·lo·cyte (meg′ă-lō-sīt) A large (i.e., 10–20 mcm) nonnucleated red blood cell. [megalo- + G. *kytos,* cell]

meg·a·lo·don·ti·a (meg′ă-lō-don′shē-ă) SYN macrodontia.

meg·a·lo·en·ce·phal·ic (meg′ă-lō-en′se-fal′ik) Denoting an abnormally large brain.

meg·a·lo·en·ceph·a·lon (meg′ă-lō-en-sef′ă-lon) An abnormally large brain. [megalo- + G. *enkephalos,* brain]

meg·a·lo·en·ceph·a·ly (meg′ă-lō-en-sef′ă-lē) Abnormal largeness of the brain. [megalo- + G. *enkephalon,* brain]

meg·a·lo·en·ter·on (meg′ă-lō-en′tĕr-on) Abnormal largeness of the intestine. SYN enteromegaly, enteromegalia. [megalo- + G. *enteron,* intestine]

meg·a·lo·gas·tri·a (meg′ă-lō-gas′trē-ă) Abnormally large size of the stomach. [megalo- + G. *gastēr,* stomach]

meg·a·lo·glos·si·a (meg′ă-lō-glos′sē-ă) SYN macroglossia. [megalo- + G. *glōssa,* tongue]

meg·a·lo·he·pat·i·a (meg′ă-lō-hē-pat′ē-ă) SYN hepatomegaly.

meg·a·lo·kar·y·o·cyte (meg′ă-lō-kar′ē-ō-sīt) SYN megakaryocyte.

meg·a·lo·ma·ni·a (meg′ă-lō-mā′nē-ă) **1.** A delusion of greatness; e.g., belief that one is Christ, God, Napoleon, a prince, or an ace athlete in all divisions of sport. **2.** Morbid verbalized over-evaluation of oneself or of some aspect of oneself. [megalo- + G. *mania,* frenzy]

meg·a·lo·ma·ni·ac, **me·ga·lo·ma·ni·a·cal** (meg′ă-lō-mā′nē-ak, -mă-nī′ă-kăl) A person exhibiting megalomania.

meg·a·lo·me·li·a (meg′ă-lō-mē′lē-ă) SYN macromelia.

meg·a·loph·thal·mos (meg′ă-lof-thal′mŏs) Abnormal largeness of the eyeball. [megalo- + G. *ophthalmos,* eye]

meg·a·lo·po·di·a (meg′ă-lō-pō′dē-ă) SYN macropodia. [megalo- + G. *podus,* foot]

meg•a•lo•sple•ni•a (meg′ă-lō-splē′nē-ă) SYN splenomegaly.

meg•a•lo•syn•dac•ty•ly, **meg•a•lo•syn•dac•tyl•i•a** (meg′ă-lō-sin-dak′ti-lē, sin′dak-til′ē-ă) Condition of webbed or fused fingers or toes of large size. [megalo- + G. *syn,* together, + *daktylos,* finger]

meg•a•lo•u•re•ter (meg′ă-lō-yur′ĕ-tĕr) An enlarged, dilated ureter.

-megaly Suffix meaning large. [G. *megas (megal-)*]

mega-oesophagus [Br.] SYN megaesophagus.

meg•a•poi•e•tin (meg′ă-poy′ĕ-tin) SYN thrombopoietin. [mega- + G. *poiētēs,* maker, + -in]

meg•a•rec•tum (meg′ă-rek′tŭm) Extreme dilation of the rectum.

meg•a•vi•ta•min ther•a•py (meg′ă-vī′tă-min thār′ă-pē) Large doses of vitamins, minerals, and amino acids that are used as medications to treat physical and psychiatric illnesses. SYN orthomolecular medicine.

meg•a•volt (mV) (meg′ă-vōlt) One million volts.

mei•bo•mi•an (mī-bō′mē-ăn) Attributed to or described by Meibom.

mei•bo•mi•an cyst (mī-bō′mē-ăn sist) SYN chalazion.

mei•bo•mi•an glands (mī-bō′mē-ăn glandz) SYN tarsal glands.

mei•bo•mi•tis, **mei•bo•mi•a•ni•tis** (mī′bō-mī′tis, -mē-ă-nī′tis) Inflammation of the meibomian glands.

Meig•e dis•ease (mezh′ĕ di-zēz′) Autosomal dominant lymphedema with onset at about the age of puberty.

Meigs syn•drome (megz sin′drōm) Fibromyoma of the ovary associated with hydroperitoneum and hydrothorax.

meio- For words beginning thus and not found here, see mio-.

mei•o•sis (mī-ō′sis) A special process of cell division comprising two nuclear divisions in rapid succession that result in four gametocytes, each containing half the number of chromosomes found in somatic cells. [G. *meiōsis,* a lessening]

mei•ot•ic (mī-ot′ik) Pertaining to meiosis.

Meis•cher syn•drome (mī′sher sin′drōm) SYN cheilitis granulomatosa.

Meiss•ner cor•pus•cle (mīs′ner kōr′pŭs-ĕl) SYN tactile corpuscle.

mel-, **melo-** Combining forms meaning **1.** Limb [G. *melos*]; **2.** a cheek [G. *mēlon*]; **3.** Honey, sugar [L. *mel, mellis,* G. *meli, melitos*]; **4.** Sheep [G. *mēlon*] SEE ALSO meli-.

melaena [Br.] SYN melena.

me•lag•ra (mĕ-lag′ră) Rheumatic or myalgic pains in the arms or legs. [G. *melos,* limb, + *agra,* seizure]

me•lal•gi•a (mĕl-al′jē-ă) Pain in a limb; specifically, burning pain in the feet extending up the leg and even to the thigh. [G. *melos,* a limb, + *algos,* pain]

melan-, **melano-** Combining forms meaning black, extreme darkness of hue. [G. *melas*]

mel•an•cho•li•a (mel-ăn-kō′lē-ă) **1.** A severe form of depression marked by anhedonia, insomnia, psychomotor changes, and guilt. **2.** A symptom occurring in other conditions, marked by depression of spirits and by a sluggish and painful process of thought. SYN melancholy. [melan- + G. *cholē,* bile. See humoral *doctrine*]

mel•an•chol•ic (mel-ăn-kol′ik) **1.** Relating to or characteristic of melancholia. **2.** Denoting a temperament characterized by irritability and a pessimistic outlook. **3.** A person who is exhibiting melancholia.

mel•an•chol•y (mel′ăn-kol-ē) SYN melancholia.

mel•an•e•de•ma (mel′ăn-ĕ-dē′mă) SYN anthracosis. SYN melanoedema. [melan- + G. *oidēma,* swelling]

mel•a•nif•er•ous (mel-ă-nif′ĕr-ŭs) Containing melanin or other black pigment. [melan- (melanin) + L. *ferro,* to carry]

mel•a•nin (mel′ă-nin) Any of the dark brown to black pigments that occur in the skin, hair, pigmented coat of the retina, and medulla and zona reticularis of the suprarenal gland. [G. *melas (melan-),* black]

mel•a•nism (mel′ă-nizm) Unusually marked, diffuse melanin pigmentation of body hair and skin (usually not affecting the iris). SEE ALSO melanosis.

mel•a•no•ac•an•tho•ma (mel′ă-nō-ak′an-thō′mă) A seborrheic keratosis with melanin pigmentation associated with proliferation of intraepidermal melanocytes. [melano- + G. *akantha,* thorn, + suffix *-ōma,* tumor]

mel•a•no•blast (mel′ă-nō-blast) A cell derived from the neural crest, which matures into a melanocyte. [melano- + G. *blastos,* germ, sprout]

mel•a•no•cyte (mel′ă-nō-sīt) A pigment-producing cell located in the basal layer of the epidermis with branching processes by means of which melanosomes are transferred to epidermal cells, resulting in pigmentation of the epidermis. [melano- + G. *kytos,* cell]

mel•a•no•cyte-stim•u•lat•ing hor•mone

(MSH) (mel′ă-nō-sīt-stim′yū-lā-ting hōr′mōn) SYN melanotropin, bioregulator.

mel•a•no•cy•to•ma (mel′ă-nō-sī-tō′mă) **1.** A pigmented tumor of the uveal stroma. **2.** Usually benign melanoma of the optic disc, appearing in markedly pigmented people as a small deeply pigmented tumor at the edge of the disc, sometimes extending into the retina and choroid. [megalo- + cyto- + G. *-oma;* tumor]

mel•a•no•der•ma (mel′ă-nō-dĕr′mă) **1.** An abnormal darkening of the skin by deposition of excess melanin. **2.** Hyperpigmentation of the skin by melanin or deposition of dark metallic substances such as silver and iron. [melano- + G. *derma,* skin]

mel•a•no•der•ma•ti•tis (mel′ă-nō-dĕr′mă-tī′tis) Excessive deposit of melanin in an area of dermatitis.

mel•a•no•der•mic (mel′ă-nō-dĕr′mik) Relating to or marked by melanoderma.

melanoedema [Br.] SYN melanedema.

me•lan•o•gen (mĕ-lan′ŏ-jen) A colorless substance that may be converted into melanin. [melanin + G. *-gen,* producing]

mel•a•no•gen•e•sis (mel′ă-nō-jen′ĕ-sis) Formation of melanin. [melanin + G. *genesis,* production]

mel•a•no•glos•si•a (mel′ă-nō-glos′ē-ă) SYN black tongue. [melano- + G. *glōssa,* tongue]

mel•a•noid (mel′ă-noyd) A dark pigment, resembling melanin, formed from glucosamines in chitin.

mel•a•no•leu•ko•der•ma (mel′ă-nō-lū′kō-dĕr′mă) Marbled, or marmorated, skin. [melano- + G. *leukos,* white, + *derma,* skin]

mel•a•no•leu•ko•der•ma col•li (mel′ă-nō-lū′kō-dĕr′mă kol′ē) SYN syphilitic leukoderma.

mel•an•o•lib•er•in (mel′ă-nō-lib′ĕr-in) A hexapeptide similar to oxytocin; it stimulates the release of melanotropin. SYN melanotropin-releasing factor, melanotropin-releasing hormone. [melanotropin + L. *libero,* to free, + -in]

mel•a•no•ma (mel′ă-nō′mă) A malignant neoplasm, derived from cells that are capable of forming melanin, arising most commonly in the skin or in the eye, and, rarely, in the mucous membranes of the genitalia, anus, oral cavity, or other sites; occurs mostly in adults and may originate de novo or from a pigmented nevus or lentigo maligna. Melanomas frequently metastasize widely; regional lymph nodes, skin, liver, lungs, and brain are likely to be involved. See page B14. [melano- + G. *-ōma,* tumor]

mel•a•no•ma in si•tu (mel′a-nō′mă in sī′tū) A melanoma limited to the epidermis and composed of nests of atypical melanocytes and scattered single cells extending into the upper epi-

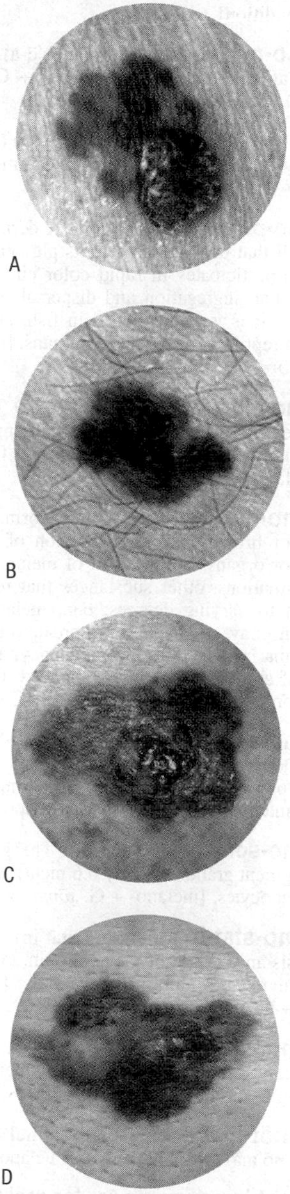

melanoma: ABCDs. (A) asymmetry; (B) borders scalloped, irregular, indistinct; (C) color variegated; (D) diameter more than 6 mm

dermis; local excision is curative although the lesion, if untreated, may soon invade the dermis. Malignant lentigo may be considered a slowly progressive type of melanoma in situ.

mel•a•no•ma•to•sis (mel′ă-nō′mă-tō′sis) A condition characterized by numerous, widespread lesions of melanoma. [melanoma + G. *-osis,* condition]

mel•a•no•nych•i•a (mel'ă-nō-nik'ē-ă) Black pigmentation of the nails. [melano- + G. *onyx* (*onych-*), nail]

mel•a•no•phage (mel'ă-nō-fāj, mĕ-lan'ō-fāj) A histiocyte that has phagocytized melanin. [melano- + G. *phagō,* to eat]

mel•a•no•phore (mel'ă-nō-fōr') A dermal pigment cell that does not secrete its pigment granules but participates in rapid color changes by intracellular aggregation and dispersal of melanosomes; it is well developed in fish, amphibians, and reptiles, but absent in humans. [melano- + G. *phoros,* bearing]

mel•a•no•pla•ki•a (mel'ă-nō-plā'kē-ă) The occurrence of pigmented patches on the tongue and buccal mucous membrane. [melano- + G. *plax,* plate, plaque]

mel•a•no•sis (mel'ă-nō'sis) Abnormal dark brown or brown-black pigmentation of various tissues or organs, as the result of melanin or, in some situations, other substances that resemble melanin to varying degrees; e.g., melanosis of the skin may occur in widespread metastatic melanoma, sunburn, during pregnancy, and as a result of chronic infections. [melano- + G. *-osis,* condition]

mel•a•no•sis co•li (mel'ă-nō'sis kō'lī) Melanosis of the large intestinal mucosa due to accumulation of pigment of uncertain composition within macrophages in the lamina propria.

mel•a•no•some (mel'ă-nō-sōm) The generally oval pigment granule (0.2 by 0.6 mcm) produced by melanocytes. [melano- + G. *sōma,* body]

mel•a•no•stat•in (mel'ă-nō-stat'in) Inhibits synthesis and release of melanotropin. SYN melanotropin release-inhibiting hormone. [melanotropin + G. *states*, stationary, + -in]

mel•a•not•ic (mel'ă-not'ik) **1.** Pertaining to the presence, normal or pathologic, of melanin. **2.** Relating to or characterized by melanosis.

mel•a•not•ic car•ci•no•ma (mel'ă-not'ik kahr'si-nō'mă) Obsolete term for melanoma.

mel•a•not•ic neu•ro•ec•to•der•mal tu•mor of in•fan•cy (mel'ă-not'ĭk nū'rō-ek'tō-dĕr-măl tū'mŏr in'făn-sē) A benign neoplasm of neuroectodermal origin that most often involves the anterior maxilla of infants in the first year of life; presents clinically as a rapidly growing blue-black lesion producing a destructive radiolucency; histologically, characterized by small, round, undifferentiated tumor cells interspersed with larger, polyhedral, melanin-producing cells arranged in an alveolar configuration.

mel•a•no•troph (mel'ă-nō-trōf) A cell of the intermediate lobe of the hypophysis that produces melanotropin. [melano- + G. *trophē,* nourishment]

mel•a•no•tro•phin (mel'ă-nō-trō'fin) SYN melanotropin. [melano- + G. *trophē,* nourishment, + -in]

mel•a•no•tro•pin (mel'ă-nō-trō'pin) A polypeptide hormone secreted by the intermediate lobe of the hypophysis in humans (in neurohypophysis in certain other species) that causes dispersion of melanin by melanophores, resulting in darkening of the skin, presumably by promoting melanin synthesis; this effect is readily demonstrated in some lower vertebrates, such as frogs and fish; α-melanotropin is an *N*-acetylated peptide with 13 amino acids; β-melanotropin has 22 amino acids. Cf. bioregulator. SYN melanocyte-stimulating hormone, melanotrophin.

mel•a•no•tro•pin re•lease-in•hib•it•ing hor•mone (MIH) (melă-nō-trō'pin rĕ'lēs-in-hib'i-ting hōr'mōn) SYN melanostatin.

mel•a•no•tro•pin-re•leas•ing fac•tor (MRF) (mel'ă-nō-trō'pin rĕ'lēs'ing fak'tŏr) SYN melanoliberin.

mel•a•no•tro•pin-re•leas•ing hor•mone (MRH) (mel'ă-nō-trō'pin rē-lēs-ing hōr'mōn) SYN melanoliberin.

mel•a•nu•ri•a (mel'ă-nyū'rē-ă) The excretion of dark-colored urine, resulting from the presence of melanin or other pigments or from the action of phenol and other coal tar derivatives. [melano- + G. *ouron,* urine]

mel•a•nu•ric (mel'ă-nyū'rik) Pertaining to or characterized by melanuria.

MELAS (mel'as) Acronym for a constellation of findings that includes mitochondrial myopathy, encephalopathy, lactic acidosis, and strokelike episodes. One of the mitochondrial disorders, this condition is usually hereditary, with a mutation at the mitochondrial genome at locus 3243.

i **me•las•ma** (mĕ-laz'mă) A patchy or generalized pigmentation of the skin. SEE ALSO chloasma. See page 963. SYN mask of pregnancy. [G. a black color, a black spot]

me•las•ma grav•i•dar•um (mĕ-laz'mă grav'i-dā'rŭm) Chloasma occurring in pregnancy.

mel•a•to•nin (mel'ă-tōn'in) A substance formed by the pineal gland that appears to depress gonadal function; serotonin is a precursor, melatonin is rapidly metabolized and is taken up by all tissues; it is involved in circadian rhythms. Cf. bioregulator. [melanophore + G. *tonos,* stretching, + -in]

me•le•na (mĕ-lē'nă) Passage of tarry stools, due to the presence of blood altered by the intestinal juices. Cf. hematochezia. SYN melaena. [G. *melaina,* fem. of *melas,* black]

Me•le•ney ul•cer (mĕ-lē'nē ŭl'sĕr) Undermining ulcer of the skin and subcutaneous tissues

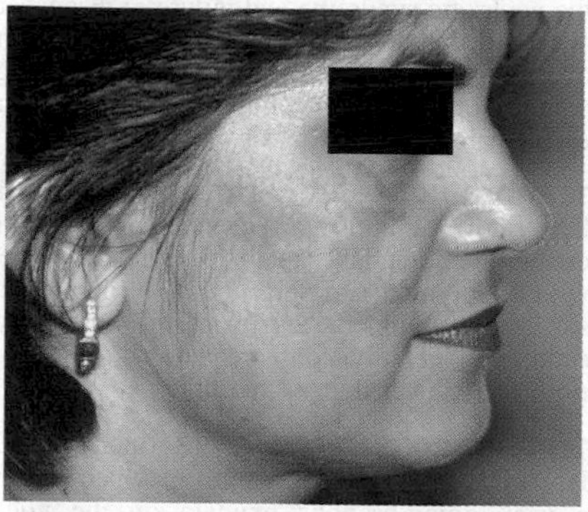

melasma: cheek

caused by a synergistic infection by microaerophilic nonhemolytic streptococci and aerobic hemolytic staphylococci.

meli- Combining form meaning honey, sugar. SEE ALSO mel-. [G. *meli*]

me•li•tis (mĕ-lī′tis) Inflammation of the cheek. [G. *mēlon,* cheek, + *-itis,* inflammation]

Mel•nick-Nee•dles os•te•o•dys•plas•ty (mel′nik-nēd′elz os′tē-ō-dis-plas′tē) A generalized skeletal dysplasia with prominent forehead and small mandible; radiographically, there are irregular ribbonlike constrictions of the ribs and tubular bones; probably X-linked. Autosomal dominant and recessive inheritance have also been suggested. SYN osteodysplasty.

mel•o•plas•ty (mel′ō-plas-tē) Surgical repair of the cheek. [melo- + G. *plastos,* formed]

mel•o•rhe•os•to•sis (mel′ō-rē-os-tō′sis) Rheostosis confined to the long bones. [G. *melos,* limb, + *rheos,* stream, + *osteon,* bone, + *-ōsis*]

me•lo•ti•a (me-lō′shē-ă) Congenital displacement of the auricle of the external ear onto the cheek. [G. *mēlon,* cheek, + *ous,* ear]

melt (melt) Denature, used to describe RNA polymerase action in decoupling DNA base pairs.

melt•ing-curve a•nal•y•sis (melt′ing kŭrv ă-nal′i-sis) A real-time polymerase chain reaction (PCR) method used to determine whether nonspecific PCR products or primer-dimers have formed. The method is also used to determine the identity of a target.

melt•ing point (Tm) (mel′ting poynt) **1.** The temperature at which a solid becomes a liquid. **2.** The temperature at which 50% of a macromolecule becomes denatured.

Melt•zer law (melt′zĕr law) All living functions are continually controlled by two opposite forces: augmentation or action on the one hand, and inhibition on the other.

mem•ber (mem′bĕr) SYN limb (1). [L. *membrum*]

mem•bra (mem′bră) [TA] Plural of membrum. [L.]

mem•bra•na, gen. and pl. **mem•bra•nae** (mem-brā′nă, -nē) [TA] SYN biomembrane, membrane (1). [L.]

mem•bra•na ad•ven•ti•ti•a (mem-brā′nă ad′vĕn-tish′ē-ă) SYN decidua capsularis.

mem•bra•na de•cid•u•a (mem-brā′nă dē-sid′yū-ă) SYN decidua.

mem•bra•na pu•pil•la•ris (mem-brā′nă pyū-pi-lā′ris) [TA] SYN pupillary membrane.

mem•bra•na re•tic•u•la•ris (mem-brā′nă re-tik-yū-lā′ris) [TA] SYN reticular membrane.

mem•bra•na ser•o•sa (mem-brā′nă ser-ō′să) **1.** SYN serosa, chorion. **2.** SYN serosa (2).

mem•bra•na syn•o•vi•a•lis (mem-brā′nă si-nō-vī-ā′lis) [TA] SYN synovial membrane.

mem•bra•na tec•to•ri•a duc•tus co•chle•a•ris (mem-brā′nă tek-tō′rē-ă dŭk′tŭs kok′lē-ār′is) [TA] SYN tectorial membrane of cochlear duct.

mem•bra•na tym•pa•ni (mem-brā′nă tim′pă-nī) [TA] SYN tympanic membrane.

mem•bra•na tym•pa•ni se•cun•dar•i•a (mem-brā′nă tim′pă-nīsek-ŭn-dā′rē-ă) [TA] SYN secondary tympanic membrane.

mem•bra•na vit•el•li•na (mem-brā′nă vī-tel′ē-nă) **1.** The membrane enveloping the yolk; specifically, the thickened cell membrane of large-yolked oocyte. SYN ovular membrane. **2.** Sometimes used to designate the zona pellucida of a mammalian oocyte. SYN yolk membrane.

mem•bra•na vi•tre•a (mem-brā′nă vit′rē-ă) [TA] SYN posterior limiting layer of cornea.

mem•brane (mem′brān) **1.** A thin sheet or layer of pliable tissue, serving as a covering or envelope, the lining of a cavity, a partition or septum, or a connection between two structures. SYN membrana [TA]. **2.** SYN biomembrane. [L. *membrana,* a skin or membrane that covers parts of the body, fr. *membrum,* a member]

mem•brane bone (mem′brān bōn) A bone that develops embryologically within a membrane of vascularized primordial mesenchymal tissue without prior formation of cartilage.

mem•brane-coat•ing gran•ule (mem′brān kōt′ing gran′yūl) SYN keratinosome.

mem•brane ex•pan•sion the•o•ry (mem′brān eks-pan′shŭn thē′ōr-ē) That adsorption of anesthetics into membranes so alters membrane volume or configuration that membrane function is affected in such a way as to produce anesthesia.

mem•brane po•ten•tial (mem′brān pŏ-ten′shăl) The potential inside a cell membrane, measured relative to the fluid just outside; it is negative under resting conditions and becomes positive during an action potential.

mem•brane rup•ture (mem′brān rŭp′chŭr) Rupture of the amnionic sac allowing the amnionic fluid to escape through the vagina.

mem•brane strip•ping (mem′brān strip′ing) Separation of gestational membranes from the lower uterine segment by insertion of a finger through the cervical os to initiate the Ferguson reflex or prostaglandin release from the decidua and hasten labor.

mem•bra•ni•form (mem-brā′ni-fōrm) Of the appearance or character of a membrane. SYN membranoid.

mem•bra•no•car•ti•lag•i•nous (mem′bră-nō-kahr′ti-laj′i-nŭs) **1.** Partly membranous and partly cartilaginous. **2.** Derived from both a mesenchymal membrane and cartilage; denoting certain bones.

mem•bra•noid (mem′bră-noyd) SYN membraniform.

mem•bra•no•pro•lif•er•a•tive glo•mer•u•lo•ne•phri•tis (mem′bră-nō′prō-lif′ĕr-ă-tiv glō-mer′yū-lō-nĕ-frī′tis) Chronic glomerulonephritis characterized by mesangial cell proliferation, increased lobular separation of glomeruli, thickening of glomerular capillary walls and increased mesangial matrix, and low serum levels of complement; occurs mainly in older children, with a variably slow progressive course, episodes of hematuria or edema, and hypertension. SYN lobular glomerulonephritis.

mem•bra•nous (mem′bră-nŭs) Relating to or of the form of a membrane.

mem•bra•nous am•pul•lae of the sem•i•cir•cu•lar ducts (mem′bră-nŭs am-pul′ē sem′ē-sĕr′kyū-lăr dŭkt) A nearly spheric enlargement of one end of each of the three semicircular ducts, anterior, posterior, and lateral, where they connect with the utricle. Each contains a neuroepithelial crista ampullaris. SYN ampulla membranacea.

mem•bra•nous cat•a•ract (mem′bră-nŭs kat′ăr-akt) A secondary cataract composed of the remains of the thickened capsule and degenerated lens fibers.

mem•bra•nous dys•men•or•rhe•a (mem′bră-nŭs dis-men-ōr-ē′ă) Dysmenorrhea accompanied by an exfoliation of the menstrual decidua.

mem•bra•nous glo•mer•u•lo•ne•phri•tis (mem′bră-nŭs glō-mer′yū-lō-nĕ-frī′tis) Glomerulonephritis characterized by diffuse thickening of glomerular capillary basement membranes, due in part to subepithelial deposits of immunoglobulins separated by spikes of basement membrane material, and clinically by an insidious onset of the nephrotic syndrome and failure of disappearance of proteinuria; the disease is most commonly idiopathic but may be secondary to malignant tumors, drugs, infections, or systemic lupus erythematosus.

mem•bra•nous lab•y•rinth (mem′bră-nŭs lab′i-rinth) A complex arrangement of communicating membranous canaliculi and sacs, filled with endolymph and surrounded by perilymph, suspended within the cavity of the bony labyrinth; its chief divisions are the cochlear labyrinth and the vestibular labyrinth.

mem•bra•nous lar•yn•gi•tis (mem′bră-nŭs lar-in-jī′tis) A form of laryngitis in which there is a pseudomembranous exudate on the vocal cords.

mem•bra•nous os•si•fi•ca•tion (mem′bră-nŭs os′i-fi-kā′shŭn) Development of osseous tissue that occurs within mesenchymal tissue without prior cartilage formation, such as occurs in the frontal and parietal bones.

mem•brum, pl. **mem•bra** (mem′brŭm, -bră) A limb; a member. [L. member]

mem•o•ry (mem′ŏ-rē) **1.** Generally, recollection of that which was once experienced or learned. **2.** The mental information processing system that receives (registers), modifies, stores, and retrieves informational stimuli; composed of three stages: encoding, storage, and retrieval. [L. *memoria*]

mem•o•ry B cells (mĕm′ō-rē selz) B lymphocytes that mediate immunologic memory; they allow for enhanced immunologic reaction when an immunologically competent organism is reexposed to an antigen.

mem•o•ry T cells (mĕm′ō-rē selz) T lymphoctyes that mediate immunologic memory; they allow for enhanced immunologic reaction when an immunologically competent organism is reexposed to an antigen.

MEN Abbreviation for multiple endocrine neoplasia.

MEN1 Abbreviation for multiple endocrine neoplasia 1.

MEN2 Abbreviation for multiple endocrine neoplasia 2.

MEN2B Abbreviation for multiple endocrine neoplasia 2B.

MEN3 Abbreviation for multiple endocrine neoplasia 3.

men•ac•me (me-nak′mē) The period of menstrual activity in a woman's life. [G. *mēn,* month, + *akmē,* prime]

Me•nan•gle vi•rus (men′ang-gĕl vī′rŭs) A virus of the family Paramyxoviridae causing infection in pigs, humans, and fruit bats in Australia; human infection has resulted in an influenzalike illness with rash. [fr. the location in Australia of the laboratory where it was first isolated]

men·a·quin·one-6 (MK-6) (men′ă-kwin′ōn) Isolated from putrified fish meal, potency is about 60% of that of phylloquinone (vitamin K_1). SYN vitamin K2, vitamin K2(30).

men·ar·che (men′ahr′kē) Establishment of the menstrual function; the time of the first menstrual period. [G. *mēn,* month, + *archē,* beginning]

Men·del-Bech·te·rew re·flex (men′dĕl bek-tĕr′yev rē′fleks) SYN Bechterew-Mendel reflex.

Men·de·lé·eff law (men′de-lā′ĕf law) The properties of elements are periodical functions of their atomic weights; i.e., if the elements are arranged in the order of their atomic weights, every element in the series will be related in respect to its properties to the eighth in order before or after it.

men·de·le·vi·um (Md) (men-dĕ-lē′vē-ŭm) An element, atomic no. 101, atomic wt. 258.1, prepared in 1955 by bombardment of einsteinium with alpha particles. [*D. Mendeléeff*]

Men·del first law (men′dĕl fĕrst law) SYN law of segregation.

men·de·li·an (men-dē′lē-ăn) Attributed to or described by Gregor Mendel; usually referring to the behavior and the mechanism of the genetic transmission of single-locus traits.

men·de·li·an in·her·i·tance (men-dē′lē-ăn in-her′i-tăns) Inheritance in which stable and undecomposable characters controlled entirely or overwhelmingly by a single genetic locus are transmitted over many generations. SEE law of segregation, law of independent assortment.

Men·de·li·an In·her·i·tance in Man (MIM) (men-dē′lē-ăn in-her′i-tăns man) A standard, comprehensive, regularly updated reference source for traits in humans that have been shown to be mendelian or that are thought on reasonable grounds to be so. Each entry has a six-digit catalog number. Those securely established (by molecular biology or by extensive clinical studies) are marked with an asterisk.

Men·del in·step re·flex (men′dĕl in′step rē′fleks) The foot being firmly supported on its inner side, a sharp tap on the dorsal tendons causes extension of the second to the fifth toes.

Men·del sec·ond law (men′dĕl sek′ŏnd law) SYN law of independent assortment.

Men·del·sohn ma·neu·ver (men′dĕl-sŏn mă-nū′vĕr) During a swallow, maintenance of the larynx for a few seconds at the highest position in the neck by voluntary muscular contraction. This laryngeal elevation results in a wider and longer esophageal opening and is a therapeutic technique for management of swallowing disorders.

Mé·né·tri·er dis·ease, Mé·né·trier syn·drome (mā-nā-trē-ā′ di-zēz′, sin′drōm) Gastric mucosal hyperplasia, either mucoid or glandular; the latter type may be associated with the Zollinger-Ellison syndrome.

Men·ge pes·sa·ry (meng′gĕ pes′ă-rē) A ring pessary with a central horizontal bar into which a detachable handle is inserted.

Mé·nière dis·ease, Mé·nière syn·drome (mĕn-yār′ di-zēz′, sin′drōm) An affliction characterized clinically by vertigo, nausea, vomiting, tinnitus, and progressive hearing loss due to hydrops of the endolymphatic duct. SYN auditory vertigo, endolymphatic hydrops, labyrinthine vertigo.

me·nin·ge·al (men′in-jē′ăl) Relating to the meninges.

me·nin·ge·al veins (men′in-jē′ăl vānz) Accompany the meningeal arteries; they communicate with venous sinuses and diploic veins and drain into regional veins outside the cranial vault.

me·nin·ge·or·rha·phy (mĕ-nin′jē-ōr′ă-fē) Suture of the cranial or spinal meninges or of any membrane. [G. *mēninx (mēning-),* membrane, + *rhaphē,* suture]

me·nin·ges (mĕ-nin′jēz) Plural of meninx.

me·nin·gi·o·ma (mĕ-nin′jē-ō′mă) A benign, encapsulated neoplasm of arachnoidal origin, occurring most frequently in adults; most frequent form consists of elongated, fusiform cells in whorls and pseudolobules with psammoma bodies frequently present; meningiomas tend to occur along the superior sagittal sinus, along the sphenoid ridge, or in the vicinity of the optic chiasm; in addition to meningothelial meningioma, angiomatous, chondromatous, osteomatous, lipomatous, melanotic, fibroblastic and transitional varieties are recognized. [mening- + G. *-oma,* tumor]

me·nin·gism (men′in-jizm) A condition in which the symptoms simulate meningitis, but in which no actual inflammation of these membranes is present.

men·in·git·ic (men′in-jit′ik) Relating to or characterized by meningitis.

men·in·git·ic streak (men′in-jit′ik strēk) A line of redness resulting from drawing a point across the skin, especially notable in cases of meningitis. SYN Trousseau spot.

i **men·in·gi·tis**, pl. **men·in·git·i·des** (men′in-jī′tis, -jit′i-dēz) Inflammation of the membranes of the brain or spinal cord. SEE ALSO arachnoiditis, leptomeningitis. See page B4. SYN cerebrospinal meningitis. [mening- + G. *itis,* inflammation]

meningo-, **mening-** Combining forms meaning the meninges. [G. *mēninx,* membrane]

me·nin·go·cele (mĕ-ning′gō-sēl) Protrusion of the meninges (membranes) of the brain or spinal cord through a defect in the cranium or vertebral column. [meningo- + G. *kēlē,* tumor]

meningococcaemia [Br.] SYN meningococcemia.

me·nin·go·coc·cal men·in·gi·tis (mĕ-ning-gō-kok′ăl men-in-jī′tis) An acute infectious disease affecting children and young adults, caused by *Neisseria meningitidis;* characterized by nasopharyngeal catarrh, headache, vomiting, convulsions, stiffness in the neck (nuchal rigidity), photophobia, constipation, cutaneous hyperesthesia, a purpuric or herpetic eruption, and the presence of Kernig sign. Fulminant form may cause Waterhouse-Friderichsen syndrome.

me·nin·go·coc·ce·mia (mĕ-ning′gō-kok-sē′mē-ă) Presence of meningococci (*N. meningitidis*) in the circulating blood. SYN meningococcaemia.

me·nin·go·coc·cus, pl. **me·nin·go·coc·ci** (mĕ-ning-gō-kok′ŭs, -kok′ī) SYN *Neisseria meningitidis.* [meningo- + G. *kokkos,* berry]

me·nin·go·cor·ti·cal (mĕ-ning-gō-kōr′ti-kăl) Relating to the meninges and the cortex of the brain.

me·nin·go·cyte (mĕ-ning′gō-sīt) A mesenchymal epithelial cell of the subarachnoid space; it may become a macrophage. [meningo- + G. *kytos,* cell]

me·nin·go·en·ceph·a·li·tis (mĕ-ning′gō-en-sef-ăl-ī′tis) An inflammation of the brain and its membranes. SYN cerebromeningitis, encephalomeningitis. [meningo- + G. *enkephalos,* brain, + *-itis,* inflammation]

me·nin·go·en·ceph·a·lo·cele (mĕ-ning′gō-en-sef′ă-lō-sēl) A protrusion of the meninges and brain through a congenital defect in the cranium, usually in the frontal or occipital region. SYN encephalomeningocele. [meningo- + G. *enkephalos,* brain, + *kēlē,* hernia]

me·nin·go·en·ceph·a·lo·my·e·li·tis (mĕ-ning′gō-en-sef′ă-lō-mī-ĕ-lī′tis) Inflammation of the brain and spinal cord together with their membranes. [meningo + G. *enkephalos,* brain, + *myelos,* marrow, + *-itis,* inflammation]

me·nin·go·en·ceph·a·lop·a·thy (mĕ-ning′gō-en-sef-ă-lop′ă-thē) Disorder affecting the meninges and the brain. SYN encephalomeningopathy. [meningo- + G. *enkephalos,* brain, + *pathos,* suffering]

me·nin·go·my·e·li·tis (mĕ-ning′gō-mī-ĕ-lī′tis) Inflammation of the spinal cord and of its enveloping arachnoid and pia mater, and less commonly also of the dura mater. [meningo- + G. *myelos,* marrow, + *-itis,* inflammation]

me·nin·go·my·e·lo·cele (mĕ-ning′gō-mī′ĕ-lō-sēl) Protrusion of the meninges and spinal cord through a defect in the vertebral column. SYN myelocystomeningocele, myelomeningocele. [meningo- + G. *myelos,* marrow, + *kēlē,* tumor]

me·nin·go·ra·dic·u·lar (mĕ-ning′gō-ră-dik′yū-lăr) Relating to the meninges covering cranial or spinal nerve roots. [meningo- + L. *radix,* root]

me·nin·go·ra·dic·u·li·tis (mĕ-ning′gō-ră-dik′yū-lī′tis) Inflammation of the meninges and roots of the nerves.

me·nin·gor·rha·chid·i·an (mĕ-ning′gō-ră-kid′ē-ăn) Relating to the spinal cord and its membranes. [meningo- + G. *rhachis,* spine]

me·nin·gor·rha·gi·a (mĕ-ning-gō-rā′jē-ă) Hemorrhage into or beneath the cerebral or spinal meninges. [meningo- + G. *rhēgnymi,* to burst forth]

men·in·go·sis (men′in-gō′sis) Membranous union of bones, as in the cranium of the newborn. [meningo- + G. *-ōsis,* condition]

me·nin·go·vas·cu·lar (mĕ-ning-gō-vas′kyū-lăr) Concerning the blood vessels in the meninges; or the meninges and blood vessels.

me·ninx, gen. **me·nin·gis**, pl. **me·nin·ges** (mē′ninks, mĕ-nin′jis, -jēz) Any membrane; specifically, one of the membranous coverings of the brain and spinal cord. SEE ALSO arachnoidea, dura mater, pia mater. See page 967. [Mod. L. fr. G. *mēninx,* membrane]

men·is·cec·to·my (men′i-sek′tŏ-mē) Excision of a meniscus, usually from the knee joint. [G. *mēniskos,* crescent (meniscus) + *ektomē,* excision]

me·nis·ci (mĕ-nis′ī) Plural of meniscus.

men·is·ci·tis (men-i-sī′tis) Inflammation of a fibrocartilaginous meniscus. [G. *mēniskos,* crescent (meniscus), + *-itis,* inflammation]

me·nis·cus, pl. **me·nis·ci** (mĕ-nis′kŭs, mĕ-nis′ī) **1.** SYN meniscus lens. **2.** [TA] Any crescent-shaped structure. **3.** A crescent-shaped fibrocartilaginous structure of the knee, the acromio- and sternoclavicular and the temporomandibular joints. **4.** The crescentic curvature of the surface of a liquid standing in a narrow vessel (e.g., pipette, burette). [G. *mēniskos,* crescent]

me·nis·cus lens (mĕ-nis′kŭs lenz) A lens having a spheric concave curve on one side and a spheric convex curve on the other. SYN meniscus (1).

me·nis·cus sign (mĕ-nis′kŭs sīn) SYN crescent sign.

Men·kes syn·drome (meng′kĕs sin′drōm) SYN kinky-hair disease.

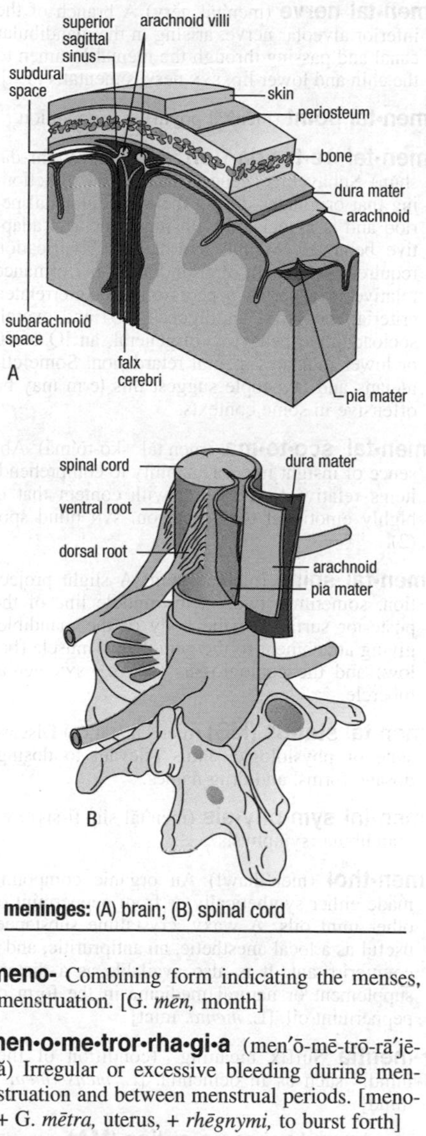

meninges: (A) brain; (B) spinal cord

meno- Combining form indicating the menses, menstruation. [G. *mēn,* month]

men·o·me·tror·rha·gi·a (men′ō-mē-trō-rā′jē-ă) Irregular or excessive bleeding during menstruation and between menstrual periods. [meno- + G. *mētra,* uterus, + *rhēgnymi,* to burst forth]

men·o·pau·sal (men′ō-paw′zăl) Associated with or occasioned by the menopause.

men·o·pause (men′ō-pawz) Permanent cessation of the menses. [meno- + G. *pausis,* cessation]

men·or·rha·gi·a (men′ō-rā′jē-ă) SYN hypermenorrhea. [meno- + G. *rhēgnymi,* to burst forth]

men·or·rhal·gi·a (men′ō-ral′jē-ă) SYN dysmenorrhea. [meno- + G. *algos,* pain]

me·nos·che·sis (me-nos′kĕ-sis) Suppression of menstruation. [meno- + G. *schesis,* retention]

men·o·stax·is (men′ō-stak′sis) SYN hypermenorrhea. [meno- + G. *staxis,* a dripping]

men·o·tro·pins (men′ō-trō′pinz) Extract of postmenopausal urine that primarily contains the follicle-stimulating hormone. SEE ALSO human menopausal gonadotropin, urofollitropin.

MENS Abbreviation for microcurrent electrical neuromuscular stimulator.

men·ses (men′sēz) A periodic physiologic hemorrhage, which occurs at approximately 4-week intervals, its source is the uterine mucous membrane; usually the bleeding is preceded by ovulation and predecidual changes in the endometrium. SEE ALSO menstrual cycle. SYN emmenia, menstrual period. [L. pl. of *mensis,* month]

men·stru·al (men′strū-ăl) Relating to the menses. SYN emmenic. [L. *menstrualis*]

men·stru·al cramps (men′strū-ăl kramps) Abdominopelvic pain accompanying menstruation.

men·stru·al cy·cle (men′strū-ăl sī′kĕl) The period in which an oocyte or ovum matures, is ovulated, and enters the uterine lumen through the uterine tube; ovarian hormonal secretions effect endometrial changes such that, if fertilization occurs, nidation will be possible; in the absence of fertilization, ovarian secretions wane, the endometrium sloughs, and menstruation begins; this cycle lasts an average of 28 days, with day 1 of the cycle designated as that day on which menstrual flow begins.

men·stru·al mo·lim·i·na (men′strū-ăl mŏ-lim′i-nă) SYN premenstrual syndrome.

men·stru·al pe·ri·od (men′strū-ăl pēr′ē-ŏd) SYN menses.

men·stru·ate (men′strū-āt) To undergo menstruation. [L. *menstruo,* pp. *-atus,* to be menstruant]

men·stru·a·tion (men′strū-ā′shŭn) Cyclic endometrial shedding and discharge of a bloody fluid from the uterus during the menstrual cycle. SEE menstruate.

men·ta de lo·bo (men′tă dā lō′bō) SYN bugleweed. [Sp., wolf's mint]

men·tal (men′tăl) **1.** Relating to the mind. [L. *mens* (*ment-*), mind] **2.** Relating to the chin. SYN genial, genian. [L. *mentum,* chin]

men·tal age (MA) (men′tăl āj) A measure, expressed in years and months, of a child's intelligence relative to age norms as determined by testing with the Stanford-Binet intelligence scale.

men·tal ar·ter·y (men′tăl ahr′tĕr-ē) *Distribution,* chin; the terminal branch of the inferior alveolar; *anastomoses,* inferior labial artery. SYN arteria mentalis [TA].

men·tal branch of in·fe·ri·or al·ve·o·lar

ar·ter·y (men′tăl branch in-fēr′ē-ŏr al-vē′ō-lăr ahr′tĕr-ē) *Distribution,* chin; the terminal branch of the inferior alveolar; *anastomoses,* inferior labial artery.

men·tal dis·ease (men′tăl di-zēz′) SEE mental illness, mental disorder.

men·tal dis·or·der (men′tăl dis-ōr′dĕr) A psychological syndrome or behavioral pattern associated with either subjective distress or objective impairment. SEE ALSO mental illness, behavior disorder.

men·tal fo·ra·men (men′tăl fōr-ā′mĕn) The anterior opening of the mandibular canal on the body of the mandible lateral to and above the mental tubercle giving passage to the mental artery and nerve.

men·tal health (men′tăl helth) Emotional, behavioral, and social maturity or normality; the absence of a mental or behavioral disorder; a state of psychological well-being in which the person has achieved a satisfactory integration of instinctual drives acceptable to both self and social milieu; an appropriate balance of love, work, and leisure pursuits.

Men·tal Health As·so·ci·a·tion (MHA) (men′tăl helth ōr′găn-ī-zā′shŭn) A state affiliate of the National Mental Health Association, the oldest and largest nonprofit organization in the United States; purpose is to address all issues related to mental health and mental illness. Goals are achieved through education, advocacy, research, and service, with initiatives such as support groups, housing services, and socialization.

men·tal hy·giene (men′tăl hī′jēn) The science and practice of maintaining and restoring mental health; a branch of early twentieth-century psychiatry that has become an interdisciplinary field including subspecialities in psychology, nursing, social work, law, and other professions.

men·tal ill·ness (men′tăl il′nes) **1.** A broadly inclusive term, generally denoting either or both a disease of the brain, with predominant behavioral symptoms; a disease of the "mind" or personality, evidenced by abnormal behavior, as in hysteria or schizophrenia. **2.** Any psychiatric illness listed in *Current Medical Information and Terminology* of the American Medical Association or in the *Diagnostic and Statistical Manual of Mental Disorders* of the American Psychiatric Association. SEE ALSO behavior disorder.

men·tal im·age (men′tăl im′ăj) A picture of an object not present, produced in the mind by memory or imagination.

men·ta·lis mus·cle (men-tā′lis mŭs′ĕl) *Origin,* incisor fossa of mandible; *insertion,* skin of chin; *action,* raises and wrinkles skin of chin, thus elevating the lower lip; *nerve supply,* facial. SYN musculus mentalis [TA].

men·tal·i·ty (men-tal′i-tē) The functional attributes of the mind; mental activity.

men·tal nerve (men′tăl nĕrv) A branch of the inferior alveolar nerve, arising in the mandibular canal and passing through the mental foramen to the chin and lower lip. SYN nervus mentalis [TA].

men·tal point (men′tăl poynt) SYN pogonion.

men·tal re·tar·da·tion (men′tăl rē′tahr-dā′shŭn) Subaverage general intellectual functioning that originates during the developmental period and is associated with impairment in adaptive behavior. Mental retardation classification requires assignment of an index for performance relative to a person's peers on two interrelated criteria: measured intelligence (IQ) and overall socioadaptive behavior. In general, an IQ of 70 or lower indicates mental retardation. Some clinicians and laypeople suggest this term may be offensive in some contexts.

men·tal sco·to·ma (men′tăl skŏ-tō′mă) Absence of insight into, or inability to comprehend, items relative to a subject with content that is highly emotional to the person. SYN blind spot (2).

men·tal spine (men′tăl spīn) A slight projection, sometimes two, in the middle line of the posterior surface of the body of the mandible, giving attachment to the geniohyoid muscle (below) and the genioglossus (above). SYN genial tubercle.

men·tal stat·us (MS) (men′tăl stat′ŭs) Disease state or physiologic status relevant to dosing, dosage forms, and drug names.

men·tal sym·phy·sis (men′tăl sim′fi-sis) SYN mandibular symphysis.

men·thol (men′thawl) An organic compound made either synthetically or from peppermint or other mint oils. A waxy, crystalline substance, useful as a local anesthetic, an antipruritic, and a counterirritant. It is also available as a dietary supplement or natural medicine in the form of peppermint oil. [L. *menta,* mint]

♻ **-mentia** Suffix meaning "(condition of the) mind," such as in dementia. [L. *mens (ment-),* mind]

men·to·an·te·ri·or po·si·tion (MA) (men′tō-an-tēr′ē-ŏr pŏ-zish′ŏn) A cephalic presentation of the fetus with its chin pointing to the right (right mentoanterior, RMA) or to the left (left mentoanterior, LMA) acetabulum of the mother.

men·ton (men′tŏn) A cephalometric landmark used in orthodontia; lowest point on the mandible (chin) as seen in a lateral radiologic view of the head. [L. *mentum,* chin]

men·to·plas·ty (men′tō-plas-tē) Surgical repair of the chin, whereby its shape or size is altered. SYN genioplasty. [L. *mentum,* chin, + G. *plastos,* formed]

men·to·pos·te·ri·or po·si·tion (MP) (men′tō-pos-tēr′ē-or pŏ-zish′ŏn) A cephalic presentation of the fetus with its chin pointing to the right (right mentoposterior, RMP) or to the left (left mentoposterior, LMP) sacroiliac articulation of the mother.

men·to·trans·verse po·si·tion (MT) (men′to-tranz′vĕrs pŏ-zish′ŏn) A cephalic presentation of the fetus with its chin pointing to the right (right mentotranverse, RMT) or to the left (left mentotransverse, LMT) iliac fossa of the mother.

men·tum, gen. **men·ti** (men′tŭm, -tī) SYN chin. [L.]

MEOS Abbreviation for microsomal ethanol-oxidizing system.

MEP Abbreviation for maximum expiratory pressure.

me·phit·ic (me-fit′ik) Foul, poisonous, or noxious. [L. *mephitis,* a noxious exhalation]

mEq, meq Abbreviation for milliequivalent.

mEq/L Abbreviation for milliequivalents per liter.

♻ **-mer** **1.** Chemical suffix attached to a prefix such as mono-, di-, poly-, tri-, etc., to indicate the smallest unit of a repeating structure; e.g., polymer. **2.** Suffix denoting a member of a particular group; e.g., isomer, enantiomer.

me·ral·gi·a (mĕ-ral′jē-ă) Pain in the thigh; specifically, meralgia paresthetica. [G. *mēros,* thigh, + *algos,* pain]

me·ral·gi·a par·a·es·thet·i·ca (mĕ-ral′jē-ă par′ă-es-thet′i-kă) Tingling, formication, itching, and other forms of paresthesia in the outer side of the lower part of the thigh in the area of distribution of the lateral femoral cutaneous nerve; there may be pain, but the skin is usually hypesthetic to the touch. SYN Bernhardt disease.

M:E ra·ti·o (rā′shē-ō) The ratio of myeloid:erythroid precursors in bone marrow; normally it varies from 2:1 to 4:1. An increased ratio is caused by infections, chronic myelogenous leukemia, or erythroid hypoplasia; a decreased ratio may mean a depression of leukopoiesis or normoblastic hyperplasia, depending on the overall cellularity of the bone marrow.

mer·cap·tan (mĕr-kap′tan) **1.** A class of substances in which the oxygen of an alcohol has been replaced by sulfur (e.g., cysteine). **2.** DENTISTRY a class of elastic impression compounds sometimes referred to as rubber base materials.

♻ **mercapto-** Prefix indicating the presence of a thiol group, –SH.

mer·cap·tu·ric ac·id (mĕr-kap′tyūr-ik as′id) A condensation product of L-cysteine with aromatic compounds, such as bromobenzene; formed in the liver and excreted in the urine.

Mer·ci·er sound (mer-sē-ā′ sownd) A catheter with a short beak bent at almost a right angle.

mer·cu·ri·al (mĕr-kyū′rē-ăl) **1.** Relating to mercury. **2.** Any salt of mercury used medicinally. **3.** Having the characteristic of rapid, changing moods.

mer·cu·ri·a·lism (mĕr-kyū′rē-ă-lizm) SYN mercury poisoning.

mer·cu·ric (mĕr-kyū′rik) Denoting a salt of mercury in which the ion of the metal is bivalent.

mer·cu·rous (mĕr-kyū′rŭs) Denoting a salt of mercury in which the ion of the metal is univalent.

mer·cu·ry (Hg) (mĕr′kyū-rē) A dense, liquid metallic element, atomic no. 80, atomic wt. 200.59; used in thermometers, barometers, manometers, and other scientific instruments; some salts and organic mercurials are used medicinally; ^{197}Hg (half-life of 2.672 days) and ^{203}Hg (half-life of 46.61 days) have been used in brain and renal scanning. [L. *Mercurius,* Mercury, the god of trade, messenger of the gods; in Mediev. L., quicksilver, mercury]

mer·cu·ry poi·son·ing (mĕr′kyū-rē poy′zŏn-ing) A disease usually caused by the ingestion of mercury or mercury compounds, which are toxic in relation to their ability to produce mercuric ions; **acute mercury poisoning** is usually associated with ulcerations of the stomach and intestine and toxic changes in the renal tubules; anuria and anemia may occur; **chronic mercury poisoning** is usually a result of industrial poisoning and causes gastrointestinal or central nervous system manifestations including stomatitis, diarrhea, ataxia, tremor, hyperreflexia, sensorineural impairment, and emotional instability (Mad Hatter syndrome). SYN hydrargyria, hydrargyrism, mercurialism.

mer·cy kill·ing (mĕr′sē kil′ing) The intentional putting to death of a person with an incurable or painful disease, intended as an act of mercy. Cf. euthanasia.

♻ **mere-, mero-** Combining forms meaning part; also indicating one of a series of similar parts. SEE ALSO -mer. [G. *mēros,* share]

Mer·en·din·o tech·nique (mer-en-dē′nō tek-nēk′) Plastic reconstruction of an incompetent mitral valve using heavy sutures to narrow the anulus in the region of the medial commissure.

Me·re·to·ja syn·drome (me-re-tōy′ah sin′drōm) A familial form of systemic amyloidosis with lattice corneal dystrophy, cranial and peripheral nerve palsies, protruding lips, masklike facies, and floppy ears.

me·rid·i·an (mĕ-rid′ē-an) **1.** A line encircling a globular body at right angles to its equator and touching both poles, or the half of such a circle extending from pole to pole. **2.** ACUPUNCTURE the lines connecting different anatomic sites. [L. *meridianus,* pertaining to midday, on the south side, southern]

me•rid•i•o•nal (mĕ-rid′ē-ō-năl) Relating to a meridian.

me•rid•i•o•nal ab•er•ra•tion (mĕ-rid′ē-ō-năl ab-ĕr-ā′shŭn) An aberration produced in the plane of a single meridian of a lens.

me•rid•i•o•nal am•bly•op•i•a (mĕ-rid′ē-ō-năl am′blē-ō′pē-ă) Amblyopia due to an uncorrected, large astigmatism during the amblyogenic period of visual development.

me•rid•i•o•nal fi•bers of ci•li•ar•y mus•cle (mĕ-rid′ē-ō-năl fī′bĕrz sil′ē-ar-ē mŭs′ĕl) The longitudinal fibers of the ciliary muscle. SYN fibrae meridionales muscularis ciliaris [TA].

Mer•kel cell car•ci•no•ma (mĕr′kĕl sel kahr′si-nō′mă) Rare and highly aggressive skin cancer, with lesions that develop on or just below the skin that are usually found on sun-exposed body areas, appear as painless, firm nodules or tumors; metastasize quickly and spread to other parts of the body, tending toward the regional lymph nodes. Twice as common in older men.

Mer•kel cor•pus•cle (mer′kel kōr′pŭs-ĕl) SYN tactile meniscus.

Mer•kel tac•tile cell (mer′kel tak′tīl sel) SYN tactile meniscus.

Mer•kel tac•tile disc (mer′kel tak′tīl disk) SYN tactile meniscus.

Mer•mis (mer′mis) Genus of long, opaque nematodes; larval stages passed in the hemocelic cavity of insects, particularly grasshoppers, whereas adults live free in soil. Accidental ingestion by humans causes infection.

Mer•mis ni•gres•cens (mer′mis nī-gres′senz) Nematode species found in soil that deposits eggs on above ground plants; normal host is the grasshopper; has been recovered from alimentary and urogenital tracts of humans (usually children) but infections are rare.

mer•o•crine gland (mer′ō-krin gland) A gland that releases only an acellular secretory product, in contrast to a holocrine gland.

mer•o•di•a•stol•ic (mer′ō-dī-ă-stol′ik) Partially diastolic; relating to a part of the diastole of the heart. [mero- + diastole]

mer•o•en•ceph•a•ly (mĕr′ō-en-sef′ă-lē) Congenital defective development of the brain in which the brain and cranium are present in rudimentary form. SYN anencephaly. [meros + G. *an-*, priv. + *enkephalos*, brain]

mer•o•gen•e•sis (mer-ō-jen′ĕ-sis) **1.** Reproduction by segmentation. **2.** Cleavage of an oocyte. [mero- + G. *genesis,* origin]

mer•o•ge•net•ic, mer•o•gen•ic (mer′ō-jĕ-net′ik, -jen′ik) Relating to merogenesis.

me•rog•o•ny (mĕ-rog′ŏ-nē) **1.** The incomplete development of an oocyte that has been disorganized. **2.** A form of asexual schizogony, typical of sporozoan protozoa, in which the nucleus divides several times before the cytoplasm divides; the schizont divides to form merozoites in this asexual phase of the life cycle. [mero- + G. *gonē,* generation]

mer•o•me•li•a (mer-ō-mē′lē-ă) Partial absence of part of a limb (exclusive of girdle); e.g., hemimelia, phocomelia. [mero- + G. *melos,* a limb]

mer•o•mi•cro•so•mi•a (mer′ō-mī-krō-sō′mē-ă) Abnormal smallness of some portion of the body; local dwarfism. [mero- + G. *mikros,* small, + *sōma,* body]

mer•o•my•o•sin (mer-ō-mī′ō-sin) A subunit of the tryptic digestion of myosin; two types are produced, H-meromyosin and L-meromyosin.

me•ros•mi•a (mĕ-roz′mē-ă) A condition in which the perception of certain odors is wanting; analogous to color blindness. [mero- + G. *osmē,* smell]

mer•o•sys•tol•ic (mer′ō-sis-tol′ik) Partially systolic; relating to a portion of the systole of the heart. [mero- + systole]

me•rot•o•my (mĕ-rot′ŏ-mē) The procedure of cutting into parts, as the cutting of a cell into separate parts to study their capacity for survival and development. [mero- + G. *tomē,* incision]

mer•o•zo•ite (mer-ō-zō′īt) The motile infective stage of sporozoan protozoa that results from schizogony or a similar type of asexual reproduction. Merozoites are responsible for the vast reproductive powers of sporozoan parasites. [mero- + G. *zōon,* animal]

me•ro•zy•gote (mer-ō-zī′gōt) MICROBIAL GENETICS an organism that, in addition to its own original genome (endogenote), contains a fragment (exogenote) of a genome from another organism; the relatively small size of the exogenote permits a diploid condition for only a limited region of the endogenote. [mero- + *zygōtos,* yoked]

MERRF (mĕrf) Acronym for myoclonic epilepsy with ragged red fiber myopathy. One of the mitochondrial disorders, this condition is caused by a point mutation of the mitochondria genome locus 8344, where transfer RNA is coded.

MES Abbreviation for microcurrent electrical stimulator.

♻ **mes-, meso-** **1.** Combining forms meaning middle, mean, intermediate. **2.** Combining forms indicating a mesentery, mesenterylike structure. **3.** Combining forms denoting a compound, containing more than one chiral center, having an internal plane of symmetry; such compounds do not exhibit optic activity (e.g., *meso*-cystine). [G. *mesos*]

me•sad (mē′sad) Passing or extending toward the median plane of the body or of a part. SYN mesiad. [G. *mesos,* middle, + L. *ad,* to]

mes·an·gi·al (mes-an′jē-ăl) Referring to the mesangium.

mes·an·gi·al ne·phri·tis (mes-an′jē-ăl nĕ-frī′tis) Glomerulonephritis with an increase in glomerular mesangial cells or matrix, or mesangial deposits.

mes·an·gi·al pro·lif·er·a·tive glo·mer·u·lo·ne·phri·tis (mes-an′jē-ăl prō-lif′ĕr-ă-tiv glō-mer′yū-lō-nĕ-frī′tis) Disorder characterized clinically by the nephrotic syndrome and histologically by diffuse glomerular increases in endocapillary and mesangial cells and in mesangial matrix; in some cases, there are mesangial deposits of IgM and complement.

mes·an·gi·um (mes-an′jē-ŭm) A central part of the renal glomerulus between capillaries; mesangial cells are phagocytic and for the most part separated from capillary lumina by endothelial cells. [mes- + G. *angeion,* vessel]

mes·a·or·ti·tis (mes′ā-ōr-tī′tis) Inflammation of the middle or muscular coat of the aorta. [mes- + aortitis]

mes·ar·ter·i·tis (mes′ahr-tĕr-ī′tis) Inflammation of the middle (muscular) coat of an artery. [mes- + arteritis]

me·sat·i·pel·lic, me·sat·i·pel·vic (mĕ-sat-i-pel′ik, mĕ-sat-i-pel′vik) Denoting a person with a pelvic index of 90–95; the superior strait has a round appearance, the transverse diameter exceeds the anteroposterior by 1 cm or less. [G. *mesatos,* midmost, + *pellis,* a bowl (pelvis)]

mes·ax·on (mes-ak′son) The plasma membrane of the neurolemma that is folded in to surround a nerve axon. In electron micrographs this double layer resembles a mesentery in appearance.

mes·ca·line (mes′kă-lin) Naturally occurring psychedelic drug in long use, especially in Native American religious ceremonies; produces visual hallucinations and radically altered states of consciousness, often experienced as pleasurable and illuminating but occasionally as anxious or revolting. Schedule I hallucinogen; considered a poisonous alkaloid. Also called *peyote*. [Sp. *mezcal*]

mes·ec·to·derm (mes-ek′tō-dĕrm) **1.** Cells in the area around the dorsal lip of the blastopore where mesoderm and ectoderm undergo a process of separation. **2.** That part of the mesenchyme derived from ectoderm, especially from the neural crest in the cephalic region in very young embryos. [mes- + ectoderm]

mes·en·ce·phal·ic (mes′en-se-fal′ik) Relating to the mesencephalon.

mes·en·ce·phal·ic flex·ure (mes′en-se-fal′ik flek′shŭr) SYN cephalic flexure.

mes·en·ce·phal·ic teg·men·tum (mes′en-se-fal′ik teg-men′tŭm) That major part of the substance of the mesencephalon or midbrain that extends from the substantia nigra to the level of the cerebral aqueduct. SYN tegmentum (2).

mes·en·ceph·a·li·tis (mes′en-sef′ă-lī′tis) Inflammation of the midbrain (mesencephalon).

mes·en·ceph·a·lon (mes′en-sef′ă-lon) [TA] That part of the brainstem developing from the middle of the three primary cerebral vesicles of the embryo. In an adult, the mesencephalon is characterized by the unique conformation of its roof plate, the lamina of the mesencephalic tectum, composed of the bilaterally paired superior and inferior colliculi, and by the massive paired prominence of the crus cerebri at its ventral surface. Prominent cell groups of the mesencephalon include the motor nuclei of the trochlear and oculomotor nerves, the red nucleus, and the substantia nigra. SYN midbrain. [mes- + G. *enkephalos,* brain]

mes·en·ceph·a·lot·o·my (mes′en-sef-ă-lot′ō-mē) **1.** The sectioning of any structure in the midbrain, especially of the spinothalamic tracts for the relief of intractable pain or the cerebral peduncle for dyskinesias. **2.** A mesencephalic spinothalamic tractotomy. [mesencephalon + G. *tomē,* incision]

me·sen·chy·mal (mes-eng′ki-măl) Relating to the mesenchyme.

mes·en·chyme (mes′eng-kīm) **1.** An aggregation of mesenchymal cells. **2.** Primordial embryonic connective tissue consisting of mesenchymal cells, usually stellate in form, supported in interlaminar jelly. [mes- + G. *enkyma,* infusion]

mes·en·chy·mo·ma (mes′eng-kī-mō′mă) Neoplasm in which there is a mixture of mesenchymal derivatives, other than fibrous tissue. A **benign mesenchymoma** may contain foci of vascular, muscular, adipose, osteoid, osseous, and cartilaginous tissue. A **malignant mesenchymoma** may also occur as a similar mixture of two or more types of mesenchymal cells that are malignant.

mes·en·ter·ic (mes′en-ter′ik) Relating to the mesentery.

mes·en·ter·i·o·pex·y (mes′en-ter-ē-ō-pek′sē) Fixation or attachment of a torn or incised mesentery. SYN mesopexy. [mesentery + G. *pēxis,* fixation]

mes·en·ter·i·or·rha·phy (mes′en-ter-ē-ōr′ă-fē) Suture of the mesentery. SYN mesorrhaphy. [mesentery + G. *rhaphē,* suture]

mes·en·te·ri·pli·ca·tion (mes′en-ter-i-pli-kā′shŭn) Reducing redundancy of a mesentery by making one or more tucks in it. [mesentery + L. *plico,* pp. *-atus,* to fold]

mes·en·ter·i·tis (mes′en-tĕr-ī′tis) Inflammation of the mesentery.

mes·en·te·ri·um (mes′en-ter′ē-ŭm) SYN mesentery, mesentery. [Mod. L.]

me•sen•ter•o•ax•i•al vol•vu•lus (mes′en-ter′ō-aks′ē-ăl vol′vyū-lŭs) A type of gastric volvulus in which the axis of twist is parallel to the line of the gastric mesentery.

mes•en•ter•y (mes′en-ter-ē) **1.** A double layer of peritoneum attached to the abdominal wall and enclosing in its fold a portion or all of one of the abdominal viscera, conveying to it its vessels and nerves. **2.** The fan-shaped fold of peritoneum encircling the greater part of the small intestines (jejunum and ileum) and attaching it to the posterior abdominal wall at the root of the mesentery (radix mesenterii). SYN mesenterium. [Mod. L. *mesenterium,* fr. G. *mesenterion,* fr. G. *mesos,* middle, + *enteron,* intestine]

MeSH (mesh) Acronym for Medical Subject Headings.

mesh graft (mesh graft) A partial or split-thickness skin graft in which multiple slits have been made so that it can be stretched to cover a lage area, usually a burn or other cutaneous defect. The slits also allow for the seepage of fluids, thus promoting the body's acceptance of the graft.

me•si•ad (mē′zē-ad) SYN mesad.

me•si•al (mē′zē-ăl) Toward the median plane following the curvature of the dental arch, in contrast to distal (2). SYN proximal (2). [G. *mesos,* middle]

me•si•al an•gle (mē′zē-ăl ang′gĕl) The angle formed by the meeting of the mesial with the labial (or buccal) or lingual surface of a tooth.

me•si•al oc•clu•sion (mē′zē-ăl ŏ-klū′zhŭn) **1.** Occlusion in which the mandibular teeth articulate with the maxillary teeth in a position anterior to normal. SYN mesioocclusion. **2.** SYN mesiocclusion.

♻ **mesio-** Combining form meaning mesial (especially in dentistry). [G. *mesos,* middle]

me•si•o•buc•cal (mē′zē-ō-bŭk′ăl) Relating to the mesial and buccal surfaces of a tooth; denoting especially the angle formed by the junction of these two surfaces.

me•si•oc•clu•sion (mē′zē-ŏ-klū′zhŭn) A malocclusion in which the mandibular arch articulates with the maxillary arch in a position mesial to normal; in Angle classification, a Class III malocclusion. SYN mesial occlusion (2).

me•si•o•cer•vi•cal (mē′zē-ō-sĕr′vi-kăl) **1.** Relating to the line angle of a cavity preparation at the junction of the mesial and cervical walls. **2.** Pertaining to the area of a tooth at the junction of the mesial surface and the cervical region.

me•si•o•dens (mē′zē-ō-denz) A supernumerary tooth located in the midline of the anterior maxillae, generally between the maxillary central incisor teeth. Surgical removal is usually indicated. [mesio- + L. *dens,* tooth]

me•si•o•dis•tal (mē′zē-ō-dis′tăl) Pertaining to both the mesial and distal surfaces of a tooth, as a diameter measured from one surface to the other.

me•si•o•gin•gi•val (mē′zē-ō-jin′ji-văl) Relating to the angle formed by the junction of the mesial surface with the gingival line of a tooth.

me•si•o•la•bi•al (mē′zē-ō-lā′bē-ăl) Relating to the mesial and labial surfaces of a tooth; denoting especially the angle formed by their junction.

me•si•o•lin•gual (mē′zē-ō-ling′gwăl) Relating to the mesial and lingual surfaces of a tooth; denoting especially the angle formed by their junction.

me•si•o•lin•guo•oc•clu•sal (mē′zē-ō-ling′gwō-ŏ-klū′zăl) Denoting the angle formed by the junction of the mesial, lingual, and occlusal surfaces of a premolar or molar tooth.

me•si•o•lin•guo•pul•pal (mē′zē-ō-ling′gwō-pŭl′păl) Relating to the angle denoting the junction of the mesial, lingual, and pulpal surfaces in a tooth cavity preparation.

me•sio•oc•clu•sal (mē′zē-ō-ŏ-klū′zăl) Denoting the angle formed by the junction of the mesial and occlusal surfaces of a premolar or molar tooth.

me•sio•oc•clu•sion (mē′zē-ō-ŏ-klū′zhŭn) SYN mesial occlusion (1).

me•si•o•ver•sion (mē′zē-ō-ver′zhŭn) Malposition of a tooth mesial to normal, in an anterior direction following the curvature of the dental arch.

mes•mer•ism (mes′mĕr-izm) A system of therapeutics from which were developed hypnotism and therapeutic suggestion.

mes•o•ap•pen•dix (mez′ō-ă-pen′diks) [TA] The short mesentery of the appendix lying behind the terminal ileum, in which the appendicular artery courses.

mes•o•bi•lane (mez′ō-bī′lān) A reduced mesobilirubin with no double bonds between the pyrrole rings and, consequently, colorless. SEE ALSO bilirubinoids. SYN mesobilirubinogen.

mes•o•bil•i•ru•bin (mez′ō-bil-i-rū′bin) A compound differing from bilirubin only in that the vinyl groups of bilirubin are reduced to ethyl groups. SEE ALSO bilirubinoids.

mes•o•bil•i•ru•bin•o•gen (mez′ō-bil-i-rū-bin′ō-jen) SYN mesobilane.

mes•o•blast (mez′ō-blast) SYN mesoderm. [meso- + G. *blastos,* germ]

mes•o•blas•te•ma (mez′ō-blas-tē′mă) All those cells that collectively constitute the early undifferentiated mesoderm. [meso- + G. *blastēma,* a sprout]

mes·o·blas·te·mic (mez′ō-blas-tē′mik) Relating to or derived from the mesoblastema.

mes·o·blas·tic (mez′ō-blas′tik) Relating to or derived from the mesoderm.

mesocaecal [Br.] SYN mesocecal.

mesocaecum [Br.] SYN mesocecum.

mes·o·car·di·a (mez′ō-kahr′dē-ă) **1.** Atypical position of the heart in a central position in the thorax, as in early embryonic life. **2.** Plural of mesocardium. [meso- + G. *kardia,* heart]

mes·o·car·di·um, pl. **mes·o·car·di·a** (mez-ō-kahr′dē-ŭm, -dē-ă) The double layer of splanchnic mesoderm supporting the embryonic heart in the pericardial cavity. It disappears before birth. [meso- + G. *kardia,* heart]

mes·o·ca·val shunt (mez′ō-kā′văl shŭnt) **1.** Anastomosis of the side of the superior mesenteric vein to the proximal end of the divided inferior vena cava, for control of portal hypertension. **2.** H-shunt anastomosis of the inferior vena cava to the superior mesenteric vein, using a synthetic conduit or autologous vein.

mes·o·ce·cal (mez′ō-sē′kăl) Relating to the mesocecum. SYN mesocaecal.

mes·o·ce·cum (mez′ō-sē′kŭm) Part of the mesocolon, supporting the cecum, which occasionally persists when the ascending colon becomes retroperitoneal during fetal life. SYN mesocaecum. [meso- + cecum]

Mes·o·ces·toi·des (mez′ō-ses-toy′dēz) Tapeworm genus found in carnivorous mammals (e.g., foxes); mites are probably intermediate hosts; a few human cases have been identified in Japan, the U.S., and China.

mes·o·col·ic (mez′ō-kol′ik) Relating to the mesocolon.

mes·o·co·lon (mez′ō-kō′lŏn) The fold of peritoneum attaching the colon to the posterior abdominal wall; ascending mesocolon (mesocolon ascendens [TA]), transverse mesocolon (mesocolon transversum [TA]), descending mesocolon (mesocolon descendens [TA]), and sigmoid mesocolon (mesocolon sigmoideum [TA]) correspond to the respective divisions of the colon; the ascending and descending portions are usually fused to the peritoneum of the posterior abdominal wall, but can be mobilized. [meso- + *kolon,* colon]

mes·o·co·lo·pex·y (mez′ō-kō′lō-pek-sē) An operation for shortening the mesocolon, for correction of undue mobility and ptosis. SYN mesocoloplication. [meso- + G. *kolon,* colon, + *pēxis,* fixation]

mes·o·co·lo·pli·ca·tion (mez′ō-kō′lō-pli-kā′shŭn) SYN mesocolopexy. [meso- + G. *kolon,* colon, + L. *plico,* pp. *-atus,* to fold]

mes·o·cord (mez′ō-kōrd) A fold of amnion that sometimes binds a segment of the umbilical cord to the placenta.

mes·o·derm (mez′ō-dĕrm) The middle of the three primary germ layers of the embryo (the others being ectoderm and endoderm); mesoderm is the origin of all connective tissues, all musculature, blood, cardiovascular and lymphatic systems, most of the urogenital system, and the lining of the pericardial, pleural, and peritoneal cavities. SYN mesoblast. [meso- + G. *derma,* skin]

mes·o·der·mic (mez′ō-dĕrm′ik) Relating to the mesoderm.

mes·o·du·o·de·nal (mez′ō-dū-ō-dē′năl) Relating to the mesoduodenum.

mes·o·du·o·de·num (mez′ō-dū′ō-dē′nŭm) The mesentery of the duodenum.

mes·o·ep·i·did·y·mis (mez′ō-ep-i-did′i-mis) An occasional fold of the tunica vaginalis binding the epididymis to the testis. [meso- + epididymis]

mes·o·gas·ter (mez′ō-gas′tĕr) SYN mesogastrium.

mes·o·gas·tric (mez′ō-gas′trik) Relating to the mesogastrium.

mes·o·gas·tri·um (mez′ō-gas′trē-ŭm) In the embryo, the mesentery of the dilated portion of the alimentary canal that is the primordium of the stomach; it gives rise to the greater omentum and consequently is involved in the formation of the omental bursa. The spleen and body of the pancreas develop within it, and thus the splenorenal and gastrosplenic ligaments are derivatives of the (dorsal) mesogastrium. SYN mesogaster. [meso- + G. *gastēr* stomach]

mes·o·gen·ic (mez′ō-jen′ik) Denoting a virus capable of inducing lethal infection in embryonic hosts, after a short incubation period, and an inapparent infection in immature and adult hosts. [meso- + G. *-gen,* producing]

me·sog·li·a (me-sog′lē-ă) Neuroglial cells of mesodermal origin. SEE ALSO microglia. SYN mesoglial cells. [meso- + G. *glia,* glue]

me·sog·li·al cells (me-sog′lē-ăl selz) SYN mesoglia.

mes·o·glu·te·al (mez′ō-glū′tē-ăl) Relating to the musculus gluteus medius.

mes·o·il·e·um (mez′ō-il′ē-ŭm) The mesentery of the ileum.

mes·o·je·ju·num (mez′ō-jĕ-jū′nŭm) The mesentery of the jejunum.

mes·o·lym·pho·cyte (mez′ō-lim′fō-sīt) A mononuclear leukocyte of medium size, probably a lymphocyte, with a deeply staining nucleus of large size but relatively smaller than that in most lymphocytes. [meso- + lymphocyte]

mes·o·me·li·a (mez′ō-mē′lē-ă) The condition of having abnormally short forearms and legs. [meso- + G. *melos,* limb]

mes·o·mel·ic dwarf·ism (mez′ō-mel′ik dwōrf′izm) Dwarfism with shortness of the forearms and legs.

mes·o·mere (mez′ō-mēr) **1.** A blastomere of a size intermediate between that of a macromere and a micromere. **2.** The zone between an epimere and a hypomere. [meso- + G. *meros,* part]

mes·o·met·a·neph·ric car·ci·no·ma (mez′ō-met-ă-nef′rik kahr′si-nō′mă) SYN mesonephroma.

mes·o·me·tri·um (mez′ō-mē′trē-ŭm) [TA] The broad ligament of the uterus, below the mesosalpinx. [meso- + G. *mētra,* uterus]

mes·o·morph (mez′ō-mōrf) A constitutional body type or build (biotype or somatotype) in which tissues that originate from the mesoderm prevail; from the morphologic standpoint, a balance exists between trunk and limbs. SEE ALSO hypomorph, ectomorph, endomorph. [meso- + G. *morphē,* form]

mes·o·mor·phic (mez′ō-mōrf′ik) Relating to a mesomorph.

me·son (mes′on) An elementary particle having a rest mass intermediate in value between the mass of an electron and that of a proton. [G. neuter of *mesos,* middle]

mes·o·neph·ric (mez′ō-nef′rik) Relating to the mesonephros.

mes·o·neph·ric duct (mez′ō-nef′rik dŭkt) A duct in the embryo draining the mesonephric tubules; in the male it becomes the ductus deferens and ureter; in the female it becomes the ureter's vestigial structures. SYN wolffian duct.

mes·o·neph·ric fold (mez′ō-nef′rik fōld) SYN mesonephric ridge.

mes·o·neph·ric ridge (mez′ō-nef′rik rij) A ridge that, in early human embryos, comprises the entire urogenital ridge; however, later in development a more medial genital ridge, the potential gonad, is demarcated from it. SEE ALSO urogenital ridge. SYN mesonephric fold.

mes·o·neph·roi (mez′ō-nef′roy) Plural of mesonephros.

mes·o·ne·phro·ma (mez′ō-ne-frō′mă) A rare malignant neoplasm of the ovary and corpus uteri, thought to originate in mesonephric structures that become misplaced in ovarian tissue during embryonic development. SYN clear cell carcinoma, mesometanephric carcinoma. [mesonephros + *-oma,* tumor]

mes·o·neph·ros, pl. **mes·o·neph·roi** (mez′ō-nef′ros, mez′ō-nef′roy) One of three excretory organs appearing in the evolution of vertebrates; in life forms with a metanephros, it is located between the regressing pronephros and the metanephros, cephalic to the latter. In young mammalian embryos, the mesonephros is well developed and briefly functional until establishment of the metanephros, the definitive kidney; in older embryos, the mesonephros undergoes regression as an excretory organ, but its duct system is retained in the male as the epididymis and ductus deferens. SYN wolffian body. [meso- + G. *nephros,* kidney]

mes·o·neu·ri·tis (mez′ō-nūr-ī′tis) Inflammation of a nerve or of its connective tissue without involvement of its sheath.

mes·o·pexy (mez′ō-pek-sē) SYN mesenteriopexy.

mes·o·phil, **mes·o·phile** (mez′ō-fil, -fīl) A microorganism with an optimal temperature between 25–40°C, but growing within the limits of 10–45°C. [meso- + G. *philos,* fond]

mes·o·phil·ic (mez′ō-fil′ik) Pertaining to a mesophil.

mes·o·phle·bi·tis (mez′ō-flĕ-bī′tis) Inflammation of the middle coat of a vein. [meso- + phlebitis]

me·soph·ry·on (mez-of′rē-on) SYN glabella (2). [meso- + Gr. *ophrys,* eyebrow]

mes·o·por·phy·rins (mez′ō-pōr′fi-rinz) Porphyrin compounds resembling the protoporphyrins except that the vinyl side chains of the latter are reduced to ethyl side chains; e.g., mesobilane.

me·sor·chi·al (mez-ōr′kē-ăl) Relating to the mesorchium.

me·sor·chi·um (mez-ōr′kē-ŭm) **1.** In the fetus, a fold of tunica vaginalis testis supporting the mesonephros and the developing testis. **2.** In the adult, a fold of tunica vaginalis testis between the testis and epididymis. [meso- + G. *orchis,* testis]

mes·o·rec·tum (mez′ō-rek′tŭm) The peritoneal investment of the rectum, covering the upper part only.

mes·or·rha·phy (mez-ōr′ă-fē) SYN mesenteriorrhaphy.

mes·o·sal·pinx (mez′ō-sal′pingks) [TA] The part of the broad ligament investing the uterine (fallopian) tube. [meso- + G. *salpinx,* trumpet]

mes·o·sig·moid (mez′ō-sig′moyd) Sigmoid mesocolon. SEE mesocolon.

mes·o·sig·moid·i·tis (mez′ō-sig-moy-dī′tis) Inflammation of the mesosigmoid.

mes·o·sig·moid·o·pex·y (mez′ō-sig-moy′dō-pek-sē) Surgical fixation of the mesosigmoid.

mes·o·some (mez′ō-som) A convoluted membranous body formed by involution of the plasma membranes of certain bacteria; functions in cellular respiration and septum formation. [meso + G. *soma*, body]

mes•o•ten•din•e•um (mez′ō-ten-din′ē-ŭm) SYN mesotendon.

mes•o•ten•don (mez′ō-ten′don) The synovial layers that pass from a tendon to the wall of a tendon sheath in certain places where tendons lie within osteofibrous canals. In most instances, the mesotendon degenerates, leaving only the vincula. SYN mesotendineum.

mes•o•the•li•a (mez′ō-thē′lē-ă) Plural of mesothelium.

mes•o•the•li•al (mez′ō-thē′lē-ăl) Relating to the mesothelium.

mes•o•the•li•o•ma (mez′ō-thē-lē-ō′mă) A rare malignant neoplasm, derived from the lining cells of the pleura and peritoneum, which grows as a thick sheet covering the viscera. [mesothelium + G. *-oma*, tumor]

mes•o•the•li•um, pl. **mes•o•the•li•a** (mez′ō-thē′lē-ŭm, mez′ō-thē′lē-ă) A single layer of flattened cells forming an epithelium that lines serous cavities; e.g., peritoneum, pleura, pericardium. [meso- + epithelium]

mes•o•tym•pan•um (mez-ō-tim′pă-nŭm) The portion of the middle ear medial to the tympanic membrane.

mes•o•va•ri•um, pl. **mes•o•va•ri•a** (mez′ō-vā′rē-ŭm, -ă) A short peritoneal fold connecting the anterior border of the ovary with the posterior layer of the broad ligament of the uterus. [meso- + L. *ovarium*, ovary]

mes•sen•ger RNA (mRNA) (mes′en-jĕr) The RNA reflecting the exact nucleoside sequence of the genetically active DNA and carrying the "message" of the latter, coded in its sequence, to the cytoplasmic areas where protein is made in amino acid sequences specified by the mRNA, and hence primarily by the DNA; viral RNA is considered to be natural messenger RNA.

MET Abbreviation for metabolic equivalent; muscle energy technique.

Met Abbreviation for the amino acid methionine. SEE methionine.

♻**meta-** **1.** Combining form denoting after, subsequent to, behind, or hindmost. Cf. post-. **2.** CHEMISTRY an italicized prefix denoting joint, action sharing. **3.** (*m-*) CHEMISTRY an italicized prefix denoting compound formed by two substitutions in the benzene ring separated by one carbon atom (i.e., linked to the first and third, second and fourth) carbon atoms of the ring. For terms beginning with *meta-*, or *m-*, see the specific name. SYN *m-*. [G. after, between, over]

met•a•a•nal•y•sis (met′ă-ă-nal′i-sis) The systematic process of using statistical methods to combine the results of different studies; systematic, organized, and structured evaluation of a problem using information, commonly in the form of statistical tables, from a number of different studies of a problem. SEE ALSO analysis.

me•tab•a•sis (mĕ-tab′ă-sis) Rarely used term for a change of any kind in symptoms or course of a disease. [G. a passing over, change, fr. *metabainō*, to pass over]

met•a•bi•o•sis (met′ă-bī-ō′sis) Dependence of one organism on another for its existence. SEE ALSO commensalism, mutualism, parasitism. [meta- + G. *biōsis*, way of life]

met•a•bi•sul•fite test (met′ă-bī-sŭl′fīt test) A test for sickle cell hemoglobin (Hb S); deoxygenation of cells containing Hb S is enhanced by addition of sodium metabisulfite to the blood, causing sickling visible on a slide; certain other abnormal hemoglobins (Hb C_{Harlem} and Hb I) also sickle in this test.

met•a•bol•ic (met′ă-bol′ik) Relating to metabolism.

met•a•bol•ic ac•i•do•sis (met′ă-bol′ik as-i-dō′sis) Decreased pH and bicarbonate concentration in the body fluids caused either by the accumulation of acids or by abnormal losses of fixed base from the body, as in diarrhea or renal disease.

met•a•bol•ic al•ka•lo•sis (met′ă-bol′ik al-kă-lō′sis) A disorder associated with an increased arterial bicarbonate concentration, resulting from an excessive intake of alkaline materials or an excessive loss of acid in the urine or through persistent vomiting; the base excess and standard bicarbonate are both elevated. SEE ALSO compensated alkalosis.

met•a•bol•ic burst (met′ă-bol′ik bŭrst) A transient increase in oxygen consumption by a neutrophil occurring immediately after phagocytosis. Also referred to as respiratory burst.

met•a•bol•ic cir•rho•sis (met′ă-bol′ik sĭr-ō′sis) Cirrhosis due to a metabolic disorder that causes the deposition of minerals in the liver, as in hemochromatosis (iron deposition) or Wilson disease (copper deposition).

met•a•bol•ic co•ma (met′ă-bol′ik kō′mă) Coma resulting from diffuse failure of neuronal metabolism, caused by such abnormalities as intrinsic disorders of neuron or glial cell metabolism, or extracerebral disorders that produce intoxication or electrolyte imbalances.

met•a•bol•ic cra•ni•op•a•thy (met′ă-bol′ik krā-nē-op′ă-thē) SYN Morgagni syndrome.

met•a•bol•ic en•ceph•a•lop•a•thy (met′ă-bol′ik en-sef′ă-lop′ă-thē) Encephalopathy characterized by memory loss, vertigo, and generalized weakness, due to metabolic brain disease including hypoxia, ischemia, hypoglycemia, or secondary to other organ failure such as liver or kidney.

met·a·bol·ic e·quiv·a·lent (MET) (met′ă-bol′ik ē-kwiv′ă-lĕnt) The oxygen cost of energy expenditure measured at supine rest (1 MET = 3.5 mL O_2 per kg of body weight per minute); multiples of MET are used to estimate the oxygen cost of activity.

met·a·bol·ic mu·ci·no·sis (met′ă-bol′ik myū si-nō′sis) SEE mucinosis.

met·a·bol·ic path·way (met′ă-bol′ik path′wā) Intercellular chemical reactions; catalyzed by enzymes; include the principal chemical reactions, mostly enzyme-dependent, that an organism needs to maintain homeostasis and to break down or build up molecules.

met·a·bol·ic res·pi·ra·tor·y quo·tient (met′ă-bol′ik res′pir-ă-tōr-ē kwō′shĕnt) SEE respiratory quotient.

met·a·bol·ic syn·drome (met′ă-bŏl′ik sin′drōm) A group of health risks that increase the chances of developing heart disease, stroke, and diabetes. The criteria for this syndrome are any 3 of these 5 risk factors: (1) BP> 130/80 mmHg; (2) abdominal obesity (men > 40 inches and women > 35 inches); (3) triglycerides > 150 mg/dL; (4) HDL cholesterol for men < 40 mg/dL and women <50 mg/dL; and (5) fasting glucose > 110mg/dL. SYN insulin-resistance syndrome, multiple metabolic syndrome, syndrome X.

me·tab·o·lism (mĕ-tab′ŏ-lizm) **1.** The sum of the chemical and physical changes occurring in tissue, consisting of anabolism, those reactions that convert small molecules into large, and catabolism, those reactions that convert large molecules into small, including both endogenous large molecules as well as biodegradation of xenobiotics. **2.** Often incorrectly used as a synonym for either anabolism or catabolism. [G. *metabolē,* change]

me·tab·o·lite (mĕ-tab′ō-līt) Any product (intermediate or final, including waste) of a metabolic process.

me·tab·o·lize (mĕ-tab′ŏ-līz) To undergo the chemical changes of metabolism.

me·tab·o·re·cep·tors (mĕ-tab′ō-rē-sep′tŏrz) Peripheral afferent nerve endings that respond to metabolites (lactate, CO_2, pH) produced by active muscle. [*metabo*lism + receptor]

met·a·car·pal (met′ă-kahr′păl) **1.** Relating to the metacarpus. **2.** Any one of the metacarpal bones (I–V).

met·a·car·pal bones [I–V] (met′ă-kahr′păl bōnz) Five long bones (numbered I–V, beginning with the bone on the radial or thumb side) forming the skeleton of the metacarpus or palm; they articulate with the bones of the distal row of the carpus and with the five proximal phalanges. SYN ossa metacarpi.

met·a·car·pec·to·my (met′ă-kahr-pek′tŏ-mē) Excision of one or all of the metacarpals. [metacarpus + G. *ektomē,* excision]

met·a·car·po·pha·lan·ge·al (MCP) (met′ă-kahr′pō-fă-lan′jē-ăl) Relating to the metacarpus and the phalanges; denoting the articulations between them.

met·a·car·po·pha·lan·ge·al joint (met′ă-kahr′pō-fă-lan′jē-ăl joynt) The spheroid synovial joints between the heads of the metacarpals and the bases of the proximal phalanges. See this page.

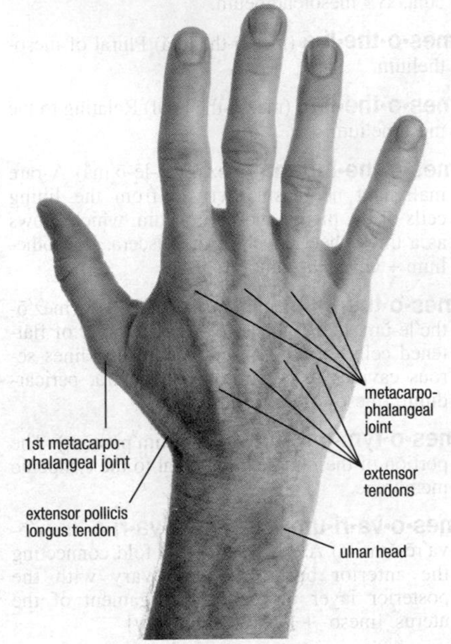

metacarpophalangeal joint

met·a·car·pus, pl. **met·a·car·pi** (met′ă-kahr′pŭs, -pī) [TA] The five bones of the hand between the carpus and the phalanges. [meta- + G. *karpos,* wrist]

met·a·cen·tric chro·mo·some (met′ă-sen′trik krō′mŏ-sōm) A chromosome with a centrally placed centromere that divides the chromosome into two arms of approximately equal length. [meta- + G. *kentron,* circle]

met·a·cer·ca·ri·a, pl. **met·a·cer·ca·ri·ae** (met′ă-sĕr-kar′ē-ă, -ē) The postcercarial encysted stage in the life history of a fluke, before transfer to the definitive host. Some cercariae attach themselves to vegetation, form metacercariae, and are ingested by herbivores; others encyst in muscles of fish or crayfish. [meta- + G. *kerkos,* tail]

met·a·chro·ma·si·a (met′ă-krō-mā′zē-ă) **1.** The condition in which a cell or tissue component takes on a color different from the dye solution with which it is stained. SYN metachromatism (2). **2.** A change in the characteristic color of certain basic thiazine dyes, such as toluidine blue, when the dye molecules are bound to tissue polyanionic polymers. [meta- + G. *chrōma*, color]

met·a·chro·mat·ic (met′ă-krō-mat′ik) Denoting cells or dyes that exhibit metachromasia. SYN metachromophil, metachromophile.

met·a·chro·mat·ic bod·ies (met′ă-krō-mat′ik bod′ēz) Concentrated deposits consisting primarily of polymetaphosphate and occurring in many bacteria as well as in algae, fungi, and protozoa; m. bodies differ in staining properties from the surrounding protoplasm. SEE metachromasia.

met·a·chro·mat·ic leu·ko·dys·tro·phy (met′ă-krō-mat′ik lū′kō-dis′trŏ-fē) A metabolic disorder, usually of infancy, characterized by myelin loss, accumulation of metachromatic lipids (galactosyl sulfatidates) in the white matter of the central and peripheral nervous systems, progressive paralysis, and mental retardation; psychosis and dementia are seen in adults.

met·a·chro·mat·ic stain (met′ă-krō-mat′ik stān) A stain (e.g., methylene blue, thionine, or azure A) that interacts chemically with certain histologic or cytologic structures, yielding a color different from that of the stain.

met·a·chro·ma·tism (met′ă-krō′mă-tizm) **1.** Any color change, whether natural or produced by basic aniline dyes. **2.** SYN metachromasia (1). [meta- + G. *chrōma*, color]

met·a·chro·mo·phil, **met·a·chro·mo·phile** (met′ă-krō′mō-fil, -fīl) SYN metachromatic. [meta- + G. *chrōma*, color, + *philos*, fond]

met·a·cone (met′ă-kōn) **1.** The distobuccal cusp of human upper molars. **2.** A cusp derived from the protocone in the evolutionary history of the molars. [meta- + G. *chronos*, time]

met·a·co·nid (met′ă-kon′id) **1.** The mesiolingual cusp of human lower molars. **2.** A cusp derived from the protoconid in the evolutionary history of the molars.

met·a·her·pet·ic ker·a·ti·tis (met′ă-hĕr-pet′ik ker′ă-tī′tis) A postinfectious corneal inflammation in herpetic keratitis leading to epithelial erosion; not due to virus replication.

met·a·ki·ne·sis, **met·a·ki·ne·si·a** (met′ă-ki-nē′sis, -sē-ă) Moving apart; the separation of the two chromatids of each chromosome and their movement to opposite poles in the anaphase of mitosis. [meta- + G. *kinēsis*, movement]

met·al (met′ăl) One of the electropositive elements, either amphoteric or basic, characterized by luster, malleability, ductility, the ability to conduct electricity and heat, and the tendency to lose rather than gain electrons in chemical reactions. [L. *metallum*, a mine, a mineral, fr. G. *metallon*, a mine, pit]

met·al fume fe·ver (me′tăl fyūm fē′ver) An occupational disorder caused by the inhalation of fumes or metallic oxides; characterized by symptoms similar to influenzas. The condition occurs among workers engaged in welding, metal fabrication, casting, and other metal-working tasks. Fresh air and treatment of symptoms usually alleviate the conditions.

met·a·lin·guis·tics (met′ă-ling-gwis′tiks) The ability to understand, organize, and interpret language (e.g., idioms, homonyms).

♻ **metallo-** Prefix meaning metal, metallic. [see metal]

me·tal·lo·en·zyme (mĕ-tal′ō-en′zīm) An enzyme containing a metal (ion) as an integral part of its active structure; e.g., cytochromes (Fe, Cu), aldehyde oxidase (Mo), catechol oxidase (Cu), carbonic anhydrase (Zn).

me·tal·lo·por·phy·rin (mĕ-tal′ō-pōr′fi-rin) A combination of a porphyrin with a metal, e.g., Fe (hematin), Mg (as in chlorophyll), Cu (in hemocyanin), Zn.

me·tal·lo·pro·tein (mĕ-tal′ō-prō′tēn) A protein with a tightly bound metal ion or ions; e.g., hemoglobin.

me·tal·lo·pro·tein·ase (mĕ-tal′ō-prō′tēn-ās) A family of protein-hydrolyzing endopeptidases that contain zinc ions as part of the active structure.

me·tal·lo·thi·o·ne·in (mĕ-tal′ō-thī′ō-nē′in) A small protein, rich in cysteinyl residues, which is synthesized in the liver and kidney in response to the presence of divalent ions (zinc, mercury, cadmium, copper) and that binds these ions tightly; of importance in ion transport and detoxification.

met·a·mer (met′ă-mĕr) An entity that is similar to, but ultimately differentiable from, another entity. [meta- + -mer]

met·a·mere (met′ă-mēr) One of a series of homologous segments in the body. SEE ALSO somite. [meta- + G. *meros*, part]

met·a·mer·ic (met-ă-mer′ik) Relating to or showing metamerism, or occurring in a metamere.

met·a·mer·ic ner·vous sys·tem (met-ă-mer′ik nĕr′vŭs sis′tĕm) The part of the nervous system that innervates body structures developed in ontogeny from the segmentally arranged somites or, in the head region, pharyngeal (branchial in fish) arches. The term implies reference to the neural mechanisms intrinsic to the spinal cord and brainstem (represented by the sensory nuclei, motoneuronal cell groups, and their associated interneurons in the reticular formation); by strict definition it should exclude the autonomic nervous system.

me·tam·er·ism (me-tam′ĕr-izm) A pattern of anatomic structure exhibiting serial repetition of homologous structures, as vertebrae, ribs, intercostal muscles, and spinal nerves.

met·a·mor·phop·si·a (met′ă-mōr-fop′sē-ă) Distortion of visual images. [meta- + G. *morphē,* shape, + *opsis,* vision]

met·a·mor·pho·sis (met′ă-mōr′fō-sis) **1.** A change in form, structure, or function. **2.** Transition from one developmental stage to another. SYN transformation (1). [G. *meta,* beyond, over, + *morphē,* form]

met·a·mor·phot·ic (met′ă-mōr-fot′ik) Relating to or marked by metamorphosis.

met·a·my·el·o·cyte (met′ă-mī′el-ō-sīt) A transitional form of myelocyte with nuclear construction that is intermediate between the mature myelocyte (myelocyte C of Sabin) and the two-lobed granular leukocyte. SYN juvenile cell. [meta- + G. *myelos,* marrow, + *kytos,* cell]

met·a·neph·ric blas·te·ma (met′ă-nef′rik blas-tē′mă) SYN metanephric mass of mesoderm.

met·a·neph·ric di·ver·tic·u·lum (met′ă-nef′rik dī′vĕr-tik′yū-lŭm) An outgrowth from the mesonephric duct that gives rise to the ureter, renal pelvis, calyces, and collecting tubules. See this page. SYN ureteric bud.

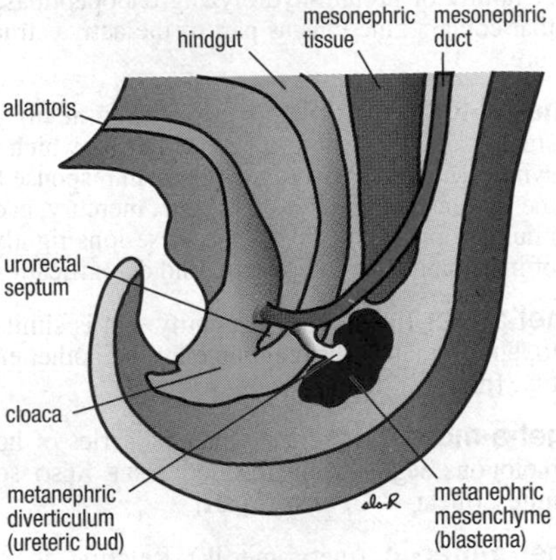

metanephric diverticulum: penetration of the metanephric mesenchyme; end of fifth week

met·a·neph·ric duct (met′ă-nef′rik dŭkt) The slender tubular portion of the metanephric diverticulum; the primordium of the epithelial lining of the ureter.

met·a·neph·ric mass of mes·en·chyme (met′ă-nef′rik mas mes′en-kīm) SYN metanephrogenic blastema.

met·a·neph·ric mass of mes·o·derm (met′a-nĕf′rik mas mez′ŏ-dĕrm) The mesoderm covering the distal end of the metanephric diverticulum; it gives rise to the nephrons in the permanent kidneys. SYN metanephric blastema.

met·a·neph·rine (met′ă-nef′rin) A metabolite of epinephrine, excreted in the urine and found in some tissues. SEE respiratory quotient.

met·a·neph·ro·gen·ic, met·a·ne·phrog·e·nous (met′ă-nef-rō-jen′ik, -nĕ-froj′ĕ-nŭs) Applied to the more caudal part of the intermediate mesoderm, which, under the inductive action of the metanephric diverticulum, has the potency to form metanephric tubules. [meta- + G. *nephros,* kidney, + *-gen,* producing]

met·a·neph·ro·gen·ic blas·te·ma (met′ă-nef′rō-jen′ik blas-tē′mă) The mesenchyme covering the distal end of the metanephric diverticulum; it gives rise to the nephrons of the permanent kidneys. SYN metanephric mass of mesenchyme.

met·a·neph·ros, pl. **met·a·neph·roi** (met′ă-nef′rŏs, met′ă-nef′roy) The most caudally located of the three excretory organs appearing in the evolution of the vertebrates (the others being the pronephros and the mesonephros); in mammalian embryos, the metanephros develops caudal to the mesonephros during its regression, becoming the permanent kidney. [meta- + G. *nephros,* kidney]

met·a·phase (met′ă-fāz) The stage of mitosis or meiosis in which the chromosomes become aligned on the equatorial plate of the cell separating the centromeres. In mitosis and in the second meiotic division, the centromeres of each chromosome divide, and the two daughter centromeres are directed toward opposite poles of the cell; in the first division of meiosis, the centromeres do not divide, but the centromeres of each pair of homologous chromosomes become directed toward opposite poles. [meta- + G. *phasis,* an appearance]

met·a·phys·i·al dys·os·to·sis (met′ă-fiz′ē-ăl dis-os-tō′sis) A rare developmental abnormality of the skeleton in which metaphyses of tubular bones are expanded by deposits of cartilage.

met·a·phys·i·al dys·pla·si·a (met′ă-fiz′ē-ăl dis-plā′zē-ă) An abnormality that occurs when new bone at the metaphyses of long bones fails to undergo remodeling to the normal tubular structure; the ends of long bones appear to be expanded and porotic, with thin cortex; there may be an associated overgrowth of cranial bones (craniometaphysial dysplasia).

met·a·phys·i·al fi·brous cor·ti·cal de·fect (met′ă-fiz′ē-ăl fī′brŭs kōr′ti-kăl dē-fekt′) A small fibrous cortical defect located in the metaphysis of a long bone.

me·taph·y·sis, pl. **me·taph·y·ses** (mĕ-taf′i-sis, -sēz) A conic segment between the epiphysis and diaphysis of a long bone. [meta- + G. *physis,* growth]

met·a·pla·si·a (met′ă-plā′zē-ă) Abnormal transformation of an adult, fully differentiated tissue of one kind into a differentiated tissue of another kind; an acquired condition, in contrast to heteroplasia. [G. *metaplasis,* transformation]

met•a•plasm (met′ă-plazm) SYN cell inclusions (1). [meta- + G. *plasma,* something formed]

met•a•plas•tic (met′ă-plas′tik) Pertaining to metaplasia or metaplasis.

met•a•plas•tic a•ne•mi•a (met′ă-plas′tik ă-nē′mē-ă) Pernicious anemia in which the various formed elements in the blood are changed, e.g., multisegmented, unusually large neutrophils (macropolycytes), immature myeloid cells, bizarre platelets. Cf. diphyllobothriasis.

met•a•plas•tic car•ci•no•ma (met′ă-plas′tik kahr′si-nō′mă) A carcinoma in which some of the tumor cells are spindle shaped, suggesting a sarcoma, or in which the stroma shows foci of bone or cartilage.

met•a•plas•tic os•si•fi•ca•tion (met′ă-plas′tik os′i-fi-kā′shŭn) The formation of irregular foci of bone (sometimes including bone marrow) in various soft structures, such as the muscles, lungs, brain, and other sites where osseous tissue is abnormal.

met•a•plas•tic pol•yp (met′ă-plas′tik pol′ip) SYN hyperplastic polyp.

met•a•psy•chol•o•gy (met′ă-sī-kol′ŏ-jē) **1.** A systematic attempt to discern and describe what lies beyond the empiric facts and laws of psychology, such as the relations between body and mind, or concerning the place of the mind in the universe. **2.** PSYCHOANALYSIS psychology concerning the fundamental assumptions of the freudian theory of the mind, which entail five points of view: 1) dynamic, concerning psychological forces; 2) economic, concerning psychological energy; 3) structural, concerning psychological configurations; 4) genetic, concerning psychological origins; 5) adaptive, concerning psychologic relations with the environment. [G. *meta,* beyond, transcending, + psychology]

met•ar•te•ri•ole (met-ahr-tēr′ē-ōl) One of the small peripheral blood vessels between the arterioles and the true capillaries that contain scattered groups of smooth muscle fibers in their walls. [meta- + arteriole]

met•a•ru•bri•cyte (met-ă-rū′bri-sīt) Orthochromatic normoblast; the oldest type of nucleated red cell. SEE normoblast.

me•tas•ta•sis, pl. **me•tas•ta•ses** (mĕ-tas′tă-sis, -sēz) **1.** The shifting of a disease or its local manifestations, from one part of the body to another, as in mumps when the symptoms referable to the parotid gland subside and the testis becomes affected. **2.** The spread of a disease process from one part of the body to another, as in the appearance of neoplasms in parts of the body remote from the site of the primary tumor; results from dissemination of tumor cells by the lymphatics or blood vessels or by direct extension through serous cavities or subarachnoid or other spaces. **3.** Transportation of bacteria from one part of the body to another, through the bloodstream (hematogenous metastasis) or through lymph channels (lymphogenous metastasis). [G. a removing, fr. *meta,* in the midst of, + *stasis,* a placing]

me•tas•ta•size (mĕ-tas′tă-sīz) To pass into or invade by metastasis.

met•a•stat•ic (met′ă-stat′ik) Relating to metastasis.

met•a•stat•ic ab•scess (met′ă-stat′ik ab′ses) A secondary abscess formed, at a distance from the primary focus, as a result of the transportation of pyogenic bacteria by the lymph or bloodstream.

met•a•stat•ic cal•ci•fi•ca•tion (met′ă-stat′ik kal′si-fi-kā′shŭn) Calcification occurring in nonosseous, viable tissue in hypercalcemia.

met•a•tar•sal (met′ă-tahr′săl) Relating to the metatarsus or to one of the metatarsal bones.

met•a•tar•sal ar•ter•y (met′ă-tahr′săl ahr′tĕr-ē) One of four dorsal or four plantar arteries coursing in relation to the metatarsal bones, each dividing distally into a medial and a lateral digital artery, serving the dorsal or plantar aspects of adjacent sides of two toes.

met•a•tar•sal (bones) [I–V] (met′ă-tahr′săl bōnz) The five long bones numbered I–V, beginning with the bone on the medial side forming the skeleton of the anterior portion of the foot, articulating posteriorly with the three cuneiform and the cuboid bones, anteriorly with the five proximal phalanges. SYN ossa metatarsi.

met•a•tar•sal•gi•a (met′ă-tahr-sal′jē-ă) Pain in the forefoot in the region of the heads of the metatarsals. [meta- + G. *algos,* pain]

met•a•tar•sec•to•my (met′ă-tahr-sek′tŏ-mē) Excision of the metatarsus. [metarsus + G. *ektomē,* excision]

met•a•tar•so•pha•lan•ge•al (MTP) (met′ă-tahr′sō-fă-lan′jē-ăl) Relating to the metatarsal bones and the phalanges; denoting the articulations between them.

met•a•tar•so•pha•lan•ge•al joints (met′ă-tahr′sō-fă-lan′jē-ăl joynts) The spheroid synovial joints between the heads of the metatarsals and the bases of the proximal phalanges of the toes.

met•a•tar•sus, pl. **me•ta•tar•si** (met′ă-tahr′sŭs, -sī′) The part of the foot between the tarsus and the toes, having as its skeleton the five long bones (metatarsal bones) articulating posteriorly with the cuboid and cuneiform bones and distally with the phalanges. [meta- + G. *tarsos,* tarsus]

met•a•tar•sus la•tus (met′ă-tahr′sŭs lā′tŭs) Deformity caused by sinking down of the transverse arch of the foot.

met•a•tar•sus val•gus (met′ă-tahr′sŭs val′

gŭs) Fixed deformity in which the forepart of the foot is rotated on the long axis of the foot, so that the plantar surface faces away from the midline of the body, whereas the heel remains straight. SYN duck walk, toeing out. [meta- + G. *tarsos,* flat surface, sole, + L. *valgus,* bent]

met•a•tar•sus var•us (met′ă-tahr′sŭs vā′rŭs) Fixed deformity in which the forepart of the foot is rotated on the long axis of the foot, so that the plantar surface faces the midline of the body. SYN intoe.

met•a•thal•a•mus (met′ă-thal′ă-mŭs) The most caudal and ventral part of the thalamus, composed of the medial and lateral geniculate bodies. [meta- + G. *thalamos,* thalamus]

me•tath•e•sis (me-tath′ĕ-sis) **1.** Transfer of a pathologic product (e.g., a calculus) from one place to another where it causes less inconvenience or injury, when it is not possible or expedient to remove it from the body. **2.** CHEMISTRY a double decomposition, wherein a compound, A-B, reacts with another compound, C-D, to yield A-C + B-D, or A-D + B-C. [meta- + G. *thesis,* a placing]

met•a•tro•phic (met′ă-trō′fik) Denoting the ability to undertake anabolism or to obtain nourishment from varied sources, i.e., both nitrogenous and carbonaceous organic matter. [meta- + G. *trophē,* nourishment]

Met•a•zo•a (met′ă-zō′ă) A subkingdom of the kingdom Animalia, including all multicellular animal organisms in which the cells are differentiated and form tissues; distinguished from the subkingdom Protozoa, or unicellular animal organisms. [meta- + G. *zōon,* animal]

met•a•zo•o•no•sis (met′ă-zō-ŏ-nō′sis) A zoonosis that requires both a vertebrate and an invertebrate host to complete the life cycle of the causative organism. [meta- + G. *zōon,* animal, + *nosos,* disease]

Metch•ni•koff the•o•ry (mech′ni-kof thē′ŏr-ē) The phagocytic theory, according to which the body is protected against infection by the leukocytes and other cells that engulf and destroy the invading microorganisms.

met•en•ce•phal•ic (met′en-se-fal′ik) Relating to the metencephalon.

met•en•ceph•a•lon (met′en-sef′ă-lon) The anterior of the two major subdivisions of the rhombencephalon (the posterior being the myelencephalon or medulla oblongata), composed of the pons and the cerebellum. [meta- + G. *enkephalos,* brain]

Me•te•nier sign (met-en-yā′ sīn) Easy eversion of the upper eyelid in Ehlers-Danlos syndrome.

me•te•or•ism (mē′tē-ŏ-rizm) SYN tympanites. [G. *meteōrismos,* a lifting up]

me•te•or•o•tro•pic (mē′tē-ŏr-ō-trō′pik) Denoting diseases affected in their incidence by the weather. [G. *meteōra,* things high in the air, + G. *tropos,* a turning]

me•ter (mē′tĕr) **1.** The fundamental unit of length in both the SI and metric system, equivalent to 39.37007874 inches. Defined to be the length of path traveled by light in a vacuum in 1/299792458 sec. **2.** A device for measuring the quantity of that which passes through it. SYN metre. [Fr. *metre;* G. *metron,* measure]

me•ter an•gle (mē′tĕr ang′gĕl) The amount of convergence required to view binocularly an object 1 meter distant and exerting 1 diopter of accommodation. SYN metre angle.

me•ter-can•dle (mē′tĕr-kan′dĕl) SYN lux. SYN metre-candle.

me•tered-dose in•hal•er (MDI) (mē-tĕrd′dōs in-hāl′ĕr) SYN inhaler. See this page.

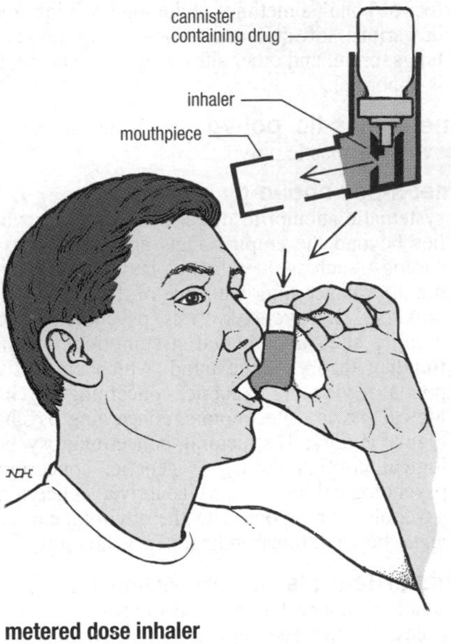

metered dose inhaler

met•es•trus, met•es•trum (met-es′trŭs, -trŭm) The period between estrus and diestrus in the estrous cycle. SYN metoestrus. [meta- + estrus]

meth-, metho- Chemical prefixes usually denoting a methyl, methoxy group.

methaemalbumin [Br.] SYN methemalbumin.

methaemalbuminaemia [Br.] SYN methemalbuminemia.

methaemoglobin [Br.] SYN methemoglobin.

methaemoglobinaemia [Br.] SYN methemoglobinemia.

methaemoglobinuria [Br.] SYN methemoglobinuria.

meth•ane (meth′ān) An odorless gas produced by the decomposition of organic matter; explosive when mixed with 7 or 8 volumes of air, constituting in such cases the firedamp in coal mines.

meth•an•o•gen (meth-an′ō-jen) Any methane-producing bacterium of the family Methanobacteriaceae.

meth•a•nol (meth′ă-nol) SYN methyl alcohol.

metHb Abbreviation for methemoglobin.

met•hem•al•bu•min (met′hēm-al-bū′min) An abnormal compound formed in the blood as a result of heme combining with plasma albumin. SYN methaemalbumin.

met•hem•al•bu•mi•ne•mi•a (met′hēm-al-bū′min-ē′mē-ă) The presence of methemalbumin in the circulating blood, indicative of hemoglobin breakdown; found in some patients with blackwater fever or paroxysmal nocturnal hemoglobinuria. SYN methaemalbuminaemia.

met•he•mo•glo•bin (metHb) (met-hē′mō-glō′bin) A transformation product of oxyhemoglobin because of the oxidation of the normal Fe^{2+} to Fe^{3+}, thus converting ferroprotoporphyrin to ferriprotoporphyrin; useless for respiration; found in bloody effusions and in the circulating blood after poisoning with acetanilid, potassium chlorate, and other substances. SYN hemiglobin, methaemoglobin.

met•he•mo•glo•bi•ne•mi•a (met-hē′mō-glō-bi-nē′mē-ă) The presence of methemoglobin in the circulating blood. SYN hemiglobinemia, methaemoglobinaemia. [methemoglobin + G. *haima,* blood]

met•he•mo•glo•bi•nu•ri•a (met-hē′mō-glō-bin-yūr′ē-ă) The presence of methemoglobin in the urine. SYN hemiglobinuria, methamoglobinuria. [methemoglobin + G. *ouron,* urine]

meth•en•a•mine sil•ver stain (me-then′ă-mēn sil′vĕr stān) A stain primarily used for cysts of *Pneumocystis jiroveci* (formerly *P. carinii*), but valid for other pathogens (e.g., fungi, helminths).

meth•i•cil•lin so•di•um (meth′i-sil′in sō′dē-ŭm) A semisynthetic penicillin salt for parenteral administration; restriction of its use to infections caused by penicillin G-resistant staphylococci is recommended; it is less effective than penicillin G in infections caused by hemolytic streptococci, pneumococci, gonococci, and penicillin G-sensitive staphylococci.

me•thi•o•nine (me-thī′ō-nēn) A nutritionally essential amino acid and the most important natural source of "active methyl" groups in the body, hence usually involved in methylations in vivo.

meth•od (meth′ŏd) The orderly sequence of events of a process or procedure. SEE ALSO fixative, operation, procedure, stain, technique. [G. *methodos;* fr. *meta,* after, + *hodos,* way]

meth•od•ol•o•gy (meth′ŏ-dol′ŏ-jē) **1.** A body of methods rules, and postulates employed by a discipline; a particular procedure or set of procedures. **2.** Analysis of the principles or procedures of inquiry in a particular field. [G. *meta,* after, + *hodos,* way, + *logos,* science]

♻ **methoxy-** Chemical prefix denoting substitution of a methoxyl group.

me•thox•yl (me-thok′sil) The group, $-OCH_3$.

meth•yl (meth′il) The radical, $-CH_3$. [G. *methy,* wine, + *hylē,* wood]

meth•yl al•co•hol (meth′il al′kŏ-hol) A flammable, toxic, mobile liquid, used as an industrial solvent and antifreeze, and in the manufacture of chemicals; ingestion may result in severe acidosis, visual impairment, and other effects on the central nervous system. SYN methanol.

meth•yl•a•tion (meth′i-lā′shŭn) Addition of methyl groups; in histochemistry, used to esterify carboxyl groups and remove sulfate groups by treating tissue sections with hot methanol in the presence of hydrochloric acid; the net effect being to reduce tissue basophilia and abolish metachromasia.

meth•yl•di•chlo•ro•ar•sine (MD) (meth′il-dī-klōr′ō-ahr′sēn) A vesicant; irritating to the respiratory tract; produces lung and eye injury; has been used in certain military operations.

meth•yl•ene (meth′i-lēn) The radical, $-CH_2-$.

meth•yl•ene blue (meth′i-lēn blū) A basic dye easily oxidized to azure, with dye mixtures; used in histology and microbiology, to stain intestinal protozoa in wet-mount preparations, to track RNA and RNase in electrophoresis, and as an antidote for methemoglobinemia; its redox indicator properties are useful in milk bacteriology.

meth•yl green (meth′il grēn) A basic triphenylmethane dye used as a chromatin stain and, in combination with pyronin, for differential staining of RNA (red) and DNA (green); also used as a tracking dye for DNA in electrophoresis.

meth•yl•ol (meth′i-lol) Hydroxymethyl; the radical, $-CH_2OH$.

meth•yl•pen•tose (meth′il-pen′tōs) A hexose (a 6-deoxyhexose) in which carbon-6 is part of a methyl group; e.g., rhamnose, fucose.

meth•yl•trans•fer•ase (meth′il-trans′fĕr-ās) Any enzyme transferring methyl groups from one compound to another. SYN transmethylase.

metMb Abbreviation for metmyoglobin.

met·my·o·glo·bin (metMb) (met-mī′ō-glō′bin) Myoglobin in which the ferrous ion of the heme prosthetic group is oxidized to ferric ion.

metoestrum [Br.] SYN metestrum.

metoestrus [Br.] SYN metestrus.

me·ton·y·my (mĕ-ton′i-mē) Imprecise or circumscribed labeling of objects or events, characteristic of the language disturbance of people with schizophrenia; e.g., the patient speaks of having had a "menu" rather than a "meal." [meta- + G. *onyma,* name]

me·top·ic (mē-top′ik) Relating to the forehead or anterior portion of the cranium. [G. *metōpon,* forehead]

me·top·ic su·ture (mē-top′ik sū′chŭr) A persistent frontal suture, sometimes discernible a short distance above sutura frontonasalis.

met·o·po·plas·ty (met′ŏ-pō-plas-tē) Surgical repair of the skin or bone of the forehead. [G. *metōpon,* forehead, + *plastos,* formed]

♻**metr-, metra-, metro-** Combining forms indicating the uterus. SEE ALSO hystero- (1), utero-. [G. *mētra*]

me·tra (mē′tră) SYN uterus. [G. uterus]

me·tral·gi·a (mē-tral′jē-ă) Tenderness or pain in the uterus. [Gk, *metra,* womb, + *algos,* pain]

me·tra·to·ni·a (mē-tră-tō′nē-ă) Atony of the uterine walls after childbirth. [metra- + G. *a-* priv. + *tonos,* tension]

me·trat·ro·phy, me·tra·tro·phi·a (mē-trat′rŏ-fē, mē-tră-trō′fē-ă) Uterine atrophy. [metra- + atrophy]

metre [Br.] SYN meter.

metre angle [Br.] SYN meter angle.

metre-candle [Br.] SYN meter-candle.

me·tri·a (mē′trē-ă) Pelvic cellulitis or other inflammatory affection in the puerperal period. [G. *mētra,* uterus]

met·ric (met′rik) Quantitative; relating to measurement. SEE metric system. [G. *metrikos,* fr. *metron,* measure]

met·ric sys·tem (met′rik sis′tĕm) A system of weights and measures, universal for scientific use, based on the meter, the gram, and the liter.

me·tri·tis (mĕ-trī′tis) Inflammation of the uterus. [G. *mētra,* uterus, + *-itis,* inflammation]

me·tro·cyte (mē′trō-sīt) SYN mother cell. [G. *mētēr,* mother, + *kytos,* a hollow (cell)]

me·tro·dyn·i·a (mē′trō-dī′nē-ă) SYN hysteralgia. [metro- + G. *odynē,* pain]

me·tro·fi·bro·ma (mē′trō-fī-brō′mă) A fibroma of the uterus.

me·trol·o·gy (mĕ-trol′ŏ-jē) **1.** The science of weights and measures. **2.** The arithmetic of pharmacy and its application to dosage, preparation, compounding, and dispensing of medication. [G. *metro,* measure, + *logos,* study]

me·tro·lym·phan·gi·tis (mē′trō-lim-fan-jī′tis) Inflammation of the uterine lymphatics. [metro- + lymphangitis]

me·tro·pa·ral·y·sis (mē′trō-pă-ral′i-sis) Flaccidity or paralysis of the uterine muscle during or immediately after childbirth. [metro- + paralysis]

me·tro·path·i·a (mē′trō-path′ē-ă) SYN metropathy. [L.]

me·tro·path·ia hem·or·rhag·i·ca (mē′trō-path′ē-ă hē-mōr′raj′ik-ă) Abnormal, excessive, often continuous uterine bleeding due to persistence and exaggeration of the follicular phase of the menstrual cycle; the endometrium is the seat of glandular hyperplasia with cyst formation.

me·tro·path·ic (mē′trō-path′ik) Relating to or caused by uterine disease.

me·trop·a·thy (mē-trop′ă-thē) Any disease of the uterus, especially of the myometrium. SYN metropathia. [metro- + G. *pathos,* suffering]

me·tro·per·i·to·ni·tis (mē′trō-per-i-tō-nī′tis) Inflammation of the uterus involving the peritoneal covering. SYN perimetritis. [metro- + peritonitis]

me·tro·phle·bi·tis (mē′trō-flĕ-bī′tis) Inflammation of the uterine veins usually following childbirth. [metro- + G. *phleps,* vein, + *-itis,* inflammation]

met·ro·plas·ty (mē′trō-plas-tē) SYN uteroplasty.

me·tror·rha·gi·a (mē′trō-rā′jē-ă) Any irregular, acyclic bleeding from the uterus between periods. [metro- + G. *rhēgnymi,* to burst forth]

me·tror·rhe·a (mē′trō-rē′ă) Discharge of mucus or pus from the uterus. SYN metrorrhoea. [metro- + G. *rhoia,* a flow]

metrorrhoea [Br.] SYN metrorrhea.

me·tro·sal·pin·gi·tis (mē′trō-sal-pin-jī′tis) Inflammation of the uterus and of one or both fallopian tubes. [metro- + G. *salpinx,* trumpet (oviduct), + *-itis,* inflammation]

me·tro·sal·pin·gog·ra·phy (mē′trō-sal-pin-gog′ră-fē) SYN hysterosalpingography. [metro- + G. *salpinx,* tube, + *graphō,* to write]

me·tro·scope (mē′trō-skōp) SYN hysteroscope. [metro- + G. *skopeō,* to view]

me·tro·stax·is (mē′trō-stak′sis) Small but continuous hemorrhage of the uterine mucous membrane. [metro- + G. *staxis,* a dripping]

me·tro·ste·no·sis (mē′trō-stĕ-nō′sis) A narrowing of the uterine cavity. [metro- + G. *stenōsis,* a narrowing]

Mev Abbreviation for 1 million electron-volts.

Mex•i•can hat cell (mek′si-kăn hat sel) SYN target cell.

Mex•i•co seed (mek′si-kō sēd) SYN castor bean.

Mey•en•burg com•plex (mī′ĕn-berg kom′pleks) Clusters of small bile ducts occurring in polycystic livers, separate from the portal areas.

Mey•en•burg dis•ease (mī′ĕn-berg di-zēz′) SYN relapsing polychondritis.

Mey•er line (mī′ĕr līn) A line through the axis of the great toe and passing the midpoint of the heel in a normal foot.

Mey•nert cells (mī′nĕrt selz) Solitary pyramidal cells found in the cortex in the region of the calcarine fissure.

MFD Abbreviation for minimal fatal dose.

Mg Symbol for magnesium.

mg Abbreviation for milligram.

MGUS Abbreviation for monoclonal gammopathy of unknown significance.

MHA Abbreviation for Mental Health Association.

MHC Abbreviation for major histocompatibility complex.

mho (mō) SYN siemens. [*ohm* reversed]

MHSS Abbreviation for Military Health Services System.

MHz Abbreviation for megahertz.

MI Abbreviation for myocardial infarction.

Mi•bel•li an•gi•o•ker•a•to•ma (mē-bel′ē an′jē-ō-ker′ă-tō′mă) A small telangiectatic papule occurring commonly on the extremities in adolescent girls.

Mi•bel•li dis•ease (mē-bel′ē di-zēz′) SYN porokeratosis.

mi•ca (mī′kă) A silicate mineral with almost perfect cleavage that occurs in thin laminated scales. It is used in paints and as an insulator in high-voltage equipment. Because of its heat resistance, it is used instead of glass in windows for stoves and kerosene heaters. [L. *mico,* to shine]

mi•ca•to•sis (mī′kă-tō′sis) A form of pneumoconiosis caused by the inhalation of and tissue reaction to mica particles. Also known as mica pneumoconiosis. SEE ALSO pneumoconiosis.

Mi•chae•lis con•stant (mi-kā′lis kon′stănt) **1.** The true dissociation constant for the enzyme-substrate binary complex in a single-substrate rapid equilibrium enzyme-catalyzed reaction (usually symbolized by K_s). **2.** The concentration of the substrate at which half the true maximum velocity of an enzyme-catalyzed reaction is achieved.

Mi•chae•lis-Men•ten hy•poth•e•sis (mi-kā′lis-men′tĕn hī-poth′ĕ-sis) That a complex is formed between an enzyme and its substrate (the O'Sullivan-Tompson hypothesis), which complex then decomposes to yield free enzyme and the reaction products (Brown hypothesis), the latter rate determining the overall rate of substrate-product conversion.

Mi•chel mal•for•ma•tion (mē-shel′ mal′fōr-mā′shŭn) Hypoplasia of the petrous pyramid and aplasia of the inner ear.

Mi•chel spur (mē-shel′ spŭr) Epithelial outgrowth of the dilator muscle of the pupil at the peripheral border of the sphincter; part of the insertion of the dilator muscle onto the iris sphincter.

-micin Suffix used to form names for some aminoglycoside antibiotics. [alteration of *-mycin,*]

mi•cra•cou•stic (mī′kră-kū′stik) **1.** Relating to faint sounds. **2.** Magnifying very faint sounds so as to make them audible. SYN microcoustic. [micro- + G. *akoustikos,* relating to hearing, fr. *akouō,* to hear]

mi•cren•ceph•a•ly (mī′kren-sef′ă-lē) Abnormal smallness of the brain. SYN microencephaly. [micro- + G. *enkephalos,* brain]

micro-, micr- **1.** Prefixes denoting smallness. **2.** Prefixes (abbrev. mc) used in the SI and metric system to signify one millionth (10^{-6}) of such unit. **3.** CHEMISTRY prefix to terms denoting chemical procedures or analyses that use minimal quantities of substance to be examined; specimen materials and reagents. **4.** Microscopic; opposite of macro-, megalo-. [G. *mikros,* small]

mi•cro•ab•scess (mī′krō-ab′ses) A small circumscribed collection of leukocytes in solid tissues.

mi•cro•ad•e•no•ma (mī′krō-ad-ĕ-nō′mă) A pituitary adenoma less than 10 mm in diameter.

mi•cro•aer•o•phil, mi•cro•aer•o•phile (mī-krō-ār′ō-fil, -fīl) **1.** An aerobic bacterium that requires oxygen, but less than is present in the air, and grows best under modified atmospheric conditions. **2.** Relating to such an organism. SYN microaerophilic. [micro- + G. *aēr,* air, + *philos,* fond]

mi•cro•aer•o•phil•ic (mī′krō-ār-ō-fil′ik) SYN microaerophil (2).

mi•cro•ag•gre•gate (mī′krō-ag′rĕ-gāt) A small loose mass (20–120 mcm) of fibrin, degenerating platelets, white blood cells, or cellular debris that forms in blood stored in the refrigerator five days or longer. Special filters can be used to separate them during administration of the blood unit.

mi·cro·al·bu·mi·nu·ri·a (mī′krō-al-bū-min-yūr′ē-ă) A slight increase in urinary albumin excretion that can be detected using immunoassays but not by means of conventional urine protein measurements; an early marker for renal disease in patients with diabetes. [micro- + albuminuria]

mi·cro·a·nas·to·mo·sis (mī′krō-ă-nas-tō-mō′sis) Anastomosis of minute structures performed under a surgical microscope.

mi·cro·a·nat·o·mist (mī′krō-ă-nat′ŏ-mist) SYN histologist.

mi·cro·a·nat·o·my (mī′krō-ă-nat′ŏ-mē) SYN histology.

mi·cro·an·eu·rysm (mī-krō-an′yūr-izm) Focal dilation of retinal capillaries occurring in diabetes mellitus, retinal vein obstruction, and absolute glaucoma, or of arteriolocapillary junctions in many organs in thrombotic thrombocytopenic purpura.

mi·cro·an·gi·og·ra·phy (mī′krō-an-jē-og′ră-fē) Radiography of the finer vessels of an organ after the injection of a contrast medium and enlargement of the resulting radiograph. [micro- + angiography]

mi·cro·an·gi·o·path·ic he·mo·lyt·ic a·ne·mi·a (mī′krō-an-jē-ō-path′ik hē′mō-lit′ik ă-nē′mē-ă) Hemolysis attributed to narrowing or obstruction of small blood vessels usually due to inflammation; causes fragmentation and distortion in the shape of red blood cells.

mi·cro·an·gi·op·a·thy (mī′krō-an-jē-op′ă-thē) SYN capillaropathy.

mi·cro-As·trup meth·od (mī′krō as′trŭp meth′ŏd) An interpolation technique for acid-base measurement, based on pH and the use of the Siggaard-Andersen nomogram.

mi·crobe (mī′krōb) Any minute organism, including both microscopic and ultramicroscopic organisms (spirochetes, bacteria, rickettsiae, and viruses). These organisms are considered to form a biologically distinctive group, in that the genetic material is not surrounded by a nuclear membrane and mitosis does not occur during replication. [Fr., fr. G. *mikros,* small, + *bios,* life]

mi·cro·bi·al (mī-krō′bē-ăl) SYN microbic.

mi·cro·bic (mī-krō′bik) Of or involving or caused by or being microbes. SEE ALSO microbe. SYN microbial. [Fr., fr. G. *micros,* small, + *bios,* life]

mi·cro·bi·ci·dal (mī-krō′bi-sī′dăl) Destructive to microbes. SYN microbicide (1).

mi·cro·bi·cide (mī-krō′bi-sīd) **1.** SYN microbicidal. **2.** An agent destructive to microbes; a germicide; an antiseptic. [microbe + L. *caedo,* to kill]

mi·cro·bi·o·log·ic (mī′krō-bī-ŏ-loj′ik) Relating to microbiology.

mi·cro·bi·ol·o·gist (mī′krō-bī-ol′ŏ-jist) One who specializes in the science of microbiology.

mi·cro·bi·ol·o·gy (mī′krō-bī-ol′ŏ-jē) The science concerned with microorganisms, including fungi, protozoa, bacteria, and viruses. [Fr. *microbiologie*]

mi·cro·blast (mī′krō-blast) A small, nucleated red blood cell. [micro- + G. *blastos,* sprout, germ]

mi·cro·bleph·a·ron (mī′krō-blef′ă-ron) Eyelids with abnormal vertical shortness. [micro + G. *blepharon,* eyelid + *ia,* condition]

mi·cro·bod·y (mī′krō-bod-ē) SYN peroxisome.

mi·cro·bra·chi·a (mī′krō-brā′kē-ă) Abnormal smallness of the upper limbs. [micro- + G. *brachiōn,* arm]

mi·cro·cal·ci·fi·ca·tions (mī′krō-kal-si-fi-kā′shŭns) Calcifications smaller than 1 mm in diameter as seen on mammography; often associated with malignant lesions when seen in clusters. [micro- + calcification]

mi·cro·car·di·a (mī′krō-kahr′dē-ă) Abnormal smallness of the heart. [micro- + G. *kardia,* heart]

mi·cro·cen·trum (mī′krō-sen′trŭm) SYN cytocentrum. [micro- + G. *kentron,* center]

mi·cro·ce·phal·ic (mī′krō-se-fal′ik) Having an abnormally small head. SYN nanocephalous, nanocephalic.

mi·cro·ceph·a·ly (mī′krō-sef′ă-lē) Abnormal smallness of the head; applied to a cranium with a capacity less than 1350 mL. Usually associated with mental retardation. SYN nanocephaly. [micro- + G. *kephalē,* head]

mi·cro·chei·li·a, mi·cro·chi·li·a (mī-krō-kī′lē-ă) Abnormal smallness of the lips. [micro- + G. *cheilos,* lip]

mi·cro·chei·ri·a, mi·cro·chi·ri·a (mī-krō-kī′rē-ă) Abnormal smallness of the hands. [micro- + G. *cheir,* hand]

mi·cro·chem·is·try (mī′krō-kem′is-trē) The use of chemical procedures involving minute quantities or reactions not visible to the unaided eye.

micro·chim·er·ism (mī′krō-kim′ĕr-izm) The presence of donor cells in a graft recipient, or of fetal cells remaining in maternal circulation, which can be detected by molecular methods but not by flow cytometry.

mi·cro·cin·e·ma·tog·ra·phy (mī′kro-sin′ĕ-mă-tog′ră-fē) The application of moving pictures taken through magnifying lenses to the study of an organ or system in motion; e.g., the circulation in living embryos. [micro- + G. *kinēma,* movement, + *graphō,* to write]

mi•cro•cir•cu•la•tion (mī′krō-sĭr-kyū-lā′shŭn) Passage of blood in the smallest vessels, namely arterioles, capillaries, and venules.

Mi•cro•coc•ca•ce•ae (mī′krō-kok-ā′sē-ē) A family of bacteria containing gram-positive spheric cells that occur singly or in pairs, tetrads, packets, irregular masses, or even chains. Free-living, saprophytic, parasitic, and pathogenic species occur. The type genus is *Micrococcus.*

mi•cro•coc•ci (mī′krō-kok′sī) Plural of micrococcus.

Mi•cro•coc•cus (mī′krō-kok′ŭs) A bacterial genus of Micrococcaceae containing gram-positive, spheric cells that occur in irregular masses, never in packets. Some species are motile or produce motile mutants. These organisms are saprophytic, facultatively parasitic, or parasitic but are not truly pathogenic. The type species is *M. luteus.* [micro- + G. *kokkos,* berry]

mi•cro•coc•cus, pl. **mi•cro•coc•ci** (mī′krō-kok′ŭs, -sī) A vernacular usage for any member of the genus *Micrococcus.*

mi•cro•co•lon (mī′krō-kō-lŏn) A small-caliber unused colon, seen in the neonate on radiographic contrast enema; usually a consequence of intestinal atresia or meconium ileus.

mi•cro•co•ri•a (mī′krō-kōr′ē-ă) A congenitally small pupil with an inability to dilate. [micro- + G. *korē,* pupil]

mi•cro•cor•ne•a (mī′krō-kōr′nē-ă) An abnormally small cornea.

mi•cro•cou•lomb (mī′krō-kū′lom) One millionth of a coulomb.

mi•cro•cou•stic (mī′krō-kū′stik) SYN micracoustic.

mi•cro•cu•rie (mcCi) (mī′krō-kyūr′ē) One millionth of a curie; a quantity of any radionuclide with 3.7×10^4 disintegrations per second.

mi•cro•cur•rent (mī′krō-kŭr′rĕnt) An electrotherapeutic modality that uses low levels of electrical current (less than 1 mAmp) to facilitate circulation and cellular healing or to reduce pain or edema. SYN low-intensity stimulator, microcurrent electrical neuromuscular stimulator, microcurrent electrical stimulator.

mi•cro•cur•rent e•lec•tri•cal neu•ro•mus•cu•lar stim•u•la•tor (MENS) (mī′krō-kŭr′ĕnt ĕ-lek′trik-ăl nūr′ō-mŭs′kyū-lăr stim′yū-lā-tŏr) SYN microcurrent.

mi•cro•cur•rent e•lec•tri•cal stim•u•la•tor (MES) (mī′krō-kŭr′ĕnt ĕ-lek′trik-ăl stim′yū-lā-tŏr) SYN microcurrent.

mi•cro•cyst (mī′krō-sist) A tiny lesion, frequently of such dimensions that a magnifying lens or microscope is required for observation.

mi•cro•cyte (mī′krō-sīt) A small (i.e., 5 mcm or less) nonnucleated red blood cell; with decreased mean corpuscular volume. SYN microerythrocyte. [micro- + G. *kytos,* cell]

microcythaemia [Br.] SYN microcythemia.

mi•cro•cy•the•mi•a (mī′krō-sī-thē′mē-ă) The presence of many microcytes in the circulating blood. SYN microcythaemia, microcytosis. [microcyte + G. *haima,* blood]

mi•cro•cyt•ic a•ne•mi•a (mī-krō-sit′ĭk ă-nē′mē-ă) Any anemia in which the average size of circulating erythrocytes is smaller than normal, i.e., the mean corpuscular volume is 80 mcm^3 or less (normal range, 82–92 μm^3). See page B3.

mi•cro•cy•tic hy•po•chro•mic a•ne•mi•a (mī′krō-sit′ik hī′pō-krō′mik ă-nē′mē-ă) Any anemia with microcytes that are reduced in size and in hemoglobin content; the most common type is iron deficiency anemia.

mi•cro•cy•to•sis (mī′krō-sī-tō′sis) SYN microcythemia. See page B3. [microcyte + G. *-osis,* condition]

mi•cro•dac•ty•ly (mī′krō-dak′ti-lē) Smallness or shortness of the fingers or toes. [micro- + G. *dactylos,* finger, toe]

mi•cro•di•al•y•sis (mī′krō-dī-al′i-sis) A method of studying extracellular fluid composition and response to exogenous agents, utilizing a tiny tubular probe with a dialysis membrane and fluid flow rates of 1–3 mcL/min, inserted into tissues.

mi•cro•dis•sec•tion (mī′krō-dī-sek′shŭn) Dissection of tissues under a microscope or magnifying glass, usually done by teasing the tissues apart by means of needles.

mi•cro•don•ti•a, **mi•cro•don•tism** (mī′krō-don′shē-ă, -tizm) A condition in which a single tooth, or pairs of teeth, or the whole dentition, is disproportionately small. [micro- + G. *odous,* tooth]

mi•cro•drip (mī′krō-drip) In intravenous therapy, an infusion system that delivers 60 drops/mL that is used when small volumes are being delivered (e.g., less than 50 mL/hour); this reduces the risk of blood clotting in the intravenous line due to slow infusion rates. When using the microdrip system, the IV drip calculation is thus: drops/minute = mL/hour. [G. *micros,* small]

mi•cro•en•ceph•a•ly (mī′krō-en-sef′ă-lē) SYN micrencephaly.

mi•cro•e•ryth•ro•cyte (mī′krō-ĕ-rith′rō-sīt) SYN microcyte.

mi•cro•fi•bril (mī′krō-fī′bril) A very small fibril

having an average diameter of 13 nm; it may be a bundle of still smaller microfilaments.

mi·cro·fil·a·ment (mī′krō-fil′ă-mĕnt) The finest filamentous element of the cytoskeleton, having a diameter of about 5 nm and consisting primarily of actin. SEE ALSO actin filament.

microfilaraemia [Br.] SYN microfilaremia.

mi·cro·fil·a·re·mi·a (mī′krō-fil-ă-rē′mē-ă) Infection of the blood with microfilariae. SYN microfilaraemia.

mi·cro·fi·lar·i·a, pl. **mi·cro·fi·lar·i·ae** (mī′krō-fi-lar′ē-ă, -ē) Term for embryos of filarial nematodes in the family Onchocercidae. SEE *Filaria.* See page B5.

mi·cro·ga·mete (mī′krō-gam′ēt) The male element in anisogamy, or conjugation of cells of unequal size; it is the smaller of the two cells and actively motile. [micro- + G. *gametēs,* husband]

mi·cro·ga·me·to·cyte (mī′krō-gă-mē′tō-sīt) The mother cell producing the microgametes, or male elements of sexual reproduction in sporozoan protozoans and fungi.

mi·cro·gas·tri·a (mī′krō-gas′trē-ă) Smallness of the stomach. [micro- + G. *gastēr,* stomach]

mi·cro·gen·i·a (mī′krō-jĕn′ē-ă) Abnormal smallness of the chin resulting from underdevelopment of the mandibular symphysis. [micro- + G. *geneion,* chin]

mi·cro·gen·i·tal·ism (mī′krō-jen′i-tăl-izm) Abnormal smallness of the external genital organs.

mi·cro·glan·du·lar ad·e·no·sis (mī′krō-glan′dyū-lăr ad′ĕ-nō′sis) Adenosis of the breast in which irregular clusters of small tubules are present in adipose or fibrous tissues, resembling tubular carcinoma but lacking stromal fibroblastic proliferation.

mi·crog·li·a (mī-krog′lē-ă) Small neuroglial cells, possibly of mesodermal origin, which may become phagocytic, in areas of neural damage or inflammation. SYN Hortega cells. [micro- + G. *glia,* glue]

mi·crog·li·a·cyte (mī-krōg′lē-ă-sīt) A cell, especially an embryonic cell, of the microglia. [micro- + G. *glia,* glue, + *kytos,* cell]

mi·cro·glos·si·a (mī′krō-glos′ē-ă) Abnormal smallness of the tongue. [micro- + G. *glōssa,* tongue]

mi·cro·gna·thi·a (mī′krog-nā′thē-ă) Abnormal smallness of the jaws, especially of the mandible. [micro- + G. *gnathos,* jaw]

mi·cro·gram (mcg) (mī′krō-gram) One millionth of a gram.

mi·cro·graph (mī′krō-graf) SYN photomicrograph. [micro- + G. *graphō,* to write]

mi·cro·gy·ri·a (mī′krō-jī′rē-ă) Abnormal narrowness of the cerebral convolutions. [micro- + G. *gyros,* convolution]

microhaematocrit concentration [Br.] SYN microhematocrit concentration.

mi·cro·he·mat·o·crit con·cen·tra·tion (mī′krō-hĕ-mat′ŏ-krit kon′sĕn-trā′shŭn) The centrifugation of whole, anticoagulated blood, using microhematocrit tubes, to obtain a buffy coat layer containing white blood cells; blood films for staining can be prepared from this layer of cells and examined for the presence of parasites (trypanosomes and intracellular leishmaniae). SYN microhaematocrit concentration.

mi·cro·he·pat·i·a (mī′krō-he-pat′ē-ă) Abnormal smallness of the liver. [micro- + G. *hepar* (*hepat-*), liver]

mi·crohm (mcΩ) (mī′krōm) One millionth of an ohm.

mi·cro·in·cis·ion (mī′krō-in-sizh′ŭn) An incision made with the aid of a microscope.

mi·cro·in·va·sion (mī′krō-in-vā′zhŭn) Invasion of tissue immediately adjacent to a carcinoma in situ, the earliest stage of malignant neoplastic invasion.

mi·cro·kat·al (mī′krō-kat′ăl) One millionth of a katal.

mi·cro·li·ter (mcL, mcl, λ) (mī′krō-lē-tĕr) One millionth of a liter. SYN microlitre.

mi·cro·lith (mī′krō-lith) A minute stone or stonelike concretion, especially a calculus fragment passed in the urine as a component of gravel. [micro- + G. *lithos,* stone]

mi·cro·li·thi·a·sis (mī′krō-li-thī′ă-sis) The formation, presence, or discharge of minute concretions, or gravel.

microlitre [Br.] SYN microliter.

mi·cro·ma·nip·u·la·tion (mī′krō-mă-nip′yū-lā′shŭn) Dissection, stimulation, and other mechanical operations performed on minute structures under the microscope.

mi·cro·me·li·a (mī′krō-mē′lē-ă) Condition of having disproportionately short or small limbs. SEE ALSO achondroplasia. SYN nanomelia. [micro- + G. *melos,* limb]

mi·cro·mel·ic dwarf·ism (mī′krō-mel′ik dwōrf′izm) Dwarfism with abnormally short or small limbs.

mi·cro·mere (mī′krō-mēr) A small blastomere (e.g., one of the blastomeres at the animal pole of an amphibian egg). [micro- + G. *meros,* a part]

mi·cro·me·tas·ta·sis (mī′krō-mĕ-tas′tă-sis) A stage of metastasis when the secondary tumors are too small to be clinically detected, as in micrometastatic disease.

mi•cro•met•a•stat•ic (mī′krō-met-ă-stat′ik) Denoting or characterized by micrometastasis, as in micrometastatic disease.

mi•crom•e•ter (mcm) (mī-krom′ĕ-tĕr) **1.** One millionth of a meter; formerly called micron. **2.** A device for measuring various objects in an accurate and precise manner. In medicine and biology, the term is usually used with reference to a glass slide or lens that is accurately marked for measuring microscopic forms. SYN micrometre. [micro- + G. *metron,* measure]

micrometre [Br.] SYN micrometer.

mi•crom•e•try (mī-krom′ĕ-trē) Measurement of objects with some type of micrometer and a microscope.

micromicro- (mcmc) Prefix formerly used to signify one trillionth (10^{-12}); replaced by pico-.

mi•cro•mo•lar (mcM, mcmol/L) (mī′krō-mō′lăr) Denoting a concentration of 10^{-6} mole per liter (10^{-6} M or 1 MCM).

mi•cro•mole (mcmol) (mī′krō-mōl) One millionth of a mole.

mi•cro•my•e•li•a (mī′krō-mī-ē′lē-ă) Abnormal smallness or shortness of the spinal cord. [micro- + G. *myelos,* marrow]

mi•cro•my•el•o•blast (mī′krō-mī′el-ō-blast) A small myeloblast, often the predominating cell in myeloblastic leukemia.

mi•cro•my•el•o•blas•tic leu•ke•mi•a (mī′krō-mī′el-ō-blast′ik lū-kē′mē-ă) A form of myelocytic leukemia in which relatively large proportions of micromyeloblasts are found in the circulating blood and in bone marrow and other tissues.

mi•cron (mī′kron) Former term for the measurement now termed a micrometer.

mi•cro•nod•u•lar (mī′krō-nod′yū-lăr) Characterized by the presence of minute nodules; denoting a somewhat coarser appearance than that of a granular tissue or substance. [G. *mikros,* small]

mi•cro•nu•cle•us (mī′krō-nū′klē-ŭs) **1.** A small nucleus in a large cell, or the smaller nuclei in cells that have two or more such structures. **2.** The smaller of the two nuclei in ciliates dividing mitotically and bearing specific inheritable material. SEE ALSO macronucleus (2).

mi•cro•nu•tri•ents (mī′krō-nū′trē-ĕnts) Essential food factors required in only small quantities by the body; e.g., vitamins, trace minerals.

mi•cro•nych•i•a (mī′krō-nik′ē-ă) Abnormal smallness of nails. [micro- + G. *onyx,* nail]

mi•cro•oph•thal•mi•a trans•crip•tion fac•tor gene (mī′krō-of-thal′mē-ă tran-skrip′shŭn fak′tŏr jēn) Gene that when mutated causes Waardenburg syndrome type 2 and Tietz syndrome in at least some subsets of families with these autosomal dominant inherited syndromes.

mi•cro•or•gan•ism (mī′krō-ōr′găn-izm) A microscopic organism (plant or animal).

mi•cro•pa•thol•o•gy (mī′krō-pă-thol′ŏ-jē) The microscopic study of disease changes. [micro- + G. *pathos,* suffering, + *logos,* study]

mi•cro•pe•nis (mī′krō-pē′nis) Abnormally small penis. SYN microphallus.

mi•cro•phage (mī′krō-fāj) A polymorphonuclear leukocyte that is phagocytic. SEE ALSO phagocyte. [micro- + phag(ocyte)]

mi•cro•phal•lus (mī′krō-fal′ŭs) SYN micropenis.

mi•cro•pho•to•graph (mī′krō-fō′tō-graf) A minute photograph of any object, as distinguished from a photomicrograph.

mi•croph•thal•mos (mī′krof-thal′mŏs) Abnormal smallness of the eye. [micro + G. *ophthalmos,* eye]

mi•cro•pleth•ys•mog•ra•phy (mī′krō-pleth-iz-mog′ră-fē) The technique of measuring minute changes in the volume of a part as a result of blood flow into or out of it.

mi•cro•po•di•a (mī′krō-pō′dē-ă) Abnormal smallness of the feet. [micro- + G. *pous,* foot]

mi•crop•si•a (mī-krop′sē-ă) Perception of objects as smaller than they are. [micro- + G. *opsis,* sight]

mi•cro•punc•ture (mī′krō-pungk-chŭr) A puncture made with the aid of a microscope.

mi•cro•re•frac•tom•e•ter (mī′krō-rē-frak-tom′ĕ-tĕr) A refractometer used in the study of blood cells.

mi•cro•res•pi•rom•e•ter (mī′krō-res-pi-rom′ĕ-tĕr) An apparatus for measuring the use of oxygen by small particles of isolated tissues or cells or particles of cells.

mi•cro•scope (mī′krŏ-skōp) An instrument that gives an enlarged image of an object or substance that is minute or not visible with the naked eye; usually denotes a compound microscope; for low magnifications the term "simple microscope," or "magnifying glass," is used. [micro- + G. *skopeō,* to view]

mi•cro•scop•ic, **mi•cro•scop•i•cal** (mī′krŏ-skop′ik, mī′krŏ-skop-i-kăl) **1.** Of minute size; visible only with the aid of the microscope. **2.** Relating to a microscope.

mi•cro•scop•ic a•nat•o•my (mī′krŏ-skop′ik ă-nat′ŏ-mē) The branch of anatomy in which the structure of cells, tissues, and organs is studied with the light microscope. SEE ALSO histology.

mi•cro•scop•ic pol•y•an•gi•i•tis (mī′krŏ-skop′ik pol′ē-an′jē-ī′tis) Systemic, nongranulomatous small-vessel vasculitis, associated with glomerulonephritis, pulmonary capillaritis, palpable purpura, and antineutrophil cytoplasmic autoantibodies.

mi•cros•co•py (mī-kros′kŏ-pē) Investigation of minute objects by means of a microscope. SEE ALSO microscope.

mi•cro•so•mal eth•a•nol-ox•i•diz•ing system (MEOS) (mī′krō-sō′măl eth′ă-nol-oks′i-dīz-ing sis′tĕm) A hepatic enzyme system that metabolizes alcohol, drugs, and other foreign substances in the blood.

mi•cro•some (mī′krō-sōm) One of the small spheric vesicles derived from the endoplasmic reticulum after disruption of cells and ultracentrifugation. [micro- + G. *sōma,* body]

mi•cro•so•mi•a (mī′krō-sō′mē-ă) Abnormal smallness of the body, as in dwarfism or as in a fetus. SYN nanocormia. [micro- + G. *sōma,* body]

mi•cro•spec•tro•pho•tom•e•try (mī′krō-spek′trō-fō-tom′ĕ-trē) A technique for characterizing and quantitating nucleoproteins in single cells or cell organelles by their natural absorption spectra (ultraviolet) or after binding stoichiometrically in selective cytochemical staining reactions, as in the Feulgen stain for DNA.

mi•cro•spec•tro•scope (mī′krō-spek′trŏ-skōp) An instrument for observing the optic spectrum of microscopic objects.

mi•cro•sphe•ro•cy•to•sis (mī′krō-sfēr′ō-sī-tō′sis) A condition of the blood seen in hemolytic icterus in which small spherocytes are predominant; the red blood cells are smaller and more globular than normal.

mi•cro•sphyg•my (mī′krō-sfig′mē) A circumstance in which the pulse is difficult to discern manually. [micro- + G. *sphygmos,* pulse]

mi•cro•sple•ni•a (mī′krō-splē′nē-ă) Abnormal smallness of the spleen.

Mi•cro•spo•rum (mī-krō-spō′rŭm) A genus of pathogenic fungi causing dermatophytosis. See page B5. [micro- + G. *sporos,* seed]

Mi•cro•spo•rum au•dou•i•ni (mī-krō-spō′rŭm ow-dū-ē′nē) Ringworm fungus that commonly causes tinea capitis in children. SYN *Audouin microsporum.*

Mi•cro•spo•rum ca•nis (mī-krō-spō′rŭm kā′nis) A zoophilic fungus common in cats and dogs; in humans, infects the scalp and skin; rarely infects nails.

Mi•cro•spo•rum gyp•se•um (mī-krō-spō′rŭm jip′sē-ŭm) A geophilic fungus; causes infections of the scalp or skin in humans.

mi•cro•steth•o•scope (mī′krō-steth′ŏ-skōp) A stethoscope that amplifies the sounds heard.

mi•cro•sto•mi•a (mī′krō-stō′mē-ă) Abnormal smallness of the mouth. [micro- + G. *stoma,* mouth]

mi•cro•sur•gery (mī′krō-sŭr′jĕr-ē) Surgical procedures performed under the magnification of a surgical microscope.

mi•cro•su•ture (mī′krō-sū′chūr) Small caliber suture material, often 9-0 or 10-0, with an attached needle of corresponding size, for use in microsurgery.

mi•cro•sy•ringe (mī′krō-si-rinj′) A hypodermic syringe that has a micrometer screw attached to the piston, allowing accurately measured minute quantities of fluid to be injected.

mi•cro•ti•a (mī-krō′shē-ă) Abnormal smallness of the auricle of the acoustic external ear with a blind or absent external auditory meatus. [micro- + G. *ous,* ear]

mi•cro•tome (mī′krō-tōm) An instrument for making sections of biological tissue for examination under the microscope. SYN histotome.

mi•crot•o•my (mī-krot′ŏ-mē) The making of thin sections of tissues for examination under the microscope. SYN histotomy. [micro- + G. *tomē,* incision]

mi•cro•trau•ma (mī′krō-traw′mă) A minor or microscopic lesion due to injury, which may become significant if often repeated. SYN cumulative trauma disorder.

Mi•cro•trom•bid•i•um (mī′krō-trom-bid′ē-ŭm) A genus of chigger or harvest mites that causes severe itching from the presence of the larval stage (chigger) in the skin. [micro- + Mod. L. *trombidium,* a timid one]

mi•cro•tu•bule (mī′krō-tūb′yūl) A cylindric cytoplasmic element that occurs widely in the cytoskeleton of plant and animal cells; microtubules increase in number during mitosis and meiosis, where they may be related to movement of the chromosomes or chromatids on the nuclear spindle during nuclear division. See page 989.

mi•cro•vil•lus, pl. **mi•cro•vil•li** (mī′krō-vil′ŭs, -ī) One of the minute projections of cell membranes greatly increasing surface area; microvilli form the striated or brush borders of certain cells.

mi•cro•volt (mcV) (mī′krō-vōlt) One millionth of a volt.

mi•cro•waves (mī′krō-wāvz) That portion of the radio wave spectrum of shortest wavelength, including the region with wavelengths of 1 mm–30 cm (1000–300,000 megacycles per second).

mi•crox•y•phil (mī-krok′si-fil) A multinuclear oxyphil leukocyte. [micro- + G. *oxys,* acid, + *philos,* fond]

mi•cro•zo•on (mī′krō-zō′on) A microscopic

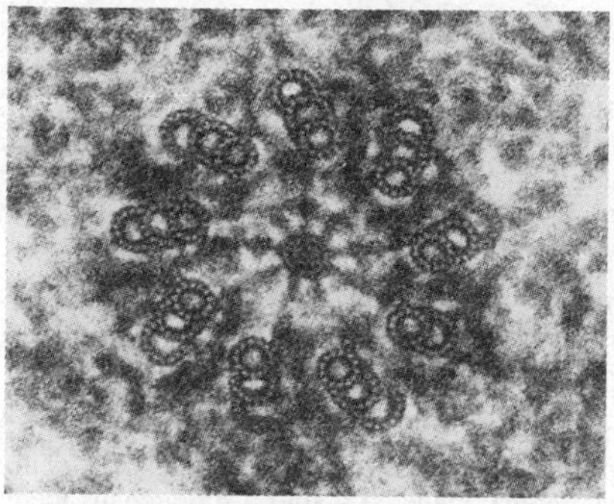

microtubules: electron micrograph (×330,000) of a centriole in transverse section; nine triplet microtubules are arranged around an axial cartwheel-like structure

form of the animal kingdom; a protozoon. [micro- + G. *zōon,* animal]

mi·crur·gi·cal (mī-krŭr′ji-kăl) Relating to procedures performed on minute structures under a microscope. [micro- + G. *ergon,* work]

mic·tion (mik′shŭn) SYN urination.

mic·tu·rate (mik′chū-rāt) SYN urinate. SEE micturition.

mic·tu·rat·ing cys·to·u·re·thro·gram (mik′chū-rā′ting sis′tō-yū-rēth′rō-gram) SYN voiding cystourethrogram.

mic·tu·ri·tion (mik-chŭr-ish′ŭn) **1.** SYN urination. **2.** The desire to urinate. **3.** Frequency of urination. [L. *micturio,* to desire to make water]

mic·tu·ri·tion re·flex (mik′chŭr-ish′ŭn rē′fleks) Relaxation of the urethral sphincter in response to increased pressure in the bladder. It normally produces a series of contractions of the urinary bladder. [L. *micturio,* to urinate, *reflectexus,* bent back]

MICU Abbreviation for medical intensive care unit.

MID Abbreviation for minimal infecting dose.

♻ **mid-** Combining form meaning middle. [A.S. *mid, midd*]

mid·ax·il·lar·y line (mid-ak′si-lar-ē līn) An imaginary division halfway between the anterior axillary line and the posterior axillary line, passing through the apex of the axilla. SYN median axillary line [TA].

mid·bod·y (mid′bod-ē) A dense stalk of residual interzonal spindle fibers (microtubules) and actin-containing filaments that is formed during anaphase of mitosis and connects daughter cells during telophase; midbodies are frequently observed between spermatids.

mid·brain (mid′brān) SYN mesencephalon.

MID-CABG Abbreviation for minimally invasive directed coronary artery bypass graft; performed through a left anterior thoracotomy without cardiopulmonary bypass.

mid·car·pal (mid-kahr′păl) **1.** Relating to the central part of the carpus. **2.** Denoting the articulation between the two rows of carpal bones. SYN mediocarpal.

mid·cla·vic·u·lar line (mid′klă-vik′yū-lăr līn) An imaginary vertical division on the anterior surface of the body, passing through the midpoint of the clavicle. SYN midclavicular plane [TA].

mid·cla·vic·u·lar plane (mid′klă-vik′yū-lăr plān) [TA] SYN midclavicular line.

mid·dle (mid′ĕl) Denoting an anatomic structure that is between two other similar structures or that is midway in position.

mid·dle a·dult (mid′ĕl ă-dŭlt′) A person in a nonspecific stage of life, being neither young nor old, but somewhere in the middle. According to Erik Erikson, between ages 40 to 65 years, with the developmental (psychological) task of generativity vs. despair. Often associated with the potential onset of midlife crisis. [AS. *middel,* + L. *adultus,* grown up]

mid·dle car·di·ac vein (mid′dĕl kahr′dē-ak vān) Begins at the apex of the heart, anastomoses with the great cardiac vein, and ascends within the posterior interventricular sulcus to the coronary sinus.

mid·dle cer·e·bel·lar pe·dun·cle (mid′ĕl ser-ĕ-bel′ăr pĕ-dŭnk′ĕl) The largest of three paired cerebellar peduncles, composed mainly of fibers that originate in the pontine nuclei, cross the midline in the ventral part of pons, and emerge on the opposite side as a massive bundle arching dorsally along the lateral side of the pontine tegmentum into the cerebellum; its fibers are distributed chiefly to the cortex of the cerebellar hemisphere.

mid·dle ce·re·bral ar·ter·y (mid′el ser′ĕ-brăl ahr′tĕr-ē) One of the two large terminal branches (with anterior cerebral artery) of the internal carotid artery; it passes laterally around the pole of the temporal lobe, then posteriorly in the depth of the lateral cerebral fissure. SYN arteria cerebri media.

mid·dle cer·vi·cal gan·gli·on (mid′ĕl sĕr′vi-kăl gang′glē-ŏn) A paravertebral small sympathetic ganglion, sometimes absent; located at the level of the cricoid cartilage.

mid·dle clu·ne·al nerves (mid′el klū′nē-ăl nĕrvz) SYN medial cluneal nerves.

mid·dle col·ic ar·ter·y (mid′ĕl kol′ik ahr′tĕr-ē) *Origin*, superior mesenteric; *distribution*, transverse colon; *anastomoses*, right and left colic.

mid•dle col•lat•er•al ar•ter•y (mid′ĕl kŏ-lat′ĕr-ăl ahr′tĕr-ē) The posterior terminal branch of the profunda brachii, anastomosing with arteries that form the articular network of the elbow. SYN arteria collateralis media, medial collateral artery.

mid•dle con•stric•tor mus•cle of phar•ynx (mid′ĕl kŏn-strik′tĕr mŭs′ĕl far′ingks) *Origin*, stylohyoid ligament, lesser cornu of the hyoid bone (chondropharyngeal part) and greater cornu of the hyoid bone (ceratopharyngeal part); *insertion*, pharyngeal raphe in the posterior wall of the pharynx; *action*, narrows pharynx in the act of swallowing; *nerve supply*, pharyngeal plexus.

mid•dle ear (mid′ĕl ēr) SEE ear. SEE ALSO tympanic cavity.

mid•dle-ear ef•fu•sion (mid′dĕl-ēr ĕ-fyū′zhŭn) A condition in which the air in the middle ear has been replaced with serous or mucoid fluid as a consequence of otitis media. SYN serous otitis media.

mid•dle fos•sa ap•proach (mid′ĕl fos′ă ă-prōch′) Surgical approach to the cerebellopontine angle through that portion of the floor of the middle cranial fossa that is the anterior surface of the petrous pyramid of the temporal bone.

mid•dle ge•nic•u•lar ar•ter•y (mid′ĕl je-nik′yū-lăr ahr′tĕr-ē) *Origin*, popliteal; *distribution*, synovial membrane and cruciate ligaments of knee joint.

mid•dle he•morr•hoid•al ar•ter•y (mid′ĕl hem′ŏr-oyd′ăl ahr′tĕr-ē) SYN middle rectal artery.

mid•dle kid•ney (mid′ĕl kid′nē) SEE mesonephros.

mid•dle la•ten•cy re•sponse (mid′ĕl lā′tĕn-sē rĕ-spons′) A response to acoustic stimulation recorded from the auditory cortex of the brain.

mid•dle mac•u•lar ar•ter•i•ole (mid′ĕl mak′yū-lăr ahr-tēr′ē-ōl) An arteriole supplying the part of the retina between the optic disc and the macula.

mid•dle me•nin•ge•al veins (mid′dĕl mĕ-nin′jē-ăl vānz) The venae comitantes of the middle meningeal artery that empty into the pterygoid plexus.

mid•dle na•sal con•cha (mid′ĕl nā′zăl kong′kă) **1.** The middle thin, spongy, bony plate with curved margins, part of the ethmoidal labyrinth, projecting from the lateral wall of the nasal cavity and separating the superior meatus from the middle meatus. **2.** The above bony plate and its thick mucoperiosteum containing a cavernous vascular bed for heat exchange.

mid•dle rec•tal ar•ter•y (mid′ĕl rek′tăl ahr′tĕr-ē) *Origin*, internal iliac; *distribution*, middle portion of rectum; *anastomoses*, inferior rectal and superior rectal. SYN arteria rectalis media, middle hemorrhoidal artery.

mid•dle rec•tal lymph node (mid′ĕl rek′tăl limf nōd) A lymph node along the middle rectal artery that receives afferents from the pararectal nodes and sends efferents to the internal iliac nodes.

mid•dle su•pra•cla•vic•u•lar nerve (mid′ĕl sū′pră-klă-vik′yū-lăr nĕrv) SYN intermediate supraclavicular nerve.

mid•dle su•pra•re•nal ar•ter•y (mid′ĕl sū′pră-rē′năl ahr′tĕr-ē) *Origin*, aorta; *distribution*, suprarenal gland. SYN arteria suprarenalis media.

mid•dle tem•po•ral vein (mid′ĕl tem′pŏr-ăl vān) It arises near the lateral angle of the eye and joins the superficial temporal veins to form the retromandibular vein.

mid•foot (mid′fut) The section of the foot between the hindfoot and forefoot; includes five of the seven tarsal bones (e.g., navicular, cuboid, and three cuneiforms).

midge (mij) The smallest of the biting flies, in the genus *Culicoides;* swarms may attack humans and other animals; vectors of filarial infections. [O.E. *mycg*]

mid•gut (mid′gŭt) **1.** The central portion of the digestive tube; the distal duodenum, small intestine, and proximal colon. **2.** The portion of the embryonic gut between the foregut and the hindgut that originally is open to the yolk sac.

mid•gut loop (mid-gut lūp) The U-shaped part of the embryonic midgut that herniates into the extraembryonic celom in the proximal part of the umbilical cord when the embryonic celom (primordial abdominal cavity) temporarily becomes too small to contain the intestinal loops. SYN umbilical intestinal loop.

mid•life (mid′līf) Middle age.

mid•life cri•sis (mid-līf krī′sis) A point in a sequence of events during the middle years of life at which certain trends of earlier and later events in one's life are pondered, generally involving an aggregate of personal, career, or sexual dissatisfactions.

mid•line e•pi•si•ot•o•my (mid′līn ĕ-piz′ē-ot′ŏ-mē) Incision of the perineum in the midline during childbirth to ease delivery. Although less painful after delivery than a mediolateral incision, it is associated with a higher risk of injury to the anal sphincter and the rectum. SYN median episiotomy.

mid•line le•thal gran•u•lo•ma (mid′līn lē′thăl gran′yū-lō′mă) Destruction of the nasal septum, hard palate, lateral nasal walls, paranasal sinuses, skin of the face, orbit, and nasopharynx by an inflammatory infiltrate with atypical lymphocytic and histiocytic cells; presumably a hypersensitivity response to an unidentified antigen in most cases. The prognosis is poor, despite radiotherapy. SYN malignant granuloma.

mid·line my·e·lot·o·my (mid′līn mī-ĕ-lot′ŏ-mē) Section of the midline transverse fibers of the spinal cord for the treatment of intractable pain. SYN commissurotomy (2).

mid·riff (mid′rif) SYN diaphragm (1). [A.S. *mid,* middle, + *hrif,* belly]

mid·sag·it·tal plane (mid-saj′i-tăl plān) SYN median plane.

mid-spec·trum a·gent (mid-spek′trŭm ā′jĕnt) A term increasingly used to refer to toxins, synthetic viruses, and genocidal agents as mass-casualty agents having features of both chemical-warfare agents and biological-warfare agents.

mid·stream ur·ine spec·i·men (MCUS) (mid-strēm yūr′in spes′i-mĕn) A urine specimen collected from the middle flow of urine after cleansing of the external genitalia. Used for microbial studies to identify infective agents and in testing antibiotic sensitivity.

mid·tar·sal (mid-tahr′săl) Relating to the middle of the tarsus.

mid·wife (mid′wīf) A person qualified to practice midwifery, having received specialized training in obstetrics and child care. SEE ALSO doula. [A.S. *mid,* with, + *wif,* wife]

mid·wif·e·ry (mid-wif′ĕ-rē) Independent care of essentially normal, healthy women and infants by a midwife, antepartally, intrapartally, postpartally, or obstetrically in a hospital, birth center, or home setting, and including normal delivery of the infant, with medical consultation, collaborative management, and referral of cases in which abnormalities develop; strong emphasis is placed on educational preparation of parents for child-bearing and child-rearing, with an orientation toward childbirth as a normal physiologic process requiring minimal intervention. SEE ALSO doula.

Mie·scher e·las·to·ma (mē′sher ē-las-tō′mă) Circinate groups of hyperkeratotic papules that become dislodged, leaving a small bloody depression; associated with pseudoxanthoma elasticum.

Mie·scher gran·u·lo·ma (mē′sher gran′yū-lō′mă) SYN actinic granuloma.

Mie·scher tube (mē′sher tūb) An elongate fusiform or cylindric body forming the encapsulated cystic intramuscular stage of the protozoan *Sarcocystis.*

mi·graine (mī′grān) A symptom complex occurring periodically and characterized by pain in the head (usually unilateral), vertigo, nausea and vomiting, photophobia, and scintillating appearances of light. Subtypes include classic migraine, common migraine, cluster headache, hemiplegic migraine, ophthalmoplegic migraine, and ophthalmic migraine. SYN hemicrania (1), sick headache. [through O. Fr., fr. G. *hēmi-krania,* pain on one side of the head, fr. *hēmi-,* half, + *kranion,* skull]

mi·graine head·ache (mī′grān hed′āk) SEE migraine.

mi·graine-re·lat·ed ves·tib·u·lop·a·thy (mī′grān′ rē-lā′tĕd ves-tib′yū-lŏp′ă-thē) A disorder characterized by movement-associated disequilibrium, unsteadiness, space and motion discomfort, and vertigo before onset of headache.

mi·grat·ing ab·scess (mī′grā-ting ab′ses) SYN perforating abscess.

mi·gra·tion (mī-grā′shŭn) **1.** Passage from one part to another, said of certain morbid processes or symptoms. **2.** SYN diapedesis. **3.** Movement of a tooth or teeth out of normal position. **4.** Movement of molecules during electrophoresis. **5.** Geographic spread of disease-causing agents, rectors, or populations. [L. *migro,* pp. *-atus,* to move from place to place]

MIH Abbreviation for melanotropin release-inhibiting hormone.

Mi·ku·licz aph·thae (mē′kū-lich af′thē) SYN aphthae major.

Mi·ku·licz dis·ease (mē′kū-lich di-zēz′) Benign swelling of the lacrimal, and usually also of the salivary, glands due to infiltration of and replacement of the normal gland structure by lymphoid tissue. SEE ALSO Mikulicz syndrome, Sjögren syndrome.

Mi·ku·licz drain (mē′kū-lich drān) A drain made of several strings of gauze held together by a single layer of gauze.

Mi·ku·licz op·er·a·tion (mē′kū-lich op-ĕr-ā′shŭn) Excision of bowel in two stages: 1) exteriorizing thc diseased area, suturing efferent and afferent limbs together, and closing the abdomen around them, after which the diseased part is excised; 2) at a later time, cutting the spur with an enterotome and closing the stoma extraperitoneally.

Mi·ku·licz syn·drome (mē′kū-lich sin′drōm) The symptoms characteristic of Mikulicz disease occurring as a complication of some other disease, such as lymphoma, leukemia, or uveoparotid fever.

Miles op·er·a·tion (mīlz op-ĕr-ā′shŭn) Combined abdominoperineal resection for carcinoma of the rectum.

mil·i·a (mil′ē-ă) Plural of milium.

mil·i·a·ri·a (mil-ē-ā′rē-ă) An eruption of minute vesicles and papules due to retention of fluid at the orifices of sweat glands. SYN miliary fever (2). [L. *miliarius,* relating to millet, fr. *milium,* millet]

mil·i·a·ri·a ru·bra (mil-ē-ā′rē-ă rū′bră) An

eruption of papules and vesicles at the orifices of sweat glands, accompanied by redness and inflammatory reaction of the skin. SYN heat rash, prickly heat, strophulus, tropical lichen, lichen tropicus.

mil•i•a•ry (mil′ē-ā-rē) **1.** Resembling a millet seed in size (about 2 mm). **2.** Marked by the presence of nodules of millet seed size on any surface. SEE miliaria.

mil•i•a•ry ab•scess (mil′ē-ā-rē ab′ses) One of several minute collections of pus, widely disseminated throughout an area or the whole body.

mil•i•a•ry em•bo•lism (mil′ē-ā-rē em′bŏ-lizm) One occurring simultaneously in a number of capillaries.

mil•i•a•ry fe•ver (mil′ē-ā-rē fē′vĕr) **1.** An infectious disease characterized by profuse sweating and the production of sudamina; formerly occurring in severe epidemics. **2.** SYN miliaria.

mil•i•a•ry pat•tern (mil′ē-ā-rē pat′ĕrn) A chest radiographic pattern of fine, rounded opacities, typical of hematogenous dissemination of tuberculosis.

mil•i•a•ry tu•ber•cu•lo•sis (mil′ē-ā-rē tū-bĕr′kyū-lō′sis) General dissemination of tubercle bacilli in the blood, resulting in the formation of miliary tubercles in various organs and tissues, and occasionally producing symptoms of profound toxemia. SYN generalized tuberculosis.

mi•lieu (mēl-yeuh′) **1.** Surroundings; environment. **2.** PSYCHIATRY the social setting of the mental patient, e.g., the family setting or a hospital unit. [Fr. *mi-*, fr. L. *medius*, middle, + *lieu*, fr. L. *locus*, place]

mil•ieu ther•a•py (mēl-yeuh′ thār′ă-pē) Psychiatric treatment employing manipulation of the social environment for the benefit of the patient.

mil•i•tar•y an•ti•shock trou•sers (MAST) (mil′i-tar-ē an′tī-shok trow′zĕrz) SYN pneumatic antishock garment.

Mil•i•tar•y Health Ser•vic•es Sys•tem (MHSS) (mil′i-tar-rē helth sĕr′vis-ez sis′tĕm) The network of hospitals and clinics that comprise the health care system of the U.S. Department of Defense. Although its primary function is to maintain the health of members of the U.S. Armed Forces, it also provides health care if space and services are available to dependents, retirees, and other participants in TRICARE, the U.S. military health benefit plan.

mil•i•um, pl. **mil•i•a** (mil′ē-ŭm, -ă) A small subepidermal keratin cyst, usually multiple and therefore commonly referred to in the plural. See page B13. SYN whitehead (1). [L. millet]

milk (milk) **1.** A white liquid, containing nutrients and other substances (e.g., proteins, sugar, and lipids), secreted by the mammary glands after birth, and serving to nourish the infant or young animal. **2.** Any whitish, milky fluid; e.g., the juice of the coconut or a suspension of various metallic oxides. **3.** A pharmacopeial preparation that is a suspension of insoluble drugs in a water medium; distinguished from gels mainly in that the suspended particles of milk are larger. **4.** SYN strip (1). [A.S. *meolc*]

milk-al•ka•li syn•drome (milk-al′kă-lī sin′drōm) A chronic disorder of the kidneys, reversible in its early stages, induced by ingestion of large amounts of calcium and alkali in the therapy of peptic ulcer; can progress to renal failure. SYN Burnett syndrome.

milk crust (milk krŭst) SYN crusta lactea.

milk den•ti•tion (milk den-tish′ŭn) SYN deciduous tooth.

milk ducts (milk dŭkts) SYN lactiferous ducts.

milk fe•ver (milk fē′vĕr) **1.** A slight elevation of temperature following childbirth, said to be due to the establishment of the secretion of milk, but probably the same as absorption fever. **2.** An afebrile metabolic disease, occurring shortly after parturition in dairy cattle, characterized by hypocalcemia and manifested by loss of consciousness and general paralysis.

milk•ing (milk′ing) A procedure used to express the contents of a tube or duct to obtain a specimen or to test for tenderness.

milk line (milk līn) SYN mammary crest.

Milk•man syn•drome (milk′man sin′drōm) Osteomalacia with multiple pseudofractures, usually bilateral and symmetric; true pathologic fractures may also develop.

milk ridge (milk rij) SYN mammary crest.

milk sug•ar (milk shug′ăr) SYN lactose.

milk tooth (milk tūth) SYN deciduous tooth.

milk vetch root (milk vech rūt) SYN *Astragalus.*

Mil•ler-Ab•bott tube (mil′ĕr ab′ŏt tūb) A tube with two lumens, one ending in a small collapsible balloon and the other in a metallic tip with numerous perforations; used for intestinal decompression. SYN Abbott tube.

Mil•ler chem•i•co•par•a•sit•ic the•o•ry (mil′ĕr kem′i-kō-par-ă-sit′ik thē′ŏr-ē) The theory that dental caries is caused by microorganisms of the mouth that ferment dietary carbohydrates and produce acids that demineralize the teeth.

mill•er's asth•ma (mil′ĕr az′mă) Asthma caused by flour or grain allergens.

milli- Prefix used in the SI and metric system to signify one thousandth (10^{-3}). [L. *mille*, one thousand]

mil•li•am•pere (ma, mA) (mil′ē-am′pēr) One thousandth of an ampere.

mil·li·am·pere-im·pulse (mAi) (mil′i-am′ pēr-im′pŭls) SYN milliampere-second.

mil·li·am·pere-sec·ond (mA-s) (mil′i-am′ pēr-sek′ŏnd) A radiologic unit denoting the product of the number of electrons applied to the cathode of the x-ray tube multiplied by the exposure time in seconds; it directly determines the amount of x-ray energy produced. SYN milliampere-impulse.

mil·li·cu·rie (mc, mCi) (mil′i-kyūr′ē) A unit of radioactivity equivalent to 3.7×10^7 disintegrations per second.

mil·li·e·quiv·a·lent (mEq, meq) (mil′i-ē-kwiv′ă-lĕnt) One thousandth equivalent; 10^{-3} mole divided by valence.

mil·li·gram (mg) (mil′i-gram) One thousandth of a gram.

mil·li·li·ter (mL, ml) (mil′i-lē′tĕr) One thousandth of a liter. SYN millilitre.

millilitre [Br.] SYN milliliter.

mil·li·me·ter (mm) (mil′i-mē′tĕr) One thousandth of a meter. SYN millimetre.

millimetre [Br.] SYN millimeter.

♻ **millimicro-** Prefix formerly used to signify one billionth (10^{-9}); now nano-.

mil·li·mi·cron (mmcm) (mil′i-mī′kron) Former term for nanometer.

mil·li·mole (mmol) (mil′i-mōl) One thousandth of a gram-molecule.

mil·li·sec·ond (msec) (mil′i-sek′ŏnd) One thousandth of a second.

mil·li·volt (mV) (mil′i-vōlt) One thousandth of a volt.

mil·pho·sis (mil-fō′sis) Loss of eyelashes. [G. *milphōsis*]

Mil·roy dis·ease (mil′roy di-zēz′) The congenital type of autosomal dominant lymphedema.

MIM (mim) Acronym for Mendelian Inheritance in Man.

mi·me·sis (mi-mē′sis) **1.** Hysteric simulation of organic disease. **2.** The symptomatic imitation of one organic disease by another. [G. *mimēsis,* imitation, fr. *mimeomai,* to mimic]

mi·met·ic (mi-met′ik) Relating to mimesis. [G. *mimētikos,* imitative]

mim·ic (mim′ik) To imitate or simulate. [G. *mimikos,* imitating, fr. *mimos,* a mimic]

MIM num·ber (mim nŭm′bĕr) The catalogue assignment for a mendelian trait in the MIM system. If the initial digit is 1, the trait is deemed autosomal dominant; if 2, autosomal recessive; if 3, then X-linked.

Mi·na·ma·ta dis·ease (min-ă-mah′tă di-zēz′) A neurologic disorder caused by methyl mercury intoxication; first described in the inhabitants of Minamata Bay, Japan, resulting from eating fish contaminated with mercury-tainted industrial waste. Characterized by peripheral sensory loss, tremors, dysarthria, ataxia, and both hearing and visual loss.

mind (mīnd) **1.** The organ or seat of consciousness and higher functions of the human brain, such as cognition, reasoning, willing, and emotion. **2.** The organized totality of all mental processes and psychic activities, with emphasis on the relatedness of the phenomena. [A.S. *gemynd*]

mind/bod·y med·i·cine (mīnd-bod′ē med′i-sin) A theory that involves the relationship between the mind and body as well as the body's innate ability to heal itself when given a positive physical and emotional environment.

min·er·al (min′ĕr-ăl) Any homogeneous inorganic material usually found in the earth's crust. [L. *mineralis,* pertaining to mines, fr. *mino,* to mine]

min·er·al·o·cor·ti·coid (min′ĕr-ăl-ō-kōr′ti-koyd) One of the steroids of the cortex of the suprarenal gland that influence salt (sodium and potassium) metabolism. Cf. bioregulator.

min·er·al wa·ter (min′ĕr-ăl waw′tĕr) Any water that contains appreciable amounts of certain salts, which give it therapeutic properties.

min·er's elbow (mī′nĕrz el′bō) Inflammation of the olecranon bursa, caused by resting the weight of the body on the elbows.

min·er's lung (mī′nĕrz lŭng) **1.** SYN anthracosis. **2.** SYN black lung.

min·i·lap·a·rot·o·my (min′ē-lap-ă-rot′ŏ-mē) Technique for sterilization by surgical ligation of the uterine tubes, performed through a small suprapubic incision.

min·im (min′im) **1.** A fluid measure, 1/60 of a fluidram; in the case of water, about one drop. **2.** Smallest; least; the smallest of several similar structures. [L. *minimus,* least]

min·i·mal brain dys·func·tion (min′i-măl brān dis-fŭngk′shŭn) SEE attention deficit disorder.

min·i·mal dose (min′i-măl dōs) The smallest amount of a drug or physical procedure that will produce a desired physiologic effect in an adult.

min·i·mal fa·tal dose (MFD) (min′i-măl fā′tăl dōs) SEE minimal lethal dose.

min·i·mal in·fect·ing dose (MID) (min′i-măl in-fekt′ting dōs) The smallest quantity of infectious material regularly producing infection; usually expressed as ID_{50}, the quantity causing infection in 50% of a suitable series of animals or cells (cell cultures).

min·i·mal le·thal dose (MLD, mld) (min′i-măl lē′thăl dōs) **1.** The minimal dose of a toxic substance or infectious agent that is lethal, as assayed in various experimental animals; when followed by a subscript (generally "MLD_{50}"), denotes the minimal dose that is lethal to a certain percentage (e.g., 50%) of animals so assayed. **2.** LD_{50}. SEE lethal dose.

min·i·mal oc·clu·ding vol·ume (MOV) (min′i-măl ŏ-klūd′ing vol′yūm) Level of pressure at which a cuff is used in ventilation therapy must be set to so as to avoid air leaks during patient's inspiration.

min·i·mal re·act·ing dose (MRD, mrd) (min′i-măl rē-akt′ting dōs) The minimal dose of a toxic substance causing a reaction, as manifested in the skin of a series of susceptible test animals; the assay is based on the development of a characteristic, minimal but definite, "standard," focal inflammation.

Mi·ni-Men·tal State Ex·am·i·na·tion (min′ē men′tăl stāt′ eg-zam′i-nā′shŭn) Widely used written assessment instrument that measures and evaluates cognitive function and mental impairment. Often given serially to gauge the effect of time on patients' condition.

min·i·mum as·sis·tance (min′i-mŭm ă-sis′tăns) Application by a caregiver of support or assitance at a single point of contact to enable a patient to perform an activity safely. The patient expends at least 75% of the effort; the caregiver, 25% or less.

min·i·mum da·ta set (MDS) (min′i-mŭm dā′tă set) Smallest number of data that can be collected and still positively identify the patient. SEE ALSO Nursing Minimum Data Set.

min·i·mum leak tech·nique (MLT) (min′i-mŭm lēk tek-nēk′) After full inflation of the occluding cuff of an endotracheal or tracheostomy tube, the withdrawal of a small volume of air or saline solution so that a slight leak is heard at the end of (positive pressure) inspiration, to avoid tracheal trauma resulting from overinflation. In respiratory therapy, a form of mechanical ventilation often used in association with tracheotomy. An invasive procedure, it carries a substantial risk of patients' aspirating of fluids.

mi·ni·thor·a·cot·omy (min′ē-thōr′ă-kot′ă-mē) Any thoracotomy involving less muscle division than the classic posterolateral thoracotomy.

Min·ne·so·ta Mul·ti·pha·sic Per·son·al·i·ty In·ven·to·ry (MMPI) (min-ĕ-sō′tă mŭl-ti-fā′zik pĕr-sŏn-al′i-tē in′vĕn-tōr-ē) A questionnaire type of psychological test for ages 16 years and older, with 550 true-false statements coded in four validity and 10 personality scales, which may be administered in either an individual or group format.

mi·nor (mī′nŏr) Smaller; lesser; denoting the smaller of two similar structures. [L.]

mi·nor ag·glu·ti·nin (mī′nŏr ă-glū′ti-nin) Immune agglutinin present in an antiserum in lesser concentration than the major agglutinin. SYN partial agglutinin.

mi·nor his·to·com·pat·i·bil·ity com·plex (mī′nŏr his′tō-kom-pat-i-bil′i-tē kom′pleks) Genes outside of MHC that are present on various chromosomes that encode antigens contributing to graft rejection.

mi·nor hys·te·ri·a (mī′nŏr his-ter′ē-ă) A mild form of hysteria characterized chiefly by subjective pains, nervousness, undue sensitiveness, and sometimes episodes of emotional excitement, but without paralysis or other such symptoms.

mi·nor sal·i·var·y glands (mī′nŏr sal′i-var-ē glandz) The smaller, largely mucous-secreting, exocrine glands of the oral cavity, consisting of the labial, buccal, molar, lingual, and palatine glands.

mi·nor sub·lin·gual ducts (mī′nŏr sŭb-ling′gwăl dŭkts) The 8–20 small ducts of the sublingual salivary gland that open into the mouth on the surface of the sublingual fold; a few join the submandibular ducts. SYN Rivinus ducts, Walther ducts.

min·ute ven·ti·la·tion (min′ŭt ven′ti-lā′shŭn) SYN minute volume.

min·ute vol·ume (min′ŭt vol′yūm) The amount of any gas or fluid moved in 1 minute (e.g., cardiac output or the respiratory minute volume). SYN minute ventilation.

♻ **mio-** Combining form meaning less. [G. *meiōn*]

mi·o·sis (mī-ō′sis) **1.** Contraction of the pupil. **2.** Incorrect alternative spelling for meiosis. [G. *meiōsis,* a lessening]

mi·o·sphyg·mi·a (mī-ō-sfig′mē-ă) Condition in which pulse beats are fewer than heart beats. [mio- + G. *sphygmos,* pulse]

mi·ot·ic (mī-ot′ik) **1.** Relating to or characterized by contraction of the pupil. **2.** An agent that causes the pupil to contract.

MIP Abbreviation for maximum inspiratory pressure; maximum intensity projection; middle interphalangeal joint.

mire (mēr) One of the test objects in the ophthalmometer; its image (also called a mire), mirrored on the corneal surface, is measured to determine the radii of curvature of the cornea. [L. *miror,* pp. *-atus,* to wonder at]

Mi·riz·zi syn·drome (mē-rēt′sē sin′drōm) Benign obstruction of the hepatic ducts due to spasm and/or fibrous scarring of surrounding connective tissue; often associated with a stone in the cystic duct and chronic cholecystitis.

mir·ror (mir′ŏr) A polished surface reflecting the rays of light reflected from objects in front of it. [Fr. *miroir,* fr. L. *miror,* to wonder at]

mir•ror-im•age cell (mir′ŏr′im′ăj sel) **1.** A cell with nuclei that have identical features and are placed in the cytoplasm in similar fashion. **2.** A binucleate form of Reed-Sternberg cell often found in Hodgkin disease; the twin nuclei are disposed in relation to an imaginary plane between them, like a single nucleus together with its image in a mirror.

mir•ror speech (mir′ŏr spēch) A reversal of the order of syllables in a word, analogous to mirror writing.

mir•yach•it (mēr-yach′it) A nervous affliction observed in Siberia. SEE jumping disease.

♻**mis-** Combining form denoting not, opposite, incorrect, improper.

mis•ad•min•i•stra•tion (mis′ad-min′i-strā′shŭn) In radiation therapy, incorrect administration of radiation by dose or treatment.

mis•an•dry (mis′an-drē) Aversion to or hatred of men. [G. *miseō,* to hate, + *anēr, andros,* male]

mis•an•thro•py (mis-an′thrŏ-pē) Aversion to or hatred of human beings. [G. *miseō,* to hate, + *anthrōpos,* man]

mis•car•riage (mis′kar-ăj) Spontaneous expulsion of the products of pregnancy before the middle of the second trimester.

mis•ci•ble (mis′i-bĕl) Capable of being mixed and remaining so after the mixing process ceases. [L. *misceo,* to mix]

mis•di•ag•no•sis (mis′dī-ag-nō′sis) A wrong or mistaken diagnosis.

mi•sog•a•my (mi-sog′ă-mē) Aversion to marriage. [G. *miseō,* to hate, + *gamos,* marriage]

mi•sog•y•ny (mi-soj′i-nē) Aversion to or hatred of women. [G. *miseō,* to hate, + *gynē,* woman]

mis•o•pe•di•a, **mis•op•e•dy** (mis-ō-pē′dē-ă, mis-op′ĕ-dē) Aversion to or hatred of children. [G. *miseō,* to hate, + *pais (paid-),* child]

missed a•bor•tion (mist ă-bōr′shŭn) Abortion in which the fetus dies but is retained in utero for 2 months or longer.

missed la•bor (mist lā′bŏr) Brief uterine contractions that do not lead to labor and expulsion of the infant, but which cease, resulting in the indefinite retention of the fetus (usually lifeless).

mis•sense mu•ta•tion (mis′sens myū-tā′shŭn) A mutation in which a base change or substitution results in a codon that causes insertion of a different amino acid into the growing polypeptide chain, giving rise to an altered protein. [missense by analogy with non-sense]

mis•sion-or•i•ent•ed pro•tec•tive pos•ture (MOPP) (mish′ŭn ōr′ē-en-tĕd prō-tek′tiv pos′chŭr) Delineation of protection afforded by clothing and equipment vs. various threats; the MOPP level number rises with the threat.

Mis•sou•ri (Kan•sas) snake•root (mi-zŭr′ē kan′zăs snāk′rūt) SYN echinacea.

Mitch•ell dis•ease (mich′ĕl di-zēz′) SYN erythromelalgia.

Mitch•ell pro•ce•dure (mich′ĕl prŏ-sē′jŭr) Surgical procedure to correct a hallux valgus by combining a bunionectomy and soft tissue correction of the first metatarsophalangeal joint with an osteotomy of the proximal portion of the first metatarsal.

Mitch•ell treat•ment (mich′ĕl trēt′mĕnt) Treatment of mental illness by rest, nourishing diet, and a change of environment.

mite (mīt) A minute arthropod of the order Acarina, a vast assemblage of parasitic and (primarily) free-living organisms. A few are of medical importance as vectors or intermediate hosts of pathogenic agents, by directly causing dermatitis or tissue damage, or by causing blood or tissue fluid loss. See page B8. [A.S.]

mite ty•phus (mīt tī′fŭs) SYN tsutsugamushi disease.

mith•ri•da•tism (mith-ri-dā′tizm) Immunity against the action of a poison produced by small, gradually increasing doses of the same. [*Mithridates,* King of Pontus (132–63 BCE), supposedly an inadvertent suicide (by poison) because of repeated small doses he took, intending to become invulnerable to assassination by poisoning]

mi•ti•ci•dal (mī-ti-sī′dăl) Destructive to mites.

mi•ti•cide (mī′ti-sīd) An agent destructive to mites. [mite + L. *caedo,* to kill]

mit•i•gate (mit′i-gāt) SYN palliate. [L. *mitigo,* pp. *-atus,* to make mild or gentle, fr. *mitis,* mild, + *ago,* to do, make]

mi•to•chon•dri•a (-ă) Plural of mitochondrion.

mi•to•chon•dri•al (mī-tō-kon′drē-ăl) Relating to mitochondria.

mi•to•chon•dri•al bi•o•gen•e•sis (mī-tō-kon′drē-ăl bī′ō-jen′ĕ-sis) The process by which mitochondria increase their ability to make adenosine triphosphate by synthesizing additional respiratory enzyme complexes.

mi•to•chon•dri•al chro•mo•some (mī-tō-kon′drē-ăl krō′mŏ-sōm) The DNA component of mitochondria, the chief function of which is synthesis of adenosine triphosphate and the management of cellular energy.

mi•to•chon•dri•al dis•or•ders (mī-tō-kon′drē-ăl dis-ōr′dĕrz) A group of diverse hereditary disorders caused by genetic mutation of mitochrondrial DNA; includes: ragged red fiber myopathy; progressive external ophthalmoplegia; Leigh syndrome; myoclonic epilepsy with ragged red fiber myopathy (MERRF); mitochondrial myopathy, encephalopathy, lactacidosis, and stroke (MELAS); and Lieber optic neuropathy.

mi•to•chon•dri•al mem•brane (mī-tō-kon′drē-ăl mem′brān) The mitochondrion has two membranes: the inner where the electron transport system is located and the outer, which acts as a gatekeeper and allows only certain molecules to enter.

mi•to•chon•dri•on, pl. **mi•to•chon•dri•a** (mī-tō-kon′drē-ŏn, -ă) An organelle of the cell cytoplasm consisting of two sets of membranes, a smooth continuous outer coat and an inner membrane arranged in tubules or more often in folds that form platelike double membranes called cristae; mitochondria are the principal energy source of the cell and contain the cytochrome enzymes of terminal electron transport and the enzymes of the citric acid cycle, fatty acid oxidation, and oxidative phosphorylation. See this page. [G. *mitos,* thread, + *chondros,* granule, grits]

mi•to•gen (mī′tō-jen) A substance that stimulates mitosis and lymphocyte transformation; includes not only lectins such as phytohemagglutinins and concanavalin A, but also substances from streptococci (associated with streptolysin S) and from strains of α-toxin-producing staphylococci. [mitosis + G. *-gen,* producing]

mi•to•gen•e•sis (mī-tō-jen′ĕ-sis) The induction of mitosis in a cell. [mitosis + G. *genesis,* origin]

mi•to•ge•net•ic (mī′tō-jĕ-net′ik) Pertaining to the factor or factors promoting cell mitosis.

mi•to•gen•ic (mī-tō-jen′ik) Causing mitosis or transformation.

mi•to•sis, pl. **mi•to•ses** (mī-tō′sis, -sēz) The usual process of somatic reproduction of cells consisting of a sequence of modifications of the nucleus (prophase, prometaphase, metaphase, anaphase, telophase) that result in the formation of two daughter cells with exactly the same chromosome and DNA content as that of the original cell. SEE ALSO cell cycle. SYN indirect nuclear division. [G. *mitos,* thread]

mi•tot•ic (mī-tot′ik) Relating to or marked by mitosis.

mi•tot•ic fig•ure (mī-tot′ik fig′yŭr) The microscopic appearance of a cell undergoing mitosis; a cell of which the chromosomes are visible by the light microscope.

mi•tot•ic rate (mī-tot′ik rāt) The proportion of cells in a tissue that are undergoing mitosis, expressed as a mitotic index or, roughly, as the number of cells in mitosis in each microscopic high-power field in tissue sections.

mi•tot•ic spin•dle (mī-tot′ik spin′dĕl) The fusiform figure characteristic of a dividing cell; it consists of microtubules (spindle fibers), some of which become attached to each chromosome at its centromere and appear to be involved in chromosomal movement; other microtubules (continuous fibers) pass from pole to pole. SYN nuclear spindle.

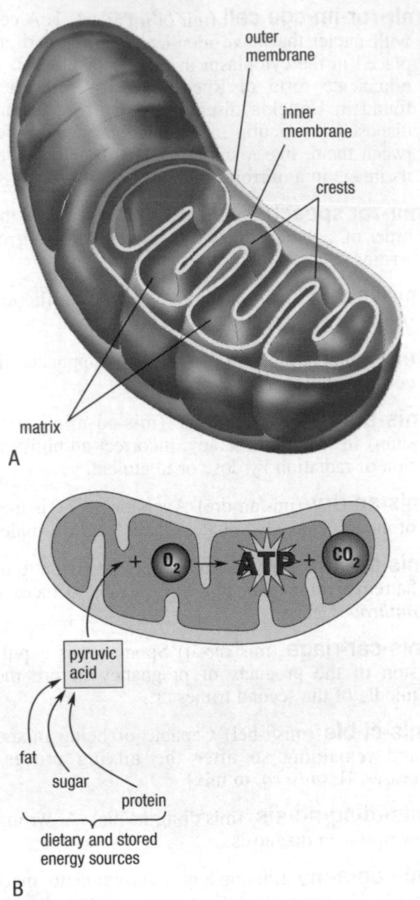

mitochondrion (A) and cellular respiration (B): adenosine 5′-triphosphate (ATP) is the energy currency that fuels biochemical reactions in cells

mi•tral (mī′trăl) **1.** Relating to the mitral or bicuspid valve. **2.** Shaped like a bishop's miter; denoting a structure resembling the shape of a headband or turban. [L. *mitra,* a coif or turban]

mi•tral a•tre•si•a (mī′trăl ă-trē′zē-ă) Congenital absence of the mitral valve between the left atrium and left ventricle, usually associated with transposition of the great vessels or hypoplastic left heart syndrome. [L. *mitra,* turban, + G. *trēsis,* perforation]

mi•tral com•mis•sur•ot•o•my (mī′trăl kom′i-shur-ot′ŏ-mē) A surgical procedure (open or closed) to repair the mitral valve, usually required as a result of valvular disease such as mitral stenosis. SYN mitral valvulotomy. [L. *mi-*

tra, turban, + *commissura,* a joining together, + G. *tomē,* incision]

mi•tral gra•di•ent (mī′trăl grā′dē-ĕnt) During diastole, difference in pressure between left atrium and left ventricle. A normal mitral valve does not impede the flow of blood from left atrium to left ventricle during (ventricular) diastole, pressures in left atrium and left ventricle during diastole will be equal.

mi•tral in•suf•fi•cien•cy (mī′trăl in′sŭ-fish′ĕn-sē) SEE valvular regurgitation.

mi•tral•i•za•tion (mī′tral′ī-zā′shŭn) Straightening of the left heart border on a chest radiograph due to prominence of the left atrial appendage or the pulmonary outflow tract; an unreliable indication of mitral valve disease.

mi•tral mur•mur (mī′trăl mŭr′mŭr) A murmur produced at the mitral valve, either obstructive or regurgitant.

mi•tral or•i•fice (mī′trăl ōr′i-fis) An atrioventricular opening that leads from the left atrium into the left ventricle of the heart.

mi•tral re•gur•gi•ta•tion (mī′trăl rē-gŭr′ji-tā′shŭn) SEE valvular regurgitation.

mi•tral ste•no•sis (MS) (mī′trăl stĕ-nō′sis) Pathologic narrowing of the orifice of the mitral valve.

mi•tral valve (mī′trăl valv) The valve closing the orifice between the left atrium and left ventricle of the heart; its two cusps are called anterior and posterior. SYN bicuspid valve.

mi•tral valve pro•lapse (MVP) (mī′trăl valv prō′laps) Excessive retrograde movement of one or both mitral valve leaflets into the left atrium during left ventricular systole, often allowing mitral regurgitation; responsible for the click-murmur of Barlow syndrome, and rarely may be due to rheumatic carditis, a connective tissue disorder such as Marfan syndrome, or ruptured chorda tendinea ("flail mitral leaflet").

mi•tral val•vu•lo•to•my (mī′trăl val′vyū-lot′ŏ-mē) SYN mitral commissurotomy.

Mit•su•o phe•nom•e•non (mit-sū′ō fĕ-nom′ĕ-non) Restoration of the normal color of the fundus with dark adaptation in Oguchi disease.

mit•tel•schmerz (mit′el-schmārtz) Abdominal pain occurring at the time of ovulation, resulting from irritation of the peritoneum by bleeding from the ovulation site. SYN intermenstrual pain (2). [Ger. *Mittelschmerz,* middle + pain]

Mit•ten•dorf dot (mit′ĕn-dōrf dot) A small spot visible on the posterior aspect of the lens capsule on ophthalmologic examination that represents a remnant of the primitive hyaloid vascular system.

mixed ag•glu•ti•na•tion re•ac•tion (mikst ă-glū′ti-nā′shŭn rē-ak′shŭn) Immune agglutination in which the aggregates contain cells of two different kinds but with common antigenic determinants; when used to identify isoantigens, the test cells are exposed to appropriate isoantibody, washed, and then mixed with indicator erythrocytes that combine with free sites on the test cell-attached isoantibody.

mixed ag•glu•ti•na•tion test (mikst ă-glū′ti-nā′shŭn test) SEE mixed agglutination reaction.

mixed a•pha•si•a (mikst ă-fā′zē-ă) SYN global aphasia.

mixed a•stig•ma•tism (mikst ă-stig′mă-tizm) A vision defect in which one meridian is hyperopic while the one at a right angle to it is myopic.

mixed con•nec•tive-tis•sue dis•ease (mikst kŏ-nek′tiv tish′ū di-zēz′) Disorder with overlapping features of various systemic connective-tissue diseases and with serum antibodies to nuclear ribonucleoprotein.

mixed ex•pired gas (mikst eks-pīrd′ gas) One or more complete breaths of expired gas coming thoroughly mixed from the dead space and the alveoli.

mixed gland (mikst gland) **1.** A gland that contains both serous and mucous secretory units. **2.** A gland that is both exocrine and endocrine, e.g., the pancreas.

mixed hear•ing loss (mikst hēr′ing laws) Combination of conductive and sensorineural hearing loss.

mixed leu•ke•mi•a, mixed cell leu•ke•mi•a (mikst lū-kē′mē-ă, mikst sel) Granulocytic leukemia with occurrence in the blood of increased numbers of cells in the myeloid series (i.e., neutrophilic, eosinophilic, and basophilic granulocytes).

mixed lym•pho•cyte cul•ture (MLC) (mikst lim′fŏ-sīt kŭl′chŭr) SEE mixed lymphocyte culture test.

mixed lym•pho•cyte cul•ture test (mikst lim′fŏ-sīt kŭl′chŭr test) An assay for histocompatibility of human leukocyte antigens in which donor and recipient lymphocytes are mixed in culture; the degree of incompatibility is indicated by the number of cells that have undergone transformation and mitosis, or by the uptake of radioactive isotope-labeled thymidine.

mixed nerve (mikst nĕrv) A nerve containing both afferent and efferent fibers.

mixed pa•ral•y•sis (mikst păr-al′i-sis) Combined motor and sensory paralysis.

mixed tu•mor (mikst tū′mŏr) A tumor composed of two or more varieties of tissue.

♻ **-mixis, -mixia, -mixy, mixo-** Combining word forms, meaning "related to reproduction" (e.g., amphimixis). [G. *mixis,* mingling, coupling]

mix·ture (miks′chŭr) **1.** A mutual incorporation of two or more substances, without chemical union, and with the physical characteristics of each of the components being retained. A **mechanical mixture** is a mixture of particles or masses distinguishable as such under the microscope or in other ways; a **physical mixture** is a more intimate mixture of molecules, as in the case of gases and many solutions. **2.** CHEMISTRY a mingling of two or more substances without the occurrence of a reaction by which they would lose their individual properties, i.e., without permanent gain or loss of electrons. **3.** PHARMACY a preparation consisting of a liquid holding an insoluble medicinal substance in suspension by means of acacia, sugar, or some other viscid material. [L. *mixtura* or *mistura*]

Mi·ya·ga·wa·nel·la (mē′yă-gah-wă-nel′ă) Formerly considered a genus of Chlamydiaceae, but now synonymous with *Chlamydia*. [Y. *Miyagawa*]

mi·zi·boc (mē′sē-bōk) SYN damiana.

MK-6 Abbreviation for menaquinone-6.

mL, ml Abbreviation for milliliter.

MLC Abbreviation for mixed lymphocyte culture.

MLD, mld Abbreviation for minimal lethal dose; manual lymph drainage.

MLEE Abbreviation for multilocus enzyme electrophoresis.

MLF Abbreviation for medial longitudinal fasciculus.

M line (līn) A fine line in the center of the A band of the sarcomere of striated muscle myofibrils. SYN M band.

MLS Abbreviation for medical language specialist.

MLST Abbreviation for multiple sleep latency test; multilocus sequence typing.

MLT Abbreviation for minimum leak technique; medical laboratory technician; multiple logical tasking.

mm Abbreviation for millimeter.

MMAD Abbreviation for mass median aerodynamic diameter.

mmcm Abbreviation for millimicron.

MMFR Abbreviation for mixed midexpiratory flow rate.

mmHg Abbreviation for millimeters of mercury. SYN torr.

MMI Abbreviation for maximum medical improvement.

M-mode (mōd) A diagnostic ultrasound presentation of the temporal changes in echoes in which the depth of echo-producing interfaces is displayed along one axis with time (T) along the second axis; motion (M) of the interfaces toward and away from the transducer is displayed.

M-mode ech·o·car·di·og·ra·phy (mōd ek′ō-kahr′dē-og′ră-fē) SEE M-mode.

mmol Abbreviation for millimole.

MMPI Abbreviation for Minnesota Multiphasic Personality Inventory.

MMR Abbreviation for measles, mumps, rubella.

MMT Abbreviation for manual muscle testing.

Mn Symbol for manganese.

M'Nagh·ten rule (mik-naw′tĕn rūl) The classic English test of criminal responsibility (1843): "to establish a defense on the ground of insanity, it must be clearly proved that, at the time of committing the act, the party accused was laboring under such a defect of reasoning, from disease of the mind, as not to know the nature and quality of the act he was doing, or if he did know it, that he did not know he was doing what was wrong."

mne·men·ic, mne·mic (nē-men′ik, nē′mik) Relating to memory.

mne·mon·ic (nē-mon′ik) SYN anamnestic (1).

mne·mon·ics (nē-mon′iks) The art of improving the memory; a system for aiding the memory. [G. *mnēmonikos,* mnemonic, pertaining to memory]

MNL Abbreviation for mononuclear leukocyte.

Mo Symbol for molybdenum.

mo·bile end (mō′bil end) For a given movement, the end of a bone that moves in response to muscle activity or gravity while the other end of the bone (the fixed end) is held stationary (as a consequence of attachment or muscular fixation). SYN punctum mobile.

mo·bi·li·za·tion (mō′bi-lī-zā′shŭn) **1.** Making movable; restoring the power of motion in a joint. **2.** The act or the result of the act of mobilizing; exciting a hitherto quiescent process into physiologic activity. [see mobilize]

Mo·bitz block (mō′bits blok) Second degree atrioventricular block in which there is a ratio of two or more atrial deflections (P waves) to ventricular responses.

Mö·bi·us sign (mō′bē-us sīn) Impairment of ocular convergence in Graves disease.

Mö·bi·us syn·drome (mō′bē-us sin′drōm) A developmental bilateral facial paralysis usually associated with oculomotor or other neurological disorders.

mo·dal fre·quen·cy (mōdăl frē′kwĕn-sē) SYN habitual pitch.

mo·dal·i·ty (mō-dal′i-tē) **1.** A form of application or employment of a therapeutic agent or regimen. **2.** Various forms of sensation, e.g., touch, vision. [Mediev. L. *modalitas,* fr. L. *modus,* a mode]

mo•dal pitch (mōdăl pich) SYN habitual pitch.

mode (mōd) In a set of measurements, that value which appears most frequently. [L. *modus,* a measure, quantity]

mod•el (mod′ĕl) **1.** A representation of something, often idealized or modified to make it conceptually easier to understand. **2.** Something to be imitated. **3.** DENTISTRY a cast. **4.** A mathematical representation of a particular phenomenon. **5.** An animal that is used to mimic a pathologic condition. [It. *modello,* fr. L. *modus,* measure, standard]

mod•el•ing (mod′ĕl-ing) **1.** LEARNING THEORY the acquiring and learning of a new skill by observing and imitating that behavior being performed by another individual. **2.** BEHAVIOR MODIFICATION a treatment procedure whereby the therapist or another significant person presents (models) the target behavior which the learner is to imitate. **3.** A continuous process by which a bone is altered in size and shape during its growth by resorption and formation of bone at different sites and rates. SYN modelling.

modelling [Br.] SYN modeling.

mod•er•ate as•sis•tance (mod′ĕr-ăt ă-sis′tăns) Application of suport or assistance at two points of contact by one or more people to enable a patient to perform a desired activity safely; caregivers supply 25–75% of needed effort.

mode of trans•mis•sion (mōd trans-mish′ŭn) The route by which an organism is transferred from one host to another.

mode of ven•ti•la•tion (mōd ven′ti-lā′shŭn) A particular breathing pattern provided by a mechanical ventilator. The mode can be described by the variable controlled by the ventilator (e.g., volume control, pressure control, or dual control) and the breath sequence (e.g., CMV, IMV, or CSV). Pressure support can be described as pressure-controlled continuous spontaneous ventilation.

mod•i•fi•ca•tion (mod′i-fi-kā′shŭn) **1.** A nonhereditary change in an organism; e.g., one that is acquired from its own activity or environment. **2.** A chemical or structural alteration in a molecule.

mod•i•fied acid-fast stain (mod′i-fīd as′id-fast stān) An acid-fast staining procedure using highly dilute acid as a decolorizer, suitable for detection of coccidia, *Cryptosporidium, Cyclospora,* and *Isospora,* which bind function stains less firmly than mycobacteria.

mod•i•fied bar•i•um swal•low (mod′i-fīd bar′ē-ŭm swah′lō) Radiologic test to assess the structure and function of the oropharynx, pharynx, larynx, and upper esophagus before, during, and after the swallow.

mod•i•fied jaw thrust (mod′i-fīd jaw thrŭst) An airway opening maneuver, used during resuscitative efforts when there is suspicion of cervical injury. The head is maintained in neutral alignment while the jaw is displaced forward at the mandibular angle: the rescuer places the tips of the fingers behind the angle of the jaw and, without moving the patient's neck, thrusts the jaw upward/forward, moving the jaw away from the back of the patient's head.

mod•i•fied rad•i•cal mas•tec•to•my (mod′i-fīd rad′i-kăl mas-tek′tŏ-mē) Excision of the entire breast including the nipple, areola, and the overlying skin, as well as the lymphatic-bearing tissue in the axilla, with preservation of the pectoral muscles.

mod•i•fied rad•i•cal mas•toid•ec•to•my (mod′i-fīd rad′i-kăl mas′toy-dek′tŏ-mē) An operation for the management of cholesteatoma that lies lateral to the remnant of the tympanic membrane and middle-ear ossicles; involves exenteration of the remaining air cells of the mastoid process and removal of the posterior and superior walls of the external auditory canal to open the mastoid and attic of the middle ear to the outside and preserve hearing.

mod•i•fied tri•chrome stain (mod′i-fīd trī′krōm stān) A reformulation of the Gomori trichrome stain with a tenfold increase of chromotype 2R dye, adapted for detection of microsporidian spores.

mod•i•fi•er (mod′i-fī′ĕr) That which alters or limits.

mo•di•o•lus, pl. **mo•di•o•li** (mō-dī′ō-lŭs, -ō-lī) **1.** The central cone-shaped core of spongy bone about which the spiral canal of the cochlea turns. **2.** SYN modiolus labii. [L., the nave of a wheel]

mo•di•o•lus la•bi•i (mō-dī′ō-lŭs lā′bē-ī) A point near the corner of the mouth where several muscles of facial expression converge. SYN modiolus (2).

mod•u•la•tion (mod-yŭ-lā′shŭn) **1.** The functional and morphologic fluctuation of cells in response to changing environmental conditions. **2.** Systematic variation in a characteristic (e.g., frequency, amplitude) of a sustained oscillation to code additional information. **3.** A change in the kinetics of an enzyme or metabolic pathway. **4.** The regulation of the rate of translation of mRNA by a modulating codon. **5.** Change in parameters of electrotherapy (e.g., frequency, amplitude). [L. *modulor,* to measure off properly]

mod•u•la•tor (mod′yŭ-lā′tōr) That which regulates or adjusts.

mo•du•lus (mod′yū-lŭs) A coefficient expressing the magnitude of a physical property by a numerical value. [L. dim. of *modus,* a measure, quantity]

MODY Abbreviation for mature onset diabetes of youth.

mohel (moyl) Ordained Jew who performs circumcisions as prescribed by Jewish customs. [Hebrew]

Mohs che•mo•sur•ger•y (mōz kē′mō-sŭr′jĕr-ē) A technique for removal of skin tumors with a minimum of normal tissue, by prior necrosis with zinc chloride paste, mapping of the tumor site, and excision and microscopic examination of frozen section of thin horizontal layers of tissue, until all of the tumor is removed. The preliminary step of chemical necrosis may be omitted.

Mohs fresh tis•sue che•mo•sur•ger•y tech•nique (mōz fresh tish′ū kē′mō-sŭr′jĕr-ē tek-nēk′) Chemosurgery in which superficial cancers are excised after fixation in vivo.

moi•e•ty (moy′i-tē) **1.** Originally indicated half; now, less precisely, a portion of something. **2.** Functional group. [M.E. *moite,* a half]

moist gan•grene (moyst gang-grēn′) SYN wet gangrene.

moist rale (moyst rahl) A bubbling rale caused by air mixing with a fluid exudate in the bronchial tubes or a cavity.

Mo•ko•la vi•rus (mō-kō′lah vī′rŭs) A rabies-related virus of the genus Lyssavirus, which has caused fatal neurologic disease.

mol Abbreviation for mole (4).

mo•lal (mō′lăl) Denoting 1 mol of solute dissolved in 1000 g of solvent; such solutions provide a definite ratio of solute to solvent molecules. Cf. molar (4).

mo•lal•i•ty (mō-lal′i-tē) Moles of solute per kilogram of solvent; the molarity is equal to $m\rho/(1 + mM)$, where m is the molality, ρ is the density of the solution, and M is the molar mass of the solute. Cf. molarity.

mo•lar (mō′lăr) **1.** Denoting a grinding, abrading, or wearing away. [L. *molaris,* relating to a mill, millstone] **2.** SYN molar tooth. **3.** Massive; relating to a mass; not molecular. [L. *moles,* mass] **4.** Denoting a concentration of 1 gram-molecular weight (1 mol) of solute per liter of solution, the common unit of concentration in chemistry. Cf. molal. **5.** Denoting specific quantity, e.g., molar volume (volume of 1 mol).

mo•lar ab•sorp•tion co•ef•fi•cient (ε) (mō′lăr ab-sōrp′shŭn kō-ĕ-fish′ĕnt) Absorbance (of light) per unit path length (usually the centimeter) and per unit of concentration (moles per liter); a fundamental unit in spectrophotometry. SYN absorbancy index (2), absorptivity (2).

mo•lar•i•ty (M) (mō-lar′i-tē) Moles per liter of solution (mol/L). Cf. molality.

mo•lar tooth (mō′lăr tūth) A tooth having a somewhat quadrangular crown with four or five cusps on the grinding surface; the root is bifid in the lower jaw, but there are three conic roots in the upper jaw; there are six molars in each jaw, three on either side behind the premolars in the permanent dentition; in the deciduous dentition there are but four molars in each jaw, two on either side behind the canines. See this page. SYN dens molaris [TA], molar (2).

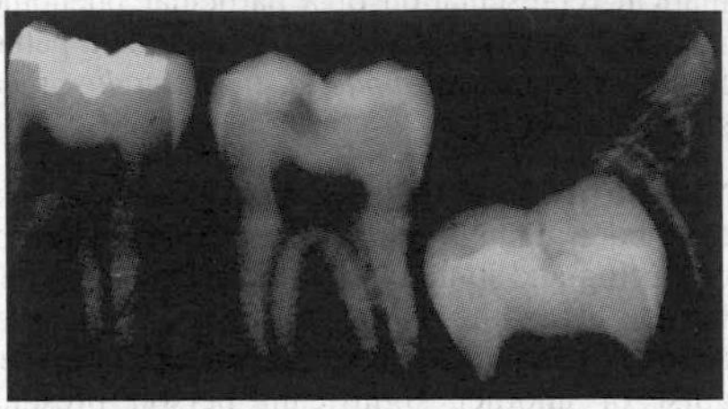

molar tooth: in this view of an unerupted third molar, the crown is formed but the roots are incomplete

mold (mōld) **1.** A filamentous fungus, generally a circular colony that may be cottony, wooly, or glabrous, but with filaments not organized into large fruiting bodies, such as mushrooms. **2.** A shaped receptacle into which wax is pressed or fluid plaster is poured in making a cast. **3.** To shape a mass of plastic material according to a definite pattern. **4.** To change in shape; denoting especially the adaptation of the fetal head to the pelvic canal. **5.** The term used to specify the shape of an artificial tooth (or teeth).

mold•ing (mōld′ing) The shaping of a baby's head to facilitate passage down the birth canal. The molding disappears after birth.

mole (mōl) **1.** SYN nevus (2). **2.** SYN nevus pigmentosus. [A.S. *māēl* (L. *macula*), a spot] **3.** An intrauterine mass formed by the degeneration of the partly developed products of conception. [L. *moles,* mass] **4. (mol)** In the SI, the unit of amount of substance, defined as that amount of a substance containing as many "elementary entities" as there are atoms in 0.0120 kg of carbon-12; elementary entities may be atoms, molecules, ions, or any describable entity or defined mixture of entities and must be specified when this term is used; in practical terms, the mole is 6.0221367 $\times 10^{23}$ "elementary entities." SEE ALSO Avogadro number.

mo•lec•u•lar (mō-lek′yū-lăr) Relating to molecules.

mo•lec•u•lar bi•ol•o•gy (mō-lek′yū-lăr bī-ol′ŏ-jē) Study of phenomena in terms of molecular interactions; it differs from biochemistry in that it emphasizes chemical interactions involved in the replication of DNA, its "transcription" into

RNA, and its "translation" into or expression in protein.

mo•lec•u•lar dis•ease (mō-lek′yū-lăr di-zēz′) A disease in which the manifestations are due to alterations in molecular structure and function.

mo•lec•u•lar epi•de•mi•ol•o•gy (mō-lek′yū-lăr ep′i-dē-mē-ol′ŏ-jē) The use in epidemiologic studies of techniques of molecular biology such as DNA typing.

mo•lec•u•lar move•ment (mō-lek′yū-lăr mūv′mĕnt) SYN brownian movement.

mo•lec•u•lar ro•ta•tion (mō-lek′yū-lăr rō-tā′shŭn) One-hundredth of the product of the specific rotation of an optically active compound and its molecular weight.

mo•lec•u•lar weight (mol wt, MW) (mō-lek′yū-lăr wāt) The sum of the atomic weights of all the atoms constituting a molecule; the mass of a molecule relative to the mass of a standard atom, now ^{12}C (taken as 12.000). Relative molecular mass (M_r) is the mass relative to the dalton and has no units. SEE ALSO atomic weight. SYN molecular weight ratio, relative molecular mass.

mo•lec•u•lar weight ra•ti•o (M_r) (mō-lek′yū-lăr wāt rā′shē-ō) SYN molecular weight.

mol•e•cule (mol′ĕ-kyūl) The smallest possible quantity of a di-, tri-, or polyatomic substance that retains the chemical properties of the substance. [Mod. L. *molecula,* dim. of L. *moles,* mass]

mo•li•men, pl. **mo•lim•i•na** (mō-lī′men, -lim′i-nă) An effort; laborious performance of a normal function. [L. an endeavor]

Mol•la•ret men•in•gi•tis (mō-lah-rā′ men′in-jī′tis) A recurrent aseptic meningitis; febrile illness accompanied by headaches, malaise, meningeal signs, and cerebrospinal fluid monocytes.

Moll glands (mol glandz) SYN ciliary glands.

mol•li•ti•es (mō-lish′ē-ēz) **1.** Characterized by a soft consistency. **2.** SYN malacia. [L. *mollis,* soft]

Mol•lusc•i•pox•vi•rus (mo-lusk′i-poks-vī′rŭs) A genus in the family Poxviridae; causes localized wartlike skin lesions.

mol•lus•cous (mo-lŭs′kŭs) Relating to or resembling molluscum.

mol•lus•cum (mo-lŭs′kŭm) A benign viral disease marked by the occurrence of soft rounded tumors of the skin. [L. *molluscus,* soft]

mol•lus•cum con•ta•gi•o•sum (mo-lŭs′kŭm kon-tā′jē-ō′sŭm) A contagious disease of the skin caused by intranuclear proliferation of a virus of the family Poxviridae and characterized by the appearance of small, pearly, umbilicated papular epidermal growths. In adults it typically occurs on or near the genitals and is sexually transmitted. See page B6.

Mo•lo•ney test (mŏ-lō′nē test) A test to detect a high degree of sensitivity to diphtheria toxoid; more than a minimal local reaction to toxoid given intradermally indicates that prophylactic toxoid should be administered in fractional doses at suitable intervals.

Mo•lo•ney vi•rus (mŏ-lō′nē vī′rŭs) A lymphoid leukemia retrovirus of mice, in the family Retroviridae, isolated originally during propagation of S 37 mouse sarcoma.

molt (mōlt) To cast off feathers, hair, or cuticle; to undergo ecdysis. [L. *muto,* to change]

mol wt (mōl) Abbreviation for molecular weight.

mo•lyb•den•ic, **mo•lyb•de•nous** (mō-lib′den-ik, mō-lib′den-ŭs) Relating to molybdenum.

mo•lyb•de•num (Mo) (mō-lib′dĕ-nŭm) A silvery white metallic element; atomic no. 42, atomic wt. 95.94; a bioelement found in a number of proteins (e.g., xanthine oxidase). SEE molybdenum target tube. [G. *molybdaina,* a piece of lead; a metal, prob. galena, fr. *molybdos,* lead]

mo•lyb•de•num tar•get tube (mō-lib′dĕ-nŭm tahr′gĕt tūb) An x-ray tube with an anode surface made of molybdenum instead of tungsten, used in mammography.

mo•men•tum (mō-men′tŭm) The tendency of an object in motion to continue in motion. [L., abridgment of *movimentum,* movement]

mo•nad (mō′nad) **1.** A univalent element or radical. **2.** A unicellular organism. **3.** In meiosis, the single chromosome derived from a tetrad after the first and second maturation divisions. [G. *monas,* the number one, unity]

monaesthetic [Br.] SYN monesthetic.

Mo•na•kow syn•drome (mō-nah′kof sin′drōm) Contralateral hemiplegia, hemianesthesia, and homonomous hemianopsia due to occlusion of the anterior choroidal artery.

mon•ar•thric (mon-ahr′thrik) SYN monarticular.

mon•ar•thri•tis (mon′ahr-thrī′tis) Arthritis of a single joint.

mon•ar•tic•u•lar (mon′ahr-tik′yū-lăr) Relating to a single joint. SYN monarthric.

mon•as•ter (mon-as′tĕr) The single star figure at the end of prophase in mitosis. [mono- + G. *astēr,* star]

mon•ath•e•to•sis (mon′ath-ĕ-tō′sis) Athetosis affecting one hand or foot.

mon•a•tom•ic (mon′ă-tom′ik) **1.** Relating to or containing a single atom. **2.** SYN monovalent (1).

mon•au•ral (mon-aw′răl) Pertaining to one ear. [mono- + L. *auris,* ear]

Mön·cke·berg ar·te·ri·o·scle·ro·sis (merng′kĕ-bĕrg ahr-tēr′ē-o-skle-rō′sis) Arterial sclerosis involving the peripheral arteries, especially of the legs of older people, with deposition of calcium in the medial coat (pipestem arteries) but with little or no encroachment on the lumen. SYN Mönckeberg calcification, Mönckeberg degeneration, Mönckeberg sclerosis.

Mön·cke·berg cal·ci·fi·ca·tion (merng′kĕ-bĕrg kal′si-fi-kā′shŭn) SYN Mönckeberg arteriosclerosis.

Mön·cke·berg de·gen·er·a·tion (merng′kĕ-bĕrg dĕ-jen′ĕr-ā′shŭn) SYN Mönckeberg arteriosclerosis.

Mön·cke·berg scle·ro·sis (merng′kĕ-bĕrg skler-ō′sis) SYN Mönckeberg arteriosclerosis.

Mon·day fe·ver (mŏn′dā fē′vĕr) Occupational hypersensitivity reaction with symptoms occurring (or recurring) at the beginning of the work week and diminishing as the week progresses and tolerance develops; most common when afflicted person exposed to cotton, dust, hemp, and flax.

Mon·de·green syn·drome (mon′dĕ-grēn′ sin′drōm) A seldom described form of auditory dysfunction and periphrasis common among youth in English-speaking countries.

Mon·di·ni dys·pla·si·a (mōn-dē′nē dis-plā′zē-ă) Congenital anomaly of osseus and membranous labyrinth characterized by aplastic cochlea, and deformity of the vestibule and semicircular canals with partial or complete loss of auditory and vestibular function; may be associated with spontaneous cerebrospinal fluid otorrhoea resulting in meningitis.

Mon·di·ni hear·ing im·pair·ment (mōn-dē′nē hēr′ing im-păr′mĕnt) The hearing impairment resulting from the structural aberration of Mondini dysplasia.

Mon·dor dis·ease (mōn′dōr di-zēz′) Thrombophlebitis of the thoracoepigastric vein of the breast and chest wall.

mon·es·thet·ic (mon-es-thet′ik) Relating to a single sense or sensation. SYN monaesthetic. [mono- + G. *aisthēsis,* sense perception]

Mon·ge dis·ease (mōn′hā di-zēz′) SYN chronic mountain sickness.

Mon·go·li·an (mon-gō′lē-ăn) Relating to a member of the Mongolian race.

mon·go·li·an spot (mon-gō′lē-ăn spot) Any of a number of dark-bluish or mulberry-colored rounded or oval spots on the skin in the sacral region due to the ectopic presence of scattered melanocytes in the dermis. These congenital lesions are frequent in black, Native American, and Asian children from 2–12 years of age after which time they gradually recede; they do not disappear on pressure and are sometimes mistaken for bruises from child abuse. SYN blue spot (2).

mo·nil·e·thrix (mō-nil′ĕ-thriks) An inherited trichodystrophy in which brittle hairs show a series of constrictions, usually without a medulla. SYN beaded hair, moniliform hair. [L. *monile,* necklace, + G. *thrix,* hair]

Mo·nil·i·a (mō-nil′ē-ă) Generic term for a group of fungi commonly known as fruit molds; the sexual state is *Neurospora.* A few closely related pathogenic organisms formerly classified in this genus are now properly termed *Candida.* [L. *monile,* necklace]

mo·nil·i·al (mō-nil′ē-ăl) Pertaining to the genus *Candida* (formerly grouped with the genus *Monilia*).

mon·i·li·a·sis (mō′ni-lī′ă-sis) SYN candidiasis.

mo·nil·i·form (mō-nil′i-fōrm) Shaped like a string of beads or beaded necklace. [L. *monile,* necklace, + *forma,* appearance]

mo·nil·i·form hair (mō-nil′i-fōrm hār) SYN monilethrix.

Mo·nil·i·for·mis (mō-nil′i-fōr′mis) A genus of thorny-headed worms. A few infections in humans have been reported. [L. *monile,* necklace, + *forma,* appearance]

i **mo·nil·i·id** (mō-nil′ē-id) Minute macular or papular lesions occurring as an allergic reaction to monilial infection.

mon·i·tor (mon′i-tŏr) **1.** A device that displays or records specified data for a given series of events, operations, or circumstances. **2.** To assess a function of the body on a close constant basis. [L., one who warns, fr. *moneo,* pp. *monitum,* to warn]

mon·i·tor·ing (mon′i-tŏr′ing) **1.** Performance and analysis of routine measurements aimed at detecting a change in the environment or health status of a population. **2.** Ongoing measurement of performance of a health service. **3.** Continuous oversight of implementation of an activity.

mon·i·tor u·nit (MU) (mon′i-tŏr yū′nit) In radiation therapy, output measurement of radiation exposure.

mon·key·pox (mŏng′kē-poks) A rare smallpox-like disease caused by the monkeypox virus transmitted by exposure to infected prairie dogs or giant rats of the Gambia. Transmission can also occur by contact with a human patient. The incubation period is 12 days and is characterized by rash and may include chills and sweats, headache, backache, lymphadenopathy, sore throat, cough, and shortness of breath. Small pox vaccine has been reported to reduce the risk of monkeypox among people previously vaccinated.

monks·hood (mŭngks′hud) SYN aconite.

mono-, mon- Combining forms indicating the

participation or involvement of a single element or part. Cf. uni-. [G. *monos,* single]

mon•o•a•me•li•a (mon-ō-ă-mē′lē-ă) Absence of one limb.

mon•o•am•ide (mon-ō-am′īd) A molecule containing one amide group.

mon•o•am•ine (mon′ō-ă-mēn′) A molecule containing one amine group.

mon•o•am•ine hy•poth•e•sis (mon′ō-ă-mēn′ hī-poth′ĕ-sis) The classical theory of the neurochemical basis of depression linking it to a deficiency of at least one of three monoamine neurotransmitters, norepinephrine, serotonin, or dopamine.

mon•o•am•ine ox•i•dase in•hib•i•tor (MAOI) (mon′ō-ă-mēn′ ok′si-dās in-hib′i-tŏr) Any of several antidepressants that inhibit enzymatic breakdown of monoamine neurotransmitters of the sympathetic/adrenergic system; not used as first-line therapy because of the risk of hypertensive crisis after consumption of foods or beverages containing pressor amines, including cheese, chocolate, beer, and wine.

mon•o•am•i•ner•gic (mon′ō-am-i-nĕr′jik) Referring to nerve cells or fibers that transmit nervous impulses by the medium of a catecholamine or indolamine. [monoamine + G. *ergon,* work]

mon•o•am•ni•ot•ic twins (mon′ō-am-nē-ot′ik twinz) Twins within a common amnion; such twins are monozygotic in origin and may be conjoined.

mon•o•ba•sic (mon′ō-bā′sik) Denoting an acid with only one replaceable hydrogen atom, or only one replaced hydrogen atom.

mon•o•blast (mon′ō-blast) An immature cell that develops into a monocyte. [mono- + G. *blastos,* germ]

mon•o•blas•tic leu•ke•mi•a (mon′ō-blast′ik lū-kē′mē-ă) SEE monocytic leukemia.

mon•o•cho•re•a (mon′ō-kō-rē′ă) Chorea affecting the head alone or only one extremity.

mon•o•cho•ri•on•ic (mon′ō-kōr-ē-on′ik) Relating to or having a single chorion; denoting monovular twins.

mon•o•cho•ri•on•ic di•am•ni•on•ic pla•cen•ta (mon′ō′kōr-ē-on′ik dī-am′nē-on′ik plă-sen′tă) SEE twin placenta.

mon•o•chro•mat•ic (mon′ō-krō-mat′ik) **1.** Having but one color. **2.** Indicating a light of a single wavelength. **3.** Relating to or characterized by monochromatism.

mon•o•chro•mat•ic ab•er•ra•tion (mon′ō-krō-mat′ik ab-ĕr-ā′shŭn) A defect in an optic image arising because of the nature of lenses; the main types are spheric, coma, curvature, and distortion aberration, and astigmatism of oblique pencils.

mon•o•chro•mat•ic ra•di•a•tion (mon′ō-krō-mat′ik rā′dē-ā′shŭn) Light rays or ionizing radiation of a very narrow band of wavelengths (ideally, of a single wavelength). Cf. characteristic radiation.

mon•o•chro•ma•tism (mon′ō-krō′mă-tizm) **1.** The state of having or exhibiting only one color. **2.** SYN achromatopsia. [mono- + G. *chrōma,* color]

mon•o•chro•mat•o•phil, mon•o•chro•mat•o•phile (mon′ō-krō-mat′ō-fil, -fīl) **1.** Taking only one stain. **2.** A cell or any histologic element staining with only one kind of dye. [mono- + G. *chrōma,* color, + *philos,* fond]

mon•o•clo•nal (mon′ō-klōn′ăl) IMMUNOCHEMISTRY pertaining to a protein from a single clone of cells, all molecules of which are the same.

mon•o•clo•nal an•ti•bod•y (mon′ō-klōn′ăl an′ti-bod-ē) An antibody produced by a clone or genetically homogeneous population of hybrid cells (i.e., hybridoma); hybrid cells are cloned to establish cell lines producing a specific antibody that is chemically and immunologically homogeneous; a mainstay of immunologic research and medical diagnosis. SEE ALSO cluster of differentiation.

mon•o•clo•nal gam•mop•athy of un•known sig•ni•fi•cance (MGUS) (mon′ō-klōn′ăl gam-mop′ă-thē ŭn′nōn sig-nif′i-kăns) A gammopathy diagnosed by electrophoresis of serum of asymptomatic old people who have no other evidence of plasma cell neoplasia; in 20% of cases, it evolves into plasma cell malignancy. SYN benign monoclonal gammopathy.

mon•o•clo•nal im•mu•no•glob•u•lin (mon′ō-klōn′ăl im′yū-nō-glob′yū-lin) A homogeneous immunoglobulin resulting from the proliferation of a single clone of plasma cells that; during electrophoresis of serum, appears as a narrow band or "spike"; it is characterized by heavy chains of a single class and subclass, and light chains of a single type. SYN paraprotein (2).

mon•o•crot•ic (mon′ō-krot′ik) Denoting a pulse the curve of which presents no notch or subsidiary wave in its descending line. [mono- + G. *krotos,* a beat]

mon•o•crot•ic pulse (mon′ō-krot′ik pŭls) SEE monocrotic, monocrotism.

mon•oc•ro•tism (mon-ok′rō-tizm) The state in which the pulse is monocrotic. [mono- + G. *krotos,* a beat]

mo•noc•u•lar (mon-ok′yū-lăr) Relating to, affecting, or visible by one eye only. [mono- + L. *oculus,* eye]

mo•noc•u•lar di•plo•pi•a (mon-ok′yū-lăr dip-lō′pē-ă) A double image or an extra ghost image produced in one eye.

mon•o•cyte (mon′ō-sīt) A relatively large mononuclear leukocyte (16–22 mcm in diameter); monocytes normally constitute 3–7% of the leukocytes of the circulating blood; normally found in lymph nodes, spleen, bone marrow, and loose connective tissue. In stained smears, monocytes have abundant pale blue or blue-gray cytoplasm that contains numerous fine red-blue granules and vacuoles; the nucleus is usually indented, or slightly folded. [mono- + G. *kytos,* cell]

mon•o•cyte che•mo•a•ttrac•tant pro•tein (mon′ō-sīt kē′mō-ă-trak′tănt prō′tēn) A cytokine involved in monocyte migration.

mon•o•cyte-de•rived neu•tro•phil che•mo•tac•tic fac•tor (mon′ō-sīt-dĕ-rīvd′ nū′trō-fil kē′mō-tak′tik fak′tŏr) SYN interleukin-8.

mon•o•cyt•ic leu•ke•mi•a (mon′ō-sit′ĭk lū-kē′mē-ă) A form of leukemia characterized by large numbers of cells that can be definitely identified as monocytes, in addition to larger, apparently related cells formed from the uncontrolled proliferation of the reticuloendothelial tissue. The disease runs an acute or subacute course in older people, and is characterized by swelling of gums, oral ulceration, bleeding in skin or mucous membranes, secondary infection, and splenomegaly.

mon•o•cy•toid cell (mon′ō-sī′toyd sel) A cell that resembles a monocyte but is nonphagocytic.

mon•o•cy•to•pe•ni•a (mon′ō-sī-tō-pē′nē-ă) A decrease in the number of monocytes in the circulating blood. [mono- + G. *kytos,* cell, + *penia,* poverty]

mon•o•cy•to•sis (mon′ō-sī-tō′sis) An abnormal increase in the number of monocytes in the circulating blood.

mon•o•dac•ty•ly, mon•o•dac•tyl•ism (mon′ō-dak′ti-lē, -lizm) The presence of a single finger on the hand, or a single toe on the foot. [mono- + G. *daktylos,* digit]

mon•o•fix•a•tion syn•drome (mon′ō-fik-sā′shŭn sin′drōm) A small-angle strabismus (fewer than 10 prism diopters) with central fixation by the preferred eye, central suppression of the deviating eye, and binocular fusion of peripheral vision

mon•o•ga•met•ic (mon′ō-gă-met′ik) SYN homogametic.

mo•nog•a•my (mon-og′ă-mē) The marriage or mating system in which each partner has but one mate. [mono- + G. *gamos,* marriage]

mon•o•gen•e•sis (mon′ō-jen′ĕ-sis) **1.** The production of similar organisms in each generation. **2.** The production of young by one parent only, as in nonsexual generation and parthenogenesis. **3.** The process of parasitizing a single host, in which the entire life cycle of the parasite is passed. [mono- + G. *genesis,* origin, production]

mon•o•ge•net•ic (mon′ō-jĕ-net′ik) Relating to monogenesis. SYN monoxenous.

mon•o•gen•ic (mon′ō-jen′ik) Relating to a hereditary disease or syndrome, or to an inherited characteristic, controlled by alleles at a single genetic locus.

mo•nog•e•nous (mŏ-noj′ĕ-nŭs) Asexually produced, as by fission, gemmation, or sporulation.

mon•o•hy•dric al•co•hol (mon′ō-hī′drik al′kŏ-hol) An alcohol containing one OH group.

mon•o•lay•ers (mon′ō-lā′ĕrz) **1.** Films, one molecule thick, formed on water by certain substances (e.g., proteins and fatty acids) characterized by molecules containing some atom groupings that are soluble in water and other atom groupings that are insoluble in water. **2.** A confluent sheet of cells, one cell deep, growing on a surface in a cell culture.

mon•o•loc•u•lar (mon′ō-lok′yū-lăr) Having one cavity or chamber. SYN unicameral, unicamerate. [mono- + L. *loculus,* a small place]

mon•o•ma•ni•a (mon′ō-mā′nē-ă) An obsession or abnormal enthusiasm for a single idea or subject; a psychosis marked by limitation of symptoms to a certain group, as the delusion in paranoia. [mono- + G. *mania,* frenzy]

mon•o•mel•ic (mon′ō-mel′ik) Relating to one limb. [mono- + G. *melos,* limb]

mon•o•mer (mon′ō-mĕr) **1.** The molecular unit that, by repetition, constitutes a large structure or polymer. **2.** The protein structural unit of a virion capsid. SEE virion. **3.** The protein subunit of a protein composed of several loosely associated such units, usually noncovalently bound together. [mono- + -mer]

mon•o•mer•ic (mon′ō-mer′ik) **1.** Consisting of a single component. **2.** GENETICS relating to a hereditary disease or characteristic controlled by genes at a single locus. **3.** Consisting of monomers. [mono- + G. *meros,* part]

mon•o•mor•phic (mon′ō-mōr′fik) Of one shape; unchangeable in shape. [mono- + G. *morphē,* shape]

mon•o•my•o•ple•gi•a (mon′ō-mī-ō-plē′jē-ă) Paralysis limited to one muscle. [mono- + G. *mys,* muscle, + *plēgē,* a stroke]

mon•o•my•o•si•tis (mon′ō-mī-ō-sī′tis) Inflammation of a single muscle.

mon•o•neu•ral, mon•o•neu•ric (mon′ō-nūr′ăl, -ik) **1.** Having only one neuron. **2.** Supplied by a single nerve.

mon•o•neu•ral•gi•a (mon′ō-nūr-al′jă) Pain along the course of one nerve.

mon•o•neu•ri•tis (mon′ō-nūr-ī′tis) Inflammation of a single nerve.

mon•o•neu•rop•a•thy (mon′ō-nūr-op′ă-thē) Disorder involving a single nerve.

mon•o•nu•cle•ar (mon′ō-nū′klē-ăr) Having only one nucleus; used especially in reference to blood cells.

mon•o•nu•cle•ar phag•o•cyte sys•tem (mon′ō-nū′klē-ăr fag′ō-sīt sis′tĕm) A widely distributed family of both free and fixed macrophages derived from bone marrow precursor cells by way of monocytes; their substantial phagocytic activity is mediated by immunoglobulin and the serum complement system. In both connective and lymphoid tissue, they may occur as free and fixed macrophages; in the sinusoids of the liver, as Kupffer cells; in the lung, as alveolar macrophages; and in the nervous system, as microglia.

mon•o•nu•cle•o•sis (mon′ō-nū-klē-ō′sis) Presence of abnormally large numbers of mononuclear leukocytes in the circulating blood, especially with reference to forms that are not normal.

mon•o•nu•cle•o•tide (mon′ō-nū′klē-ō-tīd) SYN nucleotide.

mon•o•ox•y•ge•na•ses (mon′ō-ok′si-jĕ-nās-ez) Oxidoreductases that induce the incorporation of one atom of oxygen from O_2 into the substance being oxidized.

monoparaesthesia [Br.] SYN monoparesthesia.

mon•o•pa•re•sis (mon′o-pă-rē′sis) Paresis affecting a single extremity or part of an extremity.

mon•o•par•es•the•si•a (mon′ō-par-es-thē′zē-ă) Paresthesia affecting a single region only. SYN monoparaesthesia.

mon•o•path•ic (mon′ō-path′ik) Relating to a monopathy.

mo•nop•a•thy (mon-op′ă-thē) **1.** A single uncomplicated disease. **2.** A local disease affecting only one organ or part. [mono- + G. *pathos,* suffering]

mon•o•pha•si•a (mon′ō-fā′zē-ă) Inability to speak other than a single word or sentence. [mono- + G. *phasis,* speech]

mon•o•pha•sic (mon′ō-fāz′ik) **1.** Marked by monophasia. **2.** Occurring in or characterized by only one phase or stage. **3.** Fluctuating from the baseline in one direction only.

mon•oph•thal•mos (mon′of-thal′mŏs) Failure of outgrowth of a primary optic vesicle with absence of ocular tissues; the remaining eye is often maldeveloped. [mono- + G. *ophthalmos,* eye]

mon•o•phy•let•ic (mon′ō-fī-let′ik) **1.** Having a single cell type of origin; derived from one line of descent, in contrast to polyphyletic. **2.** HEMATOLOGY relating to monophyletism. [mono- + G. *phylē,* tribe]

mon•o•ple•gi•a (mon′ō-plē′jē-ă) Paralysis of one limb. [mono- + G. *plēgē,* a stroke]

mon•o•po•di•a (mon′ō-pō′dē-ă) Malformation in which sirenomelia is accompanied by fusion of the feet into a single structure. [mono- + G. *pous,* foot]

mon•o•po•lar cau•ter•y (mon′ō-pō′lăr kaw′tĕr-ē) Electrocautery by high frequency electrical current passed from a single electrode, where the cauterization occurs, the patient's body serving as a ground.

mon•or•chid•ic, mon•or•chid (mon′ōr-kid′ik, mon-ōr′kid) **1.** Having only one testis. **2.** Having apparently only one testis, the other being absent or undescended.

mon•or•chism (mon′ōr-kizm) A condition in which only one testis is apparent, the other being absent or undescended. [mono- + G. *orchis,* testis]

mon•o•sac•cha•ride (mon′ō-sak′ă-rīd) A carbohydrate that cannot form any simpler sugar by simple hydrolysis; e.g., pentoses, hexoses.

mon•o•so•di•um glu•ta•mate (MSG) (mon′ō-sō′dē-ŭm glū′tă-māt) The monosodium salt of the naturally occurring L form of glutamic acid; used as a flavor enhancer that is a cause or contributing factor to colloquially named "Chinese restaurant" syndrome; also used intravenously as an adjunct in treatment of encephalopathies associated with hepatic disease.

mon•o•some (mon′ō-sōm) **1.** Obsolete term for ribosome. **2.** A structure consisting of a single ribosome bound to a molecule of mRNA. [mono- + chromosome]

mon•o•so•mi•a (mon′ō-sō′mē-ă) In conjoined twins, a condition in which the trunks are completely merged although the heads remain separate. SEE conjoined twins. [mono- + G. *sōma,* body]

mon•o•so•mic (mon′ō-sō′mik) Relating to monosomy.

mon•o•so•my (mon′ō-sō-mē) Absence of one chromosome of a pair of homologous chromosomes. [see monosome]

mon•o•spasm (mon′ō-spazm) Spasm affecting only one muscle or group of muscles, or a single extremity.

mon•o•stot•ic (mon′os-tot′ik) Involving only one bone. [mono- + G. *osteon,* bone]

mon•o•stra•tal (mon′ō-strā′tăl) Composed of a single layer. [mono- + L. *stratum,* layer]

mon•o•symp•to•mat•ic (mon′ō-simp-tō-mat′

ik) Denoting a disease or morbid condition manifested by only one marked symptom.

mon•o•sy•nap•tic (mon′ō-si-nap′tik) Referring to direct neural connections not involving an intermediary neuron.

mon•o•ther•mi•a (mon′ō-thĕr′mē-ă) Evenness of bodily temperature; absence of an evening rise in body temperature. [mono- + G. *thermē,* heat]

mo•not•ri•chous (mŏ-not′ri-kŭs) Denoting a microorganism possessing a single flagellum or cilium.

mon•o•un•sat•ur•at•ed fat (mon′ō-ŭn-sach′ŭr-ā-tĕd fat) A type of unsaturated fat that may help to reduce blood cholesterol levels.

mon•o•va•lence, **mon•o•va•len•cy** (mon′ō-vā′lĕns, mon′ō-vā′lĕn-sē) A combining power (valence) equal to that of a hydrogen atom. SYN univalence, univalency.

mon•o•va•lent (mon′ō-vā′lĕnt) **1.** Having the combining power (valence) of a hydrogen atom. SYN monatomic (2), univalent. **2.** Pertaining to a monovalent (specific) antiserum to a single antigen or organism.

mon•o•xe•nic cul•ture (mon′ō-zē′nik kŭl′chŭr) Culture containing a single known species.

mon•ox•e•nous (mon-oks′ĕ-nŭs) SYN monogenetic. [mono- + G. *xenos,* stranger]

mon•ox•ide (mon-ok′sīd) Any oxide having only one atom of oxygen (e.g., CO).

mon•o•zy•got•ic (MZ), **mon•o•zy•gous** (mon′ō-zī-got′ik, -zī′gŭs) SYN unigerminal. SEE monozygotic twins. [mono- + G. *zygōtos,* yoked]

mon•o•zy•got•ic twins (mon′ō-zī-got′ik twinz) Twins resulting from a single zygote that at an early stage of development becomes separated into independently growing cell aggregations giving rise to two individuals of the same sex and identical genetic constitution. SYN enzygotic twins, identical twins.

Mon•ro doc•trine (mŏn-rō′ dok′trin) A concept that states that the cranial cavity is a closed rigid box and that therefore a change in the quantity of intracranial blood can occur only through the displacement of or replacement by cerebrospinal fluid.

Mon•ro for•a•men (mŏn-rō′ fōr-ā′mĕn) SYN interventricular foramen.

mons, gen. **mon•tis**, pl. **mon•tes** (monz, mon′tis, mon′tēz) An anatomical prominence or slight elevation above the general level of the surface. [L. a mountain]

mons pu•bis (monz pyū′bis) The prominence caused by a pad of fatty tissue over the symphysis pubis in the female.

mons ve•ne•ris (monz vĕ-ner′is) SEE mons pubis.

Mon•teg•gi•a frac•ture (mon-tej′jē-ă frak′shŭr) Fracture of the proximal ulna with dislocation of the head of the radius. See page B25.

Mon•te•vi•de•o u•nit (mon′tĕ-vi-dā′ō yū′nit) A unit of uterine contraction intensity in labor, defined as the peak pressure achieved by the contraction minus the baseline tone. [fr. Montevideo, Argentina, where developed]

Mon•te•zu•ma's re•venge (mon′tĕ-zū′măz rē-venj′) A colloquial term for traveler's diarrhea contracted in Mexico. The most common causative organisms are enterotoxigenic *Escherichia coli*, *Shigella*, and *Campylobacter jejuni.* SYN turista.

Mont•gom•er•y fol•li•cles (mont-gŭm′ĕr-ē fol′i-kĕlz) SYN areolar glands.

Mont•gom•er•y straps (mont-gŭm′ĕr-ē straps) SYN Montgomery tapes.

Mont•gom•er•y tapes (mont-gŭm′ĕr-ē tāps) Adhesive straps (tape) affixed to the skin arranged opposite to each other so that gauze straps can be placed between holes of each end of the middle of the paired tapes so as to provide a method of securing a bandage and subsequently changing it without having to replace the tape each time. Most often used for abdominal incisions, requiring frequent dressing changes. SYN Montgomery straps.

Mont•gom•er•y tu•ber•cles (mont-gŭm′ĕr-ē tū′bĕr-kĕlz) Elevated reddened areolar glands, usually associated with pregnancy.

mon•tic•u•lus, pl. **mon•tic•u•li** (mon-tik′ū-lŭs, -lī) **1.** Any slight rounded projection above a surface. **2.** The central portion of the superior vermis forming a projection on the surface of the cerebellum; its anterior and most prominent portion is called the culmen, its posterior sloping portion, the declive. [L. dim. of *mons,* mountain]

mood (mūd) The pervasive feeling, tone, and internal emotional state that, when impaired, can markedly influence virtually all aspects of a person's behavior or perception of external events.

mood-con•gru•ent hal•lu•ci•na•tion (mūd-kon-grū′ent hă-lū′si-nā′shŭn) Hallucination in which the content is mood appropriate.

mood-in•con•gru•ent hal•lu•ci•na•tion (mūd-in-kon-grū′ent hă-lū′si-nā′shŭn) Hallucination that is not consistent with external stimuli; content is not consistent with either manic or depressed mood.

mood sta•bil•i•zing a•gent (mūd stā′bil-ī-zing ā′jĕnt) A functional category of drugs used to normalize mood, particularly by damping mood swings (e.g., lithium and some anticonvulsants such as carbamazepine and valproic acid).

mood swing (mūd swing) Oscillation of a person's emotional feeling between euphoria and depression.

moon face (mūn fās) The round, usually red face, with large jowls, seen in Cushing disease or in exogenous hyperadrenocorticalism.

Moon mo•lars (mūn mōl'ărz) Small dome-shaped first molar teeth occurring in congenital syphilis.

Moore light•ning streaks (mūr līt'ning strēks) Photopsia manifested by vertical flashes of light, seen usually on the temporal side of the affected eye, caused by the involutional shrinkage of vitreous humor.

Moore meth•od (mūr meth'ŏd) Treatment of aneurysm by the introduction of silver or zinc wire into the sac to induce fibrin deposition.

Moo•ren ul•cer (mō'rĕn ŭl'sĕr) Chronic inflammation of the peripheral cornea that slowly progresses centrally with corneal thinning and sometimes perforation.

MOPP (mop) Acronym for mission-oriented protective posture.

mor•al (mōr'ăl) **1.** Pertaining to the rightnss or wrongness of an act. **2.** Ethical; in accord with accepted rules of what is right. **3.** Teaching or conveying a moral (i.e., a moral lession).

Mor•ax•el•la (mōr'ak-sel'ă) A genus of obligately aerobic nonmotile bacteria containing gram-negative coccoids or short rods that usually occur in pairs. They are parasitic on the mucous membranes of man and other mammals. [V *Morax*]

mor•bid (mōr'bid) **1.** Diseased or pathologic. **2.** PSYCHOLOGY abnormal or deviant. [L. *morbidus,* ill, fr. *morbus,* disease]

mor•bid•i•ty (mōr-bid'i-tē) **1.** A diseased state. **2.** The ratio of sick to well people in a community. SEE ALSO morbidity rate. **3.** The frequency of the appearance of complications following a surgical procedure or other treatment.

mor•bid•i•ty rate (mōr-bid'i-tē rāt) The proportion of patients with a particular disease during a given year per given unit of population.

mor•bid o•be•si•ty (mōr'bid ō-bē'si-tē) Being sufficiently overweight so as to prevent normal activity or physiologic function or to cause the onset of a pathologic condition.

mor•bif•ic (mōr-bif'ik) SYN pathogenic. [L. *morbus,* disease, + *facio,* to make]

mor•bil•li (mōr-bil'ī) SYN measles (1). [Mediev. L. *morbillus,* dim. of L. *morbus,* disease]

mor•bil•li•form (mōr-bil'i-fōrm) Resembling measles (1). [see morbilli]

Mor•bil•li•vi•rus (mōr-bil'i-vī'rŭs) A genus in the family Paramyxoviridae, including measles, canine distemper, and bovine rinderpest viruses.

mor•bus (mōr'bŭs) SYN disease (1). [L. disease]

mor•cel•lat•ed neph•rec•tomy (mōr'se-lā'lĕd ne-frek'tŏ-mē) Removal of a kidney in pieces.

mor•cel•la•tion (mōr'sĕ-lā'shŭn) Division into and removal of small pieces, as of a tumor. [Fr. *morceler,* to subdivide]

mor•cel•la•tion op•er•a•tion (mōr'sĕ-lā'shŭn op-ĕr-ā'shŭn) Vaginal hysterectomy in which the uterus is removed in multiple pieces after being split or partitioned.

mor•dant (mōr'dănt) **1.** A substance capable of combining with a dye and the material to be dyed, thereby increasing the affinity or binding of the dye. **2.** To treat with a mordant. [L. *mordeo,* to bite]

Mo•rel ear (mŏ-rel' ēr) A large, misshapen, outstanding auricle, with obliterated grooves and thinned edges.

mor•gag•ni•an cyst (mōr-gahn'yē-ăn sist) SYN vesicular appendage of epoophoron.

Mor•ga•gni cat•a•ract (mōr-gahn'yē kat'ăr-akt) A hypermature cataract in which the nucleus gravitates within the capsule.

Mor•ga•gni col•umns (mōr-gahn'yē kol'ŭmz) SYN anal columns.

Mor•ga•gni dis•ease (mōr-gahn'yē di-zēz') SYN Adams-Stokes syndrome.

Mor•ga•gni for•a•men her•ni•a (mōr-gahn'yē fōr-ā'mĕn hĕr'nē-ă) A congenital anterior, retrosternal hernia of abdominal contents, most often only omentum but occasionally stomach, usually through the right retrosternal Morgagni foramen, through which the internal mammary artery passes to become the superior epigastric artery; often asymptomatic. SYN parasternal hernia.

Mor•ga•gni glands (mōr-gahn'yē glandz) Mucus-secreting glands lining the urethral lumen in males. SYN Littré glands.

Mor•ga•gni glob•ules (mōr-gahn'yē glob'yūlz) Vesicles beneath the capsule and between lens fibers in early cataract.

Mor•ga•gni pro•lapse (mōr-gahn'yē prō'laps) Chronic inflammation of laryngeal ventricle.

Mor•ga•gni ret•i•nac•u•lum (mōr-gahn'yē ret'i-nak'yū-lŭm) SYN frenulum of ileal orifice.

Mor•ga•gni si•nus (mōr-gahn'yē sī'nŭs) **1.** SYN anal sinuses (1). **2.** SYN prostatic utricle. **3.** SYN laryngeal ventricle.

Mor•ga•gni syn•drome (mōr-gahn'yē sin'drōm) Hyperostosis frontalis interna in elderly women, with obesity and neuropsychiatric disorders of uncertain cause; at least sometimes familial. SYN metabolic craniopathy.

mor•gan (mōr′găn) The standard unit of genetic distance on the genetic map: the distance between two loci such that on average one crossing over will occur per meiosis; for working purposes, the centimorgan (0.01 M) is used.

Mor•gan•el•la (mōr′gan-el′-ă) A genus of gram-negative, facultatively anaerobic, chemoorganotrophic, straight rods that are motile by peritrichous flagella. Found in feces of human beings, other animals, and reptiles. Can cause opportunistic infections of the blood, respiratory tract, wounds, and urinary tract.

Mor•gan•el•la mor•gan•i•i (mōr′gan-el′ă mōr-gan′ē-ī) Type (and only) species of the genus *Morganella*.

Mor•gan lens (mōr′găn lenz) Contact lens-like device for ocular irrigation.

morgue (mōrg) **1.** A building where unidentified dead are kept pending identification before burial. **2.** A building or room in a hospital or other facility where the dead are kept pending autopsy, burial, or cremation; often includes a laboratory to perform autopsies. SYN mortuary (2). [Fr.]

mo•ri•a (mōr′ē-ă) **1.** Rarely used term denoting foolishness or dullness of comprehension. **2.** Rarely used term for a mental state marked by frivolity, joviality, an inveterate tendency to jest, and inability to take anything seriously.

mor•i•bund (mōr′i-bŭnd) Dying; at the point of death. [L. *moribundus*, dying, fr. *morior*, to die]

Mor•mon tea (mōr′mŏn tē) SYN ephedra.

Mör•ner test (mĕr′ner test) **1.** For cysteine, which gives a brilliant purple color with sodium nitroprusside. **2.** For tyrosine, which gives a green color on boiling with sulfuric acid containing formaldehyde.

morn•ing af•ter pill (mōr′ning af′tĕr pil) An oral medication, consisting of two pills taken 12 hours apart that, when taken by a woman within 2–3 days after intercourse, reduces the probability that she will become pregnant. SYN emergency contraceptive, emergency hormonal contraception, postcoital contraception.

morn•ing sick•ness (mōr′ning sik′nĕs) The nausea and vomiting of early pregnancy. SYN nausea gravidarum.

Mo•ro re•flex (mō′rō rē′fleks) Response of infants at birth and for the first three months of life to acoustic stimuli characterized by extension and abduction of arms, hands, and fingers.

mor•phe•a (mōr-fē′ă) Cutaneous lesion(s) characterized by indurated, slightly depressed plaques of thickened dermal fibrous tissue, of a whitish or yellowish white color surrounded by a pinkish or purplish halo. SYN localized scleroderma, morphoea. [G. *morphē*, form, figure]

♻ **-morphia**, **-morphy** Suffix meaning "a condition or form." [G. *morphē*]

mor•phine (mōr′fēn) The major phenanthrene alkaloid of opium, which contains 9–14% of anhydrous morphine. It produces a combination of depression and excitation in the central nervous system and some peripheral tissues; predominance of either central stimulation or depression depends on the species and dose; repeated administration leads to the development of tolerance, physical dependence, and (in instances of abuse) psychic dependence. Used as an analgesic, sedative, and anxiolytic. Classified as a U.S. Schedule II controlled medication. [L. *Morpheus,* god of dreams or of sleep]

mor•phine sul•fate (MS) (mōr′fēn sŭl′fāt) Agent used for formulation of tablets as well as solutions for parenteral, epidural, or intrathecal injection to relieve pain.

♻ **morpho-**, **morph-** Combining forms indicating form, shape, structure. [G. *morphē*]

morphoea [Br.] SYN morphea.

mor•pho•gen•e•sis (mōr′fō-jen′ĕ-sis) **1.** Differentiation of cells and tissues in the early embryo that establishes the form and structure of the various organs and parts of the body. **2.** The ability of a molecule or group of molecules (particularly macromolecules) to assume a certain shape. [morpho- + G. *genesis,* production]

mor•pho•ge•net•ic (mōr′fō-jĕ-net′ik) Relating to morphogenesis.

mor•pho•ge•net•ic move•ment (mōr′fō-jĕ-net′ik mūv′mĕnt) The streaming of cells in the early embryo to form tissues or organs.

mor•pho•log•ic (mōr′fō-loj′ik) Relating to morphology.

mor•phol•o•gy (mōr-fol′ŏ-jē) The science concerned with the configuration or the structure of animals and plants. [morpho- + G. *logos,* study]

mor•pho•met•ric (mōr′fō-met′rik) Pertaining to morphometry.

mor•phom•e•try (mōr-fom′ĕ-trē) The measurement of the form of organisms or their parts. [morpho- + G. *metron,* measure]

mor•pho•sis (mōr-fō′sis) Mode of development of a part. [G. formation, act of forming]

mors, gen. **mor•tis** (mōrz, mōr′tis) SYN death. [L.]

mor•tal (mōr′tăl) **1.** Pertaining to or causing death. **2.** Destined to die. [L. *mortalis,* fr. *mors,* death]

mor•tal•i•ty (mōr-tal′i-tē) **1.** The state of being mortal. **2.** SYN death rate. **3.** A fatal outcome. [L. *mortalitas,* fr. *mors* (*mort-*), death]

mor•tal•i•ty rate (mōr-tal′i-tē rāt) SYN death rate.

mor·tar (mōr′tăr) A vessel with a rounded interior in which crude drugs and other substances are crushed or bruised by means of a pestle. [L. *mortarium*]

mor·ti·fi·ca·tion (mōr′ti-fi-kā′shŭn) SYN gangrene (1). [L. *mors* (*mort-*), death, + *facio,* to make]

mor·ti·fied (mōr′ti-fīd) SYN gangrenous.

mor·tise joint (mōr′tis joynt) SYN ankle joint.

Mor·ton neu·ral·gi·a (mōr′tŏn nūr-al′jē-ă) Neuralgia of an interdigital nerve, usually the anastomotic branch between the medial and lateral plantar nerves, resulting from compression of the nerve by the metatarsophalangeal joint.

Mor·ton neu·ro·ma (mōr′tŏn nūr-ō′mă) Metatarsal pain caused by compression of sensory nerves by the metatarsal heads, sometimes with neuroma formation.

Mor·ton syn·drome (mōr′tŏn sin′drōm) Congenital shortening of the first metatarsal causing metatarsalgia.

Mor·ton toe (mōr′tŏn tō) Anatomic anomaly wherein second toe is longer than the great toe.

mor·tu·a·ry (mōr′chū-ar-ē) **1.** Relating to death or to burial. **2.** SYN morgue. [L. *mortuus,* dead, part. adj. fr. *morior,* pp. *mortuus,* to die]

mor·u·la (mōr′yū-lă) The solid mass of blastomeres resulting from the early cleavage divisions of the zygote. See page B1. [Mod. L. dim. of L. *morus,* mulberry]

mor·u·la·tion (mōr-yū-lā′shŭn) Formation of the morula.

Mor·van cho·re·a (mōr-vah[n]′ kōr-ē′ă) SYN myokymia.

Mor·van dis·ease (mōr-vah[n]′ di-zēz′) SYN syringomyelia.

mo·sa·ic (mō-zā′ik) **1.** Inlaid; resembling inlaid work. **2.** The juxtaposition in an organism of genetically different tissues; it may occur normally (as in lyonization, *q.v.*), or pathologically, as an occasional phenomenon. [Mod. L. *mosaicus, musaicus,* pertaining to the Muses, artistic]

mo·sa·ic in·her·i·tance (mō-zā′ik in-her′i-tăns) Inheritance in which the paternal influence is dominant in one group of cells and the maternal in another. Cf. lyonization.

mo·sa·i·cism (mō-zā′i-sizm) Condition of being mosaic (2).

mo·sa·ic pat·tern (mō-zā′ik pat′ĕrn) On high-resolution CT scans of the lungs, a pattern of brighter and darker regions corresponding to differences in perfusion or aeration; found in some cases of chronic thromboembolism or of bronchiolitis obliterans. Cf. oligemia.

mo·sa·ic wart (mō-zā′ik wōrt) Plantar growth of numerous closely aggregated warts forming a mosaic appearance, frequently caused by human papilloma virus type 2.

Mos·ler sign (mōz′lĕr sīn) Tenderness over the sternum in a patient with acute myeloblastic anemia.

mos·qui·to, pl. **mos·qui·toes** (mŏs-kē′tō, -tōz) A blood-sucking dipterous insect of the family Culicidae. *Aedes*, *Anopheles*, *Culex*, *Mansonia*, and *Stegomyia* are genera containing most species involved in the transmission of protozoan and other disease-producing parasites. [Sp. dim. of *mosca,* fly, fr. L. *musca,* a fly]

Mos·so er·go·graph (mos′ō ĕr′gō-graf) An instrument consisting of pulleys, weights, and a recording lever, which is used to obtain a graphic record of flexion of a finger, hand, or arm.

Mos·so sphyg·mo·ma·nom·e·ter (mos′ō sfig′mō-mă-nom′e-tĕr) An apparatus for measuring the blood pressure in the digital arteries.

Moss tube (maws tūb) **1.** A triple-lumen, nasogastric, feeding-decompression tube that uses a gastric balloon to occlude the cardioesophageal junction, with simultaneous esophageal aspiration and intragastric feeding. **2.** A double-lumen, gastric lavage tube that provides continuous delivery of saline through a small bore, with simultaneous aspiration of fluid and some particles through a large bore.

Mo·tais op·er·a·tion (mō-tā′ op-ĕr-ā′shŭn) Transplantation of the middle third of the tendon of the superior rectus muscle of the eyeball into the upper lid, between the tarsus and skin, to supplement the action of the levator muscle in ptosis.

mote (mōt) A small particle; a speck. [A.S. *mot*]

moth·er (mŏth′ĕr) **1.** The female parent. **2.** Any cell or other structure from which other similar bodies are formed. [A.S. *mōdor*]

moth·er cell (mŏth′ĕr sel) A cell that, by division, gives rise to two or more daughter cells. SYN metrocyte.

moth·er cyst (mŏth′ĕr sist) A hydatid cyst from the inner, or germinal, layer, from which secondary cysts containing scoleces (daughter cysts) are developed; occurs most frequently in the liver, but may be found in other organs and tissue. SYN parent cyst.

moth·er yaw (mŏth′ĕr yaw) A large granulomatous lesion, considered to be the initial lesion in yaws, most commonly present on the hand, leg, or foot. SYN buba madre, frambesioma.

mo·tile (mō′til) **1.** Having the power of spontaneous movement. **2.** Denoting the type of mental imagery in which one learns and recalls most readily that which has been felt. Cf. audile. **3.** A person having such mental imagery.

mo•til•i•ty (mō-til′i-tē) The power of spontaneous movement.

mo•tion seg•ment (mō′shŭn seg′mĕnt) A functional unit made up of two adjacent articulating surfaces and the connecting tissues binding them together.

mo•tion sick•ness (mō′shŭn sik′nĕs) The syndrome of pallor, nausea, weakness, and malaise, which may progress to vomiting and incapacitation, caused by stimulation of the semicircular canals during travel or motion as on a boat, airplane, train, car, swing, or rotating amusement ride. SYN kinesia.

mo•ti•va•tion (mō-ti-vā′shŭn) Psychological force that moves a person to act to meet a need or achieve a goal. SEE ALSO motive.

mo•tive (mō′tiv) **1.** An acquired predisposition, need, or specific state of tension within a person that arouses, maintains, and directs behavior toward a goal. SYN learned drive. **2.** The reason attributed to or given by an individual for a behavioral act. Cf. instinct. [L. *moveo,* to move, to set in motion]

mo•to•fa•cient (mō′tō-fā′shĕnt) Causing motion; denoting the second phase of muscular activity in which actual movement is produced. [L. *motus,* motion, + *facio,* to make]

mo•to•neu•ron (mō′tō-nūr′on) SYN motor neuron.

motoneurone [Br.] SYN motor neuron.

mo•tor (mō′tŏr) **1.** ANATOMY, PHYSIOLOGY denoting those neural structures that, by the impulses generated and transmitted by them cause muscle fibers or pigment cells to contract, or glands to secrete. SEE ALSO motor cortex, motor endplate, motor neuron. **2.** PSYCHOLOGY denoting the overt reaction of an organism to a stimulus (motor response). **3.** Pertaining to a set of skills involving movement or motion. [L. a mover, fr. *moveo,* to move]

mo•tor a•lex•i•a (mō′tŏr ă-lek′sē-ă) SEE alexia.

mo•tor a•pha•si•a (mō′tŏr ă-fā′zē-ă) SYN expressive aphasia. SYN Broca aphasia (1).

mo•tor a•prax•i•a (mō′tŏr ă-prak′sē-ă) An inability to make movements or to use objects for the purpose intended.

mo•tor ar•e•a (mō′tŏr ār′ē-ă) SYN motor cortex.

mo•tor a•tax•i•a (mō′tŏr ă-tak′sē-ă) Condition developing on attempting to perform coordinated muscular movements.

mo•tor con•trol (mō′tŏr kŏn-trōl′) The process of initiating, directing, and grading purposeful voluntary movement.

mo•tor cor•tex (mō′tŏr kōr′teks) The region of the cerebral cortex most immediately influencing movements of the face, neck, trunk, arms, and leg; its effects on the motor neurons innervating the skeletal musculature are mediated by the pyramidal tract. SYN excitable area, motor area, Rolando area.

mo•tor de•cus•sa•tion (mō′tŏr dē-kŭs-ā′shŭn) SYN pyramidal decussation.

mo•tor end•plate (mō′tŏr end′plāt) The large and complex end-formation by which the axon of a motor neuron establishes synaptic contact with a striated muscle fiber (cell).

mo•tor fi•bers (mō′tŏr fī′bĕrz) Nerve fibers that transmit impulses that activate effector cells, e.g., in muscle or gland tissue.

mo•tor im•age (mō′tŏr im′ăj) The image of body movements.

mo•tor learn•ing (mō′tŏr lĕrn′ing) **1.** The process of acqiring a skill by which the learner, through practice and assimilation, refines and make automatic the desired movement. **2.** An internal neurologic process that results in the ability to produce a new motor task.

mo•tor nerve (mō′tŏr nĕrv) An efferent nerve conveying an impulse that excites muscular contraction; motor nerves in the autonomic nervous system also elicit secretions from glandular epithelia.

mo•tor neu•ron (mō′tŏr nūr′on) A nerve cell in the spinal cord, rhombencephalon, or mesencephalon characterized by an axon that leaves the central nervous system to establish a functional connection with an effector (muscle or glandular) tissue; somatic motor neurons directly synapse with striated muscle fibers by motor endplates; visceral motor neurons or autonomic motor neurons (preganglionic motor neurons), by contrast, innervate smooth muscle fibers or glands only by the intermediary of a second, peripheral, neuron (postganglionic or ganglionic motor neuron) located in an autonomic ganglion. SEE ALSO motor endplate, autonomic division of nervous system. SYN motoneuron, motoneurone.

mo•tor neu•ron dis•ease (mō′tŏr nūr′on di-zēz′) A general term comprising progressive spinal muscular atrophy (infantile, juvenile, and adult), amyotrophic lateral sclerosis, progressive bulbar paralysis, and primary lateral sclerosis; frequently a familial disease.

mo•tor pa•ral•y•sis (mō′tŏr păr-al′i-sis) Loss of the power of muscular contraction.

mo•tor plate (mō′tŏr plāt) SEE motor endplate.

mo•tor point (mō′tŏr poynt) A point on the skin where the application of an electrical stimulus, through an electrode, will cause the contraction of an underlying muscle.

mo•tor speech cen•ter (mō′tŏr spēch sen′tĕr) SYN Broca center.

mo•tor speech dis•or•der (mō′tŏr spēch dis-ōr′dĕr) Difficulty in planning or producing speech due to problems with motor planning or muscle tone (e.g., apraxia, dysarthria).

mo•tor u•nit (mō′tŏr yū′nit) A single somatic motor neuron and the group of muscle fibers innervated by it.

mo•tor ur•gen•cy (mō′tŏr ŭr′jĕn-sē) Urgency from overactive detrusor function.

MOTT (mot) Acronym used to describe mycobacteria other than *Mycobacterium tuberculosis, M. bovis,* and *M. africanum,* (*M. tuberculosis* complex).

mot•tled e•nam•el (mŏt′ĕld ĕ-nam′ĕl) Alterations in enamel structure often due to excessive fluoride ingestion during tooth formation. Mottling may also be caused by tetracycline therapy in women during the first half of pregnancy or in children whose teeth are still developing.

mot•tling (mot′ĕ-ling) An area of skin composed of macular lesions of varying shades or colors. [E. *motley,* variegated in color]

mound•ing (mownd′ing) SYN myoedema.

mount (mownt) **1.** To prepare for microscopic examination. **2.** To climb on for purposes of copulation.

moun•tain dai•sy (mown′tăn dā′zē) SYN arnica.

moun•tain sick•ness (mown′tăn sik′nĕs) SYN altitude sickness.

mouse (mows) A small rodent belonging to the genus *Mus.*

mouse-tooth for•ceps (mows-tūth fōr′seps) A forceps with one or two fine points at the tip of each blade, fitting into hollows between the points on the opposite blade.

mouth (mowth) **1.** SYN oral cavity. **2.** The opening, usually the external opening, of a cavity or canal. SEE os (2), ostium, orifice, stoma (2). See this page. [A.S. *mūth*]

mouth-to-mouth res•pi•ra•tion (mowth-mowth res′pir-ā′shŭn) A method of artificial ventilation involving an overlap of the patient's mouth (and nose in small children) with the rescuer's mouth to inflate the patient's lungs by blowing, followed by an unassisted expiratory phase brought about by elastic recoil of the patient's chest and lungs; repeated 12–16 times a minute; where the nose is not covered by the operator's mouth, the nostrils must be pinched closed.

mouth-to-mouth re•sus•ci•ta•tion (mowth-mowth rē-sŭs′i-tā′shŭn) Mouth-to-mouth respiration employed as part of emergency cardiopulmonary resuscitation.

mouth•wash (mowth′wawsh) A medicated liquid used for cleaning the mouth and treating

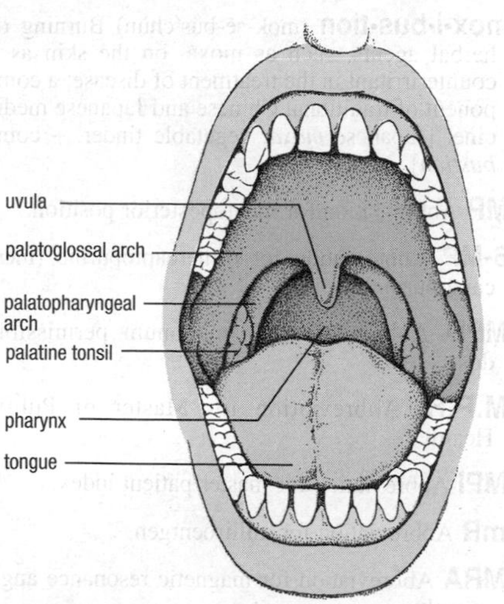

oral cavity

disorders of the oral mucosa; also called mouthrinse.

MOV Abbreviation for minimal occluding volume.

mov•a•ble joint (mūv-ă-bĕl joynt) SYN synovial joint. SYN moveable joint.

mov•a•ble spleen (mūv-ă′bĕl splēn) SYN floating spleen. SYN moveable spleen.

moveable joint [Br.] SYN movable joint.

moveable spleen [Br.] SYN movable spleen.

move•ment (mūv′mĕnt) **1.** Active change of position or location; said of the entire body or of one or more of its members or parts. **2.** SYN stool. **3.** SYN defecation. [L. *moveo,* pp. *motus,* to move]

move•ment de•com•po•si•tion (mūv′mĕnt dē-kom′pŏ-zish′ŭn) A neurologic disorder characterized by distinct jerky movements rather than a single fluid, smoothly coordinated action.

move•ment e•con•o•my (mūv′mĕnt ē-kon′ŏ-mē) SYN exercise economy.

move•ment sys•tem (mūv′mĕnt sis′tĕm) **1.** A physiologic system that functions to produce motion of the whole body or of its component parts. **2.** The functional interaction of structures that contribute to the act of moving.

move•ment time (mūv′mĕnt tīm) The time elapsed between the beginning and the end of a movement.

mov•er (mūv′ĕr) A person or thing that moves or causes to move.

Mow•ry col•loi•dal i•ron stain (mow′rē koloyd′ăl ī′ŏrn stān) A stain used for demonstrating acid mucopolysaccharides.

mox•i•bus•tion (mok-sē-bŭs′chŭn) Burning of herbal agents, such as moxa, on the skin as a counterirritant in the treatment of disease; a component of traditional Chinese and Japanese medicine. [Japanese *moxa*, vegetable tinder, + com*bustion*]

MP Abbreviation for mentoposterior position.

6-MP Abbreviation for 6-mercaptopurine (mercaptopurine).

MPD Abbreviation for maximum permissible dose.

M.P.H. Abbreviation for Master of Public Health.

MPI Abbreviation for master patient index.

mR Abbreviation for milliroentgen.

MRA Abbreviation for magnetic resonance angiography.

mrad Abbreviation for millirad.

MRD, mrd Abbreviation for minimal reacting dose.

mrem Abbreviation for millirem.

MRF Abbreviation for melanotropin-releasing factor.

MRH Abbrevation for melanotropin-releasing hormone.

MRI Abbreviation for magnetic resonance imaging.

mRNA Abbreviation for messenger RNA. SEE entries beginning with ribonucleic acid.

MRO Abbreviation for medical review officer.

MRSA Abbreviation for methicillin-resistant *Staphylococcus aureus*. SEE multidrug-resistant organisms.

MS Abbreviation for multiple sclerosis; morphine sulfate; mitral stenosis; mental status.

ms Abbreviation for millisecond. (The form msec is preferred, however.)

MSAFP test (test) Abbreviation for maternal serum alfa-fetoprotein test.

MSDS Abbreviation for Material Safety Data Sheet.

msec Abbreviation for millisecond.

MSG Abbreviation for monosodium glutamate.

MSH Abbreviation for melanocyte-stimulating hormone.

M shell (shel) The lowest energy level at which electron transitions give rise to x-rays.

MSN Abbreviation for Master of Science in Nursing.

MT Abbreviation meaning medical transcription, medical transcriptionist; mentotransverse position.

MTCC Abbreviation for medical transcription certification commission. SEE ALSO CMT.

MTP Abbreviation for metatarsophalangeal.

MU Abbreviation for monitor unit.

mu (myū) Twelfth letter of the Greek alphabet (μ). USAGE NOTE The JCAHO directs that units including the prefix *micro-* be written in full (*microgram, microliter*) instead of abbreviated (as μ*g* and μ*L*) because the Greek letter is often misread as *m*.

Much ba•cil•lus (mūk bă-sil′ŭs) An alleged non-acid-fast granular form of the tubercle bacillus; not demonstrable by the Ziehl stain, but takes a modified Gram stain; it is said to be the form present in the tuberculous skin lesion.

♻ **muci-** Combining form indicating mucous, mucin. SEE ALSO muco-. [L. *mucus*]

mu•ci•car•mine (myū′si-kahr′mīn) A red stain containing aluminum chloride and carmine; used to detect epithelial mucins and mucin-secreting adenocarcinomas; also used to demonstrate the capsule of *Cryptococcus neoformans* and other fungi.

mu•ci•form (myū′si-fōrm) Resembling mucus. SYN blennoid, mucoid (2).

mu•ci•he•ma•te•in (myū′si-hē′mă-tē-in) A violet-blue staining fluid containing aluminum chloride and hematein; used to detect connective tissue mucins.

mu•ci•lage (myū′si-lăj) A pharmacopeial preparation consisting of a solution in water of the mucilaginous principles of vegetable substances; used as a soothing application to the mucous membranes and in the preparation of official and extemporaneous mixtures. [L. *mucilago*]

mu•ci•lag•i•nous (myū′si-laj′i-nŭs) Resembling mucilage; i.e., adhesive, viscid, sticky.

mu•cin (myū′sin) A secretion containing carbohydrate-rich glycoproteins such as that from the goblet cells of the intestine, the submaxillary glands, and other mucous glandular cells; it is also present in the ground substance of connective tissue.

mu•cin•ase (myū′si-nās) Any enzyme that hydrolyzes mucopolysaccharide substances (mucins). SYN mucopolysaccharidase.

mu•cin•o•gen (myū-sin′ō-jen) A glycoprotein that forms mucin through the imbibition of water. [mucin + G. *-gen,* producing]

mu•ci•noid (myū′si-noyd) **1.** SYN mucoid (1). **2.** Resembling mucin.

mu•ci•no•sis (myū′si-nō′sis) A condition in which mucin is present in the skin in excessive amounts, or in abnormal distribution. Classified as metabolic mucinosis, secondary mucinosis, and localized mucinosis. [mucin + G. *-osis,* condition]

mu·ci·nous (myū′si-nŭs) Relating to or containing mucin. SYN mucoid (3).

mu·ci·nous car·ci·no·ma (myū′si-nŭs kahr′si-nō′mă) A variety of adenocarcinoma in which the neoplastic cells secrete conspicuous quantities of mucin; the neoplasms are glistening, sticky, and gelatinoid in consistency. SYN colloid carcinoma.

muco- Combining form meaning mucous, mucous (mucous membrane). SEE ALSO muci-. [L. *mucus*]

mu·co·cele (myū′kō-sēl) A retention cyst of the salivary gland, lacrimal sac, paranasal sinuses, appendix, or gallbladder. Most common site is the lower lip lateral to the midline. [muco- + G. *kēlē,* tumor, hernia]

mu·co·cil·i·ar·y (myū′kō-sil′ē-ar-ē) Pertaining to ciliated columnar epithelium found in the bronchial tree to the level of the terminal bronchioles, and in the uterine tubes. SEE ciliary.

mu·co·cil·i·ar·y clear·ance (myū′kō-sil′ē-ar-ē klēr′ăns) The movement of the mucous covering of the respiratory epithelium by the beating of cilia: rapid, forward (effective) stroke and slow, return (recovery) stroke.

mu·co·cil·i·ar·y clear·ance rate (myū′kō-sil′ē-ar-ē klēr′ans rāt) Velocity of movement of the mucus blanket over respiratory epithelium, usually expressed in mm/hr.

mu·co·cil·i·ar·y trans·port (myū′kō-sil′ē-ar-ē trans′pōrt) Movement of mucus and mucoid fluid through the bronchial tree by the action of cilia.

mu·co·cu·ta·ne·ous (myū′kō-kyū-tā′nē-ŭs) Relating to mucous membrane and skin; denoting the line of junction of the two at the nasal, oral, vaginal, and anal orifices.

mu·co·cu·ta·ne·ous junc·tion (myū′kō-kū-tā′nē-ŭs jŭngk′shŭn) The site of transition from epidermis to the epithelium of a mucous membrane.

mu·co·cu·ta·ne·ous leish·man·i·a·sis (myū′kō-kyū-tā′nē-ŭs lēsh′mă-nī′ă-sis) A grave disease caused by *Leishmania braziliensis* complex, endemic in Mexico and Central and South America. The organism does not invade the viscera, and the disease is limited to the skin and mucous membranes, the lesions resembling the sores of cutaneous leishmaniasis. The sores heal after a time, but some months or years later, fungating and eroding forms of ulceration may appear on the tongue and buccal or nasal mucosa. SEE ALSO espundia. SYN American leishmaniasis, nasopharyngeal leishmaniasis, New World leishmaniasis.

mu·co·cu·ta·ne·ous lymph node syn·drome (myū′kō-kyū-tā′nē-ŭs limf nōd sin′drōm) SYN Kawasaki disease.

mu·co·en·ter·i·tis (myū′kō-en-tĕr-ī′tis) **1.** Inflammation of the intestinal mucous membrane. **2.** SYN mucomembranous enteritis.

mu·co·ep·i·der·moid (myū′kō-ep-i-dĕr′moyd) Denoting a mixture of mucus-secreting and epithelial cells, as in mucoepidermoid carcinoma.

mu·coid (myū′koyd) **1.** General term for a mucin, mucoprotein, or glycoprotein. SYN mucinoid (1). **2.** SYN muciform. **3.** SYN mucinous. [mucus + G. *eidos,* appearance]

mu·coid de·gen·er·a·tion (myū′koyd dĕ-jen′ĕr-ā′shŭn) A conversion of any of the connective tissues into a gelatinous or mucoid substance. SYN myxomatosis (1).

mu·co·lyt·ic (myū′kō-lit′ik) Capable of dissolving, digesting, or liquefying mucus.

mu·co·mem·bra·nous (myū′kō-mem′bră-nŭs) Relating to a mucous membrane.

mu·co·mem·bra·nous en·ter·i·tis (myū′kō-mem′bră-nŭs en′tĕr-ī′tis) A disorder of the intestinal mucous membrane characterized by constipation or diarrhea (sometimes alternating), colic, and the passage of pseudomembranous shreds or incomplete casts of the intestine. SYN mucoenteritis (2).

mu·co·per·i·os·te·al (myū′kō-per-ē-os′tē-ăl) Relating to mucoperiosteum.

mu·co·per·i·os·te·um (myū′kō-per-ē-os′tē-ŭm) Mucous membrane and periosteum so intimately united as practically to form a single membrane, as that covering the hard palate.

mu·co·pol·y·sac·cha·ri·dase (myū′kō-pol-ē-sak′ă-ri-dās) SYN mucinase.

mu·co·pol·y·sac·cha·ride (myū′kō-pol-ē-sak′ă-rīd) General term for a protein-polysaccharide complex obtained from proteoglycans and containing as much as 95% polysaccharide; mucopolysaccharides include the blood group substances. A more modern term is glycosaminoglycan.

mu·co·pol·y·sac·cha·ri·do·sis, pl. **mu·co·pol·y·sac·cha·ri·do·ses** (myū′kō-pol-ē-sak′ă-ri-dōs′is, myū′kō-pol-ē-sak′ă-rī-dōs′ēz) Any of a group of lysosomal storage diseases that have in common a disorder in metabolism of mucopolysaccharides, as evidenced by excretion of various mucopolysaccharides in urine and infiltration of these substances into connective tissue, with resulting various defects of bone, cartilage, connective tissue, and other organs.

mu·co·pol·y·sac·cha·ri·du·ri·a (myū′kō-pol-ē-sak′ă-ri-dyūr′ē-ă) Excretion of glycosaminoglycans in urine.

mu·co·pro·tein (myū′kō-prō′tēn) General term

for a protein-polysaccharide complex, usually implying that the protein component is the major part of the complex. Mucoproteins include the α_1- and α_2-globulins of serum.

mu·co·pu·ru·lent (myū′kō-pyūr′yū-lent) Pertaining to an exudate that is chiefly purulent (pus) but contains relatively conspicuous proportions of mucous material.

Mu·cor (myū′kōr) A genus of fungi (class Zygomycetes, family Mucoraceae), most species of which are saprobic; characterized by sparsely septate hyphoe, large sporangia that contain sporangiospores but lack rhizoids. Several are pathogenic and may cause zygomycosis in humans.

Mu·cor·al·es (myū′kō-rā′lēz) An order of the fungal class Zygomycetes that contains all the species causing mucormycosis in humans. The genera include *Cunninghamella*, *Rhizopus*, *Absidia*, *Rhizomucor*, *Mucor*, *Apophysomyces*, *Saksenaea*, *Syncephalastrum*, and *Cokeromyces*. Although *Mortierella* species are included, they are of doubtful pathogenicity in humans.

mu·cor·my·co·sis (myū′kōr-mī-kō′sis) SYN zygomycosis.

mu·co·sa (myū-kō′să) A mucous tissue lining various tubular structures, consisting of epithelium, lamina propria, and, in the digestive tract, a layer of smooth muscle. SYN mucous membrane. [L. fem. of *mucosus,* mucous]

mu·co·sa-as·so·ci·at·ed lym·phoid tis·sue (MALT) (myū-kō′să-ă-sō′sē-ā-tĕd lim′foyd tish′ū) A class of lymphoid tissue comprising nodular aggregates found in association with the wet mucosal surfaces of the body such as those of the respiratory, digestive, and urinary systems.

mu·co·sal (myū-kō′săl) Relating to the mucosa or mucous membrane.

mu·co·sal wave (myū-kō′săl wāv) The movement of the mucous membrane of the vocal cord during phonation.

mu·co·san·guin·e·ous, mu·co·san·guin·o·lent (myū′kō-san-gwin′ē-ŭs, -ō-lent) Pertaining to an exudate or other fluid material that has a relatively high content of blood and mucus. [muco- + L. *sanguis,* blood]

mu·co·sec·to·my (myū′kō-sek′tŏ-mē) Excision of the mucosa, usually of the rectum before ileoanal anastomosis for treatment of ulcerative colitis. [mucosa + G. *ektomē,* excision]

mu·co·se·rous (myū′kō-sē′rŭs) Pertaining to an exudate or secretion that consists of both mucus and serum or a watery component.

mu·co·se·rous cells (myū′kō-sē′rŭs selz) Glandular cells intermediate in histologic characteristics between serous and mucous cells

mu·cous (myū′kŭs) Relating to mucus or a mucous membrane. [L. *mucosus,* mucous, fr. *mucus*]

mu·cous cell (myū′kŭs sel) A cell that secretes mucus (e.g., a goblet cell).

mu·cous co·li·tis (myū′kŭs kō-lī′tis) An affliction of the mucous membrane of the colon characterized by colicky pain, constipation, or diarrhea (sometimes alternating), and passage of mucous or slimy pseudomembranous shreds and patches.

mu·cous con·nec·tive tis·sue (myū′kŭs kŏn-ek′tiv tish′ū) A type of connective tissue little differentiated beyond the mesenchymal stage; its ground substance of glycoproteins is abundant and contains fine collagenous fibers and fibroblasts; in its most characteristic form, it appears in the umbilical cord as Wharton jelly.

mu·cous cyst (myū′kŭs sist) A retention cyst resulting from obstruction in the duct of a mucous gland.

mu·cous gland (myū′kŭs gland) A gland that secretes mucus.

mu·cous glands of au·di·to·ry tube (myū′kŭs glandz aw′di-tōr-ē tūb) Glands located principally near the pharyngeal end of the auditory tube.

mu·cous mem·brane (myū′kus mem′brān) SYN mucosa.

mu·cous plug (myū′kŭs plŭg) **1.** A mass of mucus and cells filling the cervical canal between periods or during pregnancy. **2.** A mass of mucous occluding a main or lobar bronchus.

mu·cus (myū′kŭs) The clear viscid secretion of the mucous membranes, consisting of mucin, epithelial cells, leukocytes, and various inorganic salts suspended in water. [L.]

mu·cus blan·ket (myū′kŭs blangk′ĕt) The mucous covering of respiratory epithelium.

mud fe·ver (mŭd fē′vĕr) A leptospirosis caused by the *grippotyphosa* serovar of *Leptospira interrogans*.

Muehr·cke line (myūr′kĕ līn) A white line of the nail; lines occur serially, parallel with the lunula and separated from each other by normal pink areas; associated with hypoalbuminemia; the lines do not move outward with nail growth, but disappear when the serum albumin returns to normal.

Muel·ler e·lec·tron·ic to·nom·e·ter (myū′lĕr ĕ-lek-tron′ik tō-nom′ĕ-tĕr) A Schiötz type tonometer that electronically indicates the extent of corneal indentation; may also have an attached recorder for continuous pressure readings (tonography).

Muel·ler-Hin·ton me·di·um (myū′lĕr hin′tŏn mē′dē-ŭm) The standard agar-based medium for antibacterial susceptibility tests for the most common aerobic and facultatively anaerobic bacteria. Nutritional supplements are added for fastidious organisms. The pH cation content and depth of the agar must be properly controlled because these factors affect the accuracy of the test results.

MUGA (mū′gă) Acronym for multiple-gated acquisition scan.

mug•wort (mŭg′wōrt) SYN carline thistle.

mul•ber•ry mo•lar (mŭl′ber-ē mō′lăr) A malformed molar with a crown resembling a mulberry, with hypoplasia, crenellations, and short cusps. It may be a manifestation of congenital syphilis but also occurs in other conditions.

Mules op•er•a•tion (myūlz op-ĕr-ā′shŭn) Evisceration of the eyeball followed by the insertion within the sclera of a spheric prosthesis to support an artificial eye.

mule-spin•ner's can•cer (myūl spin′ĕrz kan′sĕr) Carcinoma of the scrotum or adjacent skin exposed to oil, observed in some workers in cotton spinning mills.

mu•li•e•bri•a (mū′lē-ē′brē-ă) The female genital organs. [L. neut pl. of *muliebris,* relating to *mulier,* a woman]

Mül•ler duct, mül•le•ri•an duct (mēl′er dŭkt, myū-ler′ē-ăn) SYN paramesonephric duct.

Mül•ler fix•a•tive (mēl′er fisk′ă-tiv) A hardening fixative composed of potassium dichromate, sodium sulfate and distilled water, similar to Regaud fixative.

mül•le•ri•an in•hib•i•ting sub•stance (mē-ler′ē-ăn in-hib′i-ting sub′stăns) A 535-amino acid glycoprotein secreted by the Sertoli cells of the testis. It is related to inhibin.

Mül•ler law (mēl′er law) Each type of sensory nerve ending, however stimulated (electrically, mechanically), gives rise to its own specific sensation; moreover, each type of sensation depends not on any special character of the different nerves but on the part of the brain in which their fibers terminate.

Mül•ler ma•neu•ver (mēl′er mă-nū′vĕr) After a forced expiration, an attempt at inspiration is made with closed mouth and nose or closed glottis, whereby the negative pressure in the chest and lungs is made very subatmospheric; the reverse of Valsalva maneuver.

Mül•ler sign (mēul′er sīn) In aortic insufficiency, rhythmic pulsatory movements of the uvula, synchronous with cardiac contractions; accompanied by swelling and redness of the velum palati and tonsils.

Mül•ler tu•ber•cle (mēl′er tū′bĕr-kĕl) SYN sinual tubercle.

mul•tang•u•lar bone (mŭl-tan-gyū′lăr bōn) SEE trapezium, trapezoid bone.

♻ **multi-** Combining form meaning many. SEE ALSO pluri-. Cf. poly-. [L. *multus,* much]

mul•ti•ar•tic•u•lar (mŭl′tē-ahr-tik′yū-lăr) Relating to or involving many joints. SYN polyarthric, polyarticular. [multi- + L. *articulus,* joint]

mul•ti•ax•i•al joint (mŭl′tē-aks′ē-ăl joynt) One in which movement occurs in a number of axes. SEE ball-and-socket joint. SYN polyaxial joint.

mul•ti•col•o•ny-stim•u•lat•ing fac•tor (mŭl′tē-kol′ŏ-nē-stim′yū-lā-ting fak′tŏr) SYN interleukin-3.

mul•ti•cus•pi•date (mŭl′tē-kŭs′pi-dāt) **1.** Having more than two cusps. **2.** A molar tooth with three or more cusps or projections on the crown.

mul•ti•dis•ci•plin•a•ry (mŭl′tē-dis′i-pli-nar′ē) Collective; involving health care providers from more than one discipline. SEE ALSO interdisciplinary.

mul•ti•drug-re•sis•tant or•gan•isms (mŭl′tē′drŭg-rē-zis′tănt ōr′găn-izmz) Bacteria and other microorganisms that have develped resistance to many antimicrobial drugs (e.g., methicillin/oxacillin-resistant *Staphylococcus aureus*, vancomycin-resistant enterococci, and penicillin-resistant *Streptococcus pneumoniae*).

mul•ti•fac•to•ri•al in•her•i•tance (mŭl′tē-fak-tōr′ē-ăl in-her′i-tăns) Inheritance involving many factors, of which at least one is genetic but none is of overwhelming importance, as in the causation of a disease by multiple genetic and environmental factors.

mul•ti•fid (mŭl′ti-fid) Divided into many clefts or segments. [L. *multifidus,* fr. *multus,* much, + *findo,* to cleave]

🅸 **mul•tif•i•dus mus•cle** (mŭl-tif′i-dŭs mŭs′ĕl) *Origin,* from the sacrum, sacroiliac ligament, mammillary processes of the lumbar vertebrae, transverse processes of thoracic vertebrae, and articular processes of last four cervical vertebrae; *insertion,* into the spinous processes of all the vertebrae up to and including the axis; *action,* rotates vertebral column; *nerve supply,* dorsal primary rami of spinal nerves. See page 1016. SYN musculus multifidus lumborum [TA], musculus multifidus [TA].

🅸 **mul•ti•fo•cal** (mŭl′tē-fō′kăl) Relating to or arising from many foci. See page B19.

mul•ti•fo•cal a•tri•al tach•y•car•di•a (MAT) (mŭl′tē-fō′kăl ā′trē-ăl tak′i-kahr′dē-ă) SYN atrial chaotic tachycardia.

mul•ti•fo•cal lens (mŭl′tē-fō′kăl lenz) A lens with segments providing two or more powers; commonly, a trifocal lens.

mul•ti•form (mŭl′ti-fōrm) SYN polymorphic.

mul•ti•for•mat cam•er•a (mŭl′tē-fōr′mat kam′ĕr-ă) Photographic or laser printer for recording

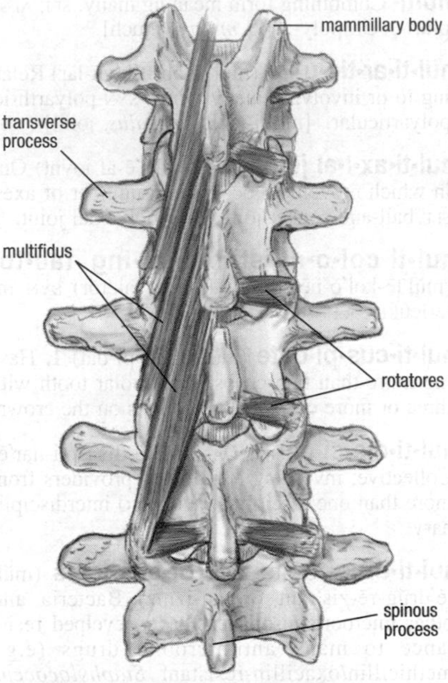

multifidus muscles: lumbar vertebrae

a variable number of video images on a sheet of film, as in computed tomography or ultrasound.

mul·ti·form lay·er of cer·e·bral cor·tex (mŭl′ti-fōrm lā′ĕr ser′ĕ-brăl kōr′teks) The innermost layer of the cerebral cortex, layer XI. SYN lamina multiformis [TA].

mul·ti·grav·i·da (mŭl′tē-grav′i-dă) A pregnant woman who has been pregnant one or more times previously. [multi- + L. *gravida,* pregnant]

mul·ti·in·fec·tion (mŭl′tē-in-fek′shŭn) Mixed infection with two or more varieties of microorganisms developing simultaneously.

mul·ti·lam·el·lar bod·y (mŭl′tē-lam′ĕ-lăr bod′ē) SYN cytosome (2).

mul·ti·lo·bar, mul·ti·lo·bate, mul·ti·lobed (mŭl′tē-lō′bahr, -lō′bāt, -lōbd′) Having several lobes.

mul·ti·lob·u·lar (mŭl′tē-lob′yū-lăr) Having many lobules.

mul·ti·lo·cal (mŭl′tē-lō′kăl) Denoting traits with an etiology comprising effects of multiple genetic loci operating together and simultaneously.

mul·ti·loc·u·lar (mŭl′tē-lok′yū-lăr) Many-celled; having many compartments or loculi.

mul·ti·loc·u·lar ad·i·pose tis·sue (mŭl′tē-lok′yū-lăr ad′i-pōs tish′ū) SYN brown fat.

mul·ti·loc·u·lar cyst (mŭl′tē-lok′yū-lăr sist) A cyst containing several compartments formed by membranous septa.

mul·ti·loc·u·lar fat (mŭl′tē-lok′yū-lăr fat) SYN brown fat.

mul·ti·lo·cus en·zyme e·lec·tro·pho·re·sis (MLEE) (mŭl′tē-lō′kŭs en′zīm ĕ-lek′trō-fŏr-ē′sis) A nonamplified strain-typing method. Proteins are isolated from the strain of interest and separated in a gel. A probe is used to detect a specific protein.

mul·ti·lo·cus se·quence typ·ing (MLST) (mŭl′tē-lō′kŭs sē′kwĕns tīp′ing) A strain typing method that uses polymerase chain reaction to amplify several different genetic loci. The resulting fragments are separated by electrophoresis and analyzed.

mul·ti·nod·u·lar, mul·ti·nod·u·late (mŭl′tē-nod′yū-lăr, -yū-lāt) Having many nodules.

mul·ti·nod·u·lar goi·ter (mŭl′tē-nod′yū-lăr goy′tĕr) Adenomatous goiter with several colloid nodules.

mul·ti·nu·cle·ar, mul·ti·nu·cle·ate (mŭl′tē-nū′klē-ăr, -āt) Having two or more nuclei. SYN polynuclear, polynucleate.

mul·tip·a·ra (mŭl-tip′ă-ră) A woman who has given birth at least twice to an infant, liveborn or not, weighing 500 g or more, or having an estimated length of gestation of at least 20 weeks. [multi- + L. *pario,* to bring forth, to bear]

mul·ti·par·i·ty (mŭl′tē-par′i-tē) Condition of being a multipara.

mul·tip·a·rous (mŭl-tip′ă-rŭs) Relating to a multipara.

mul·ti·ple chem·i·cal sen·si·tiv·i·ty (MCS) (mŭl′ti-pĕl kem′i-kăl sen′si-tiv′i-tē) SYN idiopathic environmental intolerance.

mul·ti·ple e·go states (mŭl′ti-pĕl ē′gō stāts) Various psychological organizational states reflecting different personas or life experiences.

mul·ti·ple en·do·crine de·fi·cien·cy syn·drome (mŭl′ti-pĕl en′dō-krin dĕ-fish′ĕn-sē sin′drōm) Acquired deficiency of the function of several endocrine glands, usually on an autoimmune basis.

mul·ti·ple en·do·crine ne·o·pla·si·a (MEN) (mŭl′ti-pĕl en′dō-krin nē-ō-plā′zē-ă) A group of disorders characterized by functioning tumors in more than one endocrine gland.

mul·ti·ple en·do·crine ne·o·pla·si·a 1 (MEN1) (mŭl′ti-pĕl en′dō-krin nē-ō-plā′zē-ă) Syndrome characterized by tumors of the pituitary gland, pancreatic islet cells, and parathyroid glands and may be associated with Zollinger-Ellison syndrome; autosomal dominant inheritance, caused by mutation in the MEN1 gene on chromosome 11q.

mul·ti·ple en·do·crine ne·o·pla·si·a 2 (MEN2) (mŭl′ti-pĕl en′dō-krin nē-ō-plā′zē-ă) Syndrome associated with pheochromocytoma, parathyroid adenoma, and medullary thyroid carcinoma; autosomal dominant inheritance, caused by mutation in the RET oncogene on chromosome 10q.

mul·ti·ple en·do·crine ne·o·pla·si·a 2B (MEN2B) (mŭl′ti-pĕl en′dō-krin nē-ō-plā′zē-ă) SYN multiple endocrine neoplasia 3.

mul·ti·ple en·do·crine ne·o·pla·si·a 3 (MEN3) (mŭl′ti-pĕl en′dō-krin nē-ō-plā′zē-ă) Syndrome characterized by tumors found in MEN2, tall, thin habitus, prominent lips, and neuromas of the tongue and eyelids; autosomal dominant inheritance, caused by mutation in the RET oncogene on 10q. SYN multiple endocrine neoplasia 2B.

mul·ti·ple ep·i·phys·i·al dys·pla·si·a (EDM) (mŭl′ti-pĕl ep′i-fiz′ē-ăl dis-plā′zē-ă) A dominantly inherited abnormality of epiphyses characterized by difficulty in walking, pain and stiffness of joints, stubby fingers, and often dwarfism of short-limb type; on x-ray examination, the epiphyses are mottled and irregular; ossification centers are late in appearance and may be multiple, but the vertebrae are normal. There is also an autosomal recessive form. SYN dysplasia epiphysialis multiplex.

mul·ti·ple fis·sion (mŭl′ti-pĕl fish′ŭn) Division of the nucleus into a number of daughter nuclei, followed by division of the cell body into an equal number of daughter cells, each containing a nucleus.

mul·ti·ple frac·ture (mŭl′ti-pĕl frak′shŭr) **1.** Fracture at two or more places in a bone. **2.** Fracture of several bones occurring simultaneously.

mul·ti·ple-ga·ted ac·qui·si·tion scan (MUGA) (mŭl′ti-pĕl-gāt′ĕd ak-wi-zi′shŭn skan) A nuclear medicine cardiac blood pool study collected by multiple-gated acquisition; uscd for ejection fraction and wall motion assessment. SEE ALSO radionuclide ejection fraction.

mul·ti·ple in·tes·ti·nal pol·y·po·sis (mŭl′ti-pĕl in-tes′ti-năl pol′i-pō′sis) **1.** A disorder that usually begins in late childhood; polyps increase in numbers, causing symptoms of chronic colitis, and carcinoma of the colon almost invariably develops in untreated cases; autosomal dominant inheritance. In the Gardner syndrome there are extracolonic changes (e.g., desmoid tumors). **2.** Hamartomatous polyposis of the small or large intestine, Peutz-Jeghers syndrome with melanin spots on the lips, less common.

mul·ti·ple mark·er screen (mŭl′ti-pĕl mahr′kĕr skrēn) Use of two or more markers in the maternal serum to determine the relative risk of an abnormal fetus. SEE ALSO triple screen.

mul·ti·ple me·ta·bol·ic syn·drome (mŭl′ti-pĕl met′ă-bol′ik sin′drōm) SYN metabolic syndrome.

mul·ti·ple mu·co·sal neu·ro·ma syn·drome (mŭl′ti-pĕl myū-kō′săl nūr-ō′mă sin′drōm) Multiple submucosal neuromas or neurofibromas of the tongue, lips, and eyelids in young people; sometimes associated with tumors of the thyroid or medulla of suprarenal gland, or with subcutaneous neurofibromatosis.

mul·ti·ple my·e·lo·ma, my·e·lo·ma mul·ti·plex (mŭl′ti-pĕl mī-ĕ-lō′mă, mī-ĕ-lō′mă mŭl′ti-pleks) An uncommon disease that occurs more frequently in men and is associated with anemia, hemorrhage, recurrent infections, and weakness. A malignant neoplasm that originates in bone marrow and involves chiefly the skeleton; characterized by numerous diffuse foci or nodular accumulations of abnormal or malignant plasma cells in the marrow of various bones and abnormal proteins in the serum and urine; the most frequent abnormalities in the metabolism of protein are Bence Jones proteinuria, an increase in monoclonal γ-globulin in the plasma, the formation of cryoglobulin, and a form of primary amyloidosis. SEE ALSO plasma cell myeloma. See this page. SYN plasma cell myeloma (1).

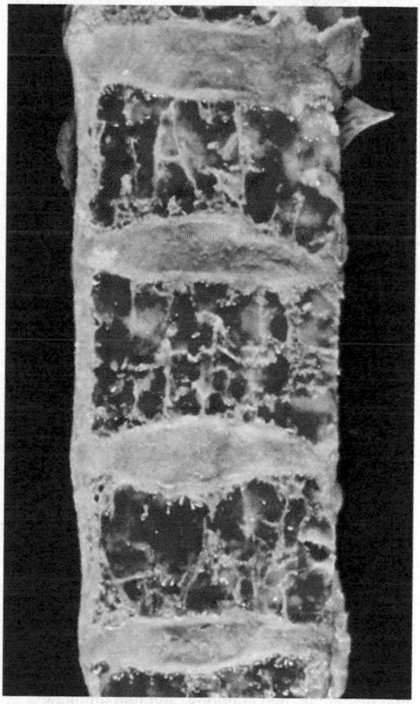

multiple myeloma: multiple lytic bone lesions present in vertebra

mul·ti·ple my·o·si·tis (mŭl′ti-pĕl mī-ō-sī′tis) The occurrence of multiple foci of acute inflammation in the muscular tissue and overlying skin in various parts of the body, accompanied by fever and other signs of systemic infection. SEE ALSO dermatomyositis.

mul·ti·ple neu·ri·tis (mŭl′ti-pĕl nūr-ī′tis) SYN polyneuropathy.

mul·ti·ple per·son·al·i·ty (mŭl′ti-pĕl pĕr-sŏn-al′i-tē) A dissociative disorder in which two or more distinct conscious personalities alternately prevail in the same person, without any personality being aware of the others.

mul·ti·ple preg·nan·cy (mŭl′ti-pĕl preg′năn-sē) Condition of bearing two or more fetuses simultaneously. See this page. SYN polycyesis.

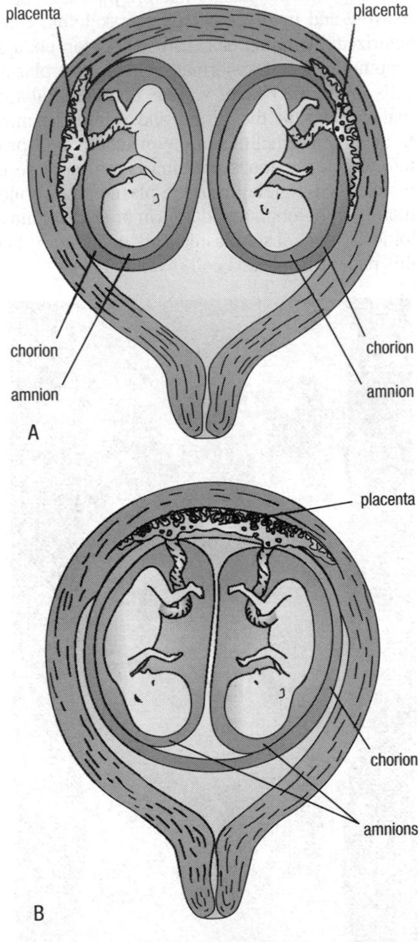

multiple pregnancy: (A) **dizygotic twins** showing two placentas, two chorions, and two amnions; (B) **monozygotic twins** with one placenta, one chorion, and two amnions

mul·ti·ple punc·ture tu·ber·cu·lin test (mŭl′ti-pĕl pungk′shŭr tū-bĕr′kyū-lin test) A kind of tine test SEE tuberculin test.

mul·ti·ple scle·ro·sis (MS) (mŭl′ti-pĕl skler-ō′sis) Common demyelinating disorder of the central nervous system, causing patches of sclerosis (plaques) in the brain and spinal cord; occurs primarily in young adults; clinical manifestations depend on the location and size of the plaques; typical symptoms include visual loss, diplopia, nystagmus, dysarthria, weakness, paresthesias, bladder abnormalities, and mood alterations; characteristically, the symptoms show exacerbations and remissions. See page B22.

mul·ti·ple sleep la·ten·cy test (MLST) (mŭl′ti-pĕl slēp lā′tĕn-sē test) Sleep study that involves 15- to 20-minute nap periods every 2 hours over 8 to 10 hours, with polysomnography during each nap.

mul·ti·ple stain (mŭl′ti-pĕl stān) A mixture of several dyes each having an independent selective action on one or more portions of the tissue.

mul·ti·ple sys·tem at·ro·phy (mŭl′ti-pĕl sis′tĕm at′rŏ-fē) Nonhereditary, neurodegenerative disease of unknown cause, characterized clinically by the development of parkinsonism, ataxia, autonomic failure, or pyramidal tract signs, in various combinations. Pathologically there are nerve cell loss, gliosis, and the accumulation of abnormal tubular structures in the cytoplasm and nucleus of oligodendrocytes and neurons in the basal ganglion, cerebellum, and intermediolateral columns of the spinal cord; can present as predominantly parkinsonism, as predominantly ataxia, or as a combination of parkinsonism, ataxia, and autonomic failure; it is a relatively rapidly progressive and fatal disorder.

mul·ti·ple vi·sion (mŭl′ti-pĕl vizh′ŭn) SYN polyopia.

mul·ti·plex PCR (mŭl′tē-pleks) A polymerase chain reaction method that uses two primer sets in the same tube. Each primer set is specific for a different target.

mul·ti·pli·ca·tive di·vi·sion (mŭl′ti-pli′kā-tiv di-vizh′ŭn) Reproduction by simultaneous division of a mother cell into a number of daughter cells. If the process occurs without fertilization of the mother cell, or encystment, the daughter cells are called merozoites; if they develop within a cyst, and usually after fertilization, they are called sporozoites.

mul·ti·po·lar (mŭl′tē-pō′lăr) Having more than two poles; denoting a nerve cell in which the branches project from several points.

mul·ti·po·lar cell (mŭl′tē-pō′lăr sel) A nerve cell with a number of dendrites arising from the cell body.

mul·ti·po·lar neu·ron (mŭl′tē-pō′lăr nūr′on) A neuron with several processes, usually an axon and three or more dendrites.

mul·ti·sy·nap·tic (mŭl′tē-si-nap′tik) SYN polysynaptic.

mul·ti·va·lence, **mul·ti·va·len·cy** (mŭl′tē-vā′lĕns, -vā′lĕn-sē) The state of being multivalent.

mul•ti•va•lent (mŭl′tē-vā′lĕnt) **1.** CHEMISTRY having a combining power (valence) of more than one hydrogen atom. **2.** Efficacious in more than one direction. **3.** An antisera specific for more than one antigen or organism. SYN polyvalent (1).

mul•ti•va•lent vac•cine (mŭl′tē-vā′lĕnt vak-sēn′) SYN polyvalent vaccine.

mum•mi•fi•ca•tion (mŭm′i-fi-kā′shŭn) **1.** SYN dry gangrene. **2.** Shriveling of a dead, retained fetus. **3.** DENTISTRY treatment of inflamed dental pulp with fixative drugs (usually formaldehyde derivatives) to retain teeth so treated for relatively short periods; generally acceptable only for deciduous teeth. [mummy + L. *facio,* to make]

i **mumps** (mŭmps) SYN epidemic parotiditis. See page B30. [dialect Eng. *mump,* a lump or bump]

mumps or•chi•tis (mŭmps ōr-kī′tis) Inflammation of the testes, caused by the mumps paramyxovirus (genus rubulavirus). The condition is more serious in teenage and adult males and can lead to infertility. Symptoms include pain and swelling of the testes. SEE ALSO epidemic parotiditis.

mumps skin test an•ti•gen (mŭmps skin test an′ti-jen) A suspension of killed mumps virus used to determine susceptibility to mumps or to confirm previous exposure.

mumps vi•rus (mŭmps vī′rŭs) A virus of the genus Paramyxovirus causing parotitis, sometimes with complications of orchitis, oophoritis, pancreatitis, meningoencephalitis and other disorders, and transmitted by infectious salivary secretions. SYN epidemic parotitis virus.

Munch•hau•sen syn•drome (mūn′chow-zĕn sin′drōm) A psychiatric disorder characterized by repeated simulation of illness to gain medical attention.

Munch•hau•sen syn•drome by prox•y (mūn′chow-zĕn sin′drōm prok′sē) Simulation of illness in a child or incompetent adult by a caregiver.

munch•ing (mŭnch′ing) An oral-motor pattern seen in children at about 6 months of age; earliest form of chewing; includes rhythmic up and down movement of the jaw that can appear as a stereotypic pattern or include movements that vary in degree of jaw opening and timing, it is elicited by stimulation of the gums or teeth.

Mun•ro mi•cro•ab•scess (mŭn-rō′ mī′krō-ab′ses) A microscopic collection of polymorphonuclear leukocytes found in the stratum corneum in psoriasis.

Mun•ro point (mŭn-rō′ poynt) A point at the right edge of the rectus abdominis muscle, between the umbilicus and the anterior superior spine of the ilium, where pressure elicits tenderness in appendicitis.

Mun•son sign (mŭn′son sīn) In keratoconus, the extra bowing of the lower eyelid caused by the misshapen cornea as the eye rotates downward.

mu•ral (myū′răl) Relating to the wall of any cavity. [L. *muralis;* fr. *murus,* wall]

mu•ral en•do•car•di•tis (myū′răl en′dō-kahr-dī′tis) Inflammation of the endocardium involving the walls of the chambers of the heart.

mu•ral throm•bo•sis (myū′răl throm-bō′sis) The formation of a thrombus in contact with the endocardial lining of a cardiac chamber, or a large blood vessel, if not occlusive.

mu•ral throm•bus (myū′răl throm′bŭs) A thrombus formed on and attached to a diseased patch of endocardium, not on a valve or on one side of a large blood vessel. SEE ALSO parietal thrombus.

mu•ram•i•dase (myū-ram′i-dās) SYN lysozyme.

mu•rine (myūr-ēn′) Relating to animals of the family Muridae. [L. *murinus,* relating to mice, fr. *mus* (*mur-*), a mouse]

mu•rine ty•phus (myūr-ēn′ tī′fŭs) A milder form of epidemic typhus caused by *Rickettsia typhi* and transmitted to humans by fleas from rats or mice. SYN endemic typhus.

mur•mur (mŭr′mŭr) An abnormal, usually periodic sound heard on auscultation of the heart or blood vessels. [L.]

Mur•phy but•ton (mĕr′fē bŭt′ŏn) A device used for intestinal anastomosis; it consists of two round, hollow cylinders that insert into each end of the transected intestine; the intestine is secured to each of the components with a suture and the ends are brought into approximation and the two cylinders joined with a locking mechanism; the apparatus is degradable and within approximately 10 days dissolves and is sloughed into the lumen of the intestine. A modification of an obsolete metal device bearing the same name.

Mur•phy drip (mĕr′fē drip) SYN proctoclysis.

Mur•phy per•cus•sion (mĕr′fē pĕr-kŭsh′ŏn) Examination for dullness by striking the chest wall directly with the fingertips of one hand successively, beginning with the fifth finger.

Mur•phy sign (mĕr′fē sīn) Pain on palpation of the right subcostal area during inspiration frequently associated with acute cholecystitis.

Mur•ray Val•ley en•ceph•a•li•tis (mĕr′ē val′ē en-sef′ă-lī′tis) A severe encephalitis with a high mortality rate occurring in the Murray Valley of Australia; the disease is most severe in children and is characterized by headache, fever, malaise, drowsiness or convulsions, and rigidity of the neck; extensive brain damage may result; it is caused by the Murray Valley encephalitis virus (genus *Flavivirus*). SYN Australian X disease.

Mus•ca (mŭs′kă) A genus of flies that includes the common housefly, *Musca domestica;* it breeds in filth and organic waste; involved in the mechanical transfer of numerous pathogens. [L. fly]

mus•cae vol•i•tan•tes (mŭs′kē vol-i-tan′tēz) Floaters; Appearance of moving spots before the eyes, arising from remnants of the embryologic hyaloid vascular system in the vitreous humor. [L. pl. of *musca,* fly; pres. ppl. of *volito,* to fly to and fro]

mus•ca•rine (mŭs′kă-rēn) A toxin with neurologic effects, first isolated from *Amanita muscaria* (fly agaric) and also present in some species of *Hebeloma* and *Inocybe*. It is a cholinergic substance with pharmacologic effects that include cardiac inhibition, vasodilation, salivation, lacrimation, bronchoconstriction, and gastrointestinal stimulation.

mus•ca•rin•ic (mŭs-kă-rin′ik) **1.** Having a muscarinelike action, i.e., producing effects that resemble postganglionic parasympathetic stimulation. **2.** An agent that stimulates the postganglionic parasympathetic receptor. SEE ALSO muscarine, nicotinic.

mus•cle (mŭs′ĕl) A primary tissue, consisting predominantly of highly specialized contractile cells, which may be classified as skeletal muscle, cardiac muscle, or smooth muscle; microscopically, the latter is lacking in transverse striations characteristic of the other two types; one of the contractile organs of the body by which movements of the various organs and parts are effected; typical musculus is a mass of musculus fibers (venter or belly), attached at each extremity, by means of a tendon, to a bone or other structure; the more proximal or more fixed attachment is called the *origin*, the more distal or more movable attachment is the *insertion;* the narrowing part of the belly that is attached to the tendon of origin is called the caput or head. For gross anatomic description, SEE musculus. SYN musculus. [L. *musculus*]

mus•cle-bound (mŭs′ĕl-bownd) Denoting a condition in which individual muscles are overdeveloped but dyssynergic in concerted action.

mus•cle con•trac•tion head•ache (mŭs′ĕl kŏn-trak′shŭn hed′āk) SYN tension headache.

mus•cle en•er•gy tech•nique (MET) (mŭs′ĕl en′ĕr-jē tek-nēk′) A massage therapy modality that works to adjust proprioceptive activity and levels of resting tension through stretches and muscle contraction with resistance. SEE ALSO proprioceptive neuromuscular facilitation. SYN strain-counterstrain.

mus•cle fa•tigue (mus′ĕl fă-tēg′) A state of exhaustion or loss of strength and/or muscle endurance following strenuous activity associated with the accumulation of lactic acid in muscles.

mus•cle fi•ber (mŭs′ĕl fī′bĕr) Classification of muscle fiber is based on contractile and metabolic characteristics. Slow-twitch (type I) fibers contract slowly and develop relatively low tension; they display high oxidative and low glycolytic capacity associated with endurance performance. Fast-twitch (type II) fibers have rapid speed of activation and develop high tension; they display low oxidative and high glycolytic capacity associated with strength and power performance.

mus•cle of heart (mŭs′ĕl hahrt) SYN cardiac muscle.

mus•cle he•mo•glo•bin (mŭs′ĕl hē′mō-glō-bin) SYN myoglobin.

mus•cle plate (mŭs′ĕl plāt) SYN myotome (2).

mus•cles of au•di•to•ry os•si•cles (mŭs′ĕlz aw′di-tōr-ē ŏs′i-kĕlz) The musculus stapedius and musculus tensor tympani.

mus•cle se•rum (mŭs′ĕl sēr′ŭm) The fluid remaining after the coagulation of muscle plasma and the separation of myosin.

mus•cles of head (mŭs′ĕlz hed) The muscles of expression, of mastication, and the suboccipital muscles in general. See this page.

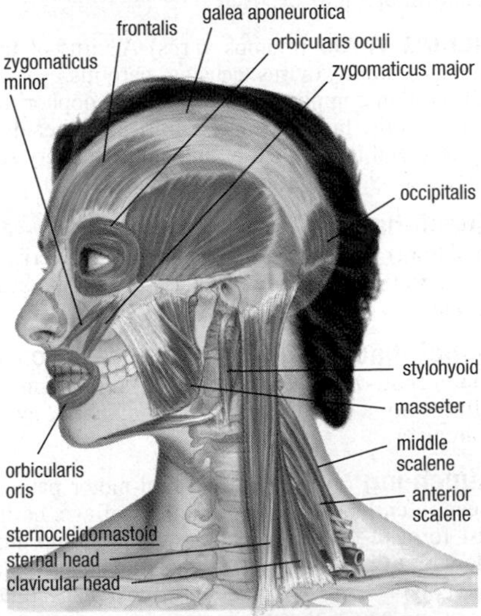

muscles of the head

mus•cles of lar•ynx (mŭs′ĕlz lar′ingks) The intrinsic muscles that regulate the length, position and tension of the vocal cords and adjust the size of the openings between the aryepiglottic folds, the ventricular folds, and the vocal folds. SYN musculi laryngis [TA].

mus•cle-spar•ing thor•a•cot•omy (mŭs′ĕl-spār′ing thōr-ă-kot′ō-mē) Any type of thoracotomy that does not involve significant division of the latissimus dorsi muscle and the serratus anterior muscle.

mus•cle spasm (mŭs′ĕl spazm) SYN spasm.

mus•cle spin•dle (mŭs′ĕl spin′dĕl) SYN neuromuscular spindle. SEE ALSO muscle spindle reflex.

mus•cle spin•dle re•flex (mŭs′ĕl spin′dĕl rē′fleks) SYN myotactic reflex. SEE ALSO neuromuscular spindle.

mus•cle tone (mŭs′ĕl tōn) **1.** The internal state of muscle-fiber tension within individual muscles and muscle groups. **2.** Degree of muscle tension or resistance during rest or in response to stretching. SEE ALSO hypertonia, hypotonia (3).

mus•cle of tra•gus (mŭs′ĕl trā′gŭs) SYN tragicus muscle.

mus•cle of u•vu•la (mŭs′ĕl yū′vyū-lă) SYN uvular muscle.

mus•cu•lar (mŭs′kyū-lăr) **1.** Relating to a muscle or the muscles. **2.** Having well-developed musculature.

mus•cu•lar as•the•no•pi•a (mŭs′kyū-lăr as′thĕ-nō′pē-ă) Asthenopia due to imbalance of the extrinsic ocular muscles.

mus•cu•lar at•ro•phy (mŭs′kyū-lăr at′rŏ-fē) Wasting of muscular tissue.

mus•cu•lar coat (mŭs′kyū-lăr kōt) The muscular, usually middle, layer of a tubular structure; for most of the gastrointestinal tract, it consists of an outer longitudinal layer of muscle and an inner circular layer.

mus•cu•lar dys•tro•phy (mŭs′kyū-lăr dis′trŏ-fē) A general term for a number of hereditary, progressive degenerative disorders affecting skeletal muscles, and often other organ systems as well. SYN myodystrophy, myodystrophia.

mus•cu•lar en•du•rance (mŭs′kyū-lăr en-dūr′ăns) Ability of muscles to exert tension over an extended period.

mus•cu•la•ris (mŭs-kyū-lā′ris) The muscular coat of a hollow organ or tubular structure. [Mod. L. muscular]

mus•cu•la•ris mu•co•sae (mŭs-kyū-lā′ris myū-kō′sē) The thin layer of smooth muscle found in most parts of the digestive tube located outside the lamina propria mucosae and adjacent to the tela submucosa.

mus•cu•lar•i•ty (mŭs′kyū-lar′i-tē) The state or condition of having well-developed muscles.

mus•cu•lar pow•er (mŭs′kyū-lăr pow′ĕr) Ability of muscles to produce force in or at a given time.

mus•cu•lar re•lax•ant (mŭs′kyū-lăr rē-laks′ănt) An agent that relaxes striated muscle; includes drugs acting at the brain or spinal cord level or directly on muscle; also called muscle relaxant.

mus•cu•lar sense (mŭs′kyū-lăr sens) SYN myesthesia.

mus•cu•lar strength train•ing (mus′kyū-lăr strength trān′ing) SYN strength training.

mus•cu•lar tis•sue (mŭs′kyū-lăr tish′ū) A tissue characterized by the ability to contract upon stimulation; its three varieties are skeletal, cardiac, and smooth. SEE muscle. SYN flesh (2).

mus•cu•lar tri•an•gle (mŭs′kyū-lăr trī′ang-gĕl) The triangle bounded by the sternocleidomastoid muscle, the superior belly of the omohyoid muscle, and the anterior midline of the neck; the infrahyoid muscles occupy most of it. SYN trigonum musculare [TA].

mus•cu•la•ture (mŭs′kyū-lă-chŭr) The arrangement of the muscles in a part or in the body as a whole.

mus•cu•li ar•rec•to•res pi•lo•rum (mŭs′kyū-lī ă-rek-tō′rēz pī-lō′rum) [TA] SYN arrector muscle of hair.

mus•cu•li in•ter•os•se•i (mŭs′kyū-lī in′tĕr-os′ē-ī) SYN interosseous muscles.

mus•cu•li in•ter•os•se•i dor•sal•es ma•nus (mŭs′kyū-lī in′tĕr-os′ē-ī dōr-sā′lēz mā′nŭs) SYN dorsal interossei (interosseous muscles) of hand.

mus•cu•li in•ter•os•se•i dor•sa•les pe•dis (mŭs′kyū-lī in′tĕr-os′ē-ī dōr-sā′lēz ped′is) SYN dorsal interossei (interosseous muscles) of foot.

mus•cu•li in•ter•spi•na•les (mŭs′kyū-lī in′tĕr-spī-nā′lēz) [TA] SYN interspinales muscles.

mus•cu•li in•ter•trans•ver•sa•ri•i (mŭs′kyū-lī in′tĕr-trans-vĕr-sā′rē-ī) [TA] SYN intertransversarii muscles.

mus•cu•li la•ryn•gis (mŭs′kyū-lī lar-in′jis) [TA] SYN muscles of larynx.

mus•cu•li lev•a•to•res cos•tar•um (mŭs′kyū-lī lev-a-tō′rēz kos-tā′rŭm) SYN levator costarum muscles.

mus•cu•li pec•ti•na•ti (mŭs′kyū-lī pek′ti-nā′tī) [TA] SYN pectinate muscles.

mus•cu•li ro•ta•to•res (mŭs′kyū-lī rō-tă-tō′rēz) [TA] SYN rotatores muscles.

mus•cu•li sub•oc•cip•i•ta•les (mŭs′kyū-lī sub′ok-sip-i-tā′lēz) SYN suboccipital muscles.

mus•cu•lo•ap•o•neu•rot•ic (mŭs′kyū-lō-ap′ō-nūr-ot′ik) Relating to muscular tissue and an aponeurosis of origin or insertion.

mus•cu•lo•cu•ta•ne•ous (mŭs′kyū-lō-kyū-tā′

nē-ŭs) Relating to both muscle and skin. SYN myocutaneous.

mus·cu·lo·cu·ta·ne·ous nerve (mŭs′kyū-lō-kyū-tā′nē-ŭs nĕrv) Arises from lateral cord of the brachial plexus, passes through the coracobrachialis muscle, and then downward between the brachialis and biceps, supplying these three muscles and being prolonged as the lateral cutaneous nerve of the forearm. SYN nervus musculocutaneus [TA].

mus·cu·lo·cu·ta·ne·ous nerve of leg (mŭs′kyū-lō-kyū-tā′nē-ŭs nĕrv leg) SYN superficial fibular nerve.

mus·cu·lo·mem·bra·nous (mŭs′kyū-lō-mem′bră-nŭs) Relating to both muscular tissue and membrane; denoting certain muscles, such as the occipitofrontalis, that are largely membranous.

mus·cu·lo·phren·ic ar·ter·y (mŭs′kyū-lō-fren′ik ahr′tĕr-ē) *Origin*, the lateral terminal branch of internal thoracic; *distribution*, diaphragm and intercostal muscles; *anastomoses*, branches of pericardiacophrenic, inferior phrenic, and posterior intercostal arteries. SYN arteria musculophrenica [TA].

mus·cu·lo·phren·ic veins (mŭs′kyū-lō-fren′ik vānz) Accompany the musculophrenic artery and drain blood from the upper abdominal wall and anterior portions of the lower intercostal spaces and the diaphragm.

mus·cu·lo·skel·e·tal (mŭs′kyū-lō-skel′ĕ-tăl) Relating to muscles and to the skeleton, as, for example, the musculoskeletal system.

mus·cu·lo·spi·ral pa·ral·y·sis (mŭs′kyū-lō-spī′răl păr-al′i-sis) Paralysis of the muscles of the forearm due to injury of the radial (musculospiral) nerve.

mus·cu·lo·ten·di·nous (mŭs′kyū-lō-ten′di-nŭs) Relating to both muscular and tendinous tissues.

mus·cu·lo·tro·pic (mŭs′kyū-lō-trō′pik) Affecting, acting on, or attracted to muscular tissue.

mus·cu·lo·tu·bal ca·nal (mŭs′kyū-lō-tū′băl kă-nal′) A canal beginning at the anterior border of the petrous portion of the temporal bone near its junction with the squamous portion, and passing to the tympanic cavity; it is divided by the cochleariform process into two semicanals: one for the auditory (eustachian) tube, the other for the tensor tympani muscle. SYN canalis musculotubarius [TA].

mus·cu·lus, gen. and pl. **mus·cu·li** (mŭs′kyū-lŭs, -lī) SYN muscle. [L. a little mouse, a muscle, fr. *mus* (*mur-*), a mouse]

mus·cu·lus ab·duc·tor hal·lu·cis (mŭs′kyū-lŭs ab-duk′tōr hal′ū-sis) [TA] SYN abductor hallucis muscle.

mus·cu·lus ab·duc·tor pol·li·cis brev·is (mŭs′kyū-lŭs ab-duk′tōr pol′i-sis brev′is) SYN abductor pollicis brevis muscle.

mus·cu·lus ab·duc·tor pol·li·cis lon·gus (mŭs′kyū-lŭs ab-duk′tōr pol′i-sis long′gŭs) SYN abductor pollicis longus muscle.

mus·cu·lus ad·duc·tor brev·is (mŭs′kyū-lŭs ad-duk′tōr brev′is) [TA] SYN adductor brevis muscle.

mus·cu·lus ad·duc·tor hal·lu·cis (mŭs′kyū-lŭs ad-duk′tōr hal′ū-sis) [TA] SYN adductor hallucis muscle.

mus·cu·lus ad·duc·tor lon·gus (mŭs′kyū-lŭs ad-duk′tōr long′gus) [TA] SYN adductor longus muscle.

mus·cu·lus ad·duc·tor mag·nus (mŭs′kyū-lŭs ad-duk′tōr mag′nŭs) [TA] SYN adductor magnus muscle.

mus·cu·lus ad·duc·tor min·i·mus (mŭs′kyū-lŭs ad-duk′tōr min′ē-mus) SYN adductor minimus muscle.

mus·cu·lus ad·duc·tor pol·li·cis (mŭs′kyū-lŭs ad-duk′tōr pol′i-sis) [TA] SYN adductor pollicis muscle.

mus·cu·lus an·co·ne·us (mŭs′kyū-lŭs an-kō′nē-us) [TA] SYN anconeus muscle.

mus·cu·lus an·ti·trag·i·cus (mŭs′kyū-lŭs an-tī′traj′i-kus) [TA] SYN antitragicus muscle.

mus·cu·lus ar·ti·cu·la·ris cu·bi·ti (mŭs′kyū-lŭs ahr-tik′yū-lār′is kyū′bi-tī) [TA] SYN articularis cubiti muscle.

mus·cu·lus ar·ti·cu·la·ris ge·nus (mŭs′kyū-lŭs ahr-tik′yū-lār′is jē′nus) [TA] SYN articularis genus muscle.

mus·cu·lus ar·y·ep·i·glot·ti·cus (mŭs′kyū-lŭs ar-ē-ep-i-glot′i-kŭs) [TA] SYN aryepiglottic muscle.

mus·cu·lus at·tol·lens au·rem, **mus·cu·lus at·tol·lens au·ric·u·lam** (mŭs′kyū-lŭs at-tol′enz aw′rem, aw-rik′yū-lam) SYN auricularis superior muscle.

mus·cu·lus at·tra·hens au·rem, **mus·cu·lus at·tra·hens au·ric·u·lam** (mŭs′kū-lŭs at′ră-henz awr′em, awr′ik′yū-lam) SYN anterior auricular muscle.

mus·cu·lus au·ric·u·lar·is an·te·ri·or (mŭs′kyū-lŭs aw-rik′yū-lā′ris an-tēr′ē-ŏr) SYN auricularis anterior muscle.

mus·cu·lus au·ric·u·lar·is pos·te·ri·or (mŭs′kyū-lŭs aw-rik′yū-lā′ris pos-tēr′ē-ŏr) SYN auricularis posterior muscle.

mus·cu·lus au·ric·u·lar·is su·pe·ri·or (mŭs′kyū-lŭs aw-rik′yū-lā′ris sŭ-pēr′ē-ŏr) SYN auricularis superior muscle.

mus•cu•lus bi•ceps bra•chi•i (mŭs′kyū-lŭs bī′seps brāk′ē-ī) [TA] SYN biceps brachii muscle.

mus•cu•lus bi•ceps fem•o•ris (mŭs′kyū-lŭs bī′seps fem′ō-ris) [TA] SYN biceps femoris muscle.

mus•cu•lus bra•chi•a•lis (mŭs′kyū-lŭs brāk′ē-ā′lis) [TA] SYN brachialis muscle.

mus•cu•lus bra•chi•o•ra•di•a•lis (mŭs′kyū-lŭs brā′kē-ō-rā-dē-ā′lis) [TA] SYN brachioradialis muscle.

mus•cu•lus buc•ci•na•tor (mŭs′kyū-lŭs buk-sin-ā′tōr) [TA] SYN buccinator muscle.

mus•cu•lus bul•bo•ca•ver•no•sus (mŭs′kyū-lŭs bul′bō-kav-ĕr-nō′sŭs) SYN bulbospongiosus muscle.

mus•cu•lus bul•bo•spon•gi•o•sus (mŭs′kyū-lŭs bul′bō-spon-jē-ō′sŭs) SYN bulbospongiosus muscle.

mus•cu•lus cap•i•tis pos•te•ri•or ma•jor (mŭs′kyū-lŭs kap′i-tis pos-tēr′ē-ŏr mā′jōr) [TA] SYN rectus capitis posterior major muscle.

mus•cu•lus cer•a•to•cri•coi•de•us (mŭs′kyū-lŭs ser′ă-tō-kri-koy′dē-ŭs) [TA] SYN ceratocricoid muscle.

mus•cu•lus cil•i•ar•is (mŭs′kyū-lŭs sil′ē-ā′ris) [TA] SYN ciliary muscle.

mus•cu•lus coc•cyg•e•us (mŭs′kyū-lŭs kok′sij′ē-ŭs) [TA] SYN coccygeus muscle.

mus•cu•lus con•stric•tor phar•yn•gis in•fe•ri•or (mŭs′kyū-lŭs kon-strik′tōr fă-rin′jis in-fēr′ē-ŏr) SYN inferior constrictor muscle of pharynx.

mus•cu•lus con•stric•tor phar•yn•gis su•pe•ri•or (mŭs′kyū-lŭs kon-strik′tōr fă-rin′jis sū-pēr′ē-ŏr) [TA] SYN superior constrictor muscle of pharynx.

mus•cu•lus con•stric•tor u•reth•rae (mŭs′kyū-lŭs kon-strik′tōr yū′rēth′rē) SYN external urethral sphincter muscle.

mus•cu•lus cor•a•co•bra•chi•a•lis (mŭs′kyū-lŭs kōr-a-kō-brāk′ē-ā′lis) [TA] SYN coracobrachialis muscle.

mus•cu•lus cor•ru•ga•tor su•per•ci•li•i (mŭs′kyū-lŭs kōr′ŭ-gā-tōr sū′pĕr-sil′ē-ī) [TA] SYN corrugator supercilii muscle.

mus•cu•lus cre•mas•ter (mŭs′kyū-lŭs krē-mas′tĕr) [TA] SYN cremaster muscle.

mus•cu•lus cri•co•ar•y•te•noid•e•us la•ter•a•lis (mŭs′kyū-lŭs krī′kō-ar′i-tē-noy′dē-ŭs lat′tĕr-ā-lis) SYN lateral cricoarytenoid muscle.

mus•cu•lus cri•co•ar•y•te•noid•e•us pos•te•ri•or (mŭs′kyū-lŭs krī′kō-ar′i-tē-noy′dē-ŭs pos-tēr′ē-ŏr) SYN posterior cricoarytenoid muscle.

mus•cu•lus cri•co•thy•roi•de•us (mŭs′kyū-lŭs krī-kō-thī-royd′ē-ŭs) [TA] SYN cricothyroid muscle.

mus•cu•lus del•toi•de•us (mŭs′kyū-lŭs del-toy′dē-ŭs) [TA] SYN deltoid muscle.

mus•cu•lus de•pres•sor an•gu•li o•ris (mŭs′kyū-lŭs dĕ-pres′ŏr ang′gyū-lī ōr′is) [TA] SYN depressor anguli oris muscle.

mus•cu•lus de•pres•sor la•bi•i in•fe•ri•o•ris (mŭs′kyū-lŭs dĕ-pres′ŏr lā′bē-ī in-fēr′ē-ōr′is) [TA] SYN depressor labii inferioris muscle.

mus•cu•lus de•pres•sor sep•ti (mŭs′kyū-lŭs dĕ-pres′ŏr sep′tī) [TA] SYN depressor septi nasi muscle.

mus•cu•lus de•pres•sor su•per•ci•li•i (mŭs′kyū-lŭs dĕ-pres′ŏr sū′pĕr-sil′ē-ī) [TA] SYN depressor supercilii muscle.

mus•cu•lus di•gas•tri•cus (mŭs′kyū-lŭs dī-gas′trik-us) [TA] SYN digastric muscle (2).

mus•cu•lus di•la•ta•tor pu•pil•lae (mŭs′kyū-lŭs dil′ă-tā-tōr pyū-pil′ē) [TA] SYN dilator pupillae muscle.

mus•cu•lus di•la•ta•tor tu•bae (mŭs′kyū-lŭs dil′ă-tā-tōr tū′bē) [TA] SYN dilator tubae muscle.

mus•cu•lus e•jac•u•la•tor sem•i•nis (mŭs′kyū-lŭs ē-jak-yū-lā′tōr sem′i-nis) SYN bulbospongiosus muscle.

mus•cu•lus ep•i•cra•ni•us (mŭs′kyū-lŭs ep′i-krā′nē-us) [TA] SYN epicranius muscle.

mus•cu•lus e•rec•tor spi•nae (mŭs′kyū-lŭs ē-rek′tōr spī′nē) [TA] SYN erector spinae muscles.

mus•cu•lus ex•ten•sor brev•is pol•li•cis (mŭs′kyū-lŭs eks-ten′sŏr brev′is pol′i-sis) SYN extensor pollicis brevis muscle.

mus•cu•lus ex•ten•sor car•pi ra•di•a•lis brev•is (mŭs′kyū-lŭs eks-ten′sŏr kahr′pī rā-dē-ā′lis brev′is) [TA] SYN extensor carpi radialis brevis muscle.

mus•cu•lus ex•ten•sor car•pi ra•di•a•lis long•us (mŭs′kyū-lŭs eks-ten′sŏr kahr′pī rā-dē-ā′lis long′gus) [TA] SYN extensor carpi radialis longus muscle.

mus•cu•lus ex•ten•sor car•pi ul•na•ris (mŭs′kyū-lŭs eks-ten′sŏr kahr′pī ul-nā′ris) [TA] SYN extensor carpi ulnaris muscle.

mus•cu•lus ex•ten•sor di•gi•ti mi•ni•mi (mŭs′kyū-lŭs eks-ten′sŏr dij′i-tī mi′ni-mī) [TA] SYN extensor digiti minimi muscle.

mus•cu•lus ex•ten•sor di•gi•to•rum (mŭs′kyū-lŭs eks-ten′sŏr dij′i-tō′rŭm) [TA] SYN extensor digitorum muscle.

mus•cu•lus ex•ten•sor di•gi•to•rum brev•is

(mŭs′kyū-lŭs eks-ten′sŏr dij′i-tō′rŭm brev′is) [TA] SYN extensor digitorum brevis muscle.

mus•cu•lus ex•ten•sor di•gi•to•rum com•mu•nis (mŭs′kyū-lŭs eks-ten′sŏr dij′i-tō′rŭm kom′yū-nis) SYN extensor digitorum muscle.

mus•cu•lus ex•ten•sor di•gi•to•rum lon•gus (mŭs′kyū-lŭs eks-ten′sŏr dij′i-tō′rum long′gus) [TA] SYN extensor digitorum longus muscle.

mus•cu•lus ex•ten•sor hal•lu•cis brev•is (mŭs′kyū-lŭs eks-ten′sŏr hal′ū-sis brev′is) [TA] SYN extensor hallucis brevis muscle.

mus•cu•lus ex•ten•sor hal•lu•cis lon•gus (mŭs′kyū-lŭs eks-ten′sŏr hal′ū-sis long′gus) [TA] SYN extensor hallucis longus muscle.

mus•cu•lus ex•ten•sor in•di•cis (mŭs′kyū-lŭs eks-ten′sŏr in′di-sis) [TA] SYN extensor indicis muscle.

mus•cu•lus ex•ten•sor os•sis me•ta•car•pi pol•li•cis (mŭs′kyū-lŭs eks-ten′sŏr os′is met′ă-kahr′pī pol′li-sis) SYN abductor pollicis longus muscle.

mus•cu•lus ex•ten•sor pol•li•cis brev•is (mŭs′kyū-lŭs eks-ten′sŏr pol′i-sis brev′is) SYN extensor pollicis brevis muscle.

mus•cu•lus ex•ten•sor pol•li•cis lon•gus (mŭs′kyū-lŭs eks-ten′sŏr pol′i-sis long′gus) SYN extensor pollicis longus muscle.

mus•cu•lus fib•u•lar•is lon•gus (mŭs′kyū-lŭs fib′yū-lā′ris long′gus) SYN fibularis longus muscle.

mus•cu•lus fib•u•lar•is ter•ti•us (mŭs′kyū-lŭs fib′yū-lā′ris tĕr′shē-ŭs) SYN fibularis tertius muscle.

mus•cu•lus flex•or car•pi ra•di•a•lis (mŭs′kyū-lŭs fleks′ōr kahr′pī rā-dē-ā′lis) [TA] SYN flexor carpi radialis muscle.

mus•cu•lus flex•or car•pi ul•na•ris (mŭs′kyū-lŭs fleks′ōr kahr′pī ŭl-nā′ris) [TA] SYN flexor carpi ulnaris muscle.

mus•cu•lus flex•or di•gi•ti mi•ni•mi brev•is ma•nus (mŭs′kyū-lŭs fleks′ōr dij′i-tī mi′ni-mī brev′is man′ŭs) [TA] SYN flexor digiti minimi brevis muscle of hand.

mus•cu•lus flex•or di•gi•ti mi•ni•mi brev•is pe•dis (mŭs′kyū-lŭs fleks′ōr dij′i-tī mi′ni-mī brev′is ped′is) [TA] SYN flexor digiti minimi brevis muscle of foot.

mus•cu•lus flex•or di•gi•to•rum brev•is (mŭs′kyū-lŭs fleks′ōr dij′i-tō′rŭm brev′is) [TA] SYN flexor digitorum brevis muscle.

mus•cu•lus flex•or di•gi•to•rum lon•gus (mŭs′kyū-lŭs fleks′ōr dij′i-tō′rŭm long′gus) [TA] SYN flexor digitorum longus muscle.

mus•cu•lus flex•or di•gi•to•rum pro•fun•dus (mŭs′kyū-lŭs fleks′ōr dij′i-tō′rŭm prō-fŭnd′dŭs) [TA] SYN flexor digitorum profundus muscle.

mus•cu•lus flex•or di•gi•to•rum su•per•fi•ci•a•lis (mŭs′kyū-lŭs fleks′ōr dij′i-tō′rŭm sū′pĕr-fish′ē-ā′lis) [TA] SYN flexor digitorum superficialis muscle.

mus•cu•lus gas•troc•ne•mi•us (mŭs′kyū-lŭs gas-trok-nē′mē-ŭs) [TA] SYN gastrocnemius muscle.

mus•cu•lus ge•mel•lus in•fe•ri•or (mŭs′kyū-lŭs je-mel′ŭs in-fēr′ē-ŏr) SYN inferior gemellus muscle.

mus•cu•lus ge•mel•lus su•pe•ri•or (mŭs′kyū-lŭs je-mel′ŭs sŭ-pēr′ē-ŏr) SYN superior gemellus muscle.

mus•cu•lus ge•ni•o•glos•sus (mŭs′kyū-lŭs jē′nē-ō-glos′ŭs) [TA] SYN genioglossus muscle.

mus•cu•lus ge•ni•o•hy•o•glos•sus (mŭs′kyū-lŭs jē′nē-ō-hī-ō-glos′ŭs) SYN genioglossus muscle.

mus•cu•lus ge•ni•o•hy•oi•de•us (mŭs′kyū-lŭs jē′nē-ō-hī-oyd′ē-ŭs) [TA] SYN geniohyoid muscle.

mus•cu•lus glu•te•us max•i•mus (mŭs′kyū-lŭs glū′tē-us maks′si-mŭs) [TA] SYN gluteus maximus muscle.

mus•cu•lus glu•te•us me•di•us (mŭs′kyū-lŭs glū′tē-us mē′dē-ŭs) [TA] SYN gluteus medius muscle.

mus•cu•lus glu•te•us mi•ni•mus (mŭs′kyū-lŭs glū′tē-us min′i-mŭs) [TA] SYN gluteus minimus muscle.

mus•cu•lus grac•i•lis (mŭs′kyū-lŭs grā′sil-is) [TA] SYN gracilis muscle.

mus•cu•lus hy•o•glos•sus (mŭs′kyū-lŭs hī′ō-glos′ŭs) [TA] SYN hyoglossus muscle.

mus•cu•lus il•i•a•cus (mŭs′kyū-lŭs il′ē-ā′kŭs) [TA] SYN iliacus muscle.

mus•cu•lus il•i•o•coc•cyg•e•us (mŭs′kyū-lŭs il′ē-ō-kok′sij′ē-ŭs) [TA] SYN iliococcygeus muscle.

mus•cu•lus il•i•o•cos•ta•lis (mŭs′kyū-lŭs il′ē-ō-kos-tā′lis) [TA] SYN iliocostalis muscle.

mus•cu•lus il•i•o•pso•as (mŭs′kyū-lŭs il′ē-ō-sō′as) [TA] SYN iliopsoas muscle.

mus•cu•lus in•fra•spi•na•tus (mŭs′kyū-lŭs in′fră-spī-nā′tŭs) [TA] SYN infraspinatus muscle.

mus•cu•lus in•ter•cos•ta•lis ex•ter•nus (mŭs′kyū-lŭs in′tĕr-kos-tā′lis eks-ter′nŭs) SYN external intercostal muscle.

mus•cu•lus in•ter•cos•ta•lis in•ti•mus (mŭs′kyū-lŭs in′tĕr-kos-tā′lis in′ti-mŭs) SYN innermost intercostal muscle.

mus·cu·lus in·ter·os·se·us pal·mar·is, pl. **mus·cu·li in·ter·os·se·i pal·ma·res** (mŭs′kyū-lŭs in′ter-os′sē-ŭs pal-mā′ris, mŭs′kyū-lī in′tĕr-os′ē-ī pal-mā′rēz) [TA] SYN palmar interosseous muscle.

mus·cu·lus in·ter·os·se·us plan·tar·is, pl. **mus·cu·li in·ter·os·se·i plan·tar·es** (mŭs′kyū-lŭs in′ter-os′sē-ŭs plan-tā′ris, mŭs′kyū-lī in′tĕr-os′ē-ī plan-tā′rēz) [TA] SYN plantar interosseous muscle.

mus·cu·lus is·chi·o·cav·er·no·sus (mŭs′kyū-lŭs is-kē-ō-kav-ĕr-nō′sŭs) [TA] SYN ischiocavernous muscle.

mus·cu·lus is·chi·o·coc·cy·ge·us (mŭs′kyū-lŭs is-kē-ō-kok-sij′ē-us) SYN coccygeus muscle.

mus·cu·lus la·ryn·go·pha·ryn·ge·us (mŭs′kyū-lŭs lă-ring′gō-fă-rin′jē-us) SYN inferior constrictor muscle of pharynx.

mus·cu·lus la·tis·si·mus dor·si (mŭs′kyū-lŭs lă-tē′si-mŭs dōr′sī) [TA] SYN latissimus dorsi muscle.

mus·cu·lus le·va·tor an·gu·li o·ris (mŭs′kyū-lŭs le-vā′tōr ang′gyū-lī ō′ris) [TA] SYN levator anguli oris muscle.

mus·cu·lus le·va·tor a·ni (mŭs′kyū-lŭs le-vā′tōr ā′nī) [TA] SYN levator ani muscle.

mus·cu·lus le·va·tor glan·du·lae thy·roi·de·ae (mŭs′kyū-lŭs le-vā′tōr glan′dyū-lē thī-royd′ē-ē) [TA] SYN levator muscle of thyroid gland.

mus·cu·lus le·va·tor la·bi·i su·pe·ri·o·ris (mŭs′kyū-lŭs le-vā′tōr lā′bē-ī sū-pēr′ē-ōr′is) [TA] SYN levator labii superioris muscle.

mus·cu·lus le·va·tor la·bi·i su·pe·ri·o·ris a·lae·que na·si (mŭs′kyū-lŭs le-vā′tōr lā′bē-ī sū-pēr′ē-ō′ris ā-lē′kwā nā′sī) [TA] SYN levator labii superioris alaeque nasi muscle.

mus·cu·lus le·va·tor pal·pe·brae su·pe·ri·o·ris (mŭs′kyū-lŭs le-vā′tōr pal-pē′brē sū-pēr′ē-ōr′is) [TA] SYN levator palpebrae superioris muscle.

mus·cu·lus le·va·tor pro·sta·tae (mŭs′kyū-lŭs le-vā′tōr pros-tā′tē) [TA] SYN levator prostatae muscle.

mus·cu·lus le·va·tor scap·u·lae (mŭs′kyū-lŭs le-vā′tōr skap′yū-lē) [TA] SYN levator scapulae muscle.

mus·cu·lus le·va·tor ve·li pa·la·ti·ni (mŭs′kyū-lŭs le-vā′tōr vē′lī pal-ă-tē′nī) [TA] SYN levator veli palatini muscle.

mus·cu·lus lon·gis·si·mus ca·pi·tis (mŭs′kyū-lŭs lon-jē-sē-mŭs kap′i-tis) [TA] SYN longissimus capitis muscle.

mus·cu·lus lon·gis·si·mus cer·vi·cis (mŭs′kyū-lŭs lon-jē-sē-mŭs ser-vī′sis) [TA] SYN longissimus cervicis muscle.

mus·cu·lus lon·gis·si·mus tho·ra·cis (mŭs′kyū-lŭs lon-jē-sē-mŭs thō-rā′sis) [TA] SYN longissimus thoracis muscle.

mus·cu·lus lon·gi·tu·di·na·lis in·fe·ri·or lin·guae (mŭs′kyū-lŭs lon-ji-tū-di-nā′lis in-fēr′ē-ōr ling′gwē) SYN inferior longitudinal muscle of tongue.

mus·cu·lus lon·gi·tu·di·na·lis su·pe·ri·or lin·guae (mŭs′kyū-lŭs lon-ji-tū-di-nā′lis sŭ-pēr′ē-ōr ling′gwē) SYN superior longitudinal muscle of tongue.

mus·cu·lus lon·gus ca·pi·tis (mŭs′kyū-lŭs long′gŭs kap′i-tis) [TA] SYN longus capitis muscle.

mus·cu·lus lon·gus col·li (mŭs′kyū-lŭs long′gŭs kol′ī) [TA] SYN longus colli muscle.

mus·cu·lus lum·bri·ca·lis ma·nus, pl. **mus·cu·li lum·bri·ca·les ma·nus** (mŭs′kyū-lŭs lum-bri-kā′lis mā′nŭs, mŭs′kyū-lī lum-brik-ā′lēz mā′nŭs) [TA] SYN lumbrical muscles of hand.

mus·cu·lus lum·bri·ca·lis pe·dis, pl. **mus·cu·li lum·bri·ca·les pe·dis** (mŭs′kyū-lŭs lum-bri-kā′lis ped′is, mŭs′kyū-lī lum-brik-ā′lēz ped′is) [TA] SYN lumbrical muscles of foot.

mus·cu·lus mas·se·ter (mŭs′kyū-lŭs mas′ē-tĕr) [TA] SYN masseter muscle.

mus·cu·lus men·ta·lis (mŭs′kyū-lŭs men-tā′lis) [TA] SYN mentalis muscle.

mus·cu·lus mul·tif·i·dus (mŭs′kyū-lŭs mŭl-ti-fī′dŭs) [TA] SYN multifidus muscle.

mus·cu·lus mul·ti·fi·dus lum·bo·rum (mŭs′kyū-lŭs mŭl-ti-fī′dŭs lum-bō′rŭm) [TA] SYN multifidus muscle.

mus·cu·lus my·lo·hy·oi·de·us (mŭs′kyū-lŭs mī′lō-hī-oy′dē-ŭs) [TA] SYN mylohyoid muscle.

mus·cu·lus na·sa·lis (mŭs′kyū-lŭs nā-sā′lis) [TA] SYN nasalis muscle.

mus·cu·lus ob·li·qu·us ca·pi·tis in·fe·ri·or (mŭs′kyū-lŭs ō-blik′yū-ŭs kap′i-tis in-fēr′ē-ŏr) SYN obliquus capitis inferior muscle.

mus·cu·lus ob·li·qu·us ca·pi·tis su·pe·ri·or (mŭs′kyū-lŭs ō-blik′yū-ŭs kap′i-tis sŭ-pēr′ē-ŏr) SYN obliquus capitis superior muscle.

mus·cu·lus ob·li·qu·us ex·ter·nus ab·do·mi·nis (mŭs′kyū-lŭs ō-blik′yū-ŭs eks-ter′nŭs ab-dom′i-nis) [TA] SYN external oblique muscle.

mus·cu·lus ob·li·qu·us in·fe·ri·or (mŭs′kyū-lŭs ō-blik′yū-ŭs in-fēr′ē-ŏr) [TA] SYN inferior oblique muscle.

mus·cu·lus ob·li·qu·us in·ter·nus ab·do·

mi•nis (mŭs′kyū-lŭs ō-blik′yū-ŭs in-ter′nŭs ab-dom′i-nis) [TA] SYN internal oblique muscle.

mus•cu•lus ob•li•qu•us su•pe•ri•or (mŭs′kyū-lŭs ō-blik′yū-ŭs sŭ-pēr′ē-ōr) [TA] SYN superior oblique muscle.

mus•cu•lus ob•tu•ra•tor•i•us ex•ter•nus (mŭs′kyū-lŭs ob-tū-rā-tō′rē-ŭs eks-ter′nŭs) [TA] SYN obturator externus muscle.

mus•cu•lus ob•tu•ra•tor•i•us in•ter•nus (mŭs′kyū-lŭs ob-tū-rā-tō′rē-ŭs in-ter′nŭs) [TA] SYN obturator internus muscle.

mus•cu•lus oc•cip•i•to•fron•ta•lis (mŭs′kyū-lŭs ok-sip′i-tō-fron-tā′lis) [TA] SYN occipitofrontalis muscle.

mus•cu•lus o•mo•hy•oi•de•us (mŭs′kyū-lŭs ō′mō-hī-oy′dē-ŭs) [TA] SYN omohyoid muscle.

mus•cu•lus op•po•nens di•gi•ti mi•ni•mi (mŭs′kyū-lŭs ō-pō′nenz dij′i-tī mi′ni-mī) [TA] SYN opponens digiti minimi muscle.

mus•cu•lus op•po•nens pol•li•cis (mŭs′kyū-lŭs ō-pō′nenz pol′li-sis) [TA] SYN opponens pollicis muscle.

mus•cu•lus or•bi•cu•la•ris oc•u•li (mŭs′kyū-lŭs ōr-bik′yū-lā′ris ok′yū-lī) [TA] SYN orbicularis oculi muscle.

mus•cu•lus or•bi•cu•la•ris o•ris (mŭs′kyū-lŭs ōr-bik′yū-lā′ris ō′ris) [TA] SYN orbicularis oris muscle.

mus•cu•lus or•bi•ta•lis (mŭs′kyū-lŭs ōr′bi-tā′lis) [TA] SYN orbitalis muscle.

mus•cu•lus pal•a•to•glos•sus (mŭs′kyū-lŭs pal-a-tō-glos′ŭs) [TA] SYN palatoglossus muscle.

mus•cu•lus pal•a•to•pha•ryn•ge•us (mŭs′kyū-lŭs pal-ă-tō-fă-rin′jē-ŭs) [TA] SYN palatopharyngeus muscle.

mus•cu•lus pal•ma•ris brev•is (mŭs′kyū-lŭs pal-mā′ris brev′is) SYN palmaris brevis muscle.

mus•cu•lus pal•mar•is lon•gus (mŭs′kyū-lŭs pal-mā′ris long′gus) SYN palmaris longus muscle.

mus•cu•lus pa•pil•la•ris (mŭs′kyū-lŭs pa-pi-lā′ris) [TA] SYN papillary muscle.

mus•cu•lus pec•ti•ne•us (mŭs′kyū-lŭs pek-tin′ē-ŭs) [TA] SYN pectineus muscle.

mus•cu•lus pec•to•ral•is ma•jor (mŭs′kyū-lŭs pek′tōr-ā′lis mā′jōr) SYN pectoralis major muscle.

mus•cu•lus pec•to•ral•is mi•nor (mŭs′kyū-lŭs pek′tōr-ā′lis mī′nŏr) SYN pectoralis minor muscle.

mus•cu•lus pe•ro•ne•us lon•gus (mŭs′kyū-lŭs per-ō-nē′ŭs long′gŭs) SYN fibularis longus muscle.

mus•cu•lus pe•ro•ne•us ter•ti•us (mŭs′kyū-lŭs per-ō-nē′ŭs ter′shē-ŭs) SYN fibularis tertius muscle.

mus•cu•lus pi•ri•for•mis (mŭs′kyū-lŭs pir′i-fōr′mis) [TA] SYN piriformis muscle.

mus•cu•lus plan•tar•is (mŭs′kyū-lŭs plan-tā′ris) [TA] SYN plantaris muscle.

mus•cu•lus pleu•ro•e•so•pha•ge•us (mŭs′kyū-lŭs plū′rō-ē-sō-fā′jē-ŭs) [TA] SYN pleuroesophageal muscle.

mus•cu•lus pop•lit•e•us (mŭs′kyū-lŭs pop-li′tē-ŭs) [TA] SYN popliteus muscle.

mus•cu•lus pro•ce•rus (mŭs′kyū-lŭs prō-sē′rŭs) [TA] SYN procerus muscle.

mus•cu•lus pro•na•tor quad•ra•tus (mŭs′kyū-lŭs prō′nā-tōr kwahd-rā′tŭs) [TA] SYN pronator quadratus muscle.

mus•cu•lus pro•na•tor te•res (mŭs′kyū-lŭs prō′nā-tōr tē′rēz) [TA] SYN pronator teres muscle.

mus•cu•lus pso•as ma•jor (mŭs′kyū-lŭs sō′as mā′jŏr) SYN psoas major muscle.

mus•cu•lus pso•as mi•nor (mŭs′kyū-lŭs sō′as mī′nŏr) SYN psoas minor muscle.

mus•cu•lus pte•ry•goi•de•us ex•ter•nus (mŭs′kyū-lŭs ter-i-goy′dē-ŭs eks-ter′nŭs) SYN lateral pterygoid muscle.

mus•cu•lus pte•ry•goi•de•us in•ter•nus (mŭs′kyū-lŭs ter-i-goy′dē-ŭs in-ter′nŭs) SYN medial pterygoid muscle.

mus•cu•lus pte•ry•goi•de•us lat•e•ra•lis (mŭs′kyū-lŭs ter-i-goy′dē-ŭs lat′tĕr-ā′lis) SYN lateral pterygoid muscle.

mus•cu•lus pte•ry•goi•de•us me•di•a•lis (mŭs′kyū-lŭs ter-i-goy′dē-ŭs mē-dē-ā′lis) SYN medial pterygoid muscle.

mus•cu•lus pu•bo•coc•cy•ge•us (mŭs′kyū-lŭs pyū′bō-kok-sij′ē-ŭs) [TA] SYN pubococcygeus muscle.

mus•cu•lus pu•bo•pros•ta•ti•cus (mŭs′kyū-lŭs pyū′bō-pros-tat′i-kŭs) [TA] SYN puboprostatic muscle.

mus•cu•lus pu•bo•rec•ta•lis (mŭs′kyū-lŭs pyū′bō-rek-tā′lis) [TA] SYN puborectalis muscle.

mus•cu•lus pu•bo•va•gi•na•lis (mŭs′kyū-lŭs pyū′bō-vaj-i-nā′lis) [TA] SYN pubovaginalis muscle.

mus•cu•lus pu•bo•ve•si•ca•lis (mŭs′kyū-lŭs pyū′bō-ves-i-kā′lis) [TA] SYN pubovesicalis muscle.

mus•cu•lus py•ra•mi•da•lis (mŭs′kyū-lŭs pir-ā-mi-dā′lis) [TA] SYN pyramidalis muscle.

mus•cu•lus py•ra•mi•da•lis au•ric•u•lae

(mŭs′kyū-lŭs pir-ā-mi-dā′lis aw-rik′yū-lē) [TA] SYN pyramidal auricular muscle.

mus•cu•lus quad•ra•tus fem•o•ris (mŭs′kyū-lŭs kwahd-rā′tŭs fem′ō-ris) [TA] SYN quadratus femoris muscle.

mus•cu•lus quad•ra•tus la•bi•i su•pe•ri•o•ris (mŭs′kyū-lŭs kwahd-rā′tŭs lā′bē-ī sū-pēr′ē-ō′ris) SYN quadratus labii superioris muscle.

mus•cu•lus quad•ra•tus lum•bo•rum (mŭs′kyū-lŭs kwahd-rā′tŭs lŭm-bō′rŭm) [TA] SYN quadratus lumborum muscle.

mus•cu•lus quad•ra•tus plan•tae (mŭs′kyū-lŭs kwahd-rā′tŭs plan′tē) [TA] SYN quadratus plantae muscle.

mus•cu•lus quad•ri•ceps fem•o•ris (mŭs′kyū-lŭs kwahd′ri-seps fem′ō-ris) [TA] SYN quadriceps femoris muscle.

mus•cu•lus rec•to•coc•cyg•e•us (mŭs′kyū-lŭs rek′tō-kok-sij′ē-us) [TA] SYN rectococcygeus muscle.

mus•cu•lus rec•to•u•re•thra•lis (mŭs′kyū-lŭs rek′tō-yū-rē-thrā′lis) [TA] SYN rectourethralis muscle.

mus•cu•lus rec•to•u•te•ri•nus (mŭs′kyū-lŭs rek′tō-yū-tĕ-rī′nŭs) [TA] SYN rectouterine muscle.

mus•cu•lus rec•to•ve•si•ca•lis (mŭs′kyū-lŭs rek′tō-ves-i-kā′lis) [TA] SYN rectovesicalis muscle.

mus•cu•lus rec•tus ab•do•mi•nis (mŭs′kyū-lŭs rek′tŭs ab-dom′i-nis) [TA] SYN rectus abdominis muscle.

mus•cu•lus rec•tus ca•pi•tis an•te•ri•or (mŭs′kyū-lŭs rek′tŭs kap′i-tis an-tēr′ē-ŏr) [TA] SYN rectus capitis anterior muscle.

mus•cu•lus rec•tus ca•pi•tis la•te•ra•lis (mŭs′kyū-lŭs rek′tŭs kap′i-tis lat′tĕr-ā′lis) [TA] SYN rectus capitis lateralis muscle.

mus•cu•lus rec•tus fem•o•ris (mŭs′kyū-lŭs rek′tŭs fem′ō-ris) [TA] SYN rectus femoris muscle.

mus•cu•lus rec•tus in•fe•ri•or (mŭs′kyū-lŭs rek′tŭs in-fēr′ē-ŏr) [TA] SYN inferior rectus muscle.

mus•cu•lus rec•tus la•te•ra•lis (mŭs′kyū-lŭs rek′tŭs lat′tĕr-ā-lis) [TA] SYN lateral rectus muscle.

mus•cu•lus rec•tus me•di•a•lis (mŭs′kyū-lŭs rek′tŭs mē-dē-ā′lis) [TA] SYN medial rectus muscle.

mus•cu•lus rec•tus su•pe•ri•or (mŭs′kyū-lŭs rek′tŭs sŭ-pēr′ē-ŏr) [TA] SYN superior rectus muscle.

mus•cu•lus re•tra•hens au•rem (mŭs′kyū-lŭs rē-trā′henz awr′em) SYN auricularis posterior muscle.

mus•cu•lus rhom•boi•de•us ma•jor (mŭs′kyū-lŭs rahm-boy′dē-ŭs mā′jŏr) SYN rhomboid major muscle.

mus•cu•lus rhom•boi•de•us mi•nor (mŭs′kyū-lŭs rahm-boy′dē-ŭs mī′nŏr) SYN rhomboid minor muscle.

mus•cu•lus ri•so•ri•us (mŭs′kyū-lŭs rī-sō′rē-ŭs) [TA] SYN risorius muscle.

mus•cu•lus sal•pin•go•pha•ryn•ge•us (mŭs′kyū-lŭs sal-ping′gō-fă-rin′jē-ŭs) [TA] SYN salpingopharyngeus muscle.

mus•cu•lus sar•to•ri•us (mŭs′kyū-lŭs sahr-tō′rē-ŭs) [TA] SYN sartorius muscle.

mus•cu•lus sca•le•nus an•te•ri•or (mŭs′kyū-lŭs skā-lē′nŭs an-tēr′ē-ŏr) SYN scalenus anterior muscle.

mus•cu•lus sca•le•nus an•ti•cus (mŭs′kyū-lŭs skā-lē′nŭs an′tē-kŭs) SYN scalenus anterior muscle.

mus•cu•lus sca•le•nus me•di•us (mŭs′kyū-lŭs skā-lē′nŭs mē′dē-ŭs) SYN scalenus medius muscle.

mus•cu•lus sca•le•nus pos•te•ri•or (mŭs′kyū-lŭs skā-lē′nŭs pos-tēr′ē-ŏr) SYN scalenus posterior muscle.

mus•cu•lus sca•le•nus pos•ti•cus (mŭs′kyū-lŭs skā-lē′nŭs pos′tē-kŭs) SYN scalenus posterior muscle.

mus•cu•lus sem•i•mem•bra•no•sus (mŭs′kyū-lŭs sem′ē-mem′bră-nō′sŭs) [TA] SYN semimembranosus muscle.

mus•cu•lus sem•i•spi•na•lis ca•pi•tis (mŭs′kyū-lŭs sem′ī-spī-nā′lis kap′i-tis) [TA] SYN semispinalis capitis muscle.

mus•cu•lus sem•i•spi•na•lis cer•vi•cis (mŭs′kyū-lŭs sem′ī-spī-nā′lis ser′vi-sis) [TA] SYN semispinalis cervicis muscle.

mus•cu•lus sem•i•spi•na•lis tho•ra•cis (mŭs′kyū-lŭs sem′ī-spī-nā′lis thō-rā′sis) [TA] SYN semispinalis thoracis muscle.

mus•cu•lus sem•i•ten•di•no•sus (mŭs′kyū-lŭs sem′ē-ten′di-nō′sŭs) [TA] SYN semitendinosus muscle.

mus•cu•lus ser•ra•tus an•te•ri•or (mŭs′kyū-lŭs ser-ā′tŭs an-tēr′ē-ŏr) [TA] SYN serratus anterior muscle.

mus•cu•lus ser•ra•tus pos•te•ri•or in•fe•ri•or (mŭs′kyū-lŭs ser-ā′tŭs pos-tēr′ē-ŏr in-fēr′ē-ŏr) SYN serratus posterior inferior muscle.

mus•cu•lus ser•ra•tus pos•te•ri•or su•pe•ri•or (mŭs′kyū-lŭs ser-ā′tŭs pos-tēr′ē-ŏr sŭ-pēr′ē-ŏr) SYN serratus posterior superior muscle.

mus•cu•lus so•le•us (mŭs′kyū-lŭs sō′lē-ŭs) [TA] SYN soleus muscle.

mus•cu•lus sphinc•ter a•ni ex•ter•nus (mŭs′kyū-lŭs sfingk′ter ā′nī eks-ter′nŭs) SYN external anal sphincter muscle.

mus•cu•lus sphinc•ter duc•tus cho•le•do•chi (mŭs′kyū-lŭs sfingk′tĕr dŭk′tŭs kō-lē-dō′kī) [TA] SYN sphincter of common bile duct.

mus•cu•lus sphinc•ter duc•tus pan•cre•a•ti•ci (mŭs′kyū-lŭs sfingk′tĕr, dŭk′tŭs pan-krē-at′i-sī) [TA] SYN sphincter of pancreatic duct.

mus•cu•lus sphinc•ter pu•pil•lae (mŭs′kyū-lŭs sfingk′tĕr pyū-pil′ē) [TA] SYN sphincter pupillae.

mus•cu•lus sphinc•ter py•lo•ri•cus (mŭs′kyū-lŭs sfingk′tĕr pī-lō′ri-kŭs) [TA] SYN pyloric sphincter.

mus•cu•lus sphinc•ter u•re•thrae (mŭs′kyū-lŭs sfingk′tĕr yū-rēth′rē) [TA] SYN sphincter urethrae.

mus•cu•lus sphinc•ter u•re•thrae exter•nus (mŭs′kyū-lŭs sfingk′tĕr yū-rēth′rē eks-ter′nŭs) SYN external urethral sphincter muscle.

mus•cu•lus sphinc•ter vag•i•nae (mŭs′kyū-lŭs sfingk′tĕr va′ji-nē) SYN bulbospongiosus muscle.

mus•cu•lus sphinc•ter ve•si•cae (mŭs′kyū-lŭs sfingk′tĕr ves′i-kē) [TA] SYN sphincter vesicae.

mus•cu•lus spi•na•lis ca•pi•tis (mŭs′kyū-lŭs spī-nā′lis kap′i-tis) [TA] SYN spinalis capitis muscle.

mus•cu•lus spi•na•lis cer•vi•cis (mŭs′kyū-lŭs spī-nā′lis ser′vi-sis) [TA] SYN spinalis cervicis muscle.

mus•cu•lus spi•na•lis tho•ra•cis (mŭs′kyū-lŭs spī-nā′lis thō-rā′sis) [TA] SYN spinalis thoracis muscle.

mus•cu•lus sple•ni•us ca•pi•tis (mŭs′kyū-lŭs splē′nē-ŭs kap′i-tis) [TA] SYN splenius capitis muscle.

mus•cu•lus sple•ni•us cer•vi•cis (mŭs′kyū-lŭs splē′nē-ŭs ser′vi-sis) [TA] SYN splenius cervicis muscle.

mus•cu•lus sta•pe•di•us (mŭs′kyū-lŭs stā-pē′dē-ŭs) [TA] SYN stapedius muscle.

mus•cu•lus ster•na•lis (mŭs′kyū-lŭs stĕr-nā′lis) [TA] SYN sternalis muscle.

mus•cu•lus ster•no•clei•do•mas•toi•de•us (mŭs′kyū-lŭs stĕr′nō-klī-do-mas-toy′dē-ŭs) [TA] SYN sternocleidomastoid muscle.

mus•cu•lus ster•no•hy•oi•de•us (mŭs′kyū-lŭs stĕr′nō-hī-oy′dē-ŭs) [TA] SYN sternohyoid muscle.

mus•cu•lus ster•no•thy•roi•de•us (mŭs′kyū-lŭs stĕr′nō-thī-roy′dē-ŭs) [TA] SYN sternothyroid muscle.

mus•cu•lus sty•lo•glos•sus (mŭs′kyū-lŭs stī′lō-glos′ŭs) [TA] SYN styloglossus muscle.

mus•cu•lus sty•lo•hy•oi•de•us (mŭs′kyū-lŭs stī′lō-hī-oy′dē-′us) [TA] SYN stylohyoid muscle.

mus•cu•lus sty•lo•pha•ryn•ge•us (mŭs′kyū-lŭs stī-lō-far-in′jē-ŭs) [TA] SYN stylopharyngeus muscle.

mus•cu•lus sub•cla•vi•us (mŭs′kyū-lŭs sŭb-klā′vē-ŭs) [TA] SYN subclavius muscle.

mus•cu•lus sub•cos•ta•lis, pl. **mus•cu•li sub•cos•ta•les** (mŭs′kyū-lŭs sŭb′kos-tā′lis, mŭs′kyū-lī sŭb′kos-tā′lēz) [TA] SYN subcostal muscle.

mus•cu•lus sub•scap•u•la•ris (mŭs′kyū-lŭs sŭb′skap-pyū-lā′ris) [TA] SYN subscapularis muscle.

mus•cu•lus su•pi•na•tor (mŭs′kyū-lŭs sū′pi-nā′tŏr) [TA] SYN supinator muscle.

mus•cu•lus su•pra•spi•na•tus (mŭs′kyū-lŭs sū-pră-spin′ă-tŭs) [TA] SYN supraspinatus muscle.

mus•cu•lus sus•pen•so•ri•us du•o•de•ni (mŭs′kyū-lŭs sus-pen-sōr′ē-ŭs dū-od′ē-nī) [TA] SYN suspensory muscle of duodenum.

mus•cu•lus tem•po•ra•lis (mŭs′kyū-lŭs tem-pō-rā′lis) [TA] SYN temporalis muscle.

mus•cu•lus tem•po•ro•pa•ri•e•ta•lis (mŭs′kyū-lŭs tem-pō-rō-pa-rī′ē-tā′lis) [TA] SYN temporoparietalis muscle. SEE ALSO anterior auricular muscle, superior auricular muscle.

mus•cu•lus ten•sor fas•ci•ae la•tae (mŭs′kyū-lŭs ten′sōr făsh′-ē-ē lā′tē) [TA] SYN tensor fasciae latae muscle.

mus•cu•lus ten•sor tym•pa•ni (mŭs′kyū-lŭs ten′sŏr tim-pan′ī) [TA] SYN tensor tympani muscle.

mus•cu•lus ten•sor ve•li pa•la•ti•ni (mŭs′kyū-lŭs ten′sōr vē′lī pal-ă-tē′nī) [TA] SYN tensor veli palati muscle.

mus•cu•lus te•res ma•jor (mŭs′kyū-lŭs tē′rēz mā′jōr) [TA] SYN teres major muscle.

mus•cu•lus te•res mi•nor (mŭs′kyū-lŭs tē′rēz mī′nōr) [TA] SYN teres minor muscle.

mus•cu•lus thy•ro•ar•y•te•noi•de•us (mŭs′kyū-lŭs thī′rō-ar-ē-tē-noy′dē-ŭs) [TA] SYN thyroarytenoid muscle.

mus•cu•lus thy•ro•ep•i•glot•ti•cus (mŭs′kyū-lŭs thī-rō-ep-i-glot′i-kŭs) [TA] SYN thyroepiglottic muscle.

mus•cu•lus thy•ro•hy•oi•de•us (mŭs′kyū-lŭs thī-rō-hī-oy′dē-ŭs) SYN thyrohyoid muscle.

mus•cu•lus tib•i•al•is pos•te•ri•or (mŭs′kyū-lŭs tib-ē-ā′lis pos-tēr′ē-ōr) [TA] SYN tibialis posterior muscle.

mus•cu•lus tib•i•o•fas•ci•a•lis an•te•ri•or, mus•cu•lus tib•i•o•fas•ci•a•lis an•ti•cus (mŭs′kyū-lŭs tib′ē-ō-fash-ē-ā′lis an-tēr′ē-ōr, an′ti-kŭs) SYN anterior tibiofascial muscle.

mus•cu•lus tra•che•a•lis (mŭs′kyū-lŭs trā-kē-ā-′lis) [TA] SYN trachealis muscle.

mus•cu•lus tra•gi•cus (mŭs′kyū-lŭs traj′i-kŭs) [TA] SYN tragicus muscle.

mus•cu•lus trans•ver•so•spi•na•lis (mŭs′kyū-lŭs tranz-ver-sō′spin-ā′lis) [TA] SYN transversospinalis muscle.

mus•cu•lus trans•ver•sus ab•do•mi•nis (mŭs′kyū-lŭs tranz-ver′sŭs ab-dom′i-nis) [TA] SYN transversus abdominis muscle.

mus•cu•lus trans•ver•sus lin•guae (mŭs′kyū-lŭs tranz-ver′sŭs ling′wē) [TA] SYN transverse muscle of tongue.

mus•cu•lus trans•ver•sus men•ti (mŭs′kyū-lŭs tranz-ver′sŭs men′tī) [TA] SYN transversus menti muscle.

mus•cu•lus trans•ver•sus nu•chae (mŭs′kyū-lŭs tranz-ver′sŭs nū′kē) [TA] SYN transversus nuchae muscle.

mus•cu•lus trans•ver•sus pe•ri•ne•i pro•fun•dus (mŭs′kyū-lŭs tranz-ver′sŭs per-ī′nē-ī prō-fun′dus) [TA] SYN deep transverse perineal muscle.

mus•cu•lus trans•ver•sus pe•ri•ne•i su•per•fi•ci•a•lis (mŭs′kyū-lŭs tranz-ver′sŭs per-ī′nē-ī sū′pĕr-fish′ē-ā′lis) [TA] SYN superficial transverse perineal muscle.

mus•cu•lus trans•ver•sus tho•ra•cis (mŭs′kyū-lŭs trans-ver′sŭs thō-rā′sis) [TA] SYN transversus thoracis muscle.

mus•cu•lus tra•pe•zi•us (mŭs′kyū-lŭs tră-pē′zē-ŭs) [TA] SYN trapezius muscle.

mus•cu•lus tri•ceps bra•chi•i (mŭs′kyū-lŭs trī′seps brā′kē-ī) [TA] SYN triceps brachii muscle.

mus•cu•lus tri•ceps su•rae (mŭs′kyū-lŭs trī′seps sū′rē) [TA] SYN triceps surae muscle.

mus•cu•lus u•vu•lae (mŭs′kyū-lŭs ū′vyū-lē) [TA] SYN uvular muscle.

mus•cu•lus ver•ti•ca•lis lin•guae (mŭs′kyū-lŭs ver-ti-kā′lis ling′gwē) [TA] SYN vertical muscle of tongue.

mus•cu•lus vo•ca•lis (mŭs′kyū-lŭs vō-kā′lis) [TA] SYN vocalis muscle.

mus•cu•lus zy•go•ma•ti•cus (mŭs′kyū-lŭs zī-gō-mat′i-kŭs) SYN zygomaticus major muscle.

mus•cu•lus zy•go•ma•ti•cus ma•jor (mŭs′kyū-lŭs zī-gō-mat′i′kŭs mā′jōr) [TA] SYN zygomaticus major muscle.

mus•cu•lus zy•go•ma•ti•cus mi•nor (mŭs′kyū-lŭs zī-gō-mat′i-kŭs mī′nōr) SYN zygomaticus minor muscle.

mush•room poi•son•ing (mŭsh-rūm poy′zŏn-ing) SEE mycetism.

mu•si•cian's ear•plugs (myū-zish′ănz ēr′plŭgz) Custom-fitted earplugs that attenuate all frequencies evenly in relation to normal hearing sensitivity; allow musicians to hear music at levels below the damage-risk level without sacrificing sound quality; must be fitted by a licensed hearing health professional.

mu•sic ther•a•py, mu•si•co•ther•a•py (myū′sĭk thār′ă-pē, myū′sik-ō-thār′ă-pē) An adjunctive treatment of mental disorders by means of music.

Mus•set sign (mū-sā′ sīn) A finding involving incompetence of the aortic valve, rhythmic nodding of the head, synchronous with ventricular contractions of the heart. SYN de Musset sign.

mus•si•ta•tion (mŭs-i-tā′shŭn) Movements of the lips as if speaking, but without sound; observed in delirium and in semicoma. [L. *mussito,* to murmur constantly, fr. *musso,* pp. *-atus,* to mutter]

mus•tard (mŭs′tĕrd) **1.** A plant of the genus *Brassica* with pungent edible seeds. **2.** A semisolid preparation of mustard seeds used as a condiment. **3.** A material having the appearance or consistency of mustard (2). [L. *mustum,*fruit juice or pulp prepared for fermentation]

mus•tard gas (mŭs′tĕrd gas) A commonly used term for the vesicating chemical-warfare agent sulfur mustard, even though sulfur mustard is usually encountered as a solid, a liquid, or a vapor and does not boil until 217°C (423°F).

Mus•tard op•er•a•tion (mŭs′tĕrd op-ĕr-ā′shŭn) Correction, at the atrial level, of hemodynamic abnormality due to transposition of the great arteries by an intraatrial baffle to direct pulmonary venous blood through the tricuspid orifice into the right ventricle and the systemic venous blood through the mitral valve into the left ventricle, allowing more oxygenated blood to be circulated systematically.

mu•ta•gen (myū′tă-jen) Any agent that promotes a mutation or causes an increase in the rate of mutational events, e.g., radioactive substances, x-rays, or certain chemicals. [L. *muto,* to change, + G. *-gen,* producing]

mu•ta•gen•e•sis (myū-tă-jen′ĕ-sis) **1.** Production of genetic alterations by using chemicals or radiation. **2.** Production of a mutation.

mu•ta•gen•ic (myū-tă-jen′ik) Promoting mutation.

mu•tant (myū′tănt) **1.** A phenotype in which a

mutation is manifested. **2.** A gene that is rare and usually harmful, in contrast to a wild-type gene, not necessarily generated recently.

mu•tant gene (myū′tănt jēn) A gene that has been changed from an ancestral type, not necessarily in the current generation. SEE ALSO mutant, mutation.

mu•tase (myū′tās) Any enzyme that catalyzes the apparent migration of groups within one molecule; sometimes the transfer is from one molecule to another.

mu•ta•tion (myū-tā′shŭn) **1.** A change in the chemistry of a gene that is perpetuated in subsequent divisions of the cell in which it occurs; a change in the sequence of base pairs in the chromosomal molecule. **2.** The sudden production of a species, as distinguished from variation. [L. *muto,* pp. *-atus,* to change]

mu•ta•tion•al fal•set•to (myū-tā′shŭn-ăl fawl-sĕt′ō) Habitual use of an abnormally high-pitched voice that persists after puberty. SYN puberphonia.

mu•ta•tion rate (myū-tā′shŭn rāt) The probability (or proportion) of progeny genes with a particular component of the genome not present in either biologic parent; usually expressed as the number of mutants per generation occurring at one gene or locus.

mute (myūt) **1.** Unable or unwilling to speak. **2.** A person who does not have the faculty of speech. [L. *mutus*]

mu•tein (myū′tēn) A protein arising as a result of a mutation. [*mut*ation + prot*ein*]

mu•ti•lat•ing ker•a•to•der•ma (myū′ti-lāt′ing ker′ă-tō-dĕr′mă) Diffuse keratoderma of the extremities, with the development during childhood of constricting fibrous bands around the middle phalanges of the fingers or toes that may lead to spontaneous amputation.

mu•ti•la•tion (myū-ti-lā′shŭn) Disfigurement or injury by removal or destruction of any conspicuous or essential part of the body. [L. *mutilatio,* fr. *mutilo,* pp. *-atus,* to maim]

mut•ism (myū′tizm) **1.** The state of being silent. **2.** Organic or functional absence of the faculty of speech. [L. *mutus,* mute]

mu•ton (myū′ton) GENETICS the smallest unit of a chromosome in which alteration can be effective in causing a mutation. [*mut*ation + -on]

mu•tu•al•ism (myū′chyū-ăl-izm) Symbiotic relationship from which both species derive benefit. Cf. commensalism, metabiosis, parasitism.

mu•tu•al•ist (myū′chū-ăl-ist) SYN symbion. [L. *mutuus,* in return, mutual]

mu•tu•al re•sis•tance (myū′chū-ăl rĕ-zis′tăns) SYN antagonism.

mV Abbreviation for millivolt; megavolt.

MVC Abbreviation for maximum voluntary contraction.

MVP Abbreviation for mitral valve prolapse.

MVV Abbreviation for maximum voluntary ventilation.

MW Abbreviation for molecular weight.

MWT Abbreviation for maintenance of wakefulness test.

MX Abbreviation for monozygotic.

myaesthesia [Br.] SYN myesthesia.

my•al•gi•a (mī-al′jē-ă) Muscular pain. SYN myodynia. [G. *mys,* muscle, + *algos,* pain]

my•al•gic as•the•ni•a (mī-al′jik as-thē′nē-ă) A condition associated with muscle pain and/or tenderness, generalized weakness, and loss of strength. [G. *mys,* muscle + *algos,* pain, + *astheneia,* weakness, fr. *a-* priv., + *sthenos,* strength]

my•al•gic en•ceph•a•lo•mye•li•tis (ME) (mī-al′jik en-sef′a-lō-mī′ĕ-lī′tis) SYN chronic fatigue syndrome.

my•as•the•ni•a (mī-as-thē′nē-ă) Muscular weakness. [G. *mys,* muscle, + *astheneia,* weakness]

my•as•the•ni•a an•gi•o•scle•ro•ti•ca (mī-as-thē′nē-ă an′jē-ō-skler-ot′i-kă) SYN intermittent claudication.

my•as•the•ni•a gra•vis (mī-as-thē′nē-ă gra′vis) Disorder of neuromuscular transmission, marked by fluctuating weakness, especially of the oculofacial muscles and the proximal limb muscles; the weakness characteristically increases with activity; due to an immunological disorder. SYN Goldflam disease.

my•as•then•ic (mī-as-then′ik) Relating to myasthenia.

my•as•then•ic fa•ci•es (mī-as-then′ik fash′ē-ēz) The facial expression in myasthenia gravis, caused by drooping of the eyelids and corners of the mouth, and weakness of the muscles of the face.

my•as•then•ic syn•drome (mī-as-then′ik sin′drōm) A disorder of neuromuscular transmission marked primarily by limb and girdle weakness, absent deep tendon reflexes, dry mouth, and impotence; due to an immunologic disorder; often, especially in males, a paraneoplastic syndrome linked to small cell carcinoma of the lung.

my•ce•li•a (mī-sē′lē-ă) Plural of mycelium.

my•ce•li•an (mī-sē′lē-ăn) Pertaining to a mycelium.

my•ce•li•um, pl. **my•ce•li•a** (mī-sē′lē-ŭm, -ă) The mass of hyphae making up a colony of fungi. [G. *mykēs,* fungus, + *hēlos,* nail, wart, excrescence on animal or plant]

mycet-, myceto- Combining forms meaning fungus. SEE ALSO myco-. [G. *mykēs,* fungus]

my·cete (mī′sēt) A fungus. [G. *mykēs,* fungus]

my·ce·tism, my·ce·tis·mus (mī′sĕ-tizm, -tiz′mŭs) Poisoning by certain species of mushrooms. [G. *mykēs,* fungus]

my·ce·to·ge·net·ic, my·ce·to·gen·ic (mī′sĕ-tō-jĕ-net′ik, -jen′ik) Caused by fungi. [G. *mykēs,* fungus, + *gennētos,* begotten]

my·ce·to·ma (mī-sĕ-tō′mă) **1.** A chronic infection involving the feet and characterized by the formation of localized lesions with tumefactions and multiple draining sinuses. The exudate contains granules that may be yellow, white, red, brown, or black, depending on the causative agent. Actinomycotic mycetoma is caused by bacterial species in the actinomycetes group; eumycotic mycetoma is caused by true fungi. SYN Madura boil, maduromycosis. **2.** Any tumor with draining sinuses produced by filamentous fungi.

my·cid (mī′sid) An allergic reaction to a remote focus of mycotic infection. [G. *mykēs,* fungus, + -id]

myco- Combining form meaning fungus. SEE ALSO mycet-. [G. *mykēs,* fungus]

my·co·bac·te·ri·a (mī′kō-bak-tēr′ē-ă) Organisms belonging to the genus *Mycobacterium.*

my·co·bac·te·ri·o·sis (mī′kō-bak-tēr-ē-ō′sis) Infection with mycobacteria.

My·co·bac·te·ri·um (mī′kō-bak-tēr′ē-ŭm) A genus of aerobic, nonmotile bacteria (family Mycobacteriaceae) containing gram-positive, acid-fast, slender, straight or slightly curved rods; slender filaments occasionally occur, but branched forms rarely are produced. Parasitic and saprophytic species occur. A number of species are associated with infections in immunocompromised people, especially those with AIDS. The type species is *M. tuberculosis.* It is the type genus of the family Mycobacteriaceae. [myco- + bacterium]

My·co·bac·te·ri·um a·vi·um (mī′kō-bak-tēr′ē-ŭm ā′vē-ŭm) A bacterial species causing tuberculosis in fowl and other birds. Recently linked to opportunistic infections in humans. SYN tubercle bacillus (3).

***My·co·bac·te·ri·um a·vi·um-in·tra·cel·lu·la·re* com·plex (MAIC)** (mī-kō-bak-tēr′ē-ŭm ā′vē-ŭm in-tră-sel′yū-lār′ē kom′pleks) Consists of *M. avium* and *M. intracellulare,* two similar species. They are commonly found in the environment but have become serious opportunistic agents in pulmonary disease in patients with AIDS. Difficult to treat because *Mycobacterium* is resistant to many antibiotics.

My·co·bac·te·ri·um bo·vis (mī′kō-bak-tēr′ē-ŭm bō′vis) A bacterial species that is the primary cause of tuberculosis in cattle; transmissible to humans and other animals, causing tuberculosis. SYN tubercle bacillus (2).

My·co·bac·te·ri·um che·lo·nae (mī′kō-bak-tēr′ē-ŭm kē-lō′nē) Rapidly growing mycobacterium that causes sporadic infection following cardiothoracic surgery, peritoneal dialysis, hemodialysis, augmentation mammaplasty, and arthroplasty, and in immunocompromised patients.

My·co·bac·te·ri·um gor·do·nae (mī′kō-bak-tēr′ē-ŭm gōr-dō′nē) A scotochromogenic bacillus found in soil and tap water; isolation from cases of meningitis in patients with ventriculoatrial shunts reported.

My·co·bac·te·ri·um hae·mo·phi·lum (mī′kō-bak-tēr′ē-ŭm hē-mof′i-lŭm) A nonchromogenic acid-fast bacillus; infections occur mainly in immunocompromised patients (e.g., those with AIDS, Hodgkin disease). Submandibular lymphadenitis, subcutaneous nodules, and ulcers that progress to abscesses and fistulae are common manifestations.

My·co·bac·te·ri·um kan·sa·si·i (mī′kō-bak-tēr′ē-ŭm kan-sas′ē-ī) A bacterial species causing a tuberculosislike pulmonary disease; also found to cause infections (and usually lesions) in meninges, spleen, liver, pancreas, testes, hip joint, knee joint, finger, wrist, and lymph nodes.

My·co·bac·te·ri·um lep·rae (mī′kō-bak-tēr′ē-ŭm lep′rē) A bacterial species that causes Hansen disease. SYN Hansen bacillus.

My·co·bac·te·ri·um ma·ri·num (mī′kō-bak-tēr′ē-ŭm mah-rē′nŭm) A bacterial species causing spontaneous tuberculosis in saltwater fish; it also occurs in other cold-blooded animals, in some swimming pools in which it may cause human cutaneous infection, in irrigation canals and ditches, and on ocean beaches. See this page.

My·co·bac·te·ri·um scro·fu·la·ce·um (mī′kō-bak-tēr′ē-ŭm skrō′fyū-lā′shē-ŭm) A bacterial

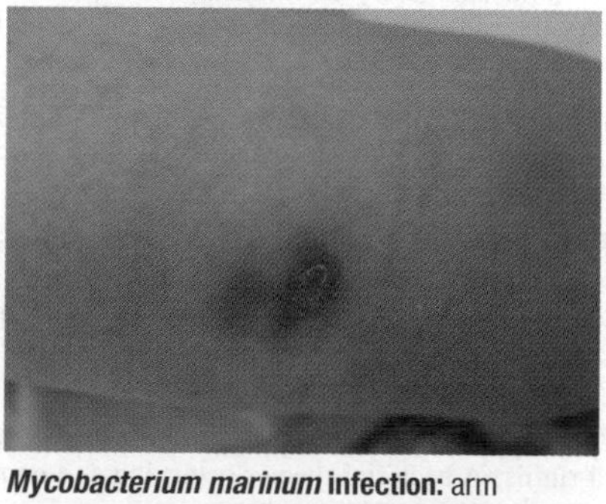

***Mycobacterium marinum* infection: arm**

species frequently associated with cervical adenitis in children.

My·co·bac·te·ri·um sim·i·ae (mī′kō-bak-tēr′ē-ŭm sim′ē-ē) A slow-growing, photochromogenic, acid-fast bacillus; rarely associated with pulmonary disease in humans.

My·co·bac·te·ri·um tu·ber·cu·lo·sis (mī′kō-bak-tēr′ē-ŭm tū-bĕr′kyū-lō′sis) A bacterial species that causes tuberculosis in humans. It is the type species of the genus *Mycobacterium*. SYN Koch bacillus, tubercle bacillus (1).

My·co·bac·te·ri·um vac·cae (mī′kō-bak-tēr′ē-ŭm vak′ē) A rapidly growing scotochromogenic, nonpathogenic bacterial species that is distributed widely in nature.

my·co·der·ma·ti·tis (mī′kō-dĕr-mă-tī′tis) A nonspecific term used to designate an eruption of mycotic (fungus, yeast, mold) origin.

my·col·o·gist (mī-kol′ŏ-jist) A person specializing in mycology.

my·col·o·gy (mī-kol′ŏ-jē) The study of fungi: their identification, classification, edibility, cultivation, and biology, including pathogenicity. [myco- + G. *logos,* study]

my·co·phage (mī′kō-fāj) A virus with a fungal host. SEE ALSO mycovirus. [myco- + G. *phagō,* to eat]

My·co·plas·ma (mī′kō-plaz′mă) A genus of aerobic to facultatively anaerobic bacteria containing gram-negative cells that do not possess a true cell wall but are bounded by a three-layered membrane. The cells are pleomorphic and, in liquid media, appear as coccoid bodies, rings, or filaments. These organisms are found in humans and other animals and are parasitic to pathogenic. [myco- + G. *plasma,* something formed (plasm)]

my·co·plas·ma, pl. **my·co·plas·ma·ta** (mī′kō-plaz-mă, -plaz′mă-tă) A vernacular term used to refer to any member of the genus *Mycoplasma.*

My·co·plas·ma hom·i·nis (mī′kō-plaz′mă hom′i-nis) A bacterial species that is an agent of pelvic inflammatory disease and other genitourinary tract infections; can also cause chorioamnionitis and postpartum fever.

my·co·plas·mal pneu·mo·ni·a (mī′kō-plaz′măl nū-mō′nē-ă) SYN primary atypical pneumonia.

My·co·plas·ma my·coi·des (mī′kō-plaz′mă mī-koy′dēz) A bacterial species that can cause contagious pleuropneumonia in cattle, sheep, and goats. It is the type species of the genus *Mycoplasma.*

My·co·plas·ma pha·ryn·gis (mī′kō-plaz′mă fă-rin′jis) A bacterial species occurring as a commensal in the human oropharynx.

My·co·plas·ma pneu·mo·ni·ae (mī′kō-plaz′mă nū-mō′nē-ē) A bacterial species causing primary atypical pneumonia in human beings. SYN Eaton agent.

My·co·plas·ma·ta·les (mī′kō-plaz-mă-tā′lēz) An order of gram-negative bacteria with cells that are bounded by a three-layered membrane but do not possess a true cell wall. Pathogenic and saprophytic species occur. These organisms reproduce through the breaking up of branched filaments into coccoid, filterable elementary bodies. The order includes the so-called pleuropneumonialike organisms (PPLO).

my·co·sis, pl. **my·co·ses** (mī-kō′sis, -sēz) Any disease caused by a fungus (filamentous or yeast). [myco- + G. *-osis,* condition]

my·co·sis fun·goi·des (mī-kō′sis fung-goyd′ēz) A chronic progressive lymphoma arising in the skin that initially simulates eczema or other inflammatory dermatoses; in advanced cases, ulcerated tumors and infiltrations of lymph nodes may occur. See this page.

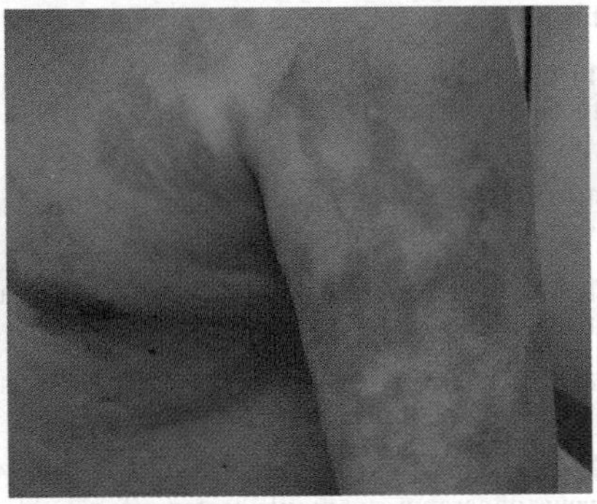

mycosis fungoides

my·cot·ic (mī-kot′ik) Relating to or caused by a fungus.

my·cot·ic an·eu·rysm (mī-kot′ik an′yūr-izm) An aneurysm caused by the growth of fungi within the vascular wall, usually following impaction of a septic embolus; also used to refer to the growth of bacteria within the vascular wall of an aneurysm; may result from impaction of septic embolus or from primary infection of the vessel wall.

my·co·tox·i·co·sis (mī′kō-tok-si-kō′sis) Poisoning due to the ingestion of preformed substances produced by the action of certain fungi on particular foodstuffs or by ingestion of the fungi themselves; e.g., ergotism. [myco- + G. *toxikon,* poison, + *-osis,* condition]

my·co·tox·in (mī′kō-tok′sin) A toxin produced by a fungus. SEE ALSO yellow rain, trichothecene mycotoxin, alimentary toxic aleukia (ATA) toxicosis.

my•co•vi•rus (mī′kō-vī′rŭs) A virus that infects fungi.

my•dri•a•sis (mi-drī′ă-sis) Dilation of the pupil. [G.]

myd•ri•at•ic (mi-drē-at′ik) **1.** Causing mydriasis or dilation of the pupil. **2.** An agent that dilates the pupil.

my•ec•to•my (mī-ek′tŏ-mē) Excision of all or part of a muscle. [G. *mys,* muscle, + *ektomē,* excision]

my•ec•to•py, my•ec•to•pi•a (mī-ek′tŏ-pē, mī-ek-tō′pē-ă) Rarely used term for dislocation of a muscle. [G. *mys,* muscle, + *ektopos,* out of place]

♻ **myel-, myelo-** Combining forms indicating bone; spinal cord and medulla oblongata; myelin sheath of nerve fibers. Cf. medullo-. [G. *myelos,* medulla, marrow]

my•el•ap•o•plex•y (mī-el-ap′ō-plek-sē) SYN hematomyelia. [myel- + G. *apoplēxia,* apoplexy]

my•el•a•te•li•a (mī′el-ă-tē′lē-ă) Developmental defect of the spinal cord. [myel- + G. *ateleia,* incompleteness]

my•el•en•ceph•a•lon (mī′el-en-sef′ă-lon) SYN medulla oblongata. [myel- + G. *enkephalos,* brain]

my•e•lin (mī′ĕ-lin) **1.** The lipoproteinaceous material of the myelin sheath, composed of alternating membranes of lipid and protein. **2.** Droplets of lipid formed during autolysis and postmortem decomposition.

my•e•li•nat•ed (mī′ĕ-li-nāt-ĕd) Having a myelin sheath. SYN medullated (2).

my•e•li•na•tion (mī′ĕ-li-nā′shŭn) The acquisition, development, or formation of a myelin sheath around a nerve fiber.

my•e•li•nol•y•sis (mī′ĕ-li-nol′i-sis) Dissolution of the myelin sheaths of nerve fibers. [myelin + G. *lysis,* dissolution]

my•e•lin sheath (mī′ĕ-lin shēth) The lipoproteinaceous envelope in vertebrates surrounding most axons of more than 0.5-μm diameter; it consists of a double plasma membrane wound tightly around the axon in a variable number of turns, and supplied by oligodendroglia cells (in the brain and spinal cord) or Schwann cells (in peripheral nerves).

my•e•lit•ic (mī′ĕ-lit′ik) Relating to or affected by myelitis.

my•e•li•tis (mī′ĕ-lī′tis) **1.** Inflammation of the spinal cord. **2.** Inflammation of the bone marrow. [myel- + G. *-itis,* inflammation]

my•e•lo•blast (mī′ĕ-lō-blast) An immature cell in the granulocytic series, occurring normally in bone marrow but not in the blood. When stained, the cytoplasm is light blue and variable in amount; the nucleus deep purple-blue with finely divided, punctate, threadlike chromatin. A few light blue nucleoli in the nucleus generally disappear as the myeloblast matures into a promyelocyte and then a myelocyte. [myelo- + G. *blastos,* germ]

myeloblastaemia [Br.] SYN myeloblastemia.

my•e•lo•blas•te•mi•a (mī′ĕ-lō-blas-tē′mē-ă) The presence of myeloblasts in the circulating blood. SYN myeloblastaemia. [myeloblast + G. *haima,* blood]

my•e•lo•blas•tic leu•ke•mi•a (mī′ĕ-lō-blas′tik lū-kē′mē-ă) A form of granulocytic leukemia in which there are large numbers of myeloblasts in various tissues and in the blood. Used synonymously for acute granulocytic leukemia. SYN acute granulocytic leukemia, acute myeloblastic leukemia.

my•e•lo•blas•to•ma (mī′ĕ-lō-blas-tō′mă) A nodular focus or fairly well-circumscribed accumulation of myeloblasts, as sometimes observed in acute myeloblastic leukemia and chlorosis. [myeloblast + G. *-oma,* tumor]

my•e•lo•blas•to•sis (mī′ĕ-lō-blas-tō′sis) The presence of unusually large numbers of myeloblasts in the circulating blood, or tissues, or both (as in acute leukemia).

my•e•lo•cele (mī′ĕ-lō-sēl) **1.** Protrusion of the spinal cord through a defect in the vertebral arch in spina bifida. [myelo- + G. *kēlē,* hernia] **2.** The central canal of the spinal cord. [G. *myelos,* marrow, + *koilia,* a hollow]

my•e•lo•cyst (mī′ĕ-lō-sist) Any cyst (usually lined with columnar or cuboidal cells) that develops from a rudimentary central canal in the central nervous system. [myelo- + G. *kystis,* bladder]

my•e•lo•cyst•ic (mī′ĕ-lō-sist′ik) Pertaining to or characterized by the presence of a myelocyst.

my•e•lo•cys•to•cele (mī′ĕ-lō-sis′tō-sēl) Spina bifida containing spinal cord substance. [myelo- + G. *kystis,* bladder, + *kēlē,* tumor]

my•e•lo•cys•to•me•ning•o•cele (mī′ĕ-lō-sis′tō-mĕ-ning′gō-sēl) SYN meningomyelocele. [myelo- + G. *kystis,* bladder, + *mēninx* (*mēning-*), membrane, + *kēlē,* hernia]

my•e•lo•cyte (mī′ĕ-lō-sīt) **1.** A young cell of the granulocytic series, occurring normally in bone marrow, but not in circulating blood. When stained, the cytoplasm is distinctly basophilic and more abundant than in myeloblasts or promyelocytes; numerous cytoplasmic granules are present in the more mature forms. The nucleus is regular in contour, i.e., not indented, and seems to be "buried" beneath the numerous cytoplasmic granules. **2.** A nerve cell of the gray matter of the brain or spinal cord. [myelo- + G. *kytos,* cell]

myelocythaemia [Br.] SYN myelocythemia.

my•e•lo•cy•the•mi•a (mī′ĕ-lō-sī-thē′mē-ă) The presence of myelocytes in the circulating blood, especially in persistently large numbers (as in myelocytic leukemia). SYN myelocythaemia. [myelocyte + G. *haima,* blood]

my•e•lo•cyt•ic (mī′ĕ-lō-sit′ik) Pertaining to or characterized by myelocytes.

my•e•lo•cyt•ic leu•ke•mi•a, my•e•lo•gen•ic leu•ke•mi•a, my•e•log•e•nous leu•ke•mi•a, my•e•loid leu•ke•mi•a (mī′ĕ-lō-sit′ik lū-kē′mē-ă, mī′ē-lō-jen′ik, mī′ĕ-loj′ĕ-nŭs, mī′ĕ-loyd) SYN granulocytic leukemia.

my•e•lo•cy•to•ma (mī′ĕ-lō-sī-tō′mă) A nodular focus or fairly well-circumscribed, relatively dense accumulation of myelocytes, as in certain tissues of people with myelocytic leukemia. [myelocyte + G. *-oma,* tumor]

my•e•lo•cy•to•ma•to•sis (mī′ĕ-lō-sī-tō′ă-tō′sis) A form of tumor involving chiefly the myelocytes.

my•e•lo•cy•to•sis (mī′ĕ-lō-sī-tō′sis) The occurrence of abnormally large numbers of myelocytes in the circulating blood, or tissues, or both. [myelocyte + G. *-osis,* condition]

my•e•lo•dys•pla•si•a (mī′ĕ-lō-dis-plā′zē-ă) **1.** An abnormality in development of the spinal cord, especially the lower part of the cord. **2.** A disorder within the bone marrow, characterized by the proliferation of abnormal stem cells, which have the potential of developing into a specific type of leukemia. [myelo- + G. *dys-,* difficult, + *plasis,* a molding]

my•e•lo•dys•plas•tic syn•drome (mī′ĕ-lō-dis-plast′ik sin′drōm) A primary, neoplastic, pluripotential stem cell disorder characterized by peripheral blood cytopenias and prominent maturation abnormalities in the bone marrow. The disease evolves progressively and may transform into leukemia. Classified by the French-American-British (FAB) system into five groups. SEE ALSO French-American-British classification system. SYN chronic erythremic myelosis, preleukemia, smoldering leukemia.

my•e•lo•fi•bro•sis (mī′ĕ-lō-fī-brō′sis) Fibrosis of the bone marrow, especially generalized, associated with myeloid metaplasia of the spleen and other organs, leukoerythroblastic anemia, and thrombocytopenia, although the bone marrow often contains many megakaryocytes. SYN myelosclerosis.

my•e•lo•gen•e•sis (mī′ĕ-lō-jen′ĕ-sis) **1.** Development of bone marrow. **2.** Development of the central nervous system. **3.** Formation of myelin around an axon.

my•e•lo•ge•net•ic, my•e•lo•gen•ic (mī′ĕ-lō-jĕ-net′ik, -jen′ik) **1.** Relating to myelogenesis. **2.** Produced by or originating in the bone marrow. SYN myelogenous.

my•e•log•e•nous (mī-ĕ-loj′ĕ-nŭs) SYN myelogenetic (2).

my•e•lo•gone, my•e•lo•go•ni•um (mī′ĕ-lō-gōn, -gō′nē-ŭm) An immature white blood cell of the myeloid series that is characterized by a large, deeply stained, reticulated nucleus and a scant amount of nongranular basophilic cytoplasm. [myelo- + G. *gonē,* seed]

my•e•lo•gram (mī′ĕ-lō-gram) Radiographic contrast study of the spinal subarachnoid space and its contents. See page B20.

my•e•log•ra•phy (mī′ĕ-log′ră-fē) Radiography of the spinal cord and nerve roots after the injection of a contrast medium into the spinal subarachnoid space. [myelo- + G. *graphē,* a drawing]

my•e•loid (mī′ĕ-loyd) **1.** Pertaining to, derived from, or manifesting certain features of the bone marrow. **2.** Sometimes used with reference to the spinal cord. **3.** Pertaining to certain characteristics of myelocytic forms, but not necessarily implying origin in the bone marrow. [myel- + -oid]

my•e•loid met•a•pla•si•a (mī′ĕ-loyd met-ă-plā′zē-ă) A syndrome characterized by anemia, enlargement of the spleen, nucleated red blood cells and immature granulocytes in the blood, and foci of extramedullary hemopoiesis in the spleen and liver; may develop in the course of polycythemia rubra vera; there is a high incidence of development of myeloid leukemia.

my•e•loi•do•sis (mī′ĕ-loy-dō′sis) General hyperplasia of myeloid tissue.

my•e•loid sar•co•ma (mī′ĕ-loyd sahr-kō′mă) SYN granulocytic sarcoma.

my•e•loid se•ries (mī′ĕ-loyd sēr′ēz) The granulocytic and the erythrocytic series.

my•e•loid tis•sue (mī′ĕ-loyd tish′ū) Bone marrow consisting of the developmental and adult stages of erythrocytes, granulocytes, and megakaryocytes in a stroma of reticular cells and fibers, with sinusoidal vascular channels.

my•e•lo•ka•thex•is (mī′ĕ-lō-kă-thek′sis) SYN kathexis.

my•e•lo•li•po•ma (mī′ĕ-lō-li-pō′mă) Nodular foci that are not neoplasms, but probably represent localized proliferation of reticuloendothelial tissue in the suprarenal glands; foci of bone marrow containing erythropoietic or myeloid cells.

my•e•lo•ma (mī′ĕ-lō′mă) **1.** A tumor composed of cells derived from hemopoietic tissues of the bone marrow. **2.** A plasma cell tumor. [myelo- + G. *-oma,* tumor]

my•e•lo•ma•la•ci•a (mī′ĕ-lō-mă-lā′shē-ă) Softening of the spinal cord. [myelo- + G. *malakia,* a softness]

my•e•lo•ma•to•sis (mī′ĕ-lō-mă-tō′sis) A disease characterized by the occurrence of myeloma in various sites.

my·e·lo·me·nin·go·cele (mī′ĕ-lō-mĕ-ning′gō-sēl) SYN meningomyelocele. [myelo- + G. *mēninx,* membrane, + *kēlē,* hernia]

my·e·lo·mere (mī′ĕ-lō-mēr) Neuromere of the brain or spinal cord. [myelo- + G. *meros,* part]

my·e·lo·neu·ri·tis (mī′ĕ-lō-nūr-ī′tis) SYN neuromyelitis.

my·e·lon·ic (mī′ĕ-lon′ik) Relating to the spinal cord. [G. *myelon,* fr. *myelos,* marrow]

my·e·lo·path·ic (mī′ĕ-lō-path′ik) Relating to myelopathy.

my·e·lop·a·thy (mī′ĕ-lop′ă-thē) **1.** Disorder of the spinal cord. **2.** A disease of the myelopoietic tissues. [myelo- + G. *pathos,* suffering]

my·e·lop·e·tal (mī′ĕ-lop′ĕ-tăl) Proceeding in a direction toward the spinal cord; said of different nerve impulses. [myelo- + L. *peto,* to seek]

my·e·loph·this·ic (mī′ĕ-lof-thiz′ik) Relating to or suffering from myelophthisis.

my·e·loph·this·ic a·ne·mi·a, my·e·lo·path·ic a·ne·mi·a (mī′ĕ-lof-thiz′ik ă-nē′mē-ă, mī′ĕ-lō-path′ik) SYN leukoerythroblastosis.

my·e·loph·thi·sis (mī′ĕ-lof′thi-sis) **1.** Wasting or atrophy of the spinal cord as in tabes dorsalis. **2.** Replacement of hemopoietic tissue in the bone marrow by abnormal tissue, usually fibrous tissue metastatic carcinomas. SYN panmyelophthisis. [myelo- + G. *phthisis,* a wasting away]

my·e·lo·plast (mī′ĕ-lō-plast) Any of the leukocytic series of cells in the bone marrow, especially young forms. [myelo- + G. *plastos,* formed]

my·e·lo·poi·e·sis (mī′ĕ-lō-poy-ē′sis) Formation of the tissue elements of bone marrow, or any of the types of blood cells derived from bone marrow; or both. [myelo- + G. *poiēsis,* a making]

my·e·lo·poi·et·ic (mī′ĕ-lō-poy-et′ik) Relating to myelopoiesis.

my·e·lo·pro·lif·er·a·tive (mī′ĕ-lō-prō-lif′ĕr-ă-tiv) Pertaining to or characterized by unusual proliferation of myelopoietic tissue.

my·e·lo·pro·lif·er·a·tive syn·dromes (mī′ĕ-lō-prō-lif′ĕr-ă-tiv sin′drōmz) A group of conditions that result from a disorder in the rate of formation of cells of the bone marrow, including chronic granulocytic leukemia, erythremia, myelosclerosis, panmyelosis, and erythremic myelosis and erythroleukemia.

my·e·lo·ra·dic·u·li·tis (mī′ĕ-lō-ră-dik′yū-lī′tis) Inflammation of the spinal cord and nerve roots. [myelo- + L. *radicula,* root, + G. *-itis,* inflammation]

my·e·lo·ra·dic·u·lo·dys·pla·si·a (mī′ĕ-lō-ră-dik′yū-lō-dis-plā′zē-ă) Congenital maldevelopment of the spinal cord and spinal nerve roots. [myelo- + L. *radicula,* root, + dysplasia]

my·e·lo·ra·dic·u·lop·a·thy (mī′ĕ-lō-ră-dik′yū-lop′ă-thē) Disease involving the spinal cord and nerve roots. SYN radiculomyelopathy. [myelo- + L. *radicula,* root, + G. *pathos,* disease]

my·e·lor·rha·gi·a (mī′ĕ-lō-rā′jē-ă) SYN hematomyelia. [myelo- + G. *rhēgnymi,* to burst forth]

my·e·lor·rha·phy (mī-ĕ-lōr′ă-fē) Suture of a wound of the spinal cord. [myelo- + G. *rhaphē,* a seam]

my·e·lo·scle·ro·sis (mī′ĕ-lō-skle-rō′sis) SYN myelofibrosis. [myelo- + G. *sklērōsis,* induration]

my·e·lo·sis (mī′ĕ-lō′sis) **1.** A condition characterized by abnormal proliferation of tissue or cellular elements of bone marrow (e.g., multiple myeloma, myelocytic leukemia, myelofibrosis). **2.** A condition in which there is abnormal proliferation of medullary tissue in the spinal cord, as in a glioma.

my·e·lo·sup·pres·sion (mī′ĕ-lō-sŭ-presh′ŭn) A reduction in the ability of the bone marrow to produce blood cells: platelets, red blood cells, and white blood cells. Typically caused by cancer chemotherapy and radiation therapy. During the period of myelosuppression, patients may be at an increased risk of infection or bleeding or may experience symptoms due to anemia. [G. *myelos,* marrow, + L. *suppressio,* pressing under]

my·e·lot·o·my (mī′ĕ-lot′ŏ-mē) Incision of the spinal cord. [myelo- + G. *tomē,* incision]

my·e·lo·tox·ic (mī′ĕ-lō-tok′sik) **1.** Inhibitory, depressant, or destructive to one or more of the components of bone marrow. **2.** Pertaining to, derived from, or manifesting the features of diseased bone marrow.

my·en·ter·ic (mī′en-ter′ik) Relating to the myenteron.

my·en·ter·ic plex·us (mē′en-ter′ik plek′sŭs) A plexus of unmyelinated fibers and postganglionic autonomic cell bodies lying in the muscular coat of the esophagus, stomach, and intestine; it communicates with the subserous and submucous plexuses, all subdivisions of the enteric plexus.

my·en·ter·on (mī-en′tĕr-on) The muscular coat, or muscularis, of the intestine. [G. *mys,* muscle, + *enteron,* intestine]

my·es·the·si·a (mī-es-thē′zē-ă) The sensation felt in muscle when it is contracting; awareness of movement or activity in muscles or joints; sense of position or movement mediated in large part by the posterior columns and medial lemniscus. SEE ALSO bathyesthesia. SYN kinesthetic sense, muscular sense, myaesthesia. [G. *mys,* muscle, + *aisthēsis,* sensation]

my·i·a·sis (mī-ī′ă-sis) Any infection due to invasion of tissues or cavities of the body by larvae of dipterous insects. [G. *myia,* a fly]

my·lo·hy·oid (mī′lō-hī′oyd) Relating to the molar teeth, or posterior portion of the lower jaw, and to the hyoid bone; denoting various structures. SEE nerve, muscle, region, sulcus. [G. *mylē,* a mill, in pl. *mylai,* molar teeth]

my·lo·hy·oid ar·ter·y (mī′lō-hī′oyd ahr′tĕr-ē) SYN mylohyoid branch of inferior alveolar artery.

my·lo·hy·oid branch of in·fe·ri·or al·ve·o·lar ar·ter·y (mī′lō-hī′oyd branch in-fēr′ē-ŏr al-vē′ŏ-lăr ahr′tĕr-ē) Branch of inferior alveolar artery to the mylohyoid muscle. SYN mylohyoid artery, ramus mylohyoideus arteriae alveolaris inferioris.

my·lo·hy·oid mus·cle (mī′lō-hī′oyd mŭs′ĕl) *Origin,* mylohyoid line of mandible; *insertion,* upper border of hyoid bone and raphe separating muscle from its fellow; *action,* elevates floor of mouth and the tongue, depresses jaw when hyoid is fixed; *nerve supply,* nerve to mylohyoid from mandibular division of trigeminal. SYN musculus mylohyoideus [TA].

my·lo·hy·oid nerve (mī′lō-hī′oyd nĕrv) SYN nerve to mylohyoid.

♻ **myo-** Combining form meaning muscle. [G. *mys,* muscle]

***myo*-in·o·si·tol** (mī′ō-in-os′i-tol) A constituent of various phosphatidylinositols and the most widely distributed form of inositol found in microorganisms, higher plants, and animals.

my·o·ar·chi·tec·ton·ic (mī′ō-ahr-ki-tek-ton′ik) Relating to the structural arrangement of muscle or of fibers in general. [myo- + G. *architektonikos,* relating to construction]

my·o·blast (mī′ō-blast) A primordial muscle cell with the potentiality of developing into a muscle fiber. SYN sarcoblast. [myo- + G. *blastos,* germ]

my·o·blas·tic (mī′ō-blas′tik) Relating to a myoblast or to the mode of formation of muscle cells.

my·o·blas·to·ma (mī′ō-blas-tō′mă) A tumor of immature muscle cells. [myo- + G. *blastos,* germ, + *-oma,* tumor]

my·o·bra·di·a (mī′ō-brā′dē-ă) Sluggish reaction of muscle to stimulation. [myo- + G. *bradys,* slow]

my·o·car·di·al (mī-ō-kahr′dē-ăl) Relating to the myocardium.

my·o·car·di·al de·pres·sant fac·tor (MDF) (mī′ō-kahr′dē-ăl dĕ-pres′ănt fak′tŏr) A toxic factor in shock that impairs cardiac contractility.

my·o·car·di·al in·farc·tion (MI) (mī′ō-kahr′dē-ăl in-fahrk′shŭn) Infarction of an area of the heart muscle, usually as a result of occlusion of a coronary artery. SYN heart attack, infarctus myocardii.

my·o·car·di·al in·suf·fi·cien·cy (mī′ō-kahr′dē-ăl in′sŭ-fish′ĕn-sē) SYN heart failure (1).

my·o·car·di·o·graph (mī′ō-kahr′dē-ō-graf) An instrument composed of a tambour with recording lever attachment, by which a tracing is made of the movements of the heart muscle. [myo- + G. *kardia,* heart, + *graphō,* to record]

my·o·car·di·op·a·thy (mī′ō-kahr-dē-op′ă-thē) SYN cardiomyopathy. [myocardium + G. *pathos,* suffering]

my·o·car·di·tis (mī′ō-kahr-dī′tis) Inflammation of the muscular walls of the heart.

my·o·car·di·um, pl. **my·o·car·di·a** (mī′ō-kahr′dē-ŭm, -ă) The middle layer of the heart, consisting of cardiac muscle. [myo- + G. *kardia,* heart]

my·o·cele (mī′ō-sēl) **1.** Protrusion of muscle substance through a tear in its sheath. [myo- + G. *kēlē,* hernia] **2.** The small cavity that appears in somites. [myo- + G. *koilia,* a cavity]

my·o·cel·lu·li·tis (mī′ō-sel-yū-lī′tis) Inflammation of muscle and cellular tissue. [myo- + Mod. L. *cellularis,* cellular (tissue), + G. *-itis,* inflammation]

my·o·ce·ro·sis (mī′ō-sē-rō′sis) Waxy degeneration of the muscles. [myo- + G. *kēros,* wax]

my·o·clo·ni·a (mī′ō-klō′nē-ă) Any disorder characterized by myoclonus. [myo- + G. *klonos,* a tumult]

my·o·clon·ic (mī′ō-klon′ik) Showing myoclonus.

my·o·clon·ic a·stat·ic ep·i·lep·sy (mī′ō-klon′ik ā-stat′ik ep′i-lep′sē) A petit mal variant characterized by atonic (drop attacks) and tonic or tonic-clonic attacks in neurologically disabled children (e.g., patients with hemiplegia, ataxia) with mental retardation; usually progresses despite medication.

my·oc·lo·nus (mī′ok′lō-nŭs) One or a series of shocklike contractions of a group of muscles, of variable regularity, synchrony, and symmetry, generally due to a central nervous system lesion. [myo- + G. *klonos,* tumult]

my·oc·lo·nus ep·i·lep·sy (mī′ok′lō-nŭs ep′i-lep′sē) A clinically diverse group of epilepsy syndromes, some benign, some progressive. Many are hereditary and all are characterized by the occurrence of myoclonus. Specific syndromes include cherry red spot myoclonus syndrome, ceroid lipofuscinosis, myoclonic epilepsy with ragged red fibers, and Baltic myoclonus. SYN localization-related epilepsy (1).

my·oc·lo·nus mul·ti·plex (mī′ok′lō-nŭs mŭl-ti-pleks) An ill-defined disorder marked by rapid and widespread muscle contractions. SYN polyclonia, polymyoclonus.

my•o•cu•ta•ne•ous (mī′ō-kyū-tā′nē-ŭs) SYN musculocutaneous. [myo- + L. *cutis,* skin]

my•o•cyte (mī′ō-sīt) A muscle cell. [myo- + G. *kytos,* cell]

my•o•cy•tol•y•sis (mī′ō-sī-tol′i-sis) Dissolution of muscle fiber. [myo- + G. *kytos,* cell, + *lysis,* a loosening]

my•o•cy•to•ma (mī′ō-sī-tō′mă) A benign neoplasm derived from muscle.

my•o•de•mi•a (mī′ō-dē′mē-ă) Fatty degeneration of muscle. [myo- + G. *dēmos,* tallow]

my•o•dyn•i•a (mī′ō-din′ē-ă) SYN myalgia. [myo- + G. *odynē,* pain]

my•o•dys•to•ny (mī′ō-dis′tō-nē) A condition of slow relaxation, interrupted by a succession of slight contractions, following electrical stimulation of a muscle. [myo- + G. *dys-,* difficult, + *tonos,* tone, tension]

my•o•dys•tro•phy, my•o•dys•tro•phi•a (mi′ō-dis′trŏ-fē, -trō′fē-ă) SYN muscular dystrophy. [myo- + G. *dys-,* difficult, poor, + *trophē,* nourishment]

my•o•e•de•ma (mī′ō-ĕ-dē′mă) A localized contraction of a degenerating muscle, occurring at the point of a sharp blow, independent of the nerve supply. SYN idiomuscular contraction, mounding, myo-oedema. [myo- + G. *oidēma,* swelling]

my•o•e•las•tic (mī′ō-ē-las′tik) Pertaining to closely associated smooth muscle fibers and elastic connective tissue.

my•o•en•do•car•di•tis (mī′ō-en′dō-kahr-dī′tis) Inflammation of the muscular wall and lining membrane of the heart. [myo- + G. *endon,* within, + *kardia,* heart, + *-itis,* inflammation]

my•o•ep•i•the•li•al (mī′ō-ep-i-thē′lē-ăl) Relating to myoepithelium.

my•o•ep•i•the•li•o•ma (mī′ō-ep′i-thē-lē-ō′mă) A benign tumor of myoepithelial cells. [myo- + epithelium, + G. *-ōma,* tumor]

my•o•ep•i•the•li•um (mī′ō-ep-i-thē′lē-ŭm) Spindle-shaped, contractile, smooth musclelike cells of epithelial origin that are arranged longitudinally or obliquely around sweat glands and the secretory alveoli of the mammary gland; stellate myoepithelial cells occur around lacrimal and some salivary gland secretory units. [myo- + epithelium]

my•o•fas•ci•al (mī′ō-fash′ē-ăl) Of or relating to the fascia surrounding and separating muscle tissue.

my•o•fas•ci•al pain-dys•func•tion syn•drome (mī′ō-fash′ē-ăl pān-dis-fŭngk′shŭn sin′drōm) A condition involving the development of regional trigger points that create pain, weakness, limited range of motion, and general dysfunction. Postural compensation for painful areas can lead to the development of additional trigger points, allowing the myofascial pain-dysfunction syndrome to progress to a more severe state. SYN temporomandibular joint pain-dysfunction syndrome.

my•o•fas•ci•tis (mī′ō-fă-sī′tis) SYN myositis fibrosa.

my•o•fi•bril (mī′ō-fī′bril) One of the fine longitudinal fibrils occurring in a skeletal or cardiac muscle fiber and consisting of many regularly overlapped ultramicroscopic thick and thin myofilaments. [myo- + Mod. L. *fibrilla,* fibril]

my•o•fi•bro•blast (mī′ō-fī′brō-blast) A cell thought to be responsible for contracture of wounds; such cells have some characteristics of smooth muscle, such as contractile properties and fibrils, and are also believed to produce, temporarily, type III collagen.

my•o•fi•bro•ma (mī′ō-fī-brō′mă) A benign neoplasm that consists chiefly of fibrous connective tissue, with variable numbers of muscle cells forming portions of the neoplasm.

my•o•fi•bro•sis (mī′ō-fī-brō′sis) Chronic myositis with diffuse hyperplasia of the interstitial connective tissue pressing upon and causing atrophy of the muscular tissue.

my•o•fi•bro•si•tis (mī′ō-fī-brō-sī′tis) Inflammation of the perimysium.

my•o•fil•a•ments (mī′ō-fil′ă-mĕnts) The ultramicroscopic threads of filamentous proteins making up myofibrils in striated muscle. Thick ones contain myosin and thin ones, actin; thick and thin myofilaments also occur in smooth muscle fibers but are not regularly arranged in discrete myofibrils and thus do not impart a striated appearance to these cells.

my•o•func•tion•al ther•a•py (mī′ō-fŭngk′shŭn-ăl thār′ă-pē) SPEECH PATHOLOGY any technique used to promote normal patterns of tongue movement and swallowing; primarily used to ameliorate tongue thrust. SEE tongue thrust. SYN tongue thrust therapy.

my•o•gen•e•sis (mī′ō-jen′ĕ-sis) Embryonic formation of muscle cells or fibers. [myo- + G. *genesis,* origin]

my•o•ge•net•ic, my•o•gen•ic (mī′ō-jĕ-net′ik, -jen′ik) **1.** Originating in or starting from muscle. **2.** Relating to the origin of muscle cells or fibers. SYN myogenous.

my•og•e•nous (mī-oj′ĕ-nŭs) SYN myogenetic.

my•o•glo•bin (MbO_2, Mb) (mī′ō-glō′bin) The oxygen-transporting and storage protein of muscle, resembling blood hemoglobin in function but with a molecular weight approximately one quarter that of hemoglobin. Serum levels of this protein are often measured to facilitate diagnosis of an acute myocardial infarction; it is released into the circulation within 2–4 hours after myocardial infarction, peaks at about 8–12 hours, and returns to normal after 18–24 hours. SEE ALSO oxymyoglobin. SYN muscle hemoglobin. [myo- + hemoglobin]

my•o•glo•bi•nu•ri•a (mī′ō-glō-bi-nyūr′ē-ă) Excretion of myoglobin in urine; results from muscle degeneration, which releases myoglobin into the blood; occurs in certain types of trauma (e.g., crush syndrome), advanced or protracted ischemia of muscle, or as a paroxysmal process of unknown etiology.

my•o•glob•u•lin (mī′ō-glob′yū-lin) Globulin present in muscle tissue.

my•o•glob•u•li•nu•ri•a (mī′ō-glob′yū-li-nūr′ē-ă) Excretion of myoglobulin in the urine.

my•o•gram (mī′ō-gram) The tracing made by a myograph. [myo- + G. *gramma,* a drawing]

my•o•graph (mī′ō-graf) A recording instrument by which tracings are made of muscular contractions. [myo- + G. *graphō,* to write]

my•o•graph•ic (mī-ō-graf′ik) Relating to a myogram, or the record of a myograph.

my•og•ra•phy (mī-og′ră-fē) **1.** The recording of muscular movements by the myograph. **2.** A description of or treatise on the muscles.

my•oid (mī′oyd) **1.** Resembling muscle. **2.** One of the fine, contractile, threadlike protoplasmic elements found in certain epithelial cells in lower animals. [myo- + G. *eidos,* appearance]

my•oid cells (mī′oyd selz) Flattened smooth musclelike cells of mesodermal origin that lie just outside the basal lamina of the seminiferous tubule. SYN peritubular contractile cells.

my•o•kin•e•sim•e•ter (mī′ō-kin-ĕ-sim′ĕ-tĕr) A device for registering the exact time and extent of contraction of the larger muscles of the lower extremity in response to electric stimulation. [myo- + G. *kinesis,* movement, + *metron,* measure]

my•o•ky•mi•a (mī′ō-kī′mē-ă) Continuous involuntary quivering or rippling of muscles at rest, caused by spontaneous, repetitive firing of groups of motor unit potentials. SYN kymatism, Morvan chorea. [myo- + G. *kyma,* wave]

my•o•li•po•ma (mī′ō-li-pō′mă) A benign neoplasm that consists chiefly of fat cells (adipose tissue), with variable numbers of muscle cells forming portions of the neoplasm.

my•ol•o•gy (mī-ol′ŏ-jē) The branch of science concerned with the muscles and their accessory parts, tendons, aponeuroses, bursae, and fasciae. [myo- + G. *logos,* study]

my•ol•y•sis (mī-ol′i-sis) Dissolution or liquefaction of muscular tissue, frequently preceded by degenerative changes such as infiltration of fat, atrophy, and fatty degeneration. [myo- + G. *lysis,* dissolution]

my•o•ma (mī-ō′mă) A benign neoplasm of muscular tissue. SEE ALSO leiomyoma, rhabdomyoma. [myo- + G. *-oma,* tumor]

my•o•ma•la•ci•a (mī′ō-mă-lā′shē-ă) Pathologic softening of muscular tissue. [myo- + G. *malakia,* softness]

my•o•ma•tous (mī-ō′mă-tŭs) Pertaining to or characterized by the features of a myoma.

my•o•mec•to•my (mī′ō-mek′tŏ-mē) Operative removal of a myoma, specifically of a uterine myoma. [myoma + G. *ektomē,* excision]

my•o•mel•a•no•sis (mī′ō-mel-ă-nō′sis) Abnormal dark pigmentation of muscular tissue. SEE ALSO melanosis. [myo- + G. *melanōsis,* becoming black]

my•o•mere (mī′ō-mēr) SYN myotome (4). [myo- + G. *meros,* a part]

my•om•e•ter (mī-om′ĕ-tĕr) An instrument for measuring the extent of a muscular contraction. [myo- + G. *metron,* measure]

my•o•me•tri•al (mī′ō-mē′trē-ăl) Relating to the myometrium.

my•o•me•tri•tis (mī′ō-mē-trī′tis) Inflammation of the muscular wall of the uterus. [myo- + G. *mētra,* uterus, + *-itis,* inflammation]

my•o•me•tri•um (mī′ō-mē′trē-ŭm) The muscular wall of the uterus. [myo- + G. *mētra,* uterus]

my•o•ne•cro•sis (mī′ō-nĕ-krō′sis) Necrosis of muscle.

my•o•neme (mī′ō-nēm) **1.** A muscle fibril. **2.** One of the contractile fibrils of certain protozoans; thought to function in an analogous fashion to metazoan muscle fibers. [myo- + G. *nēma,* thread]

my•o•neu•ral (mī′ō-nūr′ăl) Relating to both muscle and nerve; denoting specifically the synapse of the motor neuron with striated muscle fibers: myoneural junction or motor endplate. SEE ALSO neuromuscular. [myo- + G. *neuron,* nerve]

my•o•neu•ral block•ade (mī′ō-nūr′ăl blok-ād′) Inhibition of nerve impulse transmission at myoneural junctions by a drug such as curare.

my•o•neu•ral junc•tion (mī′ō-nūr′ăl jŭngk′shŭn) The synaptic connection of the axon of the motor neuron with a muscle fiber. SEE motor endplate.

myo-oedema [Br.] SYN myoedema.

my•o•pal•mus (mī′ō-pal′mŭs) Muscle twitching. [myo- + G. *palmos,* a quivering]

my•o•pa•ral•y•sis (mī′ō-pă-ral′i-sis) Muscular paralysis.

my•o•pa•re•sis (mī′ō-pă-rē′sis) Slight muscular paralysis.

my•o•path•ic (mī′ō-path′ik) Denoting a disorder involving muscular tissue.

my•op•a•thy (mī-op′ă-thē) Any abnormal condition or disease of the muscular tissues; commonly designates a disorder involving skeletal muscle. [myo- + G. *pathos,* suffering]

my•o•per•i•car•di•tis (mī′ō-per-i-kahr-dī′tis) Inflammation of the muscular wall of the heart and of the enveloping pericardium; also, perimyocarditis. [myo- + pericarditis]

my•o•pi•a (mī-ō′pē-ă) That optic condition in which parallel light rays are brought by the ocular media to focus in front of the retina. See this page. SYN nearsightedness, shortsightedness. [G. fr. *myo,* to shut, + *ōps,* eye]

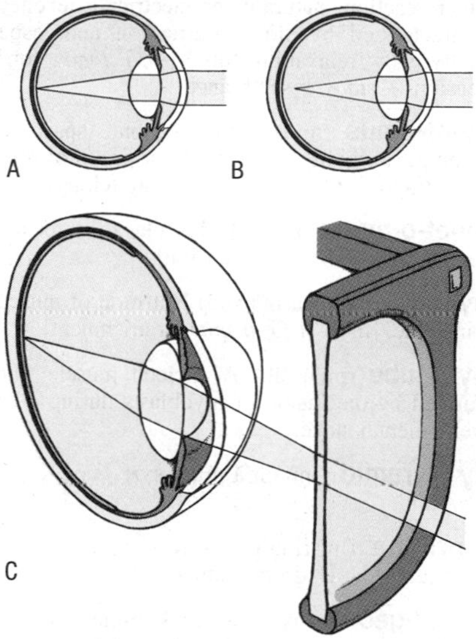

myopia: (A) normal (20/20) vision: light rays focus sharply on retina, (B) myopic (nearsighted) vision: light rays from a distance come to sharp focus in front of the retina, (C) myopia corrected by eyeglasses with concave lenses

my•op•ic (mī-op′ik) Relating to or suffering from myopia.

my•op•ic a•stig•ma•tism (mī-op′ik ă-stig′mă-tizm) An astigmatism in which both meridians are myopic.

my•op•ic cres•cent (mī-op′ik kres′ĕnt) A white or grayish white crescentic area in the fundus of the eye located on the temporal side of the optic disc; caused by atrophy of the choroid, permitting the sclera to become visible.

my•o•plasm (mī′ō-plazm) The contractile portion of the muscle cell, as distinguished from the sarcoplasm. [myo- + G. *plasma,* a thing formed]

my•o•plas•tic (mī′ō-plas′tik) Relating to surgical repair of the muscles, or to the use of muscular tissue in correcting defects.

my•o•plas•ty (mī′ō-plas-tē) Surgical repair of muscular tissue. [myo- + G. *plastos,* formed]

my•or•rha•phy (mī-ōr′ă-fē) Suture of a muscle. [myo- + G. *rhaphē,* seam]

my•or•rhex•is (mī-ō-rek′sis) Tearing of a muscle. [myo- + G. *rhēxis,* a rupture]

my•o•sal•pinx (mī′ō-sal′pingks) The muscular tunic of the uterine tube. [myo- + salpinx]

my•o•sar•co•ma (mī′ō-sahr-kō′mă) A general term for a malignant neoplasm derived from muscular tissue. SEE ALSO leiomyosarcoma, rhabdomyosarcoma.

my•o•scle•ro•sis (mī′ō-skle-rō′sis) Chronic myositis with hyperplasia of the interstitial connective tissue.

my•o•sin (mī′ō-sin) A globulin present in muscle; in combination with actin, it forms actomyosin; myosin forms the thick filaments in muscle.

my•o•sin fil•a•ment (mī′ō-sin fil′ă-mĕnt) One of the contractile elements in skeletal, cardiac, and smooth muscle fibers; in skeletal muscle, the filament is about 10 nm thick and 1.5 mcm long.

my•o•sit•ic (mī-ō-sit′ik) Relating to myositis.

my•o•si•tis (mī-ō-sī′tis) Inflammation of a muscle. SYN initis (2). [myo- + G. *-itis,* inflammation]

my•o•si•tis fi•bro•sa (mī-ō-sī′tis fī-brō′să) Induration of a muscle through an interstitial growth of fibrous tissue. SYN myofascitis.

my•o•si•tis os•si•fi•cans (mī-ō-sī′tis os-if′i-kanz) SYN heterotopic ossification. See page 1040.

my•o•spasm, **my•o•spas•mus** (mī′ō-spazm, mī-ō-spaz′mŭs) Spasmodic muscular contraction.

my•o•tac•tic (mī-ō-tak′tik) Relating to the muscular sense. [myo- + L. *tactus,* a touching]

my•o•tac•tic re•flex (mī-ō-tak′ik rē′fleks) Tonic contraction of the muscles in response to a stretching force, due to stimulation of muscle proprioceptors. SYN deep tendon reflex, muscle spindle reflex, stretch reflex.

my•ot•a•sis (mī-ot′ă-sis) Stretching of a muscle. [myo- + G. *tasis,* a stretching]

my•o•tat•ic (mī-ō-tat′ik) Relating to myotasis.

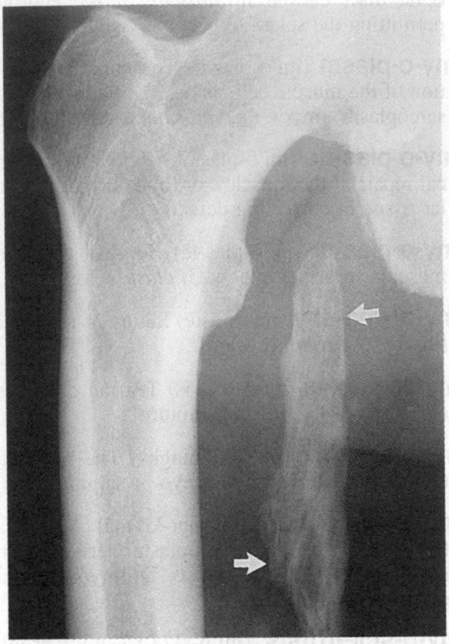

myositis ossificans: well-organized ossifying hematoma present in the adductor magnus muscle (arrows)

my·o·tat·ic con·trac·tion (mī-ō-tat′ik kŏn-trak′shŭn) A reflex contraction of a skeletal muscle that occurs as a result of stimulation of the stretch receptors in the muscle, i.e., as part of a myotatic reflex.

my·o·tat·ic ir·ri·ta·bil·i·ty (mī-ō-tat′ik ir′i-tă-bil′i-tē) The ability of a muscle to contract in response to the stimulus produced by a sudden stretching.

my·o·ten·o·si·tis (mī′ō-ten-ō-sī′tis) Inflammation of a muscle with its tendon. [myo- + G. *tenōn,* tendon, + *-itis,* inflammation]

my·o·te·not·o·my (mī′ō-te-not′ŏ-mē) Cutting through the principal tendon of a muscle, with division of the muscle itself in whole or in part. SYN tenomyotomy. [myo- + G. *tenōn,* tendon, + *tomē,* incision]

my·o·ther·a·py (mī′ō-thār′ă-pē) SYN massage therapy.

my·o·tome (mī′ō-tōm) **1.** A knife for dividing muscle. **2.** In embryos, that part of the somite that develops into skeletal muscle. SYN muscle plate. **3.** All muscles derived from one somite and innervated by one segmental spinal nerve. **4.** In primitive vertebrates, the muscular part of a metamere. SYN myomere. [myo- + G. *tomos,* a cut]

my·ot·o·my (mī-ot′ŏ-mē) **1.** Anatomy or dissection of the muscles. **2.** Surgical division of a muscle. [myo- + G. *tomē,* excision]

my·o·to·ni·a (mī-ō-tō′nē-ă) Delayed relaxation of a muscle after a strong contraction, or prolonged contraction after mechanical stimulation (as by percussion) or brief electrical stimulation; due to abnormality of the muscle membrane, specifically the ion channels. [myo- + G. *tonos,* tension, stretching]

my·o·to·ni·a con·gen·i·ta (mī′ō-tō′nē-ă kŏn-jen′i-tă) SYN amyotonia congenita. SYN Thomsen disease.

my·o·ton·ic (mī-ō-ton′ik) Pertaining to or exhibiting myotonia.

my·o·ton·ic chon·dro·dys·tro·phy (mī-ō-ton′ik kon′drō-dis′trŏ-fē) A rare congenital disease that causes myotonia, muscular hypertrophy, joint and long bone abnormalities, and weakness.

my·o·ton·ic re·sponse (mī-ō-ton′ik rĕ-spons′) Failure of muscle relaxation caused by repetitive discharge of muscle fiber action potentials.

my·ot·o·noid (mī-ot′ŏ-noyd) Denoting a muscular reaction, naturally or electrically excited, characterized by slow contraction and, especially, slow relaxation. [myo- + G. *tonos,* tone, tension, + *eidos,* resemblance]

my·ot·o·nus (mī-ot′ŏ-nŭs) A tonic spasm or temporary rigidity of a muscle or group of muscles. [myo- + G. *tonos,* tension, stretching]

my·ot·o·ny (mī-ot′ŏ-nē) Muscular tonus or tension. [myo- + G. *tonos,* tension]

my·ot·ro·phy (mī-ot′rŏ-fē) Nutrition of muscular tissue. [myo- + G. *trophē,* nourishment]

my·o·tube (mī′ō-tūb) A skeletal muscle fiber formed by the fusion of myoblasts during a developmental stage.

My Pyramid (mī pir′ă-mid) SYN Food Guide Pyramid.

my·rin·ga (mi-ring′gă) SYN tympanic membrane. [Mod. L. drum membrane]

myr·in·gec·to·my (mir-in-jek′tŏ-mē) Excision of the tympanic membrane. [myring- + G. *ektomē,* excision]

myr·in·gi·tis (mir-in-jī′tis) Inflammation of the tympanic membrane. SYN tympanitis. [myring- + G. *-itis,* inflammation]

myringo-, myring- Combining forms indicating the membrana tympani. [Mod. L. *myringa*]

my·rin·go·plas·ty (mi-ring′gō-plas′tē) Operative repair of a damaged tympanic membrane. [myringo- + G. *plassō,* to form]

my·rin·go·scle·ro·sis (mi-ring′gō-skler-ō′sis) Formation of dense connective tissue in the tympanic membrane, usually not associated with hearing loss. [myringo- + sclerosis]

my·rin·go·sta·pe·di·o·pex·y (mi-ring′gō-stā-pē′dē-ō-pek′sē) A technique of tympanoplasty in which the drum membrane or grafted drum membrane is brought into functional connection with the stapes. [myringo- + L. *stapes,* stirrup (stapes), + G. *pēxis,* fixation]

myr•in•got•o•my (mir-in-got′ŏ-mē) Paracentesis of the tympanic membrane. SYN tympanostomy, tympanotomy. [myringo- + G. *tomē,* excision]

my•rinx (mir′ingks) SYN tympanic membrane. [Mod. L. *myringa,* drum membrane]

myr•me•ci•a (mir-mē′shē-ă) A form of viral wart in which the lesion has a domed surface (i.e., an ant hill configuration). [G. *murmex,* ant]

my•so•phil•i•a (mī-sō-fil′ē-ă) Sexual interest in excretions. [G. *mysos,* defilement, + *philos,* fond]

my•so•pho•bi•a (mī-sō-fō′bē-ă) Morbid fear of dirt or defilement from touching familiar objects. [G. *mysos,* defilement, + *phobos,* fear]

myx-, myxo- Combining forms relating to mucus (e.g., myxocyte). [G. *myxa,* nasal mucus]

myx•ad•e•no•ma (miks-ad-ĕ-nō′mă) A benign neoplasm derived from glandular epithelial tissue.

myx•as•the•ni•a (miks-as-thē′nē-ă) Faulty secretion of mucus. [myx- + G. *astheneia,* weakness]

myx•e•de•ma (miks-ĕ-dē′mă) Nonpitting waxy edema of the skin, often most pronounced in the face and shins (pretibial myxedema), owing to subcutaneous deposition of mucoid material in hypothyroidism. SYN myxoedema. [myx- + G. *oidēma,* swelling]

myx•e•dem•a•toid (miks-ĕ-dem′ă-toyd) Resembling myxedema. SYN myxoedematoid.

myx•e•dem•a•tous (miks-ĕ-dem′ă-tŭs) Relating to myxedema. SYN myxoedematous.

myx•o•chon•dro•fi•bro•sar•co•ma (mik′sō-kon′drō-fī′brō-sahr-kō′mă) A malignant neoplasm derived from fibrous connective tissue in which there are foci of cartilaginous and myxomatous tissue. [myxo- + G. *chondros,* cartilage, + L. *fibra,* fiber, + G. *sarx,* flesh, + *-ōma,* tumor]

myx•o•chon•dro•ma (mik′sō-kon-drō′mă) A benign neoplasm of cartilaginous tissue in which the stroma resembles primitive mesenchymal tissue. [myxo- + G. *chondros,* cartilage, + *-ōma,* tumor]

myx•o•cyte (mik′sō-sīt) One of the stellate or polyhedral cells present in mucous tissue. [myxo- + G. *kytos,* cell]

myxoedema [Br.] SYN myxedema.

myxoedematoid [Br.] SYN myxedematoid.

myxoedematous [Br.] SYN myxedematous.

myx•o•fi•bro•ma (mik′sō-fī-brō′mă) A benign neoplasm of fibrous connective tissue that resembles primitive mesenchymal tissue. [myxo- + L. *fibra,* fiber, + G. *-ōma,* tumor]

myx•o•fi•bro•sar•co•ma (mik′sō-fī′brō-sahr-kō′mă) A malignant fibrous histiocytoma with a predominance of myxoid areas that resemble primitive mesenchymal tissue. [myxo- + L. *fibra,* fiber, + G. *sarx,* flesh, + *-ōma,* tumor]

myx•oid (mik′soyd) Resembling mucus. [myxo- + G. *eidos,* resemblance]

myx•oid cyst (mik′soyd sist) SYN ganglion (2).

myx•o•li•po•ma (mik′sō-li-pō′mă) A benign neoplasm of adipose tissue in which portions of the tumor resemble mucoid mesenchymal tissue. [myxo- + G. *lipos,* fat, + *-ōma,* tumor]

myx•o•ma (mik-sō′mă) A benign neoplasm derived from connective tissue, consisting of polyhedral and stellate cells embedded in a soft mucoid matrix; occurs in bone, skin, and muscle; when arising from cardiac muscle may encroach on the cavity of an atrium. [myxo- + G. *-ōma,* tumor]

myx•o•ma•to•sis (mik′sō-mă-tō′sis) **1.** SYN mucoid degeneration. **2.** Multiple myxomas.

myx•o•ma•tous (mik-sō′mă-tŭs) **1.** Pertaining to or characterized by the features of a myxoma. **2.** Said of tissue that resembles primitive mesenchymal tissue.

myx•o•pap•il•lar•y ep•en•dy•mo•ma (mik′sō-pap′i-lar-ē ĕ-pen′di-mō′mă) A slow-growing ependymoma of the filum terminale, occurring most often in young adults, which consists of cuboidal cells in papillary arrangement around a mucinous vascular core.

myx•o•pap•il•lo•ma (mik′sō-pap′i-lō′mă) A benign neoplasm of epithelial tissue in which the stroma resembles primitive mesenchymal tissue. [myxo- + L. *papilla,* a nipple, + G. *-ōma,* tumor]

myx•o•poi•e•sis (mik′sō-poy-ē′sis) Mucus production. [myxo- + G. *poiēsis,* a making]

myx•o•sar•co•ma (mik′sō-sahr-kō′mă) A sarcoma, usually a liposarcoma or malignant fibrous histiocytoma, with an abundant component of myxoid tissue resembling primitive mesenchyme containing connective tissue mucin. [myxo- + G. *sarx,* flesh, + *-ōma,* tumor]

MZ Abbreviation for monozygotic.

N

ν Nu. SEE nu.

N_A Abbreviation for Avogadro number.

n Abbreviation for nano- (2); reaction order.

N Abbreviation for normal concentration. SEE normal (3).

n **1.** The number in a scientific study; sample size. **2.** Refractive index.

Na Symbol for sodium.

Na•ber probe (nā′bĕr prōb) A type of periodontal tool used to evaluate bone support in the furcation areas of bifurcated and trifurcated teeth. SYN furcation probe.

na•both•i•an cyst (nă-bō′thē-ăn sist) A retention cyst that develops when a mucous gland of the cervix uteri is obstructed; of no pathologic significance. SYN nabothian follicle.

na•both•i•an fol•li•cle (nă-bō′thē-ăn fol′i-kĕl) SYN nabothian cyst.

NACCM Abbreviation for National Center for Complementary and Alternative Medicine.

***N*-a•ce•tyl•cys•teine** (ă-sē′til-sis′tēn) An agent administered orally or by inhalation to counteract acetaminophen toxicity.

na•cre•ous (nā′krē-ŭs) Lustrous, like mother-of-pearl; descriptive term for bacterial colonies. [Fr. *nacre,* mother-of-pearl]

NAD Abbreviation for nicotinamide adenine dinucleotide.

NAD^+ Abbreviation for nicotinamide adenine dinucleotide (oxidized form).

NADH Abbreviation for nicotinamide adenine dinucleotide (reduced form).

NADH de•hy•dro•gen•ase (dē-hī′drō-jen-ās) An iron-sulfur–containing flavoprotein reversibly oxidizing NADH to NAD^+; an inherited deficiency of this complex results in overwhelming acidosis.

NADP Abbreviation for nicotinamide adenine dinucleotide phosphate.

$NADP^+$ Abbreviation for nicotinamide adenine dinucleotide phosphate (oxidized form).

NADPH Abbreviation for nicotinamide adenine dinucleotide phosphate (reduced form).

Nae•ge•li syn•drome (nā′gĕ-lē sin′drōm) Reticular skin pigmentation, diminished sweating, hypodontia, and hyperkeratosis of the palms and soles.

Nae•gle•ri•a (nā-glē′rē-ă) Free-living freshwater and soil ameboflagellates that cause amebic meningitis.

naevi [Br.] SYN nevi.

naevoid [Br.] SYN nevoid.

naevose [Br.] SYN nevose.

naevous [Br.] SYN nevous.

naevus [Br.] SYN nevus.

naevus cell [Br.] SYN nevus cell.

naevus comedonicus [Br.] SYN nevus comedonicus.

naevus flammeus [Br.] SYN nevus flammeus.

naevus pigmentosus [Br.] SYN nevus pigmentosus.

naevus pilosus [Br.] SYN nevus pilosus.

naevus spilus [Br.] SYN nevus spilus.

naevus unius lateris [Br.] SYN nevus unius lateris.

naevus vascularis [Br.] SYN nevus vascularis.

naevus vasculosus [Br.] SYN nevus vasculosus.

Naff•zi•ger op•er•a•tion (naf′zig-ĕr op-ĕr-ā′shŭn) Orbital decompression for severe malignant exophthalmos by removal of the lateral and superior orbital walls.

Nä•ge•le ob•liq•ui•ty (nah′gĕ-lĕ ō-blik′wi-tē) Inclination of the fetal head in cases of flat pelvis, so that the biparietal diameter is oblique in relation to the plane of the pelvic brim, the anterior parietal bone presenting to the parturient canal.

Nä•ge•le pel•vis (nah′gĕ-lĕ pel′vis) An obliquely contracted or unilateral synostotic pelvis, marked by arrest of development of one lateral half of the sacrum, usually ankylosis of the sacroiliac joint on that side, rotation of the sacrum toward the same side, and deviation of the symphysis pubis to the opposite side.

Nä•ge•le rule (nah′gĕ-lĕ rūl) Determination of the estimated delivery date by adding 7 days to the first day of the last normal menstrual period, counting back 3 months, and adding 1 year.

Na•gel test (nā′gel test) A test for color vision in which the observer determines the relative amounts of red and green necessary to match spectral yellow; an instrument called the Nagel anomaloscope is used.

nail (nāl) **1.** One of the thin, horny, translucent plates covering the dorsal surface of the distal end of each terminal phalanx of fingers and toes. A nail consists of a visible corpus or body, and a radix or root at the proximal end concealed under a fold of skin. The under part of the nail is formed from the stratum germinativum of the epidermis, and the free surface from the stratum lucidum, with the thin cuticular fold that overlaps the lunula representing the stratum corneum. **2.** A slender rod of metal, bone, or other solid substance, used in operations to fasten together the divided extremities of a broken bone. SYN unguis [TA], nail plate, onyx. [A.S. *naegel*]

nail bed (nāl bed) The area of the corium on which the nail rests; it is extremely sensitive and presents numerous longitudinal ridges on its surface. SYN keratogenous membrane (2), matrix unguis.

nail fold (nāl fōld) The fold of skin overlapping the lateral and proximal margins of the nail.

nail ma•trix (nāl mā′triks) SYN keratogenous membrane (1). SEE nail bed.

nail pits (nāl pits) Small punctate depressions on the surface of the nail plate due to defective nail formation; seen in psoriasis and other disorders.

nail plate (nāl plāt) SYN nail.

Nair buf•fered meth•y•lene blue stain (nār bŭf′ĕrd meth′il-ēn blū stān) Procedure that shows nuclear detail of protozoan trophozoites when used at low pH (3.6–4.8).

Na•ka•ni•shi stain (nah-kah-nē′shē stān) A method for vital staining of bacteria in which a slide is treated with hot methylene blue solution until it acquires a sky-blue color, after which a drop of an emulsion of the bacteria is put on the cover glass and the latter laid on the slide; the bacteria are stained differentially, some parts more intensely than others.

na•ked vi•rus (nā′kĕd vī′rŭs) A virus consisting only of a nucleocapsid; i.e., one that does not possess an enclosing envelope.

NANB Abbreviation for non-A, non-B hepatitis.

Nance-In•sley syn•drome (nans-ins′lē sin′drōm) SYN chondrodystrophy with sensorineural deafness.

Nance-Swee•ney chon•dro•dys•pla•si•a (nans-swē′nē kon′drō-dis-plā′zhē-ă) SYN chondrodystrophy with sensorineural deafness.

NANDA (nanda) Acronym for the North American Nursing Diagnosis Association.

nan•ny•ber•ry (nan′ē-ber-ē) SYN black haw.

♻**nano-** **1.** Prefix meaning dwarfism (nanism). **2.** (n) Prefix used in the SI and metric system to signify one billionth (10^{-9}). [G. *nanos,* dwarf]

nan•o•ceph•a•lous, nan•o•ce•phal•ic (nan′ō-sef′ă-lŭs, -se-fal′ik) SYN microcephalic.

nan•o•ceph•a•ly (nan′ō-sef′ă-lē) SYN microcephaly. [nano- + G. *kephalē,* head]

nan•o•cor•mi•a (nan′ō-kōr′mē-ă) SYN microsomia. [nano- + G. *kormos,* trunk]

nan•o•gram (ng) (nan′ō-gram) One billionth of a gram (10^{-9} g).

nan•o•me•li•a (nan′ō-mē′lē-ă) SYN micromelia. [nano- + G. *melos,* limb]

nan•o•me•ter (nm) (nan′ŏ-mē-tĕr) One billionth of a meter (10^{-9} m). SYN nanometre.

nanometre [Br.] SYN nanometer.

nan•o•sec•ond (nan′ō-sek-ŏnd) One billionth of a second.

nape (nāp) SYN nucha.

naph•thol yel•low S (naf′thol yel′ō) [CI 10316] An acid dye used as a stain for basic proteins in microspectrophotometry.

nar•cis•sism (nar′si-sizm) **1.** Sexual attraction toward one's own person. **2.** A state in which the person interprets and regards everything in relation to himself or herself and not to other people or things. SYN self-love. [*Narkissos,* G. myth. char.]

♻**narco-** Prefix meaning stupor, narcosis. [G. *narkoō,* to benumb, deaden]

nar•co•a•nal•y•sis (nahr′kō-ă-nal′i-sis) Psychotherapeutic treatment under light anesthesia. SYN narcosynthesis.

nar•co•hyp•ni•a (nahr-kō-hip′nē-ă) A general numbness sometimes experienced at the moment of waking. [narco- + G. *hypnos,* sleep]

nar•co•hyp•no•sis (nahr′kō-hip-nō′sis) Stupor or deep sleep induced by hypnosis. [narco- + G. *hypnos,* sleep]

nar•co•lep•sy (nahr′kō-lep-sē) A sleep disorder that usually appears in young adulthood, consisting of recurring episodes of sleep during the day, and often disrupted nocturnal sleep; frequently accompanied by cataplexy, sleep paralysis, and hypnagogic hallucinations; a genetically determined disease. SYN Gélineau syndrome. [narco- + G. *lēpsis,* seizure]

nar•co•sis (nahr-kō′sis) General and nonspecific reversible depression of neuronal excitability, produced by a number of physical and chemical agents, usually resulting in stupor rather than in anesthesia (with which narcosis was once synonymous). [G. a benumbing]

nar•co•syn•the•sis (nahr′kō-sin′thĕ-sis) SYN narcoanalysis.

nar•co•ther•a•py (nahr′kō-thār′ă-pē) Psychotherapy conducted with the patient under the influence of a sedative or narcotic.

nar•cot•ic (nahr-kot′ik) **1.** Any drug derived from opium or opiumlike compounds with potent analgesic effects associated with both significant alteration of mood and behavior and potential for dependence and tolerance. **2.** Any drug, synthetic or naturally occurring, with effects similar to those of opium and opium derivatives. **3.** Capable of inducing a state of stuporous analgesia. [G. *narkōtikos,* benumbing]

nar•cot•ic an•al•ge•sic (nahr-kot′ik an′ăl-jē′zik) SEE narcotic.

nar•cot•ic an•tag•o•nist (nahr-kot′ik an-tag′ŏ-nist) SEE opioid antagonist.

nar•cot•ic block•ade (nahr-kot′ik blok-ād′) The use of drugs to inhibit the effects of narcotic substances, as with naloxone.

nar•cot•ic re•ver•sal (nahr-kot′ik rē-vĕr′săl) The use of narcotic antagonists, such as naloxone, to terminate the action of narcotics.

na•ris, pl. **na•res** (nā′ris, -res) SYN nostril. [L.]

NARP (nahrp) Acronym for a syndrome composed of neuropathy, ataxia, retinitis pigmentosa; one of the inherited mitochondrial disorders, caused by a point mutation resulting in the substitution of a single amino acid in the mitochondrial DNA at position 8993. A more severe expression of the same point mutation manifests clinically as Leigh disease.

nar•row-an•gle glau•co•ma (nar′rō-ang′gĕl glaw-kō′mă) SYN angle-closure glaucoma.

nar•row•band (nar′rō-band′) A limited band of sound frequencies, as opposed to the wideband of frequencies also known as white noise; used to mask hearing in the nontest ear in hearing measurement.

na•sal (nā′zăl) Relating to the nose. SYN rhinal. [L. *nasus,* nose]

na•sal bal•loon tam•pon•ade (nā′zăl bă-lūn′ tam′pŏ-nād′) A procedure to control posterior epistaxis in which a commercial nasal balloon or Foley catheter is inserted into the nasal cavity and filled with saline, putting pressure against the bleeding varices. [L. *nasus,* nose, Fr. *ballon,* ball, + *tamponner,* to plug up]

na•sal bone (nā′zăl bōn) An elongated rectangular bone which, with its fellow, forms the bridge of the nose; it articulates with the frontal bone superiorly, the ethmoid and the frontal process of the maxilla posteriorly, and its fellow medially. SYN os nasale [TA].

na•sal can•nu•la (nā′zăl kan′yū-lă) Apparatus for delivery of oxygen to the nostrils, usually at flow rates. See this page. SYN nasal prongs.

na•sal cap•sule (nā′zăl kap′sŭl) The cartilage around the developing nasal cavity of the embryo.

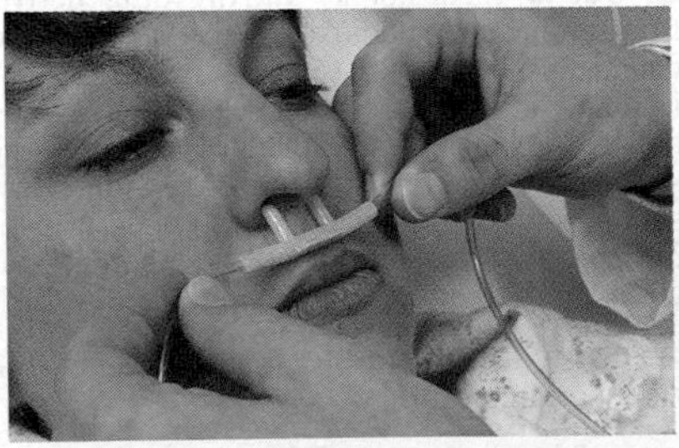
nasal cannula

na•sal car•ti•lage (nā′zăl kahr′ti-lăj) Dense connective tissue of the nose; includes the greater alar (lower lateral), the lesser alar, the lateral nasal (upper lateral), the vomeronasal, and the accessory nasal. [L. *nasus,* nose + *cartilago,* gristle]

na•sal cav•i•ty (nā′zăl kav′i-tē) The cavity on either side of the nasal septum, lined with ciliated respiratory mucosa, extending from the naris anteriorly to the choana posteriorly, and communicating with the paranasal sinuses through their orifices in the lateral wall, from which also project the three conchae; the cribriform plate, through which the olfactory nerves are transmitted, forms the roof; the floor is formed by the hard palate. See this page.

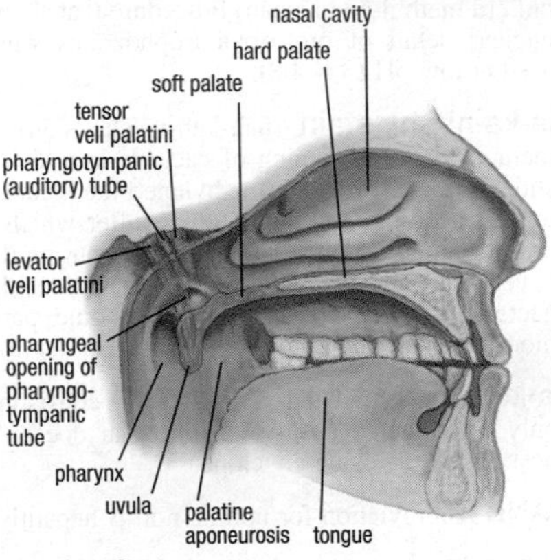

nasal cavity

na•sal crest (nā′zăl krest) The midline ridge in the floor of the nasal cavity, formed by the union of the paired maxillae and palatine bones; the vomer attaches to the crest.

na•sal e•mis•sion (nā′zăl ē-mish′ŭn) SPEECH PATHOLOGY the sound of air forcefully flowing through the nose during speech (as opposed to nasal resonance), usually due to poor valving between the oral and nasal cavities, as in cleft palate. SEE hypernasality. SYN nasal escape.

na•sal es•cape (nā′zăl es-kāp′) SYN nasal emission.

na•sa•lis mus•cle (nā-sā′lis mŭs′ĕl) Compound muscle consisting of: a transverse part (pars transversa musculi nasalis [NA], musculus compressor naris) arising from the maxilla above the root of the canine tooth on each side and forming an aponeurosis across the bridge of the nose; and an alar part (pars alaris musculi nasalis [NA], musculus dilator naris) arising from the maxilla above the lateral incisor and attaching to the wing of the nose; the alar part dilates the nostril; *nerve supply,* facial. SYN musculus nasalis [TA], nasal muscle.

na•sal me•a•tus (nā′zăl mē-ā′tŭs) The three

passages (inferior, middle, superior) in the nasal cavity formed by the projection of the conchae. SYN meatus nasi.

na•sal mus•cle (nā′zăl mŭs′ĕl) SYN nasalis muscle.

na•sal pits (nā′zăl pits) The paired depressions formed when the nasal placodes come to lie below the general external contour of the developing face as a result of the rapid growth of the adjacent nasal elevations; the pits are the primordia of the rostral portions of the nasal chambers.

na•sal point (nā′zăl poynt) SYN nasion.

na•sal prongs (nā′zăl prongz) SYN nasal cannula.

na•sal re•flex (nā′zăl rē′fleks) Sneezing caused by irritation of the nasal mucous membrane.

na•sal sep•tal car•ti•lage (nā′zăl sep′tăl kahr′ti-lăj) A thin cartilaginous plate located between vomer, perpendicular plate of the ethmoid, and nasal bones, and completing the nasal septum anteriorly.

na•sal sep•tum (nā′zăl sep′tŭm) The wall dividing the nasal cavity into halves; it is composed of a central supporting skeleton covered on each side by a mucous membrane.

na•sal spine of fron•tal bone (nā′zăl spīn frŏn′tăl bōn) A projection from the center of the nasal part of the frontal bone, which lies between and articulates with the nasal bones and the perpendicular plate of the ethmoid.

na•sal spines (nā′zăl spīnz) Anterior nasal spine, posterior nasal spine, and nasal spine of frontal bone.

nas•cent (nā′sĕnt) **1.** Beginning; being born or produced. **2.** Denoting the state of a chemical element at the moment it is set free from one of its compounds. [L. *nascor,* pres. p. *nascens,* to be born]

na•si•on (nā′zē-on) [TA] A point on the cranium corresponding to the middle of the nasofrontal suture. SYN nasal point. [L. *nasus,* nose]

naso- Combining form meaning the nose. [L. *nasus*]

na•so•an•tral (nā′zō-an′trăl) Relating to the nose and the maxillary sinus.

na•so•cil•i•ar•y nerve (nā′zō-sil′-ē-ar-ē nĕrv) A branch of the ophthalmic nerve in the superior orbital fissure, passing through the orbit, giving rise to the communicating branch to the ciliary ganglion, the long ciliary nerves, and the posterior and anterior ethmoidal nerves, and terminating as the infratrochlear and nasal branches, which supply the mucous membrane of the nose, the skin of the tip of the nose, and the conjunctiva. SYN nervus nasociliaris [TA].

na•so•fron•tal (nā′zō-frŭn′tăl) Relating to the nose and forehead, or to the nasal cavity and frontal sinuses.

na•so•fron•tal vein (nā′zō-frŭn′tăl vān) Located in the anterior medial part of the orbit that connects the superior ophthalmic vein with the angular vein.

na•so•gas•tric (nā′zō-gas′trik) Pertaining to or involving the nasal passages and the stomach, as in nasogastric intubation.

na•so•gas•tric tube (nā′zō-gas′trik tūb) A tube used for feeding or suctioning stomach contents; inserted through the nose and down the esophagus into the stomach. See this page. SYN NG tube.

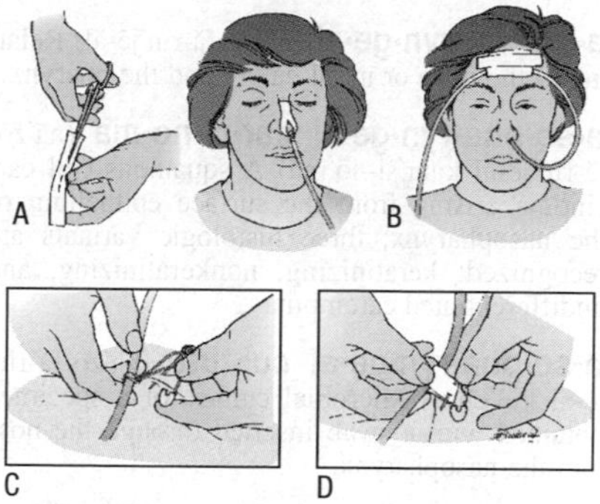

securing nasogastric and nasoenteric tubes: (A) the nasogastric tube is secured to the nose with tape to prevent injury to the nasopharyngeal passages; (B) tape is placed on the forehead and the nasoenteric tube is taped to it, thereby allowing the tube to be advanced until desired placement is achieved; (C, D) tubing is secured to the patient's gown with either an elastic band or tape attached to a safety pin to prevent tension on the line during movement

na•so•la•bi•al (nā′zō-lā′bē-ăl) Relating to the nose and upper lip. [naso- + L. *labium,* lip]

na•so•la•bi•al lymph node (nā′zō-lā′bē-ăl limf nōd) One of the facial lymph nodes located near the junction of the superior labial and facial arteries.

nasolachrymal [Br.] SYN nasolacrimal.

na•so•lac•ri•mal (nā′zō-lak′ri-măl) Relating to the nasal and the lacrimal bones, or to the nasal cavity and the lacrimal ducts. SYN nasolachrymal.

na•so•lac•ri•mal ca•nal (nā′zō-lak′ri-măl kă-nal′) The bony canal formed by the maxilla, lacrimal bone, and inferior concha, which transmits the nasolacrimal duct from the orbit to the inferior meatus of the nose. SYN canalis nasolacrimalis [TA].

na•so•lac•ri•mal duct (nā′zō-lak′ri-măl dŭkt)

The passage leading downward from the lacrimal sac on each side to the anterior portion of the inferior meatus of the nose, through which tears are conducted into the nasal cavity.

na•so-o•ral (nā′zō-ō′răl) Relating to the nose and mouth.

na•so•pal•a•tine (nā′zō-pal′ă-tīn) Relating to the nose and the palate.

na•so•pal•a•tine nerve (nā′zō-pal′ă-tīn nĕrv) A branch from the pterygopalatine ganglion, passing through the sphenopalatine foramen, crossing to and then down the nasal septum, and through the incisive foramen to supply the mucous membrane of the hard palate. SYN nervus nasopalatinus [TA], Cotunnius nerve.

na•so•pha•ryn•ge•al (nā′zō-fă-rin′jē-ăl) Relating to the nose or nasal cavity and the pharynx.

na•so•pha•ryn•ge•al car•ci•no•ma (nā′zō-fă-rin′jē-ăl kahr′si-nō′mă) A squamous cell carcinoma arising from the surface epithelium of the nasopharynx; three histologic variants are recognized: keratinizing, nonkeratinizing, and undifferentiated carcinoma.

na•so•pha•ryn•ge•al cul•ture (nā′zō-fă-rin′jē-ăl kŭl′chŭr) Microbial culture of a specimen obtained with a swab inserted through the nose into the nasopharynx.

na•so•pha•ryn•ge•al leish•man•i•a•sis (nā′zō-fă-rin′jē-ăl lēsh′mă-nī′ă-sis) SYN mucocutaneous leishmaniasis.

na•so•pha•ryn•go•la•ryn•go•scope (nā′zō-fă-ring′gō-lă-ring′gō-skōp) An instrument, often of fiberoptic type, used to visualize the upper airways and pharynx.

na•so•pha•ryn•gos•co•py (nā′zō-far-in-gos′kŏ-pē) Examination of the nasopharynx by flexible or rigid optic instruments, or with a mirror. [nasopharynx + G. *skopeō,* to view]

na•so•pha•rynx (nā′zō-far′ingks) The part of the pharynx that lies above the soft palate; anteriorly it opens into the nasal cavity; inferiorly, it communicates with the oropharynx through the pharyngeal isthmus; laterally it communicates with tympanic cavities through auditory tubes. SYN epipharynx.

na•so•si•nus•i•tis (nā′zō-sī-nŭ-sī′tis) Inflammation of the nasal cavities and of the accessory sinuses.

na•so•tra•che•al tube (nā′zō-trā′kē-ăl tūb) A tracheal tube inserted through the nasal passages.

Nas•se law (nah′sĕ law) An early statement of the pattern of X-linked recessive inheritance: hemophilia affects only boys but is transmitted through mothers and sisters.

na•sus (nā′sŭs) **1.** SYN external nose. **2.** SYN nose. [L.]

NASW Abbreviation for National Association of Social Workers.

na•tal (nā′tăl) **1.** Relating to birth. [L. *natalis,* fr. *nascor,* pp. *natus,* to be born] **2.** Relating to the buttocks or nates. [L. *nates,* buttocks]

na•tal•i•ty (nā-tal′i-tē) The birth rate; the ratio of births to the general population. SEE natal (1).

Na•tal sore (nă-tahl′ sōr) Lesion of cutaneous leishmaniasis.

na•tal tooth (nā′tăl tūth) A deciduous tooth that is in the oral cavity at birth.

na•tes (nā′tēz) [TA] SYN buttocks. [L. pl. of *natis*]

na•ti•mor•tal•i•ty (nā′ti-mōr-tal′i-tē) The perinatal death rate; the proportion of fetal and neonatal deaths to the general natality. [L. *natus,* birth, + *mortalitas,* fr. *mors,* death]

Na•tion•al Cen•ter for Com•ple•men•ta•ry and Al•ter•na•tive Med•i•cine (NCCAM) (nash′ŏ-năl sen′tĕr kom′plĕ-ment′ă-rē awl-tĕr′nă-tiv med′i-sin) A federal program established to support development and research of complementary and alternative medicines for the safety of the public.

Na•tion•al Com•mit•tee for Qual•i•ty As•su•rance (NCQA) (nash′ŏ-năl kŏ-mit′ē kwahl′i-tē ă-shŭr′ĕns) A U.S. national independent nonprofit organization that accredits managed care plans and measures their quality of care.

Na•tion•al Cor•rect Cod•ing I•ni•ti•a•tive (NCCI) (nash′ŏ-năl kŏr-ekt′ kōd′ing in-ish′ă-tiv) Software used by health care providers and insurers in the Medicare system to prevent overpayment for procedures.

Na•tion•al Counc•il Li•cen•sure Ex•am•in•a•tion–Prac•ti•cal Nurse (NCLEX-PN) (nash′ŏ-năl kown′sil lī′sĕn-shŭr eg-zam′in-ā′shŭn prak′tik-ăl nŭrs) A standardized computer administered examination that is taken by new applicants for state licensure. The test is offered in all states by the National Council of State Boards of Nursing. A passing standard is set to determine the applicant's minimum competence for safe practice.

Na•tion•al Coun•cil Li•cen•sure Ex•am•i•na•tion–Reg•is•tered Nurse (NCLEX-RN) (nash′ŏ-năl kown′sil lī′sĕn-shŭr eg-zam′in-ā′shŭn rej′is-tĕrd nŭrs) A standardized computer administered examination that is taken by new applicants for state licensure. The test is offered in all states by the National Council of State Boards of Nursing. A passing standard is set to determine the applicant's minimum competence for safe practice.

Na•tion•al For•mu•la•ry (nash′ŏ-năl fōr′myū-lar-ē) An official compendium published by the United States Pharmacopeial Convention (formerly issued by the American Pharmaceutical Association) for the purpose of providing standards and specifications that can be used to evaluate the quality of pharmaceuticals and therapeutic agents.

Na·tion·al In·ci·dent Man·age·ment Sys·tem (NIMS) (nash′ō-năl in′si-dĕnt man′āj-mĕnt sis′tĕm) The U.S. plan that sets out a common language and common procedures for all levels (local through federal) in reaction to a mass-casualty incident.

Na·tion·al In·sti·tute for Oc·cu·pa·tion·al Safe·ty and Health (NIOSH) (nash′ō-năl in′sti-tūt ok′yū-pā′shŭn-ăl sāf′tē helth) U.S. federal agency established to perform epidemiologic and laboratory research into the causes of occupational diseases and injuries and methods of preventing them; also focuses on strengthening the training of professional workers in occupational health and safety.

Na·tion·al In·sti·tutes of Health (nash′ō-năl in′sti-tūts helth) A nonregulatory U.S. federal agency that oversees research activities funded by the Institute.

Na·tion·al League of Nurs·ing (NLN) (nash′ō-năl lēg nŭrs′ing) An international federation of about 120 national professional organizations; based in Geneva, Switzerland; promotes nursing educational standards.

Na·tion·al Li·bra·ry of Med·i·cine (NLM) (nash′ō-năl lī′brar-ē med′i-sin) World's largest medical library; collects materials in all areas of biomedicine; health care; biomedical aspects of technology, humanities, and physical, life, and social sciences; collections include books, journals, technical reports, manuscripts, microfilms, photographs, and images; Web page provides access to multiple types of health care information.

Na·tion·al Pro·vi·der I·den·ti·fi·er (NPI) (nash′ō-năl prō-vī′dĕr ī-den-ti-fī′ĕr) A standard and unique identification number created by the U.S. HHS for each provider of health care services, supplies, and equipment.

Na·tion·al Re·sponse Plan (NRP) (nash′ō-năl rē-spons′ plan) The program that organizes mobilization of U.S. federal plans in response to a mass-casualty incident of national significance.

Na·tion·al School Lunch Pro·gram (nash′ō-năl skūl lŭnch prō′gram) A U.S.D.A. program that provides a nutritious lunch to children and the opportunity to make healthy choices from nutrition education in the classroom.

Na·tion·al Stu·dent Nurs·es As·so·ci·a·tion (nash′ō-năl stū′dĕnt nŭrs′ĕz ă-sō′sē-ā′shŭn) A nonprofit organization, founded in 1952, for students enrolled in all generic nursing programs as well as generic graduate nursing programs; official publication is *Imprint*, which is published five times a year and is distributed to all members. The organization also sponsors an annual convention, awards scholarships, and participates in legislative activities to promote health care and the future of nursing.

Na·tive A·mer·i·can med·i·cine (nā′tiv ă-mer′i-kăn med′i-sin) Therapy based on a spiritual view of life. Methods of healing include prayer, chanting, music, smudging (burning sage or aromatic woods), herbs, laying-on of hands, massage, counseling, imagery, fasting, harmonizing with nature, dreaming, sweat lodges, taking hallucinogens (e.g., peyote), developing inner silence, going on a shamanic journey, and partaking in ceremony.

NATO code (nā′tō kōd) A one- to three-letter designation assigned by the North Atlantic Treaty Organization to some chemical compounds (including chemical warfare agents) considered to be of significance on the battlefield.

natraemia [Br.] SYN natremia.

na·tre·mi·a, na·tri·e·mi·a (nă-trē′mē-ă, -trē-ē′mē-ă) The presence of sodium in the blood. SYN natraemia. [natrium, sodium, + G. *haima,* blood]

natriaemia [Br.] SYN natriemia.

na·trif·er·ic (nā-trif′ĕr-ik) Tending to increase sodium transport. [natrium + L. *fero,* to carry]

na·tri·um (nā′trē-ŭm) SYN sodium. [Ar. *natrūm,* fr. G. *nitron,* carbonate of soda]

na·tri·u·re·sis (nā′trē-yū-rē′sis) Urinary excretion of sodium; commonly designates enhanced sodium excretion, which may occur in certain diseases or as a result of the administration of diuretic drugs. [natrium + G. *ouron,* urine]

na·tri·u·ret·ic (nā′trē-yū-ret′ik) **1.** Pertaining to or characterized by natriuresis. **2.** A substance that increases urinary excretion of sodium, usually as a result of decreased tubular reabsorption of sodium ions from glomerular filtrate.

Nat·tras·si·a man·gi·fe·rae (na-tras′ē-ă man-gif′ĕ-rē) A dematiaceous mold, previously known as *Hendersonula toruloidea*, which causes onychomycosis and phaeohyphomycosis. *Scytalidium dimidiatum* is a synanamorph.

na·tu·ral an·ti·bod·y (na′chŭr-ăl an′ti-bod-ē) SYN normal antibody.

nat·u·ral birth (nach′ŭr-ăl bĭrth) SYN natural childbirth.

nat·u·ral child·birth (nach′ŭr-ăl chīld′bĭrth) A method of childbirth in which medical intervention is minimized and the mother often practices relaxation and breathing techniques to control pain and ease delivery. A natural birth also increases the probability of a healthier postnatal period and an easier recovery without the discomfort of an episiotomy or cesarean section incision. SYN natural birth.

na·tu·ral dye (na′chŭr-ăl dī) Dye obtained from animals or plants.

na·tu·ral im·mu·ni·ty, non·spe·cif·ic im·mu·ni·ty (na′chŭr-ăl i-myū′ni-tē, non′spĕ-sif′ik i-myū′ni-tē) SYN innate immunity.

na·tu·ral kil·ler cell leu·ke·mi·a (na′chŭr-ăl kil′ĕr sel lū- kē′mē-ă) A leukemia originating from cells of natural killer cell origin; often associated with the presence of monoclonal Epstein-Barr virus infecting tumor cells; usually indicates a leukemic subtype of poor prognosis.

na·tu·ral kill·er (NK) cells (na′chŭr-ăl kil′ĕr selz) Large granular lymphocytes that do not express markers of either T- or B-cell lineage. These cells kill target cells using antibody-dependent cell-mediated cytotoxicity. NK cells can also use perforin to kill cells in the absence of antibody. Killing may occur without previous sensitization. SYN NK cells.

na·tu·ral pitch (na′chŭr-ăl pitch) SYN optimal pitch.

na·tu·ral se·lec·tion (nă-chŭr′ăl sĕ-lek′shŭn) Colloquially, "survival of the fittest," the principle that in nature those individuals best able to adapt to their environment will survive and reproduce, whereas those less able will die without progeny, and the genes carried by the survivors will increase in frequency. This principle is heuristic rather than rigorous because it cannot be tested, the outcome being tautologous with the empiric definition of fitness.

nat·ur·o·path (nach′ŭr-ō-path) One who practices naturopathy. [L. *natura,* nature, + G. *pathos,* disease]

na·tur·o·path·ic (na′chūr-ō-path′ik) Relating to or by means of naturopathy.

na·tur·o·path·ic med·i·cine (nach′ŭr-ō-path′ik med′i-sin) A branch of health care based on recognition of the healing power of nature. It supplements conventional medical theory and practice with emphasis on understanding and treating the whole patient, avoiding potentially harmful therapies, adding education for self-care, and aiding nature to restore health and equilibrium. Methods include dietary revision, counseling for lifestyle modification, botanical medicine, physical medicine, and mind-body therapies. Naturopathic physicians are licensed in some states as primary health care providers with authority to write prescriptions.

na·tur·op·a·thy (na-chŭr-op′ă-thē) A system of therapeutics that relies on natural (nonmedicinal) forces (e.g., diet, exercise, and massage). Focus is on preventing disease and restoring function.

nau·se·a (naw′zē-ă) A feeling of being sick at the stomach; an inclination to vomit. [L. fr. G. *nausia,* seasickness, fr. *naus,* ship]

nau·se·a grav·i·dar·um (naw′zē-ă grav-i-dā′rŭm) SYN morning sickness.

nau·se·ant (naw′zē-ănt) **1.** Nauseating; causing nausea. **2.** An agent that causes nausea.

nau·se·ate (naw′zē-āt) To cause an inclination to vomit.

nau·se·at·ed (naw′zē-ā-tĕd) Affected with nausea. SYN sick (2).

nau·se·ous (naw′shŭs) Causing nausea.

Nau·ta stain (now′tă stān) A stain for degenerating axons, with which they appear as fragmented and swollen fibers.

na·vel (nā′vĕl) SYN umbilicus. [A.S. *nafela*]

na·vic·u·lar (nă-vik′yū-lăr) SYN scaphoid. [L. *navicularis,* relating to shipping]

na·vic·u·lar ab·do·men (nā-vik′yū-lăr ab′dŏ-mĕn) SYN scaphoid abdomen.

na·vic·u·lar bone (nă-vik′yū-lăr bōn) A bone of the tarsus on the medial side of the foot articulating with the head of the talus, the three cuneiform bones, and occasionally the cuboid.

na·vic·u·lar fos·sa of u·re·thra (nah-vik′yū-lăr fŏs′ă yūr-ē′thră) The terminal dilated portion of the urethra in the glans penis.

nav·i·ga·tor ech·o (nav′i-gā′tŏr ek′ō) A method of respiratory gating used in magnetic resonance imaging to limit respiratory motion artifact; a signal is derived from the top of the diaphragm, and image data are collected only when it is in a selected range.

Nb Symbol for niobium.

n.b. Abbreviation for the Latin *nota bene*, note well.

NBC Abbreviation for nuclear, biologic, chemical, as types of mass-casualty weapons.

NBNA Abbreviation for the National Black Nurses Association.

NCCAM Abbreviation for National Center for Complementary and Alternative Medicine.

NCCI Abbreviation for National Correct Coding Initiative.

NCHS Abbreviation for U.S. National Centers for Health Statistics.

NCLEX-PN Abbreviation for National Council Licensure Examination–Practical Nurse.

NCLEX-RN Abbreviation for National Council Licensure Examination–Registered Nurse.

NCQA Abbreviation for National Committee for Quality Assurance.

ND Abbreviation for Doctor of Naturopathic Medicine.

Nd Symbol for neodymium.

NDC Abbreviation for U.S. National Drug Code.

NDT Abbreviation for neurodevelopmental treatment.

Nd:YAG la•ser (lā′zĕr) Device with a beam in the infrared spectrum (1064 nm), with a greater depth of penetration than other lasers. [*Nd* (neodymium) + *Y*ttrium-*A*luminum- *G*arnet]

Ne Symbol for neon.

near in•fra•red (nēr in′fră-red) Range of light that is closest to visible light with waves ranging between 700–1500 nm.

near point (nēr poynt) That point in conjugate focus with the retina when the eye exerts maximal accommodation.

near•sight•ed•ness (nēr-sīt′ĕd-nĕs) SYN myopia.

ne•ar•thro•sis (nē-ahr-thrō′sis) A new joint (e.g., a pseudarthrosis arising in an ununited fracture, or an artificial joint resulting from a total joint replacement operation). SYN neoarthrosis. [G. *neos,* new, + *arthrōsis,* a jointing]

near ul•tra•vi•o•let (nēr ŭl′tră-vī′ō-lĕt) Range of light with wave lengths between 290–390 nm.

NEAT Abbreviation for nonexercise activity thermogenesis.

neat (nēt) Pure, distilled, or unmixed, when relating to chemical compounds. [F. *net,* clean, fr. L. *nitidus,* shining]

neb•u•la, pl. **neb•u•lae** (neb′yū-lă, -lē) **1.** A translucent foglike opacity of the cornea. **2.** A spray. [L. fog, cloud, mist]

neb•u•liz•er (neb′yū-lī-zĕr) A device used to disperse liquid medicine in a mist of extremely fine particles; useful in delivering medicine to the lower respiratory tract; used in biowarfare to disperse toxins or other harmful biologic agents. SEE ALSO atomizer, vaporizer. See this page.

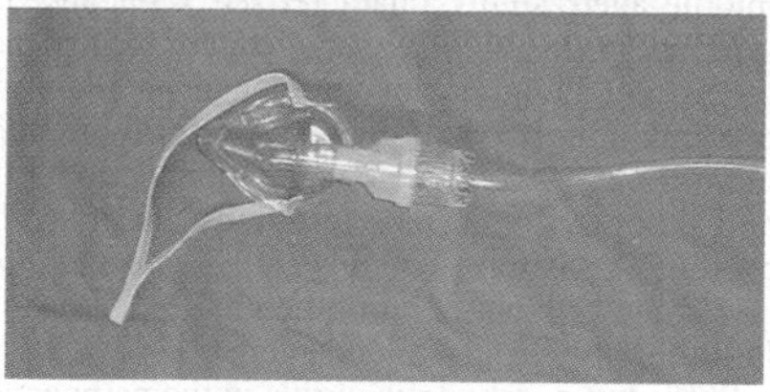

nebulizer

Ne•ca•tor (nē-kā′tōr) A genus of nematode hookworms with species that include *N. americanus*, the New World hookworm; the adults of this species attach to villi in the small intestine and suck blood, causing abdominal discomfort, diarrhea and cramps, anorexia, weight loss, and hypochromic microcytic anemia. SEE ALSO *Ancylostoma.* [L. a murderer]

ne•ca•to•ri•a•sis (nē-kā-tō-rī′ă-sis) Hookworm disease caused by *Necator*, the resulting anemia being usually less severe than that resulting from ancylostomiasis.

ne•ces•sar•y (ne′se-sar-ē) Requisite or essential. [L. *necessarius*]

neck (nek) **1.** Part of body by which the head is connected to the trunk: it extends from the base of the cranium to the top of the shoulders. **2.** In anatomy, any constricted portion having a fancied resemblance to the neck of an animal. **3.** The germinative portion of an adult tapeworm that develops the segments or proglottids; the region of cestode segmentation behind the scolex. See page A4. SYN cervix (1) [TA], collum. [A.S. *hnecca*]

neck of glans (nek glanz) A constriction behind the corona of the glans penis.

neck•lace (nek′lăs) Term used to describe a rash that encircles the neck.

neck of pan•cre•as (nek pan′krē-ăs) Segment of pancreas, approximately 2 cm long, connecting head and body of pancreas; it intervenes between the duodenum anteriorly and the junction of the splenic and superior mesenteric veins, forming the beginning of the portal vein, posteriorly. SYN collum pancreatis [TA].

neck of ur•i•nar•y blad•der (nek yūr′i-nar-ē bla′dĕr) The lowest part of the bladder formed by the junction of the fundus and the inferolateral surfaces.

necro-, **necr-** Combining forms meaning death, necrosis. [G. *nekros,* corpse]

nec•ro•bi•o•sis (nek′rō-bī-ō′sis) **1.** Physiologic or normal death of cells or tissues as a result of changes associated with development, aging, or use. **2.** Necrosis of a small area of tissue. SYN bionecrosis. [necro- + G. *biōs,* life]

nec•ro•bi•o•sis li•poi•di•ca, **nec•ro•bi•o•sis li•poi•di•ca di•a•be•ti•co•rum** (nek′rō-bī-ō′sis li-poyd′i-kă, dī-ă-bet′i-kōr′ŭm) A condition often associated with diabetes, in which one or more yellow, atrophic lesions develop on the legs.

nec•ro•bi•ot•ic (nek′rō-bī-ot′ik) Pertaining to or characterized by necrobiosis.

nec•ro•cy•to•sis (nek′rō-sī-tō′sis) Abnormal death of cells [necro- + G. *kytos,* cell, + *-osis,* condition]

nec•ro•gen•ic (nek′rō-jen′ik) Relating to, living in, or having origin in dead matter. [necro- + G. *genesis,* origin]

nec•ro•gen•ic wart (nek′rō-jen′ik wōrt) SYN postmortem wart.

ne•crol•o•gy (nĕ-krol′ŏ-jē) The science of the collection, classification, and interpretation of mortality statistics. [necro- + G. *logos,* study]

ne•crol•y•sis (nĕ-krol′i-sis) Necrosis and loosening of tissue. [necro- + G. *lysis,* loosening]

nec•ro•ma•ni•a (nek′rō-mā′nē-ă) **1.** A morbid

tendency to dwell with longing on death. **2.** A morbid attraction to dead bodies. [necro- + G. *mania,* frenzy]

ne•croph•a•gous (nĕ-krof′ă-gŭs) **1.** Living on carrion. **2.** SYN necrophilous. [necro- + G. *phagō,* to eat]

nec•ro•phil•i•a, ne•croph•i•lism (nek′rō-fil′ē-ă, nĕ-krof′i-lizm) **1.** A morbid fondness for being in the presence of dead bodies. **2.** The impulse to have sexual contact, or the act of such contact, with a dead body, usually of males with female corpses. [necro- + G. *phileō,* to love]

ne•croph•i•lous (nĕ-krof′i-lŭs) Having a preference for dead tissue; denoting certain bacteria. SYN necrophagous (2). [necro- + G. *philos,* fond]

nec•ro•pho•bi•a (nek′rō-fō′bē-ă) Morbid fear of corpses. [necro- + G. *phobos,* fear]

ne•crop•sy (nek′rop-sē) SYN autopsy. [necro- + G. *opsis,* view]

ne•crose (nek′rōs) **1.** To cause necrosis. **2.** To become the site of necrosis.

ne•cro•sis (nĕ-krō′sis) Pathologic death of one or more cells, or of a portion of tissue or organ, resulting from irreversible damage; earliest irreversible changes are mitochondrial, consisting of swelling and granular calcium deposits seen by electron microscopy; most frequent visible alterations are nuclear pyknosis and abnormally dark basophilic staining; karyolysis, swelling and abnormally pale basophilic staining; or karyorrhexis, rupture and fragmentation of the nucleus. After such changes, the outlines of individual cells are indistinct, and affected cells may become merged, sometimes forming a focus of coarsely granular, amorphous, or hyaline material. See this page. [G. *nekrōsis,* death, fr. *nekroō,* to make dead]

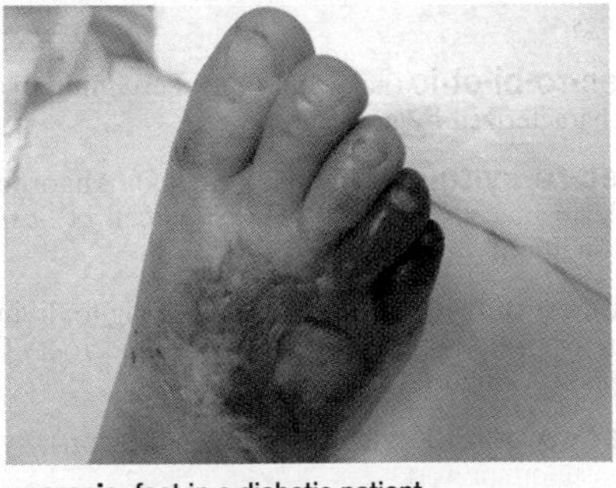

necrosis: foot in a diabetic patient

nec•ro•sper•mi•a (nek′rō-spĕr′mē-ă) A condition in which there are dead or immobile sperms in the semen. [necro- + G. *sperma,* seed]

ne•crot•ic (nĕ-krot′ik) Pertaining to or affected by necrosis.

ne•crot•ic a•rach•ni•dism (nĕ-krot′ik ă-rak′ni-dizm) Systemic poisoning caused by spiders belonging to the genus *Loxosceles;* cutaneous necrosis develops at the bite site, with slow healing and possible disfigurement.

ne•crot•ic cir•rho•sis (nĕ-krot′ik sir-ō′sis) SYN postnecrotic cirrhosis.

ne•crot•ic in•flam•ma•tion, nec•ro•tiz•ing in•flam•ma•tion (nĕ-krot′ik in′flă-mā′shŭn, nek′rō-tīz-ing) An acute inflammatory reaction in which the predominant histologic change is rapid necrosis that occurs diffusely or extensively throughout the affected tissue.

ne•crot•ic pulp (nĕ-krot′ik pŭlp) Necrosis of the dental pulp that clinically does not respond to thermal stimulation; the tooth may be asymptomatic or sensitive to percussion and palpation. SYN dead pulp, nonvital pulp.

nec•ro•tiz•ing (nek′rō-tīz-ing) That which causes the death of tissues or organisms. SEE necrosis. [G. *nekros,* dead body]

nec•ro•tiz•ing ar•ter•i•o•li•tis (nek′rō-tīz-ing ahr-tēr′ē-ō-lī′tis) Necrosis in the media of arterioles, characteristic of malignant hypertension. SYN arteriolonecrosis.

nec•ro•tiz•ing en•ter•o•co•li•tis (nek′rō-tīz-ing en′tĕr-ō-kō-lī′tis) Extensive ulceration and necrosis of the ileum and colon in premature infants.

nec•ro•tiz•ing ker•a•ti•tis (nek′rō-tīz-ing ker′ă-tī′tis) Severe inflammation and destruction of corneal tissue that may be seen in response to herpes infection.

nec•ro•tiz•ing ul•cer•a•tive gin•gi•vi•tis (NUG) (nek′rō-tīz-ing ŭl′sĕr-ă-tiv jin′ji-vī′tis) An acute or recurrent gingivitis of young and middle-aged adults characterized clinically by gingival erythema and pain, fetid odor, and necrosis and sloughing of interdental papillae and marginal gingiva that give rise to a gray pseudomembrane; fever, regional lymphadenopathy, and other systemic manifestations also may be present. A fusiform bacillus and *Treponema vincentii* can be isolated from the gingival tissues in large numbers and are considered to play a significant but poorly defined role in the pathogenesis. SYN fusospirochetal gingivitis, trench mouth, ulceromembranous gingivitis, Vincent disease, Vincent infection.

ne•crot•o•my (ne-krot′ŏ-mē) **1.** SYN dissection. **2.** Operation for the removal of a necrotic portion of bone (sequestrum). [necro- + G. *tomē,* cutting]

ne•do•cro•mil (ne-dok′ră-mil) A nonbronchodilator, antiinflammatory, antiasthmatic drug that acts on the mast cells to inhibit the release of histamine.

nee•dle (nē′dĕl) **1.** A slender, solid, usually sharp-pointed instrument used for puncturing tissues, suturing, or passing a ligature around or through a vessel. **2.** A hollow needle used for injection, aspiration, biopsy, or to guide introduction of a catheter into a vessel or other space. **3.** To separate the tissues by means of one or two needles, in the dissection of small parts. **4.** To perform discission of a cataract by means of a knife needle. [M.E. *nedle*, fr. A.S. *nǣdl*]

nee•dle bath (nē′dĕl bath) A bath in which water is projected forcibly against the body in many very fine jets.

nee•dle bi•op•sy (nē′dĕl bī′op-sē) Any method in which the specimen for biopsy is removed by aspirating it through an appropriate needle or trocar that pierces the skin, or the external surface of an organ. SYN aspiration biopsy.

nee•dle cri•co•thy•rot•o•my (nē′dĕl krī′kō-thī-rot′ŏ-mē) Cricothyrotomy performed by passing a large-bore needle percutaneously through the cricothyroid membrane into the trachea. Used as an emergency airway procedure when surgical cricothyrotomy is not possible. SYN percutaneous transtracheal ventilation.

nee•dle for•ceps (nē′dĕl fōr′seps) SYN needle-holder.

nee•dle-hold•er, nee•dle-car•ri•er, nee•dle-driv•er (nē′dĕl hōl′dĕr, kar′ē-ĕr, drī′vĕr) An instrument for grasping a needle in suturing. SYN needle forceps.

nee•dle•less sys•tem (nē′dĕl-les sis′tĕm) A type of injection using a blunt cannula attached to a syringe with medication to be delivered intravenously through a port.

nee•dle•stick (nē′dĕl-stik) Accidental puncture of a health care worker's skin with a contaminated needle. The window of vulnerability for sustaining a needlestick opens when the needle is removed for the patient and does not close until it is safely discarded.

need•ling (nēd′ĕ-ling) Discission of a soft or secondary cataract or opening of a blocked glaucoma filtering bleb with a needle puncture.

NEEP (nēp) Acronym for negative end-expiratory pressure.

Neer im•pinge•ment sign (nēr im-pinj′mĕnt sīn) Pain produced by forceful maximum forward elevation of the upper extremity.

ne•ga•tion (nĕ-gā′shŭn) SYN denial.

neg•a•tive (neg′ă-tiv) **1.** Not affirmative; refutative; not positive. **2.** MATHEMATICS having a value less than zero. **3.** PHYSICS, CHEMISTRY having an electric charge resulting from a gain or overabundance of electrons, hence able to donate (lose) electrons. **4.** MEDICINE denoting a response to a diagnostic maneuver or laboratory study that indicates the absence of the disease or condition tested for. [L. *negativus,* fr. *nego,* to deny]

neg•a•tive ac•com•mo•da•tion (neg′ă-tiv ă-kom′ŏ-dā′shŭn) The decrease of accommodation that occurs when shifting from near vision to distance vision.

neg•a•tive base ex•cess (neg′ă-tiv bās eks′es) A measure of metabolic acidosis; the amount of strong alkali that would have to be added per unit volume of whole blood to titrate it to pH 7.4 while at 37°C and at a carbon dioxide pressure of 40 mmHg.

neg•a•tive con•ver•gence (neg′ă-tiv kŏn-vĕr′jĕns) The slight divergence of the visual axes when convergence is at rest, as when observing the far point or during sleep.

neg•a•tive e•lec•trode (neg′ă-tiv ĕ-lek′trōd) SYN cathode.

neg•a•tive end-ex•pi•ra•to•ry pres•sure (NEEP) (neg′ă-tiv end-eks-pī′ră-tōr-ē presh′ŭr) A subatmospheric pressure at the airway at the end of expiration.

neg•a•tive en•er•gy bal•ance (neg′ă-tiv en′ĕr-jē bal′ăns) A depletion of the body's energy stores due to inadequate intake of energy sources.

neg•a•tive my•o•clon•ic seiz•ure (neg′ă-tiv mī′ō-klon′ik sē′zhŭr) Seizure characterized by abrupt, brief cessation of muscular activity, occasionally preceded by a single myoclonic contraction; term usually is applied to unilateral, distal muscles.

neg•a•tive ni•tro•gen bal•ance (net′ă-tiv nī′trō-jen bal′ăns) Nonphysiologic state wherein nitrogenous output is greater than nitrogen intake.

neg•a•tive pre•dic•tive val•ue (neg′a-tiv prē-dik′tiv val′yū) The probability of a negative test result indicates the absence of an analyte or a specific disease.

neg•a•tive pres•sure ven•ti•la•tion (neg′ă-tiv presh′ŭr ven′ti-lā′shŭn) A mode of mechanical ventilation in which a positive transrespiratory pressure is generated by decreasing body surface pressure below the pressure at the airway opening.

neg•a•tive sco•to•ma (neg′ă-tiv skō-tō′mă) A scotoma that appears as a blank or black patch in the visual field.

neg•a•tive stain (neg′ă-tiv stān) Stain forming an opaque or colored background against which the object to be demonstrated appears as a translucent or colorless area; in electron microscopy, an electron opaque material, such as phosphotungstic acid or sodium phosphotungstate, is used to give detail as to surface structure.

neg•a•tive symp•tom (neg′ă-tiv simp′tŏm) One of the deficit symptoms of schizophrenia that follow from diminished volition and executive function including inertia, anergia, lack of involvement with the environment, poverty of thought, social withdrawal, and blunted affect.

neg•a•tiv•ism (neg′ă-tiv-izm) A tendency to do the opposite of what one is requested to do, or to stubbornly resist for no apparent reason; seen in catatonic states and in toddlers.

neg•a•tron (neg′ă-tron) Term used for an electron to emphasize its negative charge in contradistinction to the positive charge carried by the otherwise similar positron.

ne•glect (nĕ-glekt′) **1.** Failure of a health care provider or caregiver to observe due care and diligence in performing services or delivering medicine or other products so as to avoid harming a patient. **2.** Generally, indifference or inadequate attention to one's responsibilities in regard to self-care, care of others, or other aspects of one's personal or professional life. **3.** OCCUPATIONAL THERAPY the tendency to behave as if one side of the body or one side of space does not exist, with impairment of skilled or purposeful movements and visual scanning and awareness. Types of neglect include spatial, visual, and body schema (i.e., personal). SEE ALSO hemiapraxia.

neg•li•gence (neg′li-jĕns) Failure to perform duties or activities with due diligence and attention or to meet the standards of regular care.

Ne•gri bod•ies (nā′grē bod′ēz) Eosinophilic, sharply outlined, pathognomonic inclusion bodies (2–10 mcm in diameter) found in the cytoplasm of certain nerve cells containing the virus of rabies, especially in Ammon horn of the hippocampus.

Neis•se•ri•a (nī-sē′rē-ă) A genus of aerobic to facultatively anaerobic bacteria containing gram-negative cocci that occur in pairs with the adjacent sides flattened. [A. *Neisser*]

neis•se•ri•a, pl. **neis•se•ri•ae** (nī-sē′rē-ă, -ē) A vernacular term used to refer to any member of the genus *Neisseria*.

Neis•se•ri•a gon•or•rhoe•ae (nī-sē′rē-ă gon-ō-rē-ē) A bacterial species that causes gonorrhea and other infections in humans. It is the type species of the genus *Neisseria*. See page B4. SYN gonococcus.

Neis•se•ri•a me•nin•gi•ti•dis (nī-sēr′ē-ă men-in-jit′i-dis) A species found in the nasopharynx; the causative agent of meningococcal meningitis. Virulent organisms are strongly gram-negative and occur singly or in pairs; in the latter case the cocci are elongated and are arranged with long axes parallel and facing sides kidney shaped. Groups characterized by serologically specific capsular polysaccharides are designated by capital letters (the main serogroups being A, B, C, and D). SYN meningococcus.

Neis•se•ri•a sic•ca (nī-sēr′ē-ă sik′ă) Gram-negative diplococci of the family Neisseriaceae, characterized by dry grayish or slimy white or yellow colonies; part of the normal flora of the human nasopharynx, saliva, and sputum.

NEJM Common abbreviation for *New England Journal of Medicine*.

Né•la•ton cath•e•ter (nā-lah-ton[h]′ kath′ĕ-tĕr) A flexible catheter of red rubber.

Né•la•ton line (nā-lah-ton[h]′ līn) A line drawn from the anterior superior iliac spine to the tuberosity of the ischium; normally the greater trochanter lies in this line, but in cases of iliac dislocation of the hip or fracture of the neck of the femur the trochanter is felt above the line.

Nel•son syn•drome (nel′sŏn sin′drōm) A syndrome of hyperpigmentation, third nerve damage, and enlarging sella turcica caused by pituitary adenomas presumably present before adrenalectomy for Cushing syndrome but enlarging and symptomatic afterward. SYN postadrenalectomy syndrome.

nem A nutritional unit defined as 1 g breast milk of specific nutritional components having a caloric value equivalent to 2/3 calorie. [Ger. *Nahrungseinheit Milch,* milk nutrition unit]

nema- A prefix meaning thread. [Gr. *nēma,* thread]

nem•a•to•cyst (nem′ă-tō-sist) A stinging cell of coelenterates consisting of a poison sac and a coiled barbed sting capable of being ejected and penetrating the skin of an animal on contact; of considerable consequence in large jellyfish and in the Portuguese man-of-war whose large numbers of these stinging cells can cause great pain and even death. [nemato- + G. *kystis*, bladder]

Nem•a•to•da (nem-ă-tō′dă) The roundworms, a large class of the phylum Aschelminthes that includes many of the helminths parasitic in humans. Parasitic nematodes include the intestinal roundworms and the filarial roundworms of the blood, lymphatic tissues, and viscera and some subcutaneous and migratory roundworms. [nemat- + G. *eidos,* form]

nem•a•tode (nem′ă-tōd) A common name for any roundworm of the phylum Nematoda. See page B7.

nem•a•to•di•a•sis (nem′ă-tō-dī′ă-sis) Infection with nematode parasites.

nem•a•toid (nem′ă-toyd) **1.** Resembling a thread. **2.** Relating to nematodes.

neo- Prefix meaning new, recent. [G. *neos*]

ne•o•ad•ju•vant (nē′ō-ad′jū-vănt) Chemotherapy or radiation given before cancer surgery or other phase of treatment. [neo- + adjuvant]

ne•o•an•ti•gens (nē′ō-an′ti-jenz) SYN tumor antigens.

ne•o•ar•thro•sis (nē′ō-ahr-thrō′sis) SYN nearthrosis.

ne•o•blad•der (nē′ō-blad′ĕr) Surgically constructed replacement for urinary bladder, usually using stomach or intestine.

ne•o•blas•tic (nē′ō-blas′tik) Developing in or characteristic of new tissue. [neo- + G. *blastos,* germ, offspring]

ne•o•cer•e•bel•lum (nē′ō-ser-ĕ-bel′ŭm) [TA] The larger lateral portion of the cerebellar hemisphere, receiving its dominant input from the pontine nuclei that, in turn, are dominated by afferent nerves from the cerebral cortex; phylogenetically of more recent origin than the archicerebellum and paleocerebellum the neocerebellum reaches its largest development in humans and other primates.

ne•o•cor•tex (nē′ō-kōr′teks) The newest part of the cerebral cortex, involved in higher functions such as sensory perception, generation of motor commands, spatial reasoning, conscious thought, and in humans, language; consists of gray matter surrounding the deeper white matter of the cerebrum; accounts for approximately 23% of the neurons in brains of human males and 19% of the neurons in human females. SYN neopallium. [G. *neos,* new, + L. *cortex,* bark]

ne•o•cys•tos•to•my (nē′ō-sis-tos′tŏ-mē) An operation in which the ureter is implanted into the bladder. [neo- + G. *kystis,* bladder, + *stoma,* mouth]

ne•o•cyte (nē′ō-sīt) A new cell; one recently released into the peripheral blood from the bone marrow. SEE reticulocyte. [neo- + -cyte]

ne•o•dym•i•um (Nd) (nē′ō-dim′ē-ŭm) One of the rare earth elements; atomic no. 60, atomic wt. 144.24. [*neo-,* new, + G. *didymos,* twin (of lanthanum)]

ne•o•gen•e•sis (nē′ō-jen′ĕ-sis) SYN regeneration (1). [neo- + G. *genesis,* origin]

ne•o•ge•net•ic (nē′ō-jĕ-net′ik) Pertaining to or characterized by neogenesis.

ne•o•ki•net•ic (nē′ō-ki-net′ik) Denoting one of the divisions of the motor system, the function of which is the transmission of isolated synergic movements of voluntary origin; it represents a more highly specialized form of movement than the paleokinetic function. [neo- + G. *kinētikos,* relating to movement]

ne•ol•o•gism (nē-ol′ō-jizm) A new word or phrase of the patient's own making often seen in schizophrenia (e.g., headshoe to mean hat), or an existing word used in a new sense; in psychiatry, such usages may have meaning only to the patient or be indicative of the underlying condition. [neo- + G. *logos,* word]

ne•o•mem•brane (nē′ō-mem′brān) SYN false membrane.

ne•on (Ne) (nē′on) An inert gaseous element in the atmosphere; atomic no. 10, atomic wt. 20.1797. [G. *neos,* new]

ne•o•na•tal (nē′ō-nā′tăl) Relating to the period immediately succeeding birth and continuing through the first 28 days of life. SYN newborn. [neo- + L. *natalis,* relating to birth]

ne•o•na•tal a•ne•mi•a (nē′ō-nā′tăl ă-nē′mē-ă) SYN erythroblastosis fetalis.

ne•o•na•tal con•junc•ti•vi•tis (nē′ō-nā′tăl kŏn-jungk′ti-vī′tis) SEE ophthalmia neonatorum.

ne•o•na•tal death (nē′ō-nā′tăl deth) The death of a live newborn during the first 28 days of life. An early neonatal death is considered by the World Health Organization to be a death within the first 7 days of life. [neo + L. *natalis,* relating to birth, + A.S. *dēath*]

ne•o•na•tal di•ag•no•sis (nē′ō-nā′tăl dī-ăg-nō′sis) Systematic evaluation of the newborn for evidence of disease or malformations, and the conclusion reached.

ne•o•na•tal hep•a•ti•tis (nē′ō-nā′tăl hep′ă-tī′tis) The disorder in the neonatal period attributable to a variety of causes, chiefly viral.

ne•o•na•tal her•pes (nē′ō-nā′tăl hĕr′pēz) Herpes simplex virus type 1 or 2 infection transmitted from the mother to the newborn infant, often during passage through an infected birth canal.

ne•o•na•tal hy•per•bil•i•ru•bi•ne•mi•a (nē′ō-nā′tăl, hī′pĕr-bil′i-rū-bi-nē′mē-ă) Serum bilirubin greater than 12.9 mg/dL (220 mcmol/L) or rising at a rate greater than 5 mg/dL per day; also applied to a nonphysiologic pattern of hyperbilirubinemia, i.e., jaundice in the first 24 hours of life or extending beyond the first week of life in term infants.

ne•o•na•tal in•ten•sive care u•nit (NICU) (nē′ō-nā′tăl in-ten′siv kār yū′nit) Hospital unit designated for care of critically ill premature and full-term newborns.

ne•o•na•tal med•i•cine (nē′ō-nā′tăl med′i-sin) SYN neonatology.

ne•o•na•tal mor•tal•i•ty rate (nē′ō-nā′tăl mōr-tal′i-tē rāt) The number of deaths in the first 28 days of life divided by the number of live births occurring in the same population during the same period of time.

ne•o•na•tal period (nē′ō-nā′tăl pēr′ē-ŏd) The time elapsed between birth and 28 days of age. The first 24 hours of life are the most vulnerable time for the neonate because major physiologic adjustments are needed for extrauterine life.

ne•o•na•tal tet•a•ny (nē′ō-nā′tăl tet′ă-nē) Hypocalcemic tetany occurring in neonates or young infants, due to transient functional hypoparathyroidism in consumption of cow's milk (high phosphorus content). SYN tetanism.

ne•o•nate (nē′ō-nāt) A newborn infant. SYN newborn. [neo- + L. *natus,* born, fr. *nascor,* to be born]

ne•o•na•tol•o•gist (nē′ō-nā-tol′ŏ-jist) One who specializes in neonatology.

ne•o•na•tol•o•gy (nē′ō-nā-tol′ŏ-jē) The pediatric subspecialty concerned with disorders of the neonate. SYN neonatal medicine. [neo- + L. *natus,* pp. born, + G. *logos,* theory]

ne•o•neu•rot•i•za•tion (nē′ō-nū-rot′i-zā′shŭn) Rarely observed phenomenon of return of facial motor function following deliberate transection of the facial nerve; believed to represent trigeminal reinnervation of the facial muscles.

ne•o•pal•li•um (nē′ō-pal′ē-ŭm) SYN neocortex.

ne•o•pla•si•a (nē′ō-plā′zē-ă) The pathologic process that results in the formation and growth of a neoplasm. See page B14. [neo- + G. *plasis,* a molding]

ne•o•plasm (nē′ō-plazm) An abnormal tissue that grows by cellular proliferation more rapidly than normal and continues to grow after the stimuli that initiated the new growth cease. Neoplasms show partial or complete lack of structural organization and functional coordination with the normal tissue, and usually form a distinct mass of tissue which may be either benign (benign tumor) or malignant (cancer). SYN tumor (2). [neo- + G. *plasma,* thing formed]

ne•o•plas•tic (nē′ō-plas′tik) Pertaining to or characterized by neoplasia, or containing a neoplasm.

ne•o•prene sleeve (nē′ō-prēn′ slēv) A sheath of synthetic rubber used to provide warmth and minor support to an upper or lower limb.

ne•op•ter•in (nē-op′tĕr-in) A pteridine present in body fluids; elevated levels result from immune system activation, malignant disease, allograft rejection, and viral infections (especially as in AIDS). [neo- + G. *pteron,* wing, + -in]

ne•o•stri•a•tum (nē′ō-strī-ā′tŭm) The caudate nucleus and putamen considered as one and distinguished from the globus pallidus (paleostriatum).

ne•o•thal•a•mus (nē′ō-thal′ă-mŭs) The portion of the thalamus projecting to the neocortex.

ne•o•vas•cu•lar•i•za•tion (nē′ō-vas′kyū-lar-ī-zā′shŭn) Proliferation of blood vessels in tissue not normally containing them, or proliferation of blood vessels of a different kind than usual in tissue.

ne•per (ne′pĕr) A unit for comparing the magnitude of two powers, usually in electricity or acoustics; it is one half of the natural logarithm of the ratio of the two powers. [fr. *neperus,* latinized form of (John) Napier, Scottish mathematician, 1550–1617]

neph•e•lom•e•try (nef-ĕ-lom′ĕ-trē) Estimation of the number and size of particles in suspension by measurement of light scattered from a beam passed through the solution.

ne•phral•gi•a (ne-fral′jē-ă) Pain in the kidney. [nephr- + G. *algos,* pain]

ne•phrec•to•my (ne-frek′tŏ-mē) Surgical removal of a kidney. [nephr- + G. *ektomē,* excision]

neph•rel•co•sis (nef-rel-kō′sis) Ulceration of the mucous membrane of the pelvis or calyces of the kidney. [nephr- + G. *helkōsis,* ulceration]

neph•ric (nef′rik) Relating to the kidney. SYN renal.

-nephric Suffix meaning kidneys (e.g., cardionephric). [G. *nephros,* kidney]

ne•phrit•ic (ne-frit′ik) Relating to or suffering from nephritis.

ne•phrit•ic syn•drome (ne-frit′ik sin′drōm) The clinical symptoms of acute glomerulonephritis, particularly hematuria, hypertension, and renal failure.

ne•phri•tis, pl. **ne•phrit•i•des** (nĕ-frī′tis, frit′i-dēz) Inflammation of the kidneys. [nephr- + G. *-itis,* inflammation]

ne•phrit•o•gen•ic (ne-fri′tō-jen′ik) Causing nephritis; said of conditions or agents. [nephritis + G. *genesis,* production]

nephro-, nephr- Combining forms meaning the kidney. SEE ALSO reno-. [G. *nephros,* kidney]

neph•ro•blas•to•ma (nef′rō-blast-ō′mă) SYN Wilms tumor.

neph•ro•cal•ci•no•sis (nef′rō-kal-si-nō′sis) A form of renal lithiasis characterized by diffusely scattered foci of calcification in the renal parenchyma; deposits of calcium phosphate, calcium oxalate monohydrate, and similar compounds are usually demonstrable radiologically. [nephro- + calcinosis]

neph•ro•car•di•ac (nef′rō-kahr′dē-ak) SYN cardiorenal. [nephro- + G. *kardia,* heart]

neph•ro•cele (nef′rō-sēl) **1.** Hernial displacement of a kidney. [nephro- + G. *kēlē,* hernia] **2.** In lower vertebrates, the developmental cavity connecting the myocele with the celom. [nephro- + G. *koilōma,* a hollow (celom)]

neph•ro•cys•ti•tis (nef′rō-sist-ī′tis) Inflammation of the kidney and the bladder.

neph•ro•cys•to•sis (nef′rō-sis-tō′sis) Formation of renal cysts. [nephro- + G. *kystis,* cyst, + *-osis,* condition]

neph•ro•ge•net•ic, neph•ro•gen•ic (nef′rō-jĕ-net′ik, -jen′ik) Developing into kidney tissue. [nephro- + G. *genesis,* origin]

neph•ro•gen•ic di•a•be•tes in•sip•i•dus (nef′rō-jen′ik dī-ă-bē′tēz in-sip′i-dŭs) Diabetes insipidus due to inherited inability of the kidney tubules to respond to antidiuretic hormone.

ne•phrog•e•nous (ne-froj′ĕ-nŭs) Developing from kidney tissue.

neph•ro•gram (nef′rō-gram) Radiographic examination of the kidney after the intravenous injection of a water-soluble iodinated contrast material; also, the diffuse opacification of the renal parenchyma following such injection, an indication of renal blood flow and glomerular filtration. A persistent nephrogram indicates obstruction of kidney drainage.

ne•phrog•ra•phy (ne-frog′ră-fē) Radiography of the kidney. [nephro- + G. *graphō,* to write]

neph•roid (nef′royd) Kidney-shaped; resembling a kidney. SYN reniform. [nephro- + G. *eidos,* resemblance]

neph•ro•li•thi•a•sis (nef′rō-li-thī′ă-sis) Presence of renal calculi. See this page.

neph•ro•li•thot•o•my (nef′rō-li-thot′ŏ-mē) Incision into the kidney for the removal of a renal calculus. [nephro- + G. *lithos,* stone, + *tomē,* incision]

ne•phrol•o•gy (ne-frol′ŏ-jē) The branch of medical science concerned with medical diseases of the kidneys. [nephro- + G. *logos,* study]

ne•phrol•y•sis (ne-frol′i-sis) **1.** Freeing of the kidney from inflammatory adhesions, with preservation of the capsule. **2.** Destruction of renal cells. [nephro- + G. *lysis,* dissolution]

neph•ro•lyt•ic (nef-rō-lit′ik) Pertaining to, characterized by, or causing nephrolysis. SYN nephrotoxic (2).

ne•phro•ma (ne-frō′mă) A tumor arising from renal tissue. [nephro- + G. *-oma,* tumor]

neph•ro•meg•a•ly (nef′rō-meg′ă-lē) Extreme hypertrophy of one or both kidneys. [nephro- + G. *megas,* great]

neph•ron (nef′ron) A long convoluted tubular structure in the kidney, consisting of the renal corpuscle, the proximal convoluted tubule, the nephronic loop, and the distal convoluted tubule. [G. *nephros,* kidney]

neph•ron•ic loop (nef-ron′ik lūp) SYN nephron loop.

neph•ron loop (nef′ron lūp) The U-shaped part of the nephron, extending from the proximal to the distal convoluted tubules, consisting of descending and ascending limbs, located in the renal medulla and medullary ray. SYN Henle ansa, Henle loop, nephronic loop.

neph•ro•path•i•a (nef′rō-path′ē-ă) SYN nephropathy.

ne•phrop•a•thy (ne-frop′ă-thē) Any disease of the kidney including inflammatory and degenerative conditions. SYN nephropathia, nephrosis (1). [nephro- + G. *pathos,* suffering]

neph•ro•pex•y (nef′rō-pek-sē) Operative fixation of a floating or mobile kidney. [nephro- + G. *pēxis,* fixation]

neph•roph•thi•sis (nef-rof′thi-sis) **1.** Suppurative nephritis with wasting of the substance of the organ. **2.** Tuberculosis of the kidney. [nephro- + G. *phthisis,* a wasting]

neph•rop•to•sis, neph•rop•to•si•a (nef′rop-tō′sis, -tō′sē-ă) Prolapse of the kidney. [nephro- + G. *ptōsis,* a falling]

neph•ro•py•o•sis (nef′rō-pī-ō′sis) SYN pyonephrosis. [nephro- + G. *pyōsis,* suppuration]

neph•ror•rha•phy (nef-rōr′ă-fē) Nephropexy by suturing the kidney. [nephro- + G. *rhaphē,* a suture]

neph•ro•scle•ro•sis (nef′rō-skle-rō′sis) Induration of the kidney from overgrowth and contraction of the interstitial connective tissue. [nephro- + G. *sklērōsis,* hardening]

neph•ro•scle•rot•ic (nef′rō-skle-rot′ik) Pertaining to or causing nephrosclerosis.

neph•ro•scope (ne′frō-skōp) An endoscope passed into the renal pelvis to view it. Route of access may be percutaneous (through a surgically exposed kidney) or retrograde through the ureter.

ne•phro•sis (ne-frō′sis) **1.** SYN nephropathy. **2.** Degeneration of renal tubular epithelium. **3.** SYN nephrotic syndrome. [nephro- + G. *-osis,* condition]

ne•phros•to•gram (ne-fros′tō-gram) A radiograph of the kidney after opacification of the

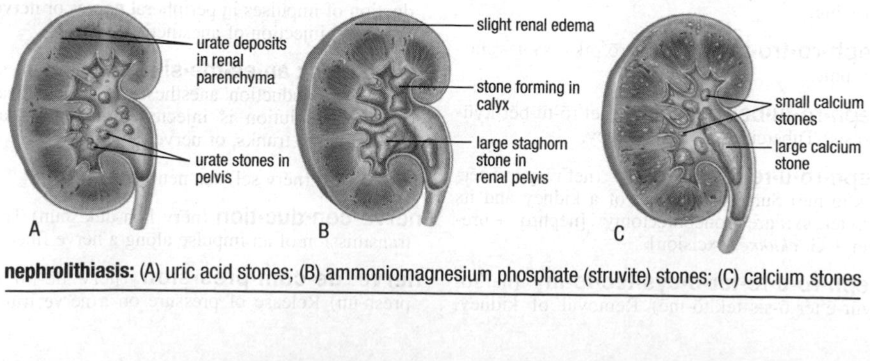

nephrolithiasis: (A) uric acid stones; (B) ammoniomagnesium phosphate (struvite) stones; (C) calcium stones

renal pelvis by injecting a contrast agent through a nephrostomy tube. [nephrostomy + G. *gramma*, writing]

ne•phros•to•my (ne-fros′tŏ-mē) Establishment of an opening between the pelvis of the kidney through its cortex to the exterior of the body. [nephro- + G. *stoma*, mouth]

ne•phros•to•my tube (ne-fros′tŏ-mē tūb) A tube placed in the renal collecting system for drainage, diagnostic tests, or removal of calculi. May be placed through a percutaneous route or during an open surgical procedure.

neph•rot•ic (nef-rot′ik) Relating to, caused by, or similar to nephrosis.

neph•rot•ic syn•drome (nef-rot′ik sin′drōm) A clinical state characterized by edema, albuminuria, decreased plasma albumin, doubly refractile bodies in the urine, and usually increased blood cholesterol; lipid droplets may be present in the cells of the renal tubules, but the basic lesion is increased permeability of the glomerular capillary basement membranes, of unknown cause or resulting from glomerulonephritis, diabetic glomerulosclerosis, systemic lupus erythematosus, amyloidosis, renal vein thrombosis, or hypersensitivity to various toxic agents. SYN nephrosis (3).

neph•ro•to•mo•gram (nef-rō-tō′mō-gram) A tomographic examination of the kidneys following the intravenous administration of water-soluble iodinated contrast material. [nephro- + G. *tomos*, a cutting + *gramma*, a writing]

neph•ro•to•mog•ra•phy (nef′rō-tō-mog′ră-fē) Tomographic examination of the kidney.

ne•phrot•o•my (ne-frot′ŏ-mē) Incision into the kidney. [nephro- + G. *tomē*, incision]

neph•ro•tox•ic (nef-rō-tok′sik) **1.** Pertaining to nephrotoxin; toxic to renal cells. **2.** SYN nephrolytic.

neph•ro•tox•ic•i•ty (nef′rō-tok-sis′i-tē) The quality or state of being toxic to kidney cells.

neph•ro•tox•in (nef′rō-tok′sin) A cytotoxin that is specific for cells of the kidney.

neph•ro•tro•phic (nef′rō-trō′fik) SYN renotrophic.

neph•ro•tro•pic (nef′rō-trō′pik) SYN renotrophic.

neph•ro•tu•ber•cu•lo•sis (nef′rō-tū-bĕr-kyū-lō′sis) Tuberculosis of the kidney.

neph•ro•u•re•ter•ec•to•my (nef′rō-yūr-ĕ-tĕr-ek′tŏ-mē) Surgical removal of a kidney and its ureter. SYN ureteronephrectomy. [nephro- + ureter + G. *ektomē*, excision]

neph•ro•u•re•ter•o•cys•tec•to•my (nef′rō-yūr-ē′tĕr-ō-sis-tek′tŏ-mē) Removal of kidney, ureter, and part or all of the bladder. [nephro- + ureter + G. *kystis*, bladder, + *ektomē*, excision]

Nep•tune gir•dle (nep′tūn gĕr′dĕl) A wet pack applied around the abdomen.

nep•tu•ni•um (Np) (nep-tū′nē-ŭm) A radioactive element; atomic no. 93; first element of the transuranian series (not found in nature); ^{237}Np has a half-life of 2.14×10^6 years. [planet, *Neptune*]

Né•ri sign (nā′rē sīn) In hemiplegia, the knee bends spontaneously when the leg is passively extended.

Nernst e•qua•tion (nernst ĕ-kwā′zhŭn) The equation relating the equilibrium potential of electrodes to ion concentrations; the equation relating the electrical potential and concentration gradient of an ion across a permeable membrane at equilibrium: $E = [RT/nF]$ [ln (C_1/C_2)], where E = potential, R = absolute gas constant, T = absolute temperature, n = valence, F = the Faraday, ln = the natural logarithm, and C_1 and C_2 are the ion concentrations on the two sides; in nonideal solutions, concentration should be replaced by activity. SEE ALSO activity (2).

nerve (nĕrv) A whitish cordlike structure composed of one or more bundles (fascicles) of myelinated or unmyelinated nerve fibers, or more often mixtures of both, coursing outside of the central nervous system, together with connective tissue within the fascicle and around the neurolemma of individual nerve fibers (endoneurium), around each fascicle (perineurium), and around the entire nerve and its nourishing blood vessels (epineurium), by which stimuli are transmitted from the central nervous system to a part of the body or the reverse. SYN nervus [TA]. [L. *nervus*]

nerve a•gent (nĕrv ā′jĕnt) Any of several highly toxic organophosphorus compounds used as chemical-warfare agents because of their ability to inhibit cholinesterase. They include the nonpersistent G agents and the persistent V agents.

nerve a•vul•sion (nĕrv ă-vŭl′shŭn) The tearing away of a peripheral nerve at its point of origin from its parent nerve due to traction.

nerve block (nĕrv block) Interruption of conduction of impulses in peripheral nerves or nerve trunks by injection of anesthetic.

nerve block an•es•the•si•a (nĕrv blok an′es-thē′zē-ă) Conduction anesthesia in which local anesthetic solution is injected around or near nerves, nerve trunks, or nerve plexuses.

nerve cell (nĕrv sel) SEE neuron.

nerve con•duc•tion (nĕrv kŏn-dŭk′shŭn) The transmission of an impulse along a nerve fiber.

nerve de•com•pres•sion (nĕrv dē-kŏm-presh′ŭn) Release of pressure on a nerve trunk by the surgical excision of constricting bands or widening of a bony canal.

nerve growth fac•tor (NGF) (nĕrv grōth fak′tŏr) A protein secreted by the neuron's target, critical for the survival and maintenance of sympathetic and sensory neurons. The movement of NGF from axon tip to soma is thought to be involved in the long-distance signaling of neurons; binds at least two receptors, which are capable of responding to this growth factor, TrkA (pronounced "Track A") and the LNGFR (for "low affinity nerve growth factor receptor") on the surface of cells.

nerve to my•lo•hy•oid (nĕrv mī′lō-hī′oyd) Small branch of inferior alveolar nerve given off posteriorly just before it enters mandibular foramen, distributed to anterior belly of digastric muscle and mylohyoid muscle. SYN nervus mylohyoideus [TA], mylohyoid nerve.

nerve plex•us (nĕrv pleks′ŭs) A plexus formed by the interlacing of nerves by means of numerous communicating branches.

nerve of pter•y•goid ca•nal (nĕrv ter′i-goyd kă-nal′) The nerve constituting the parasympathetic and sympathetic root of the pterygopalatine ganglion; it is formed in the region of the foramen lacerum by the union of the greater superficial petrosal and the deep petrosal nerves, and runs through the pterygoid canal to the pterygopalatine fossa. SYN nervus canalis pterygoidei [TA].

nerve to sta•pe•di•us mus•cle (nĕrv stă-pē′dē-us mŭs′ĕl) A branch of the facial nerve arising in the facial canal and innervating the stapedius muscle. SYN nervus stapedius [TA].

nerve of ten•sor tym•pa•ni mus•cle (nĕrv ten′sōr tim′pă-nī mŭs′ĕl) A branch of the mandibular nerve conveying fibers from the motor root of the trigeminal nerve which pass through the otic ganglion without synapse to supply the tensor tympani muscle. SYN nervus musculi tensoris tympani [TA].

nerve of ten•sor ve•li pa•la•ti•ni mus•cle (nĕrv ten′sōr vē′lī pal-ă-tē′nī mŭs′ĕl) A branch of the mandibular nerve conveying fibers from the motor root of the trigeminal nerve which pass through the otic ganglion without synapse to supply the tensor veli palatini muscle. SYN nervus tensoris veli palatini [TA].

ner•vi (nĕr′vī) Plural of nervus. [L.]

ner•vi a•nal•es in•fe•ri•or•es (nĕr′vī ā-nā′lēz in-fēr′ē-ōr′ēz) SYN inferior anal nerves.

ner•vi au•ric•u•la•res an•te•ri•o•res (nĕr′vī aw-rik-yū-lā′rēz an-tē-rē-ō′rēz) [TA] SYN anterior auricular nerves.

ner•vi car•di•a•ci tho•ra•ci•ci (nĕr′vī kahr′dē-ă′sī thō-ră′si-sī) [TA] SYN thoracic cardiac nerves.

ner•vi ca•ro•ti•ci ex•ter•ni (nĕr′vī kar-rot′i-sī eks-ter′nī) [TA] SYN external carotid nerves.

ner•vi ca•ver•no•si cli•tor•i•dis (nĕr′vī kav′ĕr-nō′sī klit-ō′ri-dis) [TA] SYN cavernous nerves of clitoris.

ner•vi ca•ver•no•si pe•nis (nĕr′vī kav-ĕr-nō′sī pē′nis) [TA] SYN cavernous nerves of penis.

ner•vi clu•ni•um in•fe•ri•or•es (nĕr′vī klū′nē-ŭm in-fēr′ē-ōr′ēz) SYN inferior cluneal nerves.

ner•vi clu•ni•um me•di•i (nĕr′vī klū′nē-ŭm mē′dē-ī) SYN medial cluneal nerves.

ner•vi clu•ni•um su•pe•ri•or•es (nĕr′vī klū′nē-ŭm sū-pēr′ē-ōr′ēz) SYN superior cluneal nerve.

ner•vi cra•ni•a•les (nĕr′vī krā-nē-ā′lēz) [TA] SYN cranial nerves.

ner•vi dig•i•ta•les dor•sa•les man•us (nĕr′vī di-ji-tā′lēz dōr-sā′lēz mā′nŭs) [TA] SYN dorsal digital nerves of hand.

ner•vi dig•i•ta•les dor•sa•les pe•dis (nĕr′vī dij-i-tā′lēz dōr-sā′lēz ped′is) [TA] SYN dorsal digital nerves of foot.

ner•vi dig•i•ta•les pal•mar•es com•mu•nes (nĕr′vī dij-i-tā′lēz pal-mā′rēz kō-myū′nēz) SYN common palmar digital nerve.

ner•vi dig•i•ta•les plan•tar•es com•mu•nes (nĕr′vī dij-i-tā′lēz plan-tā′rēz kō-myū′nēz) SYN common plantar digital nerves.

ner•vi e•ri•gen•tes (nĕr′vī e-ri-gen′tēz) SYN pelvic splanchnic nerves.

ner•vi in•ter•cos•ta•les (nĕr′vī in′tĕr-kos-tā′lēz) [TA] SYN intercostal nerves.

ner•vi in•ter•cos•to•bra•chi•a•les (nĕr′vī in′tĕr-kos-tō-brā′kē-ā′lēz) [TA] SYN intercostobrachial nerves.

ner•vi la•bi•al•es pos•te•ri•or•es (nĕr′vī lā-bē-ā′lēz pos-tēr′ē-ōr′ēz) SYN posterior labial nerves.

ner•vi lum•ba•les (nĕr′vī lŭm-bā′lēz) [TA] SYN lumbar nerves [L1–L5].

ner•vi•mo•tor (nĕr′vi-mō′tŏr) Relating to a motor nerve. SYN neurimotor.

ner•vine (nĕr-vēn′) A natural substance, such as an herb, which is calming to the nervous system.

ner•vi ol•fac•to•ri•i (nĕr′vī ol-fak-tō′rē-ī) [TA] SYN olfactory nerve [CN I].

ner•vi pa•la•ti•ni mi•no•res (nĕr′vī pal-a-tē′nī mī-nō′rēz) [TA] SYN lesser palatine nerves.

ner•vi pel•vi•ci splanch•ni•ci (nĕr′vī pel′vi-sī splangk′ni-sī) SYN pelvic splanchnic nerves.

ner•vi pe•ri•ne•al•es (nĕr′vī per-in-ē-ā′lēz) [TA] SYN perineal nerves.

ner•vi phren•i•ci ac•ces•so•ri•i (něr′vī frē-ni′sī ak-ses-sō′rē-ī) [TA] SYN accessory phrenic nerves.

ner•vi pte•ry•go•pa•la•ti•ni (něr′vī ter′i-gō-pal-ă-tē′nī) [TA] SYN ganglionic branches of maxillary nerve.

ner•vi rec•ta•les in•fe•ri•o•res (něr′vī rek-tā′lēz in-fēr′ē-ōr′ēz) [TA] SYN inferior anal nerves.

ner•vi sa•cra•les (něr′vī sā-krā′lēz) [TA] SYN sacral nerves [S1–S5].

ner•vi spi•na•les (něr′vī spī′nā-lēz) [TA] SYN spinal nerves.

ner•vi splanch•ni•ci lum•ba•les (něr′vī splangk′ni-sī lŭm-bāl′ēz) [TA] SYN lumbar splanchnic nerves.

ner•vi splanch•ni•ci sa•cra•les (něr′vī splangk′ni-sī sā-krā′lēz) [TA] SYN sacral splanchnic nerves.

ner•vi sub•scap•u•la•res (něr′vī sŭb′skap-yū-lā′rēz) SYN subscapular nerves.

ner•vi tem•po•ra•les pro•fun•di (něr′vī tem-pō-rā′lēz prō-fŭn′dī) [TA] SYN deep temporal nerves.

ner•vi ter•mi•na•les (něr′vī těr-mi-nā′lēz) [TA] SYN terminal nerves.

ner•vi tho•ra•ci•ci [T1–12] (něr′vī thō-rā′si-sī) [TA] SYN thoracic nerves [T1–T12].

ner•vi va•gi•na•les (něr′vī va′ji-nā′lēz) [TA] SYN vaginal nerves.

ner•von•ic ac•id (něr-von′ik as′id) A 24-carbon straight-chain fatty acid unsaturated between C-15 and C-16; occurs in cerebrosides such as nervone.

ner•vous (něr′vŭs) **1.** Relating to a nerve or the nerves. **2.** Easily excited or agitated; suffering from mental or emotional instability; tense or anxious. **3.** Formerly, denoting a temperament characterized by excessive mental and physical alertness, rapid pulse, excitability, often volubility, but not always fixity of purpose. [L. *nervosus*]

ner•vous blad•der (něr′vŭs blad′ěr) A bladder condition in which there is a need to urinate frequently but with failure to empty the bladder completely.

ner•vous break•down (něr′vŭs brāk′down) Nonmedical but very common term for an emotional or mental illness; often a colloquialism for a psychiatric disorder.

ner•vous in•di•ges•tion (něr′vŭs in′di-jes′chŭn) Gastrointestinal problems caused by emotional upset or stress.

ner•vous lobe of hy•poph•y•sis (něr′vŭs lōb hī-pof′i-sis) The bulbous part of the neurohypophysis attached to the hypothalamus by the infundibulum. It is composed of pituicytes, blood vessels, and terminals of nerve fibers from the supraoptic and paraventricular nuclei.

ner•vous•ness (něr′vŭs-nēs) A condition of being nervous (2).

i **ner•vous sys•tem** (něr′vŭs sis′tĕm) The entire nerve apparatus, composed of a central part, the brain and spinal cord, and a peripheral part, the cranial and spinal nerves, autonomic ganglia, and plexuses. See page A7, A15.

ner•vus, gen. and pl. **ner•vi** (něr′vŭs, -vī) [TA] SYN nerve. [L.]

ner•vus ab•du•cens [CN VI] (něr′vŭs ab-dū′senz) [TA] SYN abducent nerve [CN VI].

ner•vus ac•ces•so•ri•us [CN XI] (něr′vŭs ak-ses-sō′rē-ŭs) [TA] SYN accessory nerve [CN XI].

ner•vus al•ve•o•la•ris in•fe•ri•or (něr′vŭs al-vē-ō-lā′ris in-fēr′ē-ŏr) [TA] SYN inferior alveolar nerve.

ner•vus a•no•coc•cyg•e•us (něr′vŭs ā′nō-kok-sij′ē-ŭs) [TA] SYN anococcygeal nerve.

ner•vus au•ric•u•la•ris mag•nus (něr′vŭs aw-rik′yū-lā′ris mag′nŭs) [TA] SYN great auricular nerve.

ner•vus au•ric•u•la•ris pos•te•ri•or (něr′vŭs aw-rik′yū-lā′ris pos-tēr′ē-ŏr) [TA] SYN posterior auricular nerve.

ner•vus au•ric•u•lo•tem•po•ra•lis (něr′vŭs aw-rik′yū-lō-tem-pō-rā′lis) [TA] SYN auriculotemporal nerve.

ner•vus ax•il•la•ris (něr′vŭs ak-sil-lā′ris) [TA] SYN axillary nerve.

ner•vus buc•ca•lis (něr′vŭs bŭk-ā′lis) [TA] SYN buccal nerve.

ner•vus ca•na•lis pte•ry•goi•de•i (něr′vŭs kă-nā′lis ter-i-goy′dē-ī) [TA] SYN nerve of pterygoid canal.

ner•vus ca•ro•ti•cus in•ter•nus (něr′vŭs kă-rŏt′i-kŭs in-těr′nŭs) [TA] SYN internal carotid nerve.

ner•vus cil•i•ar•is brev•is (něr′vŭs sil′ē-ā′ris brev′is) SYN short ciliary nerve.

ner•vus cil•i•ar•is lon•gus (něr′vŭs sil′ē-ā′ris long′ŭs) SYN long ciliary nerve.

ner•vus coc•cyg•e•us (něr′vŭs kok′sij′ē-us) [TA] SYN coccygeal nerve [Co].

ner•vus cu•ta•ne•us an•te•bra•chi•i la•ter•al•is (něr′vŭs kyū-tā′nē-ŭs an-tē-brā′kē-ī lat′ĕr-ā′lis) SYN lateral cutaneous nerve of forearm.

ner•vus cu•ta•ne•us an•te•bra•chi•i me•di•a•lis (něr′vŭs kyū-tā′nē-ŭs an-tē-brā′kē-ī mē-dē-ā′lis) SYN medial cutaneous nerve of forearm.

ner•vus cu•ta•ne•us bra•chi•i me•di•a•lis (nĕr′vŭs kyū-tā′nē-ŭs brā′kē-ī mē-dē-ā′lis) SYN medial cutaneous nerve of forearm.

ner•vus cu•ta•ne•us dor•sal•is me•di•a•lis (nĕr′vŭs kyū-tā′nē-ŭs dor-sā′lis mē-dē-ā′lis) SYN medial dorsal cutaneous nerve.

ner•vus cu•ta•ne•us fem•o•ris la•ter•a•lis (nĕr′vŭs kyū-tā′nē-ŭs fem′ō-ris lat′tĕr-ā′lis) SYN lateral cutaneous nerve of thigh.

ner•vus cu•ta•ne•us fem•o•ris pos•te•ri•or (nĕr′vŭs kyū-tā′nē-ŭs fem′ō-ris pos-tēr′ē-ŏr) SYN posterior cutaneous nerve of thigh.

ner•vus dor•sa•lis cli•tor•i•dis (nĕr′vŭs dōr-sā′lis klit-ō′ri-dis) [TA] SYN dorsal nerve of clitoris.

ner•vus dor•sa•lis pe•nis (nĕr′vŭs dōr-sā′lis pē′nis) [TA] SYN dorsal nerve of penis.

ner•vus dor•sa•lis scap•u•lae (nĕr′vŭs dōr-sā′lis skap′yū-lē) [TA] SYN dorsal scapular nerve.

ner•vus eth•moi•da•lis an•te•ri•or (nĕr′vŭs eth-moy-dā′lis an-tēr′ē-ŏr) SYN anterior ethmoidal nerve.

ner•vus eth•moi•dal•is pos•te•ri•or (nĕr′vŭs eth-moy-dā′lis pos-tēr′ē-ŏr) SYN posterior ethmoidal nerve.

ner•vus fa•ci•a•lis [CN VII] (nĕr′vŭs fā-shē-ā′lis) [TA] SYN facial nerve [CN VII].

ner•vus fe•mo•ra•lis (nĕr′vŭs fem-ō-rā′lis) [TA] SYN femoral nerve.

ner•vus fib•u•lar•is com•mu•nis (nĕr′vŭs fib-yū-lā′ris ko-myū′nis) SYN common fibular nerve.

ner•vus fib•u•lar•is pro•fun•dus (nĕr′vŭs fib-yū-lā′ris prō-fŭn′dŭs) SYN deep fibular nerve.

ner•vus fib•u•lar•is su•per•fi•ci•al•is (nĕr′vŭs fib-yū-lā′ris sū′pĕr-fish′ē-ā′lis) SYN superficial fibular nerve.

ner•vus fron•ta•lis (nĕr′vŭs fron-tā′lis) [TA] SYN frontal nerve.

ner•vus gen•i•to•fe•mo•ra•lis (nĕr′vŭs jen-i-tō-fem-ō-rā′lis) [TA] SYN genitofemoral nerve.

ner•vus glos•so•pha•ryn•ge•us [CN IX] (nĕr′vŭs glos-ō-fă-rin′jē-ŭs) [TA] SYN glossopharyngeal nerve [CN IX].

ner•vus glu•te•us in•fe•ri•or (nĕr′vŭs glū′tē-ŭs in-fēr′ē-ŏr) SYN inferior gluteal nerve.

ner•vus glu•te•us su•pe•ri•or (nĕr′vŭs glū′tē-ŭs sŭ-pēr′ē-ŏr) SYN superior gluteal nerve.

ner•vus hy•po•gas•tri•cus (nĕr′vŭs hī-pō-gas′trik-ŭs) [TA] SYN hypogastric nerve.

ner•vus hy•po•glos•sus [CN XII] (nĕr′vŭs hī-pō-glos′ŭs) [TA] SYN hypoglossal nerve [CN XII].

ner•vus il•i•o•hy•po•gas•tri•cus (nĕr′vŭs il′ē-ō-hī-pō-gas′trik-ŭs) [TA] SYN iliohypogastric nerve.

ner•vus il•i•o•in•gui•na•lis (nĕr′vŭs il′ē-ō-in′gwi-nā′lis) [TA] SYN ilioinguinal nerve.

ner•vus in•fra•or•bi•ta•lis (nĕr′vŭs in-fra-ōr′bi-tā′lis) [TA] SYN infraorbital nerve.

ner•vus in•fra•troch•le•a•ris (nĕr′vŭs in-fra-trō-klē-ā′ris) [TA] SYN infratrochlear nerve.

ner•vus in•ter•me•di•us (nĕr′vŭs in′tĕr-mē′dē-ŭs) [TA] SYN intermediary nerve.

ner•vus in•ter•os•se•us an•te•bra•chi•i an•te•ri•or (nĕr′vŭs in-tĕr-os′sē-us an′tē-brā′kē-ī an-tēr′ē-ŏr) [TA] SYN anterior interosseous nerve.

ner•vus in•ter•os•se•us an•te•bra•chi•i pos•te•ri•or (nĕr′vŭs in-tĕr-os′sē-us an-tē-brā′kē-ī pos-tēr′ē-ŏr) [TA] SYN posterior interosseous nerve.

ner•vus in•ter•os•se•us cru•ris (nĕr′vŭs in′tĕr-os′ē-ŭs krūr′is) [TA] SYN crural interosseous nerve.

ner•vus is•chi•a•di•cus (nĕr′vŭs is-kē-ad′i-kŭs) [TA] SYN sciatic nerve.

ner•vus ju•gu•la•ris (nĕr′vŭs jŭg-yū-lā′ris) [TA] SYN jugular nerve.

ner•vus la•cri•ma•lis (nĕr′vŭs lak′rē-mā′lis) [TA] SYN lacrimal nerve.

ner•vus lar•yn•ge•us su•pe•ri•or (nĕr′vŭs lă-rin′jē-ŭs sŭ-pēr′ē-ŏr) SYN superior laryngeal nerve.

ner•vus lin•gua•lis (nĕr′vŭs ling-gwā′lis) [TA] SYN lingual nerve.

ner•vus man•di•bu•la•ris [CN V3] (nĕr′vŭs man-di-byū-lā′ris) [TA] SYN mandibular nerve [CN V3].

ner•vus mas•se•te•ri•cus (nĕr′vŭs mas-ĕ-ter′i-kŭs) [TA] SYN masseteric nerve.

ner•vus max•il•la•ris [CN V2] (nĕr′vŭs maks′i-lā′ris) [TA] SYN maxillary nerve [CN V2].

ner•vus men•ta•lis (nĕr′vŭs men-tā′lis) [TA] SYN mental nerve.

ner•vus mus•cu•li ten•so•ris tym•pa•ni (nĕr′vŭs mŭs′kyū-lī ten-sō′ris tim′pan-ē) [TA] SYN nerve of tensor tympani muscle.

ner•vus mus•cu•lo•cu•ta•ne•us (nĕr′vŭs mŭs′kyū-lō-kyū-tā′nē-ŭs) [TA] SYN musculocutaneous nerve.

ner•vus my•lo•hy•oi•de•us (nĕr′vŭs mī′lō-hī-oy′dē-ŭs) [TA] SYN nerve to mylohyoid.

ner•vus na•so•cil•i•a•ris (nĕr′vŭs nā′so-sil′ē-ā′ris) [TA] SYN nasociliary nerve.

ner•vus na•so•pal•a•tin•us (nĕr′vŭs nā′so-pal-ă-tī′nŭs) [TA] SYN nasopalatine nerve.

ner•vus ob•tu•ra•to•ri•us (nĕr′vŭs ob-tū-rā-tō′rē-ŭs) [TA] SYN obturator nerve.

ner•vus oc•cip•i•ta•lis mi•nor (nĕr′vŭs ok-sip-i-tā′lis mī′nŏr) SYN lesser occipital nerve.

ner•vus o•cu•lo•mo•to•ri•us [CN III] (nĕr′vŭs ok-yū-lō-mō-tō′rē-ŭs) [TA] SYN oculomotor nerve [CN III].

ner•vus ol•fac•to•ri•i [CN I] (nĕr′vŭs ol-fak-tō′rē-ī) [TA] SYN olfactory nerve [CN I].

ner•vus oph•thal•mi•cus [CN V1] (nĕr′vŭs of-thal′mi-kŭs) [TA] SYN ophthalmic nerve [CN V1].

ner•vus op•ti•cus [CN II] (nĕr′vŭs op′ti-kŭs) [TA] SYN optic nerve [CN II].

ner•vus pal•a•ti•nus ma•jor (nĕr′vŭs pa-lă-tī′nŭs mā′jŏr) [TA] SYN greater palatine nerve.

ner•vus pec•to•ral•is la•te•ra•lis (nĕr′vŭs pek′tō-rā′lis lat′tĕ-rā′lis) SYN lateral pectoral nerve.

ner•vus pec•to•ral•is me•di•a•lis (nĕr′vŭs pek′tō-rā′lis mē-dē-ā′lis) SYN medial pectoral nerve.

ner•vus pe•ro•ne•us com•mu•nis (nĕr′vŭs per-ō′nē-ŭs ko-myū′nis) SYN common fibular nerve.

ner•vus pe•ro•ne•us pro•fun•dus (nĕr′vŭs per-ō′nē-ŭs prō-fŭn′dis) SYN deep fibular nerve.

ner•vus pe•ro•ne•us su•per•fi•ci•al•is (nĕr′vŭs per-ō′nē-ŭs sū′pĕr-fish′ē-ā′lis) SYN superficial fibular nerve.

ner•vus pe•tro•sus ma•jor (nĕr′vŭs pe-trō′sŭs mā′jor) SYN greater petrosal nerve.

ner•vus pe•tro•sus mi•nor (nĕr′vŭs pe-trō′sŭs mī′nŏr) SYN lesser petrosal nerve.

ner•vus pe•tro•sus pro•fun•dus (nĕr′vŭs pe-trō′sŭs prō-fŭn′dŭs) SYN deep petrosal nerve.

ner•vus pha•ryn•ge•us (nĕr′vŭs fă-rin′jē-ŭs) SYN pharyngeal nerve.

ner•vus phre•ni•cus (nĕr′vŭs fren′i-kŭs) [TA] SYN phrenic nerve.

ner•vus plan•tar•is la•te•ra•lis (nĕr′vŭs plan-tā′ris lat′tĕr-ā′lis) SYN lateral plantar nerve.

ner•vus plan•tar•is me•di•a•lis (nĕr′vŭs plan-tā′ris mē-dē-ā′lis) SYN medial plantar nerve.

ner•vus pte•ry•goi•de•us (nĕr′vŭs ter-i-goy′dē-ŭs) [TA] SYN pterygoid nerve.

ner•vus pu•den•dus (nĕr′vŭs pū-den′dŭs) [TA] SYN pudendal nerve.

ner•vus ra•di•a•lis (nĕr′vŭs rā-dē-ā′lis) [TA] SYN radial nerve.

ner•vus sac•cu•la•ris (nĕr′vŭs sak-kyū-lā′ris) [TA] SYN saccular nerve.

ner•vus sa•phe•nus (nĕr′vŭs saf′en-ŭs) [TA] SYN saphenous nerve.

ner•vus splanch•ni•cus i•mus (nĕr′vŭs splangk′nik-ŭs ī′mŭs) [TA] SYN lowest splanchnic nerve.

ner•vus splanch•ni•cus ma•jor (nĕr′vŭs splangk′nik-ŭs māj′ŏr) [TA] SYN greater splanchnic nerve.

ner•vus splanch•ni•cus mi•nor (nĕr′vŭs splangk′nik-ŭs mī′nŏr) [TA] SYN lesser splanchnic nerve.

ner•vus sta•pe•di•us (nĕr′vŭs stā-pē′dē-us) [TA] SYN nerve to stapedius muscle.

ner•vus sub•cla•vi•us (nĕr′vŭs sŭb-klā′vē-ŭs) [TA] SYN subclavian nerve.

ner•vus sub•cos•ta•lis (nĕr′vŭs sŭb-kos-tā′lis) [TA] SYN subcostal nerve.

ner•vus sub•lin•gua•lis (nĕr′vŭs sŭb-ling-gwā′lis) [TA] SYN sublingual nerve.

ner•vus sub•oc•cip•i•ta•lis (nĕr′vŭs sŭb-ok-sip-i-tā′lis) [TA] SYN suboccipital nerve.

ner•vus su•pra•cla•vic•u•la•ris in•ter•me•di•us (nĕr′vŭs sū′pră-klă-vik-yū-lā′ris in-tĕr-mē′dē-ŭs) SYN intermediate supraclavicular nerve.

ner•vus su•pra•cla•vic•u•la•ris la•te•ra•lis (nĕr′vŭs sū′pră-klă-vik-yū-lā′ris lat′tĕr-āl′is) SYN lateral supraclavicular nerve.

ner•vus su•pra•cla•vic•u•la•ris me•di•a•lis (nĕr′vŭs sū′pră-klă-vik-yū-lā′ris mē-dē-ā′lis) SYN medial supraclavicular nerve.

ner•vus su•pra•or•bi•ta•lis (nĕr′ŭs sū′pră-ōr′bi-tā′lis) [TA] SYN supraorbital nerve.

ner•vus su•pra•scap•u•la•ris (nĕr′vŭs sū′pră-skap′yū-lā′ris) [TA] SYN suprascapular nerve.

ner•vus su•pra•troch•le•ar•is (nĕr′vŭs sū′pră-trō′klē-ā′ris) [TA] SYN supratrochlear nerve.

ner•vus su•ra•lis (nĕr′vŭs sū-rā′lis) [TA] SYN sural nerve.

ner•vus ten•so•ris ve•li pa•la•ti•ni (nĕr′vŭs ten-sō′ris vē′lī pal-ă-tē′nī) [TA] SYN nerve of tensor veli palatini muscle.

ner•vus ten•to•ri•i (nĕr′vŭs ten-tō′rē-ī) SYN tentorial nerve.

ner•vus tho•ra•ci•cus lon•gus (nĕr′vŭs thō-rā′si-kŭs long′ŭs) [TA] SYN long thoracic nerve.

ner•vus tho•ra•co•dor•sa•lis (nĕr′vŭs thō-rā-kō-dōr-sā′lis) [TA] SYN thoracodorsal nerve.

ner•vus tib•i•a•lis (nĕr′vŭs tib-ē-ā′lis) [TA] SYN tibial nerve.

ner•vus trans•ver•sus col•li (nĕr′vŭs trans-vĕr′sŭs kol′ī) [TA] SYN transverse cervical nerve.

ner•vus tri•gem•i•nus [CN V] (nĕr′vŭs trī-jem′i-nŭs) [TA] SYN trigeminal nerve [CN V].

ner•vus troch•le•ar•is [CN IV] (nĕr′vŭs trō-klē-ā′ris) [TA] SYN trochlear nerve [CN IV].

ner•vus tym•pa•ni•cus (nĕr′vŭs tim-pan′i-kŭs) [TA] SYN tympanic nerve.

ner•vus ul•na•ris (nĕr′vŭs ŭl-nā′ris) [TA] SYN ulnar nerve.

ner•vus u•tri•cu•la•ris (nĕr′vŭs ū-trik-yū-lā′ris) [TA] SYN utricular nerve.

ner•vus u•tri•cu•lo•am•pul•la•ris (nĕr′vŭs ū-trik-yū-lo-am-pyū-lā′ris) [TA] SYN utriculoampullar nerve.

ner•vus va•gus [CN X] (nĕr′vŭs vāg′ŭs) [TA] SYN vagus nerve [CN X].

ner•vus ver•te•bra•lis (nĕr′vŭs vĕr-tĕ-brā′lis) [TA] SYN vertebral nerve.

ner•vus ves•ti•bu•lo•co•chle•a•ris [CN VIII] (nĕr′vŭs ves-tib′yū-lō-kok-lē-ā′ris) [TA] SYN vestibulocochlear nerve [CN VIII].

ner•vus zy•go•ma•ti•cus (nĕr′vŭs zī′gō-mat′i-kŭs) [TA] SYN zygomatic nerve.

♻ **-ness** A suffix meaning a quality or state of being (e.g., illness). [M.E., fr. O.E.]

nest (nest) A group or collection of similar objects. SEE ALSO nidus. [A.S.]

nest•ed pol•y•mer•ase chain re•ac•tion (PCR) (nest′ĕd pŏ-lim′ĕr-ās chān rē-ak′shŭn) Use of PCR in series, so that a specified piece of DNA is amplified, and then a portion contained within the first piece is amplified further; used where extremely low amounts of DNA are present, or where there are problems with background or contaminating DNA.

net (net) SYN network (1).

Neth•er•ton syn•drome (neth′ĕr-tŏn sin′drōm) Congenital ichthyosiform erythroderma or ichthyosis linearis circumscripta associated with bamboo hair, atopy, urticaria, intermittent aminoaciduria, and mental retardation; probably an autosomal recessive trait; frequently resolves or improves in adolescence.

net ox•y•gen con•sump•tion (net ok′si-jen kŏn-sŭmp′shŭn) Consumption of oxygen beyond that necessary to sustain life at rest (i.e., oxygen consumption for a given activity less resting oxygen consumption).

net pro•tein u•ti•li•za•tion (NPU) (net prō′tēn yū′ti-lī-zā′shŭn) Measurement of the body's use of ingested protein.

Net•tle•ship-Falls al•bin•ism (net′ĕl-shop fawlz al′bi-nizm) SYN ocular albinism 1.

net•work (net′wŏrk) **1.** A structure bearing a resemblance to a woven fabric. A network of nerve fibers or small vessels. SYN rete (1) [TA], net. SEE ALSO reticulum. **2.** The people in a patient's environment, especially as significant for the course of the illness.

net•work mod•el HMO (net′wŏrk mod′ĕl) Arrangement by which an HMO contracts with group practice physicians to be providers for HMO subscribers, with the physicians retaining the option to see other patients.

net wt. (net) Abbreviation for net weight.

Neu•bau•er ar•ter•y (nū-bow′ĕr ahr′tĕr-ē) SYN thyroid ima artery.

Neu•feld cap•su•lar swell•ing (nū′feld kap′sŭ-lăr swel′ing) Increase in opacity and visibility of the capsule of capsulated organisms exposed to specific agglutinating anticapsular antibodies. SYN Neufeld reaction, quellung phenomenon, quellung reaction (1), quellung test.

Neu•feld re•ac•tion (nū′feld rē-ak′shŭn) SYN Neufeld capsular swelling.

Neu•mann law (nū′măn law) In compounds of analogous chemical constitution, the molecular heat, or the product of the specific heat and the atomic weight, is always the same.

♻ **neur-, neuri-, neuro-** Combining forms meaning nerve, nerve tissue, the nervous system. [G. *neuron*]

neu•ral (nūr′ăl) **1.** Relating to any structure composed of nerve cells or their processes, or that on further development will evolve into nerve cells. **2.** Referring to the dorsal side of the vertebral bodies or their precursors, where the spinal cord is located, as opposed to hemal (2). [G. *neuron,* nerve]

♻ **-neural, -neuric** Suffix meaning nerve or nerves (e.g., epineural). [G. *neuron,* sinew, nerve]

neu•ral arch (nūr′ăl ahrch) SYN vertebral arch.

neu•ral ca•nal (nūr′ăl kă-nal′) The ependyma-lined lumen (cavity) of the neural tube, the cerebral part of which remains patent to form the ventricles of the brain, while the spinal part forms the central canal of the spinal cord, which in the adult is often reduced to a solid strand of modified ependyma. SYN syringocele (1).

neu•ral crest (nūr′ăl krest) A band of neuroectodermal cells along either side of the line of closure of the embryonic neural groove; with the formation of the neural tube, these bands come to lie dorsolateral to the developing spinal cord and lateral to the brainstem, where they separate into clusters of cells that develop into, for example, spinal ganglion cells, autonomic ganglion cells, the chromaffin cells of the suprarenal medulla, Schwann cells, sensory ganglia of cranial nerves V, VII, VIII, IX, and X, part of the meninges, or integumentary pigment cells.

neu•ral crest syn•drome (nū′răl krest sin′drōm) Syndrome consisting of loss of pain sensibility, autonomic dysfunction, pupillary abnormalities, neurogenic anhidrosis, vasomotor instability, aplasia of dental enamel, meningeal thickening, hyperflexion, and a degree of albinism; may reflect developmental abnormalities of the neural crest.

neu•ral folds (nūr′ăl fōldz) The elevated margins of the neural groove. See page B1.

neu•ral•gi•a (nūr-al′jē-ă) Pain of a severe, throbbing, or stabbing character in the course or distribution of a nerve. SYN neurodynia. [neur- + G. *algos,* pain]

neu•ral•gi•a fa•ci•a•lis ve•ra (nūr-al′jē-ă fā-shē-ā′lis vē′ră) SYN geniculate neuralgia.

neu•ral•gic (nū-ral′jik) Relating to, resembling, or of the character of, neuralgia.

neu•ral•gic a•my•ot•ro•phy (nūr-al′jik ā′mī-ot′rŏ-fē) A neurologic disorder of unknown cause, characterized by the sudden onset of severe pain, usually about the shoulder and often beginning at night, soon followed by weakness and wasting of various forequarter muscles, particularly shoulder girdle muscles; both sporadic and familial in occurrence with the former much more common; often preceded by some antecedent event, such as an upper respiratory infection, hospitalization, vaccination, or nonspecific trauma; usually attributed to a brachial plexus lesion, because the nerve fibers involved are most often derived from the upper trunk, but actually multiple proximal mononeuropathies. SYN shoulder-girdle syndrome.

neu•ral groove (nūr′ăl grūv) The gutterlike groove formed in the midline of the dorsal surface of the embryo by the progressive elevation of the lateral margins of the neural plate; the dorsal fusion of the folds results in the formation of the neural tube.

neu•ral hear•ing loss (nūr′răl hēr′ing laws) Form of sensorineural hearing loss due to a lesion in the auditory division of the eighth cranial nerve.

neu•ral plate (nūr′ăl plāt) The unpaired neuroectodermal region on the dorsal surface of the early embryo that becomes the neural tube and neural crest. SYN medullary plate.

neu•ral ret•i•na (nūr′ăl ret′i-nă) The optic part of the retina; it contains photoreceptors that are sensitive to visual light rays.

neu•ral spine (nūr′ăl spīn) The middle point of the neural arch of the typical vertebra, represented by the spinous process.

neu•ral ther•a•py (nūr′ăl thār′ă-pē) The use of injections of anesthetics to reverse the effects of cumulative trauma to the body.

neu•ral tube de•fect (nūr′ăl tūb dē′fekt) A birth defect that may be caused by a deficiency of folate early in pregnancy, characterized by incomplete midline fusion of the developing central nervous system.

neur•a•min•ic ac•id (nūr′ă-min′ik as′id) An aldol product of D-mannosamine and pyruvic acid. The *N*- and *O*-acyl derivatives of neuraminic acid are known as sialic acids and are constituents of gangliosides and of the polysaccharide components of muco- and glycoproteins from many tissues and secretions.

neur•an•a•gen•e•sis (nūr′an-ă-jen′ĕ-sis) Regeneration of a nerve. [neur- + G. *ana,* up, again, + *genesis,* origin]

neur•a•poph•y•sis (nūr′ă-pof′i-sis) SYN lamina of vertebral arch. [neur- + G. *apophysis,* offshoot]

neur•a•prax•i•a (nūr′ă-prak′sē-ă) The mildest type of focal nerve lesion that produces clinical deficits; localized loss of conduction along a nerve without axon degeneration; caused by a focal lesion, usually demyelinating, and followed by a complete recovery. SEE ALSO axonotmesis. [neur- + G. a- priv. + *praxis,* action]

neur•as•the•ni•a (nūr′as-thē′nē-ă) An ill-defined condition, commonly accompanying or following depression, characterized by vague fatigue believed to be brought on by psychological factors. [neur- + G. *astheneia,* weakness]

neur•as•then•ic (nūr′as-then′ik) Relating to, or suffering from, neurasthenia.

neur•ax•is (nū-rak′sis) The axial, unpaired part of the central nervous system: spinal cord, rhombencephalon, mesencephalon, and diencephalon, in contrast to the paired cerebral hemispheres, or telencephalon.

neur•ec•ta•sis, neur•ec•ta•si•a, neur•ec•ta•sy (nūr-ek′tă-sis, nūr-ek-tā′zē-ă, nūr-ek′tă-sē) The operation of stretching a nerve or nerve trunk. [neur- + G. *ektasis,* extension]

neu•rec•to•my (nūr-ek′tŏ-mē) Excision of a segment of a nerve. [neur- + G. *ektomē,* excision]

neur•ec•to•pi•a, neur•ec•to•py (nūr′ek-tō′pē-ă, nūr-ek′tō-pē) **1.** Dislocation of a nerve trunk. **2.** A condition in which a nerve follows an anomalous course. [neur- + G. *ektopos,* fr. *ek,* out of, + *topos,* place]

neur•en•ter•ic cysts (nūr′en-ter′ik sists) Paravertebral cysts commonly connected to the meninges or a portion of the gastrointestinal tract that develop due to incomplete separation of endoderm from the notochord during early fetal life; often symptomatic.

neu•rer•gic (nūr-ĕr′jik) Relating to the activity of a nerve. [neur- + G. *ergon,* work]

neur•ex•er•e•sis (nūr′ek-ser′ĕ-sis) Tearing out or evulsion of a nerve. [neur- + G. *exairesis,* a taking out, fr. *haireō,* to grasp, take]

neu•ri•lem•ma (nūr′i-lem′ă) A cell that enfolds one or more axons of the peripheral nervous system; in myelinated fibers its plasma membrane forms the lamellae of myelin. SYN neurolemma, sheath of Schwann. [neuri + G. *lemma,* husk]

neu•ri•lem•ma cells (nūr′i-lem′ă selz) SYN Schwann cells.

neu•ri•lem•mo•ma (nūr′i-le-mō′mă) SYN schwannoma. [neurilemma + G. *-oma,* tumor]

neu•ri•mo•tor (nūr′i-mō′tŏr) SYN nervimotor.

neu•ri•no•ma (nūr′i-nō′mă) Obsolete term for schwannoma.

neu•rit•ic (nūr-it′ik) Relating to neuritis.

neu•rit•ic plaque (nūr-it′ik plak) SYN senile plaque.

neu•ri•tis, pl. **neu•ri•ti•des** (nūr-ī′tis, -rit′i-dēz) **1.** Inflammation of a nerve. **2.** SYN neuropathy. [neuri- + G. *-itis,* inflammation]

♻ **neuro-** Combining form meaning nerve, nerve tissue, the nervous system.

neu•ro•an•as•to•mo•sis (nūr′ō-ă-nas-tō-mō′sis) Surgical formation of a junction between nerves.

neu•ro•a•nat•o•my (nūr′ō-ă-nat′ŏ-mē) The anatomy of the nervous system, usually specific to the central nervous system.

neu•ro•ar•throp•a•thy (nūr′ō-ahr-throp′ă-thē) A joint disorder caused by loss of joint sensation. SEE Charcot joint. [neuro- + G. *arthron,* joint, + *pathos,* suffering, disease]

neu•ro•blast (nūr′ō-blast) An embryonic nerve cell. [neuro- + G. *blastos,* germ]

🅸 **neu•ro•blas•to•ma** (nūr′ō-blas-tō′mă) A malignant neoplasm characterized by immature nerve cells of embryonic type (e.g., neuroblasts) the stroma is sparse and foci of necrosis and hemorrhage are not unusual. Neuroblastomas occur frequently in infants and children in the mediastinal and retroperitoneal regions; widespread metastases to the liver, lungs, lymph nodes, cranial cavity, and skeleton are common. See page B31.

neu•ro•car•di•ac (nūr′ō-kahr′dē-ak) **1.** Relating to the nerve supply of the heart. **2.** Relating to a cardiac neurosis. [neuro- + G. *kardia,* heart]

neu•ro•car•di•o•gen•ic syn•co•pe (nūr′ō-kar′dī-ō-jen′ik sing′kŏ-pē) SYN vasodepressor syncope.

neu•ro•chem•is•try (nūr′ō-kem′is-trē) The science concerned with the chemical aspects of nervous system structure and function.

neu•ro•cho•ri•o•ret•i•ni•tis (nūr′ō-kōr′ē-ō-ret-in-ī′tis) Inflammation of the choroid, the retina, and the optic nerve.

neu•ro•cho•roi•di•tis (nūr′ō-kōr-oyd-ī′tis) Inflammation of the choroid and the optic nerve.

neu•roc•la•dism (nū-rok′lă-dizm) The outgrowth of axons from the central stump to bridge the gap in a cut nerve. [neuro- + G. *klados,* a young branch]

neu•ro•cra•ni•um (nūr′ō-krā′nē-ŭm) Those bones of the cranium enclosing the brain, as distinguished from the bones of the face. SYN brain box, braincase. [neuro- + G. *kranion,* skull]

neu•ro•cris•top•a•thy (nūr′ō-kris-top′ă-thē) Any congenital anomaly resulting from abnormal development of the neural crest. [neuro- + L. *crista,* crest, + G. *pathos,* suffering]

neu•ro•cyte (nūr′o-sīt) SYN neuron (1). [neuro- + G. *kytos,* cell]

neu•ro•cy•tol•y•sin (nūr′ō-sī-tol′i-sin) A toxic substance in the venom of some snakes (e.g., cobras, coral snakes) that causes the lysis of nerve cells. [neuro + G. *kytos,* cell, + *lysis,* dissolution]

neu•ro•cy•tol•y•sis (nūr′ō-sī-tol′i-sis) Destruction of neurons. [neuro- + G. *kytos,* cell, + *lysis,* dissolution]

neu•ro•cy•to•ma (nūr′ō-sī-tō′mă) A tumor of neuronal differentiation usually intraventricular in location, consisting of sheets of cells with uniform nuclei and occasional perivascular pseudorosette formation. [neuro- + G. *kytos,* cell, + *-oma,* tumor]

neu•ro•den•drite (nūr′ō-den′drīt) SYN dendrite (1).

neu•ro•der•ma•ti•tis (nūr′ō-dĕr-mă-tī′tis) A chronic lichenified skin lesion; loosely applied to atopic dermatitis. SYN neurodermatosis. [neuro- + G. *derma,* skin, + *-itis,* inflammation]

neu•ro•der•ma•to•sis (nūr′ō-dĕr-mă-tō′sis) SYN neurodermatitis.

neu•ro•de•vel•op•men•tal treat•ment (NDT) (nūr′ō-dĕ-vel-ŏp-men′tăl trēt′mĕnt) A therapeutic system in occupational and physical therapy that employs six methods to inhibit spasticity and promote normal movement in patients with neurologic illness. The focus is on normal movement development.

neu•ro•dy•nam•ic (nūr′ō-dī-nam′ik) Pertaining to nervous energy. [neuro- + G. *dynamis,* force]

neu•ro•dyn•i•a (nūr′ō-din′ē-ă) SYN neuralgia. [neuro- + G. *odynē,* pain]

neu•ro•ec•to•derm (nūr′ō-ek′tō-dĕrm) That

central region of the early embryonic ectoderm that on further development forms the brain and spinal cord, and also evolves into the nerve cells that become the neural crest cells and neurilemma or Schwann cells of the peripheral nervous system.

neu•ro•ec•to•der•mal (nūr′ō-ek-tō-dĕr′măl) Relating to the neuroectoderm.

neu•ro•en•ceph•a•lo•my•e•lop•a•thy (nūr′ō-en-sef′ă-lō-mī-ĕ-lop′ă-thē) Disease of the brain, spinal cord, and nerves.

neu•ro•en•do•crine (nūr′ō-en′dō-krin) **1.** Pertaining to the anatomic and functional relationships between the nervous system and the endocrine apparatus. **2.** Descriptive of cells that release a hormone into the circulating blood in response to a neural stimulus.

neu•ro•en•do•crin•ol•o•gy (nūr′ō-en′dō-krin-ol′ŏ-jē) The specialty concerned with the anatomic and functional relationships between the nervous system and the endocrine apparatus.

neu•ro•ep•i•the•li•al (nūr′ō-ep-i-thē′lē-ăl) Relating to the neuroepithelium.

neu•ro•ep•i•the•li•um (nūr′ō-ep-i-thē′lē-ŭm) Epithelial cells specialized for the reception of external stimuli, such as the hair cells of the inner ear, the receptor cells of the taste buds, and the rods and cones of the retina.

neu•ro•fi•bril (nūr′ō-fī′bril) A filamentous structure seen with the light microscope in the body, dendrites, axons, and sometimes synaptic endings of a nerve cell.

neu•ro•fi•bril•lar (nūr′ō-fī′bri-lăr) Relating to neurofibrils.

neu•ro•fi•bro•ma (nūr′ō-fī-brō′mă) A benign, encapsulated tumor resulting from proliferation of Schwann cells. SYN fibroneuroma.

neu•ro•fi•bro•ma•to•sis (nūr′ō-fī-brō-mă-tō′sis) Two distinct major hereditary disorders called type 1 and type 2. **Type 1 (peripheral) neurofibromatosis**, by far the more common, is characterized by patches of hyperpigmentation and both cutaneous and subcutaneous tumors. Hyperpigmented skin areas, present from birth, are called café-au-lait spots. The cutaneous and subcutaneous tumors, nerve sheath neoplasms called neurofibromas, can develop anywhere along the peripheral nerves. Neurofibromas can become large enough to cause disfigurement, erode bone, and compress peripheral nerves. If a hamartoma is found in the iris of affected patients, the disease is called von Recklinghausen disease. **Type 2 (central) neurofibromatosis** has few cutaneous manifestations, and consists primarily of acoustic neuromas that can cause deafness, often accompanied by other intracranial/paraspinal neoplasms, such as meningiomas and gliomas. SYN elephant man disease (2).

neu•ro•fil•a•ment (nūr′ō-fil′ă-mĕnt) A class of intermediate filaments found in neurons.

neu•ro•gang•li•on (nūr′ō-gang′lē-ŏn) SYN ganglion (1).

neu•ro•gen•e•sis (nūr′ō-jen′ĕ-sis) Formation of the nervous system. [neuro- + G. *genesis,* production]

neu•ro•gen•ic, neu•ro•ge•net•ic (nūr′ō-jen′ik, -jĕ-net′ik) **1.** Originating in, starting from, or caused by, the nervous system or nerve impulses. SYN neurogenous. **2.** Relating to neurogenesis.

neu•ro•gen•ic blad•der (nūr′ō-jen′ik blad′ĕr) SYN neuropathic bladder.

neu•ro•gen•ic clau•di•ca•tion (nūr′ō-jen′ik klaw′di-kā′shŭn) Claudication with neurologic injury, usually in association with lumbar spinal stenosis.

neu•ro•gen•ic frac•ture (nūr′ō-jen′ik frak′shŭr) A break in a bone weakened by disease of its nerve supply.

neu•ro•gen•ic shock (nūr′ō-jen′ik shok) A rare, usually transitory shock caused by decreased sympathetic control of blood vessel tone due to a defect in the vasomotor center in the brainstem or the sympathetic outflow to the blood vessels; may be due to brain injury, depressant action of drugs, general anesthesia, hypoxia, or hypoclycemia (e.g., insulin shock).

neu•rog•e•nous (nūr-oj′ĕ-nŭs) SYN neurogenic (1).

i **neu•rog•li•a** (nūr-og′lē-ă) [TA] Nonneuronal cellular elements of the central and peripheral nervous system; thought to have important metabolic functions. In central nervous tissue they include oligodendroglia cells, astrocytes, ependymal cells, and microglia cells. See page 1065. SYN glia, reticulum (2). [neuro- + G. *glia,* glue]

neu•rog•li•a•cyte (nūr-og′lē-ă-sīt) A neuroglia cell. SEE neuroglia. [neuro- + G. *glia,* glue, + *kytos,* cell]

neu•rog•li•al, neu•rog•li•ar (nūr-og′lē-ăl, -ăr) Relating to neuroglia.

neu•rog•li•o•ma•to•sis (nūr-og′lē-ō-mă-tō′sis) SYN gliomatosis.

neu•ro•gram (nūr′ō-gram) The imprint on the brain substance theoretically remaining after every mental experience, i.e., the engram or physical register of the mental experience, stimulation of which retrieves and reproduces the original experience, thereby producing memory. [neuro- + G. *gramma,* something written]

neu•ro•his•tol•o•gy (nūr′ō-his-tol′ŏ-jē) Study of the microscopic anatomy of the nervous system.

neu•ro•hor•mone (nūr′ō-hōr′mōn) A hormone

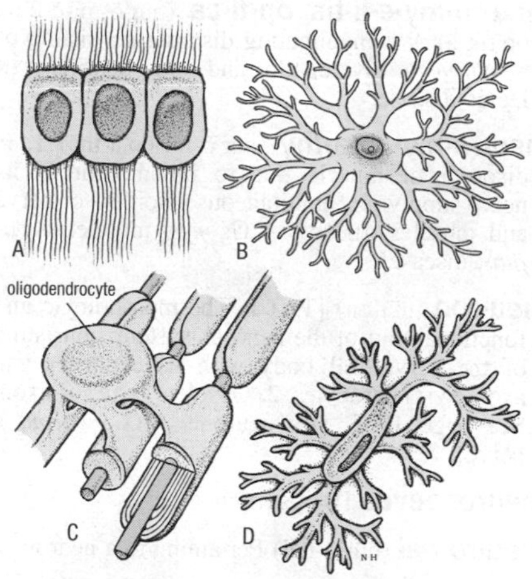

neuroglia: (A) ependymal cells, (B) astrocyte, (C) oligodendrocyte, (D) microglia

formed by neurosecretory cells and liberated by nerve impulses (e.g., norepinephrine).

neu·ro·hy·po·phys·i·al (nūr′ō-hī-pō-fiz′ē-ăl) Relating to the neurohypophysis.

neu·ro·hy·po·phys·i·al bud (nūr′ō-hī-pō-fiz′ē-ăl bŭd) SYN neurohypophysial diverticulum.

neu·ro·hy·po·phys·i·al di·ver·tic·u·lum (nūr′ō-hī-pō-fiz′ē-ăl dī′vĕr-tik′yū-lŭm) A downgrowth from the neuroectoderm of the diencephalon; it forms the neurohypophysis (nervous part of the pituitary gland). SYN infundibulum of diencephalon, neurohypophysial bud.

neu·ro·hy·poph·y·sis (nūr′ō-hī-pof′i-sis) [TA] A neuroendocrine structure suspended from the base of the hypothalamus. It is composed of the infundibulum and the posterior lobe of the hypophysis. SEE ALSO hypophysis. SYN lobus posterior hypophyseos [TA], posterior lobe of hypophysis. [neuro- + hypophysis]

neu·roid (nūr′oyd) Resembling a nerve; nervelike. [neuro- + G. *eidos,* resemblance]

neu·ro·lem·ma (nūr′ō-lem′ă) SYN neurilemma. [neuro- + G. *lemma,* husk]

neu·ro·lem·ma cells (nūr′ō-lem′ă selz) SYN Schwann cells.

neuroleptanaesthesia [Br.] SYN neuroleptanesthesia.

neu·ro·lept·an·al·ge·si·a (nūr′ō-lept-an-ăl-jē′zē-ă) An intense analgesic and amnesic state produced by administration of narcotic analgesics and neuroleptic drugs; unconsciousness may or may not occur, and cardiorespiratory function may be altered.

neu·ro·lept·an·es·the·si·a (nūr′ō-lept-an-es-thē′zē-ă) A technique of general anesthesia based on intravenous administration of neuroleptic drugs, together with inhalation of a weak anesthetic with or without neuromuscular relaxants. SYN neuroleptanaesthesia.

neu·ro·lep·tic (nūr′ō-lep′tik) **1.** Any of a class of psychotropic drugs used to treast psychosis, particularly schizophrenia; includes the phenothiazine, thioxanthene, and butyrophenone derivatives and the dihydroindolones. SYN neuroleptic agent. SEE ALSO antipsychotic agent. **2.** Denoting a condition similar to that produced by such an agent. [neuro- + G. *lēpsis,* taking hold]

neu·ro·lep·tic a·gent (nūr′ō-lep′tik ā′jĕnt) SYN neuroleptic (1).

neu·ro·lep·tic ma·lig·nant syn·drome (nūr′ō-lep′tik mă-lig′nănt sin′drōm) Hyperthermia with extrapyramidal and autonomic disturbances that may result in death, following the use of neuroleptic agents.

neu·ro·lin·guis·tic pro·gram·ming (nūr′ō-ling-gwis′tik prō′gram-ing) A branch of cognitive-behavioral psychology employing specific techniques, which use language to access the unconscious to change a client's internal states or external behaviors.

neu·ro·lin·guis·tics (nūr′ō-ling-gwis′tiks) Clinical science centered on human brain mechanisms underlying the comprehension, production, and abstract knowledge of language.

neu·ro·log·ic as·sess·ment (nūr′ō-loj′ik ă-ses′mĕnt) The appraisal of the nervous system by a health care provider.

neu·rol·o·gist (nūr-ol′ŏ-jist) A specialist in the diagnosis and treatment of disorders of the neuromuscular system: the central, peripheral, and autonomic nervous systems, the neuromuscular junction, and muscle.

neu·rol·o·gy (nūr-ol′ŏ-jē) The branch of medical science concerned with the various nervous systems (central, peripheral, and autonomic, plus the neuromuscular junction and muscle) and its disorders. [neuro- + G. *logos,* study]

neu·rol·y·sin (nūr-ol′i-sin) An antibody causing destruction of ganglion and cortical cells, obtained by the injection of brain substance. SYN neurotoxin (1).

neu·rol·y·sis (nūr-ol′i-sis) **1.** Destruction of nerve tissue. **2.** Freeing of a nerve from inflammatory adhesions. [neuro- + G. *lysis,* dissolution]

neu·ro·lyt·ic (nūr′ō-lit′ik) Relating to neurolysis.

neu·ro·ma (nūr-ō′mă) General term for any neoplasm derived from cells of the nervous system, e.g., ganglioneuroma, neurilemmoma (schwannoma), pseudoneuroma. [neuro- + G. *-oma,* tumor]

neu·ro·ma cu·tis (nūr-ō′mă kyū′tis) Neurofibroma of the skin.

neu·ro·ma·la·ci·a (nūr′ō-mă-lā′shē-ă) Pathologic softening of nervous tissue. [neuro- + G. *malakia,* softness]

neu·ro·ma tel·an·gi·ec·to·des (nūr-ō′mă tel-an′jē-ek-toyd′ēz) A neurofibroma with a conspicuous number of blood vessels, some of which have unusually large lumens (in proportion to the thickness of the walls).

neu·ro·ma·to·sis (nūr′ō-mă-tō′sis) The presence of multiple neuromas, as in neurofibromatosis.

neu·ro·mere (nūr′ō-mēr) Elevations in the wall of the developing neural tube, which divide the developing spinal cord into portions to which dorsal and ventral roots are attached. [neuro- + G. *meros,* part]

neu·ro·mus·cu·lar (nūr′ō-mŭs′kyū-lăr) Referring to the relationship between nerves and muscles, in particular to the motor innervation of skeletal muscles and its pathology (e.g., neuromuscular disorders). SEE ALSO myoneural.

neu·ro·mus·cu·lar block·ade (nūr′ō-mŭs′kyū-lăr blok-ād′) The blockage of transmission through the myoneural junction at nicotinic receptors, decreasing skeletal muscle tone and resulting in muscle weakness and/or paralysis.

neu·ro·mus·cu·lar block·ing a·gent (nūr′ō-mŭs′kyū-lăr blok′ing ā′jĕnt) A drug used to block neuromuscular transmission at the myoneural junction, which elicits paralysis of the affected skeletal muscles. This type of drug may also cause hypotension, flushing, tachycardia, and bronchospasms and should be used with caution in those with myasthenia gravis, in old and debilitated patients, and in those with renal, hepatic, and pulmonary disease.

neu·ro·mus·cu·lar spin·dle (nūr′ō-mŭs′kyū-lăr spin′dĕl) A fusiform end organ in skeletal muscle in which afferent and a few efferent nerve fibers terminate; this sensory end organ is particularly sensitive to passive stretch of the muscle in which it is enclosed. SYN muscle spindle.

neu·ro·mus·cu·lar ther·a·py (NMT) (nūr′ō-mŭs′kyū-lăr thār′ă-pē) Integrative system of bodywork designed to incorporate neurologic responses with myofascial tissue states; it addresses trigger points, hypertonicity in muscles, and postural compensation patterns to improve range of motion and reduce musculoskeletal pain and to restore balance between the nervous and musculoskeletal systems.

neu·ro·my·as·the·ni·a (nūr′ō-mī-as-thē′nē-ă) Obsolete term for muscular weakness due to a neurologic or psychological disorder. [neuro- + G. *mys,* muscle, + *a-* priv. + *sthenos,* strength]

neu·ro·my·e·li·tis (nūr′ō-mī-ĕ-lī′tis) Neuritis combined with spinal cord inflammation. SYN myeloneuritis. [neuro- + G. *myelos,* marrow, + *-itis,* inflammation]

neu·ro·my·e·li·tis op·ti·ca (nūr′ō-mī-ĕ-lī′tis op′tik-ă) A demyelinating disorder consisting of a transverse myelopathy and optic neuritis. SYN Devic disease.

neu·ro·my·op·a·thy (nūr′ō-mī-op′ă-thē) **1.** A disorder of muscle due to impairment of its nerve supply. **2.** Simultaneous disorders of nerve and muscles. [neuro- + G. *mys,* muscle, + *pathos,* disease]

neu·ron (nūr′on) [TA] **1.** The morphologic and functional unit of the nervous system, consisting of the nerve cell body with its dendrites and axon. SYN neurocyte. **2.** Obsolete term for axon. See page 1067. SYN neurone. [G. *neuron,* a nerve]

neuronaevus [Br.] SYN neuronevus.

neu·ro·nal (nūr′ō-năl) Pertaining to a neuron.

neurone [Br.] SYN neuron.

neu·ro·ne·vus (nūr′ō-nē′vŭs) A variety of intradermal nevus in adults in which nests of atrophic nevus cells in the lower dermis are hyalinized and resemble nerve bundles. SYN neuronaevus.

neu·ron·i·tis (nūr′ō-nī′tis) Inflammatory disorder of the neuron.

neu·ro·nop·a·thy (nūr-o-nop′ă-thē) Disorder, often toxic, of the neuron (1).

neu·ron·o·phage (nūr-on′ō-fāj) A phagocyte that ingests neuronal elements. SEE microglia. [neuron + G. *phagō,* to eat]

neu·ron·o·pha·gi·a, neu·ro·noph·a·gy (nūr-on′ō-fā′jē-ă, nūr′ō-nof′ă-jē) Phagocytosis of nerve cells. [neuron + G. *phagō,* to eat]

neu·ron-spe·ci·fic e·no·lase (nūr′on-spĕ-sif′ik ē′nō-lās) An isoenzyme of enolase present in neurons and glial cells; stains for this enzyme are frequently used in the differential diagnosis of neuronal or neuroendocrine tumors.

neu·ro·on·col·o·gy (nūr′ō-on-kol′ŏ-jē) The branch of medicine concerned with the direct and indirect effects of neoplasms on the nervous system, neuromuscular junction, and muscle. [neuro- + onco- + G. *logos,* study]

neu·ro·oph·thal·mol·o·gy (nūr′ō-of-thal-mol′ŏ-jē) That branch of medicine concerned with the neurologic aspects of the visual apparatus.

neu·ro·o·tol·o·gy (nūr′ō-ō-tol′ŏ-jē) The branch of medicine concerned with the nervous system related to the auditory and vestibular systems.

neu·ro·pa·ral·y·sis (nūr′ō-pă-ral′i-sis) Paralysis resulting from disease of the nerve supplying the affected part.

neu·ro·par·a·lyt·ic (nūr′ō-par-ă-lit′ik) Denoting or characterized by neuroparalysis.

neu•ro•par•a•lyt•ic ker•a•ti•tis (nūr′ō-par-ă-lit′ik ker′ă-tī′tis) SYN neurotrophic keratitis.

neu•ro•par•a•lyt•ic ker•a•top•a•thy (nūr′ō-par-ă-lit′ik ker′ă-top′ă-thē) Corneal inflammation or ulceration associated with dysfunction of the ophthalmic branch of the trigeminal nerve.

neu•ro•path•i•a (nūr′ō-pāth′ē-ă) SYN neuropathy.

neu•ro•path•ic (nūr′ō-path′ik) Relating in any way to neuropathy.

neu•ro•path•ic ar•throp•a•thy (nūr′ō-path′ik ahr-throp′ă-thē) SYN neuropathic joint.

neu•ro•path•ic blad•der (nūr′ō-path′ik blad′ĕr) Any defective functioning of bladder due to impaired innervation. SYN neurogenic bladder.

neu•ro•path•ic joint (nūr′ō-path′ik joynt) Joint disease caused by diminished proprioceptive sensation, with gradual destruction of the joint by repeated subliminal injury, commonly associated with tabes dorsalis or diabetic neuropathy. SYN Charcot joint, neuropathic arthropathy.

neu•ro•path•o•gen•e•sis (nūr′ō-path-ō-jen′ĕ-sis) The origin or causation of a disease of the nervous system. [neuro- + G. *pathos,* suffering, + *genesis,* origin]

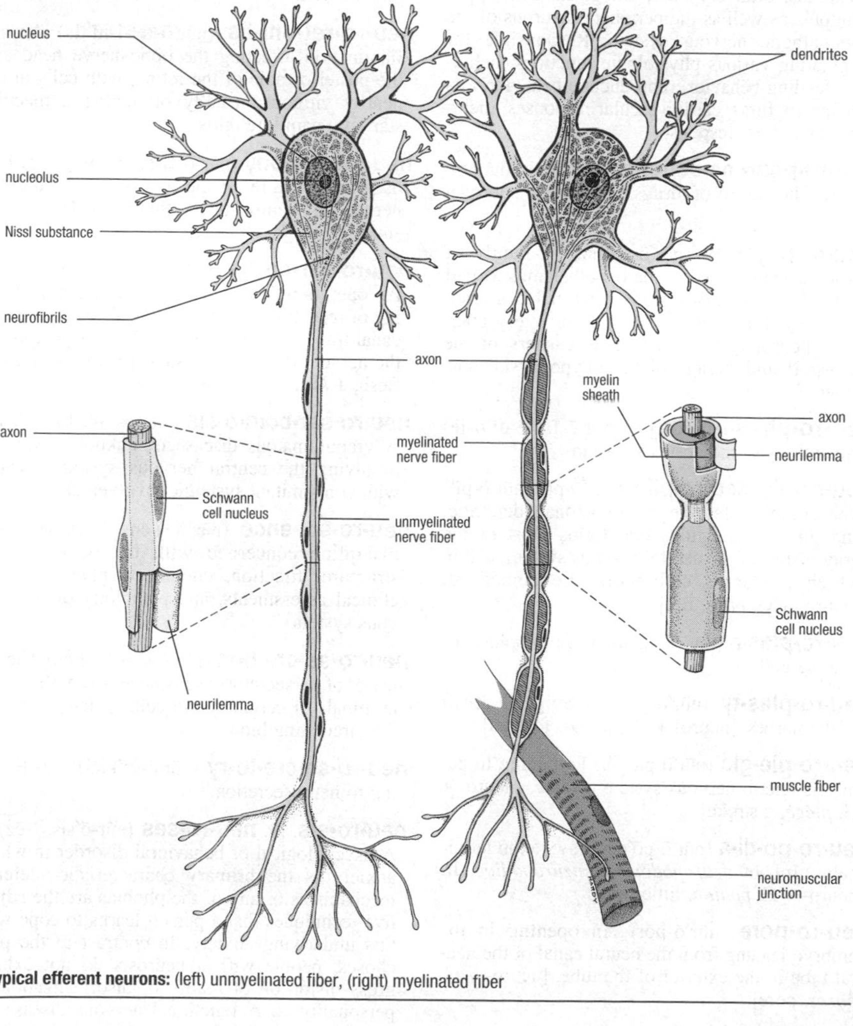

typical efferent neurons: (left) unmyelinated fiber, (right) myelinated fiber

neu•ro•pa•thol•o•gy (nūr′ō-pă-thol′ŏ-jē) **1.** Disease state involving the nervous system. **2.** That branch of pathology concerned with the nervous system.

neu•rop•a•thy (nūr-op′ă-thē) **1.** Any disorder affecting the nervous system. **2.** In contemporary usage, a disease involving the cranial nerves, or the peripheral or autonomic nervous systems. SYN neuritis (2), neuropathia. [neuro- + G. *pathos,* suffering]

neu•ro•pep•tide (nūr′ō-pep′tīd) Any of a variety of peptides found in neural tissue; e.g., endorphins, enkephalins. Cf. bioregulator.

neu•ro•pep•tide Y (NPY) (nū′rō-pep′tīd) A 36-amino acid peptide expressed in most regions of the CNS including the cortex, hypothalamus, thalamus, olfactory bulb, amygdala, and hippocampus, as well as the peripheral neurons of the sympathetic nervous system. Responsible for regulating various physiologic functions including feeding behavior, reproductive behavior, circadian rhythms, cardiovascular responses, memory, and stress response.

neu•ro•phar•ma•col•o•gy (nūr′ō-fahr′mă-kol′ŏ-jē) The study of drugs that affect neuronal tissue.

neu•ro•phys•ins (nūr′ō-fiz′inz) A family of proteins synthesized in the hypothalamus as part of the large precursor protein that includes vasopressin and oxytocin in the neurosecretory granules; neurophysins function as carriers in the transport and storage of neurohypophysial hormones.

neu•ro•phys•i•ol•o•gy (nūr′ō-fiz-ē-ol′ŏ-jē) Physiology of the nervous system.

neu•ro•pil, **neu•ro•pile** (nūr′ō-pil, nūr′ō-pīl) The complex, feltlike net of axonal, dendritic, and glial arborizations that forms most of the gray matter of the central nervous system, and in which the nerve cell bodies lie embedded. [neuro- + G. *pilos,* felt]

neu•ro•plasm (nūr′ō-plazm) The protoplasm of a nerve cell.

neu•ro•plas•ty (nūr′ō-plas-tē) Surgical repair of the nerves. [neuro- + G. *plastos,* formed]

neu•ro•ple•gic (nūr′ō-plē′jik) Pertaining to paralysis due to nervous system disease. [neuro- + G. *plēgē,* a stroke]

neu•ro•po•di•a (nūr′ō-pō′dē-ă) SYN axon terminals. [pl. of *neuropodium* or *neuropodion,* fr. neuro- + G. *podion,* little foot]

neu•ro•pore (nūr′ō-pōr) An opening in the embryo leading from the neural canal of the neural tube to the exterior of the tube. [neuro- + G. *poros,* pore]

neu•ro•psy•chi•a•try (nūr′ō-sī-kī′ă-trē) The specialty dealing with both organic and psychic disorders of the nervous system.

neu•ro•psy•cho•log•ical dis•or•der (nū′rō-sī-kŏ-loj′ik-ăl dis-ōr′dĕr) A disturbance of mental function due to brain trauma, associated with one of more of the following: neurocognitive, psychotic, neurotic, behavioral, or psychophysiologic manifestations, or mental impairment. SEE ALSO mental illness.

neu•ro•psy•chop•a•thy (nūr′ō-sī-kop′ă-thē) An emotional illness of neurologic and/or functional origin.

neu•ro•ra•di•ol•o•gy (nūr′rō-rā-dē-ol′ŏ-jē) The clinical subspecialty concerned with the diagnostic radiology of diseases of the central nervous system, head, and neck.

neu•ro•reg•u•la•tor (nūr′ō-reg′yū-lā-tŏr) A chemical factor that exerts a modulatory effect on a neuron.

neu•ro•ret•i•ni•tis (nūr′ō-ret-i-nī′tis) An inflammation affecting the optic nerve head and the posterior pole of the retina, with cells in the nearby vitreous, usually producing a macular star. SYN papilloretinitis.

neu•ror•rha•phy (nūr-ōr′ă-fē) Joining together, usually by suture, of the two parts of a divided nerve. SYN neurosuture. [neuro- + G. *rhaphē,* suture]

neu•ro•sar•co•clei•sis (nūr′ō-sahr-kō-klī′sis) An operation for the relief of neuralgia, consisting of resection of one of the walls of an osseous canal traversed by the nerve and transposition of the nerve into the soft tissues. [neuro- + G. *sarx,* flesh, + *kleisis,* closure]

neu•ro•sar•coid•o•sis (nūr′ō-sahr-koy-dō′sis) A granulomatous disease of unknown etiology involving the central nervous system, usually with concomitant systemic involvement.

neu•ro•sci•ence (nūr′ō-sī′ĕns) The scientific discipline concerned with the development, structure, function, chemistry, pharmacology, clinical assessments, and pathology of the nervous system.

neu•ro•se•cre•tion (nūr′ō-sĕ-krē′shŭn) The release of a secretory substance from the axon terminals of certain nerve cells in the brain into the circulating blood.

neu•ro•se•cre•to•ry (nūr′ō-sē′krĕ-tōr-ē) Relating to neurosecretion.

neu•ro•sis, pl. **neu•ro•ses** (nūr-ō′sis, -sēz) **1.** A psychological or behavioral disorder in which anxiety is the primary characteristic; defense mechanisms or any of the phobias are the adjustive techniques that a person learns to cope with this underlying anxiety. In contrast to the psychoses, people with a neurosis do not exhibit gross distortion of reality or disorganization of personality. **2.** A functional nervous disease, or one for which there is no evident lesion. **3.** A peculiar state of tension or irritability of the nervous system; any form of nervousness. SYN neurotic disorder, psychoneurosis. [neuro- + G. *-osis,* condition]

neu•ro•splanch•nic (nūr′ō-splangk′nik) SYN neurovisceral. [neuro- + G. *splanchnon,* a viscus]

Neu•ros•po•ra (nūr′ō-spōr′ă) A genus of fungi grown in cultures and used in research in genetics and cellular biochemistry. [neuro- + G. *spora,* seed]

neu•ro•sur•geon (nūr′ō-sŭr′jŭn) A surgeon specializing in operations on the nervous system.

neu•ro•sur•ger•y (nūr′ō-sŭr′jĕr-ē) Surgery of the nervous system.

neu•ro•su•ture (nūr′ō-sū′chūr) SYN neurorrhaphy.

neu•ro•syph•i•lis (nūr′ō-sif′i-lis) Infection of the central nervous system by *Treponema pallidum.*

neu•ro•ten•di•nous (nūr′ō-ten′di-nŭs) Relating to both nerves and tendons.

neu•ro•ten•di•nous spin•dle (nūr′ō-ten′di-nŭs spin′dĕl) SYN Golgi tendon organ.

neu•ro•ten•sin (nū′rō-ten′sin) A 13-amino acid peptide neurotransmitter found in synapsomes in the hypothalamus, amygdala, basal ganglia, and dorsal gray matter of the spinal cord.

neu•ro•the•ke•o•ma (nūr′ō-thē-kē-ō′mă) A benign myxoma of cutaneous nerve sheath origin. [neuro- + G. *thēkē,* box, sheath, + *-oma,* tumor]

neu•rot•ic (nūr-ot′ik) Relating to or suffering from a neurosis. SEE neurosis.

neu•rot•ic dis•or•der (nūr-ot′ik dis-ōr′dĕr) SYN neurosis.

neu•rot•i•za•tion (nūr′ō-tī-zā′shŭn) The acquisition of nervous substance; the regeneration of a nerve.

neu•rot•me•sis (nūr′ot-mē′sis) A type of axon loss lesion resulting from focal peripheral nerve injury in which, at the lesion site, the nerve stroma is damaged to varying degrees, as well as the axon and myelin, which degenerate from that point distally. SEE axonotmesis, neurapraxia. [neuro- + G. *tmēsis,* a cutting]

neu•rot•o•my (nūr-ot′ŏ-mē) Operative division of a nerve. [neuro- + G. *tomē,* a cutting]

neu•ro•ton•ic (nūr′ō-ton′ik) **1.** Strengthening or stimulating impaired nervous action. **2.** An agent that improves the tone or force of the nervous system.

neu•ro•tox•ic (nūr′ō-tok′sik) Poisonous to nervous substance.

neu•ro•tox•in (nūr′ō-tok′sin) **1.** SYN neurolysin. **2.** Any toxin that acts specifically on nervous tissue.

neu•ro•trans•mit•ter (nūr′ō-trans′mit-ĕr) Any specific chemical agent released by a presynaptic cell, on excitation, which crosses the synapse to stimulate or inhibit the postsynaptic cell. [neuro- + L. *transmitto,* to send across]

neu•ro•trip•sy (nūr′ō-trip′sē) Operative crushing of a nerve. [neuro- + G. *tripsis,* a rubbing]

neu•ro•tro•phic (nūr′ō-trō′fik) Relating to neurotrophy.

neu•ro•tro•phic ker•a•ti•tis (nūr′ō-trō′fik ker′ă-tī′tis) Inflammation or decreased corneal sensation of the cornea after corneal anesthesia. SYN neuroparalytic keratitis.

neu•rot•ro•phy (nū-rot′rŏ-fē) Nutrition and metabolism of tissues under nervous influence. [neuro- + G. *trophē,* nourishment]

neu•ro•tro•pic (nūr′ō-trō′pik) Having an affinity for the nervous system.

neu•rot•ro•py, neu•rot•ro•pism (nū-rot′rŏ-pē, -pizm) **1.** Affinity of basic dyes for nervous tissue. **2.** The attraction of certain pathogenic microorganisms, poisons, and nutritive substances toward the nerve centers. [neuro- + G. *tropē,* a turning]

neu•ro•tu•bule (nūr′ō-tūb′yūl) One of the microtubules, 10–20 nm in diameter, occurring in the cell body, dendrites, axon, and in some synaptic endings of neurons.

neu•ro•vac•cine (nūr′ō-vak-sēn′) A fixed or standardized vaccine virus of definite strength, obtained by continued passage through the brains of rabbits.

neu•ro•vas•cu•lar (nūr′ō-vas′kyū-lăr) Relating to both nervous and vascular systems; relating to the nerves supplying the walls of the blood vessels, the vasomotor nerves.

neu•ro•vas•cu•lar bun•dle of Walsh (nūr′ō-vas′kyū-lăr bŭn′dĕl wawsh) The anatomic structure composed of capsular arteries and veins to the prostate and cavernous nerves that provides the macroscopic landmark used during nerve-sparing radical pelvic surgery.

neu•ro•vi•rus (nūr′ō-vī′rŭs) Vaccine virus modified by means of passage into and growth in nervous tissue.

neu•ro•vis•cer•al (nūr′ō-vis′ĕr-ăl) Referring to the innervation of the internal organs by the autonomic nervous system. SYN neurosplanchnic. [neuro- + L. *viscera,* the internal organs]

neu•ru•la, pl. **neu•ru•lae** (nūr′yū-lă, -lē) Stage in embryonic development during which the neural plate forms and closes to form the neural tube. [neur- + L. *-ulus,* small one]

neu•ru•la•tion (nūr′yū-lā′shŭn) Formation of the neural plate and closure of the neural folds to form the neural tube. SEE neurula.

Neus•ser gran•ule (noy′sĕr gran′yūl) A tiny basophilic granule sometimes observed in groups forming an indistinct zone about the nucleus of a leukocyte.

neu•ter (nū′tĕr) To sterilize a male or female animal surgically. [L. neither, i.e., neither male nor female]

neu•tral (nū′trăl) **1.** Exhibiting no positive properties; indifferent. **2.** CHEMISTRY neither acid nor alkaline. [L. *neutralis,* fr. *neuter,* neither]

neu•tral fat (nū′trăl fat) Common fats of animals and plant tissues that are compounds of the higher fatty acids such as palmitic, stearic, and oleic acids with glycerol.

neutralisation [Br.] SYN neutralization.

neu•tral•i•za•tion (nū′trăl-ī-zā′shŭn) **1.** The change in reaction of a solution from acid or alkaline to neutral by the addition of just a sufficient amount of an alkaline or an acid substance, respectively. **2.** The rendering ineffective of any action, process, or potential. SYN neutralisation.

neu•tral•i•za•tion plate (nū′trăl-ī-zā′shŭn plāt) A metal plate used for the internal fixation of a long bone fracture to neutralize the forces producing displacement.

neu•tral•i•za•tion test (nū′trăl-ī-zā′shŭn test) SYN protection test.

neu•tra•liz•ing an•ti•bod•y (nū′trăl-ī-zing an′ti-bod-ē) A form of antibody that reacts with an infectious agent (usually a virus) and destroys or inhibits its infectivity and virulence.

neu•tral mu•ta•tion (nū′trăl myū-tā′shŭn) A mutation with a negligible impact on genetic fitness.

neu•tral oc•clu•sion (nū′trăl ŏ-klū′zhŭn) **1.** An arrangement of teeth such that the maxillary and mandibular first permanent molars are in normal anteroposterior relation. SYN normal occlusion (2). **2.** SYN neutroclusion.

neu•tral stain (nū′trăl stān) A compound of an acid stain and a basic stain, such as the eosinate of methylene blue, in which the anion and cation each contains a chromophore group.

♻ **neutro-, neutr-** Combining forms meaning neutral. [L. *neutralis,* fr. *neuter,* neither]

neu•tro•clu•sion (nū′trō-klū′zhŭn) Malocclusion in which there is a normal anteroposterior relationship between the maxilla and mandible; in Angle classification, a class I malocclusion. SYN neutral occlusion (2). [neutro- + occlusion]

neu•tron (nū′tron) An electrically neutral particle in the nuclei of all atoms (except hydrogen-1) with a mass slightly larger than that of a proton; in isolation, it breaks down to a proton and an electron with a half-life of about 10.3 minutes. [L. *neuter,* neither]

neu•tro•pe•ni•a (nū′trō-pē′nē-ă) Condition that occurs when neutrophil counts fall below the normal percentage in circulating blood. [neutrophil + G. *penia,* poverty]

neu•tro•phil, neu•tro•phile (nū′trō-fil, -fīl) **1.** A mature white blood cell in the granulocytic series, formed by bone marrow and released into the circulating blood, where neutrophils normally represent from 54 to 65% of the total number of leukocytes in a differential. When stained, neutrophils are characterized by: 1) a nucleus that is dark purple-blue and lobated; 2) a cytoplasm that is faintly pink and contains numerous fine pink or violet-pink granules. The precursors of neutrophils in order of increasing maturity, are: myeloblasts, promyelocytes, myelocytes, metamyelocytes, and band forms. SEE ALSO leukocyte, leukocytosis. **2.** Any cell or tissue that manifests no special affinity for acid or basic dyes, i.e., the cytoplasm stains approximately equally with either type of dye. See page B2. [neutro- + G. *philos,* fond]

neu•tro•phil-ac•ti•vat•ing fac•tor (nū′trō-fil-ak′ti-vāt-ing fak′tŏr) SYN interleukin-8.

neu•tro•phil-ac•ti•vat•ing pro•tein (nū′trō-fil-ak′ti-vāt-ing prō′tēn) Older term for interleukin-8.

neu•tro•phil•i•a (nū′trō-fil′ē-ă) An increase of neutrophils in blood or tissues.

neu•tro•phil•ic (nū′trō-fil′ik) **1.** Pertaining to or characterized by neutrophils, such as an exudate in which the predominant cells are neutrophilic granulocytes. **2.** Characterized by a lack of affinity for acid or basic dyes, i.e., staining approximately equally with either type.

neu•tro•phil•ic leu•ko•cyte (nū′trō-fil′ik lū′kō-sīt) A neutrophilic granulocyte, the most frequent of the polymorphonuclear leukocytes, and also the most active phagocyte among the various types of white blood cells; when treated with Wright stain the fairly abundant cytoplasm is faintly pink, and numerous tiny pink or violet-pink granules are recognizable in the cytoplasm; the deeply stained blue nucleus is sharply distinguished from the cytoplasm and is distinctly lobated, with thin strands of chromatin connecting the three to five lobes.

neu•tro•tax•is (nū′trō-tak′sis) A phenomenon in which neutrophilic leukocytes are stimulated by a substance in such a manner that they are either attracted and move toward it (positive neutrotaxis), or they are repelled and move away from it (negative neutrotaxis). [neutrophil + G. *taxis,* arrangement]

ne•vi (nē′vī) Plural of nevus. SYN naevi. [L.]

ne•void (nē′voyd) Resembling a nevus. SYN naevoid, nevose (2), nevous. [L. *naevus,* mole (nevus), + G. *eidos,* resemblance]

ne•vose, ne•vous (nē′vōs, -vŭs) **1.** Marked with nevi. **2.** SYN nevoid. SYN naevose.

ne•vus, pl. **ne•vi** (nē′vŭs, -vī) **1.** A circumscribed malformation of the skin, especially one that is colored by hyperpigmentation or increased vascularity; a nevus may be predominantly epidermal, adnexal, melanocytic, vascular, or mesodermal, or a compound overgrowth of these tissues. **2.** A benign localized overgrowth of melanin-forming cells of the skin at birth or appearing early in life. SYN mole (1). See this page. SYN naevus. [L. *naevus,* mole, birthmark]

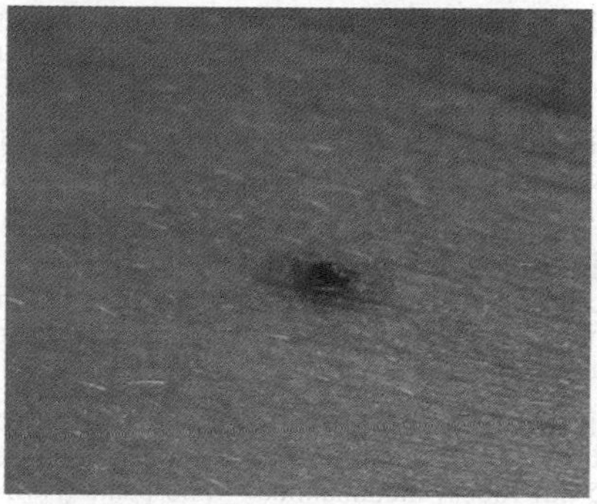

nevus

ne•vus cell (nē′vŭs sel) The cell of a pigmented cutaneous nevus that differs from a normal melanocyte in that it lacks dendrites. SYN naevus cell.

ne•vus co•me•do•ni•cus, com•e•do ne•vus (nē′vŭs kom′e-dō-nik′us, kom′ĕ-dō nē′vŭs) Congenital or childhood linear keratinous cystic invaginations of the epidermis, with failure of development of normal pilosebaceous follicles. SYN naevus comedonicus.

ne•vus flam•me•us (nē′vŭs flam′ē-ŭs) A large congenital vascular nevus having a purplish color; it is usually found on the head and neck and persists throughout life. SYN naevus flammeus, port-wine mark, port-wine stain.

ne•vus pig•men•to•sus (nē′vŭs pig-men-tō′sus) A benign pigmented melanocytic proliferation; raised or level with the skin, present at birth or arising early in life. SYN mole (2), naevus pigmentosus.

ne•vus pi•lo•sus (nē′vŭs pī-lō′sŭs) A mole covered with an abundant growth of hair. SYN hairy mole, naevus pilosus.

ne•vus spi•lus (nē′vŭs spī′lŭs) A form of (flat) nevus pigmentosus. SYN naevus spilus.

ne•vus u•ni•us la•te•ris (nē′vŭs ūn′ē-ŭs lat′ĕr-is) A congenital systematized linear nevus limited to one side of the body or to portions of the limbs on one side; lesions are often extensive, forming wavelike bands on the trunk and spiraling streaks on the limbs. SYN naevus unius lateris.

ne•vus vas•cu•la•ris, ne•vus vas•cu•lo•sus (nē′vŭs vas-kū-lā′ris, vas-kū-lō′sus) SYN capillary hemangioma. SYN naevus vascularis.

new•born (nū′bōrn) SYN neonatal, neonate.

New•cas•tle dis•ease (nū′kas-ĕl di-zēz′) Conjunctivitis, eyelid edema, and inflammation caused by infection with an avian virus; recovery is usually spontaneous and takes 10–14 days.

New•com•er fix•a•tive (nū′kŏm-ĕr fiks′ă-tiv) A fixative containing isopropanol, propionic acid, and dioxane, recommended as a substitute for Carnoy fixative in preservation of chromatin; also useful for fixing polysaccharides; small pieces of tissue must be used, although excessive shrinkage may still occur.

New Hamp•shire rule (nū-hamp′shĕr rūl) Pioneering American test of criminal responsibility (1871): "if the [criminal] act was the offspring of insanity, a criminal intent did not produce it."

new pa•tient (nū pā′shĕnt) A patient who has either never been seen or has not been seen by a given physician in the past 3 years or any physician of the same specialty within such group.

new•ton (nū′tŏn) Derived unit of force in the SI system, expressed as meters-kilograms per second squared ($m{\cdot}kg{\cdot}s^{-2}$); equivalent to 10^5 dynes in the CGS system. [I. *Newton*]

New•ton disc (nū′tŏn disk) A disc on which are seven colored sectors, each occupying proportionally the same space as the corresponding primary color in the spectrum; when the disc is rapidly rotated it appears white. [Isaac Newton, 1643–1727, English physicist]

new•to•ni•an con•stant of grav•i•ta•tion (G) (nū-tō′nē-ăn kon′stănt grav-i-tā′shŭn) A universal constant relating the gravitational force, f, attracting two masses, m_1 and m_2, toward each other when they are separated by a distance, r, in the equation: $f = G(m_1m_2/r^2)$; it has the value of 6.67259×10^{-8} dyne cm^2 g^{-2} = 6.67259×10^{-11} m^3 kg^{-1} s^{-2} in SI units.

New•ton law (nū′tŏn law) The attractive force between any two bodies is proportional to the product of their masses, and inversely proportional to the square of the distance between their centers.

new•ton-me•ter (nū′tŏn-mē′tĕr) A unit of the MKS system, expressed as energy expended, or work done, by a force of 1 newton acting through a distance of 1 meter; equal to 1 joule = 10^7 ergs.

New World leish•man•i•a•sis (nū-wŏrld lēsh′mă-nī′ă-sis) SYN mucocutaneous leishmaniasis.

New York Heart As•so•ci•a•tion clas•si•fi•ca•tion (nū-yōrk hahrt ă-sō′sē-ā′shŭn klas′i-fi-kā′shŭn) A functional classification to assess cardiovascular disability. Class I: cardiac disease without limitation of physical activity. Ordinary activity does not cause symptoms. Class II: cardiac disease with slight limitation of activity; comfortable at rest. Ordinary physical activity results in fatigue, palpitations, dyspnea or angina. Class III: cardiac disease producing marked limitation of activity: comfortable at rest. Less than ordinary physical activity causes symptoms. Class IV: cardiac disease resulting in inability to carry on any physical activity without discomfort. Symptoms may be present even at rest.

New York vi•rus (nū yŏrk vī′rŭs) A species of hantavirus in the United States causing hantavirus pulmonary syndrome.

nex•ins (neks′inz) Proteins that bridge adjacent microtubule doublets of the axoneme of cilia and flagella. [L. *nexus,* a binding, fr. *necto,* to bind + -in]

nex•us, pl. **nex•us** (neks′ŭs) SYN gap junction. [L. interconnection]

Ney•man-Pear•son test (nē′măn-pēr′sŏn test) A statistical procedure that assigns different weights to a false-positive result and a false-negative result in an experimental study so as to maximize the power of the study.

NFPA sym•bol (sim′bŏl) The National Fire Protection Agency (NFPA) label displays warnings for firefighters of the location of hazardous materials in the event of a fire. It includes a diamond-shaped symbol with four quadrants that indicate the relative danger level in four different areas: health (blue), fire (red), chemical stability (yellow), and other specific hazard types.

ng Abbreviation for nanogram.

NGF Abbreviation for nerve growth factor.

NG tube (tūb) SYN nasogastric tube.

Ni Symbol for nickel.

ni•a•cin (nī′ă-sin) SYN nicotinic acid.

ni•a•cin•a•mide (nī′ă-sin′ă-mīd) SYN nicotinamide.

Ni•ag•ar•a blue (nī-ag′ăr-ă blū) SYN Congo blue.

nib (nib) DENTISTRY the portion of a condensing instrument that comes into contact with the restorative material being condensed.

NIC (nik) Acronym for Nursing Interventions Classification.

niche (nich, nēsh) **1.** RADIOGRAPHY an eroded or ulcerated area, especially gastrointestinal or vascular, which can be detected when it fills with contrast medium. **2.** An ecologic term for the position occupied by a species in a biotic community, particularly its relationships to various other competitor, predator, prey, and parasite species. [Fr.]

nick•el (Ni) (nik′ĕl) A metallic bioelement; atomic no. 28, atomic wt. 58.6934; closely resembles cobalt and often associated with it. Protects ribosome structure against heat denaturation. A deficiency of nickel causes changes in the ultrastructure of the liver. [abbrev. fr. Ger. *kupfer-nickel,* name of copper-colored ore from which nickel was first obtained; *nickel,* the Ger. word for a dwarfish imp]

nick•ing (nik′ing) Localized constrictions in retinal blood vessels, seen at arteriovenous crossings; usually due to chronic hypertension.

Nick pro•ce•dure (nik prŏ-sē′jŭr) Enlarges the aortic anulus by incising the noncoronary sinus and the roof of the left atrium.

Ni•colle stain for cap•sules (nē-kōl′ stān kap′sūlz) Stain in a mixture of a saturated solution of gentian violet in alcohol-phenol.

nic•o•tin•a•mide (nik′ō-tin′ă-mīd) The biologically active amide of nicotinic acid, used in the prevention and treatment of pellagra. SYN niacinamide.

nic•o•tin•a•mide ad•e•nine di•nu•cle•o•tide (NAD) (nik′ō-tin′ă-mīd ad′ĕ-nēn dī-nū′klē-ō-tīd) Ribosylnicotinamide 5′-phosphate (NMN) and adenosine 5′-phosphate (AMP) linked by the two phosphoric groups; binds as a coenzyme to proteins, serves in respiratory metabolism (hydrogen acceptor and donor). See also entries under NAD and NADP. SYN diphosphopyridine nucleotide.

nic•o•tin•a•mide ad•e•nine di•nu•cle•o•tide phos•phate (NADP) (nik′ō-tin′ă-mīd ad′ĕ-nēn dī-nū′klē-ō-tīd fos′fāt) A coenzyme of many oxidases (dehydrogenases), in which the reaction $NADP^+ + 2H \rightarrow NADPH + H^+$ takes place; the third phosphoric group esterifies the 2′-hydroxyl of the adenosine moiety of NAD.

nic•o•tin•a•mide mon•o•nu•cle•o•tide (NMN) (nik′ō-tin′ă-mīd mon′ō-nū′klē-ō-tīd) A condensation product of nicotinamide and ribose 5-phosphate, a precursor in the synthesis of NAD^+.

nic•o•tine (nik′ō-tēn′) A poisonous volatile alkaloid derived from tobacco (*Nicotiana* spp.) and responsible for many of the effects of tobacco; it first stimulates (small doses), then depresses (large doses) at autonomic ganglia and myoneural junctions. It is an important tool in physiologic and pharmacologic investigation; also used as an insecticide and fumigant.

nic•o•tin•ic (nik′ō-tin′ik) Relating to the stimulating action of acetylcholine and other nicotine-like agents on autonomic ganglia, medulla of suprarenal gland, and the motor end plate of striated muscle.

nic•o•tin•ic ac•id (nik′ō-tin′ik as′id) A part of the vitamin B3 complex; used in the prevention and treatment of pellagra, as a vasodilator, and as an HDL-raising agent; taken by some people in erroneous idea it will hide drug use in urine tests; such use can elicit GI complaints, dizziness, and loss of consciousness. SYN niacin.

nic•ti•ta•tion (nik′ti-tā′shŭn) Winking. [L. *nicto,* pp. *-atus,* to wink, fr. *nico,* to beckon]

NICU Abbreviation for neonatal intensive care unit.

ni•dal (nī′dăl) Relating to a nidus, or nest.

ni•da•tion (nī-dā′shŭn) Embedding of the blastocyst in the uterine endometrium. [L. *nidus,* nest]

ni•dus, pl. **ni•di** (nī′dŭs, -dī) **1.** A nest. **2.** The nucleus or central point of origin of a nerve. **3.** A focus of infection. **4.** The coalescence of molecules or small particles that is the beginning of a crystal or similar solid deposit. **5.** The focus of reduced density at the center of an osteoid osteoma, on bone radiographs. [L. nest]

ni•dus a•vis (nī′dŭs ā′vis) A deep depression on each side of the inferior surface of the cerebellum, between the uvula and the biventral lobe, in which the tonsil rests. [L. bird's nest]

Nie•mann-Pick C1 dis•ease (NPC) (nē′mahn-pik′ di-zēz′) Rare inherited lipid storage disorder, affecting viscera and the central nervous system, inherited as an autosomal recessive. There are two types of this disease, with the same clinical manifestations and biochemical abnormalities, resulting from abnormalities in two separate genes: NPC-1, the major locus, and NPC-2, the minor locus; the two types have identical clinical and biochemical phenotypes. Cells from NPC patients are defective in the esterification and release of cholesterol from lysosomes; lysosomal sequestration of LDL-derived cholesterol, including delayed downregulation of LDL uptake and de novo synthesis, occur.

Nie•mann-Pick cell (nē′mahn pik sel) SYN Pick cell.

Nie•mann sple•no•meg•a•ly (nē′mahn splē′nō-meg′ăl-ē) Enlargement of spleen occurring in Niemann-Pick disease.

night blind•ness (nīt blīnd′nĕs) SYN nyctalopia.

night guard (nīt gahrd) A removable acrylic appliance intended to relieve temporomandibular joint pain and other effects of grinding the teeth (bruxism). Usually worn at night to prevent grinding during sleep. SYN occlusal guard.

night•mare (nīt′mār) A terrifying dream, as in which one is unable to cry for help or to escape from a seemingly impending evil. SYN incubus (2). [*A.S. nyht,* night, + *mara,* a demon]

night•shade (nīt′shād) Any of various plants of the genus *Solanum* or *Atropa*, many of which have medicinal or toxic properties.

night soil (nīt soyl) Human feces used for fertilizer.

night•stick frac•ture (nīt′stik frak′shŭr) Breakage of the ulna due to a direct blow.

night sweats (nīt swets) Excessive perspiration at night, which can be a sign of lymphoma or tuberculosis.

night ter•rors (nīt tār′ŏrz) A disorder allied to nightmare, occurring in children, in which the child awakes screaming with fright, the distress persisting for a time during a state of semiconsciousness. SYN pavor nocturnus.

night vi•sion (nīt vizh′ŭn) SYN scotopic vision.

ni•gra (nī′gră) NEUROANATOMY the substantia nigra. [L. fr. *niger,* black]

ni•gri•ti•es (nī-grish′ē-ēz) A black pigmentation. [L. blackness, fr. *niger,* black]

ni•gro•sin, ni•gro•sine (nī′grō-sin, nī′grō-sēn) [CI 50420] A mixture of blue-black aniline dyes used as a histologic stain for nervous tissue and as a negative stain for studying bacteria and spirochetes; also used to discriminate between live and dead cells in dye-exclusion staining.

ni•gro•stri•a•tal (nī′grō-strī-ā′tăl) Referring to the efferent connection of the substantia nigra with the striatum. SEE substantia nigra.

NIH Abbreviation for U.S. National Institutes of Health (an agency or operating division of the U.S. Public Health Service).

ni•hil•ism (nī′i-lizm) **1.** PSYCHIATRY the delusion of the nonexistence of everything, especially of the self or part of the self. **2.** Engagement in acts that are totally destructive to one's own purposes and those of one's group. [L. *nihil,* nothing]

Ni•ki•fo•roff meth•od (nē-kē′fōr′of meth′ŏd) The fixing of blood films by immersion for 5–15 minutes in absolute alcohol, a mixture of equal parts of alcohol and ether, or pure ether.

Ni•kol•sky sign (ni-kol′skē sīn) A peculiar vulnerability of the skin in pemphigus vulgaris; the apparently normal epidermis can be separated at the basal layer and rubbed off when pressed with a sliding motion.

nil or•al•ly (nil ōr′ă-lē) Patient is not permitted to have anything by mouth.

nil per os (NPO, n.p.o.) (nil per os) [L.] Latin for nothing by mouth; instruction often included in dietary orders for patients scheduled for surgery.

NIMS Abbreviation for National Incident Management System.

nin•hy•drin (nin-hī′drin) Triketohydrindene, an analytic reagent that reacts with free amino acids to yield CO_2, NH_3, and an aldehyde, the NH_3 produced yielding a colored product. SEE ALSO ninhydrin reaction. [Ger. trade name, fr. the chemical name]

nin•hy•drin re•ac•tion (nin-hī′drin rē-ak′shŭn) A procedure for proteins, peptones, peptides, and amino acids possessing free carboxyl and α-amino groups that is based on the reaction with triketohydrinene hydrate; a blue color reaction is used to quantitate free amino acids.

ninth cra•ni•al nerve [CN IX] (nīnth krā′nē-ăl nĕrv) SYN glossopharyngeal nerve [CN IX].

ni•o•bi•um (Nb) (nī-ō′bē-ŭm) A rare metallic element; atomic no. 41, atomic wt. 92.90638; usually found with tantalum. [*Niobe,* daughter of Tantalus]

NIOSH (nī′osh) Acronym for U.S. National Institute for Occupational Safety and Health.

Ni•pah vi•rus (nē′pă vī′rŭs) A paramyxovirus that can cause fatal disease in humans, with features of encephalitis and meningitis; the virus spreads from swine to humans. [Nipah, Malaysia, where first human case detected, 1999]

nip•ple (nip′ĕl) A blunt conic projection at the apex of the breast on the surface of which the lactiferous ducts open; it is surrounded by a circular pigmented area, the areola. SYN mammilla (2), teat (1), thelium (3). [dim. of A.S. *neb,* beak, nose]

nip•ple line (nip′ĕl līn) SYN mammillary line.

nip•ple shield (nip′ĕl shēld) A cap or dome placed over the nipple to protect it during nursing.

NIPPV Abbreviation for noninvasive positive pressure ventilation.

ni•sin (nī′sin) A polypeptide antibiotic produced by *Streptococcus lactis;* active against some streptococci, *Mycobacterium tuberculosis, Clostridium difficile,* and other bacteria.

Nis•sen fun•do•pli•ca•tion (nis′en fŭn′dō-pli-kā′shŭn) Complete (360°) surgery at the esophagogastric junction; can be done through abdominal or thoracic approach; currently most often performed laparoscopically.

Niss•l bod•ies (nis′ĕl bŏd′ēz) SYN Nissl substance.

Niss•l gran•ules (nis′ĕl gran′yūlz) SYN Nissl substance.

Niss•l stain (nis′ĕl stān) **1.** A method for staining nerve cells with basic fuchsin. **2.** A method for staining aggregates of rough endoplasmic reticulum and ribosomes in neuronal cell bodies and dendrites with basic dyes such as cresyl violet (or cresyl echt violet), thionine, toluidin blue O, or methylene blue.

Niss•l sub•stance (nis′ĕl sub′stăns) The material consisting of granular endoplasmic reticulum and ribosomes that occurs in nerve cell bodies and dendrites. SYN Nissl bodies, Nissl granules.

nit (nit) **1.** The ovum of a body, head, or crab louse; it is attached to human hair or clothing by a layer of chitin. **2.** A unit of luminance; a luminous intensity of 1 candela per square meter of orthogonally projected surface. See page B8. [A.S. *knitu*]

Ni•ta•buch mem•brane, Ni•ta•buch stri•a, Ni•ta•buch lay•er (nē′tă-būk mem′brān, strī′ă, lā′ĕr) A layer of fibrin between the boundary zone of the compact endometrium and the cytotrophoblastic shell in the placenta.

ni•trate (nī′trāt) A salt of nitric acid.

ni•tric ac•id (nī′trik as′id) A strong acid oxidant and corrosive.

ni•tric ox•ide (NO) (nī′trik ok′sīd) A colorless, free-radical gas; it reacts rapidly with O_2 to form other nitrogen oxides (e.g., $NO_2\cdot$, N_2O_3, and N_2O_4) and ultimately is converted to nitrite (NO_2^-) and nitrate (NO_3^-). Physiologically, it is a naturally occurring vasodilator formed in endothelial cells, macrophages, neutrophils, and platelets, and a mediator of cell-to-cell communication formed in bone, brain, endothelium, granulocytes, pancreatic β-cells and peripheral nerves.

ni•trid•a•tion (nī′tri-dā′shŭn) Formation of nitrides; formation of nitrogen compounds through the action of ammonia (analogous to oxidation).

ni•tride (nī′trīd) A compound of nitrogen and one other element; e.g., magnesium nitride, Mg_3N_2.

ni•tri•fi•ca•tion (nī′tri-fi-kā′shŭn) **1.** Bacterial conversion of nitrogenous matter into nitrates. **2.** Treatment of a material with nitric acid.

ni•trile (nī′tril) An alkyl cyanide. Individual nitriles are named for the acid formed on hydrolysis.

nitrilo- Prefix indicating a tervalent nitrogen atom attached to three identical groups; e.g., nitrilotriacetic acid, $N(CH_2COOH)_3$.

ni•trite (nī′trīt) A salt of nitrous acid.

ni•tri•tu•ri•a (nī-tri-tyūr′ē-ă) The presence of nitrites in the urine, as a result of the action of *Escherichia coli, Proteus vulgaris,* and other microorganisms that may reduce nitrates.

nitro- Prefix denoting the group $-NO_2$. [G. *nitron,* sodium carbonate.]

ni•tro dyes (nī′trō dīz) Dyes in which the chromophore is $-NO_2$, which is so acidic that all dyes in this group are also acidic.

ni•tro•fu•ran•to•in (nī′trō-fyūr-an′tō-in) A nitrofuran compound (*O*-[5-nitrofurfurylidene-amino]hydantoin) with antimicrobial activity against a wide spectrum of gram-positive and gram-negative bacteria.

ni·tro·gen (nī′trŏ-jĕn) **1.** A gaseous element; atomic no. 7, atomic wt. 14.00674; forms about 78.084% by volume of the dry atmosphere. **2.** The molecular form of nitrogen, N_2. **3.** Pharmaceutical grade N_2, containing not less than 99.0% by volume of N_2; used as a diluent for medicinal gases, and for air replacement in pharmaceutical preparations. [L. *nitrum,* niter, + *-gen,* to produce]

ni·tro·ge·nase (nī-troj′ĕ-nās) A term for enzyme systems that catalyze the reduction of molecular nitrogen to ammonia in nitrogen-fixing bacteria with reduced ferredoxin and ATP.

ni·tro·gen bal·ance (nī′trŏ-jĕn bal′ăns) The difference between the total nitrogen intake by an organism and its total nitrogen loss. A normal, healthy adult has a zero nitrogen balance.

ni·tro·gen cy·cle (nī′trŏ-jĕn sī′kĕl) The series of events in which the nitrogen of the atmosphere is fixed, thus made available for plant and animal life, and is then returned to the atmosphere: nitrifying bacteria convert N_2 and O_2 to NO_2^- and NO_3^-, the latter being absorbed by plants and converted to protein; if plants decay, the nitrogen is in part given up to the atmosphere and the remainder is converted by microorganisms to ammonia, nitrites, and nitrates; if the plants are eaten, the animals' excreta or bacterial decay return the nitrogen to the soil and air.

ni·tro·gen dis·tri·bu·tion (nī′trŏ-jĕn dis′tri-byū′shŭn) SYN nitrogen partition.

ni·tro·gen e·quiv·a·lent (nī′trŏ-jĕn ē-kwiv′ă-lĕnt) The nitrogen content of protein; used in calculating the protein breakdown in the body from the nitrogen excreted in the urine, 1 g of nitrogen considered as having originated in 6.25 g of protein catabolized.

ni·tro·gen group (nī′trŏ-jĕn grūp) Five trivalent or quinquivalent elements whose hydrogen compounds that are basic and with oxyacids that vary from monobasic to tetrabasic: nitrogen, phosphorus, arsenic, antimony, and bismuth.

ni·tro·gen lag (nī′trŏ-jĕn lag) The length of time after the ingestion of a given protein before the amount of nitrogen equal to that in the protein has been excreted in the urine.

ni·tro·gen mus·tards (HN) (nī′trŏ-jĕn mus′tĕrdz) A group of toxic chemicals (the NATO codes for which are HN_1, HN_2, and HN_3), developed for use as chemical-warfare agents; HN_2, also called mechlorethamine, was further investigated for its potential medical uses and became the first practical antineoplastic alkylating agent.

ni·tro·gen nar·co·sis (nī′trŏ-jĕn nahr-kō′sis) **1.** That state produced by nitrogenous materials such as occurs in certain forms of uremia and hepatic coma. **2.** The stuporous condition characterized by disorientation and by loss of judgment and skill, attributed to an increased partial pressure of nitrogen in the inspired air of deep-sea divers during underwater operations. Commonly referred to as "rapture of the deep."

ni·trog·e·nous (nī-troj′ĕ-nŭs) Relating to or containing nitrogen.

ni·tro·gen par·ti·tion (nī′trŏ-jĕn pahr-ti′shŭn) Determination of the distribution of nitrogen in the urine among the various constituents. SYN nitrogen distribution.

ni·tro·prus·side test (nī′trō-prŭs′īd test) A qualitative procedure for cystinuria; following the addition of sodium cyanide to the urine, the further addition of nitroprusside produces a red-purple color if the cyanide has reduced any cystine present to cysteine.

ni·tro·sa·mines (nī-trō′să-mēnz) Carcinogenic chemical compounds produced when nitrite, a preservative typically added to certain foods (especially beer, fish, fish byproducts, and certain types of meat and cheese products), combines with amino acids in the stomach. Nitrosamines can also be found in tobacco smoke and latex products.

♻ **nitroso-** Prefix denoting a compound containing nitrosyl. [L. *nitrosus*]

***S*-ni·tro·so·he·mo·glo·bin** (nī-trō′sō-hē′mō-glō′bin) A compound formed by the binding of nitric oxide with hemoglobin; release and uptake of the nitric oxide group produce changes in vascular resistance and blood flow, which assist in oxygen homeostasis.

ni·tro·syl (nī′trō-sil) A univalent radical or atom group, –N=O, forming the nitroso compounds.

ni·trous (nī′trŭs) Denoting a nitrogen compound containing one less atom of oxygen than the nitric compounds; one in which the nitrogen is present in its trivalent state.

ni·trous ac·id (nī′trŭs as′id) A standard biologic and clinical laboratory reagent.

ni·trous ox·ide (nī′trŭs ok′sīd) A nonflammable, nonexplosive gas that will support combustion; widely used as a rapidly acting, rapidly reversible, nondepressant, and nontoxic inhalation analgesic to supplement other anesthetics and analgesics; its anesthetic potency is inadequate to provide surgical anesthesia. SYN laughing gas.

ni·tryl (nī′tril) The radical $-NO_2$ of the nitro compounds.

NK cells (selz) SYN natural killer (NK) cells.

NLM Abbreviation for U.S. National Library of Medicine.

NLN Abbreviation for National League of Nursing.

nM Abbreviation for nanomolar (10^{-9} M).

nm Abbreviaton for nanometer.

NMDS Abbreviation for Nursing Minimum Data Set. SEE ALSO minimum data set.

NMN Abbreviation for nicotinamide mononucleotide.

NMR Abbreviation for nuclear magnetic resonance.

NMT Abbreviation for neuromuscular therapy.

NNN me•di•um (mē′dē-ŭm) Agar slant overlaid with defibrinated rabbit blood used to detect the presence of leishmania or *Trypanosoma cruzi.*

NNRTIs Abbreviation for nonnucleoside reverse transcriptase inhibitors.

NO Abbreviation for nitric oxide.

No Symbol for nobelium.

No•ack syn•drome (nō′ahk sin′drōm) SYN Pfeiffer syndrome.

no•bel•i•um (No) (nō-bel′ē-ŭm) An unstable transuranium element; atomic no. 102; atomic wt. 259.1009; prepared by bombardment of curium with carbon-12 nuclei and similar heavy ions on other elements of the transuranium series. [*Nobel* Institute for Physics and A.B. Nobel, Swedish inventor, 1833–1896]

no•ble gas•es (nō′bĕl gas′ĕz) Elements in the zero group in the periodic series: helium, neon, argon, krypton, xenon, and radon. SYN inert gases.

No•ble po•si•tion (nō′bĕl pŏ-zish′ŏn) Patient stands, bent slightly forward; useful for inspection of swelling that may occur with pyelonephritis.

No•ble stain (nō′bĕl stān) A basic fuchsin-orange G staining technique for detection of viral inclusion bodies in fixed tissues.

NOC (nok) Acronym for Nursing Outcomes Classification.

No•car•di•a (nō-kahr′dē-ă) A genus of aerobic actinomycetes (family Nocardiaceae, order Actinomycetales), higher bacteria, containing weakly acid-fast, slender rods or filaments, frequently swollen and occasionally branched, forming a mycelium. Coccus or bacillary forms are produced by these organisms, which are mainly saprophytic but may be a cause of mycetoma or nocardiosis. [E. *Nocard*]

no•car•di•a, pl. **no•car•di•ae** (nō-kahr′dē-ă, -ē) A vernacular term used to refer to any member of the genus *Nocardia.*

No•car•di•a as•ter•oi•des (nō-kahr′dē-ă as-tē-roy′dēz) A bacterial species of aerobic, gram-positive, partially acid-fast, branching organisms causing nocardiosis and possibly mycetoma in humans.

No•car•di•a bra•sil•i•en•sis (nō-kahr′dē-ă bră-zil-ē-en′sis) A bacterial species that is partially acid-fast; associated with subcutaneous skin infections such as mycetoma (actinomycotic), skin abscesses, and cellulitis. Microscopically, *Nocardia* species are gram-positive filamentous, branching bacilli.

No•car•di•a ca•vi•ae (nō-kahr′dē-ă kā′vē-ē) A bacterial species that causes mycetoma in humans.

No•car•di•a far•ci•ni•ca (nō-kahr′dē-ă far-si′ni-kă) A bacterial species causing bovine farcy. It is the type species of the genus *Nocardia.*

No•car•di•a med•i•ter•ra•ne•i (nō-kahr′dē-ă med′i-tĕr-ā′nē-ī) A bacterial species that produces rifamycin.

No•car•di•a no•va (nō-kahr′dē-ă nō′vă) A bacterial species commonly recovered from human infections.

No•car•di•a or•i•en•ta•lis (nō-kahr′dē-ă ōr-ē-en-tā′lis) A bacterial species that produces vancomycin.

No•car•di•a o•ti•ti•dis•ca•vi•a•rum (nō-kahr′dē-ă ō-tī-tī-dis-kā-vē-ā′rum) A higher bacterial species (formerly *Nocardia caviae*) living in soil; causes nocardiosis and actinomycetoma.

No•car•di•a trans•va•len•sis (nō-kahr′dē-ă trans-vā-len′sis) A bacterial aerobic actinomycete; a cause of nocardiosis.

No•car•di•op•sis (nō-kahr-dē-op′sis) A genus of higher bacteria living in soil that causes subacute or chronic pneumonia, subcutaneous infection, or disseminated disease, usually in immunosuppressed patients.

No•car•di•op•sis das•son•vil•le•i (nō-kahr-dē-op′sis das′ŏn-vil-ē-ī) An aerobic bacterial actinomycete, formerly *Nocardia dassonvillei;* a cause of actinomycetoma.

no•car•di•o•sis (nō-kahr′dē-ō′sis) A generalized disease in humans and other animals caused by *Nocardia asteroides* and *N. brasiliensis;* characterized by primary pulmonary lesions that may be subclinical or chronic with hematogenous spread, and usually with involvement of the central nervous system.

no•ce•bo (nō-sē′bō) An unpleasant effect attributable to administration of a placebo. [L. I shall harm, fr. *noceo,* to harm, by analogy with *placebo,* I shall please]

♻**noci-** Prefix meaning hurt, pain, injury. [L. *noceo*]

no•ci•cep•tive (nō′si-sep′tiv) Capable of appreciation or transmission of pain. SEE nociceptor.

no•ci•cep•tive re•flex (nō′si-sep′tiv rē′fleks) A spinal reflex intended to protect the body from harm. It is an automatic (involuntary) neuromuscular action elicited by a defined painful stimulus. SYN nociceptive withdrawal reflex.

no·ci·cep·tive stim·u·lus (nō′si-sep′tiv stim′yū-lŭs) A painful agent (stimulus) that can be injurious or detrimental (e.g., hot coals). [L. *noceo,* to hurt + *capio,* to receive, + *stimulus,* a goad]

no·ci·cep·tive with·draw·al re·flex (nō′si-sep′tiv with-draw′ăl rē′fleks) SYN nociceptive reflex.

no·ci·cep·tor (nō′si-sep′tŏr) A peripheral nerve organ or mechanism for the reception and transmission of painful or injurious stimuli. [noci- + L. *capio,* to take]

no·ci·fen·sor (nō′si-fen′sŏr) Denoting processes or mechanisms that act to protect the body from injury; specifically, a system of nerves in the skin and mucous membranes that react to adjacent injury by causing vasodilation. [noci- + L. *fendo* (only in compounds), to strike, ward off]

no·ci-in·flu·ence (nō′si-in′flū-ĕns) Injurious or harmful influence.

no·ci·per·cep·tion (nō′si-pĕr-sep′shŭn) The appreciation of injurious influences, referring to nerve centers. [noci- + perception]

♲ **noct-** Prefix meaning night, nocturnal. SEE ALSO nycto-. [L. *nox,* night]

noc·te (nok′tē) At night. [L.]

noc·tu·ri·a (nok-tyūr′ē-ă) Excessive urination at night. [noct- + G. *ouron,* urine]

noc·tur·nal (nok-tŭr′năl) Pertaining to the hours of darkness; opposite of diurnal (1). [L. *nocturnus,* of the night]

noc·tur·nal en·u·re·sis (nok-tŭr′năl en-yūr-ē′sis) Urinary incontinence during sleep. SYN bed-wetting.

noc·tur·nal my·oc·lo·nus (nok-tŭr′năl mī-ok′lō-nŭs) Frequently repeated muscular jerks occurring at the moment of dropping off to sleep.

noc·tur·nal ox·y·gen ther·a·py trial (NOTT) (nok-tŭr′năl ok′si-jĕn thār′ă-pē trī′ăl) Assessment used in patients with advanced stages of COPD that compares the effect of oxygen delivered over a 24-hour period with therapy for shorter periods.

noc·u·ous (nok′yū-ŭs) Harmful. [L. *nocuus,* fr. *noceo,* to harm]

no·dal (nō′dăl) Relating to any node.

no·dal point (nō′dăl poynt) One of two points in a compound optic system so related that a ray directed toward the first point will appear to have passed through the second point parallel to its original direction. SYN axial point.

nod·ding spasm (nŏd′ing spazm) **1.** In infants, a drop of the head on the chest due to loss of tone in the neck muscles as in epilepsia nutans, or to tonic spasm of anterior neck muscles as in West syndrome. **2.** In adults, a nodding of the head from clonic spasms of the sternomastoid muscles.

node (nōd) **1.** A knob or nodosity; a circumscribed swelling. **2.** ANATOMY a circumscribed mass of differentiated tissue, especially a lymph node. SYN nodus. [L. *nodus,* a knot]

node of Clo·quet (nōd klō-kā′) One of the deep inguinal lymph nodes located in or adjacent to the femoral canal; sometimes mistaken for a femoral hernia when enlarged.

node of Ran·vi·er (nōd rahn-vē-ā′) SYN Ranvier node.

no·di (nō′dī) Plural of nodus. [L.]

no·dose (nō′dōs) Having nodes or knotlike swellings. SYN nodous, nodular, nodulate, nodulated, nodulous. [L. *nodosus*]

no·dose rheu·ma·tism (nō′dōs rū′mă-tizm) **1.** SYN rheumatoid arthritis. **2.** An acute or subacute articular rheumatism, accompanied by the formation of nodules on the tendons, ligaments, and periosteum in the neighborhood of the affected joints.

no·dos·i·ty (nō-dos′i-tē) **1.** A node; a knoblike or knotty swelling. **2.** The condition of being nodose. [L. *nodositas*]

no·dous, nod·u·lar, nod·u·late, nod·u·lat·ed (nō′dŭs, nod′jū-lăr, nod′jū-lāt, nod′jū-lā-tĕd) SYN nodose.

nod·u·lar am·y·loi·do·sis (nod′jū-lăr am′i-loy-dō′sis) A localized form of amyloidosis in which amyloid occurs as masses or nodules beneath the skin or mucous membranes (e.g., in the larynx). SYN amyloid tumor, focal amyloidosis.

nod·u·lar lep·ro·sy (nod′jū-lăr lep′rŏ-sē) SYN tuberculoid leprosy.

nod·u·lar lym·pho·ma (nod′jū-lăr lim-fō′mă) Malignant lymphoma arising from lymphoid follicular B cells that may be small or large, growing in a nodular pattern. SYN follicular lymphoma.

nod·u·la·tion (noj′yū-lā′shŭn) The formation or the presence of nodules.

nod·ule (nod′jūl) A small node. SYN nodulus (1). [L. *nodulus,* dim. of *nodus,* knot]

nod·ule of sem·i·lu·nar valve (nod′jūl sem′ē-lū′năr valv) A nodule at the center of the free border of each semilunar valve at the beginning of the pulmonary artery and aorta.

nod·u·lous (nod′jū-lŭs) SYN nodose.

no·du·lus, pl. **no·du·li** (nod′yū-lŭs, -lī) **1.** SYN nodule. **2.** The posterior extremity of the inferior vermis of the cerebellum, forming with the posterior medullary velum the central portion of the flocculonodular lobe. SYN nodulus vermis [TA]. [L. dim. of *nodus*]

no•du•lus lym•pha•ti•cus (nod′jū-lŭs lim-fat′ik-ŭs) SYN lymph follicle.

no•du•lus ver•mis (nod′jū-lŭs vĕr′mis) [TA] SYN nodulus.

no•dus, pl. **no•di** (nō′dŭs, -dī) [TA] SYN node. [L. a knot]

no•dus lym•pha•ti•cus, pl. **no•di lym•pha•ti•ci** (nō′dŭs lim-fat′i-kŭs, nō′dī lim-fat′i-sī) [TA] SYN lymph node. [lympho- + L. *nodus*, node]

no•dus lym•phoid•e•us, pl. **no•di lym•phoid•e•i** (nō′dŭs lim-foy′dē-ŭs, nō′dī lim-foyd′ē-ī) [TA] SYN lymph node.

♻**-noia** A suffix meaning related to the mind (e.g., paranoia). [G. *nous*, mind]

noise (noyz) **1.** Unwanted sound, particularly complex sound that lacks a musical quality because the various frequencies of which it is composed are not whole or partial number multiples (harmonics) of each other. **2.** Unwanted additions to a signal not arising at its source; includes visual noise on imaging studies. SEE signal:noise ratio. **3.** Extraneous uncontrolled variables influencing the distibution of measurements in a set of data. [M.E., fr. O.Fr., fr. L.L. *nausea*, seasickness]

noise-in•duced hear•ing loss (noyz-in-dūst′ hēr′ing laws) Sensory hearing loss due to exposure to intense impulse or continuous sound. SYN boilermaker's hearing loss, industrial hearing loss, occupational hearing loss.

noise pol•lu•tion (noyz pŏ-lū′shŭn) Annoying or physiologically damaging environmental sound levels, as from automobile engines, industrial machinery, and amplified music.

NOK, **nok** Abbreviation for next of kin.

no•ma (nō′mă) Gangrenous stomatitis with conspicuous necrosis and sloughing of tissue. Several organisms are usually found in the necrotic material, but fusiform bacilli, *Borrelia* organisms, staphylococci, and anaerobic streptococci are most frequently observed. SYN stomatonecrosis. [G. *nomē,* a spreading (sore)]

♻**nomen-** A prefix meaning a name or pertaining to names (e.g., nomenclature). [L. *nomen,* name]

no•men•cla•ture (nō′mĕn-klā-chŭr) A set system of names used in any science, as of anatomic structures, organisms, and other classifications. [L. *nomenclatura*, a listing of names, fr. *nomen*, name, + *calo*, to proclaim]

nom•i•nal a•pha•si•a (nom′i-năl ă-fā′zē-ă) SYN anomic aphasia.

nom•o•gram (nōm′ō-gram) A form of line chart showing scales for the variables involved in a particular formula in such a way that corresponding values for each variable lie in a straight line intersecting all the scales. [G. *nomos,* law, + *gramma,* something written]

no•mo•top•ic (nō-mō-top′ik) Relating to, or occurring at, the usual or normal place. [G. *nomos,* law, custom, + *topos,* place]

non- A prefix meaning the reverse of something; opposite; negative.

♻**nona-** A prefix meaning the number nine e.g., nonigravida). [L. *nonus,* ninth, fr. *novem,* nine]

non-A-E hep•a•ti•tis (non hep′ă-tī′tis) An acute hepatitis not caused by any identified viral agents A through E.

non-A, non-B hep•a•ti•tis (NANB) (hep′ă-tī′tis) Hepatitis caused by any number of infectious agents not detectable by methods that reveal the presence of hepatitis viruses A and B.

non•a•vail•a•bil•i•ty state•ment (non′ă-vāl′ă-bil′i-tē stāt′mĕnt) A statement issued by the base commander to a Tricare (q.v.) patient that allows such patient or dependent to go off the base for treatment even though less than 40 miles from a military treatment facility (catchment area).

non•bac•te•ri•al ver•ru•cous en•do•car•di•tis (non′bak-tēr′ē-ăl vĕr-ū′kŭs en′dō-kahr-dī′tis) SYN Libman-Sacks endocarditis.

non•chro•mo•ge•nic (non-krō-mō-jen′ik) Nonphotoreactive; pertains to lack of pigment production when colonies are exposed to light.

non•com•mu•ni•cat•ing hy•dro•ceph•a•lus (non′kŏm-myū-ni-kā′ting hī′drō-sef′ă-lŭs) SYN obstructive hydrocephalus.

non•com•pet•i•tive in•hi•bi•tion (non′kŏm-pet′i-tiv in′hi-bish′ŭn) A type of enzyme inhibition in which the inhibiting compound does not compete with the natural substrate for the active site on the enzyme, but inhibits the reaction by combining with the enzyme-substrate complex, after the latter has been formed, and with the free enzyme.

non com•pos men•tis (non kom′pŏs men′tis) Not of sound mind; mentally incapable of managing one's affairs. [L. *non,* not, + *compos,* participating, competent, + *mens,* gen. *mentis,* mind]

non•con•ju•ga•tive plas•mid (non-kon′jū-gă-tiv plaz′mid) A plasmid that cannot effect conjugation and self-transfer to another bacterium (bacterial strain); transfer depends on mediation of another (and conjugative) plasmid.

non•con•tained disc her•ni•a•tion (non′-kon-tānd′ disk hĕr′nē-ā′shŭn) Herniated disc material that comes directly in contact with the anterior epidural space through a complete defect in the posterior anulus fibrosus and posterior longitudinal ligament; of two main types: (1) extrusions, herniated material that is in continuity with the disc space, but extends completely into the epidural space and (2) sequestered, material that has lost continuity with the disc space and becomes a free fragment in the epidural space.

non·co·va·lent bond (non′kō-vā′lĕnt bond) Bond in which electrons are not shared between atoms; e.g., electrostatic bond, hydrogen bond.

non·de·po·lar·iz·ing block (non′dē-pō-lăr-ī-zing blok) Skeletal muscle paralysis unaccompanied by changes in polarity of the motor endplate, such as occurs following administration of tubocurarine.

non·dis·junc·tion (non′dis-jŭngk′shŭn) Failure of one or more pairs of chromosomes to separate at the meiotic stage of karyokinesis, with the result that both chromosomes are carried to one daughter cell and none to the other.

non-dose-re·lat·ed ad·verse ef·fect (non-dōs rē-lā′tĕd ad-vĕrs′ e-fekt′) A drug reaction with an intensity or severity that is not proportional to dosage and typically involves an allergic reaction.

non·e·lec·tro·lyte (non′ē-lek′trō-līt) A substance with molecules that do not, in solution, dissociate to ions and therefore do not carry an electric current.

non·es·sen·tial a·mi·no ac·ids (non′ĕ-sen′shăl ă-mē′nō as′idz) Those amino acids that may be synthesized by an organism and are thus not required as such in its diet.

non·ex·er·cise-ac·tiv·i·ty ther·mo·gen·e·sis (NEAT) (non-eks′ĕr-sīz ak-tiv′i-tē thĕr′mō-jen′ĕ-sis) Energy output that does not produce useful activity or heat.

non·fen·es·trat·ed for·ceps (non-fen′ĕ-strā′tĕd fōr′seps) Obstetric forceps without openings in the blades, thus facilitating rotation of the head.

non·flu·en·cy (non-flū′en-sē) SYN dysfluency.

non·flu·ent a·pha·si·a (non-flū′ĕnt ă-fā′zē-ă) SYN expressive aphasia.

non·he·mo·ly·tic jaun·dice (non-hē′mō-lit′ik jawn′dis) Jaundice caused by an abnormality in the metabolism of bilirubin, which results in an excessive accumulation of unconjugated bilirubin in the blood (e.g., physiologic jaundice of the newborn).

non-Hodg·kin lym·pho·ma (non-hoj′kin lim-fō′mă) A lymphoma other than Hodgkin disease, classified by Rappaport into a nodular or diffuse tumor pattern and by cell type; a working or international formulation separates such lymphomas into low, intermediate, and high grade malignancy and into cytologic subtypes reflecting follicular center cell or other origin. See page B31.

non·im·mune se·rum (non′i-myūn′ sēr′ŭm) A serum from a subject that is not immune; a serum that is free of antibodies to a given antigen.

non·in·su·lin-de·pen·dent di·a·be·tes mel·li·tus (non-in′sū-lin dĕ-pen′dĕnt dī-ă-bē′tēz mel′i-tŭs) SYN Type 2 diabetes.

non·in·va·sive (non′in-vā′siv) Denoting a procedure that does not require insertion of an instrument or device through the skin or a body orifice for diagnosis or treatment.

non·in·va·sive pos·i·tive pres·sure ven·ti·la·tion (NIPPV) (non′in-vā′siv poz′i-tiv presh′ŭr ven′ti-lā′shŭn) In respiratory therapy, use of a full face mask covering both nose and mouth; often used temporarily before endotracheal intubation.

non·i·on·ic con·trast a·gent (non′ī-on′ik kon′trast ā′jĕnt) SYN low osmolar contrast agent.

non·i·so·lat·ed pro·tein·u·ri·a (non-ī′sō-lā-tĕd prō′tē-nūr′ē-ă) The urinary disorder, when associated with other abnormalities.

non·la·mel·lar bone (non′lă-mel′ăr bōn) SYN woven bone.

non·le·thal a·gent (non-lē′thăl ā′jĕnt) A common but incorrect term for incapacitation chemical agent.

non·lip·id his·ti·o·cy·to·sis SYN Letterer-Siwe disease.

non·ma·lef·i·cence (non′mal-ef′i-sens) Ethical principle of doing no harm.

non·med·ul·lat·ed fi·bers (non-med′yū-lāt-ĕd fī′bĕrz) SYN unmyelinated fibers.

non·nu·cle·o·side re·verse tran·scrip·tase in·hi·bi·tors (NNRTIs) (non-nū′klē-ō-sīd rē-vĕrs′ trans-krip′tāz in-hib′i-tŏrz) Class of medications to treat HIV infection (e.g., efavirenz, nevirapine).

non·nu·tri·tive suck·ing (non-nū′tri-tiv sŭk′ing) The sucking patterns used by infants to self-calm, regulate, organize, and explore; not associated with feeding.

non·ob·struc·tive jaun·dice (non′ob-strŭk′tiv jawn′dis) Any such hepatic disorder in which the main biliary passages are not obstructed.

non·or·al com·mu·ni·ca·tion (non-ōr′ăl kŏ-myū-ni-kā′shŭn) SYN augmentative and alternative communication.

non·os·te·o·gen·ic fi·bro·ma (non-os′tē-ō-jen′ik fī-brō′mă) SYN fibrous cortical defect.

non·ox·y·nol 9 (non-oks′i-nol) A group of compounds that are surface acting agents, used in spermicidal preparations such as contraceptive foam and diaphragm jelly.

nonPAR (non′pahr) SYN nonparticipating physician.

non•pa•ra•met•ric (non-par′ă-met′rik) A group of statistical maneuvers that can be applied effectively to data that are nonnormal or nongaussian in distribution.

non•par•ti•ci•pat•ing phy•si•cian (non′par-tis′i-pā-ting fi-zish′ŭn) In the U.S. Medicare program, a physician who does not accept assignment on all Medicare claims. SYN nonPAR.

non•path•o•gen•ic (non-path′ŏ-jen′ik) Not causing disease.

non•pen•e•trance (non-pen′ĕ-trăns) The state in which a genetic trait, although present in the appropriate genotype, fails to manifest itself in the phenotype because of nongenetic mechanisms. Cf. hypostasis.

non•pen•e•trant trait (non-pen′ĕ-trănt trāt) A genetic trait that is not phenotypically manifest because of nongenetic factors; it therefore does not include recessivity, epistasis, hypostasis, or parastasis but does include environmental factors and pure random effects such as lyonization.

non•pen•e•trat•ing wound (non-pen′ĕ-trā-ting wūnd) Injury, especially within the thorax or abdomen, produced without disruption of the surface of the body.

non•per•sis•tent a•gent (non′pĕr-sis′tĕnt ā′jĕnt) A chemical agent that under given conditions of temperature, pressure, wind, and other variables remains in the environment for less than 1 day. Removal may be by evaporation or chemical decomposition. Examples include chlorine, phosgene, cyanide, and the G-series nerve agents.

non•pit•ting e•de•ma (non-pit′ting ĕ-dē′mă) Swelling of subcutaneous tissues that cannot be indented easily by compression; usually due to metabolic abnormality, such as increased glycosaminoglycan content, like that which occurs in Graves disease (pretibial myxedema) or in early phase of scleroderma. SYN brawny edema.

non•pre•scrip•tion drug (non′prĕ-skrip′shŭn drŭg) A pharmaceutical that may be obtained without a physician's prescription. SYN over-the-counter medication.

non•prop•o•si•tion•al speech (non-prop′ă-zi′shŭn-ăl spēch) SYN automatic speech.

non•pro•pri•e•tar•y name (non′prō-prī′ĕ-tar-ē nām) A short name (often called a generic name) of a chemical, drug, or other substance that is not subject to trademark (proprietary) rights but is, in contrast to a trivial name, recognized or recommended by government agencies (e.g., The U.S. Food and Drug Administration) and by quasiofficial organizations (e.g., U.S. Adopted Names Council) for general public use. Cf. trivial name, proprietary name, systematic name.

non•pro•tein ni•tro•gen (NPN) (non-prō′tēn nī′trŏ-jĕn) The nitrogen content of other than protein bodies; e.g., about one half the nonprotein nitrogen in the blood is contained in urea.

non•rap•id eye move•ment sleep (NREM) (non-rap′id ī mūv′mĕnt slēp) Sleep during which rapid eye movement does not occur.

non•re•as•sur•ing fe•tal stat•us (non-rē′ă-shŭr′ing fē′tăl stat′ŭs) Abnormal fetal heart rate or rhythm on electronic monitoring, suggesting fetal ischemia.

non•re•breath•ing an•es•the•si•a (non′rē-brēdh′ing an′es-thē′zē-ă) A technique for inducing inhalation anesthesia in which valves exhaust all exhaled air from the circuit.

non•rig•id con•nec•tor (non-rij′id kŏ-nek′tŏr) A connector or joint that is not rigid or solid. SYN stress-broken connector, stress-broken joint.

non•se•cre•tor (non′sē-krē′tŏr) A person whose saliva does not contain antigens of the ABO blood group. SEE ALSO secretor.

non•sense (non′sens) GENETICS a mutation that causes a sequence such that the growing peptide chain terminates, often after several incorrect amino acid residues are incorporated.

non•sense trip•let (non′sens trip′lĕt) **1.** A trinucleotide (codon) in which a base change to a termination codon results in premature termination of the growing polypeptide chain and, consequently, incomplete protein molecules. **2.** A termination codon.

non•sex•u•al gen•er•a•tion (non-sek′shū-ăl jen-ĕr-ā′shŭn) SYN asexual generation.

non•shiv•er•ing ther•mo•gen•e•sis (non-shi′vĕr-ing thĕr-mō-jen′ĕ-sis) Thermogenesis resulting from the effects of the sympathetic nervous system neurotransmitters, epinephrine and norepinephrine, acting to increase the cellular metabolic rate in skeletal muscle and other tissues, thereby increasing heat production. In a specialized form of adipose tissue, brown fat, the effect of the sympathetic neurotransmitters is to increase the rate of uncoupled oxidative phosphorylation by the mitochondria, which results in heat production without formation of adenosine triphosphate.

non•spec•i•fic build•ing-re•lated ill•ness•es (non′spĕ-sif′ik bil′ding-rē-lāt′ĕd il′nes-ĕz) A heterogeneous group of work- or domicile-related symptoms without clear objective physical or laboratory findings. Cf. specific building-related illnesses.

non•spe•cif•ic pro•tein (non′spĕ-sif′ik prō′tēn) A protein substance that elicits a response not mediated by specific antigen-antibody reaction.

non•ste•roi•dal an•ti•in•flam•ma•to•ry drug (NSAID) (non′ster-oy′dăl an′tī-in-flam′ă-tōr-ē drŭg) Any one of a group of pharmacotherapeutic agents exerting antiinflammatory (and also usually analgesic and antipyretic) actions (e.g., aspirin, diclofenac, ibuprofen, and naproxen). A contrast is made with steroidal compounds (e.g., hydrocortisone or prednisone) exerting antiinflammatory activity.

non•sup•pres•si•ble in•su•lin•like ac•tiv•i•ty (non′sŭ-prĕs′;i-bĕl in′sū-lin′līk ak-tiv′i-tē) Plasma insulinlike activity not suppressed by antibodies to insulin and mostly present after pancreatectomy. Nonsuppressible insulinlike activity is mostly the action of the polypeptide insulinlike growth factors IGF-I and IGF-II.

non•throm•bo•cy•to•pe•nic pur•pu•ra (non-throm′bō-sī-tō-pēn′ik pŭr′pyŭr-ă) SYN purpura simplex.

non•tox•ic goi•ter (non′toks′ik goy′tĕr) Goiter not accompanied by hyperthyroidism.

non•trop•i•cal sprue (non-trop′ik-ăl sprū) Sprue occurring in persons away from the tropics; usually called celiac disease; due to gluten-induced enteropathy.

non•un•ion (non-yūn′yŭn) Failure of normal healing of a fractured bone.

non•va•lent (non-vā′lĕnt) Having no valency; not capable of entering into chemical composition.

non•ver•bal com•mu•ni•ca•tion (non-vĕr′băl kŏ-myū-ni-kā′shŭn) SYN augmentative and alternative communication.

non•vi•a•ble (non-vī′ă-bĕl) **1.** Incapable of independent existence; often denoting a prematurely born embryo or fetus. **2.** Denoting a microorganism or parasite incapable of metabolic or reproductive activity.

non•vi•su•al ret•i•na (non-vizh′ū-ăl ret′i-nă) An anterior continuation of the pigment layer of the retina; it is not light-sensitive.

non•vit•al pulp (non-vī′tăl pŭlp) SYN necrotic pulp.

non-weight-bear•ing ex•er•cise (non-wāt′bār-ing ek′sĕr-sīz) Exercise performed with one's body weight artificially supported (e.g., stationary cycling and swimming). SYN weight-supported exercise.

Noo•nan syn•drome (nūn′ăn sin′drōm) A syndrome found in both males and females, with a phenotype reminiscent of Turner syndrome; characterized by hypertelorism, downslanting of palpebral fissures, webbing of the neck, short stature, and congenital heart disease, especially pulmonary stenosis; normal chromosomal karyotype; autosomal dominant inheritance.

♲ **nor-** Chemical prefix denoting: **1.** elimination of one methylene group from a chain, the highest permissible locant being used. **2.** contraction of a (steroid) ring by one CH_2 unit, the locant being the capital letter identifying the ring. Elimination of two methylene groups is denoted by the prefix dinor-; three groups, by trinor-. **3.** Chemical prefix denoting "normal," i.e., unbranched chain of carbon atoms in aliphatic compounds, as opposed to branched with the same number of carbon atoms; e.g., norleucine, leucine.

nor•a•dren•a•line (nor′ă-dren′ă-lin) SYN norepinephrine.

nor•ep•i•neph•rine (nōr′ep-i-nef′rin) A catecholamine hormone, acting on α- and β-receptors; it is stored in chromaffin granules in the medulla of suprenal gland in much smaller amounts than epinephrine and secreted in response to hypotension and physical stress; used pharmacologically as a vasopressor. SYN noradrenaline.

nor•leu•cine (nōr-lū′sēn) α-amino-*n*-caproic acid; 2-aminohexanoic acid; an α-amino acid, not found in proteins; a deamination product of L-lysine, to which it is linked in collagens.

nor•ma, pl. **nor•mae** (nōr′mă, -mē) SYN profile (1). [L. a carpenter's square]

nor•mal (nōr′măl) **1.** Typical; usual; according to the rule or standard. **2.** BACTERIOLOGY nonimmune; untreated; denoting an animal, or the serum or substance contained therein, which has not been experimentally immunized against any microorganism or its products. **3.** Denoting a solution containing one equivalent of replaceable hydrogen or hydroxyl per liter. **4.** PSYCHIATRY, PSYCHOLOGY denoting a level of effective functioning that is satisfactory to both the patient and the patient's social milieu. [L. *normalis,* according to pattern]

nor•mal an•ti•bod•y (nōr′măl an′ti-bod-ē) Antibody demonstrable in the serum or plasma of various people or animals not known to have been stimulated by specific antigen, either artificially or as the result of naturally occurring contact. SYN natural antibody.

nor•mal an•ti•tox•in (nōr′măl an′tē-tok′sin) Serum that is capable of neutralizing an equivalent quantity of a normal toxin solution.

nor•mal con•cen•tra•tion (N) (nōr′măl kon-sĕn-trā′shŭn) SEE normal (3).

nor•mal dis•tri•bu•tion (nōr′măl dis′tri-byū′shŭn) SYN gaussian distribution.

nor•mal flo•ra (nōr′măl flōr′ă) Microorganisms that normally reside at a given site and under normal circumstances do not cause disease.

nor•mal hu•man plas•ma (nōr′măl hyū′măn plaz′mă) Sterile plasma obtained by pooling approximately equal amounts of the liquid portion of citrated whole blood from eight or more adult humans who have been certified as free from any disease that is transmissible by transfusion, and treating it with ultraviolet irradiation to destroy possible bacterial and viral contaminants.

nor•mal hu•man se•rum al•bu•min (nōr′măl hyū′măn sēr′ŭm al-bū′min) A sterile preparation of serum albumin obtained by fractionating blood plasma proteins from healthy people; used as a transfusion material and to treat edema due to hypoproteinemia.

normalisation [Br.] SYN normalization.

nor•ma•li•za•tion (nōr′măl-ī-zā′shŭn) **1.** Making normal or according to the standard. **2.** Reducing or strengthening of a solution to make it normal. **3.** Adjusting one curve to another by multiplication of the points of the one by some arbitrary factor. SYN normalisation.

nor•mal oc•clu•sion (nōr′măl ŏ-klū′zhŭn) **1.** The arrangement of teeth and their supporting structure usually found in health and that approaches an ideal or standard arrangement. **2.** SYN neutral occlusion (1).

nor•mal op•so•nin (nōr′măl op′sŏ-nin) That normally present in the blood without stimulation by a specific antigen; it is relatively thermolabile and reacts with various organisms.

nor•mal pres•sure hy•dro•ceph•a•lus (nōr′măl presh′ŭr hī′drō-sef′ă-lŭs) A type of hydrocephalus developing usually in older people, due to failure of cerebrospinal fluid to be absorbed by the pacchionian granulations, and characterized clinically by progressive dementia, unsteady gait, urinary incontinence, and usually, a normal spinal fluid pressure.

nor•mal range (nōr′măl rānj) SYN reference range.

nor•mal res•pir•a•tor•y se•cre•tions (NRS) (nōr′măl res′pir-ă-tōr-ē sĕ-krē′shŭnz) Clear, colorless, or white sputum.

nor•mal sa•line (nōr′măl sā′lēn) SYN normal saline (NS) solution.

nor•mal sa•line (NS) so•lu•tion (nōr′măl sā′lēn sŏ-lū′shŭn) A sterile solution of 0.9% w/v (grams of solute per mL of solution) sodium chloride in water, considered to be isotonic with blood; used IV for dehydrated patients who cannot take fluids orally. SYN normal saline.

nor•mal se•rum (nōr′măl sēr′ŭm) A nonimmune serum, usually with reference to a serum obtained before immunization.

nor•mal so•lu•tion (nōr′măl sŏ-lū′shŭn) SEE normal (3).

nor•mal-ten•sion glau•co•ma (nōr′măl ten′shŭn glaw-kō′mă) SYN low-tension glaucoma.

nor•mal val•ues (nōr′măl val′yūz) Outmoded term for a set of laboratory test values used to characterize apparently healthy people; replaced by reference values.

♻**normo-** Prefix meaning normal, usual. [L. *normalis,* according to pattern]

nor•mo•blast (nōr′mō-blast) A nucleated red blood cell, the immediate precursor of a normal erythrocyte in humans. Its four stages of development are: 1) pronormoblast, 2) basophilic normoblast, 3) polychromatic normoblast, and 4) orthochromatic normoblast. SEE ALSO erythroblast. [normo- + G. *blastos,* sprout, germ]

nor•mo•cap•ni•a (nōr-mō-kap′nē-ă) A state in which the arterial carbon dioxide pressure is normal, about 40 mmHg. [normo- + G. *kapnos,* vapor]

nor•mo•chro•mi•a (nōr-mō-krō′mē-ă) Normal color; referring to blood in which the amount of hemoglobin in the red blood cells is normal. [normo- + G. *chrōma,* color]

nor•mo•chro•mic a•ne•mi•a (nōr-mō-krōm′ik ă-nē′mē-ă) Any such hematologic disorder in which the concentration of hemoglobin in the erythrocytes is within the normal range (i.e., the mean corpuscular hemoglobin concentration is 32–36%).

nor•mo•cyte (nōr′mō-sīt) A red blood cell of normal size, shape, and color. Cf. macrocyte, microcyte. [normo + G. *kytos,* cell]

nor•mo•cyt•ic a•ne•mi•a (nōr-mō-sit′ik ă-nē′mē-ă) Any anemia in which the erythrocytes are of normal size (i.e., the mean corpuscular volume ranges from 82–92 mcm^3).

nor•mo•cy•to•sis (nōr′mō-sī-tō′sis) A normal state of the blood cell with regard to its component formed elements.

normoglycaemia [Br.] SYN normoglycemia.

normoglycaemic [Br.] SYN normoglycemic.

nor•mo•gly•ce•mi•a (nōr′mō-glī-sē′mē-ă) SYN euglycemia. SYN normoglycaemia.

nor•mo•gly•ce•mic (nōr′mō-glī-sēm′ik) SYN euglycemic. SYN normoglycaemic.

normokalaemia [Br.] SYN normokalemia.

normokalaemic periodic paralysis [Br.] SYN normokalemic periodic paralysis.

nor•mo•ka•le•mi•a, nor•mo•ka•li•e•mi•a (nōr′mō-kă-lē′mē-ă, nōr′mō-ka-lē-ē′mē-ă) A normal level of potassium in the blood. SYN normokalaemia.

nor•mo•ka•le•mic pe•ri•od•ic pa•ral•y•sis (nōr′mō-ka-lē′mik pēr′ē-od′ik păr-al′i-sis) Periodic paralysis in which the serum potassium level is within normal limits during attacks; there is often severe quadriplegia, usually improved by the administration of sodium salts. SYN normokalaemic periodic paralysis.

normokaliaemia [Br.] SYN normokaliemia.

nor•mo•ten•sive (nōr-mō-ten′siv) Indicating a normal arterial blood pressure. SYN normotonic (2).

nor•mo•ther•mi•a (nōr-mō-thĕr′mē-ă) Environmental temperature that does not cause increased or depressed activity of body cells. [normo- + G. *thermē*, heat]

nor•mo•ton•ic (nōr-mō-ton′ik) **1.** Relating to or characterized by normal muscular tone. SYN eutonic. **2.** SYN normotensive.

normovolaemia [Br.] SYN normovolemia.

nor•mo•vol•e•mi•a (nōr′mō-vō-lē′mē-ă) A normal blood volume. SYN normovolaemia. [normo- + volume, + G. *haima*, blood]

norm-re•fer•enced (nōrm-ref′ĕr-ĕnst) A psychometric property of a standardized test that compares a person's performance with those of the general population.

Nor•rie dis•ease (nōr′ē di-zēz′) Congenital bilateral masses of tissue arising from the retina or vitreous and resembling gliomas (pseudogliomas), usually with atrophy of iris and development of cataract; associated mental retardation and deafness; X-linked recessive inheritance, caused by mutation in the Norrie disease gene (NDP) on Xp.

Nor•ris cor•pus•cle (nōr′is kōr′pŭs-ĕl) A decolorized red blood cell that is invisible or almost invisible in the blood plasma, unless appropriately stained.

North A•mer•i•can blas•to•my•co•sis (nōrth ă-mer′i-kăn blas′tō-mī-kō′sis) SEE blastomycosis.

North A•mer•i•can Nurs•ing Di•ag•no•sis As•so•ci•a•tion (NANDA) (nōrth ă-mer′i-kăn nŭrs′ing dī-ăg-nō′sis ă-sō-sē-ā′shŭn) NURSING organization for development and classification of nursing diagnoses.

North•ern blot a•nal•y•sis (nōr′dhĕrn blot ă-nal′i-sis) A procedure similar to the Southern blot analysis, used mostly to separate and identify RNA fragments; typically done through transferring RNA fragments from an agarose gel to a nitrocellulose filter followed by detection with a suitable probe. [Coined to distinguish it from eponymic Southern blot a.]

Nor•ton op•er•a•tion (nor′tŏn op-ĕr-ā′shŭn) Extraperitoneal cesarean section by a paravesical approach.

Nor•walk vi•rus (nōr′wawk vī′rŭs) A virus associated with acute viral gastroenteritis and probably belonging to the calicivirus group.

Nor•wood op•er•a•tion (nor′wud op-ĕr-ā′shŭn) Surgical procedure performed in infants with subaortic stenosis and tricuspid atresia; the pulmonary artery is divided and both ends are attached to the aorta, the distal end by a prosthetic graft.

nose (nōz) That portion of the respiratory pathway above the hard palate; includes both the external nose and the nasal cavity. SYN nasus (2). [A.S. *nosu*]

nose•bleed (nōz′blēd) SYN epistaxis.

nose•piece (nōz′pēs) A microscope attachment, consisting of several objectives surrounding a central pivot.

♻ **noso-** Combining form meaning disease. SEE ALSO path-. [G. *nosos*]

no•so•ac•u•sis (nō-sō-ă-kyu′sis) Hearing loss due to disease, as opposed to aging. [noso- + G. *akousis*, hearing]

nos•o•co•mi•al (nō′sō-kō′mē-ăl) **1.** Relating to a hospital. **2.** Denoting a new disorder (not the patient's original condition) associated with being treated in a hospital, such as a hospital-acquired infection. [G. *nosokomeion*, hospital, fr. *nosos*, disease, + *komeō*, to take care of]

nos•o•gen•ic (nos-ō-jen′ik) SYN pathogenic.

nos•o•log•ic (nos-ō-loj′ik) Relating to nosology.

no•sol•o•gy (nō-sol′ŏ-jē) **1.** The science of classification of diseases. **2.** Classification of sick people into groups, whatever the criteria for the classification, and agreement as to the boundaries of the groups. SYN nosonomy, nosotaxy. [noso- + G. *logos*, study]

nos•o•ma•ni•a (nos-ō-mā′nē-ă) An unfounded morbid belief that one is suffering from some special disease. [noso- + G. *mania*, insanity]

no•son•o•my (nō-son′ŏ-me) SYN nosology. [noso- + G. *nomos*, law]

nos•o•phil•i•a (nos-ō-fil′ē-ă) A morbid desire to be sick. [noso- + G. *phileō*, to love]

nos•o•pho•bi•a (nos-ō-fō′bē-ă) An inordinate dread and fear of disease. [noso- + G. *phobos*, fear]

nos•o•poi•et•ic (nos′ō-poy-et′ik) SYN pathogenic. [noso- + G. *poiēsis*, a making]

nos•o•tax•y (nos′ō-tak′sē) SYN nosology. [noso- + G. *taxis*, arrangement]

nos•tal•gi•a (nos-tal′jē-ă) The longing to return home, to a former time in one's life, or to familiar people and surroundings. [G. *nostos*, a return (home), + *algos*, pain]

nos•tril (nos′tril) Anterior opening to either side of the nasal cavity. SYN naris, prenaris.

nos•trum (nos′trŭm) General term for a therapeutic agent, sometimes patented but usually of secret composition, offered to the general public as a specific remedy for any disease or class of diseases. [L. neuter of *noster*, our, "our own remedy"]

no•tal (nō′tăl) Relating to the back. [G. *nōtos*, the back]

no·tan·ce·pha·li·a (nō′tan-se-fā′lē-ă) Congenital absence of the occipital bone of the cranium. [G. *nōtos,* back, + *an-* priv. + *kephalē,* head]

no·tan·en·ce·pha·li·a (nō′tan-en-se-fā′lē-ă) Absence of the cerebellum. [G. *nōtos,* back, + *an-* priv. + *enkephalos,* brain]

notch (noch) **1.** An indentation at the edge of any structure. **2.** Any short, narrow, V-shaped deviation, whether positive or negative, in a linear tracing. SYN incisura [TA], incisure.

no·ten·ceph·a·lo·cele (nō′ten-sef′ă-lō-sēl) Malformation in the occipital portion of the cranium with protrusion of brain substance. [G. *nōtos,* back, + *enkephalos,* brain, + *kēlē,* hernia]

Noth·na·gel syn·drome (not′nă-gel sin′drōm) Dizziness, staggering, and rolling gait, with irregular forms of oculomotor paralysis and often nystagmus, seen in cases of tumor of the midbrain.

no·tice of non·cov·er·age (nō′tis non′kŏv′ĕr-ăj) SYN advance beneficiary notice.

No·tice of Pri·va·cy Prac·tic·es (NPP) (nō′tis prī′vă-sē prak′tis-ĕz) Printed advisory given to patients that explains the health care office's use of the patient's protected health information (PHI).

no·ti·fi·a·ble dis·ease (nō-tĭ-fī′ă-băl di-zēz′) A disease that, by statutory requirements, must be reported to public health or veterinary authorities or to law enforcement agencies. SYN reportable disease.

no·to·chord (nō′tō-kōrd) **1.** In primitive vertebrates, the primary axial supporting structure of the body, derived from the notochordal or head process of the early embryo; an important organizer for determining the final form of the nervous system and related structures. **2.** In embryos, the axial fibrocellular cord about which the vertebral primordia develop; vestiges of it persist in the adult as the nuclei pulposi of the intervertebral discs. [G. *nōtos,* back, + *chordē,* cord, string]

no·to·chor·dal (nō-tō-kōr′dăl) Relating to the notochord.

NOTT Abbreviation for nocturnal oxygen therapy trial.

nour·ish·ment (nŭr′ish-mĕnt) A substance used to feed or to sustain life and growth of an organism.

No·vy and Mac·Neal blood a·gar (nō′vē mak-nēl′ blŭd ā′gahr) A nutrient agar containing two volumes of defibrinated rabbit's blood; suitable for the cultivation of a number of trypanosomes.

nox·ious (nok′shŭs) Injurious; harmful. [L. *noxius,* injurious, fr. *noceo,* to injure]

NP Abbreviation for nurse practitioner.

Np Symbol for neptunium.

NPC Abbreviation for Niemann-Pick C1 disease.

NPH in·su·lin (in′sŭ-lin) Modified form of insulin composed of insulin, protamine, and zinc; an intermediately acting preparation used for the treatment of diabetes mellitus. SYN isophane insulin.

NPI Abbreviation for National Provider Identifier number.

NPN Abbreviation for nonprotein nitrogen.

NPO, **n.p.o.** Abbreviation for L. *non per os* or *nil per os*, nothing by mouth.

NPP Abbreviation for Notice of Privacy Practices.

NPU Abbreviation for net protein utilization.

NPY Abbreviation for neuropeptide Y.

NREM Abbreviation for nonrapid eye movement sleep.

nRNA Abbreviation for nuclear RNA.

NRP Abbreviation for National Response Plan.

NRS Abbreviation for normal respiratory secretions.

NRTIs Abbreviation for nucleoside reverse transcriptase inhibitors.

NSAID (en′sād) Acronym for nonsteroidal antiinflammatory drug.

NSNA Abbreviation for National Student Nurses Association.

NSR Abbreviation for normal sinus rhythm.

NTD Abbreviation for neural tube defect.

N ter·mi·nus (ter′mi-nŭs) SEE amino-terminal.

NTG Abbreviation for nitroglycerin.

nu (nū) **1.** Thirteenth letter of the Greek alphabet (ν). **2.** Kinematic viscosity; frequency; stoichiometric number. **3.** CHEMISTRY the position of a substituent located on the thirteenth atom from the carboxyl or other functional group.

nu·cha (nū′kă) The back of the neck. SYN nape. [Fr. *nuque*]

nu·chal (nū′kăl) Relating to the nucha.

nu·chal arm (nū′kăl ahrm) Situation in vaginal breech delivery during which one or both arms are found around the back of the neck, interfering with delivery.

nu·chal cord (nū′kăl kōrd) Loop(s) of umbilical cord around the fetal neck, posing risk of intrauterine hypoxia, fetal distress, or death.

nu·chal lig·a·ment (nū′kăl lig′ă-mĕnt) SYN ligamentum nuchae.

nu•chal plane (nū′kăl plān) The external surface of the squamous part of the occipital bone below the superior nuchal line, giving attachment to the muscles of the back of the neck.

nu•chal rig•id•i•ty (nū′kăl ri-jid′i-tē) Impaired neck flexion resulting from muscle spasm (not actual rigidity) of the extensor muscles of the neck; usually attributed to meningeal irritation.

nu•cle•ar (nū′klē-ăr) Relating to a nucleus, either cellular or atomic; in the latter sense, usually referring to radiation emanating from atomic nuclei (α, β, or γ) or to atomic fission.

nu•cle•ar ag•gre•ga•tion (nū′klē-ăr ag′rĕ-gā′shŭn) SYN syncytial knot.

nu•cle•ar cat•a•ract (nū′klē-ăr kat′ăr-akt) A cataract involving the nucleus of the lens.

nu•cle•ar:cy•to•plas•mic (N:C) ra•ti•o (nū′klē-ĕr-sī-tō-plaz′mik rā′shē-ō) The ratio of the volume of the cell's nucleus to the volume of the cytoplasm. In general, as blood cells mature, the N:C ratio decreases.

nu•cle•ar en•ve•lope (nū′klē-ăr en′vĕ-lōp) The double membrane at the boundary of the nucleoplasm; it has regularly spaced pores covered by a disclike nuclear pore complex and a space or cisterna about 150 Å wide between the two layers; the outer membrane is continuous at intervals with the endoplasmic reticulum. SYN nuclear membrane.

nu•cle•ar fac•tor-κB (nū′klē-ĕr fak′tŏr) A transcription factor associated with cytokine production.

nu•cle•ar fam•i•ly (nū′klē-ăr fam′i-lē) In genetics, two parents and their progeny in common.

nu•cle•ar in•clu•sion bod•ies (nū′klē-ăr in-klū′zhŭn bod′ēz) SEE inclusion bodies.

nu•cle•ar jaun•dice (nū′klē-ăr jawn′dis) SYN kernicterus.

nu•cle•ar mag•net•ic res•o•nance (NMR) (nū′klē-ăr mag-net′ik rez′ŏ-năns) The phenomenon in which certain atomic nuclei possessing a magnetic moment will precess around the axis of a strong external magnetic field, the frequency of precession being specific for each nucleus and the strength of the magnetic field; spinning nuclei induce their own oscillating magnetic fields and therefore emit electromagnetic radiation that can produce a detectable signal. NMR is used as a method of identifying covalent bonds and is applied clinically in magnetic resonance imaging.

i nu•cle•ar med•i•cine (nū′klē-ăr med′i-sin) The clinical discipline concerned with the diagnostic and therapeutic uses of radionuclides, excluding the therapeutic use of sealed radiation sources. See page B23.

nu•cle•ar med•i•cine tech•nol•o•gist (nū′klē-ăr med′i-sin tek-nol′ŏ-jist) Someone skilled in injecting and following the course of radioisotopes in the body in the diagnosing of disease.

nu•cle•ar mem•brane (nū′klē-ăr mem′brān) SYN nuclear envelope.

nu•cle•ar oph•thal•mo•ple•gi•a (nū′klē-ăr of-thal-mō-plē′jē-ă) Ophthalmoplegia due to a lesion of the nuclei of origin of the motor nerves of the eye.

Nu•cle•ar Reg•u•la•to•ry Com•mis•sion (nū′klē-ăr reg′yū-lă-tōr′ē kŏ-mish′ŭn) The U.S. federal commission supervising the use of radioactive by-product material for commercial and medical purposes; successor of the Atomic Energy Commission along with the U.S. Department of Energy.

nu•cle•ar RNA (nRNA) (nū′klē-ăr) RNA found in nuclei, or associated with DNA, or with nuclear structures (nucleoli).

nu•cle•ar spin•dle (nū′klē-ăr spin′dĕl) SYN mitotic spindle.

nu•cle•ar stain (nū′klē-ăr stān) A stain for cell nuclei, usually based on the binding of a basic dye to DNA or nucleohistone.

nu•cle•ase (nū′klē-ās) General term for enzymes that catalyze the hydrolysis of nucleic acid into nucleotides or oligonucleotides. Cf. exonuclease, endonuclease.

nu•cle•ate (nū′klē-āt) A salt of a nucleic acid.

nu•cle•at•ed (nū′klē-āt-ĕd) Provided with a nucleus, a characteristic of all true cells.

nu•cle•a•tion (nū′klē-ā′shŭn) Process of forming a nidus (4).

nu•cle•i (nū′klē-ī) Plural of nucleus.

nu•cle•i an•ter•i•or•es thal•a•mi (nū′klē-ī an-tēr-ē-ōr-ēz thal′ă-mī) [TA] SYN anterior nuclei of thalamus.

nu•cle•ic ac•id (nū-klē′ik as′id) A family of macromolecules found in the chromosomes, nucleoli, mitochondria, and cytoplasm of all cells, and in viruses; in complexes with proteins, they are called nucleoproteins.

nu•cle•i co•chle•a•res (nū′klē-ī kō-klē-ăr′ēz) [TA] The nucleus cochlearis dorsalis and nucleus cochlearis ventralis, located on the dorsal and lateral surface of the inferior cerebellar peduncle, in the floor of the lateral recess of the rhomboid fossa. They receive the incoming fibers of the cochlear part of the vestibulocochlear nerve and are the major source of origin of the lateral lemniscus or central auditory pathway.

nu•cle•i•form (nū′klē-i-fōrm) Shaped like or having the appearance of a nucleus. SYN nucleoid (1).

nu•cle•i of or•i•gin (nū′klē-ī ōr′i-jin) Collections of motor neurons (forming a continuous column in the spinal cord, discontinuous in the medulla and pons) giving origin to the spinal and cranial motor nerves.

♻**nucleo-, nucl-** Combining forms meaning nucleus, nuclear. SEE ALSO karyo-, caryo-. [L. *nucleus*]

nu•cle•o•cap•sid (nū′klē-ō-kap′sid) SEE virion.

nu•cle•of•u•gal (nū′klē-of′yū-găl) **1.** Moving within the cell body in a direction away from the nucleus. **2.** Moving in a direction away from a nerve nucleus; said of nerve transmission. [nucleo- + L. *fugio,* to flee]

nu•cle•o•his•tone (nū′klē-ō-his′tōn) A complex of histone and deoxyribonucleic acid, the form in which the latter is usually found in the nuclei of cells.

nu•cle•oid (nū′klē-oyd) **1.** SYN nucleiform. **2.** A nuclear inclusion body. **3.** SYN nucleus (2). [nucleo- + G. *eidos,* resemblance]

nu•cle•o•lar (nū′klē-ō′lăr) Relating to a nucleolus.

nu•cle•o•li (nū′klē-ō′lī) Plural of nucleolus.

nu•cle•o•li•form (nū′klē-ō′li-fōrm) Resembling a nucleolus. SYN nucleoloid.

nu•cle•o•loid (nū′klē-ō-loyd) SYN nucleoliform. [nucleolus + G. *eidos,* resemblance]

nu•cle•o•lo•ne•ma (nū′klē-ō′lō-nē′mă) The irregular network or rows of fine ribonucleoprotein granules or microfilaments forming most of the nucleolus. [nucleolus + G. *nēma,* thread]

nu•cle•o•lus, pl. **nu•cle•o•li** (nū-klē′ō-lŭs, nū′klē-ō′lī) A small, rounded mass within the cell nucleus where ribonucleoprotein is produced. [L. dim of *nucleus,* a nut, kernel]

nu•cle•on (nū′klē-on) **1.** One of the subatomic particles of the atomic nucleus; i.e., either a proton or a neutron. **2.** Slang term for specialist in nuclear medicine. [nucleus + -on]

nu•cle•op•e•tal (nū′klē-op′ĕ-tăl) **1.** Moving in the cell body in a direction toward the nucleus. **2.** Moving in a direction toward a nerve nucleus; said of a nervous impulse. [nucleo- + L. *peto,* to seek]

nu•cle•o•phil, **nu•cle•o•phile** (nū′klē-ō-fil, -fīl) **1.** The electron pair donor atom in a chemical reaction in which a pair of electrons is picked up by an electrophil. **2.** Relating to a nucleophil. SYN nucleophilic (1). [nucleo- + G. *philos,* fond]

nu•cle•o•phil•ic (nū′klē-ō-fil′ik) **1.** SYN nucleophil (2). **2.** A reaction involving a nucleophile.

nu•cle•o•plasm (nū′klē-ō-plazm) The protoplasm of the nucleus of a cell.

nu•cle•o•pro•tein (nū′klē-ō-prō′tēn) A complex of protein and nucleic acid, the form in which essentially all nucleic acids exist in nature; chromosomes and viruses are largely nucleoprotein.

nu•cle•or•rhex•is (nū′klē-ō-rek′sis) Fragmentation of a cell nucleus. [nucleo- + G. *rhēxis,* rupture]

nu•cle•o•si•das•es (nū′klē-ō-sī′dās-ĕz) Enzymes that catalyze the hydrolysis or phosphorolysis of nucleosides, releasing the purine or pyrimidine base.

nu•cle•o•side (nū′klē-ō-sīd) A compound of a sugar (usually ribose or deoxyribose) with a purine or pyrimidine base.

nu•cle•o•side re•verse tran•scrip•tase in•hib•i•tors (NRTIs) (nyū′klē-ō-sīd rē-vĕrs′ trans-krip′tās in-hib′i-tŏrz) Class of medications to treat HIV infection (e.g., zidovudine, lamivudine).

nu•cle•o•some (nū′klē-ō-sōm) A localized aggregation of histone and DNA that is evident when chromatin is in the uncondensed stage. [nucleo- + G. *sōma,* body]

nu•cle•o•ti•da•ses (nū′klē-ō-tī′dās-ĕz) Enzymes that catalyze the hydrolysis of nucleotides into phosphoric acid and nucleosides.

nu•cle•o•tide (nū′klē-ō-tīd) A combination of a (nucleic acid) purine or pyrimidine, one sugar (usually ribose or deoxyribose), and a phosphoric group. SYN mononucleotide.

nu•cle•o•tid•yl•trans•fer•as•es (nū′klē-ō-tī′dil-trans′fĕr-ās-ĕz) Enzymes transferring nucleotide residues (nucleotidyls) from nucleoside di- or triphosphates into dimer or polymer forms.

nu•cle•o•tox•in (nū′klē-ō-tok′sin) A toxin acting on the cell nuclei.

nu•cle•us, pl. **nu•cle•i** (nū′klē-ŭs, -ī) **1.** CYTOLOGY typically a rounded or oval mass of protoplasm within the cytoplasm of a plant or animal cell; it is surrounded by a nuclear envelope, which encloses euchromatin, heterochromatin, and one or more nucleoli and undergoes mitosis during cell division. SYN karyon. **2.** By extension, because of similar function, the genome of microorganisms (microbes), which is relatively simple in structure, lacks a nuclear membrane and does not undergo mitosis during replication. SYN nucleoid (3). SEE ALSO virion. **3.** NEUROANATOMY a group of nerve cell bodies in the brain or spinal cord that can be demarcated from neighboring groups on the basis of either differences in cell type or the presence of a surrounding zone of nerve fibers or cell-poor neuropil. **4.** Any substance (e.g., foreign body, mucus, crystal) around which a urinary or other calculus is formed. **5.** The central portion of an atom (composed of protons and neutrons) where most of the mass and all of the positive charge are concentrated. **6.** A particle on which a crystal, droplet, or bubble forms. **7.** A characteristic arrangement of atoms in a series of molecules; e.g., the benzene nucleus in a series of aromatic compounds. [L. a little nut, the kernel, stone of fruits, the inside of a thing, dim. of *nux,* nut]

nu·cle·us of the an·sa len·tic·u·lar·is (nū′klē-ŭs an′să len-tik′yū-lār′is) [TA] SEE dorsal hypothalamic area.

nu·cle·us cae·ru·le·us (nū′klē-ŭs sē-rū′lē-us) [TA] A shallow depression, colored blue in a fresh brain, lying laterally in the most rostral portion of the rhomboidal fossa near the cerebral aqueduct; it lies near the lateral wall of the fourth ventricle and consists of about 20,000 melanin-pigmented neuronal cell bodies the norepinephrine-containing axons which have a remarkably wide distribution in the cerebral cortex, dorsal thalamus, amygdaloid complex, hippocampus, mesencephalic tegmentum, cerebellar nuclei and cortex, various nuclei in the pons and medulla, and the gray matter of the spinal cord.

nu·cle·us den·ta·tus (nū′klē-ŭs den-tā′tus) [TA] SYN dentate nucleus of cerebellum.

nu·cle·us of pos·ter·i·or com·mis·sure (nū′klē-ŭs pos-tēr′ē-ŏr kom′i-shŭr) [TA] A group of cells located immediately adjacent to the posterior commissure at the mesencephalon-diencephalon junction; may be divided into pars ventralis [TA] (ventral subdivision), pars dorsalis [TA] (dorsal subdivision), and pars interstitialis [TA] (interstitial subdivision).

nu·cle·us of sol·i·tary tract (nū′klē-ŭs sol′i-tar-ē trakt) A slender cell column extending sagittally through the dorsal part of the medulla oblongata, beneath the floor of the rhomboid fossa, immediately lateral to the limiting sulcus. It is the visceral sensory (visceral afferent) nucleus of the brainstem, receiving the afferent fibers of the vagus, glossopharyngeal, and facial nerves by way of the solitary tract. The caudal two thirds of the nucleus processes impulses originating in the pharynx, larynx, intestinal and respiratory tracts, and heart and large blood vessels; its rostral one third receives impulses from the taste buds and is known as the rhombencephalic gustatory nucleus. SYN nucleus tractus solitarii [TA].

nu·cle·us tract·us so·li·ta·ri·i (nū′klē-ŭs trak′tŭs sol-i-tā′rē-ī) [TA] SYN nucleus of solitary tract.

nu·clide (nū′klīd) A particular (atomic) nuclear species with defined atomic mass and number. SEE ALSO isotope.

NUG Abbreviation for necrotizing ulcerative gingivitis.

null cells (nŭl selz) **1.** SYN killer cells. **2.** Large granular lymphocytes that lack surface markers or membrane-associated proteins of either B or T lymphocytes.

null hy·poth·e·sis (nŭl hī-poth′ĕ-sis) The statistical hypothesis that one variable has no association with another, or that experimental results do not differ from those that might be expected by the operation of chance alone.

nul·li·grav·i·da (nŭl-i-grav′i-dă) A woman who has never conceived a child. [L. *nullus,* none, + *gravida,* pregnant]

nul·lip·a·ra (nŭ-lip′ă-ră) A woman who has never borne children. [L. *nullus,* none, + *pario,* to bear]

nul·li·par·i·ty (nŭl′i-par′i-tē) Condition of having borne no children.

nul·lip·a·rous (nŭl-ip′ă-rŭs) Having never borne children.

numb chin syn·drome (nŭm chin sin′drōm) Paresthesia and sensory loss affecting one side of the chin and lower lip, resulting from neoplastic infiltration of the ipsilateral mental nerve; common causes include multiple myeloma and breast or prostate carcinoma.

num·ber (nŭm′bĕr) **1.** A symbol expressive of a certain value or of a specific quantity determined by count. **2.** The place of any unit in a series.

numb·ness (nŭm′nĕs) Imprecise term for abnormal sensation, including absent or reduced sensory perception as well as paresthesias.

num·mu·lar (nŭm′yū-lăr) **1.** Discoid or coin-shaped; denoting thick mucopurulent sputum, so called because of the disk shape assumed when it is flattened on the bottom of a sputum mug containing water or transparent disinfectant. **2.** Arranged like stacks of coins, denoting the lining up of the red blood cells into rouleaux formation. [L. *nummulus,* small coin, dim. of *nummus,* coin]

num·mu·lar ec·ze·ma (nŭm′yū-lăr ek′sĕ-mă) Discrete, coin-shaped patches of eczema. See this page.

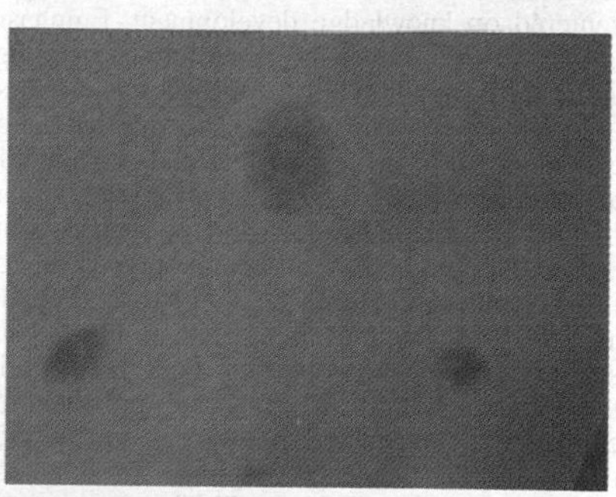

nummular eczema: back

num·mu·lar spu·tum (nŭm′yū-lăr spyūt′ŭm) A thick, coherent mass expectorated in globular shape that does not run at the bottom of the cup but forms a discoid mass that resembles a coin.

nurse (nŭrs) **1.** To breast-feed; suckle. **2.** To provide care of the sick. **3.** One who is educated in the scientific basis of nursing under defined standards of education and is concerned with the diagnosis and treatment of human responses to actual or potential health problems. [O. Fr. *nourice,* fr. L. *nutrix,* wet-nurse, nurse, fr. *nutrio,* to suckle, to tend]

nurse a•nes•the•tist (nŭrs ă-nes′thĕ-tist) A registered nurse qualified to administer anesthesia, in both inpatient and outpatient settings; in the U.S., the title "certified registered nurse anesthetist" (CRNA) is conferred on registered nurses with at least 1 year of acute care experience who complete a graduate program recognized by the American Association of Nurse Anesthetists and pass a national certification examination; CRNAs are the sole providers of anesthesia in most rural U.S. hospitals.

nurse-cli•ent re•la•tion•ship (nŭrs klī′ent rĕ-lā′shŭn-ship) A professional relationship between a patient and a nurse based on therapeutic communication. Not a social relationship.

nurse•maid's el•bow (nŭrs-mādz el′bō) Longitudinal subluxation of the radial head from the anular ligament. SYN Malgaigne luxation.

nurse prac•tice act (nŭrs prak′tis akt) Legal provisions in each U.S. state regulating nursing practice; intent is to protect public and enforce acceptable standards of practice.

nurse prac•ti•tion•er (NP) (nŭrs prak-tish′ŭn-ĕr) A registered nurse with advanced education in the primary care of particular groups of clients, who provides services, within the scope of nursing practice, in the areas of health promotion, disease prevention, therapy, rehabilitation, and support at all levels of the health care system.

nurs•ing (nŭrs′ing) **1.** A discipline, profession, and area of practice. As a discipline, nursing is centered on knowledge development. Emphasis is placed on discovering, describing, extending, and modifying knowledge for professional nursing practice. As a profession, nursing has a social mandate to be responsible and accountable to the public it serves. Nursing is an integral part of the health care system, and as such encompasses the promotion of health, prevention of illness, and care of physically ill, mentally ill, and disabled people of all ages, in all health care settings and other community contexts. Within this broad spectrum of health care, the phenomena of particular concern to nurses are individual, family, and group "responses to actual or potential health problems." The human responses range broadly from health-restoring reactions to an individual episode of illness to the development of policy in promoting the long-term health of a population. **2.** Feeding an infant at the breast; tending and caring for a young child.

nurs•ing au•dit (nŭrs′ing aw′dit) A method of evaluating nursing practice by reviewing records that document the care provided to patients.

nurs•ing care plan (nŭrs′ing kār plan) Care plan created by a nurse for patients as a result of assessment of patient needs. The plan of care is focused on nursing interventions, not medical interventions.

nurs•ing con•cep•tu•al frame•work (nŭrs′ing kŏn-sep′shū-al frām′wŏrk) A grouping of related concepts and theories that are of importance to nurses to guide nursing practice, education, and research. SYN nursing model.

nurs•ing di•ag•no•sis (nŭrs′ing dī-ăg-nō′sis) The process of assessing potential or actual health problems, including those pertaining to an individual patient, a family or community, that fall within the scope of nursing practice; a judgment or conclusion reached as a result of such assessment or derived from assessment data. SEE ALSO diagnosis.

nurs•ing ed•u•ca•tion pro•gram (nŭrs′ing ej′ū-kā′shŭn prō′gram) Planned curriculum usually with clinical practice experiences to prepare nurses; includes diploma (hospital school of nursing), at associate, baccalaureate (bachelor's), master's, and doctoral levels; also includes certificate, continuing education, and in-service programs.

nurs•ing fa•cil•i•ty (nŭrs′ing fă-sil′i-tē) Health care facility for patients who require long-term nursing or rehabilitation services; formerly known as a nursing home. SYN assisted living facility, long-term care facility.

nurs•ing his•to•ry (nŭrs′ing his′tŏr-ē) A comprehensive set of information about a patient's medical history, including the history of the present illness, as well as the person's psychosocial and spiritual history; used as the basis for nursing diagnosis and development of a care plan.

nurs•ing home (nŭrs′ing hōm) SYN extended-care facility.

nurs•ing in•for•mat•ics (nŭrs′ing in′fōr-mat′iks) **1.** Nursing specialty surrounding the use of computer technology to support nursing practice, management, research, and education. It is informed by both computer science and nursing science. **2.** Integration of data to support patient care, nurses, and other providers.

nurs•ing in•ter•ven•tion (nŭrs′ing in′tĕr-ven′shŭn) Treatments that nurses perform in all settings and in all specialties; activities nurses perform; nursing care measures.

Nurs•ing In•ter•ven•tions Clas•si•fi•ca•tion (NIC) (nŭrs′ing in-tĕr-ven′shŭnz klas′i-fi-kā′shŭn) Standardized classification of patient/client outcomes for evaluating effects of nursing interventions.

Nurs•ing Min•i•mum Da•ta Set (NMDS) (nŭrs′ing min′i-mŭm dā′tă set) **1.** Standardized set of nursing data developed to describe nursing care applicable across diverse clinical practice settings; includes data relating to nursing diagnoses, interventions, outcomes, and intensity of nursing care. **2.** Smallest amount of information necessary to define cost and quality of nursing care.

nurs·ing mod·el (nŭrs′ing mo′dĕl) SYN nursing conceptual framework.

Nurs·ing Out·comes Clas·si·fi·ca·tion (NOC) (nŭrs′ing owt′kŭmz klas′i-fi-kā′shŭn) Standardized classification of patient/client outcomes for evaluating effects of nursing interventions.

nurs·ing pro·cess (nŭrs′ing pros′es) Structured, organized, and systematic approach to developing and delivering patient care including assessment, diagnosis, planning, implementation, and evaluation; series of nursing actions for meeting patient's needs and promoting better health. This problem-solving approach has four steps: assess, plan, implement, and evaluate. Nursing theories and conceptual frameworks guide each step of the nursing process.

nurs·ing the·o·ry (nŭrs′ing thē′ŏr-ē) Set of concepts, definitions, and propositions that present a systematic view of various phenomena related to nursing's unique role; guides practice, education, and research.

nu·tans (nū′tahns) Nodding. [L.]

nu·ta·tion (nū-tā′shŭn) CHIROPRACTIC the backward rotation of the ilium on the sacrum. USAGE NOTE this concept is not shared by some medical practitioners.

nu·tra·ceu·ti·cal (nū′tră-sū′ti-kăl) A product derived from a food that is marketed in the form of medicine and is demonstrated to have a physiologic benefit or to provide protection against chronic disease. Cf. functional food. [*nutr*ient + pharm*aceutical*]

nu·tra·ge·nom·ics (nū′tră-jē-nō′miks) SYN nutrigenomics.

nu·tri·ent (nū′trē-ĕnt) A constituent of food necessary for normal physiologic function. See this page. [L. *nutriens,* fr. *nutrio,* to nourish]

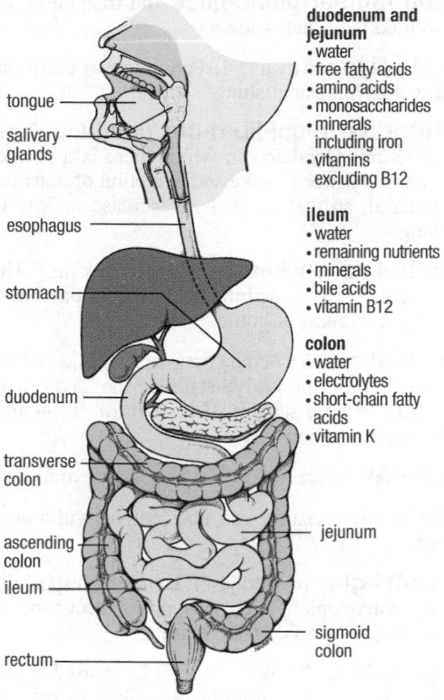

nutrient absorption: gastrointestinal tract sites

nu·tri·ent ar·ter·ies of hu·mer·us (nū′trē-ĕnt ahr′tĕr-ēz hyū′mĕr-ŭs) *Origin,* deep brachial; *distribution,* the medullary cavity of the humerus.

nu·tri·ent ar·ter·y (nū′trē-ĕnt ahr′tĕr-ē) An artery of variable origin that supplies the medullary cavity of a long bone. SYN arteria nutricia [TA], nutrient vessel.

nu·tri·ent ar·ter·y of fe·mur (nū′trē-ĕnt ahr′tĕr-ē fē′mŭr) One of two arteries, superior and inferior, arising from the first and third perforating arteries respectively (sometimes second and fourth). SYN arteria nutricia femoris [TA].

nu·tri·ent ar·ter·y of fib·u·la (nū′trē-ĕnt ahr′tĕr-ē fib′yū-lă) *Origin,* peroneal (fibular); *distribution,* fibula. SYN arteria nutricia fibulae [TA].

nu·tri·ent ca·nal (nū′trē-ĕnt kă-nal′) A canal in the shaft of a long bone or in other locations in irregular bones through which the nutrient artery enters a bone. SYN canalis nutricius [TA].

nu·tri·ent fo·ra·men (nū′trē-ĕnt fōr-ā′mĕn) The external opening of the nutrient canal in a bone.

nu·tri·ent ves·sel (nū′trē-ĕnt ves′ĕl) SYN nutrient artery.

nu·tri·ge·no·mics (nū′tri-jē-nō′miks) The study of how diet influences gene expression, and thus, health. SYN nutragenomics, nutritional genomics. [nutri- + genomics]

nu·trit·ion (nū-trish′ŭn) **1.** A function of living plants and animals, consisting in the taking in and metabolism of food material whereby tissue is built up and energy liberated. **2.** The study of the food and liquid requirements of human beings or animals for normal physiologic function, including energy, maintenance, growth, activity, reproduction, and lactation. [L. *nutritio,* fr. *nutrio,* to nourish]

nu·tri·tion·al as·sess·ment (nū-trish′ŏ-năl ă-ses′mĕnt) Measurement of the body through anthropometrics, biochemical testing, clinical examination, and dietary intake.

nu·tri·tion·al ge·no·mics (nū-trish′ŭn-ăl jē-nō′miks) SYN nutrigenomics.

nu·tri·tive (nū′tri-tiv) **1.** Pertaining to nutrition. **2.** Capable of nourishing.

nu·tri·tive e·qui·lib·ri·um (nū′tri-tiv ē′kwi-lib′rē-ŭm) Condition in which there is a perfect balance between intake and excretion of nutritive material, so that there is no increase or loss in weight.

nu·tri·tive suck·ing (nū′tri-tiv sŭk′ing) The patterns used by the infant to obtain nourishment from the breast or bottle.

nu·tri·ture (nū′tri-chŭr) State or condition of the nutrition of the body; state of the body with regard to nourishment. [L. *nutritura,* a nursing, fr. *nutrio,* to nourish]

NV, **n&v** Abbreviation for nausea and vomiting.

NWR Abbreviation for nociceptive withdrawal reflex.

nyc·tal·gi·a (nik-tal′jē-ă) Denoting especially the osteocopic pains of syphilis occurring at night. [nyct- + G. *algos,* pain]

nyc·ta·lo·pi·a (nik-tă-lō′pē-ă) Decreased ability to see in reduced illumination. Seen in patients with impaired rod function; often associated with a deficiency of vitamin A. SYN night blindness. [nyct- + G. *alaos,* obscure, + *ōps,* eye]

nyc·ter·ine (nik′tĕr-ēn) **1.** By night. **2.** Dark or obscure. [G. *nykterinos*]

nycto-, nyct- Combining forms meaning night, nocturnal. SEE ALSO noct-. [G. *nyx*]

nyc·to·hem·e·ral (nik′tō-hem′ĕr-ăl) Both daily and nightly. [nycto- + G. *hēmera,* day]

nyc·to·phil·i·a (nik-tō-fil′ē-ă) Preference for the night or darkness. SYN scotophilia. [nycto- + G. *philos,* fond]

nyc·to·pho·bi·a (nik-tō-fō′bē-ă) Morbid fear of night or of the dark. SYN scotophobia. [nycto- + G. *phobos,* fear]

nym·pha, pl. **nym·phae** (nim′fă, -fē) One of the labia minora. [Mod. L., fr. G. *nymphē,* a bride]

nym·phec·to·my (nim-fek′tŏ-mē) Surgical removal of hypertrophied labia minora. [nympha + G. *ektomē,* excision]

nym·phi·tis (nim-fī′tis) Inflammation of the labia minora. [nympha + G. *-itis,* inflammation]

nympho-, nymph- Combining forms indicating the nymphae (labia minora). [L. *nympha*]

nym·pho·ma·ni·a (nim-fō-mā′nē-ă) An insatiable impulse to engage in sexual behavior in a female; the counterpart of satyriasis in a male. [nympho- + G. *mania,* frenzy]

nym·pho·ma·ni·a·cal (nim′fō-mă-nī′ă-kăl) Pertaining to, or exhibiting, nymphomania.

nym·phon·cus (nim-fongk′ŭs) Swelling or hypertrophy of one or both labia minora. [nympho- + G. *onkos,* tumor]

nym·phot·o·my (nim-fot′ŏ-mē) Incision into the labia minora or the clitoris. [nympho- + G. *tomē,* incision]

Ny·quist the·o·rem (nī′kvist thē′ō-rĕm) That a frequency must be sampled at least twice to reproduce it reliably.

nys·tag·mic (nis-tag′mik) Relating to or suffering from nystagmus.

nys·tag·mi·form (nis-tag′mi-fōrm) SYN nystagmoid.

nys·tag·mo·graph (nis-tag′mō-graf) An apparatus for measuring the amplitude, periodicity, and velocity of ocular movements in nystagmus, by measuring the change in the resting potential of the eye as the eye moves. [nystagmus + G. *graphō,* to write]

nys·tag·mog·ra·phy (nis′tag-mog′ră-fē) The technique of recording nystagmus.

nys·tag·moid (nis-tag′moyd) Resembling nystagmus. SYN nystagmiform. [nystagmus + G. *eidos,* resemblance]

nys·tag·mus (nis-tag′mŭs) Rhythmic oscillation of the eyeballs, either pendular or jerky. See this page. [G. *nystagmos,* a nodding, fr. *nystazō,* to be sleepy, nod]

nyx·is (nik′sis) A pricking; paracentesis. [G.]

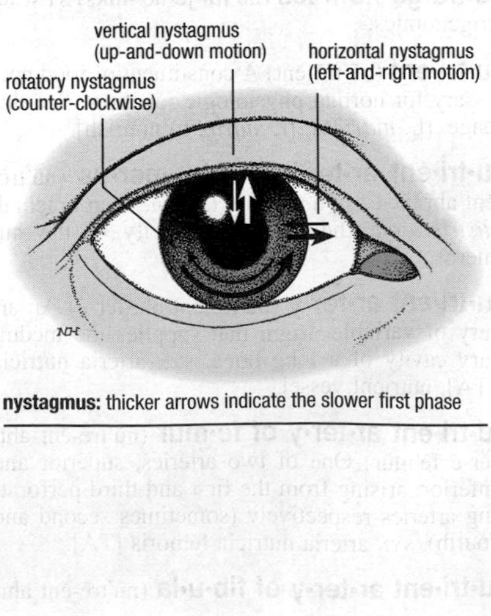

nystagmus: thicker arrows indicate the slower first phase

O

Ω, ω Omega. SEE omega.

O **1.** Symbol for oxygen; abbreviation for orotidine. **2.** Opening (in formulas for electrical reactions). **3.** A blood group in the ABO system. **4.** An abbreviation derived from *ohne Hauch* (German for "without a film"), used as a designation for: 1) antigens that occur in the bacterial cell, in contrast to those in the flagella; 2) specific antibodies for such somatic antigens; 3) the agglutinative reaction between somatic antigen and its antibody.

O_2 Abbreviation for oxygen molecule. SEE oxygen.

OA Abbreviation for occipitoanterior position.

OAE Abbreviation for otoacoustic emission.

O ag•glu•ti•nin (ă-glū′ti-nin) An agglutinin that is formed as the result of stimulation by, and that reacts with, the relatively thermostable antigen(s) in the cell bodies of microorganisms.

oak (ōk) A deciduous tree (*Quercus* spp.) that provides material in its leaves and bark to produce many forms of herbal nostrums. Used as an astringent, a therapeutic remedy for skin disorders (approved for use for this purpose in Germany), and countless other unconfirmed purposes. Because of high levels of tannic acid, it has caused death, respiratory failure, and hepatotoxicity.

O an•ti•gen (an′ti-jen) Somatic antigen of enteric gram-negative bacteria. External part of cell wall lipopolysaccharide. SEE ALSO H antigen (1).

OASIS (ō-ā′sĭs) Acronym for Outcome and Assessment Information Set.

oat cell (ōt sel) A short, bluntly spindle-shaped cell that contains a relatively large, hyperchromatic nucleus, frequently observed in undifferentiated bronchogenic carcinoma.

oat cell car•ci•no•ma (ōt sel kahr′si-nō′mă) An anaplastic, highly malignant, and usually bronchogenic carcinoma composed of small ovoid cells with very scanty cytoplasm; this carcinoma and small round cell carcinomas comprise over one-third of carcinomas of the lung. SYN small cell carcinoma (2).

OB (ob) Acronym and abbreviation for obstetrics.

ob•dor•mi•tion (ob-dōr-mi′shŭn) Numbness of an extremity, due to pressure on the sensory nerve. [L. *ob-dormio,* pp. *-itus,* to sleep]

o•be•li•ac (ō-bē′lē-ak) Relating to the obelion.

o•be•li•on (ō-bē′lē-on) A craniometric point on the sagittal suture between the parietal foramina near the lambdoid suture. [G. *obelos,* a spit]

O•ber test (ō′bĕr test) Test to evaluate a tight, contracted, or inflamed iliotibial tract; the patient lies on the uninvolved side and the involved hip is abducted by the examiner as the knee is flexed to 90°; the hip is allowed to adduct passively; the degree of abduction or the production of pain along the iliotibial tract can assist in identifying the location of the inflammation or contracture.

o•bese (ō-bēs′) Extremely fat; having a body mass index of 30 or higher. SYN corpulent. [L. *obesus,* fat, partic. adj., fr. *ob-edo,* pp. *-esus,* to eat away, devour]

o•be•si•ty (ō-bē′si-tē) An excessive accumulation of fat in the body. SYN adiposity (1), corpulence, corpulency.

o•be•si•ty-hy•per•ven•ti•la•tion syn•drome (ō-bē′si-tē hī′pĕr-ven′ti-lā′shŭn sin′drōm) SEE pickwickian syndrome.

o•be•si•ty-hy•po•ven•ti•la•tion syn•drome (ō-bē′si-tē hī′pō-ven′ti-lā′shŭn sin′drōm) Constellation of findings consisting of obesity, hypoxemia, hypercapnia, erythrocytosis, and lethargy.

o•bex (ō′beks) The point on the midline of the dorsal surface of the medulla oblongata that marks the caudal angle of the rhomboid fossa or fourth ventricle. It corresponds to a small, transverse medullary fold overhanging the calamus scriptorius. [L. barrier]

OBG Abbreviation for obstetrics and gynecology.

OB/GYN (ob-gīn′) Acronym and abbreviation for obstetrics and gynecology.

ob•ject (ob′jekt) **1.** Anything to which thought or action is directed. **2.** In psychoanalysis, that through which an instinct can achieve its aim. **3.** In psychoanalysis, often used synonymously with person.

ob•ject choice (ob′jekt choys) PSYCHOANALYSIS the object (usually a person) on which (or whom) psychic energy is centered.

ob•jec•tive (ŏb-jek′tiv) **1.** The lens or lenses in the lower end of the body tube of a microscope. **2.** Pertaining to facts, conditions, or phenomena as they actually exist, without distortion by personal viewpoint or prejudice; open to observation by oneself and by others. Cf. subjective. **3.** A goal, as in a desired outcome of treatment. [L. *ob- jicio,* pp. *-jectus,* to throw before]

ob•jec•tive as•sess•ment da•ta (ŏb-jek′tiv ă-ses′mĕnt dā′tă) Information about a patient that is observable and measurable by the nurse.

ob•jec•tive sen•sa•tion (ŏb-jeck′tiv sen-sā′shŭn) A sensation caused by a verifiable stimulus.

ob•jec•tive symp•tom (ŏb-jek′tiv simp′tŏm) A symptom that is evident to the observer.

ob•ject per•ma•nence (ob′jekt pĕr′mă-nens) Developmental term for a child's ability to understand that objects still exist even when out of sight. Infants 8 months old or younger rarely have this ability.

ob·ject re·la·tion·ship (ob′jekt rĕ-lā′shŭn-ship) BEHAVIORAL SCIENCES the emotional bond between an individual and another person (or between two groups), as opposed to the individual's or group's interest in self.

OBLA (ob′lă) Acronym for onset of blood lactate accumulation.

ob·li·gate (ob′li-gāt) Without an alternative system or pathway. [L. *ob-ligo,* pp. *-atus,* to bind to]

ob·li·gate aer·obe (ob′li-gāt ār′ōb) An organism that cannot live or grow in the absence of oxygen.

ob·li·gate an·aer·obe (ob′li-gāt an′ăr-ōb) An anaerobe that will grow only in the absence of free oxygen.

ob·li·gate par·a·site (ob′li-gāt par′ă-sīt) A parasite that cannot lead an independent non-parasitic existence, in contrast to facultative parasite.

o·blig·a·to·ry wa·ter loss (ŏ-blig′ă-tōr-ē waw′tĕr laws) Minimal volume of urine that must be produced to dispose of dissolved wastes, which amounts to about 600 mOsm/day.

ob·lique (ō-blēk′) **1.** Slanting; deviating from the perpendicular, horizontal, sagittal, or coronal plane of the body. **2.** RADIOGRAPHY a projection that is neither frontal nor lateral. [L. *obliquus*]

ob·lique am·pu·ta·tion (ō-blēk′ amp′yū-tā′shŭn) Amputation in which the line of section through an extremity is at other than a right angle; this yields an oval appearance to the cut surface.

ob·lique ban·dage (ō-blēk′ ban′dăj) A bandage in which successive turns proceed obliquely up or down a limb, in a slanting or sloping pattern.

ob·lique di·am·e·ter (ō-blēk′ dī-am′ĕ-tĕr) A measurement across the pelvic inlet from the sacroiliac joint of one side to the opposite iliopectineal eminence.

ob·lique fi·bers of mus·cu·lar la·yer of stom·ach (ō-blēk′ fī′bĕrz mŭs′kyū-lăr lā′ĕr stŏm′ăk) The smooth muscle fibers of the innermost layer of the muscular coat of the stomach; the fibers occur chiefly at the cardiac end of the stomach and spread over the anterior and posterior surfaces.

ob·lique frac·ture (ō-blēk′ frak′shŭr) A break along the line that runs obliquely to the axis of the bone.

ob·lique lie (ō-blēk′ lī) SYN oblique presentation.

ob·lique pre·sen·ta·tion (ō-blēk′ prez′ĕn-tā′shŭn) A fetal presentation in which the long axis of the fetus is oblique (i.e., slanted) with respect to the long axis of the mother. SYN oblique lie.

ob·lique ridge (ō-blēk′ rij) A crest on the occlusal surface of upper molars comprising the distal cusp ridge of the mesiolingual cusp and the triangular ridge of the distobuccal cusp.

ob·lique sec·tion (ō-blēk′ sek′shŭn) A diagonal cross section attained by slicing, actually or through imaging techniques, the body or any part of the body or anatomic structure, in any plane that does not parallel the longitudinal axis or intersect it at a right angle, i.e., which is neither longitudinal (vertical) nor transverse (horizontal).

ob·lique vein of left a·tri·um (ō-blēk′ vān left ā′trē-ŭm) A small vein on the posterior wall of the left atrium that merges with the great cardiac vein to form the coronary sinus; it is developed from the left common cardinal vein, and occasionally persists as a left superior vena cava. SYN Marshall oblique vein.

ob·liq·ui·ty (ob-lik′wi-tē) SYN asynclitism.

ob·li·quus ca·pi·tis in·fe·ri·or mus·cle (ob-lī′kwŭs kap′i-tis in-fēr′ē-ŏr mŭs′ĕl) Suboccipital muscle that, despite its name, has no attachment to skull; *origin,* spinous process of axis; *insertion,* transverse process of atlas; *action,* rotates head. SYN inferior oblique muscle of head, musculus obliquus capitis inferior.

ob·li·quus ca·pi·tis su·pe·ri·or mus·cle (ob-lī′kwŭs kap′i-tis sŭ-pēr′ē-ŏr mŭs′ĕl) Suboccipital muscle; *origin,* transverse process of atlas; *insertion,* lateral third of inferior nuchal line; *action,* rotates head; *nerve supply,* suboccipital. SYN musculus obliquus capitis superior, superior oblique muscle of head.

ob·lit·er·ans (ob-lit′ĕ-ranz) Obliterating. [L.]

ob·lit·er·a·tion (ob-lit-ĕr-ā′shŭn) **1.** Blotting out, especially by filling of a natural space or lumen by fibrosis or inflammation. **2.** RADIOLOGY disappearance of the contour of an organ when the adjacent tissue has the same x-ray absorption. [L. *oblittero,* to blot out]

o·blit·er·a·tive bron·chi·tis, **bron·chi·tis ob·li·te·rans** (ob-lit′ĕr-ă′tiv brongk′ī-tis, brongk′ī-tis ob-lit′ĕr-anz) Fibrinous bronchitis in which the exudate is not expectorated but becomes organized, obliterating the affected portion of the bronchial tubes with consequent permanent collapse of affected portions of the lung.

ob·lit·er·at·ive per·i·car·di·tis (ob-lit′ĕr-ă′tiv per′ē-kahr-dī′tis) Complete obliteration of the pericardial cavity by postinflammatory adhesions.

ob·lon·ga·ta (ob-long-gah′tă) SYN medulla oblongata. [L. fem. of *oblongatus,* from *oblongus,* rather long]

OBS Abbreviation for organic brain syndrome.

ob•ses•sion (ob-sesh′ŭn) A recurrent and persistent idea, thought, or impulse to carry out an act that is ego-dystonic, that is experienced as senseless or repugnant, and that the person cannot voluntarily suppress. [L. *obsideo,* pp. *-sessus,* to besiege, fr. *sedeo,* to sit]

ob•ses•sive-com•pul•sive (ob-ses′iv-kŏm-pŭl′siv) Having a tendency to perform certain repetitive acts or ritualistic behavior to relieve anxiety, as in obsessive-compulsive neurosis (e.g., a compulsive, ritualistic need to wash one's hands many dozens of times per day).

ob•ses•sive-com•pul•sive dis•or•der (OCD) (ob-ses′iv-kŏm-pŭl′siv dis-ōr′dĕr) A type of anxiety disorder the essential feature of which is recurrent obsessions, persistent, intrusive ideas, thoughts, impulses or images, or compulsions (repetitive, purposeful, and intentional behaviors performed in response to an obsession) sufficiently severe to cause marked distress, be time-consuming, or interfere significantly with the person's normal routine, occupational functioning, or usual social activities or relationships with others.

ob•stet•ric, ob•stet•ri•cal (ob-stet′rik, -ri-kăl) Relating to obstetrics.

ob•stet•ric bind•er (ob-stet′rik bīn′dĕr) A supporting garment covering the abdomen from the ribs to the trochanters, tightly pinned at the back, affording support after childbirth or, rarely, during childbirth.

ob•stet•ric con•ju•gate (ob-stet′rik kon′jŭ-găt) The shortest diameter through which the fetal head must pass in descending into the superior strait; as measured by x-ray, the distance from the promontory of the sacrum to a point on the inner surface of the symphysis a few millimeters below its upper margin.

ob•stet•ric for•ceps (ob-stet′rik fōr′seps) Forceps used for grasping and applying traction to or for rotation of the fetal head; the blades are introduced separately into the genital canal, permitting the fetal head to be grasped firmly but with minimal compression, and are articulated after being placed in position.

ob•stet•ri•c hand (ob-stet′rik hand) SYN accoucheur's hand.

ob•ste•tri•cian (ob-stĕ-trish′ŭn) A physician specializing in the medical care of women during pregnancy and childbirth. SEE obstetrics.

ob•stet•ric pal•sy (ob-stet′rik pawl′zē) A brachial plexus lesion sustained by an infant during delivery; three types are recognized: 1) upper plexus type, affecting the shoulder and upper arm (Erb palsy, by far the most common form); 2) total plexus type, involving the whole arm; 3) lower plexus type, involving the forearm and hand (Klumpke palsy). SYN obstetric paralysis.

ob•stet•ric pa•ral•y•sis (ob-stet′rik păr-al′i-sis) SYN obstetric palsy.

ob•stet•rics (OB) (ob-stet′riks) The specialty of medicine concerned with the care of women during pregnancy, parturition, and the puerperium. [L. *obstetrix,* a midwife, fr. *ob-sto,* to stand before, denoting the position formerly taken by the midwife]

ob•sti•nate (ob′sti-năt) **1.** Firmly adhering to one's own purpose or opinion, even when proven wrong; not yielding to argument, persuasion, or entreaty. SYN intractable (2), refractory (2). **2.** SYN refractory (1). [L. *obstinatus,* determined]

ob•sti•pa•tion (ob′sti-pā′shŭn) Intestinal obstruction; severe constipation. [L. *ob,* against, + *stipo,* pp. *-atus,* to crowd]

ob•struc•tion (ŏb-strŭk′shŭn) Blockage or clogging, e.g., by occlusion or stenosis. [L. *obstructio*]

ob•struc•tive ap•ne•a, pe•riph•e•ral ap•ne•a (ŏb-strŭk′tiv ap′nē-ă, pĕr-if′ĕr-ăl ap′nē-ă) Apnea either as the result of obstruction of the air passages or inadequate respiratory muscle activity.

ob•struc•tive dys•men•or•rhe•a (ŏb-strŭk′tiv dis-men′ōr-ē′ă) SYN mechanical dysmenorrhea.

ob•struc•tive hy•dro•ceph•a•lus (ŏb-strŭk′tiv hī′drō-sef′ă-lŭs) Hydrocephalus secondary to a block in cerebrospinal fluid flow in the ventricular system or between the ventricular system and spinal canal. SYN noncommunicating hydrocephalus.

ob•struc•tive jaun•dice (ŏb-strŭk′tiv jawn′dis) Hepatic disorder resulting from obstruction to the flow of bile into the duodenum, whether intra- or extrahepatic. SYN mechanical jaundice.

ob•struc•tive mur•mur (ŏb-strŭk′tiv mŭr′mŭr) A murmur caused by narrowing of one of the valvular orifices.

ob•struc•tive sleep ap•ne•a (OSA) (ŏb-strŭk′tiv slēp ap′nē-ă) A disorder, first described in 1965, characterized by recurrent interruptions of breathing during sleep due to temporary obstruction of the airway by lax, excessively bulky, or malformed pharyngeal tissues (soft palate, uvula, and sometimes tonsils), with resultant hypoxemia and chronic lethargy.

ob•struc•tive throm•bus (ŏb-strŭk′tiv throm′bŭs) A thrombus due to obstruction in the vessel from compression or other cause.

ob•struc•tive ur•op•a•thy (ŏb-strŭk′tiv yūr-op′ă-thē) Any pathologic condition, anatomic or functional, of the urinary tract caused by obstruction.

ob•struc•tive ven•ti•la•tory de•fect (ŏb-strŭk′tiv ven′til-ă-tōr-ē dē′fekt) Slowing of airflow during forced ventilatory maneuvers, generally expiratory.

ob•tund (ob-tŭnd′) To dull or blunt, especially to blunt sensation or deaden pain. [L. *ob-tundo,* pp. *-tusus,* to beat against, blunt]

ob•tu•rat•ing em•bo•lism (ob′tūr-ā′ting em′bō-lizm) Complete closing of the lumen of a vessel by an embolus.

ob•tu•ra•tion (ob′tūr-ā′shŭn) Obstruction or occlusion. SEE obturator.

ob•tu•ra•tor (ob′tŭr-ā-tŏr) **1.** Any structure that occludes an opening. **2.** Denoting the obturator foramen, the obturator membrane, or any of several parts in relation to this foramen. **3.** A prosthesis used to close an opening of the hard palate, usually a cleft palate. **4.** The stylus or removable plug used during the insertion of many tubular instruments. [L. *obturo,* pp. *-atus,* to occlude or stop up]

ob•tu•ra•tor ar•ter•y (ob′tŭr-ā-tŏr ahr′tĕr-ē) *Anastomoses*, iliolumbar, inferior epigastric, medial circumflex femoral; *origin*, anterior division of the internal iliac; *distribution*, ilium, pubis, obturator and adductor muscles; *branches*, pubic, acetabular, anterior, and posterior. SYN arteria obturatoria [TA].

ob•tu•ra•tor branch of pu•bic branch of in•fe•ri•or epi•gas•tric vein (ob′tŭr-ā-tŏr branch pyū′bik branch in-fēr′ē-ŏr ep′i-gas′trik vān) Branch of the pubic branch of inferior epigastric artery that descends over the pelvic brim to anastomose with the pubic branch of the obturator artery; in 20–30% of people, this branch is larger than or replaces the obturator artery.

ob•tu•ra•tor ca•nal (ob′tŭr-ā-tŏr kă-nal′) The opening in the superior part of the obturator membrane through which the obturator nerve and vessels pass from the pelvic cavity into the thigh. SYN canalis obturatorius [TA].

ob•tu•ra•tor crest (ob′tŭr-ā-tŏr krest) A ridge that extends from the pubic tubercle to the acetabular notch, giving attachment to the pubofemoral ligament of the hip joint.

ob•tu•ra•tor ex•ter•nus mus•cle (ob′tŭr-ā-tŏr eks-tĕr′nŭs mŭs′ĕl) *Origin*, lower half of margin of obturator foramen and adjacent part of external surface of obturator membrane; *insertion*, trochanteric fossa of greater trochanter; *action*, rotates thigh laterally; *nerve supply*, obturator. See this page. SYN musculus obturatorius externus [TA], external obturator muscle.

ob•tu•ra•tor fo•ra•men (ob′tŭr-ā-tŏr fōr-ā′mĕn) A large, oval or irregularly triangular aperture in the hip bone, the margins of which are formed by the pubis and the ischium; it is closed by the obturator membrane, except for a small opening for the passage of the obturator vessels and nerve. SYN foramen obturatum [TA].

ob•tu•ra•tor her•ni•a (ob′tŭr-ā-tŏr hĕr′nē-ă) Hernia through the obturator foramen.

ob•tu•ra•tor in•ter•nus mus•cle (ob′tŭr-ā-tŏr in-tĕr′nŭs mŭs′ĕl) *Origin*, pelvic surface of obturator membrane and margin of obturator foramen; *insertion*, passes out of pelvis through lesser sciatic foramen, in so doing, making a 90° turn to insert into the medial surface of greater trochanter; *action*, rotates thigh laterally; *nerve supply*, nerve to obturator internus (sacral plexus). See this page. SYN musculus obturatorius internus [TA], internal obturator muscle.

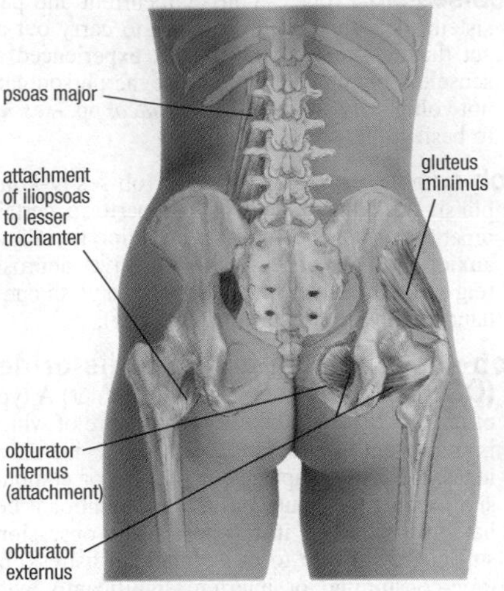

obturator externus muscle

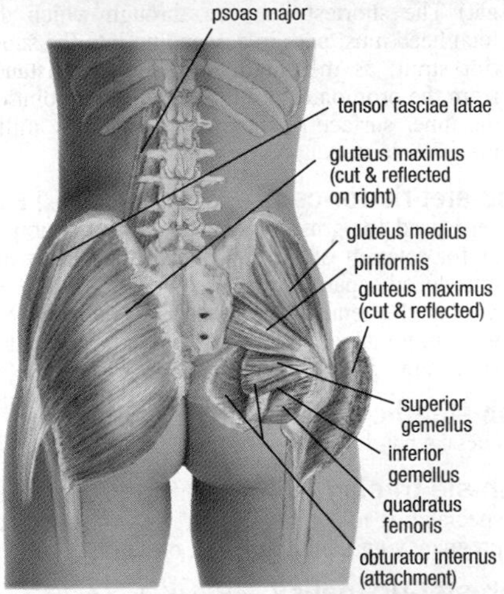

obturator internus muscle

ob•tu•ra•tor mem•brane (ob′tŭr-ā-tŏr mem′brān) The thin membrane of strong interlacing fibers filling the obturator foramen and with the surrounding bone, giving origin to the obturator externus and internus muscles.

ob•tu•ra•tor nerve (ob′tŭr-ā-tŏr nĕrv) Arises

from the second, third, and fourth lumbar nerves in the psoas muscle, crosses the brim of the pelvis, and enters the thigh through the obturator canal; it supplies muscles of the medial compartment of the thigh (adductors of thigh at the hip joint) and terminates as the cutaneous branch of the obturator nerve, supplying a small area of medial thigh above knee. SYN nervus obturatorius [TA].

ob·tu·ra·tor vein (ob′tŭr-ā-tŏr vān) Formed by the union of tributaries draining the hip joint and the obturator and adductor muscles of the thigh; it enters the pelvis by the obturator canal as venae comitantes of the obturator artery and empties into the internal iliac vein.

ob·tuse (ob-tūs′) **1.** Dull in intellect; of slow understanding. **2.** Blunt; not acute. SEE obtund.

ob·tu·sion (ob-tū′zhŭn) **1.** Dullness of sensibility. **2.** A dulling or deadening of sensibility.

OC Abbreviation for oral contraceptive.

Oc·cam's ra·zor (ok′ămz rā′zŏr) The principle of scientific parsimony. William of Occam (14th century philosopher) stated it thus: "The assumptions introduced to explain a thing must not be multiplied beyond necessity."

oc·cip·i·tal (ok-sip′i-tăl) Relating to the occiput; referring to the occipital bone or to the back of the head.

oc·cip·i·tal ar·ter·y (ok-sip′i-tăl ahr′tĕr-ē) *Origin*, external carotid; *branches*, sternocleidomastoid, meningeal, auricular, occipital, mastoid, and descending. SYN arteria occipitalis [TA].

oc·cip·i·tal bone (ok-sip′i-tăl bōn) A bone at the lower and posterior part of the skull, consisting of three parts (basilar, condylar, and squamous), enclosing a large oval hole, the foramen magnum; it articulates with the parietal and temporal bones on either side, the sphenoid anteriorly, and the atlas below. See this page. SYN os occipitale [TA].

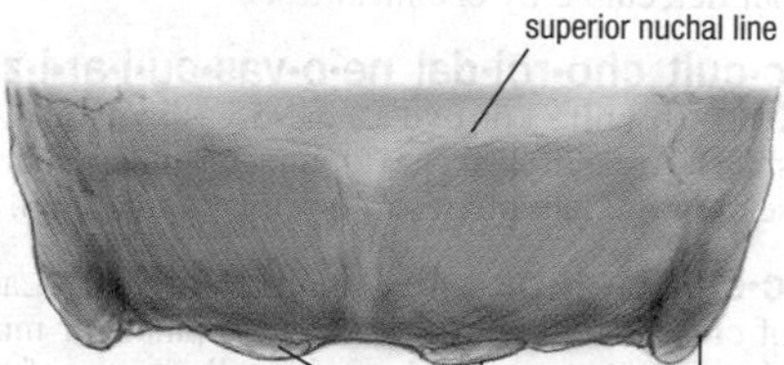

occipital bone

oc·cip·i·tal ce·re·bral veins (ok-sip′i-tăl ser′ĕ-brăl vānz) The superior cerebral veins draining the occipital cortex and emptying into the superior sagittal sinus and the transverse sinus.

oc·cip·i·tal con·dyle (ok-sip′i-tăl kon′dīl) One of two elongated oval facets on the undersurface of the occipital bone, one on each side of the foramen magnum, which articulate with the atlas.

oc·cip·i·tal·i·za·tion (ok-sip′i-tăl-ī-zā′shŭn) Bony ankylosis between the atlas and occipital bone.

oc·cip·i·tal lobe of cer·e·brum (ok-sip′i-tăl lōb ser′ĕ-brŭm) The posterior, somewhat pyramidal part of each cerebral hemisphere, demarcated by no distinct surface markings on the lateral convexity of the hemisphere from the parietal and temporal lobes, but sharply delineated from the parietal lobe by the parieto-occipital sulcus on the medial surface.

oc·cip·i·tal lobe ep·i·lep·sy (ok-sip′i-tăl lōb ep′i-lep′sē) A localization-related epilepsy where seizures originate from the occipital lobe. Symptoms commonly include visual abnormalities during seizures.

oc·cip·i·tal pole of cer·e·brum (ok-sip′i-tăl pōl ser′ĕ-brŭm) The most posterior promontory of each cerebral hemisphere; the apex of the occipital lobe.

oc·cip·i·tal si·nus (ok-sip′i-tăl sī′nŭs) An unpaired dural venous sinus commencing at the confluence of the sinuses and passing downward in the base of the falx cerebelli to the foramen magnum.

oc·cip·i·tal vein (ok-sip′i-tăl vān) Drains the occipital region and empties into the internal jugular vein or the suboccipital plexus.

occipito- Combining form indicating the occiput, occipital structures. [L. *occiput*]

oc·cip·i·to·an·te·ri·or po·si·tion (OA) (ok-sip′i-tō-an-tēr′ē-or pŏ-zish′ŏn) A cephalic presentation of the fetus with its occiput turned toward the right (right occipitoanterior, ROA) or to the left (left occipitoanterior, LOA) acetabulum of the mother.

oc·cip·i·to·fa·cial (ok-sip′i-tō-fā′shăl) Relating to the occiput and the face.

oc·cip·i·to·fron·tal (ok-sip′i-tō-frŏn′tăl) **1.** Relating to the occiput and the forehead. **2.** Relating to the occipital and frontal lobe of the cerebral cortex and association pathways that interconnect these regions.

oc·cip·i·to·fron·tal di·am·e·ter (ok-sip′i-tō-frŏn′tăl dī-am′ĕ-tĕr) The diameter of the fetal head from the external occipital protuberance to the most prominent point of the frontal bone in the midline.

oc·cip·i·to·fron·ta·lis mus·cle (ok-sip′i-tō-fron-tā′lis mŭs′ĕl) A part of musculus epicranius; the occipital belly (occipitalis muscle) arises from the occipital bone and inserts into the galea aponeurotica; the frontal belly (frontalis muscle) arises from the galea and inserts into the skin of the eyebrow and nose; *action*, to move the scalp; *nerve supply*, facial. SYN musculus occipitofrontalis [TA], occipitofrontal muscle.

oc·cip·i·to·fron·tal mus·cle (ok-sip′i-tō-frŏn′tăl mŭs′ĕl) SYN occipitofrontalis muscle.

oc·cip·i·to·men·tal (ok-sip′i-tō-men′tăl) Relating to the occiput and the chin.

oc·cip·i·to·men·tal di·am·e·ter (ok-sip′i-tō-men′tăl dī-am′ĕ-tĕr) The diameter of the fetal head from the external occipital protuberance to the midpoint of the chin.

oc·cip·i·to·pos·te·ri·or po·si·tion (OP) (ok-sip′i-tō-pos-tēr′ē-ōr pŏ-zish′ŏn) A cephalic presentation of the fetus with its occiput turned toward the right (right occipitoposterior, ROP) or to the left (left occipitoposterior, LOP) sacroiliac joint of the mother.

oc·cip·i·to·trans·verse po·si·tion (ok-sip′i-to-trans-vĕrs′ pŏ-zish′ŏn) A cephalic presentation of the fetus with its occiput turned toward the right (right occipitotransverse ROT) or to the left (left occipitotransverse, LOT) iliac fossa of the mother.

oc·ci·put, gen. **oc·cip·i·tis** (ok′si-put, ok-sip′i-tis) The back of the head. [L.]

oc·clude (ŏ-klūd′) **1.** To close, plug, obstruct, or bring together. **2.** To enclose, as in an occluded virus. SEE occlusion.

oc·clu·sal (ŏ-klū′zăl) **1.** Pertaining to occlusion or closure. **2.** DENTISTRY pertaining to the contacting surfaces of opposing occlusal units (teeth or occlusion rims), or the masticating surfaces of the posterior teeth.

oc·clu·sal ad·just·ment (ŏ-klū′zal ă-jŭst′mĕnt) Selective grinding of occlusal (i.e., masticatory) surfaces of the teeth to eliminate premature contacts and occlusal interferences. SYN adjustment (2).

oc·clu·sal a·nal·y·sis (ŏ-klū′zăl ă-nal′i-sis) A study of the relations of the occlusal surfaces of opposing teeth and their effect on related structures. SYN bite analysis.

oc·clu·sal e·quil·i·bra·tion (ŏ-klū′zăl ē-kwil-i-brā′shŭn) The modification of occlusal forms of teeth by grinding with the intent of equalizing occlusal stress, or of producing simultaneous occlusal contacts, or of harmonizing cuspal relations.

oc·clu·sal film (ŏ-klū′zăl film) Intraoral projection taken to provide a wider view of either the maxilla and palate or the mandible and floor of the mouth. Used to view eruption pattern of teeth.

oc·clu·sal force (ŏ-klū′zăl fōrs) The result of muscular force applied on opposing teeth.

oc·clu·sal guard (ŏ-klū′zăl gahrd) SYN night guard.

oc·clu·sal im·bal·ance (ŏ-klū′zăl im-bal′ăns) An inharmonious relationship between the teeth of the maxilla and mandible during closing or functional movements of the jaw.

oc·clu·sal po·si·tion (ŏ-klū′zăl pŏ-zish′ŏn) The relationship of the mandible and maxillae when the jaws are closed and the teeth are in maximum contact; may or may not coincide with centric occlusion.

oc·clu·sion (ŏ-klū′zhŭn) **1.** The act of closing or the state of being closed. **2.** In chemistry, the absorption of a gas by a metal or the inclusion of one substance within another (as in a gelatinous precipitate). **3.** Any contact between the incising or masticating surfaces of the upper and lower teeth. **4.** The relationship between the occlusal surfaces of the maxillary and mandibular teeth when they are in contact. [L. *oc- cludo,* pp. *-clusus,* to shut up, fr. *ob.*, against, + *claudo,* to close]

oc·clu·sive (ŏ-klū′siv) Serving to close; denoting a bandage or dressing that closes a wound and excludes it from the air.

oc·clu·sive dress·ing (ŏ-klū′siv dres′ing) A dressing that hermetically seals a wound.

oc·clu·sive il·e·us (ŏ-klū′siv il′ē-ŭs) Complete mechanical blocking of the intestinal lumen.

oc·clu·sive men·in·gi·tis (ŏ-klū′siv men-in-jī′tis) Leptomeningitis causing occlusion of the spinal fluid pathways.

oc·cult (ŏ-kŭlt′) **1.** Hidden; concealed; not manifest. **2.** Denoting a disease or condition (bleeding, infection) that is clinically inapparent, though it may be inferred from indirect evidence or identified by special tests. SEE occult blood. **3.** ONCOLOGY a clinically unidentified primary tumor with recognized metastases. [L. *oc-culo,* pp. *-cultus,* to cover, hide]

oc·cult blood (ŏ-kŭlt′ blŭd) Blood in the feces in amounts too small to be seen by the naked eye but detectable by chemical tests.

oc·cult cho·roi·dal ne·o·vas·cu·l·ar·i·za·tion (ŏ-kŭlt′ kōr-oyd′ăl, nē-ō-vas′kyū-lăr-ī-zā′shŭn) Area of leakage of undetermined source seen in the late phases of a retinal angiogram.

oc·cult cleft pa·late (ŏ-kŭlt′ kleft pal′ăt) Lack of closure in the bone of the hard palate or muscle of the soft palate, but with full closure of the overlying surface tissues. SYN submucous cleft palate.

oc·cult frac·ture (ŏ-kŭlt′ frak′shŭr) A condition in which there are clinical signs of fracture but no radiologic evidence; after 3–4 weeks, radiologic imaging shows new bone formation.

oc·cult PEEP (ŏ-kŭlt′ pēp) SYN auto-positive-end-expiratory-pressure.

oc·cult pos·te·ri·or la·ryn·ge·al cleft

(ŏ-kŭlt′ pos-tēr′ē-ŏr lă-rin′jē-ăl kleft) SEE laryngotracheoesophageal cleft.

oc•cu•pa•tion (ok′yū-pā′shŭn) The activity that constitutes the social contribution one makes, for which some sort of compensation may generally be received.

oc•cu•pa•tion•al dis•ease (ok′yū-pā′shŭn-ăl di-zēz′) A morbid condition resulting from exposure to an agent during the usual performance of one's occupation. Cf. industrial disease.

oc•cu•pa•tion•al hear•ing loss (ok′yū-pā′shŭn-ăl hēr′ing laws) SYN noise-induced hearing loss.

oc•cu•pa•tion•al per•for•mance (ok′yū-pā′shŭn-ăl pĕr-fōr′măns) Broadly, engagement in purposeful activity; such behavior has an organizing and integrating effect on psychological and social functioning; it is employed in occupational therapy to restore or maintain interest and self-confidence, overcome disability, or combat various features of physical or mental illness.

oc•cu•p•atio•nal pro•file (ok′yū-pā′shŭn-ăl prō′fīl) A method of systematically describing a person's occupational history, patterns of daily living, interests, values, and needs.

oc•cu•pa•tion•al role (ok′yū-pā′shŭn-ăl rōl) A set of behaviors connected to social norms that allows someone to organize and allocate time for self-care activities, work, play, social activities, leisure, and rest; examples include the roles of student, spouse, worker, and caregiver.

oc•cu•pa•tion•al sci•ence (ok′yū-pā′shŭn-ăl sī′ĕns) The study of the effects of occupation on human behavior.

oc•cu•pa•tion•al ther•a•pist (ok′yū-pā′shŭn-ăl thār′ă-pist) A degree conferred on completion of a 2-year professional course pursued by the holder of a B.A. or B.Sc. degree. Practitioners use their skills to help patients regain or continue living a normal life after illness or injury.

oc•cu•pa•tion•al ther•a•py (ok′yū-pā′shŭn-ăl thār′ă-pē) Therapeutic use of self-care, work, and recreational activities to increase independent function, enhance development, prevent disability, and achieve optimum quality of life.

oc•cur•rence (ŏ-kŭr′ĕns) Any event or incident.

OCD Abbreviation for obsessive-compulsive disorder.

***o*-chlor•o•ben•zyl•i•dene mal•o•non•i•trile** (ōr′thō-klōr-ō-bĕn-zĭl′ī -dēn măl-ō′nō-nī′trīl′) A compound (NATO code CS) widely used as a lacrimator on the battlefield and as a riot-control agent in law enforcement.

O•cho•a law (ō-chō′ah law) The content of the X-chromosome tends to be phylogenetically conserved.

och•ra•tox•in (ō-kra-toks′in) A mycotoxin produced by *Aspergillus ochraceus* growing on stored cereal grains. Affects poultry and other animals fed the grain.

och•ra•tox•in A (ō-kra-toks′in) Ochratoxin produced by some species of *Aspergillus* and *Penicillium* that can contaminate cereal grains and feeds, primarily following improper storage; a potent carcinogen in rodents.

o•chre co•don (ō′kĕr kō′don) The termination codon UAA.

Och•ro•bac•trum (ō-krō-bak′trum) A gram-negative genus of bacteria similar to *Alcaligenes* and *Pseudomonas* spp. in their distribution in environmental and water sources and their culture characteristics; have been isolated from a number of clinical sources and appear to be a cause of nosocomial bacteremia.

o•chrom•e•ter (ō-krom′ĕ-tĕr) An instrument for determining the capillary blood pressure; one of two adjacent fingers is compressed by a rubber balloon until blanching of the skin occurs, after which the force necessary to accomplish this color change is read in millimeters of mercury. [G. *ōchros,* pale yellow, + *metron,* measure]

o•chro•no•sis (ō-kron-ō′sis) A condition observed in people with alkaptonuria, characterized by pigmentation of the cartilages; also may affect the sclerae, mucous membrane of the lips, and skin of the ears, face, and hands and may cause standing urine to be dark and contain pigmented casts; pigmentation results from oxidized homogentisic acid; cartilage degeneration results in osteoarthritis. [G. *ōchros,* pale yellow, + *nosos,* disease]

o•chro•not•ic (ō-kron-ot′ik) Relating to or characterized by ochronosis.

OCN Abbreviation for oncology certified nurse.

♻ **oct-, octi-, octo-, octa-** Combining forms meaning eight. [G. *oktō,* L. *octo*]

oc•ta•fluor•o•pro•pane (ok′tă-flōr′ō-prō′pān) A drug used for contrast enhancement during ultrasound imaging.

oc•tan (ok′tan) Applied to fever, the paroxysms of which recur every eighth day, the day of a paroxysm being counted as the first in the computation. [L. *octo,* eight]

oc•u•lar (ok′yū-lăr) **1.** SYN ophthalmic. **2.** The eyepiece of a microscope, the lens or lenses at the observer end of a microscope, by means of which the image focused by the objective is viewed. [L. *oculus,* eye]

oc•u•lar al•bin•ism 1 (ok′yū-lăr al′bin-izm) Visual disorder characterized by depigmentation of the fundus and prominent choroidal vessels, nystagmus, and titubation; vision is usually impaired; caused by mutation in the OA1 gene on chromosome Xp; X-linked inheritance. SYN Nettleship-Falls albinism.

oc•u•lar al•bin•ism 2 (ok′yū-lăr al′bin-izm) Visual disorder characterized by hypoplasia of the fovea, marked impairment of vision, nystagmus, myopia, astigmatism, and protanomalous color blindness, in addition to albinism of the fundus. SYN Forsius-Eriksson albinism.

oc•u•lar al•bin•ism 3 (ok′yū-lăr al′bin-izm) Visual disorder characterized by impaired vision, translucent irides, congenital nystagmus, photophobia, albinotic fundi with hyperplasia of the fovea, and strabismus; caused by mutation in the pinkeye gene (P) on 6q; autosomal recessive inheritance.

oc•u•lar al•bi•nism (ok′yū-lăr al′bin-izm) Absence of pigment chiefly in the iris, choroid, and retinal pigment epithelium with deafness; X-linked inheritance. SYN Aland Island albinism.

oc•u•lar cic•a•tri•cial pem•phi•goid (ok′yū-lăr sik′ă-trish′ăl pem′fi-goyd) A chronic disease that produces adhesions and progressive cicatrization and shrinkage of the conjunctival, oral, and vaginal mucous membranes.

oc•u•lar dys•me•tri•a (ok′yū-lăr dis-mē′trē-ă) An abnormality of ocular movements in which the eyes overshoot on attempting to fixate on an object; usually indicating cerebellar disease; symptom of several neurologic conditions, including multiple sclerosis. [L. *oculus,* eye + dys- + G. *metron,* measure]

oc•u•lar hu•mor (ok′yū-lăr hyū′mŏr) One of the two humors of the eye: aqueous and vitreous.

oc•u•lar hy•per•tel•or•ism (ok′yū-lăr hī′pĕr-tel′ŏr-izm) Increased width between the eyes due to an enlarged sphenoid bone; other congenital anomalies and mental retardation may be associated. SYN Greig syndrome, Opitz BBB syndrome, Opitz G syndrome.

oc•u•lar•ist (ok′yū-lăr-ist) One skilled in the design, fabrication, and fitting of artificial eyes and the making of prostheses associated with the appearance or function of the eyes. [L. *oculus,* eye]

oc•u•lar lar•va mi•grans gran•u•lo•ma (ok′yū-lăr lahr′vă mī′granz gran′yū-lō′mă) Eosinophilic granulomata found surrounding dead worms (generally, *Toxocara* spp.) in the eye; may mimic retinoblastoma.

oc•u•lar ten•sion (Tn) (ok′yū-lăr ten′shŭn) Resistance of the tunics of the eye to deformation; it can be estimated digitally or measured by means of a tonometer. The pressure in the eye is measured in increased mmHg levels.

oc•u•lar ver•ti•go (ok′yū-lăr vĕr′ti-gō) Dizziness attributed to refractive errors or imbalance of the extrinsic muscles.

oc•u•li (ok′yu-lī) Plural of oculus. [L.]

oc•u•list (ok′yū-list) SYN ophthalmologist. [L. *oculus,* eye]

♻**oculo-** Combining form meaning the eye, ocular. SEE ALSO ophthalmo-. [L. *oculus*]

oc•u•lo•cu•ta•ne•ous (ok′yū-lō-kyū-tā′nē-ŭs) Relating to the eyes and the skin.

oc•u•lo•dyn•i•a (ok′yū-lō-din′ē-ă) Pain in the eyeball. [ophthalmo- + G. *algos,* pain]

oc•u•lo•fa•cial (ok′yū-lō-fā′shăl) Relating to the eyes and the face.

oc•u•log•ra•phy (ok′yū-log′ră-fē) A method of recording eye position and movements. [oculo- + G. *graphē,* a writing]

oc•u•lo•gy•ri•a (ok′yū-lō-jī′rē-ă) The limits of rotation of the eyeballs. [oculo- + G. *gyros,* circle]

oc•u•lo•gy•ric (ok′yū-lō-jī′rik) Referring to rotation of the eyeballs; characterized by oculogyria.

oc•u•lo•mo•tor (ok′yū-lō-mō′tŏr) Pertaining to the oculomotor cranial nerve. [L. *oculomotorius,* fr. oculo- + L. *motorius,* moving]

oc•u•lo•mo•tor nerve [CN III] (ok′yū-lō-mō′tŏr nĕrv) The third cranial nerve, it supplies all the extrinsic muscles of the eye, except the lateral rectus and superior oblique; it also supplies the levator palpebrae superioris and conveys presynaptic parasympathetic fibers to the ciliary ganglion for innervation of the ciliary muscle and sphincter pupillae; its origin is in the midbrain below the cerebral aqueduct; it emerges from the brain in the interpeduncular fossa, pierces the dura mater to the side of the posterior clinoid process, passes in the lateral wall of the cavernous sinus, and enters the orbit through the superior orbital fissure. SYN nervus oculomotorius [CN III] [TA], third cranial nerve [CN III].

oc•u•lo•mo•tor nu•cle•us (ok′yū-lō-mō′tŏr nū′klē-ŭs) The composite group of motor neurons innervating all of the external eye muscles except the musculus rectus lateralis and musculus obliquus superior, and including the musculus levator palpebrae superioris; the most rostral component of the nucleus is the Edinger-Westphal nucleus, which innervates the musculi sphincter pupillae and ciliaris through the ciliary ganglion. The oculomotor nucleus lies in the rostral half of the midbrain, near the midline in the most ventral part of the central gray substance; fibers of the medial longitudinal fasciculus form its lateral borders.

oc•u•lo•na•sal (ok′yū-lō-nā′zăl) Relating to the eyes and the nose. [oculo- + L. *nasus,* nose]

oc•u•lo•pha•ryn•ge•al dys•tro•phy (ok′yū-lō-fă-rin′jē-ăl dis′trŏ-fē) A dominantly inherited form of chronic progressive external ophthalmoplegia usually presenting in middle life or old age with chronic ptosis and difficulty swallowing. Many sufferers have Québecois ancestry.

oc•u•lo•pleth•ys•mog•ra•phy (ok′yū-lō-pleth-iz-mog′ră-fē) Indirect measurement of the hemodynamic significance of internal carotid artery stenosis or occlusion by demonstration of an ipsilateral delay in the arrival of ocular pressure transmitted from branches of the ophthalmic artery. [oculo- + G. *plēthymos,* increase, + *graphē,* to write]

oc•u•lo•pneu•mo•pleth•ys•mog•ra•phy (ok′yū-lō-nū′mō-pleth-iz-mog′ră-fē) A method of bilateral measurement of ophthalmic artery pressure that reflects pressure and flow in the internal carotid artery. SEE oculoplethysmography.

oc•u•lo•pu•pil•lar•y (ok′yū-lō-pyū′pi-lar-ē) Pertaining to the pupil of the eye.

oc•u•lo•sym•pa•thet•ic (ok′yū-lō-sim-pă-the′tik) Pertaining to the sympathetic pathway to the eye, damage to which produces Horner syndrome.

oc•u•lo•zy•go•mat•ic (ok′yū-lō-zī-gō-mat′ik) Relating to the orbit or its margin and the zygomatic bone.

oc•u•lus, gen. and pl. **oc•u•li** (ok′yū-lŭs, -lī) [TA] SYN eye (1). [L.]

♻ **ocy-** SEE oxy-.

OD Abbreviation for drug overdose; optic density (SEE ALSO absorbance); oculus dexter (L. right eye); Doctor of Optometry.

od (od) A force assumed to be exerted on the nervous system by magnets. [G. *hodos,* way]

o•dax•et•ic (ō′dak-set′ik) **1.** Causes formication or itching. **2.** An agent or substance that causes formication or itching. [G. *odaxēsmos,* an irritation]

OD'd (ō-dēd′) A slang abbreviation for the term overdosed. It typically refers to a person who has suffered adverse effects from taking too much of an illicit drug, such as heroin.

♻ **-odes** Suffix meaning having the form of, resembling. [G. *eidos,* form, resemblance]

♻ **odont-**, **odonto-** Prefix meaning a tooth, teeth. [G. *odous* (*odont-*)]

o•don•tal•gi•a (ō-don-tal′jē-ă) SYN toothache. [odont- + G. *algos,* pain]

o•don•tal•gic (ō-don-tal′jik) Relating to or marked by toothache.

o•don•tec•to•my (ō-don-tek′tŏ-mē) Removal of teeth by the reflection of a mucoperiosteal flap and excision of bone from around the root or roots before the application of force to effect the tooth removal. [odont- + G. *ektomē,* excision]

♻ **-odontia**, **-odontic** Combining form meaning teeth or dentistry (e.g., periodontia).

o•don•ti•a•sis (ō′don-tī′ă-sis) Teething; the eruption or "cutting" of teeth, especially deciduous teeth. [G. *odontiaō,* to cut teeth]

o•don•to•blast (ō-don′tō-blast) One of the dentin-forming cells, derived from mesenchyme of neural crest origin, lining the pulp cavity of a tooth. [odonto- + G. *blastos,* sprout, germ]

o•don•to•blas•tic lay•er (ō-don′tō-blast′ik lā′ĕr) A layer of connective tissue cells at the periphery of the dental pulp of the tooth.

o•don•to•blas•to•ma (ō-don′tō-blas-tō′mă) **1.** A tumor composed of neoplastic epithelial and mesenchymal cells that may differentiate into cells able to produce calcified tooth substances. **2.** An odontoma in its early formative stage. [odontoblast + G. *-oma,* tumor]

o•don•to•clast (ō-don′tō-klast) One of the osteoclastic cells believed to produce resorption of the roots of the deciduous teeth. [odonto- + G. *klastos,* broken]

o•don•to•dys•pla•si•a (ō-don′tō-dis-plā′zē-ă) A developmental disturbance of one or of several adjacent teeth, of unknown etiology, characterized by deficient formation of enamel and dentin that results in an abnormally large pulp chamber and imparts a ghostlike radiographic image to the teeth; such teeth exhibit delayed eruption into the oral cavity.

o•don•to•gen•e•sis (ō-don′tō-jen′ĕ-sis) The process of development of the teeth. SYN odontogeny, odontosis. [odonto- + G. *genesis,* production]

o•don•to•gen•ic cyst (ō-don′tō-jen′ĭk sist) A cyst derived from odontogenic epithelium. [odont- + G. *genos,* birth, origin, + suffix *-ic,* pertaining to]

o•don•to•gen•ic ke•ra•to•cyst (ō-don′tō-jen′ik ker′ă-tō-sist) A cyst originating in the dental lamina that has a high recurrence rate, a corrugated parakeratin surface, uniformly thin epithelium, and a palisaded basal layer; one manifestation of the basal cell nevus syndrome.

o•don•tog•e•ny (ō′don-toj′ĕ-nē) SYN odontogenesis.

o•don•to•glyph•ics (ō-don′tō-glif′iks) A method of classification of the molar grooves defined in an individually distinctive pattern like that of fingerprints. [odonto- + G. *glyphē,* carving]

o•don•toid (ō-don′toyd) **1.** Shaped like a tooth. **2.** Relating to the toothlike odontoid process of the second cervical vertebra. [odont- + G. *eidos,* resemblance]

o•don•toid pro•cess of ep•i•stro•phe•us (ō-don′toyd pros′es ep′i-strō′fē-ŭs) SYN dens (2).

o·don·tol·o·gy (ō′don-tol′ŏ-jē) The study of the teeth and their supporting structures. [odonto- + G. *logos,* study]

o·don·tol·y·sis (ō′don-tol′i-sis) SYN erosion (3). [odonto- + G. *lysis,* dissolution]

o·don·to·ma (ō′don-tō′mă) **1.** A tumor of odontogenic origin. **2.** A hamartomatous odontogenic tumor composed of enamel, dentin, cementum, and pulp tissue that may or may not be arranged in the form of a tooth. [odonto- + G. *-oma,* tumor]

o·don·to·neu·ral·gi·a (ō-don′tō-nū-ral′jē-ă) Facial neuralgia caused by a carious tooth.

o·don·ton·o·my (ō′don-ton′ŏ-mē) Dental nomenclature. [odonto- + G. *onoma,* name]

o·don·top·a·thy (ō′don-top′ă-thē) Any disease of the teeth or of their sockets. [odonto- + G. *pathos,* suffering]

o·don·to·plas·ty (ō-don′tō-plas-tē) Reshaping of a portion of a tooth; may be performed for therapeutic or cosmetic purposes. [odonto- + -plasty]

o·don·to·sis (ō′don-tō′sis) SYN odontogenesis.

o·don·tot·o·my (ō′don-tot′ŏ-mē) Cutting into the crown of a tooth. [odonto- + G. *tomē,* incision]

o·dor (ō′dŏr) Emanation from any substance that stimulates the olfactory cells in the organ of smell. SYN smell (3). [L.]

ODTS Abbreviation for organic dust toxic syndrome.

♲**odyn-, odyno-** Combining forms meaning pain. [G. *odynē*]

o·dyn·a·cu·sis (ō-din′ă-kyū′sis) Hypersensitivity of the organ of hearing, so that noises cause actual pain. [odyn- + G. *akouō,* to hear]

o·dy·nom·e·ter (ō′di-nom′ĕ-tĕr) SYN algesiometer. [odyno- + G. *metron,* measure]

o·dyn·o·pha·gi·a (ō-din′ō-fā′jē-ă) Pain on swallowing. [odyno- + G. *phagō* to eat]

♲**oe-** For words so beginning and not found here, see e-.

oedema [Br.] SYN edema.

oedematous [Br.] SYN edematous.

oe·di·pal phase (ed′i-păl fāz) PSYCHOANALYSIS a stage in the psychosexual development of the child, characterized by erotic attachment to the parent of the opposite sex, repressed because of fear of the parent of the same sex; usually seen in children aged 3–6 years.

oe·di·pism (ed′i-pizm) **1.** Self-infliction of injury to the eyes, usually an attempt at evulsion. **2.** Manifestation of the Oedipus complex. [*Oedipus,* G. myth. char.]

Oed·i·pus com·plex (ed′i-pŭs kom′pleks) A group of associated ideas, aims, instinctual drives, and fears in male children 3–6 years old; at the peak of the phallic phase of psychosexual development, the child's sexual interest is attached primarily to the mother and is accompanied by aggressive feelings toward the father; in psychoanalytic theory, it is replaced by the castration complex. [*Oedipus,* G. myth. char.]

oenology [Br.] SYN enology.

oenomania [Br.] SYN delirium tremens.

OER Abbreviation for oxygen enhancement ratio.

oer·sted (er′sted) A unit of magnetic field intensity; the magnetic field intensity that exerts a force of 1 dyne on unit magnetic pole; equal to $(1000/4\pi)\ A{\cdot}m^{-1}$.

oesophageal [Br.] SYN esophageal.

oesophageal achalasia [Br.] SYN esophageal achalasia.

oesophageal hiatus [Br.] SYN esophageal hiatus.

oesophageal lead [Br.] SYN esophageal lead.

oesophageal reflux [Br.] SYN esophageal reflux.

oesophageal speech [Br.] SYN esophageal speech.

oesophageal varices [Br.] SYN esophageal varices.

oesophageal veins [Br.] SYN esophageal veins.

oesophagectasia [Br.] SYN esophagectasia.

oesophagectasis [Br.] SYN esophagectasis.

oesophagectomy [Br.] SYN esophagectomy.

oesophagi [Br.] SYN esophagi.

oesophagism [Br.] SYN esophagism.

oesophagitis [Br.] SYN esophagitis.

oesophagocardioplasty [Br.] SYN esophagocardioplasty.

oesophagocele [Br.] SYN esophagocele.

oesophagoduodenostomy [Br.] SYN esophagoduodenostomy.

oesophagoenterostomy [Br.] SYN esophagoenterostomy.

oesophagogastrectomy [Br.] SYN esophagogastrectomy.

oesophagogastric junction [Br.] SYN esophagogastric junction.

oesophagogastroanastomosis [Br.] SYN esophagogastroanastomosis.

oesophagogastroduodenoscopy [Br.] SYN esophagogastroduodenoscopy.

oesophagogastroplasty [Br.] SYN esophagogastroplasty.

oesophagogastrostomy [Br.] SYN esophagogastrostomy.

oesophagogram [Br.] SYN esophagogram.

oesophagography [Br.] SYN esophagography.

oesophagomalacia [Br.] SYN esophagomalacia.

oesophagomyotomy [Br.] SYN esophagomyotomy.

oesophagoplasty [Br.] SYN esophagoplasty.

oesophagoplication [Br.] SYN esophagoplication.

oesophagoptosia [Br.] SYN esophagoptosia.

oesophagoptosis [Br.] SYN esophagoptosis.

oesophagoscope [Br.] SYN esophagoscope.

oesophagoscopy [Br.] SYN esophagoscopy.

oesophagospasm [Br.] SYN esophagospasm.

oesophagostenosis [Br.] SYN esophagostenosis.

oesophagostomiasis [Br.] SYN esophagostomiasis.

Oe·soph·a·gos·to·mum (ē-sof′ă-gos′tō-mŭm) A genus of nematodes (superfamily Strongyloidea), which parasitize the intestines of animals; larvae encyst in the intestinal wall.

oesophagostomy [Br.] SYN esophagostomy.

oesophagotomy [Br.] SYN esophagotomy.

oesophagus [Br.] SYN esophagus.

oestradiol [Br.] SYN estradiol.

oestriol [Br.] SYN estriol.

oestrogen [Br.] SYN estrogen.

oestrogenic [Br.] SYN estrogenic.

oestrogen receptor [Br.] SYN estrogen receptor.

oestrogen replacement therapy [Br.] SYN estrogen replacement therapy.

oestrone [Br.] SYN estrone.

oestrous cycle [Br.] SYN estrous cycle.

oestrual [Br.] SYN estrual.

oestruation [Br.] SYN estruation.

oestrus [Br.] SYN estrus.

of·fice hy·per·ten·sion (awf′is hī′pĕr-ten′shŭn) SYN white coat hypertension.

Of·fice of In·spec·tor Gen·er·al (OIG) (aw′fis in-spek′tŏr jen′ĕr-ăl) Government (federal, state) agency that investigates and prosecutes fraud in government health care programs.

Of·fice of the In·spec·tor Gen·er·al's (OIG) work plan (aw′fis in-spek′tŏr jen′ĕr-ălz wŏrk plan) The OIG's annual list of planned projects under the U.S. federal Medicare Fraud and Abuse Initiative.

of·fi·cial (ō-fish′ăl) Authoritative; denoting a drug, a chemical, or a pharmaceutical preparation recognized as standard in the Pharmacopeia. [L. *officialis,* fr. *officium,* a favor, service, fr. *opus,* work, + *facio,* to do]

of·fi·cial for·mu·la (ō-fish′ăl fōrm′yū-lă) A formula contained in the Pharmacopeia or the National Formulary.

off-la·bel in·di·ca·tion (awf-lā′bĕl in′di-kā′shŭn) Use of a medication for a purpose other than that approved by the U.S. Food and Drug Administration.

off-site tran·scrip·tion (awf′sīt tran-skrip′shŭn) System in which medical transcription is done outside of the health care facility; a satellite facility, home-based transcription, or a medical transcription service may be used. SYN remote transcription.

off-ver·ti·cal ro·ta·tion (awf-vĕr′ti-kăl rō-tā′shŭn) Rotation about an axis eccentric to the body.

O·fu·ji dis·ease (ō-fū′jē di-zēz′) SYN eosinophilic pustular folliculitis.

Og·il·vie syn·drome (ō′gil-vē sin′drōm) Pseudoobstruction, predominantly of the colon, believed to be the result of motility disturbance; without physical obstruction.

O·gi·no-Knaus rule (ō-jē′nō-naws′ rūl) The time in the menstrual period when conception is most likely to occur is at about midway between two menstrual periods; fertilization of the ovum is least likely just before or just after menstruation; the basis for the rhythm method of contraception.

Og·ston line (og′stŏn līn) A line drawn from the adductor tubercle of the femur to the intercondylar notch; a guide to resection of the medial condyle for knock-knee.

O·gu·chi dis·ease (ō-gū′chē di-zēz′) A rare congenital nonprogressive night blindness with diffuse yellow or gray coloration of fundus; after two or three hours in total darkness, fundus resumes normal color; autosomal recessive inheritance, caused by mutation in either the arrestin gene (SAG) on 2q or the rhodopsin kinase gene (RHOK) on 13q.

O·gu·ra op·er·a·tion (ō-gū′ră op-ĕr-ā′shŭn) Orbital decompression by removal of the floor of the orbit through an opening made in the supradental (canine) fossa.

O·har·a dis·ease (ō-har′ă di-zēz′) Another name for tularemia, which is caused by *Francisella tularensis* (q.v.).

OHI-S Abbreviation for Simplified Oral Hygiene Index.

ohm (Ω) (ōm) The practical unit of electrical resistance; the resistance of any conductor allowing 1 ampere of current to pass under the electromotive force of 1 volt.

Ohm law (ōm law) In an electric current passing through a wire, the intensity of the current (I) in amperes equals the electromotive force (E) in volts divided by the resistance (R) in ohms: $I = E/R$.

oh·ne Hauch (ō′nĕ howk[h]) Term used to designate the nonspreading growth of nonflagellated bacteria on agar media; also applied to somatic agglutination. SEE ALSO O antigen. [Ger. without breath]

Ohn·gren line (ōn′gren līn) A theoretic plane passing between the medial canthus of the eye and the angle of the mandible; used as an arbitrary dividing line in classifying localized tumors of the maxillary sinus; tumors above the line invade vital structures early and have a poorer prognosis, whereas those below the line have a more favorable prognosis.

OI Abbreviation for osteogenesis imperfecta.

OID Abbreviation for object-to-image distance.

-oid Combining form meaning resemblance to, joined properly to words formed from G. roots; equivalent to Eng. -form. [G. *eidos,* form, resemblance]

o·id·i·o·my·cin (ō-id′ē-ō-mī′sin) An antigen used to demonstrate cutaneous hypersensitivity in patients infected with *Candida;* one of a series of antigens used to demonstrate an immunocompromised patient's capacity to react to any cutaneous antigen. [oidium + G. *mykēs,* fungus, + -in]

OIG Abbreviation for Office of Inspector General.

oil (oyl) An inflammable liquid, of fatty consistency and unctuous feel, that is insoluble in water, soluble or insoluble in alcohol, and freely soluble in ether. Oils are variously classified as animal, vegetable, or mineral, according to their source; into fatty (fixed) and volatile oils; and into drying and nondrying (fatty) oils, the former becoming gradually thicker when exposed to air and finally drying to a varnish, the latter not drying but liable to become rancid on exposure. Many of the oils, both fixed and volatile, are used in medicine. For individual oils, see the specific names.

oil re·ten·tion en·e·ma (oyl rē-ten′shŭn en′ĕ-mă) An enema containing approximately 250 mL of an oil-based fluid, prescribed to soften a hardened fecal mass and ease its passage through the anal canal, after being retained by the patient for at least 30 minutes. SYN emollient enema, lubricating enema.

oil of vi·tri·ol (oyl vit′rē-ol) SYN sulfuric acid.

oint·ment (oynt′mĕnt) A semisolid preparation usually containing medicinal substances and intended for external application. SYN salve, unguent. [O. Fr. *oignement;* L. *unguo,* pp. *unctus,* to smear]

OKT cells (selz) Cells recognized by monoclonal antibodies to T lymphocyte antigens. Current usage favors CD designations. [*Ortho-Kung T* cell]

-ol Suffix denoting that a substance is an alcohol or a phenol.

Old·field syn·drome (ōld′fēld sin′drōm) Familial polyposis of the colon.

Old World leish·man·i·a·sis (ōld wŏrld lēsh′mă-nī′ă-sis) SYN cutaneous leishmaniasis.

-ole Combining form meaning small or little (e.g., arteriole). [L. *-olus, -ola, -olum,* dim. suffixes]

o·le·ag·i·nous (ō-lē-aj′i-nŭs) Oily or greasy. [L. *oleagineus,* pertaining to *olea,* the olive tree]

o·le·ate (ō′lē-āt) **1.** A salt of oleic acid. **2.** A pharmacopeial preparation consisting of a combination or solution of an alkaloid or metallic base in oleic acid, used as an inunction.

o·lec·ra·non (ō-lek′ră-non) [TA] The prominent curved proximal extremity of the ulna, the upper and posterior surface of which gives attachment to the tendon of the triceps muscle, the anterior surface entering into the formation of the trochlear notch. SYN elbow bone, point of elbow. [G. the head or point of the elbow, fr. *ōlenē,* ulna, + *kranion,* skull, head]

ole·fin (ō′lĕ-fin) SYN alkene.

oleo- Combining form meaning oil. SEE ALSO eleo-. [L. *oleum*]

o·le·o·sa (ō-lē-ō′să) Oily. [L.]

o·les·tra A fat substitute that is stable for frying, but that also prevents fatty acids and fat-soluble vitamins from being absorbed. Some adverse effects have been reported.

o·le·um car·i (ō′lē-ŭm kar′ī) SYN caraway. [L. *oleum,* oil, + *cari,* of caraway, fr. *carum carvi,* caraway seed]

ol·fac·tion (ōl-fak′shŭn) **1.** The sense of smell. SYN smell (2). **2.** The act of smelling. See page 1103. SYN osphresis. [L. *ol- facio,* pp. *-factus,* to smell]

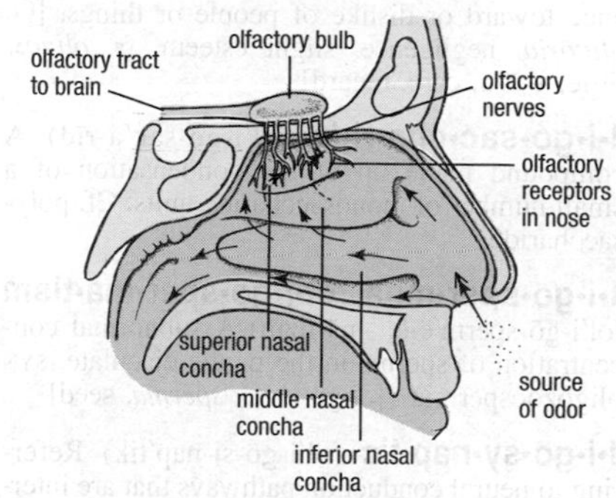

olfaction

ol·fac·to·ry (ōl-fak′tŏr-ē) Relating to the sense of smell. SEE olfaction. SYN osphretic.

ol·fac·tory ag·no·si·a (ōl-fak′tŏr-ē ag-nō′zē-ă) Inability to classify or identify an odorant, although the ability to distinguish between or recognize odorants may be normal; may be general, partial, or specific.

ol·fac·tory au·ra (ōl-fak′tŏr-ē awr′ă) Epileptic aura characterized by illusions or hallucinations of smell. SEE ALSO aura (1).

ol·fac·to·ry bulb (ōl-fak′tŏr-ē bŭlb) The grayish expanded rostral extremity of the olfactory tract, lying on the cribriform plate of the ethmoid and receiving the olfactory filaments. SYN bulbus olfactorius [TA].

ol·fac·to·ry ep·i·the·li·um (ōl-fak′tŏr-ē ep′i-thē′lē-ŭm) An epithelium of the pseudostratified type that contains olfactory, receptor, nerve cells with axons that extend to the olfactory bulb of the brain.

ol·fac·to·ry fo·ra·men (ōl-fak′tŏr-ē fōr-ā′mĕn) One of the openings in the cribriform plate of the ethmoid bone, transmitting the olfactory nerves.

ol·fac·to·ry glands (ōl-fak′tŏr-ē glandz) Branched tubuloalveolar serous secreting glands (of Bowman) in the mucous membrane of the olfactory region of the nasal cavity.

ol·fac·to·ry mem·brane (ōl-fak′tŏr-ē mem′brān) That part of the nasal mucosa having olfactory receptor cells and glands of Bowman.

ol·fac·to·ry nerve [CN I] (ōl-fak′tŏr-ē nĕrv) Collective term denoting the numerous olfactory filaments: slender fascicles each composed of the thin, unmyelinated axons of 8–12 of the bipolar olfactory receptor cells in the olfactory portion of the nasal mucosa; the olfactory filaments pass through the cribriform plate of the ethmoid bone and enter the olfactory bulb, where they terminate in synaptic contact with mitral cells, tufted cells, and granule cells. SYN nervi olfactorii [TA], nervus olfactorii [CN I] [TA], first cranial nerve [CN I].

ol·fac·to·ry re·cep·tor cells (ōl-fak′tŏr-ē rĕ-sep′tŏr selz) Very slender nerve cells, with large nuclei and surmounted by six to eight long, sensitive cilia in the olfactory epithelium at the roof of the nose; they are the receptors for smell.

ol·fac·to·ry sul·cus (ōl-fak′tŏr-ē sŭl′kŭs) The sagittal sulcus on the inferior or orbital surface of each frontal lobe of the cerebrum, demarcating the straight gyrus from the orbital gyri, and covered on the orbital surface by the olfactory bulb and tract.

o·lib·a·num (ō-lib′ă-nŭm) A gum resin from several trees of the genus *Boswellia* (family Burseraceae); used as a stimulant expectorant in bronchitis, for fumigations, and as incense. SYN frankincense, thus. [Ar. *al,* the, + *lubān,* frankincense]

oligaemia [Br.] SYN oligemia.

oligaemic [Br.] SYN oligemic.

ol·i·ge·mi·a (ol-i-jē′mē-ă) A deficiency of blood in the body or any organ or tissue. SYN oligaemia. [oligo- + G. *haima,* blood]

ol·i·ge·mic (ol-i-jē′mik) Pertaining to or characterized by oligemia. SYN oligaemic.

ol·i·go (ol′i-gō) MOLECULAR GENETICS oligonucleotide.

oligo-, olig- **1.** Combining forms meaning a few, a little; too little, too few. **2.** CHEMISTRY used in contrast to "poly-" in describing polymers (e.g., oligosaccharide). [G. *oligos,* few]

ol·i·go·am·ni·os (ol′i-gō-am′nē-os) SYN oligohydramnios. [oligo- + amnion]

ol·i·go·clo·nal band (ol′i-gō-klō′năl band) Small discrete bands in the gamma globulin region of the spinal fluid electrophoresis, indicating local central nervous system production of IgG; frequently seen in cases of multiple sclerosis but also found in other diseases of the central nervous system, including syphilis, sarcoidosis, and chronic infection or inflammation.

ol·i·go·cys·tic (ol′i-gō-sis′tik) Consisting of only a few cysts. [oligo- + G. *kystis,* bladder, cyst]

o·l·i·go·dac·ty·ly, ol·i·go·dac·tyl·i·a (ol′i-gō-dak′ti-lē, -dak-til′ē-ă) SYN hypodactyly. [oligo- + G. *daktylos,* finger or toe]

ol·i·go·den·dri·a (ol′i-gō-den′drē-ă) SYN oligodendroglia.

ol·i·go·den·dro·cyte (ol′i-gō-den′drō-sīt) A cell of the oligodendroglia.

ol·i·go·den·drog·li·a (ol′i-gō-den-drog′lē-ă) One of three types of glia cells (the other two being macroglia or astrocytes, and microglia) that, together with nerve cells, compose the tissue of the central nervous system. Oligodendroglia cells are characterized by variable numbers of veillike or sheetlike processes that are wrapped each around individual axons to form the myelin sheath of nerve fibers in the central nervous system. SYN oligodendria. [oligo- + G. *dendron,* tree, + *glia,* glue]

ol·i·go·den·dro·gli·o·ma (ol′i-gō-den′drō-glī-ō′mă) A rare, slowly growing glioma derived from oligodendrocytes that occurs most frequently in the cerebrum of adult persons. [oligo- + G. *dendron*, tree, + glia, + -oma]

ol·i·go·dip·si·a (ol′i-gō-dip′sē-ă) Abnormal lack of thirst. SEE ALSO hypodipsia. [oligo- + G. *dipsa,* thirst]

ol·i·go·don·ti·a (ol′i-gō-don′shē-ă) SYN hypodontia. [oligo- + G. *odous,* tooth]

ol·i·go·dy·nam·ic (ol′i-gō-dī-nam′ik) Active in very small quantity. [oligo- + G. *dynamis,* power]

ol·i·go·ga·lac·ti·a (ol′i-gō-gă-lak′tē-ă) Slight or scant secretion of milk. [oligo- + G. *gala,* milk]

ol·i·go-α1,6-glu·co·si·dase (ol′i-gō glū-kō′si-dās) A glucanohydrolase cleaving α-1,6 links in isomaltose and dextrins produced from starch and glycogen by α-amylase; secreted into the duodenum; a deficiency of this enzyme leads to defects in intestinal digestion of limit dextrins. SEE ALSO sucrose alpha-D-glucohydrolase.

ol·i·go·hy·dram·ni·os (ol′i-gō-hī-dram′nē-os) The presence of an insufficient amount of amniotic fluid (less than 300 mL at term). SYN oligoamnios. [oligo- + G. *hydōr,* water, + amnion]

ol·i·go·men·or·rhe·a (ol′i-gō-men-ō-rē′ă) Scanty menstruation. SYN oligomenorrhoea. [oligo- + menorrhea]

oligomenorrhoea [Br.] SYN oligomenorrhea.

oligomerisation [Br.] SYN oligomerization.

o·li·go·mer·i·za·tion (ol′i-gō-mĕr-ī-zā′shŭn) Formation of oligomers from larger or smaller molecules. SYN oligomerisation.

ol·i·go·mor·phic (ol′-i-gō-mōr′fik) Presenting few changes of form; not polymorphic. [oligo- + G. *morphē,* form]

ol·i·go·nu·cle·o·tide (ol′i-gō-nū′klē-ō-tīd) A compound made up of the condensation of a small number (typically fewer than 20) of nucleotides. Cf. polynucleotide.

ol·i·go·pep·tide (ol′igō-pep′tīd) A peptide the molecule of which contains a few amino acid residues up to about 20.

ol·i·gop·ne·a (ol′i-gop-nē′ă) SYN hypopnea. [oligo- + G. *pnoē,* breath]

ol·i·gop·ty·a·lism (ol′i-gop-tī′ă-lizm) A scanty secretion of saliva. [oligo- + G. *ptyalon,* saliva]

ol·i·gor·i·a (ol′i-gōr′ē-ă) An abnormal indifference toward or dislike of people or things. [G. *oligōria,* negligence, slight esteem, fr. *oligos,* little, + *ōra,* care, regard]

ol·i·go·sac·cha·ride (ol′i-gō-sak′ă-rīd) A compound made up of the condensation of a small number of monosaccharide units. Cf. polysaccharide.

ol·i·go·sper·mi·a, **ol·i·go·sper·ma·tism** (ol′i-gō-spĕrm′ē-ă, -mă-tizm) A subnormal concentration of sperms in the penile ejaculate. SYN oligozoospermia. [oligo- + G. *sperma,* seed]

ol·i·go·sy·nap·tic (ol′i-gō-si-nap′tik) Referring to neural conduction pathways that are interrupted by only a few synaptic junctions, i.e., made up of a sequence of only few nerve cells, in contrast to polysynaptic pathways. SYN paucisynaptic.

ol·i·go·tro·phi·a, **ol·i·got·ro·phy** (ol′i-gō-trō′fē-ă, -got′rō-fē) Deficient nutrition. [oligo- + G. *trophē,* nourishment]

ol·i·go·zo·o·sper·mi·a (ol′i-gō-zō′ō-spĕrm′ē-ă) SYN oligospermia. [oligo- + G. *zōos,* living, + *sperma,* seed, semen, + -ia]

ol·i·gu·ri·a (ol′i-gyūr′ē-ă) Scanty urine production (i.e., less than 500 mL in 24 hours); results in inefficient excretion of the products of metabolism. [oligo- + G. *ouron,* urine]

o·lis·thy (ō-lis′thē) The slippage of bone(s) from the normal anatomic site. [G. *olisthēsis,* a slipping]

o·li·va, pl. **o·li·vae** (ō-lī′vă, -vē) [TA] A smooth oval prominence of the ventrolateral surface of the medulla oblongata lateral to the pyramidal tract, corresponding to the inferior olivary nucleus. SYN corpus olivare [TA], olive (1). [L.]

ol·i·var·y (ol′i-var-ē) **1.** Relating to the oliva. **2.** Relating to or shaped like an olive.

ol·ive (ol′iv) **1.** SYN oliva. **2.** Common name for a tree of the genus *Olea* (family Oleaceae) or its fruit. [L. *oliva*]

ol·i·vif·u·gal (ol′i-vif′yū-găl) In a direction away from the olive. [oliva + L. *fugio,* to flee]

ol·i·vip·e·tal (ol′i-vip′ĕ-tăl) In a direction toward the olive. [oliva + L. *peto,* to seek]

ol·i·vo·pon·to·cer·e·bel·lar (ol′i-vō-pon′tō-ser′ĕ-bel′ăr) Relating to the olivary nucleus, basis pontis, and cerebellum.

Ol·li·er graft (ō-lē-ā′ graft) A thin split-thickness graft, usually in small pieces. SYN Ollier-Thiersch graft.

Ol·li·er the·o·ry (ō-lē-ā′ thē′ŏr-ē) A theory of compensatory growth; after resection of the articular extremity of a bone, the articular cartilage of the other bone entering into the structure of the joint takes on an increased growth.

Ol•li•er-Thiersch graft (ō-lē-ā′-tērsh′ graft) SYN Ollier graft.

Olm•sted syn•drome (ohlm′sted sin′drōm) Congenital palmar, plantar, and periorificial keratoderma leading to flexion contractures and digital spontaneous amputation.

-ology 1. Suffix denoting study of. 2. SYN -logia.

-olol Combining form meaning beta blocker (e.g., atenolol).

OM Abbreviation for otitis media.

-oma, -omata Combining forms denoting a tumor or neoplasm. [G. *-ōma*]

O•ma•ha sys•tem (ō′mă-haw sis′tĕm) Classification system for managing data involving individual patients, families, and communities. Data are organized under three components: problems, interventions, and outcomes.

o•mal•gi•a (ō-mal′jē-ă) Pain in the shoulder. [G. *ōmos,* shoulder + *algos,* pain]

o•me•ga (ō-mā′gă) 1. Twenty-fourth and last letter of the Greek alphabet (ω). 2. Ohm.

o•me•ga-6 fat•ty ac•id (ω) (ō-mā′gă fat′ē as′id) Any polyunsaturated fatty acid in which the first double bond occurs between the sixth and seventh carbon atoms from the methyl end.

o•me•ga-9 fat•ty ac•id (ω) (ō-mā′gă fat′ē as′id) Any polyunsaturated fatty acid in which the first double bond occurs between the ninth and tenth carbon atoms from the methyl end.

o•me•ga (ω)-3 fat•ty ac•ids (o-māg′ă fat′ē as′idz) A series of dietary polyunsaturated fatty acids that includes: α-linolenic acid (all-*cis*-9,12,15-octadecatrienoic acid) or 18:3 (n-3); EPA (all *cis*-5,8,11,14,17-eicosapentaenoic acid) or 20:5 (n-3); and DHA (all-*cis*-4,7,10,13,16,19-docosahexaenoic acid) or 22:6 (n-3); reportedly, they play a role in lowering cholesterol and LDL levels.

o•me•ga-ox•i•da•tion the•o•ry (ō-māg′ă oks-i-dā′shŭn thē′ŏr-ē) That the oxidation of fatty acids commences at the CH_3 group, i.e., the terminal or omega-group; beta-oxidation then proceeds at both ends of the fatty acid chain.

O•menn syn•drome (ō′men sin′drōm) A rapidly fatal immunodeficiency disease characterized by erythroderma, diarrhea, repeated infections, hepatosplenomegaly, and leukocytosis with eosinophilia; autosomal recessive inheritance, caused by mutation in either the recombination activating gene 1 (RAG1) or the adjacent RAG2 gene on chromosome 11p.

o•men•tal (ō-men′tăl) Relating to the omentum. SYN epiploic.

o•men•tal ap•pen•dices (ō-men′tăl ă-pen′di-sēz) One of a number of small processes or sacs of peritoneum filled with adipose tissue and projecting from the serous coat of the large intestine, except the rectum; they are most evident on the transverse and sigmoid colon, being most numerous along the free tenia. SYN appendices omentales [TA].

o•men•tal bur•sa (ō-men′tăl bŭr′să) An isolated portion of the peritoneal cavity lying dorsal to the stomach and extending craniad to the liver and diaphragm and caudad into the greater omentum; it opens into the general peritoneal cavity at the epiploic foramen.

o•men•tal flap (ō-men′tăl flap) A segment of omentum, with its supplying blood vessels, transplanted either with an intact pedicle or as free tissue to a distant area and revascularized by arterial and venous anastomoses. SYN omental graft.

o•men•tal for•a•men (ō-men′tăl fōr-ā′mĕn) The passage, below and behind the porta hepatis, connecting the two sacs of the peritoneum; it is bounded anteriorly by the hepatoduodenal ligament and posteriorly by a peritoneal fold over the inferior vena cava.

o•men•tal graft (ō-men′tăl graft) SYN omental flap.

o•men•tec•to•my (ō′men-tek′tŏ-mē) Resection or excision of the omentum. [omentum + G. *ektomē,* excision]

o•men•ti•tis (ō′men-tī′tis) Peritonitis involving the omentum. [L. *omentum* + G. *-itis,* inflammation]

omento-, oment- Combining forms denoting the omentum. SEE ALSO epiplo-. [L. *omentum*]

o•men•to•fix•a•tion (ō-men′tō-fik-sā′shŭn) SYN omentopexy.

o•men•to•pex•y (ō-men′tō-pek-sē) 1. Suture of the greater omentum to the abdominal wall to induce collateral portal circulation. 2. Suture of the omentum to another organ to increase arterial circulation. SEE ALSO omentoplasty. SYN omentofixation. [omento- + G. *pēxis,* fixation]

o•men•to•plas•ty (ō-men′tō-plas-tē) Use of the greater omentum to cover or fill a defect, augment arterial or portal venous circulation, absorb effusions, or increase lymphatic drainage. SEE ALSO omentopexy. [omento- + G. *plastos,* formed]

o•men•tor•rha•phy (ō′men-tōr′ă-fē) Suture of an opening in the omentum. [omento- + G. *rhaphē,* suture]

o•men•tum, pl. **o•men•ta** (ō-men′tŭm, -tă) [TA] A fold of peritoneum passing from the stomach to another abdominal organ. [L. the membrane that encloses the bowels]

o•mis•sion (ō-mi′shŭn) PHARMACY drug error in which the requisite dose is erroneously missed. SEE ALSO improper dose quantity.

OML Abbreviation for orbitomeatal line.

♻**omni-** Combining form meaning all. [L. *omnis,* all]

om·ni·fo·cal lens (ŏm′nē-fō′kal lenz) A lens for near and distant vision in which the reading portion is a continuously variable curve.

om·niv·o·rous (om-niv′ŏ-rŭs) Living on food of all kinds, on both animal and vegetable food. [L. *omnis,* all, + *voro,* to eat]

♻**omo-** Combining form denoting the shoulder (sometimes including the upper arm). [G. *ōmos,* shoulder]

o·mo·hy·oid mus·cle (ō′mō-hī′oyd mŭs′ĕl) Formed of two bellies attached to intermediate tendon; *origin,* by inferior belly from upper border of scapula between superior angle and notch; *insertion,* by superior belly into hyoid bone; *action,* depresses hyoid; *nerve supply,* upper cervical spinal nerves through ansa cervicalis. SYN musculus omohyoideus [TA].

o·mo·pha·gi·a (ō′mō-fā′jē-ă) The consumption of raw flesh, particularly raw meat and fish. [G. *ōmos,* raw, + *phagia,* eating]

♻**omphal-**, **omphalo-** Combining forms denoting the umbilicus, the navel. [G. *omphalos,* navel (umbilicus)]

om·pha·lec·to·my (om′fă-lek′tŏ-mē) Excision of the umbilicus or of a neoplasm connected with it. [omphal- + G. *ektomē,* excision]

om·phal·el·co·sis (om′fal-el-kō′sis) Ulceration at the umbilicus. [omphal- + G. *helkōsis,* ulceration]

om·phal·ic (om-fal′ik) SYN umbilical. [G. *omphalos,* umbilicus]

om·pha·li·tis (om′fă-lī′tis) Inflammation of the umbilicus and surrounding parts.

om·phal·o·cele (om-fal′ŏ-sēl) Congenital herniation of viscera into the base of the umbilical cord, with a covering membranous sac of peritoneum-amnion. SEE ALSO umbilical hernia. SYN exomphalos (3), exumbilication (3). [omphalo- + G. *kēlē,* hernia]

om·pha·lo·en·ter·ic (om′fă-lō-en-ter′ik) Relating to the umbilicus and intestine.

om·pha·lo·en·ter·ic duct (om′fă-lō-en-ter′ik dŭkt) Narrowed tubular connection between the embryonic midgut and umbilical vesicle (yolk sac). SYN omphalomesenteric duct, yolk stalk.

om·pha·lo·mes·en·ter·ic (om′fă-lō-mez-en-ter′ik) **1.** Term denoting relationship of the midgut to the umbilical vesicle (yolk stalk). As the head and tail folds of the embryo continue to form, this relationship is diminished and is represented by a narrow omphaloenteric duct (yolk stalk) or vitelline duct. **2.** Relating to the vitelline duct.

om·pha·lo·mes·en·ter·ic duct (om′fă-lō-mez-en-ter′ik dŭkt) SYN omphaloenteric duct.

om·pha·lo·phle·bi·tis (om′fă-lō-fle-bī′tis) Inflammation of the umbilical veins. [omphalo- + G. *phleps,* vein, + *-itis,* inflammation]

om·pha·lor·rha·gi·a (om′fă-lō-rā′jē-ă) Bleeding from the umbilicus. [omphalo- + G. *rhēgnymi,* to burst forth]

om·pha·lor·rhe·a (om′fă-lō-rē′ă) A serous discharge from the umbilicus. SYN omphalorrhoea. [omphalo- + G. *rhoia,* flow]

om·pha·lor·rhex·is (om′fă-lō-rek′sis) Rupture of the umbilical cord during childbirth. [omphalo- + G. *rhēxis,* rupture]

omphalorrhoea [Br.] SYN omphalorrhea.

om·pha·lo·site (om′fă-lō-sīt) Underdeveloped twin of allantoangiopagous twin; joined by umbilical vessels. [omphalo- + G. *sitos,* food]

om·pha·lo·spi·nous (om′fă-lō-spī′nŭs) Denoting a line connecting the umbilicus and the anterior superior spine of the ilium, on which lies McBurney point.

om·pha·lot·o·my (om′fă-lot′ŏ-mē) Cutting of the umbilical cord at birth. [omphalo- + G. *tomē,* incision]

o·nan·ism (ō′năn-izm) **1.** Withdrawal of the penis before ejaculation, to prevent conception. **2.** Incorrectly, masturbation. [*Onan,* son of Judah, who practiced it. Genesis 38:9]

on·cho·cer·co·ma (ong′kō-sĕr-kō′mă) In humans, nodule containing adult worms of *Onchocera volvulus*. Other species of *Onchocera* can produce onchercecomas in many other mammals, especially horses and cattle. [*Onchocerca,* taxonomic term, + -oma]

♻**onco-**, **oncho-** Combining forms indicating a tumor. [G. *onkos,* bulk, mass]

on·co·cyte (ong′kō-sīt) A large, granular, acidophilic tumor cell containing numerous mitochondria; a neoplastic oxyphil cell. [onco- + G. *kytos,* cell]

on·co·cy·tic ade·no·ma (ong′kō-sit′ik ad′ĕ-nō′mă) SYN Hürthle cell adenoma.

on·co·cy·tic car·ci·no·ma (ong′kō-sit′ik kahr′si-nō′mă) SYN Hürthle cell carcinoma.

on·co·cyt·ic hep·a·to·cel·lu·lar tu·mor (ong′kō-sit′ik he-pat′ō-sel′yū-lăr tū′mŏr) SYN fibrolamellar liver cell carcinoma.

on·co·fe·tal (ong′kō-fē′tăl) Relating to tumor-associated substances present in fetal tissue, as oncofetal antigens.

on·co·fe·tal an·ti·gens (ong′kō-fē′tăl an′ti-jenz) Tumor-associated antigens present in fetal tissue but not in normal adult tissue, including α-fetoprotein and carcinoembryonic antigen.

on•co•fe•tal mark•er (ong′kō-fē′tăl mahrk′ĕr) A tumor marker produced by tumor tissue and by fetal tissue of the same type as the tumor, but not by normal adult tissue from which the tumor arises.

on•co•gene (ong′kō-jēn) Any of a family of genes, which under normal circumstances, code for proteins involved in cell growth or regulation (e.g., protein kinases, GTPases, nuclear proteins, growth factors) but may foster malignant processes if mutated or activated by contact with retroviruses. Oncogenes often work in concert to produce cancer, and their action may be exacerbated by retroviruses, jumping genes, or inherited genetic mutations. SEE antioncogene. [onco- + gene]

on•co•gen•e•sis (ong′-kō-jen′ĕ-sis) Origin and growth of a neoplasm. [onco- + G. *genesis,* production]

on•co•gen•ic (ong′kō-jen′ik) SYN oncogenous.

on•co•gen•ic vi•rus (ong′kō-jen′ik vī′rŭs) A virus of one of the two groups that induce tumors; the RNA tumor viruses, which are well defined and rather homogeneous, or the DNA viruses, which are more diverse. SYN tumor virus.

on•cog•en•ous (ong-koj′ĕ-nŭs) Causing, inducing, or being suitable for the formation and development of a neoplasm. SYN oncogenic.

on•co•log•ic e•mer•gen•cies (ong′kŏ-loj′ik ē-mĕr′jĕn-sēz) Life-threatening medical emergencies that result from cancer or cancer therapies. The emergencies can be obstructive (e.g., superior vena cava syndrome), metabolic (e.g., hypercalcemia), or infiltrative (e.g., carotid artery rupture).

on•col•o•gist (ong-kol′ŏ-jist) A specialist in oncology.

on•col•o•gy (ong-kol′ŏ-jē) The study or science dealing with the physical, chemical, and biologic properties and features of neoplasms, including causation, pathogenesis, and treatment. [onco- + G. *logos,* study]

on•col•o•gy cer•ti•fied nurse (OCN) (on-kol′ŏ-jē sĕr′ti-fīd nŭrs) A nurse who specializes in treatment of patients with cancer and has passed a certification examination, developed and administered by the Oncology Nursing Certification Corporation (ONCC).

On•col•o•gy Nurs•ing So•ci•e•ty (ONS) (ong-kol′ŏ-jē nŭrs′ing sŏ-sī′ĕ-tē) A professional organization of registered nurses and other health care providers dedicated to excellence in patient care, education, research, and administration in oncology nursing; the largest professional oncology association in the world.

on•col•y•sis (ong-kol′i-sis) Destruction of a neoplasm; sometimes used with reference to the reduction of any swelling or mass. [onco- + G. *lysis,* dissolution]

on•co•lyt•ic (ong′kō-lit′ik) Pertaining to, characterized by, or causing oncolysis.

on•cor•na•vi•rus•es (ong-kōr′nă-vī′rŭs-ĕz) SYN Oncovirinae.

on•co•sis (ong-kō′sis) The formation of one or more neoplasms or tumors. [G. *onkōsis,* swelling, fr. *onkos,* bulk, mass]

on•cot•ic (ong-kot′ik) Relating to or caused by edema or any swelling (oncosis).

on•cot•ic pres•sure (ong-kot′ik presh′ŭr) The osmotic pressure attributed to proteins and other macromolecules.

on•co•tro•pic (ong′kō-trō′pik) Manifesting a special affinity for neoplasms or neoplastic cells. [onco- + G. *tropē,* a turning]

On•co•vir•i•nae (ong′kō-vir′i-nē) A subfamily of viruses (family Retroviridae) composed of the RNA tumor viruses that contain two identical plus stranded RNA molecules. SYN oncornaviruses.

on•co•vi•rus (ong′kō-vī′rŭs) Any virus of the subfamily Oncovirinae. SEE ALSO oncogenic virus.

On•dine curse (on-dēn′ kŭrs) Idiopathic central alveolar hypoventilation in which involuntary control of respiration is depressed, but voluntary control of ventilation is not impaired. [*Ondine,* char. in play by J. Giraudoux, based on Undine, Ger. myth. char.]

♻ **-one** Suffix indicating a ketone (–CO–) group.

one-car•bon frag•ment (wŭn-kahr′bŏn frag′mĕnt) The formyl or methyl group that takes part in transformylation or transmethylation reactions; by means of these reactions, a group containing a single carbon atom is added to a compound being biosynthesized, adding a methyl or hydroxymethyl group or closing a ring.

o•nei•ric (ō-nī′rik) **1.** Pertaining to dreams. **2.** Pertaining to the clinical state of oneirophrenia. [G. *oneiros,* dream]

o•nei•rism (ō-nī′rizm) A waking dream state. [G. *oneiros,* dream]

o•nei•ro•dyn•i•a (ō-nī′rō-din′ē-ă) Rarely used term for an unpleasant or painful dream. [G. *oneiros,* dream, + *odynē,* pain]

o•nei•ro•phre•ni•a (ō-nī′rō-frē′nē-ă) A state in which hallucinations occur, caused by such conditions as prolonged deprivation of sleep, sensory isolation, and a variety of drugs. [G. *oneiros,* dream, + *phrēn,* mind]

o•nei•ros•co•py (ō′nī-ros′kŏ-pē) The diagnosis of a patient's mental state by an analysis of the person's dreams. [G. *oneiros,* dream, + *skopeō,* to examine]

one-rep·e·ti·tion max·i·mum (1-RM) (wŭn′ rep-ĕ-tish′ŏn mak′si-mŭm) The maximum amount of weight that can be lifted once using proper form and technique (typically refers to standard sets of exercise such as bench press, leg press, one-arm curl).

on·go·ing as·sess·ment (on′gō-ing ă-ses′ mĕnt) Repeat of the focused or rapid emergency department assessment of a prehospital patient to detect changes in condition and to judge the effectiveness of treatment before or during transport. Repeated every 5 minutes for an unstable patient and every 15 minutes for a stable patient.

-onium Suffix indicating a positively charged radical; e.g., ammonium, NH_4^+.

onko- SEE onco-.

on·lay (on′lā) **1.** A metal cast restoration of the occlusal surface of a posterior tooth or the lingual surface of an anterior tooth, the entire surface of which is in dentin without side walls; retention in the anterior tooth is by pins and in the posterior by pins or boxes in retentive grooves in the buccal and lingual walls. **2.** A graft applied on the exterior of a bone, or the surface of an organ or structure.

on-off phe·nom·e·non (on-awf fĕ-nom′ĕ-non) A phase in the treatment of Parkinson disease with L-dopa, in which there is a rapid fluctuation of akinetic (off) and choreoathetotic (on) states.

on·o·mat·o·ma·ni·a (on′ō-mat-ō-mā′nē-ă) An abnormal impulse to dwell on certain words and their supposed significance, or frantically to try to recall a particular word. [G. *onoma,* name, + *mania,* frenzy]

on·o·mat·o·pho·bi·a (on′ō-mat-ō-fō′bē-ă) Abnormal dread of certain words or names because of their supposed significance. [G. *onoma,* name, + *phobos,* fear]

ONS Abbreviation for Oncology Nursing Society.

on·set of ac·tion (on′set ak′shŭn) The time from drug administration until the drug exerts an observable specific effect or response.

on·set of blood lac·tate ac·cu·mu·la·tion (OBLA) (on′set blŭd lak′tāt ă-kyū-myū-lā′shŭn) SYN lactate threshold.

on-site mas·sage (on-sīt mă-sahzh′) SYN seated massage.

on·to·gen·e·sis (on′tō-jen′ĕ-sis) SYN ontogeny.

on·to·ge·net·ic, on·to·gen·ic (on′tō-jĕ-net′ ik, -jen′ik) Relating to ontogeny.

on·tog·e·ny (on-toj′ĕ-nē) Development of the individual, as distinguished from phylogeny, which is evolutionary development of the species. SYN ontogenesis. [G. *ōn,* being, + *genesis,* origin]

on·y·chal·gi·a (on′i-kal′jē-ă) Pain in the nails. [onycho- + G. *algos,* pain]

on·ych·a·tro·phi·a, on·ych·at·ro·phy (on′ i-kă-trō′fē-ă, on′ik-at′rō-fē) Atrophy of the nails. [onycho- + G. *atrophia,* atrophy]

on·y·chaux·is (on′i-kawk′sis) Marked overgrowth of the fingernails or toenails. [onycho- + G. *auxē,* increase]

on·y·chec·to·my (on′i-kek′tŏ-mē) Ablation of a toenail or fingernail. [onycho- + G. *ektomē,* excision]

o·nych·i·a (ō-nik′ē-ă) Inflammation of the matrix of the nail. SYN onychitis. [onycho- + G. *-ia,* condition]

on·y·chi·tis (on′i-kī′tis) SYN onychia.

onycho-, onych- Combining forms denoting a fingernail or a toenail. [G. *onyx,* nail]

on·y·choc·la·sis (on′i-kok′lă-sis) Breaking of the nails. [onycho- + G. *klasis,* breaking]

on·y·cho·dys·tro·phy (on′i-kō-dis′trŏ-fē) Dystrophic changes in the nails occurring as a congenital defect or due to any illness or injury that may cause a malformed nail. [onycho- + G. *dys-,* bad, + *trophē,* nourishment]

on·y·cho·graph (on′i-kō-graf) An instrument for recording the capillary blood pressure as shown by the circulation under the nail. [onycho- + G. *graphō,* to write]

on·y·cho·gry·po·sis (on′i-kō-gri-pō′sis) Enlargement with increased thickening and curvature of the fingernails or toenails. [onycho- + G. *grypōsis,* a curvature]

on·y·cho·het·er·o·to·pi·a (on′i-kō-het′ĕr-ō-tō′pē-ă) Abnormal placement of nails.

on·y·choid (on′i-koyd) Resembling a fingernail in structure or form. [onycho- + G. *eidos,* resemblance]

on·y·chol·y·sis (on′i-kol′i-sis) Loosening of the nails, beginning at the free border, and usually incomplete. See page B12. [onycho- + G. *lysis,* loosening]

on·y·cho·ma (on′i-kō′mă) A tumor arising from the nail bed. [onycho- + G. *-ōma,* tumor]

on·y·cho·ma·de·sis (on′i-kō-mă-dē′sis) Complete shedding of the nails, usually associated with systemic disease. [onycho- + G. *madēsis,* a growing bald, fr. *madaō,* to be moist, (of hair) fall off]

on·y·cho·ma·la·ci·a (on′i-kō-mă-lā′shē-ă) Abnormal softness of the nails. [onycho- + G. *malakia,* softness]

on·y·cho·my·co·sis (on′i-kō-mī-kō′sis) Very common fungus infections of the nails, causing thickening, roughness, and splitting, often caused by *Trichophyton rubrum* or *T. mentagro-*

phytes, Candida in the immunodeficient, and various molds in the elderly. See page B12. [onycho- + G. *mykēs,* fungus, + *-ōsis,* condition]

on·y·cho·path·ic (on′i-kō-path′ik) Relating to or suffering from any disease of the nails.

on·y·chop·a·thy (on′i-kop′ă-thē) Any disease of the nails. SYN onychosis. [onycho- + G. *pathos,* suffering]

on·y·choph·a·gy, on·y·cho·pha·gi·a (on′i-kof′ă-jē, on′i-kō-fā′jē-ă) Habitual nailbiting. [onycho- + G. *phagō,* to eat]

on·y·cho·plas·ty (on′i-kō-plas-tē) A corrective or surgical operation on the nail matrix. [onycho- + G. *plastos,* formed, shaped]

on·y·chor·rhex·is (on′i-kō-rek′sis) Abnormal brittleness of the nails with splitting of the free edge. [onycho- + G. *rhēxis,* a breaking]

on·y·cho·schiz·i·a (on′i-kō-skit′sē-ă) Splitting of the nails in layers. See page B12. [onycho- + G. *schizō,* to divide, + *-ia,* condition]

on·y·cho·sis (on′i-kō′sis) SYN onychopathy.

on·y·chot·il·lo·ma·ni·a (on′i-kot′i-lō-mā′nē-ă) A tendency to pick at the nails. [onycho- + G. *tillō,* to pluck, + *mania,* insanity]

on·y·chot·o·my (on′i-kot′ŏ-mē) Incision into a toenail or fingernail. [onycho- + G. *tomē,* cutting]

on·yx (on′iks) SYN nail. [G. nail]

oo- Prefix meaning egg, ovary. SEE ALSO oophor-, ovario-, ovi-, ovo-. [G. *ōon,* egg]

oob Abbreviation for out of bed.

oobe Abbreviation for out of body experience.

o·o·cyst (ō′ō-sist) The encysted form of the fertilized macrogamete, or zygote, in coccidian Sporozoea in which sporogonic multiplication occurs; results in the formation of sporozoites, infectious agents for the next stage of the sporozoan life cycle. [G. *ōon,* egg, + *kystis,* bladder]

o·o·cyte (ō′ō-sīt) The female sex cell. When fertilized by a sperm, a gamete or zygote is capable of developing into a new individual of the same species; during maturation, the oocyte, like the sperm, undergoes a halving of its chromosomal complement so that, at its union with the male gamete, the species number of chromosomes (46 in humans) is maintained; yolk contained in the oocyte (ova in nonhuman species) varies greatly in amount and distribution, which influences the pattern of the cleavage divisions. See page B1. SYN ovum. [G. *ōon,* egg, + *kytos,* a hollow (cell)]

o·o·gen·e·sis (ō-ō-jen′ĕ-sis) Process of formation and development of the oocyte. SYN ovigenesis. [G. *ōon,* egg, + *genesis,* origin]

o·o·ge·net·ic (ō′ō-jĕ-net′ik) Producing oocytes (ova). SYN ovigenetic, ovigenic.

o·o·go·ni·um, pl. **o·o·go·ni·a** (ō-ō-gō′nē-ŭm, -nē-ă) **1.** Primordial germ cells; proliferate by mitotic division. **2.** In fungi, the female gametangium bearing one or more oospores. [G. *ōon,* egg, + *gonē,* generation]

o·o·ki·ne·sis, o·o·ki·ne·si·a (ō′ō-ki-nē′sis, -nē′zē-ă) Chromosomal movements of the oocyte during maturation and fertilization. [G. *ōon,* egg, + *kinēsis,* movement]

o·o·ki·nete (ō′ō-kī′net) The motile zygote of the malarial organism that penetrates the mosquito stomach to form an oocyst under the outer gut lining; the contents of the oocyst subsequently divide to produce numerous sporozoites. [G. *ōon,* egg, + *kinētos,* motile]

o·o·lem·ma (ō-ō-lem′ă) Plasma membrane of the oocyte. [G. *ōon,* egg, + *lemma,* sheath]

oophor-, oophoro- Combining forms meaning the ovary. SEE ALSO oo-, ovario-. [Mod. L. *oophoron,* ovary, fr. G. *ōophoros,* egg-bearing]

o·oph·or·al·gi·a (ō-of′ŏr-al′gē-ă) Pain in an ovary. [oophoor- + G. *algos,* pain]

o·oph·o·rec·to·my (ō′of-ōr-ek′tŏ-mē) SYN ovariectomy. [G. *ōon,* egg, + *phoros,* bearing, + *ektomē,* excision]

o·oph·or·i·tis (ō′of-ōr-ī′tis) Inflammation of an ovary. SYN ovaritis. [G. *ōon,* egg, + *phoros,* a bearing, + *-itis,* inflammation]

o·oph·or·o·cys·tec·to·my (ō-of′ōr-ō-sis-tek′tŏ-mē) Excision of an ovarian cyst.

o·oph·or·o·cys·to·sis (ō-of′ōr-ō-sis-tō′sis) Ovarian cyst formation.

o·oph·or·o·hys·ter·ec·to·my (ō-of′ōr-ō-his-tĕr-ek′tŏ-mē) SYN ovariohysterectomy.

o·oph·or·on (ō-of′ŏr-on) SYN ovary. [G. *ōon,* egg, + *phoros,* bearing]

o·oph·or·o·pex·y (ō-of′ŏr-ō-pek′sē) Surgical fixation or suspension of an ovary. [oophoro- + G. *pēxis,* fixation]

o·oph·or·o·plas·ty (ō-of′ŏr-ō-plas-tē) Surgical repair on an ovary. [oophoro- + G. *plastos,* formed, shaped]

o·oph·or·o·sal·pin·gec·to·my (ō-of′ŏr-ō-sal′pin-jek′tŏ-mē) The surgical removal of one or both ovaries, along with the corresponding uterine tube(s). [oophoro- + salpingo- + G. *ektomē,* excision]

o·oph·or·o·sal·pin·gi·tis (ō-of′ŏr-ō-sal′pin-jī′tis) Inflammation that involves the ovary and uterine tube. SYN ovariosalpingitis. [oophoro- + G. *salpinx,* tube + -itis, inflammation]

o•oph•or•os•to•my (ō-of′ōr-os′tŏ-mē) SYN ovariostomy. [oophoro- + G. *stoma,* mouth]

o•oph•or•ot•o•my (ō-of′ōr-ot′ŏ-mē) SYN ovariotomy. [oophoro- + G. *tomē,* incision]

o•oph•or•rha•gi•a (ō-of′ōr-rā′jē-ă) Ovarian hemorrhage. [oophoro- + G. *rhēgnymi,* to burst forth]

o•o•plasm (ō′ō-plazm) Protoplasmic portion of the oocyte. [G. *ōon,* egg, + *plasma,* a thing formed]

o•o•tid (ō′ō-tid) The nearly mature oocyte after the first meiotic division has been completed and the second initiated; in most higher mammals (including humans), the second meiotic division is not completed unless fertilization occurs. [G. *ōotidion,* a diminutive egg. See -id (2)]

OP Abbreviation for occipitoposterior position.

o•pac•i•fi•ca•tion (ō-pas′i-fi-kā′shŭn) **1.** The process of making opaque. **2.** The formation of opacities. [L. *opacus,* shady]

o•pac•i•ty (ō-pas′i-tē) **1.** A lack of transparency; an opaque or nontransparent area. **2.** On a radiograph, a more transparent area is interpreted as an opacity to x-rays in the body. **3.** Mental dullness. [L. *opacitas,* shadiness]

o•pal co•don (ō-păl kō′don) SYN umber codon.

o•pal•es•cent den•tin (ō-pă-les′ĕnt den′tin) Dentin usually associated with dentinogenesis imperfecta; gives an unusual opalescent or translucent appearance to the teeth.

o•paque (ō-pāk′) Impervious to light; not translucent or only slightly so. Cf. radiopaque. [Fr. fr. L. *opacus,* shady]

OPD Abbreviation for outpatient department.

o•pen am•pu•ta•tion (ō′pĕn amp′yū-tā′shŭn) An amputation after which the stump is left unsutured (without skin flap closure) for several weeks while débridement and antibiotic therapy are carried out. Closing the stump before the wound is free from bacteria or debris increases the risk of infection and compromises healing.

o•pen-an•gle glau•co•ma (ō′pĕn-ang′gĕl glaw-kō′mă) This most prevalent form of the disease is sometimes called 'the thief in the night.' The flow of aqueous humor is slowed or completely stopped by an obstruction in the trabecular network. SYN simple glaucoma, glaucoma simplex.

o•pen bi•op•sy (ō′pĕn bī′op-sē) Biopsy requiring a surgical incision.

o•pen chain com•pound (ō′pĕn chān kom′pownd) SYN acyclic compound.

o•pen-chain movement (ō′pĕn chān mūv′mĕnt) Kinematic chain movement in which the distal end of the body part moves freely through space.

o•pen chest mas•sage (ō′pĕn chest mă-sahzh′) Rhythmic manual compression of the ventricles of the heart with the hand inside the thoracic cavity.

o•pen-cir•cuit meth•od (ō′pĕn-sĭr′kit meth′ŏd) A process for measuring oxygen consumption and carbon dioxide production by collecting the expired gas over a known period of time and measuring its volume and composition.

o•pen-cir•cuit ni•tro•gen wash-out (ō′pĕn-sĭr′kĭt nī′trŏ-jĕn wawsh′owt) A gas-dilution technique for measuring the functional residual capacity; the patient breathes 100% oxygen to wash out the nitrogen.

o•pen-cir•cuit spi•rom•e•try (ō′pĕn-sĭr′kĭt spī-rom′ĕ-trē) Measurement of the volume and rate of respiratory air flow by a device into which the subject expels inspired room air.

o•pen com•e•do (ō′pĕn kom′ĕ-dō) A comedo with a wide opening on the skin surface capped with a melanin-containing blackened mass of epithelial debris. SYN blackhead (1).

o•pen dis•lo•ca•tion (ō′pĕn dis-lō-kā′shŭn) A dislocation complicated by a wound opening from the surface down to the affected joint. SYN compound dislocation.

o•pen drain•age (ō′pĕn drān′ăj) Drainage allowing air to enter.

o•pen drop an•es•the•si•a (ō′pĕn drop an′es-thē′zē-ă) Inhalation anesthesia achieved by vaporization of a liquid anesthetic placed drop by drop on a gauze mask covering the mouth and nose.

o•pen flap (ō′pĕn flap) SYN flat flap.

o•pen frac•ture (ō′pĕn frak′shŭr) Break in which the skin is perforated and there is an open wound down to the fracture. SYN compound fracture.

o•pen head in•ju•ry (ō′pĕn hed in′jŭr-ē) A head wound in which there is a loss of continuity of scalp or mucous membranes; the term is sometimes used to indicate a communication between the exterior and the intracranial cavity. SEE ALSO penetrating wound.

o•pen heart sur•ger•y (ō′pĕn hahrt sŭr′jĕr-ē) Operative procedure(s) performed on or within the exposed heart, usually with cardiopulmonary bypass.

o•pen hos•pi•tal (ō′pĕn hos′pi-tăl) A health care facility where all physicians, not only members of the regular staff, are permitted to send their patients and control their treatment.

o•pen•ing (ō′pĕn-ing) A gap in or entrance to an organ, tube, or cavity. SEE ALSO aperture, fossa, ostium, orifice, pore.

o•pen•ing of ex•ter•nal a•cous•tic me•a•tus (ō′pĕn-ing eks-tĕr′năl ă-kūs′tik mē-ā′tŭs)

The orifice of the external acoustic meatus in the tympanic portion of the temporal bone.

o•pen•ing of in•ter•nal a•cous•tic me•a•tus (ō′pĕn-ing in-tĕr′năl ă-kūs′tik mē-ā′tŭs) The inner opening of the internal acoustic meatus on the posterior surface of the petrous part of the temporal bone.

o•pen•ing of pul•mo•na•ry trunk (ō′pĕn-ing pul′mŏ-nār-ē trŭngk) The opening of the pulmonary trunk from the right ventricle, guarded by the pulmonary valve.

o•pen•ing snap (ō′pĕn-ing snap) A sharp, high-pitched click in early diastole, usually best heard between the cardiac apex and the lower left sternal border, related to opening of the abnormal valve in cases of mitral stenosis.

o•pen-packed po•si•tion (ō′pĕn-pakt pŏ-zish′ŏn) **1.** Joint position in which contact between the articulating structures is minimal. **2.** SYN flexion.

o•pen pneu•mo•thor•ax (ō′pĕn nū′mō-thōr′aks) A free communication between the atmosphere and the pleural space either through the lung or through the chest wall. SYN sucking chest wound, sucking wound.

o•pen re•duc•tion of frac•tures (ō′pĕn rē-duk′shŭn frak′shŭrz) Reduction by manipulation of bone, after incision in skin and muscle over the site of the fracture.

o•pen skill (ō′pĕn skil) One of a series of movement patterns performed in an unpredictable environment such that the individual must adapt movements in response to changes within the environment (e.g., playing soccer, riding a bicycle over a trail).

o•pen tu•ber•cu•lo•sis (ō′pĕn tū-bĕr-kyū-lō′sis) Pulmonary tuberculosis, tuberculous ulceration, or other form in which the tubercle bacilli are present in the excretions or secretions; in the lung, usually the result of cavity formation.

o•pen wound (ō′pĕn wūnd) A wound in which the tissues are exposed to the air.

op•er•a•ble (op′ĕr-ă-bĕl) Denoting a patient or condition on which a surgical procedure can be performed with a reasonable expectation of cure or relief.

op•er•ant (op′ĕr-ănt) In conditioning, any behavior or specific response chosen by the experimenter; its frequency is intended to increase or decrease by the judicious pairing with it of a reinforcer when it occurs. SYN target response.

op•er•ate (op′ĕr-āt) To perform a therapeutic procedure on the body with the hands or with instruments. [L. *operor,* pp. *-atus,* to work, fr. *opus,* work]

op•er•at•ing mi•cro•scope (op′ĕr-ā′ting mī′krō-skōp) SYN surgical microscope.

op•er•at•ing room tech•ni•cian (op′ĕr-āt-ing rūm tek-nish′ŭn) The member of the surgical team who assists in preparing the operating room for surgery and performing other tasks (i.e., arranging equipment, assisting doctors in passing instrument). Training programs last 1 to 2 years. At the end of the training period, students must pass an examination by the Association of Surgical Technologists to become certified. SYN surgical technician, surgical technologist.

op•er•a•tion (op-ĕr-ā′shŭn) **1.** Any surgical procedure. **2.** The act, manner, or process of functioning. SEE ALSO method, procedure, technique.

Op•er•a•tion Re•store Trust (ORT) (op-ĕr-ā′shŭn rē-stōr′trŭst) A U.S. federal pilot program designed to combat fraud, waste, and abuse in the Medicare and Medicaid programs.

op•er•a•tive (op′ĕr-ă-tiv) **1.** Relating to, or effected by means of an operation. **2.** Active or effective.

op•er•a•tive cho•lan•gi•og•ra•phy (op′ĕr-ă-tiv kō-lan′jē-og′ră-fē) Radiographic examination of the bile ducts with contrast medium during surgery to detect residual biliary calculi.

op•er•a•tor (op′ĕr-ā-tŏr) **1.** One who performs an operation or operates equipment. **2.** GENETICS a sequence of DNA that interacts with a repressor of operon to control the expression of adjacent structural genes. SEE operator gene. **3.** A symbol representing a mathematic operation. [L. worker, fr. *operor,* to work]

op•er•a•tor gene (op′ĕr-ā-tŏr jēn) A gene with the function of activating the production of messenger RNA by one or more adjacent structural loci; part of the feedback system for determining the rate of production of an enzyme.

o•per•cu•lar (ō-per′kyū-lăr) Relating to an operculum.

o•per•cu•li•tis (ō-per′kyū-lī′tis) A pericoronitis originating under an operculum. [operculum + G. *-itis,* inflammation]

o•per•cu•lum, gen. **oper•cu•li**, pl. **oper•cu•la** (ō-per′kū-lŭm, -lī, -lă) **1.** Anything resembling a lid or cover. **2.** [TA] ANATOMY the portions of the frontal, parietal, and temporal lobes bordering the lateral sulcus and covering the insula. **3.** Mucus sealing the endocervical canal of the uterus after conception has taken place. **4.** PARASITOLOGY the lid or caplike cover of the shell opening of operculated freshwater snails in the subclass Prosobranchiata, and of the eggs of certain trematode and cestode parasites. **5.** The attached flap in the tear of retinal detachment. **6.** The mucosal flap partially or completely covering a partially erupted tooth. [L. cover or lid, fr. *operio,* pp. *opertus,* to cover]

o•phi•a•sis (ō-fī′ă-sis) A form of alopecia areata in which the loss of hair occurs in bands along the scalp margin partially or completely encircling the head. [G., fr. *ophis,* snake]

oph·ri·tis (of-rī′tis) Dermatitis in the region of the eyebrows. [G. *ophrys,* eyebrow, + *-itis,* inflammation]

oph·ry·on (of′rē-on) The point on the midline of the forehead just above the glabella (1). [G. *ophrys,* eyebrow]

oph·ry·o·sis (of′rē-ō′sis) Spasmodic twitching of the upper portion of the orbicularis palpebrarum muscle causing a wrinkling of the eyebrow. [G. *ophrys,* eyebrow, + *-osis,* condition]

oph·thal·mi·a (of-thal′mē-ă) **1.** Severe, often purulent, conjunctivitis. **2.** Inflammation of the deeper structures of the eye. [G.]

oph·thal·mi·a ne·o·na·to·rum (of-thal′mē-ă nē-ō′nā-tō′rŭm) A conjunctival inflammation occurring within the first 10 days of life; causes include *Neisseria gonorrhoeae*, *Staphylococcus* sp., *Streptococcus pneumoniae*, and *Chlamydia trachomatis*. SYN infantile purulent conjunctivitis.

oph·thal·mic (of-thal′mik) Relating to the eye. SYN ocular (1). [G. *ophthalmikos*]

oph·thal·mic ar·tery (of-thal′mik ahr′tĕr-ē) *Origin*, internal carotid; *branches*, ciliary, central artery of retina, anterior meningeal, lacrimal, conjunctival, episcleral, supraorbital, ethmoidal, palpebral, dorsal nasal, and supratrochlear. SYN arteria ophthalmica [TA].

oph·thal·mic nerve [CN V1] (of-thal′mik nĕrv) A branch of the trigeminal nerve that passes forward from the trigeminal ganglion in the lateral wall of the cavernous sinus, entering the orbit through the superior orbital fissure; through its branches, frontal, lacrimal, and nasociliary, it supplies sensation to the orbit and its contents, the anterior part of the nasal cavity, and the skin of the nose and forehead. SYN nervus ophthalmicus [CN V1] [TA].

oph·thal·mic so·lu·tion (of-thal′mik sŏ-lū′shŭn) Sterile solution, free from foreign particles and suitably compounded and dispensed for instillation into the eye.

oph·thal·mic ves·i·cle (of-thal′mik ves′i-kĕl) In the embryo, one of the paired evaginations from the ventrolateral walls of the forebrain from which the sensory and pigment layers of the retina develop.

♻ **ophthalmo-, ophthalm-** Combining forms indicating a relationship to the eye. SEE ALSO oculo-. [G. *ophthalmos*]

oph·thal·mo·dy·na·mom·e·ter (of-thal′mō-dī′nă-mom′ĕ-tĕr) An instrument to measure the blood pressure in the retinal vessels. [ophthalmo- + G. *dynamis,* power, + *metron,* measure]

oph·thal·mo·dy·na·mom·e·try (of-thal′mō-dī′nă-mom′ĕ-trē) The measurement of blood pressure in the retinal vessels by means of an ophthalmodynamometer. [ophthalmo- + G. *dynamis,* power, + *metron,* measure]

oph·thal·mo·lith (of-thal′mō-lith) SYN dacryolith. [ophthalmo- + G. *lithos,* stone]

oph·thal·mol·o·gist (of′thăl-mol′ŏ-jist) A medical specialist in ophthalmology who treats diseases of the eye medically and surgically. SYN oculist.

oph·thal·mol·o·gy (of′thăl-mol′ŏ-jē) The medical specialty concerned with the eye, its diseases, and refractive errors. [ophthalmo- + G. *logos,* study]

oph·thal·mo·ma·la·ci·a (of-thal′mō-mă-lā′shē-ă) Abnormal softening of the eyeball. [ophthalmo- + G. *malakia,* softness]

oph·thal·mom·e·ter (of-thăl-mom′ĕ-tĕr) SYN keratometer. [ophthalmo- + G. *metron,* measure]

oph·thal·mo·my·co·sis (of-thal′mō-mī-kō′sis) Any disease of the eye or its appendages caused by a fungus. [ophthalmo- + G. *mykēs,* fungus, + *-osis,* condition]

oph·thal·mop·a·thy (of-thăl-mop′ă-thē) Any disease of the eyes. [ophthalmo- + G. *pathos,* suffering]

oph·thal·mo·ple·gi·a (of-thal′mō-plē′jē-ă) Paralysis of one or more of the ocular muscles. [ophthalmo- + G. *plēgē,* stroke]

oph·thal·mo·ple·gi·a ex·ter·na (of-thal′mō-plē′jē-ă eks-ter′nă) Paralysis affecting one or more of the extrinsic eye muscles. SYN external ophthalmoplegia.

oph·thal·mo·ple·gi·a in·ter·na (of-thal′mō-plē′jē-ă in-ter′nă) Paralysis affecting only the sphincter muscle of the pupil and the ciliary muscle. SYN internal ophthalmoplegia.

oph·thal·mo·ple·gic (of-thal′mō-plē′jik) Relating to or marked by ophthalmoplegia.

i **oph·thal·mo·scope** (of-thal′mŏ-skōp) A device for studying the interior of the eyeball through the pupil. See page B26. SYN funduscope. [ophthalmo- + G. *skopeō,* to examine]

oph·thal·mo·scop·ic (of′thăl-mŏ-skop′ik) Relating to examination of the interior of the eye.

oph·thal·mos·co·py (of′thăl-mos′kŏ-pē) Examination of the fundus of the eye by means of the ophthalmoscope.

oph·thal·mo·vas·cu·lar (of-thal′mō-vas′kyū-lăr) Relating to the blood vessels of the eye.

♻ **-opia** Suffix meaning vision. [G. *ōps,* eye]

o·pi·ate (ō′pē-ăt) Any preparation or derivative of opium.

o·pi·ate re·cep·tors (ō′pē-ăt rĕ-sep′tŏrz) Regions of the brain that have the capacity to bind

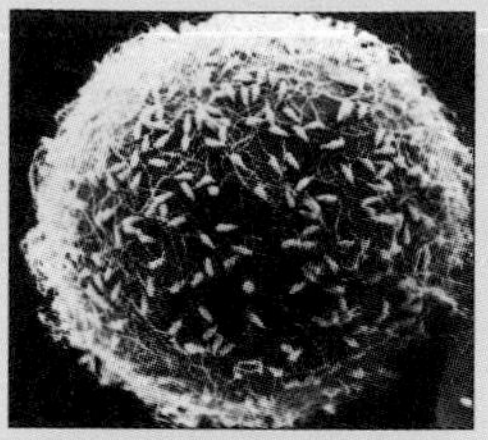

sperms binding to oocyte

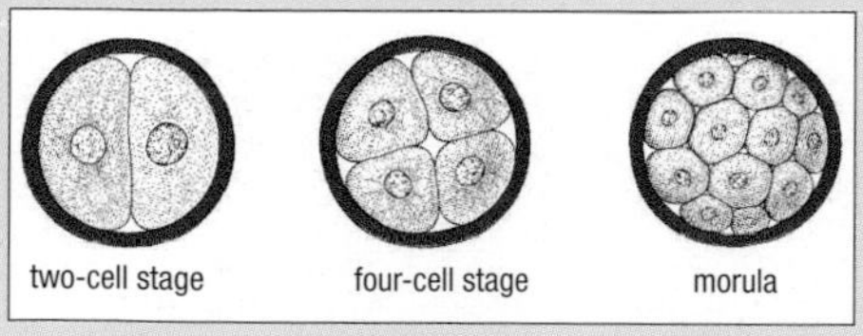

development of the zygote from two-cell to the late morula stage

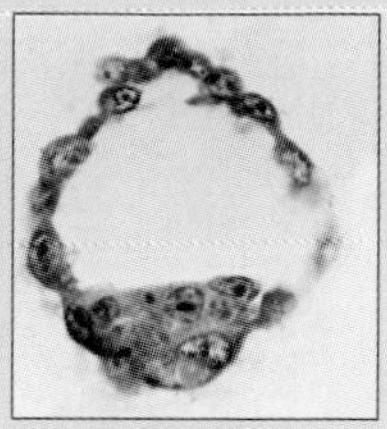

107-cell human blastocyst

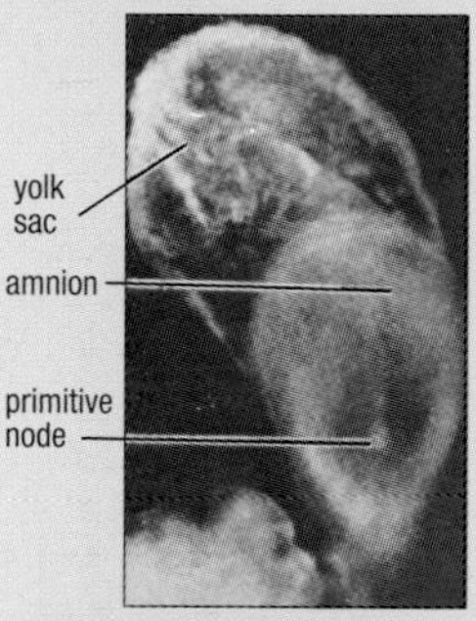

18-day human embryo

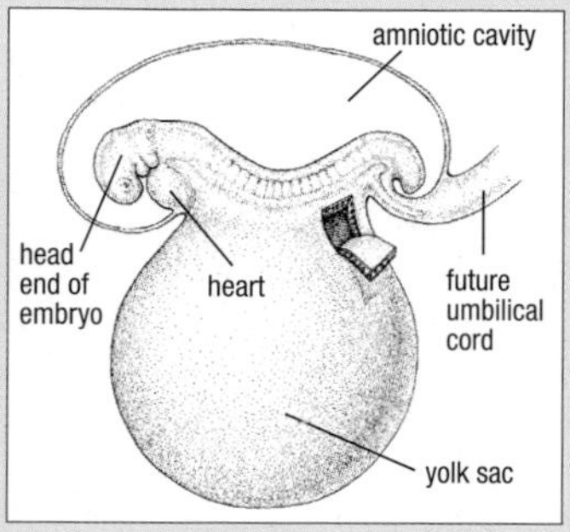

3-week human embryo

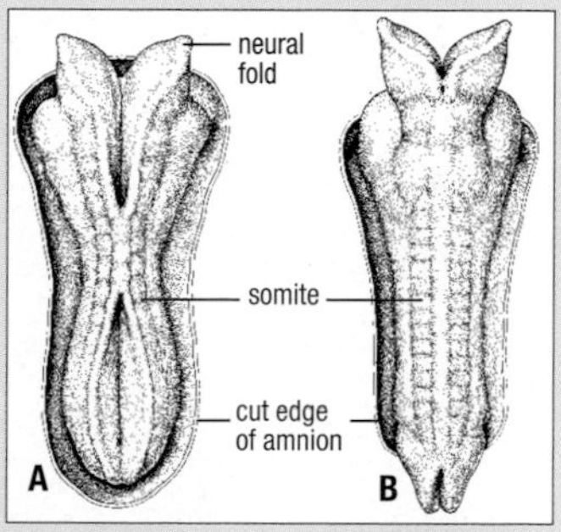

22-day (A) and 23-day (B) human embryos

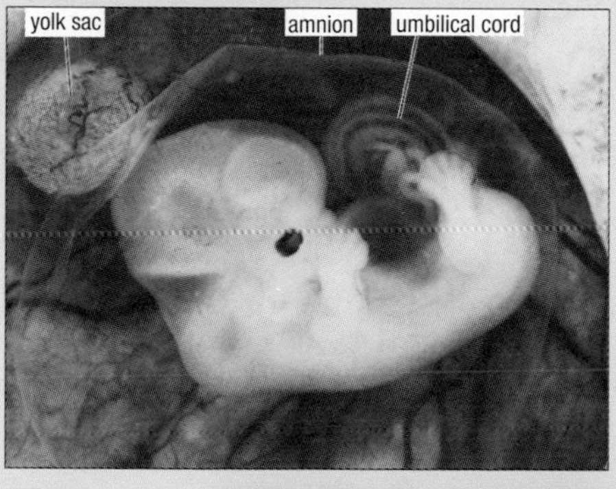

▲ 7-week human embryo

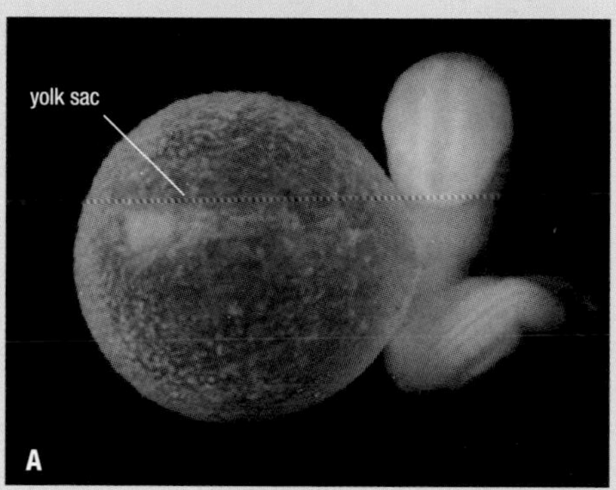

▲ 28-somite human embryo (A, B) ▶

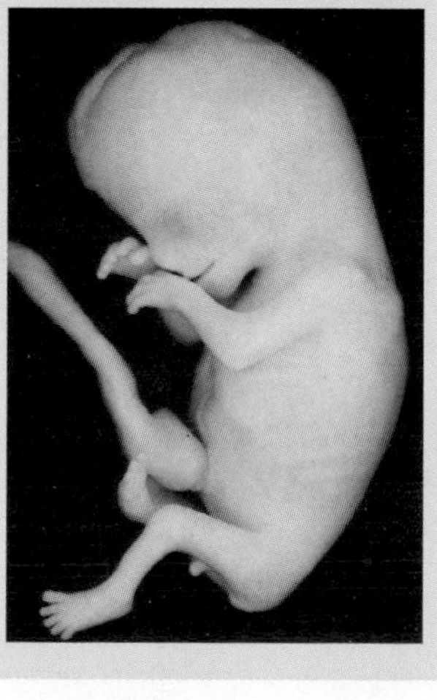

▶ 11-week fetus

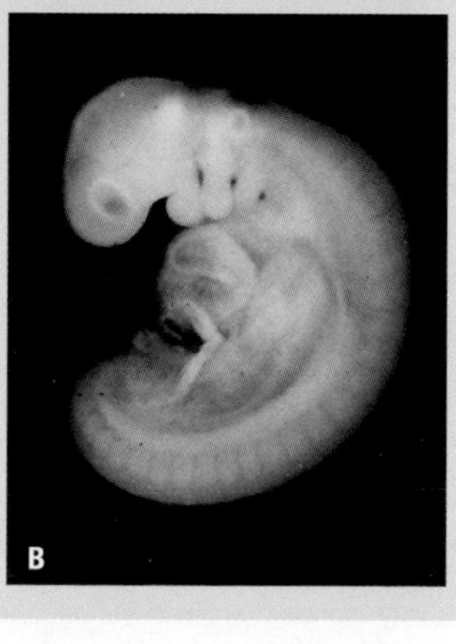

PLATE 2: BLOOD CELLS

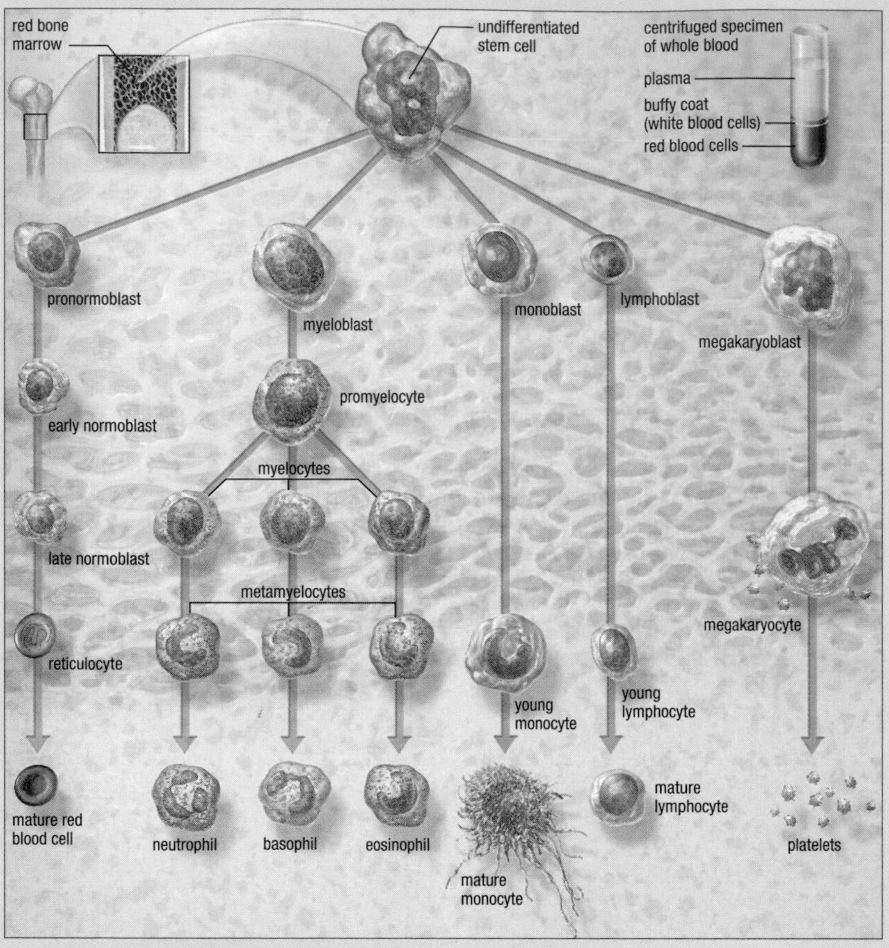

the development of blood cells

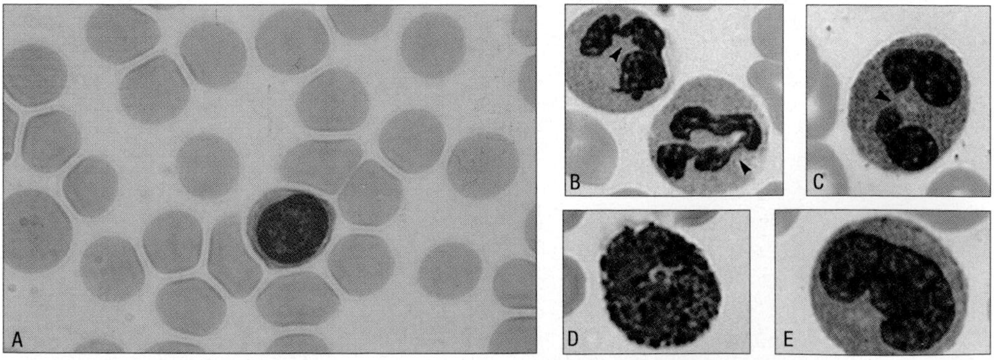

blood cells: (A) mature **lymphocyte** (size 7-15 mcm); (B) **neutrophils** showing a somewhat granular cytoplasm and lobulated nuclei (arrows); (C) **eosinophils** with large dark pink granules and sausage-shaped nuclei (arrow); (D) **basophil** with dense, dark, large granules; (E) **monocyte** characterized by large size, acentric, kidney-shaped nucleus, and lack of specific granules.

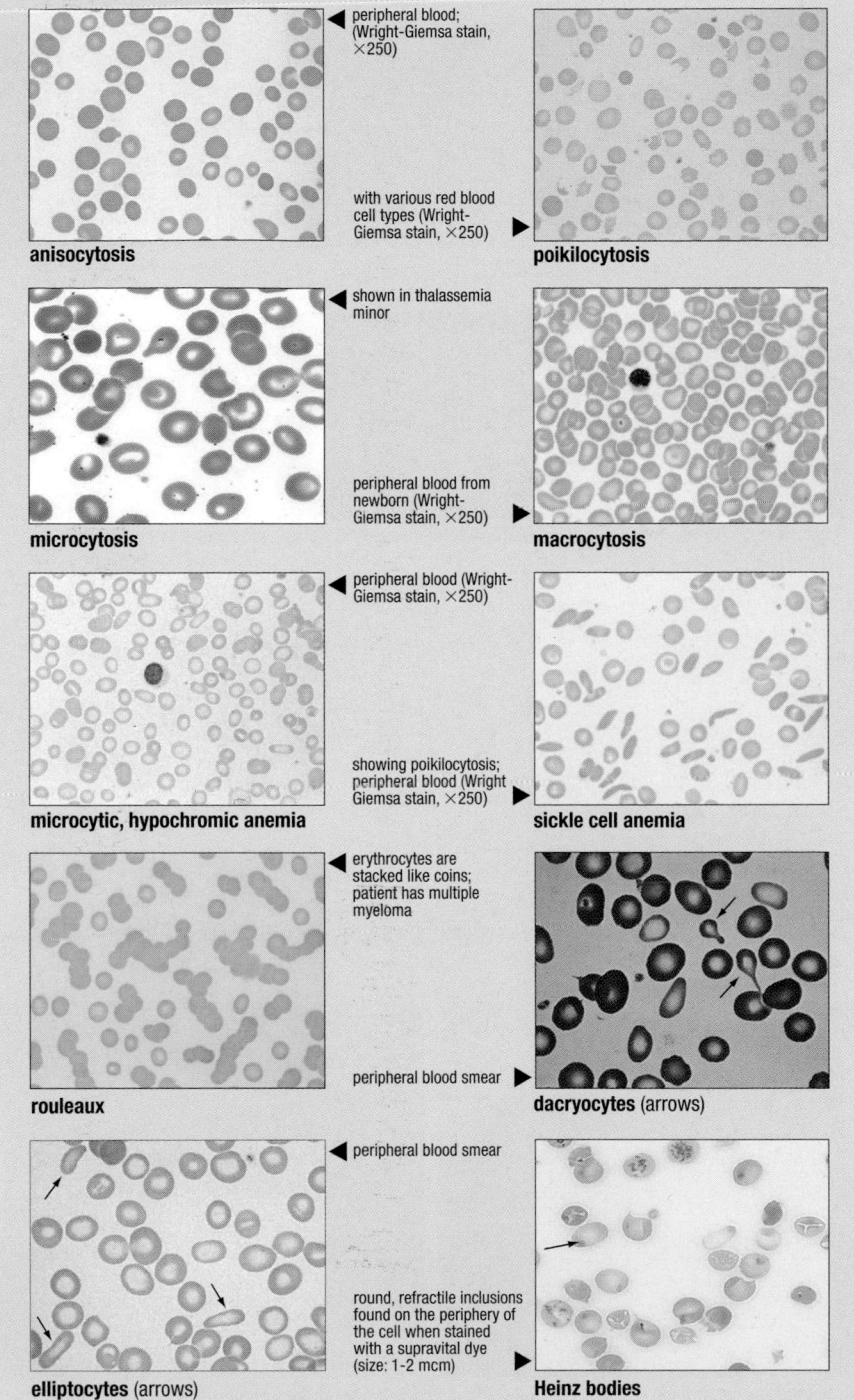

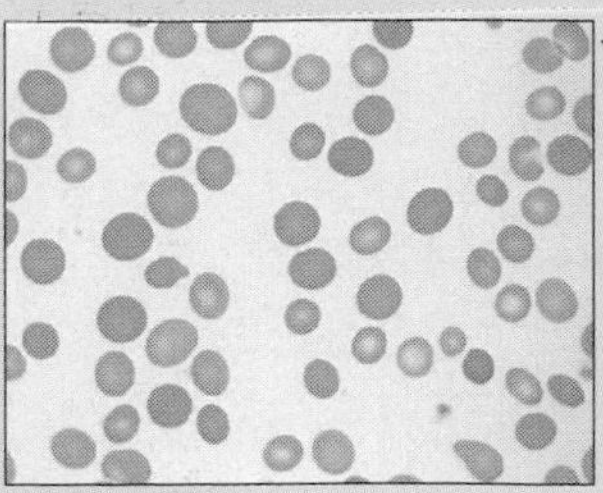

anisocytosis

peripheral blood; (Wright-Giemsa stain, ×250)

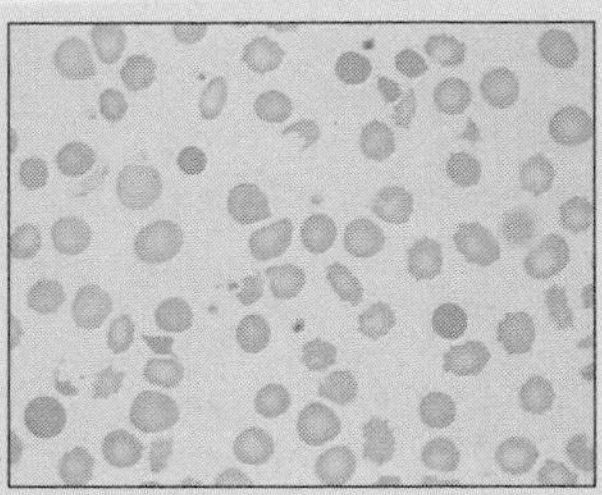

poikilocytosis

with various red blood cell types (Wright-Giemsa stain, ×250)

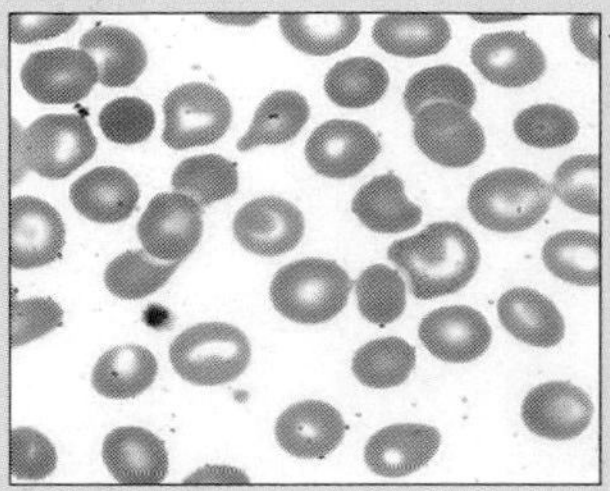

microcytosis

shown in thalassemia minor

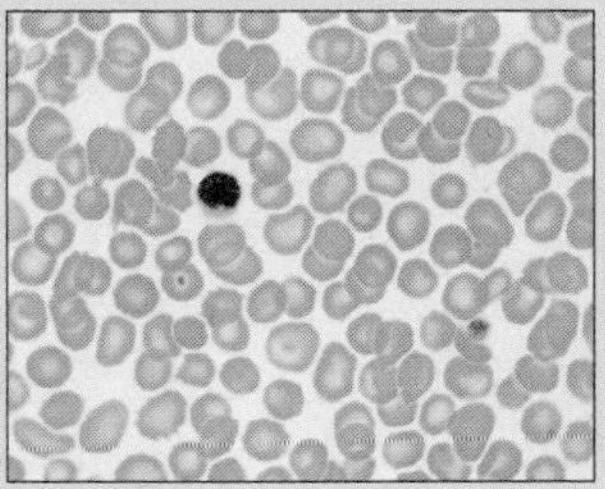

macrocytosis

peripheral blood from newborn (Wright-Giemsa stain, ×250)

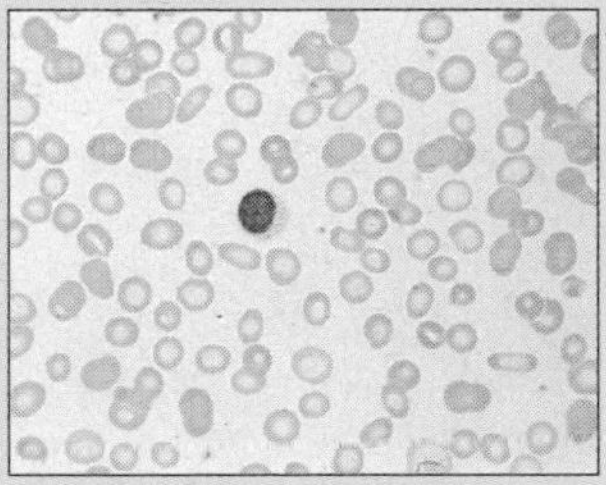

microcytic, hypochromic anemia

peripheral blood (Wright-Giemsa stain, ×250)

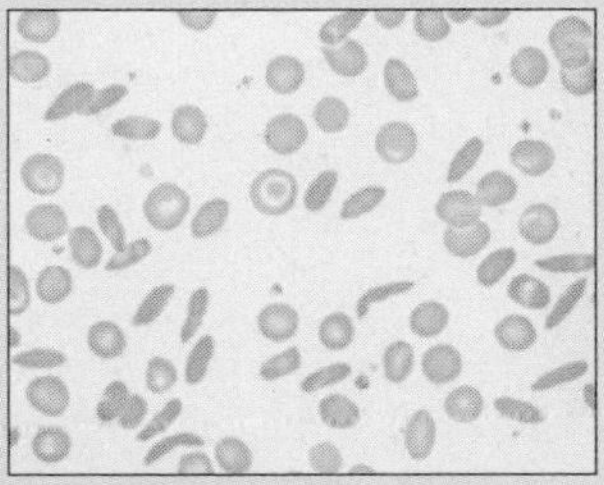

sickle cell anemia

showing poikilocytosis; peripheral blood (Wright Giemsa stain, ×250)

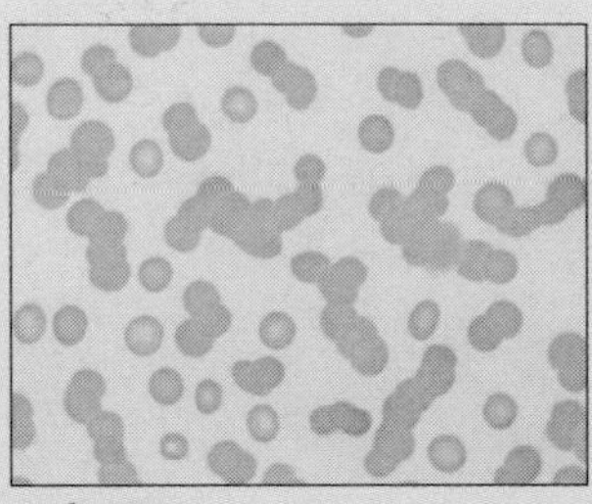

rouleaux

erythrocytes are stacked like coins; patient has multiple myeloma

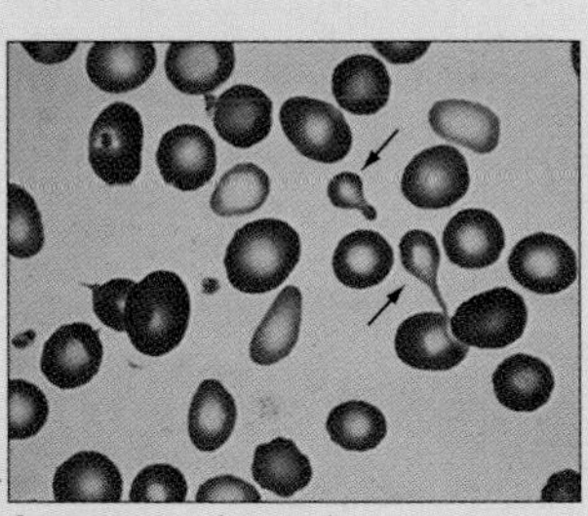

dacryocytes (arrows)

peripheral blood smear

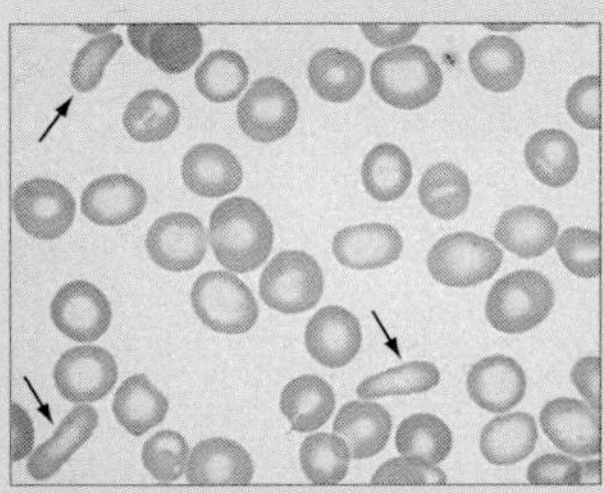

elliptocytes (arrows)

peripheral blood smear

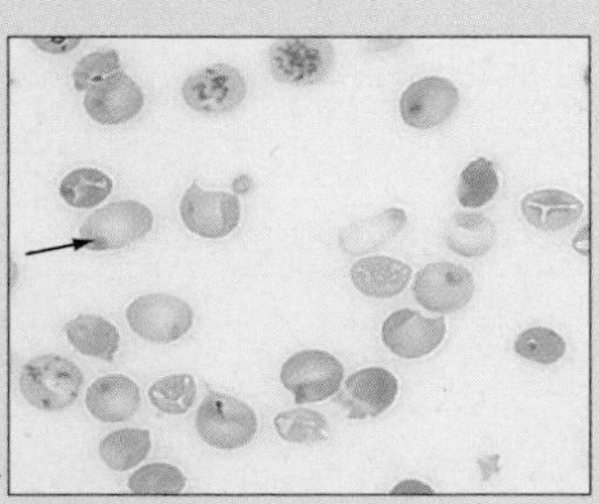

Heinz bodies

round, refractile inclusions found on the periphery of the cell when stained with a supravital dye (size: 1-2 mcm)

PLATE 4: BACTERIA AND BACTERIAL INFECTIONS

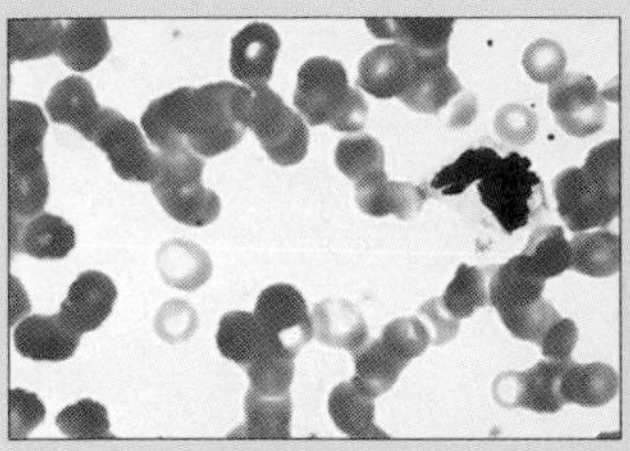

Borrelia (Wright-Giemsa stain)

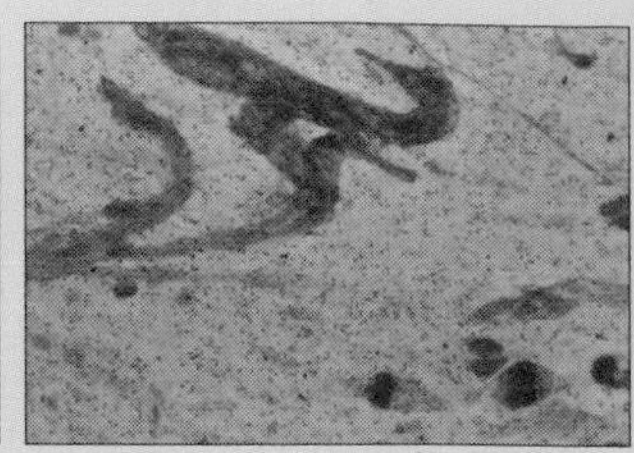

Gram stain of ***Haemophilus influenzae*** in sputum

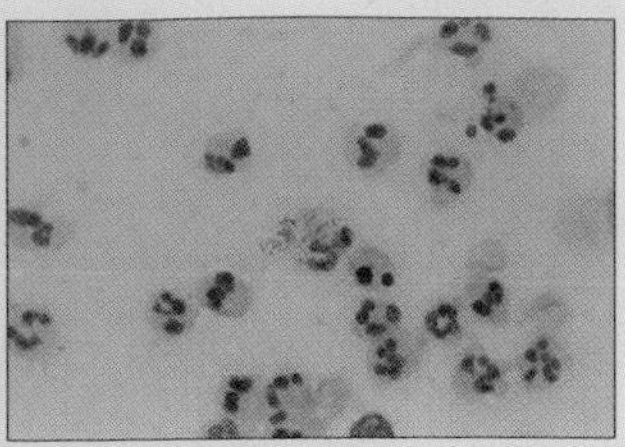

Gram stain of ***Neisseria gonorrhoeae*** in urethral exudate

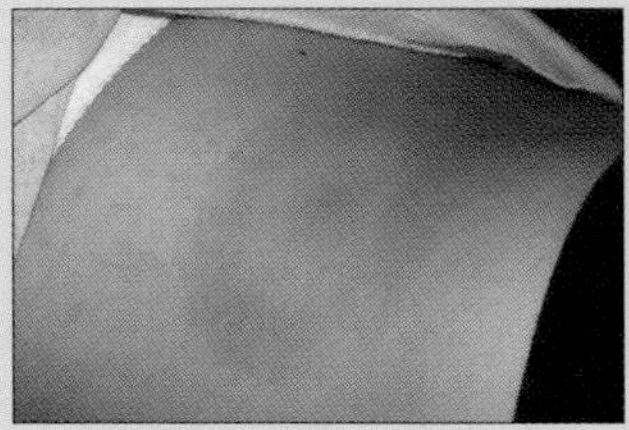

acute Lyme disease (*Borrelia* infection)

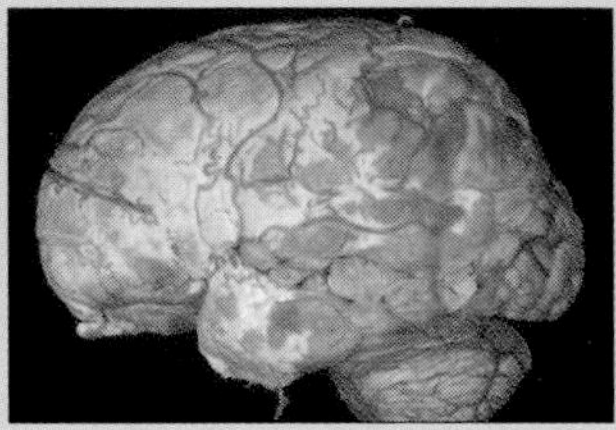

***Haemophilus influenzae* meningitis**

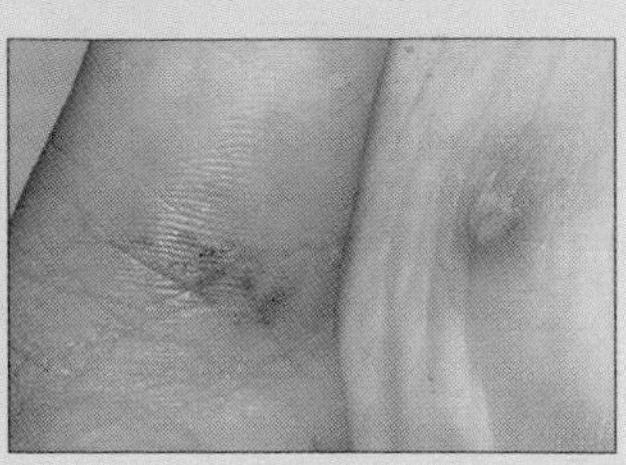

disseminated gonococcemia (*Neisseria gonorrhoeae* infection)

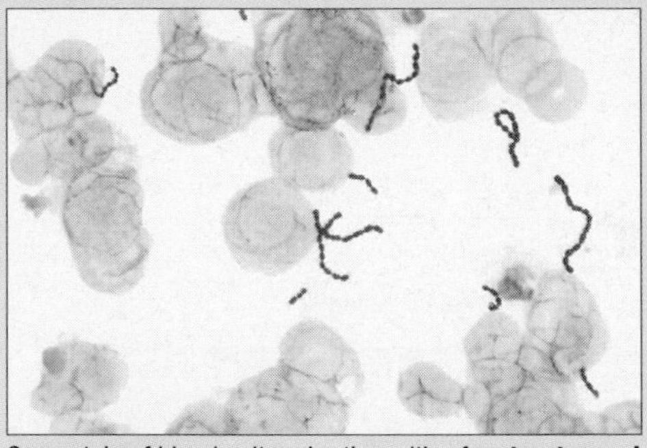

Gram stain of blood culture broth positive for **streptococci**

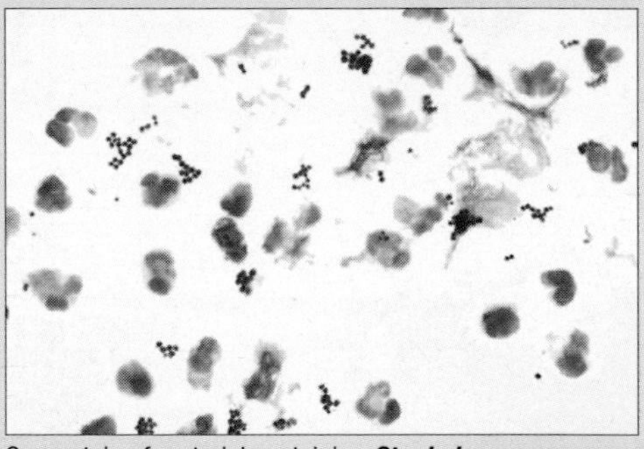

Gram stain of material containing ***Staphylococcus aureus***

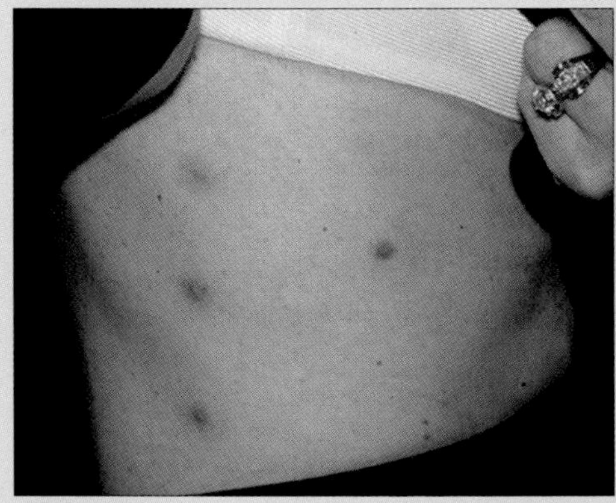

hot tub foliculitis (*Pseudomonas aeruginosa* infection)

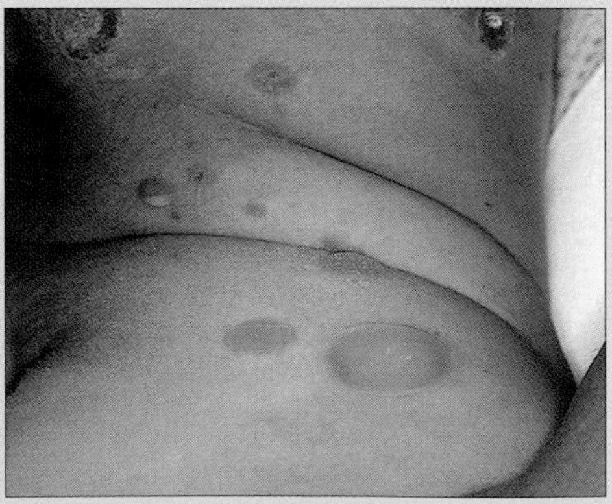

bullous impetigo (*Staphylococcus aureus* infection)

PLATE 5: FUNGI AND FUNGAL INFECTIONS

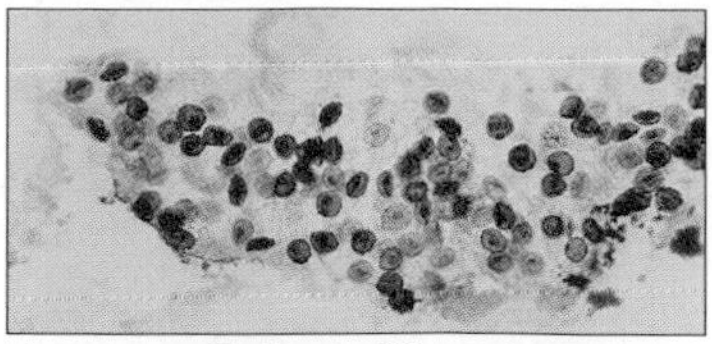

Pneumocystis jiroveci (Gomori methenamine silver stain, ×1,000)

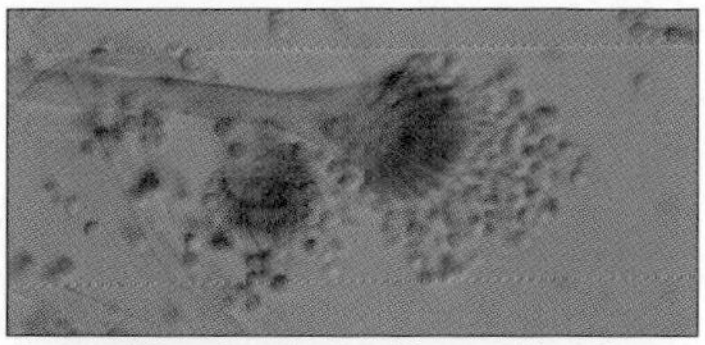

Aspergillus fumigatus (Nomarski optics, ×625)

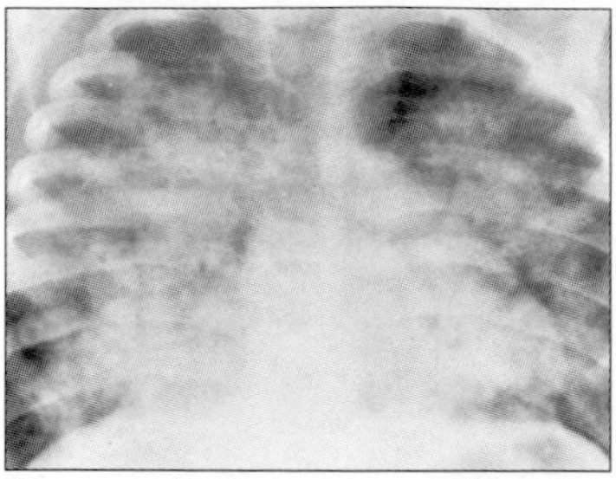

Pneumocystis jiroveci **pneumonia**

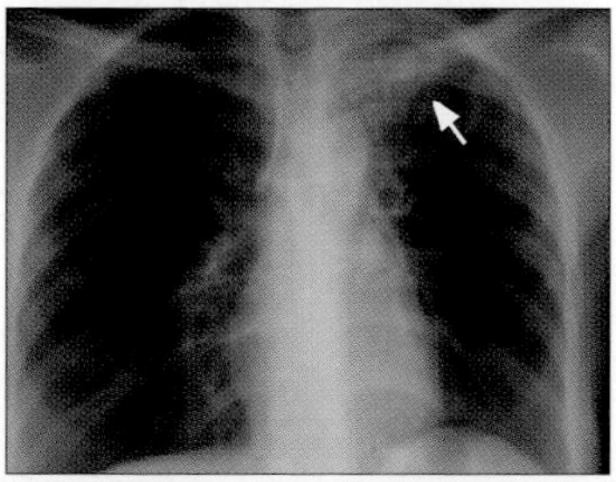

posttuberculous bronchiectasis complicated by a mycetoma (*Aspergillus fumigatus*, arrow)

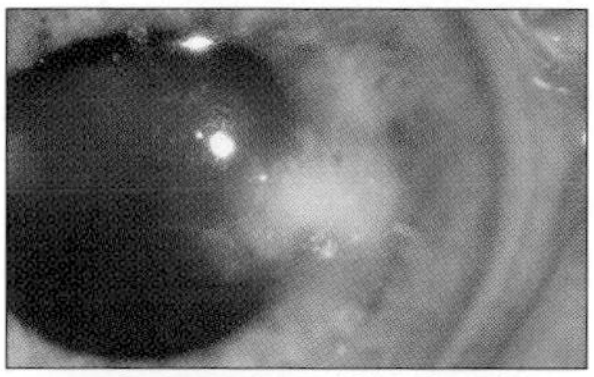

corneal ulcer caused by *Fusarium*

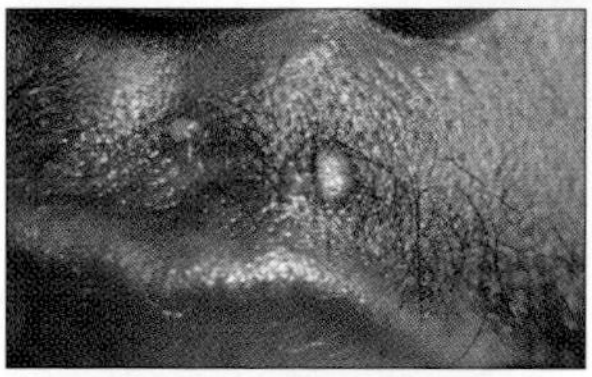

disseminated cryptococcosis

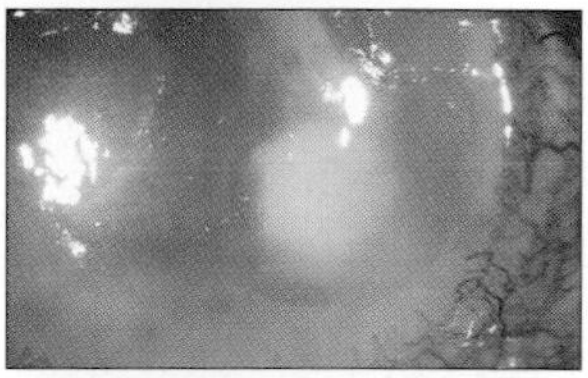

corneal ulcer caused by *Candida albicans* infection

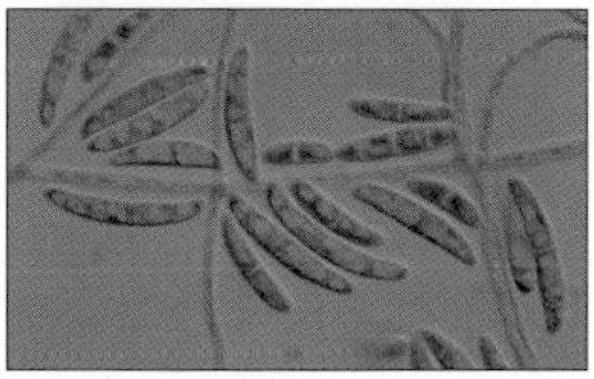

Fusarium solani (×625)

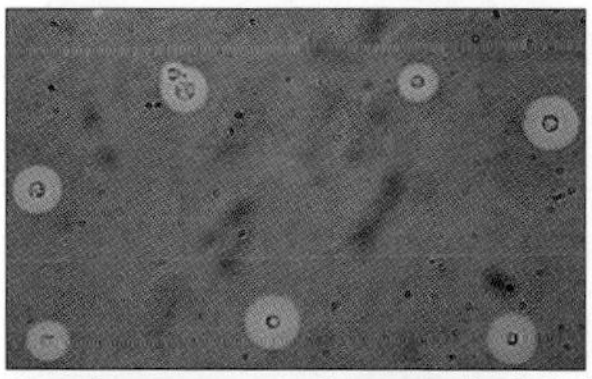

Cryptococcus neoformans (India ink, ×600)

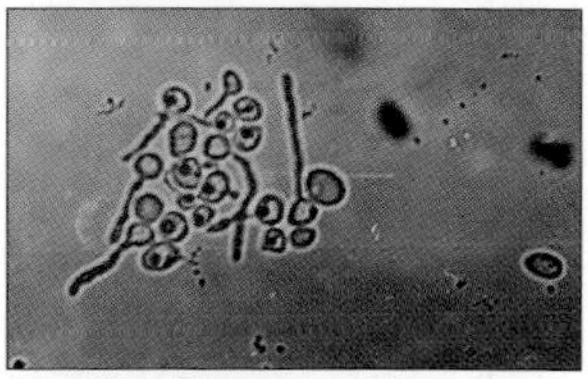

Candida albicans (×600)

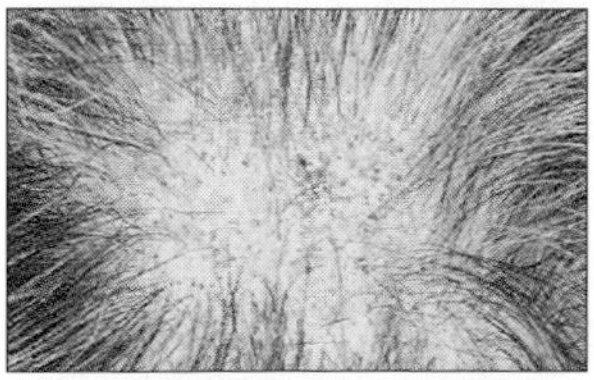

tinea capitis (black dot type) caused by *Trichophyton tonsurans*

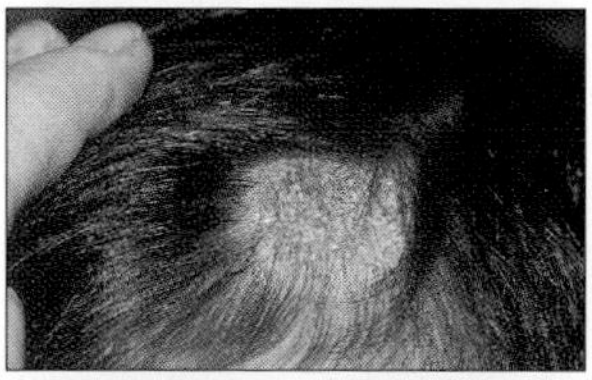

tinea capitis (gray patch type) caused by *Microsporum canis*

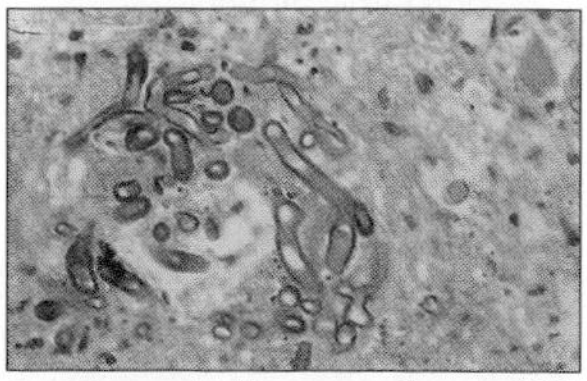

zygomycosis (tissue section, ×600)

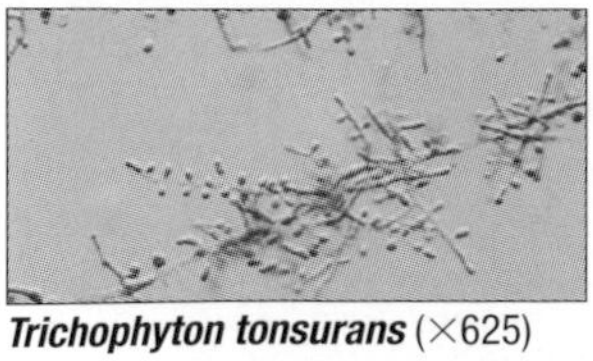

Trichophyton tonsurans (×625)

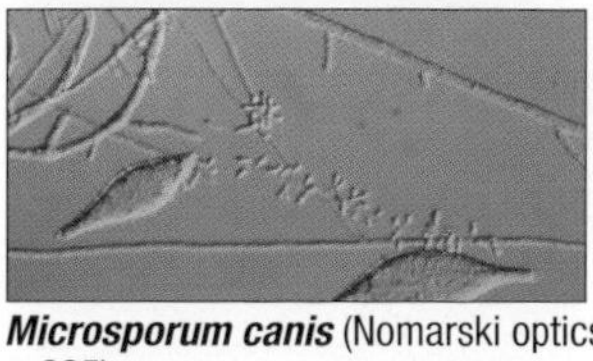

Microsporum canis (Nomarski optics, ×625)

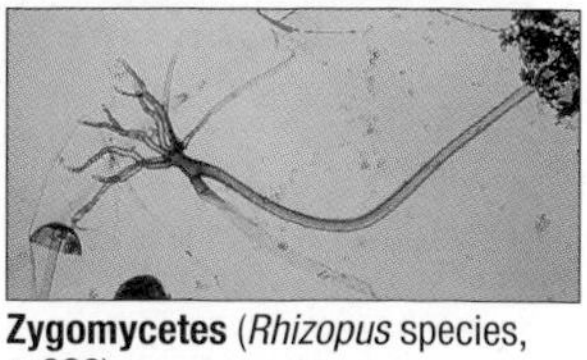

Zygomycetes (*Rhizopus* species, ×300)

PLATE 6: VIRUSES AND VIRAL INFECTIONS

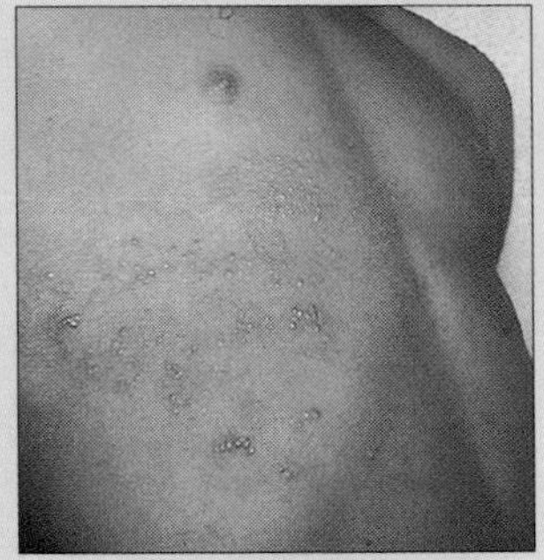

mild zoster eruption

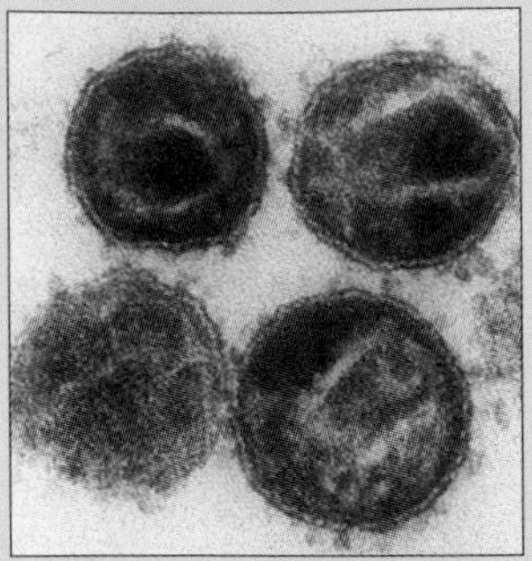

human immunodeficiency virus (HIV)

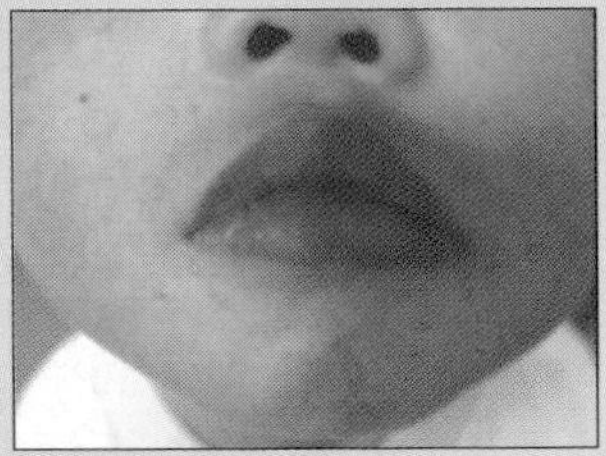

molluscum contagiosum

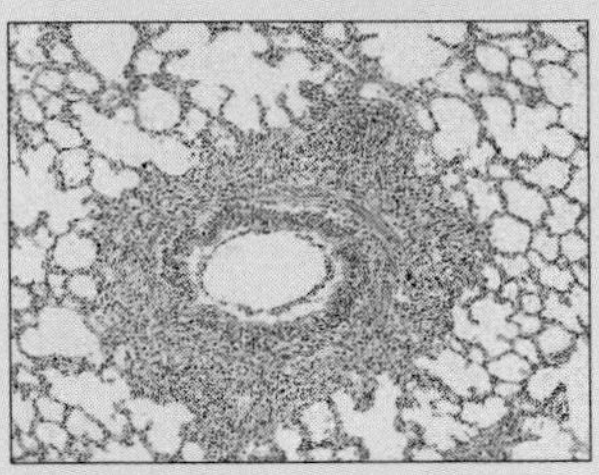

bronchiolitis due to **adenovirus**

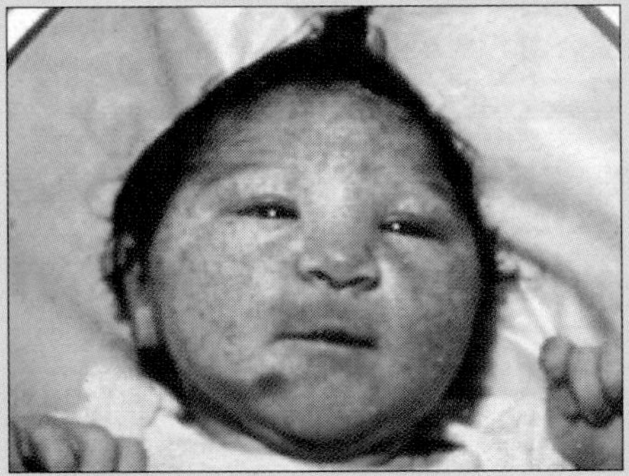

congenital cytomegalovirus

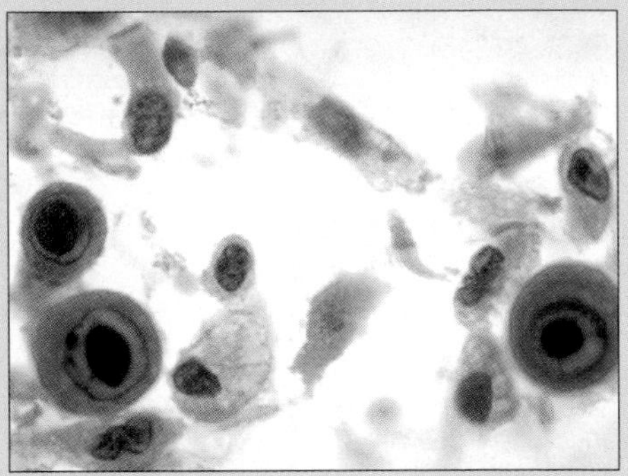

cytomegalovirus (CMV) infection in bronchial washings

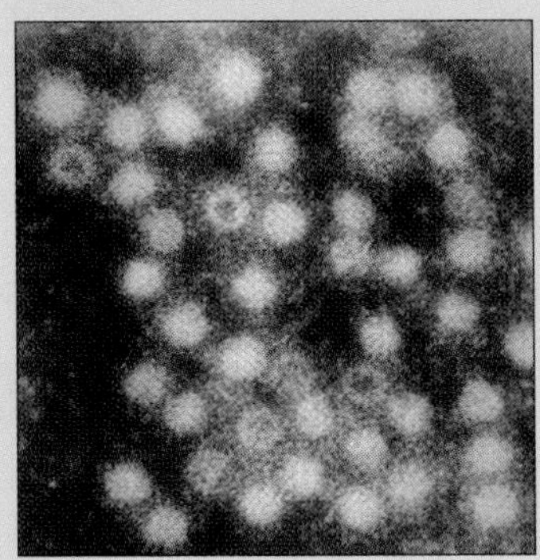

hepatitis A virus (HAV)

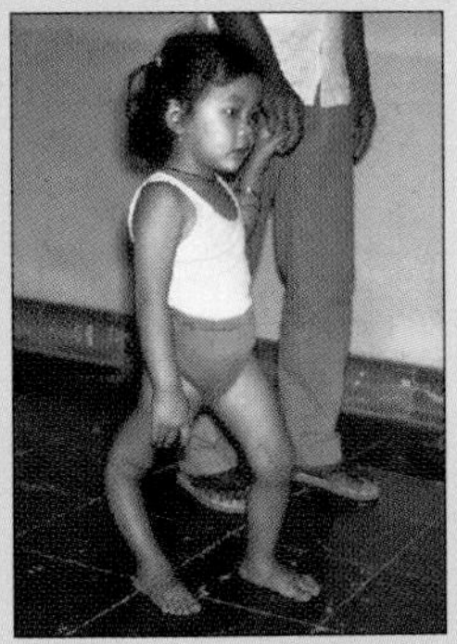

deformed leg of child due to **polio**

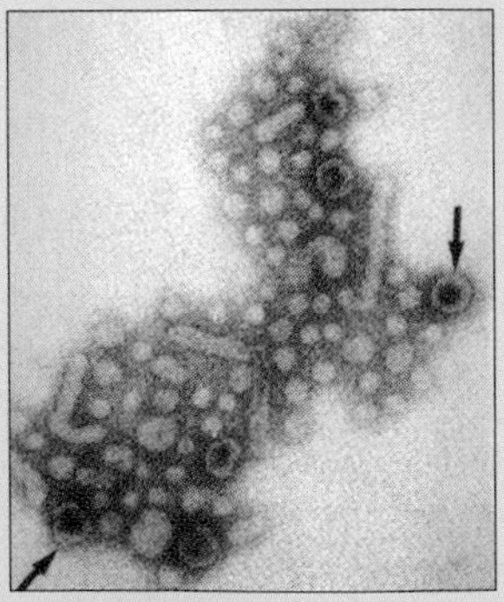

hepatitis B: Dane particles (arrows)

PLATE 7: PARASITES AND PARASITIC INFECTIONS

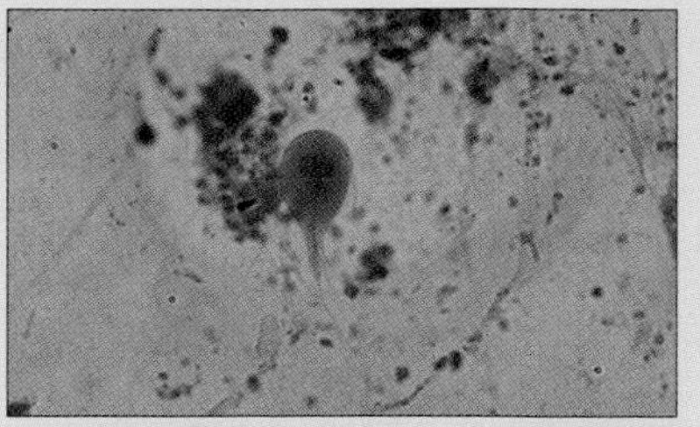

trophozoite of *G. lamblia* (trichrome, ×400)

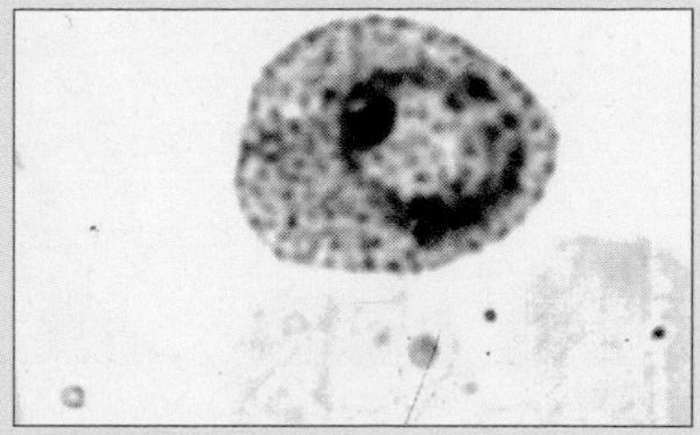

Plasmodium vivax

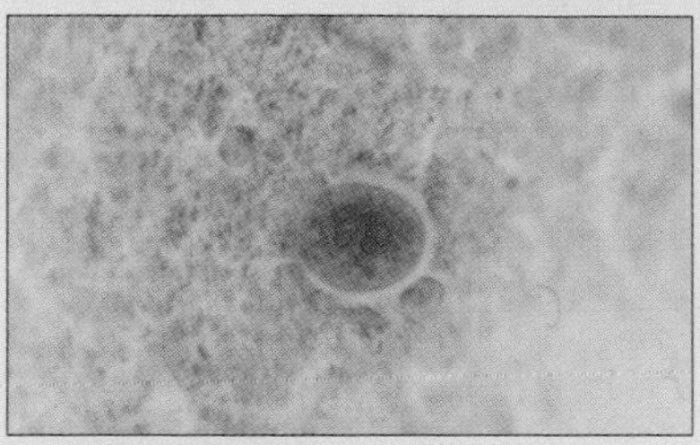

cyst of *E. coli* (unstained, ×160)

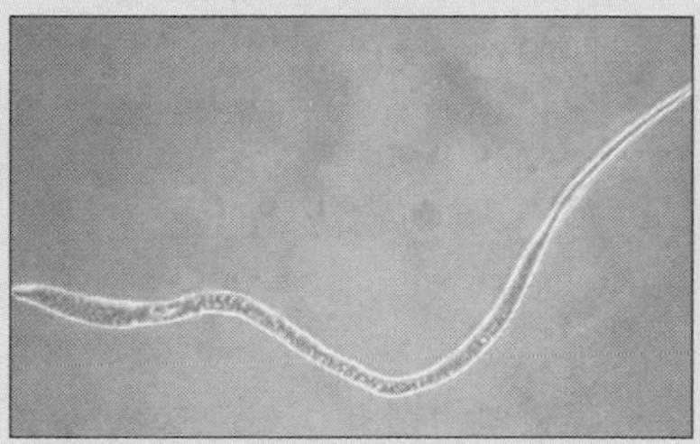

adult female worm of *Trichinella spiralis* (phase-contrast microscopy, ×32)

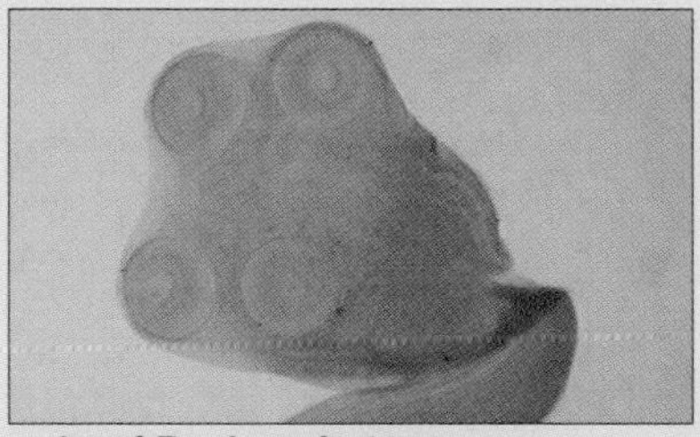

scolex of *Taenia saginata*

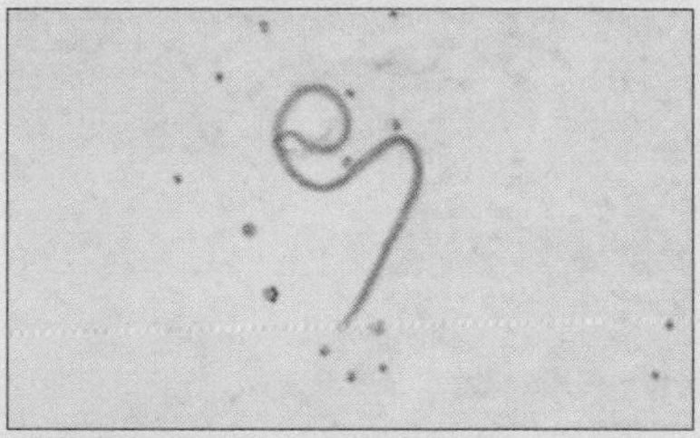

microfilaria of *W. bancrofti* (Giemsa, ×100)

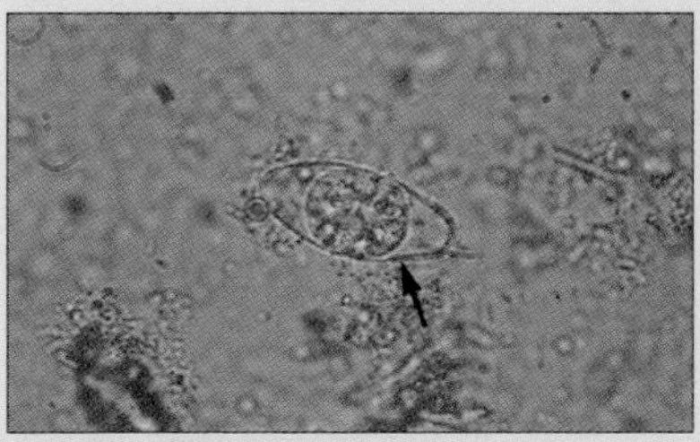

immature oocyst of *I. belli* (unstained stool wet-mount, ×400)

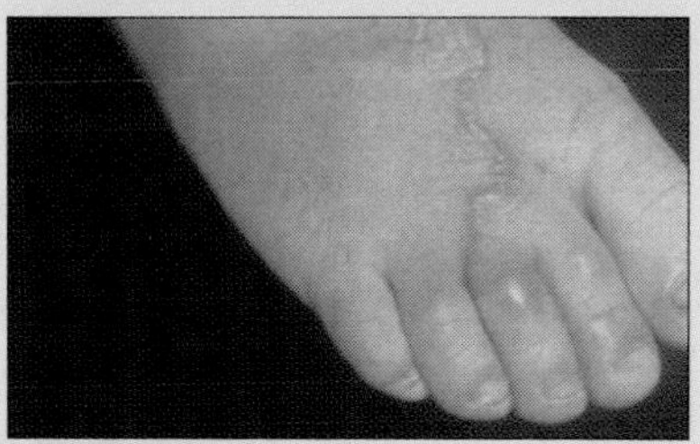

cutaneous larva migrans (creeping eruption) caused by hookworm infection

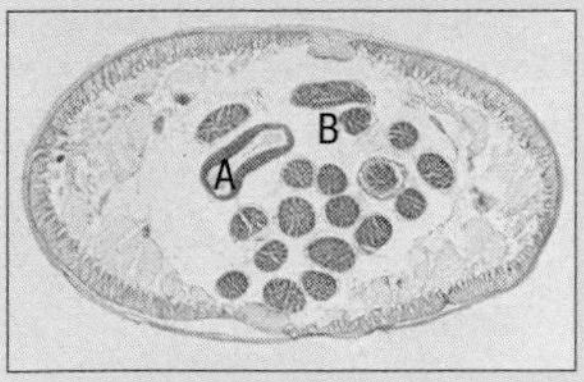

nematode (cross-section): (A) alimentary canal; (B) body cavity

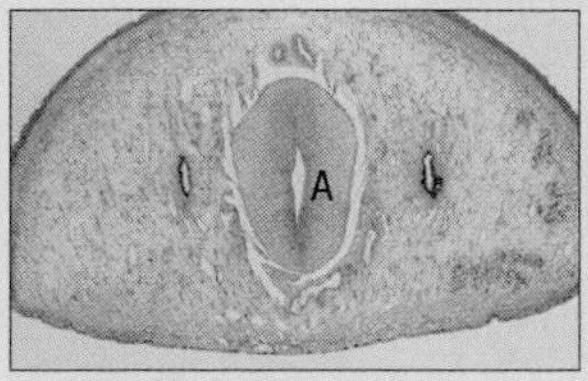

trematode (cross-section): (A) alimentary canal

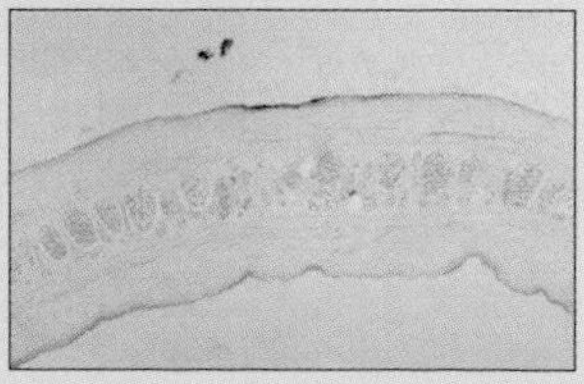

cestode (cross-section, hematoxylin and eosin, ×16)

PLATE 8: BITES, STINGS, AND INFESTATIONS

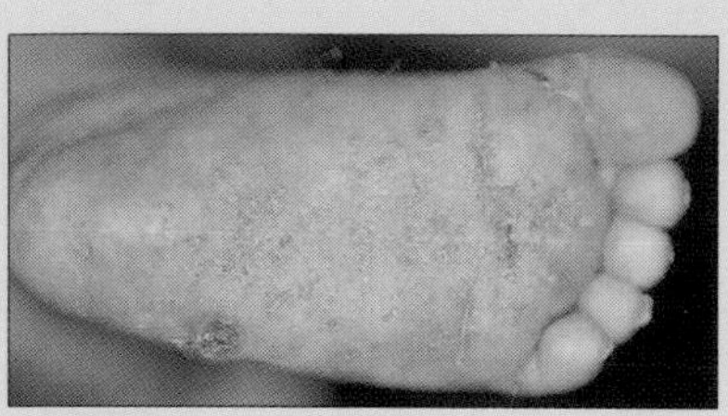

scabies

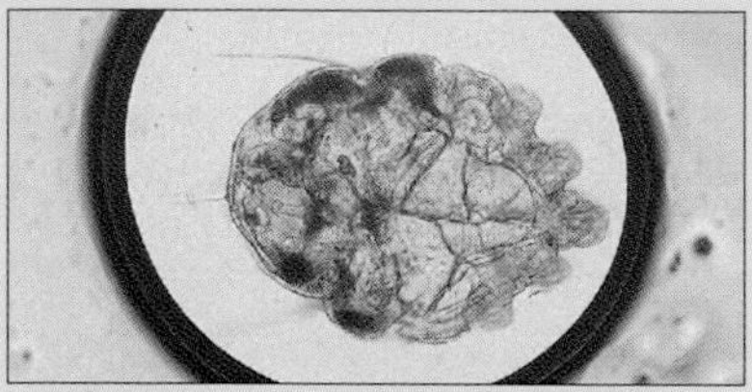

scabies mite

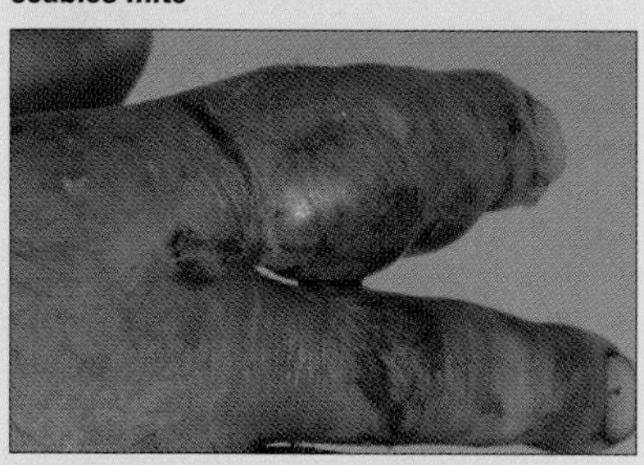

right index bleb: patient was bitten by a Western Diamondback rattlesnake and used belt around base of finger to act as a tourniquet

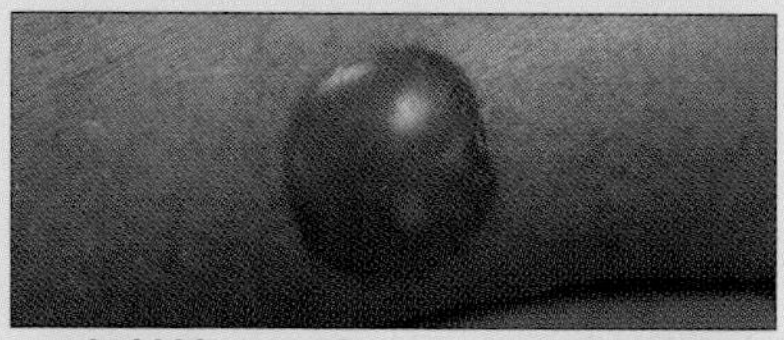

arachnid bite reaction

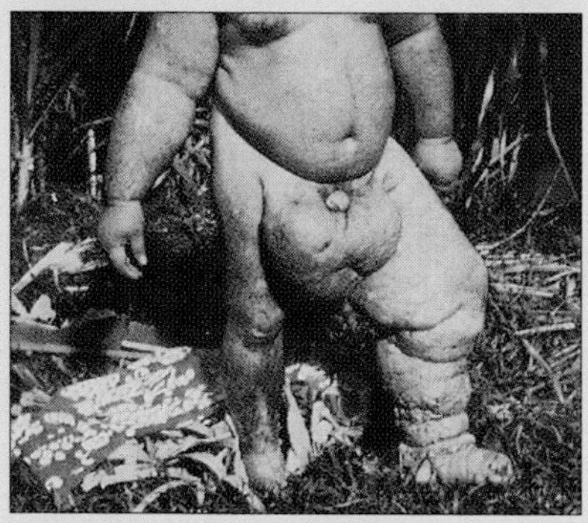

bancroftian filariasis (elephantiasis)

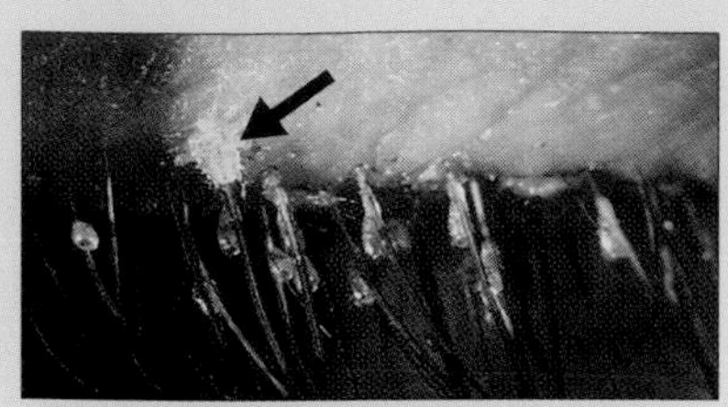

***Pthirus pubis* infestation**

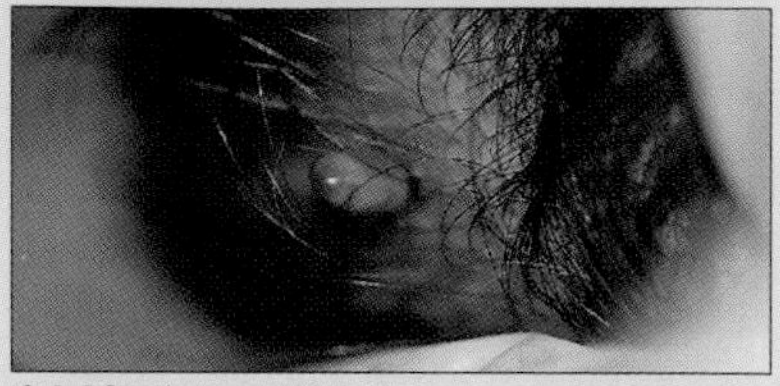

tick bite (engorged tick)

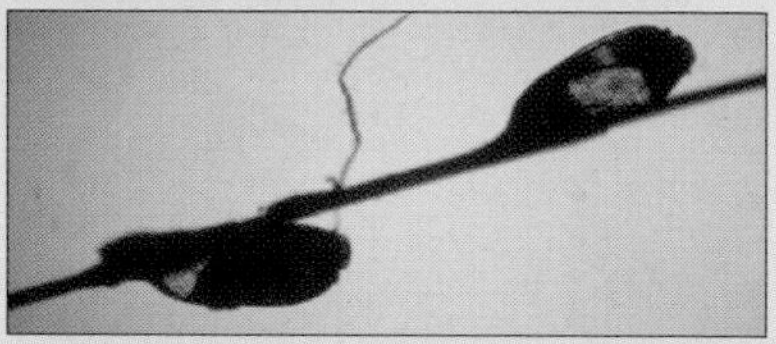

nits (egg cases) attached to hairs

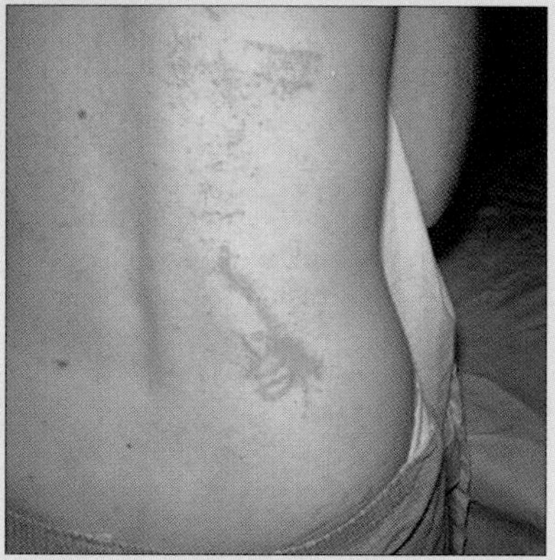

jellyfish sting

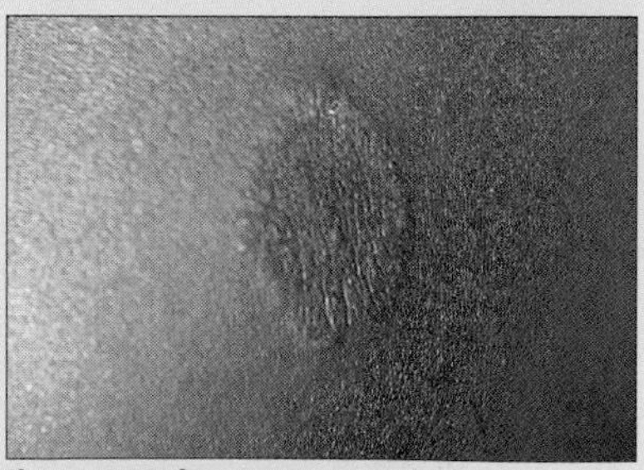

tinea corporis

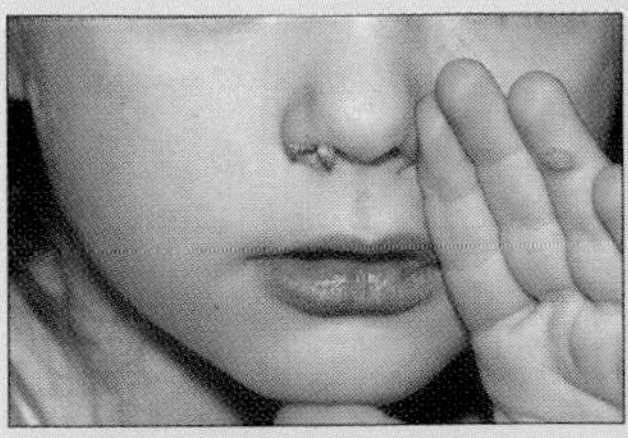

filiform (nose) and **common warts** (finger)

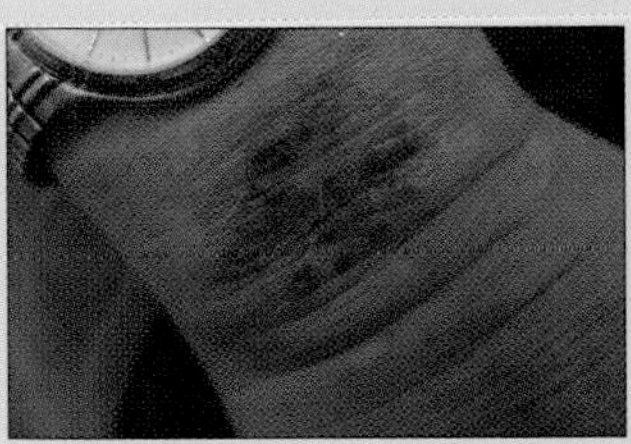

contact dermatitis (nickel on watch)

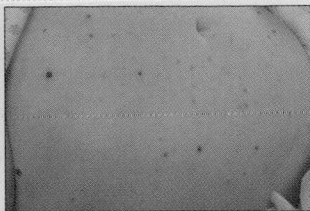

disseminated shingles (herpes zoster)

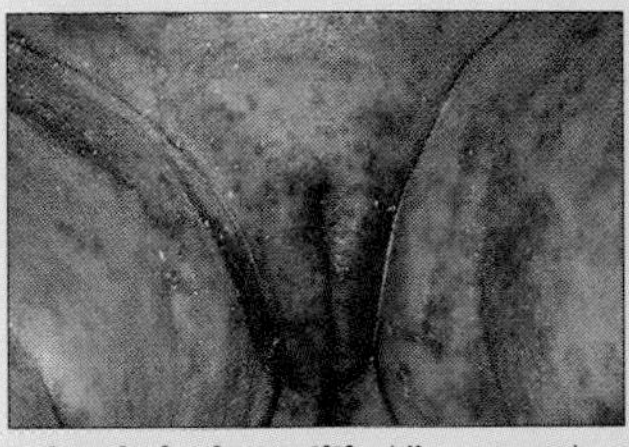

seborrheic dermatitis (diaper area)

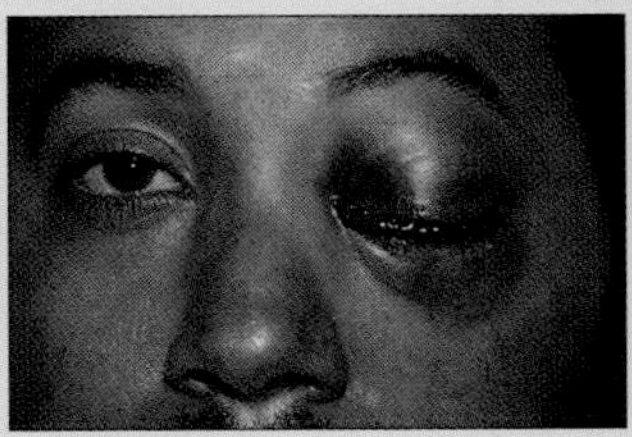

orbital cellulitis

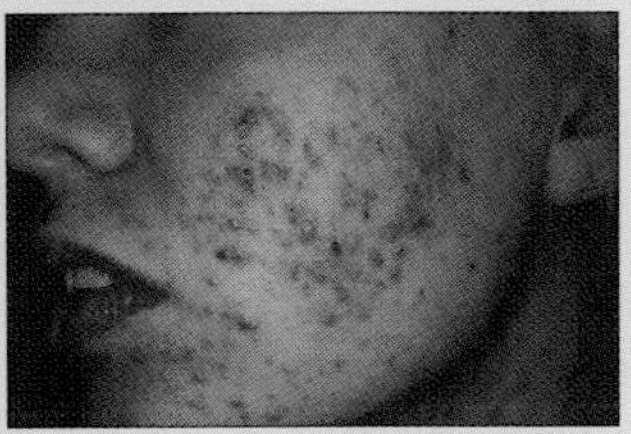

facial acne in an adolescent

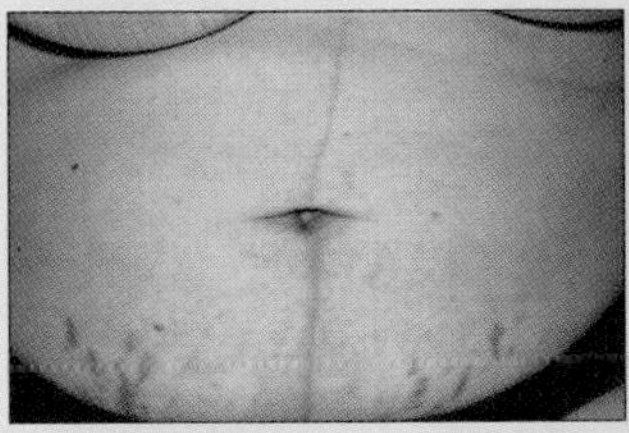

linea nigra and striae gravidarum

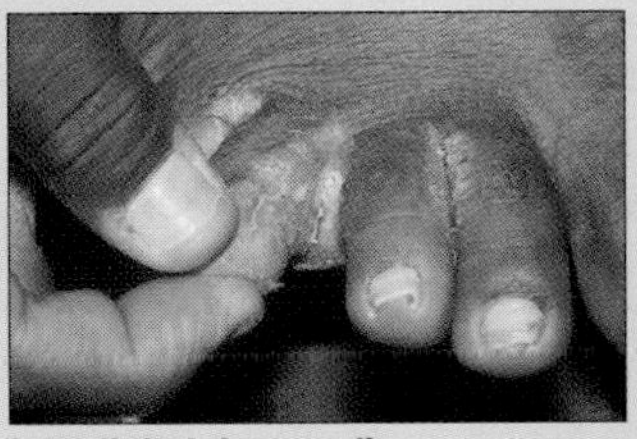

interdigital tinea pedis (toe web infection)

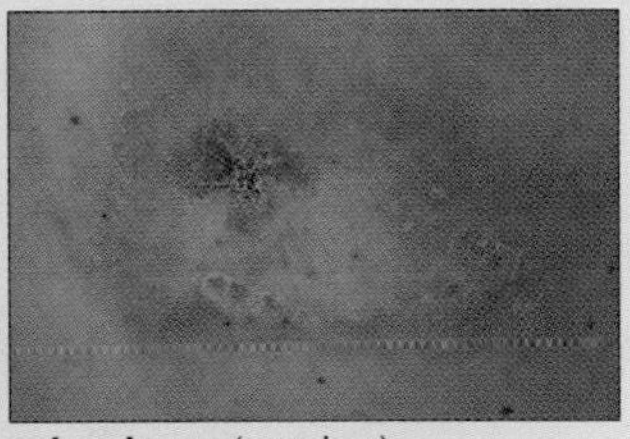

scleroderma (morphea)

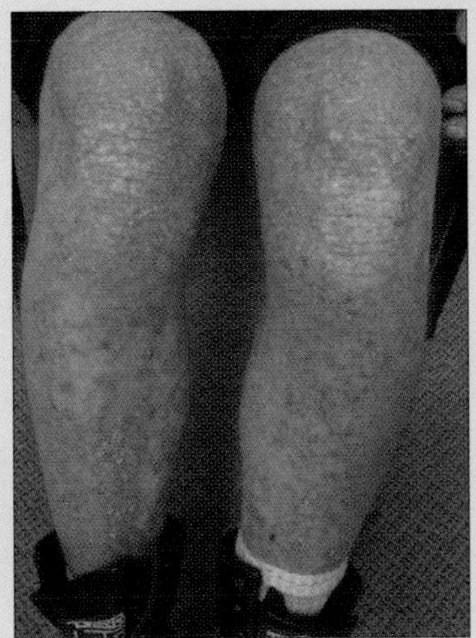

psoriasis on legs

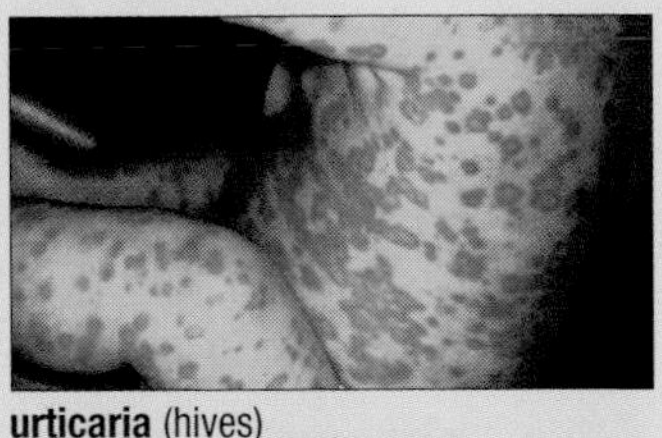

urticaria (hives)

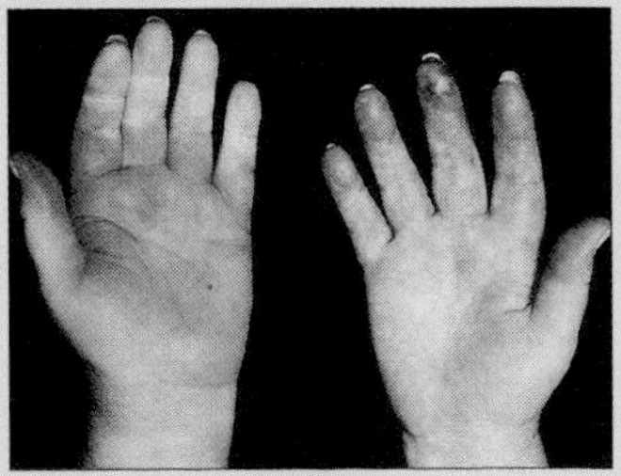

Raynaud phenomenon

PLATE 10: PRIMARY LESIONS

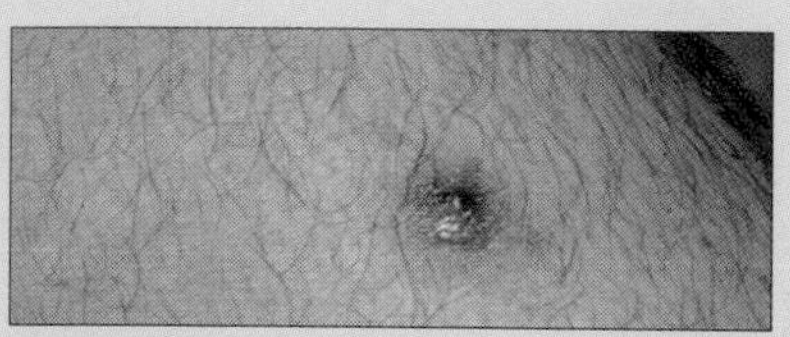

furuncle

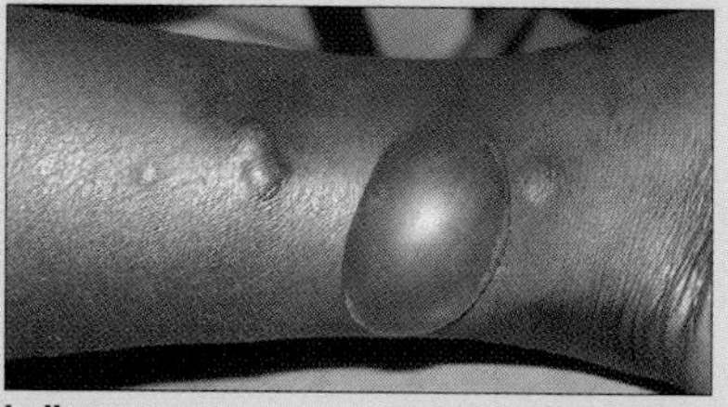

bulla

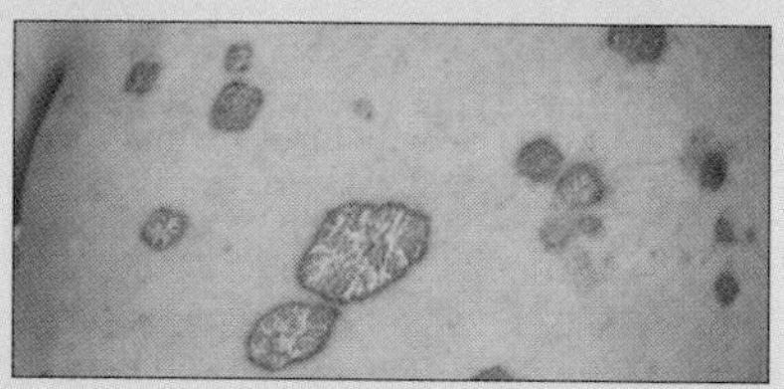

plaque

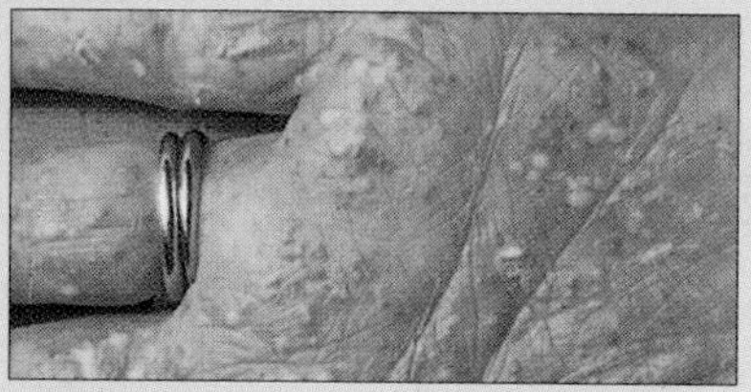

pustules (in pustular psoriasis)

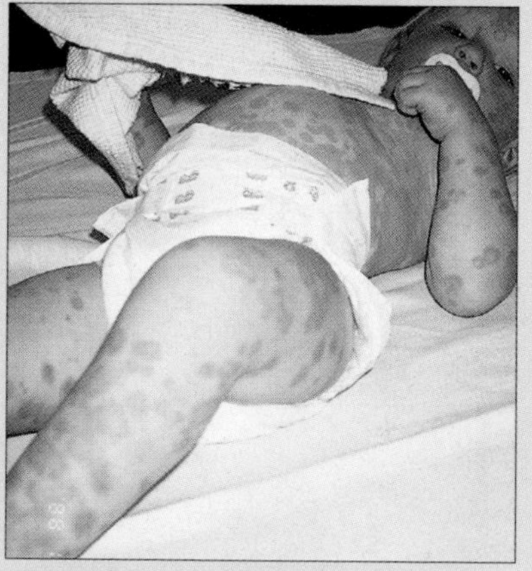

wheals (urticaria)

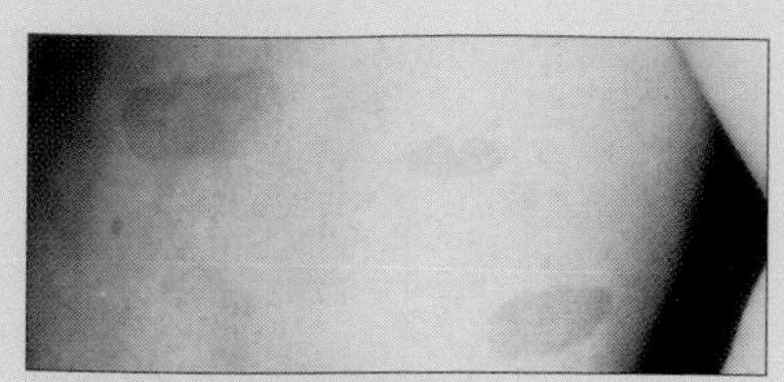

patch (café au lait spot)

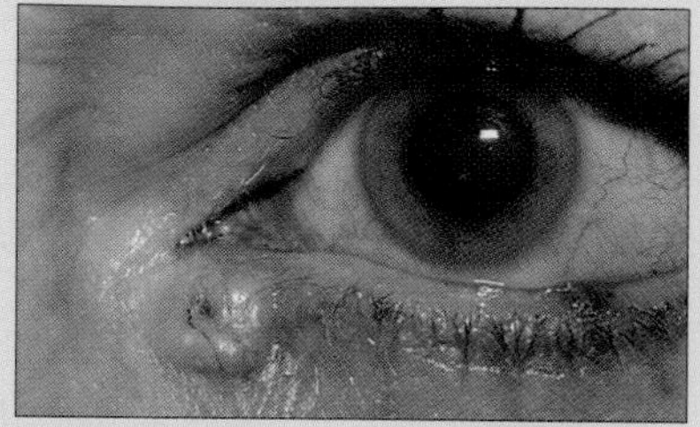

tumor

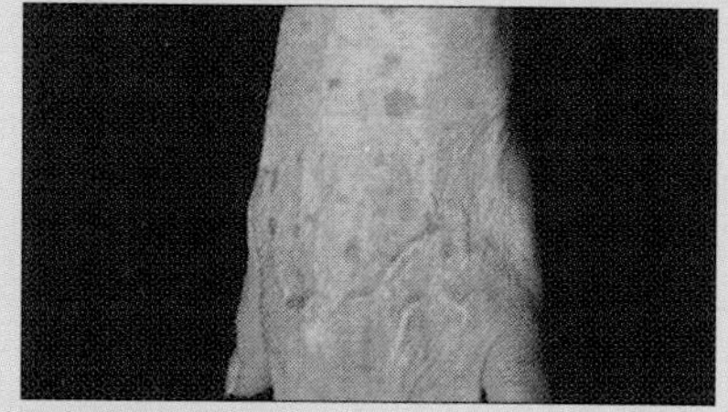

macules (actinic lentigines)

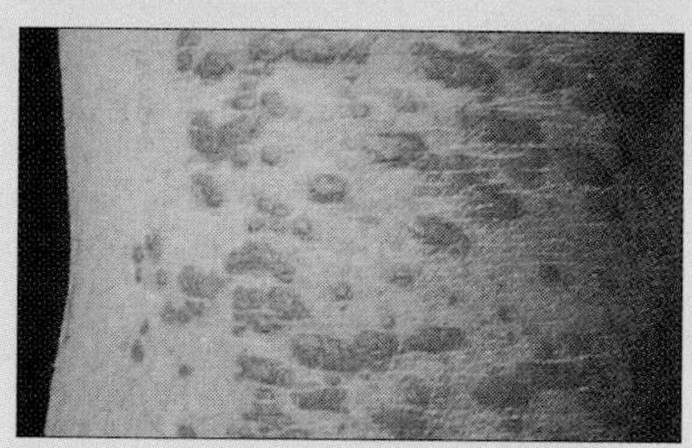

papules (in lichen planus)

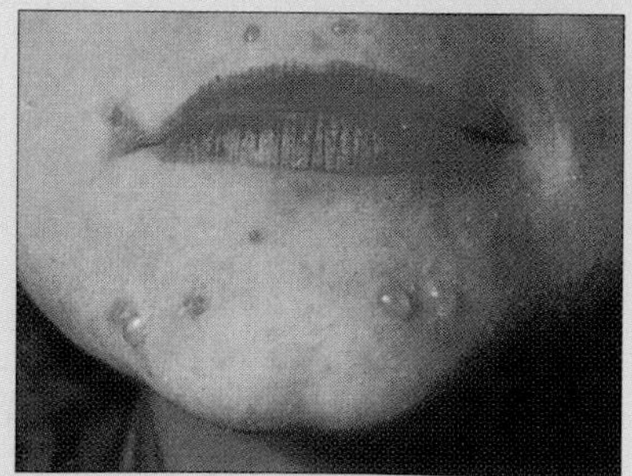

vesicles (in pemphigus)

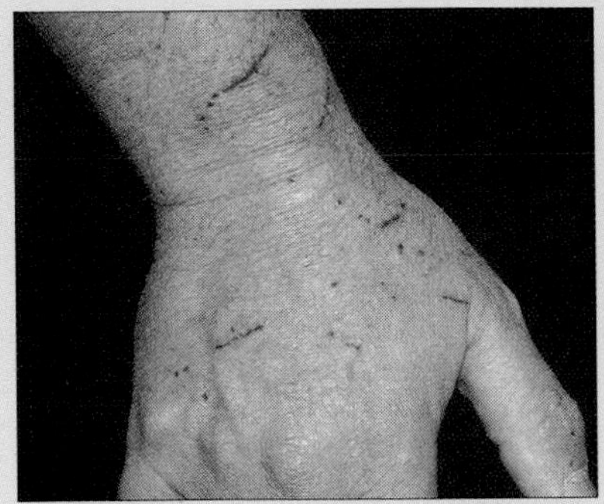

excoriation

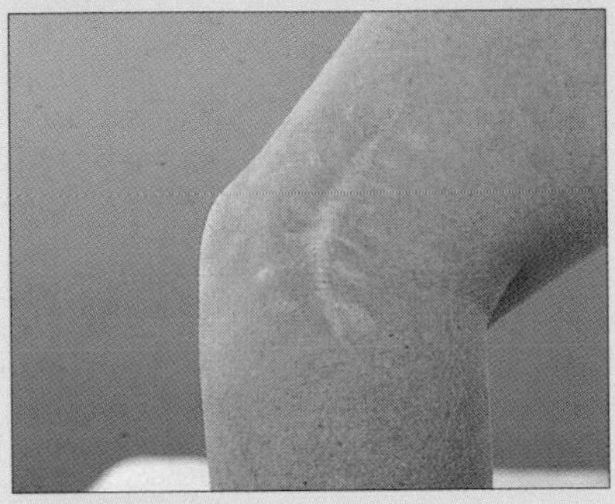

scar

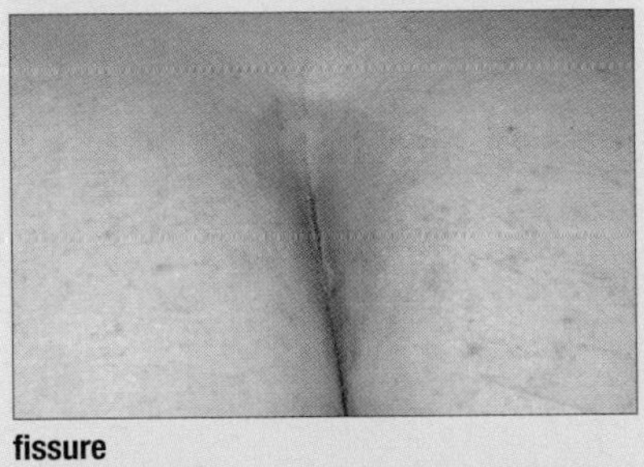

fissure

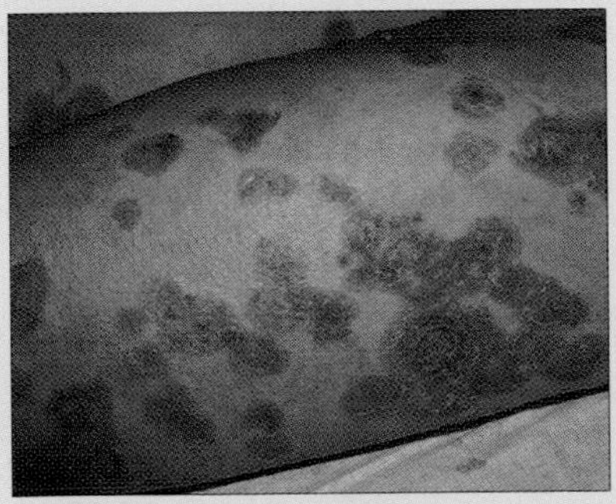

crusts (streptococcal impetigo)

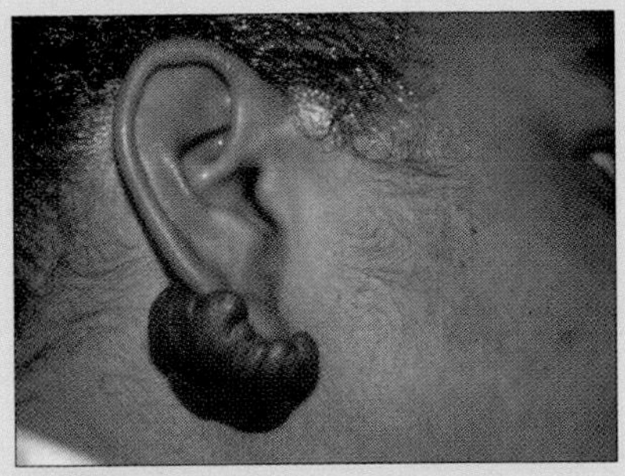

keloid

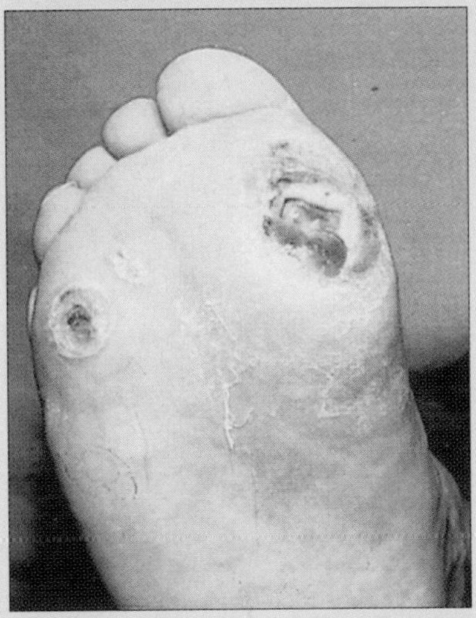

ulcers

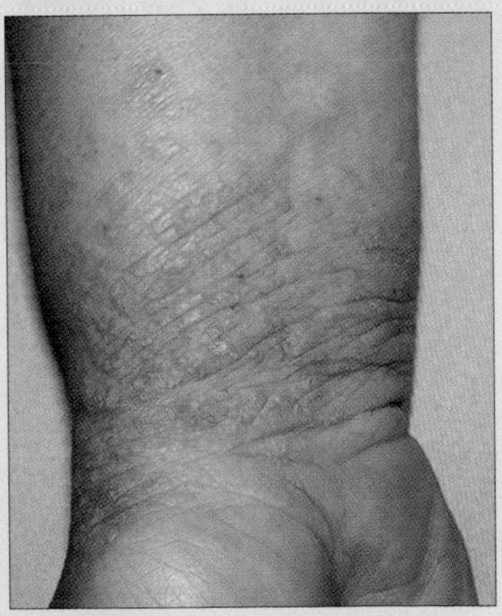

lichenification

PLATE 12: NAIL AND HAIR DISORDERS

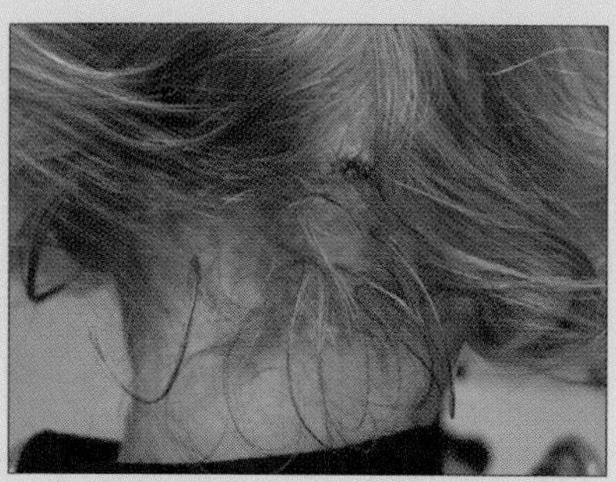

trichotillomania

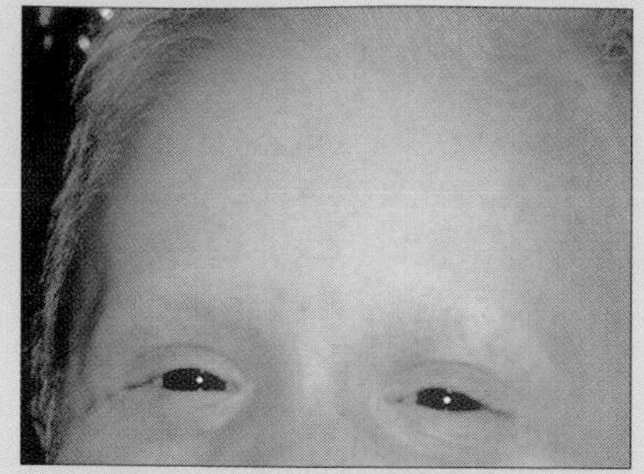

hypohidrotic ectodermal dysplasia

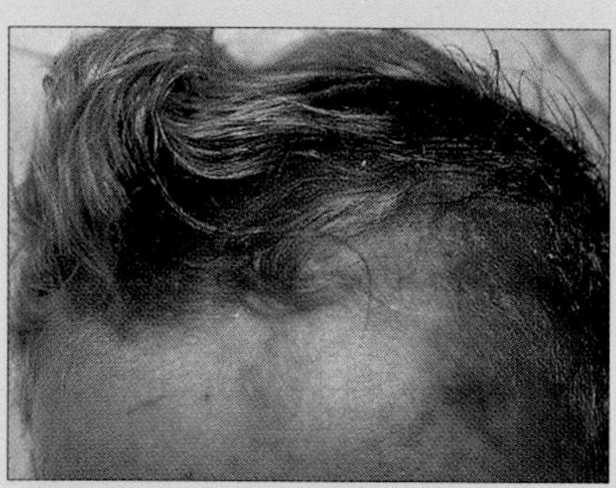

Chédiak-Higashi syndrome

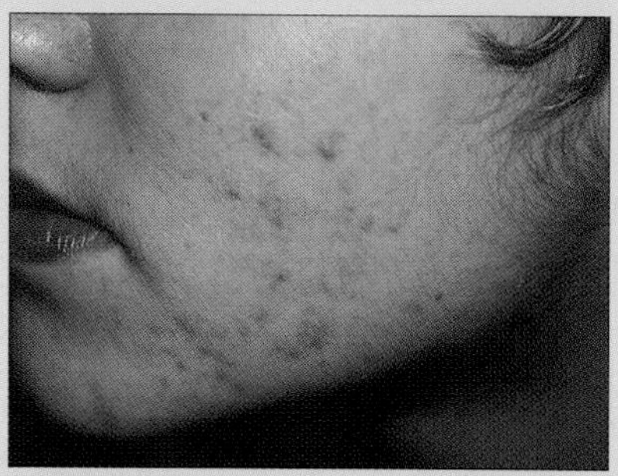

hirsutism

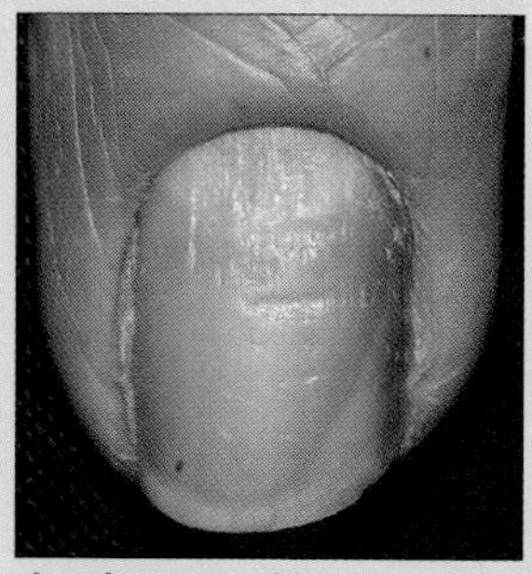

chronic paronychia

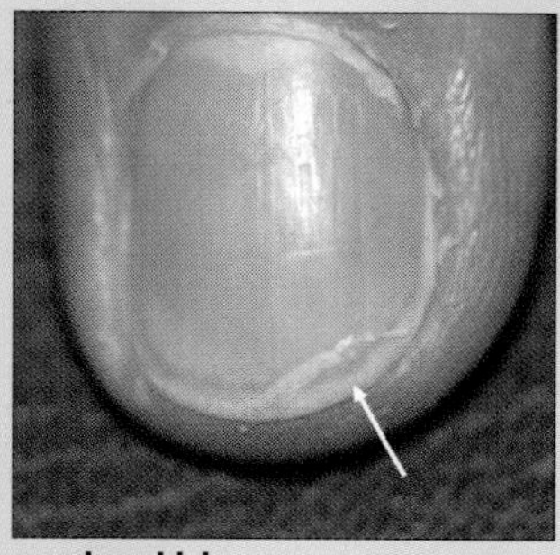

onychoschizia

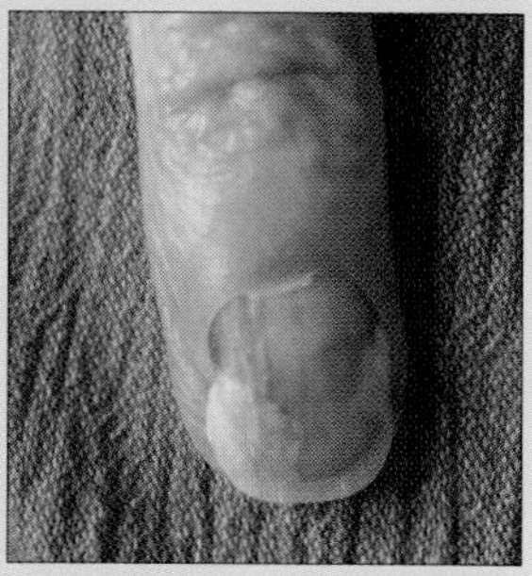

onycholysis in psoriasis

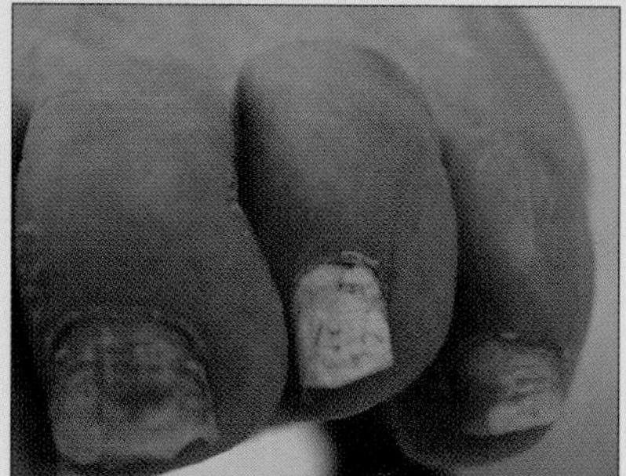

onychomycosis *(Trichophyton mentagrophytes)*

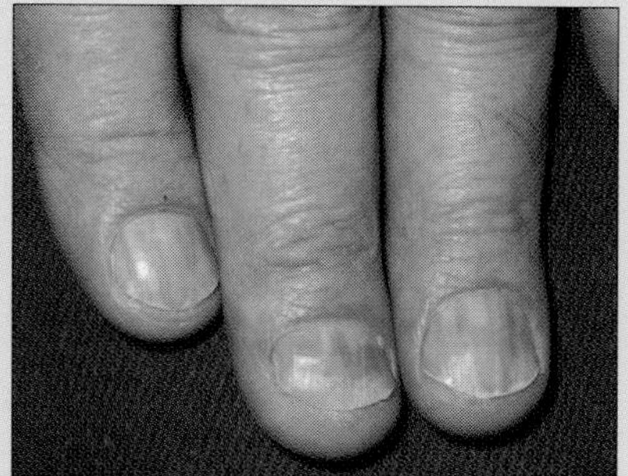

Darier disease (keratosis follicularis)

PLATE 13: VASCULAR AND SPECIALIZED PRIMARY LESIONS

Vascular Lesions

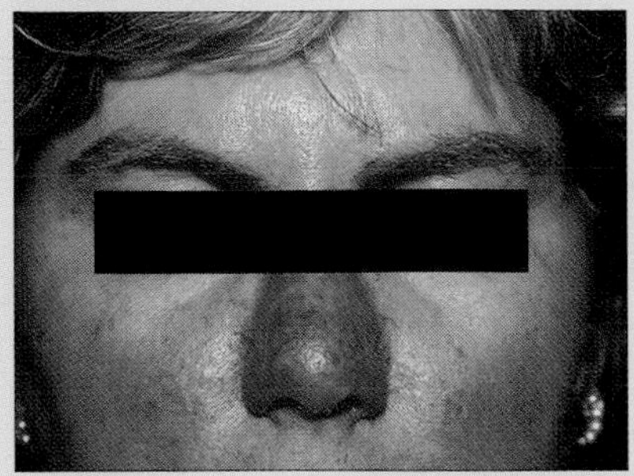

telangiectases

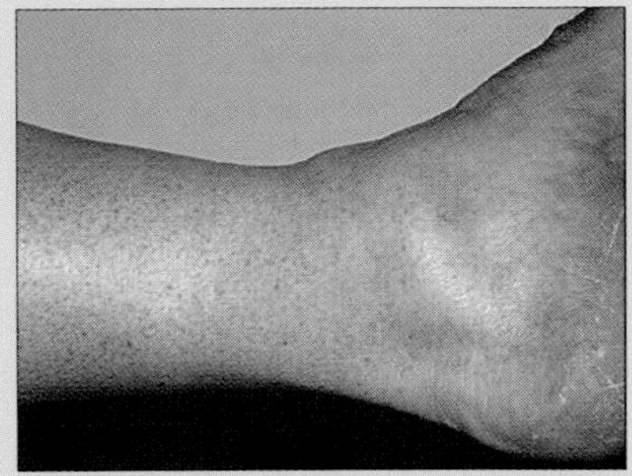

petechiae

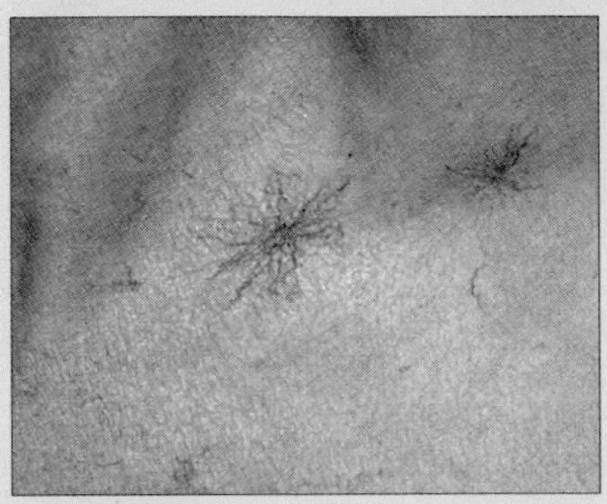

spider angioma

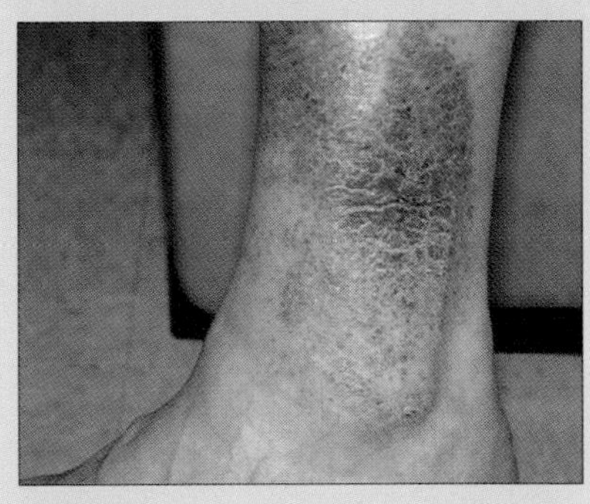

purpura

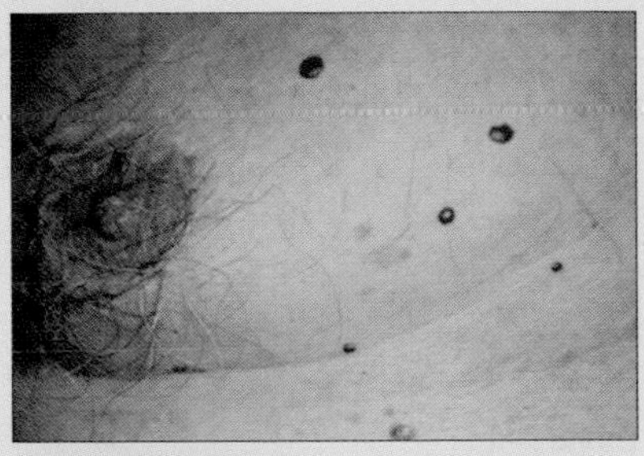

cherry angiomas

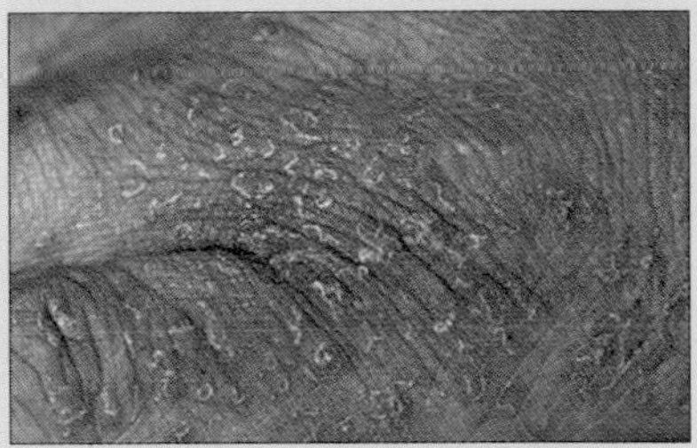

burrows

Specialized Primary Lesions

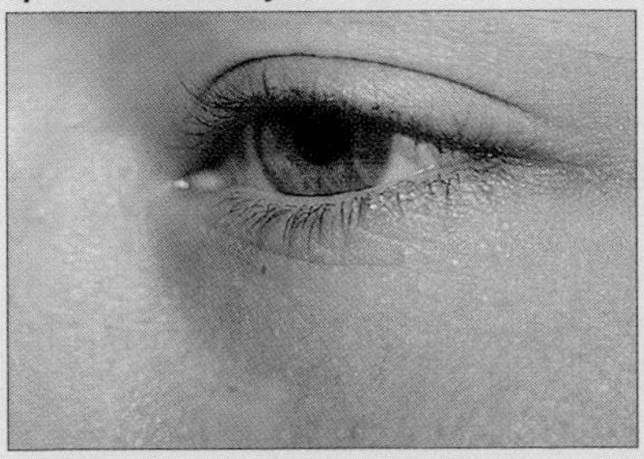

milia

comedones (open)

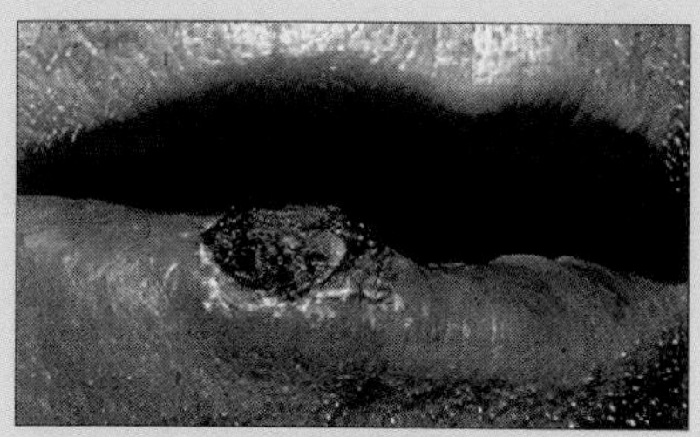
squamous cell carcinoma

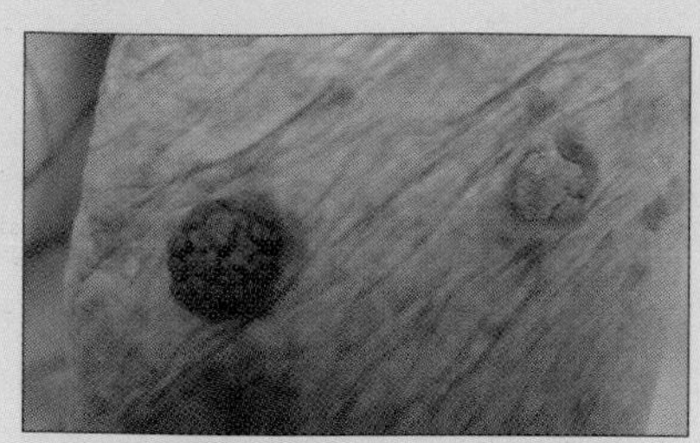
seborrheic keratoses

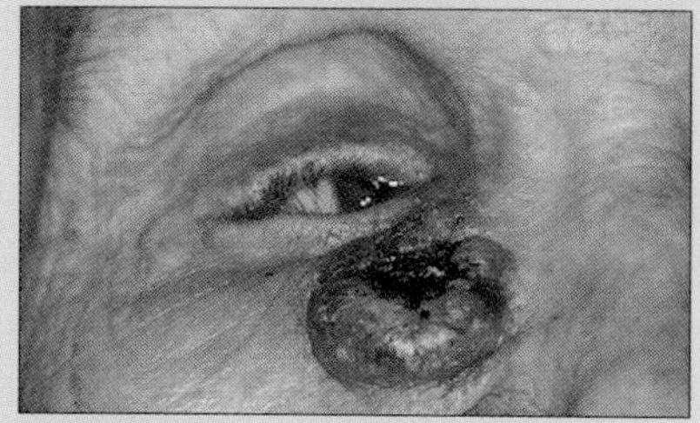
keratoacanthoma

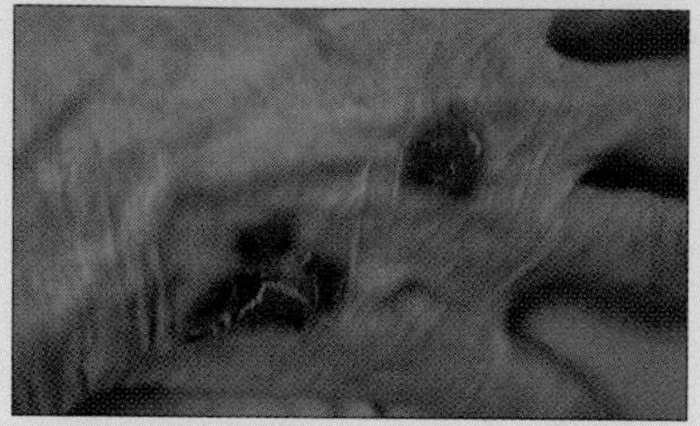
cutaneous lymphoma

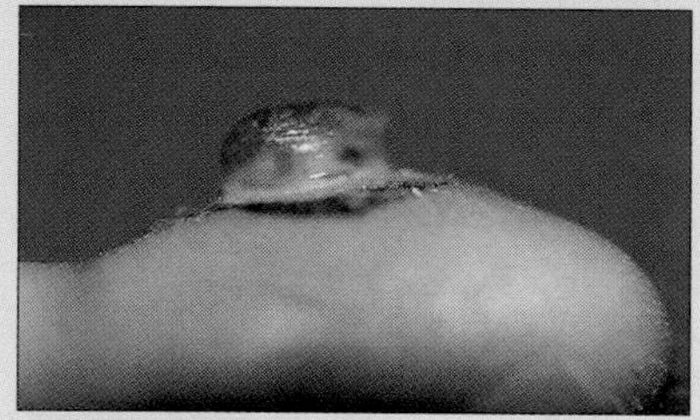
pyogenic granuloma

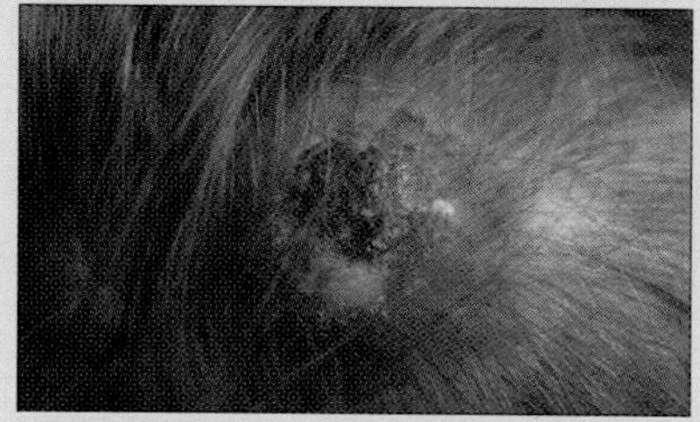
lymphoma metastatic to scalp

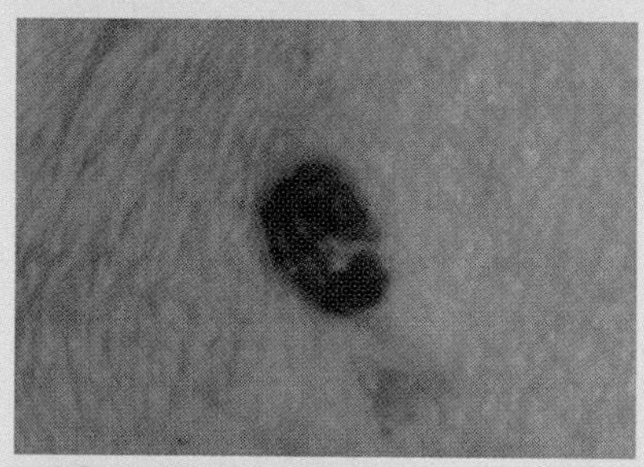
nodular malignant melanoma

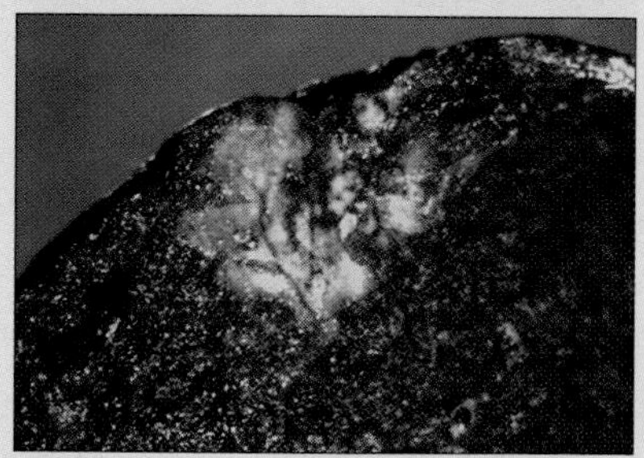
adenocarcinoma of the lung

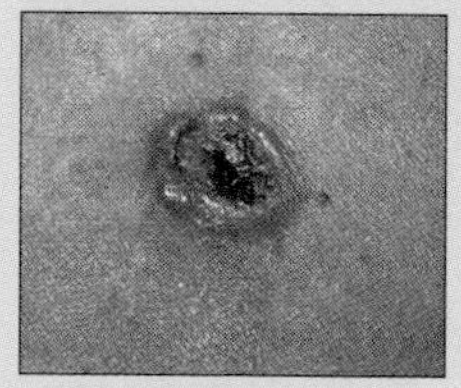
basal cell carcinoma

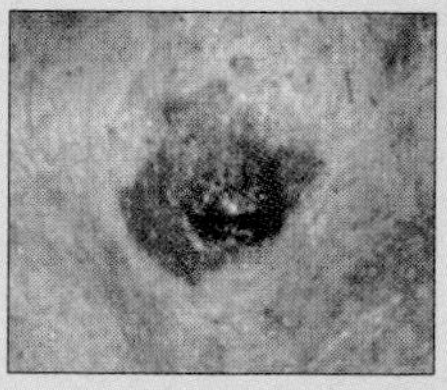
lentigo maligna melanoma

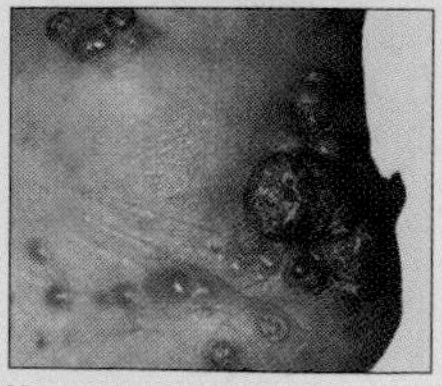
Kaposi sarcoma

PLATE 15: DISORDERS ASSOCIATED WITH THE MOUTH

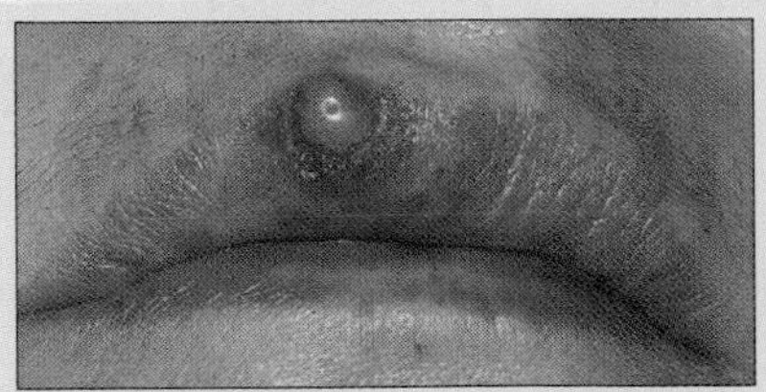

cold sore (recurrent herpes simplex)

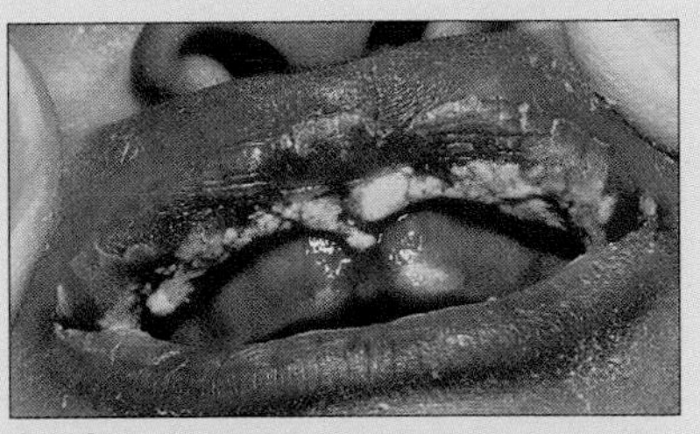

thrush

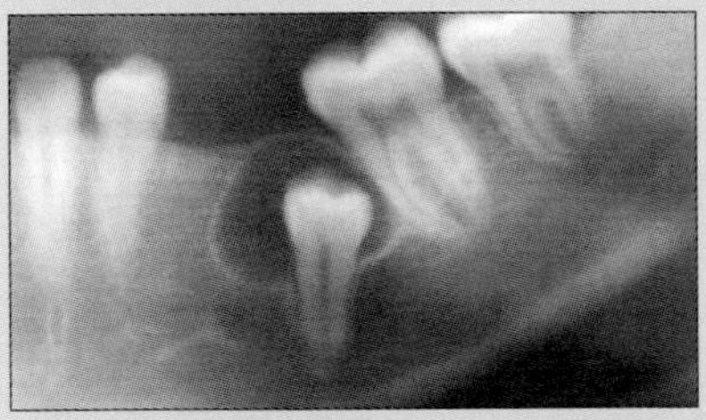

dentigerous cyst

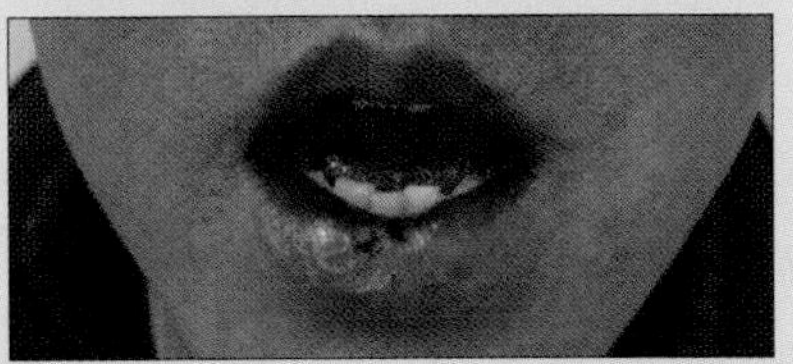

cheilitis

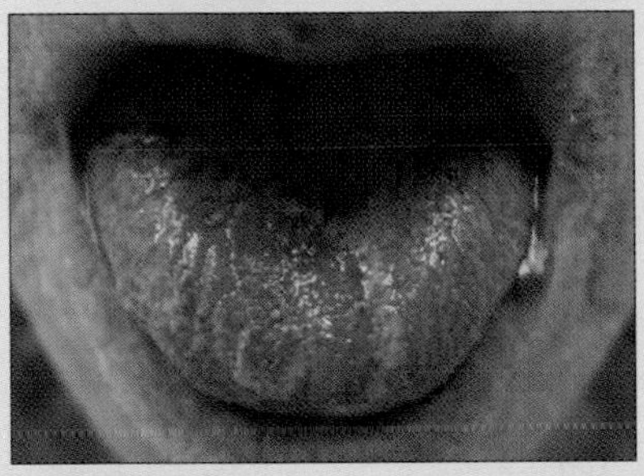

geographic tongue

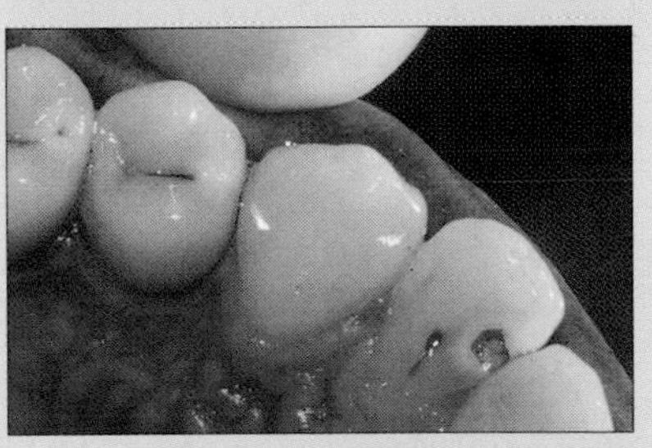

caries (class II mesial premolars; class III lateral)

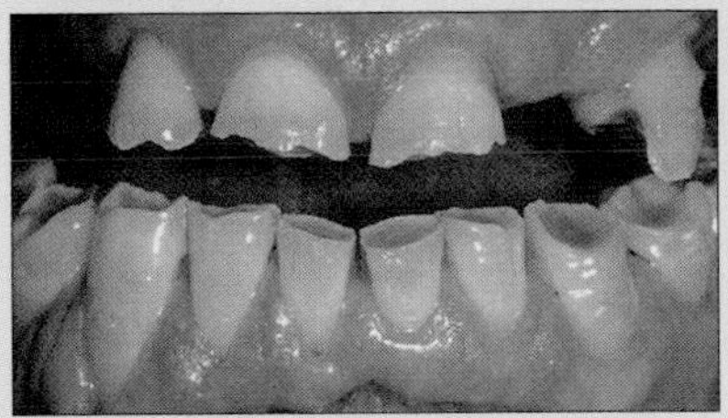

attrition

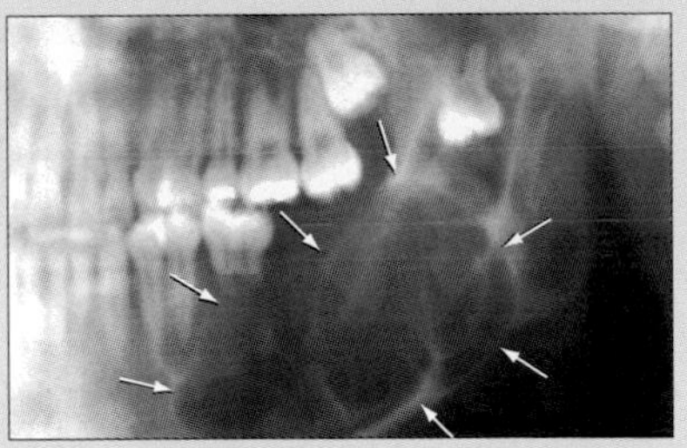

ameloblastoma

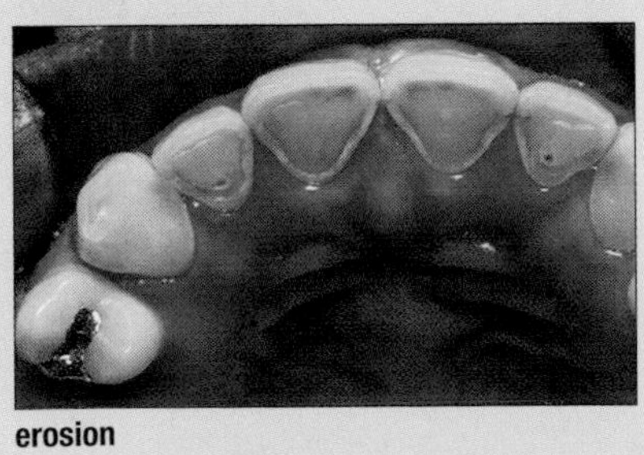

erosion

hairy tongue ▶
(glossotrichia)

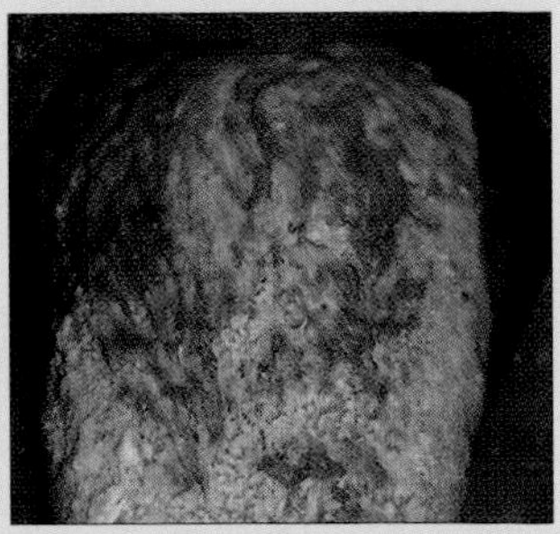

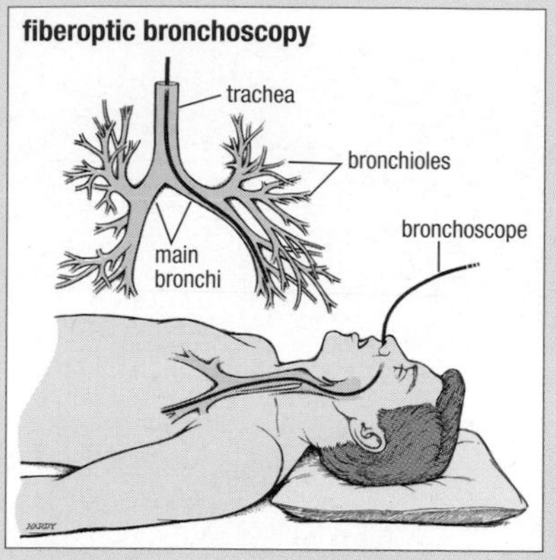

Bronchoscopy is the examination of the respiratory apparatus with a flexible bronchoscope for diagnostic or treatment purposes. The bronchoscope is introduced nasally and slowly led down the trachea until the desired level is reached. The photographs on this page were taken with a camera that attaches to the examiner's end of the instrument.

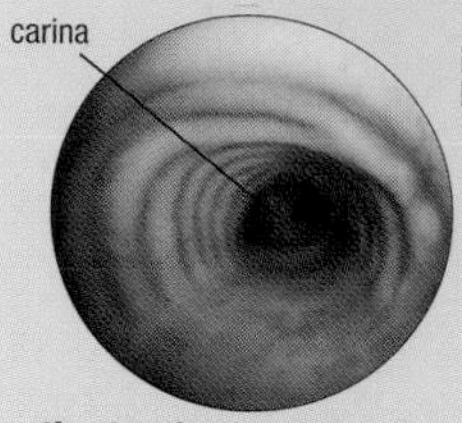

entire trachea and the carina

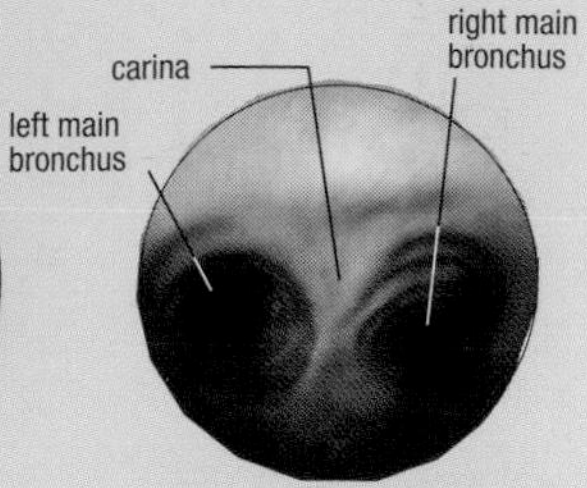

carina

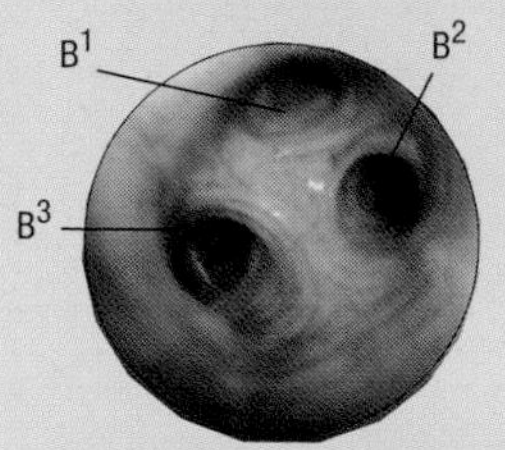

right upper lobe bronchus

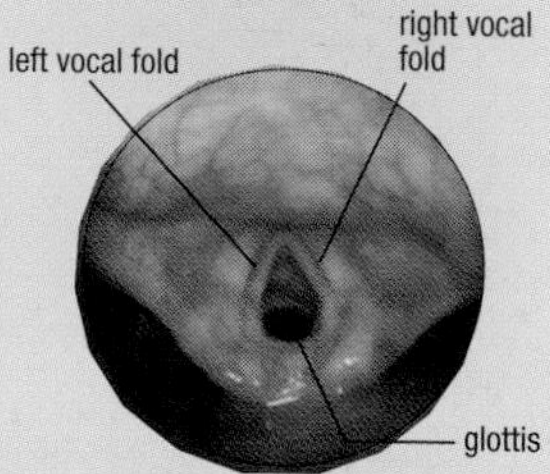

vocal folds

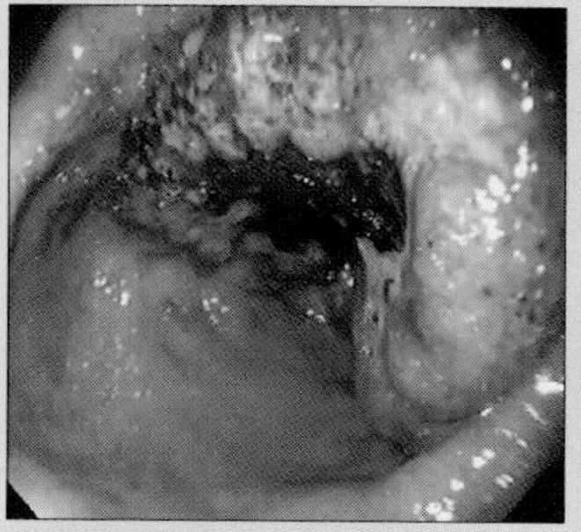

ulcerated adenocarcinoma of the gastric antrum

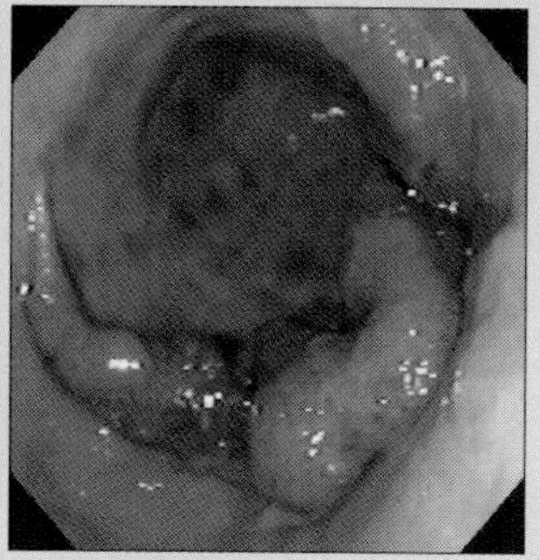

abnormal antral fold

Esophagogastroduodenoscopy is the examination of the esophagus, stomach, and upper small intestine using a flexible gastroscope. Fiberoptics in the instrument conduct bright, cool light along a curved path, allowing illumination of tissues and structures within the body. The scope often contains small instruments such as biopsy snares.

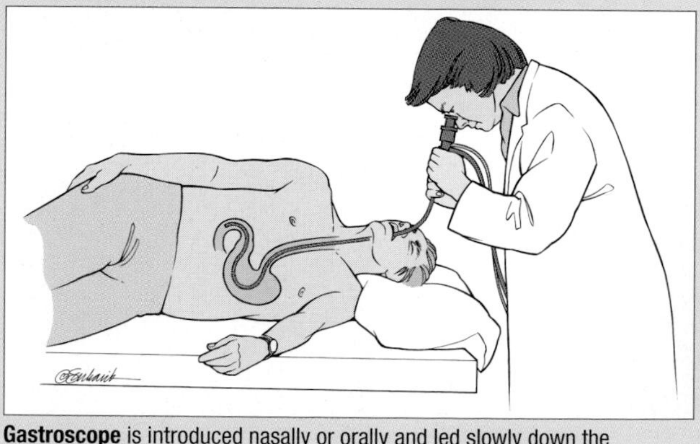

Gastroscope is introduced nasally or orally and led slowly down the esophagus and gastrointestinal tract until the desired level is reached.

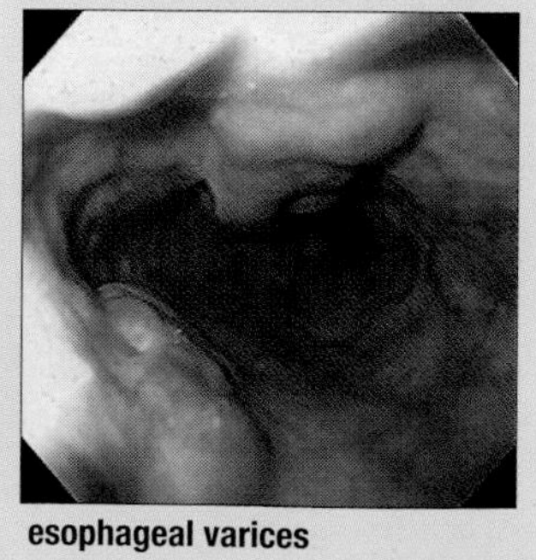

esophageal varices

PLATE 17: ENDOSCOPY

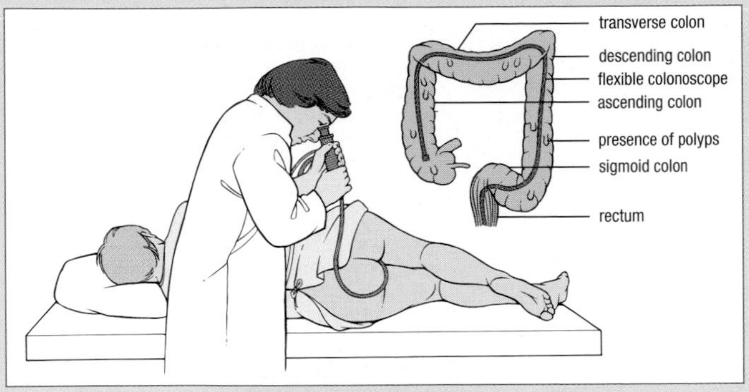

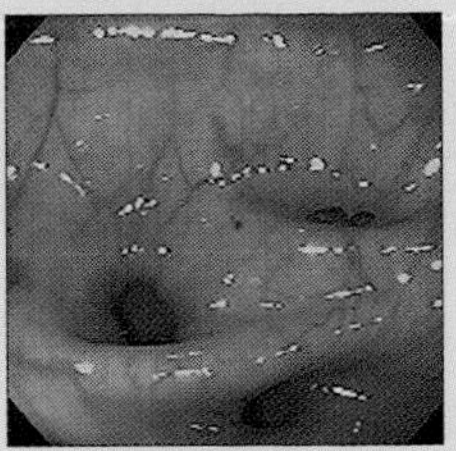

diverticulosis: multiple diverticular orifices

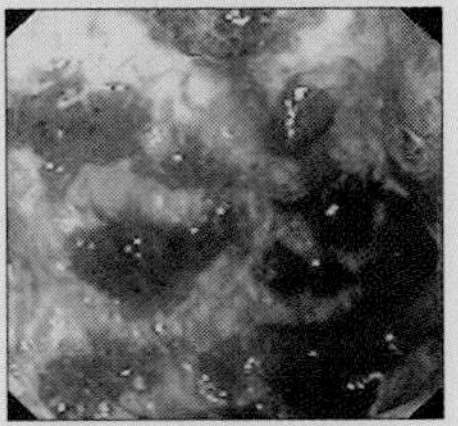

severly active ulcerative colitis

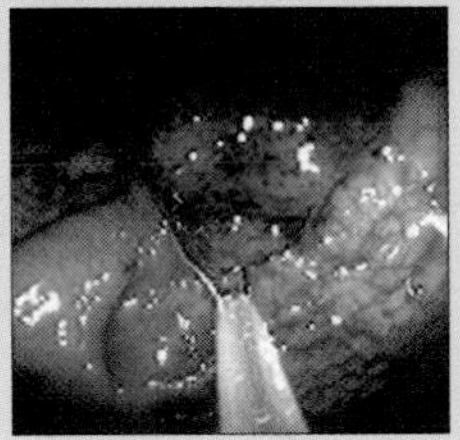

colon polypectomy

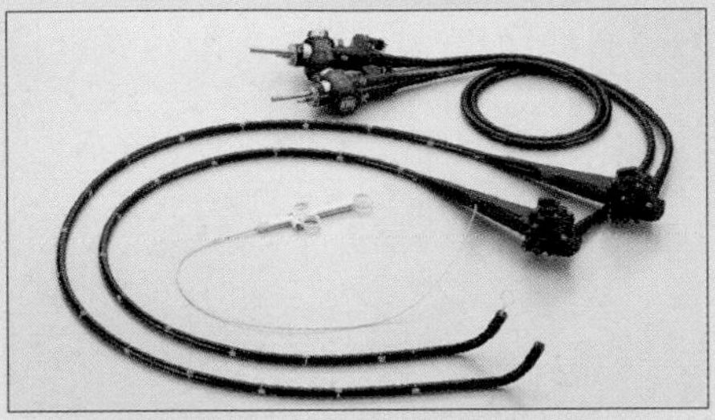

Innoflex Adjustable Stiffness Video Colonoscope

Colonoscopy is the examination and diagnosis of conditions of the colon. The flexible colonoscope passes through the rectum and sigmoid colon into the descending, transverse, and ascending colon. Small instruments can be passed through the colonoscope and used to perform minor operative procedures. The images on the right were taken by a camera attached to the colonoscope.

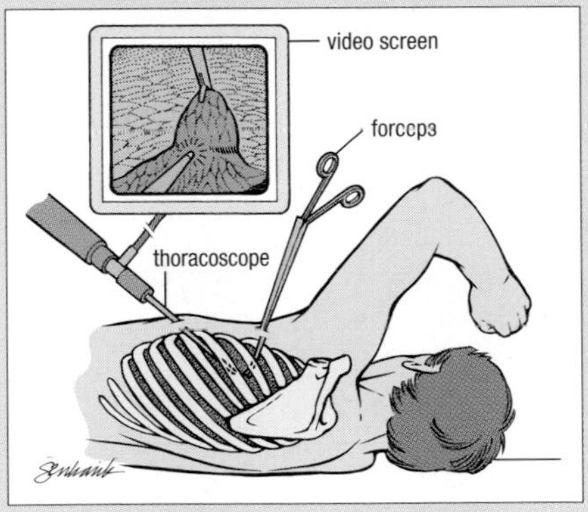

Thoracoscopy is a diagnostic procedure in which the pleural cavity is examined with an endoscope. Small incisions are made into the pleural cavity in an intercostal space. The use of fiberoptic instruments and miniature video equipment permits visualization of thoracic structures. Tissue biopsy and treatment of some thoracic conditions can be conducted.

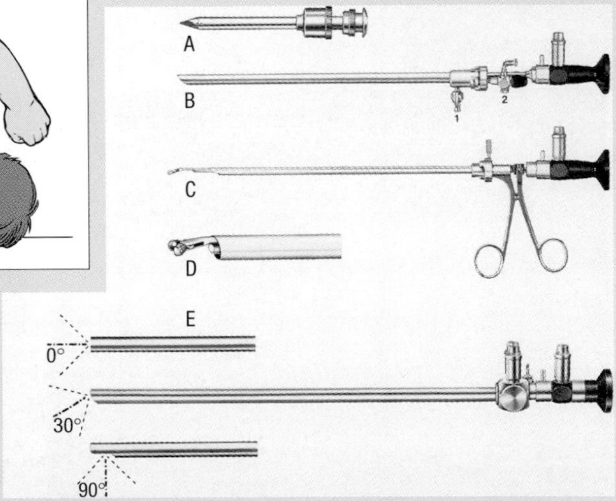

Basic instruments for **thoracoscopy:** (A) trocar obturator with integrated valve and sharp internal cannula; (B) single incision thoracoscope; (C) biopsy forceps; (D) magnification of optics and forceps in the thoracoscope shaft ready for biopsy; (E) various straight and angled vision telescopes, with adapted photograph light shaft.

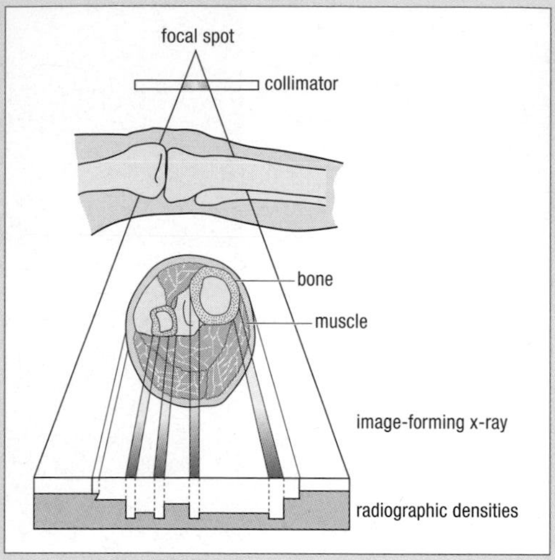

Radiography or **roentgenography** is the examination of any part of the body for diagnostic purposes by means of x-rays, with the record of findings usually impressed upon the photographic film.

◀ X-rays pass through body parts, with denser structures absorbing more x-rays and consequently appearing as lighter areas on the radiograph.

As shown in the graphic, differential absorption of x-rays depends on the composition of various tissues. Denser tissue (such as bone) absorbs more x-rays, less dense tissue (such as subcutaneous fat) transmits more x-rays. Greater absorption produces more darkening. The resultant radiographic image is essentially a "shadowgram."

The **plain chest radiology** images on this page show various pathological conditions of the chest and respiratory system.

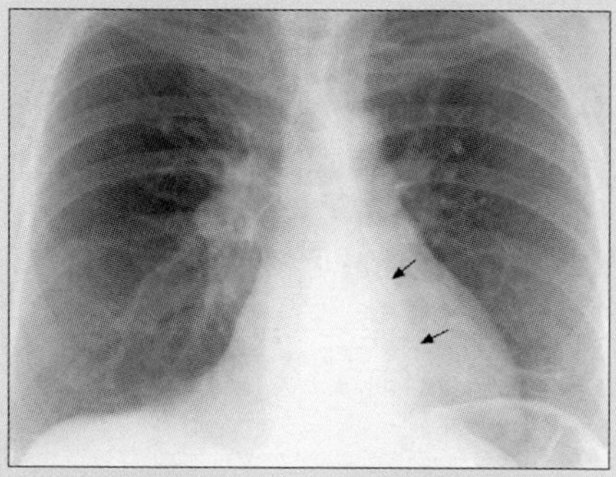

chronic left lower lobe collapse with silhouette sign (arrows)

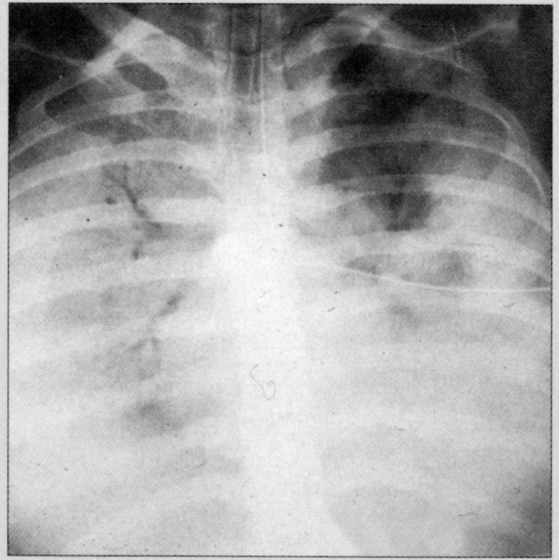

adult respiratory distress syndrome (ARDS)

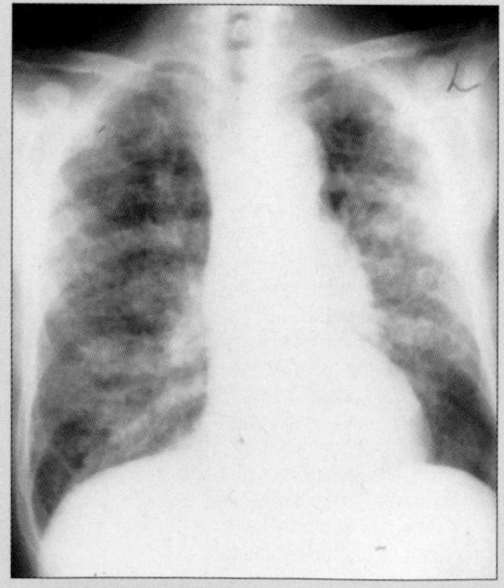

interstitial lung disease

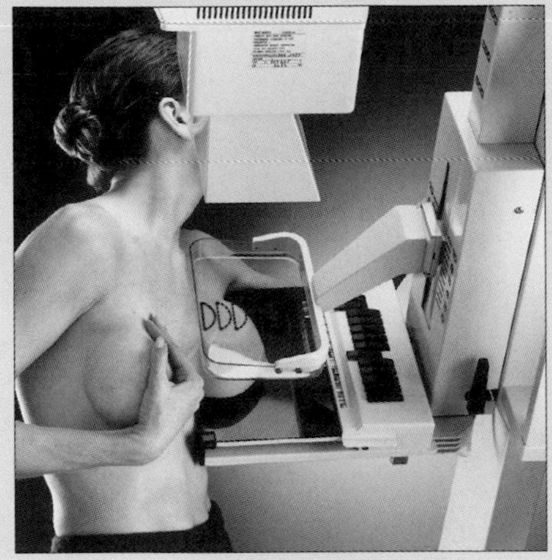

patient positioning for a mediolateral oblique (MLO) view

Mammography is the imaging examination of the breast by means of x-rays, ultrasound, and nuclear magnetic resonance, used for screening and diagnosis of breast disease. X-ray mammography has proved to have the greatest efficacy for detecting occult breast cancer.

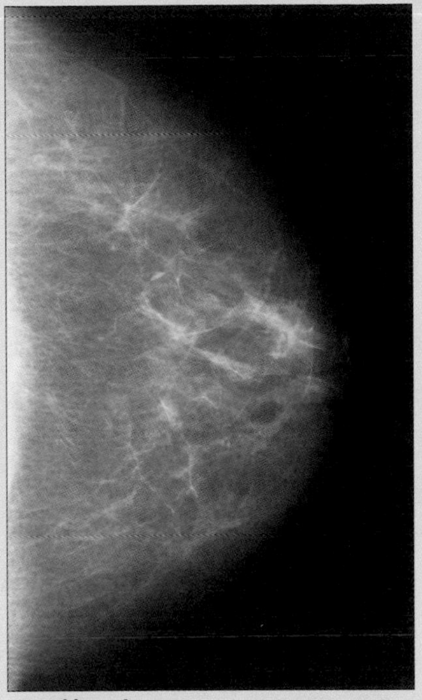

normal breast

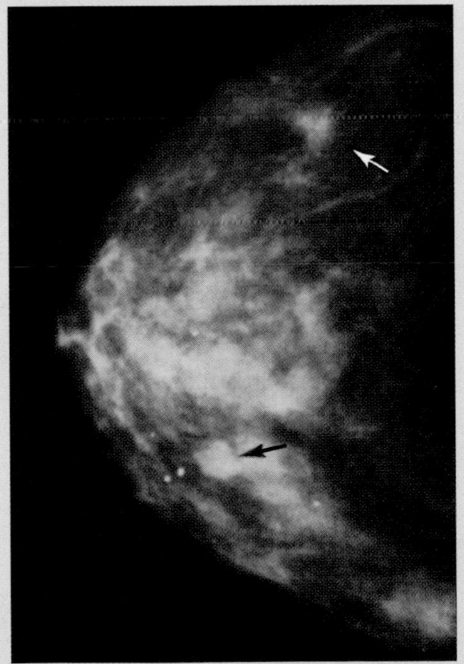

cephalocaudal film-screen mammogram: small scirrhous carcinoma (arrow) is contrasted with well-marginated fibroadenoma (arrowhead)

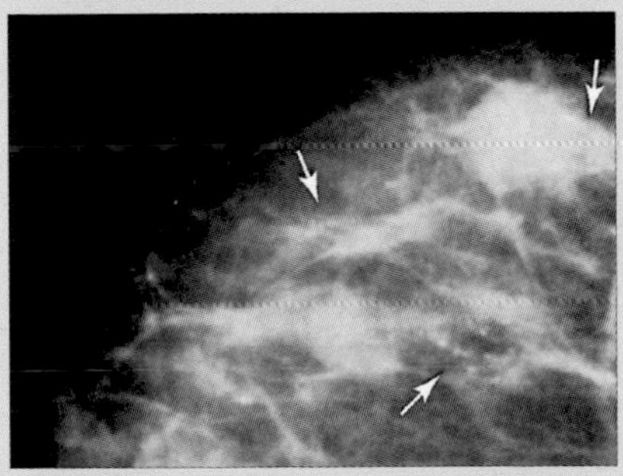

multifocal duct carcinoma: close-up shows multiple clusters of calcifications (arrows) and two masses

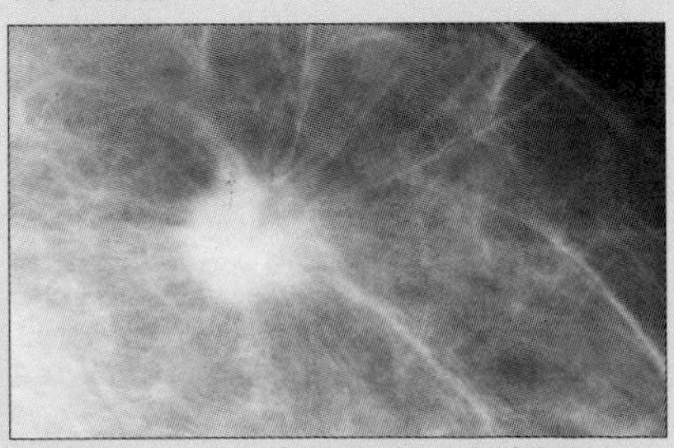

classic breast carcinoma: this spiculated breast mass is an infiltrating duct carcinoma

Computed tomography (CT) is a radiologic procedure using a machine called a scanner to examine a body site by taking a series of cross-sectional images one slice at a time in a full-circle rotation. A computer then calculates and converts the rates of absorption and density of the x-rays into a picture on a screen.

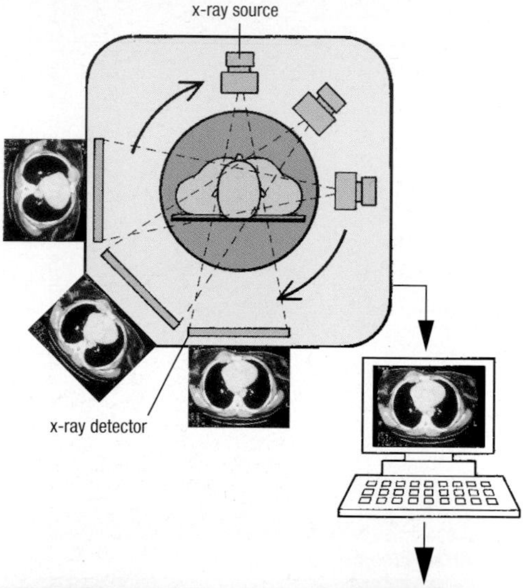

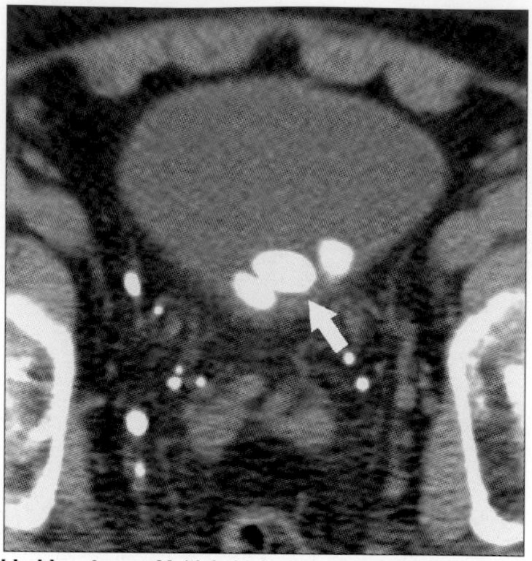

bladder stones: Multiple high-attenuation stones (arrow) are seen within the lumen of the bladder on this non-contrast CT. Contrast opacification of the bladder may obscure the presence of bladder stones. This patient has a neurogenic bladder, which has resulted in chronic urine stasis within the bladder.

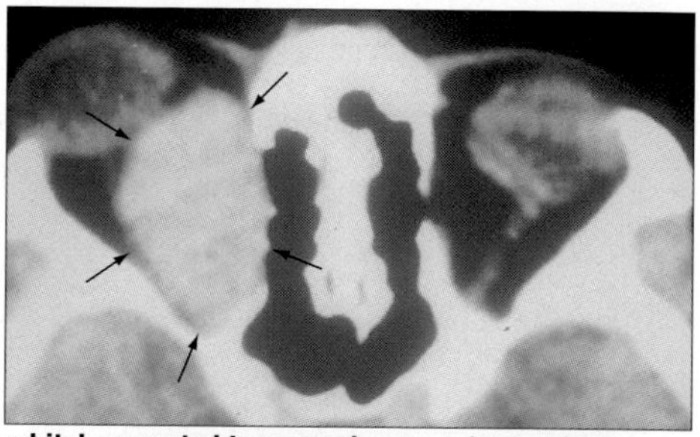

orbital computed tomography scan shows a large metastasis of carcinoid tumor in the right orbit

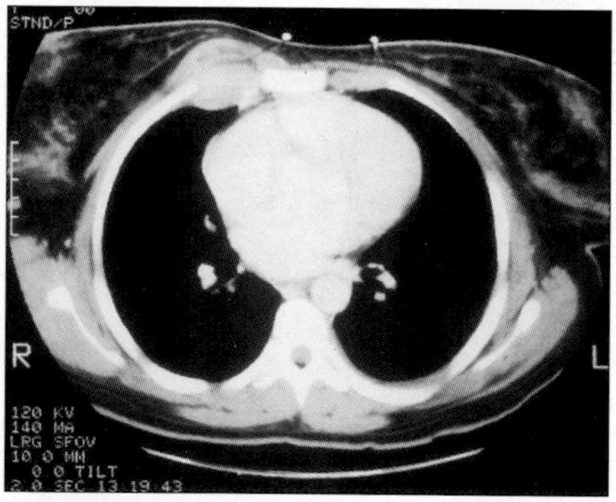

CT of bony blastomycosis involving a right anterior rib

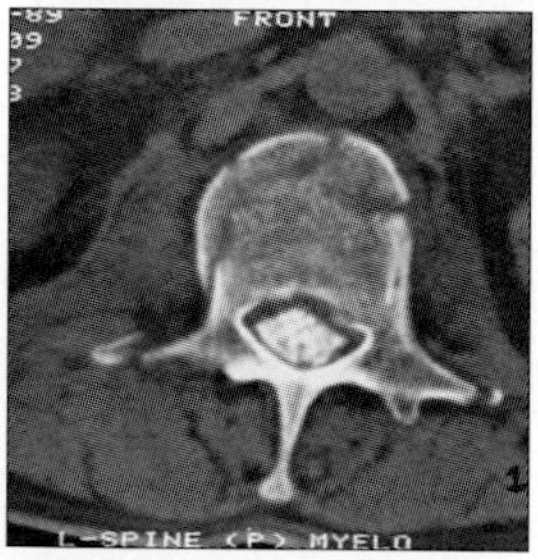

T12 compression fracture
(CT enhanced with intrathecal dye)

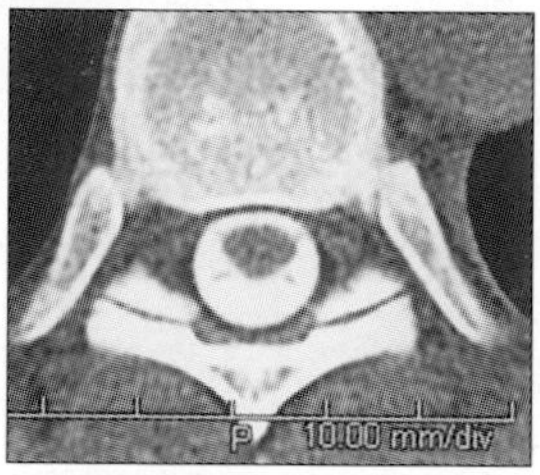

CT myelogram of transverse section of the spinal cord showing its characteristic appearance at thoracic levels (T4)

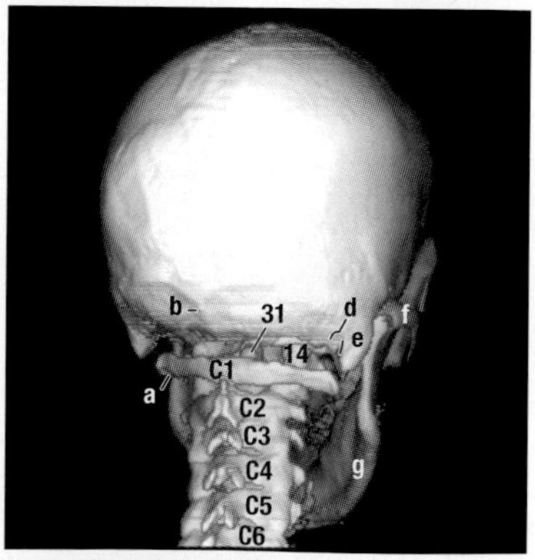

three-dimensional (3D) CT: adjacent CT slices, covering the approximately 30-cm height of the neck and head, have been used to produce surface images of the skull

PLATE 21: SONOGRAPHY

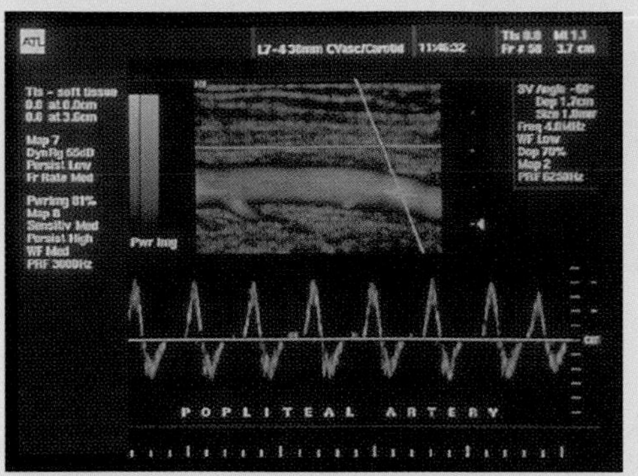

color flow duplex image of popliteal artery with normal triphasic **Doppler flow**

During **sonography,** energy in the form of high-frequency sound waves is reflected by internal organs and transformed into an image on a monitor screen.

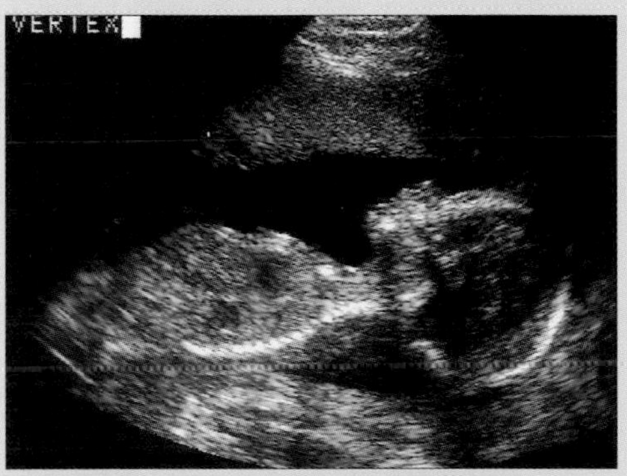

fetus in breech position (sagittal view)

In **Doppler sonography**, blood flow and other movement in the area examined alter the frequency of reflected sound waves and can be exhibited in a color display. Doppler sonography is often used to diagnose cardiac and peripheral vascular disease.

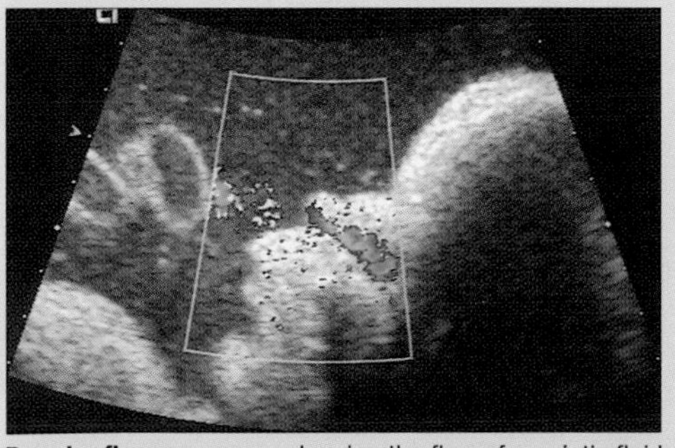

Doppler flow sonogram showing the flow of amniotic fluid into the nasal cavity of the fetus

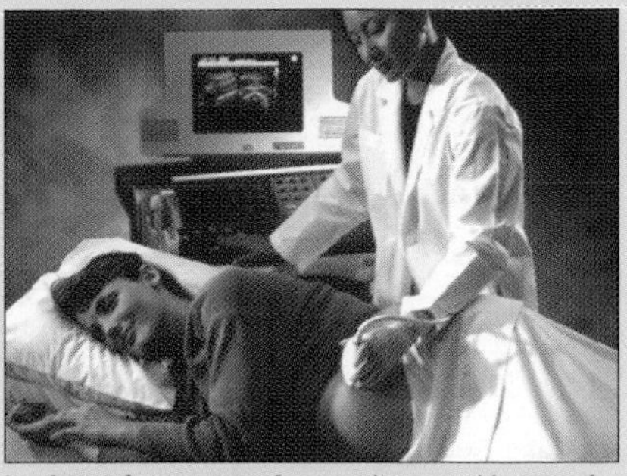

in **obstetric sonography**, an ultrasound image of the pregnant uterus and fetus is created in order to assess fetal development and well-being

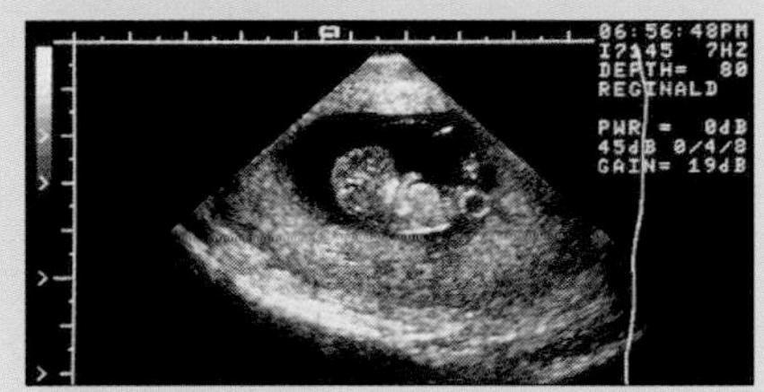

two-dimensional sonogram of 8-week embryo

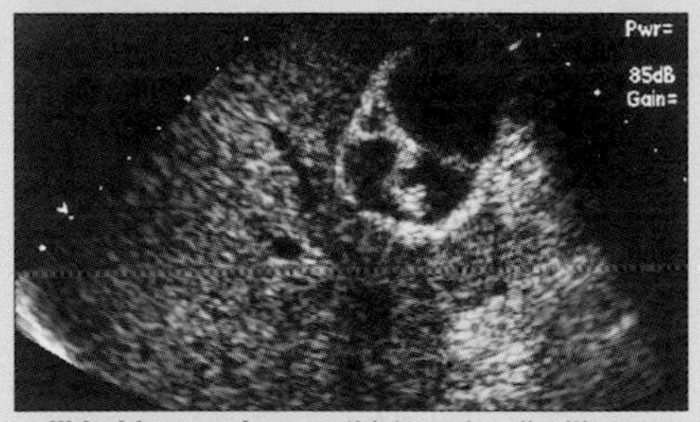

gallbladder carcinoma: thickened wall with a polypoid mass protruding into the lumen

Echocardiography uses ultrasound to investigate the structure and function of the heart and great vessels.

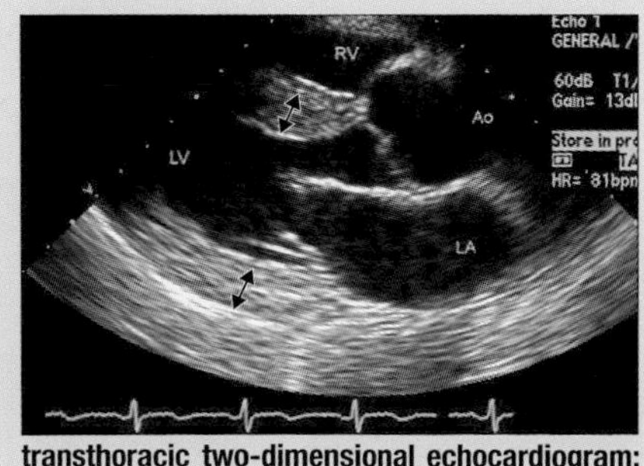

transthoracic two-dimensional echocardiogram: recorded in a parasternal long-axis view revealing the right ventricle (RV), left ventricle (LV), left atrium (LA) and proximal aorta (Ao) as well as septal and posterior wall thickness (arrows)

PLATE 22: MAGNETIC RESONANCE IMAGING

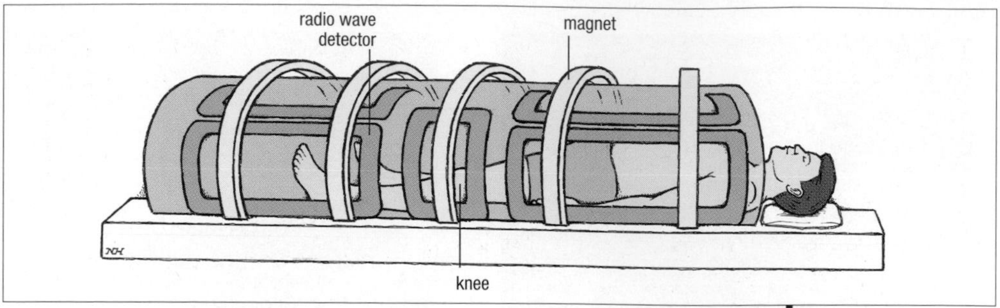

Magnetic resonance imaging (MRI) is a nonionizing (non-x-ray) technique using magnetic fields and radio frequency waves to visualize anatomic structures. It is useful in detecting joint, tendon, and vertebral disorders. The patient is positioned within a magnetic field as radio wave signals are conducted through the selected body part. Energy is absorbed by tissues and then released.

computer processes the released energy and formulates image

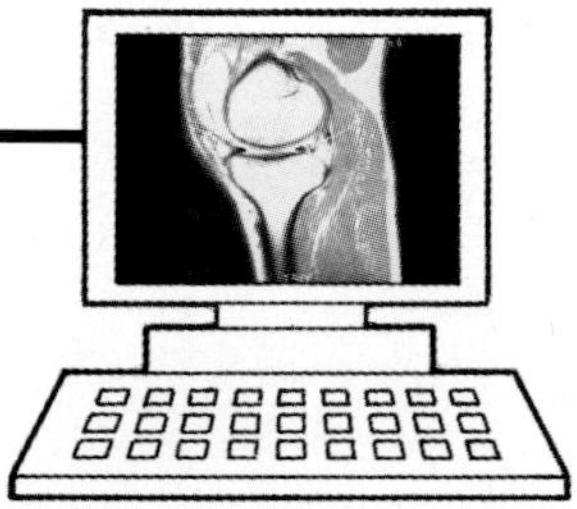

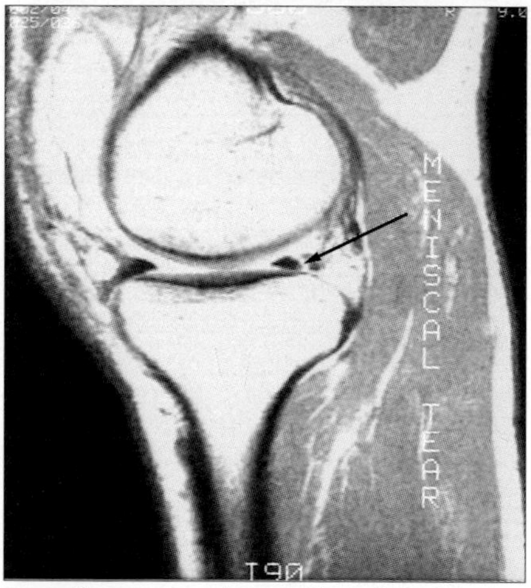

magnetic resonance image of knee (lateral view) identifying a torn meniscus

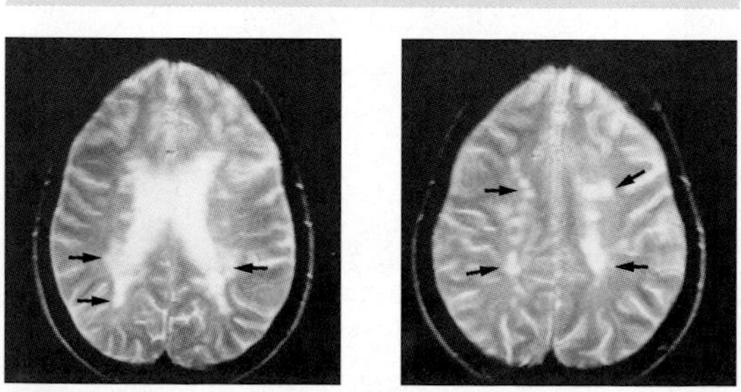

multiple sclerosis: contiguous T2-weighted MR images, showing areas of ventricular plaques of high signal (arrows)

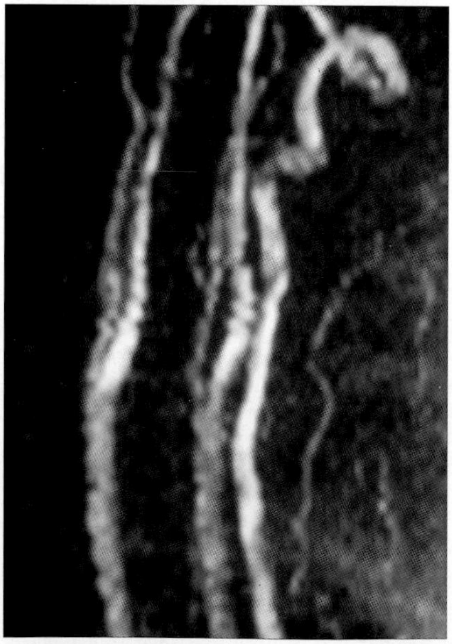

magnetic resonance angiogram revealing absence of the right vertebral artery

PLATE 23: NUCLEAR MEDICINE

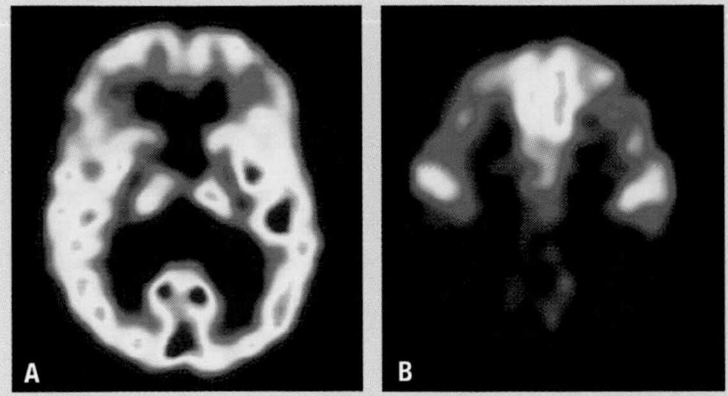

Positron emission tomography (PET) combines nuclear medicine and computed tomography to produce images of brain anatomy and corresponding physiology. Warm colors (red and yellow) indicate a higher rate of metabolism and brain activity in the normal brain (A) when compared to the brain of a patient with Alzheimer disease (B).

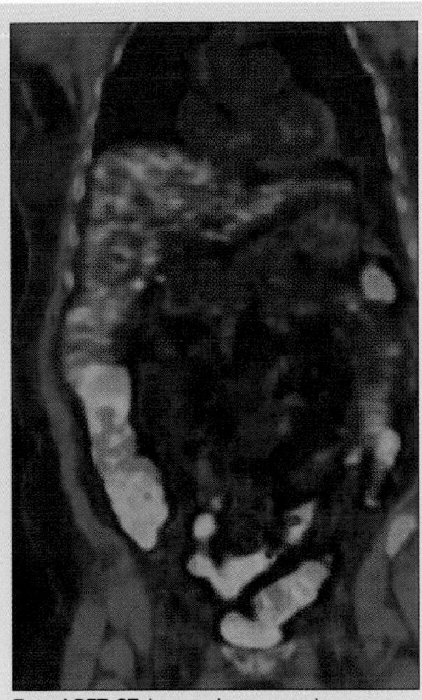

Fused PET-CT: image shows massive physiologic colon activity; note the normal heterogeneous fluorodeoxyglucose activity in the liver.

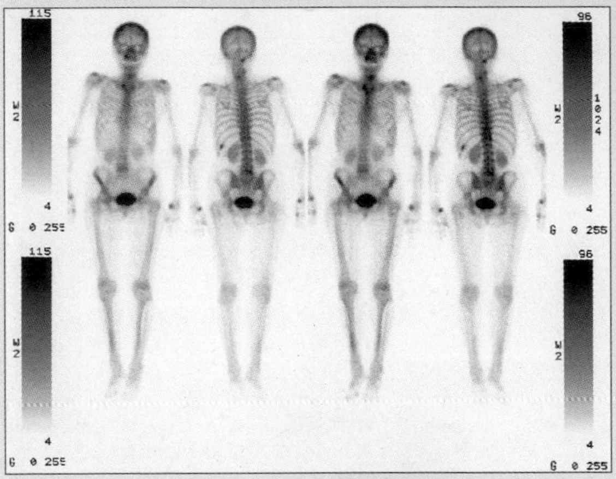

▲ **Full-body bone scan:** nuclear scan of bone tissue to detect abnormalities such as tumors and malignancies.

Nuclear medicine imaging is a diagnostic technique using injected or ingested radioactive isotopes and a gamma camera to determine size, shape, location, and function of various body parts.

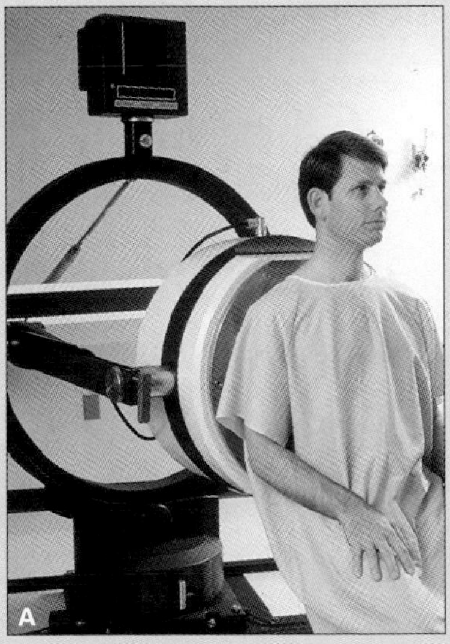

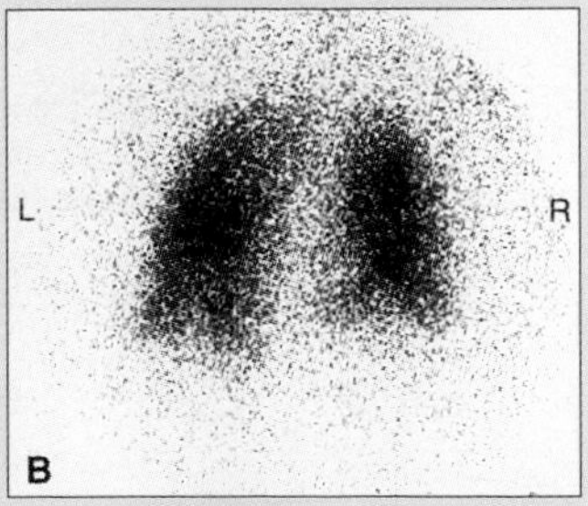

Nuclear lung scan is used ▶ to detect abnormalities of perfusion (blood flow) or ventilation (respiration), commonly called V̊/Q (ventilation/perfusion) scan. (A) gamma-camera used to produce lung scan. In this patient, a posterior lung scan shows an embolus in the right lung. Ventilation scan (B) shows a normal pattern. Absence of blood flow to the right lung is apparent on perfusion scan (C).

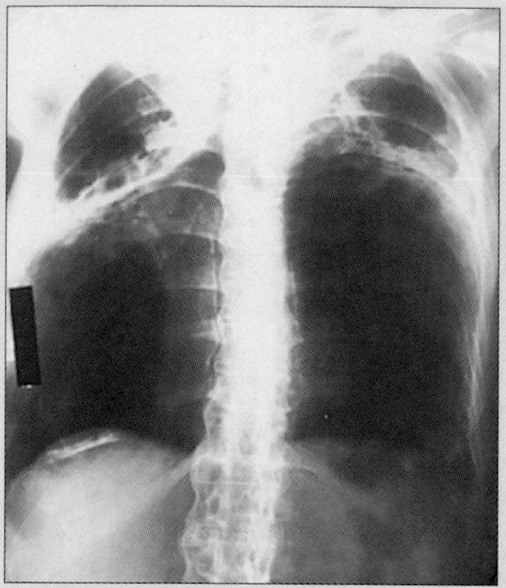

ankylosing spondylitis demonstrates "bamboo spine"

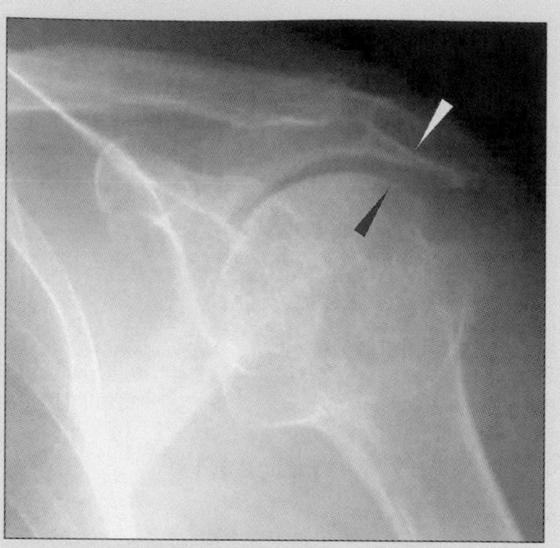

rheumatoid arthritis in the shoulder: anteroposterior view of shoulder shows that the distance between the acromion and the humeral head is diminished (arrowheads)

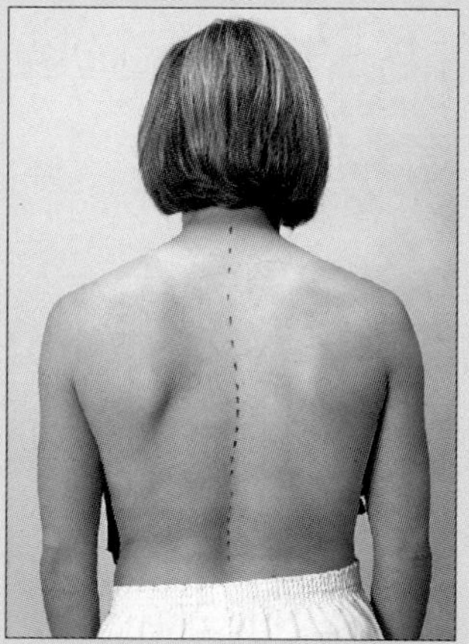

thoracic left lumbar idiopathic scoliosis

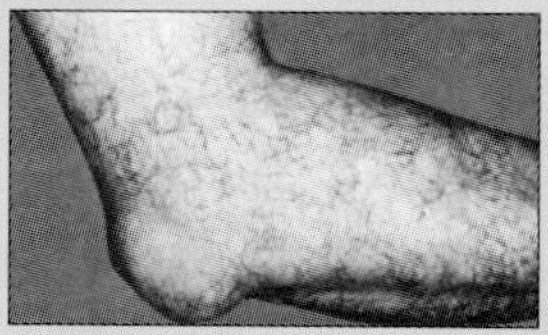

bursitis: student's elbow

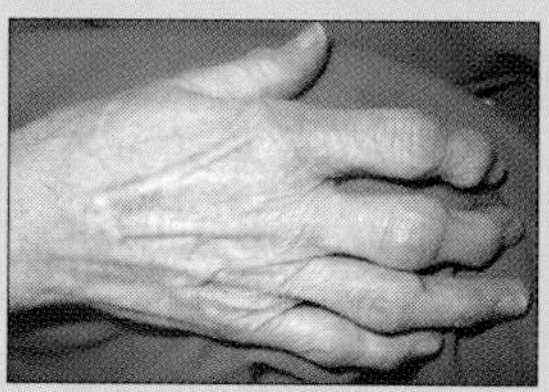

rheumatoid arthritis

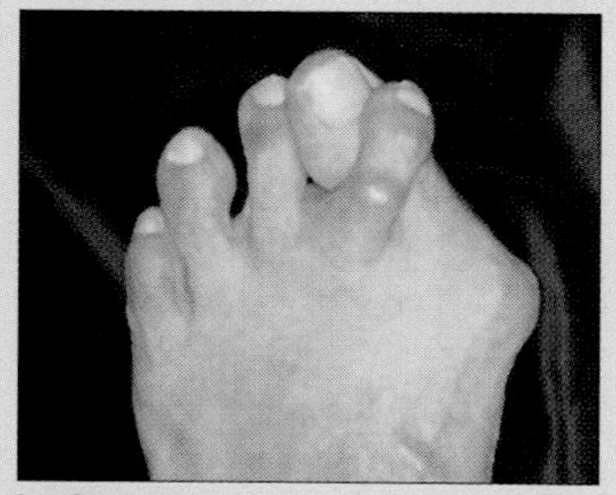

bunion: result of hallux valgus

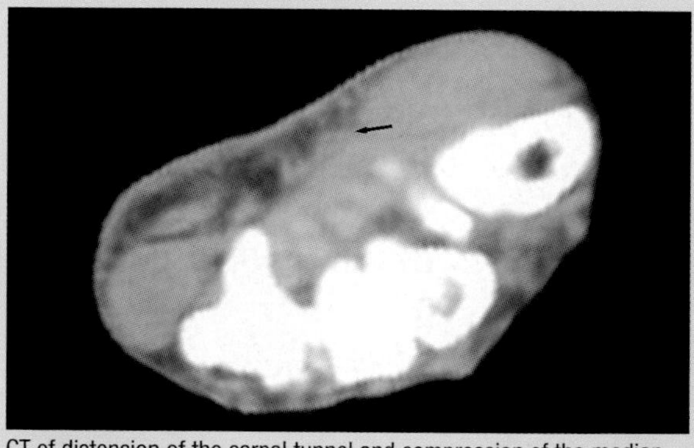

CT of distension of the carpal tunnel and compression of the median nerve (arrow) in **carpal tunnel syndrome**

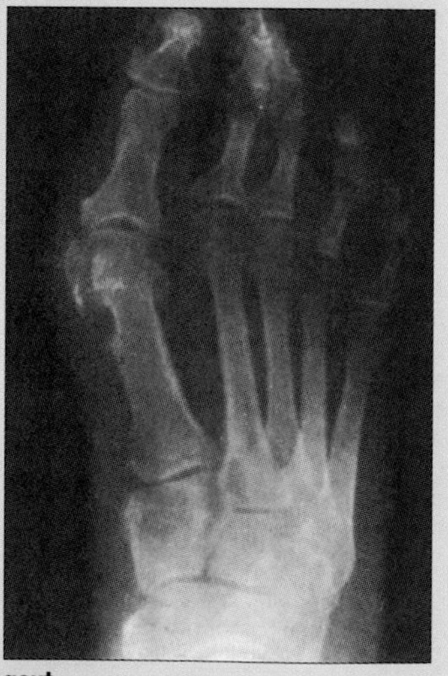

gout

PLATE 25: BONE FRACTURES

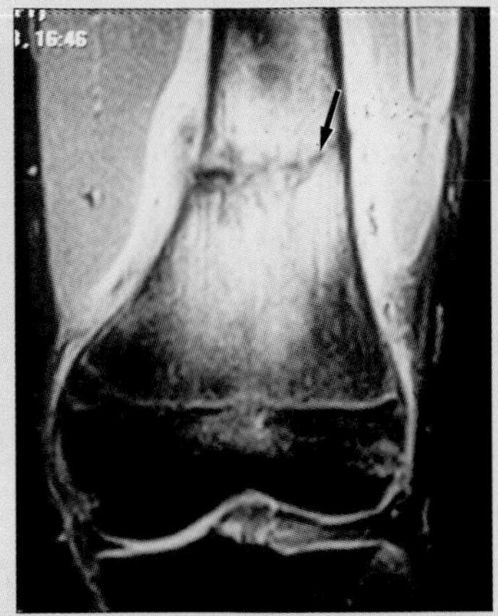

fatigue fracture (arrow)

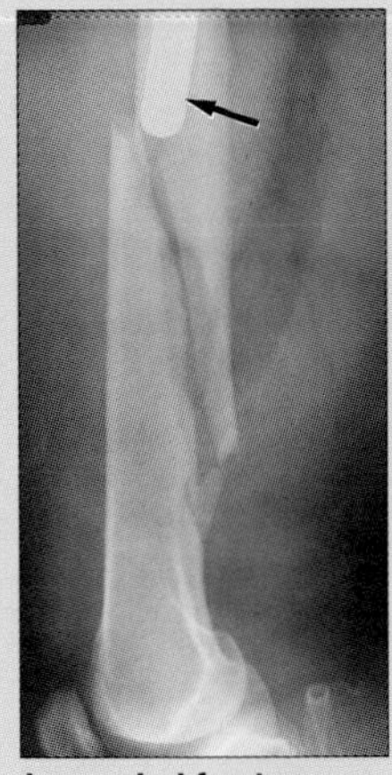

long spiral fracture; prosthesis (arrow)

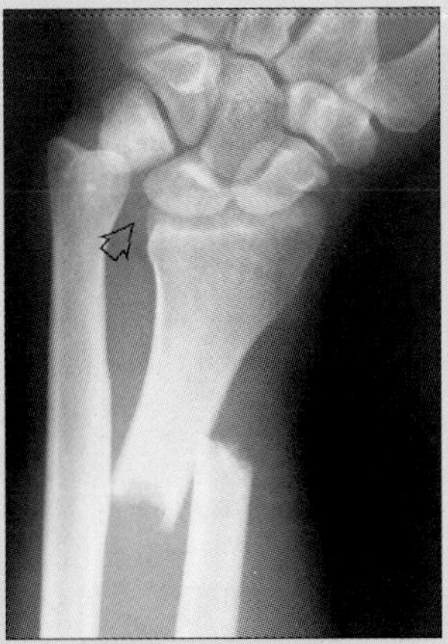

severely displaced Galeazzi fracture with distal radioulnar dislocation (open arrow)

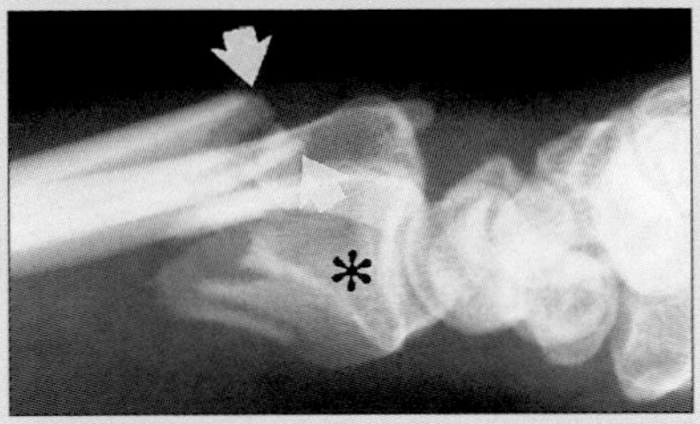

Smith fracture (arrows); displaced fragment (asterisk)

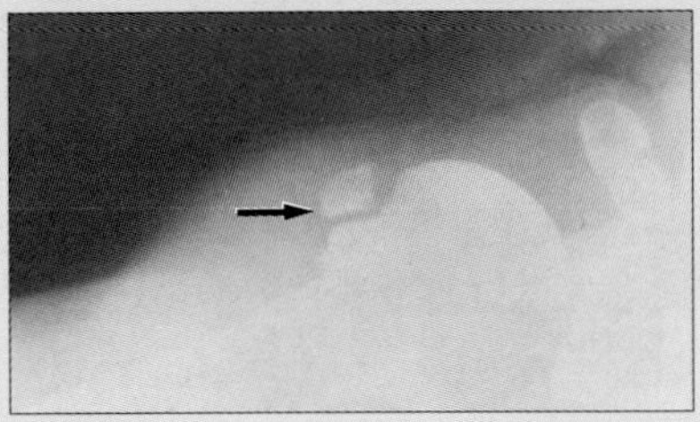

avulsion fracture of the lesser tuberosity (arrow)

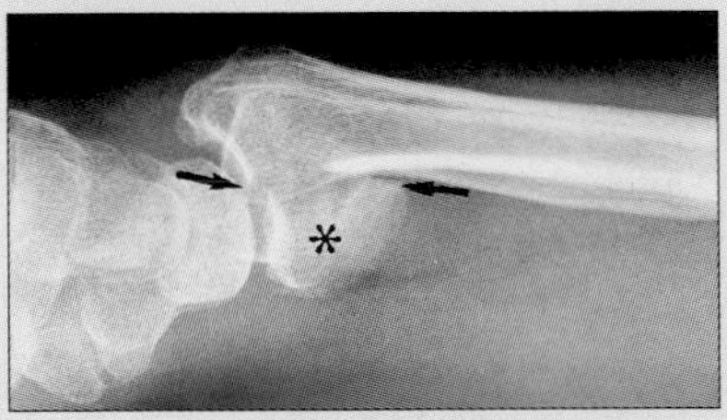

classic volar Barton fracture: fracture (arrows); displaced fragment (asterisk)

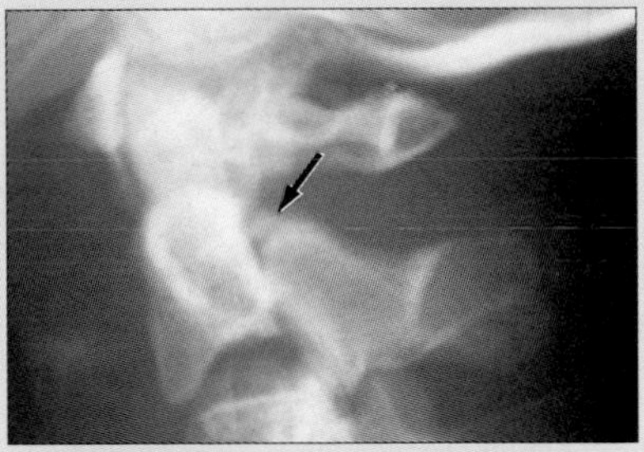

type III hangman's fracture (arrow)

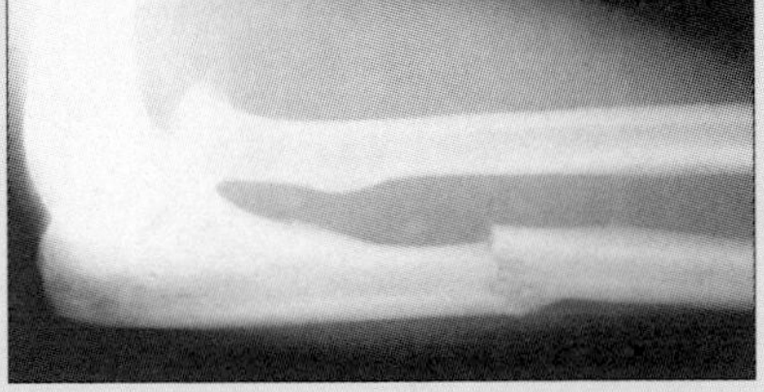

Monteggia fracture

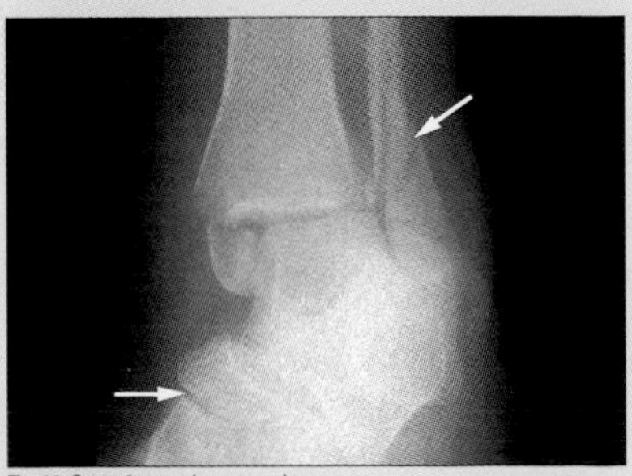

Pott fracture (arrows)

PLATE 26: OPHTHALMOLOGY

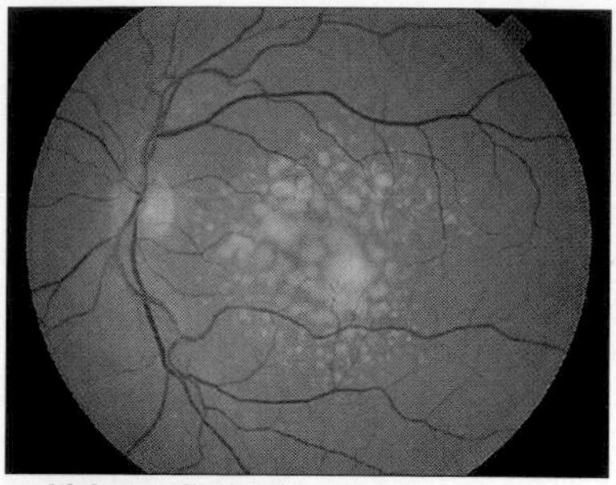

multiple, confluent drusen

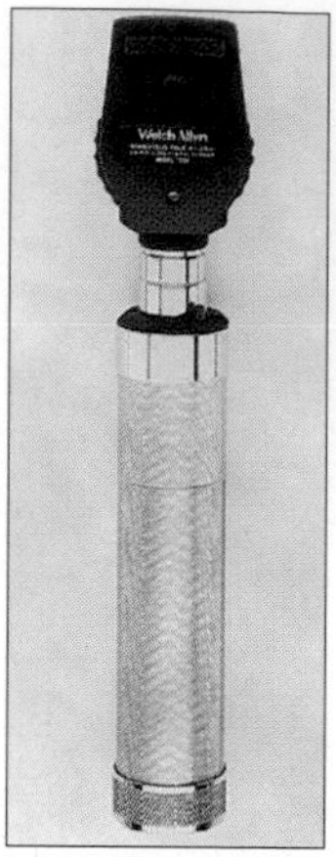

ophthalmoscope

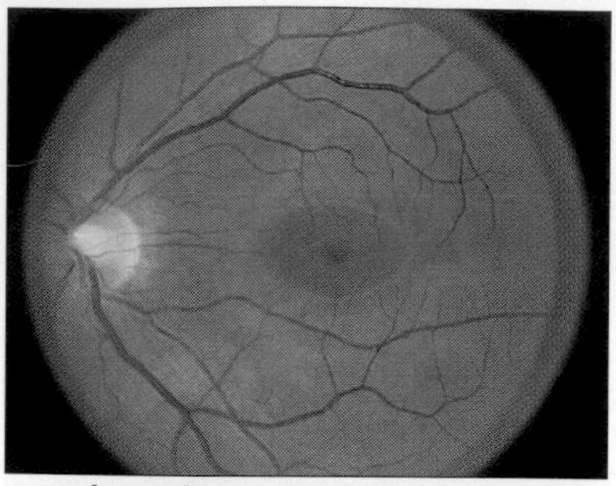

normal macula

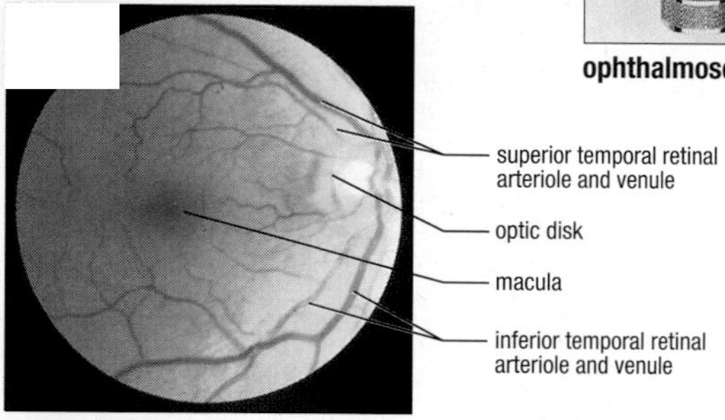

normal fundus

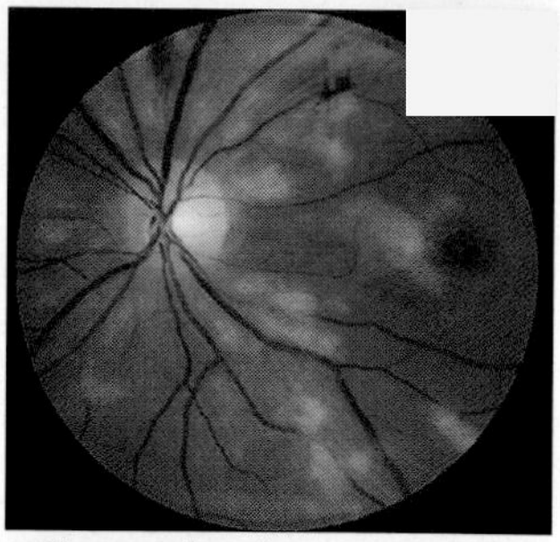

cotton-wool spots

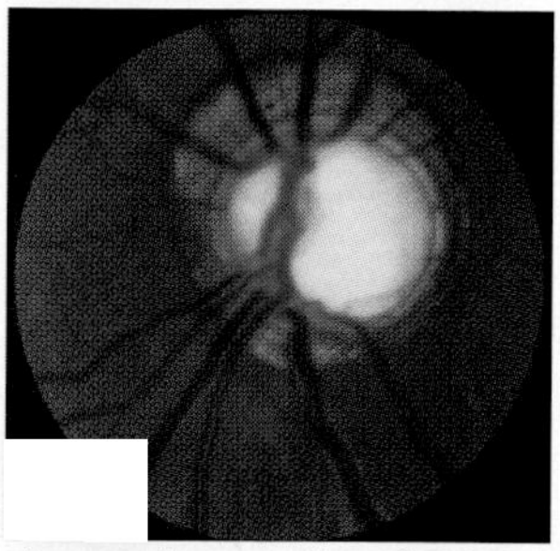

glaucomatous cupping of disk

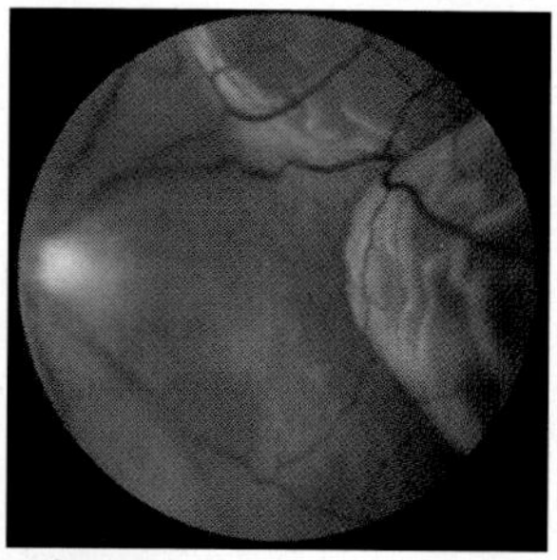

retinal detachment

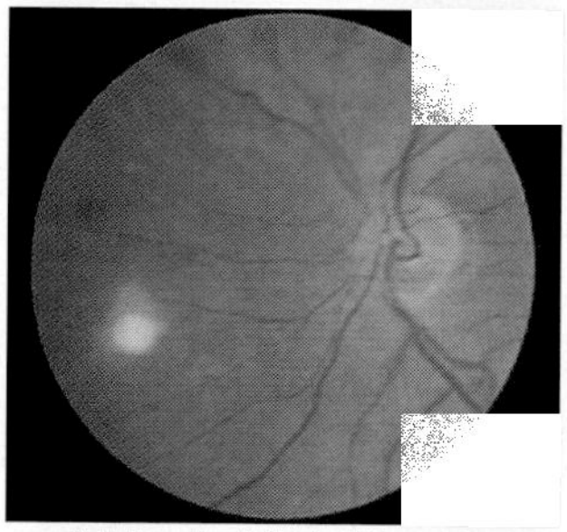

candidal endophthalmitis

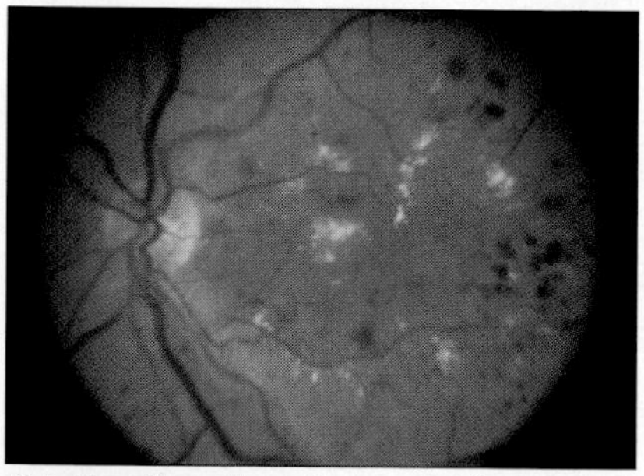

diabetic retinopathy: note several yellowish "hard" exudates

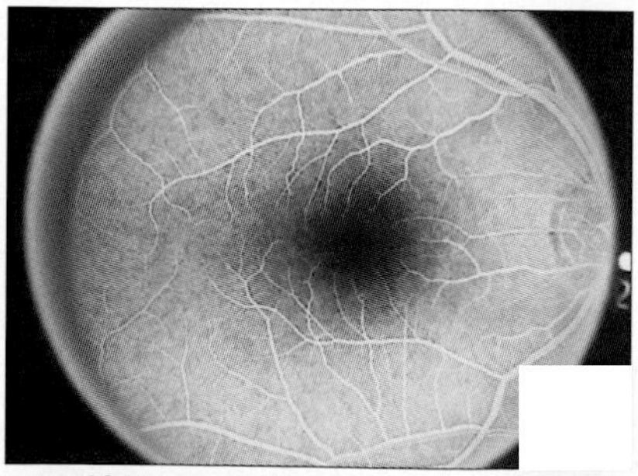

normal intravenous fluorescein angiogram

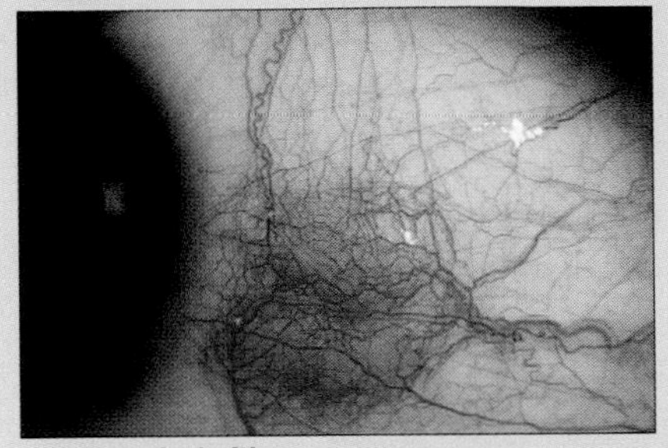
nodular episcleritis

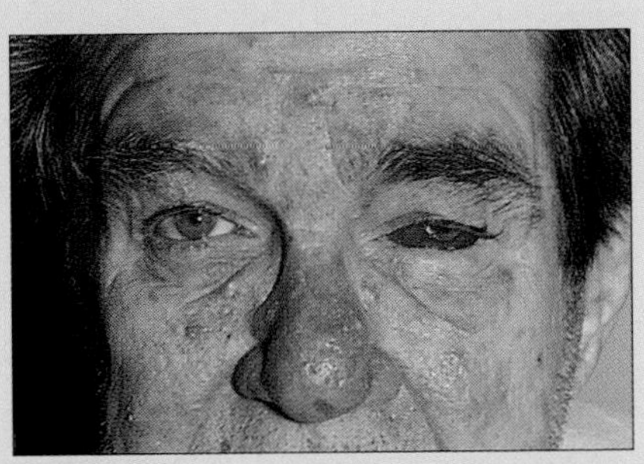
blepharitis

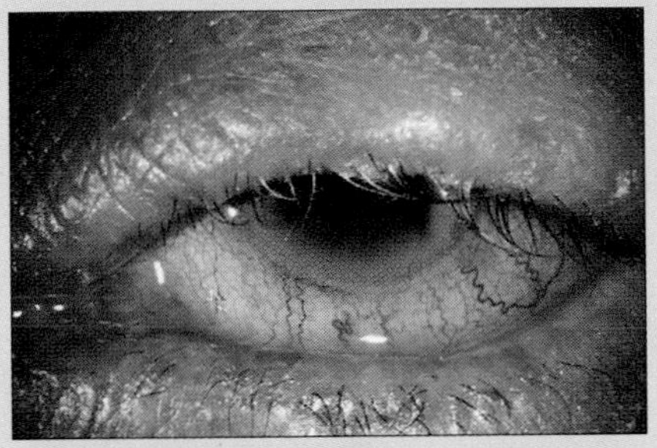
acute bacterial conjunctivitis

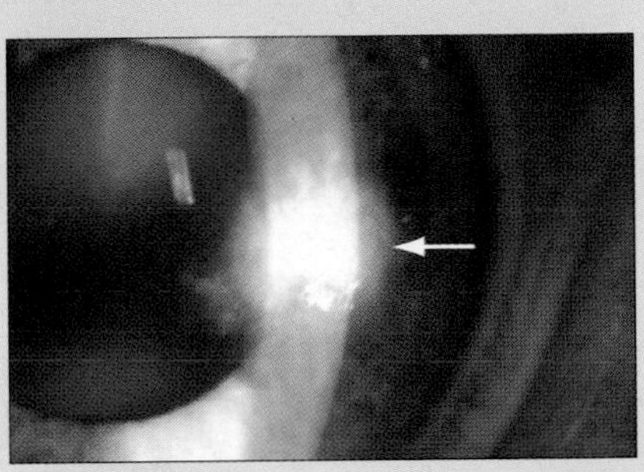
corneal ulcer

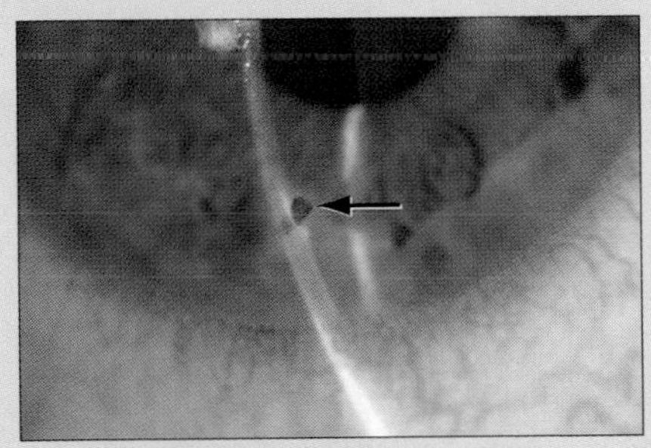
corneal foreign body

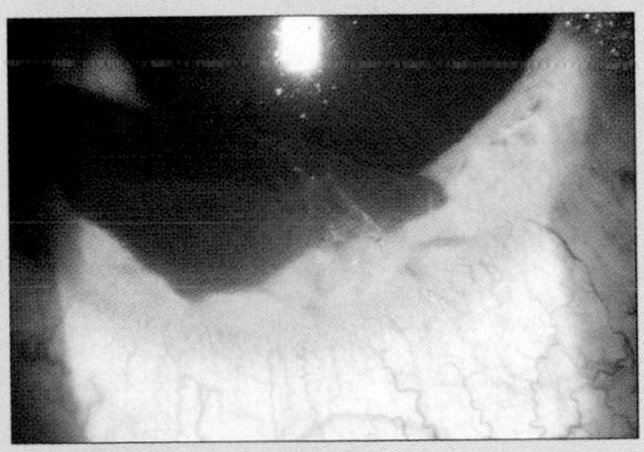
hyphema

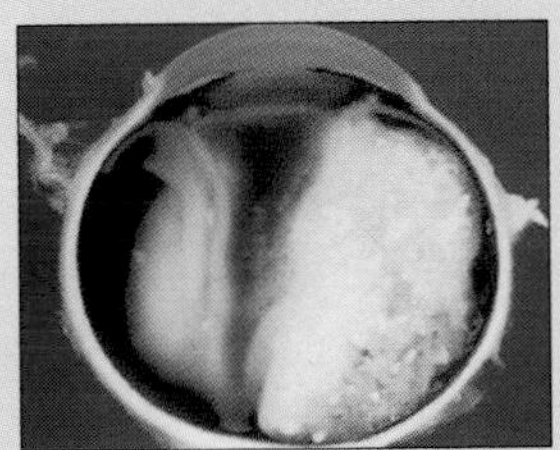
retinoblastoma

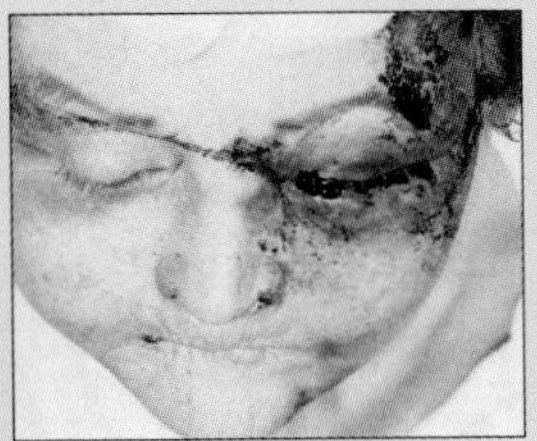
ruptured globe from blunt trauma

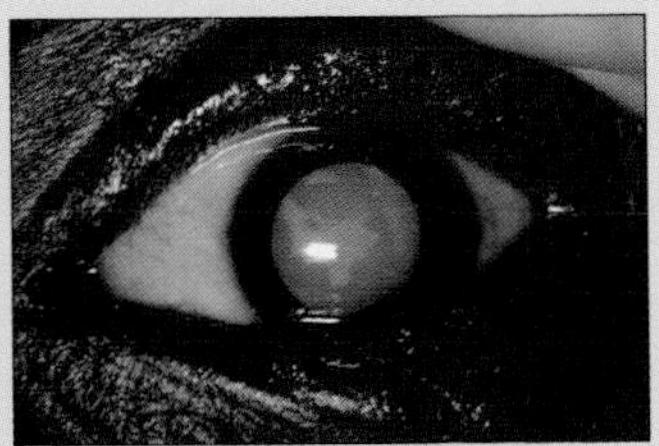
mature cataract

PLATE 28: OTOSCOPY

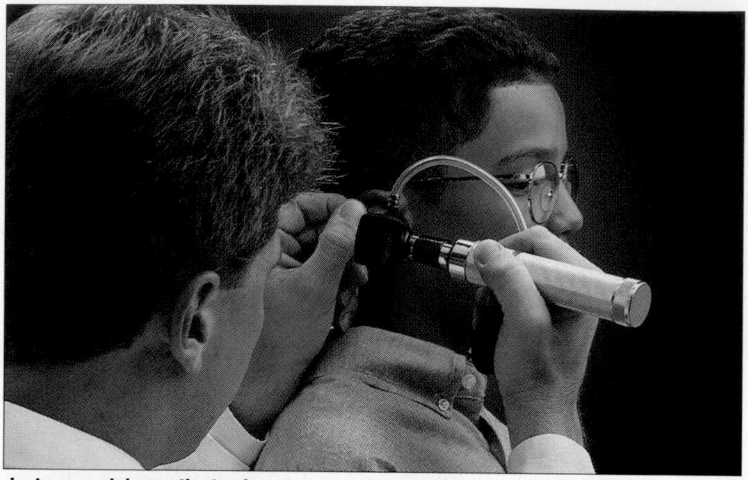

doctor examining patient using otoscope

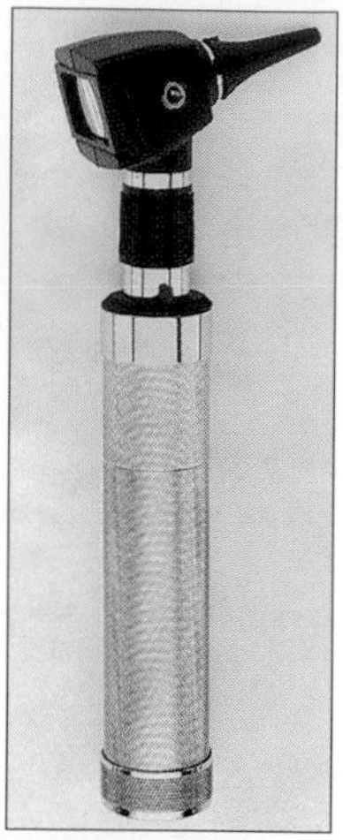

otoscope

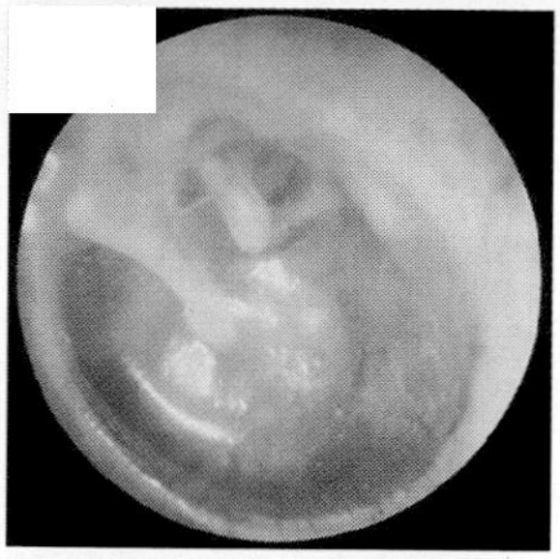

normal tympanic membrane

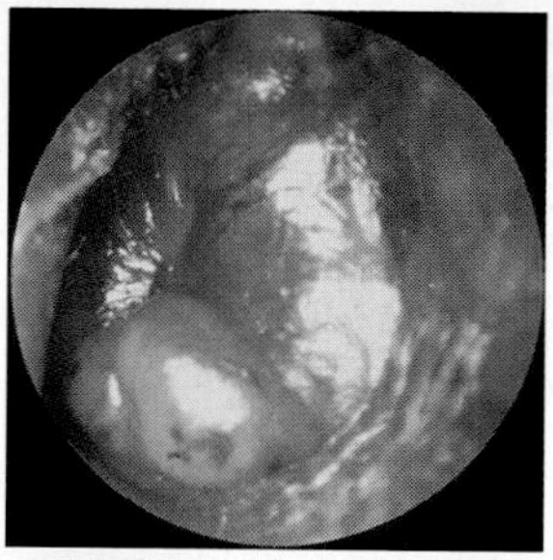

acute otitis media

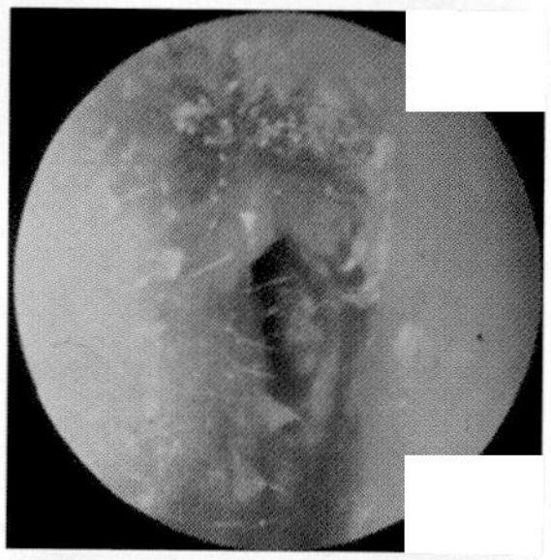

otitis externa

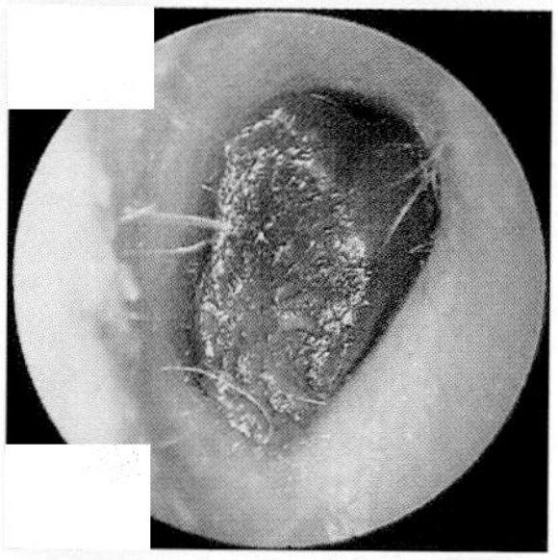

buildup of cerumen in ear canal

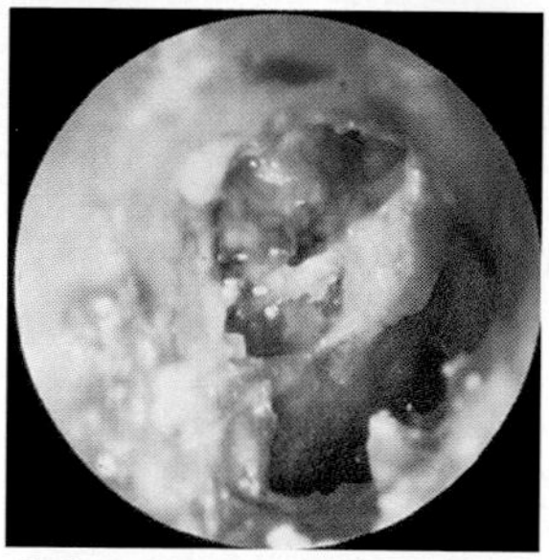

cholesteatoma

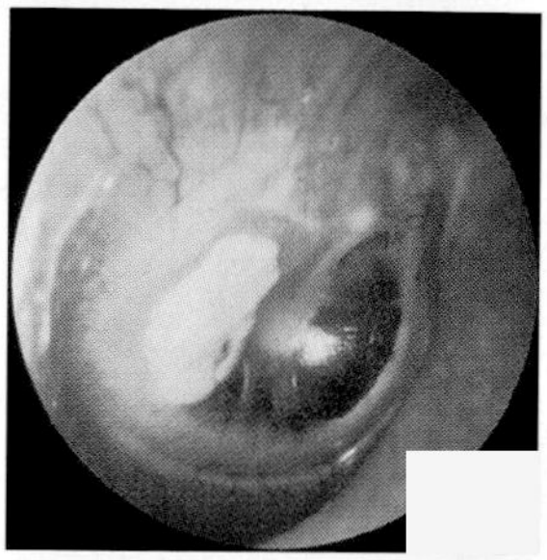

tympanosclerosis

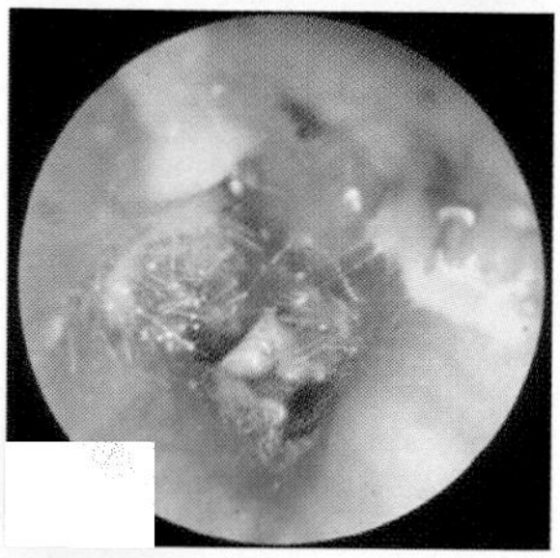

otomycosis

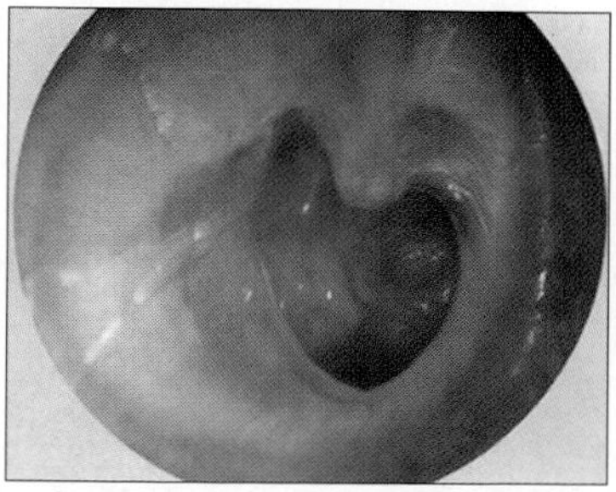

perforation

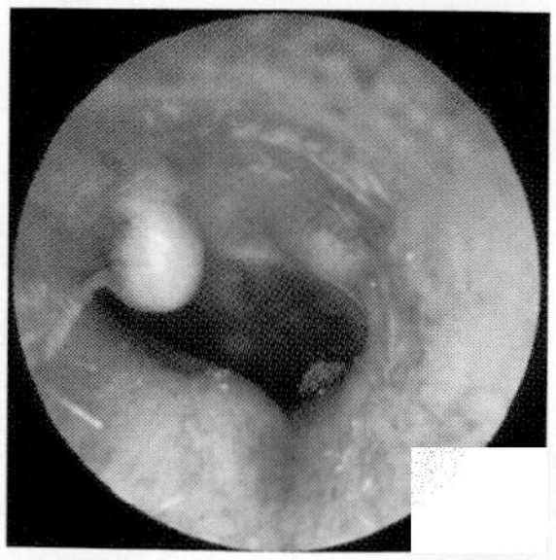

exostosis

PLATE 29: SURGICAL POSITIONS

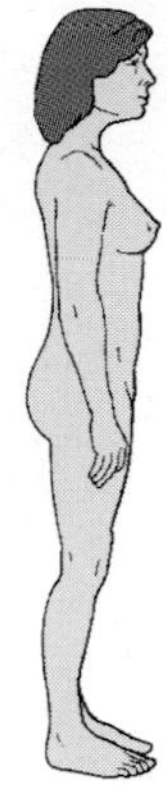
erect (standing) position

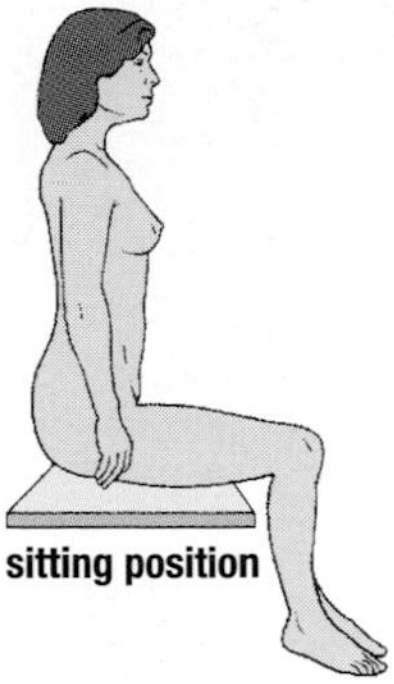
sitting position

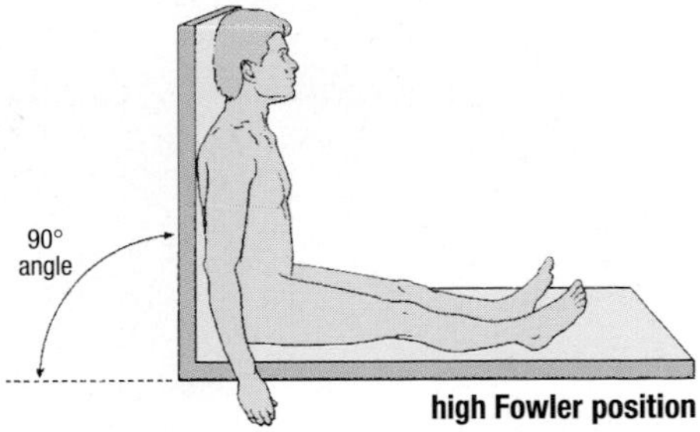

high Fowler position

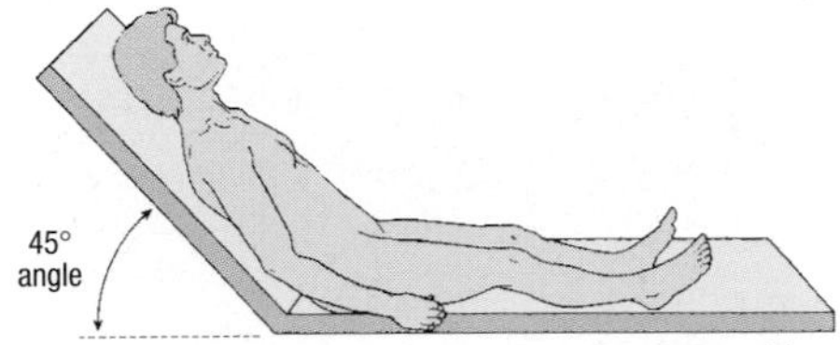

Fowler position

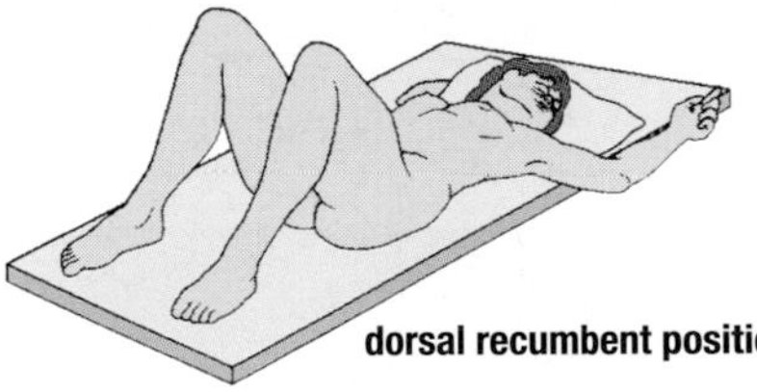
dorsal recumbent position

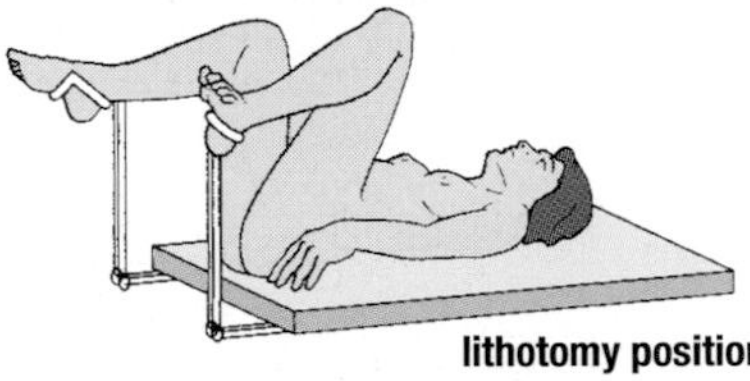
lithotomy position

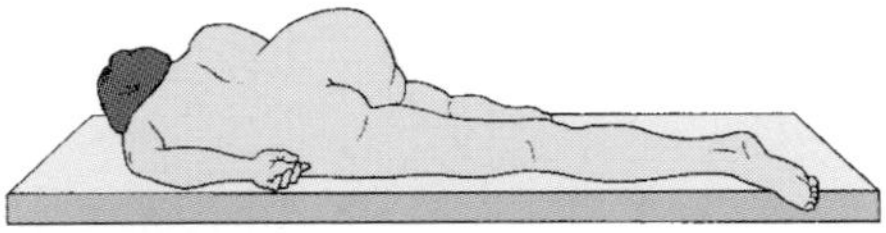
Sims position

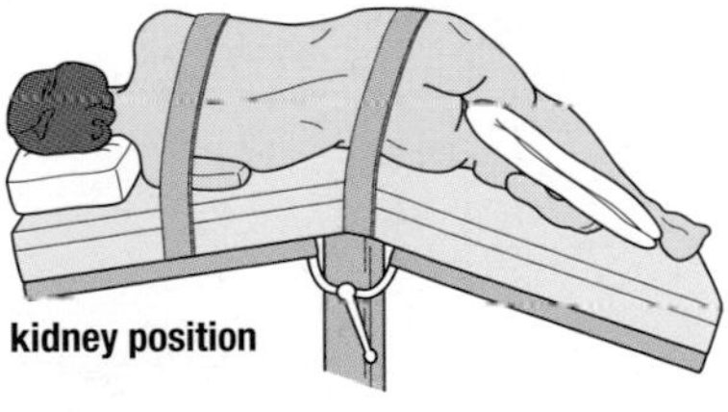
kidney position

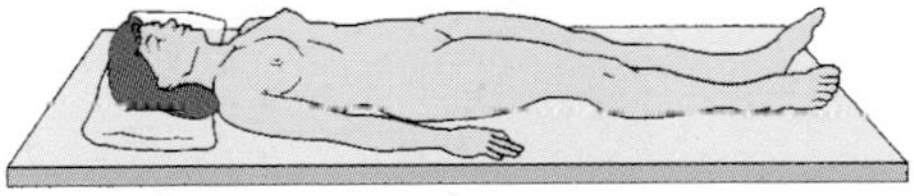
supine position

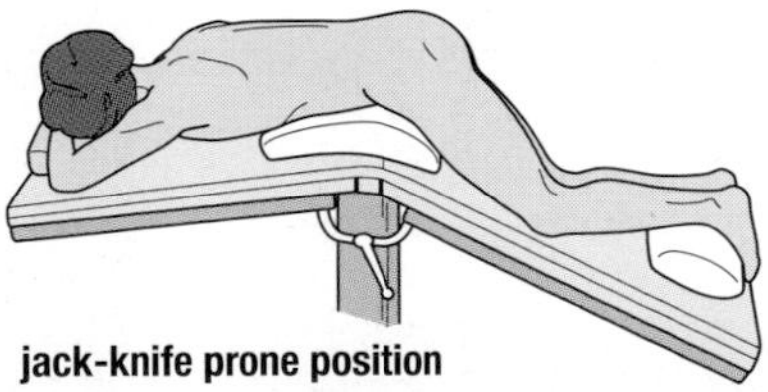
jack-knife prone position

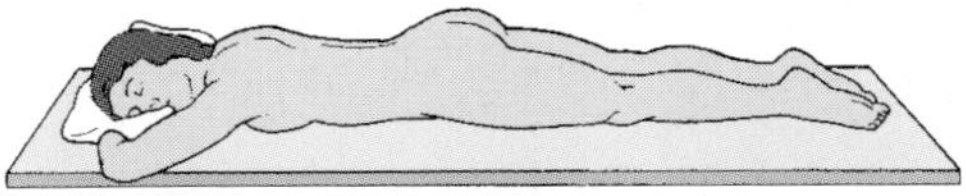
prone position

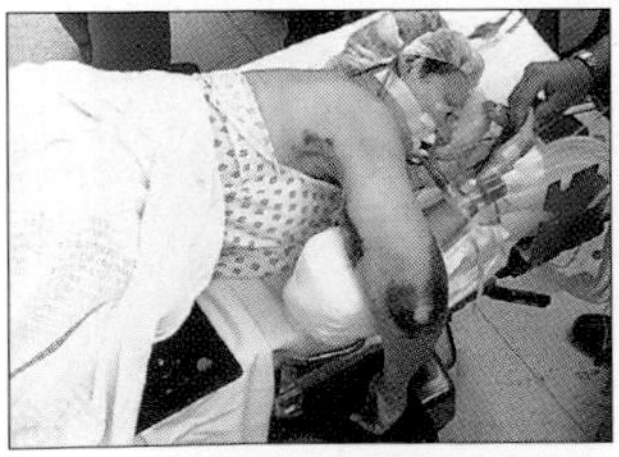
lateral decubitus position

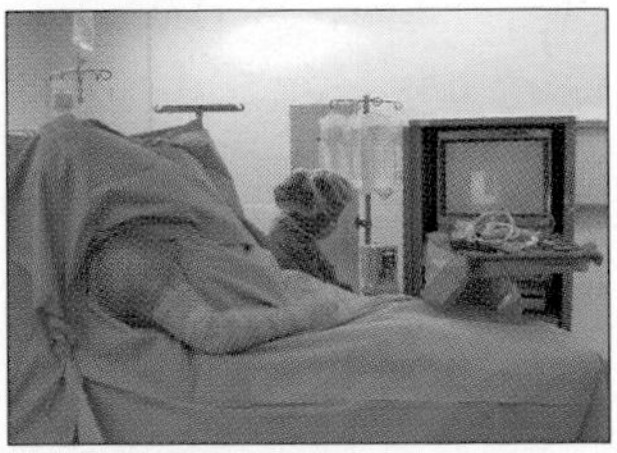
beach chair position

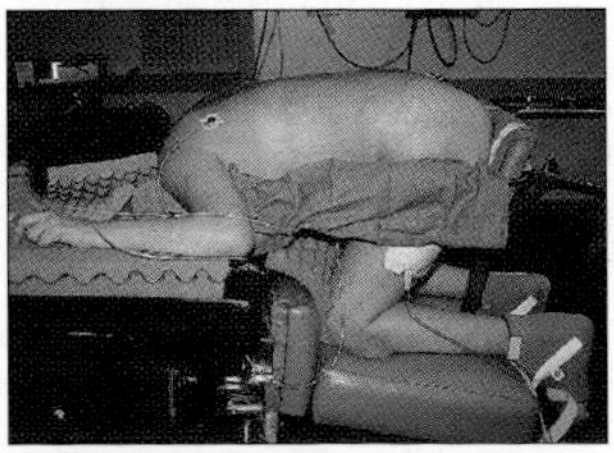
knee-chest position

PLATE 30: CHILDHOOD CONDITIONS

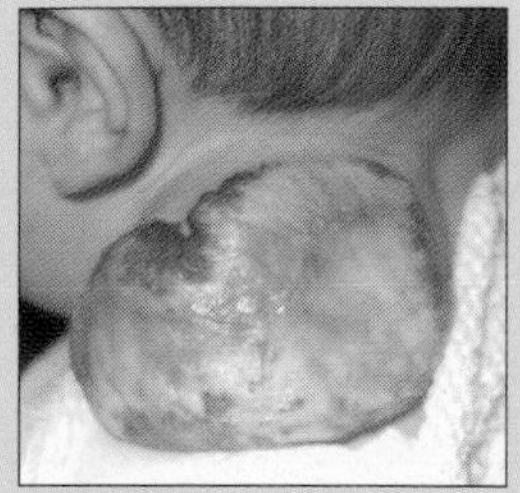

strawberry hemangioma

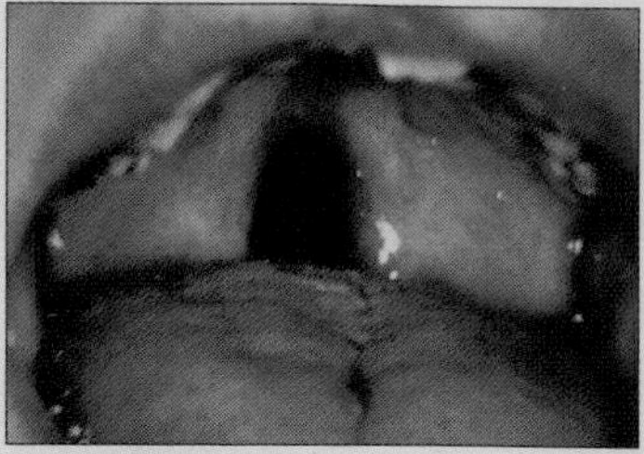

cleft soft palate

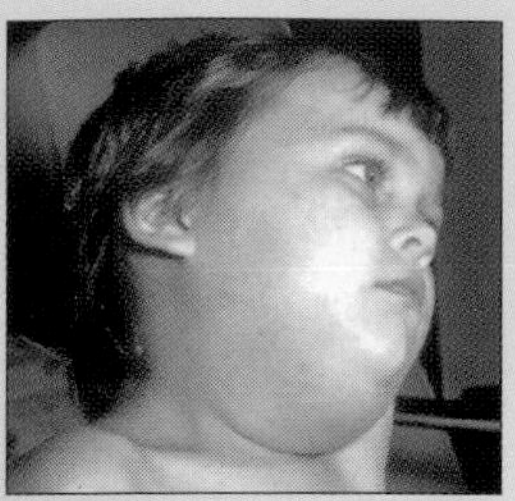

mumps

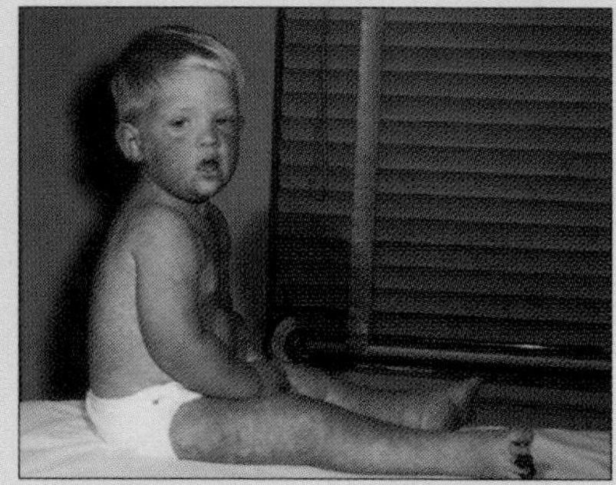

◀ **measles**

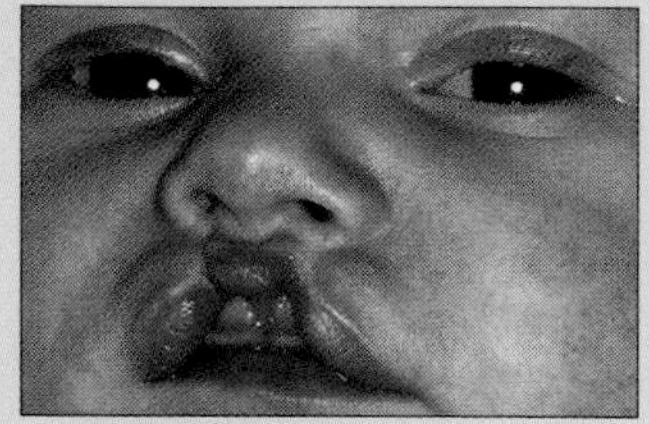

bilateral cleft lip ▶

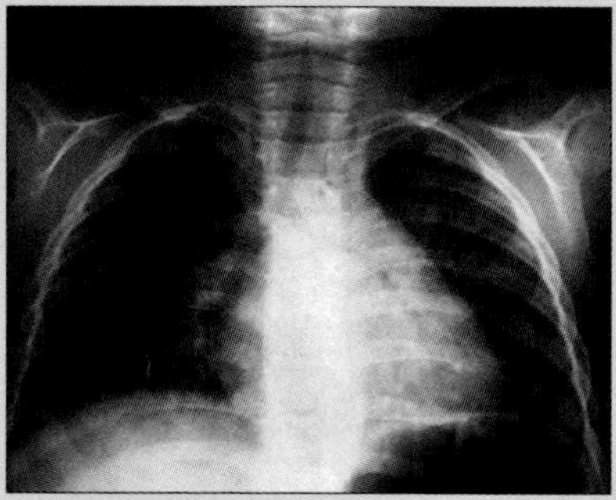

◀ **croup:** steeple sign on a soft-tissue neck radiograph

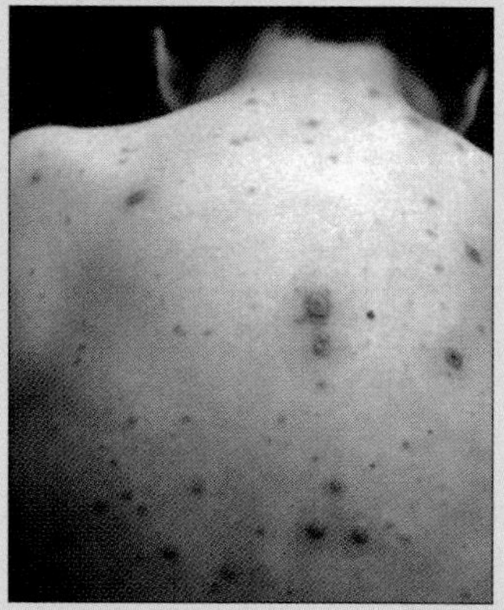

varicella (chickenpox)

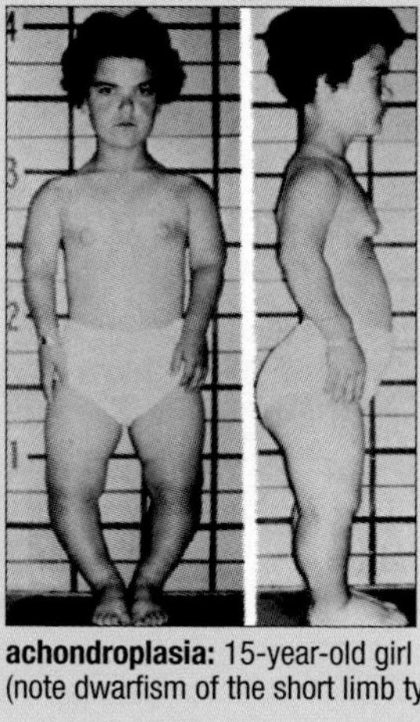

achondroplasia: 15-year-old girl (note dwarfism of the short limb type)

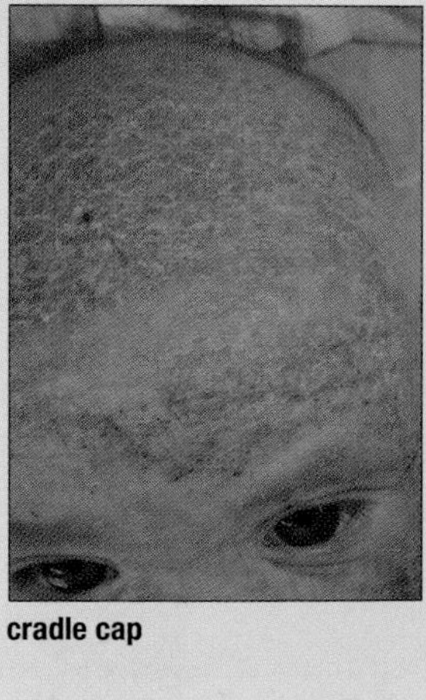

cradle cap

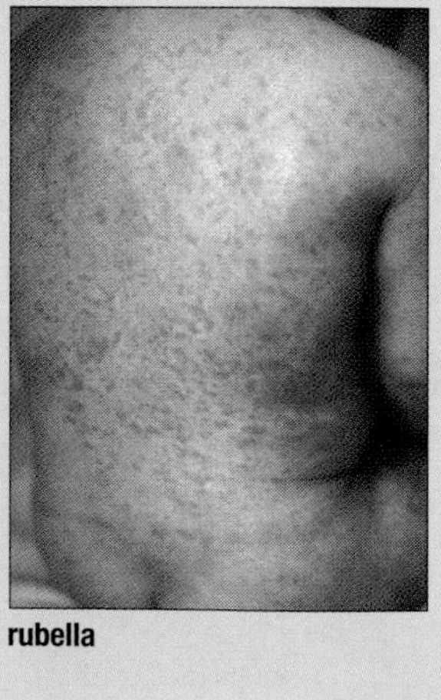

rubella

PLATE 31: CHILDHOOD CANCERS

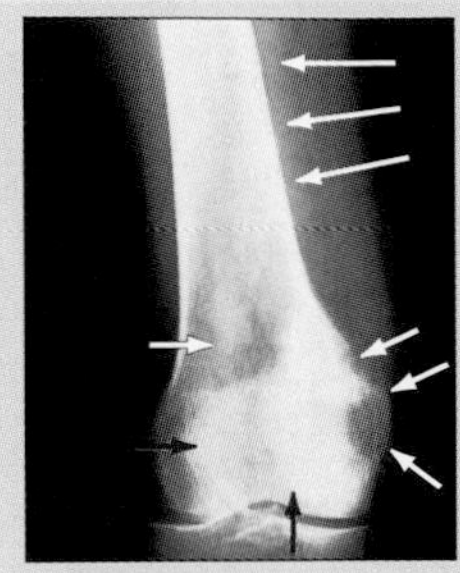

osteosarcomas of the distal femur: radiograph showing areas of bone destruction (short white arrows), sclerosis (red arrows), and periosteal calcification (long white arrows)

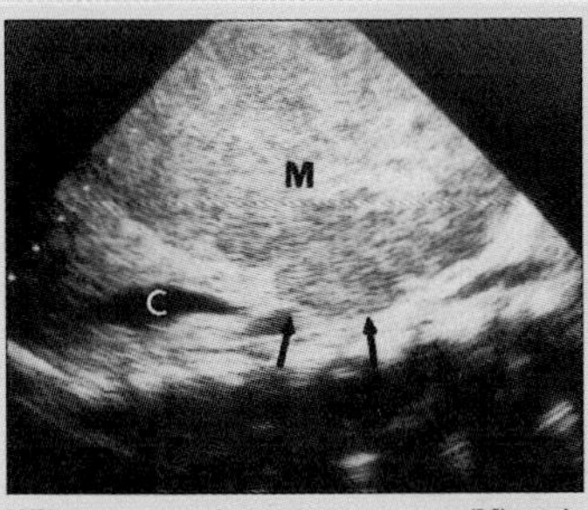

Wilms tumor: large tumor mass (M) and a tumor nodule (arrows) compressing the inferior vena cava (C)

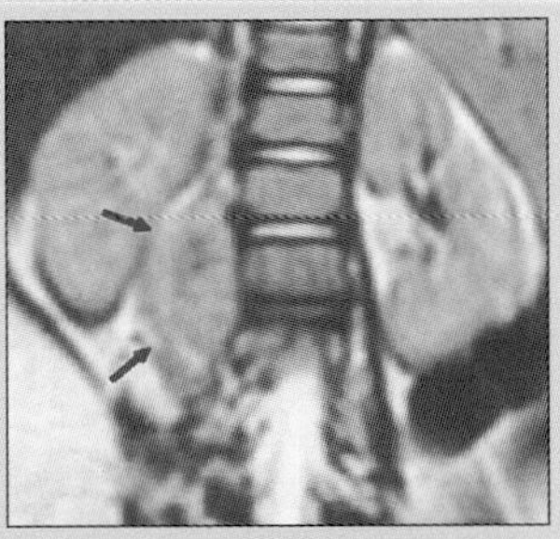

dumbbell neuroblastoma: small adrenal tumors (arrows)

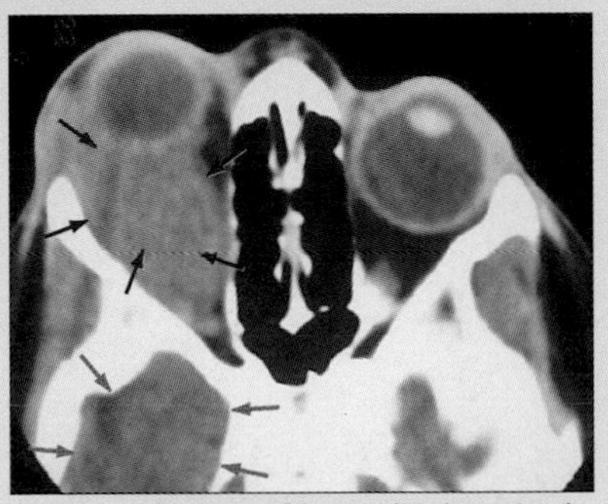

rhabdomyosarcoma: CT scan showing extensive invasion of the right orbit (red arrows) with forward displacement of the eyeball, and of the middle cranial fossa (green arrows)

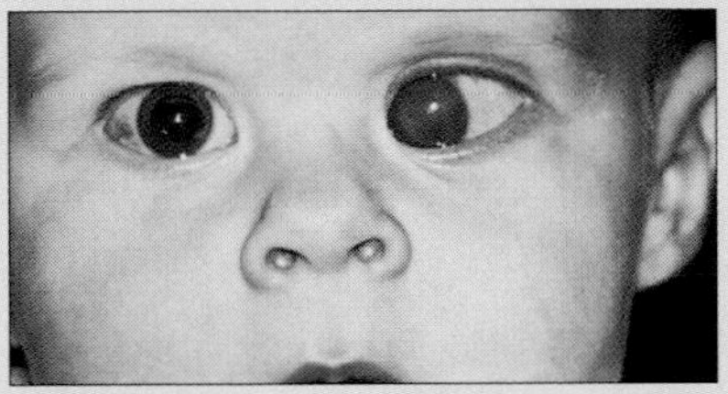

retinoblastoma causing glaucoma

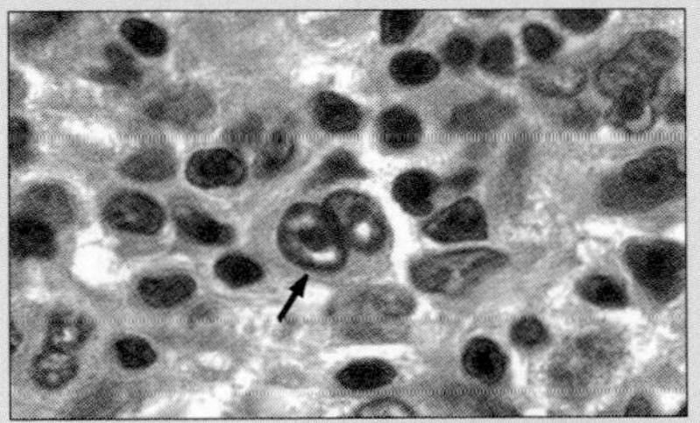

Hodgkin disease: lymph node biopsy; Reed-Sternberg cell (arrow) looks like two cells side by side, but is only one cell

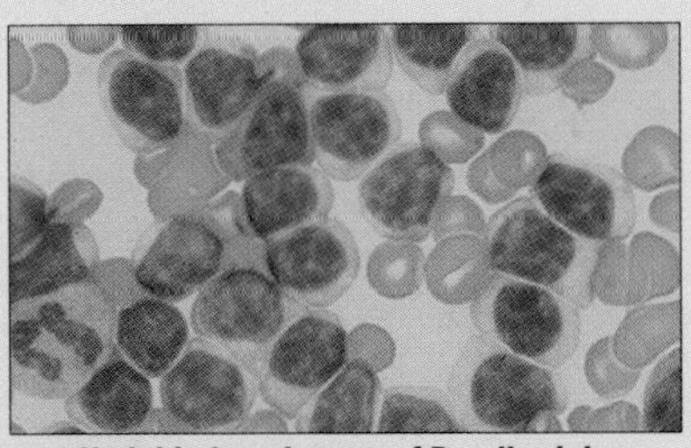

non-Hodgkin lymphomas of B-cell origin: small lymphocytic lymphoma or chronic lymphocytic leukemia

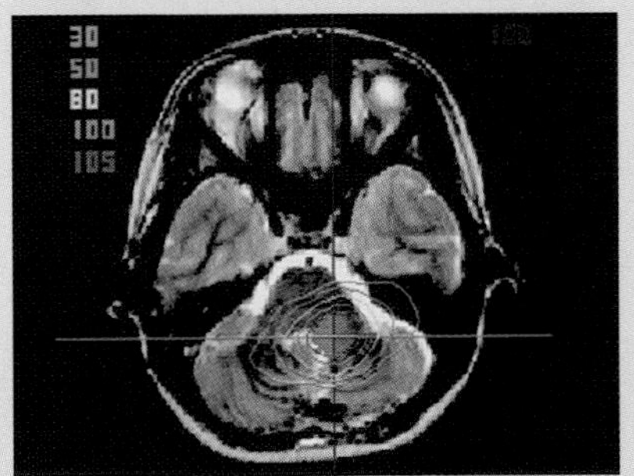

low-grade astrocytoma: MRI of posterior fossa in a 12-year-old female patient

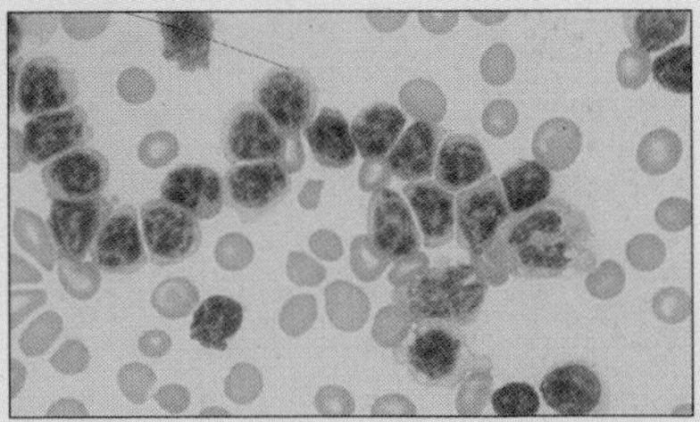

chronic lymphocytic leukemia: bone marrow smear

PLATE 32: EMERGENCY MEDICINE

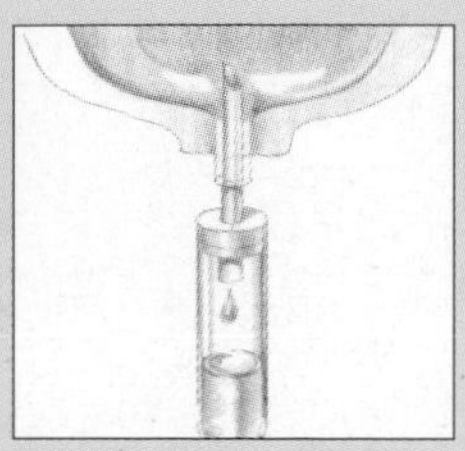

standard (macrodrip) set:
delivers 10-20 drops/mL

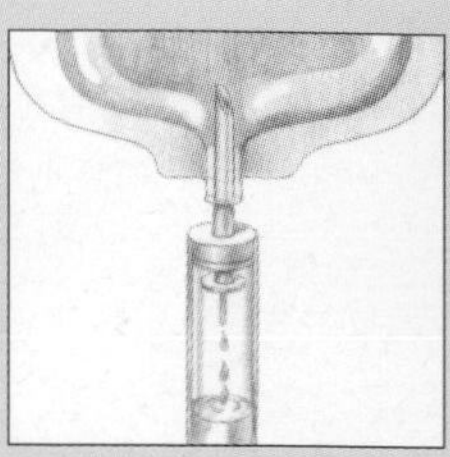

pediatric (microdrip) set:
delivers 60 drops/mL

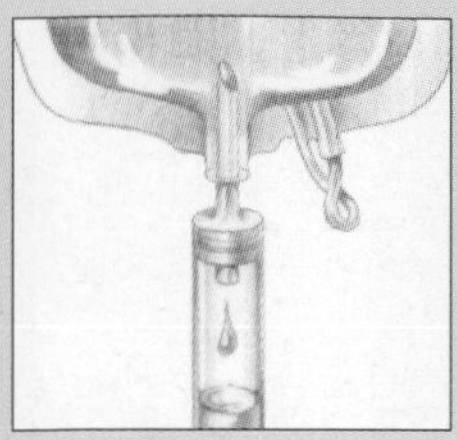

blood transfusion set:
delivers 10 drops/mL

To **calculate the flow rate**, you must know the calibration of the drip rate for each manufacturer's product. Use this formula to calculate specific drip rates:

$$\frac{\textbf{volume of infusion (in mL)}}{\textbf{time of infusion (in minutes)}} \textbf{ X drip factor (in drops/mL) = drops/minute}$$

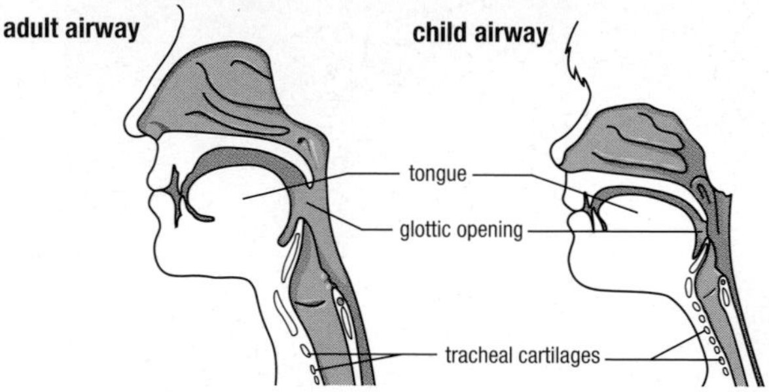

adult vs. child airways

There are many differences between the airway of an adult and that of a child. The tongue sits anteriorly and is larger in relation to the oropharynx in the child. The child's glottic opening is narrower then the adult's. The tracheal cartilages are also unformed in the child, preventing the head tilt from being performed because it would result in a closed trachea.

Inserting a nasopharyngeal airway

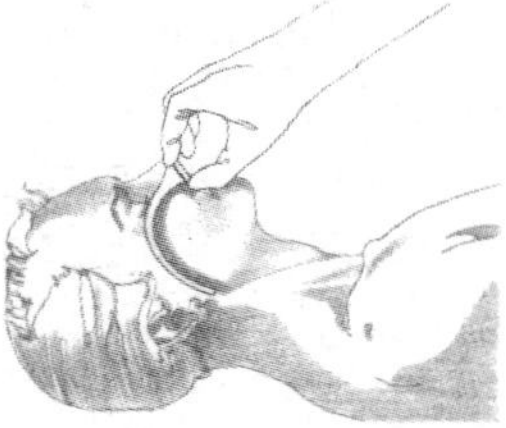

First, hold the airway beside the patient's face to make sure it's the proper size. It should be slightly smaller than the patient's nostril diameter and slightly longer than the distance from the tip of the nose to the earlobe.

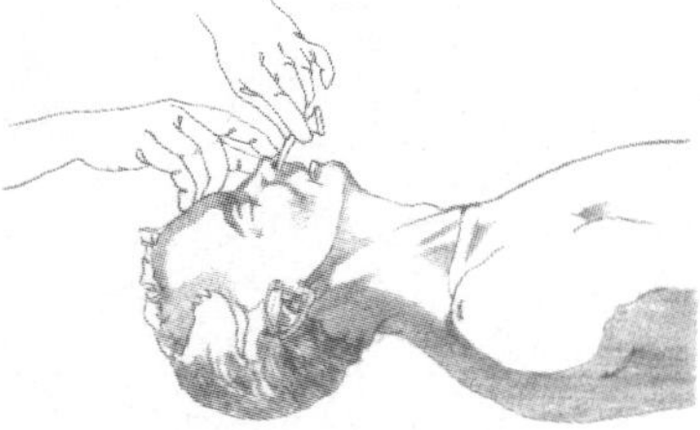

To insert airway, hyperextend the patient's neck (unless contraindicated). Push the tip of the nose and pass the airway into the nostril. Avoid pushing against any resistance to prevent tissue trauma and airway kinking.

Inserting an oral airway

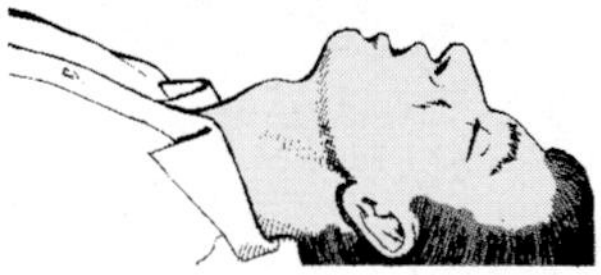

Unless this position is contraindicated, hyperextend the patient's head.

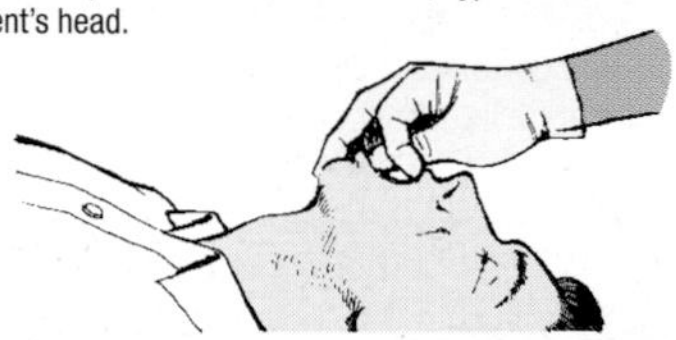

To insert an oral airway using the cross-finger method, place your thumb on the patient's lower teeth and your index finger on the upper teeth. Gently open his mouth by pushing the teeth apart.

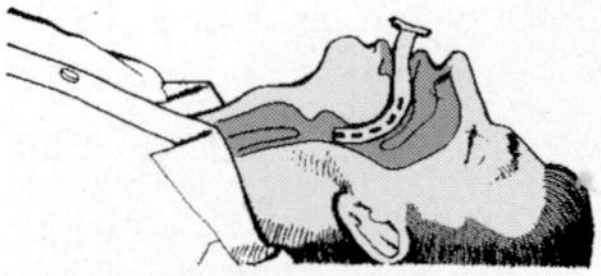

Insert the airway upside down to avoid pushing the tongue toward the pharynx, and slide it over the tongue toward the back of the mouth. Rotate the airway as it approaches the posterior wall of the pharynx so that it points downward.

morphine; some, along the aqueduct of Sylvius and in the centromedian nucleus, are in areas related to pain, but others, as in the striatum, are not related.

-opic, **-opical** Combining forms meaning a (specified) visual field. [G. *opsis,* vision]

o•pi•o•cor•tin (ō′pē-ō-kōr′tin) SYN opiomelanocortin.

o•pi•oid (ō′pē-oyd) A narcotic substance, either natural or synthetic.

o•pi•oid ant•ag•on•ist (ō′pē-oyd an-tag′ŏ-nist) Examples include naloxone and naltrexone that have high affinity for opiate receptors but do not activate these receptors. These drugs block the effects of exogenously administered opioids (e.g., morphine, heroin, meperidine, and methadone), or of endogenously released endorphins and enkephalins.

o•pi•o•mel•a•no•cor•tin (ō′pē-ō-mel′ă-nō-kōr′tin) A linear polypeptide of the pituitary gland that contains in its sequence the sequences of endorphins, MSH, ACTH, and the like, which are split off enzymically. SYN opiocortin.

o•pis•the•nar (ō-pis′thē-năr) Dorsum of the hand. [G. back of the hand, from *opisthen,* behind, + *thenar,* palm of the hand]

o•pis•thi•on (ō-pis′thē-on) [TA] The middle point on the posterior margin of the foramen magnum, opposite the basion. [G. *opisthios,* posterior]

opistho- Combining form meaning backward, behind, dorsal. [G. *opisthen,* at the rear, behind]

op•is•tho•ton•ic (ō-pis-thot′ō-nik) Relating to or characterized by opisthotonos.

op•is•thot•o•nos, **op•is•thot•o•nus** (ō-pis-thot′ō-nŭs) A tetanic spasm in which the spine and extremities are bent with convexity forward, the body resting on the head and the heels. [opistho- + G. *tonos,* tension, stretching]

O•pitz BBB syn•drome (ō′pits sin′drōm) SYN ocular hypertelorism.

O•pitz G syn•drome (ō′pits sin′drōm) SYN ocular hypertelorism.

Op•pen•heim dis•ease (op′en-hīm di-zēz′) SYN amyotonia congenita.

Op•pen•heim re•flex (op′en-hīm rē′fleks) Extension of the toes induced by scratching of the inner side of the leg or by sudden flexion of the thigh on the abdomen and the leg on the thigh; a sign of cerebral irritation.

op•po•nens di•gi•ti mi•ni•mi mus•cle (op-ō′nenz dij′i-tī mi′ni-mī mŭs′ĕl) *Origin,* hamulus of the hamate bone and transverse carpal ligament; *insertion,* shaft of fifth metacarpal; *action,* "cups" palm, drawing ulnar side of hand toward center of palm; *nerve supply,* ulnar. SYN musculus opponens digiti minimi [TA].

op•po•nens pol•li•cis mus•cle (op-ō′nenz pol′li-sis mŭs′ĕl) *Origin,* ridge of trapezium and flexor retinaculum; *insertion,* anterior surface of the full length of the shaft of the first metacarpal bone; *action,* acts at carpometacarpal joint to "cup" palm, enabling one to oppose thumb to other fingers; *nerve supply,* median. SYN musculus opponens pollicis [TA].

op•por•tun•is•tic (op′ŏr-tū-nis′tik) **1.** Denoting an organism capable of causing disease only in a host with lowered resistance; e.g., by other diseases or by drugs. **2.** Denoting a disease caused by such an organism.

op•po•si•tion•al de•fi•ant dis•or•der (op-pŏ-sish′ŭn-ăl dĕ-fī′ănt dis-ōr′dĕr) A disorder of childhood or adolescence characterized by a recurrent pattern of negativistic, hostile, and disobedient behavior toward authority figures.

op•pres•sion (ŏ-pres′shŭn) NURSING acts of subjugation or coercion related to decisions about health care.

ops-, **opto-**, **opti-**, **optico-** Combining forms meaning the eye or vision.

op•sin (op′sin) The protein portion of the rhodopsin molecule; at least three separate opsins are located in cone cells.

op•sin•o•gen (op-sin′ō-jen) A substance that stimulates the formation of opsonin, such as the antigen contained in a suspension of bacteria used for immunization. SYN opsogen. [opsonin + -gen]

op•si•u•ri•a (op-sē-yū′rē-ă) A more rapid excretion of urine during fasting than after a full meal. [G. *opsi,* late, + *ouron,* urine]

op•so•clo•nus (op′sō-klō′nus) Repetitive irregular multidirectional ocular movement associated with cerebellar or brainstem disorders. [G. *ops*, eye, + clonus]

op•so•gen (op′sō-jen) SYN opsinogen.

op•so•ma•ni•a (op′sō-mā′nē-ă) A longing for a particular article of diet, or for highly seasoned food. [G. *opson,* seasoning, + *mania,* frenzy]

op•son•ic (op-son′ik) Relating to opsonins or to their utilization.

op•son•ic in•dex (op-son′ik in′deks) A value that indicates the relative content of opsonin in the blood of a person with an infectious disease, as evaluated in vitro in comparison with presumably normal blood; the opsonic index is calculated from the following equation: phagocytic index of normal serum ÷ phagocytic index of test serum = 1 ÷ x, where x represents the opsonic index.

op•so•nin (op′sŏ-nin) A substance that binds to

antigens, enhancing phagocytosis. [G. *opson,* boiled meat, provisions, fr. *hepsō,* to boil, + -in]

opsonisation [Br.] SYN opsonization.

op·son·i·za·tion (op′sŏ-nī-zā′shŭn) The process by which bacteria are altered so that they are more readily and more efficiently engulfed by phagocytes. SYN opsonisation.

op·so·nize (op′sŏn-īz) To prepare microorganisms for phagocytosis and ultimate destruction.

op·so·no·cy·to·pha·gic (op′sŏ-nō-sī′tō-fā′jik) Pertaining to the increased efficiency of phagocytic activity of the leukocytes in blood that contains a specific opsonin. [opsonin + G. *kytos,* a hollow (cell), + *phagō,* to eat]

op·so·nom·e·try (op-sŏ-nom′ĕ-trē) Determination of the opsonic index or the opsonocytophagic activity.

op·tic, op·ti·cal (op′tik, -ti-kăl) Relating to the eye, vision, or optics. [G. *optikos*]

op·tic ab·er·ra·tion (op′tik ab-ĕr-ā′shŭn) Failure of rays from a point source to form a perfect image after traversing an optic system.

op·tic ac·tiv·i·ty (op′tik ak-tiv′ĭ-tē) The ability of a compound in solution (one possessing no plane of symmetry, usually because of the presence of one or more asymmetric carbon atoms) to rotate the plane of polarized light.

op·tic a·lex·i·a (op′tik ă-lek′sē-ă) SEE alexia.

op·tic a·tax·i·a (op′tik ă-taks′ē-ă) An inability to guide the hand toward an object using visual information; seen in Balint syndrome.

op·tic ax·is (op′tik ak′sis) The axis of the eye connecting the anterior and posterior poles; it usually diverges from the visual axis by five degrees or more.

op·tic ca·nal (op′tik kă-nal′) The short canal through the lesser wing of the sphenoid bone at the apex of the orbit that gives passage to the optic nerve and the ophthalmic artery. SYN canalis opticus [TA], optic foramen.

op·tic cap·sule (op′tik kap′sŭl) The concentrated zone of mesenchyme around the developing optic cup; the primordium of the sclera of the eye.

op·tic chi·asm (op′tik kī′azm) A flattened quadrangular body in front of the tuber cinereum and infundibulum, the point of crossing or decussation of the fibers of the optic nerves; most of the fibers cross to the opposite side, some run directly forward on each side without crossing, some pass transversely on the posterior surface between the two optic tracts and others pass transversely on the anterior surface between the two optic nerves. SYN optic decussation.

op·tic cup (op′tik kŭp) The double-walled cup formed by the invagination of the embryonic optic vesicle; its inner component becomes the neural layer of the retina; its outer layer, the pigmented layer.

op·tic de·cus·sa·tion (op′tik dē-kŭs-ā′shŭn) SYN optic chiasm.

op·tic den·si·ty (OD) (op′tik den′si-tē) SYN absorbance.

op·tic disc (op′tik disk) An oval area of the ocular fundus devoid of light receptors where the axons of the retinal ganglion cells converge to form the optic nerve head. SYN discus nervi optici [TA], blind spot (3), optic papilla.

op·tic fis·sure (op′tik fish′ŭr) SYN retinal fissure.

op·tic fo·ra·men (op′tik fōr-ā′mĕn) SYN optic canal.

op·ti·cian (op-tish′ăn) A health care professional who is trained and licensed to make corrective lenses, adjust and repair spectacles, and fit contact lenses.

op·tic im·age (op′tik im′ăj) An image formed by the refraction or reflection of light.

op·tic i·som·er·ism (op′tik ī-som′ĕr-izm) Stereoisomerism involving the arrangement of substituents about an asymmetric atom or atoms (usually carbon) so that a difference exists in the behavior of the various isomers with regard to the extent of their rotation of the plane of polarized light. Cf. stereoisomerism.

op·tic ker·a·to·plas·ty (op′tik ker′ă-tō-plas-tē) Transplantation of transparent corneal tissue to replace a leukoma or scar that impairs vision.

op·tic nerve [CN II] (op′tik nĕrv) Although classified as a cranial nerve, it is actually an extension of the forebrain; it conveys afferent fibers from the ganglion cells of the retina, it passes out of the orbit through the optic canal to the chiasm, where part of the fibers cross to the opposite side and pass through the optic tract to the geniculate bodies, superior colliculus, and the pretectum. SYN nervus opticus [CN II] [TA], second cranial nerve [CN II].

op·tic neu·ri·tis (op′tik nūr-ī′tis) Inflammation of the optic nerve. SEE ALSO neuromyelitis optica, retrobulbar neuritis, papillitis.

op·ti·co·cil·i·a·ry (op′ti-kō-sil′ē-ar-ē) Relating to the optic and ciliary nerves.

op·ti·co·pu·pil·lary (op′ti-kō-pyū′pi-lar-ē) Relating to the optic nerve and the pupil.

op·tic pa·pil·la (p) (op′tik pă-pil′ă) SYN optic disc.

op·tic ra·di·a·tion (op′tik rā′dē-ā′shŭn) The massive, fanlike fiber system passing from the lateral geniculate body of the thalamus to the visual cortex; the fibers follow the retrolenticular and sublenticular limbs of the internal capsule into the corona radiata but they curve back along the lateral wall of the temporal and occipital horns of the lateral ventricle to the striate cortex on the medial surface and pole of the occipital lobe. SYN radiatio optica.

op·tic ro·ta·tion (op′tik rō-tā′shŭn) The change in the plane of polarization of polarized light of a given wavelength on passing through optically active substances; measured in terms of specific rotation by polarimetry, an important tool in chemical structural work, especially on carbohydrates.

op·tic ro·ta·to·ry dis·per·sion (op′tik rō′tă-tōr′ē dis-pĕr′zhŭn) The change in optic rotation with the wavelength of the incident monochromatic polarized light; the displacement of the former from zero within the absorption band is known as the cotton effect.

op·tics (op′tiks) The science concerned with the properties of light, its refraction and absorption, and the refracting media of the eye in that relation. [G. *optikos,* fr. *ōps,* eye]

op·tic tract (op′tik trakt) The continuation of the optic nerve fibers beyond their hemidecussation in the optic chiasm; each of the two symmetric optic tracts is composed of fibers originating from the temporal half of the retina of the ipsilateral eye and a nearly equal number of fibers from the nasal half of the contralateral retina; it forms a compact, somewhat flattened fiber band passing caudolaterally along the base of the hypothalamus and over the basal surface of the crus cerebri; most of its fibers terminate in the lateral geniculate body; a smaller number of fibers enter the brachium of the superior colliculus, to terminate in the superior colliculus and the pretectal region. SYN tractus opticus [TA].

op·ti·mal dose (op′ti-măl dōs) The dose of a drug or radiation that will produce the desired effect with minimum likelihood of undesirable symptoms.

op·ti·mal pitch (op′ti-măl pich) The frequency of vocal fold movement that allows optimal resonance with least vocal effort. SEE ALSO habitual pitch, fundamental frequency. SYN natural pitch.

♻**opto-, optico-** Combining forms meaning optic; ocular. [G. *optikos,* optic, from *ōps,* eye]

op·to·ki·net·ic nys·tag·mus (op′tō-ki-net′ik nis-tag′mŭs) Nystagmus induced by looking at moving visual stimuli.

op·tom·e·ter (op-tom′ĕ-tĕr) An instrument for determining the refraction of the eye. [opto- + G. *metron,* measure]

op·tom·e·trist (op-tom′ĕ-trist) One who practices optometry.

op·tom·e·try (op-tom′ĕ-trē) **1.** The profession concerned with the examination of the eyes and related structures to determine the presence of vision problems and eye disorders, and with the prescription and adaptation of lenses and other optic aids or the use of visual training for maximum visual efficiency. **2.** The use of an optometer.

op·to·my·om·e·ter (op′tō-mī-om′ĕ-tĕr) An instrument for determining the relative power of the extrinsic muscles of the eye. [opto- + G. *mys,* muscle, + *metron,* measure]

OPV Abbreviation for oral poliovirus vaccine.

OR Abbreviation for operating room.

o·ra (ō′ră) Plural of L. *os,* the mouth. [L.]

o·ra, pl. **o·rae** (ō′ră, -ē) An edge or a margin. [L.]

or·ad (ōr′ad) **1.** In a direction toward the mouth. **2.** Situated nearer the mouth in relation to a specific reference point; opposite of aborad. [L. *os,* mouth, + *ad,* to]

or·al (ōr′ăl) Relating to the mouth. [L. *os* (*or-*), mouth]

or·al a·prax·i·a (ōr′ăl ă-praks′ē-ă) Reduced ability, due to cortical sensorimotor damage, to perform voluntary movements of the oral musculature, especially sequenced movements. Often occurs with apraxia of speech. SEE ALSO apraxia. SYN oral motor apraxia.

or·al au·di·tory meth·od (ōr′ăl aw′di-tōr-ē meth′ŏd) An approach to the education of deaf children that emphasizes early auditory training, speech and speech reading, and early and consistent use of high quality amplification for residual hearing. SEE ALSO manual visual method, combined methods, total communication.

or·al a·ware·ness (ōr′ăl ă-wār′nĕs) Perception of structures or conditions within one's own mouth.

or·al bi·ol·o·gy (ōr′ăl bī-ol′ŏ-jē) That aspect of biology devoted to the study of biologic phenomena associated with the oral cavity in health and disease (e.g., dental caries, mastication, periodontal disease).

or·al cav·i·ty (ōr′ăl kav′i-tē) The region consisting of the vestibulum oris, the narrow cleft between the lips and cheeks, and the teeth and gums, and the cavitas oris propria. SYN mouth (1).

or·al con·tra·cep·tive (OC) (ōr′ăl kon-tră-sep′tiv) A medication taken by mouth designed to prevent conception.

or·al de·fen·sive·ness (ōr′ăl dē-fen′siv-nĕs) Overreaction to the tastes or textures of things placed in one's mouth.

or·al hy·giene (ōr′ăl hī′jēn) Cleaning the mouth by brushing, flossing, irrigating, massaging, or the use of other devices.

o·ral·i·ty (ōr-al′i-tē) PSYCHOLOGY Freud's theory of psychic organization derived from, and characteristic of, the oral period of psychosexual development.

o·ral·ly (ōr′ă-lē) By or through the mouth. [L. *os, oris,* mouth]

or·al and max·il·lo·fa·cial sur·ge·ry (ōr′al mak′sil-ō-fā′shăl sŭr′jĕr-ē) The dental specialty that includes the surgical correction of injuries and malformations of the midface, jaws, and dentition. Cf. oral surgery.

or·al mo·tor a·prax·i·a (ōr′ăl mō′tŏr ă-prak′sē-ă) SYN oral apraxia.

or·al pa·thol·o·gy (ōr′ăl pă-thol′ŏ-jē) The branch of dentistry concerned with the etiology, pathogenesis, and clinical, gross, and microscopic aspects of oral and paraoral disease, including oral soft tissues, the teeth, jaws, and salivary glands.

or·al phase (ōr′ăl fāz) In psychoanalytic personality theory, the earliest stage in psychosexual development, lasting through the first 18 months of life, during which the oral zone is the center of the infant's needs, expression, gratification, and pleasurable erotic experiences; has a strong influence on the organization and development of the child's psyche.

or·al po·li·o·vi·rus vac·cine (OPV) (ōr-ăl pō′lē-ō vī′rŭs vak-sēn′) SEE poliovirus vaccine (2).

or·al sur·geon (ōr′ăl sŭr′jŏn) SYN dental surgeon.

or·al sur·ge·ry (ōr′ăl sŭr′jĕr-ē) A dentist who specializes in the surgical removal of teeth and surrounding oral tissues. Cf. oral and maxillofacial surgery.

or·al ves·ti·bule (ōr′ăl ves′ti-byūl) That part of the mouth bounded anteriorly and laterally by the lips and the cheeks, posteriorly and medially by the teeth and/or gums, and above and below by the reflections of the mucosa from the lips and cheeks to the gums.

or·ange-top tube (awr′ănj-top tūb) A tube of this color indicates the container has been treated with lithium heparin.

or·ange wood (awr′anj wūd) A soft wood used in dentistry for placement of bridges and crowns using pressure; also used as a burnishing point in the polishing of root surfaces.

o·ra ser·ra·ta re·ti·nae (ōr′ă sē-rā′tă ret′i-nē) The serrated extremity of the optic part of the retina, located a little behind the ciliary body and marking the limits of the percipient portion of the membrane.

or·bic·u·lar (ōr-bik′yū-lăr) Similar in form to an orb; circular in form. [L. *orbiculus,* a small disc, dim. of *orbis,* circle]

or·bic·u·la·re (ōr-bik′yū-lā′rē) SYN lenticular process of incus. [L., fr. *orbiculus,* a small disc]

or·bi·cu·la·ris oc·u·li mus·cle (ōr-bik′yū-lā′ris ok′yū-lī mŭs′ĕl) Consists of three portions: orbital part, or external portion, which arises from frontal process of maxilla and nasal process of frontal bone, encircles aperture of orbit, and is inserted near origin; palpebral part, or internal portion, which arises from medial palpebral ligament, passes through each eyelid, and is inserted into lateral palpebral raphe; lacrimal part (tensor tarsi muscle, Duverney or Horner muscle), which arises from posterior lacrimal crest and passes across lacrimal sac to join palpebral portion; *action*, closes eye, wrinkles forehead vertically; *nerve supply*, facial. SYN musculus orbicularis oculi [TA].

or·bi·cu·la·ris o·ris mus·cle (ōr-bik′yū-lā′ris ō′ris mŭs′ĕl) *Origin*, by nasolabial band from septum of the nose, by superior incisive bundle from incisor fossa of maxilla, by inferior incisive bundle from lower jaw each side of symphysis; *insertion*, fibers surround mouth between skin and mucous membrane of lips and cheeks, and are blended with other muscles; *action*, closes lips; *nerve supply*, facial. See this page. SYN musculus orbicularis oris [TA].

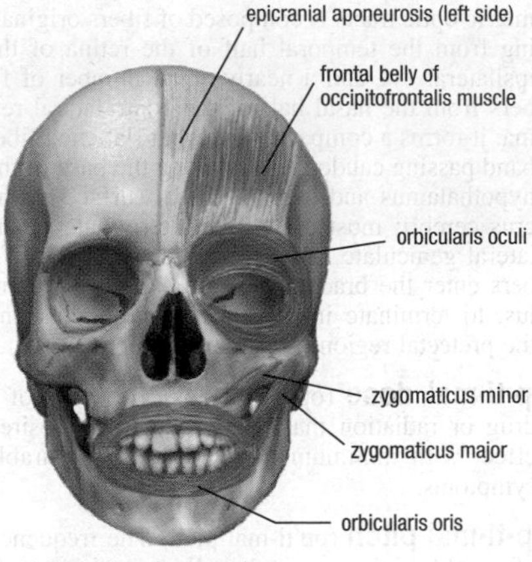

orbicularis oris muscle

or·bi·cu·lus cil·i·ar·is (ōr-bik′yū-lŭs sil′ē-ār′is) The darkly pigmented posterior zone of the ciliary body continuous with the retina at the ora serrata. SYN ciliary disc, ciliary ring, pars plana. [Mod. L.]

or·bit (ōr′bit) The bony cavity containing the eyeball and its adnexa; it is formed of parts of the frontal, maxillary, sphenoid, lacrimal, zygomatic, ethmoid, and palatine bones. See page 1117. SYN orbita [TA], orbital cavity.

or·bi·ta, gen. **or·bi·tae** (ōr′bi-tă, -tē) [TA] SYN orbit. [L. a wheel-track, fr. *orbis,* circle]

or·bi·tal (ōr′bi-tăl) Relating to the orbits.

or·bi·tal cav·i·ty (ōr′bi-tăl kav′i-tē) SYN orbit.

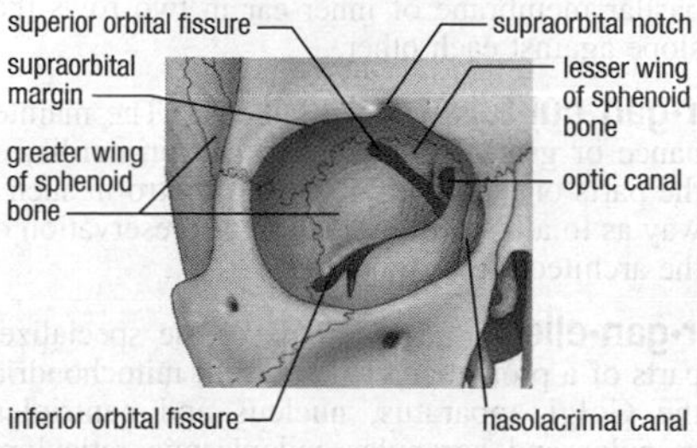

bony orbit

or•bi•tal cel•lu•li•tis (ōr′bi-tăl sel′yū-lī′tis) Cellulitis that involves the tissue layers posterior to the orbital septum. See page B9.

or•bi•ta•le (ōr-bi-tā′lē) CEPHALOMETRICS the lowermost point in the lower margin of the bony orbit that may be felt under the skin. [L. of an orbit]

or•bi•tal ex•en•te•ra•tion (ōr′bi-tăl eks-en′tĕr-ā′shŭn) Surgical removal of orbital contents, most commonly used in cases of orbital malignancy with local spread of disease.

or•bi•tal gy•ri (ōr′bi-tăl jī′rī) Small, irregular convolutions occupying the concave inferior surface of each frontal lobe of the cerebrum.

or•bi•ta•lis mus•cle (ōr-bi-tā′lis mŭs′ĕl) A rudimentary nonstriated muscle, crossing the infraorbital groove and sphenomaxillary fissure, intimately united with the periosteum of the orbit. SYN musculus orbitalis [TA], orbital muscle.

or•bi•tal mar•gin (ōr′bi-tăl mahr′jin) The mostly sharp edge of the orbital opening that is the peripheral border of the base of the pyramidal orbit. The superior half of the orbital rim is the supraorbital margin; the inferior half is the infraorbital margin. The frontal, maxillary, and zygomatic bones contribute to the orbital rim, which is generally strong to protect the orbital contents. Weak, potential fracture sites of the rim coincide with the sutures between the participating bones. SYN margo orbitalis [TA].

or•bi•tal mus•cle (ōr′bi-tăl mŭs′ĕl) SYN orbitalis muscle.

or•bi•tal plane (ōr′bi-tăl plān) The orbital surface of the maxilla, lying perpendicular to the orbitomeatal plane at the orbitale.

or•bi•tal pro•cess (ōr′bi-tăl pros′es) The anterior and larger of the two processes at the upper extremity of the vertical plate of the palatine bone, articulating with the maxilla, ethmoid, and sphenoid bones.

or•bi•tog•ra•phy (ōr-bi-tog′ră-fē) Radiographic evaluation of the orbit. [L. *orbita,* orbit, + G. *graphō,* to write]

or•bi•to•me•a•tal line (OML) (ōr′bi-tō-mē-ā′tăl līn) SYN baseline.

or•bi•to•me•a•tal plane (ōr′bi-tō-mē-ā′tăl plān) A standard craniometric reference plane passing through the right and left porion and the left orbitale; drawn on the profile radiograph or photograph from the superior margin of the acoustic meatus to the orbitale.

or•bi•to•na•sal (ōr′bi-tō-nā′zăl) Relating to the orbit and the nose or nasal cavity.

or•bi•to•nom•e•ter (ōr′bi-tō-nom′ĕ-tĕr) An instrument that measures the resistance offered to pressing the eyeball backwards into its socket. [L. *orbita,* orbit, + G. *metron,* measure]

or•bi•to•nom•e•try (ōr′bi-tō-nom′ĕ-trē) Measurement by means of the orbitonometer.

or•bi•top•a•thy (ōr′bi-top′ă-thē) Disease of the orbit and its contents.

or•bi•tot•o•my (ōr-bi-tot′ŏ-mē) Surgical incision into the orbit. [L. *orbita,* orbit, + *tomē,* a cutting]

Or•bi•vi•rus (ōr′bi-vī′rŭs) A genus of viruses of vertebrates that multiply in insects, including human Colorado tick fever virus. [L. *orbis,* ring, + virus]

or•ce•in (ōr′sē-in) A natural dye derived from orcinol that is used in various histologic staining methods.

orch•al•gi•a (ōr-kal′jē-ă) SYN orchialgia.

orchi-, orchido-, orchio- Combining forms meaning the testes. [G. *orchis,* testis]

or•chi•al•gi•a (ōr-kē-al′jē-ă) Pain in the testis. SYN orchalgia, testalgia. [orchi- + G. *algos,* pain]

or•chi•dec•to•my (ōr-ki-dek′tŏ-mē) SYN orchiectomy.

or•chid•ic (ōr-kid′ik) Relating to the testis.

or•chi•dom•e•ter (ōr-ki-dom′ĕ-tĕr) **1.** A caliper device used to measure the size of testes. **2.** A set of sized models of testes for comparison of testicular development. [orchido- + G. *metron,* measure]

or•chi•do•pex•y (ōr-kid′ō-peks′ē) SYN orchiopexy.

or•chi•ec•to•my (ōr-kē-ek′tŏ-mē) Removal of one or both testes. SYN orchidectomy, testectomy. [orchi- + G. *ektomē,* excision]

or•chi•ep•i•did•y•mi•tis (ōr′kē-ep′i-did-i-mī′tis) Inflammation of the testis and epididymis. [orchi- + epididymis, + G. *-itis,* inflammation]

or•chi•o•cele (ōr′kē-ō-sēl) A testis retained in the inguinal canal. [orchio- + G. *kēlē,* hernia, tumor]

or•chi•op•a•thy (ōr′kē-op′ă-thē) Disease of a testis. [orchio- + G. *pathos,* suffering]

or•chi•o•pex•y (ōr′kē-ō-pek′sē) Surgical treatment of an undescended testicle by freeing it and implanting it into the scrotum. SYN cryptorchidopexy, orchidopexy. [orchio- + G. *pēxis,* fixation]

or•chi•o•plas•ty (ōr′kē-ō-plas-tē) Surgical reconstruction of the testis. [orchio- + G. *plastos,* formed]

or•chi•ot•o•my (ōr′kē-ot′ŏ-mē) Incision into a testis. [orchio- + G. *tomē,* incision]

or•chis, pl. **or•chis•es** (ōr′kis, -ki-sēz) [TA] SYN testis. [G. testis, an orchid]

or•chit•ic (ōr-kit′ik) Denoting orchitis.

or•chi•tis (ōr-kī′tis) Inflammation of the testis. SYN testitis. [orchi- + G. *-itis,* inflammation]

Ord Abbreviation for orotidine.

or•der (ōr′dĕr) **1.** In biologic classification, the division just below the class (or subclass) and above the family. **2.** In a reaction, the sum of the exponents of all the concentration terms in that reaction's rate expression. [L. *ordo,* regular arrangement]

or•der of draw (ōr′dĕr draw) Recommended sequence in which blood specimens should be drawn so as to minimize interference in testing caused by carryover of additives in tubes.

or•der•ly (ōr′dĕr-lē) An attendant in a hospital unit who assists in the care of patients.

or•di•nate (ōr′di-nāt) In a cartesian plane coordinate system, the vertical axis (*y*).

Or•e•gon grape (ōr′ĕ-gon grāp) SYN barberry.

O•rem self-care de•fi•cit the•o•ry (ōr′em self-kār def′i-sit thē′ŏr-ē) Theory of nursing promulgated by the American nursing educator, Dorothea Orem (b. 1914). The focus of nursing is teaching patients self-care.

♻ **-orexia** Combining form meaning (condition of the) appetite, e.g., anorexia. [G. *orexis,* appetite]

o•rex•i•gen•ic (ŏ-rek-si-jen′ik) Appetite-stimulating.

o•rex•in (ōr-eks′in) A class of hypothalamic neuropeptide hormones that regulates sleep cycles and energy expenditure; they probably do not directly affect appetite, as was once believed.

or•gan (ōr′găn) A differentiated structure or part of a system of the body; composed of tissues and cells; exercises a specific function (e.g., respiration, secretion, digestion). SYN organum [TA], organon. [L. *organum,* fr. G. *organon,* a tool, instrument]

or•ga•na (ōr′gă-nă) Plural of organum.

or•gan of Cor•ti (ōr′găn kōr′tē) Specialized hair cells that receive sound vibrations and transmit them as impulses to the brain; located on basilar membrane of inner ear in two rows that slope against each other.

or•gan cul•ture (ōr′găn kŭl′chŭr) The maintenance or growth of tissues, organ primordia, or the parts or whole of an organ in vitro in such a way as to allow differentiation or preservation of the architecture or function.

or•gan•elle (ōr′gă-nel′) One of the specialized parts of a protozoan or tissue cell; mitochondria, the Golgi apparatus, nucleus and centrioles, granular and agranular endoplasmic reticulum, vacuoles, microsomes, lysosomes, plasma membrane, and certain fibrils, as well as plastids of plant cells. SYN organoid (3). [G. *organon,* organ, + Fr. *-elle,* dim. suffix, fr. L. *-ella*]

or•gan•ic (ōr-gan′ik) **1.** Relating to an organ. **2.** Relating to or formed by an organism. **3.** Organized; structural. **4.** SEE organic compound. **5.** Denotes agricultural production of a more ecologically beneficial type. [G. *organikos*]

or•gan•ic ac•id (ōr-gan′ik as′id) An acid composed of molecules containing organic radicals; e.g., acetic acid, citric acid, which contain the ionizable —COOH group.

or•gan•ic brain syn•drome (OBS) (ōr-gan′ik brān sin′drōm) A constellation of behavioral or psychological signs and symptoms including problems with attention, concentration, memory, confusion, anxiety, and depression caused by transient or permanent dysfunction of the brain.

or•gan•ic chem•is•try (ōr-gan′ik kem′is-trē) That branch of chemistry concerned with covalently linked atoms, centering around carbon compounds of this type; originally, and still including, the chemistry of natural products.

or•gan•ic com•pound (ōr-gan′ik kom′pownd) A compound composed of atoms (some of which are carbon) held together by covalent (shared electron) bonds. Cf. inorganic compound.

or•gan•ic con•trac•ture (ōr-gan′ik kŏn-trak′shŭr) Contracture, usually due to fibrosis within the muscle that persists whether the patient is conscious or unconscious.

or•gan•ic de•lu•sions (ōr-gan′ik dĕ-lū′zhŭnz) False beliefs experienced in the delirium associated with injury to the brain, organic change in the brain such as in Alzheimer syndrome, or cocaine or other drug intoxication.

or•gan•ic dis•ease (ōr-gan′ik di-zēz′) A disease with anatomic or pathophysiologic changes in some bodily tissue or organ, in contrast to a disorder of psychogenic origin.

or•gan•ic dust tox•ic syn•drome (ODTS) (ōr-gan′ik dŭst tok′sik sin′drōm) A noninfectious febrile illness associated with chills, malaise, myalgia, dry cough, dyspnea, headache, and nausea that occur after exposure to heavy organic dust; condition shares many clinical features with acute farmer's lung and other forms of hypersensitivity pneumonitis (e.g., presence of increased numbers of neutrophils in bronchoalveolar lavage).

or•gan•ic ev•o•lu•tion (ōr-gan′ik ev-ŏ-lū′shŭn) SYN biologic evolution.

or•gan•ic food (ōr-gan′ik fūd) Food grown or raised without the use of additives, coloring, synthetic chemicals (e.g., fertilizers, pesticides, hormones), radiation, or genetic manipulation and meet the U.S.D.A. Standard National Organic Program.

or•gan•ic hear•ing im•pair•ment (ōr-gan′ik hēr′ing im-pār′mĕnt) Deafness due to a pathologic process or an organic cause, as opposed to psychogenic hearing impairment.

or•gan•ic men•tal dis•or•der (ōr-gan′ik men′tăl dis-ōr′dĕr) A psychological, cognitive, or behavioral abnormality associated with transient or permanent dysfunction of the brain, usually characterized by the presence of an organic mental syndrome.

or•gan•ic mur•mur (ōr-gan′ik mŭr′mŭr) A murmur caused by structural change.

or•gan•ic ver•ti•go (ōr-gan′ik vĕr′ti-gō) The dizziness-related disorder due to brain damage.

or•ga•nism (ōr′gă-nizm) Any living individual, whether plant or animal, considered as a whole.

or•ga•ni•za•tion (ōr′găn-ī-zā′shŭn) **1.** An arrangement of distinct but mutually dependent parts. **2.** A facility or set of coordinated facilities that provide health care. **3.** The conversion of coagulated blood, exudate, or dead tissue into fibrous tissue.

or•ga•nize (ōr′găn-īz) To provide with, or to assume, a structure.

or•ga•niz•er (ōr′găn-ī-zĕr) **1.** A group of cells on the dorsal lip of the blastopore, which induce differentiation of cells in the embryo and control growth and development of adjacent parts. **2.** Any group of cells having such a controlling influence, the effects being brought about through the action of an evocator.

♻ **organo-** Prefix meaning organ; organic. [G. *organon*]

or•gan•o•gel (ōr-gan′ō-jel) A hydrogel with an organic liquid instead of water as the dispersion means.

or•ga•no•gen•e•sis (ōr′gă-nō-jen′ĕ-sis) Formation of organs during development. SYN organogeny. [organo- + G. *genesis,* origin]

or•ga•no•ge•net•ic, or•ga•no•gen•ic (ōr′gă-nō-jĕ-net′ik, -jen′ik) Relating to organogenesis.

or•ga•nog•e•ny (ōr-găn-oj′ĕ-nē) SYN organogenesis.

or•gan•oid (ōr′gă-noyd) **1.** Resembling in superficial appearance or in structure any of the organs or glands of the body. **2.** Composed of glandular or organic elements, and not of a single tissue; pertaining to certain neoplasms that contain cytologic and histologic elements arranged in a pattern that closely resembles that of a normal organ. SEE ALSO histoid. **3.** SYN organelle. [organo- + G. *eidos,* resemblance]

or•gan•oid tu•mor (ōr′gă-noyd tū′mŏr) A tumor of complex structure, glandular in origin, containing epithelium and connective tissue.

or•ga•no•meg•a•ly (ōr′gă-nō-meg′ă-lē) SYN visceromegaly.

or•gan•o•mer•cur•i•al (ōr′gă-nō-mĕr-kyūr′ē-ăl) Any organic mercurial compound (e.g., merbromin, thimerosal).

or•ga•no•me•tal•lic (ōr′gă-nō-mĕ-tal′ik) Denoting an organic compound containing one or more metallic atoms in its structure.

or•ga•non, pl. **or•ga•na** (ōr′gă-non, -nă) SYN organ. [G. organ]

or•ga•no•phos•phates (ōr′gă-nō-fos′fāts) SEE organophosphorous compounds.

or•gan•o•phos•phor•ous com•pounds (ōr′gă-nō-fos′fōr-ŭs kom′powndz) A group of phosphorous-containing organic compounds that produce cholinergic effects in the body by acting as anticholinesterases, i.e., by inactivating the enzyme cholinesterase. These compounds include certain insecticides ("OP insecticides") and also all of the chemical-warfare nerve agents. Also incorrectly called organaphosphates.

or•ga•no•tro•phic (ōr′gă-nō-trō′fik) **1.** Pertaining to the nourishment of an organ. **2.** Pertaining to a microorganism that uses organic sources as a reducing power. [organo- + G. *trophē,* nourishment]

or•ga•no•tro•pic (ōr′gă-nō-trō′pik) Pertaining to or characterized by organotropism.

or•ga•no•tro•pism (ōr′gă-nō-trō′pizm) The special affinity of certain drugs, pathogens, or metastatic tumors for particular organs or their component parts. Cf. parasitotropism. [organo- + G. *tropē,* a turning]

or•gan-spe•cif•ic (ōr′gan-spe-sif′ik) Denoting or pertaining to a serum produced by the injection of the cells of a certain organ or tissue that, when injected into another animal, destroys the cells of the corresponding organ.

or•gan-spe•cif•ic an•ti•gen (ōr′găn-spĕ-sif′ik an′ti-jen) A heterogenetic antigen with organ specificity; e.g., in addition to species-specific antigen, a kidney of one species contains antigen that is identical to that in a kidney of another species. SYN tissue-specific antigen.

or•ga•num, pl. **or•ga•na** (ōr′gă-nŭm, -nă) [TA] SYN organ, organ. [L. tool, instrument]

or•gasm (ōr′gazm) The peak state of excitement

in the sexual act. SYN climax (2). [G. *orgaō,* to swell, be excited]

or·gas·mic, **or·gas·tic** (ōr-gaz′mik, ōr-gas′tik) Relating to, characteristic of, or tending to produce an orgasm.

or·i·en·ta·tion (ōr-ē-ĕn-tā′shŭn) **1.** The recognition of one's temporal, spatial, and personal relationships and environment. **2.** The relative position of an atom with respect to one to which it is connected. [Fr. *orienter,* to set toward the East, fr. L. *sol oriens*, the rising sun]

Or·i·en·ti·a (ōr-ē-en′shă) A genus of the bacterial family Rickettsiaceae.

Or·i·en·ti·a rick·ett·si·a (ōr-ē-en′shă ri-ket′shă) Formerly *Rickettsia tsutsugamushi*. A bacterial species causing tsutsugamushi disease.

Or·i·en·ti·a tsut·su·ga·mu·shi (ōr-ē-en′shă sū-sū-gă-mū′shē) A bacterial species that causes tsutsugamushi disease and scrub typhus; transmitted by trombiculid mites; formerly known as *Rickettsia tsutsugamushi*.

or·i·ent·ing re·flex (ōr′ē-en-ting rē′fleks) An aspect of attending in which an organism's initial response to a change or to a novel stimulus is such that the organism becomes more sensitive to the stimulation (e.g., dilation of the pupil of the eye in response to dim light). SYN orienting response.

or·i·ent·ing re·sponse (ōr′ē-en-ting rĕ-spons′) SYN orienting reflex.

or·i·fice (ōr′i-fis) Any aperture or opening. SYN orificium. [L. *orificium*]

or·i·fi·cial (ōr-i-fish′ăl) Relating to an orifice of any kind.

or·i·fi·ci·um, pl. **or·i·fi·ci·a** (ōr-i-fish′ē-ŭm, -shē-ă) SYN orifice. [L.]

or·i·gin (ōr′i-jin) **1.** The less movable of two sites of attachment of a muscle; that which is attached to the more fixed part of the skeleton. **2.** The starting point of a cranial or spinal nerve. The former have two origins: the ental origin, deep origin, or real origin, the cell group in the brain or medulla whence the fibers of the nerve begin, and the ectal origin, superficial origin, or apparent origin, the point where the nerve emerges from the brain. [L. *origo,* source, beginning, fr. *orior,* to rise]

or·ig·i·na·tor (ŏr-ij′i-nā-tĕr) SYN author.

or·li·stat (ōr′li-stat) A lipase inhibitor that works in the gastrointestinal tract to reduce the body's absorption of fat.

Or·mond dis·ease (or′mŏnd di-zēz′) SYN retroperitoneal fibrosis.

Orn Abbreviation for ornithine or its radical.

or·ni·thine (Orn) (ōr′ni-thēn) The amino acid formed when L-arginine is hydrolyzed by arginase; an important intermediate in the urea cycle; elevated levels seen in certain defects of the urea cycle.

or·ni·thi·nu·ri·a (ōr′ni-thi-nyūr′ē-ă) Excretion of excessive amounts of ornithine in urine.

Or·ni·thod·o·ros (ōr-ni-thod′ō-rŏs) A genus of soft ticks, several species of which are vectors of pathogens of various relapsing fevers. [G. *ornis* (*ornith-*), bird, + *doros,* a leather bag]

or·ni·tho·sis (ōr-ni-thō′sis) SYN psittacosis. [G. *ornis* (*ornith-*), bird, + *-osis,* condition]

Oro Abbreviation for orotic acid or orotate.

oro- Prefix meaning the mouth. [L. *os, oris,* mouth]

or·o·dig·i·to·fa·cial (ōr′ō-dij′i-tō-fā′shăl) Relating to the mouth, fingers, and face.

or·o·fa·cial (ōr-ō-fā′shăl) Relating to the mouth and face.

or·o·lin·gual (ōr-ō-ling′gwăl) Relating to the mouth and tongue.

or·o·na·sal (ōr-ō-nā′zăl) Relating to the mouth and nose.

or·o·pha·ryn·ge·al (ōr′ō-fă-rin′jē-ăl) Relating to the oropharynx. See this page.

or·o·phar·ynx (ōr′ō-far′ingks) The portion of

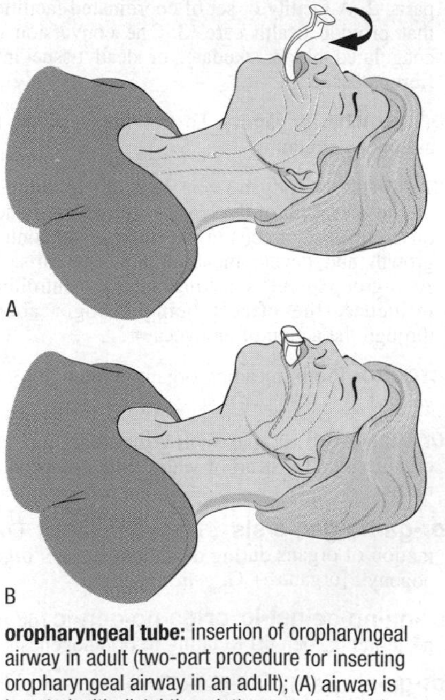

oropharyngeal tube: insertion of oropharyngeal airway in adult (two-part procedure for inserting oropharyngeal airway in an adult); (A) airway is inserted with distal tip pointing toward roof of patient's mouth; (B) rotate airway 180 degrees until flange rests on patient's lips or teeth

the pharynx that lies posterior to the mouth; it is continuous above with the nasopharynx through the pharyngeal isthmus and below with the laryngopharynx. [L. *os* (*or-*), mouth]

O•ro•pouche fe•ver (ōr′ō-pū′shĕ fē′vĕr) Acute febrile illness caused by a species of Bunyavirus.

or•o•so•mu•coid (ōr′ō-sō-myū′koyd) Increased plasma levels associated with inflammation.

or•o•tate (Oro) (ōr′ō-tāt) A salt or ester of orotic acid.

o•rot•ic ac•id (Oro) (ōr-ot′ik as′id) An important intermediate in the formation of the pyrimidine nucleotides; elevated in certain inherited defects of pyrimidine biosynthesis.

o•rot•i•dine (O, Ord) (ō-rot′i-dēn) Orotic acid-3-β-D-ribonucleoside; uridine-6-carboxylic acid; Elevated in cases of orotidinuria.

or•o•tra•che•al tube (ōr′ō-trā′kē-ăl tūb) A tracheal tube inserted through the mouth.

O•ro•ya fe•ver (ō-roy′ă fē′vĕr) A generalized, acute, febrile, endemic, and systemic form of bartonellosis; marked by high fever, rheumatic pains, progressive, severe anemia, and albuminuria. SYN Carrión disease.

or•phan dis•ease (ōr′făn di-zēz′) A disease for which no treatment has been developed because of the disorder's rarity. SEE ALSO orphan products.

or•phan drugs (ōr′făn drŭgz) SEE orphan products.

or•phan pro•ducts (ōr′făn prod′ŭkts) Drugs, biologicals, and medical devices (including diagnostic in vitro tests) that may be useful in treating rare diseases but not considered commercially viable.

or•phan re•cep•tor (ōr′făn rĕ-sep′tŏr) A nuclear receptor for which no ligand has yet been identified.

or•phan vi•rus•es (ōr′făn vī′rŭs-ĕz) Viruses (e.g., the enteric orphan viruses) that when originally found were not specifically associated with disease; several such have since been shown to be pathogenic.

♻**-orrhagia**, **-rrhagia, -rrhage** Combining forms meaning excessive flow. [G. *haimorrhagia,* hemorrhage]

♻**-orrhea**, **-rrhea** Combining forms meaning discharge or flow. [G. *rhea,* a flowing]

♻**-orrhexis, -rrhexis** Combining forms meaning to rupture. [G. *rhēxis,* breaking, bursting]

ORT Abbreviation for Operation Restore Trust.

or•the•sis (ōr-thē′sis) SYN orthosis. [ortho- + *-esis,* process]

or•thet•ics (ōr-thet′iks) SYN orthotics.

Orth fix•a•tive (orth fiks′ă-tiv) Formalin added to Müller fixative, used for bringing out chromaffin, studying early degenerative processes and necrosis, and for demonstrating rickettsiae and bacteria.

♻**ortho-**, **orth-** **1.** Combining forms meaning straight, normal, in proper order. **2.** CHEMISTRY italicized prefix denoting that a compound has two substitutions on adjacent carbon atoms in a benzene ring. For terms beginning *ortho-* or *o-*, see the specific name. [Gr. *orthos* correct]

or•tho•cho•re•a (ōr′thō-kōr-ē′ă) A form of chorea in which the spasms occur only or chiefly when the patient is in the erect posture.

or•tho•chro•mat•ic (ōr′thō-krō-mat′ik) Denoting any tissue or cell that stains the color of the dye used, i.e., the same color as the dye solution with which it is stained. [ortho- + G. *chrōma,* color]

or•tho•cy•to•sis (ōr′thō-sī-tō′sis) A condition in which all of the cellular elements in the circulating blood are mature forms, irrespective of the proportions of various types and total numbers. [ortho- + G. *kytos,* cell, + *-osis,* condition]

or•tho•de•ox•i•a (ōr′thō-dē-oks′ē-ă) Fall in arterial blood oxygen on assuming the upright posture.

or•tho•don•tics (ōr-thō-don′tiks) That branch of dentistry concerned with the correction and prevention of irregularities and malocclusion of the teeth. [ortho- + G. *odous,* tooth]

or•tho•dont•ist (ōr-thō-don′tist) A dental specialist who practices orthodontics.

or•tho•dro•mic (ōr-thō-drō′mik) Denoting the propagation of an impulse along an axon in the normal direction. Cf. antidromic. [ortho- + G. *dromos,* course]

or•thog•na•thi•a (ōr-thog-nath′ē-ă) The study of the causes and treatment of conditions related to malposition of the bones of the jaws. [ortho- + G. *gnathos,* jaw]

or•thog•nath•ic, **or•thog•na•thous** (ōr-thōg-nath′ik, -thog′nă-thŭs) **1.** Relating to orthognathia. **2.** Having a face without projecting jaw, that is one with a gnathic index less than 98. SEE ALSO prognathic. **3.** Having a normal relationship of the jaws. [ortho- + G. *gnathos,* jaw]

or•thog•o•nal ra•di•o•graphs (ōr-thog′ă-năl rā′dē-ō-grafs) Two radiographs imaged 90 degrees apart; used in the treatment planning process for radiation.

or•tho•grade (ōr′thō-grād) Walking or standing erect; denoting the posture of human beings; opposed to pronograde. [ortho- + L. *gradior,* pp. *gressus,* to walk]

or•tho•grade de•gen•er•a•tion (ōr′thō-grād dĕ-jen′ĕr-ā′shŭn) SYN wallerian degeneration.

or·tho·ker·a·tol·o·gy (ōr′thō-ker′ă-tol′ŏ-jē) A method of molding the cornea with contact lenses to improve unaided vision. [ortho- + G. *keras,* horn (cornea), + *logos,* science]

or·tho·ker·a·to·sis (ōr′thō-ker′ă-tō′sis) Formation of an anuclear keratin layer, as in the normal epidermis. [ortho- + G. *keras,* horn, + *-osis,* condition]

or·tho·me·chan·i·cal (ōr′thō-mĕ-kan′i-kăl) Pertaining to braces, prostheses, orthotic devices, and appliances. [ortho- + mechanical]

or·tho·mo·lec·u·lar (ōr′thō-mō-lek′yū-lăr) A therapeutic approach designed to provide an optimal molecular environment for body functions, with particular reference to the optimal concentrations of substances normally present in the body.

or·tho·mol·e·cu·lar me·di·cine (ōr′thō-mŏ-lek′yū-lăr med′i-sin) SYN megavitamin therapy.

Or·tho·myx·o·vir·i·dae (ōr′thō-mik′sō-vir′i-dē) The family of viruses that comprises the three groups of influenza viruses, types A, B, and C. The only recognized genus is Influenzavirus, which comprises the strains of virus types A and B, both of which are subject to mutation resulting in epidemics. Influenza virus type C differs from types A and B somewhat and probably belongs to a separate genus. SEE ALSO Influenzavirus.

or·tho·pae·dic sur·ger·y (ōr′thō-pē′dik sŭr′jĕr-ē) The branch of surgery that embraces the treatment of acute and chronic disorders of the musculoskeletal system, including injuries, diseases, dysfunction, and deformities (orig. deformities in children) in the extremities and spine. SEE ALSO orthopaedics.

or·tho·pe·dics, or·tho·pae·dics (ōr′thō-pē′diks) The medical specialty concerned with the preservation, restoration, and development of form and function of the musculoskeletal system, extremities, spine, and associated structures by medical, surgical, and physical methods. [USAGE NOTE Although this is the correct U.S. spelling according to rule and precedent, the American Academy of Orthopaedic Surgeons has officially adopted the spelling *orthopaedics*.] [ortho- + G. *pais* (*paid-*), child]

or·tho·per·cus·sion (ōr′thō-pĕr-kŭsh′ŭn) Very light percussion of the chest, used to determine the size of the heart.

or·tho·pho·ri·a (ōr-thō-fōr′ē-ă) Absence of heterophoria; the condition of binocular fixation in which the lines of sight meet at a distant or near point of reference in the absence of a fusion stimulus. [ortho- + G. *phora,* motion]

or·tho·phor·ic (ōr-thō-fōr′ik) Pertaining to orthophoria.

or·tho·phos·phate (ōr-thō-fos′fāt) A salt or ester of orthophosphoric acid.

or·tho·phos·phor·ic ac·id (ōr′thō-fos-fōr′ik as′id) Phosphoric acid, $O{=}P(OH)_3$, distinguished by ortho- from meta- and pyrophosphoric acids.

or·thop·ne·a (ōr-thop-nē′ă) Discomfort in breathing that is brought on or aggravated by lying flat. Cf. platypnea. SYN orthopnoea. [ortho- + G. *pnoē,* a breathing]

or·thop·ne·ic (or-thop-nē′ik) Relating to or characterized by orthopnea. SYN orthopnoeic.

orthopnoea [Br.] SYN orthopnea.

orthopnoeic [Br.] SYN orthopneic.

Or·tho·pox·vi·rus (ōr′thō-poks′vī′rŭs) The genus of the family Poxviridae that comprises the Alastrim, Vaccinia, Variola, Cowpox, Ectromelia, Monkeypox, and Rabbitpox viruses.

or·tho·psy·chi·a·try (ōr′thō-sī-kī′ă-trē) A cross-disciplinary science combining child psychiatry, developmental psychology, pediatrics, and family care devoted to the discovery, prevention, and treatment of mental and psychological disorders in children and adolescents.

or·thop·tic (ōr-thop′tik) Relating to orthoptics.

or·thop·tics (ōr-thop′tiks) The study and treatment of defective binocular vision, of defects in the action of the ocular muscles, or of faulty visual habits. [*ortho-* straightened + G. *optikos,* sight]

Or·tho·re·o·vi·rus (ōr′thō-rē′ō-vī′rŭs) A genus in the family Reoviridae associated with a variety of respiratory and enteric diseases, but its causal relationship is not proven.

or·tho·scope (ōr′thō-skōp) An instrument by means of which one is able to draw the outlines of the various normas of the skull. [ortho- + G. *skopeō,* to view]

or·tho·sis, pl. **or·tho·ses** (ōr-thō′sis, -sēz) An external orthopedic appliance, as a brace or splint, that prevents or assists movement of the spine or the limbs. SYN orthesis. [G. *orthōsis,* a making straight]

or·tho·stat·ic (ōr′thō-stat′ik) Relating to an erect posture or position.

orth·o·sta·tic con·ges·tion (ōr′thō-stat′ik kŏn-jes′chŭn) Pooling of blood in lower parts of the body due to upright posture.

or·tho·stat·ic de·con·di·tion·ing (ōr′thō-stat′ik dē′kŏn-dish′ŏn-ing) Negative effects of prolonged bed rest or of space flight at minimal gravity, resulting in tachycardia and hypotension in the upright position.

or·tho·stat·ic hy·po·ten·sion (ōr′thō-stat′ik hī′pō-ten′shŭn) A form of low blood pressure that occurs in a standing patient. SYN postural hypotension.

or·tho·stat·ic in·tol·er·ance (ōr′thō-stat′ik in-tol′ĕr-ăns) Decreased venous return in the upright position typically experienced by astronauts after returning to an environment subject to gravity.

or•tho•tic (ōr-thot′ik) **1.** Pertaining to orthotics. **2.** An orthotic appliance.

or•thot•ics (ōr-thot′iks) The science concerned with the making and fitting of orthopaedic appliances. SYN orthetics.

or•tho•tist (ōr-thŏt′ist) A maker and fitter of orthopaedic appliances.

or•thot•o•nos, **or•thot•o•nus** (ōr-thot′ŏ-nŭs) A form of tetanic spasm in which the neck, limbs, and body are held fixed in a straight line. [ortho- + G. *tonos,* tension]

or•tho•top•ic (ōr-thō-tō′pik) In the normal or usual position. [ortho- + G. *topos,* place]

or•tho•top•ic u•re•ter•o•cele (ōr′thō-tō′pik yū-rē′tĕr-ō-sēl) A ureterocele entirely within the bladder.

or•tho•tro•pic (ōr′thō-trō′pik) Extending or growing in a straight, especially a vertical, direction. [ortho- + G. *tropē,* a turn]

Orth stain (orth stān) A lithium carmine stain for nerve cells and their processes.

Or•to•la•ni man•eu•ver (or-tō-lah′nē mă-nū′vĕr) A maneuver for reduction of hip dislocation, using thigh flexion and abduction with anterior movement of the femoral head; reduction is accompanied by palpable reseating of the femoral head in the acetabulum.

Or•to•la•ni sign (ōr-tō-lah′nē sīn) A palpable and audible click elicited by adduction and abduction of the infant femur in congenital hip dislocation. [Marius Ortolani, 1904–1987, Italian orthopedist]

ORYX A proprietary methodology that enables standardized outcome and performance measurement for health care organizations; established by the Joint Commission on Accreditation of Healthcare Organizations.

Os (os) Symbol for osmium.

os, gen. **o•ris**, pl. **o•ra** (os, ō′ris, ō′ră) **1.** [TA] The mouth. **2.** Term applied sometimes to an opening into a hollow organ or canal, especially one with thick or fleshy edges. [L. mouth]

os, gen. **os•sis**, pl. **os•sa** (os, os′is, -ă) [TA] For histologic description, see bone. SYN bone. [L. bone]

OSA Abbreviation for obstructive sleep apnea.

♲**osche-**, **oscheo-** Combining forms meaning the scrotum. [G. *oschē*]

os•che•al (os′kē-ăl) SYN scrotal.

os•che•i•tis (os-kē-ī′tis) Inflammation of the scrotum. [osche- + G. *-itis,* inflammation]

os•che•o•hy•dro•cele (os′kē-ō-hī′drō-sēl) Scrotal hydrocele. [oscheo- + G. *hydōr,* water, + *kēlē,* tumor]

os•che•o•plas•ty (os′kē-ō-plas-tē) SYN scrotoplasty. [oscheo- + *plastos,* formed]

os•cil•lat•ing vi•sion (os′ĭl-āt′ing vizh′ŭn) SYN oscillopsia.

os•cil•la•tion (os′il-ā′shŭn) **1.** A to-and-fro movement. **2.** A stage in inflammation in which the accumulation of leukocytes in small vessels arrests the passage of blood and there is simply a to-and-fro movement at each cardiac contraction. [L. *oscillatio,* fr. *oscillo,* to swing]

os•cil•la•to•ry po•ten•tial (os′i-lă-tōr-ē pō-ten′shăl) The variable voltage in the positive deflection of the electroretinogram (B-wave) of the dark-adapted eye arising from amacrine cells.

os•cil•lom•e•ter (os-i-lom′ĕ-tĕr) An apparatus for measuring oscillations of any kind, especially those of the bloodstream in sphygmomanometry. [L. *oscillo,* to swing, + G. *metron,* measure]

os•cil•lo•met•ric (os′i-lō-met′rik) Relating to the oscillometer or the records made by its use.

os•cil•lom•e•try (os′i-lom′ĕ-trē) The measurement of oscillations of any kind with an oscillometer.

os•cil•lop•si•a (os′i-lop′sē-ă) The subjective sensation of oscillation of objects viewed. SYN oscillating vision. [L. *oscillo,* to swing, + G. *opsis,* vision]

os cox•a (os kok′să) SYN hip bone.

os•cu•lum, pl. **os•cu•la** (os′kyū-lŭm, -lă) A pore or minute opening. [L. dim. of *os,* mouth]

♲**-ose** **1.** CHEMISTRY a suffix usually indicating a carbohydrate. **2.** Suffix appended to some Latin stems, with significance of the more common suffix, -ous (2). [L. *-osus,* full of, abounding] **3.** Suffix meaning full of, having much of.

Os•good-Schlat•ter dis•ease (oz′gud shlaht′er di-zēz′) Inflammation or partial avulsion of the tibial apophysis due to traction forces. SYN Schlatter disease, Schlatter-Osgood disease.

OSHA (ō′shă) Acronym for Occupational Safety and Health Administration of the U.S. Department of Labor, responsible for establishing and enforcing safety and health standards in the workplace.

os ha•ma•tum (os hă-ma′tŭm) [TA] SYN hamate bone.

O shell (shel) The outermost shell of electrons, so called because displacement of electrons causes an emission in the visible or optic range.

os in•ci•si•vum (os in′si-sī′vŭm) The anterior and inner portion of the maxilla, which in the fetus and sometimes in the adult is a separate bone; the incisive suture runs from the incisive canal between the lateral incisor and the canine tooth. SYN incisive bone, intermaxillary bone, premaxillary bone.

os in·ter·met·a·tar·se·um (os in′tĕr-met-ă-tahr′sē-ŭm) A supernumerary bone at the base of the first metatarsal, or between the first and second metatarsal bones, usually fused with one or the other or with the medial cuneiform bone.

♻**-osis**, pl. **-os·es** Combining form meaning a process, condition, or state, usually abnormal or diseased; production of an abnormal substance, increase of a normal substance, or parasitic infestation. [G.]

Os·ler dis·ease (ōs′lĕr di-zēz′) SYN polycythemia vera.

Os·ler node (ōs′lĕr nōd) A small, tender, nodular cutaneous lesion in the pads of fingers or toes, probably of immunopathic origin, characteristic of subacute bacterial endocarditis.

Os·ler-Va·quez dis·ease (ōs′lĕr vah-kā′ di-zēz′) SYN polycythemia vera.

OSMED (os′med) Acronym for otospondylomegaepiphysial dysplasia.

os·mic ac·id (oz′mik as′id) A volatile caustic and strong oxidizing agent; colorless crystals, poorly soluble in water, but soluble in organic solvents; the aqueous solution is a fat and myelin stain and a general fixative for electron microscopy.

os·mics (oz′miks) The science of olfaction. [G. *osmē,* smell]

os·mi·dro·sis (oz-mī-drō′sis) SYN bromidrosis. [G. *osmē,* smell, + *hidrōs,* sweat]

os·mi·um (Os) (oz′mē-ŭm) A metallic element of the platinum group, atomic no. 76, atomic wt. 190.2. [G. *osmē,* smell, because of the strong odor of the tetroxide]

♻**osmo-** **1.** Prefix meaning osmosis. [G. *ōsmos,* impulsion] **2.** Prefix meaning smell, odor. [G. *osmē*]

os·mo·lal·i·ty (os′mō-lal′i-tē) The concentration of a solution expressed in osmoles of solute particles per kilogram of solvent.

os·mo·lar (os-mō′lăr) SYN osmotic.

os·mo·lar·i·ty (os′mō-lar′i-tē) The osmotic concentration of a solution expressed as osmoles of solute per liter of solution.

os·mole (os′mōl) The molecular weight of a solute, in grams, divided by the number of ions or particles into which it dissociates in solution.

os·mo·me·ter (os-mom′ĕ-tĕr) Instrument used to determine concentration of free particles in solution; usually by freezing point depression or vapor pressure. SEE ALSO osmolality, freezing point depression.

os·mom·e·try (os-mom′ĕ-trē) Technique used to determine the number of solute particles in solution by measuring changes in a colligative property. [osmo- + -metry]

os·mo·re·cep·tor (os′mō-rē-sep′tŏr, -tōr) **1.** A receptor in the central nervous system (probably the hypothalamus) that responds to changes in the osmotic pressure of the blood. [G. *osmos,* impulsion] **2.** A receptor that receives olfactory stimuli. [G. *osmē,* smell]

os·mo·reg·u·la·to·ry (os′mō-reg′yū-lă-tōr-ē) Influencing the degree and rapidity of osmosis.

os·mose (os′mōs) To move through a membrane by osmosis.

os·mo·sis (os-mō′sis) The process by which solvent tends to move through a semipermeable membrane from a solution of lower to a solution of higher osmolal concentration of the solutes to which the membrane is relatively impermeable. [G. *ōsmos,* a thrusting, an impulsion]

os·mot·ic (os-mot′ik) Relating to osmosis. SYN osmolar.

os·mot·ic di·u·ret·ics (os-mot′ik dī-yūr-et′iks) Drugs (e.g., mannitol) that by their osmotic effects, promote the elimination of water and electrolytes in the urine.

os·mot·ic fra·gil·i·ty (os-mot′ik fră-jil′i-tē) The susceptibility of erythrocytes to hemolyze when exposed to increasingly hypotonic saline solutions. SYN fragility of the blood.

os·mot·ic pres·sure (Π) (os-mot′ik presh′ŭr) The pressure that must be applied to a solution to prevent the passage into it of solvent when solution and pure solvent are separated by a membrane permeable only to the solvent.

os mult·ang·u·lum ma·jus (os mŭlt-ang′yū-lŭm mā′jŭs) SYN trapezium (bone).

os na·sale (os nă-sā′lē) [TA] SYN nasal bone.

os oc·ci·pi·ta·le (os ok′si-pi-tā′lē) [TA] SYN occipital bone.

♻**osphresio-** Prefix denoting odor; sense of smell. [G. *osphrēsis,* smell]

os·phre·sis (os-frē′sis) SYN olfaction. [G. *osphrēsis,* smell]

os·phret·ic (os-fret′ik) SYN olfactory.

os·sa (os′ă) Plural of L. *os*, bone. [L.]

os·sa cra·ni·i (os′ă kra′nē-ī-ī) [TA] SYN bones of cranium.

os·sa me·ta·car·pi (os′ă met-ă-kahr′pī) SYN metacarpal bones [I–V].

os·sa me·ta·tar·si, pl. **os·sa me·ta·tar·sa·li·a** (os′ă met′ă-tahr′sī, os′ă met-ă-tahr-sāl′ē-ă) SYN metatarsal (bones) [I–V].

os sca·phoi·de·um (os skaf-oy′dē-ŭm) SYN scaphoid (bone).

os·se·in, os·se·ine (os′ē-in, īn) SYN collagen. [L. *os,* bone]

♻**osseo-** Combining form meaning bony. SEE ALSO ossi-, osteo-. [L. *osseus*]

os·se·o·car·ti·lag·i·nous (os′ē-ō-kahr′ti-laj′i-nŭs) Relating to, or composed of, both bone and cartilage. SYN osteocartilaginous.

os·se·o·in·te·gra·tion (os′ē-ō-in′tĕ-grā′shŭn) The direct attachment to bone of an inert, alloplastic material without intervening connective tissue, as with dental implants.

os·se·o·mu·cin (os′ē-ō-myū′sin) The ground substance of bony tissue.

os·se·ous (os′ē-ŭs) Bony; of bonelike consistency or structure. SYN osteal. [L. *osseus*]

os·se·ous hy·da·tid cyst (os′ē-ŭs hī′dă-tid sist) A morphologic form of hydatid cyst caused by *Echinococcus granulosus* and found in the long bones.

os·se·ous la·cu·na (os′ē-ŭs lă-kū′nă) A cavity in bony tissue occupied by an osteocyte.

os·se·ous spi·ral lam·i·na (os′ē-ŭs spī′răl lam′i-nă) A double plate of bone winding spirally around the modiolus dividing the spiral canal of the cochlea incompletely into two, scala tympani and scala vestibuli; between the two plates of this lamina the fibers of the cochlear nerve reach the spiral organ (organ of Corti).

os·se·ous tis·sue (os′ē-ŭs tish′ū) A connective tissue, the matrix of which consists of collagen fibers and ground substance and in which are deposited calcium salts (phosphate, carbonate, and some fluoride) in the form of an apatite. SYN bone tissue.

♻**ossi-** Combining form denoting bone. SEE ALSO osseo-, osteo-. [L. *os*]

os·si·cle (os′i-kĕl) A small bone; specifically, one of the bones of the tympanic cavity or middle ear. SYN bonelet, ossiculum. [L. *ossiculum,* dim. of *os,* bone]

os·sic·u·la (ŏ-sik′yū-lă) Plural of ossiculum. [L.]

os·sic·u·la au·di·tus (ŏ-sik′yū-lă aw-dĭt′ŭs) [TA] SYN auditory ossicles.

os·sic·u·lar (ŏ-sik′yū-lăr) Pertaining to an ossicle.

os·sic·u·lar re·con·struc·tion (ŏ-sik′yū-lăr rē′kŏn-strŭk′shŭn) Generic term denoting a number of surgical techniques to restore the continuity of the ossicular chain from the tympanic membrane to the oval window for sound pressure transmission and, thereby, improved hearing.

os·sic·u·lec·to·my (os′i-kyū-lek′tŏ-mē) Removal of one or more of the ossicles of the middle ear. [L. *ossiculum,* ossicle, + G. *ektomē,* excision]

os·si·cu·lot·o·my (os′i-kyū-lot′ŏ-mē) Division of one of the processes of the ossicles of the middle ear, or of a fibrous band causing ankylosis between any two ossicles. [L. *ossiculum,* ossicle, + G. *tomē,* incision]

os·sic·u·lum, pl. **os·sic·u·la** (ŏ-sik′yū-lŭm, -lă) SYN ossicle. [L. dim. of *os,* bone]

os·sif·er·ous (ŏ-sif′ĕr-ŭs) Containing or producing bone. [ossi- + L. *fero,* to bear]

os·sif·ic (ŏ-sif′ik) Relating to a change into, or formation of, bone.

os·sif·i·cans (ŏs-if′i-kănz) Ossifying; forming or turning into bone. [L.]

os·si·fi·ca·tion (os′i-fi-kā′shŭn) **1.** The formation of bone. **2.** A change into bone. [L. *ossificatio,* fr. *os,* bone, + *facio,* to make]

os·sif·ic cen·ter (ŏ-sif′ik sen′tĕr) SYN center of ossification.

os·si·fy (os′i-fī) To form bone or convert into bone. [ossi- + L. *facio,* to make]

os·te·al (os′tē-ăl) SYN osseous. [G. *osteon,* bone]

os·te·al·gi·a (os-tē-al′jē-ă) Pain in a bone. SYN osteodynia. [osteo- + G. *algos,* pain]

os·te·al·gic (os-tē-al′jik) Relating to or marked by bone pain.

os·tec·to·my (os-tek′tŏ-mē) **1.** Surgical removal of bone. **2.** DENTISTRY resection of supporting osseous structure to eliminate periodontal pockets. [osteo- + G. *ektomē,* excision]

os·te·in, os·te·ine (os′tē-in, -īn) SYN collagen. [G. *osteon,* bone]

os·te·it·ic (os-tē-it′ik) Relating to or affected by osteitis. SYN ostitic.

os·te·i·tis (os-tē-ī′tis) Inflammation of bone. SYN ostitis. [osteo- + G. *-itis,* inflammation]

os·te·i·tis de·for·mans (os-tē-ī′tis dĕ-fōr′manz) SYN Paget disease (1).

os·te·i·tis fi·bro·sa cys·ti·ca (os-tē-ī′tis fī-brō′să sis′ti-kă) Increased osteoclastic resorption of calcified bone with replacement by fibrous tissue, due to primary hyperparathyroidism or other causes of the rapid mobilization of mineral salts. SYN Recklinghausen disease of bone.

os·te·i·tis pu·bis (os-tē-ī′tis pyū′bis) Painful inflammation of the pubic bones near the midline, sometimes due to repeated overload of the adductor muscles or repetitive stress activities.

os·te·mi·a (os-tē′mē-ă) **1.** Congestion of blood

in a bone. **2.** Hyperemia of a bone. [osteo- + G. *haima,* blood]

os tem·po·ra·le (os tem-pō-rā′lē) [TA] SYN temporal bone.

os·tem·py·e·sis (os′tem-pī-ē′sis) Suppuration in bone. [osteo- + G. *empyēsis,* suppuration]

osteo-, ost-, oste- Combining forms denoting bone. SEE ALSO osseo-, ossi-. [G. *osteon*]

os·te·o·an·a·gen·e·sis (os′tē-ō-an-ă-jen′ĕ-sis) Regeneration of bone. [osteo- + G. *ana,* again, + *genesis,* generation]

os·te·o·ar·thri·tis (os′tē-ō-ahr-thrī′tis) Arthritis characterized by erosion of articular cartilage, which becomes soft, frayed, and thinned with eburnation of subchondral bone and outgrowths of marginal osteophytes; pain and loss of function result; mainly affects weight-bearing joints, is more common in women, the overweight, and in older people. See this page. SYN degenerative joint disease, hypertrophic arthritis, osteoarthrosis.

os·te·o·ar·throp·a·thy (os′tē-ō-ahr-throp′ă-thē) A disorder affecting bones and joints. [osteo- + G. *arthron,* joint, + *pathos,* suffering]

os·te·o·ar·thro·sis (os′tē-ō-ahr-thrō′sis) SYN osteoarthritis. [osteo- + G. *arthron,* joint, + *-osis,* condition]

os·te·o·blast (os′tē-ō-blast) A bone-forming cell that is derived from mesenchymal progenitor cells and forms an osseous matrix in which it becomes enclosed as an osteocyte. [osteo- + G. *blastos,* germ]

os·te·o·blas·tic (os′tē-ō-blas′tik) Relating to the osteoblasts; describes any region of increased radiographic bone density, in particular, metastases that stimulate osteoblastic activity.

os·te·o·blas·to·ma (os′tē-ō-blas-tō′mă) An uncommon benign tumor of osteoblasts with areas of osteoid and calcified tissue, occurring most frequently in the spine of a young person.

os·te·o·car·ti·lag·i·nous (os′tē-ō-kahr-ti-laj′i-nŭs) SYN osseocartilaginous.

os·te·o·chon·dral frac·ture (os′tē-ō-kon′drăl frak′shŭr) Fracture involving the articular cartilage and underlying bone.

os·te·o·chon·dri·tis (os′tē-ō-kon-drī′tis) Inflammation of a bone and its articular cartilage. [osteo- + G. *chondros,* cartilage, + *-itis,* inflammation]

os·te·o·chon·dri·tis dis·se·cans (os′tē-ō-kon-drī′tis dis′sĕ-kanz) Complete or incomplete separation of a portion of joint cartilage and underlying bone, usually involving the knee, associated with epiphysial aseptic necrosis.

os·te·o·chon·dro·dys·tro·phy (os′tē-ō-kon-drō-dis′trŏ-fē) SYN chondroosteodystrophy.

os·te·o·chon·dro·ma (os′tē-ō-kon-drō′mă) A benign cartilaginous neoplasm that consists of a pedicle of normal bone covered with a rim of proliferating cartilage cells; multiple osteochondromas are inherited and referred to as hereditary multiple exostoses. [osteo- + G. *chondros,* cartilage, + *-oma,* tumor]

os·te·o·chon·dro·sar·co·ma (os′tē-ō-kon′drō-sahr-kō′mă) Chondrosarcoma arising in bone. Sarcomas in bone containing foci of neoplastic cartilage as well as bone are classified as osteogenic sarcomas. [osteo- + G. *chondros,* cartilage, + *sarx,* flesh, + *-oma,* tumor]

os·te·o·chon·dro·sis (os′tē-ō-kon-drō′sis) Any of a group of disorders of one or more ossification centers in children, characterized by degeneration or aseptic necrosis followed by reossification; includes the various forms of epiphysial aseptic necrosis. [osteo- + G. *chondros,* cartilage, + *-osis,* condition]

os·te·oc·la·sis, os·te·o·cla·sia (os-tē-ok′lă-sis, -ō-klā′zē-ă) Intentional fracture of a bone to correct deformity. [osteo- + G. *klasis,* fracture]

os·te·o·clast (os′tē-ō-klast) **1.** A large multinucleated cell, possibly of monocytic origin, with abundant acidophilic cytoplasm, functioning in the absorption and removal of osseous tissue.

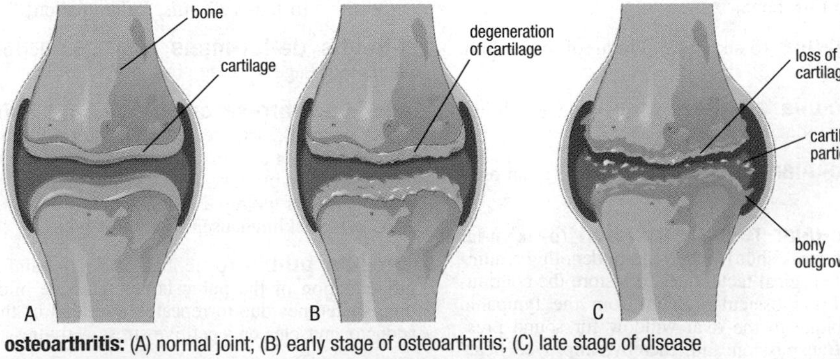

osteoarthritis: (A) normal joint; (B) early stage of osteoarthritis; (C) late stage of disease

SYN osteophage. **2.** An instrument used to fracture a bone to correct a deformity. [osteo- + G. *klastos,* broken]

os·te·o·clast ac·ti·vat·ing fac·tor (os′tē-ō-klast ak′ti-vāt-ing fak′tŏr) A lymphokine that stimulates bone resorption and inhibits bone-collagen synthesis.

os·te·o·clas·tic (os′tē-ō-klas′tik) Pertaining to osteoclasts, especially with reference to their activity in the absorption and removal of osseous tissue.

os·te·o·clas·to·ma (os′tē-ō-klas-tō′mă) SYN giant cell tumor of bone.

os·te·o·cra·ni·um (os′tē-ō-krā′nē-ŭm) The cranium of the fetus after ossification of the membranous cranium has made it firm. [osteo- + G. *kranion,* skull]

os·te·o·cys·to·ma (os′tē-ō-sis-tō′mă) SYN solitary bone cyst.

os·te·o·cyte (os′tē-ō-sīt) A cell of osseous tissue that occupies a lacuna and has cytoplasmic processes that extend into canaliculi and make contact with the processes of other osteocytes. [osteo- + G. *kytos,* cell]

os·te·o·den·tin (os′tē-ō-den′tin) **1.** In humans, the rapidly formed tertiary dentin that contains entrapped odontoblasts and few dentinal tubules, thereby superficially resembling bone. **2.** A bonelike dentin found in some marine mammals and fish. [osteo- + L. *dens,* tooth]

os·te·o·der·mi·a (os′tē-ō-dĕrm′ē-ă) SYN osteoma cutis. [osteo- + G. *derma,* skin]

os·te·o·di·as·ta·sis (os′tē-ō-dī-as′tă-sis) Separation of two adjacent bones, as of the cranium. [osteo- + G. *diastasis,* a separation]

os·te·o·dyn·i·a (os′tē-ō-din′ē-ă) SYN ostealgia. [osteo- + G. *odynē,* pain]

os·te·o·dys·plas·ty (os′tē-ō-dis-plas′tē) SYN Melnick-Needles osteodysplasty. [osteo- + G. *dys-,* bad, + *plastos,* formed]

os·te·o·dys·tro·phi·a (os′tē-ō-dis-trō′fē-ă) SYN osteodystrophy.

os·te·o·dys·tro·phy (os′tē-ō-dis′trŏ-fē) Defective formation of bone; common in dogs with chronic nephritis. SYN osteodystrophia. [osteo- + G. *dys,* difficult, imperfect, + *trophē,* nourishment]

os·te·o·ec·ta·si·a (os′tē-ō-ek-tā′zē-ă) Bowing of bones, particularly of the legs. [osteo- + G. *ektasis,* a stretching]

os·te·o·fi·bro·ma (os′tē-ō-fī-brō′mă) A benign lesion of bone, probably not a true neoplasm, consisting of connective tissue in which there are small foci of osteogenesis.

os·te·o·fi·bro·sis (os′tē-ō-fī-brō′sis) Fibrosis of bone, mainly involving red bone marrow.

os·te·o·gen (os′tē-ō-jen) A bone matrix–producing tissue or layer. [osteo- + G. *-gen,* producing]

os·te·o·gen·e·sis (os′tē-ō-jen′ĕ-sis) The formation of bone. SYN osteogeny, osteosis (2). [osteo- + G. *genesis,* production]

os·te·o·gen·e·sis im·per·fec·ta (OI) (os′tē-ō-jen′ĕ-sis im-pĕr-fek′tă) Abnormal fragility and plasticity of bone, with recurring fractures on trivial trauma; variable associated features include deformity of long bones, blueness of sclerae, laxity of ligaments, and otosclerosis. SYN brittle bones.

os·te·o·gen·e·sis im·per·fec·ta con·gen·i·ta (os′tē-ō-jen′ĕ-sis im-pĕr-fek′tă kon-jen′i-tă) Any of various genetic disorders in the biosynthesis of collagen resulting in abnormal fragility and plasticity of bone, with recurrent fractures after mild trauma; may also result in deformity of long bones, blueness of sclerae, laxity of ligaments, and otosclerosis.

os·te·o·gen·e·sis im·per·fec·ta tar·da (os-tē-ō-jen′ĕ-sis im-pĕr-fek′tă tahr′dă) A less severe form, with fractures occurring later in childhood.

os·te·o·gen·e·sis im·per·fec·ta type I (os′tē-ō-jen′ĕ-sis im-pĕr-fek′tă tīp) A mild form characterized by blue sclerae, hearing loss, easy bruising, prepubertal bone fragility, and short stature.

os·te·o·gen·e·sis im·per·fec·ta type II (os′tē-ō-jen′ĕ-sis im-pĕr-fek′tă tīp) A perinatal lethal form associated with stillbirth or lifespan less than 1 year; very fragile connective tissue, and radiographic findings of fractures in utero, large soft cranium, micromelia, tubular long bones, and beaded ribs.

os·te·o·gen·e·sis im·per·fec·ta type III (os′tē-ō-jen′ĕ-sis im-pĕr-fek′tă tīp) A progressive deforming form with severe bone fragility, easy fractures, triangular facies with relative macrocephaly, skeletal deformities with scoliosis, bowing of limbs, dwarfism, and radiographic findings of metaphyseal flaring of long bones with sutural bone formation. Most cases are autosomal dominant disorders, but autosomal recessive inheritance has also been described.

os·te·o·gen·e·sis im·per·fec·ta type IV (os′tē-ō-jen′ĕ-sis im-pĕr-fek′tă tīp) A moderately severe form, characterized by short stature, bone fragility, preambulatory fractures, and bowing of long bones.

os·te·o·ge·net·ic fi·bers (os′tē-ō-jĕ-net′ik fī′bĕrz) The fibers in the osteogenetic layer of the periosteum.

os·te·o·ge·net·ic lay·er (os′tē-ō-jĕ-net′ik lā′ĕr) The inner bone-forming layer of the periosteum.

os·te·o·gen·ic, **os·te·o·ge·net·ic** (os′tē-ō-jen′ik, -jĕ-net′ik) Relating to osteogenesis. SYN osteogenous.

os•te•o•gen•ic sar•co•ma (os′tē-ō-jen′ik sahr-kō′mă) The most common and malignant of bone sarcomas, which arises from bone-forming cells and chiefly affects the ends of long bones; its greatest incidence is in the 10–25-year-old age group. SYN osteosarcoma.

os•te•og•e•nous (os-tē-oj′ĕ-nŭs) SYN osteogenic.

os•te•og•e•ny (os-tē-oj′ĕ-nē) SYN osteogenesis.

os•te•oid (os′tē-oyd) **1.** Relating to or resembling bone. **2.** Newly formed organic bone matrix before calcification. [osteo- + G. *eidos,* resemblance]

os•te•oid os•te•o•ma (os′tē-oyd os-tē-ō′mă) A painful benign neoplasm that usually originates in one of the bones of the lower extremities, especially in adolescents and young adults; characterized by a nidus of osteoid material, vascularized osteogenic stroma, and poorly formed bone; around the nidus there is a relatively large zone of reactive thickening of the cortex.

os•te•o•kin•e•mat•ics (os′tē-o-kin-ē-mat′iks) The study of the movement of bones associated with joints.

os•te•ol•o•gy (os′tē-ol′ŏ-jē) The anatomy of the bones; the science concerned with the bones and their structure. [osteo- + G. *logos,* study]

os•te•ol•y•sis (os′tē-ol′i-sis) Softening, absorption, and destruction of bony tissue, a function of the osteoclasts. [osteo- + G. *lysis,* dissolution]

os•te•o•lyt•ic (os′tē-ō-lit′ik) Pertaining to, characterized by, or causing osteolysis.

os•te•o•ma (os′-tē-ō′mă) A benign slow-growing mass of mature, predominantly lamellar bone, usually arising from the skull or mandible. [osteo- + G. *-oma,* tumor]

os•te•o•ma cu•tis (os′tē-ō′mă kyū′tis) Cutaneous ossification in foci of degeneration in tumors or inflammatory lesions or rarely primary new bone formation with normal skin. SYN osteodermia, osteosis cutis.

os•te•o•ma•la•ci•a (os′tē-ō-mă-lā′shē-ă) A disease characterized by a gradual softening and bending of the bones with varying severity of pain; softening occurs because the bones contain osteoid tissue which has failed to calcify due to lack of vitamin D or renal tubular dysfunction. SYN adult rickets, late rickets. [osteo- + G. *malakia,* softness]

os•te•o•ma•la•cic (os′tē-ō-mă-lā′sik) Relating to, or suffering from, osteomalacia.

os•te•o•ma•la•cic pel•vis (os′tē-ō-mă-lā′sik pel′vis) A pelvic deformity in osteomalacia; the pressure of the trunk on the sacrum and lateral pressure of the femoral heads produce a pelvic aperture that is three-cornered or has the shape of a heart or a cloverleaf, whereas the pubic bone becomes beak shaped. SYN beaked pelvis.

os•te•o•ma me•dul•la•re (os′tē-ō′mă me-dyū-lā′rē) An osteoma containing spaces that are filled (or partly filled) with various elements of bone marrow.

os•te•o•ma spon•gi•o•sum (os′tē-ō′mă spŭn′jē-ō′sŭm) An osteoma that consists chiefly of cancellous bone tissue.

os•te•o•ma•toid (os′tē-ō′mă-toyd) An abnormal nodule or small mass of overgrowth of bone; lesions are not neoplasms but anomalous outpouchings of the cortex, and are more properly termed exostoses. [osteoma + G. *eidos,* appearance, form]

os•te•o•mere (os′tē-ō-mēr) One of a series of bone segments, such as the vertebrae. [osteo- + G. *meros,* a part]

os•te•o•my•e•li•tis (os′tē-ō-mī-ĕ-lī′tis) Inflammation of the bone marrow and adjacent bone. SYN central osteitis (1). [osteo- + G. *myelos,* marrow, + *-itis,* inflammation]

os•te•o•my•e•lo•dys•pla•si•a (os′tē-ō-mī′ĕ-lō-dis-plā′zē-ă) A disease characterized by enlargement of the marrow cavities of the bones, thinning of the osseous tissue, leukopenia, and irregular fever. [osteo- + G. *myelos,* marrow, + dysplasia]

os•te•on, os•te•one (os′tē-on, os′tē-ōn) A central canal containing blood capillaries and the concentric osseous lamellae around it occurring in compact bone. SYN haversian system. [G. *osteon,* bone]

os•te•o•ne•cro•sis (os′tē-ō-nĕ-krō′sis) The extensive death of bone, as distinguished from caries ("molecular death") or relatively small foci of necrosis in bone. [osteo- + G. *nekrōsis,* death]

os•te•o•path (os′tē-ō-path) SYN osteopathic physician.

os•te•o•path•i•a (os′tē-ō-path′ē-ă) SYN osteopathy (1).

osteopathia haemorrhagica infantum [Br.] SYN osteopathia hemorrhagica infantum.

os•te•o•path•i•a he•mor•rhag•i•ca in•fan•tum (os′tē-ō-path′ē-ă hĕm′mōr-raj′ik-ă in-fan′tum) SYN infantile scurvy. SYN osteopathia haemorrhagica infantum.

os•te•o•path•ic (os′tē-ō-path′ik) Relating to osteopathy.

os•te•o•path•ic med•i•cine (os′tē-ō-path′ik med′i-sin) SYN osteopathy (2).

os•te•o•path•ic phy•si•cian (os′tē-ō-path′ik fi-zish′ŭn) A practitioner of osteopathy. SYN osteopath.

os•te•op•a•thy (os′tē-op′ă-thē) **1.** Any disease

of bone. SYN osteopathia. **2.** A school of medicine based on a concept of the normal body as a vital machine capable, when in correct adjustment, of making its own remedies against infections and other toxic conditions; practitioners use the diagnostic and therapeutic measures of conventional medicine in addition to manipulative measures. SYN osteopathic medicine. [osteo- + G. *pathos,* suffering]

os•te•o•pe•ni•a (os′tē-ō-pē′nē-ă) **1.** Decreased calcification or density of bone; a descriptive term applicable to all skeletal systems in which such a condition is noted; carries no implication about causality. **2.** Reduced bone mass due to inadequate osteoid synthesis. [osteo- + G. *penia,* poverty]

os•te•o•per•i•os•ti•tis (os′tē-ō-per′ē-os-tī′tis) Inflammation of the periosteum and of the underlying bone.

os•te•o•pe•tro•sis (os′tē-ō-pĕ-trō′sis) Excessive formation of dense trabecular bone and calcified cartilage, especially in long bones, leading to obliteration of marrow spaces and to anemia, with myeloid metaplasia and hepatosplenomegaly, beginning in infancy and with progressive deafness and blindness. SYN Albers-Schönberg disease. [osteo- + G. *petra,* stone, + *-osis,* condition]

os•te•o•phage (os′tē-ō-fāj) SYN osteoclast (1). [osteo- + G. *phagō,* to eat]

os•te•o•phle•bi•tis (os′tē-ō-flĕ-bī′tis) Inflammation of the veins of a bone. [osteo- + G. *phleps,* vein, + *-itis,* inflammation]

os•te•o•phy•ma (os′tē-ō-fī′mă) SYN osteophyte. [osteo- + G. *phyma,* tumor]

os•te•o•phyte (os′tē-ō-fīt) A bony outgrowth or protuberance. See this page. SYN osteophyma. [osteo- + G. *phyton,* plant]

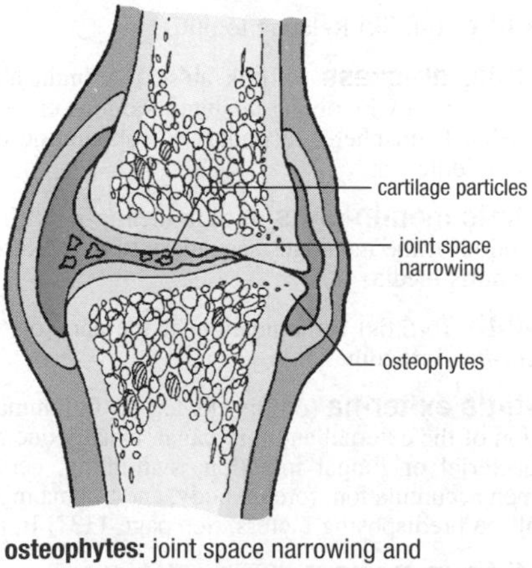

osteophytes: joint space narrowing and osteophytes (bone spurs) are characteristic of degenerative changes in joints

os•te•o•plas•tic bone flap (os′tē-ō-plas′tik bōn flap) Vascularized tissue that includes living bone, usually with attached muscle and fascia, which can be attached by its pedicle or transferred by microvascular anastomosis from one site to another.

os•te•o•plas•tic ob•lit•er•a•tion of the fron•tal si•nus (os′tē-ō-plas′tik ob-lit-ĕr-ā′shŭn frŏn′tăl sī′nŭs) Operation to remove diseased contents, including the mucous membrane, of the frontal sinus and to obliterate the sinus with a free fat graft without altering the external contour of the sinus.

os•te•o•plas•ty (os′tē-ō-plas-tē) **1.** Bone grafting; reparative or plastic surgery of the bones. **2.** DENTISTRY resection of osseous structure to achieve acceptable gingival contour. [osteo- + G. *plastos,* formed]

os•te•o•poi•ki•lo•sis (os′tē-ō-poy-ki-lō′sis) Mottled or spotted bones caused by widespread foci of compact bone in the substantia spongiosa. [osteo- + G. *poikilos,* dappled, + *-osis,* condition]

os•te•o•po•ro•sis (os′tē-ō-pŏr-ō′sis) Reduction in the quantity of bone or atrophy of skeletal tissue; occurs in postmenopausal women and elderly men, resulting in bone trabeculae that are scanty, thin, and without osteoclastic resorption. [osteo- + G. *poros,* pore, + *-osis,* condition]

os•te•o•po•rot•ic (os′tē-ō-pŏ-rot′ik) Pertaining to, characterized by, or causing a porous condition of the bones.

os•te•o•pro•gen•i•tor cell (os′tē-ō-prō-jen′i-tŏr sel) A mesenchymal cell that differentiates into an osteoblast. SYN preosteoblast.

os•te•o•pro•teg•er•in (os′tē-ō-prō-tej′ĕr-in) A secreted protein that inhibits osteoclast differentiation.

os•te•o•ra•di•ol•o•gy (os′tē-ō-rā-dē-ol′ŏ-jē) The clinical subspecialty of diagnostic bone radiology.

os•te•o•ra•di•o•ne•cro•sis (os′tē-ō-rā′dē-ō-ne-krō′sis) Bone death produced by ionizing radiation; may be planned or unplanned. [osteo- + radionecrosis]

os•te•or•rha•phy (os-tē-ōr′ă-fē) Wiring together the fragments of a broken bone. SYN osteosuture. [osteo- + G. *rhaphē,* suture]

os•te•o•sar•co•ma (os′tē-ō-sahr-kō′mă) SYN osteogenic sarcoma. See page B31.

os•te•o•scle•ro•sis (os′tē-ō-skle-rō′sis) Abnormal hardening or eburnation of bone. [osteo- + G. *sklērōsis,* hardness]

os•te•o•scle•rot•ic (os′tē-ō-skle-rot′ik) Relating to, due to, or marked by hardening of bone substance.

os•te•o•sis (os-tē-ō′sis) **1.** A morbid process in

bone. **2.** SYN osteogenesis. [osteo- + G. *-osis,* condition]

os·te·o·sis cu·tis (os-tē-ō′sis kyū′tis) SYN osteoma cutis.

os·te·o·su·ture (os′tē-ō-sū′chŭr) SYN osteorrhaphy.

os·te·o·sy·no·vi·tis (os′tē-ō-sin′ō-vī′tis) Inflammation of a synovial membrane and the surrounding bones. [osteo- + synovitis]

os·te·o·syn·the·sis (os′tē-ō-sin′thĕ-sis) Internal fixation of a fracture by means of a mechanical device, such as a pin, screw, or plate.

os·te·o·throm·bo·sis (os′tē-ō-throm-bō′sis) Thrombosis in one or more of the veins of a bone.

os·te·o·tome (os′tē-ō-tōm) An instrument for use in cutting bone. [osteo- + G. *tomē,* incision]

os·te·ot·o·my (os′tē-ot′ŏ-mē) Cutting a bone, usually by means of a saw or chisel. [osteo- + G. *tomē,* incision]

os·te·o·tribe (os′tē-ō-trīb) An instrument for crushing off bits of necrotic or carious bone. [osteo- + G. *tribō,* to bruise, to grind down]

os·te·o·trite (os′tē-ō-trīt) An instrument with conic or olive-shaped tip with a cutting surface, resembling a dental bur, used for the removal of carious bone. [osteo- + L. *tritus,* a grinding, a wearing off]

os·ti·a (os′tē-ă) Plural of ostium. [L.]

os·ti·al (os′tē-ăl) Relating to any orifice, or ostium.

os·ti·tic (os-tī′tik) SYN osteitic.

os·ti·tis (os-tī′tis) SYN osteitis.

os·ti·um, pl. **os·ti·a** (os′tē-ŭm, -ă) [TA] A small opening, especially one of entrance into a hollow organ or canal. [L. door, entrance, mouth]

os·ti·um il·e·a·le (os′tē-ŭm il-ē-āl′ē) SYN ileal orifice.

os·to·mate (os′tō-māt) Term for one who has an ostomy. [L. *ostium,* mouth]

os·to·my (os′tŏ-mē) **1.** An artificial stoma or opening into the urinary or gastrointestinal canal, or the trachea. **2.** Any operation by which a permanent opening is created between two hollow organs or between a hollow viscus and the skin externally, as in tracheostomy. [L. *ostium,* mouth]

os tra·pe·zi·um (os tră-pē′zē-ŭm) [TA] SYN trapezium (bone).

os tri·go·num (os trī-gō′nŭm) An independent ossicle sometimes present in the tarsus; usually it forms part of the talus, constituting the lateral tubercle of the posterior process. SYN triangular bone.

Ost·wald sol·u·bil·i·ty co·ef·fi·cient (λ, lamb·da) (ost′wahld sol-yū-bil′i-tē kō-e-fish′ĕnt lamb′dă) The milliliters of gas dissolved per milliliter of liquid and per atmosphere (760 mmHg) partial pressure of the gas at any given temperature. This differs from Bunsen solubility coefficient (α) in that the amount of dissolved gas is expressed in terms of its volume at the temperature of the experiment, instead of STPD. Thus, $\lambda = \alpha (1 + 0.00367t)$, where t = temperature in degrees Celsius.

os zy·go·ma·ti·cum (os zī-gō-ma′ti-kŭm) [TA] SYN zygomatic bone.

ot- Combining form denoting the ear. SEE ALSO auri-. [G. *ous*]

o·tal·gi·a (ō-tal′jē-ă) SYN earache. [ot- + G. *algos,* pain]

o·tal·gic (ō-tal′jik) **1.** Relating to otalgia, or earache. **2.** A remedy for earache.

OTC Abbreviation for over the counter (i.e., drugs, medications).

oth·er-di·rect·ed (ŭth′ĕr-di-rek′tĕd) Pertaining to a person readily influenced by the attitudes of others.

o·tic (ō′tik) Relating to the ear. [G. *otikos,* fr. *ous,* ear]

o·tic cap·sule (ō′tik kap′sŭl) The cartilage that, in the embryo, surrounds the developing otic vesicle and develops into the bony labyrinth of the internal ear. SYN auditory capsule.

o·tic gan·gli·on (ō′tik gang′glē-ŏn) An autonomic ganglion situated below the foramen ovale medial to the mandibular nerve; its postganglionic, parasympathetic fibers are distributed to the parotid gland.

o·ti·tic (ō-tit′ik) Relating to otitis.

o·ti·tic ab·scess (ō-tit′ik ab′ses) A brain abscess, usually involving the temporal lobe or cerebellar hemisphere, secondary to suppuration of the middle ear.

o·tit·ic men·in·gi·tis (ō-tit′ik men-in-jī′tis) Infection of the meninges secondary to mastoiditis or otitis media.

o·ti·tis (ō-tī′tis) Inflammation of the ear. [ot- + G. *-itis,* inflammation]

o·ti·tis ex·ter·na (ō-tī′tis eks-ter′nă) Inflammation of the external auditory canal, usually due to bacterial or fungal infection; swimming, cerumen accumulation, foreign body, and trauma may all be predisposing factors. See page 1131, B28.

o·ti·tis in·ter·na (ō-tī′tis in-ter′nă) SYN labyrinthitis.

o·ti·tis me·di·a (OM) (ō-tī′tis mē′dē-ă) Inflam-

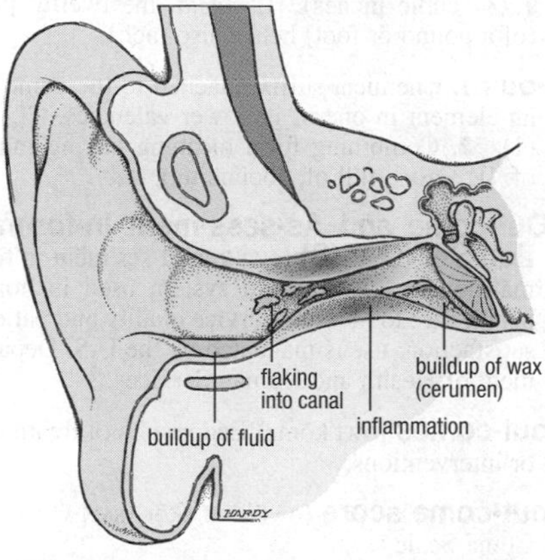

otitis externa

mation of the middle ear, or tympanum. See this page, B28.

♻ **oto-** Combining form denoting the ear. SEE ALSO auri-. [G. *ous*]

o·to·a·cous·tic e·mis·sion (OAE) (ō-tō-ă-kū′stik ē-mish′ŭn) Sounds that issue from the external acoustic meatus as a result of vibrations originating within the cochlea. SEE ALSO Kemp echo.

o·to·ceph·a·ly (ō-tō-sef′ă-lē) Malformation characterized by markedly defective development of the lower jaw (micrognathia or agnathia) and the union or close approach of the ears (synotia) on the front of the neck. [oto- + G. *kephalē,* head]

o·to·co·ni·a, sing. **o·to·co·ni·um** (ō-to-kō′nē-ă, ō-tō-kō′nē-ŭm) SYN statoliths.

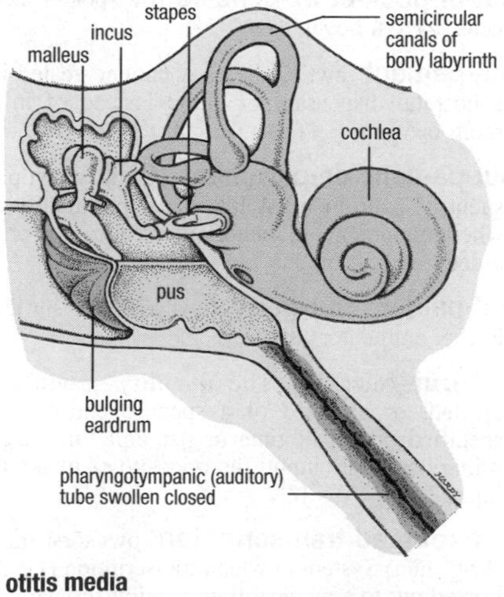

otitis media

o·to·cra·ni·al (ō-tō-krā′nē-ăl) Relating to the otocranium.

o·to·cra·ni·um (ō-tō-krā′nē-ŭm) The bony case of the internal and middle ear, consisting of the petrous portion of the temporal bone. [oto- + G. *kranion,* cranium]

o·to·dyn·i·a (ō-tō-din′ē-ă) SYN earache. [oto- + G. *odynē,* pain]

o·to·en·ceph·a·li·tis (ō′tō-en-sef-ă-lī′tis) Inflammation of the brain by extension of the process from the middle ear and mastoid cells. [oto- + G. *enkephalos,* brain, + *-itis,* inflammation]

o·to·gen·ic, **o·tog·e·nous** (ō-tō-jen′ik, ō-toj′ĕ-nŭs) Of otic origin; originating within the ear, especially from inflammation of the ear. [oto- + G. *-gen,* producing]

o·to·lar·yn·gol·o·gist (ō′tō-lar-in-gol′ŏ-jist) A physician who specializes in otolaryngology.

o·to·lar·yn·gol·o·gy (ō′tō-lar-in-gol′ŏ-jē) The combined specialties of diseases of the ear and larynx, often including upper respiratory tract and many diseases of the head and neck, tracheobronchial tree, and esophagus. [oto- + G. *larynx,* + *logos,* study]

o·to·lith·ic cri·sis (ō-tō-lith′ik krī′sis) A sudden drop attack without loss of consciousness, vertigo, auditory disturbances, or autonomic manifestations.

o·to·lith·ic or·gans (ō-to-lith′ik ōr′gănz) The utricle and saccule of the inner ear that possess otoliths and respond to linear acceleration and deceleration, including gravity.

o·to·liths (ō′tō-līths) Crystalline particles of calcium carbonate and a protein adhering to the gelatinous membrane of the maculae of the utricle and saccule. [oto- + G. *lithos,* stone]

o·to·log·ic (ō-tō-loj′ik) Relating to otology.

o·tol·o·gist (ō-tol′ŏ-jist) A specialist in otology.

o·tol·o·gy (ō-tol′ŏ-jē) The branch of medical science concerned with the study, diagnosis, and treatment of diseases of the ear and related structures. [oto- + G. *logos,* study]

o·to·mu·cor·my·co·sis (ō-tō-myū′kōr-mī-kō′sis) Mucormycosis of the ear.

♻ **-otomy** SEE -tomy.

ℹ **oto·my·co·sis** (ō′tō-mī-kō′sis) An infection due to a fungus in the external auditory canal, usually unilateral, with scaling, itching, and pain as the primary symptoms. See page B28.

o·top·a·thy (ō-top′ă-thē) Any disease of the ear. [oto- + G. *pathos,* suffering]

o·to·pha·ryn·ge·al (ō′tō-fă-rin′jē-ăl) Relating to the middle ear and the pharynx.

o•to•plas•ty (ō′tō-plas-tē) Reparative surgery of the auricle of the ear. [oto- + G. *plastos,* formed]

o•to•rhi•no•lar•yn•gol•o•gy (ō′tō-rī′nō-lar-in-gol′ŏ-jē) The combined specialties of diseases of the ear, nose, and larynx; including diseases of related structures of the head and neck. SEE ALSO otolaryngology. [oto- + G. *rhis,* nose, + *larynx,* larynx, + *logos,* study]

o•tor•rhe•a (ō-tō-rē′ă) A discharge from the ear. SYN otorrhoea. [oto- + G. *rhoia,* flow]

otorrhoea [Br.] SYN otorrhea.

o•to•scle•ro•sis (ō′tō-skle-rō′sis) A new formation of spongy bone about the stapes and fenestra vestibuli (ovalis), resulting in progressively increasing deafness, without signs of disease in the auditory tube or tympanic membrane. [oto- + G. *sklērōsis,* hardening]

o•to•scope (ō′tō-skōp) An instrument for examining the drum membrane or auscultating the ear. See page B28. [oto- + G. *skopeō,* to view]

o•tos•co•py (ō-tos′kŏ-pē) Inspection of the ear, especially of the drum membrane. See page B28. [oto- + G. *skopeō,* to view]

o•to•spon•dy•lo•me•ga•epi•phy•si•al dys•pla•si•a (ō′tō-spon′di-lō-meg′ă-ep-i-fiz′ē-ăl dis-plā′zē-ă) SYN chondrodystrophy with sensorineural deafness.

o•to•spon•gi•o•sis (ō′tō-spŭn-jē-ō′sis) A more accurately descriptive term for the pathologic changes in otosclerosis.

o•tos•te•al (ō-tos′tē-ăl) Relating to the ossicles of the ear. [oto- + G. *osteon,* bone]

o•to•tox•ic (ō′tō-tok′sik) Having a toxic action on the ear. [oto- + G. *toxikon,* poison]

o•to•tox•ic•i•ty (ō′tō-tok-sis′i-tē) The property of being ototoxic.

Ot•to dis•ease (ot′ō di-zēz′) A disease characterized by an inward bulging of the acetabulum into the pelvic cavity, resulting in protrusion of the femoral head; found in association with arthritis of the hip joints, usually rheumatoid arthritis.

Ouch•ter•lo•ny tech•nique (ok′tĕr-lō-nē tek-nēk′) A process in which both reaction partners (antigen and antibody) are allowed to diffuse to each other in a gel in a precipitation reaction.

ounce (owns) **1.** A weight containing 480 gr, or 1/12 pound troy and apothecaries' weight, or 437½ grains 1/16 pound avoirdupois. The apothecary ounce (used in the USP) contains 8 drams and is equivalent to 31.10349 gram; the avoirdupois ounce is equivalent to 28.35 g. **2.** Fluid ounce; United States: 1/128 U.S. gallon (29.57 mL, 1.804 cubic inches). British Imperial System: the volume occupied by 1 avoirdupois ounce of distilled water at 62° F (28.41 mL, 1.734 cubic inches). [L. *uncia,* the twelfth part (of a pound or foot) hence also inch]

-ous **1.** Chemical suffix attached to the name of an element in one of its lower valencies. Cf. -ic (1). **2.** Combining form meaning having much of. [L. *-osus,* full of, abounding]

Out•come and As•sess•ment In•for•ma•tion Set (OASIS) (owt′kŭm ă-ses′mĕnt in′fōr-mā′shŭn set) A standard system used in home health care to measure service quality and patient satisfaction; use is mandated by the U.S. Department of Health and Human Services.

out•comes (owt′kŏmz) End results of treatment or interventions.

out•come score (owt′kŏm skōr) SYN Glasgow Coma Scale.

out•comes man•age•ment (owt′kŏmz man′ăj-mĕnt) Use of information collected through measurement of outcomes to improve effectiveness and value of treatments and services.

out•let (owt′lĕt) An exit or opening of a passageway. SEE ALSO aperture.

out•let for•ceps de•liv•ery (owt′lĕt fōr′seps dĕ-liv′ĕr-ē) Delivery by forceps applied to the fetal head when it has reached the perineal floor and is visible between contractions.

out•li•er (owt′lī-ĕr) **1.** Deviant values or figures that are obviously from a different population than those from the rest of the sample. Deviant values are identified and eliminated because they distort the analysis of the entire sample. **2.** Additions to an estimated cost of delivered services when exceeding a fixed loss threshold.

out-of-pock•et costs (owt-pok′ĕt kawsts) SYN copayment.

out-of-pock•et ex•pens•es (owt-pok′ĕt eks-pens′ĕz) SYN copayment.

out•pa•tient (owt′pā′shĕnt) A patient treated in a hospital dispensary or clinic instead of in a room or ward.

out•pa•tient de•part•ment (OPD) (owt′pā-shĕnt dĕ-pahrt′mĕnt) A hospital department/unit where nonurgent ambulatory medical care is provided.

out•pa•tient sur•ger•y (owt′pā-shĕnt sŭr′jĕr-ē) SYN ambulatory surgery.

out•put (owt′put) The quantity produced, ejected, or excreted of a specific entity in a specified period of time or per unit time, e.g., urinary sodium output; the opposite of intake or input.

out•sourced tran•scrip•tion (owt′sōrst tran-skrip′shŭn) System in which transcription is contracted out to a medical transcription service.

out•stand•ing ear (owt-stan′ding ēr) Excessive protrusion of the auricle of the external ear from the head, usually due to failure of the antihelical fold to develop. SYN protruding ear.

o•va (ō′vă) Plural of ovum. [L.]

o•val am•pu•ta•tion (ō′văl amp′yū-tā′shŭn) **1.** Surgical removal in which the flaps are obtained by oval incisions through the skin and muscle; **2.** Rarely used term for oblique amputation.

o•val•bu•min (ōv′al-bū′min) The chief protein occurring in the white of egg and resembling serum albumin; also found in phosphorylated form. SYN albumen, egg albumin.

o•val•o•cyte (ō′val-ŏ-sīt) SYN elliptocyte. [L. *ovalis,* oval, + G. *kytos,* cell]

o•val•o•cy•to•sis (ō′val-ō-sī-tō′sis) SYN elliptocytosis.

o•val win•dow (ō′văl win′dō) SYN fenestra vestibuli.

o•va and pa•ra•site ex•am•in•a•tion (ō′vă par′ă-sīt eg-zam′i-nā′shŭn) A comprehensive review of a fecal specimen, using direct wet mounts, concentration wet mounts, and permanent stained smears, for the recovery and identification of protozoan and helminthic parasite stages such as trophozoites, cysts, oocysts, spores, eggs, and larvae.

o•var•i•al•gi•a (ō-var-ē-al′jē-ă) Pain in an ovary. [ovario- + G. *algos,* pain]

o•var•i•an (ō-var′ē-ăn) Relating to the ovary.

o•var•i•an ar•ter•y (ō-var′ē-ăn ahr′tĕr-ē) *Origin,* aorta; *distribution,* ureter, ovary, ovarian ligament and uterine tube; *anastomoses,* uterine. SYN arteria ovarica [TA].

o•var•i•an can•cer (ō-var′ē-ăn kan′sĕr) A malignancy that arises from the female reproductive organ; one of the most common gynecologic malignancies and one of the most frequent causes of cancer death in women, with 50% of all cases occurring in women older than age 65.

o•var•i•an cy•cle (ō-var′ē-ăn sī′kĕl) The normal sex cycle that includes development of an ovarian (graafian) follicle, rupture of the follicle with discharge of the ovum, and formation and regression of a corpus luteum.

o•var•i•an cyst (ō-var′ē-ăn sist) A cystic tumor of the ovary, either non-neoplastic (follicle, lutein, germinal inclusion, or endometrial) or neoplastic.

o•var•i•an fol•li•cle (ō-var′ē-ăn fol′i-kĕl) One of the spheric cell aggregations in the ovary containing an oocyte.

o•var•i•an fos•sa (ō-var′ē-ăn fos′ă) A depression in the parietal peritoneum of the pelvis; it is bounded in front by the obliterated umbilical artery, and behind by the ureter and the uterine vessels; it lodges the ovary.

o•var•i•an preg•nan•cy (ō-var′ē-ăn preg′năn-sē) Development of an impregnated oocyte in an ovarian follicle. SYN ovariocyesis.

ovar•i•ec•to•my (ō-var-ē-ek′tŏ-mē) Excision of one or both ovaries. SYN oophorectomy. [ovario- + G. *ektomē,* excision]

♻**ovario-, ovari-** Combining forms meaning ovary. SEE ALSO oo-, oophor-. [L. *ovarium*]

o•var•i•o•cele (ō-var′ē-ō-sēl) Hernia of an ovary. [ovario- + G. *kēlē,* hernia]

o•var•i•o•cen•te•sis (ō-var′ē-ō-sen-tē′sis) Puncture of an ovary or an ovarian cyst. [ovario- + G. *kentēsis,* puncture]

o•var•i•o•cy•e•sis (ō-var′ē-ō-sī-ē′sis) SYN ovarian pregnancy. [ovario- + G. *kyēsis,* pregnancy]

o•var•i•o•hys•ter•ec•to•my (ō-var′ē-ō-his-tĕr-ek′tŏ-mē) Removal of ovaries and uterus. SYN oophorohysterectomy. [ovario- + G. *hystera,* uterus, + *ektomē,* excision]

o•var•i•or•rhex•is (ō-var′ē-ō-rek′sis) Rupture of an ovary. [ovario- + G. *rhēxis,* rupture]

o•var•i•o•sal•pin•gec•to•my (ō-var′ē-ō-sal-pin-jek′tŏ-mē) Operative removal of an ovary and the corresponding oviduct. [ovario- + salpingectomy]

o•var•i•o•sal•pin•gi•tis (ō-var′ē-ō-sal′pin-jī′tis) SYN oophorosalpingitis.

o•var•i•os•to•my (ō-var-ē-os′tŏ-mē) Establishment of a temporary fistula for drainage of a cyst of the ovary. SYN oophorostomy. [ovario- + G. *stoma,* mouth]

o•var•i•ot•o•my (ō-var-ē-ot′ŏ-mē) An incision into an ovary, e.g., a biopsy or a wedge excision. SYN oophorotomy. [ovario- + G. *tomē,* incision]

o•va•ri•tis (ō-vă-rī′tis) SYN oophoritis.

ovar•i•um, pl. **ova•ri•a** (ō-var′ē-ŭm, -ă) [TA] SYN ovary. [Mod. L. fr. *ovum,* egg]

o•va•ry (ō′vă-rē) One of the paired female reproductive glands containing the oocytes (ova) or germ cells; its stroma is a vascular connective tissue containing ovarian follicles, each enclosing an oocyte; surrounding this stroma is a denser layer called the tunica albuginea. SYN ovarium [TA], oophoron. [Mod. L. *ovarium,* fr. *ovum,* egg]

o•ver•anx•ious dis•or•der (ō′vĕr-angk′shŭs dis-ōr′dĕr) A mental disorder of childhood or adolescence marked by excessive worry and fearful behavior not related specifically to separation or due to recent stress.

o•ver•bite (ō′vĕr-bīt) SYN vertical overlap.

o•ver•clo•sure (ō′vĕr-klō′zhūr) A decrease in occlusal vertical dimension.

o•ver•com•pen•sa•tion (ō′vĕr-kom-pen-sā′shŭn) **1.** An exaggeration of personal capacity by which one overcomes a real or imagined inferiority. **2.** The process in which a psychologic deficiency inspires exaggerated correction. SEE compensation.

o·ver·cor·rec·tion (ō′vĕr-kŏ-rek′shŭn) In behavior modification treatment programs, especially those involving mentally retarded people, overlearning the desired target behavior beyond the set criterion to ensure that the behavior will continue to meet the established criterion when the decrements and forgetting occur after the learning process has concluded.

o·ver the coun·ter (OTC) (ō′vĕr kown′tĕr) Denotes drugs or therapeutic aids sold to the consumer without the necessity of prescription provided by a health care professional.

o·ver·den·ture (ō′vĕr-den′chūr) SYN overlay denture.

o·ver·de·ter·mi·na·tion (o′vĕr-dē-tĕr′min-ā′shŭn) PSYCHOANALYSIS ascribing the cause of a single behavioral or emotional reaction, mental symptom, or dream to the operation of two or more forces (e.g., ascribing an emotional outburst not only to the immediate precipitant but also to a lingering inferiority complex).

o·ver·dom·i·nance (ō′vĕr-dom′i-năns) That state in which the heterozygote has greater phenotype value and perhaps is more fit than the homozygous state for either of the alleles that it comprises. Cf. balanced polymorphism.

o·ver·dom·i·nant (ō′vĕr-dom′i-nănt) Denoting heterozygous states that exhibit overdominance.

o·ver·drive (ō′vĕr-drīv) An electrophysiologic pacing technique to exceed the rate of an abnormal pacemaker and so capture the territory controlled by that pacemaker (usually atrial).

o·ver·jet, **o·ver·jut** (ō′vĕr-jĕt, ō′ver-jŭt) SYN horizontal overlap.

o·ver·lap (ō′vĕr-lap) **1.** Suturing of one layer of tissue above or under another to gain strength. **2.** An extension or projection of one tissue over another. **3.** RADIOGRAPHY use of incorrect angles to enable viewing between structures.

o·ver·lay den·ture (ō′vĕr-lā den′chŭr) A complete denture that is supported by both soft tissue and natural teeth that have been altered to permit the denture to fit over them. The altered teeth may have been fitted with short or long copings, locking devices, or connecting bars. SYN overdenture.

o·ver·load prin·ci·ple (ō′vĕr-lōd prin′si-pĕl) EXERCISE SCIENCE fundamental principle of training stating that exercise at an intensity above that normally attained will induce highly specific adaptations, enabling the body to function more efficiently. Overload is applied by manipulating combinations of training frequency, intensity, and duration.

o·ver·rid·ing (ō′vĕr-rī′ding) **1.** Slippage of the lower fragment of a broken long bone upward and next to the proximal portion. **2.** Denoting a fetal head which is palpable above the symphysis because of cephalopelvic disproportion.

o·ver·shoot (ō′vĕr-shūt) **1.** Any response to a step change in some factor that is greater than the steady-state response to the new level of that factor; common in systems in which inertia or a time lag in negative feedback outweighs any damping that may be present. **2.** Momentary reversal of the membrane potential of a cell (inside becoming positive rather than negative relative to the outside) during an action potential.

o·ver-the-coun·ter med·i·ca·tion (ō′vĕr kown′tĕr med′i-kā′shŭn) SYN nonprescription drug.

o·vert ho·mo·sex·u·al·i·ty (ō-vĕrt′ hō′mō-sek′shū-al′i-tē) Homosexual inclinations consciously experienced and expressed in actual homosexual behavior.

o·ver·train·ing syn·drome (ō′vĕr-trān′ing sin′drōm) A group of symptoms resulting from excessive physical training; includes fatigue, poor exercise performance, frequent upper-respiratory tract infections, altered mood, general malaise, weight loss, muscle stiffness and soreness, and loss of interest in high-level training. SYN burnout, staleness.

o·ver·use syn·drome (ō′vĕr-yūs sin′drōm) Injury caused by accumulated microtraumatic stress placed on a structure or body area.

o·ver·weight (ō′vĕr-wāt′) The classification of body weight that is greater than the normal range but less than the obese range; defined by the U.S. National Institutes of Health as a body mass index between 25 and 30 kg/m^2.

o·ver·win·ter·ing (ō′vĕr-win′tĕr-ing) Persistence of an infectious agent in its vector for extended periods, such as the cooler winter months, during which the vector has no opportunity to be reinfected or to infect another host.

ovi- Prefix meaning egg or oocyte. SEE ALSO oo-, ovo-. [L. *ovum*]

o·vi·ci·dal (ō′vi-sī′dăl) Causing death of the egg or oocyte. [ovi- + L. *caedo,* to kill]

o·vi·du·cal (ō-vi-dū′kăl) SYN oviductal.

o·vi·duct (ō′vi-dŭkt) SYN uterine tube. [ovi- + L. *ductus,* a leading, fr. *duco,* pp. *ductus,* to lead]

o·vi·duc·tal (ō′vi-dŭk′tăl) Relating to a uterine tube. SYN oviducal.

o·vif·er·ous (ō-vif′ĕr-ŭs) Carrying, containing, or producing oocytes (ova). [ovi- + L. *fero,* to carry]

o·vi·form (ō′vi-fōrm) SYN ovoid (2).

o·vi·gen·e·sis (ō-vi-jen′ĕ-sis) SYN oogenesis.

o•vi•ge•net•ic, **o•vi•gen•ic** (ō′vi-jĕ-net′ik, -jen′ik) SYN oogenetic.

♻ **ovo-** Prefix meaning oocyte or egg. SEE ALSO oo-, ovi-. [L. *ovum*]

o•void (ō′voyd) **1.** An oval or egg-shaped form. **2.** Resembling an egg. SYN oviform. [ovo- + G. *eidos,* resemblance]

o•voids (ō′voydz) Also known as colpostats; oval applicators that are inserted into the lateral fornices of the vagina; used in conjunction with a tandem for the treatment of gynecologic malignancies with a radioactive source. SEE ALSO tandem. SYN colpostats.

o•vo•lac•to•ve•ge•tar•i•an (ō′vō-lakt′ō-vej-e-tar′ē-ăn) One whose diet contains vegetables, eggs, and dairy products. SEE ALSO vegetarian, vegan.

o•vo•tes•tis (ō′vō-tes′tis) Gonad in which both testicular and ovarian components are present; present in some true hermaphrodites.

ovu•lar (ov′yū-lăr) Relating to an ovule.

o•vu•lar mem•brane (ov′yū-lăr mem′brān) SYN membrana vitellina (1).

o•vu•la•tion (ov′yū-lā′shŭn) Release of an oocyte from the ovarian follicle.

o•vu•la•to•ry (ov′yū-lă-tō-rē) Relating to ovulation.

o•vule (ov′yūl) **1.** The oocyte (ovum) of a mammal, especially while still in the ovarian follicle. **2.** A small beadlike structure resembling an ovule. SYN ovulum. [Mod. L. *ovulum,* dim. of L. *ovum,* egg]

o•vu•lo•cy•clic (ov′yū-lō-sīk′lik) Denoting any recurrent phenomenon associated with and occurring at a certain time within the ovulatory cycle, as, for example, ovulocyclic porphyria.

o•vu•lum, pl. **o•vu•la** (ov′yū-lŭm, -lă) SYN ovule.

o•vum, gen. **o•vi**, pl. **o•va** (ō′vŭm, -vī, -vă) SYN oocyte. [L. egg]

Ow•en lines (ō′ĕn līnz) Accentuated incremental lines in the dentin thought to be due to disturbances in the mineralization process.

Ow•ren dis•ease (ō′ren di-zēz′) A congenital deficiency of factor V, resulting in prolongation of prothrombin time; bleeding and clotting times are consistently prolonged; autosomal recessive inheritance caused by mutation in the F5 gene on chromosome 1q.

♻ **oxa-** Combining form inserted in names of organic compounds to signify the presence or addition of oxygen atom(s) in a chain or ring (as in ethers), not appended to either (as in ketones and aldehydes). SEE ALSO hydroxy-, oxo-, oxy-. [English *oxygen*]

oxalaemia [Br.] SYN oxalemia.

ox•a•late (ok′să-lāt) A salt of oxalic acid.

ox•a•late cal•cu•lus (ok′să-lāt kal′kyū-lŭs) A urinary calculus of calcium oxalate.

ox•a•le•mi•a (ok-să-lē′mē-ă) The presence of an abnormally large amount of oxalate in the blood. SYN oxalaemia. [oxalate + G. *haima,* blood]

ox•al•ic ac•id (ok-sal′ik as′id) An acid found in many plants and vegetables; used as a hemostatic in veterinary medicine, but toxic when ingested by humans; also used in the removal of ink and other stains, and as a general reducing agent; salts of oxalic acid are found in renal calculi; accumulates in cases of primary hyperoxaluria.

ox•a•lo•a•ce•tic ac•id (ok′să-lō-ă-sē′tik as′id) A ketodicarboxylic acid and important intermediate in the tricarboxylic acid cycle.

ox•a•lo•suc•cin•ic ac•id (ok′să-lō-sŭk-sin′ik as′id) An enzyme-bound intermediate of the tricarboxylic acid cycle.

ox•a•lu•ri•a (ok-sal-yūr′ē-ă) SYN hyperoxaluria. [oxalate + G. *ouron,* urine]

ox•a•lyl•u•re•a (ok′să-lil-yūr′ē-ă) The cyclic (end-to-end) amide anhydride of oxaluric acid; an oxidation product of uric acid.

ox•a•zin dyes (oks′ă-zin dīz) Similar to azin dyes except that one of the connecting N atoms is replaced by O.

ox•a•zo•lid•i•nones (oks′ă-zō-lid′i-nōnz) Any of a new class of antibacterial antibiotics.

ox heart (oks hahrt) A very large heart, usually due to chronic hypertension or, more often, to aortic valve disease. SYN cor bovinum.

ox•i•dant (ok′si-dănt) The substance that is reduced and that, therefore, oxidizes the other component of an oxidation-reduction system.

ox•i•dase (ok′si-dās) One of a group of enzymes that bring about organic reactions in which O_2 acts as an acceptor (of H or of electrons).

ox•i•da•tion (ok′si-dā′shŭn) **1.** Combination with oxygen; increasing the valence of an atom or ion by the loss from it of hydrogen or of one or more electrons. **2.** BACTERIOLOGY the aerobic dissimilation of substrates with the production of energy and water; the transfer of electrons is accomplished through the respiratory chain, which uses oxygen as the final electron acceptor.

ox•i•da•tion-re•duc•tion (ok′si-dā′shŭn rē-dŭk′shŭn) Any chemical oxidation or reduction reaction, which must, in toto, comprise both oxidation and reduction; the basis for calling all oxidative enzymes (formerly oxidases) oxidoreductases. Often shortened to “redox.”

ox•i•da•tive (ok′si-dā′tiv) Having the power to oxidize; denoting a process involving oxidation.

ox·i·da·tive phos·pho·ryl·a·tion (ok′si-dā′tiv fos′fōr-i-lā′shŭn) Formation of high energy phosphoric bonds from the energy released by the dehydrogenation (*i.e.*, oxidation) of various substrates.

ox·ide (ok′sīd) A compound of oxygen with another element or a radical.

ox·i·dize (ok′si-dīz) To combine or cause an element or radical to combine with oxygen or to lose electrons.

ox·i·do·re·duc·tase (ok′si-dō-rē-dŭk′tās) An enzyme (EC class 1) catalyzing an oxidation-reduction reaction. Trivial names for oxidoreductases include dehydrogenase, reductase, oxidase, oxygenase, peroxidase, and hydroxylase. SEE ALSO oxidase.

ox·ime (ok′sēm) A compound resulting from the action of hydroxylamine, NH_2OH, on a ketone or an aldehyde to yield the group =N–OH attached to the former carbonyl carbon atom.

ox·im·e·ter (ok-sim′ĕ-tĕr) A laboratory instrument capable of measuring the concentration of oxyhemoglobin, reduced hemoglobin, carboxyhemoglobin, and methemoglobin in a sample of blood. SYN cooximeter, hemoximeter.

ox·im·e·try (ok-sim′ă-trē) Measurement with an oximeter of the oxygen saturation of hemoglobin in a sample of blood.

♻ **oxo-** Combining form denoting addition of oxygen; used in place of keto- in systematic nomenclature. SEE ALSO hydroxy-, oxa-, oxy-

3-ox·o·ac·yl-ACP re·duc·tase (oks′ō-as′il rē-dŭk′tās) An enzyme of the fatty acid synthase complex.

3-ox·o·ac·yl-ACP syn·thase (oks′ō-as′il sin′thās) An enzyme participating in fatty acid synthesis.

17-ox·o·ste·roids (oks′ō-ster′oydz) SYN 17-ketosteroids.

ox's tongue (oks′ĕz tŭng) SYN borage.

♻ **oxy-** **1.** Combining form meaning shrill; sharp, pointed; quick (incorrectly used for ocy-, from G. *ōkys*, swift). **2.** CHEMISTRY combining form denoting the presence of oxygen, either added or substituted, in a substance. SEE ALSO hydroxy-, oxa-, oxo-. [G. *oxys*, keen]

oxyaesthesia [Br.] SYN oxyesthesia.

ox·y·ce·phal·ic, ox·y·ceph·a·lous (ok′sē-se-fal′ik, -sef′ă-lŭs) Relating to or characterized by oxycephaly. SYN acrocephalic, acrocephalous.

ox·y·ceph·a·ly (ok′sē-sef′ă-lē) A type of craniosynostosis in which there is premature closure of the lambdoid and coronal sutures, resulting in an abnormally high, peaked, or cone-shaped cranium. SYN acrocephaly, acrocephalia. [G. *oxys*, pointed, + *kephalē*, head]

ox·y·chro·mat·ic (ok′sē-krō-mat′ik) SYN acidophilic. [G. *oxys*, sour, acid, + *chrōma*, color]

11-ox·y·cor·ti·coids (ok′sē-kōr′ti-koydz) Corticosteroids bearing an alcohol or ketonic group on carbon-11; e.g., cortisone, cortisol.

ox·y·es·the·si·a (ok′sē-es-thē′zē-ă) SYN hyperesthesia. SYN oxyaesthesia. [G. *oxys*, acute, + *aisthēsis*, sensation]

ox·y·gen (O) (ok′si-jĕn) **1.** A gaseous element, atomic no. 8, atomic wt. 15.9994 on basis of ^{12}C = 12.0000; an abundant and widely distributed chemical element, which combines with most of the other elements to form oxides and is essential to animal and plant life. **2.** The molecular form of oxygen, O_2. **3.** A medicinal gas that contains not less than 99.0%, by volume, of O_2. [G. *oxys*, sharp, acid and *genes*, forming]

ox·y·gen af·fin·i·ty hy·pox·i·a (ok′si-jĕn ă-fin′i-tē hī-pok′sē-ă) Hypoxia due to a reduced capacity of hemoglobin to release oxygen.

ox·y·gen·ase (ok′si-jĕ-nās) One of a group of enzymes (EC subclass 1.13) catalyzing direct incorporation of O_2 into substrates. Cf. dioxygenase, monooxygenases.

ox·y·gen·ate (ok′si-jĕ-nāt) To accomplish oxygenation.

ox·y·gen·a·tion (ok′si-jĕ-nā′shŭn) Addition of oxygen to any chemical or physical system.

ox·y·gen ca·pac·i·ty (ok′si-jĕn kă-pas′i-tē) The maximum quantity of oxygen that will combine chemically with the hemoglobin in a unit volume of blood; normally it amounts to 1.34 mL of O_2 per g of Hb or 20 ml of O_2 per 100 mL of blood.

ox·y·gen con·cen·tra·tor (ok′si-jĕn kon′sĕn-trā′tŏr) An electrically powered device for oxygen delivery in the home; it uses a filtering mechanism to separate oxygen from room air.

ox·y·gen con·sump·tion ($\mathring{V}O_2$) (ok′si-jĕn kŏn-sŭmp′shŭn) The volume of oxygen consumed by the body in 1 minute; it is reported in liters or mL per minute at STPD. SYN oxygen uptake.

ox·y·gen con·tent (ok′si-jĕn kon′tent) The total amount of oxygen carried in the blood; equal to the amount of oxygen carried by the hemoglobin in the red blood cells plus the amount of oxygen dissolved in the plasma.

ox·y·gen debt (ok′si-jĕn det) The extra oxygen, taken in by the body during recovery from exercise, beyond the resting needs of the body; sometimes used as if synonymous with oxygen deficit.

ox·y·gen def·i·cit (ok′si-jĕn def′i-sit) The difference between oxygen uptake of the body during early stages of exercise and during a similar duration in a steady state of exercise; sometimes considered as the formation of the oxygen debt.

ox·y·gen-de·rived free rad·i·cals (ok′si-jĕn dē-rīved′ frē ra′di-kălz) An atom or atom group having an unpaired electron on an oxygen atom, typically derived from molecular oxygen. For example, one-electron reduction of O_2 produces the superoxide radical, $\bar{O}_2\cdot$; other examples include the hydroperoxyl radical (HOO·), the hydroxyl radical (HO·), and nitric oxide (NO·). These apparently have a role in reprofusion injury.

ox·y·gen de·sat·u·ra·tion (ok′si-jĕn dē-sach′ŭr-ā′shŭn) A decrease in oxygen concentration in the blood resulting from any condition that affects the exchange of carbon dioxide and oxygen. SEE ALSO oxygen debt, oxygen deficit.

ox·y·gen di·lu·tion meth·od (ok′si-jen di-lū′shŭn meth′ŏd) A technique using 100% oxygen when assessing residual lung volume.

ox·y·gen en·hance·ment ra·ti·o (OER) (ok′si-jĕn en-hans′mĕnt rā′shē-ō) Ratio of the dose of radiation necessary to produce a given biologic response in the absence of oxygen to the dose required to achieve the same response in the presence of oxygen.

ox·y·gen ex·trac·tion (ok′si-jĕn eks-trak′shŭn) The amount of oxygen removed from the blood as it passes through capillaries (the difference between the oxygen content of arterial and venous blood).

ox·y·gen pulse ($\mathring{V}O_2$ HR) (ok′si-jĕn pŭls) Volume of oxygen consumed by the body per heartbeat.

ox·y·gen sat·u·ra·tion (SaO_2) (ok-si′jĕn sach′ŭr-ā′shŭn) The percentage of oxygen-binding sites in blood that are combined with oxygen.

ox·y·gen sat·u·ra·tion test (SaO_2 test) (ok′si-jĕn sach′ŭr-ā′shŭn tĕst) Noninvasive measurement of blood oxygen saturation by differential absorption of red and infrared light beams with an oximeter applied to the skin.

ox·y·gen ther·a·py (oks′i-jĕn thār′ă-pē) A medically supervised use of pure oxygen, hydrogen peroxide, or ozone to treat a wide range of health problems. SYN biooxidative therapy.

ox·y·gen tox·ic·i·ty (ok′si-jĕn tok-sis′i-tē) A body disturbance resulting from breathing high partial pressures of oxygen; characterized by visual and hearing abnormalities, unusual fatigue while breathing, muscular twitching, anxiety, confusion, incoordination, and convulsions.

ox·y·gen up·take (ok′si-jĕn up′tāk) SYN oxygen consumption.

ox·y·geu·si·a (ok-sē-gū′sē-ă) SYN hypergeusia. [G. *oxys,* acute, + *geusis,* taste]

oxyhaeme [Br.] SYN oxyheme.

oxyhaemochromogen [Br.] SYN oxyhemochromogen.

oxyhaemoglobin [Br.] SYN oxyhemoglobin.

oxyhaemoglobin dissociation curve [Br.] SYN oxyhemoglobin dissociation curve.

ox·y·heme (ok′si-hēm) SYN hematin. SYN oxyhaeme.

ox·y·he·mo·chro·mo·gen (ok′sē-hēm′ō-krō′mō-jen) SYN hematin. SYN oxyhaemochromogen.

ox·y·he·mo·glo·bin (ok′sē-hē′mō-glō′bin) Hemoglobin in combination with oxygen; the form of hemoglobin present in arterial blood, scarlet or bright red when dissolved in water. SYN oxyhaemoglobin.

ox·y·he·mo·glo·bin dis·so·ci·a·tion curve (ok′sē-hē′mō-glōb′in di-sō′sē-ā′shŭn kŭrv) A graphic illustration of the relationship between oxygen saturation of hemoglobin and the partial pressure of arterial oxygen (PaO_2); the position and overall shape of this sigmoidal curve are affected by the hydrogen ion concentration (pH), body temperature, partial pressure of carbon dioxide (PCO_2), and organic phosphates. SYN oxyhaemoglobin dissociation curve.

ox·y·my·o·glo·bin (MbO_2) (ok′sē-mī′ō-glō′bin) Myoglobin in its oxygenated form, analogous in structure to oxyhemoglobin. SEE ALSO myoglobin.

ox·yn·tic (ok-sin′tik) Acid-forming, e.g., the parietal cells of the gastric glands. [G. *oxynō,* to sharpen, make sour, acid]

ox·yn·tic cell (ok-sin′tik sel) SYN parietal cell.

ox·y·phil, **ox·y·phile** (ok′sē-fil, -fīl) **1.** Oxyphil *cell.* **2.** SYN eosinophilic leukocyte. **3.** SYN oxyphilic. [G. *oxys,* sour, acid, + *philos,* fond]

ox·y·phil cell (ok′sē-fil sel) Cell of the parathyroid gland that increase in number with age; the cytoplasm contains numerous mitochondria and stains with eosin. Similar cells, and tumors composed of them, are found in salivary glands and the thyroid; in the latter, also called Hürthle cell.

ox·y·phil·ic (ok′sē-fil′ik) Having an affinity for acid dyes; denoting certain cell or tissue elements. SYN oxyphil (3), oxyphile.

ox·y·phil·ic car·ci·no·ma (ok′sē-fil′ik kahr′si-nō′mă) SYN Hürthle cell carcinoma.

ox·y·phil·ic leu·ko·cyte (ok′sē-fil′ik lū′kō-sīt) SYN eosinophilic leukocyte.

ox·y·pho·ni·a (ok-sē-fō′nē-ă) Shrillness or high pitch of the voice. [G. *oxys,* sharp, + *phōnē,* voice]

ox·y·ta·lan (ok-sit′ă-lan) A type of connective tissue fiber found in the periodontal ligaments of a number of animals having the same ultrastructural features as immature elastin, i.e., microfilaments without the elastin. [G. *oxys,* acid, + *talas,* suffering, resisting; coined term probably intended to mean "resistant to acid hydrolysis"]

ox·y·to·ci·a (ok′sē-tō′shē-ă) Rapid parturition. [G. *okytokos,* swift birth]

ox·y·to·cic (ok′sē-tō′sik) Hastening childbirth.

ox·y·to·cin (ok′sē-tō′sin) A nonapeptide neurohypophysial hormone that causes myometrial contractions at term and promotes milk release during lactation; used for the induction or stimulation of labor, in the management of postpartum hemorrhage and atony, and to relieve painful breast engorgement. It is produced in the posterior pituitary gland. [G. *oxytokos,* swift birth]

ox·y·to·cin chal·lenge test (ok′sē-tō′sin chal′ĕnj test) A contraction stress test accomplished by administration of intravenous dilute oxytocin solution to stimulate contractions. SYN contraction stress test.

ox·y·u·ri·a·sis (ok′sē-yūr-ī′ă-sis) Infection with nematode parasites of the genus *Oxyuris.*

ox·y·u·ri·cide (ok′sē-yūr′i-sīd) An agent that destroys pinworms. [oxyurid + L. *caedo,* to kill]

ox·y·u·rid (ok-sē-yū′rid) Common name for members of the family Oxyuridae. [see *Oxyuris*]

Ox·y·u·ri·dae (ok′sē-yū′ri-dē) A family of parasitic nematodes found in the large intestine or cecum of vertebrates and the intestine of invertebrates, especially insects and millipedes.

Ox·y·u·ris (ok′sē-yū′ris) A genus of nematodes commonly called seatworms or pinworms (although the pinworm of humans is the closely related form, *Enterobius vermicularis*). [G. *oxys,* sharp, + *oura,* tail]

♲**-oyl** Suffix denoting an acyl radical; -yl replaces -ic in acid names.

ozaena [Br.] SYN ozena.

o·ze·na (ō-zē′nă) A disease characterized by intranasal crusting, atrophy, and fetid odor. SYN ozaena. [G. *ozaina,* a fetid polyp, fr. *ozō,* to smell]

o·zone (ō′zōn) A powerful oxidizing agent; air containing a perceptible amount of O_3 formed by an electric discharge or by the slow combustion of phosphorus; also formed by the action of solar UV radiation on atmospheric O_2. [G. *ozō,* to smell]

P

π, Π Pi. SEE pi.

φ, Φ Phi. SEE phi.

Ψ Psi. SEE psi.

P_{CO_2}, pCO_2 Abbreviation for partial pressure (tension) of carbon dioxide. SEE partial pressure.

P_i Abbreviation for inorganic orthophosphate.

P_b Abbreviation for barometric pressure.

p **1.** Abbreviation for pupil, optic papilla. **2.** In polynucleotide symbolism, phosphoric ester or phosphate. **3.** Abbreviation for pico- (2); momentum (*p*). **4.** CYTOGENETICS the short arm of a chromosome. [fr. Fr. *petit,* small] **5.** In nucleic acid terminology, symbol for phosphoric residue.

p53 A tumor suppressor gene located on the short arm of chromosome 17 that encodes a nucleophosphoprotein that binds DNA and negatively regulates cell division; frequently measured as a marker of malignant diseases.

P_1 Abbreviation for parental generation.

P_2 Symbol for the second pulmonic heart sound.

PA Abbreviation for posteroanterior.

P & A **1.** Abbreviation for posterior and anterior. **2.** Abbreviation for percussion and auscultation.

Pa **1.** Abbreviation for pascal. **2.** Symbol for protactinium.

paan (pahn) SYN betel palm (nut).

Paas dis•ease (pahz di-zēz′) A familial skeletal deformation marked by coxa valga, double patella, shortening of the middle and terminal phalanges of fingers and toes, deformities of the elbows, scoliosis, and spondylitis deformans of the lumbar vertebrae; all these manifestations may be unilateral or bilateral.

PABA Abbreviation for *p*-aminobenzoic acid.

pab•lum (pab′lŭm) A precooked infant food, a mixture of wheat, oat, and corn meals, wheat embryo, alfalfa leaves, brewers' yeast, iron, and sodium chloride. SYN pabulum. [L. *pabulum,* nourishment, fr. *pasco,* to nourish]

pab•u•lum (pab′yū-lŭm) SYN pablum. [L. *pabulum,* foodstuff]

PA-C Abbreviation for physician assistant, certified.

PAC Abbreviation for premature atrial contraction.

pac•chi•o•ni•an (pahk-ē-ō′nē-ăn) Attributed to or described by Antonio Pacchioni (1665–1726).

pac•chi•o•ni•an bod•ies (pahk-ē-ō′nē-ăn bod′ēz) SYN arachnoid granulations.

pace•fol•low•er (pās′fol-ō-ĕr) Any cell in excitable tissue that responds to stimuli from a pacemaker.

pace•ma•ker (pās′mā-kĕr) **1.** Biologically, any rhythmic center that establishes a pace of activity. **2.** An artificial regulator of rate activity. **3.** CHEMISTRY the substance with a rate of reaction that sets the pace for a series of chain reactions. [L. *passus,* step, pace]

pace•ma•ker lead (pās′mā-kĕr lēd) A wire transmitting impulses from an artificial pacemaker to the heart.

pace•ma•ker rule (pās′mā-kĕr rūl) The pacemaker site with the fastest rate will control the heart.

pace•ma•ker syn•drome (pās′mā-kĕr sin′drōm) A complex of signs and symptoms that occur when AV synchrony is lost during pacing and relieved when AV synchrony is restored. Should be suspected if preimplantation symptoms recur in the presence of a properly functioning pacemaker. Symptoms may include vertigo, syncope, dyspnea, weakness, orthopnea, and postural hypotension.

Pa•che•co par•rot dis•ease vi•rus (pa-chā′kō par′ŏt di-zēz′ vī′rŭs) A virus of the family Herpesviridae, possibly related to the virus causing infectious laryngotracheitis.

Pa•chon meth•od (pah-shōn[h]′ meth′ŏd) Cardiography carried out with the patient lying on his or her left side.

Pa•chon test (pah-shōn[h]′ test) In a case of aneurysm, determination of the collateral circulation by estimation of the blood pressure.

♻**pachy-** Combining form meaning thick. [G. *pachys,* thick]

pach•y•bleph•a•ron (pak-ē-blef′ă-ron) Thickening of the tarsal border of the eyelid. [pachy- + G. *blepharon,* eyelid]

pach•y•ce•phal•ic, pach•y•ceph•a•lous (pak′ē-se-fal′ik, -sef′ă-lŭs) Relating to or marked by pachycephaly.

pach•y•ceph•a•ly (pak-ē-sef′ă-lē) Abnormal thickness of the skull. [pachy- + G. *kephalē,* head]

pach•y•chei•li•a, pach•y•chi•li•a (pak-ē-kī′lē-ă) Swelling or abnormal thickness of the lips. [pachy- + G. *cheilos,* lip]

pach•y•cho•li•a (pak′i-kō′lē-ă) An increased thickening of bile. [pachy- + -cholia, condition of bile]

pach•y•chro•mat•ic (pak-ē-krō-mat′ik) Having a coarse chromatin reticulum.

pach•y•dac•ty•ly (pak-ē-dak′ti-lē) Enlargement of the fingers or toes, especially extremities; often seen in neurofibromatosis. [pachy- + G. *daktylos,* finger or toe]

pach·y·der·ma (pak-ē-dĕr′mă) Abnormally thick skin. SEE ALSO elephantiasis. [pachy- + G. *derma,* skin]

pach·y·der·ma la·ryn·gis (pak-ē-dĕr′mă lă-rinj′is) A circumscribed connective tissue hyperplasia at the posterior commissure of the larynx.

pach·y·der·mat·o·cele (pak-ē-der-mat′ō-sēl) SYN dermatochalasis. [pachy- + G. *derma,* skin, + *kēlē,* tumor]

pach·y·der·mo·dac·ty·ly (pak-ē-dĕr′mo-dak′ti-lē) Digital swelling due to diffuse fibromatosis occurring on the proximal interphalangeal joints of the index, middle, and ring fingers (sometimes involving the fifth finger, rarely the thumb); a familial form exists.

pach·y·glos·si·a (pak-ē-glos′ē-ă) An enlarged, thick tongue. [pachy- + G. *glōssa,* tongue]

pach·y·gy·ri·a (pak-ē-jī′rē-ă) Condition in which the convolutions of the cerebral cortex are abnormally large; there are fewer sulci than normal and the amount of brain substance may be increased. [pachy- + G. *gyros,* circle]

pach·y·lep·to·men·in·gi·tis (pak-ē-lep′tō-men-in-jī′tis) Inflammation of all membranes of the brain or spinal cord. [G. *pachys,* thick, + *leptos,* thin, + *mēninx* (*mēning-*), membrane, + *-itis,* inflammation]

pach·y·men·in·gi·tis (pak′ē-men-in-jī′tis) Inflammation of the dura mater. SYN perimeningitis. [pachy- + G. *mēninx,* membrane, + *-itis,* inflammation]

pach·y·me·nin·gop·a·thy (pak′ē-mĕn-in-gop′ă-thē) Disease of the dura mater. [pachy- + G. *mēninx* (*mēning-*), membrane, + *pathos,* disease]

pach·y·me·ninx (pak-ē-mē′ningks) [TA] The dura mater. [pachy- + G. *mēninx,* membrane]

pa·chyn·sis (pă-kin′sis) Any pathologic thickening. [G. a thickening]

pa·chyn·tic (pă-kin′tic) Relating to pachynsis.

pach·y·o·nych·i·a (pak′ē-ō-nik′ē-ă) Abnormal thickness of the fingernails or toenails. [pachy- + G. *onyx,* nail]

pach·y·per·i·os·ti·tis (pak′ē-per-ē-ŏs-tī′tis) Proliferative thickening of the periosteum caused by inflammation. [pachy- + periostitis]

pach·y·per·i·to·ni·tis (pak′ē-per′i-tō-nī′tis) Inflammation of the peritoneum with thickening of the membrane. [pachy- + peritonitis]

pach·y·pleu·ri·tis (pak′ē-plū-rī′tis) Inflammation of the pleura with thickening of the membrane. [pachy- + pleura + G. *-itis,* inflammation]

pach·y·sal·pin·gi·tis (pak′ē-sal-pin-jī′tis) SYN chronic interstitial salpingitis.

pach·y·sal·pin·go-o·va·ri·tis (pak′ē-sal-pin′gō-ō-va-rī′tis) Chronic parenchymatous inflammation of the ovary and uterine (fallopian) tube. [pachy- + salpinx + Mod. L. *ovarium,* ovary, + G. *-itis,* inflammation]

pach·y·so·mi·a (pak-ē-sō′mē-ă) Pathologic thickening of the soft parts of the body, notably in acromegaly. [pachy- + G. *sōma,* body]

pach·y·tene (pak′i-tēn) The stage of prophase in meiosis in which pairing of homologous chromosomes is complete; longitudinal cleavage occurs in each chromosome to form two sister chromatids so that each homologous chromosome pair becomes a set of four intertwined chromatids. [pachy- + G. *tainia,* band, tape]

pach·y·vag·i·nal·i·tis (pak′ē-vaj-i-năl-ī′tis) Chronic inflammation with thickening of the tunica vaginalis testis. [pachy- + Mod. L. (tunica) *vaginalis,* + G. *-itis,* inflammation]

pach·y·vag·i·ni·tis (pak′ē-vaj-i-nī′tis) Chronic vaginitis with thickening and induration of the vaginal walls. [pachy- + vagina + G. *-itis,* inflammation]

pac·ing cath·e·ter (pā′sing kath′ĕ-tĕr) A cardiac catheter with one or more electrodes at its tip that can be used to artificially pace the heart; usually inserted into a patient's right ventricle.

pa·ci·ni·an (pă-chē′nē-ăn) Attributed to or described by Filippo Pacini (1812–1883).

pa·ci·ni·an cor·pus·cles (pă-chē′ē-ăn kōr′pŭs′elz) SYN lamellated corpuscles.

pack (pak) **1.** To fill, stuff, or tampon. **2.** To enwrap or envelop the body in a sheet, blanket, or other covering. **3.** To apply a dressing or covering to a surgical site. **4.** Prepackaged organized container for medications. [M.E. *pak,* fr. Germanic]

pack·age (păk′ăj) **1.** A box or container in which something can be packed for transport or storage. **2.** A parcel consisting of such a container and its contents. [pack + -age]

pack·age in·sert (pak′ăj in′sĕrt) A manufacturer's printed guideline for the use and dosing of a drug; includes the pharmacokinetics, dosage forms, and other relevant information about a drug.

packed cells (pakt selz) A blood product consisting of concentrated cells, most of the plasma having been removed; given to the patient who needs red blood cells but not increased fluid volume, e.g., the patient in congestive heart failure. SYN packed red blood cells.

packed red blood cells (pakt red blŭd selz) SYN packed cells.

pack·er (pak′ĕr) **1.** An instrument for tamponing. **2.** SYN plugger.

pack·ing (pak′ing) **1.** Filling a natural cavity, a

wound, or a mold with some material. **2.** The material so used. **3.** The application of a pack.

pack years (pak′ yērz) Person's cigarette consumption calculated as the packs of cigarettes smoked per day, multiplied by the length of consumption in years (e.g., 1.5 packs of cigarettes smoked per day for 20 years is 30 pack years).

PA con•duc•tion time (kŏn-dŭk′shŭn tīm) SEE atrioventricular conduction.

PACS (paks) Acronym for picture archive and communication system, a computer network for digitized radiologic images and reports.

PACU Abbreviation for postanesthesia care unit.

PAD Abbreviation for peripheral arterial disease.

pad (pad) **1.** A thin cushion of resilient or absorbent material applied to relieve pressure or absorb fluid. **2.** A more or less encapsulated body of fat or some other tissue serving to fill a space or act as a cushion in the body.

PADL Abbreviation for personal activities of daily living.

pad-to-pad pinch (pad pad pinch) OCCUPATIONAL THERAPY a grip between the thumb pad and the index finger pad distal to the distal interphalangeal joint.

PAE Abbreviation for postantibiotic effect.

Pae•cil•o•my•ces (pē-sil-ō-mī′sēz) A genus of saprophytic deuteromycetous fungi with conidia-bearing hyphae that superficially resemble the penicilli of *Penicillium;* occasional opportunistic human pathogen that causes pulmonary infection, keratitis, and endocarditis.

Pae•cil•o•my•ces li•la•ci•nus (pē-sil-ō-mī′sēz li-lā′si-nŭs) A mold; a rare cause of paecilomycosis; has been implicated in human eye infections due to contaminated implanted intraocular lenses; formerly *Penicillium lilacinum.*

paed- [Br.] SYN ped-.

paederasty [Br.] SYN pederasty.

paedi- [Br.] SYN pedi-.

-paedia [Br.] SYN -pedia.

paediatric [Br.] SYN pediatric.

paediatric dentist [Br.] SYN pediatric dentist.

paediatric dentistry [Br.] SYN pediatric dentistry.

paediatrician [Br.] SYN pediatrician.

paediatrics [Br.] SYN pediatrics.

paedo- [Br.] SYN pedo-.

paedodontia [Br.] SYN pedodontia.

paedodontics [Br.] SYN pedodontics.

paedodontist [Br.] SYN pedodontist.

paedomorphism [Br.] SYN pedomorphism.

paedophilia [Br.] SYN pedophilia.

paedophilic [Br.] SYN pedophilic.

PAF Abbreviation for platelet-aggregating factor.

PAGE (pāj) Acronym for polyacrylamide gel electrophoresis.

Pa•gen•stech•er cir•cle (pah′gen-stek-ĕr sĭr′kĕl) In the case of a freely movable abdominal tumor, the mass is moved throughout its entire range, its position at intervals being marked on the abdominal wall; when these points are joined, a circle is formed, the center of which marks the point of attachment of the tumor.

Pa•get cell (paj′ĕt sel) A relatively large, neoplastic epithelial cell (carcinoma cell) with a hyperchromatic nucleus and abundant palely staining cytoplasm; in Paget disease of the breast, such cells occur in neoplastic epithelium in the ducts and in the epidermis of the nipple, areola, and adjacent skin.

Pa•get dis•ease (paj′ĕt di-zēz′) **1.** A generalized skeletal disease, frequently familial, of older people in which bone resorption and formation are both increased, leading to thickening and softening of bones (e.g., the skull), and bending of weight-bearing bones; SYN osteitis deformans. **2.** A disease of elderly women, characterized by an infiltrated, somewhat eczematous lesion surrounding and involving the nipple and areola, and associated with subjacent intraductal cancer of the breast and infiltration of the lower epidermis by malignant cells. **3.** SYN extramammary Paget disease. See page 1142.

pag•et•oid cells (paj′ĕt-oyd selz) Atypical melanocytes resembling Paget cells, found in some cutaneous melanomas.

pa•go•pha•gi•a (pāg′ō-fā′jē-ă) The compulsive eating of ice, often a symptom of iron deficiency. [G. *pagos,* frost + *phagia,* eating]

-pagus Suffix indicating conjoined twins, the first element of the word denoting the parts fused. SEE ALSO -didymus, -dymus. [G. *pagos,* something fixed, fr. *pēgnymi,* to fasten together]

PAI-1 Abbreviation for plasminogen activator inhibitor-1.

pain (pān) An unpleasant sensation associated with actual or potential tissue damage, and mediated by specific nerve fibers to the brain, where its conscious appreciation may be modified by various factors. See page 1143. [L. *poena,* a fine, a penalty]

pain•ful arc sign (pān′ful ahrk sīn) Pain elicited during active abduction of the upper extremity between 60 and 120 degrees.

pain•ful heel (pān′ful hēl) A condition in which

bearing weight on the heel causes pain of varying severity. SYN calcaneodynia, calcodynia.

pain-plea•sure prin•ci•ple (pān-ple′zhŭr prin′si-pĕl) PSYCHOANALYSIS the concept that one tends to seek pleasure and avoid pain; a term borrowed by experimental psychology to denote the same tendency of an animal in a learning situation. SYN pleasure principle.

pain-spasm-is•che•mi•a cy•cle (pān-spazm-is-kē′mē-ă sī′kĕl) SYN pain-spasm-pain cycle.

pain-spasm-pain cy•cle (pān-spazm-pān sī′kĕl) A self-perpetuating cycle in which skeletal muscle spasm causes local ischemia and pain, which exacerbates the spasm, which in turn exacerbates the pain. SEE ALSO myofascial pain-dysfunction syndrome, trigger point. SYN pain-spasm-ischemia cycle.

PA in•ter•val (in′tĕr-văl) The time from onset of the P wave to the initial rapid deflection of the A wave in the His bundle electrogram (normally 25–45 msec); it represents the intraatrial conduction time.

pal•a•tal (pal′ă-tăl) Relating to the palate or the palate bone. SYN palatine.

pal•a•tal lift (pal′ă-tăl lift) A prosthetic device designed to fit against the hard palate, anchored by the teeth, with an extension along the soft palate to occlude part of the velopharyngeal opening. The device is used mainly by people with weak velopharyngeal musculature or excessively wide velopharyngeal openings, to reduce nasal resonance and airflow during speech.

pal•a•tal my•oc•lo•nus (pal′ă-tăl mī-ok′lō-nŭs) Tinnitus that may be elicited by contractions of the soft palate. It is classified as an extracochlear muscular somatosound.

pal•a•tal re•flex, pal•a•tine re•flex (pal′ă-tăl rē′fleks, pal′ă-tīn rē′fleks) Swallowing reflex induced by stimulation of the palate.

pal•ate (pal′ăt) The bony and muscular partition between the oral and nasal cavities. SYN palatum [TA]. [L. *palatum,* palate]

pal•a•tine (pal′ă-tīn) SYN palatal.

pal•a•tine ap•o•neu•ro•sis (pal′ă-tīn ap′ō-nūr-ō′sis) The expanded interlacing tendons of the tensor veli palatini muscles in the anterior two thirds of the soft palate to which the other palatine muscles attach.

pal•a•tine bone (pal′ă-tīn bōn) An irregularly shaped bone posterior to the maxilla, which enters into the formation of the nasal cavity, the orbit, and the hard palate; it articulates with the maxilla, inferior nasal concha, sphenoid, and ethmoid bones, the vomer and its fellow of the opposite side.

pal•a•tine pro•cess (pal′ă-tīn pros′es) In the embryo, medially directed shelves from the oral surface of the maxillae; they develop into the secondary palate after midline fusion.

pal•a•tine ra•phe (pal′ă-tīn rā′fē) A rather narrow, low elevation in the center of the hard palate that extends from the incisive papilla posteriorly over the entire length of the mucosa of the hard palate.

pal•a•tine spines (pal′ă-tīn spīnz) The longitudinal ridges along the palatine grooves on the

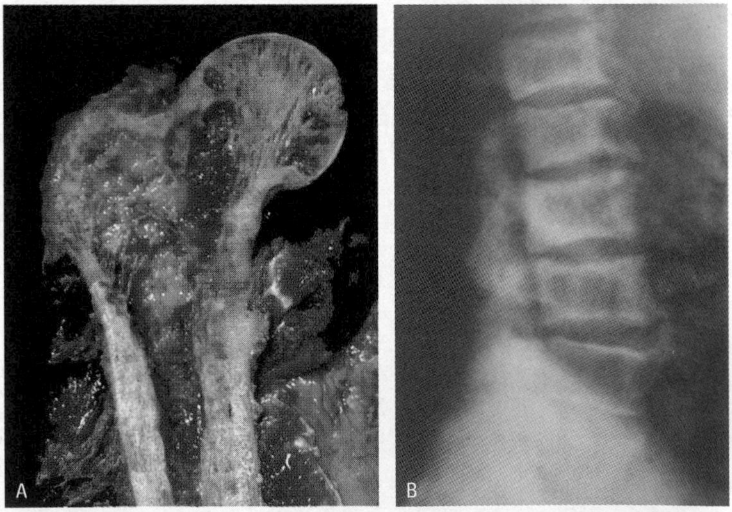

Paget disease: (A) gross specimen of proximal femur showing cortical thickening and coarse trabeculations of the femoral head and neck; (B) Paget disease of spine shows shortening and widening of lumbar vertebral bodies, cortices and endplates are thickened and have "picture-frame" appearance

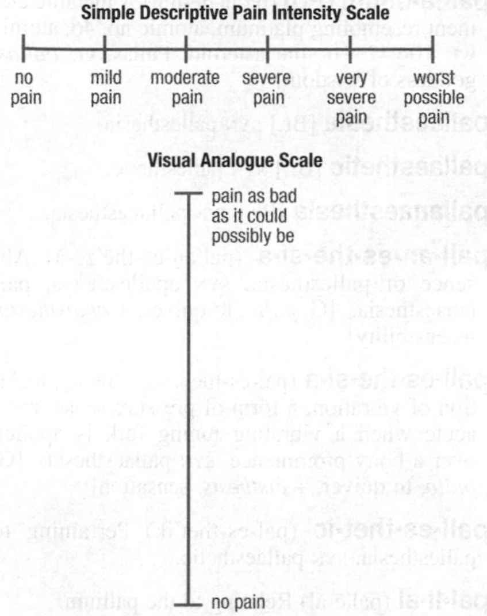

pain scales: patient indicates level of pain by marking appropriate site on scale chosen

inferior surface of the palatine process of the maxilla.

pal·a·tine ton·sil (pal′ă-tīn ton′sil) A large, oval mass of lymphoid tissue embedded in the lateral wall of the oropharynx on either side between the pillars of the fauces. SYN tonsilla palatina [TA], tonsilla [TA], faucial tonsil, tonsil (2).

pal·a·tine u·vu·la (pal′ă-tīn yū′vyū-lă) A conic projection from the posterior edge of the middle of the soft palate, composed of connective tissue containing a number of racemose glands, and some muscular fibers (musculus uvulae).

pal·a·tine vein (pal′ă-tīn vān) Drains the palatine regions and empties into the facial vein.

pal·a·ti·tis (pal-ă-tī′tis) Inflammation of the palate.

♻ **palato-** Combining form meaning palate. [L. *palatum,* palate]

pal·a·to·glos·sal (pal′ă-tō-glos′ăl) Relating to the palate and the tongue, or to the palatoglossus muscle.

pal·a·to·glos·sal arch (pal′ă-tō-glos′ăl ahrch) One of a pair of ridges or folds of mucous membrane passing from the soft palate to the side of the tongue; it encloses the palatoglossus muscle and forms the anterior margin of the tonsillar fossa. Also demarcates the oral cavity from the isthmus of fauces.

pal·a·to·glos·sus mus·cle (pal′ă-tō-glos′ŭs mŭs′ĕl) Forms anterior pillar of tonsillar fossa; *origin,* oral surface of soft palate; *insertion,* side of tongue; *action,* raises back of tongue and narrows fauces; *nerve supply,* pharyngeal plexus (cranial root of accessory nerve). SYN musculus palatoglossus [TA].

pal·a·tog·na·thous (pal-ă-tog′nă-thŭs) Having a cleft palate. [palato- + G. *gnathos,* jaw]

pal·a·to·max·il·lar·y (pal′ă-tō-mak′si-lar-ē) Relating to the palate and the maxilla.

pal·a·to·na·sal (pal′ă-tō-nā′zăl) Relating to the palate and the nasal cavity.

pal·a·to·pha·ryn·ge·al (pal′ă-tō-fă-rin′jē-ăl) Relating to the palate and the pharynx.

pal·a·to·pha·ryn·ge·al arch (pal′ă-tō-fă-rin′jē-ăl ahrch) One of a pair of ridges or folds of mucous membrane that pass downward from the posterior margin of the soft palate to the lateral wall of the pharynx. It encloses the palatopharyngeus muscle and forms the posterior margin of the tonsillar fossa. It also demarcates the isthmus of the fauces from the oropharynx.

pal·a·to·pha·ryn·ge·al mus·cle (pal′ă-tō-fă-rin′jē-ăl mŭs′ĕl) SYN palatopharyngeus muscle.

pal·a·to·pha·ryn·ge·us mus·cle (pal′ă-tō-fă-rin′jē-us mŭs′ĕl) *Origin,* soft palate; forms the posterior pillar of the fauces or tonsillar fossa; *insertion,* posterior border of thyroid cartilage and aponeurosis of pharynx; *action,* narrows fauces, depresses soft palate, elevates pharynx and larynx; *nerve supply,* pharyngeal plexus (cranial root of accessory nerve). SYN musculus palatopharyngeus [TA], palatopharyngeal muscle.

pal·a·to·pha·ryn·gor·rha·phy (pal′ă-tō-far′in-gōr′ă-fē) SYN staphylopharyngorrhaphy. [palato- + pharynx + G. *rhaphē,* suture]

pal·a·to·plas·ty (pal′ă-tō-plas-tē) Surgery of the palate to restore form and function. SYN staphyloplasty, uranoplasty. [palato- + G. *plassō,* to form]

pal·a·to·ple·gi·a (pal′ă-tō-plē′jē-ă) Paralysis of the muscles of the soft palate. [palato- + G. *plēgē,* stroke]

pal·a·tor·rha·phy (pal-ă-tōr′ă-fē) The surgical repair of a cleft palate. SYN staphylorrhaphy, uranorrhaphy. [palato- + G. *rhaphē,* suture]

pal·a·tos·chi·sis (pal-ă-tos′ki-sis) SYN cleft palate. [palato- + G. *schisis,* fissure]

pa·la·tum, pl. **pa·la·ti** (pă-lā′tŭm, -tī) [TA] SYN palate. [L.]

PALE Abbreviation for postantibiotic leukocyte enhancement.

♻ **paleo-, pale-** Combining forms meaning old, primordial, primary, early. [G. *palaios,* old, ancient]

pa·le·o·cer·e·bel·lum (pā′lē-ō-ser-ĕ-bel′ŭm) [TA] The portion of the cerebellum including most of the vermis and the adjacent zones of the cerebellar hemispheres rostral to the primary fissure, corresponding to the zone of distribution of the spinocerebellar tracts; in phylogenetic age, it is thought to be intermediate between the archicerebellum and the neocerebellum. SYN spinocerebellum [TA]. [paleo- + L. *cerebellum*]

pa•le•o•cor•tex (pā′lē-ō-kōr′teks) [TA] The oldest part phylogenetically of the cortical mantle of the cerebral hemisphere, represented by the olfactory cortex.

pa•le•o•ki•net•ic (pā′lē-ō-ki-net′ik) Denoting the primitive motor mechanisms underlying muscular reflexes and automatic, stereotyped movements. [paleo- + G. *kinētikos,* relating to movement]

pa•le•o•pa•thol•o•gy (pā′lē-ō-pă-thol′ŏ-jē) The science of disease in prehistoric times as revealed in bones, mummies, and archaeologic artifacts. [paleo- + pathology]

pa•le•o•stri•a•tal (pā′lē-ō-strī-ā′tăl) Relating to the paleostriatum.

pa•le•o•stri•a•tum (pā′lē-ō-strī-ā′tŭm) Term denoting the globus pallidus and expressing the hypothesis that this component of the striate body developed earlier in evolution than the so-called neostriatum or striatum (caudate nucleus and putamen) and that it is a diencephalic derivative. [paleo- + L. *striatum*]

pa•le•o•thal•a•mus (pā′lē-ō-thal′ă-mŭs) The intralaminar nuclei, believed to be the earliest components of the thalamus to have evolved; they lack reciprocal connections with the isocortex.

pal•i•ki•ne•si•a, **pal•i•ci•ne•si•a** (pal′i-ki-nē′zē-ă, pal′i-si-nē′zē-ă) Involuntary repetition of movements. [G. *palin,* again, + *kinēsis,* movement]

pal•i•la•li•a (pal-i-lā′lē-ă) SYN paliphrasia. [G. *palin,* again, + *lalia,* a form of speech]

pal•in•drome (pal′in-drōm) MOLECULAR BIOLOGY a self-complementary nucleic acid sequence; a sequence identical to its complementary strand, if both are “read” in the same 5′–3′ direction, or inverted repeating sequences running in opposite directions (but same 5′- to 3′-direction) on either side of an axis of symmetry; palindromes occur at sites of important reactions. [G. *palindromos,* a running back]

pal•in•dro•mi•a (pal-in-drō′mē-ă) A relapse or recurrence of a disease. [G. *palindromos,* a running back, + *-ia,* condition]

pal•in•drom•ic (pal-in-drom′ik) Recurring.

pal•i•nop•si•a (pal-i-nop′sē-ă) Abnormal recurring visual hallucinations. [G. *palin,* again, + *opsis,* vision]

pal•i•phra•si•a (pal-i-frā′zē-ă) In speech, involuntary repetition of words or sentences. SEE ALSO echolalia. SYN palilalia. [G. *palin,* again, + *phrasis,* speech]

pal•la•di•um (Pd) (pă-lā′dē-ŭm) A metallic element resembling platinum, atomic no. 46, atomic wt. 106.42. [fr. the asteroid, Pallas; G. *Pallas,* goddess of wisdom]

pallaesthesia [Br.] SYN pallesthesia.

pallaesthetic [Br.] SYN pallesthetic.

pallanaesthesia [Br.] SYN pallanesthesia.

pall•an•es•the•si•a (pal′an-es-thē′zē-ă) Absence of pallesthesia. SYN apallesthesia, pallanaesthesia. [G. *pallō,* to quiver, + *anaisthēsia,* insensibility]

pall•es•the•si•a (pal-es-thē′zē-ă) The appreciation of vibration, a form of pressure sense; most acute when a vibrating tuning fork is applied over a bony prominence. SYN pallaesthesia. [G. *pallō,* to quiver, + *aisthēsis,* sensation]

pall•es•thet•ic (pal-es-thet′ik) Pertaining to pallesthesia. SYN pallaesthetic.

pal•li•al (pal′ē-ăl) Relating to the pallium.

pal•li•ate (pal′ē-āt) To reduce the severity of; to relieve slightly. SYN mitigate. [L. *palliatus* (adj.), dressed in a *pallium,* cloaked]

pal•li•a•tive (pal′ē-ă-tiv) Reducing the severity of; denoting the alleviation of symptoms without curing the underlying disease.

pal•li•a•tive treat•ment (pal′ē-ă-tiv trēt′mĕnt) Therapy that alleviates symptoms but does not cure the disease.

pal•lid (pal′id) Pale, faint, or deficient in color. [L. *pallidus,* pale]

pal•li•dal (pal′i-dăl) Relating to the pallidum.

pal•li•dec•to•my (pal-i-dek′tŏ-mē) Excision or destruction of the globus pallidus, usually by stereotaxy. [pallidum + G. *ektomē,* excision]

pal•li•do•an•sot•o•my (pal′i-dō-an-sot′ŏ-mē) Production of lesions in the globus pallidus and ansa lenticularis.

pal•li•dot•o•my (pal-i-dot′ŏ-mē) A destructive operation on the globus pallidus, done to relieve involuntary movements or muscular rigidity. [pallidum + G. *tomē,* incision]

pal•li•dum (pal′i-dŭm) SYN globus pallidus. [L. *pallidus,* pale]

pal•li•um (pal′ē-ŭm) [TA] The cerebral cortex with the subjacent white substance. SYN mantle (2). [L. cloak]

pal•lor (pal′ŏr) Paleness, as of the skin. [L.]

palm (pahlm) The flat of the hand; the flexor or anterior surface of the hand, exclusive of the thumb and fingers; the opposite of the dorsum. SYN palma [TA]. [L. *palma*]

pal•ma, pl. **pal•mae** (pahl′mă, -mē) [TA] SYN palm, palm. [L.]

pal•mar (pahl′măr) Pertaining to the palm of the hand or the caudal aspect of the carpus on the forelimb of an animal. [L. *palmaris,* fr. *palma*]

pal•mar arch (pahl′măr ahrch) **1.** Deep palmar arch; the arterial arch located deep to the long flexor tendons in the hand, formed by the radial artery and the deep palmar branch of the ulnar artery. SYN arcus palmaris profundus [TA]. **2.** Superficial palmar arch; the arterial arch in the hand located superficial to the long flexor tendons, formed principally by the ulnar artery and usually completed by a communication with the superficial palmar branch of the radial artery. SYN arcus palmaris superficiales [TA]. SYN arcus palmaris.

pal•mar car•pal branch of ra•di•al ar•ter•y (pahl′măr kahr′păl branch rā′dē-ăl ahr′tĕr-ē) A small branch of the radial artery that passes medially across the wrist to supply the carpal joints; it anastomoses with the anterior carpal branch of the ulnar artery. SYN ramus carpalis palmaris arteriae radialis, ramus carpeus palmaris arteriae radialis.

pal•mar car•pal branch of ul•nar ar•ter•y (pahl′măr kahr′păl branch ŭl′năr ahr′tĕr-ē) A branch of the ulnar artery that supplies the carpal joints and communicates with the anterior carpal branch of the radial artery. SYN ramus carpalis palmaris arteriae ulnaris, ramus carpeus palmaris arteriae ulnaris.

pal•mar e•ry•the•ma (pahl′măr er′i-thē′mă) Reddening of the palms, associated with various physiologic as well as pathologic changes, the principal one of which is portal hypertension. It is also seen in patients with liver dysfunction and can be the result of dermatoses such as eczema or psoriasis. It may also be a normal finding, however, and has been attributed to high estrogen levels.

pal•mar grasp (pahl′măr grasp) A grasp pattern emerging in the 5th–6th month whereby the child places a pronated forearm or hand down on an object and the fingers simultaneously curl around the object, securing it in the midsection of the palm; the thumb is adducted against the radial aspect of the palm and does not assist with the grasp.

pal•mar in•ter•os•se•ous ar•ter•y (pahl′măr in-tĕr-os′ē-ŭs ahr′tĕr-ē) SYN palmar metacarpal artery.

pal•mar in•ter•os•se•ous mus•cle (pahl′măr in-tĕr-os′ē-ŭs mŭs′ĕl) Three muscles in the hand; *origin*, first: ulnar side of second metacarpal; second and third: radial sides of fourth and fifth metacarpals; *insertion*, first: into ulnar side of index; second and third: into radial sides of ring and little fingers; *action*, adducts fingers toward axis of middle finger; *nerve supply*, ulnar. See this page. SYN musculus interosseus palmaris [TA].

pal•mar•is brev•is mus•cle (pahl-măr′is brev′ĭs mŭs′ĕl) Cutaneous muscle of hand; *origin*, ulnar side of central portion of the palmar aponeurosis; *insertion*, skin of ulnar side of hand; *action*, wrinkles skin on medial side of palm; *nerve supply*, ulnar. SYN musculus palmaris brevis, short palmar muscle.

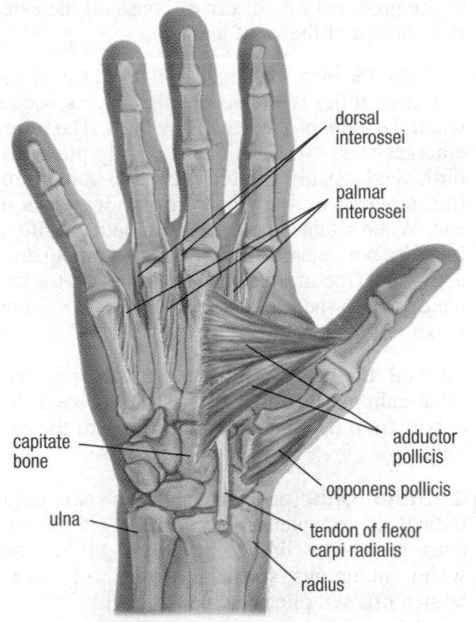

palmar interosseous muscle

pal•mar•is lon•gus mus•cle (pahl′măr-is long′gus mŭs′ĕl) Muscle of superficial layer of anterior (flexor) compartment of forearm; *origin*, medial epicondyle of humerus; *insertion*, flexor retinaculum of wrist and palmar fascia; *action*, tenses palmar fascia and flexes the hand and forearm; *nerve supply*, median. SYN long palmar muscle, musculus palmaris longus.

pal•mar met•a•car•pal ar•ter•y (pahl′măr met-ă-kahr′păl ahr′tĕr-ē) One of three arteries springing from the deep palmar arch and running in the three medial interosseous metacarpal spaces; they anastomose with the common palmar and, through perforating branches, with the dorsal metacarpal arteries. SYN arteria metacarpalis palmaris, palmar interosseous artery.

pal•mar pinch (pahl′măr pinch) OCCUPATIONAL THERAPY pinch between the pad of the thumb and the pads of the index and middle fingers. SEE ALSO pinch.

pal•mar pso•ri•a•sis (pahl′măr sōr-ī′ă-sis) Patchy, hyperkeratotic psoriasis affecting contact points of the volar surface of fingers and palms, alone or with mild psoriasis elsewhere; believed to be an isomorphic response, it may affect one palm involved in a sport or occupation.

pal•mar ra•di•o•car•pal lig•a•ment (pahl′măr rā′dē-ō-kahr′păl lig′ă-mĕnt) A strong ligament that passes from the distal end of the radius to the proximal row of carpal bones on the anterior surface of the wrist joint.

pal·mar re·flex (pahl′măr rē′fleks) One of the primitive reflexes: flexion of the fingers occurs when the palm of the hand is irritated. The reflex emerges at 11 weeks in utero, is fully present at birth, and usually inhibited by 2–3 months of life; replaced by the pincer grip at 36 weeks of age. When retained beyond 4–5 months of life, it impedes both manual dexterity and manipulatory activities. One of a group of reflexes that affect handwriting, speech, and articulation. SYN infant grasp reflex.

pal·mar ul·no·car·pal lig·a·ment (pahl′măr ŭl′nō-kahr′păl lig′ă-mĕnt) The fibrous band that passes from the ulnar styloid process to the carpal bones.

pal·mate folds (pahl′māt fōldz) The two longitudinal ridges, anterior and posterior, in the mucous membrane lining the cervix uteri, from which numerous secondary folds, or rugae, branch off. SYN plicae palmatae [TA].

Pal·mer den·tal no·men·cla·ture (pahl′mĕr den′tăl nō′mĕn-klā-chŭr) **1.** A system of identifying permanent teeth by the use of a number indicating the sequential position of a tooth distally from the midline; the number is bracketed with a right angle to identify the tooth's dental quadrant. **2.** A system for deciduous teeth analogous to the permanent tooth with letters substituted for numbers (A through E or a through e). SEE ALSO F.D.I. dental nomenclature, universal dental nomenclature. SYN Zsigmondy dental nomenclature.

palm·ic (pahl′mik) Beating; throbbing; relating to a palmus.

pal·mit·o·le·ic ac·id (pal′mi-tō-lē′ik as′id) A monounsaturated 16-carbon acid; one of the common constituents of the triacylglycerols of human adipose tissue.

pal·mus, pl. **pal·mi** (pahl′mŭs, -mī) **1.** SYN facial tic. **2.** Rhythmic fibrillary contractions in a muscle. SEE ALSO jumping disease. **3.** The heart beat. [G. *palmos,* pulsation, quivering]

pal·pa·ble (pal′pă-bĕl) **1.** Perceptible to touch; capable of being palpated. **2.** Evident; plain. SEE palpation.

pal·pate (pal′pāt) To examine by feeling and pressing with the palms of the hands and the fingers.

pal·pa·tion (pal-pā′shŭn) **1.** Examination with the hands, feeling for organs, masses, or infiltration of a part of the body, feeling the heart or pulse beat, vibrations in the chest, and other diagnostic functions. SYN touch (2). **2.** Touching, feeling, or perceiving by the sense of touch. See this page. [L. *palpatio,* fr. *palpo,* pp. *-atus,* to touch, stroke]

pal·pa·to·ry per·cus·sion (pal′pă-tōr′ē pĕr-

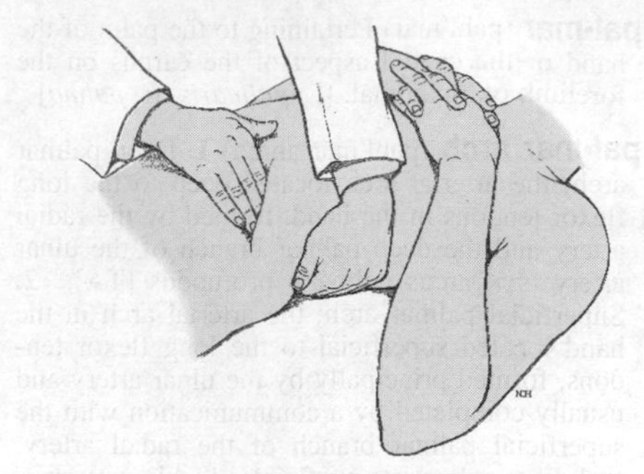

palpation technique

kŭsh′ŭn) Finger percussion in which attention is focused on the resistance and reverberation of the tissues under the finger as well as on the sound elicited.

pal·pe·bra, pl. **pal·pe·brae** (pal-pē′bră, -brē) [TA] SYN eyelid. [L.]

pal·pe·bral (pal′pĕ-brăl) Relating to an eyelid or the eyelids.

pal·pe·bral ar·ter·ies (pal′pĕ-brăl ahr′tĕr-ēz) Branches of the ophthalmic supplying the upper and lower eyelids, consisting of two sets, lateral and medial. SYN arteriae palpebrales [TA].

pal·pe·bral fis·sure (pal′pĕ-brăl fish′ŭr) SYN rima palpebrarum.

pal·pe·bral veins (pal′pĕ-brăl vānz) These drain the superior eyelid posteriorly as tributaries of the superior ophthalmic vein.

pal·pi·tate (pal′pi-tāt) **1.** To beat with excessive rapidity; throb, as in the rapid beating of the heart during periods of stress or specified heart conditions. **2.** To move with a slight tremulous motion; tremble, shake, or quiver. [L. *palpito,* to pulsate]

pal·pi·ta·tion (pal-pi-tā′shŭn) Forcible or irregular pulsation of the heart, perceptible to the patient, usually with an increase in frequency or force, with or without irregularity in rhythm. SYN trepidatio cordis. [L. *palpito,* to throb]

PALS (palz) Acronym for pediatric advanced life support.

pal·sy (pawl′zē) Paralysis or paresis. [a corruption of O. Fr. fr. L. and G. *paralysis*]

PAM (pam) Acronym for potential acuity meter.

2-PAM chlo·ride (pam klōr′īd) SYN pyridostigmine bromide.

***p*-ami·no·ben·zo·ic ac·id (PABA)** (ă-mē′nō-ben-zō′ik as′id) A factor in the vitamin B complex, a part of all folic acids and required for its formation; neutralizes the bacteriostatic effects of the sulfonamides because it furnishes an essential growth factor for bacteria, with the use of which sulfonamides interfere; used as an ultraviolet screen in lotions and creams.

pam•pin•i•form (pam-pin′i-fōrm) Having the shape of a tendril; denoting a vinelike structure. [L. *pampinus,* a tendril, + *forma,* form]

pam•pin•i•form plex•us (pam-pin′i-fōrm pleks′ŭs) A plexus formed, in the male, by veins from the testicle and epididymis, consisting of 8–10 veins lying in front of the ductus deferens and forming part of the spermatic cord; in the female the ovarian veins form this plexus between the layers of the broad ligament; in the male it is part of the thermoregulatory system of the testis, helping to keep the testis at a constant temperature slightly lower than the main body temperature.

pan- Prefix meaning all, entire (properly affixed to words derived from G. roots). SEE ALSO pant-. [G. *pas,* all]

pan•a•ce•a (pan-ă-sē′ă) A cure-all; a remedy claimed to be curative of all diseases. [G. *panakeia,* universal remedy, fr. Panacea, Aesculapius' daughter]

panaesthesia [Br.] SYN panesthesia.

pan•ag•glu•ti•nins (pan-ă-glū′ti-ninz) Agglutinins that react with all human erythrocytes. [pan + L. *agglutino,* to glue]

pan•an•gi•i•tis (pan-an-jē-ī′tis) Inflammation involving all the coats of a blood vessel. [pan- + angiitis]

pan•ar•thri•tis (pan-ahr-thrī′tis) **1.** Inflammation involving all the tissues of a joint. **2.** Inflammation of all the joints of the body.

pan•at•ro•phy (pan-at′rō-fē) **1.** Atrophy of all the parts of a structure. **2.** General atrophy of the body.

pan•cake kid•ney (pan′kāk kid′nē) A disc-shaped organ produced by fusion of both poles of the contralateral kidney primordia. SYN disc kidney.

pan•car•di•tis (pan-kahr-dī′tis) Inflammation of all the structures of the heart.

Pan•coast syn•drome (pan′kōst sin′drōm) Lower trunk brachial plexopathy and Horner syndrome due to malignant tumor in the region of the superior pulmonary sulcus.

pan•co•lec•to•my (pan′kō-lek′tŏ-mē) Extirpation of the entire colon.

pan•cre•as, pl. **pan•cre•a•ta** (pan′krē-ăs, -ā′tă) [TA] An elongated lobulated retroperitoneal gland extending from the duodenum to the spleen; it consists of a flattened head (caput) within the duodenal concavity, an elongated three-sided body extending transversely across the abdomen, and a tail in contact with the spleen. The gland secretes from its exocrine part pancreatic juice that is discharged into the intestine, and from its endocrine part the internal secretions, insulin and glucagon. See this page. [G. *pankreas,* the sweetbread, fr. *pas* (*pan*), all, + *kreas,* flesh]

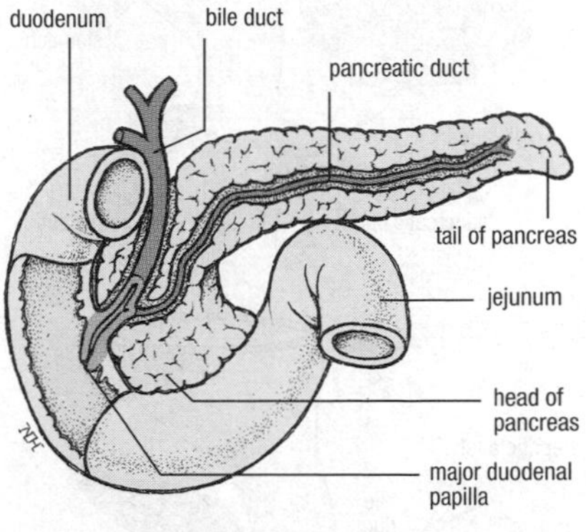

pancreas and part of duodenum

pancreat-, pancreatico-, pancreato-, pancreo- Combining forms indicating the pancreas. [G. *pankreas,* pancreas]

pan•cre•a•tal•gi•a (pan-krē-ă-tal′jē-ă) Pain arising from the pancreas or felt in or near the region of the pancreas. [pancreat- + G. *algos,* pain]

pan•cre•a•tec•to•my (pan-krē-ă-tek′tŏ-mē) Excision of the pancreas. [pancreat- + G. *ektomē,* excision]

pan•cre•at•ic (pan-krē-at′ik) Relating to the pancreas.

pan•cre•at•ic am•y•lase (pan-krē-at′ik am′i-lās) An enzyme secreted by the pancreas that digests starch.

pan•cre•at•ic buds (pan-krē-at′ik bŭdz) Outgrowths of endodermal lining of the caudal part of foregut; the ventral and dorsal buds fuse and develop into the pancreas. The ventral bud forms the uncinate process and inferior part of the head of the pancreas and the remaining part of the gland is derived from the dorsal bud. See page 1148.

pan•cre•at•ic cal•cu•lus (pan-krē-at′ik kal′kyū-lŭs) A concretion, usually multiple, in the pancreatic duct, associated with chronic pancreatitis.

pan•cre•at•ic cys•to•du•o•de•nos•to•my (pan-krē-at′ik sis′tō-dū′ō-dĕ-nos′tŏ-mē) Surgical or endoscopic drainage of pancreatic pseudocyst into duodenum. SYN duodenocystostomy (3).

pan•cre•at•ic di•ges•tion (pan-krē-at′ik di-jes′chŭn) Digestion in the intestine by the enzymes of the pancreatic juice.

pan•cre•at•ic duct (pan-krē-at′ik dŭkt) The excretory duct of the pancreas, which extends

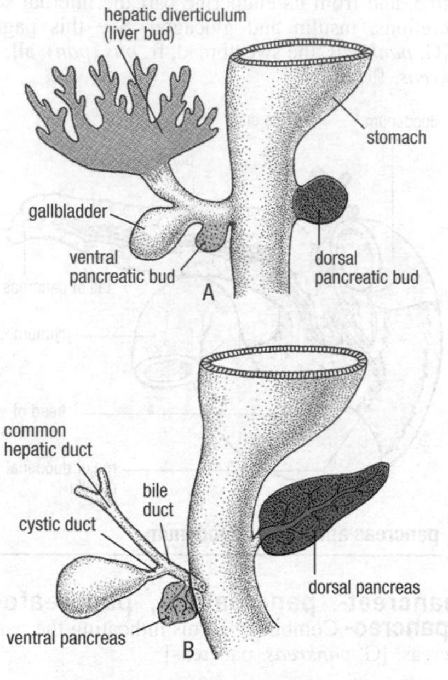

stages in development of the pancreas: (A) 30 days (approximately 5 mm); (B) 35 days (approximately 7 mm) (initially the ventral pancreatic bud lies close to the hepatic diverticulum, but later it moves posteriorly around the duodenum toward the dorsal pancreatic bud)

through the gland from tail to head, where it empties into the duodenum at the greater duodenal papilla. SYN Wirsung canal, Wirsung duct.

pan·cre·at·i·co·du·o·de·nal (pan-krē-at′i-kō-dū-ō-dē′năl) Relating to the pancreas and the duodenum.

pan·cre·at·i·co·du·o·de·nal veins (pan-krē-at′i-kō-dū-ō-dē′năl vānz) Accompany the superior and inferior pancreaticoduodenal arteries and empty into the superior mesenteric or portal vein.

pan·cre·at·ic veins (pan-krē-at′ik vānz) Drain the pancreas and empty into the splenic vein and the superior mesenteric vein.

pan·cre·at·in (pan′krē-ă-tin) A combination of specific digestive (pancreatic) enzymes obtained from swine or cattle: lipase, protease, and amylase. These enzymes aid in the digestion and absorption of fats and starches. Pancreatin is given for treatment of various pancreatic enzyme deficiencies resulting from conditions such as pancreatitis, cystic fibrosis, or complications of gastrointestinal bypass surgery. [G. *pankreas,* pancreas]

pan·cre·a·ti·tis (pan′krē-ă-tī′tis) Inflammation of the pancreas.

pan·cre·at·o·du·o·de·nec·to·my, pan·cre·at·i·co·duo·den·ec·to·my (pan-krē-at′ō-dū-ō-dĕ-nek′tŏ-mē, pan-krē-at′i-kō-dū-ō-dĕ-nek′ō-mē) Excision of all or part of the pancreas together with the duodenum. SYN Whipple operation.

pan·cre·at·o·du·o·de·nos·to·my (pan-krē-at′ō-dū-ō-dĕ-nos′tŏ-mē) Surgical anastomosis of a pancreatic duct, cyst, or fistula to the duodenum.

pan·cre·at·o·gas·tros·to·my (pan′krē-at′ō-gas-tros′tŏ-mē) Surgical anastomosis of a pancreatic cyst or fistula to the stomach.

pan·cre·a·to·gen·ic, pan·cre·a·tog·en·ous (pan-krē-ă-tō-jen′ik, -toj′ĕ-nŭs) Of pancreatic origin; formed in the pancreas. [pancreato- + G. *genesis,* origin]

pan·cre·a·tog·ra·phy (pan′krē-ă-tog′ră-fē) Radiographic demonstration of the pancreatic ducts, after retrograde injection of radiopaque material into the distal duct. [pancreato- + G. *graphō,* to write]

pan·cre·at·o·je·ju·nos·to·my (pan-krē-at′ō-jĕ′jūn-os′tŏ-mē) The surgical formation of an artificial opening between the jejunum and a pancreatic duct, cyst, or fistula.

pan·cre·at·o·li·thec·to·my (pan-krē-at′ō-li-thek′tŏ-mē) SYN pancreatolithotomy. [pancreato- + G. *lithos,* stone, + *ektomē,* excision]

pan·cre·at·o·li·thi·a·sis (pan-krē-at′ō-li-thī′ă-sis, pan′krē-ă-tō-) Stones in the pancreas, usually found in the pancreatic duct system.

pan·cre·at·o·li·thot·o·my (pan-krē-at′ō-li-thot′ŏ-mē) Removal of a pancreatic concretion. SYN pancreatolithectomy. [pancreato- + G. *lithos,* stone, + *tomē,* incision]

pan·cre·a·tol·y·sis (pan-krē-ă-tol′i-sis) Destruction of the pancreas. [pancreato- + G. *lysis,* dissolution]

pan·cre·a·to·lyt·ic (pan-krē-ă-tō-lit′ik) Denoting pancreatolysis.

pan·cre·at·o·meg·a·ly (pan-krē-at′ō-meg′ă-lē) An abnormal enlargement of the pancreas. [pancreato- + G. *megas,* great]

pan·cre·a·top·a·thy (pan-krē-ă-top′ă-thē) Any disease of the pancreas. [pancreato- + G. *pathos,* suffering]

pan·cre·a·to·re·nal syn·drome (pan-krē-at′ō-rēn′ăl sin′drōm) Acute renal failure occurring in a patient with severe acute pancreatitis; the mortality rate is high.

pan·cre·a·tot·o·my (pan′krē-ă-tot′ŏ-mē) Incision of the pancreas. [pancreato- + G. *tomē,* incision]

pan·cre·a·tro·pic (pan′krē-ă-trō′pik) Exerting an action on the pancreas. [pancreat- + G. *tropikos,* relating to a turning]

pan·cre·li·pase (pan-krē-lip′ās) A concentrate of pancreatic enzymes standardized for lipase content; a lipolytic used in substitution therapy.

pan·cy·to·pe·ni·a (pan′sī-tō-pē′nē-ă) Pronounced reduction in the number of erythrocytes, all types of leukocytes, and the blood platelets in the circulating blood. [pan- + G. *kytos,* cell, + *penia,* poverty]

pan·dem·ic (pan-dem′ik) Denoting a disease affecting or attacking the population of an extensive region, country, continent; extensively epidemic. [pan- + G. *dēmos,* the people]

pan·di·a·stol·ic (pan′dī-ă-stol′ik) SYN holodiastolic.

pan·en·ceph·a·li·tis (pan′en-sef-ă-lī′tis) A diffuse inflammation of the brain.

pan·en·do·scope (pan-en′dō-skōp) An illuminated instrument for inspection of the interior of the urethra as well as the bladder by means of a Foroblique lens system. [pan- + G. *endon,* within, + *skopeō,* to view]

pan·es·the·si·a (pan-es-thē′zē-ă) The sum of all the sensations experienced by a person at one time. SEE ALSO cenesthesia. SYN panaesthesia. [pan- + G. *aisthēsis,* sensation]

pang (păng) A sudden sharp, brief pain.

pan·hy·po·pi·tu·i·tar·ism (PHP) (pan-hī′pō-pi-tū′i-tă-rizm) A state in which the secretion of all anterior pituitary hormones is inadequate or absent. SYN hypophysial cachexia.

pan·hys·ter·ec·to·my (pan-his′ter-ek′tŏ-mē) The surgical removal of the uterus and the cervix. SEE ALSO hysterectomy. [pan- + G. *hystera,* uterus + *ektomē,* excision]

pan·ic (pan′ik) Extreme and unreasoning anxiety and fear, often accompanied by disturbed breathing, increased heart activity, vasomotor changes, sweating, and a feeling of dread. SEE anxiety. [fr. G. myth. char., *Pan*]

pan·ic at·tack (pan′ik ă-tak′) Sudden onset of intense apprehension, fear, terror, or sense of impending doom accompanied by increased autonomic nervous system activity and by various constitutional disturbances, depersonalization, and derealization.

pan·ic dis·or·der (pan′ik dis-ōr′dĕr) Recurrent panic attacks that occur unpredictably. SEE generalized anxiety disorder.

pan·im·mu·ni·ty (pan-i-myū′ni-tē) A general immunity to all infectious diseases.

pan·lo·bar (pan′lō-bahr) Pertaining to all of the lung lobe.

pan·lob·u·lar em·phy·se·ma (pan-lōb′yū-lăr em′fi-sē′mă) Emphysema affecting all parts of the lobules, in part, or usually the whole, of the lungs, and usually associated with α_1-antiprotease deficiency emphysema.

pan·my·e·loph·thi·sis (pan′mī-ĕ-lof′thi-sis) SYN myelophthisis (2).

pan·my·e·lo·sis (pan′mī-ĕ-lō′sis) Myeloid metaplasia with abnormal immature blood cells in the spleen and liver; associated with myelofibrosis. [pan- + G. *myelos,* marrow, + *-osis,* condition]

Pan·ner dis·ease (pahn′ĕr di-zēz′) Epiphysial osteonecrosis of the capitellum of the humerus.

pan·nic·u·lar her·ni·a (pă-nik′yū-lăr hĕr′nē-ă) The escape of subcutaneous fat through a gap in a fascia or an aponeurosis. SYN fatty hernia.

pan·nic·u·lec·to·my (pă-nik-yū-lek′tŏ-mē) Surgical excision of abdominal subcutaneous fat. [panniculus + G. *ektomē,* a cutting out]

pan·nic·u·li·tis (pă-nik-yū-lī′tis) Inflammation of subcutaneous adipose tissue. [panniculus + G. *-itis,* inflammation]

pan·nic·u·lus, pl. **pan·nic·u·li** (pă-nik′yū-lŭs, -lī) [TA] A sheet or layer of tissue. [L. dim. of *pannus,* cloth]

pan·ning (pan′ing) Use of plastic plates or surfaces coated with either antigen or antibody to separate or concentrate specific cells with appropriate receptors.

i **pan·nus**, pl. **pan·ni** (pan′ŭs, -ī) **1.** A membrane of granulation tissue covering a normal surface. **2.** The articular cartilages in rheumatoid arthritis and in chronic granulomatous diseases such as tuberculosis. **3.** The cornea in trachoma. SEE ALSO corneal pannus. See page 1150. [L. cloth]

pan·nus cras·sus (pan′ŭs kra′sŭs) SEE corneal pannus.

pan·nus sic·cus (pan′ŭs sik′ŭs) SEE corneal pannus.

pan·nus ten·u·is (pan′ŭs ten′yū-is) SEE corneal pannus.

i **pan·o·ram·ic ra·di·o·graph** (pan-ŏ-ram′ik rā′dē-ō-graf) Radiographic view of the maxillae and mandible extending from the left to the right glenoid fossae. See page 1151. SYN panoramic x-ray film.

pan·o·ram·ic x-ray film (pan-ŏ-ram′ik eks′rā film) SYN panoramic radiograph.

pan·o·ti·tis (pan-ō-tī′tis) General inflammation of all parts of the ear; specifically, a disease that begins as an otitis interna, the inflammation subsequently extending to the middle ear and neighboring structures. [pan- + G. *ous,* ear, + *-itis,* inflammation]

pan·si·nu·si·tis (pan-sī-nū-sī′tis) Inflammation of all the accessory sinuses of the nose on one or both sides.

pan•sys•tol•ic (pan′sis-tol′ik) Lasting throughout systole, extending from first to second heart sound. SYN holosystolic.

pan•sys•tol•ic mur•mur (pan′sis-tol′ik mŭr′mŭr) A murmur occupying the entire systolic interval, from first to second heart sounds.

pant (pant) To breathe rapidly and shallowly. [Fr. *panteler,* to gasp]

pant-, panto- Combining forms meaning entire. SEE ALSO pan-. [G. *pas,* all]

pan•tal•gi•a (pan-tal′jē-ă) Pain involving the entire body. [pant- + G. *algos,* pain]

pan•ta•loon her•ni•a (pan′tă-lūn hĕr′nē-ă) An inguinal hernia that involves both an indirect and a direct component.

Pan•to•e•a ag•glom•er•ans (pan-tō-ē′ă ă-glom′ĕ-ranz) Formerly *Enterobacter agglomerans*, member of the family Enterobacteriaceae; associated with infections acquired from contaminated intravenous fluids.

pan•to•mo•gram (pan′tō-mō-gram) A panoramic radiographic record of the maxillary and mandibular dental arches and their associated structures, obtained by a pantomograph. [pan- + tomogram]

pan•to•mo•graph (pan′tō-mō-graf) A panoramic radiographic instrument that permits visualization of the entire dentition, alveolar bone, and contiguous structures on a single extraoral film.

pan•to•mog•ra•phy (pan-tō-mog′ră-fē) A method of radiography by which a radiograph (pantomogram) of the maxillary and mandibular dental arches and their contiguous structures may be obtained on a single film.

Pan•ton-Val•en•tine leu•ko•ci•din (pan′tŏn-val′ĕn-tīn lū′kō-sī′din) A staphylococcal cytolytic toxin that can act on polymorphonuclear leukocytes.

pan•to•scop•ic tilt (pan-tō-skop′ik tilt) An oblique astigmatism caused by slanting a spheric lens so that light rays strike the lens at a nonperpendicular angle, altering the spheric and cylindric refractive power of the lens.

pan•to•the•nate (pan-tō′then-āt) A salt or ester of pantothenic acid.

pan•to•then•ic ac•id (pan-tō-then′ik as′id) The β-alanine amide of pantoic acid. A growth substance widely distributed in plant and animal tissues, and essential for growth of a number of organisms; deficiency in diet causes a dermatitis in chicks and rats and achromotrichia in the latter; a precursor to coenzyme A.

Pan•um ar•ea (pah′nŭm ār′ē-ă) Area in space surrounding the empiric horopter where single binocular vision is observed despite stimulation of noncorresponding retinal points.

pan•u•ve•i•tis (pan-yū-vē-ī′tis) SYN iridocyclochoroiditis.

PAP (pap) Acronym for peroxidase antiperoxidase complex, 3′-phosphoadenosine 5′-phosphate. SEE PAP technique.

Pa•pa•ni•co•laou (Pap) smear (pa-pă-ni′kō-lō smēr) A smear of vaginal or cervical cells obtained for cytologic study.

Pa•pa•ni•co•laou (Pap) stain (pa-pă-ni′kō-lō stān) A multichromatic stain used principally on exfoliated cytologic specimens and based on aqueous hematoxylin with multiple counterstaining dyes in 95% ethyl alcohol, giving great transparency and delicacy of detail; important in cancer screening, especially of gynecologic smears.

Pa•pa•ni•co•laou (Pap) test (pa-pă-ni′kō-lō

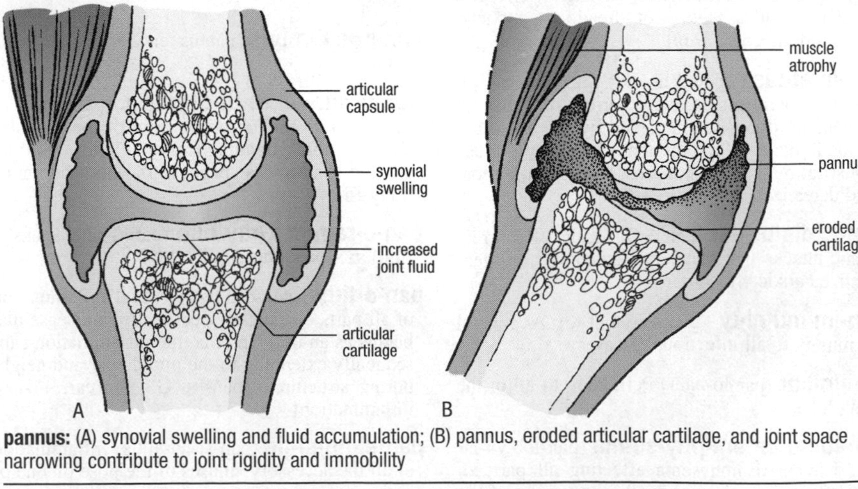

pannus: (A) synovial swelling and fluid accumulation; (B) pannus, eroded articular cartilage, and joint space narrowing contribute to joint rigidity and immobility

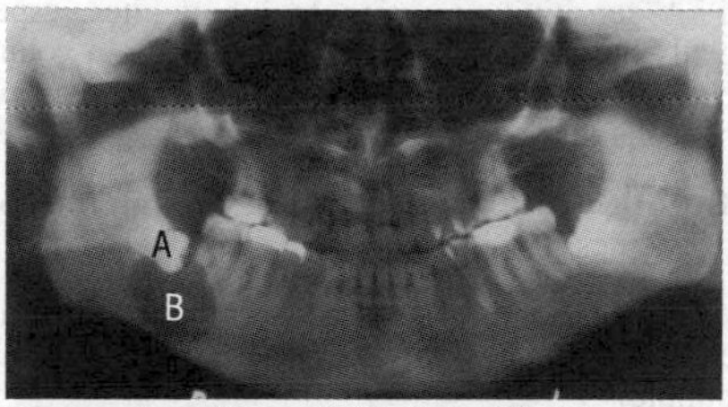

panoramic radiograph (adult dentition): (A) unerupted mandibular third molar; (B) large cyst in mandibular bone around crown of molar

test) Microscopic examination of cells exfoliated or scraped from a mucosal surface after staining with Papanicolaou stain; used especially for detection of cancer of the uterine cervix.

pa·per chro·ma·tog·ra·phy (pā′pĕr krō′mă-tog′ră-fē) Partition chromatography in which the moving phase is a liquid and the stationary phase is paper.

pa·per mill work·er's dis·ease (pā′pĕr mil work′ĕrz di-zēz′) Extrinsic allergic alveolitis caused by moldy wood pulp containing spores of *Alternaria* fungi.

pa·pil·la, pl. **pa·pil·lae** (pă-pil′ă, -ē) Any small, nipplelike process. SEE ALSO dental papilla. SYN teat (3). [L. a nipple, dim. of *papula,* a pimple]

pa·pil·la of der·mis (pă-pil′ă dĕr′mis) The superficial projections of the dermis (corium) that interdigitate with recesses in the overlying epidermis; they contain vascular loops and specialized nerve endings, and are arranged in ridgelike lines best developed in the hand and foot. SYN dermal papillae.

pa·pil·lae val·la·tae (pa-pil′ē val-ă-tē) SYN vallate papilla.

pa·pil·la pi·li (pă-pil′ă pil′ī) A knoblike indentation of the bottom of the hair follicle, on which the hair bulb fits like a cap; it is derived from the corium and contains vascular loops for the nourishment of the hair root. SYN hair papilla.

pap·il·lar·y, **pap·il·late** (pap′i-lar-ē, -i-lāt) Relating to, resembling, or provided with papillae.

pap·il·lar·y ad·e·no·car·ci·no·ma (pap′i-lar-ē ad′ĕ-nō-kahr-si-nō′mă) An adenocarcinoma containing fingerlike processes of vascular connective tissue covered by neoplastic epithelium, projecting into cysts or the cavities of glands or follicles.

pap·il·lar·y ad·e·no·ma of large in·tes·tine (pap′i-lar′ē ad′ĕ-nō′mă lahrj in-tes′tin) SYN villous adenoma.

pap·il·lar·y car·ci·no·ma (pap′i-lar-ē kahr′si-nō′mă) A malignant neoplasm characterized by the formation of numerous irregular fingerlike projections of fibrous stroma covered with a layer of neoplastic epithelial cells.

pap·il·lar·y cys·tic ad·e·no·ma (pap′i-lar-ē sis′tik ad′ĕ-nō′mă) An adenoma in which the lumens of the acini are frequently distended by fluid, and the neoplastic epithelial elements tend to form irregular, fingerlike projections.

pap·il·lar·y ducts (pap′i-lar-ē dŭkts) [TA] The largest straight excretory ducts in the kidney medulla and papillae, with openings that form the area cribrosa; they are a continuation of the collecting tubules. SYN Bellini ducts.

pap·il·lar·y hi·drad·e·no·ma (pap′i-lar-ē hī-drad′ĕ-nō′mă) A solitary benign tumor occurring in women, usually in the labia majora; cystic and papillary, and composed of epithelium resembling that of apocrine glands. SYN apocrine adenoma.

pap·il·lar·y mus·cle (pap′i-lar-ē mŭs′ĕl) One of the group of myocardial bundles that terminate in the chordae tendineae which attach to the cusps of the atrioventricular valves; each has an anterior and a posterior papillary muscle; the right ventricle sometimes has a septal papillary muscle. SYN musculus papillaris [TA].

pap·il·lar·y sta·sis (pap′i-lar-ē stā′sis) Obsolete term for papilledema.

pap·il·lar·y tu·mor (pap′i-lar-ē tū′mŏr) SYN papilloma.

pa·pil·la val·la·ta (pă-pil′ă val-ā′tă) [TA] SYN vallate papilla.

pap·il·lec·to·my (pap-i-lek′tŏ-mē) Surgical removal of any papilla. [papilla + G. *ektomē,* excision]

pa·pil·le·de·ma (pap′il-ĕ-dē′mă) Edema of the optic disc, due to increased intracranial pressure. SYN choked disc, papilloedema. [papilla + edema]

pa·pil·li·form (pă-pil′i-fōrm) Resembling or shaped like a papilla.

pap·il·li·tis (pap-i-lī′tis) **1.** Optic neuritis with swelling of the optic disc. **2.** Inflammation of the renal papilla. [papilla + G. *-itis,* inflammation]

♻ **papillo-** Combining form meaning a papilla, papillary. [L. *papilla*]

pap·il·lo·ad·e·no·cys·to·ma (pap′i-lō-ad′ĕ-nō-sis-tō′mă) A benign epithelial neoplasm characterized by glands or glandlike structures, formation of cysts, and fingerlike projections of neoplastic cells covering a core of fibrous connective tissue.

pap·il·lo·car·ci·no·ma (pap′i-lō-kar-si-nō′mă) **1.** A papilloma that has become malignant. **2.** A carcinoma that is characterized by papillary, fingerlike projections of neoplastic cells in association with cores of fibrous stroma as a supporting structure. [papilla + G. *karkinōma,* cancer]

papilloedema [Br.] SYN papilledema.

pap•il•lo•ma (pap-i-lō′mă) A circumscribed benign epithelial tumor projecting from the surrounding surface and consisting of villous or arborescent outgrowths of fibrovascular stroma covered by neoplastic cells. SYN papillary tumor, villoma. [papilla + G. *-oma,* tumor]

pap•il•lo•ma•to•sis (pap′i-lō-mă-tō′sis) **1.** The development of numerous papillomas. **2.** Papillary projections of the epidermis forming a microscopically undulating surface.

pap•il•lo•ma•tous (pap-i-lō′mă-tŭs) Relating to a papilloma.

Pa•pil•lo•ma•vi•rus (pap-i-lō′mă-vī-rŭs) A genus of viruses containing DNA and including the papilloma viruses and wart viruses of humans and other animals, some of which are associated with induction of carcinoma. More than 70 types are known to infect humans and are differentiated by DNA homology.

pap•il•lo•ret•i•ni•tis (pap′i-lō-ret-i-nī′tis) SYN neuroretinitis.

pap•il•lot•o•my (pa-pi-lot′ŏ-mē) An incision into the major duodenal papilla. [papilla + G. *tomē,* incision]

pa•poose root (pa-pūs′ rūt) SYN blue cohosh.

Pa•po•va•vir•i•dae (pă-pō′vă-vir′i-dē) A family of small, antigenically distinct viruses that replicate in nuclei of infected cells; most have oncogenic properties. The family includes the genera Papillomavirus and Polyomavirus. [*pa*pilloma + *po*lyoma + *va*cuolating]

pa•po•va•vi•rus (pă-pō′vă-vī′rŭs) Any virus of the family Papovaviridae.

Pap•pen•hei•mer bod•ies (pahp′ĕn-hī-mĕr bod′ēz) Phagosomes, containing ferruginous granules, found in red blood cells in some diseases (e.g., sideroblastic anemia, hemolytic anemia, and sickle cell disease).

PA pro•jec•tion (prŏ-jek′shŭn) A radiographic study in which x-rays travel from posterior to anterior. SYN posteroanterior projection.

PAP tech•nique (pap tek-nēk′) An unlabeled antibody peroxidase method that reacts both with the rabbit antihorseradish peroxidase antibody and free horseradish peroxidase to form a soluble complex of peroxidase antiperoxidase (i.e., PAP); a uniquely sensitive immunohistochemical method that is applicable to paraffin-embedded tissues.

pap•u•lar (pap′yū-lăr) Relating to papules.

pap•u•lar mu•ci•no•sis (pap′yū-lăr myū′si-nō′sis) SYN lichen myxedematosus.

pap•u•lar tu•ber•cu•lid (pap′yū-lăr tū-bĕr′kyū-lid) SYN lichen scrofulosorum.

pap•u•lar ur•ti•car•i•a (pap′yū-lăr ŭr′ti-kar′ē-ă) A sensitivity reaction to insect bites, especially human and pet fleas, seen mostly in young children as wheals followed by papules on exposed areas. SYN lichen urticatus.

pap•u•la•tion (pap-yū-lā′shŭn) The formation of papules.

pap•ule (pap′yūl) A small, circumscribed, solid elevation on the skin. See page B10. [L. *papula,* pimple]

papulo- Prefix meaning papule. [L. *papula,* papule]

pap•u•lo•er•y•them•a•tous (pap′yū-lō-er-i-them′ă-tŭs) Denoting an eruption of papules on an erythematous surface.

pap•u•lo•ne•crot•ic tu•ber•cu•lid (pap′yū-lō-nĕ-krot′ik tū-bĕr′kyū-lid) Dusky-red papules followed by crusting and ulceration primarily on the extremities and predominantly in young adults with a deep focus of tuberculosis or with a history of preceding infection.

pap•u•lo•pus•tu•lar (pap′yū-lō-pŭs′chū-lăr) Denoting an eruption composed of papules and pustules.

pa•pu•lo•sis (pap-yū-lō′sis) The occurrence of numerous widespread papules.

pap•u•lo•squa•mous (pap′yū-lō-skwā′mŭs) Denoting an eruption composed of both papules and scales. [papulo- + L. *squamosus,* scaly (squamous)]

pap•u•lo•ve•sic•u•lar (pap′yū-lō-ve-sik′yū-lăr) Denoting an eruption composed of papules and vesicles.

PAPVR Abbreviation for partial anomalous pulmonary venous return.

pap•y•ra•ceous (pap-i-rā′shŭs) Like parchment or paper. [L. *papyraceus,* made of papyrus]

PAR Abbreviation for par level; periodic automatic replenishment; participate.

par (pahr) A pair; specifically a pair of cranial nerves, e.g., par nonum, ninth pair, glossopharyngeal; par vagum, the vagus or tenth pair. [L. equal]

par•a (par′ă) A woman who has given birth to one or more infants. Para followed by a roman numeral or preceded by a Latin prefix (primi-, secundi-, terti-, quadri-, etc.) designates the number of times a pregnancy has culminated in a single or multiple birth; e.g., **para I**, primipara; a woman who has given birth for the first time; **para II**, secundipara; a woman who has given birth for the second time to one or more infants. Cf. gravida. [L. *pario,* to bring forth]

para- **1.** Prefix denoting a departure from the normal. **2.** Prefix denoting involvement of two like parts or a pair. **3.** Prefix denoting adjacent, beside, near. **4.** CHEMISTRY an italicized prefix denoting two substitutions in the benzene ring arranged symmetrically, i.e., linked to opposite carbon atoms in the ring. For words beginning with *para-* or *p-*, see the specific name. [G. alongside of, near]

par•a•a•or•tic bod•ies (par′ă-ā-ōr′tik bod′ēz) Small masses of chromaffin tissue found near the sympathetic ganglia along the abdominal aorta; they are more prominent during fetal life. The chromaffin cells secrete norepinephrine; chemoreceptive endings monitor levels of blood gases. SYN corpora para-aortica [TA], Zuckerkandl bodies.

par•a•bal•lism (par-ă-bahl′izm) Severe jerking movements of both legs. [para- + G. *ballismos,* jumping about]

par•a•ba•sal bod•y (par′ă-bā′săl bod′ē) Part of the giant mitochondrion of certain parasitic flagellates. The parabasal body plus the basal body were previously thought to constitute a kinetoplast, but kinetoplast is now restricted to part of the DNA giant mitochondrion.

par•a•bi•o•sis (par-ă-bī-ō′sis) **1.** The fusion of embryos, as occurs in conjoined twins. **2.** Surgical joining of the vascular systems of two organisms. [para- + G. *biōsis,* life]

par•a•bi•ot•ic (par-ă-bī-ot′ik) Relating to, or characterized by, parabiosis.

par•a•bu•li•a (par-ă-bū′lē-ă) Perversion of volition or will in which one impulse is checked and replaced by another. [para- + G. *boulē,* will]

par•a•ca•se•in (par-ă-kā′sē-in) The compound produced by the action of rennin on κ-casein, which precipitates with calcium ion as the insoluble curd.

paracenaesthesia [Br.] SYN paracenesthesia.

par•a•ce•nes•the•si•a (par′ă-sē-nes-thē′zē-ă) Deterioration in one's sense of bodily well-being (i.e., of the normal functioning of one's organs). SYN paracenaesthesia. [para- + G. *koinos,* common, + *aisthēsis,* feeling]

par•a•cen•te•sis (par′ă-sen-tē′sis) The passage into a cavity of a trocar and cannula, needle, or other hollow instrument for the purpose of removing fluid; variously designated according to the cavity punctured. SYN tapping (2). [G. *parakentēsis,* a tapping for dropsy, fr. *para,* beside, + *kentēsis,* puncture]

par•a•cen•tet•ic (par-ă-sen-tet′ik) Relating to paracentesis.

par•a•cen•tral fis•sure (par′ă-sen′trăl fish′ŭr) A curved fissure (sulcus) on the medial surface of the cerebral hemisphere, bounding the paracentral gyrus and separating it from the precuneus and the cingulate gyrus.

par•a•cer•vi•cal (par′ă-sĕr′vi-kăl) Connective tissue adjacent to the uterine cervix.

par•a•cer•vix (par′ă-sĕr′viks) The connective tissue of the pelvic floor extending from the fibrous subserous coat of the cervix of the uterus laterally between the layers of the broad ligament.

par•ac•e•tal•de•hyde (par-as′ĕt-al′dĕ-hīd) SYN paraldehyde.

par•a•chol•er•a (par′ă-kol′ĕr-ă) A disease resembling Asiatic cholera due to a vibrio species but not *Vibrio cholerae.*

par•a•chor•dal (par′ă-kōr′dăl) Denoting a position alongside the rostral portion of the notochord in the embryo; designating the bilateral cartilaginous bars that enter into the formation of the base of the cranium. [para- + G. *chordē,* cord]

par•a•chro•ma, **par•a•chro•ma•to•sis** (par′ă-krō′mă, -tō′sis) Abnormal coloration of the skin. [para- + G. *chrōma,* color]

par•a•chute mi•tral valve (par′ă-shūt mī′trăl valv) A congenital deformity of the mitral valve characterized by the presence of a single papillary muscle from which the tendinous cords or chordae tendineae of both valve leaflets divide; the condition often produces a stenosis as the combined result of the tugging action of the cords on, and the subsequent narrowing between, the leaflets.

par•a•chute re•flex (par′ă-shūt rē′fleks) SYN startle reflex (1).

par•a•ci•ca•tri•cial em•phy•se•ma (par′ă-sik-ă-trish′ăl em′fi-sē′mă) Dilated terminal air spaces adjacent to a scar in the lung.

par•a•coc•cid•i•oi•dal gran•u•lo•ma (par′ă-kok-sid-ē-oyd′ăl gran′yū-lō′mă) SYN paracoccidioidomycosis.

Par•a•coc•cid•i•oi•des bra•sil•i•en•sis (par′ă-kok-sid-ē-oy′dēz bră-sil-ē-en′sis) A dimorphic fungus that causes paracoccidioidomycosis.

par•a•coc•cid•i•oi•din (par′ă-kok-sid-ē-oy′din) Antigen prepared using the fungus *Paracoccidioides brasiliensis;* used for demonstrating present or past infection and identifying endemic areas.

par•a•coc•cid•i•oi•do•my•co•sis (par′ă-kok-sid-ē-oy′dō-mī-kō′sis) A chronic fungal disease characterized by primary pulmonary lesions with dissemination to many visceral organs, conspicuous ulcerative granulomas of the buccal and nasal mucosa with extensions to the skin, and generalized lymphangitis; caused by *Paracoccidioides brasiliensis.* SYN Almeida disease, Lutz-Splendore-Almeida disease, paracoccidioidal granuloma, South American blastomycosis.

par•a•co•li•tis (par′ă-kō-lī′tis) Inflammation of the peritoneal coat of the colon.

par•a•cone (par′ă-kōn) **1.** The mesiobuccal

cusp of human upper molars. **2.** A cusp arising from the protocone in the evolution of the molars; thought to be the first cusp to arise, rather than the protocone. [para- + G. *kōnos*, cone]

par•a•con•id (par′ă-kon′id) A cusp derived from the protoconid in the evolution of the molars; in humans, it is very small or nonexistent. [paracone + -id (2)]

par•a•crine (par′ă-krin) Relating to a kind of hormone function in which the effects of the hormone are restricted to the local environment. Cf. endocrine. [para- + G. *krinō,* to separate]

par•a•cu•sis, **par•a•cu•si•a** (par′ă-kyū′sis, -sē-ă) **1.** Impaired hearing. **2.** Auditory illusions or hallucinations. [para- + G. *akousis,* hearing]

par•a•cys•tic (par′ă-sis′tik) Beside or near a bladder, specifically the urinary bladder. [para- + G. *kystis,* bladder]

par•a•cys•ti•tis (par′ă-sis-tī′tis) Inflammation of the connective tissue and other structures about the urinary bladder. [para- + G. *kystis,* bladder, + *-itis,* inflammation]

par•a•did•y•mis, pl. **par•a•did•y•mi•des** (par-ă-did′i-mis, -mi-dēz) A small body sometimes attached to the front of the lower part of the spermatic cord above the head of the epididymis; the remnants of tubules of the mesonephros. SYN parepididymis. [para- + G. *didymos,* twin, in pl. *didymoi,* testes]

par•a•dip•si•a (par′ă-dip′sē-ă) An abnormal desire to consume fluids, without regard to bodily need. [para- + G. *dipsa,* thirst]

par•a•dox (par′ă-doks) That which is apparently, although not actually, inconsistent with or opposed to the known facts in any case. [G. *paradoxos,* incredible, beyond belief, fr. *doxa,* belief]

par•a•dox•i•c con•trac•tion (par′ă-doks′ik kŏn-trak′shŭn) A tonic contraction of the anterior tibial muscles when a sudden passive dorsal flexion of the foot is made.

par•a•dox•i•c di•a•phragm phe•nom•e•non (par′ă-doks′ik dī′ă-fram fē-nom′ĕ-non) In pyopneumothorax, hydropneumothorax, and some cases of injury, the diaphragm on the affected side rises during inspiration and falls during expiration.

par•a•dox•ic ef•fect (par′ă-dok′sik e-fekt′) As related to minimal bactericidal concentration testing, decreased bactericidal activity of an antimicrobial agent at higher concentrations, as demonstrated by growth of more colonies on subcultures at higher concentrations than at lower concentrations.

par•a•dox•ic ex•ten•sor re•flex (par′ă-doks′ik eks-ten′sŏr rē′fleks) SYN Babinski sign (1).

par•a•dox•i•c pulse (par′ă-doks′ik pŭls) A reversal of the normal variation in the pulse volume with respiration, the pulse becoming weaker with inspiration and stronger with expiration; characteristic of cardiac tamponade and rare in constrictive pericarditis. So called because these changes are independent of changes in the cardiac rate as measured directly or by electrocardiogram. SYN pulsus paradoxus.

par•a•dox•ic pu•pil•lar•y re•flex (par′ă-doks′ik pyū′pi-lar-ē rē′fleks) Constriction of pupils in darkness, the reverse of that expected.

par•a•dox•i•c re•flex (par′ă-doks′ik rē′fleks) Any reflex in which the usual response is reversed or does not conform to the pattern characteristic of the particular reflex.

par•a•dox•i•c res•pi•ra•tion (par′ă-doks′ik res′pir-ā′shŭn) Deflation of the lung during inspiration and inflation of the lung during the phase of expiration; seen in the lung on the side of an open pneumothorax.

par•a•dox•i•c sleep (par′ă-doks′ik slēp) A deep sleep, with a brain wave pattern more like that of waking states than of other states of sleep, that occurs during rapid eye movement sleep. SEE ALSO rapid eye movement sleep.

par•a•dox•i•c vo•cal cord move•ment (par′ă-doks′ik vō′kăl kōrd mūv′mĕnt) Adduction of the vocal cords on inspiration, resulting in stridor and airway obstruction.

paraesthesia [Br.] SYN paresthesia.

paraesthetic [Br.] SYN paresthetic.

par•af•fin bait tech•nique (par′ă-fin bāt tek-nēk′) Technique used to recover *Nocardia* spp. and aerobic actinomycetes from contaminated samples. It is based on the principle that these organisms can use simple carbon sources for nutrition.

par•af•fin bath (par′ă-fin bath) Warmed paraffin wax and mineral oil mixture used to coat a body part, causing heat to penetrate into the tissues; used to treat joint inflammation.

par•af•fi•no•ma (par′ă-fi-nō′mă) A tumefaction, usually a granuloma, caused by the prosthetic or therapeutic injection of paraffin into the tissues. SEE ALSO lipogranuloma.

par•a•fol•lic•u•lar cells (par′ă-fŏ-lik′yū-lăr selz) Cells present between follicles or interspersed among follicular cells; they are rich in mitochondria and are believed to be the source of thyrocalcitonin.

par•a•func•tion (par′ă-fŭngk′shŭn) **1.** Abnormal or disordered function. **2.** DENTISTRY movements of the mandible that are outside normal function (e.g., bruxism). [para- + function]

par•a•gan•gli•a (par′ă-gang′glē-ă) Plural of paraganglion.

par•a•gan•gli•o•ma (par′ă-gang-glē-ō′mă) A neoplasm usually derived from the chromoreceptor tissue of a paraganglion, such as the carotid body, or the medulla of suprarenal gland; the latter is usually termed a chromaffinoma or pheochromocytoma.

par•a•gan•gli•on, pl. **par•a•gan•gli•a** (par′ă-gang′glē-ŏn, -ă) A small, roundish body containing chromaffin cells; a number of such bodies may be found retroperitoneally near the aorta and in organs such as the kidney, liver, heart, and gonads. SYN chromaffin body.

par•a•geu•si•a (par′ă-gū′sē-ă) Disordered or abnormal sense of taste. [para- + G. *geusis,* taste]

par•a•geu•sic (par′ă-gū′sik) Relating to parageusia.

par•a•glot•tic space (par′ă-glot′ik spās) The space on each side of the glottis bounded laterally by the perichondrium of the thyroid cartilage and the cricothyroid membrane and posteriorly by the mucous membrane of the pyriform sinus; anterosuperiorly it extends into the preepiglottic space. It is an important route of transglottic and extralaryngeal spread of carcinoma of the larynx.

***Par•a•go•ni•mus* gran•u•lo•ma** (par′ă-gon′i-mŭs gran′yū-lō′mă) Lesions caused by adult worms and eggs of the lung fluke trapped in the pulmonary parenchyma.

par•a•gram•ma•tism (par′ă-gram′ă-tizm) Speech that is fluent but consists mainly of semantic and phonetic errors (paraphasias), so that grammatic structure and meaning cannot be discerned. This disorder is typical of severe receptive aphasia. SYN jargon aphasia.

par•a•graph•i•a (par′ă-graf′ē-ă) **1.** Loss of the power of writing from dictation, although the words are heard and comprehended. **2.** Writing one word when another is intended. [para- + G. *graphō,* to write]

par•a•hip•po•cam•pal gy•rus (par′ă-hip′ō-kam′păl jī′rŭs) A long convolution on the medial surface of the temporal lobe, forming the lower part of the fornicate gyrus, extending from behind the splenium corporis callosi forward along the dentate gyrus of the hippocampus from which it is demarcated by the hippocampal fissure. The anterior extreme of the gyrus curves back on itself, forming the uncus, the major location of the olfactory cortex.

par•a•hor•mone (par′ă-hōr′mōn) A substance, the product of ordinary metabolism, not produced for a specific purpose, that acts like a hormone in modifying the activity of some distant organ (e.g., the action of carbon dioxide on the control of breathing).

par•a•in•flu•en•za vi•rus•es (par′ă-in-flū-en′ ză vī′rŭs-ĕz) Viruses of the genus Paramyxovirus, of four types: **type 1** (hemadsorption virus type 2), which includes Sendai virus, causes acute laryngotracheitis in children and occasionally adults; **type 2** (croup-associated virus) is associated especially with acute laryngotracheitis or croup in young children and minor upper respiratory infections in adults; **type 3** (hemadsorption virus type 1; shipping fever virus) has been isolated from small children with pharyngitis, bronchiolitis, and pneumonia, and causes occasional respiratory infection in adults; **type 4** has been isolated from a very few children with minor respiratory illness.

par•a•ker•a•to•sis (par′ă-ker-ă-tō′sis) Retention of nuclei in the cells of the stratum corneum of the epidermis, observed in many scaling dermatoses such as psoriasis and subacute or chronic dermatitis.

par•a•ki•ne•si•a, **par•a•ki•ne•sis** (par′ă-ki-nē′zē-ă, -sis) Any motor abnormality. [para- + G. *kinēsis,* movement]

par•a•la•li•a (par′ă-lā′lē-ă) Any speech defect; especially one in which one letter is habitually substituted for another. [para- + G. *lalia,* talking]

par•al•de•hyde (par-al′dĕ-hīd) A cyclic polymer of acetaldehyde; a potent hypnotic and sedative, suitable for oral or rectal administration; its offensive odor limits its use. SYN paracetaldehyde.

par•a•lex•i•a (par′ă-lek′sē-ă) Misapprehension of written or printed words, other meaningless words being substituted for them in reading. [para- + G. *lexis,* speech]

par•al•ge•si•a (par′al-jē′zē-ă) Painful paresthesia; any disorder or abnormality of the sense of pain. [para- + G. *algēsis,* the sense of pain]

par•al•lac•tic (par′ă-lak′tik) Relating to a parallax.

par•al•lax (par′ă-laks) The apparent displacement of an object that follows a change in the position from which it is viewed. [G. alternately, fr. *par-allassō,* to make alternate, fr. *allos,* other]

par•al•lax test (par′ă-laks test) Measurement of the deviation in strabismus by the alternate cover test combined with neutralization of the deviation using prisms.

par•al•lel play (par′ă-lel plā) A developmental psychology concept in which toddlers (ages 2–3 years) play alongside each other, in similar activities, without obvious communication or interaction. Children younger than that tend to play by themselves (solitary play). Older children (preschool age) interact with each other more during group play.

par•al•ler•gic (par′ă-lĕr′jik) Denoting an allergic state in which the body becomes predisposed to nonspecific stimuli following original sensitization with a specific allergen.

par•a•lo•gi•a, **pa•ral•o•gism, pa•ral•o•gy** (par′ă-lō′jē-ă, pă-ral′ō-jizm, -jē) False reasoning, involving self-deception. [G. *paralogia,* a fallacy, fr. *para,* beside, + *logos,* reason]

pa•ral•y•sis, pl. **pa•ral•y•ses** (păr-al′i-sis,

-sēz) **1.** Loss of power of voluntary movement in a muscle through injury to or disease of its nerve supply. **2.** Loss of any function, such as sensation, secretion, or mental ability. [G. fr. para- + *lysis,* a loosening]

par·a·lyt·ic (par′ă-lit′ik) Relating to paralysis or suffering from paralysis.

par·a·lyt·ic de·men·ti·a (par′ă-lit′ik dĕ-men′shē-ă) A slow progressive mental disease with paralysis as a finding.

par·a·lyt·ic il·e·us (par′ă-lit′ik il′ē-ŭs) SYN adynamic ileus.

par·a·ly·tic in·con·ti·nence (par′ă-lit′ik in-kom′pĕ-tĕns) A form of urinary incontinence that is a symptom of neurogenic disorders involving damage to the brain or the spinal cord. Voluntary control over the sacral micturition center is lost and bladder function reverts to the type of reflex seen in babies. SYN reflex bladder.

par·a·ly·zant (pă-ral′i-zănt) **1.** Causing paralysis. **2.** Any agent, such as curare, which causes paralysis.

par·a·lyze (par′ă-līz) To render incapable of movement.

Par·a·me·ci·um (par′ă-mē′sē-ŭm) An abundant genus of freshwater holotrichous ciliates, characteristically slipper shaped and often large enough to be visible to the naked eye; commonly used for genetic and other studies. [G. *paramēkēs,* rather long, fr. *mēkos,* length]

par·a·me·di·an in·ci·sion (par′ă-mē′dē-ăn in-sizh′ŭn) An incision lateral to the midline.

par·a·med·ic (par′ă-med′ik) SYN prehospital provider.

par·a·med·i·cal (par′ă-med′i-kăl) **1.** Related to the medical profession in an adjunctive capacity (e.g., denoting allied health fields such as physical therapy, and speech pathology). **2.** Relating to a paramedic.

par·a·me·ni·a (par′ă-mē′nē-ă) Any disorder or irregularity of menstruation. [para- + G. *mēn,* month]

par·a·mes·o·neph·ric duct (par′ă-mĕz′ō-nef′rik dŭkt) Either of the two paired embryonic tubes extending along the mesonephros roughly parallel to the mesonephric duct and emptying into the urogenital sinus; in the female, the upper parts of the ducts form the uterine tubes, whereas the lower parts fuse to form the uterus; in the male, vestiges of the ducts form the prostatic utricle (vagina masculina) and the appendix of the testis. SYN Müller duct, müllerian duct.

pa·ram·e·ter (pă-ram′ĕ-tĕr) **1.** One of many dimensions or ways of measuring or describing an object or evaluating a subject **2.** MATHEMATICS an arbitrary constant that can possess different values, each value defining other expressions. **3.** STATISTICS a term used to define a characteristic of a population, in contrast to a sample from that population. **4.** PSYCHOANALYSIS any tactic, other than interpretation, used by the analyst to further the patient's progress. [para- + G. *metron,* measure]

par·a·me·tri·al (par′ă-mē′trē-ăl) Pertaining to the parametrium.

par·a·met·ric (par′ă-met′rik) Relating to the parametrium, or structures immediately adjacent to the uterus.

par·a·me·trit·ic (par′ă-me-trit′ik) Relating to parametritis.

par·a·me·tri·tis (par′ă-me-trī′tis) Inflammation of the tissue adjacent to the uterus, particularly in the broad ligament. SYN pelvic cellulitis. [parametrium + G. *-itis,* inflammation]

par·a·me·tri·um, pl. **par·a·me·tri·a** (par′ă-mē′trē-ŭm, -ă) [TA] The connective tissue of the pelvic floor extending from the fibrous subserous coat of the supracervical portion of the uterus laterally between the layers of the broad ligament. [para- + G. *mētra,* uterus]

par·a·mim·i·a (par′ă-mim′ē-ă) The use of gestures unsuited to the words that they accompany. [para- + G. *mimia,* imitation]

par·am·ne·si·a (par′am-nē′zē-ă) False recollection, as of events that have never occurred. [para- + G. *amnēsia,* forgetfulness]

par·am·y·loi·do·sis (par-am′i-loy-dō′sis) **1.** Deposition in tissues of an amyloidlike protein in primary amyloidosis or in atypical amyloidosis of multiple myeloma. **2.** Various hereditary amyloidoses (Portuguese amyloidosis, Indiana amyloidosis) characterized by progressive hypertrophic polyneuritis with sensory changes, ataxia, paresis, and muscle atrophy due to amyloid deposits in peripheral and visceral nerves.

par·a·my·o·to·ni·a (par′ă-mī-ō-tō′nē-ă) An atypical form of myotonia.

Par·a·myx·o·vir·i·dae (par′ă-mik-sō-vir′i-dē) A family of RNA-containing viruses. Three genera are recognized: Paramyxovirus, Morbillivirus, and Pneumovirus, all of which cause cell fusion and produce cytoplasmic eosinophilic inclusions.

Par·a·myx·o·vi·rus (par′ă-mik′sō-vī′rŭs) A genus of viruses that includes Newcastle disease, mumps, and the parainfluenza viruses (types 1–4).

paranaesthesia [Br.] SYN paranesthesia.

par·a·na·sal (par′ă-nā′zăl) Adjacent to the nasal cavities. [para- + L. *nasus,* nose]

par·a·na·sal si·nus·es (par′ă-nā′zăl sī′nŭs-ez) The paired air-filled cavities in the bones of the face lined by mucous membrane continuous with that of the nasal cavity; these sinuses are the frontal, sphenoidal, maxillary, and ethmoidal.

par•a•ne•o•pla•si•a (par′ă-nē-ō-plā′zē-ă) Hormonal, neurologic, hematologic, and other clinical and biochemical disturbances associated with malignant neoplasms but not directly related to invasion by the primary tumor or its metastases.

par•a•ne•o•plas•tic (par′ă-nē-ō-plas′tik) Relating to or characteristic of paraneoplasia.

par•a•ne•o•plas•tic en•ceph•a•lo•my•e•lop•a•thy (par′ă-nē-ō-plas′tik en-sef′ă-lō-mī-ĕ-lop′ă-thē) An encephalomyelopathy as a remote effect of carcinoma, most often oat cell carcinoma of the lung.

par•a•ne•o•plas•tic pem•phi•gus (par′ă-nē-ō-plas′tik pem′fi-gŭs) Painful mucosal erosions and polymorphous skin eruptions with biopsy findings resembling pemphigus vulgaris, associated with neoplasm and serum antibodies reactive with intercellular substance of all epithelia; usually rapidly fatal.

par•a•ne•o•plas•tic syn•drome (par′ă-nē-ō-plas′tik sin′drōm) A syndrome directly resulting from a malignant neoplasm, but not resulting from the presence of tumor cells in the affected parts.

par•a•neph•ric (par′ă-nef′rik) **1.** Relating to the suprarenal gland (i.e., paranephros). **2.** SYN pararenal.

par•a•neph•ros, pl. **par•a•neph•roi** (par′ă-nef′rŭs, -roy) SYN suprarenal gland. [para- + G. *nephros,* kidney]

par•an•es•the•si•a (par′an-es-thē′zē-ă) Loss of feeling or sensation (anesthesia) in the lower half of the body. SYN paranaesthesia. [para- + G. an- *priv.* + *aisthēsis,* sensation]

par•a•noi•a (par′ă-noy′ă) A disorder characterized by the presence of systematized delusions, often of a persecutory character involving being followed, poisoned, or harmed by other means, in an otherwise intact personality. SEE ALSO paranoid personality. [G. derangement, madness, fr. para- + *noeō,* to think]

par•a•noid (par′ă-noyd) **1.** Relating to or characterized by paranoia. **2.** Having delusions of persecution.

par•a•noid per•son•al•i•ty (par′ă-noyd pĕr-sŏn-al′i-tē) A personality disorder characterized by hypersensitivity, rigidity, unwarranted suspicion, jealousy, and a tendency to blame others and ascribe evil motives to them; although neither a neurosis nor psychosis, it interferes with the person's ability to maintain interpersonal relationships.

par•a•noid schiz•o•phre•ni•a (par′ă-noyd skits′ō-frē′nē-ă) A form of that mental disorder characterized predominantly by delusions of persecution and megalomania.

par•a•no•mi•a (par′ă-nō′mē-ă) A form of aphasia in which objects are named incorrectly. [para- + G. *onoma,* name]

par•a•nu•cle•ar (par′ă-nū′klē-ăr) **1.** SYN paranucleate. **2.** Outside, but near the nucleus.

par•a•nu•cle•ate (par′ă-nū′klē-āt) Relating to or having a paranucleus. SYN paranuclear (1).

par•a•nu•cle•us (par′ă-nū′klē-ŭs) An accessory nucleus or small mass of chromatin lying outside, though near, the nucleus.

par•a•op•er•a•tive (par′ă-op′ĕr-ă-tiv) SYN perioperative.

par•a•pa•re•sis (par′ă-pă-rē′sis) Weakness affecting the lower extremities. [para- + paresis]

par•a•pa•ret•ic (par′ă-pă-ret′ik) **1.** Relating to paraparesis. **2.** A person with paraparesis.

par•a•per•i•to•ne•al her•ni•a (per′ă-per′i-tō-nē′ăl hĕr′nē-ă) A vesical hernia in which only a part of the protruded organ is covered by the peritoneum of the sac.

par•a•pha•ryn•ge•al ab•scess (par′ă-fă-rin′jē-ăl ab′ses) An abscess lying lateral to the pharynx.

par•a•pha•si•a (par′ă-fā′zē-ă) A symptom of aphasia in which speech is fluent but incorrect due to word and sound substitutions. SEE ALSO paragrammatism, receptive aphasia. [para- + G. *phasis,* speech]

par•a•pha•sic (par′ă-fā′zik) Relating to paraphasia.

pa•ra•phi•a (pă-rā′fē-ă) Any disorder of the sense of touch. SYN parapsia, pseudesthesia (1). [para- + G. *haphē,* touch]

par•a•phil•i•a (par′ă-fil′ē-ă) A mental disorder characterized by socially proscribed sexual practices. [para- + G. *philos,* fond]

par•a•phi•mo•sis (par′ă-fī-mō′sis) Painful constriction of the glans penis by a phimotic foreskin that has been retracted behind the corona. It can occur after male catheterization if the foreskin is not pulled back over the corona. [para- + G. phimosis]

par•a•plec•tic (par′ă-plek′tik) SYN paraplegic. [G. *paraplēktikos,* paralyzed]

par•a•ple•gi•a (par′ă-plē′jē-ă) Paralysis of both lower extremities and, generally, the lower trunk. [para- + *plēgē,* a stroke]

par•a•ple•gic (par′ă-plē′jik) Relating to or suffering from paraplegia. SYN paraplectic.

par•a•prax•i•a (par′ă-prak′sē-ă) A condition analogous to paraphasia and paragraphia in which there is a defective performance of purposive acts (e.g., slips of the tongue, or mislaying of objects). [para- + G. *praxis,* a doing]

par•a•pro•tein (par′ă-prō′tēn) **1.** A monoclonal

immunoglobulin of the blood plasma, produced by a clone of plasma cells arising from the abnormal rapid multiplication of a single cell. Paraprotein in serum may be seen in various malignant, benign, or nonneoplastic diseases. **2.** SYN monoclonal immunoglobulin. [para + protein, fr. G. *protos*, first]

paraproteinaemia [Br.] SYN paraproteinemia.

par•a•pro•tein•e•mi•a (par′ă-prō-tēn-ē′mē-ă) The presence of abnormal proteins in the blood. SYN paraproteinaemia.

pa•rap•si•a (pă-rap′sē-ă) SYN paraphia. [para- + G. *hapsis*, touch]

par•a•pso•ri•a•sis (par′ă-sō-rī′ă-sis) A heterogenous group of skin disorders including pityriasis lichenoides and small and large plaque variants.

par•a•psy•chol•o•gy (par′ă-sī-kol′ŏ-jē) The study of extrasensory perception, such as thought transference (telepathy) and clairvoyance.

par•a•re•flex•i•a (par′ă-rē-flek′sē-ă) A condition characterized by abnormal reflexes.

par•a•re•nal (par′ă-rē′năl) Near or adjacent to the kidneys. SYN paranephric (2).

par•a•ro•san•i•lin (par′ă-rō-san′i-lin) [CI 42500] A biologic stain used in a Schiff reagent to detect cellular DNA (Feulgen stain), mucopolysaccharides (PAS stain), and proteins (ninhydrin-Schiff stain).

par•ar•rhyth•mi•a (par′ă-ridh′mē-ă) A cardiac dysrhythmia in which two independent rhythms coexist, but not as a result of A-V block; pararrhythmia thus includes parasystole and A-V dissociation (2), but not complete A-V block. [para- + G. *rhythmos*, rhythm]

par•a•si•noi•dal (par′ă-sī-noy′dăl) Near a sinus, particularly a cerebral sinus.

parasitaemia [Br.] SYN parasitemia.

par•a•site (par′ă-sīt) **1.** An organism that lives on or in another and draws its nourishment therefrom. **2.** In the case of a fetal inclusion or conjoined twins, the usually incomplete twin that derives its support from the more nearly normal autosite. [G. *parasitos*, a guest, fr. *para*, beside, + *sitos*, food]

par•a•si•te•mi•a (păr′ă-sī-tē′mē-ă) The presence of parasites in the circulating blood; used especially with reference to malarial and other protozoan forms, and microfilariae. SYN parasitaemia.

par•a•sit•ic (par′ă-sit′ik) **1.** Relating to or of the nature of a parasite. **2.** Denoting organisms that normally grow only in or on the living body of a host.

par•a•sit•ic cyst (par′ă-sit′ik sist) A cyst formed by the larva of a metazoan parasite (e.g., hydatid or trichinal cyst).

par•a•sit•i•ci•dal (par′ă-sīt-i-sī′dăl) Destructive to parasites.

par•a•sit•i•cide (par′ă-sīt′i-sīd) An agent that destroys parasites. [parasite + L. *caedo*, to kill]

par•a•sit•ic mel•a•no•der•ma (par′ă-sit′ik mel′ă-nō-dĕr′mă) Excoriations and melanoderma caused by scratching the bites of the body louse, *Pediculus corporis*. SYN vagabond's disease, vagrant's disease.

par•a•sit•ism (par′ă-sīt-izm) A symbiotic relationship in which one species (the parasite) benefits at the expense of the other (the host). Cf. mutualism, commensalism, symbiosis, metabiosis.

par•a•si•tize (par′ă-si-tīz) To invade as a parasite.

par•a•si•to•gen•ic (par′ă-sī-tō-jen′ik) **1.** Caused by certain parasites. **2.** Favoring parasitism. [parasite + G. *-gen*, producing]

par•a•si•tol•o•gist (par′ă-sī-tol′ŏ-jist) One who specializes in the science of parasitology.

par•a•si•tol•o•gy (par′ă-sī-tol′ŏ-jē) The branch of biology and of medicine concerned with all aspects of parasitism. [parasite + G. *logos*, study]

par•a•sit•o•sis (par′ă-sī-tō′sis) Infestation or infection with parasites.

par•a•si•to•tro•pic (par′ă-sī-tō-trō′pik) Pertaining to or characterized by parasitotropism.

par•a•si•tot•ro•pism (par′ă-sī-to′trō-pizm) The special affinity of particular drugs or other agents for parasites rather than for their hosts, including microparasites that infect a larger parasite. Cf. organotropism. [parasite + G. *tropē*, a turning]

par•a•som•ni•a (par′ă-som′nē-ă) Any dysfunction associated with sleep (e.g., somnambulism, pavor nocturnus, enuresis, or nocturnal seizures).

par•a•sta•sis (par′ă-stā′sis) **1.** A reciprocal relationship among causal mechanisms that can compensate for, or mask defects in, each other. **2.** GENETICS a relationship between nonalleles (classified by some as a form of epistasis). [G. standing shoulder to shoulder]

par•a•ster•nal her•ni•a (par′ă-stĕr′năl hĕr′nē-ă) SYN Morgagni foramen hernia.

par•a•sym•pa•thet•ic (par′ă-sim-pă-thet′ik) Pertaining to a division of the autonomic nervous system. SEE autonomic division of nervous system.

par•a•sym•pa•thet•ic gan•gli•a (par′ă-sim-pă-thet′ik gang′glē′ă) Those ganglia of the autonomic nervous system composed of cholinergic neurons receiving afferent fibers from preganglionic visceral motor neurons in either the brainstem or the middle sacral spinal segments (S2–S4). SEE ALSO autonomic division of nervous system.

par·a·sym·pa·thet·ic nerve (par′ă-sim-pă-thet′ik nĕrv) One of the nerves of the parasympathetic nervous system.

par·a·sym·pa·thet·ic ner·vous sys·tem (par′ă-sim′pă-thet′ik nĕr′vŭs sis′tĕm) The branch of the autonomic nervous system that sends motor signals to glandular smooth muscle, and cardiac tissue, during recovery from threat. Cf. sympathetic nervous system.

par·a·sym·pa·thet·ic re·sponse (par′ă-sim′pă-thet′ik rē-spons′) The response in glandular, smooth muscle, and cardiac tissue during relief from threat or stress; the lay term for this state is "rest and digest," as opposed to the common term for the sympathetic response, "fight or flight."

par·a·sym·pa·thet·ic root of o·tic gan·gli·on (par′ă-sim′pă-thet′ik rūt ō′tik gang′glē-ŏn) SYN lesser petrosal nerve.

par·a·sym·pa·thet·ic root of pel·vic gan·gli·a (par′ă-sim′pă-thet′ik rūt pel′vik gang′glē-ă) SYN pelvic splanchnic nerves.

pa·ra·sym·pa·thet·ic root of pte·ry·go·pal·a·tine gan·gli·on (par′ă-sim′pă-thet′ik rūt ter′i-gō-pal′ă-tīn gang′glē-ŏn) SYN greater petrosal nerve.

par·a·sym·pa·tho·lyt·ic (par′ă-sim′pă-thō-lit′ik) Relating to an agent that annuls or antagonizes the effects of the parasympathetic nervous system (e.g., atropine).

par·a·sym·pa·tho·mi·met·ic (par′ă-sim′pă-thō-mi-met′ik) SYN cholinomimetic. [para- + G. *sympatheia,* sympathy, + *mimētikos,* imitative]

par·a·sym·pa·tho·mi·met·ic drug (par′ă-sim′pă-thō-mi-met′ik drŭg) A drug that acts by stimulating or mimicking the parasympathetic nervous system (PNS); are also called cholinergics because acetylcholine (ACh) is the neurotransmitter used by the PNS.

par·a·sy·nap·sis (par′ă-si-nap′sis) Union of chromosomes side to side in the process of reduction. [para- + G. *synapsis,* a connection, junction]

par·a·sy·no·vi·tis (par′ă-si-nō-vī′tis) Inflammation of the tissues immediately adjacent to a joint. [para- + synovitis]

par·a·sys·to·le (par′ă-sis′tō-lē) A second automatic rhythm existing simultaneously with normal sinus or other dominant rhythm, the parasystolic center being protected from the dominant rhythm's impulses so that its basic rhythm is undisturbed, although it may be manifest in the ECG only at various multiples of its basic periodicity. [para- + G. *systolē,* a contracting]

par·a·tax·ic dis·tor·tion (par′ă-taks′ik dis-tōr′shŭn) An attitude toward another person based on a distorted evaluation, usually because of too close an identification of that person with other emotionally significant figures in the patient's past life.

par·a·ten·on (par′ă-ten′on) The tissue, fatty or synovial, between a tendon and its sheath. [para- + G. *tenōn,* tendon]

par·a·thy·roid (par′ă-thī′royd) **1.** Adjacent to the thyroid gland. **2.** SYN parathyroid gland.

par·a·thy·roid·ec·to·my (par′ă-thī-roy-dek′tŏ-mē) Excision of the parathyroid glands. [parathyroid + G. *ektomē,* excision]

par·a·thy·roid gland (par′ă-thī′royd gland) One of two small paired endocrine glands, superior and inferior, usually found embedded in the connective tissue capsule on the posterior surface of the thyroid gland; they secrete parathyroid hormone, which regulates the metabolism of calcium and phosphorus. The parenchyma is composed of chief and oxyphilic cells arranged in anastomosing cords. Inadvertent removal of all parathyroid glands, as during thyroidectomy, produces tetany and death. SYN parathyroid (2).

par·a·thy·roid hor·mone (PTH) (par′ă-thī′royd hōr′mōn) A peptide hormone formed by the parathyroid glands; it maintains the serum calcium level by promoting intestinal absorption and renal tubular reabsorption of calcium, and release of calcium from bone to extracellular fluid. Cf. bioregulator.

par·a·thy·roid hor·mone-re·lat·ed pep·tide (PTHrP) (par′ă-thī′royd hōr′mōn-rē-lā′tĕd pep′tīd) A hormone that can be produced by tumors, especially of the squamous cell type; massive overproduction can lead to hypercalcemia and other manifestations of hyperparathyroidism. PTHrP exerts a biologic action similar to that of parathyroid hormone (PTH), acting through the same receptor, which is expressed in many tissues but most abundantly in kidney, bone, and growth plate cartilage. It apparently has significant actions during development, but it is uncertain whether PTHrP circulates at all or has any function in normal human adults. The structure of the gene for human PTHrP is more complex than that of PTH, and varying molecular forms exist, including proteins of 141, 139, and 173 amino acids, which share a significant homology with parathyroid hormone. Cf. bioregulator.

par·a·thy·roid hor·mone test (par′ă-thī′royd hōr′mōn test) A venous blood assessment performed to determine the serum levels of a hormone (PTH) secreted by the parathyroid gland in response to low blood calcium levels.

par·a·thy·roid tet·a·ny (par′ă-thī′royd tet′ă-nē) Tetany due to a lack of parathyroid function, spontaneous or following excision of the parathyroid glands.

par·a·thy·ro·tro·pic, **par·a·thy·ro·tro·phic** (par′ă-thī-rō-trō′pik, -trō′fik) Influencing the growth or activity of the parathyroid glands. [parathyroid + G. *tropē,* a turning; *trophē,* nourishment]

par·a·tope (par′ă-tōp) That part of an antibody molecule composed of the variable regions of both the light and heavy chains that combine with the antigen. SYN antibody-combining site.

par·a·ty·phoid fe·ver, **par·a·ty·phoid** (par′ă-tī′foyd fē′vĕr) An acute infectious disease with symptoms and lesions resembling those of typhoid fever, although milder in character; associated with the presence of the paratyphoid organism, of which at least three varieties (types A, B, and C) have been described.

par·a·um·bil·i·cal veins (par′ă-ŭm-bil′i-kăl vānz) *Origin:* arise from cutaneous veins around the umbilicus running along the round ligament of the liver, and terminating as accessory portal veins in its substance; they constitute a portocaval anastomosis and are subject to varicosity during portal hypertension; varicose paraumbilical veins form the caput medusae.

par·a·u·re·thral ducts (par′ă-yū-rē′thrăl dŭkts) Inconstant ducts along the side of the female urethra that convey the mucoid secretion of Skene glands to the vestibule.

par·a·vag·i·ni·tis (par′ă-vaj-i-nī′tis) Inflammation of the connective tissue alongside the vagina.

par·a·ver·te·bral (par′ă-vĕr′tĕ-brăl) Beside or near the vertebral column.

par·a·ver·te·bral gan·gli·a (par′ă-vĕr′tĕ-brăl gang′glē-ă) SYN ganglia of sympathetic trunk.

par·ax·i·al (par-ak′sē-ăl) By the side of the axis of any body or part.

par·ax·on (par-ak′son) A collateral branch of an axon. [para- + G. *axōn,* axis]

pa·ren·chy·ma (pă-rengk′i-mă) **1.** The distinguishing or specific cells of a gland or organ, contained in and supported by the connective tissue framework, or stroma. **2.** The endoplasm of a protozoan cell. [G. anything poured in beside, fr. *parencheō,* to pour in beside]

pa·ren·chy·ma·ti·tis (par′ĕn-kim-ă-tī′tis) Inflammation of the parenchyma or differentiated substance of a gland or organ.

par·en·chym·a·tous (par′ĕn-kim′ă-tŭs) Relating to the parenchyma.

par·en·chym·a·tous de·gen·er·a·tion (par′ĕn-kim′ă-tŭs dĕ-jen′ĕr-ā′shŭn) SYN cloudy swelling.

par·en·chym·a·tous goi·ter (par′ĕn-kim′ă-tŭs goy′tĕr) A form of goiter in which there is a great increase in the follicles with proliferation of the epithelium. SYN follicular goiter.

par·en·chym·a·tous hem·or·rhage (par′ĕn-kim′ă-tŭs hem′ŏr-ăj) Bleeding into the substance of an organ.

par·en·chym·a·tous neu·ri·tis (par′ĕn-kim′ă-tŭs nūr-ī′tis) Inflammation of the nervous substance proper, the axons, and myelin.

pa·ren·tal gen·er·a·tion (P_1) (pă-ren′tăl jen-ĕr-ā′shŭn) The parents of a mating, commonly experimental, involving contrasting genotypes; the original mating of a genetic experiment; parents of the F_1 generation.

par·ent cyst (par′ĕnt sist) SYN mother cyst.

par·en·ter·al (pă-ren′tĕr-ăl) By some other means than through the gastrointestinal tract; referring particularly to the introduction of substances into an organism by intravenous, subcutaneous, intramuscular, or intramedullary injection. [para- + G. *enteron,* intestine]

par·en·ter·al nu·tri·tion (PN) (pă-ren′tĕr-ăl nū-trish′ŭn) Providing the body with nutrition intravenously. SYN intravenous alimentation.

par·en·ter·ic fe·ver (par′en-ter′ik fē′vĕr) One of a group of fevers clinically resembling typhoid and paratyphoid A and B, but caused by bacteria differing specifically from those of either of these diseases.

Pa·ren·ti-Frac·ca·ro syn·drome (pah-ren′tē-frah-kah′rō sin′drōm) SYN achondrogenesis type IB.

par·ep·i·did·y·mis (par′ep-i-did′i-mis) SYN paradidymis.

pa·re·sis (pă-rē′sis) **1.** Partial or incomplete paralysis. **2.** A disease of the brain, marked by progressive dementia, tremor, speech disturbances, and increasing muscular weakness; in a large proportion of patients there is a preliminary stage of irritability often followed by exaltation and delusions of grandeur. SYN Bayle disease. [G. a letting go, slackening, paralysis, fr. *paritēmi,* to let go]

par·es·the·si·a (par-es-thē′zē-ă) A subjective report of any abnormal sensation, could be experienced as numbness, tingling, or what is colloquially called "pins and needles." SYN paraesthesia. [para- + G. *aisthēsis,* sensation]

par·es·thet·ic (par-es-thet′ik) Relating to or marked by paresthesia; denoting numbness and tingling in an extremity that usually occurs on the resumption of the blood flow to a nerve following temporary pressure or mild injury. SYN paraesthetic.

Pa·ré su·ture (pah-rā′ sū′chŭr) The approximation of the edges of a wound by pasting strips of cloth to the surface and stitching them instead of the skin.

pa·ret·ic (pă-ret′ik) Relating to or suffering from paresis.

pa•reu•ni•a (pă-rū′nē-ă) SYN coitus. [G. *pareunos,* lying beside, fr. *para,* beside, + *eunē,* a bed]

par•fo•cal (pahr-fō′kăl) Describes a microscope with interchangeable objectives that do not require refocus. [L. *par*, equal, + focal]

par•i•es, gen. **pa•ri•e•tis**, pl. **pa•ri•e•tes** (par′ē-ēz, pă-rī′ĕ-tis, -tēz) SYN wall. [L. wall]

pa•ri•e•tal (pă-rī′ĕ-tăl) **1.** Relating to the wall of any cavity. **2.** SYN somatic (1). **3.** SYN somatic (2). **4.** Relating to the parietal bone.

pa•ri•e•tal bone (pă-rī′ĕ-tăl bōn) A flat, curved bone of irregular quadrangular shape, at either side of the vault of the cranium; it articulates, with its fellow medially, with the frontal anteriorly, the occipital posteriorly, and the temporal and sphenoid inferiorly.

pa•ri•e•tal cell (pă-rī′ĕ-tăl sel) One of the cells of the gastric glands; it lies on the basement membrane, covered by the chief cells, and secretes hydrochloric acid that reaches the lumen of the gland through fine intracellular and intercellular canals (canaliculi). SYN acid cell, oxyntic cell.

pa•ri•e•tal fis•tu•la (pă-rī′ĕ-tăl fis′chū-lă) A fistula, either blind or complete, opening on the wall of the thorax or abdomen.

pa•ri•e•tal fo•ra•men (pă-rī′ĕ-tăl fōr-ā′mĕn) An inconstant foramen in the parietal bone occasionally found bilaterally near the sagittal margin posteriorly; when present, it transmits an emissary vein to the superior sagittal sinus.

pa•ri•e•tal her•ni•a (pă-rī′ĕ-tăl her′ne-ă) A hernia in which only a portion of the wall of the intestine is engaged. SYN Littré hernia (1), Richter hernia.

pa•ri•e•tal lobe of cer•e•brum (pă-rī′ĕ-tăl lōb ser′ĕ-brŭm) The middle portion of each cerebral hemisphere, separated from the frontal lobe by the central sulcus, from the temporal lobe by the lateral sulcus in front and an imaginary line projected posteriorly, and from the occipital lobe only partially by the parietooccipital sulcus on its medial aspect.

pa•ri•e•tal lymph nodes (pă-rī′ĕ-tăl limf nōdz) The lymph nodes draining the walls of the abdomen or of the pelvis.

pa•ri•e•tal pleu•ra (pă-rī′ĕ-tăl plūr′ă) The serous membrane that lines the different parts of the wall of the pulmonary cavity; called costal, diaphragmatic, and mediastinal, according to the parts invested.

pa•ri•e•tal throm•bus (pă-rī′ĕ-tăl throm′bŭs) An arterial thrombus adhering to one side of the wall of the vessel. SEE ALSO mural thrombus.

pa•ri•e•tal wall (pă-rī′ĕ-tăl wawl) The body wall or the somatopleure from which it is formed.

♻**parieto-** Combining form denoting a wall of the body (e.g., the abdominal wall); a parietal bone. [L. *paries,* wall]

pa•ri•e•tog•ra•phy (pă-rī-ē-tog′ră-fē) Rarely used term for a radiographic examination of the wall of the stomach using a combination of pneumoperitoneum and intraluminal air and barium. [parieto- + G. *graphē,* a writing]

pa•ri•e•to•oc•cip•i•tal (pă-rī′ĕ-tō-ok-sip′i-tăl) Relating to the parietal and occipital bones or to the parts of the cerebral cortex corresponding thereto.

pa•ri•e•to•oc•cip•i•tal sul•cus (pă-rī′ĕ-tō-ok-sip′i-tăl sŭl′kŭs) A very deep, almost vertically oriented fissure on the medial surface of the cerebral cortex, marking the border between the parietal lobe and the cuneus of the occipital lobe; its lower part curves forward and fuses with the anterior extent of the calcarine fissure (sulcus calcarinus); the great depth of this combined fissure causes a bulge in the medial wall of the occipital horn of the lateral ventricle, the calcar avis.

Pa•ri•naud con•junc•ti•vi•tis (pah-ri-nō′ kŏn-jŭngk′ti-vī′tis) A chronic necrotic inflammation of the conjunctiva characterized by large, irregular, reddish follicles and regional lymphadenopathy.

Pa•ri•naud oc•u•lo•glan•du•lar syn•drome (pah-ri-nō′ ok′yū-lō-glan′dyū-lăr sin′drōm) Unilateral conjunctival granuloma with preauricular adenopathy in tularemia, chancre, tuberculosis, and cat-scratch disease.

Pa•ri•naud syn•drome, Pa•ri•naud oph•thal•mo•ple•gi•a (pah-rī-nō′ sin′drōm, of-thal′mō-plē′jē-ă) Paralysis of conjugate upward gaze caused by a lesion at the level of the superior colliculi; characterized by convergence-retraction nystagmus, light-near dissociation of the pupillary response, and lid retraction. SYN dorsal midbrain syndrome.

par•ish nur•sing (par′ish nŭrs′ing) Nursing care and spiritual counseling provided by visiting nurses to members of a spiritual community.

par•i•ty (par′i-tē) The condition of having given birth to an infant or infants, alive or dead; a multiple birth is considered as a single parous experience. [L. *pario,* to bear]

Park an•eu•rysm (pahrk an′yūr-izm) An arteriovenous aneurysm in which the brachial artery communicates with the brachial and median basilic veins.

Parkes Web•er syn•drome (pahrks vā′ber sin′drōm) A rare vascular malformation; often involves lower limbs, which enlarge; other findings include abnormal venous and arterial strictures.

Par•kin•son dis•ease (pahr′kin-sŏn di-zēz′) SYN parkinsonism (1).

Par·kin·son fa·ci·es (pahr′kin-sŏn fā′shē-ēz) The expressionless or masklike facies characteristic of parkinsonism (1). SYN masklike face.

par·kin·so·ni·an (par-kin-sō′nē-an) Relating to or the suffering from parkinsonism (1).

par·kin·so·ni·an dys·arth·ri·a (par-kin-sō′nē-ăn dis-ahr′thrē-ă) A hypokinetic dysarthria associated with parkinsonism, characterized by rigidity and reduced range of articulatory movements, monotony of pitch and loudness, reduced loudness, short rushes of speech, and rapid rate. SEE parkinsonism.

par·kin·son·ism (pahr′kin-sŏn-izm) **1.** A neurologic syndrome usually resulting from deficiency of the neurotransmitter dopamine as the consequence of degenerative, vascular, or inflammatory changes in the basal ganglia; characterized by rhythmic muscular tremors, rigidity of movement, festination, droopy posture, and masklike facies. SYN Parkinson disease. **2.** A syndrome similar to parkinsonism appearing as an adverse effect of certain antipsychotic drugs.

par level (PAR) (pahr lev′ĕl) The minimum quantity of an item stocked, which will be automatically reordered, should the level fall below a preset level.

par·ol·fac·tory sul·ci (pahr-ōl-fak′tŏr-ē sŭl′sī) Small sulci found in the parolfactory area, which is located immediately rostral to the lamina terminalis; they frequently consist of anterior and posterior sulci. SYN sulci paraolfactorii [TA].

par·om·pha·lo·cele (par-om-fal′ō-sēl) **1.** A tumor near the umbilicus. **2.** A hernia through a defect in the abdominal wall near the umbilicus. [para- + G. *omphalos,* umbilicus, + *kēlē,* tumor, hernia]

par·o·nych·i·a (par-ō-nik′ē-ă) Suppurative inflammation of the nail fold surrounding the nail plate; may be due to bacteria or fungi, most commonly staphylococci and streptococci. See this page. [para- + G. *onyx,* nail]

par·o·nych·i·al (par-ō-nik′ē-ăl) Relating to paronychia.

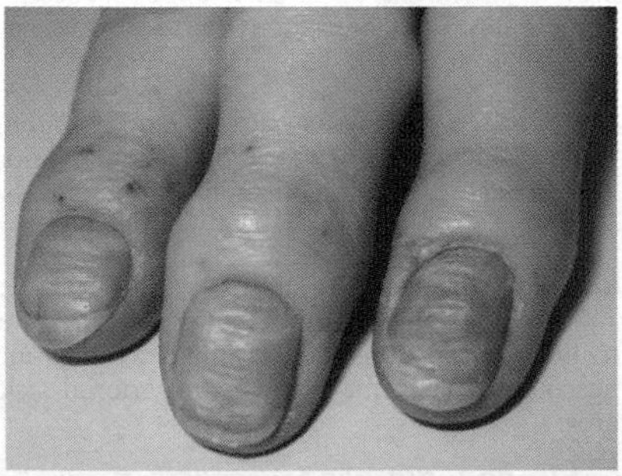

chronic paronychia

par·o·oph·o·ron (par-ō-of′ōr-on) Remnants of the tubules and glomeruli of the lower part of the mesonephros appearing as a few scattered tubules in the broad ligament between the epoöphoron and the uterus. Its equivalent in the male is the paradidymis. [para- + oophoron, ovary]

par·or·chid·i·um (par-ōr-kid′ē-ŭm) SYN ectopia testis. SYN ectopia testis. [para- + G. *orchis,* testis]

par·o·rex·i·a (par-ō-rek′sē-ă) An abnormal or disordered appetite. [para- + G. *orexis,* appetite]

par·os·mi·a (par-oz′mē-ă) Any disorder of the sense of smell, especially subjective perception of nonexistent odors. [para + G. *osmē,* sense of smell]

par·os·te·o·sis, par·os·to·sis (par′os-tē-ō′sis, -os-tō′sis) **1.** Development of bone in an unusual location, as in the skin. **2.** Abnormal or defective ossification. [para- + G. *osteon,* bone, + *-osis,* condition]

pa·rot·ic (pă-rot′ik) Near or beside the ear. [para- + G. *ous,* ear]

pa·rot·id (pă-rot′id) Situated near the ear; denoting several structures in this neighborhood. Usually refers to the parotid salivary gland. [G. *parōtis* (*parōtid-*), the gland beside the ear, fr. *para,* beside, + *ous* (*ōt-*), ear]

pa·rot·id duct (pă-rot′id dŭkt) The duct of the parotid gland opening from the cheek into the vestibule of the mouth opposite the neck of the superior second molar tooth. SYN Stensen duct, Steno duct.

pa·rot·i·dec·to·my (pă-rot′i-dek′tŏ-mē) Surgical removal of the parotid gland. [parotid + G. *ektomē,* excision]

pa·rot·id gland (pă-rot′id gland) The largest of the salivary glands, one of two compound acinous glands situated inferior and anterior to the ear, on either side, extending from the angle of the jaw to the zygomatic arch and posteriorly to the sternocleidomastoid muscle; it is subdivided into a superficial part and a deep part by emerging branches of the facial nerve, and discharges through the parotid duct.

pa·rot·i·di·tis (pă-rot-i-dī′tis) Inflammation of the parotid gland. SYN parotitis.

pa·rot·id notch (pă-rot′id noch) The space between the ramus of the mandible and the mastoid process of the temporal bone.

pa·rot·id pa·pil·la (pă-rot′id pă-pil′ă) The projection at the opening of the parotid duct into the vestibule of the mouth opposite the neck of the upper second molar tooth.

pa·rot·id veins (pă-rot′id vānz) Veins that drain part of the parotid gland and empty into the retromandibular vein.

par·o·ti·tis (par-ō-tī′tis) SYN parotiditis.

par•ous (par′ŭs) Pertaining to parity. [L. *pario,* to bear]

par•o•var•i•an (par-ō-var′ē-ăn) **1.** Relating to the paroophoron. **2.** Beside or in the neighborhood of the ovary.

par•ox•ysm (par′ok-sizm) **1.** A sharp spasm or convulsion. **2.** A sudden onset of a symptom or disease, especially one with recurrent manifestations such as the chills and rigor of malaria. [G. *paroxysmos,* fr. *paroxynō,* to sharpen, irritate, fr. *oxys,* sharp]

par•ox•ys•mal (par-ok-siz′măl) Relating to or occurring in paroxysms.

par•ox•ys•mal cold he•mo•glo•bin•u•ri•a (PCH) (par-ok-siz′măl kōld hē′mō-glō-bi-nyūr′ē-ă) An autoimmune hemolytic anemia characterized by hemolysis and subsequent hemoglobinuria on exposure to cold. The hemolysis is caused by the Donath-Landsteiner antibody, which attaches to the red cell at temperatures below 15°C. On warming, the antibody dissociates from the cell, but the terminal complement components are activated, causing cell injury and hemolysis. SEE ALSO Donath-Landsteiner antibody.

par•ox•ys•mal hy•per•ten•sion (par-ok-siz′măl hī′pĕr-ten′shŭn) SYN episodic hypertension.

par•ox•ys•mal noc•tur•nal dysp•ne•a (PND) (par-ok-siz′măl nok-tŭr′năl disp′nē-ă) Acute shortness of breath that appears suddenly at night, usually waking the patient after an hour or two of sleep; caused by pulmonary congestion that results from left-sided heart failure.

par•ox•ys•mal noc•tur•nal he•mo•glo•bin•e•mi•a (par-ok-siz′măl nok-tŭr′năl hē′mō-glo-bi-nē′mē-ă) An acquired hematopoictic stem cell disorder characterized by formation of defective platelets, granulocytes, erythrocytes, and possibly lymphocytes. The red cell abnormality causes complement-mediated intravascular lysis, which may be expressed in an irregular or even occult manner.

par•ox•ys•mal noc•tur•nal he•mo•glo•bin•u•ri•a (PNH) (par-ok-siz′măl nok-tŭr′năl hē′mō-glō-bi-nyūr′ē-ă) A hemolytic anemia in which the red blood cell membrane is abnormal, rendering the cell more susceptible to hemolysis by complement. The membrane defects include a lack of decay-accelerating factor (DAF) and C8 binding protein (C8bp) due to lack of glycosyl phosphatidyl inositol (GPI). GPI is a membrane glycolipid that attaches proteins to the cell membrane. Hemolysis is intravascular and intermittent, characterized by passage of reddish urine.

par•ox•ys•mal tach•y•car•di•a (par-ok-siz′măl tak′i-kahr′dē-ă) Recurrent attacks of tachycardia, with abrupt onset and often also abrupt termination, originating from an ectopic focus that may be atrial, A-V junctional, or ventricular.

PAR-Q Abbreviation for Physical Readiness Questionnaire.

par•rot beak tear (par′ŏt bēk tār) An injury to articular cartilage resulting in the separation of a narrow, curved wedge resembling a parrot's beak.

Par•rot dis•ease (par′ŏt di-zēz′) **1.** Pseudoparalysis in infants, due to syphilitic osteochondritis. **2.** SYN marasmus. **3.** SYN psittacosis.

par•rot fe•ver (par′ŏt fē′vĕr) SYN psittacosis.

Par•ry dis•ease (par′ē di-zēz′) SYN Graves disease.

pars, pl. **par•tes** (pahrz, pahr′tēz) A part; a portion. [L. *pars* (*part-*) a part]

pars ab•dom•i•na•lis a•or•tae (pahrz ab-dom′i-nā′lis ā-ōr′tē) SYN abdominal aorta.

pars a•mor•pha (pahrz ă-mōr′fă) The part of the nucleolus that occupies irregular spaces in the nucleolonema and contains finely filamentous substance. SEE ALSO pars granulosa.

pars as•cen•dens a•or•tae (pahrz ă-send′enz ā-ōr′tē) SYN ascending aorta.

pars gran•u•lo•sa (pahrz gran′yū-lō′să) The granular and filamentous part of the nucleolonema of the nucleolus.

pars in•ter•ar•tic•u•lar•is (pahrz in-tĕr-ahr-tik′yū-lā′ris) The region between the superior and inferior articulating facets of a vertebra; frequently the site of fracture in spondylolysis.

pars pla•na (pahrz plān′ă) SYN orbiculus ciliaris.

pars-pla•ni•tis (pahrz-plā-nī′tis) A clinical syndrome consisting of inflammation of the peripheral retina and pars plana, exudation into the overlying vitreous base, and edema of the optic disc and adjacent retina.

pars tho•ra•ci•ca a•or•tae (pahrz thōr-ras′ik-ă ā-ōr′tē) SYN thoracic aorta.

pars tym•pan•i•ca (pahrz tim-pan′i-kă) Tympanic portion of the temporal bone, forming the greater part of the wall of the external acoustic meatus.

pars u•te•ri•na pla•cen•tae (pahrz yū-tĕr-ē′nă plă-sen′tē) [TA] SYN maternal part of placenta.

par•the•no•gen•e•sis (pahr′thĕ-nō-jen′ĕ-sis) A form of nonsexual reproduction, or agamogenesis, in which the female reproduces its kind without fecundation by the male. [G. *parthenos,* virgin, + *genesis,* production]

par•tial ag•glu•ti•nin (pahr′shăl ă-glū′ti-nin) SYN minor agglutinin.

par•tial an•om•a•lous pul•mo•na•ry ve•nous con•nec•tions (pahr′shăl ă-nom′ă-lŭs pul′mŏ-nar′ē vē′nŭs kŏ-nek′shŭnz) SEE anomalous pulmonary venous connections, total or partial.

par·tial an·ti·gen (pahr′shăl an′ti-jen) SYN hapten.

par·tial cri·coid cleft (pahr′shăl krī′koyd kleft) SEE laryngotracheoesophageal cleft.

par·tial den·ture (pahr′shăl den′shŭr) A dental prosthesis that restores one or more, but not all, of the natural teeth or associated parts and is supported by the teeth or the mucosa; it may be removable or fixed. SYN bridgework.

par·tial lar·yn·gec·to·my (pahr′shăl lar-in-jek′tŏ-mē) Incomplete resection of the larynx in which the supraglottic portion is removed, preserving the vocal cords. SYN horizontal laryngectomy, supraglottic laryngectomy.

par·tial left ven·tric·u·lec·tomy (pahr′shăl left ven-trik-yū-lek′tō-mē) SYN left ventricular volume reduction surgery.

par·tial pos·te·ri·or la·ryn·ge·al cleft (pahr′shăl pos-tēr′ē-ŏr lă-rin′jē-ăl kleft) SEE laryngotracheoesophageal cleft.

par·tial pres·sure (pahr′shăl presh′ŭr) The pressure exerted by a single component of a mixture of gases, commonly expressed in mm Hg or torr; for a gas dissolved in a liquid, the partial pressure is that of a gas that would be in equilibrium with the dissolved gas. In respiratory physiology, symbolized by P, followed by subscripts denoting location and/or chemical species (e.g., P_{CO_2}, P_{O_2}, $P_{A_{CO_2}}$).

par·tial re·breath·ing mask (pahr′shăl rē-brēdh′ing mask) A face mask and a reservoir bag permitting a portion of exhaled gas to enter the bag for mixing with source gas.

par·tial sei·zure (pahr′shăl sē′zhŭr) Seizure characterized by localized cerebral ictal onset. The symptoms experienced are dependent on the cortical area of ictal onset or seizure spread.

par·tial-thick·ness burn (pahr′shăl thik′nĕs bŭrn) A burn involving the epidermis and dermis that usually forms blisters; followed by epithelial regeneration extending from the dermal appendages. SYN second-degree burn.

par·tial-thick·ness flap (pahr′shăl-thik′nĕs flap) SYN split-thickness flap.

par·tial-thick·ness graft (pahr′shăl-thik′nĕs graft) SYN split-thickness graft.

par·tial throm·bo·plas·tin time (PTT) (pahr′shăl throm-bō-plas′tin tīm) SEE activated partial thromboplastin time.

par·tial vol·ume (pahr′shăl vol′yūm) The actual volume occupied by one species of molecule or particle in a solution; the reciprocal of the density of the molecule.

par·ti·ci·pa·ting phy·si·cian or sup·pli·er (pahr-tis′i-pā-ting fi-zish′ŭn sŭ-plī′ĕr) A physician or health care supplier who agrees to accept assignment on Medicare claims, billing for Medicare deductible(s), and coinsurance amounts.

par·ti·ci·pa·tion (pahr-tis-i-pā′shŭn) OCCUPATIONAL THERAPY involvement in a life situation.

par·ti·cle (pahr′ti-kĕl) **1.** A small piece or portion of anything. **2.** An elementary particle such as a proton or electron. [L. *particula,* dim. of *pars,* part]

par·tic·u·late (pahr-tik′yū-lāt) Relating to or occurring in the form of fine particles; formed elements, discrete bodies, as contrasted with the surrounding liquid or semiliquid material (e.g., granules or mitochondria in cells).

par·tic·u·late wear de·bris (pahr-tik′yū-lăt wār dĕ-brē′) Microscopic particles produced by friction between articulating surfaces in a total joint replacement; debris can include particles of metal, polyethylene, and polymethylmethacrylate cement, and can induce osteolysis.

par·ti·tion chro·ma·tog·ra·phy (pahr-tish′ŭn krō′mă-tog′ră-fē) The separation of similar substances by repeated divisions between two immiscible liquids, so that the substances, in effect, cross the partition between the liquids in opposite directions.

par·to·gram (pahr′tō-gram) Graph of labor parameters of time and dilation with alert and action lines to prompt intervention if the curve deviates from expected. SYN Friedman curve, labor curve. [L. *partus,* childbirth, + -gram]

par·tu·ri·ent (pahr-chŭr′ē-ĕnt) Relating to or in the process of childbirth. [L. *parturio,* to be in labor]

par·tu·ri·ent ca·nal (pahr-chŭr′ē-ĕnt kă-nal′) SYN birth canal.

par·tu·ri·om·e·ter (pahr-chŭr′ē-om′ĕ-tĕr) Device for determining the force of the uterine contractions in childbirth. [L. *parturitio,* parturition, + G. *metron,* measure]

par·tu·ri·tion (pahr-chŭr-ish′ŭn) SYN childbirth. [L. *parturitio,* fr. *parturio,* to be in labor]

pa·ru·lis (pă-rū′lis) SYN gingival abscess. [G. *paroulis,* gumboil, fr. *para,* beside, + *oulon,* gum]

par·vo·cel·lu·lar (pahr-vō-sel′yū-lăr) Relating to or composed of cells of small size. [L. *parvus,* small, + Mod. L. *cellularis,* cellular]

Par·vo·vir·i·dae (pahr-vō-vir′i-dē) A family of small viruses containing single-stranded DNA. Three genera are recognized: Parvovirus, Densovirus, and Dependovirus, which includes the adeno-associated satellite virus.

Par·vo·vi·rus (pahr′vō-vī′rŭs) A genus of viruses that replicate autonomously in suitable cells. [L. *parvus,* small, + virus]

Par•vo•vi•rus B19 (pahr′vō-vī′rŭs) A single-stranded DNA virus belonging to the family Parvoviridae; the cause of erythema infectiosum (fifth disease) and aplastic crises.

pas•cal (Pa) (pas-kahl′) A derived unit of pressure or stress in the SI system, expressed in newtons per square meter; equal to 10^{-5} bar or 7.50062×10^{-3} torr. [B. *Pascal*]

Pas•cal law (pahs-kahl′ law) Fluids at rest transmit pressure equally in every direction.

Pas•sa•vant ridge (pahs′ă-vahnt rij) A prominence on the posterior wall of the nasopharynx formed by contraction of the superior constrictor muscle of the pharynx during swallowing.

Pas•sa•voy fac•tor (pas′ă-voy fak′tŏr) A clotting factor of which congenital deficiency causes a moderate bleeding diathesis in which the activated partial thromboplastin time is prolonged. SEE ALSO Hageman factor.

pas•sive (pas′iv) Not active; submissive. [L. *passivus,* fr. *patior,* to endure]

pas•sive-ag•gres•sive per•son•al•i•ty (pas′iv-ă-gres′siv pĕr-sŏn-al′i-tē) A personality disorder in which aggressive feelings are shown in passive ways, especially through mild obstructionism and stubbornness.

pas•sive an•a•phy•lax•is (pas′iv an′ă-fi-lak′sis) A reaction resulting from inoculation of antigen in an animal previously inoculated intravenously with specific antiserum from another animal, a latent period being required between the two inoculations. SYN antiserum anaphylaxis.

pas•sive at•el•ec•ta•sis (pas′iv at-ĕ-lek′tă-sis) The pulmonary collapse that occurs due to a space-occupying intrathoracic process such as pneumothorax or hydrothorax.

pas•sive clot (pas′iv klot) A clot formed in an aneurysmal sac consequent to cessation or slowing of circulation.

pas•sive con•ges•tion (pas′iv kŏn-jes′chŭn) Congestion caused by obstruction or slowing of the venous drainage, resulting in partial stagnation of blood in the capillaries and venules.

pas•sive dif•fu•sion (pas′iv di-fyū′zhŭn) Passage of molecules across a semipermeable membrane without expenditure of energy.

pas•sive he•mag•glu•ti•na•tion (pas′iv hē′mă-glū-ti-nā′shŭn) Agglutination in which erythrocytes, usually modified by treatment with chemicals, adsorb soluble antigen and then agglutinate in the presence of antiserum specific for the adsorbed antigen. SYN indirect hemagglutination test.

pas•sive hy•per•e•mi•a (pas′iv hī′pĕr-ē′mē-ă) Hyperemia due to an obstruction in the flow of blood from the affected part, the venous radicles becoming distended. SYN venous hyperemia.

pas•sive im•mu•ni•ty (pas′iv i-myūn′i-tē) SEE acquired immunity.

pas•sive move•ment (pas′iv mūv′mĕnt) Movement imparted to an organism or any of its parts by external agency; movement of any joint effected by the hand of another person, or by mechanical means, without participation of the subject.

pas•sive range of mo•tion (PROM) (păs-iv′ rānj mō′shŭn) Amount of motion at a given joint when the joint is moved by an external force or therapist.

pas•sive trans•port (pas′iv trans′pōrt) The movement of particles or ions across a semipermeable membrane without the expenditure of energy. It is directly influenced by chemical or electrical gradients: the difference in the number of particles on either side of the membrane (chemical) or a difference in charged particles or ions (electrical).

pas•siv•ism (pas′iv-izm) An attitude of submission, particularly in sexual relations. SEE ALSO passive.

Pas•sy-Mu•ir valve (pas′ē-myū′ĭr valv) One-way valvular device to facilitate ventilation and speech in patients who have undergone tracheotomy.

paste (pāst) A soft semisolid of firmer consistency than pap but soft enough to flow slowly and not retain its shape. [L. *pasta*]

Pas•teur ef•fect (pahs-tur′ e-fekt′) The inhibition of fermentation by oxygen, first observed by L. Pasteur; either not observed, or only slightly observed, in malignant tumors.

Pas•teur•el•la (pas-tur-el′ă) A genus of aerobic to facultatively anaerobic, nonmotile bacteria (family Brucellaceae) containing small, gram-negative cocci or ellipsoidal to elongated rods that, with special methods, may show bipolar staining. These organisms are parasites of humans and other animals, including birds. The type species is *P. multocida.*

pas•teu•rel•la, pl. **pas•teu•rel•lae** (pas-tur-el′ă, -ē) A vernacular term used to refer to any member of the genus *Pasteurella.*

Pas•teur•el•la aer•o•gen•es (pas-tur-el′ă ār-oj′jĕ-nēz) A bacterial species found in swine that can infect human wounds after pig bites.

Pas•teur•el•la mul•to•ci•da (pas-tur-el′ă mŭl-tō′sē-dŭh) A bacterial species that causes fowl cholera and hemorrhagic septicemia in warm-blooded animals and may infect dog or cat bites or scratches and cause cellulitis and septicemia in humans with chronic disease. The most common pathogen associated with cat and dog bites. It is the type species of the genus *Pasteurella.*

Pas·teur·el·la pseu·do·tu·ber·cu·lo·sis (pas-tur-el′ă sū′do-tū-ber-kyu-lō′sis) SYN *Yersinia pseudotuberculosis.*

pas·teur·el·lo·sis (pas′tur-ĕ-lō′sis) Infection with bacteria of the genus *Pasteurella.*

pasteurisation [Br.] SYN pasteurization.

pas·teur·i·za·tion (pas′tyur-ī-zā′shŭn) The heating of milk, wines, and fruit juice for about 30 minutes at 68°C (154.4°F), whereby living bacteria are destroyed but the flavor or bouquet is preserved; the spores are unaffected but are kept from developing by immediately cooling the liquid to 10°C (50°F) or lower. SEE ALSO sterilization. SYN pasteurisation.

Pas·ti·a sign (pahs′tē-ah sīn) The presence of pink or red transverse lines at the bend of the elbow in the preeruptive stage of scarlatina; they persist through the eruptive stage and remain as pigmented lines after desquamation. SYN Thomson sign.

pas·tille, pas·til (pas-tēl′, pas′til) **1.** A small mass of benzoin and other aromatic substances to be burned for fumigation. **2.** SYN troche. [Fr. *pastille;* L. *pastillus,* a roll (of bread), dim. of *panis,* bread]

i patch (pach) **1.** A small, circumscribed area differing in color or structure from the surrounding surface. **2.** DERMATOLOGY a flat area larger than 1.0 cm in diameter. **3.** An intermediate stage in the formation of a cap on the surface of a cell. See page B10.

patch test (pach test) A test of skin sensitiveness: a small piece of paper, tape, or a cup, wet with a dilute solution or suspension of test material, is applied to skin of the upper back or upper outer arm, and after 48 hours the area previously covered is compared with the uncovered surface; an erythematous reaction with vesicles occurs if the substance causes contact allergy. SEE ALSO photo-patch test.

pa·tel·la, gen. and pl. **pa·tel·lae** (pă-tel′ă, -ē) [TA] The large sesamoid bone that covers the anterior surface of the knee. It is formed in the tendon of the quadriceps femoris muscle and is attached to the tibia by the patellar tendon. SYN kneecap. [L. a small plate, the kneecap, dim. of *patina,* a shallow disk, fr. *pateo,* to lie open]

pa·tel·la al·ta (pă-tel′ă al′tă) Term used to describe a somewhat more proximal position of the patella than anticipated when visualized on a lateral radiograph of the knee. [patella + L. *alta,* high]

pa·tel·la ap·pre·hen·sion test (pă-tel′ă a-prē-hen′shŭn test) SYN patellar apprehension sign.

pa·tel·la ba·ja (pă-tel′ă bah′hah) Term used to describe a somewhat more distal position of the patella than anticipated when visualized on a lateral radiograph of the knee. [patella + Sp. *baja,* low]

pa·tel·lar (pă-tel′ăr) Relating to the patella.

pa·tel·lar ap·pre·hen·sion sign (pă-tel′ăr ap-prē-hen′shŭn sīn) A physical finding in which forced lateral displacement of the patella produces anxiety and resistance in patients with a history of lateral patellar instability. SYN patella apprehension test.

pa·tel·lar lig·a·ment (pă-tel′ăr lig′ă-mĕnt) A strong, flattened, fibrous band passing from the apex and adjoining margins of the patella to the tuberosity of the tibia. SYN ligamentum patellae [TA].

pa·tel·lar re·flex (pă-tel′ăr rē′fleks) A sudden contraction of the anterior muscles of the thigh, caused by a smart tap on the patellar tendon while the leg hangs loosely at a right angle with the thigh. SYN knee reflex, knee-jerk reflex, quadriceps reflex.

pat·el·lec·to·my (pat-ĕ-lek′tŏ-mē) Excision of the patella. [patella + G. *ektomē,* excision]

pa·tel·li·form (pă-tel′i-fōrm) Of the shape of the patella.

pa·tel·lo·ad·duc·tor re·flex (pă-tel′ō-ad-dŭk′tŏr rē′fleks) Crossed adduction of the leg on tapping of the quadriceps tendon.

pa·tel·lo·fem·or·al joint (pă-tel-ō-fem′ŏr-ăl joynt) The sliding articulation between the patella and the distal femur. SEE ALSO knee complex.

pa·tel·lo·fem·or·al stress syn·drome (pă-tel′ō-fem′ŏ-răl stres sin′drōm) SYN runner's knee.

pa·tel·lo·fem·or·al syn·drome (pă-tel′ō-fem′ŏ-răl sin′drōm) Degenerative condition affecting the articular cartilage of the patella caused by abnormal compression or shearing forces at the knee joint; may cause patellalgia.

pa·ten·cy (pā′tĕn-sē) The state of being freely open or exposed.

pa·tent (pā′tĕnt) Open or exposed. SYN patulous. [L. *patens,* pres. p. of *pateo,* to lie open]

pa·tent duc·tus ar·te·ri·o·sus (pā′tent dŭk′tŭs ahr-tē-rē-ō′sus) A condition in which the normal channel between the pulmonary artery and the aorta fails to close at birth. In fetal circulation, the blood bypasses the pulmonary circuit because oxygen and carbon dioxide are exchanged through the placenta. After birth, this channel normally closes in response to expansion of the lungs.

pa·tent for·a·men o·va·le (pa′tĕnt fōr-ā′mĕn ō-vā′lē) Valvular incompetence of the patent foramen ovale of the heart; a condition contrasting with probe patency of the foramen ovale in that the valve of the foramen ovale has abnormal perforations in it, or is of insufficient size to afford adequate valvular action at the foramen ovale prenatally, or effect a complete closure postnatally.

pa·tent med·i·cine (pa′tĕnt med′i-sin) An increasingly outdated term for a medication or product that was patented and marketed to the public, rather than physicians.

path (path) The route or course along which something travels. [O.E. *paeth*]

♻ **path-, -pathy, patho-, pathic** Combining forms meaning disease. [G. *pathos,* feeling, suffering, disease]

path·er·gy (path′ĕr-jē) Those reactions resulting from a state of altered activity, both allergic (immune) and nonallergic. [G. *pathos,* disease, + *ergon,* work]

♻ **-pathetic, -pathetical** Combining forms meaning emotions.

path·find·er (path′fīnd-ĕr) A filiform bougie introduced through a narrow stricture that serves as a guide for the passage of a larger sound or catheter.

♻ **-pathic** Combining form meaning disease or suffering. [G. *patheia,* suffering]

path·o·bi·ol·o·gy (path′ō-bī-ol′ŏ-jē) Pathology with emphasis more on the biologic than on the medical aspects.

path·o·bi·o·me·chan·ics (path′ō-bī′ō-mĕ-kan′iks) Postural adaptations and asymmetries; relates to imbalances of strength, mismatched forces, inappropriate actions of assistance (synergistic) muscle contractions, and excessive actions of opposing (antagonistic) muscle contractions.

path·o·clis·is (path-ō-klis′is) A specific tendency to sensitivity to special toxins; a tendency for toxins to attack certain organs. [patho- + G. *klisis,* bending, proneness]

path·o·gen (path′ŏ-jĕn) Any virus, microorganism, or other substance that causes disease. [patho- + G. *-gen,* to produce]

path·o·gen·e·sis (path′ō-jen′ĕ-sis) The pathologic, physiologic, or biochemical mechanism resulting in the development of a disease or morbid process. Cf. etiology. [patho- + G. *genesis,* production]

path·o·gen·ic, path·o·ge·net·ic (path′ō-jen′ik, -jĕ-net′ik) Causing disease or abnormality. SYN morbific, nosogenic, nosopoietic.

path·o·ge·nic·i·ty (path′ō-jĕ-nis′i-tē) The condition or quality of being pathogenic, or the ability to cause disease.

path·o·gen·ic oc·clu·sion (path′ō-jen′ik ŏ-klū′zhŭn) An occlusal relationship capable of producing pathologic changes in the supporting tissues.

path·og·no·mon·ic (path′og-nō-mon′ik) Denoting something characteristic or indicative of a disease; denoting especially one or more typical symptoms, findings, or patterns of abnormalities specific to a given disease and not found in any other condition.

path·og·no·mon·ic symp·tom (path′og-nō-mon′ik simp′tŏm) A symptom that, when present, points unmistakably to the presence of a certain definite disease.

path·o·log·ic, path·o·log·i·cal (path′ō-loj′ik, -i-kăl) **1.** Pertaining to the essential nature of disease and to the physical, functional, biochemical, and immunologic changes induced by illness. **2.** Morbid or diseased; resulting from disease.

path·o·log·ic ab·sorp·tion (path′ō-loj′ik ăb-sōrp′shŭn) Parenteral absorption of any excremental or pathologic material into the bloodstream (e.g., pus, urine, bile).

path·o·log·ic a·nat·o·my (path′ō-loj′ik ă-nat′ŏ-mē) SYN anatomic pathology.

path·o·log·ic cal·ci·fi·ca·tion (path′ō-loj′ik kal′si-fi-kā′shŭn) Calcification occurring in excretory or secretory passages as calculi, and in tissues other than bone and teeth.

path·o·log·ic frac·ture (path′ō-loj′ik frak′shŭr) A fracture occurring at a site weakened by preexisting disease, especially neoplasm or necrosis, of the bone.

path·o·log·ic mod·el (path′ō-loj′ik mod′ĕl) An animal or animal stock that by inheritance or by artificial manipulation develops a disorder similar to some disease of interest and hence directly or by analogy furnishes evidence of its pathogenesis and may be used as a model for the study of preventive or therapeutic measures.

path·o·log·ic my·o·pi·a (path′ō-loj′ik mī-ō′pē-ă) Progressive myopia marked by fundus changes, posterior staphyloma, and subnormal corrected acuity.

path·o·log·ic pro·teins (path′ō-loj′ik prō′tēnz) Incomplete monoclonal immunoglobulin occurring in association with plasma cell disorders. SEE ALSO paraprotein.

path·o·log·ic re·trac·tion ring (path′ō-loj′ik rĕ-trak′shŭn ring) A constriction located at the junction of the thinned lower uterine segment with the thick retracted upper uterine segment, resulting from obstructed labor; this is one of the classic signs of threatened rupture of the uterus. SYN Bandl ring.

pa·thol·o·gist (pa-thol′ŏ-jist) A specialist in pathology; a physician who performs, interprets, or supervises diagnostic tests, using materials removed from living or dead patients, and functions as a laboratory consultant to clinicians, or who conducts experiments or other investigations to determine the causes or nature of disease changes.

pa·thol·o·gy (pă-thol′ŏ-jē) The medical science, and specialty practice, concerned with all aspects of disease but with special reference to the essential nature, causes, and development of abnormal conditions, as well as the structural and functional changes that result from the disease processes. [patho- + G. *logos,* study, treatise]

path·o·mi·me·sis (path′ō-mī-mē′sis) Mimicry of a disease or dysfunction, whether intentional or unconscious. [patho- + G. *mimēsis,* imitation]

path·o·phys·i·ol·o·gy (path′ō-fiz-ē-ol′ŏ-jē) **1.** The study of structural and functional changes in tissue and organs that lead to disease. **2.** Derangement of function seen in disease; alteration in function as distinguished from structural defects.

pa·tho·sis (pă-thō′sis) Rarely used term for a state of disease, diseased condition, or disease entity. [patho- + G. *-osis,* condition]

path·way (path′wā) **1.** A collection of axons establishing a conduction route for nerve impulses from one group of nerve cells to another group or to an effector organ composed of muscle or gland cells. **2.** Any sequence of chemical reactions leading from one compound to another; if taking place in living tissue, usually referred to as a biochemical pathway.

pa·tient (pā′shĕnt) One who is suffering from disease, injury, an abnormal state, or a mental disorder, and is engaged in related treatment. Cf. case (1), client. [L. *patiens,* pres. p. of *patior,* to suffer]

pa·tient care tech·ni·cian (PCT) (pā′shĕnt kār tek-nish′ŭn) A health care worker who uses both nursing and medical assisting skills to provide patient care in a hospital setting.

pa·tient-con·trolled an·al·ge·si·a (PCA), pa·tient-con·trolled an·es·the·si·a (pā′shĕnt kŏn-trōld′ an′ăl-jē′zē-ă, an′es-thē′zē-ă) A method for control of pain based on use of a pump for the constant intravenous or, less frequently, epidural infusion of a dilute narcotic solution that includes a mechanism for the self-administration at predetermined intervals of the narcotic solution should the infusion fail to relieve pain.

pa·tient edu·ca·tion (pā′shĕnt ej′ū-kā′shŭn) NURSING teaching of the patient; process of assisting the patient to gain knowledge, skill, and a value or attitude related to a health problem or for health promotion.

pa·tient sat·is·fac·tion (pā′shĕnt sat-is-fak′shŭn) Patient's opinion of care received.

Pa·tient's Bill of Rights (pā′shĕnts bil rīts) Developed in 1973 by the AHA to affirm the rights of patients. Key elements are the right to respectful and considerate care, privacy, information about treatment, and prognosis, as well as the right to refuse treatment.

Pat·rick test (pat′rik test) A procedure to determine the presence or absence of sacroiliac disease; with the patient supine, the hip and knee are flexed and the external malleolus is placed above the patella of the opposite leg; this can ordinarily be done without pain, but, on depressing the knee, pain is promptly elicited in sacroiliac disease.

pat·ri·lin·e·al (pat-ri-lin′ē-ăl) Related to descent through the male line; inheritance of the Y chromosome is exclusively patrilineal. [L. *pater,* father, + *linea,* line]

pat·tern (pat′ĕrn) **1.** A design. **2.** DENTISTRY a form used in making a mold, as for an inlay or partial denture framework.

pat·tern dis·tor·tion am·bly·o·pi·a (pat′ĕrn dis-tōr′shŭn am′blē-ō′pē-ă) Amblyopia due to a blurred retinal image during the amblyogenic period of visual development.

pat·terned al·o·pe·ci·a (pat′ĕrnd al-ō-pē′shē-ă) SYN androgenic alopecia.

pat·tern ret·i·nal dys·tro·phy (pat′ĕrn ret′i-năl dis′trŏ-fē) A spectrum of autosomal dominant diseases affecting the retinal pigment epithelium, leading to mild to moderate vision loss.

pat·tern-sen·si·tive ep·i·lep·sy (păt′ĕrn-sen′si-tiv ep′i-lep′sē) A form of reflex epilepsy precipitated by viewing certain patterns.

pat·u·lous (pat′yū-lŭs) SYN patent. [L. *patulus,* fr. *pateo,* to lie open]

pau·ci·ar·ti·cu·lar (paw-sē-ahr-tik′yū-lăr) A joint condition in which only a few (1–5) joints are involved [L. *pauci,* few, + articular]

pau·ci·bac·il·lary (pa-sē-bas′i-lār-ē) Made up of, or denoting the presence of, few bacilli.

pau·ci·sy·nap·tic (paw′sē-si-nap′tik) SYN oligosynaptic. [L. *paucus,* few, + synapse]

Pau·li ex·clu·sion prin·ci·ple (pawl′ē eks-klū′zhŭn prin′si-pĕl) The theory limiting the number of electrons in the orbit or shell of an atom: that it is not possible for any two electrons to have all four quantum numbers identical.

pause sig·nal (pawz sig′năl) A DNA sequence that causes pausing of RNA polymerase transcription.

Pau·tri·er mi·cro·ab·scess (pō-trē-ā′ mī′krō-ab′ses) A microscopic lesion in the epidermis, seen in mycosis fungoides; it is composed of the same type of atypical mononuclear cells as those that form the infiltrate in the corium.

PAV Abbreviation for proportional assist ventilation.

Pav•lov re•flex (pahv′lof rē′fleks) SYN auriculopressor reflex.

pav•or noc•tur•nus (pā′vōr nok-tŭr′nŭs) SYN night terrors. [L.]

pay•ee (pā-ē′) The person receiving a payment or financial reimbursement either in written form or electronically through funds transfer.

Payne op•er•a•tion (pān op-ĕr-ā′shŭn) A jejunoileal bypass for morbid obesity utilizing end-to-side anastomosis of the upper jejunum to the terminal ileum, with closure of the proximal end of the bypassed intestine.

pay•or, **pay•er** (pā′ŏr, -ĕr) The person paying the bill, satisfying the claim, or settling a financial obligation.

Payr clamp (pīr klamp) A large, slightly curved clamp used in gastrectomy or enterectomy.

Payr sign (pīr sīn) Pain on pressure over the sole of the foot; a sign of thrombophlebitis.

PB Abbreviation for pyridostigmine bromide.

Pb Symbol for lead (plumbum).

PBG Abbreviation for porphobilinogen.

p.c. Abbreviation for L. *post cibum,* after a meal.

PCA Abbreviation for patient-controlled analgesia.

pCa A way of reporting calcium ion levels; equal to $-\log[Ca^{2+}]$.

PCH Abbreviation for paroxysmal cold hemoglobinuria.

PCI Abbreviation for percutaneous coronary intervention.

PCIRV Abbreviation for pressure-controlled inverse ratio ventilation.

PCIS Abbreviation for patient care information system, an interactive computer system used to store medical records in hospitals and other types of health care facilities.

PCM Abbreviation for protein calorie malnutrition.

P con•gen•i•ta•le (kon-jen-i-tā′lē) The P-wave pattern in the electrocardiogram seen in some cases of congenital heart disease, consisting of tall peaked P waves in leads I, II, aVF, and aVL (usually largest in lead II), with predominant positivity of diphasic waves in V1–2.

PCR Abbreviation for polymerase chain reaction.

PCr Abbreviation for phosphocreatine.

PCT Abbreviation for patient care technician.

PCWP Abbreviation for pulmonary capillary wedge pressure.

PD Abbreviation for phenyldichloroarsine; peritoneal dialysis.

Pd Symbol for palladium.

PDCAAS Abbreviation for protein digestibility corrected amino acid score.

PDLL Abbreviation for poorly differentiated lymphocytic lymphoma.

PDT Abbreviation for photodynamic therapy.

PE Abbreviation for pulmonary embolism; preeclampsia.

PEA Abbreviation for pulseless electrical activity.

peak (pēk) The top or upper limit of a graphic tracing or of any variable. [M.E. *peke, pike,* fr. Sp. *pico,* beak, fr. L. *picus,* magpie]

peak ex•pi•ra•to•ry flow rate (PEFR) (pēk ek-spīr′ă-tōr-ē flō rāt) The maximum flow at the outset of forced expiration, which is reduced in proportion to the severity of airway obstruction, as in asthma.

peak flow•me•ter (pēk flō′mē-tĕr) A portable device for measuring and displaying the highest level of expiratory flow produced by a patient; commonly used to monitor pulmonary function in patients with a reversible disease of the airways.

peak lev•el (pēk lev′ĕl) The highest concentration reached by a drug, as determined by therapeutic drug monitoring.

peak and trough spec•i•mens (pēk trawf spes′i-mĕnz) A serum sample collected to determine the changing levels of an antibiotic or other medication in the blood.

pearl (pĕrl) **1.** A concretion formed around a grain of sand or other foreign body within the shell of certain mollusks. **2.** One of a number of small, tough masses (e.g., mucus occurring in the sputum in asthma).

pearl bar•ley (pĕrl bahr′lē) SYN barley.

Pearl in•dex (pĕrl in′deks) The number of failures of a contraceptive method per 100 woman years of exposure.

peau d'or•ange (pō-dŏ-rōnzh′) A swollen, pitted skin surface overlying carcinoma of the breast in which there is both stromal infiltration and lymphatic obstruction with edema. [Fr. orange peel]

pec•cant (pek′ănt) Unhealthy; producing disease. [L. *peccans (-ant-),* pres. p. of *peccare,* to sin]

pec•ten (pek′tĕn) **1.** A structure with comblike processes or projections. **2.** SYN anal pecten. [L. comb]

pec•ten an•a•lis (pek′tĕn ā-năl′is) SYN anal pecten.

pec•ten•i•tis (pek-ten-ī′tis) Inflammation of the anal sphincter. [L. *pecten,* a comb, + G. *-itis,* inflammation]

pec•ten•o•sis (pek-ten-ō′sis) Exaggerated enlargement of the pecten band.

pec•ten pu•bis (pek′tĕn pyū′bis) The continuation on the superior ramus pubis of the linea terminalis, forming a sharp ridge.

pec•ti•nate (pek′ti-nāt) **1.** Combed; comb-shaped. SYN pectiniform. **2.** In fungi, used to describe a particular type of branching hyphae in cultures of dermatophytes.

pec•ti•nate line (pek′ti-nāt līn) The line between the simple columnar epithelium of the rectum and the stratified epithelium of the anal canal. SYN linea anocutanea [TA].

pec•ti•nate mus•cles (pek′ti-nāt mŭs′ĕlz) Prominent ridges of atrial myocardium located on the inner surface of much of the right atrium and both auricles. SYN musculi pectinati [TA].

pec•ti•nate zone (pek′ti-nāt zōn) The outer two-thirds of the basilar membrane of the cochlear duct. SYN zona pectinata.

pec•tin•e•al (pek-tin′ē-ăl) Ridged; relating to the os pubis or to any comblike structure.

pec•tin•e•al lig•a•ment (pek-tin′ē-ăl lig′ă-mĕnt) A thick, strong, fibrous band that passes laterally from the lacunar ligament along the pectineal line of the pubis. SYN ligamentum pectineale [TA].

pec•tin•e•al mus•cle (pek-tin′ē-ăl mŭs′ĕl) SYN pectineus muscle.

pec•ti•ne•us mus•cle (pek-tin′ē-ŭs mŭs′ĕl) *Origin*, crest of pubis; *insertion*, pectineal line of femur; *action*, adducts thigh and assists in flexion; *nerve supply*, obturator and femoral. SYN musculus pectineus [TA], pectineal muscle.

pec•tin•i•form (pek-tin′i-fōrm) SYN pectinate (1).

pector- Combining form meaning breast. [L. *pectus,* breast]

pec•to•ral (pek′tŏr-ăl) Relating to the chest. [L. *pectoralis;* fr. *pectus,* breast bone]

pec•to•ral•gi•a (pek′tŏr-al′jē-ă) Any pain in the chest. [pector- + G. *algos,* a pain]

pec•to•ral gir•dle (pek′tŏr-ăl gĭr′dĕl) SYN shoulder girdle.

pec•to•ra•lis ma•jor mus•cle (pek-tōr-āl′is mā′jŏr mŭs′ĕl) Superficial thoracoappendicular muscle of chest; *origin*, clavicular part [TA] (pars clavicularis [TA]), medial half of clavicle; sternocostal part [TA] (pars sternocostalis [TA]), anterior surface of manubrium and body of sternum and cartilages of first to sixth ribs; abdominal part [TA] (pars abdominalis [TA]), aponeurosis of external oblique; *insertion*, crest of greater tubercle of humerus; *action*, adducts and medially rotates arm; *nerve supply*, anterior thoracic. SYN greater pectoral muscle, musculus pectoralis major.

pec•to•ra•lis mi•nor mus•cle (pek′tōr-āl′is mī′nŏr mŭs′ĕl) Deep thoracoappendicular muscle of chest; *origin*, third to fifth ribs at costochondral articulations; *insertion*, tip of coracoid process of scapula; *action*, draws down scapula or raises ribs; *nerve supply*, medial pectoral. SYN musculus pectoralis minor, smaller pectoral muscle.

pec•to•ral re•gion (pek′tŏr-ăl rē′jŭn) The region of the chest demarcated by the outline of the pectoralis major muscle. SEE ALSO regions of chest. See this page.

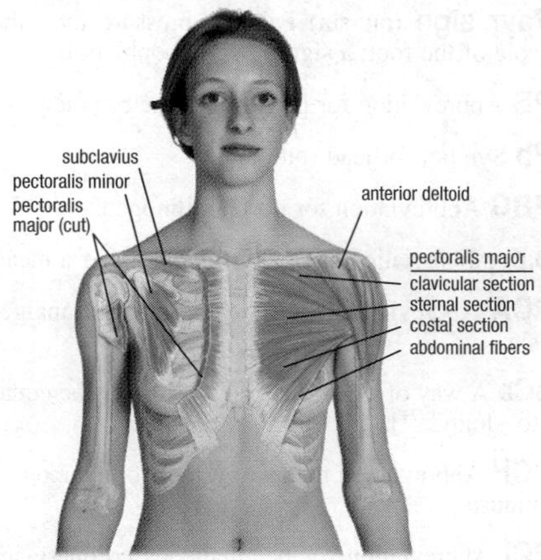

pectoral region

pec•to•ral veins (pek′tŏr-ăl vānz) Veins that drain the pectoral muscles and empty directly into the subclavian vein.

pec•to•ril•o•quy (pek-tō-ril′ŏ-kwē) Increased transmission of the voice sound through the pulmonary structures, so that it is clearly audible on auscultation of the chest; usually indicates consolidation of the underlying lung parenchyma. [L. *pectus,* chest, + *loquor,* to speak]

pec•tus, gen. **pec•to•ris**, pl. **pec•to•ra** (pek′tŭs, pek-tōr′is, -ră) [TA] SYN chest. [L.]

pec•tus ca•ri•na•tum (pek′tŭs kar′i-nā′tŭm) Flattening of the thorax (chest) on either side with forward projection of the sternum resembling the keel of a boat. SYN chicken breast.

pec•tus ex•ca•va•tum (pek′tŭs eks-kă-vā′tŭm) A hollow at the lower part of the thorax (chest) caused by a backward displacement of the xiphoid cartilage. SYN funnel breast, funnel chest.

♻ **ped-**, **pedi-**, **pedo-** **1.** Combining forms denoting child. [G. *pais,* child] **2.** Combining forms denoting foot, feet. [L. *pes,* foot] SYN paed-.

ped•al (ped′ăl) Relating to the feet, or to any structure called pes. [L. *pedalis,* fr. *pes* (*ped-*), a foot]

ped•er•as•ty (ped′ĕr-as-tē) Sexual relations between a man and a boy. SYN paederasty. [G. *paiderastia;* fr. *pais* (*paid-*), boy, + *eraō,* to long for]

Pe•der•son spec•u•lum (pē′dĕr-sŏn spek′yū-lŭm) A narrow, flat speculum used to examine a vagina with a narrow introitus.

pe•de•sis (pē-dē′sis) SYN brownian movement. [G. *pēdēsis,* a leaping]

♻ **pedia-**, **pedo-** Combining forms meaning child. [G. *pais,* child]

♻ **-pedia** Combining form meaning to educate or indicating a full list/inventory of knowledge (e.g., pharmacopedia). SYN -paedia. [G. *paideia,* a general knowledge]

pe•di•at•ric (pē-dē-at′rik) Relating to health care in children. SYN paediatric. [G. *pais* (*paid-*), child, + *iatrikos,* relating to medicine]

pe•di•at•ric ad•vanced life sup•port (PALS) (pē-dē-at′rik ad-vanst′ līf sŭ-pōrt′) Assessment and maintenance of pulmonary and circulatory function in the period before, during, and after an instance of cardiopulmonary arrest in a child.

pe•di•at•ric den•tist (pē-dē-at′rik den′tist) A health care professional concerned with the dental care and treatment of children. SYN paediatric dentist, pedodontist.

pe•di•at•ric den•tis•try (pē-dē-at′rik den′tis-trē) The branch of dentistry concerned with the dental care and treatment of children. SYN paediatric dentistry, pedodontia, pedodontics.

pe•di•a•tric•ian (pē′dē-ă-trish′ăn) A specialist in pediatrics. SYN paediatrician.

pe•di•a•tric in•ten•sive care u•nit (PICU) (pē-dē-at′rik in-ten′siv kār yū′nit) Hospital unit designated for care of critically ill children.

pe•di•at•rics (pē-dē-at′riks) The medical specialty concerned with the study and treatment of children in health and disease during development from birth through adolescence. SYN paediatrics. [G. *pais* (*paid-*), child, + *iatreia,* medical treatment]

ped•i•cel (ped′i-sel) The secondary process of a podocyte, which helps form the visceral capsule of a renal corpuscle. SYN foot process, footplate (2), foot-plate. [Mod. L. *pedicellus,* dim. of L. *pes,* foot]

ped•i•cel•late (ped′i-sel′āt) SYN pediculate.

ped•i•cel•la•tion (ped′i-sĕ-lā′shŭn) Formation of a pedicle or peduncle.

ped•i•cle (ped′i-kĕl) **1.** A constricted portion or stalk. SYN pediculus (1). **2.** A stalk by which a nonsessile tumor is attached to normal tissue. SYN peduncle (2), pedunculus. **3.** A stalk through which a flap receives nourishment until its transfer to another site results in the nourishment coming from that site. [L. *pediculus,* dim. of *pes,* foot]

ped•i•cle arch of ver•te•bra (ped′i-kĕl ahrch vĕr′tĕ-bră) Portion of vertebral arch that extends from the body to the lamina; pedicle of adjacent vertebrae create the intervertebral foramina through which spinal nerves emerge.

ped•i•cle flap (ped′i-kĕl flap) **1.** A skin flap sustained by a blood-carrying stem from the donor site during transfer; **2.** PERIODONTAL SURGERY a flap used to increase the width of attached gingiva, or to cover a root surface, by moving the attached gingiva, which remains joined at one side, to an adjacent position and suturing the free end.

pe•dic•u•lar (pĕ-dik′yū-lăr) Relating to pediculi, or lice. [L. *pedicularis*]

pe•dic•u•late (pĕ-dik′yū-lāt) Not sessile, having a pedicle or peduncle. SYN pedicellate, pedunculate. [L. *pediculatus*]

pe•dic•u•la•tion (pĕ-dik-yū-lā′shŭn) Infestation with lice. [L. *pediculus,* louse]

pe•dic•u•li (pĕ-dik′yū-lī) Plural of pediculus. [L.]

pe•dic•u•li•cide (pĕ-dik′yū-li-sīd) A chemical agent used to kill lice. [L. *pediculus,* louse + L. *caedo,* to kill]

pe•dic•u•lo•sis (pĕ-dik-yū-lō′sis) The state of being infested with lice. [L. *pediculus,* louse, + G. *-osis,* condition]

pe•dic•u•lo•sis pu•bis (pĕ-dik-yū-lō′sis pyū′bis) Infestation with the pubic or crab louse, *Pthirus pubis,* especially in pubic hair, causing pruritus and maculae ceruleae.

pe•dic•u•lous (pĕ-dik′yū-lŭs) Infested with lice.

Pe•dic•u•lus (pĕ-dik′yū-lŭs) A genus of parasitic lice that live in the hair and feed periodically on blood. Important species include *P. humanus* var. *capitis,* the human head louse; *P. humanus* var. *corporis* (also called *P. corporis*), the body louse or clothes louse, which lives and lays eggs (nits) in clothing and feeds on the human body; and *P. pubis.* [L.]

pe•dic•u•lus, pl. **pe•dic•u•li** (pĕ-dik′yū-lŭs, -lī) **1.** SYN pedicle (1). [L. pedicle] **2.** A louse. SEE *Pediculus.* [L.]

ped•i•gree (ped′i-grē) Ancestral line of descent, especially as diagrammed on a chart to show ancestral history; used in genetics to analyze inheritance. [M.E. *pedegra* fr. O.Fr. *pie de grue,* foot of crane]

ped•i•gree a•nal•y•sis (ped′i-grē ă-nal′i-sis) The formal study of the pattern of a trait in a pedigree to determine such properties as its mode of inheritance, age of onset, and variability in phenotype.

pe•do•don•ti•a (pē′dō-don′shē-ă) SYN pediatric dentistry. SYN paedodontia.

pe•do•don•tics (pē′dō-don′tiks) SYN pediatric dentistry. SYN paedodontics. [G. *pais,* child, + *odous,* tooth]

pe•do•don•tist (pē′dō-don′tist) SYN pediatric dentist. SYN paedodontist.

ped•o•dy•na•mom•e•ter (ped′ō-dī-nă-mom′ĕ-tĕr) An instrument for measuring the strength of the leg muscles. [L. *pes* (*ped-*), foot, + G. *dynamis,* force, + G. *metron,* measure]

pe•do•me•ter (pĕ-dom′ĕ-tĕr) Portable device usually attached to clothing at waist level, which mechanically registers hip elevations during walking or running. Usually measures steps taken, although some models can be calibrated to estimate distance and energy cost of walking.

pe•do•mor•phism (pē-dō-mōr′fizm) Description of adult behavior in terms appropriate to child behavior. SYN paedomorphism. [G. *pais* (*paid*), child, + *morphē,* form]

pe•do•phil•i•a (pē-dō-fil′ē-ă) An abnormal sexual attraction to children in an adult. SYN paedophilia. [G. *pais,* child, + *philos,* fond]

pe•do•phil•ic (pē-dō-fil′ik) Relating to or exhibiting pedophilia. SYN paedophilic.

pe•dun•cle (pĕ-dŭngk′ĕl) **1.** NEUROANATOMY term loosely applied to various stalklike connecting structures in the brain, composed either exclusively of white matter (e.g., cerebellar peduncle) or of white and gray matter (e.g., cerebral peduncle). **2.** SYN pedicle (2). [Mod. L. *pedunculus,* dim. of *pes,* foot]

pe•dun•cu•lar (pĕ-dŭngk′yū-lăr) Relating to a pedicle or peduncle.

pe•dun•cu•late (pĕ-dŭngk′yū-lāt) SYN pediculate.

pe•dun•cu•lot•o•my (pĕ-dŭngk′yū-lot′ŏ-mē) **1.** A total or partial section of a cerebral peduncle. **2.** A mesencephalic pyramidal tractotomy. [peduncle + G. *tomē,* incision]

pe•dun•cu•lus, pl. **pe•dun•cu•li** (pĕ-dŭngk′yū-lŭs, -lī) SYN pedicle (2). [Mod. L. dim. of *pes,* foot]

PEEP Abbreviation for positive end-expiratory pressure.

peep•ing tes•tis (pē′ping tes′tis) An undescended testis that migrates back and forth at the internal inguinal ring.

peer re•view (pēr rĕ-vyū′) Assessment of research proposals, manuscripts submitted for publication, or a physician's clinical practice by other physicians or scientists in the same field.

peer-re•view or•gan•i•za•tion (PRO) (pēr-rĕ-vyū′ ōr′găn-ī-zā′shŭn) An organization that contracts with the U.S. Centers for Medicare and Medicaid Services (which pays for health care to Medicare patients) to review the need for and quality of care given to Medicare patients, and to monitor the accuracy of assigned DRGs submitted by the health care facility as the basis for reimbursement for services provided.

PEFR Abbreviation for peak expiratory flow rate.

PEG Abbreviation for percutaneous endoscopic gastrostomy.

pegged tooth (pegd tūth) A conic tooth with sides that converge from the cervical to the incisal region.

PEG tube (peg tūb) Abbreviation for percutaneous endoscopic gastrostomy tube. Inserted under fluoroscopy for the administration of fluids or nutrition.

pei-ma (pā-mah) SYN castor bean.

Pel-Eb•stein fe•ver, **Pel-Eb•stein dis•ease** (pel eb′stīn fē′vĕr, di-zēz′) The remittent fever common in Hodgkin disease.

pe•li•o•sis (pel′ē-ō′sis) SYN purpura. [G. *peliōsis,* a livid spot, livor]

pe•li•o•sis hep•a•tis (pel′ē-ō′sis hē-pā′tis) The presence throughout the liver of blood-filled cavities that may become lined by endothelium or become organized; a feature of bacillary angiomatosis caused by *Rochalimaea henselae* in immunocompromised people.

pel•lag•ra (pĕ-lag′ră) An affection characterized by diarrhea, dermatitis, and dementia due to dietary deficiency of nicotinic acid (niacin). [It. *pelle,* skin, + *agra,* rough]

pel•lag•rous (pĕ-lag′rŭs) Relating to or suffering from pellagra.

Pel•le•gri•ni dis•ease (pel-ĕ-grē′nē di-zēz′) A calcific density in the medial collateral ligament and/or bony growth on the medial aspect of the medial condyle of the femur.

pel•let (pel′ĕt) **1.** A pilule, or very small pill. **2.** A small, rod-shaped dosage form composed essentially of pure steroid hormones in compressed form, intended for subcutaneous implantation in body tissues; serves as a depot providing for the slow release of the hormone over an extended time. [Fr. *pelote;* L. *pila,* a ball]

pel•li•cle (pel′i-kĕl) **1.** Literally and nonspecifically, a thin skin. **2.** A film or scum on the surface of a liquid. **3.** Cell boundary of sporozoites and merozoites among members of the protozoan subphylum Apicomplexa (Sporozoa), consisting of an outer unit membrane and an inner layer of two unit membranes. [L. *pellicula,* dim of *pellis,* skin]

pel•lu•cid (pĕ-lū′sid) Allowing the passage of light. [L. *pellucidus*]

pel•lu•cid mar•gi•nal cor•ne•al de•gen•er•a•tion (pĕ-lū′sid mahr′ji-năl kōr′nē-ăl dĕ-jen′ĕr-ā′shŭn) Bilateral thinning of the inferior cornea, progressing to formation of corneal ectasia.

pel•lu•cid zone (pĕ-lū′sid zōn) SYN zona pellucida.

pel•ta•tion (pel-tā′shŭn) Protection provided by inoculation with an antiserum or with a vaccine. [L. *pelta,* a light shield, fr. G. *peltē*]

pelvi-, pelvio-, pelvo- Combining forms denoting the pelvis. Cf. pyelo-. [L. *pelvis,* basin (pelvis)]

pel•vic (pel′vik) Relating to a pelvis.

pel•vic ax•is (pel′vik ak′sis) A hypothetic curved line joining the center point of each of the four planes of the pelvis, marking the center of the pelvic cavity at every level. SYN plane of pelvic canal.

pel•vic cav•i•ty (pel′vik kav′i-tē) The space bounded at the sides by the bones of the pelvis, above by the superior aperture of the pelvis, and below by the pelvic diaphragm; it contains the pelvic viscera.

pel•vic cel•lu•li•tis (pel′vik sel′yū-lī′tis) SYN parametritis.

pel•vic di•a•phragm, di•a•phragm of pel•vis (pel′vik dī′ă-fram, dī′ă-fram pel′vis) The paired levator ani and coccygeus muscles together with the fascia above and below them. See this page.

pel•vic di•rec•tion (pel′vik di-rek′shŭn) The direction of the axis of the pelvis.

pel•vi•ceph•a•lom•e•try (pel′vi-sef-ă-lom′ĕ-trē) Measurement of the female pelvic diameters in relation to those of the fetal head. [pelvi- + G. *kephalē,* head, + *metron,* measure]

pel•vic fas•ci•a (pel′vik fash′ē-ă) General term for the fascia lining the pelvic cavity (fascia pelvis parietalis) and investing the pelvic viscera (fascia pelvis visceralis).

pel•vic gan•gli•a (pel′vik gang′glē-ă) The parasympathetic ganglia scattered through the pelvic plexus on either side.

pel•vic gir•dle (pel′vik gĭr′dĕl) The bony ring formed by the hip bones and the sacrum, to which the lower limbs are attached. See page 1174.

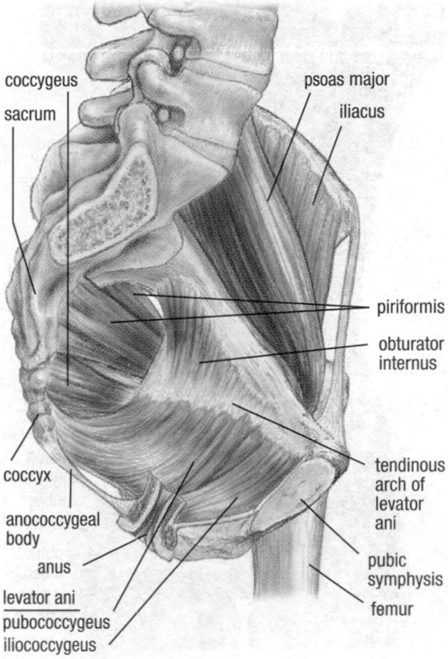

pelvic diaphragm: sagittal section

pel•vic in•flam•ma•to•ry dis•ease (PID) (pel′vik in-flam′ă-tōr-ē di-zēz′) Acute or chronic inflammation in the organs of the female pelvic cavity, particular suppurative lesions of the upper genital tract; most commonly due to infection by *Chlamydia trachomatis* or *Neisseria gonorrhoeae*, which have ascended into the uterus, uterine tubes, or ovaries from the lower genital tract as a result of childbirth or surgical procedures. The chief symptoms are pelvic pain and fever; complications include abscess formation and generalized peritonitis. Scarring may cause tubal infertility and raise the risk of ectopic pregnancy.

pel•vic per•i•to•ni•tis (pel′vik per′i-tō-nī′tis) Generalized inflammation of the peritoneum surrounding the uterus and fallopian tubes. SYN pelviperitonitis.

pel•vic plane of great•est di•men•sions (pel′vik plān grāt′ĕst di-men′shŭnz) The plane that extends from the middle of the posterior surface of the pubic symphysis to the junction of the second and third sacral vertebrae, and laterally passes through the ischial bones over the middle of the acetabulum.

pel•vic plane of least di•men•sions (pel′vik plān lēst di-men′shŭnz) The plane that extends from the end of the sacrum to the inferior border of the pubic symphysis; it is bounded posteriorly by the end of the sacrum, laterally by the ischial spines, and anteriorly by the inferior border of the pubic symphysis.

pel•vic pole (pel′vik pōl) The breech end of the fetus.

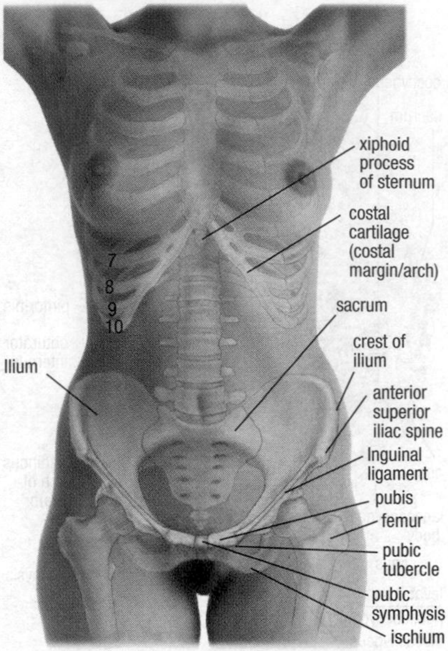

pelvic girdle

pel•vic splanch•nic nerves (pel′vik splangk′nik nĕrvz) Visceral branches from ventral primary rami of second to fourth sacral spinal nerves that join inferior hypogastric plexus to form pelvic plexuses, to and from which they convey presynaptic parasympathetic and sensory fibers, respectively. SYN nervi erigentes, nervi pelvici splanchnici, parasympathetic root of pelvic ganglia, radices parasympathicae gangliorum pelvicorum.

pel•vic tilt (pel′vik tilt) An exercise that strengthens abdominal muscles, relieves backache, and improves posture. The back is pressed to a firm, flat surface (wall or floor), flattening the spine. This can be done in supine, sitting, or standing positions. The pelvic tilt is the most commonly recommended prenatal exercise for back pain.

pel•vic ver•sion (pel′vik vĕr′zhŭn) Version by means of which a transverse or oblique presentation is converted into a pelvic presentation by manipulating the buttocks of the fetus.

pel•vi•fix•a•tion (pel′vi-fik-sā′shŭn) Surgical attachment of a floating pelvic organ to the wall of the pelvic cavity.

pel•vi•li•thot•o•my (pel′vi-li-thot′ŏ-mē) SYN pyelolithotomy. [pelvi- + G. *lithos,* stone, + *tomē,* incision]

pel•vim•e•ter (pel-vim′ĕ-tĕr) Calipers for measuring the diameters of the pelvis.

pel•vim•e•try (pel-vim′ĕ-trē) Measurement of the diameters of the pelvis. [pelvi- + G. *metron,* measure]

pel•vi•o•plas•ty (pel′vē-ō-plas-tē) **1.** Symphysiotomy or pubiotomy for enlargement of the female pelvic outlet. **2.** SYN pyeloplasty. [pelvio- + G. *plastos,* formed]

pel•vi•ot•o•my, **pel•vit•o•my** (pel′vē-ot′ŏ-mē, pel-vit′ŏ-mē) **1.** SYN symphysiotomy. **2.** SYN pubiotomy. **3.** SYN pyelotomy. [pelvio- + G. *tomē,* incision]

pel•vi•per•i•to•ni•tis (pel-vē-per-i-tō-nī′tis) SYN pelvic peritonitis.

pel•vis, pl. **pel•ves** (pel′vis, -vēz) [TA] **1.** The massive, cup-shaped ring of bone, with its ligaments, at the lower end of the trunk, formed of the hip bone (the pubic bone, ilium, and ischium) on either side and in front, and of the sacrum and the coccyx posteriorly. **2.** Any basinlike or cup-shaped cavity, as the pelvis of the kidney. [L. basin]

pel•vis jus•to ma•jor (pel′vis jus′tō maj′ŏr) A symmetric pelvis with greater than normal measurements in all diameters.

pel•vis jus•to mi•nor (pel′vis jus′tō mī′nŏr) A pelvis of the female type, but with all its diameters smaller than normal.

pel•vi•ver•te•bral an•gle (pel-vi-vĕr′tĕ-brăl ang′gĕl) The angle made by the pelvis as defined by the plane of the superior pelvic aperture with the general axis of the trunk or vertebral column.

pel•vo•ca•li•ec•ta•sis (pel′vō-kal-ē-ek-tā′sis) SYN hydronephrosis.

PEM Abbreviation for protein energy malnutrition.

pem•phi•goid (pem′fi-goyd) **1.** Resembling pemphigus. **2.** A disease resembling pemphigus but significantly distinguishable histologically (nonacantholytic) and clinically (generally benign course). [G. *pemphix,* blister, + *eidos,* resemblance]

pem•phi•gus (pem′fi-gŭs) **1.** Autoimmune bullous diseases with acantholysis: pemphigus vulgaris, pemphigus foliaceus, pemphigus erythematosus, or pemphigus vegetans. **2.** A nonspecific term for blistering skin diseases. [G. *pemphix,* a blister]

pem•phi•gus er•y•the•ma•to•sus (pem′fi-gŭs er′i-thē′mă-tō′sŭs) An eruption involving sun-exposed skin, especially the face; the lesions are scaling erythematous macules and blebs.

pem•phi•gus fo•li•a•ce•us (pem′fi-gŭs fō-lī-ā′shē-ŭs) A generally chronic form of pemphigus in which extensive exfoliative dermatitis may be present in addition to the bullae.

pem•phi•gus gan•gre•no•sus (pem′fi-gŭs gang′grē-nō′sŭs) **1.** SYN dermatitis gangrenosa infantum. **2.** SYN bullous impetigo of newborn.

pem•phi•gus vul•ga•ris (pem′fi-gŭs vul′gā′ris) A serious form of pemphigus, occurring in middle age, in which cutaneous bullae and oral erosions may be localized a few months before becoming generalized; blisters break easily and are slow to heal; results from the action of autoimmune antibodies that localize to intercellular sites of stratified squamous epithelium. See this page.

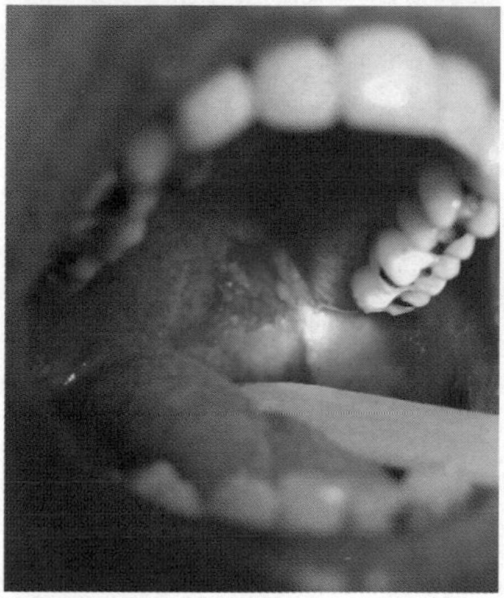

pemphigus vulgaris: oral cavity

Pen•dred syn•drome (pen′drĕd sin′drōm) Characterized by congenital sensorineural hearing impairment with goiter (usually small) due to defective organic binding of iodine in the thyroid; those afflicted are usually euthyroid; autosomal recessive inheritance, caused by mutation in the Pendred syndrome gene (PDS) encoding pendrin on chromosome 7q.

pen•du•lar nys•tag•mus (pen′jū-lăr nis-tag′mŭs) A nystagmus that has oscillations equal in speed and amplitude, usually arising from a visual disturbance.

pe•nes (pē-nēz) Plural of penis.

pen•e•trance (pen′ĕ-trăns) The frequency, expressed as a fraction or percentage, of people who are phenotypically affected, among people of an appropriate genotype; factors affecting expression may be environmental, or due to purely random variation; contrasted with hypostasis where the condition has a genetic origin and therefore tends to cause correlation in relatives.

pen•e•trat•ing wound (pen′ĕ-trā′ting wūnd) A wound with disruption of the body surface that extends into underlying tissue or into a body cavity.

-penia Suffix meaning deficiency. [G. *penia,* poverty]

pe•ni•cil•li•o•sis (pen′i-sil′ē-ō′sĭs) Invasive infection by a species of *Penicillium.*

Pen•i•cil•li•um (pen-i-sil′ē-ŭm) A genus of fungi, some species of which yield various antibiotic substances and biologicals. SEE penicillus.

pen•i•cil•lus, pl. **pe•ni•cil•li** (pen-i-sil′ŭs, -sil′ī) **1.** One of the tufts formed by the repeated subdivision of the minute arterial twigs in the spleen. **2.** In fungi, one of the branched conidiophores bearing chains of conidia in *Penicillium* species. [L. paint brush]

pe•nile (pē′nīl) Relating to the penis.

pe•nile pros•the•sis (pē′nīl pros-thē′sis) Device placed inside the penis to correct erectile failure.

pe•nile ra•phe (pē′nīl rā′fē) The continuation of the raphe of the scrotum onto the underside of the penis.

pe•nis, pl. **pe•nes** (pē′nis, pē-nēz) [TA] The organ of copulation in the male; it is formed of three columns of erectile tissue, two arranged laterally on the dorsum (corpora cavernosa penis) and one median below (corpus spongiosum); the urethra traverses the latter; the extremity (glans penis) is formed by an expansion of the corpus spongiosum, and is more or less completely covered by a free fold of skin (preputium). [L. tail]

pe•nis•chi•sis (pē-nis′ki-sis) A fissure of the penis resulting in an abnormal opening into the urethra, either above (epispadias), below (hypospadias), or to one side (paraspadias). [L. *penis* + G. *schisis,* fissure]

pen•nate (pen′āt) Feathered; resembling a feather. SYN penniform. [L. *pennatus,* fr. *penna,* feather]

pen•ni•form (pen′i-fōrm) SYN pennate. [L. *penna,* feather, + *forma,* form]

Pen•rose drain (pen′rōz drān) A soft, tube-shaped rubber drain.

penta- Combining form meaning five. [G. *pente,* five]

pen•tose (pen′tōs) A monosaccharide containing five carbon atoms in the molecule.

pen•tose phos•phate path•way (pen′tōs fos′fāt path′wā) A secondary pathway for the oxidation of D-glucose (not occurring in skeletal muscle), generating reducing power (NADPH) in the cytoplasm outside the mitochondria and synthesizing pentoses and a few other sugars. This pathway is defective in certain inherited diseases (e.g., glucose-6-phosphate dehydrogenase deficiency). SYN Dickens shunt.

pen•to•su•ri•a (pen-tō-syūr′ē-ă) The excretion of one or more pentoses in the urine.

pen·tyl (pen′til) **1.** SYN amyl. **2.** The $CH_3(CH_2)_3CH_2$– moiety.

pe·num·bra (pĕ-nŭm′bră) **1.** RADIOLOGY the blurred margin of an image. **2.** RADIATION PHYSICS the region at the edges of a radiation beam over which a rapid change in dosage rate occurs. SYN geometric unsharpness.

pep·lo·mer (pep′lō-mĕr) A part or subunit of the peplos of a virion, the assemblage of which produces the complete peplos, produced from the peplos by detergent treatment. SEE ALSO peplos.

pep·los (pep′lōs) The coat or envelope of lipoprotein material that surrounds certain virions. [G. an outer garment worn by women]

pep pills (pep pĭlz) Colloquialism for tablets containing a central nervous system stimulant, especially amphetamine.

pep·sin (pep′sin) The enzyme produced by the stomach for the digestion of protein.

pep·sin·o·gen (pep-sin′ō-jen) A proenzyme formed and secreted by the chief cells of the gastric mucosa; the acidity of the gastric juice and pepsin itself remove 42 amino acid residues from pepsinogen to form active pepsin. SYN propepsin. [pepsin + G. *-gen,* producing]

pep·tic (pep′tik) Relating to the stomach, to gastric digestion, or to pepsin A. [G. *peptikos,* fr. *peptō,* to digest]

pep·tic cell (pep′tik sel) SYN zymogenic cell.

pep·tic di·ges·tion (pep′tik di-jes′chŭn) SYN gastric digestion.

pep·tic ul·cer (pep′tik ŭl′sĕr) An ulcer of the alimentary mucosa, usually in the stomach or duodenum, that has been exposed to acid gastric secretion. See this page.

pep·ti·dase (pep′ti-dās) Any enzyme capable of hydrolyzing one of the peptide links of a peptide (e.g., carboxypeptidases, aminopeptidases).

pep·tide (pep′tīd) A compound of two or more amino acids in which a carboxyl group of one is united with an amino group of another, with the elimination of a molecule of water, thus forming a peptide bond, –CO–NH–; i.e., a substituted amide. Cf. bioregulator.

pep·tide an·ti·bi·ot·ic (pep′tīd an′ti-bī-ot′ik) An antibiotic composed of peptides; its antibacterial action is based on the physical disruption of cellular membranes.

pep·tide bond (pep′tīd bond) The common link (—CO—NH—) between amino acids in proteins, formed by elimination of H_2O between the —COOH of one amino acid and the H_2N— of another.

pep·ti·der·gic (pep-ti-dĕr′jik) Referring to nerve cells or fibers that are believed to employ small peptide molecules as their neurotransmitter. [peptide + G. *ergon,* work]

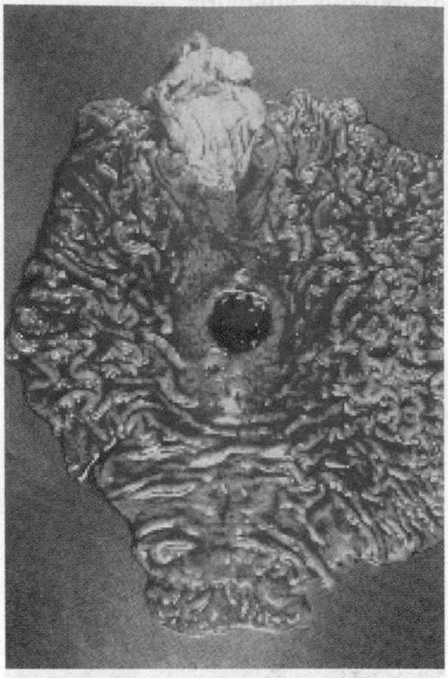

deep peptic ulcer

pep·tide YY (pep′tīd) A hormone released by the small intestine to signal the brain to stop eating.

pep·ti·do·gly·can (pep′ti-dō-glī′kan) A compound containing amino acids (or peptides) linked to sugars, with the latter preponderant. Cf. glycopeptide.

pep·ti·doid (pep′ti-doyd) A condensation product of two amino acids involving at least one condensing group other than the α-carboxyl or α-amino group, e.g., glutathione.

pep·ti·do·lyt·ic (pep′ti-dō-lit′ik) Causing the cleavage or digestion of peptides. [peptide + G. *lytikos,* solvent]

pep·ti·dyl di·pep·ti·dase A (pep′ti-dil dī-pep′ti-dās) A hydrolase cleaving C-terminal dipeptides from a variety of substrates, including angiotensin I, which is converted to angiotensin II and histidylleucine. An important step in the metabolism of certain vasopressor agents.

Pep·to·coc·cus (pep-tō-kok′ŭs) A genus of nonmotile, anaerobic, chemoorganotrophic bacteria containing gram-positive, spheric cells that occur singly, in pairs, tetrads, or irregular masses, more rarely in short chains. They are frequently found in association with pathologic conditions. The type species is *Peptococcus niger*. [G. *peptō,* to digest, + *kokkos,* berry]

pep·to·gen·ic, pep·tog·e·nous (pep-tō-jen′

ik, -toj′ĕ-nŭs) **1.** Producing peptones. **2.** Promoting digestion.

pep•tol•y•sis (pep-tol′i-sis) The hydrolysis of peptones.

pep•to•lyt•ic (pep-tō-lit′ik) **1.** Pertaining to peptolysis. **2.** Denoting an enzyme or other agent that hydrolyses peptones.

pep•tone (pep′tōn) Descriptive term applied to intermediate polypeptide products, formed in partial hydrolysis of proteins, that are soluble in water, diffusible, and not coagulable by heat; used in bacterial culture media.

pep•ton•ic (pep-ton′ik) Relating to or containing peptone.

pep•to•ni•za•tion (pep′ton-ī-zā′shŭn) Conversion by enzymic action of native protein into soluble peptone.

Pep•to•strep•to•coc•cus (pep′tō-strep-tō-kok′ŭs) A genus of nonmotile, anaerobic, chemoorganotrophic bacteria containing spheric to ovoid, gram-positive cells that occur in pairs and short or long chains. These organisms are found in normal and pathologic female genital tracts and blood in puerperal fever, in respiratory and intestinal tracts of normal humans and other animals, in the oral cavity, and in pyogenic infections, putrefactive war wounds, and appendicitis; they may be pathogenic. The type species is *P. anaerobius*. [G. *peptō,* to digest, + *streptos,* curved, + *kokkos,* berry]

PER Abbreviation for protein efficiency ratio.

per- **1.** Prefix meaning through; denoting intensity. **2.** CHEMISTRY more or most, with respect to the amount of a given element or radical contained in a compound; the degree of substitution for hydrogen, as in peroxides, peroxy acids (e.g., hydrogen peroxide, peroxyformic acid). SEE ALSO peroxy-. [L. through, throughout, extremely]

per•ac•id (per-as′id) An acid containing a peroxide group (–O–OH); e.g., peracetic acid.

per•a•cute (per′ă-kyūt′) Very acute; said of a disease. [L. *peracutus,* very sharply]

per an•um (pĕr ā′nŭm) By or through the anus. [L.]

per•cept (pĕr′sept) **1.** That which is perceived; the complete mental image, formed by the process of perception, of an object or idea. **2.** CLINICAL PSYCHOLOGY a single unit of perceptual report, such as one of the responses to an inkblot in the Rorschach test. [L. *perceptum,* a thing perceived]

per•cep•tion (pĕr-sep′shŭn) The mental process of becoming aware of or recognizing an object or idea; primarily cognitive rather than affective or conative, although all three aspects are manifested. SYN esthesia.

per•cep•tive (pĕr-sep′tiv) Relating to or having a higher than normal power of perception.

per•cep•tiv•i•ty (pĕr-sep-tiv′i-tē) The power of perception.

per•cep•tu•al nar•row•ing (pĕr-sep′shū-ăl nar′ō-ing) Tendency of an individual to narrow the attentional focus and miss certain types of information in the environment as the level of arousal increases (e.g., the novice golfer practicing on a driving range vs. playing in his or her first golf tournament).

per•cep•tu•al pro•ces•sing (pĕr-sep′shū-ăl pro′ses-ing) The organization of sensory input into meaningful patterns.

per•co•la•tion (pĕr-kō-lā′shŭn) **1.** SYN filtration. **2.** Extraction of the soluble portion of a solid mixture by passing a solvent liquid through it. **3.** Passage of saliva or other fluids into the interface between tooth structure and restoration; sometimes induced by thermal changes. [L. *percolatio,* fr. per- + *colare,* to strain]

per con•tig•u•um (pĕr kon-tig′yū-ŭm) In contiguity; denoting the mode by which an inflammation or other morbid process spreads into an adjacent contiguous structure. [per- + L. *contiguus,* touching, fr. *tango,* to touch]

per con•tin•u•um (pĕr kon-tin′yū-ŭm) In continuity; continuous; denoting the mode by which an inflammation or other morbid process spreads from one part to another through continuous tissue. [per- + L. *continuus,* holding together, continuous, fr. *teneo,* to hold]

per•cuss (pĕr-kŭs′) To perform percussion.

per•cus•sion (pĕr-kŭsh′ŭn) **1.** A diagnostic procedure designed to determine the density of a part by the sound produced by tapping the surface with the finger or a plessor; performed primarily over the chest to determine presence of normal air content in the lungs and over the abdomen to evaluate air in the loops of intestine. **2.** A form of massage, consisting of repeated blows or taps of varying force. See page 1178. [L. *percussio,* fr. *per-cutio,* pp. *-cussus,* to beat, fr. *quatio,* to shake, beat]

per•cus•sor (pĕr-kŭs′ŏr) SYN plessor.

per•cu•ta•ne•ous (pĕr-kyū-tā′nē-ŭs) Denoting the passage of substances through unbroken skin, as in absorption by inunction; also passage through the skin by needle puncture, including introduction of wires and catheters by Seldinger technique.

per•cu•ta•ne•ous co•ro•nar•y in•ter•ven•tion (PCI) (pĕr′kyū-tā′nē-yŭs kōr′ŏ-nar′ē in′tĕr-ven′shŭn) The treatment measure used during cardiac catheterization to reduce or remove occlusion within the coronary arteries and increase perfusion to the myocardium. PCIs include atherectomy, brachytherapy, stent implantation, an-

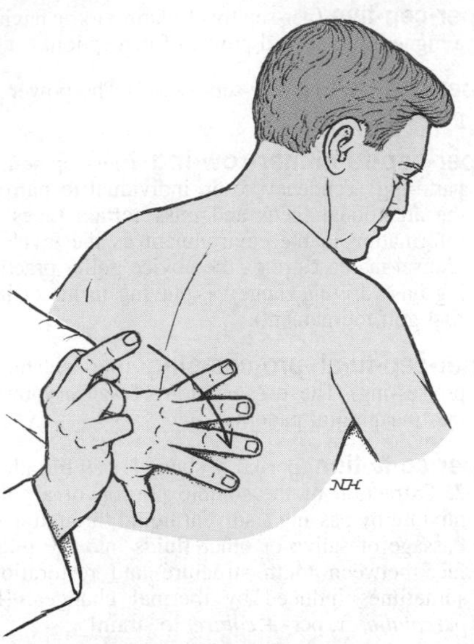

percussion: distal phalanx of finger is pressed firmly against chest wall parallel with ribs; a short, quick blow is struck at the base of the distal phalanx of the finger with the tip of finger of the opposite hand

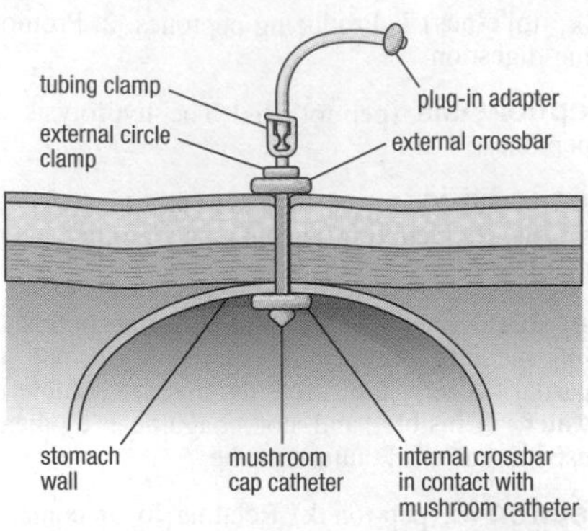

percutaneous endoscopic gastrostomy (PEG) tube: stomach placement

gioplasty, and laser revascularization. SYN intracoronary stenting.

per·cu·ta·ne·ous en·do·scop·ic gas·tros·to·my (PEG) (pĕr′kyū-tā′nē-yŭs en′dō-skop′ik gas-tros′tŏ-mē) The placement of a tube in the stomach through an opening in the abdominal wall with the aid of an endoscope, to permit enteral feeding and administration of medicine to a patient who is unable to swallow.

per·cu·ta·ne·ous en·do·scop·ic gas·tros·to·my tube (PEG tube) (pĕr′kyū-tā′nē-ŭs en′dō-skop′ik gās-tros-tŏ′mē tūb) Tube is placed through the abdominal wall with the aid of an endoscope into the stomach. Used for feeding patients unable to swallow food. See this page. SYN G-tube, gastrostomy tube.

per·cu·ta·ne·ous trans·he·pa·tic chol·an·gi·og·ra·phy (PTHC) (pĕr′kyū-tā′nē-ŭs trans′hĕ-pat′ik kō-lan′jē-og′ră-fē) Contrast radiographic examination of the biliary system performed by injection through a percutaneously placed needle inserted into an intrahepatic bile duct.

per·cu·ta·ne·ous trans·lu·mi·nal an·gi·o·plas·ty (PTA) (pĕr′kyū-tā′nē-ŭs trans-lū′mĕn-ăl an′jē-ō-plas-tē) An operation for enlarging a narrowed vascular lumen by inflating and withdrawing a balloon on the tip of an angiographic catheter through the stenotic region; may include positioning of an intravascular stent. Used in the treatmnt of atherosclerotic coronary heart disease and angina pectoris to improve circulation. See this page.

per·cu·ta·ne·ous trans·tra·che·al ven·ti·la·tion (pĕr′kyū-tā′nē-ŭs trans-trā′kē-ăl ven′ti-lā′shŭn) SYN needle cricothyrotomy.

per·en·ceph·a·ly (pĕr-en-sef′ă-lē) A condition marked by one or more cerebral cysts. [G. *pēra*, a purse, a wallet, + *enkephalos*, brain]

per·fect fun·gus (pĕr′fekt fŭng′gŭs) A fungus

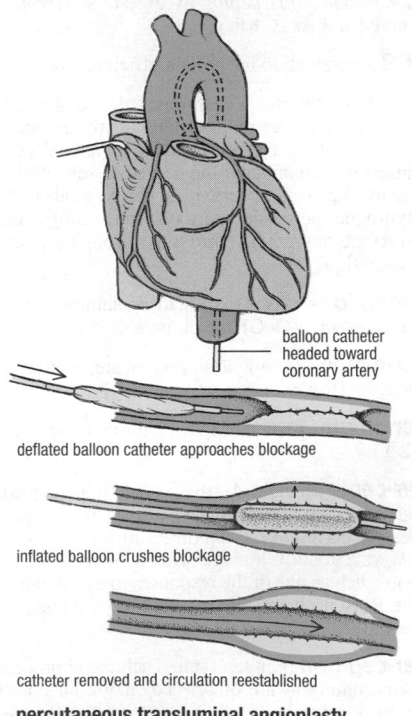

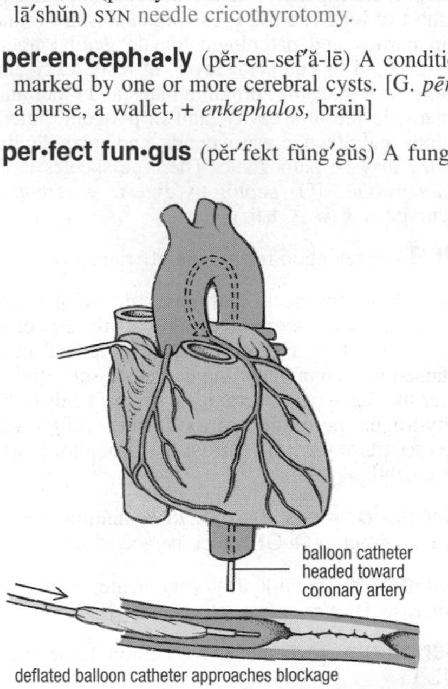

percutaneous transluminal angioplasty

possessing both sexual and asexual means of reproduction, and in which both mating forms are recognized.

per·fec·tion·ism (pĕr-fek′shŭn-izm) A tendency to set rigid high standards of performance for oneself.

per·fec·tion·is·tic per·so·na·li·ty (pĕr-fek′shŭn-is′tik pĕr-sŏn-al′i-tē) A personality characterized by rigidity, extreme inhibition, and excessive concern with conformity and adherence to often unique standards.

per·fect stage (pĕr′fekt stāj) MYCOLOGY the sexual life cycle phase of a fungus in which spores are formed after nuclear fusion.

per·fo·rat·ed (pĕr′fŏr-āt-ĕd) Pierced with one or more holes. [L. *perforatus,* fr. *per-foro,* pp. *-atus,* to bore through]

per·fo·rat·ed ul·cer (pĕr′fŏr-āt-ĕd ŭl′sĕr) An ulcer extending through the wall of an organ.

per·fo·rat·ing ab·scess (pĕr′fŏr-āt-ing ab′ses) An abscess that breaks down tissue barriers to enter adjacent areas. SYN migrating abscess, wandering abscess.

per·fo·rat·ing ar·ter·ies (pĕr′fŏr-āt-ing ahr′tĕr-ēz) *Origin,* arteria profunda femoris; *distribution,* as three or four vessels that pass through the aponeurosis of the adductor magnus to the posterior and anterior compartments of the thigh. SYN arteriae perforantes [TA].

per·fo·rat·ing fi·bers (pĕr′fŏr-āt-ing fī′bĕrz) Bundles of collagenous fibers that pass into the outer circumferential lamellae of bone or the cementum of teeth.

per·fo·rat·ing veins (pĕr′fŏr-āt-ing vāns) Accompany the perforating arteries from the profunda femoris artery; drain blood from the vastus lateralis and hamstring muscles and terminate in the profunda femoris vein.

per·fo·rat·ing wound (pĕr′fŏr-āt-ing wūnd) A wound with entrance and exit openings.

per·fo·ra·tion (pĕr′fŏr-ā′shŭn) Abnormal opening in a hollow organ or viscus. SEE ALSO perforated. See page B28. SYN tresis.

per·fo·rin (pĕr′fŏ-rin) A protein found in the cytoplasmic granules of both T-cytotoxic lymphocytes and natural killer cells, implicated in target cell lysis. [L. *per-foro,* to bore, pierce, + -in]

per·for·mance (pĕr-fōr′măns) Organized patterns of behavior that are characteristic or expected of a person in a given situation.

per·for·mance ar·e·as (pĕr-fōr′măns ār′ē-ăz) Activities of daily living, work or other productive activity, play, and leisure that determine a person's functional abilities and define human activity. SYN performance patterns.

per·for·mance com·po·nents (pĕr-fōr′măns kŏm-pō′nĕnts) Sensorimotor, cognitive, psychosocial, and psychological elements of performance required for successful engagement in performance areas.

per·for·mance con·text (pĕr-fōr′măns kon′tekst) A set of conditions, both internal and external, that mediate, support, and influence someone's performance of human activities; these conditions may include those of a cultural, physical, social, personal, temporal, spiritual, or virtual (i.e., occurring online) nature.

per·for·mance in·ten·si·ty (pĕr-fōr′măns in-ten′si-tē) The improvement in recognition of spoken words that occurs with increasing intensity of sound.

per·for·mance pat·terns (pĕr-fōr′măns pa′tĕrnz) SYN performance areas.

per·fuse (pĕr-fyūz′) To force blood or other fluid to flow from the artery through the vascular bed of a tissue or to flow through the lumen of a hollow structure (e.g., an isolated renal tubule). [L. *perfusio,* fr. per- + *fusio,* a pouring]

per·fu·sion (pĕr-fyū′zhŭn) **1.** The act of perfusing. **2.** The flow of blood or other perfusate per unit volume of tissue, as in ventilation:perfusion ratio.

peri- Prefix denoting around, about, near. Cf. circum-. [G. around]

per·i·ad·e·ni·tis (per′ē-ad-ĕ-nī′tis) Inflammation of the tissues surrounding a gland. [peri- + G. *adēn,* gland, + *-itis,* inflammation]

per·i·ad·e·ni·tis mu·co·sa ne·cro·ti·ca re·cur·rens (per′ē-ad-ĕ-nī′tis myū′kō-să ne-krot′i-kă rē-kur′enz) SYN aphthae major.

per·i·a·nal (per′ē-ā′năl) Pertaining to the area around the anus. [G. *peri,* around + L. *anus*]

per·i·a·nal ab·scess (per′ē-ā′năl ab′ses) An infection of the soft tissues surrounding the anal canal, with formation of a discrete abscess cavity.

per·i·an·gi·tis (per′ē-an-jī′tis) Inflammation of the adventitia of a blood vessel or of the tissues surrounding it or a lymphatic vessel. SEE ALSO periarteritis, periphlebitis, perilymphangitis. SYN perivasculitis. [peri- + G. *angeion,* a vessel, + *-itis,* inflammation]

per·i·a·or·ti·tis (per′ē-ā-ōr-tī′tis) Inflammation of the adventitia of the aorta and of the tissues surrounding it.

per·i·ap·i·cal (per′ē-ap′i-kăl) **1.** At or around the apex of a root of a tooth. **2.** Denoting the periapex.

per·i·ap·i·cal ce·ment·al dys·pla·si·a (per′ē-ap′i-kăl sĕ-men′tăl dis-plā′zē-ă) A benign, painless, nonneoplastic condition of the jaws that occurs almost exclusively in middle-aged black females; lesions are usually multiple, most frequently involve vital mandibular anterior teeth, surround the root apices, and are initially radiolucent (becoming more opaque as they mature).

per·i·ap·i·cal cu·ret·tage (per′ē-ap′i-kăl kūr′ĕ-tahzh′) **1.** Removal of a cyst or granuloma from its pathologic bony crypt, using a curette. **2.** The removal of tooth fragments and debris from sockets at the time of extraction or of bone sequestra subsequently.

per·i·ap·i·cal film (per′ē-ap′i-kăl film) Intraoral radiographic projection taken to include tooth apices and surrounding alveolar bone. Film sizes 0–2 made be used. SEE periapical radiograph.

per·i·ap·i·cal gran·u·lo·ma (per′ē-ap′i-kăl gran′yū-lō′mă) A proliferation of granulation tissue surrounding the apex of a nonvital tooth and arising in response to pulpal necrosis. SYN apical granuloma, dental granuloma.

per·i·ap·i·cal ra·di·o·graph (per′ē-ap′i-kăl rā′dē-ō-graf) A radiograph demonstrating tooth apices and surrounding structures in a particular intraoral area.

per·i·ap·pen·di·ce·al ab·scess (per′ē-ap′i-kăl ab′ses) SYN appendiceal abscess.

per·i·ap·pen·di·ci·tis (per′ē-ă-pen-di-sī′tis) Inflammation of the tissue surrounding the vermiform appendix.

per·i·ar·te·ri·al plex·us (per′ē-ahr-tēr′ē-ăl plek-sŭs) An autonomic plexus that accompanies an artery, surrounding it in a network of autonomic nerve fibers.

per·i·ar·te·ri·al plex·us·es of co·ro·na·ry ar·te·ries (per′ē-ahr-tēr′ē-ăl plek-sŭs′ēz kōr′ŏ-nar-ē ahr′tĕr-ēz) The continuation of the cardiac plexus onto the coronary arteries.

per·i·ar·te·ri·al sym·pa·thec·to·my (per′ē-ahr-tēr′ē-ăl sim′pă-thek′tŏ-mē) Sympathetic denervation by arterial decortication. SYN Leriche operation.

per·i·ar·te·ri·tis (per′ē-ahr-tĕr-ī′tis) Inflammation of the adventitia of an artery.

per·i·ar·te·ri·tis no·do·sa (per′ē-ahr-tĕr-ī′tis nō-dō′să) SYN polyarteritis nodosa.

per·i·ar·thri·tis (per′ē-ahr-thrī′tis) Inflammation of the parts surrounding a joint. [peri- + arthritis]

per·i·ar·tic·u·lar ab·scess (per′ē-ahr-tik′yū-lăr ab′ses) An abscess surrounding a joint, but not necessarily involving it.

per·i·bron·chi·o·li·tis (per′i-brong-kē-ō-lī′tis) Inflammation of the tissues surrounding the bronchioles.

per·i·bron·chi·tis (per′i-brong-kī′tis) Inflammation of the tissues surrounding the bronchi or bronchial tubes.

per·i·car·di·a (per′i-kahr′dē-ă) Plural of pericardium.

per·i·car·di·ac, per·i·car·di·al (per′i-kahr′dē-ak, per′i-kahr′dē-ăl) **1.** Surrounding the heart. **2.** Relating to the pericardium.

per·i·car·di·a·co·phren·ic ar·ter·y (per′i-kahr′dē-ă-kō-fren′ik ahr′tĕr-ē) *Origin*, internal thoracic; *distribution*, pericardium, diaphragm, and pleura; *anastomoses*, musculophrenic, inferior phrenic, mediastinal and pericardial branches of the internal thoracic. SYN arteria pericardiacophrenica [TA].

per·i·car·di·a·co·phren·ic veins (per′i-kahr′dē-ă-kō-fren′ik vānz) Accompany the pericardiacophrenic artery and empty into the brachiocephalic veins or superior vena cava.

per·i·car·di·al cav·i·ty (per′i-kahr′dē-ăl kav′i-tē) **1.** The potential space between the parietal and visceral layers of the serous pericardium. **2.** In the embryo, that part of the primary celom containing the heart; originally it is in open communication with the pericardioperitoneal cavities and indirectly, through them, with the peritoneal part of the celom.

per·i·car·di·al de·com·pres·sion (per′i-kahr′dē-ăl dē-kŏm-presh′ŭn) SYN cardiac decompression.

per·i·car·di·al ef·fu·sion (per′i-kahr′dē-ăl ĕ-fyū′zhŭn) Increased amounts of fluid within the pericardial sac, usually due to inflammation.

per·i·car·di·al frem·i·tus (per′i-kahr′dē-ăl frem′i-tŭs) Vibration in the chest wall produced by the friction of opposing roughened surfaces of the pericardium.

per·i·car·di·al mur·mur (per′i-kahr′dē-ăl mŭr′mŭr) A friction sound, synchronous with the heart movements, heard in some cases of pericarditis.

per·i·car·di·al sym·phy·sis (per′i-kahr′dē-ăl sim′fi-sis) Adhesion between the parietal and visceral layers of the pericardium.

per·i·car·di·al veins (per′i-kahr′dē-ăl vānz) Several small veins from the pericardium that empty into the brachiocephalic veins or superior vena cava.

per·i·car·di·cen·te·sis (per′i-kahr′dē-sen-tē′sis) Needle drainage of the pericardium, usually accompanied by placement of an indwelling catheter for continuing drainage.

per·i·car·di·ec·to·my (per′i-kahr′dē-ek′tŏ-mē) Excision of a portion of the pericardium. [pericardium + G. *ektomē*, excision]

per·i·car·di·ol·o·gy (per′i-kahr′dē-ol′ŏ-jē) The science or study of the pericardium and its physiology and diseases.

per·i·car·di·o·per·i·to·ne·al (per′i-kahr′dē-ō-per′i-tō-nē′ăl) Relating to the pericardial and peritoneal cavities.

per·i·car·di·o·per·i·to·ne·al ca·nal (per′i-kahr′dē-ō-per′i-tō-nē′ăl kă-nal′) The portion of the embryonic celom that joins the pericardial cavity to the peritoneal cavity, developing into the pleural cavities.

per·i·car·di·o·phren·ic (per′i-kahr′dē-ō-fren′ik) Relating to the pericardium and the diaphragm. [pericardium + G. *phrēn,* diaphragm]

per·i·car·di·o·pleu·ral (per′i-kahr′dē-ō-plūr′ăl) Relating to the pericardial and pleural cavities.

per·i·car·di·or·rha·phy (per′i-kahr′dē-ōr′ă-fē) Suture of the pericardium. [pericardium + G. *rhaphē,* suture]

per·i·car·di·os·to·my (per′i-kahr′dē-os′tŏ-mē) Establishment of an opening into the pericardium. [pericardium + G. *stoma,* mouth]

per·i·car·di·ot·o·my (per′i-kahr′dē-ot′ŏ-mē) Incision into the pericardium for drainage. [pericardium + G. *tomē,* incision]

per·i·car·dit·ic (per′i-kahr-dit′ik) Relating to pericarditis.

per·i·car·di·tis (per′i-kahr-dī′tis) Inflammation of the pericardium.

per·i·car·di·tis ob·li·te·rans (per′i-kahr-dī′tis ob-lit′ĕr-anz) Inflammation of the pericardium leading to adhesion of the two layers, obliterating the sac. SEE ALSO adhesive pericarditis.

per·i·car·di·tis with ef·fu·sion (per′i-kahr-dī′tis ĕ-fyū′zhŭn) Pericardial inflammation producing excess pericardial fluid.

per·i·car·di·um, pl. **per·i·car·di·a** (per′i-kahr′dē-ŭm, -dē-ă) [TA] The fibroserous membrane, consisting of mesothelium and submesothelial connective tissue, covering the heart and beginnings of the great vessels. It is a closed sac having two layers: the visceral layer (epicardium), immediately surrounding the heart, and the outer parietal layer, forming the sac, composed of strong fibrous tissue, the fibrous pericardium, lined with a serous membrane, the serous pericardium. SYN heart sac, theca cordis. [L. fr. G. *pericardion,* the membrane around the heart]

per·i·cho·lan·gi·tis (per′i-kō-lan-jī′tis) Inflammation of the tissues around the bile ducts. [peri- + G. *cholē,* bile, + *angeion,* vessel, + *-itis,* inflammation]

per·i·chon·dral, **per·i·chon·dri·al** (per′i-kon′drăl, -drē-ăl) Relating to the perichondrium.

per·i·chon·dral bone (per′i-kon′drăl bōn) In the development of a long bone, a collar or cuff of osseous tissue forms in the perichondrium of the cartilage model; the connective tissue membrane of this perichondral bone then becomes periosteum.

per·i·chon·dri·tis (per′i-kon-drī′tis) Inflammation of the perichondrium.

per·i·chon·dri·um (per′i-kon′drē-ŭm) [TA] The dense, irregular connective tissue membrane around cartilage. [peri- + G. *chondros,* cartilage]

per·i·chrome (per′i-krōm) Denoting a nerve cell in which the chromophil substance, or stainable material, is scattered throughout the cytoplasm. [peri- + G. *chrōma,* a color]

per·i·co·li·tis (per′i-kō-lī′tis) Inflammation of the connective tissue or peritoneum surrounding the colon. SYN serocolitis.

per·i·col·pi·tis (per′i-kol-pī′tis) SYN perivaginitis. [peri- + G. *kolpos,* bosom (vagina), + *-itis,* inflammation]

per·i·cor·o·ni·tis (per′i-kōr-ŏ-nī′tis) Inflammation around the crown of a tooth, usually a partially emerged one; it is commonly seen in the eruption of a third molar. [peri- + L. *corona,* crown, + G. *-itis,* inflammation]

per·i·cra·ni·tis (per′i-krā-nī′tis) Inflammation of the pericranium.

per·i·cra·ni·um (per′i-krā′nē-ŭm) The periosteum of the skull. [peri- + G. *kranion,* skull]

per·i·cys·tic (per′i-sis′tik) **1.** Surrounding the urinary bladder. **2.** Surrounding the gallbladder. **3.** Surrounding a cyst. SYN perivesical. [peri- + G. *kystis,* bladder]

per·i·cys·ti·tis (per′i-sis-tī′tis) Inflammation of the tissues surrounding a bladder, especially the urinary bladder.

per·i·cyte (per′i-sīt) One of the slender mesenchymallike cells found in close association with the outside wall of postcapillary venules; it is relatively undifferentiated and may become a fibroblast, macrophage, or smooth muscle cell. SYN adventitial cell. [peri- + G. *kytos,* cell]

per·i·cyt·ic ven·ules (per′i-sīt′ik ven′yūls) SYN postcapillary venules.

per·i·den·tal mem·brane (per′i-den′tăl mem′brān) SYN periodontal ligament.

per·i·derm, **per·i·der·ma** (per′i-dĕrm, -dĕr′mă) The outermost layer of the epidermis of the embryo and fetus up to the sixth month of intrauterine life; desquamated epitrichial cells are a considerable component of the vernix caseosa. SYN epitrichium. [peri- + G. *derma,* skin]

per·i·des·mi·tis (per′i-dez-mī′tis) Inflammation of the connective tissue surrounding a ligament. [peri- + G. *desmos,* band, + *-itis,* inflammation]

per·i·des·mi·um (per′i-dez′mē-ŭm) The connective tissue membrane surrounding a ligament. [peri- + G. *desmion (desmos),* band]

per·i·did·y·mi·tis (per′i-did-i-mī′tis) Inflammation of the perididymis.

per·i·di·ver·tic·u·li·tis (per′i-dī-vĕr-tik′yū-lī′tis) Inflammation of the tissues around an intestinal diverticulum.

per·i·du·o·de·ni·tis (per′i-dū-ō-dē-nī′tis) Inflammation around the duodenum.

per·i·du·ral an·es·the·si·a (per′i-dūr′ăl an′es-thē′zē-ă) SYN epidural anesthesia.

per·i·en·ceph·a·li·tis (per′ē-en-sef-ă-lī′tis) Inflammation of the cerebral membranes, particularly leptomeningitis or inflammation of the pia mater with involvement of the underlying cortex. [peri- + G. *enkephalos,* brain]

per·i·en·ter·i·tis (per′ē-en-tĕr-ī′tis) Inflammation of the peritoneal coat of the intestine. SYN seroenteritis.

per·i·e·soph·a·gi·tis (per′ē-ē-sof′ă-jī′tis) Inflammation of the tissues surrounding the esophagus. SYN perioesophagitis.

per·i·fol·lic·u·li·tis (per′i-fŏ-lik′yū-lī′tis) The presence of an inflammatory infiltrate surrounding hair follicles; frequently occurs in conjunction with folliculitis.

per·i·gas·tri·tis (per′i-gas-trī′tis) Inflammation of the peritoneal coat of the stomach.

per·i·glot·tis (per′i-glot′is) The mucous membrane of the tongue. [G. *periglōttis,* covering of the tongue]

per·i·hep·a·ti·tis (per′i-hep-ă-tī′tis) Inflammation of the serous, or peritoneal, covering of the liver. [peri- + G. *hēpar,* liver, + *-itis,* inflammation]

per·i·in·farc·tion block (per′ē-in-fark′shŭn blok) An electrocardiographic abnormality associated with an old myocardial infarct and caused by delayed activation of the myocardium in the region of the infarct; characterized by an initial vector directed away from the infarcted region with the terminal vector directed toward it.

per·i·je·ju·ni·tis (per′i-jĕ-jū-nī′tis) Inflammation around the jejunum.

per·i·kar·y·on, pl. **per·i·kar·y·a** (per′i-kar′ē-on, -ă) **1.** The cytoplasm around the nucleus, such as that of the cell body of nerve cells. **2.** The body of the odontoblast, excluding the dentinal fiber. **3.** The cell body of the nerve cell, as distinguished from its axon and dendrites. [peri- + G. *karyon,* kernel]

per·i·ky·ma·ta (per′i-kī′mă-tă) Shallow, horizontal furrows on the enamel of a tooth where the striae of Retzius meet the surface. [peri- + G. *kyma*, wave]

per·i·lab·y·rin·thi·tis (per′i-lab′i-rin-thī′tis) Inflammation of the parts about the labyrinth.

per·i·lymph (per′i-limf) The fluid contained within the osseous labyrinth, surrounding and protecting the membranous labyrinth; perilymph resembles extracellular fluid in composition (sodium is the predominant cation) and, via the perilymphatic duct, is in continuity with cerebrospinal fluid. SYN perilympha.

per·i·lym·pha (per′i-lim′fă) SYN perilymph. [peri- + L. *lympha,* a clear fluid (lymph)]

per·i·lym·phan·gi·tis (per′i-lim-fan-jī′tis) Inflammation of the tissues surrounding a lymphatic vessel.

per·i·lym·phat·ic (per′i-lim-fat′ik) **1.** Surrounding a lymphatic structure (node or vessel). **2.** The spaces and tissues surrounding the membranous labyrinth of the inner ear.

per·i·lym·phat·ic duct (per′i-lim-fat′ik dŭkt) A fine canal connecting the perilymphatic space of the cochlea with the subarachnoid space. SYN aqueductus cochleae [TA].

per·i·lym·pha·tic fis·tu·la (per′i-lim-fat′ik fis′chū-lă) A fistula between the vestibule of the inner ear and the middle ear through which perilymph can leak, resulting in auditory and vestibular disturbances; common sites for perilymphatic fistula are the oval window through or around the footplate of the stapes or the round window through the round window membrane.

per·i·lym·pha·tic gush·er (per′i-lim-fat′ik gŭsh′ĕr) Abnormal flow of perilymph when the footplate of the stapes is perforated; occurs in X-linked mixed deafness (DFN 3) due to a mutation of the POU3F4 gene and in other conditions.

per·i·lym·phat·ic space (per′i-lim-fat′ik spās) Space between the bony and membranous portions of the labyrinth.

per·i·men·in·gi·tis (per′i-men-in-jī′tis) SYN pachymeningitis.

pe·rim·e·ter (pĕ-rim′ĕ-tĕr) **1.** A circumference, edge, or border. **2.** An instrument, usually half a circle or sphere, used to measure the field of vision. [G. *perimetros,* circumference, fr. *peri,* around, + *metron,* measure]

per·i·met·ric (per′i-met′rik) **1.** Surrounding the uterus; relating to the perimetrium. SYN periuterine. [G. *peri,* around, + *mētra,* uterus] **2.** Relating to the circumference of any part or area. [G. *perimetros,* circumference] **3.** Relating to perimetry.

per·i·me·trit·ic (per′i-me-trit′ik) Relating to or marked by perimetritis.

per·i·me·tri·tis (per′i-me-trī′tis) SYN metroperitonitis. [perimetrium + G. *-itis,* inflammation]

per·i·me·tri·um, pl. **per·i·me·tri·a** (per′i-mē′trē-ŭm, -ă) [TA] The serous (peritoneal) coat of the uterus. [peri- + G. *mētra,* uterus]

pe·rim·e·try (pĕr-im′ĕ-trē) **1.** The determination of the limits of the visual field. **2.** The mapping of the sensitivity contours of the visual field. [G. *perimetros,* circumference]

per•i•mol•y•sis (per′i-mol′i-sis) Decalcification of the teeth from exposure to gastric acid in people with chronic vomiting. [perimylolysis, fr. peri- + G. *mylos*, molar + *lysis*, loosening, dissolving, fr. *luō*, to loosen]

per•i•my•e•li•tis (per′i-mī-ĕ-lī′tis) SYN endosteitis.

per•i•my•o•si•tis (per′i-mī-ō-sī′tis) Inflammation of the loose cellular tissue surrounding a muscle. SYN perimysiitis (2), perimysitis.

per•i•my•si•al (per′i-mis′ē-ăl) Relating to the perimysium; surrounding a muscle.

per•i•my•si•i•tis, per•i•my•si•tis (per′i-mis-ē-ī′tis, -mī-sī′tis) **1.** Inflammation of the perimysium. **2.** SYN perimyositis.

per•i•my•si•um, pl. **per•i•my•si•a** (per′i-mis′ē-ŭm, -ă) The fibrous sheath enveloping each of the primary bundles of skeletal muscle fibers. [peri- + G. *mys,* muscle]

per•i•na•tal (per′i-nā′tăl) Occurring during, or pertaining to, the periods before, during, or after the time of birth, i.e., before delivery from the 28th week of gestation through the first 7 days after delivery. [peri- + L. *natus,* pp. of *nascor,* to be born]

per•i•na•tal med•i•cine (per′i-nā′tăl med′i-sin) SYN perinatology.

per•i•na•tol•o•gist (per′i-nā-tol′ŏ-jist) An obstetrician who subspecializes in perinatology.

per•i•na•tol•o•gy (per′i-nā-tol′ŏ-jē) A subspecialty of obstetrics concerned with care of the mother and fetus during pregnancy, labor, and delivery, particularly when the mother and/or fetus is at high risk of complications. SYN perinatal medicine.

per•i•ne•al (per′i-nē′ăl) Relating to the perineum.

per•i•ne•al ar•ter•y (per′i-nē′ăl ahr′tĕr-ē) *Origin*, internal pudendal; *distribution*, superficial structures of the perineum; *anastomoses*, external pudendal arteries. SYN arteria perinealis [TA].

per•i•ne•al fas•ci•a (per′i-nē′ăl fash′ē-ă) Fascia that intimately invests the superficial perineal muscles (ischiocavernosus, bulbospongiosus, and superficial transverse perineal muscles); anteriorly it is fused to the suspensory ligament of the penis/clitoris and is continuous with the deep fascia covering the external oblique muscle of the abdomen and the rectus sheath. SYN superficial investing fascia of perineum.

per•i•ne•al her•ni•a (per′i-nē′ăl hĕr′nē-ă) A hernia protruding through the pelvic diaphragm.

per•i•ne•al mem•brane (per′i-nē′ăl mem′brān) The layer of fascia extending between the ischiopubic rami inferior to the sphincter urethrae and the deep transverse perineal muscles.

per•i•ne•al nerves (per′i-nē′ăl nĕrvz) The superficial terminal branches of the pudendal nerve, supplying most of the muscles of the perineum (deep branch) as well as the skin of that region (superficial branch). SYN nervi perineales [TA].

per•i•ne•al ra•phe (per′i-nē′ăl rā′fē) The central anteroposterior line of the perineum, most marked in the male, being continuous with the raphe of the scrotum.

per•i•ne•al sec•tion (per′i-nē′ăl sek′shŭn) Any cutting through the perineum, either lateral or median lithotomy or external urethrotomy.

♲ **perineo-** Combining form indicating the perineum. [L. fr. G. *perineos, perinaion*]

per•i•ne•o•cele (per′i-nē′ō-sēl) A hernia in the perineal region, either between the rectum and the vagina or the rectum and the bladder, or alongside the rectum. [perineo- + G. *kēlē,* hernia]

per•i•ne•o•plas•ty (per′i-nē′ō-plas-tē) Surgical repair of the perineum. [perineum + G. *plastos,* formed]

per•i•ne•or•rha•phy (per′i-nē-ōr′ă-fē) Suture of the perineum, performed in perineoplasty. [perineum + G. *rhaphē*, a sewing]

per•i•ne•o•scro•tal (per′i-nē′ō-skrō′tăl) Relating to the perineum and the scrotum.

per•i•ne•os•to•my (per′i-nē-os′tŏ-mē) Urethrostomy through the perineum. [perineo- + G. *stoma,* mouth]

per•i•ne•ot•o•my (per′i-nē-ot′ŏ-mē) Incision into the perineum to facilitate childbirth. SEE ALSO episiotomy.

per•i•ne•o•vag•i•nal (per′i-nē′ō-vaj′i-năl) Relating to the perineum and the vagina.

per•i•neph•ri•al (per′i-nef′rē-ăl) Relating to the perinephrium.

per•i•neph•ri•tis (per′i-ne-frī′tis) Inflammation of perinephric tissue.

per•i•neph•ri•um, pl. **per•i•neph•ri•a** (per′i-nef′rē-ŭm, -ă) The connective tissue and fat surrounding the kidney. [peri- + G. *nephros,* kidney]

per•i•ne•um, pl. **per•i•ne•a** (per′i-nē′ŭm, -nē′ă) **1.** The area between the thighs extending from the coccyx to the pubis and lying below the pelvic diaphragm. **2.** The external surface of the central tendon of the perineum, lying between the vulva and the anus in the female and the scrotum and the anus in the male. [L. fr. G. *perineon, perinaion*]

per•i•neu•ral an•es•the•si•a (per′i-nūr′ăl an-es-thē′zē-ă) Anesthesia produced by injection of an anesthetic agent around a nerve.

per•i•neu•ri•al (per′i-nūr′ē-ăl) Relating to the perineurium.

per•i•neu•ri•tis (per′i-nūr-ī′tis) Inflammation of the perineurium. SEE ALSO adventitial neuritis.

per•i•neu•ri•um, pl. **per•i•neu•ri•a** (per′i-nūr′ē-ŭm, -ē-ă) [TA] One of the supporting structures of peripheral nerve trunks, consisting of layers of flattened cells and collagenous connective tissue, which surround the nerve fasciculi and form the major diffusion barrier within the nerve; with the endoneurium and epineurium, composes the peripheral nerve stroma. [L. fr. peri- + G. *neuron,* nerve]

pe•ri•od (pēr′ē-ŏd) **1.** A certain duration or division of time. **2.** One of the stages of a disease, e.g., period of incubation, period of convalescence. SEE ALSO stage, phase. **3.** Colloquialism for menses. **4.** Any of the horizontal rows of chemical elements in the periodic table. [G. *periodos,* a way round, a cycle, fr. *peri,* around, + *hodos,* way]

pe•ri•od•ic (pēr′ē-od′ik) **1.** Recurring at regular intervals. **2.** Denoting a disease with regularly recurring exacerbations or paroxysms.

pe•ri•od•ic dis•ease (pēr′ē-od′ik di-zēz′) Any condition or disease in which episodes tend to recur at regular intervals; many such cases are manifestations of familial Mediterranean fever; the cause of the periodicity is usually unknown.

per•i•o•dic•i•ty (pēr′ē-ō-dis′i-tē) Tendency to recurrence at regular intervals.

per•i•od•ic limb move•ments dis•or•der (PLMD) (pēr′ē-od′ik lim mūv′mĕnts dis-ōr′dĕr) SEE restless legs syndrome.

pe•ri•od•ic neu•tro•pe•ni•a (pēr′ē-od′ik nū-trō-pē′nē-ă) Neutropenia that recurs at regular intervals, in association with various types of infectious diseases.

pe•ri•od•ic pa•ral•y•sis (pēr′ē-od′ik pă-ral′i-sis) Term for a group of diseases characterized by recurring episodes of muscular weakness or flaccid paralysis without loss of consciousness, speech, or sensation; attacks begin when the patient is at rest, and there is apparent good health between attacks. SEE hyperkalemic periodic paralysis, hypokalemic periodic paralysis, normokalemic periodic paralysis.

pe•ri•od•ic ta•ble (pēr′ē-od′ik tā′bĕl) A graphic arrangement of chemical elements by atomic number and chemical properties.

per•i•o•di•za•tion (pēr′ē-ŏd-ī-zā′shŭn) Sequenced strength-training program that varies training volume and intensity to optimize physiologic functional capacity and exercise performance by structuring training into time blocks of different duration (macrocycles, mesocycles, microcycles). The goal is to prevent staleness while peaking physiologically for competition.

per•i•o•don•tal (per′ē-ō-don′tăl) Around a tooth. [peri- + G. *odous,* tooth]

Per•i•o•don•tal In•dex (PI) (per′ē-ō-don′tăl in′deks) An index for the epidemiologic classification of periodontal disease.

per•i•o•don•tal lig•a•ment (per′ē-ō-don′tăl lig′ă-mĕnt) The connective tissue that surrounds the tooth root and attaches it to its bony socket; it consists of fibers anchored in the cementum and extending into the alveolar bone, as well as the tissues that surround and support the teeth, including the gingivae, cementum, periodontal ligament, and alveolar and supporting bone. SYN alveolodental ligament, alveolodental membrane, peridental membrane, periodontal membrane, periodontium (2).

per•i•o•don•tal mem•brane (per′ē-ō-don′tăl mem′brān) SYN periodontal ligament.

per•i•o•don•tal poc•ket (per′ē-ō-don′tal pock′ĕt) Pathologically deepened gingival sulcus, a finding in periodontal disease.

Per•i•o•don•tal Screen•ing Rec•ord (PSR) (per′ē-ō-don′tăl skrēn′ing rek′ŏrd) A modified CPITN used primarily in the United States. SEE ALSO Community Periodontal Index of Treatment Needs.

Per•i•o•don•tal Screen•ing and Re•cord•ing (PSR) (per′ē-ō-don′tăl skrēn′ing rē-kōr′ding) An early detection system of the American Dental Association for periodontal disease.

per•i•o•don•ti•a (per′ē-ō-don′shē-ă) Plural of periodontium.

per•i•o•don•tics (per′ē-ō-don′tiks) The branch of dentistry concerned with the study of the normal tissues and the treatment of abnormal conditions of the tissues immediately about the teeth. [peri- + G. *odous,* tooth]

per•i•o•don•tist (per′ē-ō-don′tist) A dentist who specializes in periodontics.

per•i•o•don•ti•tis (per′ē-ō-don-tī′tis) **1.** Inflammation of the periodontium. **2.** A chronic inflammatory disease of the periodontium occurring in response to bacterial plaque on the adjacent teeth; characterized by gingivitis, destruction of the alveolar bone and periodontal ligament, apical migration of the epithelial attachment resulting in the formation of periodontal pockets, and, ultimately, loosening and exfoliation of the teeth. [periodontium + G. *-itis,* inflammation]

per•i•o•don•ti•um, pl. **per•i•o•don•ti•a** (per′ē-ō-don′shē-ŭm, -ă) **1.** All of the tissues that invest and support the teeth. **2.** SYN periodontal ligament. [L. fr. peri- + G. *odous,* tooth]

per•i•o•don•to•cla•si•a (per′ē-ō-don-tō-klā′zē-ă) Destruction of periodontal tissues, gingiva, pericementum, alveolar bone, and cementum. [periodontium + *klasis,* breaking]

per•i•o•don•to•sis (per′ē-ō-don-tō′sis) SYN juvenile periodontitis. [periodontium + G. *-osis,* condition]

perioesophagitis [Br.] SYN periesophagitis.

per•i•o•nych•i•a (per′ē-ō-nik′ē-ă) **1.** Inflammation of the perionychium. **2.** Plural of perionychium.

per•i•o•nych•i•um, pl. **per•i•o•nych•i•a** (per′ē-ō-nik′ē-ŭm, -ă) SYN eponychium (2). [peri- + G. *onyx,* nail]

per•i•o•o•pho•ri•tis (per′ē-ō-of-ŏr-ī′tis) Inflammation of the peritoneal covering of the ovary. SYN periovaritis. [peri- + Mod. L. *oophoron,* ovary, + *-itis,* inflammation]

per•i•o•o•pho•ro•sal•pin•gi•tis (per′ē-ō-of′ŏr-ō-sal′pin-jī′tis) Inflammation of the peritoneum and other tissues around the ovary and oviduct. SYN perisalpingoovaritis. [peri- + Mod. L. *oophoron,* ovary, + *salpinx,* trumpet, + *-itis,* inflammation]

per•i•op•er•a•tive (per′ē-op′ĕr-ă-tiv) Around the time of operation. SYN paraoperative.

per•i•or•bit (per′ē-ōr′bit) SYN periorbita.

pe•ri•or•bi•ta (per′ē-ōr′bi-tă) [TA] The periosteum of the orbit. SYN periorbit. [peri- + L. *orbita,* orbit]

per•i•or•bi•tal (per′ē-ōr′bi-tăl) **1.** Relating to the periorbita. **2.** SYN circumorbital.

per•i•or•bi•tal cel•lu•li•tis (per′ē-ōr′bi-tăl sel′yū-lī′tis) SYN preseptal cellulitis.

per•i•or•chi•tis (per′ē-ōr kī′tis) Inflammation of the tunica vaginalis testis. [peri- + G. *orchis,* testis, + *-itis,* inflammation]

pe•ri•os•te•a (per′ē-os′tē-ă) Plural of periosteum.

per•i•os•te•al (per′ē-os′tē-ăl) Relating to the periosteum.

per•i•os•te•al bud (per′ē-os′tē-ăl bŭd) A vascular connective tissue bud from the perichondrium that invades the ossification center of the cartilaginous model of a developing long bone.

per•i•os•te•al el•e•va•tor (per′ē-os′tē-ăl el′ĕ-vā-tŏr) An instrument used for separating the periosteum from the bone. SYN rugine (1).

per•i•os•te•al graft (per′ē-os′tē-ăl graft) A graft of periosteum, usually placed on bare bone.

per•i•os•te•i•tis (per′ē-os-tē-ī′tis) SYN periostitis.

♻**periosteo-** Combining form indicating the periosteum. [Mod. L. *periosteum*]

per•i•os•te•o•ma (per′ē-os-tē-ō′mă) A neoplasm derived from the periosteum. SYN periosteophyte.

per•i•os•te•o•my•e•li•tis (per′ē-os′tē-ō-mī-ĕ-lī′tis) Inflammation of the entire bone, with the periosteum and marrow. [periosteo- + G. *myelos,* marrow, + *-itis,* inflammation]

per•i•os•te•o•phyte (per′ē-os′tē-ō-fīt) SYN periosteoma. [periosteo- + G. *phyton,* growth]

per•i•os•te•o•plas•tic am•pu•ta•tion (per′ē-os-tē-ō-plas′tik amp′yū-tā′shŭn) SYN subperiosteal amputation.

per•i•os•te•o•sis (per′ē-os-tē-ō′sis) The formation of a periosteoma. SYN periostosis.

per•i•os•te•ot•o•my (per′ē-os-tē-ot′ŏ-mē) The operation of cutting through the periosteum to the bone. [periosteo- + G. *tomē,* incision]

per•i•os•te•um, pl. **pe•ri•os•te•a** (per′ē-os′tē-ŭm, -ă) [TA] The thick, fibrous membrane covering the entire surface of a bone except its articular cartilage. In young bones, it consists of two layers: an inner cellular layer that is osteogenic, forming new bone tissue, and an outer fibrous connective tissue layer conveying the blood vessels and nerves supplying the bone; in older bones, the osteogenic layer is reduced. SEE ALSO perichondral bone. [Mod. L. fr. G. *periosteon,* ntr. of adj. *periosteos,* around the bones, fr. *peri,* around, + *osteon,* bone]

per•i•os•ti•tis (per′ē-os-tī′tis) Inflammation of the periosteum. SYN periosteitis.

per•i•os•to•sis, pl. **per•i•os•to•ses** (per′ē-os-tō′sis, -sēz) SYN periosteosis.

per•i•o•va•ri•tis (per′ē-ō′văr-ī′tis) SYN perioophoritis.

per•i•pach•y•men•in•gi•tis (per′i-pak′ē-men-in-jī′tis) Inflammation of the area between the dura and bony covering of the central nervous system. [peri- + pachymeninx (dura mater) + G. *-itis,* inflammation]

per•i•pan•cre•a•ti•tis (per′i-pan′krē-ă-tī′tis) Inflammation of the peritoneal coat of the pancreas.

pe•riph•e•rad (pĕr-if′ĕr-ad) In a direction toward the periphery. [G. *periphereia,* periphery, + L. *ad,* to]

pe•riph•e•ral (pĕr-if′ĕr-ăl) **1.** Relating to or situated at the periphery. **2.** Situated nearer the periphery of an organ or part of the body in relation to a specific reference point; opposite of central (centralis). SYN eccentric (3).

pe•riph•e•ral ar•te•ri•al di•sease (pĕr-if′ĕr-ăl ahr-tēr′ē-ăl di-zēz′) Any disorder involving the arteries outside of, or peripheral to, the heart.

pe•riph•e•ral fa•cial pa•ral•y•sis (pĕr-if′ĕr-ăl fā′shăl păr-al′i-sis) SYN Bell palsy.

pe•riph•er•al•ly in•sert•ed cen•tral cath•e•ter (PICC) (pĕr-if′ĕr-ăl-ē′ in-sĕr′tĕd sĕn′trăl kath′ĕ-tĕr) Tube inserted into the superior vena cava through a peripheral vein.

pe•riph•e•ral ner•vous sys•tem (PNS) (pĕr-if′ĕr-ăl nĕr′vŭs sis′tĕm) The peripheral part of the nervous system external to the brain and spinal cord from their roots to their peripheral terminations. This includes the ganglia, both sensory and autonomic, and any plexuses through which the nerve fibers run. SEE ALSO autonomic division of nervous system. SYN peripheral part of nervous system.

pe•riph•e•ral os•si•fy•ing fi•bro•ma (pĕr-if′ĕr-ăl os′i-fī-ing fī-brō′mă) A reactive focal gingival overgrowth derived histogenetically from cells of the periodontal ligament and usually developing in response to local irritants (plaque and calculus) on associated teeth; consists microscopically of a hyperplastic cellular fibrous stroma supporting deposits of bone, cementum, or dystrophic calcification.

pe•riph•e•ral part of ner•vous sys•tem (pĕr-if′ĕr-ăl pahrt nĕr′vŭs sis′tĕm) SYN peripheral nervous system.

pe•riph•er•al re•sist•ance (pĕr-if′ĕr-ăl rē-zis′tăns) Resistance to blood flow through arterioles and capillaries.

pe•riph•e•ral sco•to•ma (pĕr-if′ĕr-ăl skō-tō′mă) A scotoma outside of the central 30 degrees of the visual field.

per•iph•e•ral T-cell lym•pho•ma, un•spe•ci•fied (pĕr-if′ĕr-ăl sel lim-fō′mă un-spes′i-fīd) A heterogeneous group of T-cell neoplasms expressing typical T-cell markers such as CD2, CD3, CD5, and either T-cell α/β or γ/δ receptors.

pe•ri•phe•ral vas•cu•lar dis•ease (PVD) (pĕr-if′ĕr-ăl vas′kyū-lăr di-zēz′) Noncardiac-centered disease of blood vessels, often in extremities. Spider veins are one sign of the presence of such disease.

pe•riph•e•ral vi•sion (pĕr-if′ĕr-ăl vizh′ŭn) Vision resulting from retinal stimulation beyond the macula. SYN indirect vision.

pe•riph•e•ry (pĕr-if′ĕr-ē) **1.** The part of a body away from the center; the outer part or surface. **2.** SYN denture border. [G. *periphereia,* fr. *peri,* around, + *pherō,* to carry]

per•i•phle•bi•tis (per′i-flĕ-bī′tis) Inflammation of the outer coat of a vein or of the tissues surrounding it. [peri- + G. *phleps,* vein, + *-itis,* inflammation]

per•i•po•ri•tis (per′i-pŏr-ī′tis) Miliary papules and papulovesicles with staphylococcic infection; most frequently on the face and in infants. [peri- + G. *poros,* pore, + *-itis,* inflammation]

per•i•proc•ti•tis (per′i-prok-tī′tis) Inflammation of the areolar tissue about the rectum. SYN perirectitis.

per•i•pros•ta•ti•tis (per′i-pros-tă-tī′tis) Inflammation of the tissues surrounding the prostate.

per•i•py•le•phle•bi•tis (per′i-pī′lĕ-flĕ-bī′tis) Inflammation of the tissues around the portal vein. [peri- + G. *pylē,* gate, + *phleps,* vein, + *-itis,* inflammation]

per•i•rec•ti•tis (per′i-rek-tī′tis) SYN periproctitis.

per•i•rhi•zo•cla•si•a (per′i-rī-zō-klā′zē-ă) Inflammatory destruction of tissues immediately around the root of a tooth. [peri- + G. *rhiza,* root, -o- + *klasis,* destruction]

per•i•sal•pin•gi•tis (per′i-sal′pin-jī′tis) Inflammation of the peritoneum that covers the uterine tube. [peri- + G. *salpinx,* trumpet, + *-itis,* inflammation]

per•i•sal•pin•go•o•va•ri•tis (per′i-sal-pin′gō-ō-văr-ī′tis) SYN perioophorosalpingitis. [peri- + G. *salpinx,* trumpet, + ovary + G. *-itis,* inflammation]

per•i•sal•pinx (per′i-sal′pingks) The peritoneal covering of the uterine tube. [peri- + G. *salpinx* (*salping-*), trumpet]

per•i•scop•ic (per′i-skop′ik) Denoting that which gives the ability to see objects to one side as well as in the direct axis of vision. [peri- + G. *skopeō,* to view]

per•i•sig•moi•di•tis (per′i-sig-moy-dī′tis) Inflammation of the connective tissues surrounding the sigmoid flexure, giving rise to symptoms, referable to the left iliac fossa, similar to those of perityphlitis in the right iliac fossa.

per•i•sper•ma•ti•tis (per′i-spĕr′mă-tī′tis) Inflammation of the tissues around the spermatic cord.

per•i•splanch•ni•tis (per′i-splangk-nī′tis) Inflammation surrounding any viscus or viscera. [peri- + G. *splanchna,* viscera, + *-itis,* inflammation]

per•i•sple•ni•tis (per′i-splē-nī′tis) Inflammation of the peritoneum covering the spleen.

per•i•spon•dy•li•tis (per′i-spond′i-lī′tis) Inflammation of the tissues about a vertebra. [peri- + G. *spondylos,* vertebra, + *-itis,* inflammation]

per•i•stal•sis (per′i-stal′sis) The movement of the intestine or other tubular structure, characterized by waves of alternate circular contraction and relaxation of the tube by which the contents are propelled onward. SYN vermicular movement. [peri- + G. *stalsis,* constriction]

per•i•stal•tic (per′i-stal′tik) Relating to peristalsis.

pe•ris•to•le (pĕr-is′tŏ-lē) The tonic activity of the walls of the stomach whereby the organ contracts about its contents; contrasting with the peristaltic waves passing from the cardia toward the pylorus (peristalsis). [peri- + G. *stellō,* to contract]

per·i·stol·ic (per′i-stol′ik) Relating to peristole.

per·i·tec·to·my (per′i-tek′tŏ-mē) **1.** The removal of a paracorneal strip of the conjunctiva for the relief of corneal disease. **2.** SYN circumcision (2). [peri- + G. *ektomē,* excision]

pe·ri·ten·di·ne·um, pl. **pe·ri·ten·di·ne·a** (per′i-ten-din′ē-ŭm, -ē-ă) One of the fibrous sheaths surrounding the primary bundles of fibers in a tendon. [L. fr. peri- + G. *tenōn,* tendon]

per·i·ten·di·ni·tis (per′i-ten′di-nī′tis) Inflammation of the sheath of a tendon. SYN peritenonitis, peritenontitis.

peri·ten·on·i·tis (per′ē-ten′ŏn-ī′tis) SYN peritendinitis.

per·i·ten·on·ti·tis (per′i-ten′ŏn-tī′tis) SYN peritendinitis.

per·i·the·li·um, pl. **per·i·the·li·a** (per′i-thē′lē-ŭm, -ă) The connective tissue that surrounds smaller vessels and capillaries. [peri- + G. *thēlē,* nipple]

per·i·thy·roi·di·tis (per′i-thī′roy-dī′tis) Inflammation of the capsule or tissues surrounding the thyroid gland.

pe·rit·o·my (pĕr-it′ŏ-mē) **1.** A circumcorneal incision through the conjunctiva. **2.** SYN circumcision (1). [G. *peritomē,* fr. *peri,* around, + *tomē,* incision]

per·i·to·ne·al (per′i-tō-nē′ăl) Relating to the peritoneum.

per·i·to·ne·al cav·i·ty (per′i-tō-nē′ăl kav′i-tē) The interior of the peritoneal sac, normally only a potential space between the parietal and visceral layers of the peritoneum.

per·i·to·ne·al di·al·y·sis (PD) (per′i-tō-nē′ăl dī-al′i-sis) Removal from the body of soluble substances and water by transfer across the peritoneum, using a dialysis solution that is intermittently introduced into and removed from the peritoneal cavity.

per·i·ton·e·al in·suf·fla·tion (per′i-tō-nē′ăl in-sŭ-flā′shŭn) Administration of a gas, usually carbon dioxide, within the peritoneal cavity to facilitate laparoendoscopic procedures.

peritoneo- Combining form denoting the peritoneum. [L. *peritoneum*]

per·i·to·ne·o·cen·te·sis (per′i-tō-nē′ō-sen-tē′sis) Paracentesis of the abdomen. [peritoneum + G. *kentēsis,* puncture]

per·i·to·ne·oc·ly·sis (per′i-tō-nē-ok′li-sis) Irrigation of the abdominal cavity. [peritoneum, + G. *klysis,* a washing out]

per·i·to·ne·o·per·i·car·di·al (per′i-tō-nē′ō-per′i-kahr′dē-ăl) Relating to both the peritoneum and the pericardium.

per·i·to·ne·o·pex·y (per′i-tō-nē′ō-pek-sē) A suspension or fixation of the peritoneum. [peritoneum + G. *pēxis,* fixation]

per·i·to·ne·o·plas·ty (per′i-tō-nē′ō-plas-tē) Loosening adhesions and covering the raw surfaces with peritoneum to prevent reformation. [peritoneum + G. *plastos,* formed]

per·i·to·ne·o·scope (per′i-tō-nē′ō-skōp) SYN laparoscope. [peritoneum + G. *skopeō,* to view]

per·i·to·ne·os·co·py (per′i-tō-nē-os′kŏ-pē) Examination of the contents of the peritoneum with a peritoneoscope passed through the abdominal wall. SEE ALSO laparoscopy. SYN abdominoscopy, celioscopy, ventroscopy.

per·i·to·ne·ot·o·my (per′i-tō′nē-ot′ŏ-mē) Incision of the peritoneum. [peritoneum + G. *tomē,* incision]

per·i·to·ne·o·ve·nous shunt (pĕr′i-tō-nē′ō-vē′nŭs shŭnt) A shunt, usually by a catheter, between the peritoneal cavity and the venous system.

per·i·to·ne·um, pl. **pe·ri·to·ne·a** (per′i-tō-nē′ŭm, -ă) [TA] The serous membrane, consisting of mesothelium and connective tissue, that lines the abdominal cavity and covers most of the viscera contained therein; it forms two sacs: the peritoneal (or greater) sac and the omental bursa (lesser sac), connected by the epiploic foramen. [Mod. L. fr. G. *peritonaion,* fr. *periteinō,* to stretch over]

per·i·to·ne·um uro·gen·i·ta·le (per′i-tō-nē′ŭm yūr-ō-jen-i-tā′lē) SYN urogenital peritoneum.

per·i·to·ni·tis (per′i-tō-nī′tis) Inflammation of the peritoneum. See this page.

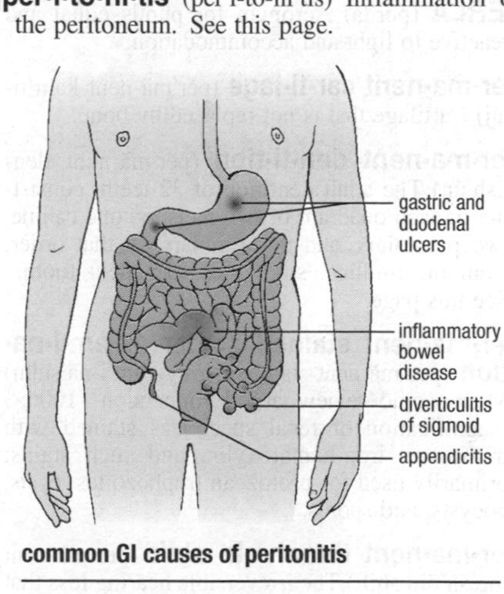

common GI causes of peritonitis

per·i·ton·sil·lar ab·scess (per′i-ton′sil-lăr ab′ses) Extension of tonsillar infection beyond the capsule with abscess formation usually above and behind the tonsil. SYN quinsy.

per·i·ton·sil·li·tis (per′i-ton′si-lī′tis) Inflammation of the connective tissue above and behind the tonsil.

pe•rit•ri•chal, pe•rit•ri•chate, per•i•trich•ic (per′i-trik′ăl, -āt, -ik) SYN peritrichous (2).

pe•rit•ri•chous (per′i-trik′ŭs) **1.** Relating to cilia or other appendicular organs projecting from the periphery of a cell. **2.** Having flagella uniformly distributed over a cell; used especially with reference to bacteria. SYN peritrichal, peritrichate, peritrichic. [peri- + G. *thrix,* hair]

per•i•tu•bu•lar con•trac•tile cells (per′i-tū′byū-lăr kon-trak′tĭl selz) SYN myoid cells.

per•i•u•re•ter•i•tis (per′ē-yū-rē-tĕr-ī′tis) Inflammation of the tissues about a ureter. [peri- + ureter + G. *-itis,* inflammation]

per•i•u•re•thri•tis (per′ē-yū-rē-thrī′tis) Inflammation of the tissues about the urethra. [peri- + urethra + G. *-itis,* inflammation]

per•i•u•ter•ine (per′ē-yū′ter-in) SYN perimetric (1).

per•i•vag•i•ni•tis (per′i-vaj-i-nī′tis) Inflammation of the connective tissue around the vagina. SYN pericolpitis.

per•i•vas•cu•li•tis (per′i-vas-kyū-lī′tis) SYN periangitis.

per•i•ves•i•cal (per′i-ves′i-kăl) SYN pericystic. [peri- + L. *vesica,* bladder]

per•i•vis•cer•i•tis (per′i-vis-ĕr-ī′tis) Inflammation surrounding any viscus or viscera. [peri- + L. *viscera,* internal organs, + G. *-itis,* inflammation]

PERLA (pĕr′lă) Acronym for pupils equal and reactive to light and accommodation.

per•ma•nent car•ti•lage (pĕr′mă-nent kahr′ti-lăj) Cartilage that is not replaced by bone.

per•ma•nent den•ti•tion (pĕr′mă-nent den-tish′ŭn) The adult dentition of 32 teeth, consisting in each quadrant of two incisors, one canine, two premolars, and three molars, in that order, from the midline. SEE ALSO permanent tooth. See this page.

per•ma•nent stained smear ex•am•i•na•tion (per-mă-nent stānd smēr eg-zam′i-nā′shŭn) Microscopic review at oil immersion (1000×) magnification of fecal specimens stained with trichrome, iron-hematoxylin, and such stains; primarily used for protozoan trophozoites, cysts, oocysts, and spores.

per•ma•nent thresh•old shift (per-mă-nent thresh′ōld shift) The irreversible hearing loss that results from exposure to intense impulse or continuous sound, as opposed to the reversible temporary threshold shift that also results from such exposure.

per•ma•nent tooth (per-mă-nent tūth) One of the 32 teeth belonging to the second, or permanent, dentition; eruption of the permanent teeth begins from the fifth to the seventh year, and is not completed until the 17–23rd year, when the last of the wisdom teeth appears. SYN dens permanens [TA], second tooth, secondary dentition.

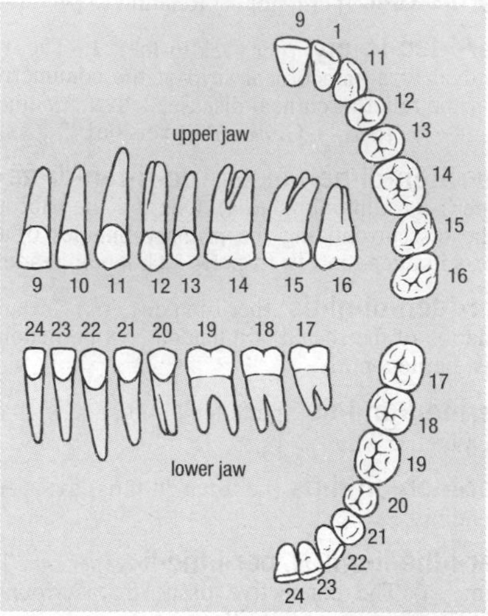

permanent dentition, half view, left side (numbering code, universal system of permanent teeth): central incisor 9, 24; lateral incisor 10, 23; canine 11, 22; first bicuspid 12, 21; second biscupid 13, 20; first molar 14, 19; second molar 15, 18; third molar 16, 17

per•me•a•bil•i•ty (pĕr′mē-ă-bil′i-tē) The property of being permeable.

per•me•a•bil•i•ty co•ef•fi•cient (pĕr′mē-ă-bil′i-tē kō-ĕ-fi′shĕnt) A coefficient associated with simple diffusion through a membrane that is proportional to the partition coefficient and the diffusion coefficient and inversely proportional to membrane thickness.

per•me•a•bil•i•ty con•stant (pĕr′mē-ă-bil′i-tē kon′stănt) A measure of the ease with which an ion can cross a unit area of membrane driven by a 1.0 M difference in concentration; usually expressed in centimeters per second. Cf. permeability coefficient.

per•me•a•ble (pĕr′mē-ă-bĕl) Permitting the passage of substances (e.g., liquids, gases), as through a membrane or other structure. SEE ALSO permeate. SYN pervious. [L. *permeabilis*]

per•me•ase (pĕr′mē-ās) Any of a group of membrane-bound carriers (enzymes) that cause transport of solute through a semipermeable membrane.

per•me•ate (pĕr′mē-āt) **1.** To pass through a membrane or other structure. **2.** That which can so pass. [L. *permeo,* to pass through]

per•me•a•tion (pĕr-mē-ā′shŭn) The process of

spreading through or penetrating, as the extension of a malignant neoplasm by proliferation of the cells continuously along the blood vessels or lymphatics. [L. *per-meo,* pp. *-meatus,* to pass through]

per•ni•cious (pĕr-nish′ŭs) Destructive; harmful; denoting a disease of severe character and usually fatal without appropriate treatment. [L. *perniciosus,* destructive, fr. *pernicies,* destruction]

per•ni•cious a•ne•mi•a (pĕr-nish′ŭs ă-nē′mē-ă) A chronic progressive anemia of older adults due to failure of absorption of vitamin B12, usually resulting from a defect of the stomach accompanied by mucosal atrophy and associated with lack of secretion of "intrinsic" factor; characterized by numbness and tingling, weakness, and a sore, smooth tongue, as well as dyspnea after slight exertion, faintness, pallor of the skin and mucous membranes, anorexia, diarrhea, loss of weight, and fever; laboratory studies usually reveal greatly decreased red blood cell counts, low levels of hemoglobin, numerous characteristically oval macrocytic erythrocytes, and hypochlorhydria or achlorhydria, in association with a predominant number of megaloblasts and relatively few normoblasts in the bone marrow; the leukocyte count in peripheral blood may be less than normal, with relative lymphocytosis and hypersegmented neutrophils; a low level of vitamin B12 is found in peripheral erythrocytes; administration of vitamin B12 results in a characteristic reticulocyte response, relief from symptoms, and an increase in erythrocytes, provided that pernicious anemia is not complicated by another disease. SEE ALSO diphyllobothriasis. SYN Addison anemia, malignant anemia

per•ni•cious vom•it•ing (pĕr-nish′ŭs vom′it-ing) Uncontrollable vomiting.

pero- Combining form meaning maimed, malformed. [G. *pēros*]

pe•ro•dac•ty•ly, **pe•ro•dac•tyl•i•a** (pē-rō-dak′ti-lē, -dak-til′ē-ă) Congenital deformity of the fingers or toes. [pero- + G. *daktylos,* finger or toe]

pe•ro•me•li•a, **pe•rom•e•ly** (pē-rō-mē′lē-ă, pĕ-rom′ĕ-lē) Severe congenital malformations of the limbs, including absence of the hand or foot. [pero- + G. *melos,* limb]

per•o•ne•al (pĕr′ō-nē′ăl) Relating to the fibula, to the lateral side of the leg, or to the muscles there present. [L. *peroneus,* fr. G. *peronē,* fibula]

per•o•ne•al ar•ter•y (pĕr′ō-nē′ăl ahr′tĕr-ē) *Origin*, posterior tibial; *distribution*, soleus, tibialis posterior, flexor longus hallucis, peroneal muscles, inferior tibiofibular articulation, and ankle joint; *anastomoses*, anterior lateral malleolar, lateral tarsal, lateral plantar, dorsalis pedis. SYN arteria peronea [TA], fibular artery.

per•o•ne•al mus•cu•lar at•ro•phy (pĕr′ō-nē′ăl mŭs′kyū-lăr at′rŏ-fē) A group of familial peripheral neuromuscular disorders, sharing the common feature of marked wasting of the distal parts of the extremities, particularly the peroneal muscle groups, resulting in "stork legs." SYN Charcot-Marie-Tooth disease.

per•o•ne•al ret•i•nac•u•lum (pĕr′ō-nē′ăl ret′i-nak′yū-lŭm) Superior and inferior fibrous bands retaining the tendons of the peroneus longus and brevis in position as they cross the lateral side of the ankle. SYN retinacula of peroneal muscles.

per•o•ne•al veins (pĕr′ō-nē′ăl vānz) Venae comitantes of the peroneal artery; they join the posterior tibial veins to enter the popliteal vein. SYN fibular veins.

pe•ro•ne•us long•us mus•cle (pĕr-ō-nē′ŭs long′gus mŭs′ĕl) SYN fibularis longus muscle.

per•o•ne•us ter•ti•us mus•cle (pĕr-ō-nē′ŭs tĕr′shē-ŭs mŭs′ĕl) SYN fibularis tertius muscle.

per•o•ral (pĕr-ō′răl) Through the mouth, denoting a method of medication or an approach. [L. *per,* through, + *os* (*or-*), mouth]

per os (PO) (pĕr os) By or through the mouth, denoting a method of medication feeding. [L.]

Pe•rout•ka syn•drome (pār-ūt′kă sin′drōm) Sneezing brought on by moving from a darker environment into a lighter one; autosomal dominant condition affecting about 25% of the U.S. population.

peroxi- SEE peroxy-.

per•ox•i•das•es (pĕr-ok′si-dās-ĕz) [EC subclass 1.11] Enzymes in animal and plant tissues that catalyze the dehydrogenation (oxidation) of various substances in the presence of hydrogen peroxide, which acts as a hydrogen acceptor, being converted to water in the process.

per•ox•ide (pĕr-ok′sīd) That oxide of any series that contains the greatest number of oxygen atoms.

per•ox•i•some (pĕr-ok′si-sōm) A membrane-bound organelle occurring in nearly all eukaryotic cells that often contains oxidative enzymes relating to the formation and degradation of H_2O_2. SYN microbody. [peroxide + G. *sōma,* body]

peroxy- Prefix denoting the presence of an extra O atom, as in peroxides and peroxy acids.

per•ox•yl (pĕr-ok′sil) One of the free radicals presumed to be formed as a result of the bombardment of tissue by high-energy radiation.

per pri•mam in•ten•ti•o•nem (pĕr prī′mam in-ten-shē-ō′nem) By first intention. SEE healing by first intention. [L.]

per rec•tum (PR) (pĕr rek′tŭm) By or through the rectum, denoting a method of examination or treatment. [L., through the rectum]

per•salt (pĕr′sawlt) CHEMISTRY any salt that contains the greatest possible amount of the acid radical.

per·sev·er·a·tion (pĕr-sĕv′ĕr-ā′shŭn) **1.** The constant repetition of a meaningless word or phrase. **2.** The duration of a mental impression, measured by the rapidity with which one impression follows another as determined by the revolving of a two-colored disc. **3.** CLINICAL PSYCHOLOGY the uncontrollable repetition of a previously appropriate or correct response, even though the repeated response has since become inappropriate or incorrect. [L. *persevero,* to persist]

per·sis·tence (pĕr-sis′tĕns) **1.** Obstinate continuation of characteristic behavior. **2.** Survival despite opposition or adverse environmental conditions. [L. *persisto,* to abide, stand firm]

per·sis·tent a·gent (pĕr-sis′tĕnt ā′jĕnt) A chemical agent that under given conditions of temperature, pressure, wind, and other variables remains in the environment for longer than 1 day. Examples include sulfur mustard, Lewisite, and the nerve agent VX.

per·sis·tent an·te·ri·or hy·per·plas·tic pri·mar·y vit·re·ous (pĕr-sis′tĕnt an-tēr′ē-ŏr hī′pĕr-plas′tik prī′măr-ē vit′rē-ŭs) A unilateral congenital abnormality occurring in full-term infants; characterized by a retrolental fibrovascular membrane formed by persistent primary vitreous with remnants of the hyaloid artery and tunica vasculosa lentis; associated with leukokoria, microphthalmos, shallow anterior chamber, and elongated ciliary processes.

per·sis·tent chron·ic hep·a·ti·tis (pĕr-sis′tĕnt kron′ik hep′ă-tī′tis) A benign chronic hepatitis that may follow acute viral hepatitis B or C infection or complicated bowel diseases; rarely progresses to cirrhosis, portal hypertension, or liver failure.

per·sis·tent clo·a·ca (pĕr-sis′tent klō-ā′kă) A condition in which the urorectal septum has failed to divide the cloaca of the embryo into rectal and urogenital portions.

per·sis·tent pos·te·ri·or hy·per·plas·tic pri·mar·y vit·re·ous (pĕr-sis′tĕnt pos-tēr′ē-ŏr hī′pĕr-plas′tik prī′mar-ē vit′rē-ŭs) A unilateral congenital anomaly in full-term infants; associated with a congenital retinal fold and a vitreous membranous stalk containing remnants of the hyaloid artery.

per·sis·tent trun·cus ar·te·ri·o·sus (pĕr-sis′tĕnt trungk′ŭs ar-tē-rē-ō′sŭs) A congenital cardiovascular anomaly resulting from failure of development of the spiral septum and consisting of a common arterial trunk opening out of both ventricles, the pulmonary arteries being given off from the ascending common trunk.

per·sis·tent veg·e·ta·tive state (PVS) (pĕr-sis′tĕnt vej′ĕ-tā-tiv stāt) Vegetative state of prolonged duration (defined in different sources as duration of longer than 1 month, 1 year, or 2 years); usually permanent. SEE ALSO vegetative.

per·so·na (pĕr-sō′nă) A term that embodies the total constellation of physical, psychological, and behavioral attributes of each unique individual; in jungian psychology, the outer aspect of character, as opposed to anima (2); the assumed personality used to mask the true one. [L. *persona,* actor's mask; character, role, prob. fr. Etruscan]

per·son·al ac·tiv·i·ties of dail·y liv·ing (PADL) (pĕr′sŏn-ăl ak-tiv′i-tēz dā′lē liv′ing) SYN instrumental activities of daily living.

per·son·al e·qua·tion (pĕr′sŏn-ăl ĕ-kwā′zhŭn) A slight error in judgment, perceptual response, or action peculiar to the person and so constant that it is usually possible to allow for it in accepting the person's statements or conclusions, thus arriving at approximate exactness.

per·son·al·i·ty (pĕr′sŏn-al′i-tē) **1.** The unique self; the organized system of attitudes and behavioral predispositions by which one feels, thinks, acts, and impresses and establishes relationships with others. **2.** An individual with a particular personality pattern.

per·son·al·i·ty dis·or·der (pĕr′sŏn-al′i-tē dis-ōr′dĕr) General term for a group of behavioral disorders characterized by usually lifelong, ingrained, maladaptive patterns of deviant behavior, lifestyle, and/or social adjustment that are different in quality from psychotic and neurotic symptoms; former designations for patients with these personality disorders were psychopath and sociopath. SEE ALSO antisocial personality disorder.

per·son·al·i·ty for·ma·tion (pĕr′sŏn-al′i-tē fōr-mā′shŭn) The life history associated with the development of individual patterns and of one's individuality.

per·son·al·i·ty pro·file (pĕr′sŏn-al′i-tē prō′fīl) **1.** A method by which the results of psychological testing are presented in graphic form. **2.** A vignette or brief personality description.

per·son·al pro·tec·tive e·quip·ment (PPE) (pĕr′sŏn-ăl prō-tek′tiv ĕ-kwip′mĕnt) Specialized clothing or equipment (e.g., gloves, lab coats, eye protection, and breathing apparatus) used by workers (e.g., EMS personnel) to protect themselves from direct exposure to blood or other potentially hazardous materials to avoid injury or disease.

per·son·al space (pĕr′sŏn-ăl spās) A term used in the behavioral sciences to denote the physical area immediately surrounding a person who is in proximity to one or more others, whether known or unknown, and which serves as a body buffer zone in such interpersonal transactions.

per·son·al train·er (pĕr′sŏn-ăl trā′nŏr) A person who is certified in developing fitness programs for all people without regard to age or level of performance.

pers•pi•ra•tion (pĕrs′pir-ā′shŭn) **1.** The excretion of fluid by the sweat glands of the skin. SYN diaphoresis, sudation, sweating. SEE ALSO sweat (2). **2.** All fluid loss through normal skin, whether by sweat gland secretion or by diffusion through other skin structures. **3.** The fluid excreted by the sweat glands; it consists of water containing sodium chloride and phosphate, urea, ammonia, ethereal sulfates, creatinine, fats, and other waste products; the average daily quantity is estimated at about 1500 g. SYN sudor. SEE ALSO sweat (1). [L. *per-spiro,* pp. *-atus,* to breathe everywhere]

per•tac•tin (pĕr-tak′tin) An antigenic material produced by *Bordetella pertussis* used to improve the effectiveness of pertussis vaccines. [*pert*ussis + act + -in]

per•tech•ne•tate (pĕr-tek′nĕ-tāt) Anionic form of technetium used widely in nuclear scanning; ^{99m}Tc04.

Per•thes test (per′tĕz test) A test for patency of the deep femoral vein; with the patient standing, a tourniquet is applied above the knee; after walking, if the deep circulation is competent, the superficial varicosities remain unchanged; if the deep circulation is occluded, the leg becomes painful.

Per•tik di•ver•tic•u•lum (per′tik dī′vĕr-tik′yū-lŭm) An abnormally deep recessus pharyngeus.

per tu•bam (pĕr tū′băm) Through a tube. [L.]

per•tus•sis (pĕr-tŭs′is) An acute infectious inflammation of the larynx, trachea, and bronchi caused by *Bordetella pertussis;* characterized by recurrent bouts of spasmodic coughing that continues until the breath is exhausted, then ends in a noisy inspiratory stridor (the "whoop") caused by laryngeal spasm. SYN whooping cough. [L. *per,* very (intensive), + *tussis,* cough]

Pe•ru•vi•an wart (pĕr-ū′vē-ăn wōrt) SYN verruga peruana.

per•va•sive de•vel•op•men•tal dis•or•der (pĕr-vā′siv dĕ-vel-ŏp-men′tăl dis-ōr′dĕr) A class of mental disorders of infancy, childhood, or adolescence characterized by distortions in the development of the multiple basic psychological functions involved in the development of social skills and language.

per vi•as na•tu•ra•les (pĕr vī′as nach-ūr-ā′lēz) Through the natural passages, e.g., denoting a normal delivery, as opposed to cesarean section, or the passage in stool of a foreign body instead of its surgical removal. [L.]

per•vi•ous (pĕr′vē-ŭs) SYN permeable. [L. *pervius,* fr. *per,* through, + *via,* a way]

pes, gen. **pe•dis**, pl. **pe•des** (pes, ped′is, -dēz) [TA] **1.** SYN foot (1). **2.** Any footlike or basal structure or part. **3.** Talipes; in this sense, pes is always qualified by a word expressing the specific type. [L.]

pes an•se•ri•nus (pes an-sĕr-ī′nŭs) **1.** SYN intraparotid plexus of facial nerve. **2.** The combined tendinous expansions of the sartorius, gracilis, and semitendinosus muscles at the medial border of the tuberosity of the tibia.

pes cav•us (pes kā′vŭs) Condition characterized by increased height of the foot's medial longitudinal arch. SYN clawfoot, claw foot.

pes pla•nus (pes plā′nŭs) SYN talipes planus.

pes•sa•ry (pes′ă-rē) **1.** An appliance of varied form, introduced into the vagina to support the uterus or to correct any displacement. **2.** A medicated vaginal suppository. [L. *pessarium,* fr. G. *pessos,* an oval stone used in certain games]

pes•ti•cide (pes′ti-sīd) General term for an agent that destroys fungi, insects, rodents, or any other pest.

pes•ti•lence (pes′ti-lĕns) **1.** SYN plague (2). **2.** A virulent outbreak of any disease. [L. *pestilentia*]

pes•ti•len•tial (pes-ti-len′shăl) Relating to or tending to produce a pestilence.

pes•tle (pes′ĕl) An instrument in the shape of a rod with one rounded and weighted extremity, used for bruising, breaking, grinding, and mixing substances in a mortar. [L. *pistillum,* fr. *pinso,* or *piso,* to pound]

PET (pĕt) Acronym for positron emission tomography.

peta- Prefix used in the SI and the metric system to signify one quadrillion (10^{15}).

-petal Suffix meaning seeking; movement toward the part indicated by the main portion of the word. [L. *peto,* to seek, strive for]

pe•te•chi•ae, sing. **pe•te•chi•a** (pe-tē′kē-ē, -ă) Minute hemorrhagic spots, of pinpoint to pinhead size, in the skin, which are not blanched by diascopy. See page B13. [Mod. L. form of It. *petecchie*]

pe•te•chi•al (pe-tē′kē-ăl) Relating to, accompanied by, or characterized by petechiae.

pe•te•chi•al hem•or•rhage (pe-tē′kē-ăl hem′ŏr-ăj) Capillary hemorrhage into the skin that forms petechiae. SYN punctate hemorrhage.

Pe•ters o•vum (pā′tĕrz ō′vŭm) An embryo with a presumptive fertilization age of about 13 days; for many years, it was one of very few young human embryos recovered in good condition, and its study furnished many facts regarding early embryonic changes.

pet•i•o•late, **pet•i•o•lat•ed** (pet′ē-ō-lāt, -ĕd) Having a stem or pedicle. [L. *petiolus*]

pe•ti•o•lus (pĕ-tē'ō-lŭs) A stem or pedicle. [L. dim. of *pes* (foot), the stalk of a fruit]

Pe•tit her•ni•a (pĕ-tē' hĕr'nē-ă) Lumbar hernia, occurring in inferior lumbar triangle.

Pe•tit her•ni•ot•o•my (pĕ-tē' her-nē-ot'ō-mē) Herniotomy without incision into the sac.

Pe•tit lum•bar tri•an•gle (pĕ-tē' lŭm'bahr trī'ang-gĕl) SYN inferior lumbar triangle.

pe•tit mal (pĕ-tē' măl) Type of seizure. [Fr. small]

Pe•tri dish cul•ture (pē'trē dish kŭl'chŭr) A combination of filter paper, fecal specimen, and tap water placed in a Petri dish; provides an environment for nematode eggs to hatch and larvae to develop.

pet•ri•fac•tion (pet-ri-fak'shŭn) Fossilization, as in conversion into stone. [L. *petra,* rock + *facio,* to make]

pé•tris•sage (pā-trē-sahzh') A movement in massage that involves the lifting of tissues away from underlying structures, with the intention of improving elasticity and stimulating blood and lymph circulation. Includes kneading, skin rolling, and wringing. [Fr. kneading]

petro- Prefix meaning stone; stonelike hardness. [L. *petra,* rock; G. *petros,* stone]

pet•ro•mas•toid (pet-rō-mas'toyd) Relating to the petrous and the squamous portions of the temporal bone, which are usually united at birth by the petrosquamosal suture.

pet•ro•oc•cip•i•tal (pet'rō-ok-sip'i-tăl) Denoting the cranial suture between the occipital bone and the petrous portion of the temporal.

pet•ro•oc•cip•i•tal fis•sure (pet'rō-ok-sip'i-tăl fish'ŭr) A fissure between the petrous part of the temporal bone and the basilar part of the occipital bone that extends anteromedially from the jugular foramen; includes the jugular foramen (at its posterior end).

pe•tro•sa, pl. **pe•tro•sae** (pe-trō'să, -sē) The petrous portion of the temporal bone. [L. fr. *petra,* rock]

pe•tro•sal (pĕ-trō'săl) Relating to the petrosa. SYN petrous (2).

pet•ro•si•tis (pet-rō-sī'tis) An inflammation involving the petrous portion of the temporal bone and its air cells.

pet•ro•sphe•noid (pet-rō-sfē'noyd) Relating to the petrous portion of the temporal bone and to the sphenoid bone.

pet•ro•squa•mo•sal, **pet•ro•squa•mous** (pet'rō-skwā-mō'săl, -skwā'mŭs) Relating to the petrous and the squamous portions of the temporal bone.

pet•ro•tym•pan•ic fis•sure (pet'rō-tim-pan'ik fish'ŭr) A fissure between the tympanic and petrous portions of the temporal bone; it transmits the chorda tympani nerve through a small patent portion, the anterior canaliculus of the chorda tympani. SYN glaserian fissure.

pet•rous (pet'rŭs) **1.** Of stony hardness. **2.** SYN petrosal. [L. *petrosus,* fr. *petra,* a rock]

pet•rous part of in•ter•nal ca•rot•id ar•ter•y (pet'rŭs pahrt in-tĕr'năl kă-rot'id ahr'tĕr-ē) The part of the internal carotid artery in the carotid canal; its branches are the carotidotympanic arteries and the artery of the pterygoid canal.

pet•rous part of tem•po•ral bone (pet'rŭs pahrt tem'pŏr-ăl bōn) The part of the temporal bone that contains the structures of the internal ear and the second part of the internal carotid artery; in prenatal life, it appears as a separate ossification center.

pet•ti•gree (pet'i-grē) SYN butcher's broom.

Petz•val sur•face (pets'vahl sŭr'făs) The curved image plane on which any extended linear object is focused by a lens; it is curved toward the edges of a convex lens and away from the edges of a concave lens. SEE ALSO barrel distortion, pincushion distortion.

pex•is (pek'sis) Fixation of substances in the tissues. [G. *pēxis,* fixation]

-pexy Suffix meaning fixation, usually surgical. [G. *pēxis,* fixation]

Pey•er patch•es (pī'ĕr pach'ĕz) Collections of many lymphoid follicles closely packed together, forming oblong elevations on the mucous membrane of the small intestine.

Pey•ro•nie dis•ease (pā-rō-nē' di-zēz') A disease in which plaques or strands of dense fibrous tissue surrounding the corpus cavernosum of the penis cause penile bending and pain on erection; sometimes associated with Dupuytren contracture.

Pey•rot tho•rax (pā-rō' thōr'aks) An obliquely oval deformity of the chest in cases of a very large pleural effusion.

PF Abbreviation for platelet factor.

Pfan•nen•stiel in•ci•sion (fahn'ĕn-shtēl in-sizh'ŭn) An incision made transversely, and through the external sheath of the recti muscles, about an inch above the pubes, the muscles being separated at the midline in the direction of their fibers.

Pfeif•fer ba•cil•lus (fī'fĕr bă-sil'ŭs) SYN *Haemophilus influenzae.*

Pfeif•fer phe•nom•e•non (fī'fĕr fĕ-nom'ĕ-non) The alteration and complete disintegration of *Vibrio cholerae* when introduced into the peritoneal cavity of an immunized guinea pig, or into that of a normal one if immune serum is injected at the same time; extended to include bacteriolysis in general.

Pfeif·fer syn·drome (fī′fĕr sin′drōm) Variable syndactyly of the fingers and toes; craniosynostosis is a variable feature. SYN Noack syndrome.

PFT Abbreviation for pulmonary function test.

pg Abbreviation for picogram.

P-gly·co·pro·tein (glī′kō-prō′tēn) Protein associated with tumor multidrug resistance; acts as an energy-requiring efflux pump for many classes of natural products and chemotherapeutic drugs.

Ph Abbreviation for phenyl.

pH Symbol for the negative logarithm of the H^+ ion concentration (measured in moles per liter); a solution with pH 7.00 is neutral at 22°C, one with a pH of more than 7.0 is alkaline, and one with a pH lower than 7.00 is acid. At a temperature of 37°C, neutrality is at a pH value of 6.8. [p (power or potency) of H^+]

PHA Abbreviation for phytohemagglutinin.

♻ **phaco-** Prefix meaning (1) lens-shaped, relating to a lens. (2) birthmark; as in phacoma tosis. [G. *phakos,* lentil (lens), anything shaped like a lentil]

phac·o·an·a·phy·lax·is (fak′ō-an-ă-fi-lak′sis) Hypersensitivity to protein of the lens of the eye.

phac·o·cele (fak′ō-sēl) Hernia of the lens of the eye through the sclera. [phaco- + G. *kēlē,* hernia]

phac·o·e·mul·si·fi·ca·tion (fak′ō-ē-mŭl-si-fi-kā′shŭn) A method of emulsifying and aspirating a cataract with a low-frequency ultrasonic needle.

phac·o·er·y·sis (fak-ō-er′i-sis) Extraction of the lens of the eye by means of a suction cup called the erysophake. [phaco- + G. *erysis,* pulling, drawing off]

phac·o·gen·ic glau·co·ma (fak′ō-jen′ik glaw-kō′mă) SYN phacomorphic glaucoma.

pha·coid (fak′oyd) Shaped like a lentil (bean). [phaco- + G. *eidos,* resemblance]

pha·col·y·sis (fă-kol′i-sis) Operative breaking down and removal of the lens. [phaco- + G. *lysis,* dissolution]

pha·co·lyt·ic (fak-ō-lit′ik) Characterized by or referring to phacolysis.

pha·co·ma (fa-kō′mă) A hamartoma found in phacomatosis; often refers to a retinal hamartoma in tuberous sclerosis. SYN phakoma. [phaco- + G. *-oma,* tumor]

pha·co·ma·la·ci·a (fak′ō-mă-lā′shē-ă) Softening of the lens, as may occur in hypermature cataract. [phaco- + G. *malakia,* softness]

phac·o·ma·to·sis (fak′ō-mă-tō′sis) A generic term for a group of hereditary diseases characterized by hamartomas involving multiple tissues (e.g., von Hippel-Lindau disease, neurofibromatosis, Sturge-Weber syndrome, tuberous sclerosis). SYN phakomatosis. [Van der Hoeve's coinage fr. G. *phakos,* mother-spot]

phac·o·mor·phic glau·co·ma (fak′ō-mōr′fik glaw-kō′mă) Secondary glaucoma caused by either excessive size or spheric shape of the lens. SYN phacogenic glaucoma.

phac·o·scope (fak′ō-skōp) An instrument in the form of a dark chamber for observing the changes in the lens during accommodation. [phaco- + G. *skopeō,* to view]

phaeo- [Br.] SYN pheo-.

phaeochrome [Br.] SYN pheochrome.

phaeochromocyte [Br.] SYN pheochromocyte.

phaeochromocytoma [Br.] SYN pheochromocytoma.

phae·o·hy·pho·my·co·sis (fē′ō-hī′fō-mī-kō′sis) A group of superficial and deep infections caused by fungi that form pigmented hyphae and yeastlike cells in tissue. [G. *phaios,* dusky, + *hyphē,* web, + mycosis]

phage (fāj) SYN bacteriophage.

♻ **-phage**, **-phagia, -phagy** Combining forms meaning eating, devouring. [G. *phagō,* to eat]

phag·e·de·na (faj-ĕ-dē′nă) An ulcer that rapidly spreads peripherally, destroying the tissues as it increases in size. [G. *phagedaina,* a canker]

phag·e·den·ic (faj-ĕ-den′ik) Relating to or having the characteristics of phagedena.

phag·e·den·ic ul·cer (faj-ĕ-den′ik ŭl′sĕr) A rapidly spreading ulcer attended by the formation of extensive sloughing.

♻ **phago-** Prefix meaning eating, devouring. [G. *phagō,* to eat]

phag·o·cyte (fag′ō-sīt) A cell possessing the property of ingesting bacteria, foreign particles, and other cells. Phagocytes are divided into two general classes: 1) microphages, polymorphonuclear leukocytes that ingest chiefly bacteria; and 2) macrophages, mononucleated cells (histiocytes and monocytes) that are largely scavengers, ingesting dead tissue and degenerated cells. [phago- + G. *kytos,* cell]

phag·o·cyt·ic (fag-ō-sit′ik) Relating to phagocytes or phagocytosis.

phag·o·cyt·ic in·dex (fag-ō-sit′ik in′deks) The average number of bacteria observed in the cytoplasm of polymorphonuclear leukocytes after mixing and incubating, at 37°C, 1) a suspension of washed, presumably normal leukocytes, 2) the serum to be tested for opsonin, and 3) a young culture of microorganisms that are causing disease in the patient.

phag•o•cyt•ic pneu•mo•no•cyte (fag-ō-sit′ik nū-mō′nō-sīt) An alveolar phagocyte containing hemosiderin, carbon, or other foreign particles.

phag•o•cy•tin (fag-ō-sī′tin) A very labile bactericidal substance that may be isolated from polymorphonuclear leukocytes.

phag•o•cy•tize (fag′ō-sī-tīz) SYN phagocytose.

phag•o•cy•tol•y•sis (fag′ō-sī-tol′i-sis) **1.** Destruction of phagocytes, or leukocytes, occurring in the process of blood coagulation or as the result of the introduction of certain antagonistic foreign substances into the body. **2.** A spontaneous breaking down of the phagocytes, preliminary to the liberation of complement. [phagocyte + G. *lysis,* dissolution]

phag•o•cy•to•lyt•ic (fag′ō-sī-tō-lit′ik) Relating to phagocytolysis.

phag•o•cy•tose (fag′ō-sī′tōs) To perform phagocytosis, denoting the action of phagocytic cells. SYN phagocytize.

phag•o•cy•to•sis (făg-ō-sī-tō′sis) The process of ingestion and digestion by cells of solid substances, e.g., other cells, bacteria, bits of necrotic tissue, foreign particles. SEE ALSO endocytosis. [phagocyte + G. *-osis,* condition]

phag•o•ly•so•some (fag-ō-lī′sō-sōm) A body formed by union of a phagosome or ingested particle with a lysosome having hydrolytic enzymes.

phag•o•some (fag′ō-sōm) A vesicle that forms around a particle (bacterial or other) within the phagocyte that engulfed it, separates from the cell membrane, then fuses with and receives the contents of cytoplasmic granules (lysosomes), thus forming a phagolysosome in which digestion of the engulfed particle occurs. [phago- + G. *sōma,* body]

phag•o•type (fag′ō-tīp) MICROBIOLOGY a subdivision of a species distinguished from other strains therein by sensitivity to a certain bacteriophage or set of bacteriophages. [phago- + G. *typos,* type]

pha•kic eye (fak′ik ī) An eye containing the natural lens.

♻ **phako-** For words so beginning and not listed here, SEE phaco-.

pha•ko•ma (fă-kō′mă) SYN phacoma.

phak•o•ma•to•sis (fă-kō′mă-tō′sis) SYN phacomatosis.

pha•lan•ge•al (fă-lan′jē-ăl) Relating to a phalanx.

phal•an•gec•to•my (fal-an-jek′tŏ-mē) Excision of one or more of the phalanges of hand or foot. [phalang- + G. *ektomē,* excision]

pha•lanx, gen. **pha•lan•gis**, pl. **pha•lan•ges** (fā′langks, fă-lan′jis, -jēz) [TA] **1.** One of the long bones of the digits, 14 in number for each hand or foot, two for the thumb or great toe, and three each for the other four digits; designated as proximal, middle, and distal, beginning from the metacarpus. **2.** One of a number of cuticular plates, arranged in several rows, on the surface of the spiral organ (of Corti), which are the heads of the outer row of pillar cells and of phalangeal cells. [L. fr. G. *phalanx* (*-ang-*), line of soldiers, bone between two joints of the fingers and toes]

Pha•len ma•neu•ver (fā′lĕn mă-nū′vĕr) Procedure in which the wrist is maintained in volar flexion; paresthesia occurring in the distribution of the median nerve within 60 seconds may be indicative of carpal tunnel syndrome. SYN Phalen test.

Pha•len test (fā′lĕn test) SYN Phalen maneuver.

♻ **phall-, phalli-, phallo-** Combining forms meaning the penis. [G. *phallos*]

phal•lec•to•my (fal-ek′tŏ-mē) Surgical removal of the penis. [phall- + G. *ektomē,* excision]

phal•lic (fal′ik) **1.** Relating to the penis. **2.** PSYCHOANALYSIS relating to the penis, especially during the phases of infantile psychosexuality. SEE ALSO phallic phase. [G. *phallos,* penis]

phal•lic phase (fal′ik fāz) In psychoanalytic personality theory, the stage in psychosexual development, occurring when a child is 2–6 years of age, during which interest, curiosity, and pleasurable experiences are centered on the penis in boys and the clitoris in girls. SEE ALSO genital phase.

phal•lo•camp•sis (fal-ō-kamp′sis) Curvature of the erect penis. SEE ALSO chordee. [phallo- + G. *kampsis,* a bending]

phal•lo•dyn•i•a (fal-ō-din′ē-ă) Pain in the penis. [phallo- + G. *odynē,* pain]

phal•loi•din (fă-loy′din) Best known of the toxic cyclic peptides produced by a poisonous mushroom, *Amanita phalloides;* closely related to amanitin.

phal•lo•plas•ty (fal′ō-plas-tē) Surgical reconstruction of the penis. [phallo- + G. *plastos,* formed]

phal•lot•o•my (fal-ot′ŏ-mē) Surgical incision into the penis. [phallo- + G. *tomē,* a cutting]

phal•lus, pl. **phal•li** (fal′ŭs, -ī) The primordium of the penis or clitoris that develops from the embryonic genital tubercle. [L.; G. *phallos*]

phan•ta•si•a (fan-tā′zē-ă) SYN fantasy. [G. appearance]

phan•tasm (fan′tazm) The mental imagery produced by fantasy. SYN phantom (1). [G. *phantasma,* an appearance]

phan•tas•ma•go•ria (fan-taz′mă-gōr′ē-ă) A fantastic sequence of haphazardly associative imagery.

phan•tom (fan′tŏm) **1.** SYN phantasm. **2.** A model, especially a transparent one, of the human body or any of its parts. **3.** RADIOLOGY a mechanical or computer-originated model for predicting irradiation dosage deep in the body. [G. *phantasma,* an appearance]

phan•tom cor•pus•cle (fan′tŏm kōr′pŭs-ĕl) SYN achromocyte.

phan•tom limb, **phan•tom limb pain** (fan′tŏm lim, pān) The sensation that an amputated limb is still present, often associated with painful paresthesia. SYN pseudesthesia (3).

phan•tom tu•mor (fan′tŏm tū′mŏr) **1.** Accumulation of fluid in the interlobar spaces of the lung, secondary to congestive heart failure, radiologically simulating a neoplasm. **2.** A muscle contraction or gaseous distortion of the intestines.

Phar.B. Abbreviation for Bachelor of Pharmacy.

Phar.D. Abbreviation for Doctor of Pharmacy.

phar•ma•ceu•tic, **phar•ma•ceu•ti•cal** (fahr-mă-sū′tik, -ti-kăl) Relating to pharmacy or to pharmaceutics. [G. *pharmakeutikos,* relating to drugs]

phar•ma•ceu•ti•cal care (fahr-mă-su′ti-kal kār) The responsible provision of drug therapy for the purpose of achieving definite outcomes that improve a patient's quality of life.

phar•ma•ceu•tics (fahr-mă-sū′tiks) **1.** SYN pharmacy (1). **2.** The science of pharmaceutic systems (i.e., preparations, dosage, forms).

phar•ma•cist (fahr′mă-sist) One who is licensed to prepare and dispense drugs and compounds and is knowledgeable concerning their properties. [G. *pharmakon,* a drug]

♻ **pharmaco-** Combining form meaning drugs. [G. *pharmakon,* medicine]

phar•ma•co•di•ag•no•sis (fahr′mă-kō-dī-ag-nō′sis) Use of drugs in diagnosis.

phar•ma•co•dy•nam•ic (fahr′mă-kō-dī-nam′ik) Relating to drug action, particularly at the receptor level.

phar•ma•co•dy•nam•ics (fahr′mă-kō-dī-nam′iks) The study of uptake, movement, binding, and interactions of pharmacologically active molecules at their tissue site(s) of action. [pharmaco- + G. *dynamis,* force]

phar•ma•co•ec•o•nom•ics (fahr′mă-kō-ek-ō-nom′iks) Science dealing with the description and analysis of the costs of drug therapy to health care systems and society.

pharm•a•co•ep•i•de•mi•ol•o•gy (fahr′mă-kō-ep-i-dē-mē-ol′ŏ-jē) The application of epidemiologic knowledge, methods, and reasoning to the study of the effects and uses of pharmacologic treatments in a defined time, space, and population. SEE ALSO epidemiology, pharmacology.

phar•ma•co•ge•net•ics, **phar•ma•co•gen•om•ics** (fahr′mă-kō-jĕ-net′iks, fahr′mă-kō-jēn-om′iks) The study of genetically determined variations in responses to drugs in humans or in laboratory organisms.

phar•ma•cog•no•sy (fahr-mă-kog′nŏ-sē) A branch of pharmacology concerned with the physical characteristics and botanic and animal sources of crude drugs. [pharmaco- + G. *gnōsis,* knowledge]

phar•ma•co•ki•net•ic (fahr′mă-kō-ki-net′ik) Relating to the disposition of drugs in the body (i.e., their absorption, distribution, metabolism, and elimination).

phar•ma•co•ki•net•ics (fahr′mă-kō-ki-net′iks) Study of the movement of drugs within biologic systems, as affected by absorption, distribution, metabolism, and excretion; particularly the rates of such movements. [pharmaco- + G. *kinēsis,* movement]

phar•ma•co•log•ic, **phar•ma•co•log•i•cal** (fahr′mă-kō-loj′ik, -i-kăl) **1.** Relating to pharmacology or to the composition, properties, and actions of drugs. **2.** PHYSIOLOGY a dose of a chemi cal agent that is so much larger or more potent than would occur naturally that it might have qualitatively different effects. Cf. homeopathic (2), physiologic (4).

phar•ma•co•log•ic stress test (fahr′mă-kō-loj′ik stres test) An assessment of cardiovascular fitness, and especially of coronary perfusion, in which the intravenous injection of a pharmacologic agent such as dobutamine, dipyridamole, or adenosine is substituted for physical exercise.

phar•ma•col•o•gist (fahr-mă-kol′ŏ-jist) A specialist in pharmacology.

phar•ma•col•o•gy (fahr-mă-kol′ŏ-jē) The science concerned with drugs and their sources, appearance, chemistry, actions, and uses. [pharmaco- + G. *logos,* study]

Phar•ma•co•pei•a, **Phar•ma•co•poe•i•a** (fahr′mă-kō-pē′ă) A work that describes therapeutic agents, standards for their strength and purity, and their formulations. The various national pharmacopeias are referred to by abbreviations, of which the most frequently encountered are *USP*, United States Pharmacopeia, and *BP*, British Pharmacopoeia. [G. *pharmakopoiia,* fr. *pharmakon,* a medicine, + *poieo,* to make]

phar•ma•co•pe•ial (fahr′mă-kō-pē′ăl) Relating

to the Pharmacopeia; denoting a drug in the list of the Pharmacopeia. SEE ALSO official. SYN pharmacopoeial.

phar•ma•co•pe•ial gel (fahr′mă-kō-pē′ăl jel) A suspension, in a water medium, of an insoluble drug in hydrated form wherein the particle size approaches or attains colloidal dimensions. SYN pharmacopoeial gel.

pharmacopoeial [Br.] SYN pharmacopeial.

pharmacopoeial gel [Br.] SYN pharmacopeial gel.

phar•ma•co•ther•a•py (fahr′mă-kō-thār′ă-pē) Treatment of disease by means of drugs. SEE ALSO chemotherapy. [pharmaco- + G. *therapeia,* therapy]

phar•ma•cy (fahr′mă-sē) **1.** The practice of preparing and dispensing drugs and the delivery of pharmaceutic care. SYN pharmaceutics (1). **2.** A facility licensed to dispense medications to the public. [G. *pharmakon,* drug]

phar•ma•cy tech•ni•cian (fahr′mă-sē tek-nishŭn) A medical professional working as an assistant to, and under the supervision of, a registered pharmacist.

phar•ma•ki•ne•tics (fahr′mă-ki-net′iks) The mathematical characterization of the disposition of a drug in the body over time. Used to facilitate understanding and interpretation of blood levels and to guide adjustments in dosage and interval for maximum therapeutic results and minimum toxic effects.

Pharm.D. SYN Doctor of Pharmacy.

pha•ryn•ge•al (făr-in′jē-ăl) Relating to the pharynx. [Mod. L. *pharyngeus*]

pha•ryn•ge•al ap•pa•rat•us (făr-in′jē-ăl ap′ă-rat′ŭs) The aggregate of pharyngeal arches, pouches, grooves, and membranes present in early embryos. SYN branchial apparatus.

pha•ryn•ge•al arch (făr-in′jē-ăl ahrch) Typically, there are six arches in embryos vertebrates; in the lower vertebrates, they bear gills; in the higher vertebrates (e.g., human embryos), they appear transiently and give rise to specialized structures in the head and neck. SYN branchial arch.

pha•ryn•ge•al arch ar•ter•ies (făr-in′jē-ăl ahrch ahr′tĕr-ēz) A series of arteries encircling the primordial embryonic pharynx in the mesenchyme of the pharyngeal arches.

pha•ryn•ge•al branch of pte•ry•go•pal•a•tine gang•li•on (făr-in′jē-ăl branch ter′i-gō-pal′ă-tīn gang′glē-ŏn) SYN pharyngeal nerve.

pha•ryn•ge•al bur•sa (făr-in′jē-ăl bŭr′să) SYN Tornwaldt cyst.

pha•ryn•ge•al cleft (făr-in′jē-ăl kleft) SYN pharyngeal groove.

pha•ryn•ge•al flap (făr-in′jē-ăl flap) Flap of tissue placed to reduce the size of the opening between the oral and nasal cavities, to mitigate insufficient velar closure. SEE ALSO hypernasality, cleft palate.

pha•ryn•ge•al groove (făr-in′jē-ăl grūv) The ectodermal groove between two pharyngeal arches in the human embryo. SYN branchial cleft, pharyngeal cleft.

pha•ryn•ge•al nerve (făr-in′jē-ăl nĕrv) Branch of pterygopalatine ganglion passing posteriorly through the pharyngeal canal to supply postsynaptic parasympathetic fibers to mucus glands of the nasopharynx. SYN Bock nerve, nervus pharyngeus, pharyngeal branch of pterygopalatine ganglion, ramus pharyngeus ganglii pterygopalatini.

pha•ryn•ge•al o•pen•ing of au•di•to•ry tube (făr-in′jē-ăl ō′pĕn-ing aw′di-tōr-ē tūb) An opening in the upper part of the nasopharynx about 1.2 cm behind the posterior extremity of the inferior concha on each side.

pha•ryn•ge•al re•flex (făr-in′jē-ăl rē′fleks) **1.** SYN swallowing reflex. **2.** SYN vomiting reflex.

pha•ryn•ge•al ton•sil (făr-in′jē-ăl ton′sil) A collection of more or less closely aggregated lymphoid nodules on the posterior wall and roof of the nasopharynx; when hypertrophic, these are called adenoids.

pha•ryn•ge•al tra•che•al lu•men air•way (făr-in′jē-ăl trā′kē-ăl lū′mĕn ār′wā) SYN pharyngeal tracheal multiple balloon system.

pha•ryn•ge•al tra•che•al mul•ti•ple bal•loon sys•tem (făr-in′jē-ăl trā-kē-al mŭl′ti-pŭl bă-lūn′ sis′tĕm) Airway management adjunct that consists of two tubes, endotracheal and esophageal. The device is inserted blindly into the oropharynx and passes either into the trachea or the esophagus. SYN esophageal tracheal airway, pharyngeal tracheal lumen airway.

pha•ryn•ge•al veins (făr-in′jē-ăl vānz) Several veins from the pharyngeal venous plexus emptying into the internal jugular vein.

pha•ryn•gec•to•my (fă-rin-jek′tŏ-mē) Resection of the pharynx. [pharyng- + G. *ektomē,* excision]

pha•ryn•ges (fă-rin′jēz) Plural of pharynx.

pha•ryn•gis•mus (fă-rin-jiz′mŭs) Spasm of the muscles of the pharynx. SYN pharyngospasm.

pha•ryn•git•ic (fă-rin-jit′ik) Relating to pharyngitis.

i **pha•ryn•gi•tis** (fă-rin-jī′tis) Inflammation of the mucous membrane and underlying parts of the pharynx. See page 1197. [pharyng- + G. *-itis,* inflammation]

♲ **pharyngo-, pharyng-** Combining forms meaning the pharynx. [Mod. L. fr. G. *pharynx*]

pha•ryn•go•cele (fă-ring′gō-sēl) A diverticulum from the pharynx. [pharyngo- + G. *kēlē,* hernia]

pha•ryn•go•con•junc•ti•val fe•ver (fă-ring′gō-kŏn-jŭngk′ti-văl fē′vĕr) A disease characterized by fever, pharyngitis, and conjunctivitis, and caused by adenoviruses, often type 3 but occasionally other types.

pha•ryn•go•ep•i•glot•tic, pha•ryn•go•ep•i•glot•tid•e•an (fă-ring′gō-ep-i-glot′ik, fă-ring′gō-ep-i-glo-tid′ē-ăn) Relating to the pharynx and the epiglottis.

pha•ryn•go•e•soph•a•ge•al (fă-ring′gō-ē-sŏf-ă′jē-ăl) Relating to the pharynx and the esophagus. SYN pharyngo-oesophageal.

pha•ryn•go•e•soph•a•ge•al di•ver•tic•u•lum (fă-ring′gō-ē-sŏf-ă′jē-ăl dī′vĕr-tik′yū-lŭm) Most common diverticulum of the esophagus; arises between the inferior pharyngeal constrictor and the cricopharyngeus muscle. SYN hypopharyngeal diverticulum, pharyngo-oesophageal diverticulum, Zenker diverticulum.

pha•ryn•go•glos•sal (fă-ring′gō-glos′ăl) Relating to the pharynx and the tongue.

pha•ryn•go•la•ryn•ge•al (fă-ring′gō-lă-rin′jē-ăl) Relating to both the pharynx and the larynx.

pha•ryn•go•lar•yn•gi•tis (fă-ring′gō-lar-in-jī′tis) Inflammation of both the pharynx and the larynx.

pha•ryn•go•lith (fă-ring′ō-lith) A concretion in the pharynx. [pharyngo- + G. *lithos,* stone]

pha•ryn•go•my•co•sis (fă-ring′gō-mī-kō′sis) Invasion of the mucous membrane of the pharynx by fungi. [pharyngo- + G. *mykēs,* a fungus]

pha•ryn•go•na•sal (fă-ring′gō-nā′săl) Relating to the pharynx and the nasal cavity.

pharyngo-oesophageal [Br.] SYN pharyngoesophageal.

pharyngo-oesophageal diverticulum [Br.] SYN pharyngoesophageal diverticulum.

pha•ryn•go•plas•ty (fă-ring′gō-plas-tē) Surgical repair of the pharynx. [pharyngo- + G. *plastos,* formed]

pha•ryn•go•ple•gi•a (fă-ring′gō-plē′jē-ă) Paralysis of the muscles of the pharynx. [pharyngo- + G. *plēgē,* stroke]

pha•ryn•go•scope (fă-ring′gŏ-skōp) An instrument like a laryngoscope, used for inspection of the mucous membrane of the pharynx. [pharyngo- + G. *skopeō,* to view]

pha•ryn•gos•co•py (far-ing-gos′kŏ-pē) Inspection and examination of the pharynx. [pharyngo- + G. *skopeō,* to view]

pha•ryn•go•spasm (fă-ring′gō-spazm) SYN pharyngismus.

pha•ryn•go•ste•no•sis (fă-ring′gō-stĕ-nō′sis) Stricture of the pharynx. [pharyngo- + G. *stenōsis,* a narrowing]

pha•ryn•got•o•my (far-ing-got′ŏ-mē) Any cutting operation on the pharynx either from without or from within. [pharyngo- + G. *tomē,* incision]

pha•ryn•go•tym•pan•ic (au•di•to•ry) tube (fă-ring′gō-tim-pan′ik aw′di-tōr-ē tūb) A tube leading from the tympanic cavity to the nasopharynx; it consists of an osseous (posterolateral) portion at the tympanic end, and a fibrocartilaginous (anteromedial) portion at the pharyngeal end; where the two portions join, in the region of the sphenopetrosal fissure, is the narrowest portion of the tube (isthmus); the auditory tube enables equalization of pressure within the tympanic cavity with ambient air pressure, referred to commonly as "popping of the ears." SYN salpinx (2) [TA], tuba auditiva [TA], auditory tube, eustachian tube, tuba auditoria.

pha•rynx, gen. **pha•ryn•gis**, pl. **pha•ryn•ges** (far′ingks, fă-rin′jis, -jēz) [TA] The upper expanded portion of the digestive tube, between

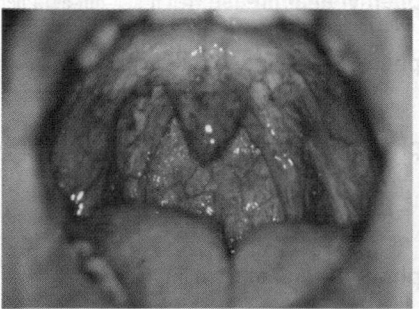

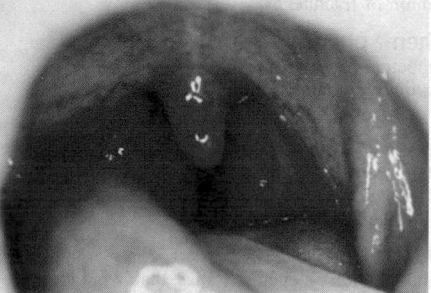

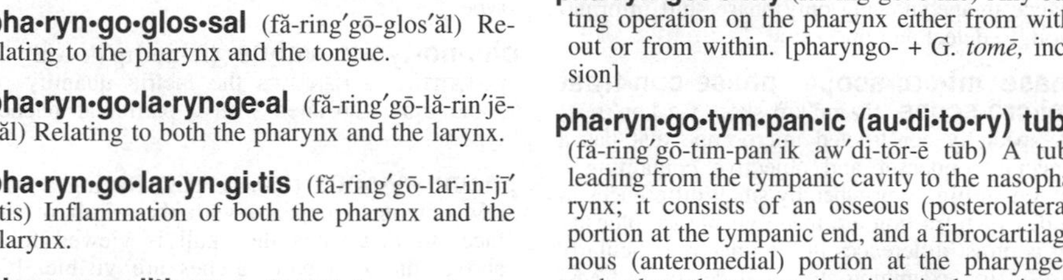

A B

pharyngitis: (A) redness and vascularity of the pillars and uvula are mild to moderate; (B) redness is diffuse and intense

the esophagus below and the mouth and nasal cavities above and in front. [Mod. L. fr. G. *pharynx* (*pharyng-*), the throat, the joint opening of the gullet and windpipe]

phase (fāz) **1.** A stage in the course of change or development. **2.** A homogeneous, physically distinct, and separable portion of a heterogeneous system; e.g., oil, gum, and water are three phases of an emulsion. **3.** The time relationship between two or more events. **4.** A particular part of a recurring time pattern or wave form. SEE ALSO stage, period. [G. *phasis,* an appearance]

phase I block (fāz blok) Inhibition of nerve impulse transmission across the myoneural junction associated with depolarization of the motor endplate, as in the muscle paralysis produced by succinylcholine.

phase II block (fāz blok) Inhibition of nerve impulse transmission across the myoneural junction unaccompanied by depolarization of the motor endplate, as in the muscle paralysis produced by tubocurarine.

phase im•age (fāz im′ăj) A magnetic resonance image showing only phase shift information, to detect motion.

phase mi•cro•scope, **phase-con•trast mi•cro•scope** (fāz mī′krŏ-skōp, fāz-kon′trast) A specially constructed microscope that has a special condenser and objective containing a phase-shifting ring whereby small differences in index of refraction are made visible as intensity or contrast differences in the image; particularly useful for examining structural details in transparent specimens such as living or unstained cells and tissues.

pha•sic bite pat•tern (fā′zik bīt pat′ĕrn) A reflexive response seen in 5–6-month-old infants; appears as a jaw opening and closing; not a functional bite.

PH con•duc•tion time (kŏn-dŭk′shŭn tīm) SEE atrioventricular conduction.

Phem•is•ter graft (fem′is-tĕr graft) An autogenous onlay bone graft used in treating delayed union of fractures.

♻**phen-, pheno-** **1.** Combining forms meaning appearance. **2.** CHEMISTRY combining forms denoting derivation from benzene (phenyl-). [fr. G. *phainō,* to appear, show forth]

phen•ac•e•tur•ic ac•id (fen′as-ĕ-tur′ik as′id) An end product of the metabolism of phenylated fatty acids with even numbers of carbon atoms. SYN phenylaceturic acid.

phe•no•cop•y (fē′nō-kop-ē) **1.** A set of clinical and laboratory characteristics that would ordinarily warrant the diagnosis of a specific genetic abnormality, but are of environmental rather than genetic etiology. **2.** A condition of environmental etiology that mimics one usually of genetic etiology. [G. *phainō,* to display, + copy]

phe•nol co•ef•fi•cient (fē′nol kō-ĕ-fish′ĕnt) SYN Rideal-Walker coefficient.

phe•nol•u•ri•a (fē-nol-yū′rē-ă) The excretion of phenols in the urine.

phe•nom•e•non, pl. **phe•nom•e•na** (fĕ-nom′ĕ-non, -nă) **1.** An occurrence or object as perceived by the senses, whether ordinary or extraordinary, in relation to a disease. **2.** Any unusual fact or occurrence. **3.** An object of perception; that noticed by mind or senses. [G. *phainomenon,* fr. *phainō,* to cause to appear]

phe•no•type (fē′nō-tīp) Manifestation of a genotype or the combined manifestation of several different genotypes. The discriminating power of the phenotype in identifying the genotype depends on its level of subtlety; thus, special methods of detecting carriers distinguish them from normal subjects from whom they are inseparable on simple physical examination. Phenotype is the immediate cause of genetic disease and object of genetic selection. [G. *phainō,* to display, + *typos,* model]

phe•no•typ•ic (fē-nō-tip′ik) Relating to phenotype.

phe•no•typ•ic val•ue (fē-nō-tip′ik val′yū) QUANTITATIVE GENETICS the metric quantity of some trait associated with a particular phenotype.

phe•no•zy•gous (fē-nō-zī′gŭs) Having a narrow cranium compared with the width of the face, so that when the skull is viewed from above, the zygomatic arches are visible. [G. *phainō,* to show, + *zygon,* yoke]

phen•yl (Ph, Φ) (fen′il) The univalent radical, C_6H_5–, of benzene.

phen•yl•a•ce•tic ac•id (fen′il-ă-sē′tik as′id) An abnormal product of phenylalanine catabolism, appearing in the urine of people with phenylketonuria.

phen•yl•a•ce•tur•ic ac•id (fen′il-as-ĕ-tyūr′ik as′id) SYN phenaceturic acid.

phen•yl•al•a•nin•ase (fen′il-al′ă-nin-ās) Phenylalanine 4-monooxygenase.

phen•yl•al•a•nine (F) (fen′il-al′ă-nēn) One of the common amino acids in proteins; a nutritionally essential amino acid.

phen•yl•al•a•nine 4-mon•o•ox•y•gen•ase (fen′il-al′ă-nēn mon-ō-ok′si-jĕn-āz) An enzyme that catalyzes the oxidation of L-phenylalanine to L-tyrosine; a deficiency results in phenylketonuria.

phen•yl•ben•zene (fen′il-ben′zēn) SYN diphenyl.

phen•yl•di•chlo•ro•ar•sine (PD) (fen′il-dī-klōr-ō-ar′sēn) A toxic liquid that has been used as a blistering and vomiting agent by certain military and police organizations; it was first used in a limited manner in World War I (1914–1918).

phen•yl•hy•dra•zine he•mol•y•sis (fen′il-hī′-drā-zin hē-mol′i-sis) An in vitro test for G6PD deficiency; hemolysis resulting from in vitro addition of phenylhydrazine to blood with red blood cells that are deficient in glucose-6-phosphate dehydrogenase (G6PD), with the appearance of Heinz-Ehrlich bodies.

phen•yl•ke•to•nu•ri•a (PKU) (fen′il-kē′tō-nyūr′ē-ă) Congenital deficiency of phenylalanine 4-monooxygenase or occasionally of dihydropherine reductase or of dihydrobiopterin synthetase; it causes inadequate formation of L-tyrosine, elevation of serum L-phenylalanine, urinary excretion of phenylpyruvic acid and other derivatives, and accumulation of phenylalanine and its metabolites, which can produce brain damage resulting in severe mental retardation, often with seizures, other neurologic abnormalities such as retarded myelination, and deficient melanin formation leading to hypopigmentation of the skin and eczema. Cf. hyperphenylalaninemia. SYN Folling disease. [phenyl + ketone + G. *ouron,* urine]

phen•yl•lac•tic ac•id (fen′il-lak′tik as′id) A product of phenylalanine catabolism, appearing prominently in the urine in people with phenylketonuria.

phe•nyl•py•ru•vic ac•id (fen′il-pī-rū′vik as′id) The transaminated product of the action of phenylalanine aminotransferase; elevated in the urine in people with phenylketonuria.

phen•yl•thi•o•hy•dan•to•in (fen′il-thī′ō-hī-dan′tō-in) The compound formed from an amino acid in the Edman method of protein degradation, in which phenylisothiocyanate reacts with the amino moiety of the *N*-terminal amino acid to form a phenylthiocarbamoyl peptide or protein, on which weak acids act to release the phenylthiohydantoin containing the *N*-terminal amino acid.

pheo- **1.** Prefix denoting the same substituents on a phorbin or phorbide (porphyrin) residue as are present in chlorophyll, excluding any ester residues and Mg. **2.** Combining form meaning gray, dark-colored. [G. *phaios,* dusky] SYN phaeo-.

phe•o•chrome (fē′ō-krōm) **1.** SYN chromaffin. **2.** Staining darkly with chromic salts. SYN phaeochrome. [G. *phaios,* dusky, + *chrōma,* color]

phe•o•chro•mo•cyte (fē′ō-krō′mō-sīt) A chromaffin cell of a sympathetic paraganglion, medulla of a suprarenal gland, or of a pheochromocytoma. SYN phaeochromocyte. [pheochrome + G. *kytos,* cell]

phe•o•chro•mo•cy•to•ma (fē′ō-krō′mō-sī-tō′mă) A functional chromaffinoma, usually benign, derived from adrenal medullary tissue cells and characterized by the secretion of catecholamines, resulting in hypertension, which may be paroxysmal and associated with attacks of palpitation, headache, nausea, dyspnea, anxiety, pallor, and profuse sweating. SEE ALSO paraganglioma. SYN phaeochromocytoma.

phe•re•sis (fĕ-rē′sis) A procedure in which blood is removed from a donor, separated, and a portion retained, with the remainder returned to the donor. SEE ALSO leukapheresis, plateletpheresis, plasmapheresis. [G. *aphairesis,* a taking away, a withdrawal]

pher•o•mones (fer′ō-mōnz) A type of ectohormone secreted by an individual and perceived by a second individual of the same species, thereby producing a change in the sexual or social behavior of that individual; first discovered as a sex attractant in insects. [G. *pherō,* to carry, + *hormaō,* to excite, stimulate]

PHI Abbreviation for protected health information.

phi (φ, Φ) (fī) **1.** The 21st letter of the Greek alphabet (φ). **2.** Phenyl; potential energy; magnetic flux (Φ). **3.** Plane angle; volume fraction; quantum yield; the dihedral angle of rotation about the $N–C_\alpha$ bond associated with a peptide bond (φ).

Phi•a•loph•o•ra (fī-ă-lof′ŏ-ră) A genus of fungi of which at least two species, *P. verrucosa* and *P. dermatitidis*, cause chromoblastomycosis. [G. *phialē,* a broad, flat vessel, + *phoreō,* to carry]

phil- Combining form meaning having an affinity or love for. [G. *philos,* loving]

-phil, -phile, -philic, -philia Combining forms denoting affinity for, craving for. [G. *philos,* fond, loving; *phileō,* to love]

Phi•la•del•phi•a chro•mo•some (fil′ă-del′fē-ă krō′mŏ-sōm) An abnormal minute chromosome. Formed by a rearrangement of chromosomes 9 and 22; found in cultured leukocytes of many patients with chronic granulocytic leukemia. See page 1200.

Phi•la•del•phi•a col•lar (fil′ă-del′fē-ă kol′ăr) Commonly used Styrofoam neck collar used for immobilization; stabilizes patients in the field for transport to a medical facility.

-philia, -phily, -philous Combining forms meaning that which has an attraction to or is stained by. [G. *philia,* love]

Phil•lips cath•e•ter (fil′ips kath′ĕ-tĕr) A catheter with a filiform guide for the urethra.

Phil•lip•son re•flex (fil′ip-sŏn rē′fleks) A contraction of the extensors of the knee when the extensors of the opposite knee are inhibited.

phil•trum, pl. **phil•tra** (fil′trŭm, -tră) **1.** A philter or love potion. **2.** [TA] The infranasal depression; the groove in the midline of the upper lip.

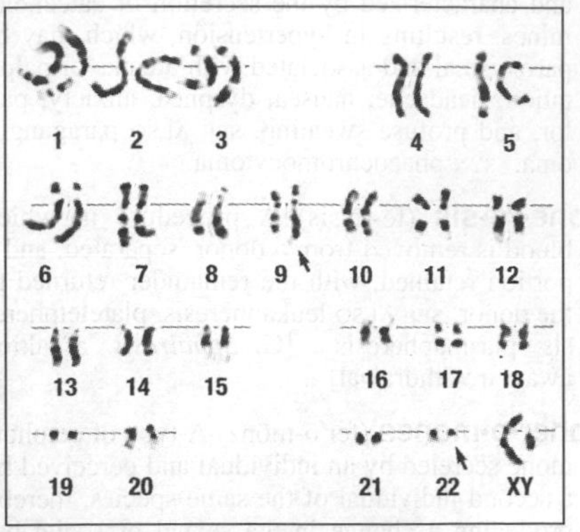

Philadelphia chromosome translocation: karyotype from a patient with chronic granulocytic leukemia showing the Philadelphia chromosome (number 22) translocation, t(9:22)(q34;q11)

[L., fr. G. *philtron,* a love-charm, depression on upper lip, fr. *phileō,* to love]

phi•mo•sis, pl. **phi•mo•ses** (fī-mō′sis, -sēz) Narrowness of the opening of the prepuce, preventing its being drawn back over the glans. [G. a muzzling, fr. *phimos,* a muzzle]

phi•mot•ic (fī-mot′ik) Pertaining to phimosis.

phleb•ec•ta•si•a (fleb′ek-tā′zē-ă) Dilation of the veins. SYN venectasia. [phlebo- + G. *ektasis,* a stretching]

phle•bec•to•my (fle-bek′tō-mē) Excision of a segment of a vein, sometimes performed to cure varicose veins. SEE ALSO strip (2). SYN venectomy. [phlebo- + G. *ektomē,* excision]

phle•bit•ic (fle-bit′ik) Relating to phlebitis.

phle•bi•tis (fle-bī′tis) Inflammation of a vein. [phlebo- + G. *-itis,* inflammation]

♻**phlebo-, phleb-** Combining forms meaning vein [G. *phleps*]

phleb•o•cly•sis (flĕ-bok′li-sis) Intravenous injection of an isotonic solution of dextrose or other substances in quantity. [phlebo- + G. *klysis,* a washing out]

phleb•o•gram (fleb′ō-gram) A tracing of the jugular or other venous pulse. SYN venogram (2). [phlebo- + G. *gramma,* something written]

phleb•o•graph (fleb′ō-graf) A venous sphygmograph; an instrument for making a tracing of the venous pulse. [phlebo- + G. *graphō,* to write]

phle•bog•ra•phy (fle-bog′ră-fē) **1.** The recording of the venous pulse. **2.** SYN venography. [phlebo- + G. *graphē,* a writing]

phleb•o•lith (fleb′ō-lith) A calcific deposit in a venous wall or thrombus; commonly seen on abdominal radiographs in the lower pelvic region. [phlebo- + G. *lithos,* stone]

phleb•o•li•thi•a•sis (fleb′ō-li-thī′ă-sis) The formation of phleboliths (stones within veins).

phle•bo•ma•nom•e•ter (fleb′ō-mă-nom′ĕ-tĕr) A manometer for measuring venous blood pressure.

phleb•o•phle•bos•to•my (fleb′ō-fle-bos′tō-mē) SYN venovenostomy.

phleb•o•plas•ty (fleb′ō-plas-tē) Repair of a vein. [phlebo- + G. *plastos,* formed]

phle•bor•rha•phy (fle-bōr′ă-fē) Suture of a vein. [phlebo- + G. *rhaphē,* seam]

phleb•o•scle•ro•sis (fleb′ō-skler-ō′sis) Fibrous hardening of the walls of the veins. SYN venosclerosis. [phlebo- + G. *sklērōsis,* hardening]

phle•bos•ta•sis (fle-bos′tă-sis) **1.** Abnormally slow motion of blood in veins, usually with venous distention. **2.** Treatment of congestive heart failure by compressing proximal veins of the extremities with tourniquets. SYN venostasis. [phlebo- + G. *stasis,* a standing still]

phleb•o•ste•no•sis (fleb′ō-sten-ō′sis) Narrowing of the lumen of a vein from any cause. [phlebo- + G. *stenōsis,* a narrowing]

phleb•o•throm•bo•sis (fleb′ō-throm-bō′sis) Thrombosis, or clotting, in a vein without primary inflammation. [phlebo- + thrombosis]

phle•bot•o•mist (fle-bot′ŏ-mist) A person trained and skilled in phlebotomy.

phle•bot•o•mize (fle-bot′ō-mīz) **1.** To draw blood from. **2.** To achieve iron overload reduction by repeated removal of blood, as in hemochromatosis.

Phle•bot•o•mus (flĕ-bot′ō-mŭs) A genus of very small bloodsucking sandflies of the subfamily Phlebotominae, family Psychodidae. [phlebo- + G. *tomos,* cutting]

phle•bot•o•my (fle-bot′ŏ-mē) Incision into a vein for the purpose of drawing blood. SYN venesection, venotomy. [phlebo- + G. *tomē,* incision]

phlegm (flem) **1.** Abnormal amounts of mucus, especially as expectorated from the mouth. **2.** One of the four humors of the body, according to the ancient Greek humoral doctrine. [G. *phlegma,* inflammation]

phleg•mat•ic (fleg-mat′ik) Relating to the heavy one of the four ancient Greek humors, phlegm, and therefore calm, apathetic, unexcitable. [G. *phlegmatikos,* relating to phlegm]

phleg•mon (fleg′mon) Obsolete term for an acute suppurative inflammation of the subcutaneous connective tissue.

phleg•mon•ous (fleg′mŏn-ŭs) Term denoting phlegmon.

phleg•mon•ous ab•scess (fleg′mŏn-ŭs ab′ses) Circumscribed suppuration characterized by an intense surrounding inflammatory reaction that produces induration and thickening of the affected area.

phlo•ri•zin gly•cos•ur•i•a, **phlo•rid•zin gly•cos•ur•i•a** (flō-riz′in glī-kō-syūr′ē-ă, flō-rid′zin) The presence of sugar in the urine after the experimental administration of phlorizin, which results in a lower renal threshold for glucose reabsorption.

phlyc•te•na, pl. **phlyc•te•nae** (flik-tē′nă, -nē) A small vesicle, especially one of a number of small blisters following a first-degree burn. [G. *phlyktaina,* a blister made by a burn]

phlyc•te•nar (flik′tĕ-năr) Relating to or marked by the presence of phlyctenae.

phlyc•te•noid (flik′tĕ-noyd) Resembling a phlyctena. [G. *phlyktaina,* blister, + *eidos,* resemblance]

phlyc•ten•u•la, pl. **phlyc•ten•u•lae** (flik-ten′yū-lă, -yū-lē) A small red nodule of lymphoid cells, with ulcerated apex, occurring in the conjunctiva. SYN phlyctenule. [Mod. L. dim. of G. *phlyktaina,* blister]

phlyc•ten•u•lar (flik-ten′yū-lăr) Relating to a phlyctenula.

phlyc•ten•u•lar ker•a•ti•tis (flik-ten′yū-lăr ker′ă-tī′tis) An inflammation of the corneal conjunctiva with the formation of small red nodules of lymphoid tissue (phlyctenulae) near the corneoscleral limbus.

phlyc•ten•ule (flik′tĕn-yūl) SYN phlyctenula.

phlyc•ten•u•lo•sis (flik-ten′yū-lō′sis) A nodular hypersensitive reaction of corneal and conjunctival epithelium to endogenous toxin.

pho•bi•a (fō′bē-ă) Any objectively unfounded morbid dread or fear that arouses a state of panic. The word is used as a combining form in many terms expressing the object that inspires the fear. [G. *phobos,* fear]

pho•bic (fō′bik) Pertaining to or characterized by phobia.

pho•bo•pho•bi•a (fō-bō-fō′bē-ă) Morbid dread of developing some phobia. [G. *phobos,* fear]

pho•co•me•li•a, **pho•com•e•ly** (fō-kō-mē′lē-ă, -kom′ĕ-lē) Defective development of the upper or lower limbs, or both, so that the hands and feet are attached close to the body, resembling the flippers of a seal. [G. *phōkē,* a seal, + *melos,* extremity]

phon (fōn) A unit of loudness of sound.

pho•nal (fō′năl) Relating to sound or to the voice. [G. *phōnē,* voice]

phon•as•the•ni•a (fō′nas-thē′nē-ă) Difficult or abnormal voice production, the enunciation being too high, too loud, or too hard. [phon- + G. *astheneia,* weakness]

pho•na•tion (fō-nā′shŭn) The utterance of sounds by means of vocal folds. [G. *phōnē,* voice]

pho•na•tor•y (fō′nă-tōr′ē) Relating to phonation.

pho•neme (fō′nēm) The smallest sound unit that, in terms of the phonetic sequences of sound, controls meaning. [G. *phōnēma,* a voice]

pho•nen•do•scope (fō-nen′dŏ-skōp) A stethoscope that intensifies the auscultatory sounds by means of two parallel resonating plates, one resting on the patient's chest or attached to a stethoscope tube, the other vibrating in unison with it. [phon- + G. *endon,* within, + *skopeō,* to view]

pho•net•ic (fŏ-net′ik) Relating to speech or to the voice. SEE ALSO phonic. [G. *phōnētikos*]

pho•net•ic ba•lance (fŏ-net′ik bal′ăns) That property by which a group of words used in the measurement of hearing has the various phonemes occurring at approximately the same frequency at which they occur in ordinary conversation in that language; phonetically balanced word lists are used in determining the discrimination score.

pho•net•ics (fŏ-net′iks) The science of speech and of pronunciation.

pho•ni•at•rics (fō-nē-at′riks) A branch of medicine concerned with the diagnosis and treatment of voice and speech disorders. [phon- + G. *iatrikos,* of the healing art]

phon•ic (fon′ik) Relating to sound or to the voice. SEE ALSO phonetic.

♻ **phono-**, **phon-** Combining forms meaning sound, speech, or voice sounds. [G. *phōnē*]

pho•no•an•gi•og•ra•phy (fō′nō-an-jē-og′ră-fē) Recording and analysis of the audible frequency-intensity components of the bruit of turbulent arterial blood flow through a stenotic lesion. [phono- + G. *angeion,* vessel, + *graphō,* to write]

pho•no•car•di•o•gram (fō-nō-kahr′dē-ō-gram) A record of the heart sounds made by means of a phonocardiograph.

pho•no•car•di•o•graph (fō-nō-kahr′dē-ō-graf) An instrument, using microphones, amplifiers, and filters, for graphically recording the heart sounds, which are displayed on an oscilloscope or analog tracing.

pho•no•car•di•og•ra•phy (fō′nō-kahr-dē-og′ră-fē) **1.** Recording of the heart sounds with a phonocardiograph. **2.** The science of interpreting phonocardiograms. [phono- + G. *kardia,* heart, + *graphō,* to record]

pho•no•cath•e•ter (fō-nō-kath′ĕ-tĕr) A cardiac catheter with a diminutive microphone housed in its tip, for recording murmurs and other sounds from within the heart and great vessels.

pho·no·gram (fō′nō-gram) A graphic curve depicting the duration and intensity of a sound. [phono- + G. *gramma,* diagram]

pho·nom·e·ter (fō-nom′ĕ-tĕr) An instrument for measuring the pitch and intensity of sounds. [phono- + G. *metron,* measure]

pho·no·my·oc·lo·nus (fō′nō-mī-ok′lŏ-nŭs) Clonic spasms of muscles in response to aural stimuli. [phono- + G. *mys,* muscle, + *klonos,* tumult]

pho·nop·a·thy (fō-nop′ă-thē) Any disease of the vocal organs affecting speech. [phono- + G. *pathos,* suffering]

pho·no·pho·re·sis (fō′nō-fŏr-ē′sĭs) Introduction of antiinflammatory drugs through the skin by the use of ultrasound. SEE ALSO iontophoresis. [phono- + G. *phorēsis,* a carrying]

pho·no·pho·tog·ra·phy (fō′nō-fŏ-tog′ră-fē) The recording on a moving photographic plate of the movements imparted to a diaphragm by sound waves. [phono- + photography]

pho·nop·si·a (fō-nop′sē-ă) A condition in which the hearing of certain sounds gives rise to a subjective sensation of color. [phono- + G. *opsis,* vision]

pho·no·re·cep·tor (fō′nō-rē-sep′tŏr) A receptor for sound stimuli.

pho·re·sis (fŏr-ē′sis) **1.** SYN electrophoresis. **2.** A biologic association in which one organism is transported by another. [G. *phorēsis,* a being borne]

phor·i·a (fōr′ē-ă) The relative directions assumed by the eyes during binocular fixation of a given object in the absence of an adequate fusion stimulus. SEE cyclophoria, esophoria, exophoria, heterophoria, hyperphoria, hypophoria, orthophoria. [G. *phora,* a carrying, motion]

♻ **phoro-, phor-** Combining forms meaning carrying, bearing; a carrier, a bearer; phobia. [G. *phoros,* carrying, bearing]

♻ **phos-** Prefix meaning light. [G. *phōs*]

phos·gene (fos′jēn) Carbonic dichloride, $COCl_2$; a colorless liquid at temperatures below 8.2°C, but an extremely poisonous gas at ordinary temperatures; more than 80% of World War I's chemical-agent fatalities were caused by this gas (NATO Code GG).

phos·gene ox·ime (fos′jēn oks′ēm) A toxic chemical-warfare agent, dichloroformoxime, CCl_2NOH, produced by Russia and other countries of the former Soviet Union. It is a crystalline solid that sublimates to produce vapor and that melts at approximately 35–40° C (95–104° F) and causes urticaria progressing to tissue necrosis (NATO Code CX). SYN dichloroformoxime.

♻ **phosph-, phospho-, phosphoro-, phosphor-** Combining forms indicating the presence of phosphorus in a compound. See phospho- for specific usage of that prefix. [G. *phōs,* light; *phoros,* carrying]

phosphataemia [Br.] SYN phosphatemia.

phos·pha·tase (fos′fă-tās) Any of a group of enzymes (EC sub-subclass 3.1.3) that liberate inorganic phosphate from phosphoric esters.

phos·phate (fos′fāt) **1.** A salt or ester (especially inorganic) of phosphoric acid. **2.** The trivalent ion, PO_4^{3-}.

phos·phate di·a·be·tes (fos′fāt dī-ă-bē′tēz) Excessive secretion of phosphate in the urine due to a defect in tubular reabsorption; usually part of a more generalized abnormality (e.g., Fanconi syndrome).

phos·pha·te·mi·a (fos-fă-tē′mē-ă) An abnormally high concentration of inorganic phosphates in the blood. SYN phosphataemia. [phosphate + G. *haima,* blood]

phos·phat·ic (fos-fat′ik) Relating to or containing phosphates.

phos·phat·i·dyl·glyc·er·ol (fos-fă-tī′dil-glis′ĕr-ol) A constituent in human amniotic fluid that denotes fetal lung maturity when present in the last trimester.

phos·pha·tu·ri·a (fos-fă-tyūr′ē-ă) Excessive excretion of phosphates in the urine. [phosphate + G. *ouron,* urine]

phos·phene (fos′fēn) Sensation of light produced by mechanical or electrical stimulation of the peripheral or central optic pathway of the nervous system. [G. *phōs,* light, + *phainō,* to show]

phos·phide (fos′fīd) A compound of phosphorus with valence –3, e.g., sodium phosphide, Na_3P.

♻ **phospho-** Prefix for *O*-phosphono-, which may replace the suffix phosphate; for instance, glucose phosphate is *O*-phosphonoglucose or phosphoglucose. SEE ALSO phosph-.

3′-phos·pho·a·den·o·sine 5′-phos·phate (PAP) (fos′fō-a-den′ō-sēn fos′fāt) A product in sulfuryl transfer reactions.

phos·pho·am·i·dase (fos′fō-am′i-dās) An enzyme catalyzing the hydrolysis of phosphorus-nitrogen bonds.

phos·pho·am·ides (fos-fō-am′īdz) Amides of phosphoric acid (phosphoramidic acids) and their salts or esters.

phos·pho·cre·a·tine (PCr) (fos′fō-krē′ă-tēn) A phosphagen; a compound of creatine with phosphoric acid; a source of energy in the contraction of vertebrate muscle, its breakdown furnishing phosphate for the resynthesis of ATP from ADP by creatine kinase. SYN creatine phosphate, N^{ω}-phosphonocreatine.

phos•pho•di•es•ter•as•es (fos′fō-dī-es′tĕr-ās-ĕz) Enzymes (EC sub-subclass 3.1.4) cleaving phosphodiester bonds, such as those in cAMP or between nucleotides in nucleic acids, liberating smaller poly- or oligonucleotide units or mononucleotides but not inorganic phosphate.

phos•pho•e•nol•pyr•u•vic ac•id (fos′fō-ē′nol-pī-rū′vik as′id) The phosphoric ester of pyruvic acid in the latter's enol form; an intermediate in the conversion of glucose to pyruvic acid and an example of a high-energy phosphate ester.

6-phos•pho-D-glu•co•no-δ-lac•tone (siks-fos′fō-dē′glū′kō-nō-del′tă-lak′tōn) An intermediate in the pentose phosphate pathway that is synthesized from D-glucose 6-phosphate.

phos•pho•glyc•er•ides (fos′fō-glis′ĕr-īdz) Acylglycerol and diacylglycerol phosphates; constituents of nerve tissue, and involved in fat transport and storage.

phos•pho•li•pase (fos′fō-lip′ās) An enzyme that catalyzes the hydrolysis of a phospholipid. SYN lecithinase.

phos•pho•lip•id (fos′fō-lip′id) A lipid containing phosphorus, thus including the lecithins and other phosphatidyl derivatives, sphingomyelin, and plasmalogens; the basic constituents of biomembranes.

phos•pho•mu•tase (fos′fō-myū′tās) One of a number of enzymes that catalyze intramolecular transfer of phosphate.

phos•pho•ne•cro•sis (fos′fō-nĕ-krō′sis) Necrosis of the osseous tissue of the jaw, as a result of poisoning by inhalation of phosphorus fumes, occurring especially in people with prolonged occupational exposure. [phosphorus + G. *nekrōsis,* death (necrosis)]

N^{ω}-phos•pho•no•cre•a•tine (fos′fō-nō-krē′ă-tēn) SYN phosphocreatine.

phos•pho•pro•tein (fos′fō-prō′tēn) A protein containing phosphoryl groups attached directly to the side chains of some of its constituent amino acids.

phos•phor (fos′fŏr) A chemical substance that transforms incident electromagnetic or radioactive energy into light, as in scintillation radioactivity determinations or radiographic intensifying screens or image amplifiers. [G. *phōs,* light, + *phoros,* bearing]

phos•pho•res•cence (fos-fō-res′ĕnts) The quality or property of emitting light with neither active combustion nor production of heat, generally as the result of prior exposure to radiation, which persists after the inciting cause is removed. [G. *phōs,* light, + *phoros,* bearing]

phos•pho•res•cent (fos′fō-res′ĕnt) Having the property of phosphorescence.

5-phos•pho-α-D-ri•bo•syl 1-py•ro•phos•phate (PRPP) (fos-fō′ā-dē-rī-bō′sil pī-rō-fos′fāt) 5-phosphoribosyl 1-diphosphate; D-ribose carrying a phosphate group on ribose carbon-5 and a pyrophosphate group on ribose carbon-1; an intermediate in the formation of the pyrimidine and purine nucleotides as well as NAD^+.

phos•phor•ic ac•id (fos-fŏr′ik as′id) A strong acid of industrial importance; dilute solutions have been used as urinary acidifiers and as dressings to remove necrotic debris. In dentistry, it comprises about 60% of the liquid used in zinc phosphate and silicate cements; solutions are used for conditioning enamel surfaces before applications of various types of resins.

phos•phor•ism (fos′fŏr-izm) Chronic poisoning with phosphorus.

phos•pho•rol•y•sis (fos-fō-rol′i-sis) A reaction analogous to hydrolysis except that the elements of phosphoric acid, rather than of water, are added in the course of splitting a bond.

phos•pho•rous (fos′fŏr-ŭs) **1.** Relating to, containing, or resembling phosphorus. **2.** Referring to phosphorus in its lower (+3) valence state.

phos•pho•rus (fos′fŏr-ŭs) A nonmetallic chemical element, atomic no. 15, atomic wt. 30.973762, occurring extensively in nature, always in chemical combination; the elemental form is extremely poisonous, causing intense inflammation and fatty degeneration; repeated inhalation of phosphorus fumes may cause necrosis of the jaw (phosphonecrosis). [G. *phōsphoros,* fr. *phōs,* light, + *phoros,* bearing]

phos•pho•rus 32 (fos′fŏr-ŭs) Radioactive phosphorus isotope; beta emitter with half-life of 14.28 days; used as tracer in metabolic studies and in the treatment of certain diseases of the osseous and hematopoietic systems.

phos•phor•y•lase (fos-fŏr′i-lās) A phosphorylated enzyme cleaving poly(1,4-α-D-glucosyl)$_n$ with inorganic phosphate to form poly(1,4-α-D-glucosyl)$_{n-1}$ and α-D-glucose 1-phosphate.

phos•phor•y•lase phos•pha•tase (fos-fŏr′i-lās fos′fă-tās) An enzyme catalyzing the conversion of one phosphorylase *a* into two phosphorylase *b*, with the release of four phosphates.

phos•pho•ryl•a•tion (fos′fŏr-i-lā′shŭn) Addition of phosphate to an organic compound, such as glucose to produce glucose monophosphate, through the action of a phosphotransferase (phosphorylase) or kinase.

phos•pho•sug•ar (fos′fō-shug′ăr) A phosphorylated saccharide; any sugar containing an alcoholic group esterified with phosphoric acid.

phos•pho•tung•stic ac•id (PTA) (fos′fō-tŭng′stik as′id) A mixture of phosphoric and tungstic acids, approximately 24 WO_3, 2 H_3PO_4, 48 H_2O; a protein precipitant and reagent for arginine, lysine, histidine, and cystine; used with hematoxylin for nuclear and muscle staining; also used in electron microscopy as a stain for collagen and as a negative stain.

phos•pho•tung•stic ac•id he•ma•tox•y•lin (PTAH) (fos′fō-tŭng′stik as′id hē′mă-toks′i-lin) A stain with broad application in cytology and histology; nuclei, mitochrondria, fibrin, neuroglial fibrils, and cross-striations of skeletal and cardiac muscle stain blue; cartilage ground substance, bone reticulum, and elastin appear in shades of yellow-orange and brownish red; also useful for demonstrating abnormal or diseased astrocytes, often in combination with periodic acid-Schiff stain and Luxol fast blue. SYN Mallory phosphotungstic acid hematoxylin stain.

pho•tal•gi•a (fō-tal′jē-ă) Light-induced pain, especially affecting the eyes. SYN photodynia. [phot- + G. *algos,* pain]

pho•tic (fō′tik) Relating to light.

pho•tic driv•ing (fō′tik drīv′ing) A normal EEG phenomenon whereby the frequency of the activity recorded over the parietooccipital regions is time locked to the flash frequency during photic stimulation.

pho•tic-sneeze re•flex (fō′tik snēz rē′fleks) SYN photoptarmosis.

pho•tism (fō′tizm) Production of a sensation of light or color by a stimulus to another sense organ (e.g., hearing, taste, or touch).

♻ **photo-, phot-** Combining forms meaning light. [G. *phōs* (*phōt-*)]

pho•to•ab•la•tion (fō′tō-ab-lā′shŭn) The process of photoablative decomposition of tissue by laser light (e.g., in photorefractive keratectomy).

pho•to•ag•ing (fō′tō-āj′ing) Damage from years of sun exposure, particularly wrinkling of skin. [photo- + aging]

pho•to•bi•ot•ic (fō′tō-bī-ot′ik) Living or flourishing only in the light. [photo- + G. *bios,* life]

pho•to•cat•a•lyst (fō′tō-kat′ă-list) A substance that helps bring about a light-catalyzed reaction, e.g., chlorophyll. [photo- + G. *katalysis,* dissolution (catalysis)]

pho•to•chem•i•cal (fō′tō-kem′i-kăl) Denoting chemical changes caused by or involving light.

pho•to•che•mo•ther•a•py (fō′tō-kēm-ō-thār′ă-pē) SYN photoradiation.

pho•to•chro•mic lens (fō′tō-krōm′ik lenz) A light-sensitive spectacle lens that reduces light transmission in sunlight and increases transmission in reduced light.

pho•to•chro•mo•gen•ic (fō′tō-krō-mŏ-jen′ik) Refers to microorganisms (e.g., *Mycobacterium kansasii*) that produce a yellow pigment when growth colonies are exposed to light.

pho•to•co•ag•u•la•tion (fō′tō-kō-ag′yū-lā′shŭn) A method by which a beam of electromagnetic energy is directed to a desired tissue under visual control; localized coagulation results from absorption of light energy and its conversion to heat or conversion of tissue to plasma (atoms stripped of electrons). [photo- + L. *coagulo,* pp. *-atus,* to curdle]

pho•to•co•ag•u•la•tor (fō′tō-kō-ag′yū-lā-tŏr) The apparatus used in photocoagulation.

pho•to•der•ma•ti•tis (fō′tō-dĕr-mă-tī′tis) Dermatitis caused or elicited by exposure to sunlight; may be phototoxic or photoallergic, and can result from topical application, ingestion, inhalation, or injection of mediating phototoxic or photoallergic material. SEE ALSO photosensitization. SYN actinic dermatitis, actinodermatitis. [photo- + G. *derma,* skin, + *-itis,* inflammation]

pho•to•de•tec•tor (fō′-tō-dĕ-tĕk-tŏr) A device in a spectrophotometer that responds to photons in a manner usually proportional to the number of photons striking its light-sensitive surface.

pho•to•dis•tri•bu•tion (fō′tō-dis-tri-byū′shŭn) Areas on the skin that receive the greatest amount of exposure to sunlight and are thereby involved in eruptions because of photosensitivity.

pho•to•dy•nam•ic sen•si•ti•za•tion (fō′tō-dī-nam′ik sen′si-tī-zā′shŭn) The action by which certain substances, notably fluorescing dyes (acridine, eosin, methylene blue, rose bengal) absorb visible light and emit the energy at wavelengths that are deleterious to microbes or other organisms in the dye-containing suspension, or selectively destroy cancer cells sensitized by intravenous porphyrin and exposed to red laser light. SYN photosensitization (2).

pho•to•dy•nam•ic ther•a•py (PDT) (fō′tō-dī-nam′ik thār′ă-pē) A surgical laser-assisted procedure to correct wet macular degeneration; excitable dye is injected into the venous system and a laser is used to treat those ocular areas that are found to be leaking dye.

pho•to•dyn•i•a (fō′tō-din′ē-ă) SYN photalgia. [photo- + G. *odynē,* pain]

pho•to•e•lec•tric (fō′tō-ĕ-lek′trik) Denoting electronic or electric effects produced by the action of light.

pho•to•fluor•og•ra•phy (fō′tō-flōr-og′ră-fē) Miniature radiographs made by contact photography of a fluoroscopic screen, formerly used in mass radiographic examination of the lungs. SYN fluorography. [photo- + L. *fluor,* a flow, + G. *graphē,* a writing]

pho•to•gas•tro•scope (fō′tō-gas′trŏ-skōp) An instrument for taking photographs of the interior of the stomach. [photo- + G. *gastēr,* stomach, + *skopeō,* to view]

pho•to•gen•ic, pho•tog•e•nous (fō′tō-jen′

ik, fō-toj′ĕ-nŭs) Denoting or capable of photogenesis.

pho·to·gen·ic ep·i·lep·sy (fō′tō-jen′ik ep′i-lep′sē) A form of reflex epilepsy precipitated by light.

pho·to·in·ac·ti·va·tion (fō′tō-in-ak-ti-vā′shŭn) **1.** Acute sensitivity to light. **2.** Inactivation by light (e.g., as in the treatment of herpes simplex by local application of a photoactive dye followed by exposure to a fluorescent lamp).

pho·to·lu·mi·nes·cent (fō′tō-lū-mi-nes′ĕnt) Having the ability to become luminescent on exposure to visible light. [photo- + L. *lumen,* light]

pho·tol·y·sis (fō-tol′i-sis) Decomposition of a chemical compound by the action of light. [photo- + G. *lysis,* dissolution]

pho·to·lyt·ic (fō′tō-lit′ik) Pertaining to photolysis.

pho·to·mi·cro·graph (fō′tō-mī′krō-graf) An enlarged photograph of an object viewed with a microscope, as distinguished from a microphotograph. SYN micrograph. [photo- + G. *mikros,* small, + *graphē,* a record]

pho·to·mi·crog·ra·phy (fō′tō-mī-krog′ră-fē) The production of a photomicrograph.

pho·to·my·oc·lo·nus (fō′tō-mī-ok′lō-nŭs) Clonic spasms of muscles in response to visual stimuli. [photo- + G. *mys,* muscle, + *klonos,* confused motion]

pho·ton (γ) (fō′ton) PHYSICS a corpuscle of energy or particle of light; a quantum of light or other electromagnetic radiation.

pho·to-patch test (fō′tō pach test) A test of contact photosensitization: After application of a patch with the suspected sensitizer for 48 hours to two sites, if there is no reaction, one area is exposed to a weak erythema dose of sunlight or ultraviolet light; if positive, a more severe reaction with vesiculation develops at the exposed patch area than the nonexposed skin patch site.

pho·to·per·cep·tive (fō′tō-pĕr-sep′tiv) Capable of both receiving and perceiving light.

pho·to·pho·bi·a (fō′tō-fō′bē-ă) Morbid dread and avoidance of light. Although often an expression of undue anxiety about the eyes, photosensitivity and photalgia, past or present, should be considered. [photo- + G. *phobos,* fear]

pho·to·pho·bic (fō′tō-fō′bik) Relating to or suffering from photophobia.

pho·toph·thal·mi·a (fō′tof-thal′mē-ă) Keratoconjunctivitis caused by ultraviolet energy, as in snow blindness, exposure to an ultraviolet lamp, arc welding, or the short circuit of a high-tension electric current. SEE ALSO photoretinopathy. [photo- + G. *ophthalmos,* eye]

pho·to·pi·a (fō-tō′pē-ă) SYN photopic vision. [photo- + G. *opsis,* vision]

pho·top·ic (fō-top′ik) Pertaining to photopic vision.

pho·top·ic ad·ap·ta·tion (fō-top′ik ad′ap-tā′shŭn) SYN light adaptation.

pho·top·ic eye (fō-top′ik ī) SYN light-adapted eye.

pho·top·ic vi·sion (fō-top′ik vizh′ŭn) Vision when the eye is adapted to light. SEE light adaptation, light-adapted eye. SYN photopia.

pho·top·si·a (fō-top′sē-ă) A subjective sensation of lights, sparks, or colors due to electrical or mechanical stimulation of the ocular system. SYN photopsy. [photo- + G. *opsis,* vision]

pho·top·sin (fō-top′sin) The protein moiety (opsin) of the pigment (iodopsin) in the cones of the retina.

pho·top·sy (fō-top′sē) SYN photopsia.

pho·top·tar·mo·sis (fō-top′tahr-mo′sis) Reflex sneezing that occurs when bright light stimulates the retina. SYN photic-sneeze reflex. [photo- + G. *ptarmos,* a sneezing, + *-osis,* condition]

pho·to·ra·di·a·tion, pho·to·ra·di·a·tion ther·a·py (fō′tō-rā′dē-ā′shŭn, thār′ă-pē) Treatment of cancer by intravenous injection of a photosensitizing agent (e.g., hematoporphyrin), followed by exposure to visible light of superficial tumors or of deep tumors by a fiberoptic probe. SYN photochemotherapy.

pho·to·re·ac·tion (fō′tō-rē-ak′shŭn) A reaction caused or affected by light, e.g., a photochemical reaction, photolysis, photosynthesis, phototropism, thymine dimer formation.

pho·to·re·ac·ti·va·tion (fō′tō-rē-ak′ti-vā′shŭn) Activation by light of something or of some process previously inactive or inactivated.

pho·to·re·cep·tive (fō′tō-rē-sep′tiv) Functioning as a photoreceptor.

pho·to·re·cep·tor (fō′tō-rē-sep′tŏr) A light-sensitive receptor (e.g., a retinal rod or cone). [photo- + L. *re-cipio,* pp. *-ceptus,* to receive, fr. *capio,* to take]

pho·to·re·cep·tor cells (fō′tō-rē-sep′tŏr selz) Rod and cone cells of the retina.

pho·to·ret·i·ni·tis (fō′tō-ret-i-nī′tis) SEE photoretinopathy.

pho·to·ret·i·nop·a·thy (fō′tō-ret-i-nop′ă-thē) A macular burn from excessive exposure to sunlight or other intense light (e.g., the flash of a short circuit); characterized subjectively by reduced visual acuity. [photo- + retina, + G. *pathos,* suffering]

pho·to·scan (fō′tō-skan) SYN scintiscan.

photosensitisation [Br.] SYN photosensitization.

pho·to·sen·si·ti·za·tion (fō′tō-sen-si-ti-zā′shŭn) **1.** Sensitization of the skin to light, usually due to the action of certain drugs, plants, or other substances; may occur shortly after administration of the drug (phototoxic sensitivity), or may occur only after a latent period of days to months (photoallergic sensitivity, or photoallergy). **2.** SYN photodynamic sensitization. SYN photosensitisation.

pho·to·sta·ble (fō′tō-stā-bĕl) Not subject to change on exposure to light.

pho·to·steth·o·scope (fō-tō-steth′ŏ-skōp) Device that converts sound into flashes of light; used for continuous observation of the fetal heart.

pho·to·syn·the·sis (fō′tō-sin′thĕ-sis) **1.** The compounding or building up of chemical substances under the influence of light. **2.** The process by which green plants, using chlorophyll and the energy of sunlight, produce carbohydrates from water and carbon dioxide, liberating molecular oxygen in the process. [photo- + G. *synthesis,* a putting together]

pho·to·tax·is (fō′tō-tak′sis) Reaction of living protoplasm to the stimulus of light, involving bodily motion of the whole organism toward (**positive phototaxis**) or away from (**negative phototaxis**) the stimulus. Cf. phototropism. [photo- + G. *taxis,* orderly arrangement]

pho·to·ther·a·peu·tic ker·a·tec·to·my (PTK) (fō′tō-thār′ă-pyū′tik ker-ă-tek′tŏ-mē) Ablation of diseased corneal tissue using an excimer laser.

pho·to·ther·a·py (fō′tō-thār′ă-pē) Treatment of disease by means of light rays. SYN light treatment.

pho·to·ther·mo·ly·sis (fō′tō-thĕrm-ol′ī-sis) Laser resurfacing; technique using laser therapy to remove fine lines and wrinkles, pigmented areas, and tattoos.

pho·to·tim·er (fō′tō-tīm-ĕr) An electronic device in radiography that measures the radiation that has passed through the patient and terminates the x-ray exposure when it is sufficient to form an image.

pho·to·tox·ic·it·y (fō′tō-tok-sis′i-tē) The condition resulting from an overexposure to ultraviolet light, or from the combination of exposure to certain wavelengths of light and a phototoxic substance. SEE ALSO photosensitization. [photo- + G. *toxikon,* poison]

pho·tot·ro·pism (fō-tot′rŏ-pizm) Movement of a part of an organism toward (**positive phototropism**) or away from (**negative phototropism**) the stimulus of light. Cf. phototaxis. [photo- + G. *tropē,* a turning]

pho·tu·ri·a (fō-tyūr′ē-ă) Passage of phosphorescent urine. [photo- + G. *ouron,* urine]

PHP Abbreviation for panhypopituitarism.

phre·nal·gi·a (fre-nal′jē-ă) **1.** SYN psychalgia (1). **2.** Pain in the diaphragm. [phren- + G. *algos,* pain]

♻**-phrenia** Suffix denoting (1) the diaphragm; (2) the mind. [G. *phrēn,* the diaphragm, mind, heart (as seat of emotions]

phren·ic (fren′ik) **1.** SYN diaphragmatic. **2.** Relating to the mind.

phren·i·cec·to·my (fren-i-sek′tŏ-mē) Exsection of a portion of the phrenic nerve, to prevent reunion such as may follow phrenicotomy. SYN phrenicoexeresis. [phreni- + G. *ektomē,* excision]

phren·ic gan·gli·a (fren′ik gang′glē-ă) Several small autonomic ganglia contained in the plexuses accompanying the inferior phrenic arteries.

phren·i·cla·si·a (fren-i-klā′zē-ă) Crushing of a section of the phrenic nerve to produce a temporary paralysis of the diaphragm. SYN phrenicotripsy. [phreni- + G. *klasis,* a breaking away]

phren·ic nerve (fren′ik nĕrv) Arises from the cervical plexus, chiefly from the fourth cervical nerve; passes downward in front of the anterior scalene muscle and enters the thorax between the subclavian artery and vein behind the sternoclavicular articulation; it then passes in front of the root of the lung to the diaphragm; it is mainly the motor nerve of the diaphragm but sends sensory fibers to the mediastinal parietal pleura, the pericardium, the diaphragmatic pleura and peritoneum, and branches (phrenicoabdominales branches) that communicate with branches from the celiac plexus. SYN nervus phrenicus [TA].

phren·i·co·ab·dom·i·nal branches of phren·ic nerve (fren′i-kō-ab-dom′i-năl branch′ĕz fren′ik nĕrv) Terminal branches of phrenic nerve providing motor innervation of diaphragm and sensory innervation to the diaphragm and the diaphragmatic pleura and peritoneum.

phren·i·co·col·ic (fren′i-kō-kol′ik) Relating to the diaphragm and the colon.

phren·i·co·col·ic lig·a·ment (fren′i-kō-kol′ik lig′ă-mĕnt) A triangular fold of peritoneum attached to the left flexure of the colon and to the diaphragm, on which rests the inferior pole or extremity of the spleen. SYN ligamentum phrenicocolicum [TA].

phren·i·co·ex·er·e·sis (fren′i-kō-ek-ser′ĕ-sis) SYN phrenicectomy. [phrenico- + G. *exairesis,* a taking out, fr. *haireō,* to take, grasp]

phren·i·co·gas·tric (fren′i-kō-gas′trik) Relating to the diaphragm and the stomach.

phren•i•co•he•pa•tic (fren′i-kō-hĕ-pa′tik) Relating to the diaphragm and the liver.

phren•i•co•pleu•ral fas•ci•a (fren′i-kō-plūr′ăl fash′ē-ă) The thin layer of endothoracic fascia intervening between the diaphragmatic pleura and the diaphragm.

phren•i•cot•o•my (fren-i-kot′ŏ-mē) Section of the phrenic nerve to induce unilateral paralysis of the diaphragm, which is then pushed up by the abdominal viscera and exerts compression on a diseased lung. [phrenico- + G. *tomē,* incision]

phren•i•co•trip•sy (fren′i-kō-trip′sē) SYN phreniclasia. [phrenico- + G. *tripsis,* a rubbing]

phreno-, phren-, phreni-, phrenico- Combining forms denoting the diaphragm; the mind; the phrenic nerve. [G. *phrēn,* diaphragm, mind, heart (as seat of emotions)]

phren•o•car•di•a (fren-ō-kahr′dē-ă) Precordial pain and dyspnea of psychogenic origin, often a symptom of anxiety neurosis. SEE cardiac neurosis. [phreno- + G. *kardia,* heart]

phren•o•ple•gi•a (fren-ō-plē′jē-ă) Paralysis of the diaphragm. [phreno- + G. *plēgē,* stroke]

phren•op•to•si•a (fren-op-tō′sē-ă) An abnormal sinking down of the diaphragm. [phreno- + G. *ptōsis,* a falling]

phryn•o•der•ma (frin-ō-dĕr′mă) A follicular hyperkeratotic eruption thought to be due to deficiency of vitamin A. [G. *phrynos,* toad, + *derma,* skin]

phy•co•my•co•sis (fī′kō-mī-kō′sis) SYN zygomycosis.

phy•lax•is (fī-lak′sis) Protection against infection. [G. a guarding, protection]

phyl•lo•qui•none (fil-ō-kwin′ōn) Compound isolated from alfalfa; also prepared synthetically; major form of vitamin K found in plants. SYN vitamin K1, vitamin K1(20).

phylo- Combining form meaning tribe, race; a taxonomic phylum. [G. *phylon,* tribe]

phy•lo•gen•e•sis (fī-lō-jen′ĕ-sis) SYN phylogeny. [phylo- + G. *genesis,* origin]

phy•lo•ge•net•ic, phy•lo•gen•ic (fī′lō-jĕ-net′ik, -jen′ik) Relating to phylogenesis.

phy•log•e•ny (fī-loj′ĕ-nē) The evolutionary development of species, as distinguished from ontogeny, development of the individual. SYN phylogenesis.

phy•lum, pl. **phy•la** (fī′lŭm, -lă) A taxonomic division below the kingdom and above the class. [Mod. L. fr. G. *phylon,* tribe]

phy•ma (fī′mă) A nodule or small rounded tumor of the skin. [G. a tumor]

phy•ma•to•sis (fī-mă-tō′sis) The growth or the presence of phymas or small nodules in the skin.

Phy•sal•i•a (fī-sā′lē-ă) A genus of the invertebrate phylum Cnidaria that includes the Portuguese man-of-war.

Phy•sal•i•a phy•sa•lis (fī-sā′-lē-ă fī-sā-lis) The Portuguese man-of-war, a jellyfishlike animal consisting of a complex colony of individual members that can inflict extremely painful stings. SYN Portuguese man-of-war.

phy•sal•i•form (fi-sal′i-fōrm) Like a bubble or small bleb. [G. *physallis,* bladder, bubble, + L. *forma,* form]

phys•a•lis (fis′ăl-is) A vacuole in a giant cell found in certain malignant neoplasms, such as chordoma. [G. *physallis,* a bladder]

phys•i•al (fis′ē-ăl) Pertaining to the physis, or growth cartilage area, separating the metaphysis and the epiphysis.

phys•i•at•rics (fiz-ē-at′riks) **1.** Old term for physical therapy. **2.** Rehabilitation management. [G. *physis,* nature, + *iatrikos,* healing]

phys•i•a•trist (fiz-ī′ă-trist) A physician who specializes in the areas of physical medicine and rehabilitation.

phys•i•a•try (fi-zī′ă-trē) SYN physical medicine.

phys•i•cal (fiz′i-kăl) Relating to the body, as distinguished from the mind. [Mod. L. *physicalis,* fr. G. *physikos*]

phys•i•cal ac•tiv•i•ty (fiz′i-kăl ak-tiv′i-tē) Any body movement produced by muscles that results in energy expenditure. SEE exercise.

phys•i•cal ac•tiv•i•ty pyr•a•mid (fiz′i-kăl aktiv′i-tē pir′ă-mid) A visual representation demonstrating how to increase physical activity until it becomes a part of daily routine.

phys•i•cal a•gent (fiz′i-kăl ā′jĕnt) A form of acoustic, aqueous, electrical, mechanical, thermal, or light energy applied to living tissues in a systematic manner to alter physiologic processes, in conjunction with or for therapeutic purposes. SEE ALSO modality.

phys•i•cal al•ler•gy (fiz′i-kăl al′ĕr-jē) Excessive response to factors in the environment such as heat or cold.

phys•i•cal con•di•tion•ing (fiz′i-kăl kŏn-di′shŭn-ing) Systematic use of regular physical activity to induce functional and structural adaptations that enhance energy capacity and exercise performance.

phys•i•cal de•mand lev•el (fiz′i-kăl dĕmand′ lev′ĕl) The U.S. Department of Labor defines five uniform levels: sedentary, light, medium, heavy, and very heavy.

phys•i•cal di•ag•no•sis (fiz′i-kăl dī-ăg-nō′sis) A diagnosis made by means of physical examination of the patient, or the process of a physical examination.

phys•i•cal fit•ness (fiz′i-kăl fit′nĕs) A set of attributes relating to one's ability to perform physical activity. SEE ALSO health-related physical fitness.

phys•i•cal map (fiz′i-kăl map) A map of a stretch of DNA with ordered landmarks a known distance from each other; the ultimate physical map would be the base sequence of the entire chromosome.

phys•i•cal med•i•cine (fiz′i-kăl med′i-sin) The study and treatment of disease mainly by mechanical and other physical methods. SYN physiatry.

Phys•i•cal Read•i•ness Ques•tion•naire (PAR-Q) (fiz′i-kăl red′ē-nĕs kwes′chŭn-ār′) A short assessment tool developed by the Canadian Society for Exercise Physiology to screen patients about to begin physical activity programs.

phys•i•cal sign (fiz′i-kăl sīn) A finding evident on inspection or elicited by auscultation, percussion, or palpation.

phys•i•cal ther•a•pist (fiz′i-kăl thār′ă-pist) A practitioner of physical therapy. SYN physiotherapist.

phys•i•cal ther•a•pist as•sis•tant (PTA) (fiz′i-kăl thār′ă-pist ă-sis′tĕnt) A paraprofessional who works under the direction of a physical therapist and assists in the application of physical therapy interventions.

phys•i•cal ther•a•py (PT) (fiz′i-kăl thār′ă-pē) **1.** Treatment of pain, disease, or injury by physical means. SYN physiotherapy. **2.** The health profession concerned with promotion of health, with prevention of physical disabilities, with evaluation and rehabilitation of people disabled by pain, disease, or injury, and with treatment by physical therapeutic measures as opposed to medical, surgical, or radiologic measures.

phy•si•cian (fi-zish′ŭn) **1.** A doctor; a person who has been educated, trained, and licensed to practice the art and science of medicine. **2.** A practitioner of medicine, as contrasted with a surgeon. [Fr. *physicien,* a natural philosopher]

phy•si•cian as•sis•tant (fi-zish′ŭn ă-sis′tĕnt) Someone certified to provide basic medical services under the supervision of a licensed medical physician.

phy•si•cian as•sis•tant, cer•ti•fied (PA-C) (fi-zish′ăn ă-sis′tănt ser′ti-fīd) A holder of a degree or certificate that requires completion of a 2-year course and successfully passing a national examination.

phy•si•cian-as•sis•ted su•i•cide (fi-zish′ŭn ă-sist′ĕd sū′i-sīd) Voluntary termination of one's own life by administration of a lethal substance with the direct or indirect assistance of a physician; distinguished from the withholding or discontinuance of life-support measures in terminal or vegetative states so that the patient dies of the underlying illness, and from administration of narcotic analgesics in terminal cancer, which may indirectly hasten death. SEE ALSO end-of-life care, advance directive.

phy•si•cian ex•ten•der (fi-zish′ŭn eks-ten′dĕr) A specially trained and licensed person who performs tasks that might otherwise be performed by physicians themselves, under the direction of a supervising physician. Examples include nurse practitioners and physician assistants.

phy•si•cian of•fice lab•o•ra•tor•y (POL) (fi-zish′ŭn awf′is lab′ră-tōr-ē) Clinical laboratory located in a physician's office for on-site testing of specimens from patients seen by the physician.

Phy•sick pouch•es (fiz′ik pow′chĕz) Proctitis with mucous discharge and burning pain, involving especially the sacculations between the rectal valves.

phys•i•co•chem•i•cal (fiz′i-kō-kem′i-kăl) Relating to the field of physical chemistry.

phys•ic root (fiz′ik rūt) SYN black root.

phys•ics (fiz′iks) The branch of science concerned with the phenomena of matter and energy and their interactions.

♻**physio-, physi-** Combining forms meaning physical, physiological; natural, relating to physics. [G. *physis,* nature]

phys•i•o•gen•ic (fiz′ē-ō-jen′ik) Related to or caused by physiologic activity. [physio- + G. *genesis,* origin]

phys•i•og•no•my (fiz′ē-og′nŏ-mē) **1.** The physical appearance of one's face, countenance, or habitus, especially regarded as an indication of character. **2.** Estimation of one's character and mental qualities by a study of the face and other external bodily features. [physio- + G. *gnōmōn,* a judge]

phys•i•o•log•ic, phys•i•o•log•i•cal (fiz′ē-ō-loj′ik, -i-kăl) **1.** Relating to physiology. **2.** Normal, as opposed to pathologic; denoting the various vital processes. **3.** Denoting something that is apparent from its functional effects rather than from its anatomic structure (e.g., a physiologic sphincter). **4.** Denoting a dose of a hormone, neurotransmitter, or other naturally occurring agent that is within the range of concentrations or potencies that would occur naturally. Cf. homeopathic (2), pharmacologic (2).

phys•i•o•log•ic an•ti•dote (fiz′ē-ō-loj′ik an′ti-dōt) An agent that produces systemic effects contrary to those of a given poison.

phys•i•o•log•i•c chem•is•try (fiz′ē-ō-loj′ik kem′is-trē) SYN biochemistry.

phys•i•o•log•ic con•ges•tion (fiz′ē-ō-loj′ik kŏn-jes′chŭn) SYN functional congestion.

phys•i•o•log•ic dead space (fiz′ē-ō-loj′ik ded spās) The sum of anatomic and alveolar dead space; the dead space calculated when the carbon dioxide pressure in systemic arterial blood is used instead of that of alveolar gas in the Bohr equation; it is a virtual or apparent volume that takes into account the impairment of gas exchange because of uneven distributions of lung ventilation and perfusion.

phys•i•o•log•i•c drives (fiz′ē-ō-loj′ik drīvz) Those drives (e.g., hunger and thirst) that stem from the biologic needs of an organism.

phys•i•o•log•ic ho•me•o•sta•sis (fiz′ē-ō-loj′ik hō′mē-ō-stā′sis) SYN Bernard-Cannon homeostasis.

phys•i•o•log•ic hy•per•tro•phy (fiz′ē-ō-loj′ik hī-pĕr′trō-fē) Temporary increase in the size of an organ or part to provide for a natural increase of function.

phys•i•o•log•ic ic•ter•us (fiz′ē-ō-loj′ik ik′tĕr-ŭs) SYN icterus neonatorum.

phys•i•o•log•ic jaun•dice (fiz′ē-ō-loj′ik jawn′dis) SYN icterus neonatorum.

phys•i•o•log•ic leu•ko•cy•to•sis (fiz′ē-ō-loj′ik lū′kō-sī-tō′sis) Any form of leukocytosis that is associated with apparently normal situations and not directly related to a pathologic condition.

phys•i•o•log•ic oc•clu•sion (fiz′ē-ō-loj′ik ŏ-klū′zhŭn) Occlusion in harmony with functions of the masticatory system.

phys•i•o•log•ic rest po•si•tion (fiz′ē-ō-loj′ik rest pŏ-zish′ŏn) SYN rest position.

phys•i•o•log•ic re•trac•tion ring (fiz′ē-ō-loj′ik rē-trak′shŭn ring) A ridge on the inner uterine surface at the boundary line between the upper and lower uterine segments that occurs in the course of normal labor.

phys•i•o•log•ic sa•line (fiz′ē-ō-loj′ik sā′lēn) An isotonic aqueous solution of salts, containing 0.9% sodium chloride.

phys•i•o•log•ic sco•to•ma (fiz′ē-ō-loj′ik skō-tō′mă) The negative scotoma in the visual field, corresponding to the optic disc. SYN blind spot (1).

phys•i•o•log•ic sphinc•ter (fiz′ē-ō-loj′ik sfingk′tĕr) A section of a tubular structure that acts as if it has a band of circular muscle to constrict it, although no such specialized structure can be found on morphologic examination. SYN radiologic sphincter.

phys•i•o•log•ic u•nit (fiz′ē-ō-loj′ik yū′nit) **1.** Spencer's concept of the ultimate (hypothetical) vital unit of protoplasm. **2.** The smallest division of an organ that will perform its function, e.g., the uriniferous tubule.

phys•i•ol•o•gist (fiz′ē-ol′ŏ-jist) A specialist in physiology.

phys•i•ol•o•gy (fiz′ē-ol′ŏ-jē) The science concerned with the normal vital processes of animal and vegetable organisms, especially as to how things normally function in the living organism rather than to their anatomic structure, their biochemical composition, or how they are affected by drugs or disease. [L. or G. *physiologia,* fr. G. *physis,* nature, + *logos,* study]

phys•i•o•ther•a•peu•tic (fiz′ē-ō-thār′ă-pyū′tik) Pertaining to physical therapy.

phys•i•o•ther•a•pist (fiz′ē-ō-thār′ă-pist) SYN physical therapist. SEE ALSO physical therapy (2).

phys•i•o•ther•a•py (fiz′ē-ō-thār′ă-pē) SYN physical therapy (1). [physio- + G. *therapeia,* treatment]

phy•sique (fi-zēk′) Constitutional type; the physical or bodily structure; the "build." [Fr.]

phys•o- Prefix meaning (1) tendency to swell or inflate; (2) relation to air or gas. [G. *physaō,* to inflate, distend]

phy•so•cele (fī′sō-sēl) **1.** A circumscribed swelling due to the presence of gas. **2.** A hernial sac distended with gas. [physo- + G. *kēlē,* tumor, hernia]

phy•so•me•tra (fī′sō-mē′tră) Distention of the uterine cavity with air or gas. [physo- + G. *mētra,* uterus]

phy•so•py•o•sal•pinx (fī′sō-pī-ō-sal′pingks) Pyosalpinx accompanied by a formation of gas in a uterine (fallopian) tube. [physo- + G. *pyon,* pus, + *salpinx,* trumpet]

phy•so•stig•mine (fī′sō-stig′mēn) A nonpolar carbamate antidote to anticholinergic compounds.

phy•tate (fī′tāt) A phosphorus-containing compound that binds with minerals in the GI tract and decreases their bioavailability.

phyto-, phyt- Combining forms meaning plants. [G. *phyton,* a plant]

phy•to•ag•glu•ti•nin (fī′tō-ă-glū′ti-nin) A lectin that causes agglutination of erythrocytes or of leukocytes.

phy•to•be•zoar (fī′tō-bē′zōr) A gastric concretion formed of vegetable fibers, with the seeds and skins of fruits, and sometimes starch granules and fat globules. SYN food ball. [phyto- + bezoar]

phy•to•chem•i•cal (fī′tō-kem′i-kăl) A biologically active but nonnutrient substance found in plants; includes antioxidants and phytosterols. SYN bioactive nonnutrient, phytoprotectant.

phy•to•der•ma•ti•tis (fī′tō-dĕr-mă-tī′tis) Dermatitis caused by various mechanisms, including mechanical and chemical injury, allergy, or photosensitization (phytophotodermatitis) at skin sites previously exposed to plants.

phy•to•es•tro•gens (fī′tō-es′trō-jenz) Plant extracts that act in the body like weak estrogens. SYN phyto-oestrogens.

phytohaemagglutinin [Br.] SYN phytohemagglutinin.

phy•to•hem•ag•glu•ti•nin (PHA) (fī′tō-hēm-ă-glū′ti-nin) A phytomitogen from plants that agglutinates red blood cells. Commonly used specifically for the lectin obtained from the red kidney bean (*Phaseolus vulgaris*), which is also a mitogen. SYN phytohaemagglutinin, phytolectin.

phy•toid (fī′toyd) Resembling a plant; denoting an animal having many of the biologic characteristics of a vegetable. [G. *phytōdēs,* fr. *phyton,* plant, + *eidos,* resemblance]

phy•tol (fī′tol) An unsaturated primary alcohol derived from the hydrolysis of chlorophyll; a constituent of vitamins E and K1.

phy•to•lec•tin (fī′tō-lek′tin) SYN phytohemagglutinin.

phy•to•med•i•cine (fī′tō-med′i-sin) SYN herbal therapy.

phy•to•mi•to•gen (fī-tō-mī′tō-jen) A mitogenic lectin causing lymphocyte transformation accompanied by mitotic proliferation of the resulting blast cells identical to that produced by antigenic stimulation (e.g., phytohemagglutinin, concanavalin A).

phyto-oestrogens [Br.] SYN phytoestrogens.

phy•to•phlyc•to•der•ma•ti•tis (fī′tō-flik′tō-dĕr-mă-ti′tis) SYN meadow dermatitis. [phyto- + G. *phlyktaina,* blister, + dermatitis]

phy•to•pho•to•der•ma•ti•tis (fī′tō-fō′tō-dĕr-mă-tī′tis) Phytodermatitis resulting from photosensitization.

phy•to•pro•tec•tant (fī′tō-prō-tek′tănt) SYN phytochemical.

phy•tos•ter•ols (fī′tō-ster′olz) Plant sterols and stanols that inhibit the absorption of cholesterol from the small intestine and, in effect, lower low-density lipoprotein cholesterol in humans.

phy•to•ther•a•py (fī′tō-thār′ă-pē) SYN herbal therapy.

phy•to•tox•ic (fī′tō-tok′sik) **1.** Poisonous to plant life. **2.** Pertaining to a phytotoxin.

phy•to•tox•in (fī′tō-tok′sin) Any toxin produced by a plant. [phyto- + G. *toxikon,* poison]

PI Abbreviation for Periodontal Index.

pI The pH value for the isoelectric point of a given substance.

pi (π, Π) (pī) **1.** The 16th letter of the Greek alphabet (π, Π). **2.** Osmotic pressure (Π). **3.** MATHEMATICS symbol for the product of a series (Π). **4.** Symbol for the ratio of the circumference of a circle to its diameter (approximately 3.14159265) (π).

pi•a (pī′ă) SYN pia mater. [L. fem. of *pius,* tender]

pi•a-a•rach•ni•tis (pī′ă-ă-rak-nī′tis) SYN leptomeningitis.

pi•a-a•rach•noid (pī′ă-ă-rak′noyd) SYN leptomeninges.

pi•al (pī′ăl) Relating to the pia mater.

pi•a mat•er (pī′ă mā′tĕr) [TA] A delicate, vasculated fibrous membrane firmly adherent to the glial capsule of the brain (**pia mater cranialis [encephali]** [TA]) and spinal cord (**pia mater spinalis** [TA] or membrana limitans gliae); following exactly the outer markings of the cerebrum and also the ependymal lining circumference of the choroid membranes and plexus, it invests the cerebellum but not so intimately as it does the cerebrum, not dipping down into all the smaller sulci. The pia mater and the arachnoid are collectively called leptomeninges, as distinguished from dura mater or pachymeninx. SYN pia. [L. tender, affectionate mother, mistransl. of Arabic *umm raqīqah,* delicate covering or protection]

pi•a ma•ter en•ceph•a•li (pī′ă mā′ter en-sef′ă-lī) [TA] SYN cranial pia mater.

pi•an (pē-an′) SYN yaws.

pi•a•no key sign (pē′ăn-ō kē sīn) A maneuver used to determine injury to the coracoclavicular ligament, whereby a downward pressure is applied on the distal end of the clavicle. The result is positive if the clavicle pops up after release of the downward pressure.

pi•a•rach•noid (pī-ă-rak′noyd) SYN leptomeninges.

pi•ca (pī′kă) An appetite for substances not fit as food or of no nutritional value (e.g., clay, dried paint, starch). [L. *pica,* magpie]

PICC Abbreviation for peripherally inserted central catheter.

Pic•chi•ni syn•drome (pĭ-kē′nē sin′drōm) A form of polyserositis involving the three great serosae in contact with the diaphragm, sometimes also the meninges, tunica vaginalis testis, synovial sheaths, and bursae, caused by a trypanosome.

Pick at•ro•phy (pik at′rŏ-fē) Circumscribed atrophy of the cerebral cortex.

Pick bod•ies (pik bod′ēz) Intracytoplasmic argentophilic neuronal inclusion bodies seen in Pick disease.

Pick cell (pik sel) A relatively large mononuclear cell with foamlike cytoplasm that contains numerous droplets of sphingomyelin; such cells are widely distributed in the spleen and other tissues in patients with Niemann-Pick disease. SYN Niemann-Pick cell.

Pick dis•ease (pik di-zēz′) Progressive circumscribed cerebral atrophy; a rare type of cerebrodegenerative disorder manifested primarily as dementia, in which there is striking atrophy of portions of the frontal and temporal lobes. [F. Pick]

Pick•les chart (pik′ĕlz chahrt) Day-by-day plots of new cases of infectious disease used to demonstrate the progress of an epidemic in a small, relatively isolated population.

pick•wick•i•an syn•drome (pik-wik′ē-ăn sin′drōm) A combination of severe, grotesque obesity, somnolence, and general debility, theoretically resulting from hypoventilation induced by the obesity; hypercapnia, pulmonary hypertension, and cor pulmonale can result. [after the "fat boy" in Dickens's *Pickwick Papers*]

♻**pico-** **1.** Prefix meaning small. **2.** **(p)** Prefix used in the SI and the metric system to signify one trillionth (10^{-12}). SYN bicro-. [It. *piccolo*]

pi•co•gram (pg) (pī′kō-gram) One trillionth of a gram.

pi•co•ka•tal (pkat) (pī′kō-kat′ăl) One trillionth of a katal (10^{-12} katal).

pi•com•e•ter (pm) (pī′kō-mē-tĕr) One trillionth of a meter. SYN bicron, picometre.

picometre [Br.] SYN picometer.

pi•co•mole (pmol) (pī′kō-mōl) One trillionth of a mole (10^{-12} mole).

Pi•cor•na•vir•i•dae (pi-kōr′nă-vir′i-dē) A family of very small viruses having a core of single-stranded RNA. Numerous species (including the polioviruses, coxsackieviruses, and echoviruses) are included in the family. There are four accepted genera: Enterovirus, Rhinovirus, Cardiovirus, and Aphthovirus. [It. *piccolo,* very small, + RNA + -viridae]

pi•cor•na•vi•rus (pi-kōr′nă-vī′rŭs) A virus of the family Picornaviridae.

pic•ro•car•mine stain, **pic•ro•car•mine** (pik′rō-kar′min stān, pik′rō-kar′min) A red crystalline powder derived from a solution of carmine, ammonia, and picric acid that is evaporated, leaving the powder (soluble in water); it produces excellent staining of keratohyaline granules.

PICU Abbreviation for pediatric intensive care unit.

PID Abbreviation for pelvic inflammatory disease.

Pid•gin Sign Eng•lish (PSE) (pij′in sīn ing′glish) A system of communication that is a manual representation of English in which American Sign Language signs are used in English word order; there are no inflectional signs, and finger spelling is used for proper names.

PIE Abbreviation for pulmonary interstitial emphysema.

pie•bald eye•lash (pī′bawld ī′lash) An isolated bundle of white eyelashes among normally pigmented eyelashes.

pie•bald•ism (pī′bawld-izm) SYN piebaldness.

pie•bald•ness (pī′bawld-nĕs) Patchy absence of the pigment of scalp hair, giving a streaked appearance; patches of vitiligo may be present in other areas due to the absence of melanocytes. May be associated with neurologic defects or eye changes. SYN piebald skin, piebaldism.

pie•bald skin (pī′bawld skin) SYN piebaldness.

pi•e•dra (pē-ā′dră) A fungal disease of the hair characterized by the formation of numerous waxy, small, firm, nodular masses on the hair shaft. [Sp. a stone]

Pi•erre Rob•in syn•drome (pē-yār′ rō-ban[h]′ sin′drōm) A complex of congenital anomalies including micrognathia and abnormal smallness of the tongue, often with cleft palate, severe myopia, congenital glaucoma, and retinal detachment. Intelligence of those affected is usually normal. SYN Robin syndrome.

pi•e•ses•the•si•a (pī-ē-ses-thē′zē-ă) SYN pressure sense. [G. *piesis,* pressure, + *aisthēsis,* sensation]

pi•e•sim•e•ter, **pi•e•som•e•ter** (pī-ĕ-sim′ĕ-ter, -som′ĕ-ter) An instrument for measuring the pressure of a gas or a fluid. [G. *piesis,* pressure]

pi•e•zo•e•lec•tric ul•tra•son•ic de•vice (pē′ā-zō-ē-lek′trik ŭl-tră-son′ik dĕ-vīs′) An electronically powered tool that uses the rapid energy vibrations of a powered instrument tip to fracture calculus from the tooth surface and clean the environment of a periodontal pocket. This device consists of a portable electronic generator, a handpiece, and instrument inserts. The instrument tip of a piezoelectric instrument vibrates at 24,000–34,000 cycles per second.

pi•e•zo•gen•ic ped•al pap•ule (pī′ā-zō-jen′ik ped′ăl pap′yūl) Pressure-induced papule of the heel, occurring probably as a result of herniation of fat tissue.

PIF Abbreviation for prolactin-inhibiting factor.

pig•bel (pig′bel) SYN enteritis necroticans.

pi•geon breast (pij′ŏn brest) SYN pigeon chest.

pi•geon chest (pij′ŏn chest) An abnormality of the thoracic cage that gives a convex appearance to the anterior chest. SYN pigeon breast.

pig•ment (pig′mĕnt) **1.** Any coloring matter, as,

for example, that of the red blood cells, hair, or iris, or the stains used in histologic or bacteriologic work, or that in paints. **2.** A medicinal preparation for external use, applied to the skin like paint or coloring agents used in paints. [L. *pigmentum,* paint]

pig·men·tar·y (pig′mĕn-tar-ē) Relating to a pigment.

pig·men·tar·y ret·i·nop·a·thy (pig′mĕn-tar-ē ret′i-nop′ă-thē) Photoreceptor degeneration associated with pigmentary changes in the retina and choroid. SEE ALSO retinitis pigmentosa.

pig·men·ta·tion (pig-mĕn-tā′shŭn) Coloration, either normal or pathologic, of the skin or tissues resulting from a deposit of pigment.

pig·ment dis·per·sion syn·drome (pig′mĕnt dis-per′zhŭn sin′drōm) Increased resistance to the flow of aqueous humor through the pupil from the anterior chamber to the posterior chamber, leading to posterior bowing of the peripheral iris against the zonules; a possible mechanism for pigmentary glaucoma.

pig·ment·ed (pig′men-tĕd) Colored as the result of a deposit of pigment.

pig·ment·ed lay·er of ret·i·na (pig′men-tĕd lā-ĕr ret′i-nă) The outer layer of the retina, consisting of pigmented epithelium.

pig·ment·ed vil·lo·nod·u·lar syn·o·vi·tis (pig′men-tĕd vil-lō′nod′yū-lăr sin′ō-vī′tis) Diffuse outgrowths of synovial membrane of a joint, usually the knee, composed of synovial villi and fibrous nodules infiltrated by hemosiderin- and lipid-containing macrophages and multinucleated giant cells; the condition may be inflammatory, although recurrence is likely to follow incomplete removal.

pig·ment·ed vil·lo·nod·u·lar ten·o·syn·o·vi·tis (pig′men-tĕd vil-ō-nod′yū-lăr ten′ō-sin′ō-vī′tis) SYN villous tenosynovitis.

pig·men·to·ly·sin (pig-men′tō-lī-sin) An antibody causing destruction of pigment. [L. *pigmentum,* pigment, + G. *lysis,* a loosening]

pig·men·tum ni·grum (pig-men′tŭm nī′grŭm) Melanin of the choroid coat of the eye.

pig·tail cath·e·ter (pig′tāl kath′ĕ-tĕr) An angiographic catheter with a tightly curled end to reduce the impact of the injectant on the vessel wall.

PIH Abbreviation for prolactin-inhibiting hormone.

pi·lar, pi·la·ry (pī′lăr, pil′ă-rē) SYN hairy. [L. *pilus,* hair]

pi·lar cyst (pī′lăr sist) A common cyst of the skin and subcutis that contains sebum and keratin; lined by pale-staining stratified epithelial cells derived from follicular trichilemma.

pi·lar tu·mor of scalp (pī′lăr tū′mŏr skalp) A benign but sometimes ulcerative solitary tumor of the scalp in elderly women.

pile (pīl) **1.** A series of plates of two different metals imposed alternately one on the other, separated by a sheet of material moistened with a dilute acid solution, used to produce a current of electricity. [L. *pila,* pillar] **2.** An individual hemorrhoidal tumor. SEE hemorrhoids. [L. *pila,* ball]

pi·le·ous (pī′lē-ŭs) SYN hairy. [L. *pilus,* hair]

pi·le·ous gland (pī′lē-ŭs gland) A sebaceous gland emptying into the hair follicle.

piles (pīlz) SYN hemorrhoids. [L. *pila,* a ball]

pi·li (pī′lī) Plural of pilus. [L.]

pi·li tor·ti (pī′lī tōr′tī) A condition in which many hair shafts are twisted on the long axis; congenital, or acquired as a result of distortion of the follicles from a scarring inflammatory process, mechanical stress, or cicatrizing alopecia; the hair shafts resemble spangles in reflected light, are brittle, and break at varying lengths, with many areas appearing bald with a dark stubble; as a developmental defect, it can be manifested in such syndromes as Björnstad, Crandall, and Menkes. SYN twisted hairs.

pill (pil) **1.** A small, globular mass of soluble material containing a medicinal substance to be swallowed; colloquially, any solid dosage form of oral medicine, including tablets and capsules. **2.** "The pill"; colloquial term for an oral contraceptive. [L. *pilula;* dim. of *pila,* ball]

pil·lar (pil′ăr) A structure or part having a resemblance to a column or pillar. [L. *pila*]

pil·lars of fau·ces (pil′lărz faw′sēz) SEE palatoglossal arch, palatopharyngeal arch.

pil·lars of for·nix (pil′lărz fōr′niks) The columna fornicis and crus fornicis.

pil·low splint (pil′ō splint) A splint that is inflatable or made from unusually bulky fabric.

pill-roll·ing trem·or (pil′rōl-ing trem′ŏr) A rhythmic circular movement of the opposed tips of the thumb and index finger, a form of tremor noted in parkinsonism, tardive dyskinesia, and other extrapyramidal syndromes.

♻ **pilo-** Combining form meaning hair. [L. *pilus*]

pi·lo·be·zoar (pī-lō-bē′zōr) SYN trichobezoar. [pilo- + bezoar]

pi·lo·car·pine i·on·to·phor·e·sis sweat chlo·ride test (pī′lō-kahr′pēn ī′ŏn-tō-fōr-ē′sis swĕt klōr′īd test) The definitive procedure for confirming the diagnosis of cystic fibrosis. The sodium and chloride levels in sweat are significantly elevated in children with cystic fibrosis. At least two positive test results are required before diagnosis is confirmed.

pi·lo·cys·tic (pi-lō-sis′tik) Denoting a dermoid cyst containing hair. [pilo- + G. *kystis,* bladder]

pi·lo·cy·tic as·tro·cy·to·ma (pī′lō-sit′ĭk as′trō-sī-tō′mă) A slowly growing astrocytoma composed histologically of elongated astrocytes; often located in the optic chiasm region of the third ventricle, hypothalamus, or cerebellum, predominantly in younger individuals.

pi·lo·e·rec·tion (pī′lō-ē-rek′shŭn) Erection of hair due to action of arrectores pilorum muscles.

pi·loid (pī′loyd) Hairlike; resembling hair. [pilo- + G. *eidos,* resemblance]

pi·lo·jec·tion (pī-lō-jek′shŭn) Process of shooting shafts of stiff mammalian hair into a saccular aneurysm in the brain to produce thrombosis. [pilo- + injection]

pi·lo·ma·trix·o·ma (pī′lō-mā-trik-sō′mă) A benign solitary hair follicle tumor containing cells resembling basal cell carcinoma and areas of epithelial necrosis. See this page. SYN Malherbe calcifying epithelioma. [pilo- + matrix + G. *-oma,* tumor]

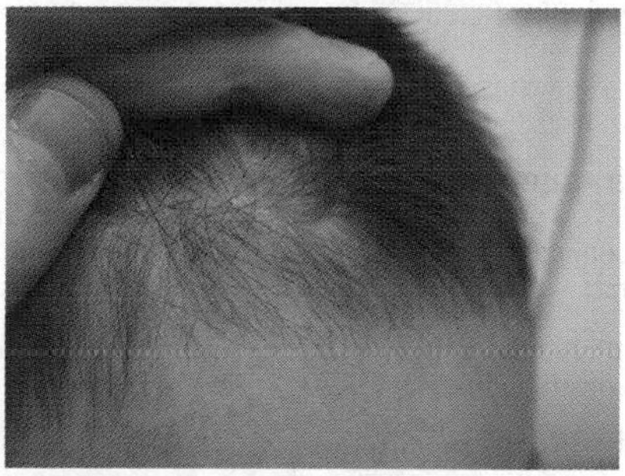

pilomatrixoma

pi·lo·mo·tor (pī′lō-mō′tŏr) Moving the hair; denoting the arrectores pilorum muscles of the skin and the postganglionic sympathetic nerve fibers innervating these small, smooth muscles. [pilo- + L. *motor,* mover]

pi·lo·mo·tor re·flex (pī′lō-mō′tŏr rē′fleks) Contraction of the smooth muscle of the skin resulting in "gooseflesh" caused by mild application of a tactile stimulus or by local cooling.

pi·lo·ni·dal (pī′lō-nī′dăl) Denoting the presence of hair in a dermoid cyst or in a sinus opening on the skin. [pilo- + L. *nidus,* nest]

pi·lo·ni·dal si·nus (pī′lō-nī′dăl sī′nŭs) A fistula or pit in the sacral region, communicating with the exterior, containing loose, broken-off body hairs that may act as a foreign body producing chronic inflammation.

pi·lose (pī′lōs) SYN hairy. [L. *pilosus*]

pi·lo·se·ba·ceous (pī′lō-sē-bā′shŭs) Relating to the hair follicles and sebaceous glands. [pilo- + L. *sebum,* suet]

pi·lus, pl. **pi·li** (pī′lŭs, -lī) **1.** One of the fine, keratinized, filamentous epidermal growths arising from the skin of the body of mammals except the palms, soles, and flexor surfaces of the joints; the full length and texture of the hair varies markedly in different body sites. **2.** A fine filamentous appendage, somewhat analogous to the flagellum, that occurs on some bacteria. SYN fimbria (2). SEE ALSO conjugative plasmid. [L.]

pi·mel·ic ac·id (pi-mel′ik as′id) An intermediate in the oxidation of oleic acid in some microorganisms; a precursor of biotin.

pimelo- Prefix meaning fat, fatty. [G. *pimelē,* soft fat, lard, fr. *piar,* fat]

pim·ple (pim′pĕl) A papule or small pustule; usually meant to denote an inflammatory lesion of acne.

PIN Abbreviation for prostatic intraepithelial neoplasia; provider identification number; personal identification number.

pin (pin) Rod used in surgical treatment of bone fractures. SEE ALSO nail. [O.E. *pinn,* fr. L. *pinna,* feather]

Pi·nard ma·neu·ver (pē-nahr′ mă-nū′vĕr) In management of a frank breech presentation, pressure on the popliteal space is made by the index finger while the other three fingers flex the leg while sliding it along the other thigh as the foot of the flexed leg is brought down and out.

pince·ment (pans-mahn[h]′) A pinching manipulation in massage. [Fr. pinching]

pin·cer grasp (pin′sĕr grasp) A grasp pattern emerging in the 10th–12th month whereby a small object is held between the distal pads of the opposed thumb and index or middle finger. The MCP and PIP joints of the index finger are slightly flexed, whereas the DIP joint is extended.

pin·cer nail (pin′sĕr nāl) Transverse overcurvature of the nail that increases distally, causing the lateral borders of the nail to pinch the soft tissue with resulting tenderness; may result from a developmental anomaly or subungual exostosis.

pinch (pinch) OCCUPATIONAL THERAPY a grip between the fingers at the most distal joints. SEE ALSO lateral pinch, pad-to-pad pinch, palmar pinch, tip pinch. See page 1214.

pinch graft (pinch graft) Small bits of skin, of partial or full thickness, removed from a healthy area and seeded in a site to be covered.

pin·cush·ion dis·tor·tion (pin-ku′shŭn dis-tōr′shŭn) Irregular image produced when axial magnification is greater than peripheral magnification. SEE Petzval surface.

pin·e·al (pin′ē-ăl) **1.** Shaped like a pinecone. SYN

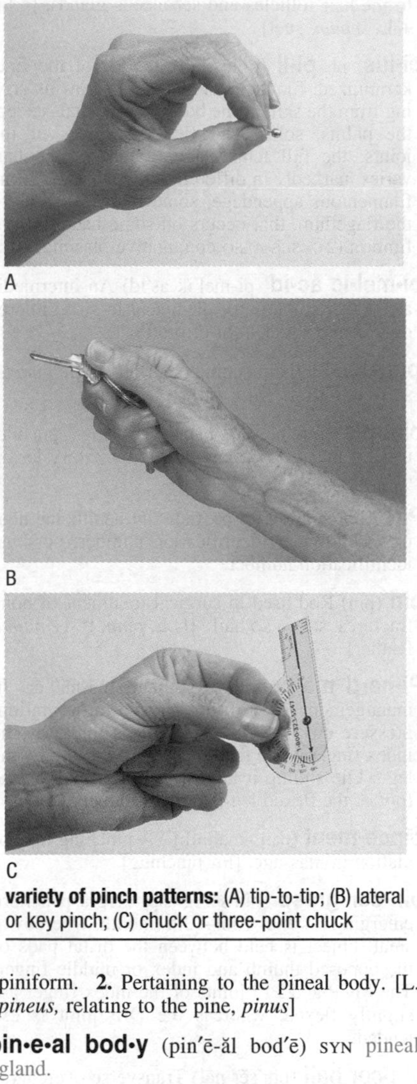

variety of pinch patterns: (A) tip-to-tip; (B) lateral or key pinch; (C) chuck or three-point chuck

piniform. **2.** Pertaining to the pineal body. [L. *pineus,* relating to the pine, *pinus*]

pin•e•al bod•y (pin′ē-ăl bod′ē) SYN pineal gland.

pin•e•al bud (pin′ē-ăl bŭd) A median evagination of the caudal part of the diencephalon; proliferation of the cells in its walls converts it into the pineal gland (body). SYN pineal diverticulum.

pin•e•al di•ver•tic•u•lum (pin′ē-ăl dī′vĕr-tik′yū-lŭm) SYN pineal bud.

pin•e•al•ec•to•my (pin′ē-ă-lek′tŏ-mē) Removal of the pineal body. [pineal + G. *ektomē,* excision]

pin•e•al gland (pin′ē-ăl gland) A small, unpaired, flattened body shaped something like a pinecone; attached at its anterior pole to the region of the posterior and habenular commissures, and lying in the depression between the two superior colliculi below the splenium of the corpus callosum. It is a glandular structure, composed of follicles containing epitheloid cells and lime concentrations called 'brain sand'; despite its attachment to the brain, it appears to receive nerve fibers exclusively from the peripheral autonomic nervous system. It produces melanin. SYN corpus pineale [TA], pineal body.

pin•e•a•lo•cyte (pin-ē′al-ō-sīt) A cell of the pineal body with long processes ending in bulbous expansions. Pinealocytes receive a direct innervation from sympathetic neurons that form recognizable synapses. [pineal + G. *kytos,* cell]

pin•e•a•lo•ma (pin′ē-ă-lō′mă) A term that has been variably used to designate germ cell tumors, pineocytomas, and pineoblastomas of the pineal gland. [pineal + G. *-oma,* tumor]

pin•e•al stalk (pin′ē-ăl stawk) The attachment of the pineal gland (body) to the roof of the third ventricle; it contains the pineal recess of the third ventricle.

Pi•nel sys•tem (pē-nel′ sis′tĕm) The abolition of forcible restraint in the treatment of the mental hospital patient.

pin•e•o•blas•to•ma (pin′ē-ō-blas-tō′mă) A poorly differentiated tumor of the pineal gland consisting of small cells with a scant amount of cytoplasms and often forming pseudorosettes. [pineal + G. *blastos,* germ, + *-oma,* tumor]

pin•guec•u•la, pin•guic•u•la (ping-gwek′yū-lă) A yellowish accumulation of protein on the conjunctiva. [L. *pinguiculus,* fattish, fr. *pinguis,* fat]

pin•hole pu•pil (pin-hōl pyū′pil) An extremely constricted pupil.

pin•i•form (pin′i-fōrm) SYN pineal (1). [L. *pinus,* pine, + *forma,* form]

pink dis•ease (pingk di-zēz′) SYN acrodynia (2).

pink•eye (pink′ī) **1.** SYN acute viral conjunctivitis. **2.** SYN infectious bovine keratoconjunctivitis. **3.** In horses, a form of equine viral arteritis.

pink-top tube (pingk-top tūb) A tube of this color indicates the container has been treated with EDTA as an anticoagulant; used for blood typing.

pin•na, pl. **pin•nae** (pin′ă, -ē) **1.** SYN auricle (1). **2.** A feather, wing, or fin. [L. *pinna* or *penna,* a feather, in pl. a wing]

pin•nal (pin′ăl) Relating to the pinna.

pin•o•cyte (pin′ō-sīt) A cell that exhibits pinocytosis. [G. *pineō,* to drink, + *kytos,* cell]

pin•o•cy•to•sis (pin′ō-sī-tō′sis) The cellular process of actively engulfing liquid, a phenomenon in which minute incuppings or invaginations are formed in the surface of the cell membrane and close to form fluid-filled vesicles; it resembles phagocytosis. [pinocyte + G. *-osis,* condition]

pin•o•some (pin′ō-sōm) A fluid-filled vacuole formed by pinocytosis. [G. *pineō,* to drink, + *sōma,* body]

Pins sign (pinz sīn) SYN Ewart sign.

Pins syn•drome (pinz sin′drōm) Dullness, diminution of vocal fremitus and of the vesicular murmur, and a slight, distant blowing sound, heard in the posteroinferior region of the chest on the left side, in cases of pericardial effusion; there is sometimes also a fine rale in this region, but all the adventitious auscultatory signs disappear when the patient assumes the knee-chest position.

pint (pīnt) A measure of quantity (U.S. liquid), containing 16 fluid ounces, 28.875 cubic inches, 473.1765 cubic centimeters. An imperial pint contains 20 British fluid ounces, 34.67743 cubic inches, 568.2615 cubic centimeters.

pin•ta (pin′tă) A disease caused by a spirochete, *Treponema carateum;* characterized by a small primary papule followed by an enlarging plaque and disseminated secondary macules of varying color called pintids that finally become white. Occurs in semiarid, warm climates (such as are found in areas of Central and South America). SYN mal del pinto. [Sp. *painted*]

pin•worm (pin′wŏrm) A member of the genus *Enterobius* or related nematodes causing intestinal parasitism in a large variety of vertebrates, including humans (*Enterobius vermicularis*, the human pinworm). SYN scatworm.

PIP Abbreviation for proximal interphalangeal joints.

Pi•per for•ceps (pī′pĕr fōr′seps) Obstetric forceps used to facilitate delivery of the head in breech presentation.

pi•pette, **pi•pet** (pī-pet′) A graduated tube (marked in mL) used to transport a definite volume of a gas or liquid in laboratory work. [Fr. dim. of *pipe,* pipe]

pir•i•form (pir′i-fōrm) Pear-shaped. [L. *pirum,* pear, + *forma,* form]

pi•ri•for•mis mus•cle (pir′i-fōrm′is mŭs′ĕl) *Origin*, margins of pelvic sacral foramina and greater sciatic notch of ilium; *insertion*, upper border of greater trochanter; *action*, rotates thigh laterally; *nerve supply*, nerve to piriformis (sciatic plexus). SYN musculus piriformis [TA], piriform muscle.

pir•i•form mus•cle (pir′i-fōrm mŭs′ĕl) SYN piriformis muscle.

pir•i•form neu•ron lay•er (pir′i-fōrm nūr′on lā′ĕr) The layer of Purkinje cells between the molecular and granular layers of the cerebellar cortex.

Pi•ro•goff am•pu•ta•tion (pēr′ō-gof amp′yū-tā′shŭn) Surgical removal of the foot; the lower articular surfaces of the tibia and fibula are sawed through and the ends covered with a portion of the os calcis, which has also been sawed through from above posteriorly downward and forward.

Pir•quet test (pēr-kvet′ test) A cutaneous tuberculin test. SEE tuberculin test.

pis•i•form (pis′i-fōrm) In the shape or size of a pea. [L. *pisum,* pea, + *forma,* appearance]

pis•i•form bone (pis′i-fōrm bōn) A small bone resembling a pea in size and shape, in the proximal row of the carpus, lying on the anterior surface of the triquetral, with which it articulates; it gives insertion to the tendon of the flexor carpi ulnaris muscle.

pit (pit) **1.** Any natural depression on the surface of the body, such as the axilla (armpit). Cf. dimple. **2.** SYN pockmark. **3.** A depression in the enamel surface of a tooth due to faulty or incomplete calcification or formed at the confluent point of two or more lobes of enamel. **4.** To indent, as by pressure of the finger on the edematous skin; to become indented, said of the edematous tissues when pressure is made with the fingertip. [L. *puteus*]

pit-1 (pit) A nuclear binding transcriptional factor found in many cells in normal human pituitary glands and expressed in a large percentage of pituitary adenomas, in particular those positive for growth hormone, or thyrotropin.

pitch (pich) Auditory perception of tone on a scale ranging from low to high, based on the frequency of vibration of the object emitting the tone. For the human voice, pitch relates to frequency of vibration of the vocal folds. SEE voice, frequency.

pitch wart (pich wōrt) A precancerous keratotic epidermal tumor, common among people working with pitch and coal tar derivatives.

pith (pith) **1.** The center of a hair. **2.** The spinal cord and medulla oblongata. **3.** To pierce the medulla of an animal with a sharp instrument introduced at the base of the skull. [A.S. *pitha*]

pith•e•coid (pith′ĕ-koyd) Resembling an ape. [G. *pithēkos,* ape, + *eidos,* resemblance]

Pi•tres sign (pē′trĕ sīn) **1.** SYN haphalgesia. **2.** Diminished sensation in the testes and scrotum in tabes dorsalis.

pit•ted ker•a•tol•y•sis (pit′tĕd ker′ă-tol′i-sis) Noninflammatory gram-positive bacterial infection of the plantar surfaces producing small depressions in the stratum corneum; associated frequently with humidity and hyperhidrosis.

pit•ting (pit′ing) DENTISTRY the formation of well-defined, relatively deep depressions in a surface, usually used in describing defects in surfaces (often golds, solder joints, or amalgam). It may arise from a variety of causes, although the clinical occurrence is often associated with corrosion. SEE ALSO pitting edema, nail pits.

pit·ting e·de·ma (pit′ing ĕ-dē′mă) Edema that retains for a time the indentation produced by pressure. See this page.

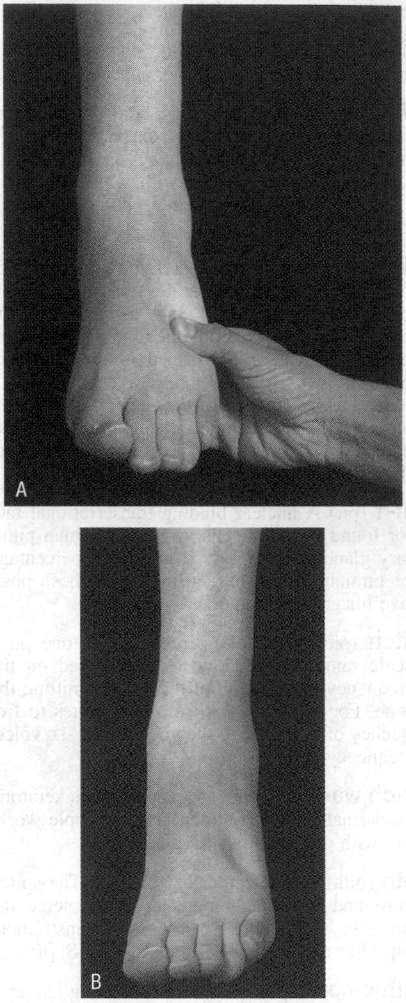

pitting edema: (A) finger pressure is applied to area near ankle; (B) when pressure is released, indentation remains in edematous tissue

Pitts·burgh pneu·mo·ni·a (pits′bŭrg nū-mō′nē-ă) A variant of Legionnaire's disease caused by *Legionella micdadei.*

Pitts·burgh pneu·mo·ni·a a·gent (pits′bŭrg nū-mō′nē-ă ā′jĕnt) SYN *Legionella micdadei.*

pi·tu·i·cyte (pi-tū′i-sīt) The primary cell of the posterior lobe of the pituitary gland, a fusiform cell closely related to neuroglia. [pituitary + G. *kytos,* cell]

pi·tu·i·cy·to·ma (pi-tū′i-sī-tō′mă) A rare gliogenous neoplasm derived from pituicytes, occurring in the posterior lobe of the pituitary gland and characterized by cells with small nuclei and long processes that form a network of cytoplasmic material, in which droplets of fat may be demonstrated. [pituicyte + G. *-oma,* tumor]

pi·tu·i·tar·ism (pi-tū′i-tar-izm) Pituitary dysfunction. SEE hyperpituitarism, hypopituitarism.

pi·tu·i·tar·y (pi-tū′i-tar-ē) Relating to the pituitary gland (hypophysis). [L. *pituita,* phlegm]

pi·tu·i·tar·y ca·chex·i·a (pi-tū′i-tar-ē kă-kek′sē-ă) SYN Simmonds disease.

pi·tu·i·tar·y di·ver·tic·u·lum (pi-tū′i-tar-ē dī′vĕr-tik′yū-lŭm) SYN hypophysial diverticulum.

pi·tu·i·tar·y dwarf·ism (pi-tū′i-tar-ē dwōrf′izm) A rare form of dwarfism caused by the absence of a functional anterior pituitary gland; may be present at birth or develop during early childhood.

pi·tu·i·tar·y dys·to·pi·a (pi-tū′i-tar-ē dis-tō′pē-ă) Failure of union of neurohypophysis and adenohypophysis.

pi·tu·i·tar·y gi·gan·tism (pi-tū′i-tar-ē jī-gant′izm) A form of gigantism caused by hypersecretion of pituitary growth hormone; a rare disorder commonly the result of a pituitary adenoma.

pi·tu·i·tar·y gland (pi-tū′i-tar-ē gland) SYN hypophysis.

pi·tu·i·tar·y go·nad·o·tro·pic hor·mone (pi-tū′i-tar-ē gō-nad′ō-trō′pik hōr′mōn) SYN anterior pituitary gonadotropin.

pi·tu·i·tar·y growth hor·mone (pi-tū′i-tar-ē grōth hōr′mōn) SYN somatotropin.

pi·tu·i·tar·y myx·e·de·ma (pi-tū′i-tar-ē mik-sĕ-dē′mă) A form of hypothyroidism resulting from inadequate secretion of the thyrotropic hormone; commonly occurs in association with inadequate secretion of other anterior pituitary hormones.

pi·tu·i·tar·y stalk (pi-tū′i-tar-ē stawk) A process comprising the tuberal part investing the infundibular stem that attaches the hypophysis to the tuber cinereum at the base of the brain.

pit·y·ri·a·sic (pit′i-rī-as′ik) Relating to or suffering from pityriasis.

pit·y·ri·a·sis (pit′i-rī′ă-sis) A dermatosis marked by branny desquamation. [G., fr. *pityron,* bran, dandruff]

pit·y·ri·a·sis al·ba (pit′i-rī′ă-sis al′bă) Patchy hypopigmentation of the skin resulting from mild dermatitis.

pit·y·ri·a·sis lin·guae (pit′i-rī′ă-sis ling′gwē) SYN geographic tongue.

pit·y·ri·a·sis ro·se·a (pit′i-rī′ă-sis rōz′ē-ă) A self-limited eruption of macules or papules involving the trunk and, less frequently, extremities, scalp, and face; the lesions are usually oval and follow the crease lines of the skin; the onset is frequently preceded by a single larger scaling lesion known as the herald patch.

pit·y·ri·a·sis ru·bra (pit′i-rī′ă-sis rū′bră) SYN exfoliative dermatitis.

pit·y·ri·a·sis ru·bra pi·la·ris (pit′i-rē′ă-sis rū-bră pi-lā′ris) An uncommon chronic pruritic eruption of the hair follicles, which become firm, red, surmounted with a horny plug, and often confluent to form scaly plaques.

pit·y·ri·a·sis ver·si·col·or (pit′i-rī′ă-sis ver′si-kŭl-ŏr) SYN tinea versicolor.

pit·y·roid (pit′i-royd) SYN furfuraceous. [G. *pityrōdēs,* branlike, fr. *pityron,* bran, + *eidos,* resemblance]

Pit·y·ro·spo·rum (pit-i-rō-spō′rŭm) A genus of fungi found in dandruff and seborrheic dermatitis. [G. *pityron,* bran, + *sporos,* seed]

PIVKA (piv′kă) Acronym for protein induced by vitamin K absence.

piv·ot joint (piv′ŏt joynt) A synovial joint in which a section of a cylinder of one bone fits into a corresponding cavity on the other. SYN rotary joint, rotatory joint, trochoid joint.

pix·el (piks′ĕl) A contraction for picture element, a two-dimensional representation of a volume element (voxel) in the display of the CT or MR image, usually 512 by 512 or 256 by 256 pixels respectively.

PJC Abbreviation for premature junctional contraction.

PJ in·ter·val (in′tĕr-văl) The time elapsing from the beginning of the P wave to the end of the QRS complex (J for junction between QRS and T wave) in the electrocardiogram.

PK Abbreviation for pyruvate kinase.

pK_a The negative decadic logarithm of the ionization constant (K_a) of an acid; equal to the pH value at which equal concentrations of the acid and conjugate base forms of a substance (often a buffer) are present.

pkat Abbreviation for picokatal.

PKU Abbreviation for phenylketonuria.

pla·ce·bo (plă-sē′bō) **1.** A medicinally inactive substance given as a medicine for its suggestive effect. **2.** An inert compound identical in appearance to material being tested in experimental research, which may or may not be known to the physician or patient, administered to distinguish between drug action and suggestive effect of the material under study. **3.** Any treatment or intervention with no intrinsic therapeutic value performed to achieve a "placebo effect." [L. I will please, future of *placeo*]

place cod·ing (plas kōd′ing) Frequency coding as determined by the activation of the spiral organ (organ of Corti) from the base to the apex of the cochlea in a gradation with higher frequencies transmitted from near the base and lower frequencies from near the apex.

pla·cen·ta (plă-sen′tă) Fetomaternal organ of metabolic interchange between embryo or fetus and mother. It has a portion of embryonic origin, derived from the outermost embryonic membrane (villous chorion), and a maternal portion formed by a modification of the part of the uterine mucosa (decidua basalis) in which the chorionic vesicle is implanted. Within the placenta, the chorionic villi, with their contained capillaries carrying blood of the embryonic circulation, are exposed to maternal blood in the intervillous spaces in which the villi lie; no direct mixing of fetal and maternal blood occurs, but the intervening tissue (the placental membrane) is sufficiently permeable to permit the absorption of nutritive materials, oxygen, and some harmful substances, such as viruses, into the fetal blood, and the release of carbon dioxide and nitrogenous waste from it. At term, the human placenta is disc shaped, about 4 cm thick and 18 cm in diameter, and averages about one sixth to one seventh the weight of the fetus; its fetal surface is smooth, being formed by the adherent amnion, with the umbilical cord usually attached near its center; the maternal surface of a detached placenta is rough because of the torn decidual tissue adhering to the chorion and shows lobular elevations called cotyledons. See page 1218. [L. a cake]

pla·cen·ta ac·cre·ta (plă-sen′tă ă-krē′tă) The abnormal adherence of the chorionic villi to the myometrium, associated with partial or complete absence of the decidua basalis and, in particular, the stratum spongiosum.

pla·cen·ta cir·cum·val·la·ta (plă-sen′tă sĕr-kŭm-val-lā′tă) A cup-shaped placenta with raised edges, having a thick, round, white, opaque ring around its periphery; a portion of the decidua separates the margin of the placenta from its chorionic plate; the remainder of the chorionic surface is normal in appearance, but the fetal vessels are limited in their course across the placenta by the ring. SEE ALSO placenta marginata, placenta reflexa.

pla·cen·ta fe·nes·tra·ta (plă-sen′tă fĕ-nes-tră′tă) A placenta in which there are sometimes areas of thinning where placental tissue is absent.

pla·cen·ta in·cre·ta (plă-sen′tă in-krē′tă) A placenta in which the chorionic villi invade the myometrium.

pla·cen·tal (plă-sen′tăl) Relating to the placenta.

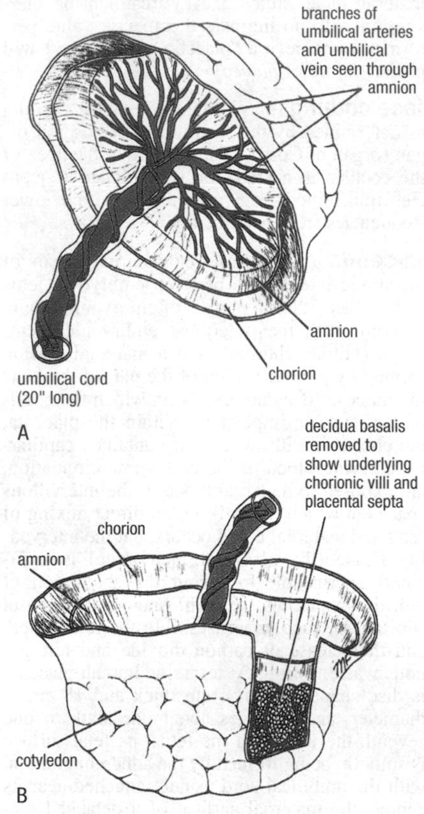

mature placenta: as seen from the fetal surface (A) and from the maternal surface (B)

pla·cen·tal ab·rup·tion (plă-sen′tăl ab-rŭp′shŭn) Premature separation of a normally situated placenta from the uterine wall after the 20th week of gestation.

pla·cen·tal bar·ri·er (plă-sen′tăl bar′ē-ĕr) SYN placental membrane.

pla·cen·tal cir·cu·la·tion (plă-sen′tăl sĭr′kyū-lā′shŭn) The circulation of fetal blood through the placenta during intrauterine life, serving the needs of the fetus for aeration, absorption, and excretion; also, there is circulation of maternal blood through the intervillous space of the placenta.

pla·cen·tal dys·to·ci·a (plă-sen′tăl dis-tō′sē-ă) Retention or difficult delivery of the placenta.

pla·cen·tal growth hor·mone (plă-sen′tăl grōth hōr′mōn) SYN human placental lactogen.

pla·cen·tal mem·brane (plă-sen′tăl mem′brān) The semipermeable layer of fetal tissue separating the maternal from the fetal blood in the placenta; composed of: 1) endothelium of the fetal tissues in the chorionic villi, 2) stromata of the villi, 3) cytotrophoblast (negligible after the fifth month of gestation), and 4) syncytiotrophoblast covering the villi; the placental membrane acts as a selective membrane regulating passage of substances from the maternal to the fetal blood. SYN placental barrier.

pla·cen·tal pre·sen·ta·tion (plă-sen′tăl prez′ĕn-tā′shŭn) SYN placenta previa.

pla·cen·tal souf·fle (plă-sen′tăl sū′fĕl) A soft humming or blowing sound produced by fetal circulation at the placenta. [Fr. *souffle,* puff]

pla·cen·tal trans·fu·sion syn·drome (plă-sen′tăl trans-fyū′zhŭn sin′drōm) In utero transfusion of blood from one twin to the other such that the donor becomes anemic and growth retarded and the recipient becomes polycythemic and develops hydrops. SEE ALSO twin-twin transfusion.

pla·cen·ta mar·gi·na·ta (plă-sen′tă mahr-ji-nā′tă) A placenta with raised edges, less pronounced than the placenta circumvallata. SEE ALSO placenta reflexa.

pla·cen·ta mem·bra·na·ce·a (plă-sen′tă mĕm′brā-nā′shē-ă) An abnormally thin placenta covering an unusually large area of the decidua basalis (uterine lining).

pla·cen·ta pre·vi·a (plă-sen′tă prē′vē-ă) The condition in which the placenta is implanted in the lower segment of the uterus, extending to the margin of the internal os of the cervix or partially or completely obstructing the os. SYN placental presentation.

pla·cen·ta re·flex·a (plă-sen′tă rē-fleks′ă) An anomaly of the placenta in which the margin is thickened so as to appear turned back on itself. SEE ALSO placenta circumvallata, placenta marginata.

pla·cen·ta spu·ri·a (plă-sen′tă spū′rē-ă) A mass of placental tissue that has no vascular connection with the main placenta.

plac·en·ta·tion (plās-en-tā′shŭn) The structural organization and mode of attachment of fetal to maternal tissues in the formation of the placenta.

plac·en·ti·tis (plās-en-tī′tis) Inflammation of the placenta.

plac·en·to·ma (plas-en-tō′mă) SYN deciduoma.

place of ser·vice (POS) (plās sĕr′vis) In health care informatics, concrete designation of the physical area wherein a service is performed (e.g., hospital, physician's office, patient's home, long-term care facility). SEE ALSO POS.

Pla·ci·do da Cos·ta disc (plah′sē-dō dah kōs′tah disk) SYN keratoscope.

plac·ode (plak′ōd) Local thickening in the embryonic ectodermal layer; the cells of the placode ordinarily constitute a primordial group from which a sense organ or ganglion develops. [G.

plakōdēs, fr. *plax,* anything flat or broad, + *eidos,* like]

pla•fond (plă-fond′) A ceiling, especially the ceiling of the ankle joint, i.e., the articular surface of the distal end of the tibia. [Fr. ceiling]

♲ **plagio-** Combining form meaning oblique, slanting. [G. *plagios*]

pla•gi•o•ce•phal•ic (plā′jē-ō-se-fal′ik) Relating to or marked by plagiocephaly.

pla•gi•o•ceph•a•ly (plā′jē-ō-sef′ă-lē) An asymmetric craniostenosis due to premature closure of the lambdoid and coronal sutures on one side; characterized by an oblique deformity of the cranium. SYN asynclitism of the skull. [G. *plagios,* oblique, + *kephalē,* head]

plague (plāg) **1.** Any disease of wide prevalence or of excessive mortality. **2.** An acute infectious disease caused by *Yersinia pestis* and marked by high fever, toxemia, prostration, a petechial eruption, lymph node enlargement, and pneumonia, or hemorrhage from the mucous membranes; primarily a disease of rodents, transmitted to humans by fleas that have bitten infected animals. In humans, the disease takes one of four clinical forms: bubonic *plague*, septicemic *plague*, pneumonic *plague*, or ambulant *plague*. SYN pestilence (1). SEE ALSO black death. [L. *plaga,* a stroke, injury]

plain film (plān film) A radiograph made without use of a contrast medium.

♲ **-plakia** Combining form meaing a plate or flat plane, usually on a mucous membrane. [G. *plakos,* plate]

plan (plan) **1.** A program or method for the achievement of an objective. **2.** A picture or diagram showing a structure or arrangement of parts. [Fr. *plant*, ground plan, fr. L. *planta*, sole of the foot]

pla•na (plā′nă) Plural of planum. [L.]

plan of care (plan kār) SYN care plan.

Planck con•stant (*h*) (plahngk kon′stănt) A constant, $6.6260755 \times 10^{-34}$ J · s (joule-seconds) or $6.6260755 \times 10^{-27}$ erg-seconds = $6.6260755 \times 10^{-34}$ J Hz^{-1} (joule per hertz).

Planck the•o•ry (plahngk thē′ŏr-ē) SYN quantum theory.

plane (plān) **1.** A flat surface. SEE ALSO planum. **2.** An imaginary surface formed by extension through any axis or two definite points, in reference to pelvimetry and especially to craniometry. [L. *planus,* flat]

plane joint (plān joynt) A synovial joint in which the opposing surfaces are nearly planes and in which there is only a slight, gliding motion, as in the intermetacarpal joints. SYN arthrodia, arthrodial joint, gliding joint.

plane of pel•vic ca•nal (plān pel′vik kă-nal′) SYN pelvic axis.

plane su•ture (plān sū′chŭr) A simple, firm apposition of two smooth surfaces of bones, without overlap, as seen in the lacrimomaxillary suture. SYN harmonic suture.

pla•nig•ra•phy (plă-nig′ră-fē) SYN tomography. [L. *planum,* plane, + G. *graphē,* a writing]

plan•ing (plān′ing) SYN dermabrasion.

plan•ning (plăn′ing) The act of formulating or drafting a plan.

♲ **plano-, plan-, plani-** Combining forms meaning **1.** A plane; flat, level. [L. *planum,* plane; *planus,* flat] **2.** Wandering.

pla•no•cel•lu•lar (plā-nō-sel′yū-lăr) Relating to or composed of flat cells. [L. *planus,* flat, + cellular]

pla•no•con•cave (plā′nō-kon′kāv) Flat on one side and concave on the other; denoting a lens of that shape.

pla•no•con•cave lens (plā′nō-kon′kāv lenz) A lens that is flat on one side and concave on the other.

pla•no•con•vex (plā′nō-kon′veks) Flat on one side and convex on the other; denoting a lens of that shape.

pla•no•con•vex lens (plā′nō-kon′veks lenz) A lens that is flat on one side and convex on the other.

pla•nog•ra•phy (plă-nog′ră-tē) SYN tomography.

pla•no•val•gus (plā′nō-val′gŭs) A condition in which the longitudinal arch of the foot is flattened and everted. [plano- + L. *valgus,* turned outward]

plan•ta, gen. and pl. **plan•tae** (plan′tă, -tē) [TA] SYN sole. [L.]

plan•tal•gi•a (plan-tal′jē-ă) Pain on the plantar surface of the foot over the plantar fascia. [L. *planta,* sole of foot, + G. *algos,* pain]

plan•tar (plan′tahr) Relating to the sole of the foot or the caudal aspect of the tarsus on the hind limb of an animal. [L. *plantaris*]

plan•tar arch (plan′tahr ahrch) **1.** The arterial arch formed by the lateral plantar artery running across the bases of the metatarsal bones and anastomosing with the dorsalis pedis artery. **2.** Either of two bony arches of the foot, longitudinal arch or transverse arch.

plan•tar cal•ca•ne•o•na•vic•u•lar lig•a•ment (plan′tahr kal-kā′nē-ō-nă-vik′yŭ-lăr lig′ă-mĕnt) A dense, fibroelastic ligament that extends from the sustentaculum tali to the plantar surface of the navicular bone; it supports the head of the talus.

plan•tar fas•ci•a (plan′tahr fash′ē-ă) Deep fascia of the sole of the foot; includes a thick central part, the plantar aponeurosis, covering the central compartment of the sole of the foot, and thinner medial and lateral parts covering the hallucis and digit minimi muscles (compartments), respectively.

plan•tar fas•ci•i•tis (plan′tahr fash′ē-ī′tis) Inflammation of the fascia of the plantar surface of the foot, usually at the calcaneal attachment.

plan•tar fi•bro•ma•to•sis (plan′tahr fī′brō-mă-tō′sis) Nodular fibroblastic proliferation in plantar fascia of one or both feet; rarely associated with contracture. SYN Dupuytren disease of the foot.

plan•tar•flex•ion (plăn-tahr-flĕk′shŭn) Extension of the ankle, pointing of the foot and toes.

plan•tar in•ter•os•se•ous mus•cle (plan′tahr in-tĕr-os′ē-ŭs mŭs′ĕl) Three intrinsic muscles of foot; *origin*, the medial side of the third, fourth, and fifth metatarsal bones; *insertion*, corresponding side of proximal phalanx of the same toes; *action*, adducts three lateral toes; *nerve supply*, lateral plantar. SYN musculus interosseus plantaris [TA].

plan•tar•is mus•cle (plan-tā′ris mŭs′ĕl) *Origin*, lateral supracondylar ridge; *insertion*, medial margin of tendo achillis and deep fascia of ankle; *action*, traditionally described as plantar flexion of foot; many investigators now believe the plantaris muscle to be primarily a proprioceptive organ; *nerve supply*, tibial nerve. SYN musculus plantaris [TA], plantar muscle.

plan•tar me•ta•tar•sal ar•ter•y (plan′tahr met-ă-tahr′săl ahr′tĕr-ē) One of four branches of the plantar arterial arch that divides into plantar digital arteries to supply the toes. SYN arteria metatarsalis plantaris [TA].

plan•tar mus•cle (plan′tahr mŭs′ĕl) SYN plantaris muscle.

plan•tar re•flex (plan′tahr rē′fleks) The response to tactile stimulation of the ball of the foot, normally plantar flexion of the toes; the pathologic response is Babinski sign (1).

plan•tar space (plan′tahr spās) One of four areas between fascial layers in the foot, where pus may be confined when the foot is infected.

plan•tar wart (plan′tahr wōrt) An often painful wart on the sole; usually caused by human papillomavirus type 1. See this page. SYN verruca plantaris.

plan•ti•grade (plan′ti-grād) Walking with the entire sole and heel of the foot on the ground, as humans and bears do. [L. *planta,* sole, + *gradior,* to walk]

pla•num, pl. **pla•na** (plā′nŭm, -nă) [TA] A plane or flat surface. SEE ALSO plane. [L. plane]

plaque (plak) **1.** A patch or small, differentiated area on a body surface (e.g., skin, mucosa, or arterial endothelium) or on the cut surface of an organ such as the brain. **2.** An area of clearing in a flat, confluent growth of bacteria or tissue cells. **3.** A sharply defined zone of demyelination characteristic of multiple sclerosis. **4.** SEE dental plaque. See page B10. [Fr. a plate]

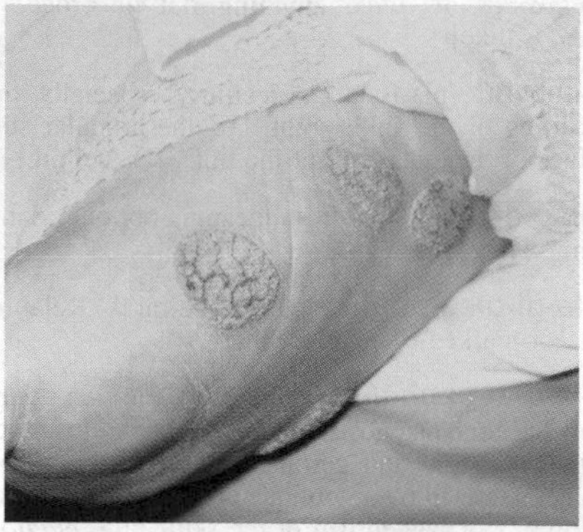

plantar warts: patient with paraplegia

-plasia Suffix denoting formation (especially of cells). SEE plasma-. [G. *plassō,* to form]

plasm (plazm) SYN plasma.

-plasm, -plasma Combining forms meaning tissue or living substance. [G. *plasma,* something formed]

plas•ma (plaz′mă) **1.** The fluid (noncellular) portion of the circulating blood, as distinguished from the serum obtained after coagulation. SYN blood plasma. **2.** The fluid portion of the lymph. **3.** A "fourth state of matter" in which, owing to elevated temperature (about 10^6 degrees), atoms have broken down to form free electrons and more or less stripped nuclei; produced in the laboratory in connection with hydrogen fusion (thermonuclear) research. SYN plasm. [G. something formed]

plasma-, plasmat-, plasmato-, plasmo- Combining forms meaning formative, organized; plasma. [G. *plasma,* something formed]

plas•ma ac•cel•er•a•tor glob•u•lin (plaz′mă ak-sel′ĕ-rā-tŏr glob′yū-lin) SYN factor V.

plas•ma•blast (plaz′mă-blast) Precursor of the plasma cell. [plasma + G. *blastos,* germ]

plas•ma cell (plaz′mă sel) An ovoid cell with an eccentric nucleus having chromatin arranged like a clock face or spokes of a wheel; the cytoplasm is strongly basophilic because of the abundant RNA in its endoplasmic reticulum; plasma cells are derived from B lymphocytes and are active in the formation of antibodies. SYN plasmacyte.

plas•ma cell leu•ke•mi•a (plaz′mă sel lū-kē′mē-ă) An unusual disease characterized by leukocytosis and other signs and symptoms that are suggestive of leukemia, in association with diffuse infiltrations and aggregates of plasma cells in the spleen, liver, bone marrow, and lymph nodes, and plasma cells in the blood.

plas•ma cell mas•ti•tis (plaz′mă sel mas-tī′tis) A condition of the breasts characterized by tumorlike indurated masses containing numerous plasma cells, usually resulting from mammary duct ectasia; although clinically resembling malignant disease (attachment to skin and enlargement of axillary lymph nodes), it is not neoplastic.

plas•ma cell my•e•lo•ma (plaz′mă sel mī-ĕ-lō′mă) **1.** SYN multiple myeloma. **2.** Plasmacytoma of bone, which is usually a solitary lesion and not associated with the occurrence of Bence Jones protein or other disturbances in the metabolism of protein (as observed in multiple myeloma).

plas•ma chol•ine•ste•rase (plaz′mă kō′lin-es′tĕr-ās) A type of cholinesterase found in plasma. SEE ALSO fluoride number. SYN butyrylcholinesterase, pseudocholinesterase.

plas•ma•crit (plaz′mă-krit) A measure of the percentage of the volume of blood occupied by plasma, in contrast to a hematocrit. [plasma + G. *krinō,* to separate]

plas•ma•crit test (plaz′mă-krit test) A serologic screening method for syphilis; heparinized blood is centrifuged in a capillary tube and the plasma thus separated with cardiolipin antigen. The presence of flocculation should not be regarded as conclusively diagnostic, but a negative result excludes the likelihood of syphilis.

plas•ma•cyte (plaz′mă-sīt) SYN plasma cell.

plas•ma•cy•to•ma (plaz′mă-sī-tō′mă) A discrete, presumably solitary mass of neoplastic plasma cells in bone or in one of various extramedullary sites; in humans, such lesions are probably the initial phase of developing plasma cell myeloma. [plasmacyte + G. *-oma,* tumor]

plas•ma•cy•to•sis (plaz′mă-sī-tō′sis) **1.** The presence of plasma cells in the circulating blood. **2.** The presence of unusually large proportions of plasma cells in the tissues or exudates. [plasmacyte + G. *-osis,* condition]

plas•ma fi•bro•nec•tin (plaz′mă fī′brō-nek′tin) A circulating α_2-glycoprotein that functions as an opsonin, mediating reticuloendothelial and macrophage clearance of fibrin microaggregates, collagen debris, and bacterial particulates, protecting microvascular perfusion and lymphatic drainage.

plas•ma•kin•ins (plaz-mă-kīn′inz) A group of highly active oligopeptides found in sera that act on smooth muscle of blood vessels, uterus, and bronchi (e.g., bradykinin, kallidin).

plas•ma•lem•ma (plaz-mă-lem′ă) SYN cell membrane. [plasma + G. *lemma,* husk]

plas•mal•o•gens (plaz-mal′ō-jenz) Generic term for glycerophospholipids in which the glycerol moiety bears a 1-alkenyl or 1-alkyl ether group.

plas•ma mem•brane (plaz′mă mem′brān) SYN cell membrane.

plas•ma•phe•re•sis (plaz′mă-fĕr-ē′sis) Removal of whole blood from the body, separation of its cellular elements by centrifugation, and reinfusion of these elements in a suspension of saline or some other plasma substitute, thus depleting the body's own plasma without depleting its cells. [plasma + G. *aphairesis,* a withdrawal]

plas•ma•phe•ret•ic (plaz′mă-fĕ-ret′ik) Relating to plasmapheresis.

plas•ma pro•teins (plaz′mă prō′tēnz) Dissolved proteins (more than 100) of blood plasma, mainly albumins and globulins (normally 6–8 g/100 mL); they hold fluid in blood vessels by osmosis and include antibodies and blood-clotting proteins.

plas•ma re•nin ac•tiv•i•ty (PRA) (plaz′mă rē′nin ak-tiv′i-tē) Estimation of renin in plasma by measurement of the rate of formation of angiotensin I or II.

plas•ma throm•bo•plas•tin an•te•ced•ent (PTA) (plaz′mă throm′bō-plas′tin an′ti-sē′dĕnt) SYN factor XI.

plas•ma throm•bo•plas•tin com•pon•ent (PTC) (plaz′mă throm′bō-plas′tin kom-po′nĕnt) SYN factor IX.

plas•mat•ic (plaz-mat′ik) Relating to plasma. SYN plasmic.

plas•mic (plaz′mik) SYN plasmatic.

plas•mid (plaz′mid) A genetic particle physically separate from the chromosome of the host cell (chiefly bacterial) that can stably function and replicate; not essential to the basic functioning of the cell. SYN extrachromosomal element, extrachromosomal genetic element. [cyto*plasm* + -id]

plas•min (plaz′min) An enzyme hydrolyzing peptides and esters of L-arginine and L-lysine, and converting fibrin to soluble products; responsible for the dissolution of blood clots. SYN fibrinase (2), fibrinolysin.

plas•min•o•gen (plaz-min′ō-jen) A precursor of plasmin; an autosomal dominant deficiency of plasminogen that may promote thrombosis. SEE ALSO plasmin.

plas•min•o•gen ac•ti•va•tor (plaz-min′ō-jen ak′ti-vā-tŏr) A proteinase that converts plasminogen to plasmin by cleavage of a single (usually Arg-Val) bond in the former. Prevents formation of fibron clots. Alteplase and streptokinase are examples of medications that promote thrombolysis by activating plasminogen. SYN urokinase.

plas•min•o•gen ac•ti•va•tor in•hib•i•tor-1 (PAI-1) (plaz-min′ō-jen ak′ti-vā-tŏr in-hib′it-tŏr) Peptide adipokine produced by visceral adipose tissue; has a regulatory role in fibrinolysis and thrombus formation.

plas•mo•di•a (plaz-mō′dē-ă) Plural of plasmodium. [L.]

plas•mo•di•al (plaz-mō′dē-ăl) **1.** Relating to a plasmodium. **2.** Relating to any species of the genus *Plasmodium*.

Plas•mo•di•um (plaz-mō′dē-ŭm) A genus of the protozoan phylum Apicomplexa and the order Haemospondia, blood parasites of vertebrates; includes the causal agents of malaria, with an asexual cycle in liver and red blood cells of vertebrates, and a sexual cycle in mosquitoes, the latter cycle resulting in the production of large numbers of infective sporozoites in the salivary glands of the vector, which are transmitted when the mosquito bites and draws blood. [Mod. L. fr. G. *plasma,* something formed, + *eidos,* appearance]

Pla•sm•od•ium fal•ci•pa•rum (plaz-mō′dē-ŭm fal-sī-pā′rum) *Laverania falciparum*, a protozoal species that is the causal agent of falciparum (malignant tertian) malaria; the species is not selective, infecting erythrocytes regardless of whether they are mature or immature or whether they are of normal, large, or contracted size; infected erythrocytes are likely to contain basophilic granules and red dots (Maurer clefts or dots); multiple infection is extremely frequent and causes bouts of fever somewhat irregularly because the parasites' cycles of multiplication are usually asynchronous.

Plas•mo•di•um ma•lar•i•ae (plaz-mō′dē-ŭm mă-lar′ē-ē) A protozoal species that is the causal agent of quartan malaria; infected erythrocytes are of normal or slightly contracted size, usually with no stippling (the two most important characteristics that distinguish infection by *P. malariae* from *P. vivax* infection), although extremely fine Ziemann dots may be observed; because multiple infection is extremely rare, bouts of fever occur fairly regularly at intervals of about 72 hours.

Plas•mo•di•um o•val•e (plaz-mō′dē-ŭm ō′val-ā) A protozoal species that is the agent of one form of human malaria; affected erythrocytes tend to be oval and show abundant early Schüffner dots; host cells are normal or only slightly enlarged, and only about 8–10 grapelike merozoites are produced; fever is tertian (every 48 hours), and relapses are infrequent.

i ***Plas•mo•di•um vi•vax*** (plaz-mō′dē-ŭm vī′vaks) A protozoal species that is the most common malarial parasite of human beings (except in West Africa); affected red blood cells are pale and enlarged and contain Schüffner dots in the later stages of growth; causes bouts of fever fairly regularly, at 48-hour intervals; multiple infection is common. See page B7.

plas•mog•a•my (plaz-mog′ă-mē) Union of two or more cells with preservation of the individual nuclei; formation of a plasmodium. [plasmo- + G. *gamos,* marriage]

plas•mol•y•sis (plaz-mol′i-sis) **1.** Dissolution of cellular components. **2.** Shrinking of plant cells by osmotic loss of cytoplasmic water. [plasmo- + G. *lysis,* dissolution]

plas•mo•lyt•ic (plaz-mō-lit′ik) Relating to plasmolysis.

plas•mon (plaz′mŏn) The total of the extrachromosomal genetic properties of the eukaryotic cell cytoplasm. [cyto*plasm* + -on]

plas•mor•rhex•is (plaz-mō-rek′sis) The splitting open of a cell from the pressure of the protoplasm.

plas•mos•chi•sis (plaz-mos′ki-sis) The splitting of protoplasm into fragments. [plasmo- + G. *schisis,* a cleaving]

plas•mo•tro•pic (plaz-mō-trō′pik) Pertaining to or manifesting plasmotropism.

plas•mot•ro•pism (plaz-mo′trō-pizm) A condition in which the bone marrow, spleen, and liver are sites for the destruction of the erythrocytes, as opposed to the circulating blood. [plasmo- + G. *tropē,* a turning]

♻ **-plast, -plastia, -plasia, -plastic** Combining forms meaning pertaining to the formation or development of, e.g., hemoplastic. [G. *plasis,* a molding]

plas•ter (plas′tĕr) **1.** A solid preparation that can be spread when heated and becomes adhesive at the temperature of the body; used to keep the edges of a wound in apposition, to protect raw surfaces, or to apply medicine topically for local or systemic effects. **2.** DENTISTRY a type of gypsum containing calcium sulfate hemihydrate and porous crystals that require more water during mixing than other such products; used in preparing study models (nonworking casts). [L. *emplastrum;* G. *emplastron,* plaster or mold]

plas•ter ban•dage (plas′tĕr ban′dăj) A roller bandage impregnated with plaster of Paris and applied moist; used to make a rigid dressing for a fracture or diseased joint.

plas•ter of Par•is (plas′tĕr par′is) Any of a group of gypsum cements, essentially hemihydrated calcium sulfate, a white powder that forms a paste when mixed with water and then hardens into a solid; used in making casts, molds, and sculpture. [L. *plastrum,* plaster + Paris, France]

plas•tic (plas′tik) **1.** Capable of being formed or molded. **2.** A material that can be shaped by pressure or heat to the form of a cavity or mold. [G. *plastikos,* relating to molding]

plas•tic en•ve•lope cul•ture (plas′tik en′vĕ-lōp kŭl′chŭr) Simplified method for transport and culture of specimens for the diagnosis of infection with *Trichomonas vaginalis;* liquid culture medium is examined microscopically through the envelope, so pipette sampling of the medium is not required.

plas•tic•i•ty (plas-tis′i-tē) The capability of being formed or molded; the quality of being plastic.

plas•tic pleu•ri•sy (plas′tik plūr′i-sē) SYN dry pleurisy.

plas•tic sur•ger•y (plas′tik sŭr′jĕr-ē) The surgical specialty or procedure concerned with the restoration, construction, reconstruction, or improvement in the shape and appearance of body structures that are missing, defective, damaged, or misshapen.

plas•tid (plas′tid) **1.** One of the differentiated structures in cytoplasm of plant cells where photosynthesis or other cellular processes are carried on; contain DNA and are self-replicating. SYN trophoplast. **2.** One of the granules of foreign or differentiated matter in cells: food particles, fat, waste material, chromatophores, and trichocysts. **3.** A self-duplicating viruslike particle that multiplies within a host cell (e.g., kappa particles in certain paramecia). [G. *plastos,* formed, + -id]

-plasty Molding, shaping or the result thereof, as of a surgical procedure. [G. *plastos,* formed, shaped]

plate (plāt) **1.** ANATOMY a thin, relatively flat structure. **2.** A metal bar, perforated for screws, applied to a fractured bone to maintain the ends in apposition. **3.** The agar layer within a Petri dish or similar vessel. **4.** To form a very thin layer of a bacterial culture by streaking it on the surface of an agar plate (usually within a Petri dish) to isolate individual organisms from each of which a colonial clone will develop. **5.** Any one of the horizontal perforated plates that make up the fractionating component of a column in fractional distillation (or, the theoretic equivalent of such a plate). [O.Fr. *plat,* a flat object, fr. G. *platys,* flat, broad]

pla•teau pres•sure (pla-tō′ presh′ŭr) The equilibrium pressure between airways and alveoli in a patient-ventilator system; considered to be an approximation of alveolar pressure.

pla•teau pulse (pla-tō′ pŭls) A slow, sustained pulse.

plate•let (plāt′lĕt) An irregularly shaped, disclike, cytoplasmic fragment of a megakaryocyte that is shed in the marrow sinus and subsequently found in the peripheral blood, where it functions in clotting. Contains granules in the central part (granulomere) and, peripherally, clear protoplasm (hyalomere), but no definite nucleus; is about one third to one half the size of an erythrocyte. SEE ALSO plate. SYN blood disc, elementary particle (1), thrombocyte, thromboplastid (1).

plate•let-ac•ti•vat•ing fac•tor (plāt′lĕt-ak′ti-vā′ting fak′tŏr) SYN platelet-aggregating factor.

plate•let-ag•gre•gat•ing fac•tor (PAF) (plāt′lĕt ag′grē-gā′ting fak′tŏr) Phospholipid mediator of platelet aggregation, inflammation, and anaphylaxis; produced in response to specific stimuli by a variety of cell types, including neutrophils, basophils, platelets, and endothelial cells. Several molecular species of PAF have been identified that vary in the length of the *O*-alkyl side chain. It is an important mediator of bronchoconstriction. SYN platelet-activating factor.

plate•let ag•gre•ga•tion (plāt′lĕt ag′rĕ-gā′shŭn) The clumping together of platelets in the blood; part of the sequence of events leading to the formation of a thrombus (clot) or hemostatic plug.

plate•let fac•tor (PF) 3 (plāt′lĕt fak′tŏr) A blood coagulation factor derived from platelets; chemically, a phospholipid lipoprotein that acts with certain plasma thromboplastin factors to convert prothrombin to thrombin.

plate•let fac•tor (PF) 4 (plāt′lĕt fak′tŏr) A cationic polypeptide synthesized by megakaryocytes and contained in platelet alpha granules; these granules, released when platelets are activated, neutralize the anticoagulant activity of heparin.

plate•let neu•tra•li•za•tion pro•ce•dure (PNP) (plāt′lĕt nū′trăl-ī-zā′shŭn prŏ-sē′jŭr) A technique based on the ability of platelets to bypass the effect of a lupus anticoagulant by correcting prolonged coagulation times in various phospholipid-dependent test systems; the disrupted platelet membranes in the freeze-thawed platelet suspension neutralize phospholipid antibodies in the plasma of patients with lupus anticoagulant; after the patient plasma is mixed with the freeze-thawed platelet suspension, the activated partial thromboplastin time will be corrected when compared with the original baseline activated partial thromboplastin time.

plate•let•phe•re•sis (plāt′lĕt-fĕ-rē′sis) Removal of blood from a donor with replacement of all blood components except platelets. [platelet + G. *aphairesis,* a withdrawal]

plate•let tis•sue fac•tor (plāt′lĕt tish′ū fak′tŏr) SYN thromboplastin.

plate•like at•el•ec•ta•sis (plāt-līk at′ĕ-lek′tă-sis) SYN subsegmental atelectasis.

-platin Combining form meaning a chemotherapeutic agent that is platinum based.

plat•i•num (Pt) (plat′i-nŭm) A metallic element, atomic no. 78, atomic wt. 195.08, used for making small parts for chemical apparatus because of its resistance to acids; in powdered form (**platinum black**), it is an important catalyst in hydrogenation. A derivative, cisplatin, is used as an antineoplastic agent. [Mod. L., originally *platina,* fr. Sp. *plata,* silver]

platy- Prefix meaning width; flatness. [G. *platys,* flat, broad]

plat·y·ba·si·a (plat′i-bā′sē-ă) A developmental anomaly of the cranium or an acquired softening of the cranial bones that allows the floor of the posterior cranial fossa to bulge upward in the region around the foramen magnum. [platy- + G. *basis,* ground]

plat·y·ceph·a·ly (plat′i-sef′ă-lē) Flatness of the cranium, a condition in which the vertical cranial index is less than 70. [platy- + G. *kephalē,* head]

plat·y·hel·minth (plat′i-hel′minth) Common name for any flatworm of the phylum Platyhelminthes; any cestode (tapeworm) or trematode (fluke). [platy- + G. *helmins,* worm]

Plat·y·hel·min·thes (plat′i-hel-min′thēz) A phylum of flatworms that are bilaterally symmetric, flattened, and acelomate. Parasitic species of medical importance are in the subclass Cestoda (the true tapeworms) of the class Cestoidea, and in the subclass Digenea (the digenetic flukes) of the class Trematoda.

plat·y·pel·lic pel·vis (plat′i-pel′ik pel′vis) Flat, oval pelvis, in which the transverse diameter is more than 3 cm longer than the anteroposterior diameter.

plat·y·pel·loid pel·vis (plat′i-pel′oyd pel′vis) Simple flat pelvis.

pla·typ·ne·a (plă-tip′nē-ă) Difficulty in breathing when erect, relieved by recumbency. Cf. orthopnea. [platy- + G. *pnoē,* a breathing]

platypnoea [Br.] SEE platypnea.

pla·tys·ma (plă-tiz′mă) [TA] SYN platysma muscle.

pla·tys·ma mus·cle (plă-tiz′mă mŭs′ĕl) *Origin*, subcutaneous layer and fascia covering pectoralis major and deltoid at level of first or second rib; *insertion*, lower border of mandible, risorius, and platysma of opposite side; *action*, depresses lower lip, forms ridges in skin of neck and upper chest when jaws are "clenched," denoting stress, anger; *nerve supply*, cervical branch of facial. See this page. SYN platysma [TA].

plat·y·spon·dyl·i·a, **plat·y·spon·dyl·i·sis** (plat′i-spon-dil′ē-ă, -i-sis) Flatness of the bodies of the vertebrae. [platy- + G. *spondylos,* vertebra]

play (plā) **1.** To perform or participate in an activity for recreation or amusement. **2.** General term for individual or group activities engaged in for fun or recreation. [O.E. *plegian*]

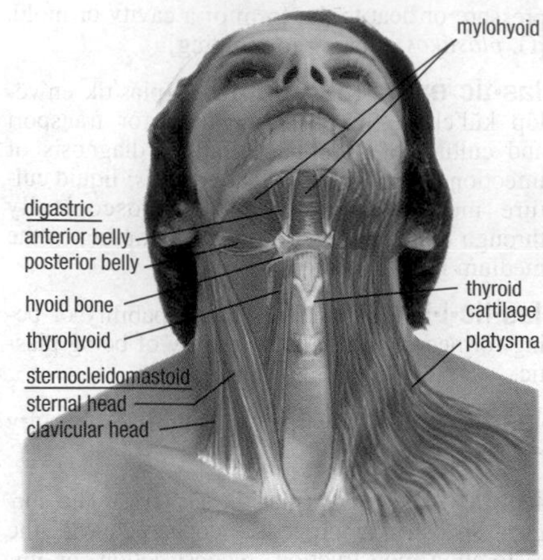

platysma muscle

play ther·a·py (plā thār′ă-pē) A type of therapy used with children in which they can express or reveal their problems and fantasies by playing with dolls or other toys, drawing, and during other activities.

plea·sure prin·ci·ple (ple′zhŭr prin′si-pĕl) SYN pain-pleasure principle.

pled·get (plej′ĕt) A tuft of wool, cotton, or lint.

-plegia Suffix meaning paralysis. [G. *plēgē,* stroke]

pleio- Rarely used alternative spelling for pleo-.

plei·o·tro·pic (plī-ō-trō′pik) Denoting, or characterized by, pleiotropy.

plei·o·tro·pic gene (plī-ō-trō′pik jēn) A gene that has multiple, apparently unrelated, phenotypic manifestations. SYN polyphenic gene.

plei·ot·ro·py, **plei·o·tro·pi·a** (plī-ot′rŏ-pē, -ō-trō′pē-ă) Production by a single mutant gene of apparently unrelated multiple effects at the clinical or phenotypic level. [pleio- + G. *tropos,* turning]

pleo- Prefix meaning more. [G. *pleiōn*]

ple·o·cy·to·sis (plē′ō-sī-tō′sis) Presence of more cells than normal, often denoting leukocytosis and especially lymphocytosis or round cell infiltration. [pleo- + G. *kytos,* cell, + *-ōsis,* condition]

ple·o·mas·ti·a, **ple·o·ma·zi·a** (plē′ō-mas′tē-ă, -mā′zē-ă) SYN polymastia. [pleo- + G. *mastos,* breast]

ple·o·mor·phic (plē′ō-mōr′fik) **1.** SYN polymorphic. **2.** Among fungi, having two or more spore forms; also used to describe a sterile mutant dermatophyte resulting from degenerative changes in culture.

ple•o•mor•phic li•po•ma (plē′ō-mōr′fik li-pō′mă) SYN atypical lipoma.

ple•o•mor•phism (plē-ō-mōr′fizm) SYN polymorphism. [pleo- + G. *morphē,* form]

ple•o•mor•phous (plē′ō-mōr′fŭs) SYN polymorphic.

ple•o•nasm (plē′ō-nazm) Excess in number or size of parts. [G. *pleonasmos,* exaggeration, excessive, fr. *pleiōn,* more]

ple•on•os•te•o•sis (plē′on-os-tē-ō′sis) Superabundance of bone formation. [pleo- + G. *osteon,* bone, + *-osis,* condition]

♻ **pless-, plessi-** Combining forms meaning a striking, especially percussion. [G. *plēssō,* to strike]

ples•sim•e•ter (ples-sim′ĕ-tĕr) An oblong flexible plate used in mediate percussion by being placed against the surface and struck with the plessor. SYN pleximeter, plexometer. [G. *plēssō,* to strike, + *metron,* measure]

ples•sor (ples′ŏr) A small hammer, usually with a soft rubber head, used to tap the part directly, or with a plessimeter, in percussion of the chest or other part. SYN percussor, plexor. [G. *plēssō,* to strike]

pleth•o•ra (pleth′ŏr-ă) **1.** SYN hypervolemia. **2.** An excess of any of the body fluids. SYN repletion (2). [G. *plēthōrē,* fullness, fr. *plēthō,* to become full]

pleth•o•ric (plĕ-thōr′ik) Relating to plethora. SYN sanguine (1), sanguineous (2).

ple•thys•mo•graph (plĕ-thiz′mō-graf) A device for measuring and recording changes in volume of a part, organ, or whole body. [G. *plēthysmos,* increase, + *graphō,* to write]

pleth•ys•mog•ra•phy (pleth-iz-mog′ră-fē) Measuring and recording changes in volume of an organ or other part of the body by a plethysmograph. [G. *plēthysmos,* increase, + *graphē,* a writing]

pleth•ys•mom•e•try (pleth-iz-mom′ĕ-trē) Measuring the fullness of a hollow organ or vessel, as of the pulse. [G. *plēthysmos,* increase, + *metron,* measure]

♻ **pleur-, pleuro-, pleura-** Combining forms meaning rib, side, pleura. [G. *pleura,* a rib, the side]

pleu•ra, gen. and pl. **pleu•rae** (plūr′ă, -ē) [TA] The serous membrane enveloping the lungs and lining the walls of the pleural cavity. [G. *pleura,* a rib, pl. the side]

pleu•ral (plūr′ăl) Relating to the pleura.

pleu•ral cav•i•ty (plūr′ăl kav′i-tē) The potential space between the parietal and visceral layers of the pleura. SYN pleural space.

pleu•ral ef•fu•sion (plūr′ăl ĕ-fyū′zhŭn) Increased amounts of fluid within the pleural cavity, usually due to inflammation.

pleu•ral flu•id (plūr′ăl flū′id) The thin film of fluid between the visceral and parietal pleurae.

pleu•ral frem•i•tus (plūr′ăl frem′i-tŭs) Vibration in the chest wall produced by the rubbing together of inflamed opposing surfaces of the pleura.

pleu•ral space (plūr′ăl spās) SYN pleural cavity.

pleu•ral tap (plūr′ăl tap) SYN thoracentesis.

pleu•ra•poph•y•sis (plūr′ă-pof′i-sis) A rib, or the process on a cervical or lumbar vertebra corresponding thereto. [pleur- + G. *apophysis,* process, offshoot]

pleur•ec•to•my (plūr-ek′tŏ-mē) Excision of pleura, usually parietal. [pleur- + G. *ektomē,* excision]

pleu•ri•sy (plūr′i-sē) Inflammation of the pleura. SYN pleuritis. [L. *pleurisis,* fr. G. *pleuritis*]

pleu•ri•sy with ef•fu•sion (plūr′i-sē ĕ-fyu′zhŭn) The inflammatory disorder accompanied by serous exudation. SYN serous pleurisy.

pleu•rit•ic (plū-rit′ik) Pertaining to pleurisy.

pleu•rit•ic rub (plū-rit′ik rŭb) A friction sound produced by the rubbing together of inflamed surfaces of the parietal and visceral pleurae.

pleu•ri•tis (plū-rī′tis) SYN pleurisy. [G. fr. *pleura,* side, + *-itis,* inflammation]

pleu•ro•cele (plūr′ō-sēl) SYN pneumonocele. [pleuro- + G. *kēlē,* hernia]

pleu•ro•cen•te•sis (plūr′ō-sen-tē′sis) SYN thoracentesis. [pleuro- + G. *kentēsis,* puncture]

pleu•ro•cen•trum (plūr′ō-sen′trŭm) One of the lateral halves of the body of a vertebra. [pleuro- + G. *kentron,* center]

pleu•roc•ly•sis (plūr-ok′li-sis) Washing out of the pleural cavity. [pleuro- + G. *klysis,* a washing out]

pleu•rod•e•sis (plūr-od′ĕ-sis) The creation of a fibrous adhesion between the visceral and parietal layers of the pleura, obliterating the pleural cavity; it is performed surgically by abrading the pleura or by inserting a sterile irritant into the pleural canal in cases of recurrent spontaneous pneumothorax, malignant pleural effusion, and chylothorax. [pleuro- + G. *desis,* a binding together]

pleu•ro•dyn•i•a (plūr-ō-din′ē-ă) **1.** Pleuritic pain in the chest. **2.** A painful affection of the tendinous attachments of the thoracic muscles, usually of one side only. SYN costalgia. [pleuro- + G. *odynē,* pain]

pleu•ro•e•soph•a•ge•al mus•cle (plūr′ō-ē-sof′ă-jē-ăl mŭs′ĕl) Muscular fasciculi, arising from the mediastinal pleura, that reinforce musculature of esophagus. SYN musculus pleuroesophageus [TA].

pleu•ro•gen•ic (plūr′ō-jen′ik) Of pleural origin; beginning in the pleura. SYN pleurogenous (1). [pleuro- + G. *-gen,* producing]

pleu•rog•e•nous (plūr-oj′ĕ-nŭs) **1.** SYN pleurogenic. **2.** In fungi, denoting spores or conidia developed on the sides of a conidiophore or hypha.

pleu•rog•ra•phy (plūr-og′ră-fē) Radiography of the pleural cavity after injection of contrast medium. [pleuro- + G. *graphō,* to write]

pleu•ro•hep•a•ti•tis (plūr′ō-hep-ă-tī′tis) Hepatitis with extension of the inflammation to the neighboring portion of the pleura. [pleuro- + G. *hēpar,* liver, + *-itis,* inflammation]

pleu•ro•lith (plūr′ō-lith) A concretion in the pleural cavity. [pleuro- + G. *lithos,* stone]

pleu•rol•y•sis (plūr-ol′i-sis) Locating pleural adhesions by the aid of an endoscope and then dividing them with the electric cautery. [pleuro- + G. *lysis,* dissolution]

pleu•ro•per•i•car•di•al (plūr′ō-per-i-kahr′dē-ăl) Relating to both pleura and pericardium.

pleu•ro•per•i•car•di•tis (plūr′ō-per′i-kahr-dī′tis) Combined inflammation of the pericardium and of the pleura. [pleuro- + pericardium + G. *-itis,* inflammation]

pleu•ro•per•i•to•ne•al (plūr′ō-per′i-tō-nē′ăl) Relating to both pleura and peritoneum.

pleu•ro•per•i•to•ne•al shunt (plūr′ō-per′i-tō-nē′ăl shŭnt) A surgically implanted catheter for transport of fluid from a pleural space into the peritoneal cavity, where it is absorbed; used mainly for treatment of malignant pleural effusions.

pleu•ro•pneu•mo•nec•to•my (plūr′ō-nū-mō-nek′tŏ-mē) Surgical resection of an entire lung along with the parietal pleura; formerly used mainly for destroyed lung due to tuberculosis; currently, a method of treating malignant mesothelioma.

pleu•ro•pneu•mo•ni•a•like or•ga•nisms (PPLO) (plūr′ō-nū-mō′nē-ă-līk ōr′gă-nizmz) The original name given to a group of bacteria that do not possess cell walls; these organisms, isolated from humans and other animals, soil, and sewage, are now assigned to the order Mycoplasmatales.

pleu•ro•pul•mo•nar•y (plūr′ō-pul′mō-nar-ē) Relating to the pleura and the lungs.

pleu•rot•o•my (plūr-ot′ŏ-mē) SYN thoracotomy. [pleuro- + G. *tomē,* incision]

pleu•ro•ve•nous shunt (plūr′ō-vē′nŭs shŭnt) A surgically implanted catheter for transport of fluid from a pleural space into the venous system; rarely used, mainly for treatment of malignant pleural effusions.

pleu•ro•vis•cer•al (plūr′ō-vis′ĕr-ăl) SYN visceropleural.

♻ **-plex, -plexus** Combining forms meaning a braid, nerve, or network. [L. *plexus,* braided]

plex•al (plek′săl) Relating to a plexus.

plex•ect•o•my (plek-sek′tŏ-mē) Surgical excision of a plexus. [plexus + G. *ektomē,* excision]

plex•i•form (plek′si-fōrm) Weblike, or resembling or forming a plexus. [plexus + L. *forma,* form]

plex•i•form neu•ro•fi•bro•ma (plek′si-fōrm nūr′ō-fī-brō′mă) A type of neurofibroma, representing an anomaly rather than a true neoplasm, in which the proliferation of Schwann cells occurs from the inner aspect of the nerve sheath; seen most frequently in neurofibromatosis. SYN plexiform neuroma.

plex•i•form neu•ro•ma (plek′si-fōrm nūr-ō′mă) SYN plexiform neurofibroma.

plex•im•e•ter (plek-sim′i-tĕr) SYN plessimeter. [G. *plēxis,* stroke]

plex•i•tis (plek-sī′tis) Inflammation of a plexus.

plex•o•gen•ic (plek′sō-jen′ik) Giving rise to weblike or plexiform structures. [plexus + G. *-gen,* producing]

plex•om•e•ter (plek-som′ĕ-tĕr) SYN plessimeter.

plex•op•a•thy (pleks-op′ă-thē) Disorder involving one of the major peripheral neural plexuses: cervical, brachial, or lumbosacral. [plexus + G. *pathos,* disease]

plex•or (plek′sŏr) SYN plessor. [G. *plēxis,* a stroke]

plex•us, pl. **plex•us**, **plex•us•es** (plek′sŭs, plek′sŭs, -ĕz) [TA] A network or interjoining of nerves and blood vessels or of lymphatic vessels. [L. a braid]

plex•us ce•li•a•cus (pleks′ŭs sē-lē-ā′kŭs) [TA] SYN celiac plexus.

plex•us gul•ae (pleks′ŭs gū′lē) SYN esophageal nervous plexus.

plex•us ner•vo•sus e•soph•a•ge•us (pleks′ŭs ner-vō′sŭs ē-sof′jē′ŭs) SYN esophageal nervous plexus.

♻ **plic-** Combining form meaning a fold or ridge. [L. *plico,* to fold]

pli•ca, gen. and pl. **pli•cae** (plī′kă, -sē) **1.** [TA] One of several anatomic structures in which there is a folding over of the parts. **2.** SYN false membrane. SEE ALSO fold. [Mod. L. a plait or fold]

pli•ca ar•y•ep•i•glot•ti•ca (plī′kă ahr′ē-ep-i-glot′i-kă) [TA] SYN aryepiglottic fold.

pli•cae cir•cu•la•res in•tes•ti•ni te•nu•is (plī′sē sĕr-kyū-lā′rēz in-tes′ti-nī ten-yū′is) [TA] SYN circular folds of small intestine.

pli•cae pal•ma•tae (plī′sē pahl′mā-tē) [TA] SYN palmate folds.

pli•cae u•re•thra•les (plī′sē yūr-ē-thrā′lēz) SYN urethral folds.

pli•ca in•ter•u•re•te•ri•ca (plī′kă in-tĕr-yūr-ĕ-ter′ik-ă) [TA] SYN interureteric fold.

pli•ca la•cri•ma•lis (plī′kă lak′rē-mā′lis) [TA] SYN lacrimal fold.

pli•ca se•mi•lu•nar•is con•junc•ti•vae (plī′kă sĕ-mē′lū-nār′is kon-jungk′ti-vē) [TA] SYN semilunar conjunctival fold.

pli•ca spi•ra•lis duc•tus cys•ti•ci (plī′kă spi-rā′lis dŭk′tŭs sis′ti-sī) [TA] SYN spiral fold of cystic duct.

pli•cate (plī′kāt) Folded; pleated; tucked.

pli•ca•tion (plī-kā′shŭn) A folding or putting together in pleats; specifically, an operation for reducing the size of a hollow viscus by taking folds or tucks in its walls. [L. *plico,* pp. *-atus,* to fold]

pli•ca ves•ti•bu•la•ris (plī′kă ves-tib-yū-lā′ris) [TA] SYN vestibular fold.

pli•ca vo•ca•lis (plī′kă vō-kāl′is) [TA] SYN vocal fold.

pli•cot•o•my (plī-kot′ŏ-mē) Division of the plica mallearis. [plica + G. *tomē,* incision]

PLMD Abbreviation for periodic limb movements disorder.

♻ **-ploid** Combining form meaning multiple in form; its combinations are used both adjectivally and substantively of a (specified) multiple of chromosomes. [G. *-plo-,* -fold, + *-ides,* in form; L. *-ploïdeus*]

ploi•dy (ploy′dē) The number of haploid sets in a cell. Gametes normally contain one; autosomal cells, two. SEE ALSO polyploidy. [-ploid + *-y,* condition]

plot (plot) A graphic representation.

plug (plŭg) Any mass filling a hole or closing an orifice.

plug•ger (plŭg′ĕr) A dental instrument used for condensing gold (foil), amalgam, or any plastic material in a tooth cavity, operated by hand or by mechanical means. SYN packer (2).

plum•bism (plŭm′bizm) SYN lead poisoning. [L. *plumbum,* lead]

plumb line (plum līn) The line that is formed when a string with a weight tied at the end is suspended vertically.

plum•bum (plŭm′bŭm) SYN lead. [L.]

Plum•mer-Vin•son syn•drome (plŭm′ĕr vin′sŏn sin′drōm) Iron deficiency anemia, dysphagia, esophageal web, and atrophic glossitis.

♻ **pluri-** Prefix meaning several, more. SEE ALSO multi-, poly-. [L. *plus, pluris*]

plu•ri•glan•du•lar (plūr′i-glan′dyū-lăr) Denoting several glands or their secretions. SYN polyglandular.

plu•rip•o•tent, plu•ri•po•ten•tial (plūr-ip′ŏ-tĕnt, plūr′ē-pŏ-ten′shăl) **1.** Having the capacity to affect more than one organ or tissue. **2.** Not fixed as to potential development.

plu•to•ni•um (Pu) (plū-tō′nē-ŭm) A transuranium artificial radioactive element, atomic no. 94, atomic wt. 244.064. The best-known α-emitting isotope is ^{239}Pu (half-life 24,110 years), which, like ^{235}U, is fissionable and can be used in atomic bombs and nuclear power plants; ^{238}Pu (half-life 87.74 years) is used as an energy source in pacemakers. Pu ions are bone seekers; ingestion is a radiation hazard as with radium and radiostrontium. [planet, *Pluto*]

PLWH Abbreviation for persons living with HIV.

ply•o•met•ric train•ing (plī′ō-met′rik trān′ing) Exercise training that exploits the stretch-recoil characteristics of skeletal muscle and neurologic modulation through the stretch or myotatic reflex; used by athletes who require specific, powerful movements (e.g., in football, volleyball, sprinting, and basketball).

Pm Symbol for promethium.

pM Abbreviation for picomolar (10^{-12} M).

pm Abbreviation for picometer.

PMDD Abbreviation for premenstrual dysphoric disorder. SEE ALSO PMS.

PMI Abbreviation for point of maximal impulse.

P mit•ra•le (mī-trā′lē) Broad, notched P waves in several or many leads of the electrocardiogram with a prominent late negative component to the P wave in lead V_1; it is characteristic of overload of the left atrium such as occurs in disease of the mitral valve. SYN P sinistrocardiale.

PML Abbreviation for progressive multifocal leukoencephalopathy.

pmol Abbreviation for picomole.

PMS Abbreviation for premenstrual syndrome.

PN Abbreviation for parenteral nutrition.

PND Abbreviation for postnasal drip; paroxysmal nocturnal dyspnea.

♻ **-pnea** Combining form denoting breath, respiration. [G. *pneō,* to breathe]

♻ **pneo-** Combining form denoting breath or respiration. SEE ALSO pneum-, pneumo-. [G. *pneō,* to breathe]

♻ **pneum-, pneuma-, pneumat-, pneumato-** Combining forms denoting presence of air or gas, the lungs, or breathing. SEE ALSO pneo-, pneumo-. [G. *pneuma, pneumatos,* air, breath]

pneu•marth•ro•gram (nū-mahrth′rō-gram) Film records of pneumarthrography.

pneu•marth•rog•ra•phy (nū′mahrth-rog′ră-fē) Radiographic examination of a joint following the introduction of air, with or without another contrast medium. SYN pneumoarthrography. [G. *pneuma,* air, + *arthron,* joint, + *graphō,* to write]

pneu•mar•thro•sis (nū′mahr-thrō′sis) Presence of air in a joint. [G. *pneuma,* air, + *arthron,* joint, + *-osis,* condition]

pneu•mat•ic (nū-mat′ik) **1.** Relating to air or gas, or to a structure filled with air. **2.** Relating to respiration. [G. *pneumatikos*]

pneu•mat•ic an•ti•shock gar•ment (nū-mat′ik an′tē-shock′ gahr′mĕnt) An inflatable suit used to apply pressure to the peripheral circulation, thus reducing blood flow and fluid exudation into tissues, to maintain central blood flow in the presence of shock. SYN military antishock trousers.

pneu•mat•ic bone (nū-mat′ik bōn) A bone that is hollow or contains many air cells, such as the mastoid process of the temporal bone. SYN hollow bone.

pneu•ma•tic di•la•tor (nū-mat′ik dī′lā-tŏr) Any of a variety of catheters fitted with distal balloons that can be inflated to desired pressures for overcoming obstructions in hollow viscera; most often used to rupture the lower esophageal sphincter to treat achalasia.

pneu•mat•ic o•tos•co•py (nū-mat′ik ō-tos′kŏ-pē) Inspection of the ear with a device capable of varying air pressure against the eardrum. Imparting movement to the tympanic membrane suggests normal middle ear compliance; the lack of movement indicates either increased impedance or eardrum perforation.

pneu•mat•ic to•nom•e•ter (nū-mat′ik tō-nom′ĕ-tĕr) A recording applanation tonometer operated by compressed gas.

pneu•mat•ic tube (nū-mat′ik tūb) A unidirectional, continuously operating vacuum system that transfers specimens in Plexiglas carriers from patient units to the laboratory.

pneu•ma•ti•za•tion (nū′mă-tī-zā′shŭn) The development of air cells such as those of the mastoid and ethmoidal bones. [G. *pneuma,* air]

pneu•ma•to•car•di•a (nū′mă-tō-kahr′dē-ă) Presence of air bubbles or gas in the blood of the heart; produced by air embolism.

pneu•mat•o•cele (nū-mat′ō-sēl) **1.** An emphysematous or gaseous swelling. **2.** SYN pneumonocele. **3.** A thin-walled cavity within the lung, one of the characteristic sequelae of staphylococcus pneumonia. [G. *pneuma,* air, + *kēlē,* tumor, hernia]

pneu•ma•tor•rha•chis (nū′mă-tōr′ă-kis) SYN pneumorrhachis. [G. *pneuma,* air, + *rhachis,* spine]

pneu•ma•to•sis (nū′mă-tō′sis) Abnormal accumulation of gas in any tissue or part of the body. [G. a blowing out]

pneu•ma•to•sis cys•toi•des in•tes•ti•na•lis (nū′mă-tō′sis sis-toyd′ēz in-tes-ti-nā′lis) A condition of unknown cause characterized by the occurrence of gas cysts in the intestinal mucous membrane; may produce intestinal obstruction. SYN intestinal emphysema.

pneu•ma•tu•ri•a (nū′mă-tyūr′ē-ă) The passage of gas or air from the urethra during or after urination, resulting from decomposition of bladder urine or, more commonly, from an intestinal fistula. [G. *pneuma,* air, + *ouron,* urine]

♻ **pneumo-, pneumon-, pneumono-** Combining forms meaning the lungs, air or gas, respiration, or pneumonia. SEE ALSO aer-, pneo-, pneum-. [G. *pneumōn, pneumonos,* lung]

pneu•mo•ar•throg•ra•phy (nū′mō-ahr-throg′ră-fē) SYN pneumarthrography.

pneu•mo•car•di•al (nū′mō-kahr′dē-ăl) SYN cardiopulmonary.

pneu•mo•cele (nū′mō-sēl) SYN pneumonocele.

pneu•mo•cen•te•sis (nū′mō-sen-tē′sis) SYN pneumonocentesis.

pneu•mo•ceph•a•lus (nū′mō-sef′ă-lŭs) Presence of air or gas within the cranial cavity. [G. *pneuma,* air, + *kephalē,* head]

pneumococcaemia [Br.] SYN pneumococcemia.

pneu•mo•coc•cal (nū′mō-kok′ăl) Pertaining to or containing the pneumococcus.

pneu•mo•coc•ce•mi•a (nū′mō-kok-sē′mē-ă) The presence of pneumococci in the blood. SYN pneumococcaemia. [pneumococcus + G. *haima,* blood]

pneu•mo•coc•ci•dal (nū′mō-kok-sī′dăl) Destructive to pneumococci. [pneumococcus + L. *caedo,* to kill]

pneu•mo•coc•co•sis (nū′mō-kok-ō′sis)

Rarely used term for infection with pneumococci.

pneu•mo•coc•co•su•ri•a (nū′mō-kok-ō-syūr′ē-ă) The presence of pneumococci or their specific capsular substance in the urine. [pneumococcus + G. *ouron,* urine]

pneu•mo•coc•cus, pl. **pneu•mo•coc•ci** (nū′mō-kok′ŭs, -kok′sī) SYN *Streptococcus pneumoniae.* [G. *pneumōn,* lung, + *kokkos,* berry (coccus)]

pneu•mo•co•ni•o•sis, pl. **pneu•mo•co•ni•o•ses** (nū′mō-kō-nē-ō′sis, -sēz) Inflammation commonly leading to fibrosis of the lungs caused by the inhalation of dust in various occupations; characterized by pain in the chest, cough with little or no expectoration, dyspnea, reduced thoracic excursion, sometimes cyanosis, and fatigue after slight exertion; degree of disability depends on the types of particles inhaled, as well as the level of exposure to them. [G. *pneumōn,* lung, + *konis,* dust, + *-osis,* condition]

pneu•mo•cra•ni•um (nū′mō-krā′nē-ŭm) Air present between the cranium and the dura mater; the term is commonly used to indicate extradural or subdural air. [G. *pneuma,* air, + -o- + *kranion,* skull]

Pneu•mo•cys•tis ji•ro•ve•ci (nū-mō-sis′tis jī-rō-vē′chē) Revised name for *Pneumocystis carinii,* the microorganism that causes interstitial plasma cell pneumonia in immunodeficient people, particularly those with AIDS. [G. *pneuma,* air, breathing, + *kystis,* bladder, pouch]

i ***Pneu•mo•cys•tis ji•ro•ve•ci* pneu•mo•ni•a** (nū-mō-sis′tis jī-rō-vē′chē nū-mō′nē-ă) Pneumonia resulting from infection with *P. jiroveci,* frequently seen in the immunologically compromised, such as people with AIDS, or steroid-treated patients, the elderly, or premature or debilitated babies. Throughout the alveolar walls and pulmonary septa there is a diffuse infiltration of mononuclear inflammatory cells, chiefly plasma cells and macrophages, as well as a few lymphocytes. Helmet-shaped organisms can be demonstrated in sputum and tissue specimens with silver stains. Patients may be only slightly febrile (or even afebrile), but are likely to be extremely weak, dyspneic, and cyanotic. This is a major cause of morbidity among patients with AIDS. See page B5. SYN interstitial plasma cell pneumonia, pneumocystosis.

pneu•mo•cys•tog•ra•phy (nū′mō-sis-tog′ră-fē) Radiography of the bladder following injection of air. [G. *pneuma,* air, + *kystis,* bladder, + *graphō,* to write]

pneu•mo•cys•to•sis (nū′mō-sis-tō′sis) SYN *Pneumocystis jiroveci* pneumonia.

pneu•mo•der•ma (nū′mō-dĕr′mă) SYN subcutaneous emphysema. [G. *pneuma,* air, + -o- + *derma,* skin]

pneu•mo•dy•nam•ics (nū′mō-dī-nam′iks) The mechanics of respiration. [G. *pneuma,* breath, + *dynamis,* force]

pneu•mo•gas•tric (nū′mō-gas′trik) Relating to the lungs and the stomach. SYN gastropulmonary. [G. *pneumōn,* lung, + *gastēr,* stomach]

pneu•mo•gas•tric nerve (nū′mō-gas′trik nĕrv) SYN vagus nerve [CN X].

pneu•mo•gram (nū′mō-gram) **1.** The record or tracing made by a pneumograph. **2.** Radiographic record of pneumography. [G. *pneumōn,* lung, + *gramma,* a drawing]

pneu•mo•graph (nū′mō-graf) Generic term for any device that records respiratory excursions from movements on the body surface. [G. *pneumōn,* lung, + *graphō,* to write]

pneu•mog•ra•phy (nū-mog′ră-fē) **1.** Examination with a pneumograph. **2.** A general term indicating radiography after injection of air. SYN pneumoradiography. [G. *pneumōn,* lung, + *graphō,* to write]

pneumohaemopericardium [Br.] SYN pneumohemopericardium.

pneumohaemothorax [Br.] SYN pneumohemothorax.

pneu•mo•he•mo•per•i•car•di•um (nū′mō-hē-mō′per-i-kahr′dē-ŭm) SYN hemopneumopericardium. SYN pneumohaemopericardium.

pneu•mo•he•mo•thor•ax (nū′mō-hē-mō-thōr′aks) SYN hemopneumothorax. SYN pneumohaemothorax.

pneu•mo•hy•dro•me•tra (nū′mō-hī-drō-mē′tră) The presence of gas and serum in the uterine cavity. [G. *pneuma,* air, + *hydōr* (*hydr-*), water, + *mētra,* uterus]

pneu•mo•hy•dro•per•i•car•di•um (nū′mō-hī′drō-per-i-kahr′dē-ŭm) SYN hydropneumopericardium.

pneu•mo•hy•dro•per•i•to•ne•um (nū′mō-hī′drō-per-i-tō-nē′ŭm) SYN hydropneumoperitoneum.

pneu•mo•hy•dro•thor•ax (nū′mō-hī′drō-thōr′aks) SYN hydropneumothorax.

pneu•mo•lith (nū′mō-lith) A calculus in the lung. [G. *pneumōn,* lung, + *lithos,* stone]

pneu•mo•li•thi•a•sis (nū′mō-li-thī′ă-sis) Formation of calculi in the lungs.

pneu•mo•me•di•as•ti•num (nū′mō-mē-dē-ă-stī′nŭm) Escape of air into mediastinal tissues, usually from interstitial emphysema or from a ruptured pulmonary bleb. [G. *pneuma,* air, + mediastinum]

pneu•mo•my•e•log•ra•phy (nū′mō-mī-ĕ-log′ră-fē) Rarely used radiographic examination of the spinal canal after injection of air or gas into the subarachnoid space. [G. *pneuma,* air, + *myelos,* marrow, + *graphō,* to write]

pneu•mo•nec•to•my (nū′mō-nek′tŏ-mē) Removal of all pulmonary lobes from a lung in one operation. [G. *pneumōn,* lung, + *ektomē,* excision]

pneu•mo•ni•a (nū-mō′nē-ă) Inflammation of the lung parenchyma characterized by consolidation of the affected part, the alveolar air spaces being filled with exudate, inflammatory cells, and fibrin. Most cases are due to infection by bacteria or viruses, a few to inhalation of chemicals or trauma to the chest wall, and a small minority to rickettsiae, fungi, yeasts, and helminths. Distribution may be lobar, segmental, or lobular; when lobular and associated with bronchitis, it is termed bronchopneumonia. SEE ALSO pneumonitis. See this page, B5. [G. fr. *pneumōn,* lung, + *-ia,* condition]

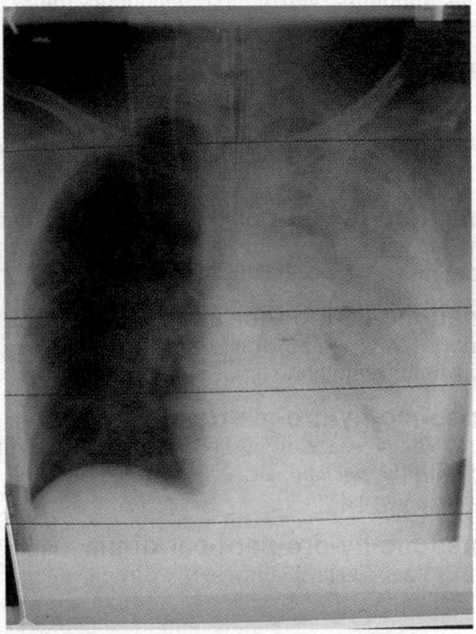

pneumonia: left lung almost entirely opacified

pneu•mon•ic (nū-mon′ik) **1.** SYN pulmonary. **2.** Relating to pneumonia.

pneu•mon•ic plague (nū-mon′ik plāg) A rapidly progressive and frequently fatal form of plague in which there are areas of pulmonary consolidation, with chills, pain in the side, bloody expectoration, and high fever. SEE ALSO *Yersinia pestis.*

pneu•mo•ni•tis (nū′mō-nī′tis) Inflammation of the lungs. SEE ALSO pneumonia. SYN pulmonitis. [G. *pneumōn,* lung, + *-itis,* inflammation]

pneu•mo•no•cele (nū-mō′nō-sēl) Protrusion of a portion of the lung through a defect in the chest wall. SYN pleurocele, pneumatocele (2), pneumocele.

pneu•mo•no•cen•te•sis (nū-mō′nō-sen-tē′sis) Rarely used term for paracentesis of the lung. SYN pneumocentesis. [G. *pneumōn,* lung, + *kentēsis,* puncture]

pneu•mo•no•coc•cal (nū′mō-nō-kok′ăl) Relating to or associated with *Streptococcus pneumoniae.*

pneu•mo•no•cyte (nū-mō′nō-sīt) Nonspecific term referring to cells lining alveoli in the respiratory part of the lung. [G. *pneumōn,* lung, + *kytos,* cell]

pneu•mo•no•pex•y (nū-mō′nō-pek-sē) Fixation of the lung by suturing the costal and pulmonary pleurae or otherwise causing adhesion of the two layers. [G. *pneumōn,* lung, + *pēxis,* fixation]

pneu•mo•nor•rha•phy (nū′mō-nōr′ă-fē) Suture of the lung. [G. *pneumōn,* lung, + *rhaphē,* suture]

pneu•mo•not•o•my (nū′mō-not′ŏ-mē) Incision of the lung. SYN pneumotomy. [G. *pneumōn,* lung, + *tomē,* incision]

pneu•mo•or•bi•tog•ra•phy (nū′mō-ōr′bi-tog′ră-fē) Radiographic visualization of the orbital contents following injection of a gas, usually air.

pneu•mo•per•i•car•di•um (nū′mō-per-i-kahr′dē-ŭm) Presence of gas in the pericardial sac. [G. *pneuma,* air, + pericardium]

pneu•mo•per•i•to•ne•um (nū′mō-per′i-tō-nē′ŭm) Presence of air or gas in the peritoneal cavity as a result of disease, or produced artificially in the abdomen to achieve exposure during laparoscopy and laporoscopic surgery for treatment of pulmonary or intestinal tuberculosis, bronchiectasis, tuberculous empyema, and certain other conditions. [G. *pneuma,* air, + peritoneum]

pneu•mo•per•i•to•ni•tis (nū′mō-per′i-tō-nī′tis) Inflammation of the peritoneum with an accumulation of gas in the peritoneal cavity. [G. *pneuma,* air, + peritonitis]

pneu•mo•pleu•ri•tis (nū′mō-plūr-ī′tis) Pleurisy with air or gas in the pleural cavity. [G. *pneuma,* air, + pleur- + *-itis,* inflammation]

pneu•mo•py•e•log•ra•phy (nū′mō-pī-ĕ-log′ră-fē) Radiography of the kidney after air or gas has been injected into the renal pelvis. [G. *pneuma,* air, + *pyelos,* pelvis, + *graphō,* to write]

pneu•mo•py•o•thor•ax (nū′mō-pī′ō-thōr′aks) SYN pyopneumothorax.

pneu•mo•ra•di•og•ra•phy (nū′mō-rā′dē-og′ră-fē) SYN pneumography (2).

pneu•mo•ret•ro•per•i•to•ne•um (nū′mō-ret′rō-per′i-tō-nē′ŭm) Escape of air into the retroperitoneal tissues.

pneu•mor•rha•chis (nū′mō-rā′kis) The presence of gas in the spinal canal. SYN pneumatorrhachis. [G. *pneuma,* air, + *rhachis,* spinal column]

pneu•mo•tach•o•gram (nū′mō-tak′ō-gram) A recording of respired gas flow as a function of time, produced by a pneumotachograph. [G. *pneuma,* air, + *tachys,* swift, + *gramma,* something written]

pneu•mo•tach•o•graph (nū′mō-tak′ō-graf) An instrument for measuring the instantaneous flow of respiratory gases. SYN pneumotachometer.

pneu•mo•ta•chom•e•ter (nū′mō-tă-kom′ĕ-tĕr) SYN pneumotachograph. [G. *pneuma,* air, + -o- + *tachys,* swift, + *metron,* measure]

pneu•mo•thor•ax (nū′mō-thōr′aks) The presence of air or gas in the pleural cavity. [G. *pneuma,* air, + thorax]

pneu•mot•o•my (nū-mot′ŏ-mē) SYN pneumonotomy.

PNF Abbreviation for proprioceptive neuromuscular facilitation.

PNH Abbreviation for paroxysmal nocturnal hemoglobinuria.

PNP Abbreviation for platelet neutralization procedure.

PNS Abbreviation for peripheral nervous system.

PO Abbreviation for per os.

Po Symbol for polonium.

pock (pok) The specific pustular cutaneous lesion of smallpox. [A.S. *poc,* a pustule]

pock•et (pok′ĕt) **1.** A cul-de-sac or pouchlike cavity. **2.** A diseased gingival attachment; a space between the inflamed gum and the surface of a tooth, limited apically by an epithelial attachment. **3.** To enclose within a confined space, as the stump of the pedicle of an ovarian or other abdominal tumor between the lips of the external wound. **4.** A collection of pus in a nearly closed sac. [Fr. *pochette*]

pock•et do•si•me•ter (pok′ĕt dō-sim′ĕ-tĕr) Small ionization chamber that provides an immediate reading of radiation exposure. SEE ALSO film badge.

pock•et•ed cal•cu•lus (pok′ĕt-ĕd kal′kyū-lŭs) SYN encysted calculus.

pock•mark (pok′mahrk) The small, depressed scar left after the healing of the smallpox pustule. SYN pit (2).

♻ **pod-, podo-** Combining forms meaning foot, foot-shaped. Cf. ped-. [G. *pous, podos*]

po•dag•ra (pō-dag′ră) Severe pain in the foot, especially that of typical gout in the great toe. [G. fr. *pous,* foot, + *agra,* a seizure]

po•dal•gi•a (pō-dal′jē-ă) Pain in the foot. SYN pododynia, tarsalgia. [pod- + G. *algos,* pain]

po•dal•ic (pō-dal′ik) Relating to the foot. [G. *pous* (*pod-*), foot]

po•dal•ic ver•sion (pō-dal′ik vĕr′zhŭn) A manual procedure that results in a podalic extraction.

pod•ar•thri•tis (pod′ahr-thrī′tis) Inflammation of any of the tarsal or metatarsal joints. [pod- + arthritis]

pod•e•de•ma (pod′ĕ-dē′mă) Edema of the feet and ankles. SYN podoedema.

po•di•a•tric (pō-dē-at′rik) Relating to podiatry.

po•di•a•tric med•i•cine (pō-dē-at′rik med′i-sin) SYN podiatry.

po•di•a•trist (pō-dī′ă-trist) A practitioner of podiatry. SYN chiropodist. [pod- + G. *iatros,* physician]

po•di•a•try (pō-dī′ă-trē) The health care specialty concerned with the diagnosis or medical, surgical, mechanical, physical, and adjunct treatment of the diseases, injuries, and defects of the human foot. SYN chiropody, podiatric medicine. [pod- + G. *iatreia,* medical treatment]

pod•o•cyte (pod′ō-sīt) An epithelial cell of the visceral layer of Bowman capsule in the renal corpuscle, attached to the outer surface of the glomerular capillary basement membrane by cytoplasmic foot processes (pedicels); believed to play a role in the ultrafiltration of blood. [podo- + G. *kytos,* a hollow (cell)]

pod•o•dy•na•mom•e•ter (pod′ō-dī′nă-mom′ĕ-tĕr) An instrument for measuring the strength of the muscles of the foot or leg. [podo- + G. *dynamis,* force, + *metron,* measure]

pod•o•dyn•i•a (pod′ō-din′ē-ă) SYN podalgia. [podo- + G. *odynē,* pain]

podoedema [Br.] SYN podedema.

pod•o•gram (pod′ō-gram) An imprint of the sole of the foot, showing the contour and the condition of the arch, or an outline tracing. [podo- + G. *gramma,* written]

pod•o•mech•a•no•ther•a•py (pod′ō-mek′ă-nō-thār′ă-pē) Treatment of foot conditions with mechanical devices, e.g., arch supports, orthoses.

poe•ci•li•a (pĕ-sil′ē-ă) Live-bearing fish including guppy and molly. Species used in cancer, neurologic, and physiologic research.

po•go•ni•on (pō-gō′nē-on) CRANIOMETRY the most anterior point on the mandible in the midline; the most anterior, prominent point on the chin. SYN mental point. [G. dim. of *pōgōn,* beard]

pOH The negative logarithm of the OH^- concentration (in moles per liter).

-poiesis Suffix meaning production; producing. [G. *poiēsis,* a making]

poikilo- Prefix meaning irregular, varied. [G. *poikilos,* many colored, varied]

poi•ki•lo•blast (poy′ki-lō-blast) A nucleated red blood cell of irregular shape. [poikilo- + G. *blastos,* germ]

poi•ki•lo•cyte (poy′ki-lō-sīt) A red blood cell of irregular shape. [poikilo- + G. *kytos,* cell]

poikilocythaemia [Br.] SYN poikilocythemia.

poi•ki•lo•cy•the•mi•a (poy′ki-lō-sī-thē′mē-ă) SYN poikilocytosis. SYN poikilocythaemia. [poikilocyte + G. *haima,* blood]

poi•ki•lo•cy•to•sis (poy′ki-lō-sī-tō′sis) The presence of poikilocytes in the peripheral blood. See page B3. SYN poikilocythemia. [poikilocyte + G. *-osis,* condition]

poi•ki•lo•der•ma (poy′ki-lō-dĕr′mă) A variegated hyperpigmentation and telangiectasia of the skin, followed by atrophy. [poikilo- + G. *derma,* skin]

poi•ki•lo•ther•mic, poi•ki•lo•ther•mal, poi•ki•lo•ther•mous (poy′ki-lō-thĕr′mik, -măl, -mŭs) **1.** Varying in temperature according to the temperature of the surrounding medium; denoting the so-called cold-blooded animals, such as the reptiles and amphibians, and the plants. **2.** Capable of existence and growth in media of varying temperature. SYN hematocryal. [poikilo- + G. *thermē,* heat]

point (poynt) **1.** SYN punctum. **2.** A sharp end or apex. **3.** A slight projection. **4.** A stage or condition reached, as the boiling point. **5.** To become ready to open, referring to an abscess or boil, the wall of which is becoming thin and is about to break. **6.** In mathematics, a dimensionless geometric element. **7.** A location or position on a graph, plot, or diagram. **8.** Decimal point. [Fr.; L. *punctum,* fr. *pungo,* pp. *punctus,* to pierce]

point A (poynt) SYN subspinale.

point an•gle (poynt ang′gĕl) The junction of three surfaces of the crown of a tooth, or of the walls of a cavity.

point B (poynt) SYN supramentale.

point of care tes•ting (poynt kār test′ing) Performance of clinical laboratory testing at the site of patient care rather than in a laboratory, and often by nonlaboratorians. SYN bedside testing.

point of el•bow (poynt el′bō) SYN olecranon.

point ep•i•dem•ic (poynt ep′i-dem′ik) An epidemic in which a pronounced clustering of cases of disease occurs within a short time (i.e., within a few days or even hours) due to exposure of persons or animals to a common source of infection such as food or water.

point of fix•a•tion (poynt fik-sā′shŭn) The point on the retina at which the rays coming from an object regarded directly are focused.

poin•til•lage (pwahn-tē-ahzh′) A massage manipulation with the tips of the fingers. [Fr. dotting, stippling]

point of max•i•mal im•pulse (poynt mak′si-măl im′pŭls) The place on the anterior chest where the apical pulse is felt most strongly. It is located in the 3rd–5th intercostal space slightly left of the mid-clavicular line. SYN apical (3).

point mu•ta•tion (poynt myū-tā′shŭn) A mutation that involves a single nucleotide; it may consist of loss of a nucleotide, substitution of one nucleotide for another, or the insertion of an additional nucleotide.

point of os•si•fi•ca•tion (poynt os′i-fi-kā′shŭn) SYN center of ossification.

poise (pwahz) In the CGS system, the unit of viscosity equal to 1 dyne-second per square centimeter and to 0.1 pascal-second. [J. *Poiseuille*]

Poi•seuille law (pwah-sē′ law) In laminar flow, the volume of a homogeneous fluid passing per unit time through a capillary tube is directly proportional to the pressure difference between its ends and to the fourth power of its internal radius, and inversely proportional to its length and to the viscosity of the fluid.

Poi•seuille space (pwah-sē′ spās) SYN still layer.

Poi•seuille vis•cos•i•ty co•ef•fi•cient (pwah-sē′ vis-kos′i-tē kō′ĕ-fish′ĕnt) An expression of viscosity as determined by the capillary tube method; the coefficient $\eta = (\pi P r^4 t / 8vl)$, where P is the pressure difference between the inlet and outlet of the tube, r the radius of the tube, l its length, and v the volume of liquid delivered in the time t. If volume is in cubic centimeters, time is in seconds, and l and r are in centimeters, then η will be in poise.

poi•son (poy′zŏn) Any substance, either taken internally or applied externally, that is injurious to health or dangerous to life. SEE ALSO toxicant, intoxicant. [Fr., fr. L. *potio,* potion, draught]

poi•son flag (poy′zŭn flag) SYN blue flag.

poi•son•ing (poy′zŏn-ing) **1.** The administering of poison. **2.** The state of being poisoned. SYN intoxication (1).

poi•son•ous (poy′zŏn-ŭs) Characterized by, having the characteristics of, or containing a poison. SYN toxic (1), venenous.

pok•er spine (pō′kĕr spīn) Stiff spine resulting from widespread joint immobility or overwhelming muscle spasm as might occur in osteomyelitis of a vertebra or a rheumatoid spondylitis.

POL Abbreviation for physician office laboratory.

Po•land syn•drome (pō′lănd sin′drōm) An anomaly consisting of absence of the pectoralis major and minor muscles, ipsilateral breast hypoplasia, and absence of two to four rib segments.

po•lar (pō′lăr) **1.** Relating to a pole. **2.** Having poles; said of certain nerve cells having one or more processes. [Mod. L. *polaris,* fr. *polus,* pole]

po•lar bod•y (pō′lăr bod′ē) One of two small cells formed by the first and second meiotic division of oocytes; the first is usually released just before ovulation, the second not until discharge of the oocyte from the ovary.

po•lar cat•a•ract (pō′lăr kat′ăr-akt) A capsular cataract limited to an area of the anterior or posterior pole of the lens.

po•lar•i•ty (pō-lar′i-tē) **1.** The property of having two opposite poles, as that possessed by a magnet. **2.** The possession of opposite properties or characteristics. **3.** The direction or orientation of positivity relative to negativity. **4.** The direction along a polynucleotide chain, or any biopolymer, or macro structure (e.g., microtubules). [Mod. L. *polaris,* polar]

po•lar•i•ty ther•a•py (pō-lar′i-tē thār′ă-pē) A bodywork modality that blends Eastern and Western medical traditions; employs gentle touch, rocking movements, and other noninvasive therapies as well as nutritional counseling and exercise; said to restore energetic balance, reduce pain, and improve overall health. SEE ALSO five-element theory, chakra.

po•lar•i•za•tion (pō′lăr-ī-zā′shŭn) **1.** ELECTRICITY coating of an electrode with a thick layer of hydrogen bubbles, with the result that the flow of current is weakened or arrested. **2.** A change effected in a ray of light passing through certain media, whereby the transverse vibrations occur in one plane only, instead of in all planes as in an ordinary light ray. **3.** Development of differences in potential between two points in living tissues, as between the inside and outside of a cell wall.

po•lar•ized light (pō′lăr-īzd līt) Light in which, as a result of reflection or transmission through certain media, the vibrations are all in one plane, transverse to the ray, instead of in all planes.

po•lar star (pō′lăr stahr) SYN daughter star.

po•lar tem•por•al ar•te•ry (pō′lăr tem′pŏr-ăl ahr′tĕr-ē) *Origin:* anterior temporal branch of middle cerebral artery; *distribution:* superomedial aspect of temporal lobe, extending to the temporal pole of cerebrum. SYN arteria polaris temporalis [TA].

pole (pōl) **1.** One of the two points at the extremities of the axis of any organ or body. **2.** Either of the two points on a sphere at the greatest distance from the equator. **3.** One of the two points in a magnet or an electric battery or cell having extremes of opposite properties; the negative pole is a cathode, the positive pole an anode. **4.** Either end of a spindle. **5.** Either of the differentiated zones at opposite ends of an axis in a cell, organ, or organism. SYN polus [TA]. [L. *polus,* the end of an axis, pole, fr. G. *polos*]

po•lice•man (pō-lēs′măn) An instrument, usually a rubber-tipped rod, for removing solid particles from a glass container.

pol•i•cy•hold•er (pol′i-sē-hōl′dĕr) The insured; a person who is covered by the insurance policy.

po•li•o (pō′lē-ō) Shortened common form of poliomyelitis.

polio- Prefix meaning gray; gray matter (substantia grisea). [G. *polios*]

po•li•o•clas•tic (pō′lē-ō-klas′tik) Destructive to gray matter of the nervous system. [polio- + G. *klastos,* broken]

po•li•o•dys•tro•phi•a (pō′lē-ō-dis-trō′fē-ă) SYN poliodystrophy.

po•li•o•dys•tro•phi•a ce•re•bri pro•gres•si•va in•fan•ti•lis (pō′lē-ō-dis-trō′fē-ă ser′ă-brī prŏ-gres′i-vă in-fan-tā′lis) Familial progressive spastic paresis of extremities with progressive mental deterioration, with development of seizures, blindness, and deafness, beginning during the first year of life, and with destruction and disorganization of nerve cells of the cerebral cortex.

po•li•o•dys•tro•phy (pō′lē-ō-dis′trŏ-fē) Wasting of the gray matter of the nervous system. SYN poliodystrophia. [polio- + G. *dys-,* bad, + *trophē,* nourishment]

po•li•o•en•ceph•a•li•tis (pō′lē-ō-en-sef′ă-lī′tis) Inflammation of the gray matter of the brain, either of the cortex or of the central nuclei; in contrast to inflammation of the white matter. [polio- + G. *enkephalos,* brain, + *-tis,* inflammation]

po•li•o•en•ceph•a•lo•me•nin•go•my•e•li•tis (pō′lē-ō-en-sef′ă-lō-mĕ-ning′gō-mī′ĕ-lī′tis) Inflammation of the gray matter of the brain and spinal cord and of the meningeal covering of the parts. [polio- + G. *enkephalos,* brain, + *mēninx,* membrane, + *myelon,* marrow, + *-itis,* inflammation]

po•li•o•en•ceph•a•lo•my•e•li•tis (pō′lē-ō-en-sef′ă-lō-mī′ĕ-lī′tis) SYN poliomyeloencephalitis.

po•li•o•en•ceph•a•lop•a•thy (pō′lē-ō-en-sef-ă-lop′ă-thē) Any disease of the gray matter of the brain. [polio- + G. *enkephalos,* brain, + *pathos,* suffering]

po•li•o•my•e•li•tis (pō′lē-ō-mī-ĕ-lī′tis) An inflammatory process involving the gray matter of the spinal cord. See page B6. [polio- + G. *myelos,* marrow, + *-itis,* inflammation]

po•li•o•my•e•li•tis vi•rus (pō′lē-ō-mī-ĕ-lī′tis vī′rŭs) The picornavirus (genus Enterovirus) causing poliomyelitis in humans; the route of infection is the alimentary tract, but the virus may enter the bloodstream and nervous system, sometimes causing paralysis of the limbs and, rarely, encephalitis; many infections are inapparent; serologic types 1, 2, and 3 are recognized, type 1 being responsible for most paralytic poliomyelitis and most epidemics. SYN poliovirus hominis.

po•li•o•my•e•lo•en•ceph•a•li•tis (pō′lē-ō-mī′ĕ-lō-en-sef′ă-lī′tis) Acute anterior poliomyelitis with pronounced cerebral signs. SYN polioencephalomyelitis. [polio- + G. *myelon,* marrow, + *enkephalos,* brain, + *-itis,* inflammation]

po•li•o•my•e•lop•a•thy (pō′lē-ō-mī-ĕ-lop′ă-thē) Any disease of the gray matter of the spinal cord. [polio- + G. *myelon,* marrow, + *pathos,* suffering]

po•li•o•sis (pō′lē-ō′sis) A patchy absence or lessening of melanin in hair of the scalp, brows, or lashes, due to lack of pigment in the epidermis; it occurs in several hereditary syndromes but may be caused by inflammation, irradiation, or infection such as herpes zoster. [G., fr. *polios,* gray]

po•li•o•vi•rus hom•i•nis (pō′lē-ō-vī′rŭs hom′i-nis) SYN poliomyelitis virus.

po•li•o•vi•rus vac•cine (pō′lē-ō-vī′rŭs vak-sēn′) **1.** Inactivated poliovirus vaccine (IPV), an aqueous suspension of inactivated strains of poliomyelitis virus (types 1, 2, and 3) used by injection. **2.** Oral poliovirus vaccine (OPV), an aqueous suspension of live, attenuated strains of poliomyelitis virus (types 1, 2, and 3) given orally for active immunization against poliomyelitis.

Po•lit•zer bag (pol′it-zĕr bag) A pear-shaped rubber bag used for forcing air through the pharyngotympanic (auditory) tube by the Politzer method.

po•litz•er•i•za•tion (pol′it-zĕr-ī-zā′shŭn) Inflation of the pharyngotympanic (auditory) tube and middle ear by the Politzer method.

Po•lit•zer lu•mi•nous cone (pol′it-zĕr lū′mi-nŭs kōn) SYN light reflex (3).

Po•lit•zer meth•od (pol′it-zĕr meth′ŏd) Inflation of the pharyngotympanic (auditory) tube and tympanum by forcing air into the nasal cavity at the instant the patient swallows.

pol•len (pol′ĕn) Microspores of seed plants carried by wind or insects prior to fertilization; important in the etiology of hay fever and other allergies. [L. fine dust, fine flour]

pol•lex, gen. **pol•li•cis**, pl. **pol•li•ces** (pol′eks, -li-sis, -sēz) [TA] SYN thumb. [L.]

pol•li•ci•za•tion (pol′i-sī-zā′shŭn) Construction of a substitute thumb. [L. *pollex,* thumb, + *-ize,* to make like, + *-ation,* state]

pol•li•no•sis, pol•le•no•sis (pol′i-nō′sis) Hay fever excited by the pollen of various plants. [L. *pollen,* pollen, + G. *-osis,* condition]

pol•lu•tant (pŏ-lū′tănt) An undesired contaminant that results in pollution. SEE ALSO pollution.

pol•lu•tion (pŏ-lū′shŭn) **1.** That which pollutes (i.e., makes unclean, impure, or unsuitable by contact or mixture with an undesirable contaminant); a pollutant. **2.** The condition of being polluted (i.e., contaminated). [L. *pollutio,* fr. *polluo,* pp. *-lutus,* to defile]

po•lo•ni•um (Po) (pŏ-lō′nē-ŭm) A radioactive element, atomic no. 84, isolated from pitchblende; the longest-lived isotope is ^{209}Po (half-life 102 years); ^{210}Po is radium F (half-life 138.38 days), the only readily accessible isotope. [L., fr. *Polonia*, Poland, native country of Marie Curie, who, with her husband, Pierre, discovered the substance]

po•lus, pl. **po•li** (pō′lŭs, -lī) [TA] SYN pole. [L. pole]

♻**poly- 1.** Prefix meaning many; multiplicity. Cf. multi-, pluri-. **2.** CHEMISTRY prefix meaning "polymer of," as in polypeptide, polysaccharide, polynucleotide; often used with symbols, as in poly(A) for poly(adenylic acid), poly(Lys) for poly(L-lysine). [G. *polys,* much, many]

pol•y•ac•ry•la•mide gel e•lec•tro•pho•re•sis (PAGE) (pol′ē-ă-kril′ă-mīd jel ĕ-lek′trō-fŏr-ē′sis) Separation of proteins or nucleic acids on the basis of both size and charge in a gel formed by cross-linking of acrylamide.

pol•y•ad•e•ni•tis (pol′ē-ad′ĕ-nī′tis) Inflammation of many lymph nodes, especially with reference to the cervical group.

pol•y•ad•e•nop•a•thy (pol′ē-ad′ĕ-nop′ă-thē) Adenopathy affecting many lymph nodes.

polyaesthesia [Br.] SYN polyesthesia.

Pól•ya gas•trec•to•my, Pól•ya op•er•a•tion (pōl′yah gas-trek′tŏ-mē, op-ĕr-ā′shŭn) Operation in which a portion of the stomach is removed and a retrocolic gastrojejunostomy is constructed in an end-to-side fashion to the entire cut end of the stomach.

pol•y(a•mine) (pol′ē-am′ēn) A polymer of an amine. SEE ALSO poly- (2).

pol•y•an•gi•i•tis (pol′ē-an′jē-ī′tis) Inflammation of many blood vessels involving more than one type of vessel, e.g., arteries and veins, or arterioles and capillaries.

pol•y•an•i•on (pol′ē-an′ī-on) Anionic sites on proteoglycans in the renal glomeruli that restrict filtration of anionic molecules and facilitate filtration of cationic proteins; loss of polyanion may cause albuminuria in lipoid nephrosis.

pol•y•ar•ter•i•tis (pol′ē-ahr-tĕr-ī′tis) Simultaneous inflammation of a number of arteries.

pol•y•ar•ter•i•tis no•do•sa (pol′ē-ahr-tĕr-ī′tis nō-dō′să) Segmental inflammation, with infiltration by eosinophils, and necrosis of medium or small arteries; most common in males, with varied symptoms related to involvement of arteries in the kidneys, muscles, gastrointestinal tract, and heart. SYN periarteritis nodosa.

pol•y•ar•thric (pol′ē-ahr′thrik) SYN multiarticular.

pol•y•ar•thri•tis (pol′ē-ahr-thrī′tis) Simultaneous inflammation of several joints. [poly- + G. *arthron,* joint, + *-itis,* inflammation]

pol•y•ar•tic•u•lar (pol′ē-ahr-tik′yū-lăr) SYN multiarticular. [poly- + L. *articulus,* joint]

pol•y•ax•i•al joint (pol′ē-aks′ē-ăl joynt) SYN multiaxial joint.

pol•y•ba•sic (pol′ē-bā′sik) Having more than one replaceable hydrogen atom; denoting an acid with a basicity greater than 1.

pol•y•blast (pol′ē-blast) One of a group of ameboid, mononucleated, wandering phagocytic cells found in inflammatory exudates. [poly- + G. *blastos,* germ]

pol•y•chon•dri•tis (pol′ē-kon-drī′tis) A widespread disease of cartilage. [poly- + G. *chondros,* cartilage, + *-itis,* inflammation]

polychromaemia [Br.] SYN polychromemia.

pol•y•chro•ma•si•a (pol′ē-krō-mā′zē-ă) SYN polychromatophilia.

pol•y•chro•mat•ic (pol′ē-krō-mat′ik) Multicolored.

pol•y•chro•mat•ic cell (pol′ē-krō-mat′ik sel) A primitive erythrocyte in bone marrow, with basophilic material as well as hemoglobin (acidophilic) in the cytoplasm. SYN polychromatophil cell.

pol•y•chro•mat•ic ra•di•a•tion (pol′ē-krō-mat′ik rā′dē-ā′shŭn) Radiation containing gamma rays of many different energies; in diagnostic radiology, typically Bremsstrahlung radiation (q.v.).

pol•y•chro•mat•o•cyte (pol′ē-krō-mat′ō-sīt) SYN polychromatophil (2).

pol•y•chro•ma•to•phil, pol•y•chro•ma•to•phile (pol′ē-krō-mat′ō-fil, -fīl) **1.** Staining readily with acid, neutral, and basic dyes; denoting certain cells, especially certain red blood cells. SYN polychromatophilic. **2.** A young or degenerating erythrocyte that manifests acidic and basic staining affinities. SYN polychromatocyte. [poly- + G. *chrōma,* color, + *phileō,* to love]

pol•y•chro•ma•to•phil cell (pol′ē-krō-mat′ō-fil sel) SYN polychromatic cell.

pol•y•chro•ma•to•phil•i•a (pol′ē-krō′mă-tō-fil′ē-ă) **1.** A tendency of certain cells, such as the red blood cells in pernicious anemia, to stain with basic and also acidic dyes. **2.** Condition characterized by the presence of many red blood cells that have an affinity for acid, basic, or neutral stains. SYN polychromasia.

pol•y•chro•ma•to•phil•ic (pol′ē-krō′mă-tō-fil′ik) SYN polychromatophil (1).

pol•y•chro•me•mi•a (pol′ē-krō-mē′mē-ă) An increase in the total amount of hemoglobin in the blood. SYN polychromaemia.

pol•y•clin•ic (pol′ē-klin′ik) A dispensary for the treatment and study of diseases of all kinds. [poly- + G. *klinē,* bed]

pol•y•clo•nal (pol′ē-klō′năl) IMMUNOCHEMISTRY pertaining to proteins from more than a single clone of cells, in contradistinction to monoclonal.

pol•y•clo•nal gam•mop•a•thy (pol′ē-klō′năl gă-mop′ă-thē) A gammopathy in which there is a heterogeneous increase in immunoglobulins involving more than one cell line; can be caused by a variety of inflammatory, infectious, or neoplastic disorders.

pol•y•clo•ni•a (pol′ē-klō′nē-ă) SYN myoclonus multiplex. [poly- + G. *klonos,* tumult]

pol•y•co•ri•a (pol′ē-kō′rē-ă) The presence of two or more pupils in one iris. [poly- + G. *korē,* pupil]

pol•y•crot•ic (pol′ē-krot′ik) Relating to or marked by polycrotism.

po•lyc•ro•tism (pol-ik′rō-tizm) A condition in which the sphygmographic tracing shows several upward breaks in the descending wave. [poly- + G. *krotos,* a beat]

pol•y•cy•e•sis (pol′ē-sī-ē′sis) SYN multiple pregnancy. [poly- + G. *kyēsis,* pregnancy]

pol•y•cys•tic (pol′ē-sis′tik) Composed of many cysts.

pol•y•cys•tic kid•ney, pol•y•cys•tic dis•ease of kid•neys (pol′ē-sis′tik kid′nē, pol′ē-sis′tik di-zēz′ kid′nēz) A progressive disease characterized by formation of multiple cysts of varying size scattered diffusely throughout both kidneys, resulting in compression and destruction of kidney parenchyma, usually with hypertension, gross hematuria, and uremia.

pol•y•cys•tic liv•er (pol′ē-sis′tik liv′ĕr) Gradual cystic dilation of intralobular bile ducts (Meyenburg complexes) that fail to involute in embryonic development of the liver; associated with polycystic kidneys and occasionally with cystic involvement of the pancreas, lungs, and other organs.

pol•y•cys•tic o•va•ry (pol′ē-sis′tik ō′văr-ē) An enlarged pearl-white, cystic ovary, with thickened tunica albuginea. SEE ALSO polycystic ovary syndrome.

pol•y•cys•tic o•va•ry syn•drome (pol′ē-sis′tik ō′văr-ē sin′drōm) A condition commonly characterized by signs of masculinization such as hirsutism, as well as obesity, menstrual abnormalities, infertility, and enlarged ovaries; thought to reflect excessive androgen secretion of ovarian origin. SEE ALSO polycystic ovary.

polycythaemia [Br.] SYN polycythemia.

polycythaemia hypertonica [Br.] SYN polycythemia hypertonica.

polycythaemia rubra [Br.] SYN polycythemia rubra.

pol•y•cy•the•mi•a (pol′ē-sī-thē′mē-ă) An abnormal increase in the number of red blood cells. SYN erythrocythemia, polycythaemia. [poly- + G. *kytos,* cell, + *haima,* blood]

pol•y•cy•the•mi•a hy•per•to•ni•ca (pol′ē-sī-thē′mē-ă hī-pĕr-ton′i-kă) Polycythemia associated with hypertension, but without splenomegaly. SYN Gaisböck syndrome, polycythaemia hypertonica.

pol•y•cy•the•mi•a ru•bra (pol′ē-sī-thē′mē-ă rū′bră) SYN polycythemia vera. SYN polycythaemia rubra.

pol•y•cy•the•mi•a ve•ra (pol′ē-sī-thē′mē-ă vē′ră) A chronic form of polycythemia of unknown cause; characterized by bone marrow hyperplasia, an increase in blood volume as well as in the number of red blood cells, redness or cyanosis of the skin, and splenomegaly. SYN erythremia, Osler disease, Osler-Vaquez disease, polycythemia rubra, Vaquez disease.

pol•y•dac•ty•ly (pol′ē-dak′ti-lē) Presence of more than five fingers or toes on hand or foot. [poly- + G. *daktylos,* finger]

pol•y•dip•si•a (pol′ē-dip′sē-ă) Excessive thirst that is relatively prolonged. [poly- + G. *dipsa,* thirst]

pol•y•dys•pla•si•a (pol′ē-dis-plā′zē-ă) Tissue development abnormal in several respects. [poly- + G. *dys-,* bad, + *plasis,* a molding]

poly•en•do•crin•op•athy (pol′ē-en′dō-kri-nop′ă-thē) A disease usually caused by insufficiency of multiple endocrine glands. SEE ALSO multiple endocrine deficiency syndrome.

pol•y•e•no•ic ac•ids (pol′ē-en-ō′ik as′idz) Fatty acids with more than one double bond in the carbon chain (e.g., linoleic, linolenic, and arachidonic acids).

pol•y•er•gic (pol′ē-ĕr′jik) Capable of acting in several different ways. [poly- + G. *ergon,* work]

pol•y•es•the•si•a (pol′ē-es-thē′zē-ă) A disorder of sensation in which a single touch or other stimulus is felt as several. SYN polyaesthesia. [poly- + G. *aisthēsis,* sensation]

pol•y•ga•lac•ti•a (pol′ē-gă-lak′shē-ă) Excessive secretion of breast milk, especially during the weaning period. [poly- + G. *gala,* milk]

pol•y•ga•lac•tu•ro•nase (pol′ē-gă-lak-tūr′ō-nās) Pectin depolymerase; an enzyme catalyzing the random hydrolysis of 1,4-α-D-galactosiduronic linkages in pectate and other galacturonans.

pol•y•gene (pol′ē-jēn) One of many genes that contribute to the phenotypic value of a measurable phenotype.

pol•y•gen•ic (pol′ē-jen′ik) Relating to a hereditary disease or normal characteristic controlled by the added effects of genes at multiple loci.

pol•y•glan•du•lar (pol′ē-glan′jū-lăr) SYN pluriglandular.

pol•y•graph (pol′ē-graf) **1.** An instrument for obtaining simultaneous tracings from several different sources (e.g., radial and jugular pulse, apex beat of the heart, phonocardiogram, electrocardiogram). The ECG is nearly always included for timing. **2.** An instrument for recording changes in respiration, blood pressure, galvanic skin response, and other physiologic changes while the subject is interviewed or asked to give associations to relevant and irrelevant words; the physiologic changes are presumed to be emotional reactions, and thus indicative of whether the subject is telling the truth. SYN lie detector. [poly- + G. *graphō,* to write]

pol•y•gy•ri•a (pol′ē-jī′rē-ă) Condition in which the brain has an excessive number of convolutions. [poly- + G. *gyros,* circle, gyre]

pol•y•hi•dro•sis (pol′ē-hī-drō′sis) SYN hyperhidrosis.

pol•y•hy•dram•ni•os (pol′ē-hī-dram′nē-ŏs) Excess amount of amniotic fluid. [poly- + G. *hydōr,* water, + amnion]

pol•y•hy•dric (pol′ē-hī′drik) Containing more than one hydroxyl group, as in polyhydric alcohols and polyhydric acids.

pol•y•i•dro•sis (pol′ē-ī-drō′sis) SYN hyperhidrosis.

pol•y•lep•tic (pol′ē-lep′tik) Denoting a disease occurring in many paroxysms, e.g., malaria, epilepsy. [poly- + G. *lēpsis,* a seizing]

pol•y•mas•ti•a (pol′ē-mas′tē-ă) In humans, a condition in which more than two breasts are present. SYN hypermastia (1), pleomastia, pleomazia. [poly- + G. *mastos,* breast]

pol•y•me•li•a (pol′ē-mē′lē-ă) A developmental defect in which there are supernumerary limbs or parts of limbs. [poly- + G. *melos,* limb]

pol•y•men•or•rhe•a (pol′ē-men′ŏr-ē′ă) Occurrence of menstrual cycles of greater than usual frequency. SYN polymenorrhoea. [poly- + G. *mēn,* month, + *rhoia,* flow]

polymenorrhoea [Br.] SYN polymenorrhea.

pol•y•mer (pol′i-mĕr) A substance of high molecular weight, made up of a chain of repeated units sometimes called "mers." SEE ALSO -mer (1).

pol•y•mer•ase (pŏ-lim′ĕr-ās) General term for any enzyme catalyzing a polymerization, as of nucleotides to polynucleotides, thus belonging to EC class 2, the transferases.

pol•y•mer•ase chain re•ac•tion (PCR) (pŏ-lim′ĕr-ās chān rē-ăk′shŭn) An enzymatic method for the repeated copying and amplification of the two strands of DNA of a particular gene sequence.

pol•y•me•ri•a (pol′ē-mēr′ē-ă) Condition characterized by an excessive number of parts, limbs, or organs of the body. [poly- + G. *meros,* part]

pol•y•mer•ic (pol′i-mer′ik) **1.** Having the properties of a polymer. **2.** Relating to or characterized by polymeria. **3.** Rarely used synonym for polygenic.

polymerisation [Br.] SYN polymerization.

po•lym•er•i•za•tion (pol′i-mĕr′ī-zā′shŭn) A reaction in which a high molecular weight product is produced by successive additions to or condensations of a simpler compound. SYN polymerisation.

po•lym•er•ize (pol′i-mĕr-īz) To bring about polymerization.

pol•y•mor•phic (pol′ē-mōr′fik) Occurring in more than one morphologic form. SYN multiform, pleomorphic (1), pleomorphous, polymorphous. [G. *polymorphos,* multiform]

pol•y•mor•phic gen•e•tic mark•er (pol′ē-mōrf′ik jĕ-net′ik mahr′kĕr) Inherited characteristic that occurs within a given population as two or more traits.

pol•y•mor•phism (pol′ē-mōr′fizm) Occurrence in more than one form; existence in the same species or other natural group of more than one morphologic type. SYN pleomorphism.

pol•y•mor•pho•cel•lu•lar (pol′ē-mōr′fō-sel′yū-lăr) Relating to or formed of cells of several different kinds. [G. *polymorphos,* multiform, + L. *cellula,* cell]

pol•y•mor•pho•nu•cle•ar (pol′ē-mōr′fō-nū′klē-ăr) Having nuclei of varied forms; denoting a variety of leukocyte. [G. *polymorphos,* multiform, + L. *nucleus,* kernel]

pol•y•mor•pho•nu•cle•ar leu•ko•cyte, pol•y•nu•cle•ar leu•ko•cyte (pol′ē-mōr′fō-nū′klē-ăr lū′kō-sīt, pol′ē-nū′klē-ăr) Common term for granulocyte or granulocytic leukocyte; includes basophilic, eosinophilic, and neutrophilic leukocytes, but generally used with special reference to the neutrophilic leukocytes.

pol•y•mor•phous (pol′ē-mōr′fŭs) SYN polymorphic.

pol•y•mor•phous light e•rup•tion (pol′ē-mōr′fŭs līt ĕr-ŭp′shŭn) A common pruritic papular eruption appearing in a few hours and lasting up to several days on skin exposed to shortwave ultraviolet light; subepidermal edema and deep perivascular lymphocytic infiltration is seen microscopically.

pol•y•mor•phous low-grade car•ci•no•ma of sal•i•var•y glands (pol′ē-mōr′fŭs lō-grād kahr′si-nō′mă sal′i-var-ē glandz) A low-grade malignant tumor of salivary glands showing several histologic patterns, such as cribriform, ductal, and papillary growth. SYN terminal duct carcinoma.

pol•y•my•al•gi•a (pol′ē-mī-al′jē-ă) Pain in several muscle groups. [poly- + G. *mys,* muscle, + *algos,* pain]

pol•y•my•oc•lo•nus (pol′ē-mī-ok′lŏ-nŭs) SYN myoclonus multiplex.

pol•y•my•o•si•tis (pol′ē-mī′ō-sī′tis) Inflammation of a number of voluntary muscles simultaneously. [poly- + G. *mys,* muscle, + *-itis,* inflammation]

pol•y•ne•sic (pol′ē-nē′sik) Occurring in many separate foci; denoting certain forms of inflammation or infection. [poly- + G. *nēsos,* island]

pol•y•neu•ral (pol′ē-nūr′ăl) Relating to, supplied by, or affecting several nerves. [poly- + G. *neuron,* nerve]

pol•y•neu•ral•gi•a (pol′ē-nūr-al′jē-ă) Neuralgia of several nerves simultaneously.

pol•y•neu•rit•ic psy•cho•sis (pol′ē-nūr-it′ik sī-kō′sis) SYN Korsakoff syndrome.

pol•y•neu•ri•tis (pol′ē-nūr-ī′tis) SYN polyneuropathy (2).

pol•y•neu•rop•a•thy (pol′ē-nūr-op′ă-thē) **1.** A disease process involving a number of peripheral nerves (literal sense). **2.** A nontraumatic generalized disorder of peripheral nerves, affecting the distal fibers most severely, with proximal shading (e.g., the feet are affected sooner or more severely than the hands), and typically symmetrically; most often affects motor and sensory fibers almost equally, but can involve either one solely or very disproportionately; classified as axon degenerating (axonal), or demyelinating; many causes, particularly metabolic and toxic; familial or sporadic in nature. SYN polyneuritis. **3.** SYN acrodynia (2). SYN multiple neuritis. [poly- + G. *neuron,* nerve, + *pathos,* disease]

pol•y•nu•cle•ar, pol•y•nu•cle•ate (pol′ē-nū′klē-ăr, -klē-āt) SYN multinuclear.

pol•y•nu•cle•o•ti•dase (pol′ē-nū′klē-ō′ti-dās) Enzyme catalyzing the hydrolysis of polynucleotides to oligonucleotides or to mononucleotides.

pol•y•nu•cle•o•tide (pol′ē-nū′klē-ō-tīd) A linear polymer containing an indefinite (usually large) number of nucleotides, linked from one ribose (or deoxyribose) to another via phosphoric residues. Cf. oligonucleotide.

pol•y•o•don•ti•a (pol′ē-ō-don′shē-ă) Presence of supernumerary teeth. [poly- + G. *odous,* tooth]

pol•y•on•co•sis, **pol•y•on•cho•sis** (pol′ē-ong-kō′sis) Formation of multiple tumors. [poly- + G. *onkos,* tumor, + *-osis,* condition]

pol•y•o•nych•i•a (pol′ē-ō-nik′ē-ă) Presence of supernumerary nails on fingers or toes. [poly- + G. *onyx,* nail]

pol•y•o•pi•a, **pol•y•op•si•a** (pol′ē-ō′pē-ă, -op′sē-ă) The perception of several images of the same object. SYN multiple vision. [poly- + G. *ōps,* eye]

pol•y•or•chism, **pol•y•or•chid•ism** (pol′ē-ōr′kizm, -kid-izm) Presence of one or more supernumerary testes. [poly- + G. *orchis,* testis]

pol•y•os•tot•ic (pol′ē-os-tot′ik) Involving more than one bone. [poly- + G. *osteon,* bone]

pol•y•o•ti•a (pol′ē-ō′shē-ă) Presence of a supernumerary auricle of the ear on one or both sides of the head. [poly- + G. *ous,* ear]

pol•y•ov•u•lar (pol′ē-ov′yū-lăr) Containing more than one oocyte (ovum).

pol•y•ov•u•la•tor•y (pol′ē-ov′yū-lă-tōr-ē) Discharging several oocytes (ova) in one ovulatory cycle.

pol•yp (pol′ip) A general descriptive term used with reference to any mass of tissue that bulges or projects outward or upward from the normal surface level, thereby being macroscopically visible as a hemispheroid, spheroid, or irregular moundlike structure growing from a relatively broad base or a slender stalk; polyps may be neoplasms, foci of inflammation, degenerative lesions, or malformations. See this page. SYN polypus. [L. *polypus;* G. *polypous,* contr. fr. G. *polys,* many, + *pous,* foot]

pol•yp•ec•to•my (pol′i-pek′tŏ-mē) Excision of a polyp. See page B17. [polyp + G. *ektomē,* excision]

pol•y•pep•tide (pol′ē-pep′tīd) A peptide formed by the union of an indefinite (usually large) number of amino acids by peptide links (–NH–CO–). Cf. bioregulator.

pol•y•pha•gi•a (pol′ē-fā′jē-ă) Excessive eating; gluttony. [poly- + G. *phagō,* to eat]

pol•y•phar•ma•cy (pol′ē-fahr′mă-sē) The administration of many drugs at the same time.

pol•y•phen•ic gene (pol′ē-fē′nik jēn) SYN pleiotropic gene.

pol•y•phe•nols (pol′ē-fē′nolz) Organic compounds containing more than one phenol group; responsible for the color and flavor of some fruits and vegetables; may have antioxidant properties.

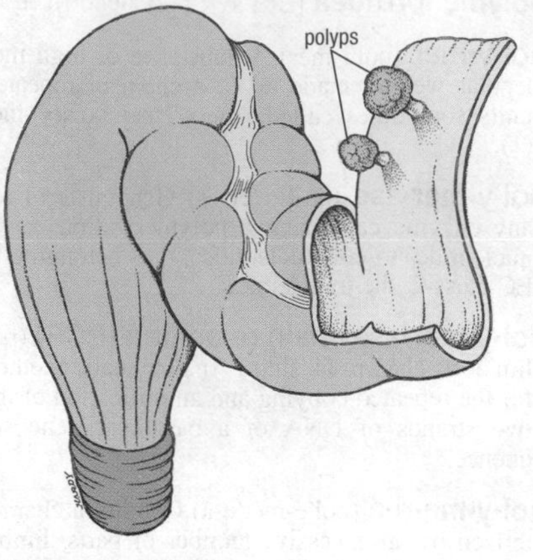

polyps: in sigmoid colon

pol•y•pho•bi•a (pol′ē-fō′bē-ă) Morbid fear of many things; a condition marked by the presence of many phobias. [poly- + G. *phobos,* fear]

pol•y•phra•si•a (pol′ē-frā′zē-ă) Extreme talkativeness. SEE ALSO logorrhea. [poly- + G. *phrasis,* speech]

pol•y•phy•let•ic (pol′ē-fī-let′ik) **1.** Derived from more than one source, or having several lines of descent, in contrast to monophyletic. **2.** HEMATOLOGY relating to polyphyletism.

pol•y•plas•tic (pol′ē-plas′tik) **1.** Formed of several different structures. **2.** Capable of assuming several forms. [poly- + G. *plastikos,* plastic]

poly•ploid (pol′ē-ployd) Characterized by or pertaining to polyploidy.

pol•y•ploi•dy (pol′ē-ploy′dē) The state of a cell nucleus containing three or more haploid sets. Cells containing three, four, five, or six multiples are referred to, respectively, as triploid, tetraploid, pentaploid, and hexaploid. [poly- + G. *ploidēs,* in form]

pol•yp•ne•a (pol′ip-nē′ă) SYN tachypnea. SYN polypnoea. [poly- + G. *pnoia,* breath]

polypnoea [Br.] SYN polypnea.

pol•yp•oid (pol′i-poyd) Resembling a polyp in gross features. [polyp + G. *eidos,* resemblance]

po•lyp•or•ous (pŏ-lip′ŏr-ŭs) SYN cribriform. [poly- + G. *poros,* pore]

pol•yp•o•sis (pol′i-pō′sis) Presence of several polyps. [polyp + G. *-osis,* condition]

pol•y•pous (pol′i-pŭs) Pertaining to, manifesting the gross features of, or characterized by the presence of a polyp or polyps.

pol•yp•tych•i•al (pol′ip-tik′ē-ăl) Folded or arranged so as to form more than one layer. [G. *polyptychos,* having many folds or layers, fr. poly- + *ptychē,* fold or layer]

pol•y•pus, pl. **po•ly•pi** (pol′i-pŭs, -pī) SYN polyp. [L.]

pol•y•ra•dic•u•li•tis (pol′ē-ră-dik′yū-lī′tis) SYN polyradiculopathy.

pol•y•ra•dic•u•lo•my•op•a•thy (pol′ē-ră-dik′yū-lō-mī-op′ă-thē) Coexisting polyradiculopathy and myopathy.

pol•y•ra•dic•u•lo•neu•ri•tis (pol′ē-ră-dik′yū-lō-nūr-ī′tis) SYN Guillain-Barré syndrome.

pol•y•ra•dic•u•lo•neu•rop•a•thy (pol-ē-ra-dik′yū-lō-nūr-op′ă-thē) Coexisting polyradiculopathy and polyneuropathy.

pol•y•ra•dic•u•lop•a•thy (pol′ē-ră-dik′yū-lop′ă-thē) Diffuse root involvement; seen with, among other disorders, diabetic neuropathy (diabetic polyradiculopathy). SYN polyradiculitis.

pol•y•ri•bo•somes (pol′ē-rī′bō-sōmz) Two or more ribosomes connected by a molecule of messenger RNA. SYN polysomes.

pol•y•sac•char•ide (pol′ē-sak′ă-rīd) A carbohydrate containing a large number of saccharide groups (e.g., starch). Cf. oligosaccharide. SYN glycan.

pol•y•sac•cha•ride con•ju•gat•ed vac•cine (pol′e-sak′a-rıd kon′jŭ-ga-tĕd vak-sēn′) A vaccine made from the capsular polysaccharide of the microorganism conjugated with a protein such as the *Haemophilus influenzae* type B vaccine against meningitis.

pol•y•ser•o•si•tis (pol′ē-sĕr′ō-sī′tis) Chronic inflammation with effusions in several serous cavities resulting in fibrous thickening of the serosa and constrictive pericarditis. SYN Bamberger disease (2), Concato disease. [poly- + L. *serum,* serum, + G. *-itis,* inflammation]

pol•y•si•nu•si•tis (pol′ē-sī′nŭ-sī′tis) Simultaneous inflammation of two or more sinuses.

pol•y•somes (pol′ē-sōmz) SYN polyribosomes.

pol•y•so•mi•a (pol′ē-sō′mē-ă) Fetal malformation involving two or more imperfect and partially fused bodies. [poly- + G. *sōma,* body]

pol•y•so•mic (pol′ē-sō′mik) Pertaining to or characterized by polysomy.

pol•y•som•no•gram (pol′ē-som′nō-gram) The recorded physiologic function(s) obtained in polysomnography. [poly- + L. *somnus,* sleep, + G. *gramma,* diagram]

pol•y•som•nog•ra•phy (pol′ē-som-nog′ră-fē) Simultaneous and continuous monitoring of relevant normal and abnormal physiologic activity during sleep. [poly- + L. *somnus,* sleep, + G. *graphō,* to write]

pol•y•so•my (pol′ē-sō′mē) State of a cell nucleus in which a specific chromosome is represented more than twice. Cells containing three, four, or five homologous chromosomes are referred to, respectively, as trisomic, tetrasomic, or pentasomic. Cf. polyploidy. [poly- + G. *sōma,* body (chromosome)]

pol•y•sper•mi•a, **pol•y•sper•mism** (pol′ē-spĕr′mē-ă, -mizm) **1.** SYN polyspermy. **2.** An abnormally profuse spermatic secretion.

pol•y•sper•my (pol′ē-spĕr′mē) The entrance of more than one sperm into the oocyte during fertilization. SYN polyspermia (1), polyspermism.

pol•y•sple•ni•a (pol′ē-splē′nē-ă) A condition in which splenic tissue is divided into nearly equal masses; there are several small spleens; congenital heart disease and malposition and maldevelopment of abdominal organs are common; may be related to situs inversus. Most cases are sporadic, although some suggest autosomal recessive inheritance. SYN Ivemark syndrome.

pol•y•stich•i•a (pol′ē-stik′ē-ă) Arrangement of the eyelashes in two or more rows. [poly- + G. *stichos,* row]

pol•y•sym•brach•y•dac•ty•ly (pol′ē-sim-brak′ē-dak′ti-lē) Malformation of the hand or foot in which the shortened fingers or toes are syndactylous and polydactylous. [poly- + symbrachydactyly]

pol•y•syn•ap•tic (pol′ē-sin-ap′tik) Referring to neural pathways formed by a chain of a large number of synaptically connected nerve cells, as distinguished from oligosynaptic conduction systems. SYN multisynaptic.

pol•y•syn•dac•ty•ly (pol′ē-sin-dak′ti-lē) Syndactyly of several fingers or toes.

pol•y•ten•di•ni•tis (pol′ē-ten′di-nī′tis) Inflammation of several tendons.

pol•y•the•li•a (pol′ē-thē′lē-ă) Presence of supernumerary nipples, either on the breast or elsewhere on the body. SYN hyperthelia. [poly- + G. *thēlē,* nipple]

pol•y•to•mog•ra•phy (pol′ē-tŏ-mog′ră-fē) Body section radiography using a machine designed to effect complex motion; images a thinner tissue plane compared with simple linear or circular tomography.

pol•y•trich•i•a (pol′ē-trik′ē-ă) Excessive hairiness. [poly- + G. *thrix* (*trich-*), hair]

pol•y•un•sat•u•ra•ted fat (pol′ē-ŭn-sach′ŭr-ā-tĕd fat) A type of unsaturated fat. Diets high in unsaturated fat produce lower cholesterol levels.

pol•y•u•ri•a (pol′ē-yūr′ē-ă) Excessive excretion of urine resulting in profuse micturition; causes include diabetes insipidus, diabetes mellitus, and hypercalcemia, but sometimes results from overhydration. [poly- + G. *ouron,* urine]

pol•y•va•lent (pol'ē-vā'lĕnt) **1.** SYN multivalent. **2.** SEE polyvalent serum.

pol•y•va•lent al•ler•gy (pol'ē-vā'lĕnt al'ĕr-jē) Allergic response manifested simultaneously for several or numerous specific allergens.

pol•y•va•lent se•rum (pol'ē-vā'lĕnt sēr'ŭm) An antiserum obtained by inoculating an animal with several antigens or species or strains of bacteria.

pol•y•va•lent vac•cine (pol'ē-vā'lĕnt vak-sēn') A vaccine prepared from cultures of two or more strains of the same species or microorganism. SYN multivalent vaccine.

po•made ac•ne (pom-ād' ak'nē) The disorder as commonly found on the forehead and temples of black people after repeated application of hair creams.

POMC Abbreviation for proopiomelanocortin.

Pom•er•oy op•er•a•tion (pom'ĕr-ōy op-ĕr-ā'shŭn) Excision of a ligated portion of the fallopian tubes.

Pom•pe dis•ease (pom'pĕ di-zēz') SYN glycogenosis type 2.

POMR Abbreviation for problem-oriented medical record.

pon•ceau de xy•li•dine (pon-sō' dĕ zī'li-dēn) [CI-16151] A monoazo acid dye originally employed as a red histologic counterstain in Masson trichrome stain.

Pon•fick shad•ow (pon'fik shad'ō) SYN achromocyte.

pons (ponz) **1.** [TA] In neuroanatomy, the pons varolii or pons cerebelli; that part of the brainstem between the medulla oblongata caudally and the mesencephalon rostrally, composed of the basilar part of pons and the tegmentum of pons. On the ventral surface of the brain the basilar part of pons, the white pontine protuberance, is demarcated from both the medulla oblongata and the mesencephalon by distinct transverse grooves. **2.** Any bridgelike formation connecting two more-or-less disjoined parts of the same structure or organ. [L. bridge]

pon•tic (pon'tik) An artificial tooth on a fixed or removable partial denture; it replaces the lost natural tooth and restores its functions, and usually occupies the space previously occupied by the natural crown.

pon•tile, pon•tine (pon'tīl, pon'tēn) Relating to a pons.

pon•tine flex•ure (pon'tēn flek'shŭr) The dorsally concave curvature of the rhombencephalon in the embryo; its appearance indicates division of rhombencephalon into myelencephalon and metencephalon. SYN basicranial flexure, transverse rhombencephalic flexure.

pon•tine nu•cle•i (pon'tēn nū'klē-ī) The massive gray matter filling the basilar pons. The nuclei are of fairly homogeneous architecture and project to the cortex of the contralateral cerebellar hemisphere by way of the middle cerebellar peduncle. Their main afferents come from the entire extent of the cerebral neocortex by way of the longitudinal pontine bundles (corticopontine fibers); thus, the pontine nuclei form a major way station in the impulse conduction from the cerebral cortex of one hemisphere to the posterior lobe of the opposite cerebellum.

pon•to•cer•e•bel•lar fi•bers (pon'tō-ser'e-bel'ăr fī'bĕrz) Those fibers arising from the nuclei of the basilar pons and primarily crossing the midline (there is a modes uncrossed projection), centering the cerebellum through the middle cerebellar peduncle and terminating as mossy fibers in the cerebellar cortex.

pon•to•med•ul•lar•y groove (pon'to-med'ū-lar-ē grūv) The transverse groove on the ventral aspect of the brainstem that demarcates the pons from the medulla oblongata; from its bottom the sixth, seventh, and eighth cranial nerves emerge.

pool (pūl) **1.** A collection of blood or other fluid in any region of the body; pool of blood results from dilation and retardation of the circulation in the capillaries and veins of the part. **2.** A combination of resources. [A.S. *pōl*]

Pool phe•nom•e•non (pūl fĕ-nom'ĕ-non) **1.** In tetany, spasm of both the quadriceps and calf muscles when the extended leg is flexed at the hip. SYN Schlesinger sign. **2.** In tetany, contraction of the arm muscles following the stretching of the brachial plexus by elevation of the arm above the head with the forearm extended; resembles the contraction resulting from stimulation of the ulnar nerve.

poor•ly dif•fer•en•ti•at•ed lym•pho•cyt•ic lym•pho•ma (PDLL) (pōr'lē dif'ĕr-en'shē-āt-ĕd lim'fō-sit'ik lim-fō'mă) A B-cell lymphoma with nodular or diffuse lymph node or bone marrow involvement by large lymphoid cells.

pop•lit•e•al (pop-lit'ē-ăl) Relating to the popliteal fossa.

pop•lit•e•al ar•ter•y (pop-lit'ē-ăl ahr'tĕr-ē) Continuation of femoral artery in the popliteal space, bifurcating (at the lower border of the popliteus muscle as it passes deep to the arcus tendineus of the soleus muscle) into the anterior and posterior tibial arteries; *branches,* lateral and medial superior genicular, middle genicular, lateral and medial inferior genicular, and sural arteries. See page B21. SYN arteria poplitea [TA].

pop•lit•e•al fos•sa (pop-lit'ē-ăl fos'ă) The diamond-shaped space posterior to the knee joint bounded superficially by the diverging biceps femoris and semimembranosus muscles above and inferiorly by the two heads of the gastrocnemius muscle; deeply, the fossa is bounded superiorly by the diverging supracondylar lines of the femur and the soleal line of the tibia inferiorly. Contents: tibial nerve, popliteal artery, vein, fat. See this page.

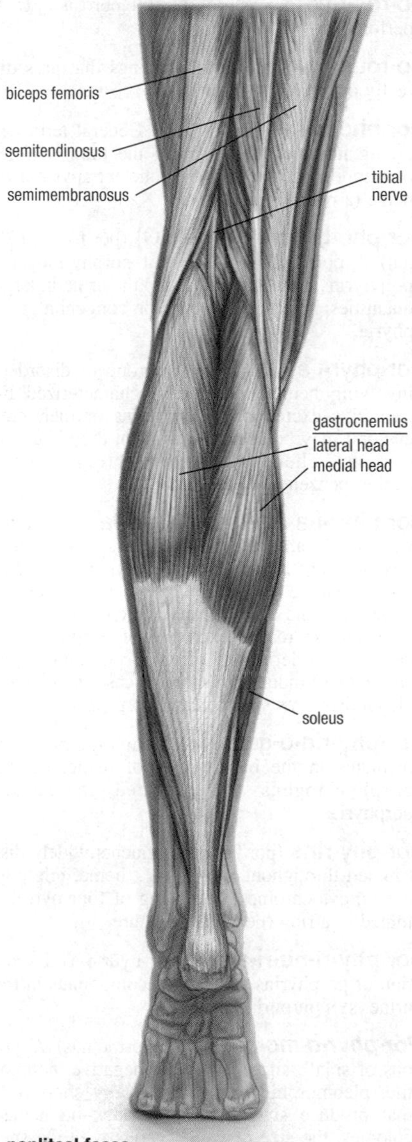

popliteal fossa

pop·lit·e·al groove (pop-lit′ē-ăl grūv) A groove on the lateral condyle of the femur between the epicondyle and the articular margin. Its anterior end gives origin to the popliteus muscle; its posterior end lodges the tendon of the muscle when the knee is fully flexed.

pop·lit·e·al mus·cle (pop-lit′ē-ăl mŭs′ĕl) SYN popliteus muscle.

pop·lit·e·al pulse (pop-lit′ē-ăl pŭls) A palpable rhythmic expansion of the popliteal artery behind the knee.

pop·lit·e·al vein (pop-lit′ē-ăl vān) Formed at the lower border of the popliteus muscle by the union of the anterior and posterior tibial veins, ascends through the popliteal space, where it receives the lesser saphenous vein and passes through the adductor hiatus, entering the adductor canal as the femoral vein.

pop·li·te·us mus·cle (pop-lit′ē-ŭs mŭs′ĕl) *Origin*, lateral condyle of femur; *insertion*, posterior surface of tibia above oblique line; *action*, from the fully extended and "locked" position, rotates the femur medially, on the fixed (planted) tibial plateau about 5 degrees, "unlocking" the knee to enable flexion to occur; *nerve supply*, tibial. See page 1242. SYN musculus popliteus [TA], popliteal muscle.

po·po·ti·llo (pō-pō-tē′yō) SYN ephedra. [Sp., fr. Nahuatl *popotl*, broom]

pop·u·la·tion (pop′yū-lā′shŭn) Statistical term denoting all the objects, events, or subjects in a particular class. Cf. sample (1). [L. *populus*, a people, nation]

pop·u·la·tion ge·net·ics (pop′yū-lā′shŭn jĕ-net′iks) The study of genetic influences on the components of cause and effect in the somatic characteristics of populations.

POR Abbreviation for problem-oriented medical record.

pore (pōr) **1.** An opening, hole, perforation, or foramen. **2.** SYN sweat pore. [G. *poros*, passageway]

por·en·ce·pha·li·a (pōr′en-sĕ-fā′lē-ă) SYN porencephaly.

por·en·ce·phal·ic (pōr′en-sĕ-fal′ik) Relating to or characterized by porencephaly. SYN porencephalous.

por·en·ceph·a·li·tis (pōr′en-sef′ă-lī′tis) Chronic inflammation of the brain, with the formation of cavities in the organ's substance. [G. *poros*, pore, + *enkephalos*, brain, + *-itis*, inflammation]

por·en·ceph·a·lous (pōr′en-sef′ă-lŭs) SYN porencephalic.

por·en·ceph·a·ly (pōr′en-sef′ă-lē) The occurrence of cavities in the brain substance, communicating usually with the lateral ventricles. SYN porencephalia. [G. *poros*, pore, + *enkephalos*, brain]

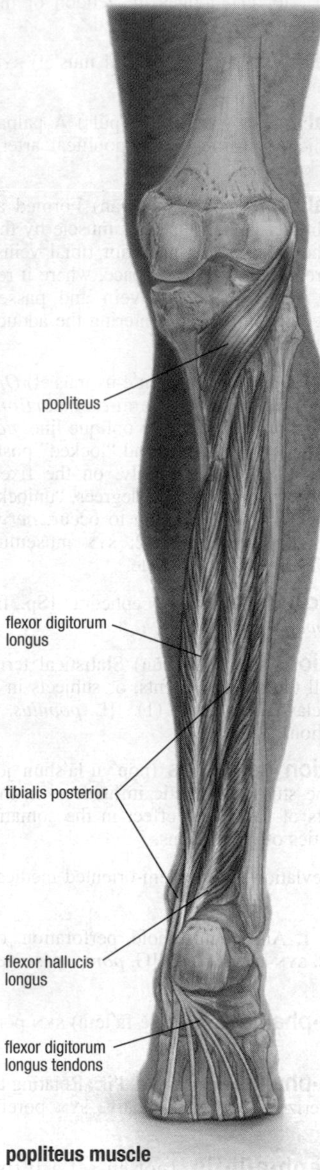

popliteus muscle

PORN (pōrn) Acronym for progressive outer retinal necrosis.

po·ro·ker·a·to·sis (pōr′ō-ker′ă-tō′sis) A rare dermatosis in which there is a thickening of the stratum corneum with an anular keratotic rim or cornoid lamella surrounding progressive centrifugal atrophy; cutaneous carcinoma has been reported to arise in the lesions. SYN Mibelli disease. [G. *poros,* pore, + keratosis]

po·ro·ma (pōr-ō′mă) **1.** SYN callosity. **2.** SYN exostosis. **3.** Induration following a phlegmon. **4.** A tumor of cells lining the skin openings of sweat glands. [G. *pōrōma,* callus, fr. *pōros,* stone]

po·ro·sis, pl. **po·ro·ses** (pōr-ō′sis, -sēz) A porous condition. SYN porosity (1). [L. *porosus,* porous]

po·ros·i·ty (pōr-os′i-tē) **1.** SYN porosis. **2.** A perforation. [G. *poros,* pore]

po·rous (pōr′ŭs) Having openings that pass directly or indirectly through the substance.

por·pho·bi·lin (pōr′fō-bī′lin) General term denoting intermediates between the monopyrrole, porphobilinogen, and the cyclic tetrapyrrole of heme (a porphin derivative).

por·pho·bi·lin·o·gen (PBG) (pōr′fō-bī-lin′ō-jen) A porphyrin precursor of porphyrinogens, porphyrins, and heme; found in the urine in large quantities in cases of acute or congenital porphyria.

por·phyr·i·a (pōr-fir′ē-ă) A group of disorders involving heme biosynthesis, characterized by excessive excretion of porphyrins or their precursors; may be acquired, as from the effects of certain chemical agents (e.g., hexachlorobenzene), or inherited.

por·phyr·i·a cu·ta·ne·a tar·da (pōr-fir′ē-ă kū-tā′nē-ă tahr′dă) Familial or sporadic porphyria characterized by liver dysfunction and photosensitive cutaneous lesions, with hyperpigmentation and sclerodermalike changes in the skin, and increased excretion of uroporphyrin; caused by a deficiency of uroporphyrinogen decarboxylase induced in sporadic cases by chronic alcoholism. SYN symptomatic porphyria.

por·phy·rin·o·gens (pōr′fir-in′ō-jenz) Intermediates in the biosynthesis of heme; certain porphyrinogens are elevated in certain porphyrias.

por·phy·rins (pōr′fir-inz) Pigments widely distributed throughout nature (e.g., heme, bile pigments, cytochromes) consisting of four pyrroles joined in a ring (porphin) structure.

por·phy·ri·nu·ri·a (pōr′fir-i-nyūr′ē-ă) Excretion of porphyrins and related compounds in the urine. SYN purpurinuria.

Por·phyr·o·mo·nas (pōr′fir-ō-mō′năs) A genus of small, anaerobic, gram-negative, nonmotile, pleomorphic cocci and usually short rods that produce smooth, gray-to-black–pigmented colonies, the size of which varies with the species. In humans, they are found as part of the normal flora in the oropharynx, including gingival crevices, and in the vaginal and intestinal tracts. The type species is *Porphyromonas asaccharolytica.*

Por·phyr·o·mo·nas a·sac·char·o·ly·ti·ca (pōr′fir-ō-mō′năs ā-săk′ă-rō-lit′i-kă) A species that rarely causes infections independently but is an important component of mixed infections associated with oral, genitourinary, and intraabdominal abscesses, as well as in infections associated with impaired circulation and diabetic gangrene.

port (pōrt) SYN portal.

por•ta, pl. **por•tae** (pōr′tă, -tē) **1.** SYN hilum (1). **2.** SYN interventricular foramen. [L. gate]

por•ta•ca•val (pōr′tă-kā′văl) Concerning the portal vein and the inferior vena cava.

por•ta•ca•val shunt (pōr′tă-kā′văl shŭnt) **1.** Surgical anastomosis between portal and systemic veins. **2.** Surgical anastomosis between the portal vein and the vena cava, as in an Eck fistula.

por•ta hep•a•tis (pōr′tă hē-pā′tis) [TA] A transverse fissure on the visceral surface of the liver between the caudate and quadrate lobes, lodging the portal vein, hepatic artery, hepatic nerve plexus, hepatic ducts, and lymphatic vessels. SYN caudal transverse fissure, portal fissure.

por•tal (pōr′tăl) **1.** Relating to any porta or hilus, specifically to the porta hepatis and the portal vein. **2.** The point of entry into the body of a pathogenic microorganism. **3.** SYN field size. SYN port. [L. *portalis,* pertaining to a porta (gate)]

por•tal ca•nals (pōr′tăl kă-nalz′) Connective tissue spaces in the substance of the liver that are occupied by preterminal ramifications of the bile ducts, portal vein, and hepatic artery, as well as nerves and lymphatics.

por•tal cir•cu•la•tion (pōr′tăl sĭr′kyū-lā′shŭn) **1.** Circulation of blood to the liver from the small intestine, the right half of the colon, and the spleen through the portal vein; sometimes specified as the hepatic portal circulation. **2.** More generally, any part of the systemic circulation in which blood draining from the capillary bed of one structure flows through a larger vessel(s) to supply the capillary bed of another structure before returning to the heart, e.g., the hypothalamohypophysial portal system.

por•tal of en•try (pōr′tăl en′trē) Refers to the process whereby a pathogen enters the body, gains access to susceptible tissues, and causes disease or infection (e.g., direct contact, ingestion, inhalation).

por•tal fis•sure (pōr′tăl fish′ŭr) SYN porta hepatis.

por•tal hy•per•ten•sion (pōr′tăl hī′pĕr-ten′shŭn) Elevation of pressure in the hepatic portal circulation due to cirrhosis or other fibrotic change in liver tissue; when pressure exceeds 10 mm Hg, a collateral circulation may develop to maintain venous return from structures drained by the portal vein; engorgement of collateral veins can lead to esophageal varices and, less often, caput medusae.

por•tal hy•po•phy•si•al cir•cu•la•tion (pōr′tăl hī′pō-fiz′ē-ăl sĭr′kyū-lā′shŭn) A capillary network that carries hormones from the hypothalamus to their sites of action in the anterior hypophysis. SEE ALSO portal circulation, hypophysis, hypothalamus. SYN hypothalamohypophysial portal system.

por•tal lob•ule of liv•er (pōr′tăl lob′yūl liv′ĕr) A conceptual unit of the liver, emphasizing its exocrine function in bile secretion, that comprises a roughly triangular cross-sectional area with a portal canal at its center and three or more venae centrales hepatis at its periphery.

por•tal sys•tem (pōr′tăl sis′tĕm) A system of vessels in which blood, after passing through one capillary bed, is conveyed through a second capillary network, as in the hepatic portal system, in which blood from the intestines passes through the liver sinusoids.

por•tal-sys•tem•ic en•ceph•a•lop•a•thy (pōr′tăl sis-tem′ik en-sef′ă-lop′ă-thē) An encephalopathy associated with cirrhosis of the liver, attributed to the passage of toxic nitrogenous substances from the portal to the systemic circulation; cerebral manifestations may include coma. SYN hepatic encephalopathy (1).

por•tal tri•ad (pōr′tăl trī′ad) Branches of the portal vein, hepatic artery, and the biliary ducts bound together in the perivascular fibrous capsule or portal tract as they ramify within the substance of the liver. SYN triad (3).

por•tal vein (pōr′tăl vān) A wide, short vein formed by the superior mesenteric and splenic vein posterior to the neck of the pancreas, ascending in front of the inferior vena cava, and dividing at the right end of the porta hepatis into right and left branches, which ramify within the liver. SYN vena portae hepatis [TA], hepatic portal vein.

por•ti•o, pl. **por•ti•o•nes** (pōr′shē-ō, -ō′nēz) [TA] A part. [L. portion]

por•tion (pōr′shŭn) Part or division.

♻**porto-** Prefix meaning portal. [L. *porta,* gate]

por•to•bil•i•o•ar•te•ri•al (pōr′tō-bil′ē-ō-ahr-tēr′ē-ăl) Relating to the portal vein, biliary ducts, and hepatic artery, which have similar distributions.

por•to•en•ter•os•to•my (pōr′tō-en′tĕr-os′tō-mē) An operation for biliary atresia in which a Roux-en-Y loop of jejunum is anastomosed to the hepatic end of the divided extravascular portal structures, including rudimentary bile ducts. SYN Kasai operation.

por•to•gram (pōr′tō-gram) Radiographic record of portography. [porto- + G. *gramma,* a writing]

por•tog•ra•phy (pōr-tog′ră-fē) Delineation of the portal circulation by roentgenograms, using radiopaque material, usually introduced into the spleen or into the portal vein at operation. [porto- + G. *graphō,* to write]

por·to·sys·tem·ic (pōr′tō-sis-tem′ik) Relating to connections between the portal and systemic venous systems.

Por·tu·guese man-of-war (pŏr′chŭ-gēz măn wōr) SYN *Physalia physalis.*

port-wine mark, port-wine stain (pōrt-wīn mahrk, pōrt-wīn stān) SYN nevus flammeus.

POS Abbrevation for place of service.

po·si·tion (pŏ-zish′ŏn) **1.** An attitude, posture, or placement. **2.** A posture or attitude assumed by a patient for comfort and to facilitate diagnostic, surgical, or therapeutic procedures. **3.** OBSTETRICS the relation of an arbitrarily chosen portion of the fetus to the right or left side of the mother; with each presentation there may be a right or left position; the fetal occiput, chin, and sacrum are the determining points of position in vertex, face, and breech presentations, respectively. Cf. presentation. See page B29. [L. *positio,* a placing, position, fr. *pono,* to place]

po·si·tion·al nys·tag·mus (pŏ-zish′ŭn-ăl nis-tag′mŭs) Nystagmus occurring only when the head is in a particular position.

po·si·tion·al ver·ti·go (pŏ-zish′ŭn-ăl vĕr′ti-gō) Vertigo occurring with a change in body position.

po·si·tion ef·fect (pŏ-zish′ŏn e-fekt′) A change in the phenotypic expression of one or more genes due to a change in physical location with respect to other genes; may result from change in chromosome structure or from crossing over.

po·si·tion sense (pŏ-zish′ŏn sens) SYN posture sense.

pos·i·tive (poz′i-tiv) **1.** Affirmative; definite; not negative. **2.** MATHEMATICS having a value more than zero. **3.** PHYSICS, CHEMISTRY having an electric charge resulting from a loss or deficit of electrons, hence able to attract or gain electrons. **4.** MEDICINE denoting a response to a diagnostic maneuver or laboratory study that indicates the presence of the disease or condition tested for. [L. *positivus,* settled by arbitrary agreement, fr. *pono,* pp. *positus,* to set, place]

pos·i·tive ac·com·mo·da·tion (poz′i-tiv ă-kom′ŏ-dā′shŭn) Increased refractivity of the eye that occurs when shifting focus from the distance to a near object.

pos·i·tive con·ver·gence (poz′i-tiv kŏn-vĕr′jĕns) Inward deviation of the visual axes even when convergence is at rest, as in cases of convergent squint.

pos·i·tive end-ex·pi·ra·to·ry pres·sure (PEEP) (poz′i-tiv end-eks-pīr′ă-tōr-ē presh′ŭr) A technique used in respiratory therapy in which airway pressure greater than atmospheric pressure is achieved at the end of exhalation by introduction of a mechanical impedance to exhalation.

pos·i·tive en·er·gy bal·ance (poz′i-tiv en′ĕr-jē bal′ăns) When energy output is less than energy consumption and results in increased body weight.

pos·i·tive-neg·a·tive pres·sure breath·ing (poz′i-tiv-neg′ă-tiv presh′ŭr brēdh′ing) Inflation of the lungs with positive pressure and deflation with negative pressure by a ventilator.

pos·i·tive ni·tro·gen bal·ance (poz′i-tiv nī′trŏ-jen bal′ăns) Nitrogen intake exceeds the sum of all nitrogen excretion.

pos·i·tive pre·dic·tive val·ue (poz′i-tiv prĕ-dik′tiv val′yū) The probability that a positive result accurately indicates that the analyte or the specific disease is present.

pos·i·tive pres·sure ven·ti·la·tion (PPV) (poz′i-tiv presh′ŭr ven′ti-lā′shŭn) A mode of mechanical ventilation in which a positive transrespiratory pressure is generated by increasing airway opening pressure above body surface pressure.

pos·i·tive sco·to·ma (poz′i-tiv skō-tō′mă) A scotoma that is perceived as a white spot within the field of vision.

pos·i·tive signs of preg·nan·cy (poz′i-tiv sīnz preg′năn-sē) Objective signs that strongly indicate pregnancy: ultrasound visualization, presence of fetal heart sounds, and fetal movements.

pos·i·tive stain (poz′i-tiv stān) Direct binding of a dye with a tissue component to produce contrast; in electron microscopy, heavy metals like uranyl and lead salts are used to bind to selective cell constituents to produce increased density to the electron beam, i.e., contrast.

pos·i·tive symp·tom (poz′i-tiv simp′tŏm) One of the acute or florid symptoms of schizophrenia, including hallucinations, delusions, thought disorder, loose associations, ambivalence, or affective lability.

pos·i·tron (β^+) (poz′i-tron) A subatomic particle of mass and charge equal to the electron but of opposite (i.e., positive) charge.

pos·i·tron e·mis·sion to·mog·ra·phy (PET) (poz′i-tron ĕ-mish′ŭn tŏ-mog′ră-fē) Tomographic images formed by computer analysis of photons detected from annihilation of positrons emitted by radionuclides incorporated into biochemical substances; the images, often quantitated with a color scale, show the uptake and distribution of the substances in the tissue, permitting analysis and localization of metabolic and physiologic function. See page B23.

po·so·log·ic (pō′sō-loj′ik) Relating to posology.

po·sol·o·gy (pō-sol′ŏ-jē) The branch of pharmacology and therapeutics concerned with a determination of the dosages of drugs; the science of dosage. [G. *posos,* how much, + *logos,* study]

post (pōst) **1.** A dental procedure in which an elongated projection is fitted and cemented within the prepared root canal; serves to strengthen and retain restorative material and/or a crown restoration. **2.** Device used in some dental implantation procedures.

♻ **post-** Prefix meaning after, behind, posterior; opposite of anti-. Cf. meta-. [L. *post*]

post·a·dre·nal·ec·to·my syn·drome (pōst′ă-drē′năl-ek′tŏ-mē sin′drōm) SYN Nelson syndrome.

post·an·ti·bi·ot·ic ef·fect (PAE) (pōst′an′ti-bī-ot′ik e-fekt′) Continual inhibition of bacterial growth after exposure to an antimicrobial agent; the time for the organism to recover from the effects of antimicrobial exposure. PAE is shown in vitro by demonstrating bacterial growth kinetics after the drug is removed.

post·an·ti·bi·ot·ic leu·ko·cyte en·hance·ment (PALE) (pōst′an′ti-bī-ot′ik lū′kō-sīt en-hans′mĕnt) Increased susceptibility of bacteria, after exposure to antibiotics, to intracellular killing or phagocytosis by leukocytes.

post·au·ri·cu·lar in·ci·sion (pōst′awr-ik′yū-lăr in-sizh′ŭn) An incision parallel and a few millimeters posterior to the retroauricular fold, made to gain access to the mastoid cortex.

post·ax·i·al (pōst-ak′sē-ăl) **1.** Posterior to the axis of the body or any limb, the latter being in the anatomic position. **2.** Denoting the portion of a limb bud that lies caudal to the axis of the limb: the ulnar aspect of the upper limb and the fibular aspect of the lower limb.

post·bra·chi·al (pōst-brā′kē-ăl) On or in the posterior part of the upper arm.

post·cap·il·lar·y ven·ules (pōst-kap′i-lar-ē ven′yūls) The microvasculature immediately following the capillaries, ranging in size from 10–50 mcm, and characterized by investment of pericytes; they are the site of extravasation of blood cells, are particularly sensitive to histamine, and are believed to be important in blood-interstitial fluid exchanges. SYN pericytic venules.

post·ca·va (pōst-kā′vă) SYN inferior vena cava.

post·ca·val (pōst-kā′văl) Relating to the inferior vena cava.

post·cen·tral ar·e·a (pōst-sen′trăl ār′ē-ă) The cortex of the postcentral gyrus.

post·cen·tral gy·rus (pōst-sen′trăl jī′rŭs) The anterior convolution of the parietal lobe, bounded in front by the central sulcus (fissure of Rolando) and posteriorly by the interparietal sulcus.

post·cen·tral sul·cus (pōst-sen′trăl sŭl′kŭs) The sulcus that demarcates the postcentral gyrus from the superior and inferior parietal lobules.

post·ci·bal (pōst-sī′băl) SYN postprandial. [L. *cibum,* food]

post·co·i·tal (pōst-kō′i-tăl) After coitus.

post·co·i·tal con·tra·cep·tion (pōst-kō′i-tăl kon-tră-sep′shŭn) SYN morning after pill.

post·co·i·tal test (pōst-kō′i-tăl test) A test on cervical mucus about time of ovulation to evaluate its receptivity to sperm.

post·co·i·tus (pōst-kō′i-tŭs) The time immediately after coitus.

post·com·mis·sur·ot·o·my syn·drome (pōst-kom′i-shŭr-ot′ŏ-mē sin′drōm) SYN postpericardiotomy syndrome.

post·con·cus·sion syn·drome (pōst′kŏn-kŭsh′ŭn sin′drōm) Delayed postconcussion signs such as headaches, blurred vision, inability to concentrate, nausea, irritability, and change of character.

post·cor·di·al (pōst-kōr′jăl) Posterior to the heart. [L. *cor* (*cord-*), heart]

post·cos·tal a·nas·to·mo·sis (pōst-kos′tăl ă-nas′tŏ-mō′sis) Longitudinal anastomosis of intersegmental arteries giving rise to the vertebral artery.

post·cu·bi·tal (pōst-kyū′bi-tăl) On or in the posterior or dorsal part of the forearm.

post·date preg·nan·cy (pōst′dāt preg′năn-sē) A pregnancy exceeding 294 days or 42 completed weeks. SYN prolonged pregnancy.

post·duc·tal (pōst-dŭk′tăl) Relating to that part of the aorta distal to the aortic opening of the ductus arteriosus.

pos·ter·i·or (pos-tēr′ē-ŏr) **1.** After, in relation to time or space. **2.** HUMAN ANATOMY denoting the back surface of the body. Often used to indicate the position of one structure relative to another, i.e., nearer the back of the body. SYN dorsal (2). **3.** Near the tail or caudal end of certain embryos. **4.** A substitute for caudal in quadrupeds; in veterinary anatomy, posterior is used only to denote some structures of the head. [L. comparative of *posterus,* following]

pos·ter·i·or al·ve·o·lar ar·ter·y (pos-tēr′ē-ŏr al-vē′ŏ-lăr ahr′tĕr-ē) SYN posterior superior alveolar artery.

pos·ter·i·or arch of at·las (pos-tēr′ē-ŏr ahrch at′lăs) The posterior arch of the atlas, which connects the lateral masses of the atlas posteriorly, forming the posterior wall of the vertebral canal at this level.

pos·ter·i·or a·syn·cli·tism (pos-tēr′ē-ŏr ā-sin′kli-tizm) SYN Litzmann obliquity.

pos·ter·i·or au·ric·u·lar ar·ter·y (pos-tēr′ē-ŏr awr-ik′yū-lăr ahr′tĕr-ē) *Origin*, posterior aspect of external carotid just above the digastric muscle; *course*, ascends first between parotid gland and styloid process, then between cartilage of auricle and the mastoid process, *branches*, muscular (digastric, stylohyoid, and sternocleidomastoid), glandular (parotid), stylomastoid, occipital, and auricular; *anastomoses*, anterior tympanic artery (through the stylomastoid artery) and occipital artery. SYN arteria auricularis posterior.

pos·ter·i·or au·ric·u·lar mus·cle (pos-tēr′ē-ŏr awr-ik′yū-lăr mŭs′ĕl) SYN auricularis posterior muscle.

pos·ter·i·or au·ric·u·lar nerve (pos-tēr′ē-ŏr awr-ik′yū-lăr nĕrv) The first extracranial branch of the facial nerve, it passes behind the ear, supplying the posterior auricular muscle and intrinsic muscles of the auricle and, through its occipital branch, innervating the occipital belly of the occipitofrontalis muscle. SYN nervus auricularis posterior [TA].

pos·ter·i·or ble·pha·ri·tis (pos-tēr′ē-ŏr blef′ă-rī′tis) SYN blepharadenitis.

pos·ter·i·or ce·re·bral ar·ter·y (pos-tēr′ē-ŏr ser′ĕ-brăl ahr′tĕr-ē) Formed by bifurcation of the basilar artery; it passes around the cerebral peduncle to reach the medial aspect of the hemisphere. SYN arteria cerebri posterior.

pos·ter·i·or ce·re·bral com·mis·sure (pos-tēr′ē-ŏr ser′ĕ-brăl kom′i-shŭr) A thin band of white matter, crossing from side to side beneath the habenula of the pineal body and over the aditus ad aqueductum cerebri; it is largely composed of fibers interconnecting the left and right pretectal regions and related cell groups of the midbrain; dorsally, it marks the junction of the diencephalon and mesencephalon. SYN commissura posterior cerebri [TA].

pos·ter·i·or cham·ber of eye·ball (pos-tēr′ē-ŏr chām′bĕr ī′bawl) The ringlike space, filled with aqueous humor, between the iris anteriorly and the lens and ciliary body posteriorly.

pos·ter·i·or cir·cum·flex hu·me·ral ar·ter·y (pos-tēr′ē-ŏr sĭr′kŭm-fleks hyū′mĕr-ăl ahr′tĕr-ē) *Origin*, axillary; *distribution*, muscles and structures of shoulder joint; *anastomoses*, anterior circumflex humeral, suprascapular, thoracoacromial, and profunda brachii. SYN arteria circumflexa humeri posterior, posterior humeral circumflex artery.

pos·ter·i·or col·umn (pos-tēr′ē-ŏr kol′ŭm) The pronounced, dorsolaterally oriented ridge of gray matter in each lateral half of the spinal cord, corresponding to the posterior or dorsal horn appearing in transverse sections of the cord. SYN posterior column of spinal cord (1).

pos·ter·i·or col·umn of spi·nal cord (pos-tēr′ē-ŏr kol′ŭm spī′năl kōrd) **1.** SYN posterior column. **2.** In clinical parlance, the term often refers to the posterior funiculus of the spinal cord.

pos·ter·i·or com·mun·i·ca·ting ar·ter·y (pos-tēr′ē-ŏr kŏ-myū′ni-kā′ting ahr′tĕr-ē) *Origin*, internal carotid; *distribution*, optic tract, crus cerebri, interpeduncular region, and hippocampal gyrus; *anastomoses* with posterior cerebral to form the cerebral arterial circle (circle of Willis). SYN arteria communicans posterior.

pos·ter·i·or com·part·ment of thigh (pos-tēr′ē-ŏr kŏm-pahrt′mĕnt thī) Posterior portion of the space enclosed by the fascia lata, separated from the medial and anterior compartments by the posterior and lateral intermuscular septa, respectively; contains the hamstring muscles (extensor of the thigh at the hip joint and flexors of the leg at the knee joint) and the short head of the biceps; all innervated by the sciatic nerve (the former by the tibial nerve portion, the latter by the fibular nerve portion).

pos·ter·i·or cord of bra·chi·al plex·us (pos-tēr′ē-ŏr kōrd brā′kē-ăl plek′sŭs) In the brachial plexus, the bundle of nerve fibers formed by the posterior divisions of the upper, middle, and lower trunks that lies posterior to the axillary artery; it gives rise to the upper and lower subscapular and thoracodorsal nerves, and ends by dividing into the axillary and radial nerves.

pos·ter·i·or cor·ne·al dys·tro·phy (pos-tēr′ē-ŏr kōr′nē-ăl dis′trŏ-fē) Opacification with primary involvement of the endothelium of the cornea.

pos·ter·i·or cri·co·ar·y·te·noid mus·cle (pos-tēr′ē-ŏr krī′kō-ar-i-tē′noyd mŭs′ĕl) Intrinsic muscle of larynx; *origin*, depression on posterior surface of lamina of cricoid; *insertion*, muscular process of arytenoid; *action*, abducts vocal folds, widening rima glottidis during deep inhalation; *nerve supply*, recurrent laryngeal. SYN musculus cricoarytenoideus posterior.

pos·ter·i·or cru·ci·ate lig·a·ment (pos-tēr′ē-ŏr krū′shē-ăt lig′ă-mĕnt) The strong, fibrous cord that extends from the posterior intercondylar area of the tibia to the anterior part of the lateral surface of the medial condyle of the femur. SYN ligamentum cruciatum posterius [TA].

pos·ter·i·or cu·tan·e·ous nerve of thigh (pos-tēr′ē-ŏr kyū-tā′nē-ŭs nĕrv thī) Arises as branch of sacral plexus, conveying fibers from ventral rami of first three sacral nerves; supplies skin of posterior surface of thigh and popliteal region (S1 and S2 component); gives off a perineal branch (S3 component) that passes to lateral aspect of scrotum or labium majus. SYN nervus cutaneus femoris posterior, posterior femoral cutaneous nerve, small sciatic nerve.

pos·ter·i·or den·tal ar·ter·y (pos-tēr′ē-ŏr den′tăl ahr′tĕr-ē) SYN posterior superior alveolar artery.

pos•ter•i•or de•scen•ding cor•o•nar•y ar•ter•y (pos-tēr′ē-ŏr dĕ-send′ing kōr′ŏ-nar′ē ahr′tĕr-ē) SYN posterior interventricular branch of right coronary artery.

pos•ter•i•or drawer test (pos-tēr′ē-ŏr drōr test) Measurement of integrity of the posterior cruciate ligament at the knee.

pos•ter•i•or e•las•tic la•mi•na of cor•ne•a (pos-tēr′ē-ŏr ĕ-las′tik lam′i-nă kōr′nē-ă) A delicate hyaline membrane lying between the substantia propria of the cornea and the corneal endothelium. SYN Descemet membrane, lamina limitans posterior corneae.

pos•ter•i•or em•bry•o•tox•on (pos-tēr′ē-ŏr em′brē-ō-tok′son) A developmental abnormality marked by a prominent white ring of Schwalbe and iris strands that partially obscure the chamber angle.

pos•ter•i•or eth•moid•al ar•ter•y (pos-tēr′ē-ŏr eth-moyd′ăl ahr′tĕr-ē) *Origin*, ophthalmic; *distribution*, posterior ethmoidal cells and upper posterior part of lateral wall of nasal cavity. SYN arteria ethmoidalis posterior.

pos•ter•i•or eth•moid•al nerve (pos-tēr′ē-ŏr eth-moyd′ăl nĕrv) Branch of nasociliary nerve providing sensory innervation to sphenoidal sinus and posterior ethmoidal air cells. SYN nervus ethmoidalis posterior.

pos•ter•i•or fem•o•ral cu•tan•e•ous nerve (pos-tēr′ē-ŏr fem′ŏr-ăl kyū-tā′nē-ŭs nĕrv) SYN posterior cutaneous nerve of thigh.

pos•ter•i•or fo•cal point (pos-tēr′ē-ŏr fō′kăl poynt) The point of a compound optic system where parallel rays entering the system are focused.

pos•ter•i•or fos•sa ap•proach (pos-tēr′ē-ŏr fos′ă ă-prōch′) Surgical approach to the cerebellopontine angle through the mastoid process of the temporal bone.

pos•ter•i•or fu•nic•u•lus (pos-tēr′ē-ŏr fyū-nik′yū-lŭs) Posterior white column of the spinal cord, the large wedge-shaped fiber bundle lying between the posterior gray column and the posterior median septum, and composed largely of dorsal root fibers.

pos•ter•i•or gas•tric ar•ter•y (pos-tēr′ē-ŏr gas′trik ahr′tĕr-ē) *Origin*, splenic artery; *distribution*, ascends retroperitoneally in the posterior wall of omental bursa toward gastric fundus to reach (and supply) the gastric wall through the gastrophrenic fold. SYN arteria gastrica posterior.

pos•ter•i•or glan•du•lar branch of su•per•i•or thy•roid ar•ter•y (pos-tēr′ē-ŏr gland′yū-lăr branch sŭ-pēr′ē-ŏr thī′royd ahr′tĕr-ē) Branch of superior thyroid artery that descends to supply the apical portion of the ipsilateral lobe of the thyroid, continuing along the posterior border of the gland to anastomose with the inferior thyroid artery.

pos•ter•i•or he•pa•tic seg•ment I (pos-tēr′ē-ŏr hĕ-pat′ik seg′mĕnt) A small lobe of the liver situated posteriorly between the sulcus for the vena cava and the fissure for the ligamentum venosum. SYN lobus caudatus, Spigelius lobe.

pos•ter•i•or horn (pos-tēr′ē-ŏr hōrn) The posterior or occipital division of the lateral ventricle of the brain, extending backward into the occipital lobe; the posterior gray column of the spinal cord as it appears in cross section. SYN cornu posterius.

pos•ter•i•or hu•mer•al cir•cum•flex ar•ter•y (pos-tēr′ē-ŏr hyū′mĕr-ăl sĭr′kŭm-fleks ahr′tĕr-ē) SYN posterior circumflex humeral artery.

pos•ter•i•or in•fe•ri•or cer•e•bell•ar ar•ter•y (pos-tēr′ē-ŏr in-fēr′ē-ŏr ser′ĕ-bĕl′lar ahr′tĕr-ē) *Origin*, intracranial part of vertebral artery; *distribution*, lateral medulla, choroid plexus of fourth ventricle, and cerebellum; *anastomoses*, superior cerebellar and anterior inferior cerebellar artery; gives rise to posterior spinal artery [TA], cerebellar tonsillar branch [TA], and choroidal branch to fourth ventricle [TA]. SYN arteria inferior posterior cerebelli.

pos•ter•i•or in•fe•ri•or na•sal bran•ches of great•er pal•a•tine nerve (pos-tēr′ē-ŏr in-fēr′ē-ŏr nā′zăl branch′ĕz grā′tĕr pal′a-tīn nĕrv) SYN posterior inferior nasal nerves.

pos•ter•i•or in•fe•ri•or nas•al nerves (pos-tēr′ē-ŏr in-fēr′ē-ŏr nā′zal nĕrvz) Branches of greater palatine nerve to posterior inferior lateral wall of nasal cavity, including posterior aspect of mucosa over posterior portion of inferior nasal concha and meatus; may arise independently from pterygopalatine ganglion. SYN posterior inferior nasal branches of greater palatine nerve, rami nasales posteriores inferiores nervi palatini majoris.

pos•ter•i•or in•ter•cos•tal ar•ter•ies 1–2 (pos-tēr′ē-ŏr in′tĕr-kos′tăl ahr′tĕr-ēz) SYN first and second posterior intercostal arteries.

pos•ter•i•or in•ter•cos•tal ar•ter•ies 3–11 (pos-tēr′ē-ŏr in′tĕr-kos′tăl ahr′tĕr-ēz) One of nine pairs of arteries arising from the thoracic aorta and distributed to the nine lower intercostal spaces, vertebral column, spinal cord, and muscles and integument of the back; they anastomose with branches of the musculophrenic, internal thoracic, superior epigastric, subcostal, and lumbar. SYN arteriae intercostales posteriores III–XI.

pos•ter•i•or in•ter•cos•tal veins (pos-tēr′ē-ŏr in′tĕr-kos′tăl vānz) Drain the intercostal spaces posteriorly; those of the first intercostal space drain into the brachiocephalic veins; from the 2nd–3rd, they drain into right and left superior intercostal veins; from the 4th–11th spaces on the right, they are tributaries of the azygos vein; on the left, they empty into either the hemiazygos or accessory hemiazygos veins. SYN venae intercostales [TA].

pos•ter•i•or in•ter•os•se•ous ar•ter•y (pos-tēr′ē-ŏr in′tĕr-os′ē-ŭs ahr′tĕr-ē) *Origin*, common interosseous artery; *distribution*, posterior compartment of forearm. SYN arteria interossea posterior, dorsal interosseous artery.

pos•ter•i•or in•ter•os•se•ous nerve (pos-tēr′ē-ŏr in′tĕr-os′ē-ŭs nĕrv) The deep terminal branch of the radial nerve; arises in the cubital region, penetrating and supplying the supinator and continuing with the posterior interosseous artery to supply all the extensor muscles in the forearm. SYN nervus interosseus antebrachii posterior [TA].

pos•ter•i•or in•ter•ven•tri•cu•lar ar•ter•y (pos-tēr′ē-ŏr in′tĕr-ven-trik′yū-lăr ahr′tĕr-ē) SYN posterior interventricular branch of right coronary artery.

pos•ter•i•or in•ter•ven•tric•u•lar branch of right cor•o•nar•y ar•ter•y (pos-tēr′ē-ŏr in′tĕr-ven-trik′yū-lar branch rīt kōr′ŏ-nar′ē ahr′tĕr-ē) Continuation of right coronary artery in posterior interventricular sulcus; descends to apex to anastomose with anterior interventricular artery; supplies most of diaphragmatic aspect of ventricles and posterior third of interventricular septum. SYN posterior descending coronary artery, posterior interventricular artery, ramus interventricularis posterior arteriae coronariae dextrae.

pos•ter•i•or la•bi•al bran•ches of in•ter•nal per•i•ne•al ar•ter•y (pos-tēr′ē-ŏr lā′bē-ăl branch′ĕz in-tĕr′năl per′i-nē′ăl ahr′tĕr-ē) Branches of the perineal artery to the posterior portion of the labium majus.

pos•ter•i•or la•bi•al branch•es of per•i•ne•al ar•te•ry (pos-tēr′ē-ŏr lā′bē-ăl branch′chĕz per′i-nē′ăl ahr′tĕr-ē) Superficial branches of the perineal artery supplying the posterior portions of the labia majora and minora.

pos•ter•i•or la•bi•al com•mis•sure (pos-tēr′ē-ŏr lā′bē-ăl kom′i-shŭr) A slight fold uniting the labia majora posteriorly in front of the anus.

pos•ter•i•or la•bi•al nerves (pos-tēr′ē-ŏr lā′bē-ăl nĕrvz) Terminal branches of superficial perineal nerve, supplying skin of posterior portion of labia and vestibule of vagina, corresponding to posterior scrotal nerves in the male. SYN nervi labiales posteriores.

pos•ter•i•or la•bi•al veins (pos-tēr′ē-ŏr lā′bē-ăl vānz) Pass posteriorly from the labia majora and minora to the internal pudendal veins.

pos•ter•i•or lac•ri•mal crest (pos-tēr′ē-ŏr lak′ri-măl krest) A vertical ridge on the orbital surface of the lacrimal bone that, together with the anterior lacrimal crest, bounds the fossa for the lacrimal sac.

pos•ter•i•or la•ryn•ge•al cleft (pos-tēr′ē-ŏr lăr-in′jē-ăl kleft) Laryngotracheoesophageal cleft (type 2 or 3).

pos•ter•i•or lat•e•ral na•sal ar•ter•ies (pos-tēr′ē-ŏr lat′ĕr-ăl nā′zăl ahr′tĕr-ēz) Branches of the sphenopalatine artery that supply the posterior parts of the conchae and lateral nasal wall. SYN arteriae nasales posteriores laterales.

pos•ter•i•or leu•ko•en•ceph•a•lop•a•thy syn•drome (pos-tēr′ē-ŏr lū′kō-en-sef′ă-lop′ă-thē sin′drōm) A reversible clinicoradiologic syndrome characterized by confusion, headaches, seizures, cortical blindness, and other visual abnormalities, emesis, and motor signs; associated with MRI or CT evidence of bilateral white matter edema involving the parietooccipital cerebral regions.

pos•ter•i•or lim•it•ing lay•er of cor•ne•a (pos-tēr′ē-ŏr lim′it-ing lā′ĕr kōr′nē-ă) A transparent homogeneous acellular layer between the substantia propria and the endothelial layer of the cornea; considered to be a highly developed basement membrane. SYN membrana vitrea [TA], vitreous membrane (1).

pos•ter•i•or lobe of hy•poph•y•sis (pos-tēr′ē-ŏr lōb hī-pof′i-sis) SYN neurohypophysis.

pos•ter•i•or na•sal spine (pos-tēr′ē-ŏr nā′zăl spīn) The sharp posterior extremity of the nasal crest of the hard palate.

pos•ter•i•or neph•rec•to•my (pos-tēr′ē-ŏr nĕ-frek′tŏ-mē) Retroperitoneal removal of a kidney through an incision in the posterior lumbar muscles, usually with the patient in a prone position.

pos•ter•i•or pan•cre•at•ic•o•du•o•den•al ar•ter•y (pos-tēr′ē-ŏr pan′krē-at′ik-ō′dū′ō-dē′năl ahr′tĕr-ē) SYN retroduodenal artery.

pos•ter•i•or pol•y•mor•phous cor•ne•al dys•tro•phy (pos-tēr′ē-ŏr pol′ē-mōr′fŭs kōr′nē-ăl dis′trŏ-fē) An autosomal dominant condition characterized by vesicular and linear abnormalities of the corneal endothelium; occasionally leads to corneal edema.

pos•te•ri•or pre•sen•ta•tion (pos-tēr′ē-ŏr prez′ĕn-tā′shŭn) SYN back labor.

pos•ter•i•or ra•mus of la•ter•al ce•re•bral sul•cus (pos-tēr′ē-ŏr rā′mŭs lat′ĕr-ăl ser′ĕ-brăl sŭl′kŭs) The long, posteriorly directed continuation of the lateral cerebral sulcus that extends between the temporal lobe inferiorly and the parietal lobe superiorly; its termination is surrounded by the supramarginal gyrus.

pos•ter•i•or ra•mus of spi•nal nerve (pos-tēr′ē-ŏr rā′mŭs spī′năl nĕrv) The smaller, posteriorly directed major terminal branch (with the anterior ramus) of all 31 pairs of mixed spinal nerves, formed at the intervertebral foramen and turning abruptly posteriorly to divide into lateral and medial branches, both of which will supply the deep (true) muscles of the back. The medial branch (ramus medialis [TA]) of the dorsal primary ramus also supplies articular branches to the zygapophysial joints and the periosteum of the vertebral arch. In the neck and upper back, the medial branch continues through the deep and superficial back muscles to supply overlying skin; in the lower back, the lateral branch does this. Terminologia Anatomica lists posterior rami (rami dorsales) for each group of spinal nerves: (1) cervical (nervorum cervicalium [TA]), (2) thoracic (nervorum thoracicorum [TA]), (3) lumbar (nervorum lumbalium [TA]), (4) sacral (nervorum sacralium [TA]), and (5) coccygeal (nervi coccygei [TA]).

pos•ter•i•or rhi•nos•co•py (pos-tēr′ē-ŏr rī-nos′kŏ-pē) Inspection of the nasopharynx and posterior portion of the nasal cavity by means of the rhinoscope, or with a nasopharyngoscope. SEE ALSO nasopharyngoscopy.

pos•ter•i•or rhi•zot•o•my (pos-tēr′ē-ŏr rī-zot′ŏ-mē) Section of posterior spinal root. SYN Dana operation.

pos•ter•i•or sag•it•tal di•am•e•ter (pos-tēr′ē-ŏr saj′i-tăl dī-am′ĕ-tĕr) Distance from the sacrococcygeal junction to the middle of an imaginary line running between the left ischial and right ischial tuberosities.

pos•ter•i•or sag test (pos-tēr′ē-ŏr sag test) Maneuver used to determine integrity of posterior cruciate ligament whereby the patient is in a supine position with the hips flexed at 45 degrees and knees flexed at 90 degrees. When viewed laterally, a loss of the tibial tubercle prominence is present in a posterior cruciate deficient knee when the tibia falls back or sags on the femur.

pos•ter•i•or sca•lene mus•cle (pos-tēr′ē-ŏr skā′lēn mŭs′ĕl) SYN scalenus posterior muscle.

pos•ter•i•or scle•ri•tis (pos-tēr′ē-ŏr skler-ī′tis) Inflammation, often monocular, of the sclera adjacent to the optic nerve, with frequent extension to the retina and choroid.

pos•ter•i•or scro•tal bran•ches of per•i•ne•al ar•ter•y (pos-tēr′ē-ŏr skrō′tăl branch′ĕz per′i-nē′ăl ahr′tĕr-ē) Branches of perineal artery supplying skin of posterior scrotal sac. SYN posterior scrotal branch of internal pudendal artery, rami scrotales posteriores arteriae perinealis, rami scrotales posteriores arteriae pudendae internae.

pos•ter•i•or scro•tal branch of in•ter•nal pu•den•dal ar•ter•y (pōs-tēr′ē-ŏr skrō′tăl branch in-tĕr′năl pū-den′dăl ahr′tĕr-ē) SYN posterior scrotal branches of perineal artery.

pos•ter•i•or seg•ment of eye•ball (pos-tēr′ē-ŏr seg′mĕnt ī′bawl) The large space between the lens and the retina; it is filled with the vitreous body.

pos•ter•i•or sep•tal ar•ter•y of nose (pos-tēr′ē-ŏr sep′tăl ahr′tĕr-ē nōz) SYN posterior septal branch of nose.

pos•ter•i•or sep•tal bran•ches of sphe•no•pal•a•tine ar•ter•y (pos-tēr′ē-ŏr sep′tăl branch′ĕz sfē′nō-pal′ă-tīn ahr′tĕr-ē) SYN posterior septal branch of nose.

pos•ter•i•or sep•tal branch of nose (pos-tēr′ē-ŏr sep′tăl branch nōz) One of the branches of the sphenopalatine artery that supplies the nasal septum and accompanies the nasopalatine nerve. SYN arteria nasalis posterior septi, posterior septal artery of nose, posterior septal branches of sphenopalatine artery, ramus septi posterioris nasalis.

pos•ter•i•or spi•nal ar•ter•y (pos-tēr′ē-ŏr spī′năl ahr′tĕr-ē) *Origin*, intracranial part of vertebral; *distribution*, medulla, spinal cord, and pia mater; *anastomoses*, spinal branches of intercostal arteries. SYN arteria spinalis posterior.

pos•ter•i•or spi•no•cer•e•bel•lar tract (pos-tēr′ē-ŏr spī′nō-ser-ĕ-bel′ăr trakt) A compact bundle of heavily myelinated, thick fibers at the periphery of the dorsal half of the lateral funiculus of the spinal cord, originating in the ipsilateral thoracic nucleus (column of Clarke) and ascending by way of the inferior cerebellar peduncle. Terminals end as mossy fibers in the granular layer of the cortex of the cerebellar vermis. The bundle conveys largely proprioceptive information originating from the anulospiral nerve endings surrounding muscle spindles and from Golgi tendon organs.

pos•ter•i•or staph•y•lo•ma (pos-tēr′ē-ŏr staf′i-lō′mă) A bulging near the posterior pole of the eyeball due to degenerative changes in severe myopia. SYN Scarpa staphyloma.

pos•ter•i•or su•per•i•or al•ve•o•lar ar•ter•y (pos-tēr′ē-ŏr sŭ-pēr′ē-ŏr al-vē′ŏ-lăr ahr′tĕr-ē) *Origin*, third part of maxillary artery within pterygopalatine fossa; *distribution*, molar and premolar teeth, gingiva, and mucous membrane of maxillary sinus. SYN arteria alveolaris superior posterior, arteria tibialis posterior, posterior alveolar artery, posterior dental artery.

pos•te•ri•or su•pe•ri•or il•i•ac spine (PSIS) (pos-tēr′ē-ŏr sŭ-pēr′ē-ŏr il′ē-ak spīn) The landmark at the posterior aspect of the ilium; palpated just lateral to the sacroiliac joint.

pos•ter•i•or su•pra•cla•vic•u•lar nerve (pos-tēr′ē-ŏr sū′pră-klă-vik′yū-lăr nĕrv) SYN lateral supraclavicular nerve.

pos•ter•i•or tem•po•ral branch of mid•dle ce•re•bral ar•te•ry (pos-tēr′ē-ŏr tem′pŏr-ăl branch mid′ĕl ser′ĕ-brăl ahr′tĕr-ē) A branch of the insular part (M2 segment) of the middle cerebral artery distributed to the cortex of the posterior part of the temporal lobe.

pos•ter•i•or tib•i•al ar•ter•y (pos-tēr′ē-ŏr tib-ē′ăl ahr′tĕr-ē) The larger and more directly continuous of the two terminal branches of the popliteal; *branches*, fibular (peroneal), nutrient of fibula, lateral and medial posterior malleolar, tibial nutrient artery, and medial and lateral plantar.

pos•ter•i•or tooth (pos-tēr′ē-ŏr tūth) Any premolar or molar tooth.

pos•ter•i•or ur•e•thral valves (pos-tēr′ē-ŏr yūr-ē′thrăl valvz) Anomalous folds occurring at the level of the seminal colliculus. SYN Amussat valvula.

pos•ter•i•or vein of left ven•tri•cle (pos-tēr′ē-ŏr vān left ven′tri-kĕl) Arises on the diaphragmatic surface of the heart near the apex, runs to the left and parallel to the posterior interventricular sulcus, and empties in the coronary sinus.

pos•ter•i•or ves•tib•u•lar branch of ves•tib•u•lo•coch•le•ar ar•te•ry (pos-tēr′ē-ŏr ves-tib′yū-lăr branch ves-tib′yū-lō-kok′lē-ăr ahr′tĕr-ē) *Origin*, terminal branch, with cochlear branch, of vestibulocochlear artery; *distribution*, utricle and (especially ampulla of) posterior semicircular duct.

pos•ter•i•or walk•er (pos-tē′rē-ŏr wawk′ĕr) Ambulatory assist device oriented with the open aspect of the device in front of the user. It promotes upright posture in children who require assistance with ambulation. SYN postural walker.

♻**postero-** Prefix meaning posterior; at the back of. [L. *posterior*]

pos•ter•o•an•te•ri•or (PA) (pos′tĕr-ō-an-tēr′ē-ŏr) A term denoting the direction of view or progression, from posterior to anterior, through a part.

pos•ter•o•an•ter•i•or pro•jec•tion (pos′tĕr-ō-an-tēr′ē-ŏr prŏ-jek′shŭn) SYN PA projection.

pos•ter•o•ex•ter•nal (pos′tĕr-ō-ek-stĕr′năl) SYN posterolateral.

pos•ter•o•in•ter•nal (pos′tĕr-ō-in-tĕr′năl) SYN posteromedial.

pos•ter•o•lat•er•al (pos′tĕr-ō-lat′ĕr-ăl) Behind and to one side, specifically to the outer side. SYN posteroexternal.

pos•ter•o•lat•er•al sul•cus (pos′tĕr-ō-lat′ĕr-ăl sŭl′kŭs) A longitudinal furrow on either side of the posterior median sulcus of the spinal cord marking the line of entrance of the posterior nerve roots. SYN dorsolateral sulcus.

pos•ter•o•la•ter•al thor•a•cot•o•my (pos′tĕr-ō-lat′ĕr-ăl thōr′ă-kot′ŏ-mē) Surgical thoracotomy, involving division of the latissimus dorsi muscle and the serratus anterior muscle.

pos•ter•o•me•di•al (pos′tĕr-ō-mē′dē-ăl) Behind and to the inner side. SYN posterointernal.

pos•ter•o•me•di•an (pos′tĕr-ō-mē′dē-ăn) Occupying a central position posteriorly.

pos•ter•o•su•pe•ri•or (pos′tĕr-ō-sŭ-pēr′ē-ŏr) Situated behind and at the upper part.

post•es•trus, **post•es•trum** (pōst-es′trŭs, -trŭm) The period in the estrus cycle following estrus; characterized by the growth of the corpus luteum and physiologic changes related to the production of progesterone. SYN postoestrus.

post•ex•tra•sys•tol•ic pause (pōst-eks′tră-sis-tol′ik pawz) The somewhat prolonged cycle immediately following an extrasystole.

post•ex•tra•sys•tol•ic T wave (pōst-eks′tră-sis-tol′ik wāv) The modified T wave of the beat immediately following an extrasystole.

post•gan•gli•on•ic (pōst′gang-glē-on′ik) Distal to or beyond a ganglion; referring to the unmyelinated nerve fibers originating from cells in an autonomic ganglion.

post•gas•trec•to•my syn•drome (pōst′gas-trek′tŏ-mē sin′drōm) SYN dumping syndrome.

post•hep•a•tit•ic cir•rho•sis (pōst′hep-ă-tit′ik sir-ō′sis) SYN active chronic hepatitis.

pos•thi•o•plas•ty (pos′thē-ō-plas-tē) Surgical reconstruction of the prepuce. [G. *posthion,* dim. form of *posthē,* prepuce, + *plastos,* formed]

pos•thi•tis (pos-thī′tis) Inflammation of the prepuce. [G. *posthē,* prepuce, + *-itis,* inflammation]

post•hu•mous (pos′chū-mŭs) Denotes occurring after a person's death. [L. *postumus,* last, corrupted by attraction to *humus,* earth, burial]

post•hyp•not•ic (pōst′hip-not′ik) Following hypnotism; denoting an act suggested during hypnosis that is to be carried out at some time after the hypnotized subject is awakened.

post•hyp•not•ic sug•ges•tion (pōst′hip-not′ik sŭg-jes′chŭn) SYN hypnotic suggestion.

post•ic•tal (pōst-ik′tăl) Following a seizure (e.g., epileptic).

post-lum•bar punc•ture syn•drome (pōst-lŭm′bahr pungk′shŭr sin′drōm) SYN spinal headache.

post•ma•lar•i•a neur•o•lo•gic syn•drome (pōst′mă-lar′ē-ă nūr-ō-loj′ik sin′drōm) A self-limited central nervous system disorder that develops soon after recovery from a severe bout of falciparum malaria, characterized principally by an acute state of confusion or psychosis, generalized convulsions, or both, lasting 1–10 days and associated with negative blood smears for malaria parasite; linked to preceding mefloquine therapy.

post•ma•ture, **post•ma•ture in•fant, post•term in•fant** (pōst′mă-chūr′, in′fănt, pōst-tĕrm) Referring to a fetus that remains in the uterus longer than the normal gestational period, i.e., longer than 42 weeks (288 days) in humans, which puts the child at risk because of inadequate placental function. The infant usually shows wrinkled skin, and sometimes more serious abnormalities.

post•men•o•pau•sal (pōst′men-ŏ-paw′zăl) Relating to the period following the menopause.

post·mor·tem (pōst-mōr′tĕm) **1.** Pertaining to or occurring during the period after death. **2.** Colloquialism for autopsy (1). [post- + L. acc. case of *mors* (*mort-*), death]

post·mor·tem de·liv·er·y (pōst-mōr′tĕm dĕ-liv′ĕr-ē) Extraction of the fetus after the death of its mother.

post·mor·tem li·ve·do, post·mor·tem li·vid·i·ty (pōst-mōr′tĕm li-vē′dō, li-vid′i-tē) A purple coloration of dependent parts, except in areas of contact pressure, appearing within 1/2–2 hours after death, as a result of gravitational movement of blood within the vessels.

post·mor·tem ri·gid·i·ty (pōst-mōr′tĕm ri-jid′i-tē) SYN rigor mortis.

post·mor·tem wart (pōst-mōr′tĕm wōrt) A tuberculous warty growth (tuberculosis cutis verrucosa) on the hand of one who performs postmortem examinations. SYN anatomic wart, dissection tubercle, necrogenic wart, verruca necrogenica.

post·na·sal (pōst-nā′zăl) **1.** Posterior to the nasal cavity. **2.** Relating to the posterior portion of the nasal cavity.

post·na·sal drip (PND) (pōst-nā′zăl drip) Term used to describe sensation of excessive mucoid or mucopurulent discharge from the posterior nares.

post·na·tal (pōst-nā′tăl) Occurring after birth. [L. *natus,* birth]

post·ne·crot·ic cir·rho·sis (pōst′nĕ-krot′ik sir-ō′sis) Hepatic disorder characterized by necrosis involving whole hepatic lobules, with collapse of the reticular framework to form large scars; regeneration nodules are also large; may follow viral or toxic necrosis, or develop as a result of ischemic necrosis. SYN necrotic cirrhosis.

postoestrum [Br.] SYN postestrum.

postoestrus [Br.] SYN postestrus.

post·op·er·a·tive (pōst-op′ĕr-ă-tiv) Following an operation.

post·o·ral (pōst-ōr′ăl) In the posterior part of, or posterior to, the mouth. [L. *os* (*or-*), mouth]

post·par·tum (pōst-pahr′tŭm) After childbirth. Cf. antepartum, intrapartum. [L. *partus,* birth (noun), fr. *pario,* pp. *partus,* to bring forth]

post·par·tum a·to·ny (pōst-pahr′tŭm at′ŏ-nē) Slackness in the uterine walls after childbirth.

post·par·tum blues (pōst-pahr′tŭm blūz) Mood disturbance (including insomnia, weepiness, depression, anxiety, and irritability) experienced by up to 50% of women the first week postpartum; apparently precipitated by progesterone withdrawal.

post·par·tum hem·or·rhage (pōst-pahr′tŭm hem′ŏr-ăj) Hemorrhage from the birth canal in excess of 500 mL after a vaginal delivery or 1000 mL after a cesarean delivery during the first 24 hours after birth.

post·par·tum psy·cho·sis (pōst-pahr′tŭm sī-kō′sis) An acute mental disorder with depression in the mother following childbirth.

post·per·i·car·di·ot·o·my per·i·car·di·tis (pōst-per′i-kahr-dē-ot′ŏ-mē per′ē-kahr-dī′tis) A syndrome characterized by fever, substernal chest pain, and pericardial rub following cardiac surgery.

post·per·i·car·di·ot·o·my syn·drome (pōst-per′i-kahr-dē-ot′ŏ-mē sin′drōm) Pericarditis, with or without fever and often in repeated episodes, weeks to months after cardiac surgery. SYN postcommissurotomy syndrome.

post·po·li·o·my·e·li·tis syn·drome (pōst-pō′lē-ō-mī′ĕ-lī′tis sin′drōm) SYN postpolio syndrome.

post·po·li·o syn·drome (PPS) (pōst-pō′lē-ō sin′drōm) A progressive weakness and deterioration in the muscles of a person previously affected by poliomyelitis. It usually affects the muscles most heavily disordered by the disease, but may affect others as well. SYN postpoliomyelitis syndrome.

post·pran·di·al (pōst-pran′dē-ăl) Following a meal. SYN postcibal. [L. *prandium,* breakfast]

post·pu·ber·al, post·pu·ber·tal (pōst-pyū′bĕr-ăl, -bĕr-tăl) SYN postpubescent.

post·pu·bes·cent (pōst′pyū-bes′ĕnt) Subsequent to the period of puberty. SYN postpuberal, postpubertal.

post·re·mal cham·ber of eye·ball (pos′trĕ-măl chām′bĕr ī′bawl) The large space between the lens and the retina; it is filled with the vitreous body. SYN camera postrema, camera vitrea.

post·ro·tar·y ny·stag·mus (pōst-rō′tă-rē ni-stag′mŭs) **1.** Reflexive movements of the eyes that occur after elicitation from a quick rotational movement (e.g., spinning) used to determine vestibular dysfunction. **2.** Involuntary oscillation of the eyes as a result of being rotated after stimulation of the vestibular system by spinning activities.

post·sphyg·mic (pōst-sfig′mik) Occurring after the pulse wave. [G. *sphygmos,* pulse]

post-steady state (pōst-sted′ē stāt) Any period of time, particularly in an enzyme-catalyzed reaction, after the steady-state interval, e.g., when the rate of product formation is declining in an enzyme-catalyzed reaction.

post·syn·ap·tic mem·brane (pōst′si-nap′tik mem′brān) That part of the plasma membrane of a neuron or muscle fiber with which an axon terminal forms a synaptic junction.

post·tib·i·al (pōst-tib′ē-ăl) Posterior to the tibia; situated in the posterior portion of the leg.

post·trans·plant lymph·o·pro·li·fer·a·tive dis·ease (pōst-trans′plant limf′ō-prō-lif′ĕr-ă-tiv di-zēz′) A complication of organ transplantation in children; characterized by a mononucleosislike syndrome, tonsillar enlargement, and Epstein-Barr virus seroconversion.

post·trau·mat·ic (pōst′traw-mat′ik) Occurring after trauma, and, by implication, caused by it.

post·trau·mat·ic de·lir·i·um (pōst′traw-mat′ik dĕ-lir′ē-ŭm) Delirium caused by a structural traumatic brain injury.

post·trau·mat·ic de·men·ti·a (pōst′traw-mat′ik dĕ-men′shē-ă) Dementia caused by traumatic brain injury.

post·trau·mat·ic ep·i·lep·sy (pōst′traw-mat′ik ep′i-lep′sē) A convulsive state following and causally related to head injury, with brain damage either manifested clinically or ascertained by special examinations such as computed tomography.

post·trau·mat·ic stress dis·or·der (PTSD) (pōst′traw-mat′ik stres dis-ōr′dĕr) Anxiety disorder that is a syndrome of responses to extremely disturbing, often life-threatening events such as combat, natural disaster, torture, maltreatment, or rape.

post·trau·mat·ic syn·drome (pōst′traw-mat′ik sin′drōm) A clinical disorder that often follows head injury, characterized by headache, dizziness, neurasthenia, hypersensitivity to stimuli, and diminished concentration.

post·trau·mat·ic ver·ti·go (pōst′traw-mat′ik vĕr′ti-gō) Sense of imbalance that follows trauma, most commonly occurring when an irritable labyrinthine focus develops during the weeks and months after the incident. Other causes of posttraumatic vertigo include vestibular lithiasis, perilymphatic fistula, and endolymphatic hydrops.

post·treat·ment mor·bid·i·ty (pōst-trēt′mĕnt mōr-bid′i-tē) Denotes the untoward signs and symptoms resulting from a treatment procedure such as surgery or chemotherapy.

pos·tu·late (pos′chū-lăt) A proposition that is taken as self-evident or assumed without proof as a basis for further analysis. SEE ALSO hypothesis, theory. [L. *postulo,* pp. *-atus,* to demand]

pos·tur·al (pos′chŭr-ăl) Relating to or affected by posture.

pos·tur·al a·lign·ment (pos′chŭr-ăl ă-līn′mĕnt) Maintenance of biomechanical integrity among body parts.

pos·tur·al con·trac·tion (pos′chŭr-ăl kŏn-trak′shŭn) Maintenance of muscular tension (usually isometric) sufficient to maintain posture.

pos·tur·al drain·age (pos′chŭr-ăl drān′ăj) Procedure to remove liquid used in bronchiectasis and lung abscess. The patient's body is positioned so that the trachea is inclined downward and below the affected chest area. See this page.

pos·tur·al Henn·e·bert test (pos′chŭr-ăl en-bār′ test) Application of air pressure to an external auditory cause with the patient standing. It measures postural destabilization, an abnormal response to pressure change of the vestibular en-

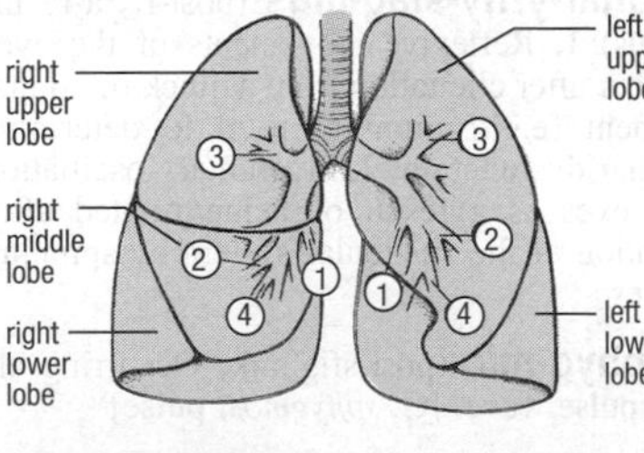

normal lung anatomy (the numbers correspond to the areas to be drained with postural drainage)

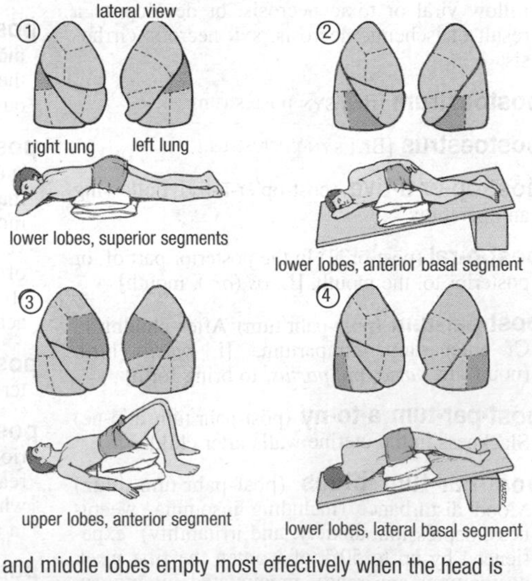

postural drainage: usually bronchi of the lower and middle lobes empty most effectively when the head is down; gravity helps drain secretions from smaller bronchial airways to the main bronchi and trachea, from which the patient is able to cough up secretions; this procedure is most effective in the early morning

dorgans (otolith organs or semicircular canals). It is often called the "platform pressure test" when performed on a force platform, which quantifies and documents the postural stabilization.

pos·tur·al hy·po·ten·sion (pos′chŭr-ăl hī′pō-tĕn′shŭn) SYN orthostatic hypotension.

pos·tur·al in·se·cur·i·ty (pos′chŭr-ăl in′sĕ-kyūr′i-tē) SYN gravitational insecurity.

pos·tur·al po·si·tion, pos·tur·al rest·ing po·si·tion (pos′chŭr-ăl pŏ-zish′ŏn, rest′ing pŏ-zish′ŏn) SYN rest position.

pos·tur·al sway re·sponse (pos′chŭr-ăl swā rĕ-spons′) The body sway induced by vestibular stimulation.

pos·tur·al syn·co·pe (pos′chŭr-ăl sing′kŏ-pē) Syncope on assuming an upright position; caused by failure of normal vasoconstrictive mechanisms.

pos·tur·al ver·ti·go (pos′chŭr-ăl vĕr′ti-gō) **1.** SYN benign positional vertigo. **2.** Light-headedness that appears particularly in elderly people with change of position, usually from lying or sitting to standing; due to orthostatic hypotension.

pos·tur·al walk·er (pos′chŭr-ăl wawk′ĕr) SYN posterior walker.

pos·ture (pos′chŭr) The position of the limbs or the carriage of the body as a whole. [L. *positura*, fr. *pono*, pp. *positus*, to place]

pos·ture sense (pos′chŭr sens) The ability to recognize the position in which a limb is passively placed, with the eyes closed. SYN position sense.

pos·tur·og·ra·phy (pos′chŭr-og′ră-fē) SYN dynamic posturography. [posture + G. *graphō*, to write]

post·vac·ci·nal en·ceph·a·lo·my·e·li·tis (pōst-vak′sĕ-năl en-sef′a-lō-mī′ĕ-lī′tis) A severe type of encephalomyelitis that can follow the rabies vaccination.

post·val·var, post·val·vu·lar (pōst-val′văr, -val′vyū-lăr) Relating to a position distal to the pulmonary or aortic valves.

po·ta·ble (pō′tă-bĕl) Drinkable; fit to drink. [L. *potabilis*, fr. *poto*, to drink]

Po·tain sign (pō-tan[h]′ sīn) In dilation of the aorta, dullness on percussion extending from the manubrium sterni toward the second intercostal space and the third costal cartilage on the right, the upper limit extending from the base of the sternum in the segment of a circle to the right.

po·tas·si·um (K) (pŏ-tas′ē-ŭm) An alkaline metallic element, atomic no. 19, atomic wt. 39.0983, occurring abundantly in nature but always in combination; its salts are used medicinally. SYN kalium. [Mod. L., fr. Eng. *potash* (fr. pot + ashes) + *-ium*]

po·tas·si·um 39 (pŏ-tas′ē-ŭm) Most abundant, nonradioactive isotope of potassium; accounts for 93.1% of natural potassium.

po·tas·si·um-spar·ing di·u·ret·ics (pō-tas′ē-ŭm spār′ing dī′yūr-et′iks) Agents that retain potassium (e.g., triamterene and amiloride). They are used in the treatment of hypertension and in congestive heart failure.

po·ten·cy (pō′tĕn-sē) **1.** Power, force, or strength; the condition or quality of being potent. **2.** Specifically, sexual potency. **3.** PHARMACY the relative pharmacologic activity of a compound. [L. *potentia*, power]

po·tent (pō′tĕnt) **1.** Possessing force, power, strength. **2.** Indicating the ability of a primordial cell to differentiate. **3.** Possessing sexual potency.

po·ten·tial (pŏ-ten′shăl) **1.** Capable of doing or being, although not yet doing or being; possible, but not actual. **2.** A state of tension in an electric source enabling it to do work under suitable conditions; in relation to electricity, potential is analogous to the temperature in relation to heat. [L. *potentia*, power, potency]

po·ten·tial a·cu·i·ty me·ter (PAM) (pŏ-ten′shăl ă-kyū′i-tē mē′tĕr) Instrument used to project an image such as Snellen test types through a cataractous lens onto the retina to predict likely visual function if the cataract were removed.

po·ten·tial di·ag·no·sis (pŏ-ten′shăl dī-ăg-nō′sis) NURSING health problem that may occur because of presence of certain risk factors; potential problem.

po·ten·tial en·er·gy (pŏ-ten′shăl en′ĕr-jē) The energy, existing in a body by virtue of its position or state of existence, that is not being exerted at the time.

po·ten·ti·a·tion (pō-ten′shē-ā′shŭn) Interaction between two or more drugs or agents resulting in a pharmacologic response greater than the sum of individual responses to each drug or agent.

po·tion (pō′shŭn) A draft or large dose of liquid medicine. [L. *potio*, *potus*, fr. *poto*, to drink]

Pott ab·scess (pot ab′ses) Tuberculous abscess of the spine.

Pott an·eu·rysm (pot an′yūr-izm) SYN aneurysmal varix.

Pott cur·va·ture (pot kŭr′vă-chŭr) SYN angular curvature.

Pott dis·ease (pot di-zēz′) SYN tuberculous spondylitis.

Pot·ter-Buck·y di·a·phragm (pot′ĕr-bŭk′ē dī′ă-fram) SYN Bucky diaphragm.

Pot·ter syn·drome (pot′ĕr sin′drōm) Renal

agenesis with hypoplastic lungs and associated neonatal respiratory distress, hemodynamic instability, acidosis, cyanosis, edema, and characteristic (Potter) facies; death usually occurs from respiratory insufficiency, which develops before uremia.

Pott frac•ture (pot frak′shŭr) Break in the lower part of the fibula and of the malleolus of the tibia, with lateral displacement of the foot. See page B25.

Pott par•a•ple•gi•a (pot par′ă-plē′jē-ă) Paralysis of the lower part of the body and the extremities, due to pressure on the spinal cord as the result of tuberculous spondylitis.

Potts clamp (pots klamp) A fine-toothed, multiple-point, vascular fixation clamp that imparts limited trauma to the vessel while securely holding it.

Potts op•er•a•tion (pots op-ĕr-ā′shŭn) Direct side-to-side anastomosis between aorta and pulmonary artery as a palliative procedure in congenital malformation of the heart.

pouch (powch) A pocket or cul-de-sac.

pouch cul•ture (powch kŭl′chŭr) Plastic culture system used for transport of specimens, culture, and examination chambers for the isolation, growth, and detection of *Trichomonas vaginalis*.

pou•drage (pū-drahzh′) **1.** Powdering; application of an irritating but nontoxic powder to the pleural space to produce pleural adhesions. **2.** SYN talc operation. [Fr.]

poul•tice (pōl′tis) A soft magma or mush prepared by wetting various powders or other absorbent substances with oily or watery fluids, sometimes medicated, and usually applied hot to the surface; it exerts an emollient, relaxing, or stimulating counterirritant effect on the skin and underlying tissues. [L. *puls* (*pult-*), a thick pap; G. *poltos*]

pound (pownd) A unit of weight, containing 12 ounces (apothecaries' weight) or 16 ounces (avoirdupois); equivalent to 2.2046 kilograms. [A.S. *pund;* L. *pondus,* weight]

Pow•as•san en•ceph•a•li•tis (pō-wah′sĕn en-sef′ă-lī′tis) An acute disease of children varying clinically from undifferentiated febrile illness to encephalitis; caused by the Powassan virus and transmitted by ixodid ticks.

pow•der (pow′dĕr) **1.** A dry mass of minute separate particles of any substance. **2.** PHARMACEUTICS a homogeneous dispersion of finely divided, relatively dry particulate matter consisting of one or more substances. **3.** A single dose of a powdered drug, enclosed in an envelope of folded paper. **4.** To reduce a solid substance to a state of very fine division. [Fr. *poudre*, fr. L. *pulvis*]

pow•er (pow′ĕr) **1.** OPTICS the refractive vergence of a lens. **2.** PHYSICS the rate at which work is done. **3.** The product of force and velocity (distance divided by time) expressed in watts.

pox (poks) **1.** An eruptive disease, usually qualified by a descriptive prefix, e.g., smallpox, cowpox, chickenpox. See the specific term. **2.** An eruption, first papular then pustular, occurring in chronic antimony poisoning. **3.** Archaic or colloquial term for syphilis (also called great pox). [var. of pl. *pocks*]

Pox•vir•i•dae (poks-vir′i-dē) A family of large, complex viruses, with a marked affinity for skin tissue, that are pathogenic for humans and other animals; a number of genera are recognized, including, Orthopoxvirus, Avipoxvirus, Capripoxvirus, Leporipoxvirus, and Parapoxvirus.

pox•vi•rus (poks′vī-rŭs) Any virus of the family Poxviridae.

PP Abbreviation for pyrophosphate.

PPA Abbreviation for primary progressive aphasia.

PPCA Abbreviation for proserum prothrombin conversion accelerator.

PPE Abbreviation for personal protective equipment.

PPI Abbreviation for patient package insert.

PPLO Abbreviation for pleuropneumonialike organisms.

ppm Abbreviation for parts per million.

PPO Abbreviation for preferred provider organization; 2,5-diphenyloxazole, a liquid scintillator.

PPPPPP A mnemonic designating the symptom complex of acute arterial occlusion (pain, pallor, paraesthesia, pulselessness, paralysis, prostration).

PPS Abbreviation for prospective payment system; postpolio syndrome; primary physician services.

P pul•mo•na•le (pul-mō-nā′lē) Tall, narrow, peaked P waves in electrocardiographic leads II, III, and aVF, and often a prominent initial positive P wave component in V_1; it is characteristic of right atrial enlargement such as occurs in pulmonary disease and tricuspid stenosis.

PPV Abbreviation for positive pressure ventilation.

PQ in•ter•val (in′tĕr-văl) SYN PR interval.

PR Abbreviation for per rectum.

Pr Abbreviation for presbyopia; praseodymium; propyl.

PRA Abbreviation for plasma renin activity; phosphoribosylamine.

prac•ti•cal nurse (prak′ti-kăl nŭrs) A nurse

who has graduated from an accredited practical nursing program, which is usually 12–16 months long. A practical nurse is licensed by a regulatory body and usually works under the supervision of a registered nurse or physician. SYN licensed vocational nurse.

prac•tice (prak′tis) **1.** Direct professional involvement in health care services. **2.** Rehearsal of a task or skill with the goal of achieving proficiency. [Mediev. L. *practica,* business, G. *praktikos,* pertaining to action]

prac•tice guide•lines (prak′tis gīd′līnz) Recommendations developed by groups of clinicians for delivery of care based on various indications.

prac•ti•tion•er (prak-tish′ŭn-ĕr) A person who practices medicine or one of the allied health care professions.

Pra•der-Wil•li syn•drome (prah′dĕr-vē′lē sin′drōm) A congenital syndrome characterized by severe obesity, mental retardation, small hands and feet, and small genitalia. More than 50% of children with this condition are missing a chromosome. Presentation in infancy includes hypotonicity and difficulty with feeding, sucking, and temperature control.

♻ **prae-** SEE pre-.

praecava [Br.] SYN precava.

praecommissure [Br.] SYN precommissure.

praecoracoid [Br.] SEE precoracoid.

praecordia [Br.] SYN precordia.

praecordial [Br.] SYN precordial.

praecordial leads [Br.] SYN precordial leads.

praecordium [Br.] SYN precordium.

praecornu [Br.] SYN precornu.

praenaris [Br.] SYN prenaris.

praenasal [Br.] SYN prenasal.

prag•mat•ics (prag-mat′iks) **1.** LINGUISTICS the set of rules that govern the use of language in context, including social conventions (e.g., eye contact, accompanying gestures, proximity between speaker and listener, and turn-taking). **2.** The effects of social setting and environment on language.

prag•ma•tism (prag′mă-tizm) A philosophy emphasizing practical applications and consequences of beliefs and theories, that the meaning of ideas or things is determined by the testability of the idea in real life. [G. *pragma* (*pragmat-*), thing done]

Prague ma•neu•ver (prahg mă-nū′vĕr) A technique for delivery of the fetus in breech position when the fetal occiput is posterior; the operator delivers the shoulders with one hand, while making pressure above the symphysis pubis with the other hand.

Prague pel•vis (prahg pel′vis) SYN spondylolisthetic pelvis.

pral•i•dox•ime chlo•ride (pral′i-dok′sēm klōr′īd) A chloride salt of the oxime pralidoxime; the salt is used as an antidote in cases of poisoning by organophosphorous anticholinesterases (including organophosphorous pesticides and nerve agents).

pran•di•al (pran′dē-ăl) Relating to a meal. [L. *prandium,* breakfast]

pra•se•o•dym•i•um (Pr) (prā′sē-ō-dim′ē-ŭm) An element of the lanthanide or "rare earth" group; atomic no. 59, atomic wt. 140.90765. [G. *prasios,* leekgreen, fr. *prason,* a leek, + *didymos,* twin]

Pratt symp•tom (prat simp′tŏm) Rarely used term for rigidity in the muscles of an injured limb, which precedes the occurrence of gangrene.

prax•is (prak′sis) OCCUPATIONAL THERAPY conception and planning of a motor act in response to an environmental demand. [G., practice, activity]

PRE Abbreviation for progressive-resistance exercise.

♻ **pre-** Prefix meaning anterior; before (in time or space). SEE ALSO ante-, pro- (1). [L. *prae*]

pre•ag•o•nal (prē-ag′ŏ-năl) Immediately preceding death. [pre- + G. *agōn,* struggle (agony)]

preanaesthetic [Br.] SYN preanesthetic.

pre•an•es•thet•ic (prē′an-es-thet′ik) Before anesthesia. SYN preanaesthetic.

pre•au•ric•u•lar pit (prē′awr-ik′yū-lăr pit) SYN preauricular sinus.

pre•au•ric•u•lar sinus (prē′awr-ik′yū-lăr sī′nŭs) Sinus tract or pit in preauricular skin, resulting from developmental defect of the first and second pharyngeal arches. SYN preauricular pit.

pre•auth•or•i•za•tion (prē′awth′ŏr-ī-zā′shun) In the U.S., authorization of medical necessity by a primary care physician before a health care service is performed. A referring health care provider must be able to document why the procedure is needed. It does not guarantee coverage. SEE ALSO assignment.

pre•au•to•mat•ic pause (prē′aw-tō′mat′ik pawz) A temporary pause in cardiac activity before an automatic pacemaker escapes. SEE ALSO escape.

pre•ax•i•al (prē-ak′sē-ăl) **1.** Anterior to the axis of the body or a limb, the latter being in the anatomic position. **2.** Denoting the portion of a limb bud that lies cranial to the axis of the limb:

the radial aspect of the upper limb and the tibial aspect of the lower limb.

pre·bi·ot·ics (prē-bī-ot′iks) Nondigestible food ingredients that target selected groups of the human colonic microflora, thus enhancing colonization of those offering health benefits, such as bifidobacteria and lactobacilli. Cf. functional food.

pre·can·cer (prē-kan′sĕr) A lesion from which a malignant neoplasm is believed to develop in a significant number of instances, and which may or may not be recognizable clinically or by microscopic changes in the affected tissue.

pre·can·cer·ous (prē-kan′sĕr-ŭs) Pertaining to any lesion that is interpreted as precancer. SYN premalignant.

pre·cap·il·lary (prē-kap′i-lar-ē) Preceding a capillary; an arteriole or venule.

pre·car·ti·lage (prē-kahr′ti-lăj) A closely packed aggregation of mesenchymal cells just before their differentiation into embryonic cartilage.

pre·ca·va (prē-kā′vă) SYN superior vena cava. SYN praecava.

pre·cen·tral ar·e·a (prē-sen′trăl ār′ē-ă) The cortex of the precentral gyrus.

pre·cen·tral gy·rus (prē-sen′trăl jī′rŭs) Bounded posteriorly by the central sulcus and anteriorly by the precentral sulcus.

pre·cen·tral sul·cus (prē-sen′trăl sŭl′kŭs) An interrupted fissure anterior to and in general parallel with the central sulcus, marking the anterior border of the precentral gyrus.

pre·cep·tor (prē′sep-tŏr) An experienced nurse, physician, or other health care professional who guides and teaches those less experienced, including students; mentor.

pre·cer·ti·fi·ca·tion (prē′sĕr-ti-fi-kā′shŭn) Verification of a procedure as a covered benefit for a third-party payer before a health care service is performed. It does not guarantee coverage.

pre·ces·sion (prē-sesh′ŭn) The secondary spin of magnetic movements around the main magnetic field.

pre·cip·i·ta·ble (prē-sip′i-tă-bĕl) Capable of being precipitated.

pre·cip·i·tant (prē-sip′i-tănt) Anything causing a precipitation from a solution.

pre·cip·i·tate **1.** (prē-sip′i-tāt) To cause a substance in solution to separate as a solid. **2.** (prē-sip′i-tăt) A solid separated out from a solution or suspension; a floc or clump, such as that resulting from the mixture of a specific antigen and its antibody. **3.** Accumulation of inflammatory cells on the corneal endothelium in uveitis (keratic precipitates). [L. *praecipito,* pp. *-atus,* to cast headlong]

pre·cip·i·tate la·bor (prē-sip′i-tăt lā′bŏr) Very rapid labor ending in delivery of the fetus.

pre·cip·i·ta·tion (prē-sip′i-tā′shŭn) **1.** The process of formation of a solid previously held in solution or suspension in a liquid. **2.** The phenomenon of clumping of proteins in serum produced by the addition of a specific precipitin. SEE ALSO precipitate.

pre·cip·i·tin (prē-sip′i-tin) An antibody that under suitable conditions combines with and causes its specific and soluble antigen to precipitate from solution.

pre·cip·i·tin·o·gen (prē-sip′i-tin′ō-jen) **1.** An antigen that stimulates the formation of specific precipitin when injected into an animal body. **2.** A precipitable soluble antigen. [precipitin + G. *-gen,* producing]

pre·cip·i·tin test (prē-sip′i-tin test) An in vitro procedure in which antigen is in soluble form and precipitates when it combines with added specific antibody in the presence of an electrolyte. SEE ALSO gel diffusion precipitin tests.

pre·ci·sion (prē-sizh′ŭn) **1.** The quality of being sharply defined or stated; one measure of precision is the number of distinguishable alternatives to a measurement. **2.** STATISTICS the inverse of the variance of a measurement or estimate. **3.** Reproducibility of a quantifiable result; an indication of the random error.

pre·clin·i·cal (prē-klin′i-kăl) **1.** Before the onset of disease. **2.** A period in medical education before the student becomes involved with patients and clinical work.

pre·co·cious (prē-kō′shŭs) Developing unusually early or rapidly. [L. *praecox,* premature]

pre·co·cious pu·ber·ty (prē-kō′shŭs pyū′bĕr-tē) Condition in which pubertal changes begin at an unexpectedly early age.

pre·coc·i·ty (prē-kos′i-tē) Unusually early or rapid development of mental or physical traits. SEE ALSO precocious.

pre·cog·ni·tion (prē′kog-nish′ŭn) Advance knowledge, by means other than the normal senses, of a future event; a form of extrasensory perception. [L. *praecogito,* to ponder before]

pre·col·lag·e·nous fi·bers (prē-kŏ-laj′i-nŭs fī′bĕrz) Immature, argyrophilic fibers.

pre·com·mis·sure (prē-kom′i-shŭr) SYN anterior commissure. SYN praecommissure.

pre·con·cep·tu·al stage (prē′kŏn-sĕp′shū-ăl stāj) PSYCHOLOGY the stage of development in an infant's life, before actual conceptual thinking, in which sensorimotor activity predominates.

pre·con·scious (prē-kon′shŭs) PSYCHOANALY-

SIS one of the three divisions of the psyche, the other two being the conscious and unconscious; includes all ideas, thoughts, past experiences, and other memory impressions that with effort can be consciously recalled. Cf. foreconscious.

pre•con•vul•sive (prē′kŏn-vŭl′siv) Denoting the stage in an epileptic paroxysm preceding convulsions (e.g., aura).

pre•cor•a•coid (prē-kōr′ă-koyd) Anterior part of coracoid in the shoulder girdle of reptiles and amphibians.

pre•cor•di•a (prē-kōr′dē-ă) The epigastrium and anterior surface of the lower part of the thorax. SYN praecordia. [L. *praecordia* (ntr. pl. only), the diaphragm, the entrails, fr. *prae,* before, + *cor* (*cord-*), heart]

pre•cor•di•al (prē-kōr′dē-ăl) Relating to the precordia. SYN praecordial.

pre•cor•di•al leads (prē-kōr′dē-ăl lēdz) SYN chest leads. SYN praecordial leads.

pre•cor•di•um (prē-kōr′dē-ŭm) Singular of precordia. SYN praecordium.

pre•cor•nu (prē-kōr′nū) SYN anterior horn. SYN praecornu.

pre•cos•tal a•nas•to•mo•sis (prē-kos′tăl ă-nas′tŏ-mō′sis) Longitudinal anastomosis of intersegmental arteries in the embryo that gives rise to the thyrocervical and costocervical trunks.

pre•cu•ne•ate (prē-kyū′nē-ăt) Relating to the precuneus.

pre•cu•ne•us (prē-kyū′nē-ŭs) A division of the medial surface of each cerebral hemisphere between the cuneus and the paracentral lobule; it lies above the subparietal sulcus and is bounded anteriorly by the marginal part of the cingulate sulcus and posteriorly by the parietooccipital sulcus. SYN quadrate lobe (3). [pre- + L. *cuneus,* a wedge]

pre•cur•sor (prē′kŭrs-ŏr) That which precedes another or from which another is derived, applied especially to a physiologically inactive substance that is converted to an active enzyme, vitamin, or hormone, or to a chemical substance that is built into a larger structure in the course of synthesizing the latter. [L. *praecursor,* fr. *prae-,* pre-, + *curro,* to run]

pre•cur•so•ry car•ti•lage (prē-kŭr′sŭr-ē kahr′ti-lăj) SYN temporary cartilage.

pre•de•cid•u•al (prē′dē-sid′yū-ăl) Relating to the premenstrual or secretory phase of the menstrual cycle.

pre•den•tin (prē-den′tin) The organic fibrillar matrix of the dentin before its calcification.

pre-De•sce•met cor•ne•al dys•tro•phy (prē′des-ĕ-mā′ kōr′nē-ăl dis′trŏ-fē) Opacification with primary involvement of the posterior stroma of the cornea.

pre•de•ter•mi•na•tion (prē′dĕ-tĕr′mi-nā′shŭn) Determination of the reimbursement amount from a third-party payor before a health care service is performed. It does not guarantee coverage.

pre•di•a•be•tes (prē′dī-ă-bē′tēz) A state of potential diabetes mellitus, with normal glucose tolerance but with an increased risk of developing diabetes (e.g., family history).

pre•di•as•to•le (prē′dī-as′tŏ-lē) The interval in the cardiac rhythm immediately preceding diastole. SYN late systole.

pre•di•a•stol•ic (prē′dī-ă-stol′ik) Late systolic, relating to the interval preceding cardiac diastole.

pre•dic•tive val•ue (prē-dik′tiv val′yū) An expression of the likelihood that a given test result will correlate with the presence or absence of disease. A positive predictive value is the ratio of patients with the disease who test positive to thc entire population of people with a positive test result; a negative predictive value is the ratio of patients without the disease who test negative to the entire population of people with a negative test result.

pre•di•ges•tion (prē′dī-jes′chŭn) The artificial initiation of digestion of proteins (proteolysis) and starches (amylolysis) before they are eaten.

pre•dis•pose (prē′dis-pōz′) To render susceptible.

pre•dis•po•si•tion (prē′dis-pō-zish′ŭn) A condition of special susceptibility to a disease.

pre•duc•tal (prē-dŭk′tăl) Relating to that part of the aorta proximal to the aortic opening of the ductus arteriosus.

pre•e•clamp•si•a (PE) (prē′ē-klamp′sē-ă) Development of hypertension with proteinuria or edema, or both, due to pregnancy or the influence of a recent pregnancy; it usually occurs after the 20th week of gestation, but may develop before this time in the presence of trophoblastic disease. [pre- + G. *eklampsis,* a shining forth (eclampsia)]

pree•mie (prē′mē) SYN preterm infant.

pre•ep•i•glot•tic space (prē-ep′i-glot′ik spās) The space anterior to the epiglottis that is bounded anteriorly by the thyrohyoid membrane and the superior parts of the lamina of the thyroid cartilage, superiorly by the hyoepiglottic ligament and inferiorly by the thyroepiglottic ligament; laterally, it extends into the paraglottic spaces. Carcinoma of the infrahyoid portion of the epiglottis often extends into the preepiglottic space.

pre•ex•ci•ta•tion (prē′ek-sī-tā′shŭn) Premature activation of part of the ventricular myocardium by an impulse that travels by an anomalous path and so avoids physiologic delay in the atrioventricular junction; an intrinsic part of the Wolff-Parkinson-White syndrome.

pre·ex·ci·ta·tion syn·drome (prē′ek-sī-tā′shŭn sin′drōm) SYN Wolff-Parkinson-White syndrome.

pre·ex·is·ting con·di·tion (prē′eg-zist′ing kŏn-di′shŭn) A health problem that existed or for which treatment was received before the effective date of a new insurance policy.

pre·ferred prac·tice pat·tern (prē-fĕrd′ prak′tis pat′ĕrn) The category of conditions used by physical therapists to diagnose and formulate a plan of care within their scope of professional practice. The categories include musculoskeletal, neuromuscular, cardiovascular-pulmonary, and integumentary.

pre·ferred pro·vi·der or·gan·i·za·tion (PPO) (prē-fĕrd′ prō-vī′dĕr ōr′găn-ī-zā′shŭn) A U.S. health care organization that negotiates set rates of reimbursement with participating health care providers for services to insured clients. This is a type of prospective payment or managed care system. SEE ALSO health maintenance organization.

pre·formed Vi·ta·min A (prē′fōrmd vī′tă-min) Retinyl esters mainly found in animal sources that are the main storage form of vitamin A.

pre·fron·tal ar·e·a (prē-frŏnt′ăl ār′ē-ă) SEE frontal cortex.

pre·gan·gli·on·ic (prē′gang-glē-on′ik) Situated proximal to or preceding a ganglion; referring specifically to the preganglionic motor neurons of the autonomic nervous system (located in the spinal cord and brainstem) and the preganglionic, myelinated nerve fibers by which they are connected to the autonomic ganglia.

preg·nan·cy (preg′năn-sē) The state of a female after conception and until the termination of the gestation. See this page. SYN gestation. [L. *praegnans* (*praegnant-*), pregnant, fr. *prae,* before, + *gnascor,* pp. *natus,* to be born]

preg·nan·cy gin·gi·vi·tis (preg′năn-sē jin′ji-vī′tis) SYN hormonal gingivitis.

preg·nan·cy-in·duced hy·per·ten·sion (preg′năn-sē-in-dūst′ hī′pĕr-ten′shŭn) SYN gestational hypertension.

preg·nane (preg′nān) Parent hydrocarbon of the progesterones, pregnane alcohols, ketones, and several adrenocortical hormones. Cf. bioregulator.

preg·nane·di·ol (preg′nān-dī′ol) The chief steroid metabolite of progesterone; it is biologically inactive and occurs as pregnanediol glucuronate in the urine. Cf. bioregulator.

preg·nane·di·one (preg′nān-dī′ōn) A metabolite of progesterone, formed in relatively small quantities that occurs in 5α and 5β isomeric forms. Cf. bioregulator.

preg·nane·tri·ol (preg′nān-trī′ol) A urinary metabolite of 17-hydroxyprogesterone and a precursor in the biosynthesis of cortisol; its excretion is enhanced in certain diseases of the cortex of suprarenal gland and following administration of corticotropin.

preg·nant (preg′nănt) Denoting a gestating female. SEE ALSO pregnancy. Cf. bioregulator. SYN gravid.

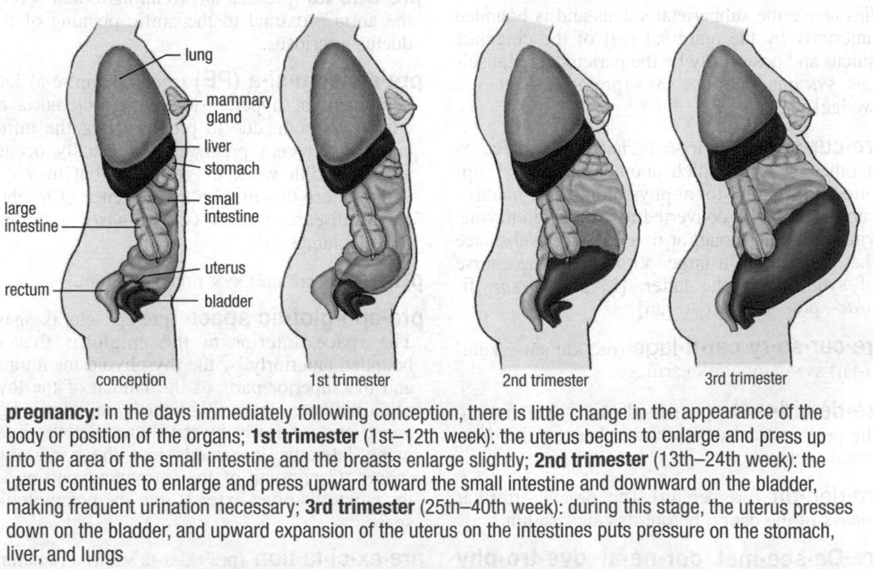

pregnancy: in the days immediately following conception, there is little change in the appearance of the body or position of the organs; **1st trimester** (1st–12th week): the uterus begins to enlarge and press up into the area of the small intestine and the breasts enlarge slightly; **2nd trimester** (13th–24th week): the uterus continues to enlarge and press upward toward the small intestine and downward on the bladder, making frequent urination necessary; **3rd trimester** (25th–40th week): during this stage, the uterus presses down on the bladder, and upward expansion of the uterus on the intestines puts pressure on the stomach, liver, and lungs

pre•hen•sile (prē-hen′sil) Adapted for taking hold of or grasping. [L. *prehendo,* pp. *-hensus,* to lay hold of, seize]

pre•hen•sion (prē-hen′shŭn) The act of grasping, or taking hold of.

pre•hor•mone (prē-hōr′mōn) A glandular secretory product, having little or no inherent biologic potency, that is converted peripherally to an active hormone. Cf. prohormone, bioregulator.

pre•hos•pi•tal care (prē-hos′pi-tăl kār) Assessment, stabilization, and care of a medical emergency or trauma victim, including transport to the appropriate receiving facility.

pre•hos•pi•tal care re•port (prē-hos′pi-tăl kār rĕ-pōrt′) An electronic or written report completed by a prehospital provider that contains demographic and medical information as well as a record of the treatment and transport of a patient. A copy of the prehospital care report often is left at the receiving facility as a medical reference and for inclusion in the patient's medical record.

pre•hos•pi•tal pro•vi•der (prē-hos′pi-tăl prō-vī′dĕr) One who provides care in case of medical emergency or trauma, most often an emergency medical technician (EMT) or paramedic. SYN emergency medical technician, paramedic.

pre•hy•per•ten•sion (prē-hī′pĕr-ten′shŭn) Classification from *The Seventh Report of the Joint National Committee on Prevention, Detection, Evaluation, and Treatment of High Blood Pressure* for blood pressure systolic reading of 120–139 mmHg and diastolic reading of 80–89 mmHg. Blood pressure in this range warrants management to prevent progression to hypertension. SEE ALSO holistic medicine.

pre•ic•tal (prē-ik′tăl) Occurring before a seizure or stroke. [pre- + L. *ictus,* a stroke]

pre•in•duc•tion (prē′in-dŭk′shŭn) A modification in the third generation resulting from the action of environment on the germ cells of one or both individuals of the grandparental generation. An effect from the action of environment on the germ cells of progenitors on their grandchildren. [L. *prae,* before, + *inductio,* a bringing in, fr. *induco,* to lead in]

pre•in•farc•tion an•gi•na (prē′in-fahrk′shŭn an′ji-nă) SYN acute coronary syndrome.

pre•kal•li•kre•in (prē′kal-i-krē′in) A plasma glycoprotein that in complex with kininogen serves as a cofactor in the activation of factor XII; also serves as the proenzyme for plasma kallikrein. SYN Fletcher factor.

preleukaemia [Br.] SYN preleukemia.

pre•leu•ke•mi•a (prē′lū-kē′mē-ă) SYN myelodysplastic syndrome. SYN preleukaemia.

pre•load (prē′lōd) **1.** The load to which a muscle is subjected before shortening. **2.** SYN ventricular preload.

pre•log•i•cal think•ing (prē-loj′ik-ăl thingk′ing) A concrete type of thinking, characteristic of children and primitives, to which schizophrenic people sometimes regress.

pre•ma•lig•nant (prē′mă-lig′nănt) SYN precancerous.

pre•ma•ture (prē′mă-chŭr′) **1.** Occurring before the usual or expected time. **2.** Denoting an infant born less than 37 weeks (8 1/2 months) after conception. [L. *praematurus,* too early, fr. *prae-,* pre-, + *maturus,* ripe (mature)]

pre•ma•ture a•tri•al con•trac•tion (PAC) (prē′mă-chŭr′ ā′trē-ăl kŏn-trak′shŭn) A premature cardiac beat arising from an ectopic atrial focus.

pre•ma•ture birth (prē′mă-chŭr′ bĭrth) Birth of an infant after viability has been achieved with gestation of at least 20 weeks or birth weight of at least 500 g, but before 37 weeks.

pre•ma•ture de•liv•er•y (prē′mă-chŭr′ dĕ-liv′ĕr-ē) Birth of a fetus before its proper time. SEE ALSO premature birth.

pre•ma•ture e•jac•u•la•tion (prē′mă-chŭr′ ē-jak′yū-lā′shŭn) During sexual intercourse, too rapid achievement of climax and ejaculation in the male relative to his own or his partner's wishes.

pre•ma•ture in•fant (prē′mă-chŭr′ in′fănt) SYN preterm infant.

pre•ma•ture junc•tion•al con•trac•tion (PJC) (prē′mă-chŭr′ jungk′shŭn-ăl kŏn-trak′shŭn) A premature cardiac beat arising from the atrioventricular junction, accompanied by normal or abnormal QRS complexes.

pre•ma•ture la•bor (prē′mă-chŭr′ lā′bŏr) Onset of labor before the 37th completed week of pregnancy dated from the last normal menstrual period.

pre•ma•ture mem•brane rup•ture (prē′mă-chŭr′ mem′brān rŭp′chŭr) Break in the membranes before the onset of labor.

pre•ma•ture men•o•pause (prē′mă-chŭr′ men′ŏ-pawz) Failure of cyclic ovarian function before age 40. SYN premature ovarian failure.

pre•ma•ture new•born (prē′mă-chŭr′ nū′bōrn) SYN preterm infant.

pre•ma•ture o•var•i•an fail•ure (prē′mă-chŭr′ ō-var′ē-ăn fāl′yŭr) SYN premature menopause.

pre•ma•ture rup•ture of mem•branes (PROM) (prē′mă-chŭr′ rŭp′chŭr mem′brānz) Rupture of the amniotic sac before onset of labor.

pre·ma·ture sys·to·le (prē′mă-chūr′ sis′tŏ-lē) SYN extrasystole.

pre·ma·ture ven·tric·u·lar con·trac·tion (PVC) (prē′mă-chūr′ ven-trik′yū-lăr kŏn-trak′shŭn) Compression within the lower cardiac chambers; such contractions may cause perception of palpitation in patient.

pre·ma·tu·ri·ty (prē′mă-chūr′i-tē) **1.** The state of being premature. **2.** DENTISTRY deflective occlusal contact.

pre·max·il·lary bone (prē-maks′i-lar′ē bōn) SYN os incisivum.

pre·med·i·ca·tion (prē′med-i-kā′shŭn) **1.** Administration of drugs before induction of general anesthesia to allay apprehension, produce sedation, and facilitate administration of anesthetic. **2.** Drugs used for such purposes.

pre·men·stru·al (prē-men′strū-ăl) Relating to the period of time preceding menstruation.

pre·men·stru·al dys·phor·ic dis·or·der (PMDD) (prē-men′strū-ăl dis-fōr′ik dis-ōr′dĕr) **1.** A pervasive pattern occurring during the last week of the luteal phase in most menstrual cycles for at least a year and remitting within a few days of the onset of the follicular phase, with some combination of depressed mood, mood lability, marked anxiety, or irritability; various specific physical symptoms; and significant functional impairment; the symptoms are comparable in severity to those seen in a major depressive episode, distinguishing this disorder from the far more common premenstrual syndrome. SEE ALSO premenstrual syndrome. **2.** A specified set of criteria in the DSM, proposed for the purpose of further research.

pre·men·stru·al syn·drome (PMS) (prē-men′strū-ăl sin′drōm) In some women of reproductive age, the regular monthly experience of physiologic and emotional distress, usually during the several days preceding menses; characterized by nervousness, depression, fluid retention, and weight gain. SYN late luteal phase dysphoria, menstrual molimina, premenstrual tension.

pre·men·stru·al ten·sion (prē-men′strū-ăl ten′shŭn) SYN premenstrual syndrome.

pre·men·stru·um (prē-men′strū-ŭm) The few days preceding menstruation. [pre- + L. *menstruum,* ntr. of *menstruus,* monthly, pertaining to menstruation]

pre·mi·um (prē′mē-ŭm) The amount that must be paid to the insurer to maintain the desired health insurance coverage.

pre·mo·lar (prē-mō′lăr) **1.** Anterior to a molar tooth. **2.** Denotes permanent teeth that replace the deciduous molars. **3.** SEE bicuspid.

pre·mo·lar tooth (prē-mō′lăr tūth) A tooth usually having two tubercles or cusps on the grinding surface and a flattened root, single in the lower jaw and upper second premolar, and furrowed in the upper first premolar. There are four premolars in each jaw, two on either side between the canine and the molars; there are no premolars in the deciduous dentition. SYN dens premolaris [TA], bicuspid tooth.

pre·mon·o·cyte (prē-mon′ō-sīt) An immature monocyte normally not seen in the circulating blood. SYN promonocyte.

pre·mor·bid (prē-mōr′bid) Preceding the occurrence of disease. [pre- + L. *morbidus,* ill, fr. *morbus,* disease]

pre·mu·ni·tion (prē′myū-nish′ŭn) A state of existing resistance of a host to infection or reinfection with a parasite; used especially in malaria epidemiology. [L. *praemunitio,* fortification in advance, fr. *prae-,* + *munio,* to fortify]

pre·mu·ni·tive (prē-myū′ni-tiv) Relating to premunition.

pre·my·e·lo·blast (prē-mī′ĕ-lō-blast) The earliest recognizable precursor of the myeloblast.

pre·my·e·lo·cyte (prē-mī′ĕ-lō-sīt) SYN promyelocyte.

pre·nar·is (prē-nā′ris) SYN nostril. SYN praenaris.

pre·na·sal (prē-nā′zăl) In front of the nose. SYN praenasal.

pre·na·tal (prē-nā′tăl) Preceding birth. SYN antenatal. [pre- + L. *natus,* born]

pre·na·tal di·ag·no·sis (prē-nā′tăl dī′ăg-nō′sis) Diagnosis using procedures available for the recognition of diseases and malformations in utero, and the conclusion reached.

pre·ne·o·plas·tic (prē-nē′ō-plas′tik) Preceding the formation of any neoplasm, benign or malignant. [pre- + G. *neos,* new, + *plastikos,* formative]

Pren·tice rule (pren′tis rūl) Each centimeter of decentration of a lens results in 1 prism diopter of deviation of light for each diopter of lens power.

pre·op·er·a·tive (prē-op′ĕr-ă-tiv) Preceding an operation.

pre·os·te·o·blast (prē-os′tē-ō-blast) SYN osteoprogenitor cell.

pre·ox·y·gen·a·tion (prē′ok-si-jĕ-nā′shŭn) Denitrogenation with 100% oxygen before induction of general anesthesia or endotracheal intubation.

prep (prep) To prepare the skin or other body surface for an operative procedure, usually by cleaning and application of antiseptic solutions. [slang for preparation or prepare]

pre·pan·cre·at·ic ar·ter·y (prē-pan-krē-at′ik

ahr′tĕr-ē) *Origin*, arises from dorsal pancreatic artery as its left terminal branch; *distribution*, often double, it runs between the neck and uncinate process of the pancreas to form an arterial arch (arcade) with the anterior superior pancreaticoduodenal artery. SYN arteria prepancreatica [TA].

pre·pa·tel·lar bur·sa (prē-pă-tel′ăr bŭr′să) A bursa between the skin and the lower part of the patella.

pre·pa·tent pe·ri·od (prē-pā′tĕnt pēr′ē-ŏd) PARASITOLOGY the period interval to the incubation period of microbial infections; it varies biologically, however, because the parasite undergoes developmental stages in the host.

pre·pon·der·ance (prē-pon′dĕr-ăns) Quality of outweighing, or exceeding in extent or importance.

pre·po·ten·tial (prē′pō-ten′shăl) A gradual rise in potential between action potentials as a phasic swing in electric activity of the cell membrane, which establishes its rate of automatic activity, as in the ureter or cardiac pacemaker.

pre·psy·chot·ic (prē′sī-kot′ik) **1.** Relating to the period before the onset of psychosis. **2.** Denoting a potential for a psychotic episode, one that appears imminent under continued stress.

pre·pu·ber·al, **pre·pu·ber·tal** (prē-pyū′bĕr-ăl, -bĕr-tăl) Before puberty.

pre·pu·bes·cent (prē′pyū-bes′ĕnt) Immediately before the commencement of puberty.

pre·puce (prē′pyūs) The free fold of skin that covers the glans penis more or less completely. SYN preputium [TA], foreskin. [L. *praeputium*, foreskin]

pre·puce of clit·o·ris (prē′pyūs klit′ŏr-is) The external fold of the labia minora, forming a cap over the clitoris.

pre·pu·ti·al (pre-pyū′shē-ăl) Relating to the prepuce.

pre·pu·ti·al cal·cu·lus (pre-pyū′shē-ăl kal′kyū-lŭs) A calculus occurring beneath the foreskin.

pre·pu·ti·al glands (pre-pyū′shē-ăl glandz) Sebaceous glands of the corona glandis and inner surface of the prepuce, which produce an odoriferous substance called smegma.

pre·pu·ti·ot·o·my (prē-pyū′shē-ot′ŏ-mē) Incision of prepuce. [preputium + G. *tomē*, incision]

pre·pu·ti·um, pl. **pre·pu·ti·a** (prē-pyū′shē-ŭm, -shē-ă) [TA] SYN prepuce. [L. *praeputium*]

pre·py·lor·ic vein (prē′pī-lōr′ik vān) A tributary of the right gastric vein that passes anterior to the pylorus at its junction with the duodenum.

pre·sac·ral fas·ci·a (prē-sā′krăl fash′ē-ă) Layer of endopelvic fascia passing between sacrum and rectum, forming the anterior boundary of the presacral (retrorectal) fascial space, in which the hypogastric nervous plexus is embedded.

pre·sa·cral neu·rec·to·my, **pre·sa·cral sym·pa·thec·to·my** (prē-sā′krăl nūr-ek′tŏ-mē, sim′pă-thek′tŏ-mē) Cutting of the presacral nerve to relieve severe dysmenorrhea. SYN Cotte operation.

♻**presby-**, **presbyo-** Combining forms denoting old age. SEE ALSO gero-. [G. *presbys,* old man]

pres·by·a·cu·sis, **pres·by·a·cu·si·a** (prez′bē-ă-kyū′sis, -kyū′sē-ă) SYN presbycusis. [presby- + G. *akousis,* hearing]

pres·by·a·sta·sis (prez′bē-ă-stā′sis) Impairment of vestibular function associated with aging. [presby- + G. *a-*, priv., + *stasis,* standing]

pres·by·cu·sis (prez′bē-kyū′sis) A usually gradual, frequently bilateral sensorineural or conductive hearing loss often related to the middle ear that gradually occurs in most people as they age; usually more pronounced for high-pitched sounds; the pattern and age of onset may vary. SYN presbyacusis, presbyacusia. [G. *presbys,* old man, + *akousis,* hearing]

pres·by·o·pi·a (Pr) (prez′bē-ō′pē-ă) The physiologic loss of accommodation in the eyes in advancing age, said to begin when the near point has receded beyond 22 cm (9 inches). [presby- + G. *ōps,* eye]

pres·by·op·ic (prez′bē-op′ik) Relating to or suffering from presbyopia.

pre·scribe (prē-skrīb′) To give directions, either orally or in writing, for the preparation and administration of a remedy to be used in the treatment of any disease. [L. *prae-scribo,* pp. *-scriptus,* to write before]

pre·scrip·tion (prē-skrip′shŭn) **1.** A written formula for the preparation and administration of any remedy. **2.** A medicinal preparation compounded according to formulated directions, consisting of four parts: 1) superscription, consisting of the word *recipe*, take, or its sign, ℞; 2) inscription, the main part of the prescription, containing the names and amounts of the drugs ordered; 3) subscription, directions for mixing the ingredients and designation of the form (pill, powder, solution) in which the drug is to be made; 4) signature, directions to the patient regarding the dose and times of taking the remedy. SEE prescribe. [L. *praescriptio;*]

pre·se·nile (prē-sen′il) Before the usual onset of senility.

pre·se·nile de·men·ti·a, **de·men·ti·a pre·se·ni·lis** (prē-sen′il dĕ-men′shē-ă, dĕ-men′shē-ă prē-sē-nā′lis) **1.** Dementia of Alzheimer disease developing before age 65. **2.** SYN Alzheimer disease.

pre•se•nil•i•ty (prē′sĕ-nil′i-tē) Premature old age; the condition of an individual, not old in years, who displays the physical and mental characteristics of old age but not to the extent of senility. [pre- + L. *senilis,* old]

pre•sent (prē-zent′) **1.** To precede or appear first at the os uteri; said of the part of the fetus first felt during examination. **2.** To appear for examination, or treatment; said of a patient. [L. *praesens (-sent-),* pres. p. of *prae-sum,* to be before, be at hand]

pre•sen•ta•tion (prez′ĕn-tā′shŭn) That part of the fetus presenting at the superior aperture of the maternal pelvis; occiput, chin, and sacrum are, respectively, the determining points in vertex, face, and breech presentation. SEE ALSO position (3), present.

pre•sep•tal cell•u•li•tis (prē-sep′tăl sel′yū-lī′tis) Infection involving the superficial tissue and periocular layers anterior to the orbital septum. SYN periorbital cellulitis.

pre•ser•va•tive (prĕ-zĕr′vă-tiv) A substance added to food products or to an organic solution to prevent chemical change or bacterial action.

pre•so•mite (prē-sō′mīt) Relating to the embryonic stage before the appearance of somites (before day 19 in human embryos).

pre•sphyg•mic (prē-sfig′mik) Preceding the pulse beat; denoting a brief interval following the filling of the ventricles with blood before their contraction forces open the semilunar valves, corresponding to the isovolumic contraction period. [pre- + G. *sphygmos,* pulse]

pres•sor (pres′ŏr) Exciting to vasomotor activity; producing increased blood pressure; denoting afferent nerve fibers that, when stimulated, excite vasoconstrictors, which increase peripheral resistance. SYN hypertensor. [L. *premo,* pp. *pressus,* to press]

pres•sor a•mine (pres′ŏr ă-mēn′) SYN pressor base.

pres•sor base (pres′ŏr bās) **1.** One of several products of intestinal putrefaction believed to cause functional hypertension when absorbed. **2.** Any alkaline substance that raises blood pressure. SYN pressor amine.

pres•so•re•cep•tive (pres′ō-rĕ-sep′tiv) Capable of detecting or responding to changes in pressure, especially changes of blood pressure. SYN pressosensitive.

pres•so•re•cep•tor (pres′ō-rĕ-sep′tŏr) SYN baroreceptor.

pres•sor fi•bers (pres′ŏr fī′bĕrz) Sensory nerve fibers, the stimulation of which causes vasoconstriction and a rise in blood pressure.

pres•sor nerve (pres′ŏr nĕrv) An afferent nerve, stimulation of which excites a reflex vasoconstriction, thereby raising the blood pressure.

pres•so•sen•si•tive (pres′ō-sen′si-tiv) SYN pressoreceptive.

pres•sure (presh′ŭr) **1.** A stress or force acting in any direction against resistance. **2.** (P, frequently followed by a subscript indicating location) PHYSICS, PHYSIOLOGY the force per unit area exerted by a gas or liquid against the walls of its container or that would be exerted on a wall immersed at that spot in the middle of a body of fluid. The pressure can be considered either relative to some reference pressure, such as that of the ambient atmosphere (gauge pressure), or relative to a perfect vacuum (absolute pressure). [L. *pressura,* fr. *premo,* pp. *pressus,* to press]

pres•sure al•o•pe•ci•a (presh′ŭr al′ō-pē′shē-ă) Loss of hair over a circumscribed area, usually on the posterior scalp, resulting from the continuous pressure on the occiput in a lengthy operative procedure, or unconsciousness following a drug overdose.

pres•sure-con•trolled in•verse ra•ti•o ven•ti•la•tion (PCIRV) (presh′ŭr kŏn-trōld′ in′vĕrs rā′shē-ō ven′ti-lā′shŭn) Mode of positive pressure ventilation used in patients with more severe respiratory disorders (e.g., ARDS) in which pressure is continuously adjusted downward as lung-compliance and gas exchange improve during inspiration.

pres•sure con•trolled ven•ti•la•tion (presh′ŭr kŏn-trōld′ ven′ti-lā′shŭn) A mode of mechanical ventilation in which the ventilator delivers a preset pressure waveform; the resultant tidal volume and inspiratory flow depend on the shape of the pressure waveform and respiratory system resistance and compliance.

pres•sure dress•ing (presh′ŭr dres′ing) A dressing by which pressure is exerted on the area covered to prevent the collection of fluids in the underlying tissues; most commonly used after skin grafting and in the treatment of burns.

pres•sure e•pi•phy•sis (presh′ŭr e-pif′i-sis) A secondary center of ossification in the articular end of a long bone.

pres•sure e•qua•li•za•tion (PE) tube (presh′ŭr ē′kwăl-ī-zā′shŭn tūb) A grommet placed through the tympanic membrane to provide continuous middle ear ventilation; most frequently used to ameliorate chronic otitis media.

pres•sure pa•ral•y•sis (presh′ŭr păr-al′i-sis) Paralysis due to compression of a nerve, nerve trunk, or spinal cord.

pres•sure point (presh′ŭr poynt) A cutaneous locus having pressure-sensitive elements that, when compressed, produce a sensation of pressure.

pres•sure pulse dif•fer•en•ti•a•tion (presh′ŭr pŭls dif′ĕr-en′shē-ā′shŭn) The processing of a pressure pulse signal so that the output depends on the rate of change of the input, yielding dP/dt (pressure) or, for noninvasively recorded pulses, dD/dt (rate of change of displacement).

pres•sure-reg•u•la•ted vol•ume con•trol (PRVC) (presh′ŭr-reg′yū-lā-tĕd vol′yūm kŏn-trōl′) A mode of mechanical ventilation.

pres•sure re•ver•sal (presh′ŭr rē-vĕr′săl) Cessation of anesthesia by hyperbaric pressure; of major importance in understanding the mode of action of anesthetics.

pres•sure sense (presh′ŭr sens) The faculty of discriminating various degrees of pressure on the surface. SYN baresthesia, piesesthesia.

pres•sure sore (presh′ŭr sōr) SYN decubitus ulcer.

pres•sure sta•sis (presh′ŭr stā′sis) SYN traumatic asphyxia.

pres•sure sup•port ven•ti•la•tion (PSV) (presh′ŭr sŭ-pōrt′ ven′ti-lā′shŭn) A mode of mechanical ventilation in which pressure is limited and flow cycled.

pres•sure tap•ping (presh′ŭr tap′ing) SYN intermittent compression (2).

pres•sure time in•dex (PTI) (presh′ŭr tīm in′deks) A calculation of the area under the diastolic component of the arterial blood pressure curve, used to determine left ventricular mass index and ventricular load in diastolic hypertension and chronic obstructive pulmonary disease.

pres•sure ul•cer (presh′ŭr ŭl′sĕr) SYN decubitus ulcer.

pres•sure ven•ti•la•tor (presh′ŭr ven′ti-lā-tŏr) A device designed to deliver pressure-controlled ventilation.

pres•sure-vol•ume in•dex (presh′ŭr-vol′yūm in′deks) Method of evaluating the cerebrospinal fluid hydrodynamics.

pres•sure wave•form (presh′ŭr wāv′fōrm) A graphic representation of intravascular or intracardiac pressure related to phases of the cardiac cycle, displayed on an oscilloscope monitor or paper copy.

pre-stead•y state (prē-sted′ē stāt) Those conditions and the time interval before establishment of steady state.

pre•sumed oc•u•lar his•to•plas•mo•sis (prē-zūmd′ ok′yū-lăr his′tō-plaz-mō′sis) Subretinal neovascularization in the macular region associated with chorioretinal atrophy and pigment proliferation adjacent to the optic disc, and peripheral chorioretinal atrophy ("histo-spots"); presumed secondary to infection by *Histoplasma capsulatum*.

pre•sump•tive signs of preg•nan•cy (prē-zŭmp′tiv sīnz preg′năn-sē) Signs and symptoms suggestive of pregnancy that may also indicate another condition. They occur early and are more subjective than other signs. The presumptive signs are amenorrhea, nausea and vomiting, frequent urination, and fatigue.

pre•sup•pu•ra•tive (prē-sŭp′yūr-ă-tiv) Denoting an early stage in an inflammation before the formation of pus.

pre•syn•ap•tic (prē′si-nap′tik) Pertaining to the area on the proximal side of a synaptic cleft.

pre•syn•ap•tic mem•brane (prē′si-nap′tik mem′brān) That part of the plasma membrane of an axon terminal that faces the plasma membrane of the neuron or muscle fiber with which the axon terminal establishes a synaptic junction. SEE ALSO synapse.

pre•sys•to•le (prē-sis′tŏ-lē) That part of diastole immediately preceding systole.

pre•sys•tol•ic (prē′sis-tol′ik) Late diastolic, relating to the interval immediately preceding systole.

pre•sys•tol•ic gal•lop (prē′sis-tol′ik gal′ŏp) Gallop rhythm in which the gallop sound is an audible fourth heart sound due to forceful ventricular filling.

pre•sys•tol•ic mur•mur (prē′sis-tol′ik mŭr′mŭr) A murmur heard at the end of ventricular diastole (during atrial systole if in sinus rhythm), usually due to obstruction at one of the atrioventricular orifices.

pre•sys•tol•ic thrill (prē′sis-tol′ik thril) A thrill immediately preceding the ventricular contraction that is sometimes felt on palpation over the apex of the heart.

pre•tar•sal (prē-tahr′săl) Denoting the anterior, or inferior, portion of the tarsus.

pre•term in•fant (prē-term in′fănt) An infant with gestational age of fewer than 37 completed weeks (259 completed days). SYN preemie, premature infant, premature newborn, preterm newborn.

pre•term mem•brane rup•ture (prē-term mem′brān rŭp′chŭr) Break in fetal membranes before term (less than 37 weeks' gestation).

pre•term new•born (prē′tĕrm nū′bōrn) SYN preterm infant.

pre•tib•i•al fe•ver (prē-tib′ē-ăl fē′vĕr) A mild disease first observed among U.S. military personnel at Fort Bragg, NC, characterized by fever, moderate prostration, splenomegaly, and a rash on the anterior aspects of the legs; due to the *autumnalis* serovar of *Leptospira interrogans*. SYN Fort Bragg fever.

pre•tib•i•al myx•e•de•ma (prē-tib′ē-ăl miks′ĕ-dē′mă) SYN circumscribed myxedema.

pre•tra•che•al lay•er of cer•vi•cal fas•ci•a (prē-trā′kē-ăl lā′ĕr sĕr′vi-kăl fash′ē-ă) The layer of fascia investing the infrahyoid muscles and contributing to the formation of the carotid sheath.

pre·treat·ment mor·bid·i·ty (prē-trēt′mĕnt mōr-bid′i-tē) The state of an illness and the degree of symptoms present immediately before the initiation of treatment.

prev·a·lence (prev′ă-lĕns) The number of cases of a disease existing in a given population at a specific period of time (i.e., period prevalence) or at a particular moment in time (i.e., point prevalence).

pre·ven·tive (prē-ven′tiv) SYN prophylactic (1). [L. *prae-venio,* pp. *-ventus,* to come before, prevent]

pre·ven·tive den·tis·try (prē-ven′tiv den′tis-trē) A philosophy and method of dental practice that seek to prevent the initiation, progression, and recurrence of dental caries.

pre·ven·tive med·i·cine (prē-ven′tiv med′i-sin) The branch of medical science concerned with the prevention of disease and with promotion of physical and mental health, through study of the etiology and epidemiology of disease processes.

pre·ven·tive nur·sing (prē-ven′tiv nŭrs′ing) Nursing interventions and care directed at health promotion and prevention of disease or injury.

pre·ver·te·bral gan·gli·a (prē-vĕr′tē-brăl gang′glē-ă) The sympathetic ganglia (celiac, aorticorenal, superior and inferior mesenteric) lying in front of the vertebral column, as distinguished from the ganglia of the sympathetic trunk (paravertebral ganglia); these ganglia occur mostly around the origins of the major branches of the abdominal aorta; all are in the abdominopelvic cavity, concerned with innervation of abdominopelvic viscera.

pre·ver·te·bral lay·er of cer·vi·cal fas·ci·a (prē-vĕr′tĕ-brăl lā′er sĕr′vi-kăl fash′ē-ă) The part of the cervical fascia that covers the bodies of the cervical vertebrae and the muscles attaching to them and to the anterior parts of their transverse processes.

pre·vi·us (prē′vē-ŭs) Obstructing; denoting anything blocking the passages in childbirth. [L. *prae,* before, + *via,* way]

Pre·vo·tel·la (prev′ō-tel′ă) Bacterial genus of gram-negative, nonmotile, non-spore-forming, obligately anaerobic, chemoorganotrophic, and pleomorphic rods; includes many species previously classified in the genus *Bacteroides.*

Pre·vo·tel·la bi·vi·a (prev′ō-tel′ă biv′ē-ă) The bacterial species of *Prevotella* in highest concentration in the human vaginal tract.

Pre·vo·tel·la den·ti·co·la (prev′ō-tel′ă den-tik′ō-lă) A bacterial species found in the human mouth; a cause of infections of the oral cavity and adjacent structures.

Pre·vo·tel·la hep·a·ri·no·lyt·ic·a (prev′ō-tel′ă hep′ă-rin′ō-lit′ik′ă) A bacterial species associated with human periodontal disease.

Pre·vo·tel·la in·ter·me·di·a (prev′ō-tel′ă in-tĕr-mē′dē-ă) A bacterial species found in gingival crevices, especially associated with gingivitis, and other oral infections.

Pre·vo·tel·la mel·a·nin·o·gen·i·ca (prev′ō-tel′ă mel′ă-nin-ō-jen′ik-ă) A species found in the mouth, feces, infections of the mouth, soft tissue, respiratory tract, urogenital tract, and intestinal tract. Implicated in periodontal disease; seen in aspiration pneumonitis. The type species of *Prevotella.*

PRF Abbreviation for prolactin-releasing factor.

PRH Abbreviation for prolactin-releasing hormone.

pri·a·pism (prī′ă-pizm) Persistent erection of the penis, accompanied by pain and tenderness, resulting from a pathologic condition rather than sexual desire.

Price-Jones curve (prīs-jōnz kŭrv) A distribution curve of the measured diameters of red blood cells.

prick·le cell (prik′ĕl sel) One of the cells of the stratum spinosum of the epidermis; so called because of shrinkage artifacts that occur in histologic preparations, resulting in intercellular bridges at points of desmosomal adhesion.

prick·le cell lay·er (prik′ĕl sel lā′ĕr) SYN stratum spinosum epidermidis.

prick·ly heat (prik′lē hēt) SYN miliaria rubra.

♲ **prim-, primi-** Combining forms meaning first. [L. *primus,* first]

pri·mal (prī′măl) **1.** First or primary. **2.** SYN primordial (2).

pri·mal scene (prī′măl sēn) PSYCHOANALYSIS the actual or fantasized observation by a child of sexual intercourse, particularly between the child's parents.

pri·mar·y (prī′mar-ē) **1.** The first or foremost, as a disease or symptoms to which others may be secondary or occur as complications. **2.** Relating to the first stage of growth or development. SEE ALSO primordial. [L. *primarius,* fr. *primus,* first]

pri·mar·y ad·he·sion (prī′mar-ē ad-hē′zhŭn) SYN healing by first intention.

pri·mar·y a·dre·no·cor·ti·cal in·suf·fi·cien·cy (prī′mar-ē ă-drē′nō-kōr′ti-kăl in′sŭ-fish′ĕn-sē) Adrenocortical insufficiency caused by disease, destruction, or surgical removal of the adrenal cortices.

pri·mar·y al·co·hol (prī′mar-ē al′kŏ-hol) An

alcohol characterized by the univalent radical —CH_2OH.

pri•mar•y al•do•ste•ron•ism (prī′mar-ē al-dos′tĕr-ōn-izm) An adrenocortical disorder caused by excessive secretion of aldosterone and characterized by headaches, nocturia, polyuria, fatigue, hypertension, potassium depletion, hypokalemic alkalosis, hypervolemia, and decreased plasma renin activity; may be associated with small, benign adrenocortical adenomas. SYN Conn syndrome, idiopathic aldosteronism.

pri•mar•y a•men•or•rhe•a (prī′mar-ē ā-men′ŏr-ē′ă) Amenorrhea in which menses has never occurred.

pri•mar•y am•ide (prī′mar-ē am′īd) SEE amide.

pri•mar•y a•mine (prī′mar-ē ă-mēn′) SEE amine.

pri•mar•y am•y•loi•do•sis (prī′mar-ē am′i-loy-dō′sis) Amyloidosis not associated with other recognized disease; tends to involve arterial walls and mesenchymal tissues in the tongue, lungs, intestinal tract, skin, skeletal muscle, and myocardium; the amyloid frequently does not manifest the usual affinity for Congo red and sometimes provokes a foreign-body type of inflammatory reaction.

pri•mar•y an•es•thet•ic (prī′mar-ē an′es-thet′ik) The compound that contributes most to loss of sensation when a mixture of anesthetics is administered.

pri•mar•y at•el•ec•ta•sis (prī′mar-ē at′ĕ-lek′tă-sis) Nonexpansion of the lungs after birth, found in all stillborn infants and in liveborn infants who die before respiration is established.

pri•mar•y a•typ•i•cal pneu•mo•ni•a (prī′mar-ē ā-tip′i-kăl-nū-mō′nē-ă) An acute systemic disease with involvement of the lungs, caused by *Mycoplasma pneumoniae* and marked by high fever, cough, relatively few physical signs, and scattered densities on x-rays; usually associated with development of cold agglutinins and antibodies to the bacteria. SYN atypical pneumonia, mycoplasmal pneumonia.

pri•mar•y blast in•jur•y (prī′mar-ē blast in′jŭr-ē) An injury, largely but not exclusively to hollow and fluid-filled organs, caused by impact of an overpressure wave from a high-grade explosive.

pri•mar•y brain ves•i•cle (prī′mar-ē brān ves′i-kĕl) SYN cerebral vesicle.

pri•mar•y bron•chi•al buds (prī′mar-ē brong′kē-ăl bŭdz) The first bronchial buds resulting from bifurcation of the tracheal bud; they give rise to the main bronchi.

pri•mar•y care (prī′mar-ē kār) Continuing, comprehensive, and preventive health care services (e.g., family practice, internal medicine, obstetrics/gynecology, or pediatrics) that are the first point of health care for a patient in an ambulatory setting.

pri•mar•y care phy•si•cian (prī′mar-ē kār fi-zish′ăn) A physician in family practice, internal medicine, obstetrics/gynecology, or pediatrics who is a patient's first contact for health care in an ambulatory setting. SEE ALSO health care provider.

pri•ma•ry cen•ter of os•si•fi•ca•tion (prī′mar-ē sen′tĕr os′i-fi-kā′shŭn) SYN primary ossification center.

pri•mar•y com•plex (prī′mar-ē kom′pleks) The typical lesions of primary pulmonary tuberculosis, consisting of a small peripheral focus of infection, with hilar or paratracheal lymph node involvement.

pri•mar•y den•tin (prī′mar-ē den′tin) Dentin that forms until the root is completed.

pri•mar•y den•ti•tion (prī′mar-ē den-tish′ŭn) SYN deciduous tooth.

pri•mar•y de•vi•a•tion (prī′mar-ē dē-vē-ā′shŭn) The ocular deviation seen in paralysis of an ocular muscle when the nonparalyzed eye is used for fixation.

pri•mar•y di•ges•tion (prī′mar-ē dī-jes′chŭn) Digestion in the alimentary tract.

pri•mar•y dis•ease (prī′mar-ē di-zēz′) A disorder that arises spontaneously and is not associated with or caused by a previous disease, injury, or event, but that may lead to a secondary disease.

pri•mar•y dye test (prī′mar-ē dī test) Assessment of lacrimal drainage following the fluorescein instillation test by attempting to recover fluorescein dye beneath the inferior turbinate using a swab. SYN Jones I test.

pri•mar•y dys•men•or•rhe•a (prī′mar-ē dis-men′ŏr-ē′ă) That condition due to a functional disturbance and not due to inflammation, new growths, or anatomic factors. SYN essential dysmenorrhea, functional dysmenorrhea, intrinsic dysmenorrhea.

pri•mar•y fis•sure of cer•e•bel•lum (prī′mar-ē fish′ŭr ser′ĕ-bel′ŭm) The deepest fissure of the cerebellum; demarcates the division of anterior and posterior lobes of the cerebellum; second to appear embryologically.

pri•mar•y gain (prī′mar-ē gān) Interpersonal, social, or financial advantages from the conversion of emotional stress directly into illness (e.g., hysterical blindness or paralysis). Cf. secondary gain.

pri•mar•y he•mo•chro•ma•to•sis (prī′mar-ē hē′mō-krō′mă-tō′sis) A specific inherited metabolic defect with increased absorption and accumulation of iron on a normal diet.

pri•mar•y hem•or•rhage (prī′mar-ē hem′ŏr-ăj) Hemorrhage immediately after an injury or operation, as distinguished from intermediate or secondary hemorrhage.

pri•mar•y her•pet•ic gin•gi•vo•sto•ma•ti•tis (prī′mar-ē hĕr-pet′ik jin′ji-vō-stō′mă-tī′tis) SYN primary herpetic stomatitis.

pri•mar•y her•pet•ic sto•ma•ti•tis (prī′mar-ē hĕr-pet′ik stō′mă-tī′tis) First infection of oral tissues with herpes simplex virus; characterized by gingival inflammation, vesicles, and ulcers. SYN primary herpetic gingivostomatitis.

pri•mar•y hy•per•ten•sion (prī′mar-ē hī′pĕr-ten′shŭn) SYN essential hypertension.

pri•mar•y im•mune re•sponse (prī′mar-ē i-myūn′ rĕ-spons′) SEE immune response.

pri•mar•y lat•er•al scle•ro•sis (prī′mar-ē lat′ĕr-ăl skler-ō′sis) Considered by many to be a subgroup of motor neuron disease; a slowly progressive degenerative disorder of the motor neurons of the cerebral cortex, resulting in widespread weakness on an upper motor neuron basis; spasticity, hyperreflexia, and Babinski sign are present, but not fasciculation potentials, nor any electrodiagnostic evidence of a lower motor neuron lesion.

pri•mar•y ly•so•somes (prī′mar-ē lī′sō-sōmz) Lysosomes produced at the Golgi apparatus where hydrolytic enzymes are incorporated; they fuse with phagosomes or pinosomes to become secondary lysosomes.

pri•mar•y non•dis•junc•tion (prī′mar-ē non′dis-jŭngk′shŭn) Nondisjunction occurring in a previously normal cell.

pri•mar•y nurs•ing (prī′mar-ē nŭrs′ing) A method of providing nursing services to inpatients whereby one nurse plans the care of specific patients for a period of 24 hours. The primary nurse provides direct care to those patients when working and is responsible for directing and supervising their care in collaboration with other health care team members.

pri•mar•y o•o•cyte (prī′mar-ē ō′ō-sīt) An oocyte during its growth phase and before it completes the first maturation division.

pri•ma•ry os•si•fi•ca•tion cen•ter (prī′mar-ē os′i-fi-kā′shŭn sen′tĕr) The first site of bone formation in the shaft of a long bone or the body of an irregular bone. SYN primary center of ossification.

pri•mar•y o•var•i•an fol•li•cle (prī′mar-ē ō-var′ē-ăn fol′i-kĕl) An ovarian follicle before the appearance of an antrum; marked by developmental changes in the oocyte and follicular cells so that the latter form one or more layers of cuboidal or columnar cells; the follicle becomes surrounded by a sheath of stroma, the theca.

pri•mar•y pre•ven•tive nur•sing (prī′mar-ē prē-ven′tiv nŭrs′ing) Nursing interventions and care directed at health promotion. The focus of primary preventive care includes promotion of a healthy lifestyle and reduction of major risk factors of health. Emphasis is on nutrition, exercise, rest, immunization, accident prevention (e.g., motor vehicle trauma, bicycles, guns, poisonings), safe environment, mental health, and abstinence from sex or safe sex. A lifestyle is promoted that reduces the risk of obesity, alcohol and substance abuse, accidents, physical or mental abuse, sexual promiscuity, and smoking.

pri•mar•y pro•cess (prī′mar-ē pros′es) PSYCHOANALYSIS the mental process directly related to the functions of the primitive life forces associated with the id and characteristic of unconscious mental activity; marked by unorganized, illogical thinking and by the tendency to seek immediate discharge and gratification of instinctual demands. Cf. secondary process.

pri•mar•y pro•gres•sive a•pha•si•a (PPA) (prī′mar-ē prŏ-gres′iv ă-fāz′ē-ă) A degenerative disorder of which the early major symptom is an aphasia that increases in severity and (usually) eventually includes dementia.

pri•mar•y pul•mo•nar•y lob•ule (prī′mar-ē pul′mŏ-nar-ē lob′yūl) SYN pulmonary acinus.

pri•mar•y se•nile de•men•ti•a (prī′mar-ē sen′il dĕ-men′shē-ă) SYN Alzheimer disease.

pri•mar•y sex char•ac•ters (prī′mar-ē seks kar′ăk-tĕrz) The sex glands (i.e., testes or ovaries) and the accessory sex organs.

pri•mar•y sper•ma•to•cyte (prī′mar-ē spĕr′mă-tō-sīt) The spermatocyte derived by a growth phase from a spermatogonium, and that undergoes the first division of meiosis.

pri•mar•y stut•ter•ing (prī′mar-ē stŭt′ĕr-ing) A pattern of dysfluency characterized by easy repetitions of words or parts of words, unaccompanied by signs of anxiety; may be a precursor of more severe stuttering.

pri•ma•ry sur•vey (prī′mar-ē sŭr′vā) SYN initial assessment.

pri•mar•y syph•i•lis (prī′mar-ē sif′i-lis) The first stage of syphilis SEE ALSO syphilis.

pri•mar•y tooth (prī′mar-ē tūth) SYN deciduous tooth.

pri•mar•y tu•ber•cu•lo•sis (prī′mar-ē tū-bĕr′kyū-lō′sis) First infection by *Mycobacterium tuberculosis*, typically seen in children but also occurring in adults, characterized in the lungs by the formation of a primary complex consisting of a small peripheral pulmonary focus with spread to hilar or paratracheal lymph nodes; may cavitate or heal with scarring, or may progress.

pri•mar•y un•ion (prī′mar-ē yūn′yŭn) SYN healing by first intention.

pri•mate (prī′māt) An individual of the order Primates. [L. *primus,* first]

prime mo•vers (prīm mū′vĕrs) Muscles that have the sole or principle responsibility for a given action or movement (e.g., biceps brachii for elbow flexion; secondary flexors are the brachioradialis and brachialis muscles).

pri•mi•grav•i•da (prī′mi-grav′i-dă) SEE gravida. [L. fr. *primus,* first, + *gravida,* a pregnant woman]

pri•ming (prīm′ing) Process of running the fluids in an IV bag through the tubing so that there is no air in the tubing.

pri•mip•a•ra (prī-mip′ă-ră) A woman who has given birth for the first time. SEE ALSO para. [L. fr. *primus,* first, + *pario,* to bring forth]

pri•mi•par•i•ty (prī′mi-par′i-tē) Condition of being a primipara.

pri•mip•a•rous (prī-mip′ă-rŭs) Denoting a primipara.

prim•i•tive (prim′i-tiv) SYN primordial (2). [L. *primitivus,* fr. *primus,* first]

prim•i•tive groove (prim′i-tiv grūv) The median depression in the primitive streak flanked by primitive ridges.

prim•i•tive gut (prim′i-tiv gŭt) SYN primordial gut.

prim•i•tive knot (prim′i-tiv not) SYN primitive node.

prim•i•tive node (prim′i-tiv nōd) A local thickening of the embryonic disc or blastoderm at the cephalic end of the primitive streak of the embryo. See page B1. SYN Hensen node, primitive knot.

prim•i•tive re•flex (prim-i′tiv rē′fleks) Any of a group of reflexes seen during gestation and infancy that typically become integrated by an early age (most by 6 months); also seen in adults who have sustained an injury or acquired a disease of the CNS.

prim•i•tive streak (prim′i-tiv strēk) An ectodermal ridge in the midline at the caudal end of the embryonic disc from which arises the intraembryonic mesoderm; achieved by inward and then lateral migration of cells; in human embryos, it appears on day 15 and gives a cephalocaudal axis to the developing embryo.

pri•mor•di•a (-ă) Plural of primordium.

pri•mor•di•al (prī-mōr′dē-ăl) **1.** Relating to a primordium. **2.** Relating to a structure in its first or earliest stage of development. SYN primal (2), primitive.

pri•mor•di•al gut (prī-mōr′dē-ăl gŭt) A flat sheet of intraembryonic endoderm that will change into a tubular gut due to the folding of embryonic body—head, tail, and lateral body folds. SYN primitive gut.

pri•mor•di•al o•var•i•an fol•li•cle (prī-mōr′dē-ăl ō-var′ē-ăn fol′i-kĕl) A follicle in which the primary oocyte is surrounded by a single layer of flattened follicular cells.

pri•mor•di•al sex cords (prī-mōr′dē-al seks kōrdz) The cellular cords arising from the epithelium of the genital ridges during the indifferent state of gonadal development; they form testicular cords in male embryos and cortical cords in female embryos. SYN germinal cords.

pri•mor•di•um, pl. **pri•mor•di•a** (prī-mōr′dē-ŭm, -ă) An aggregation of cells in the embryo indicating the first trace of an organ or structure. SYN anlage (1). [L. origin, fr. *primus,* first, + *ordior,* to begin]

prin•ceps, pl. **prin•ci•pes** (prin′seps, -si-pēz) Principal. ANATOMY term used to distinguish the largest or most important of several arteries. [L. chief, fr. *primus,* first, + *capio,* to take, choose]

prin•ceps pol•li•cis ar•te•ry (prin′seps pol′i-sis ahr′tĕr-ē) *Origin,* radial (deep palmar [arterial] arch); *distribution,* palmar surface and sides of thumb; *anastomoses,* arteries on dorsum of thumb.

prin•ci•pal di•ag•no•sis (prin′si-păl dī′ăg-nō′sis) The diagnosis that is found, after testing and study, to be the main reason for the patient's need for health care services.

prin•ci•pal op•tic ax•is (prin′si-păl op′tik ak′sis) A line passing through the center of the lens of a refracting system at right angles to its surface.

prin•ci•pal point (prin′si-păl poynt) One of two points on an optic axis so related that an object at one is exactly imaged at the other without magnification, minification, or inversion.

prin•ci•ple (prin′si-pĕl) **1.** A general or fundamental doctrine or tenet. SEE ALSO law, rule, theorem. **2.** The essential ingredient in a substance, especially one that gives it its distinctive quality or effect. [L. *principium,* a beginning, fr. *princeps,* chief]

PR in•ter•val (in′tĕr-văl) In the electrocardiogram, the time elapsing between the beginning of the P wave and the beginning of the next QRS complex; it corresponds to the a-c interval of the venous pulse and is normally 0.12–0.20 sec. SYN PQ interval.

Prinz•met•al an•gi•na (prints′met-ăl an′ji-nă) A form of angina pectoris that is characterized by pain that is not precipitated by cardiac work, is of longer duration, is usually more severe, and is associated with unusual electrocardiographic manifestations including elevated ST segments in leads that are ordinarily depressed in typical angina, and usually without reciprocal ST changes; occurring at night in bed in ECG leads in which ST segment depression occurs in typical angina. Treatment includes nitroglycerine or beta-blocker medications. SYN angina inversa, variant angina pectoris, variant angina.

pri•on (prī′on) SYN prion protein.

pri•on pro•tein (prī′on prō′tēn) Small, infectious proteinaceous particle, of nonnucleic acid composition; the causative agent of four spongiform encephalopathies in humans: kuru, Creutzfeldt-Jakob disease, Gerstmann-Straüssler-Scheinker syndrome, and fatal familial insomnia. The gene encoding for the PrP is found on chromosome 20. SYN prion.

prism (prizm) A transparent solid, with sides that converge at an angle, that deflects a ray of light toward the thickest portion (the base) and splits white light into its component colors; in spectacles, a prism corrects ocular muscle imbalance. [G. *prisma*]

pris•ma, pl. **pris•ma•ta** (priz′mă, priz′mă-tă) A structure resembling a prism. [G. something sawed, a prism]

prism bar (prizm bahr) A graduated series of prisms mounted on a frame and used in ocular diagnosis.

pri•sm di•op•ter (δ) (prizm dī-op′tĕr) The unit of measurement of the deviation of light in passing through a prism, being a deflection of 1 cm at a distance of 1 m.

pri•va•cy (prī′vă-sē) **1.** Being apart from others; seclusion; secrecy. **2.** Especially in psychiatry and clinical psychology, respect for the confidential nature of the therapist-patient relationship.

pri•vate du•ty nurse (prī′văt dū′tē nŭrs) **1.** A nurse who is not a member of a hospital staff, but is hired on a fee-for-service basis to care for a patient. **2.** A nurse who specializes in the care of patients with diseases of a particular class (e.g., surgical cases, tuberculosis, children's diseases).

pri•vate hos•pi•tal (prī′văt hos′pi-tăl) **1.** A hospital similar to a group hospital except that it is controlled by a single practitioner or by the practitioner and the associates in his or her office. **2.** A hospital operated for profit.

priv•i•leged site (priv′i-lĕjd sīt) An anatomic area lacking lymphatic drainage, such as the brain, cornea, and hamster cheek pouch, in which heterologous tumors may grow because the host does not become sensitized.

PRL Abbrevation for prolactin.

PRN Abbreviation for L. pro re nata, as needed.

PRO Abbreviation for peer-review organization.

Pro Abbreviation for proline or its radicals.

♻**pro- 1.** Prefix meaning before, forward. SEE ALSO ante-, pre-. **2.** CHEMISTRY prefix indicating precursor of. SEE ALSO -gen. [L. and G. *pro*]

pro•ac•cel•er•in (prō′ak-sel′ĕr-in) SYN factor V.

pro•ac•ro•so•mal gran•ules (prō-ak′rō-sō′măl gran′yūls) Small, carbohydrate-rich granules appearing in vesicles of the Golgi apparatus of spermatids; they coalesce into a single acrosomal granule contained within an acrosomal vesicle.

pro•ac•ti•va•tor (prō-ak′ti-vā-tŏr) A substance that, when chemically split, yields a fragment (activator) capable of rendering another substance enzymatically active.

prob•a•bil•i•ty (prob′ă-bil′i-tē) **1.** A measure, ranging from 0–1, of the degree of belief in a hypothesis or statement. **2.** The limit of the relative frequency of an event in a sequence of N random trials as N approaches infinity.

prob•a•ble signs of preg•nan•cy (prob′ă-bĕl sīnz preg′năn-sē) The probable signs are more certain than presumptive signs but are not definitive. The probable signs are elevation of basal body temperature, breast tenderness and swelling, chloasma, linea nigra, Chadwick sign, abdominal enlargement, softening of the cervix, ballotability of the uterus, quickening, and positive pregnancy test results.

pro•bac•te•ri•o•phage (prō′bak-tēr′ē-ō-fāj) The stage of a temperate bacteriophage in which the genome is incorporated into the genetic apparatus of the bacterial host. SYN prophage.

pro•band (prō′band) HUMAN GENETICS the patient or member of the family that brings a family under study. [L. *probo,* to test, prove]

probe (prōb) **1.** A slender rod of flexible material, with blunt bulbous tip, used for exploring sinuses, fistulae, other cavities, or wounds. **2.** A device or agent used to detect or explore a substance, e.g., a molecule used to detect the presence of a specific fragment of DNA or RNA or of a specific bacterial colony. **3.** To enter and explore, as with a probe. [L. *probo,* to test]

probe sy•ringe (prōb sir-inj′) A syringe with an olive-shaped tip, used in treatment of diseases of the lacrimal passages.

pro•bi•o•sis (prō′bī-ō′sis) An association of two organisms that enhances the life processes of both. Cf. antibiosis (1), symbiosis, mutualism. [pro- + G. *biōsis,* life]

pro•bi•ot•ic (prō′bī-ot′ik) Relating to probiosis.

prob•lem-o•ri•ent•ed med•i•cal rec•ord (POR, POMR) (prob′lĕm-ōr′ē-en-tĕd med′i-kăl rek′ŏrd) A medical record model designed to organize patient information by the presenting problem. The record includes the patient database, problem list, plan of care, and progress notes in an accessible format.

pro•cap•sid (prō-kap′sid) A protein shell lacking a virus genome.

pro•car•box•y•pep•ti•dase (prō′kahr-boks′ē-pep′ti-dās) Inactive precursor of a carboxypeptidase.

pro•car•y•ote (pro-kar′ē-ōt) SYN prokaryote. [pro- + G. *karyon,* kernel, nut]

pro•car•y•ot•ic (prō′kar-ē-ot′ik) SYN prokaryotic.

pro•ce•dur•al mem•o•ry (prō-sē′jūr-al mem′ŏr-ē) Knowledge needed to perform the procedures composing a given task.

pro•ce•dure (prŏ-sē′jŭr) Act or conduct of diagnosis, treatment, or operation. SEE ALSO method, operation, technique.

pro•ce•dure code (prō-sē′jĕr kōd) Numbers that identify health care services provided to a patient (required by HIPAA).

pro•ce•li•a (prō-sē′lē-ă) A lateral ventricle of the brain; the hollow of the prosencephalon. SYN procoele, procoelia. [pro- + G. *koilos,* hollow]

pro•cen•tri•ole (prō-sen′trē-ōl) The early phase in development de novo of centrioles or basal bodies from the centrosphere; procentrioles form in relation to deuterosomes (procentriole organizers).

pro•ce•phal•ic (prō-sĕ-fal′ik) Relating to the anterior part of the head. [pro- + G. *kephalē,* head]

pro•ce•rus mus•cle (prō-sē′rŭs mŭs′ĕl) *Insertion*, into frontalis; *action*, assists frontalis; *origin*, from membrane covering bridge of nose; *nerve supply*, branch of facial. SYN musculus procerus [TA].

pro•cess (pros′es) **1.** ANATOMY A projection or outgrowth. SYN processus [TA]. **2.** A method or mode of action used in the attainment of a certain result. **3.** A natural progression, development, or sequence of events, as in the progress of a disease. SEE ALSO processus. **4.** A pathologic condition or disease. **5.** DENTISTRY a series of operations that convert a wax pattern, such as that of a denture base, into a solid denture base of another material. [L. *processus,* an advance, progress, process, fr. *pro-cedo,* pp. *-cessus,* to go forward]

pro•cess con•sent (pros′es kŏn-sent′) An ongoing transactional process by which a patient or participant collaborates in making a decision about continued participation or care.

proc•es•sing (pros′es-ing) The activity of effecting a series of changes in something so as to achieve a particular result.

proc•es•sor (pros′es-sŏr) A device that converts one form of energy into another form of energy or one form of material into another form of material.

pro•cess skills (pros′es skilz) Skills used to manage and modify actions in the completing of daily living tasks, such as pacing oneself, choosing and using appropriate tools to complete a task, or organizing a task into a logical sequence for successful completion.

pro•ces•sus (prō-ses′us) [TA] SYN process (1). [L.]

pro•ces•sus ar•ti•cu•la•ris (prō-ses′us ahr-tik-yū-lā′ris) [TA] SYN articular process.

pro•ces•sus cli•noi•de•us an•te•ri•or (prō-ses′us klin-oyd′ē-ŭs an-tēr′ē-ŏr) [TA] SYN anterior clinoid process.

pro•ces•sus fal•ci•for•mis (prō-ses′us fal-si-fōr′mis) [TA] SYN falciform process.

pro•ces•sus va•gi•na•lis of per•i•to•ne•um (prō-ses′us vaj′i-nā′lis per′i-tō-nē′ŭm) A peritoneal diverticulum in the embryonic lower anterior abdominal wall that traverses the inguinal canal; in the male, it forms the tunica vaginalis testis and normally loses its connection with the peritoneal cavity; a persistent processus vaginalis in the female is known as the canal of Nuck.

pro•ces•sus xi•phoi•de•us (prō-ses′us zī-foy′dē-yŭs) [TA] SYN xiphoid process.

pro•chon•dral (prō-kon′drăl) Denoting a developmental stage prior to the formation of cartilage. [pro- + G. *chondros,* cartilage]

pro•chy•mo•sin (prō-kī′mō-sin) The precursor of chymosin. SYN prorennin, renninogen, rennogen.

pro•ci•den•ti•a (pros′i-den′shē-ă) A sinking down or prolapse of any organ or part. [L. a falling forward, fr. *procido,* to fall forward]

procoele [Br.] SYN procelia.

procoelia [Br.] SYN procelia.

pro•col•la•gen (prō-kol′ă-jen) Soluble precursor of collagen formed by fibroblasts and other cells in the process of collagen synthesis.

pro•con•ver•tin (prō′kŏn-vĕr′tin) SYN factor VII.

pro•cre•ate (prō′krē-āt′) To beget; to produce by the sexual act. [L. *pro-creo,* pp. *-creatus,* to beget]

pro•cre•a•tion (prō′krē-ā′shŭn) SYN reproduction (2).

pro•cre•a•tive (prō′krē-ā′tiv) Having the power to beget or procreate.

proc•tal•gi•a (prok-tal′jē-ă) Pain around the anus, or in the rectum. SYN proctodynia, rectalgia. [proct- + G. *algos,* pain]

proc•ta•tre•si•a (prok′tă-trē′zē-ă) SYN anal atresia. [proct- + G. *a-* priv. + *trēsis,* a boring]

proc•tec•to•my (prok-tek′tŏ-mē) Surgical resection of the rectum. SYN rectectomy. [proct- + G. *ektomē,* excision]

proc•ti•tis (prok-tī′tis) Inflammation of the mucous membrane of the rectum. SYN rectitis. [proct- + G. *-itis,* inflammation]

procto-, proct- Combining forms meaning anus; (more frequently) rectum; Cf. recto-. [G. *prōktos*]

proc·to·cele (prok′tō-sēl) Prolapse or herniation of the rectum. SYN rectocele. [procto- + G. *kēlē,* tumor]

proc·to·cly·sis (prok-tok′li-sis) Slow, continuous administration of saline solution by instillation into the rectum and sigmoid colon. SYN Murphy drip. [procto- + G. *klysis,* a washing out]

proc·to·coc·cy·pexy (prok′tō-kok′si-pek-sē) Suture of a prolapsing rectum to the tissues anterior to the coccyx. SYN rectococcypexy. [procto- + G. *kokkyx,* coccyx, + *pēxis,* fixation]

proc·to·co·lec·to·my (prok′tō-kō-lek′tō-mē) Surgical removal of the rectum together with part or all of the colon. [procto- + G. *kolon,* colon, + *ektomē,* excision]

proc·to·co·lo·nos·co·py (prok′tō-kō-lŏn-os′kŏ-pē) Inspection of the interior of the rectum and colon. [procto- + G. *kolon,* colon, + *skopeō,* to view]

proc·to·col·po·plas·ty (prok′tō-kol′pō-plas-tē) Surgical closure of a rectovaginal fistula. [procto- + G. *kolpos,* bosom (vagina), + *plastos,* formed]

proc·to·cys·to·plas·ty (prok′tō-sis′tō-plas-tē) Surgical closure of a rectovesical fistula. [procto- + G. *kystis,* bladder, + *plastos,* formed]

proc·to·cys·tot·o·my (prok′tō-sis-tot′ŏ-mē) Incision into the bladder from the rectum. [procto- + G. *kystis,* bladder, + *tomē,* incision]

proctodaeal [Br.] SYN proctodeal.

proctodaeum [Br.] SYN proctodeum.

proc·to·de·al (prok-tō′dē-ăl) Relating to the proctodeum. SYN proctodaeal.

proc·to·de·um, pl. **proc·to·de·a** (prok′tō-dē′ŭm, -dē′ă) SYN anal pit (1). SYN proctodaeum. [L. fr. G. *prōktos,* anus + *hodaios,* on the way, fr. *hodos,* a way]

proc·to·dyn·i·a (prok′tō-din′ē-ă) SYN proctalgia. [procto- + G. *odynē,* pain]

proc·to·log·ic (prok′tō-loj′ik) Relating to proctology.

proc·tol·o·gist (prok-tol′ŏ-jist) A specialist in proctology.

proc·tol·o·gy (prok-tol′ŏ-jē) Surgical specialty concerned with the anus and rectum and their diseases. [procto- + G. *logos,* study]

proc·to·pa·ral·y·sis (prok′tō-păr-al′i-sis) Paralysis of the anus, leading to incontinence of feces.

proc·to·pex·y (prok′tō-pek-sē) Surgical fixation of a prolapsing rectum. SYN rectopexy. [procto- + G. *pēxis,* fixation]

proc·to·plas·ty (prok′tō-plas-tē) Surgical repair of the anus or rectum. SYN rectoplasty. [procto- + G. *plastos,* formed]

proc·to·ple·gi·a (prok′tō-plē′jē-ă) Paralysis of the anus and rectum occurring with paraplegia. [procto- + G. *plēgē,* stroke]

proc·top·to·si·a, proc·top·to·sis (prok′top-tō′sē-ă, -tō′sis) Prolapse of the rectum and anus. [procto- + G. *ptōsis,* a falling]

proc·tor·rha·phy (prok-tōr′ă-fē) Repair by suture of a lacerated rectum or anus. [procto- + G. *rhaphē,* suture]

proc·tor·rhe·a (prok′tō-rē′ă) A mucoserous discharge from the rectum. [procto- + G. *rhoia,* a flow]

proc·to·scope (prok′tō-skōp) A rectal speculum. SYN rectoscope. [procto- + G. *skopeō,* to view]

proc·tos·co·py (prok-tos′kŏ-pē) Visual examination of the rectum and anus, as with a proctoscope.

proc·to·sig·moi·dec·to·my (prok′tō-sig′moyd-ek′tŏ-mē) Excision of the rectum and sigmoid colon. [procto- + sigmoid, + G. *ektomē,* excision]

proc·to·sig·moi·di·tis (prok′tō-sig′moyd-ī′tis) Inflammation of the sigmoid colon and rectum. [procto- + sigmoid + G. *-itis,* inflammation]

proc·to·sig·moi·dos·co·py (prok′tō-sig′moyd-os′kŏ-pē) Direct inspection through a sigmoidoscope of the rectum and sigmoid colon. [procto- + sigmoid + G. *skopeō,* to view]

proc·to·spasm (prok′tō-spazm) **1.** Spasmodic stricture of the anus. **2.** Spasmodic contraction of the rectum. [procto- + G. *spasmos,* spasm]

proc·to·ste·no·sis (prok′tō-stĕ-nō′sis) Stricture of the rectum or anus. SYN rectostenosis. [procto- + G. *stenōsis,* a narrowing]

proc·tos·to·my (prok-tos′tŏ-mē) The formation of an artificial opening into the rectum. SYN rectostomy. [procto- + G. *stoma,* mouth]

proc·tot·o·my (prok-tot′ŏ-mē) An incision into the rectum. SYN rectotomy. [procto- + G. *tomē,* incision]

proc·to·tre·si·a (prok′tō-trē′zē-ă) Operation for correction of an imperforate anus. [procto- + G. *trēsis,* a boring]

proc·to·val·vot·o·my (prok′tō-val-vot′ŏ-mē) Incision of rectal valves.

pro·cur·sive ep·i·lep·sy (prō-kŭr′siv ep′i-lep′sē) A psychomotor attack initiated by whirling or running.

pro•dro•mal (prō-drō′măl) Relating to a prodrome. SYN prodromic, prodromous.

pro•dro•mal la•bor (prō-drō′măl lā′bŏr) An early phase of labor that does not progress in a normal pattern: contractions do not increase in intensity and cervical dilatation is minimal. Cf. active labor.

pro•dro•mal stage (prō-drō′măl stāj) SYN incubation period (1).

pro•drome (prō′drōm) An early or premonitory symptom of a disease. [G. *prodromos,* a running before, fr. pro- + *dromos,* a running, a course]

pro•dro•mic, pro•dro•mous (prō-drō′mik, prod′rō-; -mŭs) SYN prodromal.

pro•drug (prō′drŭg) A class of drugs, the pharmacologic action of which results from conversion by metabolic processes within the body (biotransformation).

pro•duc•tive (prŏ-dŭk′tiv) Producing or capable of producing; denoting especially an inflammation leading to the production of new tissue with or without an exudate.

pro•duct•ive cough (prŏ-dŭk′tiv kawf) A cough accompanied by expectoration.

pro•en•zyme (prō-en′zīm) The precursor of an enzyme, requiring some change (usually the hydrolysis of an inhibiting fragment that masks an active grouping) to render it active, e.g., pepsinogen, trypsinogen, profibrinolysin. SYN zymogen.

pro•e•ryth•ro•blast (prō′ĕ-rith′rō-blast) SYN pronormoblast.

pro•e•ryth•ro•cyte (prō′ĕ-rith′rō-sīt) The precursor of a red blood cell; an immature red blood cell form with a nucleus.

pro•es•tro•gen (prō-es′trō-jen) A substance that acts as an estrogen only after it has been metabolized in the body to an active compound. SYN pro-oestrogen.

pro•es•trus (prō-es′trŭs) The period preceding estrus, characterized by heightened follicular activity and estrogen production. SYN pro-oestrus. [pro- + estrus]

pro•fes•sion•al code (prŏ-fesh′i-năl kōd) Ethical code; profession's expectations and requirements in ethical matters (e.g., Code of Ethics for Nurses with Interpretive Statements, American Medical Association Code of Medical Ethics).

pro•fes•sion•al com•po•nent (prŏ-fesh′ŭn-ăl kŏm-pō′nĕnt) In health care informatics, that portion of a service or therapy provided by a physician rather than any other health care workers.

Pro•fe•ta law (prō-fē′tă law) The subject of congenital syphilis is immune to the acquired disease.

pro•fi•bri•nol•y•sin (prō′fī-bri-nol′i-sin) SEE plasmin.

pro•fi•cien•cy sam•ples (prō-fish′ĕn-sē sam′pĕlz) Examples sent to a laboratory as unknowns to enable an external assessment of laboratory performance; a frequent practice as part of proficiency testing programs to ensure a laboratory is generating correct results. SEE ALSO proficiency testing.

pro•fi•cien•cy test•ing (prō-fish′ĕn-sē test′ing) A program in which specimens of quality control material are periodically sent to members of a group of laboratories for analysis, with each laboratory's results compared with those of its peers. SEE ALSO proficiency samples.

pro•file (prō′fīl) **1.** An outline or contour, especially one representing a side view of the human head. SYN norma. **2.** A summary, brief account, or record. **3.** BIOWARFARE set of suspected characteristics linked to a person or group allegedly responsible for a terrorist activity or other act involving the use of biologic weapons. [It. *profilo,* fr. L. *pro,* forward, + *filum,* thread, line (contour)]

pro•fun•da bra•chi•i ar•ter•y (prō-fŭn′dă brā′kē-ī ahr′tĕr-ē) *Origin,* brachial; *distribution,* humerus and muscles and integument of arm; *anastomoses,* posterior circumflex humeral, radial recurrent, recurrent interosseous, ulnar collateral, i.e., articular vascular network of elbow. SYN deep artery of arm.

pro•fun•da fem•o•ris ar•ter•y (prō-fŭn′dă fem′ŏr-is ahr′tĕr-ē) SYN deep artery of thigh.

pro•gas•trin (prō-gas′trin) Precursor of gastric secretion in the mucous membrane of the stomach.

pro•ge•ni•a (prō-jē′nē-ă) SYN prognathism. [pro- + L. *gena,* cheek]

pro•gen•i•tor (prō-jen′i-tŏr) A precursor, ancestor; one who begets. [L.]

prog•e•ny (proj′ĕ-nē) Offspring; descendants. [L. *progenies,* fr. *progigno,* to beget]

pro•ge•ri•a (prō-jēr′ē-ă) A condition in which normal development in the first year is followed by gross retardation of growth, with a senile appearance characterized by dry, wrinkled skin, total alopecia, and birdlike facies; genetics unclear. SYN Hutchinson-Gilford disease. [pro- + G. *gēras,* old age]

pro•ges•ta•tion•al (prō′jes-tā′shŭn-ăl) **1.** Favoring pregnancy; conducive to gestation; capable of stimulating the uterine changes essential for implantation and growth of a fertilized ovum. **2.** Referring to progesterone, or to a drug with progesteronelike properties.

pro•ges•ta•tion•al hor•mone (prō′jes-tā′shŭn-ăl hōr′mōn) SYN progesterone.

pro•ges•ter•one (prō-jes′tĕr-ōn) An antiestrogenic steroid, believed to be the active principle of the corpus luteum, isolated from the corpus luteum and placenta or synthetically prepared; used to correct abnormalities of the menstrual cycle, as a contraceptive, and to control habitual abortion. Cf. bioregulator. SYN luteal hormone, luteohormone, progestational hormone.

pro•gest•er•one chal•lenge test (prō-jes′tĕr-ōn chal′ĕnj test) Administration of a progestational agent in case of amenorrhea to detect the presence of an estrogen-primed endometrium.

pro•gest•er•one re•cep•tor (prō-jes′tĕr-ōn rĕ-sep′tŏr) Intracellular receptor for progesterone; often overexpressed in breast cancer.

pro•ges•tin (prō-jes′tin) **1.** A hormone of the corpus luteum. **2.** Generic term for any substance, natural or synthetic, that effects some or all of the biologic changes produced by progesterone. Cf. bioregulator. [pro- + gestation + -in]

pro•ges•to•gen (prō-jes′tō-jen) **1.** Any agent capable of producing biologic effects similar to those of progesterone; most progestogens are steroids like the natural hormones. **2.** A synthetic derivative from testosterone or progesterone that has some of the physiologic activity and pharmacologic effects of progesterone; progesterone is antiestrogenic, whereas some progestogens have estrogenic or androgenic properties in addition to progestational activity. Cf. bioregulator. [pro- + gestation + G. *-gen,* producing]

pro•glos•sis (prō-glos′is) The anterior portion, or tip, of the tongue. [pro- + G. *glōssa,* tongue]

pro•glot•tid (prō-glot′id) One of the segments of a tapeworm, containing the reproductive organs. SYN proglottis. [pro- + G. *glōssa,* tongue]

pro•glot•tis, pl. **pro•glot•ti•des** (prō-glot′is, -i-dēz) SYN proglottid.

prog•nath•ic (prog-nath′ik) **1.** Having a projecting jaw; having a gnathic index higher than 103. SEE ALSO orthognathic. **2.** Denoting a forward projection of either or both of the jaws relative to the craniofacial skeleton. SYN prognathous. [pro- + G. *gnathos,* jaw]

prog•na•thism (prog′nă-thizm) The condition of being prognathic; abnormal forward projection of one or of both jaws beyond the established normal relationship with the cranial base; the mandibular condyles are in their normal rest relationship to the temporomandibular joints. SYN progenia.

prog•na•thous (prog′nă-thŭs) SYN prognathic.

prog•no•sis (prog-nō′sis) A forecast of the probable course and/or outcome of a disease. [G. *prognōsis,* fr. *pro,* before, + *gignōskō,* to know]

prog•nos•tic (prog-nos′tik) **1.** Relating to prognosis. **2.** A symptom on which a prognosis is based, or one indicative of the likely outcome. [G. *prognōstikos*]

prog•nos•ti•cate (prog-nos′ti-kāt) To give a prognosis.

prog•nos•ti•cian (prog′nos-tish′ŭn) One skilled in prognosis.

pro•gram (prō′gram) **1.** A formal set of procedures for conducting an activity. **2.** An ordered list of instructions directing a computer to carry out a sequence of operations required to solve a problem or process data. **3.** A planned learning activity for patients, providers, or others involved in health care. SYN programme.

pro•gram•ma•ble hear•ing aid (prō-gram′ă-bĕl hēr′ing ād) Multichannel hearing aid that can use more than one level-dependent frequency response strategy.

programme [Br.] SYN program.

pro•grammed cell death (prō′gramd sel deth) SYN apoptosis.

pro•gram•ming (prō′gram-ing) Sequential instruction; a method of training in discrete segments.

pro•gran•u•lo•cyte (prō-gran′yū-lō-sīt) SYN promyelocyte.

pro•gres•sive (prŏ-gres′iv) Going forward; advancing; denoting the course of a disease, especially, when unqualified, an unfavorable course.

pro•gres•sive bul•bar pa•ral•y•sis (prŏ-gres′iv bŭl′bahr păr-al′i-sis) Progressive weakness and atrophy of the muscles of the tongue, lips, palate, pharynx, and larynx; most often caused by motor neuron disease. SYN bulbar paralysis.

pro•gres•sive cat•a•ract (prŏ-gres′iv kat′ăr-akt) A cataract in which the opacification process progresses to involve the entire lens.

pro•gres•sive chor•oi•dal a•tro•phy (prŏ-gres′iv kōr-oyd′ăl at′rŏ-fē) SYN choroideremia.

pro•gres•sive hy•per•tro•phic pol•y•neu•rop•a•thy (prŏ-gres′iv hī′pĕr-trō′fik pol′ē-nūr-op′ă-thē) SYN Dejerine-Sottas disease.

pro•gres•sive mul•ti•fo•cal leu•ko•en•ceph•a•lop•a•thy (PML) (prŏ-gres′iv mŭl′tē-fō′kăl lū′kō-en-sef′ă-lop′ă-thē) A rare, subacute, afebrile disease characterized by areas of demyelinization surrounded by markedly altered neuroglia, including inclusion bodies in glial cells; it occurs usually in people with AIDS, leukemia, lymphoma, or other debilitating diseases, or in those who have been receiving immunosuppressive treatment. Caused by JC virus, a human polyoma virus.

pro•gres•sive mus•cu•lar at•ro•phy (prŏ-gres′iv mŭs′kyū-lăr at′rŏ-fē) SYN amyotrophic lateral sclerosis.

pro•gres•sive out•er ret•i•nal ne•cro•sis (PORN) (prŏ-gres′iv owt′ĕr ret′i-năl nĕ-krō′sis) A viral syndrome occurring in AIDS patients, caused by herpesvirus and characterized by destruction of peripheral retina.

pro•gres•sive-re•sis•tance ex•er•cise (PRE) (prŏ-gres′iv-rĕ-zis′tăns ek′sĕr-sīz) The practical application of the overload principle to improve muscular strength and size. Resistance is gradually and continually increased to keep pace with strength gains as training progresses.

pro•gres•sive stain•ing (prŏ-gres′iv stān′ing) A procedure in which staining is continued until the desired intensity of coloring of tissue elements is attained.

pro•gres•sive tap•e•to•chor•oi•dal dys•tro•phy (prŏ-gres′iv tă-pē′tō-kōr-oyd′ăl dis′trŏ-fē) SYN choroideremia.

pro•hor•mone (prō-hōr′mōn) An intraglandular precursor of a hormone, e.g., proinsulin. Cf. prehormone, bioregulator.

pro•in•su•lin (prō-in′sŭ-lin) A single-chain precursor of insulin.

pro•jec•tile vom•it•ing (prō-jek′tīl vom′it-ing) Oral expulsion of the contents of the stomach with great force.

pro•jec•tion (prŏ-jek′shŭn) **1.** A pushing out; an outgrowth or protuberance. **2.** The referring of a sensation to the object producing it. **3.** PSYCHOLOGY/PSYCHIATRY A defense mechanism by which a repressed complex in the patient is denied and conceived as belonging to another person, as when faults that the person tends to commit are perceived in or attributed to others. **4.** The conception by the consciousness of a mental occurrence belonging to the self as of external origin. **5.** Localization of visual impressions in space. **6.** NEUROANATOMY the system or systems of nerve fibers by which a group of nerve cells discharges its nerve impulses ("projects") to one or more other cell groups. **7.** The image of a three-dimensional object on a plane, as in a radiograph. **8.** RADIOGRAPHY a standard x-ray study, named by body part, position, direction of the x-ray beam through the body part, or eponym. [L. *projectio;* fr. *pro-jicio,* pp. *-jectus,* to throw before]

pro•jec•tion an•gi•o•gram (prŏ-jek′shŭn an′jē-ō-gram) A digital angiogram (e.g., CT or MRI) reconstructed by computer to appear as it would in a radiographic angiogram.

pro•jec•tion fi•bers (prŏ-jek′shŭn fī′bĕrz) Nerve fibers connecting the cerebral cortex with other centers in the brain or spinal cord; fibers arising from cells in the central nervous system that pass to distant loci.

pro•jec•tive i•den•ti•fi•ca•tion (prō-jek′tiv ī-den′ti-fi-kā′shŭn) A defensive attribution of one's own psychic processes to another person.

pro•kar•y•ote (prō-kar′ē-ōt) A member of the superkingdom Prokaryotae; an organism consisting of a single cell, or a precellular organism, that lacks a nuclear membrane, paired organized chromosomes, a mitotic mechanism for cell division, microtubules, and mitochondria. SEE ALSO eukaryote. SYN procaryote.

pro•kar•y•ot•ic (prō′kar-ē-ot′ik) Pertaining to or characteristic of a prokaryote. SYN procaryotic.

pro•la•bi•um (prō-lā′bē-ŭm) **1.** The exposed carmine margin of the lip. **2.** The isolated central soft-tissue segment of the upper lip in the embryonic state and in an unrepaired bilateral cleft palate. [pro- + L. *labium,* lip]

pro•lac•tin (PRL) (prō-lak′tin) A protein hormone of the anterior lobe of the hypophysis that stimulates the secretion of milk and possibly, during pregnancy, breast growth. Cf. bioregulator. SYN lactogenic hormone. [pro- + L. *lac, lact-,* milk, + -in]

pro•lac•tin-in•hib•it•ing fac•tor (PIF) (prō-lak′tin-in-hib′i-ting fak′tŏr) SYN prolactostatin.

pro•lac•tin-in•hib•it•ing hor•mone (PIH) (prō-lak′tin-in-hib′i-ting hōr′mōn) SYN prolactostatin.

pro•lac•ti•no•ma (prō-lak′ti-nō′mă) SYN prolactin-producing adenoma.

pro•lac•tin-pro•duc•ing ad•e•no•ma (prō-lak′tin-prŏ-dūs′ing ad′ĕ-nō′mă) A pituitary adenoma composed of prolactin-producing cells; it gives rise to symptoms of nonpuerperal amenorrhea and galactorrhea (Forbes-Albright syndrome) in women and to impotence in men. SYN prolactinoma.

pro•lac•tin-re•leas•ing fac•tor (PRF) (prō-lak′tin-rĕ-lēs′ing fak′tŏr) SYN prolactoliberin.

pro•lac•tin-re•leas•ing hor•mone (prō-lak′tin-rĕ-lēs′ing hōr′mōn) SYN prolactoliberin.

pro•lac•to•lib•er•in (prō-lak′tō-lib′ĕr-in) A substance of hypothalamic origin that stimulates the release of prolactin. Cf. bioregulator. SYN prolactin-releasing factor, prolactin-releasing hormone. [prolactin + L. *libero,* to free, + -in]

pro•lac•to•stat•in (prō-lak′tō-stat′in) A substance of hypothalamic origin capable of inhibiting the synthesis and release of prolactin. Cf. bioregulator. SYN prolactin-inhibiting factor, prolactin-inhibiting hormone. [prolactin + G. *stasis,* standing still, + -in]

pro•lapse (prō′laps) **1.** To sink down; said of an organ or other part. **2.** A sinking of an organ or other part, especially its appearance at a natural or artificial orifice. SEE ALSO procidentia, ptosis. [L. *prolapsus,* a falling]

pro•lapse of um•bil•i•cal cord (prō′laps ŭm-bil′i-kăl kōrd) Presentation of part of the umbilical cord ahead of the fetus; it may cause fetal death due to compression of the cord between

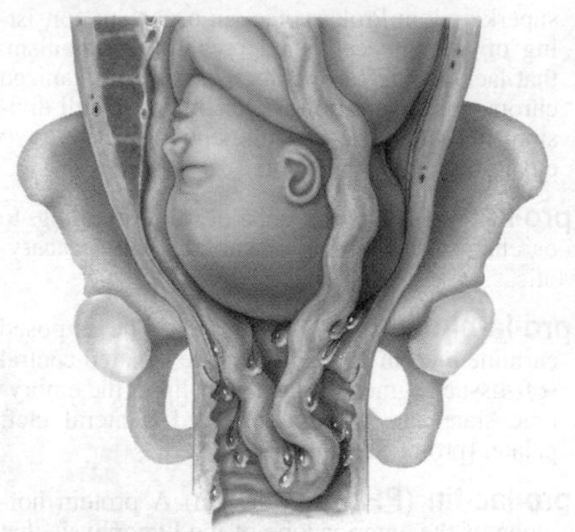

umbilical cord prolapse

the presenting part of the fetus and the maternal pelvis. See this page.

pro•lapse of u•ter•us (prō′laps yū′tĕr-ŭs) Downward movement of the uterus due to laxity and atony of the muscular and fascial structures of the pelvic floor, usually resulting from injuries of childbirth or advanced age; prolapse occurs in three forms: first-degree prolapse, second-degree prolapse, and third-degree prolapse.

pro•lec•tive (prō-lek′tiv) Number of deaths from a given cause in a specified period, per 100 or per 1000 total deaths. Pertaining to data collected by planning in advance the proportional mortality ratio. [pro- + L. *lego*, pp. *lectum*, to gather]

pro•lep•sis (prō-lep′sis) Recurrence of the paroxysm of a periodical disease at regularly shortening intervals. [G. *prolēpsis*, anticipation]

pro•lep•tic (prō-lep′tik) Relating to prolepsis.

pro•li•dase (prō′li-dās) SYN proline dipeptidase.

pro•lif•er•ate (prō-lif′ĕr-āt) To grow and increase in number by means of reproduction of similar forms. [L. *proles*, offspring, + *fero*, to bear]

pro•lif•er•at•ing cell nu•cle•ar ant•i•gen (prō-lif′ĕr-āt′ing sel nū′klē-ĕr an′ti-jen) A nuclear nonhistone protein with a molecular weight of 36 kD that plays a role in the initiation of cell proliferation by augmenting DNA polymerase; stains for proliferating cell nuclear antigen in tumors correlate with grade and mitotic activity.

pro•lif•er•a•tion (prō-lif′ĕr-ā′shŭn) Growth and reproduction of similar cells.

pro•lif•er•a•tive, **pro•lif•er•ous** (prō-lif′ĕr-ă-tiv, -ĕr-ŭs) Increasing the numbers of similar forms.

pro•lif•er•a•tive der•ma•ti•tis (prō-lif′ĕr-ă-tiv dĕr′mă-tī′tis) SYN dermatophilosis.

pro•lif•er•a•tive in•flam•ma•tion (prō-lif′ĕr-ă-tiv in′flă-mā′shŭn) An inflammatory reaction in which the distinguishing feature is an increase in the number of tissue cells, especially the reticuloendothelial macrophages, rather than of cells exuded from blood vessels. SYN hyperplastic inflammation.

pro•lif•er•a•tive ret•i•nop•a•thy (prō-lif′ĕr-ă-tiv ret′i-nop′ă-thē) Neovascularization of the retina extending into the vitreous humor. SYN retinitis proliferans.

pro•lig•er•ous (prō-lij′ĕr-ŭs) Germinating; producing offspring. [L. *proles*, offspring, + *gero*, to bear]

pro•li•nase (prō′li-nās) SYN prolyl dipeptidase.

pro•line (Pro) (prō′lēn) An amino acid found in proteins, especially the collagens.

pro•line di•pep•ti•dase (prō′lēn dī-pep′ti-dās) An enzyme cleaving aminoacyl-L-proline bonds in dipeptides containing a *C*-terminal prolyl residue; a deficiency of this enzyme results in hyperimidodipeptiduria. SYN prolidase.

pro•line im•i•no•pep•ti•dase (prō′lēn i-mē′nō-pep′ti-dās) [EC 3.4.11.5] A hydrolase cleaving L-proline residues from the *N*-terminal position in peptides.

pro•longed preg•nan•cy (prō-lawngd′ preg′năn-sē) SYN postdate pregnancy.

pro•lo•ther•a•py (prō′lō-thār′ă-pē) A technique to assist the rebuilding of damaged connective tissue structures through the injection of various substances designed to stimulate collagen proliferation.

pro•lyl (prō′lil) The acyl radical of proline.

pro•lyl di•pep•ti•dase (prō′lil dī-pep′ti-dās) An enzyme cleaving L-prolyl-amino acid bonds in dipeptides containing *N*-terminal prolyl residues. SYN prolinase.

PROM (prom) Acronym and abbreviation for premature rupture of membranes; passive range of motion.

pro•mas•ti•gote (prō-mas′ti-gōt) The flagellate stage of a trypanosomatid protozoan in which the flagellum arises from a kinetoplast in front of the nucleus and emerges from the anterior end of the organism; usually an extracellular phase, as in the insect intermediate host (or in culture) of *Leishmania* parasites. [pro- + G. *mastix*, whip]

pro•meg•a•lo•blast (prō-meg′ă-lō-blast) The earliest of four maturation stages of the megaloblast. SEE erythroblast.

pro•met•a•phase (prō-met′ă-fāz) The stage of mitosis or meiosis in which the nuclear membrane disintegrates and the centrioles reach the poles of the cell, while the chromosomes continue to contract.

pro·me·thi·um (Pm) (prō-mē′thē-ŭm) A radioactive element of the rare earth series, atomic no. 61; ^{145}Pm has the longest known half-life (17.7 years). [*Prometheus,* a Titan of G. myth who stole fire to give to mortals]

prom·i·nence (prom′i-nĕns) ANATOMY A tissue or part that projects beyond a surface. SYN prominentia. [L. *prominentia*]

prom·i·nent heel (prom′i-nĕnt hēl) A condition marked by a tender swelling on the os calcis due to a thickening of the periosteum or fibrous tissue covering the back of the os calcis.

prom·i·nen·ti·a, pl. **prom·i·nen·ti·ae** (prom′i-nen′shē-ă, -shē-ē) SYN prominence. [L. fr. *promineo,* to jut out, be prominent]

PROMM (prom) Acronym for proximal myotonic myopathy.

pro·mon·o·cyte (prō-mon′ō-sīt) SYN premonocyte.

prom·on·to·ry (prom′ŏn-tōr′ē) An eminence or projection. A projection of a part. [L. *promontorium*]

prom·on·to·ry flush (prom′ŏn-tōr′ē flŭsh) SYN Schwartze sign.

pro·mot·er (prō-mō′tĕr) **1.** CHEMISTRY a substance that increases the activity of a catalyst. **2.** MOLECULAR BIOLOGY a DNA sequence at which RNA polymerase binds and initiates transcription.

pro·mot·ing a·gent (prō-mōt′ing ā′jĕnt) SEE promotion.

pro·mo·tion (prō-mō′shŭn) Stimulation of tumor induction, following initiation, by a promoting agent which may of itself be noncarcinogenic.

pro·my·e·lo·cyte (prō-mī′ĕ-lō-sīt) **1.** The developmental stage of a granular leukocyte between the myeloblast and myelocyte, when a few specific granules appear in addition to azurophilic ones. **2.** A large mononuclear cell of bone marrow representing an undifferentiated stage in the development of a granulocyte, between myeloblast and myelocyte; contains only a few undifferentiated cytoplasmic granules; rare in circulating blood except in myelocytic leukemias. SYN premyelocyte, progranulocyte. [pro- + G. *myelos,* marrow, + *kytos,* cell]

pro·na·si·on (prō-nā′zē-on) The point of the angle between the septum of the nose and the surface of the upper lip, found at the point where a tangent applied to the nasal septum meets the upper lip. [pro- + L. *nasus,* nose]

pro·nate (prō′nāt) **1.** To assume, or to be placed in, a prone position. **2.** To perform pronation of the forearm or foot. [L. *pronatus,* fr. *prono,* pp. *-atus,* to bend forward, fr. *pronus,* bent forward]

pro·na·tion (prō-nā′shŭn) **1.** The condition of being prone; the act of assuming or of being placed in a prone position. **2.** Transverse plane motion at the radioulnar joint or transverse tarsal joint.

pro·na·tor (prō-nā′tōr) A muscle that turns a part into the prone position. SEE ALSO muscle. [L.]

pro·na·tor quad·ra·tus mus·cle (prō-nā′tōr kwa-drat′ŭs mŭs′ĕl) *Origin,* distal fourth of anterior surface of ulna; *insertion,* distal fourth of anterior surface of radius; *action,* pronates forearm; *nerve supply,* anterior interosseous. See this page. SYN musculus pronator quadratus [TA].

pro·na·tor syn·drome (prō-nā′tōr sin′drōm) Condition by which trapping of the median nerve by the pronator teres results in pain in the forearm.

pro·na·tor te·res mus·cle (prō-nā′tōr ter′ēz mŭs′ĕl) *Origin,* superficial (humeral) head (ulnar) from the common flexor origin on the medial epicondyle of the humerus, deep (ulnar) head from the medial side of the coronoid process of the ulna; *insertion,* middle of the lateral surface of the radius; *action,* pronates forearm; *nerve supply,* median. SYN musculus pronator teres [TA].

pro·na·tor te·res syn·drome (prō-nā′tōr ter′ēz sin′drōm) Entrapment or compression of the median nerve in the proximal forearm, usually where the nerve passes between the two heads of the pronator teres muscle.

prone (prōn) **1.** Denoting the position of the body when lying face downward. **2.** The position

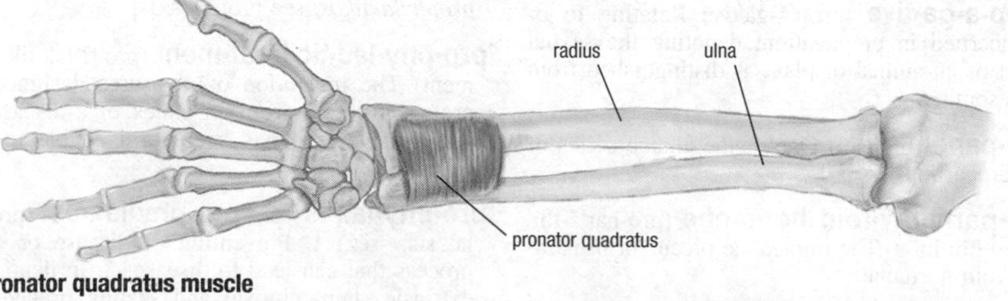

pronator quadratus muscle

of hand or foot with volar surface downward. See page B29. [L. *pronus,* bending down or forward]

pro·neph·ros, pl. **pro·neph·roi** (prō-nef′rŏs, -roy) **1.** The definitive excretory organ of primitive fishes. **2.** In the embryos of higher vertebrates, a vestigial structure consisting of a series of tortuous tubules emptying into the cloaca by way of the primordial nephric duct; in the human embryo, the pronephros is a very rudimentary, nonfunctional, and temporary structure, followed by the mesonephros and still later by the metanephros. [pro- + G. *nephros,* kidney]

prong (prawng) A fine pointed projection. [Med. L. *pronga*, fr. Germanic]

pro·nor·mo·blast (prō-nōr′mō-blast) The earliest of four stages in development of the normoblast. SEE ALSO erythroblast. SYN proerythroblast, rubriblast.

pro·nu·cle·us, pl. **pro·nu·cle·i** (prō-nū′klē-ŭs, -klē-ī) **1.** One of a pair of nuclei undergoing fusion in karyogamy. **2.** EMBRYOLOGY the nuclear material of the head of the sperm (male pronucleus) or of the oocyte (female pronucleus), after the oocyte has been penetrated by the sperm; each pronucleus normally carries a haploid set of chromosomes, so that the merging of the pronuclei in fertilization reestablishes the diploidy.

pro-oestrogen [Br.] SYN proestrogen.

pro-oestrus [Br.] SYN proestrus.

pro·o·pi·o·mel·a·no·cor·tin (POMC) (prō-ō′pē-ō-mel′ă-nō-kōr′tin) A large molecule found in the anterior and intermediate lobes of the pituitary gland, the hypothalamus, and other parts of the brain as well as in the lungs, gastrointestinal tract, and placenta; the precursor of ACTH, CLIP, β-LPH, γ-MSH, β-endorphin, and metenkephalin.

pro·o·tic (prō-ōt′ik) In front of the ear. [pro- + G. *ous,* ear]

prop·a·gate (prop′ă-gāt) **1.** To reproduce; to generate. **2.** To move along a fiber, e.g., propagation of the nerve impulse. [L. *propago,* pp. *-atus,* to generate, reproduce]

prop·a·ga·tion (prop′ă-gā′shŭn) The act of propagating.

prop·a·ga·tive (prop′ă-gā′tiv) Relating to or concerned in propagation; denoting the sexual part of an animal or plant as distinguished from the soma.

pro·pane (prō′pān) One of the alkane series of hydrocarbons.

pro·par·a·thy·roid hor·mone (prō-par′ă-thī′royd hōr′mōn) The immediate precursor of parathyroid hormone.

pro·pep·sin (prō-pep′sin) SYN pepsinogen.

pro·per·din (prō′pĕr-din) A group of proteins involved in resistance to infection that participate, in conjunction with other factors, in an alternate pathway to the activation of the terminal components of complement. SEE ALSO properdin system, component of complement. [pro- + L. *perdo,* to destroy]

pro·per·din fac·tor A (prō′pĕr-din fak′tŏr) A component of the properdin system; a hydrazine-sensitive β_1-globulin now known to be C3 (third component of complement).

pro·per·din fac·tor B (prō′pĕr-din fak′tŏr) A normal serum protein and a component of the properdin system.

pro·per·din fac·tor D (prō′pĕr-din fak′tŏr) A normal serum α-globulin required in the properdin system.

pro·per·din fac·tor E (prō′pĕr-din fak′tŏr) A serum protein required for activation of C3 (third component of complement) by cobra venom factor. SEE ALSO properdin system.

pro·per·din sys·tem (prō′pĕr-din sis′tĕm) An immunologic system that is the alternative pathway for complement, composed of several distinct proteins that react in a serial manner and activate C3 (third component of complement); the system can be activated, in the absence of specific antibody, by bacterial endotoxins, and a variety of polysaccharides and lipopolysaccharides.

prop·er pal·mar di·gi·tal ar·ter·y (prŏp′ĕr pahl′măr dij′i-tăl ahr′tĕr-ēz) Terminal branches of the common palmar digital artery that pass to the side of each finger. SYN arteria digitalis palmaris propria, collateral digital artery, digital collateral artery.

pro·phage (prō′fāj) SYN probacteriophage.

pro·phase (prō′fāz) The first stage of mitosis or meiosis, consisting of linear contraction and increase in thickness of the chromosomes (each composed of two chromatids) accompanied by migration of the two daughter centrioles and their asters toward the poles of the cell. [G. *prophasis,* from *prophainō,* to foreshadow]

pro·phy·lac·tic (prō′fi-lak′tik) **1.** Preventing disease; relating to prophylaxis. SYN preventive. **2.** An agent that acts to prevent a disease. [G. *prophylaktikos;* see prophylaxis]

pro·phy·lac·tic treat·ment (prō′fi-lak′tik trēt′mĕnt) The institution of measures designed to protect a person from an attack of a disease to which he or she has been, or is liable to be, exposed.

pro·phy·lax·is, pl. **pro·phy·lax·es** (prō′fi-lak′sis, -sēz) **1.** Prevention of disease or of a process that can lead to disease. **2.** In dentistry, extrinsic stain removal and sealing procedures done to maintain or improve oral health. [Mod.

L. fr. G. *pro-phylassō,* to guard before, take precaution]

pro·pi·o·nate (prō'pē-ō-nāt) A salt or ester of propionic acid.

Pro·pi·on·i·bac·te·ri·um (prō'pē-on-i-bak-tēr'ē-ŭm) A genus of nonmotile, non-spore-forming, anaerobic to aerotolerant bacteria containing gram-positive rods that are usually pleomorphic, diphtheroid, or club-shaped, with one end rounded, the other tapered or pointed. The cells usually occur singly, in pairs, in V and Y configurations, short chains, or clumps. These organisms occur in dairy products, on human skin, and in the intestinal tracts of humans and other animals. They may be pathogenic. The type species is *Propionibacterium freudenreichii.*

pro·pi·on·ic ac·id (prō'pē-on'ik as'id) Methylacetic acid; ethylformic acid; found in sweat.

pro·por·tion·al as·sist ven·ti·la·tion (PAV) (prŏ-pōr'shŭn-ăl ă-sist' ven'ti-lā'shŭn) Mechanical form of ventilation in which the patient controls the flow of oxygen by the amount of effort expended in breathing.

pro·por·tion·ate dwarf·ism (prō-pōr'shŭn-ăt dwōrf'izm) Inherited condition characterized by a symmetric shortening of the limbs and trunk; generally results from chemical, endocrine, nutritional, or nonosseous abnormalities.

pro·po·si·tion·al speech (prop'ŏ-zish'ŏn-ăl spēch) Intellectual, rational use of language for specific communication goals. SEE ALSO automatic speech.

pro·pos·i·tus, pl. **pro·po·si·ti** (prō-poz'i-tŭs, -tī) **1.** Proband distinguished by sex. **2.** A premise; an argument. [L. fr. *propono,* pp. *-positus,* to lay out, propound]

pro·pri·e·tar·y med·i·cine (prō-prī'ĕ-tar'ē med'i-sin) A medicinal compound for which the formula and mode of manufacture are the property of the maker.

pro·pri·e·tar·y name (prō-prī'ĕ-tar-ē nām) The protected brand name or trademark, registered with the U.S. Patent Office, under which a manufacturer markets a product. It is written with an initial capital letter, if appropriate, and is often further distinguished by a register mark (®). Cf. generic name, nonproprietary name. [L. *proprietarius*]

pro·pri·o·cep·tion (prō'prē-ō-sep'shŭn) A sense or perception, usually at a subconscious level, of the movements and position of the body and especially its limbs, independent of vision; this sense is gained primarily from input from sensory nerve terminals in muscles and tendons (muscle spindles) and the fibrous capsule of joints combined with input from the vestibular apparatus. SEE ALSO exteroceptor.

pro·pri·o·cep·tive (prō'prē-ō-sep'tiv) Capable of receiving stimuli originating in muscles, tendons, and other internal tissues. [L. *proprius,* one's own, + *capio,* to take]

pro·pri·o·cep·tive mech·a·nism (prō'prē-ō-sep'tiv mek'ă-nizm) The mechanism of sense of position and movement, by which muscular movements can be adjusted to a great degree of accuracy and equilibrium maintained.

pro·pri·o·cep·tive neu·ro·mus·cu·lar fa·cil·i·ta·tion (PNF) (prō'prē-ō-sep'tiv nūr'ō-mŭs'kyū-lăr fă-sil'i-tā'shŭn) Technique to improve range of joint motion (flexibility) by stimulating proprioceptors in muscles, joints, and tendons before joint extension. SEE ALSO muscle energy technique, Brunnstrom movement therapy.

pro·pri·o·cep·tive sen·si·bil·i·ty (prō'prē-ō-sep'tiv sens'i-bil'i-tē) SEE proprioceptive.

pro·pri·o·cep·tor (prō'prē-ō-sep'tŏr) One of a variety of sensory end organs (such as the muscle spindle and Golgi tendon organ) in muscles, tendons, and joint capsules.

prop·to·sis (prop-tō'sis) SYN exophthalmos. [G. *proptōsis,* a falling forward]

prop·tot·ic (prop-tot'ik) Referring to proptosis.

pro·pul·sion (prō-pŭl'shŭn) The tendency to fall forward; responsible for the festination in paralysis agitans. [G. *pro-pello,* pp. *-pulsus,* to drive forth]

pro·pyl (Pr) (prō'pil) The alkyl radical of propane, $CH_3CH_2CH_2$–.

pro·pyl al·co·hol (prō'pil al'kŏ-hol) A solvent for resins and cellulose esters; ethylcarbinol.

pro·py·lene (prō'pi-lēn) Methylethylene; a gaseous olefinic hydrocarbon.

pro re na·ta (PRN) (prō rā nā'tă) As the occasion arises; as necessary. [L.]

pro·ren·nin (prō-ren'in) SYN prochymosin.

pro·rhyth·mic ef·fects (prō-ridh'mik e-fekts') New or worsening arrhythmia after administration of an antiarrhythmic drug.

pro·ru·bri·cyte (prō-rū'bri-sīt) Basophilic normoblast. SEE ALSO erythroblast. [pro- + rubricyte]

pro·se·cre·tin (prō-sē-krē'tin) Unactivated secretin.

pro·sect (prō-sekt') To dissect a cadaver or any part, that it may serve for a demonstration of anatomy before a class. [L. *pro-seco,* pp. *-sectus,* to cut]

pro·sec·tor (prō'sek-tŏr) One who prosects or prepares the material for a demonstration of anatomy before a class.

pros·en·ceph·a·lon (pros'en-sef'ă-lon) The anterior primordial cerebral vesicle and the most rostral of the three primary brain vesicles of the embryonic neural tube; it subdivides to form the diencephalon and telencephalon. SYN forebrain. [G. *prosō,* forward, + *enkephalos,* brain]

pro•se•rum pro•throm•bin con•ver•sion ac•cel•er•a•tor (PPCA) (prō-sēr′ŭm prō-throm′bin kŏn-vĕr′zhŭn ak-sel′ĕr-ā-tŏr) SYN factor VIII.

pros•o•dem•ic (pros′ō-dem′ik) Denoting a disease that is transmitted directly from person to person. [G. *prosō,* forward, + *dēmos,* people]

pros•o•dy (proz′ŏ-dē) The varying rhythm, stress, and frequency of speech that aids meaning transmission.

pros•o•pag•no•si•a (pros′ō-pag-nō′sē-ă) Difficulty in recognizing familiar faces. [prosop- + G. *a-* priv. + *gnōsis,* recognition]

pros•o•pal•gi•a (pros′ō-pal′jē-ă) SYN trigeminal neuralgia. [prosop- + G. *algos,* pain]

pros•o•pal•gic (pros′ō-pal′jik) Relating to or suffering from trigeminal neuralgia.

pros•o•pla•si•a (pros′ō-plā′zē-ă) Progressive transformation, such as the change of cells of the salivary ducts into secreting cells. SEE ALSO cytomorphosis. [G. *prosō,* forward, + *plasis,* a molding]

♻**prosopo-, prosop-** Combining forms denoting the face. SEE ALSO facio-. [G. *prosōpon*]

pros•o•po•di•ple•gi•a (pros′ō-pō-di-plē′jē-ă) Paralysis affecting both sides of the face. [prosopo- + diplegia]

pros•o•po•neu•ral•gi•a (pros′ō-pō-nūr-al′jē-ă) SYN trigeminal neuralgia.

pros•o•po•ple•gi•a (pros′ō-pō-plē′jē-ă) SYN facial paralysis. [prosopo- + G. *plēgē,* stroke]

pros•o•po•ple•gic (pros′ō-pō-plē′jik) Relating to, or suffering from, facial paralysis.

pros•o•pos•chi•sis (pros′ō-pos′ki-sis) Congenital facial cleft from mouth to the medial canthus of the eye. [prosopo- + G. *schisis,* fissure]

pros•o•po•spasm (pros′ō-pō-spazm) SYN facial tic. [prosopo- + G. *spasmos,* spasm]

pro•spec•tive pay•ment (prŏs-pek′tiv pā′mĕnt) Reimbursement for services made in advance or without services having yet been performed.

pros•pec•tive pay•ment sys•tem (PPS) (prō-spek′tiv pā′mĕnt sis′tĕm) Arrangement mandated by the U.S. Tax Equity and Fiscal Responsibility Act of 1982 (TEFRA) to control Medicare costs; payment for services provided to a Medicare patient is fixed with adjustments made annually by the Centers for Medicare and Medicaid Services; payment is based on assigned diagnosis-related groups.

pros•ta•no•ic ac•id (pros′tă-nō′ik as′id) The 20-carbon acid that is the skeleton of the prostaglandins.

pros•ta•ta (pros′tă-tă) [TA] SYN prostate. [Mod. L. from G. *prostatēs,* one standing before]

pros•ta•tal•gi•a (pros′tă-tal′jē-ă) A rarely used term for pain in the area of the prostate gland. [prostat- + G. *algos,* pain]

pros•tate (pros′tāt) A chestnut-shaped body, surrounding the beginning of the urethra in the male, which consists of two lateral lobes connected anteriorly by an isthmus and posteriorly by a middle lobe lying above and between the ejaculatory ducts. In structure, the prostate consists of 3–50 compound tubuloalveolar glands between which are abundant stroma consisting of collagen and elastic fibers and many smooth muscle bundles. The secretion of the glands is a milky fluid that is discharged by excretory ducts into the prostatic urethra at the time of the emission of semen. USAGE NOTE Often mispronounced as prostrate, and so misspelled. SYN prostata [TA], prostate gland.

pros•ta•tec•to•my (pros′tă-tek′tŏ-mē) Removal of part or all of the prostate. [prostat- + G. *ektomē,* excision]

pros•tate gland (pros′tāt gland) SYN prostate.

pros•tate-spe•cif•ic an•ti•gen (PSA) (pros′tāt-spĕ-sif′ik an′ti-jen) A single-chain, 31-kD glycoprotein with 240 amino acid residues and 4 carbohydrate side-chains; a kallikrein protease produced by prostatic epithelial cells and normally found in seminal fluid and circulating blood. Elevations of serum PSA are highly organ-specific but occur in both cancer (adenocarcinoma) and benign disease (e.g., benign prostatic hyperplasia, prostatitis). A significant number of patients with organ-confined cancer have normal PSA values. SYN human glandular kallikrein 3.

pros•tat•ic (pros-tat′ik) Relating to the prostate.

pros•tat•ic bran•ches of in•fe•ri•or ves•i•cal ar•ter•y (pros-tat′ik branch′ĕz in-fēr′ē-ŏr ves′i-kăl ahr′tĕr-ē) Branches of the inferior vesicle artery that descend to the prostate, comprising its major arterial supply. SYN rami prostatici arteriae vesicalis inferioris.

pros•tat•ic bran•ches of mid•dle rec•tal ar•ter•y (pros-tat′ik branch′ĕz mid-ĕl rek′tăl ahr′tĕr-ē) Branches of the middle rectal artery that anastomose with the prostatic branches of the inferior vesicle artery and join them in supplying the prostate. SYN rami prostatici arteriae rectalis mediae.

pros•tat•ic cal•cu•lus (pros-tat′ik kal′kyū-lŭs) A concretion formed in the prostate gland, composed chiefly of calcium carbonate and phosphate (corpora amylacea).

pros•tat•ic duc•tules, pros•tat•ic ducts

(pros-tat′ik dŭkt′yūlz, pros-tat′ik dŭkts) About 20 minute canals that receive the prostatic secretion from the glandular tubules and discharge it through openings on either side of the urethral crest in the posterior wall of the urethra. SYN ductuli prostatici [TA].

pros•tat•ic flu•id (pros-tat′ik flū′id) Succus prostaticus; a whitish secretion that is one of the constituents of semen.

pros•tat•ic in•tra•ep•i•the•li•al ne•o•pla•si•a (PIN) (pros-tat′ik in-tra-ep′i-thē′lē-ăl nē′ō-plā′zē-ă) Dysplastic changes involving glands and ducts of the prostate which may be a precursor of adenocarcinoma; low grade (PIN 1), mild dysplasia with variation in nuclear size and shape and irregular cell spacing; high grade (PIN 2 and 3), moderate to severe dysplasia with nucleomegaly, nucleolomegaly, and irregular cell spacing.

pros•tat•ic mas•sage (pros-tat′ik mă-sahzh′) **1.** Manual expression of prostatic secretions by digital rectal technique. **2.** The emptying of prostatic sinuses and ducts by repeated downward compression maneuvers; used in the treatment of various congestive and inflammatory prostatic conditions.

pros•tat•ic si•nus (pros-tat′ik sī′nŭs) The groove on either side of the urethral crest in the prostatic part of the urethra into which the prostatic ducts open.

pros•tat•ic u•tri•cle (pros-tat′ik yū′tri-kĕl) A minute pouch in the prostate opening on the summit of the seminal colliculus, the analog of the uterus and vagina in the female. SYN utriculus prostaticus [TA], masculine uterus, Morgagni sinus (2), vesica prostatica.

pros•ta•tism (pros′tă-tizm) A syndrome, occurring mostly in older men, usually caused by enlargement of the prostate gland and manifested by irritative symptoms (e.g., nocturia, frequency, decreased voided volume, sensory urgency, and urgency incontinence) and obstructive symptoms (e.g., hesitancy, decreased stream, terminal dribbling, double voiding, and urinary retention).

pros•ta•ti•tis (pros′tă-tī′tis) Inflammation of the prostate. [prostat- + G. *-itis,* inflammation]

♻ **prostato-, prostat-** Combining forms indicating the prostate gland. [Med. L. *prostata* fr. G. *prostatēs,* one who stands before, protects]

pros•ta•to•cys•ti•tis (pros′tă-tō-sis-tī′tis) Inflammation of the prostate and the bladder; cystitis by extension of inflammation from the prostatic urethra. [prostato- + G. *kystis,* bladder, + *-itis,* inflammation]

pros•ta•to•li•thot•o•my (pros′tă-tō-li-thot′ŏ-mē) Incision of the prostate to remove a calculus. [prostato- + G. *lithos,* stone, + *tomē,* incision]

pros•ta•to•meg•a•ly (pros′tă-tō-meg′ă-lē) Enlargement of the prostate gland. [prostato- + G. *megas,* large]

pros•ta•tor•rhe•a (pros′tă-tō-rē′ă) Abnormal discharge of prostatic fluid. SYN prostatorrhoea. [prostato- + G. *rhoia,* a flow]

prostatorrhoea [Br.] SYN prostatorrhea.

pros•ta•tot•o•my (pros′tă-tot′ŏ-mē) An incision into the prostate. [prostato- + G. *tomē,* incision]

pros•ta•to•ve•sic•u•lec•to•my (pros′tă-tō-vĕ-sik′yū-lek′tŏ-mē) Surgical removal of the prostate gland and seminal vesicles.

pros•ta•to•ve•sic•u•li•tis (pros′tă-tō-vĕ-sik′yū-lī′tis) Inflammation of the prostate gland and seminal vesicles.

pros•the•sis, pl. **pros•the•ses** (pros-thē′sis, pros-thē′sēz) Fabricated substitute for a diseased or missing part of the body. [G. an addition]

pros•thet•ic (pros-thet′ik) **1.** Relating to a prosthesis or to an artificial part. **2.** SEE prosthetic group.

pros•thet•ic group (pros-thet′ik grūp) A nonamino acid compound attached to a protein, often in a reversible fashion, that confers new properties on the conjugated protein thus produced. SEE ALSO coenzyme.

pros•thet•ics (pros-thet′iks) The art and science of making and adjusting artificial parts of the human body.

pros•the•tist (pros′thĕ-tist) One skilled in constructing and fitting prostheses.

pros•thi•on (pros′thē-on) The most anterior point on the maxillary alveolar process in the midline. SYN alveolar point. [G. ntr. of *prosthios,* foremost]

pros•tho•don•tics (pros′thō-don′tiks) The science and art of providing suitable substitutes for the coronal portions of teeth, or for one or more lost or missing teeth and their associated parts, so that existing impaired function, appearance, comfort, and health of the patient may be restored. [L. *prosthodontia,* fr. G. *prosthesis* + *odous* (*odont-*), tooth]

pros•tho•don•tist (pros-thō-don′tist) A dentist engaged in the practice of prosthodontics.

pros•tra•tion (pros-trā′shŭn) A marked loss of strength, as in exhaustion. [L. *pro-sterno,* pp. *-stratus,* to strew before, overthrow]

♻ **prot-** SEE proteo-, proto-.

prot•ac•tin•i•um (Pa) (prō′tak-tin′ē-ŭm) A radioactive element, atomic no. 91, atomic wt. 231.03588, formed in the decay of uranium and thorium; its longest-lived isotope, ^{231}Pa, has a half-life of 32,500 years. [G. *prōtos,* first]

prot•a•mine (prō′tă-mēn) Any of a class of proteins found in fish spermatozoa in combination with nucleic acid; neutralizes anticoagulant action of heparin.

pro·ta·no·pi·a (prō-tă-nō′pē-ă) A form of dichromatism characterized by absence of the red-sensitive pigment in cones, decreased luminosity for long wavelengths of light, and confusion in recognition of red and green. [G. *prōtos,* first, + *a-* priv. + *ōps* (*ōp-*) eye]

pro·te·an (prō′tē-ăn) Changeable in form; having the power to change body form, like the ameba. [G. *Prōteus,* a god having the power to change his form]

pro·te·ase (prō′tē-ās) Descriptive term for proteolytic enzymes, both endopeptidases and exopeptidases; enzymes that hydrolyze (i.e., break) polypeptide chains.

pro·te·ase in·hib·i·tor (prō′tē-ās in-hib′i-tŏr) A class of synthetic drugs used in the treatment of HIV infection, with a mode of action different from those of formerly used antiretroviral agents including nucleoside analogues.

pro·te·ases (prō′tē-ā-sĕz) SYN proteolytic enzymes.

pro·te·a·some in·hib·i·tor (prō′tē-ă-sōm in-hib′i-tŏr) Medication to treat multiple myeloma by blocking proteasomes to disrupt growth.

pro·tec·ted health in·for·ma·tion (PHI) (prō-tek′tĕd helth in′fōr-mā′shŭn) An umbrella term embracing all data collected and stored in any medium relating to the health of the individual patient. This legal construct forbids passing along such information to a third party without the express permission of the patient or the patient's deputy.

pro·tec·ted spec·i·men brush (PSB) (prō-tek′tĕd spes′i-mĕn brŭsh) Tool used in the collection of specimen during a bronchoscopy.

pro·tec·tion test (prō-tek′shŭn test) A procedure to determine the antimicrobial activity of a serum by inoculating a susceptible animal with a mixture of the serum and the virus or other microbe being tested. SYN neutralization test.

pro·tec·tive i·so·la·tion (prō-tek′tiv ī′sō-lā′shŭn) SYN reverse isolation.

pro·tec·tive la·ryn·ge·al re·flex (prō-tek′tiv lă-rin′jē-ăl rē′fleks) Closure of the glottis to prevent entry of foreign substances into the respiratory tract.

pro·tec·tor (prō-tek′tŏr) A cover or shield. [L.L. *protectus* from pp. *protegere,* to protect, to cover over]

pro·tein (prō′tēn) Macromolecules consisting of long sequences of α-amino acids [H_2N–CHR–COOH] in peptide (amide) linkage (elimination of H_2O between the α-NH_2 and α-COOH of successive residues). Protein is three fourths of the dry weight of most cell matter and is involved in structures, hormones, enzymes, muscle contraction, immunologic response, and essential life functions. The amino acids involved are generally the 20 α-amino acids (glycine, L-alanine) recognized by the genetic code. Cross-links yielding globular forms of protein are often effected through the –SH groups of two sulfur-containing L-cysteinyl residues, as well as by noncovalent forces (e.g., hydrogen bonds, lipophilic attractions). Cf. bioregulator. [G. *prōtos,* first, + -in]

pro·tein·a·ceous (prō′tē-nā′shŭs) Resembling a protein; possessing, to some degree, the physicochemical properties characteristic of proteins.

pro·tein di·gest·i·bil·i·ty cor·rect·ed a·mi·no ac·id score (PDCAAS) (prō′tēn di-gest′ă-bil′i-tē kŏr-ek′tĕd ă-mē′nō as′id skōr) A measurement of protein quality found by multiplying the percentage of digestibility of the protein by its amino acid composition.

pro·tein ef·fi·cien·cy ra·ti·o (PER) (prō′tēn e-fish′ĕn-sē rā′shē-ō) Weight gain in grams divided by protein intake in grams.

pro·tein en·er·gy mal·nu·tri·tion (PEM) (prō′tēn en′ĕr-jē mal′nū-trish′ŭn) A deficiency of protein, energy, or both that includes marasmus (or chronic PEM) and kwashiorkor (typically, acute PEM). SYN protein kcalorie malnutrition.

pro·tein in·duced by vit·a·min K ab·sence (PIVKA) (prō′tēn in-dūst′ vī′tă-min ab′sĕns) Nonfunctional protein precursors of the prothrombin group of coagulation factors (e.g., factors II, VII, IX, X). They are synthesized in the liver in the absence of vitamin K and lack the carboxyl ($COOH^-$) group needed to bind the factor to a phospholipid surface.

pro·tein k·cal·o·rie mal·nu·tri·tion (PCM) (prō′tēn kal′ŏr-ē mal′nū-trish′ŭn) SYN protein energy malnutrition.

pro·tein ki·nase C (prō′tēn kī′nās) Any of several cytoplasmic calcium-activated kinases involved in numerous processes, including hormonal binding, platelet activation, and tumor promotion.

pro·tein-los·ing en·ter·op·a·thy (prō′tēn-lūz′ing en′tĕr-op′ă-thē) Increased fecal loss of serum protein, especially albumin, causing hypoproteinemia.

pro·tein me·tab·o·lism (prō′tēn mĕ-tab′ŏ-lizm) Decomposition and synthesis of protein in the tissues.

pro·tein·o·sis (prō′tē-nō′sis) A state characterized by disordered protein formation and distribution, particularly as manifested by the deposition of abnormal proteins in tissues. [protein + G. *-osis,* condition]

pro·tein p53 (prō′tēn) A multifunctional protein that modulates gene transcription and controls DNA repair, apoptosis, and the cell cycle.

pro•tein S (prō′tēn) A vitamin K–dependent antithrombotic protein that functions as a cofactor with activated protein C.

pro•tein turn•o•ver (prō′tēn tŭrn′ō-vĕr) The continuing breakdown and synthesis of proteins in the body, with recycling of amino acids.

pro•tei•nu•ri•a (prō′tē-nūr′ē-ă) **1.** Presence of urinary protein in concentrations greater than 0.3 g in a 24-hour urine collection or in concentrations greater than 1 g/L in a random urine collection on two or more occasions at least 6 hours apart; specimens must be clean-voided midstream (i.e., clean catch) or obtained by catheterization. **2.** SYN albuminuria. [protein + G. *ouron,* urine]

proteo-, prot- Combining forms denoting protein.

pro•te•o•gly•can ag•gre•gate (prō′tē-ō-glī′kan ag′rĕ-găt) A large aggregation of proteoglycans noncovalently bound to a long molecule of hyaluronic acid; involved in cross-linking the collagen fibrils of cartilage matrix.

pro•te•o•gly•cans (prō′tē-ō-glī′kanz) Glycoaminoglycans (mucopolysaccharides) bound to protein chains in covalent complexes; occur in the extracellular matrix of connective tissue.

pro•te•o•lip•ids (prō′tē-ō-lip′idz) A class of lipid-soluble proteins found in brain tissue, insoluble in water but soluble in chloroform-methanol-water mixtures.

pro•te•ol•y•sis (prō′tē-ol′i-sis) The decomposition of protein; primarily through hydrolysis of peptide bonds, both enzymatically and nonenzymatically. [proteo- + G. *lysis,* dissolution]

pro•te•o•lyt•ic (prō′tē-ō-lit′ik) Relating to or effecting proteolysis.

pro•te•o•ly•tic en•zymes (prō′tē-ō-lit′ik en′zīm) Enzymes that, in the opinion of some researchers, are able to break down particular proteins; forms the basis of enzyme therapy, a therapeutic modality the efficacy of which remains the subject of some controversy. SYN proteases.

pro•te•o•met•a•bol•ic (prō′tē-ō-met-ă-bol′ik) Relating to the metabolism of proteins.

pro•te•ose (prō′tē-ōs) A nondescript mixture of intermediate products of proteolysis between protein and peptone.

pro•te•o•some (prō′tē-ō-sōm) A cluster of genes that encode components of the cell cytosolic proteolytic complex, a set of proteins thought to be involved in cellular processing and transport of peptides in the formation of the major histocompatibility complex class I molecules. [proteo- + G. *sōma,* body]

Pro•te•us (prō′tē-ŭs) A genus of motile, peritrichous, non-spore-forming, aerobic to facultatively anaerobic bacteria containing gram-negative rods. The metabolism is fermentative, producing acid. *Proteus* occurs primarily in fecal matter and in putrefying materials. [G. *Prōteus,* a sea god, who had the power to change his form]

Pro•te•us mi•ra•bi•lis (prō′tē-ŭs mi-rab′i-lis) A bacterial species widely recognized as a human pathogen commonly recovered from urinary, wound, and bacteremic infections. Recognized in the laboratory by its characteristic "swarming"colony morphology on blood agar.

Pro•te•us syn•drome (prō′tē-ŭs sin′drōm) A sporadic disorder of possible genetic origin, having a variable and changing phenotype characterized by gigantism of the hands and feet, distorted abnormal growth, pigmented nevi, thickening of the palms and soles, vascular malformations, and subcutaneous lipomas; often confused with neurofibromatosis type II. SYN elephant man disease (1). [G. *Prōteus*, a sea god, who had the power to change his form]

Pro•te•us vul•ga•ris (prō′tē-ŭs vŭl-gā′ris) The type species of the genus *Proteus*, found in putrefying materials; associated with a wide variety of nosocomial infections of the respiratory and urinary tracts and other sterile sites and also with decubitus ulcers and abscesses. SEE ALSO Weil-Felix reaction.

pro•throm•bin (prō-throm′bin) A glycoprotein formed and stored in the parenchymal cells of the liver and present in blood in a concentration of approximately 20 mg/100 mL. In the presence of thromboplastin and calcium ion, prothrombin is converted to thrombin, which in turn converts fibrinogen to fibrin, resulting in coagulation of blood; a deficiency of prothrombin leads to impaired blood coagulation.

pro•throm•bin ac•cel•er•a•tor (prō-throm′bin ak-sel′ĕr-ā-tŏr) SYN factor V.

pro•throm•bin•ase (prō-throm′bi-nās) SYN factor X.

pro•throm•bin frag•ment 1.2 (F1.2) (prō-throm′bin frag′mĕnt) A peptide released when prothrombin is cleaved by factor Xa. This fragment binds to phospholipid through calcium and interacts with factor Va. Elevated plasma levels of F1.2 have been described in patients with thrombosis or in prethrombotic states.

pro•throm•bin test (prō-throm′bin test) A quantitative test for prothrombin in the blood based on the clotting time of oxalated blood plasma in the presence of thromboplastin and calcium chloride; measures the integrity of the extrinsic and common pathways of coagulation. SEE ALSO prothrombin time. SYN Quick test.

pro•throm•bin time (PT) (prō-throm′bin tīm) The time required for clotting after thromboplastin and calcium are added in optimal amounts to blood of normal fibrinogen content; if prothrombin is diminished, the clotting time increases; used to evaluate the extrinsic clotting system. SEE ALSO prothrombin test.

pro•tist (prō′tist) A member of the kingdom Protista.

Pro•tis•ta (prō-tis′tă) A kingdom of both plantlike and animallike eukaryotic unicellular organisms, either in the form of solitary organisms, e.g., protozoa, or colonies of cells lacking true tissues. [G. ntr. pl. of *prōtistos,* the first of all]

♻ **proto-, prot-** Combining forms meaning the first in a series; the highest in rank. USAGE NOTE Properly prefixed to words derived from Greek roots. [G. *prōtos,* first]

pro•to•col (prō′tŏ-kawl) **1.** A precise and detailed plan for the study of a biomedical problem or for a regimen of therapy, especially cancer chemotherapy. **2.** A record of findings in an experiment or investigation, especially an autopsy.

pro•to•cone (prō′tō-kōn) **1.** The mesiolingual cusp of human upper molars. **2.** Formerly thought to be the first upper molar cusp to develop evolutionarily. SEE ALSO protoconid. [proto- + G. *kōnos,* cone]

pro•to•con•id (prō′tō-kon′id) **1.** The mesiobuccal cusp of human lower molars. **2.** The first lower molar cusp to develop evolutionarily. SEE ALSO protocone. [protocone + -id (2)]

Pro•toc•tis•ta (prō′tok-tis′tă) A kingdom of eukaryotes incorporating the algae and the protozoans that comprise the presumed ancestral stocks of the fungi, plant, and animal kingdoms; they lack the developmental pattern stemming from a blastula (typical of animals), the pattern of embryo development (typical of plants), and development from spores as in fungi. Included are the nucleated algae and seaweeds, the flagellated water molds, slime molds and nets, and protozoa; unicellular, colonial, and multicellular organisms are included, but the complex development of tissues and organs of plants and animals is absent. [G. *prōtos,* the first, + *ktizō,* to create]

pro•to•di•a•stol•ic (prō′tō-dī′ă-stol′ik) Early diastolic, relating to the beginning of cardiac diastole.

pro•to•di•a•stol•ic gal•lop (prō′tō-dī′ă-stol′ik gal′ŏp) Rhythm in which the gallop sound is an abnormal third heart sound.

pro•to•du•o•de•num (prō′tō-dū′ō-dē′nŭm) The first part of the duodenum, which extends from the pylorus as far as the major duodenal papilla and develops from the caudal foregut of the embryo; it has no plicae circulares and is the location of the duodenal glands.

pro•ton (prō′ton) The positively charged unit of the nuclear mass; protons form part (or in hydrogen 1, the whole) of the nucleus of the atom around which the negative electrons revolve. [G. ntr. of *prōtos,* first]

pro•ton-den•si•ty weight•ing (prō′ton den′si-tē wāt′ing) Magnetic resonance image that demonstrates the differences in the proton densities of tissues.

pro•ton pump (prō′ton pŭmp) Molecular mechanism for the net transport of protons across a membrane; usually involves the activity of adenosine triphosphatase.

pro•ton pump in•hib•i•tor (prō′ton pŭmp in-hib′i-tŏr) An agent that blocks the transport of hydrogen ions into the stomach and hence is useful in the treatment of gastric hyperacidity, as observed in ulcer disease.

pro•to•nymph (prō′tō-nimf) In mites, the second instar.

pro•to•on•co•gene (prō′tō-ong′kō-jēn) A gene in the normal human genome that appears to have a role in normal cellular physiology; involved in regulation of normal cell growth or proliferation; as a result of somatic mutations, these genes may become oncogenic; products of protooncognes may have important roles in normal cellular differentiation.

pro•to•path•ic (prō′tō-path′ik) Denoting a supposedly primitive set or system of peripheral sensory nerve fibers conducting a low order of pain and temperature sensibility that is poorly localized. Cf. epicritic. [proto- + G. *pathos,* suffering]

pro•to•path•ic sen•si•bil•i•ty (prō′tō-path′ik sens′i-bil′i-tē) SEE protopathic.

pro•to•plasm (prō′tō-plazm) **1.** Living matter, the substance of which animal and vegetable cells are formed. SEE ALSO cytoplasm, nucleoplasm. **2.** The total cell material, including cell organelles. Cf. cytoplasm, cytosol, hyaloplasm. [proto- + G. *plasma,* thing formed]

pro•to•plas•mic as•tro•cyte (prō′tō-plaz′mik as′trō-sīt) One form of astrocyte, found mainly in gray matter, having few fibrils but numerous branching processes.

pro•to•plast (prō′tō-plast) A bacterial cell from which the rigid cell wall has been completely removed; the bacterium loses its characteristic form. [proto- + G. *plastos,* formed]

pro•to•por•phyr•i•a (prō′tō-pōr-fir′ē-ă) Enhanced fecal excretion of protoporphyrin.

pro•to•sty•lid (prō′tō-stī′lid) An accessory cusp found on the buccal surface of the mesiobuccal cusp of lower molars, ranging from a small groove to a cusp rivaling the mesiobuccal cusp in size. [proto- + G. *stylis, -idos,* mast, spar]

pro•to•troph (prō′tō-trōf) A bacterial strain that has the same nutritional requirements as the wild-type strain from which it was derived. [proto- + G. *trophē,* nourishment]

pro•to•type (prō′tō-tīp) The primitive form; the first form to which subsequent individuals of the class or species conform. [proto- + G. *typos,* type]

pro·to·ver·te·bra (prō′tō-vĕr′tĕ-bră) The caudal half of each sclerotomal concentration, which is the primordium of the centrum of a vertebra. SYN provertebra.

Pro·to·zo·a (prō′tō-zō′ă) Formerly considered a phylum, now regarded as a subkingdom of the animal kingdom, including all of the so-called acellular or unicellular forms. Members consist of a single functional cell unit or aggregation of nondifferentiated cells, loosely held together and not forming tissues. [proto- + G. *zōon,* animal]

pro·to·zo·al (prō′tō-zō′ăl) SYN protozoan (2).

pro·to·zo·an (prō′tō-zō′ăn) **1.** A member of the phylum Protozoa. SYN protozoon. **2.** Relating to protozoa. SYN protozoal.

pro·to·zo·i·a·sis (prō′tō-zō-ī′ă-sis) Infection with protozoans.

pro·to·zo·ol·o·gy (prō′tō-zō-ol′ŏ-jē) The science concerned with all aspects of the biology and human interest in protozoa. [protozoa + G. *logos,* study]

pro·to·zo·on, pl. **pro·to·zo·a** (prō′tō-zō′on, -zō′ă) SYN protozoan (1).

pro·to·zo·o·phage (prō′tō-zō′ō-fāj) A phagocyte that ingests protozoa. [protozoa + G. *phagō,* to eat]

pro·trac·tion (prō-trak′shŭn) **1.** DENTISTRY the extension of teeth or other maxillary or mandibular structures into a position anterior to normal. SEE ALSO protractor. **2.** Forward movement of the scapula.

pro·trac·tion (prō-trak′shŭn) Forward movement of the scapula.

pro·trac·tor (prō-trak′tōr) A muscle drawing a part forward, as antagonistic to a retractor. [L. *pro-traho,* pp. *-tractus,* to draw forth]

pro·trud·ed disc (prō-trūd′ĕd disk) SYN herniated disc.

pro·tru·ding ear (prō-trū′ding ēr) SYN outstanding ear.

pro·tru·sion (prō-trū′zhŭn) **1.** The state of being thrust forward or projected. **2.** DENTISTRY a position of the mandible forward from centric relation. [L. *protrusio*]

pro·tru·sive oc·clu·sion (prō-trū′siv ŏ-klū′zhŭn) Occlusion that results when the mandible is protruded forward from centric position.

pro·tu·ber·ance (prō-tū′bĕr-ăns) A swelling, protruding, or knoblike outgrowth or part. SYN protuberantia. [Mod. L. *protuberantia*]

pro·tu·ber·ant ab·do·men (prō-tū′bĕr-ănt ab′dō-mĕn) Unusual or prominent convexity of the abdomen, due to excessive subcutaneous fat, poor muscle tone, or an increase in intraabdominal content.

pro·tu·be·ran·ti·a (prō-tū′bĕr-an′shē-ă) SYN protuberance. SEE ALSO prominence, eminence. [Mod. L. fr. *protubero,* to swell out, fr. *tuber,* a swelling]

proud flesh (prowd flesh) Exuberant granulation tissue on the surface of a wound.

Proust space (prust spās) SYN rectovesical pouch.

pro·ver·te·bra (prō-vĕr′tĕ-bră) SYN protovertebra.

Pro·vi·den·ci·a (prov-i-den′sē-ă) A genus of motile, peritrichous, non-spore-forming, aerobic, or facultatively anaerobic bacteria containing gram-negative rods. These organisms occur particularly in urinary tract infections and in small outbreaks and sporadic cases of diarrheal disease.

Pro·vi·den·ci·a al·cal·i·fa·ci·ens (prov-i-den′sē-ă al-kal-i-fā′shē-enz) A bacterial species found in extraintestinal sources, particularly in urinary tract infections; it also has been isolated from small outbreaks and sporadic cases of diarrheal disease. It is the type species of the genus *Providencia.*

Pro·vi·den·ci·a rett·ger·i (prov-i-den′sē-ă ret′gĕr-ī) A bacterial species that is found in chicken cholera and human gastroenteritis.

Pro·vi·den·ci·a stu·ar·ti·i (prov-i-den′sē-ă stū-ahr′tē-ī) A bacterial species isolated from urinary tract infections and from small outbreaks and sporadic cases of diarrheal disease.

pro·vi·der (prō-vī′dĕr) A person or agency that supplies goods or services, particularly medical or paramedical services. [L. *pro-videre*]

pro·vid·er i·den·ti·fi·ca·tion num·ber (PIN) (prō-vī′dĕr ī-den′ti-fi-kā′shŭn num′bĕr toc) Method used to identify a health care provider in terms of relations with a specific insurance company.

pro·vi·rus (prō-vī′rŭs) The precursor of an animal virus; theoretically analogous to the prophage in bacteria, the provirus being integrated into the nucleus of infected cells.

pro·vi·ta·min (prō′vī′tă-min) An inactive form of a vitamin that needs activation before it can be used by the body.

pro·vi·ta·min A (prō′vī′tă-min) Carotenoid precursors of vitamin A found in some red and yellow fruits and vegetables.

prox·i·mad (prok′si-mad) In a direction toward a proximal part, or toward the center; not distad. [L. *proximus,* nearest, next, + *ad,* to]

prox·i·mal (prok′si-măl) **1.** Nearest the trunk or the point of origin; said of part of a limb, of an artery or a nerve, so situated. **2.** SYN mesial. **3.** DENTAL ANATOMY denoting the surface of a tooth in relation to a neighboring or adjacent tooth, whether mesial or distal, i.e., nearer to or farther from the anteroposterior median plane. [Mod. L. *proximalis,* fr. L. *proximus,* nearest, next]

prox•i•mal deep in•gui•nal lymph node (prok′si-măl dēp ing′gwi-năl limf nōd) One of those nodes located in or adjacent to the femoral canal; sometimes mistaken for a femoral hernia when enlarged. SYN Rosenmüller gland, Rosenmüller node.

prox•i•mal in•ter•pha•lan•ge•al joints (PIP) (proks′i-măl in′tĕr-fē-lan′jē-ăl joynts) The synovial joints between the proximal and middle phalanges of the fingers and of the toes.

prox•i•mal my•o•ton•ic my•o•path•y (PROMM) (proks′i-măl mī′ō-ton′ik mī-op′ă-thē) An autosomal dominant, multisystemic disorder, with onset in young adult life, characterized by proximal myotonia and weakness, muscle pain, baldness, cataracts, cardiac conduction disturbances, and testicular atrophy. In contrast to myotonic dystrophy, features of this disorder do not include facial weakness and ptosis, distal limb weakness and wasting, and trinucleotide repeat expansion at the gene loci for myotonic dystrophy.

prox•i•mal ra•di•o•ul•nar joint (prok′si-măl rā′dē-ō-ŭl′năr joynt) The pivot synovial joint between the head of the radius and the ring formed by the radial notch of the ulna and the anular ligament.

prox•i•mal sple•no•re•nal shunt (proks′i-măl splē′nō-rē′năl shŭnt) Anastomosis of the proximal end of the cut splenic vein to the side of the left renal vein for control of portal hypertension; this is considered a central or complete visceral venous shunt.

prox•i•mate (prok′si-măt) Immediate; next; proximal.

♻**proximo-, proxi-, prox-** Combining forms meaning proximal. [L. *proximus,* nearest, next (to)]

prox•i•mo•a•tax•i•a (prok′si-mō-ă-tak′sē-ă) Ataxia or lack of muscular coordination in the proximal portions of the extremities (i.e., arms and thighs). Cf. acroataxia. [proximo- + ataxia]

prox•y (proks′ē) **1.** One authorized to act as a substitute or agent for another. **2.** A document supporting such authorization. [M.E. *proccy*, fr. L. *procurare*, to take care of]

pro•zone (prō′zōn) A phenomenon in which visible agglutination and precipitation do not occur in mixtures of specific antigen and antibody because of antibody excess.

PRPP Abbreviation for 5-phospho-α-D-ribosyl 1-pyrophosphate.

PR seg•ment (seg′mĕnt) That part of the electrocardiographic curve between the end of the P wave and the beginning of the QRS complex.

pru•rig•i•nous (prūr-ij′i-nŭs) Relating to or suffering from prurigo. [L. *pruriginosus,* having the itch]

pru•ri•go (prū-rī′gō) A chronic disease of the skin marked by a persistent eruption of papules that itch intensely. [L. itch, fr. *prurio,* to itch]

pru•ri•go mi•tis (prū-rī′gō mī′tis) A mild form of a chronic dermatitis characterized by recurring, intensely itching papules and nodules, probably atopic.

pru•ri•go no•du•la•ris (prū-rī′gō nod′yū-lār′is) An eruption of hard nodules (picker's nodules) in the skin caused by rubbing and accompanied by intense itching.

pru•ri•go sim•plex (prū-rī′gō sim′pleks′) A mild form of prurigo having a pronounced tendency to relapse.

pru•rit•ic (prūr-it′ik) Relating to pruritus.

pru•rit•ic ur•ti•car•i•al pap•ules and plaques of preg•nan•cy (PUPPP) (prūr-it′ik ŭr′ti-kar′ē-ăl pap′yūlz plaks preg′năn-sē) Intensely pruritic papulovesicles that begin on the abdomen in the third trimester and spread peripherally, resolve rapidly after delivery, and do not affect the fetus.

pru•ri•tus (prū-rī′tŭs) **1.** SYN itching. **2.** SYN itch (1). [L. an itching, fr. *prurio,* to itch]

pru•ri•tus a•ni (prūr-ī′tŭs ā′nī) Itching at the anus; may be associated with seborrheic dermatitis, candidosis, or external hemorrhoids, infection by pinworms or other helminths, or systemic disease.

pru•ri•tus gra•vi•dar•um (prū-rī′tŭs grav-i-dar′ŭm) Severe pruritus without associated rash occurring during pregnancy secondary to intrahepatic cholestasis and bile salt retention.

pru•ri•tus se•ni•lis, se•nile pru•ri•tus (prū-rī′tŭs sĕ-nil′is, sen′il prūr-ī′tŭs) Itching associated with dryness of the skin in the aged.

pru•ri•tus vul•vae (prū-rī′tŭs vŭl′vē) Itching of the external female genitalia, caused by seborrheic dermatitis, allergy to local contactants, senile atrophy of the vulva, or systemic disease.

Prus•sian blue (prŭsh′ăn blū) [CI 77510] SYN Berlin blue.

PRVC Abbreviation for pressure-regulated volume control.

PSA Abbreviation for prostate-specific antigen.

♻**psammo-** Combining form denoting sand. [G. *psammos*]

psam•mo•ma (sa-mō′mă) Obsolete term for psammomatous meningioma or meningioma. [psammo- + G. *-oma,* tumor]

psam•mo•ma bo•dies (sa-mō′mă bod′ēz) **1.** Mineralized bodies occurring in the meninges, choroid plexus, and in certain meningiomas; usually composed of a central capillary surrounded by concentric whorls of meningocytes in various stages of hyaline change and mineralization; can also occur in benign and malignant epithelial tumors (often papillary) or with chronic inflammation; **2.** SYN corpora arenacea. **3.** SYN calcospherite.

psam·mo·ma·tous me·nin·gi·o·ma (sa-mō′mă-tŭs mĕ-nin′jē-ō′mă) A firm cellular neoplasm derived from fibrous tissue of the meninges, choroid plexus, and certain other structures associated with the brain, and characterized by the formation of multiple, discrete, concentrically laminated, calcareous bodies (psammoma bodies); most of these neoplasms are histologically benign, but may lead to severe symptoms as a result of compressing the brain. SYN Virchow psammoma.

psam·mous (sam′ŭs) Sandy. [G. *psammos,* sand]

PSA vel·o·ci·ty (vĕ-los′i-tē) A measure of the rapidity of change in a person's level of prostate-specific antigen.

PSB Abbreviation for protected specimen brush.

PSE Abbreviation for Pidgin Sign English.

P se·lec·tin (sĕ-lek′tin) Cell surface receptor present on endothelium that is involved with neutrophil migration into inflamed tissue.

pseud·a·graph·i·a (sū′dă-graf′ē-ă) Partial agraphia in which one can do no original writing but can copy correctly. SYN pseudoagraphia. [pseud- + G. *a-* priv. + *graphō,* to write]

Pseud·al·les·che·ri·a boy·di·i (sūd′al-es-kē′rē-ă boy′dē-ī) A species of fungus that causes eumycotic mycetoma and pseudallescheriasis; its conidial (asexual) state is *Scedosporium apiospermum.*

pseud·al·les·che·ri·a·sis (sūd′ăl-es′kĕ-rī′ă-sis) A variety of clinical diseases resulting from infection with *Pseudallescheria boydii* (e.g., pulmonary colonization, fungoma, and invasive pneumonitis), as well as mycotic keratitis, endophthalmitis, endocarditis, meningitis, sinusitis, brain abscesses, cutaneous and subcutaneous infections, and disseminated systemic infections.

pseud·an·ky·lo·sis (sūd′ang-ki-lō′sis) SYN fibrous ankylosis.

pseud·ar·thro·sis (sūd′ahr-thrō′sis) A new, false joint arising at the site of an ununited fracture. SYN false joint, pseudoarthrosis. [pseud- + G. *arthrōsis,* a joint]

pseud·es·the·si·a (sūd′es-thē′zē-ă) **1.** SYN paraphia. **2.** A subjective sensation not arising from an external stimulus. **3.** SYN phantom limb. SYN pseudoaesthesia. [pseud- + G. *aisthēsis,* sensation]

♻ **pseudo-, pseud-** Combining forms meaning false (often used about a deceptive resemblance). [G. *pseudēs*]

pseudoaesthesia [Br.] SYN pseudesthesia.

pseu·do·a·graph·i·a (sū′dō-ă-graf′ē-ă) SYN pseudagraphia.

pseu·do·al·lel·ic (sū′dō-ă-le′lik) Relating to pseudoallelism.

pseu·do·al·lel·ism (sū′dō-a-ēl′izm) Relationship of two or more loci that are difficult to distinguish from a single locus by classical genetic analysis.

pseudoanaemia [Br.] SYN pseudoanemia.

pseu·do·a·ne·mi·a (sū′dō-ă-nē′mē-ă) Pallor of the skin and mucous membranes without the blood changes of anemia. SYN false anemia, pseudoanaemia.

pseu·do·ar·thro·sis (sū′dō-ahr-thrō′sis) SYN pseudarthrosis.

pseu·do·bul·bar (sū′dō-bŭl′bahr) Denoting a supranuclear paralysis of the bulbar nerves.

pseu·do·bul·bar pal·sy (sū′dō-bŭl′bahr pawl′zē) Spastic paralysis of the bulbar musculature due to bilateral impairment of corticobulbar upper motor neuron fibers.

pseu·do·bul·bar pa·ral·y·sis (sū′dō-bŭl′bahr păr-al′i-sis) Paralysis of the lips and tongue, simulating progressive bulbar paralysis but due to supranuclear lesions with bilateral involvement of the upper motor neurons; characterized by speech and swallowing difficulties, emotional instability, and spasmodic, mirthless laughter.

pseu·do·car·ti·lage (sū′dō-kahr′ti-lij) SYN chondroid tissue (1).

pseu·do·cast (sū′dō-kast) SYN false cast.

pseu·do·chan·cre (sū′dō-shang′kĕr) A nonspecific indurated sore, usually located on the penis, resembling a chancre.

pseu·do·cho·lin·es·ter·ase (sū′dō-kō′lin-es′tĕr-ās) SYN plasma cholinesterase.

pseu·do·cho·re·a (sū′dō-kōr-ē′ă) A spasmodic disorder or extensive tic resembling chorea.

pseudochromaesthesia [Br.] SYN pseudochromesthesia.

pseu·do·chro·mes·the·si·a (sū′dō-krō′mes-thē′zē-ă) **1.** An anomaly in which each vowel in the printed word is seen as colored. SEE ALSO photism. **2.** SYN color hearing. SYN pseudochromaesthesia. [pseudo- + G. *chrōma,* color, + *aisthēsis,* sensation]

pseu·do·co·arc·ta·tion (sū′dō-kō′ahrk-tā′shŭn) Distortion, often with slight narrowing, of the aortic arch at the level of insertion of the ligamentum arteriosum.

pseu·do·cop·ro·sta·sis (sū′dō-kop′rō-stā′sis)

VETERINARY MEDICINE impaction of feces in the colon due to an external blockage of the anus, usually due to matted hair covering the anus. [pseudo- + coprostasis]

pseu·do·croup (sū′dō-krūp′) SYN laryngismus stridulus.

pseu·do·cryp·tor·chism (sū′-dō-krip′tōr-kizm) A condition in which the testes descend to the scrotum but intermittently retreat into the inguinal canal. [pseudo- + G. *kryptos,* hidden, + *orchis,* testis]

pseu·do·cy·e·sis (sū′dō-sī-ē′sis) SYN false pregnancy. [pseudo- + G. *kyēsis,* pregnancy]

pseu·do·cyl·in·droid (sū′dō-sil′in-droyd) A shred of mucus or other substance resembling a renal cast in the urine.

pseu·do·cyst (sū′dō-sist) **1.** An accumulation of fluid in a cystlike loculus, but without an epithelial or other membranous lining. SYN adventitious cyst. **2.** A cyst with a wall formed by a host cell and not by a parasite. **3.** A mass of 50 or more *Toxoplasma* bradyzoites, found within a host cell, frequently in the brain; a true cyst enclosed in its own membrane within the host cell that may rupture to release particles that form new cysts. [pseudo- + G. *kystis,* bladder]

pseu·do·de·men·ti·a (sū′dō-dĕ-men′shē-ă) A condition resembling dementia but usually due to a depressive disorder rather than brain dysfunction.

pseu·do·diph·the·ri·a (sū′dō-dif-thēr′ē-ă) SYN diphtheroid (1).

pseu·do·dom·i·nance (sū′dō-dom′i-năns) SYN quasidominance.

pseu·do·e·de·ma (sū′dō-ĕ-dē′mă) A puffiness of the skin not due to a fluid accumulation. [pseudo- + G. *oidēma,* a swelling (edema)]

pseu·do·ex·fol·i·a·tion syn·drome (sū′dō-eks-fō′lē-ā′shŭn sin′drōm) A condition, often leading to glaucoma, in which deposits on the surface of the lens resemble exfoliation of the lens capsule.

pseu·do·ex·fol·i·a·tive glau·co·ma (sū′dō-eks-fō′lē-ă′tiv glaw-kō′mă) Condition occurring in association with widespread deposition of cellular organelles on the lens capsule, ocular blood vessels, iris, and ciliary body.

pseu·do·fol·lic·u·li·tis (sū′dō-fō-lik′yū-lī′tis) Erythematous follicular papules or, less commonly, pustules resulting from close shaving of curly hair; tips of growing hairs reenter the skin, producing ingrown hairs; pseudofolliculitis of the beard area is very common in blacks.

pseu·do·frac·ture (sū′dō-frak′shŭr) A condition in which a radiograph shows formation of new bone with thickening of periosteum at the site of an injury to bone.

pseu·do·gan·gli·on (sū′dō-gang′glē-ŏn) A localized thickening of a nerve trunk having the appearance of a ganglion.

pseudogeusaesthesia [Br.] SYN pseudogeusesthesia.

pseu·do·geu·ses·the·si·a (sū′dō-gūs′es-thē′zē-ă) SYN color taste. SYN pseudogeusaesthesia. [pseudo- + G. *geusis,* taste, + *aisthēsis,* sensation]

pseu·do·geu·si·a (sū′dō-gū′sē-ă) A subjective taste sensation not produced by an external stimulus. [pseudo- + G. *geusis,* taste]

pseu·do·glan·du·lar stage of lung de·vel·op·ment (sū′dō-glan′dyū-lăr stāj lŭng dĕ-vel′ŏp-mĕnt) The period (6–16 weeks) when the lung resembles an endocrine gland; respiration is not possible during this period of embryonic growth.

pseu·do·gout (sū′dō-gowt) Acute episodes of synovitis caused by deposits of calcium pyrophosphate crystals rather than urate crystals as in true gout; associated with articular chondrocalcinosis.

pseu·do-Grae·fe phe·nom·e·non (sū′dō-grā′fē fĕ-nom′ĕ-non) Retraction of the upper eyelid on downward movement of the eyes.

pseudohaematuria [Br.] SYN pseudohematuria.

pseu·do·he·ma·tu·ri·a (sū′dō-hē′mă-tyūr′ē-ă) A red pigmentation of urine caused by certain foods or drugs, and thus not actually hematuria. SYN false hematuria, pseudohaematuria.

pseu·do·her·maph·ro·dite (sū′dō-hĕr-maf′rō-dīt) A person exhibiting pseudohermaphroditism.

pseu·do·her·maph·ro·dit·ism (sū′dō-hĕr-maf′rō-di-tizm) A state in which the person is of an unambiguous gonadal sex (i.e., possesses either testes or ovaries) but has ambiguous external genitalia. SYN false hermaphroditism.

pseudohyperkalaemia [Br.] SYN pseudohyperkalemia.

pseu·do·hy·per·kal·e·mi·a (sū′dō-hī′pĕr-kă-lē′mē-ă) A spurious elevation of the serum concentration of potassium, occurring when potassium is released in vitro from cells in a blood sample collected for a potassium measurement. May be a consequence of disease (i.e., myeloproliferative disorders with marked leukocytosis or thrombocytosis) or result from an improper collection technique with in vitro hemolysis. SYN pseudohyperkalaemia. [pseudo- + G. *hyper,* above + L. *kalium,* potassium, G. *haima,* blood]

pseu·do·hy·per·par·a·thy·roid·ism (sū′dō-hī′pĕr-par-ă-thī′roy-dizm) Hypercalcemia in a patient with a malignant neoplasm in the absence of skeletal metastases or primary hyperparathyroidism; believed to be due to formation of parathyroidlike hormone by nonparathyroid tumor tissue.

pseu•do•hy•per•tro•phic (sū′dō-hī′pĕr-trō′fik) Relating to or marked by pseudohypertrophy.

pseu•do•hy•per•tro•phy (sū′dō-hī-pĕr′trŏ-fē) Increase in size of an organ or a part, due not to increase in size or number of the specific functional elements but to that of some other tissue, fatty or fibrous.

pseu•do•hy•po•a•cu•sis (sū′dō-hī′pō-ă-kyū′sis) Apparent loss of hearing without organic disorder or with insufficient pathologic evidence to explain the extent of the loss; usually due to conversion disorder or malingering.

pseudohyponatraemia [Br.] SYN pseudohyponatremia.

pseu•do•hy•po•na•tre•mi•a (sū′dō-hī′pō-nă-trē′mē-ă) A low serum sodium concentration due to volume displacement by massive hyperlipidemia or hyperproteinemia; also used to describe the low serum sodium concentration that may occur with high blood glucose. SYN pseudohyponatraemia.

pseu•do•hy•po•par•a•thy•roid•ism (sū′dō-hī′pō-par-ă-thī′royd-izm) A disorder resembling hypoparathyroidism, with high serum phosphate and low calcium levels, but with normal or elevated serum parathyroid hormone levels; due to lack of end-organ responsiveness to parathyroid hormone.

pseu•do•ic•ter•us (sū′dō-ik′tĕr-ŭs) A yellowish discoloration of the skin resembling jaundice but due to some substance other than bile pigments. SYN pseudojaundice.

pseu•do•i•so•chro•mat•ic (sū′dō-ī′sō-krō-mat′ik) Apparently of the same color; denoting certain charts containing colored spots mixed with figures printed in confusion colors; used in testing for color vision deficiency.

pseu•do•jaun•dice (sū′dō-jawn′dis) SYN pseudoicterus.

pseu•do•lo•gi•a (sū′dō-lō′jē-ă) Pathologic lying in speech or writing. [pseudo- + G. *logos,* word]

pseu•do•lo•gi•a phan•tas•ti•ca (sū′dō-lō′jē-ă fan-tas′tik-ă) A fantastic account of a patient's exploits, which the patient appears to believe.

pseu•do•lym•pho•ma (sū′dō-lim-fō′mă) A benign infiltration of lymphoid cells or histiocytes that microscopically resembles a malignant lymphoma.

pseu•do•ma•lig•nan•cy (sū′dō-mă-lig′năn-sē) A benign tumor that appears, clinically or histologically, to be a malignant neoplasm. SEE ALSO pseudotumor.

pseu•do•ma•ni•a (sū′dō-mā′nē-ă) **1.** A factitious mental disorder. **2.** A mental disorder in which the patient falsely claims to have committed a crime. **3.** Generally, the morbid impulse to falsify or lie, as in pseudologia.

pseu•do•mem•brane (sū′dō-mem′brān) SYN false membrane.

pseu•do•mem•bra•nous (sū′dō-mem′bră-nŭs) Relating to or marked by the presence of a false membrane.

pseu•do•mem•bra•nous bron•chi•tis (sū′dō-mem′bră-nŭs brong-kī′tis) SYN fibrinous bronchitis.

pseu•do•mem•bra•nous co•li•tis (sū′dō-mem′bră-nŭs kō-lī′tis) SYN pseudomembranous enterocolitis.

pseu•do•mem•bra•nous en•ter•i•tis (sū′dō-mem′bră-nŭs en′tĕr-ī′tis) SYN pseudomembranous enterocolitis.

pseu•do•mem•bra•nous en•ter•o•co•li•tis (sū′dō-mem′bră-nŭs en′tĕr-ō-kō-lī′tis) Intestinal inflammation with the formation and passage of pseudomembranous material, due to infection by *Clostridium difficile;* it is commonly a sequel to prolonged antibiotic therapy. SYN pseudomembranous colitis, pseudomembranous enteritis.

pseu•do•mem•bra•nous gas•tri•tis (sū′dō-mem′bră-nŭs gas-trī′tis) Gastritis characterized by the formation of a false membrane.

pseu•do•mem•bra•nous in•flam•ma•tion (sū′dō-mem′bră-nŭs in′flă-mā′shŭn) A form of exudative inflammation that involves mucous and serous membranes; large quantities of fibrin in the exudate result in a tenacious membrane-like covering that is adherent to the underlying acutely inflamed tissue.

pseu•do•men•stru•a•tion (sū′dō-men′strū-ā′shŭn) Blood-tinged mucoid vaginal discharge occurring during the first week of life as a result of the withdrawal of maternal estrogen.

pseu•do•mo•nad (sū′dō-mō′nad) A vernacular term used to refer to any member of the genus *Pseudomonas.*

i ***Pseu•do•mo•nas*** (sū′dō-mō′nas) A genus of motile, polar-flagellate, non-spore-forming, strictly aerobic bacteria (family Pseudomonadaceae) containing gram-negative rods that occur singly. The metabolism is oxidative. They occur commonly in soil and in fresh-water and marine environments. Some species are plant pathogens. Others are involved in human infections. The type species is *P. aeruginosa.* See page B4. [pseudo- + G. *monas,* unit, monad]

Pseu•do•mo•nas mal•le•i (sū′dō-mō′nas mal′ē-ī) SYN *Burkholderia mallei.*

***Pseu•do•mo•nas* os•te•o•my•e•li•tis** (sū′dō-mō′nas os′tē-ō-mī-ĕ-lī′tis) SYN malignant external otitis.

pseu•do•mo•nil•e•thrix (sū′dō-mō-nil′ĕ-thriks) A nodal trichodystrophy similar to monilethrix but with fractures within the nodal swellings; autosomal dominant inheritance with late onset.

pseu•do•myx•o•ma (sū′dō-miks-ō′mă) A gelatinous mass resembling a myxoma but composed of epithelial mucus.

pseu•do•myx•o•ma pe•ri•to•ne•i (sū′dō-miks-ō′mă per′i-tō′nē-ī) The accumulation of large quantities of mucoid or mucinous material in the peritoneal cavity, either as a result of rupture of a mucocele of the appendix or rupture of benign or malignant cystic neoplasms of the ovary.

pseu•do•ne•o•plasm (sū′dō-nē′ō-plazm) SYN pseudotumor.

pseu•do•os•te•o•ma•la•cic pel•vis (sū′dō-os′tē-ō-mă-lā′sik pel′vis) An extreme degree of rachitic pelvis, resembling the puerperal osteomalacic pelvis, in which the pelvic canal is obstructed by a forward projection of the sacrum, and an approximation of the acetabula.

pseu•do•pap•il•le•de•ma (sū′dō-pap′il-ĕ-dē′mă) Anomalous elevation of the optic disc; seen in severe hyperopia and optic nerve drusen. SYN pseudopapilloedema.

pseudopapilloedema [Br.] SYN pseudopapilledema.

pseu•do•pa•ral•y•sis (sū′dō-păr-al′i-sis) Apparent paralysis due to voluntary inhibition of motion because of pain, to incoordination, or other cause, but without actual paralysis. SYN pseudoparesis (1).

pseu•do•par•a•ple•gi•a (sū′dō-par-ă-plē′jē-ă) Apparent paralysis in the lower extremities, in which the tendon and skin reflexes and the electrical reactions are normal; the condition is sometimes observed in rickets.

pseu•do•pa•re•sis (sū′dō-păr-ē′sis) **1.** SYN pseudoparalysis. **2.** A condition marked by the pupillary changes, tremors, and speech disturbances suggestive of early paresis, in which, however, the serologic test results are negative.

pseu•do•par•kin•son•ism (sū′dō-pahr′kin-sŏn-izm) Side effect of drugs that causes symptoms resembling Parkinson disease such as tremor, masklike facies, drooling, rigidity, and stiff gait.

pseu•do•pe•lade (sū′dō-pĕ-lahd′) A scarring type of alopecia; usually occurs in scattered, irregular patches; of uncertain cause. See this page. [pseudo- + Fr. *pelade,* disease that causes sporadic falling of hair]

pseu•do•plate•let (sū′dō-plāt′lĕt) Any of the fragments of neutrophils that may be mistaken for platelets, especially in peripheral blood smears of leukemic patients.

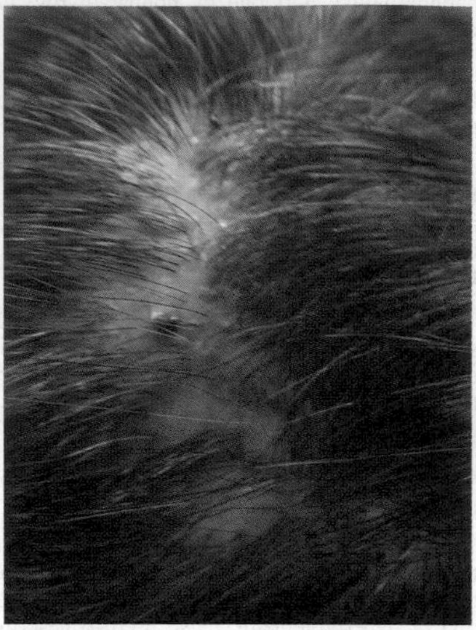

pseudopelade

pseu•do•pod (sū′dō-pod) SYN pseudopodium.

pseu•do•po•di•um, pl. **pseu•do•po•di•a** (sū′dō-pō′dē-ŭm, -pō′dē-ă) A temporary protoplasmic process, put forth by an ameboid stage or amebic protozoan for locomotion or for prehension of food. SYN pseudopod. [pseudo- + G. *pous,* foot]

pseu•do•pol•yp (sū′dō-pol′ip) A projecting mass of granulation tissue, large numbers of which may develop in ulcerative colitis; may become covered by regenerating epithelium.

pseu•do•preg•nan•cy (sū′dō-preg′năn-sē) **1.** SYN false pregnancy. **2.** A condition in which symptoms resembling those of pregnancy are present, but which is not pregnancy.

pseu•do•pte•ryg•i•um (sū′dō-tĕr-ij′ē-ŭm) Adhesion of the conjunctiva to the cornea, occurring after injury.

pseu•dop•to•sis (sū′dō-tō′sis) A condition resembling an inability to elevate the eyelid, due to blepharophimosis, blepharochalasis, or some other affliction. SYN false blepharoptosis. [pseudo- + G. *ptōsis,* a falling]

pseu•do•re•ac•tion (sū′dō-rē-ak′shŭn) A false reaction; one not due to specific causes in a given test.

pseu•do•rick•ets (sū′dō-rik′ĕts) SYN renal rickets.

pseu•do•ro•sette (sū′dō-rō-zet′) Perivascular radial arrangement of neoplastic cells around a small blood vessel. SEE ALSO rosette (2).

pseu•do•scar•la•ti•na (sū′dō-skahr′lă-tē′nă)

Erythema with fever, due to causes other than *Streptococcus pyogenes*.

pseu•dos•mi•a (sū-doz′mē-ă) Subjective sensation of an odor that is not present. [pseudo- + G. *osmē,* smell]

pseu•do•stra•bis•mus (sū′dō-stră-biz′mŭs) The appearance of strabismus when the eyes are straight, caused by epicanthal folds, abnormality in interorbital distance, or corneal light reflex not corresponding to the center of the pupil. [pseudo- + G. *strabismos,* a squinting]

pseu•do•strat•i•fied ep•i•the•li•um (sū′dō-strat′i-fīd ep′i-thē′lē-ŭm) An epithelium that gives a superficial appearance of being stratified because the cell nuclei are at different levels, but in which all cells reach the basement membrane.

pseu•do•tu•mor (sū′dō-tū′mŏr) A condition, commonly associated with obesity in young females, of cerebral edema with narrowed small ventricles but with increased intracranial pressure and frequently papilledema. SYN pseudoneoplasm, pseudotumour.

pseu•do•tu•mor cer•e•bri (sū′dō-tū′mĕr ser′ĕ-brī) A condition, commonly associated with obesity in young women, of cerebral edema with narrowed small ventricles but with increased intracranial pressure and frequently papilledema.

pseudotumour [Br.] SYN pseudotumor.

pseu•do•u•ri•dine (Ψ, Q) (sū′dō-yŭr′i-dēn) A naturally occurring isomer of uridine found in transfer ribonucleic acids; unique in that the ribosyl is attached to carbon (C-5) rather than to nitrogen; excreted in urine.

pseu•do•xan•tho•ma elas•ti•cum (sū′dō-zan-thō′mă ē-las′ti-kum) An inherited disorder of connective tissue characterized by yellowish plaques on the neck, axillae, abdomen, and thighs, associated with angioid streaks of the retina and similar elastic tissue degeneration and calcification in arteries.

psi (sī) **1.** The 23rd letter of the Greek alphabet (ψ). **2.** Abbreviation for pseudouridine; pseudo-; psychology. wave function; the dihedral angle of rotation about the C_1–C_α bond associated with a peptide bond. **3.** Wave function; the dihedral angle of rotation about the C_1–C_α bond associated with a peptide bond.

psi Abbreviation for pounds per square inch.

P sin•is•tro•car•di•a•le (sin-is′trō-kahr-dē-ā′lē) SYN P mitrale.

psi phe•nom•e•non (sī fĕ-nom′ĕ-non) A phenomenon that includes both psychokinesis and extrasensory perception; the extrasensory mental processes involved in the alleged ability to send or receive telepathic messages.

PSIS Abbreviation for posterior superior iliac spine.

psit•ta•co•sis (sit′ă-kō′sis) An infectious disease in psittacine birds and humans caused by the bacterium *Chlamydia psittaci*. Avian infections are mainly inapparent or latent, although acute disease does occur; human infections may result in mild disease with a flulike syndrome or in severe disease, with symptoms of bronchopneumonia. SYN ornithosis, Parrot disease (3), parrot fever. [G. *psittakos,* a parrot, + *-osis,* condition]

pso•as ab•scess (sō′as ab′ses) An abscess, usually tuberculous, originating in tuberculous spondylitis and extending through the iliopsoas muscle to the inguinal region.

pso•as ma•jor mus•cle (sō′as mā′jŏr mŭs′ĕl) Groin muscle; *origin*, bodies of vertebrae and intervertebral discs from twelfth thoracic to fifth lumbar, and transverse processes of lumbar vertebrae; *insertion*, forms common insertion with iliacus muscle into lesser trochanter of femur; *action*, primary flexor of hip joint; *nerve supply*, lumbar plexus (ventral rami of first, second, and usually third lumbar spinal nerves). SYN greater psoas muscle, musculus psoas major.

pso•as mi•nor mus•cle (sō′as mī′nŏr mŭs′ĕl) An inconstant muscle, absent in about 40%; *origin*, bodies of twelfth thoracic and first lumbar vertebrae and disc between them; *insertion*, iliopubic eminence through iliopectineal arch (iliac fascia); *action*, assists in flexion of lumbar spine; *nerve supply*, lumbar plexus. SYN musculus psoas minor, smaller psoas muscle.

pso•rel•co•sis (sōr′el-kō′sis) Cutaneous ulceration resulting from scabies. [G. *psōra,* itch, + *helkōsis,* ulceration]

pso•ri•a•sic (sōr′ē-as′ik) SYN psoriatic.

pso•ri•a•si•form (sōr-ī′ă-si-fōrm) Resembling psoriasis.

pso•ri•a•sis (sōr-ī′ă-sis) A common inherited condition characterized by the eruption of reddish, silvery-scaled maculopapules, predominantly on the elbows, knees, scalp, and trunk. See page 1290. [G. *psōriasis,* fr. *psōra,* the itch]

pso•ri•at•ic (sōr′ē-at′ik) Relating to psoriasis. SYN psoriasic.

pso•ri•at•ic ar•thri•tis (sōr′ē-at′ik ahr-thrī′tis) The concurrence of psoriasis and polyarthritis, resembling rheumatoid arthritis but thought to be a specific disease entity, seronegative for rheumatoid factor, and often involving the digits. See page 1291. SYN arthropathia psoriatica.

PSR Abbreviation for Periodontal Screening Record; Periodontal Screening and Recording.

PSV Abbreviation for pressure support ventilation.

psy•chal•gi•a (sī-kal′jē-ă) **1.** Distress attending a mental effort, noted especially in melancholia.

SYN phrenalgia (1). **2.** SYN psychogenic pain. [psych- + G. *algos,* pain]

psy·cha·tax·i·a (sī′kă-tak′sē-ă) Mental confusion; inability to fix one's attention or to make any continued mental effort. [psych- + G. *ataxia,* confusion]

psy·che (sī′kē) Term for the subjective aspects of the mind, self, soul; the psychological or spiritual as distinct from the bodily nature of people. [G. mind, soul]

psy·che·del·ic (sī′kĕ-del′ik) **1.** Pertaining to a category of drugs with mainly central nervous system action, said to be the expansion or heightening of consciousness (e.g., LSD, hashish, mescaline). **2.** A hallucinogenic substance, visual display, music, or other sensory stimulus having such action. SYN hallucinogenic. [psyche- + G. *dēloō,* to manifest]

psy·chi·at·ric (sī′kē-at′rik) Relating to psychiatry.

psy·chi·a·tric re·hab·i·li·ta·tion (sī′kē-at′rik rē′hă-bil′i-tā′shŭn) Service and support provided, with limited professional intervention, to people with long-term psychiatric disabilities to assist them in the performance of self-directed, self-satisfying functional life tasks.

psy·chi·a·trist (sī-kī′ă-trist) A physician who specializes in treatment of mental disorders.

psy·chi·a·try (sī-kī′ă-trē) The medical specialty concerned with the diagnosis and treatment of mental disorders. [psych- + G. *iatreia,* medical treatment]

psy·chic (sī′kik) **1.** Relating to the phenomena of consciousness, mind, or soul. **2.** A person supposedly endowed with the power of communicating with spirits. [G. *psychikos*]

psy·chic trau·ma (sī′kik traw′mă) An upsetting experience precipitating or aggravating an emotional or mental disorder.

psycho-, psych-, psyche- Combining forms denoting the mind; mental; psychological. [G. *psychē,* soul, mind]

psy·cho·ac·tive (sī′kō-ak′tiv) Possessing the ability to alter mood, anxiety, behavior, cognitive processes, or mental tension; usually applied to pharmacologic agents.

psy·cho·a·nal·y·sis (sī′kō-ă-nal′i-sis) **1.** A method of psychotherapy, originated by Sigmund Freud, designed to bring preconscious and unconscious material to consciousness primarily through the analysis of transference and resis-

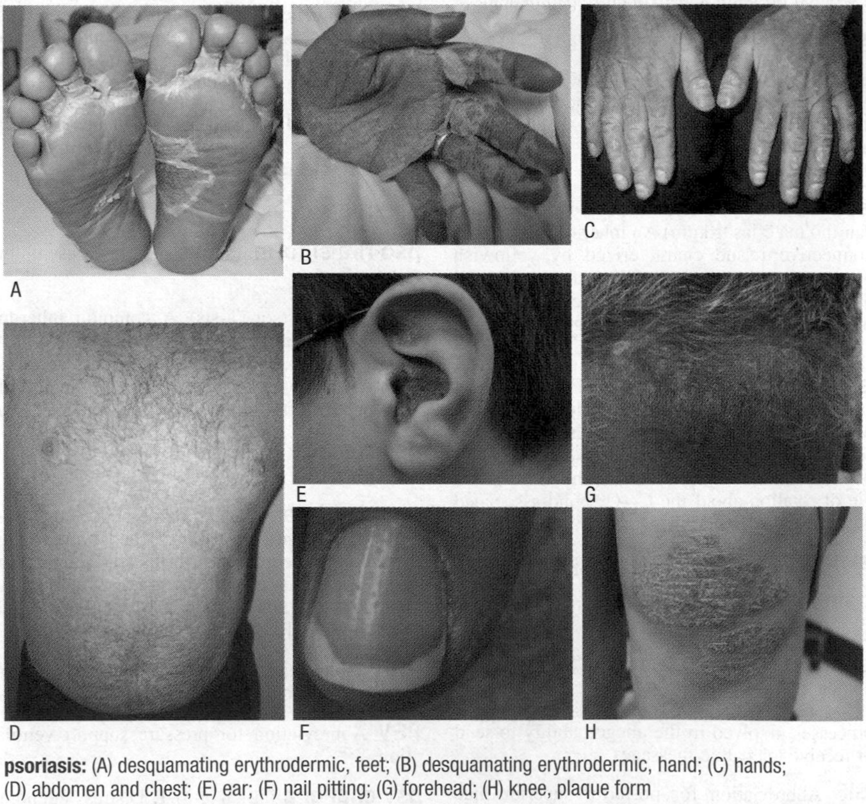

psoriasis: (A) desquamating erythrodermic, feet; (B) desquamating erythrodermic, hand; (C) hands; (D) abdomen and chest; (E) ear; (F) nail pitting; (G) forehead; (H) knee, plaque form

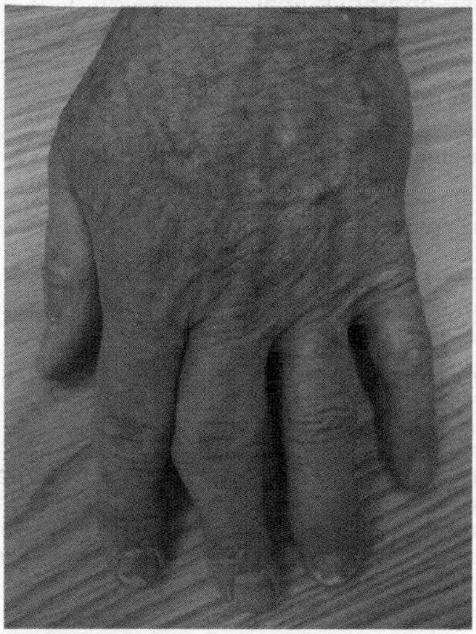

psoriatic arthritis: hand

tance. SYN psychoanalytic therapy. SEE ALSO freudian psychoanalysis. **2.** A method of investigating the total mental life, conscious and unconscious, of a person with a mental disorder, employing interpretation of resistance and transference, free association, and dream analysis. **3.** An integrated body of observations and theories on personality development, motivation, and behavior. **4.** A school of psychotherapy, as in jungian or freudian psychoanalysis. [psycho- + analysis]

psy•cho•an•a•lyst (sī'kō-an'ă-list) A psychotherapist, usually a psychiatrist or clinical psychologist, trained in psychoanalysis and employing its methods in the treatment of emotional disorders.

psy•cho•an•a•lyt•ic (sī'kō-an'ă-lit'ik) Pertaining to psychoanalysis.

psy•cho•an•a•lyt•ic psy•chi•a•try (sī'kō-an'ă-lit'ik sī-kī'ă-trē) Psychiatric theory and practice emphasizing the principles of psychoanalysis. SYN dynamic psychiatry.

psy•cho•an•a•lyt•ic ther•a•py (sī'kō-an'ă-lit'ik thār'ă-pē) SYN psychoanalysis (1).

psy•cho•bi•ol•o•gy (sī'kō-bī-ol'ŏ-jē) The study of the interrelationships of biology and psychology in cognitive functioning, including intellectual, memory, and related neurocognitive processes.

psy•cho•di•ag•no•sis (sī'kō-dī'ăg-nō'sis) **1.** Any method used to discover the factors that underlie behavior, especially maladjusted or abnormal behavior. **2.** A subspecialty within clinical psychology that emphasizes the use of psychological tests and techniques for assessing psychopathology.

psy•cho•dra•ma (sī'kō-drah'mă) A method of psychotherapy in which patients act out their personal problems by spontaneously enacting without rehearsal diagnostically specific roles in dramatic performances put on before their patient peers.

psy•cho•dy•nam•ics (sī'kō-dī-nam'iks) The systematized study and theory of the psychological forces that underlie human behavior, emphasizing the interplay between unconscious and conscious motivation and the functional significance of emotion. SEE ALSO role-playing. [psycho- + G. *dynamis,* force]

psy•cho•gen•e•sis (sī'kō-jen'ĕ-sis) The origin and development of the psychic processes, including mental, behavioral, emotional, personality, and related psychological processes. [psycho- + G. *genesis,* origin]

psy•cho•gen•ic, **psy•cho•ge•net•ic** (sī'kō-jen'ik, -jĕ-net'ik) **1.** Of mental origin or causation. **2.** Relating to emotional and related psychological development or to psychogenesis.

psy•cho•gen•ic deaf•ness (sī'kō-jen'ik def'nĕs) Hearing loss without evidence of organic cause or malingering; often follows severe psychic shock. SYN functional deafness.

psy•cho•gen•ic pain (sī'kō-jen'ik pān) Somatoform pain; pain that is associated or correlated with a psychological, emotional, or behavioral stimulus. SYN psychalgia (2).

psy•cho•gen•ic pain dis•or•der (sī'kō-jen'ik pān dis-ōr'dĕr) A disorder in which the principal complaint is pain that is out of proportion to objective findings and that is related to psychological factors.

psy•cho•gen•ic vom•it•ing (sī'kō-jen'ik vom'it-ing) Emesis associated with emotional distress and anxiety.

psy•cho•ki•ne•sis, **psy•cho•ki•ne•si•a** (sī'kō-ki-nē'sis, -nē'zē-ă) **1.** The influence of mind on matter, as the use of mental "power" to move or distort an object. **2.** Impulsive behavior. [psycho- + G. *kinēsis,* movement]

psy•cho•lin•gui•stics (sī'kō-ling-gwis'tiks) Study of a host of psychological factors associated with speech, including voice, attitudes, emotions, and grammatical rules, that affect communication and understanding of language. [psycho- + L. *lingua,* tongue]

psy•cho•log•ical (sī'kō-loj'ik-ăl) **1.** Relating to psychology. **2.** Relating to the mind and its processes. SEE ALSO psychology.

psy•chol•o•gist (sī-kol'ŏ-jist) A specialist in psychology licensed to practice professional psychology (e.g., clinical psychologist), or qualified to teach psychology as a scholarly discipline (academic psychologist), or whose scientific specialty is a subfield of psychology (research psychologist).

psy·chol·o·gy (sī-kol′ŏ-jē) Study of the behavior of humans and animals, and related mental and physiologic processes. [psycho- + G. *logos,* study]

psy·cho·met·ric prop·er·ties (sī′kō-met′rik prop′ĕr-tēz) Quantifiable attributes (e.g., validity, reliability) that relate to the statistical strength or weakness of a test or measurement. SEE ALSO reliability, validity.

psy·cho·met·rics (sī′kō-met′riks) SYN psychometry.

psy·chom·e·try (sī′kom′ĕ-trē) The discipline pertaining to psychological and mental testing, and to any quantitative analysis of a person's psychological traits or attitudes or mental processes. SYN psychometrics. [psycho- + G. *metron,* measure]

psy·cho·mo·tor (sī′kō-mō′tŏr) **1.** Relating to the psychological processes associated with muscular movement, and to the production of voluntary movements. **2.** Relating to the combination of psychic and motor events, including disturbances. [psycho- + L. *motor,* mover]

psy·cho·mo·tor ep·i·lep·sy (sī′kō-mō′tŏr ep′i-lep′sē) Attacks with elaborate and multiple sensory, motor, and psychic components, the common feature being a clouding or loss of consciousness and amnesia for the event; clinical manifestations may take the form of automatisms, emotional outbursts, or motor or psychic disturbances. SEE ALSO procursive epilepsy. SYN psychomotor seizure.

psy·cho·mo·tor sei·zure (sī′kō-mō′tŏr sē′zhŭr) SYN psychomotor epilepsy.

psy·cho·neu·ro·sis (sī′kō-nūr-ō′sis) SYN neurosis.

psy·cho·neu·rot·ic (sī′kō-nūr-ot′ik) Pertaining to or suffering from psychoneurosis.

psy·cho·path (sī′kō-path) Former designation for a person with an antisocial type of personality disorder. SEE ALSO antisocial personality disorder, sociopath. [psycho- + G. *pathos*, disease]

psy·cho·path·ic (sī′kō-path′ik) Relating to or characteristic of psychopathy.

psy·cho·pa·thol·o·gy (sī′kō-pă-thol′ŏ-jē) **1.** The science concerned with the pathology of the mind and behavior. **2.** The science of mental and behavioral disorders, including psychiatry and abnormal psychology. [psycho- + G. *pathos,* disease, + *logos,* study]

psy·cho·phar·ma·ceu·ti·cals (sī′kō-fahr′mă-sū′ti-kălz) Drugs used in the treatment of emotional disorders.

psy·cho·phar·ma·col·o·gy (sī′kō-fahr′mă-kol′ŏ-jē) **1.** The use of drugs to treat mental and psychological disorders. **2.** The science of drug-behavior relationships. [psycho- + G. *pharmakon,* drug, + *logos,* study]

psy·cho·phys·i·cal (sī′kō-fiz′i-kăl) **1.** Relating to the mental perception of physical stimuli. SEE ALSO psychophysics. **2.** SYN psychosomatic.

psy·cho·phys·ics (sī′kō-fiz′iks) The science of the relation between the physical attributes of a stimulus and the measured, quantitative attributes of the mental perception of that stimulus.

psy·cho·phys·i·o·log·ic (sī′kō-fiz′ē-ō-loj′ik) **1.** Pertaining to psychophysiology. **2.** Denoting a psychosomatic illness. **3.** Denoting a somatic disorder with significant emotional or psychological etiology.

psy·cho·phys·i·ol·o·gy (sī′kō-fiz′ē-ol′ŏ-jē) The science of the relationship between psychological and physiologic processes.

psy·cho·sen·so·ry, **psy·cho·sen·so·ri·al** (sī′kō-sen′sŏr-ē, -sen-sŏr′ē-ăl) **1.** Denoting the mental perception and interpretation of sensory stimuli. **2.** Denoting a hallucination that, with effort, the mind is able to distinguish from reality.

psy·cho·sex·u·al (sī′kō-sek′shū-ăl) Pertaining to relationships among the emotional, mental, physiologic, and behavioral components of sex or sexual development.

psy·cho·sex·u·al de·vel·op·ment (sī′kō-sek′shū-ăl dĕ-vel′ŏp-mĕnt) Maturation and development of the psychic and behavioral phases of sexuality from birth to adult life through the oral, anal, phallic, latency, and genital phases.

psy·cho·sex·u·al dys·func·tion, **sex·u·al dys·func·tion** (sī′kō-sek′shū-ăl dis-fŭngk′shŭn, sek′shū-ăl) A disturbance in sexual function (e.g., impotence, premature ejaculation, anorgasmia) presumed to be from psychological rather than physical causes.

psy·cho·sis, pl. **psy·cho·ses** (sī-kō′sis, -sēz) **1.** A mental and behavioral disorder causing gross distortion or disorganization of a person's mental capacity, affective response, and capacity to recognize reality, communicate, and relate to others to the degree of interfering with the person's capacity to cope with the ordinary demands of everyday life. **2.** Generic term for any of the major mental disorders, the most common forms being the schizophrenias. **3.** A severe emotional and behavioral disorder. SYN psychotic disorder. [G. an animating]

psy·cho·so·cial (sī′kō-sō′shăl) Involving both psychological and social aspects, e.g., age, education, marital history.

psy·cho·so·mat·ic (sī′kō-sō-mat′ik) Pertaining to the influence of the mind or higher functions of the brain (emotions, fears, desires) on the functions of the body, especially in relation to bodily disorders or disease. SEE ALSO psychophysiologic. SYN psychophysical (2). [psycho- + G. *sōma,* body]

psy·cho·so·mat·ic dis·or·der, **psy·cho·**

phys•i•o•log•ic dis•or•der (sī′kō-sō-mat′ik dis-ōr′dĕr, sī′kō-fiz′ē-ō-loj′ik dis-ōr′dĕr) A disorder characterized by physical symptoms of psychic origin, usually involving a single organ system innervated by the autonomic nervous system; physiologic and organic changes stem from a sustained disturbance.

psy•cho•so•mat•ic med•i•cine (sī′kō-sō-mat′ik med′i-sin) The study and treatment of diseases, disorders, or abnormal states in which psychological processes resulting in physiologic reactions are believed to play a prominent role.

psy•cho•so•mi•met•ic (sī′kō-sō-mi-met′ik) SYN psychotomimetic.

psy•cho•stim•u•lant (sī′kō-stim′yū-lănt) An pharmacotherapeutic agent with antidepressant or mood-elevating properties.

psy•cho•sur•ger•y (sī′kō-sŭr′jĕr-ē) The treatment of mental disorders by surgery on the brain (e.g., lobotomy).

psy•cho•ther•a•peu•tics (sī′kō-thār′ă-pyū′tiks) SYN psychotherapy.

psy•cho•ther•a•pist (sī′kō-thār′ă-pist) A person, usually a psychiatrist or clinical psychologist, professionally trained and engaged in psychotherapy. Currently, the term is also applied to social workers, nurses, and others whose state licensing practice acts include psychotherapy.

psy•cho•ther•a•py (sī′kō-thār′ă-pē) Treatment of emotional, behavioral, personality, and psychiatric disorders based primarily on verbal or nonverbal communication and interventions with the patient, in contrast to treatments using chemical and physical measures. SEE ALSO psychoanalysis, psychiatry, psychology, therapy. SYN psychotherapeutics. [psycho- + G. *therapeia,* treatment]

psy•chot•ic (sī-kot′ik) Relating to or affected by psychosis.

psy•chot•ic dis•or•der (sī-kot′ik dis-ōr′dĕr) SYN psychosis.

psy•chot•o•gen•ic (sī-kot′ō-jen′ik) Little-used term meaning capable of inducing psychosis; particularly in reference to drugs of the LSD series and similar substances.

psy•chot•o•mi•met•ic (sī-kot′ō-mi-met′ik) **1.** A drug or substance that produces psychological and behavioral changes resembling those of psychosis (e.g., LSD). **2.** Denoting such a drug or substance. SYN psychosomimetic. [psychosis + G. *mimetikos*, imitative]

psy•cho•tro•pic (sī′kō-trō′pik) Capable of affecting the mind, emotions, and behavior; denoting drugs used in the treatment of mental illnesses. [psycho- + G. *tropē,* a turning]

♻ **psychro-** Combining form denoting cold. SEE ALSO cryo-, crymo-. [G. *psychros*]

psy•chro•al•gi•a (sī′krō-al′jē-ă) A painful sensation of cold. [psychro- + G. *algos,* pain]

psy•chrom•e•try (sī-krom′ĕ-trē) The calculation of relative humidity and water vapor pressures from wet and dry bulb temperatures and barometric pressure; whereas relative humidity is the value ordinarily employed, the vapor pressure is the measurement of physiologic significance. SYN hygrometry. [psychro- + G. *metron,* measure]

psy•chro•phile, **psy•chro•phil** (sī′krō-fīl, -fil) An organism that grows best at a low temperature (0–32°C; 32–86°F), with optimal growth occurring at 15–20°C (59–68°F). [psychro- + G. *phileō,* to love]

psy•chro•phil•ic (sī′krō-fil′ik) Pertaining to a psychrophile. [psychro- + G. *phileō,* to love]

psy•chro•phore (sī′krō-fōr) A double catheter through which cold water is circulated to apply cold to the urethra or another canal or cavity. [psychro- + G. *phoros,* bearing]

psyl•li•um (sil′ē-ŭm) The husk of the psyllium seed that is used to relieve constipation and treat some other GI problems.

PT Abbreviation for physical therapy or physical therapist; prothrombin time; proficiency testing.

Pt Symbol for platinum.

PTA Abbreviation for plasma thromboplastin antecedent; phosphotungstic acid; percutaneous transluminal angioplasty; physical therapist assistant.

PTAH Abbreviation for phosphotungstic acid hematoxylin.

PT as•sis•tant (ă-sis′tănt) Abbreviation for physical therapist assistant.

PTC Abbreviation for plasma thromboplastin component.

♻ **pter-**, **ptero-** Combining forms denoting wing; feather. [G. *pteron,* wing, feather]

pte•ri•on (tĕr′ē-on) [TA] A craniometric point in the region of the sphenoid fontanelle, at the junction of the greater wing of the sphenoid, the squamous portion of the temporal, the frontal, and the parietal bones; it intersects the course of the anterior division of the middle meningeal artery. [G. *pteron,* wing]

pte•ryg•i•um (tĕr-ij′ē-ŭm) **1.** A triangular patch of hypertrophied bulbar subconjunctival tissue, extending from the medial canthus to the border of the cornea or beyond, with its apex pointing toward the pupil. **2.** Forward growth of the cuticle over the nail plate, seen most commonly in lichen planus. **3.** An abnormal skin web. [G. *pterygion,* anything like a wing, a disease of the eye, dim. of *pteryx,* wing]

♻ **pterygo-** Prefix meaning wing-shaped, usually

relating to the pterygoid process. [G. *pteryx, pterygos,* wing]

pter·y·goid (ter′i-goyd) Wing-shaped; resembling a wing; a term applied to various anatomic parts relating to the sphenoid bone. [G. *pteryx* (*pteryg-*), wing, + *eidos,* resemblance]

pter·y·goid ca·nal (ter′i-goyd kă-nal′) An opening through the base of the medial pterygoid process of the sphenoid bone through which pass the artery, vein, and nerve of the pterygoid canal. SYN canalis pterygoideus [TA].

pter·y·goid nerve (ter′i-goyd nĕrv) One of two motor branches, lateral and medial, of the mandibular nerve, supplying the lateral and medial pterygoid muscles with fibers of the motor root of the trigeminal nerve. SYN nervus pterygoideus [TA].

pter·y·goid pro·cess (ter′i-goyd pros′es) A long process extending downward from the junction of the body and greater wing of the sphenoid bone on either side; it is formed of two plates (lateral and medial), united anteriorly but separated below to form the pterygoid notch; the pterygoid fossa is formed by the divergence of these two plates posteriorly.

pter·y·go·man·dib·u·lar (ter′i-gō-man-dib′yū-lăr) Relating to the pterygoid process and the mandible.

pter·y·go·max·il·lar·y (ter′i-gō-mak′si-lar-ē) Relating to the pterygoid process and the maxilla.

pte·ry·go·men·in·ge·al ar·ter·y (ter′i-gō-mĕ-nin′jē-ăl ahr′tĕr-ē) *Origin:* maxillary or middle meningeal artery; *distribution:* traverses foramen ovale to enter cranial cavity, where it supplies the trigeminal ganglion, dura mater, and bone of the floor of the middle cranial fossa; however, its main distribution is extracranially to the pterygoid and tensor tympani muscles, the sphenoid bone, the mandibular nerve and the otic ganglion. SYN arteria pterygomeningealis [TA].

pter·y·go·pal·a·tine (ter′i-gō-pal′ă-tīn) Relating to the pterygoid process and the palatine bone.

pter·y·go·pal·a·tine ca·nal (ter′i-gō-pal′ă-tīn kă-nal′) SYN greater palatine canal.

pter·y·go·pal·a·tine gan·gli·on (ter′i-gō-pal′ă-tīn gang′glē-ŏn) A small parasympathetic ganglion in the upper part of the pterygopalatine fossa with postsynaptic fibers supplying the lacrimal, nasal, palatine, and pharyngeal glands.

PTH Abbreviation for parathyroid hormone.

PTHC Abbreviation for percutaneous transhepatic cholangiography.

i ***Pthir·us*** (thir′ŭs) A genus of lice formerly grouped in the genus *Pediculus*. The main species is *P. pubis*, the crab or pubic louse, a parasite that infests the pubes and adjacent hairy parts of the body. USAGE NOTE Often incorrectly spelled *Phthirus* or *Phthirius*. See page B8. [irreg. fr. G. *phtheir*, louse]

PTHrP Abbreviation for parathyroid hormone-related peptide.

PTI Abbreviation for pressure time index.

PTK Abbreviation for phototherapeutic keratectomy.

pto·maine (tō′mān) An indefinite term applied to poisonous substances (e.g., toxic amines) formed in the decomposition of protein by the decarboxylation of amino acids by bacterial action. [G. *ptōma,* a corpse]

ptosed (tōzd) SYN ptotic.

pto·sis, pl. **pto·ses** (tō′sis, -sēz) **1.** A sinking down or prolapse of an organ. **2.** SYN blepharoptosis. [G. *ptōsis,* a falling]

♻ **-ptosis** Suffix meaning a sinking down or prolapse of an organ. [G. *ptōsis,* a falling]

pto·tic (tot′ik) Relating to or marked by ptosis. SYN ptosed.

PTSD Abbreviation for posttraumatic stress disorder.

PTT Abbreviation for partial thromboplastin time.

pty·a·lec·ta·sis (tī′ă-lek′tă-sis) SYN sialectasis. [ptyal- + G. *ektasis,* a stretching out]

pty·a·lism (tī′ăl-izm) SYN sialism. [G. *ptyalismos,* spitting]

pty·a·lo·cele (tī′ă-lō-sēl) SYN ranula (2).

Pu Symbol for plutonium.

pu·bar·che (pyū-bahr′kē) Onset of puberty, particularly as manifested by the growth of pubic hair. [puberty + G. *archē*, beginning]

pu·ber·al, **pu·ber·tal** (pyū′bĕr-ăl, -bĕr-tăl) Relating to puberty.

pu·ber·pho·ni·a (pyū′bĕr-fō′nē-ă) SYN mutational falsetto.

pu·ber·ty (pyu′bĕr-tē) Sequence of events by which a child becomes a young adult, characterized by the beginning of gametogenesis, secretion of gonadal hormones, and development of secondary sexual characteristics and reproductive functions; sexual dimorphism is accentuated. In girls, the first signs of puberty may be evident at age 8 years with the process largely completed by age 16 years; in boys, puberty commonly begins at ages 10–12 years and is largely completed by age 18 years. Ethnic and geographic factors may influence the time at which various events typical of puberty occur. [L. *pubertas,* fr. *puber,* grown up]

pu·bes (pyū′bēz) **1.** [TA] The area above the external genitals where hair growth signals puberty. **2.** One of the pubic hairs; the hair of the pubic region. USAGE NOTE Often incorrectly called pubis. [L. *pubes,* the hair on the genitals; the genitals]

pu•bes•cence (pyū-bes′ĕns) The approach of the age of puberty or sexual maturity. [L. *pubesco,* to attain puberty]

pu•bes•cent (pyū-bes′ĕnt) Pertaining to pubescence.

pu•bic (pyū′bik) Relating to the pubes or to the pubic bone.

pu•bic an•gle (pyū′bik ang′gĕl) SYN subpubic angle.

pu•bic arch (pyū′bik ahrch) The arch formed by the symphysis and the bodies and inferior rami of the pubic bones. SEE ALSO subpubic angle.

pu•bic bone (pyū′bik bōn) The anteroinferior portion of the hip bone, distinct at birth but later becoming fused with the ilium and ischium; it consists of a body, which articulates with its fellow at the pubic symphysis, and two rami; the superior ramus enters into the formation of the acetabulum, and the inferior ramus fuses with the ramus of the ischium to form the ischiopubic ramus. See this page.

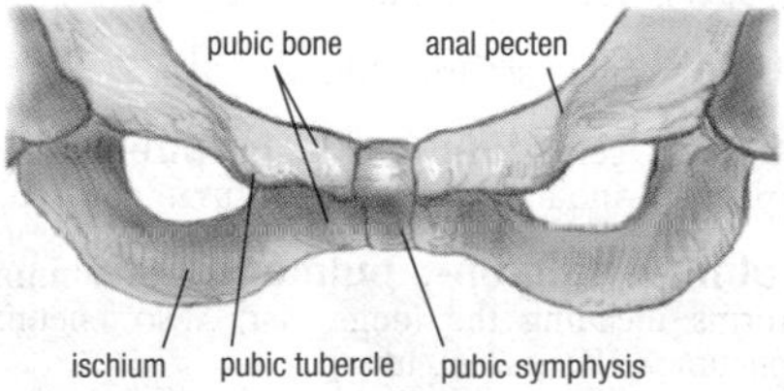

pubic bone

pu•bic crest (pyū′bik krest) The rough anterior border of the body of the pubis, continuous laterally with the pubic tubercle.

pu•bic re•gion (pyū′bik rē′jŭn) The lower central region of the abdomen below the umbilical region.

pu•bic sym•phy•sis (pyū′bik sim′fi-sis) The firm, fibrocartilaginous joint between the two pubic bones. SYN symphysis pubis.

pu•bic tu•ber•cle (pyū′bik tū′bĕr-kĕl) A small palpable projection at the anterior extremity of the crest of the pubis about 2 cm from the symphysis; site of insertion of the inguinal ligament.

pu•bi•ot•o•my (pyū′bē-ot′ŏ-mē) Severance of the pubic bone a few centimeters lateral to the symphysis, to increase the capacity of a contracted pelvis sufficiently to permit the passage of a living child. SYN pelviotomy (2), pelvitomy. [L. *pubis,* pubic bone, + G. *tomē,* incision]

pu•bis (pyū′bis) Official alternate term for os pubis, the pubic bone.

pub•lic health (pub′lik helth) The art and science of community health, concerned with statistics, epidemiology, hygiene, and the prevention and eradication of epidemic diseases; an effort organized by society to promote, protect, and restore the people's health; public health is a social institution, a service, and a practice.

pubo- Combining form meaning pubic, pubes. [L. *pubes*]

pu•bo•coc•cy•ge•al mus•cle (pyū′bō-kok-sij′ē-ăl mŭs′ĕl) SYN pubococcygeus muscle.

pu•bo•coc•cy•ge•us mus•cle (pyū′bō-kok-sij′ē-ŭs mŭs′ĕl) Fibers of the levator ani, arising from the pelvic surface of the body of the pubis and adjacent tendinous arch of obturator fascia, attaching to the coccyx. SYN musculus pubococcygeus [TA], pubococcygeal muscle.

pu•bo•pros•tat•ic (pyū′bō-pros-tat′ik) Relating to the pubic bone and the prostate.

pu•bo•pros•tat•ic mus•cle (pyū′bō-pros-tat′ik mŭs′ĕl) Smooth muscle fibers within the puboprostatic ligament. SYN musculus puboprostaticus [TA].

pu•bo•rec•tal (pyū′bō-rek′tăl) Relating to the pubic bone and the rectum.

pu•bo•rec•ta•lis mus•cle (pyū′bō-rek-tā′lis mŭs′ĕl) The medial part of the musculus levator ani (pubococcygeus muscle) that passes from the body of the pubis around the anus to form a muscular sling at the level of the anorectal junction; it contracts to increase the perineal flexure during a peristalsis to maintain fecal continence and relaxes to allow defecation. SYN musculus puborectalis [TA], puborectal muscle.

pu•bo•rec•tal mus•cle (pyū′bō-rek′tăl mŭs′ĕl) SYN puborectalis muscle.

pu•bo•va•gi•na•lis mus•cle (pyū′bō-va-ji-nā′lis mŭs′ĕl) In the female, the most medial fibers of the levator ani (pubococcygeus) muscle that extend from the pubis into the lateral walls of the vagina. SYN musculus pubovaginalis [TA], pubovaginal muscle.

pu•bo•vag•i•nal mus•cle (pyū′bō-vaj′i-năl mŭs′ĕl) SYN pubovaginalis muscle.

pu•bo•ves•i•cal (pyū′bō-ves′i-kăl) Relating to the pubic bone and the bladder.

pu•bo•ves•i•ca•lis mus•cle (pyū′bō-ves-i-kā′lis mŭs′ĕl) Smooth muscle fibers within the pubovesical ligament in the female. SYN musculus pubovesicalis [TA], pubovesical muscle.

pu•bo•ves•i•cal mus•cle (pyū′bō-ves′i-kăl mŭs′ĕl) SYN pubovesicalis muscle.

Pucht•ler-Sweat stain for base•ment mem•branes (pukt′lĕr-swet stān bās′mĕnt mĕm′brānz) A staining method using resorcin-fuchsin and nuclear fast-red solutions after Carnoy fixative; basement membranes are gray to black and nuclei pink to red.

Pucht•ler-Sweat stain for he•mo•glo•bin and he•mo•sid•er•in (pukt′lĕr-swet stān hē′mō-glō′bin hē′mō-sid′ĕr-in) A complex staining method in which, on a yellow background, hemoglobin is stained red, hemosiderin blue to green, and elastic fibers pink.

Pucht•ler-Sweat stains (pukt′lĕr-swet stāns) SEE Puchtler-Sweat stain for basement membranes, Puchtler-Sweat stain for hemoglobin and hemosiderin.

puck•ered lip breath•ing (pŭk′ĕrd lip brēdh′ing) SYN pursed-lip breathing.

pu•den•dal (pyū-den′dăl) Relating to the external genitals. SYN pudic.

pu•den•dal ca•nal (pyū-den′dăl kă-nal′) The space within the obturator internus fascia lining the lateral wall of the ischiorectal fossa that transmits the pudendal vessels and nerves. SYN canalis pudendalis [TA].

pu•den•dal cleft (pyū-den′dăl kleft) The cleft between the labia majora.

pu•den•dal nerve (pyū-den′dăl nĕrv) Formed by fibers from the ventral primary rami of the second, third, and fourth sacral spinal nerves; it exits the pelvis through the greater sciatic foramen, passes posterior to the sacrospinous ligament, and accompanies the internal pudendal artery into the perineum through the lesser sciatic foramen; it gives off inferior rectal nerves, then courses through the pudendal canal in the lateral wall of the ischiorectal fossa, terminating as the dorsal nerve of the penis or of the clitoris. SYN nervus pudendus [TA].

pu•den•dum, pl. **pu•den•da** (pyū-den′dŭm, -dă) The external genitals, especially the female genitals (vulva). Used also in the plural. [L. ntr. of *pudendus,* particip. adj. of *pudeo,* to feel ashamed]

pu•dic (pyū′dik) SYN pudendal. [L. *pudicus,* modest]

pu•er•per•a, pl. **pu•er•per•ae** (pyū-er′pĕr-ă, -per-ē) A woman who has just given birth. [L., fr. *puer,* child, + *pario,* to bring forth]

pu•er•per•al (pyū-er′pĕr-ăl) Relating to the puerperium, or period after childbirth. SYN puerperant (1).

pu•er•per•al ec•lamp•si•a (pyū-er′pĕr-ăl ĕ-klamp′sē-ă) Convulsions and coma associated with hypertension, edema, or proteinuria occurring in a woman after delivery of a child.

pu•er•per•al fe•ver (pyū-er′pĕr-ăl fē′vĕr) Postpartum sepsis with a rise in temperature after the first 24 hours following delivery, but before the eleventh postpartum day. SYN childbed fever.

pu•er•per•al sep•ti•ce•mi•a (pyū-er′pĕr-ăl sep′ti-sē′mē-ă) A severe bloodstream infection resulting from an obstetric delivery or procedure.

pu•er•per•al tet•a•nus (pyū-er′pĕr-ăl tet′ă-nŭs) Tetanus occurring during the puerperium from infection of the obstetric wound.

pu•er•per•ant (pyū-er′pĕr-ănt) **1.** SYN puerperal. **2.** A puerpera.

pu•er•pe•ri•um, pl. **pu•er•pe•ri•a** (pyū′er-pēr′ē-ŭm, -ă) Period from the termination of labor to complete involution of the uterus, usually defined as 42 days. [L. childbirth, fr. *puer,* child, + *pario,* to bring forth]

Pues•tow pro•ce•dure (pwes′tō prŏ-sē′jŭr) Longitudinal pancreaticojejunostomy for treatment of chronic pancreatitis.

Pu•lex (pyū′leks) A genus of fleas (family Pulicidae, order Siphonaptera). [L. flea]

Pul•frich phe•no•me•non (pŭl′frik fĕ-nom′ĕ-non) The binocular perception that an small target oscillating in the frontal plane is moving in an elliptic path seen when one eye is covered by a filter or in the presence of a unilateral optic neuropathy.

pu•lic•i•cide, pu•li•cide (pyū′lis′i-sīd, pyū′li-sīd) A chemical agent that kills fleas. [L. *pulex* (*pulic-*), flea, + *caedo,* to kill]

pul•ley (pul′ē) SEE trochlea.

pul•mo, gen. **pul•mo•nis**, pl. **pul•mo•nes** (pul′mō, -mō′nis, -mō′nēz) [TA] SYN lung. [L.]

♲**pulmo-, pulmon-, pulmono-** Combining forms meaning the lungs. SEE ALSO pneum-, pneumo-. [L. *pulmo,* lung]

pul•mo•a•or•tic (pul′mō-ā-ōr′tik) Relating to the pulmonary artery and the aorta.

pul•mo•nary (pul′mŏ-nār-ē) Relating to the lungs, to the pulmonary artery, or to the aperture leading from the right ventricle into the pulmonary artery. SYN pneumonic (1), pulmonic. [L. *pulmonarius,* fr. *pulmo,* lung]

pul•mo•nar•y ac•i•nus (pul′mŏ-nār-ē as′i-nŭs) That part of the airway consisting of a respiratory bronchiole and all of its branches. SYN primary pulmonary lobule.

pul•mo•nar•y ad•e•no•ma•to•sis (pul′mŏ-nār-ē ad′ĕ-nō′mă-tō′sis) A neoplastic disease in which the alveoli and distal bronchi are filled with mucus and mucus-secreting columnar epithelial cells; characterized by abundant, extremely tenacious sputum, chills, fever, cough, dyspnea, and pleuritic pain.

pul•mon•ar•y a•gent (pul′mŏ-nār-ē ā′jĕnt) A toxic chemical-warfare agent that affects the respiratory tract, especially the respiratory bronchioles, alveolar ducts, and alveoli. These agents, such as phosgene (CG), can lead to shortness of breath and pulmonary edema.

pul·mo·nar·y al·ve·o·lar mi·cro·li·thi·a·sis (pul′mŏ-năr-ē al-vē′ō-lăr mī′krō-li-thī′ă-sis) Microscopic granules of calcium or bone disseminated throughout the lungs.

pul·mo·nar·y al·ve·o·lar pro·tein·o·sis (pul′mŏ-năr-ē al-vē′ō-lăr prō′tē-nō′sis) A chronic progressive lung disease of adults, characterized by alveolar accumulation of granular proteinaceous material that is PAS positive and lipid rich, with little inflammatory cellular exudate; the cause is unknown.

pul·mo·nar·y al·ve·o·li (pul′mŏ-năr-ē al-vē′ō-lŭs) One of the thin-walled, saclike terminal dilations of the respiratory bronchioles, alveolar ducts, and alveolar sacs across which gas exchange occurs between alveolar air and the pulmonary capillaries. SYN alveolus (1) [TA], air cells (1), air vesicles, alveoli pulmonis, bronchic cell.

pul·mo·nar·y ar·ter·y (pul′mŏ-năr-ē ahr′tĕr-ē) SYN pulmonary trunk.

pul·mo·nar·y ar·ter·y a·tre·si·a (pul′mŏ-năr-ē ahr′tĕr-ē ă-trē′zē-ă) Absence of one, usually the right, pulmonary artery.

pul·mo·nar·y ar·ter·y cath·e·ter (pul′mŏ-năr-ē ahr′tĕr-ē kath′ĕ-tĕr) SYN Swan-Ganz catheter.

pul·mo·nar·y bleb (pul′mŏ-năr-ē bleb) Air-filled alveolar dilation smaller than 1 cm in diameter on the edge of the lung at the apex of upper lobe or superior segment of lower lobe; usually occurs in young people and can rupture, producing primary pneumothorax.

pul·mo·nar·y cap·il·lar·y wedge pressure (PCWP) (pul′mŏ-năr-ē kap′i-lar-ē wej presh′ŭr) The pressure obtained when a catheter is passed from the right side of the heart into pulmonary artery as far as it will go and "wedged" into an end artery. The pressure distal to the wedged catheter is an approximation of cardiac left atrial pressure. The pressure recorded with the balloon deflated is pulmonary artery pressure.

pul·mo·nar·y cir·cu·la·tion (pul′mŏ-năr-ē sĭr′kyū-lā′shŭn) The passage of blood from the right ventricle through the pulmonary artery to the lungs and back through the pulmonary veins to the left atrium. See this page.

pul·mo·nar·y col·lapse (pul′mŏ-năr-ē kŏ-laps′) Secondary atelectasis due to bronchial obsturction, pleural effusion or pneumothorax, cardiac hypertrophy, or enlargement of other structures adjacent to the lungs.

pul·mo·nar·y dys·ma·tu·ri·ty syn·drome (pul′mŏ-năr-ē dis′mă-chūr′i-tē sin′drōm) A respiratory disorder occurring in premature infants who are incapable of normal pulmonary ventilation and who often die as a result of hypoxia after an illness of 6–8 weeks; the lungs contain widespread focal emphysematous blebs and the parenchyma has thickened alveolar walls.

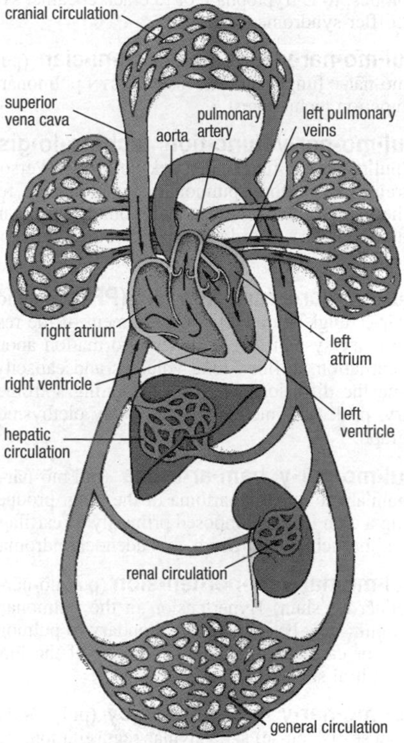

pulmonary circulation: from the right ventricle, through the lungs to the left atrium

systemic circulation: through the body, from the left ventricle to the right atrium

red: oxygenated blood

blue: deoxygenated blood

pul·mo·nar·y e·de·ma (pul′mŏ-năr-ē ĕ-dē′mă) Accumulation of extravascular fluid in lung tissues and alveoli usually resulting from mitral stenosis or left ventricular failure.

pul·mo·nar·y em·bo·lism (PE) (pul′mŏ-năr-ē em′bŏ-lizm) Embolism of pulmonary arteries, most frequently by detached fragments of thrombus from a leg or pelvic vein, commonly when thrombosis has followed an operation or confinement to bed.

pul·mo·nar·y em·phy·se·ma (pul′mŏ-năr-ē em′fi-sē′mă) SYN emphysema (2).

pul·mo·nar·y e·o·sin·o·phil·i·a (pul′mŏ-năr-ē ē′ō-sin′ō-fil′ē-ă) Eosinophilic pulmonary infiltrates, often associated with parasitic migration; also associated with reactions to some antibiotics, to L-tryptophan, or to crack cocaine. SYN Löffler syndrome.

pul•mo•nar•y func•tion tech•ni•cian (pul′mŏ-nār-ē fŭngk′shŭn tek-nish′ăn) SYN pulmonary function technologist.

pul•mo•nar•y func•tion tech•no•lo•gist (pul′mŏ-nār-ē fŭngk′shŭn tek-nol′ŏ-jist) Person trained to perform pulmonary function tests for the diagnostic assessment and monitoring of cardiopulmonary disorders. SYN pulmonary function technician.

pul•mo•nar•y func•tion test (PFT) (pul′mŏ-nār-ē fŭngk′shŭn test) An assessment of the respiratory system that provides information about ventilation, airflow, lung volumes and capacity, and the diffusion of gas incorporating spirometry, peak flow meters, and the body plethysmograph.

pul•mo•nar•y ham•ar•to•ma (pul′mŏ-nār-ē ham′ahr-tō′mă) Hamartoma of the lung, producing a coin lesion composed primarily of cartilage and bronchial epithelium. SYN adenochondroma.

pul•mo•nar•y hy•per•ten•sion (pul′mŏ-nār-ē hī′pĕr-ten′shŭn) Hypertension in the pulmonary circuit; may be primary or secondary to pulmonary or cardiac disease (e.g., fibrosis of the lung or mitral stenosis).

pul•mo•nar•y in•suf•fi•cien•cy (pul′mŏ-nār-ē in′sŭ-fish′ĕn-sē) SEE valvular regurgitation.

pul•mo•nar•y in•ter•sti•ti•al em•phy•se•ma (PIE) (pŭl′mŏ-nar-ē in′tĕr-stish′ăl em′fă-sē′mă) The presence of air in interstitial lung tissue as a result of excessive ventilatory pressure, usually seen in premature infants in whom high pressures are needed to overcome low lung compliance associated with deficiency of endogenous surfactant.

pul•mo•nar•y lig•a•ment (pul′mŏ-nār-ē lig′ă-mĕnt) Two-layered fold formed as the pleura of the mediastinum is reflected onto the lung inferior to the root of the lung. SYN ligamentum pulmonale [TA].

pul•mo•nar•y lo•bar buds (pul′mŏ-nār-ē lō′bahr bŭdz) SYN secondary bronchial buds.

pul•mo•nar•y mur•mur, pul•mon•ic mur•mur (pul′mŏ-nār-ē mŭr′mŭr, pul-mon′ik) A murmur produced at the pulmonary orifice of the heart, either obstructive or regurgitant.

pul•mo•nar•y plex•us (pul′mŏ-nār-ē plek′sŭs) One of two autonomic plexuses, anterior and posterior, at the hilus of each lung, formed by cardiopulmonary splanchnic nerves of the sympathetic trunk and bronchial branches of the vagus nerve; from them various branches accompany the bronchi and arteries into the lung.

pul•mo•nar•y re•ha•bil•i•ta•tion (pul′mŏ-nār-ē rē-hă-bil-i-tā′shŭn) SYN chest physical therapy.

pul•mo•nar•y ste•no•sis (pul′mŏ-nār-ē stĕ-nō′sis) Narrowing of the opening into the pulmonary artery from the right ventricle.

pul•mon•ar•y toi•let (pul′mŏ-nār-ē toy′lĕt) Cleansing of the trachea and bronchial tree.

pul•mo•na•ry toi•let•ing (pul′mŏ-nār-ē toy′lĕt-ing) SYN chest physical therapy.

pul•mo•nar•y trunk (pul′mŏ-nār-ē trŭngk) *Origin*, right ventricle of heart; *distribution*, it divides into the right pulmonary artery and the left pulmonary artery, which enter the corresponding lungs and branch along with the segmental bronchi. SYN truncus pulmonalis [TA], arteria pulmonalis, pulmonary artery.

pul•mo•nar•y valve (pul′mŏ-nār-ē valv) The valve at the entrance to the pulmonary trunk from the right ventricle; it consists of semilunar cusps (valvules) that are usually arranged in the adult in right anterior, left anterior, and posterior positions; however, they are named in accordance with their embryonic derivation; thus, the posteriorly located cusp is designated as the left cusp, the right anteriorly located cusp is designated the right cusp, and the left anteriorly positioned cusp is called the anterior cusp.

pul•mo•nar•y vas•cu•lar re•sis•tance (pul′mŏ-nā-rē vas′kyū-lăr rĕ-zis′tăns) The resistance to blood flow through the pulmonary circulation, which is largely influenced by the degree of tone or caliber of the pulmonary arteries and capillaries. Can be measured with the use of hemodynamic monitoring.

pul•mo•nar•y ven•ti•la•tion (pul′mŏ-nār-ē ven′ti-lā′shŭn) Respiratory minute volume, i.e., the total volume of gas per minute inspired (V_I) or expired (V_E) expressed in liters per minute; differs from alveolar ventilation in that it includes the exchange of dead space gas.

pul•mon•ic (pul-mon′ik) SYN pulmonary.

pul•mo•ni•tis (pul′mō-nī′tis) SYN pneumonitis.

pulp (pŭlp) **1.** A soft, moist, coherent solid. SYN pulpa [TA]. **2.** SYN dental pulp. **3.** SYN chyme. [L. *pulpa*, flesh]

pul•pa (pŭl′pă) [TA] SYN pulp (1). [L. pulp]

pul•pal (pŭl′păl) Relating to the pulp.

pulp am•pu•ta•tion (pŭlp amp′yū-tā′shŭn) SYN pulpotomy.

pulp ca•nal (pŭlp kă-nal′) **1.** SYN root canal of tooth. **2.** SYN root canal of tooth.

pulp cav•i•ty (pŭlp kav′i-tē) The central hollow of a tooth consisting of the crown cavity and the root canal; it contains the fibrovascular dental pulp and is lined throughout by odontoblasts.

pulp cham•ber (pŭlp chām′bĕr) The portion of the pulp cavity that is contained in the crown or body of the tooth.

pulp•ec•to•my (pŭl-pek′tō-mē) Removal of the entire pulp structure of a tooth, including the pulp tissue in the roots. [L. *pulpa,* pulp, + G. *ektomē,* excision]

pulp horn (pŭlp hōrn) A prolongation of the pulp extending toward the cusp of a tooth.

pul•pi•fac•tion (pŭlp′i-fak′shŭn) Reduction to a pulpy condition. [L. *pulpa,* pulp, + *facio,* pp. *factus,* to make]

pul•pi•tis (pŭl-pī′tis) Inflammation of the pulp of a tooth. [L. *pulpa,* pulp, + G. *-itis,* inflammation]

pulp•ot•o•my (pŭl-pot′ŏ-mē) Removal of a portion of the pulp structure of a tooth, usually the coronal portion. SYN pulp amputation. [L. *pulpa,* pulp, + G. *tomē,* incision]

pulp stone (pŭlp stōn) SYN endolith.

pulp test (pŭlp test) SYN vitality test.

pulp•y (pŭl′pē) In the condition of a soft, moist solid.

pul•sate (pŭl′sāt) To throb or beat rhythmically; said of the heart or an artery. [L. *pulso,* pp. *-atus,* to beat]

pul•sa•tile (pŭl′să-tīl) Throbbing or beating.

pul•sa•tion (pŭl-sā′shŭn) A throbbing or rhythmic beating, as of the pulse or the heart. [L. *pulsatio,* a beating]

i pulse (pŭls) Palpable rhythmic expansion of an artery, produced by the increased volume of blood pushed or forced into the vessel by the contraction of the heart. A pulse may also at times occur in a vein or a vascular organ, such as the liver. See page 1300. SYN pulsus. [L. *pulsus*]

pulse def•i•cit (pŭls def′i-sit) **1.** The absence of palpable pulse waves in a peripheral artery for one or more heartbeats, as is often seen in atrial fibrillation; the condition indicates lack of peripheral perfusion. **2.** The number of such missing pulse waves (usually expressed as heart rate minus pulse rate per minute).

pulsed las•er (pŭlst lā′zĕr) A laser in which energy output is pulsed, allowing short bursts of high energy.

pulse-field gel e•lec•tro•pho•re•sis (pŭls-fēld jel ĕ-lek′trō-fŏr-ē′sis) Gel electrophoresis in which, after electrophoretic migration has begun, the current is briefly stopped and reapplied in a different orientation; allows for the purification of long DNA molecules.

pulse gen•er•a•tor (pŭls jen′ĕr-ā-tŏr) A device that produces an electric discharge with a regular or rhythmic wave form in which the electromotive force varies in a specific pattern in relation to time; e.g., in an electronic pacemaker, it produces an electric discharge at regular intervals, and these intervals may be modified by a sensory circuit that can reset the time-base for subsequent discharge on the basis of other electrical activity, such as that produced by spontaneous cardiac beating.

pulse height an•a•lyz•er (pŭls hīt an′ă-līz-ĕr) Electronic circuitry that determines the energy of scintillations recorded by a detector, allowing use of a discriminator to select for photons of a specific type.

pulse•less dis•ease (pŭls′lĕs di-zēz′) SYN Takayasu arteritis.

pulse•less e•lec•tri•cal ac•ti•vi•ty (PEA) (pŭls′lĕs ĕ-lek′trik-ăl ak-tiv′i-tē) SYN electromechanical dissociation.

pulse ox•i•me•ter (pŭls oks-im′ĕ-tĕr) A spectrophotometric device that noninvasively estimates saturation of arterial oxyhemoglobin (SaO_2) by use of selected wavelengths of light.

pulse pres•sure (pŭls presh′ŭr) The variation in blood pressure occurring in an artery during the cardiac cycle; it is the difference between the systolic, or maximum, and diastolic, or minimum, pressures. A reading of 30–50 is considered in the normal range.

pulse rate (pŭls rāt) Rate of the pulse as observed in an artery; recorded as beats per minute. Normally, it is the same as the heart rate.

pulse se•quence (pŭls sē′kwĕns) MAGNETIC RESONANCE IMAGING a series of changes in the induced magnetic field, which includes the phase and frequency-encoding gradients and read-out functions.

pulse wave (pŭls wāv) The progressive expansion of the arteries occurring with each contraction of the left ventricle of the heart.

pulse wave du•ra•tion (pŭls wāv dūr-ā′shŭn) The interval between onset of the leading edge and the end of the trailing edge of a pulse wave.

pul•sion (pŭl′shŭn) A pushing outward or swelling. [L. *pulsio*]

pul•sion di•ver•tic•u•lum (pŭl′shŭn dī′vĕr-tik′yū-lŭm) A diverticulum formed by pressure from within, frequently causing herniation of mucosa through the muscularis.

pul•sus (pŭl′sŭs) SYN pulse. [L. a stroke, pulse]

pul•sus al•ter•nans (pŭl′sŭs awl-tĕr′nanz) SYN alternating pulse.

pul•sus bi•gem•i•nus (pŭl′sŭs bī-jem′i-nus) SYN bigeminal pulse.

pul•sus bis•fe•ri•ens (pŭl′sŭs bis-fer′ē-enz) SYN bisferious pulse.

pul•sus ce•ler (pŭl′sŭs sē′lăr) A pulse beat that is swift to rise and fall.

pul•sus dif•fer•ens (pŭl′sŭs dif′ĕr-enz) A condition in which the pulses in the two radial or other corresponding arteries differ in strength.

pul•sus par•a•dox•us (pŭl′sŭs par′ă-dok′sŭs) SYN paradoxic pulse.

pul•sus tar•dus (pŭl′sŭs tahr′dŭs) A pulse with pathologically gradual upstroke typical of severe aortic stenosis. SEE ALSO plateau pulse.

pul•sus tri•gem•i•nus (pŭl′sŭs trī-jem′i-nŭs) SYN trigeminal pulse.

pul•ta•ceous (pŭl-tā′shŭs) Macerated; pulpy. [G. *poltos,* porridge]

pul•vi•nar (pŭl-vī′năr) [TA] The expanded posterior extremity of the thalamus that forms a cushionlike prominence overlying the geniculate bodies. [L. a couch made from cushions, fr. *pulvinus,* cushion]

pump (pŭmp) **1.** An apparatus for forcing a gas or liquid from or to any part. **2.** Any mechanism for using metabolic energy to accomplish active transport of a substance.

pumped las•er (pŭmpt lā′zĕr) A laser the energy level of which is increased by the application of separate sources of electrons or photons, which may themselves be primary lasers.

pump•ing (pŭmp′ing) Vigorous opening and

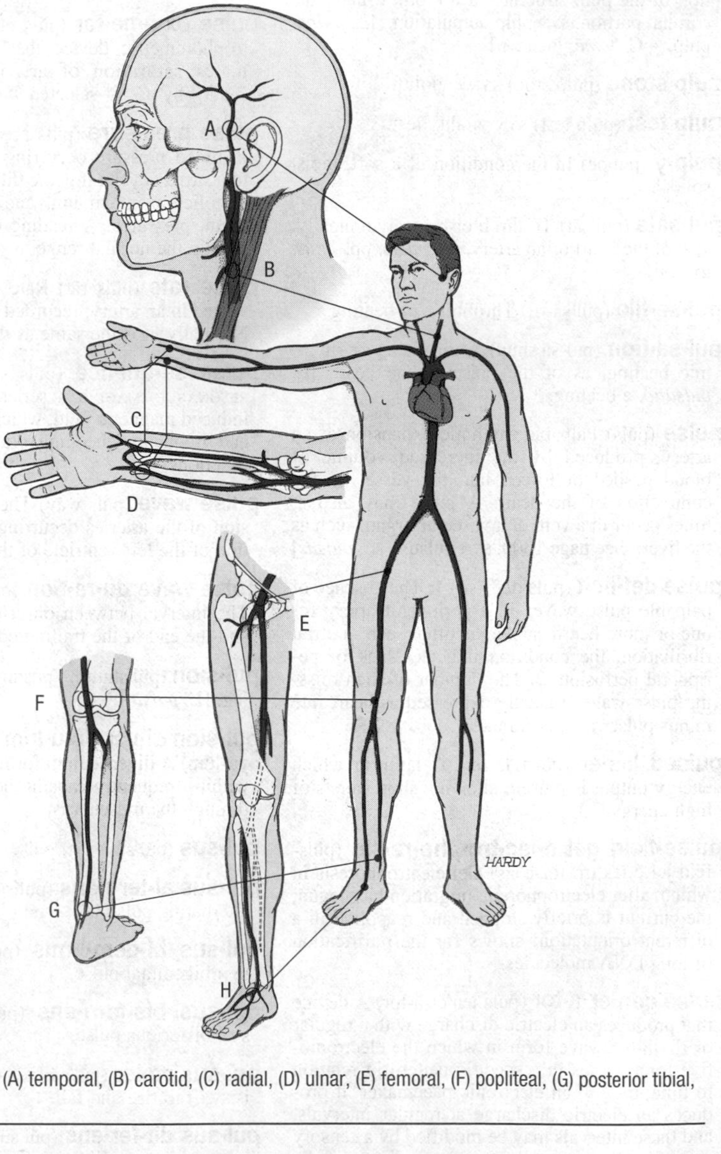

peripheral pulses: (A) temporal, (B) carotid, (C) radial, (D) ulnar, (E) femoral, (F) popliteal, (G) posterior tibial, (H) dorsalis pedis

closing of the fist to enhance filling of subcutaneous veins below a tourniquet placed around an arm in preparation for phlebotomy.

pump lung (pŭmp lŭng) SYN shock lung.

pump-ox•y•gen•a•tor (pŭmp-ok′si-jĕ-nā′tŏr) A mechanical device that can substitute for both the heart (pump) and the lungs (oxygenator) during open heart surgery.

punch bi•op•sy (pŭnch bī′op-sē) Any method that removes a small cylindric specimen for biopsy by means of a special instrument that pierces the organ directly or through the skin or a small incision in the skin.

punch•drunk syn•drome, **punch•drunk** (pŭnch′drŭngk sin′drōm) A condition seen in boxers, often years after retirement, and presumably caused by repeated cerebral injury, characterized by weakness in the lower limbs, unsteadiness of gait, slowness of muscular movements, tremors of hands, dysarthria, and slow cerebration.

punch grafts (pŭnch grafs) Small, full-thickness grafts of the scalp, removed with a circular punch and transplanted to a bald area to grow hair.

punc•ta (pŭngk′tă) Plural of punctum. [L.]

punc•tate (pŭngk′tāt) Marked with points or dots differentiated from the surrounding surface by color, elevation, or texture. [L. *punctum,* a point]

punc•tate hem•or•rhage (pŭngk′tāt hem′ŏr-ăj) SYN petechial hemorrhage.

punc•tate hy•a•lo•sis (pŭngk′tāt hī′ă-lō′sis) A condition marked by minute opacities in the vitreous.

punc•ti•form (pŭngk′ti-fōrm) Very small but not microscopic, having a diameter of less than 1 mm. [L. *punctum,* a point, + *forma,* shape]

punc•tum, gen. **punc•ti**, pl. **punc•ta** (pŭngk′tŭm, -tī, -tă) **1.** The tip of a sharp process. **2.** A minute round spot differing in color or otherwise in appearance from the surrounding tissues. **3.** The opening into the lacrimal drainage system in the upper and lower eyelids. SEE ALSO point. SYN point (1). [L. a prick, point, pp. ntr. of *pungo,* to prick, used as noun]

punc•tum ce•cum (pŭngk′tŭm sē′kŭm) The blind spot in the visual field corresponding to the location of the optic disc.

punc•tum fix•um (pŭngk′tŭm fiks′ŭm) SYN fixed end.

punc•tum mo•bi•le (pŭngk′tŭm mō′bē-lē) SYN mobile end.

punc•tum vas•cu•lo•sum (pŭngk′tŭm vas-kū-lō′sŭm) One of the minute dots seen on section of the brain, due to small drops of blood at the cut extremities of the arteries.

punc•ture (pungk′shŭr) **1.** To make a hole with a small pointed object, such as a needle. **2.** A prick or small hole made with a pointed instrument. [L. *punctura,* fr. *pungo,* pp. *punctus,* to prick]

punc•ture wound (pungk′shŭr wūnd) A wound in which the opening is relatively small as compared with the depth, as produced by a narrow pointed object.

PUO Abbreviation for pyrexia of unknown (or undetermined) origin.

pu•pa, pl. **pu•pae** (pyū′pă, -pē) The stage of insect metamorphosis following the larva and preceding the imago. [L. *pupa,* doll]

pu•pil (p) (pyū′pil) The circular orifice in the center of the iris, through which light rays enter the eye. SYN pupilla [TA]. [L. *pupilla*]

pu•pil•la, pl. **pu•pil•lae** (pyū-pil′ă, -ē) [TA] SYN pupil. [L. dim. of *pupa,* a girl or doll]

pu•pil•lar•y (pyū′pi-lār-ē) Relating to the pupil.

pu•pil•lar•y block (pyū′pi-lār-ē blok) Increased resistance to flow of aqueous humor through the pupil from the posterior chamber to the anterior chamber, leading to anterior bowing of the peripheral iris over the trabecular meshwork and to angle-closure glaucoma.

pu•pil•lar•y dis•tance (pyū′pi-lār-ē dis′tăns) The distance between the center of each pupil; the major reference points in measuring for fitting of spectacle frames and lenses.

pu•pil•lar•y mem•brane (pyū′pi-lār-ē mem′brān) Remnants of the central portion of the anterior layer of the iris stroma (the iridopupillary lamina) that occludes the pupil in fetal life, and normally atrophies about the seventh month of gestation. Failure to regress is a rare cause of congenital blindness. SYN membrana pupillaris [TA], Wachendorf membrane (1).

pu•pil•lar•y re•flex (pyū′pi-lār-ē rē′fleks) Change in diameter of the pupil as a reflex response to any type of stimulus, e.g., constriction caused by light. SYN light reflex (1).

pu•pil•lar•y-skin re•flex (pyū′pi-lār-ē-skin′ rē′fleks) Dilation of the pupil following scratching of the skin of the neck. SYN ciliospinal reflex.

♻ **pupillo-** Prefix indicating the pupils. [L. *pupilla,* pupil]

pu•pil•lom•e•ter (pyū′pi-lom′ĕ-tĕr) An instrument for measuring and recording the diameter of the pupil. [pupillo- + G. *metron,* measure]

pu•pil•lom•e•try (pyū′pi-lom′ĕ-trē) Measurement of the pupil.

pu•pil•lo•mo•tor (pyū′pi-lō-mō′tŏr) Relating to the autonomic nerve fibers that supply the smooth muscle of the iris. [pupillo- + L. *motor,* mover]

pu·pil·lo·sta·tom·e·ter (pyū′pi-lō-stă-tom′ĕ-tŏr) An instrument for measuring the distance between the centers of the pupils. [pupillo- + G. *statos,* placed, + *metron,* measure]

pu·pil·lo·to·nic pseu·do·stra·bis·mus (pyū′pil-ō-ton′ik sū′dō-stră-biz′mŭs) SYN Adie syndrome.

pu·pil re·ac·tion (pyū′pil rē-ak′shun) Constriction of the pupil in response to light rays.

PUPPP Abbreviation for pruritic urticarial papules and plaques of pregnancy, an intensely pruritic, occasionally vesicular, eruption of the trunk and arms appearing in the third trimester of pregnancy; spontaneous involution occurs within 10 days of term.

pure ab·sence (pyūr ab′sĕns) SYN simple absence.

pure au·to·no·mic fail·ure (pyūr aw′tō-nom′ik fāl′yŭr) A degenerative, sporadic neurologic disorder of adult onset, manifested principally as orthostatic hypotension and syncope, with no neurologic defects other than autonomic nervous system dysfunction evident; probably caused by selective degeneration of neurons in the sympathetic ganglia, with denervation of smooth muscle vasculature and the suprarenal glands. SYN Bradbury-Eggleston syndrome.

pure cul·ture (pyūr kŭl′chŭr) In the ordinary bacteriologic sense, a culture consisting of the descendants of a single cell.

pure tone (pyūr tōn) An audible tone that can be represented by a sine wave; an oscillation showing only one frequency of vibration, with no overtones or harmonics. SEE ALSO conduction, sine wave.

pure tone au·di·o·gram (pyūr tōn aw′dē-ō-gram) An audiogram in which the threshold for pure tone stimuli is charted in decibels of hearing level down the vertical axis, the horizontal axis being the frequency, which is usually measured in octave steps from 125 Hz–8 kHz.

pure tone av·er·age (pyūr tōn av′răj′) The average hearing threshold level for the pure tone frequencies of 500 Hz, 1 kHz, and 2 kHz. These frequencies are referred to as speech frequencies because many of the English phonemes are within this frequency range. The pure tone average is a reliable indicator of the dB level at which a listener can hear speech.

pur·ga·tion (pŭr-gā′shŭn) Evacuation of the bowels with the aid of a purgative or cathartic. SYN catharsis (1). [L. *purgatio*]

pur·ga·tive (pŭr′gă-tiv) An agent used for purging the bowels. SEE ALSO cathartic (2). [L. *purgativus,* purging]

purge (pŭrj) **1.** To cause a copious evacuation of the bowels. **2.** A cathartic remedy. [L. *purgo,* to cleanse, fr. *purus,* pure, + *ago,* to do]

pu·rine (pyūr′ēn) The parent substance of adenine, guanine, and other naturally occurring so-called purine bases; not known to exist as such in mammals.

Pur·kin·je cell lay·er (pĕr-kin′jē sel lā′yĕr) The layer of large neuron cell bodies located at the interface of molecular and granular layers in the cerebellar cortex; dendrites of these cells fan outward into the molecular layer in a plane transverse to the folium. SYN Purkinje cells, Purkinje corpuscles.

Pur·kin·je cells (pĕr-kin′jē selz) SYN Purkinje cell layer.

Pur·kin·je cor·pus·cles (pĕr-kin′jē kōr′pŭs-ĕlz) SYN Purkinje cell layer.

Pur·kin·je fi·bers (pĕr-kin′jē fī′bĕrz) SYN subendocardial branches of atrioventricular bundles.

Pur·kin·je fig·ures (pĕr-kin′jē fig′yĕrz) Shadows of the retinal vessels, seen as dark lines on a reddish field when a light enters the eye through the sclera and not the pupil.

Pur·kin·je net·work (pĕr-kin′jē net′wŏrk) The network formed by Purkinje fibers beneath the endocardium.

Pur·kin·je phe·nom·e·non (pĕr-kin′jē fē-nom′ĕ-non) In the light-adapted eye, the region of maximal brightness is in the yellow; in the dark-adapted eye, the region of maximal brightness is in the green.

Pur·kin·je-San·son im·a·ges (pŭr-kin′jē san-să-sōn[h]′ im′ăj-ĕz) The two images formed by the anterior and posterior surfaces of the cornea and the two images formed by the anterior and posterior surfaces of the lens. SYN Sanson images.

Pur·mann meth·od (pur′mahn meth′ŏd) Treatment of an aneurysm by extirpation of the sac.

pur·ple (pŭr′pĕl) A color formed by a mixture of blue and red. For individual purple dyes see specific name. [L. *purpura*]

pur·ple med·ick (pŭr′pĕl med′ik) SYN alfalfa. [L. *Medica,* fr. G. *Mēdikē,* Median]

i **pur·pu·ra** (pŭr′pyŭr-ă) A condition characterized by hemorrhage into the skin. Appearance of the lesions varies with the type of purpura, the duration of the lesions, and the acuteness of onset. The color is first red, gradually darkens to purple, fades to a brownish yellow, and usually disappears in 2–3 weeks; color of residual permanent pigmentation depends largely on the type of unabsorbed pigment of the extravasated blood; extravasations may occur also into the mucous membranes and internal organs. See page B13. SYN peliosis. [L. fr. G. *porphyra,* purple]

pur•pu•ra ful•mi•nans (pŭr′pyŭr-ă ful′mi-nanz) A severe and rapidly fatal form of purpura hemorrhagica, occurring especially in children, with hypotension, fever, and disseminated intravascular coagulation, usually following an infectious illness.

pur•pu•ra hem•or•rha•gi•ca (pŭr′pyŭr-ă hem-ō-raj′i-kă) SYN idiopathic thrombocytopenic purpura.

pur•pu•ra se•ni•lis (pŭr′pyŭr-ă sĕ-nil′is) The occurrence of petechiae and ecchymoses on the atrophic skin of the legs in aged and debilitated patients.

pur•pu•ra sim•plex (pŭr′pyŭr-ă sim′pleks) The eruption of petechiae or larger ecchymoses, usually unaccompanied by constitutional symptoms and not associated with systemic illness. SYN nonthrombocytopenic purpura.

pur•pu•ric (pŭr-pyŭr′ik) Relating to or affected with purpura.

pur•pu•ri•nu•ri•a (pŭr′pyŭr-i-nyūr′ē-ă) SYN porphyrinuria.

pursed-lip breath•ing (pŭrst lip brēdh′ing) Respirations characterized by a prolonged expiratory maneuver in which a person exhales through puckered lips. Benefits are decreased respiratory rate, increased tidal volume, and improved sense of control for oxygenation. SYN puckered lip breathing.

purse-string in•stru•ment (pŭrs′string in′strŭ-mĕnt) An intestinal clamp with jaws at an angle to the handle; when it is closed across the bowel, large grooved interdigitating serrations allow passage of a straight needle and suture through each side to form a purse-string suture.

purse-string su•ture (pŭrs′string sū′chŭr) A continuous suture placed in a circular manner either for inversion (as for an appendiceal stump) or closure (as for a hernia).

Purt•scher ret•i•nop•a•thy (pūr′cher ret′in-op′ă-thē) Transient traumatic retinal angiopathy due to a sudden rise in venous pressure, as in compression of the body from seat belt injury; ocular fundi show large white patches associated with the retinal veins about the disc or macula, hemorrhages, and retinal edema; thought to be due to fat embolism from bone marrow.

pu•ru•lence, pu•ru•len•cy (pyūr′ū-lĕns, -lĕn-sē; -sē) The condition of containing or forming pus. [L. *purulentia,* a festering, fr. *pus* (*pur-*), pus]

pu•ru•lent (pyūr′ū-lĕnt) Containing, consisting of, or forming pus.

pu•ru•lent in•flam•ma•tion (pyūr′ū-lĕnt in′flă-mā′shŭn) An acute exudative inflammation in which polymorphonuclear leukocytes cause liquefaction of the affected tissues, focally or diffusely; the purulent exudate is frequently termed pus. SYN suppurative inflammation.

pu•ru•lent oph•thal•mi•a (pyūr′ū-lĕnt of-thal′mē-ă) Purulent conjunctivitis, usually of gonorrheal origin.

pu•ru•lent pleu•ri•sy (pyūr′ū-lĕnt plūr′i-sē) Pleurisy with empyema.

pu•ru•lent syn•o•vi•tis (pyūr′ū-lĕnt sin′ō-vī′tis) SYN suppurative arthritis.

pu•ru•loid (pyū′rū-loyd) Resembling pus.

pus (pŭs) A fluid product of inflammation containing leukocytes and the debris of dead cells and tissue elements. [L.]

push (push) **1.** To apply a force that tends to move an object away from the source of the force. **2.** The power or act of applying such a force. [M.E. *pusshen,* fr. L. *pulso,* to push]

pus•tu•lar (pŭs′chū-lăr) Relating to or marked by pustules.

pus•tu•la•tion (pŭs′chū-lā′shŭn) The formation or the presence of pustules.

pus•tule (pŭs′chūl) A small, circumscribed elevation of the skin, containing purulent material. See page B10. [L. *pustula*]

pus•tu•lo•sis (pŭs′chū-lō′sis) **1.** An eruption of pustules. **2.** Term occasionally used to designate acropustulosis. [L. *pustula,* pustule, + G. *-osis,* condition]

pus•tu•lo•sis pal•mar•is et plan•tar•is (pus-chū-lō′sis pahl-mā′ris et plan-tā′ris) A sterile pustular eruption of the fingers and toes, variously attributed to dyshidrosis, pustular psoriasis, and unidentified bacterial infection. SYN acrodermatitis continua, acrodermatitis perstans, dermatitis repens.

pu•ta•men (pyū-tā′men) [TA] The outer, larger, and darker gray of the three portions into which the lenticular nucleus is divided by laminae of white fibers; it is connected with the caudate nucleus by bridging bands of gray substance that penetrate the internal capsule. Its histological structure is similar to that of the caudate nucleus; together they compose the striatum. SEE ALSO striate body. [L. that which falls off in pruning, fr. *puto,* to prune]

Put•nam-Da•na syn•drome (pŭt′năm dā′nă sin′drōm) SYN subacute combined degeneration of the spinal cord.

pu•tre•fac•tion (pyū′trĕ-fak′shŭn) Decomposition or rotting, the breakdown of organic matter, usually by bacterial action, resulting in the formation of other substances of less complex constitution with the evolution of ammonia or its derivatives and hydrogen sulfide; characterized usually by the presence of toxic or malodorous products. SYN decay (2), decomposition. [L. *putre-facio,* pp. *-factus,* to make rotten]

pu·tre·fac·tive (pyū′trĕ-fak′tiv) Relating to or causing putrefaction.

pu·tre·fy (pyū′trĕ-fī) To cause to become, or to become, putrid.

pu·tres·cence (pyū-tres′ĕns) The state of putrefaction.

pu·tres·cent (pyū-tres′ĕnt) Denoting, or in the process of, putrefaction. [L. *putresco,* to grow rotten, fr. *puter,* rotten]

pu·tres·cine (pyū-tres′ēn) A poisonous polyamine formed from the amino acid arginine during putrefaction; found in urine and feces.

pu·trid (pyū′trid) **1.** In a state of putrefaction. **2.** Denoting putrefaction. [L. *putridus*]

Put·ti-Platt op·er·a·tion (pū′tē plat op-ĕr-ā′shŭn) A procedure for recurrent dislocation of shoulder joint in which the anterior capsule and subscapularis tendon are shortened.

Pu·u·ma·la vi·rus (pū-ū′mah-lah vī′rus) A species of Hantavirus found in Europe causing hemorrhagic fever with renal syndrome.

PUVA (pū′vă) Acronym for oral administration of *p*soralen and subsequent exposure to long wavelength ultraviolet light (*uv-a*); used to treat psoriasis.

PVA fix·a·tive (fik′să-tiv) Schaudinn fixative using either a mercuric chloride, zinc sulfate, or copper sulfate base; contains polyvinyl alcohol plastic powder that is used as an adhesive for fecal specimens in the preparation of permanent smears for subsequent staining.

PVC Abbreviation for premature ventricular contraction.

PVD Abbreviation for peripheral vascular disease.

PVS Abbreviation for persistent vegetative state.

P wave (wāv) Waveform in an ECG tracing representing atrial depolarization.

pyaemia [Br.] SYN pyemia.

pyaemic [Br.] SYN pyemic.

pyaemic abscess [Br.] SYN pyemic abscess.

pyaemic embolism [Br.] SYN pyemic embolism.

py·ar·thro·sis (pī′ahr-thrō′sis) Suppurative pus within a joint cavity. [G. *pyon,* pus, + *arthron,* joint, + -osis]

♻ **pycno-** SEE pykno-.

pycnodysostosis [Br.] SYN pyknodysostosis.

pycnometer [Br.] SYN pyknometer.

py·e·lec·ta·sis, py·e·lec·ta·si·a (pī′ĕ-lek′tă-sis, -lek-tā′zē-ă) Dilation of the pelvis of the kidney. [pyel- + G. *ektasis,* extension]

py·e·lit·ic (pī′ĕ-lit′ik) Relating to pyelitis.

py·e·li·tis (pī′ĕ-lī′tis) Inflammation of the renal pelvis. [pyel- + G. *-itis,* inflammation]

♻ **pyelo-, pyel-** Combining forms meaning pelvis, usually the renal pelvis. [G. *pyelos,* trough, tub, vat]

py·e·lo·cal·y·ce·al (pī′ĕ-lō-kal′i-sē′ăl) Relating to the renal pelvis and calyces.

py·e·lo·cys·ti·tis (pī′ĕ-lō-sis-tī′tis) Inflammation of the renal pelvis and the bladder. [pyelo- + G. *kystis,* bladder, + *-itis,* inflammation]

py·e·lo·flu·o·ros·co·py (pī′ĕ-lō-flōr-os′kŏ-pē) Fluoroscopic examination of the renal pelves and ureters, following administration of contrast medium. [pyelo- + L. *fluo,* to flow, + G. *skopeō,* to view]

py·el·o·gram (pī′el-ō-gram) A radiograph or series of radiographs of the renal pelvis and ureter, following injection of contrast medium.

py·e·log·ra·phy (pī′ĕ-log′ră-fē) Radiologic study of the kidney, ureters, and usually the bladder, performed with the aid of a contrast agent injected either intravenously, or directly through a ureteral or nephrostomy catheter or percutaneously. SYN pyeloureterography, ureteropyelography. [pyelo- + G. *graphō,* to write]

py·e·lo·li·thot·o·my (pī′ĕ-lō-li-thot′ŏ-mē) Operative removal of a calculus from the kidney through an incision in the renal pelvis. SYN pelvilithotomy. [pyelo- + G. *lithos,* stone, + *tomē,* incision]

py·e·lo·ne·phri·tis (pī′ĕ-lō-nĕ-frī′tis) Inflammation of the renal parenchyma, calyces, and pelvis, particularly due to local bacterial infection. See page 1305. [pyelo- + G. *nephros,* kidney, + *-itis,* inflammation]

py·e·lo·plas·ty (pī′e-lō-plas-tē) Surgical reconstruction of the kidney pelvis to correct an obstruction. SYN pelvioplasty (2). [pyelo- + G. *plastos,* formed]

py·e·los·co·py (pī′ĕ-los′kŏ-pē) Fluoroscopic observation of the pelvis and calyces of the kidney, and the ureter, after the injection through the ureter of a radiopaque solution. [pyelo- + G. *skopeō,* to view]

py·e·los·to·my (pī′ĕ-los′tŏ-mē) Formation of an opening into the kidney pelvis to establish urinary drainage. [pyelo- + G. *stoma,* mouth]

py·e·lot·o·my (pī′ĕ-lot′ŏ-mē) Incision into the pelvis of the kidney. SYN pelviotomy (3), pelvitomy. [pyelo- + G. *tomē,* incision]

py·e·lo·u·re·ter·ec·ta·sis (pī′ĕ-lō-yūr-ē′tĕr-ek′tă-sis) Dilation of kidney pelvis and ureter, seen in hydronephrosis due to obstruction in the lower urinary tract. [pyelo- + ureter + G. *ektasis,* a stretching]

py•e•lo•u•re•ter•og•ra•phy (pī′ĕ-lō-yŭr-ē′tĕr-og′ră-fē) SYN pyelography.

py•e•lo•ve•nous (pī′ĕ-lō-vē′nŭs) Relating to the renal pelvis and renal veins. Denoting the passage of urine from the renal pelvis into the renal veins, because of increased intrapelvic pressure. [pyelo- + venous]

py•e•lo•ve•nous back•flow (pī′ĕ-lō-vē′nŭs bak′flō) Retrograde movement of fluid (urine or injected contrast materials) from the renal pelvis into the renal venous system. This occurs under conditions of distal obstruction or injection of solutions into the renal collecting system.

py•em•e•sis (pī-em′ĕ-sis) The vomiting of pus. [G. *pyon,* pus, + *emesis,* vomiting]

py•e•mi•a (pī-ē′mē-ă) Septicemia due to pyogenic organisms causing multiple abscesses. SYN pyaemia. [G. *pyon,* pus, + *haima,* blood]

py•e•mic (pī-ē′mik) Relating to or suffering from pyemia. SYN pyaemic.

py•e•mic ab•scess (pī-ē′mik ab′ses) A hematogenous abscess resulting from pyemia, septicemia, or bacteremia. SYN pyaemic abscess, septicemic abscess.

py•e•mic em•bo•lism (pī-ē′mik em′bŏ-lizm) Plugging of an artery by an embolus detached from a suppurating thrombus, producing an abscess. SYN infective embolism, pyaemic embolism.

py•en•ceph•a•lus (pī′en-sef′ă-lŭs) SYN pyocephalus. [G. *pyon,* pus, + *enkephalos,* brain]

py•e•sis (pī-ē′sis) SYN suppuration. [G. *pyon,* pus, + *-esis,* condition or process]

pyg•my (pig′mē) A physiologic dwarf, especially one of a race of similar people, such as the pygmies of central Africa. [G. *pygmaios,* dwarfish, fr. *pygmē,* fist, also a measure of length from elbow to knuckles]

pyk•nic (pik′nik) Denoting a constitutional body type characterized by well-rounded external contours and ample body cavities; virtually synonymous with endomorphic. [G. *pyknos,* thick]

♻**pykno-, pyk-** Combining forms meaning thick, dense, compact. [G. *pyknos*]

pyk•no•dys•os•to•sis (pik′nō-dis′os-tō′sis) A familial dysmorphism characterized by short stature, delayed closure of the fontanels, and hypoplasia of the terminal phalanges; autosomal recessive inheritance. SYN pycnodysostosis. [pykno- + dys- + G. *osteon,*bone, + *-osis,*condition]

pyk•nom•e•ter (pik-nom′ĕ-tĕr) A flask of standard volume, used to determine the specific gravity of fluids by weighing; a standard flask for measuring and comparing the densities of

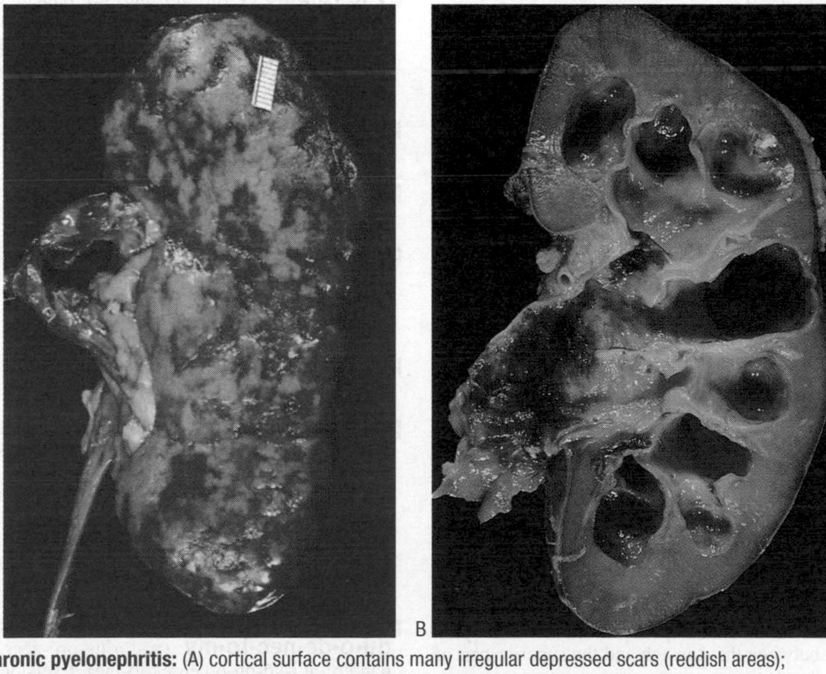

A B

chronic pyelonephritis: (A) cortical surface contains many irregular depressed scars (reddish areas); (B) marked dilation of calyces (caliectasis) caused by inflammatory destruction of papillae, with atrophy and scarring of overlying cortex

liquids. SYN pycnometer. [pykno- + G. *metron,* measure]

pyk•no•mor•phous (pik′nō-mōr′fŭs) Denoting a cell or tissue that stains deeply because the stainable material is closely packed. [pykno- + G. *morphē,* form, shape]

pyk•no•sis (pik-nō′sis) A thickening or condensation; specifically, a condensation and reduction in the size of the cell or its nucleus, usually associated with hyperchromatosis; nuclear pyknosis is a stage of necrosis. [pykno- + G. *-osis,* condition]

pyk•not•ic (pik-not′ik) Relating to or characterized by pyknosis.

py•le•phle•bi•tis (pī′lē-flĕ-bī′tis) Inflammation of the portal vein or any of its branches. [G. *pylē,* a gate, + *phleps,* vein, + *-itis,* inflammation]

py•le•throm•bo•phle•bi•tis (pī′lē-throm′bō-flĕ-bī′tis) Inflammation of the portal vein with the formation of a thrombus. [G. *pylē,* gate, + *thrombos,* a clot, + *phleps,* vein, + *-itis,* inflammation]

py•le•throm•bo•sis (pī′lē-throm-bō′sis) Thrombosis of the portal vein or its branches. [G. *pylē,* gate, + *thrombos,* a clot, + *-osis,* condition]

py•lo•rec•to•my (pī′lōr-ek′tŏ-mē) Excision of the pylorus. SYN gastropylorectomy, pylorogastrectomy. [pylor- + G. *ektomē,* excision]

py•lo•ri (pī-lōr′ī) Plural of pylorus. [L.]

py•lor•ic (pī-lōr′ik) Relating to the pylorus.

py•lor•ic an•trum (pī-lōr′ik an′trŭm) The initial portion of the pyloric part of the stomach, which may temporarily become partially or completely shut off from the remainder of the stomach during digestion by peristaltic contraction of the prepyloric "sphincter"; it is sometimes demarcated from the second part of the pyloric part of the stomach (pyloric canal) by a slight groove. SYN antrum (2).

py•lor•ic ca•nal (pī-lōr′ik kă-nal′) The segment of the stomach that succeeds the antrum and ends at the gastroduodenal junction. SYN canalis pyloricus [TA].

py•lor•ic con•stric•tion (pī-lōr′ik kŏn-strik′shŭn) A prominent fold of mucous membrane at the gastroduodenal junction overlying the pyloric sphincter.

py•lor•ic glands (pī-lōr′ik glandz) The coiled, tubular glands of the pylorus; their cells secrete mucus.

py•lor•ic or•i•fice (pī-lōr′ik ōr′i-fis) The opening between the stomach and the superior part of the duodenum.

py•lor•ic sphinc•ter (pī-lōr′ik sfingk′tĕr) A thickening of the circular layer of the gastric musculature encircling the gastroduodenal junction. SYN musculus sphincter pyloricus [TA].

py•lor•ic ste•no•sis (pī-lōr′ik stĕ-nō′sis) Narrowing of the gastric pylorus, especially by congenital muscular hypertrophy or scarring resulting from a peptic ulcer. SEE ALSO hypertrophic pyloric stenosis.

py•lor•ic vein (pī-lōr′ik vān) SYN right gastric vein.

py•lo•ri•ste•no•sis (pī-lōr′i-stĕ-nō′sis) Stricture or narrowing of the orifice of the pylorus. SYN pylorostenosis. [pylor- + G. *stenōsis,* a narrowing]

♻ **pyloro-, pylor-** Combining forms indicating the pylorus. [G. *pyloros,* gatekeeper]

py•lo•ro•du•o•de•ni•tis (pī-lōr′ō-dū-od′ĕ-nī′tis) Inflammation involving the pyloric outlet of the stomach and the duodenum. [pyloro- + duodenitis]

py•lo•ro•gas•trec•to•my (pī-lōr′ō-gas-trek′tŏ-mē) SYN pylorectomy.

py•lo•ro•my•ot•o•my (pī-lōr′ō-mī-ot′ŏ-mē) Longitudinal incision through the anterior wall of the pyloric canal to the level of the submucosa, to treat hypertrophic pyloric stenosis. SYN Fredet-Ramstedt operation, Ramstedt operation. [pyloro- + G. *mys,* muscle, + *tomē,* incision]

py•lo•ro•plas•ty (pī-lōr′ō-plas-tē) Widening of the pyloric canal and any adjacent duodenal stricture by means of a longitudinal incision closed transversely. [pyloro- + G. *plastos,* formed]

py•lo•ro•spasm (pī-lōr′ō-spazm) Spasmodic contraction of the pylorus.

py•lo•ro•ste•no•sis (pī-lōr′ō-stĕ-nō′sis) SYN pyloristenosis.

py•lo•ros•to•my (pī′lō-ros′tŏ-mē) Establishment of a fistula from the abdominal surface into the stomach near the pylorus. [pyloro- + G. *stoma,* mouth]

py•lo•rot•o•my (pī′lō-rot′ŏ-mē) Incision of the pylorus. [pyloro- + G. *tomē,* incision]

py•lo•rus, pl. **py•lo•ri** (pī-lōr′ŭs, -ī) [TA] **1.** A muscular or myovascular device to open (musculus dilator) and to close (musculus sphincter) an orifice or the lumen of an organ. **2.** The muscular tissue surrounding and controlling the aboral outlet of the stomach. [L. fr. G. *pylōros,* a gatekeeper, the pylorus, fr. *pylē,* gate, + *ouros,* a warder]

py•lor•us-pre•serv•ing pan•cre•a•tic•o•du•o•de•nec•to•my (pī-lōr′us-prē-zĕrv′ing pan′krē-at′i-kō-dū-od′ĕn-ek′tō-mē) Excision of all or part of the pancreas and the duodenum with preservation of the distal stomach and the innervated pylorus; usually limited to the head and neck of the pancreas and most often performed for pancreatic carcinoma.

pyo- Combining form meaning suppuration, accumulation of pus. [G. *pyon,* pus]

py·o·cele (pī′ō-sēl) An accumulation of pus in the scrotum. [pyo- + G. *kēlē,* tumor, hernia]

py·o·ceph·a·lus (pī′ō-sef′ă-lŭs) A purulent effusion within the cranium. SYN pyencephalus. [pyo- + G. *kephalē,* head]

py·o·che·zi·a (pī′ō-kē′zē-ă) A discharge of pus from the bowel. [pyo- + G. *chezō,* to defecate]

py·o·coc·cus (pī′ō-kok′ŭs) One of the cocci causing suppuration, especially *Streptococcus pyogenes*. [pyo- + G. *kokkos,* berry (coccus)]

py·o·col·po·cele (pī′ō-kol′pō-sēl) A vaginal tumor or cyst containing pus. [pyo- + G. *kolpos,* bosom (vagina), + *kēlē,* tumor, hernia]

py·o·col·pos (pī′ō-kol′pos) Accumulation of pus in the vagina. [pyo- + G. *kolpos,* bosom (vagina)]

py·o·cy·an·ic (pī′ō-sī-an′ik) Relating to blue pus or the organism that causes blue pus, *Pseudomonas aeruginosa*. [pyo- + G. *kyanos,* blue]

py·o·cy·a·no·gen·ic (pī′ō-sī′ă-nō-jen′ik) Causing blue pus. [pyo- + G. *kyanos,* blue, + *-gen,* producing]

py·o·cyst (pī′ō-sist) A cyst with purulent contents. [pyo- + G. *kystis,* bladder]

py·o·der·ma (pī′ō-dĕr′mă) Any pyogenic infection of the skin; may be primary, as impetigo, or secondary to a previously existing condition. [pyo- + G. *derma,* skin]

py·o·der·ma gan·gre·no·sum (pī′ō-dĕr′mă gang-grĕ-nō′sŭm) A chronic, noninfective eruption of spreading, undermined ulcers showing central healing, with diffuse dermal neutrophil infiltration; often associated with ulcerative colitis. See this page.

py·o·gen·e·sis (pī′ō-jen′ĕ-sis) SYN suppuration. [pyo- + G. *genesis,* production]

py·o·gen·ic, **py·o·ge·net·ic** (pī′ō-jen′ik, -jĕ-net′ik) Pus-forming; relating to pus formation.

py·o·gen·ic gran·u·lo·ma, **gran·u·lo·ma py·o·gen·i·cum** (pī′ō-jen′ik gran′yū-lō′mă, pī-ō-jen′i-kŭm) An acquired small, rounded mass of highly vascular granulation tissue, frequently with an ulcerated surface, projecting from the skin or mucosa; histologically, the mass resembles a capillary hemangioma. See page B14. SYN lobular capillary hemangioma.

pyohaemothorax [Br.] SYN pyohemothorax.

py·o·he·mo·tho·rax (pī′ō-hē′mō-thōr′aks) Presence of pus and blood in the pleural cavity. SYN pyohaemothorax. [pyo- + G. *haima,* blood, + thorax]

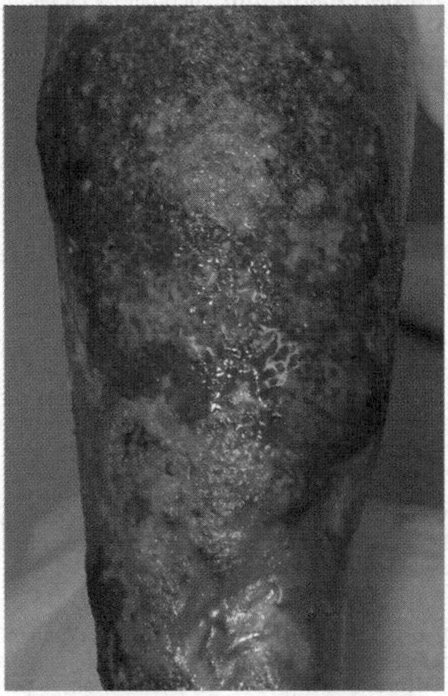

pyoderma gangrenosum: sural region

py·oid (pī′oyd) Resembling pus. [G. *pyōdēs,* fr. *pyon,* pus, + *eidos,* resemblance]

py·o·me·tra (pī′ō-mē′tră) Accumulation of pus in the uterine cavity. [pyo- + G. *mētra,* uterus]

py·o·me·tri·tis (pī′ō-mē-trī′tis) Inflammation of uterine musculature associated with pus in the uterine cavity. [pyo- + G. *mētra,* womb, + *-itis,* inflammation]

py·o·my·o·si·tis (pī′ō-mī′ō-sī′tis) Abscesses, carbuncles, or infected sinuses lying deep in muscles. [pyo- + G. *mys,* muscle, + *-itis,* inflammation]

py·o·ne·phri·tis (pī′ō-nĕ-frī′tis) Suppurative inflammation of the kidney. [pyo- + G. *nephros,* kidney, + *-itis,* inflammation]

py·o·neph·ro·li·thi·a·sis (pī′ō-nef′rō-li-thī′ă-sis) Presence in the kidney of pus and calculi. [pyo- + G. *nephros,* kidney, + *lithos,* stone, + *-iasis,* condition]

py·o·ne·phro·sis (pī′ō-nĕ-frō′sis) Distention of the pelvis and calyces of the kidney with pus, usually associated with obstruction. SYN nephropyosis. [pyo- + G. *nephros,* kidney, + *-osis,* condition]

py·o·o·va·ri·um (pī′ō-ō-var′ē-ŭm) Presence of pus in the ovary; an ovarian abscess.

py·o·per·i·car·di·tis (pī′ō-per′i-kahr-dī′tis) Suppurative inflammation of the pericardium.

py·o·per·i·car·di·um (pī′ō-per′i-kahr′dē-ŭm) An accumulation of pus in the pericardial sac.

py·o·per·i·to·ne·um (pī′ō-per′i-tō-nē′ŭm) An accumulation of pus in the peritoneal cavity. [G. *pyon,* pus]

py·o·per·i·to·ni·tis (pī′ō-per′i-tō-nī′tis) Suppurative inflammation of the peritoneum. [pyo- + peritonitis]

py·o·phy·so·me·tra (pī′ō-fī′sō-mē′tră) Presence of pus and gas in the uterine cavity. [pyo- + G. *physa,* air, + *mētra,* uterus]

py·o·pneu·mo·cho·le·cys·ti·tis (pī′ō-nū′mō-kō′lē-sis-tī′tis) Combination of pus and gas in an inflamed gallbladder caused by gas-producing organisms or by the entry of gas from the duodenum through the biliary tree. [pyo- + G. *pneuma,* air, + cholecystitis]

py·o·pneu·mo·hep·a·ti·tis (pī′ō-nū′mō-hep′ă-tī′tis) Combination of pus and gas in the liver, usually in association with an abscess. [pyo- + G. *pneuma,* air, + hepatitis]

py·o·pneu·mo·per·i·car·di·um (pī′ō-nū′mō-per′i-kahr′dē-ŭm) Presence of pus and gas in the pericardial sac. [pyo- + G. *pneuma,* air, + pericardium]

py·o·pneu·mo·per·i·to·ne·um (pī′ō-nū′mō-per′i-tō-nē′ŭm) Presence of pus and gas in the peritoneal cavity. [pyo- + G. *pneuma,* air, + peritoneum]

py·o·pneu·mo·per·i·to·ni·tis (pī′ō-nū′mō-per′i-tō-nī′tis) Peritonitis with gas-forming organisms or with gas introduced from a ruptured bowel. [pyo- + G. *pneuma,* air, + peritonitis]

py·o·pneu·mo·tho·rax (pī′ō-nū′mō-thōr′aks) The presence of gas together with a purulent effusion in the pleural cavity. SYN pneumopyothorax. [pyo- + G. *pneuma,* air, + thorax]

py·o·poi·e·sis (pī′ō-poy-ē′sis) SYN suppuration. [pyo- + G. *poiēsis,* a making]

py·o·poi·et·ic (pī′ō-poy-et′ik) Pus-producing.

py·o·py·e·lec·ta·sis (pī′ō-pī′ĕ-lek′tă-sis) Dilation of the renal pelvis with pus-producing inflammation. [pyo- + G. *pyelos,* pelvis, + *ektasis,* a stretching]

py·or·rhe·a (pī′ō-rē′ă) A purulent discharge. SYN pyorrhoea. [pyo- + G. *rhoia,* a flow]

pyorrhoea [Br.] SYN pyorrhea.

py·o·sal·pin·gi·tis (pī′ō-sal′pin-jī′tis) Suppurative inflammation of the fallopian tube. [pyo- + salpingitis]

py·o·sal·pin·go-o·oph·o·ri·tis (pī′ō-sal-ping′gō-ō-of′ŏ-rī′tis) Suppurative inflammation of the fallopian tube and the ovary. [pyo- + G. *salpinx,* trumpet (tube), + oophoritis]

py·o·sal·pinx (pī′ō-sal′pingks) Distention of a fallopian tube with pus. [pyo- + G. *salpinx,* trumpet (tube)]

py·o·sis (pī-ō′sis) SYN suppuration. [G.]

py·o·tho·rax (pī′hō-thōr′aks) Empyema in a pleural cavity.

py·o·u·ra·chus (pī′ō-yūr′ă-kŭs) A purulent accumulation in the urachus.

py·o·u·re·ter (pī′ō-yūr′ĕ-tĕr) Distention of a ureter with pus.

pyr·a·mid (pir′ă-mid) **1.** A term applied to a number of anatomic structures having a more or less pyramidal shape. SYN pyramis [TA]. **2.** An obsolete term denoting the petrous portion of the temporal bone. [G. *pyramis* (*pyramid-*), a pyramid]

py·ram·i·dal (pir-am′i-dăl) **1.** Of the shape of a pyramid. **2.** Relating to any anatomic structure called pyramid.

py·ram·i·dal au·ric·u·lar mus·cle (pir-am′i-dăl awr-ik′yū-lăr mŭs′ĕl) An occasional prolongation of the fibers of the tragicus to the spina helicis. SYN musculus pyramidalis auriculae [TA], pyramidal muscle of auricle.

py·ram·i·dal bone (pir-am′i-dăl bōn) SYN triquetral bone.

py·ram·i·dal cat·a·ract (pir-am′i-dăl kat′ăr-akt) A cone-shaped, anterior polar cataract.

py·ram·i·dal cells (pir-am′i-dăl sels) Neurons of the cerebral cortex that, in sections perpendicular to the cortical surface, exhibit a triangular shape with a long apical dendrite directed toward the surface of the cortex.

py·ram·i·dal de·cus·sa·tion (pir-am′-i-dăl dē′kŭs-ā′shŭn) The intercrossing of the bundles of the pyramidal tracts at the lower border region of the medulla oblongata. SYN decussatio pyramidum [TA], motor decussation.

py·ram·i·dal frac·ture (pir-am′i-dăl frak′shŭr) A fracture of the midfacial skeleton with the principal fracture lines meeting at an apex at or near the superior aspect of the nasal bones. SYN Le Fort II fracture.

py·ra·mi·da·lis mus·cle (pir′ă-mi-dā′lis mŭs′ĕl) *Origin*, crest of pubis; *insertion*, lower portion of linea alba; *action*, makes linea alba tense; *nerve supply*, subcostal. SYN musculus pyramidalis [TA], pyramidal muscle.

py·ram·i·dal lobe of thy·roid gland (pir-am′i-dăl lōb thī′royd gland) An inconstant narrow lobe of the thyroid gland that arises from the upper border of the isthmus and extends upward, sometimes as far as the hyoid bone; it marks the point of continuity with the thyroglossal duct.

py·ram·i·dal mus·cle (pir-am′i-dăl mŭs′ĕl) SYN pyramidalis muscle.

py·ram·i·dal mus·cle of au·ri·cle (pir-am′i-dăl mŭs′ĕl awr′i-kĕl) SYN pyramidal auricular muscle.

py•ram•i•dal ra•di•a•tion (pir-am′i-dăl rā′dē-ā′shŭn) Corticospinal fibers passing from the cortex into the pyramid. SYN radiatio pyramidalis.

py•ram•i•dal tract (pir-am′i-dăl trakt) A massive bundle of fibers originating from pyramidal cells in the precentral motor and premotor area and in the postcentral gyrus. Fibers from these cortical regions descend through the internal capsule, the middle third of the crus cerebri, and the ventral part of the pons to emerge on the ventral surface of the medulla oblongata as the pyramis. Continuing caudally, most of the fibers cross to the opposite side in the pyramidal decussation and descend in the spinal cord as the lateral pyramidal tract, which distributes its fibers to interneurons of the spinal gray matter. Interruption of the pyramidal tract at or below its cortical origin causes impairment of movement in the opposite body-half, especially severe in the arm and leg and characterized by muscular weakness, spasticity and hyperreflexia, and a loss of discrete finger and hand movements. Babinski sign is associated with this condition of hemiplegia.

pyr•a•mid of light (pir′ă-mid līt) SYN red reflex.

pyr•a•mid of me•dul•la ob•lon•ga•ta (pir′ă-mid mĕ-dŭl′ă ob-long-gā′tă) An elongated white prominence on the ventral surface of the medulla oblongata on either side along the anterior median fissure, corresponding to the pyramidal tract. SYN anterior pyramid, pyramis medullae oblongatae.

pyr•a•mid sign (pir′ă-mid sīn) Any of the symptoms indicating a morbid condition of the pyramidal tracts, such as the Babinski or Gordon sign, spastic spinal paralysis, or foot clonus.

pyr•a•mid of ver•mis (pir′ă-mid vĕr′mis) A subdivision of the inferior vermis of the cerebellum between the tuber and the uvula.

pyr•a•mis, pl. **py•ra•mi•des** (pir′ă-mis, -dēz) [TA] SYN pyramid (1). [Mod. L. fr. G. pyramid]

pyr•a•mis me•dul•lae ob•lon•ga•tae (pir′ă-mis me-dŭl′ē ob-long-gā′tē) SYN pyramid of medulla oblongata.

pyr•a•mis re•na•lis, pl. **py•ra•mi•des re•na•les** (pir′ă-mis rē-nā′lis, pi-ram′i-dēz rē-nā′lēz) SYN renal pyramid.

pyr•a•nose (pīr′ă-nōs) A cyclic form of a sugar in which the oxygen bridge forms a pyran.

py•ret•ic (pī-ret′ik) SYN febrile. [G. *pyretikos*]

pyreto- Combining form denoting fever. SEE ALSO pyro- (1). [G. *pyretos,* fever, fr. *pyr,* fire]

py•rex•i•a (pī-rek′sē-ă) SYN fever. [G. *pyrexis,* feverishness]

py•rex•i•al (pī-rek′sē-ăl) Relating to fever.

py•rex•i•a of un•known or•i•gin (pī-rek′sē-ă ŭn′nōn ōr′i-jin) SYN fever of unknown origin.

py•ri•din•i•um (pir′i-din′ē-ŭm) A breakdown product of bone collagen, excreted in urine, and assayed as a measure of osteoclast activity; increased in disease states (e.g., Paget disease, primary hyperparathyroidism, osteoporosis).

py•ri•din•o•line (pir′i-din′ŏ-lēn) Hydroxypyridinium; a breakdown product of bone collagen, assayed (as is pyridinium) to measure osteoclastic activity.

pyr•i•do•stig•mine bro•mide (PB) (pir′i-dō-stig′mēn brō′mīd) The bromide salt of a carbamate compound; the salt used as a preexposure antidotal enhancer (often incorrectly termed "pretreatment") against the nerve agent soman. SYN 2-PAM chloride.

pyr•i•do•stig•mine chlor•ide (pir′i-dō-stig′mēn klōr′ēn) The chloride salt of a carbamate anticholinesterase; the salt is used in the treatment of myasthenia gravis and also as a preexposure antidotal enhancer. SEE ALSO secondary blast injury, tertiary blast injury, quaternary blast injury.

pyr•i•dox•al 5′-phos•phate (pir-i-doks′ăl fos′fāt) A coenzyme essential to many reactions in tissue, notably transaminations and amino acid decarboxylations.

pyr•i•dox•a•mine (pir′i-dok′să-mēn) The amine of pyridoxine that has a similar physiologic action. SEE pyridoxine.

4-pyr•i•dox•ic ac•id (pir-i-dok′sik as′id) The principal product of the metabolism of pyridoxal, appearing in the urine.

pyr•i•dox•ine (pir′i-dok′sēn) The original vitamin B6; a term that now includes pyridoxal and pyridoxamine; necessary for various functions including amino acid metabolism and synthesis of heme, histamine, and dopamine. Deficiency may result in increased irritability, convulsions, and peripheral neuritis. The hydrochloride is used in pharmaceutical preparations; the chief form in plant matter.

py•rim•i•dine (pir-im′i-dēn) A heterocyclic substance, the formal parent of several "bases" present in nucleic acids (uracil, thymine, cytosine) as well as of the barbiturates.

py•rin (pī′rin) An abnormal neutrophil protein encoded by the MEFV gene in familial Mediterranean fever. SYN marenostrin.

pyro- **1.** Combining form denoting fire, heat, or fever. SEE ALSO pyreto-. **2.** CHEMISTRY combining form denoting derivatives formed by removal of water (usually by heat) to form anhydrides. SEE ALSO anhydro-. [G. *pyr,* fire]

py•ro•gen (pī′rō-jen) A fever-inducing agent; produced by bacteria, molds, viruses, and yeasts;

commonly found in distilled water. [pyro- + G. *-gen,* producing]

py·ro·gen·ic (pī′rō-jen′ik) Causing fever.

py·ro·glob·u·lins (pī′rō-glob′yū-linz) Serum proteins (immunoglobulins), usually associated with multiple myeloma or macroglobulinemia, that precipitate irreversibly when heated to 56°C.

py·rol·y·sis (pī-rol′i-sis) Decomposition of a substance by heat. [pyro- + G. *lysis,* dissolution]

py·ro·ma·ni·a (pī′rō-mā′nē-ă) A morbid impulse to set fires. [pyro- + G. *mania,* frenzy]

py·ro·nin (pī′rō-nin) A fluorescent red basic xanthene dye, used in combination with methyl green for differential staining of RNA (red) and DNA (green); also used as a tracking dye for RNA in electrophoresis.

py·ro·pho·bi·a (pī′rō-fō′bē-ă) A morbid dread of fire. [pyro- + G. *phobos,* fear]

py·ro·phos·pha·tase (pī′rō-fos′fă-tās) Any enzyme cleaving a pyrophosphate bond between two phosphoric groups, leaving one on each of the two fragments. SYN diphosphatase.

py·ro·phos·phate (PP) (pī-rō-fos′fāt) A salt of pyrophosphoric acid; accumulates in cases of hypophosphatasia; sometimes referred to as inorganic pyrophosphate (PP_i).

py·ro·sis (pī-rō′sis) A substernal pain or burning sensation, usually associated with regurgitation of acid and peptic gastric juice into the esophagus. SYN heartburn. [G. a burning]

pyr·role (pir′ōl) A heterocyclic compound found in many biologically important substances. SYN azole, imidole.

pyr·rol·i·dine (pir-ol′i-dēn) **1.** Pyrrole to which four H atoms have been added; the structural basis of proline and hydroxyproline. **2.** A class of alkaloids containing a pyrrolidine (1) moiety or a pyrrolidine derivative.

py·ru·vate (pī′rū-vāt) A salt or ester of pyruvic acid.

py·ru·vate ki·nase (PK) (pī′rū-vāt kī′nās) A phosphotransferase catalyzing the transfer of phosphate from phosphoenolpyruvate to ADP, forming ATP and pyruvate; other nucleoside phosphates can participate in the reaction; a key step in glycolysis; pyruvate kinase deficiency leads to hemolytic anemia.

py·ru·vic ac·id (pī-rū′vik as′id) An intermediate compound in the metabolism of carbohydrate; in thiamin deficiency, its oxidation is retarded and it accumulates in the tissues. SEE ALSO phosphoenolpyruvic acid.

py·u·ri·a (pī-yūr′ē-ă) Presence of pus in the urine when voided. [G. *pyon,* pus, + *ouron,* urine]

Q

Q 1. Abbreviation for coulomb; quantity; quaternary; glutamine; glutaminyl; pseudouridine; coenzyme Q; electric charge. **2.** The second product formed in an enzyme-catalyzed reaction.

$\dot{Q}$ Blood flow. SEE flow (3). [quantity + an overdot denoting the time derivative]

Q_{CO_2} Symbol for the microliters STPD of CO_2 given off per milligram of tissue per hour.

q 1. CYTOGENETICS long arm of a chromosome (in contrast to p for the short arm). **2.** Abbreviation for [L.] *quodque*, each, every. **3.** Symbol for heat.

QA Abbreviation for quality assurance.

Q-an•gle (ang′gĕl) The angle formed by the line of traction of the quadriceps tendon on the patella and the line of traction of the patellar tendon on the tibial tubercle. The area is usually larger in women than in men.

Q-band•ing stain (band′ing stān) A fluorescent stain for chromosomes that produces specific banding patterns for each pair of homologous chromosomes; the acridine dye derivative quinacrine hydrochloride or other derivatives such as quinacrine mustard dihydrochloride produce a green-yellow fluorescence at pH 4.5 in chromosome segments rich in constitutive heterochromatin with deoxyadenylate-deoxythymidilate (A-T) bases of DNA; centromeric regions of human chromosomes 3, 4, and 13 are specifically stained, as are satellites of some acrocentric chromosomes and the end of the long arm of the Y chromosome.

QC Abbreviation for quality control.

QCSW Abbreviation for Qualified Clinical Social Worker.

Q fe•ver (fē′vĕr) A febrile disease characterized by headache, myalgia, and sometimes pneumonitis or hepatitis; caused by *Coxiella burnetii;* the organism propagates in sheep and cattle, where it produces no symptoms; human infections occur when organisms in contaminated soil and dust are inhaled. [*Q,* for "query," so named because the etiologic agent was unknown]

QH_2 Abbreviation for ubiquinol.

qi (kī) SYN chi (4).

q.i.d. Four times daily. [L. *quater in die*]

QNB Abbreviation for 3-quinuclidinyl benzilate.

q.noct. Abbreviation for every night. [L. quaque nocte]

QNS Abbreviation for quantity not sufficient (amount of specimen submitted to laboratory is inadequate to perform test requested).

Q.O.L. Abbreviation for quality of life. SEE ALSO H.R.Q.O.L.

Q-probes (prōbz) An external peer comparison program sponsored by the College of American Pathologists that addresses process, outcome, and structure-oriented quality assurance issues.

QRB in•ter•val (in′tĕr-văl) The time between the onset of the Q wave of the QRS complex and the right bundle-branch potential (normally 15–20 msec) on an electrocardiogram.

QR in•ter•val (in′tĕr-văl) The time that elapses from the onset of the QRS complex to the peak of the R or the final R wave; measures the time of onset of the intrinsicoid deflection if determined in an appropriate unipolar lead tracing on an electrocardiogram.

QRNG Abbreviation for quinolone-resistant *Neisseria gonorrhoeae.*

QRS com•plex (kom′pleks) An electrocardiographic complex consisting of the Q, R, and S waves, representing propagation of a wave of depolarization over the ventricles.

q.s. ad Abbreviation for quantity sufficient to make.

QS_2 in•ter•val (in′tĕr-văl) SYN electromechanical systole.

Q-switched las•er (swicht lā′zĕr) A laser in which the quality, or energy-storage capacity, varies between very high and low values. [quality-switched]

qt. Abbreviation for quart. SEE quart. [L. *quartus,* fourth]

Q-T in•ter•val, QT in•ter•val (in′tĕr-văl) The time from Q wave (of QRS complex) to the end of the T wave as it can be measured on an electrocardiogram; corresponds to ventricular systole.

quack (kwak) SYN charlatan. [Abbreviation of quacksalver, Dutch *quack,* to boast + *salf,* cream]

quad Abbreviation for quadriceps; quadrilateral; quadrant; (slang) for quadriplegia.

quadr-, quadri- Combining forms meaning four. [L. *quattuor,* four]

qua•dran•gu•lar lob•ule (kwahd-rang′gyū-lăr lob′yūl) The main portion of the superior part of each hemisphere of the cerebellum, corresponding to the monticulus of the vermis; it is divided into two portions, the anterior and the posterior crescentic lobules, corresponding to the culmen and the declive of the vermis. SYN quadrate lobe (2).

quad•rant (quad) (kwahd′rănt) One quarter of a circle. ANATOMY roughly circular areas are divided for descriptive purposes into quadrants. The abdomen is divided into right upper and lower and left upper and lower quadrants by a horizontal and a vertical line intersecting at the umbilicus. Quadrants of the ocular fundus (superior and inferior nasal, superior and inferior temporal) are demarcated by a horizontal and a vertical line intersecting at the optic disc. The tympanic membrane is divided into anterosuperior, anteroinferior, posterosuperior, and posteroinferior quadrants by a line drawn across the diameter of the drum in the axis of the handle of the malleus and another intersecting the first at right angles at the umbo. See this page. [L. *quadrans,* a quarter]

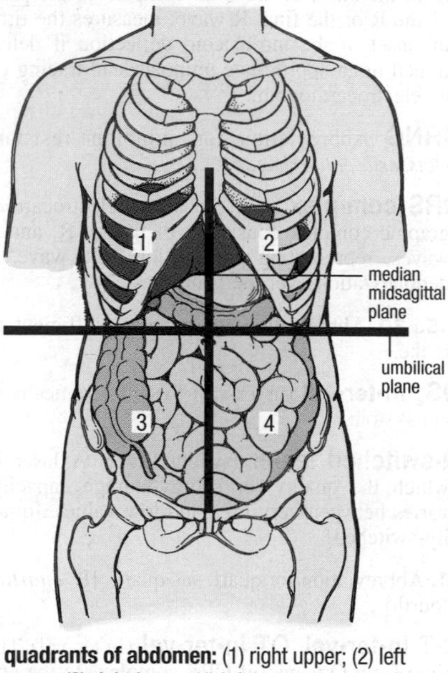

quadrants of abdomen: (1) right upper; (2) left upper; (3) right lower; (4) left lower

quad•rate (kwahd′rāt) Having four equal sides; square. [L. *quadratus,* square]

quad•rate lobe (kwahd′rāt lōb) **1.** A lobe on the inferior surface of the liver located between the fossa for the gallbladder and the fissure for the ligamentum teres; **2.** SYN quadrangular lobule. **3.** SYN precuneus.

quad•ra•tus fem•o•ris mus•cle (kwah-drā′tŭs fem′ŏr-is mŭs′ĕl) *Insertion*, intertrochanteric ridge; *origin*, lateral border of tuberosity of ischium; *action*, rotates thigh laterally; *nerve supply*, nerve to quadratus femoris (sacral plexus). SYN musculus quadratus femoris [TA].

quad•ra•tus la•bi•i su•pe•ri•or•is mus•cle (kwah-drā′tŭs lā′bē-ī sū-pēr-ē-ō′ris mŭs′ĕl) Composed of three heads usually described as three separate muscles: the caput angulare, or levator labii superioris alaeque nasi muscle; caput infraorbitale, or levator labii superioris muscle; and caput zygomaticum, or zygomaticus minor muscle. SYN musculus quadratus labii superioris.

quad•ra•tus lum•bo•rum mus•cle (kwah-drā′tŭs lŭm-bō′rŭm mŭs′ĕl) *Origin*, iliac crest, iliolumbar ligament, and transverse processes of lower lumbar vertebrae; *insertion*, twelfth rib and transverse processes of upper lumbar vertebrae; *action*, abducts trunk; *nerve supply*, ventral primary rami of upper lumbar spinal nerves. See this page. SYN musculus quadratus lumborum [TA].

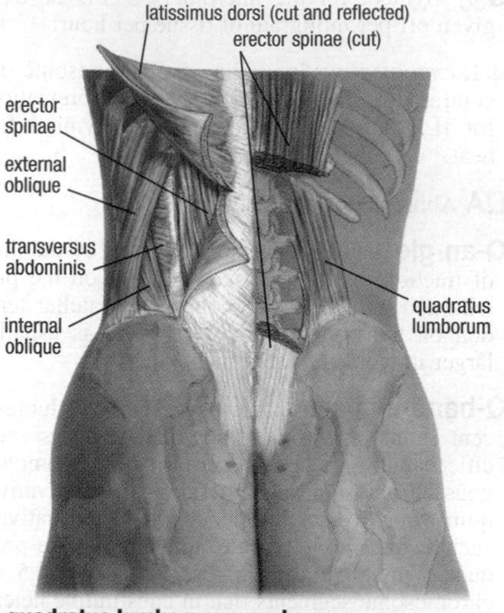

quadratus lumborum muscle

quad•ra•tus plan•tae mus•cle (kwah-drā′tŭs plan′tē mŭs′ĕl) *Origin*, by two heads from the lateral and medial borders of the inferior surface of the calcaneus; *insertion*, tendons of flexor digitorum longus; *action*, assists long flexor; *nerve supply*, lateral plantar. See page 1313. SYN musculus quadratus plantae [TA].

quadri- Prefix meaning four. [L. *quattuor*]

quad•ri•ba•sic (kwah-dri-bā′sik) Denoting an acid having four hydrogen atoms that are replaceable by atoms or radicals of a basic character.

quad•ri•ceps (quad) (kwahd′ri-seps) Having four heads; denoting a muscle of the thigh, quadriceps femoris muscle, and one of the calf, quadriceps surae muscle, or the combined gastrocnemius (with two heads), soleus, and plantaris, more commonly called triceps surae muscle, the plantaris being counted as a separate muscle. See page 1313. [L. fr. quadri- + *caput,* head]

quad•ri•ceps fem•o•ris mus•cle (kwahd′ri-seps fem′ŏr-is mŭs′ĕl) *Origin*, by four heads: rectus femoris, vastus lateralis, vastus intermedius, and vastus medialis; *insertion*, patella, and thence by ligamentum patellae to tuberosity of tibia; *action*, extends leg; flexes thigh by action of rectus femoris; *nerve supply*, femoral. SYN musculus quadriceps femoris [TA], quadriceps muscle of thigh.

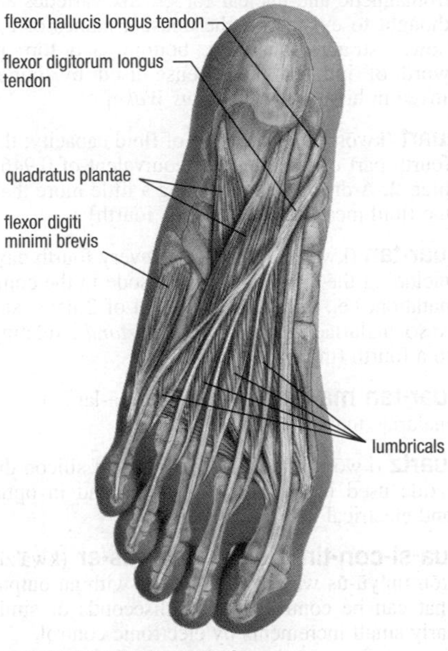

quadratus plantae muscle

quad•ri•ceps mus•cle of thigh (kwahd′ri-seps mŭs′ĕl thī) SYN quadriceps femoris muscle.

quad•ri•ceps re•flex (kwahd′ri-seps rē′fleks) SYN patellar reflex.

quad•ri•gem•i•nal (kwahd′ri-jem′i-năl) Fourfold. [quadri- + L. *geminus,* twin]

quad•ri•gem•i•nal rhythm (kwahd′ri-jem′i-năl ridh′ŭm) A cardiac arrhythmia in which the heartbeats are grouped in fours, each usually composed of one sinus beat followed by three extrasystoles, but a repetitive group of four of any composition is quadrigeminal.

quad•ri•ge•mi•num (kwahd′ri-jem′i-nŭm) One of the quadrigeminal bodies.

qua•dri•gem•i•ny (kwahd′ri-jem′i-nē) A cardiac arrhythmia in which every fourth beat is a premature contraction. [L. *quadrigeminus*, fourfold]

quad•ri•pa•re•sis (kwahd′ri-păr-ē′sis) SYN tetraparesis.

qua•dri•pe•dal ex•ten•sor re•flex (kwahd′ri-ped′ăl eks-ten′sŏr rē′fleks) Extension of the arm of a hemiplegic patient when turned prone as if on all fours. SYN Brain reflex.

quad•ri•ple•gi•a (quad) (kwahd′ri-plē′jē-ă) Paralysis of all four limbs. SYN tetraplegia. [quadri- + G. *plēgē,* stroke]

quad•ri•ple•gic (kwahd′ri-plē′jik) Pertaining to or afflicted with quadriplegia.

quad•ri•va•lent (kwahd′ri-vā′lĕnt) Having the combining power (valency) of four. SYN tetravalent.

quad•rup•let (kwahd-rŭp′let) One of four children born at one birth. [L. *quadruplus,* fourfold]

qual•i•ta•tive a•nal•y•sis (kwahl′i-tā′tiv ă-nal′i-sis) Determination of the nature, as opposed to the quantity, of each of the elements composing a substance.

qua•li•ty (kwahl′i-tē) **1.** A property or trait inherent in the nature of anything. **2.** A degree of superiority. [L. *qualitas*]

qual•i•ty as•sur•ance (QA) (kwahl′i-tē ă-shŭr′ĕns) An institutional program designed to assess the success of the total organization in achieving its goals and to ensure that quality standards are met. SEE ALSO quality control.

qual•i•ty con•trol (QC) (kwahl′i-tē′ kŏn-trōl′) Control of laboratory analytic error by the monitoring of analytic performance with control sera and maintenance of error within established limits around the mean control values, most commonly ±2 standard deviations.

qual•i•ty con•trol chart (kwahl′i-tē′ kŏn-trōl′ chahrt) A chart illustrating the allowable limits of error in laboratory test performance, the limits being a defined deviation from the mean of a control serum, most commonly ±2 standard deviations. SYN Levey-Jennings chart.

qual•i•ty fac•tor (kwah′li-tē fak′tŏr) Used in radiation protection to account for the differ-

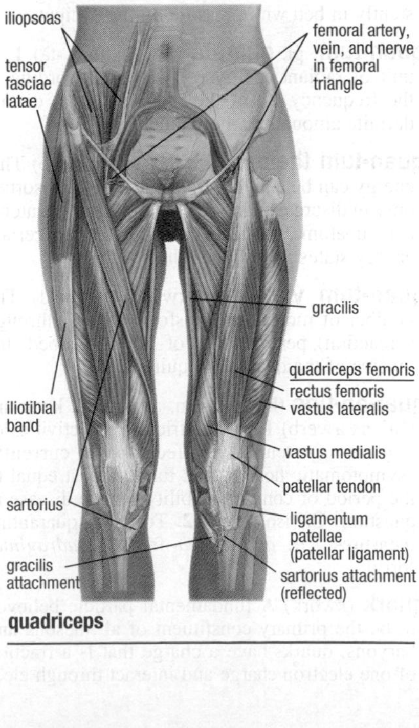

quadriceps

ences in the biological effects from various types of radiation.

qua•li•ty in•di•ca•tors (kwahl′i-tē′ in′di-kā-tŏrz) Criteria, standards, and other measures to assess the quality of health care.

qual•i•ty of life (Q.O.L.) (kwah′li-tē līf) An overall assessment of a person's well-being, which may include physical, emotional, and social dimensions, as well as stress level, sexual function, and self-perceived health status.

quan•tal ef•fect (kwahn′tăl e-fekt′) A result that can be expressed only in binary terms, as occurring or not occurring.

quan•tile (kwahn′tīl) Division or distribution into equal, ordered subgroups; deciles are tenths, quartiles are quarters, quintiles are fifths, terciles are thirds, centiles are hundredths. [L. *quantum*, how much, + *-ilis*, adj. suffix]

quan•ti•ta•tive a•nal•y•sis (kwahn′ti-ta′tiv ă-nal′i-sis) Determination of the amount, as well as the nature, of each of the elements composing a substance.

quan•ti•ty (kwahn′ti-tē) **1.** A number or amount. **2.** A measurable property of anything.

quan•ti•ty suf•fic•i•ent to make (q.s. ad) (kwahn′ti-tē sŭ-fish′ĕnt māk) Adding enough of an ingredient to achieve a specific final volume or total weight. [L. quantum sufficiat ad, however much is needed to]

Quant sign (kwahnt sīn) A T-shaped depression in the occipital bone seen in many patients with rickets, especially in infants lying constantly in bed with pressure on the occiput.

quan•tum, pl. **quan•ta** (kwahn′tŭm, -tă) **1.** A unit of radiant energy (ε) varying according to the frequency (ν) of the radiation. **2.** A certain definite amount. [L. how much]

quan•tum the•o•ry (kwahn′tŭm thē′ŏr-ē) That energy can be emitted, transmitted, and absorbed only in discrete quantities (quanta), so that atoms and subatomic particles can exist only in certain energy states. SYN Planck theory.

quan•tum yield (φ) (kwahn′tŭm yēld) The number of molecules transformed (e.g., through a reaction) per quantum of light absorbed; the inverse of the quantum requirement.

quar•an•tine (kwar′an-tēn, as a noun, kwar-an-tēn′, as a verb) **1.** The restriction of activities of contacts (potentially infected but currently asymptomatic hosts) for a time at least equal to the period of communicability for the disease in question. Cf. isolation. **2.** To apply quarantine measures. [It. *quarantina* fr. L. *quadraginta,* forty]

quark (kwŏrk) A fundamental particle believed to be the primary constituent of all mesons and baryons; quarks have a charge that is a fraction of one electron charge and interact through electromagnetic and nuclear forces. Six varieties are thought to exist, with the unusual names of up, down, strange, charmed, bottom, and top. [a word of indeterminate sense used by James Joyce in his novel *Finnegans Wake*]

quart (kwōrt) **1.** A measure of fluid capacity; the fourth part of a gallon; the equivalent of 0.9468 liter. **2.** A dry measure holding a little more than the fluid measure. [L. *quartus,* fourth]

quar•tan (kwōr′tan) Recurring every fourth day, including the first day of an episode in the computation, i.e., after a free interval of 2 days. SEE ALSO malariae malaria. [L. *quartanus,* relating to a fourth (thing)]

quar•tan ma•lar•i•a (kwōr′tan mă-lar′ē-ă) SYN malariae malaria.

quartz (kwōrts) A crystalline form of silicon dioxide used in chemical apparatus and in optic and electrical instruments.

qua•si-con•tin•u•ous wave las•er (kwā′zī-kŏn-tin′yū-ŭs wāv lā′zĕr) A laser with an output that can be controlled in milliseconds or similarly small increments by electronic control.

qua•si•dom•i•nance (kwā′zī-dom′i-năns) Simulation by a recessive trait of the pedigree of dominant inheritance (i.e., recurrence in several generations) by repeated, and often occult, consanguineous matings. SYN pseudodominance.

qua•si•dom•i•nant (kwā′zī-dom′i-nănt) Denoting a trait in an inbred pedigree that exhibits quasidominance.

qua•ter•na•ry (Q) (kwah′tĕr-nār-ē) **1.** Denoting a chemical compound containing four elements. **2.** Fourth in a series. **3.** Relating to organic compounds in which some central atom is attached to four functional groups. **4.** Referring to a level of structure of macromolecules in which more than one biopolymer is present. [L. *quaternarius,*, fr. *quaterni*, four each, fr. *quattuor,* four, + *-arius*, adj. suffix]

qua•ter•na•ry am•mo•ni•um i•on (kwah′tĕr-nar-ē ă-mō′nē-ŭm ī′on) SEE amine.

qua•ter•na•ry blast in•ju•ry (kwah′tĕr-nar-ē blast in′jŭr-ē) An injury or other condition (including burns and crush-type injury) caused by an explosion but not categorized as primary, secondary, or tertiary blast injury.

Queck•en•stedt-Stook•ey test (kvek′en-shtet stūk′ē test) Compression of the jugular vein in a healthy person causes an increase in the pressure of the spinal fluid in the lumbar region within 10–12 sec; when there is a block of subarachnoid channels, compression of the vein causes little or no increase of pressure in the cerebrospinal fluid.

quel•lung phe•nom•e•non (kvel′lung fĕ-nom′ĕ-non) SYN Neufeld capsular swelling.

quel•lung re•ac•tion (kvel′lung rē-ak′shŭn) **1.**

SYN Neufeld capsular swelling. **2.** If pneumococcal organisms, India ink, and specific antisera are mixed, the antibodies present in the sera will bind to the polysaccharide antigens of the pneumococcal capsule and the capsule will appear more opaque and swollen. [Ger. *Quellung,* swelling]

quel•lung test (kvel′lung test) SYN Neufeld capsular swelling.

quench•ing (kwench′ing) **1.** The process of extinguishing, removing, or diminishing a physical property such as heat or light. **2.** In beta liquid scintillation counting, the shifting of the energy spectrum from a true to a lower energy; it is caused by a variety of interfering materials in the counting solution. **3.** The process of stopping a chemical or enzymatic reaction. [M. E. *quenchen,* fr. O.E. *ācwencan*]

que•ry fever (kwēr′ē prōbz) The origin of Q fever, which is caused by *Coxiella burnetii.*

ques•tion•naire (kwes′chŭn-ār′) A list of questions submitted orally or in writing to obtain personal information or statistically useful data.

quick (kwik) **1.** Pregnant with a child whose fetal movements are recognizable. **2.** A sensitive part, painful to touch. [A.S. *cwic,* living]

quick•en•ing (kwik′ĕn-ing) Signs of life felt by the mother as a result of the fetal movements, usually noted from 17 to 20 weeks of pregnancy. [A.S. *cwic,* living]

Quick test (kwik test) SYN prothrombin test.

qui•es•cent (kwī-es′ĕnt) At rest or inactive.

qui•et lung (kwī′ĕt lŭng) The collapse of a lung during thoracic operations undertaken to facilitate a surgical procedure through the absence of lung movement.

Quinc•ke dis•ease (kving′kĕ di-zēz′) A well-localized edematous disorder that may variably involve the deeper skin layers and subcutaneous tissues as well as mucosal surfaces of the upper respiratory and gastrointestinal tracts; occasionally accompanied by arthralgia, purpura, or fever. SYN angioedema, angioneurotic edema (2).

Quin•cke pulse (kwing′kĕ pŭls) The capillary pulse as appreciated in the fingernails and toenails during aortic regurgitation; ebb and flow are seen; observed as alternate blanching and reddening of the skin. SYN Quincke sign.

Quinc•ke sign (kving′kĕ sīn) SYN Quincke pulse.

qui•nine (kwī′nīn) The most important of the alkaloids derived from cinchona; an antimalarial agent effective against the asexual and erythrocytic forms of the parasite but having no effect on the exoerythrocytic (tissue) forms; does not effect a radical cure of malaria produced by *Plasmodium vivax, P. malariae,* or *P. ovale,* but is used in the treatment of cerebral malaria and other severe attacks of malignant tertian malaria and in malaria produced by chloroquine-resistant strains of *P. falciparum;* also used as an antipyretic, analgesic, sclerosing agent, stomachic, and oxytocic (occasionally), and in the treatment of atrial fibrillation, myotonia congenita, and other myopathies.

quin•o•lones (kwin′ō-lōnz) A group of antimocrobial agents (e.g., norfloxacin, ciprofloxacin, levofloxacin) that block bacterial DNA synthesis.

quin•sy (kwin′zē) SYN peritonsillar abscess. [M.E. *quinsie* (*quinesie*), a corruption of L. *cynanche,* sore throat]

♻**quint-** Combining form meaning fifth or fivefold. [L. *quintus,* fifth]

quin•tan (kwin′tăn) Recurring every fifth day, including the first day of an episode in the computation, i.e., after a free interval of three days. [L. *quintus,* fifth]

quin•tup•let (kwin-tŭp′lĕt) One of five children born at one birth. [L. *quintuplex,* fivefold]

3-qui•nu•cli•din•yl ben•zi•late (QNB) (kwi-nū′kli-din′il ben′zi-lāt) An anticholinergic compound (NATO code BZ) developed for use as an incapacitating chemical-warfare agent.

qui tam ac•tion (kwē tahm ak′shŭn) A civil action brought by an informer (commonly known as a “whistle-blower”), usually against an employer, for activities alleged to be fraudulent or illegal. [L. *qui tam,* who (sues on the part of the state) as well (as for himself)]

quod•que (q) (kwod′kwā) Each, every. [L.]

quo•rum sens•ing (kwōr′ŭm sens′ing) A process whereby bacteria communicate by means of extracellular molecules called *pheromones.*

quo•tid•i•an (kwō-tid′ē-ăn) Daily; occurring every day. SEE ALSO quotidian malaria. [L. *quotidianus,* daily, fr. *quot,* as many as, + *dies,* day]

quo•tid•i•an ma•lar•i•a (kwō-tid′ē-ăn mă-lar′ē-ă) Disorder in which the paroxysms occur daily; usually a double tertian malaria, in which there is an infection by two distinct groups of *Plasmodium vivax* parasites sporulating alternately every 48 hours.

quo•tient (kwō′shĕnt) The number of times one number is contained in another. SEE ALSO index (2), ratio. [L. *quoties,* how often]

q.v. Abbreviation for [L.] as much as you wish.

Q wave (wāv) ELECTROCARDIOGRAPHY the initial deflection of the QRS complex when such deflection is negative (downward).

ρ, Ρ Rho. SEE rho.

R_f, R_F Symbol denoting movement of a substance in paper chromatography *r*elative to the solvent *f*ront; equal to the migration distance of a substance divided by the migration distance of the solvent front.

R Symbol (in italics) for molar gas constant; one of two stereochemical designations in the Cahn, Ingold, and Prelog systems; the third product formed in an enzyme-catalyzed reaction.

r, R Abbreviation for racemic, occasionally used in naming compounds in place of the more common DL- or (±)-, as "r-alanine" (more often as the prefix rac-); roentgen; radius.

RA Abbreviation for remittance advice; rheumatoid arthritis.

Ra Symbol for radium.

rab•bet•ing (rab′ĕt-ing) Making congruous stepwise cuts on apposing bone surfaces for stability after impaction. [Fr. *raboter,* to plane]

rab•bit fe•ver (rab′it fē′vĕr) SYN tularemia.

rab•id (rab′id) Relating to or suffering from rabies. [L. *rabidus,* raving, mad]

ra•bies (rā′bēz) Highly fatal infectious disease transmitted by the bite of infected animals, including dogs, cats, skunks, wolves, foxes, raccoons, and bats, and caused by a neurotropic lyssavirus that replicates in the central nervous system and the salivary glands. The symptoms are excitement, aggressiveness, and madness, followed by paralysis and death. Characteristic cytoplasmic inclusion bodies (Negri bodies) found in many of the neurons are an aid to rapid laboratory diagnosis. SYN hydrophobia. [L. rage, fury, fr. *rabio,* to rave, to be mad]

ra•bies vi•rus (rā′bēz vī′rŭs) A large, bullet-shaped virus of the genus Lyssavirus, in the family Rhabdoviridae, that is the causative agent of rabies.

♻ **rac-** Prefix meaning racemic.

rac•coon eyes (rak-ūn′ īz) Periorbital ecchymosis appearing several hours after delayed discoloration around the eyes from a fracture of the floor of the anterior cranial fossa.

rac•e•mase (rā′sĕ-mās) An enzyme capable of catalyzing racemization, i.e., inversions of asymmetric groups; when more than one center of asymmetry is present, "epimerase" is used.

rac•e•mate (rā′sĕ-māt) A racemic compound, or the salt or ester of such a compound. SEE ALSO racemic.

ra•ceme (rā-sēm′) An optically inactive chemical compound. SEE ALSO racemic.

ra•ce•mic (r, R, rad) (rā-sē′mik) Denoting a mixture of optically active compounds that is itself optically inactive, being composed of an equal number of dextrorotatory and levorotatory substances, which are separable.

rac•e•mi•za•tion (ra′sĕ-mī-zā′shŭn) Partial conversion of one enantiomorph into another (as an L-amino acid to the corresponding D-amino acid) so that the specific optic rotation is decreased, or even reduced to zero, in the resulting mixture.

rac•e•mose (ras′ĕ-mōs) Branching, with nodular terminations; resembling a bunch of grapes. [L. *racemosus,* full of clusters]

rac•e•mose an•eu•rysm (ras′ĕ-mōs an′yūr-izm) SYN cirsoid aneurysm.

rac•e•mose gland (ras′ĕ-mōs gland) A gland that has the appearance of a bunch of grapes if viewed as a three-dimensional reconstruction, e.g., a compound acinous or alveolar gland.

♻ **rachi-, rachio-** Combining forms meaning the spine. [G. *rhachis,* spine, backbone]

ra•chi•al (rā′kē-ăl) SYN spinal.

ra•chi•al•gi•a (rā′kē-al′jē-ă) Pain in the vertebral column (spine) as seen in tuberculous spondylitis (e.g., Pott disease). Formerly known as lead colic. [rachi- + G. *algos,* pain]

ra•chi•cen•te•sis (rā′kē-sen-tē′sis) SYN lumbar puncture. [rachi- + G. *kentēsis,* puncture]

ra•chid•i•al (rā-kid′ē-ăl) SYN spinal.

ra•chi•graph (rā′kē-graf) A graph for recording curves of the vertebrae. [rachi- + G. *graphō,* to write]

ra•chil•y•sis (rā-kil′i-sis) Forcible correction of lateral curvature of the spine by lateral pressure against the convexity of the curve. [rachi- + G. *lysis,* a loosening]

ra•chi•o•cen•te•sis (rā′kē-ō-sen-tē′sis) SYN lumbar puncture. [rachio- + G. *kentēsis,* puncture]

ra•chi•om•e•ter (rā′kē-om′ĕ-tĕr) An instrument for measuring the curvature of the spine, natural or pathologic, or of the spinal column. [rachio- + G. *metron,* measure]

ra•chi•ot•o•my (rā′kē-ot′ŏ-mē) SYN laminotomy. [rachio- + G. *tomē,* incision]

ra•chis, pl. **rach•i•des**, **ra•chis•es** (rā′kis, -ki-dēz, -kis-ēz) SYN vertebral column. [G. spine, backbone]

ra•chis•chi•sis (rā-kis′ki-sis) **1.** Embryologic failure of fusion of neural arches and neural tube with consequent exposure of neural tissue at the surface; spina bifida cystica with myelocele or myeloschisis. **2.** Spinal dysraphism. [G. *rhachis,* spine, + *schisis,* division]

ra•chit•ic (ră-kit′ik) Relating to or suffering from rickets (rachitis).

ra•chit•ic pel•vis (ră-kit′ik pel′vis) A contracted and deformed pelvis, most commonly flat, occurring from rachitic softening of the bones in early life.

ra•chit•ic ro•sa•ry (ră-kit′ik rō′zăr-ē) A row of beading at the junction of the ribs with their cartilages, often seen in rachitic children.

ra•chi•tis (ră-kī′tis) SYN rickets. [G. *rhachitis*]

rach•i•to•gen•ic (ră-kit′ō-jen′ik) Producing or causing rickets. [rachitis + G. *genesis,* production]

ra•cism (rā′sizm) Attitudes, practices and other factors that discriminate against people because of their race, color, or ethnicity.

rack•et am•pu•ta•tion (rak′ĕt amp′yū-tā′shŭn) A circular or slightly oval amputation, in which a long incision is made in the axis of the limb.

rad (rad) **1.** The unit for the dose absorbed from ionizing radiation, equivalent to 100 ergs per gram of tissue; 100 rad = 1 Gy. **2.** Abbreviation for radian; racemic.

ra•dec•to•my (rā-dek′tō-mē) SYN root amputation. [L. *radix,* root, + G. *ektomē,* excision]

♲**radi-** Combining form meaning root. [L. *radix,* root]

ra•di•a•bil•i•ty (rā′dē-ă-bil′i-tē) The property of being radiable.

ra•di•a•ble (rā′dē-ă-bĕl) Capable of being penetrated or examined by rays, especially by x-rays.

ra•di•ad (rā′dē-ad) In a direction toward the radial side.

ra•di•al (rā′dē-ăl) **1.** Relating to the radius (bone of the forearm), to any structures named from it, or to the radial or lateral aspect of the upper limb as compared with the ulnar or medial aspect. **2.** Relating to any radius. **3.** Radiating; diverging in all directions from any given center. SYN brachio- (2). [L. *radialis,* fr. *radius,* ray, lateral bone of the forearm]

ra•di•al ar•ter•y (rā′dē-ăl ahr′tĕr-ē) *Origin,* brachial; *branches,* radial recurrent, dorsal metacarpal, dorsal digital, princeps pollicis, radial index, palmar metacarpal, and muscular, carpal, and perforating. SYN arteria radialis [TA].

ra•di•al col•lat•er•al ar•ter•y (rā′dē-ăl kŏ-lat′ĕr-ăl ahr′tĕr-ē) The anterior terminal branch of the profunda brachii, anastomosing with the radial recurrent, forming part of the articular network of the elbow.

ra•di•al de•vi•a•tion (rā′dē-ăl dē′vē-ā′shŭn) Movement of the wrist toward the thumb side of the forearm.

ra•di•al-dig•i•tal grasp (rā′dē-ăl-dij′i-tăl grasp) A grasp pattern emerging in the 8th–9th month characterized by holding an object between an opposed thumb and fingertips with the object held toward the distal end of these digits so that a space is visible between the thumb and the fingers.

ra•di•al flex•ion (rā′dē-ăl fleks′shŭn) Flexion of the wrist accompanied by radial deviation.

ra•di•al flex•or mus•cle of wrist (rā′dē-ăl fleks′ŏr mŭs′ĕl wrist) SYN flexor carpi radialis muscle.

ra•di•al growth phase (rā′dē-ăl grōth fāz) The early pattern of growth of cutaneous malignant melanoma, in which tumor cells spread laterally in the epidermis.

ra•di•al head (rā′dē-ăl hed) The most proximal aspect of the radius bone. This area is mobile within the anular ligament and allows pronation and supination of the forearm.

ra•di•al in•dex ar•ter•y (rā′dē-ăl in′deks′ ahr′tĕr-ē) SYN radialis indicis artery.

ra•di•a•lis in•di•cis ar•ter•y (rā′dē-ā′lis in′di-sis ahr′tĕr-ē) *Origin,* radial; *distribution,* radial side of index finger. SYN arteria radialis indicis, arteria volaris indicis radialis, radial index artery.

ra•di•al ker•a•tot•o•my (rā′dē-ăl ker′ă-tot′ŏ-mē) A keratotomy with radial incisions around a clear central zone. A form of refractive keratoplasty used in the treatment of myopia.

ra•di•al nerve (rā′dē-ăl nĕrv) Arises from the posterior cord of the brachial plexus; it curves around the posterior surface of the humerus and passes down to the cubital fossa, where it divides into its two terminal branches, the superficial and deep; it supplies muscular and cutaneous branches to the posterior compartments of the arm and forearm. The radial nerve is most commonly injured by fractures of the middle third of the humerus, resulting in a loss of extension at the wrist ("wrist drop"). SYN nervus radialis [TA].

ra•di•al-pal•mar grasp (rā′dē-ăl-pawl′măr grasp) A pattern emerging in the 6th–7th month in which the index and middle fingers curl around an object with the thumb beginning to oppose and press the object into the radial side of the palm.

ra•di•al pulse (rā′dē-ăl pŭls) A palpable rhythmic expansion of the radial artery on the volar aspect of the wrist over the distal radius.

ra•di•al re•cur•rent ar•ter•y (rā′dē-ăl rē-kŭr′ĕnt ahr′tĕr-ē) *Origin,* radial; *distribution,* ascends around lateral side of elbow joint; *anastomoses,* radial collateral, interosseous recurrent.

ra•di•al tu•ber•os•i•ty (rā′dē-ăl tū′bĕr-os′i-tē) An oval projection from the medial surface of the radius just distal to the neck, giving attachment (insertion) on its posterior half to the tendon of the biceps.

ra·di·al tun·nel syn·drome (rā′dē-ăl tŭn′ĕl sin′drōm) Pain in the lateral aspect of the elbow and forearm without motor or sensory deficits, resulting from compression of the radial nerve, at any of various sites along its course, as it passes the elbow and the proximal forearm.

ra·di·al veins (rā′dē-ăl vānz) Venae comitantes of the radial artery continuing from those of the radial aspect of the deep palmar arch, draining into the venae comitantes of the brachial artery in the cubital fossa.

ra·di·an (rad) (rā′dē-ăn) A supplementary SI unit of plane angle. [L. *radius,* ray]

ra·di·ant (rā′dē-ănt) **1.** Giving out rays. **2.** A point from which light radiates to the eye.

ra·di·ant in·ten·si·ty (I) (rā′dē-ănt in-ten′si-tē) SYN luminous intensity.

ra·di·ate (rā′dē-āt) **1.** To spread out in all directions from a center. **2.** To emit radiation. [L. *radio,* pp. *-atus,* to shine]

ra·di·ate crown (rā′dē-āt krown) SYN corona radiata.

ra·di·ate lig·a·ment of head of rib (rā′dē-āt lig′ă-mĕnt hed rib) The radiate, stellate, or anterior costovertebral ligament connecting the head of each rib to the bodies of the two vertebrae with which it articulates.

ra·di·a·ti·o, pl. **ra·di·a·ti·o·nes** (rā-dē-ā′shē-ō, -ō′nēz) [TA] NEUROANATOMY a term applied to any one of the thalamocortical fiber systems that together comprise the corona radiata of the cerebral hemisphere's white matter (e.g., optic radiation, acoustic radiation.). SYN radiation (3). [L.]

ra·di·a·ti·o a·cus·ti·ca (rā-dē-ā′shē-ō ă-kū′stik-ă) [TA] SYN acoustic radiation.

ra·di·a·ti·o cor·po·ris cal·lo·si (rā-dē-ā′shē-ō kōr-pōr′is ka-lō′sī) [TA] SYN radiation of corpus callosum.

ra·di·a·tion (rā′dē-ā′shŭn) **1.** The act or condition of diverging in all directions from a center. **2.** The sending forth of light, short radio waves, ultraviolet or x-rays, or any other rays for treatment or diagnosis or for other purpose. Cf. irradiation (2). **3.** SYN radiatio. **4.** A ray. **5.** Radiant energy or a radiant beam. [L. *radiatio,* fr. *radius,* ray, beam]

ra·di·a·tion bi·ol·o·gy (rā′dē-ā′shŭn bī-ol′ŏ-jē) Science that studies the biologic effects of ionizing radiation.

ra·di·a·tion burn (rā′dē-ā′shŭn bŭrn) A burn caused by exposure to electromagnetic radiation in the form of ultraviolet rays (sunburn), ionizing rays (radiation therapy for cancer treatment), and in rarer instances, nuclear emissions or explosions.

ra·di·a·tion car·ies (rā′dē-ā′shŭn kar′ēz) Decay of the cervical regions of the teeth, incisal edges, and cusp tips due to decreased saliva production (xerostomia) induced by radiation therapy to the head and neck.

ra·di·a·tion of cor·pus cal·lo·sum (rā′dē-ā′shŭn kōr′pŭs kă-lō′sŭm) The spreading out of the fibers of the corpus callosum in the centrum semiovale of each cerebral hemisphere. SYN radiatio corporis callosi [TA].

ra·di·a·tion der·ma·ti·tis (rā′dē-ā′shŭn dĕr′mă-tī′tis) An acute or chronic inflammation of the skin caused by exposure to ionizing radiation, typically as part of cancer radiation therapy; can range from erythema to wet desquamation of the skin (tissue sloughing) in acute form; tissue atrophy, fibrosis, and permanent scarring in chronic form. Permanent changes in skin pigmentation can also occur.

ra·di·a·tion der·ma·to·sis (rā′dē-ā′shŭn dĕr′mă-tō′sis) Skin changes at the site of ionizing radiation, particularly erythema in the acute stage, temporary or permanent epilation, and chronic changes in the epidermis and dermis resembling actinic keratosis.

ra·di·a·tion ne·cro·sis (rā′dē-ā′shŭn ne-krō′sis) Death of cells or tissues resulting from the effects of radiation exposure.

ra·di·a·tion on·col·o·gy (rā′dē-ā′shŭn on-kol′ŏ-jē) **1.** The medical specialty concerned with the use of ionizing radiation in the treatment of disease. **2.** The medical specialty of radiation therapy. **3.** The use of radiation in the treatment of neoplasms. SYN therapeutic radiology.

ra·di·a·tion sick·ness (rā′dē-ā′shŭn sik′nĕs) A systemic condition caused by substantial whole-body irradiation, seen after nuclear explosions or accidents, rarely after radiotherapy. Manifestations depend on dose, ranging from anorexia, nausea, vomiting, and mild leukopenia to thrombocytopenia with hemorrhage, severe leukopenia with infection, anemia, central nervous system damage, and death.

ra·di·a·tion syn·drome (rā′dē-ā′shŭn sin′drōm) Signs and symptoms of total body exposure to radiation, most conspicuous with respect to the system most affected.

ra·di·a·tion ther·a·py (rā′dē-ā′shŭn thār′ă-pē) Treatment with x-rays or radionuclides.

ra·di·a·tion tol·e·rance dose (rā′dē-ā′shŭn tol′ĕr-ăns dōs) The amount of radiation exposure that normal tissue can tolerate and still function properly.

ra·di·a·ti·o op·ti·ca (rā-dē-ā′shē-ō op′ti-kă) SYN optic radiation.

ra·di·a·ti·o py·ra·mi·da·lis (rā-dē-ā′shē-ō pĕr′ă-mi-dā′lis) SYN pyramidal radiation.

rad·i·cal (rad′i-kăl) **1.** CHEMISTRY a group of elements or atoms usually passing intact from one compound to another, but usually incapable of prolonged existence in a free state (e.g., methyl, CH_3); in chemical formulas, a radical is often distinguished by being enclosed in parentheses or brackets. **2.** Thorough or extensive; relating or directed to the extirpation of the root or cause of a morbid process, e.g., a radical operation. **3.** Denoting treatment by extreme, drastic, or innovative, as opposed to conservative, measures. **4.** SYN free radical. [L. *radix* (*radic-*), root]

rad•i•cal dis•sec•tion (rad′i-kăl di-sek′shŭn) Surgical removal of not only the affected tissue or organ, but also the surrounding tissue in a wide margin, typically including the regional lymph nodes to remove not only the malignant tumor but also nearby tissue that may be affected to decrease the risk of recurrence or metastasis.

rad•i•cal hys•ter•ec•to•my (rad′i-kăl his′tĕr-ek′tŏ-mē) Complete removal of the uterus, upper vagina, and parametrium.

rad•i•cal mas•tec•to•my (rad′i-kăl mas-tek′tŏ-mē) Excision of the entire breast, including the nipple, areola, and overlying skin, as well as the pectoral muscles, lymphatic-bearing tissue in the axilla, and various other neighboring tissues. SYN Halsted operation (2).

rad•i•cal neck dis•sec•tion (rad′i-kăl nek di-sek′shŭn) An operation for the removal of metastases to the lymph nodes of the neck in which all of the tissue is removed between the superficial and the deep cervical fascia from the mandible to the clavicle. SEE ALSO functional neck dissection.

rad•i•cal vul•vec•to•my (rad′i-kăl vŭl-vek′tŏ-mē) Surgical removal of the entire vulva: labia majora, labia minora, clitoris, surrounding tissues, and adjacent pelvic lymph nodes; most common treatment for cancer of the vulva.

ra•di•ces (rā′di-sēz) Plural of radix.

ra•di•ces pa•ra•sym•path•i•cae gang•li•o•rum pel•vi•co•rum (rā′di-sēz par-ă-sim-path′i-sē gang′lē-ō′rŭm pel-vi-kō′rŭm) SYN pelvic splanchnic nerves.

rad•i•cle (rad′i-kĕl) A rootlet or a structure resembling one, as the radicle of a vein, a minute veinlet joining with others to form a vein, or the radicle of a nerve; a nerve fiber that joins others to form a nerve. [L. *radicula,* dim. of *radix,* root]

rad•i•cot•o•my (rad′i-kot′ŏ-mē) SYN rhizotomy. [L. *radix* (*radic-*), root, + G. *tomē,* incision]

ra•dic•u•la (ră-dik′yū-lă) A spinal nerve root. [L. dim of *radix,* root]

ra•dic•u•lal•gi•a (ră-dik′yū-lal′jē-ă) Neuralgia due to irritation of the sensory root of a spinal nerve. [radicul- + G. *algos,* pain]

ra•dic•u•lar (ră-dik′yū-lăr) **1.** Relating to a radicle. **2.** Pertaining to the root of a tooth.

ra•dic•u•lar fi•la (ră-dik′yū-lăr fī′lă) The small, individual fiber fascicles into which the roots of all the spinal nerves and several cranial nerves (hypoglossus, vagus, oculomotorius) divide in fanlike pattern before entering or leaving the spinal cord or brainstem; the spinal dorsal root may divide into 8–12 such rootlets.

ra•dic•u•lar pain (ră-dik′yū-lăr pān) Pain along the pathway of a spinal nerve.

ra•dic•u•lec•to•my (ră-dik′yū-lek′tŏ-mē) SYN rhizotomy. [radicul- + G. *ektomē,* excision]

ra•dic•u•li•tis (ră-dik′yū-lī′tis) SYN radiculopathy. [radicul- + G. *-itis,* inflammation]

♻ **radiculo-, radicul-** Combining forms meaning radicle; radicular. [L. *radicula,* radicle, dim. of *radix,* root]

ra•dic•u•lo•gang•li•o•ni•tis (ră-dik′yū-lō-gang′glē-ŏ-nī′tis) Involvement of roots and ganglia.

ra•dic•u•lo•me•nin•go•my•e•li•tis (ră-dik′yū-lō-mĕ-ning′gō-mī-ĕ-lī′tis) SYN rhizomeningomyelitis.

ra•dic•u•lo•my•e•lop•a•thy (ră-dik′yū-lō-mī′ĕ-lop′ă-thē) SYN myeloradiculopathy.

ra•dic•u•lo•neu•rop•a•thy (ră-dik′yū-lō-nūr-op′ă-thē) Disease of the spinal nerve roots and nerves.

ra•dic•u•lop•a•thy (ră-dik′yū-lop′ă-thē) Disorder of the spinal nerve roots. SYN radiculitis. [radiculo- + G. *pathos,* suffering]

ra•di•ec•to•my (rā′dē-ek′tŏ-mē) SYN root amputation. [L. *radix,* root, + G. *ektomē,* excision]

ra•di•i (rā′dē-ī) Plural of radius. [L.]

ra•di•i of lens (rā′dē-ī lenz) The 9–12 faint lines on the anterior and posterior surfaces of the lens that radiate from the poles toward the equator; they mark the lines along which the ends of lens fibers abut. SYN lens stars (1), radii lentis.

ra•di•i len•tis (rā′dē-ī len′tis) SYN radii of lens.

♻ **radio-** Prefix meaning radiation, chiefly (in medicine) gamma-ray or x-ray. [L. *radius,* ray]

ra•di•o•ac•tive (rā′dē-ō-ak′tiv) Possessing radioactivity.

ra•di•o•ac•tive con•stant (λ, lamb•da) (rā′dē-ō-ak′tiv kon′stănt) SYN decay constant.

ra•di•o•ac•tive ha•zard sym•bol (rā′dē-ō-ak′tiv haz′ărd sim′bŏl) The symbol that represents the presence of radioactive materials and the possible dangers of exposure.

ra•di•o•ac•tive i•so•tope (rā′dē-ō-ak′tiv ī′sŏ-tōp) An isotope with an unstable nuclear composition; such nuclei decompose spontaneously by emission of a nuclear electron (β particle) or helium nucleus (α particle) and radiation (γ rays), thus achieving a stable nuclear composition; used as tracers, and as radiation and energy sources. SEE ALSO half-life.

ra·di·o·ac·tiv·i·ty (rā′dē-ō-ak-tiv′i-tē) The property of some atomic nuclei of spontaneously emitting gamma rays or subatomic particles (alpha and beta rays).

ra·di·o·al·ler·go·sor·bent test (RAST) (rā′dē-ō-al′ĕr-gō-sōr′bĕnt test) A radioimmunoassay-based procedure to detect IgE-bound allergens responsible for tissue hypersensitivity: the allergen is bound to insoluble material and the patient's serum is reacted with this conjugate; if the serum contains antibody to the allergen, it will be complexed to the allergen.

ra·di·o·au·tog·ra·phy (rā′dē-ō-aw-tog′ră-fē) SYN autoradiography.

ra·di·o·bi·cip·i·tal (rā′dē-ō-bī-sip′i-tăl) Relating to the radius and the biceps muscle.

ra·di·o·bi·ol·o·gy (rā′dē-ō-bī-ol′ŏ-jē) The study of the biologic effects of ionizing radiation on living tissue. Cf. radiopathology.

ra·di·o·car·di·o·gram (rā′dē-ō-kahr′dē-ō-gram) A graphic record of the concentration of injected radioisotope within the cardiac chambers.

ra·di·o·car·di·og·ra·phy (rā′dē-ō-kahr-dē-og′ră-fē) The technique of recording or interpreting radiocardiograms.

ra·di·o·car·pal (rā′dē-ō-kahr′păl) **1.** Relating to the radius and the bones of the carpus. **2.** On the radial or lateral side of the carpus.

ra·di·o·car·pal joint (rā′dē-ō-kahr′păl joynt) SYN wrist joint.

ra·di·o·chem·is·try (rā′dē-ō-kem′is-trē) **1.** The science of using radionuclides to synthesize labeled compounds for biochemical or biologic research, or radiopharmaceuticals for clinical diagnostic studies. **2.** The study of methods of labeling compounds with radionuclides.

ra·di·o·cin·e·ma·tog·ra·phy (rā′dē-ō-si′nĕ-mă-tog′ră-fē) Taking a motion picture of the movements of organs or other structures as revealed by x-ray fluoroscopic examination. [radio- + G. *kinēma,* motion, + *graphō,* to write]

ra·di·o·cur·a·ble (rā′dē-ō-kyūr′ă-bĕl) Curable by irradiation therapy.

ra·di·o·dense (rā′dē-ō-dens′) SYN radiopaque.

ra·di·o·den·si·ty (rā′dē-ō-den′si-tē) SYN radiopacity.

ra·di·o·der·ma·ti·tis (rā′dē-ō-dĕr′mă-tī′tis) Skin disorder due to exposure to x-rays or gamma rays causing ionization of tissue water with changes resembling thermal injury.

ra·di·o·di·ag·no·sis (rā′dē-ō-dī′ăg-nō′sis) Diagnosis using x-rays; or, more broadly, diagnostic imaging, including radiology, ultrasound, and magnetic resonance.

ra·di·o·fre·quen·cy (rā′dē-ō-frē′kwĕn-sē) **1.** Radiant energy of a certain frequency range; e.g., radio and television employ radiant energy with a frequency between 10^5–10^{11} Hz, whereas diagnostic x-rays have a frequency in the range of 3×10^{18} Hz. **2.** MAGNETIC RESONANCE IMAGING the energy applied to switch or create a gradient in the magnetic field.

ra·di·o·graph (rā′dē-ō-graf) A negative image on photographic film made by exposure to x-rays that have passed through matter or tissue. [radio- + G. *graphō,* to write]

ra·di·og·ra·pher (rā′dē-og′ră-fĕr) A technologist trained to position patients and take radiographs or perform other radiodiagnostic procedures.

ra·di·o·graph·ic art·i·fact (rā′dē-ō-graf′ik ahr′ti-fakt) Blemish on a radiograph caused by heat, light, damaged screens, dust, or improper handling of the x-ray film.

ra·di·o·graph·ic con·trast (rā′dē-ō-graf′ik kon′trast) The variation of the light and dark areas on a radiograph.

ra·di·o·graph·ic den·si·ty (rā′dē-ō-graf′ik den′si-tē) The amount of blackening on an x-ray film produced by the interaction of silver halide crystals with developing agents.

ra·di·og·ra·phy (rā′dē-og′ră-fē) Examination of any part of the body for diagnostic purposes by means of x-rays with the record of the findings usually impressed on a photographic film.

ra·di·o·im·mu·ni·ty (rā′dē-ō-i-myū′ni-tē) Lessened sensitivity to radiation.

ra·di·o·im·mu·no·as·say (RIA) (rā′dē-ō-im′yū-nō-as′sā) An immunologic (immunochemical) procedure that uses the competition between radioisotope-labeled antigen (hormone) or other substance and unlabeled antigen for antiserums, resulting in quantitation of the unlabeled antigen; any method for detecting or quantitating antigens or antibodies using radiolabeled reactants.

ra·di·o·im·mu·no·dif·fu·sion (rā′dē-ō-im′yū-nō-di-fyū′zhŭn) A method for the study of antigen-antibody reactions by gel diffusion using radioisotope-labeled antigen or antibody.

ra·di·o·im·mu·no·e·lec·tro·pho·re·sis (rā′dē-ō-im′yū-nō-ĕ-lek′trō-fŏr-ē′sis) Immunoelectrophoresis in which the antigen or antibody is labeled with a radioisotope.

ra·di·o·im·mu·no·pre·cip·i·ta·tion (RIP) (rā′dē-ō-im′yū-nō-prē-sip′i-tā′shŭn) Immunoprecipitation that uses a radioisotope-labeled antibody or antigen.

ra·di·o·im·mun·o·sor·bent test (RIST) (rā′dē-ō-im′yū-nō-sōr′bĕnt test) A competition assessment, performed in vitro, used to measure

IgE specific for a particular antigen. Known amounts of radiolabeled IgE compete with the patient's unlabeled IgE to bind to a surface coated with anti-IgE. The reduction in radiolabeled IgE due to the presence of IgE in the patient's serum can be determined by comparison to known IgE standards; thus, the amount of the patient's total serum IgE can be determined.

ra•di•o•i•so•tope (rā′dē-ō-ī′sŏ-tōp) An isotope that changes to a more stable state by emitting radiation.

ra•di•o•le•sion (rā′dē-ō-lē′zhŭn) A lesion produced by ionizing radiation.

ra•di•o•li•gand (rā′dē-ō-lī′gand) A molecule with a radionuclide tracer attached; usually used for radioimmunoassay procedures. [radio- + L. *ligandus*, that which is to be bound, fr. *ligo*, to bind]

ra•di•o•log•ic, ra•di•o•log•i•cal (rā′dē-ō-loj′ik, -i-kăl) Pertaining to radiology.

ra•di•o•log•ic a•nat•o•my (rā′dē-ō-loj′ik ă-nat′ŏ-mē) The study of bodily structure by radiography and other imaging methods.

ra•di•o•log•ic dis•tor•tion (rā′dē-ō-loj′ik dis-tōr′shŭn) Misrepresentation of the true size and shape of an object being radiographed (as in magnification, elongation, and foreshortening).

ra•di•o•log•ic en•ter•o•cly•sis (rā′dē-ō-loj′ik en′tĕr-ō-klī′sis) Method of imaging the duodenum and small intestine by intubation of the duodenum and instillation of dilute barium; also known as small bowel enema.

ra•di•o•log•ic sphinc•ter (rā′dē-ō-loj′ik sfingk′tĕr) SYN physiologic sphincter.

ra•di•o•log•ic tech•no•lo•gist (rā′dē-ō-loj′ik tek-nol′ŏ-jist) A person skilled in the use of ionizing radiation to produce diagnostic images.

ra•di•ol•o•gist (rā′dē-ol′ŏ-jist) A physician trained in the diagnostic and therapeutic use of x-rays and radionuclides, radiation physics, and biology; a diagnostic radiologist is also trained in diagnostic ultrasound, magnetic resonance imaging, and applicable physics.

ra•di•ol•o•gy (rā′dē-ol′ŏ-jē) **1.** The science of high-energy radiation and of the sources and the chemical, physical, and biologic effects of such radiation; the term usually refers to the diagnosis and treatment of disease. **2.** The scientific discipline of medical imaging using ionizing radiation, radionuclides, nuclear magnetic resonance, and ultrasound. SYN diagnostic radiology. [radio- + G. *logos*, study]

ra•di•o•lu•cen•cy (rā′dē-ō-lū′sĕn-sē) The state of being radiolucent.

ra•di•o•lu•cent (rā′dē-ō-lū′sĕnt) Relatively penetrable by x-rays or other forms of radiation. Cf. radiopaque. See this page. [radio- + L. *lucens*, shining]

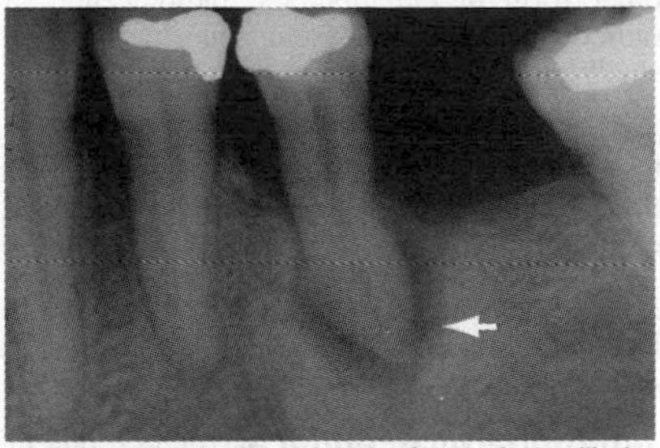

radiolucent area (arrow) around root of mandibular premolar indicating pathological process

ra•di•om•e•ter (rā′dē-om′ĕ-tĕr) A device for determining the penetrative power of x-rays. [radio- + G. *metron*, measure]

ra•di•o•mi•met•ic (rā′dē-ō-mi-met′ik) Imitating the biologic effects of radiation, as in the case of chemicals such as nitrogen mustards. [radio- + G. *mimētikos*, imitative]

ra•di•o•ne•cro•sis (rā′dē-ō-nĕ-krō′sis) Necrosis due to radiation (e.g., after excessive exposure to x-rays or gamma rays).

ra•di•o•neu•ri•tis (rā′dē-ō-nūr-ī′tis) Neuritis caused by prolonged or repeated exposure to x-rays or radium.

ra•di•o•nu•clide (rā′dē-ō-nū′klīd) An isotope of artificial or natural origin that exhibits radioactivity. Radionuclides are used in diagnostic imaging and cancer therapy.

ra•di•o•nu•clide an•gi•o•car•di•og•ra•phy (rā′dē-ō-nū′klīd an′jē-ō-kahr-dē-og′ră-fē) The display, by means of a stationary scintillation camera device, of the passage of a bolus of a rapidly injected radiopharmaceutical.

ra•di•o•nu•clide e•jec•tion frac•tion (rā′dē-ō-nū′klīd ē-jek′shŭn frak′shŭn) A nuclear medicine study for determination of ejection fraction of either ventricle; supersedes multiple-gated acquisition scan in some centers. SEE ALSO multiple-gated acquisition scan.

ra•di•o•nu•clide gen•er•a•tor (rā′dē-ō-nū′klīd jen′ĕr-ā-tŏr) A column containing a large amount of a particular radionuclide (mother radionuclide) that decays down to a second radionuclide with shorter physical half-life; the daughter radionuclide is separated from the parent by the process of elution and affords a continuing supply of relatively short-lived radionuclides for laboratory use; the elution is loosely termed "milking," with the generator referred to as a "radioactive cow."

ra•di•o•pac•i•ty (rā′dē-ō-pas′i-tē) State of being radiopaque. SYN radiodensity.

ra•di•o•paque (rā′dē-ō-pāk′) Exhibiting relative opacity to, or impenetrability by, x-rays or any other form of radiation. Cf. radiolucent. SYN radiodense. [radio- + Fr. opaque fr. L. *opacus,* shady]

ra•di•o•pa•thol•o•gy (rā′dē-ō-pă-thol′ŏ-jē) A branch of radiology or pathology concerned with the effects of radiation on cells and tissues. Cf. radiobiology.

ra•di•o•pel•vim•e•try (rā′dē-ō-pel-vim′ĕ-trē) Radiographic measurement of the pelvis. SEE ALSO pelvimetry.

ra•di•o•phar•ma•ceu•ti•cal (rā′dē-ō-fahr′mă-sū′ti-kăl) A therapeutic agent chemically bound to a radionuclide.

ra•di•o•phar•ma•ceu•ti•cal syn•o•vec•to•my (rā′dē-ō-fahr′mă-sū′tik-ăl sin′ō-vek′tŏ-mē) The treatment of abnormal synovial membranes by radiation derived from the instillation in the joint of a radiopharmaceutical, such as radiogold.

ra•di•o•pro•tec•tant (rā′dē-ō-prō-tek′tănt) Substance that prevents or lessens the effects of radiation.

ra•di•o•re•cep•tor (rā′dē-ō-rĕ-sep′tŏr) **1.** A receptor that normally responds to radiant energy such as light or heat. **2.** A receptor used as a binding agent for unlabeled and radiolabeled analyte in a type of competitive binding assay called radioreceptor assay.

ra•di•o•re•sis•tant (rā′dē-ō-rĕ-zis′tănt) Indicates cells or tissues that are less affected than average mammalian cells on exposure to radiation; when applied to neoplasms, indicates less susceptibility to damage from therapeutic radiation than the surrounding host tissues.

ra•di•o•sen•si•tive (rā′dē-ō-sen′si-tiv) Readily affected by radiation. Cf. radioresistant.

ra•di•o•sen•si•tiv•i•ty (rā′dē-ō-sen-si-tiv′i-tē) The condition of being readily affected by radiant energy.

ra•di•o•te•lem•e•try (rā′dē-ō-tĕ-lem′ĕ-trē) SEE telemetry, biotelemetry.

ra•di•o•ther•a•peu•tic (rā′dē-ō-thār-ă-pyū′tik) Relating to radiotherapy or to radiotherapeutics.

ra•di•o•ther•a•peu•tics (rā′dē-ō-thār-ă-pyū′tiks) The study and use of radiotherapeutic agents.

ra•di•o•ther•a•pist (rā′dē-ō-thār′ă-pist) One who practices radiotherapy or is versed in radiotherapeutics.

ra•di•o•ther•a•py (rā′dē-ō-thār′ă-pē) The medical specialty concerned with the use of electromagnetic or particulate radiation in the treatment of disease.

ra•di•o•ther•my (rā′dē-ō-thĕr′mē) Diathermy effected by heat from radiant sources. [radio- + G. *thermē,* heat]

radiotoxaemia [Br.] SYN radiotoxemia.

ra•di•o•tox•e•mi•a (rā′dē-ō-tok-sē′mē-ă) Radiation sickness caused by the products of disintegration produced by the action of x-rays or other forms of radioactivity and by the depletion of certain cells and enzyme systems from the organism. SYN radiotoxaemia. [radio- + G. *toxikon,* poison, + *haima,* blood]

ra•di•o•trans•par•ent (rā′dē-ō-trans-par′ĕnt) Allowing relatively free transmission of radiant energy.

ra•di•o•trop•ic (rā′dē-ō-trō′pik) Affected by radiation. [radio- + G. *tropē,* a turning]

ra•di•sec•to•my (rā′dē-sek′tŏ-mē) SYN root amputation. [L. *radix,* root, + G. *ektomē,* excision]

ra•di•um (Ra) (rā′dē-ŭm) A metallic element, atomic no. 88, extracted in minute quantities from pitchblende; an alkaline earth metal with properties similar to those of barium. Its therapeutic action is similar to that of x-rays. [L. *radius,* ray]

ra•di•us, gen. and pl. **ra•di•i** (rā′dē-ŭs, -ī) **1.** [TA] The lateral and shorter of the two bones of the forearm. **2.** A straight line passing from the center to the periphery of a circle. [L. spoke of a wheel, rod, ray]

ra•dix, gen. **ra•di•cis**, pl. **ra•di•ces** (rā′diks, -di-sis, -di-sēz′) [TA] **1.** SYN root (1). **2.** SYN root of tooth. **3.** The hypothetic size of the birth cohort in a life table, commonly 1,000 or 100,000. [L.]

ra•dix cli•ni•ca den•tis (rā′diks klin′i-kă den′tis) [TA] SYN clinical root of tooth.

ra•dix pa•ra•sym•path•i•ca gang•li•i o•ti•ci (rā′diks par′a-sim-path′i-kă gang′lē-ī ō′ti-sī) SYN lesser petrosal nerve.

ra•dix sym•path•i•ca gang•li•i pter•y•go•pal•a•ti•ni (rā′diks sim-path′i-kă gang′lē-ī ter-i-gō-pal-ah-tē′nī) SYN deep petrosal nerve.

ra•don (Rn) (rā′don) A gaseous radioactive element, atomic no. 86, resulting from the breakdown of radium; ^{222}Rn is medically significant as an alpha-emitter with a half-life of 3.8235 days; it is used in the treatment of certain malignancies. Poorly ventilated homes in some parts of the United States accumulate a dangerous amount of naturally occurring radon gas. [from radium]

RAE Abbreviation for retinol activity equivalents.

Rae•der par•a•tri•gem•i•nal syn•drome (rā′der par′ă-trī-jem′i-năl sin′drōm) A postganglionic Horner syndrome associated with trigeminal nerve dysfunction caused by involvement of the carotid sympathetic plexus, near the Meckel cave.

Rai•ney cor•pus•cles (rān′ē kōr′pŭs-ĕlz)

Rounded, ovoid, or sickle-shaped spores or bradyzoites, 12–16 by 4–9 mcm, found within the elongated cysts (Miescher tubes) of the protozoan *Sarcocystis*.

rak•ing (rāk′ing) A grasp pattern in infants emerging in the 7th–8th months characterized by the arm, hand, and loosely flexed fingers moving in unison to bring a small object into the palm.

rale (rahl) An extraneous sound heard on auscultation of breath sounds; used by some to denote rhonchus and by others for crepitation. [Fr. rattle]

ral•ox•i•fene (ral-ox′i-fēn) A selective estrogen receptor modulator (SERM) that has estrogen-agonistic effects on bone and lipid metabolism but estrogen-antagonistic effects on breast and uterus; used in the prophylaxis of osteoporosis after menopause.

ra•mal (rā′măl) Relating to a ramus.

Ram•bourg chro•mic ac•id-phos•pho•tung•stic ac•id stain (rahm′būrg krō′mik as′id fos′fō-tŭng′stik as′id stān) A stain for glycoproteins, used with an electron microscope, with which ultrathin tissue sections reveal complex carbohydrates in the same locations as shown by Rambourg periodic acid-chromic methenamine-silver stain.

Ram•bourg pe•ri•od•ic ac•id-chro•mic meth•en•a•mine-sil•ver stain (rahm′būrg pĕr′ē-od′ik as′id krō′mik meth-en′ă-mēn sil′vĕr stān) A stain for glycoproteins, used with an electron microscope, adapted from the Gomori-Jones periodic acid–methenamine-silver stain; it produces silver deposits in mature saccules of the Golgi apparatus, lysosomal vesicles, cell coat, and basement membranes.

Ram•fjord In•dex Teeth (ram′fyōrd in′deks tēth) Specific teeth used for epidemiologic studies of periodontal diseases.

ra•mi (rā′mī) Plural of ramus. [L.]

ra•mi cal•ca•ne•i (rā′mī kal-kā′nē-ī) SYN calcaneal branches.

ra•mi cu•ta•ne•i an•ter•i•or•es ner•vi fem•or•a•lis (rā′mī kyū-tā′nē-ī an-tē-rē-ō′rēz nĕr′vī fe-mō-rā′lis) SYN anterior cutaneous branches of femoral nerve.

ra•mi cu•ta•ne•i cru•ris med•i•ales ner•vi sap•he•ni (rā′mī kyū-tā′nē-ī krū′ris mē-dē-ā′lēz nĕr′vī să-fē′nī) SYN medial cutaneous nerve of leg.

ram•i•fi•ca•tion (ram′i-fi-kā′shŭn) The process of dividing into a branchlike pattern.

ram•i•fy (ram′i-fī) To split into a branchlike pattern. [L. *ramus,* branch, + *facio,* to make]

ra•mi in•ter•cos•ta•les an•ter•i•or•es (rā′mī in′tĕr-kos-tā′lēz an-tē-rē-ō′rēz) SYN anterior intercostal branches of internal thoracic artery.

ra•mi in•ter•cos•ta•les an•ter•i•or•es ar•ter•i•ae thor•ac•ic•ae in•ter•nae (rā′mī in′tĕr-kos-tā′lēz an-tē-rē-ō′rēz ahr-tē-rē′ē thō-rā′si-kē in-ter′nē) SYN anterior intercostal branches of internal thoracic artery.

ra•mi na•sal•es ex•ter•ni ner•vi in•fra•or•bit•al•is (rā′mī nā-sā′lēz eks-ter′nī nĕr′vī in′frā-ōr-bi-tā′lis) SYN external nasal branches of infraorbital nerve.

ra•mi na•sal•es pos•ter•i•or•es in•fer•i•or•es ner•vi pa•lat•i•ni ma•jor•is (rā′mī nā-sā′lēz pos-tē′rē-ōr′ēz in-fē-rē-ōr′ēz nĕr′vī pal-a-tē′nī mā-jō′ris) SYN posterior inferior nasal nerves.

ra•mi pro•sta•ti•ci ar•ter•i•ae rec•tal•is med•i•ae (rā′mī prō-stat′i-sī ahr-tē′rē-ē rek-tā′lis mēd′ē-ē) SYN prostatic branches of middle rectal artery.

ra•mi pro•sta•ti•ci ar•ter•i•ae ves•i•cal•is in•fer•i•or•is (rā′mī prō-stat′i-sī ahr-tē′rē-ē ves-i-kā′lis in-fēr′ē-ō′ris) SYN prostatic branches of inferior vesical artery.

ra•mi scro•tal•es pos•ter•i•or•es ar•ter•i•ae per•i•ne•al•is (rā′mī skrō-tā′lēz pos-tē-rē-ōr′ēz ahr-tē′rē-ē pē-ri-nē-ā′lis) SYN posterior scrotal branches of perineal artery.

ra•mi scro•tal•es pos•ter•i•or•es ar•ter•i•ae pu•den•dae in•tern•ae (rā′mī skrō-tā′lēz pos-tēr-ē-ōr′ēz ahr-tē′rē-ē pū-den′dē in-tĕr′nē) SYN posterior scrotal branches of perineal artery.

ram•i•sec•tion (ram′i-sek′shŭn) Section of the rami communicantes of the sympathetic nervous system. [L. *ramus,* branch, + L. *sectio,* section]

ram•i•tis (ram-ī′tis) Inflammation of a ramus. [L. *ramus,* branch, + G. *-itis,* inflammation]

ramp test (ramp test) A form of graded exercise test in which treadmill speed is kept constant but grade increases each minute between 1 and 4% until volitional exhaustion or other test termination criteria are achieved (e.g., Harbor protocol).

Ram•say Hunt syn•drome (ram′sē-hŭnt sin′drōm) **1.** SYN Hunt syndrome. **2.** SYN herpes zoster oticus.

Ram•stedt op•er•a•tion (rahm′shtet op-ĕr-ā′shŭn) SYN pyloromyotomy.

ram•u•lus, pl. **ram•u•li** (ram′yū-lŭs, -lī) A small branch or twig; a terminal division of a ramus. [L. dim. of *ramus,* a branch]

ra•mus, pl. **ra•mi** (rā′mŭs, -mī) **1.** [TA] SYN branch. **2.** One of the primary divisions of a nerve or blood vessel. SEE ALSO artery, nerve. **3.** A part of an irregularly shaped bone (less slender than a "process") that forms an angle with the main body (e.g., ramus of mandible). **4.** One of the primary divisions of a cerebral sulcus. [L.]

ra•mus car•pal•is dor•sal•is ar•ter•i•ae rad•i•al•is (rā′mŭs kahr-pā′lis dor-sā′lis ahr-tē′

rē-ē rā-dē-ā′lis) SYN dorsal carpal branch of radial artery.

ra•mus car•pal•is dor•sal•is ar•ter•i•ae ul•nar•is (rā′mŭs kahr-pā′lis dor-sā′lis ahr-tē′rē-ē ul-nā′ris) SYN dorsal carpal branch of ulnar artery.

ra•mus car•pal•is pal•mar•is ar•ter•i•ae rad•i•al•is (rā′mŭs kahr-pā′lis păl-mā′ris ahr-tē′rē-ē rā-dē-ā′lis) SYN palmar carpal branch of radial artery.

ra•mus car•pal•is pal•mar•is ar•ter•i•ae ul•nar•is (rā′mŭs kahr-pā′lis păl-mā′ris ahr-tē′rē-ē ul-nā′ris) SYN palmar carpal branch of ulnar artery.

ra•mus car•pe•us dor•sal•is ar•ter•i•ae rad•i•al•is (rā′mŭs kahr′pē-ŭs dor-sā′lis ahr-tē′rē-ē rā-dē-ā′lis) SYN dorsal carpal branch of radial artery.

ra•mus car•pe•us dor•sal•is ar•ter•i•ae ul•nar•is (rā′mŭs kahr′pē-ŭs dor-sā′lis ahr-tē′rē-ē ul-nā′ris) SYN dorsal carpal branch of ulnar artery.

ra•mus car•pe•us pal•mar•is ar•ter•i•ae rad•i•a•lis (rā′mŭs kahr′pē-ŭs păl-ma′ris ahr-tē′rē-ē rā-dē-ā′lis) SYN palmar carpal branch of radial artery.

ra•mus car•pe•us pal•mar•is ar•ter•i•ae ul•nar•is (rā′mŭs kahr′pē-ŭs păl-mā′ris ahr-tē′rē-ē ul-nā′ris) SYN palmar carpal branch of ulnar artery.

ra•mus cir•cum•flex•us ar•ter•i•ae cor•o•nar•i•ae sin•is•trae (rā′mŭs sir-kum-flek′sus ahr-tē′rē-ē kōr-ō-nā′rē-ē sin′is-trē) SYN circumflex branch of left coronary artery.

ra•mus dor•sal•is ner•vi ul•nar•is (rā′mŭs dor-sā′lis nĕr′vī ul-nā′ris) SYN dorsal branch of ulnar nerve.

ra•mus in•ter•ven•tri•cu•lar•is an•te•ri•or ar•ter•i•ae cor•o•nar•i•ae sin•is•trae (rā′mŭs in-tĕr-ven-trik′yū-lā′ris an-tēr′ē-ŏr ahr-tē′rē-ē kōr-ō-nā′rē-ē sin′is-trē) SYN anterior interventricular branch of left coronary artery.

ra•mus in•ter•ven•tri•cu•lar•is pos•ter•i•or ar•ter•i•ae cor•o•nar•i•ae dex•trae (rā′mŭs in-tĕr-ven-trik′yū-lā′ris pos-tēr′ē-ŏr ahr-tē′rē-ē kōr-ō-nā′rē-ē deks′trē) SYN posterior interventricular branch of right coronary artery.

ra•mus lab•i•al•is in•fe•ri•or ar•ter•i•ae fa•ci•al•is (rā′mŭs lā-bē-ā′lis in-fēr′ē-ŏr ahr-tē′rē-ē fā-shē-ā′lis) SYN inferior labial branch of facial artery.

ra•mus lab•i•al•is su•per•i•or ar•ter•i•ae fa•ci•al•is (rā′mŭs lā-bē-ā′lis sŭ-pēr′ē-ŏr ahr-tē′rē-ē fā-shē-ā′lis) SYN superior labial branch of facial artery.

ra•mus lin•gu•lar•is in•fe•ri•or (rā′mŭs ling′gyū-lā′ris in-fēr′ē-ŏr) SYN inferior lingular artery.

ra•mus lin•gu•lar•is su•per•i•or (rā′mŭs ling′gyū-lā′ris sŭ-pēr′ē-ŏr) SYN superior lingular artery.

ra•mus mar•gin•al•is dex•ter ar•ter•i•ae co•ro•na•ri•ae dex•trae (rā′mŭs mahr-jī-nā′lis deks′ter ahr-tē′rē-ē kōr-ō-nā′rē-ē deks′trē) SYN right marginal branch of right coronary artery.

ra•mus mar•gin•al•is sin•is•ter ar•ter•i•ae co•ro•na•ri•ae sin•is•trae (rā′mŭs mar-jī-nā′lis sin′is-tĕr ahr-tē′rē-ē kōr-ō-nā′rē-ē sin′is-trē) SYN left marginal artery.

ra•mus men•in•ge•us re•cur•rens ner•vi ophth•al•mi•ci (rā′mŭs mē-nin-jē′us rē-kŭr′renz nĕr′vī of-thal′mi-sī) SYN tentorial nerve.

ra•mus my•lo•hy•oi•de•us ar•ter•i•ae al•ve•o•lar•is in•fer•i•or•is (rā′mŭs mī′lō-hī-oy′dē-ŭs ahr-tē′rē-ē al-vē-ō-lā′ris in-fĕr′ē-ōr′is) SYN mylohyoid branch of inferior alveolar artery.

ra•mus no•di a•tri•o•ven•tric•u•la•ris (rā′mŭs nō′dī ā′trē-ō-ven-trik′ū-lār′is) SYN atrioventricular nodal branches.

ra•mus phar•yn•ge•us gang•li•i pter•y•go•pa•la•ti•ni (rā′mŭs fă-rin′jē-ŭs gang-glē′ī ter′i-gō-pal-ă-tē′nī) SYN pharyngeal nerve.

ra•mus pro•fund•us ner•vi rad•i•al•is (rā′mŭs prō-fŭn′dŭs nĕr′vī rā-dē-ā′lis) SYN deep branch of radial nerve.

ra•mus pro•fun•dus ner•vi ul•nar•is (rā′mŭs prō-fŭn′dŭs nĕr′vī ul-nā′ris) SYN deep branch of ulnar nerve.

ra•mus sep•ti pos•ter•i•or•is na•sal•is (rā′mŭs sep′tī pos-tēr′ē-ŏr-is nā-sā′lis) SYN posterior septal branch of nose.

ra•mus su•per•fi•ci•al•is ar•ter•i•ae trans•vers•ae col•li (rā′mŭs sū′pĕr-fish′ē-ā′lis ahr-tē′rē-ē trans-vĕr′sē kol′ī) SYN superficial cervical artery.

ra•mus su•per•fi•ci•al•is ner•vi ra•di•al•is (rā′mŭs sū′pĕr-fish′ē-ā′lis nĕr′vī rā-dē-ā′lis) SYN superficial branch of radial nerve.

ra•mus su•per•fi•ci•al•is ner•vi ul•nar•is (rā′mŭs sū′pĕr-fish′ē-ā′lis nĕr′vī ul-nā′ris) SYN superficial branch of ulnar nerve.

ra•mus ten•tor•i•i (rā′mŭs ten-tō′rē-ī) SYN tentorial nerve.

Ran•cho Los A•mi•gos Lev•els of Cog•ni•tive Func•tion•ing Scale (ranch′ō lōs ah-mē′gōs lev′ĕlz kog′ni-tiv fungk′shŭn-ing skāl) A measure used to gauge the level of cognitive function of people with head injury by close observation of behavioral signs; used to facilitate communication among health professionals and family regarding diagnosis and progress; based on patient response to therapeutic and environmental stimulation.

ran•cid (ran′sid) Having a disagreeable odor and

taste, usually characterizing fat undergoing oxidation or bacterial decomposition to more volatile odoriferous substances. [L. *rancidus,* stinking, rank]

Ran•dall plaques (ran′dăl plaks) Mineral concentrations on renal papillae.

ran•dom am•pli•fied pol•y•mor•phic DNA (RAPD) (ran′dŏm amp′li-fīd pol-ē-mōr′fik) An amplified strain-typing procedure that uses primers with random sequences that anneal to random chromosomal DNA sequences of the strain of interest.

randomisation [Br.] SYN randomization.

ran•dom•i•za•tion (ran′dŏm-ī-zā′shŭn) Assignment of the subjects of experimental research to groups by chance. SYN randomisation.

ran•dom mat•ing (ran′dŏm māt′ing) A practice of mating in a population in which at some specified locus mating patterns occur with expected frequencies predicted by the product of the frequencies of the genotypes in the population.

ran•dom pat•tern flap (ran′dŏm pat′ĕrn flap) A flap in which the pedicle blood supply is derived randomly from the network of vessels in the area, rather than from a single longitudinal artery as in an axial pattern flap.

ran•dom sam•pling (ran′dŏm sam′pling) A selection of elements by a formal randomizing device for purposes of inference about a population in such a way that the probability of each possible outcome may be precisely specified in advance; the inferences are necessarily stochastic.

ran•dom spec•i•men (ran′dŏm spes′i-mĕn) A sample that may be collected at any time.

ran•dom void•ed spec•i•men (ran′dŏm voy′dĕd spes′i-mĕn) A urine specimen, collected at any time within a 24-hour period.

range (rānj) A statistical measure of the dispersion or variation of values determined by the endpoint values themselves or the difference between them; e.g., in a group of children aged 6, 8, 9, 10, 13, and 16, the range would be from 6–16 or, alternately, 10 (16 – 6 years). [O.Fr. *rang,* line fr. Germanic]

range of ac•com•mo•da•tion (rānj ă-kom′ŏ-dā′shŭn) The distance between an object viewed with minimal refractivity of the eye and one viewed with maximal accommodation.

range of mo•tion (ROM) (rānj mō′shŭn) **1.** The measured beginning and terminal angles, as well as the total degrees of motion, traversed by a joint moved by active muscle contraction or by passive movement. **2.** Joint movement (active, passive, or a combination of both) carried out to assess, preserve, or increase the arc of joint motion.

range-of-mo•tion (ROM) ex•er•cise (rānj mō′shŭn eks′ĕr-sīz) A passive, assistive, or active exercise used to increase the range of movement in a joint or to prevent its contracture.

ra•nine (rā′nīn) **1.** Relating to the frog. **2.** Relating to the undersurface of the tongue. [L. *rana,* a frog]

Ran•kin clamp (rang′kin klamp) A three-bladed clamp used in resection of colon.

Ran•so•hoff sign (ran′sŏ-hof sīn) Yellow pigmentation in the umbilical region in rupture of the common bile duct.

ran•u•la (ran′yū-lă) **1.** Hypoglottis. **2.** Any cystic tumor of the undersurface of the tongue or floor of the mouth, especially one of the floor of the mouth due to obstruction of the duct of the sublingual glands. SYN ptyalocele, sialocele, sublingual cyst. [L. tadpole, dim. of *rana,* frog]

ran•u•lar (ran′yū-lăr) Relating to a ranula.

Ran•vi•er node (rahn-vē-ā′ nōd) A short interval in the myelin sheath of a nerve fiber, occurring between segments of the myelin sheath; at the node, the axon is invested only by short, fingerlike cytoplasmic processes of the two neighboring Schwann cells or, in the central nervous system, oligodendroglia cells. SEE ALSO myelin sheath. SYN node of Ranvier.

RAO Abbreviation for right anterior oblique, a radiographic position in which the right anterior part of the body is closest to the film.

Raoult law (rah-ūl′ law) The vapor pressure of a solution of a nonvolatile nonelectrolyte is that of the pure solvent multiplied by the mole-fraction of the solvent in the solution.

RAPD Abbreviation for random amplified polymorphic DNA.

rape (rāp) **1.** Sexual intercourse by force, duress, intimidation, or without legal consent (as with a minor). **2.** The performance of such an act. [L. *rapio,* to seize, to drag away]

ra•phe (rā′fē) The line of union of two contiguous, bilaterally symmetric structures. [G. *rhaphē,* suture, seam]

ra•phe nu•cle•i (rā′fē nū′klē-ī) Collective term denoting a variety of unpaired nerve cell groups in and along the median plane of the mesencephalic and rhombencephalic tegmentum: the nucleus centralis tegmenti superior, nucleus raphes dorsalis, nucleus raphes pontis, nucleus raphes magnus, nucleus raphes pallidus, and nucleus raphes obscurus. These nuclei include neurons characterized by their containing the neurotransmitter serotonin; their serotonin-carrying axons extend rostrally to the hypothalamus, septum, hippocampus, and cingulate gyrus and include projections to the brainstem, cerebellum, and spinal cord.

rap•id ca•ni•ti•es (rap′id kă-nish′ē-ēz) Whitening of the hair overnight or over a few days; in the latter case, may be seen in alopecia areata, when surviving pigmented hairs are preferentially shed from gray hair.

rap·id eye move·ments (REM) (rap′id ī mūv′mĕnts) Symmetric quick scanning movements of the eyes occurring many times during sleep in clusters for 5–60 minutes; associated with dreaming.

rap·id eye move·ment sleep (rap′id ī mūv′mĕnt slēp) That state of deep sleep in which rapid eye movements, alert EEG pattern, and dreaming occur; several central and autonomic functions are distinctive during this state. SEE ALSO paradoxic sleep.

ra·pid me·di·cal as·sess·ment (rap′id med′i-kăl ă-ses′mĕnt) Quick head-to-toe physical examination of an unresponsive prehospital medical patient to discover signs of disease or injury before transport.

rap·id re·sponse team (rap′id rē-spons′ tēm) Medical emergency team of clinicians with critical care expertise who intervene before cardiac or respiratory arrest occurs.

ra·pid se·quence in·tu·ba·tion (RSI) (rap′id sē′kwĕns in′tū-bā′shŭn) Endotracheal intubation performed on a patient to whom a paralytic drug has been administered. Used with prehospital care in combative or head-injured patients.

ra·pid trau·ma as·sess·ment (rap′id traw′mă ă-ses′mĕnt) Quick head-to-toe physical examination of an unresponsive prehospital trauma patient for the purpose of discovering and assessing injuries before transport.

Ra·po·port-Leu·ber·ing shunt (rap′ŏ-pōrt-loy′ber-ing shŭnt) A shunt of the glycolytic pathway in which 1,3 diphosphoglycerate (1,3-DPG) is converted to 2,3-DPG. 2,3-DPG enhances the release of oxygen from hemoglobin to the tissues.

Ra·po·port test (rap′ŏ-pōrt test) A differential ureteral catheterization assessment used to evaluate suspected renovascular hypertension; urine specimens from each kidney are obtained by bilateral ureteral catheterization, and the tubular rejection fraction ratio is determined by measuring concentrations of sodium and creatinine in the urine from each kidney.

rap·port (rap-ōr′) **1.** A feeling of relationship, especially when characterized by emotional affinity. **2.** A conscious feeling of accord, trust, empathy, and mutual responsiveness between two or more people (e.g., physician and patient) that fosters the therapeutic process. [Fr.]

rare earths (rār ĕrths) SEE lanthanides.

rar·e·fac·tion (rār′ĕ-fak′shŭn) The process of becoming light or less dense; the condition of being light; opposed to condensation. [L. *rarus,* thin, scanty + *facio,* to make]

RAS Abbreviation for reticular activating system.

rash (rash) Colloquial term for a cutaneous eruption. [O. Fr. *rasche,* skin eruption, fr. L. *rado,* pp. *rasus,* to scratch, scrape]

Ras·mus·sen an·eu·rysm (rahs′mŭ-sĕn an′yūr-izm) Aneurysmal dilation of a branch of a pulmonary artery in a tuberculous cavity, rupture of which may cause serious hemoptysis.

Ras·mus·sen en·ceph·a·li·tis (ras′mŭs-ĕn en-sef′ă-lī′tis) Encephalitis in which antibodies to a stimulatory glutamate receptor in the CNS are found; perhaps an autoimmune disease.

ras on·co·gene (ras ong′kō-jēn) Point mutations first described in rat sarcoma cells that can be shown to have transforming activity in culture, as well as in tumorigenesis models in mice; the ras gene family is composed of three closely related genes on three different chromosomes; abnormalities have been identified in a variety of human tumors.

ras·pa·to·ry (ras′pă-tōr-ē) A surgical instrument used to smooth the edges of a divided bone. [L. *raspatorium*]

RAST (rast) Acronym for radioallergosorbent test.

Ras·tel·li op·er·a·tion (rahs-te′lē op-ĕr-ā′shŭn) For "anatomic" repair of transposition of the great arteries (ventriculoarterial discordance) with ventricular septal defect and left ventricular outflow tract obstruction; conduits are used to create left ventricular to aortic continuity and right ventricular to pulmonary artery continuity. All septal defects are obliterated, as are any previously constructed palliative shunts.

rat (rat) A rodent of the genus *Rattus,* a widespread predator and pest that attacks wild and domestic animals, consumes or damages crops and stored foodstuffs, and is involved in transmission of diseases (e.g., intestinal parasites, plague, typhus, rat-bite fever) to humans; laboratory rats belong to albino strains of the Norway rat, *R. norvegicus.*

rat-bite fe·ver (rat-bīt fē′vĕr) A single designation for two bacterial diseases associated with rat bites, one caused by *Streptobacillus moniliformis* (i.e., Haverhill fever), the other by *Spirillum minus* (i.e., sodoku); both diseases are characterized by relapsing fever, chills, headache, arthralgia, lymphadenopathy, and a maculopapular rash on the extremities.

rate (rāt) **1.** A measurement of an event or process in terms of its relation to some fixed standard; expressed as the ratio of one quantity to another (e.g., velocity, distance per unit of time). **2.** A measure of the frequency of an event in a defined population; the components of a rate are: the numerator (number of events); the denominator (population at risk of experiencing the event); the specified time in which the events occur; and usually a multiplier, a power of 10, which makes it possible to express the rate as a whole number. [L. *ratum,* a reckoning (see ratio)]

rate con•stants (*k*) (rāt kon′stănts) Proportionality constants equal to the initial rate of a reaction divided by the concentration of the reactant(s); e.g., in the reaction A → B + C, the rate of the reaction equals $-d[A]/dt = k_1[A]$. The rate constant k_1 is a unimolecular rate constant, since there is only one molecular species reacting, and has units of reciprocal time (e.g., sec^{-1}). For the reverse reaction, B + C → A, the rate equals $-d[B]/dt = d[A]/dt = k_2[B][C]$. The rate constant k_2 is a bimolecular rate constant and has units of reciprocal concentration-time (e.g., M^{-1} sec^{-1}).

rate of per•ceived ex•er•tion (RPE) (rāt pĕr-sēvd′ eg-zĕr′shŭn) A scale used to measure a person's perception of the intensity of an exercise.

Rath•ke cleft cyst (raht′kĕ kleft sist) An intrasellar or suprasellar cyst lined by cuboidal epithelium derived from remnants of the Rathke pouch.

Rath•ke pock•et (raht′kĕ pok′ĕt) SYN hypophysial diverticulum.

Rath•ke pouch (raht′kĕ powch) SYN hypophysial diverticulum.

Rath•ke pouch tu•mor (raht′kĕ powch tū′mŏr) SYN craniopharyngioma.

rat•ing of per•ceived ex•er•tion (rāt′ing pĕr-sēvd′ eg-zĕr′shŭn) Subjective numeric rating (range, 6–19 or 0–10) of exercise intensity based on how a person feels in relation to levels of physiologic stress. An RPE of 13 or 14 (exercise that feels "somewhat hard") coincides with an exercise heart rate of about 70% maximum. SYN Borg scale.

ra•ti•o (rā′shē-ō) An expression of the relation of one quantity to another (e.g., of a proportion or rate). SEE ALSO index (2), quotient. [L. *ratio* (*ration-*) a reckoning, reason, fr. *reor,* pp. *ratus,* to reckon, compute]

ra•tion•al (rash′ŭn-ăl) **1.** Pertaining to reasoning or to the higher thought processes; based on objective or scientific knowledge, in contrast to empiric (1). **2.** Influenced by reasoning rather than by emotion. **3.** Having the reasoning faculties; not delirious or comatose. [L. *rationalis,* fr. *ratio,* reason]

ra•tion•al for•mu•la (rash′ŭn-ăl fōrm′yū-lă) CHEMISTRY a formula that indicates the constitution as well as the composition of a substance.

ra•tion•al•i•za•tion (ra′shŭn-ăl-ī-zā′shŭn) A psychoanalytic defense mechanism through which irrational behavior, motives, or feelings are made to appear reasonable. [L. *ratio,* reason]

ra•tion•al ther•a•py (rash′ŭn-ăl thār′ă-pē) Therapeutic procedures based on the premise that lack of information or illogical thought patterns are basic causes of a patient's difficulties.

ra•tion•ing (rash′ŭn-ing) Allotment or distribution of fixed portions. [L. *ratio,* calculation]

rat•tle•weed (rat′ĕl-wēd) SYN black cohosh.

RAV Abbreviation for Rous-associated virus.

ray (rā) **1.** A beam of light, heat, or other form of radiation. The rays from radium and other radioactive substances are produced by a spontaneous disintegration of the atom; they are electrically charged particles or electromagnetic waves of extremely short wavelength. **2.** A part or branch that extends radially from a structure. **3.** One of the grooves of the embryonic hand and foot indicating where the digital rays (e.g., hand rays) will develop. [L. *radius*]

Ray•naud phe•nom•e•non (rā-nō′ fĕ-nom′ĕ-non) Spasm of the digital arteries, with blanching and numbness or pain of the fingers, often precipitated by cold. Fingers become variably red, white, and blue. SEE ALSO Raynaud syndrome. See page B9.

Ray•naud sign (rā-nō′ sīn) SYN acrocyanosis.

Ray•naud syn•drome (rā-nō′ sin′drōm) Bilateral arterial and arteriolar cyanosis of the fingers due to vasoconstriction of uncertain cause; may be brought on by low temperatures or emotional stress. SEE ALSO Raynaud phenomenon.

R-band•ing stain (band′ing stān) A reverse Giemsa chromosome banding method that produces bands complementary to G-bands; induced by treatment with high temperature, low pH, or acridine orange staining; often used together with G-banding on human karyotype to determine whether there are deletions.

rbc, RBC Abbreviation for red blood cell; red blood count.

RBF Abbreviation for renal blood flow. SEE effective renal blood flow.

RBP Abbreviation for retinol-binding protein.

RBRVS Abbreviation for Resource-Based Relative Value Scale.

RCP Abbreviation for respiratory care practitioner.

RCS Abbreviation for registered cardiac sonographer.

RDA Abbreviation for recommended dietary allowance.

RDPA Abbreviation for right descending pulmonary artery.

RDS Abbreviation for respiratory distress syndrome of the newborn.

Re Symbol for rhenium.

re- Prefix meaning again or backward. [L.]

reach (rēch) To stretch out or put forth; to grasp or attain by extending or advancing. [O.E. *raecan*]

Reach to Re•cov•er•y (rēch rē-cŏv′ĕr-ē) An American Cancer Society-sponsored program in which breast cancer survivors, who have made a full adjustment to their breast cancer treatment, volunteer their time and services to help women who are diagnosed with breast cancer and their families.

re•act (rē-akt′) To take part in or to undergo a chemical reaction. [Mod. L. *reactus*]

re•ac•tance (X) (rē-ak′tăns) The weakening of an alternating electric current by passage through a coil of wire or a condenser.

re•ac•tant (rē-ak′tănt) A substance taking part in a chemical reaction.

re•ac•tion (rē-ak′shŭn) **1.** The response of a muscle or other living tissue or organism to a stimulus. **2.** The color change effected in litmus and certain other organic pigments by contact with substances such as acids or alkali; also the property that such substances possess to produce this change. **3.** CHEMISTRY the intermolecular action of two or more substances on each other, whereby these substances are made to disappear and new ones are formed in their place (chemical reaction). **4.** IMMUNOLOGY action of an antibody on a specific antigen in vivo or in vitro, with or without the involvement of complement or other components of the immunologic system. [L. *re-*, again, backward, + *actio,* action]

re•ac•tion of de•gen•er•a•tion (DR) (rē-ak′shŭn dĕ-jen′ĕr-ā′shŭn) The electrical reaction in a degenerated nerve and the muscles supplied by it; characterized by absence of response to both galvanic and faradic stimulus in the nerve and to faradic stimulus in the muscles.

re•ac•tion for•ma•tion (rē-ak′shŭn fōr-mā′shŭn) PSYCHOANALYSIS a postulated defense mechanism in which attitudes and behaviors that are adopted are the opposites of that which the person would ordinarily be expected to express and actually feel at an unconscious level.

re•ac•tion time (rē-ak′shŭn tīm) Interval between presentation of a stimulus and the beginning of an individual's response.

re•ac•ti•vate (rē-ak′ti-vāt) To render active once again; in particular, of an activated immune serum to which normal serum (complement) is added.

re•ac•ti•va•tion tu•ber•cu•lo•sis (rē-ak′ti-vā′shun tū-bĕr′kyū-lō′sis) SYN secondary tuberculosis.

re•ac•tive air•ways dis•ease (rē-ak′tiv ār′wāz di-zēz′) SYN asthma.

re•ac•tive chan•ges (rē-ak′tiv chānj′ĕz) Term in the Bethesda classification system for reporting cervical or vaginal cytologic diagnoses that refers to changes of a benign nature, which are associated with inflammation (including typical repair), atrophy with inflammation, radiation, an intrauterine device, and other nonspecific causes. SEE ALSO Bethesda system, AGUS, LSIL, HSIL.

re•ac•tive de•pres•sion (rē-ak′tiv dĕ-presh′ŭn) A psychological state occasioned directly by an intensely sad external situation (frequently loss of a loved person), relieved by the removal of the external situation (e.g., reunion with a loved person).

re•ac•tive hy•per•e•mi•a (rē-ak′tiv hī′pĕr-ē′mē-ă) Hyperemia following the arrest and subsequent restoration of the blood supply to a part.

re•ac•tive hy•po•gly•ce•mi•a (rē-ak′tiv hī′pō-glī-sē′mē-ă) After eating a carbohydrate meal, the affected subject overreacts and produces too much insulin in response to the food so that the glucose level decreases rapidly.

re•ac•tiv•i•ty (rē′ak-tiv′i-tē) **1.** The property of reacting, chemically or in any other sense. **2.** The process of reacting.

read•a•bil•i•ty (rēd′ă-bil′i-tē) NURSING ease with which written or printed material can be read and understood; important in assessment of patient teaching.

read•i•ness to learn (red′ē-nĕs lĕrn) NURSING time when patient, staff, and other learners demonstrate interest in learning; receptiveness to learning and willingness and ability to participate in the learning process.

read•ing (rēd′ing) **1.** The perception and understanding of the meaning of visual symbols (e.g., letters or words) by the scanning of writing or print with the eyes. **2.** Any of several alternative ways of interpreting symbols, such as Braille or the close observation of a speaker's facial movements.

read•through (rēd′thrū) MOLECULAR BIOLOGY transcription of a nucleic acid sequence beyond its normal termination sequence.

re•a•gent (rē-ā′jĕnt) Any substance added to a solution of another substance to participate in a chemical reaction. [Mod. L. *reagens*]

re•a•gin•ic an•ti•bo•dy (rē′ā-jin′ik an′ti-bod-ē) SYN homocytotropic antibody.

REAL (rēl) Acronym for Revised European-American Classification of Lymphoid Neoplasms. SEE REAL classification.

REAL clas•si•fi•ca•tion (rēl klas′i-fi-kā′shŭn) A classification of lymphoma first published in 1994 and based on the correlation of clinical features of lymphomas with their histopathology and immunophenotype and genotype of neoplastic cells; groups lymphoproliferative diseases into chronic leukemia–lymphoma, nodal or extranodal lymphoma, acute leukemia lymphoma, plasma cell disorders, and Hodgkin disease. [Revised European-American lymphoma classification]

re•al•i•ty a•ware•ness (rē-al′i-tē ă-wār′nĕs) The ability to distinguish external objects as being different from oneself.

re•al•i•ty prin•ci•ple (rē-al′i-tē prin′si-pĕl) The concept that the pleasure principle in personality development is modified by the demands of external reality; the principle or force that compels the growing child to adapt to the demands of external reality.

re•al•i•ty test•ing (rē-al′i-tē test′ing) PSYCHIATRY, PSYCHOLOGY the ego function by which the objective or real world and one's subjectively sensed relationship to it are evaluated and appreciated; the ability to distinguish internal from external events.

real-time e•cho•car•di•o•gra•phy (rēl-tīm ek′ō-kahr-dē-og′ră-fē) SYN two-dimensional echocardiography.

ream•er (rē′mĕr) A rotating finishing or drilling tool used to shape or enlarge a hole; used in dentistry for clearing or enlarging root canals. [A.S. *ryman,* to widen]

rear•foot pro•na•tion (rēr′fut prō-nā′shŭn) SYN hindfoot valgus.

rear•foot su•pi•na•tion (rēr′fut sū′pi-nā′shŭn) SYN hindfoot varus.

re•bound phe•no•me•non (rē′bownd fĕ-nom′ĕ-non) **1.** SYN Stewart-Holmes sign. **2.** Generally, any phenomenon in which a variable that has been displaced from its normal state by a disturbing influence temporarily deviates from normal in the opposite direction when the disturbing influence is suddenly removed, before finally stabilizing at its normal state.

re•bound ten•der•ness (rē′bownd ten′dĕr-nĕs) SYN Blumberg sign.

re•breath•ing (rē-brēdh′ing) Inhalation of gases, partially or completely previously exhaled.

re•breath•ing an•es•the•si•a (rē-brēdh′ing an′es-thē′zē-ă) A technique for inhalation anesthesia in which a portion or all of the gases that are exhaled are subsequently inhaled after carbon dioxide has been absorbed.

re•breath•ing tech•nique (rē-brēdh′ing tek-nēk′) Use of a breathing or anesthesia circuit in which exhaled air is subsequently inhaled either with or without absorption of CO_2 from the exhaled air.

re•breath•ing vol•ume (rē-brēth′ing vol′yūm) The volume of exhaled gas reinhaled on inspiration as a result of the presence of a breathing apparatus; this volume is also referred to as instrument dead space.

re•cal•ci•fi•ca•tion (rē-kal′si-fi-kā′shŭn) Restoration to the tissues of lost calcium salts.

re•call (rē′kawl) The process of remembering thoughts, words, and actions of a past event in an attempt to recapture actual happenings.

re•call bi•as (rē′kawl bī′ăs) Systematic error due to differences in accuracy or completeness of recall to memory of past events or experiences.

Ré•ca•mier op•er•a•tion (rā-kah-mē-ā′ op-ĕr-ā′shŭn) Curettage of the uterus.

re•ca•nal•i•za•tion (rē-kan′ăl-ī-zā′shŭn) **1.** Restoration of a lumen in a blood vessel following thrombotic occlusion, by organization of the thrombus with formation of new channels. **2.** Spontaneous restoration of the continuity of the lumen of any occluded duct or tube, as with postvasectomy recanalization.

re•ca•pi•tu•la•tion the•o•ry (rē′kă-pich′yū-lā′shŭn thē′ŏr-ē) That individuals in their embryonic development pass through stages similar in general structural plan to the stages their species passed through in its evolution; more technically phrased, the theory that ontogeny is an abbreviated recapitulation of phylogeny. SYN Haeckel law.

re•ceive band•width (rĕ-sēv′ band′width) MAGNETIC RESONANCE IMAGING range of frequencies sampled during readout.

re•cep•tac•u•lum, pl. **re•cep•tac•u•la** (rē-sĕp-tak′yū-lŭm, -lă) A receptacle. SYN reservoir. [L. fr. *re cipio,* pp. *ceptus,* to receive, fr. *capio,* to take]

re•cep•tive a•pha•si•a (rē-sĕp′tiv ă-fā′zē-ă) A condition including impairment in the comprehension of spoken and written words, associated with effortless, articulated, but paraphasic speech and writing; malformed words, substitute words, and neologisms are characteristic. When severe, and speech is incomprehensible, it is called jargon aphasia. The patient often appears unaware of this deficit. The lesion typically includes a portion of the superior temporal lobe. SYN fluent aphasia, sensory aphasia, Wernicke aphasia.

re•cep•tor (rĕ-sep′tŏr) **1.** A structural protein molecule on the cell surface or within the cytoplasm that binds to a specific factor, such as a drug, hormone, antigen, or neurotransmitter. **2.** Any one of the various sensory nerve endings in the skin, deep tissues, viscera, and special sense organs. [L. receiver, fr. *recipio,* to receive]

re•cep•tor pro•tein (rĕ-sep′tŏr prō′tēn) An intracellular protein (or protein fraction) that has an affinity for a known stimulus to cellular activity, such as a steroid hormone or adenosine 3′,5′-cyclic phosphate.

re•cess (rē′ses) A small hollow or indentation. SYN recessus [TA]. [L. *recessus*]

re•ces•sion (rĕ-sesh′ŭn) **1.** A withdrawal or retreating. SEE ALSO retraction. **2.** Surgical operation in which an extaocular muscle is detached from the globe and reattached posteriorly. **3.** Loss of gingiva on a tooth apically; measurement is made using a probe; findings are recorded as attachment loss. [L. *recessio* (see recessus)]

re•ces•sive (rĕ-ses′iv) **1.** Drawing away; receding. **2.** GENETICS denoting a trait due to a particular allele that does not manifest itself in the presence of other alleles that generate traits dominant to it.

re•ces•sive char•ac•ter (rĕ-ses′iv kar′ăk-tĕr) An inherited character expressed in the homozygous state only.

re•ces•sive in•her•i•tance (rĕ-ses′iv in-her′i-tăns) SEE dominance of traits.

re•ces•sive trait (rĕ-ses′iv trāt) SEE dominance of traits.

re•ces•sus, pl. **re•ces•sus** (rē-ses′sŭs) [TA] SYN recess. [L. a withdrawing, a receding]

re•cid•i•va•tion (rĕ-sid′i-vā′shŭn) Relapse of a disease, a symptom, or a behavioral pattern such as an illegal activity for which one was previously imprisoned. [L. *recidivus,* falling back, recurring, fr. *re- cido,* to fall back]

re•cid•i•vism (rĕ-sid′i-vizm) A tendency toward recidivation. [L. *recidivus,* recurring]

re•cid•i•vist (rĕ-sid′i-vist) A person who tends toward recidivation.

rec•i•pe (Rx) (res′i-pē) **1.** The superscription of a prescription, usually indicated by the sign ℞. **2.** A prescription or formula. [L. imperative of *recipio,* to receive]

re•cip•i•ent (rĕ-sip′ē-ĕnt) SYN beneficiary.

re•cip•ro•cal forc•es (rĕ-sip′rŏ-kăl fōr′sĕz) DENTISTRY forces whereby the resistance of one or more teeth is used to move one or more opposing teeth.

re•cip•ro•cal gait or•thot•ic (RGO) (rĕ-sip′rŏ-kăl gāt ōr-thot′ik) A hip-knee-ankle-foot orthotic (abbreviated HKAFO) that incorporates a cable system to activate hip extension and opposite hip flexion during ambulation, reducing the energy required when compared with traditional knee-ankle-foot orthotics.

re•cip•ro•cal in•hi•bi•tion (rē-sip′rŏ-kăl in′hi-bish′ŭn) The relaxation of a muscle in response to the contraction of its antagonist.

re•cip•ro•cal trans•fu•sion (rĕ-sip′rŏ-kăl trans-fyū′zhŭn) An attempt to confer immunity by transfusing blood taken from a donor into a receiver suffering from the same affection, the balance being maintained by transfusing an equal amount from the receiver to the donor.

re•cip•ro•cal trans•lo•ca•tion (rĕ-sip′rŏ-kăl tranz′lō-kā′shŭn) Translocation without demonstrable loss of genetic material.

rec•i•proc•it•y (res′i-pros′i-tē) A mutual agreement between two U.S. states whereby each agrees to grant a license to practice medicine to any person licensed by the other state.

Reck•ling•hau•sen dis•ease of bone (rek′ling-how′zen di-zēz′ bōn) SYN osteitis fibrosa cystica.

Reck•ling•hau•sen tu•mor (rek′ling-how′zen tū′mŏr) SYN adenomatoid tumor.

rec•li•na•tion (rek′li-nā′shŭn) Turning the cataractous lens over into the vitreous to displace it from the line of vision. [L. *reclino,* pp. *-atus,* to bend back]

re•clin•ing po•si•tion (rē-klīn′ing pŏ-zish′ŭn) A back lying position.

rec•luse spi•der (rek′lūs spī′dĕr) The (brown) recluse spider is a venomous representative, *Loxosceles reclusa,* of the family Sicariidae (formerly of the family Loxoscelidae); native to the United States from the southern Midwest south to the Gulf of Mexico. Most bites are minor with no necrosis, but consequences may be worse in some cases. SYN brown recluse spider.

rec•og•ni•tion fac•tors (rek′ŏg-nish′ŭn fak′tŏrs) Factors that affect "recognition" of target antigens by polymorphonuclear leukocytes; apparently the Fc portion of antibody molecules and the activated third component of complement (C3), for both of which phagocytes have receptor sites.

re•com•bi•nant (rē-kom′bi-nănt) **1.** A progeny that has received chromosomal parts from different parental strains as a result of uncorrected crossing over. **2.** Pertaining to or denoting such organisms. **3.** In linkage analysis, the change of coupling phase at two loci during meiosis. If two syntenic, nonallelic genes are inherited from the same parent, they must be in coupling.

re•com•bi•nant DNA (rē-kom′bi-nănt) Altered DNA resulting from the insertion into the chain, by chemical, enzymatic, or biologic means, of a sequence (a whole or partial chain of DNA) not originally (biologically) present in that chain.

re•com•bi•nant vec•tor (rē-kom′bi-nănt vek′tŏr) A vector into which foreign DNA has been inserted. SYN vector (5).

re•com•bi•na•tion (rē-kom′bi-nā′shŭn) **1.** The process of reuniting of parts that had become separated. **2.** The reversal of coupling phase in meiosis as gauged by the resulting phenotype. SEE ALSO recombinant.

rec•om•mend•ed di•e•tar•y al•low•ance (RDA) (rek′ŏ-mend′ĕd dī′ĕ-tār-ē ă-low′ans) The average daily intake of a nutrient judged sufficient to meet the requirements of healthy people, as categorized by gender and lifestyle.

re•con•sti•tu•tion (re-kon′sti-tū′shŭn) The process of adding a diluent to a powdered medication to prepare a solution or suspension.

re•con•struc•tion (rē′kŏn-strŭk′shŭn) The computed synthesis of one or more two-dimensional images from a series of x-ray projections in tomography, or from a large number of measurements in magnetic resonance imaging; several methods are used; the earliest was back-projection, and the most common is 2-D Fourier transformation.

re•con•struc•tive mam•ma•plas•ty (rē′kon-strŭk′tiv mam′ă-plas-tē) The making of a simulated breast by plastic surgery, to reproduce the appearance of one that has been removed.

re•con•struc•tive sur•ger•y (rē′kon-strŭk′tiv sŭr′jĕr-ē) SEE plastic surgery.

rec•ord (rek′ŏrd) **1.** A chronologic written account that includes a patient's initial complaint(s) and medical history, the physician's physical findings, the results of diagnostic tests and procedures, and any therapeutic medications or procedures. Cf. health record. **2.** DENTISTRY a registration of desired jaw relations in a plastic material or on a device to permit these relationships to be transferred to an articulator. **3.** To place in a graph (e.g., electrocardiogram) automatically. [M.E. *recorden,* fr. O.Fr. *recorder,* fr. L. *re-cordor,* to remember, fr. *re-,* back, again, + *cor,* heart]

re•cor•ded de•tail (rē-kōrd′ĕd dē′tāl) The visible sharpness of features on a radiograph (e.g., bone trabeculae or pulmonary markings).

re•cov•er•y ox•y•gen con•sump•tion (rē-kŏv′ĕr-ē ok′si-jĕn kŏn-sŭmp′shŭn) SYN excess postexercise oxygen consumption.

re•cov•er•y room (rē-kŏv′ĕr-ē rūm) Area adjacent to the operating suite used for the recovery of patients following surgery.

re•cru•des•cence (rē′krū-des′ĕns) Resumption of a morbid process or its symptoms after a period of remission. [L. *re-crudesco,* to become raw again, break out afresh, fr. *crudus,* raw, harsh]

re•cru•des•cent (rē′krū-des′ĕnt) Becoming active again, relating to a recrudescence.

re•cru•des•cent ty•phus (rē′krū-des′ĕnt tī′fŭs) SYN Brill-Zinsser disease.

re•cruit•ment (rē-krūt′mĕnt) **1.** AUDIOLOGY the unequal reaction of the ear to equal steps of increasing intensity, measured in decibels, with greater than normal increment in perceived loudness. **2.** The bringing into activity of additional motor neurons, causing greater activity in response to increased duration of the stimulus applied to a given receptor or afferent nerve. SEE ALSO irradiation. **3.** The adding of parallel channels of flow in any system. [Fr. *recrutement,* fr. L. *re-cresco,* pp. *-cretus,* to grow again]

rec•tal (rek′tăl) Relating to the rectum.

rec•tal am•pul•la (rek′tăl am-pul′lă) A dilated portion of the rectum just above the anal canal.

rec•tal an•es•the•si•a (rek′tăl an′es-thē′zē-ă) General anesthesia produced by instillation into the rectum of a solution containing a central nervous system depressant.

rec•tal col•umns (rek′tăl kol′ŭmz) SYN anal columns.

rec•tal•gi•a (rek-tal′jē-ă) SYN proctalgia.

rec•tec•to•my (rek-tek′tŏ-mē) SYN proctectomy.

rec•ti•fy (rek′ti-fī) **1.** To correct. **2.** To purify or refine by distillation; usually implies repeated distillations. [L. *rectus,* right, straight]

rec•ti•tis (rek-tī′tis) SYN proctitis.

♻**recto-, rect-** Combining forms denoting the rectum. SEE ALSO procto-. [L. *rectum,* fr. *rectus,* straight]

rec•to•cele (rek′tō-sēl) SYN proctocele. [recto- + G. *kēlē,* tumor, hernia]

rec•to•coc•cyg•e•al mus•cle (rek′tō-kok-sij′ē-ăl mŭs′ĕl) SYN rectococcygeus muscle.

rec•to•coc•cyg•e•us mus•cle (rek′tō-kok-sij′ē-ŭs mŭs′ĕl) A band of smooth muscle fibers passing from the posterior surface of the rectum to the anterior surface of second or third coccygeal segment. SYN musculus rectococcygeus [TA], rectococcygeal muscle.

rec•to•coc•cy•pexy (rek′tō-kok′si-pek-sē) SYN proctococcypexy.

rec•to•pex•y (rek′tō-pek-sē) SYN proctopexy.

rec•to•plas•ty (rek′tō-plas-tē) SYN proctoplasty.

rec•to•scope (rek′tō-skōp) SYN proctoscope.

rec•to•sig•moid (rek′tō-sig′moyd) The rectum and sigmoid colon considered as a unit; the term is also applied to the junction of the sigmoid colon and rectum.

rec•to•ste•no•sis (rek′tō-stĕ-nō′sis) SYN proctostenosis.

rec•tos•to•my (rek-tos′tŏ-mē) SYN proctostomy.

rec•tot•o•my (rek-tot′ŏ-mē) SYN proctotomy.

rec•to•u•re•thra•lis mus•cle (rek′tō-yŭr′ē-thrā′lis mŭs′ĕl) Smooth muscle fibers that pass forward from the longitudinal muscle layer of the rectum to the membranous urethra in the male. SYN musculus rectourethralis [TA].

rec•to•u•ter•ine mus•cle (rek′tō-yū′tĕr-in mŭs′ĕl) A band of fibrous tissue and smooth muscle fibers passing between the cervix of the uterus and the rectum in the rectouterine fold, on either side. SYN musculus rectouterinus [TA].

rec•to•u•ter•ine pouch (rek′tō-yū′tĕr-in powch) A pocket formed by the deflection of the peritoneum from the rectum to the uterus. SYN excavatio rectouterina [TA], cul-de-sac (2).

rec•to•vag•i•nal sep•tum (rek′tō-vaj′i-năl sep′tŭm) The fascial layer between the vagina and the lower part of the rectum.

rec•to•ve•si•ca•lis mus•cle (rek′tō-ves-i-kā′lis mŭs′ĕl) Smooth muscle fibers in the sacrogenital fold in the male; they correspond to musculus rectouterinus. SYN musculus rectovesicalis [TA], rectovesical muscle.

rec•to•ves•i•cal mus•cle (rek′tō-ves′i-kăl mŭs′ĕl) SYN rectovesicalis muscle.

rec•to•ves•i•cal pouch (rek′tō-ves′i-kăl powch) A pocket formed by the deflection of the peritoneum from the rectum to the bladder in the male. SYN excavatio rectovesicalis [TA], Proust space.

rec•to•ves•i•cal sep•tum (rek′tō-ves′i-kăl sep′tŭm) A fascial layer that extends superiorly from the central tendon of the perineum to the peritoneum between the prostate and rectum.

rec•tum, pl. **rec•tums**, **rec•ta** (rek′tŭm, -tŭmz, -tă) [TA] The terminal portion of the digestive tube, extending from the rectosigmoid junction to the anal canal. [L. *rectus,* straight, pp. of *rego,* to make straight]

rec•tus ab•do•mi•nis mus•cle (rek′tŭs ab-dom′i-nis mŭs′ĕl) Muscle of ventral abdominal wall, flanking the linea alba, and characterized by tendinous intersections separating its length into multiple bellies; *origin*, crest and symphysis of the pubis; *insertion*, xiphoid process and fifth to seventh costal cartilages; *action*, flexes lumbar vertebral column, draws thorax downward toward pubis; *nerve supply*, thoracoabdominal nerves. See this page. SYN musculus rectus abdominis [TA], rectus muscle of abdomen.

rec•tus ca•pi•tis an•te•ri•or mus•cle (rek′tŭs kap′i-tis an-tēr′ē-ŏr mŭs′ĕl) *Origin*, transverse process and lateral mass of atlas; *insertion*, basilar process of occipital bone; *action*, turns and inclines head forward; *nerve supply*, ventral primary ramus of first and second cervical spinal nerve. SYN musculus rectus capitis anterior [TA].

rec•tus ca•pi•tis la•ter•a•lis mus•cle (rek′tŭs kap′i-tis la-tĕr-ā′lis mŭs′ĕl) *Origin*, transverse process of atlas; *insertion*, jugular process of occipital bone; *action*, inclines head to one side; *nerve supply*, ventral primary ramus of first cervical spinal nerve. SYN musculus rectus capitis lateralis [TA], lateral rectus muscle of the head.

rec•tus ca•pi•tis pos•te•ri•or ma•jor mus•cle (rek′tŭs kap′i-tis pos-tē′rē-ŏr mā′jŏr mŭs′ĕl) *Origin*, spinous process of axis; *insertion*, middle of inferior nuchal line of occipital bone; *action*, rotates and draws head backward; *nerve supply*, dorsal branch of first cervical (suboccipital). SYN musculus capitis posterior major [TA], greater posterior rectus muscle of head.

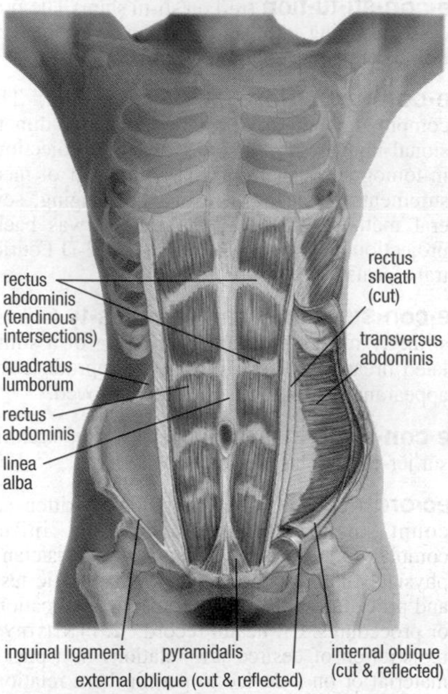

rectus abdominis muscle

rec•tus ca•pi•tis pos•te•ri•or mi•nor mus•cle (rek′tŭs kap′i-tis pos-tē′rē-ŏr mī′nŏr mŭs′ĕl) *Origin*, from posterior tubercle of atlas; *insertion*, medial third of inferior nuchal line of occipital bone; *action*, rotates head and draws it backward; *nerve supply*, dorsal branch of first cervical (suboccipital). SYN smaller posterior rectus muscle of head.

rec•tus fe•mo•ris mus•cle (rek′tŭs fem′ŏr-is mŭs′ĕl) *Origin*, anterior inferior spine of ilium and upper margin of acetabulum; *insertion*, via common tendon of quadriceps femoris into patella, and via patellar ligament to tibial tuberosity. SYN musculus rectus femoris [TA], rectus muscle of thigh.

rec•tus mus•cle of ab•do•men (rek-tŭs′ mŭs′ĕl ab′dŏ-mĕn) SYN rectus abdominis muscle.

rec•tus mus•cle of thigh (rek-tŭs′ mŭs′ĕl thī) SYN rectus femoris muscle.

re•cum•bent (rē-kŭm′bĕnt) Leaning; reclining; lying down. See page B29. [L. *recumbo,* to lie back, recline, fr. *re-*, back, + *cubo,* to lie]

re•cu•per•ate (rē-kū′pĕr-āt) To undergo recuperation. [L. *recupero* (or *recip-*), pp. *-atus,* to take again, recover]

re•cur•rence (rē-kŭr′ĕns) **1.** A return of the symptoms in the course of a disease, following improvement or remission. **2.** SYN relapse. **3.** Appearance of a genetic trait in a relative of a proband. [L. *re-curro,* to run back, recur]

re·cur·rence risk (rē-kŭr′ĕns risk) Chance or possibility that a disease will occur elsewhere in a pedigree, given that at least one member of the pedigree (the proband) exhibits the disease.

re·cur·rent (rĕ-kŭr′ĕnt) **1.** ANATOMY turning back on itself. **2.** Denoting symptoms or lesions reappearing after an intermission or remission.

re·cur·rent a·bor·tion (rĕ-kŭr′ĕnt ă-bōr′shŭn) The loss of three or more sequential pregnancies before 20 weeks' gestation.

re·cur·rent aph·thous ul·cers (rĕ-kŭr′ĕnt af′thŭs ŭl′sĕrz) SYN aphtha (2). See this page.

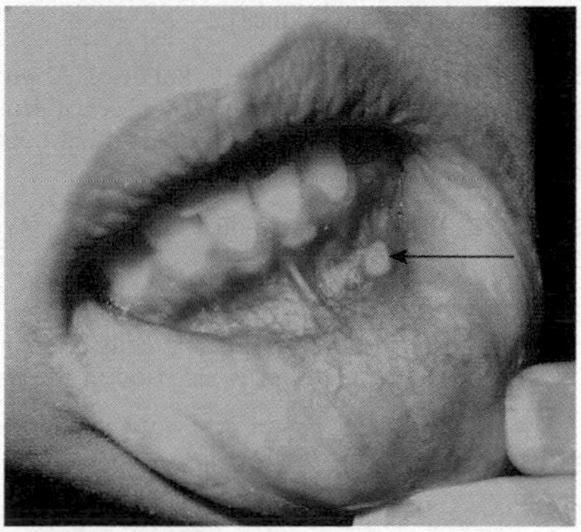

aphthous ulcer

re·cur·rent her·pet·ic sto·ma·ti·tis (rĕ-kŭr′ĕnt hĕr-pet′ik stō′mă-tī′tis) Reactivation of herpes simplex virus infection, characterized by vesicles and ulceration limited to the hard palate and attached gingiva.

re·cur·rent jaun·dice of preg·nan·cy (rĕ-kŭr′ĕnt jawn′dis preg′năn-sē) SYN intrahepatic cholestasis of pregnancy.

re·cur·rent la·ryn·ge·al nerve (rĕ-kŭr′ĕnt lă-rin′jē-ăl nĕrv) A branch of the vagus nerve curving upward, on the right side around the root of the subclavian artery, on the left side around the arch of the aorta, then passing superiorly, posterior to the common carotid artery between the trachea and the esophagus to the larynx; it supplies cardiac, tracheal, and esophageal branches and terminates as the inferior laryngeal nerve.

re·cur·rent re·spir·a·tor·y pa·pil·lo·ma·to·sis (rĕ-kŭr′ĕnt res′pir-ă-tōr-ē pap′i-lō′mă-tō′sis) A disease of the respiratory tract caused by the human papillomavirus; characterized by rapid recurrence of papillomas after surgical removal, airway obstruction, and hoarseness to aphonia when the larynx is involved. SEE ALSO laryngeal papillomatosis.

re·cur·rent ul·cer·a·tive sto·ma·ti·tis (rĕ-kŭr′ĕnt ŭl′sĕr-ă-tiv stō′mă-tī′tis) SYN aphtha (2).

re·cur·rent ul·nar ar·ter·y (rĕ-kŭr′ĕnt ŭl′năr ahr′tĕr-ē) *Origin*, ulnar artery; *distribution*, two branches, anterior and posterior, pass medially in front of and behind the elbow joint; *anastomoses*, superior and inferior ulnar collateral, i.e., with articular vascular network of elbow. SYN arteria recurrens ulnaris [TA].

re·cur·ring dig·i·tal fi·bro·ma of child·hood (rē-kŭr′ring dij′i-tăl fī-brō′mă chīld′hud) Multiple fibrous flesh-colored nodules on the extensor aspect of the terminal phalanges of adjacent digits of infants and young children that often recur after attempted excision, do not metastasize, and may spontaneously regress in 2–3 years; composed of spindle cells containing cytoplasmic inclusions believed to be derived from myofibrils.

re·cur·va·tion (rē′kŭr-vā′shŭn) A backward bending or flexure. [L. *re-curvus,* bent back]

red blood cell (rbc, RBC) (red blŭd sel) SYN erythrocyte.

red blood cell cast (red blŭd sel kast) A hyaline or granular cast that contains erythrocytes, indicative of bleeding within the kidney, as in glomerular inflammation. Seen on microscopic analysis of a urine specimen.

red blood cell count (red blŭd sel kownt) The concentration of erythrocytes in a specimen of whole blood. The count varies with age (higher in infants), time of day (lower during sleep), activity, environmental temperature, and altitude (increasing with all three). The average erythrocyte count for males is 4.7 to 6.1 million cells/mcL and for females is 4.2 to 5.4 million cells/mcL. SYN erythrocyte count.

red blood cell in·di·ces (red blŭd sel in′de-sēz) SEE erythrocyte indices.

red cell (red sel) SYN erythrocyte.

red cocks·comb (red koks′kōm) SYN amaranth.

red cor·pus·cle (red kōr′pŭs-ĕl) SYN erythrocyte.

red fire ant (red fīr ant) SYN *Solenopsis invicta.*

red hep·a·ti·za·tion (red hep′ă-tī-zā′shŭn) The first stage of hepatization, in which the exudate is blood-stained.

red in·du·ra·tion (red in′dūr-ā′shŭn) A condition observed in lungs in which there is an advanced degree of acute passive congestion, or acute pneumonitis (sometimes termed interstitial pneumonia), or a similar pathologic process.

re·din·te·gra·tion (rē′din-tē-grā′shŭn) **1.** The

restoration of lost or injured parts. **2.** Restoration to health. **3.** The recalling of a whole experience on the basis only of some item or portion of the original stimulus or circumstances of the experience. [L. *red-integro,* pp. *-atus,* to make whole again, renew, fr. *integer,* untouched, entire]

red man syn•drome (red man sin′drōm) SYN red neck syndrome.

red mite (red mīt) SEE chigger.

red mus•cle (red mŭs′ĕl) Slow-twitch muscle in which small dark "red" muscle fibers predominate; myoglobin is abundant and great numbers of mitochondria occur, characterized by slow, sustained (tonic) contraction. Contrast with white muscle.

red neck syn•drome (RNS) (red nek sin′drōm) A hypersensitivity allergic reaction most often seen when the antimicrobial, vancomycin, is adminstered too rapidly; thought to be a non-immune related release of histamine, because histamine plasma concentrations increase after administration of vancomycin; characterized by a complex of symptoms including: pruritus, urticaria, erythema, angioedema, tachycardia, hypotension, occasional muscle aches, and a maculopapular rash that usually appears on the face, neck, and upper torso. SYN red man syndrome.

red neu•ral•gi•a (red nūr-al′jē-ă) SYN erythromelalgia.

red nu•cle•us (red nū′klē-ŭs) A large, well-defined, somewhat elongated cell mass, of reddish-gray hue in the fresh brain, located in the rostral mesencephalic tegmentum. The nucleus receives a massive projection from the contralateral half of the cerebellum by way of the superior cerebellar peduncle, and an additional projection from the ipsilateral motor cortex. Projections from the anterior interposed nucleus and motor cortex to the red nucleus are somatopically organized. Its efferent connections are with the contralateral rhombencephalic reticular formation and spinal cord by way of the rubrobulbar and rubrospinal tracts. Rubrospinal fibers have somatotopic origin.

red oil (red oyl) A weakly acid diazo oil-soluble dye, used in histologic demonstration of neutral fats.

re•dox (rē′doks) Contraction of reduction-oxidation.

red pep•per (red pep′ĕr) SYN capsicum.

red puc•coon (red pŭ-kūn′) SYN blood root.

red pulp (red pŭlp) Splenic pulp seen grossly as a reddish-brown substance, due to its abundance of red blood cells, consisting of splenic sinuses and the tissue intervening between them (splenic cords).

red re•flex (red rē′fleks) Term describing reflection of light from retina in healthy eyes; abnormality in ocular media, refractive state, or retina can cause this reflex to be abnormal. SYN cone of light, light reflex (3), pyramid of light.

red•root (red′rūt) SYN blood root.

red tide (red tīd) A natural phenomenon resulting from higher than normal concentrations of the microscopic algae *Gymnodinium breve* in seawater. When the causative organism is extremely concentrated, seawater can turn a reddish-brown color.

red-top tube (plain) (red-top tūb plān) A stopper of this color indicates the container has been treated with no additives; used for serum determinations including chemistry testing, serology, and therapeutic drug monitoring.

re•duce (rē-dūs′) **1.** To perform reduction (1). **2.** CHEMISTRY to initiate reduction (2). [L. *re-duco,* to lead back, restore, reduce]

re•duced cal•o•rie (rē-dūst′ kal′ŏr-ē) A product so labeled contains, by F.D.A. order, at least 25% fewer calories than found in a similar comparison food.

re•duced hem•a•tin (rē-dūst′ hē′mă-tin) SYN heme.

re•duced he•mo•glo•bin (rē-dūst′ hē′mō-glō-bin) The form of Hb in red blood cells after the oxygen of oxyhemoglobin is released in the tissues.

re•duc•i•ble (rē-dūs′i-bĕl) Capable of being reduced.

re•duc•i•ble her•ni•a (rē-dūs′i-bĕl hĕr′nē-ă) A hernia in which the contents of the sac can be returned to their normal location.

re•duc•tant (rē-dŭk′tănt) The substance that is oxidized in the course of reduction.

re•duc•tase (rē-dŭk′tās) An enzyme that catalyzes a reduction; because all enzymes catalyze reactions in either direction, any reductase can, under the proper conditions, behave as an oxidase and vice versa; hence the term oxidoreductase.

5-α-re•duc•tase in•hib•i•tors (rē-dŭk′tās in-hib′i-tŏrs) Drugs that inhibit the action of 5α-reductase, resulting in lower levels of prostatic dihydrotestosterone, produced by the enzyme from testosterone as the primary androgen in the prostate.

re•duc•tion (rĕ-dŭk′shŭn) **1.** The restoration, by surgical or manipulative procedures, of a part to its normal anatomic relation. SYN repositioning. **2.** CHEMISTRY a reaction involving a gain of one or more electrons by a substance. **3.** Surgical procedure to reduce size. [L. *reductio,* fr. *re-duco,* pp. *ductus,* to lead back]

re•duc•tion of chro•mo•somes (rĕ-dŭk′shŭn krō′mŏ-sōmz) The process during meiosis whereby one member of each homologous pair of chromosomes is distributed to a sperm or ovum; the diploid set of chromosomes (46 in humans) is thus reduced to the haploid set in each gamete; union of the sperm and ovum restores the diploid or somatic number in the one-cell zygote.

re•duc•tion de•for•mi•ty (rĕ-dŭk′shŭn dĕ-fōrm′i-tē) Congenital absence or attenuation of one or more body parts; usually of the limbs or limb components.

re•duc•tion left ven•tri•cu•lo•plas•ty (rĕ-dŭk′shŭn left ven-trik′yū-lō-plas-tē) SYN left ventricular volume reduction surgery.

re•duc•tion mam•ma•plas•ty (rĕ-dŭk′shŭn mam′ă-plas-tē) Surgical procedure of the breast to reduce its size and (frequently) to improve its shape and position.

re•du•pli•ca•tion (rē-dū′pli-kā′shŭn) **1.** A redoubling. **2.** A duplication or doubling, as of the sounds of the heart in certain morbid states or the presence of two instead of a normally single part. **3.** A fold or duplicature. [L. *reduplicatio,* fr. *re-,* again, + *duplico,* to double, fr. *duplex,* two-fold]

Red•u•vi•i•dae (rē-dū-vī′ē-dē) A family of predatory insects, the assassin bugs; it includes the subfamily Triatominae, the kissing or cone-nosed bugs; the type genus *Triatoma* includes species that are vectors of *Trypanosoma cruzi.*

red, white, and blue sign (red wīt blū sīn) The contemporaneous occurrence of erythema, ischemia, and necrosis in a wound, as in loxoscelism.

REE Abbreviation for resting energy expenditure.

Reed-Frost mod•el (rēd-frawst mod′ĕl) Mathematical model of infectious disease transmission and herd immunity. The model gives the number of new cases of an infection that can be expected in a specified time in a closed, freely mixing population of immune and susceptible people, with varying assumptions about frequency of contact.

Reed-Stern•berg cell (rēd-stĕrn′bĕrg sel) Large transformed lymphocytes, probably B cell in origin, generally regarded as pathognomonic of Hodgkin lymphoma; a typical cell has a pale-staining acidophilic cytoplasm and one or two large nuclei showing marginal clumping of chromatin and unusually conspicuous deeply acidophilic nucleoli; binucleate Reed-Sternberg cells frequently show a mirror-image form (mirror-image cell).

reef•ing (rēf′ing) Surgically reducing the extent of a tissue by folding it and securing with sutures, as in plication.

re•en•trant mech•a•nism (rē-en′trănt mek′ă-nizm) The probable basis of most arrhythmias, requiring at least three criteria: 1. a loop circuit, 2. unidirectional block, 3. slowed conduction.

re•en•try (rē-en′trē) Return of the same impulse into a zone of heart muscle that it has recently activated, sufficiently delayed so that the zone is no longer refractory, as seen in most ectopic beats, reciprocal rhythms, and most tachycardias.

re•en•try phe•nom•e•non (rē-en′trē fĕ-nom′ĕ-non) The return of a cardiac impulse to an area of muscle that it has already activated, after the refractory period of the area has expired, resulting in one or more ectopic beats or a sustained arrhythmia.

ref•er•ence lab•o•ra•to•ry (ref′rĕns lab′ŏr-ă-tōr-ē) A large laboratory that performs miscellaneous testing not usually performed in a hospital laboratory.

ref•er•ence range (ref′rĕns rānj) The usual range of test values for a healthy population. SYN normal range.

ref•er•ence val•ues (ref′rĕns val′yūz) A set of laboratory test values obtained from an individual or group in a defined state of health; replaces the so-called normal values; based on a defined state of health.

re•ferr•al (rē-fĕr′ăl) Any health care services that are ordered or arranged.

re•ferred pain (rē-fĕrd′ pān) Unpleasant sensation at a site other than the actual location of trauma or disease.

re•ferred sen•sa•tion (rē-fĕrd′ sen-sā′shŭn) A sensation perceived in one place in response to a stimulus applied in another.

re•fine (rē-fīn′) To free from impurities.

re•flec•tance (rē-flek′tăns) A measure of reflected acoustic energy as a function of immitance, as in middle ear impedance.

re•flec•tance spec•tro•pho•to•me•try (rē-flek′tăns spek′trō-fō-tom′ĕ-trē) A quantitative spectrophotometric technique in which light is reflected from the surface of a colorimetric reaction and is then used to measure the amount of the reaction product.

re•flect•ed in•gui•nal lig•a•ment (rē-flek′tĕd ing′gwi-năl lig′ă-mĕnt) A triangular fibrous band extending from the aponeurosis of the external oblique to the pubic tubercle of the opposite side.

re•flec•tion (rē-flek′shŭn) **1.** The act of reflecting. **2.** That which is reflected. **3.** PSYCHOTHERAPY a technique in which a patient's statements are repeated, restated, or rephrased so that the patient will continue to explore and expound on emotionally significant content. [L. *reflexio,* a bending back]

re•flec•tion co•ef•fi•cient (σ) (rē-flek′shŭn kō′ĕ-fish′ĕnt) A measure of the relative permeability of a particular membrane to a particular solute; calculated as the ratio of observed osmotic pressure to that calculated from van't Hoff law.

re•flec•tor (rē-flek′tŏr) Any surface that reflects light, heat, or sound.

re•flex (rē′fleks) **1.** An involuntary reaction in response to a stimulus applied to the periphery and transmitted to the nervous centers in the brain or spinal cord. SEE ALSO phenomenon. **2.** A reflection. [L. *reflexus,* pp. of *re-flecto,* to bend back]

re•flex arc (rē′fleks ahrk) The route followed by nerve impulses in the production of a reflex act, from the peripheral receptor organ through the afferent nerve to the central nervous system synapse and then through the efferent nerve to the effector organ.

re•flex blad•der (rē′fleks blad′ĕr) SYN paralytic incontinence.

re•flex cough (rē′fleks kawf) A cough excited reflexively by irritation in some distant part, as the ear or the stomach.

re•flex ep•i•lep•sy (rē′fleks ep′i-lep′sē) Seizures that are induced by peripheral stimulation (e.g., audiogenic, laryngeal, photogenic, or other stimulation).

re•flex in•con•ti•nence (rē′fleks in-kon′ti-nĕns′) Involuntary loss of urine when a specific bladder volume is reached.

re•flex in•hi•bi•tion (rē′fleks in′hi-bish′ŭn) A situation in which sensory stimuli decrease reflex activity.

re•flex•ive squeeze grasp (rē-fleks′iv skwēz grasp) A pattern seen in the infant up to the 4th month that includes all fingers flexing when an object is placed in the palmar surface of the hand. SEE ALSO grasp pattern. SYN grasp reflex.

re•flex neu•ro•gen•ic blad•der (rē′fleks nūr-ō-jen′ik blad′ĕr) An abnormal condition of urinary bladder function whereby the bladder is cut off from upper motor neuron control, but where the lower motor neuron arc is still intact.

re•flex•o•gen•ic (rē-flek′sō-jen′ik) Causing a reflex.

re•flex•o•graph (rē-flek′sō-graf) An instrument for graphically recording a reflex. [reflex + G. *graphō,* to write]

re•flex•o•lo•gy (rē′flek-sol′ŏ-jē) A massage technique focusing on specific points on the feet, hands, and ears that are said to correspond through meridians to other organs or areas of the body. SYN reflex zone therapy.

re•flex•om•e•ter (rē′fleks-om′ĕ-tĕr) An instrument for measuring the force necessary to excite a reflex. [reflex + G. *metron,* measure]

re•flex sym•pa•thet•ic dys•tro•phy (RSD) (rē′fleks sim′pă-thet′ik dis′trŏ-fē) Diffuse persistent pain usually in an extremity often associated with vasomotor disturbances, trophic changes, and limitation or immobility of joints; frequently follows local injury. SEE ALSO causalgia.

re•flex symp•tom (rē′fleks simp′tŏm) A disturbance of sensation or function in an organ or part more or less remote from the morbid condition giving rise to it (e.g., muscle spasm due to joint inflammation).

re•flex zone ther•a•py (rē′fleks zōn thār′ă-pē) SYN reflexology.

re•flux (rē′flŭks) **1.** A backward flow. SEE ALSO regurgitation. **2.** CHEMISTRY to boil without loss of vapor because of the presence of a condenser that returns vapor as liquid. [L. *re-,* back, + *fluxus,* a flow]

re•flux e•soph•a•gi•tis, pep•tic e•soph•a•gi•tis (rē′flŭks ē-sof′ă-jī′tis, pep′tik) Inflammation of the lower esophagus resulting from regurgitation of acid gastric contents, usually due to malfunction of the lower esophageal sphincter; symptoms include substernal pain, heartburn, and regurgitation of acid juice.

re•flux o•ti•tis me•di•a (rē′flŭks ō-tī′tis mē′dē-ă) Disorder caused by passage of nasopharyngeal secretions through the auditory tube.

re•fract (rē-frakt′) **1.** To change the direction of a ray of light. **2.** To detect an error of refraction and to correct it by means of lenses. [L. *refringo,* pp. *-fractus,* to break up]

re•frac•tion (rē-frak′shŭn) **1.** The deflection of a ray of light when it passes from one medium into another of different optic density; in passing from a denser into a rarer medium, it is deflected away from a line perpendicular to the surface of the refracting medium; in passing from a rarer to a denser medium, it is bent toward this perpendicular line. **2.** The act of determining the nature and degree of the refractive errors in the eye and correction of them by lenses. SYN refringence. [L. *refractio* (see refract)]

re•frac•tion•ist (rē-frak′shŭn-ist) A person trained to measure the refraction of the eye and to determine the proper corrective lenses.

re•frac•tive (rē-frak′tiv) **1.** Pertaining to refraction. **2.** Having the power to refract. SYN refringent.

re•frac•tive in•dex (*n*) (rē-frak′tiv in′deks) The relative velocity of light in another medium compared to the velocity in air.

re•frac•tive ker•a•to•plas•ty (rē-frak′tiv ker′ă-tō-plas-tē) Any transplantation of corenal tissue to change refractive error; procedure rarely used. SEE ALSO keratophakia, keratomileusis, radial keratotomy.

re•frac•tive ker•a•tot•o•my (rē-frak′tiv ker′ă-tot′ŏ-mē) Modification of corneal curvature by means of corneal incisions to minimize hyperopia, myopia, or astigmatism. In this type of radial keratotomy surgery, performed by excimer laser, pie-shaped pieces of cornea are removed under local anesthetic. The resulting scar tissue formation reshapes the cornea.

re•frac•tiv•i•ty (rē′frak-tiv′i-tē) Refractive power.

re•frac•tom•e•ter (rē′frak-tom′ĕ-ter) An instrument for measuring the degree of refraction in translucent substances, especially the ocular media. SEE ALSO refractive index. [refraction + G. *metron,* measure]

re•frac•tom•e•try (rē′frak-tom′ĕ-trē) **1.** Measurement of the refractive index. **2.** Use of a refractometer to determine the refractive error of the eye.

re•frac•to•ry (rē-frak′tŏr-ē) **1.** Resistant to treatment, as of a disease. SYN intractable (1), obstinate (2). **2.** SYN obstinate (1). [L. *refractarius,* fr. *refringo,* pp. *-fractus,* to break in pieces]

re•frac•to•ry a•ne•mi•a (rē-frak′tŏr-ē ă-nē′mē-ă) Progressive anemia unresponsive to therapy other than transfusion.

re•frac•to•ry pe•ri•od (rē-frak′tŏr-ē pēr′ē-ŏd) **1.** The time following effective stimulation, during which excitable tissue such as heart muscle and nerve fails to respond to a stimulus of threshold intensity (i.e., excitability is depressed). **2.** A period of temporary psychophysiologic resistance to further sexual stimulation, which occurs immediately following orgasm.

re•frac•to•ry state (rē-frak′tŏr-ē stāt) Subnormal excitability immediately following a response to previous excitation; the state is divided into absolute and relative phases.

re•frac•ture (rē-frak′shŭr) Breaking a bone that has united after a previous fracture. [re- + fracture]

re•fresh (rē-fresh′) **1.** To renew; to cause to recuperate. **2.** To perform revivification (2). [O. Fr. *re-frescher*]

re•frig•er•ant (rē-frij′ĕr-ănt) **1.** Cooling; reducing slight fever. **2.** An agent that gives a sensation of coolness or relieves feverishness. [L. *re-frigero,* pp. *-atus,* pr. p. *-ans,* to make cold, fr. *frigus* (*frigor-*), cold]

re•frig•er•a•tion (rē-frij′ĕr-ā′shŭn) The act of cooling or reducing fever. [L. *refrigeratio* (see refrigerant)]

re•frig•er•a•tion an•es•the•si•a (rē-frij′ĕr-ā′shŭn an′es-thē′zē-ă) SYN cryoanesthesia.

re•frin•gence (rē-frin′jĕns) SYN refraction.

re•frin•gent (rē-frin′jĕnt) SYN refractive.

Ref•sum dis•ease (ref′sūm di-zēz′) A rare degenerative disorder due to a deficiency of phytanic acid α-hydroxylase; clinically characterized by retinitis pigmentosa, ichthyosis, demyelinating polyneuropathy, deafness, and cerebellar signs; autosomal recessive inheritance caused by mutation in the gene encoding phytanoyl-CoA hydroxylase (PAHX or PAYH) on chromosome 10p. Infantile Refsum disease is an impaired peroxisomal function with accumulation of phytanic acid and pipecolic acid; autosomal recessive inheritance caused by mutation in the PEX 1 gene on 7q.

re•fu•sal of pro•ce•dure (rē-fyū′zăl prŏ-sē′jŭr) A declining of a procedure, therapy, or treatment by the patient.

re•fu•sion (rē-fū′zhŭn) Return of the circulation of blood that has been temporarily cut off by ligature of a limb. [L. *re-fundo,* pp. *-fusus,* to pour back]

Re•gaud fix•a•tive (re-gō′ fiks′ă-tiv) A fixative containing formaldehyde and sodium dichromate, used to preserve mitochondria but not fat; requires afterchroming and extensive washing.

re•gen•er•a•tion (rē-jen′ĕr-ā′shŭn) **1.** Reproduction or reconstitution of a lost or injured part. SYN neogenesis. **2.** A form of asexual reproduction (e.g., when a worm is divided into two or more parts, each segment is regenerated into a new individual). [L. *regeneratio* (see regenerate)]

re•gen•er•a•tive pol•yp (rē-jen′ĕr-ă-tiv pol′ip) A hyperplastic polyp of the gastric mucosa.

reg•i•men (rej′i-mĕn) Any program (including drugs) that regulates aspects of one's lifestyle for a hygienic or therapeutic purpose; a program of treatment. USAGE NOTE Sometimes mistakenly called regime. [L. direction, rule]

re•gi•o, gen. **re•gi•o•nis**, pl. **re•gi•o•nes** (rē′jē-ō, -ō′nis, -ō′nēz) [TA] SYN region. [L.]

re•gion (rē′jŭn) **1.** An often arbitrarily limited portion of the surface of the body. SEE ALSO space, zone. **2.** A portion of the body having a special nervous or vascular supply, or a part of an organ having a special function. SEE ALSO area, space, spatium, zone. SYN regio [TA]. [L. *regio*]

re•gion•al (rē′jŭn-ăl) Relating to a region.

re•gion•al a•nat•o•my (rē′jŭn-ăl ă-nat′ŏ-mē) Method of anatomic study based on regions, parts, or divisions of the body (e.g., the foot or the inguinal region), emphasizing the relationships of structures (e.g., muscles, nerves, and arteries) within that area; distinguished from systemic anatomy.

re•gion•al an•es•the•si•a (rē′jŭn-ăl an′es-thē′zē-ă) Use of local anesthetic solution(s) to produce circumscribed areas of loss of sensation; a generic term including conduction, nerve block, spinal, epidural, field block, infiltration, and topical anesthesia. SYN conduction analgesia.

re•gion•al en•ter•i•tis (rē′jŭn-ăl en′tĕr-ī′tis) A chronic enteritis, of unknown cause, involving the terminal ileum and less frequently other parts of the gastrointestinal tract; characterized by patchy deep ulcers that may cause fistulas, and narrowing and thickening of the bowel by fibrosis and lymphocytic infiltration, with noncaseating tuberculoid granulomas that also may be found in regional lymph nodes; symptoms include fever, diarrhea, cramping abdominal pain, and weight loss. SYN Crohn disease, distal ileitis, regional ileitis, granulomatous enteritis.

re·gion·al gran·u·lom·a·tous lym·phad·e·ni·tis (rē′jŭn-ăl gran′yū-lō′mă-tŭs limf-ad′ĕ-nī′tis) SYN catscratch disease.

re·gion·al hy·po·ther·mi·a (rē′jŭn-ăl hī′pō-thĕr′mē-ă) Reduction of the temperature of an extremity or organ by external cold or perfusion with cold blood or solutions.

re·gi·o·nes (rē′jē-ō′nēz) Plural of regio. [L.]

re·gion of in·ter·est (rē′jŭn in′tĕr-ĕst) In computed tomography or other computerized imaging, an interactively selected portion of the image allowing individual or average pixel values to be displayed numerically.

re·gions of back (rē′jŭnz bak) The topographic regions of the back of the trunk, including the vertebral, sacral, scapular, infrascapular, and lumbar region.

re·gions of chest (rē′jŭnz chest) The topographic divisions of the chest: presternal, mammary, inframammary, and axillary. SEE pectoral region.

re·gions of face (rē′jŭnz fās) The topographic subdivisions of the face, including nasal, oral, mental, orbital, infraorbital, buccal, and zygomatic.

re·gions of head (rē′jŭnz hed) The topographic division of the cranium in relation to the bones of the cranial vault; the regions include frontal, parietal, occipital, and temporal.

re·gions of low·er limb (rē′jŭnz lō′ĕr lim) The topographic divisions of the lower limb: gluteal, thigh (or femoral), knee, leg (or crural), ankle, and foot.

re·gions of neck (rē′jŭnz nek) The topographic subdivisions of the neck.

re·gions of up·per limb (rē′jŭnz up′pĕr lim) The topographic divisions of the upper limb: deltoid, arm, elbow, forearm, carpal region, and hand.

reg·is·tered nurse (RN, R.N.) (rej′i-stĕrd nŭrs) A health care professional who has graduated from an accredited nursing program and has been licensed by public authority to practice nursing; may have advanced skills acquired through clinical master's or doctoral programs.

reg·is·tered res·pi·ra·tor·y ther·a·pist (RRT) (rej′is-tĕrd res′pir-ă-tōr-ē thār′ă-pist) Health professional who has graduated from an accredited respiratory therapy program and has passed both theoretic and practical portions of the national credentialing examination.

reg·is·tra·tion (rej′is-trā′shŭn) The reception of external stimuli; the capacity to perform this activity.

reg·is·try (rej′is-trē) A database on patients who share a particular characteristic; common registries include those for cancer, trauma, and implants; data are used to assess the quality of care, monitor trends, and do research.

re·gres·sion (rē-gresh′ŭn) **1.** A subsidence of symptoms. **2.** A relapse; a return of symptoms. **3.** Any retrograde movement or action. **4.** A return to a more primitive mode of behavior due to an inability to function adequately at a more adult level. **5.** The tendency of offspring of exceptional parents to possess characteristics closer to those of the general population. **6.** An unconscious defense mechanism by which there occurs a return to earlier patterns of adaptation. **7.** The distribution of one random variable given particular values of other variables relevant to it (e.g., a formula for the distribution of weight as a function of height and chest circumference). [L. *re-gredior,* pp. *-gressus,* to go back]

re·gres·sion a·nal·y·sis (rē-gresh′ŭn ă-nal′i-sis) The statistical method of finding the "best" mathematic model to describe one variable as a function of another.

re·gres·sive (rē-gres′iv) Relating to or characterized by regression.

re·gres·sive stain·ing (rē-gres′iv stān′ing) A type of staining in which tissues are overstained and the excess dye is then removed selectively until the desired intensity is obtained.

reg·u·lar a·stig·ma·tism (reg′yū-lăr ă-stig′mă-tizm) Ocular condition in which the curvature in each meridian is equal throughout its course, and the meridians of greatest and least curvature are at right angles to each other.

reg·u·la·tion (reg′yū-lā′shŭn) **1.** Control of the rate or manner in which a process progresses or a product is formed. **2.** EXPERIMENTAL EMBRYOLOGY the power of a pregastrula embryo to continue approximately normal development after a part or parts have been manipulated or destroyed. **3.** A rule or order issued by a regulatory agency of government or some other recognized authority (e.g., a rule on licensure of health care professionals issued by a state, province, or any other subnational jurisdiction). [L. *regula,* a rule]

reg·u·la·tor (reg′yū-lā′tŏr) A substance or process that controls another substance or process.

reg·u·la·tor gene (reg′yū-lā′tŏr jēn) A gene that produces a repressor substance that inhibits an operator gene when combined with it. It thus prevents production of a specific enzyme. When the enzyme is again in demand, a specific regulatory metabolite inhibits the repressor substance.

reg•u•la•to•ry dis•or•der (reg′yū-lă-tōr-ē dis-ōr′dĕr) A condition, first evident in infancy and early childhood, characterized by a distinct behavioral pattern that presents with a sensory, sensorimotor, or organizational processing difficulty that interferes with a child's ability to maintain positive interactions and relationships and to make daily adaptations.

reg•u•la•to•ry se•quence (reg′yū-lă-tōr-ē sē′kwĕns) Any DNA sequence that is responsible for the regulation of gene expression, such as promoters and operators.

reg•u•lon (reg′yū-lon) A set of structural genes, all with the same gene regulation, with gene products involved in the same reaction pathway.

re•gur•gi•tant (rē-gŭr′ji-tănt) Regurgitating; flowing backward.

re•gur•gi•tant mur•mur (rē-gŭr′ji-tănt mŭr′mŭr) A murmur due to leakage or backward flow at one of the valvular orifices of the heart.

re•gur•gi•tate (rē-gŭr′ji-tāt) **1.** To flow backward. **2.** To expel the contents of the stomach in small amounts, short of vomiting. [L. *re-*, back, + *gurgito,* pp. *-atus,* to flood, fr. *gurges* (*gurgit-*), a whirlpool]

re•gur•gi•ta•tion (rē-gŭr′ji-tā′shŭn) **1.** A backward flow, as of blood through an incompetent valve of the heart. **2.** SYN vomiting. [L. *regurgitatio* (see regurgitate)]

re•gur•gi•ta•tion jaun•dice (rē-gŭr′ji-tā′shŭn jawn′dis) Hepatic disorder due to biliary obstruction, in which the bile pigment has been conjugated and secreted by the hepatic cells and then reabsorbed into the bloodstream.

re•ha•bil•i•ta•tion (rē′hă-bil′i-tā′shŭn) Spontaneous or therapeutic restoration, after disease, illness, or injury, of the ability to function in a normal or near normal manner. [L. *rehabilitare,* pp. *-tatus,* to make fit, fr. *re-* + *habilitas,* ability]

re•hears•al (rē-hĕr′săl) A process associated with enhancing short-term and long-term memory wherein newly presented information, such as a name or a list of words, is repeated to oneself one or more times to avoid forgetting it.

re•hy•dra•tion (rē′hī-drā′shŭn) The return of water or other fluids to a system after its loss.

Rei•chel-Pól•ya stom•ach pro•ce•dure (rī′kel-pōl′yah stŏm′ăk prŏ-sē′jŭr) Retrocolic anastomosis of the full circumference of the open stomach to the jejunum.

Rei•chert car•ti•lage (rī′kĕrt kahr′ti-lăj) SYN second pharyngeal arch cartilage.

Reid base line (rēd bās līn) A line drawn from the inferior margin of the orbit to the auricular point (center of the orifice of the external acoustic meatus) and extending backward to the center of the occipital bone. Used as the zero plane in computed tomography.

Reif•en•stein syn•drome (rīf′ĕn-stīn sin′drōm) Partial androgen sensitivity; a familial form of male pseudohermaphroditism characterized by varying degrees of ambiguous genitalia or hypospadias, postpubertal development of gynecomastia, and infertility associated with seminiferous tubular sclerosis; cryptorchidism may be present, and Leydig cell hypofunction may lead to impotence in later years; chromosomal studies show 46,XY karyotype; X-linked recessive inheritance, caused by mutation in the androgen receptor gene (AR) on Xq.

Rei•ki (rā′kē) A healing modality developed in Japan; involves the transfer of universal energy through the laying on of hands. The Reiki practitioner, attuned to vibrations of this force, is a conduit through which the energy passes to the recipient at specific anatomic sites (e.g., chakras). SEE ALSO chi, chakra. [Jpn. universal life force]

re•im•plan•ta•tion (rē′im-plan-tā′shŭn) SYN replantation.

re•in•fec•tion (rē′in-fek′shŭn) A second infection by the same microorganism, after recovery from or during the course of a primary infection.

re•in•force•ment (rē′in-fōrs′mĕnt) **1.** An increase of force or strength; denoting specifically the increased sharpness of the patellar reflex when the patient at the same time closes the fist tightly or pulls against the flexed fingers or contracts some other set of muscles. **2.** DENTISTRY a structural addition or inclusion used to give additional strength in function (e.g., bars in plastic denture base). **3.** CONDITIONING the totality of the process in which the conditioned stimulus is followed by presentation of the unconditioned stimulus that itself elicits the response to be conditioned. SEE ALSO reinforcer.

re•in•forc•er (rē′in-fōrs′ĕr) In conditioning, a pleasant or satisfaction-yielding (positive reinforcer) or painful or unsatisfying (negative reinforcer) stimulus, object, or stimulus event that is obtained upon the performance of a desired or predetermined operant. SEE ALSO reinforcement (3). SYN reward.

Rein•ke space (rīn′kĕ spās) A potential space between the lamina propria and the external elastic lamina of the vocal fold. Edema in this space produces hoarseness in chronic inflammation.

re•in•ner•va•tion (rē-in′ĕr-vā′shŭn) Restoration of nerve control of a paralyzed muscle or other effector organ by means of regrowth of nerve fibers, either spontaneously or after anastomosis.

re•in•te•gra•tion (rē-in′tĕ-grā′shŭn) In the mental health professions, the return to well-adjusted functioning following disturbances due to mental illness.

Reis-Bück•lers cor•ne•al dys•tro•phy (rīs-bĕk′lers kōr′nē-ăl dis′trŏ-fē) An autosomal dominant disorder of Bowman membrane of the cornea, characterized by a reticular haze and associated with recurrent corneal erosions.

Reis·sei·sen mus·cles (rīs′ī-sen mŭs′ĕlz) Microscopic smooth muscle fibers in the smallest bronchial tubes.

Reiss·ner mem·brane (rīs′ner mem′brān) SYN vestibular membrane.

Rei·ter syn·drome (rī′ter sin′drōm) The association of urethritis, iridocyclitis, mucocutaneous lesions, and arthritis, sometimes with diarrhea; one or more of these conditions may recur at intervals of months or years, but the arthritis may be persistent. Pathogenesis remains unclear but is thought to represent an abnormal host response to various infectious agents.

re·jec·tion (rē-jek′shŭn) **1.** The immunologic response to incompatibility in a transplanted organ. **2.** A refusal to accept, recognize, or grant; a denial. **3.** Elimination of small ultrasonic echoes from display. [L. *rejectio,* a throwing back]

re·lapse (rē′laps) Return of the manifestations of a disease after an interval of improvement. SYN recurrence (2). [L. *re-labor,* pp. *-lapsus,* to slide back]

re·laps·ing feb·rile nod·u·lar non·sup·pur·a·tive pan·nic·u·li·tis (rē-lap′sing feb′ril noj′ū-lăr non′sŭp′yŭr-ă-tiv pă-nik′yū-lī′tis) Nodular fat necrosis of a variety of possible causes. SYN Christian disease (2), Christian syndrome, Weber-Christian disease.

re·laps·ing fe·ver (rē-lap′sing fē′vĕr) An acute infectious disease caused by any one of a number of strains of *Borrelia,* marked by febrile attacks lasting about 6 days and separated from each other by apyretic intervals of about the same length; the microorganism is found in the blood during the febrile periods but not during the intervals. There are two epidemiologic varieties: 1) the louse-borne variety, occurring chiefly in Europe, northern Africa, and India, and caused by strains of *B. recurrentis;* 2) the tick-borne variety, occurring in Africa, Asia, and North and South America, caused by various species of *Borrelia,* each of which is transmitted by a different species of *Ornithodoros,* a soft tick.

re·laps·ing pol·y·chon·dri·tis (rē-lap′sing pol′ē-kon-drī′tis) A hereditary degenerative disease of cartilage producing a bizarre form of arthritis, with collapse of the ears, the cartilaginous portion of the nose, and the tracheobronchial tree; death may occur from chronic infection or suffocation because of loss of stability in the tracheobronchial tree. SYN Meyenburg disease.

re·la·tion (rē-lā′shŭn) **1.** An association or connection between or among people or objects. SEE ALSO relationship. **2.** DENTISTRY the mode of contact of teeth or the positional relationship of oral structures. [L. *relatio,* a bringing back]

re·la·tion·ship (rĕ-lā′shŭn-ship) The state of being related, associated, or connected.

rel·a·tive ac·com·mo·da·tion (rel′ă-tiv ă-kom′ŏ-dā′shŭn) Quantity of accommodation required for single binocular vision for any specified distance, or for any particular degree of convergence.

rel·a·tive bi·o·log·ic ef·fec·tive·ness (rel′ă-tiv bī′ŏ-loj′ik e-fek′tiv-nĕs) A factor used to compare the biologic effect of absorbed doses of different types and energies of ionizing radiation. It is determined by the ratio of an absorbed dose of the particular radiation in question to the absorbed dose of a reference radiation required to produce an identical biologic effect in a specific organism, organ, or tissue.

rel·a·tive hu·mid·i·ty (rel′ă-tiv hyū-mid′i-tē) The actual amount of water vapor present in the air or in a gas, divided by the amount necessary for saturation at the same temperature and pressure; expressed as a percentage.

rel·a·tive leu·ko·cy·to·sis (rel′ă-tiv lū′kō-sī-tō′sis) An increased proportion of one or more types of leukocytes in the circulating blood, without an actual increase in the total number of white blood cells.

rel·a·tive mo·lec·u·lar mass (*M_r*) (rel′ă-tiv mŏ-lek′yū-lăr mas) SYN molecular weight.

rel·a·tive pol·y·cy·the·mi·a (rel′ă-tiv pol′ē-sī-thē′mē-ă) A relative increase in the number of red blood cells as a result of loss of the fluid portion of the blood.

rel·a·tive sco·to·ma (rel′ă-tiv skō-tō′mă) A scotoma in which there is visual depression but not complete loss of light perception.

rel·a·tive spec·i·fic·i·ty (rel′ă-tiv spes′i-fis′i-tē) The specificity of a medical screening test as determined by comparison with the same type of test (e.g., specificity of a new serologic test relative to specificity of an established serologic test).

rel·a·tive val·ue scale (RVS) (rel′ă-tiv val′yū skāl) System of assigning unit values to medical services based on the skill and time required by attending clinicians to complete a given procedure. SEE ALSO relative value unit.

rel·a·tive val·ue u·nit (RVU) (rel′ă-tiv val′yū yū′nit) A numeric factor assigned to a medical service during coding based on the skill and time required to undertake such a procedure.

re·lax·ant (rē-lak′sănt) **1.** Causing relaxation; reducing tension, especially muscular tension. **2.** An agent that reduces muscular tension or produces skeletal muscle paralysis, usually referred to as a muscle relaxant.

re·lax·ant re·ver·sal (rē-lak′sănt rē-vĕr′săl) Use of acetylcholinesterase inhibitors to terminate the action of nondepolarizing neuromuscular relaxants.

re•lax•a•tion (rē′lak-sā′shŭn) **1.** Loosening, lengthening, or lessening of tension in a muscle. **2.** MAGNETIC RESONANCE IMAGING the decay in magnetization of tissue after the direction of the surrounding magnetic field is changed; the different rates of relaxation for individual nuclei and tissues are used to provide contrast in imaging. [L. *relaxatio* (see relax)]

re•lax•a•tion su•ture (rē′lak-sā′shŭn sū′chŭr) A suture so arranged that it may be loosened if the tension of the wound becomes excessive.

re•lax•a•tion time (τ) (rē′lak-sā′shŭn tīm) The time required for the substrate in an enzymatic or chemical reaction to fall to 1/e of its initial value.

re•learn•ing (rē-lĕrn′ing) The process of regaining a skill or ability that has been partially or entirely lost; savings involved in relearning, compared with original learning, give an index of the degree of retention.

re•lease of in•for•ma•tion (rē-lēs′ in′fŏr-mā′shŭn) SYN disclosure.

re•leas•ing fac•tors (rē-lē′sing fak′tŏrz) **1.** Substances, usually of hypothalamic origin, capable of accelerating the rate of secretion of a given hormone by the anterior pituitary gland. **2.** Factors required in the termination phase of either RNA biosynthesis or protein biosynthesis. SYN liberins, releasing hormone.

re•leas•ing hor•mone (rē-lē′sing hōr′mōn) SYN releasing factors.

re•li•a•bil•i•ty (rē-lī′ă-bil′i-tē) Repeatability; ability of a test to be repeated by several testers and produce the same result.

re•lieve (rē-lēv′) To free wholly or partly from pain or discomfort, either physical or mental. [through O. Fr. fr. L. *re-levo,* to lift up, lighten]

re•lo•ca•tion test (rē′lō-kā′shŭn test) A test for anterior shoulder instability; the supine patient's humerus is abducted and rotated externally against the table edge as a fulcrum; patients with anterior stability loss become apprehensive with pressure.

REM Abbreviation for rapid eye movements.

rem Abbreviation for roentgen-equivalent-man.

Re•mak fi•bers (rā′mahk fī′bĕrz) SYN unmyelinated fibers.

Re•mak nu•cle•ar di•vi•sion (rā′mahk nū′klē-ăr di-vizh′ŏn) SYN amitosis.

Re•mak re•flex (rā′mahk rē′fleks) Plantar flexion of the first three toes and, sometimes, the foot with extension of the knee induced by stroking of the upper anterior surface of the thigh; it occurs when the conducting paths in the cord are interrupted.

Re•mak sign (rā′mahk sīn) Dissociation of the sensations of touch and of pain in tabes dorsalis and polyneuritis.

rem•e•dy (rem′ĕ-dē) An agent that cures disease or alleviates its symptoms. [L. *remedium,* fr. *re-,* again, + *medeor,* cure]

re•min•er•al•i•za•tion (rē-min′ĕr-ăl-ī-zā′shŭn) **1.** The return to the body or a local area of necessary mineral constituents lost through disease or dietary deficiencies; commonly used in referring to the content of calcium salts in bone. **2.** DENTISTRY a process enhanced by the presence of fluoride whereby partially decalcified enamel, dentin, and cementum become recalcified by mineral replacement.

rem•i•nis•cence ther•a•py (rem′i-nis′ĕns thār′ă-pē) A psychotherapeutic technique used in depressed old people to restore self-esteem and personal satisfaction with one's life accomplishments. Often used to facilitate ego integrity as defined in Erik Erikson's last developmental stage.

re•mis•sion (rē-mish′ŭn) **1.** Abatement or lessening in severity of the symptoms of a disease. **2.** The period during which such abatement occurs. [L. *remissio,* fr. *re-mitto,* pp. *-missus,* to send back, slacken, relax]

re•mit•tance (rē-mit′ĕns) A temporary amelioration, without actual cessation, of symptoms.

re•mit•tance ad•vice (RA) (rē-mit′ăns ad-vīs′) Documentation describing payment and adjustments to the health care service provider; also called explanation of benefits (EOB).

re•mit•tent (rē-mit′ĕnt) Characterized by temporary periods of abatement of the symptoms of a disease.

re•mod•el•ing (rē-mod′ĕl-ing) **1.** A cyclic process by which bone maintains a dynamic steady state through sequential resorption and formation of a small amount of bone at the same site; unlike in the process of modeling, the size and shape of remodeled bone remain unchanged. **2.** Any process of reshaping or reorganizing. **3.** Process of changing a body part, as in plastic and reconstructive surgery. SYN remodelling.

remodelling [Br.] SYN remodeling.

re•mote af•ter•load•ing bra•chy•ther•a•py (rē-mōt′ af′tĕr-lō′ding brak′ē-thār′ă-pē) Locally delivered radiotherapy that is loaded remotely into previously placed receptacles.

re•mote tran•scrip•tion (rē-mōt′ tran-skrip′shŭn) SYN off-site transcription.

re•mov•a•ble bridge (rē-mūv′ă-bĕl brij) SYN removable partial denture.

re•mov•a•ble par•tial den•ture (rē-mūv′ă-bĕl pahr′shăl den′shŭr) A partial denture that supplies teeth and associated structures on a partially edentulous jaw; can be readily removed from the mouth. SYN removable bridge.

ren, gen. **re•nis**, pl. **re•nes** (ren, rē′nis, -nēz) [TA] SYN kidney. [L.]

ren- Combining form meaning kidney. [L. *ren*, kidney]

re•nal (rē′năl) SYN nephric.

re•nal am•y•loi•do•sis (rē′năl am′i-loy-dō′sis) Renal deposits of amyloid, especially in glomerular capillary walls, which may cause albuminuria and the nephrotic syndrome. SYN amyloid nephrosis (1).

re•nal an•gi•og•ra•phy (rē′năl an′jē-og′ră-fē) Examination of the renal circulation using x-rays following the injection of a radiopaque substance.

re•nal ar•ter•y (rē′năl ahr′tĕr-ē) *Origin*, aorta; *branches*, segmental, ureteral, and inferior suprarenal; *distribution*, kidney. SYN arteria renalis [TA].

re•nal cal•cu•lus (rē′năl kal′kyū-lŭs) A stone occurring within the kidney's collecting system. SYN kidney stone.

re•nal col•ic (rē′năl kol′ik) Sharp pain in the lower back that radiates down the flank and into the groin; associated with the passage of a renal calculus through the ureter as it dilates the ureter, causing ureteral spasms as the calculus is forced along the narrow tube; usually of sudden onset, severe and colicky (intermittent), and not improved by changes in position. Nausea and vomiting are common.

re•nal col•umns (rē′năl kol′ŭmz) The prolongations of cortical substance separating the pyramids of the kidney. SYN columnae renales [TA], Bertin columns.

re•nal cor•pus•cle (rē′năl kōr′pŭs-ĕl) The tuft of glomerular capillaries and the capsula glomeruli that encloses it. SYN corpusculum renis.

re•nal cor•tex (rē′năl kōr′teks) The part of the kidney consisting of renal lobules in the outer zone beneath the capsule and the lobules of the renal columns that are extensions inward between the pyramids; contains the renal corpuscles and the proximal and distal convoluted tubules.

re•nal fail•ure (rē′năl fāl′yŭr) Impairment of renal function, either acute or chronic, with retention of urea, creatinine, and other waste products. SYN kidney failure.

re•nal fas•ci•a (rē′năl fash′ē-ă) The condensation of the fibroareolar tissue and fat surrounding the kidney to form a sheath for the organ. SYN Gerota capsule, Gerota fascia.

re•nal gan•gli•a (rē′năl gang′glē-ă) Small, scattered sympathetic ganglia along the renal plexus.

re•nal gly•co•sur•i•a (rē′năl glī′kō-syūr′ē-ă) The recurring or persistent excretion of glucose in the urine, in association with blood glucose levels in the normal range; results from the failure of proximal renal tubules to reabsorb glucose at a normal rate from the glomerular filtrate (low renal threshold); defect in the glucose carrier in the nephron.

re•nal he•ma•tu•ri•a (rē′năl hē′mă-tyūr′ē-ă) Blood in the urine resulting from extravasation of blood into the glomerular spaces, tubules, or pelves of the kidneys.

re•nal hy•per•ten•sion (rē′năl hī′pĕr-ten′shŭn) Hypertension secondary to renal disease.

re•nal hy•po•pla•si•a (rē′năl hī′pō-plā′zē-ă) An abnormally small kidney that is morphologically normal but has either a reduced number of nephrons or smaller nephrons.

re•nal lab•y•rinth (rē′năl lab′i-rinth) SYN convoluted part of kidney lobule.

re•nal me•dul•la (rē′năl mĕ-dŭl′ă) The inner, darker portion of the kidney parenchyma consisting of the renal pyramids.

re•nal (nerve) plex•us (rē′năl nĕrv plek′sŭs) The autonomic plexus surrounding the renal artery and extending with it into the substance of the kidney.

re•nal os•te•o•dys•tro•phy (rē′năl os′tē-ō-dis′trŏ-fē) Generalized bone changes resembling osteomalacia and rickets or osteitis fibrosa, occurring in chronic renal failure.

re•nal pa•pil•la (rē′năl pă-pil′ă) The apex of a renal pyramid that projects into a minor calyx; some 10–25 openings of papillary ducts occur on its tip, forming the area cribrosa.

re•nal pel•vis (rē′năl pel′vis) A flattened funnel-shaped expansion of the upper end of the ureter receiving the calyces, the apex being continuous with the ureter.

re•nal pyr•a•mid (rē′năl pir′ă-mid) One of several pyramidal masses seen on longitudinal section of the kidney; collectively, they constitute the renal medulla, and contain part of the secreting tubules and the collecting tubules. SYN malpighian pyramid, medullary pyramid, pyramis renalis.

re•nal rick•ets (rē′năl rik′ĕts) A form of rickets occurring in children in association with and apparently caused by renal disease with hyperphosphatemia. SYN pseudorickets.

re•nal si•nus (rē′năl sī′nŭs) The cavity of the kidney, containing the calyces and pelvis of the ureter and the segmental vessels embedded within a fatty matrix. The renal sinuses cause the kidneys to appear hollow or C-shaped on cross-section or medical imaging.

re•nal thresh•old (rē′năl thresh′ōld) The

plasma concentration level of a substance below which none appears in urine.

re•nal tu•bu•lar ac•i•do•sis (rē′năl tū′byū-lăr as′i-dō′sis) A clinical syndrome characterized by decreased ability to acidify urine, and by low plasma bicarbonate and high plasma chloride concentrations, often with hypokalemia.

re•nal tu•bules (rē′năl tū′byūlz) SEE convoluted tubule.

re•nal veins (rē′năl vānz) Large veins formed at the renal hilus by the merger of the segmental veins anterior to the corresponding arteries; they open at right angles into the inferior vena cava at the level of the second lumbar vertebra. The left renal vein receives the left suprarenal vein and the left gonadal vein, and passes through the angle between the abdominal aorta and superior mesenteric artery, where it may be compressed.

re•new•ing cell (rē-nū′ing sel) A type of cell found in the skin, hair, and blood that reproduces itself continuously throughout life.

ren•i•form (ren′i-fōrm) SYN nephroid.

re•nin (rē′nin) An enzyme that converts angiotensinogen to angiotensin I. SYN angiotensinogenase.

ren•in-an•gi•o•ten•sin-al•dos•ter•one sys•tem (rē′nin-an′jē-ō-ten′sin al-dos′tĕr-ōn sis′tĕm) Hormones, renin, angiotensin, and aldosterone work together to regulate blood pressure. A sustained fall in blood pressure causes the kidney to release renin. This is converted to angiotensin in the circulation. Angiotensin then raises blood pressure directly by arteriolar constriction and stimulates the suprarenal glands to produce aldosterone that promotes sodium and water retention by kidney, such that blood volume and blood pressure increase.

ren•i•por•tal (ren′i-pōr′tăl) **1.** Relating to the hilum of the kidney. **2.** Relating to the portal, or venous capillary circulation in the kidney. [reni- + L. *porta,* gate]

ren•nin (ren′in) SYN chymosin.

ren•nin•o•gen, ren•no•gen (rĕ-nin′ŏ-jen, ren′ō-jen) SYN prochymosin. [rennin + G. *-gen,* producing]

♻ **reno-, reni-** Combining forms denoting the kidney. SEE ALSO nephro-. [L. *ren*]

re•no•gen•ic (rē′nō-jen′ik) Originating in or from the kidney.

re•no•gram (rē′nō-gram) The assessment of renal function by external radiation detectors after the administration of a radiopharmaceutical that is filtered and excreted by the kidney. [reno- + G. *gramma*, something written]

re•nog•ra•phy (rē-nog′ră-fē) Radiography of the kidney.

re•no•meg•a•ly (rē′nō-meg′ă-lē) Enlargement of the kidney.

re•no•pri•val (rē′nō-prī′văl) Relating to, characterized by, or resulting from total loss of kidney function or from removal of all functioning renal tissue. [reno- + L. *privus,* deprived of]

re•no•troph•ic (rē′no-tro′fik) Relating to any agent influencing the growth or nutrition of the kidney or to the action of such an agent. SYN nephrotrophic, nephrotropic. [reno- + G. *trophē*, nourishment]

re•no•vas•cu•lar (rē′nō-vas′kyū-lăr) Pertaining to the blood vessels of the kidney, denoting especially disease of these vessels.

re•no•vas•cu•lar hy•per•ten•sion (rē′nō-vas′kyū-lăr hī′pĕr-ten′shŭn) Hypertension produced by renal arterial obstruction.

Ren•pen•ning syn•drome (ren′pen-ing sin′drōm) X-linked mental retardation with short stature and microcephaly not associated with the fragile X chromosome; occurs more frequently in males, although females may also be affected.

Ren•shaw cell (ren′shaw sel) Type of spinal cord interneuron that acts to prevent rapid repeat firing of motor neurons through a feedback circuit.

Re•o•vir•i•dae (rē-ō-vir′i-dē) A family of double-stranded RNA viruses, comprising six genera: Reovirus, Orbivirus, Rotavirus, cytoplasmic polyhidrosis virus group (Cypovirus), and two plant reovirus groups (Phytoreovirus, Fijivirus). [*R*espiratory *E*nteric *O*rphan + viridae]

Re•o•vi•rus (rē′ō-vī′rŭs) A genus of viruses recovered from children with mild fever and sometimes diarrhea, and from children with no apparent infection; a causative relationship to illness has not been proven.

rep. Abbrevation for repeat.

re•pair (rē-pār′) Restoration of diseased or damaged tissues naturally by healing processes or artificially, as by surgical means. [M.E.,fr. O.Fr.,fr. L. *re-paro,* fr. *re-*, back, again, + *paro,* prepare, put in order]

re•par•a•tive den•tin (rep′ăr-ă-tiv den′tin) SYN tertiary dentin.

re•par•a•tive gran•u•lo•ma (rep′ăr-ă-tiv gran′yū-lō′mă) Complication of stapedectomy in which a granuloma forms in the oval window around the prosthesis; results in a sensory hearing loss.

re•peat (rep.) (rē-pēt′) Prescription directions for the pharmacist. [L. repetatur, let it be repeated]

re•pel•lent (rē-pel′ĕnt) **1.** Capable of driving off or repelling; repulsive. **2.** An agent that drives away or prevents annoyance or irritation by insect pests. **3.** An astringent or other agent that reduces swelling. [L. *re-pello,* to drive back]

rep•e•ti•tion-com•pul•sion (rep′ĕ-tish′ŭn-kŏm-pŭl′shŭn) PSYCHOANALYSIS the tendency to repeat earlier experiences or actions, in an unconscious effort to achieve belated mastery over them; a morbid need to repeat a particular behavior, such as handwashing or checking to see if the door is locked.

re•pe•ti•tion max•i•mum (RM) (rep′ĕ-tish′ŭn mak′si-mŭm) Maximum load a muscle can lift for a predetermined number of repetitions to the point of fatigue.

rep•e•ti•tion time (TR) (rep′ĕ-tish′ŭn tīm) MAGNETIC RESONANCE IMAGING the time between repetitions of the pulse sequence.

re•pet•i•tive lift•ing test (rĕ-pet′i-tiv lift′ing test) A measurement of a patient's response to intermittent static effort combined with light to moderate work. SYN weight-carrying test.

re•pe•ti•tive strain dis•or•der (rĕ-pet′i-tiv strān dis-ōr′dĕr) SYN cumulative trauma disorder.

re•place•ment (rē-plās′mĕnt) **1.** Restoration. **2.** Substitution.

re•place•ment ther•a•py (rē-plās′mĕnt thār′ă-pē) Care designed to compensate for a lack or deficiency arising from inadequate nutrition, from certain dysfunctions (e.g., glandular hyposecretion), or from losses (e.g., hemorrhage); replacement may be physiologic or may entail administration of a substitute (e.g., a synthetic estrogen in place of estradiol).

re•plant (rē-plant′) **1.** To perform replantation. **2.** A part or organ so replaced or about to be so replaced.

re•plan•ta•tion (rē′plan-tā′shŭn) Replacement of an organ or part in its original site and reestablishing its circulation. SYN reimplantation. [L. *re-*, again, + *planto,* pp. *-atus,* to plant, fr. *planta,* a sprout, slip]

re•ple•tion (rē-plē′shŭn) **1.** SYN hypervolemia. **2.** SYN plethora (2). [L. *repletio,* fr. *re-pleo,* pp. *-pletus,* to fill up]

rep•li•case (rep′li-kās) Descriptive term for RNA-directed RNA polymerase (EC 2.7.7.48) associated with replication of RNA viruses.

rep•li•cate (rep′li-kāt, rep′li-kit) **1.** (-kit) One of several identical processes or observations. **2.** (kāt) To repeat; to produce an exact copy.

rep•li•ca•tion (rep-li-kā′shŭn) **1.** The execution of an experiment or study more than once so as to confirm the original findings, increase precision, and obtain a closer estimate of sampling error. **2.** Autoreproduction, as in mitosis or cellular biology. SEE ALSO autoreproduction. **3.** DNA-directed DNA synthesis. [L. *replicatio,* a reply, fr. *replico,* pp. *-atus,* to fold back]

rep•li•ca•tive form (rep′li-kă--tiv fōrm) **1.** An intermediate stage in the replication of either DNA or RNA viral genomes that is usually double stranded. **2.** The altered, double-stranded form to which single-stranded coliphage DNA is converted after infection of a susceptible bacterium, formation of the complementary ("minus") strand being mediated by enzymes that were present in the bacterium before entrance of the viral ("plus") strand.

rep•li•ca•tor (rep′li-kā-tŏr) The specific site of a bacterial genome (chromosome) at which replication begins.

rep•li•con (rep′li-kon) **1.** A segment of a chromosome (or of the DNA of a chromosome or similar entity) that can replicate, with its own initiation and termination codons, independently of the chromosome in which it may be located. **2.** The replication unit; several are found per DNA in eukaryotic systems. [*replic*ation + -on]

re•po•lar•i•za•tion (rē-pō′lăr-ī-zā′shŭn) The process whereby the membrane, cell, or fiber, after depolarization, is polarized again, with positive charges on the outer and negative charges on the inner surface.

re•port (rē-pōrt′) A formal account, oral, written, or electronic, of conditions, events, or actions. [O.Fr. *reporter,* fr. L. *re-portare,* to carry back]

re•port•a•ble dis•ease (rē-pōrt′ă-bĕl di-zēz′) SYN notifiable disease.

re•por•ting bi•as (rē-pōrt′ing bī′ăs) Selective revealing or suppression of information about past medical history (e.g., details of exposure to sexually transmitted diseases).

re•po•si•ti•o (rē-pō-zē′shē-ō) SYN reposition.

re•po•si•tion (rē′pŏ-zish′un) Movement returning palm and fingers from opposed position; opposite of opposition. SYN repositio.

re•po•si•tion•ing (rē′pŏ-zish′ŭn-ing) SYN reduction (1).

re•pos•i•tor (rē-poz′i-tŏr) An instrument used to reposition a displaced organ.

re•pressed (rē-prest′) Subjected to repression.

re•press•i•ble en•zyme (rē-pres′i-bĕl en′zīm) An enzyme that is produced continuously unless production is repressed by excess of an inhibitor (corepressor). SEE ALSO inactive repressor.

re•pres•sion (rē-presh′ŭn) **1.** PSYCHOTHERAPY the active process or defense mechanism of keeping out and ejecting, banishing from consciousness, ideas or impulses that are unacceptable to it. **2.** Decreased expression of some gene product. [L. *re-primo,* pp. *-pressus,* to press back, repress]

re•pres•sor (rē-pres′ŏr) The product of a regulator or repressor gene.

re•pres•sor gene (rē-pres′ŏr jēn) A gene that prevents a nonallele from being transcribed.

re•pro•duc•i•bil•i•ty (rē′prō-dūs′i-bil′i-tē) **1.** Ability to cause to exist again or to present again. **2.** Ability to duplicate measurements over long periods by different laboratories.

re•pro•duc•tion (rē′prō-dŭk′shŭn) **1.** The recall and presentation in the mind of the elements of a former impression. **2.** The total process by which organisms produce offspring. SYN generation (1), procreation. [L. *re-*, again, + *pro-duco,* pp. *-ductus,* to lead forth, produce]

re•pro•duc•tive cy•cle (rē′prō-dŭk′tiv sī′kĕl) The cycle that begins with conception and extends through gestation and parturition.

rep•ti•lase (rep′ti-lās) An enzyme found in the venom of *Bothrops atrox* that clots fibrinogen by splitting off its fibrinopeptide. [reptile + -ase]

re•pul•sion (rē-pŭl′shŭn) **1.** The act of repelling or driving apart, in contrast to attraction. **2.** Strong dislike; aversion; repugnance. **3.** Coupling phase of genes at linked loci that are borne on opposite chromosomes. [L. *re-pello,* pp. *-pulsus,* to drive back]

re•quire•ment (rē-kwīr′mĕnt) Anything that is obligatory or necessary; an authoritative expression of such obligation or necessity. [L. *requiro*]

res•cue (res′kyū) **1.** To save from harm, in a clinical or therapeutic sense. **2.** Describing an analgesic prescribed for breakthrough pain (e.g., opioids for cancer therapy). [M.E. *rescouen*]

res•cue breath•ing (res′kyū brēdh′ing) SYN head-tilt/chin-lift maneuver.

res•cue med•i•ca•tion (res′kyū med′i-kā′shŭn) A medicine administered to relieve an acute exacerbation of a condition (e.g., asthma, migraine) that is normally controlled with prophylactic medicine.

re•search (rē′sĕrch) **1.** The organized quest for new knowledge and better understanding (e.g., of the natural world or determinants of health and disease). Five types of research are recognized: observational (empiric), analytic, experimental, theoretic, applied. **2.** (rĕ-sĕrch′) To conduct such scientific inquiry. [O.Fr. *re-cerche,* fr. *cerchier,* to search, fr. L. *circare,* to go around, fr. *circus,* circle]

re•sect (rē-sekt′) **1.** To cut off, especially to cut off the articular ends of one or both bones, forming a joint. **2.** To excise a segment of a part. [L. *re-seco,* pp. *sectus,* to cut off]

re•sect•a•ble (rē-sek′tă-bĕl) Amenable to resection.

re•sec•tion (rē-sek′shŭn) **1.** A procedure performed for the specific purpose of removal of a significant part of an organ or bodily structure; may be partial or complete. **2.** To remove a part. **3.** SYN excision (1).

re•sec•to•scope (rē-sek′tō-skōp) A special endoscopic instrument for the transurethral electrosurgical removal of lesions involving the bladder, prostate gland, or urethra.

re•sec•to•scope e•lec•trode (rē-sek′tō-skōp ĕ-lek′trōd) A wire loop electrode that allows removal of tissue as well as cautery of the raw surface; used in endometrial ablation.

re•serve (rē-zĕrv′) Something available but held back for later use. [L. *re-servo,* to keep back, reserve]

re•serve air (rē-zĕrv′ ār) SYN expiratory reserve volume.

re•serve force (rē-zĕrv′ fōrs) The energy residing in the organism or any of its parts above that required for its normal functioning.

res•er•voir (rez′ĕr-vwahr) SYN receptaculum. [Fr.]

res•er•voir bag (rez′ĕr-vwahr bag) SYN breathing bag.

res•er•voir host (rez′ĕr-vwahr hōst) The host of an infection in which the infectious agent multiplies and develops, and on which the agent is dependent for survival in nature.

res•er•voir of in•fec•tion (rez′ĕr-vwahr in-fek′shŭn) Living or nonliving material in or on which an infectious agent multiplies and develops and is dependent on for its survival in nature. SEE ALSO fomes.

res•er•voir ox•y•gen-con•serv•ing de•vice (rez′ĕr-vwahr ok′si-jĕn-kŏn-sĕr′ving dĕ-vīs′) A device that stores oxygen in valveless expandable chambers under the nostrils or through large-bore tubing in a single valveless chamber worn on the chest; during inhalation through the nostrils, the oxygen is evacuated from the reservoir; conservation of oxygen is achieved because the constant flow of oxygen from the source can be reduced.

res•er•voir of sperms (rez′ĕr-vwahr spĕrmz) The site where sperms are stored; the distal portion of the tail of the epididymis and the beginning of the ductus deferens.

res•i•dent (rez′i-dĕnt) **1.** A house officer attached to a hospital for clinical training. **2.** A patient residing in a health care facility. [L. *resideo,* to reside]

res•i•den•tial care (rez′i-den′shăl kār) SYN extended-care facility.

re•sid•u•a (rē-zid′yu-ă) Plural of residuum.

re•sid•u•al (rē-zid′yū-ăl) Relating to or of the nature of a residue.

re•sid•u•al ab•scess (rē-zid′yū-ăl ab′ses) An abscess recurring at the site of a former abscess resulting from persistence of microbes and pus.

re•sid•u•al air (rē-zid′yū-ăl ār) SYN residual volume.

re•sid•u•al ca•pac•i•ty (rē-zid′yū-ăl kă-pas′i-tē) SYN residual volume.

re•sid•u•al dose con•tam•i•na•tion (rē-zid′yū-ăl dōs kŏn-tam′i-nā′shŭn) That portion of a chemical, biologic, or radiologic agent that remains on (external contamination) or in (internal contamination) a victim or inanimate object, especially (but not necessarily) after evaporation and absorption.

re•sid•u•al schiz•o•phre•ni•a (rē-zid′yū-ăl skits′ō-frē′nē-ă) Blunted or inappropriate affect, social withdrawal, eccentric behavior, or loose associations, but without prominent psychotic symptoms, such as the remains of former psychotic symptoms of schizophrenia.

re•sid•u•al ur•ine (rē-zid′yū-ăl yūr′in) That which remains in the bladder at the end of micturition in cases of prostatic obstruction, bladder atony, and other disorders.

re•sid•u•al vol•ume (RV) (rē-zid′yū-ăl vol′yūm) The volume of air remaining in the lungs after a maximal expiratory effort. SYN residual air, residual capacity.

res•i•due (rez′i-dū) That which remains after removal of one or more substances. SYN residuum. [L. *residuum*]

re•sid•u•um, pl. **re•sid•u•a** (re-zid′yū-ŭm, -ă) SYN residue. [L. ntr. of *residuus,* left behind, remaining, fr. *re- sideo,* to sit back, remain behind]

res•in (rez′in) **1.** An amorphous brittle substance consisting of the hardened secretion of a number of plants, probably derived from a volatile oil and similar to a stearoptene. **2.** SYN rosin. **3.** A precipitate formed by the addition of water to certain tinctures. **4.** A broad term used to indicate organic substances insoluble in water. [L. *resina*]

re•sin ce•ment (rez′in sĕ-ment′) A monomer or monomer-polymer system used as a dental luting agent; used in cementation of restorations or orthodontic brackets to the teeth.

res•in•ous (rez′i-nŭs) Relating to or derived from a resin.

res ip•sa lo•qui•tur (rĕz ip′să lō′kwē-tŭr) The thing speaks for itself; the circumstantial evidence (of malpractice) is obvious and does not require an expert witness to testify. [L.]

re•sis•tance (rĕ-zis′tăns) **1.** A passive force exerted in opposition to another active force. **2.** The opposition in a conductor to the passage of a current of electricity, whereby energy is lost and heat produced; specifically, the potential difference in volts across the conductor per ampere of current flow; unit: ohm. Cf. impedance (1). **3.** The opposition to flow of a fluid through one or more passageways; units are usually those of pressure difference per unit flow. Cf. impedance (2). **4.** PSYCHOANALYSIS a person's unconscious defense against bringing repressed thoughts to consciousness. **5.** The ability of red blood cells to resist hemolysis and to preserve their shape under varying degrees of osmotic pressure in the blood plasma. **6.** The natural or acquired ability of an organism to maintain its immunity to or to resist the effects of an antagonistic agent (e.g., pathogenic microorganism, toxin, drug). [L. *re-sisto,* to stand back, withstand]

re•sis•tance plas•mids (rĕ-zis′tăns plaz′midz) Plasmids carrying genes responsible for antibiotic (or antibacterial drug) resistance among bacteria (notably Enterobacteriaceae); they may be conjugative or nonconjugative, the former possessing transfer genes (resistance transfer factor) lacking in the latter.

re•sis•tance ther•mom•e•ter (rĕ-zis′tăns thĕr-mom′ĕ-tĕr) A device that measures temperature by changes in the electrical resistance of a metal wire.

re•sist•ance train•ing (rē-zis′tăns trān′ing) Using weights (e.g., dumbbell, barbell, machine), technique chronically loads a muscle group in an attempt to increase strength over time (some techniques include progressive resistance, isometric, and isokinetic weight training).

re•sis•tance-trans•fer fac•tor (rĕ-zis′tăns-trans′fĕr fak′tŏr) The transfer gene of the resistance plasmid.

re•sis•tant starch (rē-sis′tĕnt stahrch) Dietary starch resistant to pancreatic amylase, allowing it to escape into the large bowel, where it is fermented to short-chain fatty acids by colonic microflora.

res•o•lu•tion (rez′ŏ-lū′shŭn) **1.** The arrest of an inflammatory process without suppuration; the absorption or breaking down and removal of the products of inflammation or of a new growth. **2.** The optic ability to distinguish detail such as the separation of closely adjacent objects. SYN resolving power (3). [L. *resolutio,* a slackening, fr. *re-solvo,* pp. *-solutus,* to loosen, relax]

re•solve (rē-zawlv′) To return or cause to return to the normal, particularly without suppuration; said of a phlegmon or other form of inflammation. [L. *resolvo,* to loosen]

re•solv•ing pow•er (re-zawlv′ing pow′ĕr) **1.** Definition of a lens; in a microscope objective lens it is calculated by dividing the wavelength of the light used by twice the numerical aperture of the objective. **2.** Analogies to other modalities (e.g., two-point discrimination in neurologic examination). **3.** SYN resolution (2).

res•o•nance (rez′ŏ-năns) **1.** Sympathetic or forced vibration of air in the cavities above, below, in front of, or behind a source of sound; in speech, modification of the quality (e.g., tone) of a sound by the passage of air through the chambers of the nose, pharynx, and head, without increasing the intensity of the sound. **2.** The sound obtained on percussion of a part that can vibrate freely. **3.** The intensification and hollow character of the voice sound obtained on auscultation over a cavity. **4.** CHEMISTRY the manner in which electrons or electric charges are distributed among the atoms in compounds that are planar and symmetric, particularly those with conjugated (alternating) double bonds; the existence of resonance in the latter case reduces the energy content and increases the stability of a compound. **5.** The natural or inherent frequency of any oscillating system. **6.** SYN resonant frequency. [L. *resonantia,* echo, fr. *re-sono,* to resound, to echo]

res•o•nant fre•quen•cy (rez′ŏ-nănt frē′kwĕn-sē) The frequency at which individual magnetic nuclei absorb or emit radiofrequency energy in magnetic resonance studies. SYN resonance (6).

re•sorb (rē-sōrb′) To reabsorb; to absorb what has been excreted, as an exudate or pus. [L. *re-sorbeo,* to suck back]

re•sorp•tion (rē-sōrp′shŭn) **1.** The act of resorbing. **2.** A loss of substance by lysis, or by physiologic or pathologic means.

re•sorp•tion la•cu•nae (rē-sōrp′shŭn lă-kū′nē) SYN Howship lacunae.

Re•source-Based Rel•a•tive Val•ue Scale (rē′sōrs-bāst rel′ă-tiv val′yū skāl) A payment system mandated by U.S. federal law concerning Medicare's establishing a cost basis for Medicare services based on analysis of skill and time required by the health care provider for patient's care.

Re•source U•ti•li•za•tion Group (RUG) (rē′sōrs yū′til-ī-zā′shŭn grūp) One of 44 patient categories, each with a corresponding per diem reimbursement rate as mandated by Medicare.

res•pi•ra•ble (res′pir-ă-bĕl) Capable of being breathed.

res•pi•ra•tion (res′pir-ā′shŭn) **1.** A fundamental process of life, characteristic of both plants and animals, in which oxygen is used to oxidize organic fuel molecules, providing a source of energy as well as carbon dioxide and water. In green plants, photosynthesis is not considered respiration **2.** SYN ventilation (2). See this page. [L. *respiratio,* fr. *re-spiro,* pp. *-atus,* to exhale, breathe]

res•pi•ra•tion rate (res′pir-ā′shŭn rāt) Frequency of breathing, recorded as the number of breaths per minute.

res•pi•ra•tor (res′pir-ā′tŏr) **1.** An appliance fitting over the mouth and nose, used to exclude dust, smoke, or other irritants, or otherwise alter the air before it enters the respiratory passages. **2.** An apparatus for administering artificial respiration, especially for a prolonged period, in cases of paralysis or inadequate spontaneous ventilation. SEE ALSO ventilator.

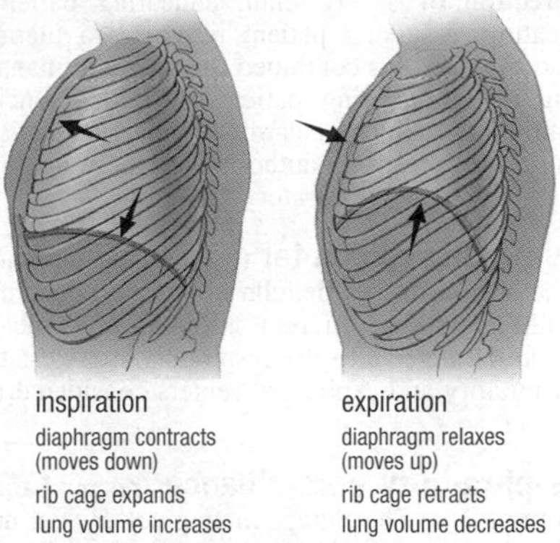

respiration: inspiration and expiration

res•pi•ra•to•ry (res′pir-ă-tōr-ē) Relating to respiration.

res•pi•ra•to•ry ac•i•do•sis (res′pir-ă-tōr-ē as′i-dō′sis) Acidosis caused by retention of carbon dioxide; due to inadequate pulmonary ventilation or hypoventilation, with decrease in blood pH unless compensated by renal retention of bicarbonate. SYN hypercapnic acidosis.

res•pi•ra•to•ry al•ka•lo•sis (res′pir-ă-tōr-ē al′kă-lō′sis) Alkalosis resulting from an abnormal loss of CO_2 produced by hyperventilation, either active or passive, with concomitant reduction in arterial bicarbonate concentration. SEE ALSO compensated alkalosis.

res•pi•ra•to•ry as•sess•ment (res′pir-ă-tōr-ē ă-ses′mĕnt) The appraisal of the patient's respiratory system by a health care provider. Performed by auscultating one region of the lung and comparing the sounds with those in the symmetric region in the other lung.

res•pi•ra•to•ry bron•chi•oles (res′pir-ă-tōr-ē brong′kē-ōlz) The smallest bronchioles (0.5 mm in diameter), which connect the terminal bronchioles to alveolar ducts; alveoli arise from part of the wall.

res•pi•ra•to•ry ca•pac•i•ty (res′pir-ă-tōr-ē kă-pas′i-tē) SYN vital capacity.

res•pi•ra•to•ry care (res′pir-ă-tōr-ē kār) An adjunctive form of health care intended to maintain or restore optimal respiratory function through the use of appropriate devices and techniques; respiratory care services, provided by qualified professionals under medical direction in a variety of settings, include diagnostic testing and monitoring, patient education, therapy, and rehabilitation.

res•pi•ra•to•ry care prac•ti•tion•er (RCP) (res′pir-ă-tōr-ē kār prak-tish′ŏn-ĕr) An allied health care professional who works under the direction of a physician, educating patients, treating, assessing patient response to therapy and the need for continued therapy, and managing and monitoring patients with deficiencies and abnormalities of cardiopulmonary function; applied by licensing authorities to those licensed to practice. SYN respiratory therapist.

res·pi·ra·to·ry cen·ter (res′pir-ă-tōr-ē sen′tĕr) The region in the medulla oblongata concerned with integrating afferent information to determine the signals to the respiratory muscles; the inspiratory and expiratory centers considered together.

res·pi·ra·to·ry com·pli·ance (res′pir-ă-tōr-ē kŏm-plī′ăns) The change in lung volume per unit change in transrespiratory pressure when the respiratory muscles are relaxed; may be static or dynamic. SYN respiratory system compliance.

res·pi·ra·to·ry dis·tress syn·drome of the new·born (res′pir-ă-tōr-ē dis-tres′ sin′drōm nū′bōrn) An acute lung condition of newborn babies, characterized by tachypnea, nasal flaring, and respiratory grunting. The condition occurs primarily in premature babies due to a lack of surfactant, causing alveolar collapse. SYN hyaline membrane disease.

res·pi·ra·to·ry di·ver·tic·u·lum (res′pir-ă-tōr-ē dī′vĕr-tik′yū-lŭm) Primordial pharynx that gives rise to the epithelial lining of the respiratory tract on glands of the bronchial tree. See this page. SYN lung bud, tracheobronchial diverticulum.

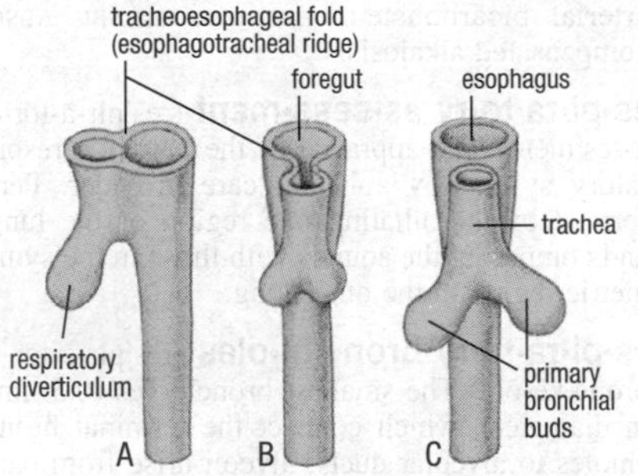

respiratory diverticulum: (A–C) successive stages in development, showing the tracheoesophageal folds and formation of the septum, splitting the foregut into esophagus and trachea with primary bronchial buds

res·pi·ra·to·ry en·ter·ic or·phan vi·rus (res′pir-ă-tōr-ē en-ter′ik ōr′făn vī′rŭs) A nonenveloped icosahedral virus with a genome that consists of double-stranded RNA, belonging to the family Reoviridae, which is frequently found in both the respiratory and enteric tracts.

res·pi·ra·to·ry en·zyme (res′pir-ă-tōr-ē en′zīm) A tissue enzyme that is part of an oxidation-reduction system accomplishing the conversion of substrates to CO_2 and H_2O and the transfer of the electrons removed to O_2.

res·pi·ra·to·ry ex·change ra·ti·o (res′pir-ă-tōr-ē eks-chānj′ rā′shē-ō) The ratio of the net output of carbon dioxide to the simultaneous net uptake of oxygen at a given site, both expressed as moles or STPD volumes per unit time.

res·pi·ra·to·ry fail·ure (res′pir-ă-tōr-ē fāl′yŭr) Loss of pulmonary function, either acute or chronic, that results in hypoxemia or hypercarbia; final common pathway for myriad respiratory disorders.

res·pi·ra·to·ry fre·quen·cy (f) (res′pir-ă-tōr-ē frē′kwĕn-sē) The number of breaths per minute.

res·pi·ra·to·ry gat·ing (res′pir-ă-tōr-ē gāt′ing) Any technique that derives a signal from breathing to trigger an electronic circuit, such as for data collection during expiration. SEE ALSO navigator echo.

res·pi·ra·tor·y in·duc·tance pleth·ys·mog·ra·phy (RIP) (res′pir-ă-tōr-ē in-dŭk′tăns pleth′iz-mog′ră-fē) A modality used in pulmonary function testing.

res·pi·ra·tor·y i·so·la·tion (res′pir-ă-tōr-ē ī′sō-lā′shŭn) Used for patients with diseases that can be spread by droplet infection. Anyone entering the patient's room must wear a mask.

res·pi·ra·to·ry min·ute vol·ume (res′pir-ă-tōr-ē mī-nūt′ vol′yūm) The minute volume of breathing; the product of tidal volume times the respiratory frequency. SEE ALSO pulmonary ventilation.

res·pi·ra·to·ry pause (res′pir-ă-tōr-ē pawz) Cessation of air flow for fewer than 10 sec. SEE ALSO sleep apnea.

res·pi·ra·to·ry pig·ments (res′pir-ă-tōr-ē pig′mĕnts) The oxygen-carrying (colored) substances in blood and tissues (e.g., hemoglobin, myoglobin, hemocyanin).

res·pi·ra·to·ry quo·tient (RQ) (res′pir-ă-tōr-ē kwō′shĕnt) The ratio of the carbon dioxide produced during tissue metabolism to the oxygen consumed; reflects net substrate oxidation; can be determined by indirect calorimetry.

res·pi·ra·to·ry rate (res′pir-ă-tōr-ē rāt) Frequency of breathing, recorded as the number of breaths per minute.

res·pi·ra·to·ry scle·ro·ma (res′pir-ă-tōr-ē skler-ō′mă) Rhinoscleroma in which the lesion involves the mucous membrane of the greater part or all of the upper respiratory tract.

res·pi·ra·to·ry sounds (res′pir-ă-tōr-ē sowndz) SYN breath sounds.

res·pi·ra·to·ry syn·cy·tial vi·rus (RSV) (res′pi-ră-tōr′ē sin-si′shăl vī′rŭs) A negative-sense RNA virus of the genus Pneumovirus, with a tendency to form syncytia in tissue culture; elicits minor respiratory infection in adults but can cause severe bronchitis and bronchopneumonia in young children. Virion is unstable in the environment and can be inactivated with soapy water and disinfectants; spread through close contact with infected people or contaminated surfaces or objects.

res•pi•ra•tor•y syn•cy•tial vi•rus im•mune glob•u•lin in•tra•ve•nous (RSV-IGIV) (res′pir-ă-tōr-ē sin-sish′ăl vī′rŭs im-yūn′ glob′yū-lin in′tră-vē′nŭs) An immunizing agent (passive) that is used to prevent infection caused by respiratory syncytial virus; given parenterally to children less than 24 months of age with breathing problems or a history of premature birth. Contraindications to the agent would be allergic reaction to human immunoglobulins or immunoglobulin A (IgA) deficiencies.

res•pi•ra•to•ry sys•tem com•pli•ance (res′pir-ă-tōr-ē sis′tĕm kŏm-plī′ăns) SYN respiratory compliance.

res•pi•ra•to•ry ther•a•pist (res′pir-ă-tōr-ē thār′ă-pist) SYN respiratory care practitioner.

res•pi•ra•to•ry ther•a•py (res′pir-ă-tōr-ē thār′ă-pē) SEE respiratory care.

res•pi•ra•to•ry tract (res′pir-ă-tōr-ē trakt) The air passages from the nose to the pulmonary alveoli, through the pharynx, larynx, trachea, and bronchi.

res•pi•rom•e•ter (res′pir-om′ĕ-tŏr) **1.** An instrument for measuring the extent of the respiratory movements. **2.** An instrument for measuring oxygen consumption or carbon dioxide production, usually of an isolated tissue. [L. *respiro,* to breathe, + G. *metron,* measure]

res•pite care (res′pit kār) Temporary or periodic care provided for a patient allowing the usual caregiver rest or time away from responsibility.

re•spon•de•at su•pe•ri•or (rē-spon′dē-at sŭ-pēr′ē-ŏr) Legal doctrine that makes an employer responsible for an employee's action; sometimes called 'captain of the ship principle' or law of agency. [L., let the superior take responsibility]

re•sponse (rĕ-spons′) **1.** The reaction of a muscle, nerve, gland, or other excitable tissue to a stimulus. **2.** Any act or behavior, or its constituents, that a living organism is capable of emitting. Reflexes are usually excluded because they are typically elicited by a specifiable (unconditioned or natural) stimulus rather than emitted under circumstances in which the stimulus was not specifiable. [L. *responsus,* an answer]

res•ponse bi•as (rĕ-spons′ bī′ăs) Systematic error due to differences in characteristics between those who choose or volunteer to take part in a study and those who do not.

rest (rest) **1.** Quiet; repose. [A.S. *raest*] **2.** To repose; to cease from work. [A.S. *raestan*] **3.** A group of poorly differentiated cells commonly believed to be cells of fetal tissue that has become displaced and lies embedded in tissue of another character. [L. *resto,* to remain] **4.** DENTISTRY an extension from a prosthesis that affords vertical support for a restoration.

re•ste•no•sis (rē′stĕ-nō′sis) Recurrence of stenosis after corrective surgery on the heart valve; narrowing of a structure (usually a coronary artery) following the removal or reduction of a previous narrowing. [re-, + G. *stenōsis,* a narrowing]

rest, ice, com•pres•sion, el•e•va•tion (RICE) (rest īs kŏm-presh′ŭn el′ĕ-vā′shŭn rīs) Mnemonic acronym for a common noninvasive way to treat acute inflammation, especially in relation to orthopedic soft-tissue injury. The affected area should be rested, ice applied, compression via support of some type (elastic bandage, laced boot), and elevation to or above heart level.

res•ti•form (res′ti-fōrm) Ropelike; rope-shaped; referring to the restiform body, the larger (lateral) part of the inferior cerebellar peduncle; contains fibers from the spinal cord (spinocerebellar) and medulla (cuneo-, olivo-, reticulocerebellar) to cerebellum. [L. *restis,* rope, + *forma,* form]

res•ti•form bo•dy (res′ti-fōrm bod′ē) A lateral (larger) subdivision of the inferior cerebellar peduncle composed of a variety of fibers including, but not limited to, olivo-, reticulo-, cuneo-, trigemino-, and dorsal spinocerebellar.

rest•ing en•er•gy ex•pen•di•ture (REE) (rest′ing en′ĕr-jē eks-pen′di-chŭr) Energy expenditure measured under resting, although not necessarily basal conditions. Cf. basal metabolic rate.

rest•ing hand splint (rest′ing hand splint) A splint intended to maintain the nonfunctional hand and wrist in a neutral position of rest so as to prevent pain and muscle contracture.

rest•ing met•a•bol•ic rate (RMR) (rest′ing met′ă-bol′ik rāt) Minimum number of calories needed to support basic functions, including breathing and circulation.

rest•ing ti•dal vol•ume (rest′ing tī′dăl vol′yūm) The volume of air inspired and expired at rest (i.e., in the absence of circumstances such as exercise that increase the rate or depth of inspirations).

rest•ing trem•or (rest′ing trem′ŏr) A coarse, rhythmic tremor, 3–5 Hz frequency, usually confined to hands and forearms, which appears when the limbs are relaxed, and disappears with active limb movements; characteristic of Parkinson disease.

rest•i•tope (res′ti-tōp) The part of the T-cell

receptor that associates with the class II major histocompatibility molecule. [*res*triction + -tope]

res•ti•tu•tion (res′ti-tū′shŭn) OBSTETRICS the return of the rotated head of the fetus to its natural relation with the shoulders after its emergence from the vulva. [L. *restitutio,* act of restoring]

rest jaw po•si•tion (rest jaw pŏ-zish′ŏn) SYN rest position.

rest•less legs syn•drome (RLS) (rest′lĕs legz sin′drōm) A sense of indescribable uneasiness, twitching, aching, burning, or restlessness that occurs in the legs after going to bed, frequently leading to insomnia, which may be relieved temporarily by walking about; thought to be caused by inadequate circulation or as an adverse effect of some SSRIs and other psychotropic medications.

Res•ton vi•rus (res′tŏn vī′rŭs) A variant of Ebola virus. SYN Ebola virus Reston.

res•to•ra•tion (res′tŏr-ā′shŭn) DENTISTRY **1.** A prosthetic restoration or appliance; a broad term applied to any inlay, crown, bridge, partial denture, or complete denture that restores or replaces lost tooth structure, teeth, or oral tissues. **2.** A plug or stopping; any substance, such as gold or amalgam, used for restoring the portion missing from a tooth as a result of the removal of decay from the tooth. See this page. [L. *restauro,* pp. *-atus,* to restore, to repair]

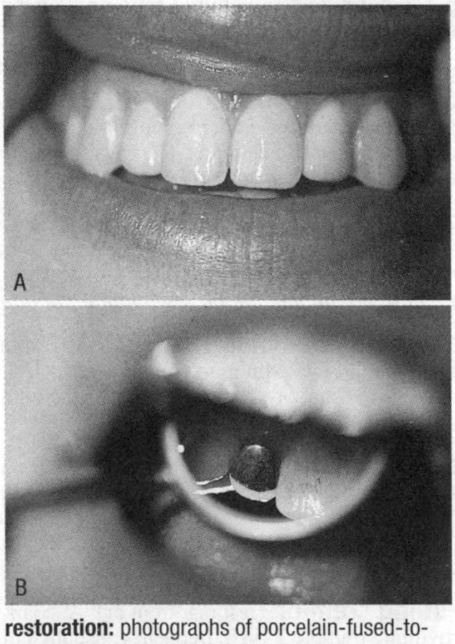

restoration: photographs of porcelain-fused-to-metal crowns restoring teeth #7 and 10; (A) labial view of both teeth; (B) lingual view of tooth #10

re•stor•a•tive (rĕ-stōr′ă-tiv) **1.** Renewing health and strength. **2.** An agent that promotes a renewal of health or strength. [L. *restauro,* to restore]

re•stor•a•tive den•tis•try (rĕ-stōr′ă-tiv den′tis-trē) Individual restoration of teeth by means of amalgam, synthetic porcelainlike materials, resins, or inlays. SEE ALSO implant, oral and maxillofacial surgery.

rest pain (rest pān) Unrelenting ischemic pain in an extremity at rest, indicating severe arterial insufficiency. SYN ischemic pain.

rest po•si•tion (rest pŏ-zish′ŏn) The usual position of the mandible when the patient is resting comfortably in an upright position and the condyles are in a neutral, unstrained position in the mandibular fossa. SYN physiologic rest position, postural position, postural resting position, rest jaw position.

re•straint (rē-strānt′) PSYCHIATRY intervention to prevent an excited or violent patient from doing harm to her- or himself or others; may involve the use of a camisole (straightjacket). [O. Fr. *restrainte*]

re•stric•tion (rĕ-strik′shŭn) **1.** The process in which foreign DNA that has been introduced into a prokaryotic cell becomes ineffective. **2.** A limitation.

re•stric•tion en•do•nu•cle•ase (rĕ-strik′shŭn en′dō-nū′klē-ās) One of many endonucleases isolated from bacteria that hydrolyze (cut) double-stranded DNA chains at specific sequences, thus inactivating a foreign (viral or other) DNA and restricting its activity; standard laboratory devices for making specific cuts in DNA as a first step in deducing sequences. SYN restriction enzyme.

re•stric•tion en•zyme (rĕ-strik′shŭn en′zīm) SYN restriction endonuclease.

re•stric•tion frag•ment length pol•y•mor•phism (RFLP) (rĕ-strik′shŭn frăg′mĕnt length pol′ē-mōrf′izm) Used in genetic analysis of populations or individual relationships. In regions of the human genome not coding for proteins there is often wide sequence variety between people that can be measured.

re•stric•tion site (rĕ-strik′shŭn sīt) A site in nucleic acid in which the bordering bases are of such a type as to leave them vulnerable to the cleaving action of an endonuclease. SYN cleavage site.

re•stric•tion-site pol•y•mor•phism (rĕ-strik′shŭn-sīt pol′ē-mōrf′izm) DNA polymorphism in which the sequence of one form of the polymorphism contains a recognition site for a particular endonuclease, but the sequence of the other form lacks such a site.

re•stric•tive ven•ti•la•to•ry de•fect (rē-strik′tiv ven′til-ă-tōr-ē dē-fekt′) Reduction in lung volumes not explainable by obstruction of the airways; most commonly characterized physiologically by a reduction in total lung capacity (TLC).

rest of Ser•res (rest sārs) Remnant of dental lamina epithelium entrapped within the gingiva.

re•sus•ci•tate (rē-sŭs′i-tāt) To perform resuscitation. [L. *re-suscito,* to raise up again, revive]

re•sus•ci•ta•tion (rē-sŭs′i-tā′shŭn) Revival from potential or apparent death. [L. *resuscitatio*]

re•tained men•stru•a•tion (rē-tānd′ men′strū-ā′shŭn) SYN hematocolpos.

re•tained pro•ducts of con•cep•tion (rē-tānd′ prod′ŭkts kŏn-sep′shŭn) Fragments of fetal, placental, or membrane tissue remaining in utero following delivery or abortion, posing an increased risk of bleeding or infection.

re•tain•er (rē-tān′ĕr) Any type of clasp, attachment, or other device used to fix or stabilize a prosthesis; an appliance used to prevent the shifting of teeth following orthodontic treatment.

re•tar•da•tion (rē′tahr-dā′shŭn) **1.** Slowness or limitation of development. **2.** An impairment associated with cognitive development.

re•tard•ed den•ti•tion (rē-tahrd′ĕd den-tish′ŭn) Dentition in which calcification, elongation, and eruption occur later than normal as a result of some systemic metabolic dysfunction (e.g., hypothyroidism).

retch (rech) To make an involuntary effort to vomit. [A.S. *hraecan,* to hawk]

retch•ing (rech′ing) Gastric and esophageal movements of vomiting without expulsion of vomitus. SYN dry vomiting, vomiturition.

re•te, pl. **re•ti•a** (rē′tē, -shē-ă) [TA] **1.** SYN network (1). **2.** A structure composed of a fibrous network or mesh. [L. a net]

re•te car•pal•e dor•sal•e (rē′tē kahr-pā′lē dōr-sā′lē) SYN dorsal carpal arterial arch.

re•te car•pi pos•ter•i•us (rē′tē kahr′pī pos-tē′rē-ŭs) SYN dorsal carpal arterial arch.

re•te cu•ta•ne•um co•ri•i (rē′tē kyū-tā′nē-ŭm kō′rē-ī) The network of vessels parallel to the surface between the corium and the tela subcutanea.

re•te mi•ra•bi•le (rē′tē mē-rab′ē-lā) [TA] A vascular network interrupting the continuity of an artery or vein, such as occurs in the glomeruli of the kidney (arterial) or in the liver (venous).

re•ten•tion (rē-ten′shŭn) **1.** The keeping in the body of what normally belongs there, especially the retaining of food and drink in the stomach. **2.** The keeping in the body of what normally should be discharged, as urine or feces. **3.** Retaining that which has been learned so that it can be used later as in recall, recognition, or, if retention is partial, relearning. SEE ALSO memory. **4.** Resistance to dislodgement. **5.** DENTISTRY a passive period following treatment when a patient is wearing an appliance or appliances to maintain or stabilize the teeth in the new position into which they have been moved. [L. *retentio,* a holding back]

re•ten•tion cyst (rē-ten′shŭn sist) A cyst resulting from some obstruction to the excretory duct of a gland.

re•ten•tion jaun•dice (rē-ten′shŭn jawn′dis) Hepatic disorder due to insufficiency of liver function or to an excess of bile pigment production; the bilirubin is unconjugated because it has not passed through the liver cells; the van den Bergh test is indirect.

re•ten•tion su•ture (rē-ten′shŭn sū′chŭr) A heavy reinforcing suture placed deep within the muscles and fasciae of the abdominal wall to relieve tension on the primary suture line and thus obviate postoperative wound disruption. SYN tension suture.

re•ten•tion vom•it•ing (rē-ten′shŭn vom′it-ing) Emesis due to mechanical obstruction, usually hours after ingestion of a meal.

re•te o•va•ri•i (rē′tē ō-var′ē-ī) A transient network of cells in the developing ovary; homologous to the rete testis.

re•te ridge (rē′tē rij) Downward thickening of the epidermis between the dermal papillae; peg is a misnomer because the dermal papillae are cylindric but the epidermal thickening between papillae is not.

re•te sub•pa•pil•la•re (rē′tē sub-pap-i-lā′re) The network of vessels between the papillary and reticular strata of the corium.

re•te tes•tis (rē′tē tes′tis) [TA] The network of canals at the termination of the straight tubules in the mediastinum testis.

re•ti•a (rē′shē-ă) Plural of rete. [L.]

re•ti•al (rē′shē-ăl) Relating to a rete.

re•tic•u•la (re-tik′yū-lă) Plural of reticulum. [L.]

re•tic•u•lar, **re•tic•u•lat•ed** (rĕ-tik′yū-lăr, -lāt′ĕd) Relating to a reticulum.

re•tic•u•lar ac•ti•vat•ing sys•tem (RAS) (rĕ-tik′yū-lăr akt′i-vā′ting sis′tĕm) A physiologic term denoting that part of the brainstem reticular formation that plays a central role in bodily and behavioral alertness; it extends as a diffusely organized neural apparatus through the central region of the brainstem into the subthalamus and the intralaminar nuclei of the thalamus; by its ascending connections it affects the function of the cerebral cortex in the sense of behavioral responsiveness; its descending (reticulospinal) connections transmit activating influence on bodily posture and reflex mechanisms (e.g., muscle tonus), in part by way of the gamma motor neurons. SEE ALSO reticular formation.

re•tic•u•lar de•gen•er•a•tion (rĕ-tik′yū-lăr dĕ-jen′ĕr-ā′shŭn) Severe epidermal edema resulting in multilocular bullae.

re•tic•u•lar dys•tro•phy of cor•ne•a (rĕ-tik′yū-lăr dis′trŏ-fē kōr′nē-ă) Bilateral, progressive, superficial degeneration of the corneal epithelium and adjacent Bowman membrane.

re•tic•u•lar fi•bers (rĕ-tik′yū-lăr fī′bĕrz) The collagen (type III) fibers forming the distinctive loose connective tissue stroma of embryonic tissues, mesenchyme, red pulp of the spleen, cortex and medulla of lymph nodes, and the hematopoietic compartments of bone marrow, and accounting for a substantial portion of the collagen fibers of the skin, blood vessels, synovial membrane, uterine tissue, and granulation tissue; characterized by its organization as a reticular meshwork of fine filaments and an affinity for silver and for periodic acid Schiff stains.

re•tic•u•lar for•ma•tion (rĕ-tik′yū-lăr fōr-mā′shŭn) A massive but vaguely delimited neural apparatus composed of gray and white matter extending throughout the central core of the brainstem into the diencephalon; the large neuronal population of the brainstem that does not compose motoneuronal cell groups or cell groups forming part of specific sensory conduction systems; its neurons generally have long dendrites and heterogeneous afferent connections; the reticular formation has complex, largely polysynaptic ascending and descending connections that play a role in the central control of autonomic (respiration, blood pressure, thermoregulation) and endocrine functions, as well as in bodily posture, skeletal muscle reflexes, and general behavioral states such as alertness and sleep. SYN formatio reticularis [TA], reticular substance (2).

re•tic•u•lar mem•brane (rĕ-tik′yū-lăr mem′brān) The membrane formed by cuticular plates of the cells of the spiral organ (organ of Corti); it appears netlike when viewed from above. SYN membrana reticularis [TA].

re•tic•u•lar sub•stance (rĕ-tik′yū-lăr sub′stăns) **1.** A filamentous plasmatic material, beaded with granules, demonstrable by means of vital staining in the immature red blood cells. **2.** SYN reticular formation.

re•tic•u•lar tis•sue, ret•i•form tis•sue (rĕ-tik′yū-lăr tish′ū, ret′i-fōrm) A tissue in which the argyrophilic collagenous fibers form a network and that usually has a network of reticular cells associated with the fibers.

re•tic•u•lat•ed bone (rĕ-tik′yū-lāt′ĕd bōn) SYN woven bone.

re•tic•u•la•tion (rĕ-tik′yū-lā′shŭn) The presence or formation of a reticulum or network, such as that observed in red blood cells during active regeneration of blood. Also used to describe a chest radiographic pattern.

re•tic•u•lin (rĕ-tik′yū-lin) The chemical substance of reticular fibers, regarded as type III collagen (with its associated proteoglygans and structural glycoproteins).

♲**reticulo-, reticul-** Combining forms meaning reticulum; reticular. [L. *reticulum,* a small net, dim. of *rete,* a net]

re•tic•u•lo•cyte (rĕ-tik′yū-lō-sīt) A young erythrocyte that contains no nucleus but has residual RNA. The RNA can be visualized as granules or filaments when the cell is stained supravitally with new methylene blue. Normally, new red cells are released from the bone marrow to the peripheral blood as reticulocytes. They mature, losing the filamentous RNA in about 2 days. Reticulocytes comprise about 1% of circulating red blood cells. Increased concentrations are associated with hemolytic anemia and blood loss. Decreased concentrations are associated with ineffective erythropoiesis, aplastic anemia, and hypocellularity of erythroid precursors in the bone marrow. SEE ALSO reticulocyte production index, erythroblast. [reticulo- + G. kytos, cell]

re•ti•cu•lo•cyte pro•duc•tion in•dex (RPI) (rĕ-tik′yū-lō-sīt prŏ-dŭk′shŭn in′deks) A calculated value that serves as an indicator of the bone marrow response in anemia. It is calculated as patient's hematocrit ÷ 0.45 L/L × reticulocyte count (%) × 1 ÷ maturation time of shift reticulocytes.

re•tic•u•lo•cy•to•pe•ni•a (rĕ-tik′yū-lō-sī′tō-pē′nē-ă) Paucity of reticulocytes in the blood. SYN reticulopenia. [reticulocyte + G. *penia,* poverty]

re•tic•u•lo•cy•to•sis (rĕ-tik′ū-lō-sī-tō′sis) An increase in the number of circulating reticulocytes above the normal, which is less than 1% of the total number of red blood cells; occurs during active blood regeneration (stimulation of red bone marrow) and in certain anemias, especially congenital hemolytic anemia. [reticulocyte + G. *-osis,* condition]

re•tic•u•lo•en•do•the•li•al (rĕ-tik′yū-lō-en′dō-thē′lē-ăl) Denoting or referring to reticuloendothelium.

re•tic•u•lo•en•do•the•li•um (rĕ-tik′yū-lō-en′dō-thē′lē-ŭm) The cells making up the reticuloendothelial system. [reticulo- + endothelium]

re•tic•u•lo•his•ti•o•cy•to•ma (rĕ-tik′yū-lō-his′tē-ō-sī-tō′mă) A solitary skin nodule composed of glycolipid-containing multinucleated large histiocytes; multiple lesions sometimes occur in association with arthritis. [reticulo- + histiocytoma]

re•tic•u•lo•pe•ni•a (rĕ-tik′yū-lō-pē′nē-ă) SYN reticulocytopenia.

re•tic•u•lo•sis (rĕ-tik′yū-lō′sis) An increase in histiocytes, monocytes, or other reticuloendothelial elements. [reticulo- + G. *-osis,* condition]

re•tic•u•lo•spi•nal tract (rĕ-tik′yū-lō-spī′năl

trakt) Collective term denoting a variety of fiber tracts descending to the spinal cord from the reticular formation of the pons and medulla oblongata. Part of these fibers conduct impulses from the neural mechanisms regulating autonomic functions to the corresponding somatic and visceral motor neurons of the spinal cord; others form links in nonpyramidal motor mechanisms affecting muscle tonus, reflex activity, and somatic movement.

re•tic•u•lum, pl. **re•tic•u•la** (rĕ-tik′yū-lŭm, -lă) **1.** A fine network formed by cells, or formed of certain structures within cells or of connective tissue fibers between cells. **2.** SYN neuroglia. **3.** The second compartment of the stomach of a ruminant, a comparatively small chamber communicating with the rumen; sometimes called the honeycomb because of the characteristic structure of its wall. [L. dim of *rete,* a net]

ret•i•form (ret′i-fōrm) Resembling a net or network. [L. *rete,* network]

ret•i•na (ret′i-nă) [TA] The light-sensitive membrane forming the innermost layer of the eyeball. Grossly, the retina consists of three parts: optic part of retina, ciliary part of retina, and iridial part of retina. The optic part, the physiologic portion that receives the visual light rays, is further divided into two parts, pigmented part (pigment epithelium) and nervous part, which are arranged in the following layers: 1) pigment epithelium; 2) layer of rods and cones; 3) external limiting lamina, actually a row of junctional complexes; 4) external nuclear lamina; 5) external plexiform lamina; 6) internal nuclear lamina; 7) internal plexiform lamina; 8) ganglionic cell lamina; 9) lamina of nerve fibers; 10) internal limiting lamina. Layers 2–10 comprise the nervous part. At the posterior pole of the visual axis is the macula, in the center of which is the fovea, the area of acute vision. Here layers 6–9 and blood vessels are absent, and only elongated cones are present. About 3 mm medial to the fovea is the optic disc, where axons of the ganglionic cells converge to form the optic nerve. The ciliary and iridial parts of the retina are forward prolongations of the pigmented layer and a layer of supporting columnar or epithelial cells over the ciliary body and the posterior surface of the iris, respectively. See this page. [Mediev. L. prob. fr. L. *rete,* a net]

ret•i•nac•u•la of ex•ten•sor mus•cles (ret′i-nak′yū-lă eks-ten′sŏr mŭs′ĕlz) SEE inferior extensor retinaculum, superior extensor retinaculum.

ret•i•nac•u•la of per•o•ne•al mus•cles (ret′i-nak′yū-lă per′ō-nē′ăl mŭs′ĕlz) SYN peroneal retinaculum.

ret•i•nac•u•lum, gen. **ret•i•nac•u•li**, pl. **ret•i•nac•u•la** (ret′i-nak′yū-lŭm, -lī, -lă) [TA] A frenum, or a retaining band or ligament. [L. a band, a halter, fr. *retineo,* to hold back]

ret•i•nac•u•lum cu•tis (ret′i-nak′yū-lŭm kyū′tis) [TA] One of the numerous small fibrous strands that extend through the superficial fascia attaching the deep surface of the dermis to the underlying deep fascia determining the mobility of the skin over the deep structures. SYN retinaculum of skin.

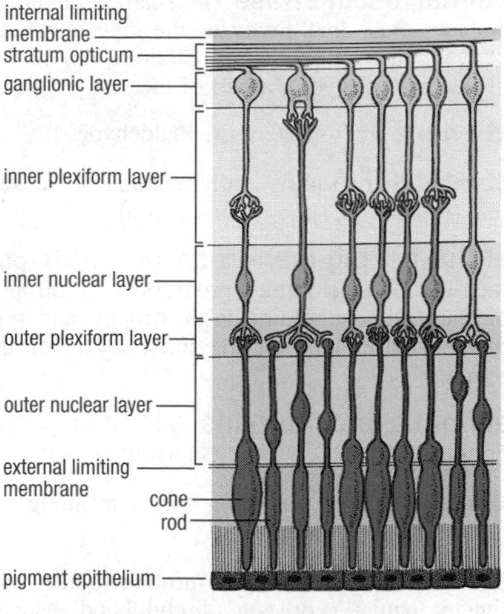

layers of the retina (innermost layer at top)

ret•i•nac•u•lum of skin (ret′i-nak′yū-lŭm skin) SYN retinaculum cutis.

ret•i•nac•u•lum ten•di•num (ret′i-nak′yū-lŭm ten-dīn′ŭm) A ligamentous structure to restrain tendons, such as the flexor or extensor retinacula, or the anular parts of the digital fibrous sheaths.

ret•i•nal (ret′i-năl) **1.** Relating to the retina. **2.** Retinaldehyde; most commonly referring to the all-*trans* form.

11-*cis*-ret•i•nal (sis′ret′i-năl) The isomer of retinaldehyde that can combine with opsin to form rhodopsin; it is formed from 11-*trans*-retinal by retinal isomerase.

ret•i•nal ad•ap•ta•tion (ret′i-năl ad′ap-tā′shŭn) Adjustment to degree of illumination.

ret•in•al•de•hyde (ret-i-nal′dĕ-hīd) Retinol oxidized to a terminal aldehyde; a carotene released (as all-*trans*-retinal[aldehyde]) in the bleaching of rhodopsin by light and the dissociation of opsin in the vision cycle. SYN retinene.

ret•i•nal de•tach•ment, de•tach•ment of ret•i•na (ret′i-năl dĕ-tach′mĕnt, ret′i-nă) Loss of apposition between the sensory retina and the retinal pigment epithelium. See page B26.

ret•i•nal fis•sure (ret′i-năl fish′ŭr) A ventral groove formed by invagination of the optic cup and its stalk by vascular mesenchyme, from which the hyaloid vessels develop. SYN choroid fissure, optic fissure.

ret·i·nal i·som·er·ase (ret′i-năl ī-som′ĕr-ās) An isomerase that catalyzes the *cis-trans*-interconversion of all-*trans*-retinal(aldehyde) to 11-*cis*-retinal(aldehyde); a part of the vision cycle.

ret·i·nene (ret′i-nēn) SYN retinaldehyde.

ret·i·ni·tis (ret′i-nī′tis) Inflammation of the retina. [retina + G. *-itis,* inflammation]

ret·i·ni·tis pig·men·to·sa (ret′i-nī′tis pig-men-tō′să) A hereditary progressive abiotrophy of the neuroepithelium, with atrophy and pigmentary infiltration of the inner layers of the retina.

ret·i·ni·tis pro·li·fer·ans (ret′i-nī′tis prō-lif′ĕr-anz) SYN proliferative retinopathy.

retino-, retin- Combining forms meaning the retina. [Med. L. *retina*]

ret·i·no·blas·to·ma (ret′i-nō-blas-tō′mă) Malignant ocular neoplasm of childhood, usually occurring before the third year of life, composed of primitive retinal small round cells with deeply staining nuclei and of elongate cells forming rosettes. In familial forms, the disease is commonly bilateral and multiple within an eye; in sporadic cases, rarely so. See page B27, B31. [retino- + G. *blastos,* germ, + *-oma,* tumor]

ret·i·no·cho·roid (ret′i-nō-kōr′oyd) SYN chorioretinal.

ret·i·no·cho·roid·i·tis (ret′i-nō-kōr′oyd-ī′tis) Inflammation of the retina extending to the choroid. [retinochoroid + G. *-itis,* inflammation]

ret·i·no·cho·roid·i·tis jux·ta·pa·pil·la·ris (ret′i-nō-kōr′oyd-ī′tis juks′tă-pap-i-lā′ris) retinochoroiditis close to the optic disc. SYN Jensen disease.

ret·i·no·ic ac·id (ret′i-nō′ik as′idz) Retinaldehyde in which the terminal –CHO has been oxidized to a –COOH; used topically in the treatment of acne; plays an important role in growth and differentiation. SYN vitamin A1 acid.

ret·i·no·ic a·cid re·cep·tor (ret′i-nō′ik as′id rĕ-sep′tŏr) Nuclear receptor for retinoic acid.

ret·i·noids (ret′i-noydz) A class of keratolytic drugs derived from retinoic acid and used for treatment of severe acne and psoriasis.

ret·i·noid X re·cep·tor (ret′i-noyd rĕ-sep′tŏr) Receptor for retinoic acids; has less affinity for retinoic acid than the retinoic acid receptors; function is not yet well understood.

ret·i·nol (ret′i-nol) An intermediate in the vision cycle, it also plays a role in growth and differentiation; a vitamin A1 alcohol.

ret·i·nol ac·tiv·i·ty e·quiv·a·lents (RAE) (ret′i-năl ak-tiv′i-tē ē-kwiv′ă-lĕns) A measure of vitamin A activity based on the capacity of the body to convert provitamin carotenoids containing at least one unsubstituted ionone ring to retinaldehyde. 1 microgram RAE = 1 mg retinol = 12 mg β-carotene = 24 mg other vitamin A precursor carotenoids.

ret·i·nol-bind·ing pro·tein (RBP) (ret′i-nol-bīnd′ing prō′tēn) A carrier protein for transporting retinols to the liver.

ret·i·nol de·hy·dro·ge·nase (ret′i-nol dē-hī-droj′ĕn-ās) An oxidoreductase-catalyzing interconversion of retinal and NADH to retinol and NAD^+.

ret·i·no·pap·il·li·tis (ret′i-nō-pap′i-lī′tis) Inflammation of the retina extending to the optic disc.

ret·i·nop·a·thy (ret′i-nop′ă-thē) Noninflammatory degenerative disease of the retina. See page B26. [retino- + G. *pathos,* suffering]

ret·i·nop·a·thy of pre·ma·tu·ri·ty (ret′i-nop′ă-thē prē′mă-chŭr′i-tē) Abnormal vasoproliferation in premature infants that may progress to fibroglial proliferative retinal detachment. SYN Terry syndrome.

ret·i·no·pex·y (ret′i-nō-pek-sē) A procedure to repair a detached retina by holding it in place, e.g., by producing chorioretinal adhesions by freezing ("retinal cryopexy"). [retino- + G. *pēxis,* fixation]

ret·i·nos·chi·sis (ret′i-nos′ki-sis) Degenerative splitting of the retina, with cyst formation between the two layers. [retino- + G. *schisis,* division]

ret·i·no·scope (ret′i-nō-skōp) An optic device used to illuminate a patient's retina during retinoscopy. [retino- + G. *skopeō,* to view]

ret·i·nos·co·py (ret′i-nos′kŏ-pē) A method of determining errors of refraction by illuminating the retina and observing the rays of light emerging from the eye. SYN shadow test, skiascopy. [retino- + G. *skopeō,* to view]

ret·i·nyl es·ters (ret′i-nil es′tĕrz) One of the storage forms of retinols that can carry retinol-binding protein (RBP) from the liver to destination points throughout the body.

re·trac·tile (rē-trak′tīl) Retractable; capable of being drawn back.

re·trac·tion (rĕ-trak′shŭn) **1.** A shrinking, drawing back, or pulling apart. **2.** Posterior movement of teeth, usually with the aid of an orthodontic appliance. [L. *retractio,* a drawing back]

re·trac·tion pock·ets (rĕ-trak′shŭn pok′ĕts) Small areas of retraction of the tympanic membrane due to chronic negative pressure in the middle ear that can lead to formation of cholesteatoma.

re·trac·tor (rē-trak′tŏr) **1.** An instrument for drawing aside the edges of a wound or for holding back structures adjacent to the operative field. **2.** A muscle that draws a part backward (e.g., the middle part of the trapezius muscle is a retractor of the scapula; the horizontal fibers of the temporalis muscle serve to retract the mandible).

re•treat from re•al•i•ty (rē-trēt′ rē-al′i-tē) Substitution of imaginary satisfactions or fantasy for relations with the real world.

re•trench•ment (rē-trench′mĕnt) The cutting away of superfluous tissue. [F. *re-*, back, + *trancher,* to cut]

re•triev•al (rē-trē′văl) The third stage in the memory process, after encoding and storage, involving mental processes associated with bringing stored information back into consciousness. SEE ALSO memory.

♻**retro-** Prefix added to words formed from L. roots, denoting backward or behind. [L. back, backward]

re•tro•au•ri•cu•lar fold (ret′rō-awr-ik′yū-lăr fōld) Skin crease made by the junction of the pinna and the postauricular skin.

ret•ro•au•ric•u•lar lymph node (ret′rō-awr-ik′yū-lăr limf nōd) One of two or three nodes in the region of the mastoid process, which receive afferent lymphatic vessels from the scalp and auricle and send efferent vessels to the superior deep cervical nodes.

ret•ro•buc•cal (ret′rō-buk′ăl) Behind the buccal region of the mouth.

ret•ro•bul•bar an•es•the•si•a (ret′rō-bŭl′bahr an′es-thē′zē-ă) Injection of a local anesthetic behind the eye to produce sensory denervation of the eye.

ret•ro•bul•bar neu•ri•tis (ret′rō-bŭl′bahr nūr-ī′tis) Optic neuritis without swelling of the optic disc.

re•tro•cal•ca•ne•al bur•sa (ret′rō-kal-kā′nē-ăl bŭr′să) SYN bursa of tendo calcaneus.

ret•ro•cal•ca•ne•o•bur•si•tis (ret′rō-kal-kā′nē-ō-bŭr-sī′tis) SYN achillobursitis. [retro- + L. *calcaneum* heel, + bursitis]

ret•ro•ce•cal (ret′rō-sē′kăl) Behind the cecum.

ret•ro•cer•vi•cal (ret′rō-sĕr′vi-kăl) Behind the cervix.

ret•ro•ces•sion (ret′rō-sesh′ŭn) **1.** A going back; a relapse. **2.** Cessation of the external symptoms of a disease followed by signs of involvement of some internal organ or part. **3.** Denoting a position of the uterus or other organ farther back than is normal. [L. *retro-cedo,* pp. *-cessus,* to go back, retire]

ret•ro•clu•sion (ret′rō-klū′zhŭn) A form of acupressure for the arrest of bleeding; the needle is passed through the tissues above the cut end of the artery, is turned around, and then is passed backward beneath the vessel to come out near the point of entrance. [retro- + L. *claudo* (*cludo*) to close]

ret•ro•co•chle•ar hear•ing loss (ret′rō-kok′lē-ăr hēr′ing laws) Term for sensorineural hearing impairment; suggesting a lesion proximal to the cochlea.

ret•ro•col•lic spasm (ret′rō-kol′ik spazm) Torticollis in which the spasm affects the posterior neck muscles. SYN retrocollis.

ret•ro•col•lis (ret′rō-kol′is) SYN retrocollic spasm.

ret•ro•cur•sive (ret′rō-kŭr′siv) Running backward. [retro- + L. *cursus,* a running]

ret•ro•cus•pid pa•pil•la (ret′rō-kŭs′pid pă-pil′ă) A normal and exceedingly common small mucosal nodule located on the mandibular gingiva lingual to the canine teeth, which regresses with age.

ret•ro•de•vi•a•tion (ret′rō-dē′vē-ā′shŭn) A backward bending or inclining.

ret•ro•dis•place•ment (ret′rō-dis-plās′mĕnt) Any backward displacement, such as retroversion or retroflexion of the uterus.

re•tro•du•o•den•al ar•ter•y (ret′rō-dū′ō-dē′năl ahr′tĕr-ē) *Origin,* one of several small branches from the gastroduodenal artery posterior to the duodenum; *distribution,* first part of duodenum. SYN arteria retroduodenalis, posterior pancreaticoduodenal artery.

ret•ro•flex•ion (ret′rō-flek′shŭn) Backward bending, as of the uterus when the corpus is bent back, forming an angle with the cervix.

ret•ro•gnath•ic (ret′rog-nath′ik) Denoting a state in which the mandible is located posterior to its normal position in relation to the maxillae.

ret•ro•gnath•ism (ret-rog′nă-thizm) A condition of facial disharmony in which one or both jaws are posterior to normal in their craniofacial relationships; usually used in reference to the mandible. [retro- + G. *gnathos,* jaw]

ret•ro•grade (ret′rō-grād) **1.** Moving backward. **2.** Degenerating; reversing the normal order of growth and development. [L. *retrogradus,* fr. retro- + *gradior,* to go]

ret•ro•grade am•ne•si•a (ret′rō-grād am-nē′zē-ă) Lack of memory about events that occurred before the trauma or disease (e.g., cerebral concussion) that caused the condition.

ret•ro•grade beat (ret′rō-grād bēt) A beat occurring as an electrical activation of a portion of a heart chamber cephalad to the chamber of origin, e.g., an atrial beat triggered by an impulse originating in the ventricle.

ret•ro•grade block (ret′rō-grād blok) Impaired conduction backward from the ventricles or A-V node into the atria.

ret•ro•grade cys•to•u•re•thro•gram (ret′rō-grād sis′tō-yūr-ē′thrō-gram) A cystourethrogram performed by injection of contrast through the urethral meatus or distal urethra.

ret•ro•grade e•jac•u•la•tion (ret′rō-grād ē-jak′yū-lā′shŭn) Delivery of semen ejaculate into the bladder; seen in neurologic disease, diabetes, and occasionally after prostate surgery.

ret•ro•grade em•bo•lism (ret′rō-grād em′bŏ-lizm) Embolism of a vein by an embolus carried in a direction opposite to that of the normal blood current, after being diverted into a smaller vein.

ret•ro•grade her•ni•a (ret′rō-grād hĕr′nē-ă) A double loop hernia the central loop of which lies in the abdominal cavity.

ret•ro•grade men•stru•a•tion (ret′rō-grād men′strū-ā′shŭn) A flow of menstrual blood back through the fallopian tubes; it sometimes carries with it endometrial cells.

ret•ro•grade ur•og•ra•phy (ret′rō-grād yūr-og′ră-fē) Radiography of the urinary tract following injection of contrast medium directly into the bladder, ureter, or renal pelvis. SYN cystoscopic urography.

ret•ro•grade VA con•duc•tion (ret′rō-grād kŏn-dŭk′shŭn) Conduction backward from the ventricles or from the AV node into and through the atria.

ret•ro•gres•sion (ret′rō-gresh′ŭn) SYN cataplasia. [L. *retrogressus*, fr. *retrogradior,* to go backwards]

ret•ro•hy•oid bur•sa (ret′rō-hī′oyd bŭr′sa) A bursa between the posterior surface of the body of the hyoid bone and the thyrohyoid membrane.

ret•ro•jec•tion (ret′rō-jek′shŭn) The washing out of a cavity by the backward flow of an injected fluid. [L. *retro,* backward, + *jacio,* to throw]

re•tro•len•tal fi•bro•pla•si•a (ret′rō-lent′ăl fī′brō-plā′zē-ă) A condition of premature infants, characterized by the presence of opaque tissue behind the lens, leading to retinal detachment and blindness; the result of an excessive concentration of oxygen.

ret•ro•man•dib•u•lar vein (ret′rō-man-dib′yū-lăr vān) Formed by the union of the superficial temporal and maxillary veins in front of the ear; runs posterior to the ramus of the mandible through the parotid gland, and unites with the posterior auricular vein to form the external jugular vein; it usually has a large communicating branch with the facial vein.

ret•ro•mo•lar pad (re′trō-mō′lăr pad) A cushioned mass of tissue, frequently pear-shaped, located on the alveolar process of the mandible behind the area of the last natural molar tooth.

ret•ro•per•i•to•ne•al fi•bro•sis (ret′rō-per-i-tō-nē′ăl fī-brō′sis) Fibrosis of retroperitoneal structures commonly involving and often obstructing the ureters; the cause is usually unknown. SYN Ormond disease.

ret•ro•per•i•to•ne•al space (ret′rō-per-i-tō-nē′ăl spās) The space between the parietal peritoneum and the muscles and bones of the posterior abdominal wall.

ret•ro•per•i•to•ne•um (ret′rō-per′i-tō-nē′ŭm) Area behind the peritoneum.

ret•ro•per•i•to•ni•tis (ret′rō-per′i-tō-nī′tis) Inflammation of the cellular tissue behind the peritoneum.

ret•ro•pha•ryn•ge•al (ret′rō-fă-rin′gē-ăl) Behind the pharynx.

ret•ro•phar•ynx (ret′rō-far′ingks) The posterior part of the pharynx.

ret•ro•pla•si•a (ret′rō-plā′zē-ă) That state of cell or tissue in which activity is decreased below that considered normal; associated with retrogressive changes (e.g., injury, degeneration, death, necrosis). [retro- + G. *plasis,* a molding]

ret•ro•posed (ret′rō-pōzd) Denoting retroposition. [retro- + L. *pono,* pp. *positus,* to place]

ret•ro•po•si•tion (ret′rō-pŏ-zish′ŭn) Simple backward displacement of a structure or organ, such as the uterus, without inclination, bending, retroversion, or retroflexion. [retro- + L. *positio,* a placing]

ret•ro•pos•on (ret′rō-pō′zon) A transposition of sequences in a DNA that does not originate in the DNA but in an mRNA that is transcribed back into the genomic DNA by reverse transcription. [retro- + L. *pono*, pp. *positum*, to place, + -on]

ret•ro•pu•bic space (ret′rō-pyū′bik spās) The area of loose connective tissue between the bladder with its related fascia and the pubis and anterior abdominal wall.

ret•ro•pul•sion (ret′rō-pŭl′shŭn) **1.** An involuntary backward walking or running, occurring in patients with parkinsonian syndrome. **2.** A pushing back of any part. [retro- + L. *pulsio,* a pushing, fr. *pello,* pp. *pulsus,* beat, drive]

re•tro•sig•moid ap•proach (ret′rō-sig′moyd ă-prōch′) A surgical approach to the cerebellopontine angle through the occipital bone posterior to the sigmoid sinus.

ret•ro•spec•tive fal•si•fi•ca•tion (ret′rō-spek′tiv fawl′si-fi-kā′shŭn) Unconscious distortion of past experience to conform to present psychological needs.

ret•ro•spec•tive pay•ment (ret′rō-spek′tiv pā′mĕnt) A payment that occurs after an action has happened or therapy provided such as in fee-for-service reimbursement.

ret•ro•spon•dy•lo•lis•the•sis (ret′rō-spon′di-lō-lis-thē′sis) Slipping posteriorly of the body of a vertebra, bringing it out of line with the adjacent vertebrae. [retro- + G. *spondylos,* vertebra, + *olisthēsis,* a slipping]

ret•ro•ver•si•o•flex•ion (ret′rō-vĕr′sē-ō-flek′shŭn) Combined retroversion and retroflexion of the uterus.

ret•ro•ver•sion (ret′rō-vĕr′zhŭn) **1.** A turning backward, as of the uterus. **2.** Condition in which the teeth are located in a more posterior position than is normal. [retro- + L. *verto,* pp. *versus,* to turn]

ret•ro•vert•ed (ret′rō-vĕr-tĕd) Denoting retroversion.

Ret•ro•vir•i•dae (ret-rō-vir′i-dē) A family of viruses grouped in three subfamilies: Oncovirinae (HTLV-I, HTLV-II RNA tumor viruses), Spumavirinae (foamy viruses), and Lentivirinae (HIV-like viruses, visna, and related agents).

ret•ro•vi•rus (ret′rō-vī′rŭs) Any virus of the family Retroviridae. A virus with RNA core genetic material; requires the enzyme reverse transcriptase to convert its RNA into proviral DNA.

re•tru•sion (rē-trū′zhŭn) **1.** Retraction of the mandible from any given point. **2.** The backward movement of the mandible. [L. *retrudo,* pp. *-trusus,* to push back]

re•tru•sive oc•clu•sion (rē-trū′siv ŏ-klū′zhŭn) **1.** A biting relationship in which the mandible is forcefully or habitually placed more distally than the patient's centric occlusion. **2.** SYN distal occlusion (1).

Rett syn•drome (ret sin′drōm) A progressive syndrome of autism, dementia, ataxia, and purposeless hand movements; associated with hyperammonemia, principally in girls.

re•turn ex•tra•sys•to•le (rĕ-tŭrn′ eks′tră-sis′tō-lē) A form of reciprocal rhythm in which the impulse having arisen in the ventricle ascends toward the atria, but before reaching the atria is reflected to the ventricles to produce a second ventricular contraction.

re•vas•cu•lar•i•za•tion (rē-vas′kyū-lăr-ī-zā′shŭn) Reestablishment of blood supply to a part.

Re•ver•din nee•dle (rev′er-dan[h] nē′dĕl) Surgical needle with an eye that can be opened and closed.

re•ver•sal (rē-vĕr′săl) **1.** A turning or changing to the opposite direction, as of a process, disease, symptom, or state. **2.** The changing of a dark line or a bright one of the spectrum into its opposite. **3.** Denoting the difficulty of some people in distinguishing the lowercase printed or written letter *p* from *q* or *g*, *b* from *d*, or *s* from *z*. **4.** PSYCHOANALYSIS the change of an instinct or affect into its opposite, as from love into hate. SYN detraining. [L. *reverto,* pp. *-versus,* to turn back or about]

re•versed co•arc•ta•tion (rē-vĕrst′ kō′ahrk-tā′shŭn) Aortic arch syndrome in which blood pressure in the arms is lower than in the legs.

re•versed per•i•stal•sis (rē′vĕrst′ per′i-stal′sis) A wave of intestinal contraction in a direction the reverse of normal, by which the contents of the intestine are forced backward. SYN antiperistalsis.

re•verse Eck fis•tu•la (rē-vĕrs′ ek fis′chū-lă) Side-to-side anastomosis of the portal vein with the inferior vena cava and ligation of the latter above the anastomosis, but below the hepatic veins; the blood from the lower part of the body is thus directed through the hepatic circulation.

re•verse i•so•la•tion (rē-vĕrs′ ī′sŏ-lā′shŭn) A form of patient isolation wherein use of protective equipment is required to prevent transmission of infection to the patient. SYN protective isolation.

re•verse os•mo•sis (rē-vĕrs′ os-mō′sis) Movement of solvent in the opposite direction from osmosis.

re•verse pas•sive he•mag•glu•ti•na•tion (rē-vĕrs′ pas′iv hē′mă-glū′ti-nā′shŭn) A diagnostic technique for virus infection using agglutination by viruses of red blood cells that previously have been coated with antibody specific to the virus.

re•verse pu•pil•lar•y block (rē-vĕrs′ pyū′pi-lar-ē blok) Increased resistance to flow of aqueous humor through the pupil from the anterior chamber to the posterior chamber, leading to posterior bowing of the peripheral iris against the zonules; a possible mechanism for pigmentary glaucoma.

re•verse tran•scrip•tase (rē-vĕrs′ tran-skrip′tās) RNA-dependent DNA polymerase, present in virions of RNA tumor viruses.

re•verse tran•scrip•tase pol•y•me•rase chain re•ac•tion (RT-PCR) (rē-vĕrs′ tran-skrip′tās pol-im′ĕr-ās chān rē-ak′shŭn) A process for specific mRNA amplification wherein reverse transcriptase added to the in vitro reaction uses mRNA as a template to produce one cDNA, which is then amplified by the usual PCR.

re•ver•si•bi•li•ty prin•ci•ple (rē-vĕr′si-bil′i-tē prin′si-pĕl) EXERCISE SCIENCE thesis stating that physiologic and performance training adaptations are lost at a relatively rapid rate when a person terminates participation in an exercise program.

re•vers•i•ble cal•ci•no•sis (rē-vĕr′si-bĕl kal′si-nō′sis) A form of calcinosis sometimes observed in patients who ingest large quantities of milk and alkaline medicines, as in the treatment of peptic ulcer.

re•ver•sion (rē-věr′zhŭn) **1.** The manifestation in an individual of certain characteristics, peculiar to a remote ancestor that have been suppressed during one or more of the intermediate generations. **2.** The return to the original phenotype, either by reinstatement of the original genotype (true reversion) or by a mutation at a site different from that of the first mutation that cancels the effect of the first mutation (suppressor mutation). [L. *reversio* (see reversal)]

re•ver•tant (rē-věr′tănt) MICROBIAL GENETICS a mutant that has reverted to its former genotype (true reversion) or to the original phenotype by means of a suppressor mutation. [L. *revertans,* pres. p. of *reverto,* to turn back]

re•view of symp•toms (ROS) (rē-vū′ simp′tŏmz) A process of gathering information about a patient's health history regardless of apparent relevance to the chief complaint.

re•vised trau•ma score (rē-vīzd′ traw′mă skōr) Assessment score based on combining the Glasgow Coma scale with cardiopulmonary data.

re•viv•i•fi•ca•tion (rē-viv′i-fi-kā′shŭn) **1.** Renewal of life and strength. **2.** Refreshening the edges of a wound by paring or scraping to promote healing. SYN vivification. [L. *re-,* again, + *vivo,* to live, + *facio,* to make]

re•vul•sion (rē-vŭl′shŭn) **1.** SYN counterirritation. **2.** SYN derivation. [L. *revulsio,* act of pulling away, fr. *revello,* pp. *-vulsus,* to pluck or pull away]

re•ward (rē-wōrd′) SYN reinforcer.

re•warm•ing (rē-wōrm′ing) Process of returing the body temperature to physiologic normal following hypothermia.

Reye syn•drome (rī sin′drōm) An acquired encephalopathy of young children that follows an acute febrile illness, usually influenza or varicella infection; characterized by recurrent vomiting, agitation, and lethargy, which may lead to coma with intracranial hypertension; ammonia and serum transaminases are elevated; death may result from edema of the brain and resulting cerebral herniation. Strongly associated with aspirin therapy. SYN hepatic encephalopathy (2).

RFLP Abbreviation for restriction fragment length polymorphism.

RFP Abbreviation for right frontoposterior position.

RFT Abbreviation for right frontotransverse position.

RGO Abbreviation for reciprocal gait orthotic.

Rh **1.** Symbol for rhodium. **2.** Abbreviation for rhesus.

♻ **rhabdo-, rhabd-** Combining forms meaning rod; rod shaped (rhabdoid). [G. *rhabdos*]

rhab•doid (rab′doyd) Rod-shaped. [rhabdo- + G. *eidos,* resemblance]

♻ **rhabdomyo-** Combining form meaning striated or skeletal muscle. [G. *rhabdos,* rod, + *mys,* muscle]

rhab•do•my•o•blast (rab′dō-mī′ō-blast) Large, round, spindle-shaped, or strap-shaped cells with deeply eosinophilic fibrillar cytoplasm that may show cross-striations; found in some rhabdomyosarcomas. [rhabdo- + G. *mys,* muscle, + *blastos,* germ]

rhab•do•my•ol•y•sis (rab′dō-mī-ol′i-sis) An acute, fulminating, potentially fatal disease of skeletal muscle that entails destruction of muscle as evidenced by myoglobinemia and myoglobinuria. [rhabdo- + G. *mys,* muscle, + *lysis,* loosening]

rhab•do•my•o•ma (rab′dō-mī-ō′mă) A benign neoplasm derived from striated muscle, occurring in the heart in children, probably as a hamartomatous process. [rhabdo- + G. *mys,* muscle, + *-oma,* tumor]

rhab•do•my•o•sar•co•ma (rab′dō-mī′ō-sahr-kō′mă) A malignant neoplasm derived from skeletal (striated) muscle, classified as embryonal alveolar (composed of loose aggregates of small round cells) or pleomorphic (containing rhabdomyoblasts). See page B31. SYN rhabdosarcoma. [rhabdo- + G. *mys,* muscle, + *sarkōma,* sarcoma]

rhab•do•sar•co•ma (rab′dō-sahr-kō′mă) SYN rhabdomyosarcoma.

Rhab•do•vir•i•dae (rab′dō-vir′i-dē) A family of rod-shaped or bullet-shaped viruses of vertebrates, insects, and plants, including rabies virus.

rhab•do•vi•rus (rab′dō-vī′rŭs) Any virus of the family Rhabdoviridae.

rha•chi•tis (rā-kī′tis) Inflammation of part of the vertebral column.

Rhad•in•o•vi•rus (ră-dē′nō-vī′rŭs) A herpesvirus genus, subfamily Gammaherpesvirinae, associated with Kaposi sarcoma.

rhag•a•des (rag′ă-dēz) Chaps, cracks, or fissures occurring at mucocutaneous junctions; seen in vitamin deficiency diseases and in congenital syphilis. SEE ALSO cheilosis. [G. *rhagas,* pl. *rhagades,* a crack]

♻ **-rhage, -rrhage, -rhagia, -rrhagia** Combining forms meaning excessive flow. [G. *haimorrhagia,* hemorrhage, bleeding]

Rh an•ti•gen in•com•pa•ti•bi•li•ty (an′ti-jen in′kŏm-pat′i-bil′i-tē) SYN erythroblastosis fetalis.

Rh blood group (blŭd grūp) SYN Rh factor.

♻ **-rhea, -rrhea** Combining forms meaning flow or discharge. SYN -rhoea. [G. *rhoia,* a flowing]

rheg•ma (reg′mă) A rent or fissure. [G. breakage]

rheg•ma•tog•e•nous (reg′mă-toj′ĕ-nŭs) Arising from a bursting or fractionating of an organ. [G. *rhēgma,* breakage, + *-gen,* producing]

rheg•ma•to•ge•nous ret•i•nal de•tach•ment (reg′mă-toj′ĕ-nŭs ret′i-năl dĕ-tach′mĕnt) An ocular insult or trauma in which a tear, hole, or rent appears in the retina that leaks fluid through the opening and thus dissects the retina from the underlying pigment epithelium.

rhe•ni•um (Re) (rē′nē-ŭm) A metallic element of the platinum group; atomic wt. 186.207, atomic no. 75. [Mod. L., fr. L. *Rhenus,* Rhine river]

♻**rheo-** Combining form meaning blood flow; electrical current. [G. *rheos,* stream, current, flow]

rhe•o•base (rē′ō-bās) The minimal strength of an electrical stimulus of indefinite duration that is able to cause excitation of a tissue, e.g., muscle or nerve. SEE ALSO chronaxie. [rheo- + G. *basis,* a base]

rhe•o•ba•sic (rē′ō-bā′sik) Pertaining to or having the characteristics of a rheobase.

rhe•ol•o•gy (rē-ol′ŏ-jē) The study of the deformation and flow of materials. [rheo- + G. *logos,* study]

rhe•om•e•try (rē-om′ĕ-trē) Measurement of electrical current or blood flow.

rhe•os•to•sis (rē-os-tō′sis) A hypertrophying and condensing osteitis that tends to run in longitudinal streaks or columns, like wax drippings on a candle, and which involves a number of the long bones. [rheo- + G. *osteon,* bone, + *-osis,* condition]

rhe•o•tax•is (rē′ō-tak′sis) A form of positive barotaxis in which a microorganism in a fluid is impelled to move against the current flow of its medium. [rheo- + G. *taxis,* orderly arrangement]

rhe•ot•ro•pism (rē-ot′rō-pizm) A movement contrary to the motion of a current, involving part of an organism, rather than the organism as a whole, as in rheotaxis. [rheo- + G. *tropos,* a turning]

Rhese pro•jec•tion (rēs prŏ-jek′shŭn) Oblique radiographic view of the skull to show the optic foramen in the lower outer quadrant of the bony orbit.

rhestocythaemia [Br.] SYN rhestocythemia.

rhes•to•cy•the•mi•a (res′tō-sī-thē′mē-ă) The presence of broken-down red blood cells in the peripheral circulation. SYN rhestocythaemia. [G. *rhaiō,* to destroy, + *kytos,* a hollow (a cell), + *haima,* blood]

Rhe•sus fac•tor (rē′sŭs fak′tŏr) SYN Rh factor.

rheum (rūm) A mucous or watery discharge. [G. *rheuma,* a flux]

rheu•mat•ic (rū-mat′ik) Relating to or characterized by rheumatism. [G. *rheumatikos,* subject to flux, fr. *rheuma,* flux]

rheu•mat•ic ar•ter•i•tis (rū-mat′ik ahr′tĕr-ī′tis) That disorder resulting from rheumatic fever; Aschoff bodies are frequently found in the adventitia of small arteries, especially in the myocardium, and may lead to fibrosis and constriction of the lumens.

rheu•mat•ic en•do•car•di•tis (rū-mat′ik en′dō-kahr-dī′tis) Endocardial involvement as part of rheumatic heart disease, recognized clinically by valvular involvement; in the acute stage, there may be tiny fibrin vegetations along the lines of closure of the valve leaflets, with subsequent fibrous thickening and shortening of the leaflets.

rheu•mat•ic fe•ver (rū-mat′ik fē′vĕr) An inflammatory disease with pyrexia following infection of the throat with group A beta-hemolytic streptococci, occurring primarily in children and young adults, and inducing an immunopathy variably associated with acute migratory polyarthritis, Sydenham chorea, subcutaneous nodules over bony prominences, myocarditis with formation of Aschoff bodies that may cause acute cardiac failure, and endocarditis (frequently followed by scarring of valves, causing stenosis or incompetence); relapses are common if streptococcal infections recur; sometimes called rheumatic heart disease.

rheu•mat•ic heart dis•ease (rū-mat′ik hahrt di-zēz′) Disease of the heart resulting from rheumatic fever, chiefly manifested by abnormalities of the valves.

rheu•mat•ic pneu•mo•ni•a (rū-mat′ik nū-mō′nē-ă) A rarely occurring pneumonia in severe acute rheumatic fever; consolidation occurs, the lungs being of a rubbery consistency, with fibrin exudate and small hemorrhages, as well as edema from left ventricle failure.

rheu•ma•tid (rū′mă-tid) Rheumatic nodules or other eruptions that may accompany rheumatism. [G. *rheuma,* flux, + -id (1)]

rheu•ma•tism (rū′mă-tizm) Indefinite term applied to various conditions with pain or other symptoms of articular origin or related to other elements of the musculoskeletal system. [G. *rheumatismos,* rheuma, a flux]

rheu•ma•toid (rū′mă-toyd) Resembling rheumatoid arthritis in one or more features. [G. *rheuma,* flux, + *eidos,* resemblance]

ℹ**rheu•ma•toid ar•thri•tis (RA)** (rū′mă-toyd ahr-thrī′tis) A systemic disease, occurring more often in women, which affects connective tissue; arthritis is the dominant clinical manifestation, involving many joints, especially those of the hands and feet, accompanied by thickening of articular soft tissue, with extension of synovial tissue over articular cartilages, which become eroded; the course is variable but often is chronic

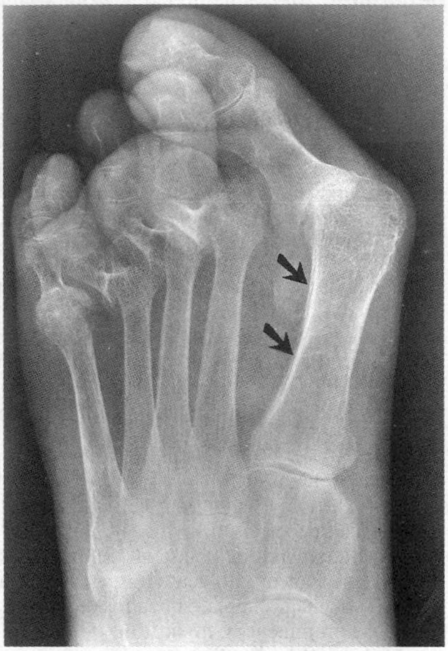

rheumatoid arthritis of the foot: radiograph showing lateral angulation and subluxation of metatarsophalangeal joints, diffuse osteoporosis with "punched out" zones of bone resorption at articular surfaces of bones, and periosteal reaction (arrows) along shaft of first metatarsal

and progressive, leading to deformities and disability. See this page, B24. SYN arthritis deformans, no-dose rheumatism (1).

rheu•ma•toid fac•tors (rū′mă-toyd fak′tōrz) Antibodies in the serum of people with rheumatoid arthritis that react with antigenic determinants or immunoglobulins that enhance agglutination of suspended particles coated with pooled human gamma-globulin; also occur in other autoimmune diseases and certain infectious diseases.

rheu•ma•toid nod•ules (rū′mă-toyd nod′yūlz) Subcutaneous nodules occurring in some patients with rheumatoid arthritis. See this page.

rheu•ma•toid po•cket (rū′mă-toyd pok′ĕt) SYN susceptibility cassette.

rheu•ma•toid spon•dy•li•tis (rū′mă-toyd spon′di-lī′tis) SYN ankylosing spondylitis.

rheu•ma•tol•o•gist (rū′mă-tol′ŏ-jist) A specialist in rheumatology.

rheu•ma•tol•o•gy (rū′mă-tol′ŏ-jē) The medical specialty concerned with the study, diagnosis, and treatment of rheumatic conditions. [G. *rheuma,* flux, + *logos,* study]

Rh fac•tor (fak′tŏr) A protein substance present in the red blood cells of most people (85%), capable of inducing intense antigenic reactions. A person who has the protein substance is called Rh-positive and a person who does not have the protein substance is called Rh-negative. Under ordinary circumstances, the presence or lack of the Rh factor has no bearing on life or health, except when the positive and negative forms commingle. The Rh factor was first identified in the blood of the rhesus monkey in 1940. SYN Rh blood group, Rhesus factor.

RhIG (rig) Abbreviation for Rh-immune globulin.

Rh-im•mune glo•bu•lin (RhIG) (im-yūn′ glob′yū-lin) A concentrated solution of IgG anti-D that is administered to an Rh-negative person who has been exposed to Rh-positive red blood cells, particularly a woman who may be carrying or has aborted an Rh-positive fetus or has delivered an Rh-negative baby, to counteract the immunizing effect of the cells.

rhin-, rhino- Combining forms denoting the nose. [G. *rhis*]

rhi•nal (rī′năl) SYN nasal.

rhi•nal•gi•a (rī-nal′jē-ă) Pain in the nose. SYN rhinodynia. [rhin- + G. *algos,* pain]

rhi•nal sul•cus (rī′năl sŭl′kŭs) The shallow rostral continuation of the collateral sulcus that delimits the rostral part of the parahippocampal

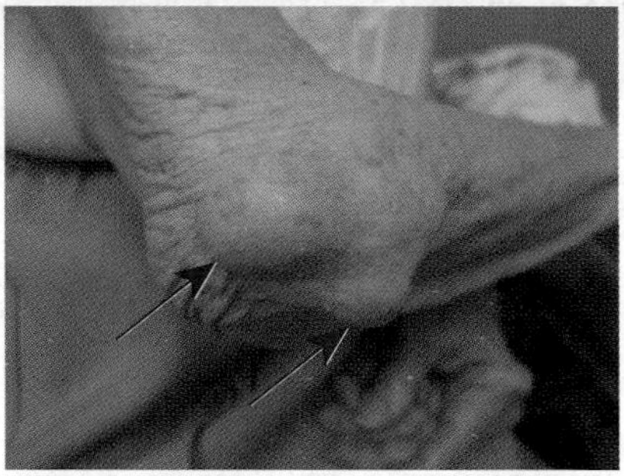

A

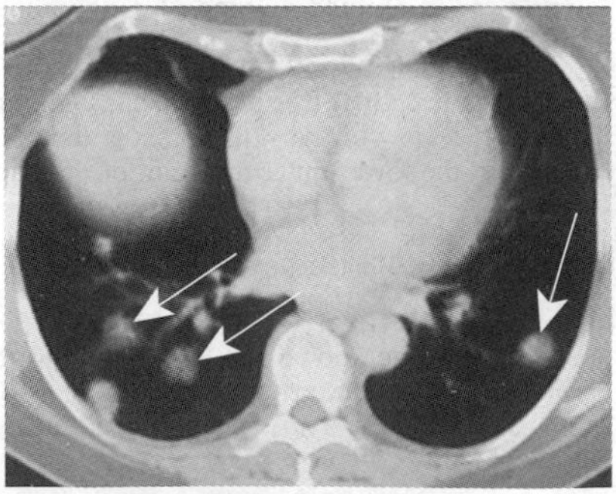

B

rheumatoid nodules: (A) elbow; (B) lower lung zones

gyrus from the fusiform or lateral occipitotemporal gyrus. One of the oldest sulci of the pallium, it marks the border between the neocortex and the allocortical (olfactory).

rhin•e•de•ma (rīn′ĕ-dē′mă) Swelling of the nasal mucous membrane. SYN rhinoedema. [rhin- + G. *oidēma,* swelling]

rhin•en•ce•phal•ic (rīn′en-sĕ-fal′ik) Relating to the rhinencephalon.

rhin•en•ceph•a•lon (rīn′en-sef′ă-lon) Collective term denoting the parts of the cerebral hemisphere directly related to the sense of smell: the olfactory bulb, olfactory peduncle, olfactory tubercle, and olfactory or piriform cortex including the cortical nucleus of the amygdala. SEE ALSO limbic system. [rhin- + G. *enkephalos,* brain]

rhi•ni•tis (rī-nī′tis) Inflammation of the nasal mucous membrane. [rhin- + G. *-itis,* inflammation]

rhi•no•an•tri•tis (rī′nō-ăn-trī′tis) Inflammation of the nasal cavities and one or both maxillary sinuses.

rhi•no•cele (rī′nō-sēl) Cavity (ventricle) of the rhinencephalon, the primordial olfactory part of the telencephalon. [rhino- + G. *koilia,* a hollow]

rhi•no•ceph•a•ly, **rhi•no•ce•pha•li•a** (rī′nō-sef′ă-lē, -se-fā′lē-ă) Rhinencephaly; a form of cyclopia in which the nose is represented by a fleshy protuberance arising above the slitlike orbits, and the rhinencephalic lobes of the telencephalon are poorly developed. [rhino- + G. *kephalē,* head]

rhi•no•chei•lo•plas•ty, **rhi•no•chi•lo•plas•ty** (rī′nō-kī′lō-plas-tē) Plastic surgery of the nose and upper lip. [rhino- + G. *cheilos,* lip, + *plastos,* formed]

Rhi•no•clad•i•el•la (rī′nō-klad′ē-el′ă) A genus of dematiaceous fungi that cause chromoblastomycosis. SEE ALSO *Phialophora.*

rhi•no•clei•sis (rī′nō-klī′sis) SYN rhinostenosis. [rhino- + G. *kleisis,* a closure]

rhi•no•dyn•i•a (rī′nō-din′ē-ă) SYN rhinalgia. [rhino- + G. *odynē,* pain]

rhinoedema [Br.] SYN rhinedema.

rhi•nog•e•nous (rī-noj′ĕ-nŭs) Originating in the nose. [rhino- + G. *-gen,* producing]

rhi•no•ky•pho•sis (rī′nō-kī-fō′sis) A humpback deformity of the nose. [rhino- + G. *kyphōsis,* humped condition]

rhi•no•la•li•a (rī′nō-lā′lē-ă) Nasalized speech. SYN rhinophonia. [rhino- + G. *lalia,* talking]

rhi•no•lith (rī′nō-lith) A calcareous concretion in the nasal cavity, often around a foreign body. [rhino- + G. *lithos,* stone]

rhi•no•li•thi•a•sis (rī′nō-li-thī′ă-sis) The presence of a nasal calculus. [rhinolith + G. *-iasis,* condition]

rhi•nol•o•gist (rī-nol′ŏ-jist) A specialist in diseases of the nose.

rhi•nol•o•gy (rī-nol′ŏ-jē) The branch of medical science concerned with the nose and its diseases. [rhino- + G. *logos,* study]

rhi•no•ma•nom•e•ter (rī′nō-mă-nom′ĕ-tĕr) A manometer used to determine the presence and amount of nasal obstruction, and the nasal air pressure and flow relationships. [rhino- + manometer]

rhi•no•ma•nom•e•try (rī′nō-mă-nom′ĕ-trē) **1.** The use of a rhinomanometer. **2.** The study and measurement of nasal air flow and pressures.

rhi•no•my•co•sis (rī′nō-mī-kō′sis) Fungus infection of the nasal mucous membranes. [rhino- + mycosis]

rhi•no•ne•cro•sis (rī′nō-nĕ-krō′sis) Necrosis of the bones of the nose. [rhino- + necrosis]

rhi•nop•a•thy (rī-nop′ă-thē) Disease of the nose. [rhino- + G. *pathos,* suffering]

rhi•no•pho•ni•a (rī′nō-fō′nē-ă) SYN rhinolalia. [rhino- + G. *phōnē,* voice]

rhi•no•phy•ma (rī-nō-fī′mă) Hypertrophy of the nose with follicular dilation, resulting from hyperplasia of sebaceous glands with fibrosis and increased vascularity. [rhino- + G. *phyma,* tumor, growth]

rhi•no•plas•ty (rī′nō-plas-tē) **1.** Repair of a defect of the nose with tissue taken from elsewhere. **2.** Plastic surgery to change the shape or size of the nose. [rhino- + G. *plastos,* formed]

rhi•nor•rhe•a (rī-nōr-ē′ă) A discharge from the nasal mucous membrane. SYN rhinorrhoea. [rhino- + G. *rhoia,* flow]

rhinorrhoea [Br.] SYN rhinorrhea.

rhi•no•sal•pin•gi•tis (rī′nō-sal-pin-jī′tis) Inflammation of the mucous membrane of the nose and auditory tube. [rhino- + G. *salpinx,* tube, + *-itis,* inflammation]

rhi•no•scle•ro•ma (rī′nō-skler-ō′mă) A chronic granulomatous process involving the nose, upper lip, mouth, and upper air passages; it may involve the external auditory meatus and is believed to be due to a specific bacterium, possibly *Klebsiella.* [rhino- + G. *sklērōma,* an induration]

rhi•no•scope (rī′nō-skōp) A small mirror attached at a suitable angle to a rodlike handle, used in posterior rhinoscopy.

rhi•no•scop•ic (rī′nō-skop′ik) Relating to the rhinoscope or to rhinoscopy.

rhi•nos•co•py (rī-nos′kŏ-pē) Inspection of the nasal cavity. [rhino- + G. *skopeō,* to view]

rhi•no•si•nus•i•tis (rī′nō-sī-nŭs-ī′tis) Inflammation of the mucous membrane of the nose and paranasal sinuses.

rhi•no•ste•no•sis (rī′nō-stĕ-nō′sis) Nasal obstruction. SYN rhinocleisis. [rhino- + G. *stenōsis,* a narrowing]

rhi•not•o•my (rī-not′ŏ-mē) **1.** Any cutting operation on the nose. **2.** Operative procedure in which the nose is incised along one side so that it may be turned away to provide full vision of the nasal passages for radical sinus operations. [rhino- + G. *tomē,* incision, cutting]

Rhi•no•vi•rus (rī′nō-vī′rŭs) [genus] A genus of acid-labile viruses associated with the common cold. There are more than 110 antigenic types.

♻**rhizo-** Combining form denoting root. [G. *rhiza*]

rhi•zoid (rī′zoyd) **1.** Rootlike. **2.** Irregularly branching, like a root; denoting a form of bacterial growth. **3.** In fungi, the rootlike hyphae that arise at the nodes of the hyphae of *Rhizopus* species. [rhizo- + G. *eidos,* resemblance]

rhi•zo•me•li•a (rī′zō-mē′lē-ă) **1.** Disproportion in the length of the most proximal segment of the limbs (arms and thighs). **2.** A disorder involving the shoulder and hip joint. [rhizo- + G. *melos,* limb]

rhi•zo•mel•ic (rī′zō-mel′ik) Of or relating to the hip joint or the shoulder joint.

rhi•zo•mel•ic chon•dro•dys•pla•si•a punc•ta•ta (rī′zō-mel′ik kon′drō-dis-plā′zē-ă pungk-tā′tă) Autosomal recessively inherited lethal chondrodysplasia caused by mutation in the PEX 7 gene encoding the peroxisomal type 2 targeting signal (PTS2) receptor on chromosomal 6q.

rhi•zo•mel•ic dwarf•ism (rī′zō-mel′ik dwōrf′izm) One of the syndromes of chondrodysplasia punctata; autosomal recessive, with variable skin keratinization disorders and variable facial, cardiac, optic, and central nervous system abnormalities; epiphysial stippling is also present. There are multiple enzymatic defects, including peroxisomal ones, and affected infants fail to thrive and usually die in infancy.

rhi•zo•me•nin•go•my•e•li•tis (rī′zō-mĕ-ning′gō-mī′ĕ-lī′tis) Inflammation of the nerve roots, the meninges, and the spinal cord. SYN radiculomeningomyelitis. [rhizo- + G. *mēninx,* membrane, + *myelon,* marrow, + *-itis,* inflammation]

Rhi•zo•mu•cor (rī′zō-myū′kōr) A genus of fungi in the family Mucoraceae; a cause of mucormycosis.

Rhi•zo•po•da (rī-zop′ō-dă) A superclass in the subphylum Sarcodina that includes the amebae of humans, having pseudopodia of various forms but without axial filaments. [rhizo + G. *pous* (*pod-*), foot]

Rhi•zo•pus (rī′zō-pŭs) A genus of fungi some species of which cause zygomycosis in humans.

rhi•zot•o•my (rī-zot′ŏ-mē) Surgical section of the spinal nerve roots for the relief of pain or spastic paralysis. SYN radicotomy, radiculectomy. [G. *rhiza,* root, + *tomē,* section]

Rh null syn•drome (nŭl sin′drōm) A lack of all Rh antigens, compensated hemolytic anemia, and stomatocytosis.

rho (ρ) (rō) **1.** 17th letter of the Greek alphabet. **2.** Population correlation coefficient. **3.** Symbol for density.

Rho•de•sian try•pan•o•so•mi•a•sis (rō-dē′zhŭn trī-pan′ō-sō-mī′ă-sis) A disease of humans caused by *Trypanosoma brucei rhodesiense* in East Africa; it is clinically similar to Gambian trypanosomiasis but of shorter duration and more acute in form; patients suffer repeated episodes of pyrexia, become anemic, and commonly die from cardiac failure. SYN acute African sleeping sickness, acute trypanosomiasis.

rho•di•um (Rh) (rō′dē-ŭm) A metallic element, atomic no. 45, atomic wt. 102.90550. [Mod. L. fr. G. *rhodon,* a rose]

Rhod•ni•us (rod′nē-ŭs) Genus of reduviid bug that is the principal vector of *Trypanosoma cruzi* in Venezuela, Colombia, French Guiana, Guyana, and Surinam.

Rhod•ni•us pro•lix•us (rod′nē-ŭs prō-lĭks′ŭs) A reduviid bug, an important vector of South American trypanosomiasis.

♻**rhodo-, rhod-** Combining forms denoting rosy, red color. [G. *rhodon,* rose]

rho•do•gen•e•sis (rō′dō-jen′ĕ-sis) The production of rhodopsin by the combination of 11-*cis*-retinal and opsin in the dark. [rhodopsin + G. *genesis,* production]

rho•do•phy•lac•tic (rō′dō-fi-lak′tik) Relating to rhodophylaxis.

rho•do•phy•lax•is (rō′dō-fi-lak′sis) The action of the pigment cells of the choroid in preserving or facilitating the reproduction of rhodopsin. [rhodopsin + G. *phylaxis,* a guarding]

rho•dop•sin (rō-dop′sin) A red thermolabile protein found in the rods of the retina; it is bleached by the action of light, which converts it to opsin and all-*trans*-retinal, and is restored in the dark by rhodogenesis; the dominant protein in the plasma membrane of rod cells. SYN visual purple.

-rhoea [Br.] SYN -rhea.

rhomb•en•ce•phal•ic isth•mus (rom-ben-sĕ-fal′ik is′mŭs) **1.** A constriction in the embryonic neural tube delineating the mesencephalon from the rhombencephalon. **2.** The anterior portion of the rhombencephalon connecting with the mesencephalon.

rhomb•en•ce•phal•ic teg•men•tum (rom-ben-sĕ-fal′ik teg-men′tŭm) The portion of the pons continuous with the mesencephalic tegmentum; it consists of reticular formation, tracts, and cranial nerve nuclei, and forms the dorsal part of the pons (pars dorsalis pontis).

rhomb•en•ceph•a•lon (rom-ben-sef′ă-lon) That part of the developing brain that is the most caudal of the three primary vesicles of the embryonic neural tube; secondarily divided into metencephalon and myelencephalon; the rhombencephalon includes the pons, cerebellum, and medulla oblongata. SYN hindbrain. [rhombo- + G. *enkephalos,* brain]

rhom•bic (rom′bik) **1.** SYN rhomboid. **2.** Relating to the rhombencephalon.

rhom•bo•cele (rom′bō-sēl) SYN rhomboidal sinus. [rhombo- + G. *koilia,* a hollow]

rhom•boid, **rhom•boid•al** (rom′boyd, -boy′dăl) Resembling a rhomb, i.e., an oblique parallelogram, but having unequal sides. SYN rhombic (1). [rhombo- + G. *eidos,* appearance]

rhom•boid•al si•nus (rom-boy′dăl sī′nŭs) A dilation of the central canal of the spinal cord in the lumbar region. SYN rhombocele.

rhom•boid fos•sa (rom′boyd fos′ă) The floor of the fourth ventricle of the brain, formed by the ventricular surface of the rhombencephalon.

rhom•boid lig•a•ment (rom′boyd lig′ă-mĕnt) SYN costoclavicular ligament.

rhom•boid ma•jor mus•cle (rŏm′boyd mā′jŏr mŭs′ĕl) Thoracoappendicular muscle; *origin*, spinous processes and corresponding supraspinous ligaments of first four thoracic vertebrae; *insertion*, medial border of scapula below spine; *action*, draws scapula toward vertebral column; *nerve supply*, dorsal nerve of scapula. SYN greater rhomboid muscle, musculus rhomboideus major.

rhom•boid mi•nor mus•cle (rŏm′boyd mī′nŏr mŭs′ĕl) Thoracoappendicular muscle; *origin*, spinous processes of sixth and seventh cervical vertebrae; *insertion*, medial margin of scapula above spine; *action*, draws scapula toward vertebral column and slightly upward; *nerve supply*, dorsal nerve of scapula. SYN lesser rhomboid muscle, musculus rhomboideus minor.

rhon•chal, **rhon•chi•al** (rong′kăl, -kē-ăl) Relating to or characteristic of a rhonchus.

rhon•chal frem•i•tus (rong′kăl frem′i-tŭs) Fremitus produced by vibrations from the passage of air in bronchial tubes partially obstructed by mucous secretion.

rhon•chus, pl. **rhon•chi** (rong′kŭs, -kī) An added sound with a musical pitch occurring during inspiration or expiration, heard on auscultation of the chest, and caused by air passing through bronchi that are narrowed by inflammation, spasm of smooth muscle, or presence of mucus in the lumen; if low-pitched, it is called sonorous rhonchus; if high-pitched, with a whistling or squeaky quality, sibilant rhonchus. [L. fr. G. *rhenchos,* a snoring]

rhythm (ridh′ŭm) **1.** Measured time or motion. **2.** The regular alternation of two or more different or opposite states. **3.** SYN rhythm method. **4.** Regular occurrence of an electrical event in the electroencephalogram. SEE ALSO wave. **5.** A regular sequence of heart beats. See page 1364. [G. *rhythmos*]

rhythm meth•od (ridh′ŭm meth′ŏd) A natural contraceptive method that spaces sexual intercourse to avoid the fertile period of the menstrual cycle. SYN rhythm (3).

rhy•tide (rī′tid) A skin wrinkle. [G. *rhytis, -idos,* wrinkle]

rhyt•i•dec•to•my (rit′i-dek′tŏ-mē) Elimination of wrinkles from, or reshaping of, the face by excising any excess skin and tightening the remainder; the so-called face-lift. SYN rhytidoplasty. [G. *rhytis* (*rhytid-*), a wrinkle, + ectomy]

rhyt•i•do•plas•ty (rit′i-dō-plas-tē) SYN rhytidectomy. [G. *rhytis,* a wrinkle, + *plastos,* formed]

rhyt•i•do•sis (rit′i-dō′sis) **1.** Wrinkling of the face to a degree disproportionate to age. **2.** Laxity and wrinkling of the cornea, an indication of approaching death. SYN rutidosis. [G. a wrinkling, fr. *rhytis,* a wrinkle, + *-osis,* condition]

RIA Abbreviation for radioimmunoassay.

rib (rib) Abbreviation for ribose.

rib•bon (rib′ŏn) A ribbon-shaped structure. [M. E. *riban*]

rib [I–XII] (rib) One of the 24 elongated curved bones forming the main portion of the bony wall of the chest. See page 1365. SYN costa (1) [TA]. [A.S. *ribb*]

ribo- **1.** Prefix denoting ribose. **2.** As an italicized prefix to the systematic name of a monosaccharide, *ribo-* indicates that the configuration of a set of three consecutive CHOH groups is that of ribose. [German *Ribose*, alt. from arabinose, fr. *gum arabic* + -ose]

ri•bo•fla•vin (rī′bō-flā-vin) A heat-stable factor of the vitamin B complex with isoalloxazine nucleotides that are coenzymes of the flavohydrogenases. SYN flavin, flavine.

ri•bo•nu•cle•ase (RNase) (rī′bō-nū′klē-ās) A transferase or phosphodiesterase that catalyzes the hydrolysis of ribonucleic acid.

ri•bo•nu•cle•ase H (rī′bō-nū′klē-ās) A ribonuclease that degrades RNA in DNA-RNA hybrids.

ri•bo•nu•cle•ic ac•id (RNA) (rī′bō-nū-klē′ik as′id) A macromolecule consisting of ribonucle-

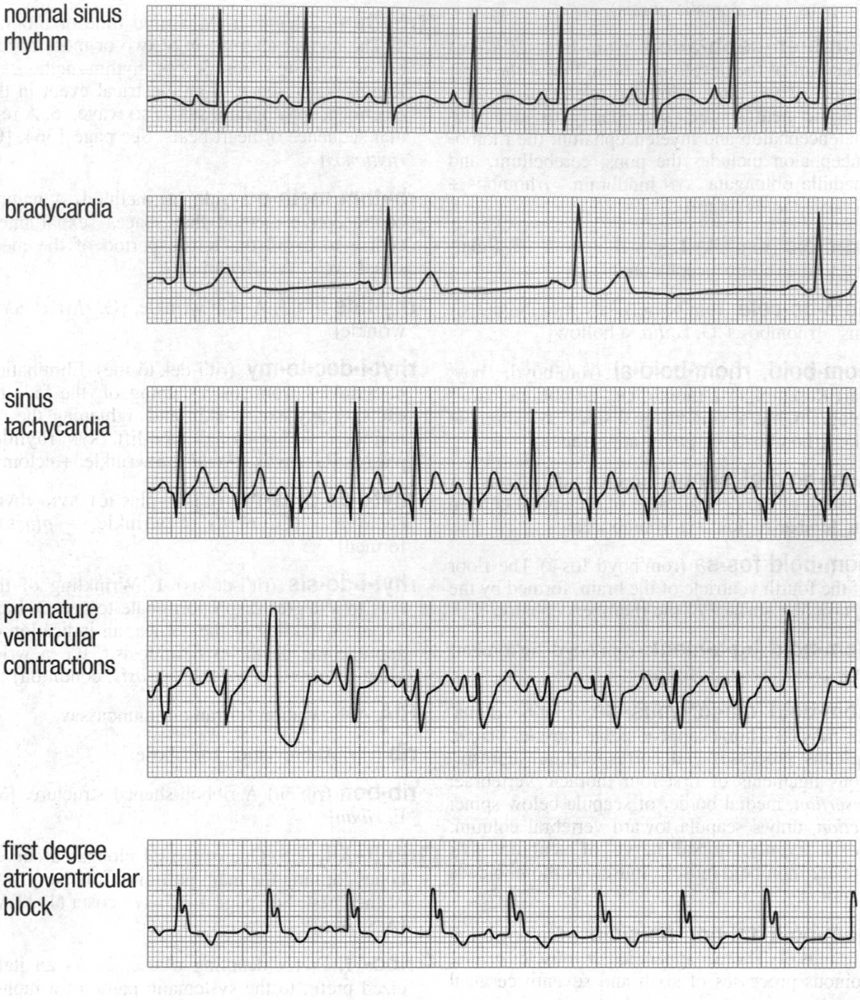

rhythm: electrocardiogram tracings showing common types of arrhythmia

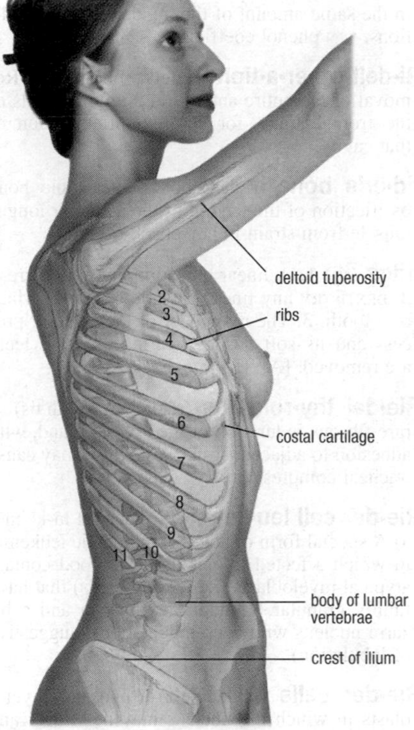

rib [II-XI]

oside residues connected by phosphate bonds, concerned in the control of cellular chemical processes, especially protein synthesis. RNA is found in all cells, in both nuclei and cytoplasm, and in many viruses.

ri•bo•nu•cle•o•pro•tein (RNP) (rī′bō-nū′klē-ō-prō′tēn) A combination of ribonucleic acid and protein.

ri•bo•nu•cle•o•side (rī′bō-nū′klē-ō-sīd) A nucleoside in which the sugar component is ribose; the common ribonucleosides of RNA are adenosine, cytidine, guanosine, and uridine.

ri•bo•nu•cle•o•tide (rī-bō-nū′klē-ō-tīd) A nucleotide (nucleoside phosphate) in which the sugar component is ribose; the major ribonucleotides of RNA are adenylic acid, cytidylic acid, guanylic acid, and uridylic acid.

ri•bose (rib) (rī′bōs) The pentose present in ribonucleic acid; epimers of D-ribose are D-arabinose, D-xylose, and L-lyxose.

ri•bose-5-phos•phate (rī′bōs fos′fāt) Ribose phosphorylated on carbon-5; an intermediate in the pentose phosphate pathway.

ri•bose-5-phos•phate i•som•er•ase (rī′bōs fos′fāt ī-som′ĕr-ās) An enzyme catalyzing interconversion of D-ribose 5-phosphate and D-ribulose 5-phosphate; of importance in ribose metabolism and in the pentose phosphate pathway.

ri•bo•som•al RNA (rī′bō-sō′măl) The RNA of ribosomes and polyribosomes.

ri•bo•some (rī′bō-sōm) A granule of ribonucleoprotein, 120–150 Å in diameter, that is the site of protein synthesis from aminoacyl-tRNAs as directed by mRNAs.

ri•bo•su•ri•a (rī′bō-syūr′ē-ă) The enhanced urinary excretion of D-ribose; commonly one manifestation of muscular dystrophy. [ribose + G. *ouron,* urine]

ri•bo•syl (rī′bō-sil) The radical formed by loss of the hemiacetal OH group from either of the two cyclic forms of ribose.

ri•bo•thy•mi•dine (T) (rī′bō-thī′mi-dēn) 5-Methyluridine; the ribosyl analogue of thymidine (deoxyribosylthymine); a nucleoside found in small amounts in ribonucleic acids.

ri•bo•thy•mi•dyl•ic ac•id (rTMP, TMP) (rī′bō-thī′mi-dil′ik as′id) Ribothymidine 5′-phosphate; the ribose analogue of thymidylic acid; a rare component of transfer RNAs.

Ri•bot law of me•mo•ry (rē-bō′ law mem′ŏr-ē) In progressive dementias, remote memories tend to be preserved whereas recent memories are lost.

Ric•co law (rē′kō law) For small images, light intensity × area = constant for the threshold.

RICE (rīs) Acronym for rest, ice, compression, elevation.

rice starch (rīs stahrch) Rice product used as a supplement in many media formulations used for the culture of intestinal protozoa (e.g., *Entamoeba histolytica*).

Rich•ter her•ni•a (rik′ter hĕr′nē-ă) SYN parietal hernia.

Rich•ter syn•drome (rik′ter sin′drōm) A high-grade lymphoma developing during the course of chronic lymphocytic leukemia; associated with cachexia, pyrexia, dysproteinemia, and lymphomas with multinucleated tumor cells.

ri•cin (rī′sin) Toxin derived from castor beans that causes inflammation of the GI mucosa and the respiratory tract. [L. *ricinus,* castor oil plant]

ric•i•nine (ris′i-nin) SEE ricin.

rick•ets (rik′ĕts) A disease due to vitamin D deficiency and characterized by overproduction and deficient calcification of osteoid tissue, with associated skeletal deformities, disturbances in growth, and hypocalcemia. SYN infantile osteomalacia, juvenile osteomalacia, rachitis. [E. *wrick,* to twist]

Rick•ett•si•a (ri-ket′sē-ă) A genus of bacteria

containing small (nonfilterable), often pleomorphic, coccoid to rod-shaped, gram-negative organisms that usually occur intracytoplasmically in lice, fleas, ticks, and mites; pathogenic species are parasitic in humans and other animals, causing epidemic typhus, murine or endemic typhus, Rocky Mountain spotted fever, tsutsugamushi disease, rickettsialpox, and other diseases; type species is *Rickettsia prowazekii*.

Rick•ett•si•a af•ri•cae (ri-ket′sē-ă af′ri-sē) A species of *Rickettsia* studied principally in Zimbabwe that appears to be carried by the tick *Amblyomma hebraeum;* a cause of spotted fever.

Rick•ett•si•a a•kar•i (ri-ket′sē-ă a-kā′rī) A species causing human rickettsialpox, a mild, acute febrile disease; transmitted by the house mouse mite *Liponyssoides sanguineus*.

Rick•ett•si•a co•no•ri•i (ri-ket′sē-ă kō-nōr′ē-ī) A widespread African species probably causing boutonneuse fever in humans; transmitted by various ticks.

Rick•ett•si•a ho•ne•i (ri-ket′sē-ă hōn′ē-ī) A bacterial species that causes Flinders Island spotted fever in Australia.

Rick•ett•si•a ja•po•ni•ca (ri-ket′sē-ă jă-pon′i-kă) A bacterial species that causes Japanese spotted fever.

rick•ett•si•al (ri-ket′sē-ăl) Pertaining to or caused by rickettsiae.

rick•ett•si•al•pox (ri-ket′sē-ăl-poks′) Bacterial infection with *Rickettsia akari*, which is spread by mites from a reservoir in mice; a benign, self-limited febrile illness.

Rick•ett•si•a pro•wa•ze•ki•i (ri-ket′sē-ă prō-vă-zek′ē-ī) A bacterial species causing epidemic and recrudescent typhus, transmitted by body lice; type species of the genus *Rickettsia*.

Rick•ett•si•a rick•ett•si•i (ri-ket′sē-ă ri-ket′sē-ī) The bacterial agent of Rocky Mountain spotted fever and its geographic variants; transmitted by infected ixodid ticks, especially *Dermacentor andersoni* and *D. variabilis*.

Rick•ett•si•a slo•va•ca (ri-ket′sē-ă slō-vah′kă) A bacterial species causing a rickettsiosis associated with local erythema and possibly meningoencephalitis; transmitted by the tick *Dermacentor marginatus*.

rick•ett•si•o•sis (ri-ket′sē-ō′sis) Infection with rickettsiae.

Rid•doch phe•no•me•non (rid′dok fĕ-nom′ĕ-non) Ability to appreciate a small moving object in an area of the visual field blind to static objects; particularly associated with occipital lobe lesions.

Rid•e•al-Walk•er co•ef•fi•cient (rid′ē-ăl waw′kĕr kō′ĕ-fish′ĕnt) A figure expressing the disinfecting power of any substance; obtained by dividing the figure indicating the degree of dilution of the disinfectant that kills a microorganism in a given time by the figure, indicating the degree of dilution of phenol that kills the organism in the same amount of time under similar conditions. SYN phenol coefficient.

Ri•dell op•er•a•tion (rī-del′ op-ĕr-ā′shŭn) Removal of the entire anterior and inferior walls of the frontal sinus, for chronic inflammation of that cavity.

rid•er's bone (rī′dĕrz bōn) Heterotopic bone ossification of the tendon of the adductor longus muscle from strain in horseback riding.

ridge (rij) **1.** A linear elevation. SEE ALSO crest. **2.** DENTISTRY any linear elevation on the surface of a tooth. **3.** The remainder of the alveolar process and its soft tissue covering after the teeth are removed. [A. S. *hrycg,* back, spine]

Rie•del thy•roid•i•tis (rē′del thī′roy-dī′tis) A rare fibrous induration of the thyroid gland, with adhesion to adjacent structures, which may cause tracheal compression.

Rie•der cell leu•ke•mi•a (rē′der sel lū-kē′mē-ă) A special form of acute granulocytic leukemia in which affected tissues and the blood contain atypical myeloblasts (i.e., Rieder cells) that have faintly granular, immature cytoplasm and a bizarre nucleus with deep indentations (suggestive of lobulation).

Rie•der cells (rē′der selz) Abnormal myeloblasts in which the nucleus may be widely and deeply indented or may actually be a bilobate or multilobate structure; frequently observed in acute leukemia.

Rie•der lym•pho•cyte (rē′der lim′fō-sīt) An abnormal form of lymphocyte that has a greatly indented (or lobed), slightly twisted nucleus; usually observed in certain examples of chronic lymphocytic leukemia.

Rie•gel pulse (rē′gel pŭls) A pulse that diminishes in volume during expiration.

Rie•ger a•nom•a•ly (rē′ger ă-nom′ă-lē) Iridocorneal mesochymal dysgenesis.

Rie•ger syn•drome (rē′ger sin′drōm) Iridocorneal mesenchymal dysgenesis combined with hypodontia or anodontia and maxillary hypoplasia; autosomal dominant; delayed sexual development and hypothyroidism are also characteristic.

Riehl mel•a•no•sis (rēl mel′ă-nō′sis) A brown pigmentary condition of the exposed portions of the skin of the neck and face with melanin pigment in dermal macrophages, thought to result from photodermatitis due to materials, such as cosmetic ingredients, or oils encountered in various occupations.

Rift Val•ley vi•rus (rift val′ē vī′rŭs) Fever-causing virus originating in livestock in Africa and transmitted to humans causing many thousands of deaths in epidemics.

Ri•ga-Fe•de dis•ease (rē′gah fā′dā di-zēz′) Ulceration of lingual frenum in infants.

right a•tri•um of heart (rīt ā′trē-ŭm hahrt) The atrium of the right side of the heart that receives the blood from the venae cavae and coronary sinus. SYN atrium cordis dextrum [TA], atrium dextrum cordis.

right au•ri•cle (rīt awr′i-kĕl) The small conic projection from the right atrium of the heart.

right col•ic ar•ter•y (rīt kol′ik ahr′tĕr-ē) *Origin*, superior mesenteric, sometimes by a common trunk with the ileocolic; *distribution*, ascending colon; *anastomoses*, middle colic, ileocolic. SYN arteria colica dextra.

right col•ic flex•ure (rīt kol′ik flek′shŭr) The bend of the colon at the juncture of its ascending and transverse portions. SYN flexura coli dextra [TA], hepatic flexure.

right cor•o•nar•y ar•ter•y (rīt kōr′ŏ-nar-ē ahr′tĕr-ē) *Origin*, right aortic sinus; *distribution*, it passes around the right side of the heart in the coronary sulcus, giving branches to the right atrium and ventricle, including the atrioventricular branches and the posterior interventricular branch. SYN arteria coronaria dextra.

right de•scen•ding pul•mo•nar•y ar•ter•y (RDPA) (rīt dĕ-send′ing pul′mŏ-nar-ē ahr′tĕr-ē) Artery supplying the right, middle, and lower lobes; comprises most of the right hilar shadow on the frontal chest radiograph.

right-foot•ed (rīt-fut′ĕd) SYN dextropedal.

right fron•to•an•ter•i•or (rīt frŏn′tō-an-tēr′ē-ŏr) SEE frontoanterior position.

right fron•to•pos•ter•i•or (rīt frŏn′tō-pos-tēr′ē-ŏr) SEE frontoposterior position.

right fron•to•trans•verse (rīt frŏn′tō-tranz-vĕrs′) SEE frontotransverse position.

right gas•tric ar•ter•y (rīt gas′trik ahr′tĕr-ē) *Origin*, hepatic; *distribution*, pyloric portion of stomach on the lesser curvature; *anastomoses*, left gastric.

right gas•tric vein (rīt gas′trik vān) It receives veins from both surfaces of the upper portion of the stomach, runs to the right along the lesser curvature of the stomach, and empties into the portal vein. SYN pyloric vein.

right-hand•ed (rīt-hand′ĕd) Denoting the habitual or more skillful use of the right hand for writing and most manual operations. SYN dextral.

right heart (rīt hahrt) The right atrium and right ventricle.

right heart by•pass (rīt hahrt bī′pas) Introduction of a circuit shunting blood from the venae cavae around the right atrium and ventricle and directly into the pulmonary artery.

right he•pat•ic duct (rīt hĕ-pat′ik dŭkt) The duct that transmits bile to the common hepatic duct from the right half of the liver and the right part of the caudate lobe.

right lat•er•al di•vi•sion of liv•er (rīt lat′ĕr-ăl di-vizh′ŭn liv′ĕr) The portion of the liver that lies to the right of the approximately vertical plane of the right hepatic vein and includes the right anterior and posterior lateral segments (hepatic segments VI and VII); it is approximately the right third of the right anatomic lobe of the liver. SYN divisio lateralis dextra hepatis [TA].

right-left dis•cri•mi•na•tion (rīt′left dis-krim′i-nā′shŭn) **1.** The process of identifying one side of the body as distinct from the other. **2.** Ability to distinguish right from left.

right and left fi•brous rings of heart (rīt left fī′brŭs ringz hahrt) Two fibrous rings that surround the atrioventricular orifices of the heart, providing attachment for the atrioventricular valve leaflets and maintaining patency of the orifices. As part of the fibrous skeleton of the heart, the fibrous rings also provide origin and insertion for the myocardium. SYN anulus fibrosus (1) [TA].

right liv•er (rīt liv′ĕr) Portion of the liver receiving blood from the right branches of the hepatic artery and portal vein, and from which bile is drained through the right hepatic duct; the plane of the middle hepatic vein separates right from left liver.

right lobe of liv•er (rīt lōb liv′ĕr) The largest lobe of the liver, separated from the left lobe above and in front by the falciform ligament and from the caudate and quadrate lobes by the sulcus for the vena cava and the fossa for the gallbladder; it contains two segments, anterior and posterior. SYN lobus hepatis dexter [TA].

right lym•phat•ic duct (rīt lim-fat′ik dŭkt) One of the two terminal lymph vessels, a short trunk, about 2 cm in length, formed by the union of the right jugular lymphatic vessel and vessels from the lymph nodes of the right superior limb, thoracic wall, and both lungs; it lies on the right side of the root of the neck and empties into the right brachiocephalic vein.

right mar•gi•nal branch of right cor•o•nar•y ar•ter•y (rīt mahr′ji-năl branch rīt kōr′ŏ-nar-ē ahr′tĕr-ē) Usually the largest of the ventricular branches of the right coronary artery; courses along the right margin of the heart, and is of sufficient caliber and length to reach the apex. SYN ramus marginalis dexter arteriae coronariae dextrae.

right me•di•al di•vi•sion of liv•er (rīt mē′dē-ăl di-vizh′ŭn liv′ĕr) The portion of the liver that lies between the approximately vertical planes of the right and middle hepatic veins and includes the right anterior and posterior medial segments (hepatic segments V and VIII); it is approximately the middle third of the anatomic right lobe of the liver. SYN divisio medialis dextra hepatis [TA].

right pul•mo•na•ry ar•ter•y (rīt pul′mō-nar-ē ahr′tĕr-ē) The longer of the two terminal branches of the pulmonary trunk, it passes transversely across the mediastinum inferior to the aortic arch to enter the hilum of the right lung. Branches are distributed with the bronchi; frequent variations occur. Typical branches to the superior lobe (rami lobi superioris [TA]) are apical (ramus apicalis [TA]), anterior ascending (rami anterior ascendens [TA]), anterior descending (ramus anterior descendens [TA]), posterior ascending (ramus posterior ascendens [TA]), and posterior descending (ramus posterior descendens [TA]); to the middle lobe (rami lobi medii [TA]) are medial (ramus medialis [TA]) and lateral (ramus lateralis [TA]), and to the inferior lobe (rami lobi inferioris [TA]) are superior (apical) branch of inferior lobe (ramus superior (apicalis) lobi inferioris [TA]), and the anterior, lateral (lateralis), medial (medialis), and posterior basal branches (rami basales).

right-to-left shunt (rīt-left shŭnt) The passage of blood from the right side of the heart into the left (as through a septal defect), or from the pulmonary artery into the aorta (as through a patent ductus arteriosus); such a shunt can occur only when the pressure on the right side exceeds that in the left.

right ven•tri•cle (rīt ven′tri-kĕl) The lower chamber on the right side of the heart that receives the venous blood from the right atrium and drives it by the contraction of its walls into the pulmonary artery.

right ven•tric•u•lar fail•ure (rīt ven-trik′yū-lăr fāl′yŭr) Congestive heart failure manifested by distention of the neck veins, enlargement of the liver, and dependent edema due to pump failure of the right ventricle.

ri•gid con•nec•tor (rij′id kŏ-nek′tŏr) DENTISTRY a connector that is solid or rigid, as a soldered joint.

ri•gid•i•ty (ri-jid′i-tē) **1.** Stiffness or inflexibility. SYN rigor (1). **2.** PSYCHIATRY, CLINICAL PSYCHOLOGY an aspect of personality characterized by a person's resistance to change. **3.** NEUROLOGY one type of increase in muscle tone at rest; characterized by increased resistance to passive stretch, independent of velocity and symmetric about joints; increases with activation of corresponding muscles in the contralateral limb. Two basic types are cogwheel rigidity and leadpipe rigidity. SEE ALSO nuchal rigidity. See this page. [L. *rigidus,* rigid, inflexible]

rig•or (rig′ŏr) **1.** SYN rigidity (1). **2.** SYN chill (2). [L. stiffness]

rig•or mor•tis (rig′ŏr mōr′tis) Stiffening of the

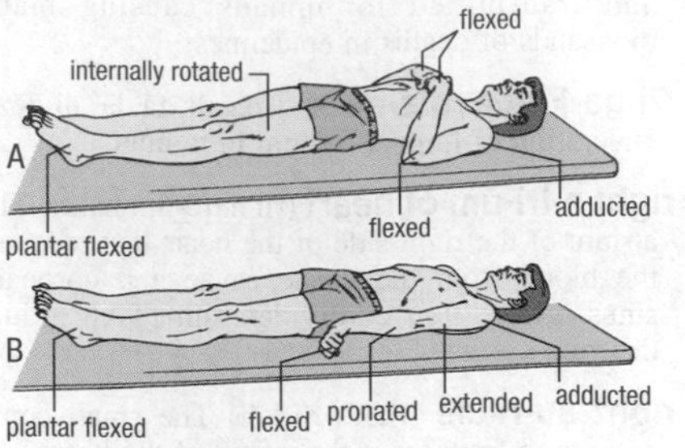

assessing the level of consciousness by rigidity: (A) flexor or decorticate posturing response; (B) extensor or decerebrate posturing

body, from 1–7 hours after death, from hardening of the muscular tissues in consequence of the coagulation of the myosinogen and paramyosinogen; it disappears after 1–6 days, or when decomposition begins. SYN postmortem rigidity.

rim (rim) A margin, border, or edge, usually circular in form.

ri•ma, gen. and pl. **ri•mae** (rī′mă, -mē) [TA] A slit or fissure, or narrow elongated opening between two symmetric parts. [L. a slit]

ri•ma glot•ti•dis (rī′mă glot′i′dis) [TA] The interval between the true vocal cords.

ri•ma o•ris (rī′mă ōr′is) [TA] The mouth slit; the aperture of the mouth.

ri•ma pal•pe•bra•rum (rī′mă pal-pē-brār′ŭm) [TA] The lid slit, or fissure between the lids of the eye. SYN palpebral fissure.

ri•ma ves•tib•u•li (rī′mă ves-tib′yū-lī) [TA] The interval between the false vocal cords or vestibular folds.

ri•mose (rī′mōs) Fissured; marked by cracks in all directions, like the crackle of porcelain. [L. *rimosus,* fr. *rima,* a fissure]

rim•u•la (rim′yū-lă) A minute slit or fissure. [L. dim. of *rima*]

ring (ring) **1.** A circular band surrounding a wide central opening; an anular or circular structure surrounding an opening or level area. SYN anulus [TA]. **2.** ANATOMY anulus. **3.** The closed chain of atoms in a cyclic compound; commonly used for "cyclic" or "cycle." **4.** A marginal growth on the upper surface of a broth culture of bacteria, adhering to the sides of the test tube in the form of a circle. [A.S. *hring*]

ring ab•scess (ring ab′ses) An acute purulent inflammation of the corneal periphery in which a necrotic area is surrounded by an anular girdle of leukocytic infiltration.

ring chro•mo•some (ring krō′mō-sōm) A chromosome with ends joined to form a circular structure. The ring form is abnormal in humans but the normal form of the chromosome in certain bacteria.

Ring·er so·lu·tion (ring'ĕr sō-lū'shŭn) **1.** A solution resembling the blood serum in its salt constituents; contains 8.6 g of NaCl, 0.3 g of KCl, and 0.33 g of $CaCl_2$ in each 1000 mL of distilled water; used as a fluid and electrolyte replenisher by intravenous infusion. SEE ALSO lactated Ringer solution. **2.** A salt solution usually used in combination with naturally occurring body substances (e.g., blood serum, tissue extracts) or more complex, chemically defined, nutritive solutions for culturing animal cells.

ring fin·ger (ring fing'gĕr) Fourth finger.

ring-knife (ring'nīf) A circular or oval ring with internal cutting edge, for shaving off tumors in the nasal and other cavities.

ring·like cor·ne·al dys·tro·phy (ring'līk kōr'nē-ăl dis'trŏ-fē) Threadlike opacities of the anterior corneal stroma, with acute, painful onset followed by decreased vision; autosomal dominant inheritance, caused by mutation in the transforming growth factor, beta-induced, gene (TGFB1) encoding keratoepithelium on chromosome 5q.

ring sco·to·ma (ring skō-tō'mă) An anular area of blindness in the visual field surrounding the fixation point in pigmentary degeneration of the retina and in glaucoma.

ring sy·ringe (ring sir-inj') SYN control syringe.

ring·worm (ring'wŏrm) SYN tinea.

Rin·ne test (rin'ĕ test) A vibrating tuning fork is held alternately with the base touching the mastoid process and with the prongs near the external ear. Normally the sound can be heard by air conduction longer than by bone conduction; the reverse phenomenon indicates conductive hearing loss in the ear tested.

Ri·o·lan a·nas·to·mo·sis (rē-ō-lon[h]' ă-nas'tŏ-mō'sis) The specific portion of the marginal artery of the colon connecting the middle and left colic arteries.

Ri·o·lan arch (rē-ō-lon[h]' ahrch) SYN marginal artery of colon.

ri·ot-con·trol a·gent (rī'ŏt kŏn-trōl' ā'jĕnt) Any of several chemical compounds used to produce temporary irritation of the eyes, throat, and upper airway in crowd-control settings. Riot-control agents are typically solids that can be dissolved in certain organic solvents and dispersed as powders, solutions, or smoke. Because they are not gases, the term "tear gas" is a misnomer for these agents. Vomiting agents (q.v.) are a subset of riot-control agents. SEE ALSO tear gas, lacrimator, vomiting agent, CA, CN, CS, CR, DM.

RIP Abbreviation for respiratory inductance plethysmography; radioimmunoprecipitation.

Ri·pault sign (rē-pō' sīn) A sign of death, consisting in a permanent change in the shape of the pupil produced by unilateral pressure on the eyeball.

Rip·stein o·per·a·tion (rip'stīn op-ĕr-ā'shŭn) An operation for rectal prolapse that involves a transabdominal approach with dissection around the rectum and placement of a mesh sling to prevent the bowel from prolapsing through the anus.

rise time (rīz tīm) The time it takes a gradient to switch on, achieve the required gradient slope, and switch off again in magnetic resonance imaging.

risk (risk) **1.** The probability that an event will occur. **2.** The possibility of adverse consequences.

risk as·sess·ment (risk ă-ses'mĕnt) Analysis of risks involved prior to action being taken.

risk of in·jur·y (risk in'jŭr-ē) A situation in which the client is at risk of injury from environmental causes. This nursing diagnosis overlaps other diagnoses: falls, trauma, suffocation, and aspiration (NANDA-approved nursing diagnosis)

Ris·ley ro·ta·ry prism (riz'lē rō'tŏr-ē prizm) A prism with a circular base that is rotated in a metal frame marked with a scale; used in examination of ocular muscle imbalance.

ri·so·ri·us mus·cle (rī-sōr'ē-ŭs mŭs'ĕl) *Origin*, from platysma and fascia of masseter; *insertion*, orbicularis oris and skin at corner of mouth; *action*, draws angle of mouth laterally, lengthening rima oris; *nerve supply*, facial. SYN musculus risorius [TA].

Riss·er cast (ris'ĕr kast) SYN clam-shell brace.

RIST Abbreviation for radioimmunosorbent test.

ri·sus ca·ni·nus (rī'sŭs kā-nī'nŭs) The semblance of a grin caused by facial spasm, especially in tetanus. SYN cynic spasm, sardonic grin. [L. *risus,* laugh + *caninus,* doglike]

Rit·gen ma·neu·ver (rit'gen mă-nū'vĕr) Delivery of a child's head by pressure on the perineum while controlling the speed of delivery by pressure with the other hand on the head.

Rit·ter dis·ease (rit'ĕr di-zēz') An exfoliative dermatitis, also known as staphylococcal scalded skin syndrome (SSSS), caused by an exfoliative toxin-producing strain of *Staphylococcus aureus* characterized by the presence of large bullae and exfoliation of the epidermal layer of the skin.

Rit·ter op·en·ing tet·a·nus (rit'ĕr ōp'ĕn-ing tet'ă-nŭs) The tetanic contraction that occasionally occurs when a strong current, passing through a long stretch of nerve, is suddenly interrupted.

rit·u·al (rich'ū-ăl) PSYCHIATRY, PSYCHOLOGY any psychomotor activity (e.g., morbid handwashing) performed by a person to relieve anxiety or forestall its development; typically seen in obsessive-compulsive disorder. [L. *ritualis,* fr. *ritus,* rite]

ri•val•ry (rī′văl-rē) Competition between two or more individuals for the same object or goal. [L. *rivalis,* competitor, rival]

Riv•ers cock•tail (riv′ĕrz kok′tāl) An intravenous slow injection of 1000–2000 mL of 10% dextrose in isotonic saline to which thiamine hydrochloride and 25 units of insulin are added; used in acute alcoholism.

Ri•vi•nus ca•nals (ri-vē′nŭs kă-nalz′) SEE major sublingual duct, minor sublingual ducts.

Ri•vi•nus ducts (ri-vē′nŭs dŭkts) SYN minor sublingual ducts.

riz•i•form (riz′i-fōrm) Resembling rice grains. [Fr. *riz,* rice]

RLE Abbreviation for right lower extremity.

RLL Abbreviation for right lower lobe (of lung).

RLQ Abbreviation for right lower quadrant (of abdomen).

RLS Abbreviation for restless legs syndrome.

RM Abbreviation for repetition maximum.

1-RM Abbreviation for one-repetition maximum. SEE ALSO dynamometer.

RMA Abbreviation for right mentoanterior position.

RML Abbreviation for right middle lobe (of lung).

RMP Abbreviation for right mentoposterior position.

RMR Abbreviation for resting metabolic rate.

RMT Abbreviation for right mentotransverse position; registered medical transcriptionist.

RN, R.N. Abbreviation for registered nurse.

Rn Symbol for radon.

RNA Abbreviation for ribonucleic acid.

RNase Abbreviation for ribonuclease.

RNase-α (ahr-en-az′ al′fă) An enzyme catalyzing endonucleolytic cleavage of *O*-methylated RNA yielding 5′-phosphomonoesters.

Rnase H Abbreviation for ribonuclease H.

RNase P An enzyme catalyzing the endonucleolytic cleavage tRNA precursors to yield 5′-phosphomonoesters.

RNA splic•ing (splīs′ing) SYN splicing (2).

RNA tu•mor vi•rus•es (tū′mŏr vī′rŭs-ĕz) Viruses of the subfamily Oncovirinae.

RNA vi•rus (vī′rŭs) A group of viruses in which the core consists of RNA; a major group of animal viruses that includes the families Picornaviridae, Reoviridae, Togaviridae, Flaviviridae, Bunyaviridae, Arenaviridae, Paramyxoviridae, Retroviridae, Coronaviridae, Orthomyxoviridae, and Rhabdoviridae.

RNP Abbreviation for ribonucleoprotein.

RNS Abbreviation for red neck syndrome.

ROA Abbreviation for right occipitoanterior position; route of administration.

Roaf syn•drome (rōf sin′drōm) Craniofacial-skeletal disorder dued to a sporadic or inheritable defect in formation of collagen II characterized by congenital or early retinal detachment, cataracts, myopia, shortened long bones, and mental retardation; progressive sensorineural hearing loss is of later onset.

ro•bert•so•ni•an trans•lo•ca•tion (rob′ĕrt-sō′nē-ăn tranz′lō-kā′shŭn) Translocation in which the centromeres of two acrocentric chromosomes appear to have fused, forming an abnormal chromosome consisting of the long arms of two different chromosomes; if the translocation is balanced, the individual is clinically normal but a carrier of the translocation; if the translocation is unbalanced, the individual is trisomic for the long arm of a chromosome. SYN centric fusion.

Rob•i•now syn•drome (rob′i-now sin′drōm) A skeletal dysplasia characterized by bulging forehead, hypertelorism, depressed nasal bridge (so-called fetal face), wide mouth, acromesomelic shortening of limbs, hemivertebrae, and hypoplastic genitalia; there is also an autosomal recessive form.

Rob•in•son in•dex (rob′in-sŏn in′deks) An index used to calculate heart work load. SEE ALSO double product.

Rob•in syn•drome (rō-ban[h]′ sin′drōm) SYN Pierre Robin syndrome.

ro•bot•ic (rō-bot′ik) Pertaining to or characteristic of a robot, an automatic mechanical device designed to duplicate a human function without direct human operation. [Czech *robot,* robot, fr. *robota,* drudgery, + -ic]

Ro•cha•li•mae•a (rō-chă-lī′mē-ă) Former designation for *Bartonella* (q.v.).

rock•er knife (rok′ĕr nīf) Knife with a curved, rocking blade designed for people with only one functioning upper limb.

rock pop•py (rok pop′ē) SYN celandine.

Rock•y Moun•tain spot•ted fe•ver (rok′ē mown′tăn spot′ĕd fē′vĕr) An acute infectious disease of high mortality, characterized by frontal and occipital headache, intense lumbar pain, malaise, a moderately high continuous fever, and a rash on wrists, palms, ankles, and soles from the second to the fifth day, later spreading to all parts of the body; it is typically contracted in the spring of the year primarily in the southeastern and the Rocky Mountain regions of the United States, although it is also endemic elsewhere in the United States, parts of Canada, Mexico, and South America. The pathogenic organism is *Rickettsia rickettsii*, transmitted by two or more tick species of the genus *Dermacentor;* in the United States it is spread by *D. andersoni* in the western states and *D. variabilis* (a dog tick) in the eastern states. SYN tick fever (4).

rod (rod) **1.** A straight, slender, cylindric structure or device. For surgical rods, see nail; pin. **2.** The photosensitive, outward-directed process of a rhodopsin-containing rod cell in the external granular layer of the retina; many millions of such rods, together with the cones, form the photoreceptive layer of rods and cones. SYN rod cell. [A.S. *rōd*]

rod cell (rod sel) SYN rod (2).

ro•den•ti•cide (rō-den′ti-sīd) An agent lethal to rodents. [rodent + L. *caedo,* to kill]

ro•dent ul•cer (rō′dĕnt ŭl′sĕr) A slowly enlarging ulcerated basal cell carcinoma, usually on the face.

rod gran•ule (rod gran′yūl) The nucleus of a retinal cell connecting with one of the rods.

roent•gen (r, R) (rent′gen) The international unit of exposure dose for x-rays or gamma rays; that quantity of radiation that will produce in 1 cm of air at STP, or 0.001293 g of air, 2.08×10^9 ions of both signs, each totaling 1 electrostatic unit (e.s.u.) of charge; in the MKS system this is 2.58×10^{-4} coulombs per kg of air. [W. K. *Roentgen*]

ro•ent•gen-e•quiv•a•lent-man (rem) (rent′gen ē-kwiv′ă-lĕnt-man) A unit of dose-equivalent quantity of ionizing radiation of any type that produces in human subjects the same biologic effect as one rad of x-rays or gamma rays; the number of rems is equal to the absorbed dose, measured in rads, multiplied by the quality factor of the radiation in question. 100 rem = 1 Sv.

roent•gen•ol•o•gist (rent′gen-ol′ŏ-jist) A person skilled in the diagnostic or therapeutic application of roentgen rays; a radiologist.

roent•gen•ol•o•gy (rent′gen-ol′ŏ-jē) The study of roentgen rays in all their applications. Radiology is the preferred term in the context of medical imaging.

ro•ent•gen ray (rent′gen rā) SYN x-ray.

Roes•ler-Dress•ler in•farct (res′ler-dres′ler in′fahrkt) Myocardial infarction in dumbbell form involving the anterior and posterior left ventricle and the left side of the ventricular septum.

Rog•er An•der•son pin fix•a•tion ap•pli•ance (roj′ĕr an′dĕr-sŏn pin fiks-ā′shŭn ă-plī′ăns) An appliance used in extraoral fixation of mandibular fractures and prognathic corrections in which pins placed in the bone segments are joined by metal connecting rods.

Ro•ger bru•it (rō-zhā′ brū-ē′) SYN Roger murmur.

Ro•ger dis•ease (rō-zhā′ di-zēz′) A congenital cardiac anomaly consisting of an asymptomatic defect of the interventricular septum, often with a loud murmur and definite thrill.

Ro•ger mur•mur (rō-zhā′ mŭr′mŭr) A loud pansystolic murmur maximal at the left sternal border, caused by a small ventricular septal defect. SYN Roger bruit.

Rog•ers sphyg•mo•ma•nom•e•ter (roj′ĕrz sfig′mō-mă-nom′ĕ-tĕr) A sphygmomanometer with an aneroid barometer gauge.

Ro•ki•tan•sky dis•ease (rō′ki-tahn′skē di-zēz′) SYN acute yellow atrophy of the liver.

Ro•ki•tan•sky her•ni•a (rō′ki-tahn′skē hĕr′nē-ă) A separation of the muscular fibers of the bowel allowing protrusion of a sac of the mucous membrane.

Ro•ki•tan•sky pel•vis (rō′ki-tahn′skē pel′vis) SYN spondylolisthetic pelvis.

Ro•ki•tan•sky syn•drome (rō′ki-tahn′skē sin′drōm) SYN Budd-Chiari syndrome.

ro•lan•dic (rō-lan′dik) Relating to or described by Luigi Rolando.

ro•lan•dic ep•i•lep•sy (rō-lan′dik ep′i-lep′sē) A benign, autosomal dominant form of epilepsy occurring in children, characterized clinically by arrest of speech, by muscular contractions of the side of the face and arm, and by epileptic discharges electroencephalographically.

Ro•lan•do ar•e•a (rō-lahn′dō ār′ē-ă) SYN motor cortex.

Ro•lan•do fiss•ure (rō-lan′dō fish′ŭr) A fissure on the lateral surface of each cerebral hemisphere, separating frontal and parietal lobes; also called fissure of Rolando and central sulcus of cerebrum.

Ro•lan•do frac•ture (rō-lan′dō frak′shŭr) Fracture to the base of the first metacarpal with vertical extension into the joint as a T or Y fracture.

role (rōl) **1.** The pattern of behavior that one exhibits in relationship to people with whom one has or had primary relationships. **2.** A socially agreed set of behaviors or accepted normative code. [Fr.]

role-play•ing (rōl-plā′ing) A psychotherapeutic method used in psychodrama to understand and treat emotional conflicts through the enactment or reenactment of stressful interpersonal events. SEE ALSO psychodrama.

rol•ler•ball e•lec•trode (rōl′ĕr-bawl ĕ-lek′trōd) A device that rolls like a paint roller over surface tissue, cauterizing it; used in endometrial ablation.

rol•ler ban•dage (rōl′ĕr ban′dăj) A strip of material, of variable width, rolled into a compact cylinder to facilitate its application.

Rol•let stro•ma (rol′et strō′mă) The colorless stroma of the red blood cells.

ROM Abbreviation for range of motion.

Ro•ma•ña sign (rō-mahn′yă sīn) Marked edema of one or both eyelids, usually a unilateral palpebral edema, thought to be a sensitization response to the bite of a triatomine bug infected with *Trypanosoma cruzi*, and a strong suggestion of acute Chagas disease.

Ro•ma•now•sky blood stain (rō-mah-nof′skē blŭd stān) Prototype of the eosin-methylene blue stains for blood smears, using aqueous solutions made of a mixture of methylene blue (saturated) and eosin. Romanowsky-type stains depend for their action on compounds formed by interaction of methylene blue and eosin; most are of no value if water is present in the alcohol because neutral dyes become precipitated.

rom•berg•ism (rom′berg-izm) SYN Romberg sign.

Rom•berg sign (rom′berg sīn) With feet approximated, the patient stands with eyes open and then closed; if closing the eyes increases the unsteadiness, a loss of proprioceptive control is indicated, and the sign is present. SYN romberg-ism.

ron•geur (rōn[h]-zhur′) A strong biting forceps for nipping away bone. [Fr. *ronger,* to gnaw]

Rønne na•sal step (rĕr′nĕ nā′zăl step) A nasal visual field defect with one margin corresponding to the retinal horizontal medium; seen in glaucoma.

roof (rūf) A covering or rooflike structure, e.g., a tectorium, tectum, tegmen, tegmentum, integument. [A.S. *hrōf*]

roof plate, **roof•plate** (rūf plāt, rūf′plāt) The thin layer of the embryonic neural tube connecting the alar plates dorsally.

room•ing-in (rūm′ing-in′) Placement of a newborn with its mother, rather than in the nursery, during the postpartum hospital stay.

root (rūt) **1.** The primary or beginning portion of any part, as of a nerve at its origin from the brainstem or spinal cord. SYN radix (1) [TA]. **2.** SYN root of tooth. **3.** The descending underground portion of a plant; it absorbs water and nutrients, provides support, and stores nutrients. [A.S. rot]

root am•pu•ta•tion (rūt amp′yū-tā′shŭn) Surgical removal of one or more roots of a multirooted tooth, the remaining root canal(s) usually being treated endodontically. SYN radectomy, radiectomy, radisectomy.

root ca•nal of tooth (rūt kă-nal′ tūth) The chamber of the dental pulp lying within the root portion of a tooth. SYN canalis radicis dentis [TA], cavity of tooth, pulp canal (1), pulp canal (2).

root car•ies in•dex (rūt kār′ēz in′deks) The ratio of the number of teeth with carious lesions of the root, and/or restorations of the root, to the number of teeth with exposed root surfaces.

root-form im•plant (rūt′fōrm im′plant) An implant shaped like the root of a tooth.

root•ing re•flex (rūt′ing rē′fleks) A reflexive movement seen in the young infant until 4–5 months of age; characterized by mouth opening and head turning in the direction of the tactile stimulus on the lips or cheeks.

root of lung (rūt lŭng) All the structures entering or leaving the lung at the hilum, forming a pedicle invested with the pleura; includes the bronchi, pulmonary artery and veins, bronchial arteries and veins, lymphatics, and nerves.

root of nail (rūt nāl) The proximal end of the nail, concealed under a fold of skin.

root of pe•nis (rūt pē′nis) The proximal attached part of the penis, including the two crura and the bulb.

root pulp (rūt pŭlp) That part of the dental pulp contained within the apical or root portion of the tooth.

root re•sec•tion (rūt rē-sek′shŭn) SYN apicoectomy.

root sheath (rūt shēth) One of the epidermic layers of the hair follicle: external root sheath is continuous with the stratum basale and stratum spinosum of the epidermis; internal root sheath comprises the cuticle of the internal roots, Huxley layer, and Henle layer.

root of tongue (rūt tŭng) The posterior attached portion of the tongue.

root of tooth (rūt tūth) That part of a tooth below the neck, covered by cementum rather than enamel, and attached by the periodontal ligament to the alveolar bone. SYN radix (2) [TA], root (2).

ROP Abbreviation for right occipitoposterior position.

Ror•schach test (rōr′shahk test) A projective psychological test of personality in which the subject reveals his or her attitudes, emotions, and personality by reporting what is seen in each of ten inkblot pictures in a standard set. SYN inkblot test.

ROS Abbreviation for review of symptoms.

ro•sa•ce•a (rō-sā′shă) Chronic vascular and follicular dilation involving the nose and contiguous portions of the cheeks with erythema, hyperplasia of sebaceous glands, deep-seated papules and pustules, and telangiectasia. SYN acne erythematosa, acne rosacea. [L. *rosaceus,* rosy]

Ro•sai-Dorf•man dis•ease (rō′zī-dorf′mĕn di-zēz′) SYN sinus histiocytosis with massive lymphadenopathy.

ro•sar•y (rō′zăr-ē) A structure consisting of bodies in linear sequence.

rose ben•gal (rōz′ beng′găl) [C.I. 45440] A fluorescein derivative used as a biologic stain.

Ro•sen•bach law (rō′zen-bahk law) **1.** In affections of the nerve trunks or nerve centers, paralysis of the flexor muscles appears later than that of the extensors. **2.** In cases of abnormal stimulation of organs with rhythmic functional periodicity, there is often a grouping of the individual acts with corresponding lengthening of the pauses, in such a way that the proportion of total rest and activity remains nearly the same.

Ro•sen•bach sign (rō′zen-bahk sīn) Loss of the abdominal reflexes in cases of acute inflammation of the viscera.

Ro•sen•mül•ler gland (rō′zen-mil-ler gland) SYN proximal deep inguinal lymph node.

Ro•sen•mül•ler node (rō′zen-mil-ler nōd) SYN proximal deep inguinal lymph node.

Ro•sen•thal ca•nal (rō′zen-tahl kă-nal′) SYN spiral canal of cochlea.

ro•se•o•la (rō′zē-ō′lă) A symmetric eruption of small, closely aggregated patches of rose-red color; caused by human herpesvirus type 6 and sometimes type 7. SEE ALSO exanthema subitum. [Mod. L. dim. of L. *roseus,* rosy]

ro•se•o•la id•i•o•path•i•ca (rō′zē-ō′lă id′ē-ō-path′i-kă) Reddish symmetric skin eruption not associated with other syndromes.

ro•se•o•la in•fan•ti•lis, **ro•se•o•la in•fan•tum** (rō′zē-ō′lă in-fan′til-is, in-fan′tŭm) SYN exanthema subitum.

Rose po•si•tion (rōz pŏ-zish′ŏn) The patient lies supine with the head falling down over the end of the table; used in operations within the mouth or pharynx.

rose spots (rōs spotz) Characteristic exanthema of typhoid fever; 10–20 small pink papules on the lower trunk lasting a few days and leaving hyperpigmentation.

ro•sette (rō-zet′) **1.** The quartan malarial parasite *Plasmodium malariae* in its segmented or mature phase. **2.** A grouping of cells characteristic of neoplasms of neuroblastic or neuroectodermal origin; a number of nuclei form a ring from which neurofibrils, which can be demonstrated by silver impregnation, extend to interlace in the center. **3.** Roselike coiling of the uterus among certain pseudophyllidean tapeworms, such as *Diphyllobothrium latum.* [Fr. a little rose]

ros•in (roz′in) The solid resin obtained after steam distillation of crude balsam from species of *Pinus;* used in plasters to render them adhesive and also in ointments to render them locally stimulating. SYN resin (2).

Ro spat•u•la (rō spach′ŭ-lă) A very small nickeled steel spatula used to transfer bits of infected material (e.g., diphtheritic membrane, to culture tubes).

Ros•so•li•mo re•flex, **Ros•so•li•mo sign** (ros-ō-lē′mō rē-fleks, sīn) Flicking the tops of the toes from the plantar surface causes flexion of the toes; a stretch reflex of the flexors of the toes seen in lesions of the pyramidal tracts. SEE ALSO Starling reflex.

Ross pro•ce•dure (raws prŏ-sē′jŭr) Therapeutic technique for aortic valve stenosis or regurgitation in which the aortic valve is replaced with the patient's own pulmonic valve (autograft) and the pulmonic valve is in turn replaced with a homograft valve.

Ross Riv•er vi•rus (raws riv′ĕr vī′rŭs) A mosquito-borne alphavirus, family Togaviridae, that causes epidemic polyarthritis.

ros•tel•lum (ros-tel′ŭm) The anterior fixed or invertible portion of the scolex of a tapeworm, frequently provided with a row (or several rows) of hooks. [L. dim. of *rostrum,* a beak]

ros•trad (ros′trad) **1.** In a direction toward any rostrum. **2.** Situated nearer a rostrum or the snout end of an organism in relation to a specific reference point; opposite of caudad (2). [L. *rostrum,* beak, + *-ad,* toward]

ros•tral (ros′trăl) Relating to any rostrum or anatomic structure resembling a beak. [L. *rostralis,* fr. *rostrum,* beak]

ros•trate (ros′trāt) Having a beak or hook. [L. *rostratus*]

ros•trum, pl. **ros•tra**, **ros•trums** (ros′trŭm, -tră, -trŭmz) Any beak-shaped structure. [L. a beak]

ROT Abbreviation for right occipitotransverse position.

rot (rot) To decay or putrify. [A.S. *rotian*]

ro•ta•mase (rō′tă-mās) Enzyme capable of altering the rotational conformation of a molecule.

ro•ta•mer (rō′tă-mĕr) An isomer differing from other conformation(s) only in rotational positioning of its parts, such as *cis-* and *trans-* forms.

ro•ta•ry chew•ing (rō′tăr-ē chū′ing) A mastication pattern seen in children by 15 months of age. It includes lateral and circular jaw movements while the tongue simultaneously moves food from side to side and across midline to the teeth surfaces for grinding and mashing of firmer foods.

ro•ta•ry joint, **ro•ta•to•ry joint** (rō′tăr-ē joynt, rō′tă-tōr′ē) SYN pivot joint.

ro•tat•ing an•ode (rō′tāt-ing an′ōd) In diagnostic radiography, modern x-ray tubes that have a mushroom-shaped anode that rotates rapidly to avoid local heat buildup from electron impact during x-ray generation.

ro•ta•tion (rō-tā′shŭn) **1.** Turning or movement around an axis. **2.** A recurrence in regular order of certain events, such as the symptoms of a periodic disease. **3.** In medical education and other health education progams, a period of time dedicated to a particular service or specialty. **4.** Practice of changing hours worked periodically; shift work. [L. *rotatio,* fr. *roto,* pp. *rotatus,* to revolve, rotate]

ro•ta•tion•al nys•tag•mus (rō′tā-shŭn-ăl nis-tag′mŭs) Jerky nystagmus arising from stimulation of the labyrinth by rotation of the head around any axis and induced by change of motion.

ro•ta•tion flap (rō-tā′shŭn flap) A pedicle flap that is rotated from the donor site to an adjacent recipient area, usually as a direct flap.

ro•ta•tor (rō′tā-tŏr) A muscle by which a part can be turned circularly. SEE ALSO rotation. [L.]

ro•ta•tor cuff of shoul•der (rō′tā-tŏr kŭf shōl′dĕr) The upper half of the capsule of the shoulder joint reinforced by the tendons of insertion of the supraspinatus, infraspinatus, teres minor, and subscapularis muscles.

ro•ta•to•res mus•cles (rō-tă-tō′rēz mŭs′ĕlz) Deepest of the three layers of transversospinalis muscles, chiefly developed in the thoracic region; they arise from the transverse process of one vertebra and are inserted into the root of the spinous process of the next two or three vertebrae above; *action*, traditionally described as a column, it is more likely that these muscles, provided with a very high density of muscle spindles, are organs of proprioception; *nerve supply*, dorsal primary rami of the spinal nerves. See this page. SYN musculi rotatores [TA].

ro•ta•to•ry nys•tag•mus (rō′tă-tōr′ē nis-tag′mŭs) A movement of the eyes around the visual axis.

Ro•ta•vi•rus (rō′tă-vī′rŭs) A genus of RNA viruses that includes the human gastroenteritis viruses (a major cause of infant diarrhea throughout the world). In May 2007, extensive outbreaks of disease were discovered in St. John's, Newfoundland. These cases were, unusually, limited almost completely to a pediatric poopulation. SYN gastroenteritis virus type B. [L. *rota,* wheel, + virus]

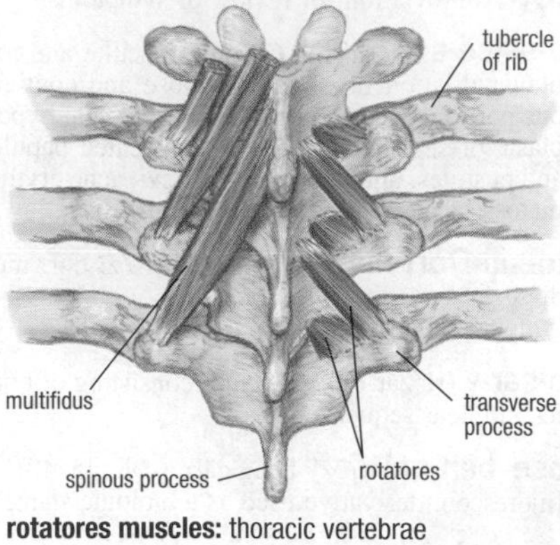

rotatores muscles: thoracic vertebrae

Rotch sign (roch sīn) In pericardial effusion, percussion dullness in the fifth intercostal space on the right.

rote learn•ing (rōt lĕrn′ing) The learning of arbitrary relationships, usually by repetition of the learning procedure through memorization and without an understanding of the relationships.

Roth•mund syn•drome (rōt′mūnd sin′drōm) Atrophy, pigmentation, and telangiectasia of the skin, usually with juvenile cataract, saddle nose, congenital bone defects, disturbance of hair growth, hypogonadism; autosomal recessive inheritance.

Roth sign (rōt sīn) SYN Bernhardt sign.

Roth spot (rōt spot) A round, white retinal spot surrounded by hemorrhage in bacterial endocarditis, and in other retinal hemorrhagic conditions.

Ro•tor syn•drome (rō-tōr′ sin′drōm) Jaundice appearing in childhood due to impaired biliary excretion; most of the plasma bilirubin is conjugated, liver function results are usually normal, and there is no hepatic pigmentation.

ro•to•sco•li•o•sis (rō′tō-skō′lē-ō′sis) Combined lateral and rotational deviation of the vertebral column. [L. *roto,* to rotate, + G. *skoliōsis,* crookedness]

ro•to•tome (rō′tō-tōm) A rotating cutting instrument used in arthroscopic surgery.

Rou•get bulb (rū-zhā′ bŭlb) A venous plexus on the surface of the ovary.

rough•age (rŭf′ăj) Anything in the diet (e.g., bran) that may act as a bulk stimulant of intestinal peristalsis.

rou•leaux for•ma•tion (rū-lō′ fōr-mā′shŭn) The arrangement of red blood cells in fluid blood (or in diluted suspensions) with their biconcave surfaces in apposition, thereby forming groups that resemble stacks of coins. See page B3. [Fr. pl. of *rouleau,* a roll]

round•ed at•el•ec•ta•sis, round at•el•ec•ta•sis (rownd′ed at′ĕ-lek′tă-sis, rownd) An area of atelectatic lung caused by parenchymal infolding due to pleural fibrosis, most often from asbestos exposure; appears as a masslike opacity and can be mistaken for lung cancer; may be associated with a comet tail sign; a high level of contrast enhancement on dynamic computed tomography aids diagnosis.

round heart (rownd hahrt) Abnormally smooth arcuate contours of the heart due either to disease of the ventricles or to a false cardiac appearance produced by excessive pericardial fluid.

round lig•a•ment of fe•mur (rownd lig′ă-mĕnt fē′mŭr) SYN ligament of head of femur.

round lig•a•ment of liv•er (rownd lig′ă-mĕnt liv′ĕr) The remains of the umbilical vein running within the free edge of the falciform ligament from the umbilicus to the liver, where it continues within the fissure for the round ligament to the origin of the left portal vein within the porta hepatis. SYN ligamentum teres hepatis [TA].

round lig•a•ment of u•ter•us (rownd lig′ă-mĕnt yū′tĕr-ŭs) A fibromuscular band that is attached to the uterus on either side in front of and below the opening of the uterine tube; it passes through the inguinal canal to the labium majus. SYN ligamentum teres uteri [TA].

round win•dow (rownd win′dō) SYN fenestra cochleae.

round win•dow mem•brane (rownd win′dō mem′brān) SYN secondary tympanic membrane.

round•worm (rownd′wŏrm) A nematode member of the phylum Nematoda, commonly confined to the parasitic forms.

Rous-as•so•ci•at•ed vi•rus (RAV) (rows ă-sō′sē-āt-ĕd vī′rŭs) A leukemia virus of the leukosis-sarcoma complex that by phenotypic mixing with a defective (noninfectious) strain of Rous sarcoma virus effects production of infectious sarcoma virus with envelope antigenicity of the RAV.

Rous sar•co•ma vi•rus (RSV) (rows sahr-kō′mă vī′rŭs) A sarcoma-producing virus of the avian leukosis-sarcoma complex identified by Rous in 1911.

Roux-en-Y a•nas•to•mo•sis (rū ōn[h] wī ă-nas′tŏ-mō′sis, rū ōn[h] ĕ′grek) Anastomosis of the distal end of the divided jejunum to the stomach, bile duct, or another structure, with implantation of the proximal end into the side of the jejunum at a suitable distance below the first anastomosis, the bowel then forming a Y-shaped pattern.

Roux meth•od (rū meth′ŏd) Division of the mandible in the median line, to facilitate the operation of ablation of the tongue.

Rov•sing sign (rov′sing sīn) Pain at the McBurney point induced in cases of appendicitis, by pressure exerted over the descending colon.

roy•al blue-top tube (roy′ăl blū-top tūb) A tube of this color indicates the container has either not been treated (plain) or has been treated with EDTA as anticoagulant. These are used in the collection of whole blood or serum for trace element analysis.

RPE Abbreviation for rate of perceived exertion.

RPF Abbreviation for renal plasma flow. SEE effective renal plasma flow.

RPI Abbreviation for reticulocyte production index.

rpm Abbreviation for revolutions per minute.

RPO Abbreviation for right posterior oblique, a radiographic position in which the right posterior side of the body is closest to the film.

R-pro•tein (prō′tēn) A protein produced by the salivary gland that is thought to protect vitamin B12 as it travels through the digestive tract.

RQ Abbreviation for respiratory quotient.

-rrhagia Suffix meaning excessive or unusual discharge. [G. *rhēgnymi,* to burst forth]

-rrhaphy Suffix meaning surgical suturing. [G. *rhaphē,* suture]

-rrhea Suffix meaning a flowing; a flux. SYN -rrhoea. [G. *rhoia,* a flow]

-rrhoea [Br.] SYN -rrhea.

rRNA Abbreviation for ribosomal ribonucleic acid.

RRT Abbreviation for registered respiratory therapist.

RSA Abbreviation for right sacroanterior position.

RSD Abbreviation for reflex sympathetic dystrophy.

RSI Abbreviation for rapid sequence intubation.

RSP Abbreviation for right sacroposterior position.

RST Abbreviation for right sacrotransverse position.

RSV Abbreviation for Rous sarcoma virus; respiratory syncytial virus..

RSV-IGIV Abbreviation for respiratory syncytial virus immune globulin intravenous.

rTMP Abbreviation for ribothymidylic acid.

RT-PCR Abbreviation for reverse transcriptase polymerase chain reaction.

RTW Abbreviation for return to work.

Ru Symbol for ruthenium.

rub (rŭb) Friction encountered in moving one body over another.

rub•ber-bulb sy•ringe (rŭb′bĕr-bŭlb′ sir-inj′) A syringe with a hollow rubber bulb and cannula provided with a check valve, used to obtain a jet of air or water.

rub•ber dam clamp for•ceps (rŭb′bĕr dam klamp fōr′seps) SYN clamp forceps.

rub•ber-shod clamp (rŭb′bĕr-shod′ klamp) A small, rubber-tipped clamp that holds sutures in place during surgery.

ru•be•do (rū-bē′dō) A temporary redness of the skin. [L. redness, fr. *ruber,* red]

ru•be•fa•cient (rū′bĕ-fā′shĕnt) **1.** Causing a reddening of the skin. **2.** A counterirritant that produces erythema when applied to the skin surface. [L. *rubi-facio,* fr. *ruber,* red, + *facio,* to make]

ru•be•fac•tion (rū′bĕ-fak′shŭn) Erythema of the skin caused by local application of a counterirritant. SEE ALSO rubefacient.

ru•bel•la (rū-bel′ă) An acute exanthematous disease caused by rubella virus (*Rubivirus*), with enlargement of lymph nodes, but usually with little fever or constitutional reaction; a high incidence of birth defects in children results from maternal infection during the first several months of fetal life (congenital rubella syndrome). See page B30. SYN epidemic roseola, German measles, third disease. [L. *rubellus,* fem. *-a,* reddish, dim. of *ruber,* red]

ru•bel•la he•mag•glu•ti•na•tion in•hi•bi•tion (HI) test (rū-bel′lă hē′mă-glū-ti-nā′shŭn in′hi-bish′ŭn test) A procedure for rubella, often performed routinely as part of a prenatal workup of a pregnant woman; the presence of any detectable HI titer in the absence of disease indicates previous infection and immunity to reinfection.

ru•bel•la ti•ter (rū-bel′ă tī′tĕr) A serum test to determine a person's state of immunity against rubella, because the disease during pregnancy carries significant risks for the fetus. Generally, a rubella titer of 1:10 or higher means that the person has developed immunity to rubella.

ru•bel•la vi•rus (rū-bel′ă vī′rŭs) An RNA virus of the genus Rubivirus; the agent causing rubella (German measles) in humans. SYN German measles virus.

ru•be•o•la (rū-bē-ō′lă) SYN measles (1). [Mod. L. dim. of *ruber,* red, reddish]

ru•be•o•la vi•rus (rū-bē-ō′lă vī′rŭs) SYN measles virus.

ru•be•o•sis (rū′bē-ō′sis) **1.** Reddish discoloration, as of the skin. **2.** Neovascularization of the iris seen in ocular ischemic diseases. [L. *ruber,* red, + G. *-osis,* condition]

ru•be•o•sis ir•i•dis di•a•be•ti•ca (rū′bē-ō′sis ī′ri-dis dī-ă-bet′i-kă) Neovascularization of the anterior surface of the iris in diabetes mellitus.

ru•bes•cent (rū-bes′ĕnt) Reddening. [L. *rubesco,* pr. p. *rubescens,* to become red]

ru•bid•i•um (rū-bid′ē-ŭm) An alkali element, atomic no. 37, atomic wt. 85.4678; its salts have been used in medicine for the same purposes as the corresponding sodium or potassium salts. [L. *rubidus,* reddish, dark red, fr. *rubeo,* to be red]

ru•bid•o•my•cin (rū-bid′ō-mī′sin) An antibiotic used as an antineoplastic; similar to doxorubicin in antitumor activity and in exhibiting cumulative cardiotoxicity. SYN daunorubicin.

Ru•bi•vi•rus (rū′bi-vī′rŭs) A genus of viruses that includes the rubella virus. [*rub*ella + virus]

Rub•ner laws of growth (rūb′ner lawz grōth) **1.** The law of constant energy consumption: The rapidity of growth is proportional to the intensity of the metabolic processes. **2.** The law of the constant growth quotient: In most young mammals, 24% of the entire food energy, or calories, is used for growth; in humans, only 5% is thus used.

ru•bor (rū′bōr) Redness of the skin or mucous membrane, as one of the four signs of hyperemia or inflammation (r., calor, dolor, tumor) enunciated by Celsus. [L.]

ru•bre•dox•ins (rū′brĕ-dok′sinz) Ferredoxins without acid-labile sulfur and with the iron in a typical mercaptide coordination.

ru•bri•blast (rū′bri-blast) SYN pronormoblast. [L. *ruber,* red, + G. *blastos,* germ]

ru•bri•cyte (rū′bri-sīt) SYN karyocyte. SEE ALSO erythroblast. [L. *ruber,* red, + *kytos,* cell]

ru•bro•spi•nal de•cus•sa•tion (rū′brō-spī′năl dē′kŭs-ā′shŭn) SEE tegmental decussations (2).

Ru•bu•la•vi•rus (rū′byū-lă-vī′rŭs) A genus in the family Paramyxoviridae; causes mumps.

ru•di•ment (rū′di-mĕnt) **1.** An organ or structure that is incompletely developed. **2.** The first indication of a structure in the course of ontogeny. SYN rudimentum. [L. *rudimentum,* a beginning, fr. *rudis,* unformed]

ru•di•men•ta•ry (rū′di-men′tăr-ē) Relating to a rudiment. SYN abortive (2).

ru•di•men•tum, pl. **ru•di•men•ta** (rū′di-men′tŭm, -tă) SYN rudiment. [L.]

Rud syn•drome (rūd sin′drōm) Ichthyosiform erythroderma associated with acanthosis nigricans, dwarfism, hypogonadism, and epilepsy;

mostly sporadic, but may be an X-linked recessive trait.

Ruf·fi·ni cor·pus·cle (rūf-ē′nē kōr′pŭs-ĕl) Sensory end-structure in the subcutaneous connective tissues of the fingers, consisting of an ovoid capsule within which the sensory fiber ends with numerous collateral knobs.

ru·fous (rū′fŭs) SYN erythristic. [L. *rufus,* reddish]

RUG Abbreviation for Resource Utilization Group.

ru·ga, pl. **ru·gae** (rū′gă, -gē) [TA] A fold, ridge, or crease; a wrinkle. [L. a wrinkle]

ru·gae of stom·ach (rū′gē stŏm′ăk) Characteristic folds of the gastric mucosa, especially evident when the stomach is contracted.

ru·gine (rū-zhēn′) **1.** SYN periosteal elevator. **2.** A raspatory. [Fr.]

ru·gose (rū′gōs) Marked by rugae; wrinkled. SYN rugous. [L. *rugosus*]

ru·gos·i·ty (rū-gos′i-tē) **1.** The state of being thrown into folds or wrinkles. **2.** A ruga.

ru·gous (rū′gŭs) SYN rugose.

Ru·he·mann pur·ple (rū′mahn pŭr′pĕl) A blue-violet dye formed in the reaction of ninhydrin with amino acids.

Ruit·er-Pom·pen dis·ease (roy′tĕr pŏm′pen di-zēz′) SYN Fabry disease.

RUL Abbreviation for right upper lobe (of lung).

rule (rūl) A criterion, standard, or guide governing a procedure, arrangement, action, or other process. SEE ALSO law, principle, theorem. [O. Fr. *reule,* fr. L. *regula,* a guide, pattern]

rule of bi·gem·i·ny (rūl bī-jem′i-nē) Statement that a ventricular premature beat will follow the beat terminating a long cycle. Sudden prolongation of the ventricular cycle, by changing the refractoriness in the conduction system, causes a peripheral region of bidirectional block to become transiently unidirectional and thus opens potential pathways for reentry to occur.

rule of nines (rūl nīnz) Method used in calculating body surface area involved in burns whereby values of 9% or 18% of surface area are assigned to specific regions as follows: head and neck, 9%; anterior thorax, 18%; posterior thorax, 18%; arms, 9% each; legs, 18% each; perineum, 1%. Somewhat different values are used with children and infants. See this page.

rule of out·let (rūl owt′lĕt) An obstetric determination of whether the pelvic outlet will permit the passage of a fetus; the sum of the posterior sagittal diameter and the transverse diameter of the outlet must equal at least 15 cm if a normal-sized baby is to pass.

Ru·mi·no·coc·cus (rū′mi-nō-kok′ŭs) A genus of anaerobic, gram-positive coccobacilli isolated from the respiratory tract of humans and the intestinal tract of humans and animals. The type species is *R. productus*, formerly *Peptostreptococcus productus*.

run (rŭn) A group of successive measurements in an analytic process or during a period of time within which the accuracy and precision of the measuring system are expected to be stable. [ME *runnen*, fr. A. S. *rinnan*, fr. O.N. *rinna*]

run·a·way pace·mak·er (run′ă-wā pās′māk-ĕr) Rapid heart rates over 140 per min. caused by electronic circuit instability in an implanted pulse generator.

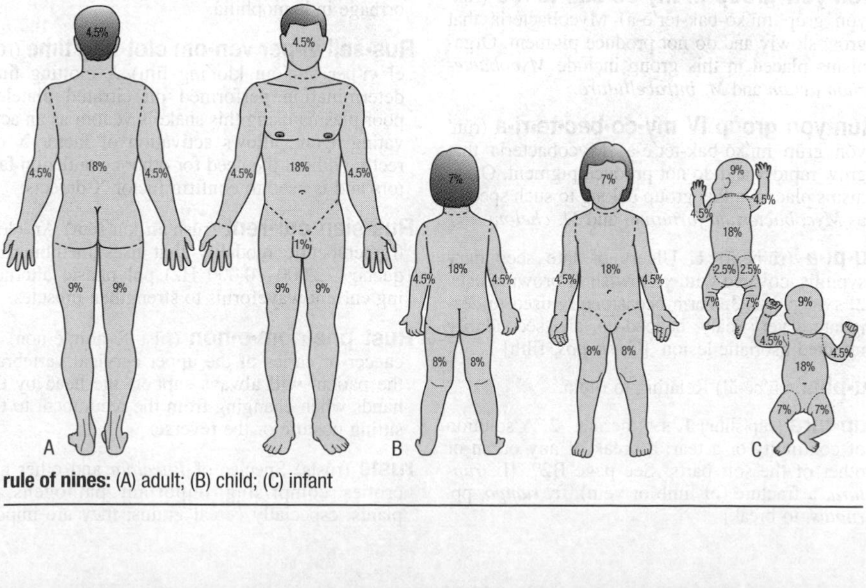

rule of nines: (A) adult; (B) child; (C) infant

Runge dis•ease (rung′ĕ di-zēz′) SYN Ballantyne disease.

run•ner's blad•der (rŭn′ĕrz blad′ĕr) Hematuria caused by running with an empty bladder.

run•ner's high (rŭn′ĕrz hī) Euphoria experienced by some runners and joggers as they near the end of a run. Believed to be associated with the release of endorphins produced by physical stress. SEE ALSO exercise high.

run•ner's knee (rŭn′ĕrz nē) An overuse syndrome of anterior knee pain associated with excessive lateral motion of the patella during activity. SYN patellofemoral stress syndrome.

Run•yon clas•si•fi•ca•tion (rŭn′yŏn klas′i-fi-kā′shŭn) A classification scheme for mycobacteria other than *Mycobacterium tuberculosis* that divides species into four categories: 1) photochromogens, which produce a yellow-to-brown carotene pigment when grown in the presence of light; 2) scotochromogens, which produce pigment in the presence or absence of light; 3) nonpigmented, which do not produce pigment; and 4) rapid growers, which grow on solid media in 5–10 days rather than 4–8 weeks. This classification has no clinical or genetic significance but remains of limited value in identification of some clinical isolates.

Run•yon group I my•co•bac•te•ri•a (rŭn′yŏn grūp mī′kō-bak-tēr′ē-ă) Mycobacteria that produce a bright yellow color when grown in the presence of light. Organisms placed in this group include *Mycobacterium kansasii.*

Run•yon group II my•co•bac•te•ri•a (rŭn′yŏn grūp mī′kō-bak-tēr′ē-ă) Mycobacteria that produce a yellow pigment even when grown in the dark; when they are grown in the light, the pigment is orange. Organisms placed in this group include *Mycobacterium scrofulaceum.*

Run•yon group III my•co•bac•te•ri•a (rŭn′yŏn grūp mī′kō-bak-tēr′ē-ă) Mycobacteria that grow slowly and do not produce pigment. Organisms placed in this group include *Mycobacterium avium* and *M. intracellulare.*

Run•yon group IV my•co•bac•te•ri•a (rŭn′yŏn grūp mī′kō-bak-tēr′ē-ă) Mycobacteria that grow rapidly and do not produce pigment. Organisms placed in this group belong to such species as *Mycobacterium fortuitum* and *M. cheloni.*

ru•pi•a (rū′pē-ă) **1.** Ulcers of late secondary syphilis, covered with yellowish or brown crusts. **2.** SYN yaws. **3.** Term occasionally used to designate a very scaly, heaped-up, and secondarily infected psoriatic lesion. [G. *rhypos,* filth]

ru•pi•al (rū′pē-ăl) Relating to rupia.

rup•ture (rŭp′shŭr) **1.** SYN hernia. **2.** A solution of continuity or a tear; a break of any organ or other of the soft parts. See page B27. [L. *ruptura,* a fracture (of limb or vein), fr. *rumpo,* pp. *ruptus,* to break]

rup•tured disc (rŭp′shŭrd disk) SYN herniated disc.

rup•ture of mem•brane (rup′shŭr mem′brān) Spontaneous tearing of the amnionic sac, with release of amnionic fluid, preceding childbirth.

RUQ Abbreviation for right upper quadrant (of abdomen).

Rus•sell bod•ies (rŭs′ĕl bod′ēz) Small, discrete, variably sized, spheric, intracytoplasmic, acidophilic, hyaline bodies that stain deeply with fuchsin; they occur frequently in plasma cells in chronic inflammation.

Rus•sell Per•i•o•don•tal In•dex (rŭs′ĕl per′ē-ō-don′tăl in′deks) An index that estimates the degree of periodontal disease present in the mouth by measuring both bone loss around the teeth and gingival inflammation; used in the epidemiologic investigation of periodontal disease.

Rus•sell sign (rŭs′ĕl sīn) Abrasions and scars on the back of the hands of people with bulimia, usually due to manual attempts to self-induce vomiting.

Rus•sell syn•drome (rŭs′ĕl sin′drōm) Failure of infants and young children to thrive due to suprasellar lesions, commonly astrocytomas of the anterior third ventricle; although the growth hormone may be elevated, the child is emaciated and has loss of body fat.

Rus•sell trac•tion (rŭs′ĕl trak′shŭn) A means of applying traction to one or both legs using 5–10 lb weights per leg. The leg is lifted off the bed in a sling.

Rus•sell vi•per ven•om (rŭs′ĕl vī′pĕr ven′ŏm) A venom derived from Russell viper (*Vipera russelli*), which acts as an intrinsic thromboplastin; used in the laboratory evaluation of deficiencies of factor X or topically to arrest local hemorrhage in hemophilia.

Rus•sell vi•per ven•om clot•ting time (rŭs′ĕl vī′pĕr ven′ŏm klot′ing tīm) A clotting time determination performed on citrated platelet-poor plasma using this snake's venom as an activating agent; allows activation of factor X directly without the need for other coagulation factors and is used to confirm factor X defects.

Rus•sian cur•rent (rŭsh′ăn kŭr′rĕnt) An electrotherapeutic modality that uses medium frequency (2,000–10,000 Hz) polyphasic alternating current waveforms to strengthen muscles.

Rust phe•nom•e•non (rūst fĕ-nom′ĕ-non) In cancer or caries of the upper cervical vertebrae, the patient will always support the head by the hands when changing from the recumbent to the sitting posture or the reverse.

rusts (rŭsts) Species of *Puccinia* and other microbes comprising important pathogens of plants, especially cereal grains; they are important allergens for humans when inhaled in large quantities, as during harvesting.

rust•y spu•tum (rŭs′tē spyū′tŭm) A reddish-brown, blood-stained expectoration characteristic of pneumonococcal lobar pneumonia.

ru•the•ni•um (Ru) (rū-thē′nē-ŭm) A metallic element of the platinum group; atomic no. 44, atomic wt. 101.07; ^{106}Ru, with a half-life of 1.020 years, has been used in the treatment of certain eye problems. [Mediev. L. *Ruthenia,* Russia, where first obtained]

ru•ti•do•sis (rū′ti-dō′sis) SYN rhytidosis.

Ruysch mem•brane (roish mem′brān) SYN choriocapillary layer.

Ruysch tube (roish tūb) A minute tubular cavity opening in the lower and anterior portion of each surface of the nasal septum.

RV Abbreviation for residual volume.

RVS Abbreviation for relative value scale.

RVU Abbreviation for relative value unit.

R wave (wāv) The first positive (upward) deflection of the QRS complex in the electrocardiogram; successive upward deflections within the same QRS complex are labeled R′, R″, and so on.

Rx Abbreviation for *recipe* (℞) in a prescription. SEE prescription (2).

ry•an•o•dine re•cep•tor (rī-an′ō-dēn rĕ-sep′tŏr) Receptor associated with a calcium conductance channel in the sarcoplasmic or endoplasmic reticulum of cells, which, when bound to ryanodine, causes the channel to remain in a subconductive state, allowing slow continuing release of calcium ions from the sarcoplasmic reticulum into the cytoplasm. The channels are normally sensitive to calcium ions and not sensitive to inositol triphosphate.

Ry•an stain (rī′ăn stān) A modified trichrome stain for microsporidian spores in which the chromotrope 2R is 10 times the normal concentration used in trichrome stains for stool specimens and the counterstain is aniline blue.

Ryle tube (rīl tūb) A thin rubber tube, with about the lumen of a no. 8 catheter, and an olive-tipped extremity, used in giving a test meal.

σ, Σ Sigma.

S **1.** Abbreviation for sacral vertebra (S1–S5); spheric lens; Svedberg unit. Siemens; sulfur; entropy in thermodynamics; substrate in the Michaelis-Menton mechanism; percentage saturation of hemoglobin (when followed by subscript O_2 or CO_2); serine; one of the two stereochemical designation (in italics) in the Cahn-Ingold-Prelog system. **2.** Designations of a rare human antigen (hemagglutinogen) related genetically to the MNSs blood group.

S100 An acidic, calcium-binding protein characterized by its partial solubility in saturated ammonium sulfate; stains for S100 are used in the differential diagnosis of melanomas, which are commonly positive for S100.

S_f Abbreviation for flotation constant.

S Abbreviation for entropy.

s Abbreviation for L. *sinister,* left; L. *semis,* half; second; as a subscript, denotes steady state.

s Abbreviation for selection coefficient; sedimentation coefficient.

S_1 Abbreviation for first heart sound.

S_2 Abbreviation for second heart sound.

S_3 Abbreviation for third heart sound.

S_4 Abbreviation for fourth heart sound.

S-A Abbreviation for sinuatrial; sinoatrial.

SA Abbreviation for sacroanterior position.

sa•ber tib•i•a, **sa•ber shin** (sā′bĕr tib′ē-ă, shin) Deformity of the tibia occurring in tertiary syphilis or yaws, the bone having a marked forward convexity as a result of the formation of gummas and periostitis.

Sa•bi•a vi•rus (sā′bē-ă vī′rŭs) An arenavirus associated with hemolytic fever.

Sa•bou•raud a•gar (sah-bū-rō′ ā′gahr) A culture medium for fungi containing neopeptone or polypeptone agar and glucose, with final pH 5.6; it is the standard, most universally used medium in mycology and is the international reference. Modified Sabouraud agar (Emmons modification) with neutral pH and less glucose is better for pigment development in the colonies.

Sa•bou•raud dex•trose a•gar (sah-bū-rō′ deks′trōs ā′gahr) A dextrose peptone medium that supports the growth of most pathogenic fungi.

Sa•bou•raud pas•tilles (sah-bū-rō′ pahs-tēlz′) Discs containing barium platinocyanide that undergo a color change when exposed to x-rays; previously used to indicate the administered dose.

sab•u•lous (sab′yū-lŭs) Sandy; gritty. [L. *sabulosus,* fr. *sabulum,* coarse sand]

sac (sak) **1.** A pouch or bursa. SYN saccus [TA]. SEE ALSO sacculus. **2.** An encysted abscess at the root of a tooth. **3.** The capsule of a tumor, or envelope of a cyst. [L. *saccus,* a bag]

sac•cade (sa-kahd′) A rapid movement of both eyes from one target to another; a sequence of such movements allows precise scanning of the field and is necessary for smooth reading. SEE ALSO saccadic movement. [Fr., twitch]

sac•cad•ic (să-kahd′ik) Jerky.

sac•cad•ic move•ment (să-kahd′ik mūv′mĕnt) **1.** A quick rotation of the eyes from one fixation point to another as in reading. **2.** The rapid correction movement of a jerky nystagmus, as in labyrinthine and optokinetic nystagmus.

sac•cate (sak′āt) Relating to a sac. [L. *saccus,* sac]

sac•cha•rides (sak′ă-rīdz) A group of carbohydrates that includes the sugars. Saccharides are classified as mono-, di-, tri-, and polysaccharides according to the number of saccharide units ($C_6H_{10}O_5$) composing them. SEE ALSO carbohydrates.

sac•cha•rif•er•ous (sak′ăr-if′ĕr-ŭs) Producing sugar.

♻ **saccharo-, sacchar-, sacchari-** Combining forms denoting sugar (saccharide). [G. *sak-charon,* sugar]

sac•cha•ro•lyt•ic (sak′ăr-ō-lit′ik) Capable of hydrolyzing or otherwise breaking down a sugar molecule. [saccharo- + G. *lysis,* loosening]

sac•cha•ro•met•a•bol•ic (sak′ăr-ō-met′ă-bol′ik) Relating to saccharometabolism.

sac•cha•ro•me•tab•o•lism (sak′ăr-ō-mĕ-tab′ŏ-lizm) Metabolism of sugar; the process of utilization of sugar in cells.

sac•cha•rose (sak′ăr-ōs) SYN sucrose.

sac•ci•form (sak′si-fōrm) Pouched; sac-shaped. SYN saccular. [L. *saccus,* sack, + *forma,* form]

sac•cu•lar (sak′yū-lăr) SYN sacciform.

sac•cu•lar an•eu•rysm, **sac•cu•lat•ed an•eu•rysm** (sak′yū-lăr an′yūr-izm, sak′yū-lā′tĕd) A saclike bulging on one side of an artery.

sac•cu•lar gland (sak′yū-lăr gland) A single alveolar gland.

sac•cu•lar nerve (sak′yū-lăr nĕrv) A branch of the vestibular nerve going to the macula of the sacculus. SYN nervus saccularis [TA].

sac•cu•la•tion (sak′yū-lā′shŭn) **1.** A structure formed by a group of sacs. **2.** The formation of a sac or pouch.

sac•cule (sak′yūl) **1.** The smaller of the two membranous sacs in the vestibule of the labyrinth, lying in the spheric recess; connected with the cochlear duct by a very short tube, the ductus reuniens, and with the utriculus by the beginning of the ductus endolymphaticus and the ductus utriculosaccularis that joins it. **2.** The immense, bag-shaped structure formed by peptidoglycans as part of the cell wall of certain microorganisms. SYN sacculus [TA]. [L. *sacculus*]

sac•cule of la•rynx (sak′yūl lar′ingks) A small diverticulum provided with mucous glands extending upward from the ventricle of the larynx between the vestibular fold and the lamina of the thyroid cartilage. SYN sacculus laryngis.

sac•cu•lo•co•chle•ar (sak′yū-lō-kok′lē-ăr) Relating to the sacculus and the membranous cochlea.

sac•cu•lus, pl. **sac•cu•li** (sak′yū-lŭs, -lī) [TA] SYN saccule. [L. dim. of *saccus,* sac]

sac•cu•lus al•ve•o•la•ris, pl. **sac•cu•li al•ve•o•la•res** (sak′yū-lŭs al-vē-ō-lā′ris, sak′yū-lī al-vē-ō-lā′rēz) [TA] SYN alveolar sac.

sac•cu•lus la•ryn•gis (sak′yū-lŭs lă-rinj′is) SYN saccule of larynx.

sac•cus, pl. **sac•ci** (sak′ŭs, -sī) [TA] SYN sac (1). [L. a bag, sack]

sac•cus con•junc•ti•va•lis (sak′ŭs kon-jungk′ti-vā′lis) [TA] SYN conjunctival sac.

sac•cus en•do•lym•phat•i•cus (sak′ŭs en-dō-lim-fat′i-kŭs) [TA] SYN endolymphatic sac.

sac•cus la•cri•ma•lis (sak′ŭs lak′rē-mā′lis) [TA] SYN lacrimal sac.

sa•crad (sā′krad) In the direction of the sacrum. [sacr- + L. *ad,* to]

sa•cral (sā′krăl) Relating to or in the neighborhood of the sacrum.

sa•cral ca•nal (sā′krăl kă-nal′) The continuation of the vertebral canal in the sacrum. SYN canalis sacralis [TA].

sa•cral crest (sā′krăl krest) One of three rough, irregular ridges on the posterior surface of the sacrum; median sacral crest; lateral sacral crests.

sa•cral flex•ure (sā′krăl flek′shŭr) SYN caudal flexure.

sa•cral flex•ure of rec•tum (sā′krăl flek′shŭr rek′tŭm) The anteroposterior curve with concavity anteriorward of the first portion of the rectum.

sa•cral fo•ra•men (sā′krăl fōr-ā′mĕn) [TA] One of the openings between the fused sacral vertebrae transmitting the sacral nerves. The anterior sacral foramina transmit ventral primary rami of the sacral nerves. The posterior sacral foramina give passage to dorsal primary rami of the sacral nerves. See this page.

sa•cral•gi•a (sā-kral′jē-ă) Pain in the sacral region. SYN sacrodynia. [sacr- + G. *algos,* pain]

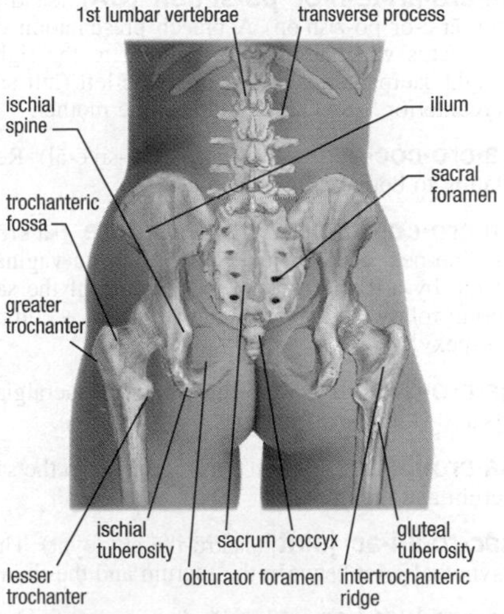

sacral foramen

sa•cral ky•pho•sis (sā′krăl kī-fō′sis) [TA] The normal, anteriorly concave curvature of the sacrum (sacral segment of the vertebral column), in which the primary curvature of the fetal embryo is maintained into maturity.

sa•cral nerves [S1–S5] (sā′krăl nĕrvz) Five nerves issuing from the sacral foramina on either side; the ventral branches of the first three enter into the formation of the sacral plexus, and the last two into the coccygeal plexus. SYN nervi sacrales [TA].

sa•cral plex•us (sā′krăl pleks′ŭs) Interconnected roots of the L4-S4 spinal nerves that innervate the lower extremities. SEE ALSO brachial plexus.

sa•cral splanch•nic nerves (sak′răl splangk′nik nĕrv) Branches from the sacral sympathetic trunk that pass to the inferior hypogastric plexus; part of the abdominopelvic (sympathetic) splanchnic nerves, but their specific function is unclear. They tend to be confused with the pelvic splanchnic nerves, which are much more significant structures. SYN nervi splanchnici sacrales [TA].

sa•cral ver•te•brae [S1–S5] (sak′răl vĕr′tĕ-brē) The segments of the vertebral column, usually five in number, that fuse to form the sacrum. SYN vertebrae sacrales [S1–S5].

sa•crec•to•my (sā-krek′tō-mē) Resection of a portion of the sacrum to facilitate an operation. [sacr- + G. *ektomē,* excision]

sa•cred bark (sā′krĕd bahrk) SYN cascara sagrada.

sacro-, sacr- Combining forms denoting muscular substance; resemblance to flesh. [L. *os sacrum,* sacred bone]

sa•cro•an•te•ri•or po•si•tion (SA) (sā′krō-an-tēr′ē-ŏr pŏ-zish′ŏn) A breech presentation of the fetus with the sacrum pointing to the right (right sacroanterior, RSA) or to the left (left sacroanterior, LSA) acetabulum of the mother.

sa•cro•coc•cyg•e•al (sā′krō-kok-sij′ē-ăl) Relating to both sacrum and coccyx.

sa•cro•col•po•pex•y pro•ce•dure (sā′krō-kol′pō-peks′ē prŏ-sē′jŭr) Supporting the vaginal vault by affixing it to the periosteum of the sacrum following a hysterectomy. [sacro- + colpo- + -pexy]

sa•cro•dyn•i•a (sā′krō-din′ē-ă) SYN sacralgia. [sacro- + G. *odynē,* pain]

sa•cro•il•i•ac (sā′krō-il′ē-ak) Relating to the sacrum and the ilium.

sac•ro•il•i•ac joint (sā′krō-il′ē-ak joynt) The synovial joint between the sacrum and the ilium.

sa•cro•lum•bar (sā′krō-lŭm′bahr) SYN lumbosacral.

sa•cro•pos•te•ri•or po•si•tion (SP) (sā′krō-pos-tēr′ē-ŏr pŏ-zish′ŏn) A breech presentation of the fetus with the sacrum pointing to the right (right sacroposterior, RSP) or to the left (left sacroposterior, LSP) sacroiliac articulation of the mother.

sa•cro•sci•at•ic (sā′krō-sī-at′ik) Relating to both sacrum and ischium.

sa•cro•spi•nal (sā′krō-spī′năl) Relating to the sacrum and the vertebral column above.

sa•cro•spi•nous lig•a•ment (sā′krō-spī′nŭs lig′ă-mĕnt) The fibrous band that passes from the ischial spine to the sacrum and coccyx.

sa•cro•spi•nous va•gi•nal vault sus•pen•sion pro•ce•dure (sā′krō-spī′nŭs vaj′i-năl vălt sŭs-pen′shŭn prŏ-sē′jŭr) Surgical repair of prolapsed vaginal vault by suturing to the sacrospinous ligament; done either vaginally or abdominally.

sa•cro•trans•verse (ST) po•si•tion (sā′krō-trans-vĕrs′ pŏ-zish′ŏn) A breech presentation of the fetus with its sacrum pointing to the right (right sacrotransverse, RST) or to the left (left sacrotransverse, LST) sacroiliac articulation of the mother.

sa•cro•tu•ber•ous lig•a•ment (sā′krō-tū′bĕr-ŭs lig′ă-mĕnt) The ligament that passes from the ischial tuberosity to the ilium, sacrum, and coccyx, transforming the sciatic notch to a large sciatic foramen, which is then further subdivided by the sacrospinous ligament.

sac•ro•u•ter•ine fold (sā′krō-yū′tĕr-in fōld) A fold of peritoneum, containing the rectouterine muscle, passing from the sacrum to the base of the broad ligament on either side, forming the lateral boundary of the rectouterine (Douglas) pouch.

sa•cro•ver•te•bral (sā′krō-vĕr′tĕ-brăl) Relating to the sacrum and the vertebrae above.

sa•crum, pl. **sa•cra** (sā′krŭm, -kră) The segment of the vertebral column forming part of the pelvis; a broad, slightly curved, spade-shaped bone, thick above, thinner below, closing in the pelvic girdle posteriorly; it is formed by the fusion of five originally separate sacral vertebrae; it articulates with the last lumbar vertebra, the coccyx, and the hip bone on either side. See this page. [L. (lit. sacred bone), neuter of *sacer* (*sacr-*), sacred]

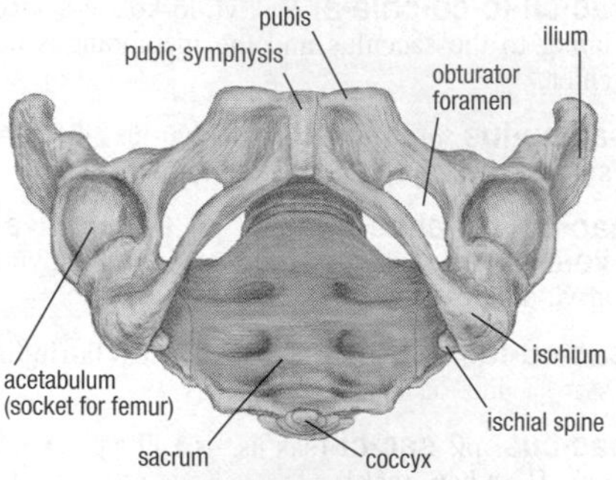

sacrum: inferior view

SAD Abbreviation for seasonal affective disorder.

sad•dle (sad′ĕl) **1.** A structure shaped like, or suggestive of, a seat or saddle as used in horseback riding. SYN sella. **2.** SYN denture base.

sad•dle•back ca•ter•pil•lar (sad′ĕl-bak kat′ĕr-pil-ĕr) *Sibine stimulea*, a cause of caterpillar dermatitis.

sad•dle block an•es•the•si•a (sad′ĕl blok an′es-thē′zē-ă) A form of spinal anesthesia limited in the area around the buttocks, perineum, and inner surfaces of the thighs.

sad•dle head (sad′ĕl hed) SYN clinocephaly.

sad•dle joint (sad′ĕl joynt) A biaxial synovial joint in which the double motion is effected by the opposition of two surfaces, each of which is concave in one direction and convex in the other.

sad•dle nose (sad′ĕl nōz) A nose with markedly depressed bridge, seen in congenital syphilis or after injury from trauma or operation.

sa•dism (sā′dizm) A form of perversion, often sexual in nature, in which a person finds pleasure in inflicting abuse and maltreatment. Cf. masochism, sadomasochism.

sa•dist (sā′dist) One who practices sadism.

sa•dis•tic (să-dis′tik) Pertaining to or characterized by sadism.

sa•do•mas•o•chism (sā′dō-mas′ŏ-kizm) A form of perversion marked by enjoyment of cruelty and humiliation, both received and dispensed. [sadism + masochism]

Sae·misch sec·tion (sā′mish sek′shŭn) Procedure of transfixing the cornea beneath an ulcer and then cutting from within outward through the base.

Sae·misch ul·cer (sā′mish ŭl′sĕr) A form of serpiginous keratitis, frequently accompanied by hypopyon.

Saen·ger op·er·a·tion (sāng′er op-ĕr-ā′shŭn) Cesarean section followed by careful closure of the uterine wound by three tiers of sutures.

Saen·ger sign (sāng′er sīn) A lost light reflex of the pupil returns after a short time in the dark; noted in cerebral syphilis but absent in tabes dorsalis.

safe sex (sāf seks) An umbrella term indicating sexual activity that has been undertaken using a latex condom to avoid sexually transmitted disease and any trasnmission of body fluids. Also called safer sex.

safe·ty lens (sāf′tē lenz) A lens that meets government specifications of impact resistance; the increased impact resistance required for safety lenses is obtained by tempering, by an ion-exchange process, or by using laminated or plastic lenses.

safe·ty mar·gin (sāf′tē mahr′jin) SYN margin of safety.

SAF fix·a·tive (fik′să-tiv) Abbreviation for sodium acetate-acetic acid-formalin fixative.

sag·it·tal (saj′i-tăl) **1.** Resembling an arrow. **2.** In an anteroposterior direction, referring to a sagittal plane or direction. [L. *sagitta,* an arrow]

sag·it·tal ax·is (saj′i-tăl ak′sis) DENTISTRY the line in the frontal plane around which the working side condyle rotates during mandibular movement.

sag·it·tal fon·ta·nelle (saj′i-tăl fon′tă-nel′) An occasional fontanellelike defect in the sagittal suture in the newborn. SYN Gerdy fontanelle.

sag·it·tal plane (saj′i-tăl plān) Originally (and strictly speaking) the sagittal plane is the median plane, and any other plane parallel to it is a parasagittal plane; in contemporary usage and in a broad sense, used for any plane parallel to the median, i.e., as a synonym for parasagittal.

sag·it·tal su·ture (saj′i-tăl sū′chŭr) Line of union between the two parietal bones. SYN interparietal suture.

sag·it·tal syn·os·to·sis (saj′i-tăl sin′os-tō′sis) SYN scaphocephaly.

sa·go spleen (sā′gō splēn) Amyloidosis in the spleen affecting chiefly the malpighian bodies.

SaH, **SAH** Abbreviation for subarachnoid hemorrhage.

Saint An·tho·ny dance, **Saint Vi·tus dance, Saint John dance** (sānt anth′ŏ-nē dans, vī′tŭs, jon) Obsolete eponyms for Sydenham chorea. [St. Anthony, Egyptian monk, about 250–350 CE]

Saint An·tho·ny fire (sānt anth′ŏ-nē fīr) **1.** SYN ergotism. **2.** Any of several inflammations or gangrenous conditions of the skin (e.g., erysipelas). [St. Anthony, Egyptian monk, about 250–350 CE]

Saint tri·ad (sānt trī′ad) The concurrence of hiatal hernia, diverticulosis, and cholelithiasis.

Sak·sen·ae·a va·si·for·mis (sak-sen′ē-ă vā-si-fōr′mis) One of the fungal species that cause zygomycosis; associated with localized bone and soft tissue infection, usually acquired as a result of traumatic injury.

sal Abbreviation for salt.

Sa·lah ster·nal punc·ture nee·dle (sah′lah stĕr′năl pungk′shŭr nē′dĕl) A wide-bore needle for obtaining samples of red marrow from the sternum.

sa·lic·y·late (să-lis′i-lāt) **1.** A salt or ester of salicylic acid. **2.** To treat foodstuffs with salicylic acid as a preservative.

sal·i·cyl·ic ac·id (sal′i-sil′ik as′id) A component of aspirin, derived from salicin and made synthetically; used externally as a keratolytic agent.

sal·i·cyl·ism (sal′i-sil′izm) Poisoning by salicylic acid or any of its compounds.

sa·line (sā′lēn) **1.** Relating to, of the nature of, or containing salt; salty. **2.** A salt solution, usually sodium chloride. [L. *salinus,* salty, fr. *sal,* salt]

sa·line ag·glu·ti·nin (sā′lēn ă-glū′ti-nin) An antibody that causes agglutination of erythrocytes when they are suspended either in saline or in a protein medium. SYN complete antibody.

sa·line so·lu·tion (sā′lēn sŏ-lū′shŭn) A solution of any salt; specifically, isotonic or physiologic sodium chloride solution; 0.9 g/100 mL water.

sa·li·va (să-lī′vă) A clear, tasteless, odorless, slightly acid (pH 6.8) viscid fluid, consisting of the secretion from the parotid, sublingual, and submandibular salivary glands and the mucous glands of the oral cavity; its function is to keep the mucous membrane of the mouth moist, to lubricate food during mastication, and to convert starch into maltose. SYN spittle. [L. akin to G. *sialon*]

sal·i·vant (sal′i-vănt) **1.** Causing a flow of saliva. **2.** An agent that increases the flow of saliva. SYN salivator.

sal·i·var·y (sal′i-var-ē) Relating to saliva. SYN sialic, sialine. [L. *salivarius*]

sal·i·var·y di·ges·tion (sal′i-var-ē di-jes′chŭn) The conversion of starch into sugar by the action of salivary amylase.

sal·i·var·y fis·tu·la (sal′i-var-ē fis′chū-lă) A pathologic communication between a salivary duct or gland and the cutaneous surface or the oral mucus.

sal·i·var·y gland (sal′i-var-ē gland) Any of the saliva-secreting exocrine glands of the oral cavity.

sa·li·va sub·sti·tute (să-lī′vă sŭb′sti-tūt) Artificial saliva is formulated to mimic natural saliva, but does not stimulate salivary gland activity. Commercially available products come in a variety of formulations including solutions, sprays, gels, and lozenges. Used to treat xerostomia (dry mouth). SYN artificial saliva.

sal·i·vate (sal′i-vāt) To cause an excessive flow of saliva.

sal·i·va·tion (sal′i-vā′shŭn) SYN sialism.

sal·i·va·tor (sal′i-vā-tŏr) SYN salivant (2).

Sal·mo·nel·la (sal′mō-nel′ă) A genus of aerobic to facultatively anaerobic bacteria containing gram-negative rods that are either motile or nonmotile. They are pathogenic for humans and other animals. The type species is *S. enterica choleraesuis*.

Sal·mo·nel·la en·ter·ic·a* ser·o·var *chol·er·ae·su·is (sal′mō-nel′ă en-ter′ik-ă sĕr′ō-vahr kōl-ĕr-ē′sū-is) A bacterial species found in pigs, in which it is an important secondary invader in the viral disease hog cholera; does not occur as a natural pathogen in other animals; occasionally causes acute gastroenteritis and enteric fever in humans; it is the type species of the genus *Salmonella*.

Sal·mo·nel·la en·ter·i·ca* ser·o·var *en·ter·i·ti·dis (sal′mō-nel′ă en-ter′ik-ă sĕr′ō-vahr en-tĕr-ī′ti-dis) A widely distributed bacterial species that can infect humans and animals, especially rodents; causes human gastroenteritis.

Sal·mo·nel·la en·ter·i·ca* se·ro·var *pa·ra·ty·phi A (sal′mō-nel′ă en-ter′ik-ă sĕr′ō-vahr par′ă-tī′fī) A bacterial species that is an important etiologic agent of enteric fever in developing countries.

Sal·mo·nel·la en·ter·i·ca* se·ro·var *pa·ra·typh·i B (sal′mō-nel′ă en-ter′ik-ă sĕr′ō-vahr par′ă-tī′fī) A bacterial species that consists of two distinct types of strains, those that produce enteric fever, found primarily in humans, and those producing gastroenteritis in humans, also found in animal species.

Sal·mo·nel·la en·ter·i·ca* se·ro·var *ty·phi·mu·ri·um (sal′mō-nel′ă en-ter′ik-ă sĕr′ō-vahr tī-fī-mŭr′ē-ŭm) A bacterial species causing food poisoning in humans; natural pathogen of all warm-blooded animals and is also found in snakes and pet turtles; worldwide, it is the most frequent cause of gastroenteritis due to *S. enterica* species.

Sal·mo·nel·la ty·phi (sal′mō-nel′ă tī′fī) A species that causes typhoid fever in humans and is transmitted in contaminated water and food. SYN typhoid bacillus.

sal·mo·nel·lo·sis (sal′mō-nĕl-ō′sis) Infection with bacteria of the genus *Salmonella*. Patients with sickle cell anemia and those with compromised immune systems are particularly susceptible. [*Salmonella* + G. *-osis,* condition]

sal·pin·gec·to·my (sal′pin-jek′tŏ-mē) Removal of the uterine tube. SYN tubectomy. [salping- + G. *ektomē,* excision]

sal·pin·ges (sal-pin′jēz) Plural of salpinx.

sal·pin·gi·an (sal-pin′jē-ăn) Relating to the uterine tube or to the auditory tube.

sal·pin·git·ic (sal′pin-jit′ik) Relating to salpingitis.

sal·pin·gi·tis (sal′pin-jī′tis) Inflammation of the uterine or the auditory tube. [salping- + G. *-itis,* inflammation]

sal·pin·gi·tis isth·mi·ca no·do·sa (sal′pin-jī′tis is′mi-kă nō-dō′să) A condition of the uterine tube characterized by nodular thickening of the tunica muscularis of the isthmic portion of the tube enclosing glandlike or cystic duplications of the lumen. SYN adenosalpingitis.

♲ **salpingo-, salping-** Combining forms denoting a tube (usually the uterine or auditory tubes). SEE ALSO tubo-. Cf. tubo-. [G. *salpinx,* trumpet (tube)]

sal·pin·go·cele (sal-ping′gō-sēl) Hernia of a uterine tube. [salpingo- + G. *kēlē,* hernia]

sal·pin·gog·ra·phy (sal′ping-gog′ră-fē) Radiography of the uterine tubes after the injection of radiopaque contrast medium. [salpingo- + G. *graphō,* to write]

sal·pin·gol·y·sis (sal′ping-gol′i-sis) Freeing the uterine tube from adhesions. [salpingo- + G. *lysis,* loosening]

sal·pin·go·ne·os·to·my (sal-ping′gō-nē-os′tŏ-mē) Surgical reopening of a uterine tube clubbed because of fimbrial adhesions. [salpingo- + neostomy]

sal·pin·go-o·oph·o·rec·to·my (sal-ping′gō-ō-of′ŏr-ek′tŏ-mē) Removal of the ovary and its uterine tube.

sal·pin·go-o·oph·o·ri·tis (sal-ping′gō-ō-of′ŏr-ī′tis) Inflammation of both uterine tube and ovary.

sal·pin·go-o·oph·o·ro·cele (sal-ping′gō-ō-of′ŏr-ō-sēl) Hernia of both ovary and uterine tube.

sal·pin·go·per·i·to·ni·tis (sal-ping′gō-per′i-tō-nī′tis) Inflammation of the uterine tube, perisalpinx, and peritoneum. [salpingo- + peritonitis]

sal·pin·go·pex·y (sal-ping′gō-pek-sē) Operative fixation of an oviduct. [salpingo- + G. *pēxis,* fixation]

sal·pin·go·phar·yn·ge·us mus·cle (sal-ping′gō-făr-in′jē-ŭs mŭs′ĕl) *Origin,* medial lamina of cartilaginous part of auditory tube; *insertion,* longitudinal muscular layer of pharynx in association with musculus palatopharyngeus; *action,* assists in elevating pharynx and, according to some, assists in opening the auditory tube during swallowing; *nerve supply,* pharyngeal plexus. SYN musculus salpingopharyngeus [TA].

sal·pin·go·plas·ty (sal-ping′gō-plas-tē) Surgical repair of the uterine tubes. SYN tuboplasty. [salpingo- + G. *plastos,* formed]

sal·pin·gor·rha·phy (sal′ping-gōr′ă-fē) Suture of the uterine tube. [salpingo- + G. *rhaphē,* stitching]

sal·pin·go·scope (sal-ping′gō-skōp) Endoscope inserted through the cervix for visual examination of the uterine tubes.

sal·pin·gos·to·my (sal′ping-gos′tŏ-mē) Establishment of an artificial opening in a uterine tube primarily as surgical treatment for an ectopic pregnancy. [salpingo- + G. *stoma,* mouth]

sal·pin·got·o·my (sal′ping-got′ŏ-mē) Incision into a uterine tube. [salpingo- + G. *tomē,* incision]

sal·pinx, pl. **sal·pin·ges** (sal′pingks, sal-pin′jēz) [TA] **1.** SYN uterine tube. **2.** SYN pharyngotympanic (auditory) tube. [G. a trumpet (tube)]

salt (sal) (sawlt) **1.** A compound formed by the interaction of an acid and a base, the ionizable hydrogen atoms of the acid being replaced by the positive ion of the base. **2.** Sodium chloride, the prototypical salt. **3.** A saline cathartic, especially magnesium sulfate, magnesium citrate, or sodium phosphate; often denoted by the plural, salts. [L. *sal*]

sal·ta·tion (sal-tā′shŭn) A dancing or leaping, as in a disease (e.g., chorea) or physiologic function (e.g., saltatory conduction). [L. *saltatio,* fr. *salto,* pp. *-atus,* to dance, fr. *salio,* to leap]

sal·ta·to·ry (sal′tă-tōr-ē) Pertaining to, or characterized by, saltation.

sal·ta·to·ry con·duc·tion (sal′tă-tōr-ē kŏn-dŭk′shŭn) Nerve conduction in which the impulse jumps from one node of Ranvier to the next.

sal·ta·to·ry ev·o·lu·tion (sal′tă-tōr-ē ev′ŏ-lū′shŭn) The theory that evolution of a new species from an older one may occur as a large jump, such as a major repatterning of chromosomes, rather than by gradual accumulation of small steps or mutations.

sal·ta·to·ry spasm (sal′tă-tōr-ē spazm) A spasmodic affection of the muscles of the lower extremities. SYN Bamberger disease (1).

Sal·ter-Har·ris frac·ture (sawl′tĕr-har′is frak′shŭr) Classification of epiphysial fracture types 1 to 5.

Sal·ter in·cre·men·tal lines (sawl′tĕr in′kră-ment′ăl līnz) Transverse lines sometimes seen in dentin; attributable to improper calcification.

salt·ing out (sawl′ting owt) The precipitation of a protein from its solution by saturation or partial saturation with such neutral salts as sodium chloride, magnesium sulfate, or ammonium sulfate.

salt-los·ing ne·phri·tis (sawlt-lū′zing nĕ-frī′tis) A rare disorder resulting from renal tubular damage of a variety of etiologies; mimics adrenocortical insufficiency in that abnormal renal loss of sodium chloride occurs, accompanied by hyponatremia, azotemia, acidosis, dehydration, and vascular collapse. SYN Thorn syndrome.

salt wast·ing (sawlt wāst′ing) Inappropriately large renal excretion of salt despite the apparent need of the body to retain it.

sa·lu·bri·ous (să-lū′brē-ŭs) Healthful, usually in reference to climate. [L. *salubris,* healthy, fr. *salus,* health]

sal·u·re·sis (sal′yūr-ē′sis) Excretion of sodium in the urine. [L. *sal,* salt, + G. *ourēsis,* uresis (urination)]

sal·u·ret·ic (sal′yūr-et′ik) Facilitating the renal excretion of sodium.

sal·u·tar·y (sal′yū-tar-ē) Healthful; wholesome. [L. *salutaris*]

salve (sav) SYN ointment. [A.S. *sealf*]

Salz·mann nod·u·lar cor·ne·al de·gen·er·a·tion (sahlts′mahn noj′ū-lăr kōr′nē-ăl dē-jen′ĕr-ā′shŭn) Large and prominent nodules of a solid, opaque material that stands out from the surface of the cornea; occurs with chronic inflammation.

sa·mar·i·um (Sm) (să-mar′ē-ŭm) A metallic element of the lanthanide group, atomic no. 62, atomic wt. 150.36. [bands indicating its presence first found in the spectrum of *samarskite,* a mineral named after Col. von Samarski, 19th-century Russian mine official]

same-day sur·ger·y (sām-dā′ sŭr′jĕr-ē) SYN ambulatory surgery.

sa·men·to (să-men′tō) SYN cat's claw.

sam·ple (sam′pĕl) **1.** A specimen of a whole entity small enough to involve no threat or damage to the whole; an aliquot. **2.** A selected subset of a population; a sample may be random or nonrandom (haphazard), representative or nonrepresentative. **3.** A piece or portion of a whole that will demonstrate the characteristics or qualities of that whole. [M.E. *ensample,* fr. L. *exemplum,* example]

sam·pling (sam′pling) The policy of inferring the behavior of a whole batch by studying a fraction of it. [MF *essample,* fr. L. *exemplum,* taking out]

sam·pling bi·as (sam′pling bī′ăs) Systematic error due to study of a nonrandom sample of a population.

Sam·ter syn·drome (sahm′ter sin′drōm) A triad of asthma, nasal polyps, and aspirin intolerance.

san·a·to·ri·um (san′ă-tōr′ē-ŭm) An institution for the treatment of chronic disorders and a place for recuperation under medical supervision. Cf. sanitarium. [Mod. L. neuter of *sanatorius,* curative, fr. *sano,* to cure, heal]

san·a·to·ry (san′ă-tōr-ē) Health-giving; conducive to health. [Mod. L. *sanatorius*]

sand (sand) The fine granular particles of quartz and other crystalline rocks, or a gritty material resembling sand. [A.S.]

Sand·hoff dis·ease (sahnd′hawf di-zēz′) An infantile form of G_{M2} gangliosidosis characterized by a defect in the production of hexosaminidases A and B; it resembles Tay-Sachs disease, but occurs predominantly (if not entirely) in non-Jewish children; accumulation of glucoside and ganglioside G_{m2}, caused by mutation in hexoaminidase B gene (HEX B) on chromosome 5q.

sands of Sa·har·a (sandz să-har′ă) SYN diffuse lamellar keratitis.

sand·wich gen·er·a·tion (sand′wich jen′ĕr-ā′shŭn) A term used to describe a generation of people who care for their aging parents or other relatives while supporting their own children: essentially "in the middle;" hence, the term sandwich.

sane (sān) Of sound mind; mentally healthy. [L. *sanus*]

San·fi·lip·po syn·drome (san-fi-lip′pō sin′drōm) An error of mucopolysaccharide metabolism, with excretion of large amounts of heparan sulfate in the urine; characterized by severe mental retardation with hepatomegaly; skeleton may be normal or may present mild changes similar to those in Hurler syndrome; several different types (A, B, C, and D) have been identified according to the enzyme deficiency; autosomal recessive inheritance.

♻ **sangui-, sanguin-, sanguino-** Combining forms denoting blood, bloody. [G. *sanguis*]

san·gui·fa·cient (sang′gwi-fā′shĕnt) SYN hemopoietic. [sangui- + L. *facio,* to make]

san·guif·er·ous (sang-gwif′ĕr-ŭs) Conveying blood. SYN circulatory (2). [sangui- + L. *fero,* to carry]

san·gui·fi·ca·tion (sang′gwi-fi-kā′shŭn) SYN hemopoiesis. [sangui- + L. *facio,* to make]

san·guine (sang′gwin) **1.** SYN plethoric. **2.** Optimistic or cheerful. SYN sanguineous (3). [L. *sanguineus*]

san·guin·e·ous (sang-gwin′ē-ŭs) **1.** Relating to blood; bloody. **2.** SYN plethoric. **3.** SYN sanguine (2). [L. *sanguineus*]

san·guin·o·lent (sang-gwin′ō-lĕnt) Bloody; tinged with blood. [L. *sanguinolentus*]

san·gui·no·pu·ru·lent (sang′gwi-nō-pyū′rū-lĕnt) Denoting exudate or matter containing blood and pus. [sanguino- + L. *purulentus,* festering (suppurative), fr. *pus,* pus]

san·guiv·or·ous (sang-gwiv′ŏr-ŭs) Bloodsucking, as applied to certain bats, leeches, and insects. [sangui- + L. *voro,* to devour]

sa·ni·es (sā′nē-ēz) A thin, blood-stained, purulent discharge. [L.]

sa·ni·o·pu·ru·lent (sā′nē-ō-pyūr′ū-lĕnt) Characterized by bloody pus. [L. *sanies,* thin, bloody matter, + *purulentus,* festering (suppurative), fr. *pus,* pus]

sa·ni·o·se·rous (sā′nē-ō-sēr′ŭs) Characterized by blood-tinged serum.

sa·ni·ous (sā′nē-ŭs) Relating to sanies; ichorous and blood-stained.

san·i·tar·i·an (san′i-tar′ē-ăn) One who is skilled in sanitation and public health. [L. *sanitas,* health, fr. *sanus,* sound]

san·i·tar·i·um (san′i-tar′ē-ŭm) A health resort. Cf. sanatorium. [L. *sanitas,* health]

san·i·tar·y (san′i-tar-ē) Healthful; conducive to health; usually in reference to a clean environment. [L. *sanitas,* health]

san·i·tar·y nap·kin (san′i-tar-ē nap′kin) Pad worn to absorb menstrual discharge.

san·i·ta·tion (san′i-tā′shŭn) Use of measures designed to promote health and prevent disease; development and establishment of conditions in the environment favorable to health. [L. *sanitas,* health]

san·i·ti·za·tion (san′i-tī-zā′shŭn) The process of making something sanitary.

san·i·ty (san′i-tē) Soundness of mind, emotions, and behavior; of a sound degree of mental health. [L. *sanitas,* health]

San Joa·quin Val·ley Fe·ver (san wah-kēn′ val′ē fē′vĕr) SYN Valley fever.

SA node SEE sinuatrial node.

San•som sign (san′sĕm sīn) In mitral stenosis, apparent duplication of the second heart sound.

San•son im•ag•es (sahn[h]-sōn[h]′ im′ăj-ĕz) SYN Purkinje-Sanson images.

San•ta Ma•ri•a (sahn′tă mă-rē′ă) SYN feverfew. [Sp., holy Mary]

San•ti•ni boom•ing sound (sahn-tē′nē būm′ ing sownd) A sonorous booming sound heard on auscultatory percussion of a hydatid cyst.

San•to•ri•ni ca•nal (sahn-tō-rē′nē kă-nal′) SYN accessory pancreatic duct.

San•to•ri•ni con•cha (sahn-tō-rē′nē kong′kă) SYN supreme nasal concha.

San•to•ri•ni duct (sahn-tō-rē′nē dŭkt) SYN accessory pancreatic duct.

San•to•ri•ni plex•us (sahn-tō-rē′nē pleks′ŭs) Venous plexus on ventral and lateral prostatic surfaces.

SaO_2 Abbreviation for oxygen saturation.

SaO_2 test (test) Abbreviation for oxygen saturation test.

sa•phe•nous (să-fē′nŭs) Relating to or associated with a saphenous vein; denoting a number of structures in the thigh and leg.

sa•phe•nous nerve (să-fē′nŭs nĕrv) A branch of the femoral, extending from the femoral triangle to the foot, becoming subcutaneous on the medial side of the knee; it supplies cutaneous branches to the skin of the leg and foot, by way of infrapatellar and medial crural branches. SYN nervus saphenus [TA].

sa•phe•nous o•pen•ing (să-fē′nŭs ō′pĕn-ing) The opening in the fascia lata inferior to the medial part of the inguinal ligament through which the saphenous vein passes to enter the femoral vein. SYN fossa ovalis (2).

sapo-, sapon- Combining forms meaning soap. [L. *sapo*]

sap•o•na•ceous (sap′ō-nā′shŭs) Soapy; relating to or resembling soap.

sa•pon•i•fi•ca•tion (să-pon′i-fi-kā′shŭn) Conversion into soap, denoting the hydrolytic action of an alkali on fat, especially on triacylglycerols. [sapo- (*sapon-*) + L. *facio,* to make]

sap•o•nins (sap′ō-ninz) Glycosides of plant origin characterized by properties of foaming in water and of lysing cells; powerful surfactants; many have antibiotic activities.

sap•phism (saf′izm) SYN lesbianism. [*Sapphō,* homosexual Greek poet, native of the island of Lesbos]

sapro-, sapr- Combining forms meaning rotten, putrid, decayed. [G. *sapros*]

sap•robe (sap′rōb) An organism that lives on dead organic material. USAGE NOTE This term is preferable to saprophyte, because bacteria and fungi are no longer regarded as plants. [sapro- + G. *bios,* life]

sa•pro•bic (să-prō′bik) Pertaining to a saprobe.

sap•ro•gen (sap′rō-jen) An organism living on dead organic matter and causing its decay. [sapro- + G. *-gen,* producing]

sap•ro•gen•ic, sa•prog•e•nous (sap′rō-jen′ ik, să-proj′ĕ-nŭs) Causing or resulting from decay.

sap•ro•phyte (sap′rō-fīt) An organism that grows on dead organic matter, plant or animal. SEE ALSO saprobe. [sapro- + G. *phyton,* plant]

sap•ro•phyt•ic (sap′rō-fit′ik) Relating to a saprophyte.

sap•ro•zo•ic (sap′rō-zō′ik) Living in decaying organic matter; especially denoting certain protozoa. [sapro- + G. *zōikos,* relating to animals]

sap•ro•zo•o•no•sis (sap′rō-zō′ŏ-nō′sis) A zoonosis the agent of which requires both a vertebrate host and a nonanimal (food, soil, plant) reservoir or developmental site for completion of its cycle. [sapro- + G. *zōon,* animal, + *nosos,* disease]

Sar•ci•na (sahr′si-nă) A genus of nonmotile, strictly anaerobic bacteria containing gram-positive cocci, which divide in three perpendicular planes, producing regular packets of eight or more cells. Saprophytic and facultatively parasitic species occur. The type species is *S. ventriculi.* [L. *sarcina,* a pack, bundle, fr. *sarcio,* to mend, patch]

sarco- Combining form denoting muscular substance or a resemblance to flesh. [G. *sarx* (*sark-*), flesh]

sar•co•blast (sahr′kō-blast) SYN myoblast. [sarco- + G. *blastos,* germ]

sar•co•car•ci•no•ma (sahr′kō-kahr′si-nō′mă) A malignant neoplasm that contains elements of carcinoma and sarcoma. SEE sinuatrial node. SEE ALSO sarcoma.

Sar•co•di•na (sahr′kō-dī′nă) The amebae; a subphylum of protozoa possessing pseudopodia or locomotive protoplasmic flow for movement. Most species are free living. [Mod. L. fr. G. *sarx,* flesh]

sar•coid (sahr′koyd) SYN sarcoidosis. [sarco- + G. *eidos,* resemblance]

sar•coid•al gran•u•lo•ma (sahr-koyd′ăl gran′ yū-lō′mă) A nonnecrotizing epithelioid cell granuloma similar to those seen in sarcoidosis.

sar•coid•o•sis (sahr′koy-dō′sis) A systemic granulomatous disease of unknown cause, especially involving the lungs with resulting fibrosis, but also involving lymph nodes, skin, liver, spleen, eyes, phalangeal bones, and parotid glands; granulomas are composed of epithelioid and multinucleated giant cells with little or no necrosis. See this page. SYN Besnier-Boeck-Schaumann disease, Boeck disease, sarcoid. [sarcoid + G. *-osis,* condition]

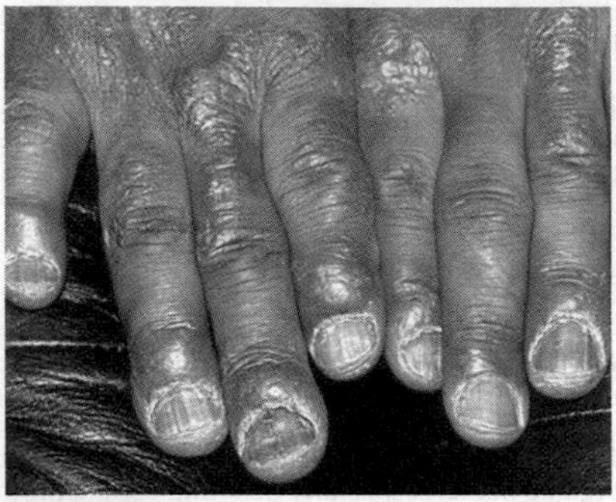

sarcoidosis

sar•co•lem•ma (sahr′kō-lem′ă) The plasma membrane of a muscle fiber; formerly, the delicate connective tissue of the endomysium was included under this term by some. [sarco- + G. *lemma,* husk]

sar•co•lem•mal, **sar•co•lem•mic, sar•co•lem•mous** (sahr′kō-lem′ăl, -lem′ik, -lem′ŭs) Relating to the sarcolemma.

sar•co•ma (sahr-kō′mă) A connective tissue neoplasm, usually highly malignant, formed by proliferation of mesodermal cells. [G. *sarkōma,* a fleshy excrescence, fr. *sarx,* flesh, + *-oma,* tumor]

sar•co•ma•toid (sahr-kō′mă-toyd) Resembling a sarcoma. [sarcoma + G. *eidos,* resemblance]

sar•co•ma•to•sis (sahr′kō-mă-tō′sis) Occurrence of several sarcomatous growths on different parts of the body. [sarcoma + G. *-osis,* condition]

sar•com•a•tous (sahr-kō′mă-tŭs) Relating to or of the nature of sarcoma.

sar•co•mere (sahr′kō-mēr) The segment of a myofibril between two adjacent Z lines, representing the functional unit of striated muscle. [sarco- + G. *meros,* part]

sar•co•pe•ni•a (sahr′kō-pē′nē-ă) Progressive reduction in muscle cross-section and mass with aging. [sarco- + G. *penia,* poverty]

sar•co•plasm (sahr′kō-plazm) The nonfibrillar cytoplasm of a muscle fiber. [sarco- + G. *plasma,* a thing formed]

sar•co•plas•mic (sahr′kō-plaz′mik) Relating to sarcoplasm.

sar•co•plas•mic re•tic•u•lum (sahr′kō-plaz′mik rĕ-tik′yū-lŭm) The endoplasmic reticulum of skeletal and cardiac muscle; the complex of vesicles, tubules, and cisternae forming a continuous structure around striated myofibrils, with a repetition of structure within each sarcomere.

sar•co•poi•et•ic (sahr′kō-poy-et′ik) Forming muscle. [sarco- + G. *poiēsis,* a making]

Sar•cop•tes sca•bi•ei (sahr-kop′tēz skā′bē-ī) The itch mite, varieties of which are distributed worldwide and affect humans and many animals. The mite burrows into the skin and lays eggs within the burrow; intense itching and rash develop near the burrow in about a month. SEE ALSO scabies, mange. [sarco- + G. *koptō,* to cut; L. *scabies,* scurf]

sar•cop•tic (sahr-kop′tik) Of, relating to, or caused by mites of the genus *Sarcoptes* or other members of the family Sarcoptidae.

sar•cop•tid (sahr-kop′tid) Common name for members of the Sarcoptidae, a family of mites that includes the genera *Sarcoptes*, *Knemidokoptes*, and *Notoedres*.

sar•co•sis (sahr-kō′sis) **1.** An abnormal increase of flesh. **2.** A multiple growth of fleshy tumors. **3.** A diffuse sarcoma involving the whole of an organ. [G. *sarkōsis,* the growth of flesh, fr. *sarx,* flesh]

sar•cos•to•sis (sahr-kos-tō′sis) Ossification of muscular tissue. [sarco- + G. *osteon,* bone, + *-osis,* condition]

sar•cot•ic (sahr-kot′ik) **1.** Relating to sarcosis. **2.** Causing an increase of flesh.

sar•co•tu•bules (sahr′kō-tū′byūlz) The continuous system of membranous tubules in striated muscle that corresponds to the smooth endoplasmic reticulum of other cells.

sar•cous (sahr′kŭs) Relating to muscular tissue; fleshy. [G. *sarx,* flesh]

sar•don•ic grin (sahr-don′ik grin) SYN risus caninus.

sar•gra•mos•tim (sahr-gram′ŏs-tim) A recombinant human granulocyte-macrophage colony-stimulating factor; used to protect against infection in the presence of acute myelogenous leukemia and in bone marrow transplants.

sa•rin (GB) (sah′rēn) A nonpersistent nerve agent developed by Germany during World War II. Its NATO code is GB, and it was used in the large-scale terrorist attack on the Tokyo subway system in 1995. SEE ALSO Adamsite, bromobenzylcyanide, CA, CN, Cr, Cs, vomiting agent.

SARS Abbreviation for severe acute respiratory syndrome.

sar•to•ri•us mus•cle (sahr-tōr′ē-ŭs mŭs′ĕl) *Origin*, anterior superior spine of ilium; *insertion*, medial border of tuberosity of tibia; *action*, flexes thigh and leg, rotates leg medially and thigh laterally; *nerve supply*, femoral. SYN musculus sartorius [TA].

Sart•well in•cu•ba•tion mo•del (sahrt′wel ing′kyū-bā′shun mod′ĕl) Mathematical model based on empiric observations, showing that incubation periods for communicable diseases have a log-normal distribution; model holds true for certain kinds of cancers that have well-defined external causes.

sat, **sat.** Abbreviation for saturated.

sat•el•lite (sat′ĕ-līt) **1.** A minor structure accompanying a more important or larger one, e.g., a vein accompanying an artery, or a small or secondary lesion adjacent to a larger one. **2.** The posterior member of a pair of gregarine gamonts in syzygy, several of which may be found in some species. [L. *satelles* (*sattelit-*), attendant]

sat•el•lite ab•scess (sat′ĕ-līt ab′ses) An abscess closely associated with a primary abscess.

sat•el•lit•o•sis (sat′ĕ-lī-tō′sis) **1.** A condition marked by an accumulation of neuroglia cells around the neurons of the central nervous system, often as a prelude to neuronophagia. **2.** The presence of satellite, smaller structures or lesions. [L. *satelles* (*satellit-*), an attendant, + G. *-ōsis,* condition]

sa•ti•a•tion (sā′shē-ā′shŭn) The state produced by fulfillment of a specific need, such as hunger or thirst. [L. *satio,* pp. *-atus,* to fill, satisfy]

sat. sol., **sat. soln.** Abbreviation for saturated solution.

Satt•ler veil (saht′ler vāl) A diffuse edema of the corneal epithelium that may develop after wearing contact lenses.

sat•u•rate (sach′ŭr-āt) **1.** To impregnate to the greatest possible extent. **2.** To neutralize; to satisfy all the chemical affinities of a substance (as by converting all double bonds to single bonds). **3.** To dissolve a substance up to that concentration beyond which the addition of more results in two phases. [L. *saturo,* pp. *-atus,* to fill, fr. *satur,* sated]

sat•u•rat•ed col•or (sach′ŭr-āt′ĕd kŏl′ŏr) A color containing a minimum amount of whiteness.

sat•u•rat•ed fat (sach′ŭr-āt′ĕd fat) A type of fat found chiefly in foods that come from animals and certain vegetable oils, which raise blood cholesterol levels and thus increase risk of atherosclerosis.

sat•u•rat•ed fat free (sach′ŭr-āt-ĕd fat frē) A product so labeled contains, by F.D.A. order, less than 0.5 g saturated fat per serving and 0.5 g trans-fatty acid per serving.

sat•u•ra•ted fat•ty ac•id (sach′ŭr-āt′ĕd fat′ē as′id) A fatty acid, the carbon chain of which contains no ethylenic or other unsaturated linkages between carbon atoms (e.g., stearic acid and palmitic acid); called saturated because it is incapable of absorbing any more hydrogen.

sat•u•rat•ed so•lu•tion (sat. sol., sat. soln.) (sach′ŭr-āt′ĕd sŏ-lū′shŭn) A solution that contains all of a solute capable of being dissolved in the solvent; a substance in equilibrium with excess undissolved substance.

sat•u•ra•tion (sach′ŭr-ā′shŭn) **1.** Impregnation of one substance by another to the greatest possible extent. **2.** Neutralization, as of an acid by an alkali. **3.** The concentration of a dissolved substance that cannot be exceeded. **4.** OPTICS SEE saturated color. **5.** Filling of all the available sites on an enzyme molecule by its substrate, or on a hemoglobin molecule by oxygen (symbol S_{O_2}) or carbon monoxide (symbol S_{CO}). [L. *saturatio*, fr. *saturo*, to fill, fr. *satis*, enough]

sat•u•ra•tion in•dex (sach′ŭr-ā′shŭn in′deks) An indication of the relative concentration of hemoglobin in the red blood cells, calculated as grams of hemoglobin per 100 mL (expressed as percent of normal) ÷ hematocrit value (expressed as percentage of normal) = saturation index.

sat•u•ra•tion sound pres•sure level (SSPL) (sach′ŭr-ā′shŭn sownd presh′ŭr lev′ĕl) A measure of the maximum output of a hearing aid.

sat•ur•nine (sat′ŭr-nīn) **1.** Relating to lead. **2.** Due to or symptomatic of lead poisoning. [Mediev. L. *saturninus,* fr. *saturnus,* lead, fr. L. *saturnus,* the god and planet Saturn]

sat•y•ri•a•sis (sat′ir-ī′ă-sis) Satyromania; excessive sexual excitement and behavior in the male; the counterpart of nymphomania in the female. [G. *satyros,* a satyr]

sau•cer•i•za•tion (saw′sĕr-ī-zā′shŭn) Excavation of tissue to form a shallow depression, performed in wound treatment to facilitate drainage from infected areas.

Sa•var•y bou•gies (sav′ăr-ē bū-zhēz′) Silastic tapered-tip bougies used over a guide wire in esophageal dilatation.

saw (saw) A metal operating instrument having an edge of sharp, toothlike projections, for dividing bone, cartilage, or plaster; edges may be attached to a rigid band, a flexible wire or chain, or a motorized oscillator. [A.S. *saga*]

sax•i•tox•in (sak′si-tok′sin) A potent neurotoxin found in shellfish, such as the mussel or the clam, produced by the dinoflagellate *Gonyaulax catenella*, which is ingested by the shellfish; the cause of poisoning due to eating California sea mussels, scallops, and Alaskan butterclams.

Sb Symbol for antimony.

SBE Abbreviation for subacute bacterial endocarditis.

SBS Abbreviation for shaken baby syndrome.

SC Abbreviation for subcutaneous.

Sc Symbol for scandium.

scab (skab) A crust formed by coagulation of blood, pus, serum, or a combination of these, on the surface of an ulcer, erosion, or other type of wound. [A.S. *scaeb*]

scab•i•ci•dal (skā′bi-sī′dăl) Destructive to scabies mites.

scab•i•cide (skā′bi-sīd) An agent lethal to scabies mites.

sca•bies (skā′bēz) A dermal eruption caused by the mite *Sarcoptes scabiei* var. *hominis;* the female of the species burrows into the skin, producing a vesicular eruption with intense pruritus between the fingers, on the male or female genitalia, on the buttocks, and elsewhere on the trunk and extremities. See this page, B8. [L. *scabo,* to scratch]

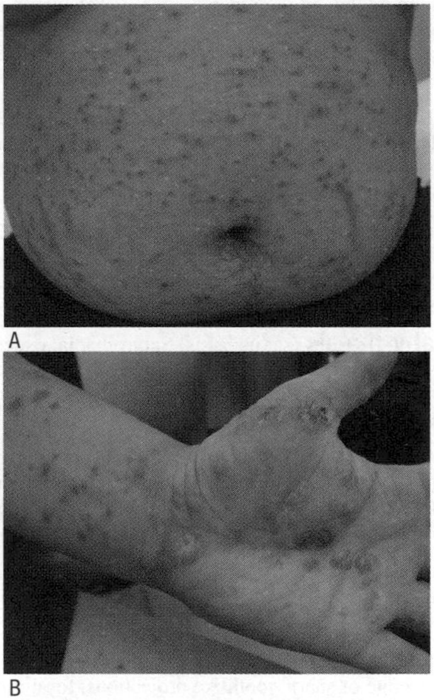

A

B

scabies: (A) abdomen; (B) arm and hand

sca•la, pl. **sca•lae** (skā′lă, -lē) One of the cavities of the cochlea winding spirally around the modiolus. [L. a stairway]

sca•la me•di•a (skā′lă mē′dē-ă) [TA] SYN cochlear duct.

sca•la tym•pa•ni (skā′lă tim′păn-ē) [TA] The division of the spiral canal of the cochlea lying on the basal side of the spiral lamina.

sca•la ves•tib•u•li (skā′lă ves-tib′yū-lī) [TA] The division of the spiral canal of the cochlea lying on the apical side of the spiral lamina and vestibular membrane. SYN vestibular canal.

scald (skawld) **1.** To burn by contact with a hot liquid or steam. **2.** The lesion resulting from such contact. [L. *excaldo,* to wash in hot water]

scald•ed mouth syn•drome (skawld′ĕd mowth sin′drōm) A syndrome in which the patient complains of a burning sensation of the tongue, lips, throat, or palate, likened to scalding caused by hot liquids; clinically the tissues appear normal; it has been associated with therapy involving angiotensin-converting enzyme inhibitors.

scale (skāl) **1.** Graduations, as on a scientific scale or instruments to mark units or divisions thereof to measure quantity. **2.** SYN squama. **3.** PSYCHOLOGY/PSYCHIATRY a standardized test for measuring psychological, personality, or behavioral characteristics. SEE ALSO test, score. **4.** A small, thin plate of horny epithelium, resembling a fish scale, cast off from the skin. **5.** To desquamate. **6.** DENTISTRY/DENTAL HYGIENE/DENTAL ASSISTING to remove calculus from the teeth. **7.** A device by which some property can be measured. [L. *scala,* a stairway]

sca•le•nec•to•my (skā′lĕ-nek′tŏ-mē) Resection of the scalene muscles. [scalene + G. *ektomē,* excision]

sca•lene mus•cles (skā′lēn mŭs′ĕlz) A group of three muscles (e.g., anterior, middle, posterior) located in the side of the neck.

sca•le•not•o•my (skā′lĕ-not′ŏ-mē) Division or section of the anterior scalene muscle. [scalene + G. *tomē,* incision]

sca•len•us an•te•ri•or mus•cle (skā-lē′nŭs an-tēr′ē-ŏr mŭs′ĕl) Lateral muscle of inferior half of neck; *origin*, anterior tubercles of transverse processes of third to sixth cervical vertebrae; *insertion*, scalene tubercle of first rib; *action*, raises first rib; *nerve supply*, cervical plexus. SYN anterior scalene muscle, musculus scalenus anterior, musculus scalenus anticus.

sca•le•nus me•di•us mus•cle (skā-lē′nŭs mē′dē-us mŭs′ĕl) *Origin*, costotransverse lamellae of transverse processes of second to sixth cervical vertebrae; *insertion*, first rib posterior to subclavian artery; *action*, raises first rib; *nerve supply*, cervical plexus. SYN musculus scalenus medius.

sca•le•nus mi•ni•mus mus•cle (skā-lē′nŭs min′i-mus mŭs′ĕl) An occasional independent muscular fasciculus between the scalenus anterior and medius, and having the same action and innervation.

sca•le•nus pos•ter•i•or mus•cle (skā-lē′nus pos-tēr′ē-ŏr mŭs′ĕl) Lateral muscle of inferior half of neck; *origin*, posterior tubercles of transverse processes of fourth to sixth cervical vertebrae; *insertion*, lateral surface of second rib; *action*, elevates second rib; *nerve supply*, cervical and brachial plexuses. SYN musculus scalenus posterior, musculus scalenus posticus, posterior scalene muscle.

scal•ing (skāl′ing) DENTISTRY removal of accretions from the crowns and roots of teeth by use of special instruments.

scal•lop•ing (skal′ŏ-ping) A series of indentations or erosions on a normally smooth margin of a structure.

scalp (skalp) The skin and subcutaneous tissue, normally hair bearing, covering the neurocranium. [M. E. fr. Scand. *skalpr,* sheath]

scal•pel (skalp′ĕl) A knife used in surgical dissection. [L. *scalpellum;* dim. of *scalprum,* a knife]

scalp hair (skalp hār) A hair of the head.

scal•prum (skal′prŭm) **1.** A large, strong scalpel. **2.** A raspatory. [L. chisel, penknife, fr. *scalpo,* pp. *scalptus,* to carve]

scal•y (skāl′ē) SYN squamous.

scan (skan) **1.** To survey by traversing with an active or passive sensing device. **2.** The image, record, or data obtained by scanning, usually identified by the technology or device employed; e.g., CT scan, radionuclide scan, ultrasound scan. **3.** Abbreviated form of scintiscan, usually identified by the organ or structure examined; e.g., brain scan, bone scan.

scan•di•um (Sc) (skan′dē-ŭm) A metallic element; atomic no. 21, atomic wt. 44.955910. [L. *Scandia,* Scandinavia, where discovered]

scan•ner (skan′ĕr) A device or instrument that scans.

scan•ning (skan′ing) The act of imaging by traversing with an active or passive sensing device, often identified by the technology or device employed.

scan•ning e•lec•tron mi•cro•scope (skan′ing ĕ-lek′tron mī′krŏ-skōp) A microscope in which the object in a vacuum is scanned in a raster pattern by a slender electron beam, generating reflected and secondary electrons from the specimen surface that are used to modulate the image on a synchronously scanned cathode ray tube; with this method a three-dimensional image is obtained, with both high resolution and great depth of focus.

scan•ning e•qual•i•za•tion ra•di•og•ra•phy (skan′ing ē′kwăl-ī-zā′shŭn rā′dē-og′ră-fē) An electronically enhanced method of radiography in which a small x-ray beam is scanned over the patient while its attenuation is measured, providing feedback to modulate beam intensity to equalize average x-ray film exposure.

scan•ning speech (skan′ing spēch) Measured or metered, often slow, speech.

scan•o•gram (skan′ō-gram) A radiographic technique for showing true dimensions by moving a narrow orthogonal beam of x-rays along the length of the structure being measured, e.g., the lower extremities. [scan- + G. *gramma,* something written]

Scan•zo•ni ma•neu•ver (skahn-tsō′nē mă-nū′vĕr) Forceps rotation and traction in a spiral course, with reapplication of forceps for delivery.

sca•pha (skā′fă) The longitudinal furrow between the helix and the antihelix of the auricle. [L. fr. G. *skaphē,* skiff]

scapho- Prefix meaning a scapha, scaphoid. [G. *skaphē,* skiff, boat]

scaph•o•ce•phal•ic (skaf′ō-sĕ-fal′ik) Denoting or relating to scaphocephaly.

scaph•o•ceph•a•lism (skaf′ō-sef′ă-lizm) SYN scaphocephaly.

scaph•o•ceph•a•ly (skaf′ō-sef′ă-lē) A form of craniosynostosis that results in a long narrow head. SYN cymbocephaly, sagittal synostosis, scaphocephalism, tectocephaly. [scapho- + G. *kephalē,* head]

scaph•oid (skaf′oyd) Boat-shaped; hollowed. SEE ALSO scaphoid (bone). SYN navicular. [scapho- + G. *eidos,* resemblance]

scaph•oid ab•do•men (skaf′oyd ab′dŏ-mĕn) A condition in which the anterior abdominal wall is sunken and presents a concave rather than a convex contour. SYN navicular abdomen.

scaph•oid (bone) (skaf′oyd bōn) The largest bone of the proximal row of the carpus on the lateral (radial) side, articulating with the radius, lunate, capitate, trapezium, and trapezoid. SYN os scaphoideum.

scaph•oid scap•u•la (skaf′oyd skap′yū-lă) A scapula in which the vertebral border below the level of the spine presents concavity instead of the normal convexity; the scaphoid type of scapula (Graves) is a scapula in which the vertebral border between the spine and the teres major process is either straight or tends toward concavity.

scap•tion (skap′shŭn) Elevation of the glenohumeral joint in the plane of the scapula, which is approximately 30 degrees of horizontal adduction from the frontal plane. [*scap*ula + eleva*tion*]

scap•u•la, gen. and pl. **scap•u•lae** (skap′yū-lă, -lē) [TA] A large, triangular, flattened bone lying over the ribs, posteriorly on either side, articulating laterally with the clavicle at the acromioclavicular joint and the humerus at the glenohumeral joint. It forms a functional joint with the chest wall, the scapulothoracic joint. See page 1392. SYN shoulder blade. [L. *scapulae,* the shoulder blades]

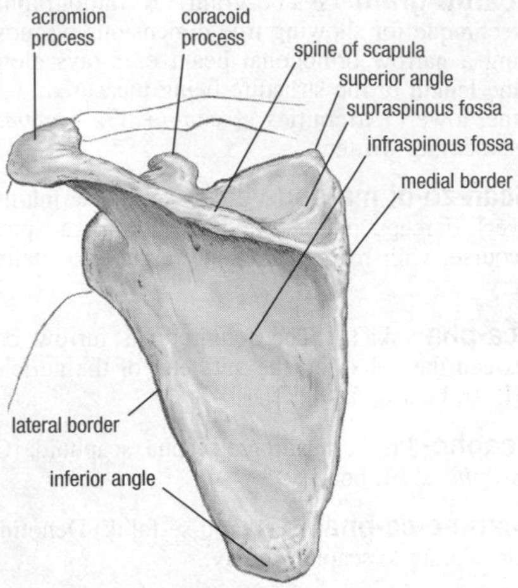

scapula: posterior view

scap•u•la a•la•ta (skap′yū-lă ă-lā′tă) SYN winged scapula.

scap•u•lar (skap′yū-lăr) Relating to the scapula.

scap•u•lar ab•duc•tion (skap′yū-lăr ab-dŭk′shŭn) Forward movement of the scapula.

scap•u•lec•to•my (skap′yū-lek′tŏ-mē) Excision of the scapula. [scapula + G. *ektomē,* excision]

scapulo- Prefix denoting scapula, scapular. [L. *scapulae,* shoulder blades]

scap•u•lo•cla•vic•u•lar (skap′yū-lō-klă-vik′yū-lăr) **1.** SYN acromioclavicular. **2.** SYN coracoclavicular.

scap•u•lo•cos•tal syn•drome (skap′yū-lō-kos′tăl sin′drōm) Pain of insidious development in the upper or posterior part of the shoulder radiating into the neck and occiput, down the arm, or around the chest; there may be numbness or tingling in the fingers; attributed to an alteration from the normal relationship between the scapula and posterior wall of the thorax.

scap•u•lo•hu•mer•al (skap′yū-lō-hyū′mĕr-ăl) Relating to both scapula and humerus. SEE ALSO glenohumeral.

scap•u•lo•hu•mer•al rhythm (skap′yū-lō-hyū′mĕr-ăl ridh′ĕm) Coordinated rotational movement of the scapula that accompanies abduction, adduction, internal and external rotation, extension, and flexion of the humerus; roughly a 2:1 ratio.

scap•u•lo•pex•y (skap′yū-lō-pek-sē) Operative fixation of the scapula to the chest wall or to the spinous process of the vertebrae. [scapulo- + G. *pēxis,* fixation]

scap•u•lo•thor•a•cic (ST) (skap′yū-lō-thōr-as′ik) Relating to the scapula and the dorsal thorax. SEE ALSO shoulder complex.

scap•u•lo•thor•a•cic joint (skap′yū-lō-thōr-as′ik joynt) The articulation between the scapula and the dorsal thorax; it is not a true anatomic joint because it lacks a synovial capsule and there are muscles between the anterior surface of the scapula and the thorax. SEE ALSO pectoral girdle, shoulder girdle.

sca•pus, pl. **sca•pi** (skā′pŭs, -pī) A shaft or stem. [L. shaft, stalk]

scar (skahr) The fibrous tissue replacing normal tissues destroyed by injury or disease. See page B11. [G. *eschara,* scab]

scar car•ci•no•ma (skahr kahr′si-nō′mă) Carcinoma of the lung, usually adenocarcinoma, arising from a peripheral lung scar or associated with interstitial fibrosis in a honeycomb lung.

scar•i•fi•ca•tion (skar′i-fi-kā′shŭn) The making of a number of superficial incisions in the skin. [L. *scarifico,* to scratch, fr. G. *skariphos,* a style for sketching]

scar•i•fi•ca•tor (skar′i-fi-kā-tŏr) An instrument for scarification, consisting of a number of concealed spring-projected cutting blades, set close together, which make superficial incisions in the skin.

scar•la•ti•na (skahr′lă-tē′nă) An acute exanthematous disease, caused by infection with streptococcal organisms producing erythrogenic toxin, marked by fever and other constitutional disturbances, and a generalized eruption of closely aggregated points or small macules of a bright red color followed by desquamation; mucous membrane of the mouth and fauces is usually also involved. SYN scarlet fever. [through It. fr. Mediev. L. *scarlatum,* scarlet, a scarlet cloth]

scar•la•ti•na hem•or•rha•gi•ca (skahr′lă-tē′nă hem′ōr-raj′i-kă) A form of scarlatina in which blood extravasates into the skin and mucous membranes, giving the eruption a dusky hue; frequent bleeding from the nose and into the intestine also occurs.

scar•la•ti•nal (skahr′lă-tē′năl) Relating to scarlatina.

scar•la•ti•ni•form (skahr′lă-tē′ni-fōrm) Resembling scarlatina, denoting a rash.

scar•let fe•ver (skahr′lĕt fē′vĕr) SYN scarlatina.

scar•let rash (skahr′lĕt rash) Bright red exanthem sometimes accompanying an infection.

Scar•pa fasc•i•a (skahr′pă fash′ē-ă) The deeper, membranous or lamellar part of the subcutaneous tissue of the lower abdominal wall; it is continuous with the superficial perineal (Colles) fascia.

Scar•pa meth•od (skahr′pă meth′ŏd) Cure of

aneurysm by ligation of the artery at some distance above the sac.

Scar·pa staph·y·lo·ma (skahr′pă staf′i-lō′mă) SYN posterior staphyloma.

Scar·pa tri·an·gle (skahr′pă trī′ang-gĕl) SYN femoral triangle.

scar·ring al·o·pe·ci·a (skahr′ing al′ō-pē′shē-ă) Skin condition in which hair follicles are irreversibly destroyed by scarring processes including trauma, burns, lupus erythematosus, lichen planopilaris, scleroderma, folliculitis decalvans, or of uncertain cause (pseudopelade). SYN cicatricial alopecia.

scataemia [Br.] SYN scatemia.

sca·te·mi·a (skă-tē′mē-ă) Intestinal autointoxication. SYN scataemia. [scato- + G. *haima,* blood]

♻ **scato-** Combining form meaning feces. SEE ALSO copro-, sterco-. [G. *skōr* (*skat-*), excrement]

scat·o·log·ic (skat′ŏ-loj′ik) Pertaining to scatology.

sca·tol·o·gy (skă-tol′ŏ-jē) **1.** The scientific study and analysis of feces, for physiologic and diagnostic purposes. SYN coprology. **2.** The study relating to the psychiatric aspects of excrement or excremental (anal) function. [scato- + G. *logos,* study]

sca·tos·co·py (skă-tos′kŏ-pē) Examination of the feces for diagnostic purposes. [scato- + G. *skopeō,* to view]

scat·ter (skat′ĕr) **1.** A change in direction of a photon or subatomic particle, as the result of a collision or interaction. **2.** The secondary radiation resulting from the interaction of primary radiation with matter.

scat·tered ra·di·a·tion (skat′tĕrd rā′dē-ā′shŭn) Radiation that has been deflected from its path by impact with matter. This form of secondary radiation is emitted diffusely by the tissues of the patient during exposure to x-radiation. SEE ALSO secondary radiation.

sca·ven·ger re·cep·tor (skav′ĕn′jĕr rĕ-sep′tŏr) A receptor on macrophages that binds preferentially to oxidized low-density lipoprotein (LDL), causing macrophages to internalize the LDL.

Sce·do·spor·i·um (sē-dō-spō′rē-ŭm) An imperfect fungus of the form-class Hyphomycetes; anamorph of *Pseudallescheria.*

Sce·do·spor·i·um ap·i·o·sper·mum (sē-dō-spō′rē-ŭm ā-pē-ō-spĕr′mŭm) The imperfect state of the fungus *Pseudallescheria boydii*, one of the fungi that cause mycetoma in humans.

Sce·do·spor·i·um pro·lif·i·cans (sē-dō-spō′rē-ŭm prō-lif′i-kanz) A mold; a rare cause of subcutaneous fungal infection. Associated with disseminated disease in bone marrow transplant patients and other immunocompromised patients.

Schäf·fer re·flex (shāf′ĕr rē′fleks) In cases of injury to the corticospinal tract, the great toe is dorsiflexed when the skin over the Achilles tendon is pinched.

Schantz dis·ease (shahnts di-zēz′) SYN Albert disease.

Scha·pi·ro sign (shă-pī′rō sīn) In myocardial weakness, no slowing of the pulse occurs when the patient lies down.

Schatz·ki ring (shots′kē ring) A narrow constriction of the distal esophagus identified by its characteristic radiographic appearance.

Schau·dinn fix·a·tive (show′din fiks′ă-tiv) A solution of mercuric chloride, sodium chloride, alcohol, and glacial acetic acid, used on wet smears for cytologic fixation.

Sche·de meth·od (shā′dĕ meth′ŏd) Filling of the defect in bone, after removal of a sequestrum or scraping away of carious material, by allowing the cavity to fill with blood that may become organized (Schede clot).

Schei·be hear·ing im·pair·ment (shī′bĕ hēr′ing im-pār′mĕnt) Auditory disorder due to cochleosaccular dysplasia; usually autosomal recessive inheritance.

Scheie syn·drome (shā sin′drōm) Allelic to Hurler syndrome but with a much milder phenotype; characterized by α-L-iduronidase deficiency, corneal clouding, deformity of the hands, aortic valve involvement, and normal intelligence; autosomal recessive inheritance, caused by mutation in the alpha-L-iduronidase gene (IUDA) on chromosome 4p.

Schei·ner ex·per·i·ment (shī′ner eks-per′i-mĕnt) A demonstration of accommodation; through two minute holes in a card, separated from each other by less than the diameter of the pupil, one looks at a pin; at a short distance from the eye the pin appears double; as it is moved from the eye a point is found where it appears single, and beyond which it remains single for the emmetropic eye, but for the myopic eye it soon again becomes double.

sche·ma, pl. **sche·ma·ta** (skē′mă, skē-mah′tă) **1.** A plan, outline, or arrangement. SYN scheme. **2.** In sensorimotor theory, the organized unit of cognitive experience. [G. *schēma,* shape, form]

scheme (skēm) SYN schema (1).

Schenck dis·ease (shengk di-zēz′) SYN sporotrichosis.

Scheu·er·mann dis·ease (shoy′ĕr-mahn di-zēz′) Epiphysial osteonecrosis of adjacent vertebral bodies in the thoracic spine. SYN juvenile kyphosis.

Schick test (shik test) An assessment for susceptibility to *Corynebacterium diphtheriae* toxin. Schick test toxin is injected into the skin; people lacking toxin-neutralizing antibodies may have a positive reaction, which consists of an area of redness.

Schiff re•a•gent (shif rē-ā′jĕnt) An aqueous solution of basic fuchsin or pararosaniline that is decolorized by sulfur dioxide; commonly prepared by addition of hydrochloric acid to a dye solution containing a metabisulphite or bisulphite salt; used for aldehydes and in histochemistry to detect polysaccharides, DNA, and proteins.

Schil•der dis•ease (shil′der di-zēz′) Term used to describe at least two separate disorders described by Schilder: 1) diffuse sclerosis or encephalitis periaxialis diffusa; a nonfamilial disorder affecting primarily children and young adults and characterized by progressive dementia, visual disturbances, deafness, pseudobulbar palsy, and hemiplegia or quadriplegia. Most patients die within a few years of onset; pathologically, there is a large, asymmetric area of myelin destruction, sometimes involving an entire cerebral hemisphere, and typically with extension across the corpus callosum. 2) the leukodystrophies. SYN encephalitis periaxialis diffusa.

Schil•ler test (shil′er test) A test for non-glycogen-containing areas of the portio vaginalis of the cervix, which may be the site of early carcinoma; such areas fail to stain dark brown with iodine solution; loss of glycogen due to erosion and other benign conditions may also give a positive result.

Schil•ling blood count (shil′ing blŭd kownt) A method of counting blood in which the polymorphonuclear neutrophils are separated into four groups according to the number and arrangement of the nuclear masses in these cells.

Schil•ling test (shil′ing test) A procedure for determining the amount of vitamin B12 excreted in the urine, using cyanocobalamin tagged with a radioisotope of cobalt.

schin•dy•le•sis (skin′di-lē′sis) [TA] SYN wedge-and-groove joint. [G. *schindylēsis,* splintering]

♻**schisto-** Prefix indicating cleft, division. SEE ALSO schizo-. [G. *schistos,* split]

schis•to•ce•li•a (skis′tō-sē′lē-ă) Congenital fissure of the abdominal wall. SYN schistocoelia. [schisto- + G. *koilia,* a hollow]

schistocoelia [Br.] SYN schistocelia.

schis•to•cor•mi•a (skis′tō-kōr′mē-ă) Congenital clefting of the trunk, the lower limbs of the fetus usually being imperfectly developed. SYN schistosomia. [schisto- + G. *kormos,* trunk of a tree]

schis•to•cyte (skis′tō-sīt) SYN keratocyte (2). [schisto- + G. *kytos,* cell]

schis•to•cy•to•sis (skis′tō-sī-tō′sis) The occurrence of many schistocytes in the blood.

schis•to•glos•si•a (skis′tō-glos′ē-ă) Congenital fissure or cleft of the tongue. [schisto- + G. *glōssa,* tongue]

Schis•to•so•ma (skis′tō-sō′mă) A genus of trematodes, including the blood flukes that cause schistosomiasis; characterized by elongatation, marked sexual dimorphism, location of adults in the smaller blood vessels of their host, and use of water snails as intermediate hosts. [schisto- + G. *sōma,* body]

Schis•to•so•ma hae•ma•to•bi•um (skis′tō-sō′mă hē-mā-tō′bē-ŭm) The vesical blood fluke, a species that occurs as a parasite in the portal system and mesenteric veins of the bladder (causing human schistosomiasis haematobium) and rectum; found throughout Africa and the Middle East; intermediate hosts are *Bulinus truncatus* and other snails.

Schis•to•so•ma ja•pon•i•cum (skis′tō-sō′mă ja-pon′ik-ŭm) The Asian or Japanese blood fluke, a species that causes schistosomiasis japonica, with extensive pathology from encapsulation of the eggs, particularly in the liver. The intermediate hosts are amphibious snails; other animals, such as pigs, oxen, cattle, and dogs, serve as reservoir hosts.

schis•to•so•mal der•ma•ti•tis (skis′tō-sōm′ăl dĕr′mă-tī′tis) A sensitization response to repeated cutaneous invasion by cercariae of bird, mammal, or human schistosomes. SYN swimmer's itch (2), water itch (2).

Schis•to•so•ma man•so•ni (skis′tō-sō′mă man-sō′nī) A common species of trematodes characterized by large eggs with a strong lateral spine and transmitted by planorbid snails of the genus *Biomphalaria;* causes schistosomiasis mansoni.

schis•to•some (skis′tō-sōm) Common name for a member of the genus *Schistosoma.*

schis•to•so•mi•a (skis′tō-sō′mē-ă) SYN schistocormia. [schisto- + G. *sōma,* body]

schis•to•so•mi•a•sis (skis′tō-sō-mī′ă-sis) Infection with a species of *Schistosoma;* manifestations of this often chronic and debilitating disease vary with the infecting species but depend in large measure on tissue reaction (granulation and fibrosis) to the eggs deposited in venules and in the hepatic portal system, the latter resulting in portal hypertension and esophageal varices, as well as liver damage leading to cirrhosis. SEE ALSO schistosomal dermatitis.

schis•to•so•mi•a•sis hae•ma•to•bi•um (skis′tō-sō-mī′ă-sis hē-mā-tō′bē-ŭm) Infection with *Schistosoma haematobium,* the eggs of which invade the urinary tract, causing cystitis and hematuria, and possibly an increased likelihood of bladder cancer. SYN endemic hematuria.

schis•to•so•mi•a•sis ja•pon•i•ca, **Jap•a•nese schis•to•so•mi•a•sis** (skis′tō-sō-mī′ă-sis ja-pon′ik-ă, jap′ă-nēz′) Infection with *Schistosoma japonicum*, characterized by dysenteric symptoms, painful enlargement of the liver and spleen, dropsy, urticaria, and progressive anemia.

schis•to•so•mi•a•sis man•so•ni (skis′tō-sō-mī′ă-sis man-sō′nī) Infection with *Schistosoma mansoni*, the eggs of which invade the wall of the large intestine and the liver, causing irritation, inflammation, and ultimately fibrosis. SYN Mansoni schistosomiasis.

schis•to•thor•ax (skis′tō-thōr′aks) Congenital cleft of the thoracic wall. [schisto- + G. *thōrax*, thorax]

schiz•am•ni•on (skiz-am′nē-on) An amnion developing, as in the human embryo, by the formation of a cavity within the embryoblast. [schiz- + amnion]

schiz•ax•on (skiz-ak′son) An axon divided into two branches. [schiz- + G. *axōn*, axis]

♻ **schizo-**, **schiz-** Combining forms denoting split, cleft, division; schizophrenia. SEE ALSO schisto-. [G. *schizō*, to split or cleave]

schiz•o•af•fec•tive (skits′ō-ă-fek′tiv) Having an admixture of symptoms suggestive of both schizophrenia and affective (mood) disorder.

schiz•o•af•fec•tive psy•cho•sis (skits′ō-ă-fek′tiv sī-kō′sis) Psychotic disturbance in which there is a mixture of schizophrenic and manic-depressive symptoms.

schiz•o•gen•e•sis (skits′ō-jen′ĕ-sis) Reproduction by fission. SYN fissiparity. [schizo- + G. *genesis*, origin]

schiz•og•o•ny (skits-og′ŏ-nē) Multiple fission in which the nucleus first divides and then the cell divides into as many parts as there are nuclei; called merogony if daughter cells are merozoites, sporogony if daughter cells are sporozoites, or gametogony if daughter cells are gametes. [schizo- + G. *gonē*, generation]

schiz•o•gy•ri•a (skits′ō-jī′rē-ă) Deformity of the cerebral convolutions marked by occasional interruptions of their continuity. [schizo- + G. *gyros*, circle (convolution)]

schiz•oid (skits′oyd) Socially isolated, withdrawn, having few (if any) friends or social relationships; resembling the personality features characteristic of schizophrenia, but in a milder form. SEE ALSO schizoid personality. [schizo-(phrenia), + G. *eidos*, resemblance]

schiz•oid per•son•al•i•ty, **schiz•oid per•son•al•i•ty dis•or•der** (skits′oyd pĕr-sŏn-al′i-tē, dis-ōr′dĕr) An enduring and pervasive pattern of behavior in adulthood characterized by social withdrawal, emotional coldness or aloofness or restriction, and indifference to others.

schiz•ont (skits′ont) A sporozoan trophozoite (vegetative form) that reproduces by schizogony, producing a varied number of daughter trophozoites or merozoites. [schizo- + G. *ōn* (*ont-*), a being]

schiz•o•nych•i•a (skits′ō-nik′ē-ă) Splitting of the nails. [schizo- + G. *onyx*, nail]

schiz•o•pha•si•a (skits′ō-fā′zē-ă) The disordered speech (word salad) of the schizophrenic patient. [schizo- + G. *phasis*, speech]

schiz•o•phre•ni•a (skits′ō-frē′nē-ă) A common type of psychosis, characterized by abnormalities in perception, content of thought, and thought processes (hallucinations and delusions), and extensive withdrawal of one's interest from other people and the outside world, the investment of it being instead in one's own mental life. [schizo- + G. *phrēn*, mind]

schiz•o•phren•ic (skits′ō-fren′ik) Relating to, characteristic of, or suffering from one of the schizophrenias.

schiz•o•trich•i•a (skits′ō-trik′ē-ă) A splitting of the hairs at their ends. [schizo- + G. *thrix*, hair]

schiz•o•typ•al per•son•al•i•ty dis•or•der, **schiz•o•typ•al per•son•al•i•ty** (skits′ō-tīp′ăl pĕr-sŏn-al′i-tē dis-ōr′dĕr) An enduring and pervasive pattern of behavior in adulthood characterized by discomfort with and reduced capacity for close relationships, cognitive or perceptual distortions, and eccentric behavior, that is people with such a disorder hold ideas that are considered unusual; have difficulty relating to others.

Schlat•ter dis•ease, **Schlat•ter-Os•good dis•ease** (shlah′ter di-zēz′, shlah′ter-oz′gud) SYN Osgood-Schlatter disease.

Schlemm ca•nal (shlem kă-nal′) SYN sinus venosus sclerae.

Schle•sing•er sign (shlā′sing-ĕr sīn) SYN Pool phenomenon (1).

Schmid•el a•nas•to•mo•ses (shmī′dĕl a-nas′tŏ-mō′sēz) Abnormal channels of communication between the caval and portal venous systems.

Schmidt-Lan•ter•man in•ci•sures (shmit lahn′ter-mahn in-sī′zhŭrz) Funnel-shaped interruptions in the regular structure of the myelin sheath of nerve fibers.

Schmidt syn•drome (shmit sin′drōm) **1.** Unilateral paralysis of a vocal cord, the velum palati, trapezius, and sternocleidomastoid. **2.** The association of primary hypothyroidism, primary adrenocortical insufficiency, and insulin-dependent diabetes mellitus.

Schmorl fer•ric-fer•ri•cy•a•nide re•duc•tion stain (shmōrl fer′ik fer′i-cī′ă-nīd rĕ-dŭk′shŭn stān) A stain to test for reducing substances in tissues, including melanin, argentaffin granules, thyroid colloid, keratin, keratohyalin, and lipofuscin pigments; ferricyanide is converted into ferrocyanide, which is converted to insoluble Prussian blue in the presence of ferric ions.

Schmorl nod•ule (shmōrl noj′yūl) Prolapse of the nucleus pulposus through the vertebral body endplate into the spongiosa of an adjacent vertebra.

Schmorl pic•ro•thi•o•nin stain (shmōrl pik′rō-thī′ŏ-nin stān) A stain for compact bone that employs thionin and picric acid solutions to produce blue to blue-black staining of bone canaliculi and cells; bone matrix is yellowish and cartilage ground substance is purple.

Schnei•der car•mine (shnī′dĕr kahr′mīn) A stain consisting of a 10% solution of carmine in 45% acetic acid, used for fresh chromosome preparations.

Schnei•der first-rank symp•toms (shnī′dĕr fīrst-rank simp′tŏms) Those symptoms that, when present, indicate that the diagnosis of schizophrenia is likely, provided that organic or toxic etiology is ruled out: delusion of control, thought broadcasting, thought withdrawal, thought insertion, hearing one's thoughts spoken aloud, auditory hallucinations that comment on one's behavior, and auditory hallucinations in which two voices carry on a conversation.

Schnitz•ler syn•drome (shnits′ler sin′drōm) Tense, generalized chronic urticaria, joint or bone pain, and monoclonal gammopathy of kappa type.

Scho•ber test (shō′ber test) A measure of lumbar spine motion in which parallel horizontal lines are drawn 10 cm above and 5 cm below the lumbosacral junction in the erect subject; with maximum forward flexion, the distance between the lines increases at least 5 cm in normal patients but far less in patients with anklylosing spondylitis.

Schön•lein pur•pu•ra (shern′līn pŭr′pŭr-ă) SYN Henoch-Schönlein purpura.

school nurse prac•ti•tion•er (skūl nŭrs prak-tish′ŭn-ĕr) A registered nurse qualified as a nurse practitioner to work in a school system, state or private.

school pho•bi•a (skūl fō′bē-ă) A young child's sudden aversion to or fear of attending school, usually considered a manifestation of separation anxiety.

Schroe•der op•er•a•tion (shrĕr′der op-ĕr-ā′shŭn) Excision of diseased endocervical mucosa.

Schu•chardt op•er•a•tion (shū′kahrt op-ĕr-ā′shŭn) A paravaginal rectal displacement incision, a surgical technique of making the upper vagina accessible for fistula closure or radical surgery through the vagina.

Schüff•ner dots (shēf′ner dots) Fine, round, uniform red or red-yellow dots (as colored with Romanowsky stains) characteristically observed in erythrocytes infected with *Plasmodium vivax* and *P. ovale*, but not ordinarily found in *P. malariae* and *P. falciparum* infections.

Schül•ler phe•nom•e•non (shēl′er fĕ-nom′ĕ-non) When patients with hemiplegia walk, if the disorder is functional they turn to the unaffected side; if it is organic, they turn to the affected side.

Schül•ler syn•drome (shēl′er sin′drōm) SYN Hand-Schüller-Christian disease.

Schultz-Charl•ton re•ac•tion (shūlts kahrl′ton rē-ak′shŭn) The specific blanching of a scarlatinal rash at the site of intracutaneous injection of scarlatina antiserum.

Schult•ze mech•a•nism (shūlt′sĕ mek′ă-nizm) Expulsion of the placenta with the fetal surface foremost.

Schult•ze phan•tom (shūlt′sĕ fan′tŏm) A model of a female pelvis used in demonstrating the mechanism of childbirth and the application of forceps.

Schult•ze pla•cen•ta (shūlt′sĕ plă-sen′tă) A placenta that appears at the vulva with the glistening fetal surface (amnion) presenting.

Schult•ze sign (shūlt′sĕ sīn) In latent tetany, tapping the tongue causes its depression with a concave dorsum.

Schwal•be line (shvahl′bĕ līn) A thin white or irregularly pigmented line observed on gonioscopy; represents the peripheral margin of the Descemet membrane.

Schwal•be ring (shvahl′bĕ ring) SYN anterior limiting ring.

Schwann cells (shwahn selz) Cells of ectodermal (neural crest) origin that compose a continuous envelope around each nerve fiber of peripheral nerves. SYN neurilemma cells, neurolemma cells.

schwan•no•ma (shwah-nō′mă) A benign, encapsulated neoplasm in which the fundamental component is structurally identical to a syncytium of Schwann cells; the neoplastic cells proliferate within the endoneurium, and the perineurium forms the capsule. The neoplasm may originate from a peripheral or sympathetic nerve, or from various cranial nerves, particularly the eighth nerve; when the nerve is small, it is usually found (if at all) in the capsule of the neoplasm; if the nerve is large, the neurilemmoma may develop within the sheath of the nerve, the fibers of which may then spread over the surface of the capsule as the neoplasm enlarges. Microscopically, neurilemmoma is composed of combinations of two patterns, Antoni types A and B, either of which may be predominant in various examples of neurilemmomas. SEE ALSO neurofibroma. SYN neurilemmoma. [Theodor *Schwann* + -oma]

schwan•no•sis (shwah-nō′sis) A nonneoplastic proliferation of Schwann cells in the perivascular spaces of the spinal cord; seen particularly in older patients, especially those with diabetes mellitus.

Schwart•ze sign (shvahrt′zĕ sīn) Vascularization of the promontory of the middle ear resulting in a rosy glow that can be seen through the tympanic membrane; a sign of otosclerosis. SEE ALSO otosclerosis. SYN promontory flush.

sci•age (sē-ahzh′) A to-and-fro, sawlike movement of the hand in massage. [Fr. *scie,* saw]

sci•at•ic (sī-at′ik) **1.** Relating to or situated in the neighborhood of the ischium or hip. Ischial or sciatic. SYN ischiadic, ischial, ischiatic. **2.** Relating to sciatica. [Mediev. L. *sciaticus,* a corruption of G. *ischiadikos,* fr. *ischion,* the hip joint]

sci•at•i•ca (sī-at′i-kă) Pain in the lower back and hip radiating down the back of the thigh into the leg, initially attributed to sciatic nerve dysfunction (hence the term), but now known to usually be due to herniated lumbar disc compromising the L5 or S1 root. SEE sciatic.

sci•a•tic bur•sa of glu•te•us max•i•mus (sī-at′ik bŭr′să glū-tē′ŭs maks′i-mŭs) The bursa between the gluteus maximus muscle and the tuberosity of the ischium.

sci•at•ic fo•ra•men (sī-at′ik fōr-ā′mĕn) Either of two foramina formed by the sacrospinous and sacrotuberous ligaments crossing the sciatic notches of the hip bone: greater sciatic foramen and lesser sciatic foramen.

sci•at•ic her•ni•a (sī-at′ik hĕr′nē-ă) Protrusion of intestine through the great sacrosciatic foramen. SYN ischiocele.

sci•at•ic nerve (sī-at′ik nĕrv) Arises from the sacral plexus, passes through the greater sciatic foramen and down the thigh, deep to the long head of biceps femoris nerve; at the apex of the popliteal fossa it divides into the common peroneal and tibial nerves, although the two may separate at higher levels. See this page. SYN nervus ischiadicus [TA].

sci•ence (sī′ĕns) **1.** The branch of knowledge that produces theoretic explanations of natural phenomena based on experiments and observations. **2.** An area of such knowledge that is restricted to explaining a limited class of phenomena. [L. *scientia,* knowledge, fr. *scio,* to know]

sci•en•ti•fic the•or•y (sī′ĕn-tif′ik thē′ŏr-ē) A proposition that can be tested and potentially disproved; failure to disprove or refute it increases confidence in it, but it cannot be considered as proven.

sci•en•to•met•rics (sī′ĕn-tō-met′riks) The measurement of scientific output, and the impact of scientific findings (e.g., on public policy). [L. *scientia,* science, knowledge, fr. *scio,* to know, + G. *metron,* measure, + -ics]

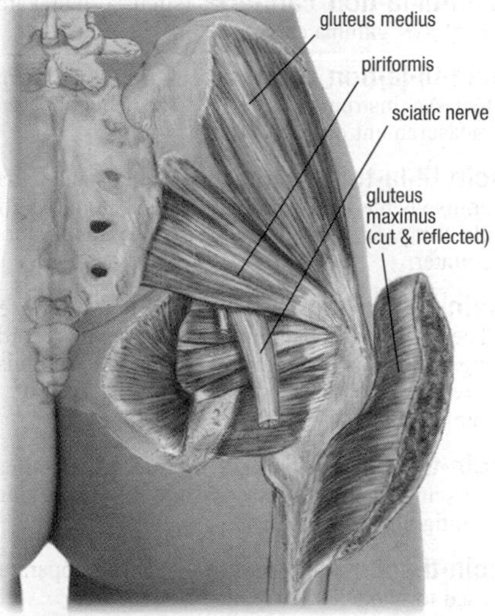

sciatic nerve

scim•i•tar sign (si′mi-tahr sīn) A curvilinear structure seen in the lung roentgenographically, associated with anomalous pulmonary venous drainage, suggesting the sickle shape of a Turkish saber; also used to refer to the scalloped shape of the sacrum in spinal dysraphism with anterior meningocele.

scin•ti•cis•tern•og•ra•phy (sin′ti-sis′tĕrn-og′ră-fē) Cisternography performed with a radiopharmaceutical and recorded with a stationary imaging device.

scin•ti•gram (sin′ti-gram) SYN scintiscan. [L. *scintilla,* spark, + G. *gramma,* something written]

scin•ti•graph•ic (sin′ti-graf′ik) Relating to or obtained by scintigraphy.

scin•tig•ra•phy (sin-tig′ră-fē) A diagnostic procedure consisting of the administration of a radionuclide with an affinity for the organ or tissue of interest, followed by recording of the distribution of the radioactivity with a stationary or scanning external scintillation camera.

scin•til•lat•ing sco•to•ma (sin′ti-lā′ting skō-tō′mă) A localized area of blindness edged by brilliantly colored shimmering lights (teichopsia); usually a prodromal symptom of migraine. SEE ALSO fortification spectrum.

scin•til•la•tion (sin′ti-lā′shŭn) **1.** Flashing or sparkling; a subjective sensation as of sparks or flashes of light. **2.** In radiation measurement, the light produced by an ionizing event in a phosphor, as in a crystal or liquid scintillator. SEE ALSO scintillation counter. [L. *scintilla,* a spark]

scin•til•la•tion cam•er•a (sin′ti-lā′shŭn kam′ ĕr-ă) SYN gamma camera.

scin•til•la•tion count•er (sin′ti-lā′shŭn kown′ tĕr) An instrument used for the detection and measurement of radioactivity.

scin•til•la•tor (sin′ti-lā-tŏr) A substance that emits visible light when hit by a subatomic particle x-ray or gamma ray. SEE ALSO scintillation counter.

scin•ti•pho•tog•ra•phy (sin′ti-fō-tog′ră-fē) The process of obtaining a photographic recording of the distribution of an internally administered radiopharmaceutical with the use of a gamma camera.

scin•ti•scan (sin′ti-skan) The record obtained by scintigraphy. SEE ALSO scan. SYN photoscan, scintigram.

scin•ti•scan•ner (sin′ti-skan′ĕr) The apparatus used to make a scintiscan.

scir•rhous (skir′ŭs) Hard; relating to a scirrhus.

scir•rhous car•ci•no•ma (skir′ŭs kahr′si-nō′ mă) A hard carcinoma, fibrous in nature, resulting from a desmoplastic reaction by the stromal tissue. See page B19. SYN fibrocarcinoma.

scis•sion (sizh′ŏn) **1.** A separation, division, or splitting, as in fission. **2.** SYN cleavage (2). [L. *scissio,* fr. *scindo,* pp. *scissus,* to cleave]

scis•sors (siz′ŏrz) An instrument with two blades, moving on a pivot, which cut against each other. SYN shears. [L. *scindo,* pp. *scissus,* to cut]

scis•sors gait (siz′ŏrz gāt) A manner of walking cross-legged, mimicking the motion of scissors; commonly associated with spastic paraplegia.

scis•su•ra, pl. **scis•su•rae** (shi-sūr′ă, -rē) **1.** Cleft or fissure. **2.** A splitting. SYN scissure. [L.]

scis•sure (sish′ŭr) SYN scissura.

scle•ra, pl. **scle•ras**, **scler•ae** (sklēr′ă, -ăz, -ē) [TA] A portion of the fibrous tunic forming the outer envelope of the eye, except for its anterior one sixth, which is the cornea. SYN sclerotica. [Mod. L. fr. G. *sklēros,* hard]

scler•ad•e•ni•tis (sklēr′ad-ĕ-nī′tis) Inflammatory induration of a gland. [scler- + G. *adēn,* gland, + *-itis,* inflammation]

scle•ral (sklēr′ăl) Relating to the sclera. SYN sclerotic (2).

scle•ral staph•y•lo•ma (sklēr′ăl staf′i-lō′mă) SYN equatorial staphyloma.

scle•ral sul•cus (sklēr′ăl sŭl′kŭs) A slight groove on the external surface of the eyeball indicating the line of union of the sclera and cornea or limbus of cornea.

scle•ral veins (sklēr′ăl vānz) Small veins draining the sclera; they are tributaries to the anterior ciliary veins.

scle•ral ve•nous si•nus (sklēr′ăl vē′nŭs sī′ nŭs) The vascular structure encircling the anterior chamber of the eye and through which the aqueous is returned to the blood circulation. SYN Lauth canal.

scle•rec•ta•si•a (sklēr′ek-tā′zē-ă) Localized bulging of the sclera. [scler- + G. *ektasis,* an extension]

scle•rec•to•my (sklĕr-ek′tŏ-mē) **1.** Excision of a portion of the sclera. **2.** Removal of the fibrous adhesions formed in chronic otitis media. [scler- + G. *ektomē,* excision]

scle•re•de•ma (sklēr′ĕ-dē′mă) Hard, nonpitting edema of the skin of the dorsal aspect of the upper body and extremities, giving a waxy appearance and no sharp demarcation. SYN scleroedema. [scler- + G. *oidēma,* a swelling (edema)]

scler•e•de•ma a•dul•tor•um (sklēr′ĕ-dē′mă ă-dŭl-tōr′ŭm) A benign spreading induration of the skin and subcutaneous tissue, possibly streptococcal in origin, which may follow a febrile illness, with thickening of the skin by collagen and mucin deposit. SYN Buschke disease, scleroedema adultorum.

scle•re•ma (sklĕr-ē′mă) Induration of subcutaneous fat. [scler- + edema]

scler•e•ma ne•o•na•to•rum (sklĕr-ē′mă nē-ō′ nā-tō′rum) Sclerema appearing at birth or in early infancy, usually in premature and hypothermic infants, as sharply demarcated and yellowish-white indurated plaques that usually involve the cheeks, buttocks, shoulders, and calves; subcutaneous fat has a high proportion of saturated fatty acids; microscopically, there is thickening of interlobular fibrous tissue and formation of triglyceride crystals and foreign body giant cells; prognosis is poor for widespread lesions, but localized lesions may resolve slowly over a period of many months.

scle•ri•tis (sklĕr-ī′tis) Inflammation of the sclera.

sclero-, **scler-** Combining forms denoting hardness (i.e., induration), sclerosis, relationship to sclera. [G. *sklēros,* hard]

scle•ro•blas•te•ma (sklēr′ō-blas-tē′mă) The embryonic tissue entering into the formation of bone. [sclero- + G. *blastēma,* sprout]

scle•ro•cho•roid•i•tis (sklēr′ō-kōr′oyd-ī′tis) Inflammation of the sclera and choroid.

scle•ro•con•junc•ti•val (sklēr′ō-kon′jŭngk-tī′ văl) Relating to the sclera and the conjunctiva.

scle•ro•cor•ne•a (sklēr′ō-kōr′nē-ă) **1.** The cornea and sclera regarded as forming together the hard outer coat of the eye, the fibrous tunic of the eye. **2.** A congenital anomaly in which the whole or part of the cornea is opaque and resembles the sclera; other ocular abnormalities are frequently present.

scle•ro•dac•ty•ly, **scle•ro•dac•tyl•i•a** (sklēr′ō-dak′ti-lē, -dak-til′ē-ă) SYN acrosclerosis. [sclero- + G. *daktylos,* finger or toe]

scle•ro•der•ma (sklēr′ō-dĕr′mă) Thickening and induration of the skin caused by new collagen formation, with atrophy of pilosebaceous follicles; either a manifestation of progressive systemic sclerosis or localized (morphea). See this page, B9. SYN dermatosclerosis, systemic scleroderma. [sclero- + G. *derma,* skin]

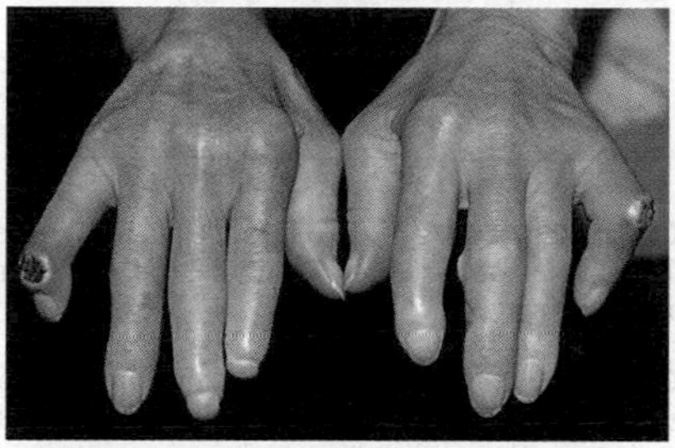

scleroderma: waxen appearance of digits of hand caused by dermal thickening resulting in deformity; note lesions on knuckles related to vasculitis

scle•ro•der•ma heart (sklēr′ō-dĕr′mă hahrt) A variably serious condition characterized by fibrosis (scarring) of the heart muscle and thickening of the small blood vessels in patients with scleroderma.

scleroedema [Br.] SYN scleredema.

scleroedema adultorum [Br.] SYN scleredema adultorum.

scle•rog•e•nous, **scle•ro•gen•ic** (sklĕr-oj′ĕ-nŭs, sklēr′ō-jen′ik) Producing hard or sclerotic tissue; causing sclerosis. [sclero- + G. *-gen,* producing]

scle•roid (sklēr′oyd) Indurated or sclerotic, of unusually firm texture, leathery, or of scarlike texture. SYN sclerosal, sclerous. [sclero- + G. *eidos,* resemblance]

scle•ro•i•ri•tis (sklēr′ō-ī-rī′tis) Inflammation of both sclera and iris.

scle•ro•ker•a•ti•tis (sklēr′ō-ker′ă-tī′tis) Inflammation of the sclera and cornea. [sclero- + G. *keras,* horn]

scle•ro•ker•a•to•i•ri•tis (sklēr′ō-ker′ă-tō-ī-rī′tis) Inflammation of sclera, cornea, and iris.

scle•ro•ma (sklēr-ō′mă) A circumscribed indurated focus of granulation tissue in the skin or mucous membrane. [G. *sklērōma,* an induration]

scle•ro•ma•la•ci•a (sklēr′ō-mă-lā′shē-ă) Degenerative thinning of the sclera, occurring in people with rheumatoid arthritis and other collagen disorders. [sclero- + G. *malakia,* a softening]

scle•ro•mere (sklēr′ō-mēr) **1.** Any metamere of the skeleton, such as a vertebral segment. **2.** Caudal half of a sclerotome. [sclero- + G. *meros,* part]

scle•ro•nych•i•a (sklēr′ō-nik′ē-ă) Induration and thickening of the nails. [sclero- + G. *onyx,* nail, + *-ia,* condition]

scle•ro-o•o•pho•ri•tis (sklēr′ō-ō-of′ŏr-ī′tis) Inflammatory induration of the ovary. [sclero- + Mod. L. *oophoron,* ovary + G. *-itis,* inflammation]

scle•roph•thal•mi•a (sklēr′of-thal′mē-ă) An abnormality in which most of the normally transparent cornea resembles the opaque sclera. [sclero- + G. *ophthalmos,* eye]

scle•ro•pro•tein (sklēr′ō-prō′tēn) SYN albuminoid (3).

scle•ro•sal (sklĕr-ō′săl) SYN scleroid.

scle•ro•sant (sklĕr-ō′sănt) An injectable irritant used to treat varices by producing thrombi in them.

scle•rose (sklĕr-ōs′) To harden; to undergo sclerosis.

scler•o•sing ad•e•no•sis (sklĕ-rō′sing ad′ĕ-nō′sis) A nodular, benign breast lesion occurring most frequently in relatively young women and consisting of hyperplastic distorted lobules of acinar tissue with increased collagenous stroma; the changes may be difficult to distinguish microscopically from carcinoma. Also, a benign nodular microscopic lesion of the prostate consisting of acinar tissue with increased stroma; the basal cell layer shows characteristic smooth muscle metaplasia. SYN adenofibrosis.

scler•o•sing he•man•gi•o•ma (sklĕ-rō′sing hē-man′jē-ō′mă) A benign lung or bronchial lesion, often subpleural, sometimes multiple, that forms hyalinized connective tissue.

scler•o•sing ker•a•ti•tis (sklĕ-rō′sing ker′ă-tī′tis) Inflammation of the cornea complicating scleritis; characterized by opacification of the corneal stroma.

scler•o•sing os•te•i•tis (sklĕ-rō′sing os′tē-ī′tis) Fusiform thickening or increased density of bones, of unknown cause. SYN Garré disease.

scle•ro•sis, pl. **scle•ro•ses** (sklĕr-ō′sis, -sēz) **1.** SYN induration (2). **2.** In neuropathy, induration of nervous and other structures by a hyperplasia of the interstitial fibrous or glial connective tissue. [G. *sklērōsis,* hardness]

scle•ro•ste•no•sis (sklēr′ō-stĕ-nō′sis) Induration and contraction of the tissues. [sclero- + G. *stenōsis,* a narrowing]

scle•ros•to•my (sklĕr-os′tŏ-mē) Surgical perforation of the sclera, as for the relief of glaucoma. [sclero- + G. *stoma,* mouth]

scle•ro•ther•a•py (sklĕr′ō-thăr′ă-pē) Treatment involving the injection of a sclerosing solution into vessels or tissues.

scle•rot•ic (sklĕr-ot′ik) **1.** Relating to or characterized by sclerosis. **2.** SYN scleral.

scle•rot•i•ca (sklĕr-ot′i-kă) SYN sclera. [Mod. L. *scleroticus,* hard]

scle•rot•ic bod•ies (sklĕr-ot′ik bod′ēz) Vegetative rounded muriform cells of dematiaceous fungi, characteristic of the causal agents of chromoblastomycosis.

scle•rot•ic ce•ment•al mass (sklĕr-ot′ik sĕ-men′tăl mas) Benign fibroosseous jaw lesions of unknown etiology, which present as large painless radiopaque masses.

scle•rot•ic den•tin (sklĕr-ot′ik den′tin) Dentin characterized by calcification of the dentinal tubules as a result of injury or normal aging. SYN transparent dentin.

scle•ro•tome (sklĕr′ō-tōm) **1.** A knife used in sclerotomy. **2.** The group of mesenchymal cells emerging from the ventromedial part of a mesodermic somite and migrating toward the notochord. Sclerotomal cells from adjacent somites become merged in intersomitically located masses that are the primordia of the centra of the vertebrae. [sclero- + G. *tomē,* a cutting]

scle•rot•o•my (sklĕr-ot′ŏ-mē) An incision through the sclera. [sclero- + G. *tomē,* incision]

scle•rous (sklĕr′ŭs) SYN scleroid. [G. *sklēros,* hard]

SCM Abbreviation for sternocleidomastoid muscle.

sco•lex, pl. **scol•e•ces, scol•i•ces** (skō′leks, -lĕ-sēz, -li-sēz) The head or anterior end of an adult tapeworm attached by suckers, and frequently by rostellar hooks, to the wall of the intestine. See page B7. [G. *skōlēx,* a worm]

scolio- Combining form meaning twisted or crooked. [G. *skolios,* curved, bent]

sco•li•o•ky•pho•sis (skō′lē-ō-kī-fō′sis) Lateral and posterior curvature of the spine. [G. *scolios,* curved, + *kyphōsis,* kyphosis]

sco•li•o•sis (skō′lē-ō′sis) Abnormal lateral curvature of the vertebral column. Depending on the etiology, there may be one curve, or primary and secondary compensatory curves; scoliosis may be "fixed" as a result of muscle and/or bone deformity or "mobile" as a result of unequal muscle contraction. See this page, B24. [G. *skoliōsis,* a crookedness]

sco•li•ot•ic (skō′lē-ot′ik) Relating to or suffering from scoliosis.

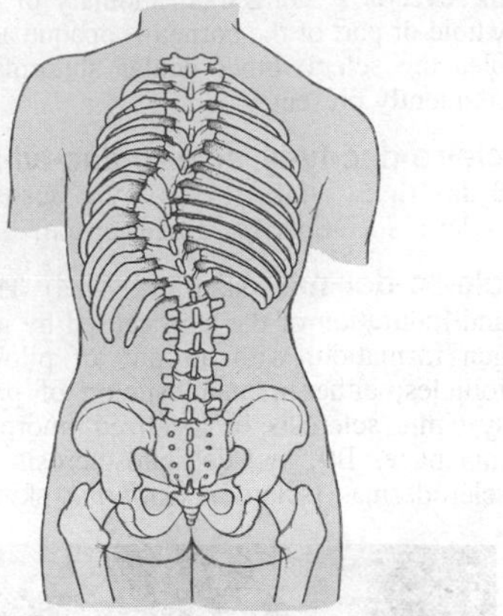

scoliosis

sco•li•ot•ic pel•vis (skō′lē-ot′ik pel′vis) A deformed pelvis associated with lateral curvature of the spine.

scom•broid poi•son•ing (skom′broyd poy′zŏn-ing) Poisoning from ingestion of heat-stable toxins produced by bacterial action on inadequately preserved dark-meat fish of the order Scombroidea (tuna, bonito, mackerel, albacore, skipjack); characterized by epigastric pain, nausea and vomiting, headache, thirst, difficulty in swallowing, and urticaria.

-scope Suffix meaning viewing, staring; an instrument for viewing but extended to include other methods of examination (e.g., stethoscope). [G. *skopeō,* to view]

sco•po•phil•i•a (skō′pō-fil′ē-ă) SYN voyeurism. [G. *skopeō,* to view, + *philos,* fond]

sco•po•pho•bi•a (skō′pō-fō′bē-ă) Morbid dread of being stared at. [G. *skopeō,* to view, + *phobos,* fear]

-scopy Suffix meaning an action or activity involving the use of an instrument for viewing. [G. *skopeō,* to view]

scor•bu•tic (skōr-byū′tik) Relating to, suffering from, or resembling scurvy.

scor•bu•ti•gen•ic (skōr-byū′ti-jen′ik) Scurvy-producing.

scor•di•ne•ma (skōr′di-nē′mă) Heaviness of the head with yawning and stretching, occurring as a prodrome of an infectious disease. [G. *skordinēma,* yawning]

score (skōr) An evaluation, usually expressed numerically, of status, achievement, or condition in a given set of circumstances. [M. E. *scor,* notch, tally]

Scotch broom (skoch brūm) SYN broom.

♻ **scoto-** Prefix meaning darkness. [G. *skotos*]

sco•to•chro•mo•gen•ic (skō′tō-krō′mō-jen′ik) Refers to microorganisms (e.g., *Mycobacterium scrofulaceum*) that produce pigment in the absence of light. Pigment may darken or be enhanced when colonies are exposed to light.

sco•to•ma, pl. **sco•to•ma•ta** (skō-tō′mă, -mă-tă) **1.** An isolated area of varying size and shape, within the visual field, in which vision is absent or depressed. **2.** A blind spot in psychological awareness. [G. *skotōma,* vertigo, fr. *skotos,* darkness]

sco•tom•a•tous (skō-tō′mă-tŭs) Relating to scotoma.

sco•tom•e•ter (skō-tom′ĕ-tĕr) An instrument for determining the size, shape, and intensity of a scotoma.

sco•tom•e•try (skō-tom′ĕ-trē) The plotting and measuring of a scotoma. [scoto- + G. *metron,* measure]

scot•o•phil•i•a (skō′tō-fil′ē-ă) SYN nyctophilia. [scoto- + G. *philos,* fond]

scot•o•pho•bi•a (skō′tō-fō′bē-ă) SYN nyctophobia. [scoto- + G. *phobos,* fear]

sco•to•pi•a (skō-tō′pē-ă) SYN scotopic vision. [scoto- + G. *opsis,* vision]

sco•top•ic (skō-top′ik) Referring to low illumination to which the eye is dark adapted. SEE ALSO scotopic vision.

sco•top•ic ad•ap•ta•tion (skō-top′ik ad′ap-tā′shŭn) SYN dark adaptation.

sco•top•ic eye (skō-top′ik ī) SYN dark-adapted eye.

sco•top•ic vi•sion (skō-top′ik vizh′ŭn) Vision when the eye is dark adapted. SEE ALSO dark adaptation, dark-adapted eye. SYN night vision, scotopia.

sco•top•sin (skō-top′sin) The protein moiety of the pigment in the rods of the retina.

Scott op•er•a•tion (skot op-ĕr-ā′shŭn) A jejunoileal bypass for morbid obesity using end-to-end anastomosis of the upper jejunum to the terminal ileum, with the bypassed intestine closed proximally and anastomosed distally to the colon.

scot•ty dog (skot′ē dawg) The fancied appearance of the articular facets on oblique radiographs of the lumbar spine; the neck of the scotty dog is the pars interarticularis, site of the most common defect in spondylolysis.

scout film (skowt film) A radiograph exposed before contrast medium is given, such as the preliminary film for an angiogram, urogram, or barium-contrast gastrointestinal examination.

scrap•ing (skrāp′ing) A specimen scraped from a lesion or specific site, for cytologic examination. SEE ALSO smear.

scratch test (skrach test) A form of skin test in which antigen is applied through a scratch in the skin.

screen (skrēn) **1.** A sheet of any substance used to shield an object from any influence (e.g., heat, light, x-rays). **2.** A sheet on which an image is projected. **3.** PSYCHOANALYSIS concealment, as one image or memory concealing another. SEE ALSO screen memory. **4.** To examine, evaluate; to process a group to select or separate certain individuals from it. **5.** A thin layer of crystals that converts x-rays to light photons to expose film; used in a cassette to produce radiographic images on film. **6.** To examine for the presence or absence of specified characteristics to determine whether further examination is needed. [Fr. *écran*]

screen•ing (skrēn′ing) **1.** To screen (5). **2.** Examination of a group of usually asymptomatic people to detect those with a high probability of having a given disease, typically by means of an inexpensive diagnostic test. **3.** MENTAL HEALTH initial patient evaluation that includes medical and psychiatric history, mental status evaluation, and diagnostic formulation to determine the patient's suitability for a particular treatment modality.

screen•ing test (skrēn′ing test) Any testing procedure designed to separate people or objects according to a fixed characteristic or property.

screen mem•o•ry (skrēn mem′ŏr-ē) PSYCHOANALYSIS a consciously tolerable memory that unwittingly serves as a cover for another associated memory that would be emotionally painful if recalled.

scro•bic•u•late (skrō-bik′yū-lăt) Pitted; marked with minute depressions. [L. *scrobiculus;* dim. of *scrobis,* a trench]

scrof•u•lo•der•ma (skrof′yū-lō-dĕr′mă) Tuberculosis resulting from extension into the skin from underlying atypical mycobacterial infection, most commonly of cervical lymph nodes. Cf. lupus vulgaris. [scrofula + G. *derma,* skin]

scro•tal (skrō′tăl) Relating to the scrotum. SYN oscheal.

scro•tal her•ni•a (skrō′tăl hĕr′nē-ă) Complete inguinal hernia, located in the scrotum.

scro•tal hy•po•spa•di•as (skrō′tăl hī′pō-spā′dē-ăs) Hypospadias with the urethral opening on the scrotal surface.

scro•tal ra•phe (skrō′tăl rā′fē) A central line, like a cord, running over the scrotum from the anus to the root of the penis; it marks the position of the septum scroti.

scro•tal sep•tum (skrō′tăl sep′tŭm) An incomplete wall of connective tissue and nonstriated muscle (dartos fascia) dividing the scrotum into two sacs, each containing a testis.

scro·tec·to·my (skrō-tek′tŏ-mē) Partial or total removal of the scrotum. [scrotum, + G. *ektomē,* excision]

scro·ti·tis (skrō-tī′tis) Inflammation of the scrotum.

scro·to·plas·ty (skrō′tō-plas-tē) Surgical reconstruction of the scrotum. SYN oscheoplasty. [scrotum + G. *plastos,* formed]

scro·tum, pl. **scro·ta**, **scro·tums** (skrō′tŭm, -tă, -tŭmz) [TA] A musculocutaneous sac containing the testes; it is formed of skin, containing a network of nonstriated muscular fibers (the dartos or dartos fascia), which also forms the scrotal septum internally. [L.]

scrub nurse (skrŭb nŭrs) A nurse who has cleansed arms and hands, donned sterile gloves and, usually, a sterile gown, and assists an operating surgeon, primarily by passing instruments.

scrub ty·phus (skrŭb tī′fŭs) SYN tsutsugamushi disease.

scru·ple (skrū′pĕl) An apothecaries' weight of 20 grains or one third of a dram. [L. *scrupulus,* a small sharp stone, a weight, the 24th part of an ounce, a scruple, dim. of *scrupus,* a sharp stone]

Scul·te·tus ban·dage (skŭl-tē′tŭs ban′dăj) A large oblong cloth, the ends of which are cut into narrow strips, that is applied to the thorax or abdomen, the strips being tied or overlapped and pinned.

Scul·te·tus po·si·tion (skŭl-tē′tŭs pŏ-zish′ŏn) A supine position on an inclined plane with head low, recommended by Scultetus for herniotomy and castration.

scurf (skŭrf) SYN dandruff. [A.S.]

scur·vy (skŭr′vē) A disease marked by inanition, debility, anemia, edema of the dependent parts, a spongy condition (sometimes with ulceration) of the gums, and hemorrhages into the skin and from the mucous membranes; attributed to a diet lacking sufficient vitamin C. [fr. A.S. *scurf*]

scute (skyūt) A thin lamina or plate. SYN scutum (1). [L. *scutum,* shield]

scu·ti·form (skyū′ti-fōrm) Shield-shaped. [L. *scutum,* shield, + *forma,* form]

scu·tu·lar (skyū′tyū-lăr) Relating to a scutulum.

scu·tu·lum, pl. **scu·tu·la** (skyū′tyū-lŭm, -lă) A yellow, saucer-shaped crust, the characteristic lesion of favus, consisting of a mass of hyphae and spores. [L. dim. of *scutum,* shield]

scu·tum, pl. **scu·ta** (skyū′tŭm, -tă) **1.** SYN scute. **2.** In ixodid (hard) ticks, a plate that largely or entirely covers the dorsum of the male and forms an anterior shield behind the capitulum of the female or immature ticks. [L. shield]

scyb·a·la (sib′ă-lă) Plural of scybalum.

scyb·a·lous (sib′ă-lŭs) Relating to scybala.

scyb·a·lum, pl. **scyb·a·la** (sib′ă-lŭm, -lă) A hard, round mass of inspissated feces. [G. *skybalon,* excrement]

scy·phoid (sī′foyd) Cup-shaped. [G. *skyphos,* cup, + *eidos,* resemblance]

SDA Abbreviation for specific dynamic action.

Se Symbol for selenium.

sea·ba·ther's e·rup·tion (sē′bādh-ĕrz ĕr-ŭp′shŭn) Pruritic rash believed to result from hypersensitivity to the venom of the larval thimble jellyfish (*Linuche unguiculata*).

sea·gull mur·mur (sē′gŭl mŭr′mŭr) A sound imitating the cooing of a seagull; nearly always due to aortic stenosis or mitral regurgitation.

sea louse (sē lows) The very small larvae of the thimble jellyfish (*Linuche unguiculata*).

sea net·tle (sē net′ĕl) SYN *Chrysaora quinquecirrha.*

search·er (sĕr′chĕr) A form of sound or exploratory probe used to determine the presence of a calculus in the bladder.

sea·sick·ness (sē′sik-nĕs) A form of motion sickness caused by the movement of a floating platform, such as a ship, boat, or raft. SYN mal de mer.

sea·son·al af·fec·tive dis·or·der (SAD) (sē′zŏn′ăl a-fek′tiv dis-ōr′dĕr) A depressive mood disorder that occurs at approximately the same time year after year and spontaneously remits at the same time each year. The most common type is winter depression, characterized by morning hypersomnia, low energy, increased appetite, weight gain, and carbohydrate craving, all of which remit in the spring.

seat·ed mas·sage (sēt′ĕd mă-sahzh′) A massage technique that is performed while the client is fully clothed and seated, often in public settings such as offices, airports, and malls. SYN on-site massage.

seat·worm (sēt′wŏrm) SYN pinworm.

sea wasp (sē wahsp) SYN *Chiropsalmus quadrumanus.*

SEB Abbreviation for staphylococcal enterotoxin B.

se·ba·ceous (sĕ-bā′shŭs) Relating to sebum; oily; fatty. [L. *sebaceus*]

se·ba·ceous ad·e·no·ma (sĕ-bā′shŭs ad′ĕ-nō′mă) A benign neoplasm of sebaceous tissue, with a predominance of mature secretory sebaceous cells.

se•ba•ceous cyst (sĕ-bā′shŭs sist) A common cyst of the skin and subcutis containing sebum and keratin, and lined by epithelium derived from the pilosebaceous follicle. SEE ALSO epidermoid cyst, pilar cyst.

se•ba•ceous ep•i•the•li•o•ma (sĕ-bā′shŭs ep′i-thē′lē-ō′mă) A benign tumor of the sebaceous gland epithelium in which small basaloid or germinative cells predominate.

se•ba•ceous fol•li•cles (sĕ-bā′shŭs fol′i-kĕlz) SYN sebaceous glands.

se•ba•ceous glands (sĕ-bā′shŭs glandz) Numerous holocrine glands in the dermis that usually open into the hair follicles and secrete an oily, semifluid sebum. SYN sebaceous follicles.

se•bif•er•ous (sĕ-bif′ĕr-ŭs) Producing sebaceous matter. [sebi- + L. *fero,* to bear]

♻ **sebo-, seb-, sebi-** Combining forms indicating sebum, sebaceous. [L. *sebum,* suet, tallow]

seb•o•lith (seb′ō-lith) A concretion in a sebaceous follicle. [sebo- + G. *lithos,* stone]

seb•or•rhe•a (seb′ōr-ē′ă) Overactivity of the sebaceous glands, resulting in an excessive amount of sebum. SYN seborrhoea. [sebo- + G. *rhoia,* a flow]

seb•or•rhe•a fa•ci•e•i, seb•or•rhe•a of face (seb′ōr-ē′ă fash′ē-ī, fās) Seborrhea oleosa affecting especially the nose and forehead. SYN seborrhoea faciei.

seb•or•rhe•a fur•fu•ra•ce•a (seb′ōr-ē′ă fŭr-fu-rā′shē-ā) SYN seborrhea sicca (1). SYN seborrhoea furfuracea.

seb•or•rhe•a o•le•o•sa (seb′ōr-ē′ă ō-lē-ō′să) Skin made greasy by excessive secretion of the sebaceous glands.

seb•or•rhe•a sic•ca (seb′ōr-ē′ă sik′ă) **1.** An accumulation on the skin, especially the scalp, of dry scales; SYN seborrhea furfuracea. **2.** SYN dandruff. SYN seborrhoea sicca.

seb•or•rhe•ic (seb′ōr-ē′ik) Relating to seborrhea. SYN seborrhoeic.

seb•or•rhe•ic bleph•a•ri•tis (seb′ōr-ē′ik blef′ăr-ī′tis) A common type of chronic inflammation of the margins of the eyelids with erythema and white scales; often with an associated seborrheic dermatitis of scalp and face. SYN seborrhoeic blepharitis.

🅸 **seb•or•rhe•ic der•ma•ti•tis, der•ma•ti•tis seb•or•rhe•i•ca** (seb′ōr-ē′ik dĕr′mă-tī′tis, seb-ōr-rē′i-kă) A common scaly macular eruption that occurs primarily on the face, scalp (dandruff), and other areas of increased sebaceous gland secretion; the lesions are covered with a slightly adherent oily scale. See this page, B9. SYN dyssebacia, dyssebacea, seborrheic dermatosis, seborrhoeic dermatitis, Unna disease.

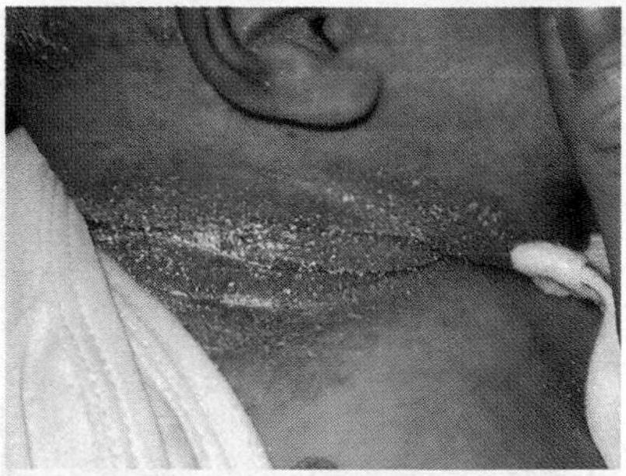

seborrheic dermatitis: neck, infant

seb•or•rhe•ic der•ma•to•sis (seb′ōr-ē′ik dĕr′mă-tō′sis) SYN seborrheic dermatitis. SYN seborrhoeic dermatosis.

🅸 **seb•or•rhe•ic ker•a•to•sis, ker•a•to•sis seb•or•rhe•i•ca** (seb′ōr-ē′ik ker′ă-tō′sis, seb-ō-rē′i-kă) **1.** A superficial, benign, verrucous, often pigmented, greasy lesion consisting of proliferating epidermal cells, resembling basal cells, enclosing horn cysts; usually occur after the third decade. **2.** SYN senile keratosis. See page 1404, B14. SYN seborrhoeic keratosis.

seborrhoea [Br.] SYN seborrhea.

seborrhoea of face [Br.] SYN seborrhea of face.

seborrhoea faciei [Br.] SYN seborrhea faciei.

seborrhoea furfuracea [Br.] SYN seborrhea furfuracea.

seborrhoea sicca [Br.] SYN seborrhea sicca.

seborrhoeic [Br.] SYN seborrheic.

seborrhoeic blepharitis [Br.] SYN seborrheic blepharitis.

seborrhoeic dermatitis [Br.] SYN seborrheic dermatitis.

seborrhoeic dermatosis [Br.] SYN seborrheic dermatosis.

seborrhoeic keratosis [Br.] SYN seborrheic keratosis.

se•bum (sē′bŭm) The secretion of the sebaceous glands. [L. tallow]

sec Abbreviation for second.

sec•ond•ar•y (sek′ŏn-dar-ē) **1.** Second in order. **2.** Caused by another condition (e.g., a secondary infection caused by antibiotic treatment for a primary infection).

sec•on•da•ry ab•dom•i•nal preg•nan•cy (sek′ŏn-dar-ē ab-dom′i-năl preg′năn-sē) A condition in which the embryo or fetus continues to grow in the abdominal cavity after its expulsion

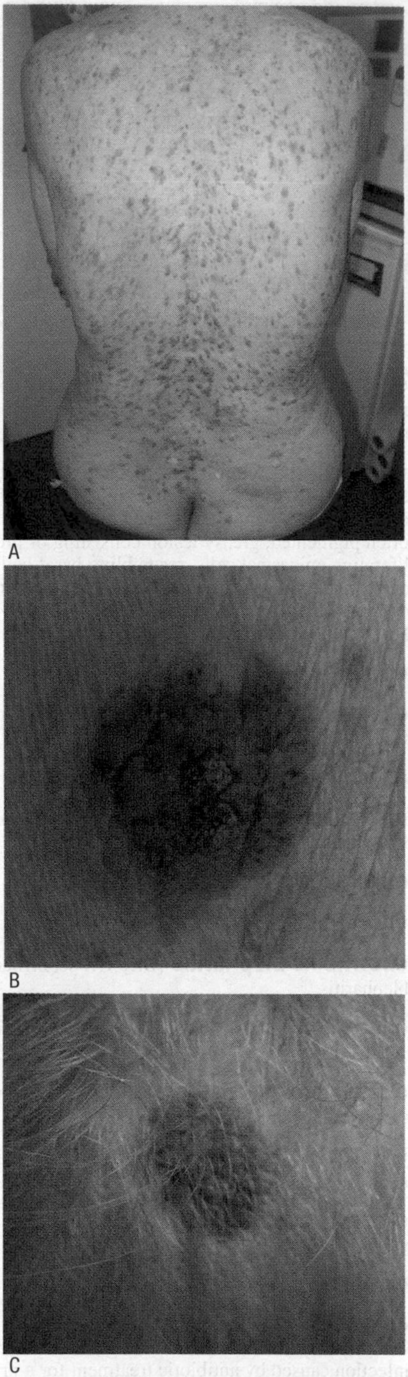
A B C
seborrheic keratoses: (A) back, diffuse type; (B) back; (C) scalp

from the uterine tube or other seat of its primary development. SYN abdominocyesis (2).

sec·on·da·ry ad·he·sion (sek′ŏn-dar-ē ad-hē′zhŭn) SYN healing by second intention.

sec·on·da·ry a·dre·no·cor·ti·cal in·suf·fi·cien·cy (sek′ŏn-dar-ē ă-drē′nō-kōr′ti-kăl in′sŭ-fish′ĕn-sē) Adrenocortical insufficiency caused by failure of ACTH secretion resulting from anterior pituitary disease or inhibition of ACTH production resulting from exogenous steroid therapy.

sec·on·da·ry al·co·hol (sek′ŏn-dar-ē al′kŏ-hol) An alcohol characterized by the bivalent atom group, —CH(OH)—.

sec·on·da·ry al·dos·te·ron·ism (sek′ŏn-dar-ē al-dos′tĕr-ōn-izm) Disorder resulting not from a defect intrinsic to the cortex of the suprarenal gland but from a stimulation of hormonal secretion caused by extra adrenal disorders; associated with increased plasma renin activity and occurs in heart failure, nephrotic syndrome, cirrhosis, and hypoproteinemia.

sec·on·da·ry a·men·or·rhe·a (sek′ŏn-dar-ē ā-men′ŏr-ē′ă) Amenorrhea in which the menses appeared at puberty but subsequently ceased.

sec·on·da·ry am·ide (sek′ŏn-dar-ē am′īd) SEE amide.

sec·on·da·ry a·mine (sek′ŏn-dar-ē ă-mēn′) SEE amine.

sec·on·da·ry am·y·loi·do·sis (sek′ŏn-dar-ē am′i-loy-dō′sis) Amyloidosis occurring in association with another chronic inflammatory disease; organs chiefly involved are the liver, spleen, and kidneys, and the adrenal glands less frequently.

sec·on·da·ry an·es·thet·ic (sek′ŏn-dar-ē an′es-thet′ik) A compound that contributes to, but is not primarily responsible for, loss of sensation when two or more anesthetics are simultaneously administered.

sec·on·da·ry at·el·ec·ta·sis (sek′ŏn-dar-ē at′ĕ-lek′tă-sis) Pulmonary collapse at any age, but particularly of infants, due to hyaline membrane disease or elastic recoil of the lungs while the patient is dying from other causes.

sec·on·da·ry ax·is (sek′ŏn-dar-ē ak′sis) Any ray passing through the optic center of a lens.

sec·ond·ar·y blast in·ju·ry (sek′ŏn-dar-ē blast in′jŭr-ē) An injury resulting from flying debris and fragments from an explosion.

sec·on·da·ry bron·chi·al buds (sek′ŏn-dar-ē brong′kē-ăl bŭdz) Buds resulting from branching of the primary bronchial buds, three on the right side and two on the left; they give rise to the lobes of the lungs. SYN pulmonary lobar buds.

sec·on·da·ry cat·a·ract (sek′ŏn-dar-ē kat′ăr-akt) **1.** A cataract that accompanies or follows some other eye disease such as uveitis; **2.** A cataract occurring in the retained lens or capsule after a cataract extraction.

sec•ond•ar•y cen•ter of os•si•fi•ca•tion (sek′ŏn-dar-ē sen′tĕr os′i-fi-kā′shŭn) SYN secondary ossification center.

sec•on•da•ry de•gen•er•a•tion (sek′ŏn-dar-ē dĕ-jen′ĕr-ā′shŭn) SYN wallerian degeneration.

sec•on•da•ry de•men•ti•a (sek′ŏn-dar-ē dĕ-men′shē-ă) Chronic dementia following and due to a psychosis or some other underlying disease process.

sec•on•da•ry den•tin (sek′ŏn-dar-ē den′tin) Dentin formed by normal pulp function after root end formation is complete.

sec•on•da•ry den•ti•tion (sek′ŏn-dar-ē den-tish′ŭn) SYN permanent tooth.

sec•on•da•ry de•vi•a•tion (sek′ŏn-dar-ē dē-vē-ā′shŭn) Ocular deviation seen in paralysis of an ocular muscle when the paralyzed eye is used for fixation.

sec•on•da•ry di•ges•tion (sek′ŏn-dar-ē di-jes′chŭn) The change in the chyle effected by the action of the cells of the body, whereby the final products of digestion are assimilated in the process of metabolism.

sec•on•da•ry dis•ease (sek′ŏn-dar-ē di-zēz′) **1.** A disease that follows and results from an earlier disease, injury, or event. **2.** A wasting disorder that follows successful transplantation of bone marrow into a lethally irradiated host, frequently severe and usually associated with fever, anorexia, diarrhea, dermatitis, and desquamation. SEE ALSO graft-versus-host disease.

sec•on•da•ry drives (sek′ŏn-dar-ē drīvz) Those urges not directly related to biologic needs; can be learned as an offshoot of a primary drive, in which case often referred to as motives. SYN acquired drives.

sec•on•da•ry dye test (sek′ŏn-dar-ē dī test) Localization of lacrimal drainage obstruction following the fluorescein instillation and primary dye tests by intubating the lower punctum and canaliculus and irrigating with saline. SYN Jones II test.

sec•on•da•ry dys•men•or•rhe•a (sek′ŏn-dar-ē dis-men′ŏr-ē′ă) Dysmenorrhea due to inflammation, infection, tumor, or anatomic factors.

sec•on•da•ry en•ceph•a•li•tis (sek′ŏn-dar-ē en-sef′ă-lī′tis) Collective term for postinfectious, postexanthem, and postvaccinal encephalitides.

sec•on•da•ry fol•li•cle (sek′ŏn-dar-ē fol′i-kĕl) SYN vesicular ovarian follicle.

sec•on•da•ry gain (sek′ŏn-dar-ē gān) Interpersonal or social advantages (e.g., assistance, attention, sympathy) gained indirectly from illness. Cf. primary gain.

sec•on•da•ry glau•co•ma (sek′ŏn-dar-ē glaw-kō′mă) Glaucoma occurring as a sequel of ocular disease or injury.

sec•on•da•ry gout (sek′ŏn-dar-ē gowt) Gout resulting from increased serum uric acid levels as a result of an antecedent disease, such as a proliferative disease of the blood and bone marrow, lead poisoning, or prolonged chronic renal failure (on dialysis).

sec•on•da•ry he•mo•chro•ma•to•sis (sek′ŏn-dar-ē hē′mō-krō′mă-tō′sis) Increased intake and accumulation of iron secondary to known cause, such as oral iron therapy or multiple transfusions.

sec•on•da•ry hem•or•rhage (sek′ŏn-dar-ē hem′ŏr-ăj) Hemorrhage at an interval after an injury or an operation.

sec•ond•ar•y hy•per•ten•sion (sek′ŏn-dar-ē hī′pĕr-ten′shŭn) Hypertension with an identifible causc (e.g., renal artery stenosis, renal failure, stress, sleep apnea, pheochromocytoma, primary hyperaldosteronism, preeclampsia). SEE ALSO hypertension.

sec•on•da•ry im•mune re•sponse (sek′ŏn-dar-ē i-myūn′ rĕ-spons′) SEE immune response.

sec•on•da•ry ly•so•somes (sek′ŏn-dar-ē lī′sō-sōmz) Lysosomes in which lysis takes place, owing to the activity of hydrolytic enzymes; they are believed to eventually become residual bodies.

sec•on•da•ry mu•ci•no•sis (sek′ŏn-dar-ē myū′si-nō′sis) SEE mucinosis.

sec•on•da•ry non•dis•junc•tion (sek′ŏn-dar-ē non′dis-jŭngk′shŭn) Nondisjunction occurring in an aneuploid cell that was the result of primary nondisjunction.

sec•on•da•ry o•o•cyte (sek′ŏn-dar-ē ō′ō-sīt) An oocyte in which the first meiotic division is completed; the second meiotic division usually stops short of completion unless fertilization occurs.

sec•ond•ar•y os•si•fi•ca•tion cen•ter (sek′ŏn-dar-ē os′i-fi-kā′shŭn sen′tĕr) Center of bone formation that appears later than the primary ossification center, usually in an epiphysis. SYN secondary center of ossification.

sec•ond•ar•y pal•ate (sek′ŏn-dar-ē pal′ăt) Portion of embryonic palate, posterior to primary palate that forms from lateral palatine processes of embryonic maxilla and develops into hard and soft palates.

se•con•da•ry pre•ven•tive nur•sing (sek′ŏn-dar-ē prē-ven′tiv nŭrs′ing) Nursing interventions and care directed at early detection and management of disease. Cancer, myocardial infarction, diabetes mellitus, obesity, infectious diseases, and glaucoma are major diseases targeted by secondary preventive nursing care.

sec•on•da•ry pro•cess (sek'ŏn-dar-ē pros'es) PSYCHOANALYSIS the mental process directly related to the learned and acquired functions of the ego and characteristic of conscious and preconscious mental activities; marked by logical thinking and by the tendency to delay gratification by regulation of the discharge of instinctual demands. Cf. primary process.

sec•on•da•ry ra•di•a•tion (sek'ŏn-dar-ē rā'dē-ā'shŭn) A form of radiation that is created when an x-ray beam interacts with matter and gives off some of its energy, forming new and less powerful wavelengths.

sec•on•da•ry sat•u•ra•tion (sek'ŏn-dar-ē sach'ŭr-ā'shŭn) A technique of nitrous oxide anesthesia consisting of an abrupt curtailment of the oxygen in the inhaled mixture to produce a deep plane of anesthesia, following which oxygen is administered to correct hypoxia.

sec•on•da•ry sex char•ac•ters (sek'ŏn-dar-ē seks kar'ăk-tĕrz) Those characters peculiar to the male or female that develop at puberty (e.g., men's beards and women's breasts).

sec•on•da•ry sper•ma•to•cyte (sek'ŏn-dar-ē spĕr-mat'ō-sīt) The spermatocyte derived from a primary spermatocyte by the first meiotic division; each secondary spermatocyte produces two spermatids by the second meiotic division.

sec•on•da•ry stut•ter•ing (sek'ŏn-dar-ē stŭt'ĕr-ing) Established stuttering behavior in which the dysfluencies are accompanied by awareness, anticipation, and resultant anxiety.

sec•ond•ar•y sur•vey (sek'ŏn-dar-ē sŭr'vā) SYN trauma assessment.

i **sec•on•da•ry syph•i•lis** (sek'ŏn-dar-ē sif'i-lis) The second stage of syphilis. SEE ALSO syphilis. See this page.

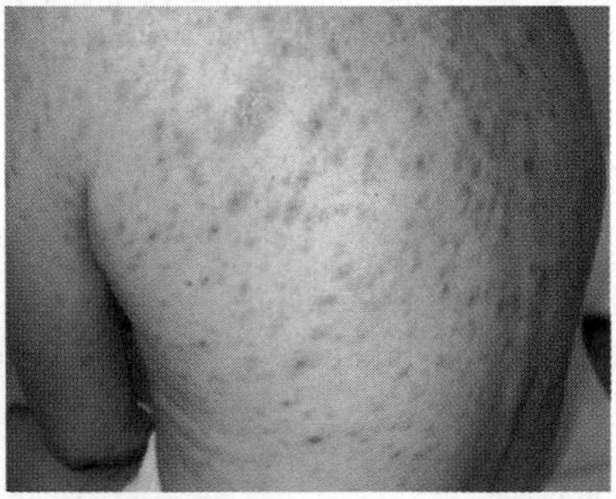

secondary syphilis: back

sec•on•da•ry tu•ber•cu•lo•sis (sek'ŏn-dar-ē tū-bĕr'kyū-lō'sis) Tuberculosis found in adults and characterized by lesions near the apex of an upper lobe, which may cavitate or heal with scarring without spreading to lymph nodes; theoretically, secondary tuberculosis may be due to exogenous reinfection or to reactivation of a dormant endogenous infection. SYN reactivation tuberculosis.

sec•on•da•ry tym•pan•ic mem•brane (sek'ŏn-dar-ē tim-pan'ik mem'brān) The membrane closing the fenestra cochleae or rotunda. SYN membrana tympani secundaria [TA], round window membrane.

sec•on•da•ry un•ion (sek'ŏn-dar-ē yūn'yŭn) SYN healing by second intention.

sec•ond cra•ni•al nerve [CN II] (sek'ŏnd krā'nē-ăl nĕrv) SYN optic nerve [CN II].

sec•ond-de•gree AV block (sek'ŏnd-dĕ-grē' blok) SEE atrioventricular block.

sec•ond-de•gree burn (sek'ŏnd-dĕ-grē' bŭrn) SYN partial-thickness burn.

sec•ond-de•gree pro•lapse (sek'ŏnd-dĕ-grē' prō'laps) Form of cervical prolapse in which the cervix is at or near the introitus.

sec•ond heart sound (S_2) (sek'ŏnd hahrt sownd) The second sound heard on auscultation of the heart; signifies the beginning of diastole and is due to closure of the semilunar valves; auscultated at base of heart.

sec•ond in•ten•tion (sek'ŏnd in-ten'shŭn) Delayed closure of two granulating surfaces. SEE ALSO first intention, third intention.

sec•ond-look op•er•a•tion (sek'ŏnd-luk op-ĕr-ā'shŭn) Exploratory celiotomy within a year after apparently curative resection of intraabdominal cancer, in patients with no sign or symptom of recurrence, to resect an occult tumor if present.

sec•ond mo•lar (sek'ŏnd mō'lăr) Seventh permanent or fifth deciduous tooth in the maxilla and mandible on either side of the midsagittal plane of the head following the arch form.

sec•ond pha•ryn•ge•al arch car•ti•lage (sek'ŏnd făr-in'jē-ăl ahrch kahr'ti-lăj) A cartilage in the mesenchyme of the second pharyngeal arch in the embryo, from which develop the stapes, styloid process, stylohyoid ligament, and lesser cornu (horn). SYN Reichert cartilage.

sec•ond toe [II] (sek'ŏnd tō) Second digit of foot.

sec•ond tooth (sek'ŏnd tūth) SYN permanent tooth.

sec•ond wind (sek'ŏnd wind) Colloquial term to describe relief from ill-defined feelings of distress that often accompany the early stages of exercise; generally related to the achievement of a steady state of pulmonary ventilation, aerobic metabolism, and thermal balance as exercise progresses.

se·cre·ta (sĕ-krē′tă) Secretions. [L. neuter pl. of *secretus,* pp. of *se-cerno,* to separate]

se·cre·ta·gogue (sĕ-krē′tă-gog) An agent that promotes secretion (e.g., acetylcholine, gastrin, secretin). [secreta + G. *agōgos,* drawing forth]

se·cre·tase (sĕ-krē′tās) A proteinase that acts on amyloid precursor protein to produce peptides that are soluble and do not precipitate to produce amyloid.

se·crete (sĕ-krēt′) To elaborate or release products of cellular metabolism (enzymes, mucus, waste products). [L. *se-cerno,* pp. *-cretus,* to separate]

se·cre·tin (sĕ-krē′tin) A hormone, formed by the epithelial cells of the duodenum under the stimulus of acid contents from the stomach, that incites secretion of pancreatic juice; used as an aid in the diagnosis of pancreatic exocrine disease and as an adjunct in obtaining desquamated pancreatic cells for cytologic examination. Cf. bioregulator. [secrete + -in]

se·cre·tion (sĕ-krē′shŭn) **1.** Production by a cell or aggregation of cells (a gland) of a physiologically active substance and its movement out of the cell or organ in which it is formed. **2.** The solid, liquid, or gaseous product of cellular or glandular activity that is stored up in or used by the organism in which it is produced. Cf. excretion. [L. *se-cerno,* pp. *-cretus,* to separate]

se·cre·to·in·hib·i·tor·y (sĕ-krē′tō-in-hib′i-tōr-ē) Restraining or curbing secretion.

se·cre·to·mo·tor, se·cre·to·mo·tor·y (sĕ-krē′tō-mō′tŏr, -mō′tŏr-ē) Stimulating secretion. [secrete = *motor,* mover]

se·cre·tor (sĕ-krē′tŏr) A person whose bodily fluids (e.g., saliva, semen, vaginal secretions) contain a water-soluble form of the antigens of the ABO blood group.

se·cre·to·ry (sē′krĕ-tōr-ē) Relating to secretion or the secretions.

se·cre·to·ry car·ci·no·ma (sē′krĕ-tōr-ē kahr′si-nō′mă) Cancer of the breast with pale-staining cells showing prominent secretory activity, as seen in pregnancy and lactation, but found mostly in children.

se·cre·to·ry nerve (sē′krĕ-tōr-ē nĕrv) A nerve conveying impulses that excite functional activity in a gland.

se·cre·to·ry o·ti·tis me·di·a (sē′krĕ-tōr-ē ō-tī′tis mē′dē-ă) SYN serous otitis.

sec·ti·o, pl. **sec·ti·o·nes** (sek′shē-ō, -ō′nēz) ANATOMY a subdivision or segment. [L.]

sec·tion (sek′shŭn) **1.** The act of cutting. **2.** A cut or division. **3.** A segment or part of any organ or structure delimited from the remainder. **4.** A cut surface. **5.** A thin slice of tissue, cells, microorganisms, or any material for examination under the microscope. [L. *sectio,* a cutting, fr. *seco,* to cut]

sec·ti·o·nes (sek′shē-ō′nēz) Plural of sectio.

Sec·tion 504 of the U.S. Re·ha·bil·i·ta·tion Act (sek′shŭn rē′hă-bil′i-tā′shŭn akt) The portion of the Rehabilitation Act of 1973 that refers to the provision of physical therapy services to children with physical disabilities enrolled in regular public education. Services are provided under a contract called the service agreement.

sec·tor·an·o·pi·a (sek′tŏr-an-ō′pē-ă) Loss of vision in a sector of the visual field. [sector + G. *an-* priv. + *opsis,* vision]

sec·tor ec·ho·car·di·o·gra·phy (sek′tŏr ek′ō-kahr′dē-og′ră-fē) Two-dimensional echocardiography with a stationary transducer.

sec·tor·i·al tooth (sek-tōr′ē-ăl tūth) SYN carnassial tooth.

sec·tor scan (sek′tŏr skan) ULTRASONOGRAPHY a system in which the transducer or transmitted ultrasound beam is rotated through an angle, resulting in a pie-shaped image.

se·cun·di·grav·i·da (sĕ-kun′di-grav′i-dă) SEE gravida.

se·cun·dines (sē-kun′dīnz) SYN afterbirth. [L. *secundinae,* the afterbirth]

se·cun·dip·a·ra (sē′kun-dip′ăr-ă) SEE para.

se·date (sĕ-dāt′) To bring under the influence of a sedative. [L. *sedatus;* see sedation]

se·da·tion (sĕ-dā′shŭn) **1.** The act of calming, especially by the administration of a sedative. **2.** The state of being calm. [L. *sedatio,* to calm, allay]

sed·a·tive (sed′ă-tiv) **1.** Calming; quieting. **2.** A drug that quiets nervous excitement; designated according to the organ or system on which specific action is exerted, e.g., cardiac, cerebral, nervous, respiratory, spinal. [L. *sedativus;* see sedation]

SEDC Abbreviation for spondyloepiphysial dysplasia congenita.

sed·en·tar·y work (sed′ĕn-tar-ē wŏrk) A physical demand level described as the exertion of up to 10 pounds of force occasionally, negligible amount of work frequently, and a negligible amount of force constantly to move objects.

sed·i·ment (sed′i-mĕnt) **1.** Insoluble material that tends to sink to the bottom of a liquid, as in hypostasis. **2.** To cause the formation of a sediment or deposit, as in the case of centrifugation or ultracentrifugation. SYN sedimentate. [L. *sedimentum,* a settling, fr. *sedeo,* to sit, settle down]

sed·i·men·tate (sed′i-mĕn-tāt) SYN sediment (2).

sed·i·men·ta·tion (sed′i-mĕn-tā′shŭn) Formation of a sediment.

sed·i·men·ta·tion co·ef·fi·cient (*s*) (sed′i-mĕn-tā′shŭn kō′ĕ-fish′ĕnt) SYN sedimentation constant.

sed·i·men·ta·tion con·stant (sed′i-mĕn-tā′shŭn kon′stănt) The constant *s* in a Svedberg equation for estimating the molecular weight of a protein from the rate of movement in a centrifugal field. The Svedberg unit (S) is arbitrarily set at 1×10^{-13} sec and is often used to describe the sedimentation rate of macromolecules (e.g., 4 S RNA). SYN sedimentation coefficient.

sed·i·men·ta·tion rate (sed. rate) (sed′i-mĕn-tā′shŭn rāt) The sinking velocity of blood cells, i.e., the degree of rapidity with which the red blood cells sink in a mass of drawn blood. It is used to detect and monitor inflammatory processes in the body: an elevated rate indicates a higher rate of inflammation.

sed·i·men·ta·tor (sed′i-mĕn-tā′tŏr) A centrifuge.

sed·i·men·tom·e·ter (sed′i-mĕn-tom′ĕ-tĕr) A photographic apparatus for the automatic recording of the blood sedimentation rate. [sediment + G. *metron,* measure]

se·dox·an·trone tri·hy·dro·chlor·ide (sē-doks′an-trōn trī-hī-drō-klōr′īd) A topoisomerase II inhibitor in cancer chemotherapy.

sed. rate (sed rāt) SEE sedimentation rate.

seed (sēd) **1.** The reproductive body of a flowering plant; the mature ovule. SYN semen (2). **2.** BACTERIOLOGY to inoculate a culture medium with microorganisms. [A.S. *soed*]

See·lig-Mül·ler sign (sē′lig-mer′ler sīn) Contraction of the pupil on the affected side in facial neuralgia.

Sees·sel pock·et (sē′sel pok′ĕt) The part of the embryonic foregut extending cephalad to the level of the buccopharyngeal membrane (oral plate) and caudal to the adenohypophysial diverticulum (Rathke pouch).

seg·ment (seg′mĕnt) **1.** A section; a part of an organ or other structure delimited naturally, artificially, or by invagination from the remainder. SYN segmentum [TA]. SEE ALSO metamere. **2.** A territory of an organ having independent function, supply, or drainage. **3.** To divide and redivide into minute, equal parts. [L. *segmentum,* fr. *seco,* to cut]

seg·men·tal an·es·the·si·a (seg-men′tăl an′es-thē′zē-ă) Loss of sensation limited to an area supplied by one or more spinal nerve roots.

seg·men·tal ar·ter·ies of kid·ney (seg-men′tăl ahr′tĕr-ēz kid′nē) The branches of the renal artery that supply the anatomic segments of kidney. Usually five in number, they are end arteries and give off interlobar, arcuate, and interlobular arteries in sequence. The latter send afferent arterioles to the glomeruli as well as branches to the kidney capsule. The segmental arteries of the kidney are identified as: (1) anterior inferior (arteriae segmenti anterioris inferioris renis [TA]); (2) anterior superior (arteriae segmenti anterioris superioris renis [TA]); (3) inferior (arteriae segmenti inferioris renis [TA]); (4) posterior (arteriae segmenti posterioris renis [TA]); and (5) superior (arteriae segmenti superioris renis [TA]).

seg·men·tal ar·ter·ies of liv·er (seg-men′tăl ahr′tĕr-ēz liv′ĕr) Anterior and posterior segmental arteries arising from the right branch of the hepatic artery, and medial and lateral segmental arteries arising from the left branch of the hepatic artery; the segmental arteries serve four of the five major divisions of the liver, and then branch in turn so that each hepatic segment receives an independent blood supply.

seg·men·tal frac·ture (seg-men′tăl frak′shŭr) A fracture in two parts of the same bone.

seg·men·tal med·ul·lar·y ar·ter·ies (seg-men′tăl mĕ-dŭl′ăr-ē ahr′tĕr-ēz) Large-caliber spinal or radicular arteries that course centrally along dorsal or ventral roots, supplying them and the surrounding meninges; continue on to reach and anastomose with anterior or posterior (longitudinal) spinal arteries. Only 4–9 of the spinal arteries are medullary spinal arteries, found mainly in the lower cervical, lower thoracic, and upper lumbar levels, the largest of which is the segmental medullary artery. SYN arteriae medullares segmentales, medullary spinal arteries.

seg·men·tal neu·ri·tis (seg-men′tăl nūr-ī′tis) **1.** Inflammation occurring at several points along the course of a nerve. **2.** Segmental demyelinating neuropathy.

seg·men·ta·tion cav·i·ty (seg′men-tā′shŭn kav′i-tē) SYN blastocele.

seg·men·ta·tion cell (seg′men-tā′shŭn sel) SEE blastomere.

seg·men·tec·to·my (seg′men-tek′tŏ-mē) Excision of a segment of any organ or gland.

seg·men·ted cell (seg′men-tĕd sel) A polymorphonuclear leukocyte matured beyond the band cell so that two or more lobes of the nucleus occur.

seg·men·ted neu·tro·phil (seg′men-tĕd nū′trō-fil) A mature and fully functional polymorphonuclear leukocyte (PMN) containing cytoplasmic granules (primary or azurophil and secondary or specific) and a lobulated chromatin-dense nucleus with no nucleolus.

seg·ments of spi·nal cord [C1–Co] (seg′mĕnts spī′năl kōrd) The 31 portions of the spinal cord, each of which gives rise to the anterior and posterior roots that combine to form a single pair of spinal nerves. These are the cervical spinal cord segments [C1–C8]; the thoracic spinal cord segments [T1–T12]; the lumbar spinal cord segments [L1–L5]; the sacral spinal cord segments [S1–S5]; and the coccygeal spinal cord segment [Co].

seg•men•tum, pl. **seg•men•ta** (seg-men′tŭm, -tă) [TA] SYN segment (1). [L. segment]

seg•re•ga•tion (seg′rĕ-gā′shŭn) **1.** Removal of certain parts from a mass (e.g., those with infectious diseases). **2.** Separation of contrasting characters in the offspring of heterozygotes. **3.** Separation of the paired state of genes, which occurs at the reduction division of meiosis; only one member of each somatic gene pair is normally included in each sperm or ovum. **4.** Progressive restriction of potencies in the zygote to the following embryo. [L. *segrego,* pp. *-atus,* to set apart from the flock, separate]

seg•re•ga•tion a•nal•y•sis (seg′rĕ-gā′shŭn ă-nal′i-sis) GENETICS the enumeration of progeny according to distinct and mutually exclusive phenotypes; used as a test of a putative pattern of inheritance (e.g., mendelian, dominant autosomal, epistatic, age dependent).

seg•re•ga•tion ra•ti•o (seg′rĕ-gā′shŭn rā′shē-ō) GENETICS the proportion of progeny of a particular genotype or phenotype from actual matings of specified genotypes. The test of a mendelian hypothesis is the comparison of the segregation rate with the mendelian rate.

Sei•del sco•to•ma (sī′del skō-tō′mă) A form of Bjerrum scotoma. SEE ALSO Seidel sign.

Sei•del sign (sī′del sīn) A sickle-shaped scotoma appearing as an upward or downward extension of the blind spot, as may be found in glaucoma.

Seip syn•drome (sīp sin′drōm) SYN congenital total lipodystrophy.

seis•mo•ther•a•py (sīz-mō-thār′ă-pē) SYN vibratory massage.

sei•zure (sē′zhŭr) **1.** An attack; the sudden onset of a disease or of certain symptoms. **2.** An epileptic attack. SYN convulsion (2). [O. Fr. *seisir,* to grasp, fr. Germanic]

sei•zure dis•or•der (sē′zhŭr dis-ōr′dĕr) SYN epilepsy.

Sel•ding•er tech•nique (sel′ding-er tek-nēk′) A method of percutaneous insertion of a catheter into a blood vessel or space, such as an abscess cavity: a needle is used to puncture the structure and a guide wire is threaded through the needle; when the needle is withdrawn, a catheter is threaded over the wire; the wire is then withdrawn, leaving the catheter in place.

se•lec•tin (sĕ-lek′tin) A cell surface molecule involved in immune adhesion and cell trafficking. [L. *se-ligo,* pp. *se-lectum,* to sort, choose, + -in]

se•lec•tion (sĕ-lek′shŭn) The combined effect of the causes and consequences of genetic factors that determine the average number of progeny of a species that attain sexual maturity. [L. *se-ligo,* to separate, select, fr. *se,* apart, + *lego,* to pick out]

se•lec•tion co•ef•fi•cient (*s*) (sĕ-lek′shŭn kō′ĕ-fish′ĕnt) The proportion of progeny or potential progeny not surviving to sexual maturity; usually defined artificially by expressing the fitness of a phenotype as a fraction of the mean or optimal fitness to give the relative fitness, and subtracting this fraction from unity. If the mean size of family in the population is 3.2 and that for a particular genotype is 2.4, then the fitness of the phenotype is 2.4/3.2 = 0.75, and the selection coefficient =1− 0.75 = .25 = 5.

se•lec•tive es•tro•gen re•cep•tor mo•du•la•tor (SERM) (sĕ-lek′tiv es′trō-jen rĕ-sep′tŏr moj′ū-lā′tŏr) Pharmaceutical agent with selective estrogen receptor affinity; current preparations have a primary effect on bone and cardiovascular tissues and less effect on endometrial, genital, and breast tissues.

se•lec•tive in•hi•bi•tion (sĕ-lek′tiv in′hi-bish′ŭn) SYN competitive inhibition.

se•lec•tive nor•ep•i•neph•rine re•up•take in•hi•bi•tor (sĕ-lek′tiv nōr-ep-i-nef′rin rē-up′tāk in-hib′i-tŏr) A class of chemical compounds that selectively, to varying degrees, inhibit reuptake of norepinephrine by the presynaptic neurons; thought to exert their antidepressant effect by this mechanism.

se•lec•tive ser•o•to•nin re•up•take in•hi•bi•tor (SSRI) (sĕ-lek′tiv ser′ŏ-tō′nin rē-up′tāk in-hib′i-tŏr) A class of drugs that selectively prevent the reuptake of serotonin and are used for the treatment of depression, e.g., fluoxetine, sertraline.

se•lec•tive stain (sĕ-lek′tiv stān) A stain that colors one portion of a tissue or cell exclusively or more deeply than the remaining portions.

se•le•ni•um (Se) (sĕ-lē′nē-ŭm) A metallic element chemically similar to sulfur; atomic no. 34, atomic wt. 78.96; an essential trace element toxic in large quantities; required for glutathione peroxidase and a few other enzymes; ^{75}Se (half-life equal to 119.78 days) is used in scintography of the pancreas and parathyroid glands. [G. *selēnē,* moon]

se•le•ni•um plate (sĕ-lē′nē-ŭm plāt) A radiation-sensitive material used in digital radiography. SEE ALSO digital radiography. SYN amorphous selenium plate.

se•le•no•cys•te•ine (sĕ-lē′nō-sis-tē′ēn) The biologically active form of selenium when attached to cysteine, an amino acid.

sel•e•noid bod•ies (sĕ-lē′noyd bod′ēz) SYN achromocyte.

se•le•no•thi•a•mine (sĕ-lē′nō-thī′ă-mēn) The

storage form of selenium when attached to thiamine.

self (self) **1.** A sum of the attitudes, feelings, memories, traits, and behavioral predispositions that make up the personality. **2.** The person as represented in his or her own awareness and in his or her environment. **3.** IMMUNOLOGY a person's autologous cell components as contrasted with nonself, or foreign, constituents; discrimination by the immune system between self and nonself protects against an attack on the host's own antigenic constituents. The mechanism of recognition of self from nonself is unknown, but serves to protect from an immunologic attack on the host's own antigenic constituents, as opposed to immune system destruction or elimination of foreign antigens.

self-a•ware•ness (self-ă-wār′nĕs) Realization of one's ongoing feeling and emotional experience; a major goal of all psychotherapy.

self-con•cept (self kon′sept) An assessment of one's own status with respect to one or several traits, using societal or personal norms as criteria.

self-con•trol (self′kŏn-trōl′) **1.** Self-regulation of one's behavior in accordance with personal beliefs, goals, attitudes, and societal expectations. **2.** Use by a person of active coping strategies to deal with problem situations, in contrast to passive conditioning strategies that do things to the person and require no response.

self-ef•fi•ca•cy (self-ef′i-kă-sē) Belief that one is capable of accomplishing a behavior or developing a competency.

self•ish DNA (sel′fish) SYN junk DNA.

self-lim•it•ed (self-lim′i-tĕd) Denoting a disease that tends to cease after a definite period (e.g., pneumonia).

self-love (self-lŏv′) SYN narcissism.

self-man•age•ment pro•gram (self-man′ăj-mĕnt prō′gram) Educational program in addtion to regular treatment and disease-specific education that helps patients cope with their health problems.

self-reg•is•ter•ing ther•mom•e•ter (self-rej′is-tĕr′ing thĕr-mom′ĕ-tĕr) A thermometer on which the maximal or minimal temperature, during a period of observation, is registered.

self-re•tain•ing cath•e•ter (self-rē-tān′ing kath′ĕ-tĕr) A catheter so constructed that it remains in urethra and bladder until removed, e.g., indwelling catheter, Foley catheter.

sel•la (sel′ă) SYN saddle (1). [L. saddle]

sel•lar (sel′ăr) Relating to the sella turcica.

sel•la tur•ci•ca (sel′ă tŭr′si-kă) A saddlelike bony prominence on the upper surface of the body of the sphenoid bone, constituting the middle part of the butterfly-shaped middle cranial fossa; it includes the tuberculum sellae anteriorly and the dorsum sellae posteriorly; with its covering of dura mater it constitutes the hypophysial fossa that accommodates the hypophysis or pituitary gland.

Sel•lick ma•neu•ver (sel′ik mă-nū′vĕr) Pressure applied to the cricoid cartilage, to prevent regurgitation or to make the vocal cords easier to visualize during tracheal intubation in the anesthetized patient.

SEM Abbreviation for standard error of measurement.

se•men, pl. **sem•i•na**, **se•mens** (sē′mĕn, -min-ă, -menz) **1.** The penile ejaculate; a thick, yellowish-white, viscid fluid containing sperms; a mixture produced by secretions of the testes, seminal glands, prostate, and bulbourethral glands. SYN seminal fluid. **2.** SYN seed (1). [L. *semen* (*semin-*), seed (of plants, men, animals)]

se•men a•nal•y•sis (sē′mĕn ă-nal′i-sis) A fluid analysis of semen done as the first step in a male infertility workup; includes measurement of semen volume, liquefaction time, sperm count, sperm morphology and motility, pH, white blood cell levels, and fructose levels.

se•men•ur•i•a (sē′mĕ-nyūr′ē-ă) The excretion of urine containing semen. SYN seminuria, spermaturia.

♻ **semi-** Prefix denoting one-half. Cf. hemi-. [L. *semis,* half]

sem•i•ca•nal (sem′ē-kă-nal′) A half canal; a deep groove on the edge of a bone that, uniting with a similar groove or part of an adjoining bone, forms a complete canal. SYN semicanalis.

sem•i•ca•na•lis, pl. **sem•i•ca•na•les** (sem′ē-kă-nal′is, -ēz) SYN semicanal. [L.]

se•mi•ca•na•lis tu•bae aud•i•tor•i•ae (sem-ē-kă-nā′lis tū′bē aw-di-tō-rī-ē) SYN canal for pharyngotympanic tube.

Sem•i•chon a•cid car•mine stain (sem′i-kon as′id kahr′mīn stān) Stain for adult trematodes.

sem•i•cir•cu•lar ca•nals of bo•ny la•by•rinth (sem′ē-sĕr′kyū-lăr kă-nalz′ bō′nē lab′ir-inth) The organ of balance; the three bony tubes in the labyrinth of the ear within which the membranous semicircular ducts are located; they lie in planes at right angles to each other and are known as anterior semicircular canal, posterior semicircular canal, and lateral semicircular canal.

sem•i•cir•cu•lar ducts (sem′ē-sĕr′kyū-lăr dŭkts) Three small, membranous tubes in the bony semicircular canals that lie within the bony labyrinth and form loops of about two thirds of a circle. The three (anterior semicircular duct, lateral semicircular duct, and posterior semicircular duct) lie in planes at right angles to each other and open into the vestibule by five openings, of which one is common to the anterior and lateral ducts. Each duct has an ampulla at one end within which filaments of the vestibular nerve terminate.

sem•i•closed an•es•the•si•a (sem′ē-klōzd an′es-thē′zē-ă) Inhalation anesthesia using a circuit in which a portion of the exhaled air is exhausted from the circuit and a portion is rebreathed following absorption of carbon dioxide.

sem•i•co•ma•tose, **sem•i•co•ma** (sem′ē-kō′mă-tōs, sem′ē-kō′ma) An imprecise term for a state of drowsiness and inaction, in which more than ordinary stimulation may be required to evoke a response, and the response may be delayed or incomplete. SYN semiconscious.

sem•i•con•scious (sem′ē-kon′shŭs) SYN semicomatose.

sem•i-Fow•ler po•si•tion (sem′ē-fowl′ĕr pŏ-zish′ŭn) Placement of the patient in the inclined position, with the head of the bed elevated approximately 30 degrees. Cf. Fowler position.

sem•i•hor•i•zon•tal heart (sem′ē-hōr′i-zon′tăl hahrt) Refers to the heart's electrical axis when this is directed at approximately 0 degrees.

sem•i•lu•nar (sem′ē-lū′năr) SYN lunar (2). [semi- + L. *luna,* moon]

se•mi•lu•nar bod•ies (sem′ē-lū′năr bod′ēz) SYN achromocyte.

sem•i•lu•nar bone (sem′ē-lū′năr bōn) Obsolete term for lunate bone.

sem•i•lu•nar car•ti•lage (sem′ē-lū′năr kahr′ti-lăj) One of the articular menisci of the knee joint.

sem•i•lu•nar con•junc•ti•val fold (sem′ē-lū′năr kŏn-jŭngk′ti-văl fōld) **1.** The semilunar fold formed by the palpebral conjunctiva at the medial angle of the eye. **2.** A fold of the conjunctival mucous membrane found in many animals; normally partially hidden in the medial canthus of the eye when at rest, it may be extended to cover part or all of the cornea in a winklike action to clean the cornea, as in birds. SYN plica semilunaris conjunctivae [TA].

sem•i•lu•nar fi•bro•car•ti•lage (sem′ē-lū′năr fī′brō-kahr′ti-lăj) SEE lateral meniscus, medial meniscus.

sem•i•lu•nar hi•a•tus (sem′ē-lū′năr hī-ā′tŭs) A deep, narrow groove in the lateral wall of the middle meatus of the nasal cavity, into which the maxillary sinus, the frontonasal duct, and the middle ethmoid cells open.

sem•i•lu•nar line (sem′ē-lū′năr līn) SYN linea semilunaris.

sem•i•lu•nar valve (sem′ē-lū′năr valv) A heart valve composed of a set of three semilunar cusps (valvules); hence, both the aortic and pulmonary valves are semilunar valves.

sem•i•mem•bran•o•sus mus•cle (sem′ē-mem′bră-nō′sŭs mŭs′ĕl) *Origin*, tuberosity of ischium; *insertion*, medial condyle of tibia and by membrane to tibial collateral ligament of knee joint, popliteal fascia, and via its reflected tendon of insertion (oblique popliteal ligament) lateral condyle of femur; *action*, flexes knee and rotates leg medially when knee is flexed, and contributes to the stability of extended knee by making capsule of knee joint tense; *nerve supply*, tibial. SYN musculus semimembranosus [TA].

sem•i•mem•bran•ous bur•sa (sem′ē-mem′bră-nŭs bŭr′să) It lies between the muscle, the head of the gastrocnemius, and the knee joint.

sem•i•nal (sem′i-năl) **1.** Relating to the semen. **2.** Original or influential of future developments.

sem•i•nal col•lic•u•lus (sem′i-năl kŏ-lik′yū-lŭs) An elevated portion of the urethral crest on which open the two ejaculatory ducts and the prostatic utricle.

sem•i•nal duct (sem′i-năl dŭkt) Any of the ducts conveying semen from the epididymis to the urethra, ductus deferens, or ejaculatory duct. SYN gonaduct (1).

sem•i•nal flu•id (sem′i-năl flū′id) SYN semen (1).

sem•i•nal gland (sem′i-năl gland) SYN seminal vesicle.

sem•i•nal gran•ule (sem′i-năl gran′yūl) One of the minute granular bodies present in the semen.

sem•i•nal lake (sem′i-năl lāk) SYN lacus seminalis.

sem•i•nal ves•i•cle (sem′i-năl ves′i-kĕl) One of two folded, sacculated, glandular diverticula of the ductus deferens; its secretion is one of the components of semen. SYN gonecyst, gonecystis, seminal gland.

sem•i•na•tion (sem′i-nā′shŭn) SYN insemination.

sem•i•nif•er•ous (sem′i-nif′ĕr-ŭs) Carrying or conducting the semen; denoting the tubules of the testis. [L. *semen,* seed (semen) + *fero,* to carry]

sem•in•if•er•ous cords (sem′i-nif′ĕr-ŭs kōrdz) The cords derived from the primordial sex cords that differentiate into seminiferous tubules during puberty.

sem•i•nif•er•ous ep•i•the•li•um (sem′i-nif′ĕr-ŭs ep′i-thē′lē-ŭm) The epithelium lining the convoluted tubules of the testis where spermatogenesis and spermiogenesis occur.

sem•i•nif•er•ous tu•bule (sem′i-nif′ĕr-ŭs tū′

byūl) One of two or three twisted, curved tubules in each lobule of the testis, in which spermatogenesis occurs. SYN tubuli seminiferi recti [TA], convoluted seminiferous tubule, tubuli contorti (2).

sem•i•nif•er•ous tu•bule dys•gen•e•sis (sem′i-nif′ĕr-ŭs tū′byūl dis-jen′ĕ-sis) A disorder in which the seminiferous tubules exhibit an abnormal cytoarchitecture and extensive hyalinization; the testes are small, and few sperms are formed; the body habitus may be eunuchoid, and gynecomastia may be present; urinary gonadotropin output is usually high, and the incidence of mental deficiency and illness increased; sex chromatin may be male or female, and androgen secretion ranges from subnormal to normal. It is a constant feature of (and is often used synonymously with) Klinefelter syndrome.

sem•i•no•ma (sem′i-nō′mă) A radiosensitive malignant neoplasm usually arising from germ cells in the testis of young male adults that metastasizes to the paraortic lymph nodes; a counterpart of dysgerminoma of the ovary. [L. *semen,* seed (semen) + G. *-oma,* tumor]

sem•in•ur•i•a (sē′mi-nyūr′ē-ă) SYN semenuria.

sem•i•o•pen an•es•the•si•a (sem′ē-ō′pĕn an′es-thē′zē-ă) Inhalation anesthesia in which a portion of inhaled gases is derived from an anesthesia circuit whereas the remainder consists of room air.

se•mi•pen•nate (sem′ē-pen′āt) Having a feather arrangement on one side; resembling one half of a feather.

sem•i•per•me•a•ble (sem′ē-pĕr′mē-ă-bĕl) Freely permeable to water (or other solvent) but relatively impermeable to solutes.

sem•i•po•lar bond (sem′ē-pō′lăr bond) A bond in which the two electrons shared by a pair of atoms belonged originally to only one of the atoms; often represented by a small arrow pointing toward the electron receiver; e.g., nitric acid, $O(OH)N{\rightarrow}O$; phosphoric acid, $(OH)_3P{\rightarrow}O$.

sem•i•re•cum•bent (sem′ē-rē-cŭm′bĕnt) Partly reclining; referring to an inclined patient position, with the head of the bed elevated 45 degrees. SYN Fowler position, semisupine position.

sem•i•spi•nal•is ca•pi•tis mus•cle (sem′ē-spī-nā′lis kap′i-tis mŭs′ĕl) *Origin,* transverse processes of five or six upper thoracic and articular processes of four lower cervical vertebrae; *insertion,* occipital bone between superior and inferior nuchal lines; *action,* rotates head and draws it backward; *nerve supply,* dorsal primary rami of cervical spinal nerves. SYN musculus semispinalis capitis [TA].

sem•i•spi•nal•is cer•vi•cis mus•cle (sem′ē-spī-nā′lis ser′vi-sis mŭs′ĕl) Continuous with musculus semispinalis thoracis; *origin,* transverse processes of second to fifth thoracic vertebrae; *insertion,* spinous processes of axis and third to fifth cervical vertebrae; *action,* extends cervical spine; *nerve supply,* dorsal primary rami of cervical and thoracic spinal nerves. SYN musculus semispinalis cervicis [TA].

sem•i•spi•nal•is tho•ra•cis mus•cle (sem′ē-spī-nā′lis thō-rā′kis mŭs′ĕl) *Origin,* transverse processes of fifth to eleventh thoracic vertebrae; *insertion,* spinous processes of first four thoracic and fifth and seventh cervical vertebrae; *action,* extends vertebral column; *nerve supply,* dorsal primary rami of cervical and thoracic spinal nerves. SYN musculus semispinalis thoracis [TA].

sem•i•sul•cus (sem′ē-sŭl′kŭs) A slight groove on the edge of a bone or other structure, which, uniting with a similar groove on the corresponding adjoining structure, forms a complete sulcus.

sem•i•su•pine po•si•tion (sem′ē-sū′pīn pŏ-zish′ŭn) SYN semirecumbent.

sem•i•syn•thet•ic (sem′ē-sin-thet′ik) Describing the process of synthesizing a particular chemical using a naturally occurring chemical as a starting material, thus obviating part of a total synthesis.

sem•i•ten•di•no•sus mus•cle (sem′ē-ten′di-nō′sus mŭs′ĕl) *Origin,* ischial tuberosity; *insertion,* medial surface of the upper fourth of shaft of tibia; *action,* extends thigh, flexes leg and rotates it medially; *nerve supply,* tibial. SYN musculus semitendinosus [TA].

sem•i•ver•ti•cal heart (sem′ē-vĕr′ti-kăl hahrt) Descriptive of the heart's electrical axis when this is directed at approximately +60 degrees.

Sem•li•ki Fo•rest vi•rus (sem′lē-kē fōr′ĕst vī′rŭs) An alphavirus in the family Togaviridae rarely associated with human disease.

se•nesc•ence (sĕ-nes′ĕns) The state of being old. [L. *senesco,* to grow old, fr. *senex,* old]

se•nes•cent (sĕ-nes′ĕnt) Growing old.

Seng•sta•ken-Blake•more tube (seng′stā-kĕn blāk′mōr tūb) A tube with three lumens, one for drainage of the stomach and two for inflation of attached gastric and esophageal balloons; used for emergency treatment of bleeding esophageal varices.

se•nile (sen′il) Relating to or characteristic of old age. [L. *senilis*]

se•nile am•y•loi•do•sis (sen′il am′i-loy-dō′sis) A common form of the disorder in very old people, usually mild and limited to the heart. SEE ALSO amyloidosis of aging.

se•nile ar•te•ri•o•scler•o•sis (sen′il ahr-tēr′ē-ō-skler-ō′sis) A disorder similar to hypertensive arteriosclerosis, but resulting from advanced age rather than hypertension.

se•nile cat•a•ract (sen′il kat′ăr-akt) A cataract occurring spontaneously in the elderly; mainly a cuneiform cataract, nuclear cataract, or posterior subcapsular cataract, alone or in combination.

se•nile de•men•ti•a (sen′il dĕ-men′shē-ă) Cognitive impairment first occurring in the seventh or eighth decade of life, usually due to Alzheimer disease or cerebrovascular impairment.

se•nile he•man•gi•o•ma (sen′il hē-man′jē-ō′mă) A red papule due to weakening of the capillary wall, seen mostly in people over 30 years of age. SYN Campbell de Morgan spots, cherry angioma, De Morgan spot.

se•nile ker•a•to•sis (sen′il ker′ă-tō′sis) Benign flat, raised, or pedunculated lesions, colored yellow to dark brown; more usual on the trunk and increase in incidence after 40 years of age; may be known as basal cell papillomas because of their cells of origin but are not neoplastic and are not related to basal cell carcinomas. SYN seborrheic keratosis (2), keratosis seborrheica. [L. senilis, *old age,* + G. *keras,* horn, + *-osis,* condition]

se•nile len•ti•go (sen′il len-tī′gō) A variably pigmented lentigo occurring on exposed skin of older white people. SYN liver spot.

se•nile mel•a•no•der•ma (sen′il mel′ă-nō-dĕr′mă) Cutaneous pigmentation occurring in the aged.

se•nile plaque (sen′il plak) A spheric mass composed primarily of amyloid fibrils and interwoven neuronal processes, frequently, although not exclusively, observed in Alzheimer disease. SYN neuritic plaque.

se•nile psy•cho•sis (sen′il sī-kō′sis) Mental disturbance occurring in old age and related to degenerative cerebral processes.

se•nile ret•i•nos•chi•sis (sen′il ret′i-nos′ki-sis) Degenerative ocular disorder occurring most often in the elderly and affecting the outer plexiform layer.

se•nile trem•or (sen′il trem′ŏr) An essential tremor that becomes symptomatic in the elderly.

se•nile vag•i•ni•tis (sen′il vaj′i-nī′tis) The atrophic form of the disorder resulting from withdrawal of estrogen stimulation of mucosa, often assuming the form of adhesive vaginitis.

se•nil•i•ty (sĕ-nil′i-tē) Old age; a general term for a variety of conditions seen in mental disorders occurring in old age, broken down into two broad categories, organic and psychological. SEE ALSO senile.

sens- Combining form meaning perception or feeling. [L. *sentio,* to feel]

sen•sate (sen′sāt) Able to perceive touch and other sensations; used in reference to patients who have had partial nerve or spinal cord injuries.

sen•sa•tion (sen-sā′shŭn) A feeling; the translation into consciousness of the effects of a stimulus exciting any of the organs of sense. [L. *sensatio,* perception, feeling, fr. *sentio,* to perceive, feel]

sen•sa•tion lev•el (sen-sā′shŭn lev′ĕl) The amount in decibels that a stimulus exceeds the hearing threshold.

sense (sens) The faculty of perceiving any stimulus. [L. *sentio,* pp. *sensus,* to feel, to perceive]

sense of e•qui•lib•ri•um (sens ē′kwi-lib′rē-ŭm) The sense that makes possible a normal physiologic posture.

sense or•gans (sens ŏr′gănz) The organs of special sense, including the eye, ear, olfactory organ, taste organs, and the accessory structures associated with these organs.

sen•si•bil•i•ty (sens′i-bil′i-tē) The consciousness of sensation; the capability of perceiving sensible stimuli. [L. *sensibilitas*]

sen•si•ble (sen′si-bĕl) **1.** Perceptible to the senses. **2.** Capable of sensation. **3.** SYN sensitive. **4.** Having reason or judgment; intelligent. [L. *sensibilis,* fr. *sentio,* to feel, perceive]

sen•si•ble pers•pir•a•tion (sen′si-bĕl pĕrs′pir-ā′shŭn) Sweat excreted in large quantity, or when there is much humidity in the atmosphere, so that it appears as moisture on the skin.

sen•si•tive (sen′si-tiv) **1.** Capable of perceiving sensations. **2.** Responding to a stimulus. **3.** Acutely perceptive of interpersonal situations. **4.** One who is readily hypnotizable. **5.** Readily undergoing a chemical change, with but slight change in environmental conditions, as a sensitive reagent. **6.** IMMUNOLOGY denoting: 1) a sensitized antigen; 2) a person (or animal) rendered susceptible to immunologic reactions by previous exposure to the antigen concerned. **7.** MICROBIOLOGY denoting a microorganism that is susceptible to inhibition or destruction by a given antimicrobial agent. SYN sensible (3).

sen•si•tiv•i•ty (sen′si-tiv′i-tē) **1.** The ability to appreciate by means of one or more of the senses. **2.** State of being sensitive. **3.** CLINICAL PATHOLOGY the proportion of patients with a given disease or condition in which a test intended to identify that disease or condition yields positive results. Sensitivity (%) = number of diseased people with a positive test result × 100 total number of diseased people tested. Cf. specificity (2). **4.** SYN susceptibility (2). [L. *sentio,* pp. *sensus,* to feel]

sen•si•ti•za•tion (sen′si-tī-zā′shŭn) Immunization, especially with reference to antigens (immunogens) not associated with infection; the induction of acquired sensitivity or of allergy.

sen•si•tize (sen′si-tīz) To render sensitive; to induce acquired sensitivity, to immunize. SEE ALSO sensitized antigen.

sen•si•tized an•ti•gen (sen′si-tīzd an′ti-jen) The complex formed when antigen combines with specific antibody; so called because the antigen, by the mediation of antibody, is rendered sensitive to the action of complement.

sen•si•tized cell (sen′si-tīzd sel) **1.** A cell that has combined with antibody to form a complex capable of reacting with complement components. **2.** A small, "committed," cell derived, by division and differentiation, from a transformed lymphocyte. **3.** A cell that has been either exposed to antigen or opsonized with antibodies and/or complement.

SENSOR (sen′sŏr) Acronym for Sentinel Event Notification System for Occupational Risks.

sen•sor (sen′sŏr) A device designed to respond to physical stimuli such as temperature, light, magnetism, or movement, and transmit resulting impulses for interpretation, recording, movement, or operating control. SEE ALSO sense.

♻**sensori-** Combining form denoting sensory. [L. *sensorius*]

sen•so•ri•al (sen-sōr′ē-ăl) Relating to the sensorium.

sen•so•ri•mo•tor (sen′sōr-i-mō′tŏr) Both sensory and motor; denoting a mixed nerve with afferent and efferent fibers.

sen•so•ri•mo•tor ar•e•a (sen′sōr-i-mō′tŏr ār′ē-ă) The precentral and postcentral gyri of the cerebral cortex.

sen•so•ri•neu•ral deaf•ness (sen′sōr-i-nūr′ăl def′nĕs) Hearing impairment due to disorders of the cochlear division of cranial nerve VII (auditory nerve), the cochlea, or the retrocochlear nerve tracts, as opposed to conductive deafness.

sen•so•ri•neu•ral hear•ing loss (sen′sōr-i-nūr′ăl hēr′ing laws) A form of hearing loss due to a lesion of the auditory division of the cranial nerve VIII or the inner ear.

sen•so•ri•um, pl. **sen•so•ri•a**, **sen•so•ri•ums** (sen-sōr′ē-ŭm, -ă, -ŭmz) **1.** An organ of sensation. **2.** The hypothetical "seat of sensation." **3.** PSYCHOLOGY consciousness; sometimes used as a generic term for the intellectual and cognitive functions. [Late L.]

sen•so•ry (sen′sŏr-ē) Relating to sensation. [L. *sensorius,* fr. *sensus,* sense]

sen•so•ry a•cu•i•ty lev•el (sen′sŏr-ē ă-kyū′i-tē lev′ĕl) A technique for determining air conduction thresholds without masking and with masking presented by bone conduction to the forehead; the change in thresholds indicates the conductive hearing loss.

sen•so•ry a•lex•i•a (sen′sŏr-ē ă-lek′sē-ă) SEE alexia.

sen•so•ry a•pha•si•a (sen′sŏr-ē ă-fā′zē-ă) SYN receptive aphasia.

sen•so•ry a•ware•ness (sen′sŏr-ē ă-wār′nĕs) The ability to receive and differentiate various types of sensory stimuli.

sen•so•ry con•flict (sen′sŏr-ē kon′flikt) A condition in which perceptions obtained through the senses of spatial orientation (e.g., visual, somatosensory) do not match. This frequently produces nausea.

sen•so•ry cor•tex (sen′sŏr-ē kōr′teks) Formerly denoting specifically the somatic sensory cortex, but now used to refer collectively to the somatic sensory, auditory, visual, and olfactory regions of the cerebral cortex.

sen•so•ry de•fen•sive•ness (sen′sŏr-ē dĕ-fens′iv-nĕs) Overreaction to a nonnoxious sensory stimulus resulting in an adverse or defensive response. Types of sensory defensiveness may be associated with tactile, oral, auditory, olfactory, visual, or movement stimuli.

sen•so•ry dep•ri•va•tion (sen′sŏr-ē dep′ri-vā′shŭn) Diminution or absence of usual external stimuli or perceptual experiences, commonly resulting in psychological distress and aberrant functioning if continued too long.

sen•so•ry ep•i•lep•sy (sen′sŏr-ē ep′i-lep′sē) Focal epilepsy initiated by a somatosensory phenomenon.

sen•so•ry gan•gli•on (sen′sŏr-ē gang′glē-ŏn) A cluster of primary sensory neurons forming a usually visible swelling in the course of a peripheral nerve or its dorsal root; such nerve cells establish the sole afferent neural connection between the sensory periphery (skin, mucous membranes of the oral and nasal cavities, muscle tissue, tendons, joint capsules, special sense organs, blood vessel walls, tissues of the internal organs) and the central nervous system; they are the cells of origin of all sensory fibers of the peripheral nervous system.

sen•so•ry hear•ing im•pair•ment (sen′sŏr-ē hēr′ing im-pār′mĕnt) Form of sensorineural hearing impairment caused by a lesion in the inner ear.

sen•so•ry im•age (sen′sŏr-ē im′ăj) An image based on one or more types of sensation.

sen•so•ry in•teg•ra•tion (SI) (sen′sŏr-ē in′tĕ-grā′shŭn) The neurologic process of organizing sensory information from one's body or the environment to make an adaptive response; a theory and method of remediation used in occupational and physical therapy.

sen•so•ry in•te•gra•tive dys•func•tion (sen′sŏr-ē in′tĕ-grā′tiv dis-fŭngk′shŭn) A disorder of the nervous system that impairs sensory integration.

sen•so•ry mod•u•la•tion (sen′sŏr-ē moj′yū-lā′shŭn) The ability to regulate and organize reactions to sensory input in a graded and adapted manner by balancing excitatory and inhibitory inputs and adapting to environmental changes.

sen•so•ry nerve (sen′sŏr-ē nĕrv) An afferent nerve conveying impulses that are processed by the central nervous system so as to become part of the organism's perception of self and its environment.

sen•so•ry neu•ron•op•a•thy (sen′sŏr-ē nūr′on-op′ă-thē) The disorder confined to dorsal root and gasserian ganglia.

sen•so•ry pa•ral•y•sis (sen′sŏr-ē păr-al′i-sis) Loss of sensation; anesthesia.

sen•so•ry phan•tom (sen′sŏr-ē fan′tŏm) A perceived sensation unrelated to or distinct from any actual stimulus, which can occur in any of the senses.

sen•so•ry pro•ces•sing (sen′sŏr-ē pros′es-ing) Interpreting and organizing varied stimuli, including those acquired by the tactile, proprioceptive, visual, vestibular, auditory, gustatory, and olfactory senses. SEE ALSO sensory integration, sensory awareness.

sen•so•ry re•gi•stra•tion (sen′sŏr-ē rej′is-trā′shŭn) The brain's ability to receive input and select that which will receive attention and that which will be inhibited from consciousness.

sen•so•ry speech cen•ter (sen′sŏr-ē spēch sen′tĕr) SYN Wernicke center.

sen•so•ry ur•gen•cy (sen′sŏr-ē ŭr′jĕn-sē) Strong need to urinate due to vesicourethral hypersensitivity.

sen•su•al (sen′shū-ăl) **1.** Relating to the body and the senses, as distinguished from the intellect or spirit. **2.** Denoting bodily or sensory pleasure, not necessarily sexual. [L. *sensualis,* endowed with feeling]

sen•su la•to (sen′sū lā′tō) In a broad sense. [L.]

sen•su stric•to (sen′sū strik′tō) In a narrow or limited sense. [L.]

sen•tient (sen′shē-ĕnt) Capable of, or characterized by, sensation. [L. *sentiens,* pres. p. of *sentio,* to feel, perceive]

sen•ti•nel e•vent (sen′ti-nĕl ē-vent′) **1.** A type of clinical indicator used to monitor and appraise the quality of care, including events that require immediate attention. **2.** NURSING any unexpected occurrence resulting in death, serious injury (e.g., physical, psychological, or other), or risk to the patient.

Sen•ti•nel E•vent No•ti•fi•ca•tion Sys•tem for Oc•cu•pa•tion•al Risks (SENSOR) (sen′ti-nĕl ē-vent′ nō′ti-fi-kā′shŭn sis′tĕm ok′yū-pā′shŭn-ăl risks) A NIOSH-sponsored program in which occupational medicine clinicians report occupational diseases to the agency for follow-up and statistical analysis.

sen•ti•nel gland (sen′ti-nĕl gland) A single enlarged lymph node in the omentum that may be an indication of an ulcer opposite to it in the greater or lesser curvature of the stomach.

sen•ti•nel lymph node (sen′ti-nĕl limf nōd) The first lymph node to receive lymphatic drainage from a malignant tumor; the sentinel node is identified as the first to take up a radionuclide or dye injected into the tumor; increasingly used in operations for melanoma and breast cancer; if the sentinel node is free of metastasis, more distal nodes are also free. SEE ALSO signal lymph node.

sen•ti•nel node bi•op•sy (sen′ti-nĕl nōd bī′op-sē) Procedure preceded by injection of a dye or radioisotope proximal to a tumor to identify for excision the primary node draining the area; used to determine the extent of spread of a malignancy.

sen•ti•nel pile (sen′ti-nĕl pīl) A circumscribed thickening of the mucous membrane at the lower end of a fissure of the anus.

sen•ti•nel tag (sen′ti-nĕl tag) Projecting edematous skin at the lower end of an anal fissure.

Seoul vi•rus (sōl vī′rŭs) A species of Hantavirus in Asia causing hemorrhagic fever with renal syndrome. [Seoul, South Korea, the city where it was first isolated.]

sep•a•ra•tion anx•i•e•ty (sep′ăr-ā′shŭn ang-zī′ĕ-tē) Apprehension or fear associated with removal from or loss of a parent or significant other.

sep•sis, pl. **sep•ses** (sep′sis, -sēz) The presence of various pus-forming and other pathogenic organisms, or their toxins, in the blood or tissues; septicemia is a common type of sepsis. [G. *sēpsis,* putrefaction]

♻ **-sepsis** Combining form meaning decay caused by a (specified) cause or of a (specified) sort. [G. *sēpsis,* decay]

sep•sis syn•drome (sep′sis sin′drōm) Clinical evidence of acute infection with hyperthermia or hypothermia, tachycardia, tachypnea, and evidence of inadequate organ function or perfusion manifested by at least one of the following: altered mental status, hypoxemia, acidosis, oliguria, or disseminated intravascular coagulation.

♻ **sept.** **1.** Combining form meaning decay. [G. *sēpsis,* decay] **2.** Combining form referring to a septum (septoplasty). [L. *septum*] [L. *septum*]] **3.** Combining form meaning seven or seventh (septigravida). [L. *septem,* seven]

♻ **sept-** SEE septi-, septico-, septo-.

sep•ta (sep′tă) Plural of septum. [L.]

sep•tal (sep′tăl) Relating to a septum.

sep•tate (sep′tāt) Having a septum; divided into compartments. [L. *saeptum,* septum]

sep•tate u•ter•us (sep′tāt yū′tĕr-ŭs) A uterus divided into two cavities by an anteroposterior septum.

sep•tec•to•my (sep-tek′tŏ-mē) Operative removal of the whole or a part of a septum, specifically of the nasal septum. [L. *saeptum,* septum, + G. *ektomē,* excision]

♻**septi-** Combining form meaning seven. [L. *septem*]

sep•tic (sep′tik) Relating to or caused by sepsis.

sep•tic a•bor•tion (sep′tik ă-bōr′shŭn) An infected abortion complicated by fever, endometritis, and parametritis.

septicaemia [Br.] SYN septicemia.

septicaemic [Br.] SYN septicemic.

septicaemic abscess [Br.] SYN septicemic abscess.

sep•ti•ce•mi•a (sep′ti-sē′mē-ă) A systemic disease caused by multiplication of microorganisms in circulating blood; formerly called "blood poisoning." SEE ALSO pyemia. SYN septic fever, septicaemia. [G. *sēpsis,* putrefaction, + *haima,* blood]

sep•ti•ce•mic (sep′ti-sē′mik) Relating to, suffering from, or resulting from septicemia. SYN septicaemic.

sep•ti•ce•mic ab•scess (sep′ti-sē′mik ab′ses) SYN pyemic abscess. SYN septicaemic abscess.

sep•tic fe•ver (sep′tik fē′vĕr) SYN septicemia.

sep•tic in•farct (sep′tik in′fahrkt) An area of necrosis resulting from vascular obstruction due to emboli composed of clumps of bacteria or infected material.

♻**septico-, septic-** Combining forms denoting sepsis, septic. [G. *sēptikos,* putrifying, fr. *sēpsis,* putrefaction]

septicopyaemia [Br.] SYN septicopyemia.

septicopyaemic [Br.] SYN septicopyemic.

sep•ti•co•py•e•mi•a (sep′ti-kō-pī-ē′mē-ă) Pyemia and septicemia occurring together. SYN septicopyaemia.

sep•ti•co•py•e•mic (sep′ti-kō-pī-ē′mik) Relating to septicopyemia. SYN septicopyaemic.

sep•tic phle•bi•tis (sep′tik flĕ-bī′tis) Inflammation of a vein due to bacterial infection.

sep•tic shock (sep′tik shok) **1.** Condition associated with sepsis and usually associated with abdominal and pelvic infection complicating trauma or operations. **2.** Condition associated with septicemia caused by gram-negative bacteria.

♻**septo-, sept-** Combining forms denoting the septum. [L. *saeptum*]

sep•to•mar•gi•nal (sep′tō-mahr′ji-năl) Relating to the margin of a septum, or to both a septum and a margin.

sep•to•na•sal (sep′tō-nā′zăl) Relating to the nasal septum.

sep•to•op•tic dys•pla•si•a (sep′tō-op′tik displā′zē-ă) Congenital, bilateral optic nerve hypoplasia associated with midline cerebral anomalies. SYN de Morsier syndrome.

sep•to•plas•ty (sep′tō-plas-tē) Surgery to correct defects or deformities of the nasal septum, often by alteration or partial removal of supporting structures. [septo- + G. *plastos,* formed]

sep•to•rhi•no•plas•ty (sep′tō-rī′nō-plas-tē) Combined surgery to repair defects or deformities of the nasal septum and of the external nasal pyramid. [septo- + G. *rhis,* nose, + *plastos,* formed]

sep•tos•to•my (sep-tos′tŏ-mē) Surgical creation of an artificial opening in a septum, particularly the interatrial septum. [septo- + G. *stoma,* mouth]

sep•tu•lum, pl. **sep•tu•la** (sep′tū-lŭm, -lă) A minute septum. [Mod. L. dim. of *septum*]

sep•tum, gen. **sep•ti**, pl. **sep•ta** (sep′tŭm, -tī, -tă) **1.** [TA] A thin wall dividing two cavities or masses of softer tissue. SEE ALSO transparent septum. **2.** In fungi, a wall; usually a cross-wall in a hypha. USAGE NOTE The plural septa is sometimes mistaken for a singular form and wrongly pluralized as septae. [L. *saeptum,* a partition]

sep•tum in•ter•a•tri•a•le (sep′tŭm in-ter′ā-trī-ā′lē) [TA] SYN interatrial septum.

sep•tum pel•lu•ci•dum (sep′tŭm pe-lū′sid-ŭm) A thin plate of brain tissue, containing nerve cells and fibers, that is stretched like a flat, vertical sheet between the column and body of fornix below, and the corpus callosum above and anteriorly.

sep•tum pe•nis (sep′tŭm pē′nis) The portion of the tunica albuginea incompletely separating the two corpora cavernosa of the penis.

sep•tup•let (sep-tŭp′lĕt) One of seven children carried through a single pregnancy and born together. [L. *septuplum,* group of seven]

se•que•la, pl. **se•que•lae** (sē-kwel′ă, -ē) A condition following as a consequence of a disease. [L. *sequela,* a sequel, fr. *sequor,* to follow]

se•quence (sē′kwĕns) The succession, or following, of one thing or event after another. [L. *sequor,* to follow]

se•quence lad•der (sē′kwĕns lad′ĕr) The array of bands, made conspicuous by labeling, formed when DNA fragmented by endonucleases is subjected to gel electrophoresis; corresponds to the nucleotide sequence.

se•quen•tial a•nas•to•mo•sis (sē-kwen′shăl ă-nas′tŏ-mō′sis) Two or more communications fashioned from a single conduit (e.g., two or more coronary arteries from a single vein graft or mammary artery).

se•ques•tra (sē-kwes′tră) Plural of sequestrum.

se•ques•tral (sē-kwes′trăl) Relating to a sequestrum.

se•ques•tra•tion (sē′kwes-trā′shŭn) **1.** Formation of a sequestrum. **2.** Loss of blood or of its fluid content into spaces within the body so that it is withdrawn from the circulating volume, resulting in hemodynamic impairment, hypovolemia, hypotension, and reduced venous return to the heart. [L. *sequestratio,* fr. *sequestro,* pp. *-atus,* to lay aside]

se•ques•trec•to•my (sē′kwes-trek′tŏ-mē) Operative removal of a sequestrum. [sequestrum + G. *ektomē,* excision]

se•ques•trum, pl. **se•ques•tra** (sē-kwes′trŭm, -tră) A piece of necrotic tissue, usually bone, which has become separated from the surrounding healthy tissue. [Mod. L. use of Mediev. L. *sequestrum,* something laid aside, fr. L. *sequestro,* to lay aside, separate]

se•quoi•o•sis (sē-kwoy-ō′sis) Extrinsic allergic alveolitis caused by inhalation of redwood sawdust containing spores of *Graphium, Aureobasidium,* and other fungi. [*Sequoia* (genus name) for *Sequoah* (George Guess), Cherokee scholar, + G. *-osis,* condition]

SER Abbreviation for somatosensory evoked response. SEE ALSO evoked response.

Ser Abbreviation for serine and its radical.

ser•al•bu•min (sēr′al-bū′min) SYN serum albumin.

Ser•gent white line (sār-zhōn[h]′ wīt līn) SYN white line (2).

se•ri•al di•lu•tion (sēr′ē-ăl di-lū′shŭn) The preparation of a graded set of solutions or suspensions, each member of the set being a fixed dilution (typically 1:2) of the preceding member; used particularly in titration of antibodies in serum.

se•ri•al ex•trac•tion (sēr′ē-ăl ek-strak′shŭn) Selective removal of certain teeth during the early years of dental development, usually with the eventual extraction of the first, or occasionally the second, premolars, to relieve crowding of anterior teeth.

se•ri•al in•ter•val (sēr′ē-ăl in′tĕr-văl) The time period between analogous phases of an infectious illness in successive cases of a chain of infection that is spread from person to person. SEE ALSO mass action principle, infection transmission parameter.

se•ri•al ra•di•og•ra•phy (sēr′ē-ăl rā′dē-og′ră-fē) Making several x-ray exposures of a single region over a period of time, as in angiography.

se•ri•al sec•tion (sēr′ē-ăl sek′shŭn) One of a number of consecutive microscopic sections.

se•ri•al skill (sēr′ē-ăl skil) One of a series of motor patterns that appear as discrete actions performed together where the sequence or order of the patterns is crucial to success (e.g., a gymnastics routine, brushing one's teeth).

se•ries, pl. **se•ries** (sēr′ēz) **1.** A succession of similar objects following one another in space or time. **2.** CHEMISTRY a group of substances, either elements or compounds, having similar properties or differing from each other in composition by a constant ratio. [L. fr. *sero,* to join together]

ser•ine (S, Ser) (sēr′ēn) One of the amino acids occurring in proteins.

SERM Abbreviation for selective estrogen receptor modulator.

♻ **sero-** Combining form denoting serum, serous. [L. *serum,* whey]

se•ro•co•li•tis (sēr′ō-kō-lī′tis) SYN pericolitis. [Mod. L. *serosa,* serous membrane, + colitis]

ser•o•con•ver•sion (sēr′ō-kŏn-vĕr′zhŭn) The process by which, after exposure to the etiologic agent of a disease, the blood changes from a negative to a positive serum marker for that specific disease.

ser•o•di•ag•no•sis (sēr′ō-dī′ăg-nō′sis) Diagnosis by means of a reaction using blood serum or other serous fluids in the body (serologic tests).

ser•o•en•ter•i•tis (sēr′ō-en′tĕr-ī′tis) SYN perienteritis. [Mod. L. *serosa,* serous membrane, + enteritis]

ser•o•ep•i•de•mi•ol•o•gy (sēr′ō-ep′i-dē′mē-ol′ŏ-jē) An epidemiologic study based on the detection of infection by serologic testing.

ser•o•fi•brin•ous (sēr′ō-fī′bri-nŭs) Denoting an exudate composed of serum and fibrin.

ser•o•fi•brin•ous pleu•ri•sy (sēr′ō-fī′bri-nŭs plūr′i-sē) The more common form of pleurisy, characterized by a fibrinous exudate on the surface of the pleura and an extensive effusion of serous fluid into the pleural cavity.

ser•o•fi•brous (sēr′ō-fī′brŭs) Relating to a serous membrane and a fibrous tissue.

ser•o•group (sēr′ō-grūp) **1.** A group of bacteria containing a common antigen, used in the classification of certain genera of bacteria. **2.** A group of viral species that are antigenically closely related.

ser•o•log•ic (sēr′ō-loj′ik) Relating to serology.

se•ro•log•ic test (sēr′ō-loj′ik test) Any diagnostic test in which serum (blood) is used.

ser•ol•o•gy (sēr-ol′ŏ-jē) The branch of science concerned with serum, especially with specific immune or lytic serums; to measure either antigens or antibodies in sera. [sero- + G. *logos,* study]

ser•o•ma (sēr-ō′mă) A mass or tumefaction caused by localized accumulation of serum within a tissue or organ. [sero- + G. *-oma,* tumor]

ser•o•mem•bra•nous (sēr′ō-mem′bră-nŭs) Relating to a serous membrane.

ser•o•mu•coid (sēr′ō-myū′koyd) General term for a mucoprotein (glycoprotein) from serum.

ser•o•mu•cous (sēr′ō-myū′kŭs) Pertaining to a mixture of watery and mucinous material, such as that of certain glands.

ser•o•mu•cous gland (sēr′ō-myū′kŭs gland) **1.** A gland in which some secretory cells are serous and others mucous. **2.** A gland with cells that secrete a fluid intermediate between a watery and a more viscous mucoid substance.

ser•o•neg•a•tive (sēr′ō-neg′ă-tiv) Lacking an antibody of a specific type in serum; denoting absence of prior infection with a specific agent, disappearance of antibodies after treatment of a disease, or absence of antibody usually found in a given syndrome.

ser•o•pos•i•tive (sēr′ō-poz′i-tiv) Containing antibody of a specific type in serum; denoting the presence of immunologic evidence of a specific infection or presence of a diagnostically useful antibody.

ser•o•pu•ru•lent (sēr-ō-pyūr′ū-lĕnt) Composed of or containing both serum and pus; denoting a discharge of thin, watery pus (seropus).

ser•o•pus (sēr′ō-pŭs) Purulent serum, i.e., pus largely diluted with serum.

ser•o•sa (sēr-ō′să) **1.** The outermost coat or serous layer of a visceral structure that lies in a body cavity (abdomen or thorax); it consists of a surface layer of mesothelium reinforced by irregular fibroelastic connective tissue. **2.** The outermost of the extraembryonic membranes, which encloses the embryo and all its other membranes; it consists of ectoderm reinforced by somatic mesoderm; the serosa of mammalian embryos is frequently called the trophoderm. SYN membrana serosa (2). SEE ALSO chorion. SYN membrana serosa (1), serous membrane. [fem. of Mod. L. *serosus,* serous]

ser•o•san•guin•e•ous (sēr′ō-sang-gwin′ē-ŭs) Denoting an exudate or a discharge composed of or containing both serum and blood.

ser•o•se•rous (sēr′ō-sēr′ŭs) **1.** Relating to two serous surfaces. **2.** Denoting a suture, as of the intestine, in which the edges of the wound are infolded so as to bring the two serous surfaces in apposition.

ser•o•si•tis (sēr′ō-sī′tis) Inflammation of a serous membrane.

ser•os•i•ty (sēr-os′i-tē) The condition of being serous or watery.

ser•o•syn•o•vi•tis (sēr′ō-sin′ō-vī′tis) Synovitis attended with a copious serous effusion.

ser•o•ther•a•py (sēr′ō-thār′ă-pē) Treatment of an infectious disease by injection of an antitoxin or serum containing specific antibody.

ser•o•to•ner•gic (sēr′ō-tō-nĕr′jik) Related to the action of serotonin or its precursor L-tryptophan. [serotonin + G. *ergon,* work]

ser•o•to•nin (ser′ŏ-tō′nin) A vasoconstrictor, liberated by platelets; inhibits gastric secretion and stimulates smooth muscle; also acts as a neurotransmitter; present in the central nervous system, many peripheral tissues and cells, and carcinoid tumors. SYN 5-hydroxytryptamine. [sero- + G. *tonos,* tone, tension, + -in]

ser•o•type (sēr′ō-tīp) SYN serovar.

se•rous (sēr′ŭs) Relating to, containing, or producing serum or a substance having a watery consistency.

se•rous cell (sēr′ŭs sel) A cell, especially of the salivary gland, that secretes a watery or thin albuminous fluid, as opposed to a mucous cell.

se•rous cyst (sēr′ŭs sist) A cyst containing clear serous fluid, such as a hygroma.

se•rous gland (sēr′ŭs gland) One that secretes a watery substance that may or may not contain an enzyme.

se•rous in•flam•ma•tion (sēr′ŭs in′flă-mā′shŭn) An exudative inflammation in which the exudate is predominantly fluid; relatively few cells are observed.

se•rous lig•a•ment (sēr′ŭs lig′ă-mĕnt) One of a number of peritoneal folds attaching certain of the viscera to the abdominal wall or to each other.

se•rous mem•brane (sēr′ŭs mem′brān) SYN serosa.

se•rous men•in•gi•tis (sēr′ŭs men′in-jī′tis) Acute form of the disease with secondary external hydrocephalus.

se•rous o•ti•tis (sēr′ŭs ō-tī′tis) Inflammation of middle ear mucosa, often accompanied by accumulation of fluid, secondary to auditory tube obstruction. SYN secretory otitis media.

se•rous o•ti•tis me•di•a (sēr′ŭs ō-tī′tis mē′dē-ă) SYN middle-ear effusion.

se•rous pleu•ri•sy (sēr′ŭs plūr′i-sē) SYN pleurisy with effusion.

se•rous syn•o•vi•tis (sēr′ŭs sin′ō-vī′tis) Inflammation of the synovial membrane with a large effusion of nonpurulent fluid.

ser•o•vac•ci•na•tion (sēr′ō-vak′si-nā′shŭn) A process for producing mixed immunity by the injection of a serum, to secure passive immunity, and by vaccination with a modified or killed culture to acquire active immunity later.

ser•o•var (sēr′ō-vahr) A subdivision of a species or subspecies distinguishable from other strains therein on the basis of antigenic character. SYN serotype. [sero- + *variant*]

ser•pig•i•nous (sĕr-pij′i-nŭs) Creeping; denoting an ulcer or other cutaneous lesion that extends with a wavy or serpentine border. [Mediev. L. *serpigo- (-gin-),* ringworm, fr. L. *serpo,* to creep]

ser•pi•go (sĕr-pī′gō) **1.** SYN tinea. **2.** SYN herpes. **3.** Any creeping or serpiginous eruption. [Mediev. L. *serpigo (-gin-)*, ringworm, fr. L. *serpo,* to creep]

ser•rate, ser•rat•ed (ser′āt, -ā′ted) Toothed. [L. *serratus,* fr. *serra,* a saw]

ser•rate su•ture (sĕr′āt sū′chŭr) One with opposing margins that present deep, sawlike indentations, as in most of the sagittal suture. SYN dentate suture.

ser•ra•tion (ser-ā′shŭn) **1.** The state of being serrated or notched. **2.** Any one of the processes in a serrate or dentate formation. [L. *serra,* saw]

ser•ra•tus an•te•ri•or mus•cle (sĕ-rā′tŭs an-tēr′ē-ŏr mŭs′ĕl) *Origin*, from center of lateral aspect of first eight to nine ribs; *insertion*, superior and inferior angles and intervening medial margin of scapula; *action*, rotates scapula and pulls it forward, elevates ribs; *nerve supply*, long thoracic from brachial plexus. See this page. SYN musculus serratus anterior [TA].

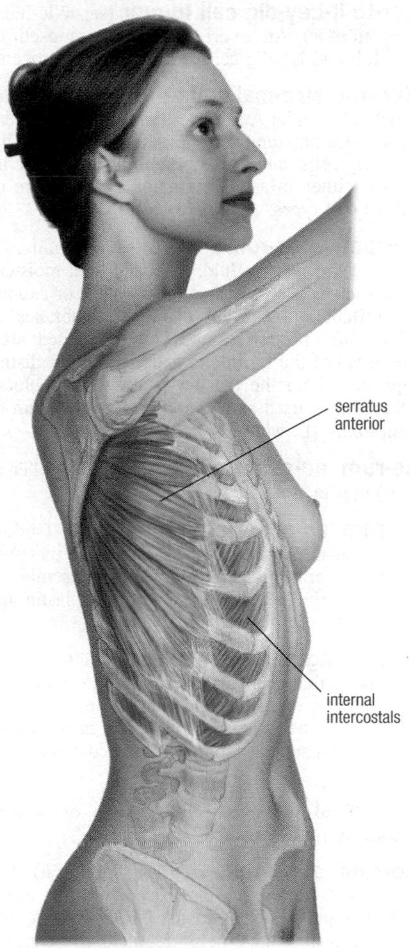

serratus anterior muscle

ser•ra•tus pos•te•ri•or in•fe•ri•or mus•cle (sĕ-rā′tŭs pos-tēr′ē-ŏr in-fēr′ē-ŏr mŭs′ĕl) Lower intermediate muscle of back; *origin*, with latissimus dorsi, from spinous processes of two lower thoracic and two upper lumbar vertebrae; *insertion*, into lower borders of last four ribs; *action*, draws lower ribs backward and downward; *nerve supply*, ninth to twelfth intercostal. SYN inferior posterior serratus muscle, musculus serratus posterior inferior.

ser•ra•tus pos•ter•i•or su•per•i•or mus•cle (sĕ-rā′t′us pos-tēr′ē-ŏr sŭ-pēr′ē-ŏr mŭs′ĕl) Upper intermediate muscle of back; *origin*, from spinous processes of two lower cervical and two upper thoracic vertebrae; *insertion*, into lateral side of angles of second–fifth ribs; *nerve supply*, first–fourth intercostals. SYN musculus serratus posterior superior, superior posterior serratus muscle.

ser•re•fine (ser-ĕ-fēn′) A small spring forceps used for approximating the edges of a wound or for temporarily closing an artery during an operation. [Fr.]

Ser•to•li-cell-on•ly syn•drome (ser-tō′lē-sel-ōn′lē sin′drōm) The absence from the seminiferous tubules of the testes of germinal epithelium, Sertoli cells alone being present; there is sterility due to azoospermia, but Leydig cells are normal; the output of gonadotrophins in the urine is increased.

Ser•to•li cells (ser-tō′lē selz) Elongated cells in the seminiferous tubules that ensheathe spermatids, providing a microenvironment that supports spermiogenesis; they secrete androgen-binding protein and establish the blood-testis barrier by forming tight junctions with adjacent Sertoli cells.

Ser•to•li cell tu•mor (ser-tō′lē sel tū′mŏr) Any neoplasm of the testis containing Sertoli cells or of the ovary containing Sertoli-like cells; malignant potential varies.

Ser•to•li-Ley•dig cell tu•mor (ser-tō′lē-lī′dig sel tū′mŏr) An ovarian tumor composed of Sertoli and Leydig cells; may secrete androgens.

Ser•to•li-stro•mal cell tu•mor (ser-tō′lē-strō′ măl sel tū′mŏr) A generic term for ovarian sex-cord stromal tumor composed of Sertoli cells, Leydig cells, and cells resembling rete epithelial cells, either in a pure form or as a mixture of these cell types.

se•rum, pl. **se•rums**, **se•ra** (sēr′ŭm, -ŭmz, -ă) **1.** A clear, watery fluid, especially that moistening the surface of serous membranes, or exuded in inflammation of any of those membranes. **2.** The fluid portion of the blood obtained after removal of the fibrin clot and blood cells, distinguished from the plasma in circulating blood. Sometimes used as a synonym for antiserum or antitoxin. [L. whey]

se•rum ac•cel•er•a•tor (sēr′ŭm ak-sel′ĕr-ā-tŏr) SYN factor VII.

se•rum ac•cel•er•a•tor glob•u•lin (sēr′ŭm ak-sel′ĕr-ā-tŏr glob′yū-lin) A substance in serum that accelerates the conversion of prothrombin to thrombin in the presence of thromboplastin and calcium.

se•rum ag•glu•ti•nin (sēr′ŭm ă-glū′ti-nin) An antibody that coats erythrocytes; the cells do not agglutinate when suspended in saline, but do agglutinate when suspended in serum or other protein media such as albumin. SYN incomplete antibody (2).

se•rum•al (sēr-ū′măl) Relating to or derived from serum.

se•rum al•bu•min (sēr′ŭm al-bū′min) The principal protein in plasma, present in blood plasma and in serous fluids. Participates in fatty acid transport and helps regulate the osmotic pressure of blood. SYN blood albumin, seralbumin.

se•rum dis•ease (sēr′ŭm di-zēz′) SYN serum sickness.

se•rum-fast (sēr′ŭm-fast) **1.** Pertaining to a serum in which there is little or no change in the titer of antibody, even under conditions of treatment or immunologic stimulation. **2.** Resistant to the destructive effect of sera.

se•rum glu•ta•mic-ox•a•lo•a•ce•tic trans•am•i•nase (SGOT) (sēr′ŭm glū-tam′ik-ok′să-lō-ă-sē′tik trans-am′i-nās) SYN aspartate aminotransferase.

se•rum glu•tam•ic-py•ru•vic trans•am•i•nase (SGPT) (sēr′ŭm glū-tam′ik-pī-rūv′ĭk trans-am′i-nās) SYN alanine aminotransferase.

se•rum hep•a•ti•tis vi•rus (sēr′ŭm hep′ă-tī′tis vī′rŭs) SYN hepatitis B virus.

se•rum ne•phri•tis (sēr′ŭm nĕ-frī′tis) Glomerulonephritis occurring in serum sickness or in animals injected with foreign serum protein.

se•rum pro•throm•bin con•ver•sion ac•cel•er•a•tor (SPCA) (sēr′ŭm prō-throm′bin kŏn-ver′zhŭn ak-sel′ĕr-ā-tŏr) SYN factor VII.

se•rum re•ac•tion (sēr′ŭm rē-ak′shŭn) SYN serum sickness.

se•rum sep•a•ra•tor tube (SST) (sēr′ŭm sep′ăr-ā′tŏr tūb) A blood collection tube containing a clot activator and a mass of gel with a density between those of serum and cells. During centrifugation, the gel comes to lie between serum and cells. Prevents contact between serum and cells.

se•rum shock (sēr′ŭm shok) Anaphylactic or anaphylactoid shock caused by the injection of antitoxic or other foreign serum.

se•rum sick•ness (sēr′ŭm sik′nĕs) An immune complex disease appearing 1–2 weeks after injection of a foreign serum or serum protein, with local and systemic reactions such as urticaria, fever, general lymphadenopathy, edema, arthritis, and occasionally albuminuria or severe nephritis. SYN serum disease, serum reaction.

ser•vice (sĕr′vis) A firm or agency that provides on-scene response, assessment, stabilization, initial treatment as directed, and transport to the appropriate receiving facility (i.e., trauma center or hospital) for medical emergency or trauma patients. [L. *servio,* to serve, fr. *servus,* slave]

ser•vice a•gree•ment (sĕr′vis ă-grē′mĕnt) A contract between a school district and a family that outlines the provision of physical therapy and other related services for children with physical disabilities who are enrolled in regular public education.

ser•vice co•ord•i•na•tor (sĕr′vis kō-ōrd′i-nā-tŏr) A person responsible for identifying, contacting, managing, and facilitating health care or developmental services provided to a patient.

ses•a•moid (ses′ă-moyd) **1.** Resembling in size or shape of a sesame seed. **2.** Denoting a sesamoid bone. [G. *sēsamoeidēs,* like sesame]

ses•a•moid bone (ses′ă-moyd bōn) A bone formed after birth in a tendon where it passes over a joint (e.g., the patella).

ses•a•moid car•ti•lage of cri•co•pha•ryn•ge•al li•ga•ment (ses′ă-moyd kahr′ti-lăj krī′kō-făr-in′jē-ăl lig′ă-mĕnt) A small nodule of elastic cartilage sometimes present on the lateral border of the arytenoid cartilage.

ses•qui•hy•drates (ses′kwi-hī′drāts) Compounds crystallizing with (nominally) 1.5 molecules of water.

ses•sile (ses′il) Having a broad base of attachment; not pedunculated. [L. *sessilis,* low-growing, fr. *sedeo,* pp. *sessus,* to sit]

set (set) **1.** To reduce a fracture, i.e., to bring the bones back into a normal position or alignment. **2.** A readiness to perceive or to respond in some way; a mindset; an attitude that affects or predetermines an outcome, e.g., prejudice or bigotry.

se•ta, pl. **set•ae** (sē′tă, -tē) A bristle or a slender, stiff, bristle like structure. [L. *saeta* or *seta*, a stiff hair or bristle]

se•ta•ceous (sē-tā′shŭs) **1.** Having bristles. **2.** Resembling a bristle. [L. *seta,* a bristle]

se•ton (sē′tŏn) A wisp of threads, a strip of gauze, a length of wire, or other foreign material passed through the subcutaneous tissues or a cyst to form a sinus or fistula. [L. *seta,* bristle]

set•point the•o•ry (set′poynt thē′ŏr-ē) A hypothesized genetically determined level of body weight controlled by the hypothalamus that varies from person to person. Only exercise and drugs have been shown to alter (lower) the setpoint.

set•ting sun sign (set′ing sŭn sīn) Retraction of the upper lid without upgaze so that the iris seems to "set" below the lower lid; suggestive of neurologic damage in the newborn, but usually clears up without sequelae.

sev•enth cra•ni•al nerve [CN VII] (sev′ĕnth krā′nē-ăl nĕrv) SYN facial nerve [CN VII].

Se•ver dis•ease (sē′vĕr di-zēz′) An osteochondrosis of the heel, probably secondary to microfractures in the bone where the Achilles tendon attaches to the posterior calcaneus; an overuse injury and a common cause of heel pain in older children. SYN calcaneal apophysitis.

se•vere a•cute res•pi•ra•tor•y syn•drome (SARS) (sĕ vēr′ ă kyūt′ res′pir-ă-tōr-ē sin′ drōm) Highly contagious, severe febrile respiratory illness caused by a coronavirus (SARS-CoV).

se•ve•ri•ty of ill•ness (sĕ-ver′i-tē il′nĕs) The degree of illness and risk of disease manifested by patients, based either on clinical data from the medical records or on hospital discharge or billing data. Outcome comparisons usually are interpreted in terms of severity of illness to ensure that meaningful data interpretations are made.

sex (seks) **1.** The biologic character or quality that distinguishes male and female from one another as expressed by analysis of the individual's gonadal, morphologic (internal and external), chromosomal, and hormonal characteristics. Cf. gender. **2.** The physiologic and psychological processes within an individual that prompt behavior related to procreation or erotic pleasure. [L. *sexus*]

sex as•sign•ment (seks ă-sīn′mĕnt) Process whereby the sex of an intersex (hermaphroditic) newborn is initially decided.

sex cell (seks sel) A sperm or an oocyte. SYN germ cell.

sex chro•ma•tin (seks krō′mă-tin) A small, condensed mass of the inactivated X-chromosome usually located just inside the nuclear membrane of the interphase nucleus; the number of sex chromatin bodies per nucleus is one less than the number of X-chromosomes; hence, normal males have none and normal females have one. For technical reasons, only about half the cells in a preparation show typical masses. SEE ALSO Lyon hypothesis. SYN Barr chromatin body.

sex chro•mo•somes (seks krō′mŏ-sōmz) The pair of chromosomes responsible for sex determination. In humans and most animals, the sex chromosomes are designated X and Y; females have two X chromosomes, males have one X and one Y chromosome.

sex de•ter•mi•na•tion (seks dĕ-tĕr′mi-nā′shŭn) Identification of the sex of a fetus in utero by identification of fetal chromosomes.

sex hor•mones (seks hōr′mōnz) A general term covering those steroid hormones that are formed by testicular, ovarian, and adrenocortical tissues, and that are androgens or estrogens.

sex-in•flu•enced (seks-in′flū-ĕnst) Denoting a class of genetic disorders in which the same genotype has differing manifestations in the two sexes. SEE ALSO sex-influenced inheritance.

sex-in•flu•enced in•her•i•tance (seks-in′flū-ĕnst in-her′i-tăns) Inheritance that is autosomal but has a different intensity of expression in the two sexes (e.g., male pattern baldness).

sex•ism (seks′izm) Attitudes and practices that place different values on, or create unequal opportunities for, people because of their gender.

sex-lim•it•ed (seks-lim′i-tĕd) Occurring in one sex only. SEE ALSO sex-limited inheritance.

sex-lim•it•ed in•her•i•tance (seks-lim′i-tĕd in-her′i-tăns) Inheritance of a trait that can be expressed in one sex only (e.g., testicular feminization).

sex link•age, **sex-linked** (seks lingk′ăj, seks′ lingkt) Inheritance of a trait or a sex chromosome or gonosome. A man receives all his sex-linked genes from his mother and transmits them all to his daughters but not to his sons; a recessive sex-linked character is much more likely to be expressed in the male. SEE ALSO sex chromosomes.

sex-linked char•ac•ter (seks′lingkt kar′ăk-tĕr) An inherited character determined by a gene on a gonosome. SEE ALSO gene.

sex-linked in•her•i•tance (seks′lingkt in-her′ i-tăns) The pattern of inheritance that may result from a mutant gene located on either the X or Y chromosome.

sex•ol•o•gy (seks-ol′ō-jē) The study of all aspects of sex and, in particular, sexual behavior. [L. *sexus,* sex, + G. *logos,* study]

sex ra•ti•o (seks rā′shē-ō) **1.** The ratio of male

to female progeny at some specified stage of the life cycle, notably at conception (primary), at birth (secondary), or at any stage between birth and death (tertiary). **2.** The ratio of the numbers of males to females affected by a particular disease or trait.

sex re·ver·sal, **sex re·as·sign·ment** (seks rĕ-vĕr′săl, seks rē′ă-sīn′mĕnt) A process whereby the sexual identity of a person is changed from one sex to the other (e.g., by a combination of surgical, pharmacologic, and psychiatric procedures); it may also occur in the life history of a pseudohermaphroditic individual whose sex at birth was uncertain; initially reared as members of one gender or sex role, such people may, on subsequent medical examination and advice, be reared thereafter as members of the opposite gender or sex role.

sex role (seks rōl) The degree to which an individual acts out a stereotypical masculine or feminine role in everyday behavior. Cf. gender role.

sex·tant (seks′tănt) One of the six divisions of the dentition, the teeth of the upper and lower jaws being divided into right posterior, left posterior, and anterior. [L. *sextus,* sixth]

sex·tup·let (seks-tŭp′lĕt) One of six children carried through a single pregnancy and born together. [L. *sextus,* sixth + -uple]

sex·u·al (sek′shū-ăl) **1.** Relating to sex. **2.** Pertaining to someone as perceived by his or her sexual attractiveness, tendencies, and overall sexuality. [L. *sexualis,* fr. *sexus,* sex]

sex·u·al a·buse (sek′shū-ăl ă-būs′) SEE domestic violence.

sex·u·al di·mor·phism (sek′shū-ăl dī-mōr′fizm) The somatic differences within species between male and female individuals that arise as a consequence of sexual maturation, including, but not restricted to, the secondary sexual characters.

sex·u·al dis·or·ders (sek′shū-ăl dis′ŏr-dĕrs) A group of behavioral and psychophysiologic conditions with symptomatic variability in sexual functioning, including either the eroticized behavior associated with sexual activity (the paraphilias) or with disturbances of desire, arousal, and orgasm.

sex·u·al gen·er·a·tion (sek′shū-ăl jen′ĕr-ā′shŭn) Reproduction by conjugation, or the union of male and female cells, as opposed to asexual generation.

sex·u·al in·fan·ti·lism (sek′shū-ăl in-fan′ti-lizm) Failure to develop secondary sexual characteristics after the normal time of puberty.

sex·u·al in·ter·course (sek′shū-ăl in′tĕr-kōrs) SYN coitus.

sex·u·al·i·ty (sek′shū-al′i-tē) **1.** The sum of a person's sexual behaviors and tendencies, and the strength of such tendencies. **2.** One's degree of sexual attractiveness. **3.** The quality of having sexual functions or implications.

sex·u·al·ly trans·mit·ted dis·ease (STD) (sek′shū-ă-lē tranz-mit′ĕd di-zēz′) Any contagious disease acquired through sexual contact (e.g., syphilis, gonorrhea, chancroid, genital warts, AIDS). SYN sexually transmitted infection, venereal disease.

sex·u·al·ly trans·mit·ted in·fec·tion (STI) (sek′shū-ăl-ē tranz-mit′ĕd in-fek′shŭn) SYN sexually transmitted disease.

sex·ual or·i·en·ta·tion (sek′shū-ăl ōr′ē-ĕn-tā′shŭn) Concept that includes permutations among body morphology, gender identity, gender role, and sexual preference.

sex·u·al pref·er·ence (sek′shū-ăl pref′ĕ-rĕns) The biologic sex preferred in one's sexual partners.

sex·u·al re·pro·duc·tion (sek′shū-ăl rē′prō-dŭk′shŭn) Reproduction by union of male and female gametes (germ cells) to form a zygote. SYN gamogenesis, syngenesis.

sex·u·al se·lec·tion (sek′shū-ăl sĕ-lek′shŭn) A form of natural selection in which, according to Darwin's theory, the male or female is attracted by certain characteristics, forms, colors, behaviors, and phenomena, in the opposite sex; thus, modifications of a special nature are brought about in the species.

Sé·zar·y cell (sā-zah-rē′ sel) An atypical mononuclear cell seen in the peripheral blood in Sézary syndrome; has a large, convoluted nucleus and scanty cytoplasm containing PAS-positive vacuoles.

SGA Abbreviation for small for gestational age.

SGOT Abbreviation for serum glutamic-oxaloacetic transaminase (obsolete, but still seen).

SGPT Abbreviation for serum glutamic-pyruvic transaminase (obsolete, but still seen).

SH Abbreviation for sulfhydryl.

shad·ow (shad′ō) **1.** A surface area defined by the interception of light or x-rays by a body. SEE ALSO density (3). **2.** PSYCHOLOGY In jungian terms, the archetype consisting of collective animal instincts. **3.** SYN achromocyte.

shad·ow test (shad′ō test) SYN retinoscopy.

shaft (shaft) An elongated rodlike structure, as the part of a long bone between the epiphysial extremities. SYN diaphysis [TA]. [A.S. *sceaft*]

sha·green skin (shă-grēn′ skin) An oval-shaped nevoid plaque, skin colored or occasionally pigmented, smooth or crinkled, appearing on the trunk or lower back in early childhood; sometimes seen with other signs of tuberous sclerosis.

sha·ken ba·by syn·drome (SBS) (shā′kĕn

bā′bē sin′drōm) A syndrome of neurologic and other injuries, of variable presentation, induced by the violent shaking of an infant.

shak•ra (shahk′ră) Point or location thought to contain an electromagnetic force indicating the state of the body. Term is used by practitioners of Reiki.

shal•low breath•ing (shal′ō brēdh′ing) Respiration with abnormally low tidal volume.

sha•man (shah′măn) The name given among indigenous people (Native Americans, Innu) to a healer, whose therapies range from chant and ritual to use of herbs.

shank (shangk) **1.** The tibia; the shin; the leg. **2.** The portion of an instrument that connects the cutting or functional portion to a handle; with rotary tools, such as burs and drills, the end that fits into the chuck. [A.S. *sceanca*]

shap•ing (shāp′ing) In operant conditioning, when the operant response is not in the organism's repertoire, a procedure in which the experimenter breaks down the response into those parts which appear most frequently, begins reinforcing them, and then slowly and successively withholds the reinforcer until more and more of the operant is emitted.

shared de•ci•sion (shārd dĕ-sizh′ŏn) A health care determination discussed and agreed on by members of the health care team. In this structure, the responsibility for the decision is placed equally on all members of the team.

shared ep•i•tope (shārd ep′i-tōp) SYN susceptibility cassette.

shared gov•er•nance (shārd gŏv′ĕr-năns) A nursing model in which staff nurses share responsibility and accountability for all aspects of patient care within the confines of the health care agency.

sharps (shahrps) Medical instruments that are sharp or may produce sharp pieces. Should be disposed of in a biohazardous sharps container. SEE ALSO blood culture, needlestick.

sharps con•tain•er (shahrps kŏn-tān′ĕr) A puncture-resistant and leak-proof container with a one-way top used to dispose of sharps.

shave bi•op•sy (shāv bī′op-sē) A biopsy technique performed with a surgical blade or a razorblade; used for lesions that are elevated above the skin level or confined to the epidermis and upper dermis, or to protrusions of lesions from internal sites.

shears (shērz) SYN scissors.

sheath (shēth) **1.** Any enveloping structure, such as the membranous covering of a muscle, nerve, or blood vessel; any sheathlike structure. SYN vagina (1). **2.** The prepuce of male animals, especially of the horse. **3.** A specially designed tubular instrument through which special obturators or cutting instruments can be passed, or through which blood clots, tissue fragments, or calculi can be evacuated. **4.** A tube used as an orthodontic appliance, usually on molars. [A.S. *scaeth*]

sheath of Schwann (shēth shwahn) SYN neurilemma.

Shee•han syn•drome (shē′an sin′drōm) Hypopituitarism developing postpartum as a result of pituitary necrosis; caused by ischemia resulting from a hypotensive episode during delivery.

sheep•ber•ry (shēp′ber-ē) SYN black haw.

sheet graft•ing (shēt graft′ing) Type of skin graft in which large strips of skin are placed over the burn as close together as possible.

shelf (shelf) ANATOMY a structure resembling a shelf.

shelf life (shelf līf) Stability of a product during storage; the maximum time during which it can be kept without undergoing change in chemical structure and properties.

shell (shel) An outer covering.

shell nail (shel nāl) Nail dystrophy accompanying clubbing of digits in bronchiectasis, with excessive longitudinal curvature of the nail plate and atrophy of the nail bed and underlying bone.

shell shock (shel shok) SYN battle fatigue.

shel•tered em•ploy•ment (shel′tĕrd em-ploy′mĕnt) An employment arrangement for people with disabilities in a self-contained work site, without integration with nondisabled workers. SEE ALSO supported employment.

Shen•ton line (shen′tŏn līn) A curved line formed by the top of the obturator foramen and the inner side of the neck of the femur, seen on an anteroposterior frontal radiograph of a normal hip joint; it is disturbed in lesions of the joint such as dislocation or fracture.

Shep•herd frac•ture (shep′ĕrd frak′shŭr) A fracture of the external tubercle (posterior process) of the talus, sometimes mistaken for a displacement of the os trigonum.

Sher•ring•ton law (sher′ing-tŏn law) Every dorsal spinal nerve root supplies a particular area of the skin, the dermatome (3), which is, however, invaded above and below by fibers from the adjacent spinal segments.

shi•at•su (shē-aht′sū) A Japanese massage technique using direct pressure, passive and active stretching, and gentle rocking movements to restore balance in the flow of energy in the body. [Jap. *shiatsuryōhō,* fr. *shi,* finger + *atsu,* pressure, + *ryōhō,* treatment]

Shib•ley sign (shib′lē sīn) On auscultation of the chest, the spoken sound "e" is heard as "ah" over an area of pulmonary consolidation or immediately above a pleural effusion.

shield (shēld) A protecting screen; lead sheet for protecting the operator and patient from x-rays. [A.S. *scild*]

shift (shift) **1.** SYN change. SEE ALSO deviation. **2.** A period of 8–12 hours during which an employee is assigned to work on a given day. Division of each 24 hours into day, evening, and night shifts is intended to maximize efficiency.

shift to the left (shift left) **1.** A marked increase in the percentage of immature neutrophils in the circulating blood. **2.** SEE maturation index.

shift to the right (shift rīt) **1.** In a differential count of white blood cells in the peripheral blood, the absence of young and immature forms. **2.** SEE maturation index.

Shi•ga-Kruse ba•cil•lus (shē′gah krūs bă-sil′ŭs) SYN *Shigella dysenteriae.*

Shi•ga•like tox•in (shē′gah-līk tok′sin) SYN vero cytotoxin.

Shi•ga tox•in (shē′gah tok′sin) The endotoxin formed by *Shigella dysenteriae* type 1.

Shi•gel•la (shē-gel′lă) A genus of nonmotile, aerobic to facultatively anaerobic bacteria containing gram-negative, non-spore-forming rods. A major cause of dysentery.

Shi•gel•la boy•di•i (shē-gel′lă boyd′ē-ī) A bacterial species found only in feces of symptomatic individuals; occurs in a low proportion of cases of bacillary dysentery.

Shi•gel•la dys•en•ter•i•ae (shē-gel′lă dis-en-ter′ē-ē) A bacterial species causing dysentery in humans and in monkeys, found only in feces of symptomatic individuals. The type species of the genus *Shigella.* SYN Shiga-Kruse bacillus.

Shi•gel•la flex•ner•i (shē-gel′lă fleks-ner′ī) A bacterial species found in the feces of symptomatic individuals and of convalescents and carriers; the most common cause of dysentery epidemics and sometimes of infantile gastroenteritis. Can be sexually transmitted, through anal intercourse. SYN Flexner bacillus.

Shi•gel•la son•ne•i (shē-gel′lă son′nē-ī) A bacterial species causing mild dysentery and also summer diarrhea in children. SYN Sonne bacillus.

shig•el•lo•sis (shig′ĕ-lō′sis) Bacillary dysentery caused by bacteria of the genus *Shigella*, often occurring in epidemic patterns; an opportunistic infection of people with AIDS.

shim•ming pro•cess (shim′ing pros′es) A method whereby the evenness of the magnetic field is optimized.

shin (shin) **1.** The anterior aspect of the leg, from knee to ankle. **2.** SYN anterior border of tibia. [A.S. *scina*]

shin bone (shin bōn) SYN tibia.

shin•gles (shing′g ĕlz) SYN herpes zoster. See this page, B9. [L. *cingulum*, girdle]

shin-splints (shin′splints) A collective term denoting tenderness and pain with induration and swelling in the anterior tibial compartment, particularly following athletic overexertion by the untrained.

ship (ship) A structure resembling the hull of a ship.

ship•yard eye (ship′yahrd ī) SYN epidemic keratoconjunctivitis virus.

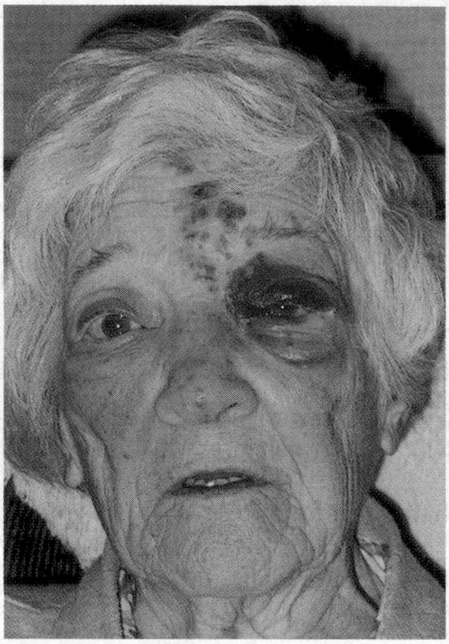

shingles (herpes zoster)

shirt-stud ab•scess (shĭrt-stŭd ab′ses) SYN collar-button abscess.

shi•ver•ing ther•mo•gen•e•sis (shiv′ĕr-ing thĕr-mō-jen′ĕ-sis) State resulting from the increase in metabolism of the skeletal muscles due to shivering.

shock (shok) **1.** A sudden physical or mental disturbance. **2.** A state of profound mental and physical depression consequent upon severe physical injury or an emotional disturbance. **3.** A severe disturbance of hemodynamics in which the circulatory system fails to maintain adequate perfusion of vital organs; may be due to reduction of blood volume (hemorrhage, dehydration), cardiac failure, or dilation of the vascular system in toxemia or septicemia. **4.** The abnormally palpable impact, appreciated by a hand on the chest wall, of an accentuated heart sound. [Fr. *choc*, fr. Germanic]

shock lung (shok lŭng) In shock, the development of edema, impaired perfusion, and reduction in alveolar space so that the alveoli collapse. SYN pump lung, wet lung (1), white lung.

shock ther·a·py, shock treat·ment (shok thār′ă-pē, trēt′mĕnt) SEE electroshock therapy.

Shone a·nom·a·ly (shōn ă-nom′ă-lē) Coarctation of the aorta, subaortic stenosis, and stenosing ring of the left atrium found in association with a parachute mitral valve.

Shone com·plex (shōn kom′pleks) An obstructive lesion of the mitral valve complex with left ventricular outflow obstruction and coarctation of the aorta.

Shone syn·drome (shōn sin′drōm) The association of obstructive lesions of the mitral valve complex, including the supravalvar ring and parachute mitral valve, with left ventricular outflow obstruction and coarctation of the aorta.

shon·ny (shon′ē) SYN black haw.

short ab·duc·tor mus·cle of thumb (shōrt ab-dŭk′tŏr mŭs′ĕl thŭm) SYN abductor pollicis brevis muscle.

short ad·duc·tor mus·cle (shōrt ă-dŭk′tŏr mŭs′ĕl) SYN adductor brevis muscle.

short bone (shōrt bōn) One with approximately equal dimensions; it consists of a layer of cortical substance enclosing spongy substance and marrow. Cf. long bone.

short-bow·el syn·drome (shōrt bow′ĕl sin′drōm) Complex of symptoms that can result whenever the absorptive surface of the small bowel is reduced, as in massive or multiple small bowel resections. Symptoms include diarrhea, weight loss, malabsorption, anemia, and vitamin, mineral, and electrolyte abnormalities. Degree of malabsorption and malnutrition depends on the site and extent of the resection. SYN short-gut syndrome.

short cil·i·ar·y nerve (shōrt sil′ē-ar-ē nĕrv) One of several branches passing from the ciliary ganglion to the eyeball, supplying the ciliary muscles, iris, and tunics of the eyeball. SYN nervus ciliaris brevis.

short ex·ten·sor mus·cle of great toe (shōrt eks-ten′sŏr mŭs′ĕl grāt tō) SYN extensor hallucis brevis muscle.

short ex·ten·sor mus·cle of thumb (shōrt eks-ten′sŏr mŭs′ĕl thŭm) SYN extensor pollicis brevis muscle.

short ex·ten·sor mus·cle of toes (shōrt eks-ten′sŏr mŭs′ĕl tōz) SYN extensor digitorum brevis muscle.

short flex·or mus·cle of great toe (shōrt fleks′ŏr mŭs′ĕl grāt tō) SYN flexor hallucis brevis muscle.

short flex·or mus·cle of lit·tle fin·ger (shōrt fleks′ŏr mŭs′ĕl lit′ĕl fing′gĕr) SYN flexor digiti minimi brevis muscle of hand.

short flex·or mus·cle of lit·tle toe (shōrt fleks′ŏr mŭs′ĕl lit′ĕl tō) SYN flexor digiti minimi brevis muscle of foot.

short flex·or mus·cle of thumb (shōrt fleks′sŏr mŭs′ĕl thŭm) SYN flexor pollicis brevis muscle.

short flex·or mus·cle of toes (shōrt fleks′ŏr mŭs′ĕl tōz) SYN flexor digitorum brevis muscle.

short gas·tric ar·ter·ies (shōrt gas′trik ahr′tĕr-ēz) Four or five small arteries that give off from the splenic, passing through the gastrosplenic ligament to the fundus of the stomach along the greater curvature, and anastomosing with the other arteries in that region.

short gas·tric veins (shōrt gas′trik vānz) Small vessels that drain the fundus and left portion of the stomach wall and empty into the splenic vein.

short-gut syn·drome (shōrt gŭt sin′drōm) SYN short-bowel syndrome.

short gy·ri of in·su·la (shōrt jī′rē in′sū-lă) Several short, radiating gyri converging toward the base of the insula, composing the anterior two thirds of the insular cortex.

short in·cre·ment sen·si·ti·vi·ty in·dex (shōrt in′krĕ-mĕnt sen′si-tiv′i-tē in′deks) A measure of the ability to detect small (1 dB) increments in intensity; with cochlear lesions, such ability exceeds normal.

short pal·mar mus·cle (shōrt pahl′măr mŭs′ĕl) SYN palmaris brevis muscle.

short pos·ter·i·or cil·i·ar·y ar·ter·y (shōrt pos-tēr′ē-ŏr sil′ē-ar-ē ahr′tĕr-ē) One of approximately seven branches of the ophthalmic artery that pass around the optic nerve to supply the eyeball. Dividing into some 15–20 branches, they penetrate the sclera adjacent to the optic nerve, supplying the choroid and ciliary processes. *Anastomoses*: with central retinal artery and long and anterior ciliary arteries (at the ora serrata). SYN arteria ciliaris posterior brevis.

short rad·i·al ex·ten·sor mus·cle of wrist (shōrt rā′dē-ăl eks-ten′sŏr mŭs′ĕl rist) SYN extensor carpi radialis brevis muscle.

short·sight·ed·ness (shōrt-sīt′ĕd-nĕs) SYN myopia.

short-term ex·po·sure lim·it (short-tĕrm eks-pō′zhŭr lim′it) The maximum concentration of a chemical to which workers may be exposed continuously for up to 15 minutes without danger to health or work efficiency and safety.

short-term mem·o·ry (STM) (shōrt-tĕrm mem′ŏr-ē) That phase of the memory process in which stimuli that have been recognized and registered are stored briefly; decay occurs rapidly, typically within seconds, but may be held indefinitely by using rehearsal as a holding process by which to recycle material over and over through STM.

shot-silk ret•i•na (shot-silk ret′i-nă) The appearance of numerous wavelike, glistening reflexes, like the shimmer of silk, observed sometimes in the retina of a young person.

shot•ty (shot′ē) Having a consistency like pieces of shot; consisting of small, firm, discrete nodules; said of lymph nodes palpated through the skin.

shoul•der (shōl′dĕr) **1.** The lateral portion of the scapular region, where the scapula joins with the clavicle and humerus and is covered by the rounded mass of the deltoid muscle. **2.** Shoulder joint. **3.** DENTISTRY the ledge formed by the junction of the gingival and axial walls in extracoronal restorative preparations. [A.S. *sculder*]

shoul•der ap•pre•hen•sion sign (shōl′dĕr ap′prē-hen′shŭn sīn) A physical finding in which placement of the humerus in the position of abduction to 90 degrees and maximum external rotation produces anxiety and resistance in patients with a history of anterior glenohumeral instability. SYN anterior apprehension test (1).

shoul•der blade (shōl′dĕr blād) SYN scapula.

shoul•der com•plex (shōl′dĕr kom′pleks) **1.** The sternoclavicular, acromioclavicular, glenohumeral, and scapulothoracic joints, together with associated muscles and connective tissue. **2.** The shoulder and the pectoral girdle. **3.** SYN shoulder girdle.

shoul•der dys•to•ci•a (shōl′dĕr dis-tō′sē-ă) Arrest of normal labor after delivery of the head by impaction of the anterior shoulder against the symphysis pubis.

shoul•der gir•dle (shōl′dĕr gĭr′dĕl) The bony ring, incomplete behind, that serves for the attachment and support of the upper limbs. It is formed by the manubrium sterni, the clavicles, and the scapulae. See this page. SYN pectoral girdle, shoulder complex (3).

shoul•der-gir•dle syn•drome (shol′dĕr-gĭr′dĕl sin′drōm) SYN neuralgic amyotrophy.

shoul•der joint (shōl′dĕr joynt) A ball-and-socket synovial joint between the head of the humerus and the glenoid cavity of the scapula. See page 1427. SYN humeral joint.

shoul•der pre•sen•ta•tion (shōl′dĕr prez′ĕn-tā′shŭn) Transverse presentation with the shoulder as the presenting part.

sho•vel-shaped in•ci•sor (shŏv′ĕl-shāpt in-sī′zŏr) An incisor in which the lingual, and occasionally the labial, marginal ridges are accentuated; highly developed in people of Asian origin.

show (shō) **1.** First appearance of blood in beginning menstruation. **2.** Sign of impending labor, characterized by the discharge from the vagina of a small amount of blood-tinged mucus representing the extrusion of the mucous plug that has filled the cervical canal during pregnancy. [A.S. *sceáwe*]

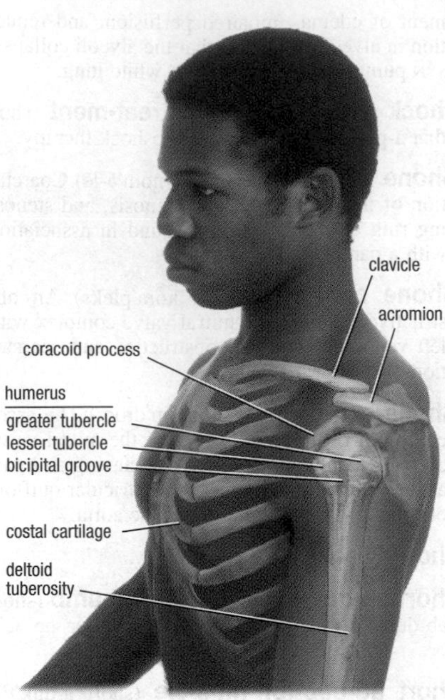

shoulder girdle

shunt (shŭnt) **1.** To bypass or divert. **2.** A bypass or diversion of fluid to another fluid-containing system by fistulation or a prosthetic device. The nomenclature commonly includes origin and terminus, e.g., atriovenous, splenorenal, ventriculocisternal. SEE ALSO bypass. [M.E. *shunten,* to flinch]

Shwartz•man phe•nom•e•non (shwērts′măn fĕ-nom′ĕ-non) A rabbit injected intradermally with a small quantity of lipopolysaccharide (endotoxin) followed by a second intravenous injection 24 hours later develops a hemorrhagic and necrotic lesion at the site of the first injection. SEE ALSO generalized Shwartzman phenomenon.

Shy-Dra•ger syn•drome (shī drā′gĕr sin′drōm) A progressive disorder involving the autonomic system, characterized by hypotension, external ophthalmoplegia, iris atrophy, incontinence, anhidrosis, impotence, tremor, and muscle wasting.

SI Abbreviation for International System of Units (Système International d'Unités); sensory integration.

Si Abbreviation for silicon.

sI Abbreviation for 6-mercaptopurine ribonucleoside (or 6-thioinosine).

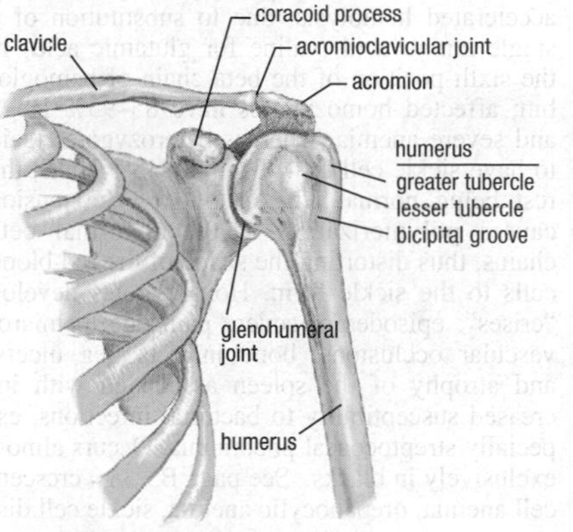

shoulder joint: anterior view

SIADH Abbreviation for syndrome of inappropriate secretion of antidiuretic hormone.

si·al·ad·e·ni·tis (sī′ăl-ad′ĕ-nī′tis) Inflammation of a salivary gland. SYN sialoadenitis. [sial- + G. *adēn,* gland, + *-itis,* inflammation]

si·al·a·gogue, **si·al·o·gogue** (sī-al′ă-gog) **1.** Promoting the flow of saliva. **2.** An agent having this action (e.g., anticholinesterase agents). [sial- + G. *agōgos,* drawing forth]

si·al·ec·ta·sis (sī′ă-lek′tă-sis) Dilation of a salivary duct. SYN ptyalectasis. [sial- + G. *ektasis,* a stretching]

si·al·em·e·sis, **si·al·e·me·si·a** (sī′al-ĕ-mē′sis, -ĕ-mē′zē-ă) Vomiting of saliva, or vomiting caused by or accompanying an excessive secretion of saliva. [sial- + G. *emesis,* vomiting]

si·al·ic (sī-al′ik) SYN salivary.

si·al·ic ac·ids (sī-al′ik as′idz) Esters and other *N*- and *O*-acyl derivatives of neuraminic acid.

si·al·i·dase (sī-al′i-dās) An enzyme that cleaves terminal acylneuraminic residues from 2,3-, 2,6-, and 2,8-linkages in oligosaccharides, glycoproteins, or glycolipids; present as a surface antigen in myxoviruses. Used in histochemistry to selectively remove sialomucins, as from bronchial mucous glands and the small intestine. A deficiency of this enzyme will result in sialidosis.

si·al·i·do·sis (sī-al′i-dō′sis) SYN cherry-red spot myoclonus syndrome.

si·a·line (sī′ă-lēn) SYN salivary.

si·a·lism, **si·a·lis·mus** (sī′ă-lizm, -liz′mŭs) An excess secretion of saliva. SYN ptyalism, salivation, sialorrhea, sialosis. [G. *sialismos*]

♻**sialo-**, **sial-** Combining forms denoting saliva, salivary glands. [G. *sialon*]

si·a·lo·ad·e·nec·to·my (sī′ă-lō-ad′ĕ-nek′tō-mē) Excision of a salivary gland. [sialo- + G. *adēn,* gland, + *ektomē,* excision]

si·a·lo·ad·e·ni·tis (sī′ă-lō-ad′ĕ-nī′tis) SYN sialadenitis.

si·a·lo·ad·e·not·o·my (sī′ă-lō-ad′ĕ-not′ō-mē) Incision of a salivary gland. [sialo- + G. *adēn,* gland, + *tomē,* incision]

si·a·lo·an·gi·ec·ta·sis (sī′ă-lō-an′jē-ek′tă-sis) Dilation of salivary ducts. [sialo- + G. *angeion,* vessel, + *ektasis,* a stretching]

si·a·lo·an·gi·i·tis (sī′ă-lō-an′jē-ī′tis) Inflammation of a salivary duct. [sialo- + G. *angeion,* vessel, + *-itis,* inflammation]

si·a·lo·cele (sī′ă-lō-sēl) SYN ranula (2). [sialo- + G. *kēlē,* tumor]

si·a·lo·do·chi·tis (sī′ă-lō-dō-kī′tis) Inflammation of the duct of a salivary gland. [sialo- + G. *dochē,* receptacle, + *-itis,* inflammation]

si·a·lo·do·cho·plas·ty (sī′ă-lō-dō′kō-plas′tē) Repair of a salivary duct. [sialo- + G. *dochē,* receptacle, + *plassō,* to fashion]

si·a·log·e·nous (sī′ă-loj′ĕ-nŭs) Producing saliva. SEE ALSO sialagogue. [sialo- + G. *-gen,* producing]

si·a·lo·gram (sī-al′ō-gram) The recorded display after sialography. [sialo- + G. *gramma,* a writing]

si·a·log·ra·phy (sī′ă-log′ră-fē) Radiography of the salivary glands and ducts after the introduction of contrast medium into the ducts. [sialo- + G. *graphō,* to write]

si·a·lo·lith (sī′ă-lō-lith) A salivary calculus. [sialo- + G. *lithos,* stone]

si·a·lo·li·thi·a·sis (sī′ă-lō-li-thī′ă-sis) The formation or presence of a salivary calculus. [sialolith + G. *-iasis,* condition]

si·a·lo·li·thot·o·my (sī′ă-lō-li-thot′ō-mē) Incision of a salivary duct or gland to remove a calculus. [sialolith + G. *tomē,* incision]

si·a·lor·rhe·a (sī′ă-lōr-ē′ă) SYN sialism. SYN sialorrhoea. [sialo- + G. *rhoia,* a flow]

sialorrhoea [Br.] SYN sialorrhea.

si·a·los·che·sis (sī′ă-los′kĕ-sis) Suppression of the secretion of saliva. [sialo- + G. *schesis,* retention]

si·a·lo·sis (sī′ă-lō′sis) SYN sialism.

si·a·lo·ste·no·sis (sī′ă-lō-stĕ-nō′sis) Stricture of a salivary duct. [sialo- + G. *stenōsis,* a narrowing]

Si·a·mese twins (sī′ă-mēz′ twinz) A much publicized pair of conjoined twins born in Thailand (then Siam) in the 19th century; this term has since come into general lay usage for any type of conjoined twins.

sib (sib) A member of a sibship. SYN sibling.

Si·be·ri·an gin·seng (sī-bēr′ē-ăn jin′seng) (*Eleutherococcus senticosus*) Herbal remedy purported of value in lowering blood pressure and increasing stamina. The latter has been ruled out by results of clinical studies. SYN touch-me-not.

sib·i·lant (sib′i-lănt) Hissing or whistling in character; denoting a form of rhonchus. [L. *sibilans* (*-ant-*), pres. p. of *sibilo,* to hiss]

sib·i·lant rale (sib′i-lănt rahl) A whistling sound caused by air moving through a viscid secretion narrowing the lumen of a bronchus.

sib·ling (sib′ling) SYN sib. [A. S. *sib,* relation, + *-ling,* diminutive]

sib·ling ri·val·ry (sib′ling rī′văl-rē) Jealous competition among children, especially for the attention, affection, and esteem of their parents; by extension, a factor in both normal and abnormal competitiveness throughout life.

sib·ship (sib′ship) **1.** The reciprocal state between individuals who have the same pair of parents. **2.** All progeny of one pair of parents. [A.S. *sib,* relationship]

sib·u·tra·mine (si-byū′tră-mēn) A serotonin and noradrenaline reuptake inhibitor used to reduce appetite to encourage weight loss.

sic·ca com·plex (sik′ă kom′pleks) Dryness of the mucous membranes, as of the eyes and mouth, in the absence of a connective tissue disease such as rheumatoid arthritis.

sic·cant (sik′ănt) **1.** Drying; removing moisture from surrounding substances. **2.** A substance with such properties. SYN siccative. [L. *siccans* (*-ant-*), pres. p. of *sicco,* pp. *-atus,* to dry]

sic·ca·tive (sik′ă-tiv) SYN siccant.

sick (sik) **1.** Unwell; suffering from disease. **2.** SYN nauseated. [A.S. *seóc*]

sick build·ing syn·drome (sik bild′ing sin′drōm) A disorder of nonspecific symptoms including fatigue, headache, dry eyes and throat, and nasal problems, occurring mostly in office workers; attributed to low-level exposures to substances used in building and interior construction; most symptoms lessen during off-work periods.

sick head·ache (sik hed′āk) SYN migraine.

sicklaemia [Br.] SYN sicklemia.

sick·le cell (sik′ĕl sel) An abnormal, crescentic erythrocyte characteristic of sickle cell anemia, resulting from an inherited abnormality of hemoglobin (hemoglobin S) that causes decreased solubility at low oxygen tension. SEE ALSO sicklemia, sickling. SYN drepanocyte.

sick·le cell a·ne·mi·a (sik′ĕl sel ă-nē′mē-ă) An autosomal dominant anemia characterized by crescentic or sickle-shaped erythrocytes and by accelerated hemolysis, due to substitution of a single amino acid (valine for glutamic acid) in the sixth position of the beta chain of hemoglobin; affected homozygotes have 85–95% Hb S and severe anemia, whereas heterozygotes (said to have sickle cell trait) have 40–45% Hb S, the rest being normal Hb A; low oxygen tension causes polymerization of the abnormal beta chains, thus distorting the shape of the red blood cells to the sickle form. Homozygotes develop "crises": episodes of severe pain due to microvascular occlusions, bone infarcts, leg ulcers, and atrophy of the spleen associated with increased susceptibility to bacterial infections, especially streptococcal pneumonia. Occurs almost exclusively in blacks. See page B3. SYN crescent cell anemia, drepanocytic anemia, sickle cell disease.

sick·le cell C dis·ease (sik′ĕl sel di-zēz′) A disorder resulting from abnormal sickle-shaped erythrocytes (containing hemoglobin C and S) that appear in response to a lowering of the partial pressure of oxygen; characterized by anemia, crises due to hemolysis or vascular occlusion, chronic leg ulcers and bone deformities, and infarcts of bone or of the spleen.

sick·le cell cri·sis (sik′ĕl sel krī′sis) SEE sickle cell anemia.

sick·le cell dac·ty·li·tis (sik′ĕl sel dak′ti-lī′tis) Painful swellings of the hands and feet seen in patients with an attack of sickle cell anemia.

sick·le cell dis·ease (sik′ĕl sel di-zēz′) SYN sickle cell anemia.

sick·le cell he·mo·glo·bin (Hb S) (sik′ĕl sel hē′mō-glō-bin) SYN hemoglobin S.

sick·le cell hep·a·top·a·thy (sik′ĕl sel hep′ă-top′ă-thē) Any liver disorder directly related to the sickling process of sickle cell disease and the transfusions required for its treatment. The direct manifestations are related primarily to vascular occlusion and include acute ischemia, sequestration, and cholestasis. Hepatitis and hepatic abscesses are also seen in acute sickle hepatic crisis.

sick·le cell ret·i·nop·a·thy (sik′ĕl sel ret′i-nop′ă-thē) A condition marked by dilation and tortuosity of retinal veins, and by microaneurysms and retinal hemorrhages; advanced stages may show neovascularization, vitreous hemorrhage, or retinal detachment.

sick·le·mi·a (sik-lē′mē-ă) Presence of sickle- or crescent-shaped erythrocytes in peripheral blood; seen in sickle cell anemia and sickle cell trait. SYN sicklaemia.

sick·le·wort (sik′ĕl-wōrt) SYN bugleweed.

sick·ling (sik′ling) Production of sickle-shaped erythrocytes in the circulation, as in sickle cell anemia.

sick•ness (sik′nĕs) SYN disease (1).

sick role (sik rōl) The familially or culturally accepted behavior pattern that one is permitted to exhibit during illness or disability, including sanctioned absence from school or work and a submissive, dependent relationship with family, health care personnel, and others.

SICU Abbreviation for surgical intensive care unit.

SID Abbreviation for source-to-image distance.

side chain (sīd chān) **1.** A chain of noncyclic atoms linked to a benzene ring, or to any cyclic chain compound. **2.** The atoms of an α-amino acid other than the α-carboxyl group, the α-amino group, the α-carbon, and the hydrogen attached to the α-carbon.

side-chain the•o•ry (sīd-chān thē′ŏr-ē) Ehrlich postulated that cells contained surface extensions or side chains (haptophores) that bind to the antigenic determinants of a toxin (toxophores); after a cell is stimulated, the haptophores are released into the circulation and become the antibodies. SEE ALSO receptor.

side ef•fect (sīd e-fekt′) A result of drug or other therapy in addition to or in extension of the desired therapeutic effect; usually, but not necessarily, connoting an undesirable effect.

♻**sidero-** Combining form meaning iron. [G. *sidēros*]

sid•er•o•blast (sid′ĕr-ō-blast) An erythroblast containing granules of ferritin stained by the Prussian blue reaction. [sidero- + G. *blastos,* germ]

sid•er•o•blas•tic a•ne•mi•a, sid•er•o•a•chres•tic a•ne•mi•a (sid′ĕr-ō-blast′ik ă-nē′mē-ă, sid′ĕr-o-ă-krest′ik) Refractory anemia characterized by the presence of sideroblasts in the bone marrow.

sid•er•o•cyte (sid′ĕr-ō-sīt) An erythrocyte containing granules of free iron, as detected by the Prussian blue reaction, in the blood of normal fetuses, where they constitute 0.10–4.5% of erythrocytes. [sidero- + G. *kytos,* cell]

sid•er•o•fi•bro•sis (sid′ĕr-ō-fī-brō′sis) Fibrosis associated with small foci in which iron is deposited.

sid•er•o•pe•ni•a (sid′ĕr-ō-pē′nē-ă) An abnormally low level of serum iron. [sidero- + G. *penia,* poverty]

sid•er•o•pe•nic (sid′ĕr-ō-pē′nik) Characterized by sideropenia.

sid•er•o•phage (sid′ĕr-ō-fāj) SYN siderophore. [sidero- + G. *phagō,* to eat]

sid•er•o•phil, sid•er•o•phile (sid′ĕr-ō-fil, -fīl) **1.** Absorbing iron. SYN siderophilous. **2.** A cell or tissue that contains iron. [sidero- + G. *philos,* fond]

sid•er•oph•i•lous (sid′ĕr-of′i-lŭs) SYN siderophil (1).

sid•er•o•phore (sid′ĕr-ō-fōr) A large, extravasated, mononuclear phagocyte containing granules of hemosiderin, found in the sputum or in the lungs of people with long-standing pulmonary congestion from left ventricular failure. SYN siderophage. [sidero- + G. *phoros,* bearing]

sid•er•o•sil•i•co•sis (sid′ĕr-ō-sil′i-kō′sis) Silicosis due to inhalation of dust containing iron and silica. SYN silicosiderosis. [sidero- + silicosis]

sid•er•o•sis (sid′ĕr-ō′sis) **1.** A form of pneumoconiosis due to the presence of iron dust. **2.** Discoloration of any part by disposition of an iron pigment; usually called hemosiderosis. **3.** An excess of iron in the circulating blood. **4.** Degeneration of the retina, lens, and uvea as a result of the deposition of iron. [sidero- + G. *-osis,* condition]

sid•er•ot•ic (sid′ĕr-ot′ik) Related to siderosis; pigmented by iron or containing an excess of iron.

sid•er•o•tic cat•a•ract (sid′ĕr-ot′ik kat′ăr-akt) A cataract resulting from deposition of iron from an iron-containing intraocular foreign body.

side•stream aer•o•sol (sīd′strēm ār′ō-sol) A system for administering an aerosol that adds the agent through a side connection into the mainstream of inspired airflow.

SIDS (sidz) Acronym for sudden infant death syndrome.

Sie•gert sign (zē′gĕrt sīn) Shortness and inward curvature of the terminal phalanges of the fifth fingers in patients with Down syndrome.

Sie•gle o•to•scope (zē′gĕl ō′tō-skōp) An otoscope with a bulb attachment by which the air pressure can be varied, thus imparting movement to the tympanic membrane, if intact, while under inspection.

sie•mens (S) (sē′mĕnz) The SI unit of electrical conductance; the conductance of a body with an electrical resistance of 1 ohm, allowing 1 ampere of current to flow per volt applied; equal to 1 mho. SYN mho.

sie•vert (Sv) (sē′vĕrt) The SI unit of ionizing radiation effective dose, equal to the absorbed dose in gray, weighted for both the quality of radiation in question and the tissue response to that radiation. The unit is the joule per kilogram and 1 Sv = 100 rem. SEE ALSO effective dose.

sight (sīt) The ability or faculty of seeing. SEE ALSO vision. [A.S. *gesihth*]

sig•ma (sig′mă) **1.** The 18th letter of the Greek alphabet (σ, Σ). **2.** (σ) reflection coefficient;

standard deviation; a factor in prokaryotic RNA initiation; surface tension. **3.** (Σ) Summation of a series.

sig•moid (sig′moyd) Resembling in outline the letter S or one of the forms of the Greek sigma. [G. *sigma,* the letter S, + *eidos,* resemblance]

sig•moid ar•ter•ies (sig′moyd ahr′tĕr-ēz) *Origin*, inferior mesenteric; *distribution*, descending colon and sigmoid flexure; *anastomoses*, left colic, superior rectal. SYN arteriae sigmoideae [TA].

sig•moid co•lon (sig′moyd kō′lŏn) The part of the colon describing an S-shaped curve between the pelvic brim and the third sacral segment; it is continuous with the rectum. SYN colon sigmoideum [TA].

sig•moid•ec•to•my (sig′moy-dek′tŏ-mē) Excision of the sigmoid colon. [sigmoid- + G. *ektomē,* excision]

sig•moid•i•tis (sig′moy-dī′tis) Inflammation of the sigmoid colon. [sigmoid- + G. *-itis,* inflammation]

♻ **sigmoido-, sigmoid-** Combining forms denoting sigmoid, usually the sigmoid colon. [G. *sigma,* the letter S, + *eidos,* resemblance]

sig•moid•o•pex•y (sig-moy′dō-pek-sē) Operative attachment of the sigmoid colon to a firm structure to correct rectal prolapse. [sigmoido- + G. *pēxis,* fixation]

sig•moid•o•proc•tos•to•my (sig-moy′dō-prok-tos′tŏ-mē) Anastomosis between the sigmoid colon and the rectum. SYN sigmoidorectostomy. [sigmoido- + G. *prōktos,* anus, + *stoma,* mouth]

sig•moid•o•rec•tos•to•my (sig-moy′dō-rek-tos′tŏ-mē) SYN sigmoidoproctostomy.

sig•moid•o•scope (sig-moy′dō-skōp) An endoscope for viewing the cavity of the sigmoid colon. [sigmoido- + G. *skopeō,* to view]

sig•moid•os•co•py (sig′moy-dos′kŏ-pē) Inspection, through an endoscope, of the interior of the sigmoid colon.

sig•moid•os•to•my (sig′moy-dos′tŏ-mē) Establishment of an artificial anus by opening into the sigmoid colon. [sigmoido- + G. *stoma,* mouth]

sig•moid•ot•o•my (sig′moy-dot′ŏ-mē) Surgical opening of the sigmoid. [sigmoido- + G. *tomē,* incision]

sig•moid si•nus (sig′moyd sī′nŭs) The S-shaped dural venous sinus lying deep to the mastoid process of the temporal bone and immediately posterior to the petrous temporal bone; it is continuous with the transverse sinus and empties into the internal jugular vein as it passes through the jugular foramen.

sig•moid veins (sig′moyd vānz) The several tributaries of the inferior mesenteric vein that drain the sigmoid colon.

sign (sīn) **1.** Any abnormality indicative of disease, discoverable on examination of a patient; an objective symptom of disease, in contrast to a symptom, which is a subjective sign of disease. **2.** An abbreviation or symbol. **3.** PSYCHOLOGY any object or artifact (stimulus) that represents a specific thing or conveys a specific idea to the person who perceives it. [L. *signum,* mark]

sig•nal (sig′năl) **1.** Something that causes an action. **2.** A DNA template sequence that alters RNA polymerase transcription. **3.** The end product observed when a specific sequence of DNA or RNA is deleted by some method.

sig•nal lymph node, **sig•nal node** (sig′năl limf nōd) A firm supraclavicular lymph node, especially on the left side, sufficiently enlarged that it is palpable from the cutaneous surface; such a lymph node is so termed because it may be the first recognized presumptive evidence of a malignant neoplasm in one of the viscera. A signal lymph node that is known to contain a metastasis from a malignant neoplasm is sometimes designated by an old eponym, Troisier ganglion. SEE ALSO sentinel lymph node. SYN jugular gland, Virchow node.

sig•nal:noise ra•ti•o (S:N) (sig′năl-noyz′ rā′shē-ō) The relative intensity of a signal to the random variation in signal intensity, or noise; used to evaluate many imaging techniques and electronic systems.

sig•nal-pro•ces•sing cir•cuits (sig′năl-pros′es-ing sĕr′kŭts) The electronic hardware of hearing aids that allows alteration in the amplification of various bands of frequencies of the acoustic signal.

sig•nal trans•duc•tion in•hib•i•tor (STI) (sig′năl trans-dŭk′shŭn in-hib′i-tŏr) Category or classification of anticancer drugs that inhibit the action of enzymes essential to the growth and survival of cancer cells while causing relatively little or no damage to noncancer cells.

sig•na•ture (sig′nă-chŭr) The part of a prescription containing the directions to the patient. [Mediev. L. *signatura,* fr. L. *signum,* a sign, mark]

Signed Eng•lish (sīnd ing′glish) A system of communication that is a semantic representation of English in which American Sign Language signs are used in English word order and additional signs are used for inflection; used principally in the education of children younger than 6 years old.

sig•net ring cells (sig′nĕt ring selz) SYN castration cells.

sign lan•guage (sīn lang′wăj) A system of manual communication used by the deaf. True sign languages such as American Sign Language (ASL) have a complete representation of morphology, semantics, and syntax.

SIH Abbreviation for somatotropin release-inhibiting hormone.

si•lent (sī′lĕnt) Producing no detectable signs or symptoms, said of certain diseases or morbid processes.

si•lent ar•e•a (sī′lĕnt ār′ē-ă) Any area of the cerebrum or cerebellum in which lesions cause no definite sensory or motor symptoms.

si•lent as•pir•a•tion (sī′lĕnt as′pir-ā′shŭn) Movement of a liquid or solid bolus into the trachea below the vocal cords, without clinical signs such as coughing, choking, color change, or change in respirations.

si•lent my•o•car•di•al in•farc•tion (sī′lĕnt mī′ō-kahr′dē-ăl in-fahrk′shŭn) Infarct that produces none of the characteristic symptoms and signs of myocardial infarction.

sil•hou•ette sign of Fel•son (sil′ō-et′ sīn fel′sŏn) In pulmonary radiology, the obliteration of a normal air-soft tissue interface, such as the cardiac silhouette, when fluid fills the adjacent part of the lung.

sil•i•ca (sil′i-kă) The chief constituent of sand, hence of glass. SYN silicon dioxide. [Mod. L. fr. L. *silex* (*silic-*), flint]

sil•i•cate rest•or•a•tion (sil′i-kăt res′tŏr-ā′shŭn) Restoration of lost tooth structure made with silicate cement.

sil•i•ca•to•sis (sil′i-kă-tō′sis) SYN silicosis.

sil•i•con (Si) (sil′i-kon) A very abundant nonmetallic element, atomic no. 14, atomic wt. 28.0855, occurring in nature as silica and silicates; in pure form, used as a semiconductor and in solar batteries; also found in certain polysaccharide structures in mammary tissue. [L. *silex,* flint]

sil•i•con di•ox•ide (sil′i-kon dī-oks′īd) SYN silica.

sil•i•cone (sil′i-kōn) A polymer of organic silicon oxides, which may be a liquid, gel, or solid, depending on the extent of polymerization; used in surgical implants, in intracorporeal tubes to conduct fluids, as dental impression material, as a grease or sealing substance, as a coating on the inside of glass vessels for blood collection, and in various ophthalmologic procedures.

sil•i•cone di•ode (sil′i-kōn dī′ōd) SYN diode.

sil•i•co•pro•tein•o•sis (sil′i-kō-prō′tēn-ō′sis) An acute pulmonary disorder, radiographically and histologically similar to pulmonary alveolar proteinosis, resulting from relatively short exposure to high concentrations of silica dust; pulmonary symptoms are of rapid onset, and the condition is invariably fatal.

sil•i•co•sid•er•o•sis (sil′i-kō-sid′ĕr-ō′sis) SYN siderosilicosis.

sil•i•co•sis (sil′i-kō′sis) A form of pneumoconiosis resulting from occupational exposure to and inhalation of silica dust over a period of years; characterized by a slowly progressive fibrosis of the lungs, which may result in impairment of lung function; silicosis predisposes to pulmonary tuberculosis. SYN silicatosis. [L. *silex,* flint, + *-osis,* condition]

sil•i•co•tu•ber•cu•lo•sis (sil′i-kō-tū-bĕr′kyū-lō′sis) Silicosis associated with tuberculous pulmonary lesions.

si•lo-fil•ler's lung (sī′lō-fil′lĕrz lŭng) Pulmonary edema usually delayed for 1–4 hours, occurring in a person exposed to silage; probably produced by nitrogen dioxide; can progress to bronchiolitis obliterans.

sil•ver (Ag) (sil′vĕr) L. argentum; a metallic element, atomic no. 47, atomic wt. 107.8682. Many salts have clinical applications. [A.S. *seolfor*]

sil•ver-am•mo•ni•ac sil•ver stain (sil′vĕr-ă-mō′nē-ăk sil′vĕr stān) A stain for the acid protein component of nucleolar regions that are active or that were transcriptionally active in the preceding interphase; uses silver nitrate, ammoniacal silver, and formalin.

sil•ver-fork frac•ture, **sil•ver-fork de•for•mi•ty** (sil′vĕr-fōrk frak′shŭr, sil′vĕr-fōrk dĕ-fōrm′i-tē) A Colles fracture of the wrist in which the deformity has the appearance of a fork in profile.

sil•ver im•preg•na•tion (sil′vĕr im′preg-nā′shŭn) Silver complexes employed to demonstrate reticulin in normal and diseased tissues, as well as neuroglia, neurofibrillae, argentaffin cells, and Golgi apparatus.

sil•ver pro•tein stain (sil′vĕr prō′tēn stān) A silver proteinate complex used in staining nerve fibers, nerve endings, and flagellate protozoa; also used to demonstrate phagocytosis in living animals by the cells of the reticuloendothelial system.

Sil•ver•sköld syn•drome (sil′ver-shŭld sin′drōm) A type of osteochondrodystrophy with only slight vertebral changes but with shortened and curved long bones of the extremities.

sim•i•an vi•rus (SV) (sim′ē-ăn vī′rŭs) Any of a number of viruses, belonging to various families, isolated from monkeys or from cultures of monkey cells.

si•mi•li•a si•mil•i•bus cur•an•tur (si-mil′ē-ă si-mil′i-bŭs kū-ran′tūr) The homeopathic formula expressing the law of similars, the doctrine that any drug capable of producing morbid symptoms in the healthy will remove similar symptoms occurring as an expression of disease. Another reading of the formula, employed by

Hahnemann, the founder of homeopathy, is *similia similibus curentur*, let likes be cured by likes. [L. likes are cured by likes]

Sim•monds dis•ease (sim′ŏndz di-zēz′) Anterior pituitary insufficiency due to trauma, vascular lesions, or tumors; usually developing postpartum as a result of pituitary necrosis caused by ischemia during a hypotensive episode during delivery; characterized clinically by asthenia, loss of weight and body hair, arterial hypotension, and manifestations of thyroid, adrenal, and gonadal hypofunction. SYN hypophysial cachexia, pituitary cachexia.

Sim•mons ci•trate me•di•um (sim′ŏnz sī′trāt mē′dē-ŭm) A diagnostic medium used in the differentiation of species of Enterobacteriaceae, based on the species' ability to use sodium citrate as the sole source of carbon.

Si•mo•nart bands (sē-mō-nahr′ bandz) **1.** SYN amnionic band. **2.** Weblike band of tissue partially filling the gap between the medial and lateral portions of a cleft lip.

Si•mo•nart lig•a•ments (sē-mō-nahr′ lig′ă-mĕnts) SYN amnionic band.

Si•mon po•si•tion (sē′mŏn pŏ-zish′ŏn) A position for vaginal examination; a supine position with hips elevated, thighs and legs flexed, and thighs widely separated.

sim•ple ab•sence (simp′ĕl ab′sĕns) A brief clouding of consciousness accompanied by the abrupt onset of 3-second spikes and waves on EEG. SYN pure absence.

sim•ple dis•lo•ca•tion (simp′ĕl dis′lō-kā′shŭn) SYN closed dislocation.

sim•ple en•do•me•tri•al hy•per•pla•si•a (simp′ĕl en′dō-mē′trē-ăl hī′pĕr-plā′zē-ă) Increase in the amount of endometrial tissue, with glands separated by abundant stroma.

sim•ple ep•i•the•li•um (simp′ĕl ep′i-thē′lē-ŭm) An epithelium having one layer of cells.

sim•ple fis•sion (simp′ĕl fish′ŭn) Division of the nucleus and then the cell body into two parts. SEE ALSO binary fission.

sim•ple frac•ture (simp′ĕl frak′shŭr) SYN closed fracture.

sim•ple glau•co•ma, glau•co•ma sim•plex (simp′ĕl glaw-kō′mă, glaw-kō′mă sim′pleks) SYN open-angle glaucoma.

sim•ple goi•ter (simp′ĕl goy′tĕr) Thyroid enlargement unaccompanied by constitutional effects, e.g., hypo- or hyperthyroidism, commonly caused by inadequate dietary intake of iodine.

sim•ple joint (simp′ĕl joynt) A joint composed of only two bones.

sim•ple mas•tec•to•my (simp′ĕl mas-tek′tō-mē) Excision of the breast including the nipple, areola, and most of the overlying skin.

sim•ple mi•cro•scope, sin•gle mi•cro•scope (simp′ĕl mī′krŏ-skōp, sing′gĕl) A microscope that has a single magnifying lens.

sim•ple pho•bi•a (simp′ĕl fō′bē-ă) SYN specific phobia.

sim•ple pro•tein (simp′ĕl prō′tēn) Protein that yields only α-amino acids or their derivatives by hydrolysis, e.g., albumins, globulins, glutelins, prolamines, albuminoids, histones, protamines. Cf. conjugated protein.

sim•ple squa•mous ep•i•the•li•um (simp′ĕl skwā′mŭs ep′i-thē′lē-ŭm) The single layer of flattened scalelike cells, such as mesothelium, endothelium, and that found in the pulmonary alveoli.

Sim•plex•vi•rus (sim′pleks-vī′rŭs) SYN herpes simplex.

Sim•pli•fied Or•al Hy•giene In•dex (OHIS) (sim′pli-fīd ōr-ăl hī′jēn in′deks) A dental survey method that scores dental calculus and plaque together.

i **Sims po•si•tion** (simz pŏ-zish′ŏn) Placement to facilitate a vaginal examination, with the patient lying on her side with the lower arm behind the back, the thighs flexed, the upper one more than the lower. See page B29. SYN lateral recumbent position.

sim•u•la•tion (sim′yū-lā′shŭn) **1.** Imitation; said of a disease or symptom that resembles another, or of the feigning of illness as in factitious illness or malingering. **2.** RADIATION THERAPY using a geometrically similar radiographic system or computer to plan the location of therapy ports. **3.** An exercise during which a hypothetical emergency is staged; the purpose is to gauge the readiness of and provide training to medical and military personnel and others involved in response to or prevention of such acts. [L. *simulatio,* fr. *simulo,* pp. *-atus,* to imitate, fr. *similis,* like]

si•mul•tan•ag•no•si•a (sī′mŭl-tān′ag-nō′sē-ă) Inability to recognize multiple elements in a visual presentation; i.e., one object or some elements of a scene can be appreciated but not the display as a whole. [simultaneous + agnosia]

si•mul•ta•ne•ous com•mu•ni•ca•tion (sī′mŭl-tān′ē-ŭs kŏ-myū′ni-kā′shŭn) SYN total communication.

SIMV Abbreviation for synchronized intermittent mandatory ventilation.

sin•cip•i•tal (sin-sip′i-tăl) Relating to the sinciput.

sin•cip•i•tal pre•sen•ta•tion (sin-sip′i-tăl prez′ĕn-tā′shŭn) SEE cephalic presentation.

sin•ci•put, pl. **sin•cip•i•ta, sin•ci•puts** (sin′

si-pŭt, sin-sip′i-tă, sin′si-pŭts) The anterior part of the head just above and including the forehead. [L. half of the head]

Sind•bis fe•ver (sind′bis fē′ver) A febrile illness of humans in Africa, Australia, and elsewhere, characterized by arthralgia, rash, and malaise; caused by the Sindbis virus, a member of the family Togaviridae, and transmitted by mosquitoes of the genus *Culex*.

Sind•bis vi•rus (sind′bis vī′rŭs) The type species of the genus Alphavirus, usually transmitted by mosquitoes of the genus *Culex*, and causative agent of Sindbis fever. [village in Egypt where first isolated]

Sind•ing-Lar•sen-Jo•hans•son syn•drome (sin′ding-lahr′sen-yō-hahn′sĕn sin′drōm) Apophysitis of the distal pole of the patella.

sin•ew (sin′yū) SYN tendon. [A.S. *sinu*]

sine wave (sīn wāv) A symmetric wave representing one complete cycle of a single-frequency oscillation; the displacement of mass over time described by using a function from trigonometry, the sine. SEE ALSO pure tone.

sing•er's no•dules (sing′ĕrz noj′yūlz) SYN vocal nodules.

sin•gle bond (sing′gĕl bond) A covalent bond resulting from the sharing of one pair of electrons; e.g., $H_3C—CH_3$ (ethane).

sin•gle nu•cle•o•tide pol•y•mor•phisms (sing′gĕl nū′klē-ō-tīd pol′ē-mōrph′izmz) Variation between two DNA sequences consisting in the difference of a single nucleotide, frequently the substitution of thymine for cytosine. Although the possession of a pair of alleles displaying such polymorphism seldom causes demonstrable abnormality or malfunction, it may influence the response to pathogens, toxins, and environmental agents and enhance susceptibility to certain conditions.

sin•gle-par•ent fam•i•ly (sing′gĕl par′ent fam′i-lē) A group in which the children live with only one parent.

sin•gle pho•ton e•mis•sion com•put•ed to•mog•ra•phy (SPECT) (sing′gĕl fō′ton ē-mi′shŭn kŏm-pyūt′ĕd tŏ-mog′ră-fē) Tomographic imaging of metabolic and physiologic functions in tissues, the image being formed by computer synthesis of photons of a single energy emitted by radionuclides administered in suitable form to the patient.

sin•gle•ton (sing′gĕl-tŏn) A fetus that develops alone.

sin•gle vi•al fix•a•tives (sing′gĕl vī′ăl fiks′ă-tivz) Proprietary and commercially available solutions used for stool fixation; from the single vial, a concentration, permanent stain, and some immunoassay procedures can be performed.

si•nis•ter (si-nis′tĕr) Left. [L.]

sin•is•trad (sin-is′trad) Toward the left side. [L. *sinister,* left, + *ad,* to]

sin•is•tral (sin′is-trăl) **1.** Relating to the left side. **2.** Denoting a left-handed person.

sin•is•tral•i•ty (sin′is-tral′i-tē) The condition of being left-handed.

♻ **sinistro-** Combining form denoting left, toward the left. [L. *sinister*]

sin•is•tro•car•di•a (sin′is-trō-kahr′dē-ă) Leftward displacement of the heart beyond its normal position. [sinistro- + G. *kardia,* heart]

sin•is•tro•ce•re•bral (sin′is-trō-ser′ĕ-brăl) Relating to the left cerebral hemisphere. [sinistro- + L. *cerebrum,* brain]

sin•is•tro•gy•ra•tion (sin′is-trō-jī-rā′shŭn) SYN sinistrotorsion. [sinistro- + L. *gyratio,* a turning around (gyration)]

sin•is•tro•man•u•al (sin′is-trō-man′yū-ăl) SYN left-handed. [sinistro- + L. *manus,* hand]

sin•is•trop•e•dal (sin′is-trop′ĕ-dăl) Denoting a person who uses the left leg by preference. SYN left-footed. [sinistro- + L. *pes* (*ped-*), foot]

sin•is•tro•tor•sion (sin′is-trō-tōr′shŭn) A turning or twisting to the left. SYN levorotation (2), levotorsion (1), sinistrogyration. [sinistro- + L. *torsio,* a twisting (torsion)]

Sin Nom•bre vi•rus (sēn nōm′brā vī′rŭs) A species of Hantavirus in North America that causes hantavirus pulmonary syndrome. SYN Four Corners virus. [Spanish, without a name]

si•no•pul•mo•nar•y (sī′nō-pul′mŏ-nar-ē) Relating to the paranasal sinuses and the pulmonary airway.

sin•u•al tu•ber•cle (sīn-yū′ăl tū′bĕr-kĕl) A median protuberance projecting into the embryonic urogenital sinus from its dorsal wall; it is formed from the fused caudal ends of the paramesonephric ducts and is the first evidence of the embryonic uterus and vagina. SYN Müller tubercle, sinusal tubercle.

si•nu•a•tri•al (S-A), si•no•a•tri•al (S-A) (sin′yū-ā′trē-ăl, sī′nō-ā′trē-ăl) Relating to the sinus venosus of the embryo, or the sinus of the venae cavae of the mature heart, and the right atrium.

si•nu•a•tri•al block, si•no•a•tri•al block (sin′yū-ā′trē-ăl blok, sī′nō-ā′trē-ăl) Blockade of an impulse leaving the sinoatrial node before it can activate atrial muscle or be propagated to the atrioventricular node. The condition is indicated on electrocardiography by the absence of some P waves.

si•nu•a•tri•al node, si•no•a•tri•al node (sin′yū-ā′trē-ăl nōd, sī′nō-ā′trē-ăl) The mass of specialized cardiac muscle fibers that normally acts as the "pacemaker" of the cardiac conduction system; it lies under the epicardium at the upper end of the sulcus terminalis.

si•nus, pl. **si•nus**, **si•nus•es** (sī′nŭs, -ĕz) **1.** A channel for the passage of blood or lymph, without the coats of an ordinary vessel, e.g., blood passages in the gravid uterus or those in the cerebral meninges. **2.** A cavity or hollow space in bone or other tissue. **3.** A dilation in a blood vessel. **4.** A fistula or tract leading to a suppurating cavity. [L. *sinus,* cavity, channel, hollow]

sin•u•sal tu•ber•cle (sī′nŭs-ăl tū′bĕr-kĕl) SYN sinual tubercle.

si•nus ar•rest (sī′nŭs ă-rest′) Cessation of sinoatrial activity; the ventricles may continue to beat under ectopic atrial, A-V junctional, or idioventricular control.

si•nus ar•rhyth•mi•a (sī′nŭs ă-ridh′mē-ă) A cyclic variation in heart rate, usually normal and linked to respiratory movements.

si•nus bra•dy•car•di•a (sī′nŭs brā′dē-kahr′dē-ă) A heart rate less than 60 beats per minute with a normal rhythm.

si•nus ca•ver•no•sus (sī′nŭs kav′ĕr-nō′sŭs) [TA] SYN cavernous sinus.

si•nus his•ti•o•cy•to•sis with mas•sive lymph•a•den•op•a•thy (sī′nŭs his′tē-ō-sī-tō′sis mas′iv limf-ad-ĕ-nop′ă-thē) A chronic disease occurring in children and characterized by massive painless cervical lymphadenopathy due to distension of the lymphatic sinuses by macrophages containing ingested lymphocytes, and by capsular and pericapsular fibrosis. SYN Rosai-Dorfman disease.

si•nu•si•tis (sī′nŭ-sī′tis) Inflammation of the lining membrane of any sinus, especially of one of the paranasal sinuses. [sinus + G. *-itis,* inflammation]

si•nu•soid (sī′nŭ-soyd) **1.** Resembling a sinus. **2.** Sinusoidal capillary; a thin-walled terminal blood vessel having a more variable and larger caliber than an ordinary capillary; its endothelial cells have large gaps and the basal lamina is either discontinuous or absent. [sinus + G. *eidos,* resemblance]

si•nu•soi•dal (sī′nŭ-soy′dăl) Relating to a sinusoid.

si•nu•sot•o•my (sī′nŭ-sot′ŏ-mē) Incision into a sinus. [sinus + G. *tomē,* incision]

si•nus pause (sī′nŭs pawz) A spontaneous interruption in the regular sinus rhythm, the pause lasting for a period that is not an exact multiple of the sinus cycle. SEE ALSO sinus arrest.

si•nus rhythm (sī′nŭs ridh′ŭm) Normal cardiac rhythm proceeding from the sinuatrial node.

si•nus tach•y•car•di•a (sī′nŭs tak′i-kahr′dē-ă) A heart rate exceeding 100 beats per minute with a normal rhythm.

si•nus of the ve•na ca•va (sī′nŭs vē′nă kā′vă) The portion of the cavity of the right atrium of the heart that receives the blood from the venae cavae; it is separated from the rest of the atrium by the crista terminalis.

si•nus ve•no•sus (sī′nŭs vē-nō′sus) The venosus sinus at the caudal end of the embryonic cardiac tube in which the veins from the intra- and extraembryonic circulatory arcs unite; in the course of development it forms the portion of the right atrium known in adult anatomy as the sinus of the vena cava or sinus venarum cavarum; the right horn of the sinus venosus forms the coronary sinus.

si•nus ve•no•sus scler•ae (sī′nŭs vē-nō′sus sklē′rē) The vascular structure encircling the anterior chamber of the eye and through which the aqueous is returned to the blood circulation. SYN circular sinus (3), Schlemm canal.

si op. sit (sī op sit) An abbreviation, in prescriptions, for L. *si opus sit,* if it should be necessary.

si•phon (sī′fŏn) A tube bent into two unequal lengths, used to remove fluid from a cavity or vessel by atmospheric pressure and gravity. [G. *siphōn,* tube]

si•phon•age (sī′fŏn-ăj) Emptying of the stomach or other cavity by means of a siphon.

Si•pho•vir•i•dae (sif′ō-vir′i-dē) A family of bacterial viruses with long, noncontractile tails and isometric or elongated heads, containing double-stranded DNA (MW 25–79 × 10^6); includes the λ temperate phage group and probably other genera. [L. *sipho,* little tube, pipe, fr. G. *siphōn,* + virus]

Sip•ple syn•drome (sip′ĕl sin′drōm) Pheochromocytoma, medullary carcinoma of the thyroid, and parathyroid adenomas; autosomal dominant inheritance, caused by mutation in the RET oncogene on chromosome 10q.

si•re•no•me•li•a (sī′rĕ-nō-mē′lē-ă) Union of the legs with partial or complete fusion of the feet. [L. *siren,* G. *seirēn,* a siren]

♻ **-sis** Combining form meaning an action, process, condition, or state. [G.]

SISI Acronym for small increment sensitivity index.

SISI test (test) The sounding of a tone 20 dB above threshold, followed by a series of 200-msec tones 1 dB louder; perception of them indicates cochlear damage.

sis•mo•ther•a•py (sis-mō-thār′ă-pē) SYN vibratory massage.

sis•ter (sis′tĕr) [Br.] **1.** The title of a head nurse in a public hospital or in a ward or the operating room of a hospital. **2.** Any registered nurse in private practice.

Sis·ter Jo·seph nod·ule (sis′tĕr-jō′sĕf noj′yūl) A malignant intraabdominal neoplasm metastatic to the umbilicus.

site (sīt) A place or location. SYN situs. [L. *situs*]

site-spe·cif·ic re·com·bi·na·tion (sīt-spĕ-sif′ik rē-kom′bi-nā′shŭn) Integration of foreign DNA into a particular site in the host genome.

♻ **sito-** Combining form denoting food, grain. [G. *sitos, sition*]

si·tot·ro·pism, si·to·tax·is (sī-tot′rŏ-pizm, sī′tō-tak′sis) Turning of living cells to or away from food. [sito- + G. *tropē,* a turning]

in si·tu (in sī′tū) In position, not extending beyond the focus or level of origin. [L. *in,* in, + *situs,* site]

sit·u·a·tion·al ho·mo·sex·u·al·i·ty (sich′ū-ā′shŭn-ăl hō′mō-sek′shū-al′i-tē) SYN circumstantial homosexuality.

sit·u·a·tion·al psy·cho·sis (si-chū′ā-shŭn-ăl sī-kō′sis) A transitory but severe emotional disorder caused in a predisposed person by a seemingly unbearable situation.

in si·tu hy·bri·di·za·tion (in sī′tū hī′brid-ī-zā′shŭn) A technique for annealing nucleic acid probes to cellular DNA for detection by autoradiography. In situ hybridization constitutes a key step in DNA fingerprinting.

si·tus (sī′tus) SYN site. [L.]

si·tus in·ver·sus (sī′tus in-vĕr′sus) Reversal of position or location, referring particularly to left-right reversal of thoracic viscera.

sitz bath (sits bath) Immersion of only the perineum and buttocks, with the legs being outside the tub. SYN hip bath. [Ger. *sitzen,* to sit]

sixth cra·ni·al nerve [CN VI] (siksth krā′nē-ăl nĕrv) SYN abducent nerve [CN VI].

sixth dis·ease (siksth di-zēz′) SYN exanthema subitum.

sixth-year mo·lar (siksth-yēr mō′lăr) The first permanent molar tooth.

si·zer (sī′zĕr) A cylinder of variable diameter, with rounded ends, used to measure the internal diameter of the bowel in preparation for stapling.

Sjö·gren syn·drome (shōr′gren sin′drōm) Keratoconjunctivitis sicca, dryness of mucous membranes, telangiectases, or purpuric spots on the face, and bilateral parotid enlargement; seen in menopausal women and often associated with rheumatoid arthritis, Raynaud phenomenon, and dental caries; there are changes in the lacrimal and salivary glands resembling those of Mikulicz disease.

SK Abbreviation for streptokinase.

skat·ole (skat′ōl) An indole derivative formed in the intestine by bacterial decomposition and found in fecal matter, to which it imparts its characteristic odor.

skat·ox·yl (skă-tok′sil) An indole derivative formed in the intestine by the oxidation of skatole; some undergoes conjugation in the body with sulfuric or gluronic acids and is excreted in the urine in conjugated form.

skel·e·tal (skel′ĕ-tăl) Relating to the skeleton.

skel·e·tal dys·pla·si·as (skel′ĕ-tăl dis-plā′zē-ăz) A heterogeneous group of disorders (more than 120 types), each of which results in numerous disturbances of the skeletal system and most of which include dwarfism. SEE ALSO chondrodystrophy.

skel·e·tal ex·ten·sion (skel′ĕ-tăl eks-ten′shŭn) SYN skeletal traction.

skel·e·tal mus·cle (skel′ĕ-tăl mŭs′ĕl) Grossly, a collection of striated muscle fibers connected at either or both extremities with the bony framework of the body; it may be an appendicular or an axial muscle; histologically, a muscle consisting of elongated, multinucleated, transversely striated skeletal muscle fibers together with connective tissues, blood vessels, and nerves; individual muscle fibers are surrounded by fine reticular and collagen fibers (endomysium); bundles (fascicles) of muscle fibers are surrounded by irregular connective tissue (perimysium); the entire muscle is surrounded, except at the muscle-tendon junction, by a dense connective tissue (epimysium). See page 1436.

skel·e·tal trac·tion (skel′ĕ-tăl trak′shŭn) Therapeutic pulling on a bone structure mediated through pin or wire inserted into the bone to reduce a fracture of long bones. SYN skeletal extension.

♻ **skeleto-** Combining form meaning skeleton. [G. *skeletos,* dried up]

skel·e·ton (skel′ĕ-tŏn) **1.** [TA] The bony framework of the body in vertebrates (endoskeleton) or the hard outer envelope of insects (exoskeleton or dermoskeleton). **2.** All the dry parts remaining after the destruction and removal of the soft parts; this includes ligaments and cartilages as well as bones. **3.** All the bones of the body taken collectively. **4.** A rigid or semirigid nonosseous structure that functions as the supporting framework of a particular structure. See page A17, A18. [G. *skeletos,* dried, ntr. *skeleton,* a mummy, a skeleton]

Skene tu·bule (skēn tū′byūl) Embryonic urethral and paraurethral glands that are the female homologue of the prostate.

♻ **skia-** Combining form meaning shadow; superseded by radio-. [G. *skia*]

ski·as·co·py (skī-as′kŏ-pē) SYN retinoscopy.

skill (skil) **1.** The ability to produce, efficiently and in a coordinated manner, movement or result on demand or desire repeatedly. **2.** Motor patterns developed as a result of practice, performed with maximum efficiency and effectiveness (e.g., playing a guitar, shooting foul shots in basketball).

skilled nurs•ing fa•cil•i•ty (SNF) (skild nŭrs′ing fă-sil′i-tē) A nursing facility providing 24-hour nonacute nursing, medical, and rehabilitative care.

skills val•i•da•tion (skilz val′i-dā′shŭn) A regularly scheduled assessment, usually annual, of the competence of nursing staff by administrative personnel of a health care institution; the purpose is to ensure delivery of safe, consistent, appropriate nursing care; both written and clinical testing may be used; nurses are tested on both generic and specialty-specific skills. SYN competence testing.

skim milk, **skimmed milk** (skim milk, skimd) The aqueous (noncream) part of milk from which casein is isolated.

skin (skin) The membranous protective covering of the body, consisting of the epidermis and corium (dermis). See page 1437. SYN cutis [TA]. [A.S. *scinn*]

skin dose (skin dōs) The quantity of radiation delivered to the skin surface.

skin•fold mea•sure•ment (skin′fōld mezh′ŭr-mĕnt) Determination of the thickness of a fold of skin and underlying subcutaneous fat using calipers. Measurements are used to assess body fat content. Standard tables are available relating skinfold thickness to body fat as a percentage of body weight according to age and sex. See page 1438.

skin ridg•es (skin rij′ĕz) SYN epidermal ridges.

skin tag (skin tag) **1.** A polypoid outgrowth of both epidermis and dermal fibrovascular tissue. **2.** Common terminology for any small benign cutaneous lesion. See page 1438. SYN acrochordon, soft wart.

skin test (skin test) A method for determining induced sensitivity (allergy) by applying an antigen (allergen) to, or inoculating it into, the skin; induced sensitivity (allergy) to the specific antigen is indicated by an inflammatory reaction of one of two general kinds: 1) immediate, appears in minutes to an hour or so and in general is dependent on circulating immunoglobulins (antibodies); 2) delayed, appears in 12–48 hours and is not dependent on these soluble substances but on cellular response and infiltration. SYN intradermal test.

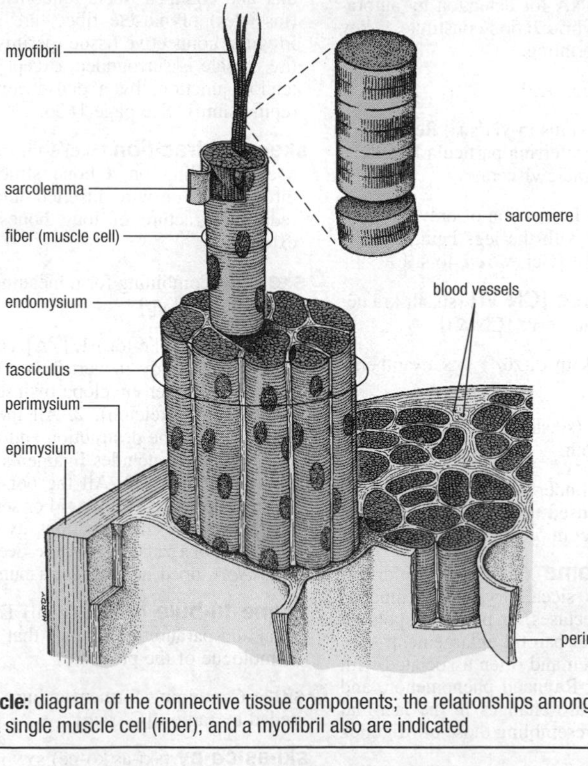

skeletal muscle: diagram of the connective tissue components; the relationships among a muscle bundle (fasciculus), a single muscle cell (fiber), and a myofibril also are indicated

skin trac•tion (skin trak′shŭn) Therapeutic modality on an extremity by means of adhesive tape or other types of strapping applied to the limb.

sko•da•ic res•o•nance (skō-dā′ik rez′ŏ-năns) A peculiar, high-pitched sound, less musical than that obtained over a cavity, elicited by percussion just above the level of a pleuritic effusion. SYN Skoda sign, Skoda tympany.

Sko•da sign (skō′dah sīn) SYN skodaic resonance.

Sko•da tym•pa•ny (skō′dah tim′pă-nē) SYN skodaic resonance.

skull (skŭl) The bones of the head collectively. In a more limited sense, the neurocranium, the bony braincase containing the brain, excluding the bones of the face (viscerocranium). See page A1, A2, A3. [Early Eng. *skulle,* a bowl]

skull base sur•ger•y (skŭl bās sŭr′jĕr-ē) Generic term to denote a specialty of surgery and a group of operations, techniques, and approaches to lesions at or involving the base of the skull or its contents.

skull•cap (skŭl′kap) SYN calvaria.

SL Abbreviation for sublingual.

slant cul•ture (slant kŭl′chŭr) A culture made on the slanting surface of a medium that has been solidified in a test tube inclined from the perpendicular so as to give a greater area than that of the lumen of the tube.

SLAP les•ion (slap lē′zhŭn) Acronymic term for the traumatic tear of the superior part of the glenoid labrum that begins posteriorly and extends anteriorly [*s*uperior *l*abrum, *a*nterior-*p*osterior].

SLE Abbreviation for systemic lupus erythematosus.

sleep (slēp) A physiologic state of relative unconsciousness and inaction of the voluntary muscles, the need for which recurs periodically. The stages of sleep have been variously defined in terms of depth (light, deep), EEG characteristics (delta waves, synchronization), physiologic characteristics (REM, NREM), and presumed anatomic level (pontine, mesencephalic, rhombencephalic, rolandic). [A.S. *slaep*]

sleep ap•ne•a (slēp ap′nē-ă) Central and peripheral apnea during sleep, associated with frequent awakening and often with daytime sleepiness.

sleep def•i•cit (slēp def′i-sit) A lack of sleep time or a relative lack of one of the stages of sleep as determined by a sleep study.

sleep•ing sick•ness (slēp′ing sik′nĕs) SEE Gambian trypanosomiasis, Rhodesian trypanosomiasis.

sleep pa•ral•y•sis (slēp păr-al′i-sis) Brief episodic loss of voluntary movement that occurs when one is falling asleep (hypnagogic sleep paralysis) or when one is awakening (hypnopompic sleep paralysis); one fourth of the narcoleptic tetrad.

slew rate (slū rāt) In electronic pacemaker function, the maximum rate of change of an amplifier

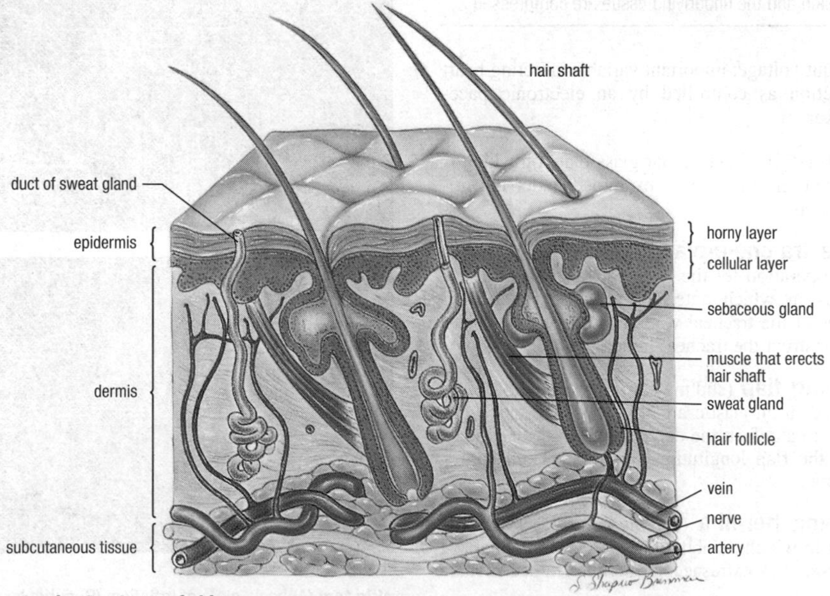

anatomic structures of skin

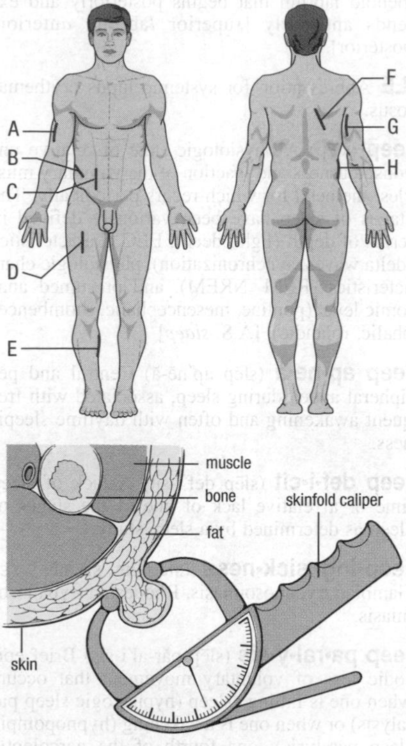

skinfold measurement sites: (A) biceps; (B) supraspinale; (C) abdominal; (D) front thigh; (E) medial calf; (F) subscapular; (G) triceps; (H) iliac crest. During measurement, a double layer of skin and the underlying tissue are compressed

output voltage; important variable affecting heart function as controlled by an electronic pacemaker.

slide (slīd) A rectangular glass plate on which is placed an object to be examined under the microscope.

slide tra·che·o·plas·ty (slīd trā′kē-ō-plas-tē) An operation for the repair of long tracheal stenosis in which anterior and posterior sliding flaps of the tracheal wall are sutured together to reconstruct the tracheal lumen.

slid·ing flap (slīd′ing flap) A rectangular area raised in an elastic area, with its free end adjacent to a defect; the defect is covered by stretching the flap longitudinally until the end comes over it.

slid·ing her·ni·a (slīd′ing hĕr′nē-ă) A condition in which an abdominal viscus forms part of the sac. SYN extrasaccular hernia, slipped hernia.

sli·ding lock (slīd′ing lok) A slot on one shank of obstetrical forceps (as in Kjelland forceps) that allows the shanks to move forward and backward independently.

sling (sling) A supporting bandage or suspensory device; especially a loop suspended from the neck and supporting the flexed forearm.

slipped her·ni·a (slipt hĕr′nē-ă) SYN sliding hernia.

slip·ping rib car·ti·lage, slip·ping rib (slip′ing rib kahr′ti-lăj) Subluxation of rib cartilage at the costochondral junction, causing pain and audible click.

slit·lamp, slit lamp (slit-lamp, slit lamp) OPHTHALMOLOGY an instrument consisting of a microscope combined with a rectangular light source that can be narrowed into a slit for examination of the eye. SYN biomicroscope, Gullstrand slitlamp.

Slo·cum draw·er test (slō′kŭm drōr test) Maneuver used to determine anterior medial rotary instability (AMRI) and anterior lateral rotary instability (ALRI) of the knee. The test is performed in the same position as anterior drawer test, but the tibia is externally rotated 15° for AMRI and internally rotated 15° for ALRI while anterior stress to the tibia is applied.

slough (slŭf) **1.** Necrosed tissue separated from the living structure. **2.** To separate from the living tissue; said of a dead or necrosed part. [M.E. *slughe*]

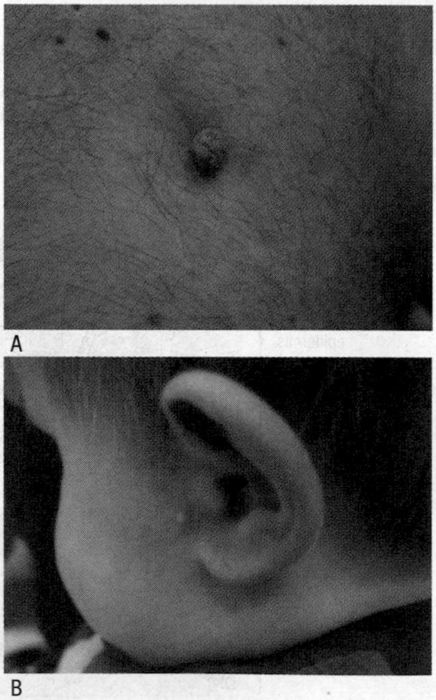

skin tag: (A) back, state of irritation; (B) auricular area, infant

slow chan•nel-block•ing a•gent (slō chan′ ĕl blok′ing ā′jĕnt) SYN calcium channel blocker.

slow code (slō kōd) Intentionally tardy response to a cardiorespiratory emergency so as to reduce the likelihood of a successful resuscitation. SYN man-made death (2).

slow com•po•nent of ny•stag•mus (slō kŏm-pō′nĕnt nis-tag′mŭs) The fundamental movement of the eyes in the vestibuloocular reflex.

slow-ox•i•da•tive (SO) fi•bers (slō ok′si-dā′ tiv fī′bĕrz) SYN slow-twitch fibers.

slow-re•act•ing sub•stance (SRS), slow-re•act•ing sub•stance of an•a•phy•lax•is (slō-rē-ak′ting sub′stăns, an′ă-fi-lak′sis) A leukotriene of low molecular weight released in anaphylactic shock that produces slower and more prolonged contraction of muscle than does histamine; it is active in the presence of antihistamines (but not epinephrine) and seems not to occur preformed in mast cells, but as a result of an antigen-antibody reaction on the granules.

slow re•lease (SR) (slō rē-lēs′) Generally used to refer to that pharmacologic property that causes medication to be spread slowly into the circulation, rather than all at once.

slow-twitch fi•bers (slō-twich fī′bĕrz) Histologically distinct skeletal muscle fibers that generate energy predominantly through the aerobic energy transfer system; are selectively recruited in aerobic activities. SYN slow-oxidative (SO) fibers, Type I fibers.

slow vi•rus (slō vī′rŭs) A virus, or a viruslike agent, etiologically associated with a disease having an incubation period of months to years with a gradual onset frequently terminating in severe illness or death.

slow-vi•rus dis•ease (slō vī′rŭs di-zēz′) **1.** An older term for any disease caused by spongiform encephalopathies, including kuru of humans and scrapie of sheep, classified as slow virus disease but now recognized as prion protein disease. **2.** A disorder that follows a slow, progressive course spanning months to years, frequently involving the central nervous system and ultimately leading to death, such as subacute sclerosing panencephalitis, seemingly caused by the measles virus.

Slu•der neu•ral•gi•a (slū′dĕr nūr-al′jē-ă) SYN sphenopalatine neuralgia.

S&M Abbreviation for sadism and masochism.

Sm Symbol for samarium.

SMA Abbreviation for spinal muscular atrophy.

small cal•o•rie (cal, c) (smawl kal′ŏr-ē) The quantity of energy required to raise the temperature of 1 g of water from 14.5–15.5°C. SYN gram calorie.

small car•di•ac vein (smawl kahr′dē-ak vān) An inconstant vessel, accompanying the right coronary artery in the coronary sulcus, from the right margin of the right ventricle, and emptying into the coronary sinus or the middle cardiac vein.

small cell (smawl sel) A short, blunt, spindle-shaped cell that contains a relatively large hyperchromatic nucleus; frequently observed in some forms of undifferentiated bronchogenic carcinoma.

small cell car•ci•no•ma (smawl sel kahr′si-nō′mă) **1.** An anaplastic carcinoma composed of small cells. **2.** SYN oat cell carcinoma.

small•er pec•tor•al mus•cle (smawl′ĕr pek′ tŏr-ăl mŭs′ĕl) SYN pectoralis minor muscle.

small•er pos•ter•i•or rec•tus mus•cle of head (smawl′ĕr pos-tēr′ē-ŏr rek′tŭs mŭs′ĕl hed) SYN rectus capitis posterior minor muscle.

small•er pso•as musc•le (smawl′ĕr sō′as mŭs′ĕl) SYN psoas minor muscle.

small for ges•ta•tion•al age (SGA) (smawl jes-tā′shŭn-ăl āj) Infant whose birth weight is below the tenth percentile for gestational age.

small in•cre•ment sen•si•tiv•i•ty in•dex (SISI) (smawl in′krĕ-mĕnt sen′si-tiv′i-tē in′deks) SEE SISI test.

small in•tes•tine (smawl in-tes′tin) The portion of the digestive tube between the stomach and the cecum or beginning of the large intestine; it consists of three portions: duodenum, jejunum, and ileum.

small•pox (smawl′poks) An acute eruptive contagious disease caused by a poxvirus (variola); characterized by chills, fever, and an eruption of papules that become umbilicated vesicles, develop into pustules, dry, and then form scabs that, when they fall off, leave permanent indentations on the skin (pockmarks). The World Health Organization initiated a global vaccination effort in 1967; no cases other than laboratory infection have been reported in the human population since 1975. Although only two legal stores of smallpox are held (one in the United States and one in Russia), evidence exists that other nations possess the virus, possibly even in biowarfare arsenals. [E. *small pocks,* or pustules]

small•pox vi•rus (smawl′poks vī′rŭs) SYN variola virus.

small sci•at•ic nerve (smawl sī-at′ik nĕrv) SYN posterior cutaneous nerve of thigh.

smear (smēr) A thin specimen for microscopic examination; usually prepared by spreading liquid or semisolid material uniformly onto a glass slide, fixing it, and staining it before examination.

smear cul•ture (smēr kŭl′chŭr) A sample obtained by spreading material presumed to be infected on the surface of a solidified medium.

smeg·ma (smeg′mă) An oily or pasty material, consisting chiefly of desquamated epidermal cells, and sebum, which accumulate around the external genitalia, particularly under the foreskin. [G. unguent]

smeg·ma·lith (smeg′mă-lith) A calcareous concretion in smegma. [smegma + G. *lithos,* stone]

smell (smel) **1.** To scent; to perceive by means of the olfactory apparatus. **2.** SYN olfaction (1). **3.** SYN odor.

Smith frac·ture (smith frak′shŭr) Reversed Colles fracture; rupture of the distal radius with displacement of the fragment toward the palmar (volar) aspect. See page B25.

Smith-In·di·an op·er·a·tion, Smith op·er·a·tion (smith-in′dē-ăn op-ĕr-ā′shŭn) A surgical technique for removal of cataract within the capsule.

Smith-Pe·ter·sen nail (smith-pē′tĕr-sĕn nāl) A fluted nail used to stabilize fractures of the femoral neck by preventing rotation of the fragments.

SMO Abbreviation for supramalleolar orthotic.

smog (smog) A hazy and often highly irritating atmosphere resulting from a mixture of fog with smoke and other air pollutants. [smoke + fog]

smol·der·ing leu·ke·mi·a (smōl′dĕr′ing lū-kē′mē-ă) SYN myelodysplastic syndrome.

smooth di·et (smūdh dī′ĕt) Consumption of food containing little roughage; used primarily in diseases of the colon.

smooth mus·cle (smūdh mŭs′ĕl) One of the muscle fibers of the internal organs, blood vessels, hair follicles; contractile elements are elongated, usually spindle-shaped cells with centrally located nuclei and a length from 20–200 mcm, or even longer in the pregnant uterus; although transverse striations are lacking, both thick and thin myofibrils occur; such fibers are bound together into sheets or bundles by reticular fibers, and frequently elastic fiber nets are also abundant. SEE ALSO involuntary muscles.

smudge cells (smŭj selz) Immature leukocytes of any type that have undergone partial breakdown during preparation of a stained smear or tissue section, because of their greater fragility; smudge cells are seen in largest numbers in chronic lymphocytic leukemia. SYN basket cell (2).

SN Abbreviation for student nurse.

S:N Abbreviation for signal:noise ratio.

Sn Symbol for tin.

sn- Prefix meaning stereospecifically numbered; a system of numbering the glycerol carbon atoms in lipids, so that the locant numbers remain constant regardless of chemical substitutions, as opposed to systematic numbering.

SNA Abbreviation for State Nurses Association.

snail track de·gen·er·a·tion (snāl trak dĕ-jen′ĕr-ā′shŭn) Circumferential line of fine white dots in the peripheral retina associated with atrophic retinal holes.

snake·root (snāk′rūt) SYN echinacea.

snake·weed (snāk′wēd) SYN bistort.

snap (snap) A click; a short, sharp sound; said especially of cardiac sounds.

snap·ping hip syn·drome (snap′ing hip sin′drōm) A phenomenon experienced during hip motions; may indicate iliotibial band syndrome.

snare (snār) An instrument for removing polyps and other projections from a surface, especially within a cavity; it consists of a wire loop passed around the base of the tumor and gradually tightened. [A.S. *snear,* a cord]

Sned·don syn·drome (sned′ŏn sin′drōm) A cerebral arteriopathy of unknown etiology, characterized by noninflammatory intimal hyperplasia of medium-sized vessels associated with diffuse cutaneous livedo reticularis.

sneeze (snēz) **1.** To expel air from the nose and mouth by an involuntary spasmodic contraction of the muscles of expiration. **2.** An act of sneezing; a reflex excited by an irritation of the mucous membrane of the nose or, sometimes, when a bright light strikes the eye. [A.S. *fneōsan*]

Snel·len E-chart (snel′ĕn chahrt) Direct visual testing tool useful in children older than 2 years but unable to read. Visual acuity is measured by showing letter Es, which are printed backward and rotated, and then having the child point to show the direction of the pointing letter.

Snel·len test type (snel′ĕn test tīp) One of a series of square black symbols employed in testing the acuity of distant vision; the letters vary in size in such a way that each one subtends a visual angle of 5′ at a particular distance.

Snell law (snel law) SYN law of refraction.

SNF Abbreviation for skilled nursing facility.

sniff test (snif test) FLUOROSCOPY a test for diaphragmatic function; paradoxic motion of a hemidiaphragm when a patient sniffs vigorously to show phrenic nerve paralysis or paresis of the hemidiaphragm. If rapid upward movement of the diaphragm occurs on brisk sniffing in the supine position, it is highly suggestive of paralysis of the diaphragm.

snore (snōr) **1.** A rough, rattling inspiratory noise produced by vibration of the pendulous palate, or sometimes of the vocal cords, during sleep or coma. SEE ALSO stertor, rhonchus. **2.** To breathe noisily, or with a snore. [A.S. *snora*]

snout re•flex (snowt rē′fleks) Pouting or pursing of the lips induced by light tapping of closed lips near the midline; seen in defective pyramidal innervation of facial musculature.

snow blind•ness (snō blīnd′nĕs) Severe photophobia secondary to ultraviolet keratoconjunctivitis.

SNP (snip) Acronym for single nucleotide polymorphisms.

snuff (snŭf) **1.** To inhale forcibly through the nose. **2.** Finely powdered tobacco used by inhalation through the nose or application to the gums. **3.** Any medicated powder applied by insufflation to the nasal mucous membrane. [echoic]

snuff•box (snŭf′boks) SEE anatomic snuffbox.

snuf•fles (snŭf′ĕlz) Obstructed nasal respiration, especially in the newborn infant, sometimes due to congenital syphilis.

Sny•der test (snī′dĕr test) A colorimetric procedure to determine dental caries activity or susceptibility based on the rate of acid production by acidogenic oral microorganisms (e.g., lactobacillus) in a glucose medium, using bromcresol green as the indicator, and producing a color change from green to yellow.

SOAP (sōp) Acronym for the conceptual device used by clinicians to organize the progress notes in the problem-oriented record; *S* stands for subjective data provided by the patient, *O* for objective data gathered by health care professionals in the clinical setting, *A* for the assessment of the patient's condition, and *P* for the plan for the patient's care.

soap (sōp) The sodium or potassium salts of long-chain fatty acids (e.g., sodium stearate); used for cleansing purposes and as an excipient in the making of pills and suppositories. [A.S. *sape,* L. *sapo,* G. *sapōn*]

So•a•ve op•er•a•tion (sō-ah′vā op-ĕr-ā′shŭn) Endorectal pull-through for treatment of congenital megacolon.

SOB Abbreviation for shortness of breath.

so•cial i•so•la•tion (sō′shăl ī′sō-lā′shŭn) A state in which the client is alone. It is usually thought of as being imposed by others and seen as negative. (NANDA-approved nursing diagnosis)

so•cial•i•za•tion (sō′shăl-ī-zā′shŭn) **1.** The process of learning attitudes and interpersonal and interactional skills that are in conformity with the values of one's society. **2.** In a group therapy setting, a way of learning to participate effectively in the group. [L. *socius,* partner, companion]

so•cial•ized med•i•cine (sō′shăl-īzd med′i-sin) **1.** The organization and control of medical practice by a government agency, the practitioners being employed by the organization from which they receive standardized compensation for their services, and to which the public contributes, usually in the form of taxation rather than fee-for-service. **2.** A system in which health care services to patients are paid for from a central financial pool created through taxation. **3.** Health care systems that use tax dollars to pay for health care services available from a nonprofit agency. **4.** Health care system in which egalitarian values are held strongly and autonomy of health care practitioners is maintained.

so•cial pho•bi•a (sō′shăl fō′bē-ă) A persistent pattern of significant fear of a social or performance situation, manifested by anxiety or panic on exposure to the situation or in anticipation of it, which the person realizes is unreasonable or excessive; it interferes significantly with the person's functioning.

so•cial psy•chi•a•try (sō′shăl sī-kī′ă-trē) An approach to psychiatric theory and practice emphasizing the cultural and sociologic aspects of mental disorders and treatment; the application of psychiatry to social problems. SEE ALSO community psychiatry.

so•cial ser•vi•ces (sō′shĕl sĕr′vi-sĕz) An agency or department that provides support and assistance to a client in resolving social issues (e.g., finances, health insurance, lodging, and employment).

♻ **socio-** Combining form denoting social, society. [L. *socius,* companion]

so•ci•o•ac•u•sis (sō′sē-ō-ă-kyū′sis) The hearing loss produced by exposure to nonoccupational noise such as small arms fire in hunting and target practice. [socio- + G. *akousis,* hearing]

so•ci•o•cen•tric (sō′sē-ō-sen′trik) Outgoing; reactive to the social or cultural milieu. [socio- + L. *centrum,* center]

so•ci•o•gen•e•sis (sō′sē-ō-jen′ĕ-sis) The origin of social behavior from past interpersonal experiences. [socio- + G. *genesis,* origin]

so•ci•o•path (sō′sē-ō-path) Former designation for a person with an antisocial personality disorder. SEE ALSO antisocial personality disorder, psychopath.

sock•et (sok′ĕt) **1.** The hollow part of a joint; the excavation in one bone of a joint that receives the articular end of the other bone. **2.** Any hollow or concavity into which another part fits (e.g., eye socket) [thr. O. Fr. fr. L. *soccus,* a shoe, a sock]

so•di•um (Na) (sō′dē-ŭm) A metallic element, atomic no. 11, atomic wt. 22.989768; an alkali metal oxidizing readily in air or water; its salts are found in natural biologic systems and are extensively used in medicine and industry. The sodium ion is the most plentiful extracellular ion in the body. SYN natrium. [Mod. L. fr. *soda*]

so·di·um ac·e·tate-a·ce·tic ac·id-form·a·lin fix·a·tive (SAF fix·a·tive) (sō′dē-ŭm as′ĕ-tāt ă-sē′tik as′id fōrm′ă-lin fiks′ă-tiv) Mixture used to fix fecal specimens for subsequent concentration and staining of smears.

so·di·um bo·rate (sō′dē-ŭm bōr′āt) Agent used in lotions, gargles, mouthwashes, and as a detergent.

so·di·um-free, salt-free (sō′dē-ŭm-frē, sawlt-) A product so-labeled contains, by F.D.A. order, no more than 5 mg of sodium per serving.

so·di·um ni·trite (sō′dē-ŭm nī′trīt) An injectable compound used immediately after inhalation of amyl nitrite in the antidotal treatment of cyanide poisoning in the U.S.

so·di·um phos·phate ^{32}P (sō-dē′ŭm fos′fāt) Anionic radioactive phosphorus in the form of a solution of sodium acid phosphate and sodium basic phosphate; a beta emitter with a half-life of 14.3 days; after administration, highest concentrations found in rapidly proliferating tissues; used in treatment of polycythemia vera, chronic myelogenous leukemia, and osseous metastases. SEE ALSO chromic phosphate ^{32}P colloidal suspension.

so·di·um pol·y·an·e·thole sul·fon·ate (SPS) (sō′dē-ŭm pol′ē-an′ĕ-thōl sŭl′fŏn-āt) An anticoagulant added to blood specimens.

so·di·um-po·tas·si·um pump (sō′dē-ŭm pō-tas′ē-ŭm pŭmp) A membrane-bound transporter that maintains high potassium and low sodium intracellular concentrations relative to the extracellular medium. This exchange is accomplished at the expense of cellular energy in the form of ATP.

so·di·um pump (sō′dē-ŭm pŭmp) A biologic mechanism that uses metabolic energy from ATP to achieve active transport of sodium across a membrane; sodium pumps expel sodium from most cells of the body, sometimes coupled with the transport of other substances, and also serve to move sodium across multicellular membranes such as renal tubule walls.

so·di·um thi·o·sul·fate (sō′dē-ŭm thī′ō-sŭl′fāt) An injectable compound used immediately after injection of sodium nitrate in the antidotal treatment of cyanide poisoning in the U.S.

sod·om·ist, sod·om·ite (sod′ŏ-mist, -mīt) One who practices sodomy. [G. *sodomitēs,* an inhabitant of the biblical city of Sodom, which was destroyed by fire because of the wickedness of its people]

sod·o·my (sod′ŏm-ē) A term denoting any one of a number of sexual practices variously considered abnormal or deviant by particular cultures, such as bestiality, oral-genital contact, and anal intercourse. SEE ALSO sodomist.

soft chan·cre (sawft shang′kĕr) SYN chancroid.

soft corn (sawft kōrn) A clavus formed by pressure between two toes; its surface is macerated and yellowish. SYN heloma molle.

soft di·et (sawft dī′ĕt) A normal diet limited to soft foods for patients who have difficulty chewing or swallowing; there are no restrictions on seasoning or method of food preparation.

soft drus·en (sawft drū′sĕn) Type of exudative structure that appears ophthalmoscopically as placoid yellow lesions characterized histopathologically by localized serous detachments of the retinal pigment epithelium from the Bruch membrane.

soft pal·ate (sawft pal′ăt) The posterior muscular portion of the palate, forming an incomplete septum between the mouth and the oropharynx, and between the oropharynx and the nasopharynx. See this page. SYN velum palatinum.

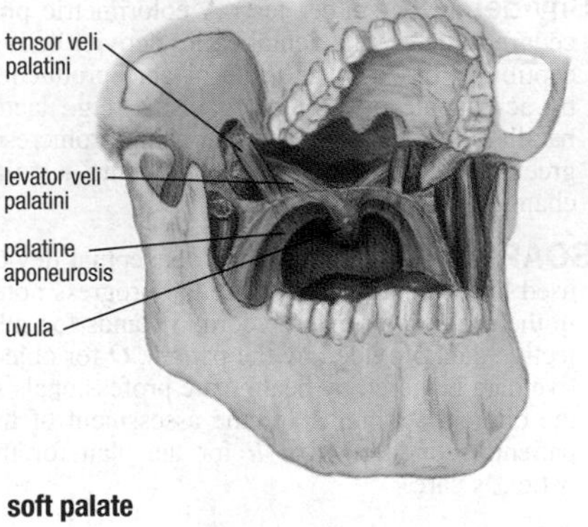

soft palate

soft tis·sue ther·a·py (sawft tish′ū thār′ă-pē) Manual therapy that affects the soft tissues of the body (e.g., muscle, fascia).

soft tu·ber·cle (sawft tū′bĕr-kĕl) A tubercle showing caseous necrosis.

soft ul·cer (sawft ŭl′sĕr) SYN chancroid.

soft wart (sawft wōrt) SYN skin tag.

soil (soyl) Dirt.

sol (sol) **1.** A collodial dispersion of a solid in a liquid. Cf. gel. **2.** Abbreviation for solution.

so·la·nine (sō′lă-nēn) A toxic alkaloid found in parts of solanaceous plants, including potato skins; plant diseases (e.g., potato blight) may raise the concentration to a harmful level.

so·lar chei·li·tis (sō′lăr kī-lī′tis) Mucosal atrophy with drying, crusting, and fissuring of the vermilion border of the lower lip, resulting from chronic exposure to sunlight; dysplastic (premalignant) changes are noted microscopically.

so·lar co·me·do (sō′lăr kom′ĕ-dō) SYN Favre-Racouchot disease.

so·lar e·las·to·sis (sō′lăr ĕ-las-tō′sis) Elastosis seen histologically in the sun-exposed skin of old people or in those who have chronic actinic damage.

so·lar plex·us (sō′lăr plek′sŭs) SYN celiac (nerve) plexus.

so·lar ther·a·py (sō′lăr thār′ă-pē) SYN heliotherapy.

so·lar ur·ti·car·i·a (sō′lăr ŭr′ti-kar′ē-ă) A form of urticaria resulting from exposure to specific light spectra (e.g., sunlight); some patients have passive-transfer antibodies, others do not.

sol·a·tion (sol-ā′shŭn) COLLOIDAL CHEMISTRY the transformation of a gel into a sol, as by melting gelatin.

sol·der·ing (sod′ĕr-ing) A laser technique to make one tissue adhere to another.

sole (sōl) The plantar surface or underside of the foot. SYN planta [TA]. [A.S.]

So·le·nop·sis (sōl-ĕ-nop′sis) The genus of fire ants, which can inflict painful burning stings that cause local and occasionally systemic reactions.

So·le·nop·sis in·vic·ta (sōl-ĕ-nop′sis in-vik′tă) The red fire ant, a species imported from South America that has spread extensively within the southeastern United States, where it has become a major pest of humans and animals; it readily stings humans, producing local swelling and pruritus with development of a pustule at the site of the sting and, in rare cases, can cause anaphylactic shock with death from respiratory or cardiac arrest. SEE ALSO *Solenopsis richteri*. SYN *red fire ant*.

So·le·nop·sis rich·ter·i (sōl-ĕ-nop′sis rik-ter′ī) The black fire ant, a species imported from South America but less extensively established in the United States than *Solenopsis invicta*. SEE ALSO *Solenopsis invicta*. SYN *black fire ant*.

so·le·us mus·cle (sō′lē-ŭs mŭs′ĕl) *Origin*, posterior surface of head and upper third of shaft of fibula, oblique line and middle third of medial margin of tibia, and a tendinous arch passing between tibia and fibula over the popliteal vessels; *insertion*, with gastrocnemius by tendo calcaneus (tendo achillis) into tuberosity of calcaneus; *action*, plantar flexion of foot; *nerve supply*, tibial. See this page. SYN musculus soleus [TA].

sol·id (sol′id) **1.** Firm; compact; not fluid; without interstices or cavities; not cancellous. **2.** A body that retains its form when not confined; one that is not fluid, neither liquid nor gaseous. [L. *solidus*]

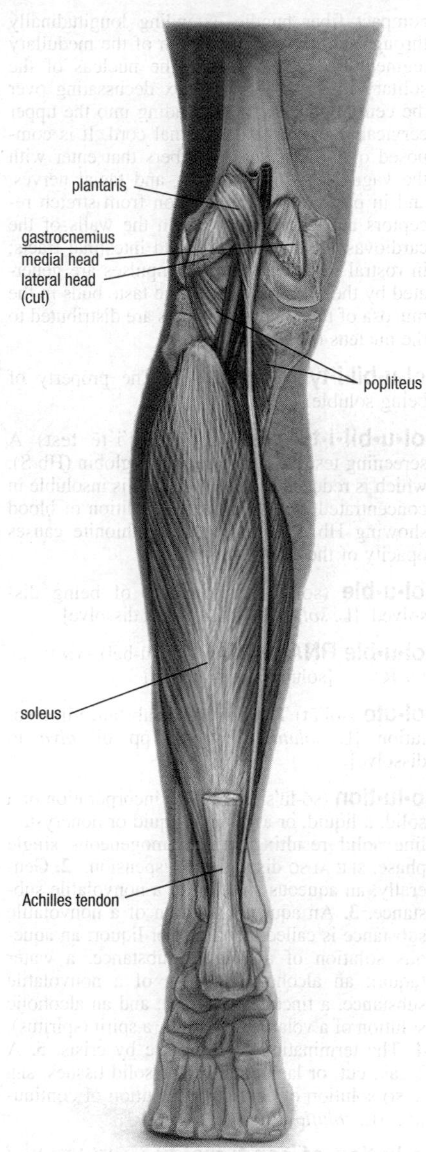

soleus muscle

sol·i·tar·y bone cyst (sol′i-tar-ē bōn sist) A unilocular cyst containing serous fluid and lined with a thin layer of connective tissue, occurring usually in the shaft of a long bone in a child. SYN osteocystoma, unicameral bone cyst.

sol·i·tar·y lym·pha·tic fol·li·cles (sol′i-tar-ē lim-fat′ik fol′i-kĕls) Minute collections of lymphoid tissue in the mucosa of the small and large intestines, being especially numerous in the cecum and appendix.

sol·i·tar·y tract (sol′i-tar-ē trakt) A slender,

compact fiber bundle extending longitudinally through the dorsolateral region of the medullary tegmentum, surrounded by the nucleus of the solitary tract, below the obex decussating over the central canal, and descending into the upper cervical segments of the spinal cord. It is composed of primary sensory fibers that enter with the vagus, glossopharyngeal, and facial nerves, and in part convey information from stretch receptors and chemoreceptors in the walls of the cardiovascular, respiratory, and intestinal tracts; in rostral parts of the tract, impulses are generated by the receptor cells of the taste buds in the mucosa of the tongue. Its fibers are distributed to the nucleus of the solitary tract.

sol•u•bil•i•ty (sol-yū-bil′i-tē) The property of being soluble.

sol•u•bil•i•ty test (sol-yū-bil′i-tē test) A screening test for sickle cell hemoglobin (Hb S), which is reduced by dithionite and is insoluble in concentrated inorganic buffer; addition of blood showing Hb S to buffer and dithionite causes opacity of the solution.

sol•u•ble (sol′yū-bĕl) Capable of being dissolved. [L. *solubilis,* fr. *solvo,* to dissolve]

sol•u•ble RNA (sRNA) (sol′yū-bĕl) SYN transfer RNA. [soluble in molar salt]

sol•ute (sol′ūt) The dissolved substance in a solution. [L. *solutus,* dissolved, pp. of *solvo,* to dissolve]

so•lu•tion (sŏ-lū′shŭn) **1.** The incorporation of a solid, a liquid, or a gas in a liquid or noncrystalline solid resulting in a homogeneous single phase. SEE ALSO dispersion, suspension. **2.** Generally, an aqueous solution of a nonvolatile substance. **3.** An aqueous solution of a nonvolatile substance is called a solution or liquor; an aqueous solution of a volatile substance, a water (aqua); an alcoholic solution of a nonvolatile substance, a tincture (tinctura); and an alcoholic solution of a volatile substance, a spirit (spiritus). **4.** The termination of a disease by crisis. **5.** A break, cut, or laceration of the solid tissues. SEE ALSO solution of contiguity, solution of continuity. [L. *solutio*]

so•lu•tion of con•ti•gu•i•ty (sŏ-lū′shŭn kon′ti-gyū′i-tē) The breaking of contiguity; a dislocation or displacement of two normally contiguous parts.

so•lu•tion of con•ti•nu•i•ty (sŏ-lū′shŭn kon′ti-nū′i-tē) Division of bones or soft parts that are normally continuous, as by a fracture, a laceration, or an incision. SYN dieresis.

sol•vent (sol′vĕnt) A liquid that holds another substance in solution, i.e., dissolves it. [L. *solvens,* pres. p. of *solvo,* to dissolve]

so•ma (sō′mă) **1.** The axial part of the body, i.e., head, neck, trunk, and tail, excluding the limbs. **2.** All of an organism with the exception of the germ cells. SEE ALSO body. **3.** The body of a nerve cell, from which axons and dendrites project. [G. *sōma,* body]

somaesthesia [Br.] SYN somesthesia.

so•man (GD) (sō′man) A nonpersistent nerve agent developed by Germany during World War II. Its NATO code is GD.

so•mas•the•ni•a (sō′măs-thē′nē-ă) SYN somatasthenia.

somataesthesia [Br.] SYN somatesthesia.

somataesthetic [Br.] SYN somatesthetic.

so•ma•tag•no•si•a (sō′mă-tag-nō′zē-ă) SYN somatotopagnosis. [somat- + G. *a-* priv. + *gnōsis,* recognition]

so•ma•tal•gi•a (sō′mă-tal′jē-ă) **1.** Pain in the body. **2.** Pain due to organic causes, as opposed to psychogenic pain. [somat- + G. *algos,* pain]

so•ma•tas•the•ni•a (sō′mat-as-thē′nē-ă) A condition of chronic physical weakness and fatigability. SYN somasthenia. [somat- + G. *astheneia,* weakness]

so•ma•tes•the•si•a (sō′mat-es-thē′zē-ă) Bodily sensation, the conscious awareness of the body. SYN somataesthesia, somesthesia. [somat- + G. *aisthēsis,* sensation]

so•mat•es•the•tic (sō′mat-es-thet′ik) Relating to somatesthesia. SYN somataesthetic.

so•mat•ic (sō-mat′ik) **1.** Relating to the soma or trunk, the wall of the body cavity, or the body in general. SYN parietal (2). **2.** Relating to or involving the skeleton or skeletal (voluntary) muscle and the innervation of the latter, as distinct from the viscera or visceral (involuntary) muscle and its (autonomic) innervation. SYN parietal (3). **3.** Relating to the vegetative, as distinguished from the generative, functions. [G. *sōmatikos,* bodily]

so•ma•tic ant•i•gen (sō-mat′ik an′ti-jen) An antigen located in the cell wall of a bacterium in contrast to one in the flagella (flagellar antigen) or in a capsule (capsular antigen).

so•mat•ic cell gene ther•a•py (sō-mat′ik sel gēn thār′ă-pē) Repair or replacement of a defective gene within somatic tissue.

so•ma•tic cells (sō-mat′ik selz) The cells of an organism other than the germ cells.

so•ma•tic cross•ing-o•ver (sō-mat′ik kraws′ing-ō′vĕr) Process that occurs during the mitosis of somatic cells, in contrast to that which occurs in meiosis.

so•ma•tic death, sys•tem•ic death (sō-mat′ik deth, sis-tem′ik) Death of the entire body, as distinguished from local death.

so•ma•tic de•lu•sion (sō-mat′ik dĕ-lū′zhŭn) A delusion having reference to a nonexistent lesion or alteration of some organ or part of the body;

sometimes indistinguishable from hypochondriasis.

so•ma•tic mo•tor nu•cle•i (sō-mat′ik mō′tŏr nū′klē-i) Collective term indicating the motor nuclei innervating the tongue musculature (hypoglossal nucleus) and the extraocular eye muscles (abducens nucleu, trochlear nucleus, and oculomotor nucleus).

so•ma•tic mu•ta•tion (sō-mat′ik myū-tā′shŭn) A change that occurs in the general body cells (as opposed to the germ cells) and hence not transmitted to progeny.

so•ma•tic mu•ta•tion the•o•ry of can•cer (sō-mat′ik myū-tā′shŭn thē′ŏr-ē kan′sĕr) The proposition that cancer is caused by a mutation or mutations in the body cells (as opposed to germ cells), especially nonlethal mutations associated with increased proliferation of the mutant cells.

so•ma•tic nerve (sō-mat′ik nĕrv) One of the nerves of parietal sensation or voluntary motion, as distinguished from the visceral sensory, involuntary motor, and secretory nerves.

so•ma•tic pain (sō-mat′ik pān) Unpleasant sensation originating in the skin, ligaments, muscles, bones, or joints.

so•ma•tic re•pro•duc•tion (sō-mat′ik rē′prō-dŭk′shŭn) Asexual reproduction by fission or budding of somatic cells.

so•ma•tic sen•so•ry cor•tex, **so•ma•to•sen•so•ry cor•tex** (sō-mat′ik sen′sŏr-ē kōr′teks, sō′mă-tō-sen′sŏr-ē) The region of the cerebral cortex receiving the somatic sensory radiation from the ventrobasal nucleus of the thalamus; it represents the primary cortical processing mechanism for sensory information originating at the body surfaces (touch) and in deeper tissues such as muscle, tendons, and joint capsules (position sense).

so•ma•tic swal•low (sō-mat′ik swahl′ō) A swallowing pattern with muscular contractions that appear to be under control of the person at a subconscious level; distinguished from visceral swallow.

so•ma•ti•za•tion (sō′mat-ī-zā′shŭn) The process by which psychological needs are expressed in physical symptoms. SEE ALSO somatization disorder.

so•ma•ti•za•tion dis•or•der (sō′mat-ī-zā′shŭn dis-ōr′dĕr) A mental disorder characterized by presentation of a complicated medical history and of physical symptoms referring to a variety of organ systems, but without a detectable or known organic basis. SEE ALSO conversion, hysteria, conversion disorder.

♻**somato-**, **somat-**, **somatico-** Combining forms meaning the body, bodily. [G. *sōma*, body]

so•ma•to•chrome (sō-mat′ō-krōm) Denoting the group of neurons or nerve cells in which there is an abundance of cytoplasm completely surrounding the nucleus. [somato- + G. *chrōma*, color]

so•ma•to•crin•in (sō′mă-tō-krin′in) Hypothalamic growth hormone-releasing hormone (GHRH). [somato- + G. *krinō*, to secrete, + -in]

so•ma•to•gen•ic (sō′mă-tō-jen′ik) **1.** Originating in the soma or body under the influence of external forces. **2.** Having origin in body cells. [somato- + G. *genesis*, origin]

so•ma•to•lib•er•in (sō′mă-tō-lib′ĕr-in) A decapeptide released by the hypothalamus, which induces the release of human growth hormone (somatotropin). Cf. bioregulator. SYN growth hormone–releasing factor, growth hormone–releasing hormone, somatotropin-releasing factor, somatotropin-releasing hormone. [somatotropin + L. *libero*, to free, + -in]

so•ma•to•mam•mo•tro•pin (sō′mă-tō-mam′ō-trō′pin) A peptide hormone, closely related to somatotropin in its biologic properties, produced by the normal placenta and by certain neoplasms. [somato- + L. *mamma*, breast, + G. tropē, a turning, + -in]

so•ma•to•me•din (sō′mă-tō-mē′din) A peptide synthesized in the liver, and probably in the kidney, capable of stimulating certain anabolic processes in bone and cartilage, such as synthesis of DNA, RNA, and protein, and the sulfation of mucopolysaccharides; secretion or biologic activity of somatomedin is known to depend on somatotropin. [*somato*tropin + *med*iator + -in]

so•ma•to•path•ic (sō′mă-tō-path′ik) Relating to bodily or organic illness, as distinguished from mental (psychological) disorder. [somato- + G. *pathos*, suffering]

so•ma•to•pause (sō′mă-tō-pawz) Decrease in growth hormone–insulinlike growth factor axis activities associated with aging.

so•ma•to•plasm (sō-mat′ō-plazm) Aggregate of all forms of specialized protoplasm entering into the composition of the body, other than germ plasm. [somato- + G. *plasma*, something formed]

so•ma•to•pleure (sō-mat′ō-plūr) Embryonic layer formed by association of the parietal layer of the lateral plate mesoderm with the ectoderm. [somato- + G. *pleura*, side]

so•ma•to•psy•chic (sō′mă-tō-sī′kik) Relating to the body-mind relationship; the study of the effects of the body on the mind, as opposed to psychosomatic, which refers to the effects of mind on body. [somato- + G. *psychē*, soul]

so•ma•to•psy•cho•sis (sō′mă-tō-sī-kō′sis) An emotional disorder associated with an organic disease. [somato- + G. *psychōsis*, an animating]

so·ma·to·sen·so·ry (sō′mă-tō-sen′sŏr-ē) Sensation relating to the body's superficial and deep parts as contrasted to specialized senses such as sight.

so·ma·to·sen·so·ry au·ra (sō′mă-tō-sen′sŏr-ē awr′ă) Epileptic aura characterized by paresthesias or abdominal somatognosia of a clearly defined regional distribution. SEE ALSO aura (1).

so·ma·to·sex·u·al (sō′mă-tō-sek′shū-ăl) Denoting the somatic aspects of sexuality as distinguished from its psychosexual aspects.

so·mat·o·sound (sō-mat′ō-sownd) A perceived tone of varying volume and pitch of which the patient is aware, although no sound is audible to anyone else. Some clinicians suggest it is a secondary manifestation of tinnitus (q.v.).

so·ma·to·stat·in (sō′mă-tō-stat′in) A tetradecapeptide capable of inhibiting release of somatotropin, insulin, and gastrin. Cf. bioregulator. SYN growth hormone–inhibiting hormone, somatotropin release-inhibiting hormone. [somatotropin + G. *stasis*, a standing still, + -in]

so·ma·to·stat·i·no·ma (sō′mă-tō-stat′i-nō′mă) A somatostatin-secreting tumor of the pancreatic islets.

so·ma·to·ther·a·py (sō′mă-tō-thār′ă-pē) **1.** Therapy directed at physical disorders. **2.** PSYCHIATRY a variety of therapeutic interventions employing chemical or physical, as opposed to psychological, methods.

so·ma·to·top·ag·no·sis (sō′mă-tō-top′ag-nō′sis) The inability to identify any part of one's own or another's body. Cf. autotopagnosia. SYN somatagnosia. [somato- + top- + G. *a-* priv. + G. *gnōsis*, knowledge]

so·ma·to·top·ic (sō′mă-tō-top′ik) Relating to somatotopy.

so·ma·tot·o·py (sō′mă-tot′ŏ-pē) The topographic association of positional relationships of receptors in the body through respective nerve fibers to their terminal distribution in specific functional areas of the cerebral cortex; the continuation of these positional relationships in all stages of the ascent of nerve fibers through the central nervous system enables the brain and spinal cord to function on a basis of spatially designated units. [somato- + G. *topos*, place]

so·ma·to·tropes (sō-mat′ō-trōps) A subclass of pituitary acidophilic cells; site of synthesis of growth hormone.

so·ma·to·troph (sō-mat′ō-trōf) A cell of the adenohypophysis that produces somatotropin.

so·ma·to·tro·pic, so·ma·to·tro·phic (sō′mă-tō-trō′pik, -trō′fik) Having a stimulating effect on body growth. [somato- + G. *tropē*, a turning]

so·ma·to·tro·pin, so·ma·to·tro·pic hor·mone (sō-mat′ō-trō′pin, -trō′pik hōr′mōn) A protein hormone of the anterior lobe of the pituitary, produced by the acidophil cells, that promotes body growth, fat mobilization, and inhibition of glucose utilization; diabetogenic when present in excess; a deficiency of somatotropin is associated with a number of types of dwarfism. Cf. bioregulator. SYN growth hormone, pituitary growth hormone. [for *somatotrophin*, fr. somato- + G. *trophē* nourishment; corrupted to *-tropin* and reanalyzed as fr. G. *tropē*, a turning]

so·ma·to·tro·pin re·lease-in·hi·bit·ing hor·mone (SIH) (sō-mat′ō-trō′pin rĕ-lēs′in-hib′i-ting hōr′mōn) SYN somatostatin.

so·ma·to·tro·pin-re·leas·ing fac·tor (sō-mat′ō-trō′pin rĕ-lēs′ing fak′tŏr) SYN somatoliberin.

so·ma·to·tro·pin-re·leas·ing hor·mone (SRH) (sō-mat′ō-trō′pin rĕ-lēs′ing hōr′mōn) SYN somatoliberin.

so·ma·to·type (sō-mat′ō-tīp) **1.** The constitutional or body type of an individual. **2.** The constitutional or body type associated with a particular personality type.

so·mat·o·visc·er·al (sō′mă-tō-vis′ĕr-ăl) Pertaining to the influence of the body framework (soma), or neuromusculoskeletal system, on the function of the internal body systems and organs.

so·ma·tro·pin (sō-mat′rō-pin) A drug identical with human growth hormone; used in the treatment of growth disturbances due to insufficient secretion of growth hormone in children or adults or associated with gonadal dysgenesis (Turner syndrome) and of growth disturbance in prepubertal children with chronic renal insufficiency.

som·es·the·si·a (sō′mes-thē′zē-ă) SYN somatesthesia. SYN somaesthesia.

so·mite (sō′mīt) One of the paired, metamerically arranged cell masses formed in the early embryonic paraxial mesoderm; commencing in the third or early fourth week in the region of the hindbrain, they develop in a caudal direction until 42 pairs are formed; their presence is considered evidence that metameric segmentation is a vertebrate characteristic. See page B1. [G. *sōma*, body, + *-ite*]

som·nam·bu·lism (som-nam′byū-lizm) **1.** A disorder of sleep involving complex motor acts that occurs primarily during the first third of the night but not during rapid eye movement sleep. **2.** A form of hysteria in which purposeful behavior is forgotten. [L. *somnus*, sleep, + *ambulo*, to walk]

som·ni·fa·cient (som′ni-fā′shĕnt) SYN soporific (1). [L. *somnus*, sleep, + *facio*, to make]

som·nif·er·ous (som-nif′ĕr-ŭs) SYN soporific (1). [L. *somnus*, sleep, + *fero*, to bring]

som·nil·o·quence, som·nil·o·quism (som-nil′ŏ-kwĕns, -kwizm) **1.** Talking or muttering in one's sleep. **2.** SYN somniloquy. [L. *somnus,* sleep, + *loquor,* to talk]

som·nil·o·quy (som-nil′ŏ-kwē) Talking under the influence of hypnotic suggestion. SYN somniloquence (2), somniloquism. [L. *somnus,* sleep, + *loquor,* to speak]

som·nip·a·thy (som-nip′ă-thē) Any sleep disorder. [L. *somnus,* sleep, + G. *pathos,* suffering]

som·no·cin·e·ma·tog·ra·phy (som′nō-sin′ĕ-mă-tog′ră-fē) The process or technique of recording movements during sleep.

som·no·lence, som·no·len·cy (som′nō-lĕns, -lĕn-sē) **1.** An inclination to sleep. **2.** A condition of obtusion. [L. *somnolentia*]

som·no·lent, som·no·les·cent (som′nō-lĕnt, som′nō-les′ĕnt) **1.** Drowsy; sleepy; inclined to sleep. **2.** In a condition of incomplete sleep; semicomatose. [L. *somnus,* sleep]

So·mog·yi ef·fect, So·mog·yi phe·no·me·non (sō-mō′jē e-fekt′, fĕ-nom′ĕ-non) A rebound phenomenon of reactive hyperglycemia following a period of relative hypoglycemia, which may be subclinical and difficult to detect; the hyperglycemia induces use of more insulin, thus aggravating the problem.

So·mog·yi u·nit (sō-mō′jē yū′nit) A measure of the level of activity of amylase in blood serum, as analyzed by means of the Somogyi method (the most frequently used procedure).

Son·der·mann ca·nal (son′der-mahn kă-nal′) A blind outpouching of Schlemm canal, extending toward, but not communicating with, the anterior chamber of the eye.

son·ic (son′ik) Of, pertaining to, or determined by sound, e.g., sonic vibration. [L. *sonus,* sound]

son·i·ca·tion (son′i-kā′shŭn) The process of disrupting biologic materials by use of sound wave energy.

son·i·fi·ca·tion (son′i-fi-kā′shŭn) The production of sound, or of sound waves.

Son·ne ba·cil·lus (son′ĕ bă-sil′ŭs) SYN *Shigella sonnei.*

son·o·gram (sŏn′ō-gram) SYN ultrasonogram. See page B21. [L. *sonus,* sound, + G. *gramma,* a drawing]

son·o·graph (son′ō-graf) SYN ultrasonograph. [L. *sonus,* sound, + G. *graphō,* to write]

so·nog·ra·pher (sŏ-nog′ră-fĕr) SYN ultrasonographer.

so·nog·ra·phy (sŏ-nog′ră-fē) SYN ultrasonography. [L. *sonus,* sound, + G. *graphō,* to write]

so·no·rous rale (son′ŏr-ŭs rahl) A cooing or snoring sound often produced by the vibration of a projecting mass of viscid secretion in a large bronchus.

so·por (sō′pŏr) An unnaturally deep sleep. [L.]

so·po·rif·ic (sop′ŏr-if′ik) **1.** Causing sleep. SYN somnifacient, somniferous. **2.** An agent that produces sleep. [L. *sopor,* deep sleep, + *facio,* to make]

sor·be·fa·cient (sōr′bĕ-fā′shĕnt) **1.** Causing absorption. **2.** An agent that causes or facilitates absorption. [L. *sorbeo,* to suck up, + *facio,* to make]

sor·des (sōr′dēz) A dark brown or blackish crustlike collection on the lips, teeth, and gums of a person with dehydration associated with a chronic debilitating disease. [L. filth, fr. *sordeo,* to be foul]

sore (sōr) **1.** Any open skin lesion (e.g., decubitus ulcer, wound, other ulcer). **2.** Painful; aching; tender. [A.S. *sār*]

sore throat (sōr thrōt) A condition characterized by pain or discomfort on swallowing; it may be due to any of a variety of inflammations of the tonsils, pharynx, or larynx.

So·ret phe·no·me·non (sō-rā′ fĕ-nom′ĕ-non) In a solution kept in a long, upright tube at room temperature, the upper part, being the warmer, is also the more concentrated.

sorp·tion (sōrp′shŭn) Adsorption or absorption.

Sors·by mac·u·lar de·gen·er·a·tion (sorz′bē mak′yū-lăr dĕ-jen′ĕr-ā-shŭn) SYN familial pseudoinflammatory macular degeneration.

Sors·by syn·drome (sorz′bē sin′drōm) Congenital macular coloboma and apical dystrophy of the extremities.

So·tos syn·drome (sō′tōs sin′drōm) Cerebral gigantism and generalized large muscles in childhood, with mental retardation and defective coordination; of unknown etiology.

souf·fle (sū′fĕl) A soft, blowing sound heard on auscultation. [Fr. *souffler,* to blow]

sound (sownd) **1.** The vibrations produced by a sounding body, transmitted by the air or other medium, and perceived by the internal ear. **2.** An elongated cylindric, usually curved, instrument of metal, used for exploring the bladder or other cavities of the body, for dilating strictures of the urethra, esophagus, or other canal, for calibrating the lumen of a body cavity, or for detecting the presence of a foreign body in a body cavity. **3.** To explore or calibrate a cavity with a sound. **4.** Whole; healthy; not diseased or injured.

sound field (sownd fēld) The environment in which sound waves are propagated. SYN acoustic surround.

source-to-im·age dis·tance (SID) (sōrs-im′ăj dis′tăns) SYN focal-film distance.

South Af·ri·can tick-bite fe·ver (sowth af′ri-kăn tik′bīt fē′vĕr) A typhuslike fever of South Africa caused by *Rickettsia africae* and usually characterized by primary eschar and regional adenitis, rigors, and maculopapular rash on the fifth day, often with severe central nervous system symptoms.

South A·mer·i·can blas·to·my·co·sis (sowth ă-mer′i-kăn blas′tō-mī-kō′sis) SYN paracoccidioidomycosis.

South A·mer·i·can try·pan·o·so·mi·a·sis (sowth ă-mer′i-kăn trī-pan′ō-sō-mī′ă-sis) Disease caused by *Trypanosoma* (or *Schizotrypanum) cruzi* and transmitted by certain species of reduviid (triatomine) bugs. In its acute form, it is seen most frequently in young children, with swelling of the skin at the site of entry, most often the face, and regional lymph node enlargement; in its chronic form it can assume several aspects, commonly cardiomyopathy, but megacolon and megaesophagus also occur; natural reservoirs include domestic, domiciliated, and wild mammals. SYN Chagas disease, Chagas-Cruz disease, Cruz trypanosomiasis.

South·ern blot a·nal·y·sis (sŭdh′ĕrn blot ă-nal′i-sis) A procedure to separate and identify DNA sequences; DNA fragments are separated by electrophoresis on an agarose gel, transferred (blotted) onto a nitrocellulose or nylon membrane, and hybridized with complementary (labeled) nucleic acid probes.

south·ern wax myr·tle (sŭdh′ĕrn waks mĭr′tĕl) SYN bayberry.

sow·ber·ry (sow′ber-ē) SYN barberry.

SP Abbreviation for sacroposterior position.

space (spās) **1.** Any demarcated portion of the body, either an area of the surface, a segment of the tissues, or a cavity. SEE ALSO area, region, zone. **2.** DENTISTRY SYN diastema. SYN spatium [TA]. [L. *spatium,* room, space]

space main·tain·er (spās mān-tān′ĕr) Prosthetic replacement for a deciduous tooth that has been lost prematurely, to prevent closure of the space before the permanent tooth erupts.

spac·er (spās′ĕr) An extension device for a metered-dose inhaler; it is designed to eliminate the need for hand-breath coordination and to reduce the deposition of large aerosol particles in the upper airway.

Spal·lan·za·ni law (spahl-lahn-tzah′nē law) The younger the individual, the greater is the regenerative power of its cells.

spal·la·tion (spaw-lā′shŭn) **1.** SYN fragmentation. **2.** Nuclear reaction in which nuclei, on being bombarded by high-energy particles, liberate a number of protons and alpha particles.

spal·la·tion pro·duct (spaw-lā′shŭn prod′ŭkt) An atomic species produced in the course of the spallation of any atom.

Span·ish in·flu·en·za (span′ish in′flū-en′ză) Disease that precipitated several waves of pandemic infection during 1918 to 1919 and resulted in more than 20 million deaths worldwide. It was caused by influenza virus A; phylogenetic analysis indicates that this strain is related to subsequently observed type A human and classic swine influenzaviruses.

spar·ing ac·tion (spār′ing ak′shŭn) The manner in which a nonessential nutritive component, by its presence in the diet, lowers the dietary requirement for an essential component.

spar·row·grass (spar′ō-gras) SYN *Asparagus.*

spasm (spazm) A sudden involuntary contraction of one or more muscle groups; includes cramps, contractures. SYN muscle spasm, spasmus. [G. *spasmos*]

♻ **spasmo-** Combining form indicating spasm. [G. *spasmos*]

spas·mod·ic (spaz-mod′ik) Relating to or marked by spasm. [G. *spasmōdes,* convulsive, fr. *spasmos,* + *eidos,* form]

spas·mo·dic dys·men·or·rhe·a (spaz-mod′ik dis-men′ŏr-ē′ă) Dysfunction of menstruation accompanied by painful contractions of the uterus.

spas·mo·dic dys·phon·i·a (spaz-mod′ik dis-fō′nē-ă) A spasmodic contraction of the intrinsic muscles of the larynx excited by attempted phonation, producing either adductor or abductor subtypes caused by a central nervous system disorder. A localized form of movement disorder. SYN spastic dysphonia.

spas·mol·y·sis (spaz-mol′i-sis) The arrest of a spasm or convulsion. [spasmo- + G. *lysis,* dissolution]

spas·mo·lyt·ic (spaz′mō-lit′ik) **1.** Relating to spasmolysis. **2.** Denoting a chemical agent that relieves smooth muscle spasms.

spas·mus (spaz′mŭs) SYN spasm. [L. fr. G. *spasmos,* spasm]

spas·mus nu·tans (spaz′mŭs nū′tanz) Head nodding and head turn with vertical, horizontal, or torsional nystagmus; appears in patients aged between 6 months and 3 years.

spas·tic (spas′tik) **1.** SYN hypertonic (1). **2.** Relating to spasm or to spasticity. [L. *spasticus,* fr. G. *spastikos,* drawing in]

spas·tic a·ba·si·a (spas′tik ă-bā′zē-ă) Inability to walk due to a spastic contraction of the muscles when an attempt is made.

spas·tic col·on (spas′tik kō′lŏn) SYN irritable bowel syndrome.

spas·tic dys·ar·thri·a (spas′tik dis-ahr′thrē-ă)

Disturbance associated with upper motor neuron disorders causing excess tone and limited range in muscle movements, characterized by imprecise consonants, monotony of pitch and reduced stress, and a labored voice quality. SEE ALSO pseudobulbar palsy.

spas·tic dys·pho·ni·a (spas′tik dis-fō′nē-ă) SYN spasmodic dysphonia.

spas·tic gait (spas′tik gāt) SYN hemiplegic gait.

spas·tic hem·i·ple·gi·a (spas′tik hem′i-plē′jē-ă) A hemiplegia with increased tone in the antigravity muscles of the affected side.

spas·tic il·e·us (spas′tik il′ē-ŭs) SYN dynamic ileus.

spas·tic·i·ty (spas-tis′i-tē) A state of increased muscular tone with exaggeration of the tendon reflexes.

spa·tial (spā′shăl) Relating to space or a space.

spa·tial an·tic·i·pa·tion (spā′shăl ăn-tis′i-pā′shŭn) Ability to predict what will happen in the environment within a performance situation, which allows the individual to organize movements in advance and to initiate the appropriate response more quickly (e.g., anticipating that one's tennis opponent is about to hit a smash to the right).

spa·tial re·la·tion (spā′shăl rē-lā′shŭn) Position of an object in relation to another.

spa·ti·um, pl. **spa·ti·a** (spā′shē-ŭm, -shē-ă) [TA] SYN space. [L.]

spat·u·la (spach′ŭ-lă) A flat blade, like that of a knife but without a sharp edge, used in pharmacy for spreading plasters and ointments and to aid in mixing ingredients with a mortar and pestle. [L. dim. of *spatha,* a broad, flat wooden instrument, fr. G. *spathē*]

spat·u·late (spach′ŭ-lāt) **1.** Shaped like a spatula. **2.** To incise the cut end of a tubular structure longitudinally and splay it open, to allow creation of an elliptic anastomosis of greater circumference than would be possible with conventional transverse or oblique (beveled) end-to-end anastomoses.

spay (spā) To remove the ovaries of an animal. [Gael. *spoth,* castrate, or G. *spadōn,* eunuch]

SPCA Abbreviation for serum prothrombin conversion accelerator.

speak·er's no·dules (spē′kĕrz noj′yūlz) SYN vocal nodules.

speak·ing tube (spēk′ing tūb) A tube with an earpiece at one end and a cone at the other to amplify speech into the cone.

spe·cial a·nat·o·my (spesh′ăl ă-nat′ŏ-mē) The anatomy of certain definite organs or groups of organs involved in the performance of special functions; descriptive anatomy dealing with the separate systems.

spe·cial·ist (spesh′ă-list) One who devotes professional attention to a particular specialty or subject area.

spe·cial·i·za·tion (spesh′ă-lī-zā′shŭn) **1.** Professional practice limited to a particular specialty or subject area. **2.** SYN differentiation (1).

spe·cial sense (spesh′ăl sens) One of the five senses related respectively to the organs of sight, hearing, smell, taste, and touch.

spe·cial·ty (spesh′ăl-tē) In health care, the particular subject area or branch of medical science to which one devotes professional attention. [L. *specialitas* fr. *specialis,* special]

spe·cial·ty re·fer·ral cen·ter (spesh′ăl-tē rē-fĕr′ăl sen′tĕr) A designated medical facility that provides specialized medical or trauma care for a particular body system by specialty or nature of injury, e.g., hand trauma center, neonatal care center.

spe·ci·a·tion (spē′shē-ā′shŭn) The evolutionary process by which diverse species of animals or plants are formed from a common ancestral stock.

spe·cies, pl. **spe·cies** (spē′shēz) **1.** A biologic division between the genus and a variety or the individual; a group of organisms that generally bear a close resemblance to one another in the more essential features of their organization, and that breed effectively, producing fertile progeny. **2.** A class of pharmaceutical preparations consisting of a mixture of dried plants, not pulverized, but in sufficiently fine division to be conveniently used in the making of extemporaneous decoctions or infusions, as a tea. [L. appearance, form, kind, fr. *specio,* to look at]

spe·cies-spe·cif·ic (spē′shēz spĕ-sif′ik) Characteristic of a given species; serum that is produced by the injection of immunogens into an animal, and that acts only on the cells or protein, of a member of the same species as that from which the original antigen was obtained.

spe·cies-spe·cif·ic ant·i·gen (spē′shēz spĕ-sif′ik an′ti-jen) Antigenic components in tissues and fluids by means of which various species may be immunologically distinguished (e.g., serum albumin of horses is immunologically different from that of humans, dogs, or sheep).

spe·cif·ic (spĕ-sif′ik) **1.** Relating to a species. **2.** Relating to an individual infectious disease, one caused by a special microorganism. **3.** A remedy having a definite therapeutic action in relation to a particular disease or symptom, as quinine in relation to malaria. [L. *specificus* fr. species + *facio,* to make]

spe·ci·fic ab·sorp·tion co·ef·fi·cient (*a*) (spĕ-sif′ik ab-sōrp′shŭn kō′ĕ-fish′ĕnt) Absorbance (of light) per unit path length (usually the centimeter) and per unit of mass concentration. Cf. molar absorption coefficient. SYN absorbancy index (1), absorptivity (1), extinction coefficient, specific extinction.

spe•ci•fic ac•tion (spĕ-sif′ik ak′shŭn) The action of a drug or a method of treatment that has a direct and especially curative effect on a disease.

spe•ci•fic ac•ti•vi•ty (spĕ-sif′ik ak-tiv′i-tē) **1.** Radioactivity per unit mass of the stated element or compound. **2.** For an enzyme, the amount of substrate consumed (or product formed) in a given time under given conditions per milligram of protein. **3.** Activity per unit mass of the stated radionuclide.

spe•ci•fic build•ing-re•lat•ed ill•nes•ses (spĕ-sif′ik bild′ing-rē-lāt′ed il′nĕs-ĕz) A group of infectious, allergic, and immunologic diseases with fairly homogeneous clinical signs with causes that can be traced to factors in buildings in which afflicted patients work or reside. Cf. nonspecific building-related illnesses.

spe•ci•fic dy•na•mic ac•tion (SDA) (spĕ-sif′ik dī-nam′ik ak′shŭn) Increase of heat production caused by the ingestion of food, especially of protein.

spe•ci•fic ex•tinc•tion (spĕ-sif′ik eks-tingk′shŭn) SYN specific absorption coefficient.

spe•ci•fic gra•vi•ty (spĕ-sif′ik grav′i-tē) The weight of any body compared with that of another body of equal volume regarded as the unit; usually the weight of a liquid compared with that of distilled water.

spe•ci•fic im•mu•ni•ty (spĕ-sif′ik i-myū′ni-tē) The immune status in which there is an altered reactivity directed solely against the antigenic determinants (infectious agent or other) that stimulated it. SEE ALSO acquired immunity.

spec•i•fic•i•ty (spes′i-fis′i-tē) **1.** The condition or state of being specific, of having a fixed relation to a single cause or to a definite result; manifested in the relation of a disease to its pathogenic microorganism, of a reaction to a certain chemical union, or of an antibody to its antigen or the reverse. **2.** CLINICAL PATHOLOGY the proportion of those who do not have a disease or condition and in whom a test intended to identify that disease or condition yields negative results. Cf. sensitivity (2).

spe•ci•fi•ci•ty of train•ing prin•ci•ple (spes′i-fis′i-tē trān′ing prin′si-pĕl) EXERCISE SCIENCE concept that specific exercise elicits specific adaptations, creating specific training effects. The effects are most effectively induced by training the specific muscles involved in the desired performance.

spe•ci•fic op•son•in (spĕ-sif′ik op′sŏ-nin) Antibodies formed in response to stimulation by a specific antigen, either as a result of an attack of a disease or injections with a suitably prepared suspension of the specific microorganism.

spe•ci•fic op•tic ro•ta•tion (spĕ-sif′ik op′tik rō-tā′shŭn) The arc through which the plane of polarized light is rotated by 1 g of a substance per milliliter of water when the length of the light path through the solution is 1 decimeter, typically using light corresponding to the D line of sodium.

spe•ci•fic par•a•site (spĕ-sif′ik par′ă-sīt) A parasite that habitually lives in its present host and is particularly adapted for the host species.

spe•ci•fic pho•bi•a (spĕ-sif′ik fō′bē-ă) A persistent pattern of significant fear of specific objects or situations, manifesting in anxiety or panic on exposure to the object or situation or in anticipation of them, which the person realizes is unreasonable or excessive and which interferes significantly with the person's functioning. SYN simple phobia.

spe•ci•fic re•ac•tion (spĕ-sif′ik rē-ak′shŭn) The phenomena produced by an agent that is identical with or immunologically related to the one that has stimulated an immune response.

spec•i•men (spes′i-mĕn) A small part or sample of any substance or material obtained for testing. [L. fr. *specio,* to look at]

SPECT (spekt) Acronym for single photon emission computed tomography.

spec•ta•cles (spek′tă-kĕlz) Lenses set in a frame that holds them in front of the eyes, used to correct errors of refraction or to protect the eyes. The parts of the spectacles are: the lenses; the bridge between the lenses, resting on the nose; the rims or frames, encircling the lenses; the sides or temples that pass on either side of the head to the ears; the bows, the curved extremities of the temples; and the shoulders, short bars attached to the rims or the lenses and jointed with the sides. SYN eyeglasses, glasses. [L. *specto,* pp. *-atus,* to watch, observe]

spec•tra (spek′tră) Plural of spectrum. [L.]

spec•tral (spek′trăl) Relating to a spectrum.

spec•trin (spek′trin) A filamentous contractile protein that together with actin and other cytoskeleton proteins forms a network that gives the red blood cell membrane its shape and flexibility; a defect or deficiency of spectrin is associated with hereditary spherocytosis and hereditary elliptocytosis; the principal component of the membrane skeleton of red blood cells.

♻ **spectro-** Combining form indicating a spectrum. [L. *spectrum,* an image]

spec•trom•e•ter (spek-trom′ĕ-tĕr) An instrument for determining the wavelength or energy of light or other electromagnetic emissions. [spectro- + G. *metron,* measure]

spec•trom•e•try (spek-trom′ĕ-trē) The procedure of observing and measuring the wavelengths of light or other electromagnetic emissions.

spec·tro·pho·tom·e·ter (spek′trō-fō-tom′ĕ-tĕr) An instrument for measuring the intensity of light of a definite wavelength transmitted by a substance or solution, giving a quantitative measure of the amount of material in the solution absorbing the light; a colorimeter with a choice of wavelengths and photometric measurements. [spectro- + photometer]

spec·tro·pho·tom·e·try (spek′trō-fō-tom′ĕ-trē) Analysis by means of a spectrophotometer.

spec·tro·scope (spek′trŏ-skōp) An instrument for resolving light from any luminous body into its spectrum, and for the analysis of the spectrum so formed; consists of a prism that refracts the light or a grating for diffraction of the light, an arrangement for rendering the rays parallel, and a telescope that magnifies the spectrum. [spectro- + G. *skopeō,* to view]

spec·tro·scop·ic (spek′trŏ-skop′ik) Relating to or performed by means of a spectroscope.

spec·tros·co·py (spek-tros′kŏ-pē) Observation and study of spectra of absorbed or emitted light by means of a spectroscope.

spec·trum, pl. **spec·tra**, **spec·trums** (spek′trŭm, -tră, -trŭmz) **1.** The range of colors presented when white light is resolved into its constituent colors by being passed through a prism or through a diffraction grating: red, orange, yellow, green, blue, indigo, and violet, arranged in increasing frequency of vibration or decreasing wavelength. **2.** The range of pathogenic microorganisms against which an antibiotic or other antibacterial agent is active. **3.** The plot of intensity versus wavelength of light emitted or absorbed by a substance, usually characteristic of the substance and used in qualitative and quantitative analysis. **4.** The range of wavelengths presented when a beam of radiant energy is subjected to dispersion and focused. [L. an image, fr. *specio,* to look at]

spec·u·lum, pl. **spec·u·la** (spek′yŭ-lŭm, -lă) An instrument for enlarging the opening of any canal or cavity to facilitate inspection of its interior. [L. a mirror, fr. *specio,* to look at]

spec·u·lum for·ceps (spek′yŭ-lŭm fōr′seps) A tubular forceps for use through a speculum.

SPEECH1 (spēch) Gene that when mutated causes motor dyspraxia.

speech (spēch) Talk; the use of the voice to communicate. [A.S. *spaec*]

speech a·ware·ness thresh·old (spēch ă-wār′nĕs thresh′ōld) The lowest sound intensity at which speech can be detected. SYN speech detection threshold.

speech bulb (spēch bŭlb) A prosthetic speech aid; a restoration used to close a cleft or other opening in the hard or soft palate, or to replace absent tissue necessary for the production of good speech.

speech cen·ters (spēch sen′tĕrz) Areas of the cerebral cortex centrally involved in speech function; one is in the left inferior frontal gyrus, a second one in the supramarginal, angular, and first and second temporal gyri. SEE ALSO Broca center, Wernicke center.

speech de·tec·tion thresh·old (spēch dĕ-tek′shŭn thresh′ōld) SYN speech awareness threshold.

speech ed·i·tor (spēch ed′i-tŏr) Medical transcriptionist who edits speech-recognized drafts to document patient care; duties may also include transcribing dictated medical reports. SYN speech recognition medical transcription editor.

speech fre·quen·cies (spēch frē′kwĕn-sēz) Acoustic sound wave frequency range in which most speech sounds occur, generally 500–3000 Hz. SEE ALSO frequency.

speech-lan·guage pa·tho·lo·gist (spēch-lang′gwăj pă-thol′ŏ-jist) A practitioner concerned with the diagnosis and rehabilitation of patients with voice, speech, and language disorders.

speech-lan·guage pa·tho·lo·gy (spēch-lang′gwăj pă-thol′ŏ-jē) SYN speech pathology.

speech me·cha·ni·sm (spēch mek′ă-nizm) Peripheral structures involved in the normal production of speech, encompassing the organs of articulation, phonation, resonance, and respiration. SEE ALSO articulation, articulators, phonation, resonance, respiration.

speech pa·tho·lo·gy (spēch pă-thol′ŏ-jē) The science concerned with functional and organic speech defects and disorders of the organs of speech. SYN speech-language pathology.

speech per·cep·tion (spēch pĕr-sep′shŭn) Identification of speech sounds, mainly from acoustic cues.

speech pro·ces·sor (spēch pros′es-sŏr) The part of a cochlear implant that converts speech into electrical impulses that are used to stimulate the neurons of the auditory division of the eighth cranial nerve.

speech read·ing (spēch rēd′ing) Use, by people with hearing impairments, of nonauditory clues as to what is being said, acquired by observing the speaker's facial expressions, lip and jaw movements, and other gestures. SYN lip reading.

speech re·cep·tion thresh·old (spēch rĕ-sep′shŭn thresh′ōld) The intensity at which speech is recognized as meaningful symbols; in speech audiometry, it is the decibel level at which 50% of spondee words can be repeated correctly by the subject.

speech rec·og·ni·tion (spēch rek′ŏg-nish′ŭn) Software program used by some medical transcription departments to translate spoken language into a draft printed format that is then edited by medical transcriptionists to create a permanent record of patient care. SYN voice recognition.

speech re·cog·ni·tion med·i·cal tran·scrip·tion ed·i·tor (spēch rek′ŏg-nish′ŏn med′i-kăl trans-krip′shŭn ed′i-tŏr) SYN speech editor.

speed (spēd) The magnitude of velocity without regard to direction. Cf. velocity.

speed play (spēd plā) SYN fartlek training.

Speed test (spēd test) Maneuver used to determine bicipital tendinitis. An attempt to flex the supinated arm forward elicits pain and tenderness. The clinician places one hand over the bicipital groove and resists forward flexion of the arm with the other hand. A positive test result shows tenderness over the bicipital groove and muscular weakness.

spell check (spel chek) Process using software that identifies incorrectly spelled or unknown words.

spell·check·er (spel′chek-ĕr) Software that identifies incorrectly spelled or unknown words; MEDICAL TRANSCRIPTION used during referencing and proofreading to ensure accuracy of transcribed reports. SEE ALSO spell check.

Spens syn·drome (spens sin′drōm) SYN Adams-Stokes syndrome.

sperm (spĕrm) The male gamete or sex cell that contains the genetic information to be transmitted by the male, exhibits autokinesia, and is able to effect zygosis with an oocyte. The human sperm is composed of a head and a tail, the tail being divisible into a neck, a middle piece, a principal piece, and an end piece; the head, 4–6 mcm in length, is a broadly oval, flattened body containing the nucleus; the tail is about 55 mcm in length. [G. *sperma,* seed]

♻ **sperma-**, **spermato-**, **spermo-** Combining forms denoting male reproductive cells, sperms. [G. *sperma,* seed]

sper·ma·cyt·ic sem·i·no·ma (spĕrm′ă-sit′ik sem′i-nō′mă) A relatively slow-growing, locally invasive type of testicular seminoma that does not metastasize and has no ovarian counterpart.

sperm-as·ter (spĕrm′as-tĕr) Cytocentrum with astral rays in the cytoplasm of an inseminated oocyte; it is brought in by the penetrating sperm and evolves into the mitotic spindle of the first cleavage division. [sperm + G. *astēr,* a star (aster)]

sper·mat·ic (spĕr-mat′ik) Relating to the sperm or semen.

sper·ma·tic cord (spĕr-mat′ik kōrd) The cord formed by the ductus deferens and its associated structures extending from the deep inguinal ring through the inguinal canal into the scrotum. SYN funiculus spermaticus [TA], testis cords.

sper·ma·tic duct (spĕr-mat′ik dŭkt) SYN ductus deferens.

sper·ma·tid (spĕr′mă-tid) A cell in a late stage of the development of the sperm; it is a haploid cell derived from the secondary spermatocyte and evolves by spermiogenesis into a sperm. [spermat- + *-id* (2)]

sper·ma·to·blast (spĕr′mă-tō-blast) SYN spermatogonium. [spermato- + G. *blastos,* germ]

sper·ma·to·cele (spĕr′mă-tō-sēl) Cyst of the epididymis containing sperm. [spermato- + G. *kēlē,* tumor]

sper·ma·to·cide (spĕr′mă-tō-sīd) SYN spermicide. [spermato- + L. *caedo,* to kill]

sper·ma·to·cy·tal (spĕr′mă-tō-sī′tăl) Relating to a spermatocyte.

sper·ma·to·cyte (spĕr-mat′ō-sīt) Parent cell of a spermatid, derived by mitotic division from a spermatogonium. [spermato- + G. *kytos,* cell]

sper·ma·to·cy·to·gen·e·sis (spĕr′mă-tō-sī′tō-jen′ĕ-sis) SYN spermatogenesis.

sper·ma·to·gen·e·sis (spĕr′mă-tō-jen′ĕ-sis) The entire process by which spermatogonial stem cells divide and differentiate into spermatozoa. SEE ALSO spermiogenesis. SYN spermatocytogenesis. [spermato- + G. *genesis,* origin]

sper·ma·to·gen·ic (spĕr′mă-tō-jen′ik) Relating to spermatogenesis; sperm-producing. SYN spermatopoietic (1).

sper·ma·to·go·ni·um (spĕr′mă-tō-gō′nē-ŭm) The undifferentiated male sex cell derived by mitotic division from a primordial germ cell; increasing several times in size, it becomes a primary spermatocyte. SEE ALSO spermatid. SYN spermatoblast. [spermato- + G. *gonē,* generation]

sper·ma·toid (spĕr′mă-toyd) **1.** Resembling a sperm, a sperm tail, or semen. **2.** A male or flagellated form of the malarial microparasite. [spermato + G. *eidos*, form]

sper·ma·tol·y·sis (spĕrm′ă-tol′i-sis) Destruction, with dissolution, of sperms. [spermato- + G. *lysis,* dissolution]

sper·ma·to·lyt·ic (spĕr′mă-tō-lit′ik) Relating to spermatolysis.

sper·ma·to·poi·et·ic (spĕr′mă-tō-poy-et′ik) **1.** SYN spermatogenic. **2.** Secreting semen. [spermato- + G. *poieō,* to make]

sper·ma·tor·rhe·a (spĕr′mă-tōr-ē′ă) An involuntary discharge of semen, without orgasm. SYN spermatorrhoea. [spermato- + G. *rhoia,* a flow]

spermatorrhoea [Br.] SYN spermatorrhea.

sper•ma•to•zo•al, **sper•ma•to•zo•an** (spĕr′mă-tō-zō′ăl, -zō′ăn) Relating to spermatozoa or sperms.

sper•ma•tu•ri•a (spĕr′mă-tyūr′ē-ă) SYN semenuria.

sper•mi•a (spĕr′mē-ă) Plural of spermium.

sper•mi•ci•dal (spĕr′mi-sī′dăl) Destructive to sperms.

sper•mi•cide (spĕr′mi-sīd) An agent destructive to sperms. SYN spermatocide.

sper•mi•duct (spĕr′mi-dŭkt) **1.** SYN ductus deferens. **2.** SYN ejaculatory duct.

sper•mi•o•gen•e•sis (spĕr′mē-ō-jen′ĕ-sis) That segment of spermatogenesis during which immature spermatids are transformed into elongated sperms. [sperm- + G. *genesis,* origin]

sper•mi•um, pl. **sper•mi•a** (spĕr′mē-ŭm, -ă) The mature male germ cell or sperm.

sper•mo•lith (spĕr′mō-lith) A concretion in the ductus deferens. [spermo- + G. *lithos,* stone]

Sper•moph•il•us (sper-mof′il-us) A genus of ground squirrel; *S. beecheyi*, *S. grammurus*, *S. pygmaeus*, *S. townsendi*, and several other species act as an important reservoir of *Yersinia pestis*.

sperm track (spĕrm trak) The path taken by a sperm through the zona pellucida surrounding an oocyte during fertilization.

SPF Abbreviation for sun protection factor.

sp. gr. Abbreviation for specific gravity.

sphac•e•late (sfas′ĕ-lāt) To become gangrenous or necrotic. [G. *sphakelos,* gangrene]

sphac•e•la•tion (sfas′ĕ-lā′shŭn) **1.** The process of becoming gangrenous or necrotic. **2.** Gangrene or necrosis. [G. *sphakelos,* gangrene]

sphac•el•ism (sfas′ĕ-lizm) The condition manifested by a sphacelus.

sphac•e•lo•der•ma (sfas′ē-lō-dĕr′mă) Gangrene of the skin. [G. *sphakelos,* gangrene, + *derma,* skin]

sphac•e•lous (sfas′ĕ-lŭs) Sloughing, gangrenous, or necrotic.

sphac•e•lus (sfas′ĕ-lŭs) A mass of sloughing, gangrenous, or necrotic matter. [G. *sphakelos,* gangrene]

Sphae•rot•i•lus (sfē-rot′i-lŭs) A genus of bacteria closely related to *Leptothrix* and found in fresh water; *S. natans* grows a thick biofilm mat in sulfite-containing water, especially that drained from paper mills.

sphe•ni•on (sfē′nē-on) The tip of the sphenoidal angle of the parietal bone; a craniometric point. [Mod. L. fr. G. *sphēn,* wedge, + dim. *-iōn*]

♻**spheno-** Combining form denoting wedge, wedge-shaped; the sphenoid bone. [G. *sphēn,* wedge]

sphe•no•bas•i•lar (sfē′nō-bas′i-lăr) Relation to the sphenoid bone and the basilar process of the occipital bone. SYN sphenooccipital.

sphe•no•ceph•a•ly (sfē′nō-sef′ă-lē) Condition characterized by a deformation of the cranium into a wedge-shaped appearance. [spheno- + G. *kephalē,* head]

sphen•o•eth•moi•dec•to•my (sfē′nō-eth′moyd-ek′tŏ-mē) An operation to remove diseased tissue from the sphenoid and ethmoid sinuses.

sphe•noid (sfē′noyd) **1.** SYN sphenoidal. **2.** SYN sphenoid bone. [G. *sphēnoeidēs,* fr. *sphēn,* wedge, + *eidos,* resemblance]

sphe•noi•dal (sfē-noy′dăl) **1.** Relating to the sphenoid bone. **2.** Wedge-shaped. SYN sphenoid (1).

sphe•noi•dal an•gle of pa•ri•e•tal bone (sfē-noyd′ăl ang′gĕl păr-ī′ĕ-tăl bōn) The anterior inferior angle of the parietal bone.

sphe•noi•dal con•chae (sfē-noy′dăl kong′kē) Paired ossicles of pyramidal shape, the spines of which are in contact with the medial pterygoid lamina, the bases forming the roof of the nasal cavity.

sphe•noi•dal si•nus (sfē noy′dăl sī′nŭs) Onc of a pair of paranasal areas in the body of the sphenoid bone communicating with the upper posterior nasal cavity or sphenoethmoidal recess.

sphe•noi•dal spine (sfē-noy′dăl spīn) A posterior and downward projection from the greater wing of the sphenoid bone on either side, located posterolateral to the foramen spinosum, which is so named for its proximity to the sphenoidal spine; gives attachment to the sphenomandibular ligament. SYN alar spine, angular spine, spinous process (2).

sphe•noid bone (sfē′noyd bōn) A bone of irregular shape occupying the base of the skull; it is described as consisting of a central portion, or body, and six processes: two greater wings, two lesser wings, and two pterygoid processes; it articulates with the occipital, frontal, ethmoid, and vomer, and with the paired temporal, parietal, zygomatic, palatine, and sphenoidal concha bones. SYN sphenoid (2).

sphe•noid crest (sfē′noyd krest) A vertical ridge in the midline of the anterior surface of the sphenoid bone that articulates with the perpendicular plate of the ethmoid bone.

sphe•noid•i•tis (sfē′noy-dī′tis) **1.** Inflammation of the sphenoid sinus. **2.** Necrosis of the sphenoid bone. [sphenoid + G. *-itis,* inflammation]

sphe•noi•dot•o•my (sfē′noy-dot′ō-mē) Any operation on the sphenoid bone or sinus. [sphenoid + G. *tomē,* a cutting]

sphe•no•oc•cip•i•tal (sfē′nō-ok-sip′i-tăl) SYN sphenobasilar.

sphe•no•pal•a•tine ar•ter•y (sfēn′ō-pal′ă-tīn ahr′tĕr-ē) *Origin,* third part of maxillary; *distribution,* posterior portion of lateral nasal wall and septum; *anastomoses,* branches of descending palatine, superior labial, and infraorbital. SYN arteria sphenopalatina [TA].

sphe•no•pal•a•tine fo•ra•men (sfēn′ō-pal′ă-tīn fōr-ā′mĕn) The foramen formed from the sphenopalatine notch of the palatine bone in articulation with the sphenoid bone; it transmits the sphenopalatine artery and accompanying nerves. SYN foramen sphenopalatinum [TA].

sphe•no•pal•a•tine neu•ral•gi•a (sfēn′ō-pal′ă-tīn nūr-al′jē-ă) Pain related to the nervous system in the lower half of the face, with pain referred to the root of the nose, upper teeth, eyes, ears, mastoid, and occiput, in association with nasal congestion and rhinorrhea occurring in infection of the nasal sinuses, and produced by lesions of the sphenopalatine ganglion; ocular hyperemia and excessive lacrimation may occur. SYN Sluder neuralgia.

sphe•no•pa•ri•e•tal si•nus (sfē′nō-păr-ī′ĕ-tăl sī′nŭs) A paired dural venous sinus beginning on the parietal bone, running along the sphenoidal ridges, and emptying into the cavernous sinus.

sphe•nor•bit•al (sfē-nōr′bi-tăl) Denoting portions of the sphenoid bone contributing to the orbits.

sphe•not•ic (sfē-not′ik) Relating to the sphenoid bone and the bony case of the ear. [spheno- + G. *ous,* ear]

sphere (sfēr) A ball or globular body. [G. *sphaira*]

spher•ic ab•er•ra•tion (sfēr′ik ab′ĕr-ā′shŭn) A monochromatic aberration occurring in refraction at a spheric surface in which the paraxial and peripheral rays focus along the axis at different points. SYN dioptric aberration.

spher•ic lens (S) (sfēr′ik lenz) A lens in which all refracting surfaces are spheric; commonly used to correct refractive errors not compounded by astigmatism.

♻ **sphero-** Combining form denoting spheric, a sphere. [G. *sphaira,* globe]

sphe•ro•cyte (sfēr′ō-sīt) A small, spheric red blood cell. [sphero- + G. *kytos,* cell]

spher•o•cy•tic a•ne•mi•a (sfēr′ō-sit′ik ă-nē′mē-ă) SYN hereditary spherocytosis.

sphe•ro•cy•to•sis (sfēr′ō-sī-tō′sis) Presence of spherelike red blood cells in the blood. [spherocyte + G. *-osis,* condition]

sphe•roid, **sphe•roi•dal** (sfēr′oyd, sfēr-oyd′ăl) Shaped like a sphere. [L. *spheroideus*]

spher•oid joint (sfēr′oyd joynt) SYN ball-and-socket joint.

sphe•ro•pha•ki•a (sfēr′ō-fā′kē-ă) A congenital bilateral aberration in which the lenses are small, spheric, and subject to subluxation; may occur as an independent anomaly or may be associated with the Weill-Marchesani syndrome. [sphero- + G. *phakos,* lens]

sphe•rule (sfēr′yūl) A thick-walled, nonbudding structure recognized as the tissue form of *Coccidioides immitis;* variable in size, it may contain endospores or granular material. When the spherule ruptures, it releases endospores into the surrounding tissues.

sphinc•ter (sfingk′tĕr) A muscle that encircles a duct, tube, or orifice in such a way that its contraction constricts the lumen or orifice; it is the closing component of a pylorus (the outer component is the musculus dilator). SYN sphincter muscle. [G. *sphinktēr,* a band or lace]

sphinc•ter•al (sfingk′tĕr-ăl) Relating to a sphincter.

sphinc•ter•al•gi•a (sfingk′tĕr-al′jē-ă) Pain in the sphincter ani muscles. [sphincter + G. *algos,* pain]

sphinc•ter of com•mon bile duct (sfingk′tĕr kom′ŏn bīl dŭkt) Smooth muscle sphincter of the common bile duct immediately proximal to the hepatopancreatic ampulla; it is this sphincter that controls the flow of bile into the duodenum. SYN musculus sphincter ductus choledochi [TA].

sphinc•ter•ec•to•my (sfingk′tĕr-ek′tŏ-mē) **1.** Excision of a portion of the pupillary border of the iris. **2.** Dissecting away any sphincter muscle. [sphincter + G. *ektomē,* excision]

sphinc•ter of hep•a•to•pan•cre•at•ic am•pul•la (sfingk′tĕr hep′ă-tō-pan′krē-at′ik am-pul′ă) The smooth muscle sphincter of the hepatopancreatic ampulla within the duodenal papilla.

sphinc•ter•is•mus (sfingk′tĕr-iz′mŭs) Spasmodic contraction of the sphincter ani muscles.

sphinc•ter•i•tis (sfingk′tĕr-ī′tis) Inflammation of any sphincter.

sphinc•ter mus•cle (sfingk′tĕr mŭs′ĕl) SYN sphincter.

sphinc•ter mus•cle of pu•pil (sfingk′tĕr mŭs′ĕl pyū′pil) SYN sphincter pupillae.

sphinct•er mus•cle of u•re•thra (sfingk′tĕr mŭs′ĕl yūr-ē′thră) SYN external urethral sphincter muscle.

sphinc•ter of Od•di (sfingk′tĕr od′ē) A valvelike muscular sheath surrounding the distal pancreatic and common bile ducts as they enter the duodenum together.

sphinc•ter of Od•di dys•func•tion (sfingk′tĕr od′ē dis-fŭngk′shŭn) Structural or functional abnormality of the sphincter of Oddi that interferes with bile drainage.

sphinc•ter•ol•y•sis (sfingk-tĕr-ol′i-sis) An operation to free the iris from the cornea in anterior synechia involving only the pupillary border. [sphincter, + G. *lysis,* loosening]

sphinc•ter•o•plas•ty (sfingk′tĕr-ō-plas-tē) Plastic surgery of any sphincter muscle. [sphincter + G. *plastos,* formed]

sphinc•ter•ot•o•my (sfingk′tĕr-ot′ŏ-mē) Incision or division of a sphincter muscle. [sphincter + G. *tomē,* incision]

sphinc•ter of pan•cre•at•ic duct (sfingk′tĕr pan′krē-at′ik dŭkt) Smooth muscle sphincter of the main pancreatic duct immediately proximal to the hepatoduodenal ampulla. SYN musculus sphincter ductus pancreatici [TA].

sphinc•ter pu•pil•lae (sfingk′tĕr pyū-pil′ē) A ring of smooth muscle fibers surrounding the pupillary border of the iris. SYN musculus sphincter pupillae [TA], sphincter muscle of pupil.

sphinc•ter u•re•thrae (sfingk′tĕr yū-rēth′rē) *Origin*, ramus of pubis; *insertion*, with fellow in median raphe behind and in front of urethra; *action*, constricts membranous urethra; *nerve supply*, pudendal. SYN musculus sphincter urethrae [TA].

sphinc•ter u•re•thrae ex•tern•us (sfingk′tĕr yū-rēth′rē eks-ter′nus) SYN external urethral sphincter muscle.

sphinc•ter vag•i•nae (sfink′tĕr vaj′i-nē) SYN bulbospongiosus muscle.

sphinc•ter ve•si•cae (sfingk′tĕr ves′i-kē) The complete collar of smooth muscle cells of the neck of the urinary bladder that extends distally to surround the preprostatic portion of the male urethra. There is no comparable structure in the neck of the female bladder; the internal urethral sphincter may exist to prevent reflux of semen into the bladder. SYN musculus sphincter vesicae [TA].

sphin•go•lip•id (sfing′gō-lip′id) Any lipid containing a long-chain base like that of sphingosine (e.g., ceramides, cerebrosides, gangliosides, sphingomyelins); a constituent of nerve tissue.

sphin•go•lip•i•do•sis, **sphin•go•lip•o•dys•tro•phy** (sfing′gō-lip′i-dō′sis, sfing′gō-lip′ō-dis′trŏ-fē) Collective designation for a variety of diseases characterized by abnormal sphingolipid metabolism, e.g., gangliosidosis, Gaucher disease, Niemann-Pick disease.

sphin•go•my•e•lin phos•pho•di•es•ter•ase (sfing′gō-mī′ĕ-lin fos′fō-dī-es′tĕr-ās) An enzyme catalyzing hydrolysis of sphingomyelin to *N*-acylsphingosine (a ceramide) and phosphocholine; a deficiency of this enzyme is associated with type I Niemann-Pick disease.

sphin•go•my•e•lins (sfing′gō-mī′ĕ-linz) A group of phospholipids, found in brain, spinal cord, kidney, and egg yolk, containing 1-phosphocholine (choline *O*-phosphate) combined with a ceramide.

sphin•go•sine (sfing′gō-sēn) The principal long-chain base found in sphingolipids.

sphyg•mic (sfig′mik) Relating to the pulse.

sphyg•mic in•ter•val (sfig′mik in′tĕr-văl) The period in the cardiac cycle when the semilunar valves are open and blood is being ejected from the ventricles into the arterial system. SYN ejection period.

♻ **sphygmo-**, **sphygm-** Combining forms denoting pulse. [G. *sphygmos*]

sphyg•mo•chron•o•graph (sfig′mō-kron′ō-graf) A modified sphygmograph that represents graphically the time relations between the beat of the heart and the pulse; one recording the character of the pulse as well as its rapidity. [sphygmo- + G. *chronos,* time, + *graphō,* to write]

sphyg•mo•gram (sfig′mō-gram) The graphic curve made by a sphygmograph. [sphygmo- + G. *gramma,* something written]

sphyg•mo•graph (sfig′mō-graf) An instrument consisting of a lever, the short end of which rests on the radial artery at the wrist, its long end being provided with a stylet, which records on a moving ribbon of paper the excursions of the pulse. [sphygmo- + G. *graphō,* to write]

sphyg•mo•graph•ic (sfig′mō-graf′ik) Relating to or made by a sphygmograph; denoting the sphygmographic tracing, or sphygmogram.

sphyg•moid (sfig′moyd) Pulselike; resembling the pulse. [sphygmo- + G. *eidos,* resemblance]

i **sphyg•mo•ma•nom•e•ter** (sfig′mō-mă-nom′ĕ-tĕr) An instrument for measuring arterial blood pressure indirectly, consisting of an inflatable cuff, inflating bulb, and a gauge showing the blood pressure. See page 1456. SYN sphygmometer. [sphygmo- + G. *manos,* thin, scanty, + *metron,* measure]

sphyg•mo•ma•nom•e•try (sfig′mō-mă-nom′ĕ-trē) Determination of the blood pressure by means of a sphygmomanometer.

sphyg•mom•e•ter (sfig-mom′ĕ-tĕr) SYN sphygmomanometer.

sphyg•mo•scope (sfig′mō-skōp) An instrument by which the pulse beats are made visible by causing fluid to rise in a glass tube, by means of a mirror projecting a beam of light, or simply by a moving lever, as in the sphygmograph. [sphygmo- + G. *skopeō,* to view]

sphyg•mos•co•py (sfig-mos′kŏ-pē) Examination of the pulse. [sphygmo- + G. *skopeō,* to view]

spi·ca ban·dage (spī′kă ban′dăj) Successive strips of material applied to the body and the first part of a limb, or to the hand and a finger, which overlap slightly in a V to resemble an ear of grain. [L. *spica,* ear of grain]

spi·ca cast (spī′kă kast) Successive strips of material applied to the body and the first part of a limb, or to the hand and a finger, which overlap slightly in a V to resemble an ear of grain.

spic·u·lar (spik′yū-lăr) Relating to or having spicules.

spic·ule (spik′yūl) A small, needle-shaped body. [L. *spiculum,* dim. of *spica,* or *spicum,* a point]

spi·der (spī′dĕr) **1.** An arthropod of the order Araneida characterized by having four pairs of legs; a cephalothorax; a globose, smooth abdomen; and a complex of spinnerets, which build the web. Among the venomous spiders are the black widow spider, *Latrodectus mactans*, and the brown recluse spider, *Loxosceles reclusus*. **2.** SYN spider angioma. [O. E. *spinnan,* to spin]

spi·der an·gi·o·ma (spī′dĕr an′jē-ō′mă) A telangiectatic arteriole in the skin with radiating capillary branches simulating the legs of a spider; characteristic, but not pathognomonic, of parenchymatous liver disease; also seen in pregnancy, often disappearing after delivery, and at times in normal persons. See page B13. SYN arterial spider, spider nevus, spider telangiectasia, spider (2), vascular spider.

spi·der-burst (spī′dĕr-bŭrst) Radiating dull red capillary lines on the skin of the leg, usually without any visible or palpable varicose veins, but nevertheless due to deep-seated venous dilation; sometimes referred to as skyrocket capillary ectasis. [*spider*web + sun*burst*]

spi·der ne·vus (spī′dĕr nē′vŭs) SYN spider angioma.

spi·der tel·an·gi·ec·ta·si·a (spī′dĕr tel-an′jē-ek-tā′zē-ă) SYN spider angioma.

Spie·gel·berg cri·te·ri·a (spē′gel-berg krī-tēr′

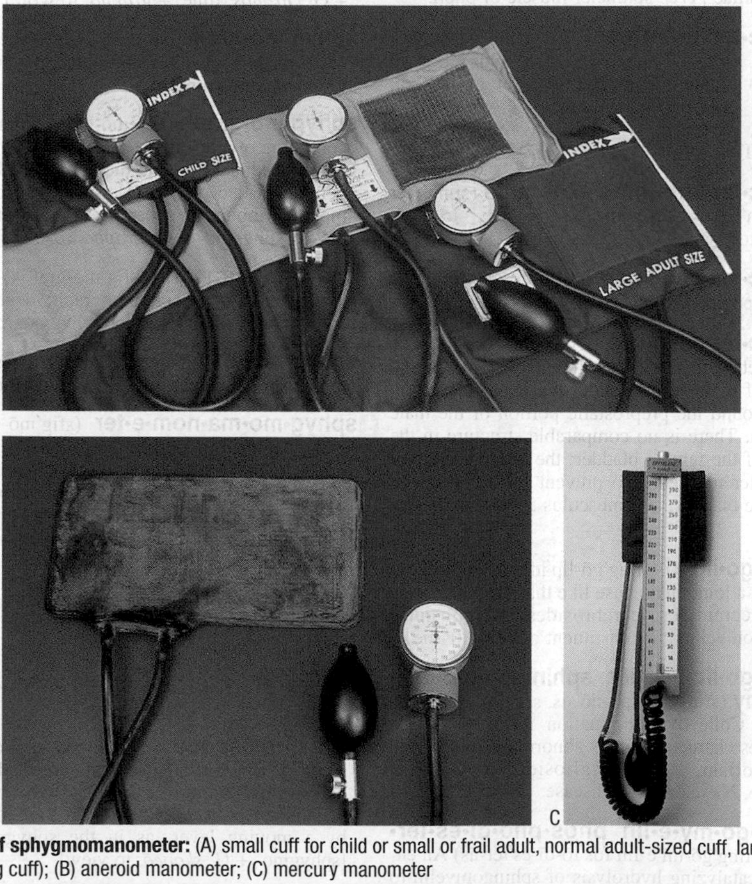

A B C

parts of sphygmomanometer: (A) small cuff for child or small or frail adult, normal adult-sized cuff, large cuff (leg cuff); (B) aneroid manometer; (C) mercury manometer

ē-ă) Used in the diagnosis of ovarian pregnancy: 1) the oviduct on the affected side must be intact; 2) the amnionic sac must occupy the position of the ovary; 3) the amnionic sac must be connected to the uterus by the ovarian ligament; and 4) ovarian tissue must be present in the wall of the amnionic sac.

Spiel•mey•er a•cute swel•ling (shpēl′mī-ĕr ă-kyūt′ swel′ing) A form of degeneration of nerve cells in which the cell body and its processes swell and stain palely and diffusely.

Spi•gel•i•us line (spi-jel′ē-us līn) SYN linea semilunaris.

Spi•ge•li•us lobe (spi-jel′ē-us lōb) SYN posterior hepatic segment I.

spike (spīk) **1.** A brief electrical event of 3–25 milliseconds that gives the appearance in the electroencephalogram of a rising and falling vertical line. **2.** ELECTROPHORESIS a sharply angled upward deflection on a densitometric tracing.

spike-and-wave com•plex (spīk wāv kom′pleks) A generalized, synchronous pattern seen on an electroencephalogram, consisting of a sharply contoured fast wave followed by a slow wave; particularly found in patients with generalized epilepsies.

spike po•ten•tial (spīk pŏ-ten′shăl) The main wave in the action potential of a nerve; it is followed by negative and positive afterpotentials.

spi•na, gen. and pl. **spi•nae** (spī′nă, -nē) SYN vertebral column. [L. a thorn, the backbone, spine]

spi•na bi•fi•da (spī′nă bif′i-dă) Embryologic failure of fusion of one or more neural arches that will become vertebral arches; subtypes of spina bifida are based on degree and pattern of deformity associated with neuroectoderm involvement. See this page.

spi•na bi•fi•da cys•ti•ca (spī′nă bif′i-dă sis′tik-ă) The condition associated with a meningeal cyst (meningocele) or a cyst containing both meninges and spinal cord (meningomyelocele), or only spinal cord (myelocele).

spi•na bi•fi•da oc•cul•ta (spī′nă bif′i-dă ō-kŭl′tă) Spina bifida in which there is a vertebral arch defect but no protrusion of the cord or its meninges, although there is often some abnormality in their development.

spi•nal (spī′năl) **1.** Relating to any spine or spinous process. **2.** Relating to the vertebral column. SYN rachial, rachidial. [L. *spinalis*]

spi•nal ad•just•ment (spī′năl ă-jŭst′mĕnt) Manual method of specific osseous movement of the vertebrae using controlled force, direction, leverage, amplitude, and velocity; typically performed by a chiropractor. SYN adjustment (1).

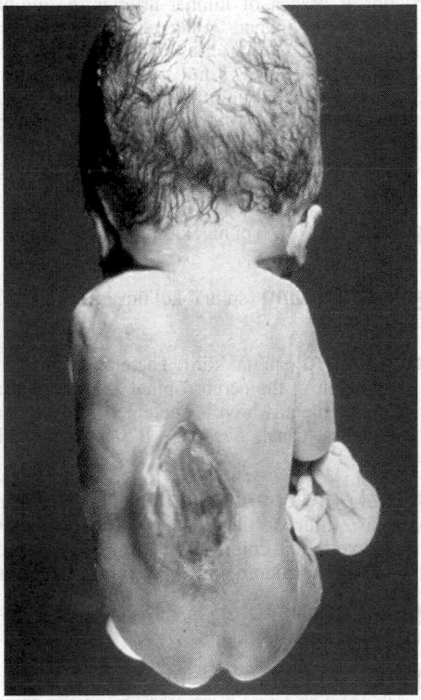

spina bifida with meningomyelocele: the deformity is evident at birth as an elliptic cutaneous defect over the lumbar spine

spi•nal an•al•ge•si•a (spī′năl an′ăl-jē′zē-ă) SEE spinal anesthesia.

spi•nal an•es•the•si•a (spī′năl an′es-thē′zē-ă) **1.** Loss of sensation produced by injection of local anesthetic solution(s) into the spinal subarachnoid space. **2.** Loss of sensation produced by disease of the spinal cord.

spi•nal a•rach•noid ma•ter (spī′năl a-rak′noyd mā′tĕr) That portion of the arachnoid that lies within the vertebral canal and surrounds the spinal cord and the vertebral portion of the subarachnoid space. It extends from the foramen magnum above to the S2 vertebral level. Given that the spinal cord ends at the L2 vertebral level, a wide separation occurs between the arachnoid and pia mater, the lumbar cistern, filled with cerebrospinal fluid in which the cauda equina is suspended.

spi•nal block (spī′năl blok) An obstruction to the flow of cerebrospinal fluid in the spinal subarachnoid space. USAGE NOTE Term sometimes used inaccurately to refer to spinal anesthesia.

spi•nal branch•es (spī′năl branch′ĕz) Branches of the following arteries that supply the meninges, the roots of the spinal nerves, and in some cases the spinal cord: 1) vertebral, 2) ascending cervical, 3) dorsal branch of posterior intercostal I to XI, 4) dorsal branch of subcostal,

5) dorsal branch of lumbar arteries, 6) lumbar branch of iliolumbar, 7) lateral sacral; all spinal arteries give rise to arteries supplying dorsal and ventral roots of spinal nerves; most are exhausted in supplying the roots as radicular arteries, but some (4–9) are large enough to reach and anastomose with the anterior and posterior spinal arteries and are designated instead as segmental medullary arteries.

spi•nal ca•nal (spī′năl kă-nal′) SYN vertebral canal.

spi•nal col•umn (spī′năl kol′ŭm) SYN vertebral column.

spi•nal cord (spī′năl kōrd) The elongated cylindric portion of the cerebrospinal axis, or central nervous system, which is contained in the spinal or vertebral canal. See page B20. SYN medulla spinalis.

spi•nal cord con•cus•sion (spī′năl kōrd kŏn-kŭsh′ŭn) Injury to the spinal cord due to a blow to the vertebral column with transient or prolonged dysfunction below the level of the lesion.

spi•nal cur•va•ture (spī′năl kŭr′vă-chŭr) SEE kyphosis, lordosis, scoliosis.

spi•nal de•com•pres•sion (spī′năl dē-kŏm-presh′ŭn) The removal of pressure on the spinal cord as created by a tumor, cyst, hematoma, herniated nucleus pulposus, abscess, or bone.

spi•nal dys•ra•phism (spī′năl dis-rāf′izm) A general term used to describe a collection of congenital abnormalities that include defects in the vertebrae and underlying spine or nerve roots.

spi•nal fu•sion, spine fu•sion (spī′năl fyū′zhŭn, spīn) A surgical procedure to accomplish bony ankylosis between two or more vertebrae. SYN spondylosyndesis.

spi•nal gan•gli•on (spī′năl gang′glē-ŏn) The ganglion of the posterior root of each spinal segmental nerve; contains the cell bodies of the pseudounipolar primary sensory neurons with peripheral axonal branches that become part of the mixed segmental nerve, while the central axonal branches enter the spinal cord as a component of the sensory posterior root.

spi•nal head•ache (spī′năl hed′āk) Headache pain, usually frontal or occipital, following dural puncture; precipitated by sitting up, relieved by lying down; due to leakage of cerebrospinal fluid from subarachnoid space through the site of the puncture. SYN post-lumbar puncture syndrome.

spi•nal in•sta•bil•i•ty (spī′năl in′stă-bil′i-tē) The inability of the spinal column, under physiologic loads, to maintain its normal configuration; may result in damage to the spinal cord or nerve roots or lead to the development of a painful spinal deformity.

spi•nal•is ca•pi•tis mus•cle (spī-nā′lis kap′i-tis mŭs′ĕl) An inconstant extension of spinalis cervicis to the occipital bone, sometimes fusing with semispinalis capitis. SYN musculus spinalis capitis [TA].

spi•nal•is cer•vi•cis mus•cle (spī-nā′lis sĕr′vi-sis mŭs′ĕl) An inconstant or rudimentary muscle; *origin*, spinous processes of sixth and seventh cervical vertebrae; *insertion*, spinous processes of axis and third cervical vertebra; *action*, extends cervical spine; *nerve supply*, dorsal primary rami of cervical. SYN musculus spinalis cervicis [TA], spinal muscle of neck.

spi•nal•is tho•ra•cis mus•cle (spī-nā′lis thō-rā′sis mŭs′ĕl) *Origin*, spinous processes of upper lumbar and two lower thoracic vertebrae; *insertion*, spinous processes of middle and upper thoracic vertebrae; *action*, supports and extends vertebral column; *nerve supply*, dorsal primary rami of thoracic and upper lumbar. SYN musculus spinalis thoracis [TA].

spi•nal ma•nip•u•la•tion (spī′năl mă-nip′yū-lā′shŭn) Manual method of osseous movement using high-velocity techniques that take the joint beyond the passive-range end barrier (without exceeding the anatomic limit) to what is known as the paraphysiologic space. SYN spinal manipulative therapy.

spi•nal ma•nip•u•la•tive ther•a•py (spī′năl mă-nip′yū-lă-tiv thār′ă-pē) SYN spinal manipulation.

spi•nal mo•tion seg•ment (spī′năl mo′shŭn seg′mĕnt) A functional unit composed of two adjacent articulating vertebrae and the connecting tissues binding them.

spi•nal mus•cle of neck (spī′năl mŭs′ĕl nek) SYN spinalis cervicis muscle.

spi•nal mus•cu•lar a•tro•phy (SMA) (spī′năl mŭs′kyū-lăr at′rŏ-fē) A heterogeneous group of degenerative diseases of the anterior horn cells in the spinal cord and motor nuclei of the brainstem; all are characterized by weakness. Upper motor neurons remain normal. These diseases include Werdnig-Hoffmann disease (SMA type 1), SMA type 2, and Kugelberg-Welander disease (SMA type 3). SEE ALSO Fazio-Londe disease.

spi•nal mus•cu•lar a•tro•phy, type I (spī′năl mŭs′kyū-lăr at′rŏ-fē tīp) The early infantile form, characterized by profound muscle weakness and wasting with onset at or shortly after birth; death occurs usually before 2 years of age. Autosomal recessive inheritance, caused by mutation in the survival motor neuron gene (SMN1) on 5q. About one half of patients are also missing both homologues of a neighboring gene that encodes neuronal apoptosis inhibitory protein (NAIP), the loss of which is thought to influence the severity of the disease. SYN Hoffmann muscular atrophy.

spi•nal mus•cu•lar a•trophy, type II (spī′

năl mŭs′kyū-lăr at′rŏ-fē tīp) A form intermediate in severity between the infantile form (SMA type I) and the juvenile form (SMA type III); characterized by proximal muscle weakness with onset usually between 3–15 months and survival until adolescence; autosomal recessive inheritance, caused by mutation in the SMN1 gene on 5q.

spi•nal mus•cu•lar a•tro•phy, type III (spī′năl mŭs′kyū-lăr at′rŏ-fē tīp) The juvenile form with onset in childhood or adolescence, characterized by progressive proximal muscular weakness and wasting, primarily in the legs, followed by distal muscle involvement, caused by degeneration of motor neurons in the anterior horns of the spinal cord; autosomal recessive inheritance, caused by mutation in the SMN1 gene on 5q.

spi•nal nerves (spī′năl nĕrvz) The nerves emerging from the spinal cord; there are 31 pairs, each attached to the cord by two roots, anterior and posterior, or ventral and dorsal; the latter is provided with a circumscribed enlargement, the dorsal root (spinal) ganglion; the two roots unite in the intervertebral foramen, and the mixed spinal nerve almost immediately divides again into ventral and dorsal primary rami, the former supplying the anterolateral trunk and the limbs, the latter the true muscles and overlying skin of the back. See page A21. SYN nervi spinales [TA].

spi•nal pa•ral•y•sis (spī′năl păr-al′i-sis) Loss of motor power due to a lesion of the spinal cord.

spi•nal pi•a ma•ter (spī′năl pī′ă mā′tĕr) The pia mater found specifically around the spinal cord; includes specializations such as the denticulate ligaments. SEE ALSO pia mater.

spi•nal re•flex (spī′năl rē′fleks) A reflex arc involving the spinal cord. SEE ALSO reflex arc.

spi•nal ste•no•sis (spī′năl stĕ-nō′sis) Abnormal narrowing of the spinal canal, often with compression of the spinal cord.

spi•nal tap (spī′năl tap) SYN lumbar puncture.

spi•nal veins (spī′năl vānz) The veins that drain the spinal cord; they form a plexus on the surface of the cord from which veins pass along the spinal roots to the internal vertebral venous plexus.

spi•nate (spī′nāt) Spined; having spines.

spin den•si•ty (spin den′si-tē) The number of nuclear dipoles per unit volume.

spin•dle (spin′dĕl) ANATOMY, PATHOLOGY any fusiform cell or structure. [A.S.]

spin•dle cell (spin′dĕl sel) A fusiform cell, such as those in the deeper layers of the cerebral cortex.

spin•dle cell car•ci•no•ma (spin′dĕl sel kahr′si-nō′mă) A carcinoma composed of elongated cells, frequently a poorly differentiated squamous cell carcinoma that may be difficult to distinguish from a sarcoma.

spin•dle cell li•po•ma (spin′dĕl sel li-pō′mă) A microscopically distinctive form of lipoma in which adipose tissue is infiltrated by fibroblasts and collagen; usually found in the shoulder or neck of elderly men.

spine (spīn) **1.** A short, sharp, thornlike process of bone; a spinous process. **2.** SYN vertebral column. **3.** The bar or stay in a horse's hoof. [L. *spina*]

spin ech•o (spin ek′ō) A commonly used technique to recover T^2 relaxation signals in magnetic resonance imaging, by using a 180° inverting pulse in the pulse sequence to compensate for loss of transverse magnetization caused by magnetic field inhomogeneities.

spine of scap•u•la (spīn skap′yū-lă) The prominent triangular ridge on the dorsal aspect of the scapula, providing attachment for the trapezius and deltoid muscles and separating the supraspinous and infraspinous fossae.

spinn•bar•keit (spin′bahr-kīt) The property of cervical mucus that permits it to be drawn out in strings; indicative of estrogenic effect, and most pronounced during the ovulatory period. [Ger. *Spinnbarkeit,* viscosity, ability to form a thread]

spino-, spin- **1.** Combining forms meaning the spine. **2.** Spinous. [L. *spina*]

spi•no•ad•duc•tor re•flex (spī′nō-ad-dŭk′tŏr rē′fleks) Contraction of the adductors of the thigh on tapping of the spinal column. SYN McCarthy reflexes.

spi•no•bul•bar (spī′nō-bŭl′bahr) SYN bulbospinal.

spi•no•ce•re•bel•lar a•tax•i•a (spī′nō-ser′ĕ-bĕl′lăr ă-tak′sē-ă) The most common hereditary ataxia, with onset in middle to late childhood, manifested as limb ataxia, nystagmus, kyphoscoliosis, and pes cavus; the major pathologic changes are found in the posterior columns of the spinal cord.

spi•no•cer•e•bel•lum (spī′nō-ser′ĕ-bel′ŭm) [TA] SYN paleocerebellum.

spi•no•cu•ne•ate fi•bers (spī′nō-kyū′nē-āt fī-bĕrz) Axons that originate from cells in the posterior horn of cervical and upper thoracic spinal levels, ascend ipsilaterally in the cuneate fasciculus, and terminate in the cuneate nucleus. These are part of the postsynaptic–dorsal column system.

spi•no•gra•cile fi•bers (spī′nō-gras′īl fī′bĕrz) Axons that originate from neurons in the posterior horn of lower thoracic and lumbosacral spinal cord levels, ascend ipsilaterally in the gracile fasciculus, and terminate in the gracile nucleus. These are part of the postsynaptic–dorsal column system.

spi•no•o•li•var•y tract (spī′nō-ol′i-var-ē trakt) A collection of axons, actually comprising several bundles, that originate from the spinal gray, ascending ipsilaterally to terminate in the accessory olivary nuclei.

spi•nous (spī′nŭs) Relating to, shaped like, or having a spine or spines.

spi•nous lay•er (spī′nŭs lā′ĕr) SYN stratum spinosum epidermidis.

spi•nous pro•cess (spīn′ŭs pros′es) **1.** The dorsal projection from the center of a vertebral arch. **2.** SYN sphenoidal spine.

spi•no•ves•ti•bu•lar tract (spī′nō-ves-tib′yū-lăr trakt) A group of axons that originate from neurons primarily in lumbosacral levels, ascend ipsilaterally and in close apposition to the posterior spinocerebellar tract, and terminate in the lateral, medial, and spinal vestibular nuclei. Some of these axons may be collaterals of posterior spinocerebellar fibers.

spi•rad•e•no•ma (spīr′ad-ĕ-nō′mă) A benign tumor of sweat glands. [G. *speira,* coil, + adenoma]

spi•ral (spī′răl) **1.** Coiled; winding around a center like a watch spring; winding and ascending like a wire spring. **2.** A structure in the shape of a coil. [Mediev. L. *spiralis,* fr. G. *speira,* a coil]

spi•ral ban•dage (spī′răl ban′dăj) An oblique bandage encircling a limb, the successive turns overlapping those preceding.

spi•ral ca•nal of coch•le•a (spī′răl kă-nal′ kok′lē-ă) The winding tube of the bony labyrinth that makes two-and-a-half turns about the modiolus of the cochlea; it is divided incompletely into two compartments by a winding shelf of bone, the bony spiral lamina. SYN Corti canal, Rosenthal canal.

spi•ral ca•nal of mo•di•o•lus (spī′răl kă-nal′ mō-dī-ō′lŭs) The space in the modiolus in which the spiral ganglion of the cochlear nerve lies. SYN canalis spiralis modioli [TA].

spi•ral fold of cys•tic duct (spī′răl fōld sis′ tik dŭkt) A series of crescentic folds of mucous membrane in the upper part of the cystic duct, arranged in a somewhat spiral manner. SYN plica spiralis ductus cystici [TA].

i spi•ral frac•ture (spī′răl frak′shŭr) A break that creates a helical line in bone. See page B25.

spi•ral gan•gli•on of coch•le•a (spī′răl gang′ glē-ŏn kok′lē-ă) An elongated ganglion of bipolar sensory nerve cell bodies on the cochlear part of the vestibulocochlear nerve in the spiral canal of the modiolus; each ganglion cell gives rise to a peripheral process that passes between the layers of the bony spiral lamina to the spiral organ (organ of Corti), and a central axon that enters the hindbrain as a component of the inferior (cochlear) root of the eighth cranial nerve.

spi•ral joint (spī′răl joynt) SYN cochlear joint.

spi•ral lig•a•ment of co•chle•a (spī′răl lig′ă-mĕnt kok′lē-ă) The thickened periosteal lining of the bony cochlea forming the outer wall of the cochlear duct to which the basal lamina attaches.

i spi•ral or•gan (spī′răl ōr′găn) A prominent ridge of highly specialized epithelium in the floor of the cochlear duct overlying the basilar membrane of cochlea, containing one inner row and three outer rows of hair cells, or cells of Corti (the auditory receptor cells innervated by the cochlear nerve), supported by various columnar cells: the pillars of Corti, cells of Hensen, and cells of Claudius; the spiral organ is partly overhung by an awninglike shelf, the tectorial membrane, the free marginal zone of which is covered by a gelatinous substance in which the stereocilia of the outer hair cells are embedded. See this page. SYN Corti organ.

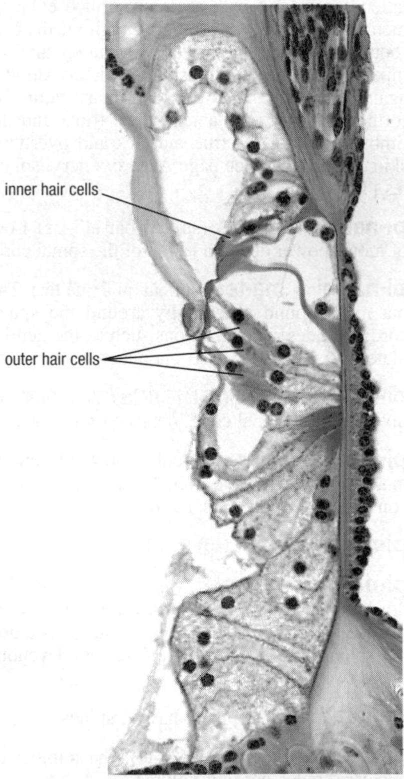

spiral organ of Corti: paraffin section, × 540

spi•ral vein of mo•di•o•lus (spī′răl vān mō-dī-ō′lŭs) The vein running a spiral course in the modiolus of the cochlea; it is tributary to both the labyrinthine vein and the vein of the cochlear canaliculus.

spi•ril•lar (spī-ril′ăr) S-shaped; referring to any bacterial cell so shaped.

Spi•ril•lum (spī-ril′ŭm) A genus of large, rigid, helical, gram-negative bacteria that are motile by means of bipolar fascicles of flagella. [Mod. L. dim. of L. *spira,* coil, fr. G. *speira*]

spi•ril•lum, pl. **spi•ril•la** (spī-ril′ŭm, -ă) A member of the genus *Spirillum.*

Spi•ril•lum mi•nus (spr-ril′ē-ŭm mī′nus) A bacterial species of uncertain taxonomic classification that causes a form of rat-bite fever (sodoku). This species has never been cultured.

spir•it (spir′it) **1.** An alcoholic liquor stronger than wine (i.e., 15%), obtained by distillation. **2.** Any distilled liquid. **3.** An alcoholic or hydroalcoholic solution of volatile substances; some spirits are used as flavoring agents; others have medicinal value. [L. *spiritus,* a breathing, soul, fr. *spiro,* to breathe]

spir•it lamp (spir′it lamp) A lamp, used mainly for heating in laboratory work, in which alcohol is burned.

spiro-, **spir-** **1.** Combining forms meaning coil, coil-shaped. [G. *speira*] **2.** Combining forms meaning breathing. [L. *spiro,* to breathe]

spirochaetaemia [Br.] SYN spirochetemia.

spi•ro•chet•e•mi•a (spī′rō-kē-tē′mē-ă) Presence of spirochetes in the blood. SYN spirochaetaemia. [spirochete + G. *haima,* blood]

spi•ro•gram (spī′rō-gram) The tracing made by the spirograph.

spi•ro•graph (spī′rō-graf) A device for representing graphically the depth and rapidity of respiratory movements. [L. *spiro,* to breathe, + G. *graphō,* to write]

spi•rom•e•ter (spī-rom′ĕ-tĕr) A gasometer used for measuring respiratory gases; usually understood to consist of a counterbalanced cylindric bell sealed by dipping into a circular trough of water. [L. *spiro,* to breathe, + G. *metron,* measure]

spi•rom•e•try (spī-rom′ĕ-trē) Making pulmonary measurements with a spirometer. See this page.

spis•si•tude (spis′i-tūd) The state of being inspissated; the condition of a fluid thickened almost to a solid by evaporation or inspissation. [L. *spissitudo,* fr. *spissus,* thick]

spit•tle (spit′ĕl) SYN saliva. [A.S. *spātl*]

Spit•zer the•o•ry (spits′er thē′ŏr-ē) An interpretation of the partitioning of the heart of mammalian embryos primarily on the basis of recapitulations of the adult structural pattern of lower forms.

Spitz ne•vus (spits nē′vŭs) A benign, slightly pigmented or red, superficial, small skin tumor composed of spindle-shaped, epithelioid, and multinucleated cells that may appear atypical; more common in children, but also appears in adults.

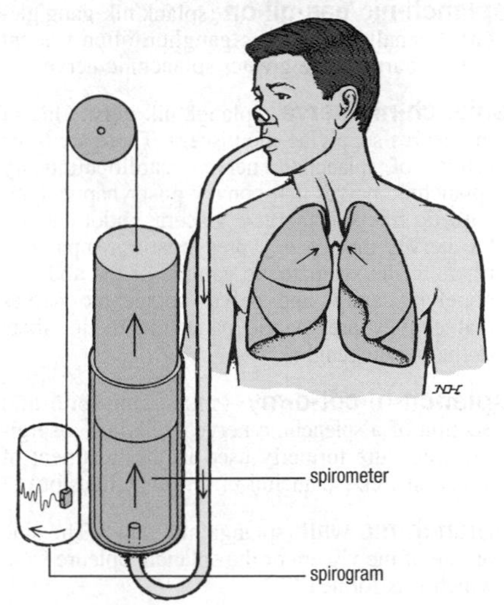

spirometry: principle of closed-circuit spirometry

splanchnaesthesia [Br.] SYN splanchnesthesia.

splanchnaesthetic sensibility [Br.] SYN splanchnesthetic sensibility.

splanch•nap•o•phys•i•al, **splanch•nap•o•phys•e•al** (splangk′nap-ō-fiz′ē-ăl) Relating to a splanchnapophysis.

splanch•na•poph•y•sis (splangk′nă-pof′i-sis) An apophysis of the typical vertebra, on the side opposite to the neural apophysis, or any bony process, giving attachment to a viscus or part of the alimentary tract. [splanchn- + G. *apophysis,* offshoot]

splanch•nec•to•pi•a (splangk′nek-tō′pē-ă) Displacement of any viscera. [splanchn- + G. *ektopos,* out of place]

splanch•nes•the•si•a (splangk′nes-thē′zē-ă) SYN visceral sense. SYN splanchnaesthesia. [splanch- + G. *aisthēsis,* sensation]

splanch•nes•the•tic sen•si•bil•i•ty (splangk′nes-thet′ik sens′i-bil′i-tē) SYN visceral sense. SYN splanchnaesthetic sensibility.

splanch•nic (splangk′nik) SYN visceral.

splanch•nic an•es•the•si•a (splangk′nik an′es-thē′zē-ă) Loss of sensation in areas of the visceral peritoneum innervated by the splanchnic nerves. SYN visceral anesthesia.

splanch•ni•cec•to•my (splangk′ni-sek′tŏ-mē) Resection of the splanchnic nerves and usually of the celiac ganglion as well. [splanchni- + G. *ektomē,* excision]

splanch•nic gan•gli•on (splank′nik gang′glē-ŏn) A small sympathetic ganglion often present in the course of the greater splanchnic nerve.

splanch•nic nerve (splangk′nik nĕrv) One of the nerves supplying the viscera. There are three groups of splanchnic nerves: cardiopulmonary splanchnic nerves that convey postsynaptic sympathetic fibers to thoracic viscera; abdominopelvic nerves that convey presynpatic sympathetic fibers to the sympathetic ganglia of the abdominopelvic cavity; and pelvic splanchnic nerves that convey presynaptic parasympathetic fibers to the pelvic ganglia.

splanch•ni•cot•o•my (splangk′ni-kot′ŏ-mē) Section of a splanchnic nerve or nerves, a surgical procedure formerly used in the treatment of hypertension. [splanchni- + G. *tomē,* incision]

splanch•nic wall (splangk′nik wawl) The side of one of the viscera or the splanchnopleure from which it is formed.

♻**splanchno-**, **splanchn-**, **splanchni-** Combining forms denoting the viscera. SEE ALSO viscero-. [G. *splanchnon,* viscus]

splanch•no•cele (splangk′nō-sēl) **1.** The primordial body cavity or celom in the embryo. [G. *koilos,* hollow] **2.** Hernia of any of the abdominal viscera. [G. *kēlē,* hernia]

splanch•nog•ra•phy (splangk-nog′ră-fē) A treatise on or description of the viscera. [splanchno- + G. *graphō,* to write]

splanch•no•lith (splangk′nō-lith) An intestinal calculus. [splanchno- + G. *lithos,* stone]

splanch•no•meg•a•ly (splangk′nō-meg′ă-lē) SYN visceromegaly. [splanchno- + G. *megas,* large]

splanch•nop•a•thy (splangk-nop′ă-thē) Any disease of the abdominal viscera. [splanchno- + G. *pathos,* disease]

splanch•no•pleure (splangk′nō-plūr) The embryonic layer formed by association of the visceral layer of the lateral plate mesoderm with the endoderm. [splanchno- + G. *pleura,* side]

splanch•nop•to•sis, **splanch•nop•to•si•a** (splangk′nop-tō′sis, -tō′sē-ă) SYN visceroptosis. [splanchno- + G. *ptōsis* a falling]

splanch•no•scle•ro•sis (splangk′nō-skle-rō′sis) Hardening, through connective tissue overgrowth, of any of the viscera. [splanchno- + G. *sklērōsis,* hardening]

splanch•no•skel•e•tal (splangk′nō-skel′ĕ-tăl) SYN visceroskeletal.

splanch•no•skel•e•ton (splangk′nō-skel′ĕ-tŏn) SYN visceroskeleton (2).

splanch•no•tribe (splangk′nō-trīb) An instrument resembling a large angiotribe used for occluding the intestine temporarily, before resection. [splanchno- + G. *tribō,* to rub, bruise]

spleen (splēn) A large vascular lymphatic organ lying in the upper part of the abdominal cavity on the left side, between the stomach and diaphragm, composed of white and red pulp; the white consists of lymphatic nodules and diffuse lymphatic tissue; the red consists of venous sinusoids between which are splenic cords; the stroma of both red and white pulp is reticular fibers and cells. A framework of fibroelastic trabeculae extending from the capsule subdivides the structure into poorly defined lobules. It is a blood-forming organ in early life and later a storage organ for red corpuscles and platelets; because of the large number of macrophages, it also acts as a blood filter, both identifying and destroying effete erythrocytes. SYN lien [TA], splen [TA]. [G. *splēn*]

splen (splen) [TA] SYN spleen.

sple•nec•to•my (splē-nek′tŏ-mē) Removal of the spleen. [splen- + G. *ektomē,* excision]

sple•nec•to•pi•a, **sple•nec•to•py** (splē′nek-tō′pē-ă, splē-nek′tō-pē) **1.** Displacement of the spleen, as in a floating spleen. **2.** The presence of rests of splenic tissue, usually in the region of the spleen. [splen- + G. *ektopos,* out of place]

splen•ic (splen′ik) Relating to the spleen. SYN lienal.

splen•ic ar•ter•y (splen′ik ahr′tĕr-ē) *Origin,* celiac trunk; *branches,* pancreatic, left gastroepiploic, short gastric, and (proper) splenic. SYN arteria lienalis [TA], lienal artery.

splen•ic flex•ure (splen′ik flek′shŭr) SYN left colic flexure.

splen•ic lymph fol•li•cles (splen′ik limf fol′i-kĕlz) Small, nodular masses of lymphoid tissue attached to the sides of the smaller arterial branches. SYN folliculi lymphatici lienales, malpighian bodies.

splen•ic pulp (splen′ik pŭlp) The soft cellular substance of the spleen.

splen•ic si•nus (splen′ik sī′nŭs) An elongated venous channel, 12–40 mcm wide, lined by rod-shaped cells.

splen•ic vein (splen′ik vān) Arises by the union of several small veins at the hilum on the anterior surface of the spleen with the short gastric and left gastroepiploic veins; passes backward through the splenorenal ligament to the left kidney, then runs behind the upper border of the pancreas to the neck of the pancreas, where it joins the superior mesenteric vein to form the portal vein.

sple•ni•tis (splē-nī′tis) Inflammation of the spleen. [splen- + G. *-itis,* inflammation]

sple•ni•um, pl. **sple•ni•a** (splē′nē-ŭm, -ă) **1.** A compress or bandage. **2.** A structure resembling a bandaged part. [Mod. L. fr. G. *splēnion,* bandage]

sple•ni•um cor•po•ris cal•lo•si (splē′nē-ŭm kōr-pō′ris kă-lō′sī) [TA] SYN splenium of corpus callosum.

sple•ni•um of cor•pus cal•lo•sum (splē′nē-ŭm kōr′pŭs kal-ō′sŭm) The thickened posterior extremity of the corpus callosum. SYN splenium corporis callosi [TA].

sple•ni•us ca•pi•tis mus•cle (splē′nē-us kap′i-tis mŭs′ĕl) *Origin*, from ligamentum nuchae of last four cervical vertebrae and supraspinous ligament of first and second thoracic vertebrae; *insertion*, lateral half of superior nuchal line and mastoid process; *action*, rotates head and extends neck; *nerve supply*, dorsal primary rami of second to sixth cervical spinal nerves. See this page. SYN musculus splenius capitis [TA], splenius muscle of head.

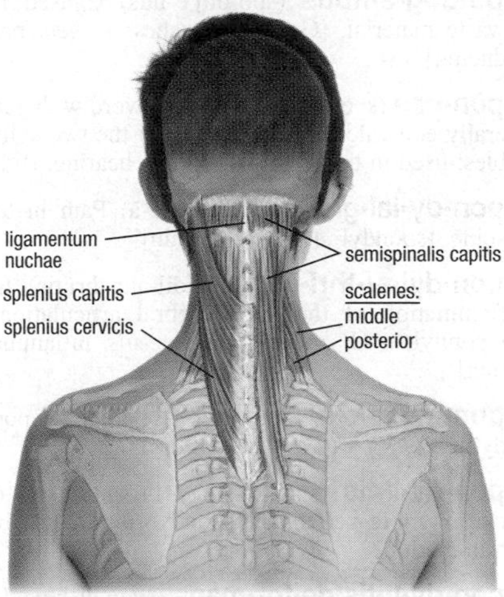

splenius capitis muscle

sple•ni•us cer•vi•cis mus•cle (splē′nē-us sĕr′vi-sis mŭs′ĕl) *Origin*, from supraspinous ligament and spinous processes of third to fifth thoracic vertebrae; *insertion*, posterior tubercles of transverse processes of first and second (sometimes third) cervical vertebrae; *action*, rotates and extends neck; *nerve supply*, dorsal primary rami of fourth to eighth cervical spinal nerves. SYN musculus splenius cervicis [TA], splenius muscle of neck.

sple•ni•us mus•cle of head (splē′nē-us mŭs′ĕl hed) SYN splenius capitis muscle.

sple•ni•us mus•cle of neck (splē-nē-us mŭs′ĕl nek) SYN splenius cervicis muscle.

spleno-, splen- Combining forms denoting the spleen. [G. *splēn*]

sple•no•cele (splē′nō-sēl) **1.** SYN splenoma. **2.** A splenic hernia. [spleno- + G. *kēlē,* tumor, hernia]

sple•no•he•pa•to•meg•a•ly, sple•no•he•pa•to•me•ga•li•a (splē′nō-hep′ă-tō-meg′ă-lē, -mĕ-gā′lē-ă) Enlargement of both spleen and liver. [spleno- + G. *hēpar,* liver, + *megas,* large]

sple•noid (splē′noyd) Resembling the spleen. [spleno- + G. *eidos,* resemblance]

sple•no•ma (splē-nō′mă) General nonspecific term for an enlarged spleen. SYN splenocele (1). [spleno- + G. *-oma,* tumor]

sple•no•ma•la•ci•a (splē′nō-mă-lā′shē-ă) Softening of the spleen. [spleno- + G. *malakia,* softness]

sple•no•med•ul•lar•y (splē′nō-med′ŭ-lar-ē) SYN splenomyelogenous. [spleno- + L. *medulla,* marrow]

sple•no•meg•a•ly, sple•no•me•ga•li•a (splē-nō-meg′ă-lē, -mĕ-gā′lē-ă) Enlargement of the spleen. See this page. SYN megalosplenia. [spleno- + G. *megas* (*megal-*), large]

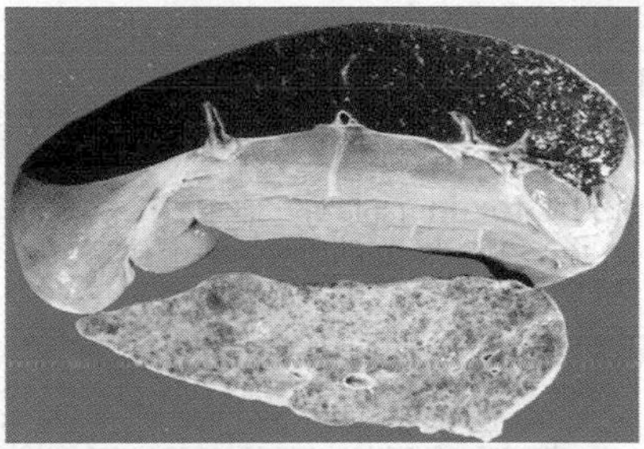

splenomegaly: abnormal enlargement of spleen (top) as sequela to cirrhosis; liver seen at bottom is normally much larger than the spleen

sple•no•my•e•log•e•nous (splē′nō-mī-ĕ-loj′ĕ-nŭs) Originating in the spleen and bone marrow, denoting a form of leukemia. SYN splenomedullary. [spleno- + G. *myelos,* marrow, + *-gen,* producing]

sple•no•my•e•lo•ma•la•ci•a (splē′nō-mī′ĕ-lō′mă-lā′shē-ă) Pathologic softening of the spleen and bone marrow. [spleno- + G. *myelos,* marrow, + *malakia,* softness]

sple•nop•a•thy (splē-nop′ă-thē) Any disease of the spleen. [spleno- + G. *pathos,* suffering]

sple•no•pex•y, sple•no•pex•i•a (splē′nō-pek-sē, -pek′sē-ă) Suturing in place an ectopic or floating spleen. SYN splenorrhaphy (2). [spleno- + G. *pēxis,* fixation]

sple•no•por•tog•ra•phy (splē′nō-pōr-tog′ră-fē) Introduction of radiopaque material into the spleen to obtain a radiologic visualization of the portal vessel of the portal circulation. [spleno- + portography]

sple·nop·to·sis, **sple·nop·to·si·a** (splē′nop-tō′sis, -tō′sē-ă) Downward displacement of the spleen, as in a floating spleen. [spleno- + G. *ptōsis,* falling]

sple·no·re·nal lig·a·ment (splē′nō-rē′năl lig′ă-mĕnt) A peritoneal fold (portion of the greater omentum) that extends from the diaphragm and the anterior aspect of the left kidney to the hilar region of the spleen, conducting the splenic vessels from the posterior body wall to the spleen. SYN ligamentum splenorenale [TA].

sple·no·re·nal shunt (splē′nō-rē′năl shŭnt) Anastomosis of the splenic vein to the left renal vein, usually end to side, for control of portal hypertension.

sple·nor·rha·gi·a (splē′nōr-ā′jē-ă) Hemorrhage from a ruptured spleen. [spleno- + G. *rhēgnymi,* to burst forth]

sple·nor·rha·phy (splē-nōr′ă-fē) **1.** Suturing of a ruptured spleen. **2.** SYN splenopexy. [spleno- + G. *rhaphē,* suture]

sple·no·sis (splē-nō′sis) Implantation and subsequent growth of splenic tissue within the abdomen as a result of disruption of the spleen.

sple·not·o·my (splē-not′ŏ-mē) **1.** Anatomy or dissection of the spleen. **2.** Surgical incision of the spleen. [spleno- + G. *tomē,* incision]

sple·no·tox·in (splē′nō-tok′sin) A cytotoxin specific for cells of the spleen. [spleno- + G. *toxikon,* poison]

splic·ing (splīs′ing) **1.** Attachment of one DNA molecule to another. SYN gene splicing. **2.** Removal of introns from mRNA precursors and the reattachment or annealing of exons. SYN RNA splicing.

splint (splint) **1.** An appliance used to prevent movement of a joint or to fixate displaced or movable parts. **2.** The splint bone, or fibula. [Middle Dutch *splinte*]

splin·ter hem·or·rhag·es (splin′tĕr hĕm′ŏr-ăj-ĕz) Multiple tiny longitudinal subungual hemorrhages undr a fingernal or toenail, typically seen in but not diagnostic of bacterial endocarditis and trichinelliasis.

split hand (split hand) SYN cleft hand.

split pel·vis (split pel′vis) A pelvis in which the symphysis pubis is absent, the pelvic bones being separated; usually associated with exstrophy of the bladder.

split-thick·ness flap (split-thik′nĕs flap) A flap of a portion of the skin (i.e., the epidermis and part of the dermis), or of part of the mucosa and submucosa, but not including the periosteum. SYN partial-thickness flap.

split-thick·ness graft (split-thik′nĕs graft) A graft of portions of the skin (i.e., the epidermis and part of the dermis), or of part of the mucosa and submucosa, but not including the periosteum. SYN partial-thickness graft.

split·ting (split′ing) CHEMISTRY the cleavage of a covalent bond, fragmenting the molecule involved.

split·ting of heart sounds (split′ing hahrt sowndz) The production of major components of the first and second heart sounds (rarely the third and fourth) due to contribution by the left-sided and right-sided valves; thus, the first heart sound would have mitral and tricuspid components and the second heart sound aortic and pulmonic components. The latter are best appreciated during respiration, with inspiration delaying the pulmonic component and producing an earlier aortic component.

spm An abbreviation meaning a gene that leads to *sup*pression and *m*utation of mutants that are unstable.

spo·dog·e·nous (spō-doj′ĕ-nŭs) Caused by waste material. [G. *spodos,* ashes, + *-gen,* producing]

spon·dee (spon′dē) A bisyllabic word with generally equivalent stress on each of the two syllables; used in the testing of speech hearing. [Fr.]

spon·dy·lal·gi·a (spond′i-lal′jē-ă) Pain in the spine. [spondyl- + G. *algos,* pain]

spon·dyl·ar·thri·tis (spon′dil-ahr-thrī′tis) Inflammation of the intervertebral articulations. [spondyl- + G. *arthron,* joint, + *-itis,* inflammation]

spon·dy·lit·ic (spond′i-lit′ik) Relating to spondylitis.

spon·dy·li·tis (spon′di-lī′tis) Inflammation of one or more vertebrae. [spondyl- + G. *-itis,* inflammation]

spon·dy·li·tis de·for·mans (spon′di-lī′tis de-fōrm′anz) Arthritis and osteitis deformans involving the spinal column; marked by nodular deposits at the edges of the intervertebral discs with ossification of the ligaments and bony ankylosis of the intervertebral articulations, it results in a rounded kyphosis with rigidity. SYN Bechterew disease, Strümpell disease (1).

♻ **spondylo-**, **spondyl-** Combining forms denoting the vertebrae. [G. *spondylos,* vertebra]

spon·dy·lo·ep·i·phys·i·al dys·pla·si·a (spon′di-lō-ep′i-fiz′ē-ăl dis-plā′zē-ă) A group of conditions characterized by growth deficiency of the vertebral column with flattening of the vertebrae or platyspondyly, lack of ossification of the epiphyses, short-trunk dwarfism with limb shortening, and sometimes other malformations; autosomal dominant, autosomal recessive, and X-linked recessive inheritance have been described.

spon·dy·lo·ep·i·phy·si·al dys·pla·si·a con·gen·i·ta (SEDC) (spon′di-lō-ep′i-fiz′ē-ăl dis-plā′zē-ă kon-jen′i-tă) A skeletal dysplasia characterized by short-trunk dwarfism with short limbs, delayed ossification of the pubic rami and femoral and tibial epiphyses, flattening of the vertebral bodies, myopia, retinal detachment, and cleft palate; autosomal dominant inheritance caused by mutation in the type II collagen gene (COL2A1) on 12q.

spon•dy•lo•e•pi•phy•si•al dys•pla•si•a tar•da (spon′di-lō-ep′i-fiz′ē-ăl dis-plā′zē-ă tahr′dă) A skeletal dysplasia of later onset, usually in the second decade, characterized by short stature, flattening of the vertebrae, epiphysial involvement with bony fusion of the hip joint, premature osteoarthritis, and distinctive radiographic findings. Autosomal dominant and X-linked recessive forms exist.

spon•dy•lo•lis•the•sis (spon′di-lō-lis-thē′sis) SYN anterolisthesis. See this page. [spondylo- + G. *olisthēsis,* a slipping and falling]

spon•dy•lo•lis•thet•ic (spon′di-lō-lis-thet′ik) Relating to or marked by spondylolisthesis.

spon•dy•lo•lis•thet•ic pel•vis (spon′di-lō-lis-thet′ik pel′vis) A pelvis with a brim that is more or less occluded by a forward dislocation of the body of one of the lower lumbar vertebrae. SYN Prague pelvis, Rokitansky pelvis.

spon•dy•lol•y•sis (spon′di-lol′i-sis) Degeneration or deficient development of the articulating part of a vertebra. [spondylo- + G. *lysis,* loosening]

spon•dy•lop•a•thy (spon′di-lop′ă-thē) Any disease of the vertebrae or spinal column. [spondylo- + G. *pathos,* suffering]

spon•dy•lo•py•o•sis (spon′di-lō-pī-ō′sis) Suppurative inflammation of one or more of the vertebral bodies. [spondylo- + G. *pyōsis,* suppuration]

spon•dy•los•chi•sis (spon′di-los′ki-sis) Embryologic failure of fusion of neural arch. SEE ALSO spina bifida. [spondylo- + G. *schisis,* fissure]

spon•dy•lo•sis (spon′di-lō′sis) Ankylosis of the vertebrae; often applied nonspecifically to any lesion of the spine of a degenerative nature. See page 1466. [G. *spondylos,* vertebra]

spon•dy•lo•syn•de•sis (spon′di-lō-sin-dē′sis) SYN spinal fusion. [spondylo- + G. *syndesis,* binding together]

sponge (spŏnj) **1.** Absorbent material (e.g., gauze or prepared cotton) used to absorb fluids. **2.** A member of the phylum Porifera, the cellular endoskeleton of which is a source of commercial natural sponges. [G. *spongia*]

sponge bath (spŏnj bath) A cleansing in which the body is washed with a wet sponge or cloth.

spon•gi•form (spŏn′ji-fōrm) SYN spongy.

spon•gi•form en•ceph•a•lop•a•thy (spŏn′ji-fōrm en-sef′a-lop′ă-thē) An encephalopathy characterized by vacuolation within nerve and glial cells.

spongio- Combining form denoting sponge, sponglike, spongy. [G. *spongia*]

spon•gi•o•blast (spŏn′jē-ō-blast) A neuroepithelial, filiform ependyma cell extending across the entire thickness of the wall of the brain or spinal cord (i.e., from the internal to the external limiting membrane); spongioblasts become neuroglial and ependymal cells. SEE ALSO glioblast. [spongio- + G. *blastos,* germ]

spon•gi•o•blas•to•ma (spŏn′jē-ō-blas-tō′mă) A glioma consisting of cells (elongated, spindle-shaped, and sometimes pleomorphic, with one or two fibrillary processes), which resembles the embryonic spongioblasts, occurring normally around the neural canal of the human embryo; it grows relatively slowly, usually originating in the brainstem, optic chiasm, or infundibulum, and infiltrates adjacent structures or causes compression of the third and fourth ventricle. [spongioblast + G. *-oma,* tumor]

spon•gi•o•cyte (spŏn′jē-ō-sīt) **1.** A neuroglial cell. **2.** A cell in the zona fasciculata of the cortex of suprarenal gland containing many droplets of lipid material that, after staining with hematoxylin and eosin, show pronounced vacuolization. [spongio- + G. *kytos,* cell]

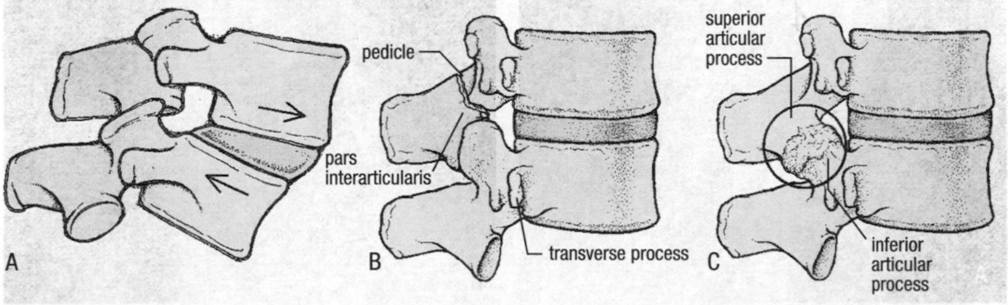

spondylolisthesis: (A) showing forward slippage of lumbar vertebra; **spondylolysis:** (B) showing fracture of pars interarticularis; **spondylosis:** (C) showing fixation of the articular processes

spon·gi·oid (spŏn′jē-oyd) SYN spongy. [spongio- + G. *eidos,* resemblance]

spon·gi·ose (spŏn′jē-ōs) Resembling or characteristic of a sponge. [L. *spongiosus*]

spon·gi·o·sis (spŏn′jē-ō′sis) Inflammatory intercellular edema of the epidermis.

spon·gi·o·si·tis (spŏn′jē-ō-sī′tis) Inflammation of the corpus spongiosum, or corpus cavernosum urethrae.

spon·gy (spŏn′jē) Resembling the commercial natural sponge; of spongelike texture or appearance. SYN spongiform, spongioid.

spon·gy bone (spŏn′jē bōn) **1.** SYN substantia spongiosa. **2.** A turbinate bone.

spon·gy sub·stance (spŏn′jē sub′stăns) SYN substantia spongiosa.

spon·ta·ne·ous a·bor·tion (spon-tā′nē-ŭs ă-bōr′shŭn) Abortion that has not been artificially induced.

spon·ta·ne·ous am·pu·ta·tion (spon-tā′nē-ŭs amp′yū-tā′shŭn) **1.** SYN congenital amputation. **2.** Amputation as the result of a pathologic process rather than external trauma.

spon·tan·e·ous breath (spon-tā′nē-ŭs breth) During mechanical ventilation, a breath for which both the timing and the size are controlled by the patient (i.e., the breath is both initiated [triggered] and terminated [cycled] by the patient).

spon·ta·ne·ous gan·grene of new·born (spon-tā′nē-ŭs gang-grēn′ nū′bōrn) The form of necrosis due to vascular occlusion of unknown cause, usually in marasmic or dehydrated infants.

spon·ta·ne·ous gen·er·a·tion (spon-tā′nē-ŭs jen′ĕr-ā′shŭn) The false concept according to which living matter can arise by the vitalization of nonliving matter. SEE ALSO biogenesis. SYN heterogenesis (3).

spon·ta·ne·ous mu·ta·tion (spon-tā′nē-ŭs myū-tā′shŭn) A mutation that arises naturally and not as a result of exposure to mutagens.

spon·ta·ne·ous pneu·mo·thor·ax (spon-tā′nē-ŭs nū′mō-thōr′aks) Air or gas in the pleural cavity occurring secondary to parenchymal lung disease, usually from an emphysematous bulla that ruptures or occasionally from a lung abscess.

spon·ta·ne·ous speech (spon-tā′nē-ŭs spēch) Spoken language that occurs without prompting or during an unstructured interview.

spon·ta·ne·ous ver·sion (spon-tā′nē-ŭs vĕr′zhŭn) Turning of the fetus effected by the unaided contraction of the uterine muscle.

spoon (spūn) An instrument with a handle and a small bowl- or cup-shaped extremity. [A.S. *spōn,* chip]

spoon nail (spūn nāl) SYN koilonychia.

spo·rad·ic (spōr-ad′ik) **1.** Denoting a temporal pattern of disease occurrence in an animal or human population in which the disease occurs only rarely and without regularity. SEE ALSO en-

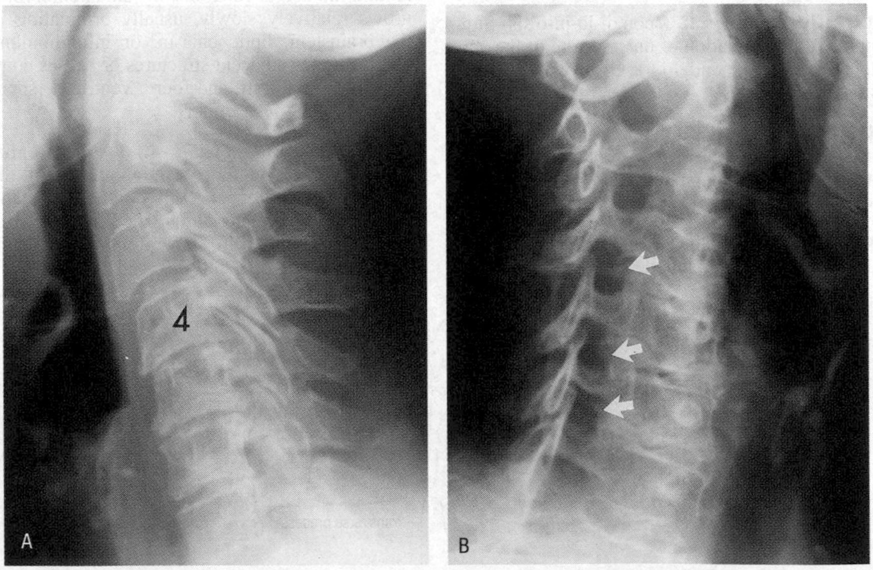

severe cervical **spondylosis:** (A) lateral radiograph shows narrowing of all the disc spaces below C4; (B) oblique view shows spurs encroaching on intervertebral foramina at several levels (arrows)

demic, epidemic, epizootic. **2.** Occurring irregularly, haphazardly. [G. *sporadikos,* scattered]

spo•ran•gi•um (spōr-anj′ē-ŭm) A saclike structure (a cell) within a fungus, in which asexual spores are borne by progressive cleavage. [L. fr. G. *sporos,* seed, + *angeion,* vessel]

spore (spōr) **1.** The asexual or sexual reproductive body of fungi or sporozoan protozoa. **2.** A cell of a plant lower in organization than the seed-bearing spermatophytic plants. **3.** A resistant form of certain species of bacteria. **4.** The highly modified reproductive body of certain protozoa, as in the phyla Microspora and Myxozoa. [G. *sporos,* seed]

spo•ri•ci•dal (spōr-i-sī′dăl) Lethal to spores. [spori- + L. *caedo,* to kill]

spo•ri•cide (spōr′i-sīd) An agent that kills spores.

spo•rid•i•um, pl. **spo•rid•i•a** (spōr-id′ē-ŭm, -ă) A protozoan spore; an embryonic protozoan organism. [Mod. L. dim., fr. G. *sporos,* seed]

♻ **sporo-, spori-, spor-** Combining forms meaning seed, spore. [G. *sporos*]

spo•ro•ag•glu•ti•na•tion (spōr′ō-ă-glū′ti-nā′shŭn) A diagnostic method in relation to the mycoses, based on the fact that the blood of patients with diseases caused by fungi contains specific agglutinins that cause clumping of the spores of these organisms.

spo•ro•blast (spōr′ō-blast) An early stage in the development of a sporocyst before differentiation of the sporozoites. SEE ALSO oocyst, sporocyst (2). [sporo- + G. *blastos,* germ]

spo•ro•cyst (spōr′ō-sist) **1.** A larval form of digenetic trematode (fluke) that develops in the body of its molluscan intermediate host, usually a snail. SEE ALSO cercaria. **2.** A secondary cyst that develops within the oocyst of Coccidia, a group of sporozoans that includes many of the most important disease agents of domestic animals and fowl. [sporo- + G. *kystis,* bladder]

spo•ro•gen•e•sis (spōr′ō-jen′ĕ-sis) SYN sporogony. [sporo- + G. *genesis,* production]

spo•rog•e•nous (spŏr-oj′ĕ-nŭs) Relating to or involved in sporogony.

spo•rog•o•ny, **spo•rog•e•ny** (spŏr-og′ŏ-nē, -oj′ĕ-nē) The formation of sporozoites in sporozoan protozoa, a process of asexual division within the sporoblast, which becomes the sporocyst within an oocyst; follows fusion of gametes (gametogony) and zygote (sporont) formation. SYN sporogenesis. [sporo- + G. *goneia,* generation]

spor•ont (spōr′ont) The zygote stage within the oocyst wall in the life cycle of coccidia; gives rise to sporoblasts, which form sporocysts, within which the infective sporozoites are produced. [sporo- + G. *ōn* (*ont*-), being]

Spo•ro•thrix (spōr′ō-thriks) A genus of dimorphic imperfect fungi, including *S. schenckii*, an organism of worldwide distribution and the causative agent of sporotrichosis in humans and animals. [Mod. L., fr. G. *sporos,* seed, + *thrix,* hair]

spo•ro•tri•cho•sis (spōr′ō-tri-kō′sis) A chronic cutaneous mycosis spread by way of the lymphatics and caused by inoculation of *Sporothrix schenckii*, typically rare in tissue sections but rapidly growing in cultures. The disease may remain localized or may become generalized, involving bones, joints, lungs, and the central nervous system; lesions may be granulomatous or suppurative, ulcerative, or draining. SYN Schenck disease.

spo•ro•zo•ite (spōr′ō-zō′īt) One of the minute elongated bodies resulting from the repeated division of the oocyst during sporogony. In the case of the malarial parasite, it is the form that is concentrated in the salivary glands and introduced into the blood by the bite of a mosquito; it enters the liver cells (exoerythrocytic cycle); its progeny, the merozoites, infect the red blood cells to initiate clinical malaria. [sporo- + G. *zōon,* animal]

sports a•ne•mi•a (spōrts ă-nē′mē-ă) SYN exercise-induced anemia.

sports mas•sage, **sports•mas•sage** (spōrts mă-sahzh′) A group of massage techniques specifically designed to aid in athletic performance. Includes preevent, interevent, and postevent massage, and maintenance and injury massage.

sports med•i•cine (spōrts med′i-sin) A field of medicine that uses a holistic, comprehensive, and multidisciplinary approach to health care for those engaged in a sporting or recreational activity.

sport-spe•ci•fic train•ing (spōrt-spĕ-sif′ik trān′ing) SYN activity grading.

spor•u•lar (spōr′yū-lăr) Relating to a spore or sporule.

spor•u•la•tion (spōr′yū-lā′shŭn) The process by which yeasts undergo meiosis and the meiotic products are encased in spore coats.

spor•ule (spōr′yūl) A spore; a small spore. [Mod. L. *sporula*, dim. of G. *sporos,* seed]

spot (spot) **1.** SYN macula. **2.** To lose a slight amount of blood through the vagina.

spot map (spot map) Graphic depiction showing the geographic location of people with a specific attribute, e.g., cases of an infectious disease.

spot•ted fe•ver (spot′ĕd fē′vĕr) Tick typhus caused by various species of the bacterial genus *Rickettsia* in North and South America, Europe, Africa, and Asia.

spot·ted this·tle (spot′ĕd this′ĕl) SYN blessed thistle.

spot test for in·fec·tious mon·o·nu·cle·o·sis (spot test in-fek′shŭs mon′ō-nū′klē-ō′sis) An assay method involving slides that is widely used for the diagnosis of infectious mononucleosis; when equine red blood cells are agglutinated by patient's serum (previously treated with guinea pig kidney, which adsorbs confounding antibodies), the presumptive diagnosis is infectious mononucleosis.

spouse a·buse, **spous·al a·buse** (spows ă-būs′, spowz′ăl) SEE domestic violence.

Sprague Daw·ley rat (sprāg daw′lē rat) Common laboratory animal used for experimentation.

sprain (sprān) **1.** An injury to a ligament when the joint is carried through a range of motion greater than normal, but without dislocation or fracture. **2.** To cause a sprain of a joint.

sprain frac·ture (sprān frak′shŭr) An avulsion break in which a small portion of adjacent bone has been pulled or pushed off.

spray (sprā) A jet of liquid in fine drops, coarser than a vapor; produced by forcing the liquid from the minute opening of an atomizer, mixed with air.

Spreng·el de·for·mi·ty (spreng′gel dĕ-fōrm′i-tē) Congenital elevation of the scapula.

spring con·junc·ti·vi·tis (spring kŏn-jŭngk′ti-vī′tis) SYN vernal conjunctivitis.

sprue (sprū) **1.** Primary intestinal malabsorption with steatorrhea. **2.** DENTISTRY wax or metal used to form the aperture(s) through which molten metal flows into a mold to make a casting; also, the metal that later fills the sprue hole(s). [D. *spruw*]

SPS Abbreviation for sodium polyanethole sulfonate.

spud (spŭd) A triangular knife used for removing foreign bodies from the cornea.

spun glass hair (spŭn glas hār) SYN uncombable hair syndrome.

spur (spŭr) SYN calcar. [A.S. *spora*]

spur cell (spŭr sel) A spiculated erythrocyte with 5–10 spiny projections of varying length distributed irregularly over the cell surface; seen in patients with liver disease and abetalipoproteinemia.

spur cell a·ne·mi·a (spŭr sel ă-nē′mē-ă) A disorder in which the red blood cells have a spiculated appearance and are destroyed prematurely, predominantly in the spleen; may be seen in patients with severe liver disease as a result of an abnormality in the cholesterol content of the red blood cell membrane.

spu·ri·ous (spyūr′ē-ŭs) False; not genuine. [L. *spurius*]

spu·ri·ous an·ky·lo·sis (spyūr′ē-ŭs ang′ki-lō′sis) SYN extracapsular ankylosis.

spu·ri·ous par·a·site (spyūr′ē-ŭs par′ă-sīt) An organism that parasitizes other hosts that pass through the human intestine and is detected in the stool after ingestion (e.g., *Capillaria* sp. eggs in animal liver).

Spurl·ing test (spŭr′ling test) Evaluation for cervical nerve root impingement in which the patient extends the neck and rotates and laterally bends the head toward the symptomatic side; an axial compression force is then applied by the examiner through the top of the patient's head; the test is considered positive when the maneuver elicits the typical radicular arm pain.

spu·tum, pl. **spu·ta** (spyū′tŭm, -tă) **1.** Expectorated matter, especially mucus or mucopurulent matter expectorated in diseases of the air passages. SEE ALSO expectoration (1). **2.** An individual mass of such matter. [L. *sputum,* fr. *spuo,* pp. *sputus,* to spit]

SQ Abbreviation for subcutaneous.

squa·la·mine lac·tate (skwā′lă-mēn lak′tāt) An antiangiogenic, noncytotoxic drug used to treat solid tumors.

squa·lene (skwā′lēn) A natural nonaromatic hydrocarbon found in plants and animals; a precursor of steroids including cholesterol. [L. *squalus,* shark]

squa·ma, pl. **squa·mae** (skwā′mă, -mē) **1.** [TA] A thin plate of bone. **2.** An epidermal scale. SYN scale (2), squame. [L. a scale]

squa·mate (skwā′māt) SYN squamous.

squame (skwām) SYN squama.

♻**squamo-** Combining form denoting squama, squamous. [L. *squama,* a scale]

squa·mo·pa·ri·e·tal su·ture (skwā′mō-păr-ī′ĕ-tăl sū′chŭr) The articulation of the parietal with the squamous portion of the temporal bone.

squa·mo·sa, pl. **squa·mo·sae** (skwā-mō′să, -sē) The squamous parts of the frontal, occipital, or temporal bone, especially the latter. [L. *squamosus,* scaly, fr. *squama,* scale]

squa·mo·sal (skwā-mō′săl) Relating especially to the squamous part of the temporal bone.

squa·mous (skwā′mŭs) Relating to or covered with scales. SYN scaly, squamate. [L. *squamosus*]

squa·mous cell (skwā′mŭs sel) A flat, scale-like epithelial cell.

🅸**squa·mous cell car·ci·no·ma** (skwā′mŭs sel kahr′si-nō′mă) A malignant neoplasm derived from stratified squamous epithelium, which may

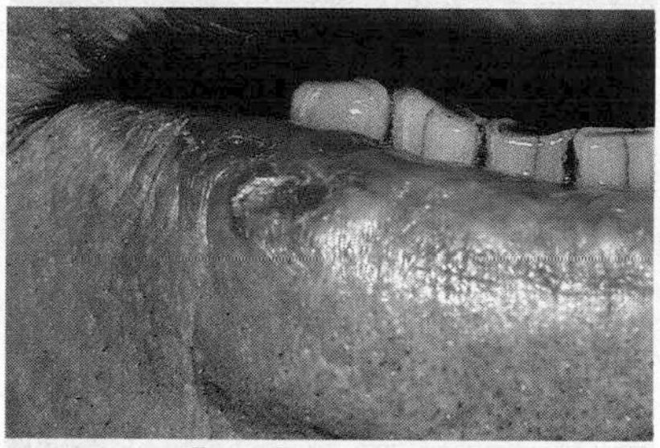

squamous cell carcinoma: indurated and raised

also occur in sites where only glandular or columnar epithelium is normally present. See this page, B14.

squa•mous ep•i•the•li•um (skwā′mŭs ep′i-thē′lē-ŭm) Epithelium consisting of a single layer of cells.

squa•mous met•a•pla•si•a (skwā′mŭs met′ă-plā′zē-ă) The transformation of glandular or mucosal epithelium into stratified squamous epithelium. SYN epidermalization.

squa•mous met•a•pla•si•a of am•ni•on (skwā′mŭs met′ă-plā′zē-ă am′nē-on) SYN amnion nodosum.

squa•mous o•don•to•gen•ic tu•mor (skwā′mŭs ō-don′tō-jen′ik tū′mŏr) A benign epithelial tumor thought to arise from the epithelial cell rests of Malassez; appears clinically as a radiolucent lesion closely associated with the tooth root and histologically as islands of squamous epithelium enclosed by a peripheral layer of flattened cells.

squa•mous su•ture (skwā′mŭs sū′chŭr) A scalelike suture, one with opposing margins that are scalelike and overlapping.

squa•mo•zy•go•mat•ic (skwā′mō-zī′gō-mat′ik) Relating to the squamous part of the temporal bone and the zygomatic process of the temporal bone.

square knot (skwār not) A double knot in which the free ends of the second loop are symmetric and in the same plane as the free ends of the first loop.

squaw root (skwaw rūt) **1.** SYN black cohosh. **2.** SYN blue cohosh.

squint (skwint) **1.** SYN strabismus. **2.** To narrow the interpalpebral openings of the eyelids to block light or improve focus.

squint•ing pa•tel•la (skwint′ing pă-tel′ă) A patella that is medially rotated.

SR Abbreviation for slow release.

Sr Symbol for strontium.

SRH Abbreviation for somatotropin-releasing hormone.

sRNA Abbreviation for soluble RNA. SEE ribonucleic acid.

SRS Abbreviation for slow-reacting substance.

SRT Abbreviation for speech recognition technology. SEE ALSO speech recognition, voice recognition.

SSA Abbreviation for sulfosalicylic acid.

SSD Abbreviation for source-to-surface distance.

SSNHL Abbreviation for sudden sensorineural hearing loss.

SSPE Abbreviation for subacute sclerosing panencephalitis.

SSPL Abbreviation for saturation sound pressure level.

SSRI Abbreviation for selective serotonin reuptake inhibitor.

SST Abbreviation for serum separator tube.

ST Abbreviation for scapulothoracic; sacrotransverse.

stab cell (stab sel) SYN band cell.

stab cul•ture (stab kŭl′chŭr) A culture produced by inserting an inoculating needle with inoculum down the center of a solid medium contained in a test tube.

stab drain (stab drān) An opening made into a cavity through a puncture made at a dependent part away from the wound of operation, so placed to prevent infection of the wound.

sta•bi•late (stā′bi-lāt) A sample of organisms preserved alive on a single occasion.

sta•bile (stā′bil) Steady; fixed; denoting: 1) certain constituents of serum unaffected by moderate heating or prolonged storage; 2) an electrode held steadily on a part during the passage of an electric current. Cf. labile. [L. *stabilis*]

sta•bil•i•ty (stă-bil′i-tē) The condition of being stable or resistant to change.

sta•bi•li•za•tion (stā′bi-lī-zā′shŭn) **1.** The accomplishment of a stable state. **2.** SYN denture stability.

sta•bi•li•za•tion ex•er•cise (stā′bi-lī-zā′shŭn eks′ĕr-sīz) Activities used to develop the ability to maintain balance or proximal control in a pain-free position. One example is sitting on an exercise ball and extending a leg without experiencing pain.

sta•ble (stā′bĕl) Steady; not varying; resistant to change. SEE ALSO stabile.

sta•ble i•so•tope (stā′bĕl ī′sŏ-tōp) A nonradioactive nuclide; an isotope that shows no tendency to undergo radioactive decomposition.

stac•ca•to speech (stă-kah′tō spēch) An abrupt utterance, each syllable being enunciated separately; noted especially in multiple sclerosis.

staff (staf) **1.** A specific group of workers. **2.** SYN director (1). [A.S. *staef*]

staff of Aes•cu•la•pi•us (staf es-kyu-lā′pē-us) A rod with a single serpent without wings encircling it; symbol of medicine and emblem of the American Medical Association, Royal Army Medical Corps (Britain), and Royal Canadian Medical Corps. SEE ALSO caduceus. [L. *Aesculapius,* G. *Asklēpios,* god of medicine]

staff cell (staf sel) SYN band cell.

staff ed•u•ca•tion (staf ej′ū-kā′shŭn) Teaching of nursing, medical, and other members of the health care team; process of assisting staff to gain knowledge, skills, values, and attitudes for maintaining and improving competencies.

staff mod•el HMO (staf mod′ĕl) Arrangement under which physician providers are salaried employees of an HMO.

stage (stāj) **1.** A period in the course of a disease; a description of the extent of involvement of a disease process or the status of a patient with a specific disease, as of the distribution and extent of dissemination of a malignant neoplastic disease; also, the act of determining the stage of a disease, especially cancer. SEE ALSO period. **2.** The part of a microscope on which the microscope slide bears the object to be examined. **3.** A particular step, phase, or position in a developmental process. [M.E. thr. O. Fr. *estage,* standing-place, fr. L. *sto,* pp. *status,* to stand]

stag•es of la•bor (staj′ĕz lā′bŏr) SEE labor.

stag•gered spon•da•ic word test (stag′ĕrd spon-dā′ik wŏrd test) A measurement of central auditory pathway integrity in which spondaic words are presented dichotically.

stag•horn cal•cu•lus (stag′hōrn kal′kyū-lŭs) A calculus occurring in the renal pelvis, with branches extending into the infundibula and calyces. See this page.

stag•ing (stāj′ing) **1.** The determination or classification of distinct phases or periods in the course of a disease or pathologic process. **2.** The determination of the specific extent of a disease process in an individual patient.

stag•nant a•nox•i•a (stag′nănt ă-nok′sē-ă) **1.** The disorder when severe enough to result in the absence of oxygen in tissues. **2.** A condition in which blood flow in the capillaries is inadequate, thus decreasing oxygen exchange; associated wtih shock and thrombosis.

stag•na•tion (stag-nā′shŭn) Retardation or cessation of blood flow in the vessels, as in passive congestion; marked slowing or accumulation in any part of a normally circulating fluid. [L. *stagnum,* a pool]

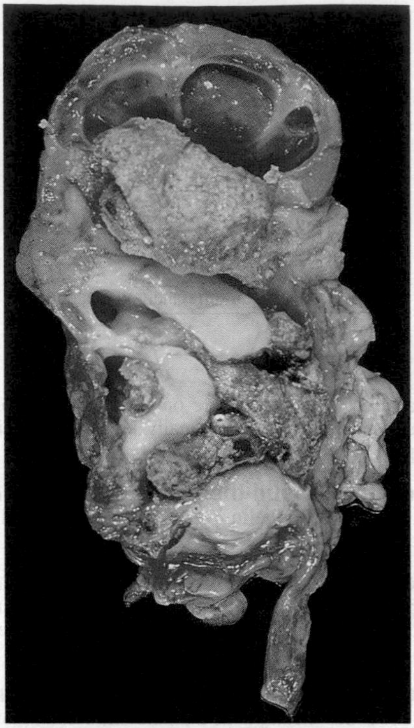

staghorn calculi: kidney shows hydronephrosis and stones that are casts of dilated calyces

Stahl ear (shtahl ēr) A deformed external ear, in which the fossa ovalis and upper portion of the scaphoid fossa are covered by the helix; previously regarded as a stigma of degenerate constitution.

stain (stān) **1.** To discolor. **2.** To color; to dye. **3.** A discoloration. **4.** A dye used in histologic and bacteriologic technique. **5.** A procedure in which a dye or combination of dyes and reagents is used to color the constituents of cells and tissues. [M.E. *steinen*]

stain•ing (stān′ing) **1.** The act of applying a stain. SEE ALSO stain. **2.** DENTISTRY modification of the color of the tooth or denture base.

stair•case (stār′kās) A series of reactions that follow one another in progressively increasing or decreasing intensity, so that a chart shows a continuous rise or fall. SEE ALSO treppe.

stair•case phe•no•me•non (stār′kās fĕ-nom′ĕ-non) SYN treppe.

stal•ag•mom•e•ter (stal′ăg-mom′ĕ-tĕr) An instrument for determining exactly the number of drops in a given quantity of liquid; used as a measure of the surface tension of a fluid (the lower the tension, the smaller the drops and, consequently, the more numerous in a given quantity of the fluid). [G. *stalagma,* a drop, + *metron,* measure]

stale•ness (stāl′nĕs) SYN overtraining syndrome.

stalk (stawk) A narrowed connection with a structure or organ.

stam•mer•ing (stam′ĕr-ing) **1.** A speech disorder characterized by hesitation and repetition of words, or by mispronunciation or transposition of certain consonants, especially *l, r,* and *s.* **2.** Sounds other than speech that are similar to stammering.

stan•dard at•mos•phere (atm) (stan′dărd at′mŏs-fēr) **1.** The pressure of the atmosphere at mean sea level, equivalent to 1,013,250 dynes/cm^2, or 101,325 Pa (N/m^2 in the SI). **2.** A standardized expression of the relation of barometric pressure, temperature, and other atmospheric variables as a function of altitude above sea level.

stan•dard bi•car•bon•ate (stan′dărd bī-kahr′bŏn-āt) The plasma bicarbonate concentration of a sample of whole blood that has been equilibrated at 37°C with a carbon dioxide pressure of 40 mmHg and an oxygen pressure greater than 100 mm Hg; abnormally high or low values indicate metabolic alkalosis or acidosis, respectively.

stan•dard of care (stan′dărd kār) The ordinary level of skill and care that any health care practitioner woud be expected to observe in caring for patients.

stan•dard de•vi•a•tion (σ) (stan′dărd dē′vē-ā′shŭn) **1.** Statistical index of the degree of deviation from central tendency, namely, of the variability within a distribution; the square root of the average of the squared deviations from the mean. **2.** A measure of dispersion or variation used to describe a characteristic of a frequency distribution.

stan•dard er•ror of dif•fer•ence (stan′dărd er′ŏr dif′ĕr-ĕns) A statistical index of the probability that a difference between two sample means is greater than zero.

stan•dard er•ror of mea•sure•ment (SEM) (stan′dărd er′ŏr mezh′ŭr-mĕnt) A test based on error with regard to reliability. The difference between the obtained test result and the hypothetical true result. SEE ALSO standard deviation.

stan•dard•i•za•tion (stan′dărd-ī-zā′shŭn) **1.** The making of a solution of definite strength so that it can be used for comparison and in tests. **2.** Any drug or other preparation made to conform to a type or standard. **3.** A set of techniques used to minimize the effects of differences in age or other confounding variables when comparing two or more populations.

stan•dard pre•cau•tions (stan′dărd prē-kaw′shŭnz) Guidelines for the prevention of infectious diseases and nosocomial infections established by the U.S. Centers for Disease Control and Prevention. Standard precautions combine universal precautions and body-substance precautions for all patients regardless of diagnosis or possible infectious status. All contact with body fluids and secretions, except sweat, are to be avoided by health care workers.

stan•dard pres•sure (stan′dărd presh′ŭr) The absolute pressure to which gases are referred under standard conditions (STPD), i.e., 760 mmHg, 760 torr, or 101,325 newtons/m^2 (i.e., 101,325 Pa).

stan•dards of nur•sing prac•tice (stan′dărdz nŭrs′ing prak′tis) Rules or definitions of competent care; guidelines for nursing.

stan•dard so•lu•tion, stan•dard•ized so•lu•tion (stan′dărd sŏ-lū′shŭn, stan′dărd-īzd) A solution of known concentration, used as a standard of comparison or analysis.

stan•dard tem•per•a•ture (stan′dărd tem′pĕr-ă-chŭr) A temperature of 0°C or 273.15° absolute (Kelvin).

stan•dard vol•ume (stan′dărd vol′yūm) The volume of an ideal gas at standard temperature and pressure, approximately 22.414 liters.

Stan•ford-Bi•net in•tel•li•gence scale (stan′fŏrd bi-nā′ in-tel′i-jĕns skāl) A standardized test for the measurement of intelligence consisting of a series of questions, graded according to the intelligence of normal children at different ages, the answers to which indicate the mental age of the person tested; primarily used with children, but also contains norms for adults standardized against adult age levels. SYN Binet scale, Binet test.

stan•nous (stan′ŭs) Relating to tin, especially when in combination in its lower valency. [L. *stannum,* tin]

stan•num (stan′ŭm) SYN tin. [L.]

sta•pe•dec•to•my (stā′pĕ-dek′tŏ-mē) Operation to remove the stapes footplate in whole or part with replacement of the stapes superstructure (crura) by metal or plastic prosthesis; used for otosclerosis with stapes fixation to overcome a conductive hearing loss. [stapes + G. *ektomē,* excision]

sta•pe•di•al (stā-pē′dē-ăl) Relating to the stapes.

sta•pe•di•al re•flex (stā-pē′dē-ăl rē′fleks) SYN acoustic reflex.

sta•pe•di•o•te•not•o•my (stā-pē′dē-ō-tĕ-not′ŏ-mē) Division of the tendon of the stapedius muscle. [stapedius + G. *tenōn,* tendon, + *tomē,* incision]

sta•pe•di•us mus•cle (stā-pē′dē-us mŭs′ĕl)

Origin, internal walls of pyramidal eminence in tympanic cavity; *insertion*, neck of the stapes; *action*, dampens vibration of stapes by drawing head of stapes backward as a result of a protective reflex stimulated by loud noise; *nerve supply*, facial. SYN musculus stapedius [TA].

sta·pe·dot·o·my (stā′pĕ-dot′ō-mē) A surgical technique for the improvement of hearing in otosclerosis: a hole is made in the footplate of the stapes bone through which is placed the piston-shaped end of a prosthesis, the other end of which is attached to the long process of the incus bone.

sta·pes, pl. **sta·pes, sta·pe·des** (stā′pēz, stā-pē′dēz) [TA] The smallest of the three auditory ossicles; its base, or footpiece, fits into the vestibular (oval) window, while its head is articulated with the lenticular process of the long limb of the incus. SYN stirrup. [Mod. L. stirrup]

sta·pes mo·bi·li·za·tion (stā′pēz mō′bi-lī-zā′shŭn) An operation to remobilize the footplate of the stapes to relieve conductive hearing impairment caused by its immobilization through otosclerosis or middle ear disease.

staph·y·lec·to·my (staf′i-lek′tŏ-mē) SYN uvulectomy. [staphyl- + G. *ektomē*, excision]

staph·yl·e·de·ma (staf′il-ĕ-dē′mă) Edema of the uvula. SYN staphyloedema. [staphyl- + G. *oidēma*, swelling (edema)]

staph·y·line (staf′i-līn) SYN botryoid.

sta·phyl·i·on (stă-fil′ē-on) The midpoint of the posterior edge of the hard palate; a craniometric point. [G. dim. of *staphylē*, a bunch of grapes]

staphylo-, staphyl- Combining forms indicating resemblance to a grape or a bunch of grapes, hence relating usually to staphylococci or to the uvula palatina. [G. *staphylē*, a bunch of grapes]

staphylococcaemia [Br.] SYN staphylococcemia.

staph·y·lo·coc·cal (staf′i-lō-kok′ăl) Relating to or caused by any organism of the genus *Staphylococcus*.

sta·phy·lo·coc·cal ble·pha·ri·tis (staf′i-lō-kok′ăl blef′ă-rī′tis) Inflammation of the eyelids characterized by brittle, hard scales along the base of the eyelashes.

sta·phy·lo·coc·cal en·ter·o·tox·in B (staf′i-lō-kok′ăl en′tĕr-ō-toks′in) A toxin produced by *Staphylococcus aureus* and developed as a military toxin agent designed to induce temporary incapacitation. Ingestion leads to a gastrointestinal syndrome, whereas respiratory effects predominate after inhalation. SEB is considered a Category B agent by the U.S. Centers for Disease Control and Prevention.

staph·y·lo·coc·ce·mi·a (staf′i-lō-kok-sē′mē-ă) The presence of staphylococci in the circulating blood. SYN staphylococcaemia. [staphylo- + G. *haima*, blood]

staph·y·lo·coc·ci (staf′i-lō-kok′sī) Plural of staphylococcus.

staph·y·lo·coc·co·sis, pl. **staph·y·lo·coc·co·ses** (staf′i-lō-kok-ō′sis, -sēz) Infection by species of the bacterium *Staphylococcus*.

Sta·phy·lo·coc·cus, pl. ***Sta·phy·lo·coc·ci*** (staf′i-lō-kok′ŭs, kok′sī) A genus of nonmotile, non-spore-forming, aerobic to facultatively anaerobic bacteria containing gram-positive, spheric cells that divide in more than one plane to form irregular clusters. Coagulase-positive strains produce a variety of toxins and therefore are potentially pathogenic and may cause food poisoning. They are found on the skin, in skin glands, on the nasal and other mucous membranes of warm-blooded animals, and in various food products. The type species is *Staphylococcus aureus*. [staphylo- + G. *kokkos*, a berry]

staph·y·lo·coc·cus, pl. **staph·y·lo·coc·ci** (staf′i-lō-kok′ŭs, kok′sī) A vernacular term used to refer to any member of the genus *Staphylococcus*.

Sta·phy·lo·coc·cus au·re·us (staf′i-lō-kok′ŭs aw-rā′ŭs) A bacterial common species found especially on nasal mucous membrane and skin (hair follicles); it causes furunculosis, cellulitis, pyemia, pneumonia, osteomyelitis, endocarditis, suppuration of wounds, other infections, and food poisoning; also a cause of infection in burn patients. Humans are the chief reservoir. The type species of the genus *Staphylococcus*. See page B4.

Sta·phy·lo·coc·cus sap·ro·phy·ti·cus (staf′i-lō-kok′ŭs sap-rō-fī′ti-kŭs) A bacterial species that has been associated with community-acquired urinary tract infections in young women who are sexually active; characterized in the laboratory as gram-positive cocci, but negative for catalase and coagulase.

***Sta·phy·lo·coc·cus* spe·cies, co·ag·u·lase-neg·a·tive** (staf′i-lō-kok′ŭs spē′shēz, kō-ag′yū-lās neg′ă-tiv) A group of bacterial species that includes a group of those present as normal flora of human skin, respiratory, and mucous membrane surfaces. Although a normal commensal, strains are prominent causes of nosocomial infections, especially in patients with implanted intravenous access devices; some strains form abscesses and cause diverse pathologic processes, such as sinusitis, wound infections, and osteomyelitis.

staph·y·lo·der·ma (staf′i-lō-dĕr′mă) Pyoderma due to staphylococci. [staphylo- + G. *derma*, skin]

staph·y·lo·der·ma·ti·tis (staf′i-lō-dĕr′mă-tī′tis) Inflammation of the skin due to the action of staphylococci.

staph·y·lo·di·al·y·sis (staf′i-lō-dī-al′i-sis) SYN

uvuloptosis. [staphylo- + G. *dialysis,* a separation]

staphyloedema [Br.] SYN staphyledema.

staph•y•lo•ki•nase (staf′i-lō-kī′nās) A microbial metalloenzyme from *Staphylococcus aureus,* with action similar to that of urokinase and streptokinase, that can convert plasminogen to plasmin but requires Ca^{2+}; separated in forms A, B, and C.

staph•y•lol•y•sin (staf′i-lol′i-sin) **1.** A hemolysin elaborated by a staphylococcus. **2.** An antibody causing lysis of staphylococci.

staph•y•lo•ma (staf′i-lō′mă) A bulging of the cornea or sclera containing uveal tissue. [staphylo- + G. *-ōma,* tumor]

staph•y•lo•ma•tous (staf′i-lō′mă-tŭs) Relating to or marked by staphyloma.

staph•y•lo•phar•yn•gor•rha•phy (staf′i-lō-far′in-gōr′ă-fē) Surgical repair of defects in the uvula or soft palate and the pharynx. SYN palatopharyngorrhaphy. [staphylo- + pharynx + G. *rhaphē,* suture]

staph•y•lo•plas•ty (staf′i-lō-plas-tē) SYN palatoplasty. [staphylo- + G. *plassō,* to form]

staph•y•lop•to•sis (staf′i-lop-tō′sis) SYN uvuloptosis. [staphylo- + G. *ptōsis,* a falling]

staph•y•lor•rha•phy (staf′i-lōr′ă-fē) SYN palatorrhaphy. [staphylo- + G. *rhaphē,* suture]

staph•y•lo•tox•in (staf′i-lō-tok′sin) The toxin elaborated by any species of *Staphylococcus.* [staphylo- + G. *toxikon,* poison]

stap•ling (stāp′ling) Use of a stapling that unites two tissues, such as the two ends of bowel, by applying a row or circle of staples.

star (stahr) Any stellate structure. SEE ALSO aster, astrosphere, stella, stellula. [A.S. *steorra*]

starch (stahrch) A high molecular weight polysaccharide built up of D-glucose residues in α-1,4 linkage, differing from cellulose in the presence of α- rather than β-glucoside linkages, that exists in most plant tissues; converted into dextrin when subjected to the action of dry heat, and into dextrin and D-glucose by amylases and glucoamylases in saliva and pancreatic juice; used as a dusting powder, an emollient, and an ingredient in medicinal tablets; chief storage carbohydrate in most higher plants. [A.S. *stearc,* strong]

star chick•weed (stahr chik′wēd) SYN chickweed.

star•flow•er (stahr′flow-ĕr) SYN borage.

Star•gardt dis•ease (stahr′gahrt di-zēz′) A hereditary macular dystrophy with macular degeneration; occurs during childhood.

Star•ling curve (stahr′ling kŭrv) A graph in which cardiac output or stroke volume is plotted against mean atrial or ventricular end-diastolic pressure; with increasing venous return and atrial pressure, the output proportionately increases until further increments overload the heart and the output falls. SYN Frank-Starling curve.

Star•ling hy•poth•e•sis (stahr′ling hī-poth′ĕ-sis) The principle that net filtration through capillary membranes is proportional to the transmembrane hydrostatic pressure difference minus the transmembrane oncotic pressure difference; although well established, it is called Starling hypothesis to distinguish it from Starling law of the heart.

Star•ling re•flex (stahr′ling rē′fleks) Tapping the volar surfaces of the fingers causes flexion of the fingers; analogous to Rossolimo reflex, for the toes.

star•tle dis•ease (stahr′tĕl di-zēz′) SYN hyperekplexia.

star•tle ep•i•lep•sy (stahr′tĕl ep′i-lep′sē) A form of reflex epilepsy precipitated by sudden noises.

star•tle re•flex (stahr′tĕl rē′fleks) **1.** The reflex response of an infant (contraction of the limb and neck muscles) when allowed to drop a short distance through the air or startled by a sudden noise or jolt. SYN parachute reflex. **2.** SYN cochleopalpebral reflex.

star•va•tion di•a•be•tes (stahr-vā′shŭn dī-ă-bē′tēz) After prolonged fasting, glycosuria following the ingestion of carbohydrate or glucose because of reduced output of insulin and/or reduced rate of glucose metabolism with a reduced ability to form glycogen.

starve (stahrv) **1.** To suffer from a lack of food. **2.** To deprive of food so as to cause suffering or death. **3.** Formerly, to die of cold. [A.S. *steorfan,* to die]

sta•sis, pl. **sta•ses** (stā′sis, -ēz) Stagnation of the blood or other fluids. [G. a standing still]

i **sta•sis der•ma•ti•tis** (stā′sis dĕr′mă-tī′tis) Erythema and scaling of the lower extremities due to impaired venous circulation; seen commonly in older women or secondary to deep vein thrombosis. See page 1474.

sta•sis ec•ze•ma (stā′sis ek′sĕ-mă) Eczematous eruption on legs due to or aggravated by venous stasis.

stat, **STAT** (stat) Referring to a diagnostic or therapeutic procedure that is to be performed immediately. [L. *statim,* immediately]

-stat Suffix denoting an agent intended to keep something from changing or moving. [G. *statēs,* stationary]

state (stāt) A condition, situation, or status. [L. *status,* condition, state]

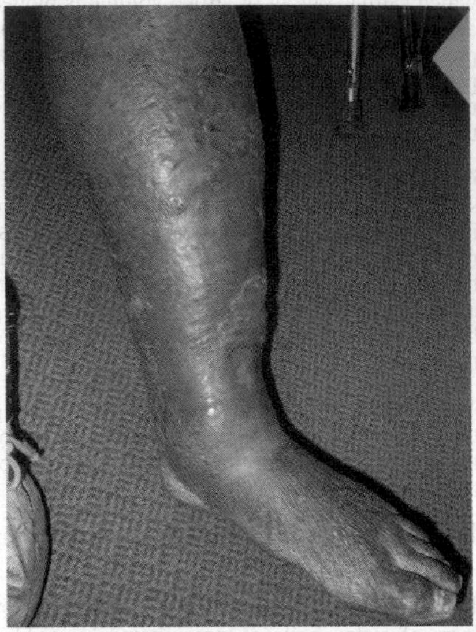

stasis dermatitis: leg

state-de•pen•dent learn•ing (stāt-dĕ-pen′dĕnt lĕrn′ing) learning during a specific state of sleep or wakefulness, or during a chemically altered state, where retrieval of learned information cannot be demonstrated unless the subject is restored to the state that originally existed during learning.

state•ment of i•den•ti•ty (stāt′mĕnt ī-den′ti-tē) A mandate of the F.D.A. that a food label prominently shall display the common name of a food.

State Nurs•es As•so•ci•a•tion (SNA) (stāt nŭrs′ĕz ă-sō′sē-ā′shŭn) An organization of the registered nurses within a state; each is a constituent of the national organization, the American Nurses Association.

sta•tic com•pli•ance (stat′ik kŏm-plī′ăns) **1.** The ratio of the change in volume of a distensible vessel to the change in distending pressure when the pressure change is measured between points in time when the system is at rest. **2.** The slope of the statically determined pressure-volume curve.

stat•ic ex•er•cise (stat′ik eks′ĕr-sīz) An exercise that passively takes a muscle to the point of tension for a short period of time or an extended period of at least 20 seconds. SYN static stretch.

stat•ic re•la•tion (stat′ik rē-lā′shŭn) Relationship between two parts that are not in motion.

stat•ic stretch (stat′ strech) SYN static exercise.

sta•tim (stā′tim) At once; immediately. [L.]

sta•tis•tics (stă-tis′tiks) **1.** A collection of numeric values, items of information, or other facts that are numerically grouped into definite classes and subject to analysis, particularly analysis of the probability that the resulting empiric findings are due to chance. **2.** The science and art of collecting, summarizing, and analyzing data that are subject to random variation.

stat•o•a•cou•stic (stat′ō-ă-kū′stik) Relating to equilibrium and hearing. SYN vestibulocochlear (2). [G. *statos,* standing, + *akoustikos,* acoustic]

stat•o•co•ni•a, sing. **stat•o•co•ni•um** (stat′ō-kō′nē-ă, -ŭm) [TA] SYN statoliths. [L. fr. G. *statos,* standing, *konis,* dust]

stat•o•ki•ne•tic re•flex (stat′ō-ki-net′ik rē′fleks) an action that, through stimulation of the receptors in the neck muscles and semicircular canals, brings about movements of the limbs and eyes appropriate to a given movement of the head in space.

stat•o•liths (stat′ŏ-liths) Crystalline particles of calcium carbonate and a protein adhering to the gelatinous membrane of the maculae of the utricle and saccule. SYN statoconia [TA], otoconia. [G. *statos,* standing, + *lithos,* stone]

stat•ure (stach′ŭr) The height of a person. [L. *statura,* fr. *statuo,* pp. *statutus,* to cause to stand]

sta•tus (stat′ŭs) A state or condition. [L. a way of standing]

sta•tus asth•ma•tic•us (stā′tus az-mat′ik-us) A condition of severe, prolonged asthma.

sta•tus ep•i•lep•tic•us (stā′tus ep-i-lep′tik-us) Repeated seizure, or a seizure prolonged for at least 30 minutes; may be convulsive (tonic-clonic), nonconvulsive (absence or complex partial), partial (epilepsia partialis continuans), or subclinical (electrographic status epilepticus).

Stauf•fer syn•drome (staw′fĕr sin′drōm) Abnormality of liver function test results, in the absence of metastatic disease, due to cholestasis in renal cell cancer patients.

stau•ri•on (stawr′ē-on) A craniometric point at the intersection of the median and transverse palatine sutures. [G. dim. of *stauros,* cross]

St. Ben•e•dict this•tle (sānt ben′ă-dikt this′ĕl) SYN blessed thistle.

STD Abbreviation for sexually transmitted disease.

stead•y state (s) (sted′ē stāt) **1.** A condition obtained in moderate muscular exercise when the removal of lactic acid by oxidation keeps pace with its production, the oxygen supply being adequate, and the muscles do not rely on energy from anaerobic sources. **2.** Any condition in which the formation or introduction of substances just keeps pace with their destruction or removal so that all volumes, concentrations, pressures, and flows remain constant. **3.** In enzyme kinetics, conditions such that the rate of change in the concentration of any enzyme species (e.g., free enzyme or the enzyme-substrate binary complex) is zero or much less than the rate of formation of product. Often subscript s or ss.

stead•y-state ex•er•cise, **stead•y-rate ex•er•cise** (sted′ē-stāt′ eks′ĕr-sīz, sted′ē-rāt′) Activity that achieves a balance between the energy required by working muscles and the rate of aerobic ATP production.

steal (stēl) Diversion of blood through alternate routes or reversed flow, from a vascularized tissue to one deprived by proximal arterial obstruction. [M.E. *stelen,* fr. A.S. *stelan*]

ste•ap•sin (stē-ap′sin) SYN triacylglycerol lipase.

ste•a•rate (stē′ă-rāt) A salt of stearic acid.

Stearns al•co•hol•ic a•men•ti•a (stĕrnz al′kŏ-hol′ik ā′men-shē-ă) A temporary alcoholic mental disorder resembling delirium tremens but lasting for a longer time and showing a greater degree of amnesia and other mental defects.

♻**stearo-**, **stear-** SYN steato-. [G. *stear,* tallow]

ste•a•ti•tis (stē′ă-tī′tis) Inflammation of adipose tissue. [G. *stear* (*steat-*), tallow, + *-itis,* inflammation]

♻**steato-** Combining form denoting fat. SYN stearo-, stear-. [G. *stear* (*steat-*), tallow]

ste•a•to•cys•to•ma (stē′ă-tō-sis-tō′mă) A cyst with sebaceous gland cells in its wall.

ste•a•tol•y•sis (stē′ă-tol′i-sis) The hydrolysis or emulsion of fat in the process of digestion. [steato- + G. *lysis,* dissolution]

ste•a•to•ly•tic (stē′ă-tō-lit′ik) Relating to steatolysis.

ste•a•to•ne•cro•sis (stē′ă-tō-nĕ-krō′sis) SYN fat necrosis. [steato- + G. *nekrōsis,* death]

ste•a•to•py•ga, **ste•a•to•py•gi•a** (stē′ă-top′i-gă, -ij′ē-ă) Excessive accumulation of fat on the buttocks. [steato- + G. *pygē,* buttocks]

ste•a•top•y•gous (stē′ă-top′i-gŭs) Having excessively fat buttocks.

ste•a•tor•rhe•a (stē′ă-tōr-ē′ă) Passage of fat in large amounts in the feces due to failure to digest and absorb it; occurs in pancreatic disease and the malabsorption syndromes; an absence of bile acids will increase steatorrhea. SYN steatorrhoea. [steato- + G. *rhoia,* a flow]

steatorrhoea [Br.] SYN steatorrhea.

ste•a•to•sis (stē′ă-tō′sis) **1.** SYN adiposis. **2.** SYN fatty degeneration. [steato- + G. *-osis,* condition]

Steell mur•mur (stēl mŭr′mŭr) SYN Graham Steell murmur.

steg•no•sis (steg-nō′sis) **1.** A stoppage of any of the secretions or excretions. **2.** A constriction or stenosis. [G. stoppage]

Stein•berg thumb sign (stīn′bĕrg thŭm sīn) In Marfan syndrome, when the thumb is held across the palm of the same hand, it projects well beyond the ulnar surface of the hand.

stein•stras•se (stīn′strah-sĕ) A complication of extracorporeal shock wave lithotripsy for urinary tract calculi in which stone fragments block the ureter to form a "stone street." [Ger. *Stein,* stone, + *Strasse,* street]

Stein test (stīn test) In cases of labyrinthine disease, the patient is unable to stand or to hop on one foot with eyes shut.

stel•la, pl. **stel•lae** (stel′ă, -ē) A star or star-shaped figure. [L.]

stel•late (stel′āt) Star-shaped. [L. *stella,* a star]

stel•late ab•scess (stel′āt ab′ses) A star-shaped necrotic area surrounded by histiocytes; seen within swollen inguinal lymph nodes in lymphogranuloma venereum.

stel•late block (stel′āt blok) Injection of local anesthetic solution in the vicinity of the stellate ganglion.

stel•late cell (stel′āt sel) A star-shaped cell, such as an astrocyte or Kupffer cell, that has many filaments extending radially.

stel•late frac•ture (stel′āt frak′shŭr) A fracture in which the lines of break radiate from a central point.

stel•late hair (stel′āt hār) Hair split in several strands at the free end.

stel•late re•tic•u•lum (stel′āt rĕ-tik′yū-lŭm) A network of epithelial cells disposed in a fluid-filled compartment in the center of the enamel organ between the outer and inner enamel epithelium.

stel•late veins (stel′āt vānz) SYN venulae stellatae.

stel•late ven•ules (stel′āt ven′yūlz) SYN venulae stellatae.

stel•lu•la, pl. **stel•lu•lae** (stel′yū-lă, -lē) A small star or star-shaped figure. [L. dim. of *stella,* star]

Stell•wag sign (stel′vahg sīn) Infrequent and incomplete blinking in Graves disease.

stem (stem) A supporting structure similar to the stalk of a plant.

stem cell (stem sel) **1.** Any precursor cell. **2.** A cell with daughter cells that may differentiate into other cell types.

stem cell fac•tor (stem sel fak′tŏr) A cytokine that promotes growth and differentiation of hematopoietic stem cells into a variety of cell lineages.

stem cell leu•ke•mi•a (stem sel lū-kē′mē-ă) A form of leukemia in which the abnormal cells are thought to be the precursors of lymphoblasts, myeloblasts, or monoblasts. SYN embryonal leukemia.

ste•ni•on (sten′ē-on) The termination in either temporal fossa of the shortest transverse diameter of the skull; a craniometric point. [G. *stenos,* narrow, + dim. *-iōn*]

steno- Combining form meaning narrowness, constriction; opposite of eury-. [G. *stenos,* narrow]

sten•o•car•dia (sten′ō-kahr′dē-ă) SYN angina pectoris. [steno- + G. *kardia,* heart]

sten•o•ceph•a•lous, **sten•o•ce•phal•ic** (sten′ō-sef′ă-lŭs, -se-fal′ik) Pertaining to, or characterized by, stenocephaly.

sten•o•ceph•a•ly (sten′ō-sef′ă-lē) Marked narrowness of the head. [steno- + G. *kephalē,* head]

sten•o•cho•ri•a (sten′ō-kōr′ē-ă) Abnormal contraction of any canal or orifice, especially of the lacrimal ducts. [G. *stenochōria,* narrowness, fr. steno- + *chōra,* place, room]

sten•o•pe•ic, **sten•o•pa•ic** (sten′ō-pē′ik, -pā′ik) Provided with a narrow opening or slit, as in stenopeic spectacles. [steno- + G. *opē,* opening]

sten•os•al mur•mur (sten-ō′săl mŭr′mŭr) An arterial murmur due to narrowing of the vessel from pressure or organic change.

ste•nosed (sten′ōst) Narrowed; contracted: strictured.

sten•os•ing ten•o•syn•o•vi•tis (sten-ō′sing ten′ō-sin-ō-vī′tis) Inflammation of a tendon and its sheath resulting in contracture of the sheath causing an obstruction of tendon gliding; can be a cause of trigger-finger conditions.

ste•no•sis, pl. **ste•no•ses** (stĕ-nō′sis, -sēz) A stricture of any canal, especially a narrowing of one of the cardiac valves. [G. *stenōsis,* a narrowing]

sten•o•sto•mi•a (sten′ō-stō′mē-ă) Narrowness of the oral cavity. [steno- + G. *stoma,* mouth]

sten•o•ther•mal (sten′ō-thĕr′măl) Thermostable through a narrow temperature range; able to withstand only slight changes in temperature. [steno- + G. *thermē,* heat]

sten•o•thor•ax (sten′ō-thōr′aks) A narrow, contracted chest. [steno- + thorax]

ste•not•ic (sten-ot′ik) Narrowed; affected with stenosis.

Ste•no•tro•pho•mo•nas (sten′ō-trō-fō-mōn′as) A genus of gram-negative bacilli that typically reside in soil and water and are not a part of normal human flora.

Ste•no•tro•pho•mo•nas mal•to•phi•li•a (sten′ō-trō-fō-mō′nas mal′tō-fil′ē-ă) An opportunistic, ocular, bacterial pathogen producing keratitis, keratopathy, and conjunctivitis; a gram-negative, non-spore-bearing rod. A nosocomial pathogen, of special importance in intensive care units in part because of its resistance to most penicillins and to cephalosporins and aminoglycosides. Formerly called *Xanthomonas maltophilia* and *Pseudomonas maltophilia.*

Sten•sen duct, **Sten•o duct** (sten′sen dŭkt, sten′ō) SYN parotid duct.

stent (stent) **1.** Device used to maintain a bodily orifice or cavity during skin grafting, or to immobilize a skin graft after placement. **2.** Slender thread, rod, or catheter, lying within the lumen of tubular structures, used to provide support during or after their anastomosis, or to assure patency of an intact but contracted lumen. See this page. [C. *Stent*]

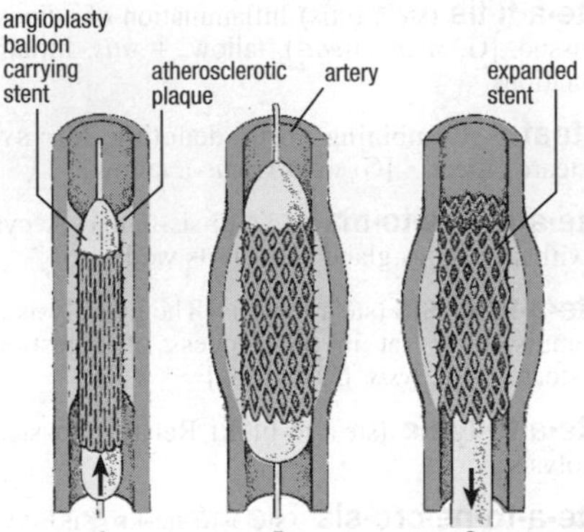

vascular stent: (A) balloon catheter positions stent at site of arterial stenosis; (B) inflation of balloon dilates artery and expands stent; (C) balloon is withdrawn, leaving expanded stent in position

stent•ing (stent′ing) Insertion or application of a stent (an appliance or material intended to support a graft or keep a passage open).

step (step) **1.** DENTISTRY a dovetailed or similarly shaped projection of a cavity prepared in a tooth into a surface perpendicular to the main part of the cavity for the purpose of preventing displacement of the restoration (filling) by the force of mastication. **2.** A change in direction resembling a stairstep in a line, a surface, or the construction of a solid body.

step-down trans•form•er (step′down trans-fōr′mĕr) Device used in radiology to decrease the voltage coming into the x-ray tube.

ste•pha•ni•al (stĕ-fā′nē-ăl) Pertaining to the stephanion.

ste•pha•ni•on (stĕ-fā′nē-on) A craniometric point where the coronal suture intersects the inferior temporal line. [G. dim. of *stephanos,* crown]

step•page gait (step′ăj gāt) A gait in which the advancing foot is lifted higher than usual so that it can clear the ground, because it cannot be dorsiflexed. Seen with peroneal neuropathies and other disorders causing foot dorsiflexion weakness. SEE ALSO high-steppage gait.

step-up trans•form•er (step′ŭp trans-fōr′mĕr) Device used in radiology to increase the voltage coming into an x-ray tube.

sterco- Combining form denoting feces. SEE ALSO copro-, scato-. [L. *stercus,* excrement]

ster•co•bi•lin (stĕr′kō-bī′lin) A brown degradation product of hemoglobin, present in the feces. SEE ALSO bilirubinoids.

ster•co•lith (stĕr′kō-lith) SYN coprolith. [sterco- + G. *lithos,* stone]

ster•co•ra•ceous, ster•co•ral, ster•co•rous (stĕr′kōr-ā′shŭs, -ăl, -ŭs) Relating to or containing feces.

ster•co•ra•ceous vom•it•ing (stĕr′kōr-ā′shŭs vom′it-ing) SYN fecal vomiting.

ster•co•ral ab•scess (stĕr′kōr-ăl ab′ses) A collection of pus and feces. SYN fecal abscess.

ster•co•ral ul•cer (stĕr′kōr-ăl ŭl′sĕr) An ulcer of the colon due to pressure and irritation of retained fecal masses.

ster•co•ro•ma (stĕr′kōr-ō′mă) SYN coproma. [sterco- + G. *-oma,* tumor]

ster•cus (stĕr′kŭs) SYN feces. [L. feces, excrement]

stereo- (ster′ē-ō) **1.** Combining form denoting a solid; a solid condition or state. **2.** Combining form denoting spatial qualities, three-dimensionality. [G. *stereos,* solid]

ster•e•o•ar•throl•y•sis (ster′ē-ō-ahr-throl′i-sis) Production of a new joint with mobility in cases of bony ankylosis. [stereo- + G. *arthron,* joint, + *lysis,* loosening]

ster•e•o•cam•pim•e•ter (ster′ē-ō-kam-pim′ĕ-tĕr) An apparatus for studying the central visual fields while the fellow eye holds fixation. [stereo- + L. *campus,* field, + G. *metron,* measure]

ster•e•o•chem•i•cal (ster′ē-ō-kem′i-kăl) Relating to stereochemistry.

ster•e•o•chem•i•cal for•mu•la (ster′ē-ō-kem′i-kăl fōrm′yū-lă) A chemical formula in which the arrangement of the atoms or atomic groupings in space is indicated.

ster•e•o•chem•is•try (ster′ē-ō-kem′is-trē) The branch of chemistry concerned with the spatial three-dimensional relations of atoms in molecules, i.e., the positions the atoms in a compound bear in relation to one another in space.

ster•e•o•e•lec•tro•en•ceph•a•log•ra•phy (ster′ē-ō-ĕ-lek′trō-en-sef′ă-log′ră-fē) Recording of electrical activity in three planes of the brain, i.e., with surface and depth electrodes.

ster•e•o•en•ceph•a•lom•e•try (ster′ē-ō-en-sef′ă-lom′ĕ-trē) Localization of brain structures by use of three-dimensional coordinates.

ster•e•o•en•ceph•a•lot•o•my (ster′ē-ō-en-sef′ă-lot′ō-mē) SYN stereotaxy. [stereo- + G. *encephalos,* brain, + *tomē,* a cutting]

ster•e•og•no•sis (ster′ē-og-nō′sis) The appreciation of the form of an object by means of touch. [stereo- + G. *gnōsis,* knowledge]

ster•e•og•nos•tic (ster′ē-og-nos′tik) Relating to stereognosis.

ster•e•o•i•so•mer (ster′ē-ō-ī′sō-mĕr) A molecule containing the same number and kind of atom groupings as another but in a different arrangement in space, in virtue of which it exhibits different optic properties, e.g., as between D and L amino acids, 5α and 5β steroids. Cf. isomer. [stereo- + G. *isos,* equal, + *meros,* part]

ster•e•o•i•so•mer•ic (ster′ē-ō-ī-sō-mer′ik) Relating to stereoisomerism.

ster•e•o•i•som•er•ism (ster′ē-ō-ī-som′ĕr-izm) Molecular asymmetry; isomerism involving different spatial arrangements of the same groups. SEE ALSO stereoisomer.

ster•e•om•e•try (ster′ē-om′ĕ-trē) **1.** Measurement of a solid object or the cubic capacity of a vessel. **2.** Determination of the specific gravity of a liquid.

ster•e•op•a•thy (ster′ē-op′ă-thē) Persistent stereotyped thinking.

ste•re•op•sis (ster′ē-op′sis) Depth perception (three-dimensional vision) provided by fusion of binocular images. SEE ALSO depth perception. SYN three-dimensional vision.

ster•e•o•ra•di•og•ra•phy (ster′ē-ō-rā′dē-og′ră-fē) Preparation of a pair of radiographs with appropriate shift of the x-ray tube or film so that the images can be viewed stereoscopically to give a three-dimensional appearance.

ster•e•o•scop•ic (ster′ē-ō-skop′ik) Relating to a stereoscope, or giving the appearance of three dimensions.

ster•e•o•scop•ic mi•cro•scope (ster′ē-ō-skop′ik mī′krō-skōp) A microscope having double eyepieces and objectives and thus independent light paths, giving a three-dimensional image.

ster•e•o•scop•ic vi•sion (ster′ē-ō-skop′ik vizh′ŭn) The single perception of a slightly different image from each eye.

ster•e•os•co•py (ster′ē-os′kŏ-pē) An optic technique by which two images of the same object are blended into one, giving a three-dimensional appearance to the single image.

ster•e•o•tac•tic, ster•e•o•tax•ic (ster′ē-ō-tak′tik, -sik) Relating to stereotaxis or stereotaxy.

ster•e•o•tac•tic bra•chy•ther•a•py (ster′ē-ō-tak′tik brak′ē-thār′ă-pē) Radiotherapy delivered with the help of CT-guided tissue localization.

ster•e•o•tac•tic in•stru•ment, ster•e•o•tax•ic in•stru•ment (ster′ē-ō-tak′tik in′strŭ-mĕnt, ster′ē-ō-tak′sik) An apparatus attached to the head, used to localize an area in the brain precisely by means of coordinates related to intracerebral structures.

ster•e•o•tac•tic sur•ger•y, ster•e•o•tax•ic sur•ger•y (ster′ē-ō-tak′tik sŭr′jĕr-ē, ster′ē-ō-tak′sik) SYN stereotaxy.

ster•e•o•tax•is (ster′ē-ō-tak′sis) **1.** Three-dimensional arrangement. **2.** Stereotropism, but applied more exactly when the organism as a whole, rather than a part only, reacts. **3.** SYN stereotaxy. [stereo- + G. *taxis,* orderly arrangement]

ster•e•o•tax•y (ster′ē-ō-tak′sē) A precise method of destroying deep-seated brain structures located by use of three-dimensional coordinates. SYN stereoencephalotomy, stereotactic surgery, stereotaxic surgery, stereotaxis (3).

ster•e•o•tro•pic (ster′ē-ō-trō′pik) Relating to or exhibiting stereotropism.

ster•e•ot•ro•pism (ster′ē-o′trō-pizm) Growth or movement of a plant or animal toward (positive stereotropism) or away from (negative stereotropism) a solid body, usually applied when a part of the organism rather than the whole reacts. [stereo- + G. *tropos,* a turning]

ster•e•o•ty•py (ster′ē-ō-tī-pē) **1.** Maintenance of one attitude for a long period. **2.** Constant repetition of certain meaningless gestures or movements, as in certain forms of schizophrenia. [stereo- + G. *typos,* impression, type]

ste•ric (ster′ik) Pertaining to stereochemistry.

ster•ile (ster′il) Relating to or characterized by sterility. [L. *sterilis,* barren]

ster•ile cyst (ster′il sist) A hydatid cyst without brood capsules or viable protoscoleces.

ste•ril•i•ty (stĕr-il′i-tē) **1.** In general, the incapability of fertilization or reproduction. **2.** Condition of being aseptic, or free from all living microorganisms and their spores. [L. *sterilitas*]

ster•il•i•za•tion (ster′i-lī-zā′shŭn) **1.** The act or process by which an individual is rendered incapable of fertilization or reproduction, as by vasectomy, partial salpingectomy, or castration. **2.** The destruction of all microorganisms in or about an object, as by steam (flowing or pressurized), chemical agents (alcohol, phenol, heavy metals, ethylene oxide gas), high-velocity electron bombardment, or ultraviolet light radiation.

ster•il•ize (ster′i-līz) To produce sterility.

ster•il•iz•er (ster′i-lī-zĕr) An apparatus for rendering objects sterile.

ster•na (stĕr′nă) Plural of sternum.

ster•nal (stĕr′năl) Relating to the sternum.

ster•nal an•gle (stĕr′năl ang′gĕl) The angle between the manubrium and the body of the sternum at the manubriosternal junction. Marks the level of the second costal cartilage (rib) for counting ribs or intercostal spaces. Denotes level of aortic arch, bifurcation of trachea, and T4-T5 intervertebral disc. SYN angulus sterni [TA], Louis angle, Ludwig angle.

ster•nal•gi•a (stĕr-nal′jē-ă) Pain in the sternum or the sternal region. SYN sternodynia. [stern- + G. *algos,* pain]

ster•na•lis mus•cle (stĕr-nā′lis mŭs′ĕl) An inconstant muscle, running parallel to the sternum across the costosternal origin of the pectoralis major, and usually connected with the sternocleidomastoid and rectus abdominis muscles due to their common development source. SYN musculus sternalis [TA], sternal muscle.

ster•nal line (stĕr′năl līn) A vertical line corresponding to the lateral margin of the sternum. SYN linea sternalis [TA].

ster•nal mus•cle (stĕr′năl mŭs′ĕl) SYN sternalis muscle.

ster•nal plane (stĕr′năl plān) A plane indicated by the front surface of the sternum.

ster•nal punc•ture (stĕr′năl pungk′shŭr) Removal of bone marrow from the manubrium by needle.

ster•ne•bra, pl. **ster•ne•brae** (stĕr′nē-bră, -brē) One of the four segments of the primordial sternum of the embryo by the fusion of which the body of the adult sternum is formed. [Mod. L. fr. stern(um) + (vert)ebra]

♻ **sterno-, stern-** Combining forms denoting the sternum, sternal. [G. *sternon,* chest]

ster•no•cla•vic•u•lar (stĕr′nō-klă-vik′yū-lăr) Relating to the sternum and the clavicle.

ster•no•cla•vic•u•lar an•gle (stĕr′nō-klă-vik′yū-lăr ang′gĕl) The angle formed by the junction of the clavicle with the sternum.

ster•no•cla•vic•u•lar joint (stĕr′nō-klă-vik′yū-lăr joynt) The synovial articulation between the medial end of the clavicle and the manubrium of the sternum and cartilage of the first rib.

ster•no•clei•do•mas•toid (stĕr′nō-klī′dō-mas′toyd) Relating to sternum, clavicle, and mastoid process.

ster•no•clei•do•mas•toid mus•cle (SCM) (stĕr′nō-klī′dō-mas′toyd mŭs′ĕl) *Origin*, by two heads from anterior surface of manubrium of the sternum and sternal end of clavicle; *insertion*, mastoid process and lateral half of superior nuchal line; *action*, turns head obliquely to opposite side; when acting together, flex the neck and extend the head; *nerve supply*, motor by accessory, sensory by cervical plexus. SYN musculus sternocleidomastoideus [TA], sternomastoid muscle.

ster•no•clei•do•mas•toid vein (stĕr′nō-klī′dō-mas′toyd vān) *Origin*, arises in the sternocleidomastoid muscle and accompanies the sternocleidomastoid branch of the occipital artery; it drains into the internal jugular or superior thyroid vein.

ster•no•cos•tal (stĕr′nō-kos′tăl) Relating to the sternum and the ribs. [L. *costa,* rib]

ster•no•dyn•i•a (stĕr′nō-din′ē-ă) SYN sternalgia. [sterno- + G. *odynē,* pain]

ster•no•glos•sal (stĕr′nō-glos′ăl) Denoting muscular fibers that occasionally pass from the sternohyoid muscle to join the hyoglossal muscle.

ster•no•hy•oid mus•cle (stĕr′nō-hī′oyd mŭs′ĕl) *Origin*, posterior surface of manubrium sterni and first costal cartilage; *insertion*, body of hyoid bone; *action*, depresses hyoid bone; *nerve supply*, upper cervical through spinal nerves (ansa cervicalis). SYN musculus sternohyoideus [TA].

ster•noid (stĕr′noyd) Resembling the sternum. [sterno- + G. *eidos,* resemblance]

ster•no•mas•toid mus•cle (stĕr′nō-mas′toyd mŭs′ĕl) SYN sternocleidomastoid muscle.

ster•no•pa•gi•a (stĕr′nō-pā′jē-ă) Condition shown by conjoined twins united at the sterna or more extensively at the ventral walls of the thorax. SEE ALSO conjoined twins. [sterno- + G. *pagos,* something fixed]

ster•no•per•i•car•di•al (stĕr′nō-per′i-kahr′dē-ăl) Relating to the sternum and the pericardium.

ster•nos•chi•sis (stĕr-nos′ki-sis) Congenital cleft of the sternum. [sterno- + G. *schisis,* a cleaving]

ster•no•thy•roid mus•cle (ster′nō-thī′royd mŭs′ĕl) *Origin*, posterior surface of manubrium of sternum and first or second costal cartilage; *insertion*, oblique line of thyroid cartilage; *action*, depresses larynx; *nerve supply*, upper cervical via spinal nerves (ansa cervicalis). SYN musculus sternothyroideus [TA].

ster•not•o•my (stĕr-not′ŏ-mē) Incision into or through the sternum. [sterno- + G. *tomē,* incision]

ster•no•ver•te•bral (stĕr′nō-vĕr′tĕ-brăl) Relating to the sternum and the vertebrae; denoting the true ribs, or the seven upper ribs on either side, which articulate with the vertebrae and with the sternum. SYN vertebrosternal.

Stern pos•ture (stĕrn pos′chŭr) A supine position with the head extended and lowered over the end of the table, by which the murmur is developed or made more distinct in cases of tricuspid insufficiency.

ster•num, gen. **ster•ni**, pl. **ster•na** (stĕr′nŭm, -nī, -nă) [TA] A long, flat bone, articulating with the cartilages of the first seven ribs and with the clavicle, that forms the middle part of the anterior wall of the thorax; it consists of three portions: the corpus or body, the manubrium, and the xiphoid process. SYN breast bone. [Mod. L. fr. G. *sternon,* the chest]

ster•nu•ta•tion (stĕr′nū-tā′shŭn) The act of sneezing. [L. *sternutatio,* fr. *sternuo (sternuto),* pp. *sternutatus,* to sneeze]

ster•oid (ster′oyd) **1.** Pertaining to the steroids. SYN steroidal. Cf. steroids. **2.** Generic designation for compounds closely related in structure to the steroids, such as sterols, bile acids, cardiac glycosides, and precursors of the D vitamins. Cf. bioregulator.

ster•oid ac•ne (ster′oyd ak′nē) Folliculitis similar to acne vulgaris, but resulting from topical or oral administration of steroids; comedones are rare.

ster•oi•dal (ster-oy′dăl) SYN steroid (1).

ster•oid cell tu•mor (ster′oyd sel tū′mŏr) A collective term used for ovarian tumors composed of cells resembling steroid-secreting lutein cells; comprises several tumors such as stromal luteoma, Leydig cell tumor, and steroid cell tumor not otherwise specified; hormonally active; may be benign or malignant.

ster•oid hor•mones (ster′oyd hor′mōnz) Those hormones possessing the steroid ring system (e.g., androgens, estrogens, adrenocortical hormones).

ster•oid•o•gen•e•sis (ster-oy′dō-jen′ĕ-sis) The formation of steroids; commonly referring to the biologic synthesis of steroid hormones, but not to the production of such compounds in a chemical laboratory. [steroid + G. *genesis,* production]

ster•oids (ster′oydz) A large family of chemical substances, comprising many hormones, body constituents, and drugs, each containing the tetracyclic cyclopenta[*a*]phenanthrene skeleton.

ster•oid ul•cer (ster′oyd ŭl′sĕr) A lesion, usually on the leg or foot, developing from a wound in patients undergoing long-term steroid therapy;

results from the wound-healing inhibitory effects characteristic of steroids.

ster·ol (ster′ol) A steroid with one OH (alcohol) group; the systematic names contain either the prefix hydroxy- or the suffix -ol, e.g., cholesterol, ergosterol.

ster·tor (stĕr′tōr) A noisy inspiration occurring in coma or deep sleep, sometimes due to obstruction of the larynx or upper airways. [L. *sterto,* to snore]

ster·to·rous (stĕr′tōr-ŭs) Relating to or characterized by stertor or snoring.

♻**stetho-, steth-** Combining forms denoting the chest. [G. *stēthos*]

steth·o·go·ni·om·e·ter (steth′ō-gō′nē-om′ĕ-tĕr) An apparatus for measuring the curvatures of the thorax. [stetho- + G. *gōnia,* angle, + *metron,* measure]

steth·o·scope (steth′ŏ-skōp) An instrument originally devised by Laënnec for aid in hearing the respiratory and cardiac sounds in the chest, but now modified in various ways and used in auscultation of any of vascular or other sounds anywhere in the body. [stetho- + G. *skopeō,* to view]

steth·o·scop·ic (steth′ŏ-skop′ik) **1.** Relating to or effected by means of a stethoscope. **2.** Relating to an examination of the chest.

ste·thos·co·py (stĕ-thos′kŏ-pē) **1.** Examination of the chest by means of auscultation, either mediate or immediate, and percussion. **2.** Mediate auscultation with the stethoscope.

steth·o·spasm (steth′ō-spazm) Spasm of the chest.

Ste·vens-John·son syn·drome (stē′vĕnz jon′sŏn sin′drōm) A bullous form of erythema multiforme that may be extensive, involving the mucous membranes and large areas of the body; it may produce serious subjective symptoms and may be fatal.

Ste·vi·o·si·de·a (stē′vē-ō-sid′ē-ă) Dietary supplement made from the leaves of *Stevia rebaudiana*, a South American shrub. It is used as an unapproved dietary sweetener.

Stew·art-Holmes sign (stū′ărt hōlmz sīn) In cerebellar disease, the inability to check a movement when passive resistance is suddenly released. SYN rebound phenomenon (1).

Stew·art test (stū′ărt test) Estimation of the amount of collateral circulation, in case of an aneurysm of the main artery of a limb, by means of a calorimeter.

Stew·art-Treves syn·drome (stū′ărt trēvz sin′drōm) Angiosarcoma arising in an arm affected by postmastectomy lymphedema.

sthe·ni·a (sthē′nē-ă) A condition of activity and apparent force, as in an acute sthenic fever. [G. *sthenos,* strength, + *-ia,* condition]

sthen·ic (sthen′ik) **1.** Active; marked by sthenia; said of a fever with strong bounding pulse, high temperature, and active delirium. **2.** Pertaining to a habitus characterized by moderate overdevelopment of skeletal muscle.

♻**stheno-** Prefix indicating strength, force, power. [G. *sthenos*]

STI Abbreviation for signal transduction inhibitor; sexually transmitted infection.

stib·i·al·ism (stib′ē-ăl-izm) Chronic antimonial poisoning. [L. *stibium,* antimony]

Stick·ler syn·drome (stik′lĕr sin′drōm) SYN hereditary progressive arthroophthalmopathy.

stick·le·wort (stik′ĕl-wōrt) SYN agrimony.

stick·y-end·ed DNA (stik′ē end′ĕd) Double-stranded DNA in which one of the strands extends beyond the other strand (i.e., has a number of unpaired bases) at one end or both.

stiff neck (stif nek) Nonspecific term for limited neck mobility, often due to muscle cramps and spasm accompanied by pain.

stiff-per·son syn·drome (stif′pĕr-sŏn sin′drōm) A rare disorder manifested clinically by the continuous isometric contraction of many of the somatic muscles; contractions are usually forceful and painful and most frequently involve the trunk musculature, although limb muscles may be involved. This is an autoimmune disease, with circulating antibodies against the GABA-synthesizing enzyme and glutamic acid decarboxylase, among other types of antibodies present.

stig·ma, pl. **stig·mas**, **stig·ma·ta** (stig′mă, -măz, -mă-tă) **1.** Visible evidence of a disease. **2.** SYN follicular stigma. **3.** Any spot or blemish on the skin. **4.** A bleeding spot on the skin, which is considered a manifestation of conversion hysteria. **5.** The orange-pigmented eyespot of certain chlorophyll-bearing protozoa, such as *Euglena viridis*, which serves as a light filter by absorbing certain wavelengths. **6.** A mark of shame or discredit. [G. a mark. fr. *stizō,* to prick]

stig·mal plates (stig′măl plāts) Area in arthropod larvae where the tracheal system opens to the outside; morphology of this area is used to identify various arthropod larvae.

stig·mat·ic (stig-mat′ik) Relating to or marked by a stigma.

stig·ma·tism (stig′mă-tizm) The condition of having a stigma. SYN stigmatization (1).

stig·ma·ti·za·tion (stig′mă-tī-zā′shŭn) **1.** SYN stigmatism. **2.** Production of stigmas, especially of a hysteric nature. **3.** Debasement of a person by the attribution of a negatively toned characteristic or other stigma.

stil•bene (stil′bēn) **1.** An unsaturated hydrocarbon, the nucleus of stilbestrol and other synthetic estrogenic compounds. **2.** A class of compounds based on stilbene (1).

stilboestrol (stil-bes′trol) [Br.] SYN diethylstilbestrol.

still•birth (stil′bĭrth) The birth of an infant who has died before delivery.

still•born (stil′bōrn) Born dead; denoting an infant dead at birth.

still•born in•fant (stil′bōrn in′fănt) A newborn who shows no evidence of life after birth. Cf. liveborn infant.

Still dis•ease (stil di-zēz′) A form of juvenile chronic arthritis (formerly juvenile rheumatoid arthritis) characterized by high fever and signs of systemic illness that can exist for months before the onset of arthritis.

still lay•er (stil lā′ĕr) The layer of the bloodstream in the capillary vessels, next to the wall of the vessel, which flows slowly and transports the white blood cells along the layer wall, whereas in the center the flow is rapid and transports the red blood cells. SYN Poiseuille space.

Still mur•mur (stil mŭr′mŭr) An innocent musical midsystolic murmur resembling the noise produced by a twanging string; almost exclusively in young children, of uncertain origin and ultimately disappearing.

stim•u•lant (stim′yū-lănt) **1.** Stimulating; exciting to action. **2.** An agent that arouses organic activity, strengthens the action of the heart, increases vitality, and promotes a sense of well-being; classified according to the parts on which it chiefly acts: cardiac, respiratory, gastric, hepatic, cerebral, spinal, vascular, or genital. SYN stimulator. SEE ALSO stimulus. [L. *stimulans,* pres. p. of *stimulo,* pp. *-atus,* to goad, incite, fr. *stimulus,* a goad]

stim•u•la•tion (stim′yŭ-lā′shŭn) **1.** Arousal of the body or any of its parts or organs to increased functional activity. **2.** The condition of being stimulated. **3.** NEUROPHYSIOLOGY the application of a stimulus to a responsive structure, such as a nerve or muscle, regardless of whether the strength of the stimulus is sufficient to produce excitation. SEE ALSO stimulant.

stim•u•la•tor (stim′yū-lā-tŏr) SYN stimulant (2).

stim•u•lus, pl. **stim•u•li** (stim′yū-lŭs, -lī) **1.** A stimulant. **2.** That which can elicit or evoke action (response) in a muscle, nerve, gland or other excitable tissue, or cause an augmenting action on any function or metabolic process. [L. a goad]

stim•u•lus con•trol (stim′yū-lŭs kŏn-trōl′) The use of conditioning techniques to bring the target behavior of an individual under environmental control.

stim•u•lus sen•si•tive my•o•clo•nus (stim′yū-lŭs sen′si-tiv mī-ok′lō-nŭs) Contractions induced by a variety of stimuli (e.g., talking, calculation, loud noises, tapping).

sting (sting) **1.** Sharp momentary pain, most commonly produced by puncture of the skin by many species of arthropods, including hexapods, myriapods, and arachnids; can also be produced by jellyfish, sea urchins, sponges, mollusks, and several species of venomous fish, such as the stingray, toadfish, rabbitfish, and catfish. SEE ALSO bites. **2.** The venom apparatus of a stinging animal, consisting of a chitinous spicule or bony spine and a venom gland or sac. **3.** To introduce (or the process of introducing) a venom by stinging. See page B8. [O.E. *stingan*]

sting•ing cat•er•pil•lar (sting′ing kat′ĕr-pil-ĕr) A caterpillar with urticarious hairs or spines that cause allergic dermatitis, e.g., the Io moth and the puss caterpillar.

stink•ing ben•ja•min (stingk′ing ben′jă-min) SYN trillium.

stip•pling (stip′ling) **1.** A speckling of a blood cell or other structure with fine dots when exposed to the action of a basic stain, due to the presence of free basophil granules in the cell protoplasm. **2.** An orange-peel appearance of the attached gingiva, which is a normal adaptive process; its absence or reduction indicates gingival disease. **3.** A roughening of the surfaces of a denture base to stimulate natural gingival stippling.

Stir•ling mod•i•fi•ca•tion of Gram stain (stĭrl′ing mod′i-fi-kā′shŭn gram stān) A stable aniline-crystal violet stain.

stir•rup (stĭr′ŭp) SYN stapes. [A.S. *stīrāp*]

stitch (stich) **1.** A sharp, sticking pain of momentary duration. **2.** A single suture. **3.** SYN suture (2). [A.S. *stice,* a pricking]

stitch ab•scess (stich ab′ses) A purulent lesion around a suture.

St. John's wort (sānt jonz wōrt) Any of various herbs or shrubs of the genus *Hypericum,* used as a treatment for mild depression in alternative medicine.

St. Lou•is en•ceph•a•li•tis vi•rus (sānt lū′is en-sef′ă-lī′tis vī′rŭs) A group B arbovirus often causing inapparent infection but sometimes encephalitis; the virus has been isolated from birds and from several mosquito species, especially *Psorophora.*

STM Abbreviation for short-term memory.

sto•chas•tic (stō-kas′tik) **1.** Random. **2.** RADIATION THERAPY pertaining to the effects of radiation seen in the person exposed to such radiation. This does not have a dose threshold, given that as the dosage increases so does the severity of the reaction. [G. *stochos,* target, guess]

stock cul•ture (stok kŭl′chŭr) A culture of a

microorganism maintained solely for the purpose of keeping the microorganism in a viable condition by subculture, as necessary, into fresh medium.

Stock·er line (stok′ĕr līn) A fine line of pigment secondary to iron deposition in the corneal epithelium near the head of a pterygium.

Stock·holm syn·drome (stok′hōlm sin′drōm) A form of bonding between a captive and captor in which the captive begins to identify with, and may even sympathize with, the captor. [*Stockholm*, Sweden, where early cases reported]

stock·ing (stok′ing) A garment worn on the leg and foot. [M.E. *stokke*]

stock·ing an·es·the·si·a (stok′ing an′es-thē′zē-ă) Loss of sensation in the distal lower extremity (i.e., the foot and toes).

stock vac·cine (stok vak-sēn′) A vaccine made from a stock microbial strain, in contradistinction to an autogenous vaccine.

Stof·fel op·er·a·tion (stof′el op-ĕr-ā′shŭn) Division of certain motor nerves for the relief of spastic paralysis.

stoi·chi·ol·o·gy (stoy′kē-ol′-ŏ-jē) [Br.] The study of the elements of any branch of knowledge.

stoi·chi·o·met·ric (stoy′kē-ō-met′rik) Pertaining to stoichiometry.

sto·i·chi·o·met·ric num·ber (v) (stoy′kē-ō-met′rik nŭm′bĕr) The number associated with a reactant or product participating in a defined chemical reaction; usually an integer.

stoi·chi·om·e·try (stoy′kē-om′ĕ-trē) Determination of the relative quantities of the substances concerned in any chemical reaction, e.g., with the laws of definite proportions in chemistry, as in the molar proportions in a reaction. [G. *stoicheion*, element, + *metron*, measure]

stoke (stōk) A unit of kinematic viscosity, that of a fluid with a viscosity of 1 poise and a density of 1 g/mL; equal to 10^{-4} square meter per second.

Stokes-Ad·ams syn·drome (stōks ad′ămz sin′drōm) SYN Adams-Stokes syndrome.

Stokes am·pu·ta·tion (stōks amp′yū-tā′shŭn) A modification of the Gritti-Stokes amputation in that the line of section of the femur is slightly higher.

Stokes law (stōks law) **1.** A muscle lying above an inflamed mucous or serous membrane is frequently the seat of paralysis. **2.** A relationship of the rate of fall of a small sphere in a viscous fluid; applicable to centrifugation of macromolecules. **3.** The wavelength of light emitted by a fluorescent material is longer than that of the radiation used to excite the fluorescence.

sto·ma, pl. **sto·mas**, **sto·ma·ta** (stō′mă, -măz, -mă-tă) **1.** A minute opening or pore. **2.** An artificial opening between two cavities or canals, or between such and the surface of the body. [G. a mouth]

sto·ma blast (stō′mă blast) Sound produced by forceful expiration of air through a tracheal stoma.

sto·ma but·ton (stō′mă bŭt′ŏn) Short plastic tube with collar inserted into a tracheal stoma to maintain or enlarge it.

stom·ach (stŏm′ăk) A large, irregularly piriform sac between the esophagus and the small intestine, lying just beneath the diaphragm. Its wall has four coats or tunics: mucous, submucous, muscular, and peritoneal; the muscular coat is composed of three layers, the fibers running longitudinally in the outer, circularly in the middle, and obliquely in the inner layer. SYN gaster [TA], ventriculus (1). [G. *stomachos*, L. *stomachus*]

stom·ach ache (stŏm′ăk āk) Pain in the abdomen, usually arising in the stomach or intestine.

stom·ach·al (stŏm′ă-kăl) Relating to the stomach.

stom·ach pump (stŏm′ăk pŭmp) An apparatus for removing the contents of the stomach by means of suction.

stom·ach tube (stŏm′ăk tūb) A flexible tube passed into the stomach for lavage or feeding.

sto·mal (stō′măl) Relating to a stoma.

sto·mal ul·cer (stō′măl ŭl′sĕr) An intestinal ulcer occurring after gastrojejunostomy in the jejunal mucosa near the opening (stoma) between the stomach and the jejunum.

sto·ma·ta (stō′mă-tă) Alternate plural of stoma.

sto·ma·tal·gi·a (stō′mă-tal′jē-ă) Pain in the mouth. SYN stomatodynia. [stomat- + G. *algos*, pain]

sto·ma·ti·tis (stō′mă-tī′tis) Inflammation of the mucous membrane of the mouth; characterized by small ulcers covered by a grayish exudate and surrounded by a longer red halo. It may be caused by mechanical or chemical trauma; may be classified as primary (i.e., aphthous stomatitis) or secondary. [stomat- + G. *-itis*, inflammation]

sto·ma·ti·tis me·di·ca·men·to·sa (stō′mă-tī′tis med-i-kă-men-tō′să) Inflammatory alterations of the oral mucosa associated with a systemic drug allergy; lesions may consist of erythema, vesicles, bullae, ulcerations, or angioedema.

♻ **stomato-, stomat-, stom-** Combining forms denoting oral cavity or mouthlike structure. [G. *stoma*]

sto•ma•to•cy•to•sis (stō′mă-tō-sī-tō′sis) A hereditary deformation of red blood cells in which they are swollen and cup shaped, causing congenital hemolytic anemia. SEE ALSO Rh null syndrome.

sto•ma•to•dyn•i•a (stō′mă-tō-din′ē-ă) SYN stomatalgia. [stomato- + G. *odynē,* pain]

sto•ma•tog•nath•ic sys•tem (stō′mă-tog-nath′ik sis′tĕm) All the structures involved in speech and in the reception, mastication, and deglutition of food.

sto•ma•to•ma•la•ci•a (stō′mă-tō-mă-lā′shē-ă) Pathologic softening of any of the structures of the mouth. [stomato- + G. *malakia,* softness]

sto•ma•to•my•co•sis (stō′mă-tō-mī-kō′sis) Disease of the mouth due to the presence of a fungus. [stomato- + G. *mykēs,* fungus, + *-osis,* condition]

sto•ma•to•ne•cro•sis (stō′mă-tō-nĕ-krō′sis) SYN noma. [stomato- + G. *nekrōsis,* death]

sto•ma•top•a•thy (stō′mă-top′ă-thē) Any disease of the oral cavity. [stomato- + G. *pathos,* suffering]

sto•ma•to•plas•tic (stō′mă-tō-plas′tik) Relating to stomatoplasty.

sto•ma•to•plas•ty (stō′mă-tō-plas-tē) Plastic surgery of the mouth. [stomato- + G. *plastos,* formed]

sto•ma•tor•rha•gi•a (stō′mă-tōr-ā′jē-ă) Bleeding from the gums or other part of the oral cavity. [stomato- + G. *rhēgnymi,* to burst forth]

sto•mo•de•al (stō′mō-dē′ăl) Relating to a stomodeum.

sto•mo•de•um (stō′mō-dē′ŭm) **1.** A midline ectodermal depression ventral to the embryonic brain and surrounded by the mandibular arch; when the buccopharyngeal membrane disappears, the stomodeum becomes continuous with the foregut and forms the mouth. **2.** The anterior portion of the insect alimentary canal. [Mod. L. fr. G. *stoma,* mouth, + *hodaios,* on the way, fr. *hodos,* a way]

-stomy Suffix denoting artificial or surgical opening. SEE ALSO stomato-. SYN caecoileostomy. [G. *stoma,* mouth]

stone (stōn) **1.** SYN calculus. **2.** A British unit of weight for the human body, equal to 14 lb. or 6.36 kg. [A.S. *stān*]

stone heart (stōn hahrt) SYN ischemic contracture of the left ventricle.

Stook•ey-Scarff op•er•a•tion (stūk′ē skahrf op-ĕr-ā′shŭn) SEE third ventriculostomy.

stool (stūl) **1.** A discharging of the bowels. **2.** The matter discharged at one movement of the bowels. SYN evacuation (2). SYN movement (2). [A.S. *stōl,* seat]

stop•ping (stop′ing) Any material used to seal a dressing in a tooth.

stop•ping rules (stop′ing rūlz) In randomized controlled trials and other systematic experiments on human subjects, regulations set out in advance that specify conditions under which the experiment will be terminated, e.g., unequivocal demonstration that one regimen in a randomized controlled trial is clearly superior to the other, or that one is clearly harmful.

stor•age (stōr′ăj) The second stage in the memory process, following encoding and preceding retrieval, involving mental processes associated with retention of stimuli that have been registered and modified by encoding. SEE ALSO memory.

stor•age dis•ease (stōr′ăj di-zēz′) Any accumulation of a specific substance within tissues, generally because of congenital deficiency of an enzyme necessary for further metabolism of the substance (e.g., glycogen-storage diseases).

STORCH (stōrch) Acronym for syndrome comprising syphilis, toxoplasmosis, other infections, rubella, cytomegalovirus infection, and herpes simplex: fetal infections that can cause congenital malformations.

stor•i•form (stōr′i-fōrm) Having a cartwheel pattern, as of spindle cells with elongated nuclei radiating from a center. [L. *storea,* woven mat, + *-formis,* form]

storm (stōrm) An exacerbation of symptoms or a crisis in the course of a disease.

STPD Symbol indicating that a gas volume has been expressed as if it were at standard temperature (0°C), standard pressure (760 mmHg absolute), and dry; under these conditions, a mole of gas occupies 22.4 liters.

stra•bis•mal (stră-biz′măl) Relating to or affected with strabismus.

stra•bis•mus (stră-biz′mŭs) A manifest lack of parallelism of the visual axes of the eyes. SYN crossed eyes, cross-eye, heterotropia, heterotropy, squint (1). [Mod. L., fr. G. *strabismos,* a squinting]

straight gy•rus (strāt jī′rŭs) A gyrus running along the medial part of the orbital surface of the frontal lobe of the cerebral hemisphere. It is bounded laterally by the olfactory sulcus.

straight sem•i•nif•er•ous tu•bule (strāt sem′i-nif′ĕr-ŭs tū′byūl) The continuation of the tubulus seminifer contortus that becomes straight just before entering the mediastinum to form the rete testis. SYN vasa recta (2).

straight si•nus (strāt sī′nŭs) An unpaired dural venous sinus in the posterior part of the falx cerebri where it is attached to the tentorium cerebelli; it is formed anteriorly by the merging of the great cerebral vein with the inferior sagittal sinus, and passes horizontally and posteriorly to the confluence of sinuses. SYN tentorial sinus.

strain (strān) **1.** A population of homogeneous organisms possessing a set of defined characters. BACTERIOLOGY the set of descendants that retains the characteristics of the ancestor; members of a strain that subsequently differ from the original isolate are regarded as belonging either to a substrain of the original strain, or to a new strain. **2.** Specific host cell(s) designed or selected to optimize production of recombinant products. [A.S. *stryand; strēon,* gain, begetting] **3.** To make an effort to the limit of one's strength. **4.** To injure by overuse or improper use. **5.** An act of straining. **6.** Injury resulting from tensile force to muscle or tendon, especially skeletal muscles. **7.** The change in shape that a body undergoes when acted on by an external stress. **8.** To filter; to percolate. [L. *stringere,* to bind]

strain-coun·ter·strain (strān-kownt′ĕr-strān) SYN muscle energy technique.

strain frac·ture (strān frak′shŭr) The tearing off, by a sudden force, of a piece of bone attached to a tendon, ligament, or capsule.

strait (strāt) A narrow passageway: **inferior strait**, apertura pelvis inferior; **superior strait**, apertura pelvis superior. [M.E. *streit* thr. O. Fr. fr. L. *strictus,* drawn together, tight]

strait·jack·et (strāt′jak′ĕt) A garmentlike device with long sleeves that can be secured to restrain a violently disturbed person.

stran·gle (strang′gĕl) To suffocate; to choke; to compress the trachea so as to prevent sufficient passage of air. [G. *strangaloō,* to choke, fr. *strangalē,* a halter]

stran·gu·lat·ed (strang′gyū-lāt-ĕd) Constricted so as to prevent sufficient passage of air, as through the trachea, or to cut off venous return or arterial air flow, as in the case of a hernia. [L. *strangulo,* pp. *-atus,* to choke, fr. G. *strangaloō,* to choke (strangle)]

stran·gu·lat·ed her·ni·a (strang′gyū-lāt-ĕd hĕr′nē-ă) An irreducible hernia in which the circulation is arrested; gangrene occurs unless relief is prompt.

stran·gu·la·tion (strang′gyū-lā′shŭn) The act of strangulating or the condition of being strangulated, in any sense.

stran·gu·ry (strang′gyūr-ē) Difficulty in micturition in which the urine is passed only drop by drop with pain and tenesmus. [G. *stranx* (*strang-*), something squeezed out, a drop, + *ouron,* urine]

strap (strap) **1.** A strip of adhesive plaster. **2.** To apply overlapping strips of adhesive plaster. [A.S. *stropp*]

strap cell (strap sel) An elongated tumor cell of uniform width that may show cross-striations; found in rhabdomyosarcoma.

stra·ta (stră′tă) Plural of stratum.

strat·i·fi·ca·tion (strat′i-fi-kā′shŭn) The process or result of separating a sample into subsamples according to specified criteria, such as age or occupational group. [L. *stratum,* layer, + *facio,* to make]

strat·i·fied (strat′i-fīd) Arranged in the form of layers or strata.

strat·i·fied ep·i·the·li·um (strat′i-fīd ep′i-thē′lē-ŭm) A type of epithelium composed of a series of layers, the cells of each varying in size and shape. It is named more specifically according to the type of cells at the surface, e.g., stratified squamous epithelium, stratified columnar epithelium, stratified ciliated columnar epithelium. SYN laminated epithelium.

stra·tig·ra·phy (stră-tig′ră-fē) SYN tomography. [L. *stratum,* layer, + G. *graphē,* a writing]

stra·tum, gen. **stra·ti**, pl. **stra·ta** (stră′tŭm, -tī, -tă) One of the layers of differentiated tissue, the aggregate of which forms any given structure, such as the retina or the skin. SEE ALSO lamina, layer. [L. *sterno,* pp. *stratus,* to spread out, strew, ntr. of pp. as noun, *stratum,* a bed cover, layer]

stra·tum ba·sa·le (stră′tŭm bā-sal′ē) **1.** The outermost layer of the endometrium, which undergoes only minimal changes during the menstrual cycle. SYN basal layer. **2.** SYN stratum basale epidermidis.

stra·tum ba·sa·le ep·i·derm·i·dis (stră′tŭm bā-sal′ē ep-i-dĕrm′i-dis) The deepest layer of the epidermis, composed of dividing stem cells and anchoring cells. SYN stratum basale (2).

stra·tum com·pac·tum (stră′tŭm kom-pak′tum) The superficial layer of decidual tissue in the pregnant uterus, in which the interglandular tissue preponderates.

stra·tum cor·ne·um ep·i·derm·i·dis (stră′tŭm kōr′nē-ŭm ep-i-dĕrm′i-dis) The outermost layer of the epidermis, consisting of nonliving, nonnucleated, fully keratinized epithelial cells about to be lost by desquamation. SYN corneal layer, horny layer.

stra·tum func·ti·o·na·le (stră′tŭm fungk-shē-ō-nā′lē) The endometrium except for the stratum basale; formerly believed to be lost during menstruation but now considered to be only partially disrupted.

stra·tum lu·ci·dum (stră′tŭm lū′sid-ŭm) A layer of lightly staining corneocytes in the deepest level of the stratum corneum; found primarily in the thick epidermis of the palmar and plantar skin. SYN clear layer of epidermis.

stra·tum spi·no·sum ep·i·derm·i·dis (stră′tŭm spī-nō′sŭm ep-i-dĕrm′i-dis) The layer of polyhedral cells in the epidermis; shrinkage artifacts and adhesion of these cells at their desmosomal junctions give a spiny or prickly appearance. SYN prickle cell layer, spinous layer.

stra•tum spon•gi•o•sum (strā′tŭm spon-jē-ō′sŭm) The middle spongy layer of the endometrium formed chiefly of dilated glandular structures; it is flanked by the stratum compacta (compact layer) on the luminal side and the stratum basalis (basal layer) on the myometrial side.

Straus sign (strows sīn) In facial paralysis, if an injection of pilocarpine is followed by sweating on the affected side later than on the other, the lesion is peripheral.

straw•ber•ry cer•vix (straw′ber-ē sĕr′viks) Macular erythema of the uterine cervix, characteristic of vaginitis due to *Trichomonas vaginalis*.

straw•ber•ry he•man•gi•o•ma (straw′ber-ē hē-man′jē-ō′mă) Hyperproliferation of immature capillary vessels, usually on the head and neck, present at birth or within the first two to three months postnatally, which commonly regresses without scar formation. SEE ALSO capillary hemangioma. See page B30.

straw•ber•ry ne•vus, straw•ber•ry mark (straw′ber-ē nē′vŭs, mahrk) A small nevus vascularis (capillary hemangioma) resembling a strawberry in size, shape, and color; it usually disappears spontaneously in early childhood. SEE ALSO capillary hemangioma.

straw•ber•ry tongue (straw′ber-ē tŭng) A tongue with a whitish coat through which the enlarged fungiform papillae project as red points; characteristic of scarlet fever and mucocutaneous lymph node syndrome.

straw itch, straw-bed itch (straw ich, straw-bed) An urticarial eruption caused by the mite, *Pyemotes ventricosus*, which can infest straw used in mattresses.

stray light (strā līt) Radiant energy that reaches the detector of a spectrophotometer and consists of wavelengths other than those selected.

streak (strēk) A line, stria, or stripe, especially one that is indistinct or evanescent. [A.S. *strica*]

streak cul•ture (strēk kŭl′chŭr) A culture produced by lightly stroking an inoculating needle or loop with inoculum over the surface of a solid medium.

stream•ing move•ment, stream•ing (strēm′ing mūv′mĕnt) The form of locomotion characteristic of the protoplasm of leukocytes, amebae, and other unicellular organisms; involves massing of the protoplasm at a point where surface pressure is lowest, extruding in the form of a pseudopod; the protoplasm may return to the body of the cell, resulting in the retraction of the pseudopod, or the entire mass may flow into the latter and thereby result in locomotion of the cell.

street drug (strēt drŭg) A controlled substance taken for nonmedical purposes; includes various amphetamines, anesthetics, barbiturates, opiates, and psychoactive drugs, and many derived from natural sources (e.g., the plants *Papaver somniferum*, *Cannibis sativa*, *Amanita pantherina*, *Lophophora williamsii*). Slang names include acid (lysergic acid diethylamide), angel dust (phencyclidine), coke (cocaine), downers (barbiturates), grass (marijuana), hash (concentrated tetrahydrocannibinol), magic mushrooms (psilocybin), cat (methamphetamines), and speed (amphetamines). During the 1980s a class of "designer drugs" arose, mostly analogues of psychoactive substances intended to escape regulation under the Controlled Substances Act. Also, crack cocaine, a potent, smokable form of cocaine, emerged as a major public health problem. In the United States, illicit use of drugs such as cocaine, marijuana, and heroin historically has occurred in cycles.

Street•er de•vel•op•men•tal ho•ri•zon(s) (strē′tĕr dĕ-vel′ŏp-ment′ăl hor-ī′zon) A term borrowed from geology and archeology by Streeter to define 23 developmental stages in human embryos, from fertilization through the first 2 months; each horizon spans 2–3 days and emphasizes specific anatomic characteristics, to avoid discrepancies in the determination of age and body dimensions of an embryo.

street vi•rus (strēt vī′rŭs) An isolate of rabies virus from a naturally infected domestic animal.

strength (strengkth) **1.** The quality of being strong or powerful. **2.** The degree of intensity. **3.** The property of materials by which they endure the application of force without yielding or breaking.

strength en•du•rance (strengkth en-dūr′ăns) SYN strength training.

strength train•ing (strengkth trān′ing) A period of training in which high levels of volume (weight resistance) with minimal rest periods resulting in muscular hypertrophy. SYN muscular strength training, strength endurance.

streph•o•sym•bo•li•a (stref′ō-sim-bō′lē-ă) **1.** Generally, the perception of objects reversed as if in a mirror. **2.** Specifically, difficulty in distinguishing written or printed letters that extend in opposite directions but are otherwise similar, such as *p* and *d*, or related kinds of mirror reversal. [G. *strephō*, to turn, + *symbolon*, a mark or sign]

strep•ta•vi•din (strep-tav′i-din) A bacterial protein used as a probe in immunologic assays because of its strong affinity and specificity for biotin; used as a bridge to link a chromogen to a biotinylated substrate specific for the substance of interest. [*strepto*coccus + avidin]

strepticaemia [Br.] SYN strepticemia.

strep·ti·ce·mi·a (strep′ti-sē′mē-ă) SYN streptococcemia. SYN strepticaemia.

strepto- Prefix meaning curved or twisted (usually relating to organisms thus described). [G. *streptos,* twisted, fr. *strephō,* to twist]

Strep·to·ba·cil·lus (strep′tō-bă-sil′ŭs) A genus of nonmotile, non-spore-forming, aerobic to facultatively anaerobic bacteria containing gram-negative, pleomorphic cells that vary from short rods to long, interwoven filaments that have a tendency to fragment into chains of bacillary and coccobacillary elements. The type species, *Streptobacillus moniliformis*, causes Haverhill fever and rat-bite fever. [strepto- + bacillus]

streptococcaemia [Br.] SYN streptococcemia.

strep·to·coc·cal (strep′tō-kok′ăl) Relating to or caused by any organism of the genus *Streptococcus.*

strep·to·coc·cal tox·ic shock syn·drome (strep′tō-kok′ăl tok′sik shok sin′drōm) A toxic syndrome characterized by hypotension and a variety of signs and symptoms indicative of multiorgan failure including cerebral dysfunction, renal failure, acute respiratory distress syndrome, toxic cardiomyopathy, and hepatic dysfunction. The syndrome is usually precipitated by local infections of skin or soft tissue by streptococci; a mortality rate of 30% has been reported.

strep·to·coc·ce·mi·a (strep′tō-kok-sē′mē-ă) The presence of streptococci in the blood. SYN strepticemia, streptococcaemia, streptosepticemia. [streptococcus + G. *haima,* blood]

strep·to·coc·ci (strep′tō-kok′sī) Plural of streptococcus. See page B4.

strep·to·coc·cic (strep′tō-kok′sik) Relating to or caused by any organism of the genus *Streptococcus.*

Strep·to·coc·cus (strep′tō-kok′ŭs) A genus of nonmotile, non-spore-forming, aerobic to facultatively anaerobic bacteria containing gram-positive, spheric, or ovoid cells that occur in pairs or short or long chains. These organisms occur regularly in the mouth and intestines of humans and other animals, in dairy products and other foods, and in fermenting plant juices. Some species are pathogenic. [strepto- + G. *kokkos,* berry (coccus)]

strep·to·coc·cus, pl. **strep·to·coc·ci** (strep′tō-kok′ŭs, -sī) A term used to refer to any member of the genus *Streptococcus.*

Strep·to·coc·cus a·gal·ac·ti·ae (strep′tō-kok′ŭs ā-gal-ak′shē-ē) A streptococcal species that possesses the Lancefield group B antigen present in the cell wall; a significant cause of bacteremia, pneumonia, and meningitis in newborns.

strep·to·coc·cus e·ryth·ro·gen·ic tox·in (strep′tō-kok′ŭs ĕ-rith-rō-jen′ik tok′sin) A culture filtrate of lysogenized group A strains of β-hemolytic streptococci, erythrogenic when inoculated into the skin of people susceptible to scarlet fever, and neutralized by antibodies that appear during scarlet fever convalescence. SYN erythrogenic toxin.

Strep·to·coc·cus in·ter·me·di·us (strep′tō-kok′ŭs in-tĕr-mē′dē-ŭs) One of a heterogenous group of streptococci, generally found in the mouth or upper respiratory tract; classification is generally established by fermentation patterns, analysis of the sugar composition of the cell wall, and use of sugar production patterns.

Strep·to·coc·cus mil·ler·i (strep′tō-kok′ŭs mil′lĕr-ī) A term used to refer to the *Streptococcus intermedius* group, which contains three distinct streptococcal species: *S. intermedius*, *S. constellatus*, and *S. anginosus*. These bacteria are found in the human oral cavity and have been associated with a variety of infections including bacteremia, endocarditis, and CNS, oral, and thoracic infections.

Strep·to·coc·cus mu·tans (strep′tō-kok′ŭs myū′tanz) A bacterial species associated with the production of dental caries in humans and in some other animals and with subacute endocarditis.

Strep·to·coc·cus pneu·mo·ni·ae (strep′tō-kok′ŭs nū-mō′nē-ē) A bacterial species of gram-positive, lancet-shaped diplococci frequently occurring in pairs or chains. Virulent forms are enclosed in type-specific polysaccharide capsules. Normal inhabitants of the respiratory tract, and the cause of lobar pneumonia, otitis media, meningitis, sinusitis, and other infections. SYN pneumococcus.

Strep·to·coc·cus py·o·ge·nes (strep′tō-kok′ŭs pī-oj′ĕ-nēz) A bacterial species found in the human mouth, throat, and respiratory tract and in inflammatory exudates, bloodstream, and lesions in human diseases; it is sometimes found in the udders of cows and in dust from sickrooms, hospital wards, schools, theaters, and other public places; it causes the formation of pus or even fatal septicemias.

Strep·to·coc·cus vi·ri·dans (strep′tō-kok′ŭs vēr′i-danz) SYN viridans streptococci.

strep·to·gram·in (strep′tō-gram′in) A mixture of two structurally distinct compounds, type A and type B, which act at the level of inhibition of translation through binding to the bacterial ribosome; separately bacteriostatic but bactericidal in appropriate ratios. Antibiotics quinupristin and dalfopristin are both streptogramins.

strep·to·ki·nase (SK) (strep′tō-kī′nās) An extracellular metalloenzyme from hemolytic streptococci that cleaves plasminogen, producing plasmin, which causes the liquefaction of fibrin; usually used in conjunction with streptodornase in the removal of clots.

strep•to•ly•sin (strep-tol′i-sin) A hemolysin produced by streptococci.

Strep•to•my•ces (strep′tō-mī′sēz) A genus of nonmotile, aerobic, gram-positive bacteria that grow in the form of a much-branched mycelium; conidia are produced in chains on aerial hyphae. These organisms (several hundred species in the genus) are predominantly saprophytic soil forms; some are parasitic on plants or animals; many produce antibiotics. The type species is *Streptomyces albus*. [strepto- + G. *mykēs,* fungus]

streptosepticaemia [Br.] SYN streptosepticemia.

strep•to•sep•ti•ce•mi•a (strep′tō-sep′ti-sē′mē-ă) SYN streptococcemia. SYN streptosepticaemia.

strep•to•thri•cho•sis (strep′tō-thri-kō′sis) SYN dermatophilosis.

strep•to•tri•chi•a•sis (strep′tō-tri-kī′ă-sis) SYN dermatophilosis.

strep•to•tri•cho•sis (strep′tō-tri-kō′sis) SYN dermatophilosis.

stress (stres) **1.** Reactions of the body to forces of a deleterious nature, infections, and various abnormal states that tend to disturb its normal physiologic equilibrium (homeostasis). **2.** DENTISTRY the forces set up in teeth, their supporting structures, and structures restoring or replacing teeth as a result of the force of mastication. **3.** The force or pressure applied or exerted between portions of a body or bodies, generally expressed in pounds per square inch. **4.** RHEOLOGY the force in a material transmitted per unit area to adjacent layers. **5.** PSYCHOLOGY a physical or psychological stimulus such as very high heat, public criticism, or another noxious agent or experience that, when impinging on a person, produces psychological strain or disequilibrium. [L. *strictus,* tight, fr. *stringo,* to draw together]

stress-bro•ken con•nec•tor, stress-bro•ken joint (stres′brō-kĕn kŏ-nek′tŏr, joynt) SYN nonrigid connector.

stress frac•ture (stres frak′shŭr) SYN fatigue fracture.

stres•sor (stres′ŏr) PSYCHIATRY any event or situation that induces emotional distress in a given patient.

stress re•ac•tion (stres rē-ak′shŭn) An acute emotional reaction related to extreme environmental stress. SYN acute situational reaction.

stress shield•ing (stres shēld′ing) Osteopenia occurring in bone as the result of removal of normal stress from the bone by an implant.

stress test (stres test) Systematic use of exercise or pharmacologic metabolic stressors to evaluate cardiovascular dynamics and evaluate the physiologic adjustments to metabolic demands that exceed the resting requirement. SEE ALSO graded exercise test, Astrand-Ryhming Cycle Ergometer Test. SYN exercise stress test.

stress ul•cer (stres ŭl′sĕr) A lesion of the duodenum in a patient with extensive superficial burns, intracranial lesions, or severe bodily injury. SYN Curling ulcer.

stress ur•i•nar•y in•con•ti•nence (SUI) (stres yŭr′i-nār-ē in-kon′ti-nĕns) Leakage of urine as a result of coughing, straining, or some sudden voluntary movement.

stretch•er (strech′ĕr) A litter, usually a sheet of canvas stretched to a frame with four handles, used for transporting the sick or injured. [A.S. *streccan,* to stretch]

stretch•ing ex•er•cise (strech′ing eks′ĕr-sīz) Exercises performed actively, passively, or with partner assistance to take a muscle to the point of tension for a period of 15–30 seconds. Used before and after exercise to prevent muscle cramps and/or injury to the muscle or joint.

stretch mark (strech mahrk) Colloquial usage for striae cutis distensae (q.v.).

stretch pain (strech pān) Myocardial pain caused by a reduction in arterial blood flow into coronary artery flow while the balloon is inflated during transluminal percutaneous coronary angioplasty.

stretch re•cep•tors (strech rĕ-sep′tŏrz) receptors that are sensitive to elongation, especially those in Golgi tendon organs and muscle spindles, but also those found in visceral organs such as the stomach, small intestine, and urinary bladder.

stretch re•flex (strech rē′fleks) SYN myotactic reflex.

stretch test (strech test) SYN Bragard sign.

stri•a, gen. and pl. **stri•ae** (strī′ă, -ē) **1.** A stripe, band, streak, or line, distinguished by color, texture, depression, or elevation from the tissue in which it is found. SYN striation (1). **2.** SYN striae cutis distensae. [L. channel, furrow]

stri•ae a•tro•phi•cae (strī′ē ă-trof′i-sē) SYN striae cutis distensae.

stri•ae cu•tis dis•ten•sae (strī′ē kyū′tis dis-ten′sē) Bands of thin, wrinkled skin, initially red but becoming purple and white, which occur commonly on the abdomen, buttocks, and thighs at puberty and/or during and following pregnancy, and result from atrophy of the dermis and overextension of the skin; also associated with ascites and Cushing syndrome. SYN lineae atrophicae, linear atrophy, stria (2), striae atrophicae.

stri•ae grav•i•dar•um (strī′ē grav-ē-dā′rŭm) Striae cutis distensae associated with pregnancy. See page B9.

stri•ae of Ret•zi•us (strī′ē rets′ē-ŭs) Incremental growth lines in enamel seen microscopically as dark bands.

stri•ate (strī′āt) Striped; marked by striae. [L. *striatus,* furrowed]

stri•ate bod•y (strī′āt bod′ē) The caudate and lentiform (lenticular) nuclei; the striate appearance on section is caused by slender fascicles of myelinated fibers. SYN corpus striatum [TA].

stri•at•ed bor•der (strī′āt-ĕd bōr′dĕr) The free surface of the columnar absorptive cells of the intestine formed by closely packed microvilli about 1 mcm long, giving the appearance of parallel striations.

stri•at•ed duct (strī′āt-ĕd dŭkt) A type of intralobular duct found in some salivary glands that modifies the secretory product; it derives its name from extensive infolding of the basal membrane.

stri•at•ed mus•cle (strī′āt-ĕd mŭs′ĕl) Skeletal or voluntary muscle in which cross-striations occur in the fibers as a result of regular overlapping of thick and thin myofilaments; contrast with smooth muscle. Although cardiac muscle is also striated in appearance, the term "striated muscle" is commonly used as a synonym for voluntary skeletal muscle.

stri•ate veins (strī′āt vānz) SYN inferior thalamostriate veins.

stri•a•tion (strī-ā′shŭn) **1.** SYN stria (1). **2.** A striate appearance. **3.** The act of streaking or making striae.

stri•a•to•ni•gral (strī′ă-tō-nī′grăl) Referring to the efferent connection of the striatum with the substantia nigra.

stri•a•tum (strī-ā′tŭm) Collective name for the caudate nucleus and putamen that together with the globus pallidus or pallidum form the striate body. [L. neut. of *striatus,* furrowed]

strict i•so•la•tion (strikt ī′sŏ-lā′shŭn) Isolation required for patients with highly contagious diseases.

stric•ture (strik′shŭr) A circumscribed narrowing or stenosis of a tube, duct, or hollow structure, such as the esophagus or urethra, usually consisting of cicatricial contracture or deposition of abnormal tissue. May be congenital or acquired. If acquired, may result from infection, trauma, muscular spasm, or mechanical or chemical irritation. [L. *strictura,* fr. *stringo,* pp. *strictus,* to draw tight, bind]

stric•tur•ot•o•my (strik′shŭr-ot′ŏ-mē) Surgical opening or division of a stricture. [stricture + G. *tomē,* incision]

stri•dor (strī′dŏr) A high-pitched, noisy respiration, like the blowing of the wind; a sign of respiratory obstruction, especially in the trachea or larynx. [L. a harsh, creaking sound]

strid•u•lous (strij′yū-lŭs) Having a shrill or creaking sound. [L. *stridulus,* fr. *strideo,* to creak, to hiss]

string sign (string sīn) PEDIATRIC GASTROINTESTINAL RADIOLOGY the narrowed pyloric canal seen with congenital pyloric stenosis; also used to describe a narrowed segment in Crohn disease on small bowel series.

stri•o•la (strī′ō-la) The narrow central area of the utricular macula where the orientations of the tallest stereocilia and kinocilia change. [L. *stria,* stripe, + *-ola,* dim. suffix]

strip (strip) **1.** To express the contents from a collapsible tube or canal, such as the urethra, by running a finger along it. SYN milk (4). **2.** Subcutaneous excision of a vein in its longitudinal axis, performed with a stripper. **3.** Any narrow piece, relatively long and of uniform width. [A.S. *strypan,* to rob]

stripe (strīp) **1.** ANATOMY a streak, line, band, or stria. **2.** RADIOGRAPHY a linear opacity differing in density from the adjacent parts of the image; usually represents the tangential image of a planar structure such as the pleura or peritoneum. [M.E.]

strip•ping (strip′ing) Removal, often of a covering.

stro•bi•la, pl. **stro•bi•lae** (strō′bi-lă, -lē) A chain of segments, less the scolex and unsegmented neck portion, of a tapeworm. [G. *stobilē,* a twist of lint]

stro•bo•scop•ic mi•cro•scope (strō′bō-skop′ik mī′krŏ-skōp) A microscope that has a light source that flashes at a constant rate so that an analysis of the motility of an object may be made; it may be used for high-speed or low-speed (time-lapse) cinephotomicrography.

stro•bos•co•py (strō-bos′kŏ-pē) Endoscopy performed with an intermittent light at a frequency that approximates the frequency of movement of the object visualized so that it appears to be motionless; useful in analyzing vocal cord structure and motion.

stroke (strōk) **1.** Any acute clinical event, related to impairment of cerebral circulation, that lasts longer than 24 hours. SEE ALSO cerebrovascular accident. **2.** A harmful discharge of lightning, particularly one that affects a human being. **3.** A pulsation. **4.** To pass the hand or any instrument over a surface. SEE ALSO stroking. **5.** A gliding movement over a surface. SYN apoplexy. [A.S. *strāc*]

stroke vol•ume (strōk vol′yūm) The volume pumped out of one ventricle of the heart in a single beat.

stroke work in•dex (strōk wŏrk in′deks) A measure of the work done by the heart with each contraction, adjusted for body surface area; equal to the stroke volume of the heart multiplied by the arterial pressure and divided by body surface area.

strok•ing (strōk′ing) The nonverbal fondling and nurturance accorded infants, or the nonverbal and verbal forms of acceptance, reassurance, and positive reinforcement accorded to children and adults either by a person to himself or herself or to another person to satisfy a basic biopsychological need of all developing humans; various psychopathologic conditions are believed to result when such stroking is absent or faulty.

stro•ma, pl. **stro•ma•ta** (strō′mă, -mă-tă) **1.** The framework, usually of connective tissue, of an organ, gland, or other structure, as distinguished from the parenchyma or specific substance of the part. **2.** Aqueous phase of chloroplasts, i.e., chloroplast matrix. [G. *strōma,* bed]

stro•mal (strō′măl) Stromatic; relating to the stroma of an organ or other structure.

strom•al cor•ne•al dys•tro•phy (strō′măl kōr′nē-ăl dis′trŏ-fē) Opacification with involvement of the middle layer of the cornea.

strom•uhr (strōm′ūr) An instrument for measuring the quantity of blood that flows per unit of time through a blood vessel. [Ger. *Strom,* stream, + *Uhr,* clock]

Stron•gy•loi•des (stron′ji-loy′dēz) The threadworm, a genus of small nematode parasites commonly found in the small intestine of mammals (particularly ruminants). Human infection is chiefly by *S. stercoralis* or *S. fuelleborn.* Fatal infection in infants produces the condition known as swollen belly disease or syndrome, which causes gross abdominal distention. [G. *strongylos,* round, + *eidos,* resemblance]

stron•gy•loi•di•a•sis (stron′ji-loy-dī′ă-sis) Infection with soil-borne nematodes of the genus *Strongyloides,* considered to be a parthenogenetic parasitic female. Larvae passed to the soil develop through four larval instars to form free-living adults or develop from first and second free-living stages into infective third-stage strongyliform or filariform larvae, which penetrate the skin or enter the buccal mucosa in drinking water. Most serious human infections and nearly all fatalities commonly follow immunosuppression by steroids, ACTH, other agents, or in AIDS.

Stron•gy•lus (stron′ji-lŭs) The palisade worm, a genus of large strongyle nematodes (subfamily Strongylinae, family Strongylidae) parasitic in horses and other equids, and the cause of strongylosis. [G. *strongylos*, round]

stron•ti•um (Sr) (stron′shē-ŭm) A metallic element; atomic no. 38, atomic wt. 87.62; one of the alkaline earth series and similar to calcium in chemical and biologic properties. Various salts of strontium are used therapeutically for their anions, e.g., strontium bromide, iodide, lactate. [*Strontian,* a town in Scotland]

stroph•u•lus (strof′yū-lŭs) SYN miliaria rubra. [Mod. L. dim. of G. *strophus,* colic]

struc•tu•ra (strŭk-tūr′ă) SYN structure.

struc•tur•al (strŭk′shŭr-ăl) Relating to the structure of a part; having a structure. SYN anatomic (2).

struc•tur•al for•mu•la (strŭk′shŭr-ăl fōrm′yū-lă) A formula in which the connections of the atoms and groups of atoms, as well as their kind and number, are indicated.

struc•tur•al gene (strŭk′shŭr-ăl jēn) A gene that codes for a specific protein or peptide.

struc•tur•al i•som•er•ism (strŭk′shŭr-ăl ī-som′ĕr-izm) Compound involving the same atoms in different arrangements.

struc•ture (strŭk′shŭr) **1.** The arrangement of the details of a part; the manner of formation of a part. **2.** A tissue or formation made up of different but related parts. **3.** CHEMISTRY the configuration and interconnections of the atoms in a given molecule. SYN structura. [L. *structura,* fr. *struo,* pp. *structus,* to build]

struc•tured ab•stract (strŭk′shŭrd ab′strakt) Summary description of a published paper, in which information about the study reported in the paper is set out in a systematic, stylized form under headings such as aims, methods, main outcome measures, results, and conclusions.

stru•ma, pl. **stru•mae** (strū′mă, -mē) SYN goiter. [L. a scrofulous tumor, fr. *struo,* to pile up, build]

stru•ma o•va•ri•i (strū′mă ō-var′ē-ī) A rare ovarian tumor, regarded as teratomatous, in which thyroid tissue has surpassed the other elements; occasionally associated with hyperthyroidism.

stru•mec•to•my (strū-mek′tŏ-mē) Surgical removal of all or a portion of a goitrous tumor. [struma + G. *ektomē,* excision]

stru•mi•form (strū′mi-fōrm) Resembling a goiter. [struma + L. *forma,* form]

stru•mi•tis (strū-mī′tis) Inflammation, with swelling, of the thyroid gland. SEE ALSO thyroiditis. [struma + G. *-itis,* inflammation]

stru•mous (strū′mŭs) Denoting or characteristic of a struma.

Strüm•pell dis•ease (strem′pel di-zēz′) **1.** SYN spondylitis deformans. **2.** SYN acute epidemic leukoencephalitis.

Strüm•pell phe•nom•e•non (strem′pel fĕ-nom′ĕ-non) Dorsal flexion of the great toe, sometimes of the entire foot, in a paralyzed limb when the extremity is drawn up against the body, flexing both knee and hip.

Strüm•pell re•flex (strem′pel rē′fleks) Stroking the abdomen or thigh causes flexion of the leg and adduction of the foot.

stru•vite cal•cu•lus (strū′vīt kal′kyū-lŭs) A calculus in which the crystalloid component consists of magnesium ammonium phosphate; usually associated with urinary tract infection caused by urease-producing bacteria.

strych•nine (strik′nīn) An alkaloid from *Strychnos nux-vomica;* colorless crystals of intensely bitter taste, nearly insoluble in water; stimulates all parts of the central nervous system; was formerly used in stomach therapy, an antidote for depressant poisons, and in the treatment of myocarditis. It blocks glycine, an inhibitory neurotransmitter, and thus can cause convulsions. It is a potent chemical capable of producing acute or chronic poisoning.

strych•nin•ism (strik′nīn-izm) Chronic strychnine poisoning, the symptoms being those that arise from central nervous system stimulation; the first signs are tremors and twitching, progressing to severe convulsions and respiratory arrest.

Stry•ker frame (strī′kĕr frām) A frame that holds the patient and permits turning in various planes without individual motion of parts.

ST seg•ment (seg′mĕnt) The part of an ECG tracing that begins at the end of a QRS complex, contains the J point, and ends at the beginning of the ensuing T wave.

Stu•art fac•tor, **Stu•art-Prow•er fac•tor** (stū′ărt fak′tŏr, prow′ĕr) SYN factor X.

stu•dent nurse (SN) (stū′dĕnt nŭrs) A student matriculated in a nursing program; may be diploma, associate degree, baccalaureate, or master's program.

Stu•dent *t*-test (stū′dĕnt test) A statistical significance test for assessing the difference between, or the equality of, two or more population means.

stud•y (stŭd′ē) Research, detailed examination, or analysis of an organism, object, or phenomenon. [L. *studium,* study, inquiry]

stump (stŭmp) **1.** The extremity of a limb left after amputation. **2.** The pedicle remaining after removal of the tumor attached to it. [M.E. *stumpe*]

stump can•cer (stŭmp kan′sĕr) Carcinoma of the stomach developing after gastroenterostomy or gastric resection for benign disease.

stun•ted (stŭnt′ĕd) Shortened; retarded, as in growth.

stu•por (stū′pŏr) A state of impaired consciousness in which the person shows a marked reduction in reactivity to environmental stimuli; only continual stimulation arouses the person. [L. fr. *stupeo,* to be stunned]

stu•por•ous (stū′pŏr-ŭs) Relating to or marked by stupor.

Sturm co•noid (stŭrm kō′noyd) OPTICS the pattern of rays formed after passage through a spherocylindric combination.

Sturm•dorf op•er•a•tion (stŭrm′dōrf op-ĕr-ā′shŭn) Conic removal of the endocervix.

Sturm in•ter•val (stŭrm in′tĕr-văl) The distance between the anterior and posterior focal lines in a spherocylindrical lens combination.

stut•ter•ing (stŭt′ĕr-ing) A phonatory or articulatory disorder, characteristically beginning in childhood, sometimes accompanied by intense anxiety about the efficiency of oral communication, characterized by hesitations, repetitions, or prolongations of sounds and syllables, interjections, broken words, circumlocutions, and words produced with excess tension. SEE ALSO dysfluency.

stut•ter test (stŭt′ĕr test) Maneuver used to detect plica syndrome. The examiner palpates the patella as the patient slowly extends the knee. A stuttering or ratcheting effect between 45–60° is a positive result.

sty, **stye**, pl. **sties**, **styes** (stī, stīz) SYN hordeolum.

sty•lette (stī-let′) **1.** A flexible metallic rod inserted in the lumen of a flexible catheter to stiffen it and give it form during its passage. **2.** A slender probe. SYN stylus (3), stilus. [It. *stilletto,* a dagger; dim. of L. *stilus* or *stylus,* a stake, a pen]

♲ **stylo-** Combining form meaning styloid (specifically the styloid process of the temporal bone). [G. *stylos,* pillar, post]

sty•lo•glos•sus mus•cle (stī′lō-glos′ŭs mŭs′ĕl) *Action,* retracts tongue; *origin,* lower end of styloid process; *insertion,* side and undersurface of tongue; *nerve supply,* hypoglossal. SYN musculus styloglossus [TA].

sty•lo•hy•al (stī′lō-hī′ăl) Relating to the styloid process of the temporal bone and to the hyoid bone.

sty•lo•hy•oid mus•cle (stī′lō-hī′oyd mŭs′ĕl) *Origin,* styloid process of temporal bone; *insertion,* hyoid bone by two slips on either side of intermediate tendon of digastric; *action,* elevates hyoid bone; *nerve supply,* facial. SYN musculus stylohyoideus [TA].

sty•loid (stī′loyd) Peg-shaped; denoting one of several slender bony processes. [stylo- + G. *eidos,* resemblance]

sty•loi•di•tis (stī-loyd-ī′tis) Inflammation of a styloid process.

sty•loid pro•cess (stī′loyd pros′es) SEE styloid process of radius, styloid process of temporal bone, styloid process of ulna.

sty•loid pro•cess of ra•di•us (stī′loyd pros′es rā′dē-ŭs) A thick, pointed, palpable projection on the lateral side of the distal extremity of the radius.

sty•loid pro•cess of tem•por•al bone (stī′loyd pros′es tem′pŏr-ăl bōn) A slender, pointed projection running downward and slightly forward from the base of the inferior surface of the petrous portion of the temporal bone where it joins the tympanic portion; it gives attachment to the styloglossus, stylohyoid, and stylopharyngeus muscles and the stylohyoid and stylomandibular ligaments.

sty•loid pro•cess of ul•na (stī′loyd pros′es ŭl′nă) A cylindric, pointed, palpable projection from the medial and posterior aspect of the head of the ulna, to the tip of which is attached the ulnar collateral ligament of the wrist.

sty•lo•mas•toid ar•ter•y (stī′lō-mas′toyd ahr′tĕr-ē) *Origin*, posterior auricular; *distribution*, external acoustic meatus, mastoid cells, semicircular canals, stapedius muscle, and vestibule; *anastomoses*, tympanic branches of internal carotid and ascending pharyngeal, and labyrinthine arteries. SYN arteria stylomastoidea [TA].

sty•lo•mas•toid for•a•men (stī′lō-mas′toyd fōr-ā′mĕn) The distal or external opening of the facial canal on the inferior surface of the petrous portion of the temporal bone, between the styloid and mastoid processes; it transmits the facial nerve and stylomastoid artery.

sty•lo•mas•toid vein (stī′lō-mas′toyd vān) Drains the tympanic cavity, traverses the facial canal exiting through the stylomastoid foramen, and empties into the retromandibular vein.

sty•lo•pha•ryn•ge•al mus•cle (stī′lō-făr-in′jē-al mŭs′ĕl) SYN stylopharyngeus muscle.

sty•lo•pha•ryn•ge•us mus•cle (stī′lō-făr-in′jē-ŭs mŭs′ĕl) *Origin*, root of styloid process; *insertion*, thyroid cartilage and wall of pharynx (becomes part of the longitudinal coat); *action*, elevates pharynx and larynx; *nerve supply*, glossopharyngeal. SYN musculus stylopharyngeus [TA], stylopharyngeal muscle.

sty•lus, sti•lus (stī′lŭs) **1.** Any pencil-shaped structure. **2.** A pencil-shaped medicinal preparation for external application. **3.** SYN stylette. [L. *stilus* or *stylus,* a stake or pen]

stype (stīp) A tampon. [G. *stypē,* tow]

styp•tic (stip′tik) **1.** Having an astringent or hemostatic effect. **2.** An astringent agent used topically to stop bleeding. [G. *styptikos,* astringent]

sub- Prefix to words formed from L. roots, denoting beneath, less than the normal or typical, inferior. Cf. hypo-. [L. *sub,* under]

sub•a•cro•mi•al bur•sa (sŭb′ă-krō′mē-ăl bŭr′să) Between the acromion and the capsule of the shoulder joint.

sub•a•cute (sŭb′ă-kyūt′) Between acute and chronic; denoting the course of a disease of moderate duration or severity.

sub•a•cute bac•ter•i•al en•do•car•di•tis (SBE) (sŭb′ă-kyūt′ bak-tēr′ē-ăl en′dō-kahr-dī′tis) Condition usually involving cardiac valves with congenital or acquired abnormalities and usually due to alpha-hemolytic streptococci.

sub•a•cute com•bined de•gen•er•a•tion of the spi•nal cord (sŭb′ă-kyūt′ kŏm-bīnd′ dĕ-jen′ĕr-ā′shŭn spī′năl kōrd) A disorder of the spinal cord, such as that occurring in vitamin B12 deficiency, characterized by gliosis with spongiform degeneration of the posterior and lateral columns. SYN Putnam-Dana syndrome, vitamin B12 neuropathy.

sub•a•cute gran•u•lom•a•tous thy•roid•i•tis (sŭb′ă-kyūt′ gran′yū-lō′mă-tŭs thī′roy-dī′tis) Thyroiditis with round cell (usually lymphocytes) infiltration, destruction of thyroid cells, epithelial giant cell proliferation, and evidence of regeneration; thought by some to be a reflection of a systemic infection and not an example of true chronic thyroiditis. SYN de Quervain thyroiditis.

sub•a•cute in•flam•ma•tion (sŭb′ă-kyūt′ in′flă-mā′shŭn) An inflammation that is intermediate in duration between that of an acute inflammation and that of a chronic inflammation, usually persisting longer than 3–4 weeks.

sub•a•cute mi•gra•to•ry pan•nic•u•li•tis (sŭb′ă-kyūt′ mī′gră-tōr-ē pă-nik′yū-lī′tis) Nonscarring plaques of changing configuration on the lateral aspect of one or both legs, of many months duration.

sub•a•cute nec•ro•tiz•ing my•e•li•tis (sŭb′ă-kyūt′ nek′rō-tīz-ing mī′ĕ-lī′tis) A disorder of the lower spinal cord in men resulting in progressive paraplegia.

sub•a•cute scler•os•ing pan•en•ceph•a•li•tis (SSPE) (sŭb′ă-kyūt′ skler-ō′sing pan′en-sef′ă-lī′tis) A rare chronic, progressive encephalitis that affects primarily children and young adults, caused by the measles virus. Characterized by a history of primary measles infection before the age of 2 years, followed by several asymptomatic years, then gradual, progressive psychoneurologic deterioration, consisting of personality change, seizures, myoclonus, ataxia, photosensitivity, ocular abnormalities, spasticity, and coma. Characteristic periodic activity is seen on EEG; pathologically, the white matter of both the hemispheres and brainstem is affected, as well as the cerebral cortex, and eosinophilic inclusion bodies are present in the cytoplasm nuclei of neurons and glial cells. Death usually occurs within 3 years. SYN Bosin disease, Dawson encephalitis.

sub•a•cute spong•i•form en•ceph•a•lop•a•thy (sŭb′ă-kyūt′ spŏn′ji-fōrm en-sef′a-lop′ă-thē) Any of various progressive and uniformly fatal prion diseases of the central nervous system in humans and other animals. SEE ALSO Creutzfeldt-Jakob disease, kuru, prion.

sub·a·or·tic ste·no·sis (sŭb'ā-ōr'tik stĕ-nō'sis) Congenital narrowing of the outflow tract of the left ventricle by a ring of fibrous tissue or by hypertrophy of the muscular septum below the aortic valve.

sub·ap·i·cal (sŭb-ap'i-kăl) Below the apex of any part.

sub·a·rach·noid bleed (sŭb'ă-rak'noyd blēd) SYN subarachnoid hemorrhage.

subarachnoid haemorrhage [Br.] SYN subarachnoid hemorrhage.

sub·a·rach·noid hem·or·rhage (SaH, SAH) (sŭb'ă-rak'noyd hem'ŏr-ăj) Bleeding between the middle membrane covering of the brain and the brain itself; 5–10% of strokes are caused by subarachnoid hemorrhage. Most common in people 20–60 years old; female predilection. SYN subarachnoid bleed, subarachnoid haemorrhage.

sub·a·rach·noid space (sŭb'ă-rak'noyd spās) The area between the arachnoidea and pia mater, traversed by delicate, fibrous trabeculae and filled with cerebrospinal fluid. Because the pia mater immediately adheres to the surface of the brain and spinal cord, the space is greatly widened wherever the brain surface exhibits a deep depression (for example, between the cerebellum and medulla); such widenings are called cisternae. The large blood vessels supplying the brain and spinal cord lie in the subarachnoid space.

sub·ar·cu·ate fos·sa (sŭb-ahr'kyū-ăt fos'ă) An irregular depression on the posterior surface of the petrous portion of the temporal bone just below its crest and above and lateral to the internal acoustic meatus. In the fetus, the flocculus of the cerebellum rests here; in the adult, a small vein enters the bone here.

sub·a·tom·ic (sŭb'ă-tom'ik) Pertaining to particles making up the intraatomic structure, e.g., protons, electrons, neutrons.

sub·ax·i·al (sŭb-ak'sē-ăl) Below the axis of the body or any part.

sub·cal·lo·sal gy·rus (sŭb'kă-lō'săl jī'rŭs) A slender, vertical, whitish band immediately anterior to the lamina terminalis and anterior commissure; contrary to its name, it is not a cortical convolution but is the ventral continuation of the transparent septum.

sub·cap·su·lar cat·a·ract (sŭb-kap'sŭl-ăr kat'ăr-akt) A cataract in which the opacities are concentrated beneath the capsule.

sub·car·ti·lag·i·nous (sŭb'kahr-ti-laj'i-nŭs) **1.** Partly cartilaginous. **2.** Beneath a cartilage.

sub·cho·ri·al space, sub·cho·ri·al lake (sŭb-kōr'ē-ăl spās, lāk) The part of the placenta beneath the chorionic plate; it joins with irregular channels to form marginal lakes.

sub·class (sŭb'klas) In biologic classification, a division between class and order.

sub·cla·vi·an ar·ter·y (sŭb-klā'vē-ăn ahr'tĕr-ē) *Origin*, right from brachiocephalic, left from arch of aorta; *branches*, vertebral, thyrocervical trunk, internal thoracic; costocervical trunk, descending scapular; it continues as the axillary artery after crossing the first rib. SYN arteria subclavia [TA].

sub·cla·vi·an mus·cle (sŭb-klā'vē-ăn mŭs'ĕl) SYN subclavius muscle.

sub·cla·vi·an nerve (sŭb-klā'vē-ăn nĕrv) A branch from the superior trunk of the brachial plexus supplying the subclavius muscle. SYN nervus subclavius [TA].

sub·cla·vi·an steal (sŭb-klā'vē-ăn stēl) Obstruction of the subclavian artery proximal to the origin of the vertebral artery; blood flow through the vertebral artery is reversed and the subclavian artery thus "steals" cerebral blood, causing symptoms of vertebrobasilar insufficiency (subclavian steal syndrome); becomes evident during vigorous use of an upper extremity.

sub·cla·vi·an vein (sŭb-klā'vē-ăn vān) The direct continuation of the axillary vein at the lateral border of the first rib; it passes medially to join the internal jugular vein and form the brachiocephalic vein on each side. SYN vena subclavia [TA].

sub·cla·vi·us mus·cle (sŭb-klā'vē-ŭs mŭs'ĕl) *Origin*, first costal cartilage; *insertion*, inferior surface of acromial end of clavicle; *action*, fixes clavicle or elevates first rib; *nerve supply*, subclavian from brachial plexus. SYN musculus subclavius [TA], subclavian muscle.

sub·clin·i·cal (sŭb-klin'i-kăl) Denoting the presence of a disease without manifest symptoms; may be an early stage in the evolution of a disease.

sub·clin·i·cal coc·ci·di·oi·do·my·co·sis (sŭb-klin'i-kăl kok-sid'ē-oyd'ō-mī-kō'sis) A form of coccidioidomycosis that does not come to medical attention because associated respiratory symptoms are mild and self-limited.

sub·clin·i·cal di·a·be·tes (sŭb-klin'i-kăl dī-ă-bē'tēz) A form of diabetes mellitus that is clinically evident only under certain circumstances, such as pregnancy or extreme stress; those so afflicted may, in time, manifest more severe forms of the disease.

sub·con·scious (sŭb-kon'shŭs) **1.** Not wholly conscious. **2.** Denoting an idea or impression that is present in the mind, even though there is at the time no conscious knowledge or realization of it.

sub·con·scious·ness (sŭb-kon'shŭs-nĕs) **1.** Partial unconsciousness. **2.** The state in which mental processes take place without the conscious perception of the person.

sub·cor·tex (sŭb-kōr′teks) Any part of the brain lying below the cerebral cortex, and not itself organized as cortex.

sub·cor·ti·cal (sŭb-kōr′ti-kăl) Relating to the subcortex; beneath the cerebral cortex.

sub·cor·ti·cal a·pha·si·a (sŭb-kōr′ti-kăl ă-fā′zē-ă) A disorder of comprehension and production of language due to damage to the basal ganglia, thalamus, or associated pathways. Symptoms vary depending on the area of subcortical damage and any related cortical damage.

sub·cost·al ar·ter·y (sŭb-kos′tăl ahr′tĕr-ē) *Origin*, thoracic aorta; *distribution*, inferior to twelfth rib in a manner similar to that of posterior intercostal arteries. SYN arteria subcostalis [TA].

sub·cost·al mus·cle (sŭb-kos′tăl mŭs′ĕl) One of a number of inconstant muscles of the posterolateral thoracic wall having the same direction as the internal intercostal muscles but extending across (deep to) one or more ribs. SYN musculus subcostalis [TA].

sub·cost·al nerve (sŭb-kos′tăl nĕrv) The ventral ramus of the twelfth thoracic nerve; it courses below the last rib, supplies parts of the abdominal muscles, and gives off cutaneous branches to the skin of the lower-most ventrolateral abdominal wall and to the superolateral gluteal region. SYN nervus subcostalis [TA].

sub·cost·al plane (sŭb-kos′tăl plān) A horizontal plane passing through the inferior limits of the costal margin (i.e., the tenth costal cartilages); it marks the boundary between the hypochondriac and epigastric regions superiorly and the lateral and umbilical regions inferiorly.

sub·crep·i·tant (sŭb-krep′i-tănt) Nearly, but not frankly, crepitant; denoting a rale.

sub·cul·ture (sŭb′kŭl-chŭr) **1.** A culture made by transferring to a fresh medium microorganisms from a previous culture; a method used to prolong the life of a particular strain where there is a tendency to degeneration in older cultures or to transfer organisms to a medium containing nutrients, reagents, dyes, or other substances to favor growth or facilitate identification. **2.** To make a fresh culture with material obtained from a previous one.

sub·cu·ta·ne·ous (SQ, SC) (sŭb′kyū-tā′nē-ŭs) Beneath the skin. SYN hypodermic. [sub- + L. *cutis*, skin]

sub·cu·ta·ne·ous em·phy·se·ma (sŭb′kyū-tā′nē-ŭs em′fi-sē′mă) The presence of air or gas in the subcutaneous tissues. SYN pneumoderma.

sub·cu·ta·ne·ous fat (sŭb-kyū-tā′nē-ŭs fat) Fat that is stored directly under the skin. Women have a higher percentage of this fat than men.

sub·cu·ta·ne·ous flap (sŭb′kyū-tā′nē-ŭs flap) A pedicle flap in which the pedicle is denuded of epithelium and buried in the subcutaneous tissue of the recipient area.

sub·cu·ta·ne·ous in·jec·tion (sŭb′kyū-tā′nē-ŭs in-jek′shŭn) Injection of fluid into loose connective tissue below the dermis. Absorption is slower than that of intramuscular injection. Common sites include outer posterior side of arm and abdomen. Usually only 0.5–1 mL fluid is given by this method.

sub·cu·ta·ne·ous mas·tec·to·my (sŭb′kyū-tā′nē-ŭs mas-tek′tŏ-mē) Excision of the breast tissues, but sparing the skin, nipple, and areola; usually followed by implantation of a prosthesis.

sub·cu·ta·ne·ous op·er·a·tion (sŭb′kyū-tā′nē-ŭs op-ĕr-ā′shŭn) An operation, as for the division of a tendon, performed without incising the skin other than by a minute opening made by the entering knife.

sub·cu·ta·ne·ous te·no·to·my (sŭb′kyū-tā′nē-ŭs te-not′ŏ-mē) Division of a tendon by means of a small pointed knife introduced through skin and subcutaneous tissue without an open operation.

sub·cu·ta·ne·ous tis·sue (sŭb′kyū-tā′nē-ŭs tish′ū) A layer of loose, irregular connective tissue immediately beneath the skin and closely attached to the corium by coarse fibrous bands, the retinacula cutis; it contains fat cells except in the auricles, eyelids, penis, and scrotum.

sub·cu·ta·ne·ous veins of ab·do·men (sŭb′kyu-ta′nē-ŭs vānz ab′dŏ-mĕn) The network of superficial veins of the abdominal wall that empty into the thoracoepigastric, superficial epigastric, or superior epigastric veins and form portocaval anastomoses through their communications with the paraumbilical veins.

sub·del·toid bur·sa (sŭb-del′toyd bŭr′să) The bursa between the deltoid muscle and the capsule of the shoulder joint. It may be combined with the subacromial bursa.

sub·duce, **sub·duct** (sŭb-dūs′, -dŭkt′) To pull or draw downward. [L. *sub-duco*, pp. *-ductus*, to lead away]

i **sub·du·ral he·ma·to·ma** (sŭb-dūr′ăl hē′mă-tō′mă) SYN subdural hemorrhage. See page 1494.

sub·du·ral hem·or·rhage (sŭb-dūr′ăl hem′ŏr-ăj) Extravasation of blood between the dural and arachnoidal membranes; acute and chronic forms occur; chronic hematomas may become encapsulated by neomembranes. SYN subdural hematoma.

sub·du·ral space (sŭb-dūr′ăl spās) An artificial space created by the separation of the arachnoid from the dura as the result of trauma or some pathologic process; in the healthy state, the arachnoid is tenuously attached to the dura and a naturally occurring subdural space is not present.

sub•en•do•car•di•al bran•ches of a•tri•o•ven•tri•cu•lar bun•dles (sŭb′en-dō-kahr′dē-ăl branch′ĕz ā′trē-ō-ven-trik′yŭ-lăr bŭn′dĕlz) Interlacing fibers formed of modified cardiac muscle cells with central granulated protoplasm containing one or two nuclei and a transversely striated peripheral portion; they are the terminal ramifications of the conducting system of the heart found beneath the endocardium of the ventricles. SEE ALSO conducting system of heart. SYN Purkinje fibers.

sub•en•do•car•di•al lay•er (sŭb′en-dō-kahr′dē-ăl lā′ĕr) The loose connective tissue layer that joins the endocardium and myocardium; in the ventricles, it contains branches of the conducting system of the heart.

sub•en•do•the•li•al lay•er (sŭb′en-dō-thē′lē-ăl lā′ĕr) The thin layer of connective tissue lying between the endothelium and elastic lamina in the intima of blood vessels.

sub•en•do•the•li•um (sŭb′en-dō-thē′lē-ŭm) The connective tissue between the endothelium and inner elastic membrane in the intima of arteries.

sub•ep•en•dy•mo•ma (sŭb′ep-en′di-mō′mă) Discrete lobulated ependymal nodules in the walls of the anterior third or posterior fourth ventricles commonly found at autopsy.

sub•fam•i•ly (sŭb′fam-i-lē) In biologic classification, a division between family and tribe or between family and genus.

sub•fer•til•i•ty (sŭb′fĕr-til′i-tē) Less than normal capacity for reproduction.

sub•ge•nus (sŭb′jē-nŭs) In biologic classification, a division between genus and species.

sub•gin•gi•val cur•et•tage (sŭb-jin′ji-văl kyūr′ĕ-tahzh′) Removal of subgingival calculus, and ulcerated epithelial and granulation tissues found in periodontal pockets.

sub•glos•sal (sŭb-glos′ăl) Below or beneath the tongue. SYN sublingual.

sub•grun•da•tion (sŭb′grŭn-dā′shŭn) The depression of one fragment of a broken cranial bone below the other. [sub- + A.S. *grund,* bottom, foundation]

su•bic•u•lum, pl. **su•bic•u•la** (sŭ-bik′yū-lŭm, -lă) **1.** A support or prop. **2.** The zone of transition between the parahippocampal gyrus and Ammon's horn of the hippocampus. [L. dim. of *subex,* support]

sub•il•i•ac (sŭb-il′ē-ak) **1.** Below the ilium. **2.** Relating to the subilium.

sub•il•i•um (sŭb-il′ē-ŭm) The portion of the ilium contributing to the acetabulum.

sub•in•fec•tion (sŭb′in-fek′shŭn) A secondary infection occurring in one exposed to and successfully resisting an epidemic of another infectious disease.

sub•in•vo•lu•tion (sŭb′in-vŏ-lū′shŭn) Arrest of the normal involution of the uterus following childbirth, with the organ remaining abnormally large.

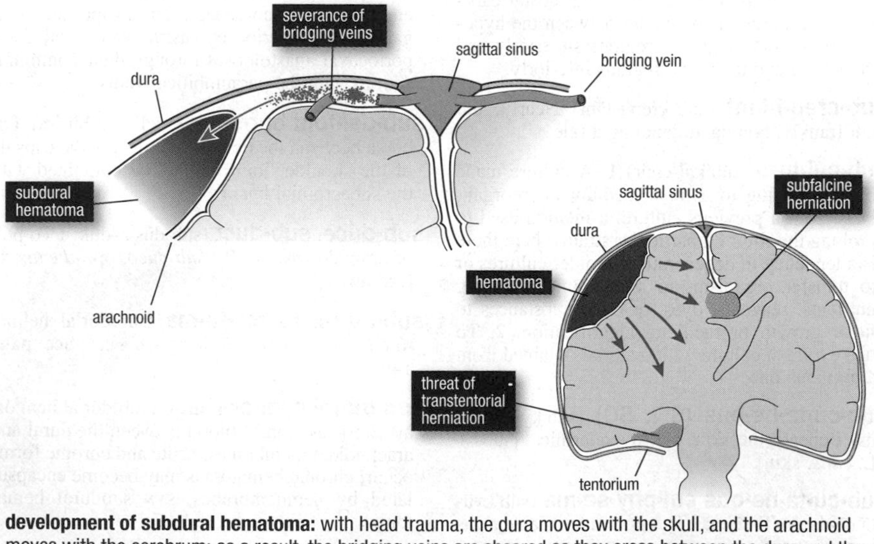

development of subdural hematoma: with head trauma, the dura moves with the skull, and the arachnoid moves with the cerebrum; as a result, the bridging veins are sheared as they cross between the dura and the arachnoid; venous bleeding creates a hematoma in the expansile subdural space; subsequent transtentorial herniation is life threatening

sub•ja•cent (sŭb-jā′sĕnt) Below or beneath another part. [L. *sub-jaceo,* to lie under]

sub•jec•tive (sŭb-jek′tiv) **1.** Perceived by the patient only and not evident to the examiner; said of certain symptoms, such as pain. **2.** Colored by one's personal beliefs and attitudes. Cf. objective (2). [L. *subjectivus,* fr. *subjicio,* to throw under]

sub•jec•tive as•sess•ment da•ta (sŭb-jek′tiv ă-ses′mĕnt dā′tă) Information presented by the patient based on his or her perception, understanding, and interpretation of his or her clinical state.

sub•jec•tive sen•sa•tion (sŭb-jek′tiv sen-sā′shŭn) A sensation not readily referable to a denotably verifiable stimulus.

sub•jec•tive symp•tom (sŭb-jek′tiv simp′tŏm) A symptom apparent only to the patient.

sub•king•dom (sŭb′king-dŏm) In biologic classification, a division between kingdom and phylum.

sub•la•tion (sŭb-lā′shŭn) Detachment, elevation, or removal of a part. [L. *sublatio,* a lifting up]

sub•le•thal (sŭb-lē′thăl) Slightly less than lethal.

subleukaemic leukaemia [Br.] SYN subleukemic leukemia.

sub•leu•ke•mic leu•ke•mi•a (sŭb′lū-kē′mik lū-kē′mē-ă) A form of leukemia in which abnormal cells are present in the peripheral blood, but the total leukocyte count is not elevated. SYN subleukaemic leukaemia.

sub•li•mate (sŭb′lim-āt) **1.** To perform or accomplish sublimation. **2.** Any substance that has been submitted to sublimation. [L. *sublimo,* pp. *-atus,* to raise on high, fr. *sublimis,* high]

sub•li•ma•tion (sŭb′li-mā′shŭn) **1.** The process of converting a solid into a gas without passing it through a liquid state; analogous to distillation. **2.** PSYCHOANALYSIS an unconscious defense mechanism in which unacceptable instinctual drives and wishes are modified into more personally and socially acceptable channels.

sub•lim•i•nal (sŭb-lim′i-năl) Below the threshold of perception or excitation; below the limit or threshold of consciousness. [sub- + L. *limen* (*limin-*), threshold]

sub•lin•gual (SL) (sŭb-ling′gwăl) SYN subglossal.

sub•lin•gual ar•ter•y (sŭb-ling′gwăl ahr′tĕr-ē) *Origin,* lingual; *distribution,* extrinsic muscles of tongue, sublingual gland, mucosa of region; *anastomoses,* the artery of opposite side and submental. SYN arteria sublingualis [TA].

sub•lin•gual cyst (sŭb-ling′gwăl sist) SYN ranula (2).

sub•lin•gual fos•sa (sŭb-ling′gwăl fos′ă) A shallow depression on either side of the mental spine, on the inner surface of the body of the mandible, superior to the mylohyoid line, lodging the sublingual gland.

sub•lin•gual gland (sŭb-ling′gwăl gland) One of two salivary glands in the floor of the mouth beneath the tongue, discharging through the sublingual ducts; most of the secretory units in the human gland are mucus secreting with serous demilunes.

sub•lin•gual nerve (sŭb-ling′gwăl nĕrv) A branch of the lingual nerve to the sublingual gland and mucous membrane of the floor of the mouth. SYN nervus sublingualis [TA].

sub•lin•gual vein (sŭb-ling′gwăl vān) Vein that accompanies the sublingual artery in the floor of the mouth, lateral to the hypoglossal nerve; it may join the deep lingual vein to form the lingual vein, or join the vena comitans nervi hypoglossi.

sub•lux•a•tion (sŭb′lŭk-sā′shŭn) An incomplete luxation or dislocation; although a relationship is altered, contact between joint surfaces remains. [sub- + L. *locatio,* luxation (dislocation)]

sub•mam•ma•ry mas•ti•tis (sŭb-mam′ŏr-rē mas-tī′tis) Inflammation of the tissues lying deep to the mammary gland.

sub•man•dib•u•lar (sŭb′man-dib′yū-lăr) Beneath the mandible or lower jaw. SYN inframandibular, submaxillary (2).

sub•man•dib•u•lar duct (sŭb′man-dib′yū-lăr dŭkt) The duct of the submandibular salivary gland; it opens at the sublingual papilla near the frenulum of the tongue. SYN Wharton duct.

sub•man•dib•u•lar fos•sa (sŭb′man-dib′yū-lăr fos′ă) The depression on the medial surface of the body of the mandible inferior to the mylohyoid line in which the submandibular gland is lodged.

sub•man•dib•u•lar gan•gli•on (sŭb′man-dib′yū-lăr gang′glē-ŏn) A small parasympathetic ganglion suspended from the lingual nerve; its postganglionic branches go to the submandibular and sublingual glands; its preganglionic fibers come from the superior salivatory nucleus by way of the chorda tympani.

sub•man•dib•u•lar gland (sŭb′man-dib′yū-lăr gland) One of two salivary glands in the neck, located in the space bounded by the two bellies of the digastric muscle and the angle of the mandible; it discharges through the submandibular duct; the secretory units are predominantly serous, although a few mucous alveoli, some with serous demilunes, occur. SYN maxillary gland.

sub·man·dib·u·lar tri·an·gle (sŭb′man-dib′yū-lăr trī′ang-gĕl) The triangle of the neck bounded by the mandible and the two bellies of the digastric muscle; it contains the submandibular gland. SYN trigonum submandibulare [TA], digastric triangle.

sub·max·il·la (sŭb′mak-sil′ă) SYN mandible.

sub·max·il·lar·y (sŭb-mak′si-lar-ē) **1.** SYN mandibular. **2.** SYN submandibular.

sub·max·i·mal ex·er·cise test·ing (sŭb-mak′si-măl eks′ĕr-sīz test′ing) A measurement to determine the heart rate response to one or more submaximal work rates and to predice VO_{2max} in patients who are asymptomatic for coronary artery disease. SEE ALSO Astrand-Ryhming Cycle Ergometer Test. SYN McMasters cycle test.

sub·men·tal ar·ter·y (sŭb-men′tăl ahr′tĕr-ē) *Origin*, facial; *distribution*, mylohyoid muscle, submandibular and sublingual glands, and structures of lower lip; *anastomoses*, inferior labial, mental branch of inferior dental and sublingual. SYN arteria submentalis [TA].

sub·men·tal vein (sŭb-men′tăl vān) Situated below the chin, this vein anastomoses with the sublingual vein, connects with the anterior jugular vein, and empties into the facial vein. SYN vena submentalis.

sub·mi·cro·scop·ic (sŭb′mī-krŏ-skop′ik) Too minute to be visible with a light microscope. SYN ultramicroscopic.

sub·mu·co·sa (sŭb′myū-kō′să) A layer of tissue beneath a mucous membrane; the layer of connective tissue beneath the tunica mucosa. SYN tela submucosa.

sub·mu·co·sal plex·us (sŭb′myū-kō′săl plek′sŭs) A gangliated plexus of unmyelinated nerve fibers, derived chiefly from the superior mesenteric plexus, ramifying in the intestinal submucosa.

sub·mu·cous cleft (sŭb-myū′kŭs kleft) SEE laryngotracheoesophageal cleft.

sub·mu·cous cleft pa·late (sŭb-myū′kŭs kleft pal′ăt) SYN occult cleft palate.

sub·mu·cous la·ryn·ge·al cleft (sŭb-myū′kŭs lăr-in′jē-ăl kleft) SEE laryngotracheoesophageal cleft.

sub·na·si·on (sŭb-nā′zē-on) The point of the angle between the septum of the nose and the surface of the upper lip.

sub·nu·cle·us (sŭb-nū′klē-ŭs) A secondary nucleus.

sub·oc·cip·i·tal mus·cles (sŭb′ok-sip′i-tăl mŭs′ĕlz) Group of muscles located immediately below the occipital bone; comprise rectus capitis anterior muscle, rectus capitis posterior major and minor muscles, rectus capitis lateralis muscle, obliquus capitis superior and inferior muscles; innervated by suboccipital nerve. SYN musculi suboccipitales.

sub·oc·cip·i·tal nerve (sŭb′ok-sip′i-tăl nĕrv) Dorsal ramus of the first cervical nerve, passing through the suboccipital triangle and sending branches to the rectus capitis posterior major and minor, obliquus capitis superior and inferior, rectus capitis lateralis, and semispinalis capitis; the first cervical spinal nerve is generally considered to have only motor fibers, but the suboccipital nerve receives sensory fibers for proprioception through a communicating branch from the second cervical spinal nerve. SYN nervus suboccipitalis [TA].

sub·oc·cip·i·to·breg·mat·ic di·am·e·ter (sŭb′ok-sip′i-tō-breg-mat′ik dī-am′ĕ-tĕr) The diameter of the fetal head from the lowest posterior point of the occipital bone to the center of the anterior fontanelle.

sub·or·der (sŭb′ōr-dĕr) In biologic classification, a division between order and family.

sub·pap·u·lar (sŭb-pap′yū-lăr) Denoting the eruption of few and scattered papules, in which the lesions are very slightly elevated, being scarcely more than macules.

sub·per·i·os·te·al am·pu·ta·tion (sŭb′per-ē-os′tē-ăl amp′yū-tā′shŭn) Form of surgical removal in which the periosteum is stripped back from the bone and replaced afterward, forming a periosteal flap over the cut end. SYN periosteoplastic amputation.

sub·phy·lum (sŭb′fī-lŭm) In biologic classification, a division between phylum and class.

sub·pu·bic an·gle (sŭb-pyū′bik ang′gĕl) The angle formed between the inferior rami of the pubic bones. In the female, the angle approximates that angle between the widely extended thumb and index finger (90°); in the male, it approximates the angle between the widely abducted index and middle fingers (60°). SEE ALSO pubic arch. SYN angulus subpubicus [TA], pubic angle.

sub·scap·u·lar ar·ter·y (sŭb-skap′yū-lăr ahr′tĕr-ē) *Origin*, axillary; *branches*, circumflex scapular, thoracodorsal; *distribution*, muscles of shoulder and scapular region; *anastomoses*, branches of transverse cervical, suprascapular, lateral thoracic, and intercostals. SYN arteria subscapularis [TA].

sub·scap·u·lar fos·sa (sŭb-skap′yū-lăr fos′ă) The concavity on the anterior (thoracic) surface of the scapula.

sub·scap·u·la·ris mus·cle (sŭb-skap-yū-lā′ris mŭs′ĕl) *Origin*, subscapular fossa; *insertion*, lesser tuberosity of humerus; *action*, rotates arm medially; *nerve supply*, upper and lower subscapular from posterior cord of brachial plexus (fifth and sixth cervical spinal nerves). See page 1497. SYN musculus subscapularis [TA], subscapular muscle.

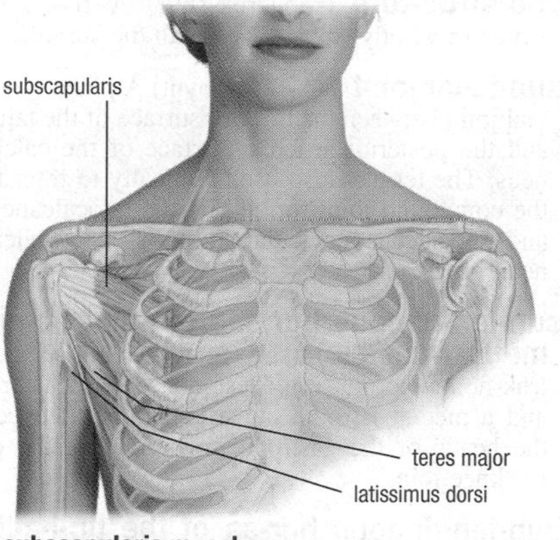

subscapularis muscle

sub•scap•u•lar mus•cle (sŭb-skap′yū-lăr mŭs′ĕl) SYN subscapularis muscle.

sub•scap•u•lar nerves (sŭb-skap′yū-lăr nĕrvz) Two branches of the posterior cord of the brachial plexus, an upper and a lower, supplying the subscapularis muscle; the lower subscapular nerve also supplies the teres major muscle. SYN nervi subscapulares.

sub•scrip•tion (sŭb-skrip′shŭn) The part of a prescription preceding the signature giving directions for compounding. [L. *subscriptio,* fr. *subscribo,* pp. *-scriptus,* to write under, subscribe]

sub•seg•men•tal at•el•ec•ta•sis (sŭb′seg-men′tăl at′ĕ-lek′tă-sis) Collapse of the portion of the lung distal to an obstructed subsegmental bronchus, manifested as a linear opacity on a chest radiograph. SEE ALSO Fleischner lines. SYN platelike atelectasis.

sub•se•ro•sa (sŭb′sēr-ō′să) The layer of connective tissue beneath a serous membrane such as that of the periconeum or pericardium.

sub•si•dence (sŭb′si-dĕns) Sinking or settling in bone, as of a prosthetic component of a total joint implant.

sub•sid•i•ar•y a•tri•al pace•mak•er (sŭb-sid′ē-ar-ē ā′trē-ăl pās′māk-ĕr) Secondary source for rhythmic control of the heart, available for controlling cardiac activity if the sinoatrial pacemaker fails; located within the crista terminalis and atrial free wall near the inferior vena cava.

sub•spi•na•le (sŭb-spī-nā′lē) CEPHALOMETRICS the most posterior midline point on the premaxilla between the anterior nasal spine and the prosthion. SYN point A.

sub•stance (sŭb′stăns) Material. SYN substantia [TA], matter. [L. *substantia,* essence, material, fr. *sub- sto,* to stand under, be present]

sub•stance a•buse (sŭb′stăns ă-būs′) Maladaptive pattern of drug or alcohol use that may lead to social, occupational, psychological, or physical problems.

sub•stance a•buse dis•or•ders (sŭb′stăns ă-byūs′ dis-ōr′dĕrz) A class of mental disorders in which behavioral and biologic changes are associated with regular use of alcohol, drugs, and related substances that affect the central nervous system and personal and social functioning.

sub•stance de•pen•dence (sŭb′stăns dĕ-pen′dĕns) A pattern of behavioral, physiologic, and cognitive symptoms due to substance use or abuse; usually indicated by tolerance to the effects of the substance and withdrawal symptoms when use of the substance is terminated.

sub•stance de•pen•dence dis•or•der (sŭb′stăns dĕ-pen′dĕns dis-ōr′dĕr) A maladaptive pattern of use of alcohol, drugs, or other substances, with tolerance or withdrawal symptoms, drug-seeking behavior, and lack of success in discontinuation of use, to the detriment of social, interpersonal, and occupational activities.

sub•stance P (sŭb′stăns) A peptide neurotransmitter composed of eleven amino acid residues normally present in minute quantities in the nervous system and intestines of humans and various animals and found in inflamed tissue; primarily involved in pain transmission and is one of the most potent compounds affecting smooth muscle (dilation of blood vessels and contraction of intestine), and thus presumed to play a role in inflammation.

sub•stan•ti•a, pl. **sub•stan•ti•ae** (sŭb-stan′shē-ă, -shē-ē) [TA] SYN substance. [L.]

sub•stan•ti•a ba•sal•is (sŭb-stan′shē-ă bā-sā′lis) [TA] SYN basal substantia.

sub•stan•ti•a com•pac•ta (sŭb-stan′shē-ă kom-pak′tă) [TA] SYN compact bone.

sub•stan•ti•a cor•ti•cal•is (sŭb-stan′shē-ă kor-ti-kā′lis) [TA] SYN cortical bone.

sub•stan•ti•a gri•se•a (sŭb-stan′shē-ă grī-sē′ă) [TA] SYN gray matter.

sub•stan•ti•a me•dul•la•ris (sŭb-stan′shē-ă med-yū-lā′ris) **1.** SYN medulla. **2.** SYN medullary substance.

sub•stan•ti•a ni•gra (sŭb-stan′shē-ă nī′gră) A large cell mass, crescentic on transverse section, extending forward over the dorsal surface of the crus cerebri from the rostral border of the pons into the subthalamic region; it is composed of a dorsal stratum of closely spaced pigmented (i.e., melanin-containing) cells, the pars compacta, and a larger ventral region of widely scattered cells, the pars reticulata; the pars compacta in particular includes numerous cells that project forward to the striatum (caudate nucleus and putamen) and contain dopamine, which acts as the transmitter substance at their synaptic endings; other, apparently nondopaminergic cells of the substantia nigra project to a rostral part of the ventral nucleus of thalamus, to the middle layers of the superior colliculus, and to restricted parts of the reticular formation of the midbrain; the nigrostriatal projection is reciprocated by a massive striatonigral fiber system with multiple neurotransmitters, chief among which is gamma-aminobutyric acid; substantia nigra receives smaller afferent projections from the subthalamic nucleus, the lateral segment of the globus pallidus, the dorsal nucleus of the raphe, and the pedunculopontine nucleus of the midbrain. The pars reticulata forms part of the output system for the striate body. The substantia nigra is involved in the metabolic disturbances associated with Parkinson disease and Huntington disease.

sub•stan•ti•a spon•gi•o•sa (sŭb-stan′shē-ă spŭn-jē-ō′să) Bone in which the spicules or trabeculae form a three-dimensional latticework (cancellus), with the interstices filled with embryonal connective tissue or bone marrow. SYN cancellous bone, spongy bone (1), spongy substance, trabecular bone.

sub•stan•tiv•i•ty (sŭb′stăn-tiv′i-tē) **1.** Property of continuing therapeutic action despite removal of vehicle. **2.** The ability of an antimicrobial agent to retain its effectiveness in the mouth for an extended period.

sub•ster•nal goi•ter (sŭb-stĕr′năl goy′tĕr) Enlargement of the thyroid gland, chiefly of the lower part of the isthmus, palpable with difficulty or not at all.

sub•sti•tute (sŭb′sti-tūt) **1.** Anything that takes the place of another. **2.** In psychology, a surrogate.

sub•sti•tu•tion (sŭb′sti-tū′shŭn) **1.** CHEMISTRY the replacement of an atom or group in a compound by another atom or group. **2.** PSYCHOANALYSIS an unconscious defense mechanism by which an unacceptable or unattainable goal, object, or emotion is replaced by one that is more acceptable or attainable; the process is more acute and direct, and less subtle, than sublimation. [L. *substitutio,* to put in place of another]

sub•sti•tu•tion pro•duct (sŭb′sti-tū′shŭn prod′ŭkt) A product obtained by replacing one atom or group in a molecule with another atom or group.

sub•sti•tu•tion ther•a•py (sŭb′sti-tū′shŭn thār′ă-pē) Replacement therapy, particularly when replacement is not physiologic but entails administration of a substitute.

sub•sti•tu•tion trans•fu•sion (sŭb′sti-tū′shŭn trans-fyū′zhŭn) SYN exchange transfusion.

sub•strate (S) (sŭb′strāt) **1.** The substance acted on and changed by an enzyme; the reactant considered to be attacked in a chemical reaction. **2.** The base on which an organism lives or grows, e.g., the substrate on which microorganisms and cells grow in cell culture. [L. *sub-sterno,* pp. *-stratus,* to spread under]

sub•struc•ture (sŭb′strŭk-shŭr) A tissue or structure wholly or partly beneath the surface.

sub•ta•lar joint (sŭb-tā′lăr joynt) A plane synovial joint between the inferior surface of the talus and the posterior articular surface of the calcaneus. The term is also used clinically to refer to the compound joint formed by the talocalcaneal and talocalcaneonavicular joints. SYN talocalcaneal joint.

sub•ten•di•nous bur•sae of gas•troc•ne•mi•us (mus•cle) (sŭb-ten′din-ŭs bŭr′sē gas′trok-nē′mē-ŭs mŭs′ĕl) These consist of a lateral and a medial [Brodie bursa (1)] bursa between the heads of the gastrocnemius and capsule of the knee joint.

sub•ten•di•nous bur•sa of the tib•i•a•lis an•te•ri•or mus•cle (sŭb-ten′din-ŭs bŭr′să tib-ē-ā′lis an-tēr′ē-ŏr mŭs′ĕl) The small bursa between the medial surface of the medial cuneiform bone and the tendon of the tibialis anterior.

sub•ten•di•nous il•i•ac bur•sa (sŭb-ten′din-ŭs il′ē-ak bŭr′să) The bursa at the attachment of the iliopsoas muscle into the lesser trochanter.

sub•tha•lam•ic (sŭb′thă-lam′ik) Related to the subthalamus region or to the subthalamic nucleus.

sub•thal•a•mus (sŭb-thal′ă-mŭs) [TA] That part of the diencephalon that lies wedged between the thalamus on the dorsal side and the cerebral peduncle ventrally, lateral to the dorsal half of the hypothalamus, from which it cannot be sharply delineated. It is composed of the subthalamic nucleus (corpus luysi), the zona incerta, and the fields of Forel; laterally, it expands in a winglike fashion into the reticular nucleus of the thalamus; caudally, it is continuous with the midbrain tegmentum.

sub•trac•tion (sŭb-trak′shŭn) A technique used to enhance detectability of opacified anatomic structures on radiographic or scintigraphic images; a negative of an image made before introduction of contrast medium or radionuclide is photographically or electronically removed from a later image; commonly used in cerebral angiography. SEE ALSO digital subtraction angiography, mask.

sub•tribe (sŭb′trīb) In biologic classification, a division between tribe and genus.

sub•un•gual, **sub•un•gui•al** (sŭb-ŭng′gwăl, -gwē-ăl) Beneath the finger or toe nail. SYN hyponychial (1). [L. *unguis,* nail]

sub•un•gual he•ma•to•ma (sŭb-ŭng′gwăl hē′mă-tō′ma) Collection of blood beneath a fingernail or toenail, usually due to trauma.

sub•un•gual mel•a•no•ma (sŭb-ŭng′gwăl mel′ă-nō′mă) A melanoma beginning in the skin at the border of or beneath the nail.

sub•u•nit vac•cine (sŭb′yū-nit vak-sēn′) A

vaccine that, through chemical extraction, is free of viral nucleic acid and contains only specific protein subunits of a given virus; such vaccines are relatively free of the adverse reactions (e.g., influenza virus) associated with vaccines containing the whole virion.

sub•vag•i•nal (sŭb-vaj′i-năl) **1.** Below the vagina. **2.** On the inner side of any tubular membrane serving as a sheath.

sub•vir•i•on (sŭb-vir′ē-on) An incomplete viral particle. [sub- + virion]

sub•vo•cal speech (sŭb-vō′kăl spēch) Slight movements of the muscles of speech related to thinking but without production of sound.

suc•ce•da•ne•ous tooth (sŭk′sē-dā′nē-ŭs tūth) **1.** A permanent tooth that succeeds an exfoliated deciduous tooth. **2.** Permanent incisors, canines, and premolars.

suc•ci•nyl-CoA (sŭk′sin-il) SYN succinyl-coenzyme A.

suc•ci•nyl-co•en•zyme A (sŭk′si-nil-kō-en′zīm) The condensation product of succinic acid and CoA; one of the intermediates of the tricarboxylic acid cycle and a precursor in the synthesis of heme. SYN succinyl-CoA.

suc•cor•rhe•a (sŭk′ōr-ē′ă) An abnormal increase in the secretion of a digestive fluid. SYN succorrhoea. [L. *succus,* juice, + G. *rhoia,* a flow]

succorrhoea [Br.] SYN succorrhea.

suc•cu•bus (sŭk′yū-bŭs) A demon, in female form, believed to have sexual intercourse with a man during sleep. Cf. incubus. [L. *succubo,* to lie under]

suc•cus•sion sound (sŭ-kŭsh′shŭn sownd) The noise made by fluid with overlying air when shaken, such as occurs with gastric dilation or with fluid and air in a pleural cavity (hydropneumothorax).

suck•ing (sŭk′ing) An oral pattern that emerges in the infant after suckling in which the tongue moves up and down but the lower jaw remains relatively stable and the lips form a firm closure around the nipple, resulting in little loss of liquid.

suck•ing blis•ter (sŭk′ing blis′tĕr) Superficial bullous skin lesion on neonate arm probably resulting from vigorous prenatal sucking.

suck•ing chest wound (sŭk′ing chest wūnd) SYN open pneumothorax.

suck•ing wound (sŭk′ing wūnd) SYN open pneumothorax.

suck•ling (sŭk′ling) An early oral intake pattern seen in infants whose lower jaw and tongue elevate as a unit and thereby place pressure on the nipple to obtain liquid nourishment. This is followed by the tongue's moving in a forward-back action drawing the liquid into the mouth and moving it back to the rear of the oral cavity for swallowing.

su•crase (sū′krās) SYN sucrose alpha-D-glucohydrolase.

sucrosaemia [Br.] SYN sucrosemia.

su•crose (sū′krōs) A nonreducing disaccharide made up of D-glucose and D-fructose obtained from sugar cane, *Saccharum officinarum* (family Gramineae), from several species of sorghum, and from the sugar beet, *Beta vulgaris* (family Chenopodiaceae); the common sweetener, table sugar, used in the manufacture of syrup and confections. SYN saccharose.

su•crose al•pha-D-glu•co•hy•dro•lase (sū′krōs al′fă glū′kō-hī′drō-lās) An enzyme hydrolyzing sucrose and maltose in a complex with isomaltase; hence, hydrolyzes both sucrose and isomaltose; found in the intestinal mucosa; a deficiency of this enzyme results in defective digestion of sucrose and linear α1,4-glucans. SYN sucrase.

su•cro•se•mi•a (sū′krō-sē′mē-ă) The presence of sucrose in the blood. SYN sucrosaemia. [sucrose + G. *haima,* blood]

su•cro•su•ri•a (sū′krō-syū′rē-ă) The excretion of sucrose in the urine. [sucrose + G. *ouron,* urine]

suc•tion cath•e•ter (sŭk′shŭn kath′ĕ-tĕr) A catheter used to remove mucus and other secretions from the upper airway, trachea, and main bronchi.

suc•tion cur•et•tage (sŭk′shŭn kyūr′ĕ-tahzh′) A form of abortion in which the cervix is dilated if necessary and the products of conception removed by use of a cannula attached to a suction source; technique used to complete a spontaneous incomplete abortion or as a form of induced abortion. SYN dilation and suction.

suc•tion drain•age (sŭk′shŭn drān′ăj) Closed drainage of a cavity, with a suction apparatus attached to the drainage tube.

suc•to•ri•al (sŭk-tōr′ē-ăl) Relating to suction, or the act of sucking; adapted for sucking.

su•da•men, pl. **su•dam•i•na** (sū-dā′men, -dam′i-nă) A minute vesicle due to retention of fluid in a sweat follicle, or in the epidermis. [Mod. L., fr. L. *sudo,* to sweat]

su•dam•i•nal (sū-dam′i-năl) Relating to sudamina.

su•dan•o•phil•ic (sū-dan′ō-fil′ik) Staining easily with Sudan dyes, usually referring to lipids in tissues.

su•dan•o•pho•bic (sū-dan′ō-fō′bik) Denoting tissue that fails to stain with a Sudan or fat-soluble dye.

Su•dan vi•rus (sū-dan′ vī′rŭs) A variant of Ebola virus. SYN Ebola virus Sudan.

Su•dan yel•low (sū-dan′ yel′ō) Metadioxy-azobenzene; a yellow stain for fats.

su•da•tion (sū-dā′shŭn) SYN perspiration (1). [L. *sudatio,* fr. *sudo,* pp. *-atus,* to sweat]

sud•den deaf•ness (sŭd′ĕn def′nĕs) A profound sensory hearing loss that develops in 24 hours or less; generally thought to be due to a viral infection in the inner ear.

sud•den death (sŭd′ĕn deth) **1.** An arrhythmogenic death in aortic stenosis, coronary disease, mesothelioma of the AV node, or single coronary artery. **2.** Unexpected death occurring within 1 hour of onset of symptoms; most often used to describe death caused by cardiac failure. SEE ALSO hypertrophic cardiomyopathy.

sud•den in•fant death syn•drome (SIDS) (sŭd′ĕn in′fănt deth sin′drōm) Abrupt and inexplicable death of an apparently healthy infant; various theories have been advanced to explain such deaths (e.g., sleep-induced apnea, laryngospasm, overwhelming infectious disease), but none have been generally accepted or demonstrated at autopsy. SYN crib death.

sud•den sen•so•ri•neu•ral hear•ing loss (SSNHL) (sud′ĕn sen-sōr′rē-nū-răl hēr′ing laws) Hearing loss that affects at least three contiguous pure tone frequencies and occurs within a time span of 72 hours. Because of its rapid onset, this type of hearing loss is frightening and may cause extreme anxiety. Causes of SSNHL include autoimmune disorders, vascular disorders, neurologic lesions, trauma, infectious diseases, and idiopathic sources.

su•do•mo•tor (sū′dō-mō′tŏr) Denoting the autonomic (sympathetic) nerves that stimulate the sweat glands to activity. [L. *sudor,* sweat, + *motor,* mover]

su•dor (sū′dōr) SYN perspiration (3). [L.]

sudor- Combining form indicating sweat, perspiration. [L. *sudor*]

su•dor•al (sū-dōr′ăl) Relating to perspiration.

su•do•re•sis (sū′dōr-ē′sis) Profuse sweating. [sudor- + G. *-ēsis,* condition]

su•do•rif•er•ous (sū′dōr-if′ĕr-ŭs) Carrying or producing sweat. [sudor- + L. *fero,* to bear]

su•do•rif•er•ous ab•scess (sū′dōr-if′ĕr-ŭs ab′ses) A collection of pus in a sweat gland.

su•do•rif•er•ous cyst (sū′dōr-if′ĕr-ŭs sist) A cyst caused by a blocked excretory duct of Moll glands. SYN apocrine hidrocystoma.

su•do•rif•ic (sū′dōr-if′ik) Causing sweat. [sudor- + L. *facio,* to make]

su•do•rip•a•rous (sū′dōr-ip′ă-rŭs) Secreting sweat. [sudor- + L. *pario,* to produce]

suf•fo•cate (sŭf′ŏ-kāt) **1.** To impede respiration; to asphyxiate or smother. **2.** To be unable to breathe; to suffer from asphyxiation. [L. *suffoco* (*subf-*), pp. *-atus,* to choke, strangle]

suf•fo•ca•tion (sŭf′ŏ-kā′shŭn) The act or condition of suffocating or of asphyxiation.

suf•fo•ca•tive goi•ter (sŭf′ŏ-kā-tiv goy′tĕr) A goiter that by pressure causes extreme dyspnea.

suf•fu•sion (sŭ-fyū′zhŭn) **1.** The act of pouring a fluid over the body. **2.** A reddening of the surface. **3.** The condition of being wet with a fluid. **4.** SYN extravasate (2). [L. *suffusio,* fr. *suffundo* (*subf-*), to pour out]

sug•ar (shug′ăr) Colloquial usage for sucrose; pharmaceutic forms include compressible sugar and confectioner's sugar. SEE ALSO sugars. [G. *sakcharon;* L. *saccharum*]

sug•ar-free (shug′ăr-frē′) A product so labeled contains, by F.D.A. order, no more than 0.5 g of sugar per serving.

sug•ars (shug′ărz) Those carbohydrates (saccharides) having the general composition $(CH_2O)_n$ and simple derivatives thereof. Sugars are generally identifiable by the ending -ose or, if in combination with a nonsugar (aglycon), -oside or -osyl. Sugars, especially D-glucose, are the chief source of energy by oxidation in nature, and they and their derivatives in polymeric form are major constituents of mucoproteins, bacterial cell walls, and plant structural material (e.g., cellulose). Sugars are often found in combination with steroids (steroid glycosides) and other aglycons.

sug•gest•i•bil•i•ty (sŭg-jes′ti-bil′i-tē) Responsiveness or susceptibility to a psychological process such as a hypnotic command whereby an idea is induced into, or adopted by, a person without argument, command, or coercion.

sug•gest•i•ble (sŭg-jes′ti-bĕl) Susceptible to suggestion.

sug•ges•tion (sŭg-jes′chŭn) The implanting of an idea in the mind of another by some word or act on one's part, the subject's conduct or physical condition being influenced to some degree by the implanted idea. SEE ALSO autosuggestion. [L. *sug-gero* (*subg-*), pp. *-gestus,* to bring under, supply]

sug•gil•la•tion (sŭg′ji-lā′shŭn) A bruise or livedo. SEE ALSO contusion. [L. *sugillo,* pp. *-atus,* to beat black and blue]

SUI Abbreviation for stress urinary incontinence.

su•i•cide (sū′i-sīd) **1.** The act of taking one's own life. **2.** A person who commits such an act. **3.** BIOWARFARE the act of taking one's own life to harm or kill one's perceived enemies (e.g., suicide bombing). [L. *sui,* self, + *caedo,* to kill]

sul•cal (sŭl′kăl) Relating to a sulcus.

sul•cate (sŭl′kāt) Grooved; furrowed; marked by a sulcus or sulci.

sul•ci par•a•ol•fac•tor•i•i (sŭl′sī par′ă-ōl-fak-tōr′ē-ī) [TA] SYN parolfactory sulci.

sul•cus, gen. and pl. **sul•ci** (sŭl′kŭs, -sī) **1.** One of the grooves or furrows on the surface of the brain, bounding the several convolutions or gyri; a fissure. SEE ALSO fissure. **2.** Any long, narrow groove, furrow, or slight depression. SEE ALSO groove. **3.** A groove or depression in the oral cavity or on the surface of a tooth. **4.** The healthy space between the marginal gingiva and a tooth; a space not exceeding 3 mm is considered healthy. SYN gingival sulcus. [L. a furrow or ditch]

sul•cus ma•tri•cis un•guis (sŭl′kŭs mā′tris-is ŭng′gwis) The cutaneous furrow in which the lateral border of the nail is situated. SYN groove of nail matrix.

sul•cus sign (sŭl′kŭs sīn) A maneuver used to determine inferior instability of the glenohumeral joint, whereby traction is applied to the humerus. If the space widens between the acromion process and humeral head to produce an indentation, a positive test result is confirmed.

sul•cus ter•mi•nal•is (sŭl′kŭs tĕr-mi-nā′lis) [TA] **1.** Sulcus terminalis linguae [NA]. A V-shaped groove, with apex pointing backward, on the surface of the tongue, marking the separation between the oral, or horizontal, and the pharyngeal, or vertical, parts. **2.** Sulcus terminalis cordis [TA]. A groove on the surface of the right atrium of the heart, marking the junction of the primitive sinus venosus with the atrium.

sul•cus test (sŭl′kŭs test) A test for multidirectional shoulder instability; the seated patient's humerus is pulled caudally, with inferior mobility indicating positive result.

♻**sulf-, sulfo-** **1.** Combining forms denoting that the compound to the name of which it is attached contains a sulfur atom. This spelling (rather than sulph-, sulpho-) is preferred by the American Chemical Society and has been adopted by the USP and NF, but not by the BP. **2.** Combining forms of sulfonic acid or sulfonate. SYN sulph-, sulpho-.

sul•fa•tase (sŭl′fă-tās) **1.** Trivial name for enzymes in EC group 3.1.6, the sulfuric ester hydrolases, which catalyze the hydrolysis of sulfuric esters (sulfates) to the corresponding alcohols plus inorganic sulfate. **2.** SYN arylsulfatase. SYN sulphatase.

sul•fa•tides (sŭl′fă-tīdz) Cerebroside sulfuric esters containing one or more sulfate groups in the sugar portion of the molecule. SYN sulphatides.

sul•fa•tion (sŭl-fā′shŭn) Addition of sulfate groups as esters to preexisting molecules. SYN sulphation.

sulf•he•mo•glo•bin (sŭlf-hē′mō-glō-bin) SYN sulfmethemoglobin. SYN sulph-haemoglobin.

sulf•he•mo•glo•bi•ne•mi•a (sŭlf-hē′mō-glō′bi-nē′mē-ă) A morbid condition due to the presence of sulfhemoglobin in the blood; it is marked by a persistent cyanosis, but the blood count does not reveal any abnormality in blood cells; thought to be caused by the action of hydrogen sulfide absorbed from the intestine. SYN sulphaemoglobinaemia.

sulf•hy•dryl (SH) (sŭlf-hī′dril) The radical –SH; contained in glutathione, cysteine, coenzyme A, lipoamide (all in the reduced state), and in mercaptans (R–SH). SYN sulph-hydryl.

sul•fide (sŭl′fīd) A compound of sulfur in which the sulfur has a valence of −2. SYN sulphide.

sul•fite ox•i•dase (sŭl′fīt ok′si-dās) A liver oxidoreductase (hemoprotein) catalyzing the reaction of inorganic sulfite ion with O_2 and water to produce sulfate ion and H_2O_2; a lower activity of this enzyme is observed in cases of molybdenum cofactor deficiency. SYN sulphite oxidase.

sulf•met•he•mo•glo•bin (sŭlf′met-hē′mō-glō′bin) The complex formed by H_2S (or sulfides) and ferric ion in methemoglobin. SYN sulfhemoglobin, sulphaemoglobin, sulphmethaemoglobin.

sul•fo•brom•oph•tha•le•in so•di•um (sŭl′fō-brō′mō-fthal′ē-in sō′dē-ŭm) A triphenylmethane derivative excreted by the liver, used in testing hepatic function, particularly of the reticuloendothelial cells. SYN bromosulfophthalein, bromsulfophthalein, sulphobromophthalein sodium.

sul•fo•nate (sŭl′fō-nāt) A salt or ester of sulfonic acid. SYN sulphonate.

sul•fone (sŭl-fōn) A compound of the general structure $R'–SO_2–R''$. SYN sulphone.

sul•fon•ic ac•id (sŭl-fon′ik as′id) Any of the compounds in which a hydrogen atom of a CH group is replaced by the sulfonic acid group $–SO_3H$; general formula: $R–SO_3H$. SYN sulphonic acid, sulphonic.

sul•fo•nyl•u•re•as (sŭl′fō-nil-yūr′ē-ăz) Derivatives of isopropylthiodiazylsulfanilamide, chemically related to the sulfonamides, which possess hypoglycemic action. Belonging to this series are acetohexamide, azepinamide, chlorpropamide, fluphenmepramide, glymidine, hydroxyhexamide, heptolamide, indylamide, thiohexamide, tolazamide, and tolbutamide. SYN sulphonylureas.

sul•fo•sal•i•cyl•ic ac•id (SSA) (sŭl′fō-sal′i-sil′ik as′id) A reagent used for semiquantitative detection of protein in urine. Protein forms a precipitate that is graded as 1+–4+.

sul•fo•trans•fer•ase (sŭl′fō-trans′fĕr-ās) Generic term for enzymes in EC sub-subclass 2.8.2 catalyzing the transfer of a sulfate group from 3′-

phosphoadenylyl sulfate (active sulfate) to the hydroxyl group of an acceptor. SYN sulphotransferase.

sulf•ox•ide (sŭl-fok′sīd) The sulfur analogue of a ketone, R′–SO–R″. SYN sulphoxide.

sul•fur (S) (sŭl′fŭr) An element, atomic no. 16, atomic wt. 32.066, that combines with oxygen to form sulfur dioxide (SO_2) and sulfur trioxide (SO_3); these combine with water to make strong acids, and with many metals and nonmetallic elements to form sulfides; used externally in the treatment of skin diseases. SYN sulphur. [L. *sulfur,* brimstone, sulfur]

sul•fur 35 (sŭl′fŭr) A radioactive sulfur isotope; a beta emitter with a half-life of 87.2 days; used as a tracer in the study of the metabolism of cysteine, cystine, methionine, and other compounds; also used to estimate, with labeled sulfate, extracellular fluid volumes. SYN sulphur 35.

sul•fur•ic ac•id (sŭl-fyūr′ik as′id) H_2SO_4; a colorless, nearly odorless, heavy, oily, corrosive liquid containing 96% of the absolute acid; used occasionally as a caustic. SYN oil of vitriol, sulphuric acid.

sul•fur mus•tard (H) (sŭl′fŭr mŭs′tărd) A vesicating chemical-warfare agent used extensively in World War I and thereafter and sometimes called "mustard gas," a misnomer because it does not boil until 217°C (423°F). The NATO code for the impure sulfur mustard prepared by the Löwenstein process used in World War I is H; the NATO code for neat, or distilled, sulfur mustard is HD.

sul•fur•yl (sŭl′fŭr-il) Bivalent radical, $–SO_2–$. SYN sulphuryl.

Sul•ko•witch test (sul′kō-vich test) Procedure used to measure the amount of calcium being excreted in urine.

♻ **sulph-, sulpho-** [Br.] SYN sulf-.

sulphaemoglobin [Br.] SYN sulfmethemoglobin.

sulphaemoglobinaemia [Br.] SYN sulfhemoglobinemia.

sulphatase [Br.] SYN sulfatase.

sulphatides [Br.] SYN sulfatides.

sulphation [Br.] SYN sulfation.

sulph-haemoglobin [Br.] SYN sulfhemoglobin.

sulph-hydryl [Br.] SYN sulfhydryl.

sulphide [Br.] SYN sulfide.

sulphite oxidase [Br.] SYN sulfite oxidase.

sulphmethaemoglobin [Br.] SYN sulfmethemoglobin.

sulpho- [Br.] SYN sulfo-.

sulphobromophthalein sodium [Br.] SYN sulfobromophthalein sodium.

sulphonate [Br.] SYN sulfonate.

sulphone [Br.] SYN sulfone.

sulphonic [Br.] SYN sulfonic acid.

sulphonic acid [Br.] SYN sulfonic acid.

sulphonylureas [Br.] SYN sulfonylureas.

sulphotransferase [Br.] SYN sulfotransferase.

sulphoxide [Br.] SYN sulfoxide.

sulphur [Br.] SYN sulfur.

sulphur 35 [Br.] SYN sulfur 35.

sul•phur•ic a•cid (sŭl-fyūr′ik as′id) SYN sulfuric acid.

sulphuryl [Br.] SYN sulfuryl.

sum•mat•ing po•ten•tials (sŭm-āt′ing pō-tĕn′shălz) Alternating current responses of the spiral organ (organ of Corti) to acoustic stimulation.

sum•ma•tion (sŭm-ā′shŭn) The aggregation of a number of similar neural impulses or stimuli. [Mediev. L. *summatio,* fr. *summo,* pp. *-atus,* to sum up, fr. L. *summa,* sum]

sum•ma•tion gal•lop (sŭm-ā′shŭn gal′ŏp) Rhythm in which the gallop sound is due to superimposition of third and fourth heart sounds; sometimes heard in normal subjects with tachycardia, but usually indicative of myocardial disease.

sum•mer di•ar•rhe•a (sŭm′ĕr dī′ă-rē′ă) Intestinal disorder of infants in hot weather, usually an acute gastroenteritis due to *Shigella* or *Salmonella.* SYN choleraic diarrhea.

Sum•ner sign (sŭm′nĕr sīn) A slight increase in tonus of the abdominal muscles, an early indication of inflammation of the appendix, stone in the kidney or ureter, or a twisted pedicle of an ovarian cyst; it is detected by exceedingly gentle palpation of the right or left iliac fossa.

sump drain (sŭmp drān) A drain consisting of an outer tube with a smaller tube within it that is attached to a suction pump; the outer tube has multiple perforations that allow fluid and air to pass into its interior and be carried away through the suction tube.

sump syn•drome (sŭmp sin′drōm) A complication of side-to-side choledochoduodenostomy in which the lower end of the common bile duct at times acts as a diverticulum, resulting in stasis, trapping of food particles, and infection.

sun•burn (sŭn′bŭrn) Erythema with or without blistering caused by exposure to critical amounts of ultraviolet light, usually within the range of 260–320 nm in sunlight (UVB).

sun•down•ing (sŭn′down-ing) The onset or exacerbation of delirium during the evening or night with improvement or disappearance during the day; most often seen in the middle and later stages of dementing disorders, such as Alzheimer disease.

sun pro•tec•tion fac•tor (SPF) (sŭn prō-tek′shŭn fak′tŏr) The ratio of the minimal ultraviolet dose required to produce erythema with and without a sunscreen; useful sunscreens require an SPF that exceeds 14.

sun•screen (sŭn′skrēn) A topical product that protects the skin from ultraviolet-induced erythema; its use also reduces formation of solar keratoses and may prevent ultraviolet-B–induced skin cancer and wrinkling.

sun•stroke, sun stroke (sŭn′strōk) A form of heatstroke resulting from undue exposure to the sun's rays, probably caused by the action of actinic rays combined with high temperature; symptoms are those of heatstroke, but often without fever.

♻ **super-** Properly only prefixed to words of L. derivation, denoting in excess, above, superior, or in the upper part of; often the same usage as L. *supra-*. Cf. hyper-. [L. *super,* above, beyond]

su•per•ac•tiv•i•ty (sū′pĕr-ak-tiv′i-tē) Abnormally great activity. SYN hyperactivity (1).

su•per•a•cute (sū′pĕr-ă-kyūt′) Extremely acute; marked by extreme severity of symptoms and rapid progress, as of the course of a disease.

su•per•cil•i•ar•y (sū′pĕr-sil′ē-ar-ē) Relating to or in the region of the eyebrow.

su•per•cil•i•ar•y arch (sū′pĕr-sil′ē-ar-ē ahrch) A fullness extending laterally from the glabella on either side, above the orbital margin of the frontal bone.

su•per•cil•i•um, pl. **su•per•cil•i•a** (sū′pĕr-sil′ē-ŭm, -ă) [TA] **1.** SYN eyebrow. **2.** An individual hair of the eyebrow. [L. fr. *super,* above, + *cilium,* eyelid]

su•per•con•duct•ing mag•net (sū′pĕr-kŏn-dŭkt′ing mag′nĕt) A magnet with coils that are cooled, usually with liquid helium, to a temperature at which the metal becomes superconducting, effectively removing all electrical resistance.

su•per•duct (sū′pĕr-dŭkt) To elevate or draw upward. [L. *super-duco,* pp. *-ductus,* to lead over]

su•per•e•go (sū′pĕr-ē′gō) PSYCHOANALYSIS one of the three components of the psychic apparatus in the freudian structural framework, the other two being the ego and the id. It is an outgrowth of the ego that has identified itself unconsciously with important people, such as parents, from early life, and results from incorporating the values and wishes of these people and subsequently societal norms as part of one's own standards to form the "conscience."

su•per•ex•ci•ta•tion (sū′pĕr-ek′sī-tā′shŭn) **1.** The act of exciting or stimulating unduly. **2.** A condition of extreme excitement or stimulation.

su•per•fi•cial (sū′pĕr-fish′ăl) **1.** Cursory; not thorough. **2.** Pertaining to or situated near the surface. **3.** SYN superficialis. [L. *superficialis,* fr. *superficies,* surface]

su•per•fi•cial bra•chi•al ar•ter•y (sū′pĕr-fish′ăl brā′kē-ăl ahr′tĕr-ē) An occasional variation in which the brachial artery lies superficial to the median nerve in the arm.

su•per•fi•cial branch of me•di•al cir•cum•flex fe•mor•al ar•ter•y (sū′pĕr-fish′ăl branch mē′dē-ăl sĭr′kŭm-fleks fem′ŏr-ăl ahr′tĕr-ē) Small branch arising from the initial portion of the medial femoral circumflex artery that passes superficially in the superomedial thigh; after giving rise to the superficial branch, the medial femoral circumflex artery continues as the deep branch.

su•per•fi•cial branch of ra•di•al nerve (sū′pĕr-fish′ăl branch rā′dē-ăl nĕrv) Cutaneous terminal branch (with deep branch) that runs under cover of brachioradialis muscle to wrist, then supplies skin of proximal portion of the dorsal aspects of thumb, index, middle, and lateral half of ring fingers and proximal portion of dorsum of hand. SYN ramus superficialis nervi radialis.

su•per•fi•cial branch of ul•nar nerve (sū′pĕr-fish′ăl branch ŭl′năr nĕrv) Branch supplying skin of palmar aspect of little finger and medial half of ring finger, portion of the palm proximal to them, and the palmaris brevis muscle. SYN ramus superficialis nervi ulnaris.

su•per•fi•cial burn (sū′pĕr-fish′ăl bŭrn) A burn involving only the epidermis and causing erythema and edema without vesiculation. SYN first-degree burn.

su•per•fi•cial cer•vi•cal ar•ter•y (sū′pĕr-fish′ăl sĕr′vi-kăl ahr′tĕr-ē) Branch of transverse cervical artery that accompanies the spinal accessory nerve on the deep surface of the trapezius muscle. Alternatively arises as a direct branch of the thyrocervical trunk, in which case it is called the superficial cervical artery. SYN ramus superficialis arteriae transversae colli.

su•per•fi•cial cir•cum•flex i•li•ac ar•ter•y (sū′pĕr-fish′ăl sĭr′kŭm-fleks il′ē-ak ahr′tĕr-ē) *Origin*, femoral; *distribution*, inguinal lymph nodes and integument of that region; sartorius and tensor fasciae latae muscles; *anastomoses*, deep circumflex iliac. SYN arteria circumflexa iliaca superficialis.

su•per•fi•cial dor•sal veins of pe•nis (sū′pĕr-fish′ăl dōr′săl vānz pē′nis) A pair of veins on the dorsum of the penis superficial to the fascia penis; they are tributaries of the external pudendal veins on each side. SYN vena dorsalis penis superficialis [TA].

su•per•fi•cial ep•i•gas•tric ar•ter•y (sū′pĕr-fish′ăl ep′i-gas′trik ahr′tĕr-ē) *Origin*, femoral;

distribution, inguinal nodes and integument of lower abdomen; *anastomoses,* inferior epigastric, superficial circumflex iliac, and external pudendal. SYN arteria epigastrica superficialis.

su·per·fi·cial ep·i·gas·tric vein (sū′pĕr-fish′ăl ep′i-gas′trik vān) Drains the lower and medial part of the anterior abdominal wall and empties into the great saphenous vein. SYN vena epigastrica.

su·per·fi·cial fa·sci·a (sū′pĕr-fish′ăl fash′ē-ă) A loose, fibrous envelope beneath the skin, containing fat in its meshes (panniculus adiposus) or fasciculi of muscular tissue (panniculus carnosus); it contains the cutaneous vessels and nerves and is in relation by its undersurface with the deep fascia. SYN hypodermis, tela subcutanea.

su·per·fi·cial fa·sci·a of per·i·ne·um (sū′pĕr-fish′ăl fash′ē-ă per′i-nē′ŭm) The membranous layer of the subcutaneous tissue in the urogenital region attaching posteriorly to the border of the urogenital diaphragm, at the sides to the ischiopubic rami, and continuing anteriorly onto the abdominal wall. SYN fascia perinei superficialis [TA].

su·per·fi·cial fib·u·lar nerve (sū′pĕr-fish′ăl fib′yū′lăr nĕrv) Branch of common fibular (peroneal) nerve that passes downward in lateral compartment of the leg to supply fibularis longus and brevis muscles and terminate as intermediate and medial dorsal cutaneous nerves supplying skin of dorsum of foot and toes (except for adjacent sides of great and second toes). SYN musculocutaneous nerve of leg, nervus fibularis superficialis, nervus peroneus superficialis, superficial peroneal nerve.

su·per·fi·cial flex·or mus·cle of fin·gers (sū′pĕr-fish′ăl fleks′ŏr mŭs′ĕl fing′gĕrs) SYN flexor digitorum superficialis muscle.

su·per·fi·cial in·gui·nal ring (sū′pĕr-fish′ăl ing′gwi-năl ring) The slitlike opening in the aponeurosis of the external oblique muscle of the abdominal wall through which the spermatic cord (round ligament in the female) and inguinal hernias emerge from the inguinal canal. SYN anulus inguinalis superficialis [TA].

su·per·fi·cial in·vest·ing fa·sci·a of per·i·ne·um (sū′pĕr-fish′ăl in-vest′ing fash′ē-ă per′i-nē′ŭm) SYN perineal fascia.

su·per·fi·ci·a·lis (sū′pĕr-fish′ē-ā′lis) Situated nearer the surface of the body in relation to a specific reference point. SYN superficial (3). [L.]

su·per·fi·cial lin·gu·al mus·cle (sū′pĕr-fish′ăl ling′gwăl mŭs′ĕl) SYN superior longitudinal muscle of tongue.

su·per·fi·cial pal·mar ar·ter·i·al arch (sū′pĕr-fish′ăl pahl′măr ahr-tēr′ē-ăl ahrch) The arterial arch in the hand located superficial to the long flexor tendons approximately at the level of a line extrapolated across the palm from the distal side of the outstretched thumb. It is formed principally by the termination of the superficial ulnar artery and is usually completed by a communication with the superficial palmar branch of the radial artery. The arch gives rise to the common palmar digital arteries. SYN arcus volaris superficialis.

su·per·fi·cial par·tial-thick·ness burn (sū′pĕr-fish′ăl pahr′shăl thik′nĕs bŭrn) Thermal injury that involves only the epidermis.

su·per·fi·cial per·o·ne·al nerve (sū′pĕr-fish′ăl per′ō-nē′ăl nĕrv) SYN superficial fibular nerve.

su·per·fi·cial re·flex (sū′pĕr-fish′ăl rē′fleks) Any reflex (e.g., the abdominal or cremasteric reflex) elicited by stimulation of the skin.

su·per·fi·cial tem·por·al ar·ter·y (sū′pĕr-fish′ăl tem′pŏr-ăl ahr′tĕr-ē) *origin,* a terminal branch of the external carotid (with maxillary artery); *branches,* transverse facial, middle temporal, orbital, parotid, anterior auricular, frontal, and parietal. SYN arteria temporalis superficialis.

su·per·fi·cial trans·verse per·i·ne·al mus·cle (sū′pĕr-fish′ăl trans-vĕrs′ per′i-nē′ăl mŭs′ĕl) An inconstant muscle; *origin,* ramus of ischium; *insertion,* central tendon of perineum; *action,* draws back and fixes the central tendon of the perineum; *nerve supply,* pudendal (perineal). SYN musculus transversus perinei superficialis [TA].

su·per·fi·cial vein (sū′pĕr-fish′ăl vān) One of a number of veins that course in the subcutaneous tissue and empty into deep veins; they form prominent systems of vessels in the limbs and are usually not accompanied by arteries.

su·per·fi·ci·es (sū′pĕr-fish′ē-ēz) Outer surface; facies. [L. the top surface, fr. *super,* above, + *facies,* figure, form]

su·per·in·duce (sū′pĕr-in-dūs′) To induce or bring on in addition to something already existing.

su·per·in·fec·tion (sū′pĕr-in-fek′shŭn) A new infection in addition to one already present.

su·per·in·vo·lu·tion (sū′pĕr-in′vŏ-lū′shŭn) An extreme reduction in size of the uterus, after childbirth, to less than the normal size of the nongravid organ. SYN hyperinvolution.

su·pe·ri·or (sŭ-pēr′ē-ŏr) **1.** Situated above or directed upward. **2.** HUMAN ANATOMY situated nearer the vertex of the head in relation to a specific reference point; opposite of inferior. SYN cranial (2). [L. comparative of *superus,* above]

su·pe·ri·or al·ve·o·lar nerves (sŭ-pēr′ē-ŏr al-vē′ŏ-lăr nĕrvz) Three branches (posterior, middle, and anterior) of the maxillary nerve (or its continuation as the infraorbital nerve) that enter the maxilla to supply the mucosa of the maxillary sinus, upper teeth, and gingiva.

su·pe·ri·or au·ric·u·lar mus·cle (sŭ-pēr′ē-ŏr

awr-ik′yū-lăr mŭs′ĕl) SYN auricularis superior muscle.

su·pe·ri·or ba·sal vein (sŭ-pēr′ē-ŏr bā′săl vān) Tributary to the common basal vein draining the lateral and anterior part of the inferior lobe of each lung.

su·pe·ri·or cer·e·bel·lar ar·ter·y (sŭ-pēr′ē-ŏr ser′ĕ-bel′ăr ahr′tĕr-ē) *Origin*, basilar; *distribution*, upper surface of cerebellum, colliculi, and most of the cerebellar nuclei; *anastomoses*, posterior inferior cerebellar.

su·pe·ri·or cer·e·bel·lar pe·dun·cle (sŭ-pēr′ē-ŏr ser′ĕ-bel′ăr pĕ-dŭngk′ĕl) A large bundle of nerve fibers that originate from the dentate and interpositus nuclei and emerges from the cerebellum in the rostral direction, along the lateral wall of the fourth ventricle. The bundle submerges from the dorsal surface of the brainstem into the mesencephalic tegmentum, where all of its fibers cross in the massive decussation of the superior cerebellar peduncles. Part of the bundle terminates in the contralateral red nucleus; the bulk of the fibers continue rostrally to parts of the ventral intermediate nucleus of thalamus, ventral posterolateral nucleus of thalamus, and central lateral nucleus of thalamus.

su·pe·ri·or ce·re·bral veins (sŭ-pēr′ē-ŏr ser′ĕ-brăl vānz) Numerous (8–10) veins that drain the dorsal convexity of the cortical hemisphere and empty into the superior sagittal sinus, curving rostrally in passing through the subdural space so as to enter the sinus at an acute forward angle. SYN venae superiores cerebri [TA].

su·pe·ri·or cer·vi·cal car·di·ac branch·es of va·gus nerve (sŭ-pēr′ē-ŏr sĕr′vi-kăl kahr′dē-ak branch′ĕz vā′gŭs nĕrv) Uppermost of the branches of vagus nerve conducting presynaptic parasympathetic fibers to, and reflex afferent fibers from, the cardiac plexus; branching from the vagi close to the base of the skull.

su·pe·ri·or cer·vi·cal car·di·ac nerve (sŭ-pēr′ē-ŏr sĕr′vi-kăl kahr′dē-ak nĕrv) The uppermost of the cardiopulmonary splanchnic nerves that arises from the lower part of the superior cervical ganglion and passes down to form, with branches of the vagus, the cardiac plexus.

su·pe·ri·or cer·vi·cal gan·gli·on (sŭ-pēr′ē-ŏr sĕr′vi-kăl gang′glē-ŏn) The most superior and the largest of the paravertebral ganglia of the sympathetic trunk, lying near the base of the skull between the internal carotid artery and the internal jugular vein. All postsynaptic sympathetic fibers distributed to the head and upper neck are derived from the cell bodies that constitute this ganglion.

su·pe·ri·or clu·ne·al nerve (sŭ-pēr′ē-ŏr klū′nē-ăl nĕrv) Terminal branches of the dorsal primary rami of the lumbar nerves, supplying the skin of the upper half of the gluteal region. SYN nervi clunium superiores.

su·pe·ri·or con·stric·tor mus·cle of phar·ynx (sŭ-pēr′ē-ŏr kŏn-strik′tŏr mŭs′ĕl far′ingks) *Origin*, medial pterygoid plate (pterygopharyngeal part), pterygomandibular raphe (buccopharyngeal part), mylohyoid line of mandible (mylopharyngeal part), and the mucous membrane of the floor of the mouth and the side of the tongue (glossopharyngeal part); *insertion*, pharyngeal raphe in the posterior wall of the pharynx; *action*, narrows pharynx; *nerve supply*, pharyngeal plexus. SYN musculus constrictor pharyngis superior [TA].

su·pe·ri·or den·tal arch (sŭ-pēr′ē-ŏr den′tăl ahrch) Those teeth supported by the alveolar process of the two maxillae, whether the 10 deciduous teeth or the 16 permanent teeth.

su·per·i·or ep·i·gas·tric ar·ter·y (sŭ-pēr′ē-ŏr ep′i-gas′trik ahr′tĕr-ē) *Origin*, the medial terminal branch of internal thoracic; *distribution*, abdominal muscles and integument, falciform ligament; *anastomoses*, inferior epigastric. SYN arteria epigastrica superior.

su·pe·ri·or ep·i·gas·tric veins (sŭ-pēr′ē-ŏr ep′i-gas′trik vānz) The venae comitantes of the artery of the same name, tributaries of the internal thoracic vein.

su·per·i·or e·so·pha·ge·al sphinc·ter (sŭ-pēr′ē-ŏr ĕ-sof′ă-jē′ăl sfingk′tĕr) SYN inferior constrictor muscle of pharynx.

su·pe·ri·or ex·ten·sor ret·i·nac·u·lum (sŭ-pēr′ē-ŏr eks-ten′sŏr ret′i-nak′yū-lŭm) The ligament that binds down the extensor tendons proximal to the ankle joint; it is continuous with a thickening of the deep fascia of the leg.

su·pe·ri·or front·al gy·rus (sŭ-pēr′ē-ŏr frŏnt′ăl jī′rŭs) A broad convolution running in an anteroposterior direction on the medial edge of the convex surface and of each frontal lobe.

su·pe·ri·or gan·gli·on of glos·so·pha·ryn·ge·al nerve (sŭ-pēr′ē-ŏr gang′glē-ŏn glos′ō-fă-rin′jē-ăl nĕrv) The upper and smaller of two ganglia on the glossopharyngeal nerve as it traverses the jugular foramen.

su·pe·ri·or gan·gli·on of va·gus nerve (sŭ-pēr′ē-ŏr gang′glē-ŏn vā′gŭs nĕrv) A small sensory ganglion on the vagus as it traverses the jugular foramen.

su·pe·ri·or ge·mel·lus mus·cle (sŭ-pēr′ē-ŏr jĕ-mel′ŭs mŭs′ĕl) *Origin*, ischial spine and margin of lesser sciatic notch; *insertion*, tendon of musculus obturator internus; *action*, rotates thigh laterally; *nerve supply*, sacral plexus. SYN musculus gemellus superior.

su·pe·ri·or glu·te·al ar·ter·y (sŭ-pēr′ē-ŏr glū′tē-ăl ahr′tĕr-ē) *Origin*, internal iliac; *distribution*, gluteal region; *anastomoses*, lateral sacral, inferior gluteal, internal pudendal, deep circumflex iliac, lateral circumflex femoral. SYN arteria glutea superior.

su·pe·ri·or glu·te·al nerve (sŭ-pēr′ē-ŏr glū′tē-ăl nĕrv) Arises from sacral plexus, conveying fibers from fourth and fifth lumbar and first sacral nerves, and supplies the gluteus medius and minimus and tensor fasciae latae muscles (abductors and medial rotators of hip joint). SYN nervus gluteus superior.

su·pe·ri·or hem·or·rhoid·al ar·ter·y (sŭ-pēr′ē-ŏr hem′ŏr-oyd′ăl ahr′tĕr-ē) SYN superior rectal artery.

su·pe·ri·or hy·po·gas·tric (nerve) plex·us (sŭ-pēr′ē-ŏr hī′pō-gas′trik nĕrv pleks′ŭs) The continuation of the aortic plexus inferior to the aortic bifurcation across the fifth lumbar vertebra into the pelvis where it divides into two hypogastric nerves at the sides of the rectum; these join the pelvic splanchnic nerves to form the inferior hypogastric plexuses supplying pelvic viscera.

su·pe·ri·or in·ter·cos·tal ar·ter·y (sŭ-pēr′ē-ŏr in′tĕr-kos′tăl ahr′tĕr-ē) SYN supreme intercostal artery.

su·pe·ri·or·i·ty com·plex (sŭ-pēr′ē-ŏr′i-tē kom′pleks) Term sometimes given to the compensatory behavior, e.g., aggressiveness, self-assertion, associated with an inferiority complex.

su·pe·ri·or la·bi·al ar·ter·y (sŭ-pēr′ē-ŏr lā′bē-ăl ahr′tĕr-ē) SYN superior labial branch of facial artery.

su·pe·ri·or la·bi·al branch of fac·ial ar·ter·y (sŭ-pēr′ē-ŏr lā′bē-ăl branch fā′shăl ahr′tĕr-ē) *Origin*, facial; *distribution*, structures of upper lip and, by a septal branch, the anterior and lower part of the nasal septum; *anastomoses*, the artery of the opposite side and the sphenopalatine. SYN arteria labialis superior, ramus labialis superior arteriae facialis, superior labial artery.

su·pe·ri·or la·bi·al vein (sŭ-pēr′ē-ŏr lā′bē-ăl vān) veins taking blood from the upper lip and discharging into the facial vein.

su·pe·ri·or lar·yn·ge·al ar·ter·y (sŭ-pēr′ē-ŏr lăr-in′jē-ăl ahr′tĕr-ē) *Origin*, superior thyroid; *distribution*, muscles and mucous membrane of larynx; *anastomoses*, cricothyroid branch of superior thyroid and terminal branches of inferior laryngeal. SYN arteria laryngea superior.

su·pe·ri·or la·ryn·ge·al nerve (sŭ-pēr′ē-ŏr lăr-in′jē-ăl nĕrv) Branch of vagus nerve at inferior ganglion; at thyroid cartilage, it divides into two branches. SYN nervus laryngeus superior.

su·pe·ri·or lim·bic ker·a·to·con·junc·ti·vi·tis (sŭ-pēr′ē-ŏr lim′bik ker′ă-tō-kŏn-jŭngk′ti-vī′tis) Inflammation of superior bulbar and palpebral conjunctivae; associated with thyroid dysfunction.

su·pe·ri·or lin·gu·lar ar·ter·y (sŭ-pēr′ē-ŏr ling′gyū-lăr ahr′tĕr-ē) Branch (of the lingular branch) of the left pulmonary artery serving the superior lingular segment of the superior lobe of the left lung. SYN arteria lingularis superior, ramus lingularis superior.

su·pe·ri·or lon·gi·tu·di·nal fa·sci·cu·lus (sŭ-pēr′ē-ŏr lon′ji-tū′di-năl fă-sik′kyū-lŭs) Long association fiber bundle lateral to the centrum ovale of the cerebral hemisphere, connecting the frontal, occipital, and temporal lobes; the fibers pass from the frontal lobe through the operculum to the posterior end of the lateral sulcus, where many fibers radiate into the occipital lobe and others turn downward and forward around the putamen and pass to anterior portions of the temporal lobe. SYN fasciculus longitudinalis superior [TA].

su·pe·ri·or long·i·tu·di·nal mus·cle of tongue (sŭ-pēr′ē-ŏr lon′ji-tū′di-năl mŭs′ĕl tŭng) An intrinsic muscle of tongue, running from base to tip on dorsum just beneath mucous membrane; *action*, shortens upper part of tongue; *nerve supply*, motor by hypoglossal, sensory by lingual. SYN musculus longitudinalis superior linguae, superficial lingual muscle.

su·pe·ri·or mac·u·lar ar·te·ri·ole (sŭ-pēr′ē-ŏr mak′yū-lăr ahr-tēr′ē-ōl) *Origin*, central artery of retina; *distribution*, upper part of macula. SYN arteriola macularis superior [TA].

su·pe·ri·or med·ul·lar·y ve·lum (sŭ-pēr′ē-ŏr med′ŭ-lar′ē vē′lŭm) The thin layer of white matter stretching between the two superior cerebellar peduncles, forming the roof of the superior recess of the fourth ventricle.

su·pe·ri·or mes·en·ter·ic ar·ter·y (sŭ-pēr′ē-ŏr mez′en-ter′ik ahr′tĕr-ē) *Origin*, abdominal aorta; *branches*, inferior pancreaticoduodenal, jejunal, ileal, ileocolic, appendicular, right colic, middle colic; *anastomoses*, superior pancreaticoduodenal and left colic. SYN arteria mesenterica superior.

su·pe·ri·or mes·en·ter·ic (nerve) plex·us (sŭ-pēr′ē-ŏr mez′en-ter′ik nĕrv pleks′ŭs) An autonomic plexus, a continuation of the abdominal aortic plexus, sending nerves to the intestines and forming with the vagus the subserous, myenteric, and submucous plexuses; this periarterial plexus is so dense that it results in the appearance of a characteristic perivascular "collar" distinguishing the superior mesenteric artery from the superior mesenteric vein in several imaging modalities such as with ultrasound.

su·pe·ri·or na·sal con·cha (sŭ-pēr′ē-ŏr nā′zăl kong′kă) **1.** The upper thin, spongy, bony plate with curved margins, part of the ethmoidal labyrinth, projecting from the lateral wall of the nasal cavity and separating the superior meatus from the sphenoethmoidal recess. **2.** The above bony plate and its thick mucoperiosteum, which is less vascular than that of the middle and inferior conchae.

su·pe·ri·or na·sal ret·i·nal ar·te·ri·ole (sŭ-pēr′ē-ŏr nā′zăl ret′i-năl ahr-tēr′ē-ōl) The branch of the central artery of the retina that passes to the upper medial, or nasal, part of the retina.

su•pe•ri•or nu•chal line (sŭ-pēr′ē-ŏr nū′kăl līn) The ridge that extends laterally from the external occipital protuberance toward the lateral angle of the occipital bone; it gives attachment to the trapezius, sternocleidomastoid, and splenius capitis muscles.

su•pe•ri•or o•blique mus•cle (sŭ-pēr′ē-ŏr ō-blēk′ mŭs′ĕl) *Origin*, above the medial margin of the optic canal; *insertion*, by a tendon passing through the trochlea, or pulley, and then reflected backward, downward, and laterally to the sclera between the superior and lateral recti; *action*, primary, intorsion; secondary, depression and abduction; *nerve supply*, trochlear nerve. SYN musculus obliquus superior [TA].

su•pe•ri•or o•blique mus•cle of head (sŭ-pēr′ē-ŏr ō-blēk′ mŭs′ĕl hed) SYN obliquus capitis superior muscle.

su•pe•ri•or or•bi•tal fis•sure (sŭ-pēr′ē-ŏr ōr′bi-tăl fish′ŭr) A cleft between the greater and lesser wings of the sphenoid establishing a channel of communication between the middle cranial fossa and the orbit, through which pass the oculomotor and trochlear nerves, the ophthalmic division of the trigeminal nerve, the abducens nerve, and the ophthalmic veins.

su•pe•ri•or pel•vic aper•ture (sŭ-pēr′ē-ŏr pel′vik ap′ĕr-chŭr) The upper opening of the true pelvis, bounded anteriorly by the pubic symphysis and the pubic crest on either side, laterally by the iliopectineal lines, and posteriorly by the promontory of the sacrum.

su•pe•ri•or phren•ic ar•ter•y (sŭ-pēr′ē-ŏr fren′ik ahr′tĕr-ē) One of a pair of small arteries given off from the thoracic aorta just superior to the diaphragm; *distribution*, diaphragm; *anastomoses*, musculophrenic, pericardiacophrenic, and inferior phrenic. SYN arteria phrenica superior.

su•per•i•or pos•ter•i•or ser•ra•tus mus•cle (sŭ-pēr′ē-ŏr pos-tēr′ē-ŏr sĕ-rā′tŭs mŭs′ĕl) SYN serratus posterior superior muscle.

su•pe•ri•or rec•tal ar•ter•y (sŭ-pēr′ē-ŏr rek′tăl ahr′tĕr-ē) *Origin*, inferior mesenteric; *distribution*, upper part of rectum; *anastomoses*, middle and inferior rectal. As a tributary of the portal vein, its anastomosis with these arteries forms a portosystemic or portocaval anastomosis. SYN arteria rectalis superior, superior hemorrhoidal artery.

su•pe•ri•or rec•tus mus•cle (sŭ-pēr′ē-ŏr rek′tŭs mŭs′ĕl) *Origin*, superior part of common tendinous ring; *insertion*, superior part of sclera of the eye; *action*, primary, elevation; secondary, adduction and intorsion; *nerve supply*, oculomotor. SYN musculus rectus superior [TA].

su•pe•ri•or sag•it•tal si•nus (sŭ-pēr′ē-ŏr saj′i-tăl sī′nŭs) An unpaired dural venous sinus in the sagittal groove, beginning at the foramen caecum and terminating at the confluence of sinuses where it merges with the straight sinus; receives the superior cerebral veins and has lateral extensions, the lateral venous lacunae.

su•pe•ri•or su•pra•re•nal ar•ter•ies (sŭ-pēr′ē-ŏr sū′pră-rē′năl ahr′tĕr-ēz) *Origin*, inferior phrenic artery; *distribution*, suprarenal gland. SYN arteriae suprarenales superiores.

su•pe•ri•or tem•por•al line (sŭ-pēr′ē-ŏr tem′pŏr-ăl līn) The upper of two curved lines on the parietal bone; the temporal fascia is attached to it.

su•pe•ri•or tem•por•al ret•i•nal ar•te•ri•ole (sŭ-pēr′ē-ŏr tem′pŏr-ăl ret′i-năl ahr-tēr′ē-ōl) The branch of the central artery of the retina that passes laterally above the macula to supply the upper lateral or temporal part of the retina.

su•pe•ri•or tem•por•al sul•cus (sŭ-pēr′ē-ŏr tem′pŏr-ăl sŭl′kŭs) The longitudinal sulcus that separates the superior and middle temporal gyri.

su•pe•ri•or thal•a•mo•stri•ate vein (sŭ-pēr′ē-ŏr thal′ă-mō-strī′āt vān) A long vein passing forward in the groove between the thalamus and caudate nucleus, covered by the lamina affixa, receiving the transverse caudate veins along its lateral side, and joining at the caudal wall of Monro foramen with the choroidal vein and vein of septum pellucidum to form the internal cerebral vein.

su•pe•ri•or thor•ac•ic ar•ter•y (sŭ-pēr′ē-ŏr thōr-as′ik ahr′tĕr-ē) *Origin*, axillary; *distribution*, muscles of superior chest; *anastomoses*, branches of suprascapular, internal thoracic, and thoracoacromial. SYN arteria thoracica superior, highest thoracic artery.

su•pe•ri•or thy•roid ar•ter•y (sŭ-pēr′ē-ŏr thī′royd ahr′tĕr-ē) *Origin*, external carotid; *branches*, infrahyoid, superior laryngeal, sternocleidomastoid, cricothyroid, and two terminal branches. SYN arteria thyroidea superior.

su•pe•ri•or ul•nar col•lat•er•al ar•ter•y (sŭ-pēr′ē-ŏr ŭl′năr kŏ-lat′ĕr-ăl ahr′tĕr-ē) *Origin*, brachial; *distribution*, elbow joint; *anastomoses*, posterior ulnar recurrent and inferior ulnar collateral, as part of the articular vascular network of the elbow. SYN arteria collateralis ulnaris superior.

su•pe•ri•or vein of ver•mis (sŭ-pēr′ē-ŏr vān vĕr′mis) A vein draining part of the superior part of the cerebellum; it runs on the superior surface of the vermis to terminate in the internal cerebral vein.

su•pe•ri•or ve•na ca•va (sŭ-pēr′ē-ŏr vē′nă kā′vă) Returns blood from the head and neck, upper limbs, and thorax to the posterosuperior aspect of the right atrium; formed in the superior mediastinum by union of the two brachiocephalic veins. SYN vena cava superior [TA], precava.

su•pe•ri•or ve•na ca•va syn•drome (sŭpĕr′ē-ŏr vē′nă kā′vă sin′drōm) Obstruction of the superior vena cava or its main tributaries by benign or malignant lesions, causing edema and engorgement of the vessels of the face, neck, and arms, nonproductive cough, and dyspnea; bluish-looking venous stars may be found in the early phases, overlying the large veins to which they are tributary, but they tend to diminish in size and disappear after collateral circulation has been reestablished.

su•pe•ri•or ver•mi•an branch (of su•pe•ri•or ce•re•bel•lar ar•te•ry) (sŭ-pēr′ē-ŏr vĕr′mē-ăn branch sū-pēr′ē-ōr ser′ĕ-bel′ăr ahr′tĕr-ē) *Origin:* medial branch of superior cerebellar artery; *distribution:* superior vermis of cerebellum.

su•pe•ri•or ves•i•cal ar•ter•y (sŭ-pēr′ē-ŏr ves′ik-ăl ahr′tĕr-ē) *Origin*, umbilical; *distribution*, bladder, urachus, ureter; *anastomoses*, other vesical branches. SYN arteria vesicalis superior.

su•per•mo•til•i•ty (sū′pĕr-mō-til′i-tē) SYN hyperkinesis.

su•per•nu•mer•ar•y (sū′pĕr-nū′mĕr-ar-ē) Exceeding the normal number. [super- + L. *numerus,* number]

su•per•nu•mer•ar•y or•gans (sū′pĕr-nū′mĕr-ar-ē ōr′gănz) Organs exceeding the normal number, which may develop from multiple foci or organization in an organ-formative field larger (originally) than that of the definitive main organ; such organs are aberrant but frequently not a cause of disease; illness may persist if they are left in the body after therapeutic removal of the main organ, e.g., accessory spleen.

su•per•o•lat•er•al (sū′pĕr-ō-lat′ĕr-ăl) At the side and above.

su•per•ox•ide (sū′pĕr-oks′īd) An oxygen free radical, O_2·, which is toxic to cells.

su•per•ox•ide dis•mu•tase (sū′pĕr-oks′īd dis′myū-tās) An enzyme that catalyzes the dismutation reaction $2O_2{\cdot}^- + 2H^+ \rightarrow H_2O_2 + O_2$; a deficiency is associated with amyotrophic lateral sclerosis.

su•per•sat•u•rate (sū′pĕr-sach′ūr-āt) To make a solution hold more of a salt or other substance in solution than it will dissolve when in equilibrium with that salt in the solid phase; such solutions are usually unstable with respect to precipitating the excess salt or substance and to becoming saturated.

su•per•sat•u•rat•ed so•lu•tion (sū′pĕr-sach′ŭr-ā-tĕd sŏ-lū′shŭn) A solution containing more of the solid than the liquid would ordinarily dissolve; it is made by heating the solvent when the substance is added, and on cooling the latter is retained without precipitation; addition of a crystal or solid of any kind usually results in precipitation of the excess solute, leaving a saturated solution.

su•per•scrip•tion (sū′pĕr-skrip′shŭn) The beginning of a prescription, consisting of the injunction *recipe*, (L., take), usually denoted by the sign ℞. [L. *super-scribo,* pp. *-scriptus,* to write on or over]

su•per•son•ic (sū′pĕr-son′ik) **1.** Pertaining to or characterized by a speed greater than the speed of sound. **2.** Pertaining to sound vibrations of high frequency, above the level of human audibility. SEE ALSO ultrasonic. [super- + L. *sonus,* sound]

su•per•struc•ture (sū′pĕr-strŭk′shŭr) A structure above the surface.

su•pi•nate (sū′pi-nāt) **1.** To assume, or to be placed in, a supine (face upward) position. **2.** To perform supination of the forearm or of the foot. [L. *supino,* pp. *-atus,* to bend backward, place on back, fr. *supinus,* supine]

su•pi•na•tion (sū′pi-nā′shŭn) **1.** The condition of being supine; the act of assuming or of being placed in a supine position. **2.** Transverse plane motion at the radioulnar joint or transverse tarsal joint.

su•pi•na•tor mus•cle (sū′pi-nā′tŏr mŭs′ĕl) *Origin*, lateral epicondyle of humerus, radial collateral and anular ligaments, and supinator ridge of ulna; *insertion*, anterior and lateral surface of radius; *action*, supinates the forearm; *nerve supply*, radial (posterior interosseous). See this page. SYN musculus supinator [TA].

su•pine (sū′pīn) **1.** Denoting the body when lying face upward; opposite of prone. **2.** Supina-

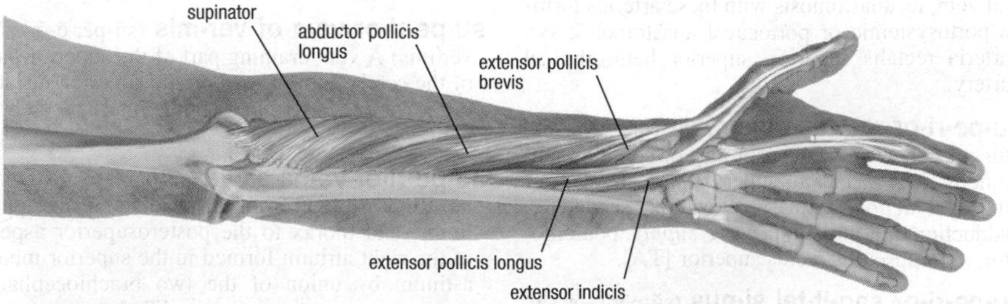

supinator muscle

tion of the forearm or of the foot. SYN dorsal recumbent position. [L. *supinus*]

su·pine po·si·tion (sū'pīn pŏ-zish'ŏn) Lying on the back. See page B29.

sup·ple·men·tal air (sŭp'plĕ-men'tăl ār) SYN expiratory reserve volume.

sup·ple·men·tal groove (sŭp'plĕ-men'tăl grūv) An indistinct linear depression, irregular in extent and direction, that does not demarcate major divisional portions of a tooth.

sup·ple·men·tal in·sur·ance (sŭp'lĕ-men'tăl in-shŭr'ăns) SYN Medigap insurance.

sup·port·ed em·ploy·ment (sŭ-pōrt'ĕd em-ploy'mĕnt) A competitive employment arrangement for people with disabilities that includes integration with nondisabled workers. SEE ALSO abduction, sheltered employment.

sup·port·ing cusp (sŭ-pōr'ting kŭsp) The buccal cusp of the lower posterior teeth and the lingual cusp of the upper posterior teeth.

sup·port sys·tem (sŭ-pōrt' sis'tĕm) NURSING resources, family, friends, and others on whom the patient relies; provides assistance to the patient; support system for family.

sup·pos·i·to·ry (sŭ-poz'i-tōr-ē) A small, solid body shaped for ready introduction into one of the orifices of the body other than the oral cavity (e.g., rectum, urethra, vagina), made of a substance, usually medicated, that is solid at ordinary temperatures but melts at body temperature. [L. *suppositorium,* fr. *suppositorius,* placed underneath]

sup·pres·sion (sŭ-presh'ŭn) **1.** Deliberate exclusion from conscious thought. Cf. repression. **2.** Arrest of the secretion of a fluid, such as urine or bile. Cf. retention (2). **3.** Checking of an abnormal flow or discharge, as in suppression of a hemorrhage. SEE ALSO epistasis. **4.** The effect of a second mutation, which overwrites a phenotypic change caused by a previous mutation at a different point on the chromosome. **5.** Inhibition of vision in one eye when dissimilar images fall on corresponding retinal points. [L. *subprimo* (*subp-*), pp. *-pressus,* to press down]

sup·pres·sion am·bly·o·pi·a (sŭ-presh'ŭn am'blē-ō'pē-ă) Suppression of the central vision in one eye when the images from the two eyes are so different that they cannot be fused into one. This may be due to: 1) faulty image formation (sensory amblyopia); 2) a large difference in refraction between the two eyes (anisometropic amblyopia); or 3) the two eyes pointing in different directions (strabismic amblyopia). Most suppression amblyopia can be reversed if appropriately treated in patients younger than 12 years old; condition may improve with better results in patients who are younger at onset of therapy.

sup·pres·sor mu·ta·tion (sū-pres'ŏr myū-tā'shŭn) **1.** A mutation that alters the anticodon in a tRNA so that it is complementary to a termination codon, thus suppressing termination of the amino acid chain. **2.** Genetic changes such that the effect of a mutation in one place can be overcome by a second mutation in another location. There are two types: intergenic suppression (occurring in a different gene) and intragenic suppression (occurring in the same gene but at a different site).

sup·pu·rate (sŭp'yŭr-āt) To form pus. [L. *suppuro* (*subp-*), pp. *-atus,* to form *pus* (*pur*), pus]

sup·pu·ra·tion (sŭp'yŭr-ā'shŭn) The formation of pus. SEE ALSO suppurate. SYN pyesis, pyogenesis, pyopoiesis, pyosis. [L. *suppuratio*]

sup·pu·ra·tive (sŭp'yŭr-ă-tiv) Forming pus.

sup·pur·a·tive ar·thri·tis (sŭp'yŭr-ă-tiv ahr-thrī'tis) Acute inflammation of synovial membranes, with purulent effusion into a joint, due to bacterial infection. SYN purulent synovitis.

sup·pur·a·tive gin·gi·vi·tis (sŭp'yŭr-ă-tiv jin'ji-vī'tis) Condition in which a purulent exudate can be expressed from the gingival surface.

sup·pur·a·tive hy·a·li·tis (sŭp'yŭr-ă-tiv hī'ă-lī'tis) Purulent vitreous humor due to exudation from adjacent structures, as in panophthalmitis.

sup·pur·a·tive in·flam·ma·tion (sŭp'yŭr-ă-tiv in'flă-mā'shŭn) SYN purulent inflammation.

sup·pur·a·tive ne·phri·tis (sŭp'yŭr-ă-tiv nĕ-frī'tis) Focal glomerulonephritis with abscess formation in the kidney.

supra- Prefix denoting a position above the part indicated by the word to which it is joined; in this sense, the same as super-; opposite of infra-. [L. *supra,* on the upper side]

su·pra·bulge (sū'pră-bŭlj) The portion of the crown of a tooth distal to its greatest circumference, with contours converging toward the occlusal surface of the tooth.

su·pra·cer·vi·cal hys·ter·ec·to·my (sū'pră-sĕr'vik-ăl his'tĕr-ek'tŏ-mē) Removal of the fundus of the uterus, leaving the cervix.

su·pra·cho·roid (sū'pră-kōr'oyd) On the outer side of the choroid of the eye.

su·pra·cla·vi·cu·lar tri·an·gle (sū'pră-klă-vik'yū-lăr trī'ang-gĕl) The triangle bounded by the clavicle, the omohyoid muscle, and the sternocleidomastoid muscle; it contains the subclavian artery and vein.

su·pra·clin·oid an·eu·rysm (sū'pră-klin'oyd an'yūr-izm) An intracranial aneurysm located immediately above the anterior clinoid process of the sphenoid bone.

su·pra·con·dy·lar pro·cess (sū'pră-kon'di-lăr pros'es) An occasional spine projecting from the anteromedial surface of the humerus about 5 cm above the medial epicondyle to which it is joined by a fibrous band. The supracondylar foramen thus formed transmits the brachial artery and median nerve.

su·pra·cos·tal (sū′pră-kos′tăl) Above the ribs.

su·pra·cris·tal (sū′pră-kris′tăl) Above or superior to a crest or ridge; specifically used to denote a line or plane across the summits of the iliac crests.

su·pra·duc·tion (sū′pră-dŭk′shŭn) The upward rotation of one eye. SYN sursumduction.

su·pra·du·o·den·al ar·ter·y (sū′pră-dū′ō-dē′năl ahr′tĕr-ē) *Origin*, gastroduodenal; *distribution*, first part of duodenum. SYN arteria supraduodenalis.

su·pra·glot·tic air·way (sū′pră-glot′ik ār′wā) Oral passageway that facilitates unobstructed access of respiratory gases to the glottic opening by displacing tissue and sealing laryngeal area.

su·pra·glot·tic la·ryn·gec·tomy (sū′pră-glot′ik lar′in-jek′tŏ-mē) SYN partial laryngectomy.

su·pra·glot·tic swal·low (sū′pră-glot′ik swahl′ō) Therapeutic technique to prevent aspiration during swallowing, involving voluntary closure of the vocal folds before and after a swallow. The patient holds her or his breath, swallows with breath held, then coughs when the swallow is finished, before inhaling again.

sup·ra·glot·ti·tis (sū′pră-glot-ī′tis) An infectious inflammation and swelling of the laryngeal tissue above the glottis, especially of the epiglottis, which becomes red and spherical leading to upper airway obstruction.

su·pra·lim·i·nal (sū′pră-lim′i-năl) More than just perceptible; above the threshhold for conscious awareness. Cf. subliminal. [supra- + L. *limen,* threshold]

su·pra·mal·le·o·lar or·thot·ic (SMO) (sū′pră-mal′ē-ō′lăr ōr-thot′ik) A foot orthotic that extends only above the malleoli, thus stabilizing the ankle-foot complex.

su·pra·mar·gin·al gy·rus (sū′pră-mahr′jin-ăl jī′rŭs) A folded convolution capping the posterior extremity of the lateral (sylvian) sulcus; together with the angular gyrus, it forms the inferior half of the parietal lobe.

su·pra·mas·toid crest (sū′pră-mas′toyd krest) The ridge that forms the posterior root of the zygomatic process of the temporal bone.

su·pra·max·il·lar·y (sū′pră-mak′si-lar-ē) Above the maxilla.

su·pra·me·a·tal tri·an·gle (sū′pră-mē-ā′tăl trī′ang-gĕl) A triangle formed by the root of the zygomatic arch, the posterior wall of the bony external acoustic meatus, and an imaginary line connecting the extremities of the first two lines; used as a guide in mastoid operations. SYN Macewen triangle.

su·pra·men·ta·le (sū′pră-men-tā′lē) CEPHALOMETRICS the most posterior midline point, above the chin, on the mandibula between the infradentale and the pogonion. SYN point B. [supra- + L. *mentum,* chin]

su·pra·nor·mal ex·cit·a·bil·i·ty (sū′pră-nōr′măl ek-sī′tă-bil′i-tē) At the end of phase 3 of the cardiac action potential, the successful stimulation threshold falls below (i.e., becomes less negative than) the level necessary to produce excitation during the rest of the phase of diastole, so that an ordinary subthreshold stimulus becomes effective.

su·pra·nu·cle·ar (sū′pră-nū′klē-ăr) Above (cranial to) the level of the motor neurons of the spinal or cranial nerves; the pathways the suprasegmental nerve fibers follow to reach the motor cell bodies in the brainstem; as used in clinical neurology, supranuclear indicates disorders of movement caused by destruction or functional impairment of brain structures other than the motor neurons, such as the motor cortex, pyramidal tract, or striate body, e.g., supranuclear palsy, as distinguished from the nuclear (or flaccid, or "lower motor neuron") paralysis that results from destruction or functional impairment of the motor neurons or their axons in a peripheral nerve.

su·pra·nu·cle·ar pa·ral·y·sis (sū′pră-nū′klē-ăr păr-al′i-sis) Disorder due to lesions above the primary motor neurons.

su·pra·oc·clu·sion (sū′pră-ŏ-klū′zhŭn) An occlusal relationship in which a tooth extends beyond the occlusal plane.

su·pra·op·tic com·mis·sures (sū′pră-op′tik kom′i-shŭrz) SYN commissurae supraopticae.

su·pra·or·bit·al ar·ter·y (sū′pră-ōr′bit-ăl ahr′tĕr-ē) *Origin*, ophthalmic; *distribution*, frontalis muscle and scalp; *anastomoses*, branches of the superficial temporal and supratrochlear. SYN arteria supraorbitalis [TA].

su·pra·or·bit·al fo·ra·men (sū′pră-ōr′bit-ăl fōr-ā′mĕn) A foramen in the supraorbital margin of the frontal bone at the junction of the medial and intermediate thirds. SYN foramen supraorbitale [TA].

su·pra·or·bi·tal groove (sū′pră-ōr′bit-ăl grūv) Depression in the frontal bone above the eyebrow.

su·pra·or·bit·al mar·gin (sū′pră-ōr′bit-ăl mahr′jin) The superior half of the orbital rim, which constitutes the curved superior border of the orbital opening, formed by the frontal bone.

su·pra·or·bit·al nerve (sū′pră-ōr′bit-ăl nĕrv) A branch of the frontal nerve leaving the orbit through the supraorbital foramen or notch and dividing into branches distributed to the forehead and scalp, upper eyelid, and frontal sinus. SYN nervus supraorbitalis [TA].

su•pra•or•bi•tal notch (sū′pră-ōr′bit-ăl noch) A groove in the orbital margin of the frontal bone, about the junction of the medial and intermediate thirds, through which pass the supraorbital nerve and artery.

su•pra•or•bit•al vein (sū′pră-ōr′bit-ăl vān) Drains the front of the scalp and unites with the supratrochlear veins to form the angular vein.

su•pra•or•bi•to•me•a•tal plane (sū′pră-ōr′bit′ō-mē-ā′tăl plān) A plane passing the superior orbital margins and the superior margin of the external acoustic meatuses; it makes an angle of approximately 25–30 degrees with the Frankfort plane and is the plane in which routine computed tomography scans of the brain are made.

su•pra•pa•tel•lar bur•sa (sū′pră-pă-tel′ăr bŭr′să) A large bursa between the lower part of the femur and the tendon of the quadriceps femoris muscle. It usually communicates with the cavity of the knee joint.

su•pra•pu•bic cath•e•ter (sū′pră-pyū′bik kath′ĕ-tĕr) Urinary drainage device inserted into the bladder through the lower abdominal wall above the symphysis pubis. Indications include urethral trauma, vaginal surgery, or long-term catheterization.

su•pra•pu•bic cys•to•to•my (sū′pră-pyū′bik sis-tot′ŏ-mē) Opening into the bladder through an incision or puncture above the symphysis pubis.

su•pra•re•nal (sū′pră-rē′năl) **1.** Above the kidney. **2.** Pertaining to the suprarenal glands.

su•pra•re•nal cor•tex (sū′pră-rē′năl kōr′teks) The outer part of the suprarenal gland, consisting of three zones from without inward: zona glomerulosa, zona fasciculata, and zona reticularis; this part of the suprarenal gland yields steroid hormones such as corticosterone, deoxycorticosterone, and estrone.

su•pra•re•nal gland (sū′pră-rē′năl gland) A flattened, roughly triangular body resting on the upper end of each kidney; an endocrine gland the medulla of which produces epinephrine and norepinephrine and cortex produces cortisol and aldosterone. SYN adrenal gland, epinephros, paranephros.

su•pra•re•nal me•dul•la (sū′pră-rē′năl mĕ-dŭl′ă) It is composed principally of anastomosing cords of cells in the core of the gland; the cells display a chromaffin reaction because of the presence of epinephrine and norepinephrine in their granules.

su•pra•scap•u•lar ar•ter•y (sū′pră-skap′yū-lăr ahr′tĕr-ē) *Origin*, thyrocervical trunk; *distribution*, clavicle, scapula, muscles of shoulder, and shoulder joint; *anastomoses*, transverse cervical circumflex scapular. SYN arteria suprascapularis [TA], transverse scapular artery.

su•pra•scap•u•lar nerve (sū′pră-skap′yū-lăr nĕrv) Arises from the upper trunk of the brachial plexus (fifth and sixth cervical spinal nerves), passes downward parallel to the cords of the brachial plexus, then through the scapular notch, supplying the supraspinatus and infraspinatus muscles, and also sending branches to the shoulder joint. It is vulnerable to injury in fractures of the middle third of the clavicle; a lesion of the suprascapular nerve results in a loss of lateral rotation at the shoulder so that when relaxed the limb rotates medially (waiter's tip position); ability to initiate abduction is also affected. SYN nervus suprascapularis [TA].

su•pra•scap•u•lar vein (sū′pră-skap′yū-lăr vān) Accompanies the suprascapular artery and empties into the external jugular vein.

su•pra•scler•al (sū′pră-skler′ăl) On the outer side of the sclera, denoting the suprascleral or perisclerotic space between the sclera and the fascia bulbi.

su•pra•spi•na•tus mus•cle (sū′pră-spī-nā′tŭs mŭs′ĕl) *Origin*, supraspinous fossa of scapula; *insertion*, greater tuberosity of humerus; *action*, initiates abduction of arm; *nerve supply*, suprascapular from fifth and sixth cervical. SYN musculus supraspinatus [TA], supraspinous muscle.

su•pra•spi•nous fos•sa (sū′pră-spī′nŭs fos′ă) The concavity on the dorsal aspect of the scapula above its spine.

su•pra•spi•nous mus•cle (sū′pră-spī′nŭs mŭs′ĕl) SYN supraspinatus muscle.

su•pra•troch•le•ar ar•ter•y (sū′pră-trō′klē-ăr ahr′tĕr-ē) *Origin*, ophthalmic; *distribution*, anterior portion of scalp; *anastomoses*, branches of supraorbital. SYN arteria supratrochlearis [TA], frontal artery.

su•pra•troch•le•ar nerve (sū′pră-trō′klē-ăr nĕrv) A branch of the frontal nerve supplying the medial part of the upper eyelid, the central part of the skin of the forehead, and the root of the nose. SYN nervus supratrochlearis [TA].

su•pra•troch•le•ar veins (sū′pră-trō′klē-ăr vānz) Several veins that drain the front part of the scalp and unite with the supraorbital vein to form the angular vein.

su•pra•vag•i•nal por•tion of cer•vix (sū′pră-vaj′i-năl pōr′shŭn sĕr′viks) The part of the cervix of the uterus lying above the attachment of the vagina.

su•pra•val•var ste•no•sis (sū′pră-val′văr stĕ-nō′sis) Narrowing of the aorta above the aortic valve by a constricting ring or shelf, or by coarctation or hypoplasia of the ascending aorta.

su•pra•ven•tric•u•lar (sū′pră-ven-trik′yū-lăr) Above the ventricles; especially applied to rhythms originating from centers proximal to the ventricles, namely in the atrium, A-V node, or A-V junction, in contrast to rhythms arising in the ventricles themselves.

su•pra•ven•tric•u•lar crest (sū′pră-ven-trik′yū-lăr krest) The internal muscular ridge that separates the conus arteriosus from the remaining part of the cavity of the right ventricle of the heart.

su•pra•ver•sion (sū′pră-vĕr′zhŭn) **1.** A turning (version) upward. **2.** DENTISTRY the position of a tooth when it is out of the line of occlusion in an occlusal direction. **3.** OPHTHALMOLOGY binocular conjugate rotation upward. [supra- + L. *verto,* pp. *versus,* to turn]

su•pra•vi•tal stain (sū′pră-vī′tăl stān) A procedure in which living tissue is removed from the body and cells are placed in a nontoxic dye solution so that their vital processes may be studied.

su•preme in•ter•cos•tal ar•ter•y (sŭ-prēm′ in′tĕr-kŏs′tăl ahr′tĕr-ē) *Origin,* costocervical trunk; *distribution,* structures of first and second intercostal spaces through its terminal branches, posterior intercostal arteries 1 and 2; *anastomoses,* anterior intercostal branches of internal thoracic. SYN arteria intercostalis suprema, highest intercostal artery, superior intercostal artery.

su•preme na•sal con•cha (sŭ-prēm′ nā′zăl kong′kă) A small concha frequently present on the posterosuperior part of the lateral nasal wall; it overlies the supreme nasal meatus. SYN concha santorini, Santorini concha.

su•ral (sūr′ăl) Relating to the calf of the leg.

sur•al ar•ter•y (sūr′ăl ahr′tĕr-ē) One of four or five arteries arising (sometimes by a common trunk) from the popliteal; *distribution,* muscles and integument of the calf; *anastomoses,* posterior tibial, medial, and lateral inferior genicular. SYN arteria suralis [TA].

sur•al nerve (sūr′ăl nĕrv) Formed by the union of the medial sural cutaneous from the tibial and the peroneal communicating branch of the common peroneal nerve, usually about the middle of the calf, although this is highly variable; thence it accompanies the small saphenous vein around the lateral malleolus to the dorsum of the foot as the lateral dorsal cutaneous nerve. SYN nervus suralis [TA].

sur•al re•gion (sūr′ăl rē′jŭn) The muscular swelling of the back of the leg below the knee, formed chiefly by the bellies of the gastrocnemius and soleus muscles. SYN calf.

sur•face (sŭr′făs) The outer part of any solid. SEE superficial. SYN facies (2) [TA], face (2). [F. fr. L. *superficius*]

sur•face-ac•tive (sŭr′făs-ak′tiv) Indicating the property of certain agents of altering the physicochemical nature of surfaces and interfaces, bringing about lowering of interfacial tension; they usually possess both lipophilic and hydrophilic groups. SEE ALSO surfactant.

sur•face a•nat•o•my (sŭr′făs ă-nat′ŏ-mē) The study of the configuration of the surface of the body, especially in its relation to deeper parts.

sur•face bi•op•sy (sŭr′făs bī′op-sē) A biopsy obtained by detaching cells from a cutaneous or mucosal surface with a spatula, cotton swab, or brush; used to diagnose cervical cancer.

sur•face coil (sŭr′făs koyl) A detector coil applied directly to a body part for high-resolution imaging; often a single loop of metal.

sur•face ep•i•the•li•um (sŭr′făs ep′i-thē′lē-ŭm) **1.** A layer of celomic epithelial cells covering the gonadal ridges as they are formed on the medial border of the mesonephroi near the root of the mesentery. **2.** The mesothelial covering of the definitive ovary.

sur•face mi•cro•sco•py (sŭr′făs mī-kros′kŏ-pē) SYN epiluminescence microscopy.

sur•face ten•sion (sŭr′făs ten′shŭn) The expression of intermolecular attraction at the surface of a liquid, in contact with air or another gas, a solid, or another immiscible liquid, tending to pull the molecules of the liquid inward from the surface; dimensional formula: mt^{-2}.

sur•face tha•lam•ic veins (sŭr′făs thă-lam′ik vānz) SYN venae directae laterales.

sur•fac•tant (sŭr-fak′tănt) **1.** A surface-active agent, including substances commonly referred to as wetting agents, surface tension depressants, detergents, dispersing agents, and emulsifiers. **2.** Those surface-active agents forming a monomolecular layer over pulmonary alveolar surfaces; lipoproteins that include lecithins and sphingomyelins that stabilize alveolar volume by reducing surface tension and altering the relationship between surface tension and surface area. [*surface active agent*]

sur•geon (sŭr′jŏn) A physician who treats disease, injury, and deformity by operation or manipulation. [G. *cheirougos;* L. *chirurgus*]

sur•geon's knot (sŭr′jŏnz not) The first loop of the knot has two throws rather than a single throw. The second loop has only one throw and is placed in a square-knot fashion, leaving the free ends in the same plane as the first loop.

sur•gery (sŭr′jĕr-ē) **1.** The branch of medicine concerned with the treatment of disease, injury, and deformity by operation or manipulation. **2.** The performance or procedures of a surgical operation. [L. *chirurgia;* G. *cheir,* hand, + *ergon,* work]

sur•gi•cal (sŭr′ji-kăl) Relating to surgery.

sur•gi•cal ab•do•men (sŭr′ji-kăl ab′dŏ-mĕn) SYN acute abdomen.

sur•gi•cal a•nat•o•my (sŭr′ji-kăl ă-nat′ŏ-mē)

Applied anatomy in reference to surgical diagnosis and treatment.

sur·gi·cal an·es·the·si·a (sŭr′ji-kăl an′es-thē′zē-ă) **1.** Any anesthesia administered for the performance of an operative procedure, as differentiated from obstetric, diagnostic, and therapeutic anesthesia. **2.** Loss of sensation with muscle relaxation adequate for an operative procedure.

sur·gi·cal di·a·ther·my (sŭr′ji-kăl dī′ă-thĕr-mē) Electrocoagulation with a high-frequency electrocautery, resulting in local tissue destruction; usually used to seal blood vessels and arrest bleeding.

sur·gi·cal em·phy·se·ma (sŭr′ji-kăl em′fi-sē′mă) Subcutaneous emphysema from air trapped in the tissues by an operation or injury.

sur·gi·cal in·ten·sive care u·nit (SICU) (sĕr′ji-kăl in-ten′siv kār yū′nit) Hospital unit designated for care of critically ill surgical patients.

sur·gi·cal mi·cro·scope (sŭr′ji-kăl mī′krŏ-skōp) A binocular microscope used to obtain good visualization of fine structures in the operating field; in the standing type of microscope, a motorized zoom lens system operated by hand or foot controls provides an adjustable working distance; in headborne models, interchangeable oculars provide the magnification needed. SYN operating microscope.

sur·gi·cal pa·tho·lo·gy (sŭr′ji-kăl pă-thol′ŏ-jē) A field in anatomic pathology concerned with examination of tissues removed from living patients for the purpose of diagnosis of disease and guidance in the care of patients.

sur·gi·cal pros·the·sis (sŭr′ji-kăl pros-thē′sis) An appliance prepared as an aid or as a part of a surgical proceeding, such as a heart valve or cranial plate.

sur·gi·cal rod (sŭr′ji-kăl rod) A cylindric implant, usually composed of metal, used to align and internally fix fractures of long bones. SEE ALSO nail, pin.

sur·gi·cal splint (sŭr′ji-kăl splint) General term for a device used to maintain tissues in a new position following surgery.

sur·gi·cal tech·ni·cian (sŭr′ji-kăl tek-nish′ăn) SYN operating room technician.

sur·gi·cal tech·no·lo·gist (sŭr′ji-kăl tek-nol′ŏ-jist) SYN operating room technician.

sur·ro·gate (sŭr′ŏ-găt) **1.** A person who functions in another's life as a substitute for some third person, such as a relative who assumes the nurturing and other responsibilities of the absent parent. **2.** A person who so reminds one of another person that one uses the first as an emotional substitute for the second. [L. *surrogo,* to put in another's place]

sur·ro·gate mo·ther (sŭr′ŏ-găt mŏdh′ĕr) A woman who is under contract to carry a pregnancy for another woman or couple.

sur·round (sŭr-ownd′) Milieu; environment.

sur·sum·duc·tion (sŭr′sŭm-dŭk′shŭn) SYN supraduction. [L. *sursum,* upward, + *duco,* pp. *-ductus,* to draw]

sur·sum·ver·sion (sŭr′sŭm-vĕr′zhŭn) The act of rotating the eyes upward. [L. *sursum,* upward, + *verto,* pp. *versus,* to turn]

sur·veil·lance (sŭr-vā′lăns) **1.** The collection, collation, analysis, and dissemination of data; a type of observational study that involves continuous monitoring of disease occurrence within a population. **2.** Ongoing scrutiny, generally using methods distinguished by practicability, uniformity, and rapidity, rather than complete accuracy. [Fr. *surveiller,* to watch over, fr. L. *super-* + *vigilo,* to watch]

sur·vey (sŭr′vā) **1.** An investigation in which information is systematically collected but in which the experimental method is not used. **2.** A comprehensive examination or group of examinations to screen for one or more findings. **3.** A series of questions administered to a sample of individuals in a population.

sus·cep·ti·bil·i·ty (sŭ-sep′ti-bil′i-tē) **1.** Likelihood of an individual to develop ill effects from an external agent, such as *Mycobacterium tuberculosis*, high altitude, or ambient temperature. **2.** Likelihood that a given pathogenic microorganism will be inhibited or killed by a given microbial agent. SYN sensitivity (4). **3.** MAGNETIC RESONANCE IMAGING the loss of magnetization signal caused by rapid phase dispersion because of marked local inhomogeneity of the magnetic field, as with the multiple air–soft tissue interfaces in the lung; susceptibility measurement can estimate calcium content in trabecular bone.

su·scep·ti·bi·li·ty cas·sette (sŭ-sep′ti-bil′i-tē kă-set′) A common sequence of amino acids in residues 70–74 in the HLA-DRB1 chains, found in alleles associated with rheumatoid arthritis. It is one of two variations: glutamine[Q]-lysine[K]-arginine[R]-alanine[A]-alanine[A] or QRRAA. These susceptibility cassettes are found in many different DRB1 alleles. The alpha and beta chains that form these antigen-presenting molecules have a configuration not unlike a trough or rain gutter; antigens are bound by sequences of amino acids in a pocket along the bottom and sides of the trough or cavity, and this complex forms a heterotrimer with the T-cell receptor on CD4+ cells. SYN rheumatoid pocket, shared epitope.

susp. Abbreviation for suspension.

sus·pend·ed an·i·ma·tion (sŭs-pend′ĕd an′i-mā′shŭn) A temporary state resembling death, with cessation of respiration; may also refer to certain forms of hibernation in animals or to endospore formation by some bacteria.

sus•pen•sion (susp.) (sŭs-pen′shŭn) **1.** Temporary interruption of any function. **2.** A hanging from a support, as used in the treatment of spinal curvatures or during the application of a plaster jacket. **3.** Fixation of an organ, such as the uterus, to other tissue for support. **4.** The dispersion through a liquid of a solid in finely divided particles of a size large enough to be detected by purely optic means; if the particles are too small to be seen by microscope but still large enough to scatter light (Tyndall phenomenon), they will remain dispersed indefinitely and are then called a colloidal suspension **5.** A class of pharmacopeial preparations of finely divided, undissolved drugs (e.g., powders for suspension) dispersed in liquid vehicles for oral or parenteral use. [L. *suspensio,* fr. *sus-pendo,* pp. *-pensus,* to hang up, suspend]

sus•pen•soid (sŭs-pen′soyd) A colloidal solution in which the dispersed particles are solid and lyophobe or hydrophobe, and are therefore sharply demarcated from the fluid in which they are suspended. [suspension + G. *eidos,* resemblance]

sus•pen•so•ry (sŭs-pen′sŏr-ē) **1.** Suspending; supporting; denoting a ligament, a muscle, or other structure that keeps an organ or other part in place. **2.** A supporter applied to uplift a dependent part, such as the scrotum or a pendulous breast.

sus•pen•sor•y ban•dage (sŭs-pen′sŏr-ē ban′dăj) A bag of expansile fabric for supporting the scrotum and its contents.

sus•pen•sor•y lig•a•ment of ax•il•la (sŭs-pen′sŏr-ē lig′ă-mĕnt ak-sil′ă) The continuation of the clavipectoral fascia downward to attach to the axillary fascia; it maintains the characteristic hollow of the armpit.

sus•pen•sor•y lig•a•ment of eye•ball (sŭs-pen′sŏr-ē lig′ă-mĕnt ī′bawl) A thickening of the inferior part of the bulbar sheath that supports the eye within the orbit; it extends between the lateral and medial orbital margins and includes the medial and lateral check ligaments.

sus•pen•sor•y lig•a•ment of lens (sŭs-pen′sŏr-ē lig′ă-mĕnt lenz) SYN ciliary zonule.

sus•pen•sor•y lig•a•ment of o•va•ry (sŭs-pen′sŏr-ē lig′ă-mĕnt ō′văr-ē) A band of peritoneum that extends upward from the upper pole of the ovary; it contains the ovarian vessels and ovarian plexus of nerves. SYN ligamentum suspensorium ovarii [TA].

sus•pen•sor•y lig•a•ments of breast (sŭs-pen′sŏr-ē lig′ă-mĕnts brest) Well-developed retinacula cutis that extend from the fibrous stroma of the mammary gland to the overlying skin. SYN ligamenta suspensoria mammae [TA].

sus•pen•sor•y mus•cle of du•o•de•num (sŭs-pen′sŏr-ē mŭs′ĕl dū′ō-dē′nŭm) A broad, flat band of smooth muscle and fibrous tissue attached to the right crus of the diaphragm and to the duodenum at its junction with the jejunum. SYN musculus suspensorius duodeni [TA].

su•stained-ac•tion tab•let (sŭs-tānd′ak′shŭn tab′lĕt) A drug in tablet form that provides the required dosage initially and then maintains or repeats it at desired intervals. SYN sustained-release tablet.

su•stained-re•lease tab•let (sŭs-tānd′rĕ-lēs′ tab′lĕt) SYN sustained-action tablet.

sus•ten•tac•u•lar (sŭs′ten-tak′yū-lăr) Relating to a sustentaculum; supporting.

sus•ten•tac•u•lum, pl. **sus•ten•tac•u•la** (sŭs′ten-tak′yū-lŭm, -lă) A structure that serves as a stay or support to another. [L. a prop, fr. *sustento,* to hold upright]

Sut•ton dis•ease (sŭt′ŏn di-zēz′) SYN aphthae major.

Sut•ton•el•la in•dol•o•ge•nes (sŭt′ŏn-el′ă in-dō-loj′en-ēz) A species that causes eye infections or endocarditis (when heart valves are present) in humans. SYN *Kingella indologenes.*

Sut•ton ne•vus (sŭt′ŏn nē′vŭs) SYN halo nevus.

Sut•ton ul•cer (sŭt′ŏn ŭl′sĕr) A solitary, deep, painful ulcer of the buccal or genital mucous membrane.

su•tu•ra, pl. **su•tu•rae** (sū-tū′ră, -rē) [TA] SYN suture (1). [L. a sewing, a suture, fr. *suo,* pp. *sutus,* to sew]

su•tur•al (sū′chŭr-ăl) Relating to a suture in any sense.

su•tur•al bones (sū′chŭr-ăl bōnz) Small, irregular bones found along the sutures of the cranium, particularly related to the parietal bone. SYN wormian bones.

su•tur•al lig•a•ment (sū′chŭr-ăl lig′ă-mĕnt) A delicate membrane binding the bones at the cranial sutures.

su•ture (sū′chŭr) **1.** A form of fibrous joint in which two bones formed in membrane are united by a fibrous membrane continuous with the periosteum. SYN sutura [TA]. **2.** To unite two surfaces by sewing. SYN stitch (3). **3.** The material (silk thread, wire, catgut) with which two surfaces are kept in apposition. **4.** The seam so formed; a surgical suture. [L. *sutura,* a seam]

su•ture ab•scess (sū′chŭr ab′ses) A purulent exudate surrounding a stitch.

su•tur•ec•to•my (sū′chŭr-ek′tŏ-mē) Removal of cranial suture.

SV Abbreviation for simian virus, numbered serially, e.g., SV1.

Sv Abbreviation for sievert.

Sved•berg of flo•ta•tion (sfed′berg flō-tā′shŭn) SYN flotation constant.

Sved•berg u•nit (S) (sfed′berg yū′nit) A sedimentation constant of 1×10^{-13} seconds.

swab (swahb) A wad of cotton, gauze, or other absorbent material attached to the end of a stick or clamp, used to apply or remove a substance from a surface.

swaged nee•dle (swājd nē′dĕl) A type of single-use surgical needle with a strand of material attached to it at the time of manufacture.

swal•low (swahl′ō) To pass anything through the fauces, pharynx, and esophagus into the stomach; to perform deglutition. See this page. [A.S. *swelgan*]

swal•low•ing re•flex (swahl′ō-ing rē′fleks) The act of swallowing (second stage) induced by stimulation of the palate, fauces, or posterior pharyngeal wall. SYN pharyngeal reflex (1).

swamp fe•ver (swahmp fē′vĕr) **1.** SYN equine infectious anemia. **2.** SYN malaria.

Swan-Ganz cath•e•ter (swahn ganz kath′ĕ-tĕr) A thin (5 Fr), flexible, flow-directed venous catheter using a balloon to carry it through the heart to a pulmonary artery; when it is positioned in a small arterial branch, pulmonary wedge pressure is measured in front of the temporarily inflated and wedged balloon. SYN pulmonary artery catheter.

swan-neck de•form•i•ty (swahn-nek dĕ-fōrm′i-tē) Deformity of a finger involving hyperextension of the proximal interphalangeal joint (PIP) and flexion of the distal interphalangeal joint (DIP).

S wave (wāv) A component of the cardiac cycle seen on ECG as a negative (downward) deflection of the QRS complex following an R wave; successive downward deflections within the same QRS complex are labeled S′, S″, and so on.

sweat (swet) **1.** Perspiration (3), especially sensible perspiration. **2.** To perspire. [*A.S. swāt*]

sweat gland car•ci•no•ma (swet gland kahr′si-nō′mă) Usually a solitary tumor, nodular and fixed to the skin and underlying structures, having slow growth for long periods followed by rapid growth and dissemination.

sweat glands (swet glandz) The coiled glands of the skin that secrete the sweat.

sweat•ing (swet′ing) SYN perspiration (1).

sweat pore (swet pōr) The surface opening of the duct of a sweat gland. SYN pore (2).

Swe•dish mas•sage (swē′dish mă-sahzh′) A massage technique that includes effleurage, pétrissage, friction, vibration, and tapotement. Swedish massage is intended to improve circulation and tissue elasticity while reducing muscle tone and creating a parasympathetic response.

Swee•ley-Kli•on•sky dis•ease (swē′lē klē-on′skē di-zēz′) SYN Fabry disease.

sweet bay (swēt bā) SYN bay.

sweet broom (swēt brūm) SYN butcher's broom.

sweet colts•foot (swēt kōlts′fut) SYN butterbur.

swell•ing (swel′ing) **1.** An enlargement, e.g., a protuberance or tumor. **2.** EMBRYOLOGY a primordial elevation that develops into a fold, ridge, prominence, or process.

Swift dis•ease (swift di-zēz′) SYN acrodynia (2).

swim•mer's ear (swim′ĕrz ēr) Otitis externa that occurs after frequent or prolonged swimming.

swim•mer's itch (swim′ĕrz ich) **1.** SYN cutaneous ancylostomiasis. **2.** SYN schistosomal dermatitis. SEE ALSO seabather's eruption.

swim•ming pool con•junc•ti•vi•tis (swim′ing pūl kŏn-jŭngk′ti-vī′tis) The disorder seen in a swimmer, which can be caused by pool chlorination, adenovirus, and rarely, *Chlamydia*.

switch•ing site (swich′ing sīt) The breakpoint in a DNA sequence at which a gene segment unites with another gene segment, as in the production of the immunoglobulins.

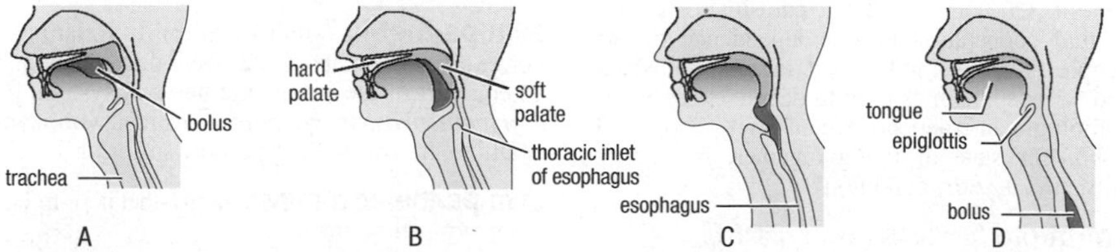

swallowing: (A) the bolus of food is pushed to the back of the mouth by pushing the tongue against the palate; (B) the nasopharynx is sealed off and the larynx is elevated, enlarging the pharynx to receive food; (C) the pharyngeal sphincters contract sequentially, squeezing food into the esophagus, the epiglottis closes the trachea; (D) the bolus of food moves down the esophagus by peristaltic contraction

Swy•er-James syn•drome (swī′ĕr jāmz sin′drōm) **1.** SYN unilateral lobar emphysema. **2.** Hyperlucency of one lung from obliterating bronchiolitis, usually caused by adenovirus infection in childhood, with decreased size and vascularity of the lung; distinguished from other causes of unilateral hyperlucency by demonstration of air trapping without central obstruction.

Swy•er syn•drome (swī′ĕr sin′drōm) Gonadal dysgenesis in phenotypic females with XY genotype.

sy•co•ma (sī-kō′mă) **1.** A pendulous, figlike growth. **2.** A large, soft wart. [G. *sykōma,* fr. *sykon,* fig, + *-oma,* tumor]

sy•co•si•form (sī-kō′si-fōrm) Resembling sycosis.

sy•co•sis (sī-kō′sis) A pustular folliculitis, particularly of the bearded area. [G. *sykōsis,* fr. *sykōn,* fig, + *-osis,* condition]

Sy•den•ham cho•re•a (sid′ĕn-ham kōr-ē′ă) A postinfectious chorea appearing several months after a streptococcal infection with subsequent rheumatic fever. The chorea typically involves the distal limbs and is associated with hypotonia and emotional lability. Improvement occurs over weeks or months, and exacerbations occur without associated infection recurrence.

Syl•vest dis•ease (sil-vest′ di-zēz′) SYN epidemic pleurodynia.

syl•vi•an (sil′vē-ăn) Relating to Franciscus or Jacobaeus Sylvius or to any of the structures described by either.

sym- SEE syn-.

sym•bal•lo•phone (sim-bal′ō-fōn) A stethoscope having two chest pieces, designed to lateralize sound and produce a stereophonic effect. [G. *symballō,* to throw together, + *phōnē,* sound]

sym•bi•on, sym•bi•ont (sim′bē-on, -ont) An organism associated with another in symbiosis. SYN mutualist, symbiote. [G. *symbion,* neut. of *symbiōs,* living together]

sym•bi•o•sis (sim′bē-ō′sis) **1.** The biologic association of two or more species to their mutual benefit. Cf. commensalism, parasitism. **2.** The mutual cooperation or interdependence of two people, such as mother and infant or husband and wife; sometimes used to denote excessive or pathologic interdependence of two people. [G. *symbiōsis,* state of living together, fr. sym- + *bios,* life, + *-osis,* condition]

sym•bi•ote (sim′bē-ōt) SYN symbion.

sym•bi•ot•ic (sim′bē-ot′ik) Relating to symbiosis.

sym•bleph•a•ron (sim-blef′ă-ron) Adhesion of one or both eyelids to the eyeball, partial or complete, resulting from burns, trauma, or cicatricial pemphigoid. SEE ALSO blepharosynechia. [sym- + G. *blepharon,* eyelid]

sym•bol•ism (sim′bŏl-izm) **1.** PSYCHOANALYSIS the process involved in the disguised representation in consciousness of unconscious or repressed contents or events. **2.** A mental state in which one regards everything that happens as symbolic of one's own thoughts. **3.** The description of the emotional life and experiences in abstract terms.

sym•bol•i•za•tion (sim′bŏ-lī-zā′shŭn) An unconscious mental mechanism whereby one object or idea is represented by another.

sym•brach•y•dac•ty•ly (sim-brak′i-dak′ti-lē) Condition in which abnormally short fingers are joined or webbed in their proximal portions. [sym- + G. *brachys,* short, + *daktylos,* finger]

Syme am•pu•ta•tion, Syme op•er•a•tion (sīm amp′yū-tā′shŭn, op-ĕr-ā′shŭn) Surgical removal of the foot at the ankle joint, the malleoli being sawed off, and a flap being made with the soft parts of the heel.

sym•me•tric fe•tal growth re•stric•tion (si-met′rik fē′tăl grōth rĕ-strik′shŭn) Proportional reduction in fetal head and body size, commonly constitutional or caused by an early intrauterine insult such as infection.

sym•met•ric gan•grene (sim-met′rik gang-grēn′) The condition affecting the extremities of both sides of the body; it is seen particularly in severe arteriosclerosis, myocardial infarction, and ball-valve thrombus.

sym•me•try (sim′ĕ-trē) Equality or correspondence in form of parts distributed around a center or an axis, at the extremities or poles, or on the opposite sides of any body. [G. *symmetria,* fr. sym- + *metron,* measure]

sympath-, sympatheto-, sympathico-, sympatho- Combining forms denoting the sympathetic part of the autonomic nervous system. SEE ALSO sympathetic.

sym•pa•thec•to•my (sim′pă-thek′tŏ-mē) Excision of a segment of a sympathetic nerve or of one or more sympathetic ganglia. [sympath- + G. *ektomē,* excision]

sym•pa•thet•ic (sim′pă-thet′ik) **1.** Relating to or exhibiting sympathy. **2.** Denoting the sympathetic part of the autonomic nervous system. [G. *sympathētikos,* fr. *sympatheō,* to feel with, sympathize, fr. *syn,* with, + *pathos,* suffering]

sym•pa•thet•ic a•mine (sim′pă-thet′ik ă-mēn′) SYN sympathomimetic amine.

sym•pa•thet•ic gan•gli•a (sim′pă-thet′ik gang′glē-ă) Those ganglia of the autonomic nervous system that receive efferent fibers originating from preganglionic visceral motor neurons in the intermediolateral cell column of thoracic and upper lumbar spinal segments (T1–L2). On the basis of their location, the sympathetic ganglia can be classified as paravertebral ganglia (ganglia trunci sympathici) and prevertebral ganglia (ganglia celiaca). SEE ALSO autonomic division of nervous system.

sym•pa•thet•ic nerve (sim′pă-thet′ik nĕrv) One of the nerves of the sympathetic nervous system.

sym•pa•thet•ic ner•vous sys•tem (sim′pă-thet′ik nĕr′vŭs sis′tĕm) **1.** In earlier usage, the entire autonomic nervous system. **2.** The branch of the autonomic nervous system that supplies motor control to glands, smooth muscle, and cardiac tissue, specifically in response to perceived threat, danger, or to stress. SEE ALSO autonomic division of nervous system. Cf. parasympathetic nervous system.

sym•pa•thet•ic oph•thal•mi•a (sim′pă-thet′ik of-thal′mē-ă) Immune inflammation in a noninfected eye after trauma to the fellow eye.

sym•pa•thet•ic re•sponse (sim′pă-thet′ik rē-spons′) The action in glandular, smooth muscle, and cardiac tissue during perceived threat or stress. Cf. parasympathetic response.

sym•pa•thet•ic root of pter•y•go•pal•a•tine gang•li•on (sim′pă-thet′ĭk rūt ter′i-gō-pal′ă-tīn gang′glē-ŏn) SYN deep petrosal nerve.

sym•pa•thet•ic trunk (sim′pă-thet′ik trŭngk) One of the two long, ganglionated nerve strands alongside the vertebral column that extend from the base of the skull to the coccyx; they are connected to each spinal nerve by gray rami and receive fibers from the spinal cord through white rami connecting with the thoracic and upper lumbar spinal nerves. See page 1518. SYN truncus sympathicus [TA].

sym•pa•thet•ic u•ve•i•tis (sim′pă-thet′ik yū′vē-ī′tis) A bilateral inflammation of the uveal tract caused by a perforating wound of one eye that injures the uvea, exposing it to the immune system.

sym•pa•thet•o•blast (sim′pă-thet′ŏ-blast) SYN sympathoblast.

sym•path•i•co•blast (sim-path′i-kō-blast) SYN sympathoblast.

sym•path•i•co•lyt•ic (sim-path′i-kō-lit′ik) SYN sympatholytic.

sym•path•i•co•mi•met•ic (sim-path′i-kō-mi-met′ik) SYN sympathomimetic.

sym•path•i•co•to•ni•a (sim-path′i-kō-tō′nē-ă) A condition in which there is increased tonus of the sympathetic system and a marked tendency to vascular spasm and high blood pressure; opposed to vagotonia. [sympathico- + G. *tonos,* tone, tension]

sym•path•i•co•ton•ic (sim-path′i-kō-ton′ik) Relating to or characterized by sympathicotonia.

sym•path•i•co•trip•sy (sim-path′i-kō-trip-sē) Operation of crushing a sympathetic ganglion. [sympathico- + G. *tripsis,* a rubbing]

sym•pa•tho•ad•re•nal (sim′pă-thō-ă-drē′năl) Relating to the sympathetic part of the autonomic nervous system and the medulla of the suprarenal gland, as the postganglionic neurons.

sym•pa•tho•blast (sim′pă-thō-blast) A primordial cell derived from the neural crest glia; with the pheochromoblasts, sympathoblasts enter into the formation of the medulla of the suprarenal gland and sympathetic ganglia. SYN sympathetoblast, sympathicoblast. [sympatho- + G. *blastos,* germ]

sym•pa•tho•go•ni•a (sim′pă-thō-gō′nē-ă) The completely undifferentiated cells of the sympathetic nervous system. [sympatho- + G. *gonē,* seed]

sym•pa•tho•lyt•ic (sim′pă-thō-lit′ik) Denoting antagonism to or inhibition of adrenergic nerve activity. SEE ALSO adrenergic blocking agent, antiadrenergic. SYN sympathicolytic. [sympatho- + G. *lysis,* a loosening]

sym•pa•tho•mi•met•ic (sim′pă-thō-mi-met′ik) Denoting mimicking of action of the sympathetic system. SEE ALSO adrenomimetic. SYN sympathicomimetic. [sympatho- + G. *mimikos,* imitating]

sym•pa•tho•mi•met•ic a•mine (sim′pă-thō-mi-met′ik ă-mēn′) An agent that evokes responses similar to those produced by adrenergic nerve activity (e.g., epinephrine, ephedrine, isoproterenol). SYN adrenomimetic amine, sympathetic amine.

sym•pa•thy (sim′pă-thē) **1.** The mutual relation, physiologic or pathologic, between two organs, systems, or parts of the body. **2.** Mental contagion, as seen in mass hysteria or in the yawning induced by seeing another person yawn. **3.** An expressed sensitive appreciation or emotional concern for and sharing of the mental and emotional state of another person. Cf. empathy (1). [G. *sympatheia,* fr. sym- + *pathos,* suffering]

sym•pha•lan•gism, **sym•pha•lan•gy** (sim-fal′ăn-jizm, -jē) **1.** SYN syndactyly. **2.** Ankylosis of the finger or toe joints. [sym- + phalanx]

sym•phys•i•al, **sym•phys•e•al** (sim-fiz′ē-ăl) Grown together; relating to a symphysis; fused.

sym•phys•i•on (sim-fiz′ē-on) A craniometric point, the most anterior point of the alveolar process of the mandible.

sym•phys•i•ot•o•my, **sym•phys•e•ot•o•my** (sim-fiz′ē-ot′ŏ-mē) Division of the pubic joint to increase the capacity of a contracted pelvis sufficiently to permit passage of a living child. SYN pelviotomy (1), pelvitomy, synchondrotomy. [symphysis + G. *tomē,* incision]

sym•phy•sis, gen. **sym•phy•ses** (sim′fi-sis, -sēz) **1.** [TA] Form of cartilaginous joint in which union between two bones is effected by means of fibrocartilage. **2.** A union, meeting

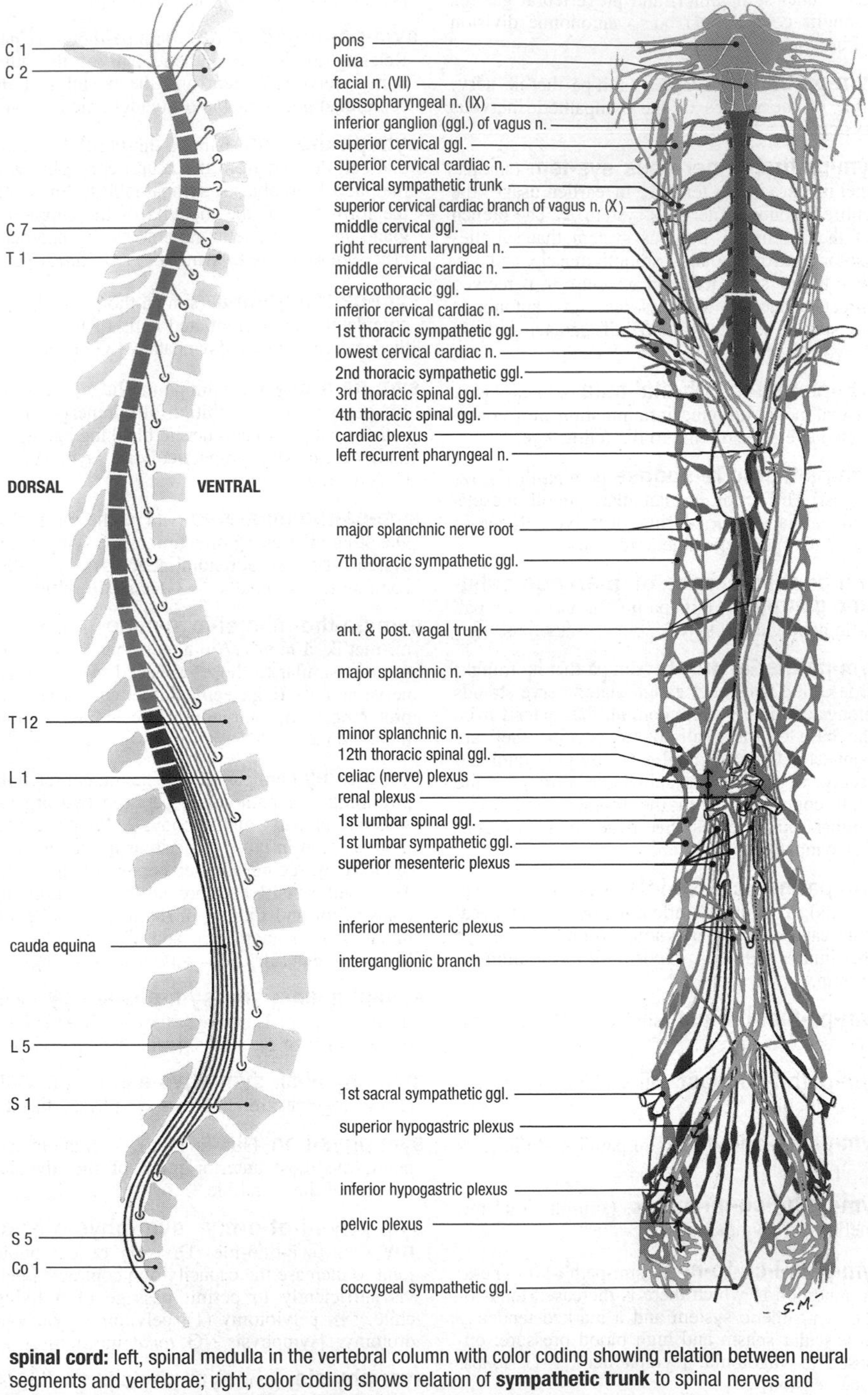

spinal cord: left, spinal medulla in the vertebral column with color coding showing relation between neural segments and vertebrae; right, color coding shows relation of **sympathetic trunk** to spinal nerves and branches; ggl. = ganglion/ganglia; n. = nerve(s)

point, or commissure of any two structures. **3.** A pathologic adhesion or growing together. [G. a growing together]

sym·phy·sis pu·bis (sim′fi-sis pyū′bis) SYN pubic symphysis.

sym·po·di·a (sim-pō′dē-ă) Condition characterized by union of the feet. SEE ALSO sirenomelia. [sym- + G. *pous,* foot]

sym·port (sim′pōrt) Coupled transport of two different molecules or ions through a membrane in the same direction by a common carrier mechanism (symporter). Cf. antiport, uniport. [sym- + L. *porto,* to carry]

symp·tom (simp′tŏm) Any morbid phenomenon or departure from the normal in structure, function, or sensation, experienced by the patient and indicative of disease. SEE ALSO phenomenon (1), reflex (1), sign (1), syndrome. [G. *symptōma*]

symp·to·mat·ic (simp′tŏ-mat′ik) Indicative; relating to or constituting the aggregate of symptoms of a disease.

symp·to·mat·ic por·phyr·i·a (simp′tŏ-mat′ik pōr-fir′ē-ă) SYN porphyria cutanea tarda.

symp·to·mat·ic pru·ri·tus (simp′tŏ-mat′ik prūr-ī′tŭs) Itching occurring as a symptom of a systemic disease.

symp·to·mat·ic re·ac·tion (simp′tŏ-mat′ik rē-ak′shŭn) An allergic response similar to the original one, but occurring after the use of a test or therapeutic dose of an allergen or atopen.

symp·tom·a·tol·o·gy (simp′tŏ-mă-tol′ŏ-jē) **1.** The science of the symptoms of disease, their production, and the indications they furnish. **2.** The aggregate of symptoms of a disease. [symptom + G. *logos,* study]

symp·to·mat·o·lyt·ic (simp′tŏ-mat′ō-lit′ik) Removing symptoms. [symptom + G. *lytikos,* dissolving]

symp·tom com·plex (simp′tŏm kom′pleks) **1.** SEE syndrome. **2.** SEE complex (1).

symp·to·sis (simp-tō′sis) A localized or general wasting of the body. [G. a falling together, collapse, fr. *syn,* together, + *ptōsis,* a falling]

♻ **syn-** Prefix meaning together, with, joined; appears as sym- before b, p, ph, or m; corresponds to L. *con-*. [G. *syn,* with, together]

synaesthesia [Br.] SYN synesthesia.

synaesthesialgia [Br.] SYN synesthesialgia.

syn·an·a·morph (sin-an′ă-mōrf) The same fungal species growing in a different form.

syn·apse, pl. **syn·aps·es** (sin′aps, -sēz) The functional membrane-to-membrane contact of the nerve cell with another nerve cell, an effector (muscle, gland) cell, or a sensory receptor cell. The synapse subserves the transmission of nerve impulses, commonly from a club-shaped axon terminal (the presynaptic element) to the circumscript patch of the plasma membrane of the receiving cell (the postsynaptic element) on which the synapse occurs. In most cases, the impulse is transmitted by means of a chemical transmitter substance (such as acetylcholine, gamma-aminobutyric acid, dopamine, norepinephrine) released into a synaptic cleft that separates the presynaptic from the postsynaptic membrane; the transmitter is stored in synaptic vesicles in the presynaptic element. In other synapses, transmission takes place by direct propagation of the bioelectrical potential from the presynaptic to the postsynaptic membrane. SYN synapsis. [syn- + G. *hapto,* to clasp]

syn·ap·sis (si-nap′sis) [TA] SYN synapse. **1.** The point-for-point pairing of homologous chromosomes during the prophase of meiosis. [G. a connection, junction]

syn·ap·tic (si-nap′tik) **1.** Relating to a synapse. **2.** Relating to synapsis.

syn·ap·tic cleft (si-nap′tik kleft) The space about 20 nm wide between the axolemma and the postsynaptic surface. SEE ALSO synapse.

syn·ap·tic con·duc·tion (si-nap′tik kŏn-dŭk′shŭn) The conduction of a nerve impulse across a synapse.

syn·ap·tic ves·i·cles (si-nap′tik ves′i-kĕlz) The small (average diameter, 30 nm), intracellular, membrane-bound vesicles near the presynaptic membrane of a synaptic junction, containing the transmitter substance that, in chemical synapses, mediates the passage of nerve impulses across the junction. SEE ALSO synapse.

syn·ap·ti·ne·mal com·plex (si-nap′ti-nē′măl kom′pleks) A submicroscopic structure interposed between the homologous chromosome pairs during synapsis.

syn·ap·to·some (si-nap′tō-sōm) Membrane-bound sac containing synaptic vesicles that breaks away from axon terminals when brain tissue is homogenized under controlled conditions; such particles can be separated from other subcellular particles by differential and density gradient centrifugation. [synapse + G. *sōma,* body]

syn·ar·thro·di·a (sin′ahr-thrō′dē-ă) SYN fibrous joint.

syn·ar·thro·di·al (sin′ahr-thrō′dē-ăl) Relating to synarthrosis; denoting an articulation without a joint cavity.

syn·ar·thro·di·al joint (sin′ahr-thrō′dē-ăl joynt) **1.** SYN fibrous joint. **2.** SYN cartilaginous joint.

syn·ar·thro·phy·sis (sin′ahr-thrō-fī′sis) The process of ankylosis. [syn- + G. *arthron,* joint, + *physis,* growth]

syn•ar•thro•sis, pl. **syn•ar•thro•ses** (sin′ahr-thrō′sis, -sēz) An immovable or nearly immovable union of rigid components of the skeletal system, including fibrous joints, cartilaginous joints, and bony unions (synostoses). SEE ALSO joint. [G. fr. *syn,* together, + *arthrōsis,* articulation]

syn•can•thus (sin-kan′thŭs) Adhesion of the eyeball to orbital structures. [syn- + L. *canthus,* wheel]

syn•ceph•a•lus (sin-sef′ă-lŭs) Conjoined twins having a single head with two bodies. [syn- + G. *kephalē,* head]

syn•ceph•a•ly (sin-sef′ă-lē) The condition exhibited by a syncephalus.

syn•chei•ri•a (sin-kī′rē-ă) A form of dyscheiria in which a stimulus applied to one side of the body is referred by the patient to both sides. [syn- + G. *cheir,* hand]

syn•chon•dro•di•al joint (sin′kon-drō′dē-ăl joynt) SYN synchondrosis.

syn•chon•dro•se•ot•o•my (sin′kon-drō′sē-ot′ŏ-mē) Operation of cutting through a synchondrosis; specifically, cutting through the sacroiliac ligaments and forcibly closing the pubic arch; used in the treatment of exstrophy of the bladder. [synchondrosis + G. *tomē,* cutting]

syn•chon•dro•sis, pl. **syn•chon•dro•ses** (sin′kon-drō′sis, -sēz) A union between two bones formed either by hyaline cartilage or fibrocartilage. SYN synchondrodial joint. [Mod. L. fr. G. *syn,* together, + *chondros,* cartilage, + *-osis,* condition]

syn•chon•dro•to•my (sin-kon-drot′ŏ-mē) SYN symphysiotomy.

syn•chro•ni•a (sin-krō′nē-ă) **1.** SYN synchronism. **2.** Origin, development, involution, or functioning of tissues or organs at the usual time for such an event. Cf. heterochronia. [syn- + G. *chronos,* time]

syn•chron•ic (sin′krō-nik) Referring to the study of the natural history of a disease by its state and distribution in a population at one time.

syn•chron•ic stud•y (sin′krō-nik stŭd′ē) SYN cross-sectional study.

syn•chro•nism (sin′krō-nizm) Occurrence of two or more events at the same time; the condition of being simultaneous. SYN synchronia (1). [syn- + G. *chronos,* time]

syn•chro•nized in•ter•mit•tent man•da•tor•y ven•ti•la•tion (SIMV) (sing′krŏ-nīzd in′tĕr-mit′ĕnt mand′ă-tōr-ē ven′ti-lā′shŭn) Intermittent mandatory ventilation in which mandatory breaths can be triggered by the patient's inspiratory effort; in the absence of patient inspiratory efforts, SIMV becomes IMV. SEE ALSO intermittent mandatory ventilation.

syn•chro•nous (sin′krō-nŭs) Occurring simultaneously. [G. *synchronos*]

syn•chy•sis (sin′ki-sis) Collapse of the collagenous framework of the vitreous humor, with liquefaction of the vitreous body. [G. a mixing together, fr. syn- + *chysis,* a pouring]

syn•chy•sis scin•til•lans (sin′ki-sis sin′til-lanz) An appearance of glistening spots in the eye, due to cholesterol crystals that are floating in a fluid vitreous.

syn•clit•ic (sin-klit′ik) Relating to or marked by synclitism.

syn•cli•tism (sin′kli-tizm) Condition of parallelism between the planes of the fetal head and of the pelvis, respectively. [G. *syn-klinō,* to incline together]

syn•clo•nus (sin′klō-nŭs) Clonic spasm or tremor of several muscles. [syn- + G. *klonos,* tumult]

syn•co•pal (sing′kŏ-păl) Relating to syncope. SYN syncopic.

syn•co•pe (sing′kŏ-pē) Loss of consciousness and postural tone caused by diminished cerebral blood flow. [G. *synkopē,* a cutting short, a swoon]

syn•cop•ic (sin-kop′ik) SYN syncopal.

syn•cy•tial (sin-sish′ăl) Relating to a syncytium.

syn•cy•tial knot (sin-sish′ăl not) A localized swelling or aggregation of syncytiotrophoblastic nuclei in the villi of the placenta during early pregnancy. SYN nuclear aggregation.

syn•cy•ti•o•tro•pho•blast (sin-sish′ē-ō-trō′fō-blast) The syncytial outer layer of the trophoblast; site of synthesis of human chorionic gonadotropin. SEE ALSO trophoblast. SYN syntrophoblast. [syncytium + trophoblast]

syn•cy•ti•um, pl. **syn•cy•ti•a** (sin-sish′ē-ŭm, -ă) A multinucleated protoplasmic mass formed by the secondary union of originally separate cells. [Mod. L. fr. syn- + G. *kytos,* cell]

syn•dac•tyl•i•a, **syn•dac•ty•lism** (sin′dak-til′ē-ă, sin-dak′ti-lizm) SYN syndactyly.

syn•dac•ty•lous (sin-dak′ti-lŭs) Having fused or webbed fingers or toes.

syn•dac•ty•ly (sin-dak′ti-lē) Any degree of webbing or fusion of fingers or toes, involving soft parts only or including bone structure. SYN symphalangism (1), symphalangy, syndactylia, syndactylism. [syn- + G. *daktylos,* finger or toe]

syn•de•sis (sin-dē′sis) SYN arthrodesis. [syn- + G. *desis,* a binding]

syn•des•mec•to•my (sin′dez-mek′tŏ-mē) Cutting away a section of a ligament. [syndesm- + G. *ektomē,* excision]

syn•des•mec•to•pi•a (sin′dez-mek-tō′pē-ă) Displacement of a ligament. [syndesm- + G. *ektopos,* out of place]

syn•des•mi•tis (sin′dez-mī′tis) Inflammation of a ligament. [syndesm- + G. *-itis,* inflammation]

♻ **syndesmo-, syndesm-** Combining forms denoting ligament, ligamentous. [G. *syndesmos,* a fastening, fr. *syndeō,* to bind]

syn•des•mo•di•al (sin′dez-mō′dē-ăl) SYN syndesmotic.

syn•des•mo•pex•y (sin-dez′mō-pek-sē) The joining of two ligaments, or attachment of a ligament in a new place. [syndesmo- + G. *pēxis,* fixation]

syn•des•mo•phyte (sin-dez′mō-fīt) An osseous excrescence attached to a ligament. [syndesmo- + G. *phyton,* plant]

syn•des•mor•rha•phy (sin′dez-mōr′ă-fē) Suture of ligaments. [syndesmo- + G. *rhaphē,* suture]

syn•des•mo•sis, pl. **syn•des•mo•ses** (sin′dez-mō′sis, -sēz) A form of fibrous joint in which opposing surfaces that are relatively far apart are united by ligaments. [syndesmo- + G. *-osis,* condition]

syn•des•mot•ic (sin′dez-mot′ik) Relating to syndesmosis. SYN syndesmodial.

syn•des•mot•o•my (sin′dez-mot′ŏ-mē) Surgical division of a ligament. [syndesmo- + G. *tomē,* incision]

syn•drome (sin′drōm) The combination of signs and symptoms associated with a particular morbid process, which together constitute the picture of a disease or inherited anomaly. SEE ALSO disease. [G. *syndromē,* a running together, tumultuous concourse; (in med.) a concurrence of signs and symptoms, fr. *syn,* together, + *dromos,* a running]

syn•drome of in•ap•pro•pri•ate se•cre•tion of an•ti•di•u•ret•ic hor•mone (SIADH) (sin′drōm in-ă-prō′prē-ăt sĕ-krē′shŭn an′tī-dī-yŭr-et′ik hōr′mōn) A condition in which ADH is in excess and causes water retention, hyponatremia, and extracellular fluid volume excess.

syn•drome X (sin′drōm) SYN metabolic syndrome.

syn•drom•ic (sin-drō′mik) Relating to a syndrome.

syn•ech•i•a, pl. **syn•ech•i•ae** (si-nek′ē-ă, -ē) Any adhesion; specifically, adhesion of an inflamed iris to the cornea (anterior synechia) or lens (posterior synechia). [G. *synecheia,* continuity, fr. *syn,* together, + *echō,* to have, hold]

syn•ech•i•ot•o•my (si-nek′ē-ot′ŏ-mē) Division of synechiae. [synechia + G. *tomē,* incision]

syn•en•ceph•a•lo•cele (sin′en-sef′ă-lō-sēl) Protrusion of brain substance through a defect in the cranium, with adhesions preventing reduction. [syn- + G. *enkephalos,* brain, + *kēlē,* hernia]

syn•er•e•sis (si-ner′ĕ-sis) **1.** The contraction of a gel, e.g., a blood clot, by which part of the dispersion medium is squeezed out. **2.** Degeneration of the vitreous humor with loss of gel consistency to become partially or completely fluid. [G. *synairesis,* a taking or drawing together]

syn•er•gism (sin′ĕr-jizm) Coordinated or correlated action of two or more structures, agents, or physiologic processes so that the combined action is greater than the sum of each acting separately. Cf. antagonism. SYN synergy. [G. *synergia,* fr. *syn,* together, + *ergon,* work]

syn•er•gist (sin′ĕr-jist) A structure, agent, or physiologic process that aids the action of another. Cf. antagonist.

syn•er•gis•tic mus•cles (sin′ĕr-jist′ik mŭs′ĕlz) Muscles having a similar and mutually helpful function or action.

syn•er•gy (sin′ĕr-jē) SYN synergism.

syn•es•the•si•a (sin′es-thē′zē-ă) A condition in which a stimulus, in addition to exciting the usual and normally located sensation, gives rise to a subjective sensation of different character or localization, e.g., color hearing, color taste. SYN synaesthesia. [syn- + G. *aisthēsis,* sensation]

syn•es•the•si•al•gi•a (sin′es-thē′zē-al′jē-ă) Painful synesthesia. SYN synaesthesialgia.

Syn•ga•mus (sin′gă-mŭs) A genus of blood-sucking, strongyle tapeworms of the family Syngamidae.

Syn•ga•mus la•ryn•ge•us (sin′gă-mŭs lă-rin′jē-ŭs) A tropical nematode that occasionally invades the larynx and trachea, causing cough, hemoptysis, foreign body sensation, and shortness of breath.

syn•ga•my (sin′gă-mē) Union of the male and female gametes. [syn- + G. *gamos,* marriage]

syn•ge•ne•ic (sin′jĕ-nē′ik) Relating to genetically identical individuals. SYN isogeneic, isogenic, isologous, isoplastic. [G. *syngenēs,* congenital]

syn•gen•e•sis (sin-jen′ĕ-sis) SYN sexual reproduction. [syn- + G. *genesis,* origin]

syn•ge•net•ic (sin′jĕ-net′ik) Relating to syngenesis.

syn•graft (sin′graft) A tissue or organ transplanted between genetically identical individuals. SYN isogeneic graft, isograft, isologous graft, isoplastic graft.

syn•i•ze•sis (sin′i-zē′sis) **1.** Closure or obliteration of the pupil. **2.** The massing of chromatin at one side of the nucleus that occurs usually at the beginning of synapsis. [G. collapse]

syn·kar·y·on (sin-kar′ē-on) The nucleus formed by the fusion of the two pronuclei in karyogamy. [syn- + G. *karyon,* kernel (nucleus)]

syn·ki·ne·sis (sin′ki-nē′sis) Involuntary movement accompanying a voluntary one, as the movement of a closed eye following that of the uncovered one, or the movement occurring in a paralyzed muscle accompanying motion in another part. [syn- + G. *kinēsis,* movement]

syn·ki·net·ic (sin′ki-net′ik) Relating to or marked by synkinesis.

syn·o·nych·i·a (sin′ō-nik′ē-ă) Fusion of two or more nails of the fingers or toes, as in syndactyly. [sin- + G. *onyx (onych-),* nail]

syn·oph·thal·mi·a (sin′of-thal′mē-ă) SYN cyclopia. [syn- + G. *ophthalmos,* eye]

syn·or·chi·dism, **syn·or·chism** (sin-ōr′ki-dizm, sin′ōr-kizm) Congenital fusion of the testes in the abdomen or scrotum. [syn- + G. *orchis,* testis]

syn·os·che·os (sin-os′kē-os) Partial or complete adhesion of the penis and scrotum, a malformation in hermaphroditism. [syn- + G. *oschē,* scrotum]

syn·os·to·sis (sin′os-tō′sis) Osseous union between the bones forming a joint. SYN bony ankylosis, true ankylosis. [syn- + G. *osteon,* bone, + *-osis,* condition]

syn·os·tot·ic (sin′os-tot′ik) Relating to synostosis.

sy·no·ti·a (si-nō′shē-ă) Fusion or abnormal approximation of the lobules (lobes) of the auricles of the external ears in otocephaly. [syn- + G. *ous,* ear]

syn·o·vec·to·my (sin′ō-vek′tŏ-mē) Excision of a portion or all of the synovial membrane of a joint. SYN villusectomy. [synovia + G. *ektomē,* excision]

syn·o·vi·a (si-nō′vē-ă) [TA] SYN synovial fluid. [Mod. L., a word coined by Paracelsus, fr. G. *syn,* together, + *ōon* (L. *ovum*), egg]

syn·o·vi·al (si-nō′vē-ăl) **1.** Relating to, containing, or consisting of synovia. **2.** Relating to the membrana synovialis.

syn·o·vi·al bur·sa (si-nō′vē-ăl bŭr′să) A sac containing synovial fluid that occurs at sites of friction, as between a tendon and a bone over which it plays, or subcutaneously over a bony prominence.

syn·o·vi·al crypt (si-nō′vē-ăl kript) A diverticulum of the synovial membrane of a joint.

syn·o·vi·al cyst (si-nō′vē-ăl sist) SYN ganglion (2).

syn·o·vi·al flu·id (si-nō′vē-ăl flū′id) A clear thixotropic fluid, the main function of which is to serve as a lubricant in a joint, tendon sheath, or bursa; consists mainly of mucin with some albumin, fat, epithelium, and leukocytes; synovial fluid also helps to nourish the avascular articular cartilage. SYN synovia [TA].

syn·o·vi·al her·ni·a (si-nō′vē-ăl hĕr′nē-ă) Protrusion of a fold of the stratum synoviale through a rent in the stratum fibrosum of a joint capsule.

syn·o·vi·al joint (si-nō′vē-ăl joynt) A joint in which (1) the opposing bony surfaces are covered with a layer of hyaline cartilage or fibrocartilage, (2) there is a joint cavity containing synovial fluid, lined with synovial membrane and reinforced by a fibrous capsule and ligaments, and (3) there is some degree of free movement possible. SYN articulatio [TA], diarthrodial joint, diarthrosis, movable joint.

syn·o·vi·al lig·a·ment (si-nō′vē-ăl lig′ă-mĕnt) One of the large synovial folds in a joint.

syn·o·vi·al mem·brane (si-nō′vē-ăl mem′brān) The connective tissue membrane that lines the cavity of a synovial joint and produces the synovial fluid; it lines all internal surfaces of the cavity except for the articular cartilage of the bones. SYN membrana synovialis [TA], synovium.

syn·o·vi·al sheath (si-nō′vē-ăl shēth) SEE synovial sheaths of fingers, synovial sheaths of toes.

syn·o·vi·al sheaths of fin·gers (si-nō′vē-al shēths fing′gĕrz) Synovial sheaths that enclose the flexor tendons of the fingers, each extending from the proximal end of the carpal ligament to the base of a distal phalanx.

syn·o·vi·al sheaths of toes (si-nō′vē-al shēths tōz) Similar in structure to the corresponding sheaths of fingers.

syn·o·vi·o·ma (si-nō′vē-ō′mă) A tumor of synovial origin involving joint or tendon sheath. [synovium + G. *-oma,* tumor]

syn·o·vi·tis (sin′ō-vī′tis) Inflammation of a synovial membrane, especially that of a joint. In general, when unqualified, the same as arthritis. [synovia + G. *-itis,* inflammation]

syn·o·vi·tis sic·ca (sin′ō-vī′tis sik′ă) SYN dry synovitis.

syn·o·vi·um (si-nō′vē-ŭm) SYN synovial membrane.

syn·ten·ic (sin-ten′ik) Pertaining to synteny.

syn·ten·y (sin′tĕ-nē) The relationship between two genetic loci (not genes) represented on the same chromosomal pair or (for haploid chromosomes) on the same chromosome; an anatomic rather than a segregational relationship. [syn- + G. *tainia,* ribbon]

syn·thase (sin′thās) Trivial name used in Enzyme Commission Report for a lyase reaction going in the reverse direction (NTP-independent). SEE ALSO synthetase.

syn•the•sis, pl. **syn•the•ses** (sin′thĕ-sis, -sēz) **1.** Generally, the process of building up, putting together, or composing. **2.** CHEMISTRY the formation of compounds by the union of simpler compounds or elements. **3.** The stage in the cell cycle in which DNA is synthesized as a preliminary to cell division. [G. fr. *syn,* together, + *thesis,* a placing, arranging]

syn•the•sis pe•ri•od (sin′thĕ-sis pēr′ē-ŏd) The period of the cell cycle when there is synthesis of DNA and histone; it occurs between gap_1 and gap_2.

syn•the•size (sin′thĕ-sīz) To make something by synthesis, i.e., synthetically.

syn•the•tase (sin′thĕ-tās) An enzyme catalyzing the synthesis of a specific substance.

syn•thet•ic (sin-thet′ik) Relating to or made by synthesis.

syn•thet•ic dyes (sin-thet′ik dīz) Organic dye compounds originally derived from coal-tar derivatives; presently produced by synthesis from benzene and its derivatives.

syn•thet•ic sen•tence i•den•ti•fi•ca•tion (sin-thet′ik sen′tĕns ī-den′ti-fi-kā′shŭn) A test of central auditory pathway integrity in which a closed set of 10 syntactically incomplete sentences are presented with a competing message for identification.

syn•ton•ic (sin-ton′ik) Having even tone or temperament; a personality trait characterized by a high degree of emotional responsiveness to the environment. [G. *syntonos,* in harmony, fr. *syn,* together, + *tonos,* tone]

syn•tro•pho•blast (sin-trō′fō-blast) SYN syncytiotrophoblast.

syn•tro•pic (sin-trō′pik) Relating to syntropy.

syn•tro•py (sin′trō-pē) **1.** The tendency sometimes seen in two diseases to coalesce into one. **2.** The state of harmonious association with others. **3.** ANATOMY a number of similar structures inclined in one general direction (e.g., the spinous processes of a series of vertebrae, the ribs). [syn- + G. *tropē,* a turning]

syph•i•lid (sif′i-lid) Any of the several kinds of cutaneous and mucous membrane lesions of secondary and tertiary syphilis, but most commonly denoting the former. [syphilis + *-id* (1)]

syph•i•lis (sif′i-lis) An acute and chronic infectious disease caused by *Treponema pallidum* subsp. *pallidum* and transmitted by direct contact, usually through sexual intercourse. After an incubation period of 12–30 days, the first symptom is a chancre (a painless, indurated ulcer), followed by slight fever and other constitutional symptoms (primary syphilis), followed by a skin eruption of various appearances with mucous patches and generalized lymphadenopathy (secondary syphilis), and subsequently by the formation of gummas, cellular infiltration, and functional abnormalities usually resulting from cardiovascular and central nervous system lesions (tertiary syphilis). [Mod. L. *syphilis* (*syphilid-*), fr. a poem, *Syphilis sive Morbus Gallicus,* by Fracastorius, *Syphilus* being a shepherd and principal character]

syph•i•lit•ic (sif′i-lit′ik) Relating to, caused by, or suffering from syphilis. SYN luetic.

sy•phi•lit•ic an•eu•rysm (sif′i-lit′ik an′yūr-izm) An aneurysm, usually involving the thoracic aorta, resulting from tertiary syphilitic aortitis.

sy•phi•lit•ic leu•ko•der•ma (sif′i-lit′ik lū′kō-dĕr′mă) A fading of the roseola of secondary syphilis, leaving reticulated depigmented and hyperpigmented areas located chiefly on the sides of the neck. SYN melanoleukoderma colli.

sy•phi•lit•ic ro•se•o•la (sif′i-lit′ik rō′zē-ō′lă) Usually the first eruption of syphilis, occurring 6–12 weeks after the initial lesion.

syphilo-, syphil-, syphili- Combining forms meaning syphilis. SEE syphilis.

syph•i•lo•ma (sif′i-lō′mă) SYN gumma. [syphilo- + G. *-oma,* tumor]

syr. Abbrevation for syrup.

syr•ing•ad•e•no•ma (sir′ing-ad-ĕ-nō′mă) A benign sweat gland tumor showing glandular differentiation typical of secretory cells. SYN syringoadenoma. [syring- + G. *adēn,* gland, + *-oma,* tumor]

sy•ringe (sir-inj′) An instrument used for injecting or withdrawing fluids. See page 1524. [G. *syrinx,* pipe or tube]

sy•rin•gec•to•my (sir′in-jek′tŏ-mē) SYN fistulectomy. [syring- + G. *ektomē,* excision]

sy•rin•gi•tis (sir′in-jī′tis) Inflammation of the auditory tube. [syring- + G. *-itis,* inflammation]

syringo-, syring- Combining forms meaning a syrinx; syringeal. [G. *syrinx,* pipe or tube]

sy•rin•go•ad•e•no•ma (si-ring′gō-ad-ĕ-nō′mă) SYN syringadenoma.

sy•rin•go•bul•bi•a (si-ring′gō-bŭl′bē-ă) A fluid-filled cavity of the brainstem, analogous to syringomyelia. [syringo- + L. *bulbus,* bulb (medulla oblongata)]

sy•rin•go•car•ci•no•ma (si-ring′gō-kahr-si-nō′mă) A malignant epithelial neoplasm that has undergone cystic change (cystic carcinoma). [syringo- + carcinoma]

sy•rin•go•cele (si-ring′gō-sēl) **1.** SYN neural canal. **2.** A meningomyelocele in which there is a

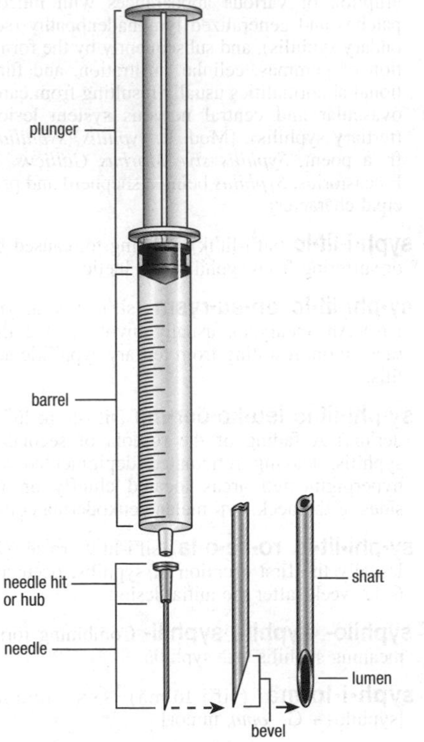

parts of needle and syringe

cavity in the ectopic spinal cord. [syringo- + G. *koilia,* a hollow]

sy•rin•go•cys•tad•e•no•ma (si-ring′gō-sis′tad-ĕ-nō′mă) A cystic benign sweat gland tumor. [syringo- + cystadenoma]

sy•rin•go•cys•to•ma (si-ring′gō-sis-tō′mă) SYN hidrocystoma. [syringo- + cystoma]

sy•rin•go•ma (sir′ing-gō′mă) A benign, often multiple, sometimes eruptive neoplasm of the sweat gland ducts composed of very small round cysts. [syringo- + G. *-ōma,* tumor]

sy•rin•go•me•nin•go•cele (si-ring′gō-mĕ-ning′gō-sēl) A form of spina bifida cystica in which the dorsal sac consists chiefly of membranes, with very little cord substance, enclosing a cavity that communicates with a syringomyelic cavity. [syringo- + meningocele]

sy•rin•go•my•e•li•a (si-ring′gō-mī-ē′lē-ă) The presence in the spinal cord of longitudinal cavities lined by dense, gliogenous tissue, which are not caused by vascular insufficiency. Syringomyelia is marked clinically by pain and paresthesia, followed by muscular atrophy of the hands and analgesia with thermoanesthesia of the hands and arms, but with the tactile sense preserved; it is later marked by painless whitlows, spastic paralysis in the lower extremities, and scoliosis of the lumbar spine. Some cases are associated with low-grade astrocytomas or vascular malformations of the spinal cord. SYN hydrosyringomyelia, Morvan disease. [syringo- + G. *myelos,* marrow]

sy•rin•go•my•e•lo•cele (si-ring′gō-mī′ĕ-lō-sēl) A form of spina bifida cystica consisting of a protrusion of the meninges and spinal cord through a dorsal defect in the vertebral column, the fluid of the syrinx of the cord being increased and expanding the cord tissue into a thin-walled sac that then expands through the vertebral defect. [syringo- + myelocele]

sy•rin•got•o•my (sir′in-got′ŏ-mē) SYN fistulotomy.

syr•inx, pl. **sy•ring•es** (sir′ingks, si-rin′jēz) **1.** A pathologic tubular cavity in the brain or spinal cord. **2.** A rarely used synonym for fistula. **3.** The lower part of the bird trachea, which produces vocal sounds. [G. a tube, pipe]

syr•up (syr.) (sir′ŭp) **1.** Refined molasses; the uncrystallizable saccharine solution left after sugar is refined. **2.** Any sweet fluid; a solution of sugar in water in any proportion. **3.** A liquid preparation of medicinal or flavoring substances in a concentrated aqueous solution of a sugar, usually sucrose; when the syrup contains a medicinal substance, it is termed a medicated syrup. [Mod. L. *syrupus,* fr. Ar. *sharāb*]

sys•tem (sis′tĕm) **1.** A consistent and complex whole composed of interrelated and interdependent parts. **2.** Any complex of structures related anatomically (e.g., the vascular system) or functionally (e.g., the digestive system). **3.** The entire organism seen as a complex organization of parts. SYN systema [TA]. **4.** A method of denoting amino acid transporters in which the word *system* is followed by one or more letters indicating the specific transporter (e.g., system N is a sodium-dependent transporter specific for amino acids such as L-glutamine, L-asparagine, and L-histidine; system y^+ is a sodium-independent transporter of cationic amino acids). **5.** An organized procedure. **6.** A way of classifying (e.g., the taxonomic system). **7.** SEE health care system. [G. *systēma,* an organized whole]

sys•te•ma (sis-tē′mă) [TA] SYN system (3). SEE ALSO system, apparatus. [L. fr. G. *systēma*]

sys•tem•a•tic name (sis′tĕ-mat′ik nām) As applied to chemical substances, a combination of specially coined or selected words or syllables, each of which has a precisely defined chemical structural meaning, so that the structure may be derived from the name.

sys•te•mat•ic re•view (sis′tĕ-mat′ik rē-vyū′) Program that integrates the results of primary research studies to identify the best available evidence on a treatment, quantitative systematic reviews use metaanalysis to combine the results of individual studies.

sys·tem·a·tized de·lu·sion (sis′tĕ-mă′tīzd dĕ-lū′zhŭn) A delusion that is logically constructed from a false premise and embraces a specific sector of the patient's life.

sys·tem·ic (sis-tem′ik) Relating to a system; specifically somatic, relating to the entire organism as distinguished from any of its individual parts.

sys·tem·ic an·a·phy·lax·is (sis-tem′ik an′ă-fi-lak′sis) SYN generalized anaphylaxis.

sys·tem·ic cap·il·lar·y leak syn·drome (sis-tem′ik kap′i-lar-ē lēk sin′drōm) A rare disorder of unknown cause presenting with episodic hypotension, hemoconcentration, and hypalbuminemia; monoclonal gammopathy is often associated.

sys·tem·ic cir·cu·la·tion (sis-tem′ik sĭr′kyū-lā′shŭn) The circulation of blood through the arteries, capillaries, and veins of the general system, from the left ventricle to the right atrium.

sys·tem·ic lu·pus er·y·the·ma·to·sus (SLE) (sis-tem′ik lū′pŭs ĕr-ith′ĕ-mă-tō′sŭs) An inflammatory connective tissue disease with variable features including fever; weakness and fatigability; joint pains or arthritis resembling rheumatoid arthritis; diffuse erythematous skin lesions on the face, neck, or upper extremities; lymphadenopathy; pleurisy or pericarditis; glomerular lesions; anemia; hyperglobulinemia; and a positive LE cell test result, with serum antibodies to double-stranded DNA and acidic nuclear protein (Sm). SYN disseminated lupus erythematosus.

sys·tem·ic scler·o·der·ma (sis-tem′ik skler′ō-dĕr′mă) SYN scleroderma.

sys·tem·ic vas·cu·lar re·sis·tance (sis-tem′ik vas′kyū-lăr rĕ-zis′tăns) An index of arteriolar compliance or constriction throughout the body; equal to the blood pressure divided by the cardiac output.

sys·to·le (sis′tŏ-lē) Contraction of the heart, especially of the ventricles, by which the blood is driven through the aorta and pulmonary artery to traverse the systemic and pulmonary circulations, respectively; its occurrence is indicated physically by the first sound of the heart heard on auscultation, by the palpable apex beat, and by the arterial pulse. [G. *systolē,* a contracting]

sys·tol·ic (sis-tol′ik) Relating to or occurring during cardiac systole.

sys·tol·ic mur·mur (sis-tol′ik mŭr′mŭr) A sound audible during ventricular systole.

sys·tol·ic pres·sure (sis-tol′ik presh′ŭr) The intracardiac pressure during or resulting from systolic contraction of a cardiac chamber; the highest arterial blood pressure reached during any given ventricular cycle.

sys·tol·ic thrill (sis-tol′ik thril) A thrill felt over the precordium or over a blood vessel during ventricular systole.

sys·trem·ma (sis-trem′ă) A muscular cramp in the calf of the leg, the contracted muscles forming a hard ball. [G. anything twisted]

τ Tau. SEE tau.

θ, Θ Theta. SEE theta.

T *Abbreviation for* **1.** Ribothymidine; tension (T+, increased tension; T–, diminished tension); tera-; tritium; threonine; torque; transmittance. **2.** As a subscript, refers to tidal volume. **3.** Thoracic vertebra (T1–T12); tocopherol. **4.** Tesla, the unit of magnetic field strength.

T1 MAGNETIC RESONANCE the time for 63% of longitudinal relaxation to occur; the value is a function of magnetic field strength and the chemical environment of the hydrogen nucleus.

T2 MAGNETIC RESONANCE the time for 63% of transverse relaxation to occur; the value is a function of magnetic field strength and the chemical environment of the hydrogen nucleus.

T Abbreviation for absolute temperature (kelvin).

Tm Abbreviation for temperature midpoint (kelvin); melting point.

t Abbreviation for metric ton; time.

t Abbreviation for temperature (Celsius); tritium.

t_m Abbreviation for temperature midpoint (Celsius).

T-2 my•co•tox•in (mī′kō-tok′sin) A type of trichothecene mycotoxin responsible for alimentary toxic aleukia (ATA) toxicosis and asserted to have been a component of yellow rain. SEE ALSO primary blast injury, secondary blast injury, quaternary blast injury, trichothecene mycotoxin, yellow rain.

TA Abbreviation for Terminologia Anatomica.

Ta Symbol for tantalum.

tab. Abbreviation for tablet.

tab•a•nid (tab′ă-nid) Common name for flies of the family Tabanidae. [L. *tabanus,* gadfly]

ta•bes (tā′bēz) Progressive wasting or emaciation. [L. a wasting away]

ta•bes•cent (tă-bes′ĕnt) Characteristic of tabes. [L. *tabesco,* to waste away, fr. *tabes,* a wasting away]

ta•bes dor•sal•is (tā′bēz dor-sā′lis) SYN tabetic neurosyphilis.

ta•bes mes•en•ter•i•ca (tā′bēz mĕz-en-ter′i-kă) Tuberculosis of the mesenteric and retroperitoneal lymph nodes.

ta•bet•ic (tă-bet′ik) Relating to or suffering from tabes, especially tabes dorsalis.

ta•bet•ic ar•throp•a•thy (tă-bet′ik ahr-throp′ă-thē) A neuropathic arthropathy that occurs with tabes dorsalis. SEE ALSO neuropathic joint.

ta•bet•ic neu•ro•sy•phi•lis (tă-bet′ik nūr′ō-sif′i-lis) Type of neurosyphilis in which the posterior roots of the spinal cord, especially in the lumbosacral area, are the principal sites of infection, resulting in ataxia, hypotonia, impotence, constipation, hypotonic bladder, areflexia, and Romberg sign; other findings include lancinating pains (most often in the legs), visceral crises, Argyll-Robertson pupils, optic atrophy, and Charcot joints. In most patients, the CSF contains antibodies to *Treponema pallidum.* SYN tabes dorsalis.

ta•bet•i•form (tă-bet′i-fōrm) Resembling tabes, especially tabes dorsalis. [irreg. formed fr. L. *tabes,* a wasting, + *forma,* form]

tab•la•ture (tab′lă-chŭr) The state of division of the cranial bones into two plates separated by the diploë. [L. *tabula,* tablet]

ta•ble (tā′bĕl) **1.** One of the two plates or laminae, separated by the diploë, into which the cranial bones are divided. **2.** An arrangement of data in parallel columns, showing the essential facts in a readily appreciable form. **3.** Any flat-surfaced structure that serves as furniture. [L. *tabula*]

ta•ble•spoon (tā′bĕl-spūn) A large spoon, used as a measure of the dose of a medicine, equivalent to about 4 fluidrams, 1/2 fluid ounce, or 15 mL.

tab•let (tab.) (tab′lĕt) A solid dosage form containing medicinal substances with or without suitable diluents. It may vary in shape, size, and weight, and may be classified according to the method of manufacture (e.g., molded tablet, compressed tablet). [Fr. *tablette*, L. *tabula*]

ta•boo, ta•bu (tab-ū′) Restricted, prohibited, or forbidden; set apart for religious or ceremonial purposes. [Tongan, set apart]

ta•bo•pa•re•sis (tā′bō-păr-ē′sis) A condition in which the symptoms of tabes dorsalis and general paresis are associated.

tab•u•lar (tab′yū-lăr) **1.** Tablelike. **2.** Arranged in the form of a table (2). [L. *tabularis,* fr. *tabula,* table]

ta•bun (GA) (tā′bŭn) A chemical-warfare agent originally developed as an insecticide. Its NATO code is GA. SEE ALSO trichothecene mycotoxin.

tache (tash) A circumscribed discoloration of the skin or mucous membrane, such as a macule or freckle. [Fr. spot]

tache noire (tahsh nwahr) Characteristic lesion (the term is French for "black spot,") that can form at the site of an arthropod bite transmitting either *Rickettsia conorii* or *Orientia tsutsugamushi* to a human host; primary lesion of boutonneuse fever.

ta•chet•ic (tă-ket′ik) Marked by bluish or brownish spots. [Fr. *tache,* spot]

ta•chom•e•ter (tak-om′ĕ-tĕr) An instrument for

measuring speed or rate, e.g., revolutions of a shaft, heart rate (cardiotachometer), arterial blood flow (hemotachometer), respiratory gas flow (pneumotachometer). [G. *tachos,* speed, + *metron,* measure]

tachy- Combining form meaning rapid. [G. *tachys,* quick,]

tach•y•ar•rhyth•mi•a (tak′ē-ă-ridh′mē-ă) Any disturbance of the heart's rhythm, regular or irregular, resulting by convention in a rate over 100 beats per minute during physical examination. [tachy- + G. *a-* priv. + *rhythmos,* rhythm]

tach•y•car•di•a (tak′i-kahr′dē-ă) Rapid beating of the heart, conventionally applied to rates over 100 beats per minute. SYN tachyrhythmia, tachysystole. [tachy- + G. *kardia,* heart]

ta•chy•car•di•a-bra•dy•car•di•a syn•drome (tak′i-kahr′dē-a-brā′di-kahr′dē-a sin′drōm) Alternating periods of slow and rapid heart beat; often associated with disturbances of both sinoatrial and atrioventricular conduction.

tach•y•car•di•ac (tak′i-kahr′dē-ak) Relating to or suffering from excessively rapid action of the heart.

ta•chy•car•di•a win•dow (tak′i-kahr′dē-ă win′dō) In paroxysmal tachycardia of the reentry type, the interval of time (the window) between the earliest and latest premature activation that can excite the paroxysm.

tach•y•crot•ic (tak′i-krot′ik) Relating to, causing, or characterized by a rapid pulse. [tachy- + G. *krotos,* a striking]

tach•yp•ne•a (tak′ip-nē′ă) Rapid breathing. SYN polypnea, tachypnoea. [tachy- + G. *pnoē* (*pnoiē*), breathing]

tachypnoea [Br.] SYN tachypnea.

tach•y•rhyth•mi•a (tak′i-ridh′mē-ă) SYN tachycardia. [tachy- + G. *rhythmos,* rhythm]

ta•chys•ter•ol (tak-is′tĕr-ol) Sterol(s) formed by ultraviolet irradiation of any 5,7-diene-3β-sterol. When it is reduced to the 5,7-diene (or 5,7,22-triene) form, antirachitic action appears.

ta•chy•sys•to•le (tak′i-sis′tŏ-lē) SYN tachycardia.

tach•y•zo•ite (tak′i-zō′īt) Motile, replicating intracellular stage of *Toxoplasma gondii.*

tack•ler's ex•o•sto•sis (tak′lĕrz eks′os-tō′sis) An exostosis of the anterolateral humerus due to repeated blunt trauma, as suffered in contact sports, especially American and Canadian football, where the injury occurs during blocking maneuvers.

tac•ti•cal e•mer•gen•cy med•i•cal ser•vice (tak′ti-kăl ē-mĕr′jĕn-sē med′i-kăl sĕr′vis) A specialized EMS unit that supports law enforcement operations.

tac•tile (tak′til) Relating to touch or to the sense of touch. [L. *tactilis,* fr. *tango,* pp. *tactus,* to touch]

tac•tile ag•no•si•a (tak′til ag-nō′zē-ă) Inability to recognize objects by touch, in the presence of intact cutaneous and proprioceptive hand sensation; caused by a lesion in the contralateral parietal lobe. SYN astereognosis.

tac•tile an•es•the•si•a (tak′til an′es-thē′zē-ă) Loss or impairment of the sense of touch.

tac•tile cor•pus•cle (tak′til kōr′pŭs-ĕl) One of numerous oval bodies found in the papillae of the skin, especially those of the fingers and toes; each consists of a connective tissue capsule in which the axon fibrils terminate around and between a pile of wedge-shaped epithelioid cells. SYN Meissner corpuscle.

tac•tile de•fen•sive•ness (tak′til dĕ-fen′siv-nĕs) Excessive reaction to tactile stimulation.

tac•tile frem•i•tus (tak′til frem′i-tŭs) Vibration palpated with the hand on the chest during vocal fremitus.

tac•tile im•age (tak′til im′ăj) An image of an object as perceived by the sense of touch.

tac•tile me•nis•cus (tak′til mĕ-nis′kŭs) A specialized tactile sensory nerve ending in the epidermis, characterized by a terminal cuplike expansion of an intraepidermal axon in contact with the base of a single modified keratinocyte. SYN Merkel corpuscle, Merkel tactile cell, Merkel tactile disc.

tac•tile pa•pil•la (tak′til pă-pil′ă) One of the papillae of the dermis containing a tactile cell or corpuscle.

tac•tile stim•u•la•tion (tak′til stim′yŭ-lā′shŭn) In the treatment of swallowing disorders, facilitation of reflexive and voluntary components of the swallow by stroking areas of the throat and tongue with a blunt probe. SEE ALSO caloric stimulation.

tac•tom•e•ter (tak-tom′ĕ-tĕr) SYN esthesiometer. [L. *tactus,* touch, + G. *metron,* measure]

tac•tual (tak′chū-ăl) Relating to or caused by touch.

TAD Abbreviation for transient acantholytic dermatosis.

Tae•ni•a (tē′nē-ă) A genus of cestodes that formerly included most of the tapeworms, but is now restricted to those species infecting carnivores with cysticerci found in tissues of various herbivores, rodents, and other animals of prey. SEE ALSO tapeworm. Cf. tenia (1). See page B7.

tae•ni•a (tē′nē-ă) **1.** A coiled, bandlike anatomic structure. SEE ALSO tenia (1). **2.** Common name for a tapeworm, especially of the genus *Taenia.* SYN tenia (2). [L., fr. G. *tainia,* band, tape, a tapeworm]

Tae•ni•a sa•gi•na•ta (tē′nē-ă saj-i-nā′tă) The beef, hookless, or unarmed tapeworm of humans, acquired by eating insufficiently cooked beef or veal infected with *Cysticercus bovis*. See page B7.

tae•ni•a•sis (tē′nē-ī′ă-sis) Infection with cestodes of the genus *Taenia*.

Tae•ni•a so•li•um (tē′nē-ă sōl′ē-ŭm) The pork, armed, or solitary tapeworm of humans, acquired by eating insufficiently cooked pork infected with *Cysticercus cellulosae;* hatching of ova within the human intestine may result in establishment of cysticerci in human tissues, resulting in cysticercosis.

tae•ni•id (tē-nē′id) Common name for a member of the family Taeniidae.

tae•ni•oid (tē′nē-oyd) Denoting members of the genus *Taenia*.

Taen•zer stain (tān′tser stān) An orcein solution used for staining elastic tissue.

TAF Abbreviation for tumor angiogenic factor.

tag (tag) **1.** SEE label, tracer. **2.** A small outgrowth or polyp.

tail (tāl) **1.** Any taillike structure, or tapering or elongated extremity of an organ or other part. **2.** VETERINARY ANATOMY a free appendage representing the caudal end of the vertebral column, covered by skin and hair, feathers, or scales. SYN cauda [TA]. [A.S. *taegl*]

tail bud (tāl bŭd) SYN caudal eminence.

tail fold (tāl fōld) The ventral folding of the caudal end of the embryonic disc.

tail of pan•cre•as (tāl pan′krē-ăs) The left extremity of the pancreas within the lienorenal ligament.

Ta•ka•ya•su ar•te•ri•tis (tah-kah-yah′sū ahr′tĕr-ī′tis) A progressive obliterative arteritis of unknown origin involving fibrosis and luminal narrowing that affects the aorta and its branches; more common in females. SEE ALSO aortic arch syndrome. SYN aortic arch syndrome, Martorell syndrome, pulseless disease.

ta•lar (tā′lăr) Relating to the talus.

talc o•per•a•tion (talk op-ĕr-ā′shŭn) An obsolete operation in which magnesium silicate (talc) powder is applied to the epicardium to create a sterile granulomatous pericarditis and thus promote pericardial anastomoses with the coronary circulation. SYN poudrage (2).

tal•co•sis (tal-kō′sis) A pulmonary disorder related to silicosis occurring in workers exposed to talc mixed with silicates; characterized by restrictive or obstructive disorders of breathing or the two in combination. [talc + G. -osis, condition]

tal•i•ped•ic (tal′i-pēd′ik) Clubfooted.

tal•i•pes (tal′i-pēz) Any deformity of the foot involving the talus. [L. *talus,* ankle, + *pes,* foot]

tal•i•pes cal•ca•ne•o•val•gus (tal′i-pēz kal-kā′nē-ō-val′gŭs) Talipes calcaneus and talipes valgus combined; the foot is dorsiflexed, everted, and abducted. SEE ALSO talipes equinovarus.

tal•i•pes cal•ca•ne•o•var•us (tal′i-pēz kal-kā′nē-ō-var′ŭs) Talipes calcaneus and talipes varus combined; the foot is dorsiflexed, inverted, and adducted. SEE ALSO talipes equinovarus.

tal•i•pes cal•ca•ne•us (tal′i-pēz kal-kā′nē-ŭs) A deformity due to weakness or absence of the calf muscles, in which the axis of the calcaneus becomes vertically oriented; commonly seen in poliomyelitis. SYN calcaneus (2).

tal•i•pes cav•us (tal′i-pēz kā′vŭs) An exaggeration of the normal arch of the foot. See this page.

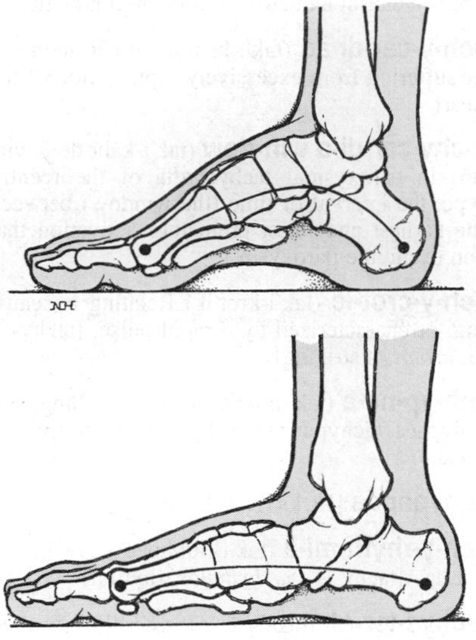

talipes cavus (top) and **talipes planus** (bottom)

tal•i•pes e•qui•no•val•gus (tal′i-pēz ē-kwī-nō-val′gŭs) Talipes equinus and talipes valgus combined; the foot is plantiflexed, everted, and abducted. SEE ALSO talipes equinovarus. SYN equinovalgus.

tal•i•pes e•qui•no•var•us (tal′i-pēz ē-kwī-nō-vā′rŭs) Talipes equinus and talipes varus combined; the foot is plantiflexed, inverted, and adducted. SYN clubfoot, club foot, equinovarus.

tal•i•pes e•qui•nus (tal′i-pēz ē-kwīn′ŭs) Permanent extension of the foot so that only the ball rests on the ground. It is commonly combined with talipes varus.

tal•i•pes pla•nus (tal′i-pēz plā′nŭs) A condition in which the longitudinal arch is broken down, the entire sole touching the ground. SYN flatfoot, pes planus.

tal•i•pes val•gus (tal′i-pēz val′gŭs) Permanent eversion of the foot, the inner side alone of the sole resting on the ground; it is usually combined with a breaking down of the plantar arch.

tal•i•pes var•us (tal′i-pēz vā′rŭs) Inversion of the foot, the outer side of the sole only touching the ground; usually some degree of talipes equinus is associated with it, and often talipes cavus.

tall let•ter writ•ing (tawl lĕt′ĕr rīt′ing) SYN tall-man letters.

tall-man let•ters (tawl-man lĕt′ĕrs) The use of writing in which medications with similar names (e.g., cephalosporins) have different distinguishing letters in capitals to prevent medication errors. Examples: cefaCLOR, cefADROxil, cefALEXin. SYN tall letter writing.

tall speed•well (tawl spēd′wel) SYN black root.

♻ **talo-** Combining form denoting the talus. [L. *talus,* ankle, ankle bone]

ta•lo•cal•ca•ne•al joint (tā′lō-kal-kā′nē-ăl joynt) SYN subtalar joint.

ta•lo•cal•ca•ne•o•na•vic•u•lar joint (tā′lō-kal-kā′nē-ō-nă-vik′kyū-lăr joynt) A ball-and-socket synovial joint, a portion of which participates in the transverse tarsal joint, formed by the head of the talus articulating with the navicular bone and the anterior part of the calcaneus.

ta•lo•cru•ral (tā′lō-krūr′ăl) Relating to the talus and the bones of the leg; denoting the ankle joint.

ta•lo•cru•ral joint (tā′lō-krūr′ăl joynt) SYN ankle joint.

tal•on (tal′ŏn) SYN hypocone. [F. heel, fr. L. *talus,* ankle]

tal•o•nid (tal′ŏ-nid) The distal portion of the human molar crown, consisting of the hypoconid, hypoconulid, and entoconid. [talon + -id (2)]

ta•lus, gen. **ta•li** (tā′lŭs, -lī) [TA] The bone of the foot that articulates with the tibia and fibula to form the ankle joint. SYN ankle bone, ankle (3), astragalus. [L. ankle bone, heel]

Tamm-Hors•fall mu•co•pro•tein (tam hōrs′fahl myū′kō-prō′tēn) The matrix of urinary casts derived from the secretion of renal tubular cells.

tam•pon (tam′pon) **1.** A cylinder or ball of cotton wool, gauze, or other loose substance; used as a plug or pack in a canal or cavity to restrain hemorrhage, absorb secretions, or maintain a displaced organ in position. **2.** To insert such a plug or pack. [O. Fr.]

tam•pon•ade, **tam•pon•age** (tam′pŏ-nād′, -nazh′) **1.** Pathologic compression of a joint. **2.** The insertion of a tampon.

tan•dem (tan′dĕm) **1.** A long narrow tube designed to fit inside the endocervical canal and uterine cavity; used in conjunction with ovoids to treat gynecologic malignancies with a radioactive source. SEE ALSO ovoids. **2.** Heel-to-toe placement, an assessment of balance with the heel of one foot against the toe of the other foot. SEE ALSO Romberg sign. SYN tandem Romberg. [L., at length]

tan•dem Rom•berg (tan′dĕm rom′berg) SYN tandem.

tan•gen•ti•al•i•ty (tan-jen′shē-al′i-tē) A disturbance in the associative thought process in which one tends to digress readily from one topic under discussion to other topics that arise in the course of associations; observed in bipolar disorder, schizophrenia, and certain types of organic brain disorders. Cf. circumstantiality. [off on a tangent, fr. L. *tangere,* to touch]

tan•gi•ble bo•dy ma•cro•phage (tanj′i-bĕl bod′ē mak′rō-fāj) A macrophage that specializes in phagocytosis of lymphoid cells.

tang-kuei (tahng-kwā) SYN Chinese angelica.

Tan•ner growth chart (tan′ĕr grōth chahrt) A series of tables showing distribution of parameters of physical development, such as stature, growth curves, and skinfold thickness, for children by sex, age, and stages of puberty.

Tan•ner stage (tan′ĕr stāj) A development level of puberty in the Tanner growth chart, based on pubic hair growth, development of genitalia in boys, and breast development in girls.

tan•ta•lum (Ta) (tan′tă-lŭm) A heavy metal of the vanadium group, atomic no. 73, atomic wt. 180.9479; used in surgical prostheses because of its noncorrosive properties. [G. mythical king of Lydia, *Tantalus*]

T ant•i•gens (an′ti-jĕnz) Tumor antigens associated with replication and transformation by certain DNA tumor viruses, including adenoviruses and papovaviruses. SEE ALSO beta (β)-hemolytic streptococci, tumor antigens.

tan-top tube (tan-top tūb) A tube of this color indicates the container has been treated with sodium heparin; used in testing for lead.

tan•trum (tan′trŭm) A fit of bad temper, especially in children.

TAP A protein that transports a peptide from the cytoplasm into the lumen of the endoplasmic reticulum.

tap (tap) **1.** To withdraw fluid from a cavity by means of a trocar and cannula, hollow needle, or catheter. **2.** To strike lightly with the finger or a hammerlike instrument in percussion or to elicit a tendon reflex. **3.** A light blow. **4.** An East Indian fever of undetermined nature. **5.** An instrument to cut threads in a hole in bone before inserting a screw. [M.E. *tappe*, fr. A.S. *taeppa*]

ta·per·ing-off (tā′pĕr-ing-awf) SYN active recovery.

ta·pe·tum, pl. **ta·pe·ta** (tă-pē′tŭm, -tă) **1.** In general, any membranous layer or covering. **2.** [TA] NEUROANATOMY a thin sheet of fibers in the lateral wall of the temporal and occipital horns of the lateral ventricle, continuous with the corpus callosum. [L. *tapeta,* a carpet]

tape·worm (tāp′wŏrm) An intestinal parasitic worm, adults of which are found in the intestine of vertebrates. Tapeworms consist of a scolex, variously equipped with spined or sucking structures by which the worm is attached to the intestinal wall of the host, and strobila having several to many proglottids that lack a digestive tract at any stage of development. The ovum, entering the intestine of an appropriate intermediate host, hatches, and the hexacanth penetrates the gut wall and develops into a specific larval form (e.g., cysticercoid, cysticercus, hydatid, strobilocercus), which develops into an adult when the intermediate host is ingested by the proper final host.

Ta·pi·a syn·drome (tah′pē-ah sin′drōm) Unilateral paralysis of the larynx, the velum palati, and the tongue, with atrophy of the latter.

ta·pir mouth (tā′pĕr mowth) Protrusion of the lips due to weakness of the orbicularis oris muscles; seen with some dystrophies.

ta·pote·ment (tă-pōt′man[h]) A group of massage movements that involve the repetitive, regular, rhythmic striking of the tissue with some part of the hand; includes beating, hacking, cupping, and tapping. SEE ALSO percussion. SYN tapping (1). [Fr. *tapoter,* to pat]

tap·ping (tap′ing) **1.** SYN tapotement. **2.** SYN paracentesis.

TAPVC Abbreviation for total anomalous pulmonary venous connection. SEE anomalous pulmonary venous connections, total or partial.

TAPVR Abbreviation for total anomalous pulmonary venous return. SEE anomalous pulmonary venous connections, total or partial.

***taq* po·lym·er·ase** (tak pol′i-mĕr-ās) A heat-stable DNA polymerase recovered from the bacterium *Thermus aquaticus*.

TAR Abbreviation for thrombocytopenia and absent radius. SEE thrombocytopenia-absent radius syndrome.

ta·ran·tu·la (tăr-anch′ū-lă) A large, hairy spider, considered highly venomous and often greatly feared; in fact, however, the bite is usually no more harmful than a bee sting.

Tar·dieu ec·chy·mos·es, Tar·dieu pe·te·chi·ae, Tar·dieu spots (tahr-dyū′ ek′ē-mō′sēz, pĕ-tē′kē-ē, spots) Subpleural and subpericardial petechiae or ecchymoses (or both), observed in the tissues of people who have been strangled or otherwise asphyxiated.

tar·dive (tahr′div) Late; delayed.

tar·dive cy·a·no·sis (tahr′div sī-ă-nō′sis) SYN cyanose tardive.

tar·dive dys·ki·ne·si·a (tahr′div dis′ki-nē′zē-ă) A neurologic disorder associated with involuntary repetitive movements of the facial muscles, tongue, limbs, and trunk; commonly associated with long-term treatment with antipsychotic medications such as phenothiazines. Can be significantly reduced by the administration of cholinergic medications.

tar·dive dys·to·ni·a (tahr′div dis-tō′nē-ă) SEE dystonia musculorum deformans.

tar·get (tahr′gĕt) **1.** An object fixed as a goal or point of examination. **2.** In the ophthalmometer, the mire. **3.** SYN target organ. **4.** Anode of an x-ray tube. SEE ALSO x-ray. **5.** In molecular diagnostic assays, the nucleic acid species being studied. The target is single-stranded and complementary to primers and/or probes. [It. *targhetta,* a small shield]

tar·get cell (tahr′gĕt sel) **1.** An erythrocyte in target cell anemia, with a dark center surrounded by a light band that again is encircled by a darker ring, thus resembling a target used in practice with firearms or archery; such cells also appear after splenectomy. **2.** A cell lysed by cytotoxic T lymphocytes, as in graft rejection. SYN codocyte, leptocyte, Mexican hat cell.

tar·get·ed sur·veil·lance (tahr′gĕt-ĕd sŭr-vāl′ăns) Monitoring of specific preidentified events of concern or importance.

tar·get gland (tahr′gĕt gland) The effector that functions when stimulated by the internal secretion of another gland or by some other stimulus.

tar·get heart rate (tahr′gĕt hahrt rāt) A range of 65–95% of age-predicted maximal heart rate or 50–85% of heart rate reserve. SEE ALSO training-sensitive zone.

tar·get heart rate range (tahr′gĕt hahrt rāt rānj) SYN training-sensitive zone.

tar·get or·gan (tahr′gĕt ōr′găn) A tissue or organ on which a hormone exerts its action; generally, a tissue or organ with appropriate receptors for a hormone. SYN target (3).

tar·get re·sponse (tahr′gĕt rĕ-spons′) SYN operant.

Tar·lov cyst (tahr′lov sist) A perineural lesion found in the proximal radicles of the lower spinal cord. It is usually productive of symptoms.

Tar·ni·er for·ceps (tahr-nē-ā′ fōr′seps) A type of axis-traction forceps.

tar·ry cyst (tahr′ē sist) A cyst or collection of

old blood with a tarry or black, sticky appearance; usually due to endometriosis.

tar·sal (tahr′săl) Relating to a tarsus in any sense.

tar·sal bones (tahr′săl bōnz) The seven bones of the instep: talus, calcaneus, navicular, three cuneiform (wedge), and cuboid.

tar·sal cyst (tahr′săl sist) SYN chalazion.

tar·sa·le, pl. **tar·sa·li·a** (tahr-sā′lē, -lē-ă) Any tarsal bone. [Mod. L. fr. G. *tarsos,* sole of the foot]

tars·al·gi·a (tahr-sal′jē-ă) SYN podalgia. [tarsus + G. *algos,* pain]

tar·sal glands (tahr′săl glandz) Sebaceous glands embedded in the tarsal plate of each eyelid, discharging at the edge of the lid near the posterior border. Their secretions create a lipid barrier along the margin of the eyelids that holds back normal secretions in the conjunctival sac by preventing the watery fluid from spilling over the barrier when the eye is open. SYN meibomian glands.

tar·sal joints (tahr′săl joynts) SYN intertarsal joints.

tar·sal si·nus (tahr′săl sī′nŭs) A hollow or canal formed by the groove of the talus and the interosseous groove of the calcaneus, which is occupied by the interosseous talocalcaneal ligament.

tar·sec·to·my (tahr-sek′tŏ-mē) Excision of the tarsus of the foot or of a segment of the tarsus of an eyelid. [tarsus + G. *ektomē,* excision]

tar·si·tis (tahr-sī′tis) **1.** Inflammation of the tarsus of the foot. **2.** Inflammation of the tarsal border of an eyelid.

♻**tarso-, tars-** Combining forms denoting a tarsus. SEE tarsus.

tar·so·cla·si·a, **tar·soc·la·sis** (tahr′sō-klā′zē-ă, tahr-sok′lă-sis) Instrumental fracture of the tarsus, for the correction of talipes equinovarus. [tarso- + G. *klasis,* a breaking]

tar·so·ma·la·ci·a (tahr′sō-mă-lā′shē-ă) Softening of the tarsal cartilages of the eyelids. [tarso- + G. *malakia,* softness]

tar·so·meg·a·ly (tahr′sō-meg′ă-lē) An uncommon developmental disorder and overgrowth of a tarsal or carpal bone. [tarso- + G. *megas,* large]

tar·so·met·a·tar·sal (TMT) (tahr′sō-met′ă-tahr′săl) Relating to the tarsal and metatarsal bones; denoting the articulations between the two sets of bones, and the ligaments in relation thereto.

tar·so·met·a·tar·sal joints (tahr′sō-met′ă-tahr′săl joynts) The three synovial articulations between the tarsal and metatarsal bones, consisting of a medial joint between the first cuneiform and first metatarsal, an intermediate joint between the second and third cuneiforms and corresponding metatarsals, and a lateral joint between the cuboid and fourth and fifth metatarsals.

tar·so·met·a·tar·sal lig·a·ments (tahr′sō-met′ă-tahr′săl lig′ă-mĕnts) The ligamentous attachments that unite tarsal and metatarsal bones; they are arranged in dorsal, interosseous, and plantar sets.

tar·so·pha·lan·ge·al (tahr′sō-fă-lan′jē-ăl) Relating to the tarsus and the phalanges.

tar·sor·rha·phy (tahr-sōr′ă-fē) The suturing together of the eyelid margins, partially or completely, to shorten the palpebral fissure or to protect the cornea in keratitis or in paralysis of the orbicularis oculi muscle. [tarso- + G. *rhaphē,* suture]

tar·sot·o·my (tahr-sot′ŏ-mē) **1.** Incision of the tarsal cartilage of an eyelid. **2.** Any operation on the tarsus of the foot. [tarso- + G. *tomē,* incision]

tar·sus, gen. and pl. **tar·si** (tahr′sŭs, -sī) [TA] **1.** As a division of the skeleton, the seven tarsal bones of the instep. SEE ALSO tarsal bones. **2.** The fibrous plates giving solidity and form to the edges of the eyelids; often erroneously called tarsal or ciliary cartilages. [G. *tarsos,* a flat surface, sole of the foot, edge of eyelid]

tar·tar (tahr′tăr) **1.** A white, brown, or yellow-brown deposit at or below the gingival margin of the teeth, chiefly hydroxyapatite in an organic matrix. SYN dental calculus (2). **2.** A crust on the interior of wine casks, consisting essentially of potassium bitartrate. [Mediev. L. *tartarum,* ult. etym. unknown]

tart cell (tahrt sel) A monocyte with an engulfed nucleus in which the structure is still well preserved.

tas·tant (tās′tănt) Any chemical that stimulates the sensory cells in a taste bud.

taste (tāst) **1.** To perceive through the medium of the gustatory nerves. **2.** The sensation produced by a suitable stimulus applied to the gustatory nerve endings in the tongue. [It. *tastare;* L. *tango,* to touch]

taste bud (tāst bŭd) One of a number of flask-shaped cell nests located in the epithelium of vallate, fungiform, and foliate papillae of the tongue and also in the soft palate, epiglottis, and posterior wall of the pharynx; it consists of sustentacular, gustatory, and basal cells between which the intragemmal sensory nerve fibers terminate.

taste cells (tāst selz) Darkly staining cells in a taste bud that have long, hairlike microvilli. SYN gustatory cells.

taste hairs (tāst hārz) Hairlike projections of

gustatory cells of taste buds; electron micrographs show them to be clusters of microvilli.

TAT Abbreviation for thematic apperception test; turnaround time.

tat•too (ta-tū′) **1.** A deliberate decorative implanting or injecting of indelible pigments into the skin or the tinctorial effect of accidental implantation. **2.** To produce such an effect. **3.** SYN amalgam tattoo. [Tahiti, *tatu*]

tau (τ) (tow) **1.** The 19th letter of the Greek alphabet (τ). **2.** Symbol for tele and relaxation time. **3.** A protein that associates with microtubules and other elements of the cytoskeleton; tau accelerates tubulin polymerization and stabilizes microtubules. Tau is also found in the plaque observed in patients with Alzheimer disease.

tau•rine (tawr′īn) **1.** An aminosulfonic acid, synthesized from L-cysteine and used in a number of roles, including in the synthesis of certain bile salts. **2.** Of or pertaining to a bull. [L. *taurinus,* of bulls, fr. *taurus,* bull, + suffiz *-inus,* pertaining to]

tau•ro•cho•lic ac•id (tawr′ō-kō′lik as′id) A compound of cholic acid and taurine, involving the carboxyl group of the former and the amino of the latter; a common bile salt in carnivores.

Taus•sig-Bing syn•drome (taw′sig bing sin′drōm) A congenital heart deformity with complete transposition of the aorta, which arises from the right ventricle, with a left-sided pulmonary artery overriding the left ventricle, and with high ventricular septal defect, right ventricular hypertrophy, anteriorly situated aorta, and posteriorly situated pulmonary artery.

tau•to•mer•ic (taw′tō-mer′ik) **1.** Relating to the same part. **2.** Relating to or marked by tautomerism. [G. *tautos,* the same, + *meros,* part]

tau•to•mer•ic fi•bers (taw′tō-mer′ik fī′bĕrz) Nerve fibers of the spinal cord that do not extend beyond the limits of the spinal cord segment in which they originate.

tau•tom•er•ism (taw-tom′ĕr-izm) A phenomenon in which a chemical compound exists in two forms of different structure (isomers) in equilibrium, the two forms differing, usually, in the position of a hydrogen atom. [G. *tautos,* the same, + *meros,* part]

tax•a (tak′să) Plural of taxon.

tax•ane (taks′ān) Any of a class of antitumor agents derived directly or semisynthetically from *Taxus brevifolius*, the Pacific yew (e.g., paclitaxel and docetaxel).

tax•is (tak′sis) **1.** Reduction of a hernia or of a dislocation of any part by means of manipulation. **2.** Systematic classification or orderly arrangement. **3.** The reaction of protoplasm to a stimulus, by virtue of which animals and plants are led to move or act in certain definite ways in relation to their environment. The various kinds of taxis are designated by a prefix denoting the stimulus governing them (e.g., chemotaxis, electrotaxis, thermotaxis). [G. orderly arrangement]

tax•on, pl. **tax•a** (tak′son, -să) The name given to a particular level or grouping in a systematic classification of living things or organisms (taxonomy). [G. *taxis,* order, arrangement, + -on]

tax•o•nom•ic (tak′sŏ-nōm′ik) Relating to taxonomy.

tax•on•o•my (taks-on′ō-mē) The systematic classification of living things or organisms. Kingdoms of living organisms are divided into groups (taxa) to show degrees of similarity or presumed evolutionary relationships, with the higher categories larger, more inclusive, and more broadly defined; the lower categories more restricted, with fewer species, and more closely related. The divisions below kingdom are, in descending order: phylum, class, order, family, genus, species, and subspecies (variety). Infra-, supra-, sub-, and super categories can be used when needed; additional categories, such as tribe, section, level, and group, are also used. [G. *taxis,* orderly arrangement, + *nomos,* law]

Tay cher•ry-red spot (tā cher′ē red spot) SYN cherry-red spot.

Tay•lor dis•ease (tā′lŏr di-zēz′) Diffuse idiopathic cutaneous atrophy.

Tay-Sachs dis•ease (tā saks di-zēz′) A lysosomal storage disease resulting from hexosaminidase-A deficiency. The monosialoganglioside is stored in central and peripheral neuronal cells. Infants present with hyperacusis and irritability, hypotonia, and failure to develop motor skills. Blindness with macular cherry-red spots and seizures are evident in the first year.

TB Abbreviation for tuberculosis.

Tb Sumbol for terbium.

TBI Abbreviation for traumatic brain injury. SEE ALSO caloric stimulation, contrecoup injury of brain.

T-bind•er (bīn′dĕr) Two strips of cloth at right angles; used for retaining a dressing, as on the perineum.

TBNA Abbreviation for transbronchial needle aspiration.

TBV Abbreviation for total blood volume.

Tc Symbol for technetium; abbreviation for T-cytotoxic cells.

TCA cy•cle (sī′kĕl) Abbreviation for tricarboxylic acid cycle.

^{99m}Tc-DTPA A radionuclide chelate complex used for renal imaging and function testing; also known as ^{99m}Tc pentatate. [*d*iethylene *t*riamine *p*enta*a*cetic *a*cid]

T cell (sel) SYN T lymphocyte.

T-cell re·cep·tor (TCR) (sel rĕ-sep′tŏr) An adhesion molecule on the membrane of T lymphocytes, which serves as the receptor for antigen bound to antigen-presenting cells (APC) through MHC molecules. It is expressed in a complex with CD3. It is in proximity to the MHC-restricted receptor (CD4 or CD8). SYN T-lymphocyte antigen receptor.

T-cell rich, B-cell lym·pho·ma (sel-rich sel lim-fō′mă) A B-cell lymphoma in which more than 90% of the cells are of T-cell origin, masking the large cells that form the neoplastic B-cell component. SEE ALSO adult T-cell lymphoma.

^{99m}Tc-glu·co·hep·ta·nate (glū-cō-hep′tă-nāt) Radiopharmaceutical possessing renal cortical-localizing and excretion-handling properties; may be used either for renal cortical imaging to determine scarring or for renal function imaging by renography.

TCM Abbreviation for traditional Chinese medicine.

TCR Abbreviation for T-cell receptor.

T-cy·to·tox·ic cells (Tc) (sī′tō-tok′sik selz) SYN killer cells.

TDD Abbreviation for telecommunications device for the deaf.

TDEE Abbreviation for total daily energy expenditure.

TDM Abbreviation for therapeutic drug monitoring.

TDP Abbreviation for ribothymidine 5′-diphosphate.

TdT Abbreviation for terminal deoxynucleotidyl transferase.

TE In magnetic resonance spin-echo pulse sequences, the time to echo, when the magnetization signal is sampled.

Te 1. ELECTRODIAGNOSIS abbreviation denoting tetanic contraction. **2.** Symbol for tellurium.

teach·ing (tēch′ing) NURSING intentional act of providing information and instruction to learner(s) based on identified learning needs; to maintain or improve knowledge, skill, value, or attitude.

teach·ing hos·pi·tal (tēch′ing hos′pi-tăl) A hospital that also functions as a formal center of learning for the training of physicians, nurses, and allied health personnel.

teach·ing plan (tēch′ing plan) NURSING outline of education to be provided to patient, family, community, and other learners; includes objectives, content, teaching methods, time frame, and evaluation.

Teale am·pu·ta·tion (tēl amp′yū-tā′shŭn) **1.** Surgical removal of the forearm in its lower half, or of the thigh, with a long posterior rectangular flap and a short anterior one. **2.** Surgical removal of the leg, with a long anterior rectangular flap and a short posterior one.

team nurs·ing (tēm nŭrs′ing) A method of providing nursing services to inpatients in which responsibility for planning and coordination of care is shared by members of a group; the team may include registered nurses, practical nurses, and other nursing personnel, but the team leader is most often a registered nurse.

tear (tār) A discontinuity in substance of a structure. Cf. laceration.

tear (tēr) Fluid secreted by the lacrimal glands by means of which the conjunctiva and cornea are kept moist. [A.S. *teăr*]

tear·drop (tēr′drop) **1.** A drop of fluid secreted by the lacrimal glands. **2.** A red blood cell with a pear shape, in which the constricted end narrows to a point. [A.S. tear, *teahor*, *taeher*, Old Norse *tar*]

tear·drop cell (tēr′drop sel) SYN dacryocyte.

tear gas (tēr gas) A common but erroneous term for compounds (e.g., acetone, benzene bromide, and xylol) that irritate the conjunctiva and cause profuse lacrimation. These compounds are typically solids dispensed either as aerosols or in solution. SEE ALSO lacrimator.

tear·ing (tēr′ing) SYN epiphora.

tear sac (tēr sak) SYN lacrimal sac.

tear stone (tēr stōn) SYN dacryolith.

tease (tēz) To separate the structural parts of a tissue by means of a needle, to prepare it for microscopic examination. [A. S. *taesan*]

tea·spoon (tē′spūn) A small spoon, holding about 1 dram (or about 5 mL) liquid; used as a measure in the dosage of fluid medicines.

teat (tēt) **1.** SYN nipple. **2.** SYN breast. **3.** SYN papilla. [A.S. *tit*]

tech-check-tech (tek-chek′tek) A system in which a trained pharmacy technician can check another technician's work on certain medications.

tech·ne·ti·um (Tc) (tek-nē′shē-ŭm) An artificial radioactive element; atomic no. 43, atomic wt. 99, produced by bombardment of molybdenum by deuterons; also a product of the fission of ^{235}U; used extensively as a radiographic tracer in imaging studies of internal organs. [G. *technetos*, artificial]

tech·ne·ti·um 99m (tek-nē′shē-ŭm) A radioisotope of technetium that decays by isomeric transition, emitting an essentially monoenergetic gamma ray of 142 keV with a half-life of 6.01 hr. It is usually obtained from a radionuclide generator of molybdenum 99 and is used to prepare radiopharmaceuticals for scanning the brain, parotid, thyroid, lungs, blood pool, liver, heart, spleen, kidney, lacrimal drainage apparatus, bone, and bone marrow.

tech•nic (tek′nik) SYN technique.

tech•ni•cal com•po•nent (tek′ni-kăl kŏm-pō′nĕnt) In health care informatics, that portion of a procedure undertaken by a technician, rather than by a physician.

tech•ni•cian (tek-nish′ŭn) SYN technologist. [G. *technē,* an art]

tech•nique (tek-nēk′) The manner of performance, or the details, of any surgical operation, experiment, or mechanical act. SEE ALSO method, operation, modality, procedure. SYN technic. [Fr., fr. G. *technikos,* relating to *technē,* art, skill]

tech•nol•o•gist (tek-nol′ŏ-jist) One trained in and using the techniques of a profession, art, or science. SYN technician.

tech•nol•o•gy (tĕk-nŏl′ŏ-jē) The application of scientific knowledge and skills for practical purposes.

tec•tal (tek′tăl) Relating to a tectum.

tec•to•ceph•a•ly (tek′tō-sef′ă-lē) SYN scaphocephaly.

tec•ton•ic ker•a•to•plas•ty (tek-ton′ik ker′ă-tō-plas-tē) Corneal transplantation performed to replace lost corneal tissue to provide support.

tec•to•ri•al (tek-tōr′ē-ăl) Relating to or characteristic of a tectorium.

tec•to•ri•al mem•brane of co•chle•ar duct (tek-tōr′ē-ăl mem′brān kok′lē-ăr dŭkt) A gelatinous membrane that overlies the spiral organ (Corti) in the inner ear. SYN membrana tectoria ductus cochlearis [TA], Corti membrane, tectorium (2).

tec•to•ri•um (tek-tōr′ē-ŭm) **1.** An overlying structure. **2.** SYN tectorial membrane of cochlear duct. [L. an overlying surface (plaster, stucco), fr. *tego,* pp. *tectus,* to cover]

tec•to•spi•nal (tek′tō-spī′năl) Denoting nerve fibers passing from the mesencephalic tectum to the spinal cord.

tec•tum, pl. **tec•ta** (tek′tŭm, -tă) Any rooflike covering or structure. [L. roof, roofed structure, fr. *tego,* pp. *tectus,* to cover]

tec•tum of mid•brain (tek′tŭm mid′brān) SYN lamina of mesencephalic tectum.

TED hose (hōz) Elastic stockings that compress the superficial veins in the lower extremities; used in postoperative patients and others immobilized by illness to prevent thrombophlebitis by shunting blood through the deep veins of the calves and thighs. TED is an abbreviation for thromboembolic disease.

teeth (tēth) Plural of tooth.

teeth•ing (tēdh′ing) Eruption or, colloquially, cutting of the teeth, especially of the deciduous teeth; inflammation of the gingival tissues during this period may cause a temporary painful condition.

teg•men, gen. **teg•mi•nis**, pl. **teg•mi•na** (teg′men, -mi-nis, -mi-nă) [TA] A structure that covers or roofs over a part. [L. a covering, fr. *tego,* to cover]

teg•men mas•toi•de•um (teg′men mas-toyd′ē-ŭm) The lamina of bone roofing over the mastoid cells.

teg•men•tal (teg-men′tăl) Relating to, characteristic of, or placed or oriented toward a tegmentum or tegmen.

teg•men•tal de•cus•sa•tions (teg-men′tăl dē′kŭs-ā′shŭnz) **1.** The dorsal tegmental decussation (fountain or Meynert decussation, decussatio fontinalis) of the left and right tectospinal and tectobulbar tracts. **2.** The ventral tegmental decussation (rubrospinal or Forel decussation) of the left and right rubrospinal and rubrobulbar tracts; both are located in the mesencephalon. SYN decussationes tegmenti.

teg•men•tal nu•cle•i (teg-men′tăl nū′klē-ī) Collective term for small round cell groups in the caudal part of the midbrain (caudal pontine tegmental nucleus, nucleus tegmenti pontis caudalis and oral pontine tegmental nucleus, nucleus tegmenti pontis oralis) associated with the mammillary body by way of the mammillary peduncle and mammillotegmental tract.

teg•men•tal syn•drome (teg-men′tăl sin′drōm) A syndrome usually caused by a vascular lesion in the tegmentum; marked by contralateral hemiplegia and ipsilateral ocular paresis.

teg•men•tum, pl. **teg•men•ta** (teg-men′tŭm, -tă) **1.** A covering structure. **2.** [TA] SYN mesencephalic tegmentum. [L. covering structure, fr. *tego,* to cover]

teg•men tym•pa•ni (teg′men tim′pan-ī) [TA] The roof of the middle ear, formed by the thinned anterior surface of the petrous portion of the temporal bone. Its anterior edge is inserted into the petrosquamous fissure so that it can be seen as a wedge of bone subdividing that fissure into a squamotympanic and a petrotympanic fissure.

teg•men ven•tric•u•li quar•ti (teg′men ven-trik′yū-lī kwahr′tī) Roof of fourth ventricle, formed in its upper part by the superior medullary velum stretching between the two brachia conjunctiva (superior cerebellar peduncles), in its lower part by the inferior medullary velum composed of the choroid membrane and choroid plexus of the fourth ventricle.

teg•u•ment (teg′yū-ment) SYN integument. [L. *tegumentum,* a collat. form of *tegmentum*]

teg•u•men•tal, **teg•u•men•ta•ry** (teg′yū-men′tăl, -tăr-ē) Relating to the integument.

Teich•mann crys•tals (tīk′mahn kris′tălz) Rhombic crystals of hemin; used in microscopic detection of blood. SEE hemin.

tei•cho•ic ac•ids (tī-kō′ik as′idz) One of two classes (the other being the muramic acids or mucopeptides) of polymers constituting the cell walls of gram-positive bacteria, but also found intracellularly.

tei•chop•si•a (tī-kop′sē-ă) The jagged, shimmering visual sensation resembling the fortifications of a walled medieval town; the scintillating scotoma of migraine. [G. *teichos,* wall, + *opsis,* vision]

tel-, tele-, telo- Combining forms meaning distance, end, other end. [G. *tēle,* distant, *telos,* end]

te•la, gen. and pl. **te•lae** (tē′lă, -lē) **1.** Any thin, weblike structure. **2.** A tissue; especially one of delicate formation. [L. a web]

te•la cho•roi•de•a of fourth ven•tri•cle (tē′lă kōr-oyd′ē-ă fōrth ven′tri-kĕl) The sheet of pia mater covering the lower part of the ependymal roof of the fourth ventricle. SYN tela choroidea ventriculi quarti [TA], tela choroidea inferior.

te•la cho•roi•de•a in•fe•ri•or (tē′lă kōr-oyd′ē-ă in-fēr′ē-ŏr) SYN tela choroidea of fourth ventricle.

te•la cho•roi•de•a su•pe•ri•or (tē′lă kōr-oyd′ē-ă sŭ-pēr′ē-ŏr) SYN tela choroidea of third ventricle.

te•la cho•roi•de•a of third ven•tri•cle (tē′lă kōr-oyd′ē-ă thērd ven′tri-kĕl) A double fold of pia mater, enclosing subarachnoid trabeculae, between the fornix above and the epithelial roof of the third ventricle and the thalami below; at each lateral margin is a vascular fringe projecting into the choroidal fissure of the lateral ventricle; on its undersurface are several small vascular projections filling the folds of the ependymal roof of the third ventricle. SYN tela choroidea superior.

te•la cho•roi•de•a ven•tri•cu•li quar•ti (tē′lă kōr-oyd′ē-ă ven-trik′yū-lī kwahr′tī) [TA] SYN tela choroidea of fourth ventricle.

te•la cho•roi•de•a ven•tri•cu•li ter•ti•i (tē′lă kōr-oyd′ē-ă ven-trik′yū-lī terts′ē-ī) [TA] SYN choroid tela of third ventricle.

tel•an•gi•ec•ta•si•a (tel-an′jē-ek-tā′zē-ă) Dilation of the previously existing small or terminal vessels of a part. [G. *telos,* end, + *angeion,* vessel, + *ektasis,* a stretching out]

tel•an•gi•ec•ta•sis, pl. **tel•an•gi•ec•ta•ses** (tel-an′jē-ek′tă-sis, -sēz) A lesion formed by a dilated capillary or terminal artery, most commonly on the skin. SEE ALSO telangiectasia. See page B13.

tel•an•gi•ec•tat•ic (tel-an′jē-ek-tat′ik) Relating to or marked by telangiectasia.

tel•an•gi•ec•tat•ic an•gi•o•ma (tel-an′jē-ek-tat′ik an′jē-ō′mă) Tumor composed of dilated vessels.

tel•an•gi•ec•tat•ic fi•bro•ma (tel-an′jē-ek-tat′ik fī-brō′mă) A benign tumor of fibrous tissue in which there are numerous small and large, frequently dilated vascular channels. SYN angiofibroma.

tel•an•gi•ec•tat•ic os•te•o•gen•ic sar•co•ma (tel-an′jē-ek-tat′ik os′tē-ō-jen′ik sahr-kō′mă) A lytic cystic variant of osteogenic sarcoma composed of aneurysmal blood-filled spaces lined by sarcoma cells producing osteoid.

tel•an•gi•ec•tat•ic wart (tel-an′jē-ek-tat′ik wōrt) SYN angiokeratoma.

tel•an•gi•o•sis (tel′an-jē-ō′sis) Any disease of the capillaries and terminal arterioles.

te•la sub•cu•ta•ne•a (tē′lă sŭb-kyū-tā′nē-ă) SYN superficial fascia.

te•la sub•mu•co•sa (tē′lă sŭb′myū-kō′să) SYN submucosa.

tel•e•can•thus (tel′ĕ-kan′thŭs) Increased distance between the medial canthi or angles of the eyelids. [G. *tēle,* distant, + *kanthos,* canthus]

te•le•com•mun•i•ca•tions de•vice for the deaf (TDD, TT) (tel′ĕ-kŏ-myū′ni-kā′shŭns dĕ-vīs′ def) Telephone accessory that transmits and receives text over standard telephone lines. Also referred to as teletypewriter (TTY) and text telephone (TT). SEE ALSO assistive listening device.

tel•e•di•ag•no•sis (tel′ĕ-dī′ăg-nō′sis) Detection of a disease by evaluation of data transmitted to a receiving station, a process normally involving patient monitoring instruments and a transfer link to a diagnostic center at some distance from the patient.

te•le•graph•ic speech (tel′ĕ-graf′ik spēch) A pattern of speech typical of expressive aphasia, in which prominent words in a sentence, usually nouns, are uttered but most other words are omitted. SEE ALSO agrammatism.

te•le•health (tel′ĕ helth) Use of telecommunications technology to deliver health care at a distance from the patient. SEE ALSO informatics.

te•lem•e•try (tĕ-lem′ĕ-trē) Process of transmitting results using radio signals. SEE ALSO biotelemetry.

tel•en•ce•phal•ic (tel′en-se-fal′ik) Relating to the telencephalon or endbrain.

tel•en•ceph•al•ic flex•ure (tel′en-se-fal′ik flek′shŭr) A flexure appearing in the embryonic forebrain region.

tel•en•ceph•a•lon (tel′en-sef′ă-lon) [TA] The anterior division of the prosencephalon, which develops into the olfactory lobes, the cortex of the cerebral hemispheres, the subcortical telencephalic nuclei, and the basal ganglia (nuclei), particularly the striatum and the amygdala. SYN endbrain. [G. *telos,* end, + *enkephalos,* brain]

te•le•nur•sing (tel′ĕ-nŭrs′ing) Use of telecommunications technology to deliver nursing care at a distance from the patient.

tel•e•o•mi•to•sis (tel′ē-ō-mī-tō′sis) A completed mitosis. [G. *teleos,* complete, + mitosis]

tel•e•op•si•a (tel′ē-op′sē-ă) An error in judging the distance of objects arising from lesions in the parietal temporal region. [G. *tēle,* distant, + *opsis,* vision]

tel•e•or•gan•ic (tel′ē-ōr-gan′ik) Manifesting life. [G. *teleos,* complete, + *organikos,* organic]

te•lep•a•thy (tĕ-lep′ă-thē) Transmittal and reception of thoughts by means other than through the normal senses, as a form of extrasensory perception. [G. *tēle,* distant, + *pathos,* feeling]

te•le•phone ear (tel′ĕ-fōn ēr) Noise-induced hearing loss due to exposure to static over telephones.

tel•e•ra•di•og•ra•phy (tel′ĕ-rā′dē-og′ră-fē) Radiography with the x-ray tube positioned about 2 m from the film, thereby securing practical parallelism of the x-rays to minimize geometric distortion; the standard configuration for chest radiography. SYN teleroentgenography. [G. *tēle,* distant, + radiography]

tel•e•ra•di•ol•o•gy (tel′ĕ-rā′dē-ol′ŏ-jē) The interpretation of digitized diagnostic images transmitted over telephone lines. [tele- + radiology]

tel•er•gy (tel′ĕr-jē) SYN automatism. [G. *tēle,* far off, + *ergon,* work]

tel•e•roent•gen•og•ra•phy (tel′ĕ-rent′gen-og′ră-fē) SYN teleradiography.

tel•e•ther•a•py (tel′ĕ-thār′ă-pē) Radiation therapy administered with the source at a distance from the body. [G. *tēle,* distant, + *therapeia,* treatment]

tel•lu•ric (tĕ-lūr′ik) **1.** Relating to or originating in the earth. **2.** Relating to the element tellurium, especially in its 6^+ valence state. [L. *tellus* (*tellur-*), the earth]

tel•lu•ri•um (Te) (tel-ūr′ē-ŭm) A rare semimetallic element, atomic no. 52, atomic wt. 127.60, belonging to the sulfur group. [L. *tellus* (*tellur-*), the earth]

tel•o•den•dron (tel′ō-den′dron) The terminal arborization of an axon. [G. *telos,* end, + *dendron,* tree]

tel•o•gen (tel′ō-jen) Resting phase of hair cycle. [G. *telos,* end, + *-gen,* producing]

tel•o•gen ef•flu•vi•um (tel′ō-jen ĕ-flū′vē-ŭm) Increased transient shedding of normal club hairs by premature development of telogen in anagen follicles, resulting from various kinds of stress (e.g., childbirth, shock, drug intake, cessation of an oral contraceptive, fever, dieting with marked weight loss). SEE ALSO anagen effluvium.

tel•o•lec•i•thal (tel′ō-les′i-thăl) Denoting an oocyte (ovum) in which a large amount of deuteroplasm accumulates at the vegetative pole, as in the eggs of birds and reptiles. [G. *telos,* end, + G. *lekithos,* yolk]

tel•o•mere (tel′ō-mēr) The distal end of a chromosome arm; telomeres undergo dramatic changes during the progression of cancer. [G. *telos,* end, + *meros,* part]

tel•o•phase (tel′ō-fāz) The final stage of mitosis or meiosis, which begins when migration of chromosomes to the poles of the cell has been completed; the chromosomes progressively lengthen, whereas the nuclear membranes of the two daughter nuclei are reconstructed and a cell membrane at the equator completes the separation of the two daughter cells. [G. *telos,* end, + *phasis,* appearance]

tem•per (tem′pĕr) **1.** Disposition; in general, any characteristic or particular state of mind. SYN temperament (2). **2.** A display of irritation or anger. SEE ALSO tantrum. **3.** To treat metal by application of heat, as in annealing or quenching.

tem•per•a•ment (tem′pĕr-ă-mĕnt) **1.** The psychological and biologic organization peculiar to the person, including one's character or personality predispositions, which influence the manner of thought and action and general views of life. **2.** SYN temper (1). [L. *temperamentum,* proper measure, moderation, disposition]

tem•per•ance (tem′pĕr-ăns) Moderation in all things; especially, abstinence from the use of alcoholic beverages. [L. *temperantia,* moderation]

tem•per•ate (tem′pĕr-ăt) Moderate; restrained in the indulgence of any appetite or activity.

tem•per•ate bac•te•ri•o•phage (tem′pĕr-ăt bak-tēr′ē-ō-fāj) A bacteria-consuming virus with a genome that incorporates with, and replicates with, that of the host bacterium; dissociation (and resultant development of vegetative bacteriophage) occurs at a slow rate resulting occasionally in lysis of a bacterium and release of mature bacteriophage, thus rendering the bacterial culture capable of inducing general lysis if transferred to a culture of a susceptible bacterial strain.

i **tem•per•a•ture** (tem′pĕr-ă-chŭr) The sensible intensity of heat of any substance; the manifestation of the average kinetic energy of the molecules making up a substance due to heat agitation. SEE ALSO scale. See page 1537. [L. *temperatura,* due measure, temperature, fr. *tempero,* to proportion duly]

tem•per•a•ture mid•point (Tm, t_m) (tem′pěr-ă-chŭr mid′poynt) The midpoint in the change in optic properties (absorbance, rotation) of a structured polymer (e.g., DNA) with increasing temperature.

The normal temperature varies from person to person, by age, and throughout the day. The rectal temperature is usually about 0.5–1°F higher than the oral, and the axillary temperature is usually about 0.5–1°F below oral.

Normal body temperature by age:	
Children 0-3 months	99.4°F
Children 3-6 months	99.5°F
Children 6 months to 1 year	99.7°F
Children 1 year to 3 years	99°F
Children 3 years to 5 years	98.6°F
Children 5 years to 9 years	98.3°F
Children 9 years to 13 years	98°F
Children 13 year to adult	97.8–99.1°F

If the reading on the thermometer is more than 1–1.5°F above the patient's normal temperature, the patient has a fever. Most fevers are a sign of infection and occur with other symptoms. Abnormally high or low temperatures can be serious, and you should consult a health care provider.

Information provided by the National Library of Medicine 2003.

tem•plate (tem′plăt) **1.** A pattern or guide that determines the shape of a substance. **2.** Metaphorically, the specifying nature of a macromolecule, usually a nucleic acid or polynucleotide, with respect to the primary structure of the nucleic acid or polynucleotide or protein made from it in vivo or in vitro. **3.** DENTISTRY a curved or flat plate used as an aid in setting teeth. **4.** An outline used to trace teeth, bones, or soft tissue to standardize their form. **5.** A pattern or guide that determines the specificity of antibody globulins. **6.** A wax impression made to assess the occlusion of the teeth. **7.** MOLECULAR BIOLOGY The target nucleic acid for molecular diagnostics assays. [Fr. *templet,* temple of a loom, fr. L. *templum,* small timber]

tem•ple (tem′pĕl) **1.** The area of the temporal fossa on the side of the head above the zygomatic arch. **2.** The part of a spectacle frame passing from the rim backward over the ear. [L. *tempus* (*tempor-*), time, the temple]

tem•po•la•bile (tem′pō-lā′bīl) Undergoing spontaneous change or destruction during the passage of time. [L. *tempus,* time, + *labilis,* perishable]

tem•po•ral (tem′pŏr-ăl) **1.** Relating to time; limited in time; temporary. **2.** Relating to the temple. [L. *temporalis,* fr. *tempus* (*tempor-*), time, temple]

tem•por•al an•tic•i•pa•tion (tem′pŏr-ăl ăn-tis′i-pā′shŭn) Predicting when an event will occur, such as anticipating when the official will throw the ball up for the jump-start to a basketball game.

tem•por•al ar•ter•i•tis (tem′pŏr-ăl ahr′tĕr-ī′tis) A subacute, granulomatous arteritis involving the external carotid arteries, especially the temporal artery; occurs in elderly people and may be manifested by constitutional symptoms, particularly severe headache, and sometimes sudden unilateral blindness. Shares many of the symptoms of polymyalgia rheumatica. SYN cranial arteritis, giant cell arteritis, Horton arteritis.

tem•por•al bone (tem′pŏr-ăl bōn) A large, irregular osseous formation situated in the base and side of the skull; it consists of three parts, squamous, tympanic, and petrous, which are distinct at birth; the petrous part contains the vestibulocochlear organ; the bone articulates with the sphenoid, parietal, occipital, and zygomatic bones, and by a synovial joint with the mandible. SYN os temporale [TA].

tem•por•al fos•sa (tem′pŏr-ăl fos′ă) The space on the side of the cranium bounded by the temporal lines and terminating below at the level of the zygomatic arch.

tem•por•a•lis mus•cle (tem-pōr-rā′lis mŭs′ĕl) *Origin*, temporal fossa; *insertion*, coronoid process of mandible and anterior border of ramus; *action*, elevates mandible (closes jaw); its posterior, nearly horizontally-oriented fibers are the primary retractors of the protruded mandible; *nerve supply*, deep temporal branches of mandibular division of trigeminal. See page 1538. SYN musculus temporalis [TA], temporal muscle.

tem•por•al lobe (tem′pŏr-ăl lōb) The long and lowest of the major subdivisions of the cortical mantle, forming the posterior two thirds of the ventral surface of the cerebral hemisphere, separated from the frontal and parietal lobes above it by the lateral sulcus arbitrarily delineated by an imaginary plane from the occipital lobe with which it is continuous posteriorly. The temporal lobe has a heterogeneous composition: in addition to a large neocortical component consisting of the superior, middle, and inferior temporal gyri and the lateral and medial occipitotemporal gyri, it includes the largely juxtallocortical parahippocampal gyrus with its paleocortical (olfactory) uncus and, beneath the latter, the amygdala. SYN lobus temporalis [TA].

tem•por•al lobe ep•i•lep•sy (tem′pŏr-ăl lōb ep′i-lep′sē) Disorder with seizures originating from the temporal lobe, most commonly the mesial temporal lobe.

tem•por•al mus•cle (tem′pŏr-ăl mŭs′ĕl) SYN temporalis muscle.

tem•por•al plane (tem′pŏr-ăl plān) A slightly depressed area on the side of the cranium, below the inferior temporal line, formed by the temporal and parietal bones, the greater wing of the sphenoid, and a part of the frontal bone.

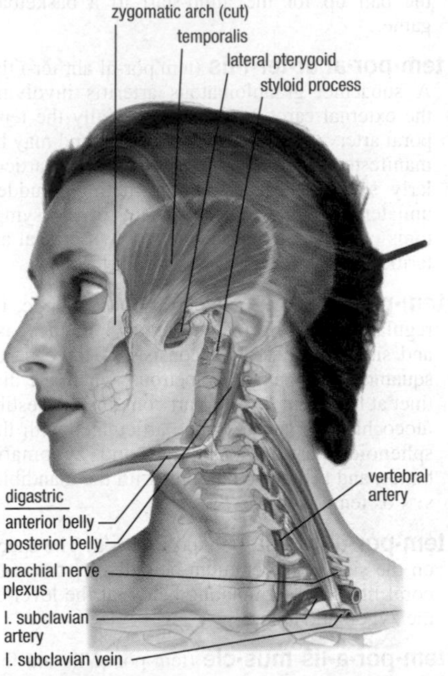

temporalis muscle

tem•por•al pole of ce•re•brum (tem′pŏr-ăl pōl ser′ĕ-brŭm) The most prominent part of the anterior extremity of the temporal lobe of each cerebral hemisphere, a short distance below the fissure of Sylvius.

tem•por•al pro•cess (tem′pŏr-ăl pros′es) The posterior projection of the zygomatic bone articulating with the zygomatic process of the temporal bone to form the zygomatic arch.

tem•po•rar•y car•ti•lage (tem′pŏ-rar-ē kahr′ti-lăj) A cartilage that is normally replaced by bone to form a part of the skeleton. SYN precursory cartilage.

tem•po•rar•y den•ture (tem′pŏ-rar-ē den′shŭr) SYN interim denture.

tem•po•rar•y par•a•site (tem′pŏ-rar-ē par′ă-sīt) An organism accidentally ingested that survives briefly in the intestine.

tem•po•rar•y thresh•old shift (tem′pŏ-rar-ē thresh′ōld shift) The reversible hearing loss that results from exposure to intense impulse or continuous sound, as opposed to the irreversible permanent threshold shift that may result from such exposure.

tem•po•rar•y tooth (tem′pŏ-rar-ē tūth) SYN deciduous tooth.

♻ **temporo-** Combining form meaning temporal (2). [L. *temporalis,* temporal]

tem•po•ro•man•dib•u•lar (tem′pŏr-ō-man-dib′yū-lăr) Relating to the temporal bone and the mandible; denoting the joint of the lower jaw. SYN temporomaxillary (2).

tem•por•o•man•di•bu•lar dis•or•der (tem′pŏr-ō-man-dib′yū-lăr dis-ōr′dĕr) An inclusive term for all functional disturbances of the masticatory system including temporomandibular joint (TMJ) syndrome, myofacial pain-dysfunction syndrome, and temporomandibular pain-dysfunction syndrome.

i **tem•por•o•man•di•bu•lar joint (TMJ)** (tem′pŏr-ō-man-dib′yū-lăr joynt) The joint between the temporal bone and the mandible. See this page. SYN mandibular joint.

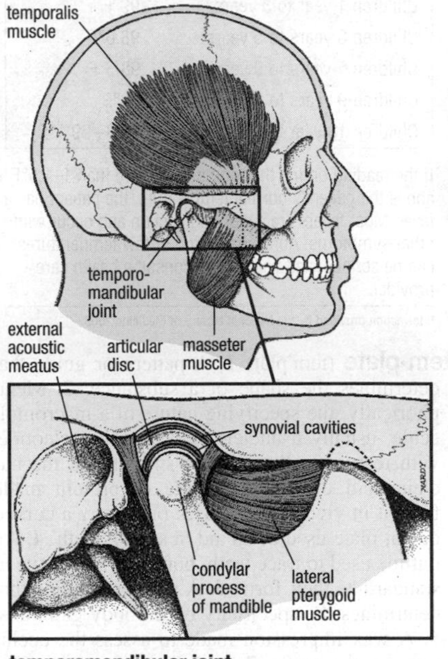

temporomandibular joint

tem•por•o•man•dib•u•lar joint pain-dys•func•tion syn•drome (TMJ syn•drome) (tem′pŏr-ō-man-dib′yū-lăr joynt pān-dis-fŭngk′shŭn sin′drōm) SYN myofascial pain-dysfunction syndrome.

tem•por•o•man•dib•u•lar nerve (tem′pŏr-ō-man-dib′yū-lăr nĕrv) SYN zygomatic nerve.

tem•po•ro•max•il•lar•y (tem′pŏ-rō-mak′si-lar-ē) **1.** Relating to the regions of the temporal and maxillary bones. **2.** SYN temporomandibular.

tem•por•o•pa•ri•e•ta•lis mus•cle (tem′pŏr-ō-pă-rī′ĕ-tā′lis mŭs′ĕl) The part of epicranius muscle that arises from the lateral part of the epicranial aponeurosis and inserts in the cartilage of the auricle. SYN musculus temporoparietalis [TA], temporoparietal muscle.

tem•por•o•pa•ri•e•tal mus•cle (tem′pŏ-rō-păr-i′ĕ-tăl mŭs′ĕl) SYN temporoparietalis muscle.

tem•por•o•pon•tine fi•bers (tem′pŏr-ō-pon′tēn fī′bĕrz) A fiber group originating in the cerebral cortex of the temporal lobe, particularly the superior and middle temporal gyri, following the sublenticular limb of the internal capsule into the lateral margin of the crus cerebri in which it descends to its termination in the pontine nuclei in the basilar part of the pons.

tem•po•ro•pon•tine tract (tem′pŏr-ō-pon′tēn trakt) SEE temporopontine fibers.

tem•po•sta•bile, **tem•po•sta•ble** (tem′pō-stā′bīl, -stā′bĕl) Not subject to spontaneous alteration or destruction. [L. *tempus,* time + *stabilis,* stable]

tem•pus, gen. **tem•po•ris**, pl. **tem•po•ra** (tem′pŭs, -pŏ-ris, -pŏ-ră) **1.** The temple. **2.** SYN time. [L. time]

TEMS (temz) Acronym for tactical emergency medical service.

TEN Abbreviation for toxic epidermal necrolysis.

te•na•cious (tĕ-nā′shŭs) Having the capacity to stick or adhere. [L. *tenax* (*tenac-*), fr. *teneo,* to hold]

te•nac•u•lum, pl. **te•nac•u•la** (tĕ-nak′yū-lŭm, -lă) A surgical clamp designed to hold or grasp tissue during dissection. [L. a holder, fr. *teneo,* to hold]

te•nac•u•lum for•ceps (tĕ-nak′yū-lŭm fōr′seps) A forceps with jaws armed each with a sharp, straight hook like a tenaculum.

te•nal•gi•a (tĕ-nal′jē-ă) Pain referred to a tendon. SYN tenodynia, tenontodynia. [G. *tenōn,* tendon, + *algos,* pain]

ten•der (ten′dĕr) Sensitive or painful as a result of pressure or contact that is not sufficient to cause discomfort in normal tissues. [L. *tener,* soft, delicate]

ten•der•ness (ten′dĕr-nĕs) The condition of being tender.

ten•der point (ten′dĕr poynt) Eighteen bilateral predefined areas in occiput, neck, shoulders, chest, elbows, gluteus, trochanter, and knees that produce painful response at 4 kg pressure; used to diagnose fibromyalgia if 11 of 18 are positive. SEE ALSO fibromyalgia.

ten•di•ni•tis (ten′di-nī′tis) Inflammation of a tendon. SYN tendonitis, tenonitis (2), tenontitis, tenositis.

ten•di•no•plas•ty (ten′din-ō-plas-tē) SYN tenontoplasty. [Mediev. L. *tendo* (*tendin-*), tendon, + G. *plastos,* formed]

ten•di•no•sis (ten′di-nō′sis) A noninflammatory condition involving a previously injured tendon that heals with weak collagenous fibers, low weight-bearing resistance, and a high risk of future injury. SEE ALSO compartment syndrome.

ten•di•no•su•ture (ten′di-nō-sū′chŭr) SYN tenorrhaphy.

ten•di•nous (ten′di-nŭs) Relating to, composed of, or resembling a tendon.

ten•di•nous arch (ten′di-nŭs ahrch) **1.** A white, fibrous band attached to bone and/or muscle, arching over and thus protecting neurovascular elements passing beneath it from injurious compression. **2.** A linear thickening of the deep fascia of a muscle that provides attachment for ligaments or muscle fibers.

ten•di•nous arch of le•va•tor a•ni mus•cle (ten′di-nŭs ahrch le-vā′tŏr ā′nī mŭs′ĕl) A thickened portion of the obturator fascia on the medial aspect of the obturator internus (muscle) that extends in an arching line from the pubis posteriorly to the ischial spine and gives origin to part of the levator ani muscle.

ten•di•nous arch of pel•vic fa•sci•a (ten′di-nŭs ahrch pel′vik fash′ē-ă) A linear thickening of the superior fascia of the pelvic diaphragm extending posteriorly from the body of the os pubis alongside the bladder (and vagina in the female) to the ischial spine and giving attachment to the supporting ligaments of the pelvic viscera.

ten•di•nous cords (ten′di-nŭs kōrdz) SYN chordae tendineae of heart.

ten•di•nous syn•o•vi•tis (ten′di-nŭs sin′ō-vī′tis) SYN tenosynovitis.

ten•do, gen. **ten•di•nis**, pl. **ten•di•nes** (ten′dō, -di-nis, -di-nēz) SYN tendon. [Mediev. L., fr. L. *tendo,* to stretch out, extend]

♻ **tendo-** [TA] Combining form meaning a tendon. SEE ALSO teno-. [L. *tendo*]

ten•do cal•ca•ne•us (ten′dō kal-kā′nē-ŭs) [TA] The tendon of insertion of the triceps surae (gastrocnemius and soleus) into the tuberosity of the calcaneus. SYN Achilles tendon, heel tendon.

ten•dol•y•sis (ten-dol′i-sis) Release of a tendon from adhesions. SYN tenolysis. [tendo- + G. *lysis,* dissolution]

ten•don (ten′dŏn) A nondistensible fibrous cord or band of variable length that is the part of the muscle that connects the fleshy (contractile) part of muscle with its bony attachment or other structure; it may unite with the fleshy part of the muscle at its extremity or may run along the side or in the center of the fleshy part for a longer or shorter distance, receiving the muscular fibers along its border; when the length of a muscle is determined, the tendon length is included as well as the fleshy part; it consists of fascicles of very densely arranged, almost parallel collagenous fibers, rows of elongated fibrocytes, and a minimum of ground substance. SYN sinew, tendo. [L. *tendo*]

ten•don cells (ten′dŏn selz) Elongated fibroblastic cells arranged in rows between the collagenous tendon fibers.

ten•don•i•tis (ten′dŏ-nī′tis) SYN tendinitis.

ten•don re•ces•sion (ten′dŏn rĕ-sesh′ŭn) Surgical displacement of the tendon of an eye muscle posterior to its anatomic insertion.

ten•don re•flex (ten′dŏn rē′fleks) A myotatic or deep reflex in which the muscle stretch receptors are stimulated by percussing the tendon of a muscle.

ten•do•plas•ty (ten′dō-plas-tē) SYN tenontoplasty.

ten•do•syn•o•vi•tis (ten′dō-sin′ō-vī′tis) SYN tenosynovitis.

ten•dot•o•my (ten-dot′ŏ-mē) SYN tenotomy.

ten•do•vag•i•nal (ten′dō-vaj′i-năl) Relating to a tendon and its sheath. [tendo- + L. *vagina,* sheath]

ten•do•vag•i•ni•tis (ten′dō-vaj-i-nī′tis) SYN tenosynovitis. [tendo- + L. *vagina,* sheath, + G. *-itis,* inflammation]

te•nec•to•my (tĕ-nek′tŏ-mē) Resection of part of a tendon. SYN tenonectomy. [G. *tenōn,* tendon, + *ektomē,* excision]

te•nes•mic (tĕ-nez′mik) Relating to or marked by tenesmus.

te•nes•mus (tĕ-nez′mŭs) A painful spasm of the anal sphincter with an urgent desire to evacuate the bowel or bladder, involuntary straining, and the passage of little fecal matter or urine. [G. *teinesmos,* ineffectual effort to defecate, fr. *teinō,* to stretch]

ten Horn sign (ten hōrn sīn) Pain caused by gentle traction on the right spermatic cord, indicative of appendicitis.

te•ni•a, pl. **te•ni•ae** (tē′nē-ă, -ē) **1.** Any anatomic bandlike structure. Cf. *Taenia.* **2.** SYN taenia (2). [L. fr. G. *tainia,* band, tape, tapeworm]

te•ni•a cho•roi•de•a (tē′nē-ă kō-royd′ē-ă) [TA] The somewhat thickened line along which a choroid membrane or plexus is attached to the rim of a brain ventricle.

te•ni•a•cide (tē′nē-ă-sīd) An agent that destroys tapeworms. [L. *taenia,* tapeworm, + *caedo,* to kill]

te•ni•ae co•li (tē′nē-ē kō′lī) [TA] The three bands in which the longitudinal muscular fibers of the large intestine, except the rectum, are collected; these are the mesocolic tenia, situated at the place corresponding to the mesenteric attachment; the free tenia, opposite the mesocolic tenia; and the omental tenia, at the place corresponding to the site of adhesion of the greater omentum to the transverse colon.

ten•i•al (tē′nē-ăl) **1.** Relating to a tapeworm. **2.** Relating to one of the structures called tenia.

te•ni•a•sis (tē-nī′ă-sis) Presence of a tapeworm in the intestine.

te•ni•o•la (tē-nē′ō-lă) A slender tenia or bandlike structure. [L. dim. of *taenia,* ribbon]

ten•nis el•bow (ten′is el′bō) SYN lateral epicondylitis.

ten•nis thumb (ten′is thŭm) Tendinitis with calcification in the tendon of the long flexor of the thumb (flexor pollicis longus) caused by friction and strain as in tennis playing, but also occurring in other exercises in which the thumb is subject to repeated pressure or strain.

teno-, tenon-, tenont-, tenonto- Combining forms meaning tendon. SEE ALSO tendo-. [G. *tenōn*]

te•no•de•sis (ten′ŏ-dē′sis) Stabilizing a joint by anchoring the tendons that move the joint. [teno- + G. *desis,* a binding]

ten•o•dyn•i•a (ten-ō-din′ē-ă) SYN tenalgia. [teno- + G. *odynē,* pain]

ten•og•ra•phy (tĕn-og-ră′fē) Radiography of a tendon after contrast material has been injected into the tendon sheath.

ten•ol•y•sis (ten-ol′i-sis) SYN tendolysis.

ten•o•my•o•plas•ty (ten-ō-mī′ō-plas-tē) SYN tenontomyoplasty.

ten•o•my•ot•o•my (ten-ō-mī-ot′ŏ-mē) SYN myotenotomy.

Te•non cap•sule (ten′on[h] kap′sŭl) SYN fascial sheath of eyeball.

ten•o•nec•to•my (ten-ō-nek′tŏ-mē) SYN tenectomy. [tenon- + G. *ektomē,* excision]

ten•o•ni•tis (ten-ō-nī′tis) **1.** Inflammation of Tenon capsule or the connective tissue within Tenon space. **2.** SYN tendinitis. [tenont- + G. *-itis,* inflammation]

ten•on•ti•tis (ten′on-tī′tis) SYN tendinitis. [tenont- + G. *-itis,* inflammation]

te•non•to•dyn•i•a (te-non′tō-din′ē-ă) SYN tenalgia.

te•non•to•my•o•plas•ty (te-non′tō-mī′ō-plas-tē) A combined tenontoplasty and myoplasty, used in the radical correction of a hernia. SYN tenomyoplasty. [tenonto- + G. *mys,* muscle, + *plastos,* formed]

te•non•to•plas•ty (te-non′tō-plas-tē) Reparative or plastic surgery of the tendons. SYN tendinoplasty, tendoplasty, tenoplasty. [tenonto- + G. *plastos,* formed]

ten•o•phyte (ten′ō-fīt) Bony or cartilaginous growth in or on a tendon. [teno- + G. *phyton,* plant]

ten•o•plas•ty (ten′ō-plas-tē) SYN tenontoplasty.

ten•o•re•cep•tor (ten′ō-rē-sep′tŏr) A receptor in a tendon, activated by increased tension.

te•nor•rha•phy (te-nōr′ă-fē) Suture of the divided ends of a tendon. SYN tendinosuture, tenosuture. [teno- + G. *rhaphē,* suture]

ten•o•si•tis (ten-ō-sī′tis) SYN tendinitis.

ten•os•to•sis (ten-os-tō′sis) Ossification of a tendon. [teno- + G. *osteon,* bone, + *-osis,* condition]

ten•o•sus•pen•sion (ten′ō-sŭs-pen′shŭn) Using a tendon as a suspensory ligament, sometimes as a free graft or in continuity.

ten•o•su•ture (ten′ō-sū′chūr) SYN tenorrhaphy.

ten•o•syn•o•vec•to•my (ten′ō-sin-ō-vek′tō-mē) Excision of a tendon sheath. [teno- + synovia + G. *ektomē,* excision]

ten•o•syn•o•vi•tis (ten′ō-sin-ō-vī′tis) Inflammation of a tendon and its enveloping sheath. SYN tendinous synovitis, tendosynovitis, tendovaginitis, tenovaginitis. [teno- + synovia + G. *-itis,* inflammation]

te•not•o•my (te-not′ŏ-mē) The surgical division of a tendon for relief of a deformity caused by congenital or acquired shortening of a muscle, as in clubfoot or strabismus. SYN tendotomy. [teno- + G. *tomē,* incision]

ten•o•vag•i•ni•tis (ten′ō-vaj-i-nī′tis) SYN tenosynovitis. [teno- + L. *vagina,* sheath, + G. *-itis,* inflammation]

TENS Abbreviation for transcutaneous electrical nerve stimulation.

ten•seg•ri•ty (ten-seg′ri-tē) A concept of muscular-skeletal relationships based on the work of architect Buckminster Fuller; refers to the forces of tension (provided by muscles, tendons, ligaments, and fascia) pulling on structure (bones and joints) that help keep the body both stable and efficient in mass and movement. [*ten*sile integ*rity*]

ten•sion (ten′shŭn) **1.** The act of stretching. **2.** The condition of being stretched or tense, or a stretching or pulling force. **3.** The partial pressure of a gas, especially that of a gas dissolved in a liquid such as blood. **4.** Mental, emotional, or nervous strain; strained relations or barely controlled hostility between people or groups. [L. *tensio,* fr. *tendo,* pp. *tensus,* to stretch]

ten•sion curve (ten′shŭn kŭrv) The direction of the trabeculae in cancellous bone tissue adapted to resist stress.

ten•sion head•ache, ten•sion-type head•ache (ten′shŭn hed′āk, ten′shŭn-tīp) Headache associated with nervous tension, anxiety, and the like, often related to chronic contraction of the scalp muscles. SYN muscle contraction headache.

ten•sion pneu•mo•per•i•car•di•um (ten′shŭn nū′mō-per′i-kahr′dē-ŭm) The presence of air under pressure in the pericardial space, with the potential for cardiac tamponade.

ten•sion su•ture (ten′shŭn sū′chŭr) SYN retention suture.

ten•sor, pl. **ten•so•res** (ten′sŏr, ten-sō′rēz) A muscle the function of which is to render a part firm and tense. [Mod. L. fr. L. *tendo,* pp. *tensus,* to stretch]

ten•sor fas•ci•ae la•tae mus•cle (ten′sōr fash′ē-ē lā′tē mŭs′ĕl) *Origin,* anterior superior spine and adjacent lateral surface of the ilium; *insertion,* iliotibial band of fascia lata; *action,* tenses fascia lata; flexes, abducts and medially rotates thigh; *nerve supply,* superior gluteal. USAGE NOTE Often mispronounced and misspelled tensor fascia lata. SYN musculus tensor fasciae latae [TA].

ten•sor mus•cle of soft pal•ate (ten′sōr mŭs′ĕl sawft pal′ăt) SYN tensor veli palati muscle.

ten•sor mus•cle of tym•pa•nic mem•brane (ten′sōr mŭs′ĕl tim-pan′ik mem′brān) SYN tensor tympani muscle.

ten•sor tym•pa•ni mus•cle (ten′sōr tim′pă-nī mŭs′ĕl) *Origin,* the cartilaginous part of the auditory (eustachian) tube and the walls of its hemicanal just above the bony portion of the auditory tube; *insertion,* handle of malleus; *action,* draws the handle of the malleus medialward, tensing the tympanic membrane to protect it from excessive vibration by loud sounds; *nerve supply,* branches of trigeminal through the otic ganglion. SYN musculus tensor tympani [TA], tensor muscle of tympanic membrane.

ten•sor tym•pa•ni re•flex (ten′sōr tim′pă-nī rē′fleks) Contraction of the tensor tympani muscle in response to intense sound, increasing impedance of the middle ear and thus protecting the inner ear from exposure.

ten•sor ve•li pa•la•ti mus•cle (ten′sōr vē′lī pal′ă-tī mŭs′ĕl) Tensor muscle of soft palate, musculus tensor palati; musculus palatosalpingeus; musculus sphenosalpingostaphylinus; dilator tubae; *origin,* scaphoid fossa of sphenoid, cartilaginous and membranous part of auditory (eustachian) tube and spine of sphenoid; *insertion,* posterior border of hard palate and aponeurosis of soft palate; *action,* tenses the soft palate; contributes to opening of auditory tube; *nerve supply,* branches of trigeminal nerve through the otic ganglion. SYN musculus tensor veli palatini [TA], tensor muscle of soft palate.

tent (tent) **1.** RESPIRATORY THERAPY canopy used to control humidity and the concentration of oxygen in inspired air. **2.** Cylinder of some material, usually absorbent, introduced into a canal or sinus to maintain its patency or to dilate it. **3.** To elevate or pick up a segment of skin, fascia, or tissue at a given point, giving it the appearance of a tent. [L. *tendo,* pp. *tensus,* to stretch]

ten•ta•cle (ten′tă-kĕl) A slender process for feeling, prehension, or locomotion in invertebrates. [Mod. L. *tentaculum,* a feeler, fr. *tento,* to feel]

tenth cra•ni•al nerve [CN X] (tĕnth krā′nē-ăl nĕrv) SYN vagus nerve [CN X].

ten•to•ri•al (ten-tōr′ē-ăl) Relating to a tentorium.

ten•tor•i•al ba•sal branch of in•ter•nal ca•ro•tid ar•ter•y (ten-tōr′ē-al bā′săl branch in-tĕr′năl kă-rot′id ahr′tĕr-ē) A small branch from the cavernous part of the internal carotid artery to the base of the tentorium.

ten•tor•i•al nerve (ten-tōr′ē-ăl nĕrv) The meningeal branch arising in a recurrent fashion from the intracranial portion of ophthalmic nerve supplying tentorium cerebelli and supratentorial falx cerebri. SYN nervus tentorii, ramus meningeus recurrens nervi ophthalmici, ramus tentorii.

ten•tor•i•al si•nus (ten-tōr′ē-ăl sī′nŭs) SYN straight sinus.

ten•to•ri•um, pl. **ten•to•ri•a** (ten-tōr′ē-ŭm, -ē-ă) A membranous cover or horizontal partition. [L. tent, fr. *tendo,* to stretch]

ten•to•ri•um ce•re•bel•li (ten-tōr′ē-ŭm ser′ĕ-bel′ī) [TA] A strong fold of dura mater roofing over the posterior cranial fossa with an anterior median opening, the tentorial notch, through which the midbrain passes; the tentorium cerebelli is attached along the midline to the falx cerebri and separates the cerebellum from the basal surface of the occipital and temporal lobes of the cerebral hemisphere.

TEP Abbreviation for tracheoesophageal puncture.

♻**tera- (T)** **1.** Prefix used in the SI and metric system to signify one trillion. **2.** Denoting a teras. SEE ALSO terato-. [G. *teras,* monster]

ter•as, pl. **ter•a•ta** (ter′as, -ă-tă) Fetus with deficient, redundant, misplaced, or grossly misshapen parts. [G.]

ter•at•ic (ter-at′ik) Relating to a teras.

ter•a•tism (ter′ă-tizm) SYN teratosis. [G. *teratisma,* fr. *teras*]

♻**terato-** Combining form indicating a teras. SEE ALSO tera- (2). [G. *teras,* monster]

ter•a•to•blas•to•ma (ter′ă-tō-blas-tō′mă) A tumor containing embryonic tissue differing from a teratoma in that not all germ layers are present.

ter•a•to•car•ci•no•ma (ter′ă-tō-kahr-si-nō′mă) **1.** A malignant teratoma, occurring most commonly in the testis. **2.** A malignant epithelial tumor arising in a teratoma.

te•rat•o•gen (ter′ă-tō-jen) A drug or other agent that can produce congenital anomalies or birth defects or increase the incidence of an anomaly in the population. [terato- + G. *-gen,* producing]

ter•a•to•gen•e•sis (ter′ă-tō-jen′ĕ-sis) The origin or mode of production of congenital anomalies; the disturbed growth processes involved in the production of a malformed neonate. [terato- + G. *genesis,* origin]

ter•a•to•gen•ic, **ter•a•to•ge•net•ic** (ter′ă-tō-jen′ik, -jĕ-net′ik) **1.** Relating to teratogenesis. **2.** Causing congenital anomalies or birth defects.

ter•a•to•ge•nic•i•ty (ter′ă-tō-jĕ-nis′i-tē) The property or capability of producing congenital anomalies. [terato- + G. *genesis,* generation]

ter•a•toid (ter′ă-toyd) Resembling a teras. [G. *teratōdēs,* fr. *teras* (*terat-*), monster, + *eidos,* resemblance]

ter•a•toid tu•mor (ter′ă-toyd tū′mŏr) SYN teratoma.

ter•a•to•log•ic (ter′ă-tŏ-loj′ik) Relating to teratology.

ter•a•tol•o•gy (ter′ă-tol′ŏ-jē) The branch of embryologic science concerned with the production, development, anatomy, and classification of malformed embryos or fetuses. SEE ALSO dysmorphology. [terato- + G. *logos,* study]

ter•a•to•ma (ter′ă-tō′mă) A neoplasm composed of multiple tissues, including tissues not normally found in the organ in which it arises. Teratomas occur most frequently in the ovary, where they are usually benign and form dermoid cysts; in the testis, where they are usually malignant; and, uncommonly, in other sites, especially the midline of the body. SYN teratoid tumor. [terato- + G. *-oma,* tumor]

ter•a•tom•a•tous (ter′ă-tō′mă-tŭs) Relating to or of the nature of a teratoma.

ter•a•to•sis (ter′ă-tō′sis) An anomaly producing a teras. SYN teratism. [terato- + G. *-osis,* condition]

ter•at•o•zo•o•sperm•i•a (ter′ă-tō-zō-ō-spĕrm′ē-ă) Condition characterized by the presence of malformed sperms in semen. [terato- + *zōos,* living, + *sperma,* seed, semen, + -ia]

ter•bi•um (Tb) (tĕr′bē-ŭm) A metallic element of the lanthanide or rare earth series, atomic no. 65, atomic wt. 158.92534. [fr. *Ytterby,* a village in Sweden]

te•res, gen. **ter•e•tis**, pl. **ter•e•tes** (tĕr′ēz, -ĕ-tis, -ĕ-tēz) Round and long; denoting certain muscles and ligaments. [L. round, smooth, fr. *tero,* to rub]

te•res ma•jor mus•cle (ter′ēz mā′jŏr mŭs′ĕl)

Origin, inferior angle and lower third of border of scapula; *insertion*, medial border of intertubercular groove of humerus; *action*, adducts and extends arm and rotates it medially; *nerve supply*, lower subscapular from posterior cord of brachial plexus (fifth and sixth cervical spinal nerves). SYN musculus teres major [TA].

te•res mi•nor mus•cle (ter′ēz mī′nŏr mŭs′ĕl) *Origin*, upper two thirds of the lateral border of scapula; *insertion*, lower facet of greater tuberosity of humerus; *action*, adducts arm and rotates it laterally; *nerve supply*, axillary (fifth and sixth cervical spinal nerves). SYN musculus teres minor [TA].

term (tĕrm) **1.** A definite or limited period. **2.** A name or descriptive word or phrase. [L. *terminus,* a limit, an end]

ter•mi•nal (tĕr′mi-năl) **1.** Relating to the end; final. **2.** Relating to the extremity or end of any body (e.g., the end of a biopolymer). **3.** A termination, extremity, end, or ending. [L. *terminus,* a boundary, limit]

ter•mi•nal ar•ter•y (tĕr′mi-năl ahr′tĕr-ē) SYN end artery.

ter•mi•nal bar (tĕr′mi-năl bahr) Dark spots or bars (depending on the plane of section) in the lateral boundary between the apical ends of columnar epithelial cells.

ter•mi•nal bou•tons, bou•tons ter•mi•naux (tĕr′mi-năl bū-tōnz′, ter-mē-nō′) SYN axon terminals.

ter•mi•nal bron•chi•ole (tĕr′mi-năl brong′kē-ōl) The end of the nonrespiratory conducting airway; the lining is simple columnar or cuboidal epithelium without mucous goblet cells; most of the cells are ciliated, but a few nonciliated serous secreting cells occur.

ter•mi•nal de•ox•y•nu•cle•o•ti•dyl trans•fer•ase (TdT) (tĕr′mi-năl dē-oks′ē-nū-klē-ō-tī′dil trans′fĕr-ās) A specialized DNA polymerase expressed in immature, pre-B, pre-T lymphoid cells, and acute lymphoblastic leukemia/lymphoma cells.

ter•mi•nal dis•in•fec•tion (tĕr′mi-năl dis-in-fek′shŭn) Application of disinfective measures after the patient has been removed, e.g., by death, or has ceased to be a source of infection.

ter•min•al duct car•ci•no•ma (tĕr′mi-năl dŭkt kahr′si-nō′mă) SYN polymorphous low-grade carcinoma of salivary glands.

ter•mi•nal fi•lum (tĕr′mi-năl fī′lŭm) A slender strand of connective tissue extending from the conus medullaris to the coccyx; its internal or pial portion lies along the nerve fibers of the cauda equina and terminates at the distal tip of the dural sac (S2 level); its tougher external or dural portion, commonly called the coccygeal ligament, anchors the dural sac to the coccyx.

ter•mi•nal hair (tĕr′mi-năl hār) A mature pigmented, coarse hair.

ter•mi•nal hinge po•si•tion (tĕr′mi-năl hinj pŏ-zish′ŏn) SYN centric relation.

ter•mi•nal in•fec•tion (tĕr′mi-năl in-fek′shŭn) An acute infection, commonly pneumonic or septic, occurring toward the end of any disease and often the cause of death.

ter•mi•nal line (tĕr′mi-năl līn) SYN linea terminalis.

ter•mi•nal nerves (tĕr′mi-năl nĕrvz) Delicate plexiform nerve strands passing parallel and medial to the olfactory tracts, distributing peripherally with the olfactory nerves and passing centrally into the anterior perforated substance; they are considered to have an autonomic function, but the exact nature of this is unknown. SYN nervi terminales [TA].

ter•mi•nal nu•cle•i (tĕr′mi-năl nū′klē-ī) Collective term indicating those nerve cell groups in the rhombencephalon and spinal cord in which the afferent fibers of the spinal and cranial nerves terminate.

ter•mi•nal sac•cu•lar per•i•od (tĕr-mi′năl sak′yū-lăr pēr′ē-ŏd) SYN terminal sac stage of lung development.

ter•mi•nal sac•cules (tĕr′mi-năl sak′yūl) The thin-walled dilations (primordial alveoli) that develop at the ends of the respiratory bronchioles and develop a close relationship with the capillaries.

ter•mi•nal sac stage of lung de•vel•op•ment (tĕr-mi′năl sak stāj lŭng dĕ-vel′ŏp-mĕnt) The period (26 weeks' gestation to birth) when many terminal sacs develop; their epithelium is very thin and capillaries bridge into the epithelial lining of the saccules, permitting adequate gas exchange for survival of the fetus if it is born prematurely. SYN terminal saccular period.

ter•mi•nal si•nus (tĕr′mi-năl sī′nŭs) The vein bounding the area vasculosa in the blastoderm.

ter•mi•nal stri•a (tĕr′mi-năl strī′ă) A slender, compact fiber bundle that connects the amygdala (amygdaloid body) with the hypothalamus and other basal forebrain regions. Originating from the amygdala, the bundle passes first caudad in the roof of the temporal horn of the lateral ventricle; it follows the medial side of the caudate nucleus forward in the floor of the central part (or body) of the ventricle until it reaches the interventricular foramen, in the posterior wall of which it curves steeply down to enter the hypothalamus, with fibers passing both rostral and caudal to the anterior commissure. Coursing caudalward in the medial part of the hypothalamus, the bundle terminates in the anterior and ventromedial hypothalamic nuclei.

ter•mi•na•tion (tĕr′mi-nā′shŭn) An end or ending. A termination or ending, particularly a nerve ending. [L. *terminatio*]

ter•mi•na•tion co•don (tĕr′mi-nā′shŭn kō′don) Trinucleotide sequence (UAA, UGA, or UAG) that specifies the end of translation or transcription. Cf. amber codon, ochre codon, umber codon. SYN termination signal.

ter•mi•na•tion sig•nal (tĕr′mi-nā′shŭn sig′năl) SYN termination codon.

Ter•mi•no•lo•gi•a An•a•to•mi•ca (TA) (tĕr-mi-nō-lō′jē-ă an-ă-tom′i-kă) A system of anatomic nomenclature, consisting of about 7500 terms, devised and approved by the International Federation of Associations of Anatomists (IFAA) and promulgated in August 1997 at São Paulo, Brazil.

ter•mi•no•ter•mi•nal a•na•sto•mo•sis (tĕr′mi-nō-tĕr′mi-năl ă-nas′tō-mō′sis) An operation by which the central end of an artery is connected with the peripheral end of the corresponding vein, and the peripheral end of the artery with the central end of the vein.

ter•mi•nus, pl. **ter•mi•ni** (ter′mi-nŭs, -nī) A boundary or limit. [L.]

ter•nar•y (tĕr′năr-ē) Denoting or composed of three compounds, elements, molecules, or anything else. [L. *ternarius,* of three]

Ter•ni•dens (tĕr′nĕ-denz) Nematode genus found in the intestine of several simian species in Africa, India, and Indonesia, and in humans in parts of Africa; differentiated from hookworms by the anteriorly directed buccal capsule guarded by a double crown of stout bristles; they inhabit the wall of the large bowel, where they may produce cystic nodules.

Ter•ni•dens di•mi•nu•tus (tĕr′nĕ-denz dī-min′yū-tŭs) Nematode species with larvae that develop in soil; probably infective for humans; life cycle not known.

ter•pene (tĕr′pēn) One of a class of hydrocarbons with an empiric formula of $C_{10}H_{16}$, occurring in essential oils and resins.

ter•race (ter′ăs) To suture in several rows, in closing a wound through a considerable thickness of tissue. [thr. O. Fr. fr. L. *terra,* earth]

Ter•ri•en mar•gin•al de•gen•er•a•tion (ter-rē-an[h]′ mahr′jin-ăl dĕ-jen′ĕr-ā′shŭn) A painless, bilateral peripheral corneal thinning disorder, characterized by intact epithelium overlying areas of thinning and by irregular astigmatism.

ter•ri•to•ri•al•i•ty (ter′i-tōr-ē-al′i-tē) **1.** The tendency of individuals or groups of people to defend a particular domain or sphere of interest or influence. **2.** The tendency of an individual animal to define a finite space as its own habitat from which it will fight off trespassing animals of its own species.

ter•ri•to•ri•al ma•trix (ter′i-tōr′ē-ăl mā′triks) SYN cartilage capsule.

Ter•ry syn•drome (ter′ē sin′drōm) SYN retinopathy of prematurity.

Ter•son syn•drome (ter-son[h]′ sin′drōm) Vitreous, retinal, and subhyaloid hemorrhages associated with subarachnoid hemorrhage.

ter•tian (tĕr′shăn) Referring to a fever that recurs at intervals of 48 hours. [L. *tertianus,* fr. *tertius,* third]

ter•ti•ar•y al•co•hol (tĕr′shē-ă-rē al′kŏ-hol) Methanol bearing three substitutes on its carbon atom.

ter•ti•ar•y a•mide (tĕr′shē-ă-rē am′īd) SEE amide.

ter•ti•ar•y a•mine (tĕr′shē-ă-rē ă-mēn′) SEE amine.

ter•ti•ar•y blast in•ju•ry (tĕr′shē-ă-rē blast in′jŭr′ē) An injury resulting when a casualty from an explosion is thrown by the blast against structures or other objects.

ter•ti•ar•y den•tin (tĕr′shē-ă-rē den′tin) Morphologically irregular dentin formed in response to an irritant. SYN irregular dentin, irritation dentin, reparative dentin.

ter•ti•ar•y pre•ven•tive nur•sing (tĕr′shē-ă-rē prē-ven′tiv nŭrs′ing) Nursing interventions and care directed at patients with incurable disease or injuries. Spinal cord injuries, multiple sclerosis, diabetes mellitus, hypertension, glaucoma, and Parkinson disease fall into this category of preventive care. Prevention of further injury or deterioriation of health is the objective of tertiary preventive nursing care.

tes•la (T) (tes′lă) SI unit of magnetic flux density expressed as kg sec^{-2} A^{-1}; equal to one weber per square meter. [N. *Tesla*]

tes•sel•lat•ed (tes′ĕ-lāt-ĕd) Made up of small squares; checkered. [L. *tessella,* a small square stone]

tes•sel•lat•ed fun•dus (tes′ĕ-lāt-ĕd fŭn′dŭs) A normal fundus to which a deeply pigmented choroid gives the appearance of dark polygonal areas between the choroidal vessels, especially in the periphery.

test (test) **1.** To prove; to try a substance; to determine the chemical nature of a substance by means of reagents. **2.** A method of examination, as to determine the presence or absence of a definite disease or dysfunction in any of the fluids, tissues, or excretions of the body, or to determine the presence or degree of a physical, psychological, or behavioral trait. **3.** A statistical procedure used to determine whether a hypothesis ought be rejected. **4.** A reagent used in undertaking a procedure. **5.** To detect, identify, or conduct a trial. SEE ALSO assay, reaction, reagent, scale, stain. **6.** SYN testa (1). [L. *testum,* an earthen vessel]

tes•ta (tes′tă) **1.** In protozoology, usually termed test; an envelope of certain forms of ameboid protozoa, consisting of various early materials cemented to a chitinous base (as in the testate rhizopods of the subclass Testacealobosia) or the calcareous, siliceous, organic, or strontium sulfate skeletons in the rhizopod subsclass Foraminifera. SYN test (6). **2.** In botany, the outer, sometimes the only, coat of a seed.

tes•tal•gi•a (tes-tal′jē-ă) SYN orchialgia. [testis + G. *algos,* pain]

test dose (test dōs) A small dose of a medication used to ascertain whether the patient is able to tolerate it.

tes•tec•to•my (tes-tek′tō-mē) SYN orchiectomy. [testis + G. G. *ektomē,* excision]

tes•tes (tes′tēz) Plural of testis. [L.]

tes•ti•cle (tes′ti-kĕl) SYN testis. [L. *testiculus,* dim. of *testis*]

tes•tic•u•lar (tes-tik′yū-lăr) Relating to the testes.

tes•tic•u•lar ar•ter•y (tes-tik′yū-lăr ahr′tĕr-ē) *Origin,* aorta; *branches,* ureteral, cremasteric, epididymal; *distribution,* testicle and parts designated by names of branches; *anastomoses,* branches of renal, inferior epigastric, deferential. SYN arteria testicularis [TA].

tes•tic•u•lar cords (tes-tik′yū-lăr kōrdz) The primordial sex cords derived from the gonad cords.

tes•tic•u•lar fe•mi•ni•za•tion syn•drome (tes-tik′yū-lăr fem′i-nī-zā′shŭn sin′drōm) A type of male pseudohermaphroditism characterized by female external genitalia, incompletely developed vagina (often with rudimentary uterus and fallopian tubes), female habitus at puberty but with scanty or absent axillary and pubic hair and amenorrhea, and testes present within the abdomen or in the inguinal canals or labia majora; epididymis and vas deferens are usually present; androgens and estrogens are formed, but target tissues are largely unresponsive to androgens; affected people are sex chromatin-negative and have a normal male karyotype; there is a defect in the androgen receptor protein. SYN complete androgen insensitivity syndrome.

tes•tic•u•lar self-ex•am•i•na•tion (TSE) (tes-tik′yū-lăr self′eg-zam′i-nā′shŭn) Procedure for detecting tumors and other abnormalities in the testes.

test•ing (test′ing) SEE test.

tes•tis, pl. **tes•tes** (tes′tis, -tēz) [TA] One of the two male reproductive glands, normally located in the cavity of the scrotum. SEE ALSO appendix of testis. SYN orchis [TA], didymus, testicle. [L.]

tes•tis cords (tes′tis kōrdz) SYN spermatic cord.

tes•ti•tis (tes-tī′tis) SYN orchitis.

test meal (test mēl) **1.** Toast and tea, or crackers and tea, or gruel or other bland food, given to stimulate gastric secretion before withdrawal of gastric contents for analysis. **2.** Administration of food containing a substance thought to be responsible for symptoms, such as an allergic reaction.

tes•tos•ter•one (tes-tos′tĕ-rōn) The most potent naturally occurring androgen, formed in greatest quantities by the interstitial cells of the testes and possibly secreted also by the ovary and adrenal cortex; used in the treatment of hypogonadism, cryptorchism, certain carcinomas, and menorrhagia. Cf. bioregulator.

tes•to•tox•i•co•sis (tes′tō-tok-si-kō′sis) A G-protein mutation disease resulting in autonomous testosterone overproduction, with precocious puberty.

test pro•file (test prō′fīl) A combination of laboratory tests ordered as a single test; usually performed by automated methods and designed to evaluate organ systems of patients on admission to a hospital or clinic.

test so•lu•tion (test sŏ-lū′shŭn) A solution of some reagent, in definite strength, used in chemical analysis or testing.

test tube (test tūb) A round-bottomed, cylindric vessel, made of plastic or transparent glass, in which laboratory tests involving liquids are performed.

test-tube ba•by (test-tūb bā′bē) Popular term for a baby born after uterine implantation of a maternal ovum fertilized in vitro.

test type (test tīp) Letters of various sizes used to test visual acuity.

test val•i•da•tion (test val-i-dā′shŭn) A continuous process of gathering information to ensure that a test is performing as expected; consists of quality control, proficiency testing, verification of employee competency, and instrument calibration.

te•tan•ic (te-tan′ik) **1.** Relating to or marked by a sustained muscular contraction, as in tetanus. **2.** An agent (e.g., strychnine) that in poisonous doses produces tonic muscular spasm. [G. *tetanikos*]

te•tan•i•form (te-tan′i-fōrm) SYN tetanoid (1).

tet•a•nig•e•nous (tet-ă-nij′ĕ-nŭs) Causing tetanus or tetaniform spasms. [tetanus + G. *-gen,* producing]

tet•a•nism (tet′ă-nizm) SYN neonatal tetany.

tet•a•ni•za•tion (tet′ă-nī-zā′shŭn) **1.** The act of tetanizing the muscles. **2.** A condition of tetaniform spasm.

tet·a·nize (tet′ă-nīz) To stimulate a muscle by a rapid series of stimuli so that the individual muscular responses (contractions) are fused into a sustained contraction; to cause tetanus (2) in a muscle.

♻**tetano-, tetan-** Combining forms denoting tetanus, tetany. [G. *tetanos,* convulsive tension]

tet·a·node (tet′ă-nōd) Denoting the quiet interval between the recurrent tonic spasms in tetanus. [G. *tetanōdēs*]

tet·a·noid (tet′ă-noyd) **1.** Resembling or of the nature of tetanus. SYN tetaniform. **2.** Resembling tetany. [tetano- + G. *eidos,* resemblance]

tet·a·no·spas·min (tet′ă-nō-spaz′min) The neurotoxin of *Clostridium tetani,* which causes the characteristic signs and symptoms of tetanus; chief action is on the anterior horn cells, and the spasms seem to be due to action at inhibitory synapses.

tet·a·nus (tet′ă-nŭs) **1.** A disease marked by painful tonic muscular contractions, caused by the neurotropic toxin (tetanospasmin) of *Clostridium tetani* acting on the central nervous system. **2.** A sustained muscular contraction caused by a series of nerve stimuli repeated so rapidly that the individual muscular responses are fused, producing a sustained tetanic contraction. SEE ALSO emprosthotonos, opisthotonos. [L. fr. G. *tetanos,* convulsive tension]

tet·a·nus ne·o·na·tor·um (tet′ă-nŭs nē-ō-nā-tō′rum) The disorder as it occurs in newborn infants, usually due to infection of the umbilical area with *Clostridium tetani,* often a result of ritualistic practices; has high fatality rate (about 60%).

tet·a·nus tox·in (tet′ă-nŭs tok′sin) The neurotropic, heat-labile exotoxin of *Clostridium tetani* and the cause of tetanus; it is one of the most poisonous substances known, and seems to function by blocking inhibitory synaptic impulses.

tet·a·ny (tet′ă-nē) A clinical neurologic syndrome characterized by muscle twitches, cramps, and carpopedal spasm, and when severe, laryngospasm and seizures; these findings reflect irritability of the central and peripheral nervous systems, usually resulting from low serum levels of ionized calcium or, rarely, magnesium. Causes include hyperventilation, hypoparathyroidism, rickets, and uremia. SYN intermittent cramp (1), intermittent tetanus. [G. *tetanos,* tetanus]

♻**tetra-** Combining form meaning four. [G. *tetra-,* four]

tet·ra·crot·ic (tet′ră-krot′ik) Denoting a pulse curve with four upstrokes in the cycle. [tetra- + G. *krotos,* a striking]

te·trad (tet′rad) **1.** A group of four things having something in common, such as a deformity with four features, e.g., Fallot tetralogy. SYN tetralogy. **2.** CHEMISTRY a quadrivalent element. **3.** GENETICS a bivalent chromosome that divides into four during meiosis. [G. *tetras* (*tetrad-*), the number four]

tet·ra·dac·tyl (tet′ră-dak′til) Having only four fingers or toes on a hand or foot. [tetra- + G. *daktylos,* finger or toe]

♻**tetrahydro-** Prefix denoting attachment of four hydrogen atoms, e.g., tetrahydrofolate, H_4folate.

tet·ra·hy·dro·fo·lic ac·id (THFA) (tet′ră-hī-drō-fō′lik as′id) The active form of folic acid, which can donate four formyl groups during DNA synthesis.

te·tral·o·gy (te-tral′ŏ-jē) SYN tetrad (1). [G. *tetralogia*]

te·tra·lo·gy of Fal·lot (te-tral′ŏ-jē fahl-ō′) A set of congenital cardiac defects including ventricular septal defect, pulmonic valve stenosis or infundibular stenosis, and dextroposition of the aorta so that it overrides the ventricular septum and receives venous as well as arterial blood. Right ventricular hypertrophy is considered part of the tetralogy, although it is reactive to the other defects. SYN Fallot tetrad.

tet·ra·mer·ic, te·tram·er·ous (tet′ră-mer′ik, tĕ-tram′ĕ-rŭs) Having four parts, or parts arranged in groups of four, or capable of existing in four forms. [tetra- + G. *meros,* part]

tet·ra·pa·re·sis (tet′ră-pă-rē′sis) Weakness of all four extremities. SYN quadriparesis.

tet·ra·pep·tide (tet′ră-pep′tīd) A compound of four amino acids in peptide linkage.

tet·ra·ple·gi·a (tet′ră-plē′jē-ă) SYN quadriplegia. [tetra- + G. *plēgē,* stroke]

tet·ra·ploid (tet′ră-ployd) SEE polyploidy. [G. *tetraploos,* fourfold, + *eidos,* form]

tet·ra·sac·cha·ride (tet′ră-sak′ă-rīd) A sugar containing four molecules of a monosaccharide.

tet·ra·so·mic (tet′ră-sō′mik) Relating to a cell nucleus in which one chromosome is represented four times, whereas all others are present in the normal number. [tetra- + chromosome]

tet·ra·va·lent (tet′ră-vā′lĕnt) SYN quadrivalent. [tetra- + L. *valentia,* strength]

tet·rose (tet′rōs) A monosaccharide containing only four carbon atoms in the main chain.

tet·ter·wort (tet′ĕr-wōrt) SYN blood root.

text blind·ness, word blind·ness (tekst blīnd′nĕs, wŏrd) SYN alexia.

tex·ti·form (teks′ti-fōrm) Weblike. [L. *textum,* something woven]

tex·tur·al (teks′chŭr-ăl) Relating to the texture of the tissues.

tex·ture (teks′chŭr) The composition or structure of a tissue or organ. [L. *textura,* fr. *texo,* pp. *textus,* to weave]

TF Abbreviation for tuning fork.

Th Symbol for thorium; T-helper cells.

thal·a·men·ceph·a·lon (thal′ă-men-sef′ă-lon) That part of the diencephalon comprising the thalamus and its associated structures. [thalamus + G. *enkephalos,* brain]

tha·lam·ic (thă-lam′ik) Relating to the thalamus.

thal·a·mic pe·dun·cle (thă-lam′ik pĕ-dŭngk′ĕl) Pedunculus thalami inferior, lateralis, and ventralis.

thalamo-, thalam- Combining forms for the thalamus. [G. *thalamos,* bedroom (thalamus)]

thal·a·mo·cor·ti·cal (thal′ă-mō-kōr′ti-kăl) Relating to the efferent connections of the thalamus with the cerebral cortex.

thal·a·mo·stri·ate veins (thal′ă-mō-strī′āt vānz) SEE inferior thalamostriate veins, superior thalamostriate vein.

thal·a·mot·o·my (thal-ă-mot′ŏ-mē) Destruction of a selected portion of the thalamus by stereotaxy for the relief of pain, involuntary movements, epilepsy, and, rarely, emotional disturbances. [thalamus + G. *tomē,* incision]

thal·a·mus, pl. **thal·a·mi** (thal′ă-mŭs, -mī) [TA] The large, ovoid mass of gray matter that forms the larger dorsal subdivision of the diencephalon; it is placed medially to the internal capsule and the body and tail of the caudate nucleus. Its medial aspect forms the dorsal half of the lateral wall of the third ventricle; its dorsal surface can be subdivided into a lateral triangle forming the floor of the body (central part) of the lateral ventricle, and a medial triangle covered by the velum interpositum; its taillike caudal part curves ventralward around the posterolateral aspect of the cerebral peduncle and ends in the lateral geniculate body. The thalamus is composed of a large number of anatomically and functionally distinct cell groups or nuclei, usually classified as: 1) sensory relay nuclei (ventral posterior nucleus, lateral and medial geniculate body) each receiving a modally specific sensory conduction system and in turn projecting each to the corresponding primary sensory area of the cortex; 2) "secondary" relay nuclei (ventral intermediate nucleus and ventral anterior nucleus) receiving fibers from the medial segment of the globus pallidus, the contralateral deep cerebellar nuclei (i.e., cerebellothalamic fibers), and the pars reticulata of the substantia nigra, which project to various regions of the motor cortex; 3) a nucleus associated with the limbic system: the composite anterior nucleus receiving the mammillothalamic tract and projecting to the fornicate gyrus; 4) association nuclei (medial dorsal nucleus, lateral nucleus including the large pulvinar), each projecting to a particular large expanse of association cortex; and 5) the midline and intralaminar nuclei or "nonspecific" nuclei (centromedian nucleus, central lateral nucleus, paracentral nucleus, nucleus reuniens). [G. *thalamos,* a bed, a bedroom]

thalassaemia [Br.] SYN thalassemia.

thalassaemia minor [Br.] SYN thalassemia minor.

thalassanaemia [Br.] SYN thalassanemia.

thal·as·se·mi·a, thal·as·sa·ne·mi·a (thal′ă-sē′mē-ă, -ă-să-nē′mē-ă) Any of a group of inherited disorders of hemoglobin metabolism in which there is impaired synthesis of one or more of the polypeptide chains of globin; several genetic types exist, and the corresponding clinical picture may vary from barely detectable hematologic abnormality to severe and fatal anemia. See this page. SYN thalassaemia. [G. *thalassa,* the sea, + *haima,* blood]

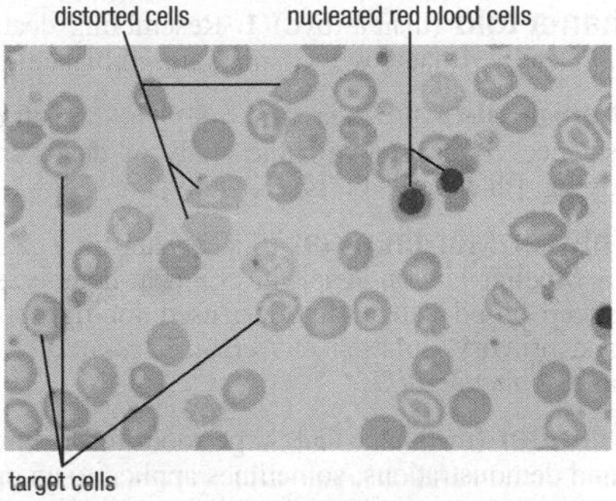

beta-thalassemia major: note the target cells, cell distortion, and nucleated red blood cells

thal·as·se·mi·a ma·jor (thal′ă-sē′mē-ă mā′jŏr) The syndrome of severe anemia resulting from the homozygous state of one of the thalassemia genes or one of the hemoglobin Lepore genes, with onset, in infancy or childhood, of pallor, icterus, weakness, splenomegaly, cardiac enlargement, thinning of inner and outer tables of the skull, and microcytic hypochromic anemia with poikilocytosis, anisocytosis, stippled cells, target cells, and nucleated erythrocytes; types of hemoglobin are variable and depend on the gene involved. SYN Cooley anemia.

thal·as·se·mi·a mi·nor (thal′ă-sē′mē-ă mī′nŏr) The heterozygous state of a thalassemia gene or a hemoglobin Lepore gene; usually asymptomatic and widely variable hematologically, with target cells, mild hypochromic microcytosis, and often slightly reduced hemoglobin level with slightly increased erythrocyte count; types of hemoglobin are variable and depend on the gene involved. SYN thalassaemia minor.

thal·lic (thal′ik) Denoting conidia produced with no enlargement or growth after delimitation by septa in the hypha (thallus); the entire parent cell becomes an arthroconidium.

thal•li•um (Tl) (thal′ē-ŭm) A white metallic element; atomic no. 81, atomic wt. 204.3833; ^{201}Tl (half-life equal to 3.038 days) is used to scan the myocardium. [G. *thallos,* a green shoot (it gives a green line in the spectrum)]

thal•lus (thal′ŭs) A simple plant or fungus body that is devoid of roots, stems, and leaves. The vegetative growth of a fungus. [G. *thallos,* a young shoot]

♻ **thanato-** Combining form meaning death. SEE ALSO necro-. [G. *thanatos,* death]

than•a•to•bi•o•log•ic (than′ă-tō-bī-ō-loj′ik) Relating to the processes involved in life and death. [thanato- + G. *bios,* life, + *logos,* study]

than•a•to•gno•mon•ic (than′ă-tog-nō-mon′ik) Of fatal prognosis, indicating the approach of death. [thanato- + G. *gnōmē,* a sign]

than•a•toid (than′ă-toyd) **1.** Resembling death. **2.** Deadly. [thanato- + G. *eidos,* resemblance]

than•a•tol•o•gy (than-ă-tol′ŏ-jē) The branch of science concerned with the study of death and dying. [thanato- + G. *logos,* study]

Thay•er-Mar•tin a•gar (thā′ĕr mahr′tin ā′gahr) A Mueller-Hinton agar with 5% heat-hemolyzed sheep blood and antibiotics, used for transport and primary isolation of *Neisseria gonorrhoeae* and *N. meningitidis.*

the•a•ter (thē′ă-tĕr) **1.** A large room for lectures and demonstrations; sometimes applied to an operating room equipped for observation by persons other than the surgical team. **2.** Any operating room or suite of such rooms. SYN theatre. [G. *theatron,* a place for seeing, theater, fr. *theomai,* to look at]

theatre [Br.] SYN theater.

the•ca, pl. **the•cae** (thē′kă, -sē) A sheath or capsule. [G. *thēkē,* a box]

the•ca cor•dis (thē′kă kōr′dis) SYN pericardium.

the•ca fol•li•cu•li (thē′kă fō-lik′yū-lī) The wall of a vesicular ovarian follicle. SEE ALSO tunica externa.

the•cal (thē′kăl) Relating to a sheath, especially a tendon sheath. SEE ALSO theca.

the•ci•tis (thē-sī′tis) Inflammation of the sheath of a tendon. [G. *thēkē,* box (sheath), + *-itis,* inflammation]

the•co•ma (thē-kō′mă) A neoplasm derived from ovarian mesenchyme, consisting chiefly of spindle-shaped cells that frequently contain small droplets of fat; may form considerable quantities of estrogen, thereby resulting in precocious development of secondary sexual features in prepubertal girls, or hyperplasia of the endometrium in older patients. [G. *thēkē,* box (theca), + *-oma,* tumor]

The•den me•thod (thē′den meth′ŏd) Treatment of aneurysms or of large sanguineous effusions by compression of the entire limb with a roller bandage.

The Guide (gīd) Colloquial usage among physical therapists meaning *The Guide to Physical Therapist Practice.*

The Guide to Phy•si•cal Ther•a•pist Prac•tice (gīd fiz′i-kăl thār′ă-pist prak′tis) A consensus document of the American Physical Therapy Association that defines the scope of physical therapy practice; identifies patterns of practice by which the physical therapist manages patients/clients.

Thei•le ca•nal (tī′lĕ kă-nal′) SYN transverse pericardial sinus.

Thei•ler mouse en•ceph•a•lo•my•e•li•tis vi•rus (tē′lĕr mows en-sef′a-lō-mī′ĕ-lī′tis vī′rŭs) A virus, genus Cardiovirus, in the family Picornaviridae.

the•lar•che (thē-lahr′kē) The beginning of development of the breasts in the female. [thel- + G. *archē,* beginning]

the•le•plas•ty (thē′lē-plas-tē) SYN mammillaplasty. [thel- + G. *plastos,* formed]

the•li•um, pl. **the•li•a** (thē′lē-ŭm, -lē-ă) **1.** A nipplelike structure. **2.** A cellular layer. **3.** SYN nipple. [Mod. L., fr. G. *thēlē,* nipple]

♻ **thelo-, thel-** Combining forms denoting the nipples. Cf. mammil-. [G. *thēlē*]

the•lor•rha•gi•a (thē′lō-rā′jē-ă) Bleeding from the nipple. [thelo- + G. *rhēgnymi,* to burst forth]

T-help•er cells (Th) (hel′pĕr selz) A subset of lymphocytes that secrete various cytokines that regulate the immune response. SYN helper cells.

T-help•er sub•set 1 cells (hel′pĕr sŭb′set selz) A subset of CD4$^+$ T cells that can secrete interferon-gamma and interleukin-2 and are responsible for cellular immunity.

T-help•er sub•set 2 cells (hel′pĕr sŭb′set selz) A subset of CD4$^+$ T cells that synthesize interleukin-4, -5, and -10 and facilitate immunoglobulin synthesis.

the•mat•ic ap•per•cep•tion test (TAT) (thē-mat′ik ap′ĕr-sep′shŭn test) A projective psychological test in which the subject is asked to tell a story about standard ambiguous pictures depicting life situations to reveal personal attitudes and feelings.

the•nar (thē′nahr) **1.** [TA] SYN thenar eminence. **2.** Applied to any structure in relation to the thenar eminence or its underlying collective components. [G. the palm of the hand]

the•nar em•i•nence (thē′nahr em′i-nĕns) The

fleshy mass on the lateral side of the palm; the radial palm; the ball of the thumb. SYN thenar (1).

the•o•rem (thē′ō-rem) A proposition that can be proved, and so is established as a law or principle. SEE ALSO law, principle, rule.

the•o•ry (thē′ŏr-ē) A reasoned explanation of known facts or phenomena that serves as a basis of investigation by which to reach the truth. SEE ALSO hypothesis, postulate. [G. *theōria,* a beholding, speculation, theory, fr. *theōros,* a beholder]

ther•a•peu•tic (thār-ă-pyū′tik) Relating to therapeutics or to the treatment, remediating, or curing of a disorder or disease. [G. *therapeutikos*]

ther•a•peu•tic a•bor•tion (thār-ă-pyū′tik ă-bōr′shŭn) Abortion induced because of the mother's physical or mental health, or to prevent birth of a deformed child or a child conceived as the result of rape or incest.

ther•a•peu•tic cri•sis (thār-ă-pyū′tik krī′sis) A turning point leading to positive or negative change in psychiatric treatment.

ther•a•peu•tic drug (thār-ă-pyū′tik drŭg) Prescription or over-the-counter medication used to treat an injury or illness.

ther•a•peu•tic drug mon•i•tor•ing (TDM) (thār-ă-pyū′tik drŭg mon′i-tĕr-ing) Clinical measurement of the effects of a drug in a specific patient rather than reliance on normative ranges (e.g., some old people need a lower dosage than their weight might suggest). Such procedures verify that therapy is as accurate as possible.

ther•a•peu•tic in•dex (thār-ă-pyū′tik in′deks) The ratio of LD_{50} to ED_{50}, used in quantitative comparisons of drugs. SYN therapeutic ratio.

ther•a•peu•tic ma•lar•i•a (thār-ă-pyū′tik mă-lar′ē-ă) Intentionally induced malaria, formerly used against neurosyphilis and certain other paralytic diseases. SYN malariotherapy.

ther•a•peu•tic phle•bot•o•my (thār-ă-pyū′tik fle-bot′ă-mē) Drawing blood for the purpose of treating a medical condition (e.g., polycythemia vera).

ther•a•peu•tic ra•di•o•lo•gy (thār-ă-pyū′tik rā′dē-ol′ŏ-jē) SYN radiation oncology.

ther•a•peu•tic range (thār-ă-pyū′tik rānj) Either the dosage range or the blood plasma or serum concentration expected to achieve therapeutic effects.

ther•a•peu•tic ra•tio (thār-ă-pyū′tik rā′shē-ō) SYN therapeutic index.

ther•a•peu•tic reg•i•men (thār-ă-pyū′tik rej′i-men) A pattern of behavior that promotes wellness or health.

ther•a•peu•tics (thār-ă-pyū′tiks) The practical branch of medicine concerned with the treatment of disease or disorder. [G. *therapeutikē,* medical practice]

ther•a•peu•tic ul•tra•sound (thār-ă-pyū′tik ŭl′tră-sownd) Therapeutic use of ultrasound to warm tissue.

ther•a•pist (thār′ă-pist) One professionally trained in the practice of a particular type of therapy.

ther•a•py (thār′ă-pē) **1.** Systematic treatment of a disease, dysfunction, or disorder. SEE ALSO therapeutics. **2.** PSYCHIATRY, CLINICAL PSYCHOLOGY psychotherapy. SEE ALSO psychotherapy, psychiatry, psychology, psychoanalysis. [G. *therapeia,* medical treatment]

thermaesthesia [Br.] SYN thermesthesia.

thermaesthesiometer [Br.] SYN thermesthesiometer.

ther•mal (thĕr′măl) Pertaining to heat.

ther•mal an•es•the•si•a, ther•mic an•es•the•si•a (thĕr′măl an′es-thē′zē-ă, thĕr′mik) Loss of temperature appreciation.

ther•mal art•i•fact (thĕr′măl ahr′ti-fakt) Distortion of microscopic structure in a tissue specimen, because of heat generated by the instrument (e.g., loop electrocautery) used to obtain the specimen.

ther•mal ca•pac•i•ty (thĕr′măl kă-pas′i-tē) SYN heat capacity.

ther•mal•ge•si•a (thĕr′măl-jē′zē-ă) High sensibility to heat; pain caused by a slight degree of heat. [therm- + G. *algēsis,* sense of pain]

ther•mal•gi•a (thĕr-mal′jē-ă) Burning pain. SEE ALSO causalgia. [therm- + G. *algos,* pain]

ther•mal stim•u•la•tion (thĕr′măl stim′yŭ-lā′shŭn) SYN caloric stimulation.

thermanaesthesia [Br.] SYN thermanesthesia.

ther•mi•o•nic e•mis•sion (thĕr-mī-on′ik ē-mish′ŭn) Sending out of free electrons by a filament that is heated by an electric current passing through it, as in an x-ray tube. SYN Edison effect.

♻**thermo-, therm-** Combining forms denoting heat. [G. *thermē,* heat; *thermos,* warm or hot]

thermoaesthesia [Br.] SYN thermoesthesia.

thermoaesthesiometer [Br.] SYN thermoesthesiometer.

thermoanaesthesia [Br.] SYN thermoanesthesia.

ther•mo•an•al•ge•si•a (ther′mō-an-ăl-jē′zē-ă) SYN thermoanesthesia.

ther•mo•an•es•the•si•a, therm•an•al•ge•si•a, therm•an•es•the•si•a (thĕr′mō-an-es-thē′zē-ă, thĕrm′an-ăl-jē′zē-ă, -es-thē′zē-ă) Loss of the temperature sense or of the ability to distinguish between heat and cold; insensibility to heat or to temperature changes. SYN thermoanaesthesia, thermoanalgesia. [thermo- + G. *an-* priv. + *aisthēsis,* sensation]

ther•mo•chem•is•try (thĕr′mō-kem′is-trē) The interrelation of chemical action and heat.

ther•mo•co•ag•u•la•tion (thĕr′mō-kō-ag′yū-lā′shŭn) The process of converting tissue into a gel by heat. SYN endocoagulation.

ther•mo•cou•ple (thĕr′mō-kŭp′ĕl) A device for measuring slight changes in temperature, consisting of two wires of different metals, one wire being kept at a certain low temperature, the other in the tissue or other material with a temperature to be measured; a thermoelectric current setup is measured by a potentiometer.

ther•mo•dif•fu•sion (thĕr′mō-di-fyū′zhŭn) Diffusion of fluids, either gaseous or liquid, as influenced by the temperature of the fluid.

ther•mo•du•ric (thĕr′mō-dyū′rik) Resistant to the effects of exposure to high temperature; used especially with reference to microorganisms. [thermo- + L. *durus,* hard, enduring]

ther•mo•dy•nam•ics (thĕr′mō-dī-nam′iks) **1.** The branch of physicochemical science concerned with heat and energy and their conversions of one into the other involving mechanical work. **2.** The study of the flow of heat. [thermo- + G. *dynamis,* force]

ther•mo•es•the•si•a, therm•es•the•si•a (thĕr′mō-es-thē′zē-ă, thĕrm′es-thē′zē-ă) The ability to distinguish differences of temperature. SYN thermoaesthesia. [thermo- + G. *aisthēsis,* sensation]

ther•mo•es•the•si•om•e•ter, therm•es•the•si•om•e•ter (thĕr′mō-es-thē-zē-om′ĕ-tĕr, thĕrm′es-thē-zē-om′ĕ-tĕr) An instrument for testing a subject's temperature sense, consisting of a metal disc with thermometer attached, by which the exact temperature of the disc at the time of application may be known. SYN thermoaesthesiometer. [thermo- + G. *aisthēsis,* sensation, + *metron,* measure]

ther•mo•ex•ci•to•ry (thĕr′mō-ek-sī′tŏ-rē) Stimulating the production of heat.

ther•mo•gen•e•sis (thĕr-mō-jen′ĕ-sis) The production of heat; specifically, the physiologic process of heat production in the body. [thermo- + G. *genesis,* production]

ther•mo•ge•net•ic, ther•mo•gen•ic (thĕr′mō-jĕ-net′ik, -jen′ik) **1.** Relating to thermogenesis. **2.** SYN calorigenic (2).

ther•mo•gram (thĕr′mō-gram) **1.** A regional temperature map of the surface of a part of the body, obtained by infrared sensing device; it measures radiant heat, and thus subcutaneous blood flow, if the environment is constant. **2.** The record made by a thermograph. [thermo- + G. *gramma,* a writing]

ther•mo•graph (thĕr′mō-graf) An instrument or device used in producing a thermogram. [thermo- + G. *graphō,* to write]

ther•mog•ra•phy (thĕr-mog′ră-fē) The technique for making a thermogram.

ther•mo•in•hib•i•to•ry (thĕr′mō-in-hib′i-tōr-ē) Inhibiting or arresting thermogenesis.

ther•mo•la•bile (thĕr′mō-lā′bīl) Subject to alteration or destruction by heat. [thermo- + L. *labilis,* perishable]

ther•mo•lu•mi•ne•scent do•si•me•ter (TLD) (thĕr′mō-lū-mi-nes′ĕnt dō-sim′ĕ-tĕr) Device resembling a film badge but that uses lithium fluoride crystals instead of film to record radiation exposure. SEE ALSO film badge.

ther•mol•y•sis (thĕr-mol′i-sis) **1.** Loss of body heat by evaporation, radiation, or other causes. **2.** Chemical decomposition by heat. [thermo- + G. *lysis,* dissolution]

ther•mo•lyt•ic (thĕr′mō-lit′ik) **1.** Relating to thermolysis. **2.** An agent promoting heat dissipation.

ther•mo•mas•sage (thĕr′mō-mă-sahzh′) Combination of heat and massage in physical therapy.

ther•mom•e•ter (thĕr-mom′ĕ-tĕr) An instrument for indicating the temperature of any substance; usually a sealed vacuum tube containing mercury, which expands with heat and contracts with cold, its level accordingly rising or falling in the tube, with the exact degree of variation of level being indicated by a scale. SEE ALSO scale. [thermo- + G. *metron,* measure]

ther•mo•met•ric (thĕr′mō-met′rik) Relating to thermometry or to a thermometer reading.

ther•mom•e•try (thĕr-mom′ĕ-trē) The measurement of temperature. [thermo- + G. *metron,* measure]

ther•mo•phile, ther•mo•phil (thĕr′mō-fīl, -fil) Any organism that thrives at a temperature of 50°C or higher. [thermo- + G. *phileō,* to love]

ther•mo•phil•ic (thĕr′mō-fil′ik) Pertaining to a thermophile.

ther•mo•phore (thĕr′mō-fōr) **1.** An arrangement for applying heat to a part; consists of a water heater, a tube conveying hot water to a coil, and another tube conducting the water back to the heater. **2.** A flat bag containing certain salts that produce heat when moistened; used as a substitute for the hot-water bag. [thermo- + G. *phoros,* bearing]

ther•mo•re•cep•tor (thĕr′mō-rē-sep′tŏr) A receptor that is sensitive to heat.

ther•mo•reg•u•la•tion (thĕr′mō-reg-yū-lā′shŭn) Temperature control, as by a thermostat.

ther•mo•sta•bile, ther•mo•sta•ble (thĕr′mō-stā′bīl, -stā′bĕl) Not readily subject to alteration or destruction by heat. [thermo- + L. *stabilis,* stable]

ther•mo•ste•re•sis (thĕr′mō-stĕ-rē′sis) The abstraction or deprivation of heat. [thermo- + G. *sterēsis,* deprivation, loss]

ther•mo•tac•tic, ther•mo•tax•ic (thĕr′mō-tak′tik, -tak′sik) Relating to thermotaxis.

ther•mo•tax•is (thĕr′mō-tak′sis) **1.** Reaction of living protoplasm to the stimulus of heat. Cf. thermotropism. **2.** Regulation of the temperature of the body. [thermo- + G. *taxis,* orderly arrangement]

ther•mo•ther•a•py (thĕr′mō-thār′ă-pē) Treatment of disease by therapeutic application of heat. [thermo- + G. *therapeia,* treatment]

ther•mo•to•nom•e•ter (thĕr′mō-tō-nom′ĕ-tĕr) An instrument for measuring the degree of thermosystaltism, or muscular contraction under the influence of heat. [thermo- + G. *tonos,* tone, tension, + *metron,* measure]

ther•mot•ro•pism (thĕr-mot′rō-pizm) The motion by a part of an organism (e.g., leaves or stems) toward or away from a source of heat. Cf. thermotaxis. [thermo- + G. *tropē,* a turning]

the•ta (θ, Θ) (thā′tă) **1.** The eighth letter in the Greek alphabet. **2.** Angle. **3.** The eighth in a series; denotes the position of a substituent located on the eighth atom from the carboxyl or other functional group.

the•ta rhythm (thā′tă ridh′ŭm) A wave pattern in the electroencephalogram in the frequency band of 4–7 Hz. SYN theta wave.

the•ta wave (thā′tă wāv) SYN theta rhythm.

THFA Abbreviation for tetrahydrofolic acid.

♲ **thia-** Combining form denoting the replacement of carbon by sulfur in a ring or chain. Cf. thio-. [G. *theion*]

thiaemia [Br.] SYN thiemia.

thi•a•min (thī′ă-min) A heat-labile and water-soluble vitamin contained in milk, yeast, and the germ and husk of grains; also artificially synthesized; essential for growth; a deficiency of thiamin is associated with beriberi and Wernicke-Korsakoff syndrome. SYN vitamin B1. [*thia-* + vitamin]

thi•a•min py•ro•phos•phate (thī′ă-min pī′rō-fos′fāt) A coenzyme that aids carboxylation and has an essential role in forming acetyl CoA from pyruvate.

thi•a•zides (thī′ă-zīdz) Abbreviated form of benzothiadiazides.

thi•a•zin (thī′ă-zin) Parent substance of a family of biologic blue dyes (e.g., methylene blue, thionine, toluidine blue).

thi•a•zin dyes (thī′ă-zin dīz) Similar to azin dyes except that one of the connecting N atoms is replaced by S; includes many important biologic stains, especially in hematology.

thick•ness (thik′nĕs) **1.** The measure of the depth of something, as opposed to its length or width. **2.** A layer or stratum.

Thie•mann syn•drome (tē′mahn sin′drōm) Avascular necrosis of the epiphyses of phalanges of fingers or toes, usually familial, beginning in childhood or adolescence, leading to deformity of the fingers; also called familial arthropathy of the fingers or toes.

thi•e•mi•a (thī-ē′mē-ă) The presence of sulfur in the circulating blood. SYN thiaemia. [G. *theion,* sulfur, + *haima,* blood]

thi•e•nyl•al•a•nine (thī′ĕ-nil-al′ă-nēn) A compound structurally similar to phenylalanine that inhibits the growth of *Escherichia coli,* presumably by competitive inhibition of enzymes for which L-phenylalanine is the substrate.

Thiersch ca•nal•ic•u•lus (tērsh kan-ă-lik′yŭ-lŭs) Any of numerous minute channels in newly formed reparative tissue permitting the circulation of nutritive fluids; precursors of new vascularization.

thigh (thī) The part of the inferior limb between the hip and the knee.

thigh bone (thī bōn) SYN femur.

thigmaesthesia [Br.] SYN thigmesthesia.

thig•mes•the•si•a (thig-mes-thē′zē-ă) Sensibility to touch. SYN thigmaesthesia. [G. *thigma,* touch, + *aisthēsis,* sensation]

thig•mo•tax•is (thig-mō-tak′sis) A form of barotaxis; denoting the reaction of plant or animal protoplasm to contact with a solid body. Cf. thigmotropism. [G. *thigma,* touch, + *taxis,* orderly arrangement]

thig•mot•ro•pism (thig-mot′rō-pizm) A movement toward or away from a touch stimulus on the part of a portion of an organism, such as leaves or tendrils. Cf. thigmotaxis. [G. *thigma,* touch, + *tropē,* a turning]

think•ing (thingk′ing) The act of reasoning.

think•ing through (thingk′ing thrū) The psychological process of understanding, with insight, one's own behavior.

thin-lay•er chro•ma•to•gra•phy (TLC) (thin-lā′ĕr krō′mă-tog′ră-fē) The investigative modality applied through a thin layer of cellulose or similar inert material supported on a glass or plastic plate.

thin sec•tion, ul•tra•thin sec•tion (thin sek′shŭn, ŭl-tră-thin) A section of tissue for electron microscopic examination; the specimen is fixed, typically in glutaraldehyde or osmium tetroxide, embedded in a plastic resin, and sectioned at less than 0.1 mcm in thickness with a glass or diamond knife in an ultramicrotome.

thio- Prefix denoting the replacement of oxygen by sulfur in a compound. Cf. thia-. [G. *theion,* sugar]

thi•o•ac•id (thī′ō-as′id) An organic acid in which one or more of the oxygen atoms have been replaced by sulfur atoms, e.g., thiosulfuric acid.

-thioic ac•id (as′id) Suffix denoting the radical –C(S)OH or –C(O)SH, the sulfur analogue of a carboxylic acid.

thi•ol•trans•a•cet•y•lase A (thī′ol-trans-ă-sē′til-as) SYN dihydrolipoamide acetyltransferase.

thi•ol•y•sis (thī-ol′i-sis) The cleavage of a chemical bond with the addition of coenzyme A to one part; analogous to hydrolysis and phosphorolysis.

-thione Suffix denoting the radical =C=S, the sulfur analogue of a ketone.

thi•on•ic (thī-on′ik) Relating to sulfur.

thi•o•nine (thī′ō-nēn) [CI 52000] Dark green powder, giving a purple solution in water; useful as a basic stain in histology for chromatin and mucin because of its metachromatic properties. SYN Lauth violet.

thi•o•sul•fate (thī′ō-sŭl′fāt) The anion of thiosulfuric acid; elevated in people with a molybdenum cofactor deficiency. SYN thiosulphate.

thi•o•sul•fur•ic ac•id (thī′ō-sŭl-fyūr′ik as′id) Sulfuric acid in which an atom of oxygen has been replaced by one of sulfur. SYN thiosulphuric acid.

thiosulphate [Br.] SYN thiosulfate.

thiosulphuric acid [Br.] SYN thiosulfuric acid.

thioxo- Prefix indicating =S in a thioketone.

third cra•ni•al nerve [CN III] (thĕrd krā′nē-ăl nĕrv) SYN oculomotor nerve [CN III].

third-de•gree burn (thĕrd-dĕ′grē bŭrn) SYN full thickness burn.

third-de•gree pro•lapse (thĕrd-dĕ-grē′ prō′laps) Form of cervical prolapse (procidentia uteri) in which the cervix protrudes well beyond the vaginal orifice.

third dis•ease (thĕrd di-zēz′) SYN rubella.

third heart sound (S_3) (thĕrd hahrt sownd) Occurs in early diastole and corresponds with the end of the first phase of rapid ventricular filling; normal in children and younger people but abnormal in others.

third in•ten•tion (thĕrd in-ten′shŭn) The slow filling of a wound cavity or ulcer by granulations, with subsequent cicatrization. SEE ALSO first intention, second intention.

third mo•lar tooth (thĕrd mō′lăr tūth) Eighth permanent tooth in maxilla and mandible on each side, making it most posterior tooth in human dentition; usually erupts between the 17th and 23rd years; roots are often fused, separation being marked only by grooves; because it tends to erupt in an anterosuperior direction, lower third molar often becomes impacted against lower second molar; common for one third molar (or more) to fail to develop. SYN dens serotinus [TA], wisdom tooth.

third-par•ty ad•mi•ni•stra•tor (thĕrd-pahr′tē ad-min′i-strā′tŏr) SYN third-party payer.

third-par•ty pay•er (thĕrd-pahr′tē pā′ĕr) An institution or company that provides reimbursement to health care providers for services rendered to a third party (i.e., the patient). SYN third-party administrator.

third per•o•ne•al mus•cle (thĕrd per′ō-nē′ăl mŭs′ĕl) SYN fibularis tertius muscle.

third spac•ing (thĕrd spās′ing) Shift of fluid from the intravascular space to a nonfunctional space (e.g., abdomen or thorax).

third toe [III] (thĕrd tō) Third digit of foot.

third ven•tri•cle (thĕrd ven′tri-kĕl) A narrow, vertically oriented, irregularly quadrilateral cavity in the midplane, extending from the lamina terminalis to the rostral opening of the mesencephalic aqueduct. This ventricle communicates at its rostrodorsal corner with each of the two lateral ventricles through the left and right interventricular foramen of Monro. Its narrow roof is formed by the tela choroidea, which is attached on either side to the tenia thalami; its lateral wall by the medial surface of the thalamus and, below the hypothalamic sulcus, by the hypothalamus, which also forms its floor. In lateral profile, the third ventricle exhibits a number of recesses: in its floor, from before backward, 1) the preoptic recess in the acute angle between the base of the lamina terminalis and the dorsum of the optic chiasm, 2) the infundibular recess extending ventrally into the infundibulum but not into the hypophysial stalk, and 3) the mammillary or inframamillary recess caused by the protrusion of the mammillary bodies into the ventricle. The pineal recess extends caudally into the pineal stalk from the dorsocaudal corner. SYN ventriculus tertius [TA].

third ven•tri•cu•los•to•my (thĕrd ven-trik′yū-los′tŏ-mē) An operation to establish an opening from the third ventricle to the prechiasmal and interpeduncular cisterns (Stookey-Scarff operation) or from the third ventricle to the interpeduncular cistern (Dandy operation).

thirst (thĕrst) A desire to drink associated with uncomfortable sensations in the mouth and pharynx. [A.S. *thurst*]

Thi·ry fis·tu·la (tē′rē fis′chū-lă) An artificial fistula for collecting the intestinal secretions of an animal for experimental purposes; a loop of intestine is isolated; its vascular and nervous connections are preserved, after the continuity of the intestinal tract is restored by an end-to-end anastomosis; one end of the isolated segment is closed, the other attached to the skin of the abdomen.

thix·o·la·bile (thik-sō-lā′bīl) Susceptible to thixotropy.

thix·o·tro·pic (thik-sō-trō′pik) Pertaining to, or characterized by, thixotropy.

thix·ot·ro·py (thik-sot′rŏ-pē) The property of certain gels of becoming less viscous when shaken or subjected to shearing forces and returning to the original viscosity on standing. [G. *thixis,* a touching, + *tropē,* turning]

thix·ot·ro·py (thik-sŏt′rō-pē) The property of certain gels (e.g., synovial fluid, connective tissue fascia) of becoming less viscous when warmed or during movement, and returning to original viscosity on standing. [G. *thixis,* touching + *tropē,* turning]

Tho·go·to·vi·rus·es (thō-gō′tō-vī′rŭs-ĕz) Any of several unclassified viruses that are similar to the Orthoviruses and share some amino acid homology with them.

Tho·ma am·pul·la (tō-mah′ am-pul′lă) A dilation of the arterial capillary beyond the sheathed artery of the spleen.

Tho·ma fix·a·tive (tō-mah′ fiks′ă-tiv) Nitric acid in 95% alcohol, used for decalcifying bone in the preparation of histologic specimens.

Tho·ma laws (tō-mah′ lawz) The development of blood vessels is governed by dynamic forces acting on their walls as follows: An increase in velocity of blood flow causes dilation of the lumen; an increase in lateral pressure on the vessel wall causes it to thicken; an increase in end pressure causes the formation of new capillaries.

Thom·as splint (tom′ăs splint) A long leg splint extending from a ring at the hip to beyond the foot, allowing traction to a fractured leg, for emergencies and transportation.

Thom·as test (tom′ăs test) Maneuver used to determine tightness of iliopsoas muscle.

Thomp·son test (tomp′sŏn test) **1.** PATHOLOGY a test for gonorrhea in which urine is passed into two glasses in succession; if gonococci and mucous threads are found only in the first glass, the probability is that the inflammation is limited to the anterior urethra. SYN two-glass test. **2.** PHYSICAL THERAPY a test to detect Achilles tendon disruption; with the patient kneeling on a chair or platform with the feet unsupported, each calf is squeezed; if the Achilles tendon is disrupted, plantarflexion of the foot will not occur.

Thom·sen dis·ease (tom′sen di-zēz′) SYN myotonia congenita.

Thom·son sign (tom′sŏn sīn) SYN Pastia sign.

tho·ra·cal·gi·a (thōr′ă-kal′jē-ă) Pain in the chest. SYN thoracodynia. [thoraco- + G. *algos,* pain]

tho·ra·cen·te·sis (thōr′ă-sen-tē′sis) Paracentesis of the pleural cavity. SYN pleural tap, pleurocentesis, thoracocentesis. [thoraco- + G. *kentēsis,* puncture]

thor·ac·ic (thōr-as′ik) Relating to the thorax.

thor·a·cic a·or·ta (thōr-as′ik ā-ōr′tă) The part of the descending aorta that supplies structures as far down as the diaphragm. SYN aorta thoracica, pars thoracica aortae, thoracic part of aorta.

thor·a·cic cage (thōr-as′ik kāj) The skeleton of the thorax consisting of the thoracic vertebrae, ribs, costal cartilages, and sternum. See this page. SYN cavea thoracis [TA].

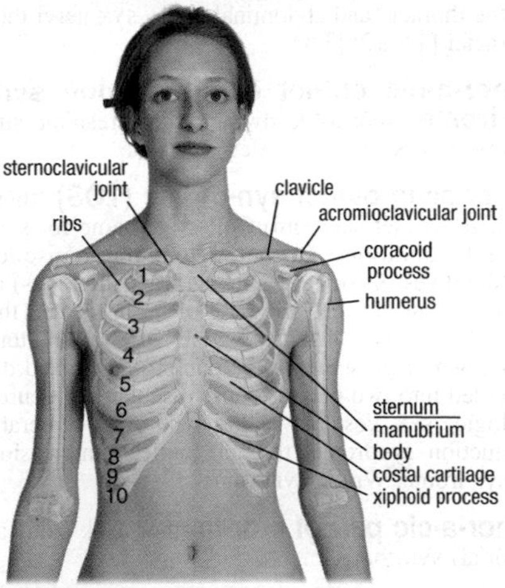

thoracic cage

thor·a·cic car·di·ac nerves (thōr-as′ik kahr′dē-ak nĕrv) That part of the cardiopulmonary splanchnic nerves from the second to fifth segments of the thoracic sympathetic trunk where they pass medially and anteriorly to enter the cardiac plexus; they convey postsynaptic sympathetic fibers to, and visceral afferent (pain) fibers from, the heart. SYN nervi cardiaci thoracici [TA].

thor·a·cic ca·vi·ty (thōr-as′ik kav′i-tē) The space within the thoracic walls, bounded below by the diaphragm and above by the neck.

thor·a·cic duct (thōr-as′ik dŭkt) The largest lymph vessel in the body, beginning at the cisterna chyli at about the level of the second lumbar vertebra; the abdominal part extends superiorly to pass through the aortic opening of the diaphragm, where it becomes the thoracic part and crosses the posterior mediastinum to form the arch of the thoracic duct and discharge into the left venous angle (origin of the brachiocephalic vein).

tho•rac•ic gan•gli•a (thōr-as′ik gang′glē-ă) Sympathetic paravertebral ganglia, with 11 or 12 on either side, at the level of the head of each rib, constituting with the interganglionic branches the thoracic part of the sympathetic trunk.

thor•a•cic ky•pho•sis (thōr-as′ik kī-fō′sis) The normal, anteriorly concave curvature of the thoracic segment of the vertebral column, in which the primary curvature of the fetal embryo is maintained into maturity.

thor•a•cic lon•gis•si•mus mus•cle (thōr-as′ik lon-jē′sē-mŭs mŭs′ĕl) SYN longissimus thoracis muscle.

thor•ac•ic nerves [T1–T12] (thōr-as′ik nĕrvz) Twelve nerves on each side, mixed motor and sensory, supplying the muscles and skin of the thoracic and abdominal walls. SYN nervi thoracici [T1–12] [TA].

thor•a•cic out•let com•pres•sion syn•drome (thōr-as′ik owt′lĕt kŏm-presh′ŭn sin′drōm) SYN thoracic outlet syndrome.

thor•ac•ic out•let syn•drome (TOS) (thōr-as′ik owt′lĕt sin′drōm) Collective name for several conditions attributed to compromise of blood vessels or nerve fibers (brachial plexus) at any point between the base of the neck and the axilla; classified on the basis of the structure known or presumed to be compromised, and divided into two main groups: vascular and neurologic. SYN costoclavicular syndrome, hyperabduction syndrome, thoracic outlet compression syndrome, Wright syndrome.

thor•a•cic part of a•or•ta (thōr-as′ik pahrt ā-ōr′tă) SYN thoracic aorta.

thor•a•cic spi•nal nerves (thōr-as′ik spī′năl nĕrvz) Twelve nerves on each side, mixed motor and sensory, supplying the muscles and skin of the thoracic and abdominal walls.

thor•a•cic splanch•nic nerves (thōr-as′ik splangk′nik nĕrvz) Splanchnic nerves arising from the thoracic portion of sympathetic trunks.

thor•ac•ic splen•o•sis (thōr-as′ik splē-nō′sis) Presence of splenic tissue in the thorax, resultant from combined thoracic and abdominal trauma followed by splenectomy.

thor•ac•ic ver•te•brae [T1–T12] (thōr-as′ik vĕr′tĕ-brē) The segments of the vertebral column, usually 12, which articulate with ribs to form part of the thoracic cage. SYN vertebrae thoracicae [TA].

thor•a•cic wall (thōr-as′ik wawl) SYN chest wall.

♲**thoraco-, thorac-, thoracico-** Combining forms denoting the chest (thorax). [G. *thōrax*]

thor•a•co•ab•dom•i•nal nerves (thōr′ă-kō-ab-dŏm′i-năl nĕrvz) Ventral primary rami of spinal nerves T7–T11 (seventh to eleventh intercostal nerves), which supply the abdominal as well as the thoracic wall; innervate intercostal, subcostal, serratus posterior inferior, transversus abdominis, external and internal oblique, and rectus abdominis muscles, and provide sensory branches to the periphery of the diaphragm, and parietal pleura and peritoneum.

thor•a•co•a•cro•mi•al (thōr′ă-kō-ă-krō′mē-ăl) Relating to the acromion and the thorax; denoting especially the thoracoacromial artery. SYN acromiothoracic.

thor•a•co•a•cro•mi•al ar•ter•y (thōr′ă-kō-ă-krō′mē-ăl ahr′tĕr-ē) *Origin*, axillary; *distribution*, muscles and skin of shoulder and upper chest; *anastomoses*, branches of superior thoracic, internal thoracic, lateral thoracic, posterior and anterior circumflex humeral, and suprascapular. SYN arteria thoracoacromialis [TA], acromiothoracic artery.

thor•a•co•a•cro•mi•al vein (thōr′ă-kō-ă-krō′mē-ăl vān) Corresponding to the artery of the same name, empties into the axillary vein, sometimes by a common trunk with the cephalic vein.

thor•a•co•ce•los•chi•sis (thōr′ă-kō-sē-los′ki-sis) A congenital fissure of the trunk involving both the thoracic and abdominal cavities. SYN thoracogastroschisis. [thoraco- + G. *koilia,* belly, + *schisis,* fissure]

thor•a•co•cen•te•sis (thōr′ă-kō-sen-tē′sis) SYN thoracentesis.

thor•a•co•cyl•lo•sis (thōr′ă-kō-si-lō′sis) A deformity of the chest. [thoraco- + G. *kyllōsis,* a crippling]

thor•a•co•cyr•to•sis (thōr′ă-kō-sĭr-tō′sis) Abnormally wide curvature of the chest wall. [thoraco- + G. *kyrtōsis,* a being crooked]

thor•a•co•dor•sal ar•ter•y (thōr′ă-kō-dōr′săl ahr′tĕr-ē) *Origin*, subscapular; *distribution*, muscles of upper part of back; *anastomoses*, branches of lateral thoracic. SYN arteria thoracodorsalis [TA].

thor•a•co•dor•sal nerve (thōr′ă-kō-dōr′săl nĕrv) Arises from the posterior cord of the brachial plexus; it contains fibers from the sixth, seventh, and eighth cervical nerves and supplies the latissimus dorsi muscle. SYN nervus thoracodorsalis [TA].

thor•a•co•dyn•i•a (thōr′ă-kō-din′ē-ă) SYN thoracalgia. [thoraco- + G. *odynē,* pain]

thor•a•co•ep•i•gas•tric vein (thōr′ă-kō-ep-i-gas′trik vān) One of two veins, sometimes a single vein, arising from the region of the superficial epigastric vein and opening into the axillary or the lateral thoracic vein, thus forming an anastomotic or collateral pathway between tributaries of the inferior and superior venae cavae.

thor•a•co•gas•tros•chi•sis (thōr′ă-kō-gas-tros′ki-sis) SYN thoracoceloschisis. [thoraco- + G. *gastēr,* belly, + *schisis,* fissure]

thor•a•co•lum•bar (thōr′ă-kō-lŭm′bahr) **1.** Relating to the thoracic and lumbar portions of the vertebral column. **2.** Relating to the origins of the sympathetic division of the autonomic nervous system. SEE ALSO autonomic division of nervous system.

thor•a•co•lum•bar fa•sci•a (thōr′ă-kō-lŭm′bahr fash′ē-ă) The fascia that covers the deep muscles of the back; it is attached to the angles of the ribs and to the spines of the thoracic, lumbar, and sacral vertebrae, to the transverse processes of the lumbar vertebrae, to the lower border of the twelfth rib and to the iliac crest, as well as to the lumbocostal, iliolumbar, intertransverse, and supraspinous ligaments. See this page.

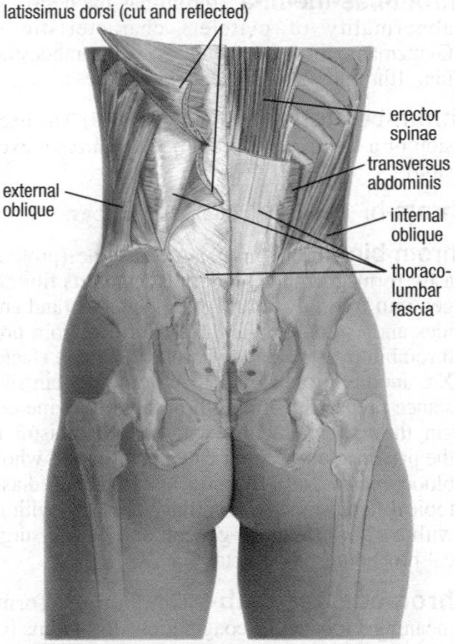

thoracolumbar fascia

thor•a•co•lum•bo•sa•cral or•tho•sis (thōr′ă-kō-lŭm′bō-sā′krăl ōr-thō′sis) An external device applied to the trunk and extending from the upper portion of the thoracic spine to the pelvis; designed to provide immobilization of the thoracic spine.

thor•a•col•y•sis (thōr-ă-kol′i-sis) Breaking up of pleural adhesions. [thoraco- + G. *lysis,* dissolution]

thor•a•com•e•ter (thōr-ă-kom′ĕ-tĕr) An instrument for measuring the circumference of the chest or its variations in respiration. [thoraco- + G. *metron,* measure]

thor•a•co•my•o•dyn•i•a (thōr′ă-kō-mī-ō-din′ē-ă) Pain in the muscles of the chest wall. [thoraco- + G. *mys,* muscle, + *odynē,* pain]

thor•a•co•plas•ty (thōr′ă-kō-plas-tē) Surgical procedure that reduces intrathoracic space. [thoraco- + G. *plastos,* formed]

thor•a•cos•chi•sis (thōr-ă-kos′ki-sis) Congenital fissure of the thoracic wall, which may result in herniation of lung tissue. [thoraco- + G. *schisis,* fissure]

tho•ra•co•scope (thō-rak′ō-skōp) A scope for viewing intrathoracic structures; may be video assisted. See page B17. [thoraco- + G. *skopeō,* to view]

thor•a•cos•co•py (thōr-ă-kos′kŏ-pē) Examination of the pleural cavity with an endoscope. See page B17. [thoraco- + G. *skopeō,* to view]

thor•a•co•ste•no•sis (thōr′ă-kō-stĕ-nō′sis) Narrowness of the chest. [thoraco- + G. *stenōsis,* narrowing]

thor•a•co•ster•no•to•my (thōr′ă-kō-stĕr-not′ŏ-mē) Chest incision combining an intercostal incision and transsection of the sternum.

thor•a•cos•to•my (thōr′ă-kos′tŏ-mē) Establishment of an opening into the chest cavity, as for the drainage of an empyema. [thoraco- + G. *stoma,* mouth]

thor•a•cot•o•my (thōr′ă-kot′ŏ-mē) Incision into the chest wall. SYN pleurotomy. [thoraco- + G. *tomē,* incision]

tho•rax, gen. **tho•ra•cis**, pl. **tho•ra•ces** (thō′raks, thō-rā′sis, -rā′sēz) [TA] The upper part of the trunk between the neck and the abdomen; it is formed by the 12 thoracic vertebrae, the 12 pairs of ribs, the sternum, and the muscles and fasciae attached to these; below, it is separated from the abdomen by the diaphragm; it contains the chief organs of the circulatory and respiratory systems. See page A9. [L. fr. G. *thōrax,* breastplate, the chest, fr. *thōrēssō,* to arm]

thor•i•um (Th) (thōr′ē-ŭm) A radioactive metallic element; atomic no. 90, atomic wt. 232.0381. ^{232}Th, the only naturally occurring nuclide, with a half-life of 14×10^9 years, is used in colloidal form in electron microscopy as a stain for acid mucopolysaccharides. [*Thor,* Norse god of thunder]

Thor•mäh•len test (tor′mā-len test) A test for melanin; the suspected liquid is treated with sodium nitroprusside, caustic potash, and acetic acid; if melanin is present, the solution takes on a deep blue color.

Thorn syn•drome (thōrn sin′drōm) SYN salt-losing nephritis.

thought (thawt) **1.** The faculty of reasoning.

2. The process or act of thinking. **3.** The result of thinking.

THR Abbreviation for total hip replacement.

Thr Abbreviation for threonine or its radical forms.

thread·ed im·plant (thred′ĕd im′plant) DENTISTRY an implant with screwlike threads that is either screwed into bone previously threaded by a tap or screwed in by self-tapping, the implant cutting threads in the bone as it is inserted into a predrilled hole.

thread·worm (thred′wŏrm) Common name for species of the genus *Strongyloides;* sometimes applied to any of the smaller parasitic nematodes.

thread·y pulse (thred′ē pŭls) A small, fine pulse, feeling like a small cord or thread under the finger.

three-di·men·sion·al vis·ion (thrē-di-men′shŭn-ăl vizh′ŭn) SYN stereopsis.

three-glass test (thrē glas test) A male patient empties his bladder into a series of 3-oz test tubes, and the contents of the first and the last are examined; the first tube contains the washings from the anterior urethra, the second, material from the bladder, and the last, material from the posterior urethra, prostate, and seminal vesicles. SEE ALSO Thompson test.

three-in·ci·sion e·so·pha·gec·to·my (thrē-in-sizh′ŭn ē-sof-ă-jek′tŏ-mē) Removal of all or part of the esophagus using laparotomy and right chest and cervical incisions.

three-jaw chuck (thrē′jaw chŭk) A grasp pattern emerging in the 10th–12th month that involves holding an object with an opposed thumb and the index and middle fingers where the interphalangeal joints are slightly flexed. The ulnar fingers are slightly flexed to stabilize the radial side of the hand.

thre·o·nine (T, Thr) (thrē′ō-nēn) One of the naturally occurring amino acids, included in the structure of most proteins and nutritionally essential in the diet of humans and other mammals.

thresh·old (thresh′ōld) **1.** The level of intensity at which a stimulus first produces a sensation. **2.** The lower limit of perception of a stimulus. **3.** The minimal stimulus that produces excitation of any structure. **4.** SYN limen. [A.S. *therxold*]

thresh·old li·mit val·ue (thresh′ōld lim′it val′yū) The maximum concentration of a chemical recommended by the American Conference of Government Industrial Hygienists for repeated exposure without adverse health effects on workers.

thresh·old sti·mu·lus (thresh′ōld stim′yū-lŭs) A stimulus of threshold strength, i.e., one just strong enough to excite. SEE ALSO adequate stimulus.

thresh·old sub·stance (thresh′ōld sub′stăns) Any material (e.g., glucose) that is excreted in the urine only when its plasma concentration exceeds a certain value, termed its threshold.

thresh·old trait (thresh′ōld trāt) A trait that falls into natural groups that originate not in categorically distinct causes but in whether the outcome attains critical values (e.g., gallstones may result from a categoric cause or from unusual levels of causal factors that themselves show no evidence of grouping).

thrill (thril) A vibration accompanying a cardiac or vascular murmur that can be palpated. SEE ALSO fremitus.

thrix (thriks) SYN hair (2). [G.]

throat (thrōt) **1.** The fauces and pharynx. SYN gullet. **2.** The anterior aspect of the neck. **3.** Any narrowed entrance into a hollow part. [A.S. *throtu*]

throb (throb) **1.** To pulsate. **2.** A beating or pulsation.

throm·bas·the·ni·a (throm-bas-thē′nē-ă) An abnormality of platelets characteristic of Glanzmann thrombasthenia. SYN thromboasthenia. [thromb- + G. *astheneia,* weakness]

throm·bec·to·my (throm-bek′tŏ-mē) The excision of a thrombus. [thromb- + G. *ektomē,* excision]

throm·bi (throm′bī) Plural of thrombus.

throm·bin (throm′bin) **1.** An enzyme (proteinase), formed in shed blood, that converts fibrinogen into fibrin by hydrolyzing peptides (and amides and esters) of L-arginine; formed from prothrombin by the action of prothrombinase (factor Xa, another proteinase). **2.** A sterile protein substance prepared from prothrombin of bovine origin through interaction with thromboplastin in the presence of calcium; causes clotting of whole blood, plasma, or a fibrinogen solution; used as a topical hemostatic for capillary bleeding with or without fibrin foam in general and plastic surgical procedures. SYN factor IIa.

thrombo-, thromb- Combining forms meaning blood clot; coagulation; thrombin. [G. *thrombos,* clot (thrombus)]

throm·bo·an·gi·i·tis (throm′bō-an-jē-ī′tis) Inflammation of the intima of a blood vessel, with thrombosis. [thrombo- + G. *angeion,* vessel, + *-itis,* inflammation]

throm·bo·an·gi·i·tis o·bli·ter·ans (throm′bō-an-jē-ī′tis ob-lit′ĕr-anz) Inflammation of the entire wall and connective tissue surrounding medium-sized arteries and veins, especially of the legs of young and middle-aged men; associated with thrombotic occlusion and commonly resulting in gangrene. See page 1557.

throm·bo·ar·te·ri·tis (throm′bō-ahr-tĕr-ī′tis) Arterial inflammation with thrombus formation.

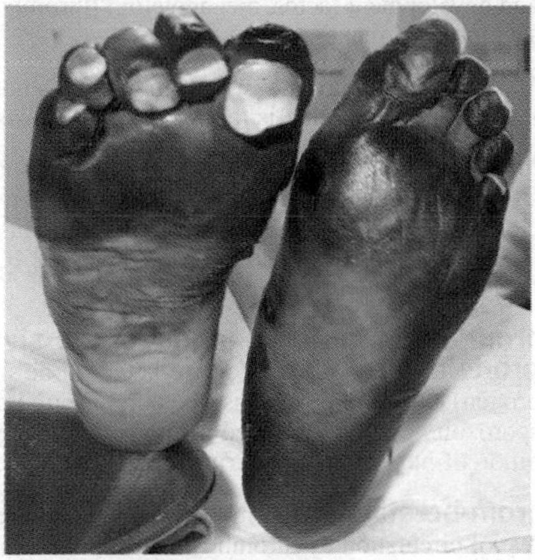

thromboangiitis obliterans: feet

throm•bo•as•the•ni•a (throm′bō-as-thē′nē-ă) SYN thrombasthenia.

throm•bo•clas•tic (throm′bō-klas′tik) SYN thrombolytic.

throm•bo•cyst, throm•bo•cys•tis (throm′bō-sist, -sis′tis) A membranous sac enclosing a thrombus. [thrombo- + G. *kystis,* a bladder]

throm•bo•cyte (throm′bō-sīt) SYN platelet. [thrombo- + G. *kytos,* cell]

thrombocythaemia [Br.] SYN thrombocythemia.

throm•bo•cy•the•mi•a (throm′bō-sī-thē′mē-ă) SYN thrombocytosis. SYN thrombocythaemia. [thrombocyte + G. *haima,* blood]

throm•bo•cy•tic ser•ies (throm′bō-sit′ik sēr′ēz) The cells of successive stages in thrombocytic (platelet) development in the bone marrow, and then into the bloodstream; examples include megakaryoblasts, romegakaryocytes, megakaryocytes, and thrombocytes.

throm•bo•cy•top•a•thy (throm′bō-sī-top′ă-thē) General term for any disorder of the coagulating mechanism that results from dysfunction of the blood platelets. [thrombocyte + G. *pathos,* suffering]

throm•bo•cy•to•pe•ni•a (throm′bō-sī-tō-pē′nē-ă) A condition in which there is a decreased number of platelets in the circulating blood. SYN thrombopenia. [thrombocyte + G. *penia,* poverty]

throm•bo•cy•to•pe•ni•a-ab•sent ra•di•us syn•drome (throm′bō-sī-tō-pē′nē-ă ab′sĕnt rā′dē-ŭs sin′drōm) Congenital absence of the radius associated with thrombocytopenia that is symptomatic in infancy but later improves; congenital heart disease and renal anomalies occur in some cases; autosomal recessive inheritance.

throm•bo•cy•to•pe•nic pur•pu•ra (throm′bō-sī′tō-pēn′ik pŭr′pyŭr-ă) SEE idiopathic thrombocytopenic purpura.

throm•bo•cy•to•poi•e•sis (throm′bō-sī-tō-poy-ē′sis) The process of formation of thrombocytes or platelets. [thrombocyte + G. *poiēsis,* a making]

throm•bo•cy•to•sis (throm′bō-sī-tō′sis) An increase in the number of platelets in the circulating blood. SYN thrombocythemia. [thrombocyte + G. *-osis,* condition]

throm•bo•e•las•to•gram (throm′bō-ĕ-las′tō-gram) Registration of the coagulation process by a thromboelastograph.

throm•bo•e•las•to•graph (throm′bō-ĕ-las′tō-graf) An apparatus for registering elastic variations of a thrombus during coagulation. [thromb- + G. *elastreō,* to push, + *graphō,* to write]

throm•bo•em•bo•lism (throm′bō-em′bŏ-lizm) Embolism from a thrombus. [thrombo- + G. *embolismos,* embolism]

throm•bo•end•ar•ter•ec•to•my (throm′bō-end′ahr-tĕr-ek′tŏ-mē) An operation that involves opening an artery, removing an occluding thrombus along with the intima and atheromatous material, and leaving a clean, fresh plane internal to the adventitia. [thrombo- + endarterectomy]

throm•bo•gen•ic (throm′bō-jen′ik) **1.** Relating to thrombogen. **2.** Causing thrombosis or coagulation of the blood.

throm•boid (throm′boyd) Resembling a thrombus. [thrombo- + G. *eidos,* resemblance]

throm•bo•ki•nase (throm′bō-kī′nās) SYN thromboplastin.

throm•bo•lym•phan•gi•tis (throm′bō-lim-fan-jī′tis) Inflammation of a lymphatic vessel with the formation of a lymph clot.

throm•bol•y•sis (throm-bol′i-sis) Liquefaction or dissolving of a thrombus. [thrombo- + G. *lysis,* a dissolving]

throm•bo•lyt•ic (throm′bō-lit′ik) Breaking up or dissolving a thrombus. SYN thromboclastic.

throm•bo•ly•tic ther•a•py (throm′bō-lit′ik thār′ă-pē) Intravenous administration of an agent intended to dissolve a clot causing acute ischemia, as in myocardial infarction, stroke, and peripheral arterial or venous thrombosis. Thrombolytic agents degrade fibrin clots by activating plasminogen, a naturally occurring modulator of hemostatic and thrombotic processes. Synthesized by the liver, plasminogen is present in circulating blood and binds to platelets, endothelium, and fibrin. At sites of vascular injury with thrombus formation, tissue plasminogen activator (TPA), produced by endothelial cells, also binds to fibrin and converts fibrin-bound plasminogen to plasmin by cleaving the arginine-valine bond in the 560–561 position of plasminogen. The resulting clot lysis is due to degradation of fibrin threads as well as of glycoproteins required for platelet adhesion and aggregation. Thrombolytic agents in current use mimic the effects of natural TPA. These include alteplase, a TPA produced by recombinant DNA technology; reteplase, a variant of the TPA molecule, also genetically engineered; urokinase, a tissue protein derived from human kidney cell cultures; streptokinase, a product of β-hemolytic streptococci that catalyzes the conversion of plasminogen to plasmin; and anistreplase, an inactive form of plasminogen that is bound to streptokinase and undergoes deacylation after administration, resulting in persistent activation of plasminogen. The latter two products are potentially antigenic and can cause systemic hypersensitivity reactions. SEE ALSO tissue plasminogen activator.

throm•bon (throm′bon) An all-inclusive term for circulating thrombocytes (blood platelets) and the cellular forms from which they arise (thromboblasts or megakaryocytes).

throm•bop•a•thy (throm-bop′ă-thē) A nonspecific term applied to disorders of blood platelets resulting in defective thromboplastin, without obvious change in the appearance or number of platelets. [thrombo- + G. *pathos,* disease]

throm•bo•pe•ni•a (throm′bō-pē′nē-ă) SYN thrombocytopenia.

throm•bo•pe•nic pur•pu•ra (throm′bō-pē′nik pŭr′pyŭr-ă) SYN idiopathic thrombocytopenic purpura.

throm•bo•phil•i•a (throm′bō-fil′ē-ă) A disorder of the hemopoietic system in which there is a tendency toward thrombosis. [thrombo- + G. *philos,* fond]

throm•bo•phle•bi•tis (throm′bō-flĕ-bī′tis) Venous inflammation with thrombus formation. [thrombo- + G. *phleps,* vein, + *-itis,* inflammation]

throm•bo•plas•tid (throm′bō-plas′tid) **1.** SYN platelet. **2.** A nucleated spindle cell in submammalian blood. [thrombo- + G. *plastos,* formed]

throm•bo•plas•tin (throm′bō-plas′tin) A substance present in tissues, platelets, and leukocytes necessary for the coagulation of blood; in the presence of calcium ions, thromboplastin is necessary for the conversion of prothrombin to thrombin, an important step in blood coagulation. SYN platelet tissue factor, thrombokinase.

throm•bo•poi•e•sis (throm′bō-poy-ē′sis) Precisely, the process of a clot forming in blood, but generally used with reference to the formation of blood platelets (thrombocytes). [thrombo- + G. *poiēsis,* a making]

throm•bo•poi•e•tin (throm′bō-poy′ĕ-tin) A cytokine that serves as a humoral regulator for the production of blood platelets through action on the receptor c-mpl. SYN megakaryocyte growth and development factor, megapoietin. [thrombo- + G. *poiētēs,* maker, + in]

throm•bosed (throm′bōst) **1.** Clotted. **2.** Denoting a blood vessel that is the seat of thrombosis.

throm•bo•sis, pl. **throm•bo•ses** (throm-bō′sis, -sēz) Formation or presence of a thrombus; clotting within a blood vessel that may cause infarction of tissues supplied by the vessel. [G. *thrombōsis,* a clotting, fr. *thrombos,* clot]

throm•bo•spon•din-re•lat•ed ad•he•sive pro•tein (throm′bō-spon′din rē-lā′tĕd ad-hē′siv prō′tēn) One of two proteins (the other is circumsporozoite protein) involved in sporozoite recognition of host cells in malaria.

throm•bo•sta•sis (throm-bos′tă-sis) Local arrest of circulation by thrombosis. [thrombo- + G. *stasis,* a standing]

throm•bot•ic (throm-bot′ik) Relating to, caused by, or characterized by thrombosis.

throm•bot•ic throm•bo•cy•to•pe•nic pur•pu•ra (throm-bot′ik throm′bō-sī′tō-pē′nik pŭr′pyŭr-ă) A rapidly fatal or occasionally protracted disease with varied symptoms in addition to dermal hemorrhage, including signs of central nervous system involvement, due to formation of fibrin or platelet thrombi in arterioles and capillaries in many organs.

throm•box•anes (throm-bok′sānz) A group of compounds, included in the eicosanoids, formally based on thromboxane, but with the terminal COOH group present; biochemically related to the prostaglandins and formed from them. Thromboxanes are so named from their influence on platelet aggregation and the formation of the oxygen-containing six-membered ring (pyran or oxane). Like the prostaglandins, individual thromboxanes (abbreviated TX) are designated by letters (A, B, C, and onward) and subscripts indicating structural features.

throm•bus (throm′bŭs) A clot in the cardiovascular system formed during life from constituents of blood; it may be occlusive or attached to the vessel or heart wall without obstructing the lumen (mural thrombus). See page 1559. SYN blood clot. [L. fr. G. *thrombos,* a clot]

through drain•age (thrū drān′ăj) Removal of liquid obtained by the passage of a perforated tube, open at both extremities, through a cavity; in addition, the cavity can be washed out by a solution passed through the tube.

through•put (thrū′put) A term applied to analytic instruments specifying the number of tests that can be performed in a given time.

thrush (thrŭsh) Infection of the oral tissues with *Candida albicans;* often an opportunistic infection in patients with AIDS or other disorders that depress the immune system. See page B15.

thrust (thrŭst) **1.** To push forward abruptly.

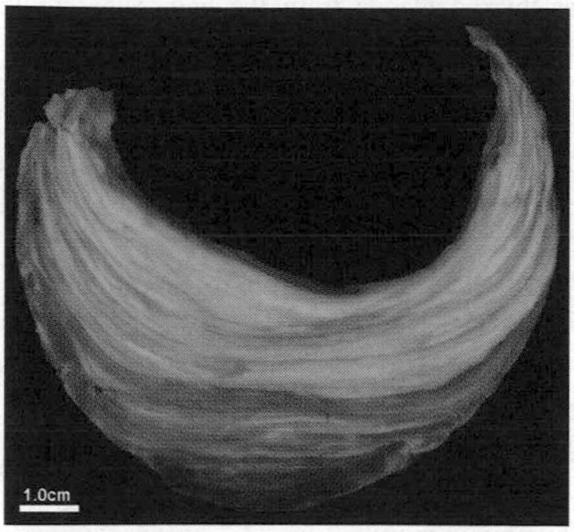

arterial thrombus: clot due to aortic aneurysm showing presence of fibrin and platelet striation known as lines of Zahn

2. The act, power, or result of thrusting. [O.N. *thrysta*]

thu•li•um (Tm) (thū′lē-ŭm) A metallic element of the lanthanide series, atomic no. 69, atomic wt. 168.93421. [L. *Thule,* the earliest name for Scandinavia]

thumb (thŭm) The first digit on the radial side of the hand. SYN pollex [TA]. [A.S. *thuma*]

thumb for•ceps (thŭm fōr′seps) A spring forceps used by compression with thumb and forefinger.

thun•der•clap head•ache (thŭn′dĕr-klap hed′āk) Sudden severe nonlocalizing head pain not associated with any abnormal neurologic findings; of varied etiology, including subarachnoid hemorrhage, migraine, carotid or vertebral artery dissection, and cavernous sinus thrombosis.

thus (thŭs) SYN olibanum.

thy•mec•to•my (thī-mek′tŏ-mē) Removal of the thymus gland. [thymus + G. *ektomē,* excision]

♻ **-thymia** Suffix denoting mind, soul, emotions. SEE ALSO thymo- (2). [G. *thymos,* the mind or heart as the seat of strong feelings or passion]

thy•mic (thī′mik) Relating to the thymus gland.

thy•mic a•lym•pho•pla•si•a (thī′mik ā-lim-fō-plā′zē-ă) Hypoplasia with absence of Hassall corpuscles and deficiency of lymphocytes in the thymus and usually in lymph nodes, spleen, and gastrointestinal tract; there is peripheral lymphopenia and often hypogammaglobulinemia and absence of plasma cells; presents in early infancy with respiratory infections and leads to death within a few months.

thy•mic cor•pus•cle (thī′mik kōr′pŭs-ĕl) Small, spheric bodies of keratinized and usually squamous epithelial cells arranged in a concentric pattern around clusters of degenerating lymphocytes, eosinophils, and macrophages; found in the medulla of the lobules of the thymus. SYN Hassall bodies, Hassall concentric corpuscle.

thy•mi•co•lym•phat•ic (thī′mi-kō-lim-fat′ik) Relating to the thymus and the lymphatic system.

thy•mic veins (thī′mik vānz) A number of small veins from the thymus emptying into the left brachiocephalic vein.

thy•mi•dine (dThd) (thī′mi-dēn) 1-(2-deoxyribosyl)thymine; one of the four major nucleosides in DNA (the others being deoxyadenosine, deoxycytidine, and deoxyguanosine). SYN deoxythymidine.

thy•mi•dine 5′-di•phos•phate (dTDP) (thī′mi-dēn dī-fos′fāt) Thymidine esterified at its 5′ position with diphosphoric acid.

thy•mine (thī′mēn) A constituent of thymidylic acid and DNA; elevated in hyperuracil-thyminuria.

thy•mi•tis (thī-mī′tis) Inflammation of the thymus gland.

♻ **thymo-, thym-, thymi-** **1.** Combining forms denoting the thymus. [G. *thymos*] **2.** Combining forms denoting mind, soul, emotions. SEE ALSO -thymia. [G. *thymos,* the mind or heart as the seat of strong feelings or passions] **3.** Combining forms denoting wart, warty. [G. *thymos, thymion*]

thy•mo•cyte (thī′mō-sīt) A cell that develops in the thymus, seemingly from a stem cell of bone marrow and of fetal liver, and is the precursor of the thymus-derived lymphocyte (T lymphocyte) that affects cell-mediated (delayed type) sensitivity. [thymus + G. *kytos,* cell]

thy•mo•gen•ic (thī′mō-jen′ik) Of affective origin. [G. *thymos,* mind, + *genesis,* origin]

thy•mo•ki•net•ic (thī′mō-ki-net′ik) Activating the thymus gland. [thymus + G. *kinēsis,* movement]

thy•mo•ma (thī-mō′mă) A neoplasm in the anterior mediastinum, originating from thymic tissue, usually benign, and frequently encapsulated; occasionally invasive, but metastases are extremely rare. [thymus + G. *-oma,* tumor]

thy•mo•pri•val, thy•mo•priv•ic, thy•mo•pri•vous (thī-mō-prī′văl, -priv′ik, -mop′ri-vŭs) Relating to or marked by premature atrophy or removal of the thymus. [thymus + L. *privus,* deprived of]

thy•mus, pl. **thy•mi**, **thy•mus•es** (thī′mŭs, -mī, -mŭs-sĕz) [TA] A primary lymphoid organ, located in the superior mediastinum and lower part of the neck, that is necessary in early life for the normal development of immunologic function. It reaches its greatest relative weight shortly after birth and its greatest absolute weight at puberty; it then begins to involute, and much of the lymphoid tissue is replaced by fat. The thymus consists of two irregularly shaped parts united by a connective tissue capsule. Each part is partially subdivided by connective tissue septa into lobules, which consist of an inner medullary portion, continuous with the medullae of adjacent lobules, and an outer cortical portion. SYN thymus gland. [G. *thymos,* excrescence, sweetbread]

thy•mus gland (thī′mŭs gland) SYN thymus.

thyro-, **thyr-** Combining forms meaning the thyroid gland. SEE ALSO thyroid.

thy•ro•a•pla•si•a (thī′rō-ă-plā′zē-ă) A congenital defect of the thyroid gland with deficiency of its secretion. [thyro- + G. *a-* priv. + *plasis,* a molding]

thy•ro•ar•y•te•noid (thī′rō-ar-i-tē′noyd) Relating to the thyroid and arytenoid cartilages. SEE ALSO thyroarytenoid muscle.

thy•ro•ar•y•te•noid mus•cle (thī′rō-ar-i-tē′noyd mŭs′ĕl) *Origin,* inner surface of thyroid cartilage; *insertion*, muscular process and outer surface of arytenoid; *action*, decreases tension on (relaxes) vocal cords, lowering the pitch of the voice tone; *nerve supply*, recurrent laryngeal. SYN musculus thyroarytenoideus [TA].

thy•ro•car•di•ac dis•ease (thī′rō-kahr′dē-ak di-zēz′) Heart disease resulting from hyperthyroidism.

thy•ro•cele (thī′rō-sēl) A tumor of the thyroid gland, such as a goiter. [thyro- + G. *kēlē*, tumor]

thy•ro•cer•vi•cal trunk (thī-rō-sĕr′vi-kăl trŭngk) A short arterial trunk arising from the subclavian artery, giving rise to the suprascapular (which may instead arise directly from the subclavian artery) and terminating by dividing into the ascending cervical and inferior thyroid arteries. SYN truncus thyrocervicalis [TA].

thy•ro•ep•i•glot•tic (thī′rō-ep-i-glot′ik) Relating to the thyroid cartilage and the epiglottis.

thy•ro•ep•i•glot•tic mus•cle, **thy•ro•ep•i•glot•ti•de•an mus•cle** (thī′rō-ep-i-glot′ik mŭs′ĕl, thī′rō-ep-i-glo-tid′ē-ăn) *Origin*, inner surface of thyroid cartilage in common with musculus thyroarytenoideus; *insertion*, aryepiglottic fold and margin of epiglottis; *action*, depresses base of epiglottis; *nerve supply*, recurrent laryngeal. SYN musculus thyroepiglotticus [TA].

thy•ro•gen•ic, **thy•rog•e•nous** (thī′rō-jen′ik, -roj′ĕ-nŭs) Of thyroid gland origin. [thyroid + G. *-gen,* producing]

thy•ro•glob•u•lin (thī′rō-glob′yū-lin) **1.** A protein that contains thyroid hormone, usually stored in the colloid within the thyroid follicles; biosynthesis of thyroid hormone entails iodination of the L-tyrosyl moieties of this protein. A defect in thyroglobulin will lead to hypothyroidism. **2.** A substance obtained by the fractionation of thyroid glands from the hog, *Sus scrofula*, containing not less than 0.7% of total iodine; used as a thyroid hormone in the treatment of hypothyroidism. Cf. bioregulator.

thy•ro•glos•sal (thī′rō-glos′ăl) Relating to the thyroid gland and the tongue, denoting especially an embryologic duct.

thy•ro•glos•sal duct (thī′rō-glos′ăl dŭkt) SYN His canal.

thy•ro•hy•al (thī′rō-hī′ăl) The greater cornu of the hyoid bone.

thy•ro•hy•oid (thī′rō-hī′oyd) Relating to the thyroid cartilage and the hyoid bone. SEE ALSO thyrohyoid muscle.

thy•ro•hy•oid mus•cle (thī′rō-hī′oyd mŭs′ĕl) Apparently a continuation of the sternothyroid; *origin*, oblique line of thyroid cartilage; *insertion*, body of hyoid bone; *action*, approximates hyoid bone to the larynx; *nerve supply*, upper cervical spinal nerves carried by hypoglossal. SYN musculus thyrohyoideus.

thy•roid (thī′royd) Resembling a shield; denoting a gland (thyroid gland) and a cartilage of the larynx (thyroid cartilage) having such a shape. See this page. [G. *thyreoeidēs*, fr. *thyreos,* an oblong shield, + *eidos,* form]

thy•roid bru•it (thī′royd brū-ē′) A vascular murmur heard over a hyperactive thyroid gland, due to increased blood flow.

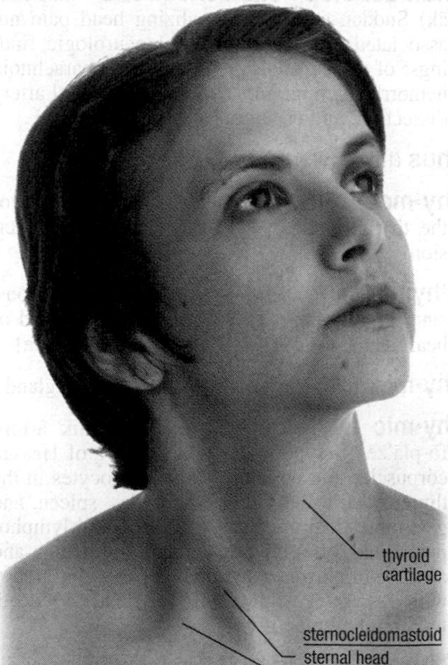

thyroid

thy·roid car·ti·lage (thī′royd kahr′ti-lăj) The largest of the cartilages of the larynx; it is formed of two approximately quadrilateral plates joined anteriorly at an angle of from 90–120°, the prominence so formed constituting the laryngeal prominence. SYN cartilago thyroidea [TA].

thy·roid·ec·to·my (thī′roy-dek′tŏ-mē) Removal of the thyroid gland. [thyroid + G. *ektomē,* excision]

thy·roid fol·li·cles (thī′royd fol′i-kĕlz) The small, spheric, vesicular components of the thyroid gland lined with epithelium and containing colloid in varying amounts; the colloid serves for storage of the thyroid hormone precursor, thyroglobulin. SYN folliculi glandulae thyroideae [TA].

thy·roid gland (thī′royd gland) An endocrine gland, consisting of irregularly spheroid follicles, lying in front and to the sides of the upper part of the trachea, of horseshoe shape, with two lateral lobes connected by a narrow central portion, the isthmus; occasionally an elongated offshoot, the pyramidal lobe, passes upward from the isthmus in front of the trachea. It is supplied by branches from the external carotid and subclavian arteries, and its nerves are derived from the middle cervical and cervicothoracic ganglia of the sympathetic system. It secretes thyroid hormone and calcitonin.

thy·roid i·ma ar·ter·y (thī′royd ī′mă ahr′tĕr-ē) An inconstant artery; *origin,* arch of aorta or brachiocephalic artery; *distribution,* thyroid gland. SYN arteria thyroidea ima, lowest thyroid artery, Neubauer artery.

thy·roid·i·tis (thī′roy-dī′tis) Inflammation of the thyroid gland. [thyroid + G. *-itis,* inflammation]

thy·roid oph·thal·mop·a·thy (thī′royd of-thăl-mop′ă-thē) SYN dysthyroid orbitopathy.

thy·roid-sti·mu·lat·ing hor·mone (thī′royd-stim′yū-lā-ting hōr′mōn) SYN thyrotropin.

thy·roid-sti·mu·lat·ing im·mu·no·glob·u·lins (TSI) (thī′royd-stim′yū-lāting im′yū-nō-glob′yū-linz) In Graves disease, the antibodies to TSH receptors in the thyroid gland. These antibodies are produced by B-lymphocytes and stimulate the receptors, causing hyperthyroidism.

thy·roid storm (thī′royd stōrm) SYN thyrotoxic crisis.

thy·ro·lib·er·in (thī′rō-lib′ĕr-in) A tripeptide hormone from the hypothalamus, which stimulates the anterior lobe of the hypophysis to release thyrotropin. Cf. bioregulator. SYN thyrotropin-releasing hormone. [thyrotropin + L. *libero,* to free, + -in]

thy·ro·meg·a·ly (thī′rō-meg′ă-lē) Enlargement of the thyroid gland. [thyro- + G. *megas,* large]

thy·ro·nine (thī′rō-nēn) An amino acid with a diphenyl ether group in the side chain; occurs in proteins only in the form of iodinated derivatives (iodothyronines), such as thyroxine.

thy·ro·par·a·thy·roid·ec·to·my (thī′rō-par-ă-thī′roy-dek′tŏ-mē) Excision of thyroid and parathyroid glands.

thy·ro·pri·val (thī′rō-prī′văl) Relating to thyroprivia, denoting hypothyroidism produced by disease or thyroidectomy. [thyro- + L. *privus,* deprived of]

thy·rop·to·sis (thī′rop-tō′sis) Downward dislocation of the thyroid gland. [thyro- + G. *ptōsis,* a falling]

thy·rot·o·my (thī-rot′ŏ-mē) **1.** Any cutting operation on the thyroid gland. **2.** SYN laryngofissure. [thyro- + G. *tomē,* a cutting]

thy·ro·tox·ic (thī′rō-tok′sik) Denoting thyrotoxicosis.

thy·ro·tox·ic cri·sis, thy·roid cri·sis (thī′rō-tok′sik krī′sis, thī′royd) The exacerbation of symptoms that occurs in severe thyrotoxicosis; marked by rapid pulse, nausea, diarrhea, fever, loss of weight, and extreme restlessness; coma and death may occur. SYN thyroid storm.

thy·ro·tox·i·co·sis (thī′rō-tok′si-kō′sis) The state produced by excessive quantities of endogenous or exogenous thyroid hormone. [thyro- + G. *toxikon,* poison, + *-osis,* condition]

thy·ro·troph (thī′rō-trōf) A cell in the anterior lobe of the pituitary that produces thyrotropin.

thy·ro·tro·phic (thī′rō-trō′fik) SYN thyrotropic. [thyro- + G. *trophē,* nourishment]

thy·rot·ro·phin (thī′rō-trō′fin) SYN thyrotropin.

thy·ro·trop·ic (thī′rō-trō′pik) Stimulating or nurturing the thyroid gland. SYN thyrotrophic. [thyro- + G. *tropē,* a turning]

thy·rot·ro·pin (thī′rō-trō′pin) A glycoprotein hormone produced by the anterior lobe of the hypophysis that stimulates the growth and function of the thyroid gland; it also is used as a diagnostic test to differentiate primary and secondary hypothyroidism. SYN thyroid-stimulating hormone, thyrotrophin. [for thyrotrophin, fr. thyro- + G. *trophē,* nourishment; corrupted to *-tropin,* and reanalyzed as fr. G. *tropē,* a turning]

thy·ro·tro·pin-re·leas·ing hor·mone (thī′rō-trō′pin rē-lēs′ing hōr′mōn) SYN thyroliberin.

thy·ro·tro·pin-re·leas·ing hor·mone (TRH) sti·mu·la·tion test (thī′rō-trō′pin rē-lēs′ing hōr′mōn stim′yŭ-lā′shŭn test) A test of pituitary response to injection of thyrotropin-releasing hormone, which normally stimulates pituitary secretion of thyroid-stimulating hormone (TSH, thyrotropin); used primarily to distinguish pituitary from hypothalamic causes of thyroid disorders; TSH does not rise in cases of pituitary dysfunction, but does rise in cases of hypothalamic disorders. Cf. bioregulator.

thy•rox•ine, **thy•rox•in** (thī-rok′sēn, -sin) The active iodine compound existing normally in the thyroid gland and extracted therefrom in crystalline form for therapeutic use; also prepared synthetically; used for the relief of hypothyroidism, cretinism, and myxedema.

TI The delay time between the inverting pulse and the "read" pulse in the inversion recovery experiment, in magnetic resonance imaging.

Ti Symbol for titanium.

TIA Abbreviation for transient ischemic attack.

TIBC Abbreviation for total iron-binding capacity.

tib•i•a, gen. and pl. **tib•i•ae** (tib′ē-ă, -ē-ē) [TA] The medial and larger of the two bones of the leg, articulating with the femur, fibula, and talus. SYN shin bone. [L. the large shinbone]

tib•i•al (tib′ē-ăl) Relating to the tibia or to any structure named from it; also denoting the medial or tibial aspect of the lower limb. [L. *tibialis*]

tib•i•al col•la•ter•al lig•a•ment (tib′ē-ăl kŏ-lat′ĕr-ăl lig′ă-mĕnt) SYN medial collateral ligament.

tib•i•al•is an•te•ri•or mus•cle (tib-ē-ā′lis an-tēr′ē-ŏr mŭs′ĕl) Medial muscle of anterior (dorsiflexor) compartment of leg; *origin*, upper two thirds of lateral surface of tibia, interosseous membrane, and overlying crural fascia; *insertion*, medial cuneiform and base of first metatarsal; *action*, dorsiflexion and inversion of foot; provides dynamic support of longitudinal and transverse arches of foot; *nerve supply*, deep peroneal. See this page.

tib•i•al•is pos•ter•i•or mus•cle (tib-ē-ā′lis pos-tēr′ē-ŏr mŭs′ĕl) Most anterior (deepest) muscle of deep posterior (plantar flexor) compartment of leg; *origin*, soleal line and posterior surface of tibia, the head and shaft of the fibula between the medial crest and interosseous border, and the posterior surface of interosseous membrane; *insertion*, navicular, three cuneiform, cuboid, and second, third, and fourth metatarsal bones; *action*, plantar flexion and inversion of foot; *nerve supply*, tibial. SYN musculus tibialis posterior [TA].

tib•i•al nerve (tib′ē-ăl nĕrv) One of the two major divisions of the sciatic nerve, it courses down the back of the leg to terminate as the medial and lateral plantar nerves in the foot; it supplies the hamstring muscles, the muscles of the back of the leg (the dorsiflexors and invertors of the foot), and the plantar aspect of the foot, as well as the skin on the back of the leg and sole of the foot. SYN nervus tibialis [TA].

tib•i•al tor•sion (tib′ē-ăl tōr′shŭn) A congenital twisting of the tibia.

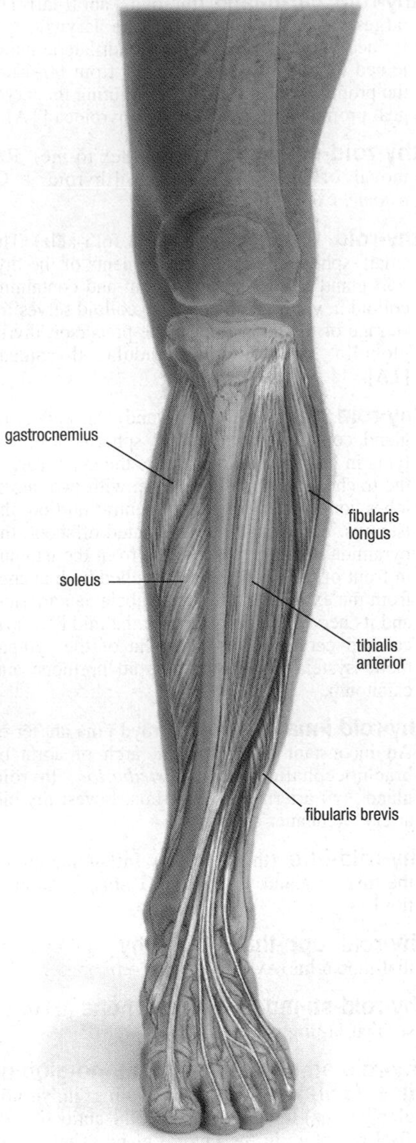

tibialis anterior muscle

tib•i•al tu•ber•os•i•ty (tib′ē-ăl tū′bĕr-os′i-tē) The protuberance at the anterior proximal tibia on which the patellar tendon inserts.

tib•i•a val•ga (tib′ē-ă val′gă) SYN genu valgum.

tib•i•a va•ra (tib′ē-ă vā′ră) SYN genu varum.

tibio- Combining form denoting the tibia. [L. *tibia,* the large shinbone]

tib•i•o•fib•u•lar joint (tib′ē-ō-fib′yū-lăr joynt) The plane synovial joint between the lateral condyle of the tibia and the head of the fibula.

tic (tik) Habitual, repeated contraction of certain muscles, resulting in stereotyped individualized actions that can be voluntarily suppressed for only brief periods (e.g., clearing the throat, sniffing, pursing the lips, excessive blinking); especially prominent when the person is under stress; there is no known pathologic substrate. SEE ALSO spasm. SYN Brissaud disease, habit spasm. [Fr.]

tic dou•lou•reux (tik dū-lū-ru′) SYN trigeminal neuralgia. [Fr. painful]

tick (tik) Any of a variety of small, bloodsucking arachnids that may have either hard (i.e., *Ixodid* ticks) or soft (i.e., *Argasid* ticks) shells. Ticks normally feed on wild birds, mammals, or reptiles, and transmit disease by feeding on an infected host (the reservoir host), then later feeding on a domestic animal or human. Ticks have a three-stage life cycle: larva, nymph (eight-legged), and adult (eight-legged), and require a blood meal at each stage before molting into the next stage or, in the case of the adult, before mating and laying eggs.

Some common tick-borne diseases are babesiosis: the black-legged and Western black-legged ticks. Colorado tick fever: Rocky Mountain wood tick. Ehrlichiosis (HGE and HME): Lone Star tick and black-legged tick. Lyme disease: black-legged tick and Western black-legged tick. The "deer tick" was once thought by scientists at Yale University to be a separate species, and was named *Ixodes dammini*. It has since been proven to be the same species as the black-legged tick, *Ixodes scapularis*. Rocky Mountain spotted fever (RMSF): American dog tick, Rocky Mountain wood tick, and Pacific Coast tick. Tick-borne relapsing fever: soft ticks (*Ornithodoros hermsi*, *O. turicata*). Tick paralysis: American dog and Rocky Mountain wood tick. Tularemia (rabbit fever): Lone Star tick, Rocky Mountain tick, Pacific Coast tick, American dog tick, black-legged tick.

tick-borne en•ceph•a•li•tis East•ern sub•type (tik′bōrn en-sef′ă-lī′tis ēst′ĕrn sŭb′tīp) A severe form of encephalitis caused by a flavivirus and transmitted by ticks (*Ixodes persulcatus* and *I. ricinus*).

tick-borne en•ceph•a•li•tis vi•rus (tik′bōrn en-sef′ă-lī′tis vī′rŭs) An arbovirus of the genus Flavivirus that occurs in Central Europe, Eastern Europe, and Eurasia, in two subtypes, causing two forms of encephalitis in humans: tick-borne encephalitis (Central European subtype) and tick-borne encephalitis (Eastern European subtype); the vectors are ticks of the genus *Ixodes*.

tick fe•ver (tik fē′vĕr) **1.** Any infectious disease of humans or other animals caused by a protozoan blood parasite, a bacterium, a rickettsia, or a virus, and transmitted by a tick. **2.** The tick-borne variety of relapsing fever. **3.** SYN bovine babesiosis. **4.** SYN Rocky Mountain spotted fever. **5.** SYN Colorado tick fever.

tick pa•ral•y•sis (tik păr-al′i-sis) An ascending paralysis caused by the continuing presence of *Dermacentor* and *Ixodes* ticks attached in the occipital region or on the upper neck of humans, often hidden under long hair.

tick ty•phus (tik tī′fŭs) SYN boutonneuse fever.

t.i.d. Three times daily. [L. *ter in die*]

ti•dal (tī′dăl) Relating to or resembling the tides, alternately rising and falling.

ti•dal air (tī′dăl ār) SYN tidal volume.

ti•dal drain•age (tī′dăl drān′ăj) Evacuation of the urinary bladder by means of an intermittent filling and emptying apparatus.

ti•dal vol•ume (tī′dăl vol′yūm) The volume of air inspired or expired in a single breath during regular breathing. SYN tidal air.

tide (tīd) An alternate rise and fall, ebb and flow, or an increase or decrease. [A.S. *tīd,* time]

Tie•tze syn•drome (tēt′sē sin′drōm) Inflammation and painful, tender, nonsuppurative swelling of a costochondral junction.

Tietz syn•drome (tētz sin′drōm) Autosomal dominant inheritance of albinism and deafness caused at least in some subsets of families by a mutation of the microophthalmia transcription factor gene.

tight junc•tion (tīt jŭngk′shŭn) An intercellular junction between epithelial cells in which the outer leaflets of lateral cell membranes fuse to form a variable number of parallel interweaving strands that greatly reduce transepithelial permeability to macromolecules, solutes, and water through the paracellular route.

tilt•ing disc valve (tilt′ing disk valv) A type of prosthetic cardiac valve that includes a caged disc.

tilt•ing disc valve pros•the•sis (tilt′ing disk valv pros-thē′sis) A low-profile artificial heart valve employing a caged disc that tilts to open during systole.

tilt test (tilt test) Any measurement of response during tilting of the body, usually head up but also head down. The test may be monitored by catheterization, echocardiography, electrophysiologic measurements, electrocardiography, or mechanocardiography. Used to study the response of the circulatory system to gravitational force.

tim•bre (tam′bĕr) The distinguishing quality of a sound, by which one may determine its source. [Fr.]

time (t) (tīm) **1.** That relation of events expressed by the terms past, present, and future, and measured by units such as minutes, hours, days, months, or years. **2.** A certain period during which something definite or determined is done. SYN tempus (2). [A.S. *tima*]

timed spec·i·men (tīmd spes′i-mĕn) A biologic specimen obtained at a certain time of day or at a certain interval after another event. Used to monitor drug therapy, blood glucose levels, and other laboratory tests.

time of flight (tīm flīt) MAGNETIC RESONANCE IMAGING Rate of flow in a given time; causes some flowing nuclei to receive only one radiofrequency pulse and therefore produce a signal void.

time of flight (TOF) an·gi·og·ra·phy (tīm flīt an′jē-og′ră-fē) Magnetic resonance imaging technique that generates vascular contrast by using the in-flow effect. SYN TOF sequence.

Time-Line ther·a·py (tīm-līn thār′ă-pē) A technique, based on the principles of neurolinguistic programming, for releasing negative emotions and revising limiting decisions, that directs the client, in a dissociated state, to return to significant past events with new resources so that negative emotions can be released or limiting decisions revised. SEE ALSO dissociation (4).

tin (Sn) (tin) A metallic element, atomic no. 50, atomic wt. 118.710. SYN stannum. [A.S., tin]

tinct. Abbreviation for tincture.

tinc·to·ri·al (tingk-tōr′ē-ăl) Relating to coloring or staining. [L. *tinctorius,* fr. *tingo,* to dye]

tinc·ture (tinct.) (tingk′shŭr) An alcoholic or hydroalcoholic solution prepared from vegetable materials or from chemical substances.

tin·e·a (tin′ē-ă) A fungus infection (dermatophytosis) of the keratin component of hair, skin, or nails. Genera of fungi causing such infection are *Microsporum*, *Trichophyton*, and *Epidermophyton*. See page 1565. SYN ringworm, serpigo (1). [L. worm, moth]

tin·e·a bar·bae (tin′ē-ă bahr′bē) A fungal infection involving the beard, occurring as a follicular infection or as a granulomatous lesion; the primary lesions are papules and pustules. SYN barber's itch, folliculitis barbae, tinea sycosis.

tin·e·a cap·i·tis (tin′ē-ă kap′i-tis) A common form of fungal infection of the scalp caused by various species of *Microsporum* and *Trichophyton* on or within hair shafts, occurring almost exclusively in children and characterized by irregularly placed and variously sized patches of apparent baldness because of hairs breaking off at the surface of the scalp, scaling, black dots, and occasionally erythema and pyoderma. See page B5.

tin·e·a circ·i·na·ta (tin′ē-ă ser′si-nā′tă) SYN tinea corporis.

tin·e·a cor·por·is (tin′ē-ă kōr-pōr′is) A well-defined, scaling, macular eruption of dermatophytosis that frequently forms anular lesions and may appear on any part of the body. See page B8. SYN tinea circinata.

tin·e·a crur·is (tin′ē-ă krūr′is) A form of tinea imbricata occurring in the genitocrural region, including the inner side of the thighs, the perineal region, and the groin. SYN eczema marginatum, jock itch.

tin·e·a im·bri·ca·ta (tin′ē-ă im-bri-kā′tă) An eruption consisting of a number of concentric rings of overlapping scales forming papulosquamous patches scattered over the body; it occurs in tropical climates and is caused by the fungus *Trichophyton concentricum.*

tin·e·a ker·i·on (tin′ē-ă ker′ē-on) An inflammatory fungus infection of the scalp and beard, marked by pustules and a boggy infiltration of the surrounding parts; most commonly caused by *Microsporum audouinii.*

tin·e·a ped·is (tin′ē-ă ped′is) Dermatophytosis of the feet, especially of the skin between the toes, caused by one of the dermatophytes, usually a species of *Trichophyton* or *Epidermophyton;* the disease consists of small vesicles, fissures, scaling, maceration, and eroded areas between the toes and on the plantar surface of the foot; other skin areas may be involved. See page B9. SYN athlete's foot.

tin·e·a sy·co·sis (tin′ē-ă sī-kō′sis) SYN tinea barbae.

tin·e·a un·gui·um (tin′ē-ă un-gwī′ŭm) Ringworm of the nails due to a dermatophyte.

tin·e·a ver·si·col·or (tin′ē-ă vĕr′si-kŏ′lōr) An eruption of tan or brown branny patches on the skin of the trunk, often appearing white, in contrast with hyperpigmented skin after exposure to the summer sun; caused by growth of *Malassezia furfur* in the stratum corneum with minimal inflammatory reaction. See page 1565. SYN pityriasis versicolor.

Ti·nel sign (tē-nel′ sīn) Distally radiating pain or paresthesia caused by tapping over the site of a superficial nerve, indicating inflammation or irritation of the nerve.

tine test (tīn test) SEE tuberculin test.

tin·ni·tus (tin′i-tŭs) A sensation of noises (ringing, whistling, booming) in the ears. [L. a jingling, fr. *tinnio,* pp. *tinnitus,* to jingle, clink]

tip (tip) **1.** A point; a more or less sharp extremity. **2.** A separate, but attached, piece of the same or another structure, forming the extremity of a part.

tip pinch (tip pinch) OCCUPATIONAL THERAPY pinch between the tips of the index finger and the thumb. SYN tip-to-tip pinch.

TIPS (tips) Abbreviation and acronym for transjugular intrahepatic portosystemic shunt.

tip-to-tip pinch (tip tip pinch) SYN tip pinch.

tir•ing (tīr′ing) SYN cerclage. [Eng. tire]

TIS Abbreviation for tumor in situ (used in staging of cancer).

tis•sue (tish′ū) An aggregation of similar cells or types of cells, together with any associated intercellular materials, adapted to perform one or more specific functions. There are four basic tissues in the body: 1) epithelium; 2) connective tissue, including blood, bone, and cartilage; 3) muscle; and 4) nerve. [Fr. *tissu,* woven, fr. L. *texo,* to weave]

tis•sue cul•ture (tish′ū kŭl′chŭr) The mainte-

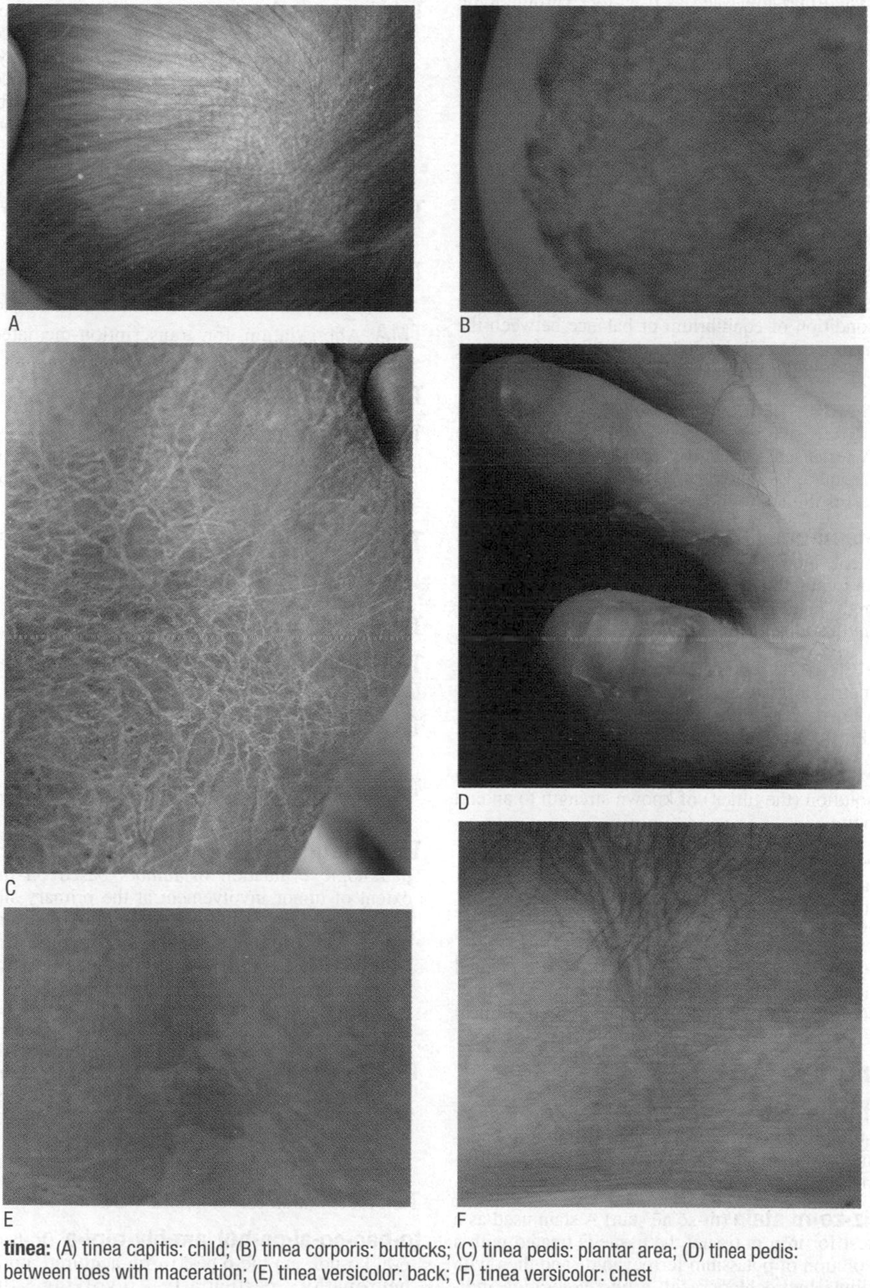

tinea: (A) tinea capitis: child; (B) tinea corporis: buttocks; (C) tinea pedis: plantar area; (D) tinea pedis: between toes with maceration; (E) tinea versicolor: back; (F) tinea versicolor: chest

nance of live tissue after removal from the body, by placing in a vessel with a sterile nutritive medium.

tis•sue lymph (tish′ū limf) True lymph (i.e., lymph derived chiefly from fluid in tissue spaces, in contrast to blood lymph).

tis•sue plas•min•o•gen ac•ti•va•tor (tPA) (tish′ū plaz-min′ō-jen ak′ti-vā-tŏr) Thrombolytic serine protease catalyzing the enzymatic conversion of plasminogen to plasmin; a genetically engineered protein used as a thrombolytic agent in patients with thrombotic occlusion of a coronary or cerebral artery.

tis•sue res•pir•a•tion (tish′ū res′pir-ā′shŭn) The interchange of gases between the blood and the tissues. SYN internal respiration.

tis•sue-spe•ci•fic ant•i•gen (tish′ū-spe-sif′ik an′ti-jen) SYN organ-specific antigen.

tis•sue ten•sion (tish′ū ten′shŭn) A theoretic condition of equilibrium or balance between the tissues and cells whereby overaction of any part is restrained by the pull of the mass.

tis•sue throm•bo•plas•tin in•hi•bi•tion time (tish′ū throm-bō-plas′tin in′hi-bish′ŭn tīm) A test used to identify lupus anticoagulant; the thromboplastin source used in the prothrombin test is diluted to increase sensitivity to inhibitors.

ti•ta•ni•um (Ti) (tī-tā′nē-ŭm) A metallic element, atomic no. 22, atomic wt. 47.88, used as an implant in dental work because of its uniquely high level of biocompatibility. [*Titans,* in G. myth., sons of Earth]

ti•ter (tī′tĕr) The standard of strength of a volumetric test solution; the assay value of an unknown measure by volumetric means. SYN titre. [Fr. *titre,* standard]

ti•trate (tī′trāt) To analyze volumetrically by a solution (the titrant) of known strength to an end point.

ti•tra•tion (tī-trā′shŭn) Volumetric analysis by addition of definite amounts of a test solution to a solution of the substance being assayed. [Fr. *titre,* standard]

ti•tra•tion dose (tī-trā′shŭn dōs) The continual adjustment of a dose based on patient response. Dosages are adjusted until the desired clinical effect is achieved.

titre [Br.] SYN titer.

tit•u•ba•tion (tit-yū-bā′shŭn) **1.** A staggering or stumbling in trying to walk. **2.** A tremor or shaking of the head, of cerebellar origin. [L. *titubo,* pp. *-atus,* to stagger]

Tiz•zo•ni stain (tit-sō′nē stān) A stain used as a test for iron in tissue; the tissue is treated with a solution of potassium ferrocyanide and then with dilute hydrochloric acid; a blue coloration indicates the presence of iron.

TKR Abbreviation for total knee replacement.

Tl Symbol for thallium.

TLC Abbreviation for thin-layer chromatography; total lung capacity.

TLD Abbreviation for thermoluminescent dosimeter.

T lym•pho•cyte (lim′fō-sīt) A thymocyte-derived lymphocyte of immunologic importance that is responsible for cell-mediated immunity. These cells have the characteristic T3 surface marker and may be further divided into subsets according to function, such as helper, suppressor, and cytotoxic. SEE ALSO B lymphocyte. SYN T cell.

T-lym•pho•cyte ant•i•gen re•cep•tor (lim′fō-sīt an′ti-jen rĕ-sep′tŏr) SYN T-cell receptor.

Tm **1.** Symbol for thulium. **2.** Abbreviation for transport maximum.

TMA Abbreviation for transcription-mediated amplification.

TMJ Abbreviation for temporomandibular joint.

TMJ syn•drome (sin′drōm) Abbreviation for temporomandibular joint pain-dysfunction syndrome. SEE myofascial pain-dysfunction syndrome.

TMP Abbreviation for ribothymidylic acid; trimethoprim; sometimes for deoxyribothymidylic acid.

TMT Abbreviation for tarsometatarsal.

T-my•co•plas•ma (mī′kō-plaz′mă) SYN *Ureaplasma.*

Tn **1.** Abbreviation for ocular tension. **2.** Abbreviation for troponin.

TNM Abbreviation for tumor-node-metastasis. SEE TNM staging.

TNM stag•ing (stāj′ing) A system of clinicopathologic evaluation of tumors based on the extent of tumor involvement at the primary site (T, followed by a number indicating size and depth of invasion), and lymph node involvement (N) and metastasis (M), each followed by a number starting at 0 for no evident metastasis; numbers used depend on the organ involved and influence the prognosis and choice of treatment.

TNTC Abbreviation for too numerous to count (indicating the finding of a large number of discrete objects, usually cells in a urine specimen, the precise enumeration of which is not practicable).

TO Abbreviation for telephone order.

to•bac•co-al•co•hol am•bly•o•pi•a (tŏ-bak′ō-al′kŏ-hol am′blē-ō′pē-ă) An acquired optic neuropathy particularly involving the maculopapillary bundle nerve fibers associated with excessive alcohol and tobacco consumption and with poor nutritional status.

to•bac•co heart (tŏ-bak′ō hahrt) Cardiac irritability marked by irregular action, palpitation, and sometimes pain, believed to occur as a result of the heavy use of tobacco.

to•cain•ide hy•dro•chlor•ide (tō-kā′nīd hī′drō-klōr′īd) An oral antiarrhythmic agent, similar in action to lidocaine, used in the treatment of ventricular arrhythmias.

♻**toco-** Combining form denoting childbirth. [G. *tokos,* birth]

toc•o•dy•na•graph (tō′kō-dī′nă-graf) A recording of the force of uterine contractions. [toco- + G. *dynamis,* force, + *graphē,* a writing]

toc•o•dy•na•mom•e•ter (tō′kō-dī-nă-mom′ĕ-tĕr) An instrument for measuring the force of uterine contractions. [toco- + G. *dynamis,* force, + *metron,* measure]

to•cog•ra•phy (tō-kog′ră-fē) The process of recording uterine contractions. [toco- + G. *graphō,* to write]

to•co•lyt•ic (tō′kō-lit′ik) Denoting any pharmacologic agent used to arrest uterine contractions; often used in an attempt to arrest premature labor contractions. [G. *tokos*, childbirth, labor, + *lysis*, loosening]

to•coph•er•ol (T) (tō-kof′ĕr-ol) **1.** A generic term for vitamin E and compounds chemically related to it, with or without biologic activity. **2.** A methylated tocol or methylated tocotrienol.

to•co•tri•enes (tō′kō-trī′ēnz) The four forms of vitamin E: alpha, beta, gamma, and delta.

tod•dler's frac•ture (tod′lĕrz frak′shŭr) A spiral fracture of the tibia seen frequently in children 1–2 years of age.

Todd pa•ral•y•sis (tod păr-al′i-sis) Temporary inability to move (normally not more than a few days) that occurs in the limb or limbs involved in jacksonian epilepsy after a seizure. SYN Todd postepileptic paralysis.

Todd post•e•pi•lep•tic pa•ral•y•sis (tod pōst-ep-ĕ-lep′tik păr-al′i-sis) SYN Todd paralysis.

toe (tō) One of the digits of the feet. [A.S. *ta*]

toe-drop (tō′drop) Inability to dorsiflex the toes, usually due to paralysis of the toe extensor muscles.

toe•ing out (tō′ing owt) SYN metatarsus valgus.

toe•nail (tō′nāl) SEE nail.

TOF se•quence (sē′kwĕns) SYN time of flight (TOF) angiography.

To•ga•vir•i•dae (tō′gă-vir′i-dē) A family of viruses that includes the following genera: Alphavirus, which includes eastern equine encephalitis; western equine encephalitis; Venezuelan equine encephalitis; and the rubella virus (*Rubivirus*).

to•ga•vi•rus (tō′gă-vī-rŭs) Any virus of the family Togaviridae. [L. *toga,* garment covering, + virus]

toi•let (toy-let′) **1.** Cleansing of the obstetric patient after childbirth or of a wound after an operation preparatory to the application of the dressing. **2.** DENTISTRY cavity débridement, the final step before placing a restoration in a tooth whereby the cavity is cleaned and all debris is removed. [Fr. *toilette*]

Toi•son stain (twa-zōn[h]′ stān) A blood diluent and leukocyte stain containing methyl violet, sodium chloride, sodium sulfate, and glycerin; also used for erythrocyte counts.

Tok•er cell (tō′ker sel) An epithelial cell with clear cytoplasm found in 10% of normal nipples; contains keratin 7, like Paget carcinoma cells, from which it must be distinguished cytologically.

♻**toko-** SEE toco-.

tol•bu•ta•mide test (tol-byū′tă-mīd test) An assay to detect insulin-producing tumors; after a 1-g intravenous dose of tolbutamide, plasma insulin and glucose are measured at intervals up to 3 hours; higher insulin responses and lower glucose values characterize patients with such tumors.

Toldt mem•brane (tōlt mem′brān) The anterior layer of the renal fascia.

tol•er•a•ble up•per in•take lev•el (tŏl′ĕr-ă-bĕl up′pĕr in′tāk lev′ĕl) The maximum level of continuing daily nutrient intake that is likely to pose no risk to the health of most of those in the age group for which it has been established.

tol•er•ance (tol′ĕr-ăns) **1.** The ability to endure or be less responsive to a stimulus, especially over a period of continued exposure. **2.** The power of resisting the action of a poison or of taking a drug continuously or in large doses without injurious effects. [L. *tolero,* pp. *-atus,* to endure]

tol•er•ance dose (tol′ĕr-ăns dōs) The largest dose of a remedy that can be accepted without the production of injurious symptoms.

tol•er•ance li•mits (tol′ĕr-ăns lim′its) Specified performance limits for allowable error for a test; the limits selected should depend on both the effect of the error on the clinical significance of a test and on what is technically achievable.

tol•er•ant (tol′ĕr-ănt) Having the property of tolerance.

tol•er•o•gen•ic (tol′ĕr-ō-jen′ik) Producing immunologic tolerance.

To•lo•sa-Hunt syn•drome (tō-lō′sah-hŭnt

sin′drōm) Cavernous sinus syndrome produced by an idiopathic granuloma.

to·lu·i·dine blue stain (tō-lū′i-dēn blū stān) A stain used for many purposes, including visualization of *Pneumocystis jiroveci* trophozoites.

To·lu·if·er·a per·e·i·rae (tō′lū-if′ĕr-ă per′ē-ī′rē) SYN balsam of Peru. [L. *(balsam of) Tolu* + -fera *bearing*]

To·ma sign (tō′mah sīn) To distinguish between inflammatory and noninflammatory ascites: in inflammatory conditions of the peritoneum, the mesentery contracts, drawing the intestines over to the right side; consequently, with the patient supine, tympany is elicited on the right side, dullness on the left.

♻ **-tome** Combining form indicating a cutting instrument (the first element in the compound usually indicating the part that the instrument is designed to cut); segment, part, section; tomography; surgery. [G. *tomos,* cutting, sharp; a cutting (section or segment)]

to·men·tum, to·men·tum ce·re·bri (tō-men′tŭm, ser′ĕ-brī) The numerous small blood vessels passing between the cerebral surface of the pia mater and the cortex of the brain. [L. a stuffing for cushions]

Tom·ma·sel·li dis·ease (tom-ĕ-sel′ē di-zēz′) Hemoglobinuria and pyrexia due to quinine intoxication.

to·mo·gram (tō′mō-gram) A radiograph obtained by tomography. [G. *tomos,* a cutting (section) + *gramma,* a writing]

to·mo·graph (tō′mō-graf) The radiographic equipment used in tomography. [G. *tomos,* a cutting (section), + *graphō,* to write]

to·mog·ra·phy (tŏ-mog′ră-fē) Making a radiographic image of a selected plane by means of reciprocal linear or curved motion of the x-ray tube and film cassette; images of all other planes are blurred ("out of focus") by being relatively displaced on the film. SYN planigraphy, planography, stratigraphy.

♻ **-tomy** Suffix indicating a cutting operation. SEE ALSO -ectomy. [G. *tomē,* incision]

tone (tōn) **1.** A musical sound. **2.** The character of the voice expressing an emotion. **3.** The tension present in resting muscles. **4.** Firmness of the tissues; normal functioning of all the organs. [G. *tonos,* tone, or a tone]

tongue (tŭng) **1.** A mobile mass of muscular tissue covered with mucous membrane, occupying the cavity of the mouth and forming part of its floor, constituting also by its posterior portion the anterior wall of the pharynx. It bears the organ of taste, assists in mastication and deglutition, and is the principal instrument of articulate speech. SYN lingua (1) [TA], glossa. **2.** A tonguelike structure. SYN lingua (2) [TA]. [A.S. *tunge*]

tongue crib (tŭng krib) An appliance used to control visceral (infantile) swallowing and tongue thrusting and to encourage the mature or somatic tongue posture and function.

tongue mo·bil·i·ty (tŭng mō-bil′i-tē) SEE ankyloglossia.

tongue re·trac·tion (tŭng rĕ-trak′shŭn) An atypical oral motor pattern whereby the tongue is pulled back or falls to the back of the mouth, making breathing and sucking difficult.

tongue-swal·low·ing (tŭng swahl′ō-ing) A slipping back of the tongue against the pharynx that causes choking.

tongue thrust (tŭng thrŭst) An atypical oral motor pattern evidenced by forceful protrusion of the tongue from the mouth; usually arrhythmic, it makes inserting a nipple or food difficult and causes food to be pushed out of the mouth.

tongue thrust ther·a·py (tŭng thrŭst thār′ă-pē) SYN myofunctional therapy.

tongue-tie (tŭng′tī) SYN ankyloglossia.

ton·ic (ton′ik) **1.** In a state of continuous unremitting action; denoting especially a muscular contraction. **2.** Invigorating; increasing physical or mental tone or strength. **3.** A remedy purported to restore enfeebled function and promote vigor and a sense of well-being, qualified, according to the organ or system on which it is presumed to act, as cardiac, digestive, hematic, vascular, nervine, uterine, general, and others. [G. *tonikos,* fr. *tonos,* tone]

ton·ic bite re·flex (ton′ik bīt rē′fleks) An atypical oral motor pattern seen when a person bites down and cannot release the position, often accompanied by increased tension throughout the face, head, and neck, which can result in shortening of muscles and connective tissue that prevents full jaw opening.

ton·ic con·trac·tion (ton′ik kŏn-trak′shŭn) Sustained contraction of a muscle, as employed in the maintenance of posture.

ton·ic con·vul·sion (ton′ik kŏn-vŭl′shŭn) A convulsion in which muscle contraction is sustained.

ton·ic ep·i·lep·sy (ton′ik ep′i-lep′sē) An attack in which the body becomes rigid.

to·nic·i·ty (tō-nis′i-tē) **1.** A state of normal tension of the tissues by virtue of which the parts are kept in shape, alert, and ready to function in response to a suitable stimulus. In the case of muscle, it refers to a state of continuous activity or tension beyond that related to the physical properties, i.e., its active resistance to stretch; in skeletal muscle, it is dependent on the efferent innervation. SYN tonus. **2.** The osmotic pressure or tension of a solution, usually relative to that of blood. SEE ALSO isotonicity. [G. *tonos,* tone]

ton•ic neck re•flex (ton′ik nek rē′fleks) A brainstem-level reflex that may produce positional changes of all limbs in response to active or passive head turning or to flexion/extension of the head.

ton•i•co•clon•ic (ton′i-kō-klon′ik) Both tonic and clonic, referring to muscular spasms. SYN tonoclonic.

ton•ic pu•pil (ton′ik pyū′pil) A general term for a pupil with delayed, slow, long-lasting contractions to light and to a near vision effort, often with light-near dissociation; due to denervation and aberrant reinnervation of the iris sphincter; seen in various autonomic neuropathies and in Adie syndrome.

ton•ic spa•sm (ton′ik spazm) A continuous involuntary muscular contraction.

ton•ic state (ton′ik stāt) Steady rigid muscle contractions with no relaxation.

tono- Combining form meaning tone, tension, pressure. [G. *tonos*]

ton•o•clon•ic (ton′ō-klon′ik) SYN tonicoclonic.

ton•o•clon•ic spa•sm (ton′ō-klon′ik spazm) Convulsive contraction of muscles.

ton•o•fi•bril (ton′ō-fī′bril) One of a system of fibers found in the cytoplasm of epithelial cells. SEE ALSO cytoskeleton.

ton•o•fil•a•ment (ton′ō-fil′ă-mĕnt) A structural cytoplasmic protein, bundles of which together form a tonofibril; tonofilaments are made up of a variable number of related proteins, keratins, and are found in all epithelial cells.

ton•o•graph (tō′nō-graf) A recording tonometer. [tono- + G. *graphō,* to write]

to•nog•ra•phy (tō-nog′ră-fē) Continuous measurement of intraocular pressure by means of a recording tonometer, to determine the facility of aqueous outflow.

to•nom•e•ter (tō-nom′ĕ-tĕr) **1.** An instrument for determining pressure or tension, especially determining ocular tension. **2.** A vessel for equilibrating a liquid (e.g., blood) with a gas, usually at a controlled temperature. [tono- + G. *metron,* measure]

to•nom•e•try (tō-nom′ĕ-trē) **1.** Measurement of the tension of a part (e.g., intravascular tension or blood pressure). **2.** Measurement of ocular tension.

ton•o•plast (tō′nō-plast) An intracellular structure or vacuole. [tono- + G. *plastos,* formed]

to•no•top•ic (tō-nō-top′ik) Denoting a spatial arrangement of structures such that certain tone frequencies are transmitted, as in the auditory pathway. [tono- + G. *topos,* place]

to•no•tro•pic (tō-nō-trō′pik) Denoting the shortening of the resting length of a muscle. [G. *tonikos, tonos,* tone, + *tropos,* a turning]

ton•sil (ton′sil) **1.** Any collection of lymphoid tissue. **2.** SYN palatine tonsil. See this page. [L. *tonsilla,* a stake, in pl. the tonsils]

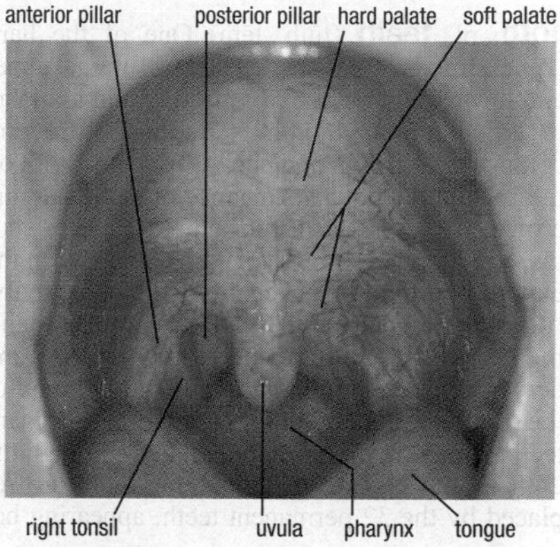

oral structures

ton•sil of ce•re•bel•lum (ton′sil ser-ĕ-bel′ŭm) A rounded lobule on the undersurface of each cerebellar hemisphere, continuous medially with the uvula of the cerebellar vermis. SYN tonsilla cerebelli [TA].

ton•sil•la, pl. **ton•sil•lae** (ton-sil′lă, -ē) [TA] SYN palatine tonsil. [L. (see tonsil)]

ton•sil•la ce•re•bel•li (ton-sil′lă ser′ă-bel′ī) [TA] SYN tonsil of cerebellum.

ton•sil•la lin•gua•lis (ton-sil′lă ling-gwā′lis) [TA] SYN lingual tonsil.

ton•sil•la pal•a•ti•na (ton-sil′lă pal′ă-tī′nă) [TA] SYN palatine tonsil.

ton•sil•lar, **ton•sil•lar•y** (ton′si-lăr, -lar-ē) Relating to a tonsil, especially the palatine tonsil.

ton•sil•lar crypt (ton′si-lăr kript) One of the variable number of deep recesses that extend into the palatine and pharyngeal tonsils from the free surface where they open at the tonsillar fossa.

ton•sil•lar fos•sa (ton′si-lăr fos′ă) The depression between the palatoglossal and palatopharyngeal arches occupied by the palatine tonsil.

ton•sil•lec•to•my (ton-si-lek′tŏ-mē) Removal of the entire tonsil. [tonsil + G. *ektomē,* excision]

ton•sil•li•tis (ton-si-lī′tis) Inflammation of a tonsil, especially of the palatine tonsil. [tonsil + G. *-itis,* inflammation]

tonsillo- Prefix meaning tonsil. [L. *tonsilla*]

ton•sil•lo•lith (ton-sil′ō-lith) A calcareous concretion in a distended tonsillar crypt. SYN tonsilolith. [tonsillo- + G. *lithos,* stone]

ton•sil•lot•o•my (ton-si-lot′ŏ-mē) The cutting away of a portion or all of a hypertrophied faucial tonsil. [tonsillo- + G. *tomē,* incision]

ton•sil•o•lith (ton-sil′ō-lith) SYN tonsillolith.

to•nus (tō′nŭs) SYN tonicity (1). [L., fr. G. *tonos*]

tooth, pl. **teeth** (tūth, tēth) One of the hard conic structures set in the alveoli of the upper and lower jaws, used in mastication and assisting in articulation. A tooth is a dermal structure composed of dentin and encased in cementum on the anatomic root and enamel on its anatomic crown. It consists of a root buried in the alveolus, a neck covered by the gum, and a crown, the exposed portion. In the center is the pulp cavity, filled with a connective tissue reticulum containing a jellylike substance, blood vessels, and nerves that enter through a canal at the apex of the root. The 20 deciduous teeth, or primary teeth, appear between the 6th and 9th through the 24th month of life; these exfoliate and are replaced by the 32 permanent teeth, appearing between the 5th and 7th years through the 17th to 23rd years. There are four kinds of teeth: incisor, canine, premolar, and molar. See this page. SYN dens (1) [TA]. [A.S. *tōth*]

tooth•ache (tūth′āk) Pain in a tooth due to the condition of the pulp or periodontal ligament resulting from caries, infection, or trauma. SYN dentalgia, odontalgia.

tooth bud (tūth bŭd) The primordial structures from which a tooth is formed; the enamel organ, the dental papilla, and the dental sac enclosing them.

tooth germ (tūth jĕrm) The enamel organ and dental papilla, constituting the developing tooth.

tooth pulp (tūth pŭlp) SYN dental pulp.

tooth sock•et (tūth sok′ĕt) An opening in the alveolar process of the maxilla or mandible, into which each tooth fits and is attached by means of the periodontal ligament. SYN alveolus (4) [TA].

topaesthesia [Br.] SYN topesthesia.

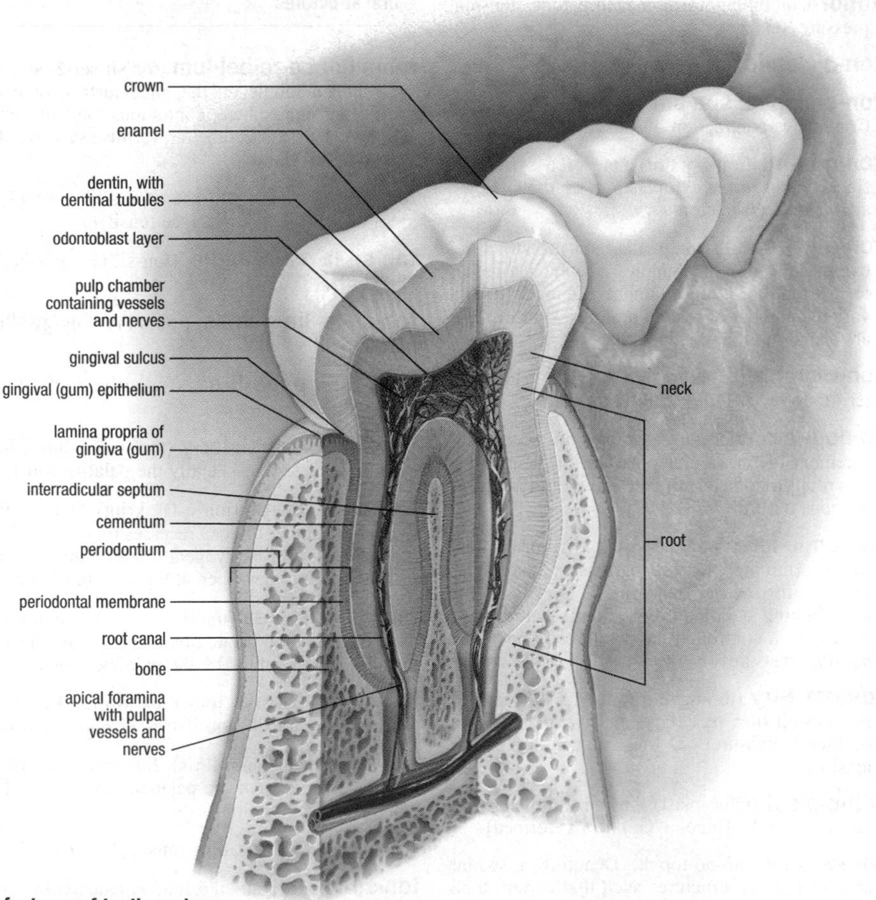

features of tooth anatomy

top•ag•no•sis (top-ag-nō′sis) Inability to localize tactile sensations. SYN topoanesthesia. [top- + G. *a-* priv. + *gnōsis,* recognition]

to•pal•gi•a (tō-pal′jē-ă) Pain localized in one spot; a symptom occurring in neuroses whereby localized pain, without evident organic basis, is experienced. [top- + G. *algos,* pain]

top-down ap•proach (top-down ă-prōch′) An up-to-date view on assessment and intervention, which is centered on the needs of the client. It begins the performance outcome as a totality rather than an assessment of level of the so-called splinter skills that contribute to the performance or the outcome.

top•es•the•si•a (top-es-thē′zē-ă) The ability to localize a light touch applied to any part of the skin. SYN topaesthesia. [top- + G. *aisthēsis,* sensation]

to•pha•ceous (tō-fā′shŭs) Sandy; gritty; pertaining to or manifesting the features of a tophus. [L. *tophaceus*]

to•pha•ceous gout (tō-fā′shŭs gowt) The condition in which deposits of uric acid and urates occur as gouty tophi. See this page.

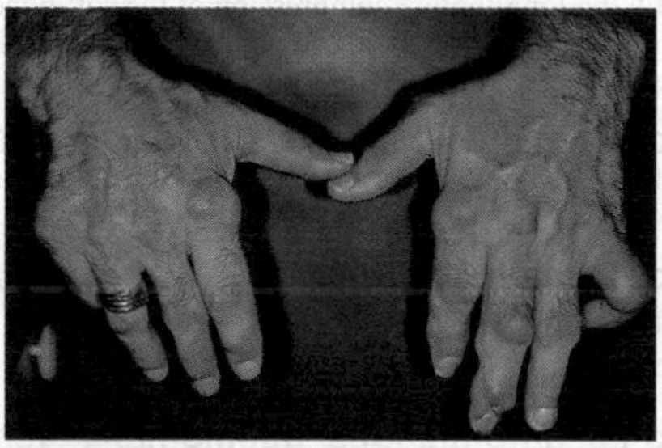

chronic tophaceous gout: hand and wrist involvement

to•phi (tō′fī) Plural of tophus.

to•phus, pl. **to•phi** (tō′fŭs, -fī) **1.** SEE gouty tophus. **2.** A salivary calculus, or tartar. [L. a calcareous deposit from springs, tufa]

top•i•cal (top′i-kăl) Relating to a definite place or locality; local. [G. *topikos,* fr. *topos,* place]

top•i•cal ad•min•i•stra•tion (top′i-kăl ad-min′i-strā′shŭn) SYN transdermal.

top•i•cal an•es•the•si•a (top′i-kăl an′es-thē′zē-ă) Superficial loss of sensation in conjunctiva, mucous membranes, or skin, produced by direct application of local anesthetic solutions, ointments, or jellies.

Top 200 Med•i•ca•tions (top med′i-kā′shŭnz) SYN Top 200 Prescriptions.

topo-, top- Combining forms meaning place, topical. [G. *topos*]

topoanaesthesia [Br.] SYN topoanesthesia.

top•o•an•es•the•si•a (top′ō-an-es-thē′zē-ă) SYN topagnosis. SYN topoanaesthesia. [topo- + anesthesia]

To•po•gra•fov vi•rus (tō-pog′rā-fov vī′rus) A Hantavirus species found in Siberia in eastern Russia.

to•po•gra•phic or•i•en•ta•tion (top-ō-graf′ik ōr′ē-ĕn-tā′shŭn) Determination of the position of objects and settings and the route to a desired location.

to•pog•ra•phy (tō-pog′ră-fē) ANATOMY the description of any part of the body, especially in relation to a definite and limited area of the surface. [topo- + G. *graphē,* a writing]

To•po•lan•ski sign (tō-pō-lan′skē sin) Congestion of the pericorneal region of the eye in Graves disease.

top•o•nar•co•sis (top′ō-nahr-kō′sis) A localized cutaneous anesthesia. [topo- + narcosis]

Top 200 Pre•scrip•tions (top prĕ-skrip′shŭnz) An annual compilation of the top 200 prescriptions dispensed in the previous year provided by NDC Health. SYN Top 200 Medications.

TORCH syn•drome (tōrch sin′drōm) A group of infections with similar clinical manifestations, although symptoms may vary in degree and time of appearance: *t*oxoplasmosis, *o*ther infections, *r*ubella, *c*ytomegalovirus infection, and *h*erpes simplex. These infections may be associated with underlying HIV infection.

Torn•waldt ab•scess (tōrn′vahlt ab′ses) Chronic suppurative infection in a Tornwaldt cyst; symptoms include purulent nasopharyngeal discharge, halitosis, sore throat, pharyngotympanic tube dysfunction, occipital headache, and cervical myalgia and stiffness. SEE ALSO Tornwaldt syndrome.

Torn•waldt cyst (tōrn′vahlt sist) An inconstant midline cleft or bursa in the posterior wall of the pharynx, lined with mucous membrane; a remnant of the embryonic communication between the anterior notochord and the pharynx. SYN pharyngeal bursa.

Torn•waldt syn•drome (tōrn′vahlt sin′drōm) Nasopharyngeal discharge, occipital headache, and stiffness of posterior cervical muscles, with halitosis due to chronic infection of the pharyngeal bursa.

to•ro•vi•rus (tōr′ō-vī′rŭs) A genus in the family Coronaviridae that causes enteric infections in animals.

tor•pid (tōr′pid) Inactive; sluggish. [L. *torpidus,* fr. *torpeo,* to be sluggish]

tor•por (tōr′pŏr) Inactivity, sluggishness. [L. sluggishness, numbness]

torque (T) (tōrk) **1.** A rotatory force. **2.** DENTISTRY a torsion force applied to a tooth to produce or maintain crown or root movement. [L. *torqueo,* to twist]

torr (tōr) SYN mmHg.

Tor•re syn•drome (tōr′ē sin′drōm) Multiple sebaceous gland adenomas associated with multiple visceral malignancies, often colorectal carcinoma.

tor•sade de pointes (tōr-sahd′ dĕ pwahnt′) Literally, "twisting of the points," a form of ventricular tachycardia nearly always due to medications and characterized by a long QT interval and a "short-long-short" sequence in the beat preceding its onset. The QRS complexes during this rhythm tend to show a series of complexes points up followed by complexes points down, often with a narrow waist between. [Fr. *torsade,* fringe, twist, or coil, + *pointe,* point or tip (euphonious for "wave burst")]

tor•sion (tōr′shŭn) **1.** A twisting or rotation of a part on its long axis. **2.** Twisting of the cut end of an artery to arrest hemorrhage. **3.** Rotation of the eye around its anteroposterior axis. SEE ALSO intorsion, extorsion, dextrotorsion, levotorsion. [L. *torsio,* fr. *torqueo,* to twist]

tor•sion•al de•for•mi•ty (tor-shŭn′ăl dĕ-fōrm′i-tē) ORTHOPEDICS a deformity caused by rotation of a portion of an extremity with relationship to the long axis of the entire extremity.

tor•sion frac•ture (tōr′shŭn frak′shŭr) A fracture resulting from twisting of the limb.

tor•sion spa•sm (tōr′shŭn spazm) SYN dystonia.

tor•si•ver•sion, **tor•so•ver•sion** (tōr-si-vĕr′zhŭn, tōr-sō-vĕr′zhŭn) A malposition of a tooth in which it is rotated on its long axis. SYN torsoclusion (2).

tor•so (tōr′sō) The trunk; the body without relation to head or extremities. [It.]

tor•so•clu•sion (tōr′sō-klū-zhŭn) **1.** Acupressure performed by entering the needle in the tissues parallel with the artery, then turning it so that it crosses the artery transversely, and passing it into the tissues on the opposite side of the vessel. **2.** SYN torsiversion. [L. *torqueo,* to twist, + *claudo* or *cludo,* to close]

tor•ti•col•lar (tōr-ti-kol′ăr) Relating to or marked by torticollis.

tor•ti•col•lis (tōr-ti-kol′is) A contraction, often spasmodic, of the muscles of the neck, chiefly those supplied by the spinal accessory nerve; the head is drawn to one side and usually rotated so that the chin points to the other side. SYN wryneck, wry neck. [L. *tortus,* twisted, + *collum,* neck]

tor•tu•ous (tōr′chū-ŭs) Having many curves; full of turns and twists. [L. *tortuosus,* fr. *torqueo,* to twist]

Tor•u•lop•sis (tōr-yū-lop′sis) A genus of yeasts with smaller blastoconidia (2–4 mm) and with a wide attachment to the parent cell; the species *T. glabrata* is the causative agent of torulopsosis, usually in immunocompromised hosts.

tor•u•lop•so•sis (tōr-yū-lop′sō-sis) A usually opportunistic infection caused by *Torulopsis glabrata* and seen in patients with severe underlying disease or in immunocompromised patients; the disease may be bronchopulmonary, genitourinary, or septicemic. SEE ALSO *Torulopsis.*

tor•u•lus, pl. **tor•u•li** (tōr′yū-lŭs, -lī) A minute elevation or papilla. [L. dim. of *torus,* a protuberance, swelling]

to•rus, pl. **to•ri** (tōr′ŭs, -rī) **1.** A geometric figure formed by the revolution of a circle around the base of any of its arcs, such as the convex molding at the base of a pillar. **2.** A rounded swelling, such as that caused by a contracting muscle. SYN elevation. [L. swelling, knot, bulge]

to•rus frac•ture (tōr′ŭs frak′shŭr) A deformity in children consisting of a local bulging caused by the longitudinal compression of the soft bone; it occurs commonly in the radius or ulna or both. SYN buckle fracture.

to•rus man•di•bu•lar•is (tōr′ŭs man-dib-yū-lā′ris) A bony protuberance on the lingual aspect of the lower jaw in the canine-premolar region.

tor•us pal•a•tin•us (tōr′ŭs pal-a-tīn′is) A bony protuberance in the midline of the hard palate.

TOS Abbreviation for thoracic outlet syndrome.

to•tal a•no•ma•lous pul•mo•nar•y ven•ous re•turn (TAPVR) (tō′tăl a-nŏm′ă-lŭs pul′mŏ-nar′ē vē′nŭs rĕ-tŭrn′) SEE anomalous pulmonary venous connections, total or partial.

to•tal a•pha•si•a (tō′tăl ă-fā′zē-ă) SYN global aphasia.

to•tal bod•y hy•po•ther•mi•a (tō′tăl bod′ē hī′pō-thĕr′mē-ă) The deliberate reduction of total body temperature, to reduce tissue metabolism.

to•tal breath•ing cy•cle time (tō′tăl brēdh′ing sī′kĕl tīm) The time necessary for a complete breath (inhalation and exhalation); the period from the beginning of inspiratory flow of one breath to the beginning of inspiratory flow for the next breath.

to•tal com•mu•ni•ca•tion (tō′tăl kŏ-myū-ni-kā′shŭn) Habilitation of patients who are deaf or hearing impaired using any or all appropriate methods to enhance communication; particularly, the combination of manual and oral techniques. SYN simultaneous communication.

to•tal cri•coid cleft (tō′tăl krī′koyd kleft) SEE laryngotracheoesophageal cleft.

to·tal dai·ly en·er·gy ex·pen·di·ture (TDEE) (tō'tăl dā'lē en'ĕr-jē ek-spen'di-chŭr) Total daily caloric expenditure, consisting of basal metabolic rate, diet-induced thermogenesis, and energy expenditure for physical activity; in the clinical setting, TDEE can be estimated by calculation or measured by indirect calorimetry.

to·tal down·time (tō'tăl down'tīm) As used in EMS parlance, temporal duration from cardiac arrest to arrival in the emergency department.

to·tal end-di·a·stol·ic di·a·me·ter (tō'tăl-end dī'ă-stol'ik dī-am'ĕ-tĕr) Cross-sectional diameter of the left ventricle, including the septum and posterior wall thicknesses in diastole.

to·tal end-sys·tol·ic di·a·me·ter (tō'tăl end-sis-tol'ik dī-am'ĕ-tĕr) Cross-sectional diameter of the left ventricle, including the septum and posterior wall thicknesses in systole.

to·tal hip re·place·ment (THR) (tō'tăl hip rē-plās'mĕnt) Surgical procedure to remove the damaged or diseased joint completely and replace it with a man-made device to replace its function.

to·tal hy·per·o·pi·a (Ht) (tō'tăl hī'pĕr-ō'pē-ă) The sum of manifest hyperopia and latent hyperopia.

to·tal i·ron-bind·ing ca·pac·it·y (TIBC) (tō'tăl ī'ŏrn bīnd'ing kă-pas'i-tē) An indirect method of determining the transferrin level in serum. Transferrin is saturated by the addition of iron to a serum specimen. Excess iron is removed, and the specimen is analyzed for iron content. The result is the total amount of iron that can be bound by transferrin. This result is helpful in differentiating anemias: high TIBC is associated with iron deficiency, low TIBC is associated with excess iron.

to·tal joint ar·thro·plas·ty (tō'tăl joynt ahr'thrō-plas'tē) Arthroplasty in which both joint surfaces are replaced with artificial materials, usually metal and high-density plastic.

to·tal knee re·place·ment (TKR) (tō'tăl nē rē-plās'mĕnt) Surgical procedure to remove the damaged or diseased joint completely and replace it with a man-made device to replace its function.

to·tal lung ca·pac·i·ty (TLC) (tō'tăl lŭng kă-pas'i-tē) The inspiratory capacity plus the functional residual capacity, i.e., the volume of air contained in the lungs at the end of a maximal inspiration; also equals vital capacity plus residual volume.

to·tal par·en·ter·al nu·tri·tion (TPN) (tō'tăl pă-ren'tĕr-ăl nū-trish'ŭn) Feeding regimen maintained entirely by intravenous injection or other nongastrointestinal route. SEE ALSO hyperalimentation.

3-in-1 to·tal par·en·ter·al nu·tri·tion (TPN) (tō'tăl par-en'tĕr-al nū-trish-ŭn) Feeding regimen with all three components of nutrition: fats, protein, and dextrose.

to·tal trans·fu·sion (tō'tăl trans-fyū'zhŭn) SYN exchange transfusion.

to·ti·po·ten·cy, **to·ti·po·tence** (tō-ti-pō'ten-sē, tō-tip'ō-tĕns) The ability of a cell to differentiate into any type of cell and thus form a new organism or regenerate any part of an organism. [L. *totus,* entire, + *potentia,* power]

to·ti·po·tent, **to·ti·po·ten·tial** (tō-tip'ŏ-tĕnt, tō'ti-pō-ten'shăl) Relating to totipotency.

touch (tŭch) **1.** The sense by which slight contact with the skin or mucous membrane is perceived. **2.** SYN palpation (1). [Fr. *toucher*]

touch-me-not (tŭch'mē-not) SYN Siberian ginseng.

Tou·pet fun·do·pli·ca·tion (tū'pā fŭn'dō-pli-kā'shŭn) A partial posterior fundoplication, in which the stomach edge is secured to the esophagus; modifications of Toupet fundoplication are commonly used for laparoscopic fundoplication.

Tou·rette dis·ease (tūr-et' di-zēz') SYN Tourette syndrome.

Tou·rette syn·drome (tūr-et' sin'drōm) A tic disorder appearing in childhood, characterized by multiple motor tics and vocal tics present for longer than 1 year. Obsessive-compulsive behavior, attention-deficit disorder, and other psychiatric disorders may be associated; coprolalia and echolalia rarely occur; autosomal dominant inheritance. SYN Gilles de la Tourette syndrome, Tourette disease.

tour·ni·quet (tūr'ni-kĕt) An instrument for temporarily arresting the flow of blood to or from a distal part by pressure applied with an encircling device. [Fr. fr. *tourner,* to turn]

Tou·ton gi·ant cell (tū-tahn[h]' jī'ănt sel) A xanthoma cell in which the multiple nuclei are grouped around a small island of nonfoamy cytoplasm.

To·vell tube (tō-vel' tūb) An armored tracheal tube with a wire spiral embedded in the wall to prevent obstruction of the lumen when the tube is compressed and kinking when the tube is bent at a sharp angle.

toxaemia [Br.] SYN toxemia.

toxaemic [Br.] SYN toxemic.

tox·e·mi·a (tok-sē'mē-ă) **1.** Clinical manifestations observed during certain infectious diseases, assumed to be caused by toxins and other noxious substances elaborated by the infectious agent. **2.** The clinical syndrome caused by toxic substances in the blood. **3.** A lay term referring to the hypertensive disorders of pregnancy. SYN toxaemia. [G. *toxikon,* poison, + *haima,* blood]

tox·e·mic (tok-sē'mik) Pertaining to, affected

by, or manifesting the features of toxemia. SYN toxaemic.

tox·ic (tok′sik) **1.** SYN poisonous. **2.** Pertaining to a toxin. [G. *toxikon,* an arrow-poison]

tox·i·cant (toks′i-kănt) SYN intoxicant. SEE ALSO toxin.

tox·ic chem·i·cal a·gent (tok′sik kem′i-kăl ā′jĕnt) In U.S. military parlance, a chemical warfare agent designed to cause death or serious injury on the battlefield. The four main classes of toxic chemical agents are lung-damaging (pulmonary) agents, so-called blood agents (cyanides), vesicants, and nerve agents.

tox·ic cir·rho·sis (tok′sik sir-ō′sis) Hepatic disorder resulting from chronic poisoning or carbon tetrachloride exposure.

tox·ic ep·i·der·mal ne·crol·y·sis (TEN) (tok′sik ep′i-dĕr′măl nĕ-krol′i-sis) A syndrome in which a large portion of the skin becomes intensely erythematous, with epidermal necrosis and flaccid bullae, resulting from drug sensitivity or of unknown cause. See this page. SYN Lyell syndrome.

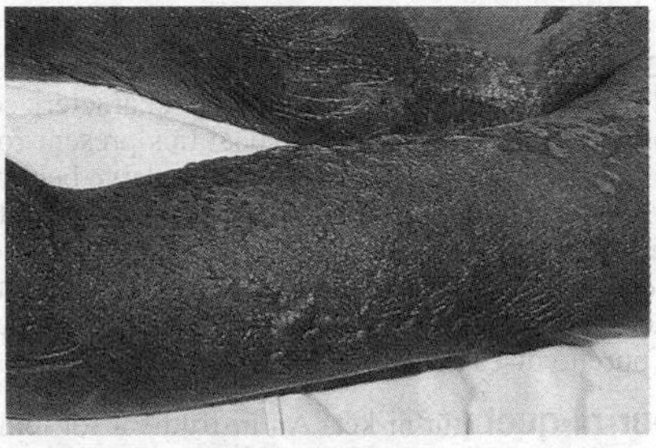

toxic epidermal necrolysis

tox·ic goi·ter (tok′sik goy′tĕr) A goiter that forms an excessive secretion, causing signs and symptoms of hyperthyroidism.

tox·ic he·mo·glo·bi·nur·i·a (tok′sik hē′mō-glō-bi-nyūr′ē-ă) The presence of hemoglobin in the urine resulting from ingestion of various poisons, certain blood diseases, and some types of infection.

tox·ic·i·ty (tok-sis′i-tē) The state of being poisonous.

tox·ic meg·a·co·lon (tok′sik meg′ă-kō-lŏn) Acute nonobstructive dilation of the colon, seen in fulminating ulcerative colitis and Crohn disease.

tox·ic ne·phro·sis (tok′sik ne-frō′sis) Acute oliguric renal failure due to chemical poisons, septicemia, or bacterial toxemia.

tox·ic neu·ri·tis (tok′sik nūr-ī′tis) Neuritis caused by an endogenous or exogenous toxin.

toxico-, tox-, toxi-, toxo- Combining forms meaning poison, toxin. [G. *toxikon,* bow, hence (arrow) poison, toxon, bow]

Tox·i·co·den·dron (tok′si-kō-den′dron) A genus of poisonous plants (also known as *Rhus*) with fruits and foliage that contain urushiol, which produces a contact dermatitis (rhus dermatitis); species include poison ivy (*T. radicans*), poison oak (*T. diversilobum*), and poison sumac (*T. vernix*). See this page. [toxico- + G. *dendron,* tree]

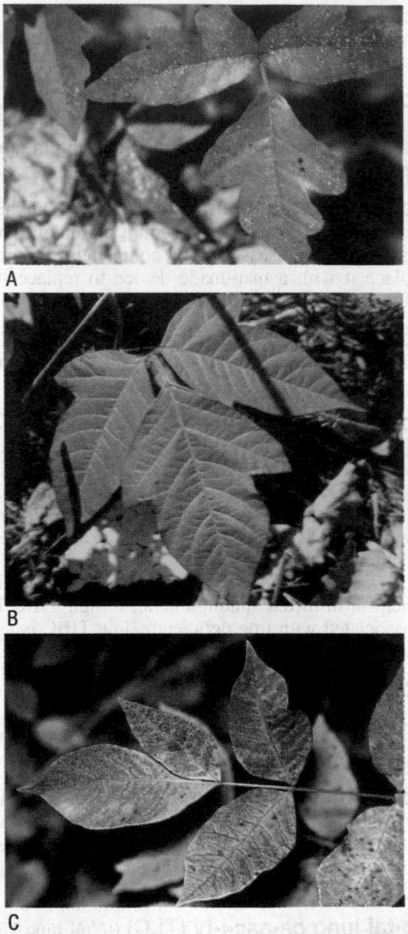

Toxicodendron: **(A) poison oak (Eastern); (B) poison ivy; (C) poison sumac**

tox·i·co·gen·ic (tok′si-kō-jen′ik) **1.** Producing a poison. **2.** Caused by a poison. [toxico- + G. *-gen,* producing]

tox·i·co·log·ic (tok′si-kō-loj′ik) Relating to toxicology.

tox·i·col·o·gist (tok′si-kol′ŏ-jist) A specialist or expert in toxicology.

tox·i·col·o·gy (tok′si-kol′ŏ-jē) The science of poisons, including their source, chemical composition, action, tests, and antidotes. [toxico- + G. *logos,* study]

tox·i·co·sis (tok′si-kō′sis) Any disease of toxic origin. [toxico- + G. *-osis,* condition]

tox·ic shock (tok′sik shok) SEE toxic shock syndrome.

tox·ic shock syn·drome (TSS) (tok′sik shok sin′drōm) Infection with toxin-producing staphylococci, occurring most often in the vagina of menstruating women using superabsorbent tampons; characterized by high fever, vomiting, diarrhea, a scarlatiniform rash followed by desquamation, and decreasing blood pressure and shock, which can result in death; hyperemia of the conjunctival, oropharyngeal, and vaginal mucous membranes also occurs.

tox·ic tet·a·nus (tok′sik tet′ă-nŭs) SYN drug tetanus.

tox·ic u·nit (tok′sik yū′nit) A unit formerly synonymous with minimal lethal dose but that, because of the instability of toxins, is now measured in terms of the quantity of standard antitoxin with which the toxin combines. SEE ALSO L doses, minimal lethal dose. SYN toxin unit.

tox·i·drome (tok′si-drōm) The constellation of clinical effects (i.e., signs and symptoms) characteristic of poisoning by a given kine of poison. SEE ALSO anticholinergic toxidrome, cholinergic toxidrome.

tox·i·gen·ic (tok′si-jen′ik) SYN toxinogenic.

tox·in (tok′sin) **1.** A noxious or poisonous substance that is formed or elaborated as an integral part of the cell or tissue, as an extracellular product (exotoxin), or as a combination of the two during the metabolism and growth of certain microorganisms and some higher plant and animal species. SEE ALSO mid-spectrum agent, biologic-warfare (BW) agent. **2.** A common misnomer for poison. SEE ALSO toxicant, chemical-warfare (CW) agent, biologic-warfare (BW) agent, mid-spectrum agent. [G. *toxikon,* poison]

tox·in·ic (tok-sin′ik) Relating to a toxin.

tox·i·no·gen·ic (tok′si-nō-jen′ik) Producing a toxin, said of an organism. SYN toxigenic. [toxin + G. *-gen,* producing]

tox·in u·nit (tok′sin yū′nit) SYN toxic unit.

tox·o·ca·ri·a·sis (tok′sō-kă-rī′ă-sis) Infection with nematodes of the genus *Toxocara;* parenterally migrating larvae, chiefly of *T. canis,* may cause visceral larva migrans; ocular involvement results in a solitary retinal granuloma, peripheral inflammatory masses, or chronic endophthalmitis.

tox·oid (tok′soyd) A toxin that has been treated (commonly with formaldehyde) so as to destroy its toxic property but retain its antigenicity, i.e., its capability of stimulating the production of antitoxin antibodies and thus of producing an active immunity. [toxin + G. *eidos,* resemblance]

tox·o·phore (tok′sō-fōr) Denoting the atomic group of the toxin molecule that carries the poisonous principle. [toxo- + G. *phoros,* bearing]

tox·oph·o·rous (tok-sof′ŏr-ŭs) Relating to the toxophore group of the toxin molecule.

Tox·o·plas·ma gon·di·i (tok-sō-plaz′mă gon′dē-ī) An abundant, widespread sporozoan species that is an intracellular, non-host-specific parasite in a great variety of vertebrates. It develops its sexual cycle, leading to oocyst production, exclusively in cats and other felids; proliferative stages (tachyzoites) and tissue cysts (containing bradyzoites) develop in a wide variety of animal species. [G. *toxon,* bow or arc, + *plasma,* anything formed]

tox·o·plas·mo·sis (tok′sō-plaz-mō′sis) A disease caused by the protozoan parasite *Toxoplasma gondii,* which can produce a variety of syndromes in humans. Prenatally acquired infection can result in abnormalities such as microcephalus or hydrocephalus at birth, jaundice with hepatosplenomegaly or meningoencephalitis in early childhood, or delayed ocular lesions such as chorioretinitis in later childhood. Postnatally acquired human infections typically remain subclinical; if clinical disease does occur, symptoms include fever, lymphadenopathy, headache, myalgia, and fatigue, with eventual recovery, except in the immunocompromised patient, in whom fatal encephalitis often develops.

tox·o·py·rim·i·dine (tok′sō-pi-rim′i-dēn) One of the products resulting from the hydrolysis of thiamin by thiaminase and appearing in the urine; a competitive inhibitor of pyridoxal.

tox screen (toks skrēn) A colloquial and jargonistic usage indicating a battery of blood tests used to determine the presence of drugs and ethanol in the bloodstream.

Toyn·bee ma·neu·ver (toyn′bē mă-nū′vĕr) Action that accomplishes pharyngotympanic (auditory) tube opening when the patient closes mouth, holds nose, and swallows. SEE ALSO Valsalva maneuver, politzerization.

Toyn·bee tube (toyn′bē tūb) A tube by which one can listen to the sounds in a patient's ear during politzerization.

tPA Abbreviation for tissue plasminogen activator.

TPN Abbreviation for total parenteral nutrition.

TPN, TPNH Abbreviation for triphosphopyridine nucleotide and its reduced form (the oxidized form is TPN^+).

TPO Abbreviation for treatment, payment, health care operations.

TR Abbreviation for repetition time.

tra•bec•u•la, gen. and pl. **tra•bec•u•lae** (tră-bek′yū-lă, -lē) [TA] **1.** One of the supporting bundles of fibers traversing the substance of a structure, usually derived from the capsule or one of the fibrous septa. **2.** A small piece of the spongy substance of bone usually interconnected with other similar pieces. **3.** HISTOPATHOLOGY a band of neoplastic tissue two or more cells wide. [L. dim. of *trabs,* a beam]

tra•bec•u•lae car•ne•ae (of right and left ven•tri•cles) (tră-bek′yū-lē kahr′nē-ē rīt left ven-tri′kĕlz) Muscular bundles on the lining walls of the ventricles of the heart.

tra•bec•u•lar (tră-bek′yū-lăr) Relating to or containing trabeculae.

tra•bec•u•lar bone (tră-bek′yū-lăr bōn) SYN substantia spongiosa.

tra•bec•u•lar re•tic•u•lum (tră-bek′yū-lăr rĕ-tik′yū-lŭm) The network of fibers (pectinate ligaments) at the iridocorneal angle between the anterior chamber of the eye and the venous sinus of the sclera; it contains spaces between the fibers that are involved in drainage of the aqueous humor, and is composed of two portions: the corneoscleral part, the part attached to the sclera, and the uveal part, the part attached to the iris.

tra•bec•u•lo•plas•ty (tră-bek′yū-lō-plas-tē) Photocoagulation of the trabecular meshwork of the eye using a laser in the treatment of glaucoma.

tra•bec•u•lot•o•my (tră-bek-yū-lot′ŏ-mē) Surgical opening of the sinus venosus sclerae (canal of Schlemm) to treat glaucoma. [trabekula + G. *tomē,* incision]

trace el•e•ments (trās el′ĕ-mĕnts) Elements present in minute amounts in the body (e.g., Zn, Se, V, Ni, Mg, Mn), many of which are essential in metabolism or for the manufacture of essential compounds.

trace min•er•als (trās min′ĕr-ălz) Minerals that are essential to the body in quantities less than 100 mg/day.

trac•er (trā′sĕr) **1.** An element or compound containing atoms that can be distinguished from their normal counterparts by physical means (e.g., radioactivity assay or mass spectrography) and can thus be used to follow (trace) the metabolism of the normal substances. **2.** A colored substance (e.g., a dye) used as a tracer to follow the flow of water. **3.** An instrument used in dissecting out nerves and blood vessels. **4.** A mechanical device with a marking point attached to one jaw and a graph plate or tracing plate attached to the other jaw; used to record the direction and extent of movements of the mandible. SEE ALSO tracing (2). [M.E. track, fr. O. Fr. *tracier*, to make one's way, fr. L. *traho*, pp. *tractum*, to draw, + *-er*, agent suffix]

tra•che•a, pl. **tra•che•ae** (trā′kē-ă, -kē-ē) [TA] The air tube extending from the larynx into the thorax (level of the fifth or sixth thoracic vertebra), where it bifurcates into the right and left main bronchi. The trachea is composed of 16–20 rings of hyaline cartilage connected by a membrane (anular ligament); posteriorly, the rings are deficient for one fifth to one third of their circumference, the interval forming the membranous wall being closed by a fibrous membrane containing smooth muscular fibers. Internally, the mucosa is composed of a pseudostratified ciliated columnar epithelium with mucous goblet cells; numerous small mixed mucous and serous glands occur, the ducts of which open to the surface of the epithelium. See page B16. SYN windpipe. [G. *tracheia artēria,* rough artery]

tra•che•al (trā′kē-ăl) Relating to the trachea.

tra•che•al car•ti•lag•es (trā′kē-ăl kahr′ti-lăj-ĕz) The 16–20 incomplete rings of hyaline cartilage forming the skeleton of the trachea; the rings are deficient posteriorly for one fifth to one third of their circumference. SYN cartilagines tracheales [TA].

tra•che•a•lis mus•cle (trā-kē-ā′lis mŭs′ĕl) The band of smooth muscular fibers in the fibrous membrane connecting posteriorly the ends of the tracheal rings. SYN musculus trachealis [TA].

tra•che•al tube (trā′kē-ăl tūb) A flexible tube inserted nasally, orally, or through a tracheotomy into the trachea to provide an airway, as in tracheal intubation. SYN endotracheal tube.

tra•che•al veins (trā′kē-ăl vānz) Several small venous trunks from the trachea, emptying into the brachiocephalic veins or the superior vena cava.

tra•che•i•tis (trā-kē-ī′tis) Inflammation of the lining membrane of the trachea. SYN trachitis. [trachea + G. *-itis,* inflammation]

trach•e•lec•to•my (trāk-ĕ-lek′tŏ-mē) SYN cervicectomy. [trachel- + G. *ektomē,* excision]

trach•e•lism, **trach•e•lis•mus** (trāk′ĕ-lizm, -liz′mŭs) A bending backward of the neck, such as sometimes ushers in an epileptic attack. [G. *trachēlismos,* a seizing by the throat]

trach•e•li•tis (trāk-ĕ-lī′tis) SYN cervicitis.

trachelo-, trachel- Combining forms denoting neck. [G. *trachēlos*]

trach•e•lo•breg•mat•ic di•a•me•ter (trāk′ĕ-lo-breg-mat′ik dī-am′ĕ-tĕr) The diameter of the fetal head from the middle of the anterior fontanelle to the neck.

trach•e•lo•dyn•i•a (trā′kĕ-lō-din′ē-ă) SYN cervicodynia. [trachelo- + G. *odynē,* pain]

trach•e•lor•rha•phy (trā′kĕ-lōr′ă-fē) Repair by suture of a laceration of the cervix uteri. SYN Emmet operation. [trachelo- + G. *rhaphē,* suture]

trach•e•lot•o•my (trā′kĕ-lot′ŏ-mē) SYN cervicotomy. [trachelo- + G. *tomē*, incision]

tracheo-, trache- Combining forms meaning the trachea. [see trachea]

tra•che•o•aer•o•cele (trā′kē-ō-ār′ō-sēl) An air cyst in the neck caused by distention of a tracheocele. [tracheo- + G. *aēr*, air, + *kēlē*, hernia]

tra•che•o•bron•chi•al (trā′kē-ō-brong′kē-ăl) Relating to both trachea and bronchi, denoting especially a set of lymph nodes.

tra•che•o•bron•chi•al di•ver•tic•u•lum (trā′kē-ō-brong′kē-ăl dī′vĕr-tik′yū-lŭm) SYN respiratory diverticulum.

tra•che•o•bron•chi•tis (trā′kē-ō-brong-kī′tis) Inflammation of the mucous membrane of the trachea and bronchi.

tra•che•o•bron•chos•co•py (trā′kē-ō-brong-kos′kŏ-pē) Inspection of the interior of the trachea and bronchi. [tracheo- + bronchus, + G. *skopeō*, to view]

tra•che•o•cele (trā′kē-ō-sēl) A protrusion of the mucous membrane through a defect in the wall of the trachea. [tracheo- + G. *kēlē*, hernia]

tra•che•o•e•soph•a•ge•al (trā′kē-ō-ē-sof-fă′jē-ăl) Relating to the trachea and the esophagus. SYN tracheo-oesophageal.

tra•che•o•e•soph•a•ge•al fis•tu•la (trā′kē-ō-ē-sof-fă′jē-ăl fis′chū-lă) Neonatal GI disorder in which a connection exists between the esophagus and the trachea. It may result in gastric juice reflux after feeding, allowing gastric acids to cross the fistula, thus irritating the trachea.

tra•che•o•e•soph•a•ge•al folds (trā′kē-ō-ē-sof-fă′jē-ăl fōldz) A pair of longitudinal folds in the laryngotracheal diverticulum that unite to form a tracheoesophageal septum, which divides the diverticulum into the esophagus and the laryngotracheal tube. SYN transesophageal folds, transesophageal ridges.

tra•che•o•e•so•pha•ge•al punc•ture (TEP), tra•che•o•e•so•pha•ge•al shunt (trā′kē-ō-ē-sof-fă′jē-ăl pungk′shŭr, shŭnt) Surgical procedure connecting the trachea and esophagus. In laryngectomies, the puncture, in combination with a prosthetic valve, allows exhaled air from the lungs to enter the esophagus for production of speech. SYN tracheo-oesophageal puncture.

tra•che•o•la•ryn•ge•al (trā′kē-ō-lă-rin′jē-ăl) Relating to the trachea and the larynx.

tra•che•o•ma•la•ci•a (trā′kē-ō-mă-lā′shē-ă) Degeneration of elastic and connective tissue of the trachea. [tracheo- + G. *malakia*, softness]

tra•che•o•meg•a•ly (trā′kē-ō-meg′ă-lē) An abnormally dilated trachea that may, like bronchiectasis, result from infection or prolonged positive pressure ventilation. [tracheo- + G. *megas* (*megal-*), large]

tracheo-oesophageal [Br.] SYN tracheoesophageal.

tracheo-oesophageal puncture [Br.] SYN tracheoesophageal puncture.

tracheo-oesophageal shunt [Br.] SYN tracheoesophageal shunt.

tra•che•o•path•i•a, tra•che•op•a•thy (trā′kē-ō-path′ē-ă, -op′ă-thē) Any disease of the trachea. [tracheo- + G. *pathos*, disease]

tra•che•o•pha•ryn•ge•al (trā′kē-ō-fă-rin′jē-ăl) Relating to both trachea and pharynx; denoting an occasional band of muscular fibers passing from the inferior constrictor of the pharynx to the trachea.

tra•che•oph•o•ny (trā′kē-of′ŏ-nē) The hollow voice sound heard in auscultating over the trachea. SEE ALSO bronchophony. [tracheo- + G. *phōnē*, voice]

tra•che•o•plas•ty (trā′kē-ō-plas-tē) Surgical repair of the trachea. [tracheo- + G. *plastos*, formed]

tra•che•or•rha•gi•a (trā′kē-ō-rā′jē-ă) Hemorrhage from the mucous membrane of the trachea. [tracheo- + G. *rhēgnymi*, to burst forth]

tra•che•os•chi•sis (trā′kē-os′ki-sis) A fissure into the trachea. [tracheo- + G. *schisis*, fissure]

tra•che•o•scop•ic (trā′kē-ō-skop′ik) Relating to tracheoscopy.

tra•che•os•co•py (trā′kē-os′kŏ-pē) Inspection of the interior of the trachea. [tracheo- + G. *skopeō*, to examine]

tra•che•o•ste•no•sis (trā′kē-ō-stĕ-nō′sis) Narrowing of the lumen of the trachea. [tracheo- + G. *stenōsis*, constriction]

tra•che•os•to•my (trā′kē-os′tŏ-mē) SYN tracheotomy. See page 1578. [tracheo- + G. *stoma*, mouth]

tra•che•os•to•my tube (trā′kē-os′tŏ-mē tūb) A curved tube used to keep the opening free after tracheotomy; may be metal or plastic.

tra•che•ot•o•my (trā′kē-ot′ŏ-mē) The operation of creating an opening into the trachea, usually intended to be temporary. SYN tracheostomy. [tracheo- + G. *tomē*, incision]

tra•che•ot•o•my tube (trā′kē-ot′ŏ-mē tūb) A curved tube used to keep the opening free after tracheotomy. May be metal or plastic.

Tra•chi•plei•stoph•or•a (trā-kē-plī-stof′ŏr-ă) A genus of microsporidia that can infect humans and cause myositis, keratoconjunctivitis, and sinusitis in the immunocompromised person.

tra•chi•tis (trā-kī′tis) SYN tracheitis.

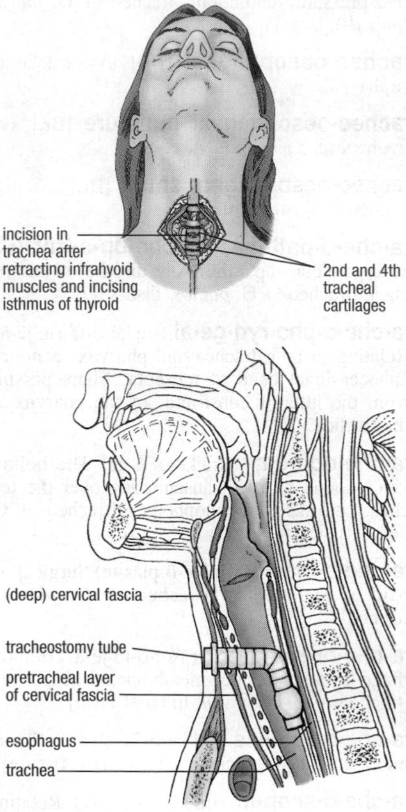

tracheostomy

tra·cho·ma (tră-kō′mă) Chronic inflammation and hypertrophy of the conjunctiva, marked by the formation of minute grayish or yellowish translucent granules, caused by *Chlamydia trachomatis*. SYN Egyptian ophthalmia, granular ophthalmia. [G. *trachōma,* fr. *trachys,* rough, harsh]

tra·cho·ma bod·ies (tră-kō′mă bod′ēz) Distinctive, complex, intracytoplasmic forms found in the conjunctival epithelial cells of patients in the acute phase of trachoma.

tra·chom·a·tous (tră-kō′mă-tŭs) Relating to or suffering from trachoma.

tra·chom·a·tous con·junc·ti·vi·tis (tră-kō′mă-tŭs kŏn-jŭngk′ti-vī′tis) A chronic infection of the conjunctiva due to *Chlamydia trachomatis*, characterized by conjunctival follicles and subsequent cicatrization. SEE ALSO trachoma. SYN granular conjunctivitis.

tra·chom·a·tous ker·a·ti·tis (tră-kō′mă-tŭs ker′ă-tī′tis) SEE pannus, corneal pannus.

trac·ing (trās′ing) **1.** A graphic reproduction of the outline or salient features of a physical object or structure. SEE ALSO curve. **2.** Any graphic display of electrical or mechanical events in normal or diseased tissues or organs, as detected or measured by diagnostic instruments. SEE ALSO curve. **3.** DENTISTRY a line or lines, inscribed on a table or plate by a pointed instrument, representing a record of movements of the mandible; may be extraoral (made outside the oral cavity) or intraoral (made within the oral cavity).

tract (trakt) An elongated area, e.g., path, track, way. SEE ALSO fascicle. SYN tractus. [L. *tractus,* a drawing out]

trac·tion (trak′shŭn) **1.** The act of drawing or pulling, as by an elastic or spring force. **2.** A pulling or dragging force exerted on a limb in a distal direction. [L. *tractio,* fr. *traho,* pp. *tractus,* to draw]

trac·tion di·ver·tic·u·lum (trak′shŭn dī′vĕr-tik′yū-lŭm) A diverticulum formed by the pulling force of contracting bands of adhesion, occurring mainly in the distal esophagus, from tuberculous hilar or mediastinal lymphadenitis.

trac·tion e·pi·phy·sis (trak′shŭn e-pif′i-sis) A secondary center of ossification at the site of attachment of a tendon.

trac·tot·o·my (trak-tot′ŏ-mē) Interruption of a nerve tract in the brainstem or spinal cord. [L. *tractus,* tract, + G. *tomē,* incision]

trac·tus, gen. and pl. **trac·tus** (trak′tŭs) SYN tract. [L. a drawing, drawing out, extent, tract, fr. *traho,* pp. *tractus,* to draw]

trac·tus il·i·o·pub·i·cus (trak′tŭs il′ē-ō-pyū′bik-ŭs) [TA] SYN iliopubic tract.

trac·tus op·ti·cus (trak′tŭs op′tik-ŭs) [TA] SYN optic tract.

tra·di·tion·al Chi·nese med·i·cine (TCM) (tră-di′shŭn-ăl chī-nēz′ med′i-sin) An ancient system (begun about 200 BCE) of healing; based on the concepts of balance, moderation, and harmony, from Taoism. Network of 12 channels carry life energy (qi) to organs. Symptoms represent disharmony in the balance of the flow of energy. Techniques used to restore harmony include herbal remedies, qi gong, massage, cupping, acupuncture, and acupressure.

tra·gal (trā′găl) Relating to the tragus.

tra·gal la·mi·na (trā′găl lam′i-nă) A longitudinal curved plate of cartilage, the beginning of the cartilaginous portion of the external acoustic meatus.

Tra·ger bod·y·work (trā′gĕr bod′ē-wŏrk) Exercise therapeutic approach that gently rocks, cradles, and moves the client's body; intended to promote relaxation, increase mobility, and accentuate mental clarity.

tra·gi (trā′jī) **1.** Plural of tragus. **2.** Hairs growing at the entrance to the external acoustic meatus.

tra·gi·cus mus·cle (trā′ji-kŭs mŭs′ĕl) A band

of vertical muscular fibers on the outer surface of the tragus of the ear. SYN musculus tragicus [TA], muscle of tragus.

tra•gus, pl. **tra•gi** (trā′gŭs, -jī) **1.** A tonguelike projection of the cartilage of the auricle in front of the opening of the external acoustic meatus and continuous with the cartilage of this canal. SYN hircus (3). **2.** SEE tragi (2). [G. *tragos,* goat, in allusion to the hairs growing on the part, like a goatee]

TRAIL A member of the tumor necrosis factor ligand family. which rapidly induces apoptosis in a variety of transformed cell lines. SYN apo-2L.

trai•ner (trā′nĕr) One who instructs, drills, corrects, or otherwise supports another in the acquisition of a skill or the performance of an activity. [Med. L. *traginare,* to direct the growth of a plant]

train•ing (trān′ing) An organized system of education, instruction, or discipline.

train•ing group (trān′ing grūp) **1.** Any group emphasizing training in self-awareness and group dynamics. **2.** BIOWARFARE group of people practicing to respond to an act of bioterrorism.

train•ing-sen•si•tive zone (trān′ing-sen′si-tiv zōn) Level of exercise heart rate, usually 65–95% of heart rate maximum or 50–85% of heart rate reserve, required to induce training improvements in aerobic fitness. Exercise heart rates below the 70% threshold are generally offset by extending exercise duration. SEE ALSO target heart rate. SYN target heart rate range.

trait (trāt) A qualitative characteristic; a discrete attribute as contrasted with metrical character. A trait is amenable to segregation rather than quantitative analysis; it is an attribute of phenotype, not of genotype. [Fr. from L. *tractus,* a drawing out, extension]

trance (trans) An altered state of consciousness as in hypnosis, catalepsy, or ecstasy. [L. *transeo,* to go across]

tran•quil•iz•er (trang′kwi-lī-zĕr) A drug that reduces anxiety without sedating or depressant effects.

trans. Abbreviation for transdermal.

♲**trans- 1.** Prefix denoting across, through, beyond; opposite of *cis-*. **2.** GENETICS denoting the location of two genes on opposite chromosomes of a homologous pair. **3.** ORGANIC CHEMISTRY a form of geometric isomerism in which the atoms attached to two carbon atoms, joined by double bonds, are located on opposite sides of the molecule. **4.** BIOCHEMISTRY a prefix to a group name in an enzyme name or a reaction denoting transfer of that group from one compound to another. [L. *trans,* through, across]

trans•a•cet•y•lase (tranz-ă-sĕt′i-lās) SYN acetyltransferase.

trans•a•cet•y•la•tion (tranz′ă-sĕt′i-lā′shŭn) Transfer of an acetyl group (CH_3CO–), from one compound to another; such reactions, usually involving formation of acetyl-CoA, occur notably in the initiation of the tricarboxylic acid cycle by the transfer of an acetyl group to oxaloacetate to form citrate.

trans•ac•tion•al a•nal•y•sis (tranz-ak′shŭn-ăl ă-nal′i-sis) A psychotherapy system, used in both individual and group treatment, involving a systematic understanding of the qualities of interpersonal interactions in the treatment sessions; includes four components: 1) structural analysis of intrapsychic phenomena; 2) transactional analysis proper, determination of the currently dominant ego state (parent, child, or adult) of each participant; 3) game analysis, identification of the games played in interactions and of the gratifications provided; 4) script analysis, uncovering of the causes of the patient's emotional problems.

trans•ac•yl•ase (tranz-as′i-lāz) SYN acyltransferase.

trans air•way pres•sure (tranz ār′wā presh′ŭr) The difference between the pressure at the airway opening and the pressure in the lungs (i.e., pressure at airway opening minus pressure in lungs).

trans•al•do•la•tion (tranz′al-dō-lā′shŭn) A reaction involving the transfer of an aldol group from one compound to another; such reactions generally involve the sugar phosphates and occur in the phosphogluconate oxidation pathway of carbohydrate catabolism.

trans•am•i•di•na•tion (tranz-am′i-di-nā′shŭn) A reaction involving the transfer of an amidine group from one compound to another; the amidine donor is generally L-arginine and the reaction is of significance in the biosynthesis of creatine.

trans•am•i•nase (tranz-am′i-nās) SYN aminotransferase.

trans•am•i•na•tion (tranz′am-i-nā′shŭn) The reaction between an amino acid and an α-keto acid through which the amino group is transferred from the former to the latter.

trans•bron•chi•al nee•dle as•pir•a•tion (TBNA) (trans-brong′kē-ăl nē′dĕl as′pir-ā′shŭn) Biopsy of a structure or region adjacent to a bronchus by means of a needle introduced through a bronchoscope. Diagnostic procedure used in cytology and histology studies of intrathoracic and respiratory disease.

trans•ca•lent (trans-kā′lent) SYN diathermanous. [trans- + L. *caleo,* to be warm]

trans•car•bam•o•y•las•es (trans-kahr-bam′ō-i-lā-sēz) SYN carbamoyltransferases.

trans•car•box•y•las•es (trans-kahr-boks′i-lās-ēz) SYN carboxyltransferases.

trans·cei·ver (tran-sē′vĕr) A coil that both transmits radiofrequency and receives the magnetic resonance signal.

trans·cell·u·lar flu·ids (tranz-sel′yū-lăr flū′idz) The fluids that are not inside cells, but are separated from plasma and interstitial fluid by cellular barriers (e.g., cerebrospinal fluid, synovial fluid, pleural fluid).

trans·cer·vi·cal thy·mec·to·my (tranz-sĕr′vik-ăl thī-mek′tŏ-mē) Removal of the thymus gland through a cervical incision.

trans·co·bal·a·mins (trans-kō-bal′ă-minz) Substances included in "R binder," the name given a family of cobalamin-binding proteins; deficiencies have been associated with low serum cobalamin levels, and can lead to megaloblastic anemia.

trans·co·chle·ar ap·proach (trans-kok′lē-ăr ă-prōch′) A surgical approach to the internal auditory canal through the cochlea.

trans·cor·ti·cal (trans-kōr′ti-kăl) **1.** Across or through the cortex of the brain, ovary, kidney, or other organ. **2.** From one part of the cerebral cortex to another; denoting the various association tracts.

trans·cor·ti·cal a·pha·si·a (trans-kōr′ti-kăl ă-fā′zē-ă) An aphasia in which the ability to imitate speech is preserved but other language abilities are impaired. In transcortical sensory aphasia, other symptoms are similar to those of receptive aphasia; in transcortical motor aphasia, other symptoms are similar to those of expressive aphasia.

trans·cor·tin (trans-kōr′tin) An α_2-globulin in blood that binds cortisol and corticosterone; the principal corticosteroid-binding protein in the plasma. SYN corticosteroid-binding globulin.

tran·script (trans′kript) Messenger RNA (mRNA), the expressed product of a gene.

tran·scrip·tase (tran-skrip′tās) A polymerase associated with the process of transcription; especially the DNA-dependent RNA polymerase. [L. *transcribo*, pp. *transcriptum*, to copy, + -ase]

tran·scrip·tion (tran-skrip′shŭn) **1.** Transfer of genetic code information from one kind of nucleic acid to another, especially with reference to the process by which a base sequence of messenger RNA is synthesized (by an RNA polymerase) on a template of complementary DNA. **2.** Process in which medical transcriptionists convert dictated health care information into a printed document.

tran·scrip·tion-based chain re·ac·tion (tran-skrip′shŭn-bāst chān rē-ak′shŭn) A technique for target amplification of DNA or RNA in which reverse transcriptase is used to produce a single-stranded DNA molecule for each DNA or RNA target; this molecule is used as a template for further amplification.

tran·scrip·tion-me·di·at·ed am·pli·fi·ca·tion (trans-krip′shŭn mē′dē-ā-tĕd amp′li-fi-kā′shŭn) An amplification assay that is similar to nucleic acid sequence-based amplification.

trans·cul·tu·ral nur·sing (trans-kŭl′chŭr-ăl nŭrs′ing) Provision of nursing care sensitive to cultural differences among members of a society.

trans·cu·ta·ne·ous blood gas mo·ni·tor (trans-kyū-tā′nē-ŭs blŭd gas mon′i-tŏr) A device that uses miniature electrodes applied to the skin to estimate blood oxygen and carbon dioxide tension; the transcutaneous carbon dioxide tension ($tcPCO_2$) provides a relatively accurate estimate of arterial carbon dioxide ($PaCO_2$) in all age groups; the estimate of transcutaneous oxygen tension ($tcPO_2$) is more accurate in neonates and small children.

trans·cu·ta·ne·ous e·lec·tri·cal nerve stim·u·la·tion (TENS) (trans-kyū′tā-nē-us ĕ-lek′trik-al nĕrv stim′yŭ-lā′shŭn) Noninvasive device that inhibits pain signals, thus reducing pain perception, as well as stimulating the body's own pain control mechanisms. Used for chronic pain and labor; can be controlled by the patient. See this page.

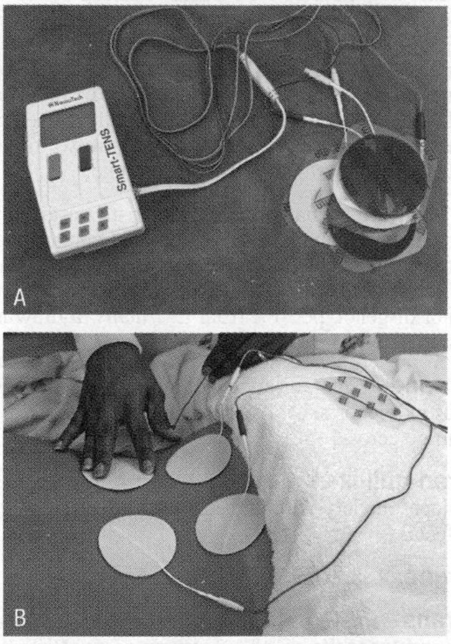

transcutaneous electrical nerve stimulation: (A) TENS unit; (B) applying TENS electrodes

trans·cy·to·sis (tranz-sī-tō′sis) A mechanism for transcellular transport in which a cell encloses extracellular material in an invagination of the cell membrane to form a vesicle (endocytosis), then moves the vesicle across the cell to eject the material through the opposite cell membrane by the reverse process (exocytosis). SYN vesicular transport.

trans•der•mal (trans.) (trans-dĕr′mal) Entering through the dermis or skin, as in administration of a drug applied to the skin in ointment or patch form. SYN topical administration.

trans•dis•cip•li•nar•y (trans-dis′ip-li-nar-ē) A unified provision of services as two or more professional disciplines work simultaneously in a single integrated plan of care.

trans•duc•er (trans-dū′sĕr) A device that converts energy from one form to another (e.g., from electrical energy into ultrasonic energy).

trans•du•cer cell (trans-dū′sĕr sel) Any cell responding to a mechanical, thermal, photic, or chemical stimulus by generating an electrical impulse synaptically transmitted to a sensory neuron in contact with the cell.

trans•duc•tion (trans-dŭk′shŭn) **1.** Transfer of genetic material (and its phenotypic expression) from one cell to another by viral infection. **2.** A form of genetic recombination in bacteria. **3.** Conversion of energy from one form to another. [trans- + L. *duco,* pp. *ductus,* to lead across]

tran•sec•tion (tran-sek′shŭn) **1.** A cross-section. **2.** Cutting across. SYN transsection. [trans- + L. *seco,* pp. *sectus,* to cut]

trans•es•oph•a•ge•al ech•o•car•di•og•ra•phy (tranz-ē-sō-fā′jē-ăl ek′ō-kahr-dē-og′ră-fē) Recording of the echocardiogram from a swallowed transducer. SYN transoesophageal echocardiography.

trans•e•soph•a•ge•al folds (tranz-ē-sō-fā′jē-ăl fōldz) SYN tracheoesophageal folds.

trans•e•soph•a•ge•al rid•ges (tranz-ē-sō-fā′jē-ăl rij′ĕz) SYN tracheoesophageal folds.

trans fat•ty ac•id (tranz fa′tē as′id) Trans form of a monounsaturated fatty acid usually produced as a result of the hydrogenation of polyunsaturated plant oils during industrial processing.

trans•fec•tion (trans-fek′shŭn) A method of gene transfer using infection of a cell with nucleic acid (as from a retrovirus) resulting in subsequent viral replication in the transfected cell. [trans- + in*fection*]

trans•fer (trans′fĕr) **1.** Process of removal or change of place. **2.** A condition in which learning in one situation influences learning in another situation; a carryover of learning that may be positive in effect, as when learning one behavior facilitates the learning of something else, or may be negative, as when one habit interferes with the acquisition of a later one. SYN transmission (1). [L. *trans-fero,* to bear across]

trans•fer•as•es (trans′fĕr-ās-ĕz) Enzymes transferring one-carbon groups, acyl and glucosyl residues, alkyl or aryl groups, nitrogenous groups, phosphorus-containing groups, and sulfur-containing groups.

trans•fer de•vic•es (trans′fĕr dĕ-vīs′ĕz) A piece of equipment used to transfer blood from a syringe to an evacuated tube with a closed system. This reduces risk of needlestick injury to the phlebotomist.

trans•fer•ence (trans-fĕr′ĕns) **1.** Conveyance of an object from one place to another. **2.** Shifting of symptoms from one side of the body to the other, as seen in certain cases of conversion hysteria. **3.** Displacement of affect from one person or one idea to another. **4.** PSYCHOANALYSIS generally applied to the projection of feelings, thoughts, and wishes onto the analyst, who has come to represent some person from the patient's past.

trans•fer•ence neu•ro•sis (trans-fĕr′ĕns nūr-ō′sis) PSYCHOANALYSIS the phenomenon of the patient's developing a strong emotional relationship with the analyst.

trans•fer fac•tor (trans′fĕr fak′tŏr) **1.** The transfer gene of a conjugative plasmid, especially of the resistance plasmid. **2.** A dialyzable extract that is obtained from the leukocytes of a person with a delayed-type sensitivity and that, following injection into the skin of a nonsensitive person, transfers the specific sensitivity to the recipient. **3.** SYN elongation factor.

trans•fer for•ceps (trans′fĕr fōr′seps) Sterile forceps used to add items to and arrange other items on a sterile tray.

trans•fer•rin (trans-fĕr′in) **1.** A nonheme β_1-globulin of the plasma, capable of associating reversibly with up to 1.25 mcg of iron per gram, and acting therefore as an iron-transporting protein. **2.** A glycoprotein, found in mammalian milk (lactoferrin) and egg white (conalbumin, ovotransferrin), that binds and transports iron (Fe^{3+}). [trans- + L. *ferrum,* iron, + -ia]

trans•fer•rin sat•ur•a•tion (trans-fĕr′in sa-chŭr-ā′shŭn) A calculation, expressed in percentages, of the amount of transferrin that is bound to iron. Determined by measuring serum iron and total iron-binding capacity (TIBC): serum iron × 100 = percentage saturation TIBC; helpful in differentiating anemias: a low transferrin saturation is associated with iron deficiency states; high with excess iron.

trans•fer RNA (tRNA) (trans′fĕr) Short-chain RNA molecules present in cells in at least 20 varieties, each variety capable of combining with a specific amino acid (see aminoacyl-tRNA). By joining (through their anticodons) with particular spots (codons) along the messenger RNA molecule and carrying their amino acyl residues along, they lead to the formation of protein molecules with a specific amino acid arrangement. SYN soluble RNA.

trans•fix•ion (trans-fik′shŭn) A maneuver in amputation in which the knife is passed from side to side through the soft parts, close to the bone, and the muscles are then divided from within in an outward direction. [L. *transfixio*]

trans•fix•ion su•ture (trans-fik′shŭn sū′chŭr) **1.** A criss-cross stitch so placed as to control bleeding from a tissue surface or small vessel when tied. **2.** A suture used to fix the columella to the nasal septum.

trans•for•ma•tion (trans-fōr-mā′shŭn) **1.** SYN metamorphosis. **2.** A change of one tissue into another, such as cartilage into bone. **3.** In metals, a change in phase and physical properties in the solid state caused by heat treatment. **4.** MICROBIAL GENETICS transfer of genetic information between bacteria by means of "naked" intracellular DNA fragments derived from bacterial donor cells and incorporated into a competent recipient cell. [L. *trans-formo,* pp. *-atus,* to transform]

trans•form•ing fac•tor (trans-fōrm′ing fak′tŏr) The DNA responsible for bacterial transformation.

trans•fuse (trans-fyūz′) To perform transfusion.

trans•fu•sion (trans-fyū′zhŭn) Transfer of blood or a blood component from one person (donor) to another (recipient). [L. *trans-fundo,* pp. *-fusus,* to pour from one vessel to another]

trans•fu•sion ne•phri•tis (trans-fyū′zhŭn nĕ-frī′tis) Renal failure and tubular damage resulting from the transfusion of incompatible blood; the hemoglobin of the hemolyzed red blood cells is deposited as casts in the renal tubules.

trans•gen•e•sis (trans-jen′ĕ-sis) Reproduction involving introduction of foreign-species DNA into an ovum.

trans•glot•tic (trans-glot′ik) Vertical crossing of the glottis, as in the spread of carcinoma from the supraglottic to the infraglottic area.

trans•he•pat•ic (trans-he-pat′ik) Through or across the liver, as an injection.

trans•hi•a•tal (trans-hī-ā′tăl) By way of a hiatus; describes a surgical procedure.

trans•hi•a•tal e•soph•a•gec•to•my (trans-hī-ā′tăl ē-sof′ă-jek′tŏ-mē) Resection of the esophagus by blunt dissection from a cervical incision from above and transhiatal approach through an abdominal incision.

tran•si•ent a•can•tho•lyt•ic der•ma•to•sis (tran′sē-ĕnt a-kan′tho-lit′ik dĕr-mă-tō′sis) A pruritic papular eruption of the chest, with scattered lesions of the back and lateral aspects of the extremities, lasting from weeks to months; seen predominantly in men older than 40 years of age. SYN Grover disease.

trans•i•ent e•voked o•to•a•cous•tic e•mis•sion (tran′sē-ĕnt ē-vōkt′ ō-tō-ă-kū′stik ē-mish′ŭn) A form in which the response is limited in time.

tran•si•ent glob•al am•ne•si•a (tran′sē-ĕnt glō′băl am-nē′zē-ă) A memory disorder seen in middle-aged and old people characterized by an episode of amnesia and bewilderment that persists for several hours; during the episode the patient has a memory defect for present and recent past events, but is fully alert, oriented, capable of high-level intellectual activity, and has a normal result on neurologic examination.

tran•si•ent ho•mo•sex•u•al•i•ty (tran′sē-ĕnt hō′mō-sek′shū-al′i-tē) SYN circumstantial homosexuality.

tran•si•ent hy•po•gam•ma•glob•u•lin•e•mi•a of in•fan•cy (tran′sē-ĕnt, hī′pō-gam′ă-glob′yū-li-nē-mē-ă in′făn-sē) A type of primary immunodeficiency that occurs in infants, probably resulting from immaturity of lymphoid tissue.

tran•si•ent is•che•mic at•tack (TIA) (tran′sē-ĕnt is-kē′mik ă-tak′) A sudden focal loss of neurologic function with complete recovery usually within 24 hours; caused by a brief period of inadequate perfusion in a portion of the territory of the carotid or vertebral basilar arteries.

trans•i•ent tach•yp•ne•a of the new•born (TTN) (tran′sē-ĕnt tă-kip′nē-ă nū′bōrn) Respiratory distress in newborn presenting in the first few hours of life, generally resolving in 12–24 hours.

tran•sil•i•ent (tran-zil′yĕnt) Jumping across; passing over; pertaining to those cortical association fibers in the brain that pass from one convolution to another, nonadjacent, one. [L. *transilio,* to leap across, fr. *salio,* to leap]

trans•il•lum•i•na•tion (tranz-i-lū′mi-nā′shŭn) Passage of light through a solid or liquid substance for diagnostic examination.

tran•si•tion•al cell car•ci•no•ma (tran-zish′ŭn-ăl sel kahr′si-nō′mă) A malignant neoplasm derived from transitional epithelium, occurring chiefly in the urinary bladder, ureters, and renal pelves.

tran•si•tion•al den•ture (tran-zish′ŭn-ăl den′shŭr) A partial denture that is to serve as a temporary prosthesis to which teeth will be added as more teeth are lost and that will be replaced after postextraction tissue changes have occurred; a transitional denture may become an interim denture when all the teeth have been removed from the affected dental arch.

tran•si•tion•al ep•i•the•li•um (tran-zish′ŭn-ăl ep′i-thē′lē-ŭm) A highly distensible pseudostratified epithelium with large polyploid superficial cells that are cuboidal in the relaxed state but broad and squamous in the distended state; occurs in the kidney, ureter, and bladder.

tran•si•tion•al gy•rus (tran-zish′ŭn-ăl jī′rŭs) A small convolution connecting two lobes or two main gyri in the depth of a sulcus.

tran•si•tion•al ob•ject (tran-zish′ŭn-ăl ob′jekt)

An object used by many children as a substitute for a parent who is absent (usually temporarily) to help them deal with separation; typically, a blanket or stuffed toy.

tran•si•tion•al zone (tran-zish′ŭn-ăl zōn) **1.** The equatorial region of the lens of the eye where the anterior epithelial cells become transformed into lens fibers. **2.** That portion of a scleral contact lens between the corneal and scleral sections.

tran•si•tion•ing (tran-zish′ŏn-ing) Moving a child or family from one governmental program to another; mandated aspect of I.D.E.A. for children with disabilities in early intervention and special education programs.

tran•si•tion mu•ta•tion (tran-zish′ŭn myū-tā′shŭn) A point mutation involving substitution of one base pair for another, i.e., replacement of one purine for another and of one pyrimidine for another pyrimidine without change in the purine-pyrimidine orientation.

trans•jug•u•lar in•tra•he•pa•tic por•to•sys•tem•ic shunt (TIPS) (trans-jŭg′yū-lăr in′tră-hĕ-pat′ik pōr′tō-sis-tem′ik shŭnt) An interventional radiology procedure to relieve portal hypertension.

trans•ke•to•la•tion (trans′kē-tō-lā′shŭn) A reaction involving the transfer of a ketole group from one compound to another.

trans•la•by•rin•thine ap•proach (trans-lab′i-rin′thīn ă-prōch′) Surgical approach to the cerebellopontine angle through the inner ear.

trans•la•tion (trans-lā′shŭn) **1.** A change or conversion into another form. **2.** The process by which messenger RNA, transfer RNA, and ribosomes effect the production of protein from amino acids. **3.** DENTISTRY the movement of a tooth through alveolar bone without change in axial inclination. [L. *translatio,* a transferring, fr. *trans- fero,* pp. *-latus,* to carry across]

trans•lo•ca•tion (trans-lō-kā′shŭn) **1.** Transposition of two segments between nonhomologous chromosomes as a result of abnormal breakage and refusion of reciprocal segments. **2.** Transport of a metabolite across a biomembrane. [trans- + L. *locatio,* placement, fr. *loco,* to place]

trans•lu•cent (trans-lū′sĕnt) Allowing light to pass through.

trans•me•at•al in•ci•sion (trans′mē-ā′tăl in-sizh′ŭn) An incision in the skin of the posterior external auditory canal that extends from just above the posterior malleolar fold to a 6 o'clock position inferiorly; for access to the posterior part of the middle ear.

trans•meth•y•lase (trans-meth′i-lās) SYN methyltransferase.

trans•meth•y•la•tion (trans′meth-i-lā′shŭn) Transfer of a methyl group from one compound to another.

trans•mi•gra•tion (trans′mī-grā′shŭn) Movement from one site to another; may entail the crossing of some usually limiting barrier, as in the passage of blood cells through the walls of the vessels (diapedesis). [L. *transmigro,* pp. *-atus,* to remove from one place to another]

trans•mis•si•ble (trans-mis′i-bĕl) Capable of being transmitted (carried across) from one person to another, as a transmissible disease, an infectious or contagious disease.

trans•mis•sion (trans-mish′ŭn) **1.** SYN transfer. **2.** The conveyance of disease from one person to another. **3.** The passage of a nerve impulse across an anatomic cleft, as in autonomic or central nervous system synapses and at neuromuscular junctions, by activation of a specific chemical mediator that stimulates or inhibits the structure across the synapse. **4.** In general, passage of energy through a material. [L. *transmissio,* a sending across]

trans•mis•sion-based pre•cau•tions (trans-mish′ŭn-bāsd prē-kaw′shŭnz) Measures established by the U.S. Centers for Disease Control and Prevention to prevent transmission of highly communicable pathogens. Extra precautions are followed, at this second level, in addition to standard precautions, based on the potential means of disease transmission: airborne, droplet, or contact.

trans•mu•ral (trans-myū′răl) Through any wall, as of the body or of a cyst or any hollow structure. [trans- + L. *murus,* wall]

trans•mu•ral pres•sure (trans-myūr′ăl presh′ŭr) The pressure difference across the chest wall; the difference between pressure in the pleural space and the pressure on the body surface (i.e., pleural pressure–body surface pressure).

trans•mu•ta•tion (trans′myū-tā′shŭn) A change; transformation. SYN conversion (1). [L. *transmuto,* pp. *-atus,* to change, transmute]

trans•na•sal fi•ber•op•tic la•ryn•gos•co•py (trans-nā′zăl fī-bĕr-op′tik lar′in-gos′kŏ-pē) Laryngoscopy performed with a fiberoptic endoscope introduced through the nose.

transoesophageal echocardiography [Br.] SYN transesophageal echocardiography.

trans•par•ent den•tin (trans-par′ĕnt den′tin) SYN sclerotic dentin.

trans•par•ent sep•tum (trans-par′ĕnt sep′tŭm) A thin plate of brain tissue, containing nerve cells and numerous nerve fibers, that is stretched like a flat, vertical sheet between the column and body of the fornix below and the corpus callosum above and anteriorly; it is usually fused in the median plane with its partner on the opposite side so as to form a thin median partition between the left and right frontal horns of the lateral ventricles; in fewer than 10% of humans there is a blind, slitlike, fluid-filled space between the two transparent septa, the cavity of septum pellucidum. The transparent septum is continuous ventralward through the interval between the corpus callosum and the anterior commissure with the precommissural septum and subcallosal gyrus.

trans•pep•ti•dase (trans-pep′ti-dās) An enzyme catalyzing a transpeptidation reaction.

trans•pep•ti•da•tion (trans′pep-ti-dā′shŭn) A reaction involving the transfer of one or more amino acids from one peptide chain to another, as by transpeptidase action, or of a peptide chain itself, as in bacterial cell wall synthesis.

trans•phos•pho•ryl•a•tion (trans′fos-fōr-i-lā′shŭn) A reaction involving the transfer of a phosphoric group from one compound to another, often with the involvement of ATP.

tran•spi•ra•tion (trans′pir-ā′shŭn) Passage of water vapor through the skin or any membrane. SEE ALSO insensible perspiration. [trans- + L. *spiro,* pp. *-atus,* to breathe]

trans•plant (trans′plant) **1.** To transfer from one part to another, as in grafting and transplantation. **2.** The tissue or organ in grafting and transplantation. SEE ALSO graft. [trans- + L. *planto,* to plant]

trans•plan•ta•tion (trans′plan-tā′shŭn) Implanting in one part a tissue or organ taken from another part or from another person. SEE ALSO graft. [L. *trans-planto,* pp. *-atus,* to transplant]

trans•port (trans′pōrt) **1.** The movement or transference of biochemical substances in biologic systems. **2.** In physical therapy, movement of patients from one area (or surface) to another. [L. *transporto,* to carry over, fr. trans- + *porto,* to carry]

trans•port max•i•mum (Tm) (trans′pōrt mak′si-mŭm) The maximal rate of secretion or reabsorption of a substance by the renal tubules.

trans•port me•di•um (trans′pōrt mē′dē-ŭm) A medium for transporting clinical specimens to the laboratory for examination.

trans•pos•a•ble el•e•ment (trans-pōz′ă-bĕl el′ĕ-mĕnt) A DNA sequence that can move from one location in the genome to another; the transposition event can involve both recombination and replication, producing two copies of the moving piece of DNA; the insertion of these DNA fragments can disrupt the integrity of the target gene, possibly causing activation of dormant genes, deletions, inversions, and a variety of chromosomal aberrations.

trans•pos•ase (trans-pōz′ās) An enzyme that is required for transposition of DNA segments. [L. *trans-pono,* pp. *trans-positum,* to set across, transfer, + -ase]

trans•pose (trans-pōz′) To transfer one tissue or organ to the place of another, and the reverse. [L. *trans-pono,* pp. *-positus,* to place across, transfer]

trans•po•si•tion (trans-pŏ-zish′ŭn) **1.** Removal from one place to another; metathesis. **2.** The condition of being transposed to the wrong side of the body, as in transposition of the viscera, in which the viscera are located opposite their normal position. **3.** Positioning of teeth out of their normal sequence in an arch.

trans•po•si•tion of the great ves•sels (trans-pŏ-zish′ŭn grāt ves′ĕlz) Congenital malformation in which the aorta arises from the morphologic right ventricle and the pulmonary artery from the morphologic left ventricle, resulting in two separate and parallel circulations. The condition is lethal unless some communication exists between the systemic and pulmonic circulation after birth; the life-sustaining communication may be an abnormal intraatrial passage or a patent ductus arteriosus.

trans•po•son (trans-pō′zon) A segment of DNA that has a repeat of an insertion sequence element at each end that can migrate from one plasmid to another within the same bacterium, to a bacterial chromosome, or to a bacteriophage. [L. *transpono,* pp. *transpositum,* to transfer, + -on]

trans•pul•mo•nar•y pres•sure (trans-pul′mŏ-nar-ē presh′ŭr) The pressure difference across the lungs; the difference between the pressure at the airway opening and the pressure on the visceral pleural surface (i.e., pressure at the airway opening – pleural pressure).

trans•res•pir•a•tor•y pres•sure (trans-res′pir-ă-tōr-ē presh′ŭr) The total pressure difference across the airways, lungs, and chest wall; the difference between the pressure at the airway opening (the mouth) and the pressure on the body surface (i.e., pressure at the airway opening – pressure at the body surface; equivalent to transairway pressure + transpulmonary pressure + transmural pressure).

trans•sec•tion (trans-sek′shŭn) SYN transection.

trans•sex•u•al (tran-sek′shū-ăl) **1.** A person with the external genitalia and secondary sexual characteristics of one sex, but whose personal identification and psychosocial configuration is that of the opposite sex; a study of morphologic, genetic, and gonadal structure may be genitally congruent or incongruent. **2.** Denoting or relating to such a person. **3.** Relating to medical and surgical procedures designed to alter a patient's external sexual characteristics so that they resemble those of the opposite sex.

trans•sex•u•al•ism (tran-sek′shū-ă-lizm) **1.** The state of being a transsexual. **2.** The desire to change one's anatomic sexual characteristics to conform physically with one's perception of self as a member of the opposite sex.

trans·syn·ap·tic de·gen·er·a·tion (tran-si-nap′tik dĕ-jen′ĕr-ā′shŭn) An atrophy of nerve cells following damage to the axons that make synaptic connection with them; noted especially in the lateral geniculate body.

trans·thor·a·cic e·soph·a·gec·to·my (trans′thōr-ās′ik ē-sof′ă-jek′tŏ-mē) Resection of the esophagus through a thoracotomy incision.

trans·tho·rac·ic re·sis·tance (trans′thōr-as′ik rē-zis′tăns) The opposition of the thoracic cavity to having a current passing through it during defibrillation.

trans·tra·che·al ox·y·gen ther·a·py (trans-trā′kē-ăl ok′si-jĕn thār′ă-pē) An oxygen delivery system in which a small-bore plastic cannula is inserted directly into the trachea through a small surgical opening. The catheter is inserted at the third or fourth tracheal cartilages and approximately 3 inches of catheter is allowed to enter the trachea.

tran·su·date (tran′sū-dāt) Any fluid (solvent and solute) that has passed through a presumably normal membrane, such as the capillary wall, as a result of imbalanced hydrostatic and osmotic forces; characteristically low in protein unless there has been secondary concentration. Cf. exudate. SYN transudation (2). [trans- + L. *sudo,* pp. *-atus,* to sweat]

tran·su·da·tion (tran′sū-dā′shŭn) **1.** Passage of a fluid or solute through a membrane by a hydrostatic or osmotic pressure gradient. **2.** SYN transudate.

trans·u·re·ter·o·u·re·ter·os·to·my (trans-yūr′ĕ-tĕr-ō-yūr′ĕ-tĕr-os′tŏ-mē) Anastomosis of the transected end of one ureter into the intact contralateral ureter, by direct or elliptic end-to-side technique. SEE ALSO ureteroureterostomy.

trans·u·re·thral re·sec·tion (trans-yŭr-ē′thrăl rē-sek′shŭn) Endoscopic removal of the prostate gland or bladder lesions, usually for relief of prostatic obstruction or treatment of bladder malignancies.

trans·va·gi·nal scan·ning (trans-vaj′i-năl skan′ing) Ultrasonography of the female pelvis with the transducer placed inside the vagina.

trans·vec·tor (trans-vek′tŏr) An animal that transmits a toxic substance that it does not produce, but that may be accumulated from animal (dinoflagellate) or plant (algae) sources.

trans·ver·sal·is fa·sci·a (trans-vĕr-săl′is fash′ē-ă) The lining fascia of the abdominal cavity, between the inner surface of the abdominal musculature and the peritoneum.

trans·verse (trans-vĕrs′) Crosswise; lying across the long axis of the body or of a part. [L. *transversus*]

trans·verse am·pu·ta·tion (trans-vĕrs′ amp′yū-tā′shŭn) Surgical removal in which the line of section through the extremity is at right angles to the long axis.

trans·verse ar·ter·y of neck (trans-vĕrs′ ahr′tĕr-ē nek) SYN transverse cervical artery.

trans·verse car·pal lig·a·ment (trans-vĕrs′ kahr′păl lig′ă-mĕnt) A strong, fibrous band crossing the front of the carpus and binding down the flexor tendons of the digits and the flexor carpi radialis tendon and the median nerve; in so doing, it creates the carpal tunnel.

trans·verse cer·vi·cal ar·ter·y (trans-vĕrs′ sĕr′vi-kăl ahr′tĕr-ē) *Origin,* thyrocervical trunk; *branches,* superficial (superficial cervical) and deep (descending scapular). SYN arteria transversa colli [TA], transverse artery of neck.

trans·verse cer·vi·cal nerve (trans-vĕrs′ sĕr′vi-kăl nĕrv) A branch of the cervical plexus that supplies the skin over the anterior triangle of the neck. SYN nervus transversus colli [TA].

trans·verse cer·vi·cal veins (trans-vĕrs′ sĕr′vi-kăl vānz) Venae comitantes of the corresponding arteries, emptying into the external jugular vein or sometimes into the subclavian vein. SYN transverse veins of neck.

trans·verse co·lon (trans-vĕrs′ kō′lŏn) The part of the colon between the right and left colic flexures. It may extend somewhat transversely across the abdomen, but more often sags centrally, frequently to subumbilical levels.

trans·ver·sec·to·my (trans′vĕr-sek′tŏ-mē) Resection of the transverse process of a vertebra. [transverse + G. *ektomē,* excision]

trans·verse di·a·me·ter (trans-vĕrs′ dī-am′ĕ-tĕr) The diameter of the pelvic inlet, measured between the terminal lines.

trans·verse fa·cial ar·ter·y (trans-vĕrs′ fā′shăl ahr′tĕr-ē) *Origin,* superficial temporal; *distribution,* parotid gland, parotid duct, masseter muscle, and overlying skin; *anastomoses,* infraorbital and buccal branches of maxillary, and buccal and masseteric branches of facial. SYN arteria transversa faciei [TA].

trans·verse fa·cial vein (trans-vĕrs′ fā′shăl vān) A tributary of the superficial temporal or retromandibular veins, anastomosing with the facial vein. SYN transverse vein of face.

trans·verse fis·sure of the right lung (trans-vĕrs′ fish′ŭr rīt lŭng) The deep fissure that separates the upper and middle lobes of the right lung.

trans·verse fo·ra·men (trans-vĕrs′ fōr-ā′mĕn) Foramen processus transversi. SYN vertebroarterial foramen.

trans·verse frac·ture (trans-vĕrs′ frak′shŭr) A fracture, the line of which forms a right angle with the axis of the bone.

trans•verse her•ma•phro•dit•ism (trans-vĕrs′ hĕr-maf′rō-dīt-izm) Pseudohermaphroditism in which the external genitalia are characteristic of one sex and the gonads characteristic of the other.

trans•verse hor•i•zon•tal ax•is (trans-vĕrs′ hōr′i-zon′tăl ak′sis) An imaginary line around which the mandible may rotate through the horizontal plane.

trans•verse lie (trans-vĕrs′ lī) That relationship in which the long axis of the fetus is transverse or at right angles to that of the mother.

trans•verse lig•a•ment of el•bow (trans-vĕrs′ lig′ă-mĕnt el′bō) A bundle of fibers running from the olecranon to the coronoid process in association with the ulnar collateral ligament.

trans•verse lig•a•ment of knee (trans-vĕrs′ lig′ă-mĕnt nē) A transverse band that passes between the lateral and medial menisci in the anterior part of the knee joint. SYN ligamentum transversum genus [TA].

trans•verse mus•cle of ab•do•men (trans-vĕrs′ mŭs′ĕl ab′dŏ-mĕn) SYN transversus abdominis muscle.

trans•verse mus•cle of chin (trans-vĕrs′ mŭs′ĕl chin) SYN transversus menti muscle.

trans•verse mus•cle of nape (trans-vĕrs′ mŭs′ĕl nāp) SYN transversus nuchae muscle.

trans•verse mus•cle of tongue (trans-vĕrs′ mŭs′ĕl tŭng) An intrinsic muscle of the tongue, the fibers of which arise from the septum and radiate to the dorsum and sides; *action*, decreases lateral dimension of the tongue; *nerve supply*, hypoglossal for motor, lingual for sensory. SYN musculus transversus linguae [TA].

trans•verse per•i•car•di•al si•nus (trans-vĕrs′ per′i-kahr′dē-ăl sī′nŭs) A passage in the pericardial sac between the origins of the great vessels (i.e., posterior to the intrapericardial portions of the pulmonary trunk and ascending aorta and anterior to the superior vena cava and superior to the atria); it is formed as a result of the flexure of the heart tube, partially approximating the great venous and arterial vessels. SYN Theile canal.

trans•verse per•i•ne•al lig•a•ment (trans-vĕrs′ per′i-nē′ăl lig′ă-mĕnt) The thickened anterior border of the urogenital diaphragm, formed by the fusion of its two fascial layers.

trans•verse plane (trans-vĕrs′ plān) A plane across the body at right angles to the coronal and sagittal planes.

trans•verse pre•sen•ta•tion (trans-vĕrs′ prez′ĕn-tā′shŭn) An abnormal presentation, neither head nor breech, in which the fetus lies transversely in the uterus across the axis of the parturient canal.

trans•verse pro•cess (trans-vĕrz′ pros′es) A bony protrusion on either side of the arch of a vertebra, from the junction of the lamina and pedicle, which functions as a lever for attached muscles.

trans•verse rec•tal folds, **trans•verse folds of rec•tum** (trans-vĕrs′ rek′tăl fōldz, rek′tŭm) The three or four crescentic folds placed horizontally in the rectal mucous membrane; the superior rectal fold is situated near the beginning of the rectum on the left side; the middle rectal fold (Nélaton fold) is most prominent and consistent and projects from the right side about 8 cm above the anus (approximately the level of the floor of the rectouterine or rectovesical pouch); the inferior rectal fold is on the left side about 5 cm above the anus.

trans•verse re•lax•a•tion (trans-vĕrs′ rē′lak-sā′shŭn) MAGNETIC RESONANCE IMAGING the rapid decay of the nuclear magnetization vector at right angles to the magnetic field after the 90° pulse is turned off; the signal is called free induction decay. SEE ALSO T2. Cf. longitudinal relaxation.

trans•verse rhomb•en•ce•phal•ic flex•ure (trans-vĕrs′ rom′ben-se-fal′ik flek′shŭr) SYN pontine flexure.

trans•verse scap•u•lar ar•ter•y (trans-vĕrs′ skap′yū-lăr ahr′tĕr-ē) SYN suprascapular artery.

trans•verse sec•tion (trans-vĕrs′ sek′shŭn) A cross-section obtained by slicing, actually or through imaging techniques, the body or any part of the body structure, in a horizontal plane, i.e., a plane that intersects the longitudinal axis at a right angle. Because actual sectioning in the transverse plane results in an inferior and a superior portion, an anatomic transverse section may be a two-dimensional view of the cut surface on the inferior aspect of the superior portion, or of the superior aspect of the inferior portion. By convention, in medical imaging, transverse sections demonstrate the former unless otherwise stated.

trans•verse si•nus (trans-vĕrs′ sī′nŭs) A paired dural venous sinus that drains the confluence of sinuses, running along the occipital attachment of the tentorium cerebelli and terminating in the sigmoid sinus.

trans•verse tar•sal joint (trans-vĕrs′ tahr′săl joynt) The synovial joints between the talus and navicular bone medially and the calcaneus and navicular bones laterally that act as a unit in allowing the front of the foot to pivot relative to the back of the foot about the longitudinal axis of the foot, contributing to the total inversion and eversion movements.

trans•verse tem•por•al gy•ri (trans-vĕrs′ tem′pŏr-ăl jī′rē) Two or three convolutions running transversely on the upper surface of the temporal lobe bordering on the lateral (sylvian) fissure, separated from each other by the transverse temporal sulci.

trans•verse thor•a•co•ster•no•to•my (trans-vĕrs′ thōr′ă-kō-stĕrn-ot′ŏ-mē) Chest incision combining an intercostal incision and transsection of the sternum.

trans•verse vein of face (trans-vĕrs′ vān fās) SYN transverse facial vein.

trans•verse veins of neck (trans-vĕrs′ vānz nek) SYN transverse cervical veins.

trans•ver•sion (trans-vĕr′zhŭn) **1.** Substitution in DNA and RNA of a pyrimidine for a purine, or vice versa, by mutation. **2.** DENTISTRY the eruption of a tooth in a position normally occupied by another; transposition of a tooth.

trans•ver•sion mu•ta•tion (trans-vĕr′zhŭn myū-tā′shŭn) A point mutation involving base substitution in which the orientation of purine and pyrimidine is reversed, in contradistinction to transition mutation.

trans•ver•so•spi•nal•is mus•cle (trans-vĕr′sō-spī-nā′lis mŭs′ĕl) The group of muscles that originate from transverse processes of vertebrae and pass to spinous processes of higher vertebrae; they act as rotators and include the semispinalis (capitis, cervicis, thoracis), multifidus, and rotatores (cervicis, thoracis, lumborum) muscles. All are innervated by dorsal primary rami of spinal nerves. SYN musculus transversospinalis [TA], transversospinal muscle.

trans•ver•so•spi•nal mus•cle (trans-vĕr′sō-spī′năl mŭs′ĕl) SYN transversospinalis muscle.

trans•ver•sus ab•do•mi•nis mus•cle (trans-vĕr′sŭs ab-dom′i-nŭs mŭs′ĕl) *Origin*, seventh to twelfth costal cartilages, lumbar fascia, iliac crest, and inguinal ligament; *insertion*, xiphoid cartilage and linea alba and, through the conjoint tendon, pubic tubercle, and pecten; *action*, compresses abdominal contents; *nerve supply*, lower thoracic. See this page. SYN musculus transversus abdominis [TA], transverse muscle of abdomen.

trans•ver•sus men•ti mus•cle (trans-vĕr′sŭs men′tī mŭs′ĕl) Inconstant fibers of the depressor anguli oris muscle continue into the neck and cross to the opposite side inferior to the chin. SYN musculus transversus menti [TA], transverse muscle of chin.

trans•ver•sus nu•chae mus•cle (trans-vĕr′sŭs nū′kē mŭs′ĕl) An occasional muscle passing between the tendons of the trapezius and sternocleidomastoid, possibly a fasciculus of the posterior auricular muscle. SYN musculus transversus nuchae [TA], transverse muscle of nape.

trans•ver•sus thor•a•cis mus•cle (trans-vĕr′sŭs thōr-ā′sis mŭs′ĕl) *Origin*, dorsal surface of xiphoid cartilage and lower portion of dorsal surface of body of sternum; *insertion*, second to sixth costal cartilages; *action*, contributes to depression of ribs, narrowing chest; *nerve supply*, intercostal. SYN musculus transversus thoracis [TA].

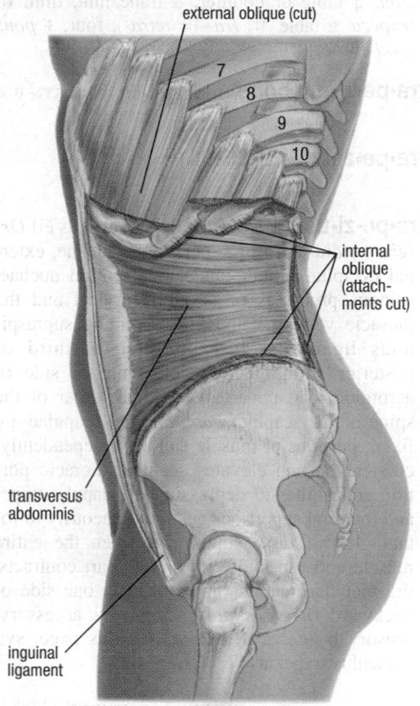

transversus abdominis muscle

trans•ves•tism (trans-ves′tizm) The practice of dressing or masquerading in the clothes of the opposite sex; especially the adoption of feminine mannerisms and costume by a male. SYN transvestitism. [trans- + L. *vestio*, to dress]

trans•ves•tite (trans-ves′tīt) A person who practices transvestism.

trans•ves•ti•tism (trans-ves′ti-tizm) SYN transvestism.

Tran•tas dots (trahn′tăs dots) Pale, grayish-red, uneven nodules of gelatinous aspect at the limbal conjunctiva in vernal conjunctivitis.

TRAP (trap) Acronym for twin reversed arterial perfusion. SEE twin reversed arterial perfusion sequence.

tra•pe•zi•al (tră-pē′zē-ăl) Relating to any trapezium.

tra•pe•zi•form (tră-pē′zi-fōrm) SYN trapezoid (1).

tra•pe•zi•um, pl. **tra•pe•zi•a**, **tra•pe•zi•ums** (tră-pē′zē-ŭm, -ă, -ŭmz) **1.** A four-sided geometric figure having no two sides parallel. **2.** The lateral (radial) bone in the distal row of the carpus; it articulates with the first and second metacarpals, scaphoid, and trapezoid bones. SYN os trapezium [TA], greater multangular bone, os multangulum majus, trapezium bone. [G. *trape-*

zion, a table or counter, a trapezium, dim. of *trapeza,* a table, fr. *tra-* (= *tetra-*), four, + *pous* (*pod-*), foot]

tra•pe•zi•um bone (tră-pē′zē-ŭm bōn) SYN trapezium.

tra•pe•zi•us (tră-pē′zē-ŭs) SYN trapezius muscle.

tra•pe•zi•us mus•cle (tră-pē′zē-ŭs mŭs′ĕl) *Origin,* medial third of superior nuchal line, external occipital protuberance, ligamentum nuchae, spinous processes of seventh cervical and the thoracic vertebrae and corresponding supraspinous ligaments; *insertion,* lateral third of posterior surface of clavicle, anterior side of acromion, and upper and medial border of the spine of the scapula; *action,* when scapulae are fixed, portions of muscle can act independently: cervical portion elevates scapula, thoracic portion contributes to depression of scapula; upper and lowermost portions act simultaneously to rotate glenoid fossa superiorly; when the entire muscle and especially its middle part contracts, the scapulae retract; draws head to one side or backward; *nerve supply,* motor by accessory, sensory by cervical plexus. See this page. SYN musculus trapezius [TA], trapezius.

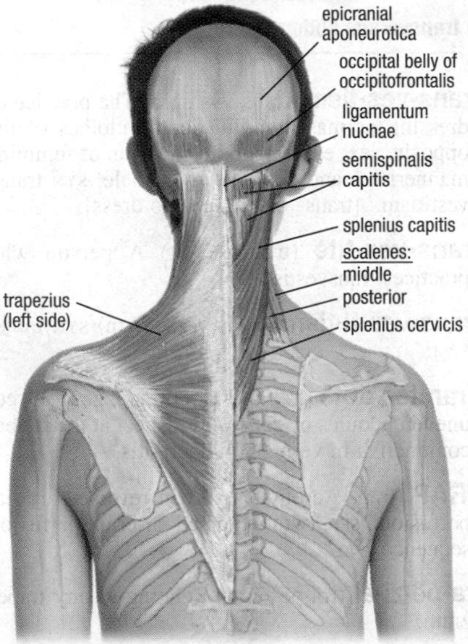

trapezius muscle

trap•e•zoid (trap′ĕ-zoyd) **1.** Resembling a trapezium. SYN trapeziform. **2.** A geometric figure resembling a trapezium except that two of its opposite sides are parallel. **3.** SYN trapezoid bone. [G. *trapeza,* table, + *eidos,* resemblance]

trap•e•zoid bone (trap′ĕ-zoyd bōn) A bone in the distal row of the carpus; it articulates with the second metacarpal, trapezium, capitate, and scaphoid. SYN trapezoid (3).

trap•e•zoid lig•a•ment (trap′ĕ-zoyd lig′ă-mĕnt) The lateral part of the coracoclavicular ligament that attaches to the trapezoid line of the clavicle. SYN ligamentum trapezoideum [TA].

trap•e•zoid line (trap′ĕ-zoyd līn) The area on the inferior surface of the clavicle near its lateral extremity on which the trapezoid ligament attaches.

Trapp factor (trahp fak′tŏr) Last two numerals of urine's specific gravity factor; multiplying by two gives parts per thousand in solids.

Trau•be bru•it (trow′bĕ brū-ē′) SYN gallop.

Trau•be cor•pus•cle (trow′bĕ kōr′pŭs-ĕl) SYN achromocyte.

Trau•be dou•ble tone (trow′bĕ dŭ′bĕl tōn) A double sound heard on auscultation over the femoral vessels in cases of aortic and tricuspid insufficiency.

Trau•be-He•ring curves, **Trau•be-He•ring waves** (trow′bĕ-her′ing kŭrvz, wāvz) Slow oscillations in blood pressure usually extending over several respiratory cycles; related to variations in vasomotor tone; rhythmic variations in blood pressure.

Trau•be sign (trow′bĕ sīn) A double sound or murmur heard in auscultation over arteries (particularly the femoral arteries) in significant aortic regurgitation.

trau•ma, pl. **trau•ma•ta**, **trau•mas** (traw′mă, -mă-tă, -măz) An injury, physical or mental. SYN traumatism. See page B27. [G. wound]

trau•ma as•sess•ment (traw′mă ă-ses′mĕnt) Evaluation of the traumatized patient after treating life threats found in the initial assessment; a full body examination of the trauma patient by EMS personnel. SYN secondary survey.

trau•ma care sys•tem (traw′mă kār sis′tĕm) A coordinated emergency medical service (EMS) system designed to provide rapid assessment of victims of severe or multisystem trauma, transport to a trauma center, and definitive care. May involve air medical transport. SEE ALSO air medical transport, emergency medical service system, trauma.

trau•ma cen•ter (traw′mă sen′tĕr) A designated medical facility for the treatment of trauma patients. Standards established by the American College of Surgeons provide for three levels of sophistication: Level I, a freestanding facility staffed 24 hours a day by surgical, specialty, and support personnel, with appropriate physical resources, conducting research, and usually associated with an academic medical center; Level II, a facility with the same capabilities as Level I but that is not required to conduct research and may be integrated with an emergency department. SEE ALSO designation.

trau•ma score (traw′mă skōr) A numeric calculation, based on the sum of a number of physiologic parameters, assigned to a trauma patient as a means of predicting outcome.

trau•mas•the•ni•a (traw′mas-thē′nē-ă) Nervous exhaustion following an injury. [traum- + G. *astheneia,* weakness]

trau•ma•ta (traw′mă-tă) Plural of trauma.

trau•mat•ic (traw-mat′ik) Relating to or caused by trauma. [G. *traumatikos*]

trau•mat•ic a•men•or•rhe•a (traw-mat′ik ā-men′ŏr-ē′ă) Absence of menses because of endometrial scarring or cervical stenosis resulting from injury or disease. SYN Asherman syndrome.

trau•mat•ic am•ne•si•a (traw-mat′ik am-nē′zē-ă) The loss or disturbance of memory following an insult or injury to the brain of the type that accompanies a head injury, or excessive use of alcohol, or following the cessation of ingestion of alcohol or other psychoactive drugs; or loss or disturbance of memory of the type seen in hysteria and other forms of dissociative disorders.

trau•mat•ic am•pu•ta•tion (traw-mat′ik amp′yū-tā′shŭn) Amputation resulting from accidental or nonsurgical injury; may be complete or incomplete.

trau•mat•ic an•es•the•si•a (traw-mat′ik an′es-thē′zē-ă) Loss of sensation resulting from nerve injury.

trau•mat•ic as•phyx•i•a (traw-mat′ik as-fik′sē-ă) Cyanotic asphyxia due to trauma; the extravasation of blood into the skin and conjunctivae, produced by a sudden mechanical increase in venous pressure, analogous to the Rumpel-Leede test; common in those who have been hanged and seen occasionally in crush injuries. SYN pressure stasis.

trau•mat•ic brain in•jur•y (TBI) (traw-mat′ik brān in′jŭr-ē) An insult to the brain as the result of physical trauma or external force, not degenerative or congenital, that may cause a diminished or altered state of consciousness and may impair cognitive, behavioral, physical, or emotional functioning. SYN acquired brain injury.

trau•mat•ic dis•cop•a•thy (traw-mat′ik dis-kop′ă-thē) An injury characterized by fissuring, laceration, or fragmentation of the disc or surrounding ligaments, with or without displacement of fragments against spinal cord, nerve roots, or ligaments.

trau•mat•ic en•ceph•a•lop•a•thy (traw-mat′ik en-sef′a-lop′ă-thē) An encephalopathy resulting from structural brain injury.

trau•mat•ic neu•ri•tis (traw-mat′ik nūr-ī′tis) Nerve lesion following an injury.

trau•mat•ic neu•ro•ma (traw-mat′ik nūr-ō′mă) The nonneoplastic proliferative mass of Schwann cells and neurites that may develop at the proximal end of a severed or injured nerve. SYN amputation neuroma, false neuroma.

trau•mat•ic neu•ro•sis (traw-mat′ik nūr-ō′sis) Any functional nervous disorder following an accident or injury. SEE ALSO posttraumatic stress disorder.

trau•mat•ic pneu•mo•thor•ax (traw-mat′ik nū′mō-thōr′aks) The presence of air in the pleural cavity caused by blunt or penetrating chest injury.

trau•mat•ic tet•a•nus (traw-mat′ik tet′ă-nŭs) The condition resulting from infection of a wound.

trau•ma•tism (traw′mă-tizm) SYN trauma.

♻ **traumato-, traumat-, traum-** Combining forms meaning wound, injury. [G. *trauma*]

trau•mat•o•gen•ic oc•clu•sion (traw′mă-tō-jen′ik ŏ-klū′zhŭn) A malocclusion capable of damaging the teeth and associated structures.

trau•ma•top•ne•a (traw′mă-top′nē-ă) Passage of air in and out through a wound of the chest wall. SYN traumatopnoea. [traumato- + G. *pnoē,* breath]

traumatopnoea [Br.] SYN traumatopnea.

trav•el•er's di•ar•rhe•a (trav′ĕl-ĕrz dī′ă-rē′ă) Of sudden onset, often accompanied by abdominal cramps, vomiting, and fever, this digestive disorder occurs sporadically in travelers usually during the first week of a trip; most commonly caused by strains of enterotoxigenic *Escherichia coli.* SYN traveller's diarrhoea.

trav•el•ing wave the•or•y (trav′ĕ-ling wāv thē′ŏr-ē) Generally held theory that a wave travels from the base to the apex of the basilar membrane of the cochlea in response to acoustic stimulation, and that the site of maximal displacement of the basilar membrane depends on the frequency of the stimulating tone, with higher frequencies causing maximal displacement near the base and lower frequencies causing maximal displacement near the apex. SYN travelling wave theory.

traveller's diarrhoea [Br.] SYN traveler's diarrhea.

travelling wave theory [Br.] SYN traveling wave theory.

tra•verse (tră-vĕrs′) COMPUTED TOMOGRAPHY one complete linear movement of the gantry across the object being scanned. [M.E., fr. O.Fr., fr. L.L. *transverso,* fr. L. *trans-verto,* to turn across]

Treach•er Col•lins syn•drome (trēch′ĕr kol′inz sin′drōm) Mandibulofacial dysostosis characterized by bone abnormalities of structures formed from the first pharyngeal arch, including downward sloping palpebral fissures, depressed cheek bones, deformed pinnae, a receding chin, and a large, fishlike mouth with dental abnormalities. Atresia of the external acoustic meatus (auditory canal), defects of the external acoustic meatus and ossicles, and cleft palate are most common. SYN mandibulofacial dysostosis.

treat (trēt) To manage a disease by medicinal, surgical, or other measures; to care for a patient medically or surgically. [Fr. *traiter,* fr. L. *tracto,* to drag, handle, perform]

treat•ment (trēt′mĕnt) Medical or surgical management of a patient. SEE ALSO therapy, therapeutics. [Fr. *traitement* (see treat)]

tre•ble in•crease at low lev•els (treb′ĕl in′krēs lō lev′ĕlz) A hearing aid signal-processing strategy to increase gradually the amplification of high-frequency sounds at low levels.

tre•ha•lose (trē-hā′lōs) A natural disaccharide occurring in some plants and in trehala, a mannalike Asian food consisting of beetle larvae; a food additive and sweetener. [*trehala,* fr. Turk. *tigala,* + -ose]

Tré•lat stools (trā-lah′ stūlz) Stools that look as if stippled with eggwhite that are also streaked with blood, as occurs in association with proctitis.

tre•ma•cam•ra (trē′mă-kam′ră) The extracellular part of the cell surface adhesion molecule ICAM-1 involved in rhinovirus attachments to mucosal cells.

Trem•a•to•da (trem′ă-tō′dă) A class in the phylum Platyhelminthes (the flatworms) consisting of flukes with a leaf-shaped body and two muscular suckers, and an acelomate parenchyma-filled body cavity. Flukes of interest to human or veterinary medicine are members of the order Digenea, with complete life cycles involving embryonic multiplication in a mollusk as their first intermediate host. [G. *trēmatōdēs,* full of holes, fr. *trēma,* a hole, + *eidos,* appearance]

i **trem•a•tode**, **trem•a•toid** (trem′ă-tōd, -ă-toyd) **1.** Common name for a fluke of the class Trematoda. **2.** Relating to a fluke of the class Trematoda. See page B7.

trem•or (trem′ŏr) **1.** Repetitive, often regular, oscillatory movements caused by alternate, or synchronous, but irregular contraction of opposing muscle groups; usually involuntary. **2.** Minute ocular movement occurring during fixation on an object. SYN trepidation (1). [L. a shaking]

trem•u•lous (trem′yū-lŭs) Characterized by tremor.

trench fe•ver (trench fē′vĕr) An uncommon rickettsial fever caused by *Bartonella quintana* and transmitted by the louse *Pediculus humanus;* first appeared as an epidemic during trench warfare in World War I (1914–1918); characterized by the sudden onset of chills and fever, myalgia (especially of the back and legs), headache, and general malaise that typically lasts 5 days but may recur.

trench•foot (trench′fut) SYN immersion foot.

trench mouth (trench mowth) SYN necrotizing ulcerative gingivitis.

Tren•del•en•burg op•er•a•tion (tren′de-len-berg op-ĕr-ā′shŭn) A pulmonary embolectomy.

Tren•de•len•burg po•si•tion (tren′de-len-berg pŏ-zish′ŏn) A supine position on the operating table, which is inclined at varying angles so that the pelvis is higher than the head; used during and after operations in the pelvis or for shock.

Tren•del•en•burg sign, **Tren•del•en•burg gait** (tren′de-len-berg sīn, gāt) A physical examination finding associated with various hip abnormalities (congenital dislocation, hip abductor weakness, rheumatic arthritis, osteoarthritis) in which the pelvis sags on the side opposite the affected side during single-leg stance on the affected side; during gait, compensation occurs by leaning the torso toward the involved side during stance phase on the affected extremity.

Tren•del•en•burg symp•tom (tren′de-len-berg simp′tŏm) A waddling gait produced by paresis of the gluteal muscles, as in progressive muscular dystrophy.

Tren•del•en•burg test (tren′de-len-berg test) A measurement of the valves of the leg veins; the leg is raised above the level of the heart until the veins are empty and is then rapidly lowered; in varicosity and incompetence of the valves the veins will at once become distended, but placement of a tourniquet around the leg will prevent distention of veins below the incompetent perforators or valves below the tourniquet.

trend of thought (trend thawt) Thinking with a tendency toward or centering on a particular idea with a particular affect.

treph•i•na•tion, **trep•a•na•tion** (tref-i-nā′shŭn, trep-ă-nā′shŭn) Removal of a circular piece ("button") of cranium by a trephine.

tre•phine, **tre•pan** (trē-fīn′, trĕ-pan′) **1.** A cylindric or crown saw used for the removal of a disc of bone, especially from the skull, or of other firm tissue as that of the cornea. **2.** To remove a disc of bone or other tissue by means of a trephine.

trep•i•dant (trep′i-dănt) Marked by tremor. [L. *trepidans,* pres. p. of *trepido,* to tremble, to be agitated]

trep•i•da•ti•o cor•dis (trep-i-dā′shē-ō kōr′dis) SYN palpitation.

trep•i•da•tion (trep-i-dā′shŭn) **1.** SYN tremor. **2.** Anxious fear. [L. *trepidatio,* fr. *trepido,* to tremble, to be agitated]

Trep•o•ne•ma (trep-ō-nē′mă) A genus of anaerobic bacteria (order Spirochaetales) consisting of cells, 3–8 mcm in length, with acute, regular, or irregular spirals and no obvious protoplasmic structure. A terminal filament may be present. They stain with difficulty except with Giemsa stain or silver impregnation. Some species are pathogenic and parasitic for humans and other animals, generally producing local lesions in tissues. [G. *trepō,* to turn, + *nēma,* thread]

Trep•o•ne•ma pal•li•dum (trep-ō-nē′mă pal′i-dŭm) A bacterial species that causes syphilis in humans.

Trep•o•ne•ma per•te•nu•e (trep-ō-nē′mă pĕr-ten′yū-ē) A bacterial species that causes yaws; patients with this disease give positive results in serologic screening tests for syphilis.

trep•o•ne•ma•to•sis (trep′ō-nē-mă-tō′sis) SYN treponemiasis.

trep•o•neme (trep′ō-nēm) A vernacular term used to refer to any member of the genus *Treponema.*

trep•o•ne•mi•a•sis (trep′ō-nē-mī′ă-sis) Infection caused by *Treponema.* SYN treponematosis.

trep•o•ne•mi•ci•dal (trep′ō-nē′mi-sī′dăl) Destructive to any species of *Treponema*, but usually with reference to *T. pallidum.* SYN antitreponemal. [*Treponema* + L. *caedo,* to kill]

tre•pop•ne•a (trē′pop-nē′ă) **1.** Dyspnea that is relieved in the lateral recumbent position. **2.** Difficult or labored breathing while lying on one side but not the other, associated with unilateral lung diseases or condtions. SEE ALSO platypnea. SYN trepopnoea. [G. *trepō,* to turn, + -pnea]

trepopnoea [Br.] SYN trepopnea.

trep•pe (trep′ĕ) A phenomenon in cardiac muscle: If a number of stimuli of the same intensity are sent into the muscle after a quiescent period, the first few contractions of the series show a successive increase in amplitude (strength). SYN staircase phenomenon. [Ger. *Treppe,* staircase]

Tre•sil•i•an sign (trē-sil′ē-ăn sīn) A reddish prominence at the orifice of Stenson duct, noted in mumps.

tre•sis (trē′sis) SYN perforation. [G. *trēsis,* a boring]

♻ **tri-** Prefix meaning three. Cf. tris-. [L. and G.]

tri•a•ce•tic ac•id (trī-ă-sē′tik as′id) A compound formed by condensation of acetyl and malonyl coenzyme A in the course of fatty acid synthesis.

tri•ac•yl•glyc•er•ol (trī-as′il-glis′ĕr-ol) Glycerol esterified at each of its three hydroxyl groups by a fatty (aliphatic) acid. SYN triglyceride.

tri•ac•yl•glyc•er•ol li•pase (trī-as′il-glis′ĕr-ol lip′ās) The fat-splitting enzyme in pancreatic juice; it hydrolyzes triacylglycerol to produce a diacylglycerol and a fatty acid anion; a deficiency of the hepatic enzyme results in hypercholesterolemia and hypertriglyceridemia. SYN steapsin.

tri•ad (trī′ad) **1.** A group of three things with something in common. **2.** The transverse tubule and the terminal cisternae on each side of it in skeletal muscle fibers. **3.** SYN portal triad. **4.** PSYCHOLOGY/PSYCHIATRY the father-mother-child relationship projectively experienced in group psychotherapy. [G. *trias* (*triad-*), the number 3, fr. *treis,* three]

tri•age (trē′ahzh) Medical screening of patients to determine their relative priority for treatment; the separation of a large number of casualties, in military or civilian disaster medical care, into three groups: 1) those who cannot be expected to survive even with treatment; 2) those who will recover without treatment; 3) the highest priority group, those who will not survive without treatment. [Fr. sorting]

tri•age tag (trē-ahzh′ tag) A tag or other method of identifying the triage level assigned to a mass-casualty victim, containing information needed for emergency and life-sustaining treatment. SEE ALSO trauma.

tri•al den•ture (trī′ăl den′shŭr) A setup of artificial teeth so fabricated that it may be placed in the patient's mouth to verify esthetics, for the making of records, or for any other operation deemed necessary before final completion of the denture.

tri•al frame (trī′ăl frām) A type of spectacle frame with variable adjustments, for holding trial lenses during refraction.

tri•al of la•bor af•ter ce•sar•e•an sec•tion (trī′ăl lā′bor af′tĕr se-zar′ē-ăn sek′shŭn) The attempt to deliver vaginally after a cesarean section; carries some risk of rupture of the uterine scar.

tri•al lens•es (trī′ăl lenz′ĕz) A series of cylindric and spheric lenses used in testing vision.

tri•an•gle (trī′ang-gĕl) ANATOMY, SURGERY a three-sided area with arbitrary or natural boundaries. SEE ALSO trigonum, region. [L. *triangulum,* fr. *tri-*, three, + *angulus,* angle]

tri•an•gle of aus•cul•ta•tion (trī′ang-gĕl aws′kŭl-tā′shŭn) Space bounded by the lower border of the trapezius, the latissimus dorsi, and the medial margin of the scapula, where the absence of musculature allows respiratory sounds to be heard clearly with a stethoscope.

tri•an•gle of safe•ty (trī′ang-gĕl sāf′tē) The area at the lower left sternal border where the pericardium is not covered by lung (pericardial notch); preferred site for aspiration of pericardial fluid.

tri·an·gu·lar ban·dage (trī-ang′gyū-lăr ban′dăj) A piece of cloth cut in the shape of a right-angled triangle, used as a sling.

tri·an·gu·lar bone (trī-ang′gyū-lăr bōn) SYN os trigonum.

tri·ang·u·lar fi·bro·car·til·age com·plex (trī-ang′gyū-lăr fī′brō′kahr-til-ăj kom′pleks) A group of structures in the wrist consisting of the disc of the ulnocarpal joint along with the ligaments attached to it.

tri·an·gu·lar mus·cle (trī-ang′gyū-lăr mŭs′ĕl) **1.** A muscle that is triangular; **2.** SYN depressor anguli oris muscle.

tri·an·gu·lar ridge (trī-ang′gyū-lăr rij) An elevation that descends from the cusp tips of premolars and molars toward the central grooves and fossae of the crown.

Tri·at·o·ma (trī-ă-tō′mă) A genus of insects that includes important vectors of *Trypanosoma cruzi*, such as *T. dimidiata*, *T. infestans*, and *T. maculata*.

tri·ba·sic (trī-bā′sik) Having three titratable hydrogen atoms; denoting an acid with a basicity of 3.

tribe (trīb) In biologic classification, an occasionally used division between the family and the genus; often the same as the subfamily. [L. *tribus*]

tri·bra·chi·a (trī-brā′kē-ă) Condition seen in conjoined twins when the fusion has merged the adjacent upper limbs to form a single one, so that there are only three upper limbs for the two bodies. SEE ALSO conjoined twins. [tri- + G. *brachiōn,* arm]

TRIC (trik) Acronym for trachoma and inclusion conjunctivitis.

tri·car·box·yl·ic ac·id cy·cle (TCA cy·cle) (trī-kahr-bok-sil′ik as′id sī′kĕl) Together with oxidative phosphorylation, the main source of energy in the mammalian body and the end toward which carbohydrate, fat, and protein metabolism is directed; a series of reactions, beginning and ending with oxaloacetic acid, during the course of which a two-carbon fragment is completely oxidized to carbon dioxide and water with the production of 12 high-energy phosphate bonds. So called because the first four substances involved (citric acid, *cis*-aconitic acid, isocitric acid, and oxalosuccinic acid) are all tricarboxylic acids; from oxalosuccinate, the others are, in order, α-ketoglutarate, succinate, fumarate, L-malate, and oxaloacetate, which condenses with acetyl-CoA (from fatty acid degradation) to form citrate (citric acid) again. SYN Krebs cycle.

TRICARE (trī′kār) Health insurance coverage provided by the U.S. Department of Defense for military personnel and their dependents when governmental medical facilities are not available: covers active or retired members of all branches of the military service plus the Public Health Service, NOAA, and dependents of military personnel killed on active duty. Formerly known as CHAMPUS/CHAMPVA (q.v.).

tri·ceps (trī′seps) Three-headed; denoting especially two muscles: triceps brachii and triceps surae. SEE ALSO muscle. [L. fr. *tri-*, three, + *caput,* head]

tri·ceps bra·chi·i mus·cle (trī′seps brā′kē-ī mŭs′ĕl) *Origin*, long or scapular head: lateral border of scapula below glenoid fossa; lateral head: lateral and posterior surface of humerus below greater tubercle; medial head: posterior surface of humerus below radial groove; *insertion*, olecranon of ulna; *action*, extends elbow; *nerve supply*, radial. See this page. SYN musculus triceps brachii [TA], triceps muscle of arm.

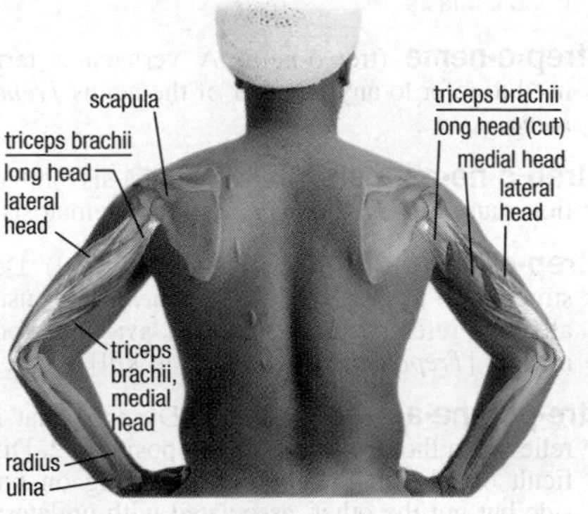

triceps brachii muscle

tri·ceps mus·cle of arm (trī′sĕps mŭs′ĕl ahrm) SYN triceps brachii muscle.

tri·ceps mus·cle of calf (trī′seps mŭs′ĕl kaf) SYN triceps surae muscle.

tri·ceps re·flex (trī′seps rē′fleks) A sudden contraction of the triceps muscle caused by a smart tap on its tendon when the forearm hangs loosely at a right angle to the arm.

tri·ceps sur·ae mus·cle (trī′seps sū′rē mŭs′ĕl) The two bellies of the gastrocnemius and soleus considered as one muscle. SYN musculus triceps surae [TA], triceps muscle of calf.

tri·ceps sur·ae re·flex (trī′seps sū′rē rē′fleks) SYN Achilles reflex.

-trichia Suffix meaning condition or type of hair. [G. *thrix* (*trich-*), hair, + *-ia,* condition]

tri·chi·a·sis (tri-kī′ă-sis) A condition in which the hair adjacent to a natural orifice turns inward and causes irritation; in inversion of an eyelid (entropion), eyelash irritation of the eye. [trich- + G. *-iasis,* condition]

trich·i·lem·mo·ma (trik′i-le-mō′mă) A benign

tumor derived from outer root sheath epithelium of a hair follicle, consisting of cells with pale-staining cytoplasm containing glycogen; multiple trichilemmomas are present on the face in Cowden disease. [trichi- + G. *lemma,* husk, + *-ōma,* tumor]

tri•chi•na, pl. **tri•chi•nae** (tri-kī′nă, -nē) A larval worm of the genus *Trichinella;* the infective form in pork. [Mod. L., fr. G. *thrix* (*trich-*), a hair]

Trich•i•nel•la (trik′i-nel′ă) A nematode genus in the aphasmid group that causes trichinosis in humans and carnivores. [Mod. L. fr. trichina + dim. suffix *ella*]

Trich•i•nel•la pseu•do•spi•ra•lis (trik′i-nel′ă sū-dō-spī-rā′lis) A nematode species with a normal life cycle in small predators; humans are an accidental host.

Trich•i•nel•la spi•ra•lis (trik′i-nel′ă spī-rā′lis) The pork or trichina worm, a species of parasites that cause trichinosis, found in most regions of the world but more frequently in the Northern Hemisphere; transmission occurs as a result of ingesting raw or inadequately cooked meat (especially pork but now often associated with game animals such as bear or walrus) that contains encysted larvae that develop into adults that survive in the jejunum and ileum for approximately 6 weeks; the female worm is viviparous, and bears approximately 1500 embryonic larvae that are laid deep in the mucosa so that they are picked up in the submucosal capillaries and are transported via the liver to the heart, lungs, and systemic circulation; eventually the larvae break out of the body capillaries, penetrate a muscle fiber, coil, and encyst, thereby inducing the strong sensitization, pain, fever, edema, and eosinophilic reaction characteristic of trichinosis. See page B7.

trich•i•no•sis (trik-i-nō′sis) The disease resulting from ingestion of raw or inadequately cooked pork or other meat that contains encysted larvae of the nematode parasite *Trichinella spiralis*. The initial symptoms are abdominal pain, cramping, and diarrhea, associated with the development of the parasites in the small intestine. After the larval parasites invade muscular tissue, a second set of symptoms is manifest, including facial and periorbital edema, myalgia, fever, pruritus, urticaria, conjunctivitis, and signs of myocarditis. [*Trichinella* (trichina) + G. *-osis,* condition]

tri•chi•no•sis gran•u•lo•ma (trik-i-nō′sis gran′yū-lō′mă) Lesions caused by cell death after penetration of migrating newborn nematode larvae.

tri•chi•nous (trik′i-nŭs) Infected with trichina worms.

tri•chi•tis (tri-kī′tis) Inflammation of the hair bulbs. [trich- + G. *-itis,* inflammation]

tri•chlo•ride (trī-klōr′īd) A chloride having three chlorine atoms in the molecule, e.g., PCl_3.

(2,4,5-tri•chlo•ro•phen•ox•y) a•ce•tic ac•id (trī-klōr′ō-fē-nok′sē ă-sē′tik as′id) A herbicide and defoliant synthesized by condensation of chloracetic acid and 2,4,5-trichlorophenol, used as the principal constituent of Agent Orange.

tricho-, trich-, trichi- Combining forms denoting the hair; a hairlike structure. [G. *thrix* (*trich-*)]

trich•o•be•zoar (trik′ō-bē′zōr) A hair cast in the stomach or intestinal tract. See this page. SYN hair ball, pilobezoar. [tricho- + bezoar]

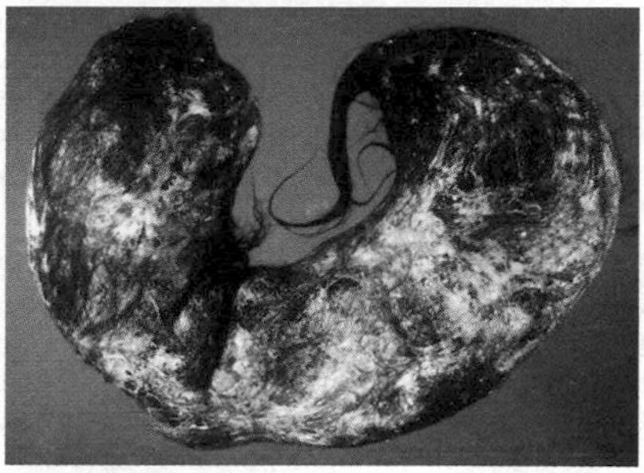

trichobezoar

trich•o•cla•si•a, **tri•choc•la•sis** (trik-ō-klā′zē-ă, tri-kok′lā-sis) SYN trichorrhexis nodosa. [tricho- + G. *klasis,* breaking off]

trich•o•dis•co•ma (trik′ō-dis-kō′mă) Elliptic parafollicular mesenchymal hamartomas. SYN haarscheibe tumor.

trich•o•ep•i•the•li•o•ma (trik′ō-ep-i-thē-lē-ō′mă) Any of numerous small benign nodules, occurring mostly on the skin of the face, derived from basal cells of hair follicles enclosing small keratin cysts. SYN Brooke tumor. [tricho- + epithelioma]

trich•o•glos•si•a (trik-ō-glos′ē-ă) SYN hairy tongue. [tricho- + G. *glōssa,* tongue]

trich•oid (trik′oyd) Hairlike. [tricho- + G. *eidos,* resemblance]

trich•o•lith (trik′ō-lith) A concretion on the hair; the lesion of piedra. [tricho- + G. *lithos,* stone]

trich•o•lo•gi•a (trik′ō-lō′jē-ă) A nervous habit of plucking at the hair. [G. *trichologeō,* to pluck hairs, fr. tricho- + *legō,* to pick out, gather]

trich•o•meg•a•ly (trik′ō-meg′ă-lē) Congenital condition characterized by abnormally long eyelashes; associated with dwarfism. [tricho- + G. *megas,* large]

trich•o•mo•na•cide (trik′ō-mō′nă-sīd) An agent that is destructive to *Trichomonas* organisms.

trich•o•mon•ad (trik′ō-mō′nad) Common name for members of the family Trichomonadidae.

tri•cho•mo•nal va•gi•ni•tis (trik′ō-mō′năl vaj′i-nī′tis) Acute vaginitis caused by infection with *Trichomonas vaginalis*, which does not invade tissues but provokes an intense local inflammatory reaction in the vagina, cervix, and sometimes the urethra; infection is sexually transmitted; symptoms include frothy green or brown discharge, vulvar itching and irritation, and dysuria.

Trich•o•mo•nas (trik-ō-mō′năs) A genus of parasitic protozoan flagellates causing trichomoniasis. [tricho- + G. *monas,* single (unit)]

Trich•o•mo•nas te•nax (trik-ō-mō′năs ten′aks) A species of parasitic protozoan flagellates that lives as a commensal in the mouth of humans and other primates, especially in the tartar around the teeth or in the defects of carious teeth.

Trich•o•mo•nas va•gi•nal•is (trik-ō-mō′năs vaj-i-nā′lis) A species of parasitic protozoan flagellates frequently found in the vagina and urethra of women, in whom it causes trichomonal vaginitis, and in the urethra and prostate gland of men.

trich•o•mo•ni•a•sis (trik′ō-mō-nī′ă-sis) Disease caused by infection with a protozoan of the genus *Trichomonas;* often used to designate trichomoniasis vaginitis.

trich•o•my•co•sis (trik′ō-mī-kō′sis) A disease of the hair caused by *Nocardia* or *Corynebacterium*. [tricho- + G. *mykēs,* fungus, + G. *-osis,* condition]

tri•cho•my•co•sis ax•il•la•ris (trik′ō-mī-kō′sis aks′i-lar′is) *Corynebacterium* infection of axillary and pubic hairs with development of yellow (flava), black (nigra), or red (rubra) concretions around the hair shafts; frequently asymptomatic. SYN lepothrix, trichonodosis.

trich•o•no•car•di•o•sis (trik′ō-nō-kahr-dē-ō′sis) An infection of hair shafts, especially of the axillary and pubic regions, with nocardiae. Yellow, red, or black concretions develop around the infected hair shafts and contain the causative agent and, frequently, micrococci. SEE ALSO trichomycosis, trichomycosis axillaris. [tricho- + *Nocardia* + G. *-osis,* condition]

trich•o•no•do•sis (trik′ō-nō-dō′sis) SYN trichomycosis axillaris. [tricho- + L. *nodus,* node (swelling), + G. *-osis,* condition]

trich•o•no•sis (trik′ō-nō′sis) SYN trichopathy.

trich•o•path•ic (trik′ō-path′ik) Relating to any disease of the hair.

tri•chop•a•thy (tri-kop′ă-thē) Any disease of the hair. SYN trichonosis, trichosis. [tricho- + G. *pathos,* suffering]

tri•choph•a•gy (tri-kof′ă-jē) Habitual biting of the hair. [tricho- + G. *phagō,* to eat]

trich•o•phyt•ic (trik′ō-fit′ik) Relating to trichophytosis.

trich•o•phy•tid (tri-kof′i-tid) An eruption remote from the site of infection, that is the expression of allergic response to *Trichophyton* infection. [tricho- + G. *phyton,* plant, + *-id* (1)]

trich•o•phy•to•be•zoar (trik′ō-fī-tō-bē′zōr) SEE bezoar. [tricho- + G. *phyton,* plant, + bezoar]

Trich•o•phy•ton (tri-kof′i-ton) A genus of pathogenic fungi causing dermatophytosis in humans and animals; species attacks the hair, skin, and nails. [tricho- + G. *phyton,* plant]

Trich•o•phy•ton con•cen•tri•cum (tri-kof′i-ton kon-sen′trik-ŭm) An anthropophilic fungal species that is the causative agent of tinea imbricata; it closely resembles the branching mycelium of *T. schoenleinii*.

Trich•o•phy•ton men•ta•gro•phy•tes (tri-kof′i-ton men′tă-grō-fī′tēz) A zoophilic small-spored ectothrix fungal species that causes infection of the hair, skin, and nails; causes ringworm in dogs, horses, rabbits, mice, rats, chinchillas, foxes, and humans (especially tinea pedis with severe inflammation and tinea cruris).

Trich•o•phy•ton ru•brum (tri-kof′i-ton rū′brŭm) A widely distributed anthropophilic fungal species that causes persistent infections of the skin, especially tinea pedis and tinea cruris and in the nails, that are unusually resistant to therapy.

Trich•o•phy•ton schoen•lei•ni•i (tri-kof′i-ton shān-līn-ē′ī) Fungal species of dermatophyte that causes favus in humans; produces tunnels within the hair shaft that are filled with air bubbles after the hyphae disintegrate.

Trich•o•phy•ton ton•sur•ans (tri-kof′i-ton ton-sū′ranz) Fungal species that causes epidemic dermatophytosis; the most common cause of tinea capitis in the United States; forms black dots where hair breaks off at the skin surface. See page B5.

Trich•o•phy•ton vi•o•la•ce•um (tri-kof′i-ton vī-ō-lā′sē-ŭm) An anthropophilic fungal species that causes black-dot ringworm or favus infection of the scalp.

trich•o•phy•to•sis (trik′ō-fī-tō′sis) Superficial fungal infection caused by species of *Trichophyton*. [tricho- + G. *phyton,* plant, + *-osis,* condition]

trich•o•pti•lo•sis (tri-kop-ti-lō′sis) A condition of splitting of the shaft of the hair, giving it a feathery appearance. [tricho- + G. *ptilōsis,* plumage, + *-osis,* condition]

trich•or•rhex•is (trik-ō-rek′sis) A condition in

which the hairs tend to break or split. [tricho- + G. *rhēxis,* a breaking]

tri·chor·rhex·is in·va·gi·na·ta (trik-ō-rek′sis in-vaj-i-nā′tă) SYN bamboo hair.

tri·chor·rhex·is no·do·sa (trik-ō-rek′sis nō-dō′să) A congenital or acquired condition in which minute nodes are formed in the hair shafts; splitting and breaking, complete or incomplete, may occur at these nodes. SYN clastothrix, trichoclasia, trichoclasis.

tri·chos·chi·sis (tri-kos′ki-sis) The presence of broken or split hairs. SEE ALSO trichorrhexis. [tricho- + G. *schisis,* a cleaving]

tri·cho·sis (tri-kō′sis) SYN trichopathy. [tricho- + G. *-osis,* condition]

Tri·chos·po·ron (trik′ō-spōr-on) A genus of imperfect fungi that possess branching septate hyphae with arthroconidia and blastoconidia; these organisms are part of the normal flora of the intestinal tract of humans. *Trichosporon beigelii* is the causative agent of white piedra or trichosporosis and fatal fungemia in immunocompromised patients. [tricho- + G. *sporos,* seed (spore)]

trich·o·sta·sis spi·nu·lo·sa (tri-kos′tă-sis spī-nyū-lō′să) A condition in which hair follicles are blocked with a keratin plug containing lanugo hairs. [tricho- + G. *stasis,* a standing; L. *spinulosus,* thorny]

tri·cho·the·cene my·co·tox·in (trī-kō-thē′sēn mī′kō-toks′in) Any fungal toxin (mycotoxin) containing a trichothecene ring (a double bond between C-9 and C-10 and an epoxide group arising from C-12 and C-13). A variety of toxins from unrelated species contain this chemical moiety. They are stable in the environment and cause multiorgan effects. One, T-2 mycotoxin, is alleged to have been used as a chemical warfare agent in the so-called yellow rain reported in Southeast Asia during the Vietnam War.

trich·o·til·lo·ma·ni·a (trik′ō-til′ō-mā′nē-ă) A compulsion to pull out one's own hair. See page B12. [tricho- + G. *tillo,* pull out, + *mania,* insanity]

tri·chro·mat·ic (trī′krō-mat′ik) **1.** Having, or relating to, the three primary colors, red, green, and blue. **2.** Capable of perceiving the three primary colors; having normal color vision. SYN trichromic.

tri·chro·ma·top·si·a (trī′krō-mă-top′sē-ă) Normal color vision; the ability to perceive the three primary colors. [tri- + G. *chrōma,* color, + *opsis,* vision]

tri·chrome stain (trī′krōm stān) Staining combinations that usually contain three dyes of contrasting colors selected to stain connective tissue, muscle, cytoplasm, and nuclei in bright colors; generally, tissue sections are first dyed in iron hematoxylin before being treated with the other dyes.

tri·chro·mic (trī-krō′mik) SYN trichromatic.

trich·u·ri·a·sis (trik′yū-rī′ă-sis) Infection with nematodes (whipworms) of the genus *Trichuris.* In humans, intestinal parasitization by *T. trichiura* is usually asymptomatic; in massive infections, it frequently induces diarrhea or rectal prolapse.

Tri·chur·is (tri-kyūr′is) A genus of aphasmid nematodes (sometimes improperly termed *Trichocephalus*) related to the trichina worm, *Trichinella spiralis,* and having a body with a slender, elongated, anterior portion that threads into the mucosa of the colon or large intestine of the host and a thick posterior portion bearing reproductive organs and their products. *Trichuris* contains about 70 species, all in mammals. [tricho- + G. *oura,* tail]

Tri·chur·is su·is (tri-kyūr′is sū′is) A nematode species found in the pig; adult worms have been found in humans.

Tri·chur·is tri·chi·u·ra (tri-kyūr′is trī-kī-yū′ră) The whipworm of humans; a species that causes trichuriasis. Its body is filiform and slender in the anterior three fifths, and more robust posteriorly. Females are 4–5 cm long, males are shorter (with coiled caudal extremity and a single eversible spicule). Eggs are barrel shaped, 50–56 by 20–22 mcm, with double shell and translucent knobs at each of the two poles. Humans are the only susceptible hosts and usually acquire infection by direct finger-to-mouth contact or by ingestion of soil, water, or food that contains larvated eggs. (Development in the soil takes 3–6 weeks under proper conditions of warmth and moisture; hence, distribution is chiefly tropical). Larvae escape from eggs in the ileum, mature in approximately 1 month, and then pass directly into the cecum without undergoing a parenteral migration such as occurs with *Ascaris lumbricoides;* adults may persist 2–7 years.

Tri·chur·is vul·pis (tri-kyūr′is vŭl′pis) A nematode species found in dogs; the sexually mature adult has been found in the human appendix.

tri·cip·i·tal (trī-sip′i-tăl) Having three heads; denoting a triceps muscle.

tri·co·no·dont (trī-kō′nō-dont) Referring to a tooth having three cones or cusps in a linear arrangement; the central one is the largest. [tri- + G. *kōnos,* cone, + *odous,* tooth]]

tri·corn pro·te·ase (trī′kōrn prō′tē-ās) A protease found in organisms lacking membrane-bound compartments that forms the core of a modular proteolytic system used to generate multicatalytic activities in a controlled manner.

tri·cor·nute (trī-kōr′nūt) Having three cornua or horns. [tri- + L. *cornutus,* horned, fr. *cornu,* a horn]

tri•crot•ic (trī-krot′ik) Thrice-beating; marked by three waves in the arterial pulse tracing. [tri- + G. *krotos,* a beat]

tri•cus•pid, tri•cus•pi•dal, tri•cus•pi•date (trī-kŭs′pid, -kŭs′pi-dăl, -kŭs′pi-dāt) **1.** Having three points, prongs, or cusps, as the tricuspid valve of the heart. **2.** Having three tubercles or cusps, as the second upper molar tooth (occasionally) and the upper third molar (usually).

tri•cus•pid a•tre•si•a (trī-kŭs′pid ă-trē′zē-ă) Congenital lack of the tricuspid orifice.

tri•cus•pid in•suf•fi•cien•cy (trī-kŭs′pid in′sŭ-fish′ĕn-sē) SEE valvular regurgitation.

tri•cus•pid mur•mur (trī-kŭs′pid mŭr′mŭr) A murmur produced at the tricuspid orifice, either obstructive or regurgitant.

tri•cus•pid or•i•fice (trī-kŭs′pid ōr′i-fis) An atrioventricular opening that leads from the right atrium into the right ventricle of the heart.

tri•cus•pid ste•no•sis (trī-kŭs′pid stĕ-nō′sis) Pathologic narrowing of the orifice of the tricuspid valve.

tri•cus•pid valve (trī-kŭs′pid valv) The valve closing the orifice between the right atrium and right ventricle of the heart; its three cusps are called anterior, posterior, and septal.

tri•den•tate (trī-den′tāt) Three-toothed; three-pronged. [tri- + L. *dentatus,* toothed]

tri•der•mic (trī-dĕr′mik) Relating to or derived from the three primary germ layers of the embryo: ectoderm, endoderm, and mesoderm. [tri- + G. *derma,* skin]

tri•fa•cial neu•ral•gi•a (trī-fā′shăl nūr-al′jē-ă) SYN trigeminal neuralgia.

tri•fid (trī′fid) Split into three. [L. *trifidus,* three-cleft]

tri•fo•cal lens (trī-fō′kăl lenz) A lens with segments of three focal powers: distant, intermediate, and near.

tri•fur•ca•tion (trī-fŭr-kā′shŭn) **1.** A division into three branches. **2.** The area where the tooth roots divide into three distinct portions. [tri- + L. *furca,* fork]

tri•gas•tric (trī-gas′trik) Having three bellies; denoting a muscle with two tendinous interruptions. [tri- + G. *gastēr,* belly]

tri•gem•i•nal cave (trī-jĕm′i-năl kāv) The cleft in the meningeal layer of dura of the middle cranial fossa near the tip of the petrous part of the temporal bone; it encloses the roots of the trigeminal nerve and the trigeminal ganglion.

tri•gem•i•nal gan•gli•on (trī-jĕm′i-năl gang′glē-ŏn) The large, flattened sensory ganglion of the trigeminal nerve lying close to the cavernous sinus along the medial part of the middle cranial fossa in the trigeminal cavity of the dura mater.

tri•gem•i•nal nerve [CN V] (trī-jĕm′i-năl nĕrv) The chief sensory nerve of the face and the motor nerve of the muscles of mastication; its nuclei are in the mesencephalon and in the pons and medulla oblongata extending down into the cervical portion of the spinal cord; it emerges by two roots, sensory and motor, from the lateral portion of the surface of the pons, and enters a cavity of the dura mater, the trigeminal cave, at the apex of the petrous portion of the temporal bone, where the sensory root expands to form the trigeminal ganglion; from there the three divisions (ophthalmic [CN V1], maxillary [CN V2], and mandibular [CN V3] nerves) arise. SYN nervus trigeminus [CN V] [TA], fifth cranial nerve [CN V].

tri•gem•i•nal neu•ral•gi•a (trī-jĕm′i-năl nūr-al′jē-ă) Severe, paroxysmal bursts of pain in one or more branches of the trigeminal nerve; often induced by touching trigger points in or about the mouth. SYN Fothergill disease (1), Fothergill neuralgia, prosopalgia, prosoponeuralgia, tic douloureux, trifacial neuralgia.

tri•gem•i•nal pulse (trī-jĕm′i-năl pŭls) A pulse in which the beats occur in trios, a pause following every third beat. SYN pulsus trigeminus.

tri•gem•i•nal rhi•zot•o•my (trī-jĕm′i-năl rī-zot′ŏ-mē) Division or section of a sensory root of the fifth cranial nerve, accomplished through a subtemporal (Frazier-Spiller operation), suboccipital (Dandy operation), or transtentorial approach.

tri•gem•i•nal rhythm (trī-jĕm′i-năl ridh′ŭm) A cardiac arrhythmia in which the beats are grouped in trios, usually composed of a sinus beat followed by two extrasystoles. SYN trigeminy.

tri•gem•i•ny (trī-jem′i-nē) SYN trigeminal rhythm. [L. *trigeminus,* threefold]

trig•ger (trig′ĕr) A substance, insect, object, or agent that initiates or stimulates an action.

trig•ger ar•e•a (trig′ĕr ār′ē-ă) SYN trigger point.

trig•ger de•lay (trig′ĕr dĕ-lā′) Waiting period after each radio wave; the time between the radio wave and the beginning of data acquisition in magnetic resonance imaging.

trig•gered ac•tiv•i•ty (trig′ĕrd ak-tiv′i-tē) One or a series of spontaneously generated heart beats originating from an action potential that produces an afterdepolarization that reaches activation threshold.

trig•ger fing•er (trig′ĕr fing′gĕr) Condition by which the finger flexors contract but are unable to reextend due to a nodule within the tendon sheath or sheath constriction.

trig•ger point (trig′ĕr poynt) Pathologic condition characterized by a small, hypersensitive area, occurring in a predictable pattern within muscles or fascia. SYN trigger area, trigger zone.

trig·ger zone (trig′ĕr zōn) SYN trigger point.

tri·glyc·er·ide (trī-glis′ĕr-īd) SYN triacylglycerol.

tri·go·na (trī-gō′nă) Plural of trigonum. [L.]

trig·o·nal (trig′ō-năl) Triangular; relating to a trigonum.

tri·gone (trī′gōn) **1.** SYN trigonum. **2.** The first three dominant cusps (protocone, paracone, and metacone), taken collectively, of an upper molar tooth. [L. *trigonum,* fr. G. *trigōnon,* triangle]

tri·gone of blad·der (trī′gōn blad′ĕr) A triangular smooth area at the base of the bladder between the openings of the two ureters and that of the urethra. SYN trigonum vesicae [TA], vesical triangle.

tri·gon·id (trī-gon′id) The first three dominant cusps, taken collectively, of a lower molar tooth. SEE ALSO trigone.

tri·go·ni·tis (trī′gō-nī′tis) Inflammation of the urinary bladder, localized in the trigone. [trigone + G. *-itis,* inflammation]

trig·o·no·ce·phal·ic (trig′ō-nō-se-fal′ik) Pertaining to trigonocephaly.

trig·o·no·ceph·a·ly (trig′ō-nō-sef′ă-lē) Malformation characterized by a triangular configuration of the cranium, due in part to premature synostosis of the cranial bones with compression of the cerebral hemispheres. [trigone + G. *kephalē,* head]

tri·go·num, pl. **tri·go·na** (trī-gō′nŭm, -nă) [TA] Any triangular area. SEE ALSO triangle. SYN trigone (1). [L., fr. G. *trigōnon,* a triangle]

tri·go·num fem·or·al·e (trī-gō′nŭm fem-ō-rā′lē) [TA] SYN femoral triangle.

tri·go·num in·gui·nal·e (trī-gō′nŭm in-gwi-nā′lē) [TA] SYN inguinal triangle.

tri·go·num lum·ba·le (trī-gō′nŭm lŭm-bā′lē) SYN lumbar triangle.

tri·go·num mus·cu·la·re (trī-gō′nŭm mŭs-kyū-lā′rē) [TA] SYN muscular triangle.

tri·go·num sub·man·dib·u·lar·e (trī-gō′nŭm sŭb-man-dib′yū-lā′rē) [TA] SYN submandibular triangle.

tri·go·num ves·i·cae (trī-gō′nŭm ves′i-sē) [TA] SYN trigone of bladder.

tri·hy·dric al·co·hol (trī-hī′drik al′kŏ-hol) Any alcohol containing three OH groups (e.g., glycerol).

tri·labe (trī′lāb) A three-pronged forceps for removal of foreign bodies from the bladder. [tri- + G. *labē,* a handle, hold]

tri·lam·i·nar (trī-lam′i-năr) Having three laminae.

tril·li·um (tril′ē-ŭm) (*T. erectum*) A member of the lily family; purported value as antiseptic and astringent; used historically in wound care. SYN beth root, coughroot, jew's harp plant, stinking benjamin. [L., fr. *tri-,* three, threefold]

tri·lo·bate, **tri·lobed** (trī-lō′bāt, trī′lōbd) Having three lobes.

tri·loc·u·lar (trī-lok′yū-lăr) Having three cavities or cells.

tril·o·gy (tril′ŏ-jē) A triad of related entities. [G. *trilogia,* fr. tri- + *logos,* study, discourse]

tril·o·gy of Fal·lot (tril′ŏ-jē fahl-ō′) A set of congenital defects including pulmonic stenosis, atrial septal defect, and right ventricular hypertrophy. SYN Fallot triad.

tri·mes·ter (trī′mes-tĕr) A period of 3 months; one third of the length of a pregnancy. [L. *trimestris,* of three-months' duration]

tri·meth·yl·am·ine (trī-meth′il-am′ēn) A degradation product, often by putrefaction, of nitrogenous plant and animal substances such as beet sugar residue or herring brine; in the body, it probably results from decomposition of choline.

tri·meth·yl·am·i·nu·ri·a (trī-meth′il-am-i-nyūr′ē-ă) Increased excretion of trimethylamine in urine and sweat, with a characteristic offensive, fishy body odor.

tri·nu·cle·o·tide (trī-nū′klē-ō-tīd) A combination of three adjacent nucleotides, free or in a polynucleotide or nucleic acid molecule; often used with specific reference to the unit (codon or anticodon) specifying a particular amino acid in expression of the genetic code.

tri·ose (trī′ōs) A three-carbon monosaccharide, e.g., glyceraldehyde and dihydroxyacetone.

tri·ose·phos·phate i·som·er·ase (trī′ōs-fos′fāt ī-som′ĕr-ās) An isomerizing enzyme that catalyzes the reversible interconversion of D-glyceraldehyde 3-phosphate and dihydroxyacetone phosphate, a reaction of importance in glycolysis and gluconeogenesis; a deficiency of this enzyme will result in hemolytic anemia and severe neurologic deficits.

tri·ox·ide (trī-oks′īd) A molecule containing three atoms of oxygen.

tri·phos·pho·pyr·i·dine nu·cle·o·tide (TPN, TPNH) (trī-fos-phō-pir′i-dēn nū′klē-ō-tīd) Former name for nicotinamide adenine dinucleotide phosphate.

Tri·pi·er am·pu·ta·tion (tri-pē-ā′ amp′yū-tā′shŭn) A modification of the Chopart amputation, in that a part of the calcaneus is also removed.

trip·le bond (trip′ĕl bond) A covalent bond resulting from the sharing of three pairs of electrons, e.g., HC≡CH (acetylene).

tri•ple•gi•a (trī-plē′jē-ă) Paralysis of an upper and a lower extremity and of the face, or of both extremities on one side and of one on the other. [tri- + G. *plēgē,* stroke]

trip•le re•peat dis•or•ders (trip′ĕl rē-pēt′ dis-ōr′dĕrz) A group of hereditary disorders in which a gene mutation on a specific chromosome produces an abnormal form of protein terminated by a long chain of amino acid glutamate repeats; includes Huntington disease, Kennedy disease, Machado-Joseph disease, myotonic dystrophy, fragile X syndrome, and some spinal cerebellar disorders.

trip•le re•sponse (trip′ĕl rĕ-spons′) The triphasic response to the firm stroking of the skin: Phase 1 is the sharply demarcated erythema that follows a momentary blanching of the skin, and is the result of release of histamine from mast cells. Phase 2 is the intense red flare extending beyond the margins of the line of pressure but in the same configuration, and is the result of arteriolar dilation. Phase 3 is the appearance of a line wheal in the configuration of the original stroking.

trip•le screen (trip′ĕl skrēn) Test of maternal serum α-fetoprotein, chorionic gonadotropin, and unconjugated estrogen for indications of increased risk of fetal abnormality, especially trisomy 21. Specimen is collected between 16 and 18 weeks' gestation.

trip•let (trip′lĕt) **1.** One of three children delivered at the same birth. **2.** A set of three similar objects, as a compound lens in a microscope, formed of three planoconvex lenses. **3.** SYN codon.

trip•le vi•sion (trip′ĕl vizh′ŭn) SYN triplopia.

trip•loid (trip′loyd) Pertaining to or characteristic of triploidy. [tri- + -ploid]

trip•loi•dy (trip′loy-dē) The presence of three haploid sets of chromosomes, instead of two, in all cells; results in fetal or neonatal death.

trip•lo•pi•a (trip-lō′pē-ă) Visual defect in which three images of the same object are seen. SYN triple vision. [G. *triploos,* triple, + *opsis,* sight]

tri•pod (trī′pod) **1.** Three-legged. **2.** A stand having three legs or supports. [G. *tripous,* fr. tri- + *pous,* foot]

tri•pod frac•ture (trī′pod frak′shŭr) A facial fracture involving the three supports of the malar prominence: the arch of the zygomatic bone, the zygomatic process of the frontal bone, and the zygomatic process of the maxillary bone.

tri•que•tral bone (trī-kwē′trăl bōn) SYN triquetrum. SYN pyramidal bone.

tri•que•trum (trī-kwē′trŭm) A bone on the medial (ulnar) side of the proximal row of the carpus, articulating with the lunate, pisiform, and hamate. SYN triquetral bone.

tris- Chemical prefix indicating three of the substituents that follow, independently linked. Cf. tri-.

tris•mus (triz′mŭs) Persistent contraction of the masseter muscles due to failure of central inhibition; often the initial manifestation of generalized tetanus. SYN lockjaw. [L. fr. G. *trismos,* a creaking, rasping]

tri•so•mic (trī-sō′mik) Relating to trisomy.

tri•so•my (trī′sō-mē) The state of an individual or cell with an extra chromosome instead of the normal pair of homologous chromosomes; in humans, the state of a cell containing 47 normal chromosomes. For various types of trisomy syndrome, see under *syndrome.* [tri- + (chromo)-some]

tri•so•my 21 syn•drome (trī′sō-mē sin′drōm) SYN Down syndrome.

tri•splanch•nic (trī-splangk′nik) Relating to the three visceral cavities: skull, thorax, and abdomen. [tri- + G. *splanchnon,* viscus]

tri•stich•i•a (trī-stik′ē-ă) Presence of three rows of eyelashes. [G. *tristichos,* in three rows, fr. *tri-,* three, + *stichos,* row]

tri•sul•cate (trī-sŭl′kāt) Marked by three grooves.

tri•ta•nom•a•ly (trī-tă-nom′ă-lē) A type of partial color blindness due to a deficiency or abnormality of blue-sensitive retinal cones. [G. *tritos,* third, + *anōmalia,* irregularity]

trit•an•o•pi•a (trī-tă-nō′pē-ă) Deficient color perception in which there is an absence of blue-sensitive pigment in the retinal cones. [G. *tritos,* third, + *an-* priv. + *ōps,* eye]

trit•i•um (T, *t*) (trit′ē-ŭm) SYN hydrogen 3.

tri•ton tu•mor (trī′tŏn tū′mŏr) A peripheral nerve tumor with striated muscle differentiation, seen most often in neurofibromatosis.

tri•tu•ber•cu•lar (trī-tū-bĕr′kyū-lăr) Referring to a tooth with three tubercles or cusps on the occlusal surface. SEE ALSO tricuspid.

trit•u•ra•ble (trit′yū-ră-bĕl) Capable of being triturated.

trit•u•rate (trit′yū-rāt) **1.** To accomplish trituration. **2.** A triturated substance.

trit•u•ra•tion (trit-yū-rā′shŭn) **1.** The act of reducing a drug to a fine powder and incorporating it thoroughly with sugar and milk by rubbing the two together in a mortar. **2.** Mixing of dental amalgam in a mortar and pestle or with a mechanical device. [L. *trituratio,* fr. *trituro,* to thresh, fr. *tero,* pp. *tritus,* to rub]

tri•va•lence, tri•va•len•cy (trī-vā′lĕns, -lĕn-sē) The property of being trivalent.

tri•va•lent (trī-vā′lĕnt) Having the combining power (valence) of 3.

triv•i•al name (triv′ē-ăl nām) A name of a chemical, no part of which is necessarily used in a systematic sense; i.e., it gives little or no indication as to chemical structure. Such names are commonly used for drugs, hormones, proteins, and other biologicals, and by the general public (e.g., water, aspirin [in the United States], chlorophyll, heme, methotrexate, folic acid, caffeine, thyroxine, epinephrine, barbital); also common abbreviations for chemically defined substances (e.g., ACTH, MSH, BAL, and DDT), which are spoken as such and not in terms of the words they represent. Trivial names often are assigned arbitrarily to chemical compounds, especially those from natural sources, before the chemical structures are known.

tRNA Abbreviation for transfer ribonucleic acid.

tro•car (trō′kahr) An instrument for withdrawing fluid from a cavity, or for use in paracentesis; it consists of a metal tube (cannula) into which fits an obturator with a sharp three-cornered tip, which is withdrawn after the instrument has been pushed into the cavity; the name trocar is usually applied to the obturator alone, the entire instrument being designated trocar and cannula. [Fr. *trocart,* fr. *trois,* three, + *carre,* side (of a sword blade)]

tro•chan•ter (trō-kan′tĕr) [TA] One of the bony prominences developed from independent osseous centers near the upper extremity of the femur; there are two in humans, three in the horse. [G. *trochantēr,* a runner, fr. *trechō,* to run]

tro•chan•ter•i•an, tro•chan•ter•ic (trō-kan-ter′ē-ăn, -ter′ik) Relating to a trochanter; especially the greater trochanter.

tro•chan•ter ma•jor (trō-kan′tĕr mā′jŏr) [TA] SYN greater trochanter.

tro•che (trō′kē) A small, disc-shaped, or rhombic body composed of solidifying paste containing an astringent, antiseptic, or demulcent drug, used for local treatment of the mouth or throat; held in the mouth until dissolved. SYN lozenge, pastille (2), pastil. [L. *trochiscus,* fr. G. *trochiskos,* a little wheel, fr. *trochos,* a wheel]

troch•le•a, pl. **troch•le•ae** (trok′lē-ă, -lē-ē) [TA] **1.** A structure serving as a pulley. **2.** A smooth articular surface of bone on which another glides. **3.** A fibrous loop in the orbit, near the nasal process of the frontal bone, through which passes the tendon of the superior oblique muscle of the eye. [L. pulley, fr. G. *trochileia,* a pulley, fr. *trechō,* to run]

troch•le•ar (trok′lē-ăr) **1.** Relating to a trochlea, especially the trochlea of the superior oblique muscle of the eye. **2.** SYN trochleiform.

troch•le•ar nerve [CN IV] (trok′lē-ăr nĕrv) Supplies the superior oblique muscle of the eye; its origin is in the midbrain below the cerebral aqueduct, and its fibers decussate in the superior medullary velum, and emerge from the brain at the side of the frenulum, the only cranial nerve to arise from the dorsal aspect of the brainstem; it therefore has the longest intracranial course, entering the dura in the free edge of the tentorium, close to the posterior clinoid process, and passing in the lateral wall of the cavernous sinus to enter the orbit through the superior orbital fissure. SYN nervus trochlearis [CN IV] [TA], fourth cranial nerve [CN IV].

tro•chle•ar notch (trok′lē-ăr noch) The deep semilunar concavity at the proximal ulna where the trochlea of the radius articulates.

troch•le•ar spine (trok′lē-ăr spīn) A spicule of bone arising from the edge of the trochlear fovea, giving attachment to the pulley of the superior oblique muscle of the eyeball.

troch•le•i•form (trok′lē-i-fōrm) Pulley-shaped. SYN trochlear (2).

tro•choid (trō′koyd) Revolving; rotating; denoting a revolving or wheellike articulation. [G. *trochōdēs,* fr. *trochos,* wheel, + *eidos,* resemblance]

tro•choid joint (trō′koyd joynt) SYN pivot joint.

Troi•si•er gan•gli•on (twah′zē-ā gang′glē-ŏn) Historical term for a lymph node immediately above the clavicle, especially on the left side, that is palpably enlarged as the result of a metastasis from a malignant neoplasm; the presence of such a node indicates that the probable site of primary involvement is in an abdominal organ. SEE ALSO signal lymph node.

Trom•bic•u•la (trom-bik′yū-lă) The chigger mite, a genus of mites the larvae of which (chiggers, red bugs) include pests of humans and other animals, and vectors of rickettsial and, probably, viral diseases.

trom•bic•u•li•a•sis (trom-bik′yū-lī′ă-sis) Infestation by mites of the genus *Trombicula.*

trom•bic•u•lid (trom-bik′yū-lid) Common name for members of the family Trombiculidae.

Trom•bic•u•li•dae (trom-bik′yū-lī′dē) A family of mites with larvae (red bugs, rougets, harvest mites, scrub mites, or chiggers) that are parasitic on vertebrates; its nymphs and adults are bright red and free living, existing on insect eggs or minute organisms in the soil. The six-legged larvae are barely visible red or orange parasites that attach to the skin for a few days to a month, producing an exceedingly irritating reaction. Chiggers of the genus *Leptotrombidium* transmit tsutsugamushi disease, caused by *Rickettsia tsutsugamushi.*

Tröm•ner re•flex (trĕrm′ner rē′fleks) A modified Rossolimo reflex in which, with the fingers of the patient partially flexed, the tapping of the volar aspect of the tip of the middle or index finger causes flexion of all four fingers and thumb; seen in pyramidal tract lesions with moderate spasticity.

troph•ec•to•derm (trof-ek′tō-dĕrm) Outermost layer of cells in the mammalian blastocyst, which will make contact with the endometrium and take part in establishing the embryo's means of receiving nutrition; the cell layer from which the trophoblast differentiates. [troph- + ectoderm]

Tro•pher•y•ma whip•pel•i•i (trō-fer′i-mă wi-pel′ē-ī) A gram-positive bacterium, related to Group B actinomycetes, which causes Whipple disease; found in tissues of infected patients and in sewage; mode of transmission unknown.

tro•phe•sic (trō-fē′sik) Pertaining to trophesy.

tro•phe•sy (trō′fĕ-sē) The results of any disorder of the trophic nerves.

tro•phic (trō′fik) **1.** Relating to or dependent on nutrition. **2.** Resulting from interruption of nerve supply. [G. *trophē,* nourishment]

♻ **-trophic** Suffix denoting nutrition. Cf. -tropic. [G. *trophē,* nourishment]

tro•phic syn•drome (trō′fik sin′drōm) Ulceration of a denervated area, frequently secondary to picking at the anesthetic surface.

tro•phic ul•cer (trō′fik ŭl′sĕr) Lesion resulting from cutaneous sensory denervation.

♻ **tropho-, troph-** Combining forms denoting food, nutrition. [G. *trophē,* nourishment]

tro•pho•blast (trō′fō-blast) The mesectodermal cell layer covering the blastocyst, which erodes the uterine mucosa and through which the embryo receives nourishment from the mother; the cells do not enter into the formation of the embryo itself, but contribute to the formation of the placenta. The trophoblast develops processes that later receive a core of vascular mesoderm and are then known as the chorionic villi; the trophoblast soon becomes two-layered, differentiating into the syncytiotrophoblast, an outer layer consisting of a multinucleated protoplasmic mass (syncytium), and the cytotrophoblast, the inner layer next to the mesoderm in which the cells retain their membranes. [tropho- + G. *blastos,* germ]

tro•pho•blas•tic (trō-fō-blas′tik) Relating to the trophoblast.

tro•pho•blas•tic la•cu•na (trō-fō-blas′tik lă-kū′nă) One of the spaces in the early syncytiotrophoblastic layer of the chorion before the formation of villi; in human embryos, maternal blood enters these spaces by the 10th day; with the differentiation of the chorionic villi they become intervillous spaces, sometimes called intervillous lacunae.

tro•pho•blas•tin (trō-fō-blas′tin) SYN interferon tau (τ).

tro•pho•blast in•ter•fer•on (trō′fō-blast in′tĕr-fēr′on) SYN interferon tau (τ).

tro•pho•der•ma•to•neu•ro•sis (trō′fō-dĕr′mă-tō-nūr-ō′sis) Cutaneous trophic changes due to neural involvement.

tro•pho•neu•ro•sis (trō′fō-nūr-ō′sis) A trophic disorder, such as atrophy, hypertrophy, or a skin eruption, occurring as a consequence of disease or injury of the nerves of the part. [tropho- + G. *neuron,* nerve, + *-osis,* condition]

tro•pho•neu•rot•ic (trō′fō-nūr-ot′ik) Relating to a trophoneurosis.

tro•pho•neu•rot•ic lep•ro•sy (trō′fō-nūr-ot′ik lep′rŏ-sē) SYN anesthetic leprosy.

tro•pho•plast (trō′fō-plast) SYN plastid (1). [tropho- + G. *plastos,* formed]

tro•pho•tax•is (trō′fō-tak′sis) SYN trophotropism. [tropho- + G. *taxis,* arrangement]

tro•pho•tro•pic (trō′fō-trō′pik) Relating to trophotropism.

tro•phot•ro•pism (trō-fot′rō-pizm) Chemotaxis of living cells in relation to nutritive material; it may be positive (toward nutritive material) or negative (away from nutritive material). SYN trophotaxis. [tropho- + G. *tropē,* a turning]

tro•pho•zo•ite (trō′fō-zō′īt) The ameboid, vegetative, asexual form of certain Sporozoea, such as the schizont of the plasmodia of malaria and related parasites. See page B7. [tropho- + G. *zōon,* animal]

♻ **-trophy** Suffix denoting food, nutrition. [G. *trophē,* nourishment]

tro•pi•a (trō′pē-ă) Abnormal deviation of the eye. SEE ALSO strabismus. [G. tropē, a turning]

♻ **-tropic** Suffix denoting a turning toward, having an affinity for. Cf. -trophic. [G. *tropē,* a turning]

trop•i•cal ab•scess (trop′ik-ăl ab′ses) SYN amebic abscess.

trop•i•cal ac•ne (trop′ik-ăl ak′nē) A severe type of acne of the entire trunk, shoulders, upper arms, buttocks, and thighs; occurs in hot, humid climates.

trop•i•cal a•ne•mi•a (trop′ik-ăl ă-nē′mē-ă) Various syndromes frequently observed in people in tropical climates, usually resulting from nutritional deficiencies or hookworm or other parasitic diseases.

trop•i•cal bu•bo (trop′ik-ăl bū′bō) SYN lymphogranuloma venereum.

trop•i•cal di•ar•rhe•a (trop′ik-ăl dī′ă-rē′ă) SYN tropical sprue.

trop•i•cal dis•eas•es (trop′ik-ăl di-zēz′ĕz) Infectious and parasitic diseases endemic to tropical and subtropical zones, including Chagas disease, leishmaniasis, leprosy, malaria, onchocerciasis, schistosomiasis, sleeping sickness, yellow fever, and others; often water- or insect-borne.

trop·i·cal e·o·sin·o·phil·i·a (trop′ik-ăl ē′ō-sin′ō-fil′ē-ă) The disorder associated with cough and asthma, often caused by occult filarial infection without evidence of microfilaremia; common in India, Southeast Asia, and parts of Latin America. Adult filaria can often be found by means of ultrasound studies of lympholytic channels.

trop·i·cal li·chen, li·chen tro·pi·cus (trop′ik-ăl lī′ken, lī′ken trop′i-kŭs) SYN miliaria rubra.

trop·i·cal med·i·cine (trop′ik-ăl med′i-sin) The branch of medicine concerned with diseases, mainly of parasitic origin, in areas having a tropical climate.

trop·i·cal sore (trop′ik-ăl sōr) SYN cutaneous leishmaniasis.

trop·i·cal sple·no·meg·a·ly syn·drome (trop′ik-ăl splē′nō-meg′ă-lē sin′drōm) SYN hyperreactive malarious splenomegaly.

trop·i·cal sprue (trop′ik-ăl sprū) A disorder that occurs in warmer climates, often associated with enteric infection and nutritional deficiency, and frequently complicated by folate deficiency with macrocytic anemia. SYN tropical diarrhea.

trop·i·cal ty·phus (trop′ik-ăl tī′fŭs) SYN tsutsugamushi disease.

trop·i·cal ul·cer (trop′ik-ăl ŭl′sĕr) **1.** The lesion occurring in cutaneous leishmaniasis. **2.** Tropical phagedenic ulceration caused by a variety of microorganisms, including mycobacteria; common in northern Nigeria.

tro·pism (trō′pizm) The phenomenon, observed in living organisms, of moving toward (positive tropism) or away from (negaive tropism) a focus of light, heat, or other stimulus; usually applied to the movement of a portion of the organism as opposed to taxis, the movement of an entire organism. [G. *tropē,* a turning]

tro·po·col·la·gen (trō′pō-kol′ă-jen) The fundamental units of collagen fibrils, consisting of three helically arranged polypeptide chains.

tro·po·my·o·sin (trō′pō-mī′ō-sin) A fibrous protein extractable from muscle; sometimes specified as tropomyosin B to distinguish it from tropomyosin A (paramyosin) prominent in mollusks.

tro·po·nin (Tn) (trō′pō-nin) A complex of three proteins, troponin-C (TnC), troponin-I (TnI), troponin-T (TnT), and present in striated muscle. Together, these proteins function as regulators of muscle contraction. Several isoforms exist. The cardiac isoform of TnT is specific for cardiac muscle; the blood level of TnT rises within 4 hours after myocardial damage and remains elevated for 10–14 days after an acute myocardial infarction (MI). Measurement of this protein is valuable in the early diagnosis of MI and in monitoring the effectiveness of thrombolytic therapy after an MI.

trough lev·el (trawf lev′ĕl) The lowest concentration reached by a drug before the next dose is administered, as determined by therapeutic drug monitoring.

trough sign (trawf sīn) An anteromedial glenoid defect that results from posterior shoulder dislocation.

Trous·seau point (trū-sō′ poynt) A painful point, in neuralgia, at the spinous process of the vertebra below which the affected nerve arises.

Trous·seau sign (trū-sō′ sīn) In latent tetany, the occurrence of carpopedal spasm accompanied by paresthesia elicited when the upper arm is compressed, as by a tourniquet or a blood pressure cuff. See this page.

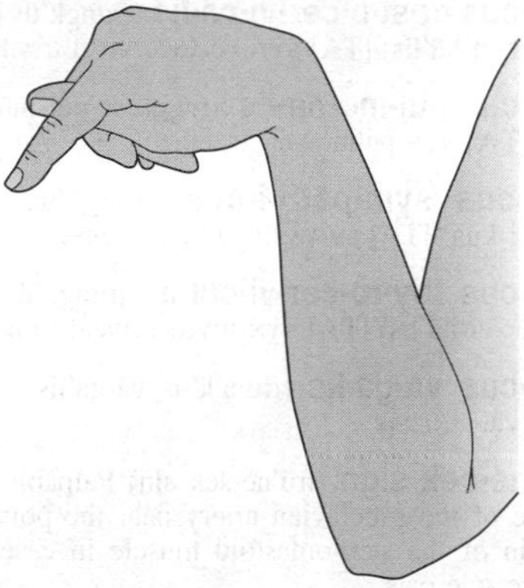

Trousseau sign: carpal spasm with hypocalcemia

Trous·seau spot (trū-sō′ spot) SYN meningitic streak.

Trous·seau syn·drome (trū-sō′ sin′drōm) Thrombophlebitis migrans associated with visceral cancer.

Trp Abbreviation for tryptophan and its radicals.

true an·ky·lo·sis (trū ang′ki-lō′sis) SYN synostosis.

true di·ver·tic·u·lum (trū dī′vĕr-tik′yū-lŭm) A term denoting a diverticulum that includes all the layers of the wall from which it protrudes.

true lu·men (trū lū′mĕn) In a dissecting aneurysm, the channel representing the actual intima-lined artery.

true pre·co·cious pu·ber·ty (trū prĕ-kō′shŭs pyū′bĕr-tē) SYN hyperovarianism.

true ribs [I–VII] (trū ribz) Seven upper ribs on

either side; their cartilages articulate directly with the sternum. SYN costae verae [TA].

true vo·cal cord (trū vō′kăl kōrd) SYN vocal fold.

trum·pe·ting (trum′pĕt-ing) A widening of the long bone metaphyses.

trun·cal (trŭng′kăl) Relating to the trunk of the body or to any arterial or nerve trunk.

trun·cate (trŭng′kāt) Truncated; cut across at right angles to the long axis, or appearing to be so cut. [L. *trunco,* pp. *-atus,* to maim, cut off]

trun·cus, gen. and pl. **trun·ci** (trungk′ŭs, -kī) [TA] SYN trunk. [L. stem, trunk]

trun·cus bra·chi·o·ce·pha·li·cus (trungk′ŭs brā′kē-ō-sef-fā′lik-ŭs) [TA] SYN brachiocephalic trunk.

trun·cus ce·li·a·cus (trungk′ŭs sē-lē-ā′kŭs) [TA] SYN celiac trunk.

trun·cus cost·o·cer·vi·ca·lis (trungk′ŭs kos-tō-sĕr-vi-kā′lis) [TA] SYN costocervical trunk.

trun·cus pul·mo·na·lis (trungk′ŭs pŭl-mō-nā′lis) [TA] SYN pulmonary trunk.

trun·cus sym·path·i·cus (trungk′ŭs sim-path′i-kŭs) [TA] SYN sympathetic trunk.

trun·cus thy·ro·cer·vi·cal·is (trungk′ŭs thī-rō-sĕr-vi-kā′lis) [TA] SYN thyrocervical trunk.

trun·cus va·ga·lis (trungk′ŭs vā-gā′lis) [TA] SYN vagal trunk.

Tru·ne·cek sign (trū′nĕ-sek sīn) Palpable impulse of the subclavian artery near the point of origin of the sternomastoid muscle in cases of aortic sclerosis.

trunk (trŭngk) **1.** The body (trunk or torso), excluding the head and extremities. **2.** A primary nerve, vessel, or collection of tissue before its division. **3.** A large collecting lymphatic vessel. SYN truncus [TA]. [L. *truncus*]

Trus·ler rule for pul·mo·nar·y ar·ter·y band·ing (trus′ler rūl pul′mŏ-nar-ē ahr′tĕr-ē band′ing) A method that gives guidance as to the correct tightness of the band; the degree of banding for a complex congenital cardiac anomaly with bidirectional shunting is less than that for simple ones.

truss (trŭs) An appliance designed to prevent the return of a reduced hernia or the increase in size of an irreducible hernia; it consists of a pad attached to a belt and kept in place by a spring or straps. [Fr. *trousser,* to tie up, to pack]

try·pan blue (trī′pan blū) SYN Congo blue.

try·pan·o·ci·dal (trī-pan′ō-sī′dăl) Destructive to trypanosomes.

try·pan·o·cide (trī-pan′ō-sīd) An agent that kills trypanosomes. [trypanosome + L. *caedo,* to kill]

Try·pan·o·so·ma (trī-pan′ō-sō′mă) A genus of asexual digenetic protozoan flagellates that are parasitic in the blood plasma of many vertebrates and as a rule have an intermediate host, a blood-sucking invertebrate such as a leech, tick, or insect; pathogenic species cause trypanosomiasis in humans. [G. *trypanon,* an auger, + *sōma,* body]

Try·pan·o·so·ma bru·ce·i gam·bi·en·se (trī-pan′ō-sō′mă brūs′ē-ī gam-bē-en′sē) A subspecies of protozoan flagellates that causes Gambian trypanosomiasis; transmitted by tsetse flies, especially *Glossina palpalis.* SYN *Trypanosoma gambiense.*

Try·pan·o·so·ma bru·ce·i rho·de·si·en·se (trī-pan′ō-sō′mă brūs′ē-ī rō-dē-zē-en′sē) A subspecies of protozoan flagellates that causes Rhodesian trypanosomiasis; it is transmitted by tsetse flies, especially *Glossina morsitans;* various game animals can act as reservoir hosts. SYN *Trypanosoma rhodesiense.*

Try·pan·o·so·ma cru·zi (trī-pan′ō-sō′mă krūz′ē) A species of protozoan flagellates that causes South American trypanosomiasis; transmission and infection are common only where the triatomine bug vector defecates while taking blood, because the bug feces contain the infective agents that are scratched into the skin or brought in contact with mucosal surfaces. Trypomastigotes are found in the blood; heart muscle and other organs are attacked.

Try·pan·o·so·ma gam·bi·en·se (trī-pan′ō-sō′mă gam-bē-en′sē) SYN *Trypanosoma brucei gambiense.*

Try·pan·o·so·ma rho·de·si·en·se (trī-pan′ō-sō′mă rō-dē-zē-en′sē) SYN *Trypanosoma brucei rhodesiense.*

try·pan·o·some (trī-pan′ō-sōm) Common name for any member of the genus *Trypanosoma* or of the family Trypanosomatidae. [G. *trypanon,* an auger, + *sōma,* body]

try·pan·o·so·mi·a·sis (trī-pan′ō-sō-mī′ă-sis) Any disease caused by a trypanosome. SYN trypanosomosis.

try·pan·o·so·mic (trī-pan′ō-sō′mik) Relating to trypanosomes, especially denoting infection by such organisms.

try·pan·o·so·mid (trī-pan′ō-sō-mid) A skin lesion caused by immunologic changes from trypanosome disease in blood and lymph of vertebrates and in vertebrates. [trypanosome + G. *-id* (1)]

try·pan·o·so·mo·sis (trī-pan′ō-sō-mō′sis) SYN trypanosomiasis.

tryp·sin (trip′sin) A proteolytic enzyme formed from trypsinogen in the small intestine by the action of enteropeptidase; a serine proteinase that hydrolyzes peptides, amides, and esters.

tryp•sin•o•gen, **tryp•so•gen** (trip-sin′ō-jen, trip′sō-jen) An inactive protein secreted by the pancreas that is converted into trypsin by the action of enteropeptidase.

tryp•tic (trip′tik) Relating to trypsin, as tryptic digestion.

tryp•to•phan (Trp, W) (trip′tō-fan) A nutritionally essential amino acid; the L-isomer is a component of proteins.

tryp•to•pha•nase (trip′tō-fă-nās) **1.** SYN tryptophan 2,3-dioxygenase. **2.** An enzyme found in bacteria that catalyzes the cleavage of L-tryptophan to indole, pyruvic acid, and ammonia; pyridoxal phosphate is a coenzyme.

tryp•to•phan 2,3-di•ox•y•gen•ase (trip′tō-fan dī-oks′ĕ-jĕn-ās) An oxidoreductase catalyzing the reaction of L-tryptophan and O_2 to produce L-*N*-formylkynurenine; an adaptive enzyme, the level (in the liver) being controlled by adrenal hormones; a step in tryptophan catabolism; also, a step in the synthesis of NAD^+ from tryptophan. SYN tryptophanase (1).

tryp•to•pha•nu•ri•a (trip′tō-fă-nyūr′ē-ă) Enhanced urinary excretion of tryptophan.

TSE Abbreviation for testicular self-examination.

tset•se (tset′sē, tsē′tsē) SEE *Glossina.*

TSI Abbreviation for thyroid-stimulating immunoglobulins.

TSS Abbreviation for toxic shock syndrome.

TSTA Abbreviation for tumor-specific transplantation antigens.

tsu•tsu•ga•mu•shi dis•ease (tsū′tsū-gă-mū′shē di-zēz′) An acute infectious disease, caused by *Orientia tsutsugamushi* and transmitted by *Trombicula akamushi* and *T. deliensis*, which occurs in harvesters of hemp in some parts of Japan; characterized by fever, painful swelling of the lymphatic glands, a small, blackish scab (on the genitals, neck, or axilla), and an eruption of large, dark red papules. SYN akamushi disease, mite typhus, scrub typhus, tropical typhus.

TT Abbreviation for text telephone. SEE telecommunications device for the deaf.

t_i:t_{tot} Abbreviation for duty cycle.

TTA Abbreviation for transtracheal aspiration.

TTN Abbreviation for transient tachypnea of the newborn.

T-tube cho•lan•gi•o•gram (tūb kō-lan′jē-ō-gram) A postoperative radiologic examination of the bile ducts that involves administration of a contrast agent through a T-tube.

T tu•bule (tū′byūl) The transverse tubule that passes from the sarcolemma across a myofibril of striated muscle; it is the intermediate tubule of the triad.

TTY Abbreviation for teletypewriter. SEE telecommunications device for the deaf.

tu•ba, gen. and pl. **tu•bae** (tū′bă, -bē) [TA] SYN tube. [L. a straight trumpet]

tu•ba au•di•ti•va (tū′bă aw-di-tī′vă) [TA] SYN pharyngotympanic (auditory) tube.

tu•ba au•di•tor•i•a (tū′bă aw-di-tō′rē-ă) SYN pharyngotympanic (auditory) tube.

tub•al (tū′băl) Relating to a tube, especially the uterine tube.

tub•al air cells of pharyn•go•tym•pan•ic tube (tū′băl ār selz fă-ring′go-tim-pan′ik tūb) Occasional small air cells in the inferior wall of the pharyngotympanic tube, near the tympanic orifice, communicating with the tympanic cavity.

tub•al li•ga•tion (tū′băl lī-gā′shŭn) Interruption of the continuity of the uterine tubes by cutting, cautery, or a plastic or metal device, to prevent future conception.

tub•al preg•nan•cy (tū′băl preg′năn-sē) Development of an impregnated ovum in the uterine tube.

tube (tūb) **1.** A hollow cylindric structure or canal. **2.** A hollow cylinder or pipe. SYN tuba [TA]. [L. *tubus*]

tu•bec•to•my (tū-bek′tŏ-mē) SYN salpingectomy. [L. *tuba,* tube, + G. *ektomē,* excision]

tubed flap (tūbd flap) A flap in which the sides of the pedicle are sutured together to create a tube, with the entire surface covered by skin. SYN Filatov flap, Filatov-Gillies flap.

tube feed•ing (tūb fēd′ing) Administering nutrition or other fluids by means of a tube inserted directly into the enteral tract. This method of administration is used when a patient is unable to swallow.

tu•ber, pl. **tu•ber•a** (tū′bĕr, -bĕr-ă) **1.** A localized swelling; a knob. **2.** A short, fleshy, thick, underground stem of plants, such as the potato. [L. protuberance, swelling]

tu•ber cin•er•e•um (tū′bĕr sī-nē′rē-ŭm) [TA] A prominence of the base of the hypothalamus, bordered caudally by the mammillary bodies, rostrally by the optic chiasm, and laterally by the optic tract, extending ventrally into the infundibulum and hypophysial stalk.

tu•ber•cle (tū′bĕr-kĕl) **1.** A nodule, especially in an anatomic, not pathologic, sense. SYN tuberculum (1) [TA]. **2.** A circumscribed, rounded, solid elevation on the skin, mucous membrane, or surface of an organ. **3.** A slight elevation from the surface of a bone giving attachment to a muscle or ligament. **4.** DENTISTRY a small elevation arising on the surface of a tooth. **5.** A granulomatous lesion due to infection by *Mycobacterium tuberculosis*. Although somewhat variable in size (0.5–3 mm in diameter) and in the proportions of various histologic components, tubercles tend to be fairly well-circumscribed, spheroid, firm lesions that usually consist of three zones: 1) an inner focus of necrosis, coagulative at first and then becoming caseous; 2) a middle zone that consists of large mononuclear phagocytes (macrophages), frequently arranged somewhat radially (with reference to the necrotic material), resembling an epithelium and hence termed epithelioid cells; multinucleated giant cells of Langhans type may also be present; and 3) an outer zone of numerous lymphocytes and a few monocytes and plasma cells. In instances in which healing has begun, a fourth zone of fibrous tissue may form at the periphery. Morphologically indistinguishable lesions may occur in diseases caused by other agents; many observers use the term nonspecifically, i.e., with reference to any such granuloma; others use "tubercle" only for tuberculous lesions and designate those of undetermined causes as epithelioid-cell granulomas. [L. *tuberculum,* dim. of *tuber,* a knob, a swelling, a tumor]

tu•ber•cle ba•cil•lus (tū′bĕr-kĕl bă-sil′ŭs) **1.** SYN *Mycobacterium tuberculosis.* **2.** SYN *Mycobacterium bovis.* **3.** SYN *Mycobacterium avium.*

tu•ber•cle of rib (tū′bĕr-kĕl rib) The knob on the posterior surface of a rib, at the junction of its neck and shaft, that articulates with the transverse process of the vertebra, which corresponds in number to the rib, forming a costotransverse joint.

tu•ber•cle of tra•pe•zi•um (tū′bĕr-kĕl tră-pē′zē-ŭm) A prominent ridge on the trapezium forming the lateral border of the groove in which runs the tendon of the flexor carpi radialis.

tu•ber•cu•la (tū-bĕr′kyū-lă) Plural of tuberculum.

tu•ber•cu•lar, tu•ber•cu•late, tu•ber•cu•lat•ed (tū-bĕr′kyū-lăr, -lāt, -lāt-ĕd) Pertaining to or characterized by tubercles or small nodules. Cf. tuberculous.

tu•ber•cu•lid (tū-bĕr′kyū-lid) A lesion of the skin or mucous membrane resulting from hypersensitivity to mycobacterial antigens disseminated from a distant site of active tuberculosis. [tubercul- + G. *-id* (1)]

tu•ber•cu•lin (tū-bĕr′kyu-lin) A glycerin-broth culture of *Mycobacterium tuberculosis* evaporated to 1/10 volume at 100°C and filtered; introduced by Robert Koch for the treatment of tuberculosis but now used chiefly for diagnostic tests; originally known as Koch old tuberculin (OT) or Koch original tuberculin

tu•ber•cu•lin test (tū-bĕr′kyū-lin test) A dermatologic procedure in which tuberculin or its purified protein derivative (PPD) is injected into the skin; the test is read on the basis of local induration occurring in 48–72 hours. See this page.

tu•ber•cu•li•tis (tū-bĕr-kyū-lī′tis) Inflammation of any tubercle. [tubercul- + G. *-itis,* inflammation]

tuberculo-, tubercul- Combining forms meaning a tubercle, tuberculosis. [L. *tuberculum,* tubercle]

tu•ber•cu•lo•cele (tū-bĕr′kyū-lō-sēl) Tuberculosis of the testes. [tuberculo- + G. *kēlē,* tumor, hernia]

tu•ber•cu•lo•fi•broid (tū-bĕr′kyū-lō-fī′broyd) A discrete, well-circumscribed, usually spheroidal, moderately to extremely firm encapsulated nodule that is formed during the process of heal-

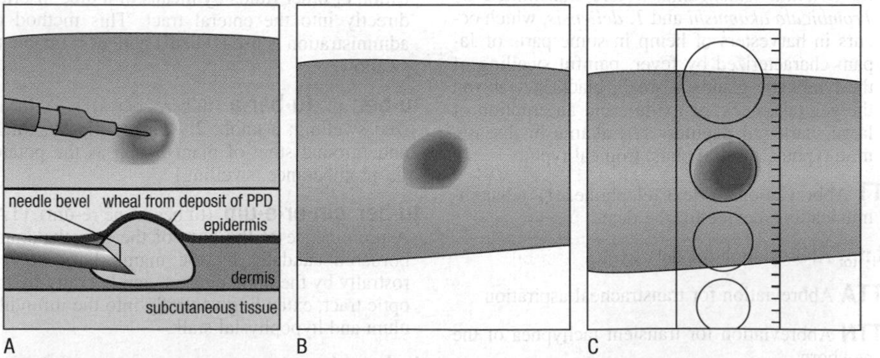

tuberculin test for tuberculosis: (A) correct technique for inserting the needle involves depositing the purified protein derivative (PPD) (of tuberculin) subcutaneously with the needle bevel facing upward; (B) the reaction to the Mantoux test usually consists of a wheal: a hivelike, firm welt; (C) to determine the extent of the reaction, the wheal is measured using a commercially prepared gauge (a wheal measuring 5 mm or more is considered significant)

ing in a focus of tuberculous granulomatous inflammation.

tu·ber·cu·loid (tū-bĕr′kyū-loyd) Resembling tuberculosis or a tubercle. [tuberculo- + G. *eidos,* resemblance]

tu·ber·cu·loid lep·ro·sy (tū-bĕr′kyū-loyd lep′rŏ-sē) A benign, stable, and resistant form of leprosy in which the lepromin reaction is strongly positive and in which the lesions are erythematous, insensitive, infiltrated plaques with distinct edges. SYN nodular leprosy.

tu·ber·cu·lo·ma (tū-bĕr′kyū-lō′mă) A rounded tumorlike but nonneoplastic mass, usually in the lungs or brain, due to localized tuberculous infection. [tuberculo- + G. *-oma,* tumor]

tu·ber·cu·lo·sis (TB) (tū-bĕr′kyū-lō′sis) A specific disease caused by *Mycobacterium tuberculosis,* which may affect almost any tissue or organ of the body, with the most common seat of the disease being the lungs; the anatomic lesion is the tubercle, which can undergo caseation necrosis; general symptoms are those of sepsis: hectic fever, sweats, and emaciation; often progressive, with high mortality if not treated. An opportunistic infection of people with compromised immune systems, including those with AIDS, are at increased risk of severe infection. A high incidence also exists among injecting drug abusers. [tuberculo- + G. *-osis,* condition]

tu·ber·cu·lo·sis cu·tis ver·ru·co·sa (tū-bĕr′kyū-lō′sis kyū′tis vĕr′rū-kō′să) A tuberculous skin lesion having a warty surface with a chronic inflammatory base. SEE ALSO postmortem wart. SYN tuberculous wart.

tu·ber·cu·lo·stat·ic (tū-bĕr′kyū-lō-stat′ik) Relating to an agent that inhibits the growth of tubercle bacilli. [tuberculo- + G. *statikos,* causing to stand]

tu·ber·cu·lous (tū-bĕr′kyū-lŭs) Relating to or affected by tuberculosis. Cf. tubercular.

tu·ber·cu·lous ab·scess (tū-bĕr′kyū-lŭs ab′ses) An abscess caused by the tubercle bacillus. SYN cold abscess (2).

tu·ber·cu·lous en·ter·i·tis (tū-bĕr′kyū-lŭs en′tĕr-ī′tis) Enteric tuberculosis that may occur in the absence of obvious pulmonary tuberculosis; may be caused by bovine tuberculosis contracted through consumption of unpasteurized milk or ingestion of tubercle bacilli expectorated from cavitary lesions in the lung.

tu·ber·cu·lous men·in·gi·tis (tū-bĕr′kyū-lŭs men-in-jī′tis) Inflammation of the cerebral leptomeninges marked by the presence of granulomatous inflammation; it is usually confined to the base of the brain (basilar meningitis, internal hydrocephalus) and is accompanied in children by an accumulation of spinal fluid in the ventricles (acute hydrocephalus).

tu·ber·cu·lous spon·dy·li·tis (tū-bĕr′kyū-lŭs spon′di-lī′tis) Tuberculous infection of the spine associated with a sharp angulation of the spine at the point of disease. SYN Pott disease.

tu·ber·cu·lous wart (tū-bĕr′kyū-lŭs wōrt) SYN tuberculosis cutis verrucosa.

tu·ber·cu·lum, pl. **tu·ber·cu·la** (tū-bĕr′kyū-lŭm, -lă) [TA] **1.** SYN tubercle (1). **2.** A circumscribed, rounded, solid elevation on the skin, mucous membrane, or surface of an organ. **3.** A slight elevation from the surface of a bone giving attachment to a muscle or ligament. [L. dim. of *tuber,* a knob, swelling, tumor]

tu·ber·cu·lum ar·thri·ti·cum (tū-bĕr′kyū-lŭm ahr-thrit′i-kŭm) **1.** SYN Heberden nodes. **2.** Any gouty concretion in or around a joint.

tu·ber·cu·lum im·par (tū-bĕr′kyū-lŭm im′pahr) SYN median lingual swelling.

tu·ber·os·i·tas (tū′bĕr-os′i-tas) SYN tuberosity. [LL., fr. L., *tuberosus,* full of lumps, fr. *tuber,* a knob]

tu·ber·os·i·ty (tū′bĕr-os′i-tē) A large tubercle or rounded elevation, especially from the surface of a bone. SYN tuberositas.

tu·ber·os·i·ty of fifth met·a·tar·sal (bone) [V] (tū′bĕr-os′i-tē fifth met′ă-tahr′săl bōn) A tubercle at the base of this bone, the posterior part of which is attached the tendon of the peroneus brevis muscle.

tu·ber·ous (tū′bĕr-ŭs) Knobby, lumpy, or nodular; presenting many tubers or tuberosities. [L. *tuberosus*]

tube tooth (tūb tūth) An artificial tooth constructed with a vertical, cylindric aperture extending from the center of the base up into the body of the tooth into which a pin may be placed or cast for the attachment of the tooth to a denture base.

♻ **tubo-** Combining form denoting tubular, a tube. SEE ALSO salpingo-. [L. *tubus, tuba,* tube]

tu·bo·ab·dom·i·nal preg·nan·cy (tū′bō-ab-dom′i-năl preg′năn-sē) Development of an ectopic pregnancy partly in the uterine tube and partly in the abdominal cavity.

tu·bo·o·var·i·an (tū′bō-ō-va′rē-ăn) Relating to the uterine (fallopian) tube and the ovary.

tu·bo·o·var·i·an ab·scess (tū′bō-ō-va′rē-ăn ab′ses) A large abscess involving a uterine tube and an adherent ovary, resulting from extension of purulent inflammation of the tube.

tu·bo·o·var·i·an preg·nan·cy (tū′bō-ō-va′rē-ăn preg′năn-sē) Development of the fertilized oocyte at the fimbriated extremity of the uterine tube and involving the ovary.

tu·bo·plas·ty (tū′bō-plas-tē) SYN salpingoplasty.

tu·bo·re·tic·u·lar struc·ture (tū′bō-rĕ-tik′yū-lar strŭk′shŭr) Tubules 20–30 nm in length that lie within cisterns of smooth endoplasmic reticulum; observed in connective tissue diseases such as SLE, and in various cancers and virus infections.

tu•bo•tor•sion (tū′bō-tōr-shŭn) Twisting of a tubular structure, such as an oviduct. [tubo- + L. *torsio,* torsion]

tu•bo•tym•pan•ic, tu•bo•tym•pa•nal (tū′bō-tim-pan′ik, -tim′pă-năl) Relating to the auditory tube and the tympanic cavity of the ear.

tu•bo•u•ter•ine (tū′bō-yū′tĕr-in) Relating to a uterine tube and the uterus.

tu•bu•lar car•ci•no•ma (tū′byū-lăr kahr′si-nō′mă) A well-differentiated form of ductal breast carcinoma with invasion of the stroma by small epithelial tubules.

tu•bu•lar cyst (tū′byū-lăr sist) SYN tubulocyst.

tu•bu•lar for•ceps (tū′byū-lăr fōr′seps) A long, slender forceps intended for use through a cannula or other tubular instrument.

tu•bu•lar gland (tū′byū-lăr gland) A gland composed of one or more tubules ending in a blind extremity.

tu•bu•lar vi•sion (tū′byū-lăr vizh′ŭn) A constriction of the visual field, as though one were looking through a hollow cylinder or tube. SYN tunnel vision.

tu•bule (tū′byūl) A small tube. SYN tubulus [TA]. [L. *tubulus,* dim. of *tubus,* tube]

tu•bu•li (tū′byū-lī) Plural of tubulus.

tu•bu•li con•tor•ti (tū′byū-lī kon-tōr′tī) **1.** SYN convoluted tubule. **2.** SYN seminiferous tubule.

tu•bu•lin (tū′byū-lin) A protein subunit of microtubules; it is a dimer composed of two globular polypeptides, α-tubulin and β-tubulin. SEE ALSO dynein.

tu•bu•li se•mi•ni•fer•i rec•ti (tū-byū′lī sem-i-nif′ĕr-ī rek′tī) [TA] SYN seminiferous tubule.

tu•bu•lo•ac•i•nar gland (tū′byū-lo-as′i-năr gland) A gland with secretory elements that are elongated acini. SYN acinotubular gland.

tu•bu•lo•cyst (tū′byū-lō-sist) A cyst formed by the dilation of any occluded canal or tube. SYN tubular cyst.

tu•bu•lo•glo•mer•u•lar feed•back (tū′byū-lō-glō-mĕr′yū-lăr fēd′bak) A blood flow control mechanism operating in the kidneys that limits changes in glomerular filtration rate.

tu•bu•lo•in•ter•sti•tial ne•phri•tis (tū′byū-lō-in-tĕr-stish′ăl nĕ-frī′tis) Inflammation affecting renal tubules and interstitial tissue, with infiltration by plasma cells and mononuclear cells; seen in lupus nephritis, allograft rejection, and methicillin sensitization.

tu•bu•lor•rhex•is (tū′byū-lō-rek′sis) A pathologic process characterized by necrosis of the epithelial lining in localized segments of renal tubules, with focal rupture or loss of the basement membrane. [tubule + G. *rhēxis,* a breaking]

tu•bu•lus, pl. **tu•bu•li** (tū′byū-lŭs, -lī) [TA] SYN tubule. [L. dim. of *tubus,* a pipe]

tu•bus, pl. **tu•bi** (tū′bŭs, -bī) A tube or canal. [L.]

tuft•ed cell (tŭf′tĕd sel) A particular type of cell in the olfactory bulb comparable to a mitral cell with respect to afferent and efferent relationships, but smaller and more superficially located.

tularaemia [Br.] SYN tularemia.

tu•la•re•mi•a (tū-lă-rē′mē-ă) A disease caused by *Francisella tularensis* and transmitted to humans from rodents through the bite of a deer fly, *Chrysops discalis,* and other bloodsucking insects; can also be acquired directly through the bite of an infected animal or through handling of an infected animal's carcass; symptoms consist of fever and swelling and suppuration of the lymph nodes draining the site of infection; rabbits are an important reservoir host. SYN deerfly fever, rabbit fever, tularaemia. [*Tulare,* Lake and County, California, + G. *haima,* blood]

Tul•li•o phe•nom•e•non (tū′lē-ō fĕ-nom′ĕ-non) Vertigo and nystagmus in response to high-intensity sounds, especially those of low frequency. SEE ALSO Hennebert sign.

Tul•li•o test (stan•dard) (tū′lē-ō test stan′dărd) A sound-evoked procedure that most often detects an abnormality in the semicircular canal. The patient is observed for abnormal eye movement phenomena during presentation of a loud sound to one ear. During the standard test, the patient is usually seated. However, it is not as useful as the postural Tullio test, which is performed with the patient standing. This latter method allows observation of possible postural destabilization, which enables detection of otolithic organ dysfunction as well.

tu•me•fac•tion (tū-mĕ-fak′shŭn) **1.** A swelling. **2.** SYN tumescence. [see tumefacient]

tu•me•fy (tū′mĕ-fī) To swell or to cause to swell.

tu•mes•cence (tū-mes′ĕns) The condition of being or becoming tumid. SYN tumefaction (2), turgescence. [L. *tumesco,* to begin to swell]

tu•mes•cent (tū-mes′ĕnt) Denoting tumescence. SYN turgescent.

tu•me•scent lip•o•suc•tion (tū-mes′ĕnt lip′ō-sŭk-shŭn) Liposuction performed after subcutaneous infusion of lidocaine solution and the use of microcannulae.

tu•mid (tū′mid) Swollen, as by congestion, edema, hyperemia. SYN turgid. [L. *tumidus*]

tum•my tuck (tŭm′ē tŭk) Colloquial usage for SYN abdominoplasty.

tu•mor (tū′mŏr) **1.** Any swelling or tumefaction. **2.** SYN neoplasm. **3.** One of the four signs of inflammation (tumor, calor, dolor, rubor) enunciated by Celsus. See page B10. SYN tumour. [L. *tumor,* a swelling]

tu•mor an•gi•o•gen•ic fac•tor (TAF) (tū′mŏr an′jē-ō-jen′ik fak′tŏr) A substance released by a solid tumor that induces formation of new blood vessels to supply the tumor. SYN tumour angiogenic factor.

tu•mor an•ti•gens (tū′mŏr an′ti-jenz) **1.** Those antigens that may be frequently associated with tumors or may be specifically found on tumor cells of the same origin (tumor specific). **2.** Tumor antigens may also be associated with replication and transformation by certain DNA tumor viruses, including adenoviruses and papovaviruses. SYN neoantigens, tumour antigens. SEE ALSO T antigens.

tu•mor blush (tū′mŏr blŭsh) Enhancement of tumor on radiologic examination by administration of contrast agents. SYN tumour blush.

tu•mor bur•den (tū′mŏr bŭr′dĕn) The total mass of tumor tissue carried by a patient with cancer. SYN tumour burden.

tu•mor•i•ci•dal (tū′mŏr-i-sī′dăl) Denoting an agent destructive to tumors. SYN tumouricidal. [tumor + L. *caedo,* to kill]

tu•mor•i•gen•e•sis (tū′mŏr-i-jen′ĕ-sis) Production of a new growth or growths. SYN tumourigenesis. [tumor + G. *genesis,* origin]

tu•mor•i•gen•ic (tū′mŏr-i-jen′ik) Causing or producing tumors. SYN tumourigenic.

tu•mor mark•er (tū′mŏr mahr′kĕr) A substance released into thc circulation by tumor tissue; its detection in the serum indicates the presence and specific type of tumor. SYN tumour marker.

tu•mor ne•cro•sis fac•tor-al•pha (α) (tū′mŏr nĕ-krō′sis fak′tŏr al′fă) A pleiotropic cytokine synthesized widely throughout the female reproductive tract.

tu•mor ne•cro•sis fac•tor-be•ta (β) (tū′mŏr nĕ-krō′sis fak′tŏr bā′tă) A cytokine that is produced by CD4 and CD8 T cells after exposure to an antigen. Adverse responses include cachexia and toxic shock syndrome.

tu•mor in si•tu (TIS) (tū′mŏr in sī′tū) A lesion that remains localized to a given site; one that has not yet metastasized.

tu•mor-spe•ci•fic trans•plan•ta•tion ant•i•gens (TSTA) (tū′mŏr-spĕ-sif′ik trans′plan-tā′shŭn an′ti-jenz) Surface antigens of DNA tumor virus–transformed cells, which elicit an immune rejection of the virus-free cells when transplanted into an animal that has been immunized against the specific cell-transforming virus. SYN tumour-specific transplantation antigens.

tu•mor stage (tū′mŏr stāj) The extent of the spread of a malignant neoplasm from its site of origin. SEE ALSO TNM staging. SYN tumour stage.

tu•mor sup•pres•sor gene (tū′mŏr sŭ-pres′ŏr jēn) **1.** A gene the function of which is to suppress cellular proliferation. Also known as an antioncogene because it suppresses neoplastic transformation. Loss of a tumor suppressor gene through chromosomal aberration leads to heightened susceptibility to neoplasia. **2.** SYN antioncogene. SYN tumour supressor gene.

tu•mor vi•rus (tū′mŏr vī′rŭs) SYN oncogenic virus. SYN tumour virus.

tumour [Br.] SYN tumor.

tumour angiogenic factor [Br.] SYN tumor angiogenic factor.

tumour antigens [Br.] SYN tumor antigens.

tumour blush [Br.] SYN tumor blush.

tumour burden [Br.] SYN tumor burden.

tumouricidal [Br.] SYN tumoricidal.

tumourigenesis [Br.] SYN tumorigenesis.

tumourigenic [Br.] SYN tumorigenic.

tumour marker [Br.] SYN tumor marker.

tumour-specific transplantation antigens [Br.] SYN tumor-specific transplantation antigens.

tumour stage [Br.] SYN tumor stage.

tumour supressor gene [Br.] SYN tumor suppressor gene.

tumour virus [Br.] SYN tumor virus.

TUNEL (tŭn′ĕl) Acronym for terminal deoxynucleotidyl transferase-mediated dUTP-biotin end labeling of fragmented DNA; uses immunohistochemistry to identify DNA fragmentation in nuclei of cells undergoing apoptosis.

Tun•ga pe•ne•trans (tŭng′ă pen′ĕ-tranz) A member of the flea family, Tungidae, commonly known as a chigger flea, sand flea, chigoe, or jigger; the minute female penetrates the skin, frequently under the toenails; as its body becomes distended with eggs, to about the size of a pea, a painful ulcer with inflammation develops at the site.

tung•sten (W) (tŭng′stĕn) A metallic element, atomic no. 74, atomic wt. 183.85. SYN wolfram, wolframium. [Swed. *tung,* heavy, + *sten,* stone]

tu•nic (tū′nik) Coat or covering; one of the enveloping layers of a part, especially one of the coats of a blood vessel or other tubular structure. SYN tunica. [L. *tunica*]

tu•ni•ca, pl. **tu•ni•cae** (tū′ni-kă, -kē) SYN tunic. [L. a coat]

tu•ni•ca ad•ven•ti•ti•a (tū′ni-kă ad-ven-tish′ē-ă) [TA] SYN adventitia.

tu•ni•ca al•bu•gin•e•a (tū′ni-kă al-byū-jin′ē-ă) A dense white collagenous tunic surrounding a structure.

tu•ni•ca al•bu•gin•e•a of tes•tis (tū′ni-kă al-byū-jin′ē-ă tes′tis) A thick white fibrous membrane forming the outer coat of the testis.

tu•ni•ca ex•ter•na (tū′ni-kă eks-ter′nă) [TA] **1.** The outer of two or more enveloping layers of any structure; **2.** Specifically, the outer fibroelastic coat of a blood or lymph vessel.

tu•ni•ca in•ti•ma (tū′ni-kă in′ti-mă) [TA] The innermost coat of a blood or lymphatic vessel; consists of endothelium, usually a thin fibroelastic subendothelial layer, and an inner elastic membrane of longitudinal fibers.

tu•ni•ca me•di•a (tū′ni-kă mē′dē-ă) The middle, usually muscular, coat of an artery or other tubular structure. SYN media (1).

tu•ni•ca pro•pri•a (tū′ni-kă prō′prē-ă) The special envelope of a part, as distinguished from the peritoneal or other investment common to several parts.

tu•ni•ca re•flex•a (tū′ni-kă rē-fleks′ă) The reflected layer of the tunica vasculosa testis that lines the scrotum.

tu•ni•ca va•gi•na•lis tes•tis (tū′ni-kă vaj-i-nā′lis tes′tis) The serous sheath of the testis and epididymis, derived from the peritoneum; it consists of outer parietal and inner visceral serous layers.

tu•ni•ca vas•cu•lo•sa (tū′ni-kă vas-kyū-lō′să) Any vascular layer.

tun•ing curve (tūn′ing kŭrv) A graph of acoustic threshold intensity at various frequencies for a single neuron.

tun•ing fork (TF) (tūn′ing fōrk) Steel or magnesium-alloy instrument roughly resembling a two-pronged fork, the vibrations of the prongs of which, when struck, give a musical tone of restricted bandwidth; used to test the hearing and vibratory sensation.

tun•nel (tŭn′ĕl) An elongated passageway, usually open at both ends.

tun•nel vi•sion (tŭn′ĕl vizh′ŭn) SYN tubular vision.

Tur•ba•trix (tŭr-bā′triks) A genus of free-living nematodes in the family Cephalobidae. [L. *turbare,* to disturb]

Tur•ba•trix a•ce•ti (tŭr-bā′triks ăs-ē′tī) A nematode species found in old vinegar, in rotting fruits and vegetables, and occasionally as a contaminant in laboratory solutions. SYN vinegar eel.

tur•bid (tŭr′bid) Clouded, as by sediment or insoluble matter in a solution. [L. *turbidus,* confused, disordered]

tur•bi•dim•e•try (tŭr-bi-dim′ĕ-trē) A method for determining the concentration of a substance in a solution by the degree of cloudiness or turbidity it causes or by the degree of clarification it induces in a turbid solution. [turbidity + G. *metron,* measure]

tur•bid•i•ty (tŭr-bid′i-tē) The quality of being turbid, of losing transparency because of sediment or insoluble matter. [L. *turbiditas,* fr. *turbidus,* turbid]

tur•bi•nate, **tur•bi•nat•ed** (tŭr′bi-nāt, -nāt-ĕd) **1.** Shaped like a top. **2.** Any of the turbinated bones. SEE ALSO inferior nasal concha, middle nasal concha, superior nasal concha, supreme nasal concha. [L. *turbinatus,*, shaped like a top]

tur•bi•nec•to•my (tŭr′bi-nek′tŏ-mē) Surgical removal of a turbinated bone. [turbinate + G. *ektomē,* excision]

tur•bi•not•o•my (tŭr′bi-not′ŏ-mē) Incision into or excision of a turbinated body. [turbinate + G. *tomē,* incision]

tur•bu•lent flow (tŭr′byū-lĕnt flō) A flow of gas characterized by a rough-and-tumble pattern; all molecules proceed at the same velocity, and resistance to flow is increased when compared with laminar flow.

Türck de•gen•er•a•tion (tērk dĕ-jen′ĕr-ā′shŭn) Degeneration of a nerve fiber and its sheath distal to the point of injury or section of the axon; usually applied to degeneration within the central nervous system.

turf burn (tŭrf bŭrn) Deep abrasion caused by friction between skin and an artificial playing surface.

turf toe (tŭrf tō) Sprain and subsequent inflammation of the first metatarsophalangeal joint.

tur•ges•cence (tŭr-jes′ĕns) SYN tumescence. [L. *turgesco,* to begin to swell, fr. *turgeo,* to swell]

tur•ges•cent (tŭr-jes′ĕnt) SYN tumescent.

tur•gid (tŭr′jid) SYN tumid. [L. *turgidus,* swollen, fr. *turgeo,* to swell]

tur•gor (tŭr′gŏr) Fullness. [L., fr. *turgeo,* to swell]

tu•ris•ta (tū-rēs′tă) SYN Montezuma's revenge. [Sp. tourist]

turn•a•round time (TAT) (tŭrn′ă-rownd tīm) The interval between the ordering of a clinical laboratory test or other diagnostic procedure and the reporting of results.

Tur•ner syn•drome (tŭr′nĕr sin′drōm) A syndrome with chromosome count 45 and only one X chromosome; buccal and other cells usually test negative for sex chromatin; anomalies include dwarfism, webbed neck, valgus of elbows, pigeon chest, infantile sexual development, and amenorrhea; the ovary has no primordial follicles and may be represented only by a fibrous streak; some patients are chromosomally mosaic, with two or more cell lines of different chromosome constitution; seen in many animal species; in the meadow vole, it is the normal female state. SYN XO syndrome.

Tur•ner tooth (tŭr′nĕr tūth) Enamel hypoplasia involving a solitary permanent tooth; related to infection in the primary tooth that preceded it or to trauma during odontogenesis.

turn•o•ver num•ber (tŭrn′ō-vĕr nŭm′bĕr) The number of substrate molecules converted into product in an enzyme-catalyzed reaction under saturating conditions per unit time per unit quantity of enzyme; e.g., $k_{cat} = V_{max}/[E_{total}]$.

tus•sal (tŭs′ăl) SYN tussive.

tus•sis (tŭs′is) A cough. [L.]

tus•sive (tŭs′iv) Relating to a cough. SYN tussal. [L. *tussis,* a cough]

tus•sive frem•i•tus (tŭs′iv frem′i-tŭs) A form of palpable vibration similar to the vocal, produced by a cough.

tus•sive syn•co•pe (tŭs′iv sing′kŏ-pē) Fainting as a result of a coughing spell, caused by persistent increased intrathoracic pressure diminishing venous return to the heart, thus lowering cardiac output; most often occurs in heavy-set male smokers who have chronic bronchitis. SYN Charcot vertigo.

Tut•tle proc•to•scope (tŭt′ĕl prok′tŏ-skōp) A tubular rectal speculum illuminated at its distal extremity; after introduction, the obturator is withdrawn and a glass window is inserted in the proximal end; then, by means of a rubber bulb and tube connected with the proctoscope, the rectal ampulla may be inflated.

TWAR (twahr) SYN *Chlamydia pneumoniae.* [Acronym derived from the laboratory designations of the first two isolates, TW-83 and AR-39]

T wave (wāv) Waveform in an ECG tracing representing ventricular repolarization.

twelfth cra•ni•al nerve [CN XII] (twelfth krā′nē-ăl nĕrv) SYN hypoglossal nerve [CN XII].

twelfth-year mo•lar (twelfth-yēr mō′lăr) The second permanent molar tooth.

twice writh•en (twīs ridh′ĕn) SYN bistort.

twi•light state (twī′līt stāt) A condition of disordered consciousness during which actions may be performed without the conscious volition of the patient and with no memory of such actions.

twin (twin) **1.** One of two children born at one birth. **2.** Double; growing in pairs. [A.S. *getwin,* double]

twinge (twinj) A sudden momentary sharp pain.

twin•ning (twin′ing) Production of equivalent structures by division; the tendency of divided parts to assume symmetric relations.

twin pla•cen•ta (twin plă-sen′tă) The placenta(s) of a twin pregnancy; if dizygotic, the placentas may be separate or fused, the latter retaining two amnionic and two chorionic sacs (dichorionic diamnionic placenta); if monozygotic, the placenta may be a monochorionic monoamnionic placenta or monochorionic diamnionic placenta, depending on the stage at which twinning took place; if twinning occurs early, there may be a fused placenta with two chorionic and two amnionic membranes.

twin re•versed ar•ter•i•al per•fu•sion se•quence (twin rē-vĕrst′ ahr-tēr′ē-ăl pĕr-fyū′zhŭn sē′kwĕns) A circulatory anomaly in monozygotic twins in whom there are placental arterioarterial and venovenous anastomoses and umbilical anomalies, with one fetus being perfused with deoxygenated blood; the recipient fetus develops as an acardiac acephalic, and the pump or donor twin is at risk for cardiac failure.

twin-twin trans•fu•sion (twin-twin trans-fyū′zhŭn) Direct vascular anastomosis, arterial or venous, between the placental circulations of twins.

twist•ed hairs (twist′ĕd hārz) SYN pili torti.

twitch (twich) **1.** To jerk spasmodically. **2.** A momentary spasmodic contraction of a muscle fiber. [A.S. *twiccian*]

two-car•bon frag•ment (tū-kahr′bŏn frag′mĕnt) The acetyl group (CH_3CO–) that takes part in transacetylation reactions with coenzyme A as carrier; commonly referred to as acetate or acetic acid, from which it is derived.

two-di•men•sion•al ech•o•car•di•og•ra•phy (tū-di-men′shŭn-ăl ek′ō-kahr-dē-og′ră-fē) That modality in which an image is reconstructed from the echoes stimulated and detected by a linear array or moving transducers. SYN real-time echocardiography.

two-di•men•sion–three-di•men•sion phe•nom•e•non (tū′dī-men′shŭn-thrē′di-men′shŭn fĕ-nom′ĕ-non) An experience in telescopic endoscopy in which a two-dimensional image appears to be three-dimensional because of the movement of the endoscope in and out of the view of the object.

two-glass test (tū-glas test) SYN Thompson test (1).

two-step ex•er•cise test (tū-step ek′sĕr-sīz test) A test used mainly for coronary insufficiency; significant depression of RS-T in the electrocardiogram is considered abnormal and suggests coronary insufficiency.

two-way cath•e•ter (tū-wā kath′ĕ-tĕr) SYN double-channel catheter.

ty•ing for•ceps (tī′ing fōr′seps) An instrument with flat, smooth tips used in ophthalmic surgery, particularly for tying sutures.

ty•lec•to•my (tī-lek′tŏ-mē) Surgical removal of a localized swelling or tumor. SEE ALSO lumpectomy. [G. *tylē,* lump, + *ektomē,* excision]

ty•lo•ma (tī-lō′mă) SYN callosity. [G. a callus]

ty•lo•sis, pl. **ty•lo•ses** (tī-lō′sis, -sēz) Formation of a callosity (tyloma). [G. a becoming callous]

ty•lot•ic (tī-lot′ik) Relating to or marked by tylosis.

tym•pa•nal (tim′pă-năl) **1.** SYN tympanic (1). **2.** Resonant. **3.** SYN tympanitic (2).

tym•pa•nec•to•my (tim-pă-nek′tŏ-mē) Excision of the tympanic membrane. [tympan- + G. *ektomē,* excision]

tym•pan•ic (tim-pan′ik) **1.** Relating to the tympanic cavity or membrane. SYN tympanal (1). **2.** Resonant. **3.** SYN tympanitic (2).

tym•pan•ic bone (tim-pan′ik bōn) SYN tympanic ring.

tym•pan•ic can•a•lic•u•lus (tim-pan′ik kan-ă-lik′yū-lŭs) A minute canal passing from the inferior surface of the petrous portion of the temporal bone between the jugular fossa and carotid canal to the floor of the tympanic cavity. Located in the wedge of bone separating the jugular canal and carotid canal, it transmits the tympanic branch of the glossopharyngeal nerve.

tym•pan•ic ca•vi•ty (tim-pan′ik kav′i-tē) An air chamber in the temporal bone containing the ossicles; it is lined with mucous membrane and is continuous with the auditory tube anteriorly and the tympanic antrum and mastoid air cells posteriorly.

tym•pan•ic gan•gli•on (tim-pan′ik gang′glē-ŏn) A small ganglion on the tympanic nerve during its passage through the petrous portion of the temporal bone.

tym•pan•ic mem•brane (tim-pan′ik mem′brān) A thin, tense covering that forms the greater part of the lateral wall of the tympanic cavity and separates it from the external acoustic meatus; it constitutes the boundary between the external and middle ear, is covered on both surfaces with epithelium, and in the tense part has an intermediate layer of outer radial and inner circular collagen fibers. See page B28. SYN membrana tympani [TA], drum membrane, drum, drumhead, eardrum, myringa, myrinx.

tym•pan•ic nerve (tim-pan′ik nĕrv) *Origin,* from the inferior ganglion of the glossopharyngeal nerve, passing through the tympanic canaliculus to the tympanic cavity, forming there the tympanic plexus that supplies the mucous membrane of the tympanic cavity, mastoid cells, and auditory tube; presynaptic parasympathetic fibers also pass through the tympanic nerve through the lesser superficial petrosal nerve to the otic ganglion, where they synapse with postsynaptic fibers that continue to supply the parotid gland. SYN nervus tympanicus [TA], Andersch nerve.

tym•pan•ic o•pen•ing of au•di•tor•y tube (tim-pan′ik ō′pĕn-ing aw′di-tōr-ē tūb) An opening in the anterior part of the tympanic cavity below the canal for the tensor tympani muscle.

tym•pan•ic plex•us (tim-pan′ik pleks′ŭs) A neural network on the promontory of the labyrinthine wall of the tympanic cavity, formed by the tympanic nerve, an anastomotic branch of the facial, and sympathetic branches from the internal carotid plexus; it supplies the mucosa of the middle ear, mastoid cells, and auditory (eustachian) tube, and gives off the lesser superficial petrosal nerve to the otic ganglion.

tym•pan•ic ring (tim-pan′ik ring) In the fetus, a more or less complete bony ring at the medial end of the cartilaginous external acoustic meatus, to which is attached the tympanic membrane. SYN anulus tympanicus [TA], tympanic bone.

tym•pan•ic si•nus (tim-pan′ik sī′nŭs) A depression in the tympanic cavity behind the tympanic promontory.

tym•pan•ic ther•mom•e•ter (tim-pan′ik thĕr-mom′ĕ-tĕr) An electronic thermometer that measures temperature by scanning the tympanic membrane. See this page.

tym•pan•ic veins (tim-pan′ik vānz) Exit from

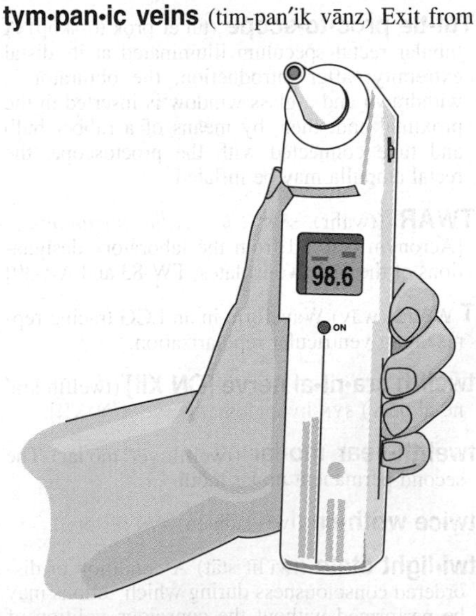

tympanic thermometer: display of core body temperature of blood vessels of tympanic membrane

the tympanic cavity through the petrotympanic fissure with the chorda tympani and empty into the retromandibular vein.

tym•pa•nism (tim′pă-nizm) SYN tympanites.

tym•pa•ni•tes (tim-pă-nī′tēz) Swelling of the abdomen due to gas in the intestinal or peritoneal cavity. SYN meteorism, tympanism. [L. fr. G. *tympanitēs,* an edema in which the belly is stretched like a drum, *tympanon*]

tym•pa•nit•ic (tim-pă-nit′ik) **1.** Referring to tympanites. SYN tympanous. **2.** Denoting the quality of sound elicited by percussing over the inflated intestine or a large pulmonary cavity. SYN tympanal (3), tympanic (3).

tym•pa•nit•ic res•o•nance (tim-pă-nit′ik rez′ ŏ-năns) SYN tympany.

tym•pa•ni•tis (tim-pă-nī′tis) SYN myringitis.

tympano-, tympan-, tympani- Combining forms denoting eardrum, tympanites, or tympanic membrane. [G. *tympanon,* drum]

tym•pa•no•cen•te•sis (tim′pă-nō-sen-tē′sis) Puncture of the tympanic membrane with a needle to aspirate middle ear fluid. [tympano- + G. *kentēsis,* puncture]

tym•pan•o•gram (tim′pă-nō-gram) A visual depiction (e.g., a printout) of the relative compliance and impedance of the structures of the middle ear in response to pressure changes in the external ear canal. See this page.

tym•pa•no•mas•toid fis•sure (tim′pă-nō-mas′toyd fish′ŭr) A fissure separating the tympanic portion from the mastoid portion of the temporal bone; it transmits the auricular branch of the vagus nerve.

tym•pa•nom•e•try (tim-pă-nom′ĕ-trē) Measurement of the pressure compliance function of the eardrum using an immitance instrument (e.g., an audiometer).

tym•pa•no•plas•ty (tim′pă-nō-plas-tē) Operative correction of a damaged middle ear. [tympano- + G. *plassō,* to form]

tym•pan•o•scler•o•sis (tim′pan-ō-skler-ō′sis) The formation of dense connective tissue in the middle ear, often resulting in hearing loss when the ossicles are involved. See page B28.

tym•pan•os•to•my (tim′pan-os′tŏ-mē) SYN myringotomy. [tympano- + G. *ostium,* mouth]

tym•pan•os•to•my tube (tim′pan-os′tŏ-mē tūb) A small tube inserted through the tympanic membrane after myringotomy to aerate the middle ear; often used as therapy for serous otitis media.

tym•pa•not•o•my (tim′pă-not′ŏ-mē) SYN myringotomy. [tympano- + G. *tomē,* incision]

tym•pa•nous (tim′pă-nŭs) SYN tympanitic (1).

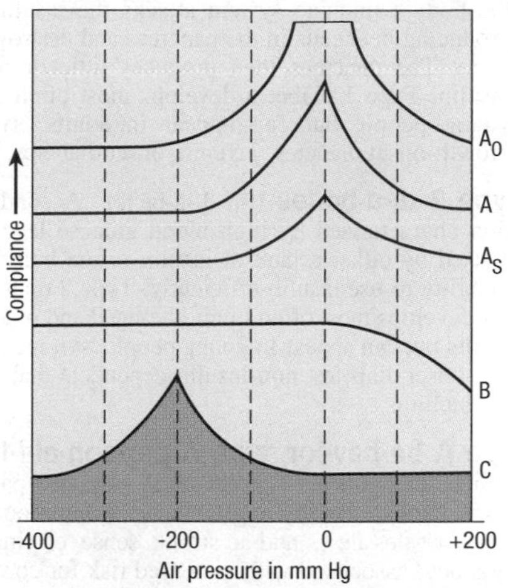

tympanogram: five tympanograms illustrating various conditions of the middle ear: type A is typical of normal middle ear; type A_S is associated with stiffness of stapes; type A_0 is associated with interruptions in the chain of bones or flaccidity of the eardrum membrane; type B suggests fluid in the middle ear; type C suggests that the pressure within the middle ear is below atmospheric pressure

tym•pan•o•ves•tib•u•lar coup•ling (tim′pă-nō-ves-tib′yū-lăr kŭp′ling) A direct or indirect coupling between the tympanic structures (e.g., tympanic membrane, ossicles, and middle ear cavity) and a vestibular end organ; results in abnormal responsiveness of the vestibular end organ to pressure changes or sound vibrations transmitted from the tympanic structures.

tym•pa•ny (tim′pă-nē) A low-pitched, resonant, drumlike note obtained by percussing the surface of a large air-containing space, such as the distended abdomen or the thorax with or without pneumothorax. SYN tympanitic resonance.

Tyn•dall phe•nom•e•non (tin′dăl fĕ-nom′ĕ-non) The visibility of floating particles in gases or liquids when illuminated by a ray of sunlight and viewed at right angles to the illuminating ray.

type (tīp) **1.** The usual form or a composite that all others of the class resemble more or less closely; a model, denoting especially a disease or a symptom complex giving the stamp or characteristic to a class. SEE ALSO constitution, habitus, personality. **2.** CHEMISTRY a substance in which the arrangement of the atoms in a molecule may be taken as representative of other substances in that class. SYN typus. [G. *typos,* a mark, a model]

Type 1 di•a•be•tes (tīp dī-ă-bē′tēz) A condition characterized by high blood glucose levels caused by a total lack of insulin. Occurs when the body's immune system attacks the insulin-producing beta cells in the pancreas and destroys them. The pancreas then produces little or no insulin. Type 1 diabetes develops most often in young people but can appear in adults. SYN growth-onset diabetes, juvenile-onset diabetes.

Type 2 di•a•be•tes (tīp dī-ă-bē′tēz) A condition characterized by high blood glucose levels caused by either a lack of insulin or the body's inability to use insulin efficiently. Type 2 diabetes develops most often in middle-aged and older adults but can appear in young people. SYN maturity-onset diabetes, non-insulin-dependent diabetes mellitus.

type A be•hav•ior, type A per•son•al•i•ty (tīp bē-hāv′yŏr, pĕr-sŏn-al′i-tē) A behavior pattern characterized by aggressiveness, ambitiousness, restlessness, and a strong sense of time urgency; associated with increased risk for coronary heart disease.

type B be•hav•ior, type B per•son•al•i•ty (tīp bē-hāv′yŏr, pĕr-sŏn-al′i-tē) A behavior pattern characterized by the absence or obverse of type A behavior characteristics.

type cul•ture (tīp kŭl′chŭr) A type strain of microorganism preserved in a culture collection as the standard or quality-control strain.

type I fa•mil•i•al hy•per•lip•o•pro•tein•e•mi•a (tīp fă-mil′ē-ăl hī′pĕr-lip′ō-prō-tēn-ē′mē-ă) Increased hematologic lipoprotein levels characterized by the presence of large amounts of chylomicrons and triglycerides in the plasma when the patient has a normal diet, and their disappearance on a fat-free diet. It is accompanied by bouts of abdominal pain, hepatosplenomegaly, pancreatitis, and eruptive xanthomas; autosomal recessive inheritance. SYN familial fat-induced hyperlipemia, familial hyperchylomicronemia, familial hypertriglyceridemia (1).

Type I fi•bers (tīp fī′bĕrz) SYN slow-twitch fibers.

type II fa•mil•i•al hy•per•lip•o•pro•tein•e•mi•a (tīp fă-mil′ē-ăl hī-pĕr-lip′ō-prō-tēn-ē′mē-ă) Increased hematologic lipoprotein levels characterized by increased plasma levels of β-lipoproteins, cholesterol, and phospholipids, but normal triglycerides levels. Homozygotes have xanthomatosis and frank clinical atherosclerosis as young adults. The primary defect is a deficiency of apoprotein of VLDL. SYN familial hypercholesterolemia.

Type II fi•bers (tīp fī′bĕrz) SYN fast-twitch fibers.

type III fa•mil•i•al hy•per•lip•o•pro•tein•e•mi•a (tīp fă-mil′ē-ăl hī-pĕr-lip′ō-prō-tēn-ē′mē-ă) Increased hematologic lipoprotein levels characterized by increased plasma levels of LDL, β-lipoproteins, pre-β-lipoproteins, cholesterol, phospholipids, and triglycerides; frequent eruptive xanthomas and atheromatosis, particularly coronary artery disease; biochemical defect lies in apolipoproteins. SYN familial hypercholesterolemia with hyperlipemia.

type IV fa•mil•i•al hy•per•lip•o•pro•tein•e•mi•a (tīp fă-mil′ē-ăl hī-pĕr-lip′ō-prō-tēn-ē′mē-ă) In people following a normal diet plasma levels of VLDL, pre-β-lipoproteins, and triglycerides are increased, but with normal levels of β-lipoproteins, cholesterol, and phospholipids; may be accompanied by abnormal glucose tolerance and susceptibility to ischemic heart disease. SYN familial hypertriglyceridemia (2).

type V fa•mil•i•al hy•per•lip•o•pro•tein•e•mi•a (tīp fă-mil′ē-ăl hī′pĕr-lip′ō-prō-tēn-ē′mē-ă) Increased hematologic lipoprotein levels characterized especially by increased plasma levels of chylomicrons, VLDL, pre-β-lipoproteins, and triglycerides; may be accompanied by bouts of abdominal pain, hepatosplenomegaly, susceptibility to atherosclerosis, and abnormal glucose tolerance.

typh•lec•ta•sis (tif-lek′tă-sis) Dilation of the cecum. [G. *typhlon*, cecum, + *ektasis*, a stretching out]

typh•lec•to•my (tif-lek′tŏ-mē) SYN cecectomy.

typh•len•ter•i•tis (tif′len-tĕr-ī′tis) SYN cecitis.

typh•li•tis (tif-lī′tis) SYN cecitis.

♻**typhlo-, typhl-** **1.** Combining forms denoting the cecum. SEE ALSO ceco-. [G. cecum] **2.** Combining forms denoting blindness. [G. *typhlos,* blind]

typh•lo•dic•li•di•tis (tif′lō-dik′li-dī′tis) Inflammation of the ileocecal valve. [G. *typhlon,* cecum, + *diklis* (*diklid-*), double-folding (of doors), + *-itis,* inflammation]

typh•lo•en•ter•i•tis (tif′lō-en-tĕr-ī′tis) SYN cecitis.

typh•lo•li•thi•a•sis (tif′lō-li-thī′ă-sis) Presence of fecal concretions in the cecum. [G. *typhlon,* cecum, + *lithos,* stone]

typh•lo•pex•y, typh•lo•pex•i•a (tif′lō-pek-sē, -pek′sē-ă) SYN cecopexy.

typh•lor•rha•phy (tif-lōr′ă-fē) SYN cecorrhaphy.

typh•lo•sis (tif-lō′sis) SYN blindness. [G. *typhlos,* blind]

typh•los•to•my (tif-los′tŏ-mē) SYN cecostomy.

typh•lot•o•my (tif-lot′ŏ-mē) SYN cecotomy.

ty•phoid (tī′foyd) **1.** Typhuslike; stuporous from fever. **2.** SYN typhoid fever. [typhus + G. *eidos,* resemblance]

ty•phoid•al (tī-foyd′ăl) Relating to or resembling typhoid fever.

ty•phoid ba•cil•lus (tī′foyd bă-sil′ŭs) SYN *Salmonella typhi.*

ty•phoid fe•ver (tī′foyd fē′vĕr) An acute infectious disease caused by *Salmonella typhi;* characterized by a continued fever, severe physical and mental depression, an eruption of rose-colored spots on the chest and abdomen, tympanites, often diarrhea, and sometimes intestinal hemorrhage or perforation of the bowel; average duration is 4 weeks, although aborted forms and relapses are not uncommon; the lesions are located chiefly in the lymph follicles of the intestines (Peyer patches), the mesenteric glands, and the spleen; antibody titer of the Widal test rises during the infection, and early positive blood and urine cultures become negative. SYN enteric fever (1), typhoid (2).

ty•phous (tī′fŭs) Relating to typhus.

ty•phus (tī′fŭs) A group of acute infectious and contagious diseases caused by rickettsiae that are transmitted by arthropods. Three main forms exist: louse borne (epidemic, recrudescent [i.e., Brill-Zinsser disease], murine (endemic), and scrub (Tsutsugamushi fever). Also called jail, camp, or ship fever. SYN camp fever (1). [G. *typhos,* smoke, stupor]

typ•i•cal dru•sen (tip′i-kăl drū′sĕn) SYN exudative drusen.

typ•ing (tīp′ing) Classification according to type. SEE ALSO type.

ty•pus (tī′pŭs) SYN type.

Tyr Abbreviation for tyrosine and its radicals.

Ty•rode so•lu•tion (tī′rōd sō-lū′shŭn) A modified Locke solution; it contains 8 g NaCl, 0.2 g KCl, 0.2 g $CaCl_2$, 0.1-g $MgCl_2$, 0.05 g NaH_2PO_4, 1 g $NaHCO_3$, 1 g D-glucose, and water to make 1000 mL; used to irrigate the peritoneal cavity, and in laboratory work.

ty•ro•ke•to•nu•ri•a (tī′rō-kē′tō-nyūr′ē-ă) The urinary excretion of ketonic metabolites of tyrosine, such as *p*-hydroxyphenylpyruvic acid.

ty•ro•ma (tī-rō′mă) A caseous tumor. [G. *tyros,* cheese, + *-ōma,* tumor]

ty•ro•sine (Tyr, Y) (tī′rō-sēn) An α-amino acid present in most proteins.

ty•ro•si•nu•ri•a (tī′rō-si-nyūr′ē-ă) The excretion of tyrosine in the urine. [tyrosine + G. *ouron,* urine]

ty•ro•sy•lu•ri•a (tī′rō-sil-yūr′ē-ă) Enhanced urinary excretion of certain metabolites of tyrosine, such as *p*-hydroxyphenylpyruvic acid; present in tyrosinosis, scurvy, pernicious anemia, and other diseases.

TYSGM-9 me•di•um (mē′dē-ŭm) Culture medium consisting of gastric mucin, nutrient broth, bovine serum, and rice starch; used to detect the presence of *Entamoeba histolytica.* SEE ALSO TY1-S-33 medium.

TY1-S-33 me•di•um (mē′dē-ŭm) Culture medium consisting of biosate peptone, dextrose, vitamins, and bovine serum; used to detect the presence of *Entamoeba histolytica.* SEE ALSO TYSGM-9 medium.

U

ʋ Upsilon.

U **1.** Abbreviation for kilurane; uranium; uridine in polymers; uracil; internal energy; urinary concentration, followed by subscripts indicating location and chemical species. **2.** Symbol for uranium.

U Internal energy.

UB-92 SYN CMS-1450.

u•bi•qui•nol (QH_2) (yū′bi-kwi′nol) The reduction product of a ubiquinone.

u•bi•qui•none (yū-bi-kwi′nōn) A 2,3-dimethoxy-5-methyl-1,4-benzoquinone with a multiprenyl side chain; a mobile component of electron transport. SEE ALSO coenzyme Q.

u•biq•ui•tin (yū-bik′kwi-tin) A small protein found in all cells of higher organisms; its structure has changed minimally during evolutionary history; involved in histone modification and intracellular protein breakdown.

u•biq•ui•tin-pro•te•ase path•way (yū-bik′ kwi-tin-prō′tē-ās path′wā) Pathway in which a small protein cofactor, ubiquitin, couples with protein substrate to catalyze proteolytic destruction by proteases; this pathway is highly selective and tightly regulated and is responsible for protein degradation seen in muscle-wasting diseases.

UDP Abbreviation for uridine 5′-diphosphate.

UDPglu•cose-hex•ose-1-phos•phate u•ri•dyl•yl•trans•fer•ase (glū′kōs-heks′ōs-fos′fāt yūr′i-dil′il-trans′fĕr-ās) An enzyme that catalyzes the reversible reaction of α-D-glucose 1-phosphate UDPgalactose to produce UDPglucose and α-D-galactose 1-phosphate.

UGI Abbreviation for upper gastrointestinal (UGI) series.

ul•cer (ŭl′sĕr) An erosive or penetrating lesion on a cutaneous or mucosal surface, usually with inflammation. Cf. erosion. See this page, B11. SYN ulcus. [L. *ulcus* (*ulcer-*), a sore, ulcer]

ul•cer•a (ŭl′sĕr-ă) Plural of ulcus.

ul•cer•ate (ŭl′sĕr-āt) To form an ulcer.

ul•cer•at•ing gran•u•lo•ma of pu•den•da (ul′sĕr-āt′ing gran′yū-lō′mă pū-den′dă) SYN granuloma inguinale.

ul•cer•a•tion (ŭl-sĕr-ā′shŭn) **1.** The formation of an ulcer. **2.** An ulcer or aggregation of ulcers.

ul•cer•a•tive (ŭl′sĕr-ă-tiv) Relating to, causing, or marked by an ulcer or ulcers.

ul•cer•a•tive co•li•tis (ŭl′sĕr-ă-tiv kō-lī′tis) A chronic disease of unknown cause characterized by ulceration of the colon and rectum, with rectal bleeding, mucosal crypt abscesses, inflammatory pseudopolyps, abdominal pain, and diarrhea; frequently causes anemia, hypoproteinemia, and electrolyte imbalance; sometimes complicated by peritonitis, toxic megacolon, or carcinoma of the colon. See page 1615, B17.

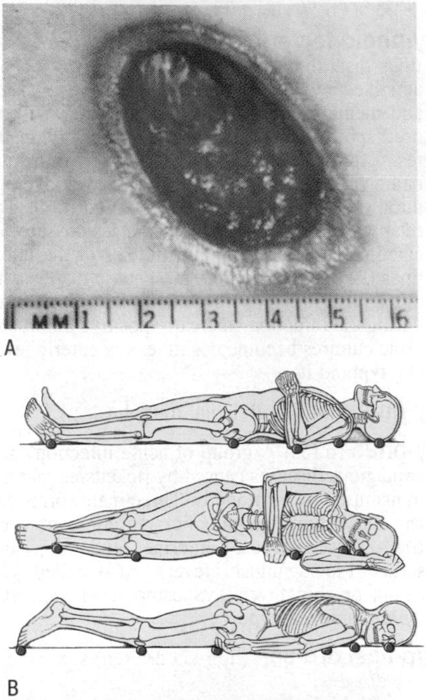

ulcers: (A) pressure ulcer (stage III): full-thickness skin loss, with damage to or necrosis of subcutaneous tissue that may extend to, but not through, underlying muscle; (B) decubitus ulcer: most common sites due to proximity of bone to skin

ul•cer•a•tive sto•ma•ti•tis (ŭl′sĕr-ă-tiv stō′mă-tī′tis) SYN aphtha (2).

ul•cer•o•mem•bra•nous gin•gi•vi•tis (ŭl′sĕr-ō-mem′bră-nŭs jin′ji-vī′tis) SYN necrotizing ulcerative gingivitis.

ul•cer•ous (ŭl′sĕr-ŭs) Relating to, affected with, or containing an ulcer. [L. *ulcerosus*]

ul•cus, pl. **ul•cer•a** (ŭl′kŭs, -sĕr-ă) SYN ulcer. [L.]

u•ler•y•the•ma (yū′ler-ith′ĕ-mă) Scarring with erythema. [G. *oulē,* scar, + *erythēma,* redness of the skin]

Ull•mann line (ūl′mahn līn) The line of displacement in spondylolisthesis.

Ull•mann syn•drome (ūl′mahn sin′drōm) A systemic angiomatosis due to multiple arteriovenous malformations.

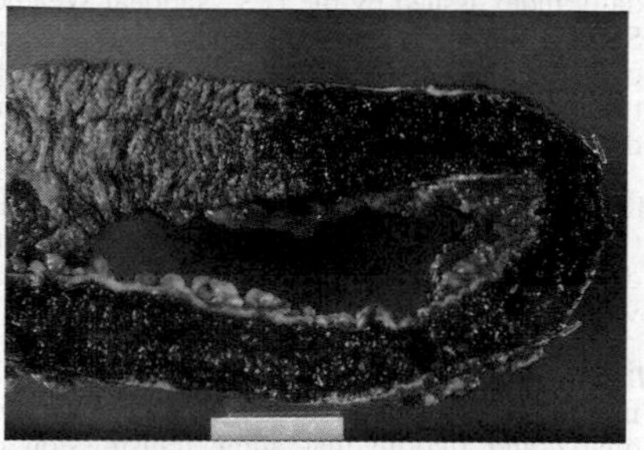

ulcerative colitis: prominent erythema and ulceration of colon begin in ascending colon and are most severe in rectosigmoid area

ul•na, gen. and pl. **ul•nae** (ŭl′nă, -nē) [TA] The medial and larger of the two bones of the forearm. SYN cubitus (2) [TA]. [L. elbow, arm, fr. G. *ōlenē*]

ul•nad (ŭl′nad) In a direction toward the ulna. [ulna + L. *ad,* to]

ul•nar (ŭl′năr) Relating to the ulna, or to any of the structures (artery, nerve) named from it; relating to the ulnar or medial aspect of the upper limb.

ul•nar ar•ter•y (ŭl′năr ahr′tĕr-ē) *Origin,* brachial; *branches,* ulnar recurrent, common interosseous, dorsal and palmar carpal, deep palmar, and superficial palmar arch with its digital branches. SYN arteria ulnaris [TA].

ul•nar de•vi•a•tion (ŭl′năr dē-vē-ā′shŭn) Movement of the wrist toward the little finger side of the forearm.

ul•nar ex•ten•sor mus•cle of wrist (ŭl′năr eks-ten′sŏr mŭs′ĕl rist) SYN extensor carpi ulnaris muscle.

ul•nar flex•ion (ŭl′năr fleks′shŭn) Flexion of the wrist combined with ulnar deviation.

ul•nar flex•or mus•cle of wrist (ŭl′năr fleks′ŏr mŭs′ĕl rist) SYN flexor carpi ulnaris muscle.

ul•nar head (ŭl′năr hed) The name applied to a head of origin of a forearm muscle arising from the ulna. *Terminologia Anatomica* lists ulnar heads (caput ulnare ...) of the following: 1) flexor carpi ulnaris [TA] (... musculi flexoris carpi ulnaris [TA]); 2) pronator teres [TA] (... musculi pronatoris teritis [TA]); and 3) extensor carpi ulnaris [TA] (... musculi extensoris carpi ulnaris [TA]).

ul•nar nerve (ŭl′năr nĕrv) Arises from medial cord of brachial plexus conveying fibers mainly from C8–T1 nerves; passes down arm, behind medial epicondyle of humerus, and down ulnar side of anterior compartment of forearm to hand; gives off muscular branches in forearm to flexor carpi ulnaris muscle and ulnar portion of flexor digitorum profundus and supplies hypothenar, interosseous, medial lumbricals, adductor pollicis, and deep head of flexor pollicis brevis, and intrinsic muscles of hand and skin of small finger and medial side of ring finger and adjacent portions of the palm of the hand. SYN nervus ulnaris [TA], cubital nerve.

ul•nar nerve com•pres•sion syn•drome (ŭl′năr nĕrv kŏm-presh′ŭn sin′drōm) SYN cyclist's palsy.

ul•nar re•cur•rent ar•ter•y (ŭl′năr rē-kŭr′ĕnt ahr′tĕr-ē) *Origin,* ulnar artery; *distribution,* two branches, anterior and posterior, pass medially in front and back of elbow joint; *anastomoses,* superior and inferior ulnar collateral, i.e., with articular vascular plexus of elbow.

ul•nar veins (ŭl′năr vānz) Venae comitantes of the ulnar artery, continuing from those of the superficial palmar arch and joining with those of the radial artery to form the brachial veins in the cubital fossa.

ulo-, ule- 1. Combining forms meaning scar, scarring. [G. *oulē*] **2.** Combining forms meaning the gums. SEE ALSO gingivo-. [G. *oulon*] **3.** Combining forms meaning curly. [G. *oulo-, ouli-,* woolly.]

u•lo•der•ma•ti•tis (yū′lō-dĕr-mă-tī′tis) Inflammation of the skin resulting in destruction of tissue and the formation of scars. [G. *oulē,* scar, + *derma,* skin, + *-itis,* inflammation]

u•loid (yū′loyd) **1.** Resembling a scar. **2.** A scarlike lesion due to a degenerative process in deeper layers of skin. [G. *oulē,* scar + *eidos,* resemblance]

ultra- Prefix meaning excess, exaggeration, beyond. [L. beyond]

ul•tra•cen•tri•fuge (ŭl′tră-sen′tri-fyūzh) A high-speed centrifuge by means of which large molecules (e.g., of protein or nucleic acids) are caused to sediment at practicable rates.

ul•tra•di•an (ŭl-tră′dē-ăn) Relating to biologic variations or rhythms occurring in cycles more frequent than every 24 hours. Cf. circadian, infradian. [ultra- + L. *dies,* day]

ul•tra•fast Pap•a•ni•co•laou (Pap) stain (ŭl′tră-fast′ pahp-ă-nē-kō-low pap stān) A modified stain suitable for use in situations in which rapid decisions are essential and frozen sections may not be sufficiently reliable or practical. SEE ALSO Papanicolaou (Pap) stain.

ul•tra•fil•tra•tion (ŭl′tră-fil-trā′shŭn) Filtration through a semipermeable membrane or any filter that separates colloid solutions from crystalloids or separates particles of different size in a colloid mixture.

ul•tra•li•ga•tion (ŭl′tră-lī-gā′shŭn) Ligation of a blood vessel beyond the point where a branch is given off.

ul•tra•mi•cro•scop•ic (ŭl′tră-mī-krŏ-skop′ik) SYN submicroscopic.

ul•tra•mi•cro•tome (ŭl′tră-mī′krō-tōm) A device used in cutting sections 0.1 mcm thick, or less, for electron microscopy.

ul•tra•short•wave di•a•ther•my (ŭl′tră-shōrt′ wāv dī′ă-thĕr′mē) Shortwave diathermy in which the wavelength is shorter than 10 m.

ul•tra•son•ic (ŭl′tră-son′ik) Relating to energy waves similar to those of sound but of higher frequencies (above 30,000 Hz). [ultra- + L. *sonus,* sound]

ul•tra•son•ic lith•o•trip•sy (ŭl′tră-son′ik lith′ ō-trip-sē) The demolition of calculi by high-frequency sound waves.

ul•tra•son•ic neb•u•liz•er (ŭl′tră-son′ik neb′ yū-lī-zĕr) A humidifier using high-frequency electricity to power a transducer that vibrates 1.35 million times per second and emits water particles 0.5–3 mcm in size; used in inhalation therapy.

ul•tra•son•ics (ŭl′tră-son′iks) The science and technology of ultrasound, its characteristics, and its phenomena.

ul•tra•son•o•gram (ŭl′tră-sŏn′ŏ-gram) The image obtained by ultrasonography. SEE ALSO echogram. SYN sonogram.

ul•tra•son•o•graph (ŭl′tră-son′ŏ-graf) Computerized instrument used to create an image using ultrasound. SYN sonograph. [ultra- + L. *sonus,* sound, + G. *graphō,* to write]

ul•tra•so•nog•ra•pher (ŭl′tră-sŏ-nog′ră-fĕr) A person who performs and interprets ultrasonographic examinations. SYN sonographer.

ul•tra•so•nog•ra•phy (ŭl′tră-sŏ-nog′ră-fē) The location, measurement, or delineation of deep structures by measuring the reflection or transmission of high-frequency or ultrasonic waves. Computer calculation of the distance to the sound-reflecting or absorbing surface plus the known orientation of the sound beam gives a two-dimensional image. SEE ALSO ultrasound. SYN echography, sonography. [ultra- + L. *sonus,* sound, + G. *graphō,* to write]

ul•tra•sound (ŭl′tră-sownd) Sound having a frequency greater than 30,000 Hz.

ul•tra•sound car•di•og•ra•phy (ŭl′tră-sownd kahr′dē-og′ră-fē) SYN echocardiography.

ul•tra•struc•tur•al a•nat•o•my (ŭl′tră-struk′ shŭr-ăl ă-nat′ŏ-mē) The ultramicroscopic study of structures too small to be seen with a light microscope.

ul•tra•vi•o•let (ŭl′tră-vī′ŏ-lĕt) Denoting electromagnetic rays at higher frequency than the violet end of the visible spectrum.

ul•tra•vio•let in•dex (ŭl′tră-vī′ŏ-lĕt in′deks) A daily index issued by the U.S. National Weather Service for many cities, forecasting the amount of dangerous ultraviolet light that will arrive at the Earth's surface about noon the following day.

ul•tra•vi•o•let ker•a•to•con•junc•ti•vi•tis (ŭl′tră-vī′ŏ-lĕt ker′ă-tō-kŏn-jŭngk′ti-vī′tis) Acute disorder resulting from exposure to intense ultraviolet irradiation.

ul•tra•vi•o•let mi•cro•scope (ŭl′tră-vī′ŏ-lĕt mī′krŏ-skōp) A microscope having optics of quartz and fluorite that allow transmission of light waves shorter than those of the visible spectrum; the image is made visible by photography, fluorescence of special glasses, or television.

ul•tra•vi•rus (ŭl′tră-vī′rŭs) SYN virus (1).

um•ber co•don (um′bĕr kō′don) The termination codon UGA. SYN opal codon.

um•bil•i•cal (ŭm-bil′i-kăl) Relating to the umbilicus. SYN omphalic.

um•bil•i•cal ar•ter•y (ŭm-bil′i-kăl ahr′tĕr-ē) Before birth, the arteria is a continuation of the internal iliac; after birth it is obliterated between the bladder and umbilicus, forming the medial umbilical ligament, the remaining portion, between the internal iliac artery and bladder, being reduced in size and giving off the superior vesical arteries. SYN arteria umbilicalis [TA].

um•bil•i•cal cord (ŭm-bil′i-kăl kōrd) The definitive connecting stalk between the embryo or fetus and the placenta; at birth it is primarily composed of mucoid connective tissue (Wharton jelly) in which the umbilical vessels are embedded. See page 1617, B1. SYN funiculus umbilicalis [TA], funis (1).

um•bil•i•cal her•ni•a (ŭm-bil′i-kăl hĕr′nē-ă) A hernia in which intestine or omentum protrudes through the abdominal wall under the skin at the umbilicus. SEE ALSO omphalocele. SYN exomphalos (2), exumbilication (2).

um•bil•i•cal in•tes•ti•nal loop (um-bil′i-kăl in-tes′ti-năl lūp) SYN midgut loop.

um•bil•i•cal ring (ŭm-bil′i-kăl ring) An opening in the linea alba through which pass the umbilical vessels in the fetus; in young embryos it is relatively nearer to the pubes, but gradually ascends to the center of the abdomen; it is closed in the adult, its site being indicated by the umbilicus or navel. SYN anulus umbilicalis [TA].

um•bil•i•cal vein (ŭm-bil′i-kăl vān) SYN left umbilical vein.

um•bil•i•cal ves•i•cle (ŭm-bil′i-kăl ves′i-kĕl) A saclike structure formed from the exocelomic cavity of a blastocyst. SYN yolk sac.

um•bil•i•cate, um•bil•i•cat•ed (ŭm-bil′i-kāt,

-kāt-ĕd) Of navel shape; pitlike; dimpled. [L. *umbilicatus*]

um•bil•i•ca•tion (ŭm-bil′i-kā′shŭn) **1.** A pit or navellike depression. **2.** Formation of a depression at the apex of a papule, vesicle, or pustule.

um•bil•i•cus, pl. **um•bil•i•ci** (ŭm-bil′i-kŭs, -sī) [TA] The pit in the center of the abdominal wall marking the site where the umbilical cord entered in the fetus. SYN navel. [L. navel]

um•bo, gen. **um•bo•nis**, pl. **um•bo•nes** (ŭm′bō, -bō-nis, -bō-nēz) **1.** A projecting point of a surface. **2.** [TA] SYN umbo of tympanic membrane. [L. boss of a shield, a knob]

um•bo of tym•pan•ic mem•brane (ŭm′bō tim-pan′ik mem′brān) The projection on the inner surface of the tympanic membrane at the end of the manubrium of the malleus; this corresponds to the most depressed point of the membrane, viewed laterally, that is commonly called the umbo. SYN umbo (2).

um•bra (ŭm′bră) RADIOLOGY an image with sharply defined margins.

UMP Abbreviation for uridine 5′-monophosphate.

♻**un-** Prefix meaning not, akin to L. *in-* and G. *a-*, *an-;* reversal, removal, release, deprivation; intensive action. [M.E.]

un•bal•anced trans•lo•ca•tion (un-băl′ănst trans-lō-kā′shŭn) Condition resulting from fertilization of a gamete containing a translocation chromosome by a normal gamete; if this abnormality is compatible with life, the person has 46 chromosomes but a segment of the translocation chromosome is represented three times in each cell and a partial or complete trisomic state exists.

un•bund•ling (ŭn-bŭnd′ling) Use of several Current Procedural Terminology codes for a service when one inclusion code is available.

un•cal (ŭngk′ăl) Denoting or relating to the uncus.

un•ci (ŭn′sī) Plural of uncus.

un•ci•form (ŭn′si-fōrm) SYN uncinate. [L. *uncus,* hook, + *forma,* form]

un•ci•form bone (ŭn′si-fōrm bōn) SYN hamate bone.

un•ci•form fas•cic•u•lus, un•ci•nate fas•cic•u•lus (ŭn′si-fōrm fă-sik′kyū-lŭs, ŭn′si-nāt) A band of long association fibers reciprocally connecting the frontal and temporal lobes of the cerebrum, running caudally through the white matter of the frontal lobe, sharply curving ventrally under the stem of the sylvian fissure, and then fanning out to the cortex of the anterior half of the superior and middle temporal gyri.

un•ci•nate (ŭn′si-nāt) **1.** Hooklike or hook-shaped. **2.** Relating to an uncus or, specifically,

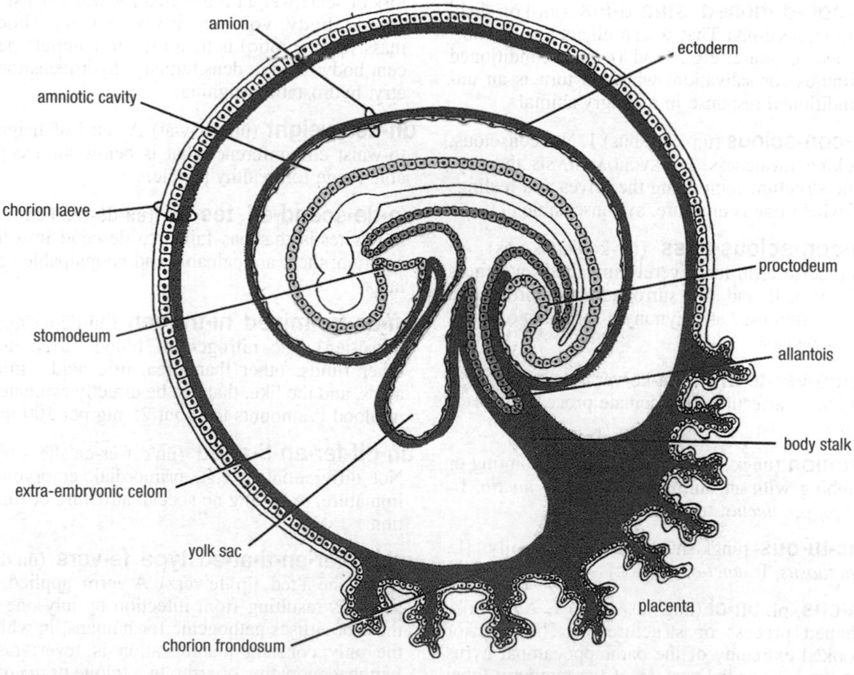

umbilical cord: simplified cross-sectional view during developmental process

to the uncinate gyrus (2) or a process of the pancreas or of a vertebra. SYN unciform. [L. *uncinatus*]

un•ci•nate gy•rus (ŭn′si-nāt jī′rŭs) SYN uncus (2).

un•comb•a•ble hair syn•drome (ŭn-kōm′ă-bĕl hār sin′drōm) A genetic disorder in which the hair, which is often silvery blond, is unruly and resists lying flat because of irregularly shaped hair shafts. SYN spun glass hair.

un•com•fort•a•ble lev•el (ŭn-kŭm′fŏr-tă-bĕl lev′ĕl) The intensity of sound that causes discomfort.

un•com•pen•sat•ed al•ka•lo•sis (ŭn-kom′pĕn-sā′tĕd al-kă-lō′sis) Disorder in which the pH of body fluids is elevated because of lack of the compensatory mechanisms of compensated alkalosis.

un•com•pe•ti•tive in•hib•i•tor (ŭn-kŏm-pet′i-tiv in-hib′i-tŏr) A type of enzyme inhibitor in which the inhibiting compound only binds to the enzyme-substrate complex.

un•con•di•tioned re•flex (ŭn-kŏn-dish′ŭnd rē′fleks) An instinctive reflex not dependent on previous learning or experience.

un•con•di•tioned re•sponse (ŭn-kŏn-dish′ŭnd rĕ-spons′) A response, such as salivation, which is part of the animal or human repertoire. Cf. conditioned response.

un•con•di•tioned stim•u•lus (ŭn-kŏn-dish′ŭnd stim′yū-lŭs) That which elicits an unconditioned response; e.g., food is an unconditioned stimulus for salivation, which in turn is an unconditioned response in a hungry animal.

un•con•scious (ŭn-kon′shŭs) **1.** Not conscious; lacking awareness. **2.** PSYCHOANALYSIS the psychic structure comprising the drives and feelings of which one is unaware. SYN insensible (1).

un•con•scious•ness (ŭn-kon′shŭs-nĕs) An imprecise term for severely impaired awareness of the self and the surrounding environment; most often used as a synonym for coma or unresponsiveness.

un•co•ver•te•bral (ŭn-kō-vĕr′tĕ-brăl) Pertaining to or affecting the uncinate process of a vertebra.

unc•tion (ŭngk′shŭn) The action of anointing or rubbing with an ointment or oil. [L. *unctio,* fr. *ungo,* pp. *unctus,* to anoint]

unc•tu•ous (ŭngk′shū-ŭs) Greasy or oily. [L. *unctuosus,* fr. *unctio,* unction]

un•cus, pl. **un•ci** (ŭng′kŭs, ŭn′sī) **1.** Any hook-shaped process or structure. **2.** The anterior hooked extremity of the parahippocampal gyrus on the basomedial surface of the temporal lobe; the anterior face of the uncus corresponds to the olfactory cortex, its ventral surface to the entorhinal area; deep to the uncus lies the amygdala (amygdaloid body). SYN uncinate gyrus. [L. a hook, fr. G. *onkos*]

un•der•bite (ŭn′dĕr-bīt) A nontechnical term applied to mandibular underdevelopment or to excessive maxillary development.

un•der•drive pac•ing (ŭn′dĕr-drīv pās′ing) Electrical stimulation of the heart at a rate lower than that of an existing tachycardia; designed to capture the heart between beats, i.e., to interrupt a reentry pathway in order to terminate the tachycardia.

un•der•nu•tri•tion (ŭn′dĕr-nū-trish′ŭn) An inadequate intake of nutrients that can result in poor health.

un•der•shoot (ŭn′dĕr-shūt) A temporary decrease below the final steady-state value that may occur immediately following the removal of an influence that had been raising that value, i.e., overshoot in a negative direction.

un•der•wa•ter seal drain•age (un-dĕr-waw′tĕr sēl drān′ăj) Connected to an intercostal catheter, a drain is placed underwater, thus creating a seal and allowing for lung reexpansion through the removal of air, or drainage of pus, blood or other fluid, while preventing reentry of air into the space.

un•der•wat•er weigh•ing (ŭn′dĕr-waw′tĕr wā′ing) Assessment of body volume by measuring a person's weight in air and again under water; loss of scale weight (corrected for water density) equals body volume. Body density (body mass:volume ratio) is then used to compute percent body fat. SYN densitometry, hydrodensitometry, hydrostatic weighing.

un•der•weight (ŭn′dĕr-wāt) A ratio of height-to-waist circumference that is below an acceptable range for healthy people.

un•de•scend•ed tes•tis (ŭn-dĕ-send′ĕd tes′tis) A testis that has failed to descend into the scrotum; there are palpable and nonpalpable variants.

un•de•ter•mined ni•tro•gen (ŭn-dē-tĕr′mind nī′trŏ-jĕn) The nitrogen of blood, urine, and other fluids, other than urea, uric acid, amino acids, and the like, that can be directly estimated; in blood it amounts to about 25 mg per 100 mL.

un•dif•fer•en•ti•at•ed (ŭn′dif-ĕr-en′shē-ā-tĕd) Not differentiated, e.g., primordial, embryonic, immature, or having no special structure or function.

un•dif•fer•en•ti•at•ed type fe•vers (ŭn′dif-fĕr-en′shē-ā′ted tīp fē′vĕrz) A term applied to illnesses resulting from infection by any one of the arboviruses pathogenic for humans, in which the only constant manifestation is fever; rash, lymphadenopathy, or arthralgia (alone or in combination) may occur in some affected people but not in others; some arboviruses may induce infections in which undifferentiated type fever is the only manifestation, whereas other arboviruses may induce in some people only undifferentiated fever, and in other persons similar fever followed by secondary manifestations, e.g., a hemorrhagic fever or encephalitis.

un•du•lant fe•ver (ŭn′dyū-lănt fē′vĕr) SYN brucellosis. [referring to the wavy appearance of the long temperature curve]

un•du•late (ŭn′dyū-lāt) Having an irregular, wavy border; denoting the shape of a bacterial colony. [Mod. L. *undula,* dim. of *unda,* wave]

un•du•lat•ing mem•brane, **un•du•la•to•ry mem•brane** (ŭn′dyū-lāt′ing mem′brān, ŭn′dyū-lă-tōr′ē) A locomotory organelle of certain flagellate (trypanosome and trichomonad) parasites, consisting of a finlike extension of the limiting membrane with the flagellar sheath; wavelike rippling of the undulating membrane produces a characteristic movement.

un•du•lat•ing pulse (ŭn′dyū-lāt′ing pŭls) A pulse in which there is a succession of waves rather than discrete pulsations.

un•du•li•po•di•um, pl. **un•du•li•po•di•a** (ŭn′dū-li-pō′dē-ŭm, -ă) A flexible, whiplike intracellular extension of many eukaryotic cells, with a characteristic arrangement of nine paired peripheral microtubules and one central pair; it appears to grow out from a basal body (kinetosome) in the cell. Both the cilium and the eukaryotic flagellum (not the bacterial flagellum, which lacks the 9 + 2 pattern) are considered undulipodia. [LL. *undulo*, to move in waves, fr. L. *unda*, wave, + Mod.L. *podium*, fr. G. *podion*, dim. of *pous*, foot]

un•e•rup•ted (un′ĕ-rŭp′tĕd) Condition of teeth that have not yet penetrated into the oral cavity.

un•gual (ŭng′gwăl) Relating to a nail or the nails. SYN unguinal. [L. *unguis,* nail]

un•guent (ŭng′gwĕnt) SYN ointment. [L. *unguentum*]

un•gui•nal (ŭng′gwi-năl) SYN ungual.

un•guis, pl. **un•gues** (ŭng′gwis, -gwēz) [TA] SYN nail. [L.]

♻**uni-** Prefix meaning one, single, not paired; corresponds to G. *mono-*. [L. *unus*]

u•ni•ax•i•al joint (yū′nē-aks′ē-ăl joynt) One in which movement is around one axis only.

u•ni•cam•er•al, **uni•cam•er•ate** (yū′ni-kam′ĕr-ăl, -kam′ĕ-rāt) SYN monolocular.

u•ni•cam•er•al bone cyst (yū′ni-kam′ĕr-ăl bōn sist) SYN solitary bone cyst.

u•ni•cel•lu•lar (yū′ni-sel′yū-lăr) Composed of but one cell, as in the protozoa (or protozoans). For such unicellular organisms capable of undertaking life processes independently of other cells, the term "acellular" is also used.

u•ni•cel•lu•lar gland (yū′ni-sel′yū-lăr gland) A single secretory cell such as a mucous goblet cell.

u•ni•cor•nous (yū′ni-kōr′nŭs) Having but one horn, or cornu. [L. *unicornis,* fr. uni- + *cornu,* horn]

u•ni•corn u•ter•us (yū′ni-kōrn yū′tĕr-ŭs) A uterus in which only one lateral half exists, the other half being undeveloped or absent.

u•ni•fo•cal (yū′ni-fō′kal) Located in a single site or arising from a single source (e.g., series of ectopic cardiac beats).

u•ni•ger•mi•nal (yū′ni-jĕr′mi-năl) Relating to a single germ, oocyte, or zygote, e.g., monozygotic. SYN monozygotic, monozygous.

u•ni•glan•du•lar (yū′ni-gland′yū-lăr) Involving, relating to, or containing but one gland.

u•ni•lat•e•ral (yū′ni-lat′ĕ-răl) Confined to one side only.

u•ni•lat•e•ral an•es•the•si•a (yū′ni-lat′ĕ-răl an′es-thē′zē-ă) SYN hemianesthesia.

u•ni•lat•e•ral her•maph•ro•dit•ism (yū′ni-lat′ĕ-răl hĕr-maf′rō-dīt′izm) Condition in which the doubling of sex characteristics occurs on one side only: ovotestis on one side and either ovary or testis on the other.

u•ni•lat•er•al hy•per•lu•cent lung (yū′ni-lat′ĕr-ăl hī′pĕr-lū′sĕnt lŭng) Chronic bronchiolitis obliterans predominating on one side. SEE ALSO unilateral lobar emphysema.

u•ni•lat•e•ral lo•bar em•phy•se•ma (yū′ni-lat′ĕr-ăl lō′bahr em′fi-sē′mă) A state in which the roentgenographic density of one lung (or one lobe) is markedly less than the density of the other(s) because of the presence of air trapped during expiration. SYN Macleod syndrome, Swyer-James syndrome (1).

u•ni•lo•bar (yū′ni-lō′bahr) Having but one lobe.

u•ni•lo•cal (yū′ni-lō′kăl) Strictly, denoting a trait in which the genetic component is contributed exclusively by one locus; in practice, any trait in which the contribution from one locus is so large that the data are readily interpreted as mendelian.

u•ni•loc•u•lar (yū′ni-lok′yū-lăr) Having but one compartment or cavity, as in a fat cell. [uni- + L. *loculus,* compartment]

u•ni•loc•u•lar cyst (yū′ni-lok′yū-lăr sist) A cyst having a single sac.

u•ni•loc•u•lar joint (yū′ni-lok′yū-lăr joynt) One in which an intraarticular disc is incomplete or absent, the joint having but a single cavity.

u•ni•mo•lec•u•lar (yū′ni-mŏ-lek′yū-lăr) Denoting a single molecule.

un•in•hib•i•ted neu•ro•gen•ic blad•der (un-in-hib′i-tĕd nūr′ō-jen′ik blad′ĕr) A condition, either congenital or acquired, of abnormal urinary bladder function in which normal inhibitory control of detrusor function by the central nervous system is impaired or underdeveloped, resulting in precipitate or uncontrolled micturition and/or anuresis.

un•in•ter•rupt•ed su•ture (un′in-tĕr-ŭp′tĕd sū′chŭr) SYN continuous suture.

un•ion (yūn′yŭn) **1.** The joining or amalgamation of two or more bodies. **2.** The structural adhesion or growing together of the edges of a wound. [L. *unus,* one]

u•ni•pen•nate (yū′ni-pen′āt) **1.** Having a featherlike arrangement on one side; resembling one half of a feather. **2.** Denoting certain muscles with fibers running at an acute angle from one side of a tendon. [uni- + L. *penna,* feather]

u•ni•po•lar (yū′ni-pō′lăr) **1.** Having but one pole; denoting a nerve cell from which the branches project from one side only. **2.** Situated at one extremity only of a cell.

u•ni•po•lar leads (yū′ni-pō′lăr lēdz) Those in which the exploring electrode is on the chest in the vicinity of the heart or on one of the limbs, whereas the other or indifferent electrode is the central terminal.

u•ni•po•lar neu•ron (yū′ni-pō′lăr nūr′on) A neuron with a cell body that gives off a single axonal process resulting from the fusion of two polar processes during development; at a variable distance from the cell body, the process divides into a peripheral axon branch extending outward as a peripheral afferent (sensory) nerve fiber, and a central axon branch that enters into synaptic contact with neurons in the spinal cord or brainstem.

u•ni•port (yū′ni-pōrt) Transport of a molecule or ion through a membrane by a carrier mechanism (uniporter), without known coupling to any other molecule or ion transport. Cf. antiport, symport. [uni- + L. *porto,* to carry]

u•nit (yū′nit) **1.** One; a single person or thing. **2.** A standard of measure, weight, or any other quality, by multiplications or fractions of which a scale or system is formed. **3.** A group of people or things considered as a whole because of mutual activities or functions. **4.** SYN international unit. [L. *unus,* one]

u•nit-dose pack•age (yū′nit-dōs pak′ăj) The repackaging of a bulk medication into smaller single-use systems for ease of dispensing to patients in hospitals or long-term care facilities.

U•ni•ted States A•dopt•ed Names (USAN) (yū-nī′tĕd stāts ă-dop′tĕd nāmz) Designation for nonproprietary names (for drugs) adopted by the USAN Council in cooperation with the manufacturers concerned; the designation USAN is applicable only to nonproprietary names coined since June 1961.

U•ni•ted States Phar•ma•co•pe•ia (USP) (yū-nī′tĕd stāts fahr′mă-kō-pē′ă) SEE Pharmacopeia.

U•ni•ted States Pub•lic Health Ser•vice (USPHS) (yū-nī′tĕd stāts pŭb′lik helth sĕr′vis) A bureau of the U.S. Department of Health and Human Services, served by a corps of medical officers presided over by the Surgeon General, concerned with scientific research, domestic and insular quarantine, administration of government hospitals, publication of sanitary reports, and statistics; associated with it are the National Institutes of Health, the Centers for Disease Control and Prevention, and other agencies.

u•nit mem•brane (yū′nit mem′brān) The trilaminar structure of the plasmalemma and other intercellular membranes, when seen in cross-section with the electron microscope, composed of two electron-dense laminae separated by a less dense lamina.

u•nit of pen•i•cil•lin (in•ter•na•tion•al) (yū′nit pen′i-sil′in in′tĕr-nash′ŭn-ăl) The penicillin activity of 0.6 mcg of penicillin G.

u•nit rec•ord (yū′nit rek′ŏrd) A single, comprehensive collection of all health care data for all episodes of care for a patient.

u•ni•va•lence, uni•va•len•cy (yū′ni-vā′lĕns, -vā′lĕn-sē) SYN monovalence.

u•ni•va•lent (yū′ni-vā′lĕnt) SYN monovalent (1).

u•ni•va•lent an•ti•bod•y (yū′ni-vā′lĕnt an′ti-bod-ē) An "incomplete" form of antibody that may coat antigen, but which according to the "lattice theory" does not have a second receptor for attachment to another molecule of antigen; in the case of Rh+ erythrocytes, such an anti-Rh antibody may coat the cells but not cause them to agglutinate in saline; however, agglutination does occur when such coated cells are suspended in serum or other protein media, such as albumin, therefore called serum agglutinin. SYN incomplete antibody (1).

u•ni•ver•sal cuff (yū′ni-vĕr′săl kŭf) A device commonly used by people with spinal cord injuries who have weak-to-absent finger flexion or gross grasp. This device is adapted to hold smaller items (e.g., pencil, toothbrush, comb).

u•ni•ver•sal cu•rette (yū′ni-vĕr′săl kyūr-et′) A periodontal instrument used to remove calculus from the crowns and roots of teeth. The working end of a universal curette has a rounded back, rounded toe, and two working cutting edges, and is semicircular in cross-section. One of the most frequently used and versatile periodontal débridement instruments.

u•ni•ver•sal den•tal no•men•cla•ture (yū′

ni-vĕr′săl den′tăl nō′mĕn-klā-chŭr) **1.** A North American system of identifying teeth by assigning a sequential number to each permanent tooth beginning with the upper right third molar (1) and continuing to the upper left third molar (16), then continuing in the lower arch and finishing with the lower right third molar (32). **2.** A system for deciduous teeth analogous to the permanent one using Arabic letters (A through T). SEE ALSO F.D.I. dental nomenclature, Palmer dental nomenclature.

u•ni•ver•sal do•nor (yū′ni-vĕr′săl dō′nŏr) In blood grouping, a person belonging to group O, i.e., one whose erythrocytes contain neither agglutinogen A nor B and are Rh negative.

U•ni•ver•sal Pre•cau•tions (yū′ni-vĕr′săl prē-kaw′shŭns) (in full, Universal Blood and Body Fluid Precautions). A set of procedural directives and guidelines published in August 1987 by the U.S. Centers for Disease Control and Prevention (CDC) (as *Recommendations for Prevention of HIV Transmission in Health-Care Settings*) to prevent parenteral, mucous membrane, and nonintact skin exposures of health care workers to bloodborne pathogens. In December 1991, the U.S. Occupational Safety and Health Administration (OSHA) promulgated its *Occupational Exposure to Bloodborne Pathogens Standard*, incorporating universal precautions and imposing detailed requirements on employers of health care workers, including engineering controls, provision of protective barrier devices, standardized labeling of biohazards, mandatory training of employees in the Universal Precautions, management of accidental parenteral exposure incidents, and availability to employees of immunization against hepatitis B virus.

un•my•e•li•nat•ed (ŭn-mī′ĕ-li-nā-tĕd) Denoting nerve fibers (axons) lacking a myelin sheath. SYN amyelinated, amyelinic.

un•my•e•li•nat•ed fi•bers (ŭn-mī′ĕ-li-nā-tĕd fī′bĕrz) In the CNS, a fiber having no myelin covering; a naked axon; in the PNS, represented by all axons lying in troughs in a single Schwann cell (Schwann cell unit); a slow conducting fiber. SYN gray fibers, nonmedullated fibers, Remak fibers.

Un•na dis•ease (ū′nah di-zēz′) SYN seborrheic dermatitis.

Un•na ne•vus (ū′nah nē′vŭs) Capillary stain on nape of neck; persistent form of nevus flammeus nuchae. SYN erythema nuchae.

Un•na stain (ū′nah stān) **1.** An alkaline methylene blue stain for plasma cells. **2.** A polychrome methylene blue stain with which mast cells stain red (metachromatic).

un•of•fi•cial (ŭn′ŏ-fish′ăl) Denoting a drug that is not listed in the U.S. Pharmacopeia or the National Formulary.

un•phys•i•o•log•ic (ŭn-fiz′ē-ō-loj′ik) Pertaining to conditions in the organism that are abnormal; can be used to refer to subjecting the body to abnormal amounts of substances normally present.

un•san•i•tar•y (ŭn-san′i-tar-ē) SYN insanitary.

un•sat•ur•at•ed (ŭn-sach′ŭr-āt-ĕd) **1.** Not saturated; denoting a solution in which the solvent is capable of dissolving more of the solute. **2.** Denoting a chemical compound in which all the affinities are not satisfied, so that still other atoms or radicals may be added to it. **3.** ORGANIC CHEMISTRY denoting compounds containing double and/or triple bonds.

un•sat•ur•at•ed fat (ŭn-sach′ŭr-āt-ĕd fat) Fat containing a high proportion of unsaturated fatty acids, i.e., fatty acids with double or triple bonds between carbon atoms. May have a healthy effect on the heart when used in moderation by lowering cholesterol levels.

un•sat•ur•at•ed fat•ty ac•id (ŭn-sach′ŭr-āt-ĕd fat′ē as′id) A fatty acid, the carbon chain of which possesses one or more double or triple bonds (e.g., oleic acid, with one double bond in the molecule, and linoleic acid, with two); called unsaturated because it is capable of absorbing additional hydrogen.

un•sta•ble an•gi•na (ŭn-stā′bĕl an′ji-nă) SYN acute coronary syndrome.

un•sta•ble lie (ŭn-stā′bĕl lī) Oblique orientation of the fetus that is neither transverse nor longitudinal, but that converts to one or the other before or during labor.

un•stri•at•ed (ŭn-strī′āt-ĕd) Without striations; not striped; denoting the structure of the smooth or involuntary muscles.

un•sys•tem•a•tized de•lu•sion (ŭn-sis′tĕ-mă′tīzd dĕ-lū′zhŭn) One of a group of apparently discrete, disconnected delusions.

Un•ver•richt dis•ease (ūn′fer-ikt di-zēz′) A progressive myoclonic epilepsy; one of the degenerative gray matter disorders characterized by myoclonus and generalized seizures, with progressive neurologic and intellectual decline; age of onset 8–13 years; autosomal recessive inheritance, caused by mutation in the cystatin B gene (CSTB) on 21q22.

un•weigh•ted (ŭn-wā′tĕd) Referring to a type of exercise in which weight bearing is reduced by application of counter-force, typically using a harness. SEE ALSO kinematic chain, weight-supported exercise.

UPIN Abbreviation for unique provider identification number.

UPJ Abbreviation for ureteropelvic junction.

up•per air•way (ŭp′ĕr ār′wā) The portion of the respiratory tract that extends from the nares or mouth to and including the larynx.

up•per ex•trem•i•ty (ŭp′ĕr eks-trem′i-tē) SYN upper limb.

up•per gas•tro•in•tes•tin•al (UGI) ser•ies (ŭp′ĕr gas′trō-in-tes′ti-năl sēr′ēz) A fluoroscopic-radiographic examination of the esophagus, stomach, and duodenum; a contrast medium, usually barium sulfate, is introduced. See this page.

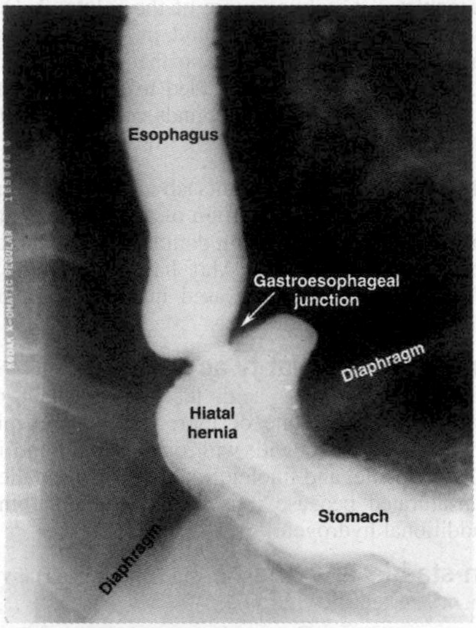

upper gastrointestinal series: radiograph showing hiatal hernia

up•per limb (ŭp′ĕr lim) The shoulder, arm, forearm, wrist, and hand. SYN upper extremity.

up•per res•pir•a•tor•y in•fec•tion (URI) (ŭp′ĕr res′pir-ă-tōr-ē in-fek′shŭn) SYN cold.

up•per res•pir•a•tor•y tract in•fec•tion (URTI) (ŭp′ĕr res′pir-ă-tōr-ē trakt in-fek′shŭn) SYN cold.

up•reg•u•la•tion (ŭp′reg-yū-lā′shŭn) Opposite of downregulation.

up•reg•u•la•tion-down•reg•u•la•tion hy•poth•e•sis (ŭp′reg-yū-lā′shŭn-down′reg-yū-lā′shŭn hī-poth′ĕ-sis) A theory of the neurochemical basis of depression (an elaboration of the monoamine hypothesis) linking it to an increase in number (upregulation) of postsynaptic monoamine receptors, which are then effectively decreased in number (downregulation) as a result of antidepressant activity. SEE ALSO monoamine hypothesis.

up•si•lon (υ) (ŭp′si-lon) **1.** The 20th letter in the Greek alphabet. **2.** Symbol for kinematic viscosity.

up•take (ŭp′tāk) The absorption by a tissue of some substance (e.g., food material, mineral) or its permanent or temporary retention.

u•ra•chal (yūr′ă-kăl) Relating to the urachus.

u•ra•chus (yūr′ă-kŭs) That portion of the allantois between the apex of the bladder and the umbilicus; becomes the median umbilical ligament. [G. *ourachos,* the urinary canal of a fetus]

u•ra•cil (U) (yūr′ă-sil) A pyrimidine (base) present in ribonucleic acid.

uraemia [Br.] SYN uremia.

uraemic [Br.] SYN uremic.

uraemic coma [Br.] SYN uremic coma.

uraemigenic [Br.] SYN uremigenic.

u•ra•ni•um (U) (yŭr-ā′nē-ŭm) A radioactive metallic element, atomic no. 92, atomic wt. 238.0289, occurring mainly in pitchblende and notable for its two isotopes: ^{238}U and ^{235}U (99.2745% and 0.720%, respectively, the rest being made up by ^{234}U), ^{235}U being the first substance ever shown capable of supporting a self-sustaining chain reaction. [G. myth. character, *Uranus*]

urano-, uranisco- Combining forms denoting the hard palate. [G. *ouranos,* sky vault, *ouraniskos,* roof of mouth (palate)]

u•ra•no•plas•ty (yūr′ă-nō-plas-tē) SYN palatoplasty.

u•ra•nor•rha•phy (yūr′ă-nōr′ă-fē) SYN palatorrhaphy. [urano- + G. *rhaphē,* suture]

u•ra•nos•chi•sis (yūr′ă-nos′ki-sis) Cleft of the hard palate. [urano- + G. *schisis,* fissure]

u•ra•no•staph•y•los•chi•sis (yūr′ă-nō-staf′i-los′ki-sis) Cleft of the soft and hard palates. [urano- + G. *staphylē,* uvula, + *schisis,* fissure]

u•ra•nyl (yūr′ă-nil) The ion, UO_2^{2+}; uranyl acetate is used in electron microscopy.

u•rar•thri•tis (yūr′ahr-thrī′tis) Gouty inflammation of a joint. [urate + arthritis]

urataemia [Br.] SYN uratemia.

ur•ate (yūr′āt) A salt of uric acid.

u•ra•te•mi•a (yūr′ă-tē′mē-ă) The presence of urates, especially sodium urate, in the blood. SYN urataemia. [urate + G. *haima,* blood]

ur•ate ox•i•dase (yūr′āt ok′si-dās) A copper-containing, oxygen-requiring oxidoreductase that oxidizes uric acid; used in the clinical diagnosis of increased uric acid levels. SYN uricase.

u•ra•to•sis (yūr′ă-tō′sis) Any morbid condition due to the presence of urates in the blood or tissues.

u•ra•tu•ri•a (yūr′ă-tyūr′ē-ă) The passage of an increased amount of urates in the urine. [urate + G. *ouron,* urine]

Ur•ban op•er•a•tion (ŭr′băn op-ĕr-ā′shŭn) Extended radical mastectomy, including en bloc resection of internal mammary lymph nodes, part of the sternum, and costal cartilages.

Urd Abbreviation for uridine.

ur·de·fens·es (ŭr′dĕ-fens′ĕz) Fundamental beliefs essential to human psychological integrity (e.g., religion, science). [Ger. *ur-*, primitive, earliest, + defenses]

ure-, urea-, ureo- Combining forms denoting urea; urine. SEE ALSO urin-, uro-. [G. *ouron,* urine]

u·re·a (yūr-ē′ă) The chief end product of nitrogen metabolism in mammals, formed in the liver, by means of the Krebs-Henseleit cycle, and excreted in normal adult human urine in the amount of about 32 g a day (about 89% of the nitrogen excreted from the body); used as a diuretic in kidney function tests and topically for various dermatitides. [G. *ouron,* urine]

u·re·a clear·ance (yūr-ē′ă klēr′ăns) *C* with a subscript indicating the substance removed; volume of plasma (or blood) that would be completely cleared of urea by 1 minute's excretion of urine.

u·re·a cy·cle (yūr-ē′ă sī′kĕl) The sequence of chemical reactions, occurring primarily in the liver, which results in the production of urea. SYN Krebs-Henseleit cycle, Krebs ornithine cycle, Krebs urea cycle.

u·re·a frost, u·re·mic frost (yūr-ē′ă frawst, yūr-ē′mik) Powdery deposits on the skin, especially the face, of urea and uric acid salts due to excretion of nitrogenous compounds in the sweat; seen in severe uremia.

u·re·a·gen·e·sis (yūr-ē′ă-jen′ĕ-sis) Formation of urea, usually referring to the metabolism of amino acids to urea. SYN ureapoiesis. [urea + G. *genesis,* production]

u·re·a ni·tro·gen (yūr-ē′ă nī′trŏ-jĕn) The portion of nitrogen in a biologic sample, such as blood or urine, which derives from its content of urea. SEE ALSO blood urea nitrogen.

U·re·a·plas·ma (yūr-ē′ă-plaz-mă) A genus of microaerophilic to anaerobic, nonmotile bacteria containing gram-negative, predominantly coccoidal to coccobacillary elements that are approximately 0.3 mcm in diameter, which frequently grow in short filaments. These organisms hydrolyze urea with production of ammonia and are found in the human genitourinary tract, occasionally in the pharynx and rectum. In males, they are associated with nongonococcal urethritis and prostatitis; in females, with genitourinary tract infections and reproductive failure. The type species is *U. urealyticum.* SYN T-mycoplasma.

u·re·a·poi·e·sis (yūr-ē′ă-poy-ē′sis) SYN ureagenesis. [urea + G. *poiēsis,* a making]

u·re·ase (yūr′ē-ās) An enzyme that catalyzes the hydrolysis of urea to carbon dioxide and ammonia; used as an antitumor enzyme; it is present in intestinal bacteria and accounts for most of the ammonia generated from urea in mammals.

u·re·de·ma (yūr′ĕ-dē′mă) Swelling due to infiltration of urine into subcutaneous tissues. SYN uroedema. [G. *ouron,* urine, + *oidēma,* swelling]

u·re·i·do·suc·cin·ic ac·id (yūr-ē′i-dō-sŭk-sin′ik as′id) A precursor of the pyrimidines. SYN *N*-carbamoylaspartic acid.

u·rel·co·sis (yūr′el-kō′sis) Ulceration of any part of the urinary tract. [G. *ouron,* urine, + *helkōsis,* ulceration]

u·re·mi·a (yūr-ē′mē-ă) **1.** An excess of urea and other nitrogenous waste in the blood. **2.** The complex of symptoms due to severe persisting renal failure that can be relieved by dialysis. SYN azotemia, uraemia. [G. *ouron,* urine, + *haima,* blood]

u·re·mic (yūr-ē′mik) Relating to uremia. SYN uraemic.

u·re·mic co·ma (yūr-ē′mik kō′mă) A metabolic encephalopathy caused by renal failure. SYN uraemic coma.

u·re·mi·gen·ic (yūr-ē′mi-jen′ik) **1.** Of uremic origin or causation. **2.** Causing or resulting in uremia. SYN uraemigenic.

uresiaesthesia [Br.] SYN uresiesthesia.

u·re·si·es·the·si·a (yūr-ē′sē-es-thē′zē-ă) The desire to urinate. SYN uresiaesthesia, uriesthesia. [G. *ourēsis,* a urinating, + *aisthēsis,* sensation]

u·re·sis (yūr-ē′sis) SYN urination. [G. *ourēsis*]

u·re·ter (yūr′ĕ-tĕr) [TA] The thick-walled tube that conducts the urine from the renal pelvis to the bladder; it consists of abdominal and pelvic parts, is lined with transitional epithelium surrounded by smooth muscle, both circular and longitudinal, and is covered externally by a tunica adventitia. [G. *ourētēr,* urinary canal]

u·re·ter·al (yūr-ē′tĕr-ăl) Relating to the ureter. SYN ureteric.

u·re·ter·al ec·top·i·a (yūr-ē′tĕr-ăl ek-tō′pē-ă) Abnormal termination of ureter within the bladder, the urethra, or outside the urinary tract.

u·re·ter·al·gi·a (yūr-ē′tĕr-al′jē-ă) Pain in the ureter. [ureter + G. *algos,* pain]

u·re·ter·al re·im·plan·ta·tion (yūr-ē′tĕr-ăl rē′im-plan-tā′shŭn) SYN ureteroneocystostomy.

u·re·ter·cys·to·scope (yūr-ē′tĕr-sis′tŏ-skōp) SYN ureterocystoscope.

u·re·ter·ec·ta·si·a (yūr-ē′tĕr-ek-tā′zē-ă) Dilation of a ureter. [ureter + G. *ektasis,* a stretching out]

u·re·ter·ec·to·my (yūr-ē′tĕr-ek′tō-mē) Excision of a segment or all of a ureter. [ureter + G. *ektomē,* excision]

u·re·ter·ic (yūr′ē-ter′ik) SYN ureteral.

u·re·ter·ic bud (yūr′ē-ter′ik bŭd) SYN metanephric diverticulum.

u·re·ter·ic or·i·fice (yūr′ē-ter′ik ōr′i-fis) The opening of the ureter in the bladder, situated one at each lateral angle of the trigone; wide gaping of the ostium usually indicates vesicoureteral reflux.

u·re·ter·i·tis (yūr-ē′tĕr-ī′tis) Inflammation of a ureter.

♻ **uretero-** Combining form denoting the ureter. [G. *ourētēr,* urinary canal]

u·re·ter·o·cele (yū-rē′tĕr-ō-sēl) Saccular dilation of the terminal portion of the ureter that protrudes into the lumen of the urinary bladder, probably due to a congenital stenosis of the ureteral meatus. [uretero- + G. *kēlē,* hernia]

u·re·ter·o·ce·lor·ra·phy (yūr-ē′tĕr-ō-sē-lōr′ă-fē) Excision and suturing of a ureterocele performed through an open cystotomy incision. [ureterocele + G. *raphē,* suture]

u·re·ter·o·co·los·to·my (yūr-ē′tĕr-ō-kō-los′tō-mē) Implantation of the ureter into the colon. [uretero- + G. *kolon,* colon, + *stoma,* mouth]

u·re·ter·o·cys·to·plas·ty (yūr-ē′tĕr-ō-sist′tō-plas-tē) Augmentation of the bladder using a native dilated ureter.

u·re·ter·o·cys·to·scope (yūr-ē′tĕr-ō-sis′tō-skōp) A cystoscope with an attachment for catheterization of the ureters; the catheter is passed into the ureter when its orifice is brought into view with the cystoscope. SYN uretercystoscope. [uretero- + G. *kystis,* bladder, + *skopeō,* to view]

u·re·ter·o·cys·tos·to·my (yūr-ē′tĕr-ō-sis-tos′tō-mē) SYN ureteroneocystostomy. [uretero- + G. *kystis,* bladder, + *stoma,* mouth]

u·re·ter·o·en·ter·os·to·my (yūr-ē′tĕr-ō-en′tĕr-os′tō-mē) Formation of an opening between a ureter and the intestine. [uretero- + G. *enteron,* intestine, + *stoma,* mouth]

u·re·ter·og·ra·phy (yūr-ē′tĕr-og′ră-fē) Radiography of the ureter after the direct injection of contrast medium. [uretero- + G. *graphē,* a writing]

u·re·ter·o·il·e·al a·nas·to·mo·sis (yūr-ē′tĕr-ō-il′ē-ăl ă-nas′tō-mō′sis) Communication between the ureter and an isolated segment of ileum. SEE ALSO Bricker operation.

u·re·ter·o·il·e·o·ne·o·cys·tos·to·my (yūr-ē′tĕr-ō-il′ē-ō-nē′ō-sis-tos′tō-mē) Restoration of the continuity of the urinary tract by anastomosis of the upper segment of a partially destroyed ureter to a segment of ileum, the lower end of which is then implanted into the bladder. SYN ileal ureter. [uretero- + ileum + G. *neos,* new, + *hystis,* bladder, + *stoma,* mouth]

u·re·ter·o·il·e·os·to·my (yūr-ē′tĕr-ō-il′ē-os′tō-mē) Implantation of a ureter into an isolated segment of ileum that drains through an abdominal stoma. [uretero- + ileum + G. *stoma,* mouth]

u·re·ter·o·li·thi·a·sis (yūr-ē′tĕr-ō-li-thī′ă-sis) The formation or presence of a calculus or calculi in one or both ureters. SEE ALSO renal calculus. [uretero-lith + G. -iasis, condition]

u·re·ter·o·li·thot·o·my (yūr-ē′tĕr-ō-li-thot′ō-mē) Removal of a stone lodged in a ureter. [ureterolith + G. *tomē,* incision]

u·re·ter·ol·y·sis (yūr-ē′tĕr-ol′i-sis) Surgical freeing of the ureter from surrounding disease or adhesions. [uretero- + G. *lysis,* a loosening]

u·re·ter·o·ne·o·cys·tos·to·my (yūr-ē′tĕr-ō-nē′ō-sis-tos′tō-mē) An operation whereby a ureter is implanted into the bladder. SYN ureteral reimplantation, ureterocystostomy. [uretero- + G. *neos,* new, + *kystis,* bladder, + *stoma,* mouth]

u·re·ter·o·ne·phrec·to·my (yūr-ē′tĕr-ō-nĕ-frek′tō-mē) SYN nephroureterectomy. [uretero- + G. *nephros,* kidney, + *ektomē,* excision]

u·re·ter·o·pel·vic junc·tion (UPJ) (yūr-ē′tĕr-ō-pel′vik jŭngk′shŭn) Site of origin of the ureter from the renal pelvis, a common location of congenital or acquired obstruction.

u·re·ter·o·pel·vic junc·tion ob·struc·tion (yūr-ē′tĕr-ō-pel′vik jŭngk′shŭn ŏb-strŭk′shŭn) An impediment to drainage of urine from kidney usually due to partial or intermittent blockage of the renal collecting system at the junction of renal pelvis and ureter.

u·re·ter·o·plas·ty (yūr-ē′tĕr-ō-plas-tē) Surgical reconstruction of the ureters. [uretero- + G. *plastos,* formed]

u·re·ter·o·py·e·li·tis (yūr-ē′tĕr-ō-pī′ē-lī′tis) Inflammation of the pelvis of a kidney and its ureter. [uretero- + G. *pyelos,* pelvis, + *-itis,* inflammation]

u·re·ter·o·py·e·log·ra·phy (yūr-ē′tĕr-ō-pī′ē-log′ră-fē) SYN pyelography.

u·re·ter·o·py·e·lo·plas·ty (yūr-ē′tĕr-ō-pī′ē-lō-plas-tē) Surgical reconstruction of the ureter and of the pelvis of the kidney, usually for congenital ureteropelvic junction obstruction. [uretero- + G. *pyelos,* pelvis, + *plastos,* formed]

u·re·ter·o·py·e·los·to·my (yūr-ē′tĕr-ō-pī′ē-los′tō-mē) Formation of a junction of the ureter and the renal pelvis. [uretero- + pelvis, + *stoma,* mouth]

u·re·ter·o·py·o·sis (yūr-ē′tĕr-ō-pī-ō′sis) An accumulation of pus in the ureter. [uretero- + G. *pyōsis,* suppuration]

u•re•ter•o•re•nal re•flux (yūr-ē′tĕr-ō-rēn′ăl rē′flŭks) Backward flow of urine from ureter into renal pelvis.

u•re•ter•or•rha•gi•a (yūr-ē′tĕr-ō-rā′jē-ă) Hemorrhage from a ureter. [uretero- + G. *rhēgnymi,* to burst forth]

u•re•ter•or•rha•phy (yūr-ē′tĕr-ōr′ă-fē) Suture of a ureter. [uretero- + G. *rhaphē,* suture]

u•re•ter•o•sig•moid•os•to•my (yūr-ē′tĕr-ō-sig′moy-dos′tŏ-mē) Implantation of the ureter into the sigmoid colon.

u•re•ter•os•to•my (yūr-ē′tĕr-os′tŏ-mē) Establishment of an external opening into the ureter. [uretero- + G. *stoma,* mouth]

u•re•ter•ot•o•my (yūr-ē′tĕr-ot′ŏ-mē) Incision and stenting of a narrow ureter. [uretero- + G. *tomē,* incision]

u•re•ter•o•u•re•ter•os•to•my (yūr-ē′tĕr-ō-yūr-ē′tĕr-os′tŏ-mē) Establishment of an anastomosis between the two ureters or between two segments of the same ureter. SEE ALSO transureteroureterostomy.

u•re•ter•o•ves•i•cal junc•tion (yūr-ē′tĕr-ō-ves′i-kăl jŭngk′shŭn) The site of entry of the ureter into the bladder, with an oblique angulation through the detrusor to avoid reflux. SEE ALSO vesicoureteral reflux.

u•re•ter•o•ves•i•cos•to•my (yūr-ē′tĕr-ō-ves′i-kos′tŏ-mē) Surgical joining of a ureter to the bladder. [uretero- + L. *vesica,* bladder, + *stoma,* mouth]

u•re•thra (yūr-ē′thră) A canal leading from the bladder, discharging the urine externally. SYN urogenital canal. [G. *ourēthra*]

urethraemorrhagia [Br.] SYN urethremorrhagia.

u•re•thral (yūr-ē′thrăl) Relating to the urethra.

u•re•thral ar•ter•y (yūr-ē′thrăl ahr′tĕr-ē) *Origin*, perineal artery; *distribution*, membranous urethra. SYN arteria urethralis [TA].

u•re•thral ca•run•cle (yūr-ē′thrăl kar′ŭng-kĕl) A small, fleshy, sometimes painful protrusion of the mucous membrane at the meatus of the female urethra.

u•re•thral crest (yūr-ē′thrăl krest) Longitudinal mucosal fold in the dorsal wall of the urethra.

u•re•thral folds (yūr-ē′thrăl fōldz) Primordia of the external genitalia derived from the cloacal folds; in males, they close over the urethral plate and fuse to form the spongy urethra and ventral aspect of the penis; in females, the unfused urogenital folds develop into the labia minora. SYN plicae urethrales, urogenital folds.

u•re•thral•gi•a (yūr′ē-thral′jē-ă) Pain in the urethra. SYN urethrodynia. [urethr- + G. *algos,* pain]

u•re•thral glands (yūr-ē′thrăl glandz) SEE glands of the female urethra, glands of the male urethra.

u•re•thral groove (yūr-ē′thrăl grūv) The groove on the ventral surface of the embryonic penis that normally closes to form the penile portion of the urethra. SYN genital furrow, genital groove.

u•re•thral he•ma•tu•ri•a (yūr-ē′thrăl hē′mă-tyūr′ē-ă) Condition in which the site of bleeding is in the urethra.

u•re•thral pa•pil•la, pa•pil•la u•re•thra•lis (yūr-ē′thrăl pă-pil′ă, yū-rēth-rā′lis) The slight projection often present in the vestibule of the vagina marking the urethral orifice.

u•re•thral valves (yūr-ē′thrăl valvz) Folds in the urethral mucous membrane.

u•re•threc•to•my (yūr′ē-threk′tŏ-mē) Excision of a segment or of the entire urethra. [urethr- + G. *ektomē,* excision]

u•re•threm•or•rha•gi•a (yūr′ē-threm-ōr-ā′jē-ă) Bleeding from the urethra. SYN urethraemorrhagia, urethrorrhagia. [urethr- + G. *haima,* blood, + *rhēgnymi,* to burst forth]

u•re•thrism, ure•thris•mus (yūr′ĕ-thrizm, -thriz′mŭs) Irritability or spasmodic stricture of the urethra. SYN urethrospasm.

u•re•thri•tis (yūr′ĕ-thrī′tis) Inflammation of the urethra. [ureth- + G. *-itis,* inflammation]

u•re•thri•tis pet•ri•fi•cans (yūr′ĕ-thrī′tis pĕ-trif′i-kanz) Urethritis, sometimes of gouty origin, in which there is a deposit of calcareous matter in the wall of the urethra.

♲ **urethro-, urethr-** Combining forms denoting the urethra. [G. *ourēthra*]

u•re•thro•bul•bar (yūr-ē′thrō-bŭl′bahr) SYN bulbourethral.

u•re•thro•cele (yūr-ē′thrō-sēl) Prolapse of the female urethra. [urethro- + G. *kēlē,* tumor, hernia]

u•re•thro•cu•tan•e•ous fis•tu•la (yūr-ē′thrō-kyū-tā′nē-ŭs fis′chū-lă) Passage between urethra and penile skin; most often a complication of hypospadias repair.

u•re•thro•cys•tom•e•try (yūr-ē′thrō-sis-tom′ĕ-trē) A procedure that simultaneously measures pressures in urinary bladder and urethra. [urethro- + G. *kystis,* bladder, + *metron,* measure]

u•re•thro•dyn•i•a (yūr-ē′thrō-din′ē-ă) SYN urethralgia. [urethro- + G. *odynē,* pain]

u•reth•ro•per•i•ne•o•scro•tal (yū-rē′thrō-per′i-nē′ō-skrō′tăl) Relating to the urethra, perineum, and scrotum.

u•re•thro•plas•ty (yūr-ē′thrō-plas-tē) Surgical

repair of the urethra, as performed to correct hypospadias, epispadias, or the effects of trauma. [urethro- + G. *plastos,* formed]

u•re•thror•rha•gi•a (yūr-ē′thrō-rā′jē-ă) SYN urethremorrhagia.

u•re•thror•rha•phy (yūr′ĕ-thrōr′ă-fē) Suture of the urethra. [urethro- + G. *rhaphē,* suture]

u•re•thror•rhe•a (yūr′ĕ-thrō-rē′ă) An abnormal discharge from the urethra. SYN urethrorrhoea. [urethro- + G. *rhoia,* a flow]

urethrorrhoea [Br.] SYN urethrorrhea.

u•re•thro•scope (yūr-ē′thrŏ-skōp) An instrument for viewing the interior of the urethra. [urethro- + G. *skopeō,* to view]

u•re•thro•scop•ic (yūr-ē′thrō-skop′ik) Relating to the urethroscope or to urethroscopy.

u•re•thros•co•py (yūr′ĕ-thros′kŏ-pē) Inspection of the urethra with a urethroscope.

u•re•thro•spasm (yūr-ē′thrō-spazm) SYN urethrism.

u•re•thro•stax•is (yūr-ē′thrō-stak′sis) The oozing of blood from the urethra. [urethro- + G. *staxis,* trickling]

u•re•thro•ste•no•sis (yūr-ē′thrō-stĕ-nō′sis) Stricture of the urethra. [urethro- + G. *stenōsis,* a narrowing]

u•re•thros•to•my (yūr′ĕ-thros′tŏ-mē) Surgical formation of a permanent opening between the urethra and the skin. [urethro- + G. *stoma,* mouth]

u•re•throt•o•my (yūr′ĕ-throt′ŏ-mē) Surgical incision of a stricture of the urethra. [urethro- + G. *tomē,* incision]

u•re•thro•vag•i•nal fis•tu•la (yūr-ē′thrō-vaj′i-năl fis′chū-lă) A fistula between the urethra and the vagina.

u•re•thro•ves•ic•al ang•le (yūr-ē′thrō-ves′i-kăl ang′gĕl) The angle between the female urethra and the posterior vesical wall, normally about 90°; narrowing of this angle in cystocele predisposes to stress incontinence.

u•re•thro•ves•i•co•pex•y (yūr-ē′thrō-ves′i-kō-pek-sē) Surgical suspension of the urethra and the base of the bladder from the posterior surface of the pubic symphysis (or anterior abdominal wall or Cooper ligament) for correction of urinary stress incontinence. [urethro- + L. *vesica,* bladder, + G. *pexis,* fixation]

♻ **-uretic** Suffix denoting urine. [G. *ourētikos,* relating to the urine]

urge in•con•ti•nence, ur•gen•cy in•con•ti•nence (ŭrj in-kon′ti-nĕns, ŭr′jĕn-sē) Leakage of urine in the presence of a strong desire to void.

ur•gen•cy (ŭr′jĕn-sē) A strong desire to void or urinate.

ur•gent care (ŭr′jĕnt kār) Care provided for a sudden illness or injury that needs immediate attention but is not life-threatening.

ur•hi•dro•sis (yūr′hī-drō′sis) SYN uridrosis.

URI Abbreviation for upper respiratory infection.

♻ **uri-, uric-, urico-** Combining forms denoting uric acid. [G. *ouron,* urine]

uriaesthesia [Br.] SYN uriesthesia.

ur•ic (yūr′ik) Relating to urine.

ur•ic ac•id (yūr′ik as′id) White crystals, poorly soluble, contained in solution in the urine of mammals; sometimes solidified in small masses as stones or crystals or in larger concretions as calculi; with sodium and other bases it forms urates; elevated levels associated with gout.

ur•i•case (yūr′i-kās) SYN urate oxidase.

ur•i•col•y•sis (yūr′i-kol′i-sis) Decomposition of uric acid. [urico- + G. *lysis,* a loosening]

ur•i•co•lyt•ic (yūr′i-kō-lit′ik) Relating to or effecting the hydrolysis of uric acid.

ur•i•co•su•ri•a (yūr′i-kō-syūr′ē-ă) Excessive amounts of uric acid in the urine. [urico- + G. *ouron,* urine]

ur•i•dine (Urd) (yūr′i-dēn) Uracil ribonucleoside; one of the major nucleosides in RNA; as the pyrophosphate (e.g., UDP, UDPG), uridine is active in sugar metabolism.

ur•i•dine 5′-di•phos•phate (UDP) (yūr′i-dēn dī-fos′fāt) A condensation product of uridine and pyrophosphoric acid.

ur•i•dine 5′-mo•no•phos•phate (UMP) (yūr′i-dēn mon′ō-fos′fāt) SYN uridylic acid.

ur•i•dine 5′-tri•phos•phate (UTP) (yūr′i-dēn trī-fos′fāt) The nucleoside esterified with triphosphoric acid at its 5′-position; the immediate precursor of uridylic acid residues in RNA.

ur•i•dro•sis (yūr′i-drō′sis) The excretion of urea or uric acid in the sweat. SYN urhidrosis. [uri- + G. *hidrōs,* sweat]

u•ri•dyl•ic ac•id (yūr′i-dil′ik as′id) Uridine esterified by phosphoric acid, precursor of the biosynthesis of other pyrimidine nucleotides. SYN uridine 5′-monophosphate.

u•ri•es•the•si•a (yūr′ē-es-thē′zē-ă) SYN uresiesthesia. SYN uriaesthesia.

♻ **urin-, urino-** Combining forms denoting urine. SEE ALSO ure-, uro-. [G. *ouron*]

ur•in•al (yūr′in-ăl) A vessel into which urine is passed.

ur•i•nal•y•sis (yūr′in-al′i-sis) Analysis of urine.

ur·i·nar·y (yūr′i-nar-ē) Relating to urine.

ur·i·nar·y blad·der (yūr′i-nar-ē blad′ĕr) A musculomembranous elastic bag serving as a storage place for the urine. SYN vesica urinaria [TA], bladder (2).

ur·i·nar·y cal·cu·lus (yūr′i-nar-ē kal′kyū-lŭs) A calculus in the kidney, ureter, bladder, or urethra.

ur·i·nar·y ni·tro·gen (yūr′i-nar-ē nī′trŏ-jĕn) Any nitrogenous substance (e.g., urea, amino acids, uric acid) excreted in the urine; 1 g of urinary nitrogen indicates the breakdown in the body of 6.25 g of protein. SEE ALSO nitrogen equivalent.

ur·i·nar·y sand (yūr′i-nar-ē sand) Multiple small calculous particles passed in the urine of patients with nephrolithiasis; each particle is usually too small to cause significant symptoms or to be identified as a true calculus.

ur·i·nar·y stut·ter·ing (yūr′i-nar-ē stŭt′ĕr-ing) Frequent involuntary interruption occurring during the act of urination.

u·ri·na·ry sys·tem (yūr′i-nar-ē sis′tĕm) Structures concerned in the production and transport of urine: kidneys, ureters, bladder, and urethra. See page A27.

ur·i·nar·y tract (yūr′i-nar-ē trakt) The passage from the pelvis of the kidney to the urinary meatus through the ureters, bladder, and urethra.

ur·i·nar·y tract in·fec·tion (UTI) (yūr′i-nar-ē trakt in-fek′shŭn) Microbial infection, usually bacterial, of any part of the urinary tract.

ur·i·nate (yūr′i-nāt) To pass urine. SYN micturate.

ur·i·na·tion (yūr′i-nā′shŭn) The passing of urine. SYN miction, micturition (1), uresis.

ur·ine (yūr′in) The fluid and dissolved substances excreted by the kidney. [L. *urina;* G. *ouron*]

ur·i·nog·e·nous (yūr′i-noj′ĕ-nŭs) **1.** Producing or excreting urine. **2.** Of urinary origin. SYN urogenous.

ur·i·no·ma (yūr′i-nō′mă) A cystic collection of extravasated urine.

ur·i·nom·e·ter (yūr′i-nom′ĕ-tĕr) Instrument used to measure specific gravity in urine, now largely replaced by the dipstick method. SEE ALSO specific gravity. SYN urogravimeter, urometer.

ur·i·nom·e·try (yūr′i-nom′ĕ-trē) The determination of the specific gravity of the urine.

ur·i·nos·co·py (yūr′i-nos′kŏ-pē) SYN uroscopy.

uro- Combining form denoting urine. SEE ALSO ure-, urin-. [G. *ouron*]

ur·o·bi·lin (yūr′ō-bī′lin) A uroporphyrin; an acyclic tetrapyrrole that is one of the natural breakdown products of heme; a urinary pigment that gives a varying orange-red coloration to urine. SYN urohematin.

urobilinaemia [Br.] SYN urobilinemia.

ur·o·bi·li·ne·mi·a (yūr′ō-bil-i-nē′mē-ă) The presence of urobilins in the blood. SYN urobilinaemia.

ur·o·bi·lin·o·gen (yūr′ō-bi-lin′ō-jen) Precursor of urobilin.

ur·o·bi·li·nur·i·a (yūr′ō-bil′i-nyū′rē-ă) Excess urobilin in urine, formed mainly from hemoglobin.

ur·o·can·ate (yūr′ō-kan′āt) A salt or ester of urocanic acid.

ur·o·can·ate hy·dra·tase (yūr′ō-kan′āt hī′dră-tās) An enzyme catalyzing the reaction of water with urocanic acid, a step in L-histidine catabolism; this enzyme is absent in cases of urocanic aciduria.

ur·o·can·ic ac·id (yūr′ō-kan′ik as′id) Derived from the oxidative deamination of L-histidine; present in sweat; elevated levels are observed in cases of urocanate hydratase deficiency.

u·ro·cele (yūr′ō-sēl) Extravasation of urine into the scrotal sac. [uro- + G. *kēlē,* hernia]

ur·o·che·si·a (yūr′ō-kē′zē-ă) Passage of urine from the anus. [uro- + G. *chezō,* to defecate]

ur·o·chrome (yūr′ō-krōm) The principal pigment of urine, a compound of urobilin and a peptide of unknown structure.

ur·o·dyn·i·a (yūr′ō-din′ē-ă) Pain on urination. [uro- + G. *odynē,* pain]

uroedema [Br.] SYN uredema.

ur·o·fla·vin (yūr′ō-flā′vin) A fluorescent product of riboflavin catabolism, or perhaps riboflavin itself, found in mammalian urine and feces.

ur·o·fol·li·tro·pin (yūr′ō-fol′i-trō′pin) A preparation of gonadotropin extracted from the urine of postmenopausal women, used in conjunction with human chorionic gonadotropin to induce ovulation. SEE ALSO menotropins.

ur·o·gas·trone (yūr′ō-gas′trōn) A fluorescent pigment extracted from urine; an inhibitor of gastric secretion and motility. Cf. enterogastrone, bioregulator.

ur·o·gen·i·tal (yūr′ō-jen′i-tăl) SYN genitourinary.

ur·o·gen·i·tal ca·nal (yūr′ō-jen′i-tăl kă-nal′) SYN urethra.

ur·o·gen·i·tal di·a·phragm (yūr′ō-jen′i-tăl dī′ă-fram) A triangular sheet of muscle between the ischiopubic rami; composed of the sphincter urethrae and the deep transverse perineal muscles.

ur•o•gen•i•tal folds (yūr′ō-jen′i-tăl fōldz) SYN urethral folds.

ur•o•gen•i•tal per•i•to•ne•um (yūr′ō-jen′i-tăl per′i-tō-nē′ŭm) Peritoneum of the pelvic cavity, including the folds and fossae formed by it. SYN peritoneum urogenitale.

ur•o•gen•i•tal ridge (yūr′ō-jen′i-tăl rij) One of the paired longitudinal ridges developing in the dorsal body wall of the embryo on either side of the dorsal mesentery; the ridge is formed at first by the growing mesonephros and later by the mesonephros and the gonad.

ur•o•gen•i•tal sin•us a•nom•a•ly (yūr′ō-jen′i-tăl sī′nŭs ă-nom′ă-lē) SYN hypospadias.

ur•o•gen•i•tal sys•tem (yūr′ō-jen′i-tăl sis′tĕm) All organs concerned with reproduction and in the formation and discharge of urine. See page A13, A14.

ur•og•e•nous (yūr-oj′ĕ-nŭs) SYN urinogenous.

ur•o•gram (yūr′ō-gram) The radiographic record obtained by urography. See this page.

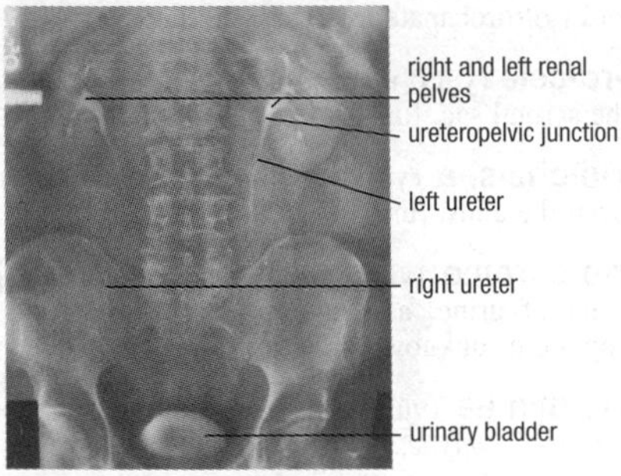

intravenous urogram: view showing the renal pelves, ureters, and urinary bladder

ur•og•ra•phy (yūr-og′ră-fē) Radiography of any part (kidneys, ureters, or bladder) of the urinary tract. SEE ALSO pyelography. [uro- + G. *graphō,* to write]

ur•o•gra•vim•e•ter (yūr′ō-gră-vim′ĕ-tĕr) SYN urinometer.

urohaematin [Br.] SYN urohematin.

ur•o•hem•a•tin (yūr′ō-hē′mă-tin) SYN urobilin. SYN urohaematin.

ur•o•ki•nase (yūr′ō-kī′nās) SYN plasminogen activator.

ur•o•li•thi•a•sis (yūr′ō-li-thī′ă-sis) Presence of calculi in the urinary system.

ur•o•lith•ic (yūr′ō-lith′ik) Relating to urinary calculi.

ur•o•log•ic, ur•o•log•i•cal (yūr′ō-loj′ik, -i-kăl) Relating to urology.

ur•ol•o•gist (yūr-ol′ŏ-jist) A specialist in urology. SYN genitourinary surgeon.

ur•ol•o•gy (yūr-ol′ŏ-jē) The medical specialty concerned with the study, diagnosis, and treatment of diseases of the genitourinary tract. [uro- + G. *logos,* study]

ur•om•e•ter (yūr-om′ĕ-tĕr) SYN urinometer.

ur•on•cus (yūr-ong′kŭs) A urinary cyst; a circumscribed area of extravasation of urine. [uro- + G. *onkos,* mass (tumor)]

ur•o•ne•phro•sis (yūr′ō-nĕ-frō′sis) SYN hydronephrosis.

ur•op•a•thy (yūr-op′ă-thē) Any disorder involving the urinary tract. [uro- + G. *pathos,* suffering]

ur•o•phan•ic (yūr′ō-fan′ik) Appearing in urine; denoting any constituent, normal or pathologic, of urine. [uro- + G. *phainō,* to appear]

ur•o•poi•e•sis (yūr′ō-poy-ē′sis) The production or secretion and excretion of urine. [uro- + G. *poiēsis,* a making]

ur•o•poi•e•tic (yūr′ō-poy-et′ik) Relating or pertaining to uropoiesis.

ur•o•por•phy•rin (yūr′ō-pōr′fi-rin) **1.** Porphyrin excreted in the urine in porphyrinuria. **2.** Class name for all porphyrins containing four acetic acid groups and four propionic acid groups in positions 1 through 8. SEE ALSO porphyrinogens.

ur•o•por•phy•rin•o•gen (yūr′ō-pōr′fir-in′ō-jen) SEE porphyrinogens.

ur•o•ra•di•ol•o•gy (yūr′ō-rā′dē-ol′ŏ-jē) The study of the radiology of the urinary tract.

ur•os•che•sis (yūr-os′kĕ-sis) **1.** Retention of urine. **2.** Suppression of urine. [uro- + G. *schesis,* a checking]

ur•o•scop•ic (yūr′ō-skop′ik) Relating to uroscopy.

u•ros•co•py (yūr-os′kŏ-pē) Examination of the urine, usually by means of a microscope. SYN urinoscopy. [uro- + G. *skopeō,* to view]

ur•o•sep•sis (yūr′ō-sep′sis) **1.** Sepsis resulting from the decomposition of extravasated urine. **2.** Sepsis from obstruction of infected urine. [uro- + G. *sēpsis,* decomposition]

ur•os•tom•y (yūr-os′tŏ-mē) Surgically created opening in the abdominal wall that diverts urine away from the bladder and into a collecting device outside the body.

ur•o•the•li•al car•ci•no•ma (yūr′ō-thē′lē-ăl kahr′si-nō′mă) A malignant neoplasm derived from transitional epithelium, occurring chiefly in the urinary bladder, ureters, or renal pelves (especially if well differentiated); frequently papillary; these carcinomas are graded according to the degree of anaplasia. So-called transitional cell carcinoma of the upper respiratory tract is more properly classified as squamous cell carcinoma. Transitional cell carcinoma is also a rare tumor of the ovary.

ur·o·the·li·al pap·il·lo·ma (yūr′ō-thē′lē-ăl pap′i-lō′mă) A benign papillary tumor of urothelium.

ur·o·the·li·um (yūr′ō-thē′lē-ŭm) The epithelial lining of the urinary tract. [uro- + epithelium]

ur·o·thor·ax (yūr′ō-thōr′aks) The presence of urine in the thoracic cavity, usually following complex multiple organ injuries.

URTI Abbreviation for upper respiratory tract infection.

ur·ti·cant (ŭr′ti-kănt) Producing a wheal or other similar itching agent. [L. *urtica,* nettle; see urtica]

ur·ti·car·i·a (ŭr′ti-kar′ē-ă) An eruption of itching wheals, usually of systemic origin; it may be due to a state of hypersensitivity to foods or drugs, foci of infection, physical agents (e.g., exercise, heat, cold, light, friction), or psychic stimuli. See page B9. SYN hives (1), urtication (3). [L. *urtica*]

ur·ti·car·i·a en·de·mi·ca, **ur·ti·car·i·a ep·i·dem·i·ca** (ŭr′ti-kar′ē-ă en-dem′i-kă, ep-i-dem′i-kă) Condition caused by the nettling hairs of certain caterpillars.

ur·ti·car·i·al, **ur·ti·car·i·ous** (ŭr′ti-kar′ē-ăl, -kar′ē-ŭs) Relating to or marked by urticaria.

ur·ti·car·i·a me·di·ca·men·to·sa (ŭr′ti-kar′ē-ă med-i-kă-men-tō′să) An urticarial form of drug eruption.

ur·ti·car·i·a pig·men·to·sa (ŭr′ti-kar′ē-ă pig-men-tō′să) Cutaneous mastocytosis resulting from an excess of mast cells in the superficial dermis, producing a chronic eruption characterized by flat or slightly elevated brownish papules that urticate when stroked.

ur·ti·cate (ŭr′ti-kāt) **1.** To perform urtication. **2.** Marked by the presence of wheals. [L. *urticatus*]

ur·ti·cat·ing a·gent (ŭr′ti-kāt-ing′ ā′jĕnt) Any toxic chemical-warfare agent that produces urticaria. In U.S. military parlance, this kind of agent is grouped with vesicating agents.

ur·ti·ca·tion (ŭr′ti-kā′shŭn) **1.** Whipping with nettles to induce counterirritation, formerly used in the treatment of peripheral paralysis. **2.** A burning sensation resembling that produced by urticaria or resulting from nettle poisoning. **3.** SYN urticaria. [L. *urticatio*]

USAN Abbreviation for U.S. Adopted Names.

U.S. De·part·ment of Health and Hu·man Serv·i·ces (HHS) (dĕ-pahrt′mĕnt helth hyū′măn sĕrv′i-sĕz) The "parent" of Centers for Medicare and Medicaid Services that administers many of the social programs dealing with the health and welfare of U.S. citizens.

U.S. Drug En·force·ment Ad·min·is·tra·tion (DEA) (drŭg en-fōrs′mĕnt ad-min′i-strā′shŭn) A division of the U.S. federal Department of Justice that is charged with the interdiction of the flow of illegal drugs or those restricted in sale by the Controlled Substances Act.

Ush·er syn·drome (ŭsh′ĕr sin′drōm) Autosomal recessive inheritance with genetic heterogeneity; the three forms are distinguishable by linkage data: Type 1 causes sensorineural hearing loss, loss of vestibular function, and retinitis pigmentosa; types 2 and 3 are characterized by hearing loss and retinitis pigmentosa.

U.S. Na·tion·al Cen·ters for Health Sta·tis·tics (NCHS) (na′shŭn-ăl sen′tĕrz helth stă-tis′tiks) A federal agency within the U.S. Centers for Disease Control and Prevention that collects, analyzes, and distributes health care statistics; its database is derived from and supports the U.S. healthcare infrastructure. NCHS also maintains the ICD-9-CM codes (ICD-10 is in preparation.).

U.S. Na·tion·al Drug Code (NDC) (na′shŭn-ăl drŭg kōd) A standard code used to identify drugs and biologicals that have been approved by the FDA.

U.S. Na·tion·al In·sti·tutes of Health (NIH) (na′shŭn-al in′sti-tūts helth) The agency within the U.S. Department of Health and Human Service responsible for medical and behavioral research.

USP Abbreviation for U.S. Pharmacopeia. SEE Pharmacopeia.

USP/DI Abbreviation for United States Pharmacopeia/Drug Index.

USPHS Abbreviation for U.S. Public Health Service.

USP u·nit (yū′nit) A unit as defined and adopted by the *United States Pharmacopeia.*

u·su·al in·ter·sti·tial pneu·mo·ni·a of Lie·bow (yū′zhū-ăl in′tĕr-stish′ăl nu-mō′nē-ă lē′bō) A progressive inflammatory condition starting with diffuse alveolar damage and resulting in fibrosis and honeycombing over a variable time period; also a common feature of collagen-vascular diseases.

u·ter·ine (yū′tĕr-in) Relating to the uterus.

u·ter·ine ar·ter·y (yū′tĕr-in ahr′tĕr-ē) *Origin,* internal iliac; *distribution,* uterus, upper part of vagina, round ligament, and medial part of uterine (fallopian) tube; *anastomoses,* ovarian, vaginal, inferior epigastric. Supplies maternal circulation to the placenta during pregnancy. SYN arteria uterina [TA].

u•ter•ine a•ton•y (yū′tĕr-in at′ŏ-nē) Failure of the myometrium to contract after delivery of the placenta; associated with excessive bleeding from the placental implantation site.

u•ter•ine cal•cu•lus (yū′tĕr-in kal′kyū-lŭs) A calcified myoma of the uterus.

u•ter•ine cav•i•ty, cav•i•ty of u•ter•us (yū′tĕr-in kav′i-tē, yū′tĕr-ŭs) The space within the uterus extending from the cervical canal to the openings of the uterine tubes.

u•ter•ine con•trac•tion (yū′tĕr-in kŏn-trak′shŭn) Rhythmic activity of the myometrium associated with menstruation, pregnancy, or labor.

u•ter•ine glands (yū′tĕr-in glandz) Numerous simple tubular glands in the uterine mucosa that secrete a glycogen-rich mucous fluid during the luteal phase of the menstrual cycle.

u•ter•ine os•ti•um of u•ter•ine tubes (yū′tĕr-in os′tē-ŭm yū′tĕr′in tūbz) The uterine opening of the oviduct.

u•ter•ine seg•ments (yū′tĕr-in seg′mĕnts) **1.** Lower: the isthmus of the uterus, the lower extremity of which joins with the cervical canal and, during pregnancy, expands to become the lower part of the uterine cavity. **2.** Upper: the main portion of the body of the gravid uterus, the contraction of which furnishes the chief expulsive force in labor.

u•ter•ine si•nus (yū′tĕr-in sī′nŭs) A small, irregular vascular channel in the endometrium, of a type that forms during pregnancy.

u•ter•ine souf•fle (yū′tĕr-in sū′fĕl) A blowing sound, synchronous with the cardiac systole of the mother, heard on auscultation of the pregnant uterus.

u•ter•ine tube (yū′tĕr-in tūb) One of the tubes leading on either side from the upper or outer extremity of the ovary, which is largely enveloped by its expanded infundibulum, to the fundus of the uterus; it consists of infundibulum, ampulla, isthmus, and uterine parts. SYN salpinx (1) [TA], fallopian tube, gonaduct (2), oviduct.

u•ter•ine veins (yū′tĕr-in vānz) Two veins on each side that arise from the uterine venous plexus, pass through a part of the broad ligament and then through a peritoneal fold, and empty into the internal iliac vein. SYN venae uterinae [TA].

♻ **utero-, uter-** Combining forms denoting the uterus. SEE ALSO hystero- (1), metr-. [L. *uterus*]

u•ter•o•cys•tos•to•my (yū′tĕr-ō-sis-tos′tŏ-mē) Formation of a communication between the uterus (cervix) and the bladder. [utero- + G. *kystis,* bladder, + *stoma,* mouth]

u•ter•o•fix•a•tion (yū′tĕr-ō-fik-sā′shŭn) SYN hysteropexy.

u•ter•o•glob•in (yū′tĕr-ō-glō′bin) Steroid-inducible, evolutionarily conserved, homodimeric secreted protein with many biologic activities including a proinflammatory effect, inhibition of soluble lipoprotein-lipase A_2, and chemotaxis of neutrophils and monocytes. It binds to several putative receptors on several cell types and inhibits cellular invasion of the extracellular matrix. It is found in blood and urine, the uterus, and numerous other tissues, but not the kidneys. In mice, uteroglobin has been shown to bind to fibronectin (Fn), preventing Fn self-aggregation and subsequent abnormal tissue deposition, especially in glomeruli. It is essential to normal renal function in mice. Cf. bioregulator. SYN bastokinin.

u•ter•o•glob•in-ad•du•cin (yū′tĕr-ō-glō′bin ad-dū′sin) An α/β heterodimeric protein found in renal tubule cells, thought to regulate ion transport through channels in the actin cytoskeleton. A mutant allele has been found in some patients with hypertension, and it may be associated with the salt-sensitive form of essential hypertension. Cf. bioregulator.

u•ter•om•e•ter (yū′tĕr-om′ĕ-tĕr) SYN hysterometer.

u•ter•o•pex•y (yū′tĕr-ō-pek-sē) SYN hysteropexy.

u•ter•o•pla•cen•tal si•nuses (yū′tĕr-ō-plă-sen′tĕl sī′nŭs-ĕz) Irregular vascular spaces in the zone of the chorionic attachment to the decidua basalis.

u•ter•o•plas•ty (yū′tĕr-ō-plas-tē) Plastic surgery of the uterus. SYN hysteroplasty, metroplasty. [utero- + G. *plastos,* formed]

u•ter•o•sal•pin•gog•ra•phy (yū′tĕr-ō-sal′ping-gog′ră-fē) SYN hysterosalpingography.

u•ter•o•scope (yū′tĕr-ō-skōp) SYN hysteroscope.

u•ter•os•co•py (yū′tĕr-os′kŏ-pē) SYN hysteroscopy.

u•ter•ot•o•my (yū′tĕr-ot′ŏ-mē) SYN hysterotomy.

u•ter•o•ton•ic (yū′tĕr-ō-ton′ik) **1.** Giving tone to the uterine muscle. **2.** An agent that overcomes relaxation of the muscular wall of the uterus. [utero- + G. *tonos,* tone, tension]

u•ter•o•tu•bog•ra•phy (yū′tĕr-ō-tū-bog′ră-fē) SYN hysterosalpingography.

u•ter•o•ves•i•cal lig•a•ment (yū′tĕr-ō-ves′i-kăl lig′ă-mĕnt) A peritoneal fold extending from the uterus to the posterior portion of the bladder.

u•ter•o•ves•i•cal pouch (yū′tĕr-ō-ves′i-kăl powch) A pocket formed by the deflection of the peritoneum from the bladder to the uterus in the female.

u•ter•us, pl. **u•ter•i** (yū′tĕr-ŭs, -ī) [TA] The hollow muscular organ in which the blastocyst develops into a fetus; it consists of a main portion (body) with an elongated lower part (cercix), at the extremity of which is the opening (os). The upper rounded portion of the uterus, opposite the os, is the fundus, at each extremity of which is the horn marking the part where the uterine tube joins the uterus and through which the morula reaches the uterine cavity after leaving the uterine tube. The organ is supported in the pelvic cavity by the broad ligaments, round ligaments, cardinal ligaments, and rectouterine and vesicouterine folds or ligaments. SYN metra, womb. [L.]

u•ter•us bi•cor•nis bi•col•lis (yū-tĕr-ŭs bī-kōr′nis bī-kol′is) SEE bicornate uterus.

u•ter•us bi•cor•nis u•ni•col•lis (yū-tĕr-ŭs bī-kōr′nis yū-ni-kol′is) SEE bicornate uterus.

u•ter•us di•del•phys (yū′tĕr-ŭs dī-del′fis) Double uterus with double cervix and double vagina; due to failure of the paramesonephric ducts to unite during embryonic development. [G. *di-*, two, + *delphys,* womb]

UTI Abbreviation for urinary tract infection.

UTP Abbreviation for uridine 5′-triphosphate.

u•tri•cle (yū′tri-kĕl) **1.** A small sac or pouch. **2.** The larger of the two membranous sacs in the vestibule of the membranous labyrinth of the internal ear, lying in the elliptic recess; from it arise the semicircular ducts. SYN utriculus [TA].

u•tric•u•lar (yū-trik′yū-lăr) Relating to or resembling a utricle.

u•tric•u•lar nerve (yū-trik′yū-lăr nĕrv) A branch of the utriculoampullar nerve, supplying the macula of the utricle. SYN nervus utricularis [TA].

u•tric•u•li (yū-trik′yū-lī) Plural of utriculus.

u•tric•u•li•tis (yū-trik′yū-lī′tis) **1.** Inflammation of the internal ear. **2.** Inflammation of the prostatic utricle. [utriculus + G. *-itis,* inflammation]

u•tric•u•lo•am•pul•lar nerve (yū-trik′yū-lō-am-pul′lăr nĕrv) A division of the vestibular part of the eighth cranial nerve; it gives off branches to the macula of the utricle (utricular nerve) and to the cristae of the ampullae of the anterior and lateral semicircular ducts (anterior and lateral ampullary nerves). SYN nervus utriculoampullaris [TA].

u•tric•u•lo•sac•cu•lar (ū-trik′yū-lō-sak′yū-lăr) Relating to the utricle and the saccule of the labyrinth, denoting especially a duct connecting the two structures.

u•tric•u•lus (yū-trik′yū-lŭs) [TA] SYN utricle. SEE ALSO vestibular organ. [L. dim. of *uter,* leather bag]

u•tric•u•lus pros•tat•i•cus (yū-trik′yū-lŭs pros-tat′i-kŭs) [TA] SYN prostatic utricle.

UV, uv Abbreviation for ultraviolet.

u•va-ur•si (yū′vă-ŭr′sē) SYN bearberry. [L. *uva,* berry, + *ursi,* of a bear]

u•ve•a (yū′vē-ă) The middle coat of the eyeball between the sclera and retina. It includes the iris and ciliary body (the anterior uvea) and the choroid.

u•ve•al (yū′vē-ăl) Relating to the uvea.

u•ve•it•ic (yū′vē-it′ik) Relating to the uvea.

u•ve•i•tis, pl. **u•ve•i•ti•des** (ū-vē-ī′tis, -it′i-dēz) Inflammation of the uveal tract: iris, ciliary body, and choroid. [uvea + G. *-itis,* inflammation]

u•ve•o•en•ceph•a•lit•ic syn•drome (yū′vē-ō-en-sef′ă-lit′ik sin′drōm) SYN Behçet syndrome.

u•ve•o•pa•rot•id fe•ver (yū′vē-ō-păr-ot′id fē′vĕr) Chronic enlargement of the parotid glands and inflammation of the uveal tract accompanied by a long-continued fever of low degree; a form of sarcoidosis. SYN Heerfordt disease.

u•ve•o•scle•ri•tis (yū′vē-ō-skler-ī′tis) Inflammation of the sclera involved by extension from the uvea.

u•vi•form (yū′vi-fōrm) SYN botryoid. [L. uva, grape, + *forma,* form]

u•vit•ex 2B (yū′vi-teks) A fluorescent stain that reacts with chitin; useful in the diagnosis of microsporidian or cryptosporidium infections.

u•vu•la, pl. **u•vu•lae** (yū′vyū-lă, -lē) [TA] An appendant fleshy mass; a structure bearing a fancied resemblance to the palatine uvula. [Mod. L. dim. of L. *uva,* a grape, the uvula]

u•vu•la of blad•der (yū′vyū-lă blad′ĕr) A slight projection into the cavity of the bladder, usually more prominent in old men, just behind the urethral opening, marking the location of the middle lobe of the prostate.

u•vu•la cer•e•bel•li (yū′vyū-lă ser-e-bel′ī) SYN uvula of cerebellum.

u•vu•la of cer•e•bel•lum (yū′vyū-lă ser-ĕ-bel′ŭm) A triangular elevation on the vermis of the cerebellum, lying between the two tonsils anterior to the pyramis. SYN uvula cerebelli, uvula vermis.

u•vu•lar (ū′vyū-lăr) Relating to the uvula.

u•vu•lar mus•cle (ū′vyū-lăr mŭs′ĕl) *Origin,* posterior nasal spine; *insertion,* forms chief bulk of the uvula; *action,* raises the uvula; *nerve supply,* pharyngeal plexus. SYN musculus uvulae [TA], muscle of uvula.

u•vu•la ver•mis (yū′vyū-lă vĕr′mis) SYN uvula of cerebellum.

u•vu•lec•to•my (yū′vyū-lek′tŏ-mē) Excision of the uvula. SYN staphylectomy. [uvula + G. *ektomē,* excision]

u•vu•li•tis (yū′vyū-lī′tis) Inflammation of the uvula. Common causes include infection and allergic reaction.

u•vu•lop•to•sis (yū′vyū-lop-tō′sis) Relaxation or elongation of the uvula. SYN staphylodialysis, staphyloptosis. [uvulo- + G. *ptōsis,* a falling]

u•vu•lot•o•my (yū′vyū-lot′ŏ-mē) Any cutting operation on the uvula. [uvulo- + G. *tomē,* a cutting]

U wave (wāv) Waveform in an ECG tracing sometimes following the T wave and representing the completion of ventricular repolarization.

V

V **1.** Abbreviation for vision; volt; valine; volume, frequently with subscripts denoting location, chemical species, and/or conditions; with numeric subscript, abbreviation for unipolar electrocardiogram leads. **2.** Symbol for vanadium.

v **1.** Abbreviation for gas flow, frequently with subscripts indicating location and chemical species. SEE flow (3). **2.** Abbreviation for ventilation (3), frequently with a subscript. [volume + overdot denoting time derivative]

$\dot{V}_A$ Abbreviation for alveolar ventilation.

V_{max} Abbreviation for maximum velocity.

V Abbreviation for volume.

v **1.** Abbreviation for volt; initial rate velocity; velocity; *vel* [L, or]. **2.** As a subscript, refers to venous blood.

$\bar{v}$ As a subscript, refers to mixed venous (pulmonary arterial) blood.

V-A, VA Abbreviation for ventriculoatrial.

vac•ci•nal (vak′si-năl) Relating to vaccine or vaccination.

vac•ci•nate (vak′si-nāt) To administer a vaccine.

vac•ci•na•tion (vak′si-nā′shŭn) The act of administering a vaccine.

vac•cine (vak-sēn′) Any preparation intended for active immunologic prophylaxis, e.g., preparations of killed microbes of virulent strains or living microbes of attenuated (variant or mutant) strains, or microbial, fungal, plant, protozoal, or metazoan derivatives or product. [L. *vaccinus,* relating to a cow]

vac•cine lymph, **vac•cin•i•a lymph** (vak-sēn′ limf, vak-sin′ē-ă) That collected from the vesicles of vaccinia infection, and used for active immunization against smallpox.

vac•cin•i•a vi•rus (vak-sin′ē-ă vī′rŭs) Virus of the genus Orthopoxvirus used in immunization against smallpox.

VACTERL syn•drome (vak-tĕrl′ sin′drōm) Acronymic term for abnormalities of *v*ertebrae, *a*nus, *c*ardiovascular tree, *t*rachea, *e*sophagus, *r*enal system, and *l*imb buds associated with administration of sex steroids during early pregnancy.

vac•u•o•lar (vak′yū-ō′lăr) Relating to or resembling a vacuole.

vac•u•o•late, **vac•u•o•lat•ed** (vak′yū-ō-lāt, -lāt′ĕd) Having vacuoles.

vac•u•o•la•tion, **vac•u•o•li•za•tion** (vak′yū-ō-lā′shŭn, -lī-zā′shŭn) **1.** Formation of vacuoles. **2.** The condition of having vacuoles.

vac•u•ole (vak′yū-ōl) **1.** A minute space in any tissue. **2.** A clear space in the substance of a cell, sometimes degenerative in character, sometimes surrounding an englobed foreign body and serving as a temporary cell stomach for the digestion of the body. [Mod. L. *vacuolum,* dim. of L. *vacuum,* an empty space]

vac•u•tome (vak′yū-tōm) Electrodermatome that applies suction to the skin to raise it before an advancing blade, usually for taking a split-thickness skin graft. [vacuum + G. *tomē,* a cutting]

va•cu•um (vak′yūm) An empty space, one practically exhausted of air or gas. [L. ntr. of *vacuus,* empty]

va•cu•um pack tech•nique (vak′yūm pak tek-nēk′) A temporary closing of the abdomen by using a fenestrated plastic sheet over the intestine but under the anterior abdominal wall followed by the placement of moistened pads with a suction catheter within the wound. The entire defect is then covered by a nonporous plastic sheet; permits drainage of the abdominal cavity by suction while maintaining anterior abdominal wall rigidity.

VAD Abbreviation for vascular access device.

vag. Abbreviation for vaginal.

vag•a•bond's dis•ease (vag′ă-bondz di-zēz′) SYN parasitic melanoderma.

va•gal (vā′găl) Relating to the vagus nerve.

va•gal nerve stim•u•la•tion (vā′găl nĕrv stim′yū-lā′shŭn) An adjunctive treatment for patients with intractable epilepsy, particularly complex partial or secondarily generalized seizures; stimulation is delivered to the left vagus nerve in the neck, usually in 30-second bursts every 5-1/2 minutes by a stimulator implanted in the anterior chest wall.

va•gal trunk (vā′găl trŭngk) One of the two nerve bundles, anterior and posterior, into which the esophageal plexus continues as it passes through the diaphragm. SYN truncus vagalis [TA].

V agents (ā-jĕnts) Abbreviation for V-series nerve agents.

va•gi (vā′jī) Plural of vagus.

va•gi•na, gen. and pl. **va•gi•nae** (vă-jī′nă, -nē) **1.** [TA] SYN sheath (1). **2.** [TA] The genital canal in the female, extending from the uterus to the vulva. [L. sheath, the vagina]

va•gi•na ca•rot•i•ca (vă-jī′nă kă-rot′i-kă) [TA] SYN carotid sheath.

vag•i•nal (vag.) (vaj′i-năl) Relating to the vagina or to any sheath. [Mod. L. *vaginalis*]

vag•i•nal ar•ter•y (vaj′i-năl ahr′tĕr-ē) *Origin,* internal iliac; *distribution,* vagina, base of bladder, rectum; *anastomoses,* uterine, internal pudendal. SYN arteria vaginalis [TA].

vag·i·nal a·tre·si·a (vaj′i-năl ă-trē′zē-ă) Congenital or acquired imperforation or occlusion of the vagina, or adhesion of the walls of the vagina. SYN colpatresia.

vag·i·nal ce·li·ot·o·my (vaj′i-năl sē′lē-ot′ŏ-mē) Opening the peritoneal cavity through the vagina.

vag·i·nal cuff (vaj′i-năl kŭf) The portion of the vaginal vault remaining open to the peritoneum following hysterectomy.

vag·i·nal gland (vaj′i-năl gland) One of the mucous glands in the mucous membrane of the vagina.

vag·i·nal hys·ter·ec·to·my (vaj′i-năl his′tĕr-ek′tŏ-mē) Removal of the uterus through the vagina.

vag·i·nal in·tra·epi·the·li·al ne·o·plas·i·a (vaj′i-năl in′tră-ep′i-thē′lē-ăl nē′ō-plā′zē-ă) Preinvasive squamous cell carcinoma (carcinoma in situ) limited to vaginal epithelium; like vulvar or cervical intraepithelial neoplasia, graded histologically on a scale from 1–3 or subdivided into low-grade and high-grade intraepithelial malignancy; usually related to human papillomavirus infection; may progress to invasive carcinoma.

vag·i·nal nerves (vaj′i-năl nĕrvz) Several nerves passing from the uterovaginal plexus to the vagina. SYN nervi vaginales [TA].

vag·i·nal or·i·fice (vaj′i-năl ōr′i-fis) The narrowest portion of the canal, in the floor of the vestibule posterior to the urethral orifice.

vag·i·nal por·tion of cer·vix (vaj′i-năl pōr′shŭn sĕr′viks) The part of the cervix uteri contained within the vagina.

vag·i·nal pouch (vaj′i-năl powch) SYN vaginal ring.

vag·i·nal ring (vaj′i-năl ring) A silicon ring impregnated with a drug (e.g., estrogen) designed for sustained release. SYN vaginal pouch.

vag·i·nal ru·gae (vaj′i-năl rū′gē) A number of transverse ridges in the mucous membrane of the vagina.

vag·i·nate (vaj′i-nāt) **1.** To ensheathe; to enclose in a sheath. **2.** Ensheathed; provided with a sheath.

vag·i·nec·to·my (vaj′i-nek′tŏ-mē) Excision of the vagina or a segment thereof. SYN colpectomy. [vagina + G. *ektomē,* excision]

vag·i·nis·mus (vaj′i-niz′mŭs) Painful spasm of the vagina preventing intercourse. [vagina + L. *-ismus,* action, condition]

vag·i·ni·tis, pl. **vag·i·ni·ti·des** (vaj′i-nī′tis, -nit′i-dēz) Inflammation of the vagina. [vagina + G. *-itis,* inflammation]

♲**vagino-, vagin-** Combining forms denoting the vagina. SEE ALSO colpo-. [L. *vagina,* sheath]

vag·i·no·cele (vaj′i-nō-sēl) SYN colpocele (1).

vag·i·no·dyn·i·a (vaj′i-nō-din′ē-ă) Vaginal pain. SYN colpodynia.

vag·i·no·fix·a·tion (vaj′i-nō-fik-sā′shŭn) Suturing a relaxed and prolapsed vagina to the abdominal wall. SYN colpopexy, vaginopexy.

vag·i·no·my·co·sis (vaj′i-nō-mī-kō′sis) Vaginal fungal infection.

vag·i·nop·a·thy (vaj′i-nop′ă-thē) Any diseased condition of the vagina. [vagino- + G. *pathos,* suffering]

vag·i·no·per·i·ne·o·plas·ty (vaj′i-nō-per′i-nē′ō-plas-tē) Surgical repair of the perineum involving the vagina. SYN colpoperineoplasty. [vagino- + perineum, + G. *plastos,* formed]

vag·i·no·per·i·ne·or·rha·phy (vaj′i-nō-per′i-nē-ōr′ă-fē) Repair of a lacerated vagina and perineum. SYN colpoperineorrhaphy. [vagino- + perineum, + G. *rhaphē,* suture]

vag·i·no·per·i·ne·ot·o·my (vaj′i-nō-per′i-nē-ot′ŏ-mē) Division of the posterior aspect of the vagina and adjacent portion of the perineum to facilitate childbirth. [vagino- + perineum, + G. *tomē,* incision]

vag·i·no·pex·y (vaj′i-nō-pek-sē) SYN vaginofixation.

vag·i·no·plas·ty (vaj′i-nō-plas-tē) Surgical repair of the vagina. SYN colpoplasty. [vagino- + G. *plastos,* formed]

vag·i·nos·co·py (vaj′i-nos′kŏ-pē) Inspection of the vagina, usually with an instrument.

vag·in·o·sis (vaj′i-nō′sis) Disease of the vagina.

vag·i·not·o·my (vaj′i-not′ŏ-mē) A cutting operation in the vagina. SYN colpotomy.

va·gi·tus u·ter·i·nus (va-jī′tŭs yū-tĕr-ī′nŭs) Crying of the fetus while still within the uterus, possible when the membranes have been ruptured and air has entered the uterine cavity. [L. fr. *vagio,* to squall; L. fr. *uterus,* womb]

♲**vago-** Combining form denoting the vagus nerve. [L. *vagus*]

va·gol·y·sis (vā-gol′i-sis) Surgical destruction of the vagus nerve. [vago- + G. *lysis,* a loosening]

va·go·lyt·ic (vā′gō-lit′ik) **1.** Pertaining to or causing vagolysis. **2.** A therapeutic or chemical agent that has inhibitory effects on the vagus nerve. **3.** Denoting an agent having such effects.

va·go·mi·met·ic (vā′gō-mi-met′ik) Mimicking the action of the efferent fibers of the vagus nerve.

va•got•o•my (vā-got′ŏ-mē) Division of the vagus nerve. [vago- + G. *tomē,* incision]

va•go•tro•pic (vā′gō-trō′pik) Attracted by, hence acting on, the vagus nerve. [vago- + G. *tropos,* turning]

va•go•va•gal (vā′gō-vā′găl) Pertaining to a process that uses both afferent and efferent vagal nerve fibers.

va•grant's dis•ease (vā′grănts di-zēz′) SYN parasitic melanoderma.

va•gus, gen. and pl. **va•gi** (vā′gŭs, -jī) SYN vagus nerve [CN X]. [L. wandering, so-called because of the wide distribution of the nerve]

va•gus nerve [CN X] (vā′gŭs nĕrv) A mixed nerve that arises by numerous small roots from the side of the medulla oblongata, between the glossopharyngeal above and the accessory below; it leaves the cranial cavity by the jugular foramen and passes down to supply the pharynx, larynx, trachea, lungs, heart, and the gastrointestinal tract as far as the left colic (splenic) flexure; the only cranial nerve that does not arise from the brain, but is classified as such because it exits from the cranium. SYN nervus vagus [CN X] [TA], pneumogastric nerve, tenth cranial nerve [CN X], vagus.

va•gus pulse (vā′gŭs pŭls) A slow pulse due to the inhibitory action of the vagus nerve on the heart.

Val Abbreviation for valine and its radicals.

va•lence, **va•len•cy** (vā′lĕns, -lĕn sē) The combining power of one atom of an element (or a radical), that of the hydrogen atom being the unit of comparison, determined by the number of electrons in the outer shell of the atom (v. electrons); e.g., in HCl, chlorine is monovalent; in H_2O, oxygen is bivalent; in NH_3, nitrogen is trivalent. [L. *valentia,* strength]

Val•en•tine po•si•tion (val′ĕn-tīn pŏ-zish′ŏn) A supine position on a table with double inclined plane so as to cause flexion at the hips; used to facilitate urethral irrigation.

va•le•ri•an (vă-lēr′ē-ăn) An herb that is used to treat anxiety, insomnia, sleep disorders, and restlessness due to nervous disorders.

val•gus (val′gŭs) Descriptive of any of the paired joints of the extremities with a static angular deformity in which the bone distal to the joint deviates laterally from the longitudinal axis of the proximal bone, and from the midline of the body, when the subject is in anatomic position. The adjective valgus is attached sometimes to the name of the joint (cubitus valgus) and sometimes to the name of the part just distal to the joint (hallux valgus). The gender of the adjective matches that of the Latin noun to which it is joined; thus, cubitus, hallux, metatarsus, pes, talipes *valgus;* coxa, manus, talipomanus *valga;* genu *valgum.* [Mod. L. turned outward, fr. L. bowlegged]

val•gus lax•i•ty (val′gŭs laks′i-tē) Abnormal flexibility on the medial side of a joint upon lateral movement of the distal segment.

va•lid•i•ty (vă-lid′i-tē) Truthfulness; the ability of a test to measure correctly as intended.

va•line (Val, V) (vā-lēn′) 2-Amino-3-methylbutanoic acid; the L-isomer is a constituent of most proteins; a nutritionally essential amino acid.

val•late (val′āt) Bordered with an elevation, as a cupped structure; denoting especially certain lingual papillae. SEE ALSO circumvallate. [L. *vallo,* pp. *-atus,* to surround with, fr. *vallum,* a rampart]

val•late pa•pil•la (val′āt pă-pil′ă) One of eight or ten projections from the dorsum of the tongue forming a row anterior to and parallel with the sulcus terminalis; each papilla is surrounded by a circular trench (fossa) having a slightly raised outer wall (vallum); on the sides of the vallate papilla and the opposed margin of the vallum are numerous taste buds. SYN papilla vallata [TA], circumvallate papillae, papillae vallatae.

val•lec•u•la, pl. **val•lec•u•lae** (vă-lek′yū-lă, -lē) [TA] **1.** A crevice or depression on any surface. **2.** A sinus located between the base of the tongue and the epiglottis. [L. dim. of *vallis,* valley]

Val•leix points (vahl′ē poynts) Various points in the course of a nerve, pressure on which is painful in cases of neuralgia; these points are: 1) where the nerve emerges from the bony canal; 2) where it pierces a muscle or aponeurosis to reach the skin; 3) where a superficial nerve rests on a resisting surface where compression is easily made; 4) where the nerve gives off one or more branches; and 5) where the nerve terminates in the skin.

Val•ley fe•ver (val′ē fē′vĕr) Primary coccidioidomycosis; common in the San Joaquin Valley of California and other areas in the southwestern United States. SYN San Joaquin Valley Fever.

Val•sal•va leak point pres•sure (VLPP) (vahl-sahl′vă lēk poynt presh′ŭr) Abdominal pressure at which urinary incontinence may occur.

Val•sal•va ma•neu•ver (vahl-sahl′vă mă-nū′vĕr) Any forced expiratory effort ("strain") against a closed airway, whether at the nose and mouth or at the glottis; because high intrathoracic pressure impedes venous return to the right atrium, this maneuver is used to study cardiovascular effects of raised peripheral venous pressure and decreased cardiac filling and cardiac output.

val•ue (val′yū) A particular quantitative determination. [M.E., fr. O.Fr., fr. L. *valeo,* to be of value]

val•va, pl. **val•vae** (val′vă, -vē) [TA] SYN valve. [L. one leaf of a double door]

val•val, **val•var** (val′văl, -văr) Relating to a valve.

val•vate (val′vāt) Relating to or provided with a valve. SYN valvular.

valve (valv) **1.** A fold of the lining membrane of a canal or other hollow organ serving to retard or prevent a reflux of fluid. **2.** Any reduplication of tissue or flaplike structure resembling a valve. SEE ALSO valvule, plica. See this page. SYN valva [TA]. [L. *valva*]

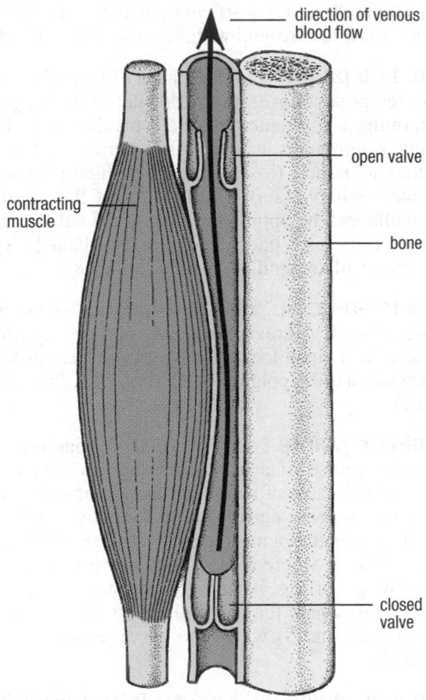

venous valves: principle of venous blood flow

valve of cor•o•nar•y si•nus (valv kōr′ŏ-nar-ē sī′nŭs) A delicate fold of endocardium at the opening of the coronary sinus into the right atrium.

val•vec•to•my (val-vek′tŏ-mē) Surgical removal of a valve.

val•vo•plas•ty (val′vō-plas-tē) Surgical reconstruction of a deformed cardiac valve, to relieve stenosis or incompetence. SYN valvuloplasty. [valve + G. *plastos,* formed]

val•vot•o•my (val-vot′ŏ-mē) **1.** Cutting through a stenosed cardiac valve to relieve the obstruction. SYN valvulotomy. **2.** Incision of a valvular structure. [valve + G. *tomē,* incision]

val•vu•la, pl. **val•vu•lae** (val′vyū-lă, -lē) SYN valvule. [Mod. L. dim. of *valva*]

val•vu•lar (val′vyū-lăr) SYN valvate.

val•vu•lar en•do•car•di•tis (val′vyū-lăr en′dō-kahr-dī′tis) Inflammation confined to the endocardium of the valves.

val•vu•lar in•suf•fi•cien•cy (val′vyū-lăr in′sŭ-fish′ĕn-sē) SYN valvular regurgitation.

val•vu•lar re•gur•gi•ta•tion (val′vyū-lăr rē-gŭr′ji-tā′shŭn) A leaky state of one or more of the cardiac valves, in which the valve does not close tightly and blood therefore regurgitates through it. SYN valvular insufficiency.

val•vule (val′vyūl) A valve, especially a small one. SYN valvula. [L. *valvula*]

val•vu•li•tis (val′vyū-lī′tis) Inflammation of a valve, especially a heart valve. [Mod. L. *valvula,* valve, + G. *-itis,* inflammation]

val•vu•lo•plas•ty (val′vyū-lō-plas-tē) SYN valvoplasty.

val•vu•lot•o•my (val′vyū-lot′ŏ-mē) SYN valvotomy (1).

va•na•di•um (V) (vă-nā′dē-ŭm) A metallic element, atomic no. 23, atomic wt. 50.9415; a bioelement; its deficiency can result in abnormal bone growth and a rise in cholesterol and triglyceride levels. [*Vanadis,* Scand. goddess]

va•na•di•um group (vă-nā′dē-ŭm grūp) Those elements resembling vanadium in chemical and metallurgic properties; included with vanadium are niobium and tantalum.

van Buch•em syn•drome (vahn bū′kem sin′drōm) An osteosclerosing skeletal dysplasia, characterized by mandibular enlargement, thickening of the diaphyses and calvaria, and increased serum alkaline phosphatase; autosomal recessive inheritance.

van•co•my•cin-re•sis•tant en•ter•o•coc•cus (VRE) (van′kō-mī′sin-rē-zis′tănt en′tĕr-ō-kahk′ŭs) A strain of enterococci bacteria that resists therapy with vancomycin.

van der Hoev•e syn•drome (vahn der hō′vĕ sin′drōm) A subtype of osteogenesis imperfecta in which progressive conductive hearing loss begins in childhood because of stapedial fixation.

van der Waals forc•es (vahn der valz fōrs′ĕz) Attractions first postulated by J.D. van der Waals in 1873 to explain deviations from ideal gas behavior seen in real gases; the attractive forces between atoms or molecules other than electrostatic (ionic), covalent (sharing of electrons), or hydrogen bonding (sharing a proton); generally ascribed to dipolar and dispersion effects, π-electrons, and other factors; these relatively nondescript forces contribute to the mutual attraction of organic molecules.

van Er•men•gen stain (vahn er′men-gen stān) A method for staining flagella that uses glacial acetic acid, osmic acid, tannic acid, silver nitrate, gallic acid, and potassium acetate.

van Gie•son stain (van gē′sŏn stān) A mixture of acid fuchsin in saturated picric acid solution, used in collagen staining.

va•nil•lism (vă-nil′izm) **1.** Symptoms of irritation of the skin, nasal mucous membrane, and conjunctiva that workers with vanilla sometimes suffer. **2.** Infestation of the skin by sarcoptiform mites found in vanilla pods.

van•il•lyl•man•del•ic ac•id (VMA) (vă-nil′il-man-del′ik as′id) The major urinary metabolite of adrenal and sympathetic catecholamines; elevated in most patients with pheochromocytoma.

van•ish•ing lung syn•drome (van′i-shing lŭng sin′drōm) Progressive decrease of radiographic opacity of the lung caused by accelerated development of emphysema or rapid cystic destruction of the lung from infection.

Van Lo•hui•zen syn•drome (vahn lō-hwē′zen sin′drōm) SYN cutis marmorata telangiectatica congenita.

van't Hoff e•qua•tion (vahnt hof ĕ-kwā′zhŭn) **1.** Calculation for osmotic pressure of dilute solutions. SEE ALSO van't Hoff law. **2.** For any reaction, d(ln K_{eq}/d(1/T) equals $-\Delta H/R$, where K_{eq} is the equilibrium constant, T the absolute temperature, R the universal gas constant, and ΔH the change in enthalpy; thus, plotting ln K_{eq} *vs.* 1/T allows the determination of ΔH.

van't Hoff law (vahnt hof law) **1.** STEREOCHEMISTRY all optically active substances have one or more multivalent atoms united to four different atoms or radicals so as to form in space an asymmetric arrangement. **2.** The osmotic pressure exerted by any substance in very dilute solution is the same that it would exert if present as gas in the same volume as that of the solution; or, at constant temperature, the osmotic pressure of dilute solutions is proportional to the concentration (number of molecules) of the dissolved substance; i.e., the osmotic pressure, Π, in dilute solutions is $\Pi = RT\Sigma c_i$, where R is the universal gas constant, T is the absolute temperature, and c_i is the molar concentration of solute i. **3.** The rate of chemical reactions increases between twofold and threefold for each 10°C rise in temperature.

van't Hoff the•o•ry (vahnt hof thē′ŏr-ē) That substances in dilute solution obey the gas laws. Cf. van't Hoff law.

va•por (vā′pŏr) **1.** The gaseous phase of a substance that can be compressed into a liquid or a solid at the temperature of the vapor. **2.** The gaseous phase of a solid or liquid at any temperature below its boiling point. **3.** (obsolete) A medicinal preparation designed to be administered by inhalation. **4.** A common but incorrect term for a liquid aerosol (a visible suspension of fine liquid droplets in the atmosphere). SYN vapour. [L. steam]

va•por•i•za•tion (vā′pŏr-ī-zā′shŭn) **1.** The change of a solid or liquid to a state of vapor. **2.** The therapeutic application of a vapor.

va•por•ize (vā′pŏr-īz) **1.** To convert a solid or liquid into a vapor. **2.** To apply a vapor therapeutically.

va•por•iz•er (vā′pŏr-īz-ĕr) **1.** An apparatus for reducing medicated liquids to a gaseous state suitable for inhalation or application to accessible mucous membranes. SEE ALSO nebulizer, atomizer. **2.** A device for volatilizing liquid anesthetics.

vapour [Br.] SYN vapor.

VAPS Abbreviation for volume assured pressure support.

Va•quez dis•ease (vah-kā′ di-zēz′) SYN polycythemia vera.

var•i•a•ble (var′ē-ă-bĕl) **1.** That which is inconstant, which can or does change, as contrasted with a constant. **2.** Deviating from the type in structure, form, physiology, or behavior. [L. *vario,* to vary, change, differ]

var•i•ab•le re•sis•tance train•ing (var′ē-ă-bĕl rĕ-zis′tăns trān′ing) Resistance training with equipment that uses a lever arm, cam, hydraulic system, or pulley to alter the resistance to match increases and decreases in a muscle's force capacity as it moves through the range of motion.

var•i•ance (var′ē-ăns) **1.** The state of being variable, different, divergent, or deviate; a degree of deviation. **2.** A measure of the variation shown by a set of observations, defined as the sum of squares of deviations from the mean, divided by the number of degrees of freedom in the set of observations.

var•i•ant (var′ē-ănt) **1.** That which, or one who, is variable. **2.** Having the tendency to alter or change, exhibit variety or diversity, not conform, or differ from the usual type.

var•i•ant an•gi•na (var′ē-ănt an′ji-nă) SYN Prinzmetal angina.

var•i•ant an•gi•na pec•to•ris (var′ē-ănt an′ji-nă pek′tŏr-is) SYN Prinzmetal angina.

var•i•a•tion (var′ē-ā′shŭn) Deviation from the type, especially the parent type, in structure, form, physiology, or behavior. [L. *variatio,* fr. *vario,* to change, vary]

var•i•ca•tion (var′i-kā′shŭn) Formation or presence of varices.

var•i•ce•al (var′i-sē′ăl) Of or pertaining to a varix.

var•i•cel•la (var′i-sel′ă) An acute contagious

disease, usually occurring in children, caused by the varicella-zoster virus and marked by a sparse eruption of papules, which become vesicles and then pustules, usually with mild constitutional symptoms; incubation period is about 14–17 days. See page B30. SYN chickenpox. [Mod. L. dim. of *variola*]

var·i·cel·la en·ceph·a·li·tis (var′i-sel′ă en-sef′ă-lī′tis) The disease occurring as a complication of chickenpox.

var·i·cel·la-zos·ter vi·rus (var′i-sel′ă-zos′tĕr vī′rŭs) A herpesvirus, morphologically identical to herpes simplex virus, that causes varicella (chickenpox) and herpes zoster; varicella results from a primary infection, herpes zoster from secondary invasion or by reactivation of infection that has been latent for years. SYN chickenpox virus, herpes zoster virus, human herpesvirus 3, Varicellovirus.

var·i·cel·li·form (var′i-sel′i-fōrm) Resembling varicella.

Var·i·cel·lo·vi·rus (var′ē-sel′ō-vī′rus) SYN varicella-zoster virus.

var·i·ces (var′i-sēz) Plural of varix.

var·i·ci·form (var-is′i-fōrm) Resembling a varix.

varico- Combining form denoting a varix, varicose, varicosity. [L. *varix,* a dilated vein]

var·i·co·bleph·a·ron (var′i-kō-blef′ă-ron) A varicosity of the eyelid. [varico- + G. *blepharon,* eyelid]

var·i·co·cele (var′i-kō-sēl) A condition manifested by abnormal dilation of the veins of the spermatic cord, caused by incompetent valves in the internal spermatic vein, and resulting in impaired drainage of blood into the spermatic cord veins when the patient assumes the upright position. [varico- + G. *kēlē,* tumor, hernia]

var·i·co·ce·lec·to·my (var′i-kō-sĕ-lek′tŏ-mē) Operation for the correction of a varicocele by ligature and excision and by ligation of the dilated veins. [varicocele + G. *ektomē,* excision]

var·i·cog·ra·phy (var′i-kog′ră-fē) Radiography of the veins after injection of contrast medium into varicose veins. [varico- + G. *graphō,* to write]

var·i·com·pha·lus (var′i-kom′fă-lŭs) A swelling formed by varicose veins at the umbilicus. [varico- + G. *omphalos,* navel]

var·i·co·phle·bi·tis (var′i-kō-flĕ-bī′tis) Inflammation of varicose veins. [varico- + G. *phleps,* vein, + *-itis,* inflammation]

var·i·cose (var′i-kōs) Relating to, affected with, or characterized by varices or varicosis.

var·i·cose an·eu·rysm (var′i-kōs an′yūr-izm) A blood-containing sac, communicating with both an artery and a vein.

var·i·cose ul·cer (var′i-kōs ŭl′sĕr) The loss of skin surface in the drainage area of a varicose vein, usually in the leg, resulting from stasis and infection. SYN venous ulcer.

var·i·cose vein (var′i-kōs vān) Permanent dilation and tortuosity of a vein, most commonly seen in the legs, probably as a result of congenitally incomplete valves; there is a predisposition to varicose veins among persons in occupations requiring long periods of standing, and in pregnant women.

var·i·co·sis, pl. **var·i·cos·es** (var′i-kō′sis, -sēz) A dilated or varicose state of a vein or veins. See this page. [varico- + G. *-osis,* condition]

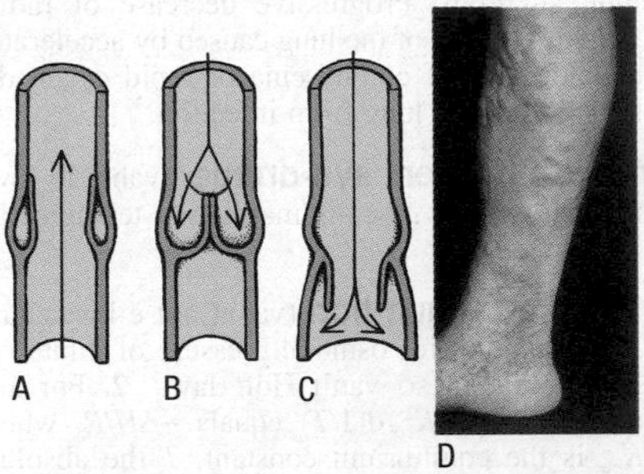

varicosis: in a healthy vein the valves allow blood to travel toward heart (A) while keeping blood from flowing back away from heart (B); valves in varicose veins (C) no longer function properly, thus allowing blood to travel back toward extremities, (D) photograph of leg with varicose veins

var·i·cos·i·ty (var′i-kos′i-tē) A varix or varicose condition.

var·i·cot·o·my (var′i-kot′ŏ-mē) An operation for varicose veins by subcutaneous incision. [varico- + G. *tomē,* a cutting]

var·i·cule (var′i-kyūl) A small varicose vein ordinarily seen in the skin; may be associated with venous stars, venous lakes, or larger varicose veins. [L. *varicula,* dim. of *varix*]

var·ie·gate por·phyr·i·a (var′ĕ-gāt pōr-fir′ē-ă) Condition characterized by abdominal pain and neuropsychiatric abnormalities, by dermal sensitivity to light and mechanical trauma, by increased fecal excretion of proto- and coproporphyrin, and by increased urinary excretion of δ-aminolevulinic acid, porphobilinogen, and porphyrins; due to a deficiency of protoporphyrinogen oxidase.

va·ri·o·la (var-ī′ō-lă) **1.** Species type of the genus Orthopoxvirus that causes human smallpox. **2.** Smallpox. [Med. L. dim of L. *varius,* spotted]

va•ri•o•la ma•jor (var-ī′ō-lă mā′jŏr) Severe form of smallpox.

va•ri•o•la mi•nor (var-ī′ō-lă mī′nŏr) A milder form of smallpox.

va•ri•o•lar (var-ī′ō-lăr) Relating to smallpox. SYN variolous.

var•i•o•late (var′ē-ō-lāt) **1.** To inoculate with smallpox. **2.** Pitted or scarred, as if by smallpox.

va•ri•o•la vi•rus (var-ī′ō-lă vī′rŭs) A poxvirus of the genus Orthopoxvirus, the pathogen of smallpox in humans. SYN smallpox virus.

var•i•ol•i•form (var′ē-ō′li-fōrm) SYN varioloid. [variola + L. *forma,* form]

va•ri•o•loid (var-ī′ō-loyd) Resembling smallpox. SYN varioliform. [variola + G. *eidos,* resemblance]

va•ri•o•lous (var-ī′ō-lŭs) SYN variolar.

var•ix, pl. **va•ri•ces** (var′iks, -i-sēz) **1.** A dilated vein. **2.** An enlarged and tortuous vein, artery, or lymphatic vessel. [L. *varix* (*varic-*), a dilated vein]

var•us (var′ŭs) Descriptive of any of the paired joints of the extremities with a static angular deformity in which the bone distal to the joint deviates medially from the longitudinal axis of the proximal bone, and toward the midline of the body, when the subject is in the anatomic position. The adjective varus is attached sometimes to the name of the joint (cubitus varus) and sometimes to the name of the body part just distal to the joint (hallux varus). The gender of the adjective matches that of the Latin noun to which it is joined; thus, cubitus, hallux, metatarsus, pes, talipes *varus;* coxa, manus, talipomanus *vara;* genu *varum.* Cf. valgus. [Mod. L. bent inward, fr. L. knock-kneed]

va•rus lax•i•ty (var′ŭs laks′i-tē) Abnormal flexibility on the lateral side of a joint on medial movement of the distal segment.

VAS Abbreviation for visual analogue scale.

vas (vas) [TA] A duct or canal conveying any liquid, such as blood, lymph, chyle, or semen. SEE ALSO vessel. [L. a vessel, dish]

♻ **vas-** (vas) Combining form indicating a vas, blood vessel. SEE ALSO vasculo-, vaso-. [L. *vas*]

va•sa (vā′să) Plural of vas.

va•sal (vā′săl) Relating to a vas or to vasa.

va•sa lym•phat•ic•a (vā′să lim-fat′i-kă) SYN lymph vessels.

va•sa pre•vi•a (vā′să prē′vē-ă) Umbilical vessels presenting in advance of the fetal head, usually traversing the membranes and crossing the internal cervical os.

va•sa rec•ta (vā′să rek′tă) **1.** Straight vessels into which the efferent arteriole of the juxtamedullary glomeruli breaks up; they form a leash of vessels that, arising at the bases of the pyramids, run through the renal medulla toward the apex of each pyramid, then reverse direction in a hairpin turn, and run straight back again toward the base of the pyramid as venae rectae. **2.** SYN straight seminiferous tubule.

va•sa va•so•rum (vā′să vā′sō-rŭm) Small arteries distributed to the outer and middle coats of the larger blood or lymph vessels, and their corresponding veins.

vas•cu•lar (vas′kyū-lăr) Relating to or containing blood vessels. [L. *vasculum,* a small vessel, dim. of *vas*]

vas•cu•lar ac•cess de•vice (VAD) (vas′kyū-lăr ak′ses dĕ-vīs′) Tubing inserted into a main vein or artery, used primarily to administer fluids and medications, monitor pressures, and collect blood.

vas•cu•lar cat•a•ract (vas′kyū-lăr kat′ăr-akt) Congenital cataract in which the degenerated lens is replaced with mesodermal tissue.

vas•cu•lar cir•cle of op•tic nerve (vas′kyū-lăr sĭr′kĕl op′tik nĕrv) A network of branches of the short ciliary arteries on the sclera around the point of entrance of the optic nerve. SYN Haller circle (1).

vas•cu•lar de•men•ti•a (vas′kyū-lăr dĕ-men′shē-ă) A steplike deterioration in intellectual functions with focal neurologic signs, as the result of multiple infarctions of the cerebral hemispheres.

vas•cu•lar•i•ty (vas′kyū-lar′i-tē) The condition of being vascular.

vas•cu•lar•i•za•tion (vas′kyū-lăr-ī-zā′shŭn) The formation of new blood vessels in a part.

vas•cu•lar•ized (vas′kyū-lăr-īzd) Rendered vascular by the formation of new vessels.

vas•cu•lar•ized graft (vas′kyū-lăr-īzd graft) The state of a graft after the recipient vasculature has been connected with the vessels in the graft.

vas•cu•lar la•cu•na (vas′kyū-lăr lă-kū′nă) The medial compartment beneath the inguinal ligament, for the passage of the femoral vessels; it is separated from the muscular lacuna by the iliopectineal arch.

vas•cu•lar lam•i•na of cho•roid (vas′kyū-lăr lam′i-nă kōr′oyd) The outer portion of the choroid of the eye containing the largest blood vessels.

vas•cu•lar lei•o•my•o•ma (vas′kyū-lăr lī′ō-mī-ō′mă) A benign neoplasm arising from the smooth muscle of blood vessels and characterized by marked vascularity.

vas•cu•lar nerve (vas′kyū-lăr nĕrv) A small

nerve filament that supplies the wall of a blood vessel.

vas•cu•lar pol•yp (vas′kyū-lăr pol′ip) A bulging or protruding angioma of the nasal mucous membrane.

vas•cu•lar ring (vas′kyū-lăr ring) Anomalous arteries (embryonic pharyngeal arch arteries) congenitally encircling the trachea and esophagus, at times producing pressure symptoms.

vas•cu•lar spi•der (vas′kyū-lăr spī′dĕr) SYN spider angioma.

vas•cu•lar sys•tem (vas′kyū-lăr sis′tĕm) The cardiovascular and lymphatic systems collectively.

vas•cu•lar tu•nic of eye (vas′kyū-lăr tū′nik ī) The vascular, pigmentary, or middle coat of the eye, comprising the choroid, ciliary body, and iris.

vas•cu•la•ture (vas′kyū-lă-chŭr) The vascular network of an organ.

vas•cu•li•tis (vas′kyū-lī′tis) SYN angiitis.

vasculo- Combining form indicating a blood vessel. SEE ALSO vas-, vaso-. [L. *vasculum,* a small vessel, dim. of *vas*]

vas•cu•lo•my•e•li•nop•a•thy (vas′kyū-lō-mī′ĕ-lin-op′ă-thē) Small cerebral vessel vasculopathy with subsequent perivascular demyelination, presumably due to circulating immune complexes.

vas•cu•lop•a•thy (vas′kyū-lop′ă-thē) Any disease affecting blood vessels. [vasculo- + G. *pathos,* disease]

vas def•er•ens, pl. **va•sa def•er•en•ti•a** (vas def′ĕr-enz, vā′să def′ĕr-en′shē-ă) SYN ductus deferens.

va•sec•to•my (vas-ek′tŏ-mē) Excision of a segment of the vas deferens, performed in association with prostatectomy, or to produce sterility. See this page. SYN deferentectomy, gonangiectomy. [vas- + G. *ektomē,* excision]

vas ef•fe•rens, pl. **va•sa ef•fer•en•ti•a** (vas ef′ĕr-enz, vā′să ef′ĕr-en′shē-ă) [TA] **1.** A vein carrying blood away from a part. **2.** SYN efferent glomerular arteriole.

vas•i•fac•tion (vas′i-fak′shŭn) SYN angiopoiesis.

vas•i•fac•tive (vas′i-fak′tiv) SYN angiopoietic.

vas•i•form (vas′i-fōrm) Having the shape of a vas or tubular structure.

vas•i•tis (vă-sī′tis) SYN deferentitis.

vaso- Combining form indicating vas, blood vessel. SEE ALSO vas-, vasculo-. [L. *vas,* a vessel]

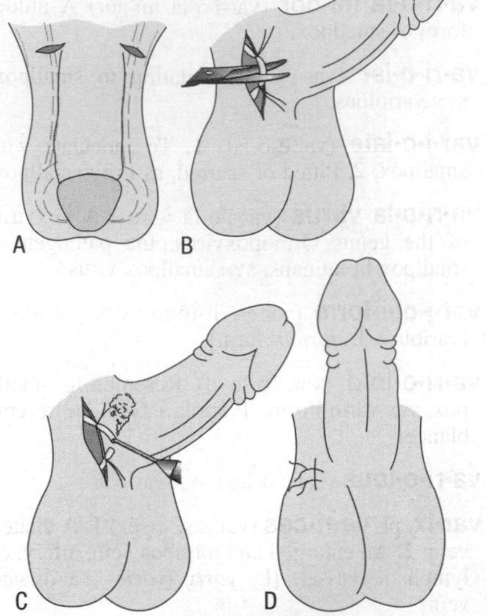

vasectomy: (A) site of vasectomy incisions; (B) the vas deferens being cut with surgical scissors; (C) cut ends of the vas deferens are cauterized to ensure complete blockage of the passage of sperm; (D) final skin suture

va•so•ac•tive (vā′sō-ak′tiv) Influencing the tone and caliber of blood vessels.

va•so•ac•tive a•mine (vā′sō-ak′tiv ă-mēn′) A substance, such as histamine or serotonin, that contains amino groups and is pharmacologically characterized by its action on the blood vessels (altering vascular caliber or permeability).

va•so•ac•tive in•tes•ti•nal pol•y•pep•tide (VIP) (vā′sō-ak′tiv in-tes′ti-năl pol′ē-pep′tīd) A polypeptide hormone secreted by the infesting non-beta islet cell tumors of the pancreas. VIP inhibits gastric acid secretion, stimulates intestinal secretions, and replaces most gastrointestinal sphincters. Cf. bioregulator.

va•so•con•stric•tion (vā′sō-kŏn-strik′shŭn) Reduction in the caliber of a blood vessel due to contraction of smooth muscle fibers in the tunica media leading to decreased blood flow to a part.

va•so•con•stric•tive (vā′sō-kŏn-strik′tiv) **1.** Causing narrowing of the blood vessels. **2.** SYN vasoconstrictor (1).

va•so•con•stric•tor (vā′sō-kŏn-strik′tŏr) **1.** An agent that causes narrowing of the blood vessels. SYN vasoconstrictive (2). **2.** A nerve, stimulation of which causes vascular constriction.

va•so•de•pres•sion (vā′sō-dĕ-presh′ŭn) Reduction of tone in blood vessels with vasodilation and resulting lowered blood pressure.

va•so•de•pres•sor (vā′sō-dĕ-pres′ŏr) **1.** Producing vasodepression. **2.** An agent that produces vasodepression.

va•so•de•pres•sor syn•co•pe (vā′sō-dĕ-pres′ŏr sing′kŏ-pē) SYN vasovagal syncope. SYN neurocardiogenic syncope.

va•so•dil•a•ta•tion (vā′sō-dil-ă-tā′shŭn) SYN vasodilation.

va•so•di•la•tion (vā′sō-dī-lā′shŭn) Increase in the caliber of a blood vessel due to relaxation of smooth muscle fibers in the tunica media. This increases blood flow but decreases systemic vascular resistance. SYN vasodilatation.

va•so•di•la•tive (vā′sō-dī-lā′tiv) **1.** Causing dilation of the blood vessels. **2.** SYN vasodilator (1).

va•so•di•la•tor (vā′sō-dī′lā-tŏr) **1.** An agent that causes dilation of the blood vessels. SYN vasodilative (2). **2.** A nerve that stimulates dilation of the blood vessels.

va•so•ep•i•did•y•mos•to•my (vā′sō-ep′i-did′i-mos′tŏ-mē) Surgical anastomosis of the vasa deferentia to the epididymis, to bypass an obstruction at the level of the mid- to distal epididymis or proximal vas. [vaso- + epididymis + G. *stoma,* mouth]

va•so•for•ma•tion (vā′sō-fōr-mā′shŭn) SYN angiopoiesis.

va•so•for•ma•tive (vā′sō-fōr′mă-tiv) SYN angiopoietic.

va•so•for•ma•tive cell (vā′sō-fōr′mă-tiv sel) SYN angioblast (1).

va•so•gan•gli•on (vā′sō-gang′glē-ŏn) A mass of blood vessels.

va•sog•ra•phy (vā-sog′ră-fē) Radiography of the vas deferens to determine patency, by injecting contrast medium into its lumen either transurethrally or by open vasotomy. [vas + G. *graphō,* to write]

va•so•hy•per•ton•ic (vā′sō-hī′pĕr-ton′ik) Relating to increased arteriolar tension or vasoconstriction. [vaso- + G. *hyper,* over, + *tonos,* tone]

va•so•hy•po•ton•ic (vā′sō-hī′pō-ton′ik) Relating to reduced arteriolar tension or vasodilation. [vaso- + G. *hypo,* under, + *tonos,* tone]

va•so•in•hib•i•tor (vā′sō-in-hib′i-tŏr) An agent that restricts or prevents the functioning of the vasomotor nerves.

va•so•in•hib•i•to•ry (vā′sō-in-hib′i-tōr-ē) Restraining vasomotor action.

va•so•li•ga•tion (vā′sō-lī-gā′shŭn) Ligation of the vas deferens, usually after its division.

va•so•mo•tion (vā′sō-mō′shŭn) Change in caliber of a blood vessel. SYN angiokinesis.

va•so•mo•tor (vā′sō-mō′tŏr) **1.** Causing dilation or constriction of the blood vessels. **2.** Denoting the nerves that have this action. SYN angiokinetic.

va•so•mo•tor im•bal•ance (vā′sō-mō′tŏr im-bal′ăns) SYN autonomic imbalance.

va•so•mo•tor nerve (vā′sō-mō′tŏr nĕrv) A motor nerve effecting or inhibiting contraction of the blood vessels.

va•so•mo•tor pa•ral•y•sis (vā′sō-mō′tŏr păr-al′i-sis) SYN vasoparesis.

va•so•mo•tor rhi•ni•tis (vā′sō-mō′tŏr rī-nī′tis) Congestion of nasal mucosa without infection or allergy.

va•so•neu•rop•a•thy (vā′sō-nūr-op′ă-thē) Any disease involving both the nerves and blood vessels. [vaso- + G. *neuron,* nerve, + *pathos,* suffering]

va•so•or•chi•dos•to•my (vā′sō-ōr′ki-dos′tŏ-mē) Reestablishment of the interrupted seminiferous channels by uniting the tubules of the epididymis or of the rete testis to the divided end of the vas deferens. [vaso- + G. *orchis,* testis, + *stoma,* mouth]

va•so•pa•ral•y•sis (vā′sō-păr-al′i-sis) Paralysis, atonia, or hypotonia of blood vessels.

va•so•pa•re•sis (vā′sō-păr-ē′sis) A mild degree of vasoparalysis. SYN vasomotor paralysis. [vaso- + G. *paresis,* weakness]

va•so•pres•sin (vā′sō-pres′in) A nonapeptide neurohypophysial hormone related to oxytocin and vasotocin; synthetically prepared or obtained from the posterior lobe of the pituitary of healthy domestic animals. In pharmacologic doses, vasopressin causes contraction of smooth muscle, notably that of all blood vessels; large doses may produce cerebral or coronary arterial spasm. Cf. bioregulator. SYN antidiuretic hormone. [vaso- + L. *premo*, pp. *pressum*, to press down, + -in]

va•so•pres•sor (vā′sō-pres′ŏr) **1.** Producing vasoconstriction and a rise in systemic arterial pressure. **2.** An agent that has this effect.

va•so•punc•ture (vā′sō-pŭngk′shŭr) The act of puncturing a vessel with a needle.

va•so•re•flex (vā′sō-rē′fleks) Any reflex that influences the caliber of blood vessels.

va•so•re•lax•a•tion (vā′sō-rē-lak-sā′shŭn, vas-ō) Reduction in tension of the walls of the blood vessels.

va•so•sec•tion (vā′sō-sek′shŭn) SYN vasotomy.

va•so•sen•so•ry (vā′sō-sen′sŏr-ē) **1.** Relating to sensation in the blood vessels. **2.** Denoting sensory nerve fibers innervating blood vessels.

va•so•spasm (vā′sō-spazm) Contraction or hypertonia of the muscular coats of the blood vessels. SYN angiospasm.

va•so•spas•tic (vā′sō-spas′tik) Relating to or characterized by vasospasm. SYN angiospastic.

va•so•stim•u•lant (vā′sō-stim′yū-lănt) **1.** Exciting vasomotor action. **2.** An agent that excites the vasomotor nerves to action. **3.** SYN vasotonic (2).

va•sos•to•my (vă-sos′tŏ-mē) Establishment of an artificial opening into the deferent duct. [vaso- + G. *stoma,* mouth]

va•sot•o•my (vă-sot′ŏ-mē) Incision into or division of the vas deferens. SYN vasosection. [vaso- + G. *tomē,* incision]

va•so•to•ni•a (vā′sō-tō′nē-ă) The tone of blood vessels, particularly the arterioles. SYN angiotonia. [vaso- + G. *tonos,* tone]

va•so•ton•ic (vā′sō-ton′ik) **1.** Relating to vascular tone. **2.** An agent that increases vascular tension. SYN vasostimulant (3).

va•so•troph•ic (vā′sō-trō′fik) Relating to the nutrition of the blood vessels or the lymphatics. [vaso- + G. *trophē,* nourishment]

va•so•tro•pic (vā′sō-trō′pik) Tending to act on the blood vessels. [vaso- + G. *tropē,* a turning]

va•so•va•gal (vā′sō-vā′găl) Relating to the action of the vagus nerve on the blood vessels.

va•so•va•gal syn•co•pe (vā′sō-vā′găl sing′kŏ-pē) Faintness or loss of consciousness due to increased vagus nerve (parasympathetic) activity. SYN vasodepressor syncope.

va•so•va•sos•to•my (vā′sō-vă-sos′tŏ-mē) Surgical anastomosis of vasa deferentia to restore fertility in previously vasectomized men. [vaso- + vaso- + G. *stoma,* mouth]

va•so•ve•sic•u•lec•to•my (vā′sō-vĕ-sik′yū-lek′tŏ-mĕ) Excision of the vas deferens and seminal vesicles. [vaso- + L. *vesicula,* vesicle, + G. *ektomē,* excision]

vas•to•my (vas′tŏ-mē) Section of the vas deferens, usually with ligation. [vas + G. *tomē,* a cutting]

vas•tus in•ter•me•di•us mus•cle (vas′tŭs in′tĕr-mē′dē-ŭs mŭs′ĕl) *Origin,* upper three quarters of anterior surface of shaft of femur; *insertion,* tibial tuberosity by way of common tendon of quadriceps femoris and patellar ligament; *action,* extends leg; *nerve supply,* femoral. SYN intermediate vastus muscle.

i vas•tus lat•er•a•lis mus•cle (vas′tŭs lat-ĕr-ā′lis mŭs′ĕl) *Origin,* lateral lip of linea aspera as far as great trochanter; *insertion,* tibial tuberosity by way of common tendon of quadriceps femoris and patellar ligament; *action,* extends leg; *nerve supply,* femoral. See this page. SYN lateral vastus muscle.

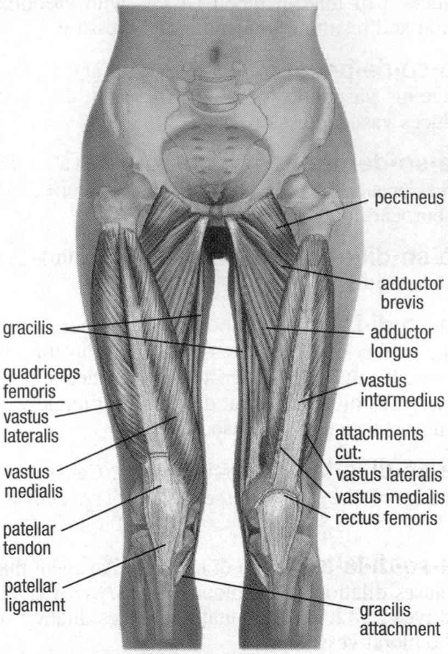

vastus lateralis muscle

vas•tus me•di•a•lis mus•cle (vas′tŭs mē-dē-ā′lis mŭs′ĕl) *Origin,* medial lip of linea aspera; *insertion,* tibial tuberosity by way of common tendon of quadriceps femoris and ligamentum patellae; *action,* extends leg; *nerve supply,* femoral. SYN medial vastus muscle.

vault (vawlt) A part resembling an arched roof or dome: e.g., the pharyngeal vault or fornix, the nonmuscular upper part of the nasopharynx; the palatine vault, arch of the plate; or vault of the vagina, fornix of vagina. [thr. O. Fr., fr. L. *volvo,* pp. *volutus,* to turn round]

VBAC Abbreviation for vaginal birth after cesarean section.

VC Abbreviation for colored vision; vital capacity.

$\mathring{V}CO_2$ Abbreviation for carbon dioxide production.

V code (kōd) In health care informatics, assignment of a numeric code used for visits to a health care professional for purposes other than for sickness (e.g., physicals, immunizations, pregnancies).

VCUG Abbreviation for voiding cystourethrogram.

VDRL Abbreviation for Venereal Disease Research Laboratories. SEE VDRL test.

VDRL test (test) A flocculation test for syphilis,

using cardiolipin-lecithin-cholesterol antigen as developed by the Venereal Disease Research Laboratory of the U.S. Public Health Service.

vec•tion (vek′shŭn) Transference of the agents of disease from an infected to an uninfected individual by a vector. [L. *vectio,* conveyance]

vec•tor (vek′tŏr) **1.** An invertebrate animal (e.g., tick, mite, mosquito, bloodsucking fly) capable of transmitting an infectious agent among vertebrates. **2.** Anything (e.g., velocity, mechanical force, electromotive force) having magnitude and direction; can be represented by a straight line of appropriate length and direction. **3.** The net electrical axis of any ECG wave (usually QRS), the length of which is proportional to the magnitude of the electrical force: Its direction gives the direction of the force, and its tip represents the positive pole of the force. **4.** DNA (e.g., a chromosome or plasmid) that autonomously replicates in a cell to which another DNA segment may be inserted and be itself replicated, as in cloning. **5.** SYN recombinant vector. **6.** Recombinant DNA systems especially suited for production of large quantities of specific proteins in bacterial, yeast, insect, or mammalian cell systems. [L. *vector,* a carrier]

vec•tor-borne in•fec•tion (vek′tŏr-bōrn in-fek′shŭn) Class of infections transmitted by an insect or animal vector. The vector may merely be a passive carrier of the infectious agent, but many kinds of infectious agents undergo a stage in biologic development in the vector, so that the vector and the human host are both essential to the survival of the infectious agent.

vec•tor•car•di•o•gram (vek′tŏr-kahr′dē-ō-gram) A graphic representation of the magnitude and direction of the heart's action currents in the form of vector loops.

vec•tor•car•di•og•ra•phy (vek′tŏr-kahr′dē-og′ră-fē) **1.** A variant of electrocardiography in which the heart's activation currents are represented by vector loops. **2.** The study and interpretation of vectorcardiograms.

vec•tor•i•al (vek-tōr′ē-ăl) Relating in any way to a vector.

veg•an (vē′găn) A strict vegetarian, one who consumes no animal or dairy products of any type. Cf. vegetarian.

veg•e•ta•ble (vej′ĕ-tă-bĕl) **1.** A plant, specifically one used for food. **2.** Relating to plants, as distinguished from animals or minerals. SYN vegetal (1). [M.E., fr. L. *vegetabilis* (see vegetation)]

veg•e•ta•ble an•ti•mo•ny (vej′ĕ-tă-bĕl an′ti-mō-nē) SYN boneset.

veg•e•tal (vej′ĕ-tăl) **1.** SYN vegetable (2). **2.** Denoting the vital functions common to plants and animals, such as respiration, metabolism, growth, and generation, distinguished from those peculiar to animals, such as conscious sensation and the mental faculties.

veg•e•tal pole, veg•e•ta•tive pole (vej′ĕ-tăl pōl, vej′ĕ-tā-tiv) The part of a telolecithal egg where the bulk of the yolk is situated.

veg•e•tar•i•an (vej′ĕ-tar′ē-ăn) One whose diet is restricted to foods of vegetable origin, excluding most animal meats. Cf. vegan.

veg•e•ta•tion (vej′ĕ-tā′shŭn) **1.** The process of growth in plants. **2.** A condition of sluggishness, comparable to the inactivity of plant life. **3.** A growth or excrescence of any sort. **4.** Specifically, a clot, composed largely of fused blood platelets, fibrin, and sometimes microorganisms, adherent to a diseased heart orifice or valve, and often initiated by infection of the structures involved. [Mod. L. *vegetatio,* growth]

veg•e•ta•tive (vej′ĕ-tā-tiv) **1.** Growing or functioning involuntarily or unconsciously, after the assumed manner of vegetable life; denoting especially a state of grossly impaired consciousness, as after severe head trauma or brain disease, in which a person is incapable of voluntary or purposeful acts and only responds reflexively to painful stimuli. **2.** Resting; not active; denoting the stage of a cell or its nucleus in which the process of karyokinesis is quiescent.

veg•e•ta•tive bac•te•ri•o•phage (vej′ĕ-tā-tiv bak-tēr′ē-ō-fāj) The form of bacteriophage in which the bacteriophage nucleic acid (lacking its coat) multiplies freely within the host bacterium, independently of bacterial multiplication.

veg•e•ta•tive en•do•car•di•tis, ver•ru•cous en•do•car•di•tis (vej′ĕ-tā-tiv en′dō-kahr-dī′tis, vĕr-ū′kŭs) Disorder associated with the presence of fibrinous clots (vegetations) forming on the ulcerated surfaces of the valves.

veg•e•ta•tive state (vej′ĕ-tā-tiv stāt) A clinical condition in which there is complete absence of awareness of the self and the environment, accompanied by sleep-wake cycles, but with either partial or complete preservation of hypothalamic and brainstem autonomic functions; may be transient or permanent. There are multiple causes, all involving the brain, including traumatic and nontraumatic injuries, metabolic and degenerative disorders, and congenital malformations.

ve•hi•cle (vē′i-kĕl) **1.** An excipient or a menstruum; a substance, usually without therapeutic action, used as a medium to give bulk for the administration of medicines. **2.** An inanimate substance (e.g., food, milk, dust, clothing, instrument) by or on which an infectious agent passes from an infected to a susceptible host. [L. *vehiculum,* a conveyance, fr. *veho,* to carry]

veil (vāl) **1.** SYN velum (1). **2.** SYN caul (1). [L. *velum*]

Veil•lo•nel•la (vā′yō-nel′ă) A genus of nonmotile, non-spore-forming, anaerobic bacteria containing small gram-negative cocci that occur as diplococci and in masses. These organisms are parasitic in the mouth and in the intestinal and respiratory tracts of humans and other animals.

vein (vān) A blood vessel carrying blood toward the heart; all the veins except the pulmonary carry dark or deoxygenated blood. SYN vena [TA]. [L. *vena*]

vein of bulb of pe•nis (vān bŭlb pē′nis) A tributary of the internal pudendal vein that drains the bulb of the penis.

vein of co•chle•ar can•a•lic•u•lus (vān kok′lē-ăr kan′ă-lik′yū-lŭs) Drains the cochlea, sacculus, and part of the utricles; empties into the superior bulb of the jugular vein by accompanying the perilymphatic duct through the cochlear canaliculus.

vein of pter•y•goid ca•nal (vān ter′i-goyd kă-nal′) A vein accompanying the nerve and artery through the pterygoid canal and emptying into the pharyngeal venous plexus.

veins of kid•ney (vānz kid′nē) The tributaries of the renal vein that drain the kidney; they parallel the arteries in the kidney and consist of interlobular, arcuate, and interlobar veins.

veins of knee (vānz nē) The veins that accompany the genicular arteries; they drain blood from the structures around the knee, terminating in the popliteal vein.

veins of tem•po•ro•man•dib•u•lar joint (vānz tem′pŏr-ō-man-dib′yū-lăr joynt) Several small tributaries to the retromandibular vein from the temporomandibular joint.

vein strip•ping (vān strip′ing) Surgical procedure to alleviate symptoms of varicose veins.

veins of ver•te•bral col•umn (vānz vĕr′tē-brăl kol′ŭm) Includes the internal and external vertebral venous plexuses, the basivertebral veins, and the anterior and posterior spinal veins.

vein of ves•tib•u•lar aq•ue•duct (vān ves-tib′yū-lăr ahk′wă-dŭkt) A small vein accompanying the endolymphatic duct; it drains much of the vestibular portion of the labyrinth and terminates in the inferior petrosal sinus.

vein of ves•tib•u•lar bulb (vān ves-tib′yū-lăr bŭlb) Drains the bulb of the vestibule; a tributary of the internal pudendal vein.

ve•la (vē′lă) Plural of velum.

ve•la•men, pl. **ve•lam•i•na** (vĕ-lā′men, -lam′i-nă) SYN velum (1). [L. a veil]

vel•a•men•tous (vel′ă-men′tŭs) Expanded in the form of a sheet or veil.

ve•lar (vē′lăr) Relating to any velum, especially the velum palatinum.

vel•lus (vel′ŭs) **1.** Fine, nonpigmented hair covering most of the body. **2.** Any structure that is fleecy, soft, and woolly. [L. fleece]

ve•loc•i•ty (v) (vĕ-los′i-tē) Rate and direction of movement; specifically, distance traveled or quantity converted per unit time in a given direction. [L. *velocitas,* fr. *velox (veloc-),* quick, swift]

vel•o•pha•ryn•ge•al (vē′lō-făr-in′jē-ăl) Pertaining to the soft palate (velum palatinum) and the posterior nasopharyngeal wall.

vel•o•pha•ryn•ge•al in•suf•fi•cien•cy (vē′lō-făr-in′jē-ăl in′sŭ-fish′ĕn-sē) Anatomic or functional deficiency in the soft palate or superior constrictor muscle, resulting in the inability to achieve velopharyngeal closure.

Vel•peau ban•dage (vel-pō′ ban′dăj) A bandage that serves to immobilize an arm to the chest wall, with the forearm positioned obliquely across and upward on the front of the chest.

Vel•peau her•ni•a (vel-pō′ hĕr′nē-ă) Femoral hernia in which the intestine is in front of the blood vessels.

ve•lum, pl. **ve•la** (vē′lŭm, -lă) **1.** Any structure resembling a veil or curtain. SYN veil (1), velamen. **2.** SYN caul (1). **3.** SYN greater omentum. **4.** Any serous membrane or membranous envelope or covering. [L. veil, sail]

ve•lum pa•la•ti•num (vē′lŭm pal′ă-tī′nŭm) SYN soft palate.

ve•na, gen. and pl. **ve•nae** (vē′nă, -nē) [TA] SYN vein. [L.]

ve•na ca•va su•per•i•or (vē′nă kā′vă sŭ-pēr′ē-ŏr) [TA] SYN superior vena cava.

ve•na•ca•vog•ra•phy (vē′nă-kā-vog′ră-fē) Angiography of a vena cava. SYN cavography.

ve•na cen•tral•is glan•du•lae su•pra•re•na•lis (vē′nă sen-trā′lis glan′dyū-lē sū-pră-rē-nā′lis) [TA] SYN central vein of suprarenal gland.

ve•na cen•tra•lis ret•i•nae (vē′nă sen-trā′lis ret′i-nē) [TA] SYN central vein of retina.

ve•na ceph•al•ic•a ac•ces•sor•i•a (vē′nă se-fal′i-kă ak-ses-ōr′ē-ă) [TA] SYN accessory cephalic vein.

ve•na dor•sa•lis pe•nis su•per•fi•ci•a•lis (vē′nă dor-sā′lis pē′nis sū′pĕr-fish′ē-ā′lis) [TA] SYN superficial dorsal veins of penis.

ve•na dor•sa•lis pro•fun•da cli•tor•i•dis (vē′nă dor-sā′lis prō-fŭn′dă kli-tōr′i-dis) [TA] SYN deep dorsal vein of clitoris.

ve•na dor•sa•lis pro•fun•da pe•nis (vē′nă dor-sā′lis prō-fŭn′dă pē′nis) [TA] SYN deep dorsal vein of penis.

ve•nae bra•chi•o•ceph•a•li•cae (vē′nē brā′kē-ō-sef-ā′li-sē) [TA] SYN brachiocephalic veins.

ve•nae com•i•tan•tes (vē′nē kom-i-tan′tēz) A pair (or occasionally more) of veins that closely accompany an artery in such a manner that the pulsations of the artery aid venous return.

ve•nae di•rec•tae la•ter•al•es (vē′nē di-rek′tē lat′ĕr-rā′lēz) [TA] One or more veins running a subependymal course in a coronal plane over the thalamus, terminating in the internal cerebral vein. SYN surface thalamic veins.

ve•nae in•ter•cos•ta•les (vē′nē in′tĕr-kos-tā′lēz) [TA] SYN posterior intercostal veins.

ve•nae in•ter•nae cer•e•bri (vē′nē in-ter′nē ser′ĕ-brī) [TA] SYN internal cerebral veins.

ve•na ep•i•gas•tri•ca (vē′nă ep-i-gas′tri-kă) SYN superficial epigastric vein.

ve•nae pro•fun•dae cer•e•bri (vē′nē prō-fŭn′dē ser′ĕ-brī) [TA] SYN deep cerebral veins.

ve•nae su•pe•ri•o•res ce•re•bri (vē′nē sū-pēr′ē-ō′rēz ser′ĕ-brī) [TA] SYN superior cerebral veins.

ve•nae u•ter•i•nae (vē′nē yū-tĕr-ī′nē) [TA] SYN uterine veins.

ve•na fem•o•ral•is (vē′nă fem′ō-rā′lis) [TA] SYN femoral vein.

ve•na hem•i•a•zy•gos ac•ces•sor•i•a (vē′nă hem′ē-ă-zī′gos ak′ses-sōr′ē-ă) [TA] SYN accessory hemiazygos vein.

ve•na il•i•o•lum•ba•lis (vē′nă il′ē-ō-lŭm-bāl′is) [TA] SYN iliolumbar vein.

ve•na por•tae he•pa•tis (vē′nă pōr′tē hē-pā′tis) [TA] SYN portal vein.

ve•na sub•clav•i•a (vē′nă sŭb-klā′vē-ă) [TA] SYN subclavian vein.

ve•na sub•men•tal•is (vē′nă sub′men-tā′lis) SYN submental vein.

ve•na um•bil•i•cal•is (vē′nă ŭm-bil-i-kā′lis) [TA] SYN left umbilical vein.

ve•na ver•te•bral•is ac•ces•sor•i•a (vē′nă vĕr-te-brā′lis ak′ses-sōr′ē-ă) [TA] SYN accessory vertebral vein.

vene- **1.** Combining form meaning the veins, venous. SEE ALSO veno-. [L. *vena,* vein] **2.** Combining form meaning venom. [L. *venenum,* poison]

ve•nec•ta•si•a (vē′nek-tā′zē-ă) SYN phlebectasia.

ve•nec•to•my (vē-nek′tŏ-mē) SYN phlebectomy.

ve•neer (vĕ-nēr′) **1.** A thin surface layer laid over a base of common material. **2.** DENTISTRY a layer of tooth-colored material, usually porcelain or acrylic resin, attached to and covering the surface of a metal crown or natural tooth structure. [Fr. *fournir,* to furnish]

ven•e•na•tion (ven′ĕ-nā′shŭn) Poisoning, as from a sting or bite. [L. *veneno,* pp. *-atus,* to poison, fr. *venenum,* poison]

ven•e•nous (ven′ĕ-nŭs) SYN poisonous. [L. *venenosus*]

ve•ne•re•al (vĕ-nēr′ē-ăl) Relating to or resulting from sexual intercourse. [L. *Venus* (*vener-*), goddess of love]

ve•ne•re•al bu•bo (vĕ-nēr′ē-ăl bū′bō) An enlarged gland in the groin associated with any sexually transmitted disease, especially chancroid.

ve•ne•re•al dis•ease (vĕ-nēr′ē-ăl di-zēz′) SYN sexually transmitted disease.

ve•ne•re•al ul•cer (vĕ-nēr′ē-ăl ŭl′sĕr) SYN chancroid.

ve•ne•re•al wart (vĕ-nēr′ē-ăl wōrt) SYN condyloma acuminatum.

ven•e•sec•tion (ven′ĕ-sek′shŭn) SYN phlebotomy. [L. *vena,* vein, + *sectio,* a cutting]

Ven•e•zue•lan hem•or•rhag•ic fe•ver (ven′ĕ-zwā′lăn hem′ŏr-aj′ik fē′vĕr) A febrile disease caused by the Guanarito virus in Venezuela; characterized by headache, arthralgia, pharyngitis, leukopenia, thrombocytopenia, and hemorrhagic manifestations.

ven•i•punc•ture (ven′i-pŭngk′shŭr) The puncture of a vein, usually to withdraw blood or inject a solution. See page 1646.

veno-, veni- Combining forms denoting the veins. SEE ALSO vene- (1). [L. *vena*]

ve•no•gram (vē′nō-gram) **1.** Radiograph of opacified veins. **2.** SYN phlebogram. [veno- + G. *gramma,* a writing]

ve•nog•ra•phy (vē-nog′ră-fē) Radiographic demonstration of a vein, after the injection of contrast medium. Used to demonstrate blockage of a vein. SYN phlebography (2). [veno- + G. *graphō,* to write]

ven•om (ven′ŏm) A toxin secreted by snakes, spiders, scorpions, and other cold-blooded animals. [M. Eng. and O. Fr. *venim,* fr. L. *venenum,* poison]

ve•no•mo•tor (vē′nō-mō′tŏr) Altering the caliber of a vein. [veno- + L. *motor,* a move]

ve•no•oc•clu•sive dis•ease of the liv•er (vē′nō-ŏ-klū′siv di-zēz′ liv′ĕr) Obliterating endophlebitis of small hepatic vein radicles, described in Jamaican children, associated with ingestion of toxic plant substances in bush tea; causes ascites, which may progress to cirrhosis.

ve•no•scle•ro•sis (vē′nō-skler-ō′sis) SYN phlebosclerosis.

ve•nos•i•ty (vē-nos′i-tē) **1.** A venous state; a condition in which the bulk of the blood is in the veins at the expense of the arteries. **2.** The unaerated condition of venous blood.

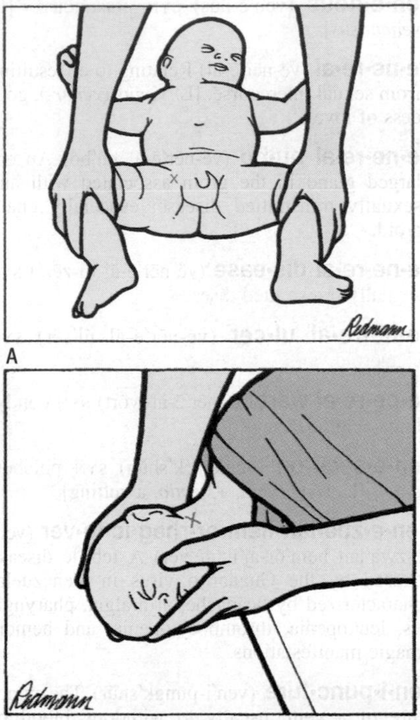

A

B

venipuncture: (A) femoral venipuncture in infant: infant shown lying supine with legs restrained in frog-leg position by two adult hands; (B) jugular venipuncture in infant: head of infant shown restrained between two adult hands (child's head is extended over edge of table)

ve•no•spasm (vē′nō-spasm) Sudden constriction of a vein.

ve•nos•ta•sis (vē′nō-stā′sis) SYN phlebostasis. [veno- + G. *stasis,* a standing]

ve•nos•to•my (vē-nos′tŏ-mē) SYN cutdown.

ve•not•o•my (vē-not′ŏ-mē) SYN phlebotomy.

ve•nous (vē′nŭs) Relating to a vein or to the veins. [L. *venosus*]

ve•nous ad•mix•ture (vē′nŭs ad′miks-chŭr) The mingling in the pulmonary circulation of arterial blood and desaturated blood resulting from ventilation-perfusion mismatching (reduced ventilation with full perfusion).

ve•nous an•gi•o•ma (vē′nŭs an′jē-ō′mă) Vascular anomaly composed of anomalous veins. SYN venous malformation.

ve•nous an•gle (vē′nŭs ang′gĕl) **1.** The junction of the internal jugular and subclavian veins, toward which converge the external and the anterior jugular and the vertebral veins, the thoracic duct in the left angle, and the right lymphatic duct in the right angle. **2.** NEURORADIOLOGY the angle of union of the superior thalamostriate vein (vena terminalis) with the internal cerebral vein, usually closely behind the interventricular foramen (Monro foramen).

ve•nous blood (vē′nŭs blŭd) That which has passed through the capillaries of various tissues, except the lungs, and found in the veins, the right chambers of the heart, and the pulmonary arteries; usually dark red as a result of a lower oxygen content.

ve•nous cap•il•lar•y (vē′nŭs kap′i-lar-ē) A capillary opening into a venule.

ve•nous hum (vē′nŭs hŭm) Brief or continuous noise originating from the neck veins that may be confused with cardiac murmurs, particularly with the continuous murmur of patent ductus arteriosus.

ve•nous hy•per•e•mi•a (vē′nŭs hī′pĕr-ē′mē-ă) SYN passive hyperemia.

ve•nous in•suf•fi•cien•cy (vē′nŭs in′sŭ-fish′ĕn-sē) Inadequate drainage of venous blood from a part, resulting in edema or dermatosis; most often seen in veins in the lower extremities.

ve•nous mal•for•ma•tion (vē′nŭs mal′fōr-mā′shŭn) SYN venous angioma.

ve•nous pulse (vē′nŭs pŭls) A pulsation occurring in the veins, especially the internal jugular vein.

ve•nous re•turn (vē′nŭs rĕ-tŭrn′) The blood returning to the heart through the great veins and coronary sinus; also used to describe venous drainage of a part of the body or particular organ.

ve•nous si•nus•es (vē′nŭs sī′nŭs-ĕz) SYN dural venous sinuses.

ve•nous star (vē′nŭs stahr) A small, red nodule formed by a dilated vein in the skin; caused by increased venous pressure.

ve•nous ul•cer (vē′nŭs ŭl′sĕr) SYN varicose ulcer.

ve•no•ve•nos•to•my (vē′nō-vē-nos′tŏ-mē) The formation of an anastomosis between two veins. SYN phlebophlebostomy. [veno- + veno- + G. *stoma,* mouth]

vent (vent) An opening into a cavity or canal, especially one through which the contents of such a cavity are discharged, as the anus. [O. Fr. *fente,* a chink, cleft]

ven•ter (ven′tĕr) **1.** SYN abdomen. **2.** SYN belly (2). **3.** One of the great cavities of the body. **4.** The uterus. [L. *venter* (*ventr-*), belly]

ven•ti•late (ven′ti-lāt) To aerate, or oxygenate, the blood in the pulmonary capillaries. SYN air

(2). [L. *ventilo,* pp. *-atus,* to fan, fr. *ventus,* the wind]

ven•ti•la•tion (ven′ti-lā′shŭn) **1.** Replacement of air or other gas in a space by fresh air or gas. **2.** Movement of gases into and out of the lungs. SYN respiration (2). **3. (v)** PHYSIOLOGY the tidal exchange of air between the lungs and the atmosphere that occurs in breathing. SEE ALSO respiration.

ven•ti•la•tion:per•fu•sion ra•ti•o ($\dot{V}_A$:$\dot{Q}$) (ven-ti-lā′shŭn-pĕr-fyū′zhŭn rā′shē-ō) The ratio of alveolar ventilation to simultaneous alveolar capillary blood flow in any part of the lung; because both ventilation and perfusion are expressed per unit volume of tissue and per unit of time, which cancel, the units become liters of gas per liter of blood.

ven•ti•la•tion-per•fu•sion scan (ven′ti-lā′shŭn-pĕr-fyū′zhŭn skan) A lung function test, especially useful in the diagnosis of pulmonary embolism, employing an inhaled radionuclide for ventilation and an intravenous radionuclide for perfusion; their respective distributions in the lung are recorded scintigraphically. See page B23.

ven•til•a•tor (ven′til-ā-tŏr) A mechanical device designed to perform part or all of the work of respiration, i.e., of moving gas into and out of the lungs.

ven•til•a•to•ry thresh•old (ven′til-ă-tōr-ē thresh′ōld) Point during exercise training at which pulmonary ventilation becomes disproportionately high with respect to oxygen consumption; believed to reflect onset of anaerobiosis and lactate accumulation.

ven•trad (ven′trad) Toward the ventral aspect; opposed to dorsad. [L. *venter,* belly, + *ad,* to]

ven•tral (ven′trăl) **1.** Pertaining to the belly or to any venter. **2.** SYN anterior (1). **3.** VETERINARY ANATOMY the undersurface of an animal; often used to indicate the position of one structure relative to another (i.e., situated nearer the undersurface of the body). [L. *ventralis*]

ven•tral ap•ron pre•puce (ven′trăl ā′prŏn prē′pyūs) The incomplete foreskin seen in epispadias.

ven•tral horn (ven′trăl hōrn) SYN anterior horn.

ven•tral plate (ven′trăl plāt) SYN floor plate.

ven•tral root (ven′trăl rūt) The motor root of a spinal nerve.

ven•tral tha•lam•ic pe•dun•cle (ven′trăl thă-lam′ik pĕ-dŭngk′ĕl) The massive system of fiber bundles emerging through the ventral, lateral, and anterior borders of the thalamus to join the internal capsule and parts of the corona radiata; contains the fibers reciprocally connecting the ventral thalamic nuclei with the precentral and postcentral gyri of the cerebral cortex.

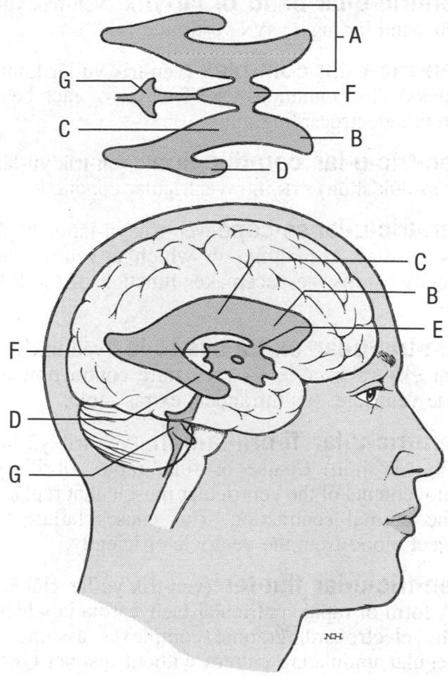

ventricles of the brain (superior and lateral views): (A) left lateral ventricle; (B) anterior horn of right lateral ventricle; (C) lateral ventricle; (D) inferior horn of right lateral ventricle; (E) interventricular foramen; (F) third ventricle; (G) fourth ventricle

ven•tri•cle (ven′tri-kĕl) A normal cavity, as of the brain or heart. See this page. SYN ventriculus (2). [L. *ventriculus,* dim. of *venter,* belly]

ven•tric•u•lar (ven-trik′yū-lăr) Relating to a ventricle, in any sense.

ven•tric•u•lar af•ter•load (ven-trik′yū-lăr af′tĕr-lōd) The sum total of the forces, both hemodynamic and mechanical, that the left ventricle of the heart must pump against to send oxygenated blood out into the body.

ven•tric•u•lar ar•ter•ies (ven-trik′yū-lăr ahr′tĕr-ēz) Branches of the right and left coronary arteries distributed to the muscle of the ventricles. SYN arteriae ventriculares [TA].

ven•tric•u•lar as•sist de•vice (ven-trik′yū-lăr ă-sist′ dĕ-vīs′) A device that supports or replaces the function of a ventricle (LVAD or RVAD indicates which ventricle, i.e., LV=left ventricle, RV right). The device is used in patients with potentially salvageable myocardium, where centrifugal or pneumatic devices can be placed in either heterotopic or orthotopic positions (the latter is termed a total artificial heart). The function of either the left, right, or both ventricles can thus be supported for days to weeks. Either recovery of heart function or need for transplantation then becomes apparent.

ven•tric•u•lar band of lar•ynx (ven-trik′yū-lăr band lar′ingks) SYN vestibular fold.

ven•tric•u•lar com•plex (ven-trik′yū-lăr kom′pleks) The continuous QRST waves of each beat in the electrocardiogram.

ven•tric•u•lar con•duc•tion (ven-trik′yū-lăr kŏn-dŭk′shŭn) SYN intraventricular conduction.

ven•tric•u•lar es•cape (ven-trik′yū-lăr es-kāp′) A cardiac arrhythmia in which a ventricular focus usurps the pacemaker function of the SA node.

ven•tric•u•lar ex•tra•sys•to•le (ven-trik′yū-lăr eks′tră-sis′tŏ-lē) A premature contraction of the ventricle. SYN infranodal extrasystole.

ven•tric•u•lar fi•bril•la•tion (ven-trik′yū-lăr fib′ri-lā′shŭn) Coarse or fine, rapid, fibrillary movements of the ventricular muscle that replace the normal contraction. This causes failure to eject blood from the ventricle efficiently.

ven•tric•u•lar flut•ter (ven-trik′yū-lăr flŭt′ĕr) A form of rapid ventricular tachycardia in which the electrocardiographic complexes assume a regular undulating pattern without distinct QRS and T waves.

ven•tric•u•lar fold (ven-trik′yū-lăr fōld) SYN vestibular fold.

ven•tric•u•lar fu•sion beat (ven-trik′yū-lăr fyū′zhŭn bēt) A fusion beat that occurs when the ventricles are activated partly by the descending sinus or A-V junctional impulse and partly by an ectopic ventricular impulse.

ven•tric•u•lar pho•na•tion (ven-trik′yū-lăr fō-nā′shŭn) Voice produced by vibration of the ventricular (vestibular) folds, just above the vocal folds. This may occur as a substitute for, or in addition to, vocal fold vibration, and creates a hoarse, low-pitched voice. SYN vestibular phonation.

ven•tric•u•lar pre•load (ven-trik′yū-lăr prē′lōd) The pressure stretching the ventricular walls at the onset of ventricular contraction, expressed in terms of the wall stress at this moment, related to the tension per unit cross-sectional area in the ventricular muscle fibers that balances this transmural pressure at the moment before contraction begins. SYN preload (2).

ven•tric•u•lar re•duc•tion sur•ger•y (ven-trik′yū-lăr rĕ-dŭk′shŭn sŭr′jĕr-ē) SYN left ventricular volume reduction surgery.

ven•tric•u•lar rhythm (ven-trik′yū-lăr ridh′ŭm) SYN idioventricular rhythm.

ven•tric•u•lar sep•tal de•fect (VSD) (ven-trik′yū-lăr sep′tăl dē-fekt′) A congenital defect in the interventricular septum, usually resulting from failure of the spiral septum to close the interventricular foramen.

ven•tric•u•lar stand•still (ven-trik′yū-lăr stand′stil) Cessation of ventricular contractions, marked by absence of ventricular complexes in the electrocardiogram.

ven•tric•u•lar tach•y•car•di•a (ven-trik′yū-lăr tak′i-kahr′dē-ă) A heart rate exceeding 100 beats per minute driven by an ectopic ventricular focus.

ven•tric•u•li•tis (ven-trik′yū-lī′tis) Inflammation of the ventricles of the brain. [ventricle + G. *-itis,* inflammation]

♻ **ventriculo-** Prefix denoting a ventricle. [L. *ventriculus*]

ven•tric•u•lo•a•tri•al (V-A, VA) (ven-trik′yū-lō-ā′trē-ăl) Relating to both ventricles and atria, especially to the sequential passage of conduction in the retrograde direction from ventricle to atrium.

ven•tric•u•lo•a•tri•al shunt (ven-trik′yū-lō-ā′trē-ăl shŭnt) Surgical procedure for hydrocephalus; a drain implanted in the lateral cerebral ventricle passes excess cerebrospinal fluid to the right atrium. SYN ventriculoatriostomy.

ven•tric•u•lo•a•tri•os•to•my (ven-trik′yū-lō-ā′trē-os′tŏ-mē) SYN ventriculoatrial shunt.

ven•tric•u•lo•cis•ter•nos•to•my (ven-trik′yū-lō-sis′tĕr-nos′tŏ-mē) An artificial opening between the ventricles of the brain and the cisterna magna. SEE ALSO shunt (2). [ventriculo- + L. *cisterna,* cistern, + G. *stoma,* mouth]

ven•tric•u•log•ra•phy (ven-trik′yū-log′ră-fē) **1.** Demonstration of the contractility of the cardiac ventricles by recording serially the distribution of intravenously injected radionuclide or that of radiographic contrast medium injected through an intracardiac catheter. **2.** Visualization by roentgenography of a cardiac ventricle by injection of radiopaque contrast material. [ventriculo- + G. *graphē,* a writing]

ven•tric•u•lo•mas•toid•os•to•my (ven-trik′yū-lō-mast′oyd-os′tŏ-mē) Establishment of a communication between the lateral cerebral ventricle and the mastoid antrum by means of a polythene tube for the relief of hydrocephalus. SEE ALSO shunt (2). [ventriculo- + mastoid, + G. *stoma,* mouth]

ven•tric•u•lo•nec•tor (ven-trik′yū-lō-nek′tŏr) SYN atrioventricular bundle. [ventriculo- + L. *necto,* to join]

ven•tric•u•lo•per•i•to•ne•al shunt (ven-trik′yū-lō-per′i-tō-nē′ăl shŭnt) Surgical procedure for hydrocephalus; a drain implanted into the lateral cerebral ventricle passes excess cerebrospinal fluid to the peritoneal cavity. See page 1649. SYN ventriculoperitoneostomy.

ven•tric•u•lo•per•i•to•ne•os•to•my (ven-trik′yū-lō-per′i-tō-nē-os′tŏ-mē) SYN ventriculoperitoneal shunt.

ven•tric•u•lo•plas•ty (ven-trik′yū-lō-plas-tē)

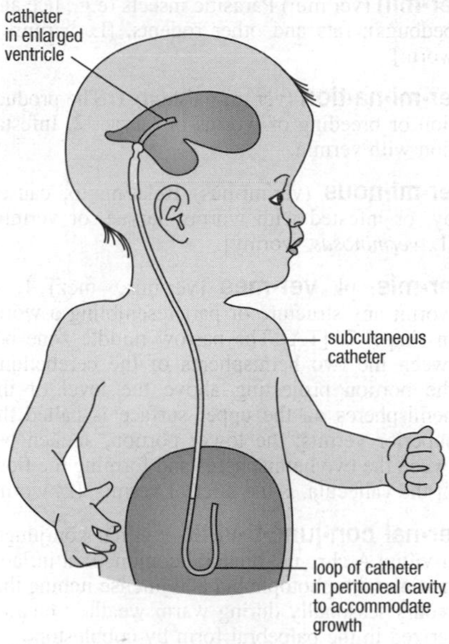

ventriculoperitoneal shunt: used to remove excess cerebrospinal fluid from the ventricles and shunt it to the peritoneal cavity

Any surgical procedure to repair a defect of one of the ventricles of the heart. [ventriculo- + G. *plastos,* formed]

ven·tric·u·lo·punc·ture (ven-trik′yū-lō-pŭngk′shŭr) Insertion of a needle into a ventricle.

ven·tric·u·los·co·py (ven-trik′yū-los′kŏ-pē) Direct inspection of a ventricle with an endoscope. [ventriculo- + G. *skopeō,* to view]

ven·tric·u·los·to·my (ven-trik′yū-los′tŏ-mē) Establishment of an opening in a ventricle, usually from the third ventricle to the subarachnoid space to relieve hydrocephalus. SEE ALSO shunt (2). [ventriculo- + G. *stoma,* mouth]

ven·tric·u·lo·sub·a·rach·noid (ven-trik′yū-lō-sŭb′ă-rak′noyd) Relating to the space occupied by the cerebrospinal fluid. [ventriculo- + subarachnoid]

ven·tric·u·lot·o·my (ven-trik′yū-lot′ŏ-mē) Incision into a ventricle of the heart or the brain. [ventriculo- + G. *tomē,* incision]

ven·tric·u·lus, pl. **ven·tric·u·li** (ven-trik′yū-lŭs, -lī) **1.** SYN stomach. **2.** [TA] SYN ventricle. [L. dim. of *venter,* belly]

ven·tri·cu·lus ter·ti·us (ven-trik′yū-lŭs ter′shē-ŭs) [TA] SYN third ventricle.

ven·tri·duc·tion (ven′tri-dŭk′shŭn) Drawing toward the abdomen or abdominal wall.

♻**ventro-** Prefix denoting ventral. [L. *venter,* belly]

ven·tros·co·py (ven-tros′kŏ-pē) SYN peritoneoscopy. [ventro- + G. *skopeō,* to view]

ven·trot·o·my (ven-trot′ŏ-mē) SYN celiotomy. [ventro- + G. *tomē,* incision]

Ven·tu·ri mask (ven-tyūr′ē mask) Oxygen delivery system that allows for the delivery of accurate oxygen concentrations. See this page.

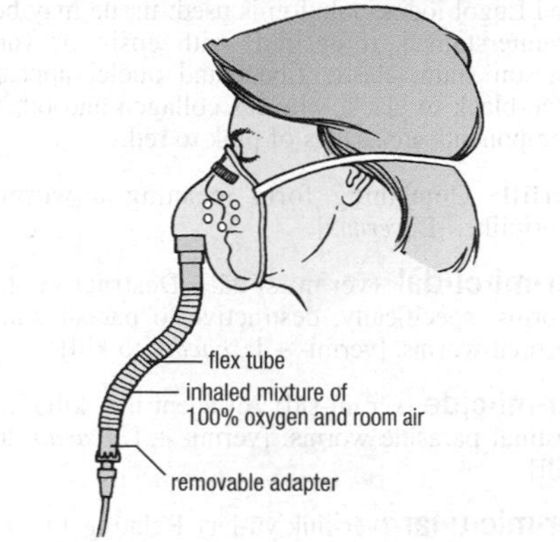

Venturi mask: constant high concentrations of oxygen can be delivered

ven·u·la, pl. **ven·u·lae** (ven′yū-lă, -lē) [TA] SYN venule. [L. dim. of *vena,* vein]

ven·u·lae stel·la·tae (ven′yū-lē stel-lā′tē) The star-shaped groups of venules in the renal cortex. SYN stellate veins, stellate venules.

ven·u·lar (ven′yū-lăr) Pertaining to venules.

ven·ule (ven′yūl) A venous radicle continuous with a capillary. SYN venula [TA], capillary vein.

ver·bal a·prax·i·a (vĕrb′ăl ă-prak′sē-ă) SYN apraxia of speech. SEE ALSO apraxia, oral apraxia, developmental apraxia of speech.

ver·bal au·top·sy (vĕrb′ăl aw′top-sē) Method of obtaining as much information as possible about a deceased person by asking questions of family and others who can describe the mode of death and circumstances preceding it; used especially in developing countries and in settings and situations in which postmortem pathologic examination is not feasible.

ver·bal dys·prax·i·a (vĕrb′ăl dis-prak′sē-ă) SYN apraxia of speech.

ver·ba·tim trans·crip·tion (vĕr-bā′tim trans-krip′shŭn) Rarely used process in which a medical transcriptionist transcribes exactly what is dictated (i.e., transcribes word for word).

ver·big·er·a·tion (vĕr-bij′ĕr-ā′shŭn) Constant repetition of meaningless words or phrases; seen in schizophrenia. SYN cataphasia. [L. *verbum,* word, + *gero,* to carry about]

verge (vĕrj) An edge or margin.

ver•gence (vĕr′jĕns) A disjunctive movement of the eyes in which the fixation axes are not parallel, as in convergence or divergence. [L. *vergo,* to incline, to turn]

Ver•hoeff e•las•tic tis•sue stain (ver′hef ĕ-las′tik tish′ū stān) A stain for tissue sections in which a mixture of hematoxylin, ferric chloride, and Lugol iodine solution is used; tissue may be counterstained, if desired, with eosin or van Gieson stain; elastic fibers and nuclei appear blue-black to black, whereas collagen and other components are shades of pink to red.

vermi- Combining form meaning a worm; wormlike. [L. *vermis*]

ver•mi•ci•dal (vĕr′mi-sī′dăl) Destructive to worms; specifically, destructive to parasitic intestinal worms. [vermi- + L. *caedo,* to kill]

ver•mi•cide (vĕr′mi-sīd) An agent that kills intestinal parasitic worms. [vermi- + L. *caedo,* to kill]

ver•mic•u•lar (vĕr-mik′yū-lăr) Relating to, resembling, or moving like a worm. [L. *vermiculus,* dim. of *vermis,* worm]

ver•mic•u•lar move•ment (vĕr-mik′yū-lăr mūv′mĕnt) SYN peristalsis.

ver•mic•u•lar pulse (vĕr-mik′yū-lăr pŭls) A small, rapid pulse, giving a wormlike sensation to the finger.

ver•mic•u•la•tion (vĕr-mik′yū-lā′shŭn) A wormlike movement, as in peristalsis.

ver•mic•u•lose, **ver•mic•u•lous** (vĕr-mik′yū-lōs, -lŭs) **1.** Wormy; infected with worms or larvae. **2.** Wormlike. SEE ALSO vermiform.

ver•mi•form (vĕr′mi-fōrm) Worm-shaped; resembling a worm in form, denoting especially the appendix of the cecum. SEE ALSO lumbricoid. [vermi- + L. *forma,* form]

ver•mi•form ap•pen•dix (vĕr′mi-fōrm ă-pen′diks) A wormlike intestinal diverticulum extending from the blind end of the cecum; it varies in length and ends in a blind extremity. SYN appendix vermiformis [TA].

ver•mil•ion bor•der (vĕr-mil′yŏn bōr′dĕr) The red margin of the upper and lower lips, which commences at the exterior edge of the intraoral labial mucosa ("moist line") and extends outward, terminating at the extraoral labial cutaneous junction; a thinly keratinized type of stratified squamous epithelium deeply penetrated by well-vascularized dermal papillae that show through the translucent epidermis to impart the typical red appearance of the lips.

ver•mil•ion•ec•to•my (vĕr-mil′yŏn-ek′tō-mē) Excision of the vermilion border. [vermilion border + G. *ektomē,* cutting out]

ver•min (vĕr′min) Parasitic insects (e.g., lice and bedbugs); rats and other rodents. [L. *vermis,* a worm]

ver•mi•na•tion (vĕr′mi-nā′shŭn) **1.** The production or breeding of worms or larvae. **2.** Infestation with vermin.

ver•mi•nous (vĕr′mi-nŭs) Relating to, caused by, or infested with worms, larvae, or vermin. [L. *verminosus,* wormy]

ver•mis, pl. **ver•mes** (vĕr′mis, -mēz) **1.** A worm; any structure or part resembling a worm in shape. **2.** [TA] The narrow middle zone between the two hemispheres of the cerebellum; the portion projecting above the level of the hemispheres on the upper surface is called the superior vermis; the lower portion, sunken between the two hemispheres and forming the floor of the vallecula, is the inferior vermis. [L. worm]

ver•nal con•junc•ti•vi•tis (vĕr′năl kŏn-jŭngk′ti-vī′tis) A chronic, bilateral conjunctival inflammation with photophobia and intense itching that recurs seasonally during warm weather; characterized in the palpebral form by cobblestone papillae in the upper palpebral conjunctiva and in the bulbar form by gelatinous nodules adjacent to the corneoscleral limbus. SYN spring conjunctivitis.

Ver•net syn•drome (ver-nā′ sin′drōm) A syndrome characterized by paralysis of the motor components of the glossopharyngeal, vagus, and accessory cranial nerves as they lie in the posterior fossa; it is most commonly the result of head injury.

ver•nix (vĕr′niks) SYN dental varnish. [Mod. L.]

ver•nix ca•se•o•sa (vĕr′niks kā-sē-ō′să) The fatty cheesy substance, consisting of desquamated epithelial cells, lanugo (downy hairs), and sebaceous matter, which covers the skin of the fetus and provides a waterproof protective cover.

ve•ro cy•to•tox•in (ver′ō sī′tō-tok′sin) A cell cytotoxin produced by enterohemorrhagic *Escherichia coli* that appears to contribute to the occurrence of hemorrhagic colitis and hemolytic uremic syndrome. SYN Shigalike toxin.

ve•ron•i•ca (vĕr-on′i-kă) SYN black root. [feminine name]

ver•ru•ca, pl. **ver•ru•cae** (vĕr-ū′kă, -kē) A flesh-colored growth characterized by circumscribed hypertrophy of the papillae of the corium, with thickening of the malpighian, granular, and keratin layers of the epidermis, caused by human papillomavirus; also applied to epidermal verrucous tumors of nonviral etiology. Cf. verruga peruana. See page 1651. SYN verruga, wart. [L.]

ver•ru•ca nec•ro•ge•ni•ca (vĕr-ū′kă nek′rō-gen′i-kă) SYN postmortem wart.

ver•ru•ca per•u•an•a, **ver•ru•ca pe•ru•vi•**

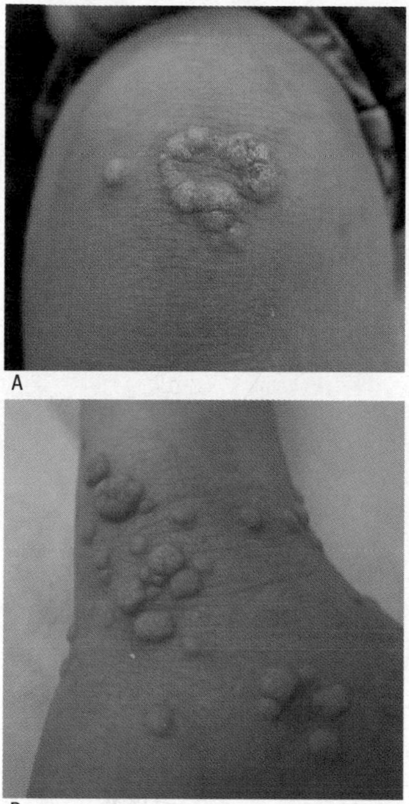

A

B

verruca: (A) knee; (B) wrist

an•a (věr-ū′kă per-ū-ahn′ă, pe-rū-vē-ahn′ă) SYN verruga peruana.

ver•ru•ca pla•na (věr-ū′kă plā′nă) A smooth, flat, flesh-colored wart of small size, occurring in groups, seen especially on the face of the young; often associated with common warts of the hands, due to human papilloma virus, commonly, types 3 and 10. SYN flat wart.

ver•ru•ca plan•tar•is (věr-ū′kă plan-tār′ris) SYN plantar wart.

ver•ru•ci•form (věr-ū′si-fōrm) Wart-shaped. [L. *verruca,* wart, + *forma,* form]

ver•ru•cose (věr-ū′kōs) Resembling a wart; denoting wartlike elevations. [L. *verrucosus*]

ver•ru•cous he•man•gi•o•ma (ver-ū′kŭs hē-man′jē-ō′mă) A variant of the angiomatous nevus, appearing at birth or in early childhood, situated on the lower extremities with bluish-red nodules and warty surface; they enlarge and sometimes have satellite lesions.

ver•ru•cous ne•vus (ver-ū′kŭs nē′vŭs) A skin-colored (or darker), wartlike, often linear, lesion appearing at birth or in early childhood, and occurring in various sizes and locations, single or multiple.

ver•ru•cous xan•tho•ma (ver-ū′kŭs zan-thō′mă) Histocytosis Y; a papilloma of the oral mucosa and skin in which squamous epithelium covers connective tissue papillae filled with large, foamy histiocytes.

ver•ru•ga (věr-ū′gă) SYN verruca. [Sp.]

ver•ru•ga per•u•an•a (věr-ū′gă per-ū-ahn′ă) A late, eruptive stage of bartonellosis, characterized by soft conic or pedunculated vascular papules on the skin or mucous membranes; resolves without scars after a few months. Cf. Oroya fever. SYN Peruvian wart, verruca peruana, verruca peruviana.

ver•sion (ver′zhŭn) **1.** Displacement of the uterus, in which the entire organ tilts without bending upon itself; such displacement may be anteversion, retroversion, or lateroversion. **2.** Change of position of the fetus in the uterus, occurring spontaneously or effected by manipulation. **3.** SYN inclination. **4.** Conjugate rotation of the eyes in the same direction; such rotation may be dextroversion, levoversion, supraversion, or infraversion. [L. *verto,* pp. *versus,* to turn]

ver•te•bra, gen. and pl. **ver•te•brae** (věr′tē-bră, -brē) [TA] One of the segments of the spinal column; in human beings there are usually 33 vertebrae: 7 cervical, 12 thoracic, 5 lumbar, 5 sacral (fused into one bone, the sacrum), and 4 coccygeal (fused into one bone, the coccyx). [L. joint, fr. *verto,* to turn]

ver•te•bra C1 (věr′tě-bră) SYN atlas.

ver•te•bra C2 (věr′tě-bră) SYN axis (5).

ver•te•bra den•ta•ta (věr′tě-bră den-tā′tă) SYN axis (5).

ver•te•brae cer•vic•al•es [C1–C7] (věr′tě-brē ser-vi-kā′lēz) [TA] SYN cervical vertebrae [C1–C7].

ver•te•brae coc•cyg•e•ae [Co1–Co4] (věr′tě-brē kok-sij′ē-ē) [TA] SYN coccygeal vertebrae Co1–Co4.

ver•te•brae lum•ba•les [L1–L5] (věr′tě-brē lŭm-bā′lēz) SYN lumbar vertebrae [L1–L5].

ver•te•brae sac•ra•les [S1–S5] (věr′tě-brē sā-krā′lēz) SYN sacral vertebrae [S1–S5].

ver•te•brae tho•ra•ci•cae (věr′tě-brē thō-rā′sis-ē) [TA] SYN thoracic vertebrae [T1–T12].

ver•te•bral (věr′tě-brăl) Relating to a vertebra or the vertebrae.

ver•te•bral arch (věr′tě-brăl ahrch) The posterior projection from the body of a vertebra that encloses the vertebral foramen; it consists of paired pedicles and laminae; the spinous, transverse, and articular processes arise from the arch. In aggregate, the venous arches, and the ligamenta flava that unite them, form the posterior wall of the vertebral (spinal) canal. SYN neural arch.

ver•te•bral ar•ter•y (vĕr′tĕ-brăl ahr′tĕr-ē) The first branch of the subclavian artery; for descriptive purposes, divided into four parts: 1) prevertebral part, the portion before it enters the foramen of the transverse process of the sixth cervical vertebra; 2) transversarial part, the portion in the transverse foramina of the first six cervical vertebrae; 3) suboccipital (atlantic) part, the portion running along the posterior arch of the atlas; and 4) intracranial part, the portion within the cranial cavity to its union with the artery from the other side to form the basilar artery. SYN arteria vertebralis [TA].

ver•te•bral bod•y (vĕr′tĕ-brăl bod′ē) The main portion of a vertebra anterior to the vertebral canal, as distinct from the arches. USAGE NOTE the term "centrum" is frequently erroneously used as a synonym for vertebral body — however the developmental centrum is less than the body, which also includes parts of the developmental neural arches.

ver•te•bral ca•nal (vĕr′tĕ-brăl kă-nal′) The canal that contains the spinal cord, spinal meninges, and related structures. It is formed by the vertebral foramina of successive vertebrae of the articulated vertebral column. SYN canalis vertebralis [TA], spinal canal.

ver•te•bral col•umn (vĕr′tĕ-brăl kol′ŭm) The series of vertebrae that extend from the cranium to the coccyx, providing support and forming a flexible bony case for the spinal cord. See this page. SYN columna vertebralis [TA], backbone, rachis, spina, spinal column, spine (2).

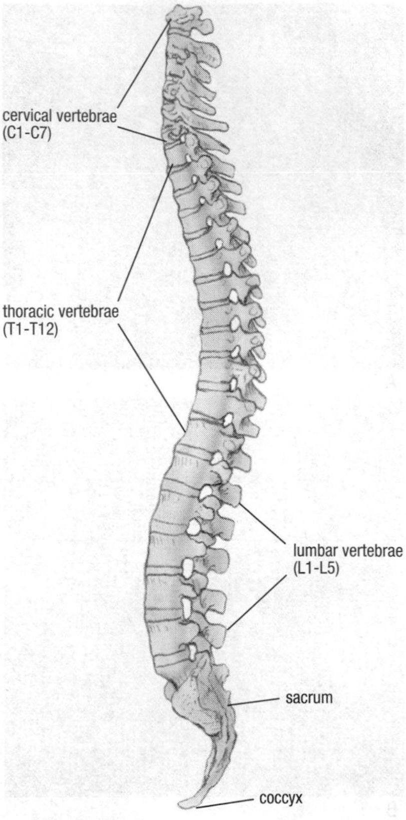

vertebral column

ver•te•bral fo•ra•men (vĕr′tĕ-brăl fōr-ā′mĕn) The foramen formed by the union of the vertebral arch with the body; in the articulated vertebral column, the vertebral foramina collectively form the vertebral column.

ver•te•bral for•mu•la (vĕr′tĕ-brăl fōrm′yū-lă) A formula indicating the number of vertebrae in each segment of the spinal column; for humans it is C. 7, T. 12, L. 5, S. 5, Co. 4 = 33, the letters standing for cervical, thoracic, lumbar, sacral, and coccygeal.

ver•te•bral nerve (vĕr′tĕ-brăl nĕrv) A branch from the stellate ganglion that ascends along the vertebral artery to the level of the axis or atlas, giving branches to the cervical nerves and meninges. SYN nervus vertebralis [TA].

ver•te•bral ribs (vĕr′tĕ-brăl ribz) SYN floating ribs [XI–XII].

ver•te•bral sub•lux•a•tion com•plex (vĕr′tĕ-brăl sŭb′lŭk-sā′shŭn kom′pleks) Theoretic model of vertebral motion segment dysfunction (subluxation) that incorporates the complex interaction of pathologic changes in nerves, and muscles, and in ligamentous, vascular, and connective tissues.

ver•te•bral vein (vĕr′tĕ-brăl vān) A vein derived from tributaries (venae comitantes) that run through the foramina in the transverse processes of the first six cervical vertebrae and form a plexus around the vertebral artery; it empties as a single trunk into the brachiocephalic veins.

ver•te•bra pla•na (vĕr′tĕ-bră plā′nă) Spondylitis with reduction of vertebral body to a thin disc.

Ver•te•bra•ta (vĕr′tĕ-brā′tă) The vertebrates, a major division of the phylum Chordata, consisting of those animals with a dorsal hollow nerve cord enclosed in a cartilaginous or bony spinal column; includes several classes of fishes, and the amphibians, reptiles, birds, and mammals. [L. *vertebratus,* jointed]

ver•te•brate (vĕr′tĕ-brāt) **1.** Having a vertebral column. **2.** An animal having vertebrae.

ver•te•brat•ed cath•e•ter (vĕr′tĕ-brāt-ĕd kath′ĕ-tĕr) A device composed of several segments moving on each other like the links of a chain.

ver•te•brec•to•my (vĕr′tĕ-brek′tŏ-mē) Resection of a vertebral body. [vertebra + G. *ektomē,* excision]

vertebro- Combining form denoting a vertebra, vertebral. [L. *vertebra*]

ver•te•bro•ar•te•ri•al fo•ra•men (vĕr′tĕ-brō-ahr-tēr′ē-ăl fōr-ā′mĕn) SYN transverse foramen.

ver•te•bro•chon•dral (vĕr′tĕ-brō-kon′drăl) Denoting the three false ribs (eighth, ninth, and tenth), which are connected with the vertebrae at one extremity and the costal cartilages at the other; those cartilages not articulating directly with the sternum. SYN vertebrocostal (2). [vertebro- + G. *chondros,* cartilage]

ver•te•bro•cos•tal (vĕr′tĕ-brō-kos′tăl) **1.** SYN costovertebral. **2.** SYN vertebrochondral. [vertebro- + L. *costa,* rib]

ver•te•bro•cos•tal tri•gone (vĕr′tĕ-brō-kos′tăl trī′gōn) A triangular area in the diaphragm near the lateral arcuate ligament that is devoid of muscle fibers; it is covered by pleura superiorly and by peritoneum inferiorly.

ver•te•bro•ster•nal (vĕr′tĕ-brō-stĕr′năl) SYN sternovertebral.

ver•tex, pl. **ver•ti•ces** (vĕr′teks, -ti-sēz) **1.** The topmost point of the vault of the cranium, a landmark in craniometry. **2.** OBSTETRICS the portion of the fetal head bounded by the planes of the trachelobregmatic and biparietal diameters, with the posterior fontanel at the apex. [L. whirl, whorl]

ver•tex pre•sen•ta•tion (vĕr′teks prez′ĕn-tā′shŭn) SEE cephalic presentation.

ver•ti•cal (vĕr′ti-kăl) **1.** Relating to the vertex, or crown of the head. **2.** Perpendicular. **3.** Denoting any plane or line that passes longitudinally through the body in the anatomic position.

ver•ti•cal band•ed gas•tro•plas•ty (vĕr′ti-kăl band′ĕd gas′trō-plas-tē) A surgical intervention for treatment of morbid obesity in which an upper gastric pouch is formed by a vertical staple line, with a cloth band applied to prevent dilation at the outlet into the main pouch. See this page.

ver•ti•cal growth phase (vĕr′ti-kăl grōth fāz) Spread of melanoma cells from the epidermis into the dermis and later the subcutis, from which site metastasis may take place.

ver•ti•cal heart (vĕr′ti-kăl hahrt) Descriptive of the heart's electrical axis when this is directed at approximately +90 degrees.

ver•ti•cal in•te•gra•tion (vĕr′ti-kăl in′tĕ-grā′shŭn) A system that provides primary care, specialty care, or hospitalization, as necessary, through interdisplinary and specialty collaboration.

ver•ti•cal lam•in•ar flow hood (vĕr′ti-kăl lam′i-năr flō hud) A laminar flow hood in which the air is pushed through a filter vertically to protect the user from exposure to harmful materials.

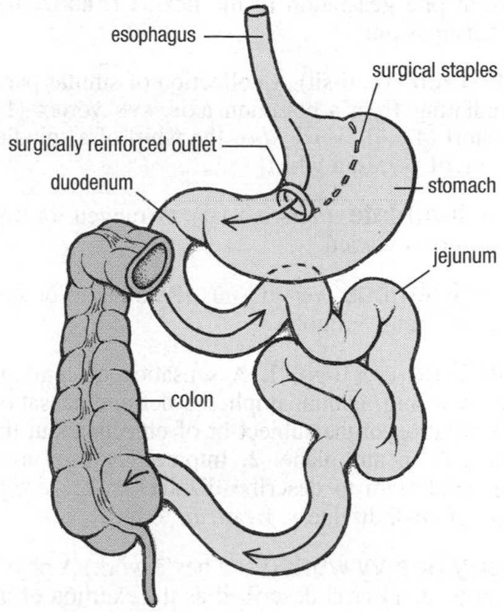

vertical banded gastroplasty: in this procedure, staples and a band are used to reduce gastric capacity, which leads to early satiety and encourages consumption of smaller amounts of food

ver•ti•cal mus•cle of tongue (vĕr′ti-kăl mŭs′ĕl tŭng) An intrinsic muscle of the tongue, consisting of fibers that pass from the aponeurosis of the dorsum to the aponeurosis of the inferior surface; *action,* decreases the superior to inferior dimension of (i.e., flattens) the tongue; *nerve supply,* hypoglossal for motor, lingual for sensory. SYN musculus verticalis linguae [TA].

ver•ti•cal nys•tag•mus (vĕr′ti-kăl nis-tag′mŭs) An up-and-down oscillation of the eyes.

ver•ti•cal o•ver•lap (vĕr′ti-kăl ō′vĕr-lap) **1.** The extension of the upper teeth over the lower teeth in a vertical direction when the opposing posterior teeth are in contact in centric occlusion. **2.** The distance that teeth lap over their antagonists vertically. **3.** The relationship of the maxillary incisors to the mandibular incisors when the incisal edges pass each other in centric occlusion. SYN overbite.

ver•ti•cal stra•bis•mus (vĕr′ti-kăl stră-biz′mŭs) A form of strabismus in which the visual axis of one eye deviates upward (strabismus sursum vergens) or downward (strabismus deorsum vergens).

ver•ti•cal trans•mis•sion (vĕr′ti-kăl trans-mish′ŭn) **1.** Passing a virus (e.g., RNA tumor virus) by means of the genetic apparatus of a cell in which the viral genome is integrated. **2.** For infectious agents in general, transmission of an agent from an individual to its offspring. i.e., from one generation to the next. Cf. horizontal transmission.

ver·ti·cil (vĕr′ti-sil) A collection of similar parts radiating from a common axis. SYN vortex (1), whorl (4). [L. *verticillus,* the whirl of a spindle, dim. of *vertex,* a whirl]

ver·ti·cil·late (vĕr-tis′i-lāt) Arranged in the form of a verticil.

ver·tig·i·nous (vĕr-tij′i-nŭs) Relating to or suffering from vertigo.

ver·ti·go (vĕr′ti-gō) **1.** A sensation of spinning or whirling motion; implies a definite sensation of rotation of the subject or of objects about the subject in any plane. **2.** Imprecisely used as a general term to describe dizziness. [L. *vertigo* (*vertigin-*), dizziness, fr. *verto,* to turn]

ver·y hea·vy work (ver′ē hev′ē wŏrk) A physical demand level described as the exertion of up to 100+ pounds of force occasionally, or up to 50+ pounds of force frequently, or 20+ pounds of force constantly to move objects.

ver·y low birth weight (VLBW) (ver′ē lō bĭrth wāt) Infant weighing less than 1500 g at birth. Can be due to a range of factors including interference with intrauterine growth or premature birth.

ver·y-low-cal·or·ie di·ets (VLCD) (ver′ē lō kal′ŏr-ē dī′ĕts) Therapeutic diets used for weight loss in cases of morbid obesity, in which daily energy intake is less than 800 kcal.

ver·y low so·di·um (ver′ē lō sō′dē-ŭm) A product so labeled contains, by F.D.A. order, no more than 35 mg of sodium per serving.

ve·si·ca, gen. and pl. **ve·si·cae** (ves′i-kă, -kē) **1.** [TA] SYN bladder. **2.** Any hollow structure or sac, normal or pathologic, containing a serous fluid. [L.]

ve·si·ca bil·i·ar·is (ves′i-kă bil′ē-ā′ris) [TA] SYN gallbladder.

ves·i·cal (ves′i-kăl) Relating to any bladder, but usually the urinary bladder.

ves·i·cal cal·cu·lus (ves′i-kăl kal′kyū-lŭs) A urinary calculus formed or retained in the bladder.

ves·i·cal di·ver·tic·u·lum (ves′i-kăl dī′vĕr-tik′yū-lŭm) A diverticulum of the bladder wall; may be either true or false type.

ves·i·cal he·ma·tu·ri·a (ves′i-kăl hē′mă-tyūr′ē-ă) Bleeding in the urinary bladder.

ves·i·cal tri·an·gle (ves′i-kăl trī′ang-gĕl) SYN trigone of bladder.

ves·i·cal veins (ves′i-kăl vānz) These drain the vesical venous plexus and join the internal iliac veins.

ves·i·cant (ves′i-kănt) An agent that produces a vesicle.

ve·si·ca pros·tat·i·ca (ves′i-kă pros-tat′ik-ă) SYN prostatic utricle.

ves·i·ca·ting a·gent (ves′i-kāt-ing ā′jĕnt) A toxic chemical-warfare agent that causes vesicles and bullae. Vesicating agents include sulfur mustards, the nitrogen mustards, and Lewisite (L). Phosgene oxime (CX), although technically an urticating agent rather than a vesicant, is sometimes grouped with vesicating agents.

ves·i·ca·tion (ves′i-kā′shŭn) SYN vesiculation (1).

ve·si·ca u·ri·na·ri·a (ves′i-kă yū-ri-nār′ē-ă) [TA] SYN urinary bladder.

ves·i·cle (ves′i-kĕl) [TA] **1.** SYN vesicula. **2.** A small, circumscribed elevation of the skin containing fluid. SEE ALSO bleb, blister, bulla. **3.** A small sac containing liquid or gas. See page B10. [L. *vesicula,* a blister, dim. of *vesica,* bladder]

ves·i·cle her·ni·a (ves′i-kĕl hĕr′nē-ă) Protrusion of a segment of the bladder through the abdominal wall or into the inguinal canal and into the scrotum.

ves·i·co-, vesic- Combining forms denoting a vesica, vesicle. SEE ALSO vesiculo-. [L. *vesica,* bladder]

ves·i·co·cele (ves′i-kō-sēl) SYN cystocele.

ves·i·coc·ly·sis (ves′i-kok′li-sis) Washing out, or lavage, of the urinary bladder. [vesico- + G. *klysis,* a washing out]

ves·i·co·pus·tu·lar (ves′i-kō-pŭs′chū-lăr) Pertaining to a vesicopustule. SYN vesiculopustular (1).

ves·i·co·rec·tos·to·my (ves′i-kō-rek-tos′tŏ-mē) Surgical urinary tract diversion by anastomosis of the posterior bladder wall to the rectum. SYN cystorectostomy. [vesico- + rectum + G. *stoma,* mouth]

ves·i·co·sig·moid·os·to·my (ves′i-kō-sig′moyd-os′tŏ-mē) Operative formation of a communication between the bladder and the sigmoid colon. [vesico- + sigmoid + G. *stoma,* mouth]

ves·i·co·spi·nal (ves′i-kō-spī′năl) Relating to the urinary bladder and the spinal cord; denoting the neural mechanisms that control retention and evacuation of urine by the bladder; located in the second lumbar and second sacral segment, respectively, of the spinal cord.

ves·i·cos·to·my (ves′i-kos′tŏ-mē) SYN cystostomy. [vesico- + G. *stoma,* mouth]

ves·i·cot·o·my (ves′i-kot′ŏ-mē) SYN cystotomy.

ve·sic·o·ur·e·ter·al re·flux (ves′i-kō-yŭr-ē′

tĕr-ăl rē′flŭks) Backward flow of urine from bladder into ureter.

ve•sic•o•ur•e•ter•al valve (ves′i-kō-yŭr-ē′tĕr-ăl valv) A lock mechanism in the wall of the intravesical portion of the ureter that normally prevents urinary reflux.

ve•sic•o•u•ter•ine fis•tu•la (ves′i-kō-yū′tĕr-in fis′chū-lă) A fistula between the bladder and the uterus.

ve•sic•u•la, gen. and pl. **ve•sic•u•lae** (vĕ-sik′yū-lă, -lē) A small bladder or bladderlike structure. SYN vesicle (1) [TA]. [L. blister, vesicle, dim. of *vesica,* bladder]

ve•sic•u•lar (vĕ-sik′yū-lăr) **1.** Relating to a vesicle. **2.** Characterized by or containing vesicles. SYN vesiculate (2), vesiculous.

ve•sic•u•lar ap•pen•dage of ep•o•oph•o•ron (vĕ-sik′yū-lăr ă-pend′ăj ep′ō-of′ŏr-on) A small, fluid-filled cyst attached by a slender stalk to the fimbriated end of the uterine tube; a vestigial remnant of the embryonic mesonephric duct. SYN morgagnian cyst.

ve•sic•u•lar mur•mur (vĕ-sik′yū-lăr mŭr′mŭr) SYN vesicular respiration.

ve•sic•u•lar o•var•i•an fol•li•cle (vĕ-sik′yū-lăr ō-var′ē-ăn fol′i-kĕl) A follicle in which the oocyte attains its full size and is surrounded by an extracellular glycoprotein layer (zona pellucida) that separates it from a peripheral layer of follicular cells permeated by one or more fluid-filled antra; the theca of the follicle develops into internal and external layers. SYN antral follicle, graafian follicle, secondary follicle.

ve•sic•u•lar res•o•nance (vĕ-sik′yū-lăr rez′ŏ-năns) The sound obtained by percussion over the normal lung.

ve•sic•u•lar res•pi•ra•tion (vĕ-sik′yū-lăr res′pir-ā′shŭn) The respiratory murmur heard on auscultation over the normal lung. SYN vesicular murmur.

ve•sic•u•lar trans•port (vĕ-sik′yū-lăr trans′pōrt) SYN transcytosis.

ve•sic•u•late (vĕ-sik′yū-lāt) **1.** To become vesicular. **2.** SYN vesicular (2).

ve•sic•u•la•tion (vĕ-sik′yū-lā′shŭn) **1.** The formation of vesicles. SYN blistering, vesication. **2.** SYN inflation. **3.** Presence of a number of vesicles.

ve•sic•u•lec•to•my (vĕ-sik′yū-lek′tŏ-mē) Resection of a portion or all of each of the seminal vesicles. [L. *vesicula,* vesicle, + G. *ektomē,* excision]

ve•sic•u•li•form (vĕ-sik′yū-li-fōrm) Resembling a vesicle.

ve•sic•u•li•tis (vĕ-sik′yū-lī′tis) Inflammation of any vesicle, especially of a seminal vesicle. [L. *vesicula,* vesicle, + G. *-itis,* inflammation]

vesiculo- Combining form indicating a vesicle. [L. *vesicula,* vesicle, dim. of *vesica,* bladder]

ve•sic•u•lo•cav•er•nous (vĕ-sik′yū-lō-kav′ĕr-nŭs) Both vesicular and cavernous denoting: **1.** An auscultatory sound having both a vesicular and a cavernous, quality. **2.** The structure of certain neoplasms.

ve•sic•u•log•ra•phy (vĕ-sik′yū-log′ră-fē) Radiographic contrast study of the seminal vesicles. [vesiculo- + G. *graphō,* to write]

ve•sic•u•lo•pap•u•lar (vĕ-sik′yū-lō-pap′yū-lăr) Pertaining to or consisting of a combination of vesicles and papules, or of papules becoming increasingly edematous with sufficient collection of fluid to form vesicles.

ve•sic•u•lo•pros•ta•ti•tis (vĕ-sik′yū-lō-pros′tă-tī′tis) Inflammation of the bladder and prostate. [vesiculo- + prostate + G. *-itis,* inflammation]

ve•sic•u•lo•pus•tu•lar (vĕ-sik′yū-lō-pŭs′chū-lăr) **1.** SYN vesicopustular. **2.** Pertaining to a mixed eruption of vesicles and pustules.

ve•sic•u•lot•o•my (vĕ-sik′yū-lot′ŏ-mē) Surgical incision of the seminal vesicles. [vesiculo- + G. *tomē,* incision]

ve•sic•u•lo•tu•bu•lar (vĕ-sik′yū-lō-tū′byū-lăr) Denoting an auscultatory sound with both vesicular and tubular qualities. Cf. vesiculotympanic.

ve•sic•u•lo•tym•pan•ic (vĕ-sik′yū-lō-tim-pan′ik) Denoting a percussion sound with both vesicular and tympanic qualities. Cf. vesiculotubular.

ve•sic•u•lo•tym•pa•nit•ic res•o•nance (vĕ-sik′yū-lō-tim′pă-nit′ik rez′ŏ-năns) A peculiar, partly tympanitic, partly vesicular sound, obtained on percussion in cases of pulmonary emphysema.

ve•sic•u•lous (vĕ-sik′yū-lŭs) SYN vesicular (2).

ves•sel (ves′ĕl) A structure conveying or containing a fluid, especially a liquid. SEE ALSO vas. [O. Fr. fr. L. *vascellum,* dim. of *vas*]

ves•tib•u•la (ves-tib′yū-lă) Plural of vestibulum.

ves•tib•u•lar (ves-tib′yū-lăr) **1.** Relating to a vestibule, especially the vestibule of the ear. **2.** Interpreting stimuli from the inner ear receptors regarding head position and movement.

ves•tib•u•lar ca•nal (ves-tib′yū-lăr kă-nal′) SYN scala vestibuli.

ves•tib•u•lar crest, **crest of ves•ti•bule** (ves-tib′yū-lăr krest, ves′ti-byūl) An oblique ridge on the inner wall of the vestibule of the labyrinth, bounding the spheric recess above and posteriorly.

ves•tib•u•lar fold (ves-tib′yū-lăr fōld) One of

the pair of folds of mucous membrane stretching across the laryngeal cavity from the angle of the thyroid cartilage to the arytenoid cartilage; they enclose a space called the rima vestibuli or false glottis. SYN plica vestibularis [TA], false vocal cord, ventricular band of larynx, ventricular fold.

ves•tib•u•lar gan•gli•on (ves-tib′yū-lăr gang′glē-ŏn) A collection of bipolar nerve cell bodies forming a swelling on the vestibular part of the vestibulocochlear nerve in the internal acoustic meatus; consists of a superior part and an inferior part connected by a narrow isthmus.

ves•tib•u•lar hy•per•a•cu•sis (ves-tib′yū-lăr hī′pĕr-ă-kyū′sis) Abnormal sensitivity to noise in which the discomfort experienced is vestibular (e.g., vertigo, imbalance, nausea). The mechanism is thought to involve altered specificity of certain vestibular endorgans whereby they are abnormally receptive to pressure change and sound.

ves•tib•u•lar mech•a•no•re•cep•tors (ves-tib′yū-lăr mek′ă-nō-rē-sep′tŏrz) The semicircular canals and the otolith organs (utricle and saccule), which are organic transducers that respond to specific physical factors (e.g., angular acceleration or linear acceleration).

ves•tib•u•lar mem•brane (ves-tib′yū-lăr mem′brān) That which separates the cochlear duct from the vestibular canal; it consists of squamous epithelial cells with microvilli toward the ductus, a basement membrane, and a thin layer of connective tissue toward the scala. SYN Reissner membrane.

ves•tib•u•lar nerve (ves-tib′yū-lăr nĕrv) The part of the vestibulocochlear nerve peripheral to the vestibular root; it is composed of the central processes of bipolar neurons that have the terminals of their peripheral processes on the hair cells in the ampullae of the semicircular ducts and the maculae of the saccule and utricle and in the cell bodies of the vestibular ganglion.

ves•tib•u•lar nerve sec•tion (ves-tib′yū-lăr nĕrv sek′shŭn) Surgical transection of the vestibular branch of the vestibulocochlear nerve (CN VIII) designed to eliminate all vestibular input from that side permanently.

ves•tib•u•lar neu•rec•to•my (ves-tib′yū-lăr nūr-ek′tŏ-mē) Transection of the vestibular division of the vestibulocochlear nerve.

ves•tib•u•lar neu•ron•i•tis (ves-tib′yū-lăr nūr′ō-nī′tis) A paroxysmal attack of severe vertigo, not accompanied by deafness or tinnitus, that affects young to middle-aged adults, often following a nonspecific upper respiratory infection; due to unilateral vestibular dysfunction. SYN Gerlier disease.

ves•tib•u•lar nu•cle•i (ves-tib′yū-lăr nū′klē-ī) A group of four main nuclei that are located in the lateral region of the hindbrain beneath the floor of the rhomboid fossa. These nuclei are the inferior vestibular nucleus, medial vestibular nucleus (Schwalbe nucleus), lateral vestibular nucleus (Deiter nucleus), and superior vestibular nucleus (Bechterew nucleus). The inferior nucleus contains a group of large cells, the magnocellular part of inferior vestibular nucleus or cell group F (pars magnocellularis nuclei vestibularis inferioris [TA]), located caudally in the nucleus. A group of medium-sized neurons is located in lateral portions of the lateral nucleus, the parvocellular part or cell group I (pars parvocellularis [TA]). These nuclei receive primary fibers of the vestibular nerve, are reciprocally connected with the flocculonodular lobe of the cerebellum, and project by way of the medial longitudinal fasciculus to the abducens, trochlear, and oculomotor nuclei and to the ventral horn of the spinal cord. The lateral vestibular nucleus projects to the ipsilateral ventral horn of the spinal cord by the vestibulospinal tract.

ves•tib•u•lar nys•tag•mus (ves-tib′yū-lăr nis-tag′mŭs) Condition resulting from physiologic stimuli to the labyrinth that may be rotatory, caloric, compressive, or galvanic, or due to labyrinthal lesions. SYN labyrinthine nystagmus.

ves•tib•u•lar oc•u•lar re•flex (ves-tib′yū-lăr ok′yū-lăr rē′fleks) SYN vestibuloocular reflex.

ves•tib•u•lar or•gan (ves-tib′yū-lăr ōr′găn) Collective term for the utricle, saccule, and semicircular ducts of the membranous labyrinth; each has a patch of ciliated receptor epithelium innervated by the vestibular nerve.

ves•tib•u•lar pho•na•tion (ves-tib′yū-lăr fō-nā′shŭn) SYN ventricular phonation.

ves•tib•u•lar schwan•no•ma (ves-tib′yū-lăr shwah-nō′mă) A benign but life-threatening tumor arising from Schwann cells, usually of the vestibular division of the vestibulocochlear nerve; produces hearing loss; tinnitus; vestibular disturbances; early and cerebellar, brainstem, and other cranial nerve signs; and increased intracranial pressure in late stages.

ves•tib•u•lar veins (ves-tib′yū-lăr vānz) Drain the saccule and utricle; they are tributaries of both the labyrinthine veins and the vein of the vestibular aqueduct.

ves•ti•bule (ves′ti-byūl) **1.** A small cavity or a space at the entrance of a canal. **2.** Specifically, the central, somewhat ovoid, cavity of the osseous labyrinth communicating with the semicircular canals posteriorly and the cochlea anteriorly. SYN vestibulum. [L. *vestibulum*]

ves•ti•bule of nose (ves′ti-byūl nōz) The anterior part of the nasal cavity, especially that portion enclosed by cartilage.

ves•ti•bule of va•gi•na (ves′ti-byūl vă-jī′nă) The space behind the glans clitoridis and between the labia minora, containing the openings of the vagina, urethra, and ducts of the greater vestibular glands.

♻ **vestibulo-** Combining form indicating vestibule, vestibulum. [L. *vestibulum*]

ves·tib·u·lo·co·chle·ar (ves-tib′yū-lō-kok′lē-ăr) **1.** Relating to the vestibulum and cochlea of the ear. **2.** SYN statoacoustic.

ves·tib·u·lo·coch·le·ar nerve [CN VIII] (ves-tib′yū-lō-kok′lē-ăr nĕrv) A composite sensory nerve innervating the receptor cells of the membranous labyrinth; it consists of two major anatomically and functionally distinct components, each of which has different central connections: the vestibular nerve and the cochlear nerve. SYN nervus vestibulocochlearis [CN VIII] [TA], acoustic nerve, eighth cranial nerve [CN VIII].

ves·tib·u·lo·coch·le·ar nu·cle·i (ves-tib′yū-lō-kok′lē-ăr nū′klē-ī) The combined cochlear and vestibular nuclei in the brainstem that receive the incoming fibers of the vestibulocochlear nerve.

ves·tib·u·lo·oc·u·lar re·flex (VOR) (ves-tib′yū-lō-ok′yū-lăr rē′fleks) Reflexive adjustment of eye position that ensures a steady image when the head or body is moving. SYN vestibular ocular reflex.

ves·tib·u·lop·a·thy (ves-tib′yū-lōp′ă-thē) Any abnormality of the vestibular apparatus (e.g., Ménière disease).

ves·tib·u·lo·plas·ty (ves-tib′yū-lō-plas-tē) Any of a series of surgical procedures designed to restore alveolar ridge height by lowering muscles attaching to the buccal, labial, and lingual aspects of the jaws. [vestibulo- + G. *plassō,* to form]

ves·tib·u·lo·spi·nal re·flex (ves-tib′yū-lō-spī′năl rē′fleks) The influence of vestibular stimulation on body posture.

ves·tib·u·lot·o·my (ves-tib′yū-lot′ŏ-mē) Operation for an opening into the vestibule of the labyrinth. [vestibulo- + G. *tomē,* incision]

ves·tib·u·lum, pl. **ves·tib·u·la** (ves-tib′yū-lŭm, -lă) SYN vestibule. [L. antechamber, entrance court]

ves·tige (ves′tij) A trace or a rudimentary structure; the degenerated remains of any structure that occurs as an entity in the embryo or fetus. [L. *vestigium*]

ves·tig·i·al (ves-tij′ē-ăl) Relating to a vestige.

ves·tig·i·al or·gan (ves-tij′ē-ăl ōr′găn) A rudimentary structure in humans corresponding to a functional structure or organ in lower animals.

vet·e·rin·ar·i·an (vet′ĕr-in-ar′ē-ăn) A person who holds an academic degree in veterinary medicine; a licensed practitioner of veterinary medicine. SEE ALSO veterinary.

vet·e·rin·ar·y (vet′ĕr-in-ar-ē) Relating to the diseases of animals. [L. *veterinarius,* fr. *veterina,* beast of burden]

vet·e·rin·ar·y med·i·cine (vet′ĕr-in-ar-ē med′i-sin) The field concerned with the diseases and health of all animal species other than humans.

vet·e·rin·ar·y tech·ni·cian spec·ial·ist (VTS) (vet′ĕr-in-ar-ē tek-nish′ŭn spesh′ă-list) A veterinary technician who has advanced academic training and credentials in a specialty of veterinary technology. Denoted by the initials VTS followed by the specialty in parentheses, such as: emergency and critical care.

VHDL Abbreviation for very high density lipoprotein. SEE lipoprotein.

vi·a·bil·i·ty (vī′ă-bil′i-tē) Capability of living; the state of being viable; usually connotes a fetus that has reached 500 g in weight and 20 gestational weeks (i.e., 18 weeks after fertilization). [Fr. *viabilité* fr. L. *vita,* life]

vi·a·ble (vī′ă-bĕl) Capable of living; denoting a fetus sufficiently developed to live outside the uterus. [Fr. fr. *vie,* life, fr. L. *vita*]

vi·bra·ting line (vī′brāt-ing līn) The imaginary line across the posterior part of the palate, marking the division between the movable and immovable tissues.

vi·bra·tion (vī-brā′shŭn) A group of movements in massage that involve fine or coarse rhythmic shaking of various structures, with or without compression or traction.

vi·bra·to·ry mas·sage (vī′bră-tōr-ē mă-sahzh′) Rapid topping of a surface using a soft-tipped device. SYN seismotherapy, sismotherapy, vibrotherapeutics.

Vib·ri·o (vib′rē-ō) A genus of motile (in some instances nonmotile), non-spore-forming, aerobic to facultatively anaerobic, gram-negative bacteria containing short curved or straight rods that occur singly or are occasionally united into S shapes or spirals. Some of these organisms are saprophytes in water and soil; others are parasites or pathogens. The type species is *V. cholerae*. [L. *vibro,* to vibrate]

vib·ri·o (vib′rē-ō) A member of the genus *Vibrio*.

Vib·ri·o al·gi·no·lyt·i·cus (vib′rē-ō al-ji-nō-lit′i-kŭs) A bacterial species associated with wound and ear infections, and with bacteremia in immunocompromised and burn patients.

Vib·ri·o cho·ler·ae (vib′rē-ō kol′ĕ-rē) A bacterial species that produces a soluble exotoxin and is the cause of cholera in humans; it is the type species of the genus *Vibrio*. SYN comma bacillus.

Vib·ri·o fe·tus (vib′rē-ō fē′tŭs) Former name for *Campylobacter fetus.*

Vib·ri·o flu·vi·al·is (vib′rē-ō flū-vī-ā′lis) A bacterial species similar to strains of *Aeromonas*, associated with diarrheal disease in humans.

Vib·ri·o fur·nis·si·i (vib′rē-ō fŭr-nis′ē-ī) An

aerogenic strain of bacteria, similar to *V. fluvialis*, associated with diarrheal disease and outbreaks of gastroenteritis.

Vib•ri•o mi•mi•cus (vib′rē-ō mim′i-kŭs) A bacterial species similar to *V. cholerae*, isolated from human stool in diarrheal disease and from human ear infections.

Vib•ri•o pa•ra•hae•mo•ly•ti•cus (vib′rē-ō par-ă-hē-mō-lit′i-kŭs) A marine bacterial species that causes gastroenteritis and bloody diarrhea, usually from eating contaminated shellfish.

vib•ri•o•sis, pl. **vib•ri•o•ses** (vib′rē-ō′sis, -sēz) Infection caused by bacteria of the genus *Vibrio*.

vi•bri•o•stat•ic (vib′rē-ō-stat′ik) Pertains to the ability of the compound O/129 to inhibit the growth of *Vibrio* species; vibriostatic agent O/129 helps distinguish *Vibrio* species that are susceptible to the agent from closely related species that are resistant.

Vib•ri•o vul•nif•i•cus (vib′rē-ō vŭl-nif′i-kŭs) A bacterial species capable of causing cutaneous lesions in an immunocompromised patient; usually contracted from contaminated oysters; also a cause of wound infections.

vi•bris•sa, gen. and pl. **vi•bris•sae** (vī-bris′ă, -ē) One of the hairs growing at the nares, or vestibule of the nose. [L. found only in pl. *vibrissae,* fr. *vibro,* to quiver]

vi•bro•car•di•o•gram (vī′brō-kahr′dē-ō-gram) A graphic record of chest vibrations produced by hemodynamic events of the cardiac cycle; the record provides an indirect, externally recorded measurement of isovolumic contraction and ejection times. [L. *vibro,* to shake, + G. *kardia,* heart, + *gramma,* a drawing]

vi•bro•ther•a•peu•tics (vī′brō-thār′ă-pū-tiks) SYN vibratory massage.

vi•car•i•ous (vī-kar′ē-ŭs) Acting as a substitute; assumption of function or character of another person or thing. [L. *vicarius,* from *vicis,* supplying place of]

vi•car•i•ous hy•per•tro•phy (vī-kar′ē-ŭs hī-pĕr′trō-fē) Enlargement of an organ following failure of another organ because of a functional relationship between them, e.g., enlargement of the pituitary gland, after destruction of the thyroid.

vi•car•i•ous men•stru•a•tion (vī-kar′ē-ŭs men′strū-ā′shŭn) Bleeding from any surface other than the mucous membrane of the uterine cavity, occurring periodically at the time when the normal menstruation should take place.

vi•cious cir•cle (vish′ŭs sĭr′kĕl) **1.** The mutually accelerating action of two independent diseases or phenomena, or of a primary and secondary affection. **2.** The passage of food, after a gastroenterostomy, from the artificial opening through the intestinal loop by antiperistaltic action and back into the stomach again by the pyloric orifice, or the reverse.

vi•cious un•ion (vish′ŭs yūn′yŭn) Attachment of the ends of a broken bone resulting in a deformity or a crooked limb; frequently used interchangeably with faulty union.

vid•e•o•end•o•scope (vid′ē-ō-end′ŏ-skōp) An endoscope fitted with a video camera.

vid•e•o•en•dos•co•py (vid′ē-ō-en-dos′kŏ-pē) Endoscopy performed with an endoscope fitted with a video camera.

Vi•er•ra sign (vē-er′ă sīn) Yellowing and canalization of the nail in the disorder fogo selvagem.

Vieth-Mül•ler cir•cle (vēth-mil′er sĭr′kĕl) A geometric circle passing through the optic centers of two eyes by which points adjacent to the point of fixation, both lying on the circle, theoretically fall on corresponding retinal points.

view (vyū) RADIOGRAPHY a standard diagnostic x-ray study, named according to the image as it appears on film or other receptor.

vig•i•lam•bu•lism (vij-i-lam′byū-lizm) A condition of unconsciousness regarding one's surroundings, with automatism, resembling somnambulism but occurring in the waking state. [L. *vigil,* awake, alert, + *ambulo,* to walk about]

vil•li (vil′ī) Plural of villus.

vil•lo•ma (vil-ō′mă) SYN papilloma.

vil•lose (vil′ōs) SYN villous (2).

vil•lo•si•tis (vil′ō-sī′tis) Inflammation of the villous surface of the placenta. [villous + G. *-itis* inflammation]

vil•los•i•ty (vi-los′i-tē) Shagginess; an aggregation of villi.

vil•lous (vil′ŭs) **1.** Relating to villi. **2.** Shaggy; covered with villi. SYN villose.

vil•lous ad•e•no•ma (vil′ŭs ad′ĕ-nō′mă) A solitary sessile, often large, tumor of colonic mucosa composed of mucinous epithelium covering delicate vascular projections; malignant change occurs frequently. SYN papillary adenoma of large intestine.

vil•lous car•ci•no•ma (vil′ŭs kahr′si-nō′mă) A form of carcinoma in which there are numerous closely packed papillary projections of neoplastic epithelial tissue.

vil•lous chor•i•on (vil′us kōr′ē-on) That part of chorion where the chorionic villi have persisted to form the fetal part of the placenta. SYN bushy chorion, chorion frondosum.

vil•lous ten•o•syn•o•vi•tis (vil′ŭs ten′ō-sin′ō-vī′tis) A condition resembling pigmented villonodular synovitis but arising in periarticular soft tissue rather than in joint synovia; occurs most commonly in the hands. SYN pigmented villonodular tenosynovitis.

vil•lus, pl. **vil•li** (vil′ŭs, -ī) **1.** A projection from the surface, especially of a mucous membrane. If the projection is minute, as from a cell surface, it is termed a microvillus. **2.** An elongated dermal papilla projecting into an intraepidermal vesicle or cleft. SEE ALSO festooning. [L. shaggy hair (of beasts)]

vil•lus•ec•to•my (vil′ŭs-ek′tŏ-mē) SYN synovectomy. [villus + G. *ektomē,* excision]

vi•men•tin (vī-men′tin) The major polypeptide that copolymerizes with other subunits to form the intermediate filament cytoskeleton of mesenchymal cells; may have a role in maintaining the internal organization of certain cells.

Vin•cent an•gi•na (van[h]-sawn[h]′ an′ji-nă) An ulcerative infection of the oral soft tissues, including the tonsils and pharynx, caused by fusiform and spirochetal organisms; it is usually associated with necrotizing ulcerative gingivitis and may progress to noma. Death from suffocation or sepsis may occur. SEE ALSO noma.

Vin•cent ba•cil•lus (van[h]-sawn[h]′ bă-sil′ŭs) SYN *Fusobacterium nucleatum.*

Vin•cent dis•ease (van[h]-sawn[h]′ di-zēz′) SYN necrotizing ulcerative gingivitis.

Vin•cent in•fec•tion (van[h]-sawn[h]′ in-fek′shŭn) SYN necrotizing ulcerative gingivitis.

Vin•cent spi•ril•lum (van[h]-sawn[h]′ spī-ril′ŭm) The spirillum or spirochete found in association with Vincent bacillus. *Fusobacterium nucleatum* is frequently the only bacillus isolated.

Vin•cent ton•sil•li•tis (van[h]-sawn[h]′ ton′si-lī′tis) Angina limited chiefly to the tonsils, caused by Vincent organisms (bacillus and spirillum).

vin•cu•la of ten•dons (ving′kyū-lă ten′dŏnz) Fibrous bands that extend from the flexor tendons of the fingers and toes to the capsules of the interphalangeal joints and to the phalanges; they convey small vessels to the tendons.

vin•cu•lum, pl. **vin•cu•la** (ving′kyū-lŭm, -lă) [TA] A frenum, frenulum, or ligament. [L. a fetter, fr. *vincio,* to bind]

vin•e•gar (vin′ĕ-găr) Impure dilute acetic acid, made from fermented wine, cider, or malt. [Fr. *vinaigre,* fr. *vin,* wine, + *aigre,* sour]

vin•e•gar eel (vin′ĕ-găr ēl) SYN *Turbatrix aceti.*

vi•nyl (vī′nil) Hydrocarbon radical CH_2=CH–. SYN ethenyl.

vi•o•let (vī′ŏ-lĕt) The color evoked by wavelengths of the visible spectrum shorter than 450 nm. [L. *viola*]

VIP Abbreviation for vasoactive intestinal polypeptide. Cf. bioregulator.

VIP•o•ma (vi-pō′mă) An endocrine tumor, usually originating in the pancreas, that produces a vasoactive intestinal polypeptide believed to cause profound cardiovascular and electrolyte changes with vasodilatory hypotension, watery diarrhea, hypokalemia, and dehydration. [*v*asoactive *i*ntestinal *p*olypeptide + G. *-ōma,* tumor]

Vi•pond sign (vē-pōn[h]′ sīn) A generalized adenopathy occurring during the period of incubation of various of the exanthemas of childhood, affording an early diagnostic sign in a case of known exposure.

viraemia [Br.] SYN viremia.

vi•ral (vī′răl) Of, pertaining to, or caused by a virus.

vi•ral dys•en•ter•y (vī′răl dis′ĕn-ter′ē) Profuse watery diarrhea due to, or thought to be due to, infection by a virus.

vi•ral en•ve•lope (vī′răl en′vĕ-lōp) The outer structure that encloses the nucleocapsids of some viruses; may contain host material.

vi•ral he•mag•glu•ti•na•tion (vī′răl hē′mă-glū-ti-nā′shŭn) The nonimmune agglutination of suspended red blood cells by certain of a wide range of otherwise unrelated viruses, usually by the virion itself but in some instances by products of viral growth, the species of erythrocyte agglutinated varying with the different viruses.

vi•ral hep•a•ti•tis (vī′răl hep′ă-tī′tis) **1.** Liver disorder caused or exacerbated by any one of at least seven immunologically unrelated viruses: hepatitis A–E and G, and the TT virus (TTV); the existence of hepatitis F virus remains unconfirmed. **2.** Hepatitis caused by a viral infection, including infection by Epstein-Barr virus, cytomegalovirus, and other herpesviruses.

vi•ral hep•a•ti•tis type A (vī′răl hep′ă-tī′tis tīp) A virus disease with a short incubation period (usually 15–50 days), caused by hepatitis A virus (family Picornaviridae, genus Hepatovirus) and often transmitted by the fecal-oral route; may be inapparent, mild, severe, or occasionally fatal, and occurs sporadically or in epidemics, commonly in school-age children and young adults; necrosis of periportal liver cells with lymphocytic and plasma cell infiltration is characteristic, and jaundice is a common symptom. SYN hepatitis A.

vi•ral hep•a•ti•tis type B (vī′răl hep′ă-tī′tis tīp) A virus disease with a long incubation period (usually 50–160 days), caused by hepatitis B virus (family Hepadnaviridae, genus Orthohepadnavirus); transmitted by blood or blood products, contaminated needles or instruments, or sexual contact; differs from hepatitis A in having a higher mortality rate and in the possibility of progression to a chronic disease, a carrier state, or both. Superinfection with hepatitis D can greatly exacerbate the effect of hepatitis B. SYN hepatitis B.

vi•ral hep•a•ti•tis type C (vī′răl hep′ă-tī′tis) (NANB); principal cause of non-A, non-B posttransfusion hepatitis caused by an RNA virus that is classified with the Flaviviridae family. The incubation period is 6–8 weeks with about 75% of infections subclinical and giving rise to chronic persistent infection. A high percentage of these develop chronic liver disease leading to cirrhosis and possible hepatocellular carcinoma.

vi•ral hep•a•ti•tis type D (vī′răl hep′ă-tī′tis tīp) Acute or chronic hepatitis caused by the hepatitis delta virus, a defective RNA virus requiring HBV for replication. The acute type occurs in two forms: 1) coinfection, the simultaneous occurrence of hepatitis B virus and hepatitis delta virus infections; 2) superinfection, the appearance of hepatitis delta virus infection in a hepatitis B virus carrier. SYN delta hepatitis.

vi•ral hep•a•ti•tis type E (vī′răl hep′ă-tī′tis) Hepatitis caused by a nonenveloped, single-stranded, positive-sense RNA virus 27–34 nm in diameter, unrelated to other hepatitis and belonging to the family Caliciviridae; it is the principal cause of enterically transmitted, waterborne, epidemic NANB hepatitis occurring primarily in Asia, Africa, and South America.

vi•ral ker•a•to•con•junc•ti•vi•tis (vī′răl ker′ă-tō-kŏn-jŭngk′ti-vī′tis) SYN epidemic keratoconjunctivitis.

vi•ral load (vī′răl lōd) The plasma level of viral RNA, as determined by various techniques including target amplification assay by reverse transcriptase polymerase chain reaction and branched DNA technology with signal amplification. Because levels of detection vary with method, results of testing by different methods are not comparable.

vi•ral spong•i•form en•ceph•a•lop•a•thy (vī′răl spŏn′ji-fōrm en-sef′a-lop′ă-thē) Progressive vacuolation in dendritic and axonal processes and in neuronal cell bodies, associated with slow virus infections.

vi•ral tro•pism (vī′răl trō′pizm) The specificity of a virus for a particular host tissue, determined in part by the interaction of viral surface structures with host cell-surface receptors.

Vir•chow node (fēr′kō nōd) SYN signal lymph node.

Vir•chow psam•mo•ma (fēr′kō sam-ō′mă) SYN psammomatous meningioma.

vi•re•mi•a (vī-rē′mē-ă) The presence of a virus in the bloodstream. SYN viraemia. [virus + G. *haima,* blood]

vir•gin (vĭr′jin) **1.** A person who has never had sexual intercourse. **2.** Unused; uncontaminated. SYN virginal (2). [L. *virgo* (*virgin-*), maiden]

vir•gin•al (vĭr′ji-năl) **1.** Relating to or having the characteristics of a virgin. **2.** SYN virgin (2). [L. *virginalis*]

vir•gin•i•ty (vĭr-jin′i-tē) The virgin state. [L. *virginitas*]

♻ **-viridae** Suffix meaning a virus family. [L. *vir,* fr. *virus,* venom]

vir•i•dans strep•to•coc•ci (ver′i-danz strep-tō-kok′sī) A name applied not to a distinct species but rather to the group of α-hemolytic streptococci as a whole; viridans streptococci have been isolated from the mouth and intestines of humans, the intestines of horses, the milk and feces of cows, milk products, and the sputum and lungs. SYN *Streptococcus viridans.*

vir•ile (vir′il) **1.** Relating to the male sex. **2.** Manly, strong, masculine. **3.** Possessing masculine traits. [L. *virilis,* masculine, fr. *vir,* a man]

vir•i•les•cence (vir′i-les′ĕns) Assumption of male characteristics by a female.

vir•il•ism (vir′i-lizm) Possession of mature masculine somatic characteristics by a girl, woman, or prepubescent male; may be present at birth or may appear later; commonly the result of gonadal or adrenocortical dysfunction or of androgenic therapy. [L. *virilis,* masculine]

vi•ril•i•ty (vir-il′i-tē) The condition or quality of being virile. [L. *virilitas,* manhood, fr. *vir,* man]

vir•il•i•za•tion (vir′i-lī-zā′shŭn) Production or acquisition of virilism.

vir•il•iz•ing (vir′i-līz-ing) Causing virilism.

♻ **-virinae** Suffix used in naming a subfamily of viruses.

vi•ri•on (vī′rē-on) The complete virus particle that is structurally intact and infectious.

vi•rol•o•gist (vī-rol′ŏ-jist) A specialist in virology.

vi•rol•o•gy (vī-rol′ŏ-jē) The study of viruses and of viral disease. [virus + G. *logos,* study]

vir•tu•al en•dos•co•py (vĭr′chū-ăl en-dos′kŏ-pē) Computed tomographic data reconstructed in three dimensions to give information similar to that obtained with endoscopy.

vi•ru•ci•dal (vī′rŭ-sī′dăl) Destructive to a virus.

vi•ru•cide (vī′rŭ-sīd) An agent active against virus infections. [virus + L. *caedo,* to kill]

vir•u•lence (vir′yū-lĕns) The disease-evoking power of a pathogen; numerically expressed as the ratio of the number of cases of overt infection to the total number infected, as determined by immunoassay. [L. *virulentia,* fr. *virulentus,* poisonous]

vir•u•lent (vir′yū-lĕnt) Extremely toxic, denoting a markedly pathogenic microorganism. [L. *virulentus,* poisonous]

vir•u•lent bac•ter•i•o•phage (vir′yū-lĕnt bak-tĕr′ē-ō-fāj) A bacteriophage that regularly causes lysis of the bacteria that it infects.

vir•u•lif•er•ous (vir′yū-lif′ĕr-ŭs) Conveying a virus.

vir•u•ri•a (vīr-yūr′ē-ă) Presence of viruses in the urine. [virus + G. *ouron,* urine]

vi•rus, pl. **vi•rus•es** (vī′rŭs, -ĕz) **1.** Specifically, a term for a group of infectious agents that with few exceptions are capable of passing through fine filters that retain most bacteria, are usually not visible through the light microscope, lack independent metabolism, and are incapable of growth or reproduction apart from living cells. They have a prokaryotic genetic apparatus but differ sharply from bacteria in other respects. The complete particle usually contains either DNA or RNA, not both, and is usually covered by a protein shell or capsid that protects the nucleic acid. They range in size from 15 nm up to several hundred. Classification of viruses depends on physiochemical characteristics of virions as well as on mode of transmission, host range, symptomatology, and other factors. SYN ultravirus. **2.** Relating to or caused by a virus, as a virus disease. [L. poison]

♻ **-virus** Suffix indicating a genus of viruses.

vi•rus•oid (vī′rŭs-oyd) A plant pathogen resembling a viroid but having a much larger circular or linear RNA segment and a capsid. [virus + G. *eidos,* resembling]

vi•rus shed•ding (vī′rŭs shed′ing) Excretion of virus by any route from the infected host; route and duration of excretion vary according to the pathogenesis of the infection or disease.

vi•rus-trans•formed cell (vī′rus-trans-fōrmd′ sel) A cell that has been genetically changed to a tumor cell, the change being subsequently transmitted to all descendent cells; cells transformed by oncornaviruses continue to produce virus in high concentration without being killed; DNA tumor virus-transformed cells develop (along with other changes) tumor-associated antigens and rarely produce virus.

vis•cer•a (vis′ĕr-ă) Plural of viscus. SYN vitals.

vis•cer•ad (vis′ĕr-ad) In a direction toward the viscera. [viscera + L. *ad,* to]

vis•cer•al (vis′ĕr-ăl) Relating to the viscera. SYN splanchnic.

visceral anaesthesia [Br.] SYN visceral anesthesia.

vis•cer•al an•es•the•si•a (vis′ĕr-ăl an′es-thē′zē-ă) SYN splanchnic anesthesia. SYN visceral anaesthesia.

vis•cer•al cleft (vis′ĕr-ăl kleft) Any cleft or groove between two pharyngeal arches in the embryo.

vis•cer•al fasc•i•a (vis′ĕr-ăl fash′ē-ă) A thin, fibrous membrane that envelops various organs and glands, binding structures together in some cases and forming partitions between them in other cases. USAGE NOTE *Terminologia Anatomica* [TA] has recommended that the terms "superficial fascia" and "deep fascia" not be used generically in an unqualified way because of variation in their meanings internationally. The recommended terms are "subcutaneous tissue" (tela subcutanea [TA]) for the former superficial fascia and "muscular fascia" or "visceral fascia" (fascia musculorum or fascia visceralis [TA]) in place of deep fascia.

vis•cer•al•gi•a (vis′ĕr-al′jē-ă) Pain in any viscus. [viscero- + G. *algos,* pain]

vis•cer•al lay•er (vis′ĕr-ăl lā′ĕr) The inner layer of an enveloping sac or bursa, which lines the outer surface of the enveloped structure, as opposed to the parietal layer, which lines the walls of the occupied space or cavity. The visceral layer is usually thin, delicate, and not apparent as being separate, but rather appears to be the outer surface of the structure itself. SYN lamina visceralis [TA].

vis•cer•al lay•er of se•rous per•i•car•di•um (vis′ĕr-ăl lā′ĕr sēr′ŭs per′i-kahr′dē-ŭm) The inner part of the serous pericardium applied directly on the heart.

vis•cer•al leish•ma•ni•a•sis (vis′ĕr-ăl lēsh′mă-nī′ă-sis) A chronic tropical disease caused by *Leishmania donovani* and transmitted by the bite of a species of sandfly of the genus *Phlebotomus* or *Lutzomyia* (less commonly *Leishmania* sp; e.g., *Leishmania tropica*); the organisms grow and multiply in macrophages, which eventually causes them to burst and liberate amastigote parasites, which then invade other macrophages; proliferation of macrophages in the bone marrow causes crowding out of erythroid and myeloid elements, which results in leukopenia, as well as anemia, splenomegaly, and hepatomegaly, which are characteristic, along with enlargement of lymph nodes; fever, fatigue, malaise, and secondary infections also occur. SYN kala azar.

vis•cer•al lymph nodes (vis′ĕr-ăl limf nōdz) The lymph nodes draining the viscera of the abdomen or of the pelvis.

vis•cer•al pain (vis′ĕr-ăl pān) Discomfort resulting from injury or disease in an organ in the thoracic or abdominal cavity.

vis•cer•al sense (vis′ĕr-ăl sens) The perception of the existence of the internal organs. SYN splanchnesthesia, splanchnesthetic sensibility.

vis•cer•al swal•low (vis′ĕr-ăl swahl′ō) The immature swallowing pattern of an infant or a person with tongue thrust, resembling peristaltic wavelike muscular contractions observed in the gut; adult or mature swallowing is more volitional and therefore somatic.

♻ **viscero-** Combining form denoting the viscera.

SEE ALSO splanchno-. [L. *viscus,* pl. *viscera,* the internal organs]

vis•cer•o•cra•ni•um (vis′ĕr-ō-krā′nē-ŭm) That part of the cranium derived from the embryonic pharyngeal arches; comprises the facial bones.

vis•cer•o•gen•ic (vis′ĕr-ō-jen′ik) Of visceral origin; denoting a number of sensory and other reflexes. [viscero- + G. *-gen,* producing]

vis•cer•o•in•hib•i•tor•y (vis′ĕr-ō-in-hib′i-tōr-ē) Restricting or arresting the functional activity of the viscera.

vis•cer•o•meg•a•ly (vis′ĕr-ō-meg′ă-lē) Abnormal enlargement of the viscera, such as may be seen in acromegaly and other disorders. SYN organomegaly, splanchnomegaly. [viscero- + G. *megas,* large]

vis•cer•o•mo•tor (vis′ĕr-ō-mō′tŏr) **1.** Relating to or controlling movement in the viscera; denoting the autonomic nerves innervating the viscera, especially the intestines. **2.** Denoting a movement having a relation to the viscera; referring to reflex muscular contractions of the abdominal wall in cases of visceral disease.

vis•cer•o•pleu•ral (vis′ĕr-ō-plūr′ăl) Relating to the pleural and the thoracic viscera. SYN pleurovisceral.

vis•cer•op•to•sis, vis•cer•op•to•si•a (vis′ĕr-op-tō′sis, -tō′sē-ă) Descent of the viscera from their normal positions. SYN splanchnoptosis, splanchnoptosia. [viscero- + G. *ptōsis,* a falling]

vis•cer•o•sen•sor•y (vis′ĕr-ō-sen′sŏr-ē) Relating to the sensory innervation of internal organs.

vis•cer•o•skel•e•tal (vis′ĕr-ō-skel′ĕ-tăl) Relating to the visceroskeleton. SYN splanchnoskeletal.

vis•cer•o•skel•e•ton (vis′ĕr-ō-skel′ĕ-tŏn) **1.** Any bony or cartilaginous formation in an organ, as in the cartilaginous rings of the trachea and bronchi. **2.** The bony framework protecting the viscera, such as the ribs and sternum, the pelvic bones, and the anterior portion of the cranium. SYN splanchnoskeleton.

vis•cer•o•so•mat•ic (vis′ĕr-ō-sō-mat′ik) Relating to the viscera and the body. [viscero- + G. *sōma,* body]

vis•cer•o•troph•ic (vis′ĕr-ō-trō′fik) Relating to any trophic change determined by visceral conditions. [viscero- + G. *trophē,* nourishment]

vis•cer•o•trop•ic (vis′ĕr-ō-trō′pik) Affecting the viscera. [L. *viscera* internal organs, + G. *tropē,* a turning]

vis•cid (vis′id) Sticky; glutinous. [L. *viscidus,* stick, fr. *viscum,* birdlime]

vis•cid•i•ty (vi-sid′i-tē) Stickiness; adhesiveness.

visc•o•can•nu•los•to•my (visk′ō-kan′yū-los′tŏ-mē) A procedure to treat glaucoma in which viscoelastic is used to open the aqueous drainage channels.

vis•cos•i•ty (vis-kos′i-tē) In general, the resistance to flow or alteration of shape by any substance as a result of molecular cohesion; most frequently applied to liquids as the resistance of a fluid to flow because of a shearing force. [L. *viscositas,* fr. *viscosus,* viscous]

vis•cous (vis′kŭs) Sticky; marked by high viscosity.

vis•cus, pl. **vis•cer•a** (vis′kŭs, vis′ĕr-ă) An organ of the digestive, respiratory, urogenital, and endocrine systems as well as the spleen, the heart, and great vessels; hollow and multilayered walled organs studied in splanchnology. [L. the soft parts, internal organs]

vis•i•ble spec•trum (viz′i-bĕl spek′trŭm) That part of electromagnetic radiation that is visible to the human eye; it extends from extreme red, 7606 Å (760.6 nm), to extreme violet, 3934 Å (393.4 nm).

vi•sion (vizh′ŭn) The act of seeing. SEE ALSO sight. See this page. [L. *visio,* fr. *video,* pp. *visus,* to see]

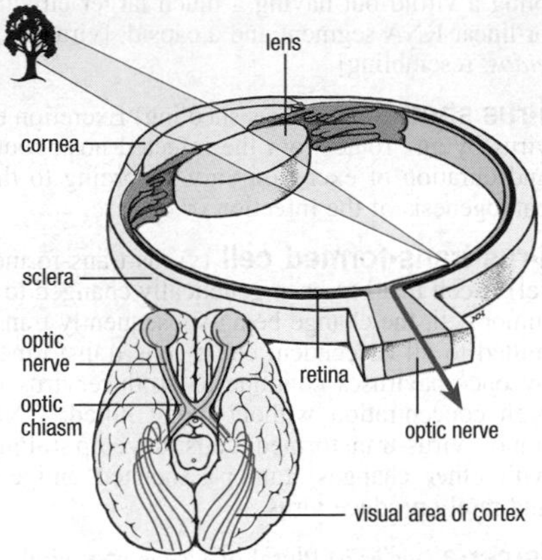

vision: light passes through the cornea and is focused onto the retina by the lens; cells in the retina then transmit this information through the optic nerve to the visual area of the cortex

vis•u•al (vizh′ū-ăl) **1.** Relating to vision. **2.** Denoting a person who learns and remembers more readily through sight than through hearing. [Late L. *visualis,* fr. *visus,* vision]

vis•u•al a•cu•i•ty (vizh′ū-ăl ă-kyū′i-tē) Sharpness or clarity of vision, measured as the ability to distinguish letters or other images of various sizes at a fixed distance, usually with a Snellen chart. Normal rating by such means is 20/20 vision.

vis•u•al ag•no•si•a (vizh′ū-ăl ag-nō′zē-ă) Inability to recognize objects by sight; usually caused by bilateral parietooccipital lesions.

vis•u•al a•lex•i•a (vizh′ū-ăl ă-lek′sē-ă) SEE alexia.

vis•u•al an•a•logue scale (VAS) (vizh′ū-ăl an′ă-lawg skāl) A graphic scale that helps a patient to quantify pain, depression, and other subjective and otherwise unmeasurable states or conditions.

vis•u•al an•gle (vizh′ū-ăl ang′gĕl) The angle formed at the retina by the meeting of lines drawn from the periphery of the object seen.

vis•u•al a•pha•si•a (vizh′ū-ăl ă-fā′zē-ă) **1.** SYN alexia. **2.** USAGE NOTE Sometimes improperly used as a synonym for anomia.

vis•u•al ar•e•a (vizh′ū-ăl ār′ē-ă) SYN visual cortex.

vis•u•al au•ra (vizh′ū-ăl awr′ă) Epileptic aura characterized by visual illusions or hallucinations, formed or unformed, including scintillations, and teichopsia. SEE ALSO aura (1).

vis•u•al ax•is (vizh′ū-ăl ak′sis) The straight line extending from the object seen, through the center of the pupil, to the macula lutea of the retina.

vis•u•al clo•sure (viz′ū-ăl klō′zhŭr) Identification of forms or objects from incomplete presentation.

vis•u•al con•fron•ta•tion (vizh′ū-ăl kon-frŭn-tā′shŭn) SYN confrontation test.

vis•u•al cor•tex (vizh′ū-ăl kōr′teks) The region of the cerebral cortex occupying the entire surface of the occipital lobe, and composed of Brodmann areas 17–19. Area 17 (which is also called the striate cortex or area because the line of Gennari is grossly visible on its surface) is the primary visual cortex, receiving the visual radiation from the lateral geniculate body of the thalamus. The surrounding Brodmann areas 18 (parastriate cortex or area) and 19 (peristriate cortex or area) are probably involved in subsequent steps of visual information processing; area 18 is referred to as the secondary visual cortex. SYN visual area.

vis•u•al dis•crim•i•na•tion (vizh′ū-ăl dis-krim′i-nā′shŭn) A general term for visual skills that require the ability to detect specific features of an object to recognize it, to match or duplicate it, and to categorize it.

vis•u•al e•voked po•ten•tial (vizh′ū-ăl ē-vōkt′ pŏ-ten′shăl) Voltage fluctuations that may be recorded from the occipital area of the scalp as the result of retinal stimulation by a light flashing at quarter-second intervals; commonly summated and averaged by computer.

vis•u•al field (F) (vizh′ū-ăl fēld) The area simultaneously visible to one eye without movement; often measured by means of a bowl perimeter located 330 mm from the eye.

vis•u•al fix•a•tion (vizh′ū-ăl fik-sā′shŭn) An optic skill that allows one to sustain gaze at a stationary object.

vis•u•al in•at•ten•tion (vizh′ū-ăl in′ă-ten′shŭn) Decreased visual screening and regard to visual stimuli. SEE ALSO visual neglect.

vis•u•al in•spec•tion with a•cet•ic ac•id (vizh′ū-ăl in-spek′shŭn ă-sē′tik as′id) SYN acetowhitening.

vis•u•al-kin•et•ic dis•soc•i•a•tion (vizh′ū-ăl ki-net′ik di-sō′sē-ā′shŭn) The neurolinguistic programming process of removing a synesthesia from a person's internal experience. SEE ALSO neurolinguistic programming.

vis•u•al mem•or•y (vizh′ū-ăl mem′ŏr-rē) Retained memory of objects when the visual stimulus is no longer present.

vis•u•al-mo•tor con•trol (vizh′ū-ăl-mō′tŏr kŏn-trōl′) Use of visual information to perform smooth, coordinated, and precise movements. SYN eye-hand coordination, visual motor coordination.

vis•u•al mo•tor co•or•di•na•tion (vizh′ū-ăl mō′tŏr kō-ōr′dĭ-nā′shŭn) SYN visual-motor control.

vis•u•al ne•glect (vizh′ū-ăl nĕ-glekt′) Inattention to visual stimuli occurring in the space on the involved side of the body.

vis•u•al or•i•en•ta•tion (vizh′ū-ăl ōr′ē-ĕn-tā′shŭn) Awareness of the location of objects in the environment and their relationship to one another and to the person viewing them.

vis•u•al pig•ments (vizh′yū-ăl pig′mĕnts) The photopigments in the retinal cones and rods that absorb light and initiate the visual process.

vis•u•al pur•ple (vizh′ū-ăl pŭr′pĕl) SYN rhodopsin.

vis•u•al re•cep•tor cells (vizh′ū-ăl rĕ-sep′tŏr selz) The rod and cone cells of the retina.

vis•u•al ver•ti•go (vizh′ū-ăl vĕr′ti-gō) That finding induced by visual stimuli.

vis•u•al vi•o•let (vizh′ū-ăl vī′ŏ-lĕt) SYN iodopsin.

vis•u•og•no•sis (vizh′ū-og-nō′sis) Recognition and understanding of visual impressions. [L. *visus,* vision, + G. *gnōsis,* knowledge]

vis•u•o•mo•tor (vizh′ū-ō-mō′tŏr) Denoting the ability to synchronize visual information with physical movement, e.g., driving a car.

vis•u•o•sen•sor•y (vizh′ū-ō-sen′sŏr-ē) Pertaining to the perception of visual stimuli.

vis•u•o•spa•tial (viz′ū-ō-spā′shăl) Denoting the

ability to comprehend and conceptualize visual representations and spatial relationships in learning and performing a task.

vit·al (vī′tăl) Relating to life. [L. *vitalis,* fr. *vita,* life]

vit·al ca·pac·i·ty (VC) (vī′tăl kă-pas′i-tē) The greatest volume of air that can be exhaled from the lungs after a maximum inspiration. SYN respiratory capacity.

vit·al in·dex (vī′tăl in′deks) The ratio of births to deaths within a population during a given time.

vi·tal·i·ty (vī-tal′i-tē) Vital force or energy.

vi·tal·i·ty test (vī-tal′i-tē test) A group of thermal and electrical tests used to aid in assessment of dental pulp health. SYN pulp test.

vit·a·lom·e·ter (vī′tă-lom′ĕ-tĕr) An electrical device for determining the vitality of the tooth pulp.

vit·al pulp (vī′tăl pŭlp) A pulp composed of viable tissue, either normal or diseased, that responds to electric stimuli and to heat and cold.

vit·al red (vī′tăl red) [C.I. 23570] Trisodium salt of a sulfonated diazo dye, used as a vital stain.

vit·als (vī′tălz) SYN viscera.

vit·al signs (vī′tăl sīnz) Objective measurements of temperature, pulse, respirations, and blood pressure as a means of assessing general health and cardiorespiratory function.

vit·al stain (vī′tăl stān) A stain applied to cells or parts of cells while they are still alive.

vit·al sta·tis·tics (vī′tăl stă-tis′tiks) Systematically tabulated information concerning births, marriages, divorces, separations, and deaths, based on the numbers of official registrations of these vital events; the branch of statistics concerned with such data.

vi·ta·mer (vī′tă-mĕr) One of two or more similar compounds capable of fulfilling a specific vitamin function in the body, e.g., niacin, niacinamide.

vit·a·min (vīt′ă-min) One of a group of organic substances, present in minute amounts in natural foodstuffs, that are essential to normal metabolism; insufficient amounts in the diet may cause deficiency diseases. [L. *vita,* life, + amine]

vit·a·min A (vīt′ă-min) **1.** Any β-ionone derivative, except provitamin A carotenoids, possessing qualitatively the biologic activity of retinol; deficiency interferes with the production and resynthesis of rhodopsin, thereby causing night blindness, and produces a keratinizing metaplasia of epithelial cells that may result in xerophthalmia, keratosis, susceptibility to infections, and retarded growth. **2.** The original vitamin A, now known as retinol.

vit·a·min A1 ac·id (vīt′ă-min as′id) SYN retinoic acid.

vit·a·min A2 (vī′tă-min) Fat-soluble vitamin occurring chiefly in the livers of freshwater fish and having about 40% of the biologic activity of vitamin A1. SEE ALSO leukoplakia.

vit·a·min B (vīt′ă-min) A group of water-soluble substances originally considered as one vitamin.

vit·a·min B1 (vīt′ă-min) SYN thiamin.

vit·a·min B2 (vī′tă-min) SEE riboflavin.

vit·a·min B6 (vīt′ă-min) Pyridoxine and related compounds (pyridoxal; pyridoxamine).

vit·a·min B12 (vīt′ă-min) Generic descriptor for compounds exhibiting the biologic activity of cyanocobalamin. The physiologically active vitamin B12 coenzymes are methylcobalamin and deoxyadenosinecobalamine. A deficiency of vitamin B12 causes megaloblastic anemia with or without peripheral neuropathy, and is often associated with certain methylmalonic acidurias. SEE ALSO pernicious anemia.

vit·a·min B12 neu·rop·a·thy (vīt′ă-min nūr-op′ă-thē) SYN subacute combined degeneration of the spinal cord.

vit·a·min B com·plex (vīt′ă-min kom′pleks) A pharmaceutical term applied to drug products containing a mixture of the B vitamins, usually B1 (thiamine), B2 (riboflavin), B3 (nicotinamide), and B6 (pyridoxine).

vit·a·min C (vīt′ă-min) SYN ascorbic acid.

vit·a·min D (vīt′ă-min) Generic descriptor for all steroids exhibiting the biologic activity of ergocalciferol or cholecalciferol, the antirachitic vitamins. They promote the proper use of calcium and phosphorus, thereby favoring proper bone and tooth formation and maintenance in children.

vit·a·min D2 (vīt′ă-min) SYN ergocalciferol.

vit·a·min D3 (vīt′ă-min) SYN cholecalciferol.

vit·a·min D–bind·ing pro·tein (vīt′ă-min bīnd′ing prō′tēn) A plasma protein that binds vitamin D.

vit·a·min D milk (vīt′ă-min milk) Cow's milk to which vitamin D has been added, so as to provide 400 USP units of vitamin D per quart.

vit·a·min D–re·sis·tant rick·ets (vīt′ă-min rĕ-zis′tănt rik′ĕts) A group of disorders characterized by hypophosphatemic osteomalacia; heritable renal tubular disorders and abnormalities in vitamin D metabolism occur in some patients.

vit·a·min E (vīt′ă-min) Generic descriptor of tocol and tocotrienol derivatives possessing the biologic activity of α-tocopherol; contained in various oils (wheat germ, cottonseed, palm, rice) and whole grain cereals, where it constitutes the nonsaponifiable fraction, also in animal tissue (liver, pancreas, heart) and leafy vegetables; deficiency produces resorption or abortion in female rats and sterility in males.

vit•a•min K (vīt′ă-min) Generic descriptor for compounds with the biologic activity of phylloquinone; fat-soluble, thermostable compounds found in alfalfa, pork liver, fish meal, and vegetable oils, essential for the formation of normal amounts of prothrombin.

vit•a•min K1, **vit•a•min K1(20)** (vīt′ă-min) SYN phylloquinone.

vit•a•min K2, **vit•a•min K2(30)** (vīt′ă-min) SYN menaquinone-6.

vi•tel•li•form ret•i•nal dys•tro•phy (vī-tel′i-fōrm ret′i-năl dis′trŏ-fē) SYN Best disease.

vi•tel•line (vī-tel′ēn) Relating to the vitellus.

vi•tel•line pole (vī-tel′ēn pōl) Pole of an oocyte or ovum.

vi•tel•lo•in•tes•ti•nal cyst (vī-tel′ō-in-tes′ti-năl sist) A small, red, sessile or pedunculated tumor at the umbilicus in an infant; it is due to the persistence of a segment of the vitellointestinal duct.

vi•tel•lus (vī-tel′ŭs) SYN yolk (1). [L.]

vit•i•a•tion (vish′ē-ā′shŭn) A change that impairs use or reduces efficiency. [L. *vitiatio* fr. *vitio,* pp. *vitiatus,* to corrupt, fr. *vitium,* vice]

vit•i•lig•i•nes (vit′i-lij′i-nēz) Plural of vitiligo.

vit•i•lig•i•nous (vit′i-lij′i-nŭs) Relating to or characterized by vitiligo.

vit•i•lig•i•nous chor•oid•i•tis (vit′i-lij′i-nŭs kōr′oyd-ī′tis) SYN bird shot retinochoroiditis.

vit•i•li•go, pl. **vit•i•lig•i•nes** (vit′i-lī′gō, -lij′i-nēz) The appearance on otherwise normal skin of nonpigmented white patches of varied sizes; hair in the affected areas is usually white. Epidermal melanocytes are completely lost in depigmented areas by an autoimmune process. See this page. [L. a skin eruption, fr. *vitium,* blemish, vice]

vi•trec•to•my (vi-trek′tŏ-mē) Removal of the vitreous by means of an instrument that simultaneously removes vitreous by suction and cutting and replaces it with saline or some other fluid. [vitreous + G. *ektomē,* excision]

vit•re•i•tis (vit′rē-ī′tis) Inflammation of the corpus vitreum. SYN hyalitis. [L. *vitreus,* glassy, + G. *-itis,* inflammation]

vitreo- Combining form denoting vitreous. [L. *vitreus,* glassy]

vit•re•o•den•tin (vit′rē-ō-den′tin) Dentin of a particularly brittle character.

vit•re•o•ret•i•nal (vit′rē-ō-ret′i-năl) Pertaining to the retina and the vitreous body.

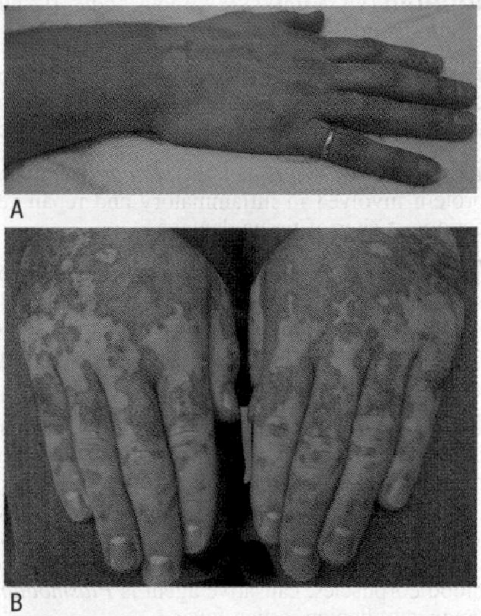

vitiligo: (A) forearm and hand; (B) repigmentation

vit•re•o•tap•e•to•ret•i•nal dys•tro•phy (vit′rē-ō-tă-pē′tō-ret′i-năl dis′trŏ-fē) Autosomal recessive bilateral peripheral and central retinoschisis with pigmentary degeneration of the retina, chorioretinal atrophy, vitreous degeneration, and night blindness. SYN Favre dystrophy.

vit•re•ous (vit′rē-ŭs) **1.** Glassy; resembling glass. **2.** SYN vitreous body. [L. *vitreus,* glassy, fr. *vitrum,* glass]

vit•re•ous bod•y (vit′re-ŭs bod′e) A transparent jellylike substance filling the interior of the eyeball behind the lens; it is composed of a delicate network (vitreous stroma) enclosing in its meshes a watery fluid (vitreous humor). SYN corpus vitreum [TA], hyaloid body, vitreous (2), vitreum.

vit•re•ous de•tach•ment (vit′rē-ŭs dĕ-tach′mĕnt) Separation of the peripheral vitreous humor from the retina.

vit•re•ous her•ni•a (vit′rē-ŭs hĕr′nē-ă) Prolapse of the vitreous humor into the anterior chamber; may follow removal or displacement of the lens from the lenticular space.

vit•re•ous hu•mor (vit′rē-ŭs hyū′mŏr) The fluid component of the vitreous body. USAGE NOTE Often erroneously equated with the vitreous body.

vit•re•ous la•mel•la (vit′rē-ŭs lă-mel′ă) SYN lamina basalis choroideae.

vit•re•ous mem•brane (vit′rē-ŭs mem′brān) **1.** SYN posterior limiting layer of cornea. **2.** A condensation of fine collagen fibers in places in the cortex of the vitreous body; formerly thought to form a membrane or capsule at its periphery. **3.** SYN lamina basalis choroideae.

vit•re•um (vit′rē-ŭm) SYN vitreous body. [L. ntr. of *vitreus,* glassy]

vit•ri•fi•ca•tion (vit′ri-fi-kā′shŭn) Conversion of dental porcelain to a glassy substance by heat and fusion. [L. *vitrium,* glassy, + *facio,* to make]

vit•ro•nec•tin (vit′rō-nek′tin) A plasma glycoprotein involved in inflammatory and repair reactions at sites of tissue damage.

Vit•ta•for•ma (vit′ă-fōr′mă) A genus of microsporidia that can infect humans and can cause keratitis in the immunocompetent and disseminated infection in the immunocompromised; formerly *Nosema.*

vi•vax ma•lar•i•a (vī′vaks mă-lar′ē-ă) A malarial fever with paroxysms that, having synchronized, recur every 48 hours or every other day (every third day, reckoning the day of the paroxysm as the first); the fever is induced by release of merozoites and their invasion of new red blood corpuscles; causative agent is *Plasmodium vivax.* SYN benign tertian fever.

♻**vivi-** Combining form denoting living. [L. *vivus,* alive]

viv•i•fi•ca•tion (viv′i-fi-kā′shŭn) SYN revivification (2). [L. *vivifico,* pp. *-atus,* fr. *vivus,* alive, + *facio,* to make]

vi•vip•a•rous (vī-vip′ă-rŭs) Giving birth to living young, in distinction to oviparous, or egg-laying. [vivi- + L. *pario,* to bear]

viv•i•sec•tion (viv′i-sek′shŭn) Any cutting operation on a living animal for purposes of experimentation; often extended to denote any form of animal experimentation. [vivi- + section]

viv•i•sec•tion•ist, viv•i•sec•tor (viv′i-sek′shŭn-ist, -sek′tŏr) One who practices vivisection.

viz. That is, namely. SEE ALSO editing. [L. *videlicet*]

VLBW Abbreviation for very low birth weight.

VLCD Abbreviation for very-low-calorie diets.

VLDL Abbreviation for very low-density lipoprotein. SEE lipoprotein.

VLPP Abbreviation for Valsalva leak point pressure.

VMA Abbreviation for vanillylmandelic acid.

VO Abbreviation for vocal order.

VO_{2max} SYN maximal oxygen consumption.

$\dot{V}O_2$ Abbreviation for oxygen consumption.

vo•cal (vō′kăl) Pertaining to the voice or the organs of speech. [L. *vocalis*]

🅸**vo•cal fold** (vō′kăl fōld) The sharp edge of a fold of mucous membrane overlying the vocal ligament and stretching along either wall of the larynx from the angle between the laminae of the thyroid cartilage to the vocal process of the arytenoid cartilage; the vocal folds are the agents concerned in voice production. See page B16. SYN plica vocalis [TA], true vocal cord.

vo•cal frem•i•tus (vō′kăl frem′i-tŭs) The palpable vibration in the chest wall, produced by the spoken voice.

vo•cal fry (vō′kăl frī) Phonation at an unnaturally low frequency resulting in low-frequency popping and ticking sounds. SYN glottalization.

vo•ca•lis mus•cle (vō-kā′lis mŭs′ĕl) *Origin,* depression between the two laminae of thyroid cartilage; *insertion,* portions of vocal process of arytenoid; *action,* shortens and relaxes vocal cords; *nerve supply,* recurrent laryngeal; a number of the deeper and finer fibers of the thyroarytenoid muscle attached directly to the outer side of the true vocal cord. SYN musculus vocalis [TA], vocal muscle.

vo•cal lig•a•ment (vō′kăl lig′ă-mĕnt) The band that extends on either side from the thyroid cartilage to the vocal process of the arytenoid cartilage; it is the thickened, free upper border of the conus elasticus of the larynx. SYN ligamentum vocale [TA].

vo•cal mus•cle (vō′kăl mŭs′ĕl) SYN vocalis muscle.

vo•cal nod•ules (vō′kăl noj′ūlz) Small, circumscribed, bilateral, beadlike enlargements on the vocal folds caused by overuse or abuse of the voice. SYN singer's nodules, speaker's nodules.

vo•cal pro•cess of ar•y•te•noid car•ti•lage (vō′kăl pros′es ar-i-tē′noyd kahr′ti-lăj) The lower end of the anterior margin of the arytenoid cartilage to which the vocal cord is attached.

vo•cal res•o•nance (VR) (vō′kăl rez′ŏ-năns) The voice sounds as heard on auscultation of the chest.

vo•cal spec•trum (vō′kăl spek′trŭm) The frequency and intensity ranges of the voice.

vo•cal tract (vō′kăl trakt) The air passages above the glottis (including the pharynx, oral and nasal cavities, and paranasal sinuses) that contribute to the quality of the voice.

vo•ca•tion•al re•ha•bil•i•ta•tion (vō-kā′shŭn-ăl rē′hă-bil′i-tā′shŭn) Programs conducted by state vocational rehabilitation agencies operating under the U.S. Rehabilitation Act of 1973. Services are intended to help people with disabilities to acquire, reacquire, and maintain employment.

Vo•gel law (vō′gĕl law) When a phenotype may be transmitted by various modes of mendelian inheritance, the dominant will have the least deleterious phenotype, the recessive the most, and the X-linked intermediate between the two.

$\dot{V}O_2$ HR (ox•y•gen pulse) (ok′si-jĕn pŭls) Abbreviation for oxygen pulse.

voice (voys) The sound made by air passing out through the larynx and upper respiratory tract, the vocal folds being approximated. [L. *vox*]

voice fa•tigue syn•drome (voys fă-tēg′ sin′drōm) Weakness and loss of the voice usually toward the end of the day because of abuse by using it too long and too loudly.

voice pros•the•sis (voys pros-thē′sis) Any device used to produce a sound source for the voice; usually used by patients who have undergone laryngectomy or tracheostomy.

voice rec•og•ni•tion (voys rek′ŏg-nish′ŭn) SYN speech recognition.

void (voyd) To evacuate urine or feces.

voi•ding cys•to•gram (voy′ding sis′tō-gram) SYN cystourethrogram.

voi•ding cys•to•u•reth•ro•gram (VCUG) (voy′ding sis′tō-yūr-ē′thrō-gram) An x-ray image made during voiding with the bladder and urethra filled with contrast medium to demonstrate the urethra. SYN micturating cystourethrogram.

vo•la (vō′lă) Palm of the hand or sole of the foot. [L.]

vo•lar (vō′lăr) Referring to the vola; denoting either the palm of the hand or sole of the foot.

vo•lar in•ter•os•se•ous ar•ter•y (vō′lăr in′tĕr-os′ē-ŭs ahr′tĕr-ē) SYN anterior interosseous artery.

vo•lar plate (vōl′ăr plāt) A tough ligamentous band bridging the volar aspect of the proximal interphalangeal joint in fingers II–V and opposing hyperextension. Rupture of the volar plate due to injury or disease permits recurrent hyperextension and can lead to swan-neck deformity.

vol•a•tile (vol′ă-til) **1.** Tending to evaporate rapidly. **2.** Tending toward violence, explosiveness, or rapid change. [L. *volatilis*, fr. *volo*, to fly]

vol•a•tile oil (vol′ă-til oyl) A substance of oily consistency and feel, derived from a plant and containing the principles to which the odor and taste of the plant are due (essential oil); in contrast to a fatty oil, a volatile oil evaporates when exposed to the air and thus is capable of distillation. SYN ethereal oil.

vol•a•til•i•za•tion (vol′ă-til-ī-zā′shŭn) SYN evaporation. [fr. L. *volatilis,* volatile, fr. *volo,* pp. *volatus,* to fly]

vo•li•tion (vō-lish′ŭn) The conscious impulse to perform any act or to abstain from its performance; voluntary action. [L. *volo*, to wish]

vo•li•tion•al (vō-lish′ŭn-ăl) Done by an act of will; relating to volition.

vo•li•tion•al trem•or (vō-lish′ŭn-ăl trem′ŏr) **1.** A tremor that can be arrested by a strong effort of the will. **2.** SYN intention tremor.

Volk•mann chei•li•tis (fōlk′mahn kī-lī′tis) SYN cheilitis glandularis.

Volk•mann con•trac•ture (fōlk′mahn kŏn-trak′shŭr) Ischemic contracture resulting from irreversible necrosis of muscle tissue, produced by a compartment syndrome; classically involves the forearm flexor muscles.

Volk•mann spoon (fōlk′mahn spūn) A sharp spoon for scraping away carious bone or other diseased tissue.

vol•ley (vol′ē) A synchronous group of impulses induced simultaneously by artificial stimulation of either nerve fibers or muscle fibers. [Fr. *volée,* fr. L. *volo,* to fly]

volt (v, V) (vōlt) The unit of electromotive force; the electromotive force that will produce a current of 1 ampere in a circuit that has a resistance of 1 ohm, i.e., joule per coulomb.

vol•tage (vōl′tăj) Electromotive force, pressure, or potential expressed in volts.

volt•am•pere (vōlt′am′pēr) A unit of electrical power; the product of 1 volt by 1 ampere; equivalent to 1 watt or 1/1000 kilowatt.

volt•me•ter (vōlt′mē-tĕr) An instrument that measures differences in electrical potential.

Vol•to•li•ni dis•ease (vōl-tō-lē′nē di-zēz′) Infectious disease of the labyrinth, leading to meningitis in young children.

vol•ume (V, *V*) (vol′yūm) Space occupied by matter, usually expressed in units such as cubic millimeters, cubic centimeters, and liters. SEE ALSO capacity, water. [L. *volumen,* something rolled up, scroll, fr. *volvo,* to roll]

vol•ume as•sured pres•sure sup•port (VAPS) (vol′yūm ă-shŭrd′ presh′ŭr sŭ-pōrt′) A mode of mechanical ventilation.

vol•ume at ATPS (vol′yūm) A volume of gas at ambient (A) temperature (T) (room temperature) and barometric pressure (P) saturated (S) with water vapor.

vol•ume at BTPS (vol′yūm) A volume of gas saturated (S) with water vapor at 37°C (body [B] temperature ([T]) and the ambient environmental barometric pressure (P).

vol•ume at STPD (vol′yūm) A volume of gas, at the standard (S) temperature (T) of 0°C and a barometric pressure (P) of 760 mmHg, and in a dry state (D).

vol•ume coil (vol′yūm koyl) MAGNETIC RESONANCE IMAGING a device that transmits and receives signals over a large volume of the patient.

vol•ume-con•trolled ven•ti•la•tion (vol′yūm-kŏn-trōld′ ven′ti-lā′shŭn) A mode of mechanical ventilation in which the ventilator delivers a preset volume waveform; the resultant airway pressure waveform depends on the shape of the flow waveform and respiratory system resistance and compliance.

vol•ume in•dex (vol′yūm in′deks) An indication of the relative size (e.g., volume) of erythrocytes, calculated as follows: Hematocrit value, expressed as the percentage of normal ÷ red blood cell count, expressed as percentage of normal = volume index.

vol•u•met•ric (vol′yū-met′rik) Relating to measurement by volume.

vol•u•met•ric a•nal•y•sis (vol′yū-met′rik ă-nal′i-sis) Quantitative analysis by the addition of graduated amounts of a standard test solution to a solution of a known amount of the substance analyzed, until the reaction is just at an end; depends on the stoichiometric nature of the reaction between the test solution and the unknown.

vol•u•met•ric so•lu•tion (VS) (vol′yū-met′rik sŏ-lū′shŭn) A solution made by mixing measured volumes of the components.

vol•ume ven•til•a•tor (vol′yūm ven′til-ā-tŏr) A device designed to deliver volume-controlled ventilation.

vol•un•tar•y (vol′ŭn-tar-ē) Relating or acting in obedience to the will; not obligatory. [L. *voluntarius,* fr. *voluntas,* will, fr. *volo,* to wish]

vol•un•tar•y mus•cle (vol′ŭn-tar-ē mŭs′ĕl) One with an action that is under the control of the will; all the striated muscles, except the heart, are voluntary muscles.

vo•lute (vō-lūt′) Rolled up; convoluted. [L. *voluta,* a scroll, fr. *volvo,* pp. *volutus,* to roll]

vol•vu•lus (vol′vyū-lŭs) A twisting of the intestine that causes obstruction; if left untreated, may result in vascular compromise of the involved intestine. See this page. [L. *volvo,* to roll]

vo•mer, gen. **vo•mer•is** (vō′mĕr, -mĕr-is) [TA] A flat bone of trapezoidal shape forming the inferior and posterior portion of the nasal septum; it articulates with the sphenoid, ethmoid, two maxillae, and two palatine bones. [L. ploughshare]

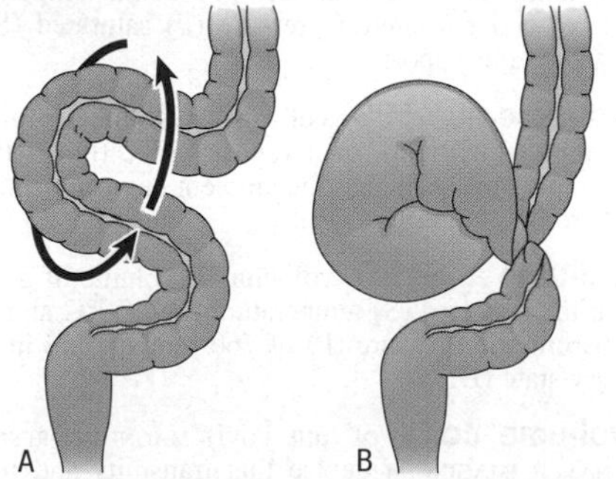

volvulus of the sigmoid colon: (A) the unattached loop of bowel twists; (B) the bowel lumen is obstructed, leading to inability of stool to pass and to compression of the blood supply to the looped bowel segment

vo•mer•ine (vō′mĕr-ēn) Relating to the vomer.

vo•mer•o•na•sal car•ti•lage, **vo•mer•ine car•ti•lage** (vō′mĕr-ō-nā′zăl kahr′ti-lăj, vō′mĕr-ēn) A narrow strip of cartilage located between the lower edge of the cartilage of the nasal septum and the vomer. SYN cartilago vomeronasalis [TA].

vom•it (vom′it) **1.** To eject matter from the stomach through the mouth. **2.** Vomitus; the matter so ejected. SYN vomitus. [L. *vomo,* pp. *vomitus,* to vomit]

vom•i•ting (vom′it-ing) The ejection of matter from the stomach through the esophagus and mouth. SYN emesis (1), regurgitation (2).

vom•i•ting a•gent (vom′it-ing ā′jĕnt) A riot-control agent that, in addition to irritating the eyes and the upper respiratory tract, induces vomiting. SEE ALSO Adamsite.

vom•i•ting of preg•nan•cy (vom′it-ing preg′năn-sē) Emesis occurring in the early months of pregnancy.

vom•i•ting re•flex (vom′it-ing rē′fleks) Emesis (contraction of the abdominal muscles with relaxation of the cardiac sphincter of the stomach and of the muscles of the throat) elicited by a variety of stimuli, especially one applied to the region of the fauces. SYN pharyngeal reflex (2).

vom•i•tu•ri•tion (vom′i-tyūr-ish′ŭn) SYN retching.

vom•i•tus (vom′i-tŭs) SYN vomit (2). [L. a vomiting, vomit]

von Gier•ke dis•ease (vahn gēr′kē di-zēz′) SYN glycogenosis type 1.

von Grae•fe sign (vahn grā′fĕ sīn) SYN Graefe sign.

von Spee curve (vahn shpē kŭrv) SYN curve of Spee.

von Wil•le•brand dis•ease (vahn vil′ĕ-brahnt di-zēz′) A hemorrhagic diathesis characterized by a tendency to bleed primarily from mucous membranes, prolonged bleeding time, normal platelet count, normal clot retraction, partial and variable deficiency of factor VIIIR, and possibly a morphologic defect of platelets; autosomal dominant inheritance with reduced penetrance and variable expressivity, caused by mutation in the von Willebrand factor gene (VWF) on 12p. Type III von Willebrand disease is a more severe disorder with markedly reduced factor VIIIR levels. A recessive version of this disease has a remarkable property in that it represents a mutation at the same locus as the dominant form.

VOR Abbreviation for vestibuloocular reflex.

vor•tex, pl. **vor•ti•ces** (vōr′teks, -ti-sēz) **1.** SYN verticil. **2.** SYN whorl (5). **3.** SYN vortex lentis. [L. whirlpool, whorl, fr. *verto* or *vorto,* to turn around]

vor•tex cor•ne•al dys•tro•phy (vōr′teks kōr′nē-ăl dis′trŏ-fē) A swirling pattern of abnormally pigmented corneal epithelial cells, seen in Fabry disease and in response to certain medications (including chloroquine, chlorpromazine, and amiodarone).

vor•tex of heart (vōr′teks hahrt) A spiral arrangement of muscular fibers at the apex of the heart. SYN whorl (2).

vor•tex len•tis (vōr′teks len′tis) One of the stellar figures on the surface of the lens of the eye. SYN vortex (3).

vor•tex veins (vōr′teks vānz) Several veins (usually four) from the vascular tunic formed of veins accompanying the posterior ciliary arteries and the ciliary body; these drain into the superior or inferior ophthalmic vein. SYN vorticose veins.

vor•ti•cose veins (vōr′ti-kōs vānz) SYN vortex veins.

Vos•si•us len•tic•u•lar ring (fos′ē-ŭs len-tik′yŭ-lăr ring) An anular opacity found on the anterior lens capsule after contusion of the eye, due to pigment and blood.

vox•el (vok′sel) A contraction for volume element, which is the basic unit of CT or MR reconstruction; represented as a pixel in the display of the CT or MR image.

voy•eur (vwah-yur′) One who practices voyeurism.

voy•eur•ism (vwah′yur-izm) The practice of obtaining sexual pleasure by looking at the naked body or genitals of another or at erotic acts between others. SYN scopophilia. [Fr. *voir,* to see]

V-pat•tern es•o•tro•pi•a (pă′tĕrn ē′sō-trō′pē-ă) Convergent strabismus greater in downward than in upward gaze.

V-pat•tern ex•o•tro•pi•a (pă′tĕrn ek′sō-trō′pē-ă) Divergent strabismus greater in upward than in downward gaze.

$\dot{V}_A$:$\dot{Q}$ Abbreviation for ventilation:perfusion ratio.

VR Abbreviation for vocal resonance.

VRE Abbreviation for vancomycin-resistant enterococcus.

VS Abbreviation for volumetric solution.

VSD Abbreviation for ventricular septal defect.

V-se•ries nerve a•gents (sēr′ēz nĕrv ā′jĕnts) Persistent nerve agents synthesized after World War II and assigned NATO codes beginning with V. The most familiar compound of this class is VX.

VTS Abbreviation for veterinary technician specialist.

vul•ga•ris (vul-gā′ris) Ordinary; of the usual type. [L. fr. *vulgus,* a crowd]

vul•ner•a•bil•i•ty (vŭl′nĕr-ă-bil′i-tē) Susceptibility or weakness; often associated with a particular situation (e.g., illiness, poverty, illiteracy).

vul•ner•a•ble phase (vŭl′nĕr-ă′bĕl fāz) A period in the cardiac cycle during which an ectopic impulse may lead to repetitive activity such as flutter or fibrillation of the affected chamber.

Vul•pi•an at•ro•phy (vūl-pē-an[h]′ at′rŏ-fē) Progressive spinal muscular wasting beginning in the shoulder.

vul•sel•la, vul•sel•lum (vŭl-sel′ă, -lŭm) SYN vulsella forceps. [L. pincers, fr. *vello,* pp. *vulsus,* to pluck]

vul•sel•la for•ceps, vul•sel•lum for•ceps (vŭl-sel′ă fōr′seps, vŭl-sel′ŭm) A forceps with hooks at the tip of each blade. SYN vulsella, vulsellum.

vul•va, pl. **vul•vae** (vŭl′vă, -vē) [TA] The external genitalia of the female, composed of the mons pubis, the labia majora and minora, the clitoris, the vestibule of the vagina and its glands, and the opening of the urethra and of the vagina. [L. a wrapper or covering, seed covering, womb, fr. *volvo,* to roll]

vul•var, vul•val (vŭl′văr, -văl) Relating to the vulva.

vul•var dys•tro•phy (vŭl′văr dis′trŏ-fē) SEE dystrophy.

vul•var in•tra•epi•the•li•al ne•o•pla•si•a (vŭl′văr in′tră-ep′i-thē′lē-ăl nē′ō-plā′zē-ă) Preinvasive squamous cell carcinoma (carcinoma in situ) limited to vulvar epithelium; like vaginal or cervical intraepithelial neoplasia, graded histologically on a scale from 1–3 or subdivided into low-grade and high-grade intraepithelial malignancy; usually related to human papillomavirus infection; may progress to invasive carcinoma.

vul•var leu•ko•pla•ki•a (vŭl′văr lū′kō-plā′kē-ă) A possibly precancerous condition in which thickened white patches of epithelial tissue occur.

vul•vec•to•my (vŭl-vek′tŏ-mē) Excision (either partial, complete, or radical) of the vulva. [vulva + G. *ektomē,* excision]

vul•vi•tis (vŭl-vī′tis) Inflammation of the vulva. [vulva + G. *-itis,* inflammation]

♲ **vulvo-** Combining form denoting the vulva. [L. *vulva*]

vul•vo•vag•i•ni•tis (vŭl′vō-vaj-i-nī′tis) Inflammation of both vulva and vagina.

V wave (wāv) A large pressure wave visible in recordings from either atrium or its incoming veins, normally produced by venous return but becoming very large when blood regurgitates through the A-V valve beyond the chamber from which the recording is made.

VX NATO code for an extremely toxic persistent nerve agent synthesized in Great Britain in World War II and developed in the United States. It has no common chemical name. SEE ALSO chemical-warfare (CW) agent, nerve agent.

V-Y plas•ty (plas′tē) A surgical method for lengthening tissues in one direction by cutting in the lines of a V, sliding the two segments apart, and closing in the lines of a Y.

W

W Abbreviation for tungsten; watt; tryptophan.

Waar•den•burg syn•drome (vahr′den-burg sin′drōm) Congenital craniofacial dysmorphism characterized by white forelock, lateral displacement of medial canthi, iris bicolored or blue, prominence of the root of the nose, hyperplasia of medial portion of eyebrows, and congenital deafness.

Wa•chen•dorf mem•brane (vahk′en-dōrf mem′brān) **1.** SYN pupillary membrane. **2.** SYN cell membrane.

waist (wāst) The portion of the trunk between the ribs and the pelvis. [A.S. *waext*]

waist:hip ra•ti•o (wāst′hip rā′shē-ō) Waist circumference divided by hip circumference; indicator of abdominal (visceral) obesity, and predictor of health risk independent of total percentage of body fat. Ratio that exceeds 0.80 for women and 0.95 for men correlates with increased risk of death, even after controlling for body mass index.

Wal•den•ström mac•ro•glob•u•lin•e•mi•a (vahl′den-strem mak′rō-glob′yū-li-nē′mē-ă) Macroglobulinemia occurring in old people, characterized by proliferation of cells resembling lymphocytes or plasma cells in the bone marrow, anemia, an increased sedimentation rate, and hyperglobulinemia with a narrow peak in γ-globulin or β_2-globulin at about 19 S units. The spleen, liver, or lymph nodes are often enlarged, and there is frequently purpura or mucosal bleeding.

Wal•dey•er sheath (vahl′dī-er shēth) The tubular space between the bladder wall and the intramural portion of the ureter as it courses obliquely through this structure; actually a space and not a true sheath.

Wal•dron test (wawl′drŏn test) Crepitation at the patellofemoral articulation on passive extension and flexion of the knee in chondromalacia patellae.

walk (wawk) **1.** To move on foot. **2.** The characteristic manner in which one moves on foot. SEE ALSO gait. [M.E. *walken*, fr. O.E. *wealcen*, to roll]

walk•er (wawk′ĕr) A light, portable framework used for support and assistance in walking by a person with a gait impairment for which a cane or crutches are inadequate.

Walk•er chart (wawk′ĕr chahrt) A system of plotting the relative fetal and placental sizes.

walk•ing (wawk′ing) Characterized by sequential movement or progression in steps. SEE ALSO gait.

walk•ing wound•ed (wawk′ing wūn′dĕd) Category of patients attending an emergency department who are ambulant, without life-threatening injuries or conditions.

walk out re•ceipt (wawk owt rē-sēt′) A printed report given to a patient or caregiver after services are completed.

walk-through an•gi•na (wawk′thrū an′ji-nă) A circumstance in which, despite continuing activity such as walking, the pain of angina pectoris diminishes or disappears.

wall (wawl) An investing part enclosing a cavity such as the thorax or abdomen, or covering a cell or any anatomic unit. A wall, as of the thorax, abdomen, or any hollow organ. SYN paries. [L. *vallum*]

wal•ler•i•an (waw-ler′ē-ăn) Relating to or described by A.V. Waller.

wal•ler•i•an de•gen•er•a•tion (waw-ler′ē-ăn dĕ-jen′ĕr-ā′shŭn) The degenerative changes observed in the distal segment of a peripheral nerve fiber (axon and myelin) when its continuity with its cell body is interrupted by a focal lesion. SYN orthograde degeneration, secondary degeneration.

wall-eye (wawl′ī) SYN exotropia.

wall-eyed bi•lat•er•al in•ter•nu•cle•ar oph•thal•mo•ple•gi•a (WEBINO) (wawl′īd bī-lat′ĕr-ăl in′tĕr-nū′klē-ăr of-thal′mō-plē′jē-ă) A disorder of ocular motility due to lesions involving both medial longitudinal fasciculus and a brainstem convergence center; characterized by bilateral adduction weakness and exotropia.

Walsh pro•ce•dure (wawlsh prŏ-sē′jŭr) Anatomic (nerve-sparing) radical retropubic prostatectomy.

Wal•thard cell rest (vahl′tahrd sel rest) A nest of epithelial cells occurring in the peritoneum of the uterine tubes or ovary; when neoplastic, possibly comprising one of the components of the Brenner tumor.

Wal•ther di•la•tor (vahl′ter dī′lā-tĕr) A gently curved instrument that tapers to an increased diameter, used to dilate the female urethra.

Wal•ther ducts (vahl′ter dŭkts) SYN minor sublingual ducts.

Wal•ther gan•gli•on (vahl′ter gang′glē-ŏn) SYN ganglion impar.

waltzed flap (wawltst flap) SYN caterpillar flap.

wan•der•ing (wahn′dĕr-ing) Moving about; not fixed; abnormally motile. [A.S. *wandrian*, to wander]

wan•der•ing ab•scess (wahn′dĕr-ing ab′ses) SYN perforating abscess.

wan•der•ing cell (wahn′dĕr-ing sel) SYN ameboid cell.

wan•der•ing goi•ter (wahn′dĕr-ing goy′tĕr) SYN diving goiter.

wan•der•ing kid•ney (wahn′dĕr-ing kid′nē) SYN floating kidney.

wan•der•ing pace•mak•er (wahn′dĕr-ing pās′ māk′ĕr) A disturbance of the normal cardiac rhythm in which the site of the controlling pacemaker shifts from beat to beat, usually between the sinus and A-V nodes, often with gradual sequential changes in P waves between upright and inverted in a given ECG lead.

Wang•i•el•la (wang′gē-el′ă) A dematiaceous genus of fungi; *W. dermatitidis* is an etiologic agent of phaeohyphomycosis.

War•burg ap•pa•ra•tus (vahr′berg ap′ă-rat′ŭs) An apparatus for measuring the oxygen consumption of incubated tissue slices by manometric measurement of changes in gas pressure produced by oxygen absorption in an enclosed flask.

War•burg the•o•ry (vahr′berg thē′ŏr-ē) That the development of cancer is due to irreversible damage to the respiratory mechanism of cells, leading to the selective multiplication of cells with increased glycolytic metabolism, both aerobic and anaerobic.

ward (wōrd) A large room or hall in a hospital containing a number of beds. SEE ALSO unit. [A.S. *weard*]

Ward•rop meth•od (wōrd′rŏp meth′ŏd) Treatment of aneurysm by ligation of the artery at some distance beyond the sac, leaving one or more branches of the artery between the sac and the ligature.

Ward tri•an•gle (wōrd trī′ang-gĕl) An area of diminished density in the trabecular pattern of the neck of the femur evident by x-ray as well as by direct inspection of a specimen.

warm-up (wōrm-ŭp) A program of gradually increasing activity to raise muscle temperature and heart rate in preparation for more strenuous exercise; may be general (e.g., calisthenics) or specific (e.g., large muscle movements), to provide rehearsal of an activity (e.g., swinging a golf club).

warm-up phe•nom•e•non (wōrm′ŭp fĕ-nom′ĕ-non) Progressive diminution of the myotonic response of a muscle during repeated contraction of the muscle.

war neu•ro•sis (wōr nūr-ō′sis) A stress condition or mental disorder induced by conditions existing in warfare. SEE ALSO battle fatigue, posttraumatic stress disorder. SYN battle neurosis.

i **wart** (wōrt) SYN verruca. See page B9.

War•ten•berg symp•tom (vahr′ten-berg simp′tŏm) **1.** Flexion of the thumb when the patient attempts to flex the four fingers against resistance, a "pyramid sign." **2.** Intense pruritus of the tip of the nose and nostrils in cases of cerebral tumor.

wash (wawsh) A solution used to clean or bathe a part.

wash-out (wawsh′owt) A technique for eliminating (washing out) a specific substance.

was•tage (wās′tăj) Decay, loss, or diminution of something.

wast•ing (wāst′ing) **1.** SYN emaciation. **2.** Denoting a disease characterized by emaciation.

wast•ing syn•drome (wāst′ing sin′drōm) Progressive involuntary weight loss seen in patients with HIV infection; may be due to a number of factors acting alone or in combination, including inadequate oral intake of food, altered metabolic state, and/or malabsorption. Does not respond to increased caloric intake. Defined as profound involuntary weight loss of greater than 10% of baseline body weight, plus either chronic diarrhea (at least two loose stools per day for more than 30 days) or chronic weakness and documented fever (for more than 30 days, intermittent or constant) in the absence of concurrent illness or condition other than HIV infection that could explain the findings (e.g., cancer, tuberculosis, cryptosporidiosis, or other specific enteritis). SYN HIV wasting syndrome.

wa•ter (H_2O) (waw′tĕr) **1.** A clear, odorless, tasteless liquid, solidifying at 32°F (0°C and R), and boiling at 212°F (100°C, 80°R), which is present in all animal and vegetable tissues and dissolves more substances than any other liquid. SEE ALSO volume. **2.** Euphemism for urine. **3.** A pharmacopeial preparation of a clear, saturated aqueous solution (unless otherwise specified) of volatile oils, or other aromatic or volatile substances, prepared by processes involving distillation or solution (agitation followed by filtration). [A.S. *waeter*]

wa•ter of crys•tal•li•za•tion (waw′tĕr kris′tăl-ī-zā′shŭn) Water of constitution that unites with certain salts and is essential to their arrangement in crystalline form, e.g., $CuSO_4 \cdot 5H_2O$.

wa•ter•fall (waw′tĕr-fawl) A term used to describe flow in vascular beds where lateral pressure tending to collapse vessels greatly exceeds venous pressure. Flow is independent of venous pressure and occurs only when arterial pressure exceeds lateral pressure.

wa•ter-ham•mer pulse (waw′tĕr ham′ĕr pŭls) A jerky pulse with forcible impulse but immediate collapse, characteristic of aortic insufficiency. SEE ALSO Corrigan sign, Corrigan pulse. SYN cannonball pulse.

Wa•ter•house-Frid•er•ich•sen syn•drome (waw′tĕr-hows frē′der-ik-sen sin′drōm) A condition due to meningococcemia, occurring mainly in children younger than 10 years of age, characterized by vomiting, diarrhea, extensive purpura, cyanosis, tonoclonic convulsions, and circulatory collapse, usually with meningitis and hemorrhage into the suprarenal glands.

wa•ter for in•jec•tion (waw′tĕr in-jek′shŭn) Sterile water used to dissolve or dilute materials for injection.

wa•ter in•tox•i•ca•tion (waw′tĕr in-toks′i-kā′shŭn) Nonphysiologic state caused by excessive water intake during exercise resulting in headache, nausea, and cramping. In severe cases, it may cause seizures and even death.

wa•ter itch (waw′tĕr ich) **1.** SYN cutaneous ancylostomiasis. **2.** SYN schistosomal dermatitis.

wa•ter of me•tab•o•lism (waw′tĕr mĕ-tab′ŏ-lizm) The water formed in the body by oxidation of the hydrogen of the food, the greatest amount being produced in the metabolism of fat (about 117 g/100 g of fat).

wa•ter plan•tain (waw′tĕr plan-tān′) SYN alisma.

wa•ters (waw′tĕrz) Colloquialism for amniotic fluid.

wa•ter sham•rock (waw′tĕr sham′rok) SYN bog bean.

wa•ter•shed (waw′tĕr-shed) **1.** The area of marginal blood flow at the extreme periphery of a vascular bed. **2.** Slopes in the abdominal cavity, formed by projections of the lumbar vertebrae and the pelvic brim, which determine the direction in which a free effusion will gravitate when the body is in a supine position.

wa•ter•shed in•farc•tion (waw′tĕr-shed in-fahrk′shŭn) Cortical infarction in an area where the distributions of major cerebral arteries meet or overlap.

Wa•ters op•er•a•tion (waw′tĕrz op-ĕr-ā′shŭn) An extraperitoneal cesarean section with a supravesical approach.

Wa•ters pro•jec•tion (waw′tĕrz prŏ-jek′shŭn) A posteroanterior radiographic view of the skull made with the orbitomeatal line at an angle of 37° from the plane of the film, to show the orbits and maxillary sinuses.

wa•ter-trap stom•ach (waw′tĕr-trap stŭm′ăk) A ptotic and dilated stomach, having a relatively high (although normally placed) pyloric outlet that is held up by the gastrohepatic ligament.

Wat•son-Crick he•lix (waht′sŏn-krik hē′liks) The helical structure assumed by two strands of deoxyribonucleic acid, held together throughout their length by hydrogen bonds between bases on opposite strands, referred to as Watson-Crick base pairing. SEE ALSO base pair. SYN DNA helix, double helix.

watt (W) (waht) The SI unit of electrical power; the power available when the current is 1 ampere and the electromotive force is 1 volt; equal to 1 joule (10^7 ergs) per second or 1 voltampere.

wave (wāv) **1.** A movement of particles in an elastic body, whether solid or fluid, whereby an advancing series of alternate elevations and depressions, or expansions and condensations, is produced. **2.** The elevation of the pulse, felt by the finger, or represented graphically in the curved line of the sphygmograph. **3.** The complete cycle of changes in the level of a source of energy that is repetitively varying with respect to time; in the electrocardiogram and the electroencephalogram, the wave is essentially a voltage-time graph. SEE ALSO rhythm. [A.S. *wafian,* to fluctuate]

wave•form (wāv′fōrm) The form of a pulse (e.g., an arterial pressure or displacement wave), or of the pacemaker pulse as demonstrated on the oscilloscope under a specified load.

wave•length (λ) (wāv′length) The distance from one point on a wave (frequently shaped like a sine curve) to the next point in the same phase; i.e., from peak to peak or from trough to trough.

wax (waks) **1.** A thick, tenacious substance, plastic at room temperature, secreted by bees for building the cells of their honeycomb. **2.** Any substance with physical properties similar to those of beeswax, of animal, vegetable, or mineral origin (oils, lipids, or fats that are solids at room temperature). SEE ALSO cerumen. **3.** Esters of high molecular weight fatty acids with monohydric or dihydric alcohols (aliphatic or cyclic) that are solid at room temperature. Often accompanied by free fatty acids. [A.S. *weax*]

wax•ber•ry (waks′ber-ē) SYN bayberry.

wax•ing, wax•ing-up (waks′ing, -ŭp′) The contouring of a pattern in wax, generally applied to the shaping in wax of the contours of a trial denture or a crown prior to casting in metal.

wax•y cast (waks′ē kast) A microscopic formed element found in the urine in renal disease.

wax•y de•gen•er•a•tion (waks′ē dĕ-jen′ĕr-ā′shŭn) **1.** SYN amyloid degeneration. **2.** SYN Zenker degeneration.

wax•y kid•ney (waks′ē kid′nē) SYN amyloid kidney.

wax•y spleen (waks′ē splēn) Amyloidosis of the spleen.

way•thorn (wā′thōrn) SYN buckthorn.

Wb Abbreviation for weber.

WBC Abbreviation for white blood cell.

WC Abbreviation for workers' compensation. SEE ALSO workers' compensation law.

WDLL Abbreviation for well-differentiated lymphocytic lymphoma.

weak•ness (wēk′nĕs) **1.** Lack of strength or potency. **2.** Inability to perform normally.

wean (wēn) To implement weaning. [A.S. *wenian*]

wean•ing (wēn′ing) **1.** Permanent deprivation of breast milk and commencement of nourishment with other food. **2.** Gradual withdrawal of a patient from dependence on a life-support system or other form of therapy.

wea•pons of mass de•struc•tion (WMD) (wep′ŏnz mas dĕ-strŭk′shŭn) **1.** Weapons capable of producing widespread damage to buildings, facilities, and equipment. These weapons include high explosives and nuclear bombs using fission and fusion. **2.** A legal term referring to high explosives, to nuclear weapons, but also misleadingly, to nondestructive unconventional mass casualty weapons to include biologic warfare agents, chemical warfare agents, and point sources of radiation. SEE ALSO mass-casualty weapons.

wear-and-tear pig•ment (wār-tār pig′mĕnt) Lipofuscin that accumulates in aging or atrophic cells as a residue of lysosomal digestion.

web (web) A tissue or membrane bridging a space. SEE ALSO tela. [A.S.]

webbed fin•gers (webd fing′gĕrs) Two or more fingers united and enclosed in a common sheath of skin.

webbed neck (webd nek) The broad neck due to lateral folds of skin extending from the clavicle to the head but containing no muscles, bones, or other structures; occurs in Turner and Noonan syndromes.

web•bing (web′ing) Congenital condition apparent when adjacent structures are joined by a broad band of tissue not normally present to such a degree.

we•ber (Wb) (vā′bĕr) SI unit of magnetic flux, equal to volt-seconds (V·s).

Web•er-Chris•tian dis•ease (web′ĕr-kris′chăn di-zēz′) SYN relapsing febrile nodular nonsuppurative panniculitis.

We•ber-Cock•ayne syn•drome (web′ĕr-kok-ān′ sin′drōm) A form of epidermolysis bullosa with only the hands and feet affected. Cf. epidermolysis bullosa.

We•ber-Fech•ner law (vā′ber-fek′nĕr law) The intensity of a sensation varies by a series of equal increments (arithmetically) as the strength of the stimulus is increased geometrically; if a series of stimuli is applied and so adjusted in strength that each stimulus causes a just-perceptible change in intensity of the sensation, then the strength of each stimulus differs from the preceding one by a constant fraction. SYN Fechner-Weber law, Weber law.

We•ber law (vā′bĕr law) SYN Weber-Fechner law.

We•ber par•a•dox (vā′bĕr par′ă-doks) If a muscle is loaded beyond its power to contract, it may elongate.

We•ber stain (web′ĕr stān) A modified trichrome stain for microsporidian spores in which the chromotrope 2R is 10 times the normal concentration used in trichrome stains for stool specimens and the counterstain is fast green.

We•ber syn•drome (web′ĕr sin′drōm) Midbrain tegmentum lesion characterized by ipsilateral oculomotor nerve paresis and contralateral paralysis of the extremities, face, and tongue.

We•ber test for hear•ing (vā′bĕr test hēr′ing) The application of a vibrating tuning fork to one of several points in the midline of the head or face, to ascertain in which ear the sound is heard by bone conduction, that ear being the affected one if the sound-conducting mechanism of the middle ear is at fault, but the normal one if there is a sensorineural hearing loss in the other ear.

We•ber tri•an•gle (vā′bĕr trī′ang-gĕl) On the sole of the foot, an area indicated by the heads of the first and fifth metatarsal bones and the center of the plantar surface of the heel.

WEBINO (web-ē′nō) Acronym for wall-eyed bilateral internuclear ophthalmoplegia.

Wechs•ler in•tel•li•gence scales (weks′lĕr in-tel′i-jĕns skālz) Continuously revised and updated standardized scales for the measurement of general intelligence in preschool children (Wechsler preschool and primary scale of intelligence), in children (Wechsler intelligence scale for children), and in adults (Wechsler adult intelligence scale).

wedge-and-groove joint (wej grūv joynt) A form of fibrous joint in which the sharp edge of one bone is received in a cleft in the edge of the other. SYN schindylesis [TA], wedge-and-groove suture.

wedge-and-groove su•ture (wej grūv sū′chŭr) SYN wedge-and-groove joint.

wedge bone (wej bōn) SYN intermediate cuneiform bone, lateral cuneiform bone, medial cuneiform bone.

wedge frac•ture (wej frak′shŭr) Compression fracture of the anterior part of a vertebral body, resulting in a wedge shape that is narrower anteriorly.

wedge pres•sure (wej presh′ŭr) The intravascular pressure reading obtained when a fine catheter is advanced until it completely occludes a small blood vessel or is sealed in place by inflation of a small cuff; commonly measured in the lung to estimate left atrial pressure.

wedge re•sec•tion (wej rē-sek′shŭn) Removal of a wedge-shaped portion of the ovary; used in the treatment of virilizing disorders of ovarian origin, such as the polycystic ovarian syndrome.

Weeks ba•cil•lus (wēks bă-sil′ŭs) SYN *Haemophilus influenzae.*

Week·sel·la (wēk-sel′ă) A bacterial genus of nonoxidative, aerobic, gram-negative rods.

Week·sel·la zo·o·hel·cum (wēk-sel′ă zō-ō-hel′kŭm) A bacterium that produces infections in bites and scratches from dogs and cats.

We·ge·ner gran·u·lo·ma·to·sis (vā′ge-ner gran′yū-lō′mă-tō′sis) A disease, occurring mainly in the fourth and fifth decades, characterized by necrotizing granulomas and ulceration of the upper respiratory tract, with purulent rhinorrhea, nasal obstruction, and sometimes with otorrhea, hemoptysis, pulmonary infiltration and cavitation, and fever; exophthalmos, involvement of the larynx and pharynx, and glomerulonephritis may occur; the underlying condition is a vasculitis affecting small vessels, and is possibly due to an immune disorder.

Wei·gert i·o·dine so·lu·tion (vī′gert ī′ō-dīn sō-lū′shŭn) An iodine-potassium iodide mixture used as a reagent to alter crystal and methyl violet so that they are retained by certain bacteria and fungi.

Wei·gert i·ron he·ma·tox·y·lin stain (vī′gert ī′ŏrn hē′mă-toks′i-lin stān) A nuclear staining solution containing hematoxylin, ferric chloride, and hydrochloric acid; useful in combination with van Gieson stain, especially for demonstrating connective tissue elements or *Entamoeba histolytica* in sections.

Wei·gert law (vī′gert law) The loss or destruction of a part or element in the organic world is likely to result in compensatory replacement and overproduction of tissue during the process of regeneration or repair (or both), as in the formation of callus when a fractured bone heals.

Wei·gert stain for *Ac·ti·no·my·ces* (vī′gert stān ak′ti-nō-mī′sēz) A staining method using immersion in a dark red orsellin solution in alcohol, then staining in crystal-violet solution.

Wei·gert stain for e·las·tin (vī′gert stān ĕ-las′tin) A staining solution of fuchsin, resorcin, and ferric chloride; elastic fibers stain blue-black.

Wei·gert stain for fi·brin (vī′gert stān fī′brin) A staining method using solutions of aniline-crystal violet and iodine-potassium iodide, then decolorizing in aniline oil and xylol; the fibrin is stained dark blue.

Wei·gert stain for my·e·lin (vī′gert stān mī′ĕ-lin) A staining method using ferric chloride and hematoxylin; myelin stains deep blue, degenerated portions a light yellowish color.

Wei·gert stain for neu·rog·li·a (vī′gert stān nūr-og′lē-ă) A complicated process in which the final treatment is like that for staining fibrin; neuroglia and nuclei stain blue.

weight (wāt) The product of the force of gravity, defined internationally as 9.81 (m/sec)/sec, × the mass of the body. [A.S. *gewiht*]

weight-bear·ing ex·er·cise (wāt′bār-ing eks′ĕr-sīz) Exercise that puts stress on muscle and bone, thereby increasing muscle mass and bone strength.

weight-car·ry·ing test (wāt-kar′ē-ing test) SYN repetitive lifting test.

weight-sup·por·ted ex·er·cise (wāt′sŭ-pōr′tĕd eks′ĕr-sīz) SYN non-weight-bearing exercise.

Weil dis·ease (vīl di-zēz′) A form of leptospirosis generally caused by *Leptospira interrogans* serogroup *icterohaemorrhagiae*, believed to be acquired by contact with the urine of infected rats; characterized clinically by fever, jaundice, muscular pains, conjunctival congestion, and albuminuria; agglutinins regularly appear in the serum.

Weil-Fe·lix test, **Weil-Fe·lix re·ac·tion** (vīl-fā′liks test, rē-ak′shŭn) A test for the presence and type of rickettsial disease based on the agglutination of X-strains of *Proteus vulgaris* with suspected rickettsia in a patient's blood serum.

Weill-Mar·che·sa·ni syn·drome (vīl′mahr-kĕ-sah′nē sin′drōm) Ectopia lentis (lens abnormally round and small), short stature, and brachydactyly; recessive autosomal inheritance.

Wein·berg re·ac·tion (vīn′berg rē-ak′shŭn) A complement fixation test of the presence of hydatid disease.

Weiss sign (vīs sīn) SYN Chvostek sign.

Welch ba·cil·lus (welch bă-sil′ŭs) SYN *Clostridium perfringens.*

well-ba·by vis·it (wel-bā′bē viz′it) Routine health maintenance examinations for infants at specified ages.

well-dif·fer·en·ti·at·ed lym·pho·cyt·ic lym·pho·ma (WDLL) (wel dif′ĕr-en′shē-ā-tĕd lim′fō-sit′ik lim-fō′mă) Essentially the same disease as chronic lymphocytic leukemia, except that lymphocytes are not increased in the peripheral blood; lymph nodes are enlarged, and other lymphoid tissue or bone marrow is infiltrated by small lymphocytes.

well·ness (wel′nĕs) A philosophy of life and personal hygiene that views health as not merely the absence of illness but the fullest realization of one's physical and mental potential, as achieved through positive attitudes, fitness training, a diet low in fat and high in fiber, and the avoidance of unhealthful practices (smoking, drug and alcohol abuse, overeating).

welt (welt) SYN wheal. [O.E. *waelt*]

Wenc·ke·bach block (veng′ke-bahk blok) A first-degree atrioventricular block in which there is a progressive lengthening of conduction, as manifested in prolonged P-Q interval on electrocardiography, until one QRS complex and T wave are missed.

Wenc•ke•bach pe•ri•od (veng′ke-bahk pēr′ē-ŏd) A sequence of cardiac cycles in the electrocardiogram ending in a dropped beat due to A-V block, the preceding cycles showing progressively lengthening P-R intervals; the P-R interval following the dropped beat is again shortened.

Werl•hof dis•ease (verl′hof di-zēz′) Former term for idiopathic thrombocytopenic purpura.

Wer•ner syn•drome (ver′ner sin′drōm) A premature aging disorder consisting of sclerodermalike skin changes, bilateral juvenile cataracts, progeria, hypogonadism, and diabetes mellitus; autosomal recessive inheritance, caused by mutation in the WRN gene, which encodes a helicase protein on chromosome 8p.

Wer•nic•ke a•pha•si•a (ver′ni-kĕ ă-fā′zē-ă) SYN receptive aphasia.

Wer•nic•ke cen•ter (ver′ni-kĕ sen′tĕr) The region of the cerebral cortex thought to be essential for understanding and formulating coherent, propositional speech; it encompasses a large region of the parietal and temporal lobes near the lateral sulcus of the left cerebral hemisphere; corresponding approximately to Brodmann areas 40, 39, and 22. SYN sensory speech center.

Wer•nic•ke-Kor•sa•koff en•ceph•a•lop•a•thy (ver′ni-kĕ-kōr′sĕ-kof en-sef′a-lop′ă-thē) SEE Wernicke syndrome, Korsakoff syndrome.

Wer•nic•ke-Kor•sa•koff syn•drome (ver′ni-kĕ-kōr′sĕ-kof sin′drōm) The coexistence of Wernicke and Korsakoff syndromes.

Wer•nic•ke re•ac•tion (ver′ni-kĕ rē-ak′shŭn) In hemianopia, a reaction due to damage of the optic tract, consisting of loss of pupillary constriction when the light is directed to the blind side of the retina; pupillary constriction is maintained when light stimulates the normal side. This sign cannot be seen with a bright light because of intraocular scatter onto the seeing half of the retina.

Wer•nic•ke syn•drome (ver′ni-kĕ sin′drōm) A condition frequently encountered in patients with long-term alcoholism, largely due to thiamin deficiency and characterized by disturbances in ocular motility, pupillary alterations, nystagmus, and ataxia with tremors; an organic-toxic psychosis is often an associated finding, and Korsakoff syndrome often coexists; characteristic cellular pathology found in several areas of the brain.

Wert•heim op•er•a•tion (vārt′hīm op-ĕr-ā′shŭn) A radical operation for carcinoma of the uterus in which as much as possible of the vagina is excised and there is wide lymph node excision.

West•berg space (vest′berg spās) The space surrounding the origin of the aorta that is invested with the pericardium.

Wes•ter•gren meth•od (ves′ter-gren meth′ŏd) A procedure for estimating the sedimentation rate in fluid blood by mixing venous blood with an aqueous solution of sodium chloride and allowing it to stand in an upright pipette; the fall of the red blood cells, in millimeters, is observed in 1 hour; the normal rate for men is 0–15 mm (average, 4 mm), and for women, 0–20 mm (average, 5 mm).

Wes•ter•mark sign (ves′ter-mahrk sīn) In chest radiography, decreased lung markings from oligemia caused by pulmonary embolism.

Wes•tern blot, **Wes•tern blot•ting** (wes′tĕrn blot, blot′ing) SYN Western blot analysis.

Wes•tern blot a•nal•y•sis (wes′tĕrn blot ă-nal′i-sis) A procedure in which proteins separated by electrophoresis in polyacrylamide gels are transferred (blotted) onto nitrocellulose or nylon membranes and identified by specific complexing with antibodies that are either pre- or post-tagged with a labeled secondary protein. SEE ALSO immunoblot. SYN Western blot, Western blotting. [Coined to distinguish it from eponymic Southern blot a.]

Wes•tern blot test (wes′tĕrn blot test) A serum electrophoretic analysis used to identify proteins.

West•ern colts•foot (west′ĕrn kōlts′fut) SYN butterbur.

Wes•tern e•quine en•ceph•a•lo•my•e•li•tis (wes′tĕrn ē′kwīn en-sef′ă-lō-mī′ĕ-lī′tis) An equine encephalomyelitis found in the western United States and parts of South America, transmitted by mosquitoes and caused by the western equine encephalomyelitis virus; the infection is similar to but milder than eastern equine encephalomyelitis in humans and is, as a rule, inapparent, but some cases with central nervous system involvement have been fatal.

West•gard rules (west′gahrd rūlz) A quality control protocol that allows detection of random and systematic error. The protocol includes the 12-s, 13-s, 22-s, R-4s, 4-1s, and 10 × rules.

West Nile fe•ver (west nīl fē′vĕr) Infection by West Nile virus. This virus is spread by mosquitoes. In mild infections, fever, headache, and muscle ache may last a few days. In severe infections, encephalitis, hyperpyrexia, stiff neck, convulsions, paralysis, and coma may last several weeks, and resulting deficits may become permanent.

West Nile vir•us (west nīl vī′rŭs) A flavivirus found in Africa, West Asia, the Middle East, and, since 1999, the United States. The virus can infect humans, birds, mosquitoes, horses, and some other mammals. West Nile fever is usually a mild disease characterized by flulike symptoms lasting only a few days and does not appear to cause any long-term health effects. Occasionally may cause encephalitis, meningitis, or meningoencephalitis.

West•phal pu•pil•lar•y re•flex (vest′fahl pyū′pi-lar-ē rē′fleks) SYN eye-closure pupil reaction.

West•phal sign (vest′fahl sīn) SYN Erb-Westphal sign.

West•phal-Strüm•pell dis•ease (vest′fahl-shtrem′pel di-zēz′) SYN Wilson disease (1).

West syn•drome (west sin′drōm) An encephalopathy in infancy characterized by infantile spasms, arrest of psychomotor development, and hypsarrhythmia.

wet-bulb ther•mom•et•er (wet′bŭlb thĕr-mom′ĕ-tĕr) Ambient air thermometer with a bulb enclosed by a wet wick. With high relative humidity, little evaporative cooling occurs, and the reading is similar to that of a dry-bulb thermometer. On a dry day, significant evaporation occurs from the wetted bulb, which maximizes the difference between the two thermometer readings.

wet gan•grene (wet gang-grēn′) Ischemic necrosis of an extremity with bacterial infection, producing cellulitis adjacent to the necrotic areas. SYN moist gangrene.

wet lung, white lung (wet lŭng, wīt) **1.** SYN shock lung. **2.** SYN adult respiratory distress syndrome.

wet nurse (wet nŭrs) A woman who breastfeeds someone else's child.

wet-tech•nique lip•o•suc•tion (wet-tek-nēk′ lip′ō-sŭk-shŭn) Liposuction performed after subcutaneous infusion of dilute epinephrine solution.

wet-to-dry dres•sing (wet-drī dres′ing) A dressing that is applied moist with saline and allowed to dry before it is removed.

WF Abbreviation for Working Formulation for Clinical Usage.

Whar•ton duct (wōr′tŏn dŭkt) SYN submandibular duct.

Whar•ton jel•ly (wōr′tŏn jel′ē) The mucoid connective tissue of the umbilical cord.

wheal (wēl) A circumscribed, evanescent papule or irregular plaque of edema of the skin, appearing as an urticarial lesion, slightly reddened, often changing in size and shape and extending to adjacent areas, and usually accompanied by intense itching; produced by intradermal injection or test, or by exposure to allergenic substances in those susceptible. See this page, B10. SYN hives (2), welt. [A.S. *hwēle*]

wheal-and-er•y•the•ma re•ac•tion (wēl er′i-thē′mă rē-ak′shŭn) The characteristic immediate reaction observed in the skin test; within 10–15 minutes after injection of antigen (allergen), an irregular, blanched, elevated wheal appears, surrounded by an area of erythema (flare). SYN wheal-and-flare reaction.

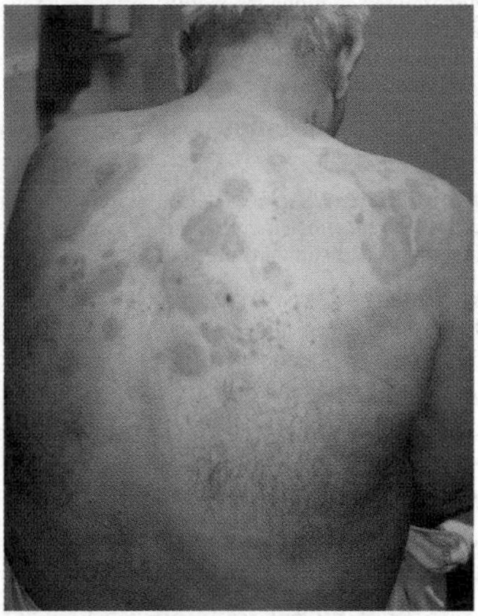

wheal: urticarial type

wheal-and-flare re•ac•tion (wēl flār rē-ak′shŭn) SYN wheal-and-erythema reaction.

Wheat•stone bridge (wēt′stōn brij) An apparatus for measuring electrical resistance; four resistors are connected to form the four sides or "arms" of a square; a voltage is applied to one diagonal pair of connections, while the voltage between the other diagonal pair is measured, e.g., by a galvanometer; the bridge is "balanced" when the measured voltage is zero; then, the ratios of the two pairs of adjoining resistances must be identical.

wheeze (wēz) **1.** To breathe with difficulty and noisily. **2.** A whistling, squeaking, musical, or puffing sound made by air passing through the fauces, glottis, or narrowed tracheobronchial airways in difficult breathing. [A.S. *hwēsan*]

whiff test (wif test) Procedure to find the fishy odor detectable when potassium hydroxide is applied to a sample of vaginal discharge in case of bacterial vaginosis.

whip•lash (wip′lash) SEE whiplash injury.

whip•lash in•ju•ry (wip′lash in′jŭr-ē) An imprecise term for various injuries resulting from sudden and violent hyperextension of the head on the trunk, followed by hyperflexion, as in a motor vehicle collision. Can include fractures, subluxations, sprains, muscle strains, and cerebral concussion. SYN acceleration-deceleration injury.

whip•lash ret•i•nop•a•thy (wip′lash ret′i-nop′ă-thē) An injury to the retina caused by a sudden acceleration-deceleration injury.

Whip•ple dis•ease (wip′ĕl di-zēz′) A rare disease characterized by steatorrhea, frequently generalized lymphadenopathy, arthritis, fever, and cough; many "foamy" macrophages are found in the jejunal lamina propria; caused by *Tropheryma whipplei*.

Whip•ple op•er•a•tion (wip′ĕl op-ĕr-ā′shŭn) SYN pancreatoduodenectomy.

whis•tle•blo•wing (wis′ĕl-blōw′ing) An employee's report of an employer's violation of the law. SEE ALSO standard precautions.

Whit•a•ker test (wit′ă-kĕr test) A pressure-perfusion test in the upper urinary tract to demonstrate impediment of flow.

white (wīt) The color resulting from commingling of all the rays of the spectrum; the color of chalk or of snow. SYN albicans (1). [A.S. *hwīt*]

white birch (wīt bĭrch) SYN birch.

white blood cell (WBC) (wīt blŭd sel) SYN leukocyte.

white coat hy•per•ten•sion (wīt kōt hī′pĕr-ten′shŭn) Frequent or continuous elevations of blood pressure in clinical settings that exceed those measured during ambulatory monitoring of the patient. SYN office hypertension.

white cor•pus•cle (wīt kōr′pŭs-ĕl) Any type of leukocyte.

white fi•ber (wīt fī′bĕr) **1.** White mammalian muscle fibers; larger in diameter than red fibers, they have less myoglobin, sarcoplasm, and mitochondria, and contract more quickly. **2.** SYN collagen fiber.

white gan•grene (wīt gang-grēn′) Death of a part accompanied by the formation of grayish-white sloughs.

white graft (wīt graft) Rejection of a skin allograft so acute that vascularization never occurs.

white•head (wīt′hed) **1.** SYN milium. **2.** SYN closed comedo.

White•head op•er•a•tion (wīt′hed op-ĕr-ā′shŭn) Excision of hemorrhoids by two circular incisions above and below involved veins, allowing normal mucosa to be pulled down and sutured to anal skin.

white in•farct (wīt in′fahrkt) **1.** SYN anemic infarct. **2.** In the placenta, intervillous fibrin with ischemic necrosis of villi.

white lim•bal gir•dle of Vogt (wīt lim′băl gĭr′dĕl fōkt) Symmetric arcuate yellow-white deposits in the peripheral cornea often seen in patients older than age 40 years.

white line (wīt līn) **1.** SYN linea alba. **2.** A pale streak appearing within 30–60 seconds after stroking of the skin with a fingernail, and lasting for several minutes; regarded as a sign of diminished arterial tension. SYN Sergent white line.

white line of a•nal ca•nal (wīt līn ā′năl kă-nal′) A bluish-pink, narrow, wavy zone in the mucosa of the anal canal below the pectinate line at the level of the interval between the subcutaneous part of the external sphincter and the lower border of the internal sphincter, said to be palpable.

white mat•ter (wīt mat′ĕr) Those regions of the brain and spinal cord that are largely or entirely composed of nerve fibers and contain few or no neuronal cell bodies or dendrites. SYN alba, white substance.

white mus•cle (wīt mŭs′ĕl) A rapid or fast-twitch muscle in which pale, large "white" fibers predominate; mitochondria and myoglobin are relatively sparse compared with red muscle; involved in phasic contraction.

whit•en•ing (wīt′ĕn-ing) Lightening of the teeth to a whiter color by use of dental bleaching materials.

white noise (wīt noyz) A complex sound consisting of many frequencies over a wide band of frequencies; often used for masking of hearing in the nontest ear in the measurement of hearing.

white pi•e•dra (wīt pē-ā′dră) Fungal disease of the beard, moustache, and genital areas, as well as the scalp, caused by *Trichosporon beigelii* and found in South America, Europe, and Japan; characterized by soft, mucilaginous, white-to-light-brown nodules within, as well as on, the hairs.

white pulp (wīt pŭlp) That part of the spleen that consists of nodules and other lymphatic concentrations.

white sub•stance (wīt sŭb′stăns) SYN white matter.

white-top tube (wīt-top tūb) This color indicates that the tube contains EDTA and a special polyester material—used for the collection of plasma for molecular (i.e., PCR) tests.

whit•low (wit′lō) SYN felon. [M.E. *whitflawe*]

Whit•man frame (wit′măn frām) A frame similar to the Bradford frame, but with curved sides.

WHO Abbreviation for World Health Organization.

whole blood (hōl blŭd) That drawn from a selected donor under rigid aseptic precautions; contains citrate ion or heparin as an anticoagulant; used as a blood replenisher.

whole-bod•y coun•ter (hōl-bod′ē kown′tĕr) Shielding and instrumentation, usually involving more than one detector, designed to evaluate the total-body burden of various gamma-emitting nuclides.

whole grains (hōl grānz) Grains that have not been processed to take away the outer layer where many nutrients lie.

whoop (hūp) The loud, sonorous inspiration in pertussis with which the paroxysm of coughing terminates, due to spasm of the larynx (glottis).

whoo•ping cough (hūp′ing kawf) SYN pertussis.

WHO probe (prōb) SYN World Health Organization probe.

whorl (wŏrl) **1.** A turn of the spiral cochlea of the ear. **2.** SYN vortex of heart. **3.** A turn of a concha nasalis. **4.** SYN verticil. **5.** An area of hair growing in a radial manner suggesting whirling or twisting. SYN vortex (2). SEE ALSO hair whorls. **6.** One of the distinguishing patterns in the Galton system of classification of fingerprints.

whorled (wŏrld) Marked by or arranged in whorls. SEE ALSO turbinate, verticillate.

whor•tle•ber•ry (wŏr′tĕl-ber-ē) SYN bilberry.

Wick•ham stri•a (wik′ăm strī′ă) A fine whitish line, appearing as part of a network on the surface of a lichen planus papule.

wide•band (wīd-band) A broad array of sound frequencies as opposed to a narrow array of frequencies.

wide dy•na•mic range com•pres•sion (wīd dī-nam′ik rānj kŏm-presh′ŭn) A hearing aid circuit in which amplification is increased across the frequency range at low input levels.

Wil•brand knee (wil′brand nē) Bundle of inferior nasal optic nerve fibers subserving the superior temporal visual field and crossing in the anterior optic chiasm, briefly entering the contralateral posterior optic nerve [CN II] before proceeding into the contralateral optic tract. Research indicates that this may be an artifact of retinal degeneration and not present in the normal anatomy.

Wil•der•muth ear (vil′der-mūt ēr) An ear in which the helix is turned backward and the anthelix is prominent.

Wil•der sign (wīl′dĕr sīn) A slight twitch of the eyeball when changing its movement from abduction to adduction or the reverse, noted in Graves disease.

Wil•der stain for re•tic•u•lum (wīl′dĕr stān rĕ-tik′yū-lŭm) A silver impregnation technique in which reticulum appears as black, well-defined fibers without beading and with a relatively clear background.

Wilde tri•an•gle (wīld trī′ang-gĕl) SYN light reflex (3).

wild go•bo (wīld gō′bō) SYN burdock.

wild type (wīld tīp) A gene, phenotype, or genotype that is overwhelmingly common among those possible at a locus of interest, and therefore presumably not harmful.

Wil•kie ar•ter•y (wil′kē ahr′tĕr-ē) The right colic artery when it occasionally crosses the duodenum.

Wil•liams-Beu•ren syn•drome (wil′yămz-byur′en sin′drōm) SYN Williams syndrome.

Wil•liams stain (wil′yămz stān) A stain for Negri bodies that uses picric acid, fuchsin, and methylene blue; Negri bodies are magenta, granules and nerve cells blue, and erythrocytes yellowish.

Wil•liams syn•drome (wil′yăms sin′drōm) Disorder characterized by distinctive facies with shallow supraorbital ridges, medial eyebrow flare, stellate patterning of the irises, small nose with anteverted nares, malar hypoplasia with droopy cheeks, full lips, supravalvar aortic stenosis, neonatal hypocalcemia, mild mental retardation, and loquacious personality. Autosomal dominant inheritance; this is a contiguous gene deletion syndrome and one of the genes mutated is the elastin gene (ELN) on chromosome 7q. SYN elfin facies syndrome, Williams-Beuren syndrome.

Wil•lis cords (wil′is kōrdz) Several fibrous cords crossing the superior sagittal sinus.

Wil•lis•ton law (wil′is-tŏn law) As the vertebrate scale is ascended, the number of bones in the cranium is reduced.

Wilms tu•mor (vilmz tū′mŏr) A malignant renal tumor of young children, composed of small spindle cells and various other types of tissue, including tubules and, in some cases, structures resembling fetal glomeruli, and striated muscle and cartilage. Often inherited as an autosomal dominant trait. See page B31. SYN nephroblastoma.

Wil•son block (wil′sŏn blok) The commonest form of right bundle-branch block, on electrocardiogram characterized in lead I by a tall, slender R wave followed by a wider S wave of lower voltage.

Wil•son dis•ease (wil′sŏn di-zēz′) **1.** A disorder of copper metabolism characterized by cirrhosis, basal ganglia degeneration, neurologic manifestations, and deposition of green or golden-brown pigment in the periphery of the cornea; the plasma levels of copper and ceruloplasmin are decreased, urinary excretion of copper is increased, and the amounts of copper in the liver, brain, kidneys, and lenticular nucleus are unusually high, while cytochrome oxidase is reduced; autosomal recessive inheritance caused by mutation in the copper-transporting ATPase gene (ATP7B) on chromosome 13q. SYN hepatolenticular degeneration (2), Westphal-Strümpell disease. SEE ALSO Kayser-Fleischer ring. **2.** SYN exfoliative dermatitis.

Wil•son meth•od (wil′sŏn meth′ŏd) A simple saline flotation method for concentrating helminth eggs in the feces. SEE ALSO flotation method. SYN Hung method.

Wil·son mus·cle (wil′sŏn mŭs′ĕl) SYN external urethral sphincter muscle.

Winck·el dis·ease (vink′el di-zēz′) SYN epidemic hemoglobinuria.

wind·burn (wind′bŭrn) Erythema of the face due to exposure to wind.

wind·chill in·dex (wind′chil in′deks) Measure of the environment's potential to cause cold injury, based on ambient air temperature and wind velocity.

win·dow (win′dō) SYN fenestra.

wind·pipe (wind′pīp) SYN trachea.

wind-suck·ing (wind′sŭk-ing) EQUINE VETERINARY MEDICINE a more severe form of crib-biting in which air is ingested abnormally and forcefully by swallowing. SEE ALSO aerophagia.

wing (wing) **1.** The anterior appendage of a bird. **2.** ANATOMY ala (q.v.).

Win·gate test (win′gāt test) Test of maximal anaerobic power output during 30 seconds of all-out exercise on either arm-crank or leg-cycle ergometer; a measure of maximal power output and capacity of immediate (ATP-PCRATP and PCr) and short-term (glycolytic) energy systems. [Test developed at Wingate Institute, Israel.]

wing-beat·ing tre·mor (wing′bēt-ing trem′ŏr) A coarse, irregular shaking movement that is most prominent when the limbs are held outstretched, reminiscent of a bird's flapping its wings; due to up-and-down excursion of arm at abducted shoulder. Seen mainly in Wilson disease.

winged cath·e·ter (wingd kath′ĕ-tĕr) A soft rubber catheter with little flaps at each side of the beak to retain it in the bladder.

winged in·fu·sion kit (wingd in-fyū′zhŭn kit) A fine-gauge needle with two flexible rubber wings for handling and a short piece of plastic tubing with an adapter instead of a hub; used for IV infusion and phlebotomy, especially in infants; used on a syringe or evacuated tube system for venipunctures. Also known as a butterfly needle.

winged scap·u·la (wingd skap′yū-lă) Condition in which the medial border of the scapula protrudes away from the thorax; the protrusion is posterior and lateral, as the scapula rotates out; caused by paralysis of the serratus anterior muscle. SYN scapula alata.

wing of nose (wing nōz) SYN ala of nose.

Wi·ni·war·ter-Man·teuf·fel-Buer·ger dis·ease (vē′nī-vahr-ter mahn-toy′fil bĕr′ger di-zēz′) SYN Buerger disease.

wink (wingk) To close and open the eyes rapidly; an involuntary act by which the tears are spread over the conjunctiva, keeping it moist. [A.S. *wincian*]

wink re·flex (wingk rē′fleks) General term for reflex closure of eyelids caused by any stimulus.

Win·ter·bot·tom sign (win′tĕr-bot′ŏm sīn) Swelling of the posterior cervical lymph nodes, characteristic of early stages of African trypanosomiasis; useful for surveys or control of migrations from endemic areas of people with preclinical infections.

Win·ter·nitz sound (vin′ter-nits sownd) A double-current catheter in which water at any desired temperature circulates.

wire (wīr) Slender and pliable rod or thread of metal.

wir·ing (wīr′ing) Fastening together the ends of a broken bone by wire sutures.

Wir·sung ca·nal, **Wir·sung duct** (vēr′sung kă-nal′, dŭkt) SYN pancreatic duct.

wir·y (wīr′ē) Resembling or having the feel of a wire; filiform and hard; denoting a variety of pulse.

wir·y pulse (wīr′ē pŭls) A small, fine, incompressible pulse.

wis·dom tooth (wiz′dŏm tūth) SYN third molar tooth.

Wis·sler-Fan·co·ni syn·drome (vis′ler-fahn-kō′nē sin′drōm) SYN Wissler syndrome.

Wis·sler sub·sep·sis al·ler·gi·ca (vis′ler sŭb-sep′sis a-lĕr′ji-kă) SYN Wissler syndrome.

Wis·sler syn·drome (vis′ler sin′drōm) High intermittent fever; irregularly recurring macular and maculopapular eruption of the face, chest and limbs; leukocytosis; arthralgia; occasionally eosinophilia; and raised erythrocyte sedimentation rate. Condition occurs in children and adolescents, with varying duration. In early stages, it is difficult to differentiate from septicemia. SYN Wissler subsepsis allergica, Wissler-Fanconi syndrome.

witch's milk (wich′ĕz milk) A secretion of colostrumlike milk sometimes occurring in the glands of newborn infants of either sex 3–4 days after birth and lasting 1–2 weeks due to endocrine stimulation from the mother before birth.

with·draw·al (with-draw′ăl) **1.** The act of removal or retreat. **2.** A psychological and physical syndrome caused by the abrupt cessation of the use of a drug in a habituated person. **3.** The therapeutic process of discontinuing a drug so as to avoid withdrawal (2). **4.** A pattern of behavior observed in schizophrenia and depression, characterized by a pathologic retreat from interpersonal contact and social involvement and leading to self-preoccupation. **5.** SYN coitus interruptus.

with·draw·al symp·toms (with-draw′ăl simp′tŏmz) A group of morbid symptoms, predominantly erethistic, occurring in an addict who is deprived of the accustomed dose of the addicting agent.

with·draw·al syn·drome (with-draw′ăl sin′drōm) A substance-specific syndrome that follows the cessation of, or reduction in, intake of a psychoactive substance previously used regularly. The syndrome that develops varies according to the psychoactive substance used. Common symptoms include anxiety, restlessness, irritability, insomnia, and impaired attention.

WLU Abbreviation for workload unit.

WMD Abbreviation for weapons of mass destruction.

wob·ble (wob′ĕl) MOLECULAR BIOLOGY unorthodox pairing between the base at the 5′ end of an anticodon and the base that pairs with it (in the 3′ position of the codon).

wolf bane (wulf bān) SYN arnica.

Wolfe graft (wulf graft) A full-thickness skin graft without any subcutaneous fat.

wolff·i·an (vōlf′ē-ăn) Relating to or described by Kaspar Wolff.

wolff·i·an body (vōlf′ē-ăn bod′ē) SYN mesonephros.

wolff·i·an cyst (vōlf′ē-ăn sist) A cyst in the broad ligament of the uterus and arising from remnants of the mesonephric ducts.

wolff·i·an duct (vōlf′ē-ăn dŭkt) SYN mesonephric duct.

wolff·i·an rest (vōlf′ē-ăn rest) Remnants of the wolffian duct in the female genital tract that give rise to cysts; e.g., Gartner duct cyst.

Wolff law (vōlf law) **1.** Every change in the form and the function of a bone is followed by changes in the bone's internal architecture and secondary alterations in its external conformation; these changes usually represent responses to alterations in weight-bearing stresses. **2.** Bone forms in areas of stress and is resorbed in areas of nonstress.

Wolff-Par·kin·son-White syn·drome (wulf′park′in-sŏn-wīt′ sin′drōm) An electrocardiographic pattern sometimes associated with paroxysmal tachycardia; it consists of a short P-R interval (usually 0.1 second or less; occasionally normal) together with a prolonged QRS complex with a slurred initial component (delta wave). SYN preexcitation syndrome.

wolf·ram, wolf·ram·i·um (wulf′răm, -ram′ē-ŭm) SYN tungsten. [from *wolframite*]

Wolf·ram syndrome (wulf′răm sin′drōm) A disorder consisting of diabetes insipidus, diabetes mellitus, optic atrophy, and deafness; the genetic abnormality is located on chromosome 4p; autosomal recessive inheritance.

Wol·las·ton dou·blet (wol′ăs-tŏn dŭb′lĕt) A combination of two planoconvex lenses in the eyepiece of a microscope designed to correct the chromatic aberration.

Wol·man dis·ease (wōl′mahn di-zēz′) SYN cholesterol ester storage disease.

Wol·man xan·tho·ma·to·sis (wōl′mahn zan′thō-mă-tō′sis) SYN cholesterol ester storage disease.

womb (wūm) SYN uterus. [A.S. the belly]

Wood glass (wud glas) A glass containing nickel oxide, used in a Wood lamp.

Wood lamp (wud lamp) An ultraviolet lamp with a nickel oxide filter that only passes light with a maximal wavelength of about 3660 Å; used to detect by fluorescence hairs infected with species of *Microsporum audouinii*, *M. canis*, var. *distortum*, or *M. ferrugineum*, which fluoresce greenish-yellow.

Wood light (wud līt) Ultraviolet light produced by a Wood lamp.

wood sour (wud sowr) SYN barberry.

word deaf·ness (wŏrd def′nĕs) SYN auditory aphasia.

word sal·ad (wŏrd sal′ăd) A jumble of meaningless and unrelated words emitted by people with certain kinds of schizophrenia.

work (wŏrk) Effort or activity performed to achieve a goal or produce something. [O.E. *weorc*]

work·a·hol·ic (wŏrk′a-hol′ik) A person who manifests a compulsive need to work, even at the expense of family responsibilities, social life, and health. [by analogy with *alcoholic*]

work of breath·ing (wŏrk brēdh′ing) The total expenditure of energy necessary to accomplish the act of breathing; may be computed in terms of the pulmonary pressure multiplied by the change in pulmonary volume, or in terms of the oxygen cost of breathing (i.e., the O_2 consumption above basal metabolic O_2 use attributable to breathing).

Work-Ca·pac·i·ty E·val·u·a·tion (wŏrk-kă-pas′i-tē ē-val′yū-ā′shŭn) SYN functional capacity evaluation.

work con·di·tion·ing (wŏrk kŏn-dish′ŏn-ing) A treatment program focused on functional requirements of a job or employment setting, incorporating the basic components of physical conditioning such as strength, endurance, flexibility, and coordination. A component of an industrial therapy program that serves as a precursor to a work hardening program; it is undertaken after acute care or basic rehabilitation treatment has been completed.

work·ers' com·pen·sa·tion (WC) (wŏr′kĕrz kom′pĕn-sā′shŭn) The U.S. social insurance system for industrial and work injuries regulated at a state level. Sometimes called workman's compensation.

work·ers' com·pen·sa·tion law (wŏr′kĕrz kom′pĕn-sā′shŭn law) A U.S. statute imposing liability on employers to pay benefits and furnish care to job-injured employees and to pay benefits to dependents of employees killed in the course of, and because of, their employment.

work hard·en·ing (wŏrk hahr′dĕn-ing) A multidisciplinary progam where actual work tasks are performed to rehabilitate an injured worker. The focus of therapy is to stimulate a regular work routine where therapy is regimented as a precursor to return to work. SEE ALSO work conditioning.

Work·ing Form·u·la·tion for Clin·ic·al Us·age (WF) (wŏrk′ing for′myū-lā′shŭn klin′i-kăl yū′săj) Classification of malignant lymphomas introduced by the National Cancer Institute in 1982, based on the correlation of clinical and histopathologic features of various lymphomas; widely used in clinical practice.

work·ing out (wŏrk′ing owt) PSYCHOANALYSIS the stage in the treatment process in which the patient's personal history and psychodynamics are uncovered.

work·ing side (wŏrk′ing sīd) The segment of a denture or dentition toward which the lower jaw is moved, the functioning side of the dentition. Cf. balancing side.

work·ing through (wŏrk′ing thrū) PSYCHOANALYSIS the process of obtaining additional insight and personality changes in a patient through repeated and varied examination of a conflict or problem; the interactions between free association, resistance, interpretation, and working out are the chief parts of this process.

work·load u·nit (WLU) (wŏrk′lōd yū′nit) A unit of work used to calculate productivity (e.g., billable procedures or patient visits).

World Health Or·gan·i·za·tion (WHO) (wŏrld helth ōr′găn-ī-zā′shŭn) A unit of the United Nations devoted to international health problems.

World Health Or·gan·i·za·tion probe (wŏrld helth ōr′găn-ī-zā′shŭn prōb) A periodontal probe developed by the World Health Organization and used with the Periodontal Screening and Recording (PSR) System for periodontal assessment. The WHO probe has a colored band (called the reference marking) located 3.5–5.5 mm from the probe tip. This colored reference marking is used when performing a PSE screening examination on dental patients. SYN WHO probe.

worm (wŏrm) **1.** ANATOMY any structure resembling a worm, e.g., the midline part of the cerebellum in the forms of "vermis" and "lumbrical." **2.** Term once used to designate any member of the invertebrate group or former subkingdom Vermes, a collective term no longer used taxonomically; now commonly used to designate any member of the separate phyla Annelida (the segmented or true worms), Nematoda (roundworms), and Platyhelminthes (flatworms). Important species include *Dracunculus medinensis* (dragon, guinea, Medina, or serpent worm), *Enterobius vermicularis* (seat worm or pinworm), *Loa loa* (African eye worm), *Moniliformis* (phylum Acanthocephala, thorny-headed worms), *Oxyspirura mansoni* (Manson eye worm), *Pentastomida* (tongue worm), *Strongylus* (palisade worm), *Thelazia* (eye worm), and *Trichinella spiralis* (pork or trichina worm). [A.S. *wyrm*]

wor·mi·an (wŏrm′ē-ăn) Relating to or described by Ole Worm.

wor·mi·an bones (wŏrm′ē-ăn bōnz) SYN sutural bones.

worm·wood (wŏrm′wud) SYN absinthe.

Worth am·bly·o·scope (wŏrth am′blē-ō-skōp) A hand-held amblyoscope consisting of angled tubes that can be swiveled to any degree of convergence or divergence.

Woulfe bot·tle (wulf bot′ĕl) A bottle with two or three necks, used in a series, connected with tubes, for working with gases (washing, drying, absorbing).

wound (wūnd) **1.** Trauma to any of the tissues of the body, especially that caused by physical means and with interruption of continuity. **2.** A surgical incision. See page 1683. [O.E. *wund*]

wound clip (wūnd klip) A metal clasp or device for surgical approximation of skin incisions.

wound i·so·la·tion (wūnd ī′sŏ-lā′shŭn) Isolation used to protect the medical worker when a patient has an open wound; also known as "skin isolation."

wo·ven bone (wō′vĕn bōn) Bony tissue characteristic of the embryonal skeleton, in which the collagen fibers of the matrix are arranged irregularly in the form of interlacing networks. SYN nonlamellar bone, reticulated bone.

W-plas·ty (plas′tē) Surgery to prevent the contracture of a straight-line scar; the edges of the wound are trimmed in the shape of a W, or a series of Ws, and closed in a zig-zag manner.

Wright stain (rīt stān) A staining mixture of eosinates of polychromed methylene blue used in staining of blood smears.

Wright syn·drome (rīt sin′drōm) SYN thoracic outlet syndrome.

Wright ver·sion (rīt vĕr′zhŭn) A cephalic version employed in cases of shoulder presentation

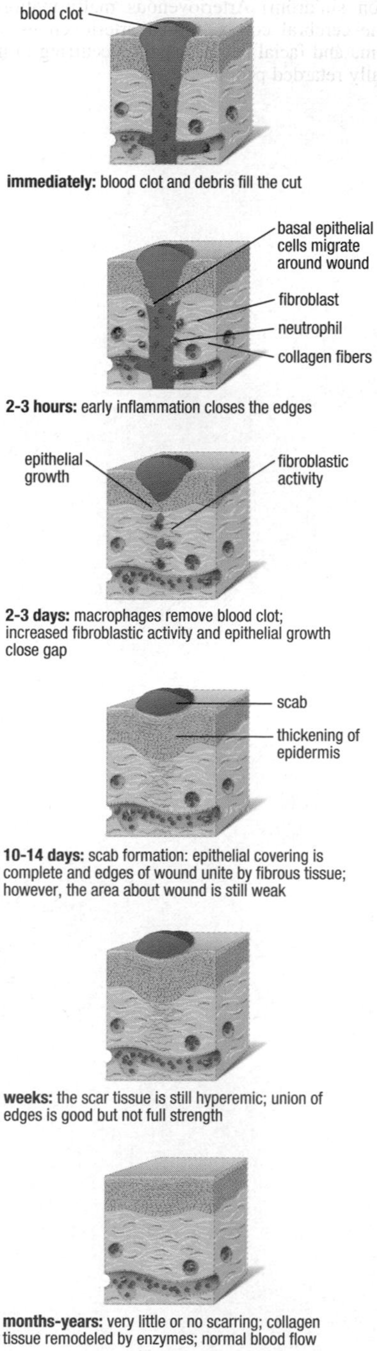
blood clot
immediately: blood clot and debris fill the cut
basal epithelial cells migrate around wound
fibroblast
neutrophil
collagen fibers
2-3 hours: early inflammation closes the edges
epithelial growth
fibroblastic activity
2-3 days: macrophages remove blood clot; increased fibroblastic activity and epithelial growth close gap
scab
thickening of epidermis
10-14 days: scab formation: epithelial covering is complete and edges of wound unite by fibrous tissue; however, the area about wound is still weak
weeks: the scar tissue is still hyperemic; union of edges is good but not full strength
months-years: very little or no scarring; collagen tissue remodeled by enzymes; normal blood flow

wound healing

when the shoulders are pushed upward while the breech is moved toward the center of the uterus by the other hand; the head is then guided into the pelvis.

Wris•berg nerve (ris′berg nĕrv) SYN medial cutaneous nerve of forearm.

wrist (rist) The proximal segment of the hand consisting of the carpal bones and the associated soft parts. See page A8. SYN carpus (1) [TA]. [A.S. wrist joint, ankle joint]

wrist-drop (rist drop) Paralysis of the extensors of the wrist and fingers; most often caused by lesion of the radial nerve. SYN drop hand.

wrist-hand or•tho•sis (rist-hand ōr-thō′sis) A device that begins at the fingers, crosses the wrist, and terminates on the distal portion of the forearm; used to provide grasp and release despite some degree of hand paralysis.

wrist joint (rist joynt) The synovial articulation between the distal end of the radius and its articular disc and the proximal row of carpal bones with the exception of the pisiform bone. SYN carpal joints (2), radiocarpal joint.

wrist sign (rist sīn) In Marfan syndrome, when the wrist is gripped with the opposite hand, the thumb and fifth finger overlap appreciably.

write off (rīt awf) An amount deducted from a patient's account balance due to a contracted negotiation or other factor (e.g., pro bono work).

writ•ing (rīt′ing) **1.** The act of forming letters to produce a visible and intelligible body of coherent language. **2.** The product of such activity.

writ•ing hand (rīt′ing hand) A contraction of the hand muscles in parkinsonism, bringing the fingers somewhat into the position of holding a pen.

wry•neck, **wry neck** (rī-nek′, rī nek) SYN torticollis.

Wu•cher•e•ri•a (vū-kĕr-ē′rē-ă) A genus of filarial nematodes characterized by adult forms that live chiefly in lymphatic vessels and produce large numbers of embryos or microfilariae that circulate in the bloodstream (microfilaremia), often appearing in the peripheral blood at regular intervals. The extreme form of this infection (wuchereriasis or filariasis) is elephantiasis or pachydermia.

Wu•cher•e•ri•a ban•crof•ti (vū-kĕr-ē′rē-ă ban-krof′tī) The bancroftian filaria, transmitted to humans (apparently the only definitive host) by mosquitoes, especially *Culex quinquefasciatus* and *Aedes pseudoscutellaris*, but also by several other species of *Culex*, *Aedes*, *Anopheles*, and *Mansonia*, depending on the specific geographic area; adults are white, threadlike worms, and the microfilariae are ensheathed, with rounded anterior end and tapered, nonnucleated tail; the adult worms inhabit the larger lymphatic vessels (e.g., in the extremities, breasts, spermatic cord, and retroperitoneal tissues) and the sinuses of lymph nodes, where they sometimes cause temporary obstruction of lymph flow and slight or moderate inflammation. See page B7.

wu•cher•e•ri•a•sis (vū′kĕr-ē-rī′ă-sis) Infection with worms of the genus *Wuchereria*. SEE ALSO filariasis.

Wy•burn-Ma•son syn•drome (wī′bŭrn-mā′sŏn sin′drōm) Arteriovenous malformation on the cerebral cortex, retinal arteriovenous angioma and facial nevus, usually occurring in mentally retarded people.

X Abbreviation for reactance; xanthosine; halogen atom; unspecified amino acid; reactance.

xanthaemia [Br.] SYN xanthemia.

xan•the•las•ma (zan-thĕ-laz′mă) SYN xanthelasma palpebrarum. [xanth- + G. *elasma,* a beaten metal plate]

xan•the•las•ma pal•pe•bra•rum (zan-thĕ-laz′mă pal-pē-brā′rŭm) Soft, yellow-orange plaques on the eyelids or medial canthus, the most common form of xanthoma; may be associated with low-density lipoproteins, especially in younger adults. See this page. SYN xanthelasma.

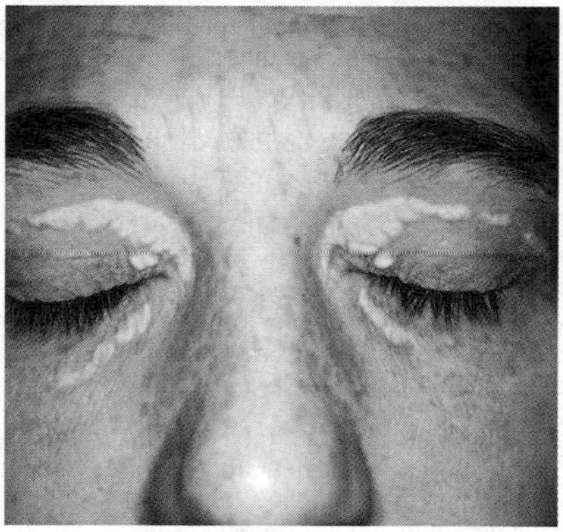

xanthelasma palpebrarum

xan•the•mi•a (zan-thē′mē-ă) SYN carotenemia. SYN xanthaemia. [xanth- + G. *haima,* blood]

xan•thene dye (zan′thēn dī) Derivative of the compound xanthene.

xan•thic (zan′thik) **1.** Yellow or yellowish in color. **2.** Relating to xanthine.

xan•thine (zan′thēn) Oxidation product of guanine and hypoxanthine, precursor of uric acid; occurs in many organs and in the urine, occasionally forming urinary calculi.

xan•thism (zan′thizm) A pigmentary anomaly in some black people, characterized by red or yellow-red hair color, copper-red skin, and often dilution of iris pigment. [G. *xanthos,* yellowish]

xantho-, xanth- Combining forms meaning yellow, yellowish. [G. *xanthos*]

xan•tho•chro•mat•ic (zan′thō-krō-mat′ik) Yellow-colored. SYN xanthochromic.

xan•tho•chro•mi•a (zan′thō-krō′mē-ă) The occurrence of patches of yellow color in the skin, resembling xanthoma, but without the nodules or plates. SYN xanthoderma (1). [xantho- + G. *chrōma,* color]

xan•tho•chro•mic (zan′thō-krō′mik) SYN xanthochromatic.

xan•tho•der•ma (zan′thō-dĕr′mă) **1.** SYN xanthochromia. **2.** Any yellow coloration of the skin. [xantho- + G. *derma,* skin]

xan•tho•gran•u•lo•ma (zan′thō-gran′yū-lō′mă) A peculiar infiltration of retroperitoneal tissue by lipid macrophages, occurring more commonly in women. See this page.

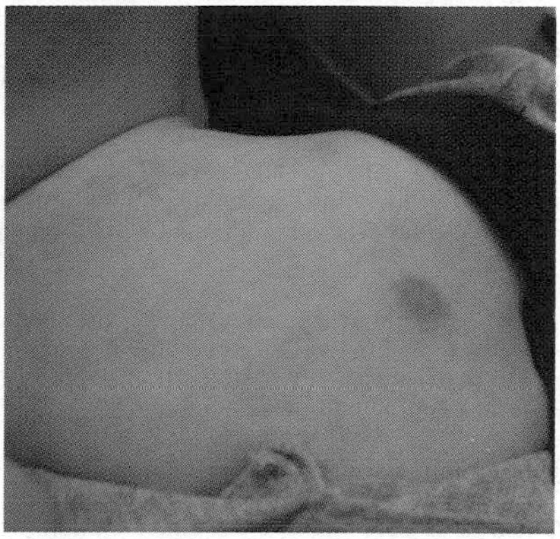

xanthogranuloma: scapular area, juvenile patient

xan•tho•ma (zan-thō′mă) A yellow nodule or plaque, especially of the skin, composed of lipid-laden histiocytes. [xantho- + G. *-oma,* tumor]

xan•tho•ma dis•sem•i•na•tum (zan-thō′mă dis-sem′i-nā′tŭm) A rare benign normolipemic disorder of adults with coalescent cutaneous xanthomas composed of non-X histiocytes on flexural surfaces, often with mild diabetes insipidus.

xan•tho•ma mul•ti•plex (zan-thō′mă mul′tē-pleks) SYN xanthomatosis.

xan•tho•ma pla•num (zan-thō′mă plā′num) A form marked by the occurrence of yellow, flat bands or minimally palpable rectangular plates in the corium, either normolipemic or associated with type IIa or III hyperlipoproteinemia.

xan•tho•ma•to•sis (zan′thō-mă-tō′sis) Widespread xanthomas, especially on the elbows and knees, that sometimes affect mucous membranes and are sometimes associated with metabolic disturbances. SYN lipid granulomatosis, lipoid granulomatosis, xanthoma multiplex.

xan•tho•ma•to•sis bul•bi (zan′thō-mă-tō′sis bŭl′bī) Ulcerative fatty degeneration of the cornea after injury.

xan•tho•ma•tous (zan-thō′mă-tŭs) Relating to xanthoma.

xan•tho•ma tu•ber•o•sum (zan-thō′mă tū-bĕr-ō′sum) Xanthomatosis associated with familial type II, and occasionally type III, hyperlipoproteinemia.

xan·tho·phyll (zan′thō-fil) Oxygenated derivative of carotene; a yellow plant pigment, occurring also in egg yolk and corpus luteum. SYN lutein (2).

xan·thop·si·a (zan-thop′sē-ă) A condition in which objects appear yellow; may occur in picric acid and santonin poisoning, in jaundice, and in digitalis intoxication. [xantho- + G. *opsis,* vision]

xan·tho·sine (X, Xao) (zan′thō-sēn) The deamination product of guanosine (O replacing $-NH_2$).

xan·tho·sis (zan-thō′sis) A yellowish discoloration of degenerating tissues, especially seen in malignant neoplasms. [xantho- + G. *-osis,* condition]

Xao Abbreviation for xanthosine.

X chro·mo·some, Y chro·mo·some (krō′mŏ-sōm) SEE sex chromosomes.

Xe Symbol for xenon.

xe·nic cul·ture (zen′ik kŭl′chŭr) Cultures of parasites grown in association with unknown microbiota. [G. *xenikos,* alien, foreign, fr. *xenos,* guest, stranger]

♻**xeno-** Combining form meaning strange; foreign material; parasite. SEE ALSO hetero-, allo-. [G. *xenos,* guest, host, stranger, foreign]

xen·o·bi·ot·ic (zen′ō-bī-ot′ik) A pharmacologically, endocrinologically, or toxicologically active substance not endogenously produced and therefore foreign to an organism.

xen·o·di·ag·no·sis (zen′ō-dī′ăg-nō′sis) **1.** A method of diagnosing acute or early *Trypanosoma cruzi* infection (Chagas disease) in humans. Infection-free triatomine insects are permitted to feed on the person thought to be infected, and the trypanosome is identified by microscopic examination of the intestinal contents of the insect after a suitable incubation period. **2.** A similar method of biologic diagnosis based on experimental exposure of a parasite-free normal host capable of allowing the organism in question to multiply, enabling it to be more easily and reliably detected.

xen·o·ge·ne·ic (zen′ō-jĕ-nē′ik) Heterologous, with respect to tissue grafts, especially when donor and recipient belong to widely separated species. SYN xenogenic (2), xenogenous (2). [xeno- + G. *-gen,* producing]

xen·o·gen·ic (zen′ō-jen′ik) **1.** Originating outside the organism, or from a foreign substance that has been introduced into the organism. SYN xenogenous (1). **2.** SYN xenogeneic. [xeno- + G. *-gen,* producing]

xe·nog·e·nous (zĕ-noj′ĕ-nŭs) **1.** SYN xenogenic (1). **2.** SYN xenogeneic.

xen·o·graft (zen′ō-graft) A graft transferred from an animal of one species to one of another species. SYN heterograft, heterologous graft.

xe·non (Xe) (zē′non) A gaseous element, atomic no. 54, atomic wt. 131.29, present in minute proportion in the atmosphere; produces general anesthesia in concentrations of 70 vol.%. [G. *xenos,* a stranger]

xe·non 133 (zē′non) A radioisotope of xenon with a gamma emission at 81 keV and a physical half-life of 5.243 days; used in the study of pulmonary function and organ blood flow.

xen·o·par·a·site (zen′ō-par′ă-sīt) An ecoparasite that becomes pathogenic in consequence of weakened resistance on the part of its host.

xen·o·pho·bi·a (zen′ō-fō′bē-ă) Morbid fear of strangers or foreigners. [xeno- + G. *phobos,* fear]

Xen·op·syl·la (zen′op-sil′ă) A genus of fleas parasitic on the rat and involved in the transmission of bubonic plague. *Xenopsylla cheopis* serves as a potent vector of *Yersinia pestis; X. astia* and *X. braziliensis* are also efficient vectors of plague. [xeno- + G. *psylla,* flea]

xen·o·tro·pic vi·rus (zen′ō-trō′pik vī′rŭs) A retrovirus that does not produce disease in its natural host and replicates only in tissue culture cells derived from a different species.

♻**xero-** Prefix meaning dry. [G. *xeros*]

xe·ro·chi·li·a (zēr′ō-kī′lē-ă) Dryness of lips. [xero- + G. *cheilos,* lip]

xe·ro·der·ma (zēr′ō-dĕr′mă) A mild form of ichthyosis characterized by excessive dryness of the skin due to slight increase of the horny layer and diminished water content of the stratum corneum from decreased perspiration, wind, or low humidity; seen with aging, atopic dermatitis, and vitamin A deficiency. [xero- + G. *derma,* skin]

xe·ro·der·ma pig·men·to·sum (zēr′ō-dĕr′mă pig-men-tō′sŭm) An eruption of exposed skin occurring in childhood and characterized by photosensitivity with severe sunburn in infancy and the development of numerous pigmented spots resembling freckles, larger atrophic lesions eventually resulting in glossy white thinning of the skin surrounded by telangiectases, and multiple solar keratoses that undergo malignant change at an early age. Severe ophthalmic and neurologic abnormalities are also found.

xe·ro·ma (zēr-ō′mă) SYN xerophthalmia.

xer·oph·thal·mi·a (zēr′of-thal′mē-ă) Excessive dryness of the conjunctiva and cornea, which lose their luster and become keratinized; may be due to local disease or to a systemic deficiency of vitamin A. SYN xeroma. [xero- + G. *ophthalmos,* eye]

xe•ro•sis (zēr-ō′sis) Pathologic dryness of the skin (xeroderma), the conjunctiva (xerophthalmia), or mucous membranes. See this page. [xero- + G. *-osis,* condition]

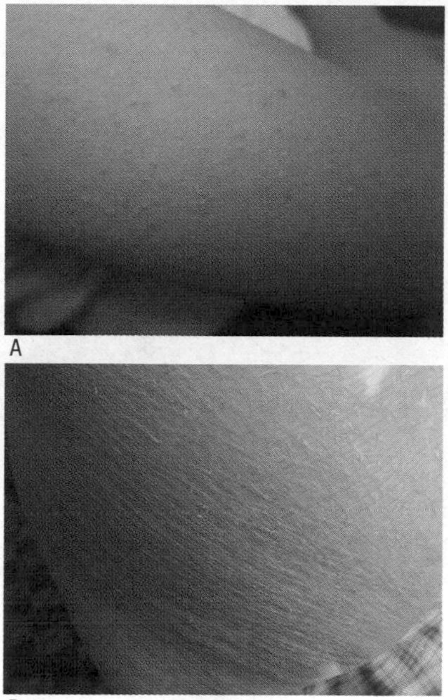

A
B
xerosis: (A) arm; (B) buttocks

xe•ro•sto•mi•a (zēr′ō-stō′mē-ă) A dryness of the mouth, having a varied etiology, resulting from diminished or arrested salivary secretion, or asialism. [xero- + G. *stoma,* mouth]

xe•rot•ic (zēr-ot′ik) Dry; affected with xerosis.

X-in•ac•ti•va•tion (in-ak′ti-vā′shŭn) SYN lyonization.

xiph•i•ster•nal (zif′i-stĕr′năl) Relating to the xiphoid process.

xiph•i•ster•num (zif′i-stĕr′nŭm) SYN xiphoid process. [xiphoid + G. *sternon,* chest]

xipho-, xiph-, xiphi- Combining forms meaning xiphoid, usually the processus xiphoideus. [G. *xiphos,* sword]

xi•phoid (zī′foyd) Sword-shaped; applied especially to the xiphoid process. SYN ensiform. [xipho- + G. *eidos,* appearance]

xi•phoid car•ti•lage (zī′foyd kahr′ti-lăj) SYN xiphoid process.

xi•phoid•i•tis (zī′foyd-ī′tis) Inflammation of the xiphoid process of the sternum. [xiphoid + G. *-itis,* inflammation]

xi•phoid pro•cess (zī′foyd pros′es) The cartilage at the lower end of the sternum. SYN processus xiphoideus [TA], ensiform process, xiphisternum, xiphoid cartilage.

xi•phoid pro•cess of ster•num (zī′foyd pros′es stĕr′nŭm) The cartilage at the lower end of the sternum.

X-linked (lingkt) Pertaining to genes borne on the X chromosome. Commonly but erroneously used synonymously with sex-linked, which would also comprise Y-linked traits.

X-linked gene (lingkt jēn) A gene located on an X chromosome.

X-linked hy•po•gam•ma•glob•u•lin•e•mi•a, X-linked in•fan•tile hy•po•gam•ma•glob•u•lin•e•mi•a (lingkt hī′pō-gam′ă-glob′yū-li-nē′mē-ă, in′făn-tīl) A congenital, X-linked recessive, primary immunodeficiency characterized by decreased numbers (or absence) of circulating B-lymphocytes with corresponding decrease in immunoglobulins; associated with marked susceptibility to infection by pyogenic bacteria after loss of maternal antibodies.

X-linked lym•pho•pro•lif•er•a•tive syn•drome (lingkt lim′fō-prō-lif′ĕr-ă-tiv sin′drōm) An X-linked recessive immunodeficiency and lymphoproliferative disease caused by mutation in the SH2 domain protein 1A gene (SH2D1A) on Xq; characterized by defective cellular or humoral immune response to Epstein-Barr virus; manifestations include fulminant infectious mononucleosis, B-cell malignancies, and hypogammaglobulinemia. SYN Duncan disease.

X-linked re•ces•sive bul•bo•spi•nal neur•on•op•a•thy (lingkt rĕ-ses′iv bŭl′bō-spī′năl nūr′on-op′ă-thē) SYN Kennedy disease.

XO syn•drome (sin′drōm) SYN Turner syndrome.

X-pat•tern es•o•tro•pi•a (pat′ĕrn ē′sō-trō′pē-ă) Decreasing convergence from the primary position in both upward and downward gaze.

X-pat•tern ex•o•tro•pi•a (pat′ĕrn ek′sō-trō′pē-ă) Increasing divergence from the primary position in both upward and downward gaze.

x-ray (rā) **1.** The ionizing electromagnetic radiation emitted from a highly evacuated tube, resulting from the excitation of the inner orbital electrons by the bombardment of the target anode with a stream of electrons from a heated cathode. **2.** Ionizing electromagnetic radiation produced by the excitation of the inner orbital electrons of an atom by other processes, such as nuclear delay and its sequelae. **3.** A radiograph. SYN roentgen ray.

x-ray mi•cro•scope (rā mī′krŏ-skōp) A microscope in which images are obtained by using x-rays as an energy source that are recorded on a very fine-grained film, or the image is enlarged by projection; if film is used, it may be examined with the light microscope at fairly high magnifications.

XXY syn•drome (sin′drōm) SYN Klinefelter syndrome.

xy•lose (zī′lōs) An aldopentose, isomeric with ribose, obtained by fermentation or hydrolysis of carbohydrate.

xy•lu•lose (zī′lyū-lōs) *Threo*-pentulose; a ketopentose that appears in the urine in cases of essential pentosuria; it is also an intermediate in the glucuronate pathway.

xys•ma (zis′mă) Membranous shreds in the feces. [G. filings, shavings, fr. *xyō,* to scrape]

XYY syn•drome (sin′drōm) Aneuploidy with a supernumerary Y chromosome; associated with increased stature, aggressiveness, hyperactive behavior, mental retardation, and acne.

Y

Y 1. Symbol for yttrium. 2. Abbreviation for tyrosine; pyrimidine nucleoside.

y⁺ SEE system (5).

YAG (yag) Acronym for yttrium-aluminum-garnet.

Yan·kau·er suc·tion cath·e·ter (yang′kow-ĕr sŭk′shŭn kath′ĕ-tĕr) A form of rigid catheter. See this page.

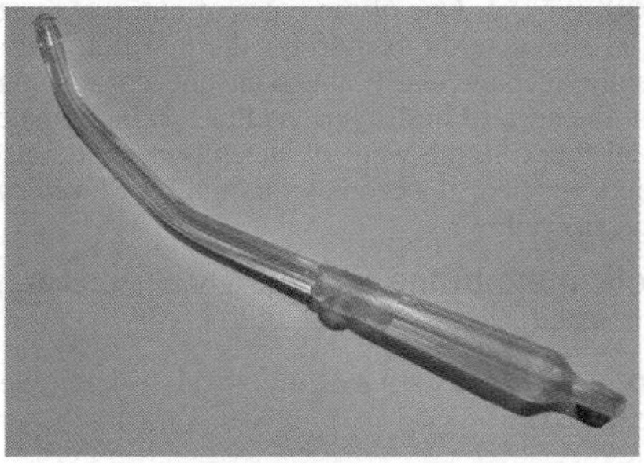

Yankauer suction catheter

yaw (yaw) An individual lesion of the eruption of yaws.

yawn (yawn) 1. To gape. 2. An involuntary opening of the mouth, usually accompanied by a movement of respiration; it may be a sign of drowsiness or of vital depression, as after hemorrhage, but is often caused by suggestion. [A.S. *gānian*]

yaws (yawz) An infectious tropical disease caused by *Treponema pertenue* characterized by the development of crusted granulomatous ulcers on the extremities; may involve bone, but, unlike syphilis, does not produce central nervous system or cardiovascular pathology. SYN boubas, bubas, frambesia, granuloma tropicum, pian, rupia (2). [of Caribbean origin; similar to Calinago *yaya*, the disease]

Yb Symbol for ytterbium.

Y car·ti·lage, Y-shaped car·ti·lage (kahr′ti-lăj, shāpt) The connecting cartilage for the ilium, ischium, and pubis; it extends through the acetabulum.

years of po·ten·tial life lost (yērz pŏ-ten′shăl līf lawst) Measure of the relative impact of various diseases and lethal forces on society, computed by estimating the number of years that people would have lived if they had not died prematurely.

yeast (yēst) A general term denoting true fungi of the family Saccharomycetaceae that are widely distributed in substrates that contain sugars (such as fruits), and in soil, animal excreta, and the vegetative parts of plants. Because of their ability to ferment carbohydrates, some yeasts are important to the brewing and baking industries. [A.S. *gyst*]

yel·low a·tro·phy of the liv·er (yel′ō at′rŏ-fē liv′ĕr) SEE acute yellow atrophy of the liver.

yel·low and black-top tube (yel′ō blak-top tūb) A container so colored is used for mycobacteria, fungal, or AFB blood cultures.

yel·low car·ti·lage (yel′ō kahr′ti-lăj) SYN elastic cartilage.

yel·low fe·ver (yel′ō fē′vĕr) A tropical mosquito-borne viral hepatitis, caused by one of the yellow fever viruses, with an urban form transmitted by *Aedes aegypti* and a rural, jungle, or sylvatic form from tree-dwelling mammals by various mosquitoes of the *Haemagogus* species complex; characterized clinically by fever, slow pulse, albuminuria, jaundice, congestion of the face, and hemorrhages, especially hematemesis; immunity to reinfection accompanies recovery.

yel·low fi·bers (yel′ō fī′bĕrz) SYN elastic fibers.

yel·low gin·seng (yel′ō jin′seng) SYN blue cohosh.

yel·low hep·a·ti·za·tion (yel′ō hep′ă-tī-zā′shŭn) The final stage of hepatization, in which the exudate is becoming purulent.

yel·low lead·er (yel′ō lē′dĕr) SYN *Astragalus.*

yel·low paint (yel′ō pānt) SYN goldenseal.

yel·low puc·coon (yel′ō pŭ-kūn′) SYN goldenseal.

yel·low rain (yel′ō rān) A smoke, mist, or powder of various colors reported in Southeast Asia during the Vietman War and variously alleged to contain T-2 mycotoxin or to consist only of bee pollen.

yel·low-top tube (yel′ō-top tūb) A tube of this color indicates the container has been treated with ACD, which is used for the collection of whole blood for special tests including flow cytometry and tissue typing assays.

yer·ba ma·té (yĕr′bă mah′tā) (*Ilex paraguariensis*) A popular beverage in South America, infusions of this herb are alleged to have value as an analgesic, antidepressant, cathartic, and diuretic. Approved for use in Germany as a stimulant. Adverse reactions include hepatotoxicity, nervousness and irritability, neurologic disorders, and increased cancer risk with prolonged consumption. SYN Bartholomew's tea, gaucho tea, yi-yi. [Sp. *yerbe,* herb, + *mate,* maté]

Yer·ga·son test (yĕr′gă-sŏn test) Maneuver to diagnose bicipital tendinitis. With the elbow flexed at 90°, and while the forearm is pronated, the patient supinates the forearm, flexes the elbow, and externally rotates the humerus while the examiner resists these movements and applies downward traction to the elbow. The test result is positive if it elicits pain over the bicipital groove or if the tendon snaps out of the groove.

Yer·sin·i·a (yĕr-sin′ē-ă) A genus of motile and nonmotile, non-spore-forming bacteria containing gram-negative, unencapsulated, ovoid to rod-shaped cells. These organisms are parasitic on humans and other animals. The type species is *Yersinia pestis.*

Yer·sin·i·a en·ter·o·col·i·tic·a (yĕr-sin′ē-ă en′tĕr-ō-kō-lit′i-kă) A bacterial species that causes yersiniosis in humans; it is found in the feces and lymph nodes of sick and healthy animals, including humans, and in material contaminated with feces.

Yer·sin·i·a pes·tis (yĕr-sin′ē-ă pes′tis) A bacterial species that causes plague in humans, rodents, cats, and many other mammals; it is transmitted from rat to rat and from rat to human host by as many as 30 species of flea, including the rat flea *Xenopsylla;* the bacterium can also be transmitted by aerosol droplets dispersed by humans or animals (especially cats) manifesting a pneumonic form of plague, or by deliberate dissemination by means of an aerosol mechanism by individual people or organizations with bioterroristic intent; the bacterium is the type species of the genus *Yersinia.* SYN Kitasato bacillus.

Yer·sin·i·a pseu·do·tu·ber·cu·lo·sis (yĕr-sin′ē-ă sū′dō-tū-bĕr′kyū-lō′sis) A bacterial species causing pseudotuberculosis in birds, rodents, and rarely in humans. SYN *Pasteurella pseudotuberculosis.*

yer·sin·i·o·sis (yĕr-sin′ē-ō′sis) A common human infectious disease caused by *Yersinia enterocolitica* and marked by diarrhea, enteritis, pseudoappendicitis, ileitis, erythema nodosum, and sometimes septicemia or acute arthritis.

yield (yēld) The amount or quantity produced or returned, often measured as a percentage of the starting material; e.g., a yield in an enzyme preparation is equal to the units of enzyme activity recovered at the end of the preparation divided by the total units observed in the starting material.

yin/yang (yin-yang) In traditional Chinese medicine, the concept of opposing but complementary forces thought to underlie concepts of good health (e.g., heat/cold, hard/soft).

yi-yi (yē-yē) SYN yerba maté.

-yl Chemical suffix signifying that the substance is a radical by loss of an H atom (e.g., alkyl, methyl, phenyl) or OH group (e.g., acyl, acetyl, carbamoyl).

-ylene Chemical suffix denoting a bivalent hydrocarbon radical (e.g., methylene, $–CH_2–$) or possessing a double bond (e.g., ethylene, $CH_2{=}CH_2$).

Y-link·age (lingk′ăj) The state of a genetic factor (gene) being borne on the Y chromosome. This idea is analogous to X-linkage, but inasmuch as the Y chromosome does not fully take part in chiasma formation and recombination, it not amenable to analysis by conventional linkage methods.

Y-linked gene (lingkt jēn) A gene located on a Y chromosome. SYN holandric gene.

yoke (yōk) SYN jugum (1). [A.S. *geoc*]

yolk (yōk) **1.** One of the types of nutritive material stored in the oocyte for the nutrition of the embryo; particularly abundant and conspicuous in the eggs of birds. SYN vitellus. **2.** Fatty material found in the wool of sheep; when extracted and purified, it becomes lanolin. [A.S. *geolca; geolu,* yellow]

yolk mem·brane (yōk mem′brān) SYN membrana vitellina.

yolk sac (yōk sak) SYN umbilical vesicle. See page B1.

yolk stalk (yōk stawk) SYN omphaloenteric duct.

Yorke au·to·lyt·ic re·ac·tion (yōrk aw′tō-lit′ik rē-ak′shŭn) A test for paroxysmal hemoglobinuria; serum is placed in an ice chest and kept at 0°C for 5–7 minutes, then in an incubator at 37°C with erythrocytes for 1 hour, at which time, if the reaction is positive, hemolysis occurs; if the serum is kept at 1°C for an hour and then placed in the incubator with erythrocytes, there is little hemolysis.

Young-Helm·holtz the·o·ry of col·or vi·sion (yŭng helm′hōlts thē′ŏr-ē kŏl′ŏr vizh′ŭn) A theory that there are three color-perceiving elements in the retina: red, green, and blue. Perception of other colors arises from the combined stimulation of these elements; deficiency or absence of any one of these elements results in inability to perceive that color and a misperception of any other color of which it forms a part.

Young mo·du·lus (yŭng moj′yū-lŭs) A type of modulus of elasticity that specifies the force applied to a body in one direction, per unit cross-sectional area of the body perpendicular to that direction, divided by the fractional change in length of the body in that direction.

yo-yo di·et (yō′yō dī′ĕt) The cyclic action of an individual who loses weight and then regains the amount lost; also called yo-yo syndrome.

Y-shaped lig·a·ment (shāpt lig′ă-mĕnt) SYN iliofemoral ligament.

yt·ter·bi·um (Yb) (i-tĕr′bē-ŭm) A metallic element of the lanthanide group; atomic no. 70, atomic wt. 173.04. ^{169}Yb, with a half-life of 32.03 days, has been used in cisternography and in brain scans. [*Ytterby,* village in Sweden]

yt•tri•um (Y) (it′rē-ŭm) A metallic element, atomic no. 39, atomic wt. 88.90585. [*Ytterby,* village in Sweden]

Z

Z 1. Abbreviation for benzyloxycarbonyl; atomic number; carbobenzoxy. **2.** Symbol for an amino acid that is either glutamic acid, glutamine, or a substance that yields glutamic acid on acid hydrolysis of peptides.

z Abbreviation for zepto-.

Zahn in•farct (tsahn in′fahrkt) A pseudoinfarct of the liver, consisting of an area of congestion with parenchymal atrophy but no necrosis; due to obstruction of a branch of the portal vein.

Za•ire vi•rus (zī-ēr′ vī′rŭs) A variant of Ebola virus. SYN Ebola virus Zaire.

Zar•it bur•den in•ter•view (zar′it bŭr′dĕn in′tĕr-vyū) A structured verbal interaction used to evaluate levels of stress in family members or caregivers of Alzheimer patients.

Za•va•nel•li ma•neu•ver (zah-vah-nel′ē mă-nū′vĕr) SYN cephalic replacement.

Z band (band) SYN Z line.

Z-DNA A form of DNA in which the helix is left-handed, and the overall appearance is elongated and slim.

ZDV Abbreviation for zidovudine.

ZEEP (zēp) Acronym for zero end-expiratory pressure.

Zeis glands (tsīs glandz) Sebaceous glands opening into the follicles of the eyelashes.

Zeit•geist (zīt′gīst) PSYCHOLOGY the climate of opinion, conventions of thought, covert influences, and unquestioned assumptions that are implicit in a given culture, the arts, or science at any time, and in which the individual person operates and thus is influenced. [Ger. *Zeit,* time, + *Geist,* spirit]

Zen•ker de•gen•er•a•tion (tsen′ker dĕ-jen′ĕr-ā′shŭn) A form of severe hyaline degeneration or necrosis in skeletal muscle, occurring in severe infections. SYN waxy degeneration (2).

Zen•ker di•ver•tic•u•lum (tsen′ker dī′vĕr-tik′yū-lŭm) SYN pharyngoesophageal diverticulum.

Zen•ker fix•a•tive (tsen′ker fiks′ă-tiv) A rapid fixative consisting of mercuric chloride, potassium dichromate, sodium sulfate, glacial acetic acid, and water, useful for trichrome stains; must be washed to remove potassium dichromate and treated with iodine solution to remove mercuric chloride; tissues tend to become brittle if left in the fixative for more than 24 hours.

Zen•ker pa•ral•y•sis (tsen′ker păr-al′i-sis) Paresthesia and paralysis in the area of the external popliteal nerve.

zep•to- (z) Prefix used in the SI and metric system to signify 10^{-21}.

ze•ro (zēr′ō) **1.** The figure 0, indicating the absence of magnitude, or nothing. **2.** THERMOMETRY the point from which the figures on the scale start in one or the other direction; in the Celsius and Réaumur scales, zero indicates the freezing point for distilled water; in the Fahrenheit scale, it is 32° below the freezing point of water. [Sp. fr. Ar. *sifr,* cipher]

ze•ro end-ex•pi•ra•to•ry pres•sure (ZEEP) (zēr′ō end-ek-spīr′ă-tōr-ē presh′ŭr) Airway pressure that, at the end of expiration, equals atmospheric pressure.

ze•ta (zāt′ă) **1.** Sixth letter of the Greek alphabet, ζ. **2.** CHEMISTRY the sixth in a series, e.g., the sixth carbon from a functional group. **3.** Electrokinetic potential.

ze•ta•crit (zā′tă-krit) The packed cell volume produced by vertical centrifugation of blood in capillary tubes, allowing controlled compaction and dispersion of red blood cells; read with a hematocrit to produce the zeta sedimentation ratio.

ze•ta sed•i•men•ta•tion ra•ti•o (zā′tă sed′i-mĕn-tā′shŭn rā′shē-ō) The ratio of the zetacrit to the hematocrit, normally 0.41–0.54 (41–54%); it is a sensitive indicator of the erythrocyte sedimentation rate (ESR) and is unaffected by anemia.

Z fil•a•ment (fil′ă-mĕnt) The thin zig-zag structure at the Z line of striated muscle fibers to which the actin filaments attach.

Zick•el nail (zik′ĕl nāl) Orthopedic device used in fixation of subtrochanteric fracture.

zi•dov•u•dine (ZDV) (zī-dō′vyū-dēn) A thymidine analogue that is an inhibitor of in vitro replication of HIV virus; also used in pharmacotherapeutic management of AIDS.

Ziehl stain (tsēl stān) A carbol-fuchsin solution of phenol and basic fuchsin used to demonstrate bacteria and cell nuclei.

Zie•mann dot (tsē′mahn dot) Any of numerous fine dots seen in erythrocytes in malariae malaria.

zig•zag plas•ty (zig′zag plast′ē) SYN Z-plasty.

Zim•mer•lin at•ro•phy (tsim′er-lin at′rŏ-fē) A variety of hereditary progressive muscular atrophy in which the atrophy begins in the upper half of the body.

zinc (zingk) A metallic element, atomic no. 30, atomic wt. 65.39; an essential bioelement; a number of salts of zinc are used in medicine; a cofactor in many proteins. [Ger. *Zink*]

zinc 65 (zingk) A radioactive zinc isotope that decays mainly by K-capture with a half-life of 243.8 days; used as a tracer in studies of zinc metabolism.

zinc sul•fate flo•ta•tion con•cen•tra•tion

(zingk sŭl′fāt flō-tā′shŭn kon′sĕn-trā′shŭn) A method using saturated zinc sulfate to separate parasitic elements from fecal debris through differences in specific gravity; most parasite cysts, oocysts, spores, eggs, and larvae can be found in the surface film after centrifugation.

Zinn zon•ule (tsin zō′nyūl) SYN ciliary zonule.

zir•co•ni•um (Zr) (zĭr-kō′nē-ŭm) A metallic element, atomic no. 40, atomic wt. 91.224; widely distributed in nature, but never found in quantity in any one place. [*zircon,* a mineral, fr. Ar. *zarkūn,* cinnabar, Pers, *zargun,* goldlike]

Z line (līn) A cross-striation bisecting the I band of striated muscle myofibrils and serving as the anchoring point of actin filaments at either end of the sarcomere. SYN Z band.

zm Abbreviation for zeptometer.

zo•ac•an•tho•sis (zō′ak-ăn-thō′sis) A cutaneous eruption due to introduction into the human skin of hair, bristles, or stingers, or other lower animal structures. [G. *zōon,* animal, + acanthosis]

zo•an•throp•ic (zō′ăn-throp′ik) Relating to or marked by zoanthropy.

zo•an•thro•py (zō-an′thrŏ-pē) A delusion that one is an animal (e.g., a dog). [G. *zōon,* animal, + *anthrōpos,* man]

Zol•lin•ger-El•li•son syn•drome (zol′in-jĕr-el′i-sŏn sin′drōm) Peptic ulceration with gastric hypersecretion and non-beta cell tumor of the pancreatic islets, sometimes associated with familial polyendocrine adenomatosis.

Zöll•ner lines (tserl′ner līnz) Figures devised to show the possibility of optic illusions; a common one consists of two parallel lines that are met by numerous short lines obliquely placed; the parallel lines then seeming to converge or diverge.

zo•na, pl. **zo•nae** (zō′nă, -nē) **1.** SYN zone. **2.** SYN herpes zoster. [L. fr. G. *zōnē,* a girdle, one of the zones of the sphere]

zo•na ar•cu•a•ta (zō′nă ahr′kyū-ā′tă) SYN arcuate zone.

zonaesthesia [Br.] SYN zonesthesia.

zo•na fasc•i•cu•la•ta (zō′nă fash-ik′yū-lā′tă) The layer of radially arranged cell cords in the cortex of the suprarenal gland, between the zona glomerulosa and zona reticularis; secretes cortisol and dehydroepiandrosterone.

zo•na glo•mer•u•lo•sa (zō′nă glō-mĕr-yū-lō′să) The outer layer of the cortex of the suprarenal gland just beneath the capsule; secretes aldosterone.

zo•nal ne•cro•sis (zō′năl nĕ-krō′sis) Necrosis predominantly affecting or limited to an anatomic zone, especially parts of the hepatic lobules defined according to proximity to either the portal tracts or central (hepatic) veins.

zo•na oph•thal•mic•a (zō′nă of-thal′mik-ă) Herpes zoster in the distribution of the ophthalmic nerve.

zo•na or•bi•cu•la•ris (zō′nă ōr-bik-yū-lār′is) Fibers of the articular capsule of the hip joint encircling the neck of the femur.

zo•na pec•ti•na•ta (zō′nă pek-ti-nā′tă) SYN pectinate zone.

zo•na pel•lu•cid•a (zō′nă pel-lū′sid-ă) An extracellular coat surrounding the oocyte; it consists of a layer of microvilli of the oocyte, cellular processes of follicular cells, and an intervening substance rich in glycoprotein; it appears homogeneous and translucent under the light microscope. SYN pellucid zone.

zo•na re•tic•u•la•ris (zō′nă re-tik′yū-lār′is) The inner layer of the cortex of the suprarenal gland, where the cell cords anastomose in a netlike fashion.

zo•na tec•ta (zō′nă tek′tă) SYN arcuate zone.

zone (zōn) A segment; any encircling or beltlike structure, either external or internal, longitudinal or transverse. SEE ALSO area, band, region, space, spot. SYN zona (1). [L. *zona*]

zone of e•quiv•a•lence (zōn ē-kwiv′ă-lens) Portion of a precipitin or agglutination curve when antibody and antigen concentrations are optimal for lattice formation.

zone of in•hi•bi•tion (zōn in′hi-bish′ŭn) The area around an antibiotic disc that contains no bacterial growth.

zo•nes•the•si•a (zōn′es-thē′zē-ă) A sensation as if a cord were drawn around the body, constricting it. SYN girdle sensation, zonaesthesia. [G. *zōnē,* girdle, + *aisthēsis,* sensation]

zo•nif•u•gal (zō-nif′yŭ-găl) Passing from within any region outward; as in mapping out an area of disturbed sensation, when the stimulus is first applied to the affected region and is carried into the area where sensation is normal. [L. *zona,* zone, + *fugio,* to flee]

zon•ing (zōn′ing) The occurrence of a stronger reaction in a lesser amount of suspected serum, observed sometimes in serologic tests used in the diagnosis of syphilis, and probably the result of high antibody titer.

zo•nip•e•tal (zō-nip′ĕ-tăl) Passing from without toward and into any region, as in mapping out an area of disturbed sensation, when the stimulus begins in a normal area and is carried into the affected region. [L. *zona,* zone, + *peto,* to seek]

zo•nog•ra•phy (zō-nog′ră-fē) A form of tomography with a relatively thick plane of focus; especially used in renal radiography. [zone + G. *graphō,* to write]

zo·nu·la, pl. **zo·nu·lae** (zōn′yū-lă, -lē) SYN zonule. [L. dim. of *zona*, zone]

zo·nu·la cil·i·ar·is (zō′nyū-lă sil′ē-ār′is) [TA] SYN ciliary zonule.

zo·nu·lar (zō′nyū-lăr) Relating to a zonula.

zo·nu·lar cat·a·ract (zō′nyū-lăr kat′ăr-akt) SYN lamellar cataract.

zo·nu·lar spac·es (zō′nyū-lăr spās′ĕz) The spaces between the fibers of the ciliary zonule at the equator of the lens of the eye.

zo·nule (zō′nyūl) A small zone. SYN zonula.

zo·nu·li·tis (zō′nyū-lī′tis) Inflammation of the zonule of Zinn, or suspensory ligament of the lens of the eye. [zonule + G. *-itis,* inflammation]

zo·nu·lol·y·sis, **zo·nu·ly·sis** (zō′nyū-lol′i-sis, -nyū-lī′sis) Dissolution of the zonula ciliaris by enzymes (α-chymotrypsin) to facilitate surgical removal of a cataract. SYN Barraquer method. [zonule + G. *lysis,* dissolution]

zoo-, **zo-** Combining forms denoting animal, animal life. [G. *zōon*]

zoo blot a·nal·y·sis (zū blot ă-nal′i-sis) A procedure using Southern blot analysis to test the ability of a nucleic acid probe from one species to hybridize with the DNA fragment of another species.

zo·o·e·ras·ti·a (zō′ō-ĕ-ras′tē-ă) SYN bestiality. [zoo- + G. *erastēs,* lover]

zo·o·graft (zō′ō-graft) A graft of tissue from an animal to a human.

zo·o·graft·ing (zō′ō-graft′ing) SYN zooplasty.

zo·oid (zō′oyd) **1.** Resembling an animal; an organism or object with an animalian appearance. **2.** An animal cell capable of independent existence or movement, as the ovum or a spermatozoon, or the segment of a tapeworm. **3.** An individual of a colonial invertebrate, such as a coral. [G. *zoōdēs,* fr. *zōon,* animal, + *eidos,* resemblance]

zo·o·lag·ni·a (zō′ō-lag′nē-ă) Sexual attraction toward animals. [zoo- + G. *lagneia,* lust]

zo·o·no·sis (zō′ō-nō′sis) An infection or infestation shared in nature by humans and other animals that are the normal or usual host; a disease of humans acquired from an animal source. SEE ALSO anthropozoonosis, metazoonosis, saprozoonosis. [zoo- + G. *nosos,* disease]

zo·o·not·ic cu·ta·ne·ous leish·ma·ni·a·sis (zo′ō-not′ik kyū-tā′nē-ŭs lēsh′mă-nī′ă-sis) A form of cutaneous leishmaniasis characterized by rural distribution of human cases near infected rodents, particularly communal ground squirrels; characterized by rapidly developing dermal lesions that become severely inflamed, with moist necrotizing sores or ulcers that heal in 2–8 months (after a 2–4 month incubation period).

zo·o·not·ic po·ten·tial (zo′ō-not′ik pŏ-ten′shăl) The possibility for infections of subhuman animals to be transmissible to humans.

zo·o·par·a·site (zō′ō-par′ă-sīt) An animal parasite; an animal existing as a parasite.

zo·o·phil·ic (zō′ō-fil′ik) Refers to microorganisms that prefer an animal other than humans as a host or reservoir.

zo·oph·i·lism (zō-of′i-lizm) Fondness for animals, especially to an extravagant degree.

zo·o·pho·bi·a (zō′ō-fō′bē-ă) Morbid fear of animals. [zoo- + G. *phobos,* fear]

zo·o·plas·ty (zō′ō-plas-tē) Grafting of tissue from an animal to a human. SYN zoografting.

zo·o·tox·in (zō′ō-tok′sin) A substance, resembling the bacterial toxins in its antigenic properties, found in the fluids of certain animals, e.g., in snake venom, the secretions of poisonous insects, eel blood.

zos·ter (zos′tĕr) SYN herpes zoster. [G. *zōstēr,* a girdle]

zos·ter·oid (zos′tĕr-oyd) Resembling herpes zoster. [zoster + G. *eidos,* resemblance]

Z-plas·ty (plas′tē) Surgery to elongate a contracted scar or to rotate tension 90°; the middle line of a Z-shaped incision is made along the line of greatest tension or contraction, and triangular flaps are raised on opposite sides of the two ends and transposed. SYN zigzag plasty.

Z-pro·tein (prō′tēn) A fatty acid–binding protein that participates in the intracellular movement of fatty acids. SYN fatty acid–binding protein.

Zr Symbol for zirconium.

Zsig·mon·dy den·tal no·men·cla·ture (tsig′mawn-dē den′tăl nō′mĕn-klā-chŭr) SYN Palmer dental nomenclature.

Z-track meth·od (trak meth′ŏd) A method of intramuscular injection used to prevent injected medicine from leaking back to the surface of the skin; the skin is pushed to one side and held in place while the medicine is injected; after the needle is withdrawn, the skin is returned to its original position. See page 1695.

Zuc·ker·kan·dl bod·ies (tsuk′er-kahn-del bod′ēz) SYN paraaortic bodies.

zwit·ter hy·poth·e·sis (zvit′ĕr hī-poth′ĕ-sis) That an amphoteric molecule (e.g., an amino acid) has, at its isoelectric point, equal numbers of positive and negative charges, thus becoming a zwitterion (dipolar ion).

zwit·ter·i·ons (zvit′ĕr-ī′onz) SYN dipolar ions. SEE ALSO zwitter hypothesis. [Ger. *Zwitter,* hermaphrodite, mongrel + ion]

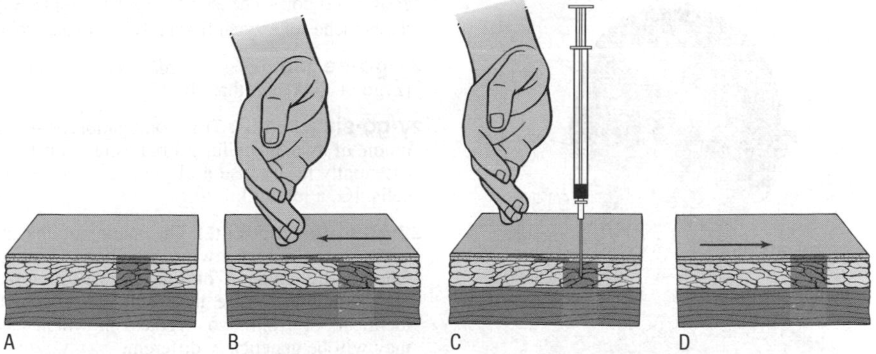

Z-track method: (A) normal skin and tissues; (B) moving skin to one side; (C) needle is inserted at 90-degree angle, aspirate for blood; (D) once needle is withdrawn, displaced tissue is allowed to return to its normal position, preventing solution from escaping from muscle tissue

zy·gal (zī′găl) Relating to or shaped like a zygon or yoke; H-shaped.

zy·ga·po·phy·si·al joint (zī′gă-pō-fiz′ē-ăl joynt) SYN facet joint.

zyg·a·poph·y·sis, zyg·a·poph·y·ses, pl. **zyg·a·poph·y·ses** (zī′gă-pof′i-sis, -sēz, -sēz) SYN articular process. [G. *zygon,* yoke, + *apophysis,* offshoot]

zygo-, zyg- Combining forms meaning a yoke, a joining. [G. *zygon,* yoke, *zygōsis,* a joining]

zy·go·ma (zī-gō′mă) **1.** SYN zygomatic bone. **2.** SYN zygomatic arch. [G. a bar, bolt, the os jugale, fr. *zygon,* yoke]

zy·go·mat·ic (zī′gō-mat′ik) Relating to the zygomatic bone.

zy·go·mat·ic arch (zī′gō-mat′ik ahrch) The arch formed by the temporal process of the zygomatic bone as it joins the zygomatic process of the temporal bones. SYN zygoma (2).

zy·go·mat·ic bone (zī′gō-mat′ik bōn) A quadrilateral bone that forms the prominence of the cheek; it articulates with the frontal, sphenoid, temporal, and maxillary bone. SYN os zygomaticum [TA], jugal bone, mala (2), malar bone, zygoma (1).

zy·go·mat·ic nerve (zī′gō-mat′ik nĕrv) A branch of the maxillary nerve in the inferior orbital fissure through which it passes; it gives rise to two sensory branches, the zygomaticotemporal and zygomaticofacial, which supply the skin of the temporal and zygomatic regions, and is continued as the communicating branch of the lacrimal nerve with the zygomatic nerve. SYN nervus zygomaticus [TA], temporomandibular nerve.

zy·go·mat·i·co·au·ric·u·lar·is (zī′gō-măt′i-kō-awr-ik′yū-lar′is) SYN auricularis anterior muscle.

zy·go·mat·i·co·fa·cial fo·ra·men (zī′gō-mat′i-kō-fā′shăl fōr-ā′mĕn) The opening on the lateral surface of the zygomatic bone below the orbital margin that transmits the zygomaticofacial nerve. SYN foramen zygomaticofaciale [TA].

zy·go·mat·i·co·or·bi·tal ar·ter·y (zī′gō-mat′i-kō-ōr′bi-tăl ahr′tĕr-ē) *Origin,* superficial temporal, sometimes middle temporal; *distribution,* orbicularis oculi muscle and portions of the orbit; *anastomoses,* lacrimal and palpebral branches of ophthalmic. SYN arteria zygomatico-orbitalis [TA].

zy·go·mat·i·co·or·bi·tal fo·ra·men (zī′gō-mat′i-kō-ōr′bi-tăl fōr-ā′mĕn) The common opening on the orbital surface of the zygomatic bone of the canals transmitting the zygomaticofacial and zygomaticotemporal nerves; sometimes each of these canals has a separate opening on the orbital surface. SYN foramen zygomaticoorbitale [TA].

zy·go·mat·i·co·tem·po·ral fo·ra·men (zī′gō-mat′i-kō-tem′pŏr-ăl fōr-ā′mĕn) The opening, on the temporal surface of the zygomatic bone, of the canal that gives passage to the zygomaticotemporal nerve. SYN foramen zygomaticotemporale [TA].

zy·go·mat·ic pro·cess of max·il·la (zī′gō-mat′ik pros′es mak-sil′ă) The rough projection from the maxilla that articulates with the zygomatic bone.

zy·go·mat·i·cus ma·jor mus·cle (zī′gō-mat′i-kŭs mā′jŏr mŭs′ĕl) Facial muscle of anterior cheek extending to upper lip; *origin,* zygomatic bone anterior to temporozygomatic suture; *insertion,* muscles at angle of mouth; *action,* draws upper lip upward and laterally; *nerve supply,* facial. See page 1696. SYN musculus zygomaticus major [TA], greater zygomatic muscle, musculus zygomaticus.

zy·go·mat·i·cus mi·nor mus·cle (zī′gō-mat′i-kŭs mī′nŏr mŭs′ĕl) Facial muscle of anterior

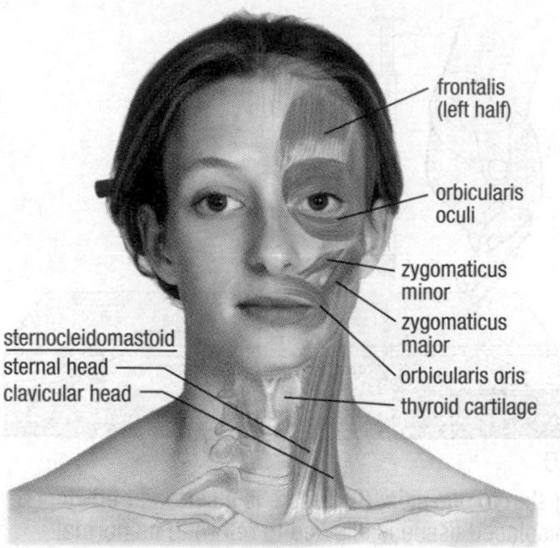

zygomaticus major muscle

cheek extending to upper lip; *origin*, zygomatic bone posterior to zygomaticomaxillary suture; *insertion*, orbicularis oris of upper lip; *action*, draws upper lip upward and outward; *nerve supply*, facial. SYN caput zygomaticum quadrati labii superioris, lesser zygomatic muscle, musculus zygomaticus minor.

zy·go·max·il·la·re (zī′gō-mak′si-lar-ē) A craniometric point located externally at the lowest extent of the zygomaticomaxillary suture. SYN zygomaxillary point.

zy·go·max·il·la·ry point (zī′gō-mak′si-lar-ē poynt) SYN zygomaxillare.

Zy·go·my·ce·tes (zī′gō-mī-sē′tēz) A class of fungi characterized by sexual reproduction resulting in the formation of a zygospore, and asexual reproduction by means of nonmotile spores called sporangiospores or conidia. See page B5. [zygo- + G. *mykēs* (*mykēt-*), fungus]

zy·go·my·co·sis (zī′gō-mī-kō′sis) A fungal infection associated with genera of the class Zygomycetes, e.g., *Absidia*, *Mortierella*, *Mucor*, *Rhizopus*. The genera *Conidiobolus* and *Basidiobolus* have species that are also causative agents. See page B5. SYN mucormycosis, phycomycosis.

zy·gon (zī′gon) The short crossbar connecting the branches of a zygal fissure. [G. crossbar, yoke]

zy·go·ne·ma (zī′gō-nē′mă) SYN zygotene. [zygo- + G. *nēma,* thread]

zy·go·sis (zī-gō′sis) True conjugation or sexual union of two unicellular organisms, consisting essentially in the fusion of the nuclei of the two cells. [G. a joining]

zy·gos·i·ty (zī-gos′i-tē) The nature of the zygotes from which twins are derived; e.g., whether by division of one zygote (monozygotic), in which case they will be genetically identical, or from two zygotes, in which case they will be genetically different.

zy·gote (zī′gōt) **1.** The diploid cell resulting from union of a sperm and an oocyte. Cf. conceptus. **2.** The early embryo that develops from a fertilized oocyte. See page B1. [G. *zygōtos,* yoked]

zy·go·tene (zī′gō-tēn) The stage of prophase in meiosis in which precise point-for-point pairing of homologous chromosomes begins. SYN zygonema. [zygo- + G. *tainia* (L. *taenia*), band]

zy·got·ic (zī-got′ik) Pertaining to a zygote, or to zygosis.

zymo-, zym- Combining forms denoting fermentation, enzymes. [G. *zymē,* leaven]

zy·mo·deme (zī′mō-dēm) An isoenzyme pattern, as identified by isoenzyme electrophoresis. [zymo- + G. *dēmos,* populace]

zy·mo·gen (zī′mō-jen) SYN proenzyme.

zy·mo·gen·e·sis (zī′mō-jen′ĕ-sis) Transformation of a proenzyme (zymogen) into an active enzyme. [zymo- + G. *genesis,* production]

zy·mo·gen·ic (zī′mō-jen′ik) **1.** Relating to a zymogen or to zymogenesis. **2.** Causing fermentation.

zy·mo·gen·ic cell (zī′mō-jen′ik sel) A cell that secretes an enzyme; specifically a chief cell of a gastric gland or an acinar cell of the pancreas. SYN peptic cell.

Contents: The Appendices

Weights and Measures

Scale of the Metric System and International System of Units (SI)

Prefix	Symbol	Power
yotta-	Y	10^{24}
zetta-	Z	10^{21}
exa-	E	10^{18}
peta-	P	10^{15}
tera-	T	10^{12}
giga-	G	10^{9}
mega-	M	10^{6}
kilo-	k	10^{3}
hecto-	h	10^{2}
deca-	da	10^{1}
base unit	—	1
deci-	d	10^{-1}
centi-	c	10^{-2}
milli	m	10^{-3}
micro-	mc	10^{-6}
nano-	n	10^{-9}
pico-	p	10^{-12}
femto-	f	10^{-15}
atto-	a	10^{-18}
zepto-	z	10^{-21}
yocto-	y	10^{-24}

SI Base Units

Quantity	Name	Symbol
length	meter	m
mass*	kilogram†	kg
time	second	s
electric current	ampere	A
thermodynamic temperature	kelvin‡	K
luminous intensity	candela	cd
amount of substance	mole	mol

*In commercial and everyday use, *weight* usually means *mass* (e.g., when speaking of a person's weight, the quantity referred to is *mass*).

†For historical reasons, *kilogram* is the only base unit with a prefix. Multiples and submultiples of the kilogram are formed by attaching the appropriate prefix to the stem *-gram* (e.g., *milligram*) and the appropriate prefix symbol to the symbol *g* (e.g., *mg*).

‡The degree Celsius (°C) is still widely accepted usage for expressing temperature and temperature intervals. Celsius (formerly centigrade) *temperature* is converted to Kelvin (K) thermodynamic temperature by adding 273.16 to the Celsius scale. For *temperature interval,* 1°C equals K.

Some SI-Derived Units Expressed in Terms of Base Units

Quantity	Name	Symbol
area	square meter	m^2
volume*	cubic meter	m^3
specific volume	cubic meter per kilogram	m^3/kg
speed, velocity	meter per second	m/s
acceleration	meter per second squared	m/s^2
mass density	kilogram per cubic meter	kg/m^3
concentration	mole per cubic meter	mol/m^3
luminance	candela per square meter	cd/m^2

*Liter (L, l). 10^{-3} m^3 is used as a special name for the cubic decimeter.

Some SI-Derived Units with Special Names

Quantity	Name	Symbol	Expression
frequency	hertz	Hz	s^{-1}
force	newton	N	$m\ kg\ s^{-2}$
pressure, stress	pascal	Pa	$m^{-1}\ kg\ s^{-2}$
energy	joule	J	$m^2\ kg\ s^{-2}$
power	watt	W	$m^2\ kg\ s^{-3}$
quantity of electricity, electric charge	coulomb	C	s A
electric potential, electromotive force	volt	V	$m^2\ kg\ s^{-3}A^{-1}$
capacitance	farad	F	$m^{-2}\ kg^{-1}\ s^4A^{-2}$
electrical resistance	ohm	Ω	$m^2\ kg^{-2}\ A^{-2}$
electrical conductance	siemens	S	$m^{-2}kg\ s^{-2}A^{-1}$
magnetic flux	weber	Wb	$m^2\ kg\ s^{-2}A^{-1}$
magnetic flux density	tesla	T	$kg\ s^{-2}A^{-1}$
activity of radionuclide	becquerel*	Bq	s^{-1}
absorbed dose of radiation	gray†	Gy	$m^2\ s^{-2}$
exposure (x and γ radiation)	coulomb per kilogram‡	C kg	kg^{-1} s A

*Replacing the curie (Ci), $3.7 \times 10^{10}\ s^{-1}$. †Replacing the rad, $10^{-2}\ J\ kg^{-1}$. ‡Replacing the roentgen (R), $2.58 \times 10^{-4}\ C\ kg^{-1}$.

Measures of Length

Micrometers	Millimeters	Centimeters	Meters	Kilometers	Miles	Yards	Feet	Inches
1	0.001	10^{-4}						0.000039
10^3	**1**	10^{-1}					.00328	0.03937
10^4	10	**1**	0.01			0.0109	.03281	0.3937
254,000	25.4	2.54	0.0254			0.0278	.0833	**1**
	304.8	30.48	0.3048			0.333	**1**	12
10^6	10^3	10^2	**1**	0.001	0.0006213	1.0936	3.2808	39.37
914,400	914.40	91.44	0.9144	0.009	0.0005681	**1**	3	36
10^9	10^6	10^5	10^3	**1**	0.6215	1093.6121	3280.8	
			1609.0	1.609	**1**	1760.0	5280.0	

To convert:

Millimeters to inches: divide by 25.4
Inches to millimeters: multiply by 25.4

Meters to yards: multiply by 1.09375
Yards to meters: multiply by 0.9143

Centimeters to feet: divide by 30.7
Feet to centimeters: multiply by 30.7

Kilometers to miles: multiply by 0.625
Miles to kilometers: multiply by 1.6

Measures of Mass (Weight)

Avoirdupois Weights						
				Metric Equivalents		
Grains	Drams	Ounces	Pounds	Milligrams	Grams	Kilograms
1	0.0366	0.0023	0.00014	64.8	0.0648	0.000065
27.34	**1**	0.0625	0.0039		1.772	0.001772
437.5	16	**1**	0.0625		28.350	0.028350
7,000	256	16	**1**		453.5924	0.453592
0.0154				**1**	0.001	
15.4324	0.5648	0.0353	0.002205	1000	**1**	0.001
15,432.358	564.32	35.27	2.2046		1000	**1**

To convert (approximately):

Kilograms to pounds: multiply by 2.2

Pounds to kilograms: multiply by 0.454

Grams to ounces: multiply by 0.03527

Ounces to grams: multiply by 28.35

Apothecaries' Weights							
					Metric Equivalents		
Grains	Scruples	Drams	Ounces	Pounds	Milligrams	Grams	Kilograms
1	0.05	0.0167	0.0021	0.00017	64.8	0.0648	0.000065
20	1	0.333	0.042	0.0035		1.296	0.001296
60	3	1	0.125	0.0104		3.888	0.000389
480	24	8	1	0.0833		31.103	0.031103
5,760	288	96	12	1		373.2417	0.373242
0.0154					1	0.001	
15.4324		0.2572	0.0322	0.0027	1000	1	0.001
15,432.358		257.2	32.15	2.6792		1000	1

Measures of Capacity

Apothecaries' Measures							
					Metric Equivalents		
Minims	Fluid Drams	Fluid Ounces	Pints	Quarts	Gallons	Liters	Milliliters
1	0.0167	0.002	0.00013			0.0006	0.06161
60	**1**	0.125	0.0078	0.0039		0.0037	3.6967
480	8	**1**	0.0625	0.0312	0.0078	0.0296	29.5737
7,680	128	16	**1**	0.5	0.125	0.4732	473.166
15,360	256	32	2	**1**	0.25	0.9464	946.358
61,440	1024	128	8	4	**1**	3.7854	3785.434
16,230	270.52	33.8418	2.1134	1.0567	0.2642	**1**	1000
16.23	0.2705	0.0338	0.00212	0.00106	0.000265	0.001	**1**

To convert (approximately)

1 British imperial gallon = 1.201 U.S. gallon
1 U.S. gallon = 0.8327 British imperial gallon

Liters to gallons: multiply by 0.264
Gallons to liters: multiply by 3.788

Liters to pints: multiply by 2.1
Pints to liters: multiply by 0.4732

Approximate Household Measures and Weights*

Teaspoons	Tablespoons	Cups or Glasses†	Drams	Fluid Ounces	Milliliters	Grams
1			**1**	0.125	5	5
3	**1**		4	0.50	15	15
48	16‡	**1**	64	8	237	240

*A drop is a measure of uncertain quantity, depending on the nature of the liquid as well as the shape of the container and of the opening from which the liquid falls. One drop of water is roughly equivalent to 1 minim.

†"Tumbler or glass" generally means 8 fluid ounces.

‡For dry measure, 12 tablespoons equal 1 cup.

Temperature Equivalents

Celsius to Fahrenheit

°C	°F	°C	°F
−50	−58.0	49	120.0
−40	−40.0	50	122.0
−35	−31.0	51	123.8
−30	−22.0	52	125.6
−25	−13.0	53	127.4
−20	−4.0	54	129.2
−15	5.0	55	131.0
−10	14.0	56	132.8
−5	23.0	57	134.6
0	**32.0**	58	136.4
1	33.8	59	138.2
2	35.6	60	140.0
3	37.4	61	141.8
4	39.2	62	143.6
5	41.0	63	145.4
6	42.8	64	147.2
7	44.6	65	149.0
8	46.4	66	150.8
9	48.2	67	152.6
10	50.0	68	154.4
11	51.8	69	156.2
12	53.6	70	158.0
13	55.4	71	159.8
14	57.2	72	161.6
15	59.0	73	163.4
16	60.8	74	165.2
17	62.6	75	167.0
18	64.4	76	168.8
19	66.2	77	170.6
20	68.0	78	172.4
21	69.8	79	174.2
22	71.6	80	176.0
23	73.4	81	177.8
24	75.2	82	179.6
25	77.0	83	181.4
26	78.8	84	183.2
27	80.6	85	185.0
28	82.4	86	186.8
29	84.2	87	188.6
30	86.0	88	190.4
31	87.8	89	192.2
32	89.6	90	194.0
33	91.4	91	195.8
34	93.2	92	197.6
35	95.0	93	199.4
36	96.8	94	201.2
37	**98.6**	95	203.0
38	100.4	96	204.8
39	102.2	97	206.6
40	104.0	98	208.4
41	105.8	99	210.2
42	107.6	**100**	**212.0**
43	109.4	101	213.8
44	111.2	102	215.6
45	113.0	103	217.4
46	114.8	104	219.2
47	116.6	105	221.0
48	118.4	106	222.8

Fahrenheit to Celsius

°F	°C	°F	°C	°F	°C
−50	−46.7	99	37.2	157	69.4
−40	−40.0	100	37.7	158	70.0
−35	−37.2	101	38.3	159	70.5
−30	−34.4	102	38.8	160	71.1
−25	−31.7	103	39.4	161	71.6
−20	−28.9	104	40.0	162	72.2
−15	−26.6	105	40.5	163	72.7
−10	−23.3	106	41.1	164	73.3
−5	−20.6	107	41.6	165	73.8
0	−17.7	108	42.2	166	74.4
1	−17.2	109	42.7	167	75.0
5	−15.0	110	43.3	168	75.5
10	−12.2	111	43.8	169	76.1
15	−9.4	112	44.4	170	76.6
20	−6.6	113	45.0	171	77.2
25	−3.8	114	45.5	172	77.7
30	−1.1	115	46.1	173	78.3
31	−0.5	116	46.6	174	78.8
32	**0**	117	47.2	175	79.4
33	0.5	118	47.7	176	80.0
34	1.1	119	48.3	177	80.5
35	1.6	120	48.8	178	81.1
36	2.2	121	49.4	179	81.6
37	2.7	122	50.0	180	82.2
38	3.3	123	50.5	181	82.7
39	3.8	124	51.1	182	83.3
40	4.4	125	51.6	183	83.8
41	5.0	126	52.2	184	84.4
42	5.5	127	52.7	185	85.0
43	6.1	128	53.3	186	85.5
44	6.6	129	53.8	187	86.1
45	7.2	130	54.4	188	86.6
46	7.7	131	55.0	189	87.2
47	8.3	132	55.5	190	87.7
48	8.8	133	56.1	191	88.3
49	9.4	134	56.6	192	88.8
50	10.0	135	57.2	193	89.4
55	12.7	136	57.7	194	90.0
60	15.5	137	58.3	195	90.5
65	18.3	138	58.8	196	91.1
70	21.1	139	59.4	197	91.6
75	23.8	140	60.0	198	92.2
80	26.6	141	60.5	199	92.7
85	29.4	142	61.1	200	93.3
86	30.0	143	61.6	201	93.8
87	30.5	144	62.2	202	94.4
88	31.0	145	62.7	203	95.0
89	31.6	146	63.3	204	95.5
90	32.2	147	63.8	205	96.1
91	32.7	148	64.4	206	96.6
92	33.3	149	65.0	207	97.2
93	33.8	150	65.5	208	97.7
94	34.4	151	66.1	209	98.3
95	35.0	152	66.6	210	98.8
96	35.5	153	67.2	211	99.4
97	36.1	154	67.7	**212**	**100.0**
98	36.6	155	68.3	213	100.5
98.6	**37.0**	156	68.8	214	101.1

Fahrenheit–Celsius Conversion Formulas

To convert Fahrenheit to Celsius (exceeding 32°F) or Celsius to Fahrenheit (above 0° C):

F to C: Subtract 32, multiply by 5, divide by 9 OR subtract 32, divide by 1.8.
Example: 63° F to Celsius: $63 - 32 = 31 \times 5 = 155 \div 9 = 17.2$°C

C to F: Multiply by 9, divide by 5, add 32 OR multiply by 1.8, add 32.
Example: 37 °C to Fahrenheit: $37 \times 9 = 333 \div 5 = 66.6 + 32 = 98.6$° F

Medical Prefixes, Suffixes, and Combining Forms: The Building Blocks of Medical Language

a- not, without, less
ab- from, away from, off
abs- from, away from, off
acantho- thorn
acou- hearing
acro- extremity
acu- hearing
ad- increase, adherence, motion toward, very
-ad toward, in the direction of, -ward
adeno- gland
adip- fat
adipo- fat
-agogue promoter, stimulator
aidoio- genitals
-al pertaining to
alb- white
albo- white
alge- pain
algesi- pain
algio- pain
algo- pain
allo- other, different
ambi- around, on (both) sides, on all sides, both
ambly- dull
amblyo- dull
amyl- starch, polysaccharide
amylo- starch, polysaccharide
an- not, without, -less
ana- up, toward, apart
andro- male
angi- vessel
angio- vessel
ankylo- crooked
ante- before
anthraco- coal, carbon
anti- **1** against, opposing, **2** curative, **3** antibody
apo- separated from, derived from
aque- water
aqueo- water
-ar pertaining to
-arche beginning
arteri- artery
arterio- artery
arthr- joint, articulation
arthro- joint, articulation
-ary pertaining to
-ase an enzyme
-ate a salt or ester of an "-ic" acid
athero- pasty, fatty
atto- one quintillionth (10^{-18})
audi- hearing
audio- hearing
aur- ear
auri- ear
auro- ear
aut- self, same
auto- self, same
bacteri- bacteria
bacterio- bacteria
balano- penis
bi- twice, double
bio- life
blasto- budding by cells or tissue
blephar- eyelid
blepharo- eyelid
brachi- arm
brachio- arm
brachy- short
bronch- bronchus
bronchi- bronchus
broncho- bronchus
carcin- cancer
carcino- cancer
cardi- **1** heart, **2** esophageal opening of stomach
cardio- **1** heart, **2** esophageal opening of stomach
carpo- wrist
cata- down
caud- tail, lower part of body
caudo- tail, lower part of body
-cele hernia, swelling
celio- abdomen
-centesis surgical puncture
centi- one hundredth (10^{-2})
cephal- the head
cephalo- the head
cervic- **1** neck, **2** uterine cervix
cervico- **1** neck, **2** uterine cervix
cheil- lip
cheilo- lip
cheir- hand
cheiro- hand
chem- **1** chemistry, **2** drug
chemo- **1** chemistry, **2** drug
chir- hand
chiro- hand
chlor- **1** green, **2** chlorine

chloro- 1 green, **2** chlorine
chol- bile
chondrio- 1 cartilage, **2** granular, **3** gritty
chondro- 1 cartilage, **2** granular, **3** gritty
chrom- color
chromat- color
chromo- color
chron- time
chrono- time
-cidal killing, destroying
-cide killing, destroying
cis- on this side, on the near side
-clast breaker
-clysis washing
co- with, together, in association, very, complete
col- with, together, in association, very, complete
colp- vagina
colpo- vagina
com- with, together, in association, very, complete
con- with, together, in association, very, complete
conio- dust
cor- with, together, in association, very, complete
coreo- pupil
cost- rib
costo- rib
crani- cranium
cranio- cranium
-crine secretion
cry- cold
cryo- cold
crypt- hidden
crypto- hidden
culdo- cul-de-sac
cyan- 1 blue, **2** cyanide
cyano- 1 blue, **2** cyanide
cycl- 1 circle, cycle, **2** ciliary body
cyst- 1 bladder, **2** cyst, **3** cystic duct
cysti- 1 bladder, **2** cyst, **3** cystic duct
cysto- 1 bladder, **2** cyst, **3** cystic duct
cyt- cell
-cyte cell
cyto- cell
dacry- tears
dacryo- tears
dactyl- finger, toe
dactylo- finger, toe
de- away from, cessation
deca- ten
deci- one tenth (10^{-1})
deka- ten
dent- tooth
denti- tooth
derm- skin
derma- skin
dermat- skin
dermato- skin
dermo- skin
-desis binding
dextr- right, toward or on the right side
dextro- right, toward or on the right side
di- separation, taking apart, reversal, not, un-
dif- separation, taking apart, reversal, not, un-
dipso- thirst
dir- separation, taking apart, reversal, not, un-
dis- separation, taking apart, reversal, not, un-
duo- two
duodeno- duodenum
-dynia pain
dynamo- force, energy
dys- bad, difficult
ect- outer, on the outside
-ectasia dilation, stretching
-ectasis dilation, stretching
ecto- outer, on the outside
-ectomy excision
-emphraxis obstruction
encephal- brain
encephalo- brain
end- within, inner
endo- within, inner
enter- intestine
entero- intestine
ent- inner, within
ento- inner, within
epi- upon, following, subsequent to
ergo- work
erythr- red, redness
erythro- red, redness
eso- inward
esthesio- sensation, perception
eu- good, well
ex- out of, from, away from
exo- exterior, external, outward
extra- outside of, without
ferri- ferric ion (Fe^{3+})
ferro- 1 metallic iron, **2** ferrous ion (Fe^{2+})
fibr- fiber
fibro- fiber
-form in the form or shape of
galact- milk
galacto- milk
gastr- 1 stomach, **2** belly
gastro- 1 stomach, **2** belly
-gen 1 producing, coming to be, **2** precursor
gen- 1 producing, coming to be, **2** precursor

giga- one billion (10^9)

gingiv- gums

gingivo- gums

gloss- tongue

glosso- tongue

gluco- glucose

glyco- sugars

gnath- jaw

gnatho- jaw

gon- seed, semen

gonio- angle

gono- seed, semen

-gram a recording

granul- granular, granule

granulo- granular, granule

-graph recording instrument

gyn- woman

gyne- woman

gyneco- woman

gyno- woman

hecto- one hundred (10^{10})

hem- blood

hema- blood

hemat- blood

hemato- blood

hemi- one half

hemo- blood

hepat- liver

hepatico- liver

hepato- liver

hept- seven

hepta- seven

hidr- sweat

hidro- sweat

hist- tissue

histio- tissue

histo- tissue

homeo- same, constant

hydr- water, hydrogen

hydro- water, hydrogen

hyper- excessive, above normal

hypo- beneath, diminution, deficiency, the lowest

hyster- 1 uterus, hysteria, **2** late, following

hystero- 1 uterus, hysteria, **2** late, following

-ia a condition

-iasis condition, state

-ic pertaining to

-ics organized knowledge, practice, treatment

ileo- ileum

ilio- ilium

in- 1 in, **2** not

-in chemical suffix

-ine chemical suffix

infra- below

inguino- groin

inter- between, among

intra- within

intro- within

irid- iris

irido- iris

ischi- ischium

ischio- ischium

-ism 1 condition, disease, **2** practice, doctrine

-ismus spasm, contraction

iso- 1 equal, like, **2** isomer, **3** sameness

-ite the nature of, resembling

-ites -y, -like

-itides plural of -itis

-itis inflammation

kal- potassium

kali- potassium

karyo- nucleus

kerat- cornea

kerato- cornea

kilo- one thousand (10^3)

kin- movement

kine- movement

kinesi- motion

kinesio- motion

kineso- motion

kino- movement

labio- lip

lacrim- tears

lacrimo- tears

lact- milk

lacti- milk

lacto- milk

laparo- abdomen, abdominal wall

laryng- larynx

laryngo- larynx

lateri- lateral, to one side, side

latero- lateral, to one side, side

-lepsis seizure

-lepsy seizure

lepto- light, slender, thin, frail

leuk- white

leuko- white

linguo- tongue

lip- fat, lipid

lipo- fat, lipid

lith- stone, calculus, calcification

litho- stone, calculus, calcification

-log speech, words

log- speech, words

logo- speech, words

-logy 1 study of, **2** collecting

lymph- lymph

lympho- lymph

lys- lysis, dissolution

lyso- lysis, dissolution
macr- large, long
macro- large, long
mal- bad, deficient
-malacia softening
mamm- breast
mamma- breast
mammo- breast
mast- breast
masto- breast
meg- large, oversize
mega- **1** large, oversize, **2** one million (10^6)
megal- large
megalo- large
-megaly, enlargement
melan- black
melano- black
men- menstruation
mening- meninges
meningo- meninges
meno- menstruation
ment- chin
mento- chin
-mer member of a series
mes- **1** middle, mean, intermediate, **2** attaching membrane
meso- **1** middle, mean, intermediate, **2** attaching membrane
meta- **1** after, behind, **2** joint action, sharing
-meter measurement, measuring device
metr- uterus
metro- uterus
micr- small, microscopic
micro- **1** small, microscopic, **2** one-millionth (10^{-6})
milli- one-thousandth (10^{-3})
mon- single
mono- single
morph- form, shape, structure
morpho- form, shape, structure
my- muscle
myo- muscle
myel- **1** bone marrow, **2** spinal cord
myelo- **1** bone marrow, **2** spinal cord
myring- tympanic membrane
myringo- tympanic membrane
myx- mucus
myxo- mucus
nano- **1** dwarf, **2** one billionth (10^{-9})
nas- nose
naso- nose
natr- sodium
natri- sodium
necr- death, necrosis
necro- death, necrosis
neo- new
nephr- kidney
nephro- kidney
neur- nerve, nervous system
neuri- nerve, nervous system
neuro- nerve, nervous system
norm- normal
normo- normal
octo- eight
oculo- eye, ocular
odont- tooth
odonto- tooth
odyn- pain
odyno- pain
-oid resemblance to
olig- few, little
oligo- few, little
-oma tumor, neoplasm
-omata plural of -oma
oncho- onco-
onco- tumor, bulk, volume
-one ketone (–CO– group)
onych- fingernail, toenail
onycho- fingernail, toenail
oo- egg, ovary
oophor- ovary
oophoro- ovary
ophthalm- eye
ophthalmo- eye
-opia vision
-opsia vision
or- mouth
orchi- testis
orchido- testis
orchio- testis
ori- mouth
oro- mouth
-ose sugar
-oses plural of -osis
-osis process, condition, state
ossi- bone
osseo- bony
ost- bone
oste- bone
osteo- bone
ovari- ovary
ovario- ovary
ovi- egg
ovo- egg
oxa- oxygen
oxo- oxygen
oxy- **1** sharp, acid, **2** acute, shrill, quick, **3** oxygen
pachy- thick
pan- all, entire

pant- all, entire
panto- all, entire
para- **1** abnormal, **2** involvement of two like parts
pari- equal
path- disease
patho- disease
-pathy disease
ped- **1** child, **2** foot
pedi- **1** child, **2** foot
pedo- **1** child, **2** foot
-penia deficiency
penta- five
per- through, thoroughly, intensely
peri- around, about
-pexy fixation, usually surgical
phaco- lens
-phage eating, devouring
-phagia eating, devouring
phago- eating, devouring
-phagy eating, devouring
phako- lens
phanero- visible, evident
pharmaco- drugs, medicine
pharyng- pharynx
pharyngo- pharynx
phil- **1** attraction, **2** chemical affinity
-philia **1** attraction, **2** chemical affinity
philo- **1** attraction, **2** chemical affinity
phleb- vein
phlebo- vein
-phobia fear
phon- sound, speech
phono- sound, speech
phor- carrying, bearing
phoro- carrying, bearing
phos- light
phot- light
photo- light
phren- **1** diaphragm, **2** mind, **3** phrenic
phreni- **1** diaphragm, **2** mind, **3** phrenic
-phrenia of mind
phrenico- **1** diaphragm, **2** mind, **3** phrenic
phreno- **1** diaphragm, **2** mind, **3** phrenic
-phylaxis protection
phyll- leaf
phyllo- leaf
physi- **1** physical, **2** natural
physio- **1** physical, **2** natural
physo- **1** swelling, inflation, **2** air, gas
phyt- plants
phyto- plants
pico- one trillionth (10^{-12})
plan- flat
plani- flat
plano- flat
-plasia formation
plasma- plasma
plasmat- plasma
plasmato- plasma
plasmo- plasma
platy- wide, flat
-plegia paralysis
pleo- more
plesio- near, similar
pleur- rib, side, pleura
pleura- rib, side, pleura
pleuro- rib, side, pleura
pluri- several, more
-pnea breath, respiration
pneo- breath, respiration
pneum- **1** air, gas, **2** lung, **3** breathing
pneuma- **1** air, gas, **2** lung, **3** breathing
pneumat- **1** air, gas, **2** lung, **3** breathing
pneumato- **1** air, gas, **2** lung, **3** breathing
pod- foot, foot-shaped
-pod foot, foot-shaped
podo- foot, foot-shaped
-poiesis production
poikilo- irregular, variable
polio- gray
poly- **1** multiplicity, **2** polymer
post- after, behind, posterior
pre- anterior, before
presby- old
pro- **1** before, forward, **2** precursor
proct- anus, rectum
procto- anus, rectum
prot- first
proto- first
pseud- false
pseudo- false
psych- mind
psyche- mind
psycho- mind
-ptosis sagging, falling
pyel- (renal) pelvis
pyelo- (renal) pelvis
pykn- dense, compact
pykno- dense, compact
pyo- suppuration, pus
pyreto- fever
pyro- fire, heat, fever
quadr- four
quadri- four
rachi- spinal column
rachio- spinal column
radio- **1** radiation, x-ray, **2** radius
re- again, backward
rect- rectum, straight

recto- rectum, straight
ren- kidney
reno- kidney
retro- backward, behind
rhin- nose
rhino- nose
-rrhagia discharge
-rrhaphy surgical suturing
-rrhea flow
-rrhexis rupture
salping- tube
salpingo- tube
sarco- flesh, muscle
schisto- split, cleft
schiz- split, cleft, division
schizo- split, cleft, division
scler- hardness (induration), sclerosis, ocular sclera
sclero- hardness (induration), sclerosis, ocular sclera
scolio- crooked
-scope instrument for viewing
-scopy viewing
scot- shadow, darkness
scoto- shadow, darkness
semi- one-half, partly
sept- **1** seven, **2** septum, **3** sepsis, infection
septi- seven
septo- **1** seven, **2** septum, **3** sepsis, infection
sial- saliva, salivary gland
sialo- saliva, salivary gland
sider- iron
sidero- iron
sigmoid- **1** S-shaped, **2** sigmoid colon
sigmoido- **1** S-shaped, **2** sigmoid colon
sin- sinus
sino- sinus
sinu- sinus
sito- food, grain
somat- body, bodily
somato- body, bodily
somatico- body, bodily
somno- sleep
son- **1** sound, **2** ultrasound
sono- **1** sound, **2** ultrasound
spasmo- spasm
spermato- semen, sperm
spermo- semen, sperm
sperma- semen, sperm
sphygmo- pulse
spir- breathing
spiro- breathing
splanchn- viscera
splanchni- viscera
splanchno- viscera
splen- spleen
spleno- spleen
staphyl- grape, bunch of grapes, staphylococci
staphylo- grape, bunch of grapes, staphylococci
-stasis stopping
-stat arresting change or movement
steno- narrowness, constriction
stereo- solid
stheno- strength, force, power
stom- mouth
stoma- mouth
stomat- mouth
stomato- mouth
sub- beneath, less than normal, inferior
super- in excess, above, superior, in the upper part
supra- above
sy- together
syl- together
sym- together
syn- together
sys- together
tachy- rapid
tel- distant
tele- distant
ten- tendon
tendin- tendon
teno- tendon
tenont- tendon
tenonto- tendon
tera- one quadrillion (10^{15})
tetra- four
thel- nipple
thelo- nipple
therm- heat
thermo- heat
thorac- chest, thorax
thoracico- chest, thorax
thoraco- chest, thorax
thromb- blood clot
thrombo- blood clot
thyr- thyroid gland
thyro- thyroid gland
toco- childbirth
-tome **1** cutting instrument, **2** segment, section
-tomy cutting operation
tono- tone, tension, pressure
top- place, topical
topo- place, topical
tox- toxin, poison
toxi- toxin, poison
toxico- toxin, poison
toxo- toxin, poison
trache- trachea

tracheo- trachea
trans- across, through, beyond
tri- three
trich- hair
trichi- hair
-trichia hair
tricho- hair
tris- three
-trophic food, nutrition
tropho- food, nutrition
-trophy food, nutrition
-tropia turning
-tropic turning toward, affinity
ultra- beyond
uni- one, single
uri- uric acid
-uria urine, urination
uric- uric acid
urico- uric acid
uro- 1 urine, **2** urinary tract
vas- duct, blood vessel
vasculo- blood vessel
vaso- duct, blood vessel
vesic- urinary bladder, vesicle
vesico- urinary bladder, vesicle
xanth- yellow, yellowish
xantho- yellow, yellowish
xero- dry
zo- 1 animal, **2** life
zoo- 1 animal, **2** life
zym- fermentation, enzymes
zymo- fermentation, enzymes

Common Medical Abbreviations and Acronyms

α alpha: Bunsen solubility coefficient; first in a series; specific rotation term; heavy chain class corresponding to IgA
α-h the right-handed helical form assumed by many proteins
α-T α-tocopherol
a (specific) absorption (coefficient) (USUALLY ITALIC); (total) acidity; area; (systemic) arterial (blood) (SUBSCRIPT); asymmetric; atto-
A absorbance
A adenosine (or adenylic acid); alveolar gas (SUBSCRIPT); ampere
Å angstrom; Ångström unit
aa [G.] ana of each (USED IN PRESCRIPTIONS)
AA amino acid; aminoacyl
a.c. [L.] ante cibum, before a meal
A:G R albumin:globulin ratio
Ab antibody
AB abortion
ABG arterial blood gas
ABI ankle-brachial index
abl Abelson murine leukemia virus
ABLB alternate binaural loudness balance (test)
ABR abortus Bang ring (test); auditory brainstem response (audiometry)
γ-Abu-γ aminobutyric acid
ABVD Adriamycin (doxorubicin), bleomycin, vinblastine, and dacarbazine
ac, Ac acetyl; actinium
aC arabinosylcytosine
AC acetate; acromioclavicular; air conduction; alternating current; atriocarotid
AC:A accommodation convergence accommodation (ratio)
ACE angiotension-converting enzyme
ACEI angiotensin-converting enzyme inhibitor
AcG accelerator globulin
ac-g accelerator globulin
ACh, Ach acetylcholine
aCL anticardiolipin (antibody)
ACP acyl carrier protein
ACTH adrenocorticotropic hormone (corticotropin)
AD Alzheimer disease
⃠ **AD** [L.] *auris dextra*, right ear
ADD attention deficit disorder
ad lib. [L.] ad libitum, freely, as desired
Ade adenine
ADH antidiuretic hormone
ADHD attention deficit hyperactivity disorder
ADLs activities of daily living
Ado adenosine
ADP adenosine 5′ diphosphate
ADR adverse drug reaction
A-E above the elbow (amputation)
AECB acute exacerbation of chronic bronchitis
AED automated external defibrillator
AFB acid fast bacillus
AFORMED alternating failure of response, mechanical, to electrical depolarization
AFP α-fetoprotein
Ag antigen; [L.] argentum, silver
AHF antihemophilic factor
AHG antihemophilic globulin
AID artificial insemination donor
AIDS acquired immunodeficiency syndrome
AIH artificial insemination by husband; artificial insemination, homologous
A-K above the knee (amputation)
Al aluminum
Ala alanine (or its monoradical or diradical)
ALA δ-aminolevulinic acid
ALD adrenoleukodystrophy
ALL acute lymphocytic leukemia
ALS advanced life support; amyotrophic lateral sclerosis; antilymphocyte serum
ALT alanine aminotransferase
Am americium
AML acute myelogenous leukemia
AMP adenosine monophosphate (adenylic acid)
amu atomic mass unit
ANA antinuclear antibody
ANF antinuclear factor
ANOVA analysis of variance
ANS autonomic nervous system
ANUG acute necrotizing ulcerative gingivitis
AP anteroposterior
APA antipernicious anemia (factor)
APAP acetaminophen
A-P-C adenoidal pharyngeal conjunctival (virus)
APC antigen presenting cell
aPS antiphospholipid antibody syndrome

The symbol indicating forbidden (⃠) appears opposite abbreviations prohibited by the Joint Commission on Accreditation of Healthcare Organizations (JCAHO).

APTT activated partial thromboplastin time
Ar argon
araC arabinosylcytosine (cytarabine)
ARDS adult *or* acute respiratory distress syndrome
ARF acute renal failure; acute rheumatic fever
Arg arginine (or its monoradical or diradical)
AROM active range of motion
⦸**AS** [L.] *auris sinistra,* left ear
As arsenic
ASA acetylsalicylic acid (aspirin)
ASCP American Society of Clinical Pathologists
ASC-US atypical squamous cells of undetermined significance
ASHD arteriosclerotic heart disease
Asn asparagine (or its mono- or diradical)
ASO antistreptolysin O
Asp aspartic acid (or its radical forms)
AST aspartate aminotransferase
At astatine
at. wt. atomic weight
ATFL anterior talofibular ligament
ATL adult T-cell leukemia; adult T-cell lymphoma
atm (standard) atmosphere
ATP adenosine 5′ triphosphate
ATPase adenosine triphosphatase
ATPD ambient temperature and pressure, dry
ATPS ambient temperature and pressure, saturated (with water vapor)
⦸**AU** [L.] *auris utraque,* each ear, both ears
Au [L.] *aurum,* gold
AUC area under the curve
AV arteriovenous
A-V arteriovenous; atrioventricular
AVM arteriovenous malformation
AVN atrioventricular node
AVP antiviral protein
AW atomic weight
ax. axis
AZT azidothymidine (zidovudine)
B barometric (pressure) (SUBSCRIPT); boron
b blood (SUBSCRIPT)
β second in a series
Ba barium
BADLs basic activities of daily living
BAER brainstem auditory evoked response
BAL British anti-Lewisite (dimercaprol); bronchoalveolar lavage
BALB binaural alternate loudness balance (test)
BBB blood brain barrier; bundle branch block
BBT basal body temperature
BCG bacille bilié de Calmette Guérin (vaccine)
BE barium enema
B-E below the elbow (amputation)
Be beryllium
Bi bismuth
b.i.d. [L.] *bis in die,* twice a day
BIDS brittle hair, impaired intelligence, decreased fertility, and short stature (syndrome)
BIPAP bilevel positive airway pressure
Bk berkelium
BM bowel movement
BMD bone mineral density
BMI body mass index
BNEd Bachelor of Nursing Education
BNP brain natriuretic peptide
BNSc Bachelor of Nursing Science
bp base pair
BP blood pressure; boiling point; *British Pharmacopoeia*
BPF bronchopleural fistula
BPH Bachelor of Public Health
BPH benign prostatic hyperplasia
Bq becquerel (SI unit of radionuclide activity)
Br bromine
BRAT (diet) banana, rice cereal, applesauce, toast
BS, BSc Bachelor of Science (Baccalaureus Scientiae)
BSA body surface area
BSE breast self-examination
BSER brainstem evoked response (audiometry)
BSN Bachelor of Science in Nursing
BSO bilateral salpingo-oophorectomy
BT bleeding time
BTPS body temperature, ambient pressure, saturated (with water vapor)
BTU British thermal unit
BTX botulinum toxin
BUN blood urea nitrogen
BUS Bartholin glands, urethra, Skene glands

The symbol indicating forbidden (⦸) appears opposite abbreviations prohibited by the Joint Commission on Accreditation of Healthcare Organizations (JCAHO).

BVMS Bachelor of Veterinary Medicine and Surgery
Bx biopsy
c calorie (small); capillary (blood); centi
C calorie (large); carbon; Celsius; centigrade; clearance (rate, renal) (AS SUBSCRIPT) $_C$; compliance; concentration; cylindric (lens); cytidine
c̄ [L.] *cum*, with
C&S culture and sensitivity
C.C. chief complaint
c/o complains of
ca. [L.] *circa*, about, approximately
c-a cardioarterial
Ca calcium; cathodal; cathode
CA cancer; carcinoma; cardiac arrest; chronologic age; contrast angiography; croup associated (virus); cytosine arabinoside
CABG coronary artery bypass graft
CAD coronary artery disease
cal calorie (small)
Cal calorie (large)
CAM complementary and alternative medicine
cAMP cyclic adenosine monophosphate
CAO conscious, alert, oriented
cap capsule
CAP catabolite (gene) activator protein; community-acquired pneumonia
CAPD continuous ambulatory peritoneal dialysis
CAT computerized axial tomography (obsolete)
CBC complete blood (cell) count
CBG corticosteroid binding globulin
CBT cognitive-behavioral therapy
Cbz carbobenzoxy (chloride)
⃠**cc, c.c.** cubic centimeter
CCK cholecystokinin
CCNU chloroethylcyclohexyl-nitrosourea (lomustine)
CCU coronary care unit; critical care unit
cd candela
Cd cadmium
CD compact disc
CDA Certified Dental Assistant
CDC (U.S) Centers for Disease Control and Prevention
cDNA complementary DNA
CDP cytidine 5′ diphosphate
Ce cerium
CEA carcinoembryonic antigen; carotid endarterectomy
CELO chicken embryo lethal orphan (virus)
CEP congenital erythropoietic porphyria
CEU continuing education unit
Cf californium
CF complement fixation; cystic fibrosis; coupling factor
CG chorionic gonadotropin
CGA catabolite gene activator
cGMP cyclic guanosine monophosphate
cgs, CGS centimeter-gram-second (system, unit)
Ch¹ Christchurch (chromosome)
ChB Bachelor of Surgery (Chirurgiae Baccalaureus)
ChD, Chir Doct Doctor of Surgery (Chirurgiae Doctor)
CHF congestive heart failure
ChM Master of Surgery (Chirurgiae Magister)
CHO carbohydrate
Ci curie
CI color index; *Colour Index*; confidence interval
CIE counterimmunoelectrophoresis
CIN cervical intraepithelial neoplasia
CIQ cognitive laterality quotient
CIU chronic idiopathic urticaria
CJD Creutzfeldt-Jakob disease
CK creatine kinase
CK-MB creatine kinase MB isoenzyme
Cl chlorine
CL cardiolipin
CLA(ASCP) Clinical Laboratory Assistant (American Society of Clinical Pathologists)
CLIA Clinical Laboratory Improvement Amendments
CLL chronic lymphocytic leukemia
cm centimeter
cM centimorgan
Cm curium
CMA Certified Medical Assistant
CMC carpometacarpal
CME continuing medical education
CMI cell mediated immunity
CML chronic myelogenous leukemia
CMO Chief Medical Officer
CMP cytidine 5′ phosphate (or any cytidine monophosphate)
CMT Certified Medical Transcriptionist
CMV controlled mechanical ventilation; cytomegalovirus
CNM Certified Nurse-Midwife
CNP Community Nurse Practitioner

The symbol indicating forbidden (⃠) appears opposite abbreviations prohibited by the Joint Commission on Accreditation of Healthcare Organizations (JCAHO).

CNS central nervous system
Co cobalt
CoA coenzyme A
COG center of gravity
conA concanavalin A
COPD chronic obstructive pulmonary disease
COS Chief of Staff
CP cerebral palsy; costophrenic
CPAP continuous (or constant) positive airway pressure
CPD cephalopelvic disproportion
CPK creatine phosphokinase
CPM continuous passive motility
CPPB continuous (or constant) positive pressure breathing
CPPV continuous positive pressure ventilation
CPR cardiopulmonary resuscitation
cps cycles per second
CPT Current Procedural Terminology
Cr chromium; creatinine
CR Chief Resident; conditioned reflex; crown rump (length)
CRD chronic respiratory disease
CRH corticotropin releasing hormone
CRL crown rump length
CRNA Certified Registered Nurse Anesthetist
CRNP Certified Registered Nurse Practitioner
CRP cross-reacting protein
CRST calcinosis cutis, Raynaud phenomenon, sclerodactyly, and telangiectasia (syndrome)
CRT Certified Respiratory Therapist
Cs cesium
CS cesarean section; Chief of Staff
CSD catscratch disease
CSF cerebrospinal fluid; colony-stimulating factor
CT computed tomography
CTP cytidine 5′ triphosphate
CTR cardiothoracic ratio
Cu [L.] cuprum, copper
CV cardiovascular
CVA cerebral vascular (cerebrovascular) accident, costovertebral angle
CVP central venous pressure
CVS cardiovascular system
CXR chest x-ray
Cyd cytidine
cyl cylinder; cylindric (lens)
CYP cytochrome P-450 (enzyme)
Cys cysteine
Cyt cytosine
Δ delta; change; heat
δ delta; heavy chain class corresponding to IgD
D & C dilatation and curettage
D & E dilatation and evacuation
D Dalton, dead (space gas) (SUBSCRIPT); deciduous; deuterium; diffusing (capacity); dihydrouridine (in nucleic acids); diopter; [L.] dexter, right (opposite of left); vitamin D potency of cod liver oil
d deci-; day
D- prefix indicating that a molecule is sterically analogous to D glyceraldehyde
da deca
dA deoxyadenosine
Da dalton
DA developmental age
dAdo deoxyadenosine
dAMP deoxyadenylic acid
DANS 1-dimethylaminonaphthalene 5 sulfonic acid
db, dB decibel
DC Dental Corps; Doctor of Chiropractic; direct current
⃠ **D/C** discharge; discontinue
DCG dacryocystography
DCh Doctor of Surgery (Doctor Chirurgiae)
DCI dichloroisoproterenol
dCMP deoxycytidylic acid
DDS Doctor of Dental Surgery
DDT dichlorodiphenyl trichloroethane (chlorophenothane)
def decayed, extracted, or filled (deciduous teeth)
DEF decayed, extracted, or filled (permanent teeth)
DES diethylstilbestrol
DET diethyltryptamine
DEV duck embryo vaccine; duck embryo virus
DEXA dual energy x-ray absorptiometry
df decayed and filled (deciduous teeth)
DF decayed and filled (permanent teeth)
Df deficiency (absence or inactivation of a gene)
dGMP deoxyguanosine monophosphate (deoxyguanylic acid)
DH Dental Hygienist
DHEA dehydro-3-epiandrosterone
DIC disseminated intravascular coagulation
DIF direct immunofluorescence
DIP desquamative interstitial pneumonia; distal interphalangeal (joint)

The symbol indicating forbidden (⃠) appears opposite abbreviations prohibited by the Joint Commission on Accreditation of Healthcare Organizations (JCAHO).

DJD degenerative joint disease
dk deca-, deka-
DKA diabetic ketoacidosis
dL deciliter
dM decimorgan
DM diabetes mellitus
DMARD disease-modifying antirheumatic drug
DMD Doctor of Dental Medicine; Duchenne muscular dystrophy
DME Director of Medical Education
dmf decayed, missing, or filled (deciduous teeth)
DMF decayed, missing, or filled (permanent teeth)
DMSO dimethyl sulfoxide
DMT *N,N* dimethyltryptamine
DMV Doctor of Veterinary Medicine
DN dibucaine number
DNA deoxyribonucleic acid
DNB Diplomate of the National Board (of Medical Examiners)
DNE Director of Nursing Education; Doctor of Nursing Education
DNP deoxyribonucleoprotein; 2,4 dinitrophenol
DNR do not resuscitate
DNS Director of Nursing Service(s)
DO Doctor of Osteopathy
DOA dead on arrival
DOB date of birth
DOC deoxycholic acid; deoxycorticosterone
DOE dyspnea on exertion
DOM 2,5-dimethoxy-4-methylamphetamine
DON Director of Nursing
DOT directly observed therapy
DP Doctor of Pharmacy; Doctor of Podiatry
Dp duplication of a gene or chromosomal segment
2,3 DPG 2,3 diphosphoglycerate
DPH Doctor of Public Health; Doctor of Public Hygiene
DPharm Doctor of Pharmacy
DPI dry powder inhaler
DPM Doctor of Physical Medicine; Doctor of Podiatric Medicine
DPN diphosphopyridine nucleotide
DPT dipropyltryptamine; diphtheria, pertussis, and tetanus (vaccines)
dr dram
DR degeneration reaction, reaction of degeneration
Dr Med Doctor of Medicine
DRE digital rectal examination
DRG diagnosis-related group
DrPH Doctor of Public Health; Doctor of Public Hygiene
DRVVT dilute Russell viper venom test
D-S Doerfler Stewart (test)
DSA digital subtraction angiography
DSc Doctor of Science
DSD dry sterile dressing
dsDNA double-stranded DNA
DSM *Diagnostic and Statistical Manual of Mental Disorders of the American Psychiatric Association*
dT deoxythymidine
DT delirium tremens; duration of tetany
dTDP deoxythymidine 5 diphosphate
dThd thymidine
DTIC dimethyltrizenoimidazole carboxamide (dacarbazine)
dTMP deoxythymidylic acid
DTP diphtheria and tetanus toxoids and pertussis vaccine; distal tingling on percussion (Tinel sign)
DTPA diethylenetriamine pentaacetic acid
DTR deep tendon reflex
dTTP deoxythymidine 5′ triphosphate
DVM Doctor of Veterinary Medicine
DVT deep vein thrombosis
Dx diagnosis
Dy dysprosium
ε epsilon; molar absorption coefficient; heavy chain class corresponding to IgE
E exa; extraction (ratio)
EBV Epstein-Barr virus
ECF extended care facility; extracellular fluid
ECF-A eosinophilic chemotactic factor of anaphylaxis
ECG electrocardiogram
ECHO enterocytopathogenic human orphan (virus)
ECM erythema chronicum migrans
ECMO extracorporeal membrane oxygenation
ECS electrocerebral silence
ECT electroconvulsive therapy
ED eating disorder; effective dose; emergency department; erectile dysfunction
EDC expected date of confinement
EDTA ethylenediaminetetraacetic acid (edathamil, edetic acid)
EEG electroencephalogram
EENT eye, ear, nose, and throat
EIA enzyme immunoassay
EKG [German] *Elektrokardiogramme*, electrocardiogram
EKY electrokymogram
ELISA enzyme-linked immunosorbent assay
EMC encephalomyocarditis (virus)

EMF electromotive force
EMG electromyogram; exomphalos, macroglossia, and gigantism (syndrome)
EMS eosinophilia-myalgia syndrome
EMT Emergency Medical Technician
ENG electronystagmography
ENT ear, nose, and throat
EOG electrooculography
EOM extraocular muscle(s)
EPAP expiratory positive airway pressure
EPO erythropoietin
ER endoplasmic reticulum; emergency room
Er erbium
ERBF effective renal blood flow
ERCP endoscopic retrograde cholangiopancreatography
ERG electroretinogram
ERPF effective renal plasma flow
ERT estrogen replacement therapy
ERV expiratory reserve volume
Es einsteinium
ESEP extreme somatosensory evoked potential
ESP extrasensory perception
ESR electron spin resonance; erythrocyte sedimentation rate
ESRD end stage renal disease
ESWL extracorporeal shock-wave lithotripsy
EtOH ethyl alcohol
Eu europium
ev, eV electron volt
F Fahrenheit; faraday (constant); fertility (factor); field (of vision); fluorine; force; fractional (concentration); free (energy)
f femto-; (respiratory) frequency

F_1 first filial generation
F1.2 (prothrombin) fragment 1.2
FAAN Fellow of the American Academy of Nursing
FAAP Fellow of the American Academy of Pediatrics
Fab fragment of antibody molecule involved in antigen binding
FACA Fellow of the American College of Anesthesiology
FACAL Fellow of the American College of Allergy
FACC Fellow of the American College of Cardiologists
FACD Fellow of the American College of Dentists
FACFP Fellow of the American College of Family Physicians
FACO Fellow of the American College of Otolaryngology
FACOG Fellow of the American College of Obstetricians and Gynecologists
FACOS Fellow of the American College of Orthopaedic Surgeons
FACP Fellow of the American College of Physicians
FACR Fellow of the American College of Radiology
FACS Fellow of the American College of Surgeons
FAD flavin(e) adenine dinucleotide; familial Alzheimer disease
FAMA Fellow of the American Medical Association
FANA fluorescent antinuclear antibody (test)

FAP familial adenomatous polyposis
FB foreign body
FBS fasting blood sugar
Fc constant fragment of an antibody molecule
FDA (U.S.) Food and Drug Administration
Fe [L.] ferrum, iron
FEF forced expiratory flow
FET forced expiratory time
FEV forced expiratory volume
FF filtration fraction
FFD focus film distance
FHR fetal heart rate
FHT fetal heart tones
FIA fluorescent immunoassay
FIGLU formiminoglutamic (acid)
FISH fluorescent in situ hybridization
Fm fermium
FMN flavin(e) mononucleotide
FNA fine-needle aspiration
fps, FPS foot pound second (system, unit)
Fr francium; French (gauge, scale)
FRC functional residual capacity (of lungs)
French (catheter gauge)
FRF follicle stimulating hormone releasing factor
FRS first rank symptom
Fru fructose
FSH follicle stimulating hormone
FSH-RF follicle stimulating hormone releasing factor
FSH-RH follicle stimulating hormone releasing hormone
FTA-ABS fluorescent treponemal antibody absorption (test)
FU fluorouracil
F/U follow-up
FUO fever of unknown origin
FVC forced vital capacity

Fw F wave (fibrillary wave, flutter wave)
Fx fracture
γ gamma; Ostwald solubility coefficient; the third in a series; heavy chain class corresponding to IgG
G1 gap 1
G2 gap 2
G giga-; glucose; gravitation (newtonian constant of); guanosine (or guanylic acid) residues in polynucleotides; gravida (obstetric history)
g gram
G6P glucose 6 phosphate
Ga gallium
GABA γ-aminobutyric acid
GABHS group-A β-hemolytic *Streptococcus*
Gal galactose
GC gonococcus, gonorrhea
GCS Glasgow coma scale
Gd gadolinium
Ge germanium
GERD gastroesophageal reflux disease
GFR glomerular filtration rate
GGT γ-glutamyl transferase
GH glenohumeral; growth hormone
GHB γ-hydroxybutyrate
GHRF growth hormone releasing factor
GH-RF growth hormone releasing factor
GHRH growth hormone releasing hormone
GI gastrointestinal; Gingival Index
GIP gastric inhibitory polypeptide
GLC gas liquid chromatography
Gln glutamine; glutaminyl
Glu glutamic acid; glutamyl
Gly glycine; glycyl
GMO General Medical Officer

GMP guanosine monophosphate (guanylic acid)
GMS Gomori (or Grocott) methenamine silver (stain)
GN Graduate Nurse
GnRH gonadotropin releasing hormone
GOT glutamic oxaloacetic transaminase (aspartate aminotransferase)
GPI Gingival Periodontal Index
GPT glutamic pyruvic transaminase (alanine aminotransferase)
gr grain
GSH reduced glutathione
GSR galvanic skin response
GSSG oxidized glutathione
GSW gunshot wound
gt. [L.] *gutta*, a drop
GTP guanosine 5′ triphosphate
gtt. [L.] *guttae*, drops
GTT glucose tolerance test
GU genitourinary
Guo guanosine
GVHD graft versus host disease
Gy gray (unit of absorbed dose of ionizing radiation)
GYN gynecology
h hecto-
^{1}H hydrogen-1 (protium, light hydrogen)
^{2}H hydrogen-2 (deuterium, heavy hydrogen)
^{3}H hydrogen-3 (tritium, radioactive hydrogen)
H henry; hydrogen; hyperopia; hyperopic
h Planck constant
H & E hematoxylin and eosin (stain)
H & H hematocrit and hemoglobin
H^+ hydrogen ion
Ha hahnium
HA hyaluronic acid; hemagglutinin

HAART highly active antiretroviral therapy
HAV hepatitis A virus
Hb hemoglobin
HbA adult hemoglobin
HbA_1 major component of adult hemoglobin
HbA_2 minor fraction of adult hemoglobin
HbAS heterozygosity for hemoglobin A and hemoglobin S (sickle cell trait)
HB_cAg Hepatitis B core antigen
HbCO carboxyhemoglobin
HB_e Hepatitis B early antigen
HB_eAb Hepatitis B early antibody
Hb_eAg Hepatitis B early antigen
HbF fetal hemoglobin
Hbg hemoglobin
HBIG hepatitis B immune globulin
HBO hyperbaric oxygen
HbO_2 oxyhemoglobin, oxygenated hemoglobin
HbS sickle cell hemoglobin
HB_sAb hepatitis B surface antibody
HB_sAg hepatitis B surface antigen
HBV hepatitis B virus
HCFA Health Care Financing Administration
HCG human chorionic gonadotropin
HCl hydrochloric acid; hydrochloride
HCS human chorionic somatomammotropin (human placental lactogen)
Hct hematocrit
HCV Hepatitis C virus
h. d. [L.] *hora decubitus*, at bedtime
HDL high-density lipoprotein
HDRV human diploid (cell strain) rabies vaccine

He helium
HEMPAS hereditary erythroblastic multinuclearity associated with positive acidified serum
Hf hafnium
HFJV high frequency jet ventilation
HFOV high frequency oscillatory ventilation
HFPPV high frequency positive-pressure ventilation
HFV high frequency ventilation
Hg [L.] *hydrargyrum*, mercury
Hgb hemoglobin
HGE human granulocytic ehrlichiosis
HGH human (pituitary) growth hormone
HGSIL high-grade squamous intraepithelial lesion
HI hemagglutination inhibition (test, titer)
5-HIAA 5-hydroxy-indoleacetic acid
HIDA hepatobiliary iminodi-acetic acid (scan)
HIPAA Health Insurance Portability and Accountability Act
His histidine
-His histidino
His- histidyl
HIV human immuno-deficiency virus
Hl hyperopia, latent
HLA human lymphocyte antigen, human leukocyte antigen
Hm hyperopia, manifest (hypermetropia)
HME human monocytic ehrlichiosis
HMG CoA 3-hydroxy-3 methylglutaryl coenzyme A
HMG human menopausal gonadotropin
HMO Health Maintenance Organization
HMWK high molecular weight kininogen (Fletcher factor)
Ho holmium
h/o history of
HPF high power field
HPI history of present illness
HPL human placental lactogen
HPLC high performance liquid chromatography
HPV human papillomavirus
HRCT high-resolution computed tomography
⦸**h. s., HS [L.]** hora somni, at bedtime
HSV herpes simplex virus
5-HT 5-hydroxytryptamine (serotonin)
Ht hyperopia, total
HTLV human T-cell lymphocytotrophic virus; human T-cell lymphoma/leukemia virus
HTN hypertension
HVL half value layer
Hx (medical) history
Hyp hydroxyproline
Hz hertz
^{125}I iodine 125
^{131}I iodine 131
^{123}I iodine 123 (radioisotope)
I inspired (gas) (SUBSCRIPT); iodine
I & D incision and drainage
I & O (fluid) intake and output
IADLs instrumental activities of daily living
IAP intermittent acute porphyria
IBD inflammatory bowel disease
IBS irritable bowel syndrome
IBW ideal body weight
ICA internal carotid artery
ICD *International Classification of Diseases of the World Health Organization*; implantable cardioverter-defibrillator
ICDA *International Classification of Diseases, Adapted for Use in the United States*
ICF intracellular fluid
ICP intracranial pressure
ICSH interstitial cell stimulating hormone
ICU intensive care unit
ID infective dose
IDU idoxuridine; injecting/injection drug user
IF initiation factor; intrinsic factor
IFN interferon
Ig immunoglobulin
IGF insulinlike growth factor
IL interleukin
ILA insulinlike activity
Ile isoleucine
IM internal medicine; intra-muscular(ly); infectious mononucleosis
IMP inosine monophosphate (inosinic acid)
IMS Indian Medical Service
IMV intermittent mandatory ventilation
In indium
IND investigational new drug
Ino inosine
INR international normalized ratio
IOML infraorbitomeatal line
IP interphalangeal; intraperitoneal(ly)

The symbol indicating forbidden (⦸) appears opposite abbreviations prohibited by the Joint Commission on Accreditation of Healthcare Organizations (JCAHO).

IPAP inspiratory positive airway pressure
IPPB intermittent positive pressure breathing
IPPV intermittent positive pressure ventilation
IPV inactivated poliovirus vaccine
IQ intelligence quotient
Ir iridium
IRB institutional review board
IRV inspiratory reserve volume
ISI International Sensitivity Index
ITP idiopathic thrombocytopenic purpura; inosine 5′ triphosphate
IU International Unit
IUCD intrauterine contraceptive device
IUD intrauterine device
IV intravenous(ly); intraventricular(ly)
IVDA intravenous drug abuse(r)
IVF in vitro fertilization
IVP intravenous pyelogram
J flux (density)
J joule
JMS Junior Medical Student
JVD jugular venous distention
K [Mod. L.] *kalium*, potassium; kelvin
k kilo
kat katal
kb kilobase
kc kilocycle
kcal kilocalorie
KCT kaolin clotting time
kDa kilodalton
kg kilogram
KJ knee jerk
K_M Michaelis constant
KOH potassium hydroxide
KP keratic precipitate
Kr krypton
17-KS 17-ketosteroid
KS Kaposi sarcoma
KUB kidneys, ureters, bladder
kv kilovolt
kVp kilovolt peak
KW Kimmelstiel Wilson (disease); Keith Wagener (retinal changes)
l liter (use of CAPITAL letter preferred)
L inductance; left; [L.] limes, boundary, limit; liter
L- prefix indicating that a molecule is sterically analogous to L-glyceraldehyde
L:S R lecithin:sphingomyelin ratio
La lanthanum
LA lupus anticoagulant
LAD left anterior descending (coronary artery)
LAO left anterior oblique (coronary artery)
LAP leucine aminopeptidase
LATS long-acting thyroid stimulator
LBT lupus band test
LBW low birth weight
LC lethal concentration
LCA left coronary artery
LCAT lecithin cholesterol acyltransferase
LCM left costal margin; lymphocytic choriomeningitis (virus)
LD lethal dose
LDH lactate dehydrogenase
LDL low-density lipoprotein
LE left eye; lupus erythematosus
LEEP loop electrosurgical excision procedure
LES lower esophageal sphincter
LETS large external transformation sensitive (fibronectin)
Leu leucine
LFA left frontoanterior (fetal position)
LFP left frontoposterior (fetal position)
LFT left frontotransverse (fetal position); liver function test
LGSIL low-grade squamous intraepithelial lesion
LGV lymphogranuloma venereum
LH luteinizing hormone
LH/FSH-RF luteinizing hormone/follicle stimulating hormone releasing factor
LH-RF luteinizing hormone releasing factor
LH-RH luteinizing hormone releasing hormone
Li lithium
LLQ left lower quadrant
LM Licentiate in Midwifery
LMA left mentoanterior (fetal position)
LMP last menstrual period; left mentoposterior (fetal position)
LMT left mentotransverse (fetal position)
LNPF lymph node permeability factor
LOA left occipitoanterior (fetal position)
LOC level of consciousness; loss of consciousness
LOP left occipitoposterior (fetal position)
LOT left occipitotransverse (fetal position)
LP lumbar puncture
LPF low power field
LPH lipotropic pituitary hormone (lipotropin)
LPN Licensed Practical Nurse
Lr lawrencium
LRCP Licentiate of the Royal College of Physicians
LRCS Licentiate of the Royal College of Surgeons
LRH luteinizing hormone releasing hormone

LSA left sacroanterior (fetal position)
LSD lysergic acid diethylamide
LSP left sacroposterior (fetal position)
LST left sacrotransverse (fetal position)
LTH luteotropic hormone
LTM long-term memory
LTR long terminal repeat
Lu lutetium
LUQ left upper quadrant
LV left ventricle
LVEF left ventricular ejection fraction
LVET left ventricular ejection time
LVH left ventricular hypertrophy
LVN Licensed Visiting Nurse; Licensed Vocational Nurse
Lw former symbol for lawrencium (now Lr)
Lys lysine (or its radicals in peptides)
⃠ **μ** mu; micro-; heavy chain class corresponding to IgM
⃠ **μg** microgram
⃠ **μl, μL** microliter
⃠ **μm** micrometer
⃠ **μμ** micromicro
M + Am compound myopic astigmatism
m mass; meter; milliminim; molar
m- *meta*
M mega , meg ; molar; moles (per liter); morgan; myopic; myopia
M molar; moles (per liter)
m moles (per liter)
mA milliampere
MA Master of Arts (Magister Artium); Medical Assistant; mental age
MAA macroaggregated albumin
MAb monoclonal antibody
MAC *Mycobacterium avium* complex
MAI *Mycobacterium avium-intracellulare*
MAO monoamine oxidase
MAOI monoamine oxidase inhibitor
MAP morning after pill
mA-S milliampere second
MAST military antishock trousers
Mb myoglobin
MBC maximum breathing capacity
MbCO carbon monoxided myoglobin
MbO_2 oxymyoglobin
MC Medical Corps
MCH mean corpuscular hemoglobin
MCHC mean corpuscular hemoglobin concentration
mCi millicurie
MCL midclavicular line
mcm millimicron
MCP metacarpophalangeal
MCV mean corpuscular volume
MD [L.] *Medicinae Doctor*, Doctor of Medicine
Md mendelevium
MDF myocardial depressant factor
MDI metered dose inhaler
MDR multidrug-resistant
ME Medical Examiner
Me methyl
Med Tech Medical Technician; Medical Technologist
MEDLARS Medical Literature Analysis and Retrieval System
MEP maximal expiratory pressure
meq, mEq milliequivalent
MeSH Medical Subject Headings
Met methionine
MET metabolic equivalent of task
metHb methemoglobin
metMb metmyoglobin
MEV million electron volts (10^6 ev)
mg milligram
Mg magnesium
MHC major histocompatibility complex
mho siemens unit
MHz megahertz
MI mitral insufficiency; myocardial infarction
MID minimal infecting dose
MIP maximum inspiratory pressure
MK menaquinone (vitamin K2)
mks, MKS meter kilogram second (system, unit)
ml, mL milliliter
MLC mixed lymphocyte culture (test)
MLD minimal lethal dose
mm millimeter
mmHg millimeters of mercury (torr)
mmol millimole
MMPI Minnesota Multiphasic Personality Inventory (test)
MMR measles-mumps-rubella (vaccine)
MMSE Mini-Mental State Examination
Mn manganese
Mo molybdenum
MO Medical Officer; mineral oil
MOC Medical Officer on Call

The symbol indicating forbidden (⃠) appears opposite abbreviations prohibited by the Joint Commission on Accreditation of Healthcare Organizations (JCAHO).

MOD Medical Officer of the Day
mol mole
mol wt molecular weight
MOPP Mustargen (mechlorethamine hydrocholoride), Oncovin (vincristine sulfate), procarbazine hydrochloride, and prednisone
MPD maximal permissible dose
MPH Master of Public Health
MPS mononuclear phagocyte system
MR milk ring (test); mitral regurgitation
M_r molecular (weight) ratio
MRA magnetic resonance augiography
MRCP Member of the Royal College of Physicians
MRCS Member of the Royal College of Surgeons
mrd, MRD minimal reacting dose
MRI magnetic resonance imaging
mRNA messenger ribonucleic acid
MRSA methicillin-resistant *Staphylococcus aureus*
MS Master of Science
MS I, II, III, IV medical student: first, second, third, and fourth year
⃠**MS** multiple sclerosis; magnesium sulfate; morphine sulfate
msec millisecond
m/sec meters per second
MSG monosodium glutamate
MSH melanocyte stimulating hormone
MSM men who have sex with men
MSN Master of Science in Nursing
MT Medical Technologist; Medical Transcriptionist; Monitor Technician
mtDNA mitochondrial DNA
MTP metatarsophalangeal (joint)
Mu Mache unit
MUGA multiple gated acquisition (imaging)
mV millivolt
Mv mendelevium
MVA motor vehicle accident
MVE Murray Valley encephalitis (virus)
MVV maximal voluntary ventilation
MW molecular weight
My myopia
ν nu; kinematic viscosity
n index of refraction; nano
N newton; nitrogen; normal (concentration)
N normal (SMALL CAPS)
Na [Modern L.] *natrium*, sodium
NA *Nomina Anatomica*
NAD nicotinamide adenine dinucleotide; no apparent (or acute) distress
NAD+ nicotinamide adenine dinucleotide (oxidized form)
NADH nicotinamide adenine dinucleotide (reduced form)
NADP nicotinamide adenine dinucleotide phosphate
NADP+ nicotinamide adenine dinucleotide phosphate (oxidized form)
NADPH nicotinamide adenine dinucleotide phosphate (reduced form)
NAME nevi, atrial myxoma, myxoid neurofibromas, and ephelides (syndrome)
NANDA North American Nursing Diagnosis Association
Nb niobium
NCV nerve conduction velocity
Nd neodymium
Nd:YAG neodymium:yttrium-aluminum-garnet (laser)
NDA New Drug Application
Ne neon
NE norepinephrine; not examined
NEEP negative end expiratory pressure
NF National Formulary
ng nanogram
NGF nerve growth factor (antigen)
Ni nickel
NIH National Institutes of Health
NK natural killer (cell)
NKA no known allergies
NLM National Library of Medicine
nm nanometer
NMN nicotinamide mononucleotide
No nobelium
NP Nurse Practitioner
Np neptunium
NPO [L.] *nihil per os*, nothing by mouth
NREM nonrapid eye movement (sleep)
nRNA nuclear RNA
NS normal saline
NSAID nonsteroidal antiinflammatory drug
NSR normal sinus rhythm
NUG necrotizing ulcerative gingivitis
Ω omega; ohm
o- *ortho*
O [L.] *oculus*, eye; opening (in formulas for electrical reactions); oxygen

---

The symbol indicating forbidden (⃠) appears opposite abbreviations prohibited by the Joint Commission on Accreditation of Healthcare Organizations (JCAHO).

O & P ova and parasites
OAV oculoauriculovertebral (dysplasia, syndrome)
OB obstetrics
OB/GYN obstetrics (and) gynecology
OBS organic brain syndrome
OC oral contraceptive
OCD obsessive compulsive disorder
OD Doctor of Optometry; Officer of the Day; overdose
⦸**OD** [L.] *oculus dexter*, right eye
ODD oculodentodigital (dysplasia, syndrome)
Oe oersted (centimeter-gram-second unit of magnetic field strength)
OFD orofaciodigital (dysostosis, syndrome)
OKT Ortho-Kung T cell
OML orbitomeatal line
OMM ophthalmomandibulomelic (dysplasia, syndrome)
OMS organic mental syndrome
OP osmotic pressure; outpatient
OPV oral poliovirus vaccine
OR operating room
ORD optical rotatory dispersion
ORIF open reduction and internal fixation
Orn ornithine (or its radical)
Oro orotate; orotic acid
Os osmium
⦸**OS** [L.] *oculus sinister,* left eye
OSA obstructive sleep apnea
OSHA Occupational Safety and Health Administration
OT occupational therapy; Koch old tuberculin
OTC over-the-counter (nonprescription) drug
⦸**OU** [L.] *oculus uterque*, each eye (both eyes)
OXT oxytocin
oz ounce
p pico; pupil
***p*-** para
P partial (pressure); peta-; phosphorus, phosphoric (residue); plasma (concentration); pressure; para- (obstetric history)
^{32}P phosphorus-32
P_1 first parental generation
PA Physician Assistant; posteroanterior
Pa pascal; protactinium
PA Physician's Assistant; posteroanterior; pulmonary artery
PABA para-aminobenzoic acid
PAF platelet-aggregating (or platelet-activating) factor
PAH paraaminohippuric (acid)
PAo_2 partial pressure of arterial oxygen
PAS paraaminosalicylic (acid), periodic acid Schiff (reagent)
PASA paraaminosalicylic acid
PAT paroxysmal atrial tachycardia
Pb [L.] *plumbum*, lead
PBG porphobilinogen
p.c. [L.] *post cibum*, after a meal
PCB polychlorinated biphenyl
Pco_2 partial pressure of carbon dioxide
PCP phencyclidine; plasma cell pneumonia (*Pneumocystis carinii* [former name for *Pneumocystis jiroveci*] pneumonia), primary care provider
PCR polymerase chain reaction
PCT percutaneous transhepatic cholangiography
PCWP pulmonary capillary wedge pressure
Pd palladium
PD prism diopter
PDA patent ductus arteriosus; posterior descending artery
PDGF platelet-derived growth factor
PDLL poorly differentiated lymphocytic lymphoma
PDR *Physicians' Desk Reference*
PEEP positive end expiratory pressure
PEG polyethylene glycol
PET positron emission tomography
PF_4 platelet factor 4
PFT pulmonary function test
pg picogram
PG prostaglandin
PGA prostaglandin A
PGB prostaglandin B
PGE prostaglandin E
PGF prostaglandin F
pH hydrogen ion concentration; p (power) of $[H^+]_{10}$
Ph phenyl
Ph^1 Philadelphia (chromosome)
PHA phytohemagglutinin (antigen)
Pharm D Doctor of Pharmacy (Pharmaciae Doctor)
PhD [L.] *Philosophiae Doctor*, Doctor of Philosophy
Phe phenylalanine (or its radical)
PhG [L.] *Pharmacopoeia Germanica*, German Pharmacopeia

The symbol indicating forbidden (⦸) appears opposite abbreviations prohibited by the Joint Commission on Accreditation of Healthcare Organizations (JCAHO).

PhG Graduate in Pharmacy
PHN Public Health Nurse; postherpetic neuralgia
PICC peripherally inserted central catheter
PID pelvic inflammatory disease
PIF prolactin inhibiting factor
PIP proximal interphalangeal (joint)
pK negative logarithm of the ionization constant (Ka) of an acid
PK pyruvate kinase
PKU phenylketonuria
pm picometer
Pm promethium
PM post mortem
PMI point of maximum intensity
PMN polymorphonuclear (leukocyte)
PMS premenstrual syndrome
PN Practical Nurse
PND paroxysmal nocturnal dyspnea; postnasal drip
PNP platelet neutralization procedure
PNPB positive-negative pressure breathing
PNS peripheral nervous system
Po polonium
PO [L.] per os, by mouth
PO_2, Po_2 partial pressure of oxygen
POEMS polyneuropathy, organomegaly, endocrinopathy, monoclonal protein, and skin changes (syndrome)
POMP prednisone, Oncovin (vincristine sulfate), methotrexate, and Purinethol (6-mercaptopurine)
POR problem-oriented (medical) record
PP pyrophosphate
PPCA proserum prothrombin conversion accelerator
PPD purified protein derivative (of tuberculin)
PPLO pleuropneumonia-like organism
ppm parts per million
PPPPP pain, pallor, pulselessness, paresthesia, paralysis
PPPPPP pain, pallor, pulselessness, paresthesia, paralysis, prostration
PPV positive pressure ventilation
Pr praseodymium; presbyopia
PR per rectum
PRA plasma renin activity
PRF prolactin releasing factor
PRL prolactin
p.r.n. PRN, [L.] *pro re nata,* as needed
Pro proline (or its radicals)
PROM passive range of motion; premature rupture of membranes
psi pounds per square inch
PSV pressure-supported ventilation
PT physical therapy; prothrombin time
Pt platinum
PTA plasma thromboplastin antecedent; phosphotungstic acid; prior to admission
PTAH phosphotungstic acid hematoxylin
PTCA percutaneous transluminal coronary angioplasty
PTH parathyroid hormone
PTT partial thromboplastin time
PTU prophylthiouracil
Pu plutonium
PUO pyrexia of unknown origin
PUPPP pruritic urticarial papules and plaques of pregnancy
PUVA (oral administration of) psoralen (and subsequent exposure to) ultraviolet light of A wavelength (UV A)
PVC polyvinyl chloride; premature ventricular contraction
PVL plasma viral load
PVP polyvinylpyrrolidone (povidone)
q [L.] *quisque*, every
Q coulomb; volume of blood flow
Qco_2 microliters CO_2 given off per milligram of dry-weight of tissue per hour
⃠ **q.d.** [L.] *quaque die*, every day
q.i.d. [L.] *quater in die*, four times a day
QNS quantity not sufficient
Qo oxygen consumption
Qo_2 oxygen consumption
⃠ **q.o.d.** every other day
q. s. [L.] *quantum satis*, as much as is enough; [L.] *quantum sufficiat*, as much as may suffice; quantity sufficient
r racemic; roentgen
R gas constant (8.315 joules); (organic) radical; Réaumur (scale) ; [L.] recipe, take; resistance determinant (plasmid); resistance (electrical); resistance (unit) (in the cardiovascular system); resolution; respiration; respiratory (exchange ratio); roentgen
Ra radium
RA rheumatoid arthritis

The symbol indicating forbidden (⃠) appears opposite abbreviations prohibited by the Joint Commission on Accreditation of Healthcare Organizations (JCAHO).

rad radian
RAD reactive airways disease
RAS reticular activating system
RAST radioallergosorbent test
RAV Rous-associated virus
RAW resistance, airway
Rb rubidium
rbc red blood cell; red blood (cell) count
RBC red blood cell; red blood (cell) count
RBF renal blood flow
RCM right costal margin
RD reaction of degeneration; reaction of denervation; Registered Dietitian
RDA recommended daily allowance
RDH Registered Dental Hygienist
rDNA ribosomal DNA
RDS respiratory distress syndrome
RDW red (blood cell) diameter (or distribution) width
Re rhenium
RE right ear; right eye
rem roentgen equivalent, man
REM rapid eye movement (sleep); reticular erythematous mucinosis
rep roentgen equivalent, physical
RF release factor; rheumatoid factor
RFA right frontoanterior (fetal position)
RFLP restriction-fragment length polymorphism
RFP right frontoposterior (fetal position)
RFT right frontotransverse (fetal position)
Rh Rhesus (Rh blood group); rhodium
RH releasing hormone
RIA radioimmunoassay
Rib ribose
RLL right lower lobe
RLQ right lower quadrant
RMA right mentoanterior (fetal position)
RML right middle lobe
RMP right mentoposterior (fetal position)
RMT right mentotransverse (fetal position)
Rn radon
RN Registered Nurse
RNA Registered Nurse Anesthetist; ribonucleic acid
RNase ribonuclease
RNC Registered Nurse, Certified
RNP Registered Nurse Practitioner
RNP ribonucleoprotein
R/O rule out
ROA right occipitoanterior (fetal position)
ROM range of motion
ROP right occipitoposterior (fetal position)
ROS review of systems
ROT right occipitotransverse (fetal position)
RP retinitis pigmentosa
RP, RPh Registered Pharmacist
RPF renal plasma flow
RPh Registered Pharmacist
rpm revolutions per minute
RPR rapid plasma reagin (test)
RQ respiratory quotient
rRNA ribosomal ribonucleic acid
RR relative risk
RRR relative-risk reduction
Rs resolution
RS respiratory syncytial (virus)
RSA right sacroanterior (fetal position)
RSD reflex sympathetic dystrophy
RSP right sacroposterior (fetal position)
RST right sacrotransverse (fetal position)
RSV Rous sarcoma virus; respiratory syncytial virus
RT Radiologic Technologist; Registered Technologist; Respiratory Therapist
RTE renal tubular epithelium
rTMP ribothymidylic acid
Ru ruthenium
RUL right upper lobe
RUQ right upper quadrant
RV residual volume; right ventricle
RVEF right ventricular ejection fraction
RVH right ventricular hypertrophy
℞ recipe, (the first word on a prescription), take; prescription; treatment
σ sigma; reflection coefficient; standard deviation; 1 millisecond (0.001 sec)
s [L.] *semis*, half; steady state (SUBSCRIPT); [L.] sinister, left
s sine, without
s/s signs and symptoms
S [L.] *sinister*, left; saturation of hemoglobin (percentage of) (followed by subscript O_2 **or** CO_2); siemens; spheric; spheric (lens); sulfur; Svedberg (unit)
S_1 first selfing generation
SA, S-A sinuatrial
SAD seasonal affective disorder
Sa_{O_2} oxygen saturation (of) arterial (oxyhemoglobin)
SARS severe acute respiratory syndrome
Sb [L.] *stibium*, antimony
SBE subacute bacterial endocarditis
sc subcutaneous(ly)
Sc scandium
SC sternoclavicular; subcutaneous(ly)
ScD Doctor of Science

SCID severe combined immunodeficiency
SD standard deviation; streptodornase
SDA specific dynamic action
Se selenium
Ser serine
SERM selective estrogen receptor modulator
Sf Svedberg flotation (constant, unit)
SGA small for gestational age
SGOT serum glutamic-oxaloacetic transaminase (aspartate aminotransferase)
SGPT serum glutamic-pyruvic transaminase (alanine aminotransferase)
SH serum hepatitis
SI [French] Système International d'Unités; International System of Units
Si silicon
s.i.d. [L.] *semel in die*, once daily
SID source-to-image (-receptor) distance
SIDS sudden infant death syndrome
sig. [L.] *signa*, affix a label, inscribe
SIMV spontaneous intermittent mandatory ventilation; synchronized intermittent mandatory ventilation
SIRD source-to-image-receptor distance
SISI small increment sensitivity index (test)
SK streptokinase
SL sublingual(ly)
SLE systemic lupus erythematosus
SLR straight leg raising
Sm samarium
SMS Senior Medical Student
Sn [L.] *stannum*, tin
SN Student Nurse
SOAP subjective data, objective data, assessment, and plan (problem oriented medical record)
SOB short(ness) of breath
sol., soln. solution
SP Speech Pathologist
S/P status post
sp. gr. specific gravity
sp. species
SPA single proton absorptiometry
SPCA serum prothrombin conversion accelerator (factor VII)
SPECT single photon emission computed tomography
SPF sun protection (or protective) factor
sph spheric (lens)
spm suppression and mutation
spp. species (plural)
SQ subcutaneous(ly)
Sr strontium
SRF somatotropin releasing factor
SRF-A slow reacting factor of anaphylaxis
SRIF somatotropin release inhibiting factor
sRNA soluble RNA
SRS slow-reacting substance (of anaphylaxis)
SRS-A slow-reacting substance of anaphylaxis
ssDNA single-stranded DNA
ssp. subspecies
SSRI selective serotonin reuptake inhibitor
ST scapulothoracic
stat; STAT [L.] *statim*, immediately, at once
STD sexually transmitted disease
STEL short-term exposure limit
STH somatotropic hormone
STI sexually transmitted infection
STM short-term memory
STPD standard temperature (0° C) and pressure (760 mmHg absolute), dry
STS serologic test for syphilis
Sv sievert (unit)
SV sievert (unit)
SVT supraventricular tachycardia
Sz seizure
t metric ton
t temperature (Celsius); tritium
T temperature, absolute (Kelvin); tension (intraocular); tera ; tesla; tetanus (toxoid); tidal (volume) (SUBSCRIPT); tocopherol; transverse (tubule); tritium; tumor (antigen)
T absolute temperature (Kelvin)
T! decreased tension (pressure)
T+ increased tension (pressure)
T_3 3,5,5′ triiodothyronine
T_4 tetraiodothyronine (thyroxine)
T & A tonsillectomy and adenoidectomy
T & C type and cross-match
Ta tantalum
TA Terminologia Anatomica
tab tablet
TAC transient aplastic crisis
TAD transient acantholytic dermatosis
TAF tumor angiogenesis factor
TAH total abdominal hysterectomy
TAR thrombocytopenia with absent radii (syndrome)
TAT thematic apperception test
Tb terbium
TB tuberculosis
TBG thyroid-binding globulin
TBP thyroxine-binding protein

TBV total blood volume
Tc technetium
^{99m}Tc technetium 99m
TCA tricarboxylic acid; trichloracetic acid
TCN talocalcaneonavicular (joint)
Td tetanus-diphtheria (toxoids, adult type)
TDP ribothymidine 5′ diphosphate
Te tellurium
TEDD total end-diastolic diameter
TEN toxic epidermal necrolysis
TESD total end-systolic diameter
TFCI transient focal cerebral ischemia
Th thorium
THC tetrahydrocannabinol
Thr threonine (or its radicals)
Ti titanium
t_i/t_{tot} duty cycle
TIA transient ischemic attack
TIBC total iron-binding capacity
t.i.d. [L.] *ter in die*, three times a day
tinct. tincture
TITh 3,5,3′ triiodothyronine
TKO to keep (venous infusion line) open
Tl thallium
TLC thin layer chromatography; total lung capacity; tender, loving care
TLV threshold-limit value
t_m temperature midpoint (Celsius)
T_m temperature midpoint (Kelvin)
Tm thulium; tubular maximal (excretory capacity of kidneys)
TM transport maximum
TMJ temporomandibular joint
TMP ribothymidine 5′ monophosphate
TMT tarsometatarsal
TMV tobacco mosaic virus
Tn (ocular) tension; (intraocular) tension normal
TNF tumor necrosis factor
TNM tumor, node, metastasis (tumor staging)
TORCH toxoplasmosis, other, rubella, cytomegalovirus, and herpes simplex (maternal infections)
t-PA, TPA tissue plasminogen activator
TPHA *Treponema pallidum* hemagglutination (test)
TPI *Treponema pallidum* immobilization (test)
TPN total parenteral nutrition
TPR temperature, pulse, and respirations
tr. tincture
TRH thyrotropin releasing hormone (stimulation test)
TRIC trachoma inclusion conjunctivitis (organism)
tRNA transfer RNA
Trp tryptophan (and its radicals)
TSH thyroid stimulating hormone
TSS toxic shock syndrome
TSTA tumor-specific transplantation antigen
TTP thrombotic thrombocytopenic purpura
TU toxic unit, toxin unit
TUR transurethral resection
TVUS transvaginal ultrasound
Tx treatment
Tyr tyrosine (and its radicals)
U uranium; uridine (in polymers); urinary (concentration)
⃠**U** unit
UA urinalysis
UDP uridine diphosphate
UDPG uridine diphosphate glucose
UGIS upper gastrointestinal series
UMP uridine monophosphate (uridylic acid)
u-PA urokinase
UPJ ureteropelvic junction
Urd uridine
URI upper respiratory infection
US ultrasound
USAN United States Adopted Names (Council)
USP *United States Pharmacopeia*
USPHS United States Public Health Service
UTI urinary tract infection
UTP uridine triphosphate
UV ultraviolet
UVB ultraviolet B
UVJ ureterovesical junction
v venous (blood); volt
V vanadium; vision; visual (acuity); volt; volume (frequently with subscripts denoting location, chemical species, and conditions)
$\dot{V}$ ventilation; gas flow (frequently with subscripts indicating location and chemical species); ventilation;
V_A alveolar ventilation
$\dot{V}a/\dot{Q}$ ventilation/perfusion ratio
V_1CV_6 unipolar precordial electrocardiogram chest leads
VA viral antigen
V-A ventriculoatrial
Val valine (and its radicals)

The symbol indicating forbidden (⃠) appears opposite abbreviations prohibited by the Joint Commission on Accreditation of Healthcare Organizations (JCAHO).

VATER vertebral defects, imperforate anus, tracheoesophageal fistula with esophageal atresia, and radial and renal dysplasia (complex)
VBAC vaginal birth after cesarean
VC vision, color; vital capacity
VCE vagina, (ecto)cervix, endocervical canal
V_D (physiologic) dead space
VDRL Venereal Disease Research Laboratory (test)
VHDL very high density lipoprotein
VIP vasoactive intestinal polypeptide
VLDL very low density lipoprotein
VMA vanillylmandelic acid (test)
V_{max} maximal velocity
VN Visiting Nurse, Vocational Nurse
VO vocal order
VP vasopressin
VR vocal resonance
VS vital signs; volumetric solution
V_T tidal volume
VZIG varicella-zoster immune globulin
W watt; [German] *Wolfram*, tungsten
Wb weber
WBC white blood cell; white blood (cell) count
WC Ward Clerk
WD well-developed
WDLL well-differentiated lymphocytic (or lymphatic) lymphoma
WEE western equine encephalomyelitis
WHO World Health Organization
WN well-nourished
WNV West Nile virus
X xanthosine
Xao xanthosine
Xe xenon
XU excretory urogram
Y yttrium
YAG yttrium-aluminum-garnet (laser)
Yb ytterbium
Z carbobenzoxy (chloride)
ZEEP zero end-expiratory pressure
ZES Zollinger-Ellison syndrome
Zn zinc
^{65}Zn zinc 65
Zr zirconium
ZSR zeta sedimentation ratio

Common Abbreviations Used in Medication Orders

a or a.	before
a.c.	before meals
ad lib	as desired
alt. h.	alternate hours
AM	in the morning; before noon
aq.	water
bid	twice a day
c̄	with
cap., caps.	capsule
dil.	dilute
dist.	distilled
DS	double strength
EC	enteric coated
elix.	elixir
ext.	external, extract
fl, fld	fluid
g	gram
gr	grain
gtt	drop
H	hypodermic
h, hr	hour
IDU	injecting/injection drug user
IM	intramuscular
inj.	injection
IV	intravenous
IVDU	intravenous drug user
IVP	IV push
IVPB	IV piggyback
kg	kilogram
L	liter
lb	pound
liq.	liquid
mcg	microgram
mEq	milliequivalent
mg	milligram
mL	milliliter
noct.	night
om	on morning
on	on night
oz	ounce
p or p.	after, per
p.c.	after meals
PO	by mouth
PM	afternoon, evening
prn	as needed, according to necessity
q	each, every
qh	every hour
qid, Qqds	four times a day
q1h	every 1 hour
q2h	every 2 hours
q3h	every 3 hours
q4h	every 4 hours
q6h	every 6 hours
q8h	every 8 hours
q12h	every 12 hours
qs	as much as needed, quantity, sufficient
qt	quart
R. or PR	rectally, per rectum
Rx	take, prescription
S, Sig	give the following directions
s̄	without
sid	once daily [Br.]
sol. or soln.	solution
SQ, SC	subcutaneous
stat.	immediately, at once
tab.	tablet
tbsp, T	tablespoon
tds, tid	three times a day
tinct., tr	tincture
tsp, t	teaspoon
ung.	ointment

Modified from Craven RF, Hirnle CJ, eds. Fundamentals of nursing: human health and function, 5th ed. Philadelphia: Lippincott Williams & Wilkins, 2007.

Common Abbreviations Not to Be Used in Medication Orders

The Joint Commission on Accreditation of Healthcare Organizations' list of dangerous abbreviations, acronyms, and symbols not to be used was originally created in 2004 and updated May 2005.

Joint Commission on Accreditation of Healthcare Organizations (JCAHO): www.jcaho.org

As of May 2005, the survey and scoring of this requirement applies to all orders and all medication-related documentation that is handwritten (including free-text computer entry) or on preprinted forms.

Official "Do Not Use" List

Abbreviation	Potential Problem	Preferred Term
U (for unit)	Mistaken as 0 (zero), 4 (four), or cc.	Write "unit".
IU (for international unit)	Mistaken as IV (intravenous) or 10 (ten).	Write "international unit".
Q.D., QD, q.d., qd (daily) Q.O.D., QOD, q.o.d, qod (every other day)	Mistaken for each other. Period after the Q mistaken for "I" and the "O" mistaken for "I".	Write "daily". Write "every other day".
Trailing zero (X.0 mg), lack of leading zero (.X mg)	Decimal point is missed.	Never write a zero by itself after a decimal point (X mg)*. Always use a zero before a decimal point (0.X mg).
MS, MSO_4 and $MgSO_4$	Can mean morphine sulfate or magnesium sulfate. Confused for one another.	Write "morphine sulfate". Write "magnesium sulfate".

An abbreviation on the "do not use" list should not be used in any of its forms—upper or lower case, with or without periods. For example, if Q.D. is on your list, you cannot use QD or qd. Any of those variations may be confusing and could be misinterpreted.

* Exception: a "trailing zero" may be used only where required to demonstrate the level of precision of the value being reported, such as for laboratory results, imaging studies that report size of lesions, or catheter/tube sizes. It may not be used in medication orders or other medication-related documentation.

Additional Abbreviations, Acronyms, and Symbols

Organizations may consider adding any or all of these to their own list of abbreviations not to use. The following items will be reviewed annually by JHACO for possible future inclusion on the official "do not use" list.

Abbreviation	Potential Problem	Preferred Term
> (greater than), < (less than)	Mistaken for 7 (seven) or the letter "L". Confused for one another.	Write "greater than" or "less than".
Abbreviations for drug names	Misinterpreted due to similar abbreviations for multiple drugs.	Write drug names in full.
Apothecary units	Unfamiliar to many practitioners. Confused with metric units.	Use metric units.
@	Mistaken for 2 (two).	Write "at".
cc (for cubic centimeter)	Mistaken for U (units) when poorly written.	Write "ml" or "milliliters".
µg (for microgram)	Mistaken for mg (milligrams), resulting in one thousand-fold overdose.	Write "mcg" or "micrograms".

Institute for Safe Medication Practices (ISMP) List of Error-Prone Abbreviations, Symbols, and Dose Designations

Abbreviations	Intended Meaning	Misinterpretation	Correction
μg	Microgram	Mistaken as "mg"	Use "mcg" or "microgram"
AD, AS, AU	Right ear, left ear, each ear	Mistaken as OD, OS, OU (right eye, left eye, each eye)	Use "right ear," "left ear," or "each ear"
OD, OS, OU	Right eye, left eye, each eye	Mistaken as AD, AS, AU (right ear, left ear, each ear)	Use "right eye," "left eye," or "each eye"
BT	Bedtime	Mistaken as "BID" (twice daily)	Use "bedtime"
cc	Cubic centimeters	Mistaken as "u" (units)	Use "mL"
D/C	Discharge or discontinue	Premature discontinuation of medications if D/C (intended to mean "discharge") has been misinterpreted as "discontinued" when followed by a list of discharge medications	Use "discharge" and "discontinue"
IJ	Injection	Mistaken as "IV" or "intrajugular"	Use "injection"
IN	Intranasal	Mistaken as "IM" or "IV"	Use "intranasal" or "NAS"
HS	Half-strength	Mistaken as bedtime	Use "half-strength" or "bedtime"
hs	At bedtime, hours of sleep	Mistaken as half-strength	Use "at bedtime"
IU*	International unit	Mistaken as IV (intravenous) or 10 (ten)	Use "units"
o.d. or OD	Once daily	Mistaken as "right eye" (OD-oculus dexter), leading to oral liquid medications administered in the eye	Use "daily"
OJ	Orange juice	Mistaken as OD or OS (right or left eye); drugs meant to be diluted in orange juice may be given in the eye	Use "orange juice"
Per os	By mouth, orally	The "os" can be mistaken as "left eye" (OS—oculus sinister)	Use "PO," "by mouth," or "orally"
q.d. or QD*	Every day	Mistaken as q.i.d., especially if the period after the "q" or the tail of the "q" is misunderstood as an "i"	Use "daily"
qhs	At bedtime	Mistaken as "qhr" or every hour	Use "at bedtime"
qn	Nightly	Mistaken as "qh" (every hour)	Use "nightly"
q.o.d. or QOD*	Every other day	Mistaken as "q.d." (daily) or "q.i.d. (four times daily) if the "o" is poorly written	Use "every other day"
q1d	Daily	Mistaken as q.i.d. (four times daily)	Use "daily"
q6PM, etc.	Every evening at 6 PM	Mistaken as every 6 hours	Use "6 PM nightly" or "6 PM daily"
SC, SQ, sub q	Subcutaneous	SC mistaken as SL (sublingual); SQ mistaken as "5 every;" the "q" in "sub q" has been mistaken as "every" (e.g., a heparin dose ordered "sub q 2 hours before surgery" misunderstood as every 2 hours before surgery)	Use "subcut" or "subcutaneously"
ss	Sliding scale (insulin) or ½ (apothecary)	Mistaken as "55"	Spell out "sliding scale;" use "one-half" or "½"
SSRI	Sliding scale regular insulin	Mistaken as selective-serotonin reuptake inhibitor	Spell out "sliding scale (insulin)"
SSI	Sliding scale insulin	Mistaken as Strong Solution of Iodine (Lugol's)	Spell out "sliding scale (insulin)"
t/d	One daily	Mistaken as "tid"	Use "1 daily"
TIW or tiw	3 times a week	Mistaken as "3 times a day" or "twice in a week"	Use "3 times weekly"
U or u*	Unit	Mistaken as the number 0 or 4, causing a tenfold overdose or greater (e.g., 4U seen as "40" or 4u seen as "44"); mistaken as "cc" so dose given in volume instead of units (e.g., 4u seen as 4cc)	Use "unit"

*Identified abbreviations above are also included on the JCAHO's "minimum list" of dangerous abbreviations, acronyms and symbols that must be included on an organization's "Do Not Use" list, effective January 1, 2004. An updated list of frequently asked questions about this JCAHO requirement can be found on their website at *www.jcaho.org*.

Dose Designations and Other Information	Intended Meaning	Misinterpretation	Correction
Trailing zero after decimal point (e.g., 1.0 mg)*	1 mg	Mistaken as 10 mg if the decimal point is not seen	Do not use trailing zeros for doses expressed in whole numbers
No leading zero before a decimal dose (e.g., .5 mg)*	0.5 mg	Mistaken as 5 mg if the decimal point is not seen	Use zero before a decimal point when the dose is less than a whole unit
Drug name and dose run together (especially problematic for drug names that end in "L" such as Inderal40 mg; Tegretol300 mg)	Inderal 40 mg Tegretol 300 mg	Mistaken as Inderal 140 mg Mistaken as Tegretol 1300 mg	Place adequate space between the drug name, dose, and unit of measure
Numeric dose and unit of measure run together (e.g., 10mg, 100mL)	10 mg 100 mL	The "m" is sometimes mistaken for a zero or two zeros, risking a 10- to 100-fold overdose	Place adequate space between the dose and unit of measure
Abbreviations such as mg. or mL. with a period following the abbreviation	mg mL	The period is unnecessary and could be mistaken as the number 1 if written poorly	Use mg, mL, and such abbreviations without a terminal period
Large doses without properly placed commas (e.g., 100000 units; 1000000 units)	100,000 units 1,000,000 units	100000 has been mistaken as 10,000 or 1,000,000; 1000000 has been mistaken as 100,000	Use commas for dosing units at or above 1,000, or use words such as 100 "thousand" or 1 "million" to improve readability

Drug Name Abbreviations	Intended Meaning	Misinterpretation	Correction
ARA A	vidarabine	Mistaken as cytarabine (ARA C)	Use complete drug name
AZT	zidovudine (Retrovir)	Mistaken as azathioprine or aztreonam	Use complete drug name
CPZ	Compazine (prochlorperazine)	Mistaken as chlorpromazine	Use complete drug name
DPT	Demerol-Phenergan-Thorazine	Mistaken as diphtheria-pertussis-tetanus (vaccine)	Use complete drug name
DTO	Diluted tincture of opium, or deodorized tincture of opium (Paregoric)	Mistaken as tincture of opium	Use complete drug name
HCl	hydrochloric acid or hydrochloride	Mistaken as potassium chloride (The "H" is misinterpreted as "K")	Use complete drug name unless expressed as a salt of a drug
HCT	hydrocortisone	Mistaken as hydrochlorothiazide	Use complete drug name
HCTZ	hydrochlorothiazide	Mistaken as hydrocortisone (seen as HCT250 mg)	Use complete drug name
$MgSO_4$*	magnesium sulfate	Mistaken as morphine sulfate	Use complete drug name
MS, MSO_4*	morphine sulfate	Mistaken as magnesium sulfate	Use complete drug name
MTX	methotrexate	Mistaken as mitoxantrone	Use complete drug name
PCA	procainamide	Mistaken as Patient Controlled Analgesia	Use complete drug name
PTU	propylthiouracil	Mistaken as mercaptopurine	Use complete drug name
T3	Tylenol with codeine No. 3	Mistaken as liothyronine	Use complete drug name
TAC	triamcinolone	Mistaken as tetracaine, Adrenalin, cocaine	Use complete drug name
TNK	TNKase	Mistaken as "TPA"	Use complete drug name
$ZnSO_4$	zinc sulfate	Mistaken as morphine sulfate	Use complete drug name

*Identified abbreviations above are also included on the JCAHO's "minimum list" of dangerous abbreviations, acronyms and symbols that must be included on an organization's "Do Not Use" list, effective January 1, 2004. An updated list of frequently asked questions about this JCAHO requirement can be found on their website at *www.jcaho.org.*

Stemmed Drug Names	Intended Meaning	Misinterpretation	Correction
"Nitro" drip	nitroglycerin infusion	Mistaken as sodium nitroprusside infusion	Use complete drug name
"Norflox"	norfloxacin	Mistaken as Norflex	Use complete drug name
"IV Vanc"	intravenous vancomycin	Mistaken as Invanz	Use complete drug name
Symbols Abbreviations	**Intended Meaning**	**Misinterpretation**	**Correction**
ʒ ♏	Dram Minim	Symbol for dram mistaken as "3" Symbol for minim mistaken as "mL"	Use the metric system
x3d	For 3 days	Mistaken as "3 doses"	Use "for three days"
> and <	Greater than and less than	Mistaken as opposite of intended; mistakenly use incorrect symbol; "< 10" mistaken as "40"	Use "greater than" or "less than"
/ (slash mark)	Separates two doses or indicates "per"	Mistaken as the number 1 (e.g., "25 units/10 units" misread as "25 units and 110" units)	Use "per" rather than a slash mark to separate doses
@	At	Mistaken as "2"	Use "at"
&	And	Mistaken as "2"	Use "and"
+	Plus or and	Mistaken as "4"	Use "and"
°	Hour	Mistaken as a zero (e.g., $q2^{\circ}$ seen as q 20)	Use "hr," "h," or "hour"

Reprinted with permission from ISMP Medication Safety Alert. 2003; 8:3–4.

Symbols

Angles, Triangles, and Circles

$\wedge$	above
	diastolic blood pressure (anesthesia records)
	elevated
	enlarged
	improved
	increased
	superior (position)
	upper
$\vee$	below
	decreased
	deficiency
	deficit
	depressed
	deteriorated
	diminished
	down
	inferior (position)
	lower
	systolic blood pressure (anesthesia records)
$>$	causes
	demonstrates
	distal
	followed by
	derived from
	greater than*
	indicates
	leads to
	more severe than
	produces
	radiates to
	radiating to
	results in
	reveals
	shows
	to
	toward
	worse than
	yields
$<$	caused by
	derived from
	less severe than
	less than*
	produced by
	proximal
$\angle$	angle
	flexion
	flexor
$\angle_{E}$	angle of entry
$\angle_{X}$	angle of exit
└	factorial product
┘	right lower quadrant
┐	right upper quadrant
┌	left upper quadrant
└	left lower quadrant
Δ	anion gap
	centrad prism
	change
	delta gap
	heat
	increment
	occipital triangle
	prism diopter
	temperature (anesthesia records)
Δ+	time interval
ΔA	change in absorbance
Δ dB	difference in decibels
Δ P	change in (intraocular) pressure
Δ pH	change in pH
Δ t	time interval
Δ H, H Δ	Hesselbach triangle

*Do not use in written patient records (JCAHO).

○	respiration (anesthesia records)
♀	female female sex
♂	male male sex
Ⓐ, ⓐⓧ	axilla (temperature)
Ⓗ, ⓗ	hypodermic hypodermically
(IM)	intramuscular intramuscularly
(IV)	intravenous intravenously
Ⓛ	left
Ⓜ	murmur
ⓜ	by mouth mouth (temperature) murmur
√ⓜ	factitial murmur
Ⓞ	by mouth oral orally
Ⓡ	rectal rectally rectum (temperature) right
Ⓧ	end of anesthesia (anesthesia records) end of operation

Arrows

↑	above elevated elevation enlarged gas greater than improved increase increased increases more than rising superior (position) up upper
↑g	increasing rising
↑V	increase due to in vivo effect (laboratory)
↓	below decrease decreased deficiency deficit depressed depression deteriorated deteriorating diminished diminution down falling inferior (position) less than low normal plantar reflex precipitate precipitates slower

↓g	decreasing diminishing falling lowering
↓V	decrease due to in vivo effect (laboratory)
↗	deviated displaced increasing
↘	decreasing
→	approaches limit of causes, demonstrates direction of flow or reaction distal due to followed by indicates leads to produces radiating to results in reveals shows to to right toward yields
←	caused by derived from direction of flow or reaction due to produced by proximal resulting from secondary to to left
⇈	extensor response (up bilaterally, positive Babinski sign) testes undescended
⇊	plantar response (down bilaterally, normal Babinski sign) testes descended
⇵	reversible reaction up and down
⇄, ⇌	reversible (chemical) reaction

Genetic Symbols

□	male
○	female
◇	sex unspecified
□ ○	normal individuals
■ ● ◆	affected individual (with ≥ 2 conditions, the symbol is partioned and shaded with a different fill defined in a key or legend)
[5] (5) ◇5	multiple individuals, number known (number of siblings written inside symbol)
[n] (n) ◇n	multiple individuals, number unknown ("n" used in place of specific number)
□–○	mating
□=○	consanguinity

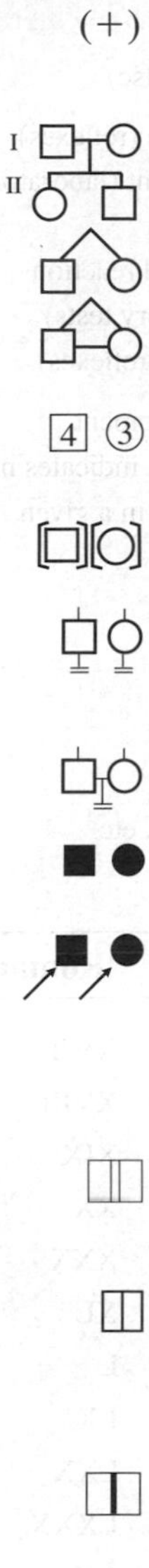

- uncommon or uncertain mode of inheritance
- parents and offspring, in generations
- dizygotic twins
- monozygotic twins
- number of children of sex indicated
- adopted individuals
- individual died without leaving offspring
- no issue
- affected individuals
- proband or propositus (first affected family member coming to medical attention)
- examined professionally normal for trait
- not examined dubiously reported to have trait
- not examined reliably reported to have trait

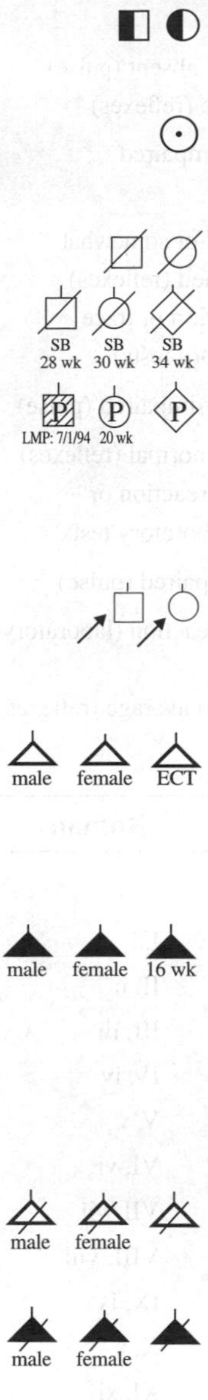

- heterozygotes for autosomal recessive
- carrier of sex-linked recessive
- death
- stillbirth (SB)
- pregnancy (P); gestational age and karyotype (if known) below symbol
- consultand (individual seeking genetic counseling/testing)
- spontaneous abortion (SAB); ECT below symbol indicates ectopic pregnancy
- affected spontaneous abortion (gestational age, if known, below symbol, and key or legend used to define shading)
- termination of pregnancy
- affected termination of pregnancy (key or legend used to define shading)

Source: Genetic symbols are public domain; we credit and gratefully acknowledge the *American Journal of Human Genetics* (56:746–747, 1995) as our source for these symbols.

Numbers

0	completely absent (pulse) no response (reflexes)	+4, 4+	normal (pulse)
+1, 1+	markedly impaired (pulse)	4+	hyperactive (reflexes) large amount (laboratory tests) pronounced reaction (laboratory tests)
1+	low normal or somewhat diminished (reflexes) slight reaction or trace (laboratory tests)	•	very brisk (reflexes)
+2, 2+	moderately impaired (pulse)	$\overline{1}$	bowel movement (numeral indicates number of stools in a given period)
2+	average or normal (reflexes) noticeable reaction or trace (laboratory tests)	1×	once o††ne time
+3, 3+	slightly impaired (pulse)	2×, ×2	twice two times
3+	moderate reaction (laboratory tests) brisker than average (reflexes)	3×, ×3	three times, etc.

Arabic	Roman	Arabic	Roman
0		17	XVII
1	I, i	18	XVIII
2	II, ii	19	XIX
3	III, iii	20	XX
4	IV, iv	30	XXX
5	V, v	40	XL
6	VI, vi	50	L
7	VII, vii	60	LX
8	VIII, viii	70	LXX
9	IX, ix	80	LXXX
10	X, x	90	XC
11	XI, xi	100	C
12	XII, xii	1,000	M
13	XIII, xiii	5,000	$\overline{V}$
14	XIV, xiv	10,000	$\overline{X}$
15	XV	100,000	$\overline{C}$
16	XVI	1,000,000	$\overline{M}$

Pluses, Minuses, and Equivalencies

+	acid (reaction)
	added to*
	convex lens
	decreased or diminished (reflexes)
	excess
	less than 50% inhibition of hemolysis, Wassermann
	low normal (reflexes)
	markedly impaired (pulse)
	mild (severity)
	plus*
	positive (laboratory tests)
	present
	slight reaction or trace (laboratory tests)
	sluggish (reflexes)
	somewhat diminished (reflexes)
(+)	significant
(+)ive	positive
+ to ++	slight pain
++	average (reflexes)
	50% inhibition of hemolysis, Wassermann
	moderate (pain, severity)
	moderately impaired (pulse)
	normally active (reflexes)
	noticeable reaction or trace (laboratory tests)
+++	increased reflexes
	75% inhibition of hemolysis, Wassermann
	moderate amount
+++	moderate reaction (laboratory tests)
	moderately hyperative (reflexes)
	moderately severe (pain, severity)
	brisker than average (reflexes)
	slightly impaired (pulse)
++++	complete inhibition of hemolysis, Wassermann
	large amount (laboratory tests)
	markedly hyperactive (reflexes)
	markedly severe (pain, severity)
	normal (pulse)
	pronounced reaction (laboratory tests)
	very brisk (reflexes)
−	absent
	alkaline (reaction)
	concave lens
	deficiency
	deficient
	minus
	negative (laboratory test)
	none
	subtract
	without
(−)	insignificant
±	doubtful
	either positive or negative
	equivocal (reflexes, qualitative tests)
	flicker (reflexes)
	indefinite
	more or less
	plus or minus
±	possibly significant
	questionable
	suggestive

*Do not use in written patient records (JCAHO).

	variable
	very slight (reaction, severity, trace)
	with or without
(±)	possibly significant
± to +	minimal pain
∓	minus or plus
‡	moderate (severity)
	normally active (reflexes)
#	fracture
	gauge
	number
	pound(s)
	weight
~	about
	approximate
	approximately
	proportionate to
≈	approximately equal to
=	equal to
≠	not equal to
⊂	combined with

≎	equivalent
≭	not equivalent to
≡	identical
	identical with
≢	not identical
	not identical with
≒	nearly equal to
÷	approximately equal
≅	approximately
	approximately equal to
	congruent to
≐	approaches
=	equilateral
≜	equiangular
>	greater than*
≯	not greater than
<	less than*
≮	not less than
≥, ⩾	greater than or equal to
≤, ⩽	less than or equal to

Primes, Checks, Dots, Roots, and Other Symbols

?	doubtful
	equivocal (reflexes)
	flicker (reflexes)
	not tested (severity)
	possible
	questionable
	question of
	suggested
	suggestive (severity)
	unknown

!	factorial product
†	death
	deceased
/	divided by
	either meaning
	extension
	extensors fraction
	of
	per*
	to
	ratio

*Do not use in written patient records (JCAHO).

′	foot hour univalent
″	bivalent ditto inch minute second (1/60 degree)
‴	line (1/12 inch) trivalent
√	check observe for urine voided (urine)
·√·	urine and defecation voided and bowels moved
√c̄	check with
√d	checked observed
√g, √ing	checking
√qs	voided quantity sufficient
$\sqrt{\ }$	radical root
$\sqrt[2]{\ }$	square root
$\sqrt[3]{\ }$	cube root
*	birth multiplication sign (genetics) not verified presumed supposed
°	degree, measurement (1/360 of circle) severity (burns, wounds) temperature time (hour)*
:	is to
...	no data (in given category)
∴	therefore
∵	because since
::	as equality between ratios proportion proportionate to

Statistical Symbols

α	probability of Type I error significance level
β	probability of Type II error
$1-\beta$	power of statistical test
$n^{C}k;\left(\frac{n}{k}\right)$	binomial coefficient number of combination of *n* things taken *k* at a time
χ^2	chi-squared statistic
E	expected frequency in cell of contingency table
$E(X)$	expected value of random variable *X*
F	*F* statistic (variance ratio)
f	frequency
H_0	null hypothesis
H_1	alternative hypothesis
μ	population mean
N	population size

*Do not use in written patient records (JCAHO).

n	sample size
$n!$	n factorial
O	observed frequency in a contingency table
ϕ	ability continuum phi coefficient
P	probability
p	probability of success in independent trials
$P(A)$	probability that event A occurs
$P(A \backslash B)$	conditional probability that A occurs given that B has occurred
r	sample correlation coefficient, usually the Pearson product-moment correlation
r^2	coefficient of determination
r_s	Spearman rank correlation coefficient
ρ	population correlation coefficient
s	sample standard deviation
s^2	sample variance
SE	standard error of estimate
σ	population standard deviation
σ^2	population variance
σdiff.	standard error of difference between scores
σest.	standard error of estimate
σmeas.	standard error of measurement
t	Student t statistic Student test variable
θ	latent trait
U	Mann-Whitney rank sum statistic
W	Wilcoxon rank sum statistic
$\overline{X}$	sample mean
$\lvert x \rvert$	absolute value of x
$\sqrt{x}$	square root of x
z	standard score
∞	infinity

Muscles of the Human Body

Muscle(s)	Origin	Insertion	Innervation	Main Action(s)
Abductor digiti minimi of foot	Medial and lateral tubercles of tuberosity of calcaneus, plantar aponeurosis, intermuscular septa	Lateral side of base of proximal phalanx of 5th toe	Lateral plantar nerve (S2 and S3)	Abducts and flexes 5th toe
Abductor digiti minimi of hand	Pisiform, pisohamate ligament, flexor retinaculum	Medial side of base of proximal phalanx of 5th finger	Deep branch of ulnar nerve (C8 and T1)	Abducts 5th finger
Abductor hallucis	Medial tubercle of tuberosity of calcaneus, flexor plantar retinaculum, plantar aponeurosis	Medial side of base of proximal phalanx of 1st toe	Medial plantar nerve (S2 and S3)	Abducts and flexes 1st toe, (great toe, hallux)
Abductor pollicis brevis	Flexor retinaculum and tubercles of scaphoid and trapezium	Lateral side of base of proximal phalanx of thumb	Recurrent branch of median nerve (C8 and T1)	Abducts thumb and helps oppose it
Abductor pollicis longus	Posterior surfaces of ulna, radius, interosseous membrane	Base of 1st metacarpal	Posterior interosseous nerve (C7 and C8), continuation of deep branch of radial nerve	Abducts longus of thumb and extends it at carpometacarpal joint
Adductor brevis	Body and inferior ramus of pubis	Pectineal line and proximal part of linea aspera of femur	Obturator nerve branch of (L2–L4), anterior division	Adducts thigh and to some extent flexes it
Adductor hallucis	Oblique head: bases of metatarsals 2–4 Transverse head: plantar ligaments of metatarsophalangeal joints	Tendons of both heads attach to lateral side of base of proximal phalanx of great toe	Deep branch of lateral plantar nerve (S2 and S3)	Adducts great toe; assists in maintaining transverse arch of foot
Adductor longus	Body of pubic bone inferior to pubic crest	Middle third of linea aspera of femur	Obturator nerve, branch of anterior division (L2–L4)	Adducts thigh
Adductor magnus	Proximal part: inferior ramus of pubis, ramus of ischium Ischial tuberosity	Proximal part: gluteal tuberosity, linea aspera, medial supracondylar line Adductor tubercle of femur	Proximal part: obturator nerve (L2–L4), branches of posterior division Tibial part of sciatic nerve (L4)	Adducts thigh Proximal part: flexes thigh Extends thigh
Adductor minimus	Inferior pubic ramus	Medial lip, uppermost linea aspera of femur	Obturator nerve (L2–L4)	Adducts and rotates thigh laterally
Adductor pollicis	Oblique head: bases of 2nd and 3rd metacarpals, capitate, adjacent carpals Transverse head: anterior surface of body of 3rd metacarpal	Medial side of base of proximal phalanx of thumb	Deep branch of ulnar nerve (C8 and T1)	Adducts thumb toward middle digit
Anconeus	Lateral epicondyle of humerus	Lateral surface of olecranon and superior part of posterior surface of ulna	Radial nerve (C7, C8, and T1)	Assists triceps in extending forearm; stabilizes elbow joint; abducts ulna during pronation

Muscle(s)	Origin	Insertion	Innervation	Main Action(s)
Articularis cubiti	Distal portion of posterior aspect of shaft of humerus	Posterior fibrous capsule of elbow joint	Radial nerve (C7, C8)	Retracts posterior joint capsule during extension of elbow
Articularis genus	Distal portion of anterior aspect of shaft of femur	Synovial membrane of suprapatellar bursa of knee joint	Femoral nerve (L2–L4)	Retracts synovial membrane during extension of knee
Arytenoid, transverse and oblique	Posterolateral border of one arytenoid cartilage	Posterolateral border of opposite arytenoid cartilage	Recurrent laryngeal nerve (branch of vagus [CN X])	Closes intercartilaginous portion of rima glottidis
Auricularis, anterior, posterior, and superior	Epicranial aponeurosis and mastoid part of temporal bone	Auricle (external ear)	Facial nerve (CN VII)	Protraction, retraction, elevation of auricle on side of head
Biceps brachii	Short head: tip of coracoid process of scapula Long head: supraglenoid tubercle of scapula	Tuberosity of radius and fascia of forearm by bicipital aponeurosis	Musculocutaneous nerve (C5, C6)	Supinates forearm and, when supine, flexes forearm
Biceps femoris	Long head: ischial tuberosity Short head: linea aspera and lateral supracondylar line of femur	Lateral side of head of fibula; tendon split at this site by fibular collateral ligament of knee	Long head: tibial division of sciatic nerve (L5, S1, and S2) Short head: common fibular (peroneal) division of sciatic nerve (L5, S1, and S2)	Flexes leg and rotates it laterally when knee is flexed; extends thigh (e.g., when starting to walk)
Brachialis	Distal two thirds of anterior surface of humerus	Coronoid process and tuberosity of ulna	Musculocutaneous nerve (C5 and C6)	Flexes forearm in all positions
Brachioradialis	Proximal two thirds of lateral supracondylar ridge of humerus	Lateral surface of distal end of radius	Radial nerve (C5–C7)	Flexes forearm
Buccinator	Mandible, pterygomandibular raphe, and alveolar processes of maxilla and mandible	Angle of mouth	Facial nerve (CN VII)	Presses cheek against molar teeth, thereby aiding chewing; expels air from oral cavity, as when a wind instrument is played; draws mouth to one side when acting unilaterally
Bulbospongiosus	Male: median raphe, ventral surface of bulb of penis, and perineal body Female: perineal body	Male: corpora spongiosa and cavernosa and fascia of bulb of penis Female: fascia of corpora cavernosa	Deep branch of perineal nerve, a branch of pudendal nerve (S2, S3, and S4)	Works with external anal sphincter to support/fix perineal body Male: compresses bulb of penis to expel last drops of urine or semen; assists erection by pushing blood into body of penis and compressing outflow veins Female: "sphincter" of vagina; assists in erection of clitoris
Ciliary	Scleral spur	Meridional, radial, and circular fibers intrinsic to ciliary body	Parasympathetic fibers of oculomotor nerve and ciliary ganglion	Relieves tension on lens of eye, allowing it to become more convex for near vision

Muscle(s)	Origin	Insertion	Innervation	Main Action(s)
Coccygeus (ischiococcygeus)	Ischial spine	Inferior end of sacrum	Branches of S4 and S5 nerves	Forms small part of pelvic diaphragm that supports pelvic viscera; flexes coccyx
Coracobrachialis	Tip of coracoid process of scapula of humerus	Middle third of medial surface of humerus (C5–C7)	Musculocutaneous nerve	Helps to flex and adduct arm
Corrugator supercilii	Medial end of superciliary arch of frontal bone	Skin above middle of eyebrow	Facial nerve (CN VII)	Draws eyebrow medially and inferiorly, producing vertical wrinkles above nose
Cremaster	Internal oblique muscle and inguinal ligament	Spermatic cord and tunica vaginalis	Genital branch of genitofemoral nerve (L1–L2)	Elevation of testis
Cricopharyngeus	Posterolateral cricoid cartilage on one side	Posterolateral cricoid cartilage of other side	Vagus nerve (CN X)	Serves as upper esophageal sphincter
Cricothyroid	Anterolateral part of cricoid cartilage	Inferior margin and inferior horn of thyroid cartilage	External laryngeal nerve	Stretches and tenses vocal fold
Deep transverse perineal muscle	Internal surface of ischiopubic ramus and ischial tuberosity	Median raphe, perineal body, and external anal sphincter	Deep branch of perineal nerve, a branch of pudendal nerve (S2, S3, and S4)	Support and fix perineal body (pelvic floor) to support abdominopelvic viscera and resist increased intra-abdominal pressure
Deltoid	Lateral third of clavicle, acromion, and spine of scapula	Deltoid tuberosity of humerus	Axillary nerve (C5, C6)	Anterior part: flexes and medially rotates arm Middle part: abducts arm Posterior part: extends and laterally rotates arm
Depressor labii inferioris/anguli oris	Anterolateral aspect of body of mandible	Lower lip/angle of mouth	Marginal mandibular branch of facial nerve (CN VII)	Depresses and/or everts lower lip; pulls angle of mouth and modiolus inferiorly
Depressor septi nasi	Incisor fossa of maxilla	Mobile part of nasal septum	Facial nerve (CN VII)	Helps to dilate nostril during deep inspiration and depresses nasal septum
Diaphragm	Xiphoid process, inferior 6 costal cartilages and adjoining ribs, arcuate ligaments, anterior longitudinal ligaments and bodies and discs of lumbar vertebrae 1–3	Central tendon of diaphragm	Phrenic nerve (C3–C5)	Diaphragm descends, decreasing intrathoracic pressure and thus resulting in inhalation and assisting return of venous blood to heart
Digastric	Anterior belly: digastric fossa of mandible Posterior belly: mastoid notch of temporal bone	Intermediate tendon to body and greater horn of hyoid bone	Anterior belly: mylohyoid nerve, a branch of inferior alveolar nerve Posterior belly: facial nerve (CN VII)	Depresses mandible; raises hyoid bone and steadies it during swallowing and speaking
Dorsal interossei (4 muscles) of foot	Adjacent sides of metatarsals 1–5	1st: medial side of proximal phalanx of 2nd toe 2nd–4th: lateral sides of 2nd–4th toes	Lateral plantar nerve (S2, S3)	Abduct toes (2–4) and flex metatarsophalangeal joints

Muscle(s)	Origin	Insertion	Innervation	Main Action(s)
Dorsal interossei 1–4 of hand	Adjacent sides of 2 metacarpals (bipennate muscles)	Extensor expansions and bases of proximal phalanges of digits 2–4	Deep branch of ulnar nerve (C8, T1)	Abduct digits from axial line and act with lumbricals to flex metacarpophalangeal joints and extend interphalangeal joints
Erector spinae	Arises by a broad tendon from posterior part of iliac crest, posterior surface of sacrum, sacral and inferior lumbar spinous processes, and supraspinous ligament	Iliocostalis—lumborum, thoracis, cervicis: fibers run superiorly to angles of lower ribs and cervical transverse processes Longissimus—thoracis, cervicis, capitis: fibers run superiorly to ribs between to tubercles and angles, to transverse processes in thoracic and cervical regions, and to mastoid process of temporal bone Spinalis—thoracis, cervicis, capitis: fibers run superiorly to spinous processes in upper thoracic region and to skull	Posterior rami of spinal nerves	Acting bilaterally, extend vertebral column and head; as back is flexed, control movement by gradually lengthening fibers; acting unilaterally, laterally bend vertebral column
Extensor carpi radialis brevis	Lateral epicondyle of humerus	Base of 3rd metacarpal bone	Deep branch of radial nerve (C7, C8)	Extend and abduct hand at wrist joint
Extensor carpi radialis longus	Lateral supracondylar ridge of humerus	Base of 2nd metacarpal bone	Radial nerve (C6, C7)	Extend and abduct hand at wrist joint
Extensor carpi ulnaris	Lateral epicondyle of humerus and posterior border of ulna	Base of 5th metacarpal bone	Posterior interosseous nerve (C7, C8), continuation of deep branch of radial nerve	Extends and adducts hand at wrist joint
Extensor digiti minimi	Lateral epicondyle of humerus	Extensor expansion of 5th digit	Posterior interosseous nerve (C7, C8), continuation of deep branch of radial nerve	Extends 5th digit at metacarpophalangeal and interphalangeal joints
Extensor digitorum	Lateral epicondyle of humerus	Extensor expansions of medial 4 digits	Posterior interosseous nerve (C7, C8), continuation of deep branch of radial nerve	Extends medial 4 digits at metacarpophalangeal joints; extends hand at wrist joint
Extensor digitorum brevis	Anteriormost portions of lateral and superior surfaces of calcaneus	Lateral side of long extensor tendons, with slips to proximal phalanges of 2nd–4th toes	Deep fibular (peroneal) nerve (L5, S1)	Assists in extending middle 3 toes
Extensor digitorum longus	Lateral condyle of tibia and superior three fourths of medial surface of fibula and interosseous membrane	Middle and distal phalanges of lateral 4 digits	Deep fibular (peroneal) nerve (L5, S1)	Extends lateral 4 digits and dorsiflexes ankle
Extensor hallucis brevis	Anteriormost portion of superior surface of calcaneus	Dorsal aspect of base of proximal phalanx of great toe (hallux)	Deep fibular (peroneal) nerve (L5, S1)	Extends great toe

Muscle(s)	Origin	Insertion	Innervation	Main Action(s)
Extensor hallucis longus	Middle part of anterior surface of fibula and interosseous membrane	Dorsal aspect of base of distal phalanx of great toe (hallux)	Deep fibular (peroneal) nerve (L5, S1)	Extends great toe and dorsiflexes ankle
Extensor indicis	Posterior surface of ulna and interosseous membrane	Extensor expansion of 2nd digit	Posterior interosseous nerve (C7, C8), continuation of deep branch of radial nerve	Extends 2nd digit and helps to extend wrist
Extensor pollicis brevis	Posterior surface of radius and interosseous membrane	Base of proximal phalanx of thumb	Posterior interosseous nerve (C7, C8), continuation of deep branch of radial nerve	Extends proximal phalanx of thumb at carpometacarpal joint
Extensor pollicis longus	Posterior surface of middle third of ulna and interosseous membrane	Base of distal phalanx of thumb	Posterior interosseous nerve (C7, C8), continuation of deep branch of radial nerve	Extends distal phalanx of thumb at metacarpophalangeal and interphalangeal joints
External anal sphincter	Skin and fascia surrounding anus and coccyx via anococcygeal ligament	Perineal body	Inferior anal nerve	Closes anal canal; works with bulbospongiosus to support and fix perineal body
External intercostal	Inferior border of ribs, from tubercle to costochondral junction	Superior border of ribs below	Intercostal nerves	Elevate ribs (when upper ribs are fixed by scalene and sternocleidomastoid muscles)
External oblique	External surfaces of 5th–12th ribs	Linea alba, pubic tubercle, anterior half of iliac crest	Thoracoabdominal nerves (inferior 6 thoracic nerves) and subcostal nerve	Compress and support abdominal viscera; flex and rotate trunk
External urethral sphincter	Internal surface of ischiopubic ramus and ischial tuberosity	Surrounds urethra; in males, also ascends anterior aspect of prostate; in females, some fibers also enclose vagina (urethrovaginal sphincter)	Deep branch of perineal nerve, a branch of pudendal nerve (S2–S4)	Compresses urethra to maintain urinary continence; in females, urethrovaginal sphincter portion also compresses vagina
Fibularis (peroneus) brevis	Inferior two thirds of lateral surface of fibula	Dorsal surface of tuberosity on lateral side of base of 5th metatarsal	Superficial fibular (peroneal) nerve (L5, S1, S2)	Everts foot and weakly plantarflexes ankle
Fibularis (peroneus) longus	Head and superior two thirds of lateral surface of fibula	Base of 1st metatarsal and medial cuneiform	Superficial fibular (peroneal) nerve (L5, S1, S2)	Everts foot and weakly plantarflexes ankle
Fibularis (peroneus) tertius	Inferior third of anterior surface of fibula and interosseous membrane	Dorsum of base of 5th metatarsal	Deep fibular (peroneal) nerve (L5, S1)	Dorsiflexes ankle and aids in eversion of foot
Flexor carpi radialis	Medial epicondyle of humerus	Base of 2nd metacarpal bone	Median nerve (C6, C7)	Flexes and abducts hand (at wrist) radially
Flexor carpi ulnaris	Humeral head: medial epicondyle of humerus Ulnar head: olecranon and posterior border of ulna	Pisiform bone, hook of hamate bone, and 5th metacarpal bone	Ulnar nerve (C7, C8)	Flexes and adducts hand (at wrist) ulnarly
Flexor digiti minimi brevis of foot	Base of 5th metatarsal	Base of proximal phalanx of 5th digit	Superficial branch of lateral plantar nerve (S2, S3)	Flexes proximal phalanx of 5th digit, thereby assisting with its flexion

Muscle(s)	Origin	Insertion	Innervation	Main Action(s)
Flexor digiti minimi brevis of hand	Hook of hamate and flexor retinaculum	Medial side of base of proximal phalanx of little finger	Deep branch of ulnar nerve (C8, T1)	Flexes proximal phalanx of 5th digit
Flexor digitorum brevis	Medial tubercle of tuberosity of calcaneus, plantar aponeurosis, intermuscular septa	Both sides of middle phalanges of lateral 4 digits	Medial plantar nerve (S2, S3)	Flexes lateral 4 digits
Flexor digitorum longus	Medial part of posterior surface of tibia inferior to soleal line and by a broad tendon to fibula	Bases of distal phalanges of lateral 4 digits	Tibial nerve (S2, S3)	Flexes lateral 4 digits and plantarflexes ankle; supports longitudinal arch of foot
Flexor digitorum profundus	Proximal three fourths of medial and anterior surfaces of ulna and interosseous membrane	Bases of distal phalanges of medial 4 digits	Medial part: ulnar nerve (C8, T1). Lateral part: median nerve (C8, T1)	Flexes distal phalanges at distal interphalangeal joints of medial 4 digits; assists with flexion of hand
Flexor digitorum superficialis	Humeroulnar head: medial epicondyle of humerus, ulnar collateral ligament, and coronoid process of ulna Radial head: superior half of anterior border of radius	Bodies of middle phalanges of medial 4 digits	Median nerve (C7, C8, T1)	Flexes middle phalanges at proximal interphalangeal joints of medial 4 digits; acting more strongly, also flexes proximal phalanges at metacarpophalangeal joints and hand at wrist
Flexor hallucis brevis	Plantar surfaces of cuboid and lateral cuneiforms	Both sides of base of proximal phalanx of 1st digit	Medial plantar nerve (S2, S3)	Flexes proximal phalanx of 1st digit
Flexor hallucis longus	Inferior two thirds of posterior surface of fibula and inferior part of interosseous membrane	Base of distal phalanx of great toe (hallux)	Tibial nerve (S2, S3)	Flexes great toe at both joints and weakly plantarflexes ankle; supports medial longitudinal arches of foot
Flexor pollicis brevis	Flexor retinaculum and tubercles of scaphoid and trapezium	Lateral side of base of proximal phalanx of thumb	Recurrent branch of median nerve (C8, T1)	Flexes thumb
Flexor pollicis longus	Anterior surface of radius and adjacent interosseous membrane	Base of distal phalanx of thumb	Anterior interosseous nerve from median (C8, T1)	Flexes phalanges of 1st digit (thumb)
Gastrocnemius	Lateral head: lateral aspect of lateral condyle of femur Medial head: popliteal surface of femur superior to medial condyle	Posterior surface of calcaneus by calcaneal tendon	Tibial nerve (S1, S2)	Plantarflexes ankle when knee is extended, raises heel during walking, flexes leg at knee joint
Gemelli, superior and inferior	Superior: ischial spine Inferior: ischial tuberosity	Medial surface of greater trochanter (trochanteric fossa) of femur	Superior gemellus: nerve to obturator internus (L5, S1) Inferior gemellus: nerve to quadratus femoris (L5, S1)	Laterally rotate extended thigh and abduct flexed thigh; keep femoral head steady in acetabulum

Muscle(s)	Origin	Insertion	Innervation	Main Action(s)
Genioglossus	Superior part of mental spine of mandible	Dorsum of tongue and body of hyoid bone	Hypoglossal nerve (CN XII)	Depresses tongue; posterior part pulls tongue anteriorly for protrusion
Geniohyoid	Inferior mental spine of mandible	Body of hyoid bone	C1 through hypoglossal nerve	Pulls hyoid bone anterosuperiorly; shortens floor of mouth; widens pharynx
Gluteus maximus	Ilium posterior to posterior gluteal line, dorsal surface of sacrum and coccyx, and sacrotuberous ligament	Most fibers end in iliotibial tract that inserts into lateral condyle of tibia; some fibers insert on gluteal tuberosity of femur	Inferior gluteal nerve (L5, S1, S2)	Extends thigh (especially from flexed position) and assists in its lateral rotation; steadies thigh and assists in rising from sitting position
Gluteus medius	External surface of ilium between anterior and posterior gluteal lines	Lateral surface of greater trochanter of femur	Superior gluteal nerve (L5, S1)	Abducts and medially rotates thigh; keeps pelvis level when opposite leg is raised off ground
Gluteus minimus	External surface of ilium between anterior and inferior gluteal lines	Anterior surface of greater trochanter of femur	Superior gluteal nerve (L5, S1)	Abducts and medially rotates thigh; keeps pelvis level when opposite leg is raised off ground
Gracilis	Body and inferior ramus of pubis	Superior part of medial surface of tibia	Obturator nerve (L2, L3)	Adducts thigh; flexes leg, helps rotate it medially
Hyoglossus	Body and greater horn of hyoid bone	Side and inferior aspect of tongue	Hypoglossal nerve (CN XII)	Depresses and retracts tongue
Iliacus	Iliac crest, superior two thirds of iliac fossa, ala of sacrum, and anterior sacroiliac ligaments	Lesser trochanter of femur and shaft inferior to it, and to psoas major tendon	Femoral nerve (L2–L4)	Flexes thigh and stabilizes hip joint; acts with psoas major
Inferior constrictor of pharynx	Oblique line of thyroid cartilage and side of cricoid cartilage	Median raphe of pharynx	Cranial root of accessory nerve (CN XI) plus branches of external and recurrent laryngeal nerves of vagus (CN X)	Constricts wall of pharynx during swallowing
Inferior longitudinal muscle of tongue	Root of tongue and body of hyoid bone	Apex of tongue	Hypoglossal nerve (CN XII)	Curls tip of tongue inferiorly and shortens tongue
Inferior oblique	Anterior part of floor of orbit	Sclera deep to lateral rectus muscle	Oculomotor nerve (CN III)	Abducts, elevates, and laterally rotates eyeball
Inferior rectus	Common tendinous ring	Sclera just posterior to cornea	Oculomotor nerve (CN III)	Depresses, adducts, and rotates eyeball medially
Infraspinatus	Infraspinous fossa of scapula	Middle facet on greater tubercle of humerus	Suprascapular nerve (C5, C6)	Laterally rotates arm; helps to hold humeral head in glenoid cavity of scapula

Muscle(s)	Origin	Insertion	Innervation	Main Action(s)
Innermost intercostal	Inner surfaces of ribs, from angles to costochondral junction	Superior borders of ribs below	Intercostal nerves	Probably depress ribs
Internal intercostal	Inferior borders of ribs	Superior border of ribs below	Intercostal nerves	Depress ribs
Internal oblique	Thoracolumbar fascia, anterior two thirds of iliac crest, and lateral half of inguinal ligament	Inferior borders of 10th–12th ribs, linea alba, and pecten pubis through conjoint tendon	Thoracoabdominal (anterior rami of inferior 6 thoracic) and 1st lumbar nerves	Compresses and supports abdominal viscera; flexes and rotates trunk
Interspinales	Superior surfaces of spinous processes of cervical and lumbar vertebrae	Inferior surfaces of spinous processes of vertebrae superior to vertebrae of origin	Posterior rami of spinal nerves	Aid in extension and rotation of vertebral column
Intertransversarii	Transverse processes of cervical and lumbar vertebrae	Transverse processes of adjacent vertebrae	Posterior and anterior rami of spinal nerves	Aid in lateral bending of vertebral column; acting bilaterally, stabilize vertebral column
Ischiocavernosus	Internal surface of ischiopubic ramus and ischial tuberosity	Crus of penis or clitoris	Deep branch of perineal nerve, a branch of pudendal nerve (S2–S4)	Maintains erection of penis or clitoris by compressing outflow veins and pushing blood into body of penis or clitoris
Lateral cricoarytenoid	Arch of cricoid cartilage	Muscular process of arytenoid cartilage	Recurrent laryngeal nerve (branch of vagus [CN X])	Adducts vocal fold (interligamentous portion)
Lateral pterygoid	Superior head: infratemporal surface and infratemporal crest of greater wing of sphenoid bone Inferior head: lateral surface of lateral pterygoid plate	Neck of mandible (pterygoid fovea); articular disc and capsule of temporomandibular joint	Mandibular nerve (CN V3) through lateral pterygoid nerve from anterior trunk, which enters its deep surface	Acting together, protrude mandible and depress chin; acting alone and alternately, produce side-to-side movements of mandible
Lateral rectus	Common tendinous ring	Sclera just posterior to cornea	Abducent nerve (CN VI)	Abducts eyeball
Latissimus dorsi	Spinous processes of inferior 6 thoracic vertebrae, thoracolumbar fascia, iliac crest, and inferior 3 or 4 ribs	Floor of intertubercular groove of humerus	Thoracodorsal nerve (C6–C8)	Extends, adducts, and medially rotates humerus; raises body toward arms during climbing
Levator anguli oris	Canine fossa of maxilla	Orbicularis oris and skin at angle of mouth	Facial nerve (CN VII)	Raises angle of mouth, as in smiling
Levator ani (pubococcygeus, puborectalis, and iliococcygeus)	Body of pubis, tendinous arch of obturator fascia, and ischial spine	Perineal body, coccyx, anococcygeal ligament, walls of prostate or vagina, rectum, and anal canal	Nerve to levator ani (branches of S4) and inferior anal (rectal) nerve and coccygeal plexus	Helps support pelvic viscera and resists increases in intraabdominal pressure
Levatores costarum	Tips of transverse processes of C7 and T1–T11 vertebrae	Pass inferolaterally and insert on subjacent rib between its tubercle and angle	Posterior rami of C8–T11 spinal nerves	Elevate ribs, assisting inspiration; assist with lateral bending of vertebral column
Levator labii superioris	Frontal process of maxilla and infraorbital region	Skin of upper lip and alar cartilage of nose	Facial nerve (CN VII)	Elevates lip, dilates nostril, and raises angle of mouth

Muscle(s)	Origin	Insertion	Innervation	Main Action(s)
Levator palpebrae superioris	Lesser wing of sphenoid bone, superior and anterior to optic canal	Tarsal plate and skin of superior (upper) eyelid	Oculomotor nerve (CN III); deep layer (superior tarsal muscle) is supplied by sympathetic fibers	Elevates superior (upper) eyelid
Levator scapulae	Posterior tubercles of transverse processes of C1–C4 vertebrae	Superior part of medial border or scapula	Dorsal scapular (C5) and cervical (C3 and C4) nerves	Elevates scapula and tilts its glenoid cavity inferiorly by rotating scapula
Levator veli palatini	Cartilage of pharyngotympanic (auditory) tube and petrous part of temporal bone	Palatine aponeurosis	Cranial part of CN XI through pharyngeal branch of vagus nerve (CN X) through pharyngeal plexus	Elevates soft palate during swallowing and yawning
Longus capitis	Basilar part of occipital bone	Anterior tubercles of C3–C6 transverse processes	Anterior rami of C1–C3 spinal nerves	Flexes head
Longus colli	Anterior tubercle of C1 vertebra (atlas); bodies of C1–C3 and transverse processes of C3–C6 vertebrae	Bodies of C5–T3 vertebrae, transverse processes of C3–C5 vertebrae	Anterior rami of C2–C6 spinal nerves	Flexes neck with rotation (torsion) to opposite side if acting unilaterally
Lumbricals of foot	Tendons of flexor digitorum longus	Medial aspects of bases of proximal phalanges of lateral 4 toes	Medial 1: medial plantar nerve (S2, S3) Lateral 3: lateral plantar nerve (S2, S3)	Flex proximal phalanges and extend middle and distal phalanges of lateral 4 digits
Lumbricals 1 and 2 of hand	Lateral 2 tendons of flexor digitorum profundus (unipennate muscles)	Lateral sides of extensor expansions of 2nd and 3rd digits	Median nerve (C8, T1)	Flex digits at metacarpophalangeal joints and extend interphalangeal joints
Lumbricals 3 and 4 of hand	Medial 3 tendons of flexor digitorum profundus (bipennate muscles)	Lateral sides of extensor expansions of 4th and 5th digits	Deep branch of ulnar nerve (C8 and T1)	Flex digits at metacarpophalangeal joints and extend interphalangeal joints
Masseter	Inferior border and medial surface of zygomatic arch	Lateral surface of ramus of mandible and its coronoid process	Mandibular nerve (CN V3) through masseteric nerve, which enters its deep surface	Elevates and protrudes mandible, thus closing jaws; deep fibers allow retrusion
Medial pterygoid	Deep head: medial surface of lateral pterygoid plate and pyramidal process of palatine bone Superficial head: tuberosity of maxilla	Medial surface of ramus of mandible, inferior to mandibular foramen	Mandibular nerve (CN V3) through medial pterygoid nerve	Acting bilaterally, elevates mandible, closing jaws; assists in protruding mandible; acting alone, assists in protruding same side of jaw; acting alternately, produces a grinding motion
Medial rectus	Common tendinous ring	Sclera just posterior to cornea	Oculomotor nerve (CN III)	Adducts eyeball
Mentalis	Incisive fossa of mandible	Skin of chin	Facial nerve (CN VII)	Elevates and protrudes lower lip
Middle constrictor of pharynx	Stylohyoid ligament and superior (greater) and inferior (lesser) horns of hyoid bone	Median raphe of pharynx	Cranial root of accessory nerve (CN XI); branches of external and recurrent laryngeal nerves of vagus (CN X)	Constricts wall of pharynx during swallowing

Muscle(s)	Origin	Insertion	Innervation	Main Action(s)
Mylohyoid	Mylohyoid line of mandible	Raphe and body of hyoid bone	Mylohyoid nerve, a branch of inferior alveolar nerve of CN V3	Elevates hyoid bone, floor of mouth, and tongue during swallowing and speaking
Nasalis	Superior part of canine ridge of maxilla	Nasal cartilages	Facial nerve (CN VII)	Draws ala (side) of nose toward nasal septum
Obliquus capitis inferior	Spinous process of axis (C2 vertebra)	Transverse process of atlas (C1 vertebra)	Suboccipital nerve	Rotation of head at atlantoaxial joint
Obliquus capitis superior	Spinous process of atlas (C1 vertebra)	Lateral third of inferior nuchal line of occipital bone	Suboccipital nerve	Rotation of head at atlantoaxial joint
Obturator externus	Margins of obturator foramen and obturator membrane	Trochanteric fossa of femur	Obturator nerve (L3, L4)	Laterally rotates thigh; steadies head of femur in acetabulum
Obturator internus	Pelvic surface of obturator membrane and surrounding bones	Medial surface of greater trochanter (trochanteric fossa) of femur	Nerve to obturator internus (L5, S1)	Laterally rotates extended thigh and abducts flexed thigh; steadies femoral head in acetabulum
Occipitofrontalis (occipital belly/frontal belly)	Lateral two thirds of superior nuchal line and mastoid temporal bone/epicranial aponeurosis	Epicranial aponeurosis/ skin of forehead and eyebrows	Posterior branch/ temporal branch of facial nerve (CN VII)	Retracts scalp/ elevates eyebrows and skin of forehead
Omohyoid	Superior border of scapula near suprascapular notch	Inferior border of hyoid bone	C1–C3 by a branch of ansa cervicalis	Depresses, retracts, and steadies hyoid bone
Opponens digiti minimi	Hook of hamate and flexor retinaculum	Medial border of 5th metacarpal	Deep branch of ulnar nerve (C8, T1)	Draws 5th metacarpal anteriorly and rotates it, bringing digit 5 into opposition with thumb
Opponens pollicis	Flexor retinaculum and tubercles of scaphoid and trapezium	Lateral side of 1st metacarpal	Recurrent branch of median nerve (C8, T1)	Draws 1st metacarpal bone laterally to oppose thumb toward center of palm and rotates it medially
Orbicularis oculi	Medial orbital margin, medial palpebral ligament, and lacrimal bone	Skin around margin of orbit; tarsal plate	Facial nerve (CN VII)	Closes eyelids; palpebral part closes lids gently; orbital part gently closes lids tightly
Orbicularis oris	Some fibers arise near median plane of maxilla superiorly and mandible inferiorly; others arise from deep surface of skin	Mucous membrane of lips	Facial nerve (CN VII)	As sphincter of oral opening, compresses and protrudes lips (e.g., purses them during whistling and sucking)
Palatoglossus	Palatine aponeurosis	Side of tongue	Cranial part of accessory nerve (CN XI) through pharyngeal branch of vagus nerve (CN X) by way of pharyngeal plexus	Elevates posterior part of tongue and draws soft palate onto tongue
Palatopharyngeus	Hard palate and palatine aponeurosis	Lateral wall of pharynx	Cranial part of accessory nerve (CN XI) through pharyngeal branch of vagus nerve (CN X) by way of pharyngeal plexus	Tenses soft palate and pulls walls of pharynx superiorly, anteriorly, and medially during swallowing

Muscle(s)	Origin	Insertion	Innervation	Main Action(s)
Palmar interossei 1–3	Palmar surfaces of 2nd, 4th, and 5th metacarpals (unipennate muscles)	Extensor expansions of digits and bases of proximal phalanges of 2nd, 4th, and 5th digits	Deep branch of ulnar nerve (C8, T1)	Adduct digits toward axial line and assist lumbricals in flexing metacarpophalangeal joints and extending interphalangeal joints
Palmaris brevis	Ulnar side of central portion of palmar aponeurosis	Skin of ulnar side of hand	Superficial ulnar nerve (T1)	Wrinkles skin on palmar side of hand
Palmaris longus	Medial epicondyle of humerus	Distal half of flexor retinaculum and palmar aponeurosis	Median nerve (C7, C8)	Flexes hand (at wrist) and tightens palmar aponeurosis
Pectineus	Superior ramus of pubis	Pectineal line of femur, just inferior to lesser trochanter	Femoral nerve (L2, L3); may receive a branch from obturator nerve	Adducts and flexes thigh; assists with medial rotation of thigh
Pectoralis major	Clavicular head: anterior surface of medial half of clavicle. Sternocostal head: anterior surface of sternum, superior 6 costal cartilages, aponeurosis of external oblique muscle	Lateral lip of intertubercular groove of humerus	Lateral and medial pectoral nerves; clavicular head (C5, C6), sternocostal head (C7, C8, T1)	Adducts and medially rotates humerus; draws scapula anteriorly and inferiorly; acting alone: clavicular head flexes humerus and sternocostal head extends it
Pectoralis minor	3rd–5th ribs near their costal cartilages	Medial border and superior surface of coracoid process of scapula	Medial pectoral nerve (C8, T1)	Stabilizes scapula by drawing it inferiorly and anteriorly against thoracic wall
Piriformis	Anterior surface of sacrum and sacrotuberous ligament	Superior border of greater trochanter of femur	Branches of anterior rami of S1, S2	Laterally rotate extended thigh and abduct flexed thigh; steady femoral head in acetabulum
Plantar interossei 1–3	Bases and medial sides of 3rd–5th metatarsals	Medial sides of bases of proximal phalanges of 3rd–5th digits	Lateral plantar nerve (S2, S3)	Adduct 2nd–4th digits and flex metatarsophalangeal joints
Plantaris	Inferior end of lateral supracondylar line of femur and oblique popliteal ligament	Posterior surface of calcaneus through calcaneal tendon	Tibial nerve (S1, S2)	Weakly assists gastrocnemius in plantarflexing ankle and flexing knee
Platysma	Superficial fascia of deltoid and pectoral regions	Mandible, skin of cheek, angle of mouth, and orbicularis oris	Facial nerve (CN VII)	Depresses mandible and tenses skin of lower face and neck
Popliteus	Lateral surface of lateral condyle of femur and lateral meniscus	Posterior surface of tibia, superior to soleal line	Tibial nerve (L4, L5, S1)	Weakly flexes knee and unlocks it
Posterior cricoarytenoid	Posterior surface of lamina of cricoid cartilage	Muscular process of arytenoid cartilage	Recurrent laryngeal nerve (branch of vagus [CN X])	Abducts vocal fold
Procerus	Aponeurosis covering bridge of nose	Skin of lower forehead between eyebrows	Facial nerve (CN VII)	Depresses medial end of eyebrow; produces transverse wrinkles over bridge of nose; produces look of concentration

Muscle(s)	Origin	Insertion	Innervation	Main Action(s)
Pronator quadratus	Distal fourth of anterior surface of ulna	Distal fourth of anterior surface of radius	Anterior interosseous nerve from median (C8, T1)	Pronates forearm; deep fibers bind radius and ulna together
Pronator teres	Medial epicondyle of humerus and coronoid process of ulna	Middle of lateral surface of radius	Median nerve (C6, C7)	Pronates and flexes forearm (at elbow)
Psoas major	Sides of T12–L5 vertebrae and discs between them; transverse processes of all lumbar vertebrae	Lesser trochanter of femur	Anterior rami of lumbar nerves (L1–L3)	Flexes and rotates thigh laterally at hip joint; when thigh is fixed, flexes lumbar vertebrae anteriorly and laterally
Psoas minor	Sides of T12–L1 vertebrae and intervertebral discs	Pectineal line, iliopectineal eminence via iliopectineal arch	Anterior rami of lumbar nerves (L1, L2)	Acts conjointly with psoas major to flex thigh at hip joint and stabilize this joint
Pyramidalis	Crest of pubis	Lower portion of linea alba	Subcostal nerve	Tenses linea alba
Quadratus femoris	Lateral border of ischial tuberosity	Quadrate tubercle on intertrochanteric crest of femur and area inferior to it	Nerve to quadratus femoris (L5, S1)	Laterally rotates thigh; steadies femoral head in acetabulum
Quadratus lumborum	Medial half of inferior border of 12th rib and tips of lumbar transverse processes	Iliolumbar ligament and internal lip of iliac crest	Ventral branches of T12 and L1–L4 nerves	Extends and laterally flexes vertebral column; fixes 12th rib during inspiration
Quadratus plantae	Medial surface and lateral margin of plantar surface of calcaneus	Posterolateral margin of tendon of flexor digitorum longus	Lateral plantar nerve (S2, S3)	Assists flexor digitorum longus in flexing lateral 4 digits
Rectus abdominis	Pubic symphysis and pubic crest	Xiphoid process and 5th–7th costal cartilages	Thoracoabdominal nerves (anterior rami of inferior 6 thoracic nerves)	Flexes trunk (lumbar vertebrae) and compresses abdominal viscera (indirectly opposing diaphragm)
Rectus capitis anterior	Anterior surface of lateral mass of C1 vertebra (atlas)	Base of skull, just anterior to occipital condyle	Branches from loop between C1 and C2 spinal nerves	Flexes head at atlantooccipital joint
Rectus capitis lateralis	Transverse process of C1 vertebra (atlas)	Jugular process of occipital bone	Branches from loop between C1 and C2 spinal nerves	Flexes head and helps to stabilize it
Rectus capitis posterior major	Spinous process of C2 vertebra (axis)	Middle of inferior nuchal line of occipital bone	Suboccipital nerve	Extends head at atlantooccipital joint
Rectus capitis posterior minor	Dorsal tubercle of C1 vertebra (atlas)	Medial third of inferior nuchal line of occipital bone	Suboccipital nerve	Extends head at atlantooccipital joint
Rectus femoris	Anterior inferior iliac spine and ilium superior to acetabulum	Base of patella and by patellar ligament to tibial tuberosity	Femoral nerve (L2–L4)	Extend leg at knee joint; rectus femoris also steadies hip joint and helps iliopsoas to flex thigh
Rhomboid minor and major	Minor: nuchal ligament and spinous processes of C7 and T1 vertebrae Major: spinous processes of T2–T5 vertebrae	Medial border of scapula from level of spine to inferior angle	Dorsal scapular nerve (C4, C5)	Retract scapula and rotate it to depress glenoid cavity; fix scapula to thoracic wall

Muscle(s)	Origin	Insertion	Innervation	Main Action(s)
Risorius	Platysma and fascia of masseter	Orbicularis oris, skin of corner of mouth, modiolus	Facial nerve (CN VII)	Retracts angle of mouth, lengthening rima oris
Salpingopharyngeus	Cartilaginous part of auditory tube	Blends with palatopharyngeus	Cranial root of accessory nerve through pharyngeal branch of vagus and pharyngeal plexus	Elevates (shortens and widens) pharynx and larynx during swallowing and speaking
Sartorius	Anterior superior iliac spine and superior part of notch inferior to it	Superior part of medial surface of tibia	Femoral nerve (L2, L3)	Flexes, abducts, and laterally rotates thigh at hip joint; flexes leg at knee joint
Scalenus anterior	Transverse processes of C4–C6 vertebrae	1st rib	Cervical spine nerves (C4–C6)	Elevates 1st rib; flexes and rotates neck laterally
Scalenus medius	Posterior tubercles of transverse processes of C4–C6 vertebrae	Superior surface of 1st rib, posterior groove for subclavian artery	Anterior rami of cervical spinal nerves	Flexes neck laterally; elevates 1st rib during forced inspiration
Scalenus posterior	Posterior tubercles of transverse processes of C4–C6 vertebrae	External border of 2nd rib	Anterior rami of cervical nerves C7 and C8	Flexes neck laterally; elevates 2nd rib during forced inspiration
Semimembranosus	Ischial tuberosity	Posterior part of medial condyle of tibia; reflected attachment forms oblique popliteal ligament (to lateral femoral condyle)	Tibial division of sciatic nerve (L5, S1, S2)	Extends thigh; flexes leg and, when knee is flexed, rotates it medially; when hip is flexed and knee is extended, can raise trunk against gravity
Semitendinosus	Ischial tuberosity	Medial surface of superior part of tibia	Tibial division of sciatic nerve (L5, S1, S2)	Extends thigh; flexes leg and, when knee is flexed, rotates it medially; when hip is flexed and knee is extended, can raise trunk against gravity
Serratus anterior	External surfaces of lateral parts of 1st–8th ribs	Anterior surface of medial border of scapula	Long thoracic nerve (C5, C6, C7)	Protracts scapula and holds it against thoracic wall; rotates scapula
Serratus posterior inferior	Spinous processes of vertebrae	Inferior borders of 8th–12th ribs near their angles	Anterior rami of 9th–12th thoracic spinal nerves	Depresses ribs
Serratus posterior superior	Ligamentum nuchae, spinous processes of C7–T3 vertebrae	Superior borders of 2nd–4th ribs	2nd–5th intercostal nerves	Elevates ribs
Soleus	Posterior aspect of head of fibula, superior fourth of posterior surface of fibula, soleal line, and medial border of tibia	Posterior surface of calcaneus via calcaneal tendon	Tibial nerve (S1, S2)	Plantarflexes ankle independently of position of knee and steadies leg on foot
Splenius capitis et cervicis	Arises from inferior half of ligamentum nuchae and spinous processes of C7–T3 or T4 vertebrae	Splenius capitis: fibers run superolaterally to mastoid process of temporal bone and lateral third of superior nuchal line of occipital bone	Posterior rami of spinal nerves	Acting alone, laterally bend and rotate head to side of active muscles; acting together, extend head and neck

Muscle(s)	Origin	Insertion	Innervation	Main Action(s)
Splenius capitis et cervicis *(cont.)*		Splenius cervicis: posterior tubercles of transverse processes of C1–C3 or C4 vertebrae		
Stapedius	Internal walls of pyramidal eminence of posterior wall of tympanic cavity	Neck of stapes	Facial nerve (CN VII)	Damps vibrations of stapes reflexively in response to loud noise
Sternocleidomastoid	Lateral surface of mastoid process of temporal bone and lateral half of superior nuchal line	Sternal head: anterior surface of manubrium of sternum Clavicular head: superior surface of medial third of clavicle	Spinal root of accessory nerve (CN XI) (motor) and C2 and C3 nerves (pain and proprioception)	Tilts head to one side, i.e., laterally; flexes neck and rotates it so face is turned superiorly toward opposite side; acting together, the right and left sternocleidomastoid muscles flex neck so chin is thrust forward
Sternohyoid	Manubrium of sternum and medial end of clavicle	Body of hyoid bone	C1–C3 by a branch of ansa cervicalis	Depresses hyoid bone after it has been elevated during swallowing
Sternothyroid	Posterior surface of manubrium of sternum	Oblique line of thyroid cartilage	C2 and C3 by a branch of ansa cervicalis	Depresses hyoid bone and larynx
Styloglossus	Styloid process and stylohyoid ligament	Side and inferior aspect of tongue	Hypoglossal nerve (CN XII)	Retracts tongue and draws it up to create a trough for swallowing
Stylohyoid	Styloid process of temporal bone	Body of hyoid bone	Cervical branch of facial nerve (CN VII)	Elevates and retracts hyoid bone, thereby elongating floor of mouth
Stylopharyngeus	Styloid process of temporal bone	Posterior and superior borders of thyroid cartilage with palatopharyngeus	Glossopharyngeal nerve (CN IX)	Elevates (shortens and widens) pharynx and larynx during swallowing and speaking
Subclavius	Junction of 1st rib and its costal cartilage	Inferior surface of middle third of clavicle	Nerve to subclavius (C5, C6)	Anchors and depresses clavicle
Subcostal	Internal surfaces of lower ribs near their angles	Superior borders of 2nd or 3rd ribs below	Intercostal nerves	Elevates ribs
Subscapularis	Subscapular fossa	Lesser tubercle of humerus	Upper and lower subscapular nerves (C5–C7)	Rotates arm medially and adducts it; helps to hold humeral head in glenoid cavity
Superficial transverse perineal muscle	Ramus of ischium	Perineal body	Deep branch of perineal nerve, branch of pudendal nerve (S2–S4)	Supports and fixes perineal body (pelvic floor) to support abdominopelvic viscera and to resist increased intraabdominal pressure
Superior constrictor of pharynx	Pterygoid hamulus, pterygomandibular raphe, posterior end of mylohyoid line of mandible and side of tongue	Median raphe of pharynx and pharyngeal tubercle on basilar part of occipital bone	Cranial root of accessory nerve through pharyngeal branch of vagus and pharyngeal plexus	Constricts wall of pharynx during swallowing

Muscle(s)	Origin	Insertion	Innervation	Main Action(s)
Superior longitudinal muscle of tongue	Submucous fibrous layer and median fibrous septum	Margins of tongue and mucous membrane	Hypoglossal nerve (CN XII)	Curls tip and sides of tongue superiorly and shortens tongue
Superior oblique	Body of sphenoid bone	Its tendon passes through a fibrous ring or trochlea, changes its direction, and inserts into sclera deep to superiorrectus muscle	Trochlear nerve (CN IV)	Abducts, depresses, and rotates eyeball medially
Superior rectus	Common tendinous ring	Sclera just posterior to cornea	Oculomotor nerve (CN III)	Elevates, adducts, and rotates eyeball medially
Supinator	Lateral epicondyle of humerus, radial collateral and anular ligaments, supinator fossa, and crest of ulna	Lateral, posterior, and anterior surfaces of proximal third of radius	Deep branch of radial nerve (C5, C6)	Supinates forearm (i.e., rotates radius to turn palm anteriorly)
Supraspinatus	Supraspinous fossa of scapula	Superior facet on greater tubercle of humerus	Suprascapular nerve (C4–C6)	Initiates and assists deltoid in abduction of arm and acts with rotator cuff muscles
Temporalis	Floor of temporal fossa and deep surface of temporal fascia	Tip and medial surface of coronoid process and anterior border of ramus of mandible	Deep temporal branches of mandibular nerve (CN V3)	Elevates mandible, closing jaws; its posterior fibers retract mandible after protrusion (SEE ALSO masseter)
Tensor fascia latae	Anterior superior iliac spine and anterior part of iliac crest	Iliotibial tract that attaches to lateral condyle of tibia	Superior gluteal (L4, by L5)	Abducts, medially rotates, and flexes thigh; helps to keep knee extended; steadies trunk on thigh
Tensor tympani	Canal for tensor tympani of petrous part of temporal bone and cartilage of pharyngotympanic (auditory) tube	Handle of malleus	Branch of mandibular nerve (CN V3) by otic ganglion	Tenses tympanic membrane to damp excessive vibration caused by loud noise
Tensor veli palatini	Scaphoid fossa of medial pterygoid plate, spine of sphenoid bone, and cartilage of pharyngotympanic (auditory) tube	Palatine aponeurosis	Medial pterygoid nerve (a branch of mandibular nerve—CN V3) by otic ganglion	Tenses soft palate and opens mouth of auditory tube during swallowing and yawning
Teres major	Dorsal surface of inferior angle of scapula	Medial lip of intertubercular groove of humerus	Lower subscapular nerve (C6, C7)	Adducts and medially rotates arm
Teres minor	Superior part of lateral border of scapula	Inferior facet on greater tubercle of humerus	Axillary nerve (C5, C6)	Laterally rotate arm; help to hold humeral head in glenoid cavity of scapula
Thyroarytenoid	Posterior surface of thyroid cartilage	Muscular process of arytenoid cartilage	Recurrent laryngeal nerve	Relaxes vocal fold
Thyrohyoid	Oblique line of thyroid cartilage	Inferior border of body and greater horn of hyoid bone	C1 by hypoglossal nerve	Depresses hyoid bone and elevates larynx

Muscle(s)	Origin	Insertion	Innervation	Main Action(s)
Tibialis anterior	Lateral condyle and superior half of lateral surface of tibia and interosseous membrane	Medial and inferior surfaces of medial cuneiform and base of 1st metatarsal	Deep fibular (peroneal) nerve (L4, L5)	Dorsiflexes ankle and inverts foot
Tibialis posterior	Interosseous membrane, posterior surface of tibia inferior to soleal line, and posterior surface of fibula	Tuberosity of navicular, cuneiform, and cuboid and bases of 2nd, 3rd, and 4th metatarsals	Tibial nerve (L4, L5)	Plantarflexes ankle and inverts foot
Transverse muscle of tongue	Median fibrous septum	Fibrous tissue at margins of tongue	Hypoglossal nerve (CN XII)	Narrows and elongates tongue; acts simultaneously to protrude tongue
Transversospinalis	Transverse processes: Semispinalis arises from transverse processes of C4–T12 vertebrae Multifidus arises from sacrum and ilium, transverse processes of T1–T3, and articular processes of C4–C7 Rotatores arise from transverse processes of vertebrae; are most highly developed in thoracic region	Spinous processes: Semispinalis—thoracis, cervicis, and capitis: fibers run superomedially to occipital bone and spinous processes in thoracic and cervical regions, spanning 4–6 segments Multifidus: fibers pass superomedially to spinous processes of vertebrae above, spanning 2–4 segments Rotatores: pass superomedially to attach to junction of lamina and transverse process, or spinous process, of vertebra above their origin, spanning 1–2 segments	Posterior rami of spinal nerves	Extend head and thoracic and cervical regions of vertebral column and rotate them contralaterally; stabilize vertebrae during local movements of vertebral column; stabilize vertebrae and assist with local extension and rotary movements of vertebral column; may function as organs of proprioception
Transversus abdominis	Internal surfaces of 7th–12th costal cartilages, thoracolumbar fascia, iliac crest, and lateral third of inguinal ligament	Linea alba with aponeurosis of internal oblique, pubic crest, and pecten pubis through conjoint tendon	Intercostal nerves 7–12, iliohypogastric nerve, ilioinguinal nerve	Compresses and supports abdominal viscera
Transversus thoracis	Posterior surface of lower sternum	Internal surface of costal cartilages 2–6	Intercostal nerves	Depress ribs
Trapezius	Medial third of superior nuchal line; external occipital protuberance, nuchal ligament, and spinous processes of C7–T12 vertebrae	Lateral third of clavicle, acromion, and spine of scapula	Spinal root of accessory nerve (CN XI) (motor) and cervical nerves (C3, C4) (pain and proprioception)	Elevates, retracts, and rotates scapula; superior fibers elevate, middle fibers retract, and inferior fibers depress scapula; superior and inferior fibers act together in superior rotation of scapula

Muscle(s)	Origin	Insertion	Innervation	Main Action(s)
Triceps brachii	Long head: infraglenoid tubercle of scapula Lateral head: posterior surface of humerus, superior to radial groove Medial head: posterior surface of humerus, inferior to radial groove	Proximal end of olecranon of ulna and fascia of forearm	Radial nerve (C6–C8)	Chief extensor of forearm at elbow; long head steadies head of abducted humerus
Uvula muscle	Posterior nasal spine and palatine aponeurosis	Mucosa of uvula	Cranial part of CN XI through pharyngeal branch of vagus nerve (CN X) via pharyngeal plexus	Shortens uvula and pulls it superiorly
Vastus intermedius	Anterior and lateral surfaces of body of femur	Base of patella and by patellar ligament to tibial tuberosity	Femoral nerve (L2–L4)	Extend leg at knee joint
Vastus lateralis	Greater trochanter and lateral lip of linea aspera of femur	Base of patella and by patellar ligament to tibial tuberosity	Femoral nerve (L2–L4)	Extend leg at knee joint
Vastus medialis	Intertrochanteric line and medial lip of linea aspera of femur	Base of patella and by patellar ligament to tibial tuberosity	Femoral nerve (L2–L4)	Extend leg at knee joint
Vertical muscle of tongue	Superior surface of borders of tongue	Inferior surface of borders of tongue	Hypoglossal nerve (CN XII)	Flattens and broadens tongue; acts simultaneously to protrude tongue
Vocalis	Vocal process of arytenoid cartilage	Vocal ligaments	Recurrent laryngeal nerve (branch of vagus [CN X])	Relaxes posterior vocal ligament while maintaining (or increasing) tension of anterior part
Zygomaticus major and zygomaticus minor	Zygomatic bone anterior/posterior to temporozygomatic suture	Muscles at angle of mouth and orbicularis oris of upper lip	Facial nerve (CN VII)	Elevate and evert upper lip

Arteries of the Human Body

Artery/Arteries	Origin	Course	Branches/ Distribution
Abdominal aorta	Continuation of thoracic aorta	Runs on anterior aspect of bodies of lumbar vertebrae	Visceral branches: celiac, superior and inferior mesenteric, renal, middle suprarenal, gonadal Parietal branches: lumbar, median sacral
Angular	Terminal branch of facial artery	Passes to medial angle (canthus) of eye	Superior part of cheek and lower eyelid
Anterior cerebral	Terminal branch (with middle cerebral) of internal carotid artery	Passes anteriorly, loops around genu of corpus callosum, then passes posteriorly in interhemispheric fissure	A1 segment: thalamus and corpus striatum A2 segment: cortex of medial aspects of frontal and parietal lobes
Anterior ciliary	Muscular (rectus) branches of ophthalmic artery	Pierces sclera at attachments of rectus muscles and forms network in iris and ciliary body	Iris and ciliary body
Anterior communicating	Anterior cerebral artery	Connects anterior cerebral arteries in prechiasmatic to complete cerebral arterial circle	Anteromedial central perforating arteries
Anterior division of internal iliac	Internal iliac	Passes anteriorly along lateral wall of lesser pelvis in hypogastric sheath and divides into visceral and parietal branches	Parietal branch: obturator artery Visceral branches: umbilical artery, inferior vesical, uterine, vaginal, middle rectal, and pudendal
Anterior ethmoidal	Ophthalmic artery	Passes through anterior ethmoidal foramen to anterior cranial fossa and into nasal cavity, sending branches to skin of nose	Supplies anterior and middle ethmoidal cells, dura of anterior cranial fossa, anterosuperior nasal cavity, and skin on dorsum of nose
Anterior inferior cerebellar	Lower (initial) part of basilar artery	Runs posterolaterally, often looping in and out of internal acoustic meatus	Supplies inferior aspect of lateral lobes of cerebellum, inferolateral pons, and choroid plexus in cerebellopontine angle; usually gives rise to labyrinthine artery
Anterior intercostal (branches)	Internal thoracic (intercostal spaces 1–6) and musculophrenic arteries (intercostal spaces 7–9)	Pass between intenal and innermost intercostal muscles	Intercostal muscles, overlying skin, underlying parietal pleura
Anterior interventricular (branch)	Left coronary artery	Passes along anterior interventricular groove to apex of heart	Walls of right and left ventricles including most of interventricular septum and contained atrioventricular bundle and branches (conducting tissue)
Anterior spinal	Superiorly, by a merger of intracranial branches, one from each vertebral artery; it is continued inferiorly by bifurcations of anterior segmental medullary arteries at various levels	Forms a continuous anastomotic chain that descends length of spinal cord in entrance to anterior median fissure	Supplies anterior portion of spinal cord by means of sulcal branches, which extend into anterior median fissure, and pial plexus, which ramifies over surface of cord
Anterior superior alveolar	Infraorbital artery	Arises within infraorbital canal and ascends through anterior alveolar canals	Supplies mucosa of maxillary sinus, maxillary superior incisor, and canine teeth

Artery/Arteries	Origin	Course	Branches/ Distribution
Anterior tibial	Terminal branch (with posterior tibial) of popliteal artery	Passes between tibia and fibula into anterior compartment through gap in superior part of interosseous membrane and descends on this membrane between tibialis anterior and extensor digitorum longus	Anterior compartment of leg
Appendicular	Ileocolic artery	Passes between layers of mesoappendix	Vermiform appendix
Arch of aorta	Continuation of ascending aorta	Arches posteriorly on left side of trachea and esophagus and superiorly to root of left lung	Brachiocephalic, left common carotid, and left subclavian
Arcuate (of foot)	Continuation of dorsalis pedis	Passes laterally, dorsal to bases of metatarsals	2nd, 3rd, and 4th dorsal metatarsal arteries
Artery of bulb of penis or vestibule of vagina	Internal pudendal artery	Pierces perineal membrane to reach bulb of penis or vestibule of vagina	Supplies bulb of penis or vestibule and bulbourethral gland (male) and greater vestibular gland (female)
Artery to ductus deferens	Inferior (or superior) vesical to ductus deferens	Runs retroperitoneally	Ductus deferens
Artery of pterygoid canal	3rd part of maxillary artery, or from greater palatine	Passes posteriorly through pterygoid canal	Mucosa of uppermost pharynx (pharyngeal recess), pharyngotympanic (auditory) tube, and tympanic cavity
Ascending aorta	Aortic orifice of left ventricle	Ascends approximately 5 cm to level of sternal angle where it becomes arch of aorta	Right and left coronary arteries
Ascending cervical	Terminal branch (with inferior thyroid artery) of thyrocervical trunk	Ascends on prevertebral fascia	Supplies anterior prevertebral muscles; anastomoses widely with other arteries of neck
Ascending palatine	Facial artery	Ascends next to and crosses over superior border of superior constrictor of pharynx to reach soft palate and tonsillar fossa	Supplies lateral wall of pharynx, tonsils, pharyngotympanic (auditory) tube, and soft palate
Ascending pharyngeal	Medial aspect of external carotid artery	Ascends between internal carotid artery and pharynx to cranial base, sending branches through jugular foramen and hypoglossal canal	Supplies pharyngeal wall, palatine tonsil, soft palate, and dura of posterior cranial fossa
Atrioventricular nodal (branch)	Right coronary artery near origin of posterior interventricular artery	Runs anteriorly in uppermost part of interventrical septum to atrioventricular node	Atrioventricular node
Axillary	Continuation of subclavian artery after crossing 1st rib	Runs inferolaterally through axillary fossa, changing to brachial artery when it crosses inferior border of teres major; parts are medial (1st), posterior (2nd), and lateral (3rd) to pectoralis minor	1st part: superior thoracic 2nd part: thoracoacromial and lateral thoracic arteries 3rd part: subclavian and anterior and posterior circumflex humeral arteries
Basilar	Formed by intracranial union of vertebral arteries	Ascends clivus in pontine cistern; terminates by bifurcating into posterior cerebral arteries	Branches: anterior inferior cerebellar, labyrinthine, pontine, mesencephalic, and superior cerebellar arteries

Artery/Arteries	Origin	Course	Branches/ Distribution
Brachial	Continuation of axillary artery past inferior border of teres major	Courses in medial intermuscular septum with median nerve; ends by bifurcating into radial and ulnar arteries in cubital fossa	Main artery of arm branches: deep artery of arm, muscular and nutrient branches, superior and inferior ulnar collateral
Brachiocephalic (trunk)	1st and largest branch of arch of aorta	Ascends posterolaterally to right, running anterior and then to right of trachea; deep to sternoclavicular joint, it bifurcates into terminal branches	Right common carotid and right subclavian arteries
Bronchial (1–2 branches)	Anterior aspect of 1st part of thoracic aorta or 3rd right posterior intercostal artery	Run on posterior aspects of primary bronchi and follow tracheobronchial tree	Bronchial and peribronchial tissue, visceral pleura
Buccal	Maxillary artery	Runs anterolaterally with buccal nerve, emerging from beneath anterior border of ramus of mandible	Supplies buccinator muscle, overlying skin, and underlying oral mucosa; anastomoses with branches of facial and infraorbital arteries
Carpal branches, dorsal and palmar	Radial and ulnar arteries at level of wrist	Anastomose with corresponding branches of counterpart artery (ulnar or to form dorsal and palmar carpal arches)	Provide collateral circulation at wrist
Celiac trunk	Abdominal aorta just distal to aortic hiatus of diaphragm	Runs a short course (1.25 cm), giving rise to left gastric, and bifurcating into splenic and common hepatic arteries	Supplies inferiormost esophagus, stomach, duodenum (proximal to bile duct), liver and biliary apparatus, and pancreas
Central artery of retina	Ophthalmic artery	Runs in dural sheath of optic nerve and pierces nerve near eyeball; ramifying from center of optic disc into retinal arterioles	Supplies optic retina (except cones and rods); branches: macular, nasal, and temporal retinal arterioles
Circumflex (branch)	Left coronary artery	Passes to left in atrioventricular groove and runs to posterior surface of heart	Primarily left atrium and left ventricle branches: left ventricular, atrial, and marginal
Circumflex humeral, anterior and posterior	3rd part of axillary artery, typically opposite origin of subscapular artery	Arteries anastomose to form a circle around surgical neck of humerus; larger posterior circumflex humeral artery passes through quadrangular space with axillary nerve	Supply shoulder joint and muscles of proximal arm: deltoid, teres major and minor, and long and lateral heads of triceps
Circumflex scapular artery	Terminal branch (with thoracodorsal artery) of subscapular artery	Curves around axillary border of scapula and enters infraspinous fossa	Supplies subscapular and infraspinatus muscles; joins collateral anastomosis of shoulder around scapula
Common carotid, left and right	Left: 2nd branch of arch of aorta Right: terminal branch (with right subclavian) of brachiocephalic artery	Ascend from/pass deep to sternoclavicular joint in carotid sheath under cover of sternocleidomastoid to level of C4 vertebra (or hyoid bone)	Terminal branches: internal and external carotid arteries
Common hepatic	Terminal branch (with splenic artery) of celiac artery (trunk)	Passes to right along superior border of pancreas, running anterior to portal vein	Terminal branches: hepatic artery proper and gastroduodenal artery
Common iliac, left and right	Terminal branches of abdominal aorta	Begin anterior to L4 vertebral body, diverging as they descend to terminate at L5-S1 level, anterior to sacroiliac joints	Terminal branches: external and internal iliac arteries

Artery/Arteries	Origin	Course	Branches/ Distribution
Common interosseous	Ulnar artery, just distal to bifurcation of brachial artery in cubital fossa	Passes deep to bifurcate into terminal branches after a short course	Terminal branches: anterior and posterior interosseous arteries
Common palmar digital	Superficial palmar arch	Pass distally anterior to lumbricals to bifurcate proxmal to webbings between digits	Receive palmar metacarpal arteries from deep palmar arch Terminal branches: proper palmar digital arteries
Common plantar digital	Terminal portions of plantar metatarsal	Short segments distal to transverse head of adductor hallucis proximal to webs between toes	Terminal branches: plantar digital arteries proper
Costocervical (trunk)	2nd part of subclavian artery	Short artery passes posteriorly superior to cervical pleura to neck of 1st rib and bifurcates into terminal branches	Terminal branches: supreme intercostal and deep cervical arteries
Cremasteric	Inferior epigastric	Accompanies spermatic cord through inguinal canal and into scrotal sac	Supplies cremaster muscle and other coverings of cord in males; round ligament in females
Cystic	Right hepatic artery	Arises within hepatoduodenal ligament	Gallbladder and cystic duct
Deep artery of penis or clitoris	Terminal branch of internal pudendal artery	Pierces perineal membrane to reach erectile bodies of clitoris or penis (corpora cavernosa)	Terminations (helicine arteries) uncoil to engorge erectile sinuses with arterial blood
Deep artery of thigh	Femoral artery in femoral triangle (about 4 cm distal to inguinal ligament)	Passes inferiorly on medial intermuscular septum, deep to adductor longus	Perforating branches pass through adductor magnus muscle to posterior and lateral part of anterior compartments of thigh
Deep auricular	1st part of maxillary artery	Ascends in parotid gland posterior to temporomandib-ular joint, piercing wall of external acoustic meatus	Supplies temporomandibular joint and skin of external acoustic meatus and tym-panic membrane
Deep cervical	Costocervical trunk	Passes posteriorly between transverse process of C7 and neck of 1st rib and ascends between semispinalis cervicis and capitis to C2 level	Supplies deep posterior muscles of neck and anasto-moses with descending branch of occipital artery and branches of vertebral artery
Deep circumflex iliac	External iliac artery	Runs on deep aspect of anterior abdominal wall, parallel to inguinal ligament	Supplies iliacus muscle and inferior part of anterolateral abdominal wall
Deep lingual	Continuation (3rd part of) lingual artery	Turns superiorly near anterior border of hyoglossus and flanking, then passes anter-iorly frenulum just deep to mucosa	Supplies genioglossus, inferior longitudinal muscle, and mucosa of underside of tongue, and of the tongue tip
Deep palmar arch	Direct continuation of radial artery, completed on medial side by deep branch of ulnar artery	Curves medially, deep to long flexor tendons in contact with bases of metacarpals	Branches: palmar metacarpal arteries
Deep plantar arch	Continuation of lateral plantar artery	Courses anteromedially, between 3rd and 4th layers of muscles of sole of foot; anastomoses with dorsalis pedis through deep plantar artery between 1st and 2nd metatarsal bases	Branches: plantar metatarsal arteries

Artery/Arteries	Origin	Course	Branches/ Distribution
Deep temporal, anterior and posterior	2nd part of maxillary artery	Ascend between temporalis and bone of temporal fossa	Supplies temporalis muscle, periosteum, and bone
Descending genicular	Femoral artery, in adductor canal	Descends in vastus medialis, just anterior to tendon of adductor magnus to anastomose with superior medial genicular artery	Branches: saphenous branch, accompanying saphenous nerve to medial skin of leg; muscular branches to vastus medialis and adductor magnus
Descending palatine	3rd part of maxillary artery	Arises in pterygopalatine fossa; descends in palatine canal	Branches: greater and lesser palatine arteries
Dorsal artery of penis or clitoris	Terminal branch of internal pudendal artery	Pierces perineal membrane and passes through suspensory ligament of penis or clitoris to run on dorsum of penis or clitoris	Skin of penis and erectile tissue of penis or clitoris
Dorsal carpal arch	Radial and ulnar arteries	Arches within fascia on dorsum of hand	Branches: dorsal metacarpal arteries
Dorsal digital arteries (of fingers)	Dorsal metacarpal arteries	Run distally on the posterolateral aspects of the proximal 1-1/2 phalanges	Supply dorsal aspects of proximal 1-1/2 phalanges of fingers
Dorsal digital arteries (of toes)	Dorsal metatarsal arteries	Run distally on posterolateral aspects of proximal 1-1/2 phalanges	Supply dorsal aspects of proximal 1-1/2 phalanges of toes
Dorsal metacarpal	Dorsal carpal arch	Run on 2nd–4th dorsal interossei	Bifurcate into dorsal digital arteries; supply skin, muscle, and bone of dorsum of hand and fingers to center of middle phalanx
Dorsal metatarsal	1st: termination of dorsalis pedis; 2nd, 3rd, and 4th: arcuate artery	Run distally on the superficial aspect of the corresponding dorsal interosseous muscles	Branches: dorsal digital arteries (of toes)
Dorsal nasal	Ophthalmic artery	Courses along dorsal aspect of nose and supplies its surface	Courses along dorsal aspect of nose and supplies its surface
Dorsal pancreatic	Splenic artery	Descends posterior to pancreas, dividing into right and left branches	Supplies middle portion of pancreas
Dorsal scapular (variation: in 1 of 3 cases, it is replaced by a deep branch of the transverse cervical artery)	3rd (or 2nd) part of subclavian artery	Passes laterally through brachial plexus then deep to levator scapulae; joins dorsal scapular nerve running along vertebral border of scapula, deep to rhomboid muscles	Supplies branches to trapezius, rhomboids, latissimus dorsi; participates in anastomoses around scapula (shoulder)
Dorsalis pedis	Continuation of anterior tibial artery distal to inferior extensor retinaculum	Descends anteromedially to 1st interosseous space and divides into plantar and arcuate arteries	Muscles on dorsum of foot; pierces 1st dorsal interosseous muscle (as deep plantar artery) to contribute to formation of plantar arch
Esophageal (4–5 branches) aorta	Anterior aspect of thoracic	Run anteriorly to esophagus	Esophagus
External carotid	Common carotid artery at superior border of thyroid cartilage	Ascends slightly anteriorly and then inclines posteriorly and laterally, passing between mastoid process and mandible; enters substance of parotid gland, bifurcating into terminal branches deep to neck of mandible	Anterior branches: superior thyroid, facial and ingual arteries Posterior branches: occipital and posterior auricular arteries Medial branch: ascending pharyngeal Terminal branches: maxillary and superficial temporal arteries

Artery/Arteries	Origin	Course	Branches/ Distribution
External pudendal, superficial, and deep branches	Femoral artery	Pass medially across thigh to reach scrotum or labia majora	Skin of mons pubis and anterior labia (female) or root of penis and anterior scrotum (male)
Facial	External carotid artery	Ascends deep to submandibular gland, winds around inferior border of mandible and enters face, ascending obliquely across cheek and side of nose to medial angle of eye	Branches: ascending palatine, tonsillar, glandular, submental, inferior and superior labial, and lateral nasal Terminal branch (continuation): angular artery
Femoral	Continuation of external iliac artery distal to inguinal ligament	Descends through femoral triangle, traverses adductor canal, and changes name to "popliteal" at adductor hiatus	Supplies anterior and anteromedial surfaces of thigh
Gastroduodenal	Hepatic artery	Descends retroperitoneally, posterior to gastroduodenal junction	Stomach, pancreas, 1st part of duodenum, and distal part of bile duct
Gastroepiploic	Gastroduodenal artery	Passes between layers of greater omentum to greater curvature of stomach	Right portion of greater curvature of stomach
Genicular (superior lateral and medial, inferior lateral, medial, and middle)	Popliteal	Arise and run to "four corners" of knee joint (viewed anteriorly) around the patella and femoral and tibial condyles; middle genicular pierces oblique popliteal ligament in posterior center of joint capsule	Form, with participation also of descending genicular, descending branch of lateral circumflex femoral, circumflex fibular and recurrent tibial arteries, and the genicular articular anastomosis
Greater pancreatic	Splenic artery	Penetrates left portion of pancreas, splitting into right and left branches, which parallel pancreatic duct	Anastomoses with other pancreatic branches; supplies primarily tail of pancreas and contained duct
Hepatic artery proper	Celiac trunk	Passes retroperitoneally to reach hepatoduodenal ligament and passes between its layers to porta hepatis; bifurcates into right and left hepatic arteries	Branches: right gastric, supraduodenal, right and left hepatic arteries; supplies liver and gallbladder, stomach, pancreas, duodenum
Ileocolic	Terminal branch of superior mesenteric artery	Runs along root of mesentery and divides into ileal and colic branches	Ileum, cecum, and ascending colon
Iliolumbar	Posterior division of internal iliac	Ascends anterior to sacroiliac joint and posterior to common iliac vessels and psoas major	Psoas major, iliacus, and quadratus lumborum muscles and cauda equina in vertebral canal
Inferior alveolar	1st part of maxillary artery	Descends posterior to inferior alveolar nerve between ramus of mandible to enter mandibular canal through mandibular foramen	Branches: mylohyoid branch, dental branches, mental medial pterygoid and branch; supplies muscles of floor of mouth, mandible and lower teeth, and soft tissue of chin
Inferior epigastric	External iliac artery	Runs superiorly and enters rectus sheath; runs deep to rectus abdominis	Rectus abdominis and medial part of anterolateral abdominal wall

Artery/Arteries	Origin	Course	Branches/ Distribution
Inferior gluteal	Anterior division of internal iliac	Exits pelvis to enter gluteal region through greater sciatic foramen inferior to piriformis and descends on medial side of sciatic nerve; anastomoses with superior gluteal artery and participates in cruciate anastomosis of thigh, involving 1st perforating artery of deep femoral and medial and lateral circumflex femoral arteries	Pelvic diaphragm (coccygeus and levator ani), piriformis, quadratus femoris, uppermost hamstrings, gluteus maximus, and sciatic nerve
Inferior labial	Facial artery near angle of mouth	Runs medially in lower lip	Lower lip and chin
Inferior mesenteric	Abdominal aorta	Descends retroperitoneally to left of abdominal aorta	Supplies part of gastrointestinal tract derived from hindgut
Inferior pancreaticoduodenal, anterior and posterior	Superior mesenteric artery	Ascends retroperitoneally on head of pancreas	Distal portion of duodenum and inferior head and uncinate process of pancreas
Inferior phrenic	As 1st branches of abdominal aorta (sometimes through a common stem or from celiac trunk)	Ascend crus to underside of domes; medial branches anastomose with each other and pericardiacophrenic arteries; lateral branches approach thoracic wall, anastomose with posterior intercostal and musculophrenic arteries	Branches: superior suprarenal arteries Supplies: diaphragm, inferior vena cava (right branch), esophagus (left branch), suprarenal glands
Inferior rectal	Internal pudendal artery	Leaves pudendal canal and crosses ischioanal fossa to anal canal	Distal portion of anal canal (mainly inferior to pectinate line)
Inferior suprarenal	Renal	Ascends vertically to gland	Posterior and inferior of aspects suprarenal gland
Inferior thyroid	Terminal branch (with ascending cervical artery) of thyrocervical trunk	Ascends anteriorly to anterior scalene, turns medially passing between vertebral vessels and carotid sheath, then descends on longus colli to lower border of thyroid gland	Branches: inferior laryngeal artery, pharyngeal, tracheal, esophageal, and inferior and ascending glandular (latter to parathyroid to glands); main visceral artery of neck
Inferior vesicle (male)	Anterior division of internal iliac	Passes retroperitoneally to inferior aspect of male urinary bladder	Inferior aspect of urinary bladder, ductus deferens, seminal vesicle, and prostate
Infraorbital	3rd part of maxillary artery	Passes along infraorbital groove and foramen to face	Supplies inferior rectus and oblique muscles, inferior eyelid, lacrimal sac, maxillary sinus, maxillary incisor and canine teeth, and anterior cheek
Internal carotid	Common carotid artery at superior border of thyroid cartilage	Ascends vertically in neck to enter carotid canal, becomes horizontal and runs anteromedially through cavernous sinus, makes a 180-degree turn under anterior clinoid process, bifurcates into anterior and middle cerebral arteries	Gives branches to walls of cavernous sinus, pituitary gland, and trigeminal ganglion; provides primary blood supply to the orbit/eyeball, upper nasal cavity/nose, and brain

Artery/Arteries	Origin	Course	Branches/ Distribution
Internal iliac	Common iliac	Passes over pelvic brim to reach pelvic cavity	Main blood supply to pelvic organs, gluteal muscles, and perineum
Internal pudendal	Anterior division of internal iliac	Leaves pelvis through greater sciatic foramen; hooks around ischial spine and enters perineum by way of lesser sciatic foramen and runs in pudendal canal to urogenital triangle	Main artery to perineum, including muscles and skin of anal and urogenital triangles; erectile bodies (does not supply branches to gluteal region)
Internal thoracic	Inferior surface of subclavian artery	Descends, inclining antero-medially, posterior to sternal end of clavicle and costal cartilages, lateral to sternum, and anterior to slips of transversus thoracis; divides at level of 6th costal cartilage into superior epigastric and musculophrenic arteries	Sternum and skin anterior to it by way of anterior intercostal arteries to 1st to 6th inter-costal spaces by way of perforating arteries, to medial aspect of breast
Interosseous, anterior and posterior	Common interosseous artery	Pass to anterior and posterior sides of interosseous membrane	Anterior and posterior compartments of forearm; anterior interosseous artery supplies both anterior and posterior compartments in distal forearm; posterior interosseous artery gives off recurrent interosseous artery, which participates in arterial anastomoses around the elbow
Ileal and jejunal ($n = 15–18$)	Superior mesenteric artery	Passes between two layers of mesentery	Jejunum and ileum
Labyrinthine	Basilar or through a common trunk with anterior inferior cerebellar	Exits cranial cavity through internal acoustic meatus; enters bony labyrinth	Membranous labyrinth
Lacrimal	Ophthalmic artery	Passes along superior border of lateral rectus muscle to supply lacrimal gland	Terminal branches to eyelids and conjunctiva
Lateral circumflex femoral	Deep artery of thigh; may arise from femoral artery	Passes laterally deep to sartorius and rectus femoris and divides into three branches	Ascending branch supplies anterior part of gluteal region; transverse branch winds around femur; descending branch descends to knee and joins genicular anastomoses
Lateral nasal branch (facial)	Facial artery as it ascends alongside nose	Passes to ala of nose	Skin on ala and dorsum of nose
Lateral plantar	Terminal branch (with medial plantar artery) of posterior tibial artery	Forms medially to calcaneus, courses anterolaterally between 1st and 2nd muscle layers of sole of foot to base of 5th metatarsal, then passes anteromedially between 3rd and 4th layers as deep plantar arch	Branches: muscular, to muscles of 1st and 2nd layers; superficial, to skin and subcutaneous tissue of lateral sole; anastomotic, with lateral tarsal and arcuate arteries; calcaneal, to calcaneus

Artery/Arteries	Origin	Course	Branches/ Distribution
Lateral sacral, superior and inferior	Posterior division of internal iliac	Runs on anteromedial aspect of piriformis to send branches into pelvic sacral foramina	Piriformis, structures in sacral canal, erector spinae and overlying skin
Lateral thoracic	2nd part of axillary artery	Descends along axillary border of pectoralis minor and follows it onto thoracic wall	Lateral chest wall (pectoral muscles, serratus anterior, intercostals) and breast
Left colic	Inferior mesenteric artery retroperitoneally to descending colon	Passes leftward	Descending colon
Left coronary	Left aortic sinus	Runs in atrioventricular groove and gives off anterior interventricular and circumflex branches	Most of left atrium and ventricle, interventricular septum, and atrioventricular bundles; may supply atrioventricular node
Left gastric	Celiac trunk	Ascends retroperitoneally to esophageal hiatus, where it passes between layers of hepatogastric ligament	Distal portion of esophagus and lesser curvature of stomach
Left gastroomental (gastroepiploic)	Splenic artery in hilum of spleen	Passes between layers of gastrosplenic ligament to greater curvature of stomach	Left portion of greater curvature of stomach
Left marginal (branch)	Circumflex branch	Follows left border of heart	Left ventricle
Left pulmonary	Pulmonary trunk	Joins left bronchus and pulmonary veins to form root of left lung; descends in lung	Supplies left lung Branches: (ductus arteriosus in fetus), superior and inferior lobar arteries (in turn give rise to segmental arteries)
Lesser palatine	Descending palatine	Descend inferoposteriorly through lesser palatine foramen	Supply soft palate
Lingual	External carotid artery	Loops over greater horn of hyoid, passes hyoglossus medially, and ascends to run along side of tongue	Branches: suprahyoid branch, dorsal lingual arteries and sublingual artery; continues as deep lingual artery
Lingular, inferior and superior	Superior lobar artery (of left lung), in oblique fissure	Descends anteriorly to lingula	Lingular division (superior [S4] and inferior [S5] bronchopulmonary segments) of left lung
Long posterior ciliaries	Ophthalmic artery	Pierce sclera to supply ciliary body and iris	Pierce sclera to supply ciliary body and iris
Lumbar	Abdominal aorta	Run in horizontal courses posteriorly around sides of lumbar vertebrae and then laterally on posterior abdominal wall	Branches: dorsal, to deep muscles of back and overlying skin; spinal, to vertebrae, contents of vertebral canal, roots, and some (as segmented medullary arteries) to spinal cord
Marginal artery (of colon)	Formed by anastomoses (arcades) between right, middle, and left colic and sigmoid arteries	Rarely interrupted anastomotic channel parallels colon at its mesenteric border	Branches passing to anterior and posterior aspects of colon
Masseteric	2nd part of maxillary artery	Passes posterior to temporalis tendon accompanying masseteric nerve through mandibular notch	Supplies masseter and temporomandibular joint; anastomoses with facial and transverse facial arteries

Artery/Arteries	Origin	Course	Branches/ Distribution
Maxillary	Terminal branch (with superficial temporal artery) of external carotid	Passes posterior and medial to neck of mandible (1st part), superficial or deep to inferior head of lateral pterygoid (2nd part), and into pterygopalatine fossa (3rd part)	1st part: deep auricular, anterior tympanic, middle meningeal, accessory meningeal, inferior alveolar; 2nd part: deep temporal, pterygoid (branches), masseteric, buccal; 3rd part: posterior superior alveolar, descending palatine, artery of pterygoid canal, pharyngeal, sphenopalatine, infraorbital
Medial circumflex femoral	Deep artery of thigh; may arise from femoral artery	Passes medially and posteriorly between pectineus and iliopsoas, enters gluteal region, and bifurcates	Supplies most blood to head and neck of femur; transverse branch takes part in cruciate anastomosis of thigh; ascending branch joins inferior gluteal artery
Medial plantar	Terminal branch (with lateral plantar artery) of posterior tibial artery	Arises medial to calcaneus, passes distally along medial side of foot between 1st and 2nd layers of plantar muscles	Branches: muscular, to flexor hallucis brevis and abductor hallucis; superficial, to skin and subcutaneous tissue of medial sole; superficial digital, that join 1st–3rd plantar metatarsals
Median sacral	Posterior aspect of abdominal aorta	Descends in median line over L4 and L5 vertebrae, sacrum, and coccyx	Lower lumbar vertebrae, sacrum, and coccyx
Mental (branch) of inferior alveolar artery	Terminal branch of inferior alveolar artery	Emerges from mental foramen and passes to chin	Facial muscles and skin of chin
Middle cerebral	Larger terminal branch (with anterior cerebral artery) of internal carotid artery	Runs in lateral cerebral sulcus, then posterosuperiorly on insula	Insula and most of lateral surface of cerebral hemispheres
Middle colic	Superior mesenteric artery	Ascends retroperitoneally and passes between layers of transverse mesocolon	Transverse colon
Middle collateral	Deep artery of arm	Descends to anastomose with recurrent interosseous artery	Part of collateral pathway around elbow; supplies lateral and medial heads of triceps
Middle meningeal	1st part of maxillary artery	Ascends vertically through foramen spinosum into middle cranial fossa; runs laterally, dividing into frontal and parietal branches, which in turn ramify, ascending lateral walls in cranial dura mater	Branches: ganglionic branches, petrosal branches, superior tympanic artery, temporal branches, anastomotic branch to lacrimal artery; most blood is distributed to perisoteum, bone, and red bone marrow
Middle rectal	Anterior division of internal iliac	Descends in pelvis to lower part of rectum	Seminal vesicles and lower part of rectum
Middle suprarenal	Abdominal aorta	Arise at level of superior mesenteric artery; run very short course over crura of diaphgram	Supply suprarenal glands; anastomose with suprarenal branches of inferior phrenic and renal arteries
Musculophrenic	Terminal branch (with superior epigastric) of internal thoracic artery	Arising in 6th intercostal space descends inferolaterally, paralleling costal margin	Branches: anterior intercostal arteries of 7th–9th intercostal spaces; also supplies upper abdominal muscles and pericardium

Artery/Arteries	Origin	Course	Branches/ Distribution
Mylohyoid (branch)	Inferior alveolar (before it enters mandibular foramen)	Pierces sphenomandibular ligament to run anteroinferiorly with nerve in groove on medial aspect of ramus of mandible	Muscles of floor of mouth; anastomoses with submental artery
Obturator	Anterior division of internal iliac	Runs anteroinferiorly on lateral pelvic wall to exit pelvis through obturator canal	Pelvic muscles, nutrient artery to ilium, head of femur, muscles of medial compartment of thigh
Occipital	External carotid artery	Passes medially to posterior belly of digastric and mastoid process; accompanies occipital nerve in occipital region	Scalp of back of head, as far as vertex
Ophthalmic	Internal carotid artery	Traverses optic foramen to reach orbital cavity	Traverses optic foramen to reach orbital cavity
Ovarian	Abdominal aorta, inferior to renal arteries	Run inferolaterally on psoas major, then pass medially to cross pelvic brim and descend in suspensory ligament of ovary	Branches: ureteric, tubal (to uterine tubes) and ovarian; latter 2 anastomose branches of uterine artery of same name
Palmar metacarpal	Deep palmar arch (from radial artery)	Run distally on plane between adductor pollicis and interosseus muscle	Anastomose distally with common palmar digital arteries
Pericardiacophrenic	Internal thoracic artery	Descends parallel to phrenic nerve between mediastinal parietal pleura and pericardium	Supplies mediastinal parietal pleura and pericardium; anastomoses with phrenic and musculophrenic arteries
Perineal	Internal pudendal artery	Leaves pudendal canal and enters superficial perineal space	Supplies superficial perineal muscles and scrotum or labia
Peroneal	Posterior tibial	Descends in posterior compartment adjacent to posterior intermuscular septum	Posterior compartment of leg: perforating branches supply lateral compartment of leg
Plantar metatarsal	1st: junction between lateral plantar and dorsalis pedis arteries; 2nd–4th: deep plantar arch	Extend distally between metatarsal bones on plantar aspect of interosseous muscles	Branches: perforating branches, common plantar digital arteries
Popliteal	Continuation of femoral artery at adductor hiatus in adductor magnus	Passes through popliteal fossa to leg; ends at lower border of popliteus muscle by dividing into anterior and posterior tibial arteries	Superior, middle, and inferior genicular arteries to both lateral and medial aspects of knee
Posterior auricular	External carotid artery	Passes posteriorly, deep to parotid, along styloid process between mastoid process and ear	Branches: auricular, occipital, stylomastoid; to middle ear, mastoid cells, auricle, parotid gland
Posterior cerebral	Terminal branch of basilar artery	Passes laterally, winding around cerebral peduncle to reach tentorial cerebral surface	Inferior aspect of temporal lobe and occipital lobe of cerebrum
Posterior communicating	Anastomosis between internal carotid and posterior cerebral arteries	Passes superior to oculomotor nerve (CN III)	Optic tract, cerebral peduncle, internal capsule, and thalamus
Posterior division of iliac	Internal iliac	Passes posteriorly and gives rise to parietal branches	Pelvic wall and gluteal region
Posterior ethmoidal	Ophthalmic artery	Passes through posterior ethmoidal foramen to posterior ethmoidal cells	Meningeal and nasal branches

Artery/Arteries	Origin	Course	Branches/ Distribution
Posterior gastric	Splenic artery	Ascends retroperitoneally (in posterior wall of omental bursa) to pass to gastric fundus through gastrophrenic fold (ligament)	Posterior wall of stomach
Posterior inferior cerebellar	Intracranial portion of vertebral artery	Passes posteriorly around side of medulla to reach inferior aspect of cerebellum	Supplies medial portion of inferior aspect of cerebellum (cerebellar tonsil and dentate nucleus), posterolateral medulla oblongata and choroid plexus of 4th ventricle
Posterior intercostals	Superior intercostal artery (intercostal spaces 1 and 2) and thoracic aorta (intercostal spaces 3 through 7)	Pass between internal and innermost intercostal muscles	Muscular and cutaneous branches to anterior and posterior thorax
Posterior interventricular	Right coronary artery	Runs from posterior interven-tricular groove to apex of heart	Right and left ventricles and interventricular septum
Posterior lateral nasal	Sphenopalatine artery	Ramify over conchae and meatuses; anastomoses with nasal branches of ethmoidal and greater palatine arteries	Supplies lateral walls of posteroinferior nasal cavity, contributing also to supply of ethmoidal cells and maxillary and sphenoidal paranasal sinuses
Posterior scrotal or labial	Terminal branches of perineal artery	Runs in superficial fascia of posterior scrotum or labium majus	Skin of scrotum or labium majus
Posterior septal	Sphenopalatine artery	Crosses inferior surface of body of sphenoid to reach nasal septum, courses anteroinferiorly on vomer to incisive canals	Supplies nasal septum; anastomoses with greater palatine artery and septal branch of superior labial artery
Posterior spinal	Superiorly from an intracranial branch of vertebral artery; continued inferiorly by bifurcations of posterior segmental medullary arteries at various levels	Forms continuous anasto-motic chain that descends length of spinal cord in posterolateral sulcus, adjacent to emerging dorsal roots (rootlets) of spinal nerves	Supplies posterolateral apect of spinal cord, through pial plexus and its peripheral branches
Posterior superior alveolar	3rd part of maxillary artery	Exits from pterygopalatine fossa through pterygomax-illary fissure; ramifies and penetrates infratemporal surface of maxilla, with some branches entering alveolar canals and others continuing over alveolar process	Supplies mucosa of maxillary sinus, maxillary molar and premolar teeth, adjacent gingiva
Posterior tibial	Popliteal	Passes through posterior compartment of leg, terminates distal to flexor retinaculum by dividing into medial and lateral plantar arteries	Posterior and lateral compartments of leg; circumflex fibular branch joins anastomoses around knee; nutrient artery passes to tibia
Princeps pollicis	Radial artery as it turns into palm	Descends on palmar aspect of 1st metacarpal, divides at the base of proximal phalanx into 2 branches that run along sides of thumb	Thumb

Artery/Arteries	Origin	Course	Branches/ Distribution
Profunda brachii	Brachial artery near its origin	Accompanies radial nerve through radial groove in humerus; terminal branches take part in anastomosis	Branches: deltoid, muscular (to head of triceps) and nutrient (to humerus) Terminal branches: middle around elbow joint and radial collateral arteries
Proper palmar digitals	Common palmar digital arteries	Run along sides of digits 2–5; at base of middle phalanx, gives rise to dorsal branch, which replaces dorsal digital arteries	All of palmar and distal part (including nail beds) of dorsal aspect of fingers
Prostatic (branches)	Inferior vesical artery	Descends on posterolateral aspect of prostate	Prostate
Radial	Smaller terminal division (with ulnar artery) of brachial artery in cubital fossa	Runs inferolaterally under cover of brachioradialis and distally lies lateral to flexor carpi radialis tendon; winds around lateral aspect of radius and crosses floor of anatomic snuffbox to pierce fascia; ends by forming deep palmar arch	Supplies muscles of lateral portions of both anterior and posterior compartments of forearm, lateral aspect of wrist, skin of dorsum hand and proximal portions of digits, deep muscles of palm
Radial collateral	Terminal branch (with middle collateral artery) of deep artery of arm	Perforates lateral inter-muscular septum with radial nerve, runs between brachialis and brachioradialis to anastomose with radial recurrent, anterior to lateral epicondyle of humerus	Forms part of cubital anastomosis; supplies upper brachialis and brachioradialis and anterolateral aspect of elbow joint
Radial recurrent	Lateral side of radial artery, just distal to its origin	Ascends on supinator and then passes between brachioradialis and brachialis to anastomose with radial collateral, anterior to lateral epicondyle of humerus	Forms part of cubital anastomosis; supplies supinator, lower brachialis and brachioradialis, and anterolateral aspect of elbow joint
Radialis indicis	Radial artery, but may arise from princeps pollicis artery	Passes along lateral side of index finger to its distal end	Entire lateral palmar and distal part (including nail bed) of dorsal aspect of index finger
Radicular, anterior and posterior	Spinal branches of segmental arteries (vertebral, posterior intercostal, lumbar and sacral arteries)	Course along anterior and posterior roots of spinal nerves, exhausting before reaching the longitudinal anterior and posterior spinal arteries	Supply anterior and posterior roots of spinal nerves and coverings (dural sheaths and arachnoid)
Renal, left and right	Posterolateral aspect of abdominal aorta, usually at L2 vertebral level	Run horizotally and laterally across crura of diaphragm and psoas major, lying posterior to renal vein, bifurcating into anterior and posterior divisions or ramifying into segmental arteries near renal hilus	Source of blood to kidneys Branches: inferior suprarenal, capsular branches, an anterior division giving rise to superior, anterior superior, anterior inferior, and inferior segmental arteries; posterior division becomes posterior segmental artery
Retroduodenal	Gastroduodenal artery	Arise and run posteriorly to 1st part of duodenum	Supply 1st part of duode-num, (common) bile duct, and head of pancreas

Artery/Arteries	Origin	Course	Branches/ Distribution
Right colic	Superior mesenteric artery	Passes retroperitoneally to reach ascending colon	Ascending colon
Right coronary	Right aortic sinus	Follows coronary (atrioventricular) groove between atria and ventricles	Right atrium, sinuatrial and atrioventricular nodes, and posterior part of interventricular septum
Right gastric	Hepatic artery	Runs between layers of hepatogastric ligament	Right portion of lesser curvature of stomach
Right marginal	Right coronary artery heart and apex	Passes to inferior margin of of heart	Right ventricle and apex
Right pulmonary	Pulmonary trunk	Passes beneath arch of aorta to join right bronchus and pulmonary veins to form root of right lung; descends in lung	Supplies right lung Branches: superior, middle, and inferior lobar arteries (in turn give rise to segmental arteries)
Segmental arteries of kidney (superior, anterior superior, anterior inferior, inferior, and posterior)	Anterior and posterior divisions (or directly from) renal arteries	Arise at hilum, course through perirenal fat of renal sinus around renal pelvis to reach renal segment	Renal segment (segmental arteries are endarteries; no significant anastomoses occur between segments)
Segmental arteries of liver (right anterior, right posterior, left medial, and left lateral)	Left and right branches of hepatic artery proper	Arise within liver; right and left branches course horizontally, right branch giving rise to anterior and posterior segmental arteries, left to medial and lateral segmental arteries	Each segmental artery serves a division of liver that, except for medial division, is further subdivided into 2 hepatic segments; both right and left branches of hepatic artery send an artery to caudate lobe
Segmental arteries of lung	Lobar arteries	Arise within lung as tertiary branches of right and left pulmonary arteries	Each segmental artery serves a bronchopulmonary segment of lung
Segmental medullary, anterior and posterior	Spinal branches of segmental arteries (vertebral, posterior intercostal, lumbar, and sacral arteries)	Course along anterior and posterior roots of spinal nerves, continue medially to anastomose with longitudinal anterior and posterior spinal arteries	Dorsal and ventral roots of certain spinal nerves and spinal cord; major anterior segmental medullary artery is largest, occurring at lower thoracic, upper lumbar level, on left side about 65% of time
Short gastric (n = 4–5)	Splenic artery in hilum of spleen	Pass between layers of gastrosplenic ligament to fundus of stomach	Fundus of stomach
Short posterior ciliaries	Ophthalmic artery	Pierce sclera at periphery of optic nerve	Supply choroid and ciliary processes
Sigmoid (n = 3–4)	Inferior mesenteric artery	Passes retroperitoneally toward left to descending colon	Descending and sigmoid colon
Sinuatrial nodal	Right coronary artery near its origin (in 60%); circumflex branch of left coronary (in 40%)	Winds around right (60%) or left (40%) side of ascending aorta and ascends to sinuatrial node	Left atrium and sinuatrial node
Sphenopalatine	3rd part of maxillary artery	Passes medially through sphenopalatine foramen, dividing immediately into septal and posterior lateral nasal arteries	Mucosa of posteroinferior half of nasal cavity, ethmoidal cells, and maxillary and sphenoidal paranasal sinuses

Artery/Arteries	Origin	Course	Branches/ Distribution
Splenic	Celiac trunk	Runs retroperitoneally along superior border of pancreas, then passes between layers of splenorenal ligament to hilum of spleen	Body of pancreas, spleen, greater curvature of stomach
Stylomastoid	Posterior auricular	Enters stylomastoid foramen and ascends facial canal, running with (and supplying) facial nerve	Branches: posterior tympanic tympanic artery (to membrane); mastoid (to mastoid cells) and stapedial (to stapedius, stapes, and secondary tympanic membrane) branches
Subclavian	Left: aortic arch Right: brachiocephalic trunk	Arises or passes posterior to sternoclavicular joint, arches over cervical pleura anterior to apex of lung, crosses 1st rib posterior to anterior scalene, becoming axillary artery at rib's outer edge	Branches: 1st part: vertebral, internal thoracic, thyrocervical (and costocervical on right side); 2nd part: dorsal scapular (and costocervical on left side) [parts: medial (1st), posterior (2nd), and lateral (3rd) to scalenus anterior muscle]
Subcostal	Thoracic aorta	Courses along inferior border of 12th rib	Muscles of anterolateral abdominal wall
Sublingual	Terminal branch (with deep lingual artery) of lingual artery	Runs on genioglossus muscle superiorly to mylohoid	Supplies muscles and mucous membrane of floor of mouth, and anterior lingual gingiva
Submental	Facial artery, distal to submandibular gland in submental triangle	Courses along inferior aspect of mylohyoid, adjacent to attachment to mandible, to mandibular symphysis	Supplies mylohyoid, anterior belly of digastric, submental lymph nodes and, through its anastomoses with inferior labial and mental arteries, lower lip
Subscapular	3rd part of axillary artery	Largest (but short—4 cm) branch of axillary artery, it descends along lateral border of subscapularis and axillary border of scapula to bifurcate at level of inferior angle	Through its terminal branches, circumflex scapular and thoracodorsal arteries, it supplies muscles on both sides of scapula, latissimus dorsi, and posterior chest wall
Superficial cervical (variant, replacing superficial branch of transverse cervical artery)	Thyrocervical trunk	Passes laterally between sternocleidomastoid and anterior scalene, across brachial plexus and posterior triangle of neck, to bifurcate and run with accessory nerve on deep aspect of trapezius	Anterior scapene, sternocleidomastoid, brachial plexus, muscles of posterior triangle of neck, and (primarily) the trapezius
Superficial circumflex iliac	Femoral artery	Runs in superficial fascia along inguinal ligament	Subcutaneous tissue and skin over inferior part of anterolateral abdominal wall
Superficial epigastric	Femoral artery	Runs in superficial fascia toward umbilicus	Subcutaneous tissue and skin over suprapubic region
Superficial palmar arch	Direct continuation of ulnar artery; completed on lateral side by superficial branch of radial artery or another of its branches	Curves laterally deep to palmar aponeurosis and superficially to long flexor tendons; curve of arch lies across palm at level of distal border of extended thumb	Branches: 3 common palmar digital arteries

Artery/Arteries	Origin	Course	Branches/ Distribution
Superficial temporal	Smaller terminal branch of external carotid artery	Ascends anterior to ear to temporal region and ends in scalp	Facial muscles and skin of frontal and temporal regions
Superior cerebellar	Upper (terminal) part of basilar artery	Curves around cerebral peduncle	Supplies superior aspect of cerebellum, colliculi, and most cerebellar nuclei; pons; pineal body; superior medullary velum; and choroid plexus of 3rd ventricle
Superior epigastric	Internal thoracic artery	Descends in rectus sheath deep to rectus abdominis	Rectus abdominis and superior part of anterolateral abdominal wall
Superior gluteal	Posterior division of internal iliac	Enters gluteal region through greater sciatic foramen superior to piriformis and divides into superficial and deep branches; anastomoses with inferior gluteal and medial circumflex femoral arteries	Piriformis muscle Superficial branch: supplies guteus maximus Deep branch: runs between gluteus medius and minimus muscles, supplying both, as well as tensor of fascia lata
Superior labial	Facial artery near angle of mouth	Runs medially in upper lip	Upper lip and ala (side) and septum of nose
Superior laryngeal	Superior thyroid	Runs deep to thyrohyoid to pierce thyrohyoid membrane with internal laryngeal nerve	Supplies larynx
Superior mesenteric	Abdominal aorta	Runs in root of mesentery to ileocecal junction	Part of gastrointestinal tract derived from midgut
Superior pancreaticoduodenal, anterior and posterior	Gastroduodenal artery	Descends on head of pancreas	Proximal portion of duodenum and head of pancreas
Superior phrenic (vary in number)	Anterior aspects of thoracic aorta	Arise at aortic hiatus and pass to superior aspect of diaphragm	Supply diaphragm and diaphragmatic parts of pericardium and parietal pleura
Superior rectal	Terminal branch (continuation of) inferior mesenteric artery	Crosses left common iliac vessels and descends into pelvis between layers of sigmoid mesocolon	Upper part of rectum; anastomoses with middle and inferior rectal arteries
Superior suprarenal	Inferior phrenic	Short, multiple branches arising from trunks of inferior phrenic arteries as they ascend diaphragmatic crura, running along superomedial aspect of gland	Superior part of suprarenal glands
Superior thoracic	Only branch of 1st part of axillary artery	Runs anteromedially along superior border of pectoralis minor, then passes between it and pectoralis major to thoracic wall	Helps to supply 1st and 2nd intercostal spaces and superior part of serratus anterior
Superior thyroid	1st branch from anterior aspect of external carotid artery	Passes inferomedially deep to infrahyoid muscles to superior pole of thyroid gland; anastomosis with inferior thyroid artery provides an important collateral pathway between external carotid and subclavian arteries	Branches: superior laryngeal artery, infrahyoid, sternocleidomastoid, cricothyroid, and anterior, posterior, and lateral glandular branches
Superior vesical	Patent (proximal) part of umbilical	Usually multiple, pass to superior aspect of urinary bladder	Superior aspect of urinary bladder, pelvic portion of ureter

Artery/Arteries	Origin	Course	Branches/ Distribution
Supraduodenal arteries	Gastroduodenal, hepatic, right gastric, or retroduodenal duodenum	Often double, pass(es) superiorly to 1st part of of duodenum	Supplies upper proximal portion of superior part
Supraorbital	Terminal branch of ophthalmic artery	Passes superiorly and posteriorly from supraorbital foramen to forehead and scalp	Supplies muscles and skin of most of forehead and anterior scalp (to vertex)
Suprascapular	Thyrocervical trunk	Passes inferolaterally over anterior scalene muscle and phrenic nerve, crosses subclavian artery and brachial plexus, runs laterally posterior and parallel to clavicle, then passes superiorly to transverse scapular ligament into supraspinous fossa, then under acromion to infraspinsous fossa	Supplies supraspinatus and infraspinatus muscles and participates in anastomosis around scapula
Supratrochlear	Terminal branch (with supraorbital artery) of ophthalmic artery	Passes from supratrochlear notch to medial forehead and anterior scalp	Skin and muscles of medial part of forehead and adjacent scalp
Supreme intercostal	Costocervical trunk	Descends between pleura and necks of first 2 ribs; anastomoses with 3rd posterior intercostal artery	Branches: 1st and 2nd posterior intercostal arteries, to muscles of and ribs bounding 1st and 2nd intercostal spaces
Sural, right and left	Popliteal	Large branches arise at level of femoral condyles and pass directly to heads of gastrocnemius, sending branches on to soleus	Supply medial and lateral heads of gastrocnemius, plantaris, and soleus muscles
Testicular	Abdominal aorta, inferior to renal arteries	Descend inferolaterally across psoas muscles, pass through inguinal canal as part of spermatic cord, reach testes in scrotum	Abdominal part provides branches and arterial blood to ureters, iliac lymph nodes; inguinal and scrotal part supplies cremaster and other coverings of cord and testes
Thoracic aorta	Continuation of arch of aorta	Descends in posterior mediastinum to left of vertebral column; gradually shifts to right to lie in median plane at aortic hiatus	Posterior intercostal arteries, subcostal, some phrenic arteries and visceral branches (tracheal and esophageal)
Thoracoacromial	2nd part of axillary artery deep to pectoralis minor	Curls around superomedial border of pectoralis minor, pierces clavipectoral fascia and divides into 4 branches	Branches: acromial, clavicular, pectoral, and deltoid
Thoracodorsal	Subscapular artery	Continues course of subscapular artery; accompanies thoracodorsal nerve to latissimus dorsi	Latissimus dorsi
Thyrocervical trunk	Anterior aspect of 1st part of subclavian artery	Ascends as a short, wide trunk near medial border of anterior scalene and posterior to carotid sheath	Branches from trunk: transverse cervical (or superficial cervical) and suprascapular Terminal branches: ascending cervical and inferior thyroid arteries
Thyroid ima	Brachiocephalic trunk or arch of aorta	Ascends on anterior aspect of trachea to thyroid gland	Supplies medial aspect of both lobes of thyroid

Artery/Arteries	Origin	Course	Branches/ Distribution
Transverse cervical (variant: may be replaced by superficial cervical and dorsal scapular arteries)	Thyrocervical trunk	Runs across anterior scalene, brachial plexus, and posterior triangle of neck and passes deep to trapezius, dividing into deep and superficial branches	Superficial branch bifurcates into ascending and descending branches that run with accessory nerve on underside of trapezius; deep branch runs with dorsal scapular nerve, deep to rhomboids
Transverse facial	Superficial temporal artery within parotid gland	Crosses face superficial to and inferior to zygomatic arch	Parotid gland and duct, muscles, and skin of face
Ulnar	Larger terminal branch of brachial artery in cubital fossa	Passes inferomedially and then directly inferiorly, deep to pronator teres, palmaris longus, and flexor digitorum superficialis to reach medial side of forearm; passes superficial to flexor retinaculum at wrist and gives a deep palmar branch to deep arch and continues as superficial palmar arch	Supplies medial (ulnar) part of anterior compartment of forearm, wrist, and hand; supplies superficial structures of central palm, and most of palmar and distal dorsal aspects of fingers
Ulnar collateral (superior and inferior)	Superior ulnar collateral arises from brachial near middle of arm; inferior ulnar collateral arises from brachial just superior to elbow	Superior ulnar collateral accompanies ulnar nerve to posterior aspect of elbow; inferior ulnar collateral divides into anterior and posterior branches; both ulnar collateral arteries take part in anastomosis around elbow joint	Anastomose distally with anterior and posterior ulnar recurrent arteries
Ulnar recurrent, anterior and posterior	Ulnar artery, just distal to elbow joint	Anterior ulnar recurrent passes superiorly and posterior ulnar collateral passes posteriorly	Anastomose with anterior and posterior ulnar collateral
Umbilical	Anterior division of internal iliac	Obliterates becoming medial umbilical ligament after running a short pelvic course during which it gives rise to superior vesical	Superior aspect of urinary bladder (through superior vesical arteries); occasionally artery to ductus deferens (males)
Uterine	Anterior division of internal iliac	Runs medially in base of broad ligament superior to cardinal ligament, crossing superior to ureter, to sides of uterus	Uterus, ligaments of uterus, uterine tube, and vagina
Vaginal	Uterine artery	Arises lateral to ureter and descends inferior to it to lateral aspect of vagina	Vagina; branches to inferior part of urinary bladder and termination of ureter
Vertebral	1st part of subclavian artery	Ascends vertically through the transverse foramina of vertebrae C6–C2, passes laterally to traverse that of C1, then runs horizontal and medial to enter foramen magnum; intracranially, merges with contralateral artery to form basilar artery	Cervical branches: spinal (giving rise to radicular and segmental medullary arteries) and muscular (to suboccipital muscles) Intracranial branches: meningeal, anterior, and posterior spinal, posterior inferior cerebellar, medial and lateral medullary

Nerves of the Human Body

Nerve(s)/Nerve Branch(es)	Origin	Course	Structures Innervated
Abdominopelvic splanchnic	Lower thoracic and lumbar segments of sympathetic trunk	Pass medially and inferiorly to prevertebral ganglion of paraaortic plexus	Motor: presynaptic sympathetics for innervation of abdominopelvic blood vessels and viscera
Abducent (CN VI)	Pons	Become intradural on clivus; traverse cavernous sinus and superior orbital fissure to enter orbit	Motor: lateral rectus
Accessory (CN XI)	Cranial root: medulla Spinal root: cervical spinal cord	Spinal root ascends into cranial cavity through foramen magnum, exits through jugular foramen, traverses posterior triangle of neck	Motor: sternocleidomastoid and trapezius
Ansa cervicalis	Superior root: hypoglossal nerve (C1–C2 fibers) Inferior root: cervical plexus (C2–C3 fibers)	Descends on external surface of carotid sheath and sternothyroid	Motor: omohyoid, sternohyoid
Anterior ethmoidal	Nasociliary nerve (CN V1)	Arises in orbit, passes through anterior ethmoidal foramen to cranial cavity, then through cribriform plate of ethmoid to nasal cavity	Sensory: dural of anterior cranial fossa; mucous membranes of sphenoidal sinus, ethmoidal cells, and upper nasal cavity
Anterior femoral cutaneous	Femoral nerve (L2–L3 fibers)	Arise in femoral triangle and pierce fascia lata of thigh along path of sartorius muscle	Sensory: skin on medial and anterior aspects of thigh
Anterior interosseous	Median nerve in distal part of cubital fossa	Passes inferiorly on interosseous membrane	Motor: flexor digitorum profundus, flexor pollicis longus, and pronator quadratus
Auriculotemporal	Mandibular nerve (CN V3)	From posterior division of CN V3, it passes between neck of mandible and external acoustic meatus to accompany superficial temporal artery	Sensory: skin anterior to auricle and posterior temporal region, tragus and part of helix of auricle, and roof of exterior acoustic meatus and upper tympanic membrane
Axillary	Terminal branch of posterior cord of brachial plexus (C5–C6 fibers)	Passes to posterior aspect of arm through quadrangular space in company with posterior circumflex humeral artery and then winds around surgical neck of humerus; gives rise to lateral brachial cutaneous nerve	Motor: teres minor and deltoid Sensory: shoulder joint and skin over inferior part of deltoid
Buccal	Mandibular nerve (CN V3)	From the anterior division of CN V3 in infratemporal fossa, it passes anteriorly to reach cheek	Sensory: skin and mucosa of cheek, buccal gingiva adjacent to 2nd and 3rd molar teeth
Calcaneal branches	Tibial and sural nerves	Pass from distal part of posterior aspect of leg to skin on heel	Sensory: skin of heel
Cardiac plexus	Cervical and cardiac branches of vagus nerve and cardiopulmonary splanchnic nerves from sympathetic trunk	From arch of aorta and posterior surface of heart, fibers extend along coronary arteries and to sinoatrial node	Sinuatrial nodal tissue and coronary arteries; parasympathetic fibers slow rate, reduce force of heart beat, and constrict arteries; sympathetic fibers have opposite effect

Nerve(s)/Nerve Branch(es)	Origin	Course	Structures Innervated
Cardiopulmonary splanchnic	Cervical and upper thoracic ganglia of sympathetic trunk	Descend anteromedially to cardiac, pulmonary, and esophageal plexuses	Motor: convey postsynaptic sympathetic fibers to nerve plexuses of thoracic viscera
Cavernous nerves of penis and clitoris	Parasympathetic fibers of prostatic nerve plexus	Perforates perineal membrane to reach erectile bodies of penis	Motor: helicine arteries of cavernous bodies; stimulation produces engorgement at arterial pressure (erection)
Cervical splanchnic	Cervical ganglia of sympathetic trunk	Pass medially and inferiorly to cardiac and pulmonary plexuses	Conducting tissue (sinuatrial and atrioventricular nodes) and coronary arteries
Chorda tympani	Facial nerve (CN VII) within facial canal	Traverses tympanic cavity, passing between incus and malleus; exits temporal bone through petrotympanic fissure to enter infratemporal fossa where it merges with lingual nerve	Motor: submandibular and sublingual (salivary) glands Sensory: taste sensation from anterior two thirds of tongue
Ciliary (long, short)	Long ciliary: nasociliary nerve (CN V1) Short ciliary: ciliary ganglion	Pass to posterior aspect of eyeball	Sensory: cornea, conjunctiva Motor: ciliary body and iris
Cluneal (superior, middle, and inferior)	Superior: posterior rami of L1, L2, and L3 Middle: posterior rami of S1, S2, and S3 Inferior: posterior cutaneous nerve of thigh	Superior nerves cross iliac crest; middle nerves exit through posterior sacral foramina and enter gluteal region; inferior nerves curve around inferior border of gluteus maximus	Sensory: skin of buttocks or gluteal region as far as greater trochanter
Coccygeal	Conus medullaris of spinal cord	Anterior and posterior rami join adjacent rami of S4 and S5; anterior rami form coccygeal plexus, which gives rise to anococcygeal nerve	Sensory: skin over coccyx
Cochlear nerve	As a division of the vestibulocochlear nerve (CN VIII)	Traverses internal acoustic meatus, entering modiolus with spiral ganglia and peripheral processes in spiral lamina	Sensory: spiral organ (for hearing)
Common fibular (peroneal)	Terminal branch (with tibial nerve) of sciatic nerve (L4–S2 fibers)	Begins at apex of popliteal fossa; follows medial border of biceps femoris muscle to posterior aspect of head of fibula; bifurcates into superficial and deep fibular nerves as it winds around neck of fibula	Sensory: skin on lateral part of posterior aspect of leg through its branch, lateral sural cutaneous nerve; knee joint through its articular branch Motor: short head of biceps femoris
Common palmar digital	Median and superficial branches of ulnar nerves	Run distally between long flexor tendons of palm, bifurcating in distal palm	Branches: proper palmar digital nerves, supplying skin and joints of palmar and distal dorsal aspect of fingers
Common plantar digital	Median and lateral plantar nerves	Run anteriorly in sole of foot between flexor tendons, bifurcating in distal sole	Branches: proper plantar digital nerves, supplying skin and joints of plantar and distal dorsal aspect of toes
Deep branch of radial nerve	Radial nerve just distal to elbow	Winds around neck of radius in supinator; enters posterior compartment of forearm becoming posterior interosseous nerve	Motor: extensor carpi radialis brevis and supinator

Nerve(s)/Nerve Branch(es)	Origin	Course	Structures Innervated
Deep branch of ulnar nerve	Ulnar nerve at wrist as it passes between pisiform and hamate bones (T1 fibers)	Passes deep between muscles of hypothenar eminence, then across palm with deep palmar (arterial) arch	Motor: hypothenar muscles (abductor, flexor, and opponens digiti minimi), lumbricals of 4th and 5th digits, all interossei, adductor pollicis, and deep head of flexor pollicis brevis
Deep fibular (peroneal)	Common fibular (peroneal) nerve	Arises between fibularis longus and neck of fibula; passes through extensor digitorum longus and descends on interosseous membrane; passes deep to extensor retinaculum, crosses distal end of tibia, and enters dorsum of foot	Motor: muscles of anterior compartment of leg and dorsum of foot Sensory: skin of 1st interdigital cleft (i.e., skin on adjacent sides of 1st and 2nd toes); sends articular branches to joints it crosses
Deep petrosal	Internal carotid plexus	Traverses cartilage of foramen lacerum to join greater petrosal nerve at entrance to pterygoid canal	Conveys the postsynaptic sympathetic fibers destined for lacrimal gland and mucosa of nasal cavity, palate, and upper pharynx
Deep temporal	Mandibular nerve (CN V3)	Ascend temporal fossa deep to temporalis muscle	Motor: temporalis Sensory: periosteum of temporal fossa
Dorsal branch of ulnar nerve	Ulnar nerve about 5 cm proximal to flexor retinaculum	Passes distally deep to flexor carpi ulnaris, then dorsally to perforate deep fascia and course along medial side of dorsum of hand, dividing into 2 to 3 dorsal digital nerves	Sensory: skin of medial aspect of dorsum of hand and proximal portions of 5th and medial half of 4th digit (occasionally also adjacent sides of proximal portions of 4th and 3rd fingers)
Dorsal scapular	Anterior ramus of C5 with frequent contribution from C4	Pierces scalenus medius, descends deep to levator scapulae, and enters deep surface of rhomboids	Motor: rhomboids; occasionally supplies levator scapulae
Esophageal plexus	Vagus nerve, sympathetic ganglia, greater splanchnic nerve	Distal to tracheal bifurcation, vagus and sympathetic nerves form a plexus around esophagus	Vagal (parasympathetic) and sympathetic fibers to smooth muscle and glands of inferior two thirds of esophagus
External nasal	Anterior ethmoidal nerve (CN V1)	Runs in nasal cavity and emerges on face between nasal bone and lateral nasal cartilage	Sensory: skin on dorsum of nose, including tip of nose
Facial (CN VII)	Posterior border of pons	Runs through internal acoustic meatus and facial canal of petrous part of temporal bone, exiting through stylomastoid foramen; main trunk forms intraparotid plexus	Motor: stapedius, posterior belly of digastric, stylohyoid, facial, and scalp muscles Sensory: some skin of external acoustic meatus SEE ALSO intermediate nerve
Femoral	Lumbar plexus (L2–L4 fibers)	Passes deep to midpoint of inguinal ligament, lateral to femoral vessels, and divides into muscular and cutaneous branches	Motor: anterior thigh muscles Sensory: hip and knee joints; skin on anteromedial side of thigh and leg

Nerve(s)/Nerve Branch(es)	Origin	Course	Structures Innervated
Frontal	Ophthalmic nerve (CN V1)	Crosses orbit on superior aspect of levator palpebrae superioris; divides into supraorbital and supratrochlear branches	Sensory: skin of forehead, scalp, upper eyelid, and nose; conjunctiva of upper lid and mucosa of frontal sinus
Genitofemoral	Lumbar plexus (L1–L2 fibers)	Descends on anterior surface of psoas major and divides into genital and femoral branches	Motor: genital branch to cremaster muscle Sensory: femoral branch supplies skin over femoral triangle; genital branch supplies scrotum or labia majora
Glossopharyngeal (CN IX)	Glossopharyngeal (CN IX)	Exits cranium through jugular foramen, passes between superior and middle constrictors of pharynx to tonsillar fossa; enters posterior third of tongue	Motor: somatic to stylopharyngeus; visceral (presynaptic parasympathetic) to parotid gland Sensory: posterior two thirds of tongue (including taste), pharynx, tympanic cavity, auditory tube, carotid body, and sinus
Great auricular	Cervical plexus (C2–C3 fibers)	Ascends vertically over sternocleidomastoid anterior and parallel to external jugular vein	Sensory: skin of auricle, adjacent scalp, and over angle of jaw; parotid sheath
Greater occipital	As medial branch of posterior ramus of spinal nerve C2	Pierces deep muscles of neck and trapezius to ascend posterior scalp to vertex	Motor: multifidus cervicis, semispinalis capitis Sensory: posterior scalp
Greater palatine	Branch of pterygopalatine ganglion (maxillary nerve)	Passes inferiorly through greater palatine canal and foramen	Motor: postsynaptic parasympathetics to palatine glands Sensory: mucosa of hard palate
Greater petrosal	Genu of facial nerve (CN VII)	Exits facial canal through hiatus for greater petrosal nerve; courses across tegmen tympani and passes through cartilage of foramen lacerum to join deep petrosal nerve at opening of pterygoid canal	Motor: presynaptic parasympathetics to pterygopalatine ganglion for innervation of lacrimal and nasal, palatine, and upper pharyngeal mucous glands
Greater splanchnic	5th–6th through 9th–10th thoracic sympathetic ganglia	Highest abdominopelvic splanchnic nerve; passes anteromedially on bodies of thoracic vertebrae, piercing diaphragm to converge on root of celiac trunk	Motor: conveys presynaptic sympathetics to celiac ganglia for innervation of celiac arteries and derivatives, and of that portion of gut they supply
Hypogastric	As continuation of superior hypogastric plexus into pelvis	Courses anteriorly to sacrum within hypogastric sheath to merge with pelvic splanchnic nerves in inferior hypogastric plexus	Motor: conveys presynaptic and postsynaptic sympathetic fibers destined for pelvic viscera Sensory: conveys pain fibers from intraperitoneal pelvic viscera (e.g., fundus, body of uterus)
Hypoglossal (CN XII)	Between pyramid and olive of myencephalon	Passes through hypoglossal canal, then runs inferiorly and anteriorly, passing medially to angle of mandible and between mylohyoid and hyoglossus to reach muscles of tongue	Motor: intrinsic and extrinsic muscles of tongue (exception: palatoglossus)

Nerve(s)/Nerve Branch(es)	Origin	Course	Structures Innervated
Iliohypogastric	Lumbar plexus (L1 fibers)	Parallels iliac crest; pierces transverse abdominal muscle; branches pierce external oblique aponeurosis to reach inguinal and pubic regions	Motor: internal oblique and transverse abdominal muscles Sensory: lateral cutaneous branch supplies superolateral quadrant of buttocks, skin over iliac crest, and hypogastric region
Ilioinguinal	Lumbar plexus (L1 fibers)	Passes between 2nd and 3rd layers of abdominal muscles, passes through inguinal canal, and divides into femoral and scrotal or labial branches	Motor: lowermost part of internal oblique and transverse abdominal muscles Sensory: femoral branch supplies skin over femoral triangle; genital branch supplies mons pubis and adjacent skin of labia majora or scrotum
Inferior alveolar	As terminal branch (with lingual nerve) of posterior trunk of mandibular nerve (CN V3)	Descends between lateral and medial pterygoid muscles of infratemporal fossa to enter mandibular canal of mandible	Sensory: lower teeth, periodontium, periosteum, and gingiva of lower jaw. SEE ALSO nerve to mylohyoid, mental nerve
Inferior anal (rectal)	Pudendal nerve (S2–S4 fibers)	Arises at entry to pudendal canal (ischial spine), courses medially through ischioanal fat pad to anal canal	Motor: external anal sphincter Sensory: anoderm, perianal skin
Inferior gluteal	Sacral plexus (L5–S2 fibers)	Leaves pelvis through greater sciatic foramen inferior to piriformis and divides into several branches	Motor: gluteus maximus
Infraorbital	Terminal branch of maxillary nerve (CN V2)	Runs in floor of orbit and emerges at infraorbital foramen	Sensory: skin of cheek, lower lid, lateral side of nose and inferior septum and upper lip, upper premolar incisors and canine teeth, mucosa of maxillary sinus and upper lip
Infratrochlear	Nasociliary nerve (CN V1)	Follows medial wall of orbit to upper eyelid	Sensory: skin and conjunctiva (lining) of upper eyelid
Intercostals	Anterior rami of T1–T11 nerves	Run in intercostal spaces between internal and innermost layers of intercostal muscles	Motor: intercostal muscles; lower nerves supply muscles of anterolateral abdominal wall Sensory: skin overlying and pleura and peritoneum deep to muscles innervated
Intermediary	From the pons as a smaller root of the facial nerve (CN VII)	Traverses internal acoustic meatus, merging at its distal end with larger (root of) facial nerve	Motor: presynaptic parasympathetics destined for pterygopalatine and submandibular ganglia through greater petrosal nerve and chorda tympani respectively Sensory: taste from anterior two thirds of tongue and soft palate
Lacrimal	Ophthalmic nerve (CN V1)	Passes through palpebral fascia of upper eyelid near lateral angle (canthus) of eye	Sensory: a small area of skin and conjunctiva of lateral part of upper eyelid

Nerve(s)/Nerve Branch(es)	Origin	Course	Structures Innervated
Lateral branch of median nerve	Median nerve as it enters palm of hand	Runs laterally to palmar thumb and radial side of index finger	Motor: 1st lumbrical Sensory: skin of palmar and distal dorsal aspects of thumb and radial half of index finger
Lateral cutaneous nerve of forearm	Continuation of musculocutaneous nerve (C6–C7 fibers)	Descends along lateral border of forearm to wrist	Sensory: skin of lateral aspect of forearm
Lateral cutaneous nerve of thigh	Lumbar plexus (L2–L3 fibers)	Passes deep to inguinal ligament, 2–3 cm medial to anterior superior iliac spine	Sensory: skin on anterior and lateral aspects of thigh
Lateral pectoral	Lateral cord of brachial plexus (C5–C7 fibers)	Pierces clavipectoral fascia to reach deep surface of pectoral muscles	Motor: primarily pectoralis major but sends a loop to medial pectoral nerve that innervates pectoralis minor
Lateral plantar	Smaller terminal branch of the tibial nerve (S1–S2 fibers)	Passes laterally in foot between quadratus plantae and flexor digitorum brevis muscles and divides into superficial and deep branches	Motor: quadratus plantae, abductor digiti minimi, flexor digiti minimi brevis; deep branch supplies plantar and dorsal interossei, lateral three lumbricals, and adductor hallucis Sensory: skin on sole lateral to a line splitting 4th digit
Least splanchnic	12th (lowest) thoracic ganglion of sympathetic trunk	Passes through diaphragm with sympathetic trunk and ends in renal plexus	Motor: presynaptic sympathetic to renal arteries and derivatives
Lesser occipital	Cervical plexus (C2–C3 fibers)	Ascends posterosuperiorly, parallel to anterosuperior border of sternocleidomastoid	Sensory: skin of posterior surface of auricle and adjacent scalp
Lesser palatine	Pterygopalatine ganglion (maxillary nerve—CN V2)	Passes inferiorly through palatine canal and lesser palatine foramen	Motor: postsynaptic parasympathetics to glands of soft palate Sensory: mucosa of soft palate
Lesser petrosal	Tympanic plexus (glossopharyngeal nerve—CN IX)	Perforates tegmen tympani to exit tympanic cavity into middle cranial fossa; runs anteriorly to descend through sphenopetrosal fissure or foramen ovale	Motor: conveys presynaptic parasympathetic fibers to otic ganglion for secretomotor innervation of parotid gland
Lesser splanchnic	10th and 11th thoracic ganglia of sympathetic trunk	Descends anteromedially to perforate diaphragm to reach aorticorenal ganglion	Motor: presynaptic sympathetics to prevertebral ganglia Sensory: visceral afferents from upper gastrointestinal tract
Lingual	Terminal branch (with inferior alveolar nerve) of posterior trunk of mandibular nerve (CN V3)	Joined by chorda tympani in infratemporal fossa; passes anteroinferiorly between lateral and medial pterygoid muscles, and above mylohyoid to enter oral cavity	Motor: presynpatic parasympathetic fibers to submandibular ganglion for submandibular and sublingual salivary glands Sensory: anterior two thirds of tongue, floor of mouth, and lingual mandibular gingiva
Long thoracic	Anterior rami of C5–C7	Descends posterior to C8 and T1 rami and passes distally on external surface of serratus anterior	Motor: serratus anterior

Nerve(s)/Nerve Branch(es)	Origin	Course	Structures Innervated
Lower subscapular	Posterior cord of brachial plexus (C5–C6 fibers)	Passes inferolaterally, deep to subscapular artery and vein to subscapularis and teres major	Motor: inferior portion of subscapularis and teres major
Lumbar splanchnic	Lumbar ganglia of sympathetic trunks	Pass anteromedially on bodies of lumbar vertebrae to prevertebral ganglia of paraaortic plexus	Motor: presynaptic sympathetics for lower abdominal and pelvic viscera Sensory: visceral afferents from same
Mandibular (CN V3)	Trigeminal ganglion (motor root from pons)	Descends through foramen ovale into infratemporal fossa; divides into anterior and posterior trunks, anterior ramifying immediately into several smaller branches, posterior bifurcating into lingual and inferior alveolar nerves	Motor: muscles of mastication, mylohyoid, anterior belly of digastric, tensor tympani, and tensor veli palatini Sensory: skin overlying mandible (except angle), lower half of mouth (including teeth, gingiva, mucosa of floor and vestibule, and anterior two thirds of tongue), and temporomandibular joint
Masseteric	Anterior trunk of mandibular nerve (CN V3)	Passes laterally through mandibular notch	Motor: masseter Sensory: temporomandibular joint
Maxillary (CN V2)	Trigeminal ganglion	Runs anteriorly through foramen rotundum into pterygopalatine fossa, sending sensory roots to the pterygopalatine ganglion (branches of the ganglion are considered branches of the maxillary nerve); main trunk continues anteriorly through infraorbital fissure as infraorbital nerve	Motor: no motor fibers initially; branches of pterygopalatine ganglion distribute postsynaptic parasympathetic fibers to lacrimal gland and mucosal glands of nasal cavity, palate, and upper pharynx Sensory: skin overlying maxilla, mucosa of posteroinferior nasal cavity and maxillary sinus; upper half of mouth (including teeth, gingiva, and mucosa of palate, vestibule, and cheek)
Medial branch of median nerve	Median nerve as it enters palm of hand	Runs medially to adjacent sides of index, middle, and ring fingers	Motor: 2nd lumbrical Sensory: skin of palmar and distal dorsal aspects of adjacent sides of the 2nd, 3rd, and 4th digits
Medial cutaneous nerve of arm	Medial cord of brachial plexus (C8 and T1 fibers)	Runs along the medial side of axillary vein and communicates with intercostobrachial nerve	Sensory: skin on medial side of arm
Medial cutaneous nerve of forearm	Medial cord of brachial plexus (C8 and T1 fibers)	Runs between axillary artery and vein	Sensory: skin over medial side of forearm
Medial cutaneous nerve of leg	Saphenous nerve	Descends medial side of leg with greater saphenous vein	Skin of anteromedial side of leg and medial side of foot
Medial dorsal cutaneous nerve	Superficial fibular (peroneal) nerve	Descends across ankle anteriorly running onto medial aspect of dorsum of foot	Supplies most of skin of dorsum of foot; proximal portion of toes, except for web between great and 2nd toes

Nerve(s)/Nerve Branch(es)	Origin	Course	Structures Innervated
Medial pectoral	Medial cord of brachial plexus (C8 and T1 fibers)	Passes between axillary artery and vein and enters deep surface of pectoralis minor	Motor: pectoralis minor and part of pectoralis major
Medial plantar	Larger terminal branch of the tibial nerve (L4 and L5 fibers)	Passes distally in foot between abductor hallucis and flexor digitorum brevis and divides into muscular and cutaneous branches	Motor: abductor hallucis, flexor digitorum brevis, flexor hallucis brevis, and 1st lumbrical Sensory: skin of medial side of sole of foot and sides of 1st 3 digits
Median	Arises by two roots, one from the lateral cord of brachial plexus (C6–C7 fibers) and one from medial cord (C8 and T1 fibers); roots join lateral to axillary artery	Over length of arm, crosses to medial side of brachial artery; exits cubital fossa between heads of pronator teres, running between intermediate and deep layers of anterior forearm compartment; becomes superficial proximal to wrist and passes deep to flexor retinaculum (transverse carpal ligament) as it passes through carpal tunnel to the hand	Motor: flexor muscles in forearm (except flexor carpi ulnaris, ulnar half of flexor digitorum profundus); thenar muscles (except adductor pollicis and deep head of flexor pollicis brevis), lateral lumbricals (for 2nd and 3rd) digits Sensory: skin of the palmar and distal dorsal aspects of the lateral (radial) 3-1/2 digits and adjacent palm
Mental	Terminal branch of inferior alveolar nerve (CN V3)	Emerges from mandibular canal at mental foramen	Sensory: skin of chin; skin and mucosa of lower lip
Musculocutaneous	Lateral cord of brachial plexus (C5–C7 fibers)	Enters deep surface of coracobrachialis and descends between biceps brachii and brachialis	Motor: flexor muscles of arm (coracobrachialis, biceps brachii, and brachialis) Sensory: continues as lateral antebrachial cutaneous nerve
Nasociliary	Ophthalmic nerve (CN V1)	Arises in superior orbital fissure, passes anteromedially across retrobulbar orbit, providing sensory root to ciliary ganglion and terminating as infratrochlear nerve and nasal branches	Motor: no motor fibers initially; branches of ciliary ganglion (short ciliary nerves) convey postsynaptic sympathetics and parasympathetics to ciliary body and iris Sensory: tactile sensation from eyeball (conjunctiva and cornea); mucous membrane of ethmoidal cells and anterosuperior nasal cavity; skin of root, dorsum, and apex of nose
Nasopalatine	Pterygopalatine ganglion (maxillary nerve—CN V2)	Exits pterygopalatine fossa through sphenopalatine foramen; crossing to and then running anteroinferiorly across nasal septum; passes through incisive foramen to palate	Motor: postsynaptic parasympathetics to mucosal glands of nasal septum Sensory: mucosa of nasal septum, anteriormost hard palate
Nerves to lateral/medial pterygoid	Anterior trunk of mandibular nerve (CN V3)	Arise in infratemporal fossa immediately inferior to foramen ovale	Motor: lateral and medial pterygoid muscles
Nerve to mylohyoid	Inferior alveolar nerve	Arises from posterior aspect of inferior alveolar nerve immediately outside mandibular foramen; descends in bony groove on medial aspect of ramus of mandible	Motor: mylohyoid and anterior belly of digastric muscle

Nerve(s)/Nerve Branch(es)	Origin	Course	Structures Innervated
Nerve to obturator internus	Sacral plexus (L5, S1, andS2)	Enters gluteal region through greater sciatic foramen inferior to piriformis; descends posteriorly to ischial spine; enters lesser sciatic foramen and passes to obturator internus	Motor: superior gemellus and obturator internus
Nerve of pterygoid canal	Formed by merger of greater and deep petrosal nerves	Traverses pterygoid canal to reach pterygopalatine ganglion in pterygopalatine fossa	Motor: conveys postsynaptic sympathetic and presynaptic parasympathetic fibers to pterygopalatine ganglion
Nerve to quadratus femoris	Sacral plexus (L5, S1, and S2)	Leaves pelvis through greater sciatic foramen deep to sciatic nerve	Motor: inferior gemellus and quadratus femoris Sensory: hip joint
Nerve to stapedius muscle	Facial nerve (CN VII)	Arises as facial nerve descends posterior to muscle in facial canal	Motor: stapedius
Nerve to tensor tympani muscle	Otic ganglion (mandibular nerve—CN V3)	Courses along cartilaginous portion of pharyngotympanic (auditory) tube to hemicanal for tensor tympani	Motor: tensor tympani
Nerve to tensor veli palatini muscle	Anterior trunk of mandibular nerve—(CN V3)	Arises as a branch of nerve to medial pterygoid	Motor: tensor veli palatini
Obturator	Lumbar plexus (L2–L4 fibers)	Enters thigh through obturator foramen and divides; its anterior branch descends between adductor longus and adductor brevis; its posterior branch descends between adductor brevis and adductor magnus	Motor: anterior branch supplies adductor longus, adductor brevis, gracilis, and pectineus; posterior branch supplies obturator externus and adductor magnus Sensory: skin of medial thigh above knee
Oculomotor (CN III)	Interpeduncular fossa of mesencephalon	Pierces dura lateral to posterior clinoid process, runs in lateral wall of cavernous sinus, enters orbit through superior fissure and divides into superior and inferior branches	Motor: somatic: all extraocular muscles except superior oblique and lateral rectus; presynaptic paraorbital sympathetic fibers to ciliary ganglion for ciliary body and sphincter pupillae
Olfactory (CN I)	Olfactory cells in olfactory epithelium (mucosa) of roof of nasal cavity plate	Approximately 20 bundles of nerve fibers ascend through foramina of cribriform of ethmoid to reach olfactory bulbs (anterior cranial fossa)	Sensory: olfactory mucosa (sense of smell)
Ophthalmic (CN V1)	Trigeminal ganglion	Passes anteriorly in lateral wall of cavernous sinus to enter orbit through superior orbital fissure, branching into frontal, nasociliary, and lacrimal nerves	Sensory: general sensation from eyeball (conjunctiva and cornea); mucous membrane of ethmoidal cells and frontal sinus, dura of anterior cranial fossa, falx cerebri and tentorium cerebelli, anterosuperior nasal cavity; skin of forehead, upper lid; root, dorsum, and apex of nose
Optic (CN II)	Ganglion cells of retina	Exits orbit through optic canals; fibers from nasal half of retina cross to contralateral side at chiasm; fibers pass through optic tracts to geniculate bodies, superior colliculus, and pretectal area	Sensory: vision from retina

Nerve(s)/Nerve Branch(es)	Origin	Course	Structures Innervated
Palmar cutaneous branch of median nerve	Arises from median nerve just proximal to flexor retinaculum	Passes between tendons of palmaris longus and flexor carpi radialis and runs superficially to flexor retinaculum	Sensory: skin of central palm
Palmar cutaneous branch of ulnar nerve	Arises from ulnar nerve near middle of forearm	Descends on ulnar artery and perforates deep fascia in the distal third of forearm	Sensory: skin at base of medial palm, overlying medial carpals
Pelvic splanchnic	Sacral plexus (S2–S4 fibers)	Run anteriorly and inferiorly to merge with inferior hypogastric plexus	Motor: presynaptic parasympathetic fibers for pelvic viscera, descending and sigmoid colon Sensory: visceral afferent fibers from subperitoneal pelvic viscera (cervix of uterus and upper vagina, floor of bladder, rectum and upper anal canal; prostate)
Perineal	Terminal branch (with dorsal nerve of penis or clitoris) of pudendal nerve (S2–S4 fibers)	Separates from pudendal nerve on exit from pudendal canal; runs to superficial perineum dividing into a superficial cutaneous branch (posterior labial/scrotal) and a deep motor branch	Motor: muscles of urogenital triangle (superficial and deep perineal muscles) Sensory: skin of posterior urogenital triangle (posterior portion of labia majora and minora, vestibule of vagina; posterior aspect of scrotum)
Pharyngeal	Pterygopalatine ganglion	Passes posteriorly through palatovaginal canal	Supplies mucosa of nasopharynx posterior to pharyngotympanic (auditory) tubes
Phrenic	Cervical plexus (C3–C5 fibers)	Passes through superior thoracic aperture and runs between mediastinal pleura and pericardium	Motor: diaphragm Sensory: pericardial sac, mediastinal and diaphragmatic pleura, and diaphragmatic peritoneum
Posterior auricular	As first extracranial branch of facial nerve (CN VII)	Passes posterior to ear, sending branch to occipital region	Motor: posterior auricular muscle and intrinsic auricular muscles, occipital belly of occipitofrontalis (epicranius)
Posterior cutaneous nerve of arm	Radial nerve (C5–C8 fibers)	Emerges from under posterior border of deltoid, between long and lateral heads of triceps brachii	Sensory: skin of posterior aspect of arm
Posterior cutaneous nerve of forearm	Arises in arm from radial nerve (C5–C8 fibers)	Perforates lateral head of triceps and descends along lateral side of arm and posterior aspect of forearm to wrist	Sensory: skin of distal posterior arm, posterior aspect of forearm
Posterior cutaneous nerve of thigh	Sacral plexus (S1–S3 fibers)	Leaves pelvis through greater sciatic foramen inferior to piriformis, runs deep to gluteus maximus, and emerges from its inferior border	Sensory: skin of buttocks through inferior cluneal branches and skin over posterior aspect of thigh and calf; lateral perineum, upper medial thigh through perineal branch
Posterior ethmoidal	Nasociliary	Leaves orbit through posterior ethmoidal foramen	Supplies ethmoidal and sphenoidal paranasal sinuses
Posterior inferior nasal	Greater palatine	Arise in greater palatine canal, pierce through perpendicular plate of palatine bone	Mucosa of inferior nasal concha and walls of inferior and middle nasal meatus

Nerve(s)/Nerve Branch(es)	Origin	Course	Structures Innervated
Posterior interosseous	Terminal branch of deep branch of radial nerve (continuation of deep radial after emerging from supinator)	Runs between superficial and deep layers of posterior forearm, then passes between extensor pollicis longus and interosseous membrane	Motor: extensor carpi ulnaris, extensors of digits (including thumb), and abductor pollicis longus
Posterior labial	Perineal nerve	Emerge from pudendal canal and ramify in subcutaneous tissue	Skin of posterior portion of labium majus
Pudendal	Sacral plexus (S2–S4)	Enters gluteal region through greater sciatic foramen inferior to piriformis; descends posteriorly to sacrospinous ligament; enters perineum through lesser sciatic foramen	Supplies most motor and sensory innervation to perineum (supplies no structures in gluteal region)
Pulmonary plexus	Vagus nerve and cardio-pulmonary splanchnic nerves from sympathetic trunk	Forms on primary bronchi and extends along root of lung and bronchial subdivisions	Motor: parasympathetic fibers constrict bronchioles; sympathetic fibers dilate them
Radial	Terminal branch of posterior cord of brachial plexus (C5–C8 and T1 fibers)	Descends posterior to axillary artery; enters radial groove with deep brachial artery to pass between long and medial heads of triceps; bifurcates in cubital fossa into superficial and deep radial nerves	Motor: proximal to bifurcation, innervates triceps brachii, anconeus, brachioradialis, and extensor carpi radialis longus muscles Sensory: skin on posterior aspect of arm and forearm via posterior cutaneous nerves of arm and forearm
Recurrent (thenar) branch of median nerve	Median nerve immediately distal to flexor retinaculum	Loops around distal border of flexor retinaculum and enters thenar muscles	Motor: abductor pollicis brevis, opponens pollicis, and superficial head of flexor pollicis brevis
Recurrent laryngeal	Vagus nerve (CN X)	Loops around subclavian on right; on left runs around arch of aorta and ascends in tracheoesophageal groove	Motor: intrinsic muscles of larynx (except cricothyroid) Sensory: inferior to level of vocal folds
Saphenous	Femoral nerve	Descends with femoral vessels through femoral triangle and adductor canal, then descends with great saphenous vein	Sensory: skin on medial side of leg and foot
Sciatic	Sacral plexus (L4–S3 fibers)	Enters gluteal region through greater sciatic foramen inferiorly to piriformis, descends along posterior aspect of thigh, and divides proximally to knee into tibial and common fibular peroneal nerves	Motor: hamstrings by tibial division (except for short head of biceps femoris, which is innervated by its common fibular division) Sensory: provides articular branches to hip and knee joints
Subclavian nerve	Superior trunk of brachial plexus (C5–C6; often C4 as well)	Descends posterior to clavicle and anterior to brachial plexus and subclavian artery	Motor: subclavius Sensory: sternoclavicular joint
Subcostal	Anterior ramus of T12 spinal nerve	Courses along inferior border of 12th rib in same manner as intercostal nerves	Motor: muscles of anterolateral abdominal wall Sensory: lateral cutaneous branch supplies skin inferior to anterior iliaccrest

Nerve(s)/Nerve Branch(es)	Origin	Course	Structures Innervated
Suboccipital	Posterior ramus of C1 spinal nerve	Emerges between occipital bone and atlas, inferior to transverse part of vertebral artery, into suboccipital triangle; communicates with occipital nerve (C2)	Motor: suboccipital muscles (rectus capitis major and minor, obliquus capitis inferior and superior)
Superficial branch of radial nerve	Continuation of radial nerve after deep branch is given off in cubital fossa	Passes distally, anterior to pronator teres and deep to brachioradialis; emerging to pierce deep fascia at wrist and pass onto dorsum of hand	Sensory: skin of lateral (radial) half of dorsum of hand and thumb, proximal portions of dorsal aspects of 2nd and 3rd digits, and of lateral (radial) half of 4th digit
Superficial branch of ulnar nerve	Arise from ulnar nerve at wrist as they pass between pisiform and hamate bones	Passes palmaris brevis and divides into 2 common palmar digital nerves	Motor: palmaris brevis Sensory: skin of palmar and distal dorsal aspects of 5th digit and of medial (ulnar) side of 4th digit and proximal portion of palm
Superficial fibular (peroneal)	Common fibular (peroneal) nerve	Arises between fibularis longus and neck of fibula and descends in lateral compartment of leg; pierces deep fascia at distal third of leg to become cutaneous and send branches to foot and digits	Motor: fibularis (peroneus) longus and brevis Sensory: skin on distal third of anterior surface of leg and dorsum of foot and all digits, except lateral side of 5th and adjoining sides of 1st and 2nd digits
Superior alveolar	Maxillary nerve (CN V2) or its continuation as infra-orbital nerve	Posterior: emerges from pterygomaxillary fissure into infratemporal fossa; pierces posterior aspect of maxilla Middle and anterior: arises from infraorbital nerve in roof of maxillary sinus, descends walls of sinus	Sensory: mucosa of maxillary sinus, maxillary teeth, and gingiva
Superior gluteal	Sacral plexus (L4–S1 fibers)	Leaves pelvis through greater sciatic foramen superior to piriformis and runs between gluteus medius and minimus	Motor: gluteus medius, gluteus minimus, and tensor fasciae latae
Superior laryngeal	Vagus (CN X)	Descends in parapharyngeal space; lateral to thyroid cartilage divides into internal and external laryngeal nerves; former pierces thyrohyoid membrane; latter runs inferomedially to gap between cricoid and thyroid cartilages	Motor: cricothyroid muscle (external laryngeal nerve) Sensory: supraglottic
Supraclavicular (lateral, intermediate, medial)	Cervical plexus (C3 and C4 fibers)	Arise from a common trunk that emerges at center of posterior border of sterno-cleidomastoid; fan out as they descend onto lower neck, upper thorax, and shoulder	Sensory: skin of lower anterolateral neck, upper-most thorax, and shoulder
Supraorbital	Continuation of frontal nerve (CN V1)	Emerges through supra-orbital notch, or foramen, and breaks up into small branches	Sensory: mucous mem-brane of frontal sinus and conjunctiva (lining) of upper eyelid; skin of forehead as far as vertex

Nerve(s)/Nerve Branch(es)	Origin	Course	Structures Innervated
Suprascapular	Superior trunk of brachial plexus (C5–C6; often C4 also)	Passes laterally across posterior triangle of neck, through scapular notch under superior transverse scapular ligament	Motor: supraspinatus, infraspinatus muscles Sensory: superior and posterior glenohumeral (shoulder) joint
Supratrochlear	Frontal nerve (CN V1)	Passes superiorly on medial of supraorbital nerve and divides into 2 or more branches	Sensory: skin in middle of forehead to hairline
Sural	Usually arises from merging of medial and lateral sural cutaneous nerves from tibial and common fibular (peroneal) nerves, respectively	Descends between heads of gastrocnemius and becomes superficial at middle of leg; descends with small saphenous vein and passes posterior to lateral malleolus to lateral side of foot	Sensory: skin on posterior and lateral aspects of leg and lateral side of foot
Tentorial	Intracranial portion of ophthalmic nerve (CN V1)	Arises as recurrent branch passing abruptly posteriorly around margins of tentorial notch onto superior aspect of tentorium cerebelli and ascending posterior limb of falx cerebri	Sensory: supratentorial dura mater (superior aspect of tentorium cerebri and falx cerebri)
Thoracic splanchnic	Thoracic ganglia of sympathetic trunk	Pass anteromedially on bodies of thoracic vertebrae as lower cardiopulmonary splanchnic nerves to thoracic autonomic plexuses (cardiac, pulmonary, and esophageal) and as upper abdominopelvic splanchnic nerves to prevertebral ganglia of paraaortic plexus	Motor: splanchnic nerves from 1st through 5th thoracic ganglia convey postsynaptic sympathetic fibers to heart, lungs, and esophagus; those from 6th through 12th thoracic ganglia (i.e., greater, lesser, and least splanchnic nerves) convey presynaptic sympathetic fibers to prevertebral ganglia
Thoracoabdominal	Continuation of lower intercostal nerves (T7–T11)	Cross costal margin to run between 2nd and 3rd layers of abdominal muscles	Motor: anterolateral abdominal muscles Sensory: overlying skin, underlying peritoneum, and periphery of diaphragm
Thoracodorsal	Posterior cord of brachial plexus (C6–C8 fibers)	Arises between upper and lower subscapular nerves and runs inferolaterally along posterior axillary wall to latissimus dorsi	Motor: latissimus dorsi
Tibial	Sciatic nerve (L4–S3 fibers)	Forms as sciatic bifurcates at apex of popliteal fossa; descends through popliteal fossa and lies on popliteus; runs inferiorly on tibialis posterior with posterior tibial vessels; terminates beneath flexor retinaculum by dividing into medial and lateral plantar nerves	Motor: muscles of posterior compartment of thigh (except short head of biceps), popliteal fossa, posterior compartment of leg, and sole of foot Sensory: knee joint; skin of leg (through medial sural), and sole of foot (through medial and lateral plantar nerves)
Transverse cervical	Cervical plexus (C2 and C3 fibers)	Emerges from middle of posterior border of sternocleidomastoid muscle; runs anteriorly across muscle	Sensory: skin overlying anterior triangle of neck

Nerve(s)/Nerve Branch(es)	Origin	Course	Structures Innervated
Trigeminal (CN V)	Lateral surface of pons by 2 roots: motor and sensory	Roots cross medial part of crest of petrous part of temporal bone, entering trigeminal cave of dura mater lateral to body of sphenoid and cavernous sinus; sensory root leads to trigeminal ganglion; motor root bypasses ganglion, becoming part of mandibular nerve (CN V3)	Motor: somatic: muscles of mastication, mylohyoid, anterior belly of digastric, tensor tympani, and tensor veli palatini; visceral: distributes postsynaptic parasympathetic fibers of head to their destinations Sensory: dura of anterior and middle cranial fossae, facial skin, teeth, gingiva, mucosa, nasal cavity, paranasal sinuses, and mouth
Trochlear (CN IV)	Dorsolateral aspect of mesencephalon below inferior colliculus (only cranial nerve to emerge from dorsal aspect of brainstem)	Runs longest intracranial course, passing around brainstem to enter dura in free edge of tentorium close to posterior clinoid process; runs in lateral wall of cavernous sinus, entering orbit via superior orbital fissure	Motor: superior oblique muscle
Tympanic	As 1st extracranial branch of glossopharyngeal nerve (CN IX), from inferior (petrosal) glossopharyngeal ganglion	Passes in recurrent manner into tympanic canaliculus, entering tympanic cavity and ramifying on promontory of labyrinthine wall as tympanic plexus	Motor: conveys presynaptic parasympathetic fibers that will reach otic ganglion for secretomotor innervation of parotid gland Sensory: mucosa of tympanic cavity, mastoid cells, and pharyngotympanic (auditory) tube
Ulnar	Terminal branch of medial cord of brachial plexus (C8 and T1 fibers; often also receives C7 fibers)	Terminal branch of medial cord of brachial plexus (C8 and T1 fibers; often also receives C7 fibers)	Motor: most intrinsic muscles of hand (hypothenar, interosseous, adductor pollicis, and deep head of flexor pollicis brevis, plus medial lumbricals [for 4th and 5th digits]) Sensory: skin of palmar and distal dorsal aspects of medial (ulnar) 1-1/2 digits and adjacent palm
Upper subscapular	Branch of posterior cord of brachial plexus (C5 and C6 fibers)	Passes posteriorly and enters subscapularis	Motor: superior portion of subscapularis
Vagus (CN X)	Through 8–10 rootlets from medulla of brainstem	Enters superior mediastinum posteriorly to sternoclavicular joint and brachiocephalic vein; gives rise to recurrent laryngeal nerve; continues into abdomen	Motor: voluntary muscle of larynx and upper esophagus; involuntary muscle and glands of tracheobronchial tree, gut (to left colic flexure), and heart through pulmonary plexus, esophageal plexus, and cardiac plexus Sensory: pharynx, larynx, reflex afferents from same areas as above
Vestibular	As a division of vestibulocochlear nerve (CN VIII)	Traverses internal acoustic meatus to reach vestibular ganglion at fundus; branches pass to vestibule of bony labyrinth	Sensory: cristae of ampullae of semicircular ducts, maculae of saccule and utricle (for sense of equilibration)

Nerve(s)/Nerve Branch(es)	Origin	Course	Structures Innervated
Vestibulocochlear (CN VIII)	Groove between pons and myencephalon	Traverses internal acoustic meatus, dividing into cochlear and vestibular nerves	Sensory: spiral organ (for sense of hearing) and cristae of ampullae of semicircular ducts, maculae of saccule and utricle (for sense of equilibration)
Zygomatic	Maxillary nerve (CN V2)	Arises in floor of orbit, divides into zygomaticofacial and zygomaticotemporal nerves, which traverse foramina of same name; communicating branch joins lacrimal nerve	Sensory: skin over zygomatic arch and anterior temporal region Motor: conveys secretory postsynaptic parasympathetic fibers from pterygopalatine ganglion to lacrimal gland

Ligaments and Tendons of the Human Body

Shoulder/Upper Arm

Latin name	English name	Articulation
Lm. acromioclaviculare	acromioclavicular l.	Connects acromion to clavicle; strengthens articular capsule
Lm. anulare radii	anular l. of radius	Connects head of radius in radial notch
Lm. collaterale ulnare	collateral ulnar l.	Connects medial epicondyle to humerus and coronoid process of ulna and olecranon
Lm. conoideum	conoid l.	Connects coracoid process of scapula to clavicle
Lm. coracoacromiale	coracoacromial l.	Connects coracoid process to acromion
Lm. coracoclaviculare	coracoclavicular l.	Connects coracoid process of scapula to clavicle
Lm. coracohumerale	coracohumeral l.	Connects coracoid process of scapula to humerus
Lm. costoclaviculare	costoclavicular l.	Connects 1st costal cartilage to clavicle
Lm. glenohumeralia	glenohumeral ligs.	Connects articular capsule of humerus to glenoid cavity and anatomic neck of humerus
Lm. interclaviculare	interclavicular l.	Connects clavicle to opposite clavicle
Lm. orbiculare radii	anular l. of radius	Encircles and holds the head of the radius in the radial notch of the ulna
Lm. sternoclaviculare anterius	anterior sternoclavicular l.	Fibrous band that reinforces the sternoclavicular joint anteriorly
Lm. sternoclaviculare posterius	posterior sternoclavicular l.	Fibrous band that reinforces the sternoclavicular joint posteriorly
Lm. suspensorium axillae	suspensory l.	Connects between the clavipectoral fascia downward to the axillary fascia
Lm. transversum humeri	transverse humeral l.	Connects obliquely from the greater to the lesser tuberosity of the humerus
Lm. transversum scapulae inferius	inferior transverse scapular l.	Connects scapula to glenoid cavity; creates foramen of scapula for vessels/nerves
Lm. transversum scapulae superius	superior transverse scapular l.	Connects coracoid process to scapular notch of scapula
Lm. trapezoideum	trapezoid l.	Connects coracoid process to clavicle

Abbreviations used: l., ligament; La. ligamenta; Lm., ligamentum; ligs., ligaments.

Hand/Forearm

Latin name	English name	Articulation
Lm. anulare radii	anular l. of radius	Connects radius to ulna
Lm. carpi radiatum	radiate carpal l.	Multiple fibrous bands on palmar surface of metacarpal joint
Lm. carpi transversum	flexor retinaculum of hand	Continuous with antebrachial fascia
Lm. carpi volare	flexor retinaculum of hand	Reinforcing fibers in antebrachial fascia, palmar surface of wrist
La. carpometacarpalia dorsalia	dorsal carpometacarpal ligs.	Join carpal bones to bases of metacarpals
La. carpometacarpalia palmaria	carpometacarpal (palmar) metacarpals	Join carpal bones to metacarpals ligs.
La. collateralia articulationum interphalangealium manus	collateral ligs.	Fibrous bands on each side of interphalangeal joints of fingers
La. collateralia articulationes metacarpophalangealieae	collateral ligs.	Fibrous bands on sides of each metacarpophalangeal joint
Lm. collaterale carpi radiale	radial collateral l.	Connects styloid process of radius to scaphoid
Lm. collaterale carpi ulnare	ulnar collateral ligament of wrist joint	Connects the styloid process of the ulna to the pisiform and triquetrum bones
Lm. collaterale radiale	collateral radial l.	Connects lateral epicondyle of humerus to anular l. of radius
Lm. intercarpalia dorsalia interossea	dorsal intercarpal ligs.	Connect carpal bones
Lm. intercarpalia interossea	interosseous intercarpal ligs.	Connect various carpal bones
Lm. intercarpalia palmaria	palmar intercarpal ligs.	Connect various carpal bones
La. metacarpalia dorsalia	dorsal metacarpal ligs.	Interconnects bases of metacarpal bones
La. metacarpalia interossea	interosseous metacarpal ligs.	Interconnects bases of metacarpal bones
La. metacarpalia palmaria	palmar metacarpal ligs.	Interconnects bases of metacarpals
La. metacarpeum transversum profundum	deep transverse metacarpal l.	Interconnects heads of metacarpals
Lm. metacarpale transversum superficiale	superficial transverse metacarpal l.	Between longitudinal bands of palmar aponeurosis
Lm. natatorium	superficial transverse metacarpal l.	Thickening of the deep fascia in most distal part of the base of the triangular palmar
La. palmaria	palmar ligs.	Connect anterior aspect of each metacarpophalangeal and interphalangeal joint of the hand
La. palmaria articulationis interphalangeae manus	palmar ligs. of interphalangeal joints of the hand	Interphalangeal articulations of hand between collateral articulations
La. palmaria articulationis metacarpophalangeae	palmar ligs. of metacarpal joints	Connects metacarpophalangeal joints to the collateral ligs.
Lm. pisohamatum	pisohamate l.	Connects pisiform bone to hook of hamate bone
Lm. pisometacarpale	pisometacarpal l.	Connects pisiform bone to bases of metacarpals
Lm. quadratum	quadrate l.	Connects radial notch of ulna to neck of radius
Lm. radiocarpale dorsale	dorsal radiocarpal l.	Connects radius to carpal bones
Lm. radiocarpale palmare	palmar radiocarpal l.	Connects radius to lunate, triquetral, capitate, and hamate bones
Lm. ulnocarpale palmare	palmar ulnocarpal l.	Connects styloid process of ulna to carpal bones

Abbreviations used: l., ligament; La. ligamenta; Lm., ligamentum; ligs., ligaments.

Spine

Latin name	English name	Articulation
La. alaria	alar l.	Connects axis to occiput; limits rotation of head
Lm. apicis dentis axis	apical dental l.	Connects axis to occiput
La. atlantooccipitale laterale	lateral atlantooccipital l.	Connects occiput to atlas
Lm. capitis costae intraarticulare	interarticular l. of head of rib	Connects crest of rib to intervertebral disc
Lm. capitis costae radiatum	radiate l. of head of rib	Connects head of rib to adjacent vertebrae/discs
Lm. caudale integumenti communis	caudal retinaculum	Forms coccygeal foveola
Lm. costotransversarium	costotransverse l.	Connects neck of rib to transverse process of corresponding vertebra
Lm. costotransversarium laterale	lateral costotransverse l.	Connects transverse process of vertebra to corresponding rib
Lm. costotransversarium superius	superior costotransverse l.	Connects neck of rib to transverse process of vertebra above
Lm. cruciforme atlantis	cruciform l. of atlas	Connects transverse l. of atlas to longitudinal fascicles
La. flava	yellow ligs.	Joins laminae of two adjacent vertebrae
Lm. iliofemorale	iliofemoral l.	Connects anterior/inferior iliac spine and intertrochanteric femur
Lm. iliolumbale	iliolumbar l.	Connects L4-L5 to iliac crest
Lm. interspinale	interspinous l.	Interconnect spinous processes
Lm. intertransversarium	intertransverse l.	Interconnect vertebral transverse processes
Lm. longitudinale anterius	anterior longitudinal l.	Extends from occiput/atlas to sacrum
Lm. longitudinale posterius	posterior longitudinal l.	Extends from occiput to coccyx
Lm. lumbocostale	lumbocostal l.	Connects 12th rib to transverse processes of L1-L2
Lm. nuchae	nuchal l.	Connects head of each rib to bodies of the two vertebrae with which it articulates
Lm. sacrococcygeum anterius	anterior sacrococcygeal l.	Connects sacrum to coccyx
Lm. sacrococcygeum laterale	lateral sacrococcygeal l.	Connects 1st coccygeal vertebra to sacrum; completes foramen of S5
Lm. sacrococcygeum posterius profundum	deep posterior sacrococcygeal l.	Terminal portion of posterior longitudinal l.; unites S5 and profundum coccyx
Lm. sacrococcygeum posterius ´superficiale	superficial posterior sacrococcygeal l.	Connects sacral hiatus to coccyx superficiale
La. sacroiliacum anterius	anterior sacroiliac ligs.	Connects sacrum to ilium
La. sacroiliacum interosseum	interosseous sacroiliac ligs.	Numerous bundles connecting tuberosities of sacrum to those of ilium
La. sacroiliacum posterius	posterior sacroiliac ligs.	Connects ilium and iliac spines to sacrum
Lm. sacrospinale	sacrospinous l.	Connects ischium to lateral margins of sacrum
Lm. sacrotuberale	sacrotuberous l.	Connects ischial tuberosity to sacrum and coccyx and iliac spine
Lm. supraspinale	supraspinous l.	Interconnects tips of spinous processes of vertebrae
Lm. transversum atlantis	transverse l. of atlas	Horizontal portion of cruciform l. of atlas

Abbreviations used: l., ligament; La. ligamenta; Lm., ligamentum; ligs., ligaments.

Abdominal/Pelvic

Latin name	English name	Articulation
Lm. arcuatum laterale	lateral arcuate l.	Connects first lumbar vertebrae and 12th rib to diaphragm
Lm. arcuatum mediale	medial arcuate l.	Connects body of first lumbar vertebra to transverse process
Lm. arcuatum pubis	inferior pubic l.	Arches across pubic symphysis
Lm. falciforme	falciform process of sacrotuberous l.	Passes from ischial tuberosity to ilium, sacrum, and coccyx
Lm. laterale vesicae	lateral l. of bladder	Passes from one side of the bladder to blend with the pelvic fascia
Lm. pectineum	pectineal l.	A strong fibrous band that passes laterally from the lacunar l. along the pectineal line of the pubis
Lm. pubicum inferius	inferior pubic l.	Arches across the inferior aspect of the pubic symphysis
Lm. pubicum superius	superior pubic l.	Passes transversely above the pubic symphysis
Lm. pubofemorale	pubofemoral l.	Connects from the superior ramus of the pubis to the intertrochanteric femur
Lm. sacrodurale	sacrodural l.	Connects between the midline of the inferior part of the dorsal sac to the posterior longitudinal l. of the sacrum.
Lm. sacroiliacum posterius	posterior sacroiliac ligs.	Connects from the ilium to the sacrum posterior to the sacroiliac joint
Lm. sacrospinale	sacrospinous l.	Connects between the ischial spine and the sacrum and coccyx

Hip/Thigh

Latin name	English name	Articulation
Lm. capitis femoris	l. of head of femur	Connects femur, acetabular notch, and transverse l. of acetabulum
Lm. inguinale	inguinal l.	Connects ilium to pubis
Lm. ischiofemorale	ischiofemoral l.	Connects ischium to femur
Lm. transversum acetabuli	transverse acetabular l.	Connects acetabular lip of hip joint to acetabular notch

Knee/Calf

Latin name	English name	Articulation
Lm. capitis fibulae anterius	anterior l. of fibular head	Connects head of fibula to lateral condyle of tibia
Lm. capitis fibulae posterius	posterior l. of fibular head	Connects head of fibula to lateral condyle of tibia
Lm. collaterale fibulare	fibular collateral l.	Connects lateral epicondyle of femur to head of fibula
Lm. collateral tibiale	tibial collateral l.	Connects medial epicondyle of femur to medial meniscus and tibia
Lm. cruciatum anterius genus	anterior cruciate l. of knee	Connects lateral condyle of femur to condylar eminence of tibia

(continued)

Abbreviations used: l., ligament; La. ligamenta; Lm., ligamentum; ligs., ligaments.

Latin name	English name	Articulation
La. cruciata genus	cruciate ligs. of knee	Bundles in knee joint between condyles of femur
Lm. cruciatum posterius genus	posterior cruciate l. of knee	Connects medial condyle of femur to intercondylar area of tibia
Lm. menisci lateralis	posterior meniscofemoral l.	Connects between the medial condyle of the femur to the posterior crus of the lateral meniscus
Lm. meniscofemorale anterius	anterior meniscofemoral l.	Connects lateral meniscus to posterior cruciate l.
Lm. meniscofemorale posterius	posterior meniscofemoral l.	Connects lateral meniscus to medial condyle of femur
Lm. patellae	patellar l.	Connects patella to tibial tuberosity
Lm. popliteum arcuatum	arcuate popliteal l.	Connects fibula to articular capsule
Lm. popliteum obliquum	oblique popliteal l.	Connects medial condyle of tibia to lateral epicondyle of femur
Lm. teres femoris	l. of head of femur	Connects from the fovea in the head of the femur to the borders of the acetabular notch
Lm. tibiofibulare anterius	anterior tibiofibular l.	Connects tibia to fibula
Lm. tibiofibulare posterius	posterior tibiofibular l.	Connects tibia to distal fibula
Lm. tibionaviculare	tibionavicular part of medial l. of ankle joint	Connects from medial malleolus of the tibia downward to the tarsal bones
Lm. transversum genus	transverse l. of knee	Connects lateral meniscus to medial meniscus

Foot and Ankle

Latin name	English name	Articulation
Lm. bifurcatum	bifurcate l.	Dorsum of foot; comprises calcaneo-navicular and calcaneocuboid ligs.
Lm. calcaneocuboideum	calcaneocuboid l.	Connects calcaneus to cuboid
Lm. calcaneocuboideum plantare	plantar calcaneocuboid l., short plantar l.	Connects calcaneus to cuboid
Lm. calcaneofibulare	calcaneofibular l.	Connects fibula to calcaneus
Lm. calcaneonaviculare	calcaneonavicular l.	Connects calcaneus to navicular bone
Lm. calcaneonaviculare dorsale	dorsal calcaneonavicular l.	Connects calcaneus to navicular bone
Lm. calcaneonaviculare plantare	plantar calcaneonavicular l.	Connects sustentaculum tali to navicular; supports talus
Lm. calcaneotibiale	tibiocalcaneal part of medial ligament of ankle joint	Connect medial malleolus to sustentaculum tali of calcaneus
Lm. collateralia articulationum	collateral ligs. of metatarsophalangeal articulations	Fibrous bands on sides of each meta-tarsophalangeal joint
Lm. cruciatum cruris	inferior extensor retinaculum	Joins malleolus to dorsum of foot
Lm. cuboideonaviculare dorsale	dorsal cuboideonavicular l.	Connects cuboid and navicular bones
La. cuboideonaviculare plantaria	plantar cuboideonavicular ligs.	Connect cuboid and navicular bones
Lm. cuneocuboideum dorsale	dorsal cuneocuboid l.	Connects cuboid and lateral cuneiform bones
Lm. cuneocuboideum interossea	interosseus cuneocuboid l.	Connects cuboid and lateral cuneiform bones
Lm. cuneocuboideum plantare	plantar cuneocuboid l.	Connects cuboid and lateral cuneiform bones

(continued)

Abbreviations used: l., ligament; La. ligamenta; Lm., ligamentum; ligs., ligaments.

Latin name	English name	Articulation
La. cuneometatarsalia interossea	interosseous cuneometatarsal ligs.	Connects cuneiform and metatarsal bones
La. cuneonavicularia dorsalia	dorsal cuneonavicular ligs.	Connects navicular and cuneiform bones
La. cuneonavicularia plantaria	plantar cuneonavicular ligs.	Connects navicular to cuneiform bones
La. intercuneiformia dorsalia	dorsal intercuneiform l.	Connects dorsal surfaces of cuneiform bones
La. intercuneiformia interossea	interosseous intercuneiform ligs.	Connects adjacent cuneiform bones
La. intercuneiformia plantaria	plantar intercuneiform ligs.	Joins plantar surfaces of cuneiform bones
Lm. laterale articulationis talocruralis	lateral l. of ankle joint	Lateral side of ankle joint
Lm. mediale articulationis talocruralis	medial l. of ankle joint	Connects medial malleolus of tibia to tarsal bones
La. meniscofemoralia	meniscofemoral ligs.	Connects from posterior part of lateral meniscus to the lateral surface of the medial meniscus
Lm. metatarsale transversum profundum	deep transverse metatarsal l.	Joins heads of metatarsals
Lm. metatarsale transversum superficiale	superficial transverse metatarsal l.	Lies on sole of foot beneath heads of metatarsals
La. metatarsalia dorsalia	dorsal metatarsal ligs.	Interconnects bases of metatarsal bones
La. metatarsalia interossea	interosseous metatarsal ligs.	Interconnects bases of metatarsal bones
La. metatarsalia plantaria	plantar metatarsal ligs.	Plantar surface of metatarsal bones
La. plantaria articulationum interphalangealium pedis	plantar ligs. of interphalangeal articulations	Interphalangeal articulations of foot between collateral ligs.
La. plantaria articulationis metatarsophalangeae	plantar ligs. of metatarsophalangeal joints	Plantar surface of metatarsophalangeal articulations between collateral ligs.
Lm. plantare longum	long plantar l.	Connects calcaneus to bases of metatarsal bones
Lm. talocalcaneum	talocalcaneal l.	Connects talus to calcaneus
Lm. talocalcaneum laterale	lateral talocalcaneal l.	Connects talus to calcaneus
Lm. talocalcaneum mediale	medial talocalcaneal l.	Connects tubercle of talus to sustentaculum tali of calcaneus
La. talocalcaneare interosseum	talocalcaneal interosseous l.	Connects calcaneus to talus
Lm. talofibulare anterius	anterior talofibular l.	Connects lateral malleolus of fibula to posterior process of talus
Lm. talonaviculare	talonavicular l.	Connects neck of talus to navicular bone
Lm. talotibiale	medial tibiotalar l.	Connects downward from the medial malleolus of the tibia of the tarsal bones
La. tarsi	tarsal ligs.	Connects bones of tarsus
La. tarsi dorsalia	dorsal tarsal ligs.	Collectively, bifurcate, dorsal cuboideonavicular, cuneocuboid, cuneonavicular, intercuneiform, and talonavicular ligs.
La. tarsi interossea	tarsal interosseous ligs.	Collectively, interosseous, cuneocuboid, intercuneiform, and talocalcaneal ligs.
La. tarsi plantaria	plantar tarsal ligs.	Inferior ligs. of foot (long plantar, plantar calcaneocuboid, calcaneonavicular, cuneonavicular, cuboideonavicular, intercuneiform, cuneocuboid)
La. tarsometatarsalia dorsalia	dorsal tarsometatarsal ligs.	Connects bases of metatarsals to dorsal cuboid and cuneiform bones

(continued)

Abbreviations used: l., ligament; La. ligamenta; Lm., ligamentum; ligs., ligaments.

Latin name	English name	Articulation
La. tarsometatarsalia plantaria	plantar tarsometatarsal ligs.	Connects metatarsal bones to cuboid and cuneiform bones
Lm. transversum cruris	superior extensor retinaculum	Connects tibia to fibula; holds extensor tendons in place
Tendo calcaneus	calcaneal tendon	Connects triceps surae muscle to tuberosity of calcaneus

Abbreviations used: l., ligament; La. ligamenta; Lm., ligamentum; ligs., ligaments.

Radiographic Anatomy and Positioning

Anatomic Planes

A plane is a flat surface formed by making a cut (imaginary or real) through the body or a part of it. In radiography, various planes are used as points of reference that assist in localizing areas of the body to permit specific centering guidelines. The major anatomic planes used in radiographic positioning are:

Longitudinal plane	Running lengthwise; in the direction of the long axis of the body or any of its parts or sections.
Transverse plane	Placed across the body at right angles to the frontal and sagittal planes. Transverse planes are perpendicular to the long axis of the body or limbs, regardless of the position of the body or limb; in the anatomic position, transverse planes are horizontal; otherwise the two terms are *not* synonymous.
Median (midsagittal) plane	A plane vertical in the anatomic position, through the midline of the body that divides the body into right and left halves.
Sagittal plane	Plane parallel to the median plane; sagittal planes are vertical planes in the anatomic position.
Frontal (coronal) plane	A vertical plane at right angles to the sagittal plane, dividing the body into anterior and posterior portions, or any plane parallel to the central frontal plane.
Transpyloric plane	A transverse plane midway between the superior margins of the manubrium of the sternum and the symphysis pubis; the pylorus may be located on this plane in the supine or prone positions, but in the erect (anatomic) position it descends to a lower level.
Subcostal plane	A transverse plane passing through the inferior limits of the costal margin (i.e., the 10th costal cartilages); it delimits the boundary between the hypochondriac and epigastric regions superiorly and the lateral and umbilical regions inferiorly.

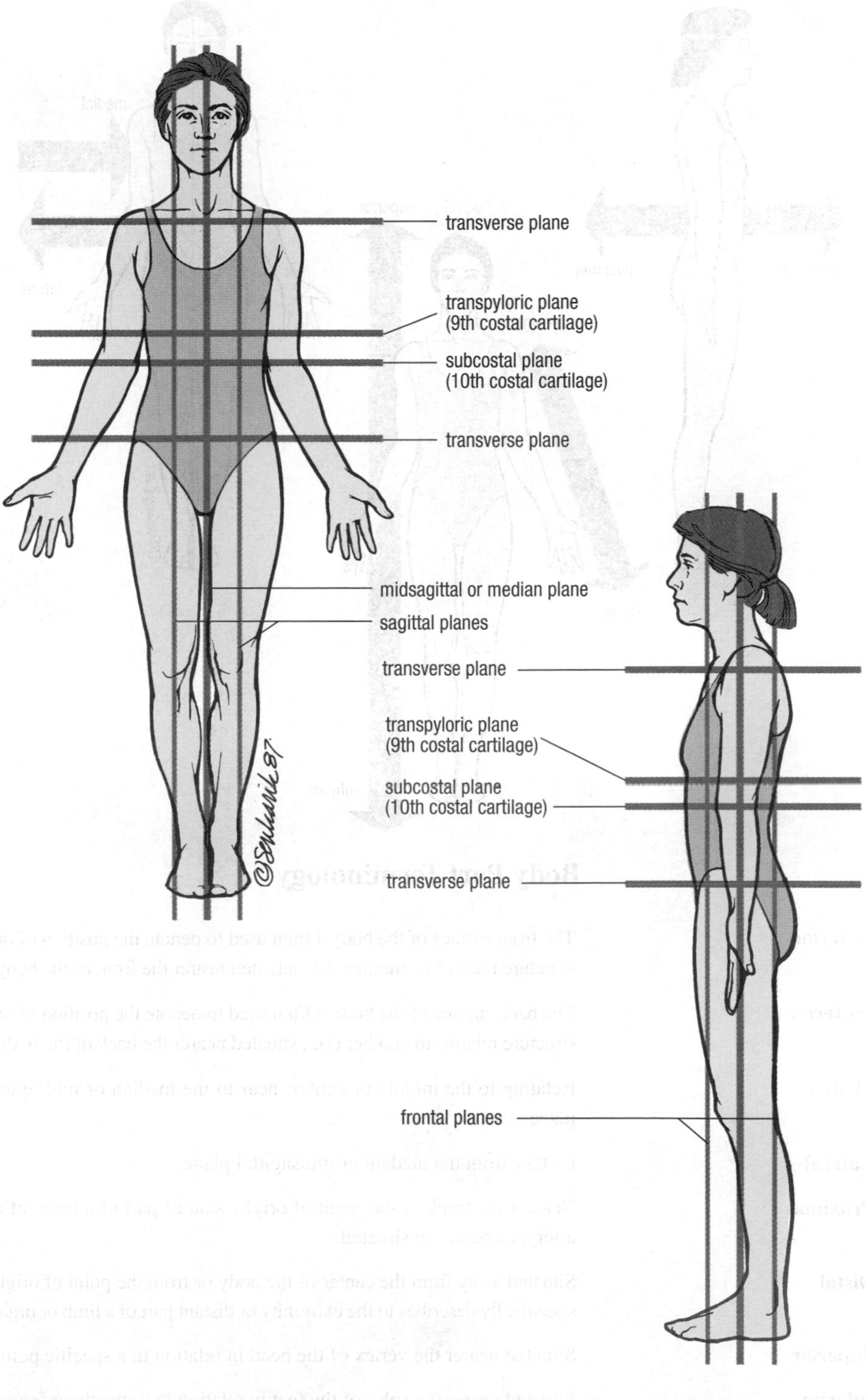
transverse plane
transpyloric plane
(9th costal cartilage)
subcostal plane
(10th costal cartilage)
transverse plane
midsagittal or median plane
sagittal planes
©Senkarik 87
transverse plane
transpyloric plane
(9th costal cartilage)
subcostal plane
(10th costal cartilage)
transverse plane
frontal planes

Anatomic Planes

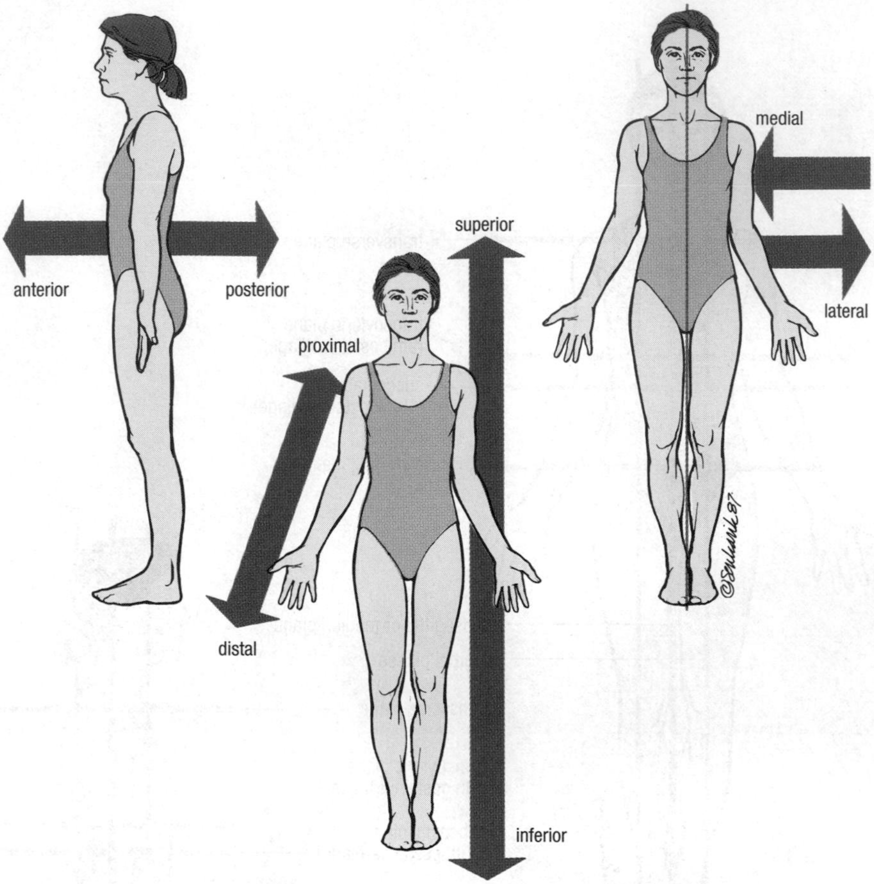

Body Part Terminology

Anterior The front surface of the body. Often used to denote the position of one structure relative to another (i.e., situated nearer the front of the body).

Posterior The back surface of the body. Often used to denote the position of one structure relative to another (i.e., situated nearer the back of the body).

Medial Relating to the middle or center; near to the median or midsagittal plane.

Lateral Farther from the median or midsagittal plane.

Proximal Nearest the trunk or the point of origin, said of part of a limb, of an artery, or nerve, so situated.

Distal Situated away from the center of the body or from the point of origin; specifically describes to the extremity or distant part of a limb or organ.

Superior Situated nearer the vertex of the head in relation to a specific point.

Inferior Situated nearer the soles of the feet in relation to a specific reference point.

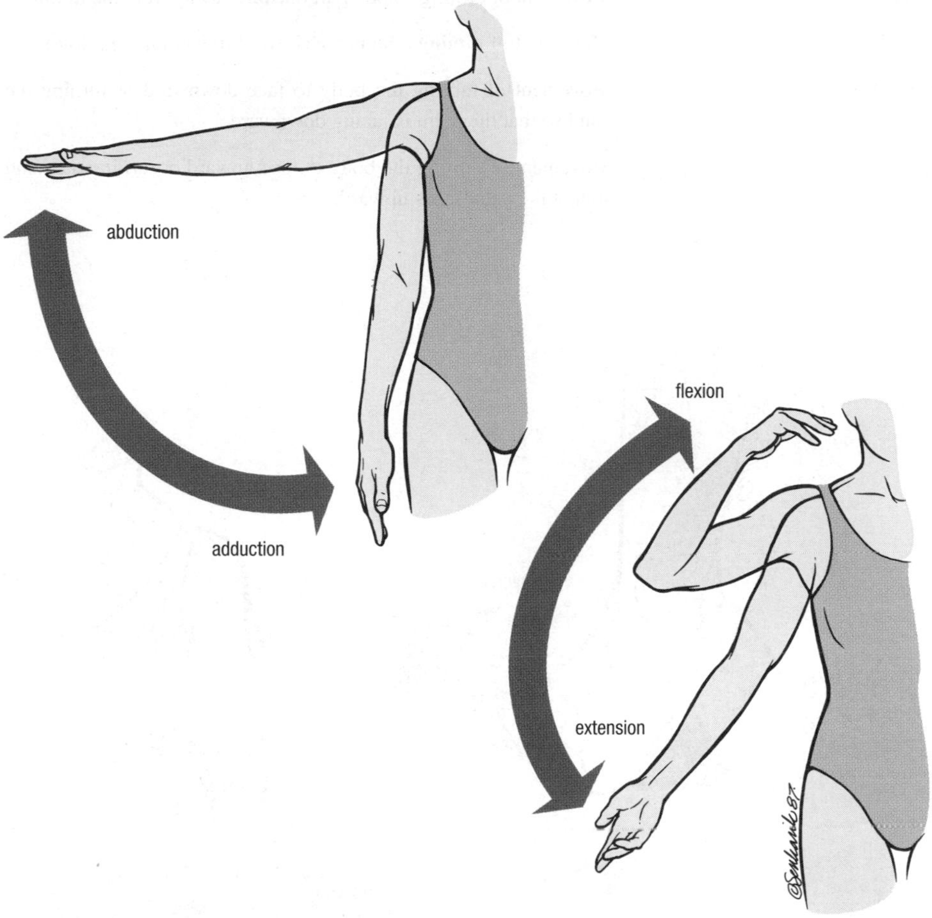

Body Movement

Abduction — Movement of a limb or body part farther from or away from the midline of the body.

Adduction — Movement of a limb or body part closer to or toward the midline of the body.

Extension — Straightening of a joint or extremity so that the angle between contiguous (adjoining) bones is increased.

Flexion — Bending of a joint or extremity so that the angle between contiguous (adjoining) bones is decreased.

Eversion Movement of turning a body part outward (away from the midline).

Inversion Movement of turning a body part inward (toward the midline).

Pronation Movement of turning the body to face downward or turning the hand so that the palm is facing downward.

Supination Movement of turning the body to face upward or turning the hand so that the palm faces upward.

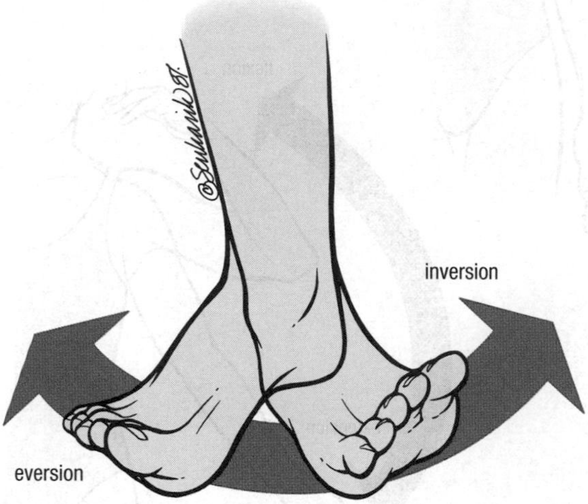

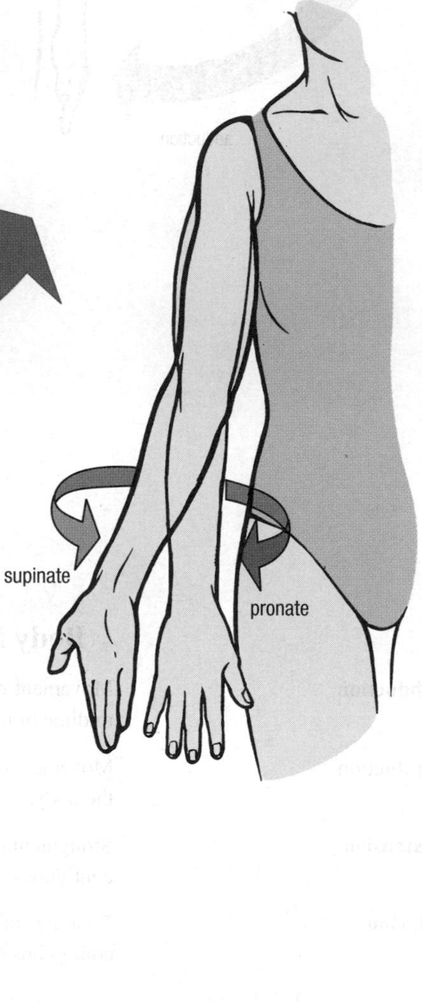

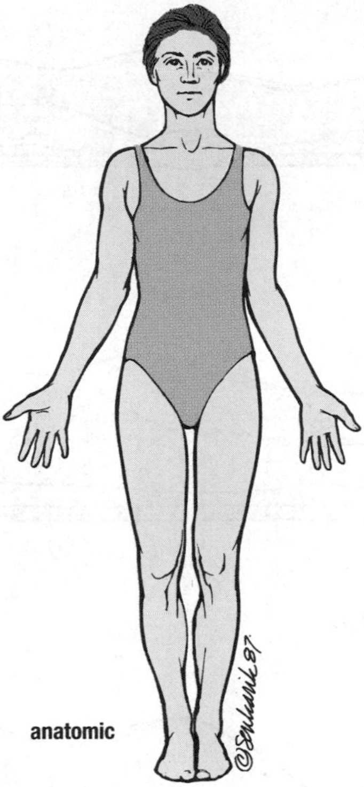

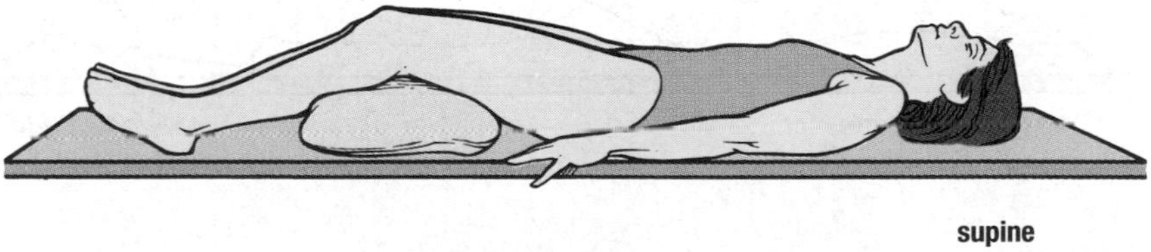

Positioning Terminology

Anatomic position Position of the body when the subject is facing the front in the erect position with the arms and legs fully extended. The palms of the hands are facing forward and the feet are together. In radiography, this term is used as the reference position of the body to describe various positions.

Supine position Position in which the subject is lying on the back with the face up. Sometimes referred to as the *dorsal recumbent* (lying down) or *dorsal decubitus* position, because the back (dorsal surface) of the body is dependent (nearer the table).

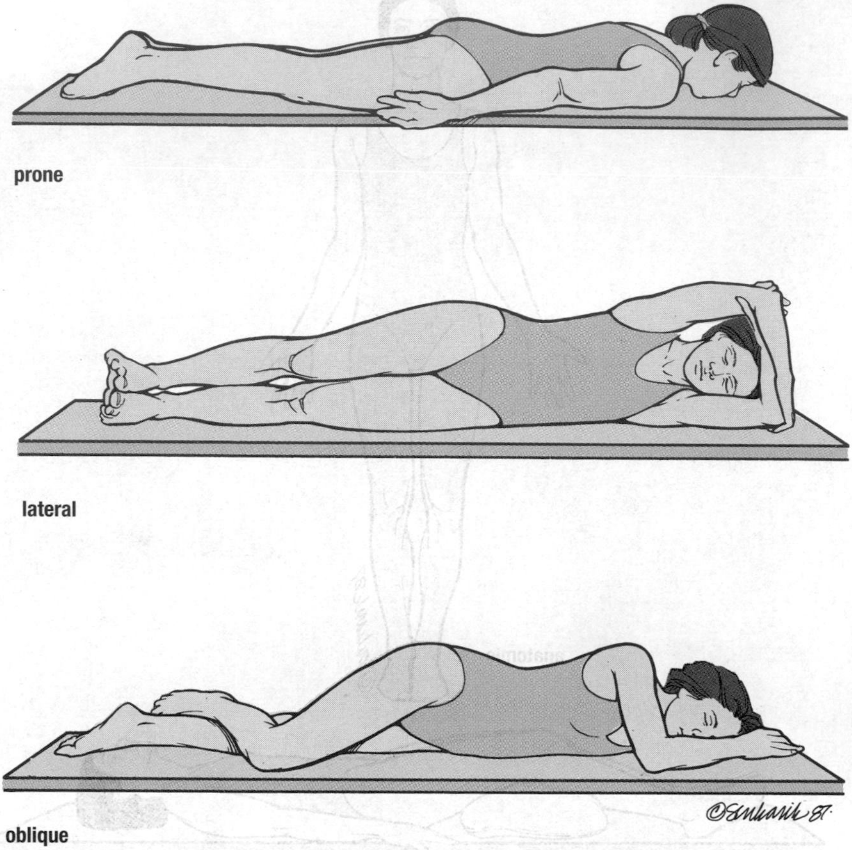

Prone position

Position in which the subject is lying face down on the front of the body. Sometimes referred to as the *ventral recumbent* or *ventral decubitus* position, because the front (ventral surface) of the body is dependent (nearer the table).

Lateral position

Position in which the side of the subject is next to the film. A lateral position is named by the side of the subject that is situated adjacent to the film. Sometimes referred to as an *erect lateral* if the subject is sitting or standing, and a *lateral recumbent* or *lateral decubitus* if the subject is lying down.

Oblique position

Position in which the subject is neither prone nor supine, but rotated somewhere between. In radiographic terminology, the subject is in a *posterior oblique position* if some part of the posterior surface of the body is closer to the film, and in an *anterior oblique position* if some part of the anterior surface of the body is closer to the film.

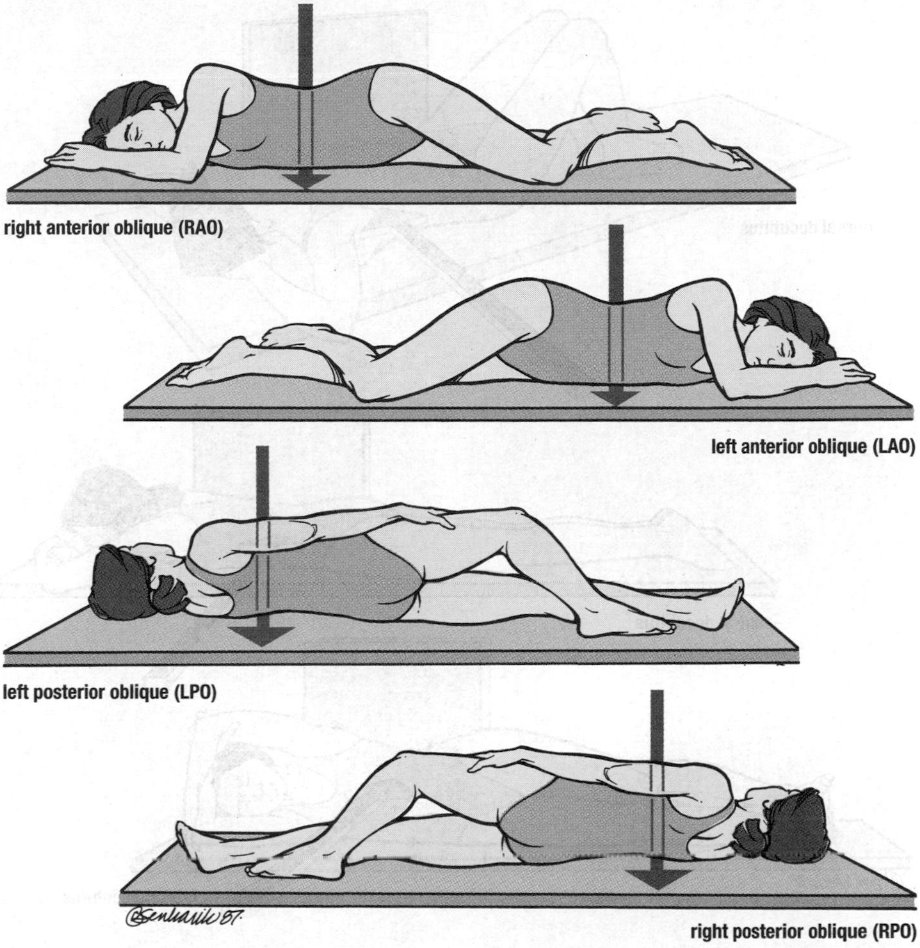

Right anterior oblique (RAO) Patient is lying semiprone (face down) on the radiographic table or standing facing a vertical grid device with the *right* side closer to the film.

Left anterior oblique (LAO) Patient is lying semiprone (face down) on the radiographic table or standing facing a vertical grid device with the *left* side closer to the film.

Left posterior oblique (LPO) Patient is lying semisupine (face up) on the radiographic table or standing with the back against a vertical grid device with the *left* side closest to the film.

Right posterior oblique (RPO) Patient is lying semisupine (face up) on the radiographic table or standing facing away from a vertical grid device with the *right* side closest to the film.

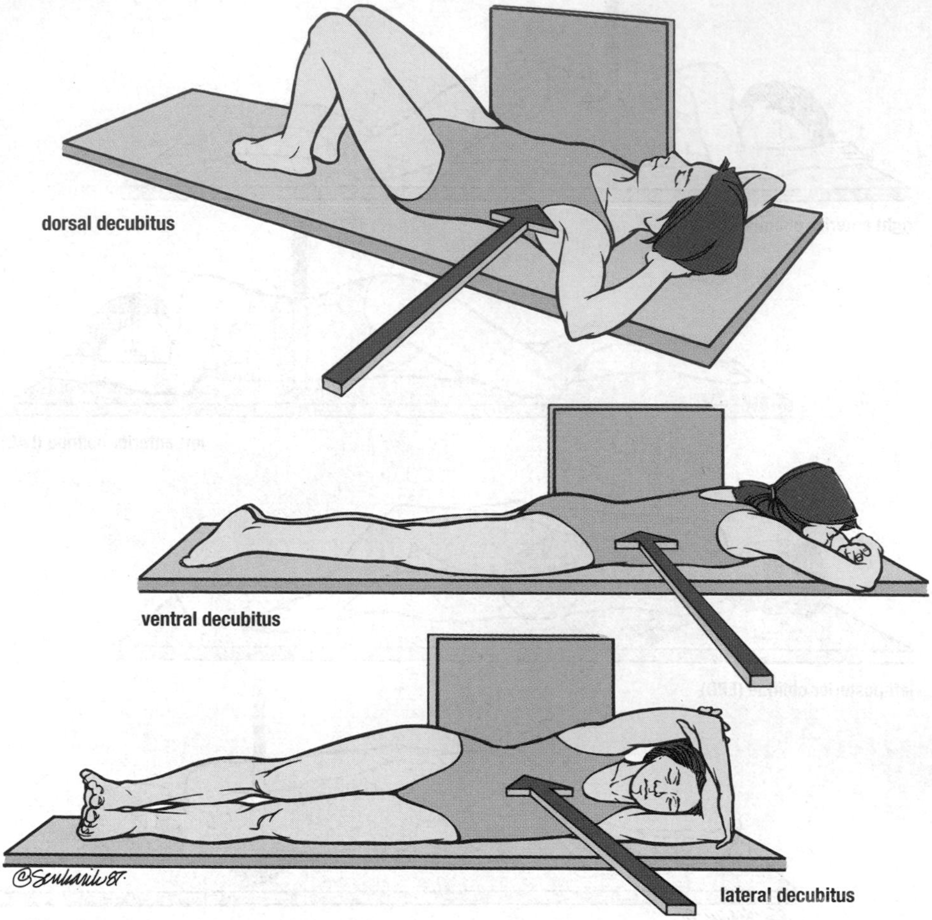

Decubitus position	Patient is lying down, and the central ray is horizontal (parallel to the floor).
Dorsal decubitus	Patient is lying supine (face up) on the radiographic table or on a stretcher placed next to a vertical grid device. The x-ray beam enters from one side of the patient and exits the other.
Ventral decubitus	Patient is lying prone (face down) on the radiographic table or on a stretcher placed next to a vertical grid device. The x-ray beam enters from one side of the patient and exits the other.
Lateral decubitus	Patient is lying on either side on the radiographic table or on a stretcher placed next to a vertical grid device. For a *left* lateral decubitus, the patient is lying on the *left* side with the *right* side up, whereas for a *right* lateral decubitus, the patient is lying on the *right* side with the *left* side up. The x-ray beam passes through the patient from front to back or back to front, depending on whether the patient is facing toward or away from the radiographic tube.

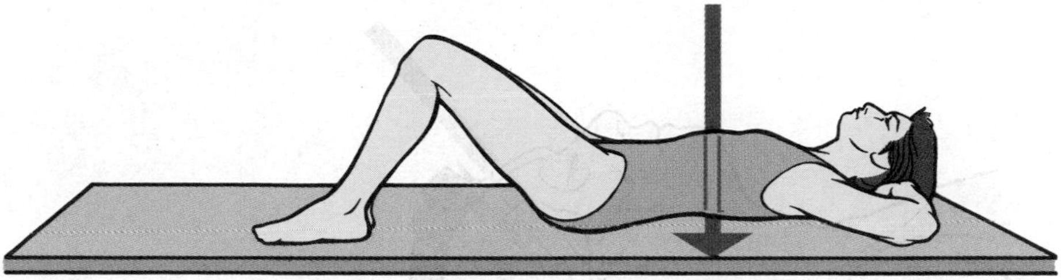

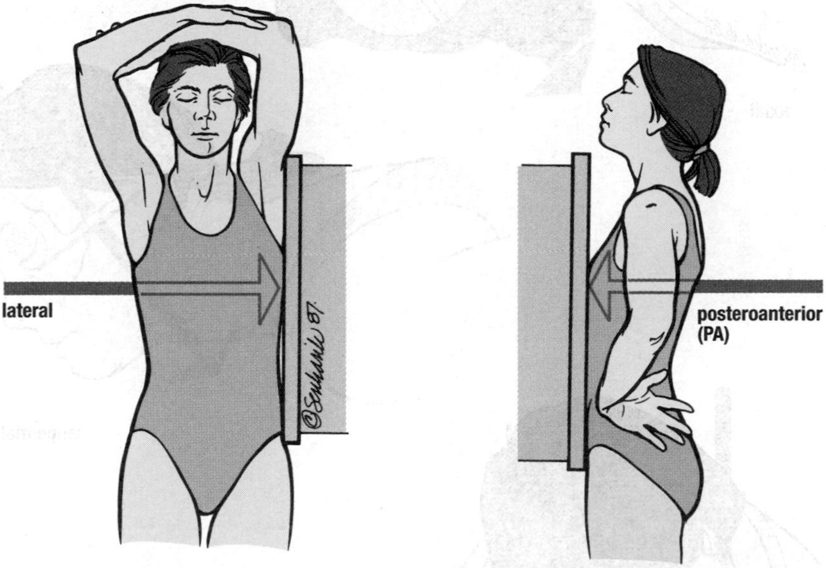

Radiographic Projections

In radiography, the term *projection* describes the path along which the x-rays travel from the radiographic tube through the subject to the image receptor.

Anteroposterior (AP) projection — Patient is either supine (face up) on the radiographic table (dorsal decubitus) or erect with the back against a vertical grid device. The x-ray beam enters the front (anterior) surface of the body and exits the back (posterior) surface.

Posteroanterior (PA) projection — Patient is either prone (face down) on the radiographic table (ventral decubitus) or erect facing a vertical grid device. The x-ray beam enters the back (posterior) surface of the body and exits the front (anterior) surface.

Lateral projection — Patient is lying on either side on the radiographic table (lateral decubitus) or standing with either side against a vertical grid device. The lateral projection is always named by the side of the patient that is placed next to the film.

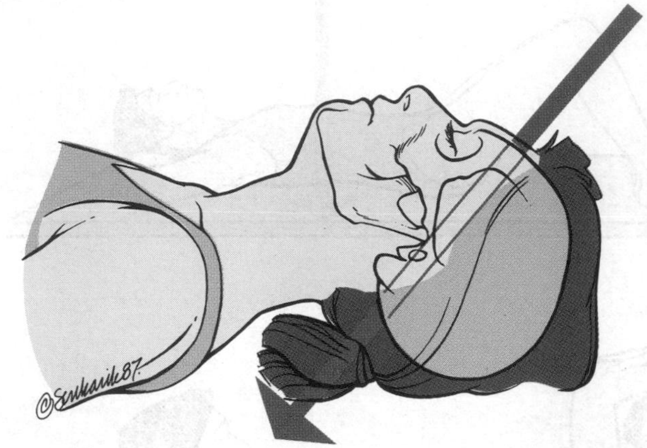

axial

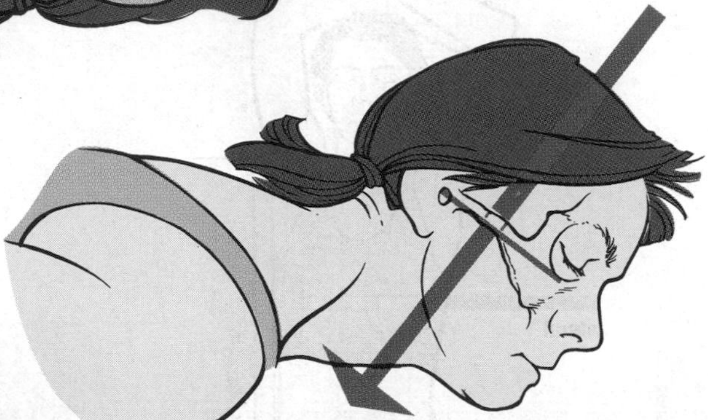

tangential

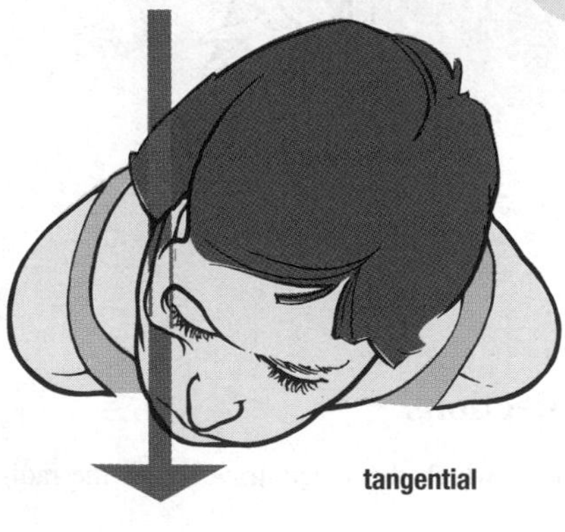

tangential

Oblique projection — Patient is rotated into a position that does not produce either a frontal (AP or PA) or lateral projection.

Axial projection — Any projection in which there is longitudinal angulation of the central ray with respect to the long axis of the body part.

Tangential projection — Any projection in which the central ray passes between or passes by (skims) body parts to project an anatomic structure in profile and free of superimposition.

Adapted from Eisenberg RL, Dennis CA, May CR. Radiographic positioning, 2nd ed. Boston: Little, Brown & Co., 1995.

Anatomy Words (English-Latin)

Arteries

accessory obturator artery	*arteria obturatoria accessoria*
acetabular branch	*arteria acetabuli*
anterior basal segmental artery	*arteria segmentalis basalis anterior pulmonis (dextri et sinistri)*
anterior cecal artery	*arteria cecalis anterior*
anterior cerebral artery	*arteria cerebri anterior*
anterior choroidal artery	*arteria choroidea anterior*
anterior ciliary arteries	*arteriae ciliares anteriores*
anterior circumflex humeral artery	*arteria circumflexa humeri anterior*
anterior communicating artery	*arteria communicans anterior*
anterior conjunctival artery	*arteria conjunctivalis anterior*
anterior ethmoidal artery	*arteria ethmoidalis anterior*
anterior inferior cerebellar artery	*arteria inferior anterior cerebelli*
anterior interosseous artery	*arteria interossea anterior*
anterior labial branches of deep external pudendal artery	*arteriae labiales anteriores*
anterior lateral malleolar artery	*arteria malleolaris anterior lateralis*
anterior medial malleolar artery	*arteria malleolaris anterior medialis*
anterior meningeal branch (of anterior ethmoidal artery)	*arteria meningea anterior*
anterior parietal artery	*arteria parietalis anterior*
anterior perforating arteries	*arteriae perforantes anteriores*
(anterior and posterior) radicular arteries	*arteriae radiculares (anterior et posterior)*
(anterior and posterior) superior pancreaticoduodenal artery	*arteria pancreaticoduodenalis superior (anterior et posterior)*
anterior spinal artery	*arteria spinalis anterior*
anterior superior alveolar arteries	*arteriae alveolares superiores anteriores*
anterior temporal branch	*arteria temporalis anterior*
anterior tibial artery	*arteria tibialis anterior*
anterior tibial recurrent artery	*arteria recurrens tibialis anterior*
anterior tympanic artery	*arteria tympanica anterior*
anterior vestibular artery	*arteria vestibularis anterior*
anterolateral central arteries	*arteriae centrales anterolaterales*
aorta	*arteria aorta*
appendicular artery	*arteria appendicularis*
arcuate arteries of kidney	*arteriae arcuatae renis*
arcuate artery (of foot) (inconstant)	*arteria arcuata (pedis)*
arteries of brain	*arteriae encephali*
arteries of lower limb	*arteriae membri inferioris*
arteries of upper limb	*arteriae membri superioris*
artery of bulb of penis	*arteria bulbi penis*
artery of bulb of vagina	*arteria bulbi vaginae*
artery of bulb of vestibule	*arteria bulbi vestibuli*
artery of caudate lobe	*arteria lobi caudati*
artery of central sulcus	*arteria sulci centralis*

artery of postcentral sulcus	*arteria sulci postcentralis*
artery of precentral sulcus	*arteria sulci precentralis*
artery of pterygoid canal	*arteria canalis pterygoidei*
artery of round ligament of uterus	*arteria ligamenti teretis uteri*
artery of tuber cinereum	*arteria tuberis cinerei*
artery to ductus deferens	*arteria deferentialis*
artery to sciatic nerve	*arteria comitans nervi ischiadici*
artery to tail of pancreas	*arteria caudae pancreatis*
ascending artery	*arteria intermesenterica*
ascending cervical artery	*arteria cervicalis ascendens*
ascending palatine artery	*arteria palatina ascendens*
ascending pharyngeal artery	*arteria pharyngea ascendens*
atrial anastomotic branch of circumflex branch of left coronary artery	*arteria anastomotica auricularis magna*
atrial arteries	*arteriae atriales*
axillary artery	*arteria axillaris*
basilar artery	*arteria basilaris*
brachial artery	*arteria brachialis*
branch to angular gyrus	*arteria angularis*
buccal artery	*arteria buccalis*
calcarine branch of medial occipital artery	*arteria calcarina*
callosomarginal artery	*arteria callosomarginalis*
caroticotympanic arteries (of internal carotid artery)	*arteriae caroticotympanicae (arteriae carotidis internae)*
celiac (arterial) trunk	*arteria celiaca*
central retinal artery	*arteria retinae centralis*
cervicovaginal artery	*arteria cervicovaginalis*
circumflex scapular artery	*arteria circumflexa scapulae*
collicular artery	*arteria collicularis*
common carotid artery	*arteria carotis communis*
common cochlear artery	*arteria cochlearis communis*
common hepatic artery	*arteria hepatica communis*
common iliac artery	*arteria iliaca communis*
common interosseous artery	*arteria interossea communis*
common plantar digital artery	*arteria digitalis plantaris communis*
cortical radiate arteries	*arteriae corticales radiatae*
cremasteric artery	*arteria cremasterica*
cystic artery	*arteria cystica*
deep artery of clitoris	*arteria profunda clitoridis*
deep artery of penis	*arteria profunda penis*
deep artery of thigh	*arteria profunda femoris*
deep auricular artery	*arteria auricularis profunda*
deep cervical artery	*arteria cervicalis profunda*
deep circumflex iliac artery	*arteria circumflexa iliaca profunda*
deep lingual artery	*arteria profunda linguae*
deep plantar artery	*arteria plantaris profundus*
deep temporal artery	*arteria temporalis profunda (anterior et posterior)*
descending genicular artery	*arteria descendens genus*

descending palatine artery	*arteria palatina descendens*
dorsal artery of clitoris	*arteria dorsalis clitoridis*
dorsal artery of penis	*arteria dorsalis penis*
dorsal digital artery	*arteria digitalis dorsalis*
dorsal metacarpal arteries	*arteriae metacarpale dorsale*
dorsal metatarsal arteries	*arteriae metatarsale dorsale*
dorsal nasal artery	*arteria nasi externa*
dorsal pancreatic artery	*arteria pancreatica dorsalis*
dorsal scapular artery	*arteria scapularis dorsalis*
dorsalis pedis artery	*arteria dorsalis pedis*
episcleral artery	*arteria episcleralis*
external carotid artery	*arteria carotis externa*
external iliac artery	*arteria iliaca externa*
facial artery	*arteria facialis*
femoral artery	*arteria femoralis*
femoral nutrient artery	*arteria nutriciae femoris*
fibular artery	*arteria fibularis*
first and second posterior intercostal arteries	*arteriae intercostales posteriores prima et secunda*
gastroduodenal artery	*arteria gastroduodenalis*
gastroepiploic arteries	*arteriae gastroepiploicae*
gastroomental arteries	*arteriae gastroomentales*
great segmental medullary artery	*arteria radicularis magna*
greater palatine artery	*arteria palatina major*
greater pancreatic artery	*arteria pancreatica magna*
helicine arteries of penis	*arteriae helicinae penis*
helicine arteries of the uterus	*arteriae helicinae uteri*
hepatic artery proper	*arteria hepatica propria*
humeral nutrient arteries	*arteriae nutriciae humeri*
hyaloid artery	*arteria hyaloidea*
ileal arteries	*arteriae ileales*
ileocolic artery	*arteria ileocolica*
iliolumbar artery	*arteria iliolumbalis*
inferior alveolar artery	*arteria alveolaris inferior*
inferior epigastric artery	*arteria epigastrica inferior*
inferior gluteal artery	*arteria glutea inferior*
inferior hypophysial artery	*arteria hypophysialis inferior*
inferior labial branch of facial artery	*arteria labialis inferior*
inferior laryngeal artery	*arteria laryngea inferior*
inferior lateral genicular artery	*arteria inferior lateralis genus*
inferior lingular artery	*arteria lingularis inferior*
inferior medial genicular artery	*arteria genus inferior medialis*
inferior mesenteric artery	*arteria mesenterica inferior*
inferior pancreatic artery	*arteria pancreatica inferior*
inferior pancreaticoduodenal artery	*arteria pancreaticoduodenalis inferior*
inferior phrenic artery	*arteria phrenica inferior*
inferior rectal artery	*arteria rectalis inferior*
inferior suprarenal artery	*arteria suprarenalis inferior*
inferior thyroid artery	*arteria thyroidea inferior*

inferior tympanic artery	*arteria tympanica inferior*
inferior ulnar collateral artery	*arteria collateralis ulnaris inferior*
inferior vesical artery	*arteria vesicalis inferior*
infraorbital artery	*arteria infraorbitalis*
insular arteries	*arteriae insulares*
interlobar arteries of kidney	*arteriae interlobares renis*
interlobular arteries of liver	*arteria interlobulares (hepatis)*
internal carotid artery	*arteria carotis interna*
internal iliac artery	*arteria iliaca interna*
internal pudendal artery	*arteria pudenda interna*
internal thoracic artery	*arteria thoracica interna*
intrarenal arteries	*arteriae intrarenales*
jejunal arteries	*arteriae jejunales*
labyrinthine artery	*arteria labyrinthi*
lacrimal artery	*arteria lacrimalis*
(lateral and medial) palpebral arteries	*arteriae palpebrales (laterales et mediales)*
(lateral and medial) parietal arteries	*arteriae parietales (laterales et mediales)*
lateral basal segmental artery	*arteria segmentalis basalis lateralis pulmonis (dextri et sinistri)*
lateral circumflex femoral artery	*arteria circumflexa femoris lateralis*
lateral frontobasal artery	*arteria frontobasalis lateralis*
lateral malleolar branch [of fibular (peroneal) artery]	*arteriae malleolares posteriores laterals*
lateral occipital artery	*arteria occipitalis lateralis*
lateral orbofrontal artery	*arteria orbofrontalis lateralis*
lateral plantar artery	*arteria plantaris lateralis*
lateral sacral arteries	*arteriae sacrales laterales*
lateral tarsal artery	*arteria tarsalis lateralis*
lateral thoracic artery	*arteria thoracica lateralis*
left colic artery	*arteria colica sinistra*
left coronary artery	*arteria coronaria sinistra*
left gastric artery	*arteria gastrica sinistra*
left gastroomental artery	*arteria gastroomentalis sinistra*
left pulmonary artery	*arteria pulmonalis sinistra*
lesser palatine arteries	*arteriae palatinae minores*
lingual artery	*arteria lingualis*
long posterior ciliary arteries	*arteriae ciliares posteriores longae*
lowest lumbar arteries	*arteriae lumbales imae*
lumbar arteries	*arteriae lumbales*
mammillary arteries	*arteriae mammillares*
marginal artery of colon	*arteria marginalis coli*
masseteric artery	*arteria masseterica*
maxillary artery	*arteria maxillaris*
medial basal segmental artery	*arteria segmentalis basalis medialis pulmonis (dextri et sinistri)*
medial circumflex femoral artery	*arteria circumflexa femoris medialis*
medial collateral artery	*arteria collateralis media*
medial frontobasal artery	*arteria frontobasalis medialis*

medial malleolar branches (of posterior tibial artery)	*arteriae malleolares posteriors mediales*
medial occipital artery	*arteria occipitalis medialis*
medial plantar artery	*arteria plantaris medialis*
medial striate artery	*arteria striata medialis distalis*
medial tarsal arteries	*arteria tarsalis medialis*
median artery	*arteria comitans nervi mediani*
median callosal artery	*arteria callosa mediana*
median commissural artery	*arteria commissuralis mediana*
median sacral artery	*arteria sacralis mediana*
mental branch (of inferior alveolar artery)	*arteria mentalis*
metatarsal artery	*arteria metatarsalis*
middle cerebral artery	*arteria cerebri media*
middle colic artery	*arteria colica media*
middle genicular artery	*arteria genus media*
middle meningeal artery	*arteria meningea media*
middle rectal artery	*arteria rectalis media*
middle suprarenal artery	*arteria suprarenalis media*
middle temporal artery	*arteria temporalis media*
muscular arteries (of ophthalmic artery)	*arteriae musculares (arteriae opthalmicae)*
musculophrenic artery	*arteria musculophrenica*
nutrient artery of radius	*arteria radii nutricia*
nutrient artery of ulna	*arteria nutricia ulnae*
nutrient artery	*arteria nutricia*
obturator artery	*arteria obturatoria*
occipital artery	*arteria occipitalis*
ophthalmic artery	*arteria ophthalmica*
ovarian artery	*arteria ovarica*
palmar metacarpal arteries	*arteriae metacarpale palmare*
paracentral branches (of pericallosal artery)	*arteria paracentralis*
parieto-occipital branches of pericallosal artery	*arteriae parieto-occipitales*
perforating arteries (of deep femoral artery)	*arteriae perforantes arteriae*
perforating arteries of penis	*arteriae perforantes penis*
perforating radiate arteries (of kidney)	*arteriae perforantes radiatae (renis)*
pericallosal artery	*arteria pericallosa*
pericardiacophrenic artery	*arteria pericardiacophrenica*
perineal artery	*arteria perinealis*
plantar metatarsal arteries	*arteriae metatarsale plantare*
polar frontal artery	*arteria polaris frontalis*
polar temporal artery	*arteria polaris temporalis*
pontine arteries	*arteriae pontis*
popliteal artery	*arteria poplitea*
posterior auricular artery	*arteria auricularis posterior*
posterior cecal artery	*arteria cecalis posterior*
posterior cerebral artery	*arteria cerebri posterior*
posterior choroidal artery	*arteria choroidea posterior*
posterior circumflex	*arteria circumflexa humerihumeral artery*
posterior communicating artery	*arteria communicans posterior*
posterior conjunctival artery	*arteria conjunctivalis posterior*

posterior ethmoidal artery	*arteria ethmoidalis posterior*
posterior gastric artery	*arteria gastrica posterior*
posterior inferior cerebellar artery	*arteria inferior posterior cerebelli*
posterior intercostal arteries 3–11	*arteriae intercostales posteriores III–XI*
posterior interosseous artery	*arteria interossea posterior*
posterior lateral nasal arteries	*arteriae nasales posteriores laterales*
posterior meningeal artery	*arteria meningea posterior*
posterior parietal artery	*arteria parietalis posterior*
posterior septal branch of nose	*arteria nasalis posterior septi*
posterior spinal artery	*arteria spinalis posterior*
posterior superior alveolar artery	*arteria alveolaris superior posterior*
posterior temporal branch of middle cerebral artery	*arteria temporalis posterior*
posterior tibial artery	*arteria tibialis posterior*
posterior tibial recurrent artery	*arteria recurrens tibialis posterior*
posterior tympanic artery	*arteria tympanica posterior*
posterolateral central arteries	*arteriae centrales posterolaterales*
posteromedial central arteries	*arteriae centrales posteriomediales*
precuneal branches of anterior pericallosal artery	*arteria precunealis*
prepancreatic artery	*arteria prepancreatica*
princeps pollicis artery	*(arteria) princeps pollicis*
profunda brachii artery	*arteria profunda brachii*
proper cochlear artery	*arteria cochlearis propria*
proper palmar digital arteries	*arteriae digitales palmares propriae*
proximal medial striate arteries	*arteria centralis brevis*
pterygomeningeal artery	*arteria pterygomeningealis*
pulmonary trunk	*arteria pulmonalis*
radial artery	*arteria radialis*
radial collateral artery	*arteria collateralis radialis*
radial recurrent artery	*arteria recurrens radialis*
radialis indicis artery	*arteria radialis indicis*
recurrent interosseous artery	*arteria interossea recurrens*
renal artery	*arteria renalis*
retroduodenal artery	*arteria retroduodenalis*
right colic artery	*arteria colica dextra*
right coronary artery	*arteria coronaria dextra*
right flexural artery	*arteria flexurae dextrae*
right gastric artery	*arteria gastrica dextra*
right gastroomental artery	*arteria gastroomentalis dextra*
right pulmonary artery	*arteria pulmonalis dextra*
segmental arteries of kidney	*arteriae renis*
segmental arteries of liver	*arteriae segmenti hepaticae*
segmental medullary arteries	*arteriae medullares segmentales*
short circumferential arteries	*arteriae circumferentiales breves*
short gastric arteries	*arteriae gastricae breves*
short posterior ciliary artery	*arteria ciliaris posterior brevis*
sigmoid arteries	*arteriae sigmoideae*
sphenopalatine artery	*arteria sphenopalatina*
splenic artery	*arteria splenica*

stylomastoid artery	*arteria stylomastoidea*
subclavian artery	*arteria subclavia*
subcostal artery	*arteria subcostalis*
sublingual artery	*arteria sublingualis*
submental artery	*arteria submentalis*
subscapular artery	*arteria subscapularis*
superficial brachial artery	*arteria brachialis superficialis*
superficial cervical artery	*arteria cervicalis superficialis*
superficial circumflex iliac artery	*arteria circumflexa iliaca superficialis*
(superficial and deep) external pudendal arteries	*arteriae pudendae externae (superficiales et profundae)*
superficial epigastric artery	*arteria epigastrica superior*
superficial temporal artery	*arteria temporalis superficialis*
superior cerebellar artery	*arteria superior cerebelli*
superior epigastric artery	*arteria epigastrica superficialis*
superior gluteal artery	*arteria glutea superior*
superior hypophysial artery	*arteria hypophysialis superior*
superior labial branch of facial artery	*arteria labialis superior*
superior laryngeal artery	*arteria laryngea superior*
superior lateral genicular artery	*arteria superior lateralis genus*
superior lingular artery	*arteria lingularis superior*
superior medial genicular artery	*arteria superior medialis genus*
superior mesenteric artery	*arteria mesenterica superior*
superior phrenic arteries	*arteriae phrenicae superiores*
superior rectal artery	*arteria rectalis superior*
superior suprarenal arteries	*arteriae suprarenales superiores*
superior thoracic artery	*arteria thoracica superior*
superior thyroid artery	*arteria thyroidea superior*
superior tympanic artery	*arteria tympanica superior*
superior ulnar collateral artery	*arteria collateralis ulnaris superior*
superior vesical arteries	*arteriae vesicales superiores*
suprachiasmatic artery	*arteria suprachiasmatica*
supraduodenal artery	*arteria supraduodenalis*
supraoptic artery	*arteria supraoptica*
supraorbital artery	*arteria supraorbitalis*
suprascapular artery	*arteria suprascapularis*
supratrochlear artery	*arteria supratrochlearis*
supreme intercostal artery	*arteria intercostalis suprema*
sural arteries	*arteriae surales*
testicular artery	*arteria testicularis*
thoracoacromial artery	*arteria thoracoacromialis*
thoracodorsal artery	*arteria thoracodorsalis*
thyroid ima artery	*arteria thyroidea ima*
tibial nutrient artery	*arteria nutricia tibiae*
transverse cervical artery	*arteria transversa colli*
transverse facial artery	*arteria transversa faciei*
ulnar artery	*arteria ulnaris*
ulnar recurrent artery	*arteria recurrens ulnaris*
umbilical artery	*arteria umbilicalis*

uncal artery	*arteria uncalis*
urethral artery	*arteria urethralis*
uterine artery	*arteria uterina*
vaginal artery	*arteria vaginalis*
ventricular arteries	*arteriae ventriculares*
vertebral artery	*arteria vertebralis*
vestibulocochlear artery	*arteria vestibulocochlearis*
vitelline artery	*arteria vitellina*
zygomatico-orbital artery	*arteria zygomatico-orbitalis*

Bones

atlas	*atlas*
axis	*axis*
basilar bone	*os basilare*
bones of cranium	*ossa cranii*
bones of digits	*ossa digitorum*
bones of foot	*ossa pedis*
bones of lower limb	*ossa membri inferioris*
calcaneus	*os calcis*
capitate	*os capitatum*
carpal bones	*ossa carpi*
clavicle	*clavicula*
coccyx	*os coccygis*
compact bone	*substantia compacta*
cortical bone	*substantia corticalis*
cribriform plate of ethmoid bone	*lamina cribrosa ossis ethmoidalis*
cuboid (bone)	*os cuboideum*
distal phalanx of foot	*phalanx distalis pedis*
distal phalanx of hand	*phalanx distalis manus*
ethmoid (bone)	*os ethmoidale*
facial bones	*ossa faciei*
femur	*femur*
fibula	*fibula*
flat bone	*os planum*
frontal bone	*os frontale*
hamate (bone)	*(os) hamatum*
hip bone	*os coxae*
humerus	*humerus*
hyoid bone	*os hyoideum*
ilium	*os ilium*
incisive bone	*os incisivum*
incus	*incus*
inferior nasal concha	*concha nasalis inferior*
interalveolar septa	*septa interalveolaria mandibulae et maxillae*
intermediate cuneiform (bone)	*os cuneiforme intermedium*
interparietal bone	*os interparietale*
irregular bone	*os irregulare*
ischium	*os ischii*
lacrimal bone	*os lacrimale*

lateral cuneiform (bone)	*os cuneiforme laterale*
long bone	*os longum*
lunate (bone)	*os lunatum*
malleus	*malleus*
mandible	*mandibula*
mastoid process	*processus mastoideus*
maxilla	*maxilla*
medial cuneiform (bone)	*os cuneiforme mediale*
metacarpal (bones) [I–V]	*ossa metacarpi*
metatarsal (bones) [I–V]	*ossa metatarsi*
middle phalanges of foot and hand	*phalanges media pedis et manus*
nasal bone	*os nasale*
navicular (bone)	*os naviculare*
occipital bone	*os occipitale*
palatine bone	*os palatinum*
parietal bone	*os parietale*
patella	*patella*
petrous part of temporal bone	*pars petrosa ossis temporalis*
pisiform (bone)	*os pisiforme*
pneumatized bone	*os pneumaticum*
proximal phalanx of foot	*phalanx proximalis pedis*
proximal phalanx of hand	*phalanx proximalis manus*
pubis	*os pubis*
radius	*radius*
rib	*os costae*
sacrum	*os sacrum*
scaphoid (bone)	*os scaphoideum*
scapula	*scapula*
sesamoid bone	*os sesamoideum*
short bone	*os breve*
sphenoid (bone)	*os sphenoidale*
stapes	*stapes*
sternum	*sternum*
substantia spongiosa	*substantia spongiosa*
suprasternal bones	*ossa suprasternalia*
sutural bones	*os suturarum*
talus	*talus*
temporal bone	*os temporale*
tibia	*tibia*
trapezium (bone)	*os trapezium*
trapezoid bone (wrist)	*os trapezoideum*
triangular bone	*os trigonum*
triquetrum (bone)	*(os) triquetrum*
tympanic ring	*anulus tympanicus*
ulna	*ulna*
vertebrae, cervical	*vertebrae cervicales*
vertebrae, coccygeal	*vertebrae coccygeae*
vertebrae, lumbar	*vertebrae lumbales*
vertebrae, sacral	*vertebrae sacrales*

vertebrae, thoracic (dorsal)	*vertebrae thoracicae*
vesalianum	*os vesalianum*
vomer (bone)	*vomer*
zygomatic bone	*os zygomaticum*

Ligaments

acromioclavicular ligament	*ligamentum acromioclaviculare*
anterior cruciate ligament	*ligamentum cruciatum anterius*
anterior ligament of fibular head	*ligamentum capitis fibulae anterius*
anterior ligament of malleus	*ligamentum mallei anterius*
anterior longitudinal ligament	*ligamentum longitudinal anterius*
anterior meniscofemoral ligament	*ligamentum meniscofemorale anterius*
anterior sacrococcygeal ligament	*ligamentum sacrococcygeum anterius*
anterior sacroiliac ligaments	*ligamenta sacroiliaca anteriora*
anterior sternoclavicular ligament	*ligamentum sternoclaviculare anterius*
anterior talofibular ligament	*ligamentum talofibulare anterius*
anterior tibiofibular	*ligamentum tibiofibulare anterius*
anular ligament of radius	*ligamentum anulare radii*
anular ligament of stapes	*ligamentum anulare stapedis*
anular ligament of trachea	*ligamentum anularia trachealia*
anular ligament	*ligamentum anulare*
apical ligament of dens	*ligamentum apicis dentis*
arcuate popliteal ligament	*ligamentum popliteum arcuatum*
arterial ligament	*ligamentum arteriosum*
auricle ligament	*ligamenta auricularia*
bifurcate ligament	*ligamentum bifurcatum*
broad ligament of the uterus	*ligamentum latum uteri*
calcaneocuboid ligament	*ligamentum calcaneocuboideum*
calcaneofibular ligament	*ligamentum calcaneofibulare*
calcaneonavicular ligament	*ligamentum calcaneonaviculare*
capsular ligament	*ligamentum capsulare*
cardinal ligament	*ligamentum cardinale*
carpometacarpal ligaments (dorsal and palmar)	*ligamentum latum uteri (dorsalia/palmaria)*
ceratocricoid ligament	*ligamentum ceratocricoideum*
collateral ligaments	*ligamentum collaterale*
conoid ligament	*ligamentum conoideum*
coracoacromial ligament	*ligamentum coracoacromiale*
coracoclavicular ligament	*ligamentum coracoclaviculare*
coracohumeral ligament	*ligamentum coracohumerale*
coronary ligament of liver	*ligamentum coronarium hepatis*
costoclavicular ligament	*ligamentum costoclaviculare*
costotransverse ligament	*ligamentum costotransversarium*
costoxiphoid ligaments	*ligamenta costoxiphoidea*
cricoarytenoid ligament	*ligamentum cricoarytenoideum posterius*
cricopharyngeal ligament	*ligamentum cricopharyngeum*
cricotracheal ligament	*ligamentum cricotracheale*
cruciate ligament of the atlas	*ligamentum cruciatum atlantis*
cruciate ligaments of knee	*ligamenta cruciata genus*
cuboideonavicular ligaments	*ligamenta cuboideonavicular*

cuneocuboid interosseous ligament	*ligamentum cuneocuboideum interosseum*
cuneocuboid ligaments	*ligamentum cuneocuboideum*
cuneometatarsal interosseous ligaments	*ligamenta cuneometatarsalia interossea*
deep posterior sacrococcygeal ligament	*ligamentum sacrococcygeum posterius profundum*
deep transversc metatarsal ligament	*ligamentum metatarsale transversum profundum*
deltoid ligament	*ligamentum deltoideum*
denticulate ligament	*ligamentum denticulatum*
dorsal carpometacarpal ligaments	*ligamenta carpometacarpalia dorsalia*
dorsal cuboideonavicular ligament	*ligamentum cuboideonaviculare dorsale*
dorsal cuneocuboid ligament	*ligamentum cuneocuboideum dorsale*
dorsal cuneonavicular ligaments	*ligamenta cuneonavicularia dorsalia*
dorsal metacarpal ligaments	*ligamenta metacarpalia dorsalia*
dorsal metatarsal ligaments	*ligamenta metatarsalia dorsalia*
dorsal radiocarpal ligament	*ligamenta radiocarpale dorsale*
dorsal tarsal ligaments	*ligamenta tarsi dorsalia*
dorsal tarsometatarsal ligaments	*ligamenta tarsometatarsalia dorsalia*
duodenorenal ligament	*ligamentum duodenorenale*
extracapsular ligaments	*ligamenta extracapsularia*
falciform ligament of liver	*ligamentum falciforme hepatis*
fibular collateral ligament	*ligamentum collaterale fibulare*
fundiform ligament of clitoris	*ligamentum fundiforme clitoridis*
fundiform ligament of penis	*ligamenta fundiforme penis*
gastrocolic ligament	*ligamentum gastrocolicum*
gastrophrenic ligament	*ligamentum gastrophrenicum*
gastrosplenic ligament	*ligamentum gastrosplenicum*
genitoinguinal ligament	*ligamentum genitoinguinale*
glenohumeral ligaments	*ligamenta glenohumeralia*
hepatocolic ligament	*ligamentum hepatocolicum*
hepatoduodenal ligament	*ligamentum hepatoduodenale*
hepatoesophageal ligament	*ligamentum hepatoesophageum*
hepatogastric ligament	*ligamentum hepatogastricum*
hepatorenal ligament	*ligamentum hepatorenale*
hyalocapsular ligament	*ligamentum hyaloideocapsular*
hyoepiglottic ligament	*ligamentum hyoepiglotticum*
iliofemoral ligament	*ligamentum iliofemorale*
iliolumbar ligament	*ligamentum iliolumbale*
iliopectineal arch	*ligamentum iliopectinale*
inferior ligament of epididymis	*ligamentum epididymidis inferius*
inferior pubic ligament	*ligamentum pubicum inferius*
inferior transverse scapular ligament	*ligamentum transversum scapulae inferius*
inguinal ligament	*ligamentum inguinale*
intercarpal ligaments	*ligamenta intercarpalia*
interclavicular ligament	*ligamentum interclaviculare*
intercuneiform ligaments	*ligamenta intercuneiformia*
interfoveolar ligament	*ligamentum interfoveolare*
interosseous metacarpal ligaments	*ligamenta metacarpalia interossea*
interosseous sacroiliac ligaments	*ligamenta sacroiliaca interossea*

interspinous ligament	*ligamentum interspinale*
intertransverse ligament	*ligamentum intertransversarium*
intraarticular ligament of head of rib	*ligamentum capitis costae intraarticulare*
intraarticular sternocostal ligament	*ligamentum sternocostale intraarticulare*
intrascapular ligaments	*ligamenta intracapsularia*
ischiofemoral ligament	*ligamentum ischiofemorale*
lacunar ligament	*ligamentum lacunare*
lateral arcuate ligament	*ligamentum arcuatum laterale*
lateral costotransverse ligament	*ligamentum costotransversarium*
lateral ligament of ankle	*ligamentum collaterale laterale*
lateral ligament of bladder	*ligamentum laterale vesicae*
lateral ligament of malleus	*ligamentum mallei laterale*
lateral ligament of temporomandibular joint	*ligamentum laterale articulationis temporomandibularis*
lateral palpebral ligament	*ligamentum palpebrale laterale*
lateral sacrococcygeal ligament	*ligamentum sacrococcygeum laterale*
lateral talocalcaneal ligament	*ligamentum talocalcaneum laterale*
lateral thyrohyoid ligament	*ligamentum thyrohyoideum laterale*
laterial puboprostatic ligament	*ligamentum laterale puboprostaticum*
left triangular ligament of liver	*ligamentum triangulare sinistrum*
lienorenal ligament	*ligamentum lienorenale*
ligament of head of femur	*ligamentum capitis femoris*
ligament of left vena cava	*ligamentum venae cavae sinistrae*
ligament of ovary	*ligamentum ovarii proprium*
ligaments of auditory ossicles	*ligamenta ossiculorum auditorium*
ligaments of epididymis (inferior and superior)	*ligamenta epididymidis (inferius et superius)*
long plantar ligament	*ligamentum plantare longum*
longitudinal ligaments	*ligamenta longitudinalia*
lumbocostal ligament	*ligamentum lumbocostale*
medial arcuate ligament	*ligamentum arcuatum mediale*
medial ligament of ankle joint	*ligamentum collaterale mediale*
medial ligament of temporomandibular joint	*ligamentum mediale articulationis temporomandibularis*
medial palpebral ligament	*ligamentum palpebral mediale*
medial talocalcaneal ligament	*ligamentum talocalcaneum mediale*
median arcuate ligament	*ligamentum arcuatum medianum*
median thyrohyoid ligament	*ligamentum thyrohyoideum medianum*
median umbilical ligament	*ligamentum umbilicale medianum*
meniscofemoral ligaments	*ligamenta meniscofemoralia*
metatarsal interosseous ligaments	*ligamenta metatarsalia interossea*
nuchal ligament	*ligamentum nuchae*
oblique popliteal ligament	*ligamentum popliteum obliquum*
palmar carpometacarpal ligaments	*ligamenta carpometacarpalia palmaria*
palmar ligaments of interphalangeal joints of hand	*ligamenta palmaria articulationis interphalangeae manus*
palmar ligaments of metacarpophalangeal joints	*ligamenta palmaria articulationis metacarpophalangeae*
palmar ligaments	*ligamenta palmaria*
palmar metacarpal ligaments	*ligamenta metacarpalia palmaria*

palmar radiocarpal ligament	*ligamentum radiocarpale palmare*
palmar ulnocarpal ligament	*ligamentum ulnocarpale palmare*
patellar ligament	*ligamentum patellae*
pectineal ligament	*ligamentum pectineum*
phrenicocolic ligament	*ligamentum phrenicocolicum*
phrenicosplenic ligament	*ligamentum phrenicosplenicum*
pisohamate ligament	*ligamentum pisohamatum*
pisometacarpal ligament	*ligamentum pisometacarpale*
plantar calcaneocuboid ligament	*ligamentum calcaneocuboideum plantare*
plantar calcaneonavicular ligament	*ligamentum calcaneonaviculare plantare*
plantar cuboideonavicular ligaments	*ligamenta cuboideonavicularia plantaria*
plantar cuneonavicular ligaments	*ligamenta cuneonavicularia plantaria*
plantar ligaments of interphalangeal joints of foot	*ligamenta plantaria articulationis interphalangeae pedis*
plantar ligaments of metatarsophalangeal joints	*ligamenta plantaria articulationis metatarsophalangeae*
plantar ligaments	*ligamenta plantaria*
plantar metatarsal ligaments	*ligamenta metatarsalia plantaria*
plantar tarsal ligaments	*ligamenta tarsi plantaria*
plantar tarsometatarsal ligaments	*ligamenta tarsometatarsalia plantaria*
posterior cruciate ligament	*ligamentum cruciatum posterius*
posterior ligament of fibular head	*ligamentum capitis fibulae posterius*
posterior ligament of incus	*ligamentum incudis posterius*
posterior longitudinal ligament	*ligamentum longitudinale posterius*
posterior meniscofemoral ligament	*ligamentum meniscofemorale posterius*
posterior sacroiliac ligaments	*ligamenta sacroiliaca posteriora*
posterior sternoclavicular ligament	*ligamentum sternoclaviculare posterius*
posterior talocalcaneal ligament	*ligamentum talocalcaneum posterius*
posterior talofibular ligament	*ligamentum talofibulare posterius*
posterior tibiofibular ligament	*ligamentum tibiofibulare posterius*
pterygospinous ligament	*ligamentum pterygospinale*
pubofemoral ligament	*ligamentum pubofemorale*
puboprostatic ligament	*ligamentum puboprostaticum*
pubovesical ligament (of female)	*ligamentum pubovesicale (feminum)*
pubovesical ligament (of male)	*ligamentum pubovesicale (masculinum)*
pulmonary ligament	*ligamentum pulmonale*
quadrate ligament	*ligamentum quadratum*
radial collateral ligament of elbow joint	*ligamentum collaterale radiale articulationis cubiti*
radial collateral ligament of wrist joint	*ligamentum collaterale carpi radiale articulationis radiocarpalis*
radiate carpal ligament	*ligamentum carpi radiatum*
radiate ligament of head of rib	*ligamentum capitis costae radiatum*
radiate sternocostal ligaments	*ligamenta sternocostalia radiata*
reflected inguinal ligament	*ligamentum reflexum*
right triangular ligament of liver	*ligamentum triangulare dextrum hepatis*
round ligament of liver	*ligamentum teres hepatis*
round ligament of uterus	*ligamentum teres uteri*
sacrodural ligament	*ligamentum sacrodurale*
sacrospinous ligament	*ligamentum sacrospinale*

sacrotuberous ligament	*ligamentum sacrotuberale*
serous ligament	*ligamentum serosum*
sphenomandibular ligament	*ligamentum sphenomandibulare*
spiral ligament of cochlear duct	*ligamentum spirale ductus cochlearis*
splenorenal ligament	*ligamentum splenorenale*
spring ligament	*ligamentum calcaneonaviculare plantare*
sternoclavicular ligaments	*ligamenta sternoclavicularia*
sternopericardial ligaments	*ligamenta sternopericardiaca*
stylohyoid ligament	*ligamentum stylohyoideum*
stylomandibular ligament	*ligamentum stylomandibulare*
superficial posterior sacrococcygeal ligament	*ligamentum sacrococcygeum posterius superficiale*
superficial transverse metacarpal ligament	*ligamentum metacarpale transversum superficiale*
superficial transverse metatarsal ligament	*ligamentum metatarsal transversum superficiale*
superior costotransverse ligament	*ligamentum costotransversarium superius*
superior ligament of epididymis	*ligamentum epididymidis superius*
superior ligament of incus	*ligamentum incudis superius*
superior ligament of malleus	*ligamentum mallei superius*
superior pubic ligament	*ligamentum pubicum superius*
superior transverse scapular ligament	*ligamentum transversum scapulae superius*
supraspinous ligament	*ligamentum supraspinale*
suspensory ligament of axilla	*ligamentum suspensorium axillae*
suspensory ligament of clitoris	*ligamentum suspensorium clitoridis*
suspensory ligament of eyeball	*ligamentum suspensorium bulbi*
suspensory ligament of ovary	*ligamentum suspensorium ovarii*
suspensory ligament of penis	*ligamentum suspensorium penis*
suspensory ligament of thyroid gland	*ligamentum suspensorium glandulae thyroideae*
suspensory ligaments of breast	*ligamenta suspensoria mammaria*
suspensory retinaculum of breast	*retinaculum cutis mammae*
talocalcaneal interosseous ligament	*ligamentum talocalcaneare interosseum*
talonavicular ligament	*ligamentum talonaviculare*
tarsal interosseous ligaments	*ligamenta tarsi interossea*
tarsal ligaments	*ligamenta tarsi*
tarsometatarsal ligaments	*ligamenta tarsometatarsalia*
thyroepiglottic ligament	*ligamentum thyroepiglotticum*
tibial collateral ligament	*ligamentum collaterale tibiale*
transverse acetabular ligament	*ligamentum transversum acetabuli*
transverse cervical ligament	*ligamentum transversale cervicis*
transverse humeral ligament	*ligamentum transversum humeri*
transverse ligament of knee	*ligamentum transversum genus*
transverse ligament of the atlas	*ligamentum transversum atlantis*
transverse perineal ligament	*ligamentum transversum perinei*
trapezoid ligament	*ligamentum trapezoideum*
ulnar collateral ligament of elbow joint	*ligamentum collaterale ulnare articulationis cubiti*
ulnar collateral ligament of wrist joint	*ligamentum collaterale carpi ulnare*
uterovesical ligament	*plica uterovesicalis*

vestibular ligament	*ligamentum vestibulare*
vocal ligament	*ligamentum vocale*

Muscles

abductor digiti minimi (muscle) of foot	*musculus abductor digiti minimi pedis*
abductor digiti minimi (muscle) of hand	*musculus abductor digiti minimi manus*
abductor hallucis (muscle)	*musculus abductor hallucis*
abductor pollicis brevis (muscle)	*musculus abductor pollicis brevis*
abductor pollicis longus (muscle)	*musculus abductor pollicis longus*
adductor brevis (muscle)	*musculus adductor brevis*
adductor longus (muscle)	*musculus adductor longus*
adductor magnus (muscle)	*musculus adductor magnus*
adductor minimus (muscle)	*musculus adductor minimus*
adductor pollicis (muscle)	*musculus adductor pollicis*
anconeus muscle	*musculus anconeus*
anorectoperineal muscles	*musculi rectourethrales*
anterior cervical intertransversarii (muscles)	*musculi intertransversarii anteriores cervicis/colli*
antitragus (muscle)	*musculus antitragicus*
arrector muscle of hair	*musculus arrector pili*
articular muscle	*musculus articularis*
articularis cubiti (muscle)	*musculus articularis cubiti*
articularis genus (muscle)	*musculus articularis genus*
auricularis anterior (muscle)	*musculus auricularis anterior*
auricularis posterior (muscle)	*musculus auricularis posterior*
auricularis superior (muscle)	*musculus auricularis superior*
biceps brachii (muscle)	*musculus biceps brachii*
biceps femoris (muscle)	*musculus biceps femoris*
Bochdalek muscle	*musculus triticeoglossus*
brachialis (muscle)	*musculus brachialis*
brachioradialis (muscle)	*musculus brachioradialis*
bronchoesophageus (muscle)	*musculus bronchoesophageus*
buccinator (muscle)	*musculus buccinator*
bulbospongiosus (muscle)	*musculus bulbospongiosus*
ceratocricoid (muscle)	*musculus ceratocricoideus*
chondroglossus muscle	*musculus chondroglossus*
ciliary muscle	*musculus ciliaris*
coccygeus muscle	*musculus coccygeus*
coracobrachialis muscle	*musculus coracobrachialis*
corrugator cutis muscle of anus	*musculus corrugator cutis ani*
corrugator supercilii (muscle)	*musculus corrugator supercilii*
cremaster muscle	*musculus cremaster*
cricopharyngeus muscle	*musculus cricopharyngeus*
cricothyroid muscle	*musculus cricothyroideus*
cruciate muscle	*musculus cruciatus*
cutaneous muscle	*musculus cutaneus*
dartos muscle	*musculus dartos*
deep transverse perineal muscle	*musculus transversus perinei profundus*
deltoid (muscle)	*musculus deltoideus*
depressor anguli oris (muscle)	*musculus depressor anguli oris*

depressor labii inferioris (muscle)	*musculus depressor labii inferioris*
depressor septi nasi	*musculus depressor septi nasi*
depressor supercilii (muscle)	*musculus depressor supercilii*
detrusor (muscle)	*musculus detrusor vesicae*
diaphragm	*musculus diaphragma*
digastric (muscle)	*musculus biventer*
dilator (muscle) of ileocecal sphincter	*musculus dilatator pylori ilealis*
dilator (muscle) of pylorus	*musculus dilatator pylori gastroduodenalis*
dilator muscle	*musculus dilatator*
dilator pupillae muscle	*musculus dilatator pupillae*
dorsal interossei (interosseous muscles) of hand	*musculi interossei dorsale manus*
dorsal interossei (interosseus muscles) of foot	*musculi interossei dorsale pedis*
dorsal sacrococcygeal muscle	*musculus sacrococcygeus dorsalis*
epicranius (muscle)	*musculus epicranius*
erector spinae (muscles)	*musculus erector spinae*
extensor carpi radialis brevis (muscle)	*musculus extensor carpi radialis brevis*
extensor carpi radialis longus (muscle)	*musculus extensor carpi radialis longus*
extensor carpi ulnaris (muscle)	*musculus extensor carpi ulnaris*
extensor digiti minimi (muscle)	*musculus extensor digiti minimi*
extensor digitorum brevis (muscle) of hand	*musculus extensor digitorum brevis manus*
extensor digitorum brevis (muscle)	*musculus extensor digitorum brevis*
extensor digitorum longus (muscle)	*musculus extensor digitorum longus*
extensor digitorum muscle	*musculus extensor digitorum*
extensor hallucis brevis (muscle)	*musculus extensor hallucis brevis*
extensor hallucis longus (muscle)	*musculus extensor hallucis longus*
extensor indicis (muscle)	*musculus extensor indicis*
extensor pollicis brevis (muscle)	*musculus extensor pollicis brevis*
extensor pollicis longus (muscle)	*musculus extensor pollicis longus*
external intercostal (muscle)	*musculus intercostales externi*
external oblique (muscle)	*musculus obliquus externus abdominis*
extraocular muscles	*musculi externi bulbi oculi*
facial muscles	*musculi faciei*
fibularis brevis (muscle)	*musculus fibularis brevis*
fibularis longus (muscle)	*musculus fibularis longus*
fibularis tertius (muscle)	*musculus fibularis tertius*
flexor accessorius (muscle)	*musculus flexor accessories*
flexor carpi radialis (muscle)	*musculus flexor carpi radialis*
flexor carpi ulnaris (muscle)	*musculus flexor carpi ulnaris*
flexor digiti minimi brevis (muscle) of foot	*musculus flexor digiti minimi brevis pedis*
flexor digiti minimi brevis (muscle) of hand	*musculus flexor digiti minimi brevis manus*
flexor digitorum brevis (muscle)	*musculus flexor digitorum brevis*
flexor digitorum longus (muscle)	*musculus flexor digitorum longus*
flexor digitorum profundus (muscle)	*musculus flexor digitorum profundus*
flexor digitorum superficialis (muscle)	*musculus flexor digitorum superficialis*
flexor hallucis brevis (muscle)	*musculus flexor hallucis brevis*
flexor hallucis longus (muscle)	*musculus flexor hallucis longus*
flexor pollicis brevis (muscle)	*musculus flexor pollicis brevis*
flexor pollicis longus (muscle)	*musculus flexor pollicis longus*

fusiform muscle	*musculus fusiformis*
gastrocnemius muscle	*musculus gastrocnemius*
genioglossus (muscle)	*musculus genioglossus*
geniohyoid muscle	*musculus geniohyoideus*
gluteal medius (muscle)	*musculus gluteus medius*
gluteus minimus (muscle)	*musculus gluteus minimus*
gluteus maximus (muscle)	*musculus gluteus maximus*
gracilis muscle	*musculus gracilis*
helices minor (muscle)	*musculus helicis minor*
Houston muscle	*compressor venae dorsalis penis*
hyoglossus (muscle)	*musculus hyoglossus*
iliacus minor (muscle)	*musculus iliacus minor*
iliacus muscle	*musculus iliacus*
iliococcygeus (muscle)	*musculus iliococcygeus*
iliocostalis cervicis (muscle)	*musculus iliocostalis cervicis/colli*
iliocostalis lumborum (muscle)	*musculus saccrolumbalis*
iliocostis (muscle)	*musculus iliocostalis*
iliopsoas (muscle)	*musculus iliopsoas*
inferior constrictor (muscle) of pharynx	*musculus constrictor pharyngis inferior*
inferior gemellus (muscle)	*musculus gemellus inferior*
inferior longitudinal muscle of tongue	*musculus longitudinalis inferior linguae*
inferior oblique (muscle)	*musculus obliquus inferior (bulbi)*
inferior rectus (muscle)	*musculus rectus inferior*
inferior tarsal muscle	*musculus tarsalis inferior*
infrahyoid muscles	*musculi infrahyoidei*
infraspinatus (muscle)	*musculus infraspinatus*
innermost intercostal (muscle)	*musculus intercostalis intimus*
internal intercostal (muscle)	*musculus intercostalis internus*
internal oblique (muscle)	*musculus obliquus internus abdominis*
interosseous muscles	*musculi interossei*
interspinales (muscles)	*musculi interspinales*
interspinales cervicis (muscles)	*musculus interspinalis cervicis/colli*
interspinalis lumborum (muscles)	*musculus interspinalis lumborum*
interspinalis thoracis (muscles)	*musculus interspinalis thoracis*
intertransversarii (muscles)	*musculi intertransversarii*
ischiocavernosus (muscle)	*musculus ischiocavernosus*
lateral cricoarytenoid (muscle)	*musculus cricoarytenoideus lateralis*
lateral lumbar intertransversarii (muscles)	*musculi intertransversarii laterales lumborum*
lateral pterygoid muscle	*musculus pterygoideus lateralis*
lateral rectus (muscle)	*musculus rectus lateralis*
latissimus dorsi (muscle)	*musculus latissimus dorsi*
levator anguli oris (muscle)	*musculus levator anguli oris*
levator ani (muscle)	*musculus levator ani*
levator labii superioris (muscle)	*musculus levator labii superioris*
levator labii superioris alaeque nasi (muscle)	*musculus levator labii superioris alaeque nasi*
levator palpebrae superioris (muscle)	*musculus levator palpebrae superioris*
levator scapulae (muscle)	*musculus levator scapulae*
levator veli palatini (muscle)	*musculus levator veli palatini*
levatores costarum (muscles)	*musculi levatores costarum*

longissimus capitis (muscle)	*musculus longissimus capitis*
longissimus cervicis (muscle)	*musculus longissimus cervicis*
longissimus muscle	*musculus longissimus*
longissimus thoracis (muscle)	*musculus longissimus thoracis*
longus capitis (muscle)	*musculus longus capitis*
longus colli (muscle)	*musculus longus colli*
lumbricals (lumbrical muscles) of foot	*musculi lumbricales pedis*
lumbricals (lumbrical muscles) of hand	*musculi lumbricales manus*
masseter (muscle)	*musculus masseter*
medial lumbar intertransversarii (muscles)	*musculi intertransversarii mediales lumborum*
medial pterygoid (muscle)	*musculus pterygoideus mediales*
medial rectus (muscle)	*musculus rectus medialis (bulbi)*
mentalis (muscle)	*musculus mentalis*
middle constrictor (muscle) of pharynx	*musculus constrictor pharyngis medius*
multifidus (muscle)	*musculus multifidus*
multipennate muscle	*musculus multipennatus*
muscle of terminal notch	*musculus incisurae helicis*
muscle of uvula	*musculus uvulae*
muscles of abdomen	*musculi abdominis*
muscles of auditory ossicles	*musculi ossiculorum auditorium*
muscles of back proper	*musculi dorsi proprii*
muscles of back	*musculi dorsi*
muscles of head	*musculi capitis*
muscles of larynx	*musculi laryngis*
muscles of neck	*musculi colli*
muscles of soft palate and fauces	*musculi palati mollis et faucium*
muscles of thorax	*musculi thoracis*
muscles of tongue	*musculi linguae*
muscles of urogenital triangle	*musculi regionis urogenitalis*
mylohyoid (muscle)	*musculus mylohyoideus*
nasalis (muscle)	*musculus nasalis*
oblique arytenoid muscle	*musculus arytenoideus obliquus*
oblique capitis inferior (muscle)	*musculus obliquus capitis inferior*
oblique capitis superior (muscle)	*musculus obliquus capitis superior*
oblique muscle of auricle	*musculus obliquus auriculae*
obturator externus (muscle)	*musculus obturator externus*
obturator internus (muscle)	*musculus obturator internus*
occipitofrontalis (muscle)	*musculus occipitofrontalis*
omohyoid (muscle)	*musculus omohyoideus*
opponens digiti minimi (muscle)	*musculus opponens digiti minimi*
opponens pollicis (muscle)	*musculus opponens pollicis*
orbicular muscle	*musculus orbicularis*
orbicularis oculi (muscle)	*musculus orbicularis oculi*
orbicularis oris (muscle)	*musculus orbicularis oris*
orbitalis (muscle)	*musculus orbitalis*
palatoglossus (muscle)	*musculus palatoglossus*
palatopharyngeus (muscle)	*musculus palatopharyngeus*
palmar interossei (interosseous muscles)	*musculus interosseus palmaris*

palmaris longus (muscle)	*musculus palmaris longus*
papillary muscle	*musculus papillaris cordis*
pectinate muscles	*musculi pectinati atrii*
pectineus (muscle)	*musculus pectineus*
pectoralis major (muscle)	*musculus pectoralis major*
pectoralis minor (muscle)	*musculus pectoralis minor*
pennate muscle	*musculus bipennatus*
perineal muscles	*musculi perinei*
peroneus brevis (muscle)	*musculus peroneus brevis*
peroneus longus (muscle)	*musculus peroneus longus*
peroneus tertius (muscle)	*musculus peroneus tertius*
piriformis (muscle)	*musculus piriformis*
plantar interossei (interosseous muscles)	*musculus interosseus plantaris*
plantaris (muscle)	*musculus plantaris*
platysma (muscle)	*musculus platysma yoides*
pleuroesophageus (muscle)	*musculus pleuroesophageus*
popliteus (muscle)	*musculus popliteus*
posterior cervical intertransversarii (muscles)	*musculi intertransversarii posteriores (laterales et mediales) cervicis*
posterior cricoarytenoid (muscle)	*musculus cricoarytenoideus posterior*
procerus (muscle)	*musculus procerus*
pronator quadratus (muscle)	*musculus pronator quadratus*
pronator teres (muscle)	*musculus pronator teres*
psoas major (muscle)	*musculus psoas major*
psoas minor (muscle)	*musculus psoas minor*
pubococcygeus (muscle)	*musculus pubococcygeus*
puboprostaticus (muscle)	*musculus puboprostaticus*
puborectalis (muscle)	*musculus puborectalis*
pubovaginalis (muscle)	*musculus pubovaginalis*
pubovesicalis (muscle)	*musculus pubovesicalis*
pyramidal muscle of auricle	*musculus pyramidalis auriculae*
quadrate muscle of upper lip	*musculus quadratus labii superioris*
quadrate muscle	*musculus quadratus*
quadratus femoris (muscle)	*musculus quadratus femoris*
quadratus lumborum (muscle)	*musculus quadratus lumborum*
quadratus plantae (muscle)	*musculus quadratus plantae*
rectococcygeus (muscle)	*musculus rectococcygeus*
rectouterinus (muscle)	*musculus rectouterinus*
rectovesicalis (muscle)	*musculus rectovesicalis*
rectus abdominis (muscle)	*musculus rectus abdominis*
rectus capitis anterior (muscle)	*musculus rectus capitis anterior*
rectus capitis lateralis (muscle)	*musculus rectus capitis lateralis*
rectus capitis posterior major (muscle)	*musculus rectus capitis posterior major*
rectus capitis posterior minor (muscle)	*musculus rectus capitis posterior minor*
rectus femoris (muscle)	*musculus rectus femoris*
rhomboid major (muscle)	*musculus rhomboideus major*
rhomboid minor (muscle)	*musculus rhomboideus minor*
risorius (muscle)	*musculus risorius*
rotatores (muscles)	*musculi rotatores*

rotatores cervicis (muscles)	*musculi rotatores cervicis/colli*
rotatores lumborum (muscles)	*musculi rotatores lumborum*
rotatores thoracis (muscles)	*musculi rotatores thoracis*
salpingopharyngeus (muscle)	*musculus salpingopharyngeus*
sartorius (muscle)	*musculus sartorius*
scalenus anterior (muscle)	*musculus scalenus anterior*
scalenus medius (muscle)	*musculus scalenus medius*
scalenus minimus (muscle)	*musculus scalenus minimus*
scalenus posterior (muscle)	*musculus scalenus posterior*
second tibial muscle	*musculus tibialis secundus*
semimembranous (muscle)	*musculus semimembranosus*
semipennate muscle	*musculus semipennatus*
semispinalis (muscle)	*musculus semispinalis*
semispinalis capitis (muscle)	*musculus semispinalis capitis*
semispinalis cervicis (muscle)	*musculus semispinalis cervicis*
semispinalis thoracis (muscle)	*musculus semispinalis thoracis*
semitendinosus (muscle)	*musculus semitendinosus*
serratus anterior (muscle)	*musculus serratus anterior*
serratus posterior inferior (muscle)	*musculus serratus posterior inferior*
serratus posterior superior (muscle)	*musculus serratus posterior superior*
skeletal muscle	*musculus skeleti*
soleus (muscle)	*musculus soleus*
spinalis (muscle)	*musculus spinalis*
spinalis capitis (muscle)	*musculus spinalis capitis*
spinalis cervicis (muscle)	*musculus spinalis cervicis*
spinalis thoracis	*musculus spinalis thoracis*
splenius capitis (muscle)	*musculus splenius capitis*
splenius cervicis (muscle)	*musculus splenius cervicis*
stapedius (muscle)	*musculus stapedius*
sternalis (muscle)	*musculus sternalis*
sternochondroscapular muscle	*musculus sternochondroscapularis*
sternoclavicular muscle	*musculus sternoclavicularis*
sternocleidomastoid (muscle)	*musculus sternocleidomastoideus*
sternohyoid (muscle)	*musculus sternohyoideus*
sternothyroid (muscle)	*musculus sternothyroideus*
styloauricular (muscle)	*musculus styloauricularis*
styloglossus (muscle)	*musculus styloglossus*
stylohyoid (muscle)	*musculus stylohyoideus*
stylopharyngeus (muscle)	*musculus stylopharyngeus*
subclavius (muscle)	*musculus subclavius*
subcostal muscle	*musculus subcostalis*
suboccipital muscles	*musculi suboccipitales*
subscapularis (muscle)	*musculus subscapularis*
superficial transverse perineal muscle	*musculus transversus perinei superficialis*
superior gemellus (muscle)	*musculus gemellus superior*
superior longitudinal muscle of tongue	*musculus longitudinalis superior linguae*
superior oblique (muscle)	*musculus obliquus superior (bulbi)*
superior pharyngeal constrictor (muscle)	*musculus constrictor pharyngis superior*
superior rectus (muscle)	*musculus rectus superior (bulbi)*

superior tarsal muscle	*musculus tarsalis superior*
supinator (muscle)	*musculus supinator*
supraclavicular muscle	*musculus supraclavicularis*
suprahyoid muscles	*musculi suprahyoidei*
supraspinalis (muscle)	*musculus supraspinalis*
supraspinatus (muscle)	*musculus supraspinatus*
suspensory muscle of duodenum	*musculus suspensorius duodeni*
temporalis (muscle)	*musculus temporalis*
temporoparietalis (muscle)	*musculus temporoparietalis*
tensor fasciae latae (muscle)	*musculus tensor fasciae latae*
tensor tympani (muscle)	*musculus tensor tympani*
tensor veli palati (muscle)	*musculus tensor veli palatini*
Teres major (muscle)	*musculus teres major*
Teres minor (muscle)	*musculus teres minor*
thoracic intertransversarii (muscles)	*musculi intertransversarii thoracis*
thyroarytenoid (muscle)	*musculus thyroarytenoideus (externus)*
thyrohyoid muscle	*musculus thyrohyoideus*
tibialis anterior (muscle)	*musculus tibialis anterior*
tibialis posterior (muscle)	*musculus tibialis posterior*
trachealis (muscle)	*musculus trachealis*
tracheloclavicular muscle	*musculus tracheloclavicularis*
tragicus (muscle)	*musculus tragicus*
transverse arytenoid (muscle)	*musculus arytenoideus transversus*
transverse muscle of auricle	*musculus transversus auriculae*
transverse muscle of tongue	*musculus transversus linguae*
transversospinales (muscles)	*musculi transversospinales*
transversus abdominis (muscle)	*musculus transversus abdominis*
transversus menti (muscle)	*musculus transversus menti*
transversus nuchae (muscle)	*musculus transversus nuchae*
transversus thoracis (muscle)	*musculus transversus thoracis*
trapezius (muscle)	*musculus trapezius*
triangular muscle	*musculus triangularis*
triceps brachii (muscle)	*musculus triceps brachii*
triceps coxae (muscle)	*musculus triceps coxae*
triceps surae (muscle)	*musculus triceps surae*
trigonal muscles (superficial and deep)	*musculi trigoni vesicae (superficialis et profunda)*
vastus intermedius (muscle)	*musculus vastus intermedius*
vastus lateralis (muscle)	*musculus vastus lateralis*
vastus medialis (muscle)	*musculus vastus medialis*
ventral sacrococcygeus (muscle)	*musculus sacrococcygeus ventralis*
vertical muscle of tongue	*musculus verticalis linguae*
vocalis (muscle)	*musculus vocalis*
zygomaticus major (muscle)	*musculus zygomaticus major*
zygomaticus minor (muscle)	*musculus zygomaticus minor*

Nerves

abducent nerve (CN VI)	*nervus abducens*
accessory nerve (CN XI)	*nervus accessorius*
accessory phrenic nerves	*nervi phrenici accessorii*
anococcygeal nerve	*nervus anococcygeus*
anterior ampullary nerve	*nervus ampullaris anterior*
anterior auricular nerves	*nervi auriculares anteriores*
anterior ethmoidal nerve	*nervus ethmoidalis anterior*
anterior interosseous nerve	*nervus interosseous antibrachii anterior*
anterior labial nerves	*nervi labiales anteriores*
anterior scrotal nerves	*nervi scrotales anteriores*
articular nerve	*nervus articularis*
auricular nerve of vagus nerve	*ramus auricularis nervi vagi*
auriculotemporal nerve	*nervus auriculotemporalis*
autonomic nerve	*nervus autonomicus*
axillary nerve	*nervus axillaris*
buccal nerve	*nervus buccalis*
caroticotympanic nerves	*nervi caroticotympanici*
cavernous nerves of clitoris	*nervi cavernosi clitoridis*
cavernous nerves of penis	*nervi cavernosi penis*
cervical nerves	*nervi cervicales*
coccygeal nerve	*nervus coccygeus*
cochlear nerve	*nervus cochlearis*
common fibular nerve	*nervus fibularis communis*
common palmar digital nerves	*nervi digitales palmares communes*
common plantar digital nerves	*nervi digitales plantares communes*
cranial nerves	*nervi craniales*
crural interosseous nerve	*nervus interosseus cruris*
cutaneous nerve	*nervus cutaneus*
deep fibular nerve	*nervus fibularis profundus*
deep temporal nerves	*nervi temporales profundi*
dorsal digital nerves of foot	*nervi digitales dorsales pedis*
dorsal digital nerves of hand	*nervi digitales dorsalis manus*
dorsal nerve of clitoris	*nervus dorsalis clitoridis*
dorsal nerve of penis	*nervus dorsalis penis*
dorsal scapular nerve	*nervus dorsalis scapulae*
external carotid nerves	*nervi carotici externi*
facial nerve (CN VII)	*nervus facialis*
femoral nerve	*nervus femoralis*
fourth lumbar nerve (L4)	*nervus furcalis*
frontal nerve	*nervus frontalis*
genitofemoral nerve	*nervus genitofemoralis*
glossopharyngeal nerve (CN IX)	*nervus glossopharyngeus*
great auricular nerve	*nervus auricularis magnus*
greater occipital nerve	*nervus occipitalis major*
greater palatine nerve	*nervus palatinus major*
greater petrosal nerve	*nervus petrosus major*
greater splanchnic nerve	*nervus splanchnicus major*
hypogastric nerve	*nervus hypogastricus*

hypoglossal nerve (CN XII)	*nervus hypoglossus*
iliohypogastric nerve	*nervus iliohypogastricus*
ilioinguinal nerve	*nervus ilioinguinalis*
inferior alveolar nerve	*nervus alveolaris inferior*
inferior ampullary nerve	*nervus ampullaris inferior*
inferior anal nerves	*nervi rectales inferiores*
inferior cervical cardiac nerve	*nervus cardiacus cervicalis inferior*
inferior cluneal nerves	*nervi clunium inferiores*
inferior gluteal nerve	*nervus gluteus inferior*
inferior laryngeal nerve	*nervus laryngeus inferior*
inferior lateral cutaneous nerve of arm	*nervus cutaneus brachii lateralis inferior*
infraorbital nerve	*nervus infraorbitalis*
infratrochlear nerve	*nervus infratrochlearis*
intercostal nerves	*nervi intercostales*
intercostobrachial nerves	*nervi intercostobrachiales*
intermediate dorsal cutaneous nerve	*nervus cutaneus dorsalis intermedius*
intermediate nerve	*nervus intermedius*
jugular nerve	*nervus jugularis*
lacrimal nerve	*nervus lacrimalis*
lateral ampullary nerve	*nervus ampullaris lateralis*
lateral cutaneous nerve forearm	*nervus cutaneus antebrachii of lateralis*
lateral cutaneous nerve of thigh	*nervus cutaneus femoris laterales*
lateral dorsal cutaneous nerve	*nervus cutaneus dorsalis lateralis*
lateral pectoral nerve	*nervus pectoralis lateralis*
lateral plantar nerve	*nervus plantaris lateralis*
lateral supraclavicular nerve	*nervus supraclavicularis lateralis*
lateral sural cutaneous nerve	*nervus cutaneus surae lateralis*
least splanchnic nerve	*nervus splanchnicus imus*
lesser occipital nerve	*nervus occipitalis minor*
lesser palatine nerves	*nervi palatini minores*
lesser petrosal nerve	*nervus petrosus minor*
lesser splanchnic nerve	*nervus splanchnicus minor*
lingual nerve	*nervus lingualis*
long ciliary nerve	*nervus ciliaris longus*
long thoracic nerve	*nervus thoracicus longus*
lumbar nerves	*nervi lumbales*
lumbar splanchnic nerves	*nervi splanchnici lumbales*
mandibular nerve (CN V3)	*nervus mandibularis*
masseteric nerve	*nervus massetericus*
maxillary nerve (CN V2)	*nervus maxillaris*
medial cutaneous nerve of arm	*nervus cutaneus antebrachii medialis*
medial cutaneous nerve of forearm	*nervus cutaneus antebrachii medialis*
medial cutaneous nerve of leg	*rami cutanei cruris mediales nervi sapheni*
medial dorsal cutaneous nerve	*nervus cutaneus dorsalis medialis*
medial pectoral nerve	*nervus pectoralis medialis*
medial plantar nerve	*nervus plantaris medialis*
medial supraclavicular nerve	*nervus supraclavicularis medialis*
medial sural cutaneous nerve	*nervus cutaneus surae medialis*
median nerve	*nervus medianus*

mental nerve	*nervus mentalis*
middle cervical cardiac nerve	*nervus cardiacus cervicalis medius*
middle cluneal nerves	*nervi clunium medii*
mixed nerve	*nervus mixtus*
motor nerve	*nervus motorius*
musculocutaneous nerve	*nervus musculocutaneus*
nasociliary nerve	*nervus nasociliaris*
nasopalatine nerve	*nervus nasopalatinus*
nerve of pterygoid canal	*nervus canalis pterygoidei*
nerve to external acoustic meatus	*nervus meatus acustici externi*
nerve to mylohyoid	*nervus mylohyoideus*
nerve to quadratus femoris	*nervus musculi quadrati femoris*
nerve to stapedius muscle	*nervus stapedius*
nerve to tensor tympani muscle	*nervus musculi tensoris tympani*
nerve to tensor veli palatini muscle	*nervus musculi tensoris veli palatini*
obturator nerve	*nervus obturatorius*
oculomotor nerve (CN II)	*nervus oculomotorius*
olfactory nerves (CN I)	*nervi olfactorii*
ophthalmic nerve	*nervus ophthalmicus*
optic nerve (CN II)	*nervus opticus*
pelvic splanchnic nerves	*nervi splanchnici pelvici*
perforating cutaneous nerve	*nervus cutaneus perforans*
perineal nerves	*nervi perineales*
phrenic nerve	*nervus phrenicus*
posterior ampullary nerve	*nervus ampullaris posterior*
posterior auricular nerve	*nervus auricularis posterior*
posterior cutaneous nerve of arm	*nervus cutaneus brachii posterior*
posterior cutaneous nerve of forearm	*nervus cutaneus antebrachii posterior*
posterior cutaneous nerve of thigh	*nervus cutaneus femoris posterior*
posterior ethmoidal nerve	*nervus ethmoidalis posterior*
posterior interosseous nerve	*nervus interosseus posterior*
posterior labial nerves	*nervi labiales posteriores*
posterior scrotal nerves	*nervi scrotales posteriores*
proper palmar digital nerves	*nervi digitales palmares proprii*
proper plantar digital nerves	*nervi digitales plantares proprii*
pterygoid nerve	*nervus pterygoideus*
pudendal nerve	*nervus pudendus*
radial nerve	*nervus radialis*
recurrent laryngeal nerve	*nervus laryngeus recurrens*
saccular nerve	*nervus saccularis*
sacral nerve	*nervus sacralis*
sacral splanchnic nerves	*nervi splanchnici sacrales*
saphenous nerve	*nervus saphenus*
sciatic nerve	*nervus ischiadicus*
sensory nerve	*nervus sensorius*
sensory root of pterygopalatine canal	*nervi pterygopalatini*
short ciliary nerve	*nervus ciliaris brevis*
spinal nerve	*nervus spinalis*
splanchnic nerve	*nervus splanchnicus*

subclavian nerve	*nervus subclavius*
subcostal nerve	*nervus subcostalis*
sublingual nerve	*nervus sublingualis*
suboccipital nerve	*nervus suboccipitalis*
subscapular nerves	*nervi subscapulares*
superficial fibular nerve	*nervus fibularis superficialis*
superior alveolar nerves	*nervi alveolares superiores*
superior cervical cardiac nerve	*nervus cardiacus cervicalis superior*
superior cluneal nerves	*nervi clunium superiores*
superior gluteal nerve	*nervus gluteus superior*
superior laryngeal nerve	*nervus laryngeus superior*
supraorbital nerve	*nervus supraorbitalis*
suprascapular nerve	*nervus suprascapularis*
supratrochlear nerve	*nervus supratrochlearis*
sural nerve	*nervus suralis*
tentorial nerve	*ramus meningeus recurrens tentorii nervi ophthalmici*
terminal nerve	*nervus terminalis*
third occipital nerve	*nervus occipitalis tertius*
thoracic cardiac nerves	*nervi cardiaci thoracici*
thoracic nerves (T1–T12)	*nervi thoracici*
thoracodorsal nerve	*nervus thoracodorsalis*
tibial nerve	*nervus tibialis*
transverse cervical nerve	*nervus transversus colli*
trigeminal nerve (CN V)	*nervus trigeminus*
trochlear nerve (CN IV)	*nervus trochlearis*
tympanic nerve	*nervus tympanicus*
ulnar nerve	*nervus ulnaris*
upper lateral cutaneous nerve of arm	*nervus cutaneus brachii lateralis superior*
utricular nerve	*nervus utricularis*
utriculoampullar nerve	*nervus utriculoampullaris*
vaginal nerves	*nervi vaginales*
vagus nerve (CN X)	*nervus vagus*
vascular nerves	*nervus vasorum*
vertebral nerve	*nervus vertebralis*
vestibular nerve	*nervus vestibularis*
vestibulochoclear nerve (CN VIII)	*nervus vestibulocochlearis*
zygomatic nerve	*nervus zygomaticus*

Veins

(anterior and posterior) vestibular veins	*venae vestibulares (anterius et posterius)*
(left and right) brachiocephalic veins	*venae brachiocephalicae (dextrae et sinistrae)*
accessory cephalic vein	*vena cephalica accessoria*
accessory hemiazygos vein	*vena hemiazygos accessoria*
accessory saphenous vein	*vena saphena accessoria*
accessory vertebral vein	*vena vertebralis accessoria*
accompanying vein	*vena comitans*
angular vein	*vena angularis*
anterior auricular vein	*vena auricularis anterior*

anterior basal vein	*vena basalis anterior*
anterior cardiac veins	*venae cardiacae anteriores*
anterior cerebral veins	*venae anteriores cerebri*
anterior ciliary veins	*venae ciliares anteriores*
anterior circumflex vein	*vena circumflexa humeri anterior*
anterior intercostal veins	*venae intercostales anteriores*
anterior jugular vein	*vena jugularis anterior*
anterior labial veins	*venae labiales anteriores*
anterior pontomesencephalic vein	*vena pontomesencephalica anterior*
anterior scrotal veins	*venae scrotales anteriores*
anterior tibial veins	*venae tibiales anteriores*
anterior vein of septum pellucidum	*vena anterior septi pellucidi*
anterior vertebral vein	*vena vertebralis anterior*
apical vein	*vena apicalis*
apicoposterior vein	*vena apicoposterior*
appendicular vein	*vena appendicularis*
arterial vein	*vena arteriosa*
ascending lumbar vein	*vena lumbalis ascendens*
axillary vein	*vena axillaris*
azygos vein	*vena azygos*
basal vein	*vena basalis*
basilic vein	*vena basilica*
basivertebral veins	*venae basivertebrales*
brachial veins	*venae brachiales*
bronchial vein	*venae bronchiales*
cavernous veins of penis	*venae cavernosae penis*
central retinal vein	*vena centralis retinae*
central vein of suprarenal gland	*vena centralis glandulae suprarenalis*
central veins of liver	*venae centrales hepatis*
cephalic vein of forearm	*vena cephalica antebrachii*
cephalic vein	*vena cephalica*
cerebellar veins	*venae cerebelli*
common basal vein	*vena basalis communis*
common facial vein	*vena facialis communis*
common iliac vein	*vena iliaca communis*
common modiolar vein	*vena communis modioli*
condylar emissary vein	*venae emissaria condylaris*
conjunctival veins	*venae conjunctivales*
cystic vein	*vena cystica*
deep cerebral veins	*venae profundae cerebri*
deep cervical vein	*vena cervicales profunda*
deep circumflex iliac vein	*vena circumflexa ilium profunda*
deep dorsal vein of clitoris	*vena dorsalis clitoridis profunda*
deep dorsal vein of penis	*vena dorsalis penis profunda*
deep facial vein	*vena profunda faciei*
deep lingual vein	*vena profunda linguae*
deep middle cerebral vein	*vena media profunda cerebri*
deep temporal veins	*venae temporales profundae*
deep veins of clitoris	*venae profundae clitoridis*

deep veins of penis	*venae profundae penis*
diploic vein	*vena diploica*
direct lateral veins	*venae directae laterales*
dorsal digital veins of foot	*venae digitales dorsales pedis*
dorsal lingual vein	*vena dorsales linguale*
dorsal metacarpal veins	*vena metacarpeae dorsales*
dorsal metatarsal veins	*venae metatarsals dorsales*
dorsal scapular vein	*vena scapularis dorsalis*
emissary vein	*vena emissaria*
episcleral vein	*venae episclerales*
ethmoidal veins	*venae ethmoidales*
external iliac vein	*vena iliaca externa*
external jugular vein	*vena jugularis externa*
external nasal veins	*venae nasales externae*
external palatine vein	*vena palatina externa*
external pudendal veins	*venae pudendae externae*
facial vein	*vena facialis*
femoral vein	*vena femoralis*
fibular veins	*venae fibulares*
genicular veins	*venae geniculares*
great cardiac vein	*vena cardiaca magna*
great cerebral vein of Galen	*vena magna cerebri*
hemiazygos vein	*vena hemiazygos*
hepatic portal vein	*vena portae hepatis*
hepatic veins	*venae hepaticae*
ileocolic vein	*vena ileocolica*
iliolumbar vein	*vena iliolumbalis*
inferior anastomotic vein	*vena anastomotica inferior*
inferior basal vein	*vena basalis inferior*
inferior cerebral veins	*venae inferiores cerebri*
inferior choroid vein	*vena choroidea inferior*
inferior epigastric vein	*vena epigastrica inferior*
inferior gluteal veins	*venae gluteae inferiores*
inferior labial vein	*vena labialis inferior*
inferior laryngeal vein	*vena laryngea inferior*
inferior mesenteric vein	*vena mesenterica inferior*
inferior ophthalmic vein	*vena ophthalmica inferior*
inferior palpebral veins	*venae palpebrales inferiores*
inferior phrenic vein	*vena phrenica inferior*
inferior rectal veins	*venae rectales inferiores*
inferior thalamostriate veins	*venae thalamostriatae inferiores*
inferior thyroid vein	*vena thyroideae inferior*
inferior vein of vermis	*vena inferior vermis*
inferior veins of cerebellar hemisphere	*venae inferiores cerebelli*
inferior ventricular vein	*vena ventricularis inferior*
intercapitular veins	*venae intercapitulares*
interlobar veins of kidney	*venae interlobares renis*
interlobular veins of kidney	*venae interlobulares renis*
interlobular veins of liver	*venae interlobulares hepatis*

intermediate basilic vein	*vena intermedia basilica*
intermediate cephalic vein	*vena intermedia cephalica*
intermediate hepatic veins	*venae hepaticae intermediae*
internal cerebral veins	*venae internae cerebri*
internal iliac vein	*vena iliaca interna*
internal jugular vein	*vena jugularis interna*
internal pudendal vein	*vena pudenda interna*
internal thoracic vein	*vena thoracica interna*
lateral thoracic vein	*vena thoracica lateralis*
left colic vein	*vena colica sinistra*
left gastric vein	*vena gastrica sinistra*
left hepatic vein	*venae hepaticae sinistrae*
left inferior pulmonary vein	*vena pulmonalis inferior sinistra*
left ovarian vein	*vena ovarica sinistra*
left superior intercostal vein	*vena intercostalis superior sinistra*
left superior pulmonary vein	*vena pulmonalis superior sinistra*
left suprarenal vein	*vena suprarenalis sinistra*
left umbilical vein	*vena umbilicalis*
lingual vein	*vena lingualis*
lumbar veins	*venae lumbales*
mastoid emissary vein	*vena emissaria mastoidea*
maxillary vein	*vena maxillaris*
medial vein of lateral ventricle	*vena medialis ventriculi lateralis*
median antebrachial vein	*vena mediana antebrachii*
median cubital vein	*vena intermedia cubiti*
median sacral vein	*vena sacralis mediana*
mediastinal vein	*vena mediastinales*
meningeal veins	*venae meningeae*
mesencephalic veins	*venae mesencephalicae*
middle cardiac vein	*vena cardiaca media*
middle colic vein	*vena colica media*
middle lobe vein of right lung	*vena lobi medii pulmonis dextra*
middle meningeal veins	*venae meningeae*
middle rectal veins	*venae rectales mediae*
middle temporal vein	*vena temporalis media*
middle thyroid vein	*vena thyroidea media*
musculophrenic veins	*venae musculophrenicae*
nasofrontal vein	*vena nasofrontalis*
oblique vein of left atrium	*vena obliqua atrii sinistri*
obturator veins	*vena obturatoria*
occipital cerebral veins	*venae encephali occipitales*
occipital emissary vein	*vena emissaria occipitalis*
occipital vein	*vena occipitalis*
palmar digital veins	*venae digitales palmares*
palmar metacarpal veins	*venae metacarpales palmares*
palpebral veins	*venae palpebrales*
pancreatic veins	*venae pancreaticae*
pancreaticoduodenal veins	*venae pancreaticoduodenales*
paraumbilical veins	*venae paraumbilicales*

parietal emissary vein	*vena emissaria parietales*
parietal veins	*venae parietales*
parotid veins	*venae parotideae*
pectoral veins	*venae pectorales*
peduncular veins	*venae pedunculares*
perforating veins	*venae perforantes*
pericardial veins	*venae pericardiacae*
pharyngeal veins	*venae pharyngeae*
plantar digital veins	*venae digitales plantares*
plantar metatarsal vein	*vena metatarsales plantares*
pontine veins	*venae pontis*
popliteal vein	*vena poplitea*
posterior auricular vein	*vena auricularis posterior*
posterior circumflex humeral vein	*vena circumflexa humeri posterior*
posterior intercostal veins	*venae intercostales posteriores*
posterior labial veins	*venae labiales posteriores*
posterior scrotal veins	*venae scrotales posteriores*
posterior tibial veins	*venae tibiales posteriores*
posterior vein of septum pellucidum	*vena posterior septi pellucidi*
posterior veins of left ventricle	*venae posteriores ventriculi sinistri*
precentral cerebellar vein	*vena precentralis cerebelli*
prefrontal veins	*venae prefrontales*
prepyloric vein	*vena prepylorica*
profunda femoris vein	*vena profunda femoris*
pulmonary veins	*venae pulmonales*
radial veins	*venae radiales*
renal veins	*venae renales*
retromandibular vein	*vena retromandibularis*
retroperitoneal veins	*venae retroperitoneales*
right colic vein	*vena colica dextra*
right gastric vein	*vena gastrica dextra*
right gastroomental vein	*vena gastroomentalis dextra*
right hepatic vein	*vena hepaticae dextrae*
right inferior pulmonary vein	*vena pulmonalis inferior dextra*
right ovarian vein	*vena ovarica dextra*
right superior intercostal vein	*vena intercostalis superior dextra*
right superior pulmonary vein	*vena pulmonalis superior dextra*
right suprarenal vein	*vena suprarenalis dextra*
right testicular vein	*vena testicularis dextra*
scleral veins	*venae sclerales*
short gastric veins	*venae gastricae breves*
sigmoid veins	*venae sigmoideae*
small cardiac vein	*vena cardiaca parva*
small saphenous vein	*vena saphena parva*
smallest cardiac vein	*vena cardiacae minimae*
spinal veins	*venae spinales*
splenic vein	*vena splenica*
sternocleidomastoid vein	*vena sternocleidomastoidea*
stylomastoid vein	*vena stylomastoidea*

subclavian vein	*vena subclavia*
subcutaneous veins of abdomen	*venae subcutaneae abdominis*
sublingual vein	*vena sublingualis*
submental vein	*vena submentalis*
superficial cerebral veins	*venae superficiales cerebri*
superficial circumflex iliac vein	*vena circumflexa ilium superficialis*
superficial dorsal veins of clitoris	*venae dorsales clitoridis superficialis*
superficial dorsal veins of penis	*venae dorsales penis superficiales*
superficial epigastric vein	*vena epigastrica superficialis*
superficial middle cerebral vein	*vena media superficialis cerebri*
superficial temporal veins	*venae temporales superficialis*
superficial vein	*vena cutanea*
superior anastomotic vein	*vena anastomotica superiore*
superior basal vein	*vena basalis superior*
superior cerebral veins	*vena superiores cerebri*
superior choroid vein	*vena choroidea superior*
superior epigastric vein	*vena epigastricae superiores*
superior gluteal veins	*venae gluteae superiores*
superior labial vein	*vena labialis superior*
superior laryngeal vein	*vena laryngea superior*
superior mesenteric vein	*vena mesenterica superior*
superior ophthalmic vein	*vena ophthalmica superior*
superior palpebral veins	*venae palpebrales superiores*
superior phrenic veins	*venae phrenicae superiores*
superior rectal vein	*vena rectalis superior*
superior thalamostriate vein	*vena thalamostriata superior*
superior thyroid vein	*vena thyroidea superior*
superior vein of vermis	*vena superior vermis*
superior veins of cerebellar hemisphere	*venae hemispherii cerebelli superiores*
supraorbital vein	*vena supraorbitalis*
suprascapular vein	*vena suprascapularis*
supreme intercostal vein	*vena intercostalis suprema*
thoracoacromial vein	*vena thoracoacromialis*
thoracoepigastric vein	*vena thoracoepigastrica*
thymic veins	*venae thymicae*
tracheal veins	*venae tracheales*
transverse cervical veins	*venae transversae cervicis*
transverse facial vein	*vena transversa faciei*
tympanic veins	*venae tympanicae*
ulnar veins	*venae ulnares*
uterine veins	*vena uterinae*
vein of bulb of penis	*vena bulbi penis*
vein of bulb of vestibule	*vena bulbi vestibuli*
vein of cochlear canaliculus	*vena aqueductus cochleae*
vein of cochlear window	*vena fenestrae cochleae*
vein of olfactory gyrus	*vena gyri olfactorii*
vein of posterior horn	*vena cornus posterioris*
vein of pterygoid canal	*vena canalis pterygoidei*
vein of scala tympani	*vena scalae tympani*

vein of scala vestibuli	*vena scalae vestibuli*
vein of uncus	*vena uncalis*
vein of vestibular aqueduct	*vena aqueductus vestibuli*
veins of caudate nucleus	*venae nuclei caudati*
veins of heart	*venae cordis*
veins of medulla oblongata	*venae medullae oblongatae*
veins of semicircular ducts	*venae ductuum semicircularium*
veins of spinal cord	*venae medullae spinalis*
veins of temporomandibular joint	*venae articulares temporomandibulares*
veins of upper limb	*vena membri superioris*
veins of vertebral column	*vena columnae vertebralis*
vertebral vein	*vena vertebralis*
vesical veins	*venae vesicales*
vitelline vein	*vena vitellina*
vorticose veins	*venae vorticosae*

Blood Groups

Linda A. Smith, PhD, CLS(NCA)
Associate Professor and Graduate Program Director
Department of Clinical Laboratory Sciences
University of Texas Health Science Center
San Antonio, TX

In this appendix, and in the related terms defined in the dictionary proper, the term *blood group* is used to refer to an entire group system consisting of heritable antigens whose specificity is controlled by a series of allelic genes. Traditionally, *blood group* is used in reference to erythrocyte antigens; however, most blood components, including erythrocytes, leukocytes, and platelets, possess heritable antigens identified as belonging to systems. The term *blood type* or *phenotype* is used to refer to a specific reaction pattern to the testing of antisera within a system. The term *blood group factor* is used to refer to a specific antigen within a system; however, this usage is not universal. It should be noted that in the current literature, a single system may be referred to in the plural (e.g., ABO blood groups) and the term *blood group* may be assigned to a single phenotype (e.g., blood group A).

Each blood group is defined in terms of reaction to the original antisera with which the system was discovered. Changes in and additions to a system occur by the discovery of additional antisera proven to be related to the same system. A new blood group antigen or factor can be defined by demonstrating that it is detected by an antiserum with reactions different from those of previously known antisera. If it is shown that the new antigen is genetically independent of known blood group systems, it may qualify as a prototype antigen for a new blood group system. Alternatively, if it can be shown that the new antigen is controlled by a gene allelic to one of the known blood group genes, it is assigned to the blood group system of its alleles.

In the blood group definitions, emphasis has been placed on identification of symbols for genes, antigens, antisera, and phenotypes. The general convention that symbols for genes and genotypes are set in italics, whereas symbols for gene products or antigens, antisera, and phenotypes are set in roman type, is followed here. In the Rh-Hr terminology for the Rh blood group, roman type is used to designate antigen substances, and boldface type is used to designate serological factors and their corresponding antibodies. These formats are in wide use but are not consistently followed by all authors.

Nomenclature

The designation of blood group systems and antigens has been based upon alphabetical assignment of names or initials of first antibody producer, reactive or nonreactive red cell source, or derivation of name, location or discovering institution. The International Society of Blood Transfusion (ISBT) developed a Working Party on Terminology of Red Cell Surface Antigens to establish a uniform nomenclature, while maintaining historical designations and guidelines. Part of the Working Party's charge is to conduct periodic reviews of the available data and report additions, alterations, or deletions to those blood group antigens considered extinct. In addition, the Working Party has developed a nomenclature coding system, based on order of discovery of the blood group systems, to aid in the computerization of data. Reports of the Working Party and updates are published in *Vox Sanguinis* (1990; 58:152–169, 1991; 61:52–57, 1993; 65:77–80, 1995; 69:265–279, 1996; 71:246–248, 1999; 61:158–160).

The ISBT classifies all antigens into one of four classifications: systems, collections, high-incidence antigens, and low-incidence antigens. Currently, there are 29 blood group systems. Each system is serologically, immunochemically, and genetically proven to be a product of distinct independent genes. Although 52 Rh antigens have been identified, some have been removed from the system since initial identification; consequently, the system currently has 45 antigens. Other systems (e.g., P, Xg, Hh, and Kx systems) have only one antigen associated with them. The table accompanying this essay lists the approved system names, abbreviated symbols, and numerical designations developed by the ISBT.

For clinical considerations, the ABO and Rh are of the most importance; others are useful for genetic linkage or red cell membrane protein studies.

In addition to the defined blood group system, there are other blood group antigens that fail, as of yet, to fit the system criteria. Some are genetically related or loosely associated by serological and immunochemical reactivity, but insufficient data exist to classify them as a system. Hence they are referred to as *collections*. There are now six collections recognized by the ISBT.

The remaining classifications of high-incidence and low-incidence antigens contain antigens that cannot be included in either a system or a collection. Antigens occurring with a high incidence in the random population are collectively referred to as *high-incidence antigens* or *public antigens*. These occur in almost all individuals. Antibodies to these antigens usually have been found in the serum of patients who lack the antigen and who have become immunized by transfusion or pregnancy. There are 12 distinct high-incidence antigens, and some of the symbols applied to public antigens include Vel, Lan, At^a, Jr^a, and JMH.

Other erythrocyte antigens are uncommon and may be found only in members of a very few families. Because of their rarity, they are often referred to as *low-incidence antigens* or *private antigens*. Antibodies to these antigens usually have been found in the serum of patients who have received transfusions or in mothers of infants with hemolytic disease of the newborn (HDN). They are often named for the family in which they were first discovered. There are 34 distinct low-incidence antigens, and some of the symbols assigned to the private antigens are By, Sw^a, Bi, NFLD, RASM, HJK, and ELO.

Designation of Blood Group Systems

No.	Name	Symbol	No. of Antigens	Gene name(s)	Chromosome
001	ABO	ABO	4	*ABO*	9
002	MNS	MNS	43	*GYPA, GYPB, GYPE*	4
003	P	P1	1	*P1*	22
004	Rh	RH	49	*RHD, RHCE*	1
005	Lutheran	LU	19	*LU*	19
006	Kell	KEL	25	*KEL*	7
007	Lewis	LE	6	*FUT3*	19
008	Duffy	FY	6	*DARC*	1
009	Kidd	JK	3	*SLC14A1*	18
010	Diego	DI	21	*SLC4A1*	17
011	Yt	YT	2	*ACHE*	7
012	Xg	XG	2	*XG, MIC2*	X/Y
013	Scianna	SC	5	*ERMAP*	1
014	Dombrock	DO	5	*ART4*	12
015	Colton	CO	3	*AQP1*	7
016	Landsteiner–Wiener	LW	3	*ICAM4*	19
017	Chido/Rodgers	CH/RG	9	*C4A, C4B*	6
018	Hh	H	1	*FUT1*	19
019	Kx	XK	1	*XK*	X
020	Gerbich	GE	8	*GYPC*	2
021	Cromer	CROM	13	*CD55*	1
022	Knops	KN	8	*CR1*	1
023	Indian	IN	2	*CD44*	11
024	Ok	OK	1	*BSG*	19
025	Raph	RAPH	1	*CD151*	11
026	John Milton Hagen	JMH	1	*SEMA7A*	15
027	I	I	1	*GCNT2*	6
028	Globoside	GLOB	1	*B3GALNT1*	3
029	Gill	GIL	1	*AQP3*	9

From Daniels G, Bromilow I. *Essential Guide to Blood Groups*. Blackwell Publishing, 2006.

Infection Surveillance, Prevention, and Control

Background

Surveillance, defined as the ongoing, systematic collection, analysis, interpretation, and dissemination of data regarding a health-related event for use in public health action to reduce morbidity and mortality and to improve health, is an essential tool for health care–associated infection (HAI). Prevention of HAI, providing protection for patients, the community, and health care personnel has evolved since the previous guidelines were published. Control issues, such as precautions and other practices, to curtail antimicrobial resistance and the spread of bloodborne infections, remain key elements for hospitals and other health care settings.

Three areas requiring understanding to facilitate prevention and control of health care associated infections are:

- Transmission of infection
- Types of health care settings
- Epidemiologically important pathogens

TRANSMISSION OF INFECTION

Understanding of transmission of infection within a health care facility underlies the rationale for recommended preventive practices.

Source or reservoir of infectious agents

Infectious agents transmitted during health care delivery derive from human and inanimate sources. Human sources include patients, health care personnel, household members, and other visitors. Among these classes are people with active infection; those who are asymptomatic and/or incubating an infectious disease; those who are transiently or chronically colonized by an infectious agent, particularly of the respiratory and gastrointestinal tracts; and the endogenous flora of the above. Inanimate sources include indwelling devices, urinary catheters, endotracheal tubes, central venous and arterial catheters, synthetic implants, environmental factors in a health care facility, other equipment and surfaces, and contaminated medications and supplies.

Susceptible host with portal of entry

Infection is the result of a complex interrelationship between the potential host and infectious agents, and most factors that influence infection, occurrence, and severity of disease are related to the host. The characteristics of the host-agent interaction as it relates to pathogenicity, virulence, and antigenicity are also important, as are the infectious dose, mechanisms of disease production, and route of exposure. There is a spectrum of possible outcomes following exposure to an infectious agent. Some people never develop symptomatic disease whereas others become severely ill and even die, and still others become transiently or permanently colonized by the pathogen, remaining asymptomatic, although some people may progress from colonization to symptomatic disease, either immediately or in the future. A person's immune state at the time of exposure, the interaction between pathogens, and the intrinsic virulence factors of the agent are important predictors of the outcome.

Host factors that may render an individual more susceptible to infection include:

- extremes of age
- underlying diseases, such as HIV/AIDS or malignancy
- transplants
- surgical procedures and radiation therapy impair defenses of the skin and other involved organ systems
- in-dwelling devices, such as urinary catheters, central arterial and venous lines, synthetic implants
- medications that alter the normal flora, such as antimicrobial agents, gastric acid suppressants, corticosteroids, antirejection drugs, antineoplastic agents, immunosuppressive drugs

Routes of transmission

Modes of transmission vary by type of organism, some are transmitted by more than one route, and of most importance, not all infectious agents are transmitted from person to person. Classes of pathogens that can cause infection include bacteria, viruses, fungi, parasites, and prions. The three principal routes of transmission are contact, which can be direct or indirect; droplet; and airborne.

Examples of **direct contact** include:

- blood or blood-containing body fluids transmitted to mucous membranes or breaks in skin
- mites from a scabies-infested patient during ungloved contact by health care worker
- herpetic whitlow on health care worker after ungloved oral care to patient with herpes simplex virus
- herpes simplex virus transmitted to the patient from herpetic whitlow on a health care worker's ungloved hand

Indirect contact transmission involves the transfer of an infectious agent through a contaminated intermediate object or person. Contaminated hands of health care personnel are important contributors to indirect contact transmission. Documented examples of opportunities for indirect contact transmission include:

- hands of health care personnel may transmit pathogens after touching a patient's infected or colonized body site or a contaminated inanimate object, if hand hygiene is not performed before another patient is touched
- patient-care devices such as electronic thermometers and glucose monitoring devices, if devices contaminated with blood or body fluids are shared among patients without cleaning and disinfecting between patients
- shared toys may transmit respiratory viruses, such as respiratory syncytial virus, *Pseudomonas aeruginosa*, or other pathogenic bacteria, among pediatric patients
- surgical or endoscopic instruments that are inadequately cleaned or sterilized, or that may have manufacturing defects that interfere with the effectiveness of reprocessing and recycling
- clothing, uniforms, laboratory coats, or isolation gowns used as personal protective equipment may become contaminated with potential pathogens after care of a patient colonized or infected with an infectious agent, such as methicillin-resistant *Staphylococcus aureus* (MRSA), vancomycin-resistant *Enterococcus* (VRE), and *Clostridium difficile*.

Droplets are transmitted by coughing, sneezing, talking, suctioning, and bronchoscopy, and are traditionally defined as being >5 mcm in size, although droplets up to 30 mcm or more can remain suspended in the air. Although respiratory syncytial virus may be transmitted by the droplet route, direct contact with infected respiratory secretions is the most important determinant of transmission. Consistent adherence to Standard Precautions plus Contact Precautions prevents transmission in health care settings.

Rarely, pathogens that are not transmitted routinely by the droplet route are dispersed into the air over short distances. For example, although *S. aureus* is transmitted most frequently by contact, viral upper respiratory tract infection has been associated with increased dispersal of *S. aureus* from the nose into the air for a distance of 4 feet under both outbreak and experimental conditions and is known as the "cloud baby" and "cloud adult" phenomenon.

Airborne transmission involves *airborne dust particles* and *droplet nuclei,* which are particles arising from desiccation of suspended droplets <5 mcm; however, size parameters are being reconsidered. Airborne transmission occurs by dissemination of either airborne droplet nuclei or small particles in the respirable size range containing infectious agents that remain infective over time and distance. Microorganisms carried in this manner may be dispersed over long distances by air currents and may be inhaled by susceptible individuals who have not had face-to-face contact with (or been in the same room with) an infectious person. Preventing the spread of pathogens that are transmitted by the airborne route requires the use of special air handling and ventilation systems such as airborne infection isolation room (AIIR) to contain and then safely remove the infectious agent.

In addition to better known organisms, (e.g., *Mycobacterium tuberculosis*, rubeola virus [measles], varicella-zoster virus [chickenpox]), published data suggest the possibility that variola virus (smallpox) may also be transmitted over long distances through the air under unusual circumstances and airborne infection isolation rooms are recommended for this agent as well; however, droplet and contact routes are the more frequent modes of transmission for smallpox. For certain other respiratory infectious agents, such as influenza and rhinovirus, and even some gastrointestinal viruses (e.g., norovirus, rotavirus) some evidence suggests that the pathogen may be transmitted via small-particle aerosols, under natural and experimental conditions, over distances >3 feet but within a defined air space (e.g., patient's room), suggesting that it is unlikely that these agents remain viable on air currents that travel long distances. Airborne infection isolation rooms are not routinely required to prevent transmission of these agents.

Emerging issues that challenge the previously held notions of isolation are the airborne transmission of infectious agents include transmission from patients, as in the outbreak of severe acute respiratory syndrome (SARS) of 2002, monkeypox in the United States in 2003, and the emergence of avian influenza. In addition to the strict interpretation for airborne route of transmission, short-distance transmission by small particles occurs during specific procedures (e.g., endotracheal intubation). Aerosolized particles <100 mcm can remain suspended in air when room air current velocities exceed the terminal settling velocities of the particles.

SARS-coronavirus transmission has been associated with endotracheal intubation, noninvasive positive pressure ventilation, and cardiopulmonary resuscitation. Although the most frequent routes of transmission of noroviruses are direct contact and food and waterborne routes, several reports suggest that noroviruses may be transmitted through aerosolization of infectious particles from vomitus or fecal matter.

The SARS outbreak also provides new definitions involving airborne transmission of infectious agents:

- *Obligate:* under natural conditions, disease occurs following transmission of the agent only through inhalation of small particle aerosols (e.g., tuberculosis)
- *Preferential:* natural infection results from transmission through multiple routes, but small-particle aerosols are the predominant route (e.g., measles, varicella)
- *Opportunistic:* agents that naturally cause disease through other routes, but under special circumstances may be transmitted via fine particle aerosols

Concerns about unknown or possible routes of transmission of agents associated with severe disease without known treatment often result in more extreme prevention strategies than may be absolutely necessary; therefore, recommended precautions could change as the epidemiology of an emerging infection is defined and controversial issues are resolved.

Airborne transmission from environmental sources of respiratory pathogens (e.g., *Legionella*) transmitted to humans through a common aerosol source is distinct from direct patient-to-patient transmission. Some airborne infectious agents are derived from the environment and do not usually involve person-to-person transmission. In particular, spores inhaled into the respiratory tract, such as finely milled anthrax spores aerosolized from contaminated environmental surfaces and spores of ubiquitous environmental fungi (e.g., *Aspergillus* spp.). As a rule, neither of these organisms is subsequently transmitted from infected patients, although there is at least one well-documented report of person-to-person transmission of *Aspergillus* spp. in an intensive care unit that was most likely due to the aerosolization of spores during wound debridement.

Environmental and vector-borne routes of transmission

Transmission of infection from sources other than infectious people include those associated with *common environmental sources or vehicles* (e.g., contaminated food, water, medications, intravenous fluids), and in the case of *Aspergillus* spp., hospital water systems. The role of water as a reservoir for illness in immunosuppressed patients remains uncertain. *Vector-borne transmission* of infectious agents from mosquitoes, flies, rats, and other vermin also can occur in health care settings. Prevention against vector-borne transmission is not addressed in this document.

Numerous factors influence differences in transmission risks among the various health care settings. These include the population characteristics (e.g., increased susceptibility to infections, type, and prevalence of in-dwelling devices), intensity of care, exposure to environmental sources, length of stay, and frequency of interaction between patients/residents with each other and with health care workers. These factors, as well as organizational priorities, goals, and resources influence how different health care agencies adapt transmission-prevention guidelines to meet their specific needs. Infection control management decisions are informed by data regarding institutional experience/epidemiology, trends in community and institutional health care–associated infection, local, regional, and national epidemiology, and emerging infectious disease threats.

Hospitals. Infection transmission risks are present in all hospital settings. However, certain hospital settings and patient populations have unique conditions that predispose patients to infection and merit special mention. These are often sentinel sites for the emergence of new transmission risks that may be unique to that setting or present opportunities for transmission to other settings in the hospital.

Intensive Care Units (ICUs) by their nature serve the most severely ill, easily compromised patients receiving the most invasive procedures with infections acquired in these units accounting for >20% of all health care–associated infection.

Burn Units. Burn wounds can provide optimal conditions for colonization, infection, and transmission of pathogens, infection that is in turn a frequent cause of morbidity and mortality; burn injuries involving >30% of the total body surface area represent the greatest risk of infection. Smaller total body surface area burn infections are commonly associated with invasive devices. Burn wound infections are caused by environmental molds, even those liberated in construction dust and debris. Hydrotherapy equipment is an environmental reservoir of gram-negative organisms. Operating room excision of burn wounds is the preferred treatment method. Advances in burn care, specifically early excision and grafting of the burn wound, use of topical antimicrobial agents, and institution of early enteral feeding, have led to decreased complications due to infection. Other advances in current practices have not been studied; prospective studies to define the most effective combination of infection control precautions in burn settings are needed

Pediatrics presents unique infection control issues. Interpatient variability factors, such as immaturity of the neonatal immune system, lack of previous natural infection, prevalence of patients with congenital or acquired immune deficiencies, congenital anatomic anomalies, and use of life-saving invasive devices in neonatal and pediatric intensive care units increase the likelihood of health care–associated infection. These patients, not yet immune by either vaccination or natural infection, are at risk for community-acquired infections due to increased numbers of patients and siblings presenting, especially during seasonal epidemics. Close physical contact between health care personnel and pediatric patients, congregation of children in play areas where toys and bodily secretions are easily shared, and family members rooming-in with pediatric patients can further increase the risk. Innovative practices, such as cobedding used to improve developmental outcomes, theoretically increase transmission risk, although infection risks may actually be reduced among infants receiving so-called kangaroo care in which infants, often preterm, share skin-to-skin contact with their mothers. Children in child care centers and pediatric rehabilitation units may increase the overall burden of antimicrobial resistance by contributing to the reservoir of community-associated methicillin-resistant *S. aureus*. Children in long-term care facilities may have increased rates of colonization with resistant gram-negative bacteria and may be sources of introduction of resistant organisms to short-term care settings. These patients are hospitalized frequently and can transfer pathogens between the long-term care facility and other health care facilities.

Medium and longer term nonhospital settings include long-term care facilities, homes for the developmentally disabled, settings where behavioral health services are provided, rehabilitation centers, and hospices. In addition, health care may be provided in nonhealth care settings such as workplaces with occupational health clinics, adult day care centers, assisted living facilities, homeless shelters, jails and prisons, school clinics, and infirmaries. Each of these settings has unique circumstances and population risks to consider when designing and implementing an infection control program.

The term **long-term care facility** encompasses a variety of residential settings, ranging from institutions for the developmentally disabled to nursing homes for the elderly and pediatric long-term care facilities. Long-term care facilities are different from other health care settings in that patients at increased risk for infection are brought together in one setting and remain in the facility for extended periods; for most elderly residents, it *is* their home. An atmosphere of community is fostered and residents share common eating and living areas and participate in various facility-sponsored activities, thus making control of organism or disease transmission challenging. Residents who are colonized or infected with certain microorganisms can be restricted to their rooms; but, because of the associated psychosocial risks, it has been recommended that psychosocial needs be balanced with infection control needs in the long-term care facility setting. Pathogens that lead to substantial mortality, morbidity, and increased medical costs include influenzavirus, rhinovirus, adenovirus (conjunctivitis), norovirus, and bacteria, including multiple-drug-resistant organisms (MDROs) and *Clostridium difficile,* requiring prompt detection and control. Because residents of long-term care facilities are hospitalized frequently, they can transfer pathogens between long-term care facilities and health care facilities in which they receive care.

Ambulatory care is provided in hospital-based outpatient clinics, nonhospital-based clinics and physicians' offices, public health clinics, free standing dialysis centers, ambulatory surgical centers, urgent care centers, and many others, which now account for most patient encounters with the health care system. In these settings, adapting transmission prevention guidelines is challenging because patients remain in common areas for prolonged periods waiting to be seen by a health care provider or awaiting admission to the hospital. Examination or treatment rooms are turned around quickly with limited cleaning, and infectious patients may not be immediately recognized. Immunocompromised patients often receive chemotherapy in infusion rooms where they stay for extended periods along with other types of patients. There are few data on the risk of health care–associated infection, except for hemodialysis centers, where contaminated solutions, equipment and bloodborne transmission cause infection, at times having involved hundreds of patients.

Home care is provided by 20,000 agencies that include home health agencies, hospices, durable medical equipment providers, home infusion therapy services, personal care and support services providers. Services are provided to patients of all ages with both acute and chronic diseases or disabilities. The scope of services offers a wide range of possible modes of transmission and includes both contact and invasive procedures. Risks of infection in this setting, other than those associated with infusion therapy, is not well-studied. Draft definitions for home care-associated infections have been developed. MDRO transmission has been a very challenging issue in the home care industry; practice has been inconsistent and frequently not based on evidence. Home health care also may contribute to antimicrobial resistance.

Other sites of health care delivery include facilities that are not primarily health care settings but in which health care is delivered, such as clinics in correctional facilities and shelters that have suboptimal features, including crowding and poor ventilation. Poor people and homeless people may have chronic illnesses and health care problems related to alcoholism, injection drug use, poor nutrition, and/or inadequate shelter; they often receive primary health care in such locations. Infectious diseases of special concern for transmission include tuberculosis, scabies, respiratory infections (e.g., *Neisseria meningitides, Streptococcus pneumoniae*), sexually transmitted and bloodborne diseases, hepatitis A virus, diarrheal agents such as norovirus, and foodborne diseases, with a high index of suspicion for tuberculosis and community-associated methicillin-resistant *S. aureus*.

EPIDEMIOLOGICALLY IMPORTANT ORGANISMS

Concerns about health care–associated infections have been expanded to include epidemiologically important organisms. These are not only the better known organisms and their evolution and the multiple-drug-resistant organisms but also emerging pathogens and agents of bioterrorism or bioweapons. Evaluation of the emerging pathogens and bioweapons is included in the 2007 guidelines because experience with these agents has broadened the understanding of modes of transmission and effective preventive measures, preparedness planning, and effective response.

Infectious Organisms

The characteristics of an epidemiologically important infectious organism are:

1. A propensity for transmission within health care facilities based on published reports and the occurrence of temporal or geographic clusters of > 2 patients (*C. difficile*, norovirus, respiratory syncytial virus, influenza, rotavirus, *Enterobacter* spp., *Serratia* spp., group A streptococcus) **or** a single case of health care–associated invasive disease caused by certain pathogens (group A streptococcus postoperatively, in burn units and long-term care facilities; *Legionella* and *Aspergillus*). These are an indication for investigation and enhanced control measures because of the associated risk of additional cases and severity of illness.
2. Antimicrobial resistance:
   - Resistance to first-line therapies (MRSA, vancomycin-intermediate *S. aureus* [VISA], vancomycin-resistant *S. aureus* [VRSA], VRE, extended-spectrum beta lactamase–producing organisms).
   - Common and uncommon microorganisms with unusual patterns of resistance within a facility (the first isolate of *Burkholderia cepacia* complex or *Ralstonia* spp. in patients who do not have cystic fibrosis or a quinolone-resistant strain of *Pseudomonas aeruginosa* in a health care facility).
   - Difficult to treat because of innate or acquired resistance to multiple classes of antimicrobial agents (*Stenotrophomonas maltophilia, Acinetobacter* spp.).
   - Association with serious clinical disease, increased morbidity and mortality (e.g., MRSA and methicillin-susceptible *S. aureus*, group A streptococcus)
   - A newly discovered or reemerging pathogen

Agents of Bioterrorism (Bioweapons)

Health care facilities confront a different set of issues when dealing with a suspected bioterrorism event as compared with other communicable diseases. The response is likely to differ for exposures resulting from an intentional release compared with naturally occurring disease because of the large number of people who can be exposed at the same time and because of possible differences in pathogenicity.

Category A (high priority) agents that are easily disseminated environmentally and/or readily transmitted from person to person include anthrax, smallpox, plague, tularemia, viral hemorrhagic fevers, and botulism. Consult the U.S. Centers for Disease Control and Prevention's (CDC) Emergency Preparedness and Response Site (www.bt.cdc.gov) for additional updated information on Category A, B, and C agents, the latter of which are important but are not as readily disseminated and cause lower morbidity and mortality. Many other sources offer guidance for the management of those exposed to the most likely agents of bioterrorism. U.S. federal agency websites and www.usamriid.army.mil/publicationspage.html, along with state and county health department web sites, should be consulted for the most up-to-date information on bioweapons.

Emerging Organisms

Prions: The infectious variety are isoforms of a host-encoded glycoprotein known as the prion protein, believed to cause Creutzfeldt-Jakob disease (CJD). Approximately 5% of CJD cases are iatrogenic, transmitted via treatment with human cadaveric pituitary-derived growth hormone or gonadotropin, implantation of contaminated human dura mater grafts or corneal transplants, and are linked to the use of contaminated neurosurgical instruments or stereotactic electroencephalographic electrodes. Ingestion of animal products infected with bovine spongiform encephalopathy (BSE) is believed to cause the variant form, vCJD. Similar to sporadic CJD, there have been no reported cases of direct human-to-human transmission of vCJD by casual or environmental contact, droplet, or airborne routes. Ongoing blood safety surveillance in the U.S. has not detected sporadic CJD transmission through blood transfusion. However, bloodborne transmission of vCJD is believed to have occurred in two patients in the United Kingdom. The U.S. Food and Drug Administration's website provides information on measures that are being taken in the United States to protect the blood supply from CJD and vCJD: www.fda.gov/cber/blood/vcjdrisk.htm.

Severe Acute Respiratory Syndrome (SARS) is caused by the SARS coronavirus (SARS-CoV). The illness is difficult to distinguish initially from other common respiratory infections. Outbreaks in health care settings, with transmission to large numbers of health care personnel and patients have been a striking characteristic of SARS. Undiagnosed infectious patients and visitors were important vectors of these outbreaks. The relative contribution of potential modes of transmission is not precisely known. Ample evidence exists for droplet and contact transmission; however, opportunistic airborne transmission cannot be excluded. Breaches in recommended laboratory practices have allowed transmission of SARS-CoV. The greatest risk of transmission is to those who have close contact, are not properly trained in use of protective infection control procedures and/or do not consistently use personal protective equipment. N95 or higher level respirators may offer additional protection to those exposed to aerosol-generating procedures and high-risk activities. Control of SARS requires a coordinated dynamic response by multiple disciplines in a health care setting. Early detection of cases is accomplished by screening those with symptoms of a respiratory infection for history of travel to areas experiencing community transmission or contact with SARS patients, followed by implementation of Respiratory Hygiene/Cough Etiquette and physical separation from other patients in common waiting areas. The precise combination of precautions to protect health care personnel has not been determined. At the time of this publication (June 22, 2007), the CDC recommends Standard Precautions, with emphasis on the use of hand hygiene, Contact Precautions with emphasis on environmental cleaning, and Airborne Precautions, including use of fit-tested NIOSH-approved N95 or higher level respirators, and eye protection. Guidance for SARS-specific infection control precautions in various settings is available at www.cdc.gov/ncidod/sars.

Noroviruses, formerly referred to as Norwalk-like viruses, are members of the Caliciviridae family, transmitted via contaminated food or water and from person-to-person, that cause explosive outbreaks of gastrointestinal disease. Environmental contamination also has been documented as a contributing factor in ongoing transmission. Outbreaks in hospitals, long-term care facilities, cruise ships, hotels, schools, and large crowded shelters established for hurricane evacuees demonstrate their highly contagious nature, the disruptive impact they have in health care facilities and the community, and the difficulty of controlling outbreaks in settings where people share common facilities and space. The epidemiology of norovirus outbreaks shows that even though primary cases may result from exposure to fecally contaminated food or water, secondary and tertiary cases often result from person-to-person transmission that is facilitated by contamination of fomites and dissemination of infectious particles, especially during the process of vomiting. Widespread, persistent, and inapparent contamination of the environment and fomites can make outbreaks extremely difficult to control. Consultation on outbreaks of gastroenteritis is available through CDC's Division of Viral and Rickettsial Diseases.

Hemorrhagic fever viruses (HFV) are a mixed group of viruses that cause serious disease with high fever, skin rash, bleeding diathesis, and in some cases, high mortality; the disease caused is referred to as viral hemorrhagic fever (VHF). Ebola and Marburg viruses (Filoviridae), Lassa virus (Arenaviridae),

Crimean-Congo hemorrhagic fever and Rift Valley Fever virus (Bunyaviridae), and dengue and yellow fever viruses (Flaviviridae) are the more commonly known HFVs. These viruses are transmitted to humans via contact with infected animals or via arthropod vectors. Although none of these viruses is endemic in the United States, outbreaks in affected countries provide potential opportunities for importation by infected humans and animals. Furthermore, there are concerns that some of these agents could be used as bioweapons. Person-to-person transmission, including to health care personnel, is documented for Ebola, Marburg, Lassa, and Crimean-Congo hemorrhagic fever viruses. This transmission is associated primarily with direct blood and body fluid contact. Percutaneous exposure to contaminated blood carries a particularly high risk for transmission and increased mortality. Postmortem handling of infected bodies is an important risk for transmission. In less developed countries, outbreaks of VHFs have been controlled with basic hygiene, barrier precautions, safe injection practices, and safe burial practices. When a patient with a syndrome consistent with hemorrhagic fever also has a history of travel to an endemic area, precautions are initiated on presentation and then modified as more information is obtained. Further recommendations are available from CDC.

TYPES OF PRECAUTIONS:

The successful experience with Standard Precautions, first recommended in the 1996 guideline, has led to a reaffirmation of this approach as the foundation for preventing transmission of infectious agents in all health care settings.

Recommendations

These recommendations are designed to prevent transmission of infectious agents among patients and health care personnel in all settings where health care is delivered. As in other CDC/Hospital Infection Control Practices Advisory Committee (HICPAC) guidelines, each recommendation is categorized on the basis of existing scientific data, theoretical rationale, applicability, and when possible, economic impact. The CDC/HICPAC system for categorizing recommendations is as follows:

Category IA Strongly recommended for implementation and strongly supported by well-designed experimental, clinical, or epidemiologic studies.

Category IB Strongly recommended for implementation and supported by some experimental, clinical, or epidemiologic studies and a strong theoretical rationale.

Category IC Required for implementation, as mandated by federal and/or state regulation or standard.

Category II Suggested for implementation and supported by suggestive clinical or epidemiologic studies or a theoretic rationale.

No recommendation Unresolved issue. Practices for which insufficient evidence or no consensus regarding efficacy exists.

I. Administrative Responsibilities

Health care organization administrators should ensure the implementation of recommendations in this section.

A. Incorporate preventing transmission of infectious agents into the objectives of the organization's patient and occupational safety programs (IB/IC).

B. Make preventing transmission of infectious agents a priority for the health care organization. Provide administrative support, including fiscal and human resources, for maintaining infection control programs (IB/IC).

   1. Assure that individuals with training in infection control are employed by or are available by contract to all health care facilities so that the infection control program is managed by one or more qualified individuals (IB/IC).

      a. Determine the specific infection control full-time equivalents (FTEs) according to the scope of the infection control program, the complexity of the health care facility or system, the characteristics of the patient population, the unique or urgent needs of the facility and community, and proposed staffing levels based on survey results and recommendations from professional organizations (IB).

2. Include prevention of health care–associated infections (HAI) as one determinant of bedside nurse staffing levels and composition, especially in high-risk units (IB).
3. Delegate authority to infection control personnel or their designees for making infection control decisions concerning patient placement and assignment of Transmission-Based Precautions (IC).
4. Involve infection control personnel in decisions on facility construction and design, determination of airborne infection isolation room (AIIR) and Protective Environment capacity needs and environmental assessments (IB/IC).
   a. Provide ventilation systems required for a sufficient number of AIIRs (as determined by a risk assessment) and Protective Environments in health care facilities that provide care to patients for whom such rooms are indicated, according to published recommendations (IB/IC).
5. Involve infection control personnel in the selection and postimplementation evaluation of medical equipment and supplies and changes in practice that could affect the risk of HAI (IC).
6. Ensure availability of human and fiscal resources to provide clinical microbiology laboratory support, including a sufficient number of medical technologists trained in microbiology, appropriate to the health care setting, for monitoring transmission of microorganisms, planning and conducting epidemiologic investigations, and detecting emerging pathogens. Identify resources for performing surveillance cultures, rapid diagnostic testing for viral and other selected pathogens, preparation of antimicrobial susceptibility summary reports, trend analysis, and molecular typing of clustered isolates (performed either on-site or in a reference laboratory) and use these resources according to facility-specific epidemiologic needs, in consultation with clinical microbiologists (IB).
7 Provide human and fiscal resources to meet occupational health needs related to infection control (IB/IC).
8. In all areas where health care is delivered, provide supplies and equipment necessary for the consistent observance of Standard Precautions, including hand hygiene products and personal protective equipment (IB/IC).
9. Develop and implement policies and procedures to ensure that reusable patient care equipment is cleaned and reprocessed appropriately before use on another patient (IA/IC).

C. Develop and implement processes to ensure oversight of infection control activities appropriate to the health care setting and assign responsibility for oversight of infection control activities to an individual or group within the health care organization that is knowledgeable about infection control (II).

D. Develop and implement systems for early detection and management of potentially infectious persons at initial points of patient encounter in outpatient settings and at the time of admission to hospitals and long-term care facilities (LTCF) (IB).

E. Develop and implement policies and procedures to limit patient visitation by persons with signs or symptoms of a communicable infection. Screen visitors to high-risk patient care areas for possible infection (IB).

F. Identify performance indicators of the effectiveness of organization-specific measures to prevent transmission of infectious agents (Standard and Transmission-Based Precautions), and establish processes to monitor adherence to those performance measures and provide feedback to staff members (IB).

II. Education and Training

A. Provide job- or task-specific education and training on preventing transmission of infectious agents associated with health care during orientation to the health care facility; update information periodically during ongoing education programs. Target all health care personnel for education and training, including but not limited to medical, nursing, clinical technicians, laboratory staff; property service (housekeeping), laundry, maintenance and dietary workers; students, contract staff, and volunteers. Document competency initially and repeatedly, as appropriate, for the specific staff positions.

Develop a system to ensure that health care personnel employed by outside agencies meet these education and training requirements through programs offered by the agencies or by participation in the health care facility's program designed for full-time personnel (IB).

1. Include in education and training programs, information concerning use of vaccines as an adjunctive infection control measure (IB).
2. Enhance education and training by applying principles of adult learning, using reading level and language appropriate material for the target audience, and using online educational tools available to the institution (IB).

B. Provide instructional materials for patients and visitors on recommended hand hygiene and Respiratory Hygiene/Cough Etiquette practices and the application of Transmission-Based Precautions (II).

III. Surveillance

A. Monitor the incidence of epidemiologically important organisms and targeted HAI that have substantial impact on outcome and for which effective preventive interventions are available; use information collected through surveillance of high-risk populations, procedures, devices, and highly transmissible infectious agents to detect transmission of infectious agents in the health care facility (IA).

B. Apply the following epidemiologic principles of infection surveillance (IB).

1. Use standardized definitions of infection.
2. Use laboratory-based data (when available).
3. Collect epidemiologically-important variables.
4. Analyze data to identify trends that may indicate increased rates of transmission.
5. Provide feedback information on trends in the incidence and prevalence of HAI, probable risk factors, and prevention strategies and their impact to the appropriate health care providers, organization administrators, and as required by local and state health authorities.

C. Develop and implement strategies to reduce risks for transmission and evaluate effectiveness (IB).

D. When transmission of epidemiologically-important organisms continues despite implementation and documented adherence to infection prevention and control strategies, obtain consultation from persons knowledgeable in infection control and health care epidemiology to review the situation and recommend additional measures for control (IB).

E. Review periodically information on community or regional trends in the incidence and prevalence of epidemiologically important organisms including those in other health care facilities that may have an impact transmission of organisms within the facility (II).

IV. Standard Precautions

Assume that every person is potentially infected or colonized with an organism that could be transmitted in the health care setting and apply the following infection control practices during the delivery of health care.

A. Hand Hygiene

See *"Guideline for Hand Hygiene in Health Care Settings"* appendix (APP 187– APP 189).

B. Personal protective equipment (PPE)

1. Observe the following principles of use:
   a. Wear PPE, when the nature of the anticipated patient interaction indicates that contact with blood or body fluids may occur (IB/IC).

b. Prevent contamination of clothing and skin during the process of removing PPE (II).

c. Before leaving the patient's room or cubicle, remove and discard PPE (IB/IC).

2. Gloves

a. Wear gloves when it can be reasonably anticipated that contact with blood or other potentially infectious materials, mucous membranes, nonintact skin, or potentially contaminated intact skin could occur (IB/IC).

b. Wear gloves with fit and durability appropriate to the task (IB).

i. Wear disposable medical examination gloves for providing direct patient care.

ii. Wear disposable medical examination gloves or reusable utility gloves for cleaning the environment or medical equipment.

c. Remove gloves after contact with a patient and/or the surrounding environment (including medical equipment) using proper technique to prevent hand contamination. Do not wear the same pair of gloves for the care of more than one patient. Do not wash gloves for the purpose of reuse because this practice has been associated with transmission of pathogens (IB).

d. Change gloves during patient care if the hands will move from a contaminated body-site to a clean body-site (II).

3. Gowns

a. Wear a gown, which is appropriate to the task, to protect skin and prevent soiling or contamination of clothing during procedures and patient-care activities when contact with blood, body fluids, secretions, or excretions is anticipated (IB/IC).

i. Wear a gown for direct patient contact if the patient has uncontained secretions or excretions (IB/IC).

ii. Remove gown and perform hand hygiene before leaving the patient's environment (IB/IC).

b. Do not reuse gowns, even for repeated contacts with the same patient (II).

c. Routine donning of gowns on entrance into a high risk unit is not indicated (IB).

4. Mouth, nose, and eye protection

a. Use PPE to protect the mucous membranes of the eyes, nose, and mouth during procedures and patient-care activities that are likely to generate splashes or sprays of blood, body fluids, secretions, and excretions. Select masks, goggles, face shields, and combinations of each according to the need anticipated by the task performed (IB/IC).

5. During aerosol-generating procedures in patients who are not suspected of being infected with an agent for which respiratory protection is otherwise recommended (e.g., *M. tuberculosis*, SARS–related Coronavirus or hemorrhagic fever viruses), wear one of the following:

a. a face shield that fully covers the front and sides of the face

b. a mask with attached shield

c. or a mask and goggles (in addition to gloves and gown) (IB)

C. Respiratory Hygiene/Cough Etiquette

1. Educate health care personnel on the importance of source control measures to contain respiratory secretions to prevent droplet and fomites-related transmission of respiratory pathogens, especially during seasonal outbreaks of viral respiratory tract infections in communities (IB).

2. Implement the following measures to contain respiratory secretions in patients and accompanying individuals who have signs and symptoms of a respiratory infection, beginning at the point of initial encounter in a health care setting.

a. Post signs at entrances and in strategic places within ambulatory and inpatient settings with instructions to patients and other persons with symptoms of a respiratory infection to cover their mouths/noses when coughing or sneezing, use and dispose of tissues, and perform hand hygiene after hands have been in contact with respiratory secretions (II).

b. Provide tissues and no-touch receptacles for disposal of tissues (II).

c. Provide resources and instructions for performing hand hygiene in or near waiting areas in ambulatory and inpatient settings; provide conveniently located dispensers of alcohol-based hand rubs and, where sinks are available, supplies for handwashing (IB).

d. During periods of increased prevalence of respiratory infections in the community, offer masks to coughing patients and other symptomatic persons on entry into the facility or medical office and encourage them to maintain special separation, ideally a distance of at least 3 feet, from others in common waiting areas (IB).

i. Some facilities may find it logistically easier to institute this recommendation year-round as a standard of practice (II).

D. Patient placement

1. Include the potential for transmission of infectious agents in patient placement decisions. Place patients who pose a risk for transmission to others in a single-patient room when available (IB).

2. Determine patient placement based on the following principles:

Route(s) of transmission of the known or suspected infectious agent

Risk factors for transmission in the infected patient

Risk factors for adverse outcomes resulting from an HAI in other patients in the area or room being considered for patient placement

Availability of single-patient rooms

Patient options for room-sharing (e.g., cohorting patients sick with the same infection) (II).

E. Patient-care equipment and instruments/devices.

1. Establish policies and procedures for containing, transporting, and handling patient-care equipment and instruments/devices that may be contaminated with blood or body fluids (IB/IC).

2. Remove organic material from critical and semicritical instrument/devices, using recommended cleaning agents, before high level disinfection and sterilization to enable effective disinfection and sterilization processes (IA).

3. Wear PPE according to the level of anticipated contamination when handling visibly soiled patient-care equipment and instruments/devices or that may have been in contact with blood or body fluids (IB/IC).

F. Care of the environment.

1. Establish policies and procedures for routine and targeted cleaning of environmental surfaces as indicated by the level of patient contact and degree of soiling (II).

2. Clean and disinfect surfaces that are likely to be contaminated with pathogens, including those that are in close proximity to the patient and frequently touched surfaces in the patient care environment on a more frequent schedule compared with that for other surfaces (IB).

3. Use EPA-registered disinfectants registered as providing microbiocidal activity against the pathogens most likely to contaminate the patient-care environment. Use in accordance with manufacturer's instructions (IB/IC).

a. Review the efficacy of in-use disinfectants when evidence of continuing transmission of an infectious agent may indicate resistance to the in-use product and change to a more effective disinfectant as indicated (II).

4. In facilities that provide health care to pediatric patients or have waiting areas with children's toys, establish policies and procedures for cleaning and disinfecting toys at regular intervals (IB). Use the following principles in developing this policy and procedures: (II)
   a. Select play toys that can be easily cleaned and disinfected.
   b. Do not permit use of stuffed furry toys if they will be shared.
   c. Clean and disinfect large stationary toys (e.g., climbing equipment) at least weekly and whenever visibly soiled.
   d. If toys are likely to be mouthed, rinse with water after disinfection; alternatively wash in a dishwasher.
   e. When a toy requires cleaning and disinfection, do so immediately or store in a designated labeled container separate from toys that are clean and ready for use.
5. Include multiuse electronic equipment in policies and procedures for preventing contamination and for cleaning and disinfection, especially those items that are used by patients, those used during delivery of patient care, and mobile devices that are moved in and out of patient rooms frequently (IB).

G. Textiles and laundry
1. Handle used textiles and fabrics with minimum agitation to avoid contamination of air, surfaces, and other people (IB/IC).
2. If laundry chutes are used, ensure that they are properly designed, maintained, and used in a manner to minimize dispersion of aerosols from contaminated laundry (IB/IC).

H. Safe injection practices: The following recommendations apply to the use of needles, cannulas that replace needles, and, where applicable, intravenous delivery systems
1. Use aseptic technique to avoid contamination of sterile injection equipment (IA).
2. Do not administer medications from a syringe to multiple patients, even if the needle or cannula on the syringe is changed. Needles, cannulas, and syringes are sterile, single-use items; they should not be reused for another patient nor to access a medication or solution that might be used for a subsequent patient (IA).
3. Use fluid infusion and administration sets for one patient only and dispose appropriately after use. Consider a syringe or needle/cannula contaminated after it has been used to enter or connect to a patient's intravenous infusion bag or administration set (IB).
4. Use single-dose vials for parenteral medications whenever possible (IA).
5. Do not administer medications from single-dose vials or ampules to multiple patients or combine leftover contents for later use (IA).
6. If multidose vials must be used, both the needle or cannula and syringe used to access the multidose vial must be sterile (IA).
7. Do not keep multidose vials in the immediate patient treatment area and store in accordance with the manufacturer's recommendations; discard if sterility is compromised or questionable (IA).
8. Do not use bags or bottles of intravenous solution as a common source of supply for multiple patients (IB).

I. Infection control practices for special lumbar puncture procedures: Wear a surgical mask when placing a catheter or injecting material into the spinal canal or subdural space (IB).

J. Worker safety

Adhere to federal and state requirements for protection of health care personnel from exposure to bloodborne pathogens (IC).

V. Transmission-Based Precautions

A. General principles

1. In addition to Standard Precautions, use Transmission-Based Precautions for patients with documented or suspected infection or colonization with highly transmissible or epidemiologically important pathogens for which additional precautions are needed to prevent transmission (IA).
2. Extend duration of Transmission-Based Precautions for immunosuppressed patients with viral infections due to prolonged shedding of viral agents that may be transmitted to others (IA).

B. Contact Precautions

1. Use Contact Precautions for patients with known or suspected infections or evidence of syndromes that represent an increased risk for contact transmission. For specific recommendations for use of Contact Precautions for colonization or infection with MDROs, see "Multidrug-Resistant Organisms Control and Prevention" section of this appendix.
2. Patient placement
   a. In *acute care hospitals,* place patients who require Contact Precautions in a single-patient room when available (IB).
      When single-patient rooms are in short supply, apply the following principles for making decisions on patient placement:
         Prioritize patients with conditions that may facilitate transmission for single-patient room placement (II).
         Place together in the same room (or cohort) patients who are infected or colonized with the same pathogen and are suitable roommates (IB).
      If it becomes necessary to place a patient who requires Contact Precautions in a room with a patient who is not infected or colonized with the same infectious agent:
         Avoid placing patients on Contact Precautions in the same room with patients who have conditions that may increase the risk of adverse outcome from infection or that may facilitate transmission (II).
         Ensure that patients are physically separated (i.e., >3 feet apart) from each other. Draw the privacy curtain between beds to minimize opportunities for direct contact (II).
         Change protective attire and perform hand hygiene between contact with patients in the same room, regardless of whether one or both patients are on Contact Precautions (IB).
   b. In *long-term care and other residential settings*, make decisions regarding patient placement on a case-by-case basis, balancing infection risks to other patients in the room, the presence of risk factors that increase the likelihood of transmission, and the potential adverse psychological impact on the infected or colonized patient (II).
   c. In *ambulatory settings*, place patients who require Contact Precautions in an examination room or cubicle as soon as possible (II).
3. Use of personal protective equipment
   a. Gloves: Wear gloves whenever touching the patient's intact skin or surfaces and articles in close proximity to the patient. Don gloves on entry into the room or cubicle (IB).
   b. Gowns
      i. Wear a gown whenever it is expected that clothing will have direct contact with the patient or potentially contaminated environmental surfaces or equipment in close proximity to the patient. Don gown on entry into the room or cubicle. Remove gown and follow hand hygiene before leaving the patient-care environment (IB).

ii. After gown removal, ensure that clothing and skin do not contact potentially contaminated environmental surfaces that could result in possible transfer of microorganisms to other patients or environmental surfaces (II).

4. Patient transport
   a. In *acute care hospitals and long-term care and other residential settings*, limit transport and movement of patients outside of the room to medically necessary purposes (II).
   b. When transport or movement in any health care setting is necessary, ensure that infected or colonized areas of the patient's body are contained and covered (II).
   c. Remove and dispose of contaminated PPE and perform hand hygiene prior to transporting patients on Contact Precautions (II).
   d. Don clean PPE to handle the patient at the transport destination (II).
5. Patient-care equipment and instruments/devices
   a. Handle patient-care equipment and instruments/devices according to Standard Precautions (IB/IC).
   b. In *acute care hospitals and long-term care and other residential settings,* use disposable noncritical patient-care equipment or implement patient-dedicated use of such equipment. If common use of equipment for multiple patients is unavoidable, clean and disinfect such equipment before use on another patient (IB).
   c. In *home care settings*
      i. Limit the amount of nondisposable patient-care equipment brought into the home of patients on Contact Precautions. Whenever possible, leave patient-care equipment in the home until discharge from home care services (II).
      ii. If noncritical patient-care equipment cannot remain in the home, clean and disinfect items before taking them from the home using a low- to intermediate-level disinfectant. Alternatively, place contaminated reusable items in a plastic bag for transport and subsequent cleaning and disinfection (II).
   d. In *ambulatory settings*, place contaminated reusable noncritical patient-care equipment in a plastic bag for transport to a utility area for soiled items for reprocessing (II).
6. Environmental measures: Ensure that rooms of patients on Contact Precautions are prioritized for frequent cleaning and disinfection with a focus on frequently touched surfaces and equipment in the immediate vicinity of the patient (IB).
7. Discontinue Contact Precautions after signs and symptoms of the infection have resolved or according to pathogen-specific recommendations (IB).

C. Droplet Precautions

1. Use Droplet Precautions as recommended for patients known or suspected to be infected with pathogens transmitted by respiratory droplets (i.e., large-particle droplets >5mcm in size) that are generated by a patient who is coughing, sneezing, or talking (IB).
2. Patient placement
   a. In acute care hospitals, place patients who require Droplet Precautions in a single-patient room when available (II). When single-patient rooms are in short supply, apply the following principles for making decisions on patient placement:
      i. Prioritize patients who have excessive cough and sputum production for single-patient room placement (II).
      ii. Place together in the same room (or cohort) patients who are infected the same pathogen and are suitable roommates (IB).

iii. If it becomes necessary to place patients who require Droplet Precautions in a room with a patient who does not have the same infection:

- Avoid placing patients on Droplet Precautions in the same room with patients who have conditions that may increase the risk of adverse outcome from infection or that may facilitate transmission (II).
- Ensure that patients are physically separated (i.e., >3 feet apart) from each other. Draw the privacy curtain between beds to minimize opportunities for close contact (IB).
- Change protective attire and perform hand hygiene between contact with patients in the same room, regardless of whether one patient or both patients are on Droplet Precautions (IB).

b. In *long-term care and other residential settings*, make decisions regarding patient placement on a case-by-case basis after considering infection risks to other patients in the room and available alternatives (II).

c. In *ambulatory settings*, place patients who require Droplet Precautions in an examination room or cubicle as soon as possible. Instruct patients to follow recommendations for Respiratory Hygiene/Cough Etiquette (II).

3. Use of personal protective equipment

a. Don a mask on entry into the patient room or cubicle (IB).

b. No recommendation about routinely wearing eye protection, in addition to a mask, for close contact with patients who require Droplet Precautions (Unresolved issue).

c. For patients with suspected or confirmed SARS, avian influenza, or pandemic influenza, refer to the following websites for the most current recommendations:
www.cdc.gov/ncidod/sars/
www.cdc.gov/flu/avian/
www.pandemicflu.gov/

4. Patient transport

a. In *acute care hospitals and long-term care and other residential settings*, limit transport and movement of patients outside of the room to medically necessary purposes (II).

b. If transport or movement in any health care setting is necessary, instruct patient to wear a mask and follow Respiratory Hygiene/Cough Etiquette (IB).

c. No mask is required for persons transporting patients on Droplet Precautions (II).

d. Discontinue Droplet Precautions after signs and symptoms have resolved or according to pathogen-specific recommendations (IB).

D. Airborne Precautions

1. Use Airborne Precautions as recommended for patients known or suspected to be infected with infectious agents transmitted person-to-person by the airborne route (IA/IC).

2. Patient placement

a. In *acute care hospitals and long-term care settings*, place patients who require Airborne Precautions in an AIIR that has been constructed in accordance with current guidelines (IA/IC).

i. Provide at least six (existing facility) or 12 (new construction/renovation) air changes per hour.

ii. Direct exhaust of air to the outside. If it is not possible to exhaust air from an AIIR directly to the outside, the air may be returned to the air-handling system or adjacent spaces if all air is directed through high-efficiency particulate (HEPA) filters.

iii. Whenever an AIIR is in use for a patient on Airborne Precautions, monitor air pressure daily with visual indicators, regardless of the presence of differential pressure sensing devices.

iv. Keep the AIIR door closed when not required for entry and exit.

b. When an AIIR is not available, transfer the patient to a facility that has an available AIIR (II).

c. In the event of an outbreak or exposure involving large numbers of patients who require Airborne Precautions:

i. Consult infection control professionals before patient placement to determine the safety of alternative rooms that do not meet engineering requirements for an AIIR.

ii. Place together (cohort) patients who are presumed to have the same infection (based on clinical presentation and diagnosis when known) in areas of the facility that are away from other patients, especially patients who are at increased risk for infection.

iii. Use temporary portable solutions to create a negative pressure environment in the converted area of the facility. Discharge air directly to the outside, away from people and air intakes, or direct all the air through HEPA filters before it is introduced to other air spaces (II).

d. In *ambulatory settings:*

i. Develop systems to identify patients with known or suspected infections that require Airborne Precautions upon entry into ambulatory settings (IA).

ii. Place the patient in an AIIR as soon as possible. If an AIIR is not available, place a surgical mask on the patient and place him/her in an examination room. After the patient leaves, the room should remain vacant for the appropriate time, generally 1 hour, to allow for a full exchange of air (IB/IC).

iii. Instruct patients with a known or suspected airborne infection to wear a surgical mask and observe Respiratory Hygiene/Cough Etiquette. After placement in an AIIR, the mask may be removed; the mask should remain on if the patient is not in an AIIR (IB/IC).

3. Personnel restrictions

Restrict susceptible health care personnel from entering the rooms of patients known or suspected to have measles (rubeola), varicella (chickenpox), disseminated herpes zoster, or smallpox if other immune health care personnel are available (IB).

4. Use of PPE

a. Wear a fit-tested NIOSH-approved N95 or higher level respirator for respiratory protection when entering the room or home of a patient when the following diseases are suspected or confirmed:

i. Infectious pulmonary or laryngeal tuberculosis or when infectious tuberculosis skin lesions are present and procedures that would aerosolize viable organisms are performed (IB).

ii. Smallpox (vaccinated and unvaccinated). Respiratory protection is recommended for all health care personnel, including those with a documented "take" after smallpox vaccination due to the risk of a genetically engineered virus against which the vaccine may not provide protection, or of exposure to a very large viral load (II).

b. No recommendation is made regarding the use of PPE by health care personnel who are presumed to be immune to measles (rubeola) or varicella-zoster based on history of disease, vaccine, or serologic testing when caring for an individual with known or suspected measles, chickenpox or disseminated herpes zoster, due to difficulties in establishing definite immunity (Unresolved issue).

c. No recommendation is made regarding the type of personal protective equipment to be worn by susceptible health care personnel who must have contact with patients with known or suspected measles, chickenpox, or disseminated herpes zoster (Unresolved issue).

5. Patient transport

a. In *acute care hospitals and long-term care and other residential settings*, limit transport and movement of patients outside the room to medically necessary purposes (II).

b. If transport or movement outside an AIIR is necessary, instruct patients to wear a surgical mask, if possible, and observe Respiratory Hygiene/Cough Etiquette (II).

c. For patients with skin lesions associated with varicella or smallpox or draining skin lesions caused by *M. tuberculosis*, cover the affected areas to prevent aerosolization or contact with the infectious agent in skin lesions (II).

d. Health care personnel transporting patients who are on Airborne Precautions do not need to wear a mask or respirator during transport if the patient is wearing a mask and infectious skin lesions are covered (II).

6. Exposure management

a. Immunize or provide the appropriate immune globulin to susceptible persons as soon as possible following unprotected contact to a patient with measles, varicella, or smallpox (IA):

b. Administer measles vaccine to exposed susceptible persons within 72 hours after the exposure or administer immune globulin within 6 days of the exposure event for high-risk persons in whom vaccine is contraindicated.

c. Administer varicella vaccine to exposed susceptible persons within 120 hours after the exposure or administer varicella immune globulin (VZIG or alternative product), when available, within 96 hours for high-risk persons in whom vaccine is contraindicated.

d. Administer smallpox vaccine to exposed susceptible persons within 4 days after exposure.

7. Discontinue Airborne Precautions according to pathogen-specific recommendations (IB).

8. Consult CDC's *"Guidelines for Preventing the Transmission of* Mycobacterium tuberculosis *in Health-Care Settings, 2005"* and the *"Guideline for Environmental Infection Control in Health Care Facilities"* for additional guidance on environment strategies for preventing transmission of tuberculosis in health care settings. The environmental recommendations in these guidelines may be applied to patients with other infections that require Airborne Precautions.

VI. Protective Environment

A. Place allogeneic hemopoietic stem cell transplant (HSCT) patients in a Protective Environment as described in the *"Guideline to Prevent Opportunistic Infections in HSCT Patients,"* the *"Guideline for Environmental Infection Control in Health-Care Facilities"*, and the *"Guidelines for Preventing Health-Care-Associated Pneumonia, 2003"* to reduce exposure to environmental fungi (e.g., *Aspergillus* spp.) (IB).

B. No recommendation for placing patients with other medical conditions that are associated with increased risk for environmental fungal infections in a Protective Environment (Unresolved issue).

C. For patients who require a Protective Environment, implement the following:

1. Environmental controls

a. Filtered incoming air using central or point-of-use HEPA filters capable of removing 99.97% of particles >0.3 mcm in diameter (IB).

b. Directed room airflow with the air supply on one side of the room that moves air across the patient bed and out through an exhaust on the opposite side of the room (IB).

c. Positive air pressure in room relative to the corridor (pressure differential of >12.5 Pa [0.01 in water gauge]) (IB).

i. Monitor air pressure daily with visual indicators (IA).

d. Well-sealed rooms that prevent infiltration of outside air (IB).

e. At least 12 air changes per hour (IB).

2. Lower dust levels by using smooth nonporous surfaces and finishes that can be scrubbed, rather than textured material. Wet dust horizontal surfaces whenever dust is detected and routinely clean crevices and sprinkler heads where dust may accumulate (II).

3. Avoid carpeting in hallways and patient rooms in areas (IB).

4. Prohibit dried and fresh flowers and potted plants (II).

D. Minimize the length of time that patients who require a Protective Environment are outside their rooms for diagnostic procedures and other activities (IB).

E. During periods of buiding construction, to prevent inhalation of respirable particles that could contain infectious spores, provide respiratory protection (e.g., N95 respirator) to patients who are medically fit to tolerate a respirator when they are required to leave the Protective Environment (II).

F. Use of Standard and Transmission-Based Precautions in a Protective Environment.

1. Use Standard Precautions as recommended for all patient interactions (IA).

2. Implement Droplet and Contact Precautions as recommended for specific diseases. Transmission-Based precautions for viral infections may need to be prolonged because of the patient's immunocompromised state and prolonged shedding of viruses (IB).

3. Barrier precautions are not required for health care personnel in the absence of suspected or confirmed infection in the patient or if they are not indicated according to Standard Precautions (II).

4. Implement Airborne Precautions for patients who require a Protective Environment room and who also have an airborne infectious disease (IA).

a. Ensure that the Protective Environment is designed to maintain positive pressure (IB).

b. Use an anteroom to further support the appropriate air-balance relative to the corridor and the Protective Environment; provide independent exhaust of contaminated air to the outside or place a HEPA filter in the exhaust duct if the return air must be recirculated (IB).

c. If an anteroom is not available, place the patient in an AIIR and use portable, industrial-grade HEPA filters in the room to enhance filtration of spores (II).

SAFE DONNING AND REMOVAL OF PERSONAL PROTECTIVE EQUIPMENT (PPE)

Donning PPE

GOWN

- Fully cover torso from neck to knees, arms to end of wrist, and wrap around the back.

Mask or Respirator

- Secure ties or elastic band at middle of head and neck.
- Fit flexible band to nose bridge.
- Fit snug to face and below chin.
- Fit-check respirator.

Goggles/Face Shield
- Put on face and adjust to fit.

Gloves
- Use nonsterile gloves for isolation.
- Select according to hand size.
- Extend to cover wrist of isolation gown.

Safe Work Practices
- Keep hands away from face.
- Work from clean to dirty.
- Limit surfaces touched.
- Change when torn or heavily contaminated.
- Perform hand hygiene.

Removing PPE
Remove PPE at doorway before leaving patient room or in anteroom
Gloves
- Remember outside of gloves are contaminated!
- Grasp outside of glove with opposite gloved hand; peel off.
- Hold glove removed in gloved hand.
- Slide fingers of ungloved hand under remaining glove at wrist.

Goggles/Face Shield
- Remember outside of goggles or face shield are contaminated!
- To remove, handle by "clean" head band or ear pieces.
- Place in designated receptacle for reprocessing or in waste container.

Gown
- Remember gown front and sleeves are contaminated!
- Unfasten neck, then waist ties.
- Remove gown using a peeling motion; pull gown from each shoulder toward the same hand.
- Gown will turn inside out.
- Hold removed gown away from body, roll into a bundle, and discard into waste or linen receptacle.

Mask or Respirator
- Remember front of mask/respirator is contaminated—DO NOT TOUCH!
- Grasp ONLY bottom then top ties/elastics and remove.
- Discard in waste container.

Hand Hygiene
Perform hand hygiene immediately after removing all PPE!

Adapted extensively from Siegel JD, Rhinehart E, Jackson M, Chiarello L, and the Healthcare Infection Control Practices Advisory Committee, *2007 Guideline for Isolation Precautions: Preventing Transmission of Infectious Agents in Health care Settings,* June 22, 2007 (http://www.cdc.gov/ncidod/dhqp/pdf/guidelines/Isolation2007.pdf).

MULTIDRUG-RESISTANT ORGANISMS CONTROL AND PREVENTION

Multidrug-resistant organisms (MDROs) including methicillin-resistant *Staphylococcus aureus* (MRSA), vancomycin-resistant enterococci (VRE), and certain gram-negative bacilli (GNB) have important infection control implications that either have not been addressed or received only limited consideration in previous isolation guidelines. Although transmission of MDROs is most frequently documented in acute care facilities, all health care settings are affected by the emergence and transmission of antimicrobial-resistant microbes. The severity and extent of disease caused by these pathogens vary by the population(s) affected and by the institution(s) in which they are found. Institutions, in turn, vary widely in physical and functional characteristics, ranging from long-term care facilities (LTCFs) to specialty units (e.g., intensive care units [ICUs], burn units, neonatal ICUs [NICUs]) in teritary care facilities. Because of this, the approaches to prevention and control of these pathogens need to be tailored to the specific needs of each population and individual institution. The prevention and control of MDROs are a national priority—one that requires all health care facilities and agencies assume responsibility.

MDRO Definition

For epidemiologic purposes, MDROs are defined as microorganisms, predominantly bacteria, that are resistant to one or more classes of antimicrobial agents. Although the names of certain MDROs describe resistance to only one agent (e.g., MRSA, VRE), these pathogens are frequently resistant to most available antimicrobial agents. These highly resistant organisms deserve special attention in health care facilities. Certain GNB, including those producing extended spectrum beta-lactamases (ESBLs) and others that are resistant to multiple classes of antimicrobial agents, are of particular concern:

- *Escherichia coli*
- *Klebsiella pneumoniae*
- Strains of *Acinetobacter baumannii* resistant to all antimicrobial agents, or all except imipenem
- *Stenotrophomonas maltophilia*
- *Burkholderia cepacia*
- *Ralstonia pickettii*
- *Streptococcus pneumoniae* (MDRSP) resistant to penicillin, macrolides, and fluoroquinolones, in long-term care facilities (LTCFs)
- Strains of *Staphylococcus aureus* that have intermediate susceptibility or are resistant to vancomycin (i.e., vancomycin-intermediate *S. aureus* [VISA], vancomycin-resistant *S. aureus* [VRSA]) in hemodialysis patients.

Clinical Importance of MDROs

- Increased lengths of stay, costs, and mortality have been associated with MDROs.
- In most instances, MDRO infections have clinical manifestations that are similar to infections caused by susceptible pathogens.
- Options for treating patients with these infections are often extremely limited.
- Antimicrobials are now available for treatment of MRSA and VRE infections, but resistance to each new agent has already emerged in clinical isolates.

Therapeutic options are limited for:

- ESBL-producing isolates of gram-negative bacilli
- Strains of *Acinetobacter baumannii* resistant to all antimicrobial agents except imipenem
- Intrinsically resistant *Stenotrophomonas* spp.

These limitations may influence antibiotic usage patterns in ways that suppress normal flora and create a favorable environment for development of colonization when exposed to potential MDR pathogens (i.e., selective advantage).

MRSA may behave differently from other MDROs.

Compared with MSSA patients, MRSA-colonized patients more frequently develop symptomatic infections and have higher case fatality rates in bacteremia, poststernotomy mediastinitis, and surgical site infections.

These outcomes may be a result of:

- Delays in the administration of vancomycin
- The relative decrease in the bactericidal activity of vancomycin, or
- Persistent bacteremia associated with intrinsic characteristics of certain MRSA strains
- Mortality may be increased further by *S. aureus* with reduced vancomycin susceptibility

Important Concepts in Transmission

After MDROs have been introduced into a health care setting, transmission and persistence of the resistant strain are determined by:

- The availability of vulnerable patients
- Selective pressure exerted by antimicrobial use
- Increased potential for transmission from larger numbers of colonized or infected patients ("colonization pressure")
- The impact of implementation and adherence to prevention efforts

Patients vulnerable to colonization and infection include those with:

- Severe disease, especially those with compromised host defenses from underlying medical conditions
- Recent surgery
- Indwelling medical devices (e.g., urinary catheter or endotracheal tubes)
- Hospitalized patients, especially ICU patients, tend to have more risk factors than nonhospitalized patients, and also have the highest infection rates
- Increasing numbers of infections with MDROs also have been reported in the non-ICU areas of hospitals

Ample epidemiologic evidence suggests that MDROs are carried from one person to another via the hands of health care providers. Without adherence to published recommendations for hand hygiene and glove use, health care providers are more likely to transmit MDROs to patients. Thus, strategies to increase and monitor adherence are important components of MDRO control programs.

Opportunities for transmission of MDROs beyond the acute care hospital result from:

- Patients receiving care at multiple health care facilities
- Moving between acute-care, ambulatory, and/or chronic care, and long-term care environments

Role of Colonized Health Care Provider in MDRO Transmission

Factors implicated in transmission include:

- Chronic sinusitis
- Upper respiratory infection
- Dermatitis

Rarely, a Health Care Provider may introduce an MDRO into a patient care unit. Occasionally, Health Care Providers may become persistently colonized with an MDRO, but these Health Care Providers have a limited role in transmission, unless other factors are present.

MDRO Surveillance

Surveillance is a critically important component of any MDRO control program:

- Allows detection of newly emerging pathogens
- Monitors epidemiologic trends
- Measures the effectiveness of interventions

Multiple MDRO surveillance strategies have been employed, ranging from surveillance of clinical microbiology laboratory results obtained as part of routine clinical care to use of active surveillance culture (ASC) to detect asymptomatic colonization.

Adapted extensively from *Management of Multidrug-Resistant Organisms in Healthcare Settings, 2006* (www.cdc.gov/ncidod/dhqp/pdf/ar/mdroGuideline2006.pdf).

MDRO Control

The CDC Campaign to Prevent Antimicrobial Resistance provides 4 strategies compartmented into 12 steps specific to each of 5 target populations: Long-Term Care (LTC), Surgical Patients, Dialysis Patients, Hospitalized Children, and Hospitalized Adults.

Strategies:

- **Prevent Infection**
- **Diagnose and Treat Infection Effectively**
- **Use Antimicrobials Wisely**
- **Prevent Transmission**

Long-Term Care Residents

Prevent Infection

Step 1. Vaccinate

- Give influenza and pneumococcal vaccinations to residents
- Promote vaccination among all staff

Step 2. Prevent Conditions That Lead to Infection

- Prevent aspiration
- Prevent pressure ulcers
- Maintain hydration

Step 3. Get the Unnecessary Devices Out

- Insert catheters and devices only when essential and minimize duration of exposure
- Use proper insertion and catheter-care protocols
- Reassess catheters regularly
- Remove catheters and other devices when no longer essential

Diagnose and Treat Infection Effectively

Step 4. Use Established Criteria for Diagnosis of Infection

- Target empiric therapy to likely pathogens
- Target definitive therapy to known pathogens
- Obtain appropriate cultures and interpret results with care
- Consider *C. difficile* in patients with diarrhea who received antibiotic therapy

Step 5. Use Local Resources

- Consult infectious disease experts for complicated infections and potential outbreaks
- Know your local and/or regional data
- Get previous microbiology data for transfer residents

Use Antimicrobials Wisely

Step 6. Know When to Say "No"

- Minimize use of broad-spectrum antibiotics
- Avoid long-term antimicrobial prophylaxis
- Develop a system to monitor antibiotic use and provide feedback to appropriate personnel

Step 7. Treat Infection, Not Colonization or Contamination

- Perform proper antisepsis with culture collection
- Reevaluate the need for continued therapy after 48 to 72 hours
- Do not treat asymptomatic bacteriuria

Step 8. Stop Antimicrobial Treatment

- When cultures are negative and infection in unlikely
- When infection has resolved

Prevent Transmission

Step 9. Isolate the Pathogen

- Use Standard Precautions
- Contain infectious body fluids (use approved droplet and contact isolation precautions)

Step 10. Break the Chain of Contagion

- Follow CDC recommendations for work restrictions and stay home when sick
- Cover your mouth when you cough or sneeze
- Educate staff, residents, and families
- Promote wellness in staff and residents

Step 11. Perform Hand Hygiene

- Use alcohol-based handrubs or wash your hands
- Encourage staff and visitors to do the same

Step 12. Identify Residents with Multidrug-Resistant Organisms (MDROs)

- Identify both new admissions and existing residents with MDROs
- Follow standard recommendations for MDRO case management

Surgical Patients

Prevent Infection

Step 1. Prevent Surgical Site Infections

- Monitor and maintain normal glycemia
- Maintain normothermia
- Perform proper skin preparation using appropriate antiseptic agent and, when necessary, hair removal techniques
- Think "outside the wound" to stop surgical site infections

Step 2. Prevent Device-Related Infections: Get the Devices Out

- Use catheters only when essential

- Use proper insertion and catheter-care protocols
- Use drains appropriately
- Remove catheters and drains when they are no longer essential

Step 3. Prevent Hospital-Acquired Pneumonia
- Wean from the ventilator when appropriate
- Elevate head of bed to 30 degrees
- Drain circuit/tubing condensate away from patient
- Prevent contamination of respiratory therapy equipment, ventilator circuits, and respiratory medications

Diagnose and Treat Infection Effectively

Step 4. Target the Pathogen
- Target empiric antimicrobial therapy to likely pathogens
- Obtain appropriate cultures
- Target definitive antimicrobial therapy to known pathogens
- Optimize timing, regimen, dose, route, and duration of antimicrobial therapy
- Practice safe source control (e.g. débridement, or open wound as indicated)

Step 5. Access the Experts
- Consult the appropriate expert for complicated infections: surgeons, infectious disease experts, and clinical pharmacists

Use Antimicrobials Wisely

Step 6. Start Prophylactic Antimicrobials Promptly
- Give the initial dose within 1 hour preceding incision
- Use the appropriate antimicrobial and dosage
- Repeat the dose during surgery as needed to maintain blood levels

Step 7. Stop Prophylactic Antimicrobials Within 24 Hours
- Discontinue use even when catheters or drains are still in place

Step 8. Use Local Data
- Know your antibiogram
- Know your formulary
- Know your patient population

Step 9. Know When to Say "No" to Vancomycin
- Vancomycin should be used to treat known infections, not for routine prophylaxis
- Treat staphylococcal infection, not contaminants or colonization
- Consider other antimicrobials in treating MRSA

Step 10. Treat Infection, not Contamination or Colonization
- Use proper antisepsis for drawing blood cultures
- Get at least one peripheral vein blood culture, if possible
- Avoid culturing vascular catheter tips
- Treat bacteremia, not the catheter tip

Prevent Transmission

Step 11. Contain Your Contaminant and Contagion
- Follow infection control precautions
- Consult infection control teams

Step 12. Practice Hand Hygiene
- Set an example
- Wash your hands or use an alcohol-based handrub
- Do not operate with open sores on hands
- Do not operate with artificial nails
- Promote good hygiene habits for the entire surgical team

Dialysis Patients

Prevent Infection

Step 1. Vaccinate Staff and Patients
- Get influenza vaccine
- Give influenza and pneumococcal vaccine to patients in addition to routine vaccines (e.g., hepatitis B)

Step 2. Get the Catheters Out

Hemodialysis
- Use catheters only when essential
- Maximize use of fistulae/grafts
- Remove catheters when they are no longer essential

Peritoneal Dialysis
- Remove/replace infected catheters

Step 3. Optimize Access Care
- Follow established Kidney Disease Outcomes Quality Initiative and CDC Guidelines for access care
- Use proper insertion and catheter-care protocols
- Remove access device when infected
- Use the correct catheter

Diagnose and Treat Infection Effectively

Step 4. Target the Pathogen
- Obtain appropriate cultures
- Target empiric therapy to likely pathogens
- Target definitive therapy to known pathogens
- Optimize timing, regimen, dose, route, and duration

Step 5. Access the Experts
- Consult the appropriate expert for complicated infections

Use Antimicrobials Wisely

Step 6. Use Local Data
- Know your local antibiogram
- Get previous microbiology results when patients transfer to your facility

Step 7. Know When To Say "No" To Vancomycin
- Follow CDC guidelines for vancomycin use
- Consider 1st generation cephalosporins instead of vancomycin

Step 8. Treat Infection, Not Contamination or Colonization

- Use proper antisepsis for drawing blood cultures
- Get one peripheral vein blood culture, if possible
- Avoid culturing vascular catheter tips
- Treat bacteremia, not the catheter tip

Step 9. Stop Antimicrobial Treatment

- When infection is treated
- When infection is not diagnosed

Prevent transmission

Step 10. Follow Infection Control Precautions

- Use standard infection control precautions for dialysis centers
- Consult local infection control experts

Step 11. Practice Hand Hygiene

- Wash your hands or use an alcohol-based handrub
- Set an example

Step 12. Partner with Your Patients

- Educate on access care and infection control measures
- Reeducate regularly

<u>**Hospitalized Children**</u>

Prevent Infection

Step 1. Vaccinate Hospitalized Children and Staff

- Vaccinate according to recommendations from the American Academy of Pediatrics Advisory Committee on Immunization Practices and the American Academy of Family Physicians
- Review immunization records and catch-up with routine vaccinations
- Give influenza vaccine to at-risk infants and children
- Give influenza vaccine to all health care personnel

Step 2. Get the Devices Out

- Insert catheters and devices only when essential
- Use proper insertion techniques and follow guidelines for catheter care
- Remove catheters and other devices when no longer essential

Diagnose and Treat Infection Effectively

Step 3. Use Appropriate Methods for Diagnosis

- Order appropriate laboratory tests
- Obtain appropriate specimens

Step 4. Target the Pathogen

- Target empiric antimicrobial therapy to likely pathogens
- Target definitive antimicrobial therapy to known pathogens

Step 5. Access the Experts

- Consult infectious disease experts for complicated infections

Use Antimicrobials Wisely

Step 6. Practice Antimicrobial Control

- Optimize timing, regimen, dose, route, and duration of antimicrobial treatment and prophylaxis
- Follow policies and protocols in your institution

Step 7. Use Local Data

- Know your regional, institutional, and high-risk unit-specific antibiograms
- Know your formulary
- Know your patient population (birth weight, age, and setting)

Step 8. Treat Infection, Not Contamination or Colonization

- Use proper antisepsis for drawing blood cultures
- Avoid routine culturing of catheter tips
- Treat bacteremia, not catheter colonization or contamination

Step 9. Know When To Say "No"

- Avoid routine use of vancomycin, extended-spectrum cephalosporins, (third [ceftriaxone, cefotaxime] and fourth [cefepime] generation cephalosporins), carbapenems, oral quinolones, and linezolid
- Follow antimicrobial prescribing guidelines from CDC, American Academy of Pediatrics, and other professional societies

Step 10. Stop Treatment

- When infection is unlikely
- When culture results indicate no clinical need for antimicrobials
- When infection is cured

Prevent Transmission

Step 11. Practice Infection Control

- Restrict visitors with symptoms of respiratory or gastrointestinal tract infections from contact with your patients

Step 12. Practice Hand Hygiene

- Wash your hands or use an alcohol-based hand rub before and after patient contact
- Set an example

<u>Hospitalized Adults</u>

Prevent Infection

Step 1. Vaccinate

- Give influenza/pneumococcal vaccine to at-risk patients before discharge
- Get influenza vaccine annually

Step 2. Get the Catheters Out

- Use catheters only when essential
- Use the correct catheter
- Use proper insertion and catheter-care protocols
- Remove catheters when they are no longer essential

Diagnose and Treat Infection Effectively

Step 3. Target the Pathogen

- Culture the patient
- Target empiric therapy to likely pathogens and local antibiogram
- Target definitive therapy to known pathogens and antimicrobial susceptibility test results

Step 4. Access the Experts

- Consult infectious diseases experts for patients with serious infections

Use Antimicrobials Wisely

Step 5. Practice Antimicrobial Control

- Engage in local antimicrobial control efforts

Step 6. Use Local Data

- Know your antibiogram
- Know your patient population

Step 7. Treat Infection, Not Contamination

- Use proper antisepsis for blood and other cultures
- Culture the blood, not the skin or catheter hub
- Use proper methods to obtain and process all cultures

Step 8. Treat Infection, Not Colonization

- Treat pneumonia, not the tracheal aspirate
- Treat bacteremia, not the catheter tip or hub
- Treat urinary tract infection, not the indwelling catheter

Step 9. Know When to Say "No" to Vancomycin

- Treat infection, not contaminants or colonization
- Fever in a patient with an intravenous catheter is not a routine indication for vancomycin

Step 10. Stop Antimicrobial Treatment:

- When infection is cured
- When cultures are negative and infection is unlikely
- When infection is not diagnosed

Prevent Transmission

Step 11. Isolate the Pathogen

- Use standard infection control precautions
- Contain infectious body fluids (follow airborne, droplet, and contact precautions)
- When in doubt, consult infection control experts

Step 12. Break the Chain of Contagion

- Stay home when you are sick
- Keep your hands clean
- Set an example

Adapted from http://www.cdc.gov/drugresistance/healthcare/default.htm.

Notifiable Infectious Diseases

AUSTRALIA

Acquired immunodeficiency syndrome (AIDS)
Anthrax
Australian bat lyssavirus
Barmah Forest virus infection
Botulism
Brucellosis
Campylobacteriosis (not notified in New South Wales)
Chlamydial infection
Cholera
Congenital rubella syndrome
Congenital syphilis
Creutzfeldt-Jakob disease (CJD)
Creutzfeldt-Jakob disease variant (vCJD)
Cryptosporidiosis
Dengue virus
Diphtheria
Donovanosis
Flavivirus infection, unspecified or not otherwise classified
Gonococcal infection
Haemolytic uraemic syndrome (HUS)
Haemophilus influenzae serotype b (Hib) (invasive only)
Hepatitis A
Hepatitis B newly acquired hepatitis B unspecified
Hepatitis C newly acquired hepatitis C unspecified
Hepatitis D
Hepatitis E
Hepatitis–not otherwise specified (not notified in Western Australia)
Human immunodeficiency virus (HIV) infection –individuals less than 18 months of age
Human immunodeficiency virus (HIV) infection –newly acquired
Human immunodeficiency virus (HIV) infection– unspecified individuals over 18 months of age
Influenza laboratory–confirmed
Japanese encephalitis virus infection
Kunjin virus infection
Legionellosis
Leprosy (Hansen disease)
Leptospirosis
Listeriosis
Lyssavirus unspecified
Malaria
Measles
Meningococcal disease (invasive)
Mumps
Murray Valley encephalitis virus infection (notified as Australian arboencephalitis in Victoria)
Pertussis (whooping cough)
Plague
Pneumococcal disease (invasive)
Poliomyelitis—wild type and vaccine-associated
Psittacosis (ornithosis)
Q fever
Rabies
Ross River virus infection
Rubella
Salmonellosis
Severe acute respiratory syndrome (SARS)
Shiga toxin and verocytotoxin-producing *Escherichia coli* (STEC/VTEC)
Shigellosis
Smallpox
Syphilis—infectious (primary, secondary and early latent), less than 2 years duration
Syphilis—more than 2 years or unknown duration
Tetanus
Tuberculosis
Tularemia
Typhoid
Varicella infection (chickenpox)
Varicella infection (unspecified)
Varicella zoster infection
Viral haemorrhagic fevers (quarantinable)
Yellow fever

Adapted from Australian National Notifiable Diseases List and Case Definitions (http://www.health.gov.au/internet/wcms/publishing.nsf/Content/cda_surveil-nndss-dislist.htm#dislist).

CANADA

Diseases Preventable by Routine Vaccination/Maladies évitables par une vaccination systématique

Acute flaccid paralysis/paralysie flasque aiguë
Diphtheria/Diphtérie
Invasive *Haemophilus influenzae* type b disease /Maladie invasive due à *Haemophilus influenzae* type b
Hepatitis B/Hépatite B
Measles/Rougeole
Mumps/Oreillons
Pertussis/Coqueluche
Poliomyelitis/Poliomyélite
Rubella/Rubéole
Congenital rubella syndrome/Rubéole congénitale
Tetanus/Tétanos

Sexually Transmitted and Bloodborne Pathogens/Pathogènes transmis sexuellement et pathogènes à diffusion hématogène

AIDS/Sida
Chlamydial infection, genital/Chlamydiose génitale
Creutzfeld-Jakob Disease (CJD) /Maladie de Creutzfeldt-Jakob (MCJ)
Gonorrhea/Gonorrhée
Hepatitis C/Hépatite
Human immunodeficiency virus (HIV) Infection/ Virus de l'immunodéficience humaine (VIH)
Syphilis, congenital/Syphilis, congénitale
Syphilis, infectious (includes syphilis primary, secondary and early latent /Syphilis infectieuse (incluent syphilis primaire, secondaire et latente précose)
Syphilis, other/Syphilis, autres

Diseases Transmitted by Direct Contact and Respiratory Routes/Maladies transmises par contact direct et par voie

Chickenpox/Varicelle
Group B streptococcal disease of the newborn/Maladie streptococcique groupe B chez les nouveauxnés
Hantavirus pulmonary syndrome/Syndrome pulmonaire à hantavirus
Influenza, laboratory confirmed/Grippe confirmée en laboratoire
Invasive group A streptococcal disease/Maladie streptococcique invasive groupe A
Invasive pneumococcal disease/Pneumococcie invasive
Legionellosis/Légionellose
Leprosy/Lèpre
Invasive meningococcal disease/Méningococcie invasive
Tuberculosis/Tuberculose

Enteric, Food and Waterborne Diseases/Entéropagies et maladies d'origine hydrique et alimentaire

Botulism/Botulisme
Campylobacteriosis/Campylobactériose
Cholera/Choléra
Cryptosporidiosis/Cryptosporidiose
Cyclosporiasis/Cyclosporiase
Giardiasis/Giardiase
Hepatitis A/Hépatite A
Salmonellosis/Salmonellose
Shigellosis/Shigellose
Typhoid/Typhoïde
Verotoxigenic *Escherichia coli/Escherichia coli* vérotoxigènes

Vectorborne and Other Zoonotic Diseases/Maladies à transmission vectorielle et autres zoönoses

Brucellosis/Brucellose
Malaria/Paludisme
Plague /Peste
Rabies/Rage
Yellow Fever/Fièvre jaune

Bioterrorism Agents/Agents bioterroristes

Anthrax/Charbon
Smallpox/Variole
Tularemia/Tularémie
Viral hemorrhagic fevers/Fièvres hémorrhagiques virales

Reporting and notification options available at Public Health Agency Canada Notifiable Diseases On-Line: http://dsol-smed.phac-aspc.gc.ca/dsol-smed/ndis/index_e.html.

Adapted from Public Health Agency of Canada, Notifiable Disease Monthly Report, December, 2006 (http://www.phac-aspc.gc.ca/bid-bmi/dsd-dsm/ndmr-rmmdo/pdf/2006/dec06.pdf).

UNITED KINGDOM

Acute encephalitis
Acute poliomyelitis
Anthrax
Cholera
Diphtheria
Dysentery
Food poisoning
Leptospirosis
Malaria
Measles
Meningitis
- meningococcal
- pneumococcal
- *Haemophilus influenzae*
- viral
- other specified
- unspecified

Meningococcal septicaemia (without meningitis)
Mumps
Ophthalmia neonatorum
Paratyphoid fever
Plague
Rabies
Relapsing fever
Rubella
Scarlet fever
Smallpox
Tetanus
Tuberculosis
Typhoid fever
Typhus fever
Viral haemorrhagic fever
Viral hepatitis
- hepatitis A
- hepatitis B
- hepatitis C
- other

Whooping cough
Yellow fever
Leprosy is also notifiable, but directly to the Health Protection Agency Centre for Infections, Information and Technology Department

Adapted from Diseases Notifiable (to Local Authority Proper Officers) under the Public Health (Infectious Diseases) Regulations 1988 [Reviewed on 18 January 2006] (http://www.hpa.org.uk/infections/topics_az/noids/noidlist.htm).

UNITED STATES

Acquired immunodeficiency syndrome (AIDS)
Anthrax
Arboviral neuroinvasive and nonneuroinvasive diseases
- California serogroup virus disease
- Eastern equine encephalitis virus disease
- Powassan virus disease
- St. Louis encephalitis virus disease
- West Nile virus disease
- Western equine encephalitis virus disease

Botulism
- botulism, foodborne
- botulism, infant
- botulism, other (wound and unspecified)

Brucellosis
Chancroid
Chlamydia trachomatis genital infections
Cholera
Coccidioidomycosis
Cryptosporidiosis
Cyclosporiasis
Diphtheria
Ehrlichiosis
- ehrlichiosis, human granulocytic
- ehrlichiosis, human monocytic
- ehrlichiosis, human, other or unspecified agent

Giardiasis
Gonorrhea
Haemophilus influenzae, invasive disease
Hansen disease (leprosy)
Hantavirus pulmonary syndrome
Hemolytic uremic syndrome, postdiarrheal
Hepatitis, viral, acute
- hepatitis A, acute
- hepatitis B, acute
- hepatitis B virus, perinatal infection
- hepatitis, C, acute

Hepatitis, viral, chronic
- chronic Hepatitis B
- hepatitis C virus infection (past or present)

HIV infection
- HIV infection, adult(≥13 years)
- HIV infection, pediatric (<13 years)

Influenza-associated pediatric mortality
Legionellosis
Listeriosis
Lyme disease
Malaria
Measles
Meningococcal disease
Mumps
Novel influenza A virus infections
Pertussis
Plague
Poliomyelitis, paralytic
Poliovirus infection, nonparalytic
Psittacosis
Q Fever
Rabies
- rabies, animal
- rabies, human

Rocky Mountain spotted fever
Rubella
- rubella, congenital syndrome

Salmonellosis
Severe acute respiratory syndrome-associated coronavirus (SARS-CoV) disease
Shiga toxin-producing *Escherichia coli* (STEC)
Shigellosis
Smallpox
Streptococcal disease, invasive, group A
Streptococcal toxic-shock syndrome
Streptococcus pneumoniae, drug resistant, invasive disease *Streptococcus pneumoniae*, invasive in children <5 years
Syphilis
- syphilis, primary
- syphilis, secondary
- syphilis, latent
- syphilis, early latent
- syphilis, late latent
- syphilis, latent, unknown duration
- neurosyphilis
- syphilis, late, nonneurologic
- syphilitic stillbirth
- syphilis, congenital

Tetanus
Toxic-shock syndrome (other than streptococcal)
Trichinellosis (trichinosis)
Tuberculosis
Tularemia
Typhoid fever
Vancomycin-intermediate *Staphylococcus aureus* (VISA)
Vancomycin-resistant *Staphylococcus aureus* (VRSA)
Varicella (morbidity)
- varicella (deaths only)

Vibriosis
Yellow fever

Adapted from Nationally Notifiable Infectious Diseases, United States, 2007, Revised (http://www.cdc.gov/epo/dphsi/PHS/infdis2007r.htm).

OCCUPATIONAL EXPOSURE TO BLOOD

Health care personnel (HCP) may be exposed to hepatitis B virus (HBV), hepatitis C virus (HCV), and human immunodeficiency virus (HIV). Most exposures do not result in infection. Your employer should have in place a system for reporting exposures in order to quickly evaluate the risk of infection, inform you about the treatments available to help prevent infection, monitor you for side effects of treatments, and determine if infection occurs. Your blood and the blood of the source may be tested to properly evaluate and recommend postexposure treatment.

An exposure that might place HCP at risk for HIV infection is defined as a percutaneous injury (e.g., a needlestick or cut with a sharp object) or contact of mucous membrane or nonintact skin (e.g., exposed skin that is chapped, abraded, or afflicted with dermatitis) with blood, tissue, or other body fluids that are potentially infectious. In addition to blood and visibly bloody body fluids, semen and vaginal secretions also are considered potentially infectious. Although semen and vaginal secretions have been implicated in the sexual transmission of HIV, they have not been implicated in occupational transmission from patients to HCP.

The following fluids also are considered potentially infectious:

- cerebrospinal fluid
- synovial fluid
- pleural fluid
- peritoneal fluid
- pericardial fluid
- amniotic fluid

The risk for transmission of HIV infection from these fluids is unknown; the potential risk to HCP from occupational exposures has not been assessed by epidemiologic studies in health care settings.

Feces, nasal secretions, saliva, sputum, sweat, tears, urine, and vomitus are not considered potentially infectious unless they are visibly bloody; the risk for transmission of HIV infection from these fluids and materials is low.

PREVENTING OCCUPATIONAL EXPOSURES

Many needlesticks and other cuts can be prevented by:

Using safer techniques

- Do not recap needles by hand
- Dispose of used needles in appropriate sharps disposal containers
- Use medical devices with safety features designed to prevent injuries

Using appropriate barriers can prevent many exposures to eyes, nose, mouth, or skin:

- Gloves
- Eye and face protection
- Gowns

VACCINATION

All health care personnel who have a reasonable chance of exposure to blood or body fluids should receive hepatitis B vaccine, ideally during the training period. Personnel then should be tested 1 to 2 months after the series completion to make sure the vaccination has provided immunity. No vaccination exists for HCV or HIV.

If an Exposure Occurs

FIRST: (immediately following an exposure to blood)

- Wash needlesticks and cuts with soap and water
- Flush splashes to the nose, mouth, or skin with water
- Irrigate eyes with clean water, saline, or sterile irrigants

(No scientific evidence shows that using antiseptics or squeezing the wound will reduce transmission of a bloodborne pathogen. Using a caustic agent such as bleach is not recommended.)

SECOND:

- Promptly report the exposure to the established department (e.g., infection control or occupational health) responsible for managing exposures to discuss the possible risks of acquiring infection and the need for postexposure treatment.

Treatment for Exposure

HBV: Hepatitis B immune globulin (HBIG) alone or in combination with vaccine (if not previously vaccinated) is effective in preventing HBV infection after exposure. The decision to begin treatment is based on whether:

- The source individual is positive for hepatitis B surface antigen
- You have been vaccinated
- The vaccine provided immunity

HCV: There is no vaccine against hepatitis C and no treatment after an exposure to prevent infection. Neither immune globulin nor antiviral therapy is recommended after exposure. For these reasons, ***preventing percutaneous injuries is imperative.***

HIV: There is no vaccine against HIV. Postexposure prophylaxis (PEP) provides adequate treatment, and there are expanded drug therapies available. The designated occupational exposure department will provide pros and cons of each regimen based on individual exposure, medical conditions, and drug sensitivities and interactions:

Monitoring and Management of PEP Toxicity

- HCP should be monitored for drug toxicity by testing at baseline and again 2 weeks after starting PEP.
- The scope of testing should be based on medical conditions in the exposed person and the toxicity of drugs included in the PEP regimen.
- Minimally, laboratory monitoring for toxicity should include a complete blood count and renal and hepatic function tests.
- Monitoring for evidence of hyperglycemia should be included for HCP whose regimens include any protease inhibitors (PI); if the exposed person is receiving indinavir, monitoring for crystalluria, hematuria, hemolytic anemia, and hepatitis also should be included.
- If toxicity is noted, modification of the regimen should be considered after expert consultation; further diagnostic studies might be indicated.
- Exposed HCP who choose to take PEP should be advised of the importance of completing the prescribed regimen.
- Information should be provided about potential drug interactions and drugs that should not be taken with PEP, side-effects of prescribed drugs, measures to minimize side-effects, and methods of clinical monitoring for toxicity during the follow-up period.

- HCP should be advised that evaluation of certain symptoms (e.g., rash, fever, back or abdominal pain, pain on urination or blood in the urine, or symptoms of hyperglycemia such as increased thirst or frequent urination) should not be delayed.
- HCP often fail to complete the recommended regimen often because they experience side-effects (e.g., nausea or diarrhea). These symptoms often can be managed with antimotility and antiemetic agents or other medications that target specific symptoms without changing the regimen. In other situations, modifying the dose interval (i.e., administering a lower dose of drug more frequently throughout the day, as recommended by the manufacturer) might facilitate adherence to the regimen.
- Serious adverse events should be reported to the U.S. Food and Drug Administration's MedWatch program.
- Although recommendations for follow-up testing, monitoring, and counseling of exposed HCP are unchanged from those published previously, greater emphasis is needed on improving follow-up care provided to exposed HCP. This might result in increased adherence to HIV PEP regimens, better management of associated symptoms with ancillary medications or regimen changes, improved detection of serious adverse effects, and serologic testing among a larger proportion of exposed personnel to determine whether infection is transmitted after occupational exposures.
- Closer follow-up should in turn reassure HCP who become anxious after these events.
- The psychological impact on HCP of needlesticks or exposure to blood or body fluid should not be underestimated.
- Providing HCP with psychologic counseling should be an essential component of the management and care of exposed HCP.

Follow-up After Exposure

HBV

- Because postexposure treatment is highly effective, CDC does not recommend routine follow-up after treatment.
- Any symptoms suggesting hepatitis, such as yellow eyes or skin, loss of appetite, nausea, vomiting, fever, stomach or joint pain, and/or extreme tiredness should be reported to your provider.
- If you receive hepatitis B vaccine, you should be tested 1 to 2 months after completing the vaccine series to determine whether you have responded to the vaccine and are protected.
- Any reaction or adverse health event after getting hepatitis B vaccine should be reported to your health care provider.

HCV

- You should be tested for HCV antibody and liver enzyme levels (alanine aminotransferase) as soon as possible after the exposure. This is the baseline.
- Then another check at 4 to 6 months after exposure.
- If infection is suspected, you can be tested for the virus, HCV RNA, at 4 to 6 weeks after exposure.
- Report any symptoms suggesting hepatitis, as listed here for HBV, to your provider.

HIV

- HCP exposed to a known HIV-positive source should be advised to use precautions (e.g., avoid blood or tissue donations, breast-feeding, or pregnancy) to prevent secondary transmission, especially during the first 6 to 12 weeks postexposure.

- Consider reevalution of exposed HCP 72 hours postexposure, especially after additional information about the exposure or source person becomes available.
- HCP with occupational exposure to HIV should receive follow-up counseling, postexposure testing, and medical evaluation regardless of whether they receive PEP. HIV-antibody testing by enzyme immunoassay should be used to monitor HCP for seroconversion for >6 months after occupational HIV exposure.
- After baseline testing at the time of exposure, follow-up testing could be performed at 6 weeks, 12 weeks, and 6 months after exposure.
- Extended HIV follow-up (e.g., for 12 months) is recommended for HCP who become infected with HCV after exposure to a source coinfected with HIV and HCV.
- Whether extended follow-up is indicated in other circumstances (e.g., exposure to a source coinfected with HIV and HCV in the absence of HCV seroconversion or for exposed persons with a medical history suggesting an impaired ability to mount an antibody response to acute infection) is unclear.
- Although rare instances of delayed HIV seroconversion have been reported, the infrequency of this does not warrant adding to exposed persons' anxiety by routinely extending the duration of postexposure followup. This should not preclude a decision to extend follow-up in a particular situation based on the clinical judgment of a person's health care provider.
- The routine use of direct virus assays (e.g., HIV p24 antigen EIA or tests for HIV ribonucleic acid) to detect infection among exposed HCP usually is not recommended. Despite the ability of direct virus assays to detect HIV infection a few days earlier than EIA, the infrequency of occupational seroconversion and increased costs of these tests do not warrant their routine use in this setting.
- In addition, the relatively high rate of false-positive results of these tests in this setting could lead to unnecessary anxiety or treatment.
- Nevertheless, HIV testing should be performed on any exposed person who has an illness compatible with an acute retroviral syndrome, regardless of the interval since exposure. A person in whom HIV infection is identified should be referred for medical management to a specialist with expertise in HIV treatment and counseling.
- Health care providers caring for persons with occupationally acquired HIV infection can report these cases to CDC at telephone 800-893-0485 or to their state health departments.

HBV-HCV-HIV PEP Resources

PEPline (the National Clinicians' Postexposure Prophylaxis Hotline) is a 24-hour, 7-day-a-week consultation service for clinicians managing occupational exposures. This service is supported by the Health Resources and Services Administration Ryan White CARE Act and the AIDS Education and Training Centers and CDC. PEPline can be contacted by phone at (888) 448-4911 (toll free).

Adapted from Centers for Disease Control and Prevention, National Center for Infectious Diseases, Division of Healthcare Quality Promotion and Division of Viral Hepatitis, National Institute for Occupational Safety and Health, *Exposure to Blood, What Healthcare Personnel Need to Know* (http://www.cdc.gov/ncidod/dhqp/pdf/bbp/Exp_to_Blood.pdf).
Adapted from Centers for Disease Control and Prevention, National Center for Infectious Diseases, Division of Healthcare Quality Promotion, *Updated U.S. Public Health Service Guidelines for the Management of Occupational Exposures to HIV and Recommendations for Postexposure Prophylaxis,* MMWR Recommendations and Reports, September 30, 2005 / 54(RR09);1-17 (http://www.cdc.gov/mmwr/preview/mmwrhtml/rr5409a1.htm).

Guideline for Hand Hygiene in Health Care Settings

Categories

These recommendations are designed to improve hand-hygiene practices of health care workers (HCWs) and to reduce transmission of pathogenic microorganisms to patients and personnel in health-care settings. This guideline and its recommendations are not intended for use in food processing or food-service establishments, and are not meant to replace guidance provided by FDA's Model Food Code.

As in previous CDC/HICPAC guidelines, each recommendation is categorized on the basis of existing scientific data, theoretical rationale, applicability, and economic impact. The CDC/HICPAC system for categorizing recommendations is as follows:

Category IA. Strongly recommended for implementation and strongly supported by well-designed experimental, clinical, or epidemiologic studies.

Category IB. Strongly recommended for implementation and supported by certain experimental, clinical, or epidemiologic studies and a strong theoretical rationale.

Category IC. Required for implementation, as mandated by federal or state regulation or standard.

Category II. Suggested for implementation and supported by suggestive clinical or epidemiologic studies or a theoretical rationale.

No recommendation. Unresolved issue. Practices for which insufficient evidence or no consensus regarding efficacy exist.

Recommendations

1. Indications for handwashing and hand antisepsis
   A. When hands are visibly dirty or contaminated with proteinaceous material or are visibly soiled with blood or other body fluids, wash hands with either a non-antimicrobial soap and water or an antimicrobial soap and water (IA).
   B. If hands are not visibly soiled, use an alcohol based hand rub for routinely decontaminating hands in all other clinical situations described in items 1C–J (IA). Alternatively, wash hands with an antimicrobial soap and water in all clinical situations described in items 1C–J (IB).
   C. Decontaminate hands before having direct contact with patients (IB) (68,400).
   D. Decontaminate hands before donning sterile gloves when inserting a central intravascular catheter (IB).
   E. Decontaminate hands before inserting indwelling urinary catheters, peripheral vascular catheters, or other invasive devices that do not require a surgical procedure (IB).
   F. Decontaminate hands after contact with a patient's intact skin (e.g., when taking a pulse or blood pressure, and lifting a patient) (IB).
   G. Decontaminate hands after contact with body fluids or excretions, mucous membranes, nonintact skin, and wound dressings if hands are not visibly soiled (IA).
   H. Decontaminate hands if moving from a contaminated-body site to a clean-body site during patient care (II).
   I. Decontaminate hands after contact with inanimate objects (including medical equipment) in the immediate vicinity of the patient (II).
   J. Decontaminate hands after removing gloves (IB).
   K. Before eating and after using a restroom, wash hands with a non-antimicrobial soap and water or with an antimicrobial soap and water (IB).
   L. Antimicrobial-impregnated wipes (i.e., towelettes) may be considered as an alternative to washing hands with non-antimicrobial soap and water. Because they are not as effective as alcohol-based hand rubs or washing hands with an antimicrobial soap and water for reducing

bacterial counts on the hands of HCWs, they are not a substitute for using an alcohol-based hand rub or antimicrobial soap (IB).

M. Wash hands with non-antimicrobial soap and water or with antimicrobial soap and water if exposure to *Bacillus anthracis* is suspected or proven. The physical action of washing and rinsing hands under such circumstances is recommended because alcohols, chlorhexidine, iodophors, and other antiseptic agents have poor activity against spores (II).

N. No recommendation can be made regarding the routine use of nonalcohol-based hand rubs for hand hygiene in health-care settings. Unresolved issue.

2. Hand-hygiene technique
   A. When decontaminating hands with an alcohol-based hand rub, apply product to palm of one hand and rub hands together, covering all surfaces of hands and fingers, until hands are dry (IB). Follow the manufacturer's recommendations regarding the volume of product to use.
   B. When washing hands with soap and water, wet hands first with water, apply an amount of product recommended by the manufacturer to hands, and rub hands together vigorously for at least 15 seconds, covering all surfaces of the hands and fingers. Rinse hands with water and dry thoroughly with a disposable towel. Use towel to turn off the faucet (IB). Avoid using hot water, because repeated exposure to hot water may increase the risk of dermatitis (IB).
   C. Liquid, bar, leaflet or powdered forms of plain soap are acceptable when washing hands with a non-antimicrobial soap and water. When bar soap is used, soap racks that facilitate drainage and small bars of soap should be used (II).
   D. Multiple-use cloth towels of the hanging or roll type are not recommended for use in health-care settings (II).

3. Surgical hand antisepsis
   A. Remove rings, watches, and bracelets before beginning the surgical hand scrub (II).
   B. Remove debris from underneath fingernails using a nail cleaner under running water (II).
   C. Surgical hand antisepsis using either an antimicrobial soap or an alcohol-based hand rub with persistent activity is recommended before donning sterile gloves when performing surgical procedures (IB).
   D. When performing surgical hand antisepsis using an antimicrobial soap, scrub hands and forearms for the length of time recommended by the manufacturer, usually 2–6 minutes. Long scrub times (e.g., 10 minutes) are not necessary (IB).
   E. When using an alcohol-based surgical hand-scrub product with persistent activity, follow the manufacturer's instructions. Before applying the alcohol solution, prewash hands and forearms with a non-antimicrobial soap and dry hands and forearms completely. After application of the alcohol-based product as recommended, allow hands and forearms to dry thoroughly before donning sterile gloves (IB).

4. Selection of hand-hygiene agents
   A. Provide personnel with efficacious hand-hygiene products that have low irritancy potential, particularly when these products are used multiple times per shift (IB). This recommendation applies to products used for hand antisepsis before and after patient care in clinical areas and to products used for surgical hand antisepsis by surgical personnel.
   B. To maximize acceptance of hand-hygiene products by HCWs, solicit input from these employees regarding the feel, fragrance, and skin tolerance of any products under consideration. The cost of hand-hygiene products should not be the primary factor influencing product selection (IB).
   C. When selecting non-antimicrobial soaps, antimicrobial soaps, or alcohol-based hand rubs, solicit information from manufacturers regarding any known interactions between products used to clean hands, skin care products, and the types of gloves used in the institution (II).

D. Before making purchasing decisions, evaluate the dispenser systems of various product manufacturers or distributors to ensure that dispensers function adequately and deliver an appropriate volume of product (II).
E. Do not add soap to a partially empty soap dispenser. This practice of "topping off" dispensers can lead to bacterial contamination of soap (IA).

5. Skin care
   A. Provide HCWs with hand lotions or creams to minimize the occurrence of irritant contact dermatitis associated with hand antisepsis or handwashing (IA).
   B. Solicit information from manufacturers regarding any effects that hand lotions, creams, or alcohol-based hand antiseptics may have on the persistent effects of antimicrobial soaps being used in the institution (IB).
6. Other Aspects of Hand Hygiene
   A. Do not wear artificial fingernails or extenders when having direct contact with patients at high risk (e.g., those in intensive-care units or operating rooms) (IA).
   B. Keep natural nails tips less than 1/4-inch long (II).
   C. Wear gloves when contact with blood or other potentially infectious materials, mucous membranes, and nonintact skin could occur (IC).
   D. Remove gloves after caring for a patient. Do not wear the same pair of gloves for the care of more than one patient, and do not wash gloves between uses with different patients (IB).
   E. Change gloves during patient care if moving from a contaminated body site to a clean body site (II).
   F. No recommendation can be made regarding wearing rings in health-care settings. Unresolved issue.
7. Health-care worker educational and motivational programs
   A. As part of an overall program to improve hand-hygiene practices of HCWs, educate personnel regarding the types of patient-care activities that can result in hand contamination and the advantages and disadvantages of various methods used to clean their hands (II).
   B. Monitor HCWs' adherence with recommended hand-hygiene practices and provide personnel with information regarding their performance (IA).
   C. Encourage patients and their families to remind HCWs to decontaminate their hands (II).
8. Administrative measures
   A. Make improved hand-hygiene adherence an institutional priority and provide appropriate administrative support and financial resources (IB).
   B. Implement a multidisciplinary program designed to improve adherence of health personnel to recommended hand-hygiene practices (IB).
   C. As part of a multidisciplinary program to improve hand-hygiene adherence, provide HCWs with a readily accessible alcohol-based hand-rub product (IA).
   D. To improve hand-hygiene adherence among personnel who work in areas in which high workloads and high intensity of patient care are anticipated, make an alcohol-based hand rub available at the entrance to the patient's room or at the bedside, in other convenient locations, and in individual pocket-sized containers to be carried by HCWs (IA).
   E. Store supplies of alcohol-based hand rubs in cabinets or areas approved for flammable materials (IC).

Adapted from Centers for Disease Control and Prevention. Guidelines for Hand Hygine in Health-Care Settings. MMWR 2002; 51(No. RR-16). Available at http://www.cdc.gov/mmwr/preview/mmwrhtml/rr5116a1.htm.

Laboratory Reference Range Values

Michael L. Bishop, MS, MT (ASCP)
Director of Educational Services
Wyndgate Technologies
El Dorado Hills, California

Rebecca J. Laudicina, PhD, Professor
Division of Clinical Laboratory Science
University of North Carolina at Chapel Hill
Chapel Hill, North Carolina

Reference range values are for presumably healthy individuals and frequently overlap significantly with the values for those who are sick. Actual values may vary significantly due to differences in preanalytical variables, assay methodologies, and standardization. Laboratories usually determine their own reference ranges based on the laboratory procedures and methods for their particular patient population; thus, regional (i.e., geographic) differences may occur. Consequently, values reported by individual laboratories may differ from those listed in this appendix. Normally, the local laboratory references range is stated in parenthesis after the patient's individual result.

All values are given in conventional and SI units. However, for those analytes in which SI units have not been widely accepted, conventional units are used. In the case of the heterogeneous nature of the materials of the materials measured or uncertainty about the exact molecular weight of compounds, SI measurements cannot be used, so that mass per volume remains as the unit of concentration.

Abbreviations

ACD, acid-citrate-dextrose; **CHF,** congestive heart failure; **Cit,** citrate; **Cl,** chloride; **CNS,** central nervous system; **CSF,** cerebrospinal fluid; **cyclic AMP,** adenosine 3′, 5′-cyclic phosphate; **EDTA,** ethylenediaminetetraacetic acid; **HDL,** high-density lipoprotein; **Hep,** heparin; **LDL-C,** low-density lipoprotein-cholesterol; **Ox,** oxalate; **RBC,** red blood cell(s); **RIA,** radioimmunoassay, **SD,** standard deviation, **WBC,** white blood cell(s).

References

Beutler E, Lichtman MA, Coller BS, Kipps TJ, Seligsohn U. *Williams Hematology*, 6th ed. New York: McGraw-Hill, 2001.

Bishop ML, Fody EP, Schoeff L. *Clinical Chemistry: Principles, Procedures, Correlations*, 5th ed. Philadelphia: Lippincott Williams & Wilkins, 2004.

Burtis CA, Ashwood ER, eds. *Tietz Textbook of Clinical Chemistry*, 3rd ed. Philadelphia: WB Saunders, 1998.

Children's Hospital, St. Louis, The Department of Clinical Laboratories. High Density Lipoprotein Lipid Panel: Cholesterol, HDL, Cholesterol, LDL (calculated), Cholesterol, Total, Triglycerides. Parathyroid Hormone (PTH). Available at: http://webserver01.bjc.org/slch/pro/Professional.htm?http://webserver01.bjc.org/labtest guide /Lab%20Test%20Guidebook/guide.htm. Accessed April 20, 2004.

Clinical chemistry laboratory: Reference range values in clinical chemistry. Professional services manual. Baltimore: Department of Pathology, University of Maryland Medical System, 1999.

Daniels, R. *Delmar's Guide to Laboratory and Diagnostic Tests*. Albany, NY: Delmar, 2002.

Department of Health and Human Services, National Institute of Health, National Heart, Lung and Blood Institute, National Cholesterol Education Project website, Cholesterol Guidelines–Adult Treatment Panel III (ATP III), http://www.nhlbi.nih.gov/health/pubs/pub_prof.htm#chol

Diagnostic Tests: A Prescriber's Guide to Test Selection and Interpretation. Philadelphia: Lippincott Williams & Wilkins, 2004.

Fischback, FT. *A Manual of Laboratory and Diagnostic Tests*, 7th ed. Philadelphia: Lippincott Williams & Wilkins, 2004.

Harmening DM, ed. *Hematologic Values in Clinical Hematology and Fundamentals of Hemostasis*, 2nd ed. Philadelphia: FA Davis, 1992.

Laboratory Corporation of America. Erythrocyte Sedimentation Rate, Westergren. Available at: http://www.labcorp.com/datasets/labcorp/html/chapter/mono/he005000.htm. Accessed April 20, 2004.

Laboratory Corporation of America. Fecal Fat, Quantitative. Available at: http://www.labcorp.com/datasets/labcorp/html/chapter/mono/sc008000.htm. Accessed April 20, 2004.

McKenzie SB. *Clinical Laboratory Hematology.* Upper Saddle River, NJ: Pearson Education, 2004.

National cholesterol education program: Report of the expert panel on detection, evaluation, and treatment of high blood cholesterol in adults. *Arch Intern Med* 1988;148:36–99.

Triglyceride, high density lipoprotein, and coronary heart disease. National Institute of Health Consensus Statement, NIH Consensus Development Conference, 1992;10.

University of Texas Health Center at San Antonio. Neonatal Bilirubin. Available at: http://labs-sec.uhs-sa.com/clinical_ext/dols/soprefrange.asp. Accessed April 20, 2004.

University of Texas Medical Branch. Erythrocyte Sedimentation Rate, Wintrobe. Available at: http://www.utmb.edu/lsg/LabSurvivalGuide/hem/Sedimentation_Rate.htm. Accessed April 20, 2004.

University of Virginia Children's Medical Center. Therapy Review: Warfarin (Coumadin®). Pediatric Pharmacotherapy. January 1995;1. Available at: http://www.people.virginia.edu/~smb4v/cmchome.html. Accessed April 20, 2004.

Warfarin Therapy in Children Who Require Long-Term Total Parenteral Nutrition. *Pediatrics* [electronic article]. November 2003;112:386. Available at: http://pediatrics.aappublications.org/cgi/content/full/112/5/e386. Accessed April 20, 2004.

Wu HB. *Tietz Clinical Guide to Laboratory Tests*, 4th ed. St. Louis: Saunders-Elsevier, 2006.

Test	Conventional Units	SI Units
Acetaminophen, serum or plasma (Hep or EDTA)		
Therapeutic	10–30 mcg/mL	66–199 mcmol/L
Toxic	>200 mcg/mL	>1324 mcmol/L
Acetone		
Serum		
Qualitative	Negative	Negative
Quantitative	0.3–2.0 mg/dL	0.05–0.34 mmol/L
Urine		
Qualitative	Negative	Negative
Acid hemolysis test	<5% lysis	<0.05 lysed fraction
Acid phosphatase, serum		
Male	2.5–11.7 U/L	4.2–19.5 $\times 10^{-8}$ kat/L
Female	0.3–9.2 U/L	0.5–15.4 $\times 10^{-8}$ kat/L
Adrenocorticotropin, plasma		
8 AM	<120 pg/mL	<26 pmol/L
Midnight (supine)	<10 pg/mL	<2.2 pmol/L
*Alanine aminotransferase, serum	6–37 U/L	1–62 $\times 10^{-7}$ kat/L
Albumin		
Serum		
Adult	3.5–5.2 g/dL	35–52 g/L
>60 y	3.2–4.6 g/dL	32–46 g/L
	Avg. of 0.3 g/dL higher in patients in upright position	Avg. of 3 g/L higher in patients in upright position
Urine		
Qualitative	Negative	Negative
Quantitative	50–80 mg/24 h	50–80 mg/24 h
CSF	10–30 mg/dL	100–300 mg/L
*Aldolase, serum	1.0–7.5 U/L (30°C)	0.02–0.13 mckat/L (30°C)
Aldosterone		
Serum		
Supine	3–16 ng/dL	80–444 pmol/L
Standing	7–30 ng/dL	190–832 pmol/L
Urine	3–19 mcg/24 h	8–51 nmol/24 h
Alkaline phosphatase, serum	30–90 U/L	30–95 U/L (Bowers and McComb)
Alpha$_1$ antitrypsin, serum	110–200 mg/dL	1.10–2.0 g/L
Alprazolam serum, plasma		
Therapeutic	10–50 mg/L	32–150 mmol/L
Toxic	>100 mg/L	>524 mmol/L
Amikacin, serum or plasma (EDTA)		
Therapeutic		
Peak	25–35 mcg/mL	43–60 mcmol/L
Trough		
Less severe infection	1–4 mcg/mL	1.7–6.8 mcmol/L
Life-threatening infection	4–8 mcg/mL	6.8–13.7 mcmol/L
Toxic		
Peak	>35–40 mcg/mL	>60–68 mcmol/L
Trough	>10–15 mcg/mL	>17–26 mcmol/L
∂-Aminolevulinic acid, urine	1.3–7.0 mg/24 h	10–53 mcmol/24 h
Amitriptyline, serum or plasma (Hep or EDTA); trough (≥12 h after dose)		
Therapeutic	80–250 ng/mL	289–903 nmol/L
Toxic	>500 ng/mL	>1805 nmol/L
Ammonia (EDTA)	<50–ng/dL	<36 nmol/L

*Test values depend on laboratory methods.

Test	Conventional Units	SI Units
Ammonia		
Plasma (Hep)	7–27 mcmol/L	7–27 mcmol/L
*Amylase		
Serum	27–131 U/L	0.46–2.23 mckat/L
Urine	1–17 U/h	0.017-0.29 mckat/h
Amylase:creatinine clearance ratio	<3%	<.03
Androstenedione, serum		
Male	75–205 ng/dL	2.6–7.2 nmol/L
Female	85–275 ng/dL	3.0–9.6 nmol/L
Anion gap ([Na + K] − [Cl + HCO_3])	10–20 mEq/L	10–20 mmol/L
α_1-Antitrypsin, serum	78–200 mg/dL	0.78–2.00 g/L
Apolipoprotein A-1		
Male	94–178 mg/dL	0.94–1.78 g/L
Female	101–199 mg/dL	1.01–1.99 g/L
Apolipoprotein B		
Male	63–133 mg/dL	0.63–1.33 g/L
Female	60–126 mg/dL	0.60–1.26 g/L
Arsenic		
Whole blood (Hep)	0.2–2.3 mcg/dL	0.03–0.31 mcmol/L
Chronic poisoning	10–50 mcg/dL	1.33–6.65 mcmol/L
Acute poisoning	60–930 mcg/dL	7.98–124 mcmol/L
Urine, 24 h	5–50 mcg/d	0.07–0.67 mcmol/d
Ascorbic acid, plasma (Ox, Hep, EDTA)	0.4–1.5 mg/dL	23–85 mcmol/L
*Aspartate aminotransferase (SGOT) serum	5–30 U/L	8.3–50 x 10^{-8} kat/L
Base excess, blood (Hep)	22 to +3 mEq/L	22 to +3 mmol/L
Bicarbonate,		
serum (venous)	22–29 mEq/L	22–29 mmol/L
plasma (arterial)	22–25 mEq/L	22–25 mmol/L
†*Bilirubin		
Bilirubin, direct		
Birth–death	0.0–0.4 mg/dL	
Bilirubin, total		
Birth–1 day	1.0–6.0 mg/dL	
1–2 days	6.0–7.5 mg/dL	
2–5 days	4.0–13.5 mg/dL	
5 days–death	0.2–1.2 mg/dL	
Total bilirubin, neonatal (full term infant)		
Birth–1 day	1.0–6.0 mg/dL	
1–2 days	6.0–7.5 mg/dL	
2–5 days	4.0–6.0 mg/dL	
5 days–1 month	0.0–1.8 mg/dL	
1 month–death	0.0–1.8 mg/dL	
Bone marrow, differential cell count		
Adult		
Undifferentiated cells	0–1%	0–0.01
Myeloblast	0–2%	0–0.02
Promyelocyte	0-4%	0–0.04
Myelocytes		
Neutrophilic	5–20%	0.05–0.20
Eosinophilic	0–3%	0–0.03
Basophilic	0–1%	0–0.01
Metamyeolocytes and bands		
Neutrophilic	5–35%	0.05–0.35
Eosinophilic	0–5%	0–0.05
Basophilic	0–1%	0–0.01

*Test values depend on laboratory methods.

†Bilirubin data—Source: http://labs-sec.uhs-sa.com/clinical_ext/dols/soprefrange.asp

Test	Conventional Units	SI Units
Bone marrow, differential cell count (continued)		
Segmented neutrophils	5–15%	0.05–0.15
Pronormoblast	0–1.5%	0–0.015
Basophilic normoblast	0–5%	0–0.05
Polychromatophilic normoblast	5–30%	0.05–0.30
Orthochromatic normoblast	5–10%	0.05–0.10
Lymphocytes	10–20%	0.10–0.20
Plasma cells	0–2%	0–0.02
Monocytes	0–5%	0–0.05
CA-125, serum	<35 U/mL	<35 kU/L
CA 15-3, serum	<25 U/mL	<30 kU/L
CA 19-9, serum	<37 U/mL	<37 kU/L
Cadmium, whole blood (Hep)	0.1–0.5 mcg/dL	8.9–44.5 nmol/L
Toxic	10–300 mcg/dL	0.89–26.70 mcmol/L
Cadmium, urine, 24 h	<15 mcg/d	<0.13 mcmol/d
Calcitonin, serum or plasma		
Male	≤100 pg/mL	≤100 ng/L
Female	≤30 pg/mL	≤30 ng/L
Calcium, serum	8.6–10.0 mg/dL	2.15–2.50 mmol/L
Child	8.6–10.6 mg/dL	2.5–2.65 mmol/L
Calcium, ionized, serum	4.64–5.28 mg/dL	1.16–1.32 mmol/L
Calcium, neonate, serum	4.8–5.9 mg/dL	1.20–1.48 mmol/L
Calcium, urine		
Low calcium diet	50–150 mg/24 h	1.25–3.75 mmol/24 h
Usual diet; trough	100–300 mg/24 h	2.50–7.50 mmol/24 h
Carbamazepine, serum or plasma (Hep or EDTA), trough		
Therapeutic	4–12 mcg/mL	17–51 mmol/L
Toxic	>15 mcg/mL	>63 mmol/L
Carbon dioxide, total, serum/ plasma (Hep)	22–28 mmol/L	22–28 mmol/L
Carbon dioxide (PCO_2), blood, arterial	Male 35–48 mmHg Female 32–45 mmHg	4.66–6.38 kPa 4.26–5.99 kPa
Carbon monoxide as carboxyhemoglobin whole blood (EDTA)		
Nonsmokers	0.5–1.5% total Hb	0.005–0.015 HbCO fraction
Smokers		
1–2 packs/d	4–5% total Hb	0.04–0.05 HbCO fraction
>2 packs/d	8–9% total Hb	0.08–0.09 HbCO fraction
Toxic	>20% total Hb	>0.20 HbCO fraction
Lethal	>50% total Hb	>0.5 HbCO fraction
Carotene, serum	10–85 mcg/dL	0.19–1.58 mcmol/L
Catecholamines, plasma (EDTA)		
Dopamine	< 30 pg/mL	<196 pmol/L
Epinephrine	<110 pg/mL	<680 pmol/L
Norepinephrine	<1700 pg/mL	<10,047 pmol/L
Catecholamines, urine		
Dopamine	65–400 mcg/24 h	425–2610 nmol/24 h
Epinephrine	0–20 mcg/24 h	0–109 nmol/24 h
Norepinephrine	15–80 mcg/24 h	89–473 nmol/24 h
CEA, serum		
Nonsmokers	<5.0 ng/mL	<5.0 mcg/L

Test	Conventional Units		SI Units
Cell counts, adult			
Erythrocytes			
Male	$4.5–5.5 \times 10^{6}$/mcL		$4.5–5.5 \times 10^{12}$/L
Female	$4.0–5.0 \times 10^{6}$/mcL		$4.2–5.0 \times 10^{12}$/L
Leukocytes			
Total	$4.5–11.0 \times 10^{3}$/mcL		$4.5–11.0 \times 10^{9}$/L
Leukocyte differential	Percentage	Absolute	Absolute (SI)
Myelocytes	0	0/mcL	0/L
Neutrophils			
Band	3–5%	$0.0–0.7 \times 10^{3}$/mcL	$0.0–0.7 \times 10^{9}$/L
Segmented	40–80%	$1.8–7.0 \times 10^{3}$/mcL	$1.8–7.0 \times 10^{9}$/L
Lymphocytes	25–35%	$1.0–4.8 \times 10^{3}$/mcL	$1.0–4.8 \times 10^{9}$/L
Monocytes	2–10%	$0.0–0.8 \times 10^{3}$/mcL	$0.0–0.8 \times 10^{9}$/L
Granulocytes	42.2–75.2%	$1.4–6.5 \times 10^{3}$/mcL	$1.4–6.5 \times 10^{9}$/L
Eosinophils	0–5%	$0.0–0.4 \times 10^{3}$/mcL	$0.0–0.4 \times 10^{9}$/L
Basophils	0–0.2%	$0.0–0.2 \times 10^{3}$/mcL	$0.0–0.2 \times 10^{9}$/L
Platelets	$150–450 \times 10^{3}$/mcL		$150–450 \times 10^{9}$/L
Reticulocytes	0.5–2.5% RBCs		0.005–0.015 of RBCs
	18,000–158,000/mcL		$18–158 \times 10^{9}$/L
Cells, CSF	<5 lymphocytes/mm^3		<5 lymphocytes/mm^3
	0 RBC/mm^3		0 RBC/mm^3
Ceruloplasmin, serum	20–60 mg/dL		0.2–0.6 g/L
Chloramphenicol, serum or plasma (Hep or EDTA); trough			
Therapeutic	10–25 mcg/mL		31–77 mcmol/L
Toxic	>25 mcg/mL		>77 mcmol/L
Chloride			
Serum or plasma (Hep)	98–107 mmol/L		98–107 mmol/L
Sweat			
Normal	5–35 mmol/L		5–35 mmol/L
Cystic fibrosis	60–200 mmol/L		60–200 mmol/L
Urine, 24 h (vary greatly with Cl intake)			
Infant	2–10 mmol/24 h		2–10 mmol/24h
Child	15–40 mmol/24 h		15–40 mmol/24h
Adult	110–250 mmol/24 h		110–250 mmol/24 h
CSF	118–132 mmol/L (20 mmol/L higher than serum)		118–132 mmol/L (20 mmol/L higher than serum)
Chlorpromazine serum, plasma (EDTA)			
Therapeutic			
Child	40–80 ng/m/L		126–251 nmol/L
Adult	50–300 ng/mL		157–942 nmol/L
Toxic	>1000 ng/mL		>3140 nmol/L
Cholesterol, serum			
Adult desirable	<200 mg/dL		<5.2 mmol/L
borderline	200–239 mg/dL		5.2–6.2 mmol/L
high-risk	≥240 mg/dL		≥6.2 mmol/L
*Cholinesterase, serum	4.9–11.9 U/mL		4.9–11.9 kU/L
Dibucaine inhibition	79–84%		0.79–0.84
Fluoride inhibition	58–64%		0.58–0.64
*Chorionic gonadotropin, intact			
Serum or plasma (EDTA)			
Male and nonpregnant female	<5.0 mIU/mL		<5.0 IU/L
Pregnant female	Varies with gestational age		
Urine, qualitative			
Male and nonpregnant female	Negative		Negative
Pregnant female	Positive		Positive

*Test values depend on laboratory methods.

Test	Conventional Units	SI Units
Clonazepam, serum or plasma (Hep or EDTA); trough		
Therapeutic	5–70 ng/mL	55–222 nmol/L
Toxic	>70 ng/mL	>222 nmol/L
Coagulation tests		
Activated partial thromboplastin time (APTT)	21–35 sec	
Activated protein C resistance	>2.1	
Antithrombin (AT)		
Activity	80–120%	
Antigen	22–40 mg/dL	
Bleeding time, template	3.0–10.0 min	
D-dimer	<250 ng/L	<1.37 nmol/L
Dilute Russell viper venom test (dRVVT)	<40 sec	
Euglobin lysis time	No lysis of plasma clot at 37°C in 60–120 min	
Factor II	80–120%	
Factor V	50–150%	
Factor VII	65–140%	
Factor VIII	55–145%	
Factor IX	60–140%	
Factor X	45–155%	
Factor XI	65–135%	
Factor XII	50–150%	
Fibrin degradation products (FDP)	Negative at 1:4 dilution or <10 mg/L	2.0–4.0 G/L
Fibrinogen	200–400 mg/dL	
International normalized ratio (INR)	2.0–3.0, varies by specific disorder	
Lupus anticoagulant	Negative	
Plasminogen activity		
Females	65–153%	
Males	76–124%	
Plasminogen activator inhibitor-1 (PAI-1)		
Activity	78–142%	
Antigen	4–43 mcg/mL	
Protein C		
Activity	70–140%	
Antigen	65–150%	
Protein S		
Activity	70–140%	
Antigen, free & total	70–160%	
Prothrombin time (PT)	11.0–13.0 sec	
Reptilase time	18–22 sec	
Thrombin time	7.0–12.0 sec	
von Willebrand factor		
Activity	42–139%	
Antigen	60–150%	
Cocaine (whole blood oxalate flouride)		
Therapeutic	100–500 ng/mL	330–1650 nmol/L
Toxic	>1000 ng/mL	>3300 nmol/L
Urine	Negative	Negative
Cold hemolysin test (Donath-Landsteiner)	No hemolysis	No hemolysis
Complement components		
Total hemolytic complement activity, plasma (EDTA)	40–90 U/mL	0.4–0.9 kU/L

Test	Conventional Units	SI Units
Complement components (continued)		
Total complement decay rate	10–20%	Fraction decay rate: 0.10–0.20
(functional), plasma (EDTA)	Deficiency: >50%	>0.50
C1q, serum	14.9–22.1 mg/dL	149–221 mg/L
C1r, serum	2.5–10.0 mg/dL	25–100 mg/L
C1s (C1 esterase), serum	5.0–10.0 mg/dL	50–100 mg/L
C2, serum	1.6–3.6 mg/dL	16–36 mg/L
C3, serum	90–180 mg/dL	0.9–1.8 g/L
C4, serum	10–40 mg/dL	0.1-0.4 g/L
C5, serum	5.5–11.3 mg/dL	55–113 mg/L
C6, serum	17.9–23.9 mg/dL	179–239 mg/L
C7, serum	2.7–7.4 mg/dL	27–74 mg/L
C8, serum	4.9–10.6 mg/dL	49–106 mg/L
C9, serum	3.3–9.5 mg/dL	33–95 mg/L
Coombs test		
Direct	Negative	Negative
Indirect	Negative	Negative
Copper		
Serum		
Male	70–140 mcg/dL	11–22 mcmol/L
Female	80–155 mcg/dL	13–24 mcmol/L
Urine	3–35 mcg/24 h	0.05–0.55 mcmol/24 h
Corpuscular values of erythrocytes		
Erythrocyte Indices		
MCV	86–94 fL	
MCH	28–34 pg	
MCHC	32–36 g/dL	
Cortisol, serum		
Plasma (Hep, EDTA, Ox)		
8 AM	9–35 mcg/dL	250–650 nmol/L
4 PM	3–12 mcg/dL	80–330 nmol/L
10 PM	<50% of 8 AM value	<0.5 of 8 AM value
Free, urine	<50 mcg/24 h	<138 mmol/24 h
*C-Peptide, serum	0.78–1.89 ng/mL	0.26–0.62 nmol/L
C-Reactive protein, serum	<0.5 mg/dL	<5 mg/L
*†Creatine kinase, serum		
Male	15–105 U/L (30°C)	0.26–1.79 mckat/L (30°C)
Female	10–80 U/L (30°C)	0.17–1.36 mckat/L (30°C)
Note: Strenuous exercise or intramuscular injections may elevate transient levels of creatine kinase.		
*Creatine kinase MB isoenzyme, serum	0–7 ng/mL	0–7 mcg/L
*Creatinine		
Serum or plasma, adult		
Male	0.7–1.3 mg/dL	62–115 mcmol/L
Female	0.6–1.1 mg/dL	53–97 mcmol/L
Urine		
Male	14–26 mg/kg body weight/24 h	124–230 mcmol/kg body weight/24 h
Female	11–20 mg/kg body weight/24 h	97–177 mcmol/kg body weight/24 h
*Creatinine clearance, serum or plasma and urine		
Male	94–140 mL/min/1.73 m2	0.91–1.35 mL/s/m2
Female	72–110 mL/min/1.73 m2	0.69–1.06 mL/s/m2
Cryoglobulins, serum	Negative	Negative
Cyanide		
Serum		
Nonsmokers	0.004 mg/L	0.15 mcmol/L

*Test values depend on laboratory methods.

†Actual therapeutic range should be adjusted for individual patient.

Test	Conventional Units	SI Units
Cyanide (continued)		
Smokers	0.006 mg/L	0.23 mcmol/L
Nitroprusside therapy	0.01–0.06 mg/L	0.38–2.30 mcmol/L
Toxic	>0.1 mg/L	>3.84 mcmol/L
Whole blood (Ox)		
Nonsmokers	0.016 mg/L	0.61 mcmol/L
Smokers	0.041 mg/L	1.57 mcmol/L
Nitroprusside therapy	0.05–0.5 mg/L	1.92–19.20 mcmol/L
Toxic	>1 mg/L	>38.40 mcmol/L
Cyclic AMP		
Plasma (EDTA)		
Male	4.6–8.6 ng/mL	14–26 nmol/L
Female	4.3–7.6 ng/mL	13–23 nmol/L
Urine, 24 h	0.3–3.6 mg/d or 0.29–2.1 mg/g creatinine	1.0–10.9 mcmol/d or 100–723 mcmol/mol creatinine
Cystine or cysteine, urine, qualitative	Negative	Negative
*†Cyclosporine, whole blood		
Therapeutic, trough	100–200 ng/mL	83–166 nmol/L
Dehydroepiandrosterone serum		
Male	180–1250 ng/dL	6.2–43.3 nmol/L
Female	130–980 ng/dL	4.5–34.0 nmol/L
Dehydroepiandrosterone sulfate serum or plasma (Hep, EDTA)		
Male	59–452 mcg/mL	1.6–12.2 mcmol/L
Female		
Premenopausal	12–379 mcg/mL	0.8–10.2 mcmol/L
Postmenopausal	30–260 mcg/mL	0.8–7.1 mcmol/L
Desipramine, serum or plasma (Hep or EDTA); trough (12 h after dose)		
Therapeutic	75–300 ng/mL	281–1125 nmol/L
Toxic	>400 ng/mL	>1500 nmol/L
Diazepam, serum or plasma (Hep or EDTA); trough		
Therapeutic	200–1500 ng/mL	0.70–5.27 mmol/L
Toxic	>3000 ng/mL	>10.53 mmol/L
Digoxin (serum)		
Therapeutic	0.8–1.5 ng/mL	1.0–1.9 mmol/L
Toxic	> 2.5 /mL	> 3.2 mmol/L
Digitoxin, serum or plasma (Hep or EDTA); 7.8 h after dose		
Therapeutic	10–30 ng/mL	13–39 nmol/L
Toxic	>45 ng/mL	>59 nmol/L
Digoxin, serum or plasma (Hep or EDTA); ≥12 h after dose		
Therapeutic		
CHF	0.8–1.5 ng/mL	1.0–1.9 nmol/L
Arrhythmias	1.5–2.0 ng/mL	1.9–2.6 nmol/L
Toxic		
Adult	>2.5 ng/mL	>3.2 nmol/L
Child	>3.0 ng/mL	>3.8 nmol/L

*Test values depend on laboratory methods.
†Actual therapeutic range should be adjusted for individual patient.

Test	Conventional Units	SI Units
Disopyramide, serum or plasma (Hep or EDTA); trough		
Therapeutic arrhythmias		
Atrial	2.8–3.2 mcg/mL	8.3–9.4 mcmol/L
Ventricular	3.3–7.5 mcg/mL	9.7–22 mcmol/L
Toxic	>7 mcg/mL	>20.7 mcmol/L
Doxepin, serum or plasma (Hep or EDTA); trough (≥12 h after dose)		
Therapeutic	150–250 ng/mL	537–895 nmol/L
Toxic	>500 ng/mL	>1790 nmol/L
*Estradiol, serum		
Adult		
Male	10–50 pg/mL	37–184 pmol/L
Female	Varies with menstrual cycle	
Ethanol (alcohol), whole blood (Ox) or serum		
Depression of CNS	>100 mg/dL	>21.7 mmol/L
Fatalities reported	>400 mg/dL	>86.8 mmol/L
Ethosuximide, serum or plasma (Hep or EDTA); trough		
Therapeutic	40–100 mcg/mL	283–708 mcmol/L
Toxic	>150 mcg/mL	>1062 mcmol/L
Euglobin lysis	No lysis of plasma clot at 37°C in 60–120 min	No lysis of plasma clot at 37°C in 60–120 min
α-Fetoprotein, serum	<15 ng/mL	<15 mcg/L
†Fat, fecal, F, 72 h		
Infant, breast-fed	<1 g/d	
Pediatrics (0–6 y)	<2 g/d	
Adult	<7 g/d	
Adult (fat-free diet)	<4 g/d	
††Fatty acids, total, serum	190–240 mg/dL	7–15 mmol/L
Nonesterified, serum	8–25 mg/dL	0.28–0.89 mmol/L
Ferritin, serum		
Male	20–300 ng/mL	20–300 mcg/L
Female	20–120 ng/mL	20–120 mcg/L
Ferritin values of <20 ng/mL (20 mcg/L) have been reported to be generally associated with depleted iron stores.		
Fibrin degradation products	<10 mcg/mL	<10 mg/L
*Fibrinogen, plasma (NaCit)	200–400 mg/dL	2–4 g/L
Fluoride		
Plasma (Hep)	0.01–0.2 mcg/mL	0.5–10.5 mcmol/L
Urine	0.2–3.2 mcg/mL	10.5–168 mcmol/L
Urine, occupational exposure	<8 mcg/mL	<421 mcmol/L
*Folate, Serum	3–20 ng/mL	7–45 nmol/L
Erythrocytes	140–628 ng/mL RBC	317–1422 nmol/L RBC
*Follicle-stimulating hormone serum and plasma (Hep)		
Male	5–20 mIU/mL	5–20 IU/L
Female	5–20 mIU/mL	5–20 IU/L
Follicular phase	1–10 mIU/mL	1–10 IU/L
Midcycle	5–20 mIU/mL	5–20 IU/L
Luteal phase	5–15 mIU/mL	5–15 IU/L
Postmenopausal	5–100 mIU/mL	5–100 IU/L

* Test values depend on laboratory methods.

† Reference values vary from laboratory to laboratory, but are generally found within the range of 5–7 g/d. It should be noted that children, especially infants, cannot ingest the 100 g/d of fat that is suggested for the test. Therefore, a fat retention coefficient is determined by measuring the difference between ingested fat and fecal fat, and expressing that difference as a percentage. The figure, called the fat retention coefficient, is 95% or greater in healthy children and adults. A low value indicates steatorrhea. http://www.labcorp.com/datasets/labcorp/html/chapter/mono/sc008000.htm

††"Fatty acids" include a mixture of different aliphatic acids of varying molecular weight; a mean molecular weight of 284 D has been assumed.

Test	Conventional Units	SI Units
*Free thyroxine index (FTI), serum	4.2–13	4.2–13
Free thyroxine, serum	0.9–2.3 ng/dL	10–30 nmol/L
Free triiodothyronin, serum	0.2–0.6 ng/dL	0.003–0.009 nmol/L
Gastrin, serum	50–150 pg/mL	50–150 ng/L
Gentamicin, serum or plasma (EDTA)		
Therapeutic		
Peak		
Less severe infection	5–8 mcg/mL	10.5–16.7 mcmol
Severe infection	8–10 mcg/mL	16.7–20.9 mcmol/L
Trough		
Less severe infection	<1 mcg/mL	<2.1 mcmol/L
Moderate infection	<2 mcg/mL	<4.2 mcmol/L
Severe infection	<2–4 mcg/mL	<4.2–8.4 mcmol/L
Toxic		
Peak	>10–12 mcg/mL	>21–25 mcmol/L
Trough	>2–4 mcg/mL	>4.2–8.4 mcmol/L
Glucose (fasting)		
Blood	70–110 mg/dL	3.9–6.0 mmol/L
Plasma or serum	74–106 mg/dL	4.1–5.9 mmol/L
Glucose, 2 h postprandial, serum	<140 mg/dL	<7.8 mmol/L
Glucose, urine		
Quantitative	<500 mg/24 h	<2.8 mmol/24 h
Qualitative	Negative	Negative
Glucose, CSF	50–80 mg/dL	2.8–4.4 mmol/L
*Glucose-6-phosphate dehydrogenase in erythrocytes, whole blood (ACD, EDTA, or Hep)	12.1 ± 2.1 U/g Hb (SD) 351 ± 60.6 U/10^{12} RBC 4.11 ± 0.71 U/mL RBC	0.78 ± 0.13 mU/mol Hb 0.35 ± 0.06 nU/RBC 4.11 ± 0.71 kU/L RBC
γ-Glutamyltransfersae serum		
Males	6–45 U/L (37°C)	10–75 × 10^{-8} kat/L (37°C)
Females	5–30 U/L (37°C)	8–50 × 10^{-8} kat/L (37°C)
Glutethimide, serum		
Therapeutic	2–6 mcg/mL	9–28 mcmol/L
Toxic	>5 mcg/mL	>23 mcmol/L
Glycated hemoglobin (Hemoglobin A1c), whole blood (EDTA)	4.2% – 5.9%	0.042–0.059
Growth hormone, serum		
Male	<0–4 ng/mL	0–4 mcg/L
Female	<0.8–18 ng/mL	0–18 mcg/L
Haptoglobin, serum	40–180 mg/dL	0.4–1.8 g/L
HDL-lipid panel		
Cholesterol, HDL	>40 mg/dL	
Cholesterol, LDL (calculated)		
optimal	<100 mg/dL	
near optimal	100–129 mg/dL	
borderline high	130–159 mg/dL	
high	>160 mg/dL	
very high	>190 mg/dL	
Cholesterol, total		
0–1 year	50–120 mg/dL	
1–2 years	70–190 mg/dL	
2–16 years	120–220 mg/dL	
>16 years	0–199 mg/dL	

*Test values depend on laboratory methods.

Test	Conventional Units	SI Units
HDL-lipid panel (continued)		
desirable	<200 mg/dL	
borderline	200–239 mg/dL	
high	>240 mg/dL	
*Tryglycerides		
desirable	<250 mg/dL	
borderline high	250–500 mg/dL	
high	>500 mg/dL	
Hematocrit		
Males	42–52%	0.42–0.52 L/L
Females	36–46%	0.36–0.46 L/L
Hemoglobin (Hb)		
Males	14.0–17.4 g/dL	140–170 g/L
Females	12.0–16.0 g/dL	120–160 g/L
Hemoglobin, fetal	≥1 y old: <2% of total Hb	≥1 y old: <0.02% of total Hb
Hemoglobin, plasma	<3 mg/dL	<0.47 mcmol/L
Hemoglobin and myoglobin, urine, qualitative	Negative	Negative
Hemoglobin electrophoresis, whole blood (EDTA, Cit, or Hep)		
HbA	>95%	
HbA_2	1.5–3.7%	
HbF	<2%	
Homogentisic acid, urine, qualitative	Negative	Negative
β-Hydroxybutyric acid, serum, plasma	0.21–2.81 mg/dL	20–270 mcmol/L
17-Hydroxycorticosteroids		
Urine		
Males	4.5–12 mg/24 h	12.4–33.1 mcmol/24 h (as cortisol)
Females	2.5–10 mg/24 h	6.9–27.6 mcmol/24 h (as cortisol)
5-Hydroxyindoleacetic acid, urine		
Qualitative	Negative	Negative
Quantitative	2–7 mg/24 h	10.4–36.6 mcmol/24 h
Imipramine, serum or plasma (Hep or EDTA); trough (≥12 h after dose)		
Therapeutic	150–250 ng/mL	536–893 nmol/L
Toxic	>500 ng/mL	>1785 nmol/L
Immunoglobulins, serum		
IgG	800–1200 mg/dL	8–12 g/L
IgA	80–312 mg/dL	0.7–3.12 g/L
IgM	50–280 mg/dL	0.5–2.8 g/L
IgD	0.5–2.8 mg/dL	0.005–0.2 mg/L
IgE	0.01–0.06 mg/dL	0.1–0.6 mg/L
Immunoglobulin G (IgC), CSF	0.5–6.1 mg/dL	0.5–6.1 g/L
Insulin, plasma (fasting)	0–35 mcU/mL	14.4–243 pmol/L
†Iron, serum		
Males	65–175 mcg/dL	11.6–31.3 mcmol/L
Females	50–170 mcg/dL	9.0–30.4 mcmol/L
Iron binding capacity, serum, total	300–310 mcg/dL	54–64 mcmol/L

*If the triglyceride value is >400 mg/dL, the LDL calculation is invalid. http://webserver01.bjc.org/slch/pro/Professional.htm?http://webserver01.bjc.org/labtestguide/Lab%20Test%20Guidebook/slchlabsiteonline.htm

† Test values depend on laboratory methods.

Test	Conventional Units	SI Units
Iron saturation, serum		
Male	20–50%	0.2–0.5
Female	15–50%	0.15–0.5
Iron total binding capacity (serum)	300–360 ng/dL	54–64 nmol/K
17-Ketogenic steroids, urine		
Males	4–14 mg/24 h	13–49 mcmol/24 h
Females	2–12 mg/24 h (decreases with age)	7–42 mcmol/24 h (decreases with age)
L-Lactate		
Plasma (NaF)		
Venous	4.5–19.8 mg/dL	0.5–2.2 mmol/L
Arterial	4.5–14.4 mg/dL	0.5–1.6 mmol/L
Whole blood (Hep), at bed rest		
Venous	8.1–15.3 mg/dL	0.9–1.7 mmol/L
Arterial	<11.3 mg/dL	<1.3 mmol/L
Urine, 24 h	496–1982 mg/d	5.5–22 mmol/d
CSF	10–22 mg/dL	1.1–2.4 mmol/L
*Lactate dehydrogenase		
Total (L→P), 37°C, serum		
Newborn	290–775 U/L	4.9–13.2 mckat/L
Neonate	545–2000 U/L	9.3–34 mckat/L
Infant	180–430 U/L	3.1–7.3 mckat/L
Child	110–295 U/L	1.9–5 mckat/L
Adult	100–190 U/L	1.7–3.2 mckat/L
>60 y	110–210 U/L	1.9–3.6 mckat/L
*Isoenzymes, serum by agarose gel electrophoresis		
Fraction 1	14–26% of total	0.14–0.26 fraction of total
Fraction 2	29–39% of total	0.29–0.39 fraction of total
Fraction 3	20–26% of total	0.20–0.26 fraction of total
Fraction 4	8–16% of total	0.08–0.16 fraction of total
Fraction 5	6–16% of total	0.06–0.16 fraction of total
*Lactate dehydrogenase, CSF	10% of serum value	0.10 fraction of serum value
LDL-cholesterol, serum or plasma (EDTA)		
Adult desirable	<130 mg/dL	<3.36 mmol/L
borderline	130–159 mg/dL	3.37–4.11 mmol/L
high risk	≥160 mg/dL	≥4.13 mmol/L
Lead		
Whole blood (Hep)	<25 mcg/dL	<0.48 mcmol/L
Urine, 24 h	<80 mcg/d	<0.39 mcmol/d
Lecithin: sphingomyelin ratio, amniotic fluid	2.0–5.0 indicates probable fetal lung maturity; >3.5 in diabetic patients	2.0–5.0 indicates probable fetal lung maturity; >3.5 in diabetic patients
Lidocaine, serum or plasma (Hep or EDTA); 45 min after bolus dose		
Therapeutic	2.0–6.0 mcg/mL	6.4–25.6 mcmol/L
Toxic		
CNS, cardiovascular depression	6–8 mcg/mL	26–34.2 mcmol/L
Seizures, obtundation, decreased cardiac output	>8 mcg/mL	>34.2 mcmol/L
*Lipase, serum	<160 U/L	<2.72 nkat/L (37°C)
Lithium, serum or plasma (Hep or EDTA); 12 h after last dose		
Therapeutic	0.6–1.2 mEq/L	0.6–1.2 mmol/L
Toxic	>2 mEq/L	>2 mmol/L
Lorazepam, serum or plasma (Hep or EDTA),		
Therapeutic	50–240 ng/mL	156–746 nmol/L
Toxic	>300 ng/mL	>933 nmol/L

*Test values depend on laboratory methods.

Test	Conventional Units	SI Units
*Luteinizing hormone, serum or plasma (Hep)		
Male	5–20 mIU/mL	5–20 IU/L
Female		
Follicular phase	5–15.0 mIU/mL	5–15.0 IU/L
Mid-cycle peak	30–60 mIU/mL	30–60 IU/L
Luteal phase	5–15 mIU/mL	5–15 IU/L
Postmenopausal	5-100 mIU/mL	5-100 IU/L
Magnesium		
Serum	1.3–2.1 mEq/L	0.65–1.07 mmol/L
Urine	6.0–10.0 mEq/24 h	3.0–5.0 mmol/24 h
Mercury		
Whole blood (EDTA)	0.6–59 mcg/L	<0.29 mcmol/L
Urine, 24 h	<20 mcg/d	<0.1 mcmol/d
Toxic	>150 mcg/d	>0.75 mcmol/d
Metanephrines, total, urine	0.1–1.6 mg/24 h	0.5–8.1 mcmol/24 h
Methemoglobin (hemoglobin), whole blood (EDTA, Hep or ACD)	0.06–0.24 g/dL	9.3–37.2 mcmol/L
Methotrexate, serum or plasma (Hep or EDTA)		
Therapeutic	Variable	Variable
Toxic		
1–2 wk after low dose therapy	≥0.02 mcmol/L	≥0.02 mcmol/L
post IV infusion 24 h	≥5 mcmol/L	≥5 mcmol/L
48 h	≥0.5 mcmol/L	≥0.5 mcmol/L
72 h	≥0.05 mcmol/L	≥0.05 mcmol/L
Myelin basic protein, CSF	<2.5 ng/mL	<2.5 mcg/L
Myoglobin, serum	30–70 ng/mL	30–70 mcg/mL
Nortriptyline, serum or plasma (Hep or EDTA); trough (≥12 h after dose)		
Therapeutic	50–150 ng/mL	190–570 nmol/L
Toxic	>500 ng/mL	>1900 nmol/L
*5´-Nucleotidase, serum	2–17 U/L	0.034–0.29 mckat/L
N-Acetylprocainamide, serum or plasma (Hep or EDTA); trough		
Therapeutic	5–30 mcg/mL	18–108 mcmol/L
Toxic	>40 mcg/mL	>144 mcmol/L
Occult blood, feces, random	Negative (<2 mL blood/150 g stool/d)	Negative (<13.3 mL blood/kg stool/d)
Qualitative, urine, random	Negative	Negative
Osmolality		
Serum	275–295 mOsm/kg serum water	275–295 mmol/kg serum water
Urine	300–900 mOsm/kg water	300–900 mmol/kg water
Ratio, urine:serum	1.0–3.0	1.0–3.0
	3.0–4.7 after 12 h fluid restriction	3.0–4.7 after 12 h fluid restriction
Osmotic fragility of erythrocytes	Begins in 0.5–0.45% NaCl Complete in 0.33–0.30% NaCl	
Oxazepam, serum or plasma (Hep or EDTA),		
therapeutic	0.2–1.4 mcg/mL	0.70–4.9 mcmol/L
toxic	>2.0 mcg/mL	>6.98 mcmol/L
Oxygen, blood		
Capacity	16–24 vol% (varies with hemoglobin)	7.14–10.7 mmol/L (varies with hemoglobin)

*Test values depend on laboratory methods.

Test	Conventional Units	SI Units
Oxygen, blood (continued)		
Content		
Arterial	15–23 vol%	0.15–0.25 mmol/L
Venous	10–16 vol%	4.46–7.14 mmol/L
Saturation		
Arterial and capillary	95–98% of capacity	0.95–0.98 of capacity
Venous	60–85% of capacity	0.60–0.85 of capacity
Tension		
pO_2 arterial and capillary	83–108 mmHg	11.1–14.4 kPa
Venous	35–45 mmHg	4.6–6.0 kPa
P50, blood	25–29 mmHg (adjusted to pH 7.4)	3.33–3.86 kPa
Partial thromboplastin time activated	<35 sec	<35 sec
Pentobarbital, serum or plasma (Hep or EDTA); trough		
Therapeutic		
Hypnotic	1–5 mcg/mL	4–22 mcmol/L
Therapeutic coma	20–50 mcg/mL	88–221 mcmol/L
Toxic	>10 mcg/mL	>44 mcmol/L
pH		
Blood, arterial	7.35–7.45	7.35–7.45
Urine	4.6–8.0 (depends on diet)	Same
Phenacetin, plasma (EDTA)		
Therapeutic	5–20 mcg/mL	6–167 mcmol/L
Toxic	50–250 mcg/mL	279–1395 mcmol/L
Phenobarbital, serum or plasma (Hep or EDTA); trough		
Hypnotic	1–5 mcg/mL	4–22 mcmol/L
Therapeutic	15–40 mcg/mL	65–172 mcmol/L
Toxic	20–50 mcg/mL	88–227 mcmol/L
Phenolsulfonphthalein (PSP) excretion, urine	28–51% in 15 min 13–24% in 30 min 9–17% in 60 min 3–10% in 2 h (After injection of 1 mL PSP intravenously)	0.28–0.51 in 15 min 0.13–0.24 in 30 min 0.09–0.17 in 60 min 0.03–0.10 in 2 h (After injection of 1 mL PSP intravenously)
Phenylalanine, serum	0.8–1.8 mg/dL	48–109 mcmol/L
Phenytoin, serum or plasma (Hep or EDTA); trough		
Therapeutic	10–20 mcg/mL	40–79 mcmol/L
Toxic	>20 mcg/mL	>79 mcmol/L
*Phosphatase, acid, prostatic, serum		
radioimmunoassay	<3.0 ng/mL	<3.0 mcg/L
*Phosphatase, alkaline, total, serum	30–90 U/L (30°C)	30–90 U/L (Bowers and McComb)
Phosphate, inorganic, serum		
Adults	2.7–4.5 mg/dL	0.87–1.45 mmol/L
Children	4.5–5.5 mg/dL	1.45–1.78 mmol/L
Phosphatidylglycerol, amniotic fluid		
Fetal lung immaturity	absent	absent
Fetal lung maturity	present	present
Phospholipids, serum	150–250 mg/dL	1.5–2.55 g/L
Phosphorus, urine	0.4–1.3 g/24 h	12.9–42 mmol/24 h
Porphobilinogen, urine		
Qualitative	Negative	Negative
Quantitative	<2.0 mg/24 h	<9 mcmol/24 h

*Test values depend on laboratory methods.

Test	Conventional Units	SI Units
Porphyrins, urine		
Coproporphyrin	34–230 mcg/24 h	52–351 nmol/24 h
Uroporphyrin	27–52 mcg/24 h	32–63 nmol/24 h
Potassium, plasma (Hep)		
Males	3.5–4.5 mEq/L	3.5–4.5 mmol/L
Females	3.4–4.4 mEq/L	3.4–4.4 mmol/L
Potassium		
Serum		
Premature		
Cord	5.0–10.2 mEq/L	5.0–10.2 mmol/L
48 h	3.0–6.0 mEq/L	3.0–6.0 mmol/L
Newborn, cord	5.6–12.0 mEq/L	5.6–12.0 mmol/L
Newborn	3.7–5.9 mEq/L	3.7–5.9 mmol/L
Infant	4.1–5.3 mEq/L	4.1–5.3 mmol/L
Child	3.4–4.7 mEq/L	3.4–4.7 mmol/L
Adult	3.5–5.1 mEq/L	3.5–5.1 mmol/L
Urine, 24 h	25–125 mEq/d, varies with diet	25–125 mmol/d; varies with diet
CSF	70% of plasma level or 2.5–3.2 mEq/L; rises with plasma hyperosmolality	0.70 of plasma level or 2.5–3.2 mmol/L; rises with plasma hyperosmolality
Prealbumin (transthyretin), serum	10–40 mg/dL	100–400 mg/L
Primidone, serum or plasma (Hep or EDTA); trough		
Therapeutic	5–12 mcg/mL	23–55 mcmol/L
Toxic	>15 mcg/mL	>69 mcmol/L
Procainamide, serum or plasma (Hep or EDTA); trough		
Therapeutic	4–8 mcg/mL	17–42 mcmol/L
Toxic (also consider effect of metabolite, i.e., NAPA)	>10–12 mcg/mL	>42–51 mcmol/L
*Progesterone, plasma		
Adult		
Male	13–97 ng/dL	0.4–3.1 nmol/L
Female		
Follicular phase	<150 ng/dL	<5 nmol/L
Luteal phase	300–1200 ng/dL	10–40 nmol/L
Pregnancy	Varies with gestational week	
1st Trimester	15000–5000 ng/dL	50–160 nmol/L
2nd and 3rd Trimesters	8000–20,000 ng/dL	250–650 nmol/L
*Prolactin, serum		
Males	Undetectable to 23 ng/mL	Undetectable to 23 mcg/L
Females	2.5–19.0 ng/mL	2.5–19.0 mcg/L
Propoxyphene, plasma (EDTA)		
Therapeutic	0.1–0.4 mcg/mL	0.3–1.2 mcmol/L
Toxic	>0.5 mcg/mL	>1.5 mcmol/L
Propranolol, serum or plasma (Hep or EDTA); trough		
Therapeutic	50–100 ng/mL	193–386 nmol/L
*Prostate-specific antigen, serum		
Male <60 years	<4.0 ng/mL	<4.0 mcg/L
Male >60 years	<7.5 ng/mL	<7.5 mcg/L
*Protein, serum		
Total		
Albumin	6.5–8.3 g/dL	65–83 g/L
Globulin	3.5–5.5 g/dL	35–55 g/L
$\alpha 1$	0.2–0.4 g/dL	2–4 g/L
$\alpha 2$	0.4–0.8 g/dL	4–8 g/L
β	0.5–1.0 g/dL	5–10 g/L
γ	0.6–1.3 g/dL	6–13 g/L

*Test values depend on laboratory methods.

Test	Conventional Units	SI Units
*Protein, serum (continued)		
Urine		
Qualitative	Negative	Negative
Quantitative	50–80 mg/24 h (at rest)	Same
CSF, total	15–50 mg/dL	0.15–0.5 g/dL
Prothrombin time-international normalized ratio	INR: 2.0–3.0	
Protoporphyrin, total, WB	<60 mcg/dL	<600 mcg/L
Pyruvate, blood	0.3–0.9 mg/dL	34–103 mcmol/L
Quinidine, serum or plasma (Hep or EDTA); trough		
Therapeutic	2–5 mcg/mL	6–15 mcmol/L
Toxic	>6 mcg/mL	>18 mcmol/L
Ranitidine, serum, plasma		
Heparin, EDTA		
Peptic ulcer disease	36–94 ng/mL	114–299 nmol/L
Hypersecretory disease	71–376 ng/mL	226–1196 nmol/L
Salicylates, serum or plasma (Hep or EDTA); trough		
Therapeutic	150–300 mcg/mL	1.09–2.17 mmol/L
Toxic	>500 mcg/mL	.3.62 mmol/L
*Sedimentation rate, erythrocyte		
Westergren		
Male: 0–50 y	0–15 mm/h	
Male: >50 y	0–20 mm/h	
Female: 0–50 y	0–20 mm/h	
Female: >50 y	0–30 mm/h	
Sodium		
Serum or plasma (Hep)		
Premature		
Cord	116–140 mEq/L	116–140 mmol/L
48 h	128–148 mEq/L	128–148 mmol/L
Newborn, cord	126–166 mEq/L	126–166 mmol/L
Newborn	133–146 mEq/L	133–146 mmol/L
Infant	139–146 mEq/L	139–146 mmol/L
Child	138–145 mEq/L	138–145 mmol/L
Adult	136–145 mEq/L	136–145 mmol/L
Urine, 24 h	40–220 mEq/d (diet dependent)	40–220 mmol/d (diet dependent)
CSF	138–150 mEq/L	138–150 mmol/L
Sweat		
Normal	8–43 mEq/L	8–43 mmol/L
Cystic fibrosis	70–190 mEq/L	70–190 mmol/L
Specific gravity, urine	1.002–1.030	1.002–1.030
†Testosterone, serum		
Male	300–1200 ng/dL	1.04–41.6 nmol/L
Female	20–80 ng/dL	0.7–2.8 nmol/L
Pregnancy	3–4 × normal	3–4 × normal
Postmenopausal	8–35 ng/dL	0.28–1.22 nmol/L
Theophylline, serum or plasma (Hep or EDTA)		
Therapeutic		
Bronchodilator	10–20 mcg/mL	46–111 mcmol/L
Prem. apnea	6–13 mcg/mL	33–72 mcmol/L
Toxic	>20 mcg/mL	>110 mcmol/L

*http://www.labcorp.com/datasets/labcorp/html/chapter/mono/he005000.htm; http://www.utmb.edu/lsg/LabSurvivalGuide/hem/Sedimentation_Rate.htm

† Test values depend on laboratory methods.

Test	Conventional Units	SI Units
Thiocyanate		
Serum or plasma (EDTA)		
Nonsmoker	1–4 mcg/mL	17–69 mcmol/L
Smoker	3–12 mcg/mL	52–206 mcmol/L
Therapeutic after nitroprusside infusion	6–29 mcg/mL	103–499 mcmol/L
Urine		
Nonsmoker	1–4 mg/d	17–69 mcmol/d
Smoker	7–17 mg/d	120–292 mcmol/d
Thiopental, serum or plasma (Hep or EDTA); trough		
Hypnotic	1.0–5.0 mcg/mL	4.1–20.7 mcmol/L
Coma	30–100 mcg/mL	124–413 mcmol/L
Anesthesia	7–130 mcg/mL	29–536 mcmol/L
Toxic concentration	>10 mcg/mL	>41 mcmol/L
*Thyroid-stimulating hormone (TSH), serum	0.5–5.0 mcU/mL	0.5–5.0 mU/L
Thyroxine serum	4.5–13 mcg/dL (varies with age, higher in children and pregnant women)	58–167 nmol/L (varies with age, higher in children and pregnant women)
*Thyroxine, free, serum	0.8–2.7 ng/dL	10.3–35 pmol/L
Thyroxine binding globulin (TBG), serum	16–32 ng/dL	120–180 mg/mL
Tobramycin, serum or plasma (Hep or EDTA)		
Therapeutic		
Peak		
Less severe infection	5–8 mcg/mL	11–17 mcmol/L
Severe infection	8–10 mcg/mL	17–21 mcmol/L
Trough		
Less severe infection	<1 mcg/mL	<2 mcmol/L
Moderate infection	<2 mcg/mL	<4 mcmol/L
Severe infection	<2–4 mcg/mL	<4–9 mcmol/L
Toxic		
Peak	>10–12 mcg/mL	>21–26 mcmol/L
Trough	>2–4 mcg/mL	>4–9 mcmol/L
Transferrin, serum		
Newborn	130–275 mg/dL	1.30–2.75 g/L
Adult	200–400 mg/dL	2–4 g/L
>60 yr	190–375 mg/dL	1.9–3.75 g/L
Triglycerides, serum, fasting		
Desirable	<250 mg/dL	<2.83 mmol/L
Borderline high	250–500 mg/dL	2.83–5.67 mmol/L
Hypertriglyceridemia	>500 mg/dL	>5.65 mmol/L
*Triiodothyronine, total (T_3) serum	80–200 ng/mL	1.3–3.8 nmol/L
*Troponin-I, cardiac, serum	<0.4 ng.mL	undetectable
Troponin-T, cardiac, serum	<0.1 ng.mL	undetectable
Urea nitrogen, serum	8–20 mg/dL	2.9–7.1 mmol urea/L
Urea nitrogen:creatinine ratio, serum	12:1 to 20:1	48–80 urea:creatinine mole ratio
*Uric acid		
Serum, enzymatic		
Male	3.5–7.2 mg/dL	208–428 nmol/L
Female	2.6–6.0 mg/dL	155–357 nmol/L
Child	2.0–5.5 mg/dL	0.12–0.32 mmol/L
Urine	250–750 mg/24 h (with normal diet)	1.48–4.43 mmol/24 h (with normal diet)
Urobilinogen, urine	0.1–0.8 Ehrlich unit/2 h 0.5–4.0 Eu/d	0.1-0.8 Eu/2h 0.5–4.0 Eu/d

*Test values depend on laboratory methods.

Test	Conventional Units	SI Units
Valproic acid, serum or plasma (Hep or EDTA); trough		
Therapeutic	50–100 mcg/mL	347–693 mcmol/L
Toxic	>100 mcg/mL	>693 mcmol/L
Vancomycin, serum or plasma (Hep or EDTA);		
Therapeutic		
Peak	20–40 mcg/mL	14–28 mcmol/L
Trough	5–10 mcg/mL	3–7 mcmol/L
Toxic	>80–100 mcg/mL	>55–69 mcmol/L
Vanillylmandelic acid, urine (4-hydroxy-3-methoxymandelic acid)	1.4–6.5 mg/24 h	7–33 mcmol/d
Viscosity, serum	1.00–1.24 cP	1.00–1.24 cP
Vitamin A, serum	16–85 mcg/dL	0.19–2.58 mcmol/L
Vitamin B12, serum	200–900 pg/mL	148–664 pmol/L
Vitamin E, serum		
Normal	5.5–18 mcg/mL	12–42 mcmol/L
Therapeutic	30–50 mcg/mL	69.6–116 mcmol/L
Zinc, serum	70–120 mcg/dL	10.7–18.4 mcmol/L

Normal Range of Motion (in Degrees) According to Various Authors*

Joint	AAOS	Boone & Azen	Clark	CMA	Daniels & Worthingham	Dorinson & Wagner	Esch & Lepley	Gerhardt & Russe	Hoppenfeld	JAMA	Kapandji	Kendall & McCreary	Wiechec & Krusen
Shoulder													
Flexion	180	167	130	170	—	180	170	170	—	150	180	180	180
Extension	60	62	80	30	50	45	60	50	45	40	50	45	45
Abduction	180	184	180	170	—	180	170	170	180	150	180	180	180
Internal rotation	70	69	90†	60†	90	90	80	80	55	40†	95	70	90
External rotation	90	104	40†	80†	90	90	90	90	45	90†	80	90	90
Horizontal abduction	—	45	—	—	—	—	—	30	—	—	—	—	—
Horizontal adduction	135	140	—	—	—	—	—	135	—	—	—	—	—
Elbow													
Flexion	150	143	150	135	160	145	150	150	150	150	145	145	135
Radioulnar													
Pronation	80	76	50	75	90	80	90	80	90	80	85	90	90
Supination	80	82	90	85	90	70	90	90	90	80	90	90	90
Wrist													
Flexion	80	76	80	70	90	80	90	60	80	70	85	80	60
Extension	70	75	70	65	90	55	70	50	70	60	85	70	55
Radial deviation	20	22	15	20	25	20	20	20	20	20	15	20	35
Ulnar deviation	30	36	30	40	65	40	30	30	30	30	—	35	75
Hip													
Flexion	120	122	120	110	125	125	130	125	135	100	120	125	120
Extension	30	10	20	30	15	50	45	15	30	30	30	10	45
Abduction	45	46	55	50	45	45	45	45	50	40	30	45	45
Adduction	30	27	45	30	0	20	15	15	30	20	30	10	—
Internal rotation	45	47	20	35	45	30	33	45	35	40	30	45	—
External rotation	45	47	45	50	45	50	36	45	45	50	60	45	—
Knee													
Flexion	135	143	145	135	130	140	135	130	135	120	160	140	135
Ankle													
Plantar flexion	50	56	50	50	45	45	65	45	50	40	50	45	55
Dorsiflexion	20	13	15	15	—	20	10	20	20	20	30	20	30

Joint	AAOS	Boone & Azen	Clark	CMA	Daniels & Worthing-ham	Dorinson & Wagner	Esch & Lepley	Gerhardt & Russe	Hoppen-feld	JAMA	Kapandji	Kandall & McCreary	Wiechec & Krusen
Subtalar Joint													
Inversion	35	37	—	35	—	50	30	40	—	30	52	35	—
Eversion	15	26	—	20	—	20	15	20	—	20	30	20	—

*References for the normal values: American Academy of Orthopaedic Surgeons. Joint motion: Method of measuring and recording. Chicago: AAOS, 1965; Boone DC, Azen SP. Normal range of motion in male subjects. *J Bone Joint Surg (Am)* 1979; 61:756; Clark WA. A system of joint measurement. J Orthop Surg 1920;2:687; Commission of California Medical Association (CMA) and The Industrial Accident Commission of the State of California: Evaluation of industrial disability. New York: Oxford University Press, 1960; Daniels L, Worthingham C. Muscle testing: Techniques of manual examination. 3rd ed. Philadelphia: WB Saunders, 1972; Dorinson SM, Wagner ML. An exact technique for clinically measuring and recording joint motion. 1948; Arch Phys Med 29:468; Esch D, Lepley M. Evaluation of joint motion: Methods of measurement and recording. Minneapolis: University of Minnesota Press, 1974; Gerhardt JJ, Russe OA. International SFTR method of measuring and recording joint motion. Bern: Huber, 1975; Hoppenfeld S. Physical examination of the spine and extremities. New York: Appleton-Century-Crofts, 1976; Journal of the American Medical Association: A guide to the evaluation of permanent impairment of the extremities and back. *JAMA 1958* (special edition), 1; Kapandji LA. Physiology of the joints. Vols. 1 and 2, 2nd ed. London: Churchill Livingstone, 1970; Kendall FP, McCreary EK. Muscles, testing and function, 3rd ed. Baltimore: Williams & Wilkins, 1983; Wiechec FJ, Krusen FH. A new method of joint measurement and a review of the literature. *Am J Surg* 1939; 43:659.

†Measurements obtained with shoulder in 0 degrees of abduction.

From Rothstein JM, Roy SH, Wolf SL. *The Rehabilitation Specialist's Handbook,* 2nd ed. Philadelphia: FA Davis, 1998.

Blood Gas Normal Values

Arterial Blood Gas

Abbreviation	Description	Normal Lab Value	
pH	alkalinity or acidity	adult pediatric	7.35–7.45 7.32–7.42
$PaCO_2$ (also PCO_2)	partial pressure of carbon dioxide	adult pediatric	35–45 mmHg 30–40 mmHg
PaO_2 (also PO_2)	partial pressure of oxygen	adult pediatric	80–105 mmHg 80–100 mmHg
HCO_3	plasma bicarbonate, indicator of metabolic acid/base status	22–28 mEq/L	
SaO_2 (also SO_2)	saturation, arterial, of oxygen	95–98%	
O_2	oxygen	15–23 vol%	
BE	base excess	0 to + or - 2 mmol/L	
ctO_2	concentration of total oxygen, arterial	female male	15.8–19.9 mL/dL 18.8–22.3 mL/dL
CaO_2	arterial blood oxygen content	16–22 mL O_2/dL blood	
metHb	methemoglobin	0.0–1.5%	

Venous Blood Gas

Abbreviation	Description	Normal Lab Value	
pH	alkalinity or acidity	7.30–7.42	
$PvCO_2$	partial pressure, venous, carbon dioxide	40–52 mmHg	
PvO_2	partial pressure, venous, oxygen	25–40 mmHg	
HCO_3	plasma bicarbonate, indicator of metabolic acid/base status	22–28 mEq/L	
SvO_2	saturation, venous, of oxygen	60–85%	
O_2	oxygen	15–23 vol%	
CvO_2	mixed venous blood oxygen content	12–17 mL O_2/dL blood	
CO as COHb	carbon monoxide as carboxyhemoglobin (mixed venous)	nonsmokers smokers 1–2 packs/day >2 packs/day toxic	0.5–1.5 % total Hb 4–5% total Hb 8–9% total Hb >20% of total Hb

Blood Gas Critical Care Parameters

Abbreviation	Description	Normal Lab Value	
AV O_2	arterial-venous oxygen difference (calculated by $C(a\text{-}v)O_2$)	3.5–5.5 ml O_2/dL blood	
Aa	alveolar-arterial gradient	room air 100% O_2	< 22mmHg 150 mmHg
ctHb (also ctO_2 Hb)	concentration of total hemoglobin in blood	female male	12–16 g/dL 13.5–17.5 g/dL
O_2Hb	oxyhemoglobin (oxygenated hemoglobin)	94–98%	
HHb	deoxyhemoglobin (deoxygenated hemoglobin)	<2%	
P O_2	oxygen pressure, room air, arterial (adult range, declines with age)	83–108 mmHg	
P_{50}	partial pressure of oxygen at 50% saturation	25.0–29.0 mmHg	

All values are reference normal ranges. These may vary according to laboratory used or proprietary test methods or in-house standards.

DuBois Body Surface Area Chart: Estimating Body Surface Area of Adults and Children

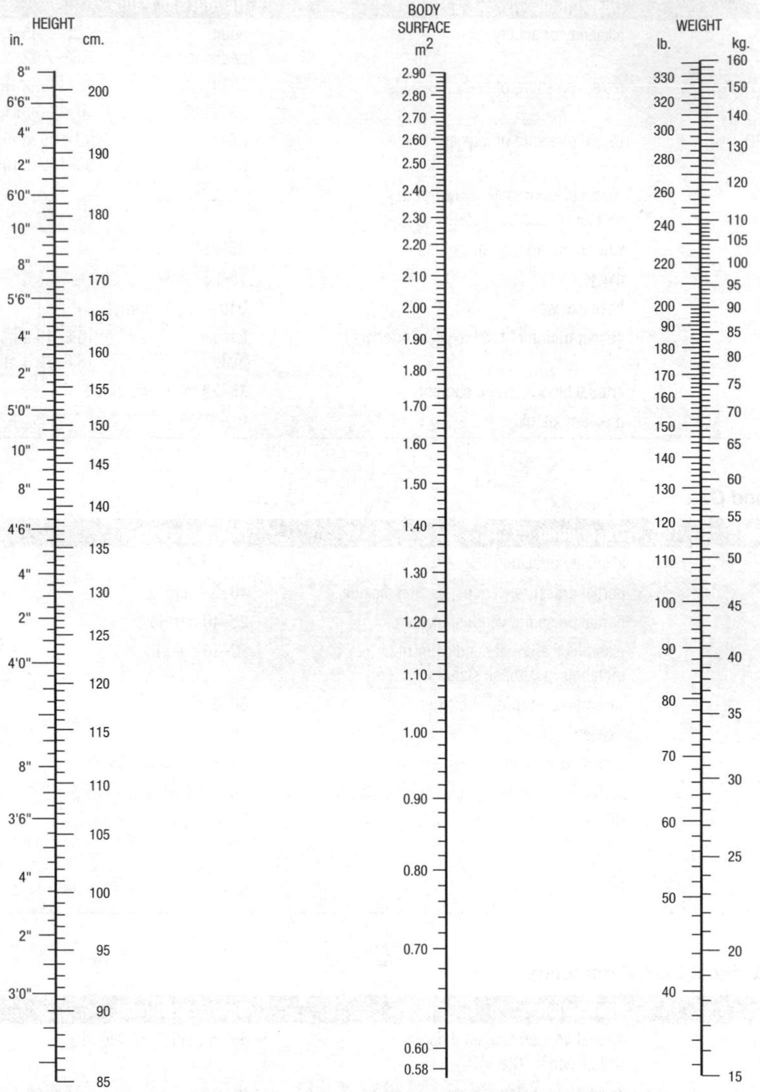

To determine body surface, draw a straight line from the point on the height scale indicating the subject's height to the point on the weight scale indicating the subject's weight. The point where the line crosses the body surface area scale will indicate the subject's body surface area. For example, for a subject 170 cm tall and weighing 75 kg, body surface area will total 1.90 square meters (m^2).

From DuBois EF, Basal metabolism in health and disease. Philadelphia: Lea & Febiger, 1936.

Nomogram: Estimating Surface Area of Infants and Young Children

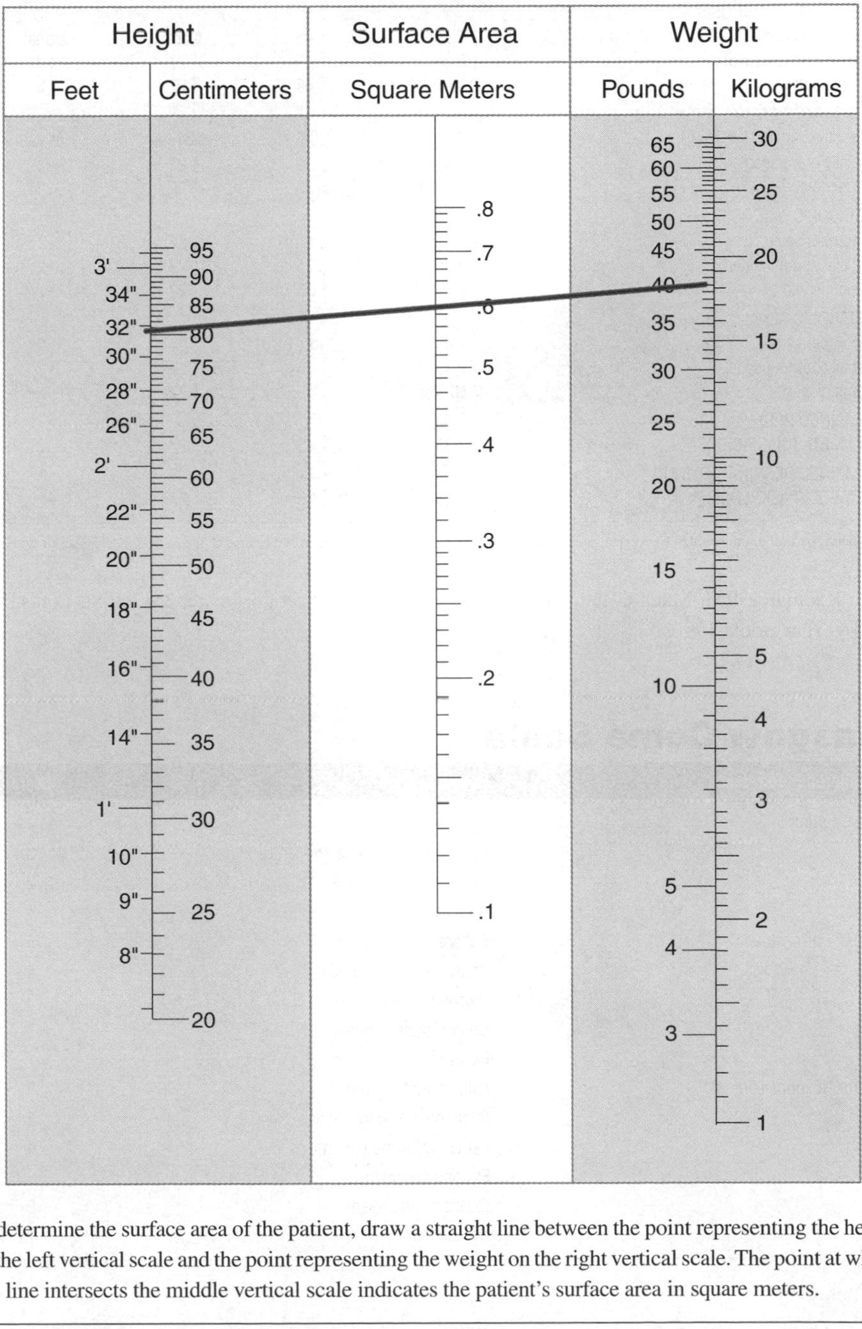

To determine the surface area of the patient, draw a straight line between the point representing the height on the left vertical scale and the point representing the weight on the right vertical scale. The point at which this line intersects the middle vertical scale indicates the patient's surface area in square meters.

From Molle EA, Kronenberger J, Durham LS, West-Stack C, Howe B. *LWW's Comprehensive Medical Assisting*, 2nd Edition. Baltimore: Lippincott Williams & Wilkins, 2005.

Classic Textbook Method of Blood Gas Interpretation

Status	pH	$PaCO_2$	HCO_3^-	BE
RESPIRATORY ACIDOSIS				
Uncompensated	↓7.35	↑45	Normal	Normal
Partially compensated	↓7.35	↑45	↑27	↑+2
Compensated	7.35–7.45	↑45	↑27	↑+2
RESPIRATORY ALKALOSIS				
Uncompensated	↑7.45	↓35	Normal	Normal
Partially compensated	↑7.45	↓35	↓22	↓−2
Compensated	7.40–7.45	↓35	↓22	↓−2
METABOLIC ACIDOSIS				
Uncompensated	↓7.35	Normal	↓22	↓−2
Partially compensated	↓7.35	↓35	↓22	↓−2
Compensated	7.35–7.40	↓35	↓22	↓−2
METABOLIC ALKALOSIS				
Uncompensated	↑7.45	Normal	↑27	↑+2
Partially compensated*	↑7.45	↑45	↑27	↑+2
Compensated*	7.40–7.45	↑45	↑27	↑+2
COMBINED RESPIRATORY AND METABOLIC ACIDOSIS	↓7.35	↑45	↓22	↓−2
COMBINED RESPIRATORY AND METABOLIC ALKALOSIS	↑7.45	↓35	↑27	↑+2

*In general, partially compensated or compensated metabolic alkalosis is rarely seen clinically because of the body's mechanism to prevent hypoventilation.

From Kacmarek RM, Mack CW, Dimas S. The essentials of respiratory care, 3rd ed. St. Louis, MO: Mosby-Year Book, 1990.

Glasgow Coma Scale

Monitored Performance	Reaction	Score
Eye Opening	Spontaneous	4
	Open when patient is spoken to	3
	Open at pain stimulus	2
	No reaction	1
Verbal Performance	Coherent	5
	Confused, disoriented	4
	Disconnected words	3
	Unintelligible sounds	2
	No verbal reaction	1
Motor Responsiveness	Follows instructions	6
	Intentional pain avoidance	5
	Large motor movement	4
	Flexor synergism	3
	Extensor synergism	2
	No reaction	1

Common Tests with Descriptions

Name/Synonyms	Indication(s)	Description/Specimen
Abdominal aorta sonogram; ultrasonography	To detect and measure suspected abdominal aortic aneurysm	Ultrasound waves sent into the body with a small transducer; sound waves are transformed into a visual display on a monitor
Acid-fast bacilli (AFB)	To identify *Mycobacterium* spp. in sputum specimens	Sputum sent for Gram stain
Adrenocorticotropic hormone (ACTH); corticotropin	To evaluate adrenal cortical dysfunction	Blood sample
Alanine aminotransferase (ALT); formerly serum glutamic-pyruvic transaminase (SGPT)	To monitor liver damage	Blood sample
Aldosterone	To diagnose primary and secondary aldosteronism	Blood and urine samples
Alkaline phosphatase (ALP)	To measure serum levels of alkaline phosphatase, an enzyme that is increased in bone growth, liver disease, biliary obstruction, osteogenic sarcoma, or breast or prostate cancer with metastases to the bone	Blood sample
Allergen-specific IgE antibody; radioallergosorbent test (RAST); allergy screen	To test for allergies to allergens	Blood sample
Alpha-fetoprotein (AFP)	To test for neural tube defects in the fetus such as spina bifida and anencephaly	Blood sample
Ambulatory electrocardiography; ambulatory monitoring; event monitoring; Holter monitoring	To monitor electrical activity of the heart and to detect arrhythmias which occur sporadically	Electrodes are applied to the skin, monitor and case are positioned, and the recorder is turned on
Ammonia	To assess for accumulation of ammonia in the bloodstream	Blood sample
Amylase	To assess for pancreatitis, diabetic ketoacidosis, cirrhosis, hepatitis, cholelithiasis, hyperthyroidism, or other conditions	Blood or urine sample
Angiotensin-converting enzyme (ACE); serum angiotensin-converting enzyme	To assess for diabetic retinopathy, Gaucher disease, hyperthyroidism, liver disease, or sarcoidosis	Blood sample
Anion gap	To determine causes of metabolic acidosis including those associated with renal failure, diabetic ketoacidosis, or lactic acidosis	Blood sample
Anti-DNA antibody test	Detects presence of antibodies to native or double-stranded DNA, indicating some type of autoimmune disease	Blood sample
Antinuclear antibody test (ANA)	Used to rule out systemic lupus erythematosus, endocarditis, cirrhosis, connective tissue diseases, and chronic autoimmune hepatitis	Blood sample
Arterial blood gas (ABG) analysis; blood gases	For information regarding the acid-base status of the patient	Blood sample
Arteriography of the lower extremities; lower extremity angiography	Visualization of blood vessels	Contrast dye is injected through a catheter into an artery; radiographic films are then taken of the artery

Name/Synonyms	Indication(s)	Description/Specimen
Arthrocentesis; synovial fluid analysis	To diagnose arthritis, to investigate joint effusion, or to remove excess fluid from the joint	Synovial fluid sample
Arthrogram	To assess for joint damage and/or cartilage tears	Injection of radiopaque dye or air into the joint; radiographs are taken as the joint is manipulated
Arthroscopy	To directly visualize joint structures and to perform biopsy and simple repairs	The arthroscope is inserted into the joint spaces; the joint is manipulated as it is visualized
Aspartate aminotransferase (AST); formerly serum glutamic oxaloacetic transaminase (SGOT)	To assess for heart muscle damage as in myocardial infarction; to assess for liver damage	Blood sample
Barium enema; large-bowel study; lower GI series	Fluoroscopic examination of the large intestines for lower abdominal pain, changes in bowel habits, stools containing blood or mucus, visualizing polyps, diverticula or tumors	The entire intestine is filled with barium from the rectum to the ileocecal valve; the area is observed on a fluoroscopic screen with films taken periodically
Barium swallow; esophageal radiography; esophagography	To evaluate dysphagia or regurgitation, hiatal hernia, diverticula, achalasia, esophagitis, polyps, and/or strictures	Patient swallows a thick barium mixture for fluoroscopic examination of the pharynx and esophagus; part of upper GI series
Bilirubin, direct (conjugated); indirect bilirubin (unconjugated); total bilirubin	To assess for choledocholithiasis, cirrhosis, hepatitis, myocardial infarction, pernicious anemia, and/or septicemia	Blood sample
Bleeding time; aspirin tolerance test; Duke bleeding time; ivy bleeding time; modified ivy; template bleeding time	To screen for disorders involving platelet function and vascular defects that interfere with clotting	A standard skin incision is made usually just below the crease of the elbow; blood drops are blotted every 30 seconds; time is stopped when bleeding ceases
Blood alcohol; ethanol; ethyl alcohol (ETOH)	To screen for alcohol ingestion	Blood sample
Blood culture and sensitivity	To screen for bacteria in the blood	Blood sample
Blood smear; peripheral blood smear; red blood cell smear (RBC smear)	Examines cells in terms of size, shape, color, and structure	Blood sample
Blood typing; ABO typing; ABO red cell groups; blood groups; Rh typing; type and crossmatch (T&C); type and screen	To determine an individual's blood type, Rh factors in the blood, and compatibility in donor blood	Blood sample
Bone marrow biopsy; bone marrow aspiration	To screen for cancer, depressed hematopoiesis, granuloma, infection, iron-deficiency anemia, leukemia, multiple myeloma, polycythemia vera, thalassemia or bone marrow transplantation donor and/or recipient	A large-bore needle is advanced through the subcutaneous tissue cortex of bone to aspirate a sample of bone marrow
Bone scan	To detect metastatic cancer of the bone and monitor the progression of degenerative bone disorders; to detect fractures in patients with continued pain when x-rays have been negative; also see DXA scan	A radionuclide is injected intravenously; scintillation camera takes radioactivity reading from the body and transforms them into two-dimensional pictures of the skeleton; also see DXA scan
Brain scan (cerebral blood flow)	To assess for brain abscess, tumors, contusions, hematomas or cerebrovascular accidents (CVAs); interruption of the blood-brain barrier	A radionuclide is injected intravenously; scintillation camera takes radioactivity reading from the head and transforms them into two-dimensional pictures of the brain
Brain natriuretic peptide (BNP); NT-proBNP	Assess cardiac risk; monitor congestive heart failure (CHF)	Blood specimen
Breast biopsy	To assess for malignancy	Needle biopsy: a sample of tissue is aspirated into a syringe for examination Open biopsy: an excision is made over the breast mass, which is excised in its entirety for testing

Name/Synonyms	Indication(s)	Description/Specimen
Bronchoscopy	To visualize abnormalities found on radiography, obtain sputum specimens, remove foreign bodies, conduct endobronchial radiation, or obliterate neoplastic obstruction	The bronchoscope is introduced through the mouth or nose; the anatomy of the trachea and bronchi are inspected
CA 15-3, CA 19-9, CA-125, tumor markers/antigens	To assess for the presence of cancer	Blood sample
Calcitonin; thyrocalcitonin	To assess for hypercalcemia	Blood sample
Calcium	To assess calcium level	Blood or urine sample
Candida antibody test	To assess for *Candida* infection	Blood sample
Carboxyhemoglobin; carbon monoxide (CO)	To assess for carbon monoxide poisoning	Blood sample
Carcinoembryonic antigen (CEA)	To assess carcinoembryonic antigen levels for malignancy	Blood sample
Cardiac catheterization; angiocardiography, coronary angiography; coronary arteriography; heart catheterization	Visualization of the blood vessels to assess for heart size, structure, movement, wall thickness, blood flow, valve motion, and/or coronary vasculature	A catheter is inserted through an artery into the correct position and dye is inserted; radiographic films are taken of the artery
Carotid duplex scanning; carotid phonoangiography (CPA)	To assess for plaque, stenosis, or partial occlusion of arteries	A transducer is placed on the skin; sound waves are transformed into a visual display on a monitor
Cerebral angiography; cerebral arteriography	To detect cerebrovascular abnormalities such as aneurysm or arteriovenous malformation, to study vascular displacement, or to evaluate postoperative status of blood vessels	A catheter is inserted through an artery into the correct position and dye is inserted; radiographic films are taken of the artery
Cerebrospinal fluid (CSF) analysis; cisternal puncture; lumbar puncture (LP); spinal tap; ventricular puncture	To assist in the diagnosis of a wide variety of central nervous system diseases, including infectious diseases	A sample of cerebrospinal fluid is collected using a spinal needle
Chemistry profile; basic metabolic profile (BMP); sequential multichannel autoanalysis (SMA, SMAC)	To assess multiple organ systems to determine overall health and wellness	May include alanine aminotransferase (ALT); alkaline phosphatase (ALP); aspartate aminotransferase (AST); bilirubin; calcium; carbon dioxide; chloride; cholesterol; creatinine kinase (CK); creatinine; gamma-glutamyl transferase (GGT); glucose; lactic dehydrogenase (LDH); phosphorus; potassium; protein; sodium; urea nitrogen; and uric acid tests
Chest x-ray (CXR); chest radiography	To identify abnormalities of the lungs and other structures of the thorax including heart, ribs, and diaphragm	X-ray of the chest
Chlamydia	To assess for *Chlamydia trachomatis,* trachoma, or sexually transmitted disease (STD)	Titer: Blood sample Eye culture: Swab of inner canthus or lower conjunctiva Cervical culture: Swab of the cervix
Chloride	To evaluate the chloride level in the blood or kidneys	Blood or urine sample
Cholecystography; gallbladder radiography; gallbladder series; oral cholecystogram	To assess for gallbladder disease	After ingestion of a contrast medium, films are taken of the right upper quadrant in three positions
Cholesterol	To evaluate LDL and HDL and risk potential for atherosclerosis and heart disease	Blood sample
Clostridium difficile (*C. difficile*) toxin assay; clostridial toxin assay	To evaluate for pseudomembranous colitis	Stool specimen

Name/Synonyms	Indication(s)	Description/Specimen
Coagulation factor assay; factor assay; clotting factors	To assess for congential or acquired deficiency of blood clotting factor	Blood sample
Coagulation studies (coags)	To evaluate coagulation disorders	Include antithrombin III; bleeding time; clot retraction; coagulation factors; D-dimer; euglobulin lysis time; fibrin degradation; fibrinogen; partial thromboplastin time; plasminogen; protein C; protein S; prothrombin time; and thrombin clotting time tests
Colonoscopy	To assess lower GI bleeding, change in bowel habits, high risk for colon cancer due to polyps, or ulcerative colitis or history	Direct visualization of the large intestine through the use of a flexible fiberoptic endoscope
Colposcopy; endometrial biopsy	To identify the area of cellular dysplasia	Direct visualization of the cervix and vagina with a colposcope with magnifying lens and light; for endometrial biopsy, small tube is inserted into cervix and sample of lining is removed by gentle suction
Complete blood cell count with differential (CBC with diff)	To evaluate red blood cell counts (RBCs), white blood cell counts (WBCs), and platelets	Includes blood smear; hematocrit; hemoglobin; platelets; RBC count; RBC indices (MCV, MCH, MCHC); WBC count; and differential, the quality and type of WBCs present
Computed tomography (CT) of the abdomen; CT scan of the abdomen; computerized axial tomography (CAT) of the abdomen	To diagnose pathologic conditions of the abdominal organs including inflammation, cysts, tumors of the liver, gallbladder, pancreas, spleen, kidneys, and pelvic organs and trauma or foreign body	When indicated, contrast dye is given by IV injection; films are taken in the body scanner
Computed tomography (CT) of the brain; CT scan of the head; computerized axial tomography (CAT) of the head	To diagnose pathologic conditions such as neoplasms, cerebral infarctions, aneurysm, and intracranial hemorrhage and trauma or foreign body	When indicated, contrast dye is given by IV injection; films are taken in the body scanner
Computed tomography (CT) of the chest; CT scan of the chest; computerized axial tomography (CAT) of the chest	To diagnose pathologic conditions, including inflammation, cysts, and tumors of the lungs, esophagus, and lymph nodes and trauma or foreign body	When indicated, contrast dye is given by IV injection; films are taken in the body scanner
Coombs test, direct; direct antiglobulin test; red blood cell (RBC) antibody screen	To assess if antibodies are attached to the red blood cells, indicating infectious mononucleosis or systemic lupus erythematosus; to detect red blood cell sensitization to drugs or blood transfusions	Blood sample
Coombs test, indirect; antibody screening test	To detect unexpected circulating antibodies that may react against transfused red blood cells, other than those of the ABO groups	Blood sample
Cortisol	To assess for normal function of the anterior pituitary gland	Blood or urine sample
C-reactive protein test (CRP)	To assess for inflammatory process	Blood sample
Creatine kinase (CK) and isoenzymes; formerly creatine phosphokinase (CPK)	To assess for myocardial infarction	Blood sample
Creatinine; creatinine clearance	To evaluate renal function	Blood and/or urine sample
Cystometry; cystometrography (CMG)	To evaluate detrusor instability and cause of bladder dysfunction	Instillation of fluid and/or air into the bladder, assessment of neurologic and muscular responses to this filling, and assessment of patient's voiding for abnormalities
Cystourethrography	To evaluate chronic urinary tract infections (UTIs)	Instillation of contrast medium into the bladder through a urethral catheter; x-ray films are taken as the bladder fills and as the patient voids

Name/Synonyms	Indication(s)	Description/Specimen
Cystourethroscopy; cystoscopy; urethroscopy	Calculi removal, diagnosis; therapeutic procedures other than calculi removal: obstruction, urothelial carcinoma, filling defects, unilateral gross hematuria, malignant cytology, surveillance, passage of ureteral catheter for obstruction of fistula, foreign body, resection/fulguration of selected tumors, and dilation/incision of strictures	Passing of cystoscope into the bladder to visualize the urinary tract
Disseminated intravascular coagulation screening (DIC screening)	To assess when both clotting and bleeding occur at abnormally high levels	See coagulation studies
Doppler study; Doppler ultrasonography	To evaluate blood flow in the major veins and arteries of the legs, arms, and neck	Ultrasound waves are sent into the body with a small transducer pressed against the skin
DXA (dual x-ray absorptiometry), DEXA (dual-energy x-ray absorptiometry), BMD (bone mineral density)	To screen for osteoporosis in hip and spine	Patient lies on scan table, transducer passed over hip and spine; dual-energy x-ray transducer relays data to computer. Two separate levels of x-ray energy are compared to determine bone mineral density
Echocardiography; echo; heart sonogram	To assess heart chambers, valves, blood flow or muscle	Ultrasound waves are sent into the body with a small transducer pressed against the skin
Electrocardiography, electrocardiogram (ECG)	To record the electrical current generated by the heart	Monitoring electrodes are placed on the body
Electroencephalography (EEG)	To record the electrical activity of the brain	Monitoring electrodes are placed on the scalp
Electromyography, electromyelography (EMG)	To record the electrical activity in the skeletal muscle groups	Insertion of needle electrodes into the muscle
Electroneurography, electromyoneurography (ENG)	To assess for peripheral nerve disease or injury	Electrodes over a nerve initiate electrical impulse at the proximal site; time is recorded for the impulse to reach a distal site on the same nerve
Endoscopic retrograde cholangiopancreatography (ERCP)	To assess for obstructive jaundice, cancer, calculi, or stenosis	Radiographic viewing of the pancreatic ducts and hepatobiliary tree through an endoscope
Erythrocyte sedimentation rate (ESR), sedimentation rate (sed rate); Westergren; Wintrobe	To assess for inflammatory and necrotic conditions	Blood sample
Esophageal manometry; acid reflux test; Bernstein test; esophageal function studies	To assess the esophagus for normal contractile activity	Manometric catheter is placed at various levels in the esophagus; baseline pressure measurements are taken as the patient swallows
Esophagogastroduodenoscopy (EGD); esophagoscopy; gastroscopy; upper gastrointestinal (GI) endoscopy	To assess the esophagus, stomach, and upper duodenum via direct visualization	The endoscope is inserted through the mouth to inspect anatomy, remove tissue specimen, and/or remove foreign bodies
Estradiol receptor and progesterone receptor (ER/PR) in breast cancer; ER/PR assay	To assess whether breast cancer tissue would respond to treatment to reduce the hormone level	Specimen of breast tissue is removed by excision or needle biopsy
Estrogen; estrogen total; estrogen fractions; estradiol; estriol	To evaluate adrenal cortex, ovaries, and testes function	Blood sample
Evoked potential studies (EP studies); evoked responses; auditory brainstem-evoked potentials; somatosensory evoked potentials; visual evoked potentials	To diagnose lesions of the nervous system by evaluating integrity of the visual, somatosensory, and auditory nerve pathways	Electrodes are placed in appropriate positions and recordings measured

Name/Synonyms	Indication(s)	Description/Specimen
Exercise electrocardiography (exercise ECG); graded exercise tolerance test; stress testing; treadmill test	Measures the efficiency of the heart during physical activity	Electrocardiography and blood pressure monitoring while the patient walks a treadmill; pharmacological stress through adenosine, dipyridamole and dobutamine rather than exercise
Fecal fat	To evaluate for steatorrhea in Crohn disease, cystic fibrosis, or Whipple disease and for chronic pancreatitis, neoplasia, stone obstruction, atrophy of malnutrition, celiac disease and sprue	Stool samples for three days
Ferritin	To evaluate the size of iron storage compartments; to diagnose anemia or hemochromatosis	Blood sample
Folic acid; folate	To diagnose macrocytic anemia and monitor levels during pregnancy	Blood sample
Follicle-stimulating hormone (FSH)	To diagnose hypogonadism, infertility, menstrual disorders, or precocious puberty	Blood sample
Free erythrocyte protoporphyrin (FEP)	To detect iron-deficiency anemia	Blood sample
Gallbladder scan; hepatobiliary imaging; HIDA scan	To assess for cholecystitis or obstruction of the cystic duct	Injection of a radionuclide compound; visualization of the biliary system using a scintillation camera
Gallium scan; body scan	To detect primary neoplasms, metastatic lesions, and inflammatory processes	Injection of radioactive gallium citrate; a scintillation camera is used to scan the entire body
Gamma-glutamyl transferase (GGT); gamma-glutamyl transpeptidase (GGTP)	To assist in the diagnosis of liver problems	Blood sample
Glucose tolerance test (GTT); oral glucose tolerance test (OGTT)	To assess the rate at which glucose is removed from the bloodstream	Blood and urine sample
Glucose, postprandial; 2-hour post-prandial blood sugar (2-hour PPBS); 2-hour p.c. glucose	To assess response of the body to ingestion of a meal with a standard amount of carbohydrates; to assess for effective-ness of insulin therapy	Blood sample
Glucose; blood sugar; fasting blood sugar (FBS); fasting plasma glucose (FPG)	To assess for problems with glucose metabolism	Blood sample
Glycosylated hemoglobin (G-Hb); glycated Hgb; glycohemoglobin; hemoglobin A1c (HbA1c, HgbA1c)	To determine the average blood glucose level for the previous two to three months	Blood sample
Gonorrhea culture	To test for *Neisseria gonorrhoeae*	Endocervical culture: swab of cervical mucus Urethral culture: swab from 2–3 cm within the urethra Rectal culture: swab from 1 inch within the anal canal Oral culture: swab of the pharynx and tonsillar crypts
Heart scan; cardiac nuclear scanning; multiple gated acquisition (MUGA) scan; myocardial scan; nitro-glycerin scan; pyrophosphate (PYP) heart scan; thallium scan; thallium stress testing	To assess for occurrence, extent, and prognosis of myocardial infarction; to monitor effectiveness of angioplasty coronary artery grafts; to assess myo-cardial wall abnormalities; to assess effect of nitroglycerin on ventricular function	Injection of radiopharmaceutical followed by nuclear imaging
Hematocrit (Hct); crit; packed cell volume (PCV)	To assess the extent of blood loss and of normal hydration levels	Blood sample
Hemoglobin electrophoresis (Hgb electrophoresis)	To identify abnormal types or amounts of hemoglobin	Blood sample

Name/Synonyms	Indication(s)	Description/Specimen
Hepatitis antigens and antibodies; hepatitis A; hepatitis B; hepatitis C; Deltavirus	To assess for inflammation of the liver caused by virus, bacteria, or toxic substance	Blood sample
Herpes simplex antibody; herpes genitalis; herpes simplex virus (HSV); herpesvirus	To assess for the herpes simplex virus	Blood sample
High-density lipoprotein (HDL)	To assess for high-density lipoprotein in the blood	Blood sample
Human immunodeficiency virus (HIV) testing; acquired immunodeficiency syndrome (AIDS) test; AIDS serology; ELISA for HIV and antibody; HIV antibody test; Western blot for HIV and antibody	To assess for human immunodeficiency virus	Blood sample
Human leukocyte antigen test (HLA test); HLA typing; tissue typing	To determine tissue compatibility (organ transplantation) and paternity testing	Blood sample
5-hydroxyindoleacetic acid (5-HIAA)	To identify the presence of carcinoid tumors of the intestine	Urine sample
Immunoelectrophoresis; antibodies; gamma globulins; immunoglobulins (IgA, IgD, IgE, IgG, IgM)	To measure immunoglobulins in the blood	Blood sample
Immunoglobulin light chain; Bence Jones protein	To assess for multiple myeloma and amyloidosis	Urine sample
Insulin; insulin assay; serum insulin	To assess the level of insulin in the serum	Blood sample
Iron (Fe)	To assess for anemia or hemochromatosis	Blood sample
Kidneys, ureters, and bladder (KUB) radiography; flat plate x-ray of the abdomen; scout film	To provide an overall view of the lower abdomen; to assess for renal enlargement or displacement, congenital anomalies, renal or ureteral calculi, or ascites and gas in the intestine	X-ray film
Lactic acid; blood lactate	To assess for liver disease	Blood sample
Lactic dehydrogenase and isoenzymes; lactate dehydrogenase (LDH, LD)	To assess for myocardial infarction, biliary obstruction, bone metastases, cancer of prostate, hepatitis, liver damage, macrocytic anemia, pneumonia, muscular dystrophy, shock, or trauma	Blood sample
Lactose tolerance test	To assess for lactose intolerance	Blood sample
Laparoscopy; gynecologic laparoscopy; pelvic endoscopy; pelviscopy; peritoneoscopy	To assess pelvic pain for carcinoma, ectopic pregnancy, endometriosis, pelvic inflammatory disease (PID), and pelvic masses; to view fallopian tubes; to perform lysis of adhesions, ovarian biopsy and tubal ligation	Insertion of a laparoscope through a small subumbilical incision for visualization and performance of procedures
Lipase	To assess abdominal pain	Blood sample
Lipid profile	To evaluate coronary heart disease risk	Usually includes high-density lipoprotein cholesterol, low-density lipoprotein cholesterol, triglycerides, and total cholesterol tests
Liver and pancreatobiliary system ultrasonography; gallbladder and biliary system sonogram; liver sonogram; pancreas sonogram	To assess for jaundice, hepatomegaly, abdominal trauma, cholecystectomy, metastatic tumors of the liver, or pancreatic carcinoma; to guide needle biopsy	Ultrasound waves are sent into the body with a small transducer pressed against the skin
Liver biopsy; percutaneous liver biopsy; percutaneous needle biopsy of the liver	To assess for disease of the liver, elevated liver enzymes, jaundice, hepatomegaly, or possible rejection of a transplanted liver	An aspirated sample of liver tissue
Low-density lipoprotein (LDL)	To assess for low-density lipoprotein in the blood	Blood sample
Lung biopsy	To determine malignancy of a lung mass	An aspirated sample of lung mass tissue

Name/Synonyms	Indication(s)	Description/Specimen
Lung scan; lung perfusion scan; lung ventilation scan; ventilation/perfusion scanning	To detect pulmonary emboli and assess arterial perfusion of the lungs	Perfusion: A radiopharmaceutical is injected; scintillation camera is positioned over the chest Ventilation: Radioactive gas is inhaled through a face mask and the chest is scanned
Lupus erythematosus test (LE test); LE cell prep	To assess for lupus erythematosus	Blood sample
Luteinizing hormone (LH)	To determine whether ovulation occurred; to assess amenorrhea and infertility	Blood sample
Lyme disease antibody test	To evaluate for *Borrelia burgdorferi* infection	Blood sample
Lymphangiography; lymphography	To detect and stage lymphomas and assist in diagnosis	Injection of contrast medium, fluoroscopic visualization, and radiographic films
Magnesium	To assess magnesium level in the blood	Blood sample
Magnetic resonance imaging (MRI)	To evaluate cerebral infarct, abnormalities of the brain and spine, knee injuries, arteriovenous malformation, congenital heart disease, dementia, glomerulonephritis, hydronephrosis, multiple sclerosis, osteomyelitis, seizures, or spinal cord injuries	Imaging while in the MRI cylinder
Mammography	Routine screening for tumors	X-ray film of the breast
Mediastinoscopy	To assess for lymphoma, sarcoidosis, staging of lung cancer	Direct visualization of the contents of the mediastinum via a mediastinoscope inserted at the suprasternal notch
Mononucleosis test; Epstein-Barr virus (EBV) antibody test; heterophil antibody titer (HAT); infectious mononucleosis testing; Monospot test	To assess for infectious mononucleosis	Blood sample
Marker test, triple screen, quad screen; human chorionic gonadotropin (hCG), estriol, alpha fetoprotein (AFP); occasionally inhibin-A	First trimester screen for Down syndrome and neural tube defects	Blood is drawn from mother; analysis of hCG, AFP, estriol and inhbin-A plus mother's age, weight, ethnicity, diabetic status, and twinning/multiple gestation are considered in making recommendations
Myelography	To assess the subarachnoid space of the spinal column for tumors, bone structure changes, or herniations of intervertebral discs	Injection of contrast dye; visualization via fluoroscopy
Osmolality; serum/urine osmolality	To assess fluid and electrolyte imbalance, fluid requirements, urine concentration, and antidiuretic hormone (ADH) secretion, and for toxicology workups	Blood or urine sample
Oximetry; ear oximetry; pulse oximetry (pulsox); oxygen saturation (SaO_2)	To monitor the oxygen saturation of arterial blood	A sensor emits beams of light through the skin tissue; rate and amount of absorption is converted to percentage of oxygen saturation present in the blood and is shown on monitor
Papanicolaou smear (Pap smear); exfoliative cytologic study; Pap test	To detect cervical cancer	Vaginal speculum is used to collect secretions from the cervix and endocervical canal
Paracentesis; abdominal paracentesis; abdominal tap; peritoneal fluid analysis; peritoneal tap	To determine cause of ascites or to remove ascites; to check for abdominal bleeding	Sample of fluid obtained through incision or needle
Parathyroid hormone (PTH); parathormone	To assist in differential diagnosis of parathyroid disorder	Blood sample
Partial thromboplastin time (PTT); activated partial thromboplastin time (APTT)	To detect bleeding disorders	Blood sample
Phosphorus (P); phosphate (PO4)	To assess phosphorus level	Blood sample

Name/Synonyms	Indication(s)	Description/Specimen
Platelet count; thrombocyte count	To assess for thrombocytopenia, thrombocytosis, and platelet production	Blood sample
Pleural biopsy	To determine the nature of pleural tissue	Pleural tissue aspirated through a needle
Positron emission tomography (PET); single photon emission computed tomography (SPECT)	To study blood flow and metabolic changes in organs or regions of body tissues	A radionuclide is administered via IV or inhalation while the patient is in the PET scanner
Potassium	To assess potassium level in the blood	Blood or urine sample
Pregnancy test; human chorionic gonadotropin (hCG)	To determine pregnancy	Blood sample
Proctosigmoidoscopy; anoscopy; proctoscopy; sigmoidoscopy	To assess lower abdominal pain, change in bowel habits, and passage of blood, mucus, or pus in the stool	The sigmoidoscope is inserted into the anus and advanced into the distal sigmoid colon; the sigmoid colon, rectum, and anus are visualized
Progesterone	To assess the level of progesterone in the blood	Blood sample
Prostate-specific antigen (PSA)	To assess for prostate cancer, monitor its progression, or monitor response to prostate cancer treatment	Blood sample
Protein C (PC)	To evaluate severe thrombosis	Blood sample
Protein electrophoresis; serum protein electrophoresis (SPEP)	To evaluate albumin and each of the globulins	Blood sample
Protein; total protein (TP); albumin; alpha globulins; beta globulins; gamma globulins	To assess level of protein in the blood	Blood sample
Prothrombin time (PT); PT-INR; pro time	To evaluate the coagulation process	Blood sample
Pulmonary function tests (PFTs); spirometry	To measure pulmonary volume and capacity	Mouth-breathing into a spirometer as directed for readings of lung capacity and volume
Pyruvate kinase (PK)	To assess the level of pyruvate kinase in the blood; to assess for hemolytic anemia	Blood sample
Red blood cell count (RBC count); erythrocyte count	To measure the number of red blood cells per cubic millimeter of blood	Blood sample
Red blood cell indices (RBC indices); blood indices; mean corpuscular hemoglobin (MCH); mean corpuscular hemoglobin concentration (MCHC); mean corpuscular volume (MCV)	To determine normal size and amount of red blood cells	Blood sample
Renal biopsy; kidney biopsy	To assist in diagnosis of renal parenchymal disease	Renal tissue sample obtained through surgical incision or needle aspiration
Renal scan; kidney scan	To detect renal infarct, renal arterial atherosclerosis, renal trauma, renal tumor or cyst, or primary renal disease	Radiopharmaceutical administered by injection; scintillation camera is positioned over the right upper quadrant
Reticulocyte count (retic count)	To assist in differential diagnosis of anemia	Blood sample
Retrograde pyelography; pyelography	To assess for bladder tumor, hydronephrosis, polycystic kidney disease, ureteral calculi, or renal cysts	Radiopaque iodine-based contrast medium is injected through a catheter into each kidney; radiographic films are taken of the ureters
Rheumatoid factor (RF); rheumatoid arthritis (RA) factor	To assess for rheumatoid arthritis	Blood test
Scrotal ultrasound; ultrasound of testes	To assess for scrotal masses and infection; to evaluate scrotal pain; to locate undescended testicles	A transducer is placed on the skin and moved as needed to provide visualization of the scrotal contents
Semen analysis; seminal cytology; sperm count	Used in fertility workup	Semen specimen

Name/Synonyms	Indication(s)	Description/Specimen
Skeletal x-ray; bone x-ray; sella turcica x-ray; skeletal radiography; skull x-ray; spinal x-ray; vertebral x-ray	To assess for bone deformities, fractures, dislocations, tumors, or metabolic abnormalities	Radiographic films of specific area
Sodium	To assess sodium level in the blood	Blood or urine sample
Sputum culture and sensitivity (sputum C&S)	To diagnose bacterial, fungal, or nonbacterial lower respiratory tract pneumonia	Sputum sample
Stool culture; stool for ova and parasites	To identify pathogens in the GI tract	Stool sample
Stool for occult blood; Hematest; Hemoccult (guaiac)	To identify blood in the GI tract	Stool sample
Syphilis serology; fluorescent treponemal antibody absorption (FTA-ABS); microhemagglutination-*Treponema pallidum* (MHA-TP); rapid plasma reagin (RPR); Venereal Disease Research Laboratory (VDRL)	To assess for *Treponema pallidum*	Blood sample
T- and B-cell lymphocyte counts; acquired immunodeficiency syndrome (AIDS) T-lymphocyte cell markers; CD4 marker; T- and B-cell lymphocyte surface markers	To assess for viral infection, human immunodeficiency virus (HIV) infection, risk of AIDS, measles, Hodgkin disease, or autoimmune processes	Blood sample
Testosterone	To assess testosterone level in blood	Blood sample
Thoracentesis; pleural fluid analysis; pleural tap	To determine the cause of fluid production in the lungs	Aspiration of pleural fluid via a needle
Throat culture and sensitivity	To assess for pathogens	Swab of the tonsillar area and posterior pharynx
Thyroid scan	To assess size, shape, position, and function of the thyroid gland	IV administration of radioactive trace; scanning with scintillation camera
Thyroid-stimulating hormone (TSH); thyrotropin	To assess thyroid hormone levels	Blood sample
Thyroxine (T_4); total T_4	To assess thyroid hormone levels	Blood sample
Thyroxine, free; free T_4 (FT_4)	To assess thyroid hormone levels	Blood sample
Total carbon dioxide content; carbon dioxide content (CO_2 content)	To assess carbon dioxide level in the blood	Blood sample
Total iron-binding capacity (TIBC)	To assess the maximum amount of iron that can be bound to transferrin	Blood sample
Toxicology screen; drug screen	To determine cause of drug toxicity, monitor compliance, and detect presence of drugs for employment or legal purposes	Blood or urine specimen
Transesophageal echocardiography (TEE)	To evaluate thoracic, aortic, and cardiac disorders	Gastroscope introduced into the mouth and advanced to the level of the right atrium of the heart; sound waves from the transducer on the gastroscope are transformed into a visual display
Transferrin; iron-binding protein; siderophilin	To assess the level of transferrin	Blood sample
Triglycerides	To assess triglyceride levels	Blood sample
Triiodothyronine (T_3); total T_3	To assess thyroid hormone levels	Blood sample
Triiodothyronine uptake test (T_3 uptake); T_3 resin uptake	To assess thyroid hormone levels	Blood sample
Troponin, TnI, TnT; cardiac-specific troponin I and T	Rule out myocardial infarction	Serial blood tests, 2 or 3 times in 12 to 16 hours
Tuberculin (TB) skin test; Mantoux test; purified protein derivative (PPD) skin test; tine test	To screen for previous infection by *Mycobacterium tuberculosis*	Intradermal injection of purified protein derivatives (PPDs)

Name/Synonyms	Indication(s)	Description/Specimen
Upper gastrointestinal and small bowel series; gastric radiography; small bowel study; stomach x-ray; upper GI series	To assess dysphagia, regurgitation, burning epigastric pain, hematemesis, melena, or weight loss	Barium is ingested while fluoroscopic films are taken of the esophagus, stomach, and small intestine
Urea nitrogen; blood urea nitrogen (BUN); urinary urea nitrogen	To assess the level of urea nitrogen	Blood or urine sample
Uric acid	To assess for uric acid	Blood or urine sample
Urinalysis (UA); routine urinalysis	Routine screening in physical examination, preoperative testing, hospital admission for diagnosis of infection of the kidneys and urinary tract, and diseases unrelated to the urinary system	Urine sample
Urine culture and sensitivity (urine for C&S)	To identify the specific bacterial organism present in the urine	Urine sample
Uroflowmetry; urine flow studies; urodynamic studies	To detect dysfunctional voiding patterns	Urination into a flowmeter to measure duration, amount, and rate
Urography; infusion pyelogram; intravenous pyelogram (IVP)	To demonstrate normal anatomy and wide range of abnormalities involving the urinary tract	IV administration of contrast material, which is excreted by the kidneys; radiographs are exposed for evaluation of the morphology and function of the urinary tract
Vanillylmandelic acid and catecholamines (VMA); dopamine; epinephrine; norepinephrine; metanephrine; normetanephrine	To assess for neuroblastoma, stress, idiopathic orthostatic hypertension, and pheochromocytoma	Urine sample
Vitamin B12; cyanocobalamin; extrinsic factor	To assess for macrocytic anemia	Blood sample
White blood cell (WBC) count and differential; basophil count; eosinophil count; leukocyte count; lymphocyte count; monocyte count; neutrophil count	To assess the total number of white blood cells and percentage of differentiation	Blood sample
Wound culture and sensitivity	To identify the specific bacterial organism present in the wound	Swab of the wound site

Laboratory Tests

Common Abbreviations

A:G	albumin:globulin ratio
A1AT	alpha-1 antitrypsin
A1C	(hemoglobin) A1C
ABG	arterial blood gas
ABO	blood group
ABO-Rh	ABO blood group, rhesus antigen
ACE	angiotensin converting enzyme
ACT	activated coagulation time
ACTH	adrenocorticotropic hormone
ADH	alcohol dehydrogenase
ADN-B	antideoxyribonuclease B
AFB	acid-fast bacteria
AFP	alpha-fetoprotein
AH	acetylhydrolase
Al	aluminum
ALA	δ-aminolevulinic acid
ALP, alkphos	alkaline phosphatase
ALT	alanine aminotransferase
AMA	antimitochondrial antibody
ANA	antinuclear antibody
ANCA	antineutrophil cytoplasmic antibodies
ANP	atrial natriuretic peptide
APC	activated protein C resistance (factor V Leiden)
APLA	antiphospholipid antibodies
APO	apolipoprotein (A, B, E)
aPTT	activated partial thromboplastin time
ASA	antisperm antibodies
ASMA	antismooth muscle antibody
ASO	allele-specific oligonucleotide hybridization
ASO	antistreptolysin O
AST	aspartate aminotransferase
ATPase	adenine triphosphatase
BAL	bronchial alveolar lavage
BEI	beta endorphin immunoreactivity
BMP	basic metabolic panel (chem-7, SMA-7)
BNP	B-type natriuretic peptide
BSFR	basal secretory flow rate
BUN	blood urea nitrogen
BUN:Cr	blood urea nitrogen: creatinine ratio
C&S	culture and sensitivity
C. diff	*Clostridium difficile*
Ca	calcium
cAMP	cyclic adenosine monophosphate
CBC	complete blood count
CCK	cholecystokinin
CD	cluster of differentiation (membrane protein on leukocytes)
CEA	carcinoembryonic antigen
CF	cystic fibrosis (gene)
CFTR	cystic fibrosis transmembrane regular (gene)
CH	congestive heart failure
CI	Colour Index
CIC	circulating immune complex
CK	creatinine kinase
CK-MB	creatinine kinase muscle-brain
CMP	comprehensive metabolic panel (chem-12, SMA-12)
CMV	cytomegalovirus
CNS	central nervous system
CO2	carbon dioxide
CRH	corticotropin releasing hormone
CRP	C-reactive protein
CSF	cerebrospinal fluid
DA	direct agglutination
D-dimer	fibrin degradation product
DFA	direct fluorescence antigen
DIC	disseminated intravascular coagulation
DLDL	direct low-density lipoprotein
DNA	deoxyribonucleic acid
DNase	deoxyribonuclease
EAC	erythrocyte antibody complement
EBNA	Epstein-Barr nuclear antigen
EBV	Epstein-Barr virus
EGFR	epidermal growth factor receptor
eGFR	estimated glomerular filtration rate

EIA	enzyme immunoassay
ELISA	enzyme-linked immunoassay
EM	electron microscopy
EP	electrophysiology
ER	estrogen receptor
ESR	electron spin resonance
ESR	erythrocyte sedimentation rate
EtOH	ethanol
FANA	fluorescent antinuclear antibody
Fe	iron
FEP	free erythrocyte protoporphyrin
fFN	fetal fibronectin
FIGLU	formiminoglutamic acid
FISH	fluorescence in situ hybridization
FNA	fine-needle aspiration
FOBT	fecal occult blood test
FSH	follicle-stimulating hormone
FSH-RH	follicle-stimulating hormone releasing hormone
FT4I	free thyroxine T4 index
FTA-ABS	fluorescent treponemal antibody-absorption
G6PD	glucose-6-phosphate dehydrogenase
GERD	gastroesophageal reflux disease
GFR	glomerular filtration rate
GGT, GGPT	gamma glutamyl transpeptidase
GI	gastrointestinal
GTT	glucose tolerance test
H&H	hemoglobin and hematocrit
H. pylori	*Helicobacter pylori*
HAMA	human antimouse antibody
HB	hepatitis B
Hb, Hbg	hemoglobin
hCG	human chorionic gonadotropin
HCT	hematocrit
HDL	high density lipoprotein
HER-2/neu	human epidermal growth factor receptor (gene)
Hg	mercury
HHV	human herpesvirus
HIV	human immunodeficiency virus
HLA	human leukocyte antigen
HPA	hypothalamic pituitary axis
HPV	human papillomavirus
HSV	herpes simplex virus
HVA	homovanillic acid
ICG	indocyanine green
IGF	insulinlike growth factor
IgG	immunoglobulin G
IgM	immunoglobulin M
IM	infectious mononucleosis
IMA	ischemia modified albumin
IMViC	indole, methyl red, Voges-Proskauer, citrate
INR	International Normalized Ratio (prothrombin time)
ISI	International Sensitivity Index
K	potassium
KOH	potassium hydroxide
L:S	lecithin:sphingomyelin ratio
LA	lupus antibody, lupus anticoagulant
LAP	leucine aminopeptidase
LATS	long-acting thyroid stimulator
LDH	lactate dehydrogenase
LDL	low-density lipoprotein
LE	lupus erythematosus cell
LFB	Luxol fast blue
LH	luteinizing hormone
Li	lithium
LMWH	low molecular weight heparin
Lp(a)	lipoprotein a
lytes	electrolytes
M:C	microalbumin:creatinine ratio
MCH	mean corpuscular hemoglobin
MCHC	mean corpuscular hemoglobin concentration
MCV	mean corpuscular volume
Mg	magnesium
MGP	methyl green pyronin
MHA	microhemagglutination
MIC	minimum inhibitory concentration
MLC	mixed lymphocyte culture
MMA	methylmalonic acid
mono	infectious mononucleosis
MOST	modified sperm stress test
MRSA	methicillin-resistant *Staphylococcus aureus*
Na	sodium
NAIT	neonatal alloimmune thrombocytopenia
NBT	nitroblue tetrazolium
NK	natural killer (cell)
NT-pro-BNP	N-terminal probrain natriuretic peptide

O&P	ova and parasites
P	blood group (PI antigen)
P&P	prothrombin and proconvertin
P	phosphorus
p24	HIV antibody
PAB	Alcian blue-periodic acid-Schiff
Pap	Papanicolaou smear
PAS	periodic acid-Schiff
Pb	lead
PCR	polymerase chain reaction
PKU	phenylketonuria
PNH	paroxysmal nocturnal hemoglobinuria
PPLO	pleuropneumonialike organism
PR	progesterone receptor
pro time	prothrombin time
PSA	prostate-specific antigen
PSEN1	presinilin 1
PT 20210	activated protein C resistance, factor V Leiden
PTH	parathyroid hormone
PT-INR	prothrombin time international normalized ratio
PTT	partial thromboplastin time
PUD	peptic ulcer disease
PVP	polyvinylpyrrolidone
RA	rheumatoid arthritis
RBC	red blood cell
RDW	red (blood cell) distribution width
Rh	rhesus antigen
RhD	rhesus antigen D typing
RIA	radioimmunoassay
RISA	radioiodinated serum albumin
RISA	radioimmunosorbent assay
RPR	rapid plasma reagin
RSV	respiratory syncytial virus
SCAT	sheep cell agglutination
SeHCAT	selenium-labeled homocholic acid taurine
SHBG	sex-hormone binding globulin
SMAC	sequential multi analyzer computer, sequential multichannel autoanalyzer
SOD	superoxide dismutase
SPCA	serum prothrombin conversion accelerator
T3	triiodothyronine
T4	thyroxine
tauAβ	amyloid beta 42 peptide and tau protein (Alzheimer marker)
TB	tuberculosis
TIBC	total iron-binding capacity
TnI	troponin I
TnT	troponin T
TORCH	toxoplasmosis, other infections, rubella, cytomegalovirus, herpes simplex
TPH, TPHA	*Treponema pallidum* hemaglutination
TPI	*Treponema pallidum* immobilization
TRH	thyroid releasing hormone
TSH	thyroid stimulating hormone
TUNEL	terminal deoxynucleotidyl transferase-mediated dUTP-biotin end labeling
TWAR	*Chlamydia pneumoniae*, from isolates TW-83 and AR-39
UA	urinalysis
UHF	unfractionated heparin
UTI	urinary tract infection
VCE	vagina, ectocervix, endocervix
VDRL	Venereal Disease Research Laboratory
VMA	vanillylmandelic acid
VP	Voges-Proskauer
VZV	varicella zoster virus
WBC	white blood cell
WNV	West Nile virus
ZPP	zinc protoporphyrin
ZSR	zeta sedimentation rate

Test Names with Description of Purpose

NOTE: The bold type indicates the name of test, roman type is brief description. Some do not have a description because the name is self-evident

Abbé test plate, evaluate microscope objectives
Abbott stain, for spores
abscess aerobic or anaerobic culture
absolute eosinophil count, for allergic or parasitic disease
absorbency index, protein identification
abuse screen (drugs of)
acetaminophen assay
Acetest, dipstick for urine ketones
acetic acid and potassium ferrocyanide test, for Bence Jones protein
acetoacetic acid test, for urine ketones
acetone test, for urine ketones
acetylcholinesterase (AcHase) assay, specialized test with reflex to fetal hemoglobin to evaluate false-positive AFP
acid elution test (Kleihauer-Betke), for fetal hemoglobin
acid-fast stain, for *Mycobacterium* spp.
acid-fast bacillus (AFB) culture, smear, stain, for *Mycobacterium*
acid hemolysin, acid serum, acidified serum test(Ham test), for paroxysmal nocturnal hemoglobinuria
acidified glycerol lysis test, for spherocytosis
acidity reduction test, for gastroesophageal reflux disease (GERD)
acid perfusion test (Bernstein test), for GERD
acid phosphatase assay or test (Gomori stain), for semen
acid phosphatase, prostatic, marker for metastatic prostate cancer
acid phosphatase tartrate test, for leukemic reticuloendotheliosis (hairy cell leukemia)
acid reflux test, for GERD
acid-Schiff, periodic acid-Schiff stain method (PAF), for histology
acquired immune deficiency syndrome (AIDS) virus culture, serology
Actinomyces culture, to identify bacteria
activated clotting time, activated coagulation time (ACT), for coagulopathy and/or antiplatelet therapy
activated partial thromboplastin time (APTT) test, for measuring common coagulation pathway and/or antiplatelet therapy
adenovirus antibody serology, titer, culture
adhesion test, for strength of dental adhesive bond or immune adhesion phenomenon
adrenal antibody, for Addison disease
adrenal function test, for cortisol or ACTH
adrenocorticotropic hormone (ACTH) infusion test, for cortisol, blood pressure, endocrine function
adrenocorticotropic hormone (ACTH) stimulation test, for adrenocortical inhibition test
adrenocorticotropic hormone (ACTH) suppression test, for adrenal excess or deficiency; Cushing disease, Addison disease, hypopituitarism
adult polycystic kidney disease inheritance determination, genetic evaluation
advanced semen analysis, to monitor intrauterine insemination
aerobic and anaerobic bacteria blood culture, for sepsis and other bacterial infections
aerobic bacterial culture, for bacteria identification
agar plate count, for quantitative microorganisms in milk, dairy, and sterile rooms
agglutination test, for presence of antibody or antigen in body fluids

agglutination titer, quantitative antibody or antigen in body fluids
aggregometer test, platelet function test
air-dried smear, for cytologic studies
alanine aminotransferase (ALT) test, for liver function
albumin suspension test, for blood grouping, microbicidal activity
albumin test, for liver or kidney function
albumin:creatinine ratio (A:Cr), for microalbuminuria
albumin:globulin ratio (A:G), for nutritional status, liver or kidney function
Alcian blue stain, for histology
Alcian blue-periodic acid-Schiff (PAB) stain, for histology
alcohol assay, for ethanol in body fluids
alcohol dehydrogenase (ADH) assay, for ethanol detection
aldolase assay, test for fructose intolerance
aldosterone assay, for aldosteronism, blood pressure
aldosterone stimulation test, for primary aldosteronism, aldosterone-producing tumor
aldosterone suppression test, for hyperaldosteronism, sodium
alimentary tract smear, for cytologic study
alizarin test, pH dye indicator
alizarin stain for calcium, calcium deposition, kidney stones
alkali denaturation test, for fetal hemoglobin
alkaline phosphatase (ALP) assay, test, for molecular biology, label for EIA, hypo- or hyperphosphatasemia
alkaloid test, for presence of alkaloids in plants or body fluids
allele-specific oligonucleotide (ASO) hybridization, for sickle cell anemia and alpha-1-antitrypsin deficiency
Allen-Doisy test, estrogen content
allergen profile, screen, multiple methods and tests
alloantigen-D antibody, for Rh-D protein
alpha amino nitrogen (alpha-AAN) test, for amino acid metabolism
alpha-1-antiprotease (A1AP) phenotype, for emphysema susceptibility
alpha-1-antitrypsin (A1AT) phenotype, for genetic evaluation for A1AT deficiency
alpha-fetoprotein (AFP) test, for neural tube defects
amebiasis antigen test, serology, to rule in/out amebiasis
American Type Culture Collection (ATCC), repository and distributor of cell lines and type cultures
amino acid screen for amino acids, inborn errors of metabolism
aminolevulinic acid (ALA) test, for porphyria, tyrosinemia
ammonium chloride loading test, for renal tubule function
amniotic fluid analysis, for various developmental and congenital conditions, erythroblastosis fetalis (hemolytic disease of newborn)
amniotic fluid karyotype, for genetic testing
amniotic fluid phospholipid profile, for fetal lung maturity
amniotic fluid spectral analysis, for fetal neural tube, sensitization conditions
amplification of genetic material, specific for various microorganisms, DNA chip technology for genotyping
amylase test, with lipase, pancreatic function; in urine, with creatinine, kidney function
amylase:creatinine clearance ratio (A:CrC), for kidney function
anaerobic bacteria culture, for bacterial identification
analytic cytology, identification and various antibodies

arsenic stain (Osborne arsenic stain), arsenic contact or ingestion
androstenedione test, for hirsutism and virilization
angiotensin I, II test, for hypertension
angiotensin-converting enzyme (ACE), sarcoidosis and response to therapy
anion gap test, for hydration status
antibiotic sensitivity test, for antimicrobial effectiveness
antibiotic-associated colitis toxin test, for *Clostridium difficile*
antibody detection, identification, stain, titer, quantitative and qualitative antibody measurements
alpha-1-antichymotrypsin test, immunologic test for deficiency
anticardiolipin antibodies (ACA), for antiphospholipid syndrome
anticytoplasmic antibody (ACPA) test, for Wegener granulomatosis
antideoxyribonuclease-B (ADN-B) assay, titer, test, for rheumatic fever
antifactor Xa assay, for heparin therapy
antigen detection, for various microorganisms and autoimmune states
antiglobulin test (Coombs test), for hemolytic anemias
antiglobulin-augmented lymphotoxicity assay, lupus-associated thrombocytopenia
antihuman globulin reagent (Coombs reagent), for antiglobulin antibodies in hemolytic anemias
antihyaluronidase (AH) assay, titer, *Streptococcus* antibody test
aPL (antiphospholipid) antibody test, for antiphospholipid syndrome
antimicrobial susceptibility testing, for effective antimicrobial therapy
antimitochondrial antibody assay, for primary biliary cirrhosis
antineutrophil cytoplasmic antibody (ANCA), for inflammatory small-vessel disease
antinuclear antibody (ANA) assay, for systemic lupus erythematosus
antiparietal cell antibody assay, for anemias
antiphospholipid antibody (APLA), for unexplained thrombotic episode, recurrent fetal loss, thrombocytopenia and/or prolonged partial thromboplastin time
anti-Rh titer, for rhesus antigen
anti-Smith (anti-Sm) antibody, for systemic lupus erythematosus
antismooth muscle antibody (ASMA) assay, immune system reactions
antispermatozoal antibody test, for fertility
antistreptococcal DNase-B titer, inflammatory conditions
antistreptolysin-O (ASO) test, titer, *Streptococcus* antibody test
antithrombin I, II, III, IV test, for hypercoagulable disorders
anti-*Toxoplasma* antibody test, for *Toxoplasma* infection
antitrypsin test, (SEE alpha-1-antitrypsin test)
antitryptic index, for protease identification
anti-Xa assay, (SEE heparin anti-Xa assay)
apoptosis assay, as diagnostic and to monitor therapies
Apt-Downey test, for maternal-fetal blood differentiation
arboviral encephalitis serology, for arbovirus encephalitis
arbovirus serology, titer, for arbovirus infection
arginine-insulin tolerance test, for growth hormone secretion
Arneth count, index, formula, for percentage of distribution of neutrophils
arterial blood gas, saturation of oxygen and carbon dioxide
arterial line culture, for microorganisms
arterial-ascitic fluid pH gradient, for peritonitis
arthropod identification, for possible envenomation
ascariasis serologic test, for roundworm infestation
ascitic fluid analysis, cytology, for cause of ascites, cancer, liver failure

Ascoli test, reaction, thermoprecipitation for anthrax
ascorbic acid test, for vitamin C status
aspartate aminotransferase (AST) test, liver function
***Aspergillus* antibody test, serology,** for fungal infection
aspirin tolerance test, assess hereditary platelet disorder
astrocyte stain (Cajal astrocyte stain), for brain histology
atrial natriuretic peptide (ANP), heart failure assessment
atypical *Mycobacterium* smear, differentiate organism and assess antitubercular therapy
autohemolysis test, hereditary spherocytosis
auramine-rhodamine stain (fluorescent), to diagnose presence of *Mycobacterium*
automated cell image analysis, automated cytophotometry
automated differential, for types/quantities of white blood cells
automated multiphasic screening, standard blood tests
automated reagin test (ART), for syphilis
Autopath QC test, computerized Papanicolaou smear evaluator
autosomal-dominant polycystic kidney disease DNA detection

***Babesia* serologic test,** for babesiosis
Bachman-Pettit test, modification of Kober test, estradiol in urine
bacitracin disc test, microbial sensitivity
bacteremia detection, buffy coat micromethod
bacterial antigen detection method
bacterial culture, genotyping, serology, stain, for identification
bacteriologic index, assessment of infection or antimicrobial therapy
bacteriophage typing, for identifying and tracking microbes
Barr chromatin body test, sex determination
***Bartonella* culture, titer, serology,** for catscratch fever
basal secretory flow rate (BSFR) test, experimental method
basic metabolic panel (BMP), standard blood screen, also called chem-7 or SMAC-7
basophil degranulation test, allergies and drug sensitivity
BCR-ABL1 kinase domain mutation analysis, measures resistance to antileukemic therapy
Beaver direct smear method, for *Ascaris* and other worm infestations
Becker antigen, stain, for spirochetes
bedside testing, out-of-laboratory test method
Bence Jones protein test, urine test for neoplastic processes
bentiromide test, pancreatic enzyme function
Bernstein test (esophageal acid perfusion test), for GERD
Berry spot test, for mucopolysaccharidosis screen
beta-hemolytic *Streptococcus* culture
beta-lactamase test, microbial identification, sensitivity, resistance
Bethesda assay, for factor VIII:C inhibitors in hemophilia A
Bethesda Papanicolaou smear, for cervical and vaginal cytology
Betke-Kleihauer test (acid elution test), for fetal hemoglobin
Beutler test (Beutler-Baluda test), infant screen for galactosemia
Bielschowsky stain, for senile plaques
bicarbonate test (CO_2), for acidosis, part of electrolyte panel
bile acid tolerance test, for liver disease
bile esculin agar (hydrolysis) test, positive for group D *Streptococcus*
bile salt breath test, for blind loop syndrome

biliary drainage examination, for gallstones
biliary sludge examination, for biliary microlithiasis
biochemical profile (chemistry panel, SMAC), electrolytes, calcium, phosphate, renal function, glucose, protein, albumin, liver function tests
biotin-streptavidin detection method, technology used to augment antigen-antibody reactions
bipolar staining (safety pin), characteristic pattern, *Yersinia pestis*
biuret test, for serum proteins
bladder washing cytology, bladder abnormalities, neoplasia
Blastomycosis dermatitidis **antibody titer, serology,** for blastomycosis
bleeding time, to assess coagulopathy
blood cell count, determine type and quantity of blood cells
blood clot lysis time, for coagulopathy
blood culture, for bacteria
blood gas analysis, oxygen and carbon dioxide in blood
blood grouping and Rh typing, for fetomaternal incompatibility
blood karyotype, determine genetic blood type; transplant, anemias, fetomaternal incompatibility
blood smear, number and types of blood cells by visual examination
blood spot screen for galactose/galactose-1 phosphate, neonatal screen for galactosemia
blood typing, determine blood group for transfusion, fetomaternal incompatibility
blood urea nitrogen (BUN), for kidney function
Bodian copper-protargol stain, for neural tissue
body cavity fluid cytology, for infection, cancer
body fluid aerobic culture, for infection
body fluid amylase, pancreatitis and other reasons for abnormal elevation
body fluid analysis, for infection and other indications
body fluid cytology, for cancer
body fluid pH, effusions, acid-base balance
body fluid specific gravity, measures homeostasis and function
bone marrow aspiration and biopsy, evaluate for hematopoietic disease and/or transplant
bone marrow chromosome analysis, engraftment analysis
bone marrow culture, for microorganism identification
bone marrow differential count, evaluate hematopoiesis
bone marrow iron stain, evaluate hematopoiesis
bone marrow karyotype, for anemias and myelodysplasias
Bordetella pertussis **culture, serology, smear, titer,** for whooping cough
Borrelia burgdorferi **DNA assay, DNA probe test, PCR,** a polymerase chain reaction test for Lyme disease
bovine cervical mucus penetration test (human or bovine cervical mucus), fertility sperm test
Boyden chamber assay device (cell-migration assay, filter membrane migration assay, trans-well migration assay), for leukocyte chemotaxis
branched-chain DNA assay, for hepatitis B
breakpoint analysis, genetics
breath analysis test, alcohol intoxication, hepatic and intestinal absorption
breath hydrogen analysis, for lactose tolerance
breath testing, for *Helicobacter pylori*
Breed smear, quantitative bacteria
bronchial alveolar lavage (BAL) culture, cytology, washings to identify microorganisms, infection, cancer
bromocriptine suppression test, for growth hormone response

bromphenol test, reagent strips for protein, albumin, and globulin in urine
bronchial brushing or washing cytology, for infection, cancer, bronchial disease
bronchoscopic smear, for bacterial or fungal infection
***Brucella* agglutination test, culture,** for brucellosis
B-type natriuretic peptide (BNP), heart failure assessment
buccal smear, for sex chromatin (Barr body) evaluation
buffy coat smear, biologic test material preparation

^{13}C-labeled ketoisocaproate breath test, liver function
^{13}C lactose test, for lactase deficiency
C3, C4 (total complement), monitor autoimmune disease
C1q immune complex detection, immune complex test for rheumatic, infectious, neoplastic disorders
Cache Valley virus, antibody test, primarily veterinary
calcitonin assay, for medullary carcinoma of thyroid
calcium ionized assay, for effects of calcium
calcium oxalate test, for kidney stones
calcium stimulation test, for insulinoma, hyperinsulinism
California encephalitis virus serology, titer
***Campylobacter pylori* serology,** for *Campylobacter pylori* infection
***Campylobacter pylori* urease test and culture,** for *Campylobacter pylori* infection
***Campylobacter*-like organism test,** *proprietary,* for *Campylobacter pylori* infection
***Candida* culture, precipitin test, serology,** for candidiasis
capillary fragility test (Göthlin), for vitamin C deficiency or thrombocytopenia
capillary tube test, pediatric hematocrit, zetacrit, equipment/method for variety of laboratory tests
captopril test, for renal hypertension
carbamazepine assay, therapeutic monitoring
carbohydrate fermentation test, for identification of *Neisseria*
carbohydrate metabolism index, metabolic syndrome
carbohydrate utilization test, for *Neisseria gonorrhoeae*
carboxyhemoglobin assay, for carbon monoxide poisoning
carcinoembryonic antigen (CEA) assay, breast cancer monitoring
Cardiac T Rapid assay, *proprietary*, coronary artery disease/myocardial infarction
cardiac troponin, for myocardial infarction
Carr-Price test, quantitative vitamin A
catscratch bacterial culture, for *Bartonella* spp.
catatorulin test, for vitamin B1
catecholamine test, for pheochromocytoma
C-banding stain, centromere banding stain, genetics
Cefinase testing, for bacterial strain beta-lactamase
centromere banding stain, C-banding stain, genetics
cephalin-cholesterol flocculation test, liver function test
cephalosporinase production testing, antimicrobial sensitivity
cerebrospinal fluid analysis, assay, for infection, autoimmune disease
cerebrospinal fluid bacterial antigen testing, identify bacterial CNS infection
cerebrospinal fluid cryptococcal latex agglutination
cerebrospinal fluid culture, for meningitis, encephalitis
cerebrospinal fluid cytology, for tumor, infection
cerebrospinal fluid glucose, for tumor, infection, CNS conditions
cerebrospinal fluid glutamine, for tumor assessment

cerebrospinal fluid glycine, nonketotic hyperglycinemia
cerebrospinal fluid immunoglobulin G (IgG) index, infection, encephalitis, meningitis
cerebrospinal fluid India ink preparation, for *Cryptococcus neoformans*
cerebrospinal fluid lactate dehydrogenase, hematooncologic disease
cerebrospinal fluid methotrexate, for therapy evaluation
cerebrospinal fluid *Mycobacterium* culture, for CNS tuberculosis
cerebrospinal fluid oligoclonal bands, for multiple sclerosis
cerebrospinal fluid protein electrophoresis, for infection, tumor, neurodegenerative disease
cerebrospinal fluid Venereal Disease Research Laboratories (VDRL), neurosyphilis
cerebrospinal fluid virus culture, presence/identification in meningitis, encephalitis
ceruloplasmin test, copper storage/metabolism disorders
cervical culture, for microorganisms
cervical mucus interaction, cross-hostility test
cervical mucus sperm penetration test (Penetrak), *proprietary,* fertility testing
cervical smear, for Papanicolaou test, microorganisms
cervical/vaginal cytology, hormone evaluation, infection, cancer
chemical inhibition isoamylase test, pancreatitis
chemiluminescence test, detection method
chemistry profile (basic metabolic panel, biophysical profile, SMAC), basic tests of blood chemistry
Chemstrip, *proprietary*, dipstick product chenodeoxycholic acid test, bile acids
chickenpox culture, titer for herpes zoster infection
***Chlamydia* culture, serology, titer, smear,** for either bronchopneumonia *(C. pneumoniae)* or sexually transmitted infection *(C. trachomatis)*
chloride:phosphorus ratio (Cl:P), hyperparathyroidism
chlormerodrin accumulation test, for renal function
cholecystokinin test, biliary disease
cholesterol test, heart disease risk analysis
cholesterol-lecithin flocculation test, parasitic disease
cholinesterase test, pesticide and toxin exposure
chorionic gonadotropin test, pregnancy
chorionic villus biopsy, sampling, for genetic disorders
Christie-Atkins-Munch-Petersen (CAMP) test, for group B *Streptococcus*
chromaffin reaction test, for pheochromocytoma and other catecholamine-producing tumors
chromate stain, for lead exposure/toxicity
^{51}C red blood cell (RBC) survival test, GI bleeding
chromogenic cephalosporin test, beta-lactamase-producing microorganisms
chromogenic enzyme substrate test, bacterial identification test
chromosome and genetic abnormality analysis
chromosome instability test, genetic conditions and susceptibility
Ciaccio stain, for insoluble intracellular lipids
***Cimex* identification,** for bedbugs
circulating anticoagulant screen, dysproteinemias and anticoagulant therapy
circulation time, cardiopulmonary function
cis-trans test, genetic mutations
citrate test, bacterial identification
citrulline antibody, for rheumatoid arthritis
Clauberg test, progestational activity
clean-catch urine culture, for urinary tract infection
Clinitest, *proprietary*, agents, various

clomiphene citrate (Clomid) challenge test, fertility assessment
clonidine suppression test, pheochromocytoma
***Clostridium difficile* toxin assay, culture,** for pseudomembranous colitis
clot retraction time, bleeding disorders
clotting time, bleeding disorders
coagglutination test, for group A *Streptococcus*
coagulase test, *Staphylococcus* strain differentiation
coagulation factor assay, for coagulopathies
coagulation time test, coagulopathies and anticlotting therapies
coagulogram, for coagulopathies
cocaine metabolite assay, for drugs of abuse
coccidioidin test, coccidioidomycosis serology, for coccidioidomycosis
cold agglutinin screen, test, titer autoimmune hemolytic anemia, some infections
cold hemolysin test (Donath-Landsteiner), for paroxysmal cold hemoglobinuria
colony-forming unit-culture, evaluation of peripheral blood and bone marrow stem cells
Colour Index (CI), chemistry of dyes
Coloscreen Self test, *proprietary*, fecal occult blood test
combined pituitary function test, anterior pituitary function
competitive protein-binding assay, various therapeutic agent evaluation
complement binding assay, for immune complex
complement fixation (CF) antibody titer, *Histoplasma, Mycoplasma,* other infections
complement fixation (CF) test, various infections
complement lysis sensitivity test, paroxysmal nocturnal hematuria
complete blood count (CBC), basic screening test
computer-assisted semen, sperm analysis
conglutinating complement absorption test, viral and other infections
Congo red, dye for amyloidosis and free hydrochloric acid in gastric contents
conjunctival culture, conjunctival smear cytology, for eye infection
consumptive coagulopathy, screen for DIC and coagulopathies
continuous flow culture, bacterial cultivation, continuous flow of fresh medium to maintain bacterial growth in logarithmic phase
Coombs indirect test (indirect antiglobulin test), for antibodies against red blood cell antigens
Coombs test (antihuman globulin), antibody test
copper reduction tablet test (Clinitest, Clinistix, Benedict test), urine glucose, ketones,
copper-binding protein test, liver function
coproporphyrin assay, test, for porphyrias
cord blood screen, for hemoglobin and blood abnormalities
corneal culture, cytology, for corneal infection and conditions
cornification count, cervical cytology
corrected reticulocyte count, for bone marrow productivity
corticotropin-releasing hormone stimulation test, for Cushing disease
cortisol assay, adrenal function
cortisone-glucose tolerance test (cortisone-primed oral glucose tolerance test), diabetes and other endocrine disorders
cough plate culture for pertussis, evaluate for *Bordetella pertussis*
Covalink MicroElisa culture plate, *proprietary*, ELISA equipment
Coxsackievirus A and/or B titer, culture, type A causes herpangina and hand-foot-and-mouth disease; type B viruses cause epidemic pleurodynia; both viral types may cause aseptic meningitis, myocarditis and pericarditis, and Type 1 diabetes.

C-reactive protein assay, test, for acute inflammation
creatine kinase test, muscle damage
creatinine clearance test, kidney function
cryocrit, for cryoglobulinemia
cryohemolysis test, hereditary spherocytosis
***Cryptococcus* antigen or antibody titer,** current or previous cryptococcal infection
crystal examination, synovial fluid for gout, deposition disease, infection
cul-de-sac smear, for ovarian cancer evaluation
culture and sensitivity (C&S) test, urinary tract infection and antimicrobial therapy
^{13}C-xylose breath test, small-bowel bacterial overgrowth
cyanide-ascorbate test, hemolysis evaluation
***Cyclospora cayetanensis* detection,** for cyclosporiasis
cyst aspiration cytology, cyst fluid analysis, chemistry, cytology, methods of evaluating cysts
cystic fibrosis (CF) sweat test, for cystic fibrosis presence
cystic fibrosis transmembrane regulator (CFTR) gene mutation analysis, genetic test
cysticercosis serology, titer, for *Taenia solium*
cytologic screening, early disease detection
Cytomegalovirus (CMV) antibody, antigen detection, cytology, DNA detection, PCR, serology, smear, titer, evidence of Cytomegalovirus inclusion disease or infection with Cytomegalovirus
cytometric image analysis, cellular DNA content
cytometry, analytic cytology
Cyto-Rich cervical cytology monolayer system, *proprietary*, system for cervical cancer screen
cytospin analysis, mechanical dissociation method

dark-field examination, leptospirosis, syphilis
D-dimer assay, test for hypercoagulability
DeBakey-type aortic dissection assay, immunoassay of monoclonal antibodies to smooth muscle myosin heavy chain
deferoxamine mesylate infusion test, chelating agent, iron overload, heavy metals
dehydroepiandrosterone (DHEA) test, fetoplacental unit status, hormonal status
deoxyribonuclease B antibody, recent *Streptococcus* infection
deoxyuridine suppression test, vitamin B12 or folate deficiency
dermatophyte fungus culture, for skin, hair, nails fungal infection
dexamethasone suppression test, for Cushing syndrome
dibucaine number, for pseudocholinesterase deficiency
diepoxybutane stress test, anemias and blood cancers
differential agglutination titer, for toxoplasmosis
dihydrotestosterone (DHT) test, male hormone evaluation
differential renal function test, for renal hypertension
differential white blood cell (WBC) count, types and quantities of white blood cells
Diff-Quik smear, *proprietary*, histologic stain
direct agglutination (DA) test, for microorganisms, infection
direct antiglobulin test (DAT) (direct Coombs test), for anemias, jaundice, hemolysis
direct bilirubin test, for hemolysis, liver function
direct Coombs test (direct antiglobulin test [DAT]), for anemias, jaundice, hemolysis
direct fluorescent antibody, direct fluorescent assay (DFA) test, presence of microorganisms
direct fluorescent antibody-*Treponema pallidum* (DFA-TP) test, for syphilis
direct low-density lipoprotein (DLDL), heart disease risk
direct Shiga toxin test, for shigellosis *Shigella dysenteriae* type 1

disaccharide tolerance test, for lactose intolerance and other GI disease
disc diffusion test (Kirby-Bauer test), microorganism antibiotic susceptibility
DM1 gene mutation analysis, for myotonic dystrophy
DNA analysis for parentage evaluation, genetic determination of individuals biological parents
DNA content, hybridization, index, ploidy, probe assay, multiple methodologies microorganism and/or genetic testing
DNA fingerprint, individual identification, criminal justice, and other applications
dot blot test, microorganism identification
double antibody immunoassay, microorganisms, hormones, therapeutic evaluation
double antibody precipitation, microorganism
double antibody sandwich assay, ELISA method for microorganism detection
double (gel) diffusion precipitin test in one dimension, antigen-antibody test
double (gel) diffusion precipitin test in two dimensions (Ouchterlony test, method), antigen-antibody test
drug abuse screen, identify common drugs of abuse
drug screening assay, therapeutic evaluation
Duchenne/Becker muscular dystrophy carrier, PCR gene test
Duffy antibodies (to antigens Fya, Fyb), for blood phenotype
Duke bleeding time test, earlobe incision
duodenal drainage examination, pancreatitis, other GI tract disorders
duodenal smear, for cancer detection
D-xylose absorption (tolerance) test, enterogenous malabsorption syndromes

ear culture, for isolation of aerobic bacteria
Eastern equine encephalitis virus serology, titer, presence or course of encephalitis
Eaton agent *(Mycoplasma pneumoniae)* titer, presence or course of infection
echinococcosis serology, taeniid tapeworm, echinococcosis
echovirus culture, alternate to immunofluorescent assay
ectoparasite identification, various methods for skin, nails, hair lice, fungus, other parasites
effusion cytology, quantitative/qualitative for cells in effusion
ehrlichiosis serology, for rickettsiae infection
elastic van Gieson stain, for connective tissue
elastic-Weigert resorcin-fuchsin stain method, for connective tissue
electroblot analysis, immunologic and microorganism identification
electrolyte panel, routine or specific for acid-base balance; Na, Cl, K, CO_2
electron microscopy, for exquisite detail, millions times magnification
electron spin resonance (ESR) assay, identification and differentiation of various chemicals
electropherogram, plot of fluorescent units over time; for various DNA analyses
electrophoresis (EP) test, separate and purify molecules
electrophoretogram, record of results of electrophoresis
Ellsworth-Howard test, for pseudohypoparathyroidism
encephalitis viral serology, determine presence and type of virus
endocervical culture, for infection
endocervical smear, for cancer and/or infection determination
endometrial smear (endometrial cytology), for cancer and/or infection determination
endometrium anaerobic culture, for endometritis
***Entamoeba histolytica* serologic test,** for amebic dysentery
enterovirus RNA detection (enterovirus genome detection, enterovirus molecular probe assay), for presence/identification of enterovirus

enzyme deficiency analysis, genetic enzyme deficiency diseases
enzyme immunoassay, anemias, antigen/antibody
enzyme-linked antibody test, anemias, antigen/antibody
enzyme-linked immunosorbent assay (ELISA), immunology for antigen and/or antibody
eosinophil count, for allergy, parasites, other conditions
eosinophil smear (Hansel stain, Wright stain for eosinophils), allergy, parasites, interstitial nephritis, GI disorders
epidermal growth factor receptor (EGFR, EGFR HER-1, erB-1), solid tumor receptor assessment
Epstein-Barr nuclear antigen (EBNA), acute infection
Epstein-Barr virus antibody assay, acute or resolving mononucleosis
Epstein-Barr virus culture, serology, titer, acute or resolving mononucleosis
erythrocyte adherence test, detection of neoplasia and microorganisms
erythrocyte count, SEE red blood cell count
erythrocyte enzyme deficiency screen, various genetic enzyme abnormalities
erythrocyte fragility test, red blood cell resistance to hemolysis in hypotonic saline solutions
erythrocyte index, hemopoiesis
erythrocyte sedimentation rate (ESR) assay, acute and chronic inflammation
erythrocyte, antibody, complement (EAC), immune status, leukemias
erythropoietin test, anemias evaluation
esophageal brushing and/or washing cytology, evaluation for cancer
esophageal smear, cytology, evaluation of cells for infection, cancer
(leukocyte) esterase test, urinary tract infection
estimated glomerular filtration rate (eGFR), for kidney function
estradiol test, fertility testing
estrogen (ER) and progesterone receptor (PR) assay, for breast cancer
estrogen receptor assay, for breast cancer
ethanol gelation test, for fibrinolysis
euglobulin clot lysis time, for venous thrombosis, bleeding disorders
exfoliative cytology, shed cells for disease states
extrinsic allergic alveolitis serology (farmer's lung), pneumonitis evaluation and identification of thermophilic actinomycetes
eye culture, for infection
eye smear for cytology, quantitative/qualitative
eye swab, bacterial culture

factor VIII-related antigen test (von Willebrand factor test), hemorrhagic disease
farmer's lung disease serology (extrinsic allergic alveolitis serology), pneumonitis evaluation and identification of thermophilic actinomycetes
Farr test (double-stranded DNA autoantibodies), for systemic lupus erythematosus
fasting bilirubin test, for liver function
fat absorption test (fecal), for GI tract function
febrile agglutination test (Widal reaction), for typhoid fever
fecal lactoferrin, for inflammatory bowel disease
fecal leukocyte count, for inflammatory bowel disease
fecal occult blood test (FOBT), colorectal cancer screen
fecal pancreatic elastase 1, for exocrine pancreas function
fecal pH, colorectal cancer risk assessment
fecal smear for eosinophils, allergy or parasites
female genital tract (FGT) cytologic smear, cancer screen

fermentation test (oxidation-fermentation test), identification of microorganisms
fern test, ovulation detection
ferric chloride test, for alkaptonuria
ferric ferricyanide reduction test (Schmorl stain), method of reducing multiple substances in tissues
ferritin assay, anemia evaluation
fetal fibronectin (fFN), to monitor preterm delivery risk
fetal hemoglobin test, evaluate persistence of fetal hemoglobin and other hemoglobinopathies
Feulgen cytometry, Feulgen-stained nuclei for chromatin, pattern and nuclear distribution of DNA
fibrin degradation products method, for DIC and hypercoagulation
fibrin titer, hypercoagulation
fibrinogen method, for thrombosis detection
fibrinogen titer test, excessive bleeding, DIC, thrombosis
fibrin-split products, DIC test
fibrin-stabilizing factor test (factor XIII), presence of factor XIII
filter paper microscopic test, for syphilis, *Strongyloides,* malaria
fine-needle aspiration (FNA) biopsy, minimally invasive, cancer and infection screen
fine-needle aspiration (FNA) biopsy cytology, analysis of cells in sample
fine-needle aspiration (FNA) culture, for microorganisms
fingerstick blood collection, method
Finn Chamber patch test, for contact dermatitis, allergy testing
Fishberg concentration test, for renal water conservation
flask culture, method of growing microorganisms
flocculation test, serologic test in which flocculent agglomerate is formed
fluorescent antibody darkfield, microorganism identification
fluorescent antibody technique or test, for microorganism detection
fluorescent treponemal antibody-absorption (FTA-ABS), for *Treponema pallidum*
fluorescent antinuclear antibody (FANA or ANA) test, for autoimmune/rheumatoid disease
fluorescent cytoprint assay, in vitro chemosensitivity
fluorescent gonorrhea test cytologic smear, for *Neisseria gonorrhoeae*
fluorescent in situ hybridization (FISH) assay, cytogenetic analysis
fluorescent rabies antibody test, detection of rabies
flow cytometry, technique for counting, examining, sorting microscopic particles suspended in a stream of fluid
fluid cytology, examination of fluids removed from body (pleural, ascitic, washings)
foam stability test, for fetal lung maturity
follicle-stimulating hormone (FSH) assay, fertility testing
formiminoglutamic acid (FIGLU) excretion test, folic acid in pregnancy
follicle-stimulating hormone:luteinizing hormone ratio (FSH:LH), distinguish primary from hypothalamic/pituitary cause of gonadal failure; menstrual disturbances and amenorrhea, menopause; fertility evaluation in women; testicular dysfunction in men
follicle-stimulating hormone-releasing hormone, for hypothalamic-pituitary-gonadal dysfunction evaluation
Fontana-Masson stain for melanin (melanin bleach), melanin deposits in skin, eye, substantia nigra, and malignant melanoma
Forssman antigen-antibody reaction, specific for infectious mononucleosis
Foshay test, intradermal test for *Francisella tularensis* and catscratch fever
Fouchet stain, for bilirubin in feces, urine, serum
four-marker test, pregnancy screen for Down syndrome; free alpha-hCG, free beta-hCG, alpha-fetoprotein (AFP), unconjugated estriol

Franklin-Dukes agglutination test, for sperm autoantibodies
Fraser-Lendrum stain for fibrin, multistaining method
free erythrocyte protoporphyrin (FEP), monitor lead exposure
free T3 (triiodothyronine), thyroid function
free T4 (thyroxine), thyroid function
fractional inhibitory concentration (FIC), interaction coefficient indicating combined
inhibitory/bacteriostatic effect of drugs as synergistic, additive or antagonistic
fragile X carrier, mutation, prenatal, DNA, genetic testing
fragility test, SEE erythrocyte fragility
frozen section, for microscopic diagnosis of tissue specimen
fructose assay, presence of fructose in body fluids
FMR1 mutation analysis, genetic testing for X-linked mental retardation
fungal antibody screen, presence of fungal infection
folded-cell index, vaginal cytology, evaluate imminent labor
fungal culture, stain, smear, presence, and identification of fungi
fungus susceptibility testing, for antimicrobial therapy

Gaddum and Schild test, sensitive method for identification of epinephrine in tissue or other material
galactose breath test, galactose tolerance test, for galactosemia
gamma glutamyltransferase (GGT) assay, liver function
gastric acid stimulation test, gastric function, PUD, gastritis, Zollinger-Ellison syndrome
gastric analysis, nocturnal acid output, for ulcer disease
gastric aspirate cell count, infection, aspiration of gastric contents into lungs
gastric emptying time, gastroparesis, diabetes mellitus, GI tract function
gastric function test, PUD, other GI tract disease
gastric smear, for cancer
gastrin assay, for Zollinger-Ellison syndrome and pernicious anemia
gastrin-secretin stimulation test, for Zollinger-Ellison syndrome
Gastroccult test, *proprietary*, test for occult blood
gastrointestinal blood loss test, for anemia, cancer
gastrointestinal protein loss test, for infection, roundworm, hookworm
gastrointestinal tract brushing/washing, for cytology
gastrointestinal tract cytology, for cancer
G-banding stain, for chromosome testing
gel diffusion precipitin tests in one dimension, antigen-antibody reactions
gel diffusion precipitin tests in two dimensions (Ouchterlony test), antigen-antibody reactions
gelation assay, for hereditary spherocytosis
Gendre fluid, histologic stain
gene frequency, to determine occurrence of an allele in relation to that of other alleles of same gene in a population
gene mapping, genetic mapping, to establish details of genes to specific locations on chromosomes
genetic abnormality analysis, markers for disease and genetic counseling
genetic linkage analysis, evaluation of jointly inherited alleles
genetic marker (genetic determinant), antigenic determinant or identifying characteristic, particularly those of allotypes
genetic screening, blood and tissue testing for genetic diseases
gestational diabetes screening test, for pregnant women
Gibson-Cooke sweat test, for cystic fibrosis
Giemsa (modified May-Grünwald) stain, for hemopoietic tissue

Giemsa stain, demonstrates Negri bodies, *Tunga* spp., spirochetes, protozoans, differential staining of blood smear, and chromosome G-bands
glial fibrillary acidic protein, glial scarring, neurodegenerative disease, Alexander disease
glomerular filtration rate (GFR), to assess kidney function
glucagon test, assessment of growth hormone/pituitary function, glycogen metabolism
glucose oxidase paper strip test culture, to identify variety of microorganisms and chemicals
glucose suppression test, for growth hormone assessment
glucose-6-phosphate dehydrogenase (G6PD) test, for G6PD deficiency
glutathione stability test, red blood cell function, anemia, G6PD deficiency
glycerol lysis test, for hereditary spherocytosis
glycine assay, for alkaline phosphatase
glycogen storage test, for glycogen storage disease
glycosylated hemoglobin test (hemoglobin A1C), for diabetes status
Gofman test, for cholesterol-containing serum lipoproteins
Gomori aldehyde fuchsin stain, specialized stain for body tissues
Gomori chrome alum hematoxylin-phloxine stain, for cytoplasmic granules
Gomori-Jones periodic acid–Schiff, for renal histopathology
Gomori methenamine-silver stain, for argentaffin cells
Gomori nonspecific acid phosphatase stain, histologic preparation
Gomori silver impregnation stain, for reticulin, diagnostic aid in neoplasm and early cirrhosis
gonadotropin test, for hypogonadotropic hypogonadism
gonorrhea culture, to isolate *Neisseria gonorrhoeae*
Gram iodine, solution of iodine and potassium iodide
Gram stain, differential staining of bacteria
granulocyte agglutination test, for granulocytopenia
granulocyte immunofluorescence test, for granulocytopenia
Gridley stain for fungi
Grimelius argyrophil stain (Pascual method), histologic staining
Grocott-Gomori methenamine silver stain, modification of Gomori stain for fungi
group A beta-hemolytic *Streptococcus*, for vasculitis, infection of respiratory tract and skin, scarlatina
guaiac test, for occult blood
guinea pig kidney absorption test, miscellaneous immune reactions
gunshot wound culture, to identify microorganisms
Günzberg test, for hydrochloric acid
Guthrie test, phenylketonuria (PKU) screen in infants

Hale colloidal iron stain, for mucopolysaccharides
Ham test (acid hemolysin test), for paroxysmal nocturnal hemoglobinuria
Hanger test, a cephalin cholesterol flocculation test
hanging-block culture, propagation of cells or microbes in block of solidified agar suspended from slide
hanging-drop culture, propagation of cells or microbes in drop suspended from slide
hantavirus serology, for infection
haptoglobin test, for hemolytic anemia
hepatic iron index, for hereditary hemochromatosis
heat instability test, for unstable hemoglobins
heavy metal screen, for heavy metal poisoning/exposure
Heinz body test, for G6PD-deficient red blood cells
***Helicobacter pylori* serology,** for peptic ulcer disease
***Helicobacter pylori* urease test and culture,** for peptic ulcer disease

hemizona binding assay, test measuring capacity of sperm to bind to zona pellucida
hemadsorption virus test, quantitative method to detect hemaglutinating viruses
hemagglutination inhibition assay, for virus identification and for antibody determination
hemagglutination assay, test, titer, measures certain antigens, antibodies, or viruses, using their ability to agglutinate certain erythrocytes
hematology profile (heme profile, CBC, SMAC), basic blood testing
Hemoccult test, *proprietary,* fecal occult blood
hemochromatosis DNA test, genetic testing
hemoglobin and hematocrit (H&H), anemia screen
hemoglobin F assay, for fetal hemoglobin
hemolytic index, hemoglobin concentration
hemosiderin, for anemias
hemosiderinuria test, for paroxysmal nocturnal hemoglobinuria
heparin anti-Xa assay, for hemostasis and thrombosis
hepatic function (liver function) tests, include bilirubin, albumin, alkaline phosphatase, transaminases (ALT, AST), PTT, gamma-glutamyl transpeptidase test, lactic dehydrogenase test, 5-nucleotidase test, alpha fetoprotein, mitochondrial antibodies
hepatitis A, B, C, D serology, to determine infection and type of hepatitis virus
herpes simplex virus antigen detection, culture, isolation, for herpesvirus infection
herpes smear, for detection/identification of human herpesviruses (HHV)
herpes zoster serology, for chickenpox, shingles
heterologous ovum penetration test, assessment of sperm penetration, fertility
heterophil antibody, antigen reaction test, for infectious mononucleosis
high-density lipoprotein (HDL) cholesterol assay, for atherosclerosis risk
histamine flare test, for allergic response
histamine test, for pheochromocytoma and scombrotoxins
histocompatibility testing, for transplantation
histoplasmin-latex test, for *Histoplasma capsulatum*
histoplasmosis serology, for *Histoplasma capsulatum*
Hoesch test, bedside screening for urinary porphobilinogen
Hoffmann test, sedimentation concentration test for *Strongyloides stercoralis* infection
Hofmeister test, for leucine
Holzer glial fiber stain¸ for neural tissue
homocystinuria test, for homocystinuria
homogentisic acid test, for alkaptonuria
homovanillic acid (HVA) test, tumor detection
Hooker-Forbes test, for compounds of progestational activity
Hopkins-Cole test, for tryptophan
Hoppe-Seyler test, for carbon monoxide in blood
Hortega pineal stain, histologic nerve tissue
Huhner test (postcoital test), for cervical mucus around time of ovulation to evaluate its receptivity to sperm
human antimouse antibody (HAMA), presence due to exposure to mice or monoclonal antibody testing or therapy
human epidermal growth factor (HER2/neu, c-erB-2), breast cancer tumor marker, for treatment and progress
human chorionic gonadotropin injection test, to trigger ovulation, stimulate testosterone production in men
human erythrocyte agglutination test, to assess various immune and autoimmune states

human herpesvirus 6 (HHV6) culture, detection, for presence of HHV6
human immunodeficiency virus (HIV) antibody, culture, serology, titer, for AIDS
human leukocyte antigen (HLA) typing, for major histocompatibility groups, allotransplantation, transfusion, immune response, autosomal dominant inheritance
human papillomavirus DNA probe test, for genital warts
Huntington disease gene mutation analysis, for Huntington disease
hyaluronidase digestion for Alcian blue stain, tissue and microorganism differentiation
hydroxybutyric test, analysis for drug(s) of abuse
hydroxyproline index, for nutrition status
hyperalimentation line culture, to isolate and identify organisms
hypercoagulable state coagulation screen (hypercoagulation panel), for blood coagulation disorders, including DIC, thrombus, systemic lupus erythematosus
hyperphenylalaninemia screen, for PKU and other phenylalanine dysfunction
hypersensitivity pneumonitis serology (farmer's lung), for thermophilic actinomycetes
hypertonic cryohemolysis test, for hereditary spherocytosis
hypoosmotic swelling test, male fertility test

idiogram (karyotype), diagrammatic representation of chromosome morphology characteristic of a species or population
image cytometry, for qualitative tests such as antibody density
immune assay, for infections, autoimmune status, hormone levels, cancers, drug levels
immunoassay (immunochemical assay), quantitative determination of antigenic substances
immunoblot test, viral assay technique
immunocapture test, for viral identification
immunoconcentration assay, for microorganism identification
immunocytochemistry, methods of determining cell types
immunodeficiency profile (acquired immunodeficiencies profile, AIDS profile, CD4:CD8, helper:suppressor ratio, T4:T8, T-helper:T-suppressor, absolute T-cell count, CD3 count, CD4 count, CD8 count, T-cell subsets), tests of immune function in AIDS
immunoenzymometric assay, method of determining tissue types
immunofluorescence assay, skin biopsy, for antibodies in sera or tissue
immunoglobulin A, D, G, M test, determine inflammation and hyper- and hypogammaglobulinemia
immunoglobulin G (IgG) index, in CSF, infection of CNS
immunoglobulin G (IgG) synthesis rate, inflammatory CNS conditions
immunoglobulin G (IgG):albumin ratio, to determine local CNS versus systemic inflammation
immunohistochemistry, localizing proteins in cells of a tissue by antibody-antigen binding
immunologic pregnancy test, various methods of measuring human chorionic gonadotrophin (hCG)
immunomicroscopy, for pathology
immunoperoxidase stain, for antibodies
immunoradiometric assay, radiolabeling method for antibodies
immunostain, for histology
implantation test, pregnancy evaluation
in vivo cervical mucus penetration test, fertility evaluation
in vivo cervical mucus postcoital test, fertility evaluation
in vivo compatibility test, for blood donor and transplantation analysis
inborn errors of metabolism screen, neonatal screening for common conditions
inclusion body cytology¸ herpesvirus infection, pemphigus, and vesiculobullous skin or mucosal disorders
India ink preparation, for *Cryptococcus* and other fungi

indirect antiglobulin test (Coombs indirect test), for antibodies against red blood cell antigens
indirect bilirubin test, for unconjugated bilirubin, liver function
indirect fluorescent antibody test, for microorganisms
indirect hemagglutination test, for anemias, infections
indole, methyl red, Voges-Proskauer, citrate (IMViC), differentiate *Escherichia coli* from *Enterobacter aerogenes* and related species
indophenol method, for quantitative vitamin C in tissue
infectious mononucleosis screen, serology, for infection with Epstein-Barr virus and/or cytomegalovirus
influenza A and B antigen, culture, titer, serology, for influenza virus infection
insulin clearance test, for glucose metabolism
insulin sensitivity test, to measure hormone response
insulin tolerance test, to measure hormone response
insulin-induced hypoglycemia test, to measure hormone response
International Normalized Ratio (INR) (International Sensitivity Index [ISI]), prothrombin time
intradermal test (skin test), method for skin reaction to antibodies
intraesophageal pH test, for GERD
intraoral needle aspiration, for cancer or infection
intravenous glucose tolerance test, for diabetes
intravenous tolbutamide tolerance test, assess for liver function, diabetes mellitus
intravital stain, living cells uptake after parenteral administration of dye
iodine test, for presence of starch based on its reaction with iodine
^{131}I (iodine-131) uptake test, for thyroid function
ionogram (ionopherogram) (electropherogram), density or color patterns on electrophoresis
iron profile (iron and TIBC), iron stores evaluation
iron stain (Prussian blue), acid potassium ferrocyanide to demonstrate presence of iron, as in siderocytes
iron stain (Turnbull blue), double cyanide of ferrous and ferric iron
islet cell antibody screening test, screen for diabetes mellitus
isocitrate dehydrogenase test, various uses
isoform ratio, molecular determination
isoniazid phenotype test, determine isoniazid disposition or resistance
Ivy bleeding time test, sphygmomanometer and arm incision method

Jerne plaque assay (hemolytic plaque assay), enumerates individual antibody-forming cells
joint fluid analysis, for infection, deposition disease, arthritis
Jones I test (primary dye), lacrimal drainage
Jones II test, secondary dye, localization of lacrimal drainage
Jones test, fluorescein instillation test for water flow

kala-azar serologic test
kaolin clotting time, screen for antiphospholipid antibodies and lupus anticoagulant
kaolin partial thromboplastin time, screen for first-stage plasma clotting deficiencies
kappa light chain analysis by flow cytometry, immunoglobulin determination in neoplasm, autoimmunity
karyopyknotic index, hormonal status index by exfoliated vaginal cell morphology
Katayama test, qualitative colorimetric test for carboxyhemoglobin in blood
ketogenic corticoids test, for adrenocortical tumors, Addison disease, or panhypopituitarism
ketone bodies test, measurement for ketones in blood, diabetes management
kidney profile, assess levels of blood urea nitrogen (BUN) and creatinine

kidney stone analysis, to determine chemical makeup
Kleihauer-Betke test, acid elution test for fetal hemoglobin
Klinger-Ludwig acid-thionin stain for sex chromatin, to differentiate Barr bodies
KOH (potassium hydroxide) preparation, test, for fungus
Kováts retention index, for gas chromatographic data
Kremer sperm-penetration test, for cervical mucus
Kurzrok-Ratner test, for estrogen in urine
Kveim test (Kveim-Stilzbach test), for sarcoidosis

lactic dehydrogenase test, for heart attack, liver disease, anemia
lactose tolerance test, for lactase deficiency
Laki-Lorand factor, factor XIII
lambda light chain analysis by flow cytometry, immunoglobulin chain, immune status
lamellar body count(lamellar body density count), amniotic fluid for fetal lung maturity
Laquer stain for alcoholic hyalin, histologic stain
large vessel hematocrit, hemodilution
lateral vaginal wall smear, for cytohormonal evaluation
latex agglutination test (latex fixation test), antibody-antigen test for microorganisms, immunity, pregnancy
latex agglutination-inhibition test, antibody-antigen assessment for microorganisms, immunity, drug screen
latex screen, for specific antibodies
latex slide agglutination test, antigen-antibody for microorganisms, immunity, drugs
lavage cytology, cells obtained by washing
lead excretion ratio, for lead poisoning
lead mobilization test, for lead poisoning
lecithin:sphingomyelin ratio (L:S), for fetal lung maturity
Lee-White clotting test, time, bleeding time
***Legionella* direct fluorescent antibody smear,** presence of *Legionella*
***Legionella* indirect fluorescent antibody titer,** presence of quantitative assessment *Legionella*
***Legionella pneumophila* culture, direct FA smear,** specific for Legionnaires' disease
Leitz image analysis system, *proprietary*, automated quantitative cytology
lepromin skin test, for *Mycobacterium leprae*
Leptospira culture, DNA amplification method, serodiagnosis, for leptospirosis
leucine aminopeptidase (LAP) test, liver function test
leukemia analysis by flow cytometry
leukocyte adherence assay test, cell-mediated antitumor immunity
leukocyte alkaline phosphatase (LAP) test, for differential diagnosis of myeloproliferative disease
leukocyte bactericidal assay test, for cell-killing ability
leukocyte cytochemistry, for evaluating white blood cell abnormalities
leukocyte differential count, qualitative and quantitative for types of white blood cells
leukocyte esterase test, for urinary tract infection
leukocyte immunophenotyping, for immune status
leukopenic index, food allergy test, decrease in white blood cell count
leukotactic assay, for inflammatory response
Levinson test, precipitation test for tuberculous meningitis
levulose tolerance test, for liver function
lice identification
light chain analysis by flow cytometry, immunoglobulin determination

Liley test, amniotic fluid analysis
***Limulus* amebocyte lysate assay,** gram-negative bacterial meningitis using *Limulus polyphemus* blood cell amebocyte lysate
lipase test, for pancreatitis
lipid profile, test for cholesterol determination
lipoprotein electrophoresis test, electrophoretic separation of plasma lipoproteins
lipoprotein phenotyping, to evaluate hyperlipidemia by determining abnormal lipoprotein distribution and concentration in the serum
liquid-based thin-layer prep gynecologic cytology, method for evaluating cervical cells
liver battery, function test, panel, profile, screen, ALT, ALP, AST, bilirubin, albumin, total protein
liver biopsy, evaluate liver tissue
liver iron concentration, evaluate for hemochromatosis
liver needle aspiration cytology, evaluate liver cells for neoplasm
long-acting thyroid-stimulating (LATS) hormone assay, test, to evaluate thyroid stimulating hormone
low-density lipoprotein (LDL) cholesterol assay, evaluate hyper/hypocholesterolemia
low-density lipoprotein (LDL) to high-density lipoprotein (HDL) ratio (LDL:HDL), coronary disease risk evaluation
low-density lipoprotein cholesterol (LDLC) to high-density lipoprotein cholesterol (HDLC) ratio (LDLC:HDLC), coronary disease risk evaluation
lower respiratory tract smear, for cytologic study of lung cancer and disease
lumbar puncture, to obtain spinal fluid for evaluation
lung needle aspiration cytology, to obtain lung cells for evaluation
lupus band test, immunofluorescence test for systemic lupus erythematosus, determines immunoglobulin and complement deposits in dermal-epidermal junction
lupus erythematosus cell test, determines presence of LE cells
Luxol fast blue stain, for myelin in nerve fibers
Lyme borreliosis serology, antibody detection, culture, DNA detection, PCR, various methods to determine infection with *Borrelia burgdorferi*
lymph node and solid tumor karyotype, genetic changes in cancers
lymph node aspiration cytology, biopsy, methods for determining metastases or infection
lymphocyte immunophenotyping, for immune deficiency, lymphocytosis, lymphoid malignancy
lymphocyte microcytotoxicity assay, for transplant crossmatch
lymphocyte mitogen response test, immune status
lymphocyte transfer test, transplant evaluation
lymphocyte transformation test, allergy and hypersensitivity
lymphocyte series (lymphoid series), stages of white blood cell development
lymphocytotoxic antibody screening, pretransplant screening
lymphocytotoxicity assay, for adverse drug reactions and conditions affecting lymphocytes
lymphogranuloma venereum culture, titer, for *Chlamydia trachomatis*
lymphoma analysis by flow cytometry, classification of type of lymphoma
lysozyme test, for sicca syndrome

Machado-Guerreiro test, complement-fixation test for infection with *Trypanosoma cruzi*
Machado-Joseph disease (MJD) DNA test, gene mutation analysis
macrophage migration inhibition test, for macrophage inhibition factor
magnesium test, screen for hyper- and hypomagnesemia
magnesium:creatinine ratio (Mg:Cr)
magnesium-loading test, for magnesium deficiency

malaria film test, smear, identify/differentiate malaria
male ASA (antisperm antibodies) test, male fertility test
Mallory stain for *Actinomyces*
Mallory stain for hemofuchsin
Mantoux skin test, tuberculin test
maturation index, vaginal hormonal evaluation
Maximow stain, for bone marrow, hematopoietic histology
Mazzotti test, for onchocerciasis
mean circulation time, for vascular capacitance
mean circulatory hematocrit, to assess vascular capacitance
mean corpuscular hemoglobin (MCH), calculated value of hemoglobin content of the average red blood cell
mean corpuscular hemoglobin concentration (MCHC), ratio of hemoglobin to hematocrit
mean corpuscular volume (MCV), calculated value of the average volume of red blood cells
melanin bleach (Fontana-Masson method), melanin deposits in skin, eye, substantia nigra, and malignant melanoma
melanin test (Thormahlen test), assessment of urine for melanoma
melanogen test, for melanoma
metabisulfite test, for sickle-cell hemoglobin
metabolic screen for amino acids, for inborn errors of metabolism
metanephrine test, for catecholamines
metanephrine:creatinine ratio, for pheochromocytoma
methanol test, for methanol poisoning
methionine loading test, for hyperhomocysteinemia
methylmalonic acid (MMA), for vitamin B12 deficiency
methyl green pyronin (MGP) stain, for assessing DNA and RNA
methyl red test, pH indicator
methyl violet stain for Heinz bodies, for G6PD deficiency, anemia
methylene blue test, histology preparation, intestinal protozoa, milk bacteriology, RNA tracking
metrotrophic test, for estrogenic substances
microalbumin, for kidney disease
microalbumin:creatinine ratio (M:C), for kidney disease
microbiologic assay, to detect microorganisms
microdeletion study, genetic testing
microdiffusion analysis, chemical analysis method
microhemagglutination assay, method to detect microorganisms
microhemagglutination *Treponema pallidum* (MHA-TP) test, for syphilis
microhematocrit, pediatric anemia screen
microlymphocytotoxicity assay, pretransplant antibody evaluation
microsomal thyroid antibody test, thyroid function, autoimmune thyroid disease
***Microsporidia* immunofluorescent assay,** for protozoan infection
microtoxicity assay, for transplant evaluation
middle ear culture, evaluate for microorganisms/infection of middle ear
midnight-to-morning urinary cortisol increment, for HPA axis function
minimum inhibitory concentration (MIC), point at which bacteria neither increase nor decrease
mite identification, determine appropriate therapy
mitomycin-C stress test, for anemias
mitosis-karyorrhexis index, tumor progression/regression

mitotic index, proliferation of cell population
mixed agglutination test, for microorganisms, proteins
mixed lymphocyte (leukocyte) culture reaction, transplantation and fetomaternal compatibility
modified elastic van Gieson stain, for connective tissue
modified Bethesda assay, detecting factor VIII:C inhibitor for hemophilia A
modified glycerol lysis test, for hereditary spherocytosis
modified thioflavin S stain, for senile plaques
molecular assay, for microorganism detection
molecular cytogenetics, identification of cells for infection, cancer, and other purposes
monocyte function test, for monocyte-mediated antibody-dependent cellular cytotoxicity
monohistiocytic series, cell development
monolayer prep gynecologic cytology, method for cervical cells
Mörner test, for cysteine
Mosenthal test, for renal concentration ability
modified sperm stress test (MOST), for male fertility
motility test, for microorganisms
Motulsky dye reduction test, for G6PD deficiency
mucicarmine stain, for microorganisms and histology
mucopolysaccharide test, for mucopolysaccharidoses
mucoprotein (Tamm-Horsfall) test, for renal tubular cell casts
multimer assay, for von Willebrand factor
multiphasic screening, simultaneous multiple laboratory tests on groups
multiple marker screening test, for genetic disease or cancer
multiple stain, for selective tissue staining
multiple-puncture tuberculin test, to assess for *Mycobacterium* infection
mumps antibody titer, culture, sensitivity, serology, active or resolving mumps virus infection
Murayama test, for hemoglobin
Murphy-Pattee test, for thyroxine
muscle biopsy, to evaluate for muscle disease
mutagenicity test, effect of chemicals
mutation test for Duchenne/Becker muscular dystrophy, genetic test
mutation test for trinucleotide repeat disorder, determine one of several genetic diseases
mutation testing, determine genetic disease
***Mycobacterium* culture, DNA detection, DNA probe susceptibility,** presence/type of *Mycobacterium* infection
***Mycoplasma pneumoniae* (Eaton agent) serology,** evaluate current or resolving infection
myeloid series, stages of blood cell development
myocardial infarct panel, CPK, troponin, myoglobin to evaluate heart muscle damage
myoglobin screen, test, muscle damage, particularly heart
myotonic dystrophy DNA test, for genetic muscular disease

Nantucket fever serologic test, for arthropod-borne disease
nasal smear, fungal and bacterial infection identification
nasopharyngeal culture, fungal and bacterial identification
National Institute on Drug Abuse (NIDA) screen, for common drugs of abuse
***Neisseria gonorrhoeae* culture, smear,** for gonorrhea
neonatal (newborn) screening, for genetic disorders, inborn errors of metabolism
nephelometric inhibition assay, method of immunoassay
nephrolithiasis analysis, for composition of kidney stones

neutral stain, compound of acid and basic dyes
neutralization test, for antiserum to microorganisms
neutron activation analysis, qualitative/quantitative trace element
newborn aneuploidy detection, genetic testing
newborn/maternal antibody workup, for fetomaternal incompatibility
Nickerson-Kveim test (Kveim test), for sarcoidosis
Nicolle stain, immersion test for capsules
Nile blue stain, for fat
ninhydrin-Schiff stain, for proteins
nipple discharge cytology, identify infection or neoplasm
Nissl stain, for neuronal cell bodies, nerve cells
nitrate reduction test, for microorganism identification
nitrate utilization test, for microorganism identification
nitroprusside screening, test, for cysteine
nitroso-indole-nitrate test, for indole and skatole
***Nocardia* culture,** diagnose nocardiosis or granulomatous disease
nonpermissive culture media, under which a conditional mutation displays its mutant phenotype
normal lymphocyte transfer test, for transplant, grafting suitability
Northern blot analysis, test, variation of Southern blot analysis, DNA identification
nuclear labeling index, for apoptosis, cancer
nucleoplasmic index, quotient of nuclear volume divided by cytoplasmic volume

off-site testing, tests sent to specialty laboratory
oil red O stain, for lung fat embolus
oleic acid uptake test, assess dietary fatty acids
oligodendroglia stain, histopathology preparation, several stains
o-nitrophenyl-beta-D-galactosidase (ONPG) test, screening for bacteria
opsonic index, ratio of phagocytized bacteria in serums of affected and normal individuals
Optochin susceptibility test, microorganism (pneumococcus) differentiation
oral cavity cytology, for infection or cancer
oral direct smear, analysis for infection or cancer
oral glucose tolerance test, for diabetes screen
oral lactose tolerance test, for lactase deficiency
oral scraping cytology, for infection or cancer
orcein stain, for histology preparation
organ culture, for infection
organ donor tissue typing, for transplant incompatibility
Orth fixative, for early degenerative processes and necrosis, rickettsiae and bacteria
Orth stain, for nerve cells and their processes
osazone test, for detecting sugars
osmotic fragility test, SEE erythrocyte fragility
Ouchterlony test (double [gel] diffusion precipitin in two dimensions), for antibody-antigen reactions
outer ear culture, for bacteria, fungi
ova and parasites (O&P) test, fecal test for parasites
ovarian ascorbic acid depletion test, for luteinizing hormone
ovarian cyst fluid cytology, for identification and in vitro fertilization
oxygen saturation, oxygen content of blood, respiratory status
oxygen dissociation assay, for detecting a high-affinity hemoglobin as a cause of erythrocytosis
oxyhemogram, graphic representation of oxygen content of blood
oxytocin challenge test, contraction test for fetal condition, late pregnancy (nonstress test)

p24 antigen detection, HIV detection
packed cell volume (hematocrit), red blood cell volume percentage
Padykula-Herman stain for myosin ATPase, muscle histology
Paget test, serum alkaline phosphatase, for bone disease
p-aminohippurate clearance test, for Type 1 diabetes
pancervical smear, for cancer detection
pancreas needle aspiration cytology, for pancreatitis, cancer
pancreatic cyst fluid cytology, for pancreatitis, cancer
pancreatic islet cell antibody test, for diabetes
pancreozymin-secretin test, for pancreas exocrine function
Pandy test, for proteins in cerebrospinal fluid
Papanicolaou (Pap) smear, test, cervical cancer screen
paper radioimmunosorbent test, method of protein separation/identification
paracentesis fluid analysis, cytology, for cancer identification
paracoagulation test, for DIC
parasite screen, parasitology examination, rule in/out parasitic infection
parathyroid hormone (PTH) assay, for calcium metabolism
paroxysmal cold hemoglobinuria test (Donath-Landsteiner)
paroxysmal nocturnal hemoglobinuria (PNH) test (Ham test)
partial thromboplastin time (PTT) test, to determine blood clotting time, screen for clotting abnormalities
parvovirus B19 DNA, serology, assess for erythema infectiosum and aplastic anemia
passive cutaneous anaphylaxis test, for allergy determination
passive hemagglutination test, for anemias, clotting disorders
patch drug detection test, method of drugs of abuse screening
patch test, for contact dermatitis, allergy, tuberculin
paternity testing by DNA testing
Paul-Bunnell te st (Paul-Bunnell-Davidsohn) (Forssman antigen), for heterophile bodies in infectious mononucleosis
pemphigus smear, identify blistering skin causes
penicillinase test, identify bacteria
penicillinase-producing organism susceptibility, determine appropriate antimicrobial
pentagastrin stimulation test, for Zollinger-Ellison disease
pepsinogen A:C ratio, for atrophic body gastritis
pepsinogen I, II, III, for peptic ulcer disease
pericardial fluid analysis, cytology, examination, evaluate for infection, cancer, causes of effusion
periodic acid-Schiff (PAS) method, reaction, stain, technique, test, staining methods for histology
periodic acid-Schiff digested stain (PAS-D), for glycogen
peripheral blood preparation, smear, for blood cell analysis
peripheral differential, for quantitative/qualitative analysis of blood cells
peritoneal fluid analysis, cytology, evaluate cells for infection, cancer
peritoneal washing cytology, evaluate cells for infection, cancer
permissive culture media, in which a conditional mutation displays a wild-type phenotype
pertussis culture, serology, for identification of *Bordetella pertussis* (whooping cough)
Petri dish culture, a combination of filter paper, fecal specimen, and tap water in a Petri dish, for nematodes
phagocytic cell immunocompetence profile, for granulomatous disease
phagocytic index, average number of bacteria ingested per white blood cell of the patient's blood
phenylalanine screening test, tolerance index, PKU test, for phenylketonuria

phenylpyruvic acid test, for phenylketonuria
phosphate excretion index, assess renal function, vitamin D metabolism, bone health
phospholipid test, assess fetal lung maturity, antiphospholipid syndrome
photopatch test, for allergy, photoallergy
phytohemagglutinin assay, chromosome analysis, cancer identification
pinworm preparation, method for detection of nematode species
Pirquet test, cutaneous tuberculin test
pituitary function test, for endocrine disorders
placental and fetoplacental function tests (DHEA loading test), evaluate complicated pregnancy, fetal distress
plaque-forming cell assay, immune status. thyroid function
plasma clotting time, monitor heparin therapy
plasma hemoglobin test, for hemolytic anemia, DIC
plasma iron disappearance time, evaluate hemochromatosis and therapy
plasminogen activator inhibitor assay, thrombosis, clotting disorders
plastic section stain, technique for electron microscopy
plate culture, agar or gelatin in Petri dish
platelet adhesion test, adhesiveness test, for platelet function evaluation
platelet aggregation test, for platelet function evaluation, clotting disorders
platelet count, quantitative evaluation of platelets
platelet index, for clotting evaluation
platelet retention test, for skin healing; diagnose von Willebrand factor
platelet serology, for thrombocytopenia due to neonatal alloimmune thrombocytopenia (NAIT), posttransfusion purpura (PTP), autoimmune idiopathic thrombocytopenic purpura (AITP), heparin-associated antibody
pleural fluid cytology, examination, pH, pulmonary disease
pleuropneumonia like organism (PPLO) titer, for organisms of order Mycoplasmatales
ploidy analysis, tumor grading
point-of-care testing, out-of-laboratory testing
polyethylene glycol precipitation assay, for circulating immune complexes
porphyrin test, to diagnose and monitor porphyria
Porter-Silber chromogens test, for plasma cortisol concentrations and the levels of urinary output of 17-hydroxycorticoid
postmortem examination, autopsy, to discover cause of death, pathologic changes, (in forensics, cause and manner)
postprandial glucose, for diabetes management
potassium hydroxide (KOH) preparation, test, for fungus
precipitation test, precipitin test, antibody reaction, for infection, immune complex
prenatal screening, serology, testing, for Down syndrome, genetic disease, infection, fetomaternal incompatibility
presenilin (PSEN1), mutation marker for early-onset Alzheimer disease
pretransfusion testing, for blood type compatibility
primed lymphocyte typing, for class II HLA antigens
progesterone receptor assay, breast cancer classification
prolactin test, prolactinoma, female infertility, male infertility/testosterone
proliferative index, for cancer evaluation
prometaphase study, for Prader-Willi syndrome
promyelocytic leukemia assay, evaluation of leukemia, therapy
prophase study, cytogenetics

prostaglandin test, readiness for labor evaluation
prostate-specific antigen (PSA) density, velocity, prostate cancer screening
prostatic fluid culture, for prostatitis, prostate cancer
protamine titration test, for reversal of heparin therapy
protein test, urine or blood screening tests for abnormal protein production
protein to creatinine ratio, for proteinuria, nephrosis
prothrombin and proconvertin (P&P) test, for hypercoagulability, antiphospholipid antibody, antiplatelet therapy
prothrombin consumption test, time for hypercoagulability, antiphospholipid antibody, antiplatelet therapy
prothrombin time (PT), screening for bleeding and antiplatelet therapies
prothrombokinase factor, test for factor V, factor VIII
protoporphyrin test, iron deficiency, lead exposure
provocative chelation test, heavy metal exposure
PSA free:total ratio, prostate cancer screen
pseudomembranous colitis toxin assay, for *Clostridium difficile*
psittacosis serology, titer, for exposure/infection with *Chlamydophila psittaci (Chlamydia psittaci),* parrot fever
Puchtler-Sweat stain for basement membranes, histology preparation
Puchtler-Sweat stain for hemoglobin and hemosiderin, histology preparation
pulmonary cytology series, evaluate pulmonary disease or cancer
pulmonary function test, evaluate lung function
pulse oximetry, noninvasive oxygen saturation
pulsed-field gel electrophoresis genotyping, method of separating proteins for analysis
puncture wound culture, to identify microorganisms and sensitivity to antimicrobial therapy
pure culture, cells or multicellular organisms growing in absence of other species/types
purified protein derivative (PPD) of tuberculin, test for tuberculosis
pyruvate kinase assay, for muscle disease

Q fever serology, titer, infection with *Coxiella burnetii*
Q-banding stain (quinacrine chromosome banding stain), for identifying Y-chromosome and certain DNA polymorphisms
qualitative analysis, nature of elements of substances
quantitative analysis, quantity of elements of substances
quantitative nuclear morphometry, evaluation of cancer cells
quantitative tip culture, for catheter-related infections
Quick test, for prothrombin
quinine carbacrylic resin test, for gastric anacidity
Quinlan test, for bile

Radford nomogram, tidal volume for artificial respiration
radioactive iodine (^{131}I) (RAI) uptake test, thyroid function
radioactive vitamin B12 absorption test with or without intrinsic factor (Schilling test), two-part test to evaluate vitamin B12 deficiency from intestines or lack of intrinsic factor
radioallergosorbent assay (RAST), RIA for IgE, hypersensitivity
radioenzymatic assay, for catalytic activity of an enzyme using radioactive substrate
radioimmunoprecipitation assay (RIPA), radioactive tracer for antigen-antibody reactions
radioimmunosorbent assay (RIST), a competition test, performed in vitro, to measure IgE specific for a particular antigen

radioisotopic culture, method of microorganism detection/identification
radioligand assay, radioactive tracer method of radioimmunoassay
radioreceptor assay, An assay employing a radioactively labelled receptor protein as a tracer
Raji cell radioimmune assay, detection of immune complexes
rapid testing, methods giving more immediate results, wide application
rapid plasma reagin (RPR) test, screening test for syphilis
Rapoport test, differential ureteral catheterization for renovascular hypertension
R-banding stain (reverse Giemsa), for chromosome deletion
reactone red test, for amylase
recombinant antigen immunoblot assay, method of immunoblotting
rectal swab culture, evaluate for microorganisms
red blood cell count, RBC volume, number of cells per volume of blood
red blood cell distribution width (RDW), calculation of variation in size, for anemias
red blood cell enzyme deficiency screen, blood markers for metabolic disorder
red blood cell fragility, SEE erythrocyte fragility
red blood cell indices, calculations from CBC to aid in diagnosis and classification of anemia
red blood cell morphology, evaluate for blood diseases
red blood cell adherence test, antigen-antibody determination
red blood cell survival test, for hereditary spherocytosis
red blood cell smear, preparation for red blood cell count
red blood cells:platelets ratio, a method for platelet count determination
Rees-Ecker fluid, sodium citrate, sucrose, and brilliant cresyl blue used in platelet counts
reference interval, range, index, standard expected results, normal versus abnormal values
Reid index, ratio of thickness of mucous gland layer to thickness of wall between epithelium and cartilage
renal function test, kidney function tests such as blood urea nitrogen and creatinine
renal pelvis washing cytology, to evaluate disease of renal pelvis
renal venous renin assay, for hypertensive disease
renin assay, for hypertensive disease
resolving time (nuclear analytic chemistry), time interval for measuring data accurately
resorcinol (Selivanoff) test, for fructosuria
respiratory syncytial virus (RSV) antibody, antigen, culture, DFA, serology, evaluate current and resolving infection
respiratory tract cytology, evaluate for disease, cancer
reticulated platelet count, for thrombocytopenia
reticulin stain, for connective tissue
reticulocyte count, assess bone marrow function
reticulocyte hemoglobin content, for pediatric iron deficiency
reticulocyte maturity index, evaluation of anemias
reticulocytic production index, evaluation of anemias
retinoblastoma gene DNA detection, used in cancer assessment
Reuss test, test for atropine
Rh blocking test, genotype, typing, for rhesus antigen
rheumatoid arthritis (RA) latex fixation test, reaction, for rheumatoid arthritis
ring precipitin test, antigen-antibody test, forms ring at optimal antibody ratio
ristocetin-induced platelet aggregation assay, for von Willebrand factor
Rocky Mountain spotted fever antibody test, serology, for current or resolving infection
Ropes test (mucin clot test), for variety of inflammatory arthritic conditions

rosette assay, erythrocyte rosette assay, active rosette test, active E-rosette test, for allergy, immune status, fetomaternal hemorrhage
rotavirus antigen detection, serology, for current or resolving infection
rotavirus detection by electron microscopy (EM), for current or resolving infection
Rothera nitroprusside test, for ketone bodies
Rous test, for hemosiderin
routine test, screening for health/disease conditions
rubella antibody test, culture, hemagglutination inhibition, serology, methods for current or resolving infection
rubeola antibody, serology, methods for current or resolving infection
Rumpel-Leede test, capillary fragility test
Russell viper (RV) venom clotting time, deficiencies of prothrombin, factor V, or factor X

Sabin-Feldman dye test, for antitoxoplasma antibody in serum with methylene blue
saline agglutination test, form of agglutination test to detect antibodies
***Salmonella* titer,** for infection
San Joaquin fever serology, for infection with *Coccidioides immitis*
saturation analysis, a competitive binding assay
saturation index, relative concentration of hemoglobin in red blood cells
Schiller test, for early vaginal cancer detection
Schilling blood count, index, polymorphonuclear neutrophils grouped according to number and arrangement of nuclear masses
Schilling test, two-part test to evaluate B12 deficiency from intestines or lack of intrinsic factor
Schirmer test, filter paper in eye to assess tear production
Schlichter test (serum bactericidal activity), antimicrobial efficacy
Schmorl (ferric-ferricyanide reduction stain), method of reducing substances in tissues
Schultz-Dale test, animal tissues used for antigen detection
Schumm test, spectroscopic method of detection of methemalbumin in blood, intravascular hemolysis
scintillation count, method of detection of radioactivity
Scotch tape test, for pinworms
scratch test, for allergy
screen, routine test to rule out disease
secretin-pancreozymin test, for pancreatic disease
secretin test, for pancreatic disease
secretin-CCK stimulation test, for pancreatic disease
sedimentation index, rate, test, screen for inflammation
selective stain, that which colors one tissue or cell exclusively or more deeply
selenium-labeled homocholic acid taurine (SeHCAT) test, for inflammatory bowel disease
Selivanoff test (resorcinol test), for fructosuria
semen analysis, cytology, male fertility testing
sentinel lymph node biopsy, evaluate for metastasis
Sequential Multiple Analyzer Computer (SMAC), equipment for automated blood tests, used to refer to tests performed with it, chemistry profiles; e.g., SMA-7, SMAC-12
serial cardiac isoenzyme assay, to evaluate myocardial infarction
serodiagnosis, diagnosis based on serologic tests
serology, tests to measure either antigens or antibodies in sera
serotonin release assay, for heparin-induced thrombocytopenia
serous effusion analysis, cytology, determine cause of effusion

serum tests, variety of tests performed on blood serum
serum lysis, for infection, immune response
serum osmolality, for antidiuretic hormone evaluation
serum prothrombin conversion accelerator (SPCA), for factor VII
serum protein electrophoresis test, evaluates specific proteins for disease
serum viscosity, evaluate monoclonal gammopathies, autoimmune disease
sex chromatin test, evaluation of sexual dysgenesis and other sex-related disorders
shake culture, method of growing microorganisms
sheep cell agglutination test (SCAT), any agglutination test with sheep erythrocytes
shingles culture, for varicella zoster
shrimp sensitivity, allergy test
Sia (sialic acids euglobulin precipitation) test, for parasite infection
sickle cell solubility test, sickle cell test, for sickling hemoglobin
Siggaard-Andersen alignment nomogram, acid-base, blood
silver nitroprusside test (Spaeth and Barber modification of Brand cyanide nitroprusside), for homocystinuria
Sims-Huhner test, for rheumatoid factor
single (gel) diffusion precipitin test in one dimension (1D), antigen-antibody reaction
single (gel) diffusion precipitin test in two dimensions (2D) (Ouchterlony test), antigen-antibody reaction
single-fiber electromyographic test, for neuromuscular junction disorder
skeletal muscle biopsy, muscle tissue for evaluation of disease
skin biopsy, skin for evaluation of disease
skin test, culture, allergy, bacterial or fungus infection, tuberculin
skin window test, method for analyzing drugs, allergens
skin-puncture test, for Behçet syndrome
slide platelet aggregation test
smear, preparation for cytology, histology
sodium test, quantitative for sodium in blood or urine
soft tissue mass aspiration, method of obtaining specimen
solid phase red blood cell adherence assay, method of blood typing
solubility test, screening test for hemoglobin S, sickle cell
soluble liver antigen antibody, for autoimmune hepatitis
Southern blot analysis, test, procedure to separate and identify DNA sequences
spectral karyotyping, fluorescent dye chromosome identification
sperm count, examination, for male fertility
sperm morphology study, for male fertility
sperm mucus penetration assay, test, for male fertility
sperm-cervical mucus interaction, for male fertility
sperm-oolemma binding test, for male fertility
S-phase analysis, DNA analysis method
spinal fluid analysis, culture, cytology, electrophoresis, leukocyte, to determine microorganisms in infection, for antibodies or autoimmune disease
spirochete stain (Steiner & Steiner method), for *Legionella* infection
spironolactone test, for primary aldosteronism
split renal function test, compare one kidney with the other
spodogram, ash residue of tissue specimen
sporotrichosis serology
sputum culture, cytology, smear, to detect bacteria or fungi

squamous cell index, cancer determinations
sickle screen, sickle cell test, blood test for hemoglobin S
St. Louis encephalitis virus serology
stab culture, method of growing cells
stain for intracellular pigment, multiple varieties, purposes, colors
Stamey test, fractionated urine culture
standard acid reflux test (SART), for GERD
standing plasma test, plasma stored upright, chylomicrons form creamy layer
staphylococcal clumping test, for fibrin degradation products
***Staphylococcus aureus* nasopharyngeal culture**
starch tolerance test, for pancreatic disease
steatocrit, fecal fat content
stem cell assay, culture medium for growing cells
steroid protein activity index, monitor steroid therapy or anabolic steroid use
Stirling modification of Gram stain, for bacteria
stock culture, standardized strain of microorganisms or cells
Stoll dilution egg count technique, for parasites in stool
stool culture, to determine infecting microorganisms
stool guaiac test, for occult blood
stool meat fiber test, for digestive enzyme analysis
streak culture, method of inoculation for growing cells
streptococcal antigen test, group A streptococcal pharyngitis, group B streptococcal infections in infants
streptozyme test, streptococcal antibodies for infection
succinylcholine sensitivity test, for pseudocholinesterase deficiency
sucrose hemolysis test, for paroxysmal nocturnal hematuria
Sudan black B stain, for fat or lipochrome
sugar water test screen, for paroxysmal nocturnal hematuria
Sulkowitch test, reagent for calcium in urine
superoxide dismutase (SOD) assay, for neurodegenerative disease, amyotrophic lateral sclerosis, Alzheimer and Huntington diseases, and Parkinsonism
surfactant:albumin ratio, for fetal lung maturity
surgical wound culture, for identification of infecting organisms
susceptibility test, to determine correct antimicrobial therapy
suspension array technology, protein and genomic analysis
swab specimen, method of obtaining specimen
Swan-Ganz tip culture, isolation of catheter-associated infection
sweat test, for cystic fibrosis
synovial fluid analysis, culture, cytology, evaluation of infection and other joint conditions
synovial fluid hyaluronate concentration, diagnosis of joint disease
synovial fluid mucin clot test (Rope test), differential diagnosis of joint disease
synovial fluid Ropes test (synovial fluid), to assess inflammatory disease
synovial fluid viscosity, for degenerative joint disease
syphilis enzyme immunoassay, for *Treponema pallidum* infection

T-and B-lymphocyte subset assay, T/B lymphocyte assay
T-method stain, for terminal end of chromosome
tanned red blood cell hemagglutination inhibition test, fibrin/fibrinogen determination
tartrate-resistant acid phosphatase (TRAP) test, diagnose hairy-cell leukemia
tau protein, fraction, in neuronal tissue, especially for Alzheimer disease

telomeric R-banding stain, method of strongly staining telomeres with faint R-bands on rest of chromosome
Tes-Tape, *proprietary*, urine glucose test
testing photopeak detection efficiency, nuclear medicine
tetanus antibody, for immune status
tetrazolium test, reagent in oxidative enzyme histochemistry
Thayer-Martin test, for *Neisseria gonorrhoeae*
thermal death time, time for bacterial death at specific temperature
thermostable opsonin test, for opsonic activity in absence of effect of heat-labile complement
thin-layer preparation, method for histology, cytology
thin-needle biopsy, fine-needle method of obtaining specimen
thioflavin S stain, for amyloid in tissue
thiopurine-S-methyltransferase (TPMT), screen for sensitivity to thiopurine drugs
Thompson test (two-glass test), for gonorrhea
thoracentesis fluid analysis, cytology, pH, evaluation of fluid production in lungs
Thormählen test, for melanin
throat culture, identify microorganisms
thrombin clotting time, coagulopathy screening
thrombocyte count, quantitative platelet count
thrombocytic series, stages of development of platelets in bone marrow
thromboelastogram, a recording of the coagulation process made by a thromboelastograph
thrombophilia panel, homocysteine, antithrombin II, factor VIIIC, protein C, free protein S, lupus anticoagulant, direct Russell viper venom time, lupus anticoagulant, and/or laboratory-specific tests
thromboplastin activation, generation, substitution, assess blood coagulation
thrombotic disease screen, antithrombin activity, plasminogen, protein C, protein S
thymidine-labeling index, cancer tissue evaluation
thyroid function tests (TFT), T3, T4, TSH, TRH
thyroid hormone binding ratio (triiodothyronine [T3] uptake test), for thyroid function
thyroid microsomal antibody test, for thyroid function, autoimmune thyroid disease
thyroid screen for newborn, for thyroid function
thyroid suppression test, for thyroid function
triiodothyronine (T3) uptake test, for thyroid function
thyroid-stimulating hormone (TSH) assay, for thyroid function
thyroid-stimulating hormone (TSH) stimulation, for thyroid function
thyrotropin-releasing hormone (TRH), for thyroid function
thyroxine (T4) assay, for thyroid function
thyroxine-binding globulin (TBG) assay, evaluate for benign X-linked disorder
thyroxine-binding index (TBI) test, for thyroid function
thyroxine-binding protein electrophoresis, evaluate for benign X-linked disorder
tick identification, evaluate for infection with disease-causing ticks
tissue culture, examination, for infection, tumor, abnormalities
tissue thromboplastin inhibition time, to identify lupus anticoagulant
tissue typing, for transplant compatibility
titratable acidity test, number of mL of NaOH to neutralize 24-hour urine specimen, for kidney function
T-lymphocyte analysis by flow cytometry, assess adult respiratory distress syndrome
tolbutamide tolerance test, insulin sensitivity
Tollen reagent, ammoniacal silver nitrate, test for aldehydes
toluidine blue stain, for mast cells

Tormahlen test (melanin test), for melanoma
total (fingertip) ridge count, for polygenic traits
total body hematocrit, evaluate for compartment syndrome
total cell count, quantitative, blood or tissue
total hemolytic complement, assess several disease states
total iron-binding capacity (TIBC) test (transferrin), for iron overload, hemochromatosis
total radical absorbing parameter (TRAP), antioxidant capacity of serum
total serum protein, albumin and globulin, for liver and renal function
total thyroxine (T4), assess thyroid function
toxicology screen, for ingestion of drugs or other toxins
toxoplasmosis serology, titer, for exposure to *Toxoplasma gondii*
toxoplasmosis, other infections, rubella, cytomegalovirus, and herpes simplex (TORCH) screen, titer, newborn infection screen
transaminases test, ALT and AST, for liver function
transbronchial aspiration biopsy, method of obtaining specimen
transcutaneous bilirubinometry, noninvasive bilirubin measurement
transferred antigen, transferred antibody, for fetomaternal incompatibility
transferrin test (total iron-binding capacity test), for iron overload, hemochromatosis
transfusion complication or reaction workup, laboratory-specific sequence of steps to determine cause
transjugular needle biopsy of liver, method of obtaining specimen
transmission electron microscopy, for minute evaluation of specimens
transplant tissue typing, for tissue compatibility
***Treponema pallidum* hemagglutination (TPH),** for syphilis
***Treponema pallidum* immobilization (TPI) assay, test,** for syphilis
trichinellosis, trichinosis serology, for infestation with *Trichinella spiralis*
trichrome stain (Masson), histology preparation
triiodothyronine (T3) uptake test (thyroid binding hormone ratio), for thyroid function
triiodothyronine (T3) suppression test, for hyperthyroidism, thyroid function
triple screen test, alpha fetoprotein (AFP), human chorionic gonadotropin (hCG), estriol, for fetal abnormalities
trypsin G-banding stain, for Down syndrome, other genetic conditions
trypsin test, cystic fibrosis screen in newborns
tryptophan load test, nutritional status, vitamin B6 deficiency, nicotinic acid deficiency (pellagra)
tube culture, method of growing cells, microorganisms
tube dilution test, for antimicrobial resistance
tubeless gastric analysis test, chemical method for cancer, Zollinger-Ellison syndrome, hyper- and hypoacidity
tuberculin test, tuberculosis skin test, for tuberculosis
tularemia serology, evaluate for exposure/infection *Francisella tularensis*
two-stage PT (prothrombin time) test, alternative method of PT test
tympanocentesis culture, evaluate infection of middle ear
type and crossmatch, blood evaluation for transfusion
type and screen, blood evaluation for possible blood transfusion
type culture, representative sample of microorganism for research/testing
typhus antibody test, for rickettsial diseases
typing, identification of tissue types and markers, for blood transfusion, organ transplant, pregnancy
tyramine test, putative marker for depressive illness
tyrosine test, for tyrosinemia, tyrosinuria, PKU nutritional status
Tzanck test, for herpesviruses and pemphigus vulgaris

Uffelmann test, for lactic acid
ultrasensitive thyroid-stimulating hormone (TSH), special thyroid function test
ultrasound-guided fine needle aspiration (FNA), method of obtaining specimen
ultrastructural study, form of electron microscopy
umbilical arterial blood gas (UAMB), fetal acidemia
umbilical cord blood tests, for fetal status
undulant fever culture, for *Brucellosis* spp.
unheated serum reagin test, quantitative test for syphilis
unsaturated vitamin B12 binding capacity (UBBC), for myeloproliferative and other diseases
unstable hemoglobin, for anemia evaluation
urate crystal stain, for gout and kidney stones
urea clearance test, to measure kidney function
***Ureaplasma urealyticum* genital culture,** newborn infection
urease test, for bacterial identification
ureteral washing cytology, for urinary tract disease, cancer
uric acid to creatinine ratio, for uric acid nephropathy
uricolytic index, percentage of uric acid oxidized to allantoin before excretion
urinalysis, urine analysis (UA), for screening kidney disease or infection
urinary concentration test, for renal tubular function
urinary sugar test, for diabetes
urinary tract cytology, for evaluation of infection, disease, cancer
urinary tract infection (UTI) screen, determination of infection and what further testing required
urine acetone test, for ketones, fatty-acid breakdown, and/or diabetes
urine calcium:creatinine ratio, for hyperparathyroidism, hematuria
urine concentration test, for kidney function
urine culture, for microorganisms
urine cytology, evaluate urinary tract for disease or infection
urine for glucose tolerance, for diabetes
urine osmolality, for fluid balance
urine osmolar gap, evaluate kidney function, electrolyte and water balance, syndrome of inappropriate secretion of antidiuretics hormone, diabetes insipidus, dehydration, amyloidosis, neonatal testing
urine protein electrophoresis, evaluate proteinuria
urine protein:creatinine ratio, determine nephrotic range
urine screen for albumin, evaluate proteinuria
urine screen for protein, evaluate type of proteinuria
urine specific gravity, kidney function, fluid balance
urine:serum osmolality ratio, kidney function, polyuria
urobilinogen test, liver function
uroporphyrin test, for porphyria

vagina, ectocervix, and endocervix (VCE) smear, for cancer screen
vaginal culture, for infection
vaginal cytology, for infection, disease, cancer
valley fever serology, for infection with *Coccidioides immitis*
van der Velden test, assess levels of free hydrochloric acid
vanillylmandelic acid (VMA) test, for catecholamine-secreting tumors, pheochromocytoma, neuroblastoma
varicella-zoster virus (VZV) antibody test, culture, DNA, serology, for chickenpox, shingles
vasopressin concentration test, renal concentrating capacity

Venereal Disease Research Laboratory (VDRL), test for syphilis
venous hematocrit, neonatal, compartment syndrome
ventricular fluid culture, analysis for brain infection, disease
verotoxin detection, for *Escherichia coli*
vesicle viral culture, find causative organism
viable cell count (colony count), enumeration of bacteria in given substance
viral antigen detection, culture, for virus identification, infection
ViraPap test, *proprietary*, for human papilloma virus (HPV)
ViraType test, *proprietary*, for human papilloma virus (HPV)
vitamin B12 absorption test (Schilling test), two-part test to evaluate B12 deficiency from intestines or lack of intrinsic factor
voided urine cytology, evaluate for disease, cancer of urinary tract
von Kossa stain for calcium, histology preparation
von Willebrand factor assay, for hemorrhagic diathesis
vulvar cytology, for cancer, other diseases

Wachstein-Meissel stain for calcium-magnesium-ATPase, for cellular enzyme activity
Wagner test, diabetic foot wound classification
Wako nonesterified fatty acid (NEFA) test kit, *proprietary*, for free fatty acids
Waldenström test, for porphobilinogen or urobilinogen in urine
Wang needle biopsy, transbronchial needle aspiration biopsy
washing cytology, specimen obtained by washing
Watson-Schwartz test, screen for acute intermittent porphyria
Webster test, for trinitrotoluene in urine
Weiger stain for actinomyces, demonstrate microorganism
Weigert stain for elastin, for connective tissue
Weigert stain for fibrin, for connective tissue
Weigert stain for myelin, for nerve tissue
Weigert stain for neuroglia, for brain tissue
Weil-Felix test, presence and type of rickettsial disease
Werner test, thyroid suppression test
Westergren sedimentation rate, method of ESR, indicator of inflammation
Western blot analysis, immunoblot test, separate and identify antibodies
Western equine encephalitis virus serology, for arbovirus infection
West Nile virus serology, test for viral infection
wheal reaction time, for allergy testing
wheal-and-erythema skin tests, for allergy testing
whiff test, for bacterial vaginosis
white blood cell (WBC) crossmatch, for transplantation, transfusion
white blood cell (WBC) morphology, evaluate for infection, leukemias
white blood cell (WBC) count, screening, evaluate for infection, leukemia, other blood disease
whole-blood clotting time, method for thrombotic disease, clotting disorders
whooping cough culture, identification of *Bordetella pertussis*
Widal test, febrile agglutination reaction, diagnosis of typhoid
Wilder stain for reticulum, for hemopoietic system
Wormley test, for alkaloids by picric acid
wound culture, identify microorganisms

xylose absorption, tolerance test, for small-intestine digestive disorders
xylose concentration test, for small-intestine digestive disorders, celiac disease

yellow fever antibody titer, detect and monitor infection with yellow fever virus

zeta sedimentation rate (ZSR), replacement for ESR, screen for inflammation and clotting disorders
zetacrit, method of determining hematocrit
Ziehl-Neelsen acid-fast stain, for *Mycobacterium leprae* and *Nocardia* spp.
Zimmermann test, reaction, basis of 17-ketogenic steroid assay
zinc protoporphyrin (ZPP), monitor lead exposure
zinc protoporphyrin to heme ratio, evaluate lead poisoning
Zollinger-Ellison test (secretin provocation test), for peptic ulceration with gastric hypersecretion and gastrinoma of the pancreas or duodenum
zona-free hamster egg penetration test, male fertility test
zoster titer, evaluate infection with herpes zoster virus, chickenpox, or shingles
zygosity Rh, phenotyping
zymogram, representation on paper or gels of enzymes after electrophoresis

Profiles of Common Medical Conditions

ALCOHOL USE DISORDERS

Any pattern of alcohol use causing significant physical, mental, or social dysfunction; key features are tolerance, withdrawal, and persistent use despite problems.

Synonyms: Alcoholism, alcohol abuse, alcohol dependence.

Treatment: Benzodiazepines reduce incidence of delirium tremens (DTs) and seizures and are the drugs of choice for palliation of symptoms of alcohol withdrawal. Carbamazepine is efficacious for mild-to-moderate withdrawal and less sedating than benzodiazepines. Phenobarbital may be safer during pregnancy.

Adjuncts to detoxification: Beta-blockers for tachycardia or comorbid coronary artery disease. Clonidine for autonomic hyperactivity. Haloperidol for psychosis, agitation; may lower seizure threshold.

Adjuncts to rehabilitation: Naltrexone: Opiate antagonist reduces craving and chance of heavy drinking with relapse; may improve abstinence rate. Acomprosate beginning after completion of withdrawal reduces relapse of drinking. Topiramate enhances abstinence.

Supplements: Thiamine, folic acid, multivitamin. Magnesium sulfate IM/IV if history of DTs or withdrawal seizure.

ALZHEIMER DISEASE

Chronic degeneration of cerebral cortex with progressive intellectual deterioration and dementia, usually occurring after age 65. Diagnosis is made clinically after ruling out treatable disorders with similar characteristics. Functional impairments, by year: Cognition 0–5, financial management 1–5, behavior 2–12, self-bathing 4–7, urinary continence 5–8. Death in 3–8 years (6–8 if diagnosed before age 65).

Synonyms: Presenile dementia, senile dementia of the Alzheimer type, primary degenerative dementia.

Diagnosis: Lumbar puncture; neuropsychological battery if clinical picture is confusing.

To rule out other causes of dementia: CBC, chemistry panel, thyroid function studies, folate and B12 levels, syphilis serology, erythrocyte sedimentation rate, HIV antibody (selected cases).

Head CT/MRI: Moderate cortical atrophy, ventricular enlargement (rule out infarcts, subdural hematomas, normal pressure hydrocephalus, neoplasm).

Pathological Findings: *Gross:* Diffuse cerebral atrophy in association areas, hippocampus, amygdala, and some subcortical nuclei. *Microscopic:* Pyramidal cell loss, decreased cholinergic innervation, neuritic senile plaques, degeneration of locus ceruleus and basal forebrain nuclei of Meynert, neurofibrillary tangles, amyloid angiopathy common, inflammatory cells present.

Treatment: No specific drug therapy available. Use as few drugs as possible. No drugs are helpful for wandering, restlessness, fidgeting, uncooperativeness, hoarding, and irritability. Use behavioral techniques and environmental modification. For depression, which occurs in one third of patients, use selective serotonin reuptake inhibitor. Start with half the usual adult dose.

Insomnia: Trazodone, zolpidem, zaleplon, ramelteon.

Severe aggressive agitation, especially if psychotic features present (delusions, hallucinations): Risperidone, olanzapine, other newer atypical antipsychotic agents. Attempt periodic dose reductions or discontinuation, especially in a long-term care facility patient.

Memory enhancement: Anticholinesterase inhibitors: donepezil, rivastigmine, or galantamine. Memantine, first of new class of N-methyl-D-aspartate receptor antagonists, can be used as monotherapy or in combination with acetylcholinesterase inhibitors to enhance or preserve memory. Anticholinesterase inhibitors provide only modest benefit for 1–2 years, after which decline continues at somewhat slower rate than placebo. No change in patient over 6–12 months is evidence of efficacy.

Angina Pectoris

Symptom complex resulting from acute myocardial ischemia. *Classic angina:* A sense of choking or of pressure or heaviness in the chest, usually brought on by exertion or anxiety and relieved by rest.

Anginal equivalent: Exertional dyspnea or exertional fatigue, which results from myocardial ischemia and is relieved by rest or nitroglycerin.

Variant angina: Also called Prinzmetal angina: occurs at rest or in atypical patterns (e.g., after exercise or nocturnally); is caused by coronary artery spasm and is associated with ECG changes (usually ST elevation) during symptoms.

Unstable angina: Pain that is new or is changed in character (more frequent, more severe, or both).

Diagnosis: ECG may show evidence of ischemia or prior myocardial infarction. Other findings are nonspecific and are frequently normal. Bundle branch block, Wolff-Parkinson-White syndrome, or intraventricular conduction delay may make the ECG findings unreliable. Exercise stress testing. *Imaging:* Radionuclide scintigraphy, stress echocardiography, stress scintigraphy, coronary angiography.

Treatment: Aspirin. Beta-blockers (atenolol, metoprolol, bisoprolol) are effective in reducing heart rate and thereby decreasing oxygen consumption and preventing angina. Nitroglycerin sublingually is the most effective therapy for acute anginal episodes. Long acting nitrates (mononitrates or transdermal nitrates) act through preload reduction and coronary vasodilatation. Side effects, which include headaches and hypotension, tend to clear with continued usage. Long acting calcium channel blockers (verapamil, diltiazem, nifedipine, or amlodipine) decrease incidence of symptomatic coronary artery disease and reduce both myocardial infarction and death from MI. Low-molecular-weight heparin in patients hospitalized with unstable angina. Combination therapy may be used (especially nitrates plus calcium antagonists with or without beta blockers).

Arteriosclerotic Heart Disease

A group of diseases characterized by myocardial ischemia caused by thickening and loss of elasticity of coronary arterial walls. Atherosclerosis is the most common form of coronary arteriosclerosis. Process is chronic, occurring over many years, and is the most common cause of cardiovascular disability and death.

Synonyms: Coronary artery disease, coronary heart disease, coronary arteriosclerosis.

Diagnosis: ECG may be normal or may show ST-segment elevation/depression and/or T-wave inversion. Exercise stress test: positive. *Lab:* Elevated triglycerides, elevated total cholesterol, elevated LDLs, decreased HDLs, elevated cholesterol/HDL ratio. *Imaging:* Angiography shows narrowed coronary arteries. Echocardiography shows wall-motion abnormalities. Pharmacologic stress test results (dobutamine, dipyridamole, adenosine) positive. Stress thallium test result positive.

Treatment: Aspirin. Cholesterol-lowering agents: HMG-CoA reductase inhibitors (atorvastatin, fluvastatin, lovastatin, pravastatin, simvastatin, rosuvastatin), bile acid sequestrants (cholestyramine, colestipol), Omega-3 acid ethyl esters, niacin, gemfibrozil, fenofibrate.

ARTHRITIS, RHEUMATOID (RA)

Chronic systemic inflammatory disease of unknown cause that typically involves joints. Articular inflammation may be remitting, but if continued, usually results in joint damage and disability. Characteristic extraarticular manifestations include rheumatoid nodules, arteritis, neuropathy, scleritis, pericarditis, and splenomegaly. Associated Conditions: Sjögren syndrome, Felty syndrome, increased incidence of infections, renal impairment, lymphomas, secondary amyloidosis, and cardiovascular disease.

Treatment: Early treatment with disease-modifying antiarthritic drugs (DMARDs) currently recommended. No one DMARD is consistently better than others, but methotrexate, hydroxychloroquine, sulfasalazine, and leflunomide are preferred over gold, D-penicillamine, azathioprine, and cyclosporine, because of adverse effects. Combinations of DMARDs may be more effective than individual drugs. Early disease or acute/chronic inflammation: Aspirin or other nonsteroidal antiinflammatory drugs, celecoxib.

BREAST CANCER

Malignant neoplasm arising in the breast. Classified as noninvasive (in situ) or invasive (infiltrating); approximately 70% of all breast cancers possess a component of invasion. Age-specific incidence of breast cancer increases sharply until menopause and continues to increase at a slower rate in the geriatric population.

Diagnosis: Bone scan if symptoms suggest bony metastasis, alkaline phosphatase levels elevated, or widespread disease is suspected. CT or ultrasound of abdomen if widespread or recurrent disease is suspected. *Lab:* CBC, liver function tests, pathologic review of biopsy, estrogen- and progesterone-receptor determination, and HER-2 status. *Imaging:* Bilateral mammography ± ultrasound. Mammography detects 80% of breast cancers and is the best technique for the detection of minimal (<0.5 cm) breast cancer. Most common abnormality representing cancer is an irregular mass. Microcalcifications can be the only sign of malignancy in 35% of breast cancers. Approximately 10–20 % of palpable cancers have normal mammograms. Ultrasound may confirm whether a suspicious lump is solid or cystic and help define its size and extent.

Treatment: Metastatic disease is considered incurable, but treatable with remissions occurring in 30–40% of the patients. Chemotherapy reduces the risk of recurrence 22–37% and death 14–27%. Combination chemotherapy is preferred over single agents. High-dose chemotherapy with bone marrow transplant does not appear to improve survival rates. Tamoxifen reduces the risk of recurrence and death for women of all ages. Treatment should be continued for 5 years. Probably no benefit to women with estrogen receptor negative tumors. Except for tiny localized tumors, all estrogen- and/or progesterone-receptor positive tumors should be treated with tamoxifen and/or an aromatase inhibitor: exemestane, anastrozole, or letrozole. Treatment regimen depends on whether patient is pre- or post-menopausal. Fulvestrant is an estrogen-receptor antagonist that can be effective in patients failed by other hormonal therapies. Treatment with tamoxifen for 5 years in receptor-positive postmenopausal women reduces the risk of recurrence by 42% and the risk of cancer-related death by 22%. The use of aromatase inhibitor for 5 years after a course of tamoxifen reduces the risk of recurrence by 43%. Tamoxifen increases risk of endometrial cancer and thrombosis. Hormonal therapy increases the risk of osteoporosis.

CARPAL TUNNEL SYNDROME

Pain and paresthesia in the hand due to compression of the median nerve as it traverses the carpal tunnel in the wrist. Symptoms tend to affect the dominant hand, but more than half of patients experience bilateral symptoms.

Diagnosis: Electromyographyis abnormal in >85% of cases. Prolonged distal latency of the median motor nerves may be seen. The most sensitive indicator is the median sensory distal latency, which is prolonged.

Treatment: Nonsteroidal antiinflammatory agents such as ibuprofen or naproxen sodium provide significant relief in many patients. Refractory symptoms or evidence of distal muscle atrophy are indications for surgical release of the nerve.

CATARACT

Any opacity of the lens, either localized or generalized. Largest cause of blindness in the world. Types: age-related ("senile"): 90%; congenital: 0.4% of newborns, 10–38% of childhood blindness; toxic/nutritional; systemic or metabolic disease (myotonic dystrophy, atopic dermatitis, diabetes mellitus, hypocalcemia, Wilson disease); complicated, due to other diseases (uveitis, juvenile rheumatoid arthritis, sarcoidosis, occult tumor [melanoma, retinoblastoma]); traumatic, due to heat (infrared), electrical shock, radiation, concussion, perforating eye injuries, or intraocular foreign body.

Diagnosis: Visual quality assessment: Glare testing, contrast sensitivity are sometimes indicated. (Hyperglycemic state as in poor diabetic control creates osmotic change within lens and may alter measurement of visual acuity and refractive state.) Retinal/macular function assessment: Potential acuity meter testing and fluorescein retinal angiography sometimes required.

Treatment: Lens extraction by phacoemulsification and replacement with a plastic lens implant.

CONGESTIVE HEART FAILURE (CHF)

A group of syndromes due to inefficiency of pumping action in the right ventricle, left ventricle, or both. Systolic failure results in reduction of emptying during ventricular systole. Diastolic failure denotes inability of the ventricle to dilate for filling during diastole. Most patients have findings consistent with both mechanisms. CHF is the principal complication of heart disease.

Diagnosis: *Lab:* Elevated creatinine, hyperbilirubinemia, dilutional hyponatremia, respiratory alkalosis, mild azotemia, decreased erythrocyte sedimentation rate, proteinuria. B-type natriuretic peptide is a marker of ventricular dysfunction; a reading >100 is consistent with CHF. *Imaging:* Echocardiographic studies are most useful. Nuclear imaging to evaluate left and right ventricular size and systolic function. Radiography shows cardiomegaly, interstitial edema, Kerley B lines, perivascular edema, pleural effusions.

Treatment: Diuretics: Furosemide metolazone, spironolactone. Angiotensin-converting enzyme inhibitors to decrease afterload. Beta-blockers: Carvedilol, bisoprolol. Digoxin improves contractility and slows ventricular rate in atrial fibrillation. Vasodilators: IV nitroglycerin may be of short-term benefit to decrease preload, afterload, and systemic resistance.

Deep Vein Thrombophlebitis (DVT)

Development of one or more clots in the deep veins of the lower limbs or pelvis, usually accompanied by inflammation of the vessel wall. The major clinical consequence is embolization, usually to the lung, which is frequently life threatening. Associated Conditions: Malignant neoplasm (20% of all venous thromboembolic disease), hyperhomocysteinemia, inherited thrombophilias, antiphospholipid antibody syndrome, Chiari syndrome (hepatic vein thrombosis), renal vein thrombosis.

Diagnosis: *Lab:* Baseline CBC, platelet count, aPTT, prothrombin time by international normalized ratio (INR). D-dimer sensitive but not specific for DVT; has a high negative predictive value. Thromboembolic disease panel: Factor V Leiden, G20210A prothrombin, serum homocysteine, factor VIII level, lupus anticoagulant, protein C and S antigen levels, antithrombin activity, and anticardiolipin antibodies. *Imaging:* Compression ultrasonography (noninvasive, highly sensitive, and specific for popliteal and femoral thrombi), contrast venography, impedance plethysmography (IPG), magnetic resonance venography, ^{125}I fibrinogen scan.

Treatment: Uncomplicated DVT: Low molecular weight heparin (enoxaparin, dalteparin). Complicated DVT: Heparin IV bolus followed by continuous infusion; or enoxaparin. Maintenance therapy: Warfarin.

Diabetes Mellitus, Type 2

Nonketosis-prone hyperglycemia and glucose intolerance; accounts for 80% of diabetic cases.

Diagnosis: *Lab:* Criteria for diagnosis (any one is sufficient): Symptoms of diabetes (polyuria, polydipsia, weight loss) plus casual (random) plasma glucose >200 mg/dL (11.1 mmol/L) or fasting plasma glucose >126 mg/dL (7.0 mmol/L) on two occasions or 2-hour plasma glucose >200 mg/dL (11.1 mmol/L) during oral glucose tolerance test with 75 g glucose load.

Treatment: Biguanides: Metformin. Sulfonylureas: Glimepiride, glipizide, glyburide. Thiazolidinediones: Pioglitazone, rosiglitazone. α-Glucosidase inhibitors: Acarbose, miglitol. Combinations: Fixed-dose combinations of metformin with glipizide, glyburide, and rosiglitazone are available. Insulin may be used in combination with oral agents. Most often required in late stages of Type 2 diabetes mellitus when oral agents fail to control blood glucose. Rapid-acting insulin: Aspart, glulisine, lispro. Short-acting insulin: Regular. Long-acting insulin: Glargine, ultralente. Home glucose monitoring (1–4 times/day) recommended for most patients taking insulin.

Fibromyalgia

A chronic syndrome of widespread pain and stiffness in skeletal muscles of the neck and trunk. Pain is reproduced by pressure on "trigger points."

Treatment: Education, graded exercise. Sleep restorative without interfering with stage IV sleep: Zolpidem, eszopiclone, zaleplon, temazepam.

Gastroesophageal Reflux Disease (GERD)

Reflux of gastroduodenal contents into the esophagus, larynx, or lungs with or without resultant esophageal inflammation. Associated Conditions: Reflux esophagitis (classified as erosive or nonerosive), asthma, aspiration, chronic cough, laryngitis, vocal cord granuloma, sinusitis, otitis media, Barrett syndrome, esophageal adenocarcinoma.

Diagnosis: Treated empirically if no dysphagia, odynophagia, weight loss, early satiety, anemia, or new onset in a male >45 years. 24-hour pH monitoring records number of reflux episodes, number that occur supine or upright. Esophageal manometry records pressure of lower esophageal sphincter and effectiveness of peristalsis. *Lab:* Check for anemia due to bleeding esophageal erosions. *Imaging:* Barium swallow: Presence of a sliding hiatal hernia appears to be a predictor of reflux esophagitis. Mucosal irregularity due to inflammation and edema.

Treatment: Lifestyle and diet modifications, H2 blocker (cimetidine, ranitidine, famotidine, nizatidine) at prescription dosage, protein pump inhibitor (omeprazole, lansoprazole, pantoprazole, rabeprazole, esomeprazole), antacids, metoclopramide.

Hypothyroidism, Adult

Clinical state resulting from decreased circulating levels of free thyroid hormone or from resistance to hormone action.

Synonym: Myxedema

Diagnosis: *Lab:* Primary hypothyroidism: thyroid-stimulating hormone (TSH) elevated, serum free thyroxine (T4) decreased. Central hypothyroidism: TSH low, serum free T4 decreased, impaired TSH response to TRH. Severe hypothyroidism: Anemia, elevated cholesterol, elevated CPK, LDH, AST; hyponatremia. Subclinical hypothyroidism: TSH elevated; serum free T4 normal.

Treatment: Levothyroxine. Dosage requirements may vary with age, sex, residual secretory capacity of thyroid gland, other drugs being taken by patient, intestinal function. Elderly patients may require about two thirds of dose used in young adults because renal clearance is decreased.

Irritable Bowel Syndrome

A condition characterized by a chronic abdominal pain associated with alteration in bowel habits in the absence of organic pathology. May be characterized as diarrhea predominant or constipation predominant or may alternate between diarrhea and constipation.

Synonyms: Mucous colitis, spastic colon, irritable colon.

Treatment: For patients with alternating diarrhea and constipation, fiber supplements. Constipation predominant: Teagaserod (approved for women only). Diarrhea predominant: Loperamide, diphenoxylate-atropine, dicyclomine, chlordiazepoxide-clidinium, hyoscyamine, phenobarbital-scopolamine-hyoscyamine-atropine. Flatulence: Simethicone. Lactose intolerance: Lactase.

Myocardial Infarction (MI)

The rapid development of myocardial necrosis resulting from a severe and sustained reduction of blood flow to a portion of the myocardium, usually due to thrombosis in an atherosclerotic coronary artery. Clinical consequences depend on the size and location of the infarction and the rapidity with which blood flow can be reestablished. After total occlusion, myocardial necrosis is complete in 4–6 hours. Flow to ischemic area must remain above 40% of preocclusion levels for that area to survive. Infarctions can be divided into Q wave and non-Q wave categories, with the former being transmural and associated with a totally obstructed infarct-related artery, and the latter being nontransmural and associated with a patent but highly narrowed infarct-related artery. Total occlusion of the left main coronary artery, which usually supplies 70% of the left ventricular mass, is catastrophic and results in death in minutes.

Synonyms: Coronary thrombosis, coronary occlusion, heart attack.

Diagnosis: *Electrocardiography (ECG):* ST segment elevation in a regional pattern in acute transmural ischemia. ST segment depression with T-wave inversions in subendocardial ischemia. New or presumably new bundle branch block, ST segment elevation, and depression are early findings of myocardial ischemia. A significant percentage of patients have nonspecific findings, such as peaked T waves and ST-segment elevation <0.1 mV. A small percentage of patients with transmural infarction present with normal ECG results. Q waves representing transmural myocardial necrosis appear within 24–48 hours. *Imaging:* Two-dimensional and M-mode echocardiography useful in evaluating wall motion abnormalities in MI, overall left ventricular function, and mechanical complications (mitral valve rupture, ventricular septal defect, mural thrombus). Chest radiography: Findings depend on severity of MI. Radionuclide studies: Thallium accumulates in viable myocardium.

Treatment: Coronary reperfusion with aspirin, alteplase, heparin, or low molecular weight heparin. Nitrates, oxygen, sedation (oxazepam, lorazepam, morphine), metoprolol. Stool softener (milk of magnesia, docusate sodium). Lidocaine IV for ventricular arrhythmias (not for arrhythmia prophylaxis). Post MI: Beta-blockers reduce mortality rates. Nitrates may be needed for angina. Angiotensin-converting enzyme inhibitors prevent adverse remodeling and may improve longevity.

OBESITY

A condition of increased adipose tissue (consisting of both lean and fat components) that leads to increased morbidity and mortality. *Android obesity* (male pattern or abdominal obesity) poses higher risk, gynecoid obesity (female pattern or *gluteal obesity*) lower risk, of long-term health problems.

Synonyms: Overweight, adiposis, adiposity.

Diagnosis: Body-mass index (BMI) = body weight (kg) divided by square of body height (m): Overweight is BMI = 25–29.9 kg/m^2; obesity is BMI >30 kg/m^2. Determine fat distribution pattern by measuring waist circumference: Waist circumference >40 inches (102 cm) for men or 35 inches (88 cm) for women is associated with increased risk of most obesity-related medical conditions

Treatment: National Institutes of Health (NIH) guidelines suggest nonpharmacologic treatment for 6 months and drug treatment for insufficient weight loss in those with a BMI >30 or a BMI >27 with associated risk factors such as coronary heart disease, diabetes, sleep apnea, hypertension, hyperlipidemia (high low-density lipoprotein or low high-density lipoprotein cholesterol). Drug therapy is recommended as part of a program that includes diet, physical activity, and behavior therapy. Sibutramine is a serotonin and norepinephrine reuptake inhibitor classified as an appetite suppressant. Orlistat is a lipase inhibitor that decreases absorption of dietary fat.

OSTEOARTHRITIS

Degenerative joint disease with progressive loss of articular cartilage and reactive changes at joint margins and in subchondral bone.

Treatment: For management of pain and inflammation: Acetaminophen. If not effective, nonacetylated salicylates (salsalate, choline-magnesium salicylate) or low-dose ibuprofen. Cyclo-oxygenase-2 specific inhibitors are less likely to cause GI ulcers and work as well as NSAIDs in reducing arthritis inflammation and pain. They are much more expensive and should be reserved for patients who are at higher risk for stomach ulcers and bleeding. Opioid analgesics (e.g., codeine, oxycodone, propoxyphene) should be restricted for treatment of acute episodes of pain. Intraarticular injections of corticosteroids for selected acute flare-ups of joints. Injections of hyaluronic acid preparation into a painful knee may provide relief of pain and improve function. Local application of capsaicin cream for pain relief; most effective in small joints of hand.

Peptic Ulcer Disease

Mucosal ulceration in a part of the alimentary canal containing acidic gastric juice (hydrochloric acid and pepsin). Duodenum is most common site. Gastric ulcer much less common than duodenal ulcer in absence of NSAIDs; commonly located along lesser curvature of the antrum near the incisura and in the antepyloric area. Esophageal ulcers in the distal esophagus may be part of a Barrett epithelial change. Ectopic gastric mucosal ulceration may develop in patients with Meckel diverticula or other sites of ectopic gastric mucosa.

Diagnosis: Helicobacter pylori *diagnostic tests:* Histology: Steiner stain of gastric biopsy for direct visualization of organism. Rapid urease test: Conducted on gastric biopsies. Serology antibody: Most commonly used for testing in primary care but cannot be used to identify persistent infection. Urea breath test: Used for posttreatment testing. Stool antigen: Can be used for screening and posttreatment testing.

Treatment: Acid suppression: H2 blockers (ranitidine, nizatidine, cimetidine, famotidine), proton pump inhibitors (PPI) (omeprazole, lansoprazole, rabeprazole, esomeprazole, pantoprazole). *H. pylori* eradication regimens: Triple therapy: 2 antibiotics plus a PPI for 14 days (omeprazole or lansoprazole plus metronidazole or amoxicillin plus clarithromycin). Alternative triple therapy regimen: Ranitidine bismuth citrate plus clarithromycin or metronidazole plus tetracycline or amoxicillin. Bacterial resistance: Clarithromycin 10%, amoxicillin 1.4%, metronidazole 37%. For treatment failures: Bismuth quadruple therapy for 14 days (bismuth subsalicylate, metronidazole, tetracycline), H2 blocker for 28 days or PPI for 14 days. Alternative second-line therapy: Levofloxacin, amoxicillin, PPI.

Pleural Effusion

The presence of excessive fluid in the pleural space. Under normal conditions, there is a small volume of pleural fluid in the pleural space that functions as a lubricant. Effusions are classified as either transudates or exudates. Transudates result from imbalance between hydrostatic and oncotic pressures (cirrhosis, congestive heart failure, nephrotic syndrome, obstruction of the superior vena cava). Exudates are due to a disturbance of the systems regulating pleural fluid formation and absorption/drainage (bacterial, viral, or fungal infection, rheumatologic disease, or malignancy).

Diagnosis: Antinuclear antibody titer, rheumatoid factor, pancreatic enzymes, cancer antigens 125 and 19-9, creatinine, or blood urea nitrogen. Aerobic/anaerobic blood cultures. Cultures of pleural fluid. Transudates and exudates must be distinguished. A transudate has none of the following characteristics, however an exudate must meet one of the following criteria: pleural fluid protein/serum protein >0.5; pleural fluid lactate dehydrogenase/serum lactate dehydrogenase >0.6; pleural fluid lactate dehydrogenase exceeds 2/3 upper limit of that in serum. All exudates must be evaluated with differential cell count, amylase level, glucose level, comprehensive microbiologic culturing, and Gram staining. If infection is suspected, the effusion should be evaluated for aerobic and anaerobic bacteria, mycobacteria, protozoa, fungi, and parasites, as appropriate. Effusions in tuberculosis (TB) may be associated with elevations in lysozyme and adenosine deaminase. Cytology for tumor cells. Triglyceride levels >110 mg/dL are consistent with chylothorax. Additional studies: pH, erythrocyte count (hemorrhagic effusion if >100,000/mL; consider trauma as cause for effusion).

Treatment: Antimicrobial therapy according to culture and sensitivity studies. Chemical pleurodesis with doxycycline, bleomycin, or talc in a slurry, as indicated. If pleurodesis fails, the patient may be offered pleural abrasion, even though this is not commonly performed. Chemotherapy according to current oncologic protocols. Corticosteroids and NSAIDs for rheumatologic and inflammatory causes. Diuresis as appropriate for effusions due to cardiac failure.

Posttraumatic Stress Disorder (PTSD)

In response to a highly traumatic event, a set of physical and emotional symptoms including reexperiencing the trauma (nightmares, flashbacks), avoidance, dissociation, emotional numbing, persistent increased physical arousal (hypervigilance, insomnia). Associated Conditions: Mood disorders, substance abuse/dependency, anxiety, panic disorder, agoraphobia, obsessive-compulsive disorder, social phobia, specific phobia, somatoform disorder, eating disorders (in women).

Treatment: Antidepressants are the standard treatment. They reduce symptoms, especially when combined with talk therapy. Initial treatment should be 12 months with longer courses if needed. Many patients will relapse after discontinuing medicine. Benzodiazepines are not recommended; no proven benefit for PTSD-specific symptoms (numbing, reexperiencing) and carry risk of dependence, withdrawal, and rebound anxiety. Selective serotonin reuptake inhibitors (SSRIs) (citalopram, escitalopram, fluoxetine, fluvoxamine, paroxetine, sertraline): Improvement in all symptom groups (reexperiencing, avoidance, hyperarousal); also appropriate for frequently comorbid depression, panic, borderline personality disorder, impulsiveness.

Prostatic Cancer

Malignant disease arising in the prostate gland; 95% of prostate cancers are acinic cell adenocarcinomas.

Diagnosis: *Lab:* Prostate specific antigen (PSA) elevated, free PSA low in cancer, alkaline phosphatase elevated with metastasis. *Imaging:* Bone scan, skeletal survey, lymph node aspiration, CT of pelvic lymph nodes positive with metastasis. Prostatic ultrasound. Biopsy, fine needle aspiration or core, ultrasound, lymph node aspiration, lymph node biopsy.

Treatment: In androgen-dependent tumors, a reduction in serum testosterone achieved by orchiectomy or medical castration (leuprolide, goserelin, nonsteroidal antiandrogens) is helpful in reducing tumor size, bone pain, and for improving survival. Radiation therapy, chemotherapy, radical prostatectomy, cryosurgery.

Pulmonary Edema

Pulmonary interstitial and/or alveolar fluid accumulation that results when the forces moving fluid out of the pulmonary capillary exceed the forces opposing that process.

Diagnosis: Arterial blood gases, ECG, pulmonary function tests, mixed venous oxygen saturation.

Treatment: Acute cardiogenic pulmonary edema: Morphine sulfate IV, furosemide IV, nitroglycerin paste. In selected cases nitroglycerin IV, nitroprusside IV, dobutamine. Long-term management of cardiogenic pulmonary edema: Furosemide, angiotensin-converting enzyme (ACE) inhibitors (captopril, lisinopril, enalapril). Digoxin, carvedilol, isosorbide dinitrate, hydrochlorothiazide, spironolactone. Noncardiogenic pulmonary edema: Oxygen, selected cardiovascular drugs to optimize tissue oxygen delivery.

Renal Failure, Acute (ARF)

A syndrome of rapid reduction in renal function. May or may not be associated with oliguria; results in failure to excrete nitrogenous wastes and maintain normal volume and electrolyte homeostasis, with rising creatinine and blood urea nitrogen levels.

Diagnosis: *Lab:* Creatinine clearance, decreased azotemia, hyperphosphatemia, hyperkalemia, acidemia (increased anion gap), decreased serum bicarbonate, decreased hemoglobin/hematocrit, increased magnesium, uric acid, amylase, lipase, hyponatremia, hypocalcemia, increased bleeding time. Urinalysis: Proteinuria, hematuria. Urine sediment: Brown granular urinary casts, urinary renal tubular epithelial cells, coarse granular casts, renal tubular epithelial cells, eosinophils (acute interstitial nephritis), red blood cell or hemoglobin casts (RPGN), crystals (lithiasis, obstruction). Urine electrolytes/osmolality: Increased urine sodium, increased fractional excretion of sodium. *Imaging:* Ultrasound identifies kidney presence and size, hydronephrosis, nephrolithiasis; Doppler flow useful for renal artery stenosis and thrombosis. Abdominal plain radiograph useful for identification of renal calculi. Radionuclide renal scan evaluates renal flow, renal function, and extravasation. Angiography: Vascular disorders, including renal artery stenosis, systemic vasculitides. MRI: An increase in T2-weighted signal may be seen in acute tubulointerstitial nephritis.

Treatment: IV expansion with normal saline followed by mannitol and calcium channel blockers. Volume expansion alone is beneficial in contrast injury.

Seizure Disorders

A seizure is a sudden change in cortical electrical activity, manifested through motor, sensory, or behavioral changes, with or without an alteration in consciousness.

Synonyms: Convulsions, epilepsy, fits, spells, attacks.

Diagnosis: *Electroencephalography:* A negative electroencephalogram does not rule out a seizure disorder. Sleep deprivation is helpful prior to electroencephalogram to identify positive spike wave formations. Video electroencephalogram monitoring is helpful in differentiating psychomotor nonepileptiform seizures. *Lab:* Serum glucose, sodium, potassium, calcium, phosphorus, magnesium, blood urea nitrogen, ammonia. Anticonvulsant levels: Inadequate level of anticonvulsant medication is the most common cause of recurrent seizures in children and many adults. Drug and toxic screens, including alcohol. CBC helpful in evaluating infection. *Imaging:* MRI of brain: Superior in evaluation of the temporal lobes. CT scan of brain indicated routinely in workup of tonic-clonic seizures

Treatment: Selection of medications from following groups, with attention toward potential side-effects, is preferred, as is monotherapy whenever possible. Generalized seizures—Tonic-clonic: Phenytoin, carbamazepine, valproic acid. Generalized seizures—absence: Ethosuximide, valproic acid. Partial seizures: Phenytoin, carbamazepine, phenobarbital.

Stroke (Brain Attack)

The sudden onset of a focal neurological deficit resulting from either infarction or hemorrhage within the brain. Adults <45 years old most likely to have a cardiac source of embolism.

Synonyms: Cerebrovascular accident (CVA), reversible ischemic neurological accident.

Diagnosis: *Lab:* Prothrombin time (PT), partial thromboplastin time (PTT), antiphospholipid antibodies, cardiac enzymes. *Imaging:* Duplex carotid ultrasonography, cerebral angiography, transthoracic echocardiogram, transesophageal echocardiogram, Holter monitoring, EEG for suspected seizure.

Treatment: IV tissue plasminogen activator in selected cases within 3 hours of ischemic stroke. Enteric-coated aspirin or dipyridamole-aspirin, clopidogrel, warfarin (international normalized ratio-adjusted dose) for patients with atrial fibrillation and cardioembolic stroke.

TRANSIENT ISCHEMIC ATTACK (TIA)

Sudden onset of focal and transient (<24 hours) neurologic deficit due to brain ischemia.

Synonym: Ministroke.

Diagnosis: Duplex carotid ultrasonography, ECG, cerebral angiography, transthoracic echocardiogram, transesophageal echocardiogram, Holter monitoring, CT of head. Acute phase: Brain MRI, include diffusion-weighted imaging. MR angiography: Brain and blood vessels. EEG, if seizure suspected.

Treatment: Enteric coated aspirin, dipyridamole-aspirin, or clopidogrel; warfarin (international normalized ratio-adjusted dose) for patients with atrial fibrillation and cardioembolic stroke.

URINARY TRACT INFECTION (UTI) IN FEMALES

Inflammation of the bladder mucosa due to infection.

Synonym: Cystitis.

Diagnosis: Some recent research suggests the most cost-effective approach is empiric treatment without laboratory tests in nonpregnant premenopausal women with symptoms of UTI and no risks for complicated infection.

Treatment: Fluoroquinolone or trimethoprim-sulfamethoxazole (TMP-SMX). Increasing resistance to TMP-SMX in pathogens is reported, but it is the preferred treatment if local sensitivity patterns indicate low resistance rates. New studies show 3-day therapy may be used in children. Postcoital: Single-dose TMP-SMX or cephalexin may reduce frequency of UTI in sexually active women. Pregnant patients: 10–14-day or longer treatment with pregnancy-safe antibiotic chosen on basis of culture/sensitivity results. May begin with cephalosporin, amoxicillin, or other antibiotic while awaiting culture/sensitivity results. All other patients: 10–14-day treatment with antibiotic chosen on basis of culture/sensitivity results. May begin with fluoroquinolone, TMP-SMX, cephalosporin, or other antibiotic while awaiting culture/sensitivity results. Change the antibiotic if it is indicated by the culture/sensitivity results.

URINARY TRACT INFECTION (UTI) IN MALES

Bacterial infection of the lower urinary tract, usually resulting from a single gram-negative enteric organism.

Synonyms: Cystitis.

Diagnosis: Urologic investigations are necessary to rule out other disorders.

Treatment: Acute infection, first infection, no risk factors for treatment: Prescribe 7–10 days of oral antibiotic, either empirically or based on culture and sensitivity results. For empiric therapy, trimethoprim-sulfamethoxazole or a fluoroquinolone. Complicated or recurrent infection: Prescribe 14–21 days of antibiotic based on antimicrobial sensitivities with repeat urine check after treatment.

Adapted from Domino FJ. *The 5-Minute Clinical Consult 2007*. Philadelphia: Lippincott Williams & Wilkins, 2007.

Pain Glossary

algesthesia	hypersensitivity to pain
allodynia	condition in which ordinarily nonpainful stimuli evoke pain
analgesia	neurologic or pharmacologic state in which painful stimuli are so moderated that, though still perceived, they are no longer painful
anesthesia dolorosa	severe spontaneous pain occurring in an anesthetic area
causalgia	persistent severe burning pain, usually following injury of a peripheral nerve (especially median and tibial) or the brachial plexus, accompanied by trophic changes
central pain syndrome	neurological condition caused by damage to or dysfunction of the central nervous system, which includes the brain, brainstem, and spinal cord
dysesthesia	impairment of sensation short of anesthesia; a condition in which a disagreeable sensation is produced by ordinary stimuli, caused by lesions of the sensory pathways, peripheral or central; abnormal sensations experienced in the absence of stimulation
hypalgesia	decreased sensibility to pain
hyperalgesia	extreme sensitivity to painful stimuli
hyperesthesia	abnormal acuteness of sensitivity to touch, pain, or other sensory stimuli
hyperpathia	exaggerated subjective response to painful stimuli, with a continuing sensation of pain after the stimulation has ceased
hypesthesia	diminished sensitivity to stimulation
intractable pain	pain resistant or refractory to ordinary analgesic agents
neuralgia	pain of a severe, throbbing, or stabbing character in the course or distribution of a nerve
neuritis	inflammation of a nerve
neuropathy	a disease involving the cranial nerves or the peripheral or autonomic nervous system
nociceptor	a peripheral nerve organ or mechanism for the reception and transmission of painful or injurious stimuli
noxious stimulus	stimulus that is potentially or actually damaging to body tissue
pain	unpleasant sensation associated with actual or potential tissue damage and mediated by specific nerve fibers to the brain where its conscious appreciation may be modified by various factors
pain threshold	the smallest intensity of a painful stimulus at which the individual perceives pain
pain tolerance	the greatest intensity of painful stimulation that an individual is able to tolerate
paralgesia	painful paresthesia; any disorder or abnormality of the sense of pain
paralgia	abnormal or unusual pain
paresthesia	an abnormal sensation, such as of burning, pricking, tickling, or tingling
rest pain	pain occurring, usually in the extremities, during rest in the sitting or lying position
telalgia	referred pain

Pain Management Techniques

I. Pharmacologic Therapy
- A. Nonsteroidal Antiinflammatory Drugs (NSAIDs)
- B. Opioids
- C. Adjuvant analgesics
  1. Anticonvulsants
  2. Local anesthetics
  3. Corticosteroids
  4. Antispasmodics
  5. Clonidine
  6. Topical agents
- D. Psychopharmacology
- E. Antidepressants
- F. Antipsychotics
- G. Mood stabilizers
- H. Anxiolytics
- I. Psychostimulants

II. Nonpharmacologic Therapy
- A. Blocks
  1. Epidural steroid injections
  2. Central nerve blocks
  3. Sympathetic nerve blocks
  4. Visceral nerve blocks
  5. Peripheral nerve blocks
  6. Facet joint blocks
  7. Sacroiliac joint blocks
  8. Trigger point injections
- B. Intravenous lidocaine injection
- C. Intravenous phentolamine infusion
- D. Intravenous regional sympathetic blocks (Bier blocks)

III. Interventional Therapy
- A. Spinal cord stimulation
- B. Intrathecal therapy
- C. Discography
- D. Intradiscal electrothermal therapy
- E. Vertebroplasty
- F. Cryosurgery
- G. Angiogenesis inhibitor therapy
- H. Bone marrow transplantation
- I. Gene therapy
- J. Hyperthermia
- K. Laser therapy
- L. Photodynamic therapy
- M. Target cancer therapy

IV. Neurosurgical Therapy
- A. Ablative procedures
- B. Augmentation procedures

V. Physical Therapy
- A. Stretching exercises
- B. Strengthening exercises
- C. Endurance exercises
- D. Electrical stimulation
- E. Ultrasound
- F. Local heat
- G. Local cooling
- H. Joint mobilization
- I. Soft-tissue mobilization

VI. Acupuncture

VII. Radiotherapy and Radiopharmaceuticals for Cancer Pain
- A. Palliative treatment
- B. Radiation therapy for bone metastases
- C. Chemotherapy for reduction of tumor size
- D. Hemibody irradiation
- E. Systemic radioisotopes

Pain Assessment Tools

Initial Pain Assessment Tool

Date ____________

Patient's name ____________ Age ______ Room ______

Diagnosis ____________ Physician ____________

Nurse ____________

1. LOCATION: Patient or nurse marks drawing.

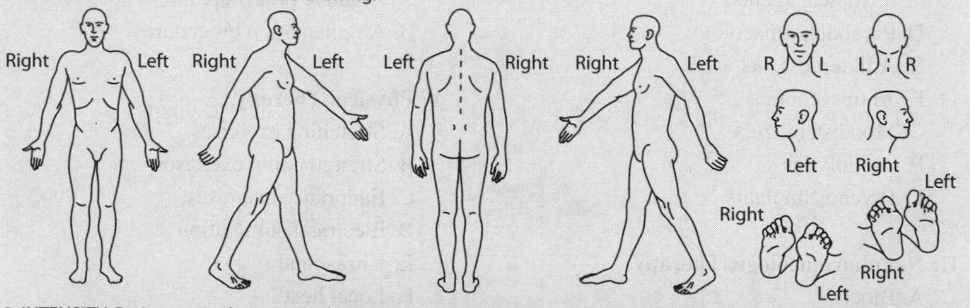

2. INTENSITY: Patient rates the pain. Scale used ____________
   - Present: ____________
   - Worst pain gets: ____________
   - Best pain gets: ____________
   - Acceptable level of pain: ____________

3. QUALITY: (Use patient's own words, e.g., prick, ache, burn, throb, pull, sharp) ____________

4. ONSET, DURATION, VARIATION, RHYTHMS: ____________

5. MANNER OF EXPRESSING PAIN: ____________

6. WHAT RELIEVES THE PAIN? ____________

7. WHAT CAUSES OR INCREASES THE PAIN? ____________

8. EFFECTS OF PAIN: (Note decreased function, decreased quality of life.)
   - Accompanying symptoms (e.g., nausea) ____________
   - Sleep ____________
   - Appetite ____________
   - Physical activity ____________
   - Relationship with others (e.g., irritability) ____________
   - Emotions (e.g., anger, suicidal, crying) ____________
   - Concentration ____________
   - Other ____________

9. OTHER COMMENTS: ____________

10. PLAN: ____________

Adapted from McCaffery M, Pasero C. *Pain: Clinical Manual.* 2nd ed. St. Louis, MO: C. V. Mosby; 1999.

Wong-Baker FACES Pain Rating Scale

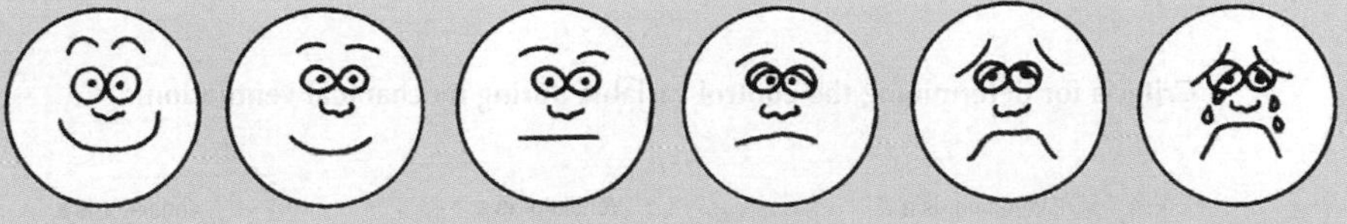

1. Explain to the child that each face is for a person who feels happy because he or she has no pain (hurt, or whatever word the child uses) or feels sad because he or she has some or a lot of pain.
2. Point to the appropriate face and state, "This face . . .":
   0—"is very happy because he [or she] doesn't hurt at all."
   1—"hurts just a little bit."
   2—"hurts a little more."
   3—"hurts even more."
   4—"hurts a whole lot."
   5—"hurts as much as you can imagine, although you don't have to be crying to feel this bad."
3. Ask the child to choose the face that best describes how he or she feels. Be specific about which pain (eg, "shot" or incision) and what time (eg, Now? Earlier before lunch?)

From Hockenberry MJ. *Wong's Essentials of Pediatric Nursing.* 7th ed. St. Louis, MO: C. V. Mosby; 2005.

Mechanical Ventilation Criteria in Respiratory Care

Criteria for determining the control variable during mechanical ventilation

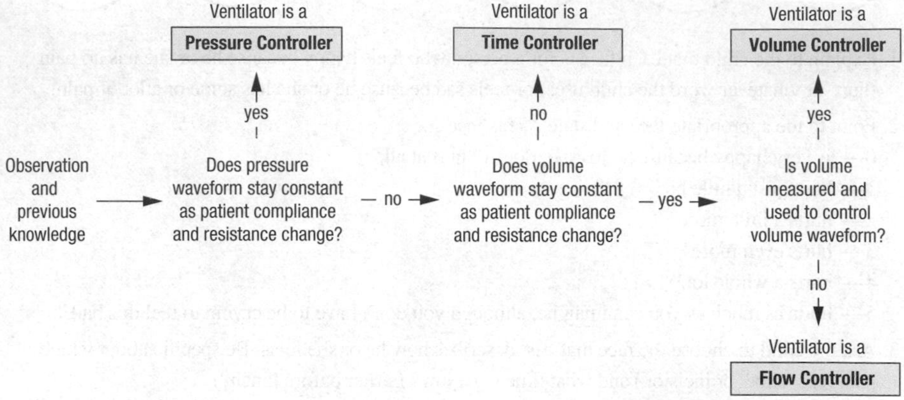

Criteria for determining the phase variables during mechanical ventilation

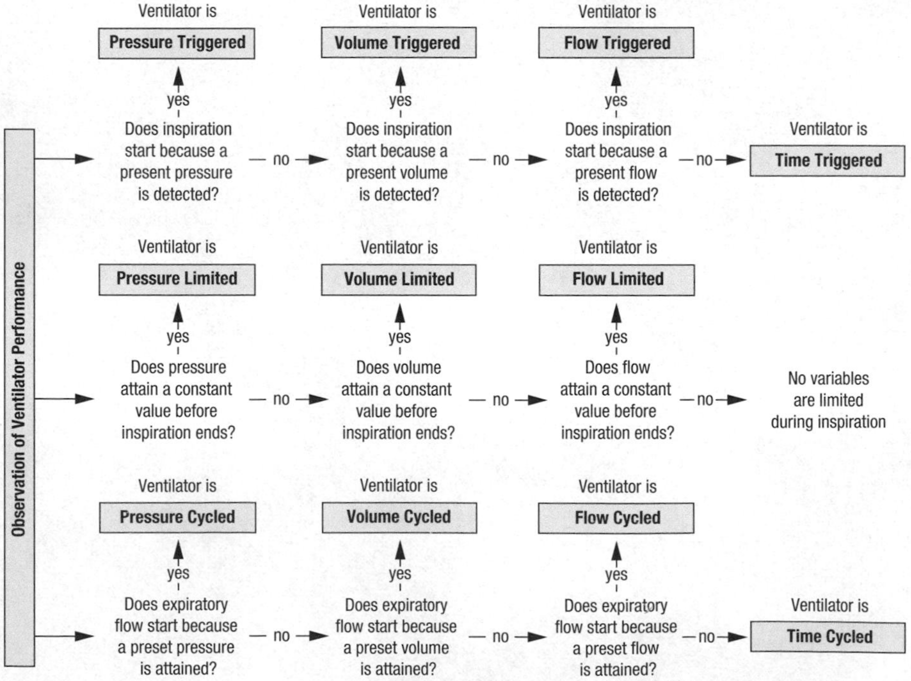

Levels of Alzheimer Disease

Levels	Description
I and II	Presenile dementia may end here with no further progression. Brain changes are not significant, and the only remarkable symptom may be forgetfulness. Patients at this level perform all activities of daily living (ADLs) with reasonable ease.
III	At this level, ability to remember facts, faces, and names decreases. The patient will still have enough awareness to recognize the problem and will become increasingly frustrated and angry. Most ADLs are still performed reasonably well.
IV	Late confusional or mild Alzheimer. The patient at this level begins to misplace things, has increasing difficulty remembering, and neglects ADLs. Most patients are aware a problem exists but deny it is a concern.
V	Early dementia or moderate Alzheimer. By this level, the patient must have custodial care. There will be severe lapses in memory, disorientation, anger, and great frustration.
VI	Middle dementia or moderately severe Alzheimer. The patient now has severe memory loss, is incapable of self-care at any level, and is disoriented most of the time. Immense anger, hostility, and combativeness are present, as well as a fear of water.
VII	Late dementia. The patient requires full-time care and is rarely seen in a medical office. Unless home care is an option, the physician will probably make calls to the long-term care facility. The patient at this state rarely speaks and almost never speaks intelligibly. There will be incontinence, and the patient may require tube feeding.

From Hosley JB, Molle-Matthews EA, eds. Lippincott's textbook for clinical medical assisting. Baltimore: Lippincott Williams & Wilkins, 1999.

Overview of Major Nursing Theories

Theorist	Purpose	Views of Components
Florence Nightingale (1860) *Notes on Nursing: What It Is Not*	To help those responsible for caring for sick to "think how to nurse." Theory addresses fundamental needs of the sick and basic principles of good health care.	**Person:** Individual with vital reparative processes to deal with disease. **Environment:** External conditions that affect life and the individual's development. Focus is on ventilation, warmth, odors, and light. **Health:** Focus is on the reparative process of getting well. **Nursing:** Goal is to place the patient in the best condition for good health care.
Hildegard E. Peplau (1952) *Interpersonal Relations in Nursing*	To develop an interpersonal interaction between client and nurse.	**Person:** An organism striving to reduce tension generated by needs. **Environment:** Implicitly defined; the interpersonal process is always included, and the psychodynamic milieu receives attention, with emphasis on the client's culture and mores. **Health:** Ongoing human process that implies forward movement of personality and other ongoing human processes in the direction of creative, constructive, productive, personal, and community living. **Nursing:** Interpersonal therapeutic process that "functions cooperatively with other human processes that make health possible for individuals in communities. Nursing is an educative instrument, a maturing force that aims to promote forward movement of personality."
Virginia Henderson (1955) *The Nature of Nursing*	To assist the client in gaining independence as rapidly as possible.	**Person:** Individual requiring assistance to achieve health and independence or a peaceful death. Mind and body are inseparable. **Environment:** All external conditions and influences that affect life and development. **Health:** Equated with independence, viewed in terms of the client's ability to perform 14 components of nursing care unaided: breathing, eating, drinking, maintaining comfort, sleeping, resting, clothing, maintaining body temperature, ensuring safety, communicating, worshiping, working, recreation, and continuing development. **Nursing:** Assists and supports the individual in life activities and the attainment of independence.
Faye Glenn Abdellah (1960) *Patient-Centered Approaches to Nursing*	To deliver nursing care for the whole individual.	**Person:** The recipient of nursing care; having physical, emotional, and sociologic needs that may be overt or covert. **Environment:** Not clearly defined. Some discussion indicates that clients interact with their environment, of which the nurse is a part.

Theorist	Purpose	Views of Components
Faye Glenn Abdellah (*cont.*)		**Health:** Implicitly defined as a state when the individual has no unmet needs and no anticipated or actual impairments. **Nursing:** Broadly grouped in "21 nursing problems," which center around needs for hygiene, comfort, activity, rest, safety, oxygen, nutrition, elimination, hydration, physical and emotional health promotion, interpersonal relationships, and development of self-awareness. Nursing care is doing something for a individual.
Ida Jean Orlando (1961) *The Dynamic Nurse-Patient Relationship*	To interact with clients to meet immediate needs by identifying client behaviors, nurse's reactions, and nursing actions to take.	**Person:** Unique individual behaving verbally and nonverbally. Assumption is that individuals are at times able to meet their own needs and at other times are unable to do so. **Environment:** Not defined. **Health:** Not defined. Assumption is that being without emotional or physical discomfort and having a sense of well-being contribute to a healthy state. **Nursing:** Professional nursing is conceptualized as finding out and meeting the client's immediate need for help. Medicine and nursing are viewed as distinctly different.
Lydia E. Hall (1964) *Nursing: What Is It?*	To provide professional nursing care to people past the acute stage of illness.	**Person:** Client is composed of body, pathology, and person. People set their own goals and are capable of learning and growing. **Environment:** Should facilitate achievement of the client's personal goals. **Health:** Development of a mature self-identity that assists in the conscious selection of actions that facilitate growth. **Nursing:** Caring is the nurse's primary function. Professional nursing is most important during the recuperative period.
Ernestine Weldenbach (1964) *Clinical Nursing—A Helping Art*	To assist individuals in overcoming obstacles that prevent meeting health care needs.	**Person:** Any individual who is receiving help (care, instruction, or advice) from a member of the healthcare profession or from a worker in the field of health. **Environment:** Not specifically addressed. **Health:** Not defined. Concepts of nursing, client, and need for help and their relationships imply health-related concerns in the nurse-client relationship (Marriner-Tomey & Alligood, 2002, p. 245). **Nursing:** Functioning human being who acts, thinks, and feels. All actions, thoughts, and feelings underlie what the nurse does.
Myra Estrin Levin (1973) *Conservation Model*	To use conservation activities aimed at optimal use of client's resources.	**Person:** A holistic being. **Environment:** Broadly, includes all the individual's experiences. **Health:** The maintenance of the client's unity and integrity. **Nursing:** A discipline rooted in the organic dependency of the individual human being on her or his relationships with others.

APP

Theorist	Purpose	Views of Components
Dorothy E. Johnson (1980) *The Behavioral System Model for Nursing*	To reduce stress so the client can recover as quickly as possible.	**Person:** A system of interdependent parts with patterned, repetitive, and purposeful ways of behaving. **Environment:** All forces that affect the person and that influence the behavioral system. **Health:** Focus on person, not illness. Health is a dynamic state influenced by biologic, psychological, and social factors. **Nursing:** Promotion of behavioral system, balance, and stability. An art and a science providing external assistance before and during system balance disturbances.
Martha E. Rogers (1970) *The Science of Unitary Man*	To assist the client in achieving a maximum level of wellness.	**Person:** Unitary man, a four-dimensional energy field. **Environment:** Encompasses all that is outside any given human field. Person exchanging matter and energy. **Health:** Not specifically addressed, but emerges out of interaction between human and environment, moves forward, and maximizes human potential. **Nursing:** A learned profession that is both science and art. The professional practice of nursing is creative and imaginative and exists to serve people.
Dorothea E. Orem (1971) *Nursing: Concepts of Practice*	To provide care and to assist the client to attain self-care.	**Person:** Biopsychosocial being capable of self-care. Includes physical, psychological, interpersonal, and social aspects of human functioning. **Environment:** Internal and external stimuli. Requisites for self-care have their origins in human beings and the environment. **Health:** State of wholeness or integrity of human beings, including physical, mental, and social well-being. **Nursing:** A creative effort of one human being to help another human being. Consists of three nursing systems: wholly compensatory, partially compensatory, and supportive/educative.
Imogene M. King (1971) *Open Systems Model*	To use communication to help the client reestablish a positive adaptation to his or her environment.	**Person:** Biopsychosocial being. **Environment:** Internal and external environment continually interact to assist in adjustments to change. **Health:** A dynamic life experience with continued goal attainment and adjustment to stressors. **Nursing:** Perceiving, thinking, relating, judging, and acting with someone who comes to a nursing situation.
Joyce Travelbee (1971) *Interpersonal Aspects of Nursing*	To assist individuals, families, communities, and groups to prevent or cope with illness and regain health.	**Person:** A unique, irreplaceable individual who is in a continuous process of becoming, evolving, and changing. **Environment:** Not explicitly defined. **Health:** Health includes the individual's perceptions of health and the absence of disease.

Theorist	Purpose	Views of Components
Joyce Travelbee (*cont.*)		**Nursing:** An interpersonal process whereby the professional nurse practitioner assists an individual, family, or community to prevent or to cope with the experience of illness and suffering and, if necessary, to find meaning in these experiences.
Betty Neuman (1972) *The Neuman Systems Model*	To address the effects of stress and reactions to it on the development and maintenance of health.	**Person:** A client system composed of physiologic, psychological, sociocultural, and environmental variables. **Environment:** Internal and external forces surrounding humans at any time. **Health:** Health or wellness exists if all parts and subparts are in harmony with the whole person. **Nursing:** A unique profession concerned with all variables affecting an individual's response to stressors.
Sister Callista Roy (1970) *Roy Adaptation Model*	To identify the type of demands placed on a client and the client's adaptation to the demands.	**Person:** A biopsychosocial being and the recipient of nursing care. **Environment:** All conditions, circumstances, and influences surrounding and affecting the development of an organism or groups of organisms. **Health:** The person encounters adaptation problems in changing environments. **Nursing:** A theoretical system of knowledge that prescribes a process of analysis and action related to the care of the ill or potentially ill person.
Jean Watson (1979) *Nursing: Human Science and Human Care*	To focus on curative factors derived from a humanistic perspective and from scientific knowledge.	**Person:** A valued being to be cared for, respected, nurtured, understood, and assisted; a fully functional, integrated self. **Environment:** Social environment, caring, and the culture of caring affect health. **Health:** Physical, mental and social well-being. **Nursing:** A human science of people and human health; illness experiences that are mediated by professional, personal, scientific, aesthetic, and ethical human care transactions.
Rosemarie Rizzo Parse (1981) *Man–Living–Health: Theory of Nursing*	To focus on humans as living unity and humans' qualitative participation with health experience.	**Person:** A major reason for nursing's existence, evidenced by a "pattern of patterns of relating." **Environment:** "Man and environment interchange energy to create what is in the world, and man chooses the meaning given to the situations he creates." **Health:** A lived experience that is a process of being and becoming. **Nursing:** "Nursing practice is directed toward illuminating and mobilizing family interrelationships in light of the meaning assigned to health and its possibilities as language in the cocreated patterns of relating."

From Craven RF, Hirnle CJ, eds. *Fundamentals of Nursing: Human Health and Function*, 5th ed. Philadelphia: Lippincott Williams & Wilkins, 2007.

References

Abdellah FG. *Patient-centered approaches to nursing.* New York: Macmillan, 1960.

Hall LE. Nursing: What is it? *Can Nurse* 1964;60:150–154.

Henderson V. *The nature of nursing.* New York: Macmillan, 1955.

Johnson DE. The behavioral system model for nursing. In: Riehl JP, Roy C, eds. *Conceptual models for nursing practice.* New York: Appleton-Century-Crofts, 1980.

King IM. *Toward a theory of nursing.* New York: Wiley, 1971.

Levine ME. *An introduction to clinical nursing,* 2nd ed. Philadelphia: FA Davis, 1973.

Marriner-Tomey A, Alligood MR. Nursing theorists and their work, 5th ed. St. Louis, MO: Mosby, 2002.

Neuman B. *The Neuman systems model: Application to nursing education and practice.* New York: Appleton-Century-Crofts, 1972.

Nightingale F. *Notes on nursing: What it is and what it is not.* London: Harrison, 1860.

Orem DE. *Nursing: Concepts of practice,* 3rd ed. New York: McGraw-Hill, 1971.

Orlando IJ. *The dynamic nurse-patient relationship: Function, process, and principles.* New York: Putnam, 1961.

Parse RR. *Man–living–health: Theory of nursing.* New York: John Wiley and Sons, 1981.

Peplau HE. *Interpersonal relations in nursing.* New York: Putnam, 1952.

Rogers ME. *An introduction to the theoretical basis of nursing.* Philadelphia: FA Davis, 1970.

Roy C. Adaption: A conceptual framework for nursing. *Nursing Outlook.* 1970; 18:42-45.

Travelbee J. *Interpersonal aspects of nursing.* Philadelphia: FA Davis, 1971.

Weidenbach E. *Clinical nursing—A helping art.* New York: Springer, 1964.

Diagnosis-Related Groups (DRGs)

DRG	DRG Description
001.	Craniotomy, Age Greater than 17, with CC
002.	Craniotomy for Trauma, Age Greater than 17, with CC
003.	Craniotomy, Age 0–17
004.	No Longer Valid
005.	No Longer Valid
006.	Carpal Tunnel Release
007.	Peripheral and Cranial Nerve and Other Nervous System Procedures with CC
008.	Peripheral and Cranial Nerve and Other Nervous System Procedures without CC
009.	Spinal Disorders and Injuries
010.	Nervous System Neoplasms with CC
011.	Nervous System Neoplasms without CC
012.	Degenerative Nervous System Disorders
013.	Multiple Sclerosis and Cerebellar Ataxia
014.	Intracranial Hemorrhage with Infarction
015.	Nonspecific Cerebrovascular and Precerebral Occlusion without Infarction
016.	Nonspecific Cerebrovascular Disorders with CC
017.	Nonspecific Cerebrovascular Disorders without CC
018.	Cranial and Peripheral Nerve Disorders with CC
019.	Cranial and Peripheral Nerve Disorders without CC
020.	Nervous System Infection Except Viral Meningitis
021.	Viral Meningitis
022.	Hypertensive Encephalopathy
023.	Nontraumatic Stupor and Coma
024.	Seizure and Headache, Age Greater than 17 with CC
025.	Seizure and Headache, Age Greater than 17 without CC
026.	Seizure and Headache, Age 0–17
027.	Traumatic Stupor and Coma, Coma Greater than One Hour
028.	Traumatic Stupor and Coma, Coma Less than One Hour, Age Greater than 17 with CC
029.	Traumatic Stupor and Coma, Coma Less than One Hour, Age Greater than 17 without CC
030.	Traumatic Stupor and Coma, Coma Less than One Hour, Age 0–17
031.	Concussion, Age Greater than 17 with CC
032.	Concussion, Age Greater than 17 without CC
033.	Concussion, Age 0–17
034.	Other Disorders of Nervous System with CC
035.	Other Disorders of Nervous System without CC
036.	Retinal Procedures
037.	Orbital Procedures
038.	Primary Iris Procedures
039.	Lens Procedures with or without Vitrectomy
040.	Extraocular Procedures Except Orbit, Age Greater than 17
041.	Extraocular Procedures Except Orbit, Age 0–17
042:	Intraocular Procedures Except Retina, Iris, and Lens
043.	Hyphema
044.	Acute Major Eye Infections
045.	Neurological Eye Disorders
046.	Other Disorders of the Eye, Age Greater than 17 with CC
047.	Other Disorders of the Eye, Age Greater than 17 without CC
048.	Other Disorders of the Eye, Age 0–17
049.	Major Head and Neck Procedures
050.	Sialoadenectomy
051.	Salivary Gland Procedures Except Sialoadenectomy
052.	Cleft Lip and Palate Repair
053.	Sinus and Mastoid Procedures, Age Greater than 17
054.	Sinus and Mastoid Procedures, Age 0–17
055.	Miscellaneous Ear, Nose, Mouth, and Throat Procedures
056.	Rhinoplasty
057.	T and A Procedures Except Tonsillectomy and/or Adenoidectomy Only, Age Greater than 17
058.	T and A Procedures Except Tonsillectomy and/or Adenoidectomy Only, Age 0–17
059.	Tonsillectomy and/or Adenoidectomy Only, Age Greater than 17
060.	Tonsillectomy and/or Adenoidectomy Only, Age 0–17
061.	Myringotomy with Tube Insertion, Age Greater than 17
062.	Myringotomy with Tube Insertion, Age 0–17
063.	Other Ear, Nose, Mouth, and Throat OR Procedures
064.	Ear, Nose, Mouth and Throat Malignancy
065.	Dysequilibrium
066.	Epistaxis
067.	Epiglottitis
068.	Otitis Media and URI, Age Greater than 17 with CC
069.	Otitis Media and URI, Age Greater than 17 without CC
070.	Otitis Media and URI, Age 0–17
071.	Laryngotracheitis
072.	Nasal Trauma and Deformity
073.	Other Ear, Nose, Mouth, and Throat Diagnoses, Age Greater than 17
074.	Other Ear, Nose, Mouth, and Throat Diagnoses, Age 0–17
075.	Major Chest Procedures
076.	Other Respiratory System OR Procedures with CC
077.	Other Respiratory System OR Procedures without CC
078.	Pulmonary Embolism
079.	Respiratory Infections and Inflammations, Age Greater than 17 with CC
080.	Respiratory Infections and Inflammations, Age Greater than 17 without CC
081.	Respiratory Infections and Inflammations, Age 0–17
082.	Respiratory Neoplasms
083.	Major Chest Trauma with CC
084.	Major Chest Trauma without CC
085.	Pleural Effusion with CC
086.	Pleural Effusion without CC

DRG	DRG Description
087.	Pulmonary Edema and Respiratory Failure
088.	Chronic Obstructive Pulmonary Disease
089.	Simple Pneumonia and Pleurisy, Age Greater than 17 with CC
090.	Simple Pneumonia and Pleurisy, Age Greater than 17 without CC
091.	Simple Pneumonia and Pleurisy, Age 0–17
092.	Interstitial Lung Disease with CC
093.	Interstitial Lung Disease without CC
094.	Pneumothorax with CC
095.	Pneumothorax without CC
096.	Bronchitis and Asthma, Age Greater than 17 with CC
097.	Bronchitis and Asthma, Age Greater than 17 without CC
098.	Bronchitis and Asthma, Age 0–17
099.	Respiratory Signs and Symptoms with CC
100.	Respiratory Signs and Symptoms without CC
101.	Other Respiratory System Diagnoses with CC
102.	Other Respiratory System Diagnoses without CC
103.	Heart Transplant or Implant of Heart Assist System
104.	Cardiac Valve and Other Major Cardiothoracic Procedures with Cardiac Catheterization
105.	Cardiac Valve and other Major Cardiothoracic Procedures without Cardiac Catheterization
106.	Coronary Bypass with PTCA
107.	No Longer Valid
108.	Other Cardiothoracic Procedures
109.	No Longer Valid
110.	Major Cardiovascular Procedures with CC
111.	Major Cardiovascular Procedures without CC
112.	No Longer Valid
113.	Amputation for Circulatory System Disorders Except Upper Limb and Toe
114.	Upper Limb and Toe Amputation for Circulatory System Disorders
115.	No Longer Valid
116.	No Longer Valid
117.	Cardiac Pacemaker Revision Except Device Replacement
118.	Cardiac Pacemaker Device Replacement
119.	Vein Ligation and Stripping
120.	Other Circulatory System OR Procedures
121.	Circulatory Disorders with Acute Myocardial Infarction and Major Complications, Discharged Alive
122.	Circulatory Disorders with Acute Myocardial Infarction without Major Complications, Discharged Alive
123.	Circulatory Disorders with Acute Myocardial Infarction, Expired
124.	Circulatory Disorders Except Acute Myocardial Infarction with Cardiac Catheterization and Complex Diagnosis
125.	Circulatory Disorders Except Acute Myocardial Infarction with Cardiac Catheterization without Complex Diagnosis
126.	Acute and Subacute Endocarditis
127.	Heart Failure and Shock
128.	Deep Vein Thrombophlebitis
129.	Cardiac Arrest, Unexplained
130.	Peripheral Vascular Disorders with CC
131.	Peripheral Vascular Disorders without CC
132.	Atherosclerosis with CC
133.	Atherosclerosis without CC
134.	Hypertension
135.	Cardiac Congenital and Valvular Disorders, Age Greater than 17 with CC
136.	Cardiac Congenital and Valvular Disorders, Age Greater than 17 without CC
137.	Cardiac Congenital and Valvular Disorders, Age 0–17
138.	Cardiac Arrhythmia and Conduction Disorders with CC
139.	Cardiac Arrhythmia and Conduction Disorders without CC
140.	Angina Pectoris
141.	Syncope and Collapse with CC
142.	Syncope and Collapse without CC
143.	Chest Pain
144.	Other Circulatory System Diagnoses with CC
145.	Other Circulatory System Diagnoses without CC
146.	Rectal Resection with CC
147.	Rectal Resection without CC
148.	Major Small and Large Bowel Procedures with CC
149.	Major Small and Large Bowel Procedures without CC
150.	Peritoneal Adhesiolysis with CC
151.	Peritoneal Adhesiolysis without CC
152.	Minor Small and Large Bowel Prooedures with CC
153.	Minor Small and Large Bowel Procedures without CC
154.	Stomach, Esophageal, and Duodenal Procedures, Age Greater than 17 with CC
155.	Stomach, Esophageal, and Duodenal Procedures, Age Greater than 17 without CC
156.	Stomach, Esophageal, and Duodenal Procedures, Age 0–17
157.	Anal and Stomal Procedures with CC
158.	Anal and Stomal Procedures without CC
159.	Hernia Procedures Except Inguinal and Femoral, Age Greater than 17 with CC
160.	Hernia Procedures Except Inguinal and Femoral, Age Greater than 17 without CC
161.	Inguinal and Femoral Hernia Procedures, Age Greater than 17 with CC
162.	Inguinal and Femoral Hernia Procedures, Age Greater than 17 without CC
163.	Hernia Procedures, Age 0–17
164.	Appendectomy with Complicated Principal Diagnosis with CC
165.	Appendectomy with Complicated Principal Diagnosis without CC
166.	Appendectomy without Complicated Principal Diagnosis with CC
167.	Appendectomy without Complicated Principal Diagnosis without CC

DRG	DRG Description
168.	Mouth Procedures with CC
169.	Mouth Procedures without CC
170.	Other Digestive System OR Procedures with CC
171.	Other Digestive System OR Procedures without CC
172.	Digestive Malignancy with CC
173.	Digestive Malignancy without CC
174.	GI Hemorrhage with CC
175.	GI Hemorrhage without CC
176.	Complicated Peptic Ulcer
177.	Uncomplicated Peptic Ulcer with CC
178.	Uncomplicated Peptic Ulcer without CC
179.	Inflammatory Bowel Disease
180.	GI Obstruction with CC
181.	GI Obstruction without CC
182.	Esophagitis, Gastroenteritis, and Miscellaneous Digestive Disorders, Age Greater than 17 with CC
183.	Esophagitis, Gastroenteritis, and Miscellaneous Digestive Disorders, Age Greater than 17 without CC
184.	Esophagitis, Gastroenteritis, and Miscellaneous Digestive Disorders, Age 0–17
185.	Dental and Oral Diseases Except Extractions and Restorations, Age Greater than 17
186.	Dental and Oral Diseases Except Extractions and Restorations, Age 0–17
187.	Dental Extractions and Restorations
188.	Other Digestive System Diagnoses, Age Greater than 17 with CC
189.	Other Digestive System Diagnoses, Age Greater than 17 without CC
190.	Other Digestive System Diagnoses, Age 0–17
191.	Pancreas, Liver, and Shunt Procedures with CC
192.	Pancreas, Liver, and Shunt Procedures without CC
193.	Biliary Tract Procedures Except Only Cholecystectomy with or without Common Duct Exploration with CC
194.	Biliary Tract Procedures Except Only Cholecystectomy with or without Common Duct Exploration without CC
195.	Cholecystectomy with Common Duct Exploration with CC
196.	Cholecystectomy with Common Duct Exploration without CC
197.	Cholecystectomy Except by Laparoscope without Common Duct Exploration with CC
198.	Cholecystectomy Except by Laparoscope without Common Duct Exploration without CC
199.	Hepatobiliary Diagnostic Procedure for Malignancy
200.	Hepatobiliary Diagnostic Procedure for Nonmalignancy
201.	Other Hepatobiliary or Pancreas OR Procedures
202.	Cirrhosis and Alcoholic Hepatitis
203.	Malignancy of Hepatobiliary System or Pancreas
204.	Disorders of Pancreas Except Malignancy
205.	Disorders of Liver Except Malignancy, Cirrhosis, and Alcoholic Hepatitis with CC
206.	Disorders of Liver Except Malignancy, Cirrhosis, and Alcoholic Hepatitis without CC
207.	Disorders of the Biliary Tract with CC
208.	Disorders of the Biliary Tract without CC
209.	No Longer Valid
210.	Hip and Femur Procedures Except Major Joint, Age Greater than 17 with CC
211.	Hip and Femur Procedures Except Major Joint, Age Greater than 17 without CC
212.	Hip and Femur Procedures Except Major Joint, Age 0–17
213.	Amputation for Musculoskeletal System and Connective Tissue Disorders
214.	No Longer Valid
215.	No Longer Valid
216.	Biopsies of Musculoskeletal System and Connective Tissue
217.	Wound Débridement and Skin Graft Except Hand for Musculoskeletal and Connective Tissue Disorders
218.	Lower Extremity and Humerus Procedures Except Hip, Foot, and Femur, Age Greater than 17 with CC
219.	Lower Extremity and Humerus Procedures Except Hip, Foot, and Femur, Age Greater than 17 without CC
220.	Lower Extremity and Humerus Procedures Except Hip, Foot, and Femur, Age 0–17
221.	No Longer Valid
222.	No Longer Valid
223.	Major Shoulder/Elbow Procedures or Other Upper Extremity Procedures with CC
224.	Shoulder, Elbow, or Forearm Procedures Except Major Joint Procedures without CC
225.	Foot Procedures
226.	Soft Tissue Procedures with CC
227.	Soft Tissue Procedures without CC
228.	Major Thumb or Joint Procedures or Other Hand or Wrist Procedures with CC
229.	Hand or Wrist Procedures, Except Major Joint Procedures without CC
230.	Local Excision and Removal of Internal Fixation Devices of Hip and Femur
231.	No Longer Valid
232.	Arthroscopy
233.	Other Musculoskeletal System and Connective Tissue OR Procedures with CC
234.	Other Musculoskeletal System and Connective Tissue OR Procedures without CC
235.	Fractures of Femur
236.	Fractures of Hip and Pelvis
237.	Sprains, Strains, and Dislocations of Hip, Pelvis, and Thigh
238.	Osteomyelitis
239.	Pathological Fractures and Musculoskeletal and Connective Tissue Malignancy
240.	Connective Tissue Disorders with CC
241.	Connective Tissue Disorders without CC
242.	Septic Arthritis

DRG	DRG Description
243.	Medical Back Problems
244.	Bone Diseases and Specific Arthropathies with CC
245.	Bone Diseases and Specific Arthropathies without CC
246.	Nonspecific Arthropathies
247.	Signs and Symptoms of Musculoskeletal System and Connective Tissue
248.	Tendonitis, Myositis, and Bursitis
249.	Aftercare, Musculoskeletal System and Connective Tissue
250.	Fractures, Sprains, Strains, and Dislocations of Forearm, Hand, and Foot, Age Greater than 17 with CC
251.	Fractures, Sprains, Strains, and Dislocations of Forearm, Hand, and Foot, Age Greater than 17 without CC
252.	Fractures, Sprains, Strains, and Dislocations of Forearm, Hand, and Foot, Age 0–17
253.	Fractures, Sprains, Strains, and Dislocations of Upper Arm and Lower Leg Except Foot, Age Greater than 17 with CC
254.	Fractures, Sprains, Strains, and Dislocations of Upper Arm and Lower Leg Except Foot, Age Greater than 17 without CC
255.	Fractures, Sprains, Strains, and Dislocations of Upper Arm and Lower Leg Except Foot, Age 0–17
256.	Other Musculoskeletal System and Connective Tissue Diagnoses
257.	Total Mastectomy for Malignancy with CC
258.	Total Mastectomy for Malignancy without CC
259.	Subtotal Mastectomy for Malignancy with CC
260.	Subtotal Mastectomy for Malignancy without CC
261.	Breast Procedure for Nonmalignancy Except Biopsy and Local Excision
262.	Breast Biopsy and Local Excision for Nonmalignancy
263.	Skin Graft and/or Débridement for Skin Ulcer or Cellulitis with CC
264.	Skin Graft and/or Débridement for Skin Ulcer or Cellulitis without CC
265.	Skin Graft and/or Débridement Except Skin Ulcer or Cellulitis with CC
266.	Skin Graft and/or Débridement Except Skin Ulcer or Cellulitis without CC
267.	Perianal and Pilonidal Procedures
268.	Skin, Subcutaneous Tissue, and Breast Plastic Procedures
269.	Other Skin, Subcutaneous Tissue, and Breast Procedures with CC
270.	Other Skin, Subcutaneous Tissue, and Breast Procedures without CC
271.	Skin Ulcers
272.	Major Skin Disorders with CC
273.	Major Skin Disorders without CC
274.	Malignant Breast Disorders with CC
275.	Malignant Breast Disorders without CC
276.	Nonmalignant Breast Disorders
277.	Cellulitis, Age Greater than 17 with CC
278.	Cellulitis, Age Greater than 17 without CC
279.	Cellulitis, Age 0–17
280.	Trauma to Skin, Subcutaneous Tissue, and Breast, Age Greater than 17 with CC
281.	Trauma to Skin, Subcutaneous Tissue, and Breast, Age Greater than 17 without CC
282.	Trauma to Skin, Subcutaneous Tissue, and Breast, Age 0–17
283.	Minor Skin Disorders with CC
284.	Minor Skin Disorders without CC
285.	Amputation of Lower Limb for Endocrine, Nutritional, and Metabolic Disorders
286.	Adrenal and Pituitary Procedures
287.	Skin Grafts and Wound Débridement for Endocrine, Nutritional, and Metabolic Disorders
288.	OR Procedures for Obesity
289.	Parathyroid Procedures
290.	Thyroid Procedures
291.	Thyroglossal Procedures
292.	Other Endocrine, Nutritional, and Metabolic OR Procedures with CC
293.	Other Endocrine, Nutritional, and Metabolic OR Procedures without CC
294.	Diabetes, Age Greater than 35
295.	Diabetes, Age 0–35
296.	Nutritional and Miscellaneous Metabolic Disorders, Age Greater than 17 with CC
297.	Nutritional and Miscellaneous Metabolic Disorders, Age Greater than 17 without CC
298.	Nutritional and Miscellaneous Metabolic Disorders, Age 0–17
299.	Inborn Errors of Metabolism
300.	Endocrine Disorders with CC
301.	Endocrine Disorders without CC
302.	Kidney Transplant
303.	Kidney and Ureter Procedures for Neoplasm
304.	Kidney and Ureter Procedures for Nonneoplasms with CC
305.	Kidney and Ureter Procedures for Nonneoplasms without CC
306.	Prostatectomy with CC
307.	Prostatectomy without CC
308.	Minor Bladder Procedures with CC
309.	Minor Bladder Procedures without CC
310.	Transurethral Procedures with CC
311.	Transurethral Procedures without CC
312.	Urethral Procedures, Age Greater than 17 with CC
313.	Urethral Procedures, Age Greater than 17 without CC
314.	Urethral Procedures, Age 0–17
315.	Other Kidney and Urinary Tract OR Procedures
316.	Renal Failure
317.	Admission for Renal Dialysis
318.	Kidney and Urinary Tract Neoplasms with CC
319.	Kidney and Urinary Tract Neoplasms without CC

DRG	DRG Description
320.	Kidney and Urinary Tract Infections, Age Greater than 17 with CC
321.	Kidney and Urinary Tract Infections, Age Greater than 17 without CC
322.	Kidney and Urinary Tract Infections, Age 0–17
323.	Urinary Stones with CC and/or ESW Lithotripsy
324.	Urinary Stones without CC
325.	Kidney and Urinary Tract Signs and Symptoms, Age Greater than 17 with CC
326.	Kidney and Urinary Tract Signs and Symptoms, Age Greater than 17 without CC
327.	Kidney and Urinary Tract Signs and Symptoms, Age 0–17
328.	Urethral Stricture, Age Greater than 17 with CC
329.	Urethral Stricture, Age Greater than 17 without CC
330.	Urethral Stricture, Age 0–17
331.	Other Kidney and Urinary Tract Diagnoses, Age Greater than 17 with CC
332.	Other Kidney and Urinary Tract Diagnoses, Age Greater than 17 without CC
333.	Other Kidney and Urinary Tract Diagnoses, Age 0–17
334.	Major Male Pelvic Procedures with CC
335.	Major Male Pelvic Procedures without CC
336.	Transurethral Prostatectomy with CC
337.	Transurethral Prostatectomy without CC
338.	Testes Procedures, For Malignancy
339.	Testes Procedures, For Nonmalignancy, Age Greater than 17
340.	Testes Procedures, For Nonmalignancy, Age 0–17
341.	Penis Procedures
342.	Circumcision, Age Greater than 17
343.	Circumcision, Age 0–17
344.	Other Male Reproductive System OR Procedures for Malignancy
345.	Other Male Reproductive System OR Procedures Except for Malignancy
346.	Malignancy of Male Reproductive System with CC
347.	Malignancy of Male Reproductive System without CC
348.	Benign Prostatic Hypertrophy with CC
349.	Benign Prostatic Hypertrophy without CC
350.	Inflammation of the Male Reproductive System
351.	Sterilization, Male
352.	Other Male Reproductive System Diagnoses
353.	Pelvic Evisceration, Radical Hysterectomy, and Radical Vulvectomy
354.	Uterine and Adnexal Procedures for Nonovarian/Adnexal Malignancy with CC
355.	Uterine and Adnexal Procedures for Nonovarian/Adnexal Malignancy without CC
356.	Female Reproductive System Reconstructive Procedures
357.	Uterine and Adnexal Procedures for Ovarian or Adnexal Malignancy
358.	Uterine and Adnexal Procedures for Nonmalignancy with CC
359.	Uterine and Adnexal Procedures for Nonmalignancy without CC
360.	Vagina, Cervix, and Vulva Procedures
361.	Laparoscopy and Incisional Tubal Interruption
362.	Endoscopic Tubal Interruption
363.	D&C, Conization, and Radioimplant for Malignancy
364.	D&C, Conization Except for Malignancy
365.	Other Female Reproductive System OR Procedures
366.	Malignancy, Female Reproductive System with CC
367.	Malignancy, Female Reproductive System without CC
368.	Infections, Female Reproductive System
369.	Menstrual and Other Female Reproductive System Disorders
370.	Cesarean Section with CC
371.	Cesarean Section without CC
372.	Vaginal Delivery with Complicating Diagnoses
373.	Vaginal Delivery without Complicating Diagnoses
374.	Vaginal Delivery with Sterilization and/or D&C
375.	Vaginal Delivery with OR Procedures Except Sterilization and/or D&C
376.	Postpartum and Postabortion Diagnoses without OR Procedures
377.	Postpartum and Postabortion Diagnoses with OR Procedures
378.	Ectopic Pregnancy
379.	Threatened Abortion
380.	Abortion without D&C
381.	Abortion with D&C, Aspiration Curettage, or Hysterotomy
382.	False Labor
383.	Other Antepartum Diagnoses with Medical Complications
384.	Other Antepartum Diagnoses without Medical Complications
385.	Neonates, Died or Transferred to Another Acute Care Facility
386.	Extreme Immaturity or Respiratory Distress Syndrome, Neonate
387.	Prematurity with Major Problems
388.	Prematurity without Major Problems
389.	Full-Term Neonate with Major Problems
390.	Neonate with Other Significant Problems
391.	Normal Newborn
392.	Splenectomy, Age Greater than 17
393.	Splenectomy, Age 0–17
394.	Other OR Procedures of the Blood and Blood-Forming Organs
395.	Red Blood Cell Disorders, Age Greater than 17
396.	Red Blood Cell Disorders, Age 0–17
397.	Coagulation Disorders
398.	Reticuloendothelial and Immunity Disorders with CC
399.	Reticuloendothelial and Immunity Disorders without CC
400.	No Longer Valid
401.	Lymphoma and Nonacute Leukemia with Other OR Procedure with CC

DRG	DRG Description
402.	Lymphoma and Nonacute Leukemia with Other OR Procedure without CC
403.	Lymphoma and Nonacute Leukemia with CC
404.	Lymphoma and Nonacute Leukemia without CC
405.	Acute Leukemia without Major OR Procedure, Age 0–17
406.	Myeloproliferative Disorders or Poorly Differentiated Neoplasms with Major OR Procedures with CC
407.	Myeloproliferative Disorders or Poorly Differentiated Neoplasms with Major OR Procedures without CC
408.	Myeloproliferative Disorders or Poorly Differentiated Neoplasms with Other OR Procedures
409.	Radiotherapy
410.	Chemotherapy without Acute Leukemia as Secondary Myeloproliferative Diagnosis
411.	History of Malignancy without Endoscopy
412.	History of Malignancy with Endoscopy
413.	Other Myeloproliferative Disorders or Poorly Differentiated Neoplasm Diagnoses with CC
414.	Other Myeloproliferative Disorders or Poorly Differentiated Neoplasm Diagnoses without CC
415.	OR Procedure for Infections and Parasitic Diseases
416.	Septicemia, Age Greater than 17
417.	Septicemia, Age 0–17
418.	Postoperative and Posttraumatic Infections
419.	Fever of Unknown Origin, Age Greater than 17 with CC
420.	Fever of Unknown Origin, Age Greater than 17 without CC
421.	Viral Illness, Age Greater than 17
422.	Viral Illness and Fever of Unknown Origin, Age 0–17
423.	Other Infections and Parasitic Diseases Diagnoses
424.	OR Procedure with Principal Diagnoses of Mental Illness
425.	Acute Adjustment Reactions and Psychosocial Dysfunction
426.	Depressive Neuroses
427.	Neuroses Except Depressive
428.	Disorders of Personality and Impulse Control
429.	Organic Disturbances and Mental Retardation
430.	Psychoses
431.	Childhood Mental Disorders
432.	Other Mental Disorder Diagnoses
433.	Alcohol/Drug Abuse or Dependence, Left Against Medical Advice
434.	No Longer Valid
435.	No Longer Valid
436.	No Longer Valid
437.	No Longer Valid
438.	No Longer Valid
439.	Skin Grafts for Injuries
440.	Wound Débridements for Injuries
441.	Hand Procedures for Injuries
442.	Other OR Procedures for Injuries with CC
443.	Other OR Procedures for Injuries without CC
444.	Traumatic Injury, Age Greater than 17 with CC
445.	Traumatic Injury, Age Greater than 17 without CC
446.	Traumatic Injury, Age 0–17
447.	Allergic Reactions, Age Greater than 17
448.	Allergic Reactions, Age 0–17
449.	Poisoning and Toxic Effects of Drugs, Age Greater than 17 with CC
450.	Poisoning and Toxic Effects of Drugs, Age Greater than 17 without CC
451.	Poisoning and Toxic Effects of Drugs, Age 0–17
452.	Complications of Treatment with CC
453.	Complications of Treatment without CC
454.	Other Injury, Poisoning, and Toxic Effect Diagnoses with CC
455.	Other Injury, Poisoning, and Toxic Effect Diagnoses without CC
456.	No Longer Valid
457.	No Longer Valid
458.	No Longer Valid
459.	No Longer Valid
460.	No Longer Valid
461.	OR Procedures with Diagnoses of Other Contact with Health Services
462.	Rehabilitation
463.	Signs and Symptoms with CC
464.	Signs and Symptoms without CC
465.	Aftercare with History of Malignancy as Secondary Diagnosis
466.	Aftercare without History of Malignancy as Secondary Diagnosis
467.	Other Factors Influencing Health Status
468.	Extensive OR Procedure Unrelated to Principal Diagnosis
469.	Principal Diagnosis Invalid as Discharge Diagnosis
470.	Ungroupable
471.	Bilateral or Multiple Major Joint Procedures of Lower Extremity
472.	No Longer Valid
473.	Acute Leukemia without Major OR Procedure, Age Greater than 17
474.	No Longer Valid
475.	Respiratory System Diagnosis with Ventilator Support
476.	Prostatic OR Procedure Unrelated to Principal Diagnosis
477.	Nonextensive OR Procedure Unrelated to Principal Diagnosis
478.	No Longer Valid
479.	Other Vascular Procedures without CC
480.	Liver Transplant and/or Intestinal Transplant
481.	Bone Marrow Transplant
482.	Tracheostomy for Face, Mouth, and Neck Diagnoses
483.	No Longer Valid
484.	Craniotomy for Multiple Significant Trauma
485.	Limb Reattachment, Hip and Femur Procedures for Multiple Significant Trauma
486.	Other OR Procedures for Multiple Significant Trauma

DRG	DRG Description
487.	Other Multiple Significant Trauma
488.	HIV with Extensive OR Procedure
489.	HIV with Major Related Condition
490.	HIV with or without Other Related Condition
491.	Major Joint and Limb Reattachment Procedures of Upper Extremity
492.	Chemotherapy with Acute Leukemia or with Use of High-Dose Chemotherapy Agent
493.	Laparoscopic Cholecystectomy without Common Duct Exploration with CC
494.	Laparoscopic Cholecystectomy without Common Duct Exploration without CC
495.	Lung Transplant
496.	Combined Anterior/Posterior Spinal Fusion
497.	Spinal Fusion Except Cervical with CC
498.	Spinal Fusion Except Cervical without CC
499.	Back and Neck Procedures Except Spinal Fusion with CC
500.	Back and Neck Procedures Except Spinal Fusion without CC
501.	Knee Procedures with Principal Diagnosis of Infection with CC
502.	Knee Procedures with Principal Diagnosis of Infection without CC
503.	Knee Procedures without Principal Diagnosis of Infection
504.	Extensive Burns or Full Thickness Burn with Mechanical Ventilation 96+ Hours with Skin Graft
505.	Extensive Burns or Full Thickness Burn with Mechanical Ventilation 96+ hours without Skin Graft
506.	Full Thickness Burn with Skin Graft or Inhalation Injuries with CC or Significant Trauma
507.	Full Thickness Burn with Skin Graft or Inhalation Injuries without CC or Significant Trauma
508.	Full Thickness Burn without Skin Graft or Inhalation Injuries with CC or Significant Trauma
509.	Full Thickness Burn without Skin Graft or Inhalation Injuries without CC or Significant Trauma
510.	Nonextensive Burns with CC or Significant Trauma
511.	Nonextensive Burns without CC or Significant Trauma
512.	Simultaneous Pancreas/Kidney Transplant
513.	Pancreas Transplant
514.	No Longer Valid
515.	Cardiac Defibrillator Implant without Cardiac Catheterization
516.	No Longer Valid
517.	No Longer Valid
518.	Percutaneous Cardiovascular Procedures without Coronary Artery Stent or Acute Myocardial Infarction
519.	Cervical Spinal Fusion with CC
520.	Cervical Spinal Fusion without CC
521.	Alcohol/Drug Abuse or Dependence with CC
522.	Alcohol/Drug Abuse or Dependence with Rehabilitation Therapy without CC
523.	Alcohol/Drug Abuse or Dependence without Rehabilitation Therapy without CC
524.	Transcient Ischemia
525.	Other Heart Assist System Implant
526.	No Longer Valid
527.	No Longer Valid
528.	Intracranial Vascular Procedure with Principal Diagnosis of Hemorrhage
529.	Ventricular Shunt Procedures with CC
530.	Ventricular Shunt Procedures without CC
531.	Spinal Procedures with CC
532.	Spinal Procedures without CC
533.	Extracranial Vascular Procedures with CC
534.	Extracranial Vascular Procedures without CC
535.	Cardiac Defibrillator Implant with Cardiac Catheterization with Acute Myocardial Infarction, Heart Failure, or Shock
536.	Cardiac Defibrillator Implant with Cardiac Catheterization without Acute Myocardial Infarction, Heart Failure, or Shock
537.	Local Excision and Removal of Internal Fixation Devices Except Hip and Femur with CC
538.	Local Excision and Removal of Internal Fixation Devices Except Hip and Femur without CC
539.	Lymphoma and Leukemia with Major OR Procedure with CC
540.	Lymphoma and Leukemia with Major OR Procedure without CC
541	ECMO or Tracheostomy with Mechanical Ventilation 96+ Hours or Principal Diagnosis Except Face, Mouth & Neck with Major OR
542	Tracheostomy with Mechanical Ventilation 96+ Hours or Principal Diagnosis Except Face, Mouth & Neck without Major OR
543	Craniotomy with Major Device Implant or Acute Complex Central Nervous System Principal Diagnosis
544	Major Joint Replacement or Reattachment of Lower Extremity
545	Revision of Hip or Knee Replacement
546	Spinal Fusion Except Cervical with Curvature of the Spine or Malignancy
547	Coronary Bypass with Cardiac Catheterization with Major Cardiovascular Diagnosis
548	Coronary Bypass with Cardiac Catheterization without Major Cardiovascular Diagnosis
549	Coronary Bypass without Cardiac Catheterization with Major Cardiovascular Diagnosis
550	Coronary Bypass without Cardiac Catheterization without Major Cardiovascular Diagnosis
551	Permanent Cardiac Pacemaker Implant with Major Cardiovascular Diagnosis or AICD Lead or Generator
552	Other Permanent Cardiac Pacemaker Implant without Major Cardiovascular Diagnosis
553	Other Vascular Procedures with CC with Major Cardiovascular Diagnosis
554	Other Vascular Procedures with CC without Major Cardiovascular Diagnosis
555	Percutaneous Cardiovascular Procedure with Major Cardiovascular Diagnosis

DRG	DRG Description
556	Percutaneous Cardiovascular Procedure with Non-Drug-Eluting Stent without Major Cardiovascular Diagnosis
557	Percutaneous Cardiovascular Procedure with Drug-Eluting Stent with Major Cardiovascular Diagnosis
558	Percutaneous Cardiovascular Procedure with Drug-Eluting Stent without Major Cardiovascular Diagnosis
559	Acute Ischemic Stroke with Use of Thrombolytic Agent
560	Bacterial & Tuberculous Infections of Nervous System
561	Non-Bacterial Infections of Nervous System Except Viral Meningitis
562	Seizure, Age Greater than 17 with CC
563	Seizure, Age Greater than 17 without CC
564	Headaches, Age Greater than 17
565	Respiratory System Diagnosis with Ventilator Support, 96+ Hours
566	Respiratory System Diagnosis with Ventilator Support, Less than 96 Hours
567	Stomach, Esophageal & Duodenal Procedure, Age Greater than 17 with CC with Major Gastrointestinal Diagnosis
568	Stomach, Esophageal & Duodenal Procedure, Age Greater than 17 with CC without Major Gastrointestinal Diagnosis
569	Major Small & Large Bowel Procedures with CC with Major Gastrointestinal Diagnosis
570	Major Small & Large Bowel Procedures with CC without Major Gastrointestinal Diagnosis
571	Major Esophageal Disorders
572	Major Gastrointestinal Disorders and Peritoneal Infections
573	Major Bladder Procedures
574	Major Hematologic/Immunologic Diagnosis Except Sickle Cell Crisis & Coagulopathy
575	Septicemia with Mechanical Ventilation 96+ Hours, Age Greater than 17
576	Septicemia without Mechanical Ventilation 96+ Hours, Age Greater than 17
577	Carotid Artery Stent Procedure
578	OR Procedure with Principal Diagnosis Except Postoperative or Posttraumatic Infection
579	OR Procedure with Principal Diagnosis of Postoperative or Posttraumatic Infection

NANDA's Nursing Diagnoses: Definitions and Classification

ACTIVITY INTOLERANCE

Definition

Insufficient physiological or psychological energy to endure or complete required or desired daily activities

Defining Characteristics

- Abnormal blood pressure response to activity
- Abnormal heart rate response to activity
- Electrocardiographic changes reflecting arrhythmias
- Electrocardiographic changes reflecting ischemia
- Exertional discomfort
- Exertional dyspnea
- Verbal report of fatigue
- Verbal report of weakness

Related Factors

Bed rest
Generalized weakness
Imbalance between oxygen supply/demand
Immobility
Sedentary lifestyle

RISK FOR ACTIVITY INTOLERANCE

Definition

At risk for experiencing insufficient physiological or psychological energy to endure or complete required or desired daily activities

Risk Factors

Deconditioned status
History of previous intolerance
Inexperience with the activity
Presence of circulatory problems
Presence of respiratory problems

INEFFECTIVE AIRWAY CLEARANCE

Definition

Inability to clear secretions or obstructions from the respiratory tract to maintain a clear airway

Defining Characteristics

- Absent cough
- Adventitious breath sounds
- Changes in respiratory rate
- Changes in respiratory rhythm
- Cyanosis
- Difficulty vocalizing
- Diminished breath sounds

- Dyspnea
- Excessive sputum
- Ineffective cough
- Orthopnea
- Restlessness
- Wide-eyed

Related Factors

Environmental

Second-hand smoke
Smoke inhalation
Smoking

Obstructed airway

Airway spasm
Excessive mucus
Exudate in the alveoli
Foreign body in airway
Presence of artificial airway
Retained secretions
Secretions in the bronchi

Physiological

Allergic airways
Asthma
Chronic obstructive pulmonary disease
Hyperplasia of the bronchial walls
Infection
Neuromuscular dysfunction

LATEX ALLERGY RESPONSE

Definition

A hypersensitive reaction to natural latex rubber products

Defining Characteristics

Life-Threatening Reactions Occurring <1 Hour After Exposure to Latex Protein

- Bronchospasm
- Cardiac arrest
- Contact urticaria progressing to generalized symptoms
- Dyspnea
- Edema of the lips
- Edema of the throat
- Edema of the tongue
- Edema of the uvula
- Hypotension
- Respiratory arrest
- Syncope
- Tightness in chest
- Wheezing

Orofacial Characteristics

- Edema of eyelids
- Edema of sclera
- Erythema of the eyes
- Facial erythema
- Facial itching
- Itching of the eyes
- Oral itching
- Nasal congestion
- Nasal erythema
- Nasal itching
- Rhinorrhea
- Tearing of the eyes

Gastrointestinal Characteristics

- Abdominal pain
- Nausea

Generalized Characteristics

- Flushing
- Generalized discomfort
- Generalized edema
- Increasing complaint of total body warmth
- Restlessness

Type 1V Reactions

Occurring >1 hour after exposure to latex protein

- Discomfort reaction to additives such as thiurams & carbamates
- Eczema
- Irritation
- Redness

Related Factors

Hypersensitivity to natural latex rubber protein

References

American Society of Anesthesiologists. (2005). *Natural rubber latex allergy: Considerations for anesthesiologists* (a practice guideline). Park Ridge, IL: Author.

AORN. (2004). AORN latex guideline. In *AORN standards, recommended practices and guidelines* (pp. 103 – 118). Denver, CO: Author.

Sussman, G.L. (2000) Latex allergy: An overview. *Canadian Journal of Allergy and Clinical Immunology, 5,* 317 – 321.

RISK FOR LATEX ALLERGY RESPONSE

Definition

Risk of hypersensitivity to natural latex rubber products

Risk Factors

Allergies to avocados
Allergies to bananas
Allergies to chestnuts
Allergies to kiwi
Allergies to poinsettia plants
Allergies to tropical fruits

History of allergies
History of asthma
History of reactions to latex
Multiple surgical procedures, especially from infancy
Professions with daily exposure to latex

References

American Society of Anesthesiologists. (2005). *Natural rubber latex allergy: Considerations for anesthesiologists* (a practice guideline). Park Ridge, IL: Author.

AORN. (2004). AORN latex guideline. In *AORN standards, recommended practices and guidelines* (pp. 103 – 118). Denver, CO: Author.

Sussman, G.L. (2000) Latex allergy: An overview. *Canadian Journal of Allergy and Clinical Immunology, 5*, 317 – 321.

ANXIETY

Definition

Vague uneasy feeling of discomfort or dread accompanied by an autonomic response (the source often non-specific or unknown to the individual); a feeling of apprehension caused by anticipation of danger. It is an alerting signal that warns of impending danger and enables the individual to take measures to deal with threat.

Defining Characteristics

Behavioral

- Diminished productivity
- Expressed concerns due to change in life events
- Extraneous movement
- Fidgeting
- Glancing about
- Insomnia
- Poor eye contact
- Restlessness
- Scanning
- Vigilance

Affective

- Apprehensive
- Anguish
- Distressed
- Fearful
- Feelings of inadequacy
- Focus on self
- Increased wariness
- Irritability
- Jittery
- Overexcited
- Painful increased helplessness
- Persistent increased helplessness
- Rattled
- Regretful
- Scared
- Uncertainty
- Worried

Physiological

- Facial tension
- Hand tremors
- Increased perspiration
- Increased tension
- Shakiness
- Trembling
- Voice quivering

Sympathetic

- Anorexia
- Cardiovascular excitation
- Diarrhea
- Dry mouth
- Facial flushing
- Heart pounding
- Increased blood pressure
- Increased pulse
- Increased reflexes
- Increased respiration
- Pupil dilation
- Respiratory difficulties
- Superficial vasoconstriction
- Twitching
- Weakness

Parasympathetic

- Abdominal pain
- Decreased blood pressure
- Decreased pulse
- Diarrhea
- Faintness
- Fatigue
- Nausea
- Sleep disturbance
- Tingling in extremities
- Urinary frequency
- Urinary hesitancy
- Urinary urgency

Cognitive

- Awareness of physiologic symptoms
- Blocking of thought
- Confusion
- Decreased perceptual field
- Difficulty concentrating
- Diminished ability to learn
- Diminished ability to problem solve
- Fear of unspecified consequences
- Forgetfulness
- Impaired attention

- Preoccupation
- Rumination
- Tendency to blame others

Related Factors

Change in
- Economic status
- Environment
- Health status
- Interaction patterns
- Role function
- Role status

Exposure to toxins
Familial association
Heredity
Interpersonal contagion
Interpersonal transmission
Maturational crises
Situational crises
Stress
Substance abuse
Threat of death
Threat to
- Economic status
- Environment
- Health status
- Interaction patterns
- Role function
- Role status

Threat to self-concept
Unconscious conflict about essential goals of life
Unconscious conflict about essential values
Unmet needs

Death Anxiety

Definition

Vague uneasy feeling of discomfort or dread generated by perceptions of a real or imagined threat to one's existence

Defining Characteristics

- Reports concerns of over-working the caregiver
- Reports deep sadness
- Reports fear of developing terminal illness
- Reports fear of loss of mental abilities when dying
- Reports fear of pain related to dying
- Reports fear of premature death
- Reports fear of the process of dying
- Reports fear of prolonged dying
- Reports fear of suffering related to dying
- Reports feeling powerless over dying

- Reports negative thoughts related to death and dying
- Reports worry about the impact of one's own death on significant others

Related Factors

Anticipating adverse consequences of general anesthesia
Anticipating impact of death on others
Anticipating pain
Anticipating suffering
Confronting reality of terminal disease
Discussions on topic of death
Experiencing dying process
Near-death experience
Nonacceptance of own mortality
Observations related to death
Perceived proximity of death
Uncertainty about an encounter with a higher power
Uncertainty about the existence of a higher power
Uncertainty about life after death
Uncertainty of prognosis

References

Abdel-Khalek, A., & Tomàs-Sàbado, J. (2005). Anxiety and death anxiety in Egyptian and Spanish nursing students. *Death Studies, 29,* 157–169.

Bay, E., & Algase, D. (1999). Fear and anxiety: A simultaneous concept analysis. *Nursing Diagnosis, 10,* 103–11.

Kastenbaum, R. (1992). *The psychology of death.* New York: The Guliford Press.

RISK FOR ASPIRATION

Definition

At risk for entry of gastrointestinal secretions, oropharyngeal secretions, solids, or fluids into tracheobronchial passages

Risk Factors

Decreased gastrointestinal motility
Delayed gastric emptying
Depressed cough
Depressed gag reflex
Facial surgery
Facial trauma
Gastrointestinal tubes
Incompetent lower esophageal sphincter
Increased gastric residual
Increased intragastric pressure
Impaired swallowing
Medication administration
Neck trauma
Neck surgery
Oral surgery
Oral trauma
Presence of endotracheal tube
Presence of tracheostomy tube
Reduced level of consciousness

Situations hindering elevation of upper body
Tube feedings
Wired jaws

Risk for Impaired Parent/Infant/Child Attachment

Definition

Disruption of the interactive process between parent/significant other and child/infant that fosters the development of a protective and nurturing reciprocal relationship

Risk Factors

Anxiety associated with the parent role
Ill infant/child who is unable to effectively initiate parental contact due to altered behavioral organization
Inability of parents to meet personal needs
Lack of privacy
Parental conflict due to altered behavioral organization
Physical barriers
Premature infant who is unable to effectively initiate parental contact due to altered behavioral organization
Separation
Substance abuse

Autonomic Dysreflexia

Definition

Life-threatening, uninhibited sympathetic response of the nervous system to a noxious stimulus after a spinal cord injury at T7 or above

Defining Characteristics

- Blurred vision
- Bradycardia
- Chest pain
- Chilling
- Conjunctival congestion
- Diaphoresis (above the injury)
- Headache (a diffuse pain in different portions of the head and not confined to any nerve distribution area)
- Horner's syndrome
- Metallic taste in mouth
- Nasal congestion
- Pallor (below the injury)
- Paresthesia
- Paroxysmal hypertension
- Pilomotor reflex
- Red splotches on skin (above the injury)
- Tachycardia

Related Factors

Bladder distention
Bowel distention
Deficient caregiver knowledge
Deficient patient knowledge
Skin irritation

Risk for Autonomic Dysreflexia

Definition

At risk for life-threatening, uninhibited response of the sympathetic nervous system, post spinal shock, in an individual with spinal cord injury or lesion at T6 or above (has been demonstrated in patients with injuries at T7 and T8)

Risk Factors

An injury at T6 or above or a lesion at T6 or above AND at least one of the following noxious stimuli:

Cardiac/Pulmonary Problems

- Deep vein thrombosis
- Pulmonary emboli

Gastrointestinal Stimuli

- Bowel distention
- Constipation
- Difficult passage of feces
- Digital stimulation
- Enemas
- Esophageal reflux
- Fecal impaction
- Gallstones
- Gastric ulcers
- GI system pathology
- Hemorrhoids
- Suppositories

Musculoskeletal-Integumentary Stimuli

- Cutaneous stimulation (e.g., pressure ulcer, ingrown toenail, dressings, burns, rash)
- Fractures
- Heterotrophic bone
- Pressure over bony prominences
- Pressure over genitalia
- Range-of-motion exercises
- Spasm
- Sunburns
- Wounds

Neurological Stimuli

- Irritating stimuli below level of injury
- Painful stimuli below level of injury

Regulatory Stimuli

- Extreme environmental temperatures
- Temperature fluctuations

Reproductive Stimuli

- Ejaculation
- Labor and delivery
- Menstruation
- Ovarian cyst
- Pregnancy
- Sexual intercourse

Situational Stimuli

- Constrictive clothing (e.g., straps, stockings, shoes)
- Drug reactions (e.g., decongestants, sympathomimetics, vasoconstrictors)
- Narcotic withdrawal
- Positioning
- Surgical procedure

Urological Stimuli

- Bladder distention
- Bladder spasm
- Calculi
- Catheterization
- Cystitis
- Detrusor sphincter dysynergia
- Epididymitis
- Instrumentation
- Surgery
- Urethritis
- Urinary tract infection

RISK-PRONE HEALTH BEHAVIOR*

Definition

Inability to modify lifestyle/behaviors in a manner consistent with a change in health status

Defining Characteristics

- Demonstrates nonacceptance of health status change
- Failure to achieve optimal sense of control
- Failure to take action that prevents health problems
- Minimizes health status change

Related Factors

Inadequate comprehension
Inadequate social support
Low self-efficacy
Low socioeconomic status
Multiple stressors
Negative attitude toward health care

* *Previously titled "Impaired Adjustment"*

References

Kiefe C.L., Heudebert G., Box J.B., Farmer R.M., Micahel M., & Clancy C.M. (1999). Compliance with post-hospitalization follow-up visits: Rationing by inconvenience? *Ethnicity & Disease, 19*, 387–395.

Koenigsberg, M., Barlett, D., & Carmer, J. (2004). Facilitating treatment adherence with lifestyle changes in diabetes. *American Family Physician, 69*, 309–316, 319–320, 323–324.

Shemesh, E. (2004). Non-adherence to medications following pediatric liver transplantation. *Pediatric Transplantation, 8*, 600–605.

DISTURBED BODY IMAGE

Definition

Confusion in mental picture of one's physical self

Defining Characteristics

- Behaviors of acknowledgment of one's body
- Behaviors of avoidance of one's body
- Behaviors of monitoring one's body
- Nonverbal response to actual change in body (e.g., appearance, structure, or function)
- Nonverbal response to perceived change in body (e.g., appearance, structure, or function)
- Verbalization of feelings that reflect an altered view of one's body (e.g., appearance, structure, function)
- Verbalization of perceptions that reflect an altered view of one's body in appearance

Objective

- Actual change in function
- Actual change in structure
- Behaviors of acknowledging one's body
- Behaviors of monitoring one's body
- Change in ability to estimate spatial relationship of body to environment
- Change in social involvement
- Extension of body boundary to incorporate environmental objects
- Intentional hiding of body part
- Intentional overexposure of body part
- Missing body part
- Not looking at body part
- Not touching body part
- Trauma to nonfunctioning part
- Unintentional hiding of body part
- Unintentional overexposing of body part

Subjective

- Depersonalization of loss by impersonal pronouns
- Depersonalization of part by impersonal pronouns
- Emphasis on remaining strengths
- Fear of reaction by others
- Fear of rejection by others
- Focus on past appearance
- Focus on past function
- Focus on past strength
- Heightened achievement
- Negative feelings about body (e.g., feelings of helplessness, hopelessness, or powerlessness)
- Personalization of loss by name
- Personalization of part by name
- Preoccupation with change
- Preoccupation with loss
- Refusal to verify actual change
- Verbalization of change in lifestyle

Related Factors

Biophysical
Cognitive
Cultural
Developmental changes
Illness
Illness treatment

Injury
Perceptual
Psychosocial
Spiritual
Surgery
Trauma

RISK FOR IMBALANCED BODY TEMPERATURE

Definition

At risk for failure to maintain body temperature within normal range

Risk Factors

Altered metabolic rate
Dehydration
Exposure to cold/cool environments
Exposure to warm/hot environments
Extremes of age
Extremes of weight
Illness affecting temperature regulation
Inactivity
Inappropriate clothing for environmental temperature
Medications causing vasoconstriction
Medications causing vasodilation
Sedation
Trauma affecting temperature regulation
Vigorous activity

BOWEL INCONTINENCE

Definition

Change in normal bowel habits characterized by involuntary passage of stool

Defining Characteristics

- Constant dribbling of soft stool
- Fecal odor
- Fecal staining of bedding
- Fecal staining of clothing
- Inability to delay defecation
- Inability to recognize urge to defecate
- Inattention to urge to defecate
- Recognizes rectal fullness but reports inability to expel formed stool
- Red perianal skin
- Self-report of inability to recognize rectal fullness
- Urgency

Related Factors

Abnormally high abdominal pressure
Abnormally high intestinal pressure
Chronic diarrhea
Colorectal lesions
Dietary habits

Environmental factors (e.g., inaccessible bathroom)
General decline in muscle tone
Immobility
Impaired cognition
Impaired reservoir capacity
Incomplete emptying of bowel
Laxative abuse
Loss of rectal sphincter control
Lower motor nerve damage
Medications
Rectal sphincter abnormality
Impaction
Stress
Toileting self-care deficit
Upper motor nerve damage

Effective Breastfeeding

Definition

Mother-infant dyad/family exhibits adequate proficiency and satisfaction with breastfeeding process

Defining Characteristics

- Adequate infant elimination patterns for age
- Appropriate infant weight pattern for age
- Eagerness of infant to nurse
- Effective mother/infant communication patterns
- Infant content after feeding
- Maternal verbalization of satisfaction with the breastfeeding process
- Mother able to position infant at breast to promote a successful latching-on response
- Regular and sustained suckling at the breast
- Regular and sustained swallowing at the breast
- Signs of oxytocin release
- Symptoms of oxytocin release

Related Factors

Basic breastfeeding knowledge
Infant gestational age >34 weeks
Maternal confidence
Normal breast structure
Normal infant oral structure
Support source

Ineffective Breastfeeding

Definition

Dissatisfaction or difficulty a mother, infant, or child experiences with the breastfeeding process

Defining Characteristics

- Inadequate milk supply
- Infant arching at the breast
- Infant crying at the breast

- Infant inability to latch on to maternal breast correctly
- Infant exhibiting crying within the first hour after breastfeeding
- Infant exhibiting fussiness within the first hour after breastfeeding
- Insufficient emptying of each breast per feeding
- Insufficient opportunity for suckling at the breast
- No observable signs of oxytocin release
- Nonsustained suckling at the breast
- Observable signs of inadequate infant intake
- Perceived inadequate milk supply
- Persistence of sore nipples beyond first week of breastfeeding
- Resisting latching on
- Unresponsive to other comfort measures
- Unsatisfactory breastfeeding process

Related Factors

Infant anomaly
Infant receiving supplemental feedings with artificial nipple
Interruption in breastfeeding
Knowledge deficit
Maternal ambivalence
Maternal anxiety
Maternal breast anomaly
Nonsupportive family
Nonsupportive partner
Poor infant sucking reflex
Prematurity
Previous breast surgery
Previous history of breastfeeding failure

INTERRUPTED BREASTFEEDING

Definition

Break in the continuity of the breastfeeding process as a result of inability or inadvisability to put baby to breast for feeding

Defining Characteristics

- Infant receives no nourishment at the breast for some or all feedings
- Lack of knowledge regarding expression of breast milk
- Lack of knowledge regarding storage of breast milk
- Maternal desire to eventually provide breast milk for infant/child's nutritional needs
- Maternal desire to maintain breastfeeding for infant/child's nutritional needs
- Maternal desire to provide breast milk for infant/child's nutritional needs
- Separation of mother and infant

Related Factors

Contraindications to breastfeeding
Infant illness
Maternal employment
Maternal illness
Need to abruptly wean infant
Prematurity

Ineffective Breathing Pattern

Definition

Inspiration and/or expiration that does not provide adequate ventilation

Defining Characteristics

- Alterations in depth of breathing
- Altered chest excursion
- Assumption of 3-point position
- Bradypnea
- Decreased expiratory pressure
- Decreased inspiratory pressure
- Decreased minute ventilation
- Decreased vital capacity
- Dyspnea
- Increased anterior-posterior diameter
- Nasal flaring
- Orthopnea
- Prolonged expiration phase
- Pursed-lip breathing
- Tachypnea
- Timing ratio
- Use of accessory muscles to breathe metabolic demands of the body

Related Factors

Anxiety
Body position
Bony deformity
Chest wall deformity
Cognitive impairment
Fatigue
Hyperventilation
Hypoventilation syndrome
Musculoskeletal impairment
Neurological immaturity
Neuromuscular dysfunction
Obesity
Pain
Perception impairment
Respiratory muscle fatigue
Spinal cord injury

Decreased Cardiac Output

Definition

Inadequate blood pumped by the heart to meet metabolic demands of the body

Defining Characteristics

Altered Heart Rate/Rhythm

- Arrhythmias
- Bradycardia

- EKG changes
- Palpitations
- Tachycardia

Altered Preload

- Edema
- Decreased central venous pressure (CVP)
- Decreased pulmonary artery wedge pressure (PAWP)
- Fatigue
- Increased central venous pressure (CVP)
- Increased pulmonary artery wedge pressure (PAWP)
- Jugular vein distention
- Murmurs
- Weight gain

Altered Afterload

- Clammy skin
- Dyspnea
- Decreased peripheral pulses
- Decreased pulmonary vascular resistance (PVR)
- Decreased systemic vascular resistance (SVR)
- Increased pulmonary vascular resistance (PVR)
- Increased systemic vascular resistance (SVR)
- Oliguria
- Prolonged capillary refill
- Skin color changes
- Variations in blood pressure readings

Altered Contractility

- Crackles
- Cough
- Decreased ejection fraction
- Decreased left ventricular stroke work index (LVSWI)
- Decreased stroke volume index (SVI)
- Decreased cardiac index
- Decreased cardiac output
- Orthopnea
- Paroxysmal nocturnal dyspnea
- S3 sounds
- S4 sounds

Behavioral/Emotional

- Anxiety
- Restlessness

Related Factors

Altered heart rate
Altered rhythm

Altered Stroke Volume

Altered afterload
Altered contractility
Altered preload

Caregiver Role Strain

Definition

Difficulty in performing family caregiver role

Defining Characteristics

Caregiving Activities

- Apprehension about care receiver's care if caregiver unable to provide care
- Apprehension about the future regarding care receiver's health
- Apprehension about the future regarding caregiver's ability to provide care
- Apprehension about possible institutionalization of care receiver
- Difficulty completing required tasks
- Difficulty performing required tasks
- Dysfunctional change in caregiving activities
- Preoccupation with care routine

Caregiver Health Status

Physical

- Cardiovascular disease
- Diabetes
- Fatigue
- GI upset
- Headaches
- Hypertension
- Rash
- Weight change

Emotional

- Anger
- Disturbed sleep
- Feeling depressed
- Frustration
- Impaired individual coping
- Impatience
- Increased emotional lability
- Increased nervousness
- Lack of time to meet personal needs
- Somatization
- Stress

Socioeconomic

- Changes in leisure activities
- Low work productivity
- Refuses career advancement
- Withdraws from social life

Caregiver-Care Receiver Relationship

- Difficulty watching care receiver go through the illness
- Grief regarding changed relationship with care receiver
- Uncertainty regarding changed relationship with care receiver

Family Processes

- Concerns about family members
- Family conflict

Related Factors

Care Receiver Health Status

Addiction
Codependency
Cognitive problems
Dependency
llness chronicity
Illness severity
Increasing care needs
Instability of care receiver's health
Problem behaviors
Psychological problems
Unpredictability of illness course

Caregiver Health Status

Addiction
Codependency
Cognitive problems
Inability to fulfill one's own expectations
Inability to fulfill other's expectations
Marginal coping patterns
Physical problems
Psychological problems
Unrealistic expectations of self

Caregiver-Care Receiver Relationship

History of poor relationship
Mental status of elder inhibiting conversation
Presence of abuse
Presence of violence
Unrealistic expectations of caregiver by care receiver

Caregiving Activities

24-hour care responsibilities
Amount of activities
Complexity of activities
Discharge of family members to home with significant care needs
Ongoing changes in activities
Unpredictability of care situation
Years of caregiving

Family Processes

History of family dysfunction
History of marginal family coping

Resources

Caregiver is not developmentally ready for caregiver role
Deficient knowledge about community resources

Difficulty accessing community resourses
Emotional strength
Formal assistance
Formal support
Inadequate community resources (e.g., respite services, recreational resources)
Inadequate equipment for providing care
Inadequate physical environment for providing care (e.g., housing, temperature, safety)
Inadequate transportation
Inexperience with caregiving
Informal assistance
Informal support
Insufficient finances
Insufficient time
Lack of caregiver privacy
Lack of support
Physical energy

Socioeconomic

Alienation from others
Competing role commitments
Insufficient recreation
Isolation from others

RISK FOR CAREGIVER ROLE STRAIN

Definition

Caregiver is vulnerable for felt difficulty in performing the family caregiver role

Risk Factors

Addiction
Amount of caregiving tasks
Care receiver exhibits bizarre behavior
Care receiver exhibits deviant behavior
Caregiver's competing role commitments
Caregiver health impairment
Caregiver is female
Caregiver is spouse
Caregiver isolation
Caregiver not developmentally ready for caregiver role
Codependency
Cognitive problems in care receiver
Complexity of caregiving tasks
Congenital defect
Developmental delay of the care receiver
Developmental delay of the caregiver
Discharge of family member with significant home care needs
Duration of caregiving required
Family dysfunction prior to the caregiving situation
Family isolation
Illness severity of the care receiver

Inadequate physical environment for providing care (e.g., housing, transportation, community services, equipment)
Inexperience with caregiving
Instability in the care receiver's health
Lack of recreation for caregiver
Lack of respite for caregiver
Marginal caregiver's coping patterns
Marginal family adaptation
Past history of poor relationship between caregiver and care receiver
Premature birth
Presence of abuse
Presence of situational stressors that normally affect families (e.g., significant loss, disaster or crisis, economic vulnerability, major life events)
Presence of violence
Psychological problems in care receiver
Retardation of the care receiver
Retardation of the caregiver
Unpredictable illness course

READINESS FOR ENHANCED COMFORT

Definition

A pattern of ease, relief, and transcendence in physical, psychospiritual, environmental, and/or social dimensions that can be strengthened

Defining Characteristics

- Expresses desire to enhance comfort
- Expresses desire to enhance feeling of contentment
- Expresses desire to enhance relaxation
- Expresses desire to enhance resolution of complaints

References

Duggleby, W., & Berry, P. (2005). Transitions in shifting goals of care for palliative patients and their families. *Clinical Journal of Oncology Nursing, 9,* 425–428.

Kolcaba, K. (1994). A theory of holistic comfort for nursing. *Journal of Advanced Nursing, 19,* 1178–1184.

Malinowski, A., & Stamler, L.L. (2002). Comfort: Exploration of the concept in nursing. *Journal of Advanced Nursing, 39,* 599–606.

IMPAIRED VERBAL COMMUNICATION

Definition

Decreased, delayed, or absent ability to receive, process, transmit, and/or use a system of symbols

Defining Characteristics

- Absence of eye contact
- Cannot speak
- Difficulty in comprehending usual communication pattern
- Difficulty expressing thoughts verbally (e.g., aphasia, dysphasia, apraxia, dyslexia)
- Difficulty forming sentences
- Difficulty forming words (e.g., aphonia, dyslalia, dysarthria)
- Difficulty in maintaining usual communication pattern
- Difficulty in selective attending

- Difficulty in use of body expressions
- Difficulty in use of facial expressions
- Disorientation to person
- Disorientation to space
- Disorientation to time
- Does not speak
- Dyspnea
- Inability to speak language of caregiver
- Inability to use body expressions
- Inability to use facial expressions
- Inappropriate verbalization
- Partial visual deficit
- Slurring
- Speaks with difficulty
- Stuttering
- Total visual deficit
- Verbalizes with difficulty
- Willful refusal to speak

Related Factors

Absence of significant others
Altered perceptions
Alteration in self-concept
Alteration in self-esteem
Alteration of central nervous system
Anatomical defect (e.g., cleft palate, alteration of the neuromuscular visual system, auditory system, phonatory apparatus)
Brain tumor
Cultural differences
Decrease in circulation to brain
Differences related to developmental age
Emotional conditions
Environmental barriers
Lack of information
Physical barrier (e.g., tracheostomy, intubation)
Physiological conditions
Psychological barriers (e.g., psychosis, lack of stimuli)
Side effects of medication
Stress
Weakening of the musculoskeletal system

READINESS FOR ENHANCED COMMUNICATION

Definition

A pattern of exchanging information and ideas with others that is sufficient for meeting one's needs and life's goals, and can be strengthened

Defining Characteristics

- Able to speak a language
- Able to write a language
- Expresses feelings

- Expresses satisfaction with ability to share ideas with others
- Expresses satisfaction with ability to share information with others
- Expresses thoughts
- Expresses willingness to enhance communication
- Forms phrases
- Forms sentences
- Forms words
- Interprets nonverbal cues appropriately
- Uses nonverbal cues appropriately

Decisional Conflict

Definition

Uncertainty about course of action to be taken when choice among competing actions involves risk, loss, or challenge to values and beliefs

Defining Characteristics

- Delayed decision making
- Physical signs of distress or tension (e.g., increased heart rate, increased muscle tension, restlessness)
- Questioning moral principles while attempting a decision
- Questioning moral rules while attempting a decision
- Questioning moral values while attempting a decision
- Questioning personal beliefs while attempting a decision
- Questioning personal values while attempting a decision
- Self-focusing
- Vacillation among alternative choices
- Verbalizes feeling of distress while attempting a decision
- Verbalizes uncertainty about choices
- Verbalizes undesired consequences of alternative actions being considered

Related Factors

Divergent sources of information
Interference with decision making
Lack of experience with decision making
Lack of relevant information
Moral obligations require performing action
Moral obligations require not performing action
Moral principles support mutually inconsistent courses of action
Moral rules support mutually inconsistent courses of action
Moral values support mutually inconsistent courses of action
Multiple sources of information
Perceived threat to value system
Support system deficit
Unclear personal beliefs
Unclear personal values

References

Beauchamp, T., & Childress, J. (2001). *Principles of biomedical ethics* (5th ed.). New York: Oxford University Press.

Kopala, B., & Burkhart, L. (2005). Ethical dilemma and moral distress: Proposed new NANDA diagnoses. *International Journal of Nursing Terminologies and Classifications, 16,* 3–13.

Webster, G., & Baylis, F. (2000). Moral residue. In S. Rubin & L. Zoloth (Eds.), *Margin of error. The ethics of mistakes in the practice of medicine* (pp. 217–230). Hagerstown, MD: University Publishing.

Parental Role Conflict

Definition

Parent experience of role confusion and conflict in response to crisis

Defining Characteristics

- Anxiety
- Demonstrated disruption in caretaking routines
- Expresses concern about perceived loss of control over decisions relating to their child
- Fear
- Parent(s) express(es) concern(s) about changes in parental role
- Parent(s) express(es) concern(s) about family (e.g., functioning, communication, health)
- Parent(s) express(es) concern(s) of inadequacy to provide for child's needs (e.g., physical, emotional)
- Parent(s) express(es) feeling(s) of inadequacy to provide for child's needs (e.g., physical, emotional)
- Reluctant to participate in usual caretaking activities even with encouragement and support
- Verbalizes feelings of frustration
- Verbalizes feelings of guilt

Related Factors

Change in marital status
Home care of a child with special needs
Interruptions of family life due to home care regimen (e.g., treatments, caregivers, lack of respite)
Intimidation with invasive modalities (e.g., intubation)
Intimidation with restrictive modalities (e.g., isolation)
Separation from child due to chronic illness
Specialized care center

Acute Confusion

Definition

Abrupt onset of reversible disturbances of consciousness, attention, cognition, and perception that develop over a short period of time

Defining Characteristics

- Fluctuation in cognition
- Fluctuation in level of consciousness
- Fluctuation in psychomotor activity
- Hallucinations
- Increased agitation
- Increased restlessness
- Lack of motivation to follow through with goal-directed behavior
- Lack of motivation to follow through with purposeful behavior
- Lack of motivation to initiate goal-directed behavior
- Lack of motivation to initiate purposeful behavior
- Misperceptions

Related Factors

Alcohol abuse
Delirium
Dementia
Drug abuse
Fluctuation in sleep-wake cycle
Over 60 years of age

References

Schor, J., Levkoff, S., Lipsitz, L., Reilly, C., Cleary, P., Rowe, J., et al. (1992). Risk factors for delirium in hospitalized elderly. *JAMA*, 267, 827–831.

Inouye, S., & Charpentier, P. (1996). Precipitating factors for delirium in hospitalized elderly persons: Predictive model and inter-relationship with baseline vulnerability. *JAMA, 275*, 852–857.

Inouye, S., Viscoli, C., Horwitz, R., Hurst, L., & Tinetti, M. (1993). A predictive model for delirium in hospitalized elderly medical patients based on admission characteristics. *Archives of Internal Medicine, 119,* 474–481.

Chronic Confusion

Definition

Irreversible, long-standing, and/or progressive deterioration of intellect and personality characterized by decreased ability to interpret environmental stimuli; decreased capacity for intellectual thought processes; and manifested by disturbances of memory, orientation, and behavior

Defining Characteristics

- Altered interpretation
- Altered personality
- Altered response to stimuli
- Clinical evidence of organic impairment
- Impaired long-term memory
- Impaired short-term memory
- Impaired socialization
- Long-standing cognitive impairment
- No change in level of consciousness
- Progressive cognitive impairment

Related Factors

Alzheimer's disease
Cerebral vascular attack
Head injury
Korsakoff's psychosis
Multi-infarct dementia

Risk for Acute Confusion

Definition

At risk for reversible disturbances of consciousness, attention, cognition, and perception that develop over a short period of time

Risk Factors

Alcohol use
Decreased mobility
Decreased restraints
Dementia
Fluctuation in sleep-wake cycle
History of stroke
Impaired cognition
Infection
Male gender

Medication/Drugs
– Anesthesia
– Anticholinergics
– Diphenhydramine
– Multiple medications
– Opioids
– Psychoactive drugs
Metabolic abnormalities
– Azotemia
– Decreased hemoglobin
– Dehydration
– Electrolyte imbalances
– Increased BUN/Creatinine
– Malnutrition
Over 60 years of age
Pain
Sensory deprivation
Substance abuse
Urinary retention

References

Schor, J., Levkoff, S., Lipsitz, L., Reilly, C., Cleary, P., Rowe, J., et al. (1992). Risk factors for delirium in hospitalized elderly. *JAMA, 267,* 827–831.

Inouye, S., & Charpentier, P. (1996). Precipitating factors for delirium in hospitalized elderly persons: Predictive model and interrelationship with baseline vulnerability. *JAMA, 275,* 852–857.

Inouye, S., Viscoli, C., Horwitz, R., Hurst, L., & Tinetti, M. (1993). A predictive model for delirium in hospitalized elderly medical patients based on admission characteristics. *Archives of Internal Medicine, 119,* 474–481.

Constipation

Definition

Decrease in normal frequency of defecation accompanied by difficult or incomplete passage of stool and/or passage of excessively hard, dry stool

Defining Characteristics

- Abdominal pain
- Abdominal tenderness with palpable muscle resistance
- Abdominal tenderness without palpable muscle resistance
- Anorexia
- Atypical presentations in older adults (e.g., change in mental status, urinary incontinence, unexplained falls, elevated body temperature)
- Borborygmi
- Bright red blood with stool
- Change in bowel pattern
- Decreased frequency
- Decreased volume of stool
- Distended abdomen
- Feeling of rectal fullness
- Feeling of rectal pressure
- Generalized fatigue
- Hard, formed stool
- Headache

- Hyperactive bowel sounds
- Hypoactive bowel sounds
- Increased abdominal pressure
- Indigestion
- Nausea
- Oozing liquid stool
- Palpable abdominal mass
- Palpable rectal mass
- Presence of soft, paste-like stool in rectum
- Percussed abdominal dullness
- Pain with defecation
- Severe flatus
- Straining with defecation
- Unable to pass stool
- Vomiting

Related Factors

Functional

Abdominal muscle weakness
Habitual denial
Habitual ignoring of urge to defecate
Inadequate toileting (e.g., timeliness, positioning for defecation, privacy)
Irregular defecation habits
Insufficient physical activity
Recent environmental changes

Psychological

Depression
Emotional stress
Mental confusion

Pharmacological

Aluminum-containing antacids
Anticholinergics
Anticonvulsants
Antidepressants
Antilipemic agents
Bismuth salts
Calcium carbonate
Calcium channel blockers
Diuretics
Iron salts
Laxative overdose
Nonsteroidal antiinflammatory agents
Opiates
Phenothiazines
Sedatives
Sympathomimetics

Mechanical

Electrolyte imbalance
Hemorrhoids
Hirschsprung's disease
Neurological impairment
Obesity
Postsurgical obstruction
Pregnancy
Prostate enlargement
Rectal abscess
Rectal anal fissures
Rectal anal stricture
Rectal prolapse
Rectal ulcer
Rectocele
Tumors

Physiological

Change in eating patterns
Change in usual foods
Decreased motility of gastrointestinal tract
Dehydration
Inadequate dentition
Inadequate oral hygiene
Insufficient fiber intake
Insufficient fluid intake
Poor eating habits

PERCEIVED CONSTIPATION

Definition

Self-diagnosis of constipation and abuse of laxatives, enemas, and suppositories to ensure a daily bowel movement

Defining Characteristics

- Expectation of a daily bowel movement
- Expectation of passage of stool at same time every day
- Overuse of laxatives
- Overuse of enemas
- Overuse of suppositories

Related Factors

Cultural health beliefs
Family health beliefs
Faulty appraisal
Impaired thought processes

RISK FOR CONSTIPATION

Definition

At risk for a decrease in normal frequency of defecation accompanied by difficult or incomplete passage of stool and/or passage of excessively hard, dry stool

Risk Factors

Functional

Habitual denial/ignoring of urge to defecate
Recent environmental changes
Inadequate toileting (e.g., timeliness, positioning for defecation, privacy)
Irregular defecation habits
Insufficient physical activity
Abdominal muscle weakness

Psychological

Depression
Emotional stress
Mental confusion

Physiological

Change in usual eating patterns
Change in usual foods
Decreased motility of gastrointestinal tract
Dehydration
Inadequate dentition
Inadequate oral hygiene
Insufficient fiber intake
Insufficient fluid intake
Poor eating habits

Pharmacological

Aluminum-containing antacids
Anticholinergics
Anticonvulsants
Antidepressants
Antilipemic agents
Bismuth salts
Calcium carbonate
Calcium channel blockers
Diuretics
Iron salts
Laxative overuse
Nonsteroidal antiinflammatory agents
Opiates
Phenothiazines
Sedatives
Sympathomimetics

Mechanical

Electrolyte imbalance
Hemorrhoids
Hirschsprung's disease
Neurological impairment
Obesity
Postsurgical obstruction
Pregnancy

Prostate enlargement
Rectal abscess
Rectal anal fissures
Rectal anal stricture
Rectal prolapse
Rectal ulcer
Rectocele
Tumors

CONTAMINATION

Definition

Exposure to environmental contaminants in doses sufficient to cause adverse health effects

Defining Characteristics

(Defining characteristics are dependent on the causative agent. Agents cause a variety of individual organ responses as well as systemic responses.)

Pesticides

- Dermatological effects of pesticide exposure
- Gastrointestinal effects of pesticide exposure
- Neurological effects of pesticide exposure
- Pulmonary effects of pesticide exposure
- Renal effects of pesticide exposure

(Major categories of pesticides: insecticides, herbicides, fungicides, antimicrobials, rodenticides. Major pesticides: organophosphates, carbamates, organochlorines, pyrethrium, arsenic, glycophosphates, bipyridyls, chlorophenoxy.)

Chemicals

- Dermatological effects of chemical exposure
- Gastrointestinal effects of chemical exposure
- Immunologic effects of chemical exposure
- Neurological effects of chemical exposure
- Pulmonary effects of chemical exposure
- Renal effects of chemical exposure

(Major chemical agents: petroleum-based agents, anticholinesterases. Type I agents act on proximal tracheobronchial portion of the respiratory tract, Type II agents act on aveoli, Type III agents produce systemic effects.)

Biologics

- Dermatological effects of exposure to biologics
- Gastrointestinal effects of exposure to biologics
- Pulmonary effects of exposure to biologics
- Neurological effects of exposure to biologics
- Renal effects of exposure to biologics (toxins from living organisms ([bacteria, viruses, fungi])

Pollution

- Neurological effects of pollution exposure
- Pulmonary effects of pollution exposure

(Major locations: air, water, soil. Major agents: asbestos, radon, tobacco, heavy metal, lead, noise, exhaust.)

Waste

- Dermatological effects of waste exposure
- Gastrointestinal effects of waste exposure
- Hepatic effects of waste exposure
- Pulmonary effects of waste exposure

(Categories of waste: trash, raw sewage, industrial waste)

Radiation

- Immunologic effects of radiation exposure
- Genetic effects of radiation exposure
- Neurological effects of radiation exposure
- Oncologic effects of radiation exposure

(Categories: Internal—exposure through ingestion of radioactive material [e.g., food/water contamination]; External—exposure through direct contact with radioactive material)

Related Factors

External

Chemical contamination of food
Chemical contamination of water
Exposure to bioterrorism
Exposure to disaster (natural or man-made)
Exposure to radiation (occupation in radiography, employment in nuclear industries and electrical generating plants, living near nuclear industries and electrical generating plants)
Flaking, peeling paint in presence of young children
Flaking, peeling plaster in presence of young children
Flooring surface (carpeted surfaces hold contaminant residue more than hard floor surfaces)
Geographic area (living in area where high level of contaminants exist)
Household hygiene practices
Inadequate municipal services (trash removal, sewage treatment facilities)
Inappropriate use of protective clothing
Lack of breakdown of contaminants once indoors (breakdown is inhibited without sun and rain exposure)
Lack of protective clothing
Living in poverty (increases potential for multiple exposure, lack of access to health care, and poor diet)
Paint, lacquer, etc. in poorly ventilated areas
Paint, lacquer, etc. without effective protection
Personal hygiene practices
Playing in outdoor areas where environmental contaminants are used
Presence of atmospheric pollutants
Use of environmental contaminants in the home (e.g., pesticides, chemicals, environmental tobacco smoke)
Unprotected contact with heavy metals or chemicals (e.g., arsenic, chromium, lead)

Internal

Age (children less than 5 years, older adults)
Concomitant exposures
Developmental characteristics of children
Female gender
Gestational age during exposure
Nutritional factors (e.g., obesity, vitamin and mineral deficiencies)
Pre-existing disease states

Pregnancy
Previous exposures
Smoking

References

Berkowitz, G.S., Obel, J., Deych, E., Lapinski, R., Godbold, J., & Liu, Z. (2003). Exposure to indoor pesticides during pregnancy in a multiethnic, urban cohort. *Environmental Health Perspectives, 111,* 79 – 84.

Center for Disease Control and Prevention. (2005). Third national report on human exposure to environmental chemicals: Executive summary (NCEH Pub # 05-0725). Atlanta, GA: Author.

McCauley, L.A., Michaels, S., Rothlein, J., Muniz, J., Lasarev, M., & Ebbert, C. (2003). Pesticide exposure and self-reported home hygiene. *AAOHN Journal, 51,* 113 – 119.

RISK FOR CONTAMINATION

Definition

Accentuated risk of exposure to environmental contaminants in doses sufficient to cause adverse health effects

Risk Factors

External

Chemical contamination of food
Chemical contamination of water
Exposure to bioterrorism
Exposure to disaster (natural or man-made)
Exposure to radiation (occupation in radiography, employment in nuclear industries and electrical generating plants, living near nuclear industries and electrical generating plants)
Flaking, peeling paint in presence of young children
Flaking, peeling plaster in presence of young children
Flooring surface (carpeted surfaces hold contaminant residue more than hard floor surfaces)
Geographic area (living in area where high level of contaminants exist)
Household hygiene practices
Inadequate municipal services (e.g., trash removal, sewage treatment facilities)
Inappropriate use of protective clothing
Lack of breakdown of contaminants once indoors (breakdown is inhibited without sun and rain exposure)
Lack of protective clothing
Living in poverty (increases potential for multiple exposure, lack of access to health care, and poor diet)
Paint, lacquer, etc. in poorly ventilated areas
Paint, lacquer, etc. without effective protection
Personal hygiene practices
Playing in outdoor areas where environmental contaminants are used
Presence of atmospheric pollutants
Use of environmental contaminants in the home (e.g., pesticides, chemicals, environmental tobacco smoke)
Unprotected contact with heavy metals or chemicals (e.g., arsenic, chromium, lead)

Internal

Age (children less than 5 years, older adults)
Concomitant exposures
Developmental characteristics of children
Female gender
Gestational age during exposure
Nutritional factors (e.g., obesity, vitamin and mineral deficiencies)

Pre-existing disease states
Pregnancy
Previous exposures
Smoking

References

Centers for Disease Control and Prevention. (2005). *Third national report on human exposure to environmental chemicals: Executive summary* (NCEH Pub # 05-0725). Atlanta: Author.

Chalupka, S.M. (2001). Essentials of environmental health. Enhancing your occupational health nursing practice (Part II). *AAOHN Journal, 49,* 194–213.

McCauley, L.A., Michaels, S., Rothlein, J., Muniz, J., Lasarev, M., & Ebbert, C. (2003). Pesticide exposure and self-reported home hygiene. *AAOHN Journal, 51,* 113–119.

COMPROMISED FAMILY COPING

Definition

Usually supportive primary person (family member or close friend) provides insufficient, ineffective, or compromised support, comfort, assistance, or encouragement that may be needed by the client to manage or master adaptive tasks related to his/her health challenge

Defining Characteristics

Objective

- Significant person attempts assistive behaviors with unsatisfactory results
- Significant person attempts supportive behaviors with unsatisfactory results
- Significant person displays protective behavior disproportionate to client's abilities
- Significant person displays protective behavior disproportionate to client's need for autonomy
- Significant person enters into limited personal communication with client
- Significant person withdraws from client

Subjective

- Client expresses a complaint about significant other's response to health problem
- Client expresses a concern about significant other's response to health problem
- Significant person expresses an inadequate knowledge base, which interferes with effective supportive behaviors
- Significant person expresses an inadequate understanding, which interferes with supportive behaviors
- Significant person describes preoccupation with personal reaction (e.g., fear, anticipatory grief, guilt, anxiety) to client's need

Related Factors

Coexisting situations affecting the significant person
Developmental crises the significant person may be facing
Exhaustion of supportive capacity of significant people
Inadequate information by a primary person
Inadequate understanding of information by a primary person
Incorrect information by a primary person
Incorrect understanding of information by a primary person
Lack of reciprocal support
Little support provided by client, in turn, for primary person
Prolonged disease that exhausts supportive capacity of significant people
Situational crises the significant person may be facing
Temporary family disorganization

Temporary family role changes
Temporary preoccupation by a significant person

DEFENSIVE COPING

Definition

Repeated projection of falsely positive self-evaluation based on a self-protective pattern that defends against underlying perceived threats to positive self-regard

Defining Characteristics

- Denial of obvious problems
- Denial of obvious weaknesses
- Difficulty establishing relationships
- Difficulty maintaining relationships
- Difficulty in perception of reality
- Difficulty in perception of reality testing
- Grandiosity
- Hostile laughter
- Hypersensitivity to criticism
- Hypersensitivity to slight
- Lack of follow-through in therapy
- Lack of follow-through in treatment
- Lack of participation in therapy
- Lack of participation in treatment
- Projection of blame
- Projection of responsibility
- Rationalization of failures
- Ridicule of others
- Superior attitude toward others

Related Factors

To be developed

Note. This diagnosis will retire from the NANDA-I Taxonomy in the 2009–2010 edition unless additional work is done to bring it to a LOE of 2.1 or higher.

DISABLED FAMILY COPING

Definition

Behavior of significant person (family member or other primary person) that disables his/her capacities and the client's capacities to effectively address tasks essential to either person's adaption to the health challenge

Defining Characteristics

- Abandonment
- Aggression
- Agitation
- Carrying on usual routines without regard for client's needs
- Client's development of dependence
- Depression
- Desertion
- Disregarding client's needs
- Distortion of reality regarding client's health problem

- Family behaviors that are detrimental to well-being
- Hostility
- Impaired individualization
- Impaired restructuring of a meaningful life for self
- Intolerance
- Neglectful care of client in regard to basic human needs
- Neglectful care of client in regard to illness treatment
- Neglectful relationships with other family members
- Prolonged overconcern for client
- Psychosomaticism
- Rejection
- Taking on illness signs of client

Related Factors

Arbitrary handling of family's resistance to treatment
Dissonant coping styles for dealing with adaptive tasks by the significant person and client
Dissonant coping styles among significant people
Highly ambivalent family relationships
Significant person with chronically unexpressed feelings (e.g., guilt, anxiety, hostility, despair)

Ineffective Coping

Definition

Inability to form a valid appraisal of the stressors, inadequate choices of practiced responses, and/or inability to use available resources

Defining Characteristics

- Abuse of chemical agents
- Change in usual communication patterns
- Decreased use of social support
- Destructive behavior toward others
- Destructive behavior toward self
- Fatigue
- High illness rate
- Inability to meet basic needs
- Inability to meet role expectations
- Inadequate problem solving
- Lack of goal-directed behavior/resolution of problem, including inability to attend to and difficulty organizing information
- Poor concentration
- Risk taking
- Sleep disturbance
- Use of forms of coping that impede adaptive behavior
- Verbalization of inability to ask for help
- Verbalization of inability to cope

Related Factors

Disturbance in pattern of appraisal of threat
Disturbance in pattern of tension release
Gender differences in coping strategies
High degree of threat
Inability to conserve adaptive energies

Inadequate level of confidence in ability to cope
Inadequate level of perception of control
Inadequate opportunity to prepare for stressor
Inadequate resources available
Inadequate social support created by characteristics of relationships
Maturational crisis
Situational crisis
Uncertainty

INEFFECTIVE COMMUNITY COPING

Definition

Pattern of community activities for adaptation and problem solving that is unsatisfactory for meeting the demands or needs of the community

Defining Characteristics

- Community does not meet its own expectations
- Deficits in community participation
- Excessive community conflicts
- Expressed community powerlessness
- Expressed vulnerability
- High illness rates
- Increased social problems (e.g., homicides, vandalism, arson, terrorism, robbery, infanticide, abuse, divorce, unemployment, poverty, militancy, mental illness)
- Stressors perceived as excessive

Related Factors

Deficits in community social support services
Deficits in community social support resources
Natural disasters
Man-made disasters
Inadequate resources for problem solving
Ineffective community systems (e.g., lack of emergency medical system, transportation system, or disaster planning systems)
Nonexistent community systems

READINESS FOR ENHANCED COPING

Definition

A pattern of cognitive and behavioral efforts to manage demands that is sufficient for well-being and can be strengthened

Defining Characteristics

- Acknowledges power
- Aware of possible environmental changes
- Defines stressors as manageable
- Seeks knowledge of new strategies
- Seeks social support
- Uses a broad range of emotion-oriented strategies
- Uses a broad range of problem-oriented strategies
- Uses spiritual resources

Readiness for Enhanced Community Coping

Definition

Pattern of community activities for adaptation and problem solving that is satisfactory for meeting the demands or needs of the community but can be improved for management of current and future problems/stressors

Defining Characteristics

- One or more characteristics that indicate effective coping:
  - – Active planning by community for predicted stressors
  - – Active problem solving by community when faced with issues
  - – Agreement that community is responsible for stress management
  - – Positive communication among community members
  - – Positive communication between community/aggregates and larger community
  - – Programs available for recreation
  - – Programs available for relaxation
  - – Resources sufficient for managing stressors

Related Factors

Community has a sense of power to manage stressors
Resources available for problem solving
Social supports available

Readiness for Enhanced Family Coping

Definition

Effective management of adaptive tasks by family member involved with the client's health challenge, who now exhibits desire and readiness for enhanced health and growth in regard to self and in relation to the client

Defining Characteristics

- Individual expresses interest in making contact with others who have experienced a similar situation
- Family member attempts to describe growth impact of crisis
- Family member moves in direction of enriching lifestyle
- Family member moves in direction of health promotion
- Chooses experiences that optimize wellness

Related Factors

Adaptive tasks effectively addressed to enable goals of self-actualization to surface
Needs sufficiently gratified to enable goals of self-actualization to surface

Risk for Sudden Infant Death Syndrome

Definition

Presence of risk factors for sudden death of an infant under 1 year of age

Risk Factors

Modifiable

Delayed prenatal care
Infant overheating
Infant overwrapping
Infants placed to sleep in the prone position

Infants placed to sleep in the side-lying position
Lack of prenatal care
Postnatal infant smoke exposure
Prenatal infant smoke exposure
Soft underlayment (loose articles in the sleep environment)

Potentially Modifiable

Low birth weight
Prematurity
Young maternal age

Nonmodifiable

Ethnicity (e.g., African American or Native American)
Male gender
Seasonality of SIDS deaths (e.g., winter and fall months)
Infant age of 2–4 months

READINESS FOR ENHANCED DECISION MAKING

Definition

A pattern of choosing courses of action that is sufficient for meeting short and long term health-related goals and can be strengthened

Defining Characteristics

- Expresses desire to enhance decision making
- Expresses desire to enhance congruency of decisions with personal values and goals
- Expresses desire to enhance congruency of decisions with sociocultural values and goals
- Expresses desire to enhance risk benefit analysis of decisions
- Expresses desire to enhance understanding of choices for decision making
- Expresses desire to enhance understanding of the meaning of choices
- Expresses desire to enhance use of reliable evidence for decisions

References

O'Connor, A.M., Stacey, D., Entwistle, V., Llewllyn-Thomas, H., Rovner, D., Homes-Rovner, M., et al. (2005). Decision aids for people facing health treatment or screening decisions. *The Cochrane Library, Vol 3., CD-ROM Computer file.* London: BMJ Publishing Group.

Paterson, B.L., Russell, C., & Thorne, S. (2001). Critical analysis of everyday self-care decision making in chronic illness. *Journal of Advanced Nursing, 35,* 335–341.

Tunis, S.R. (2005). Perspective: A clinical research strategy to support shared decision-making. *Health Affairs, 24,* 180–184.

INEFFECTIVE DENIAL

Definition

Conscious or unconscious attempt to disavow the knowledge or meaning of an event to reduce anxiety/fear, but leading to the detriment of health

Defining Characteristics

- Delays seeking health care attention to the detriment of health
- Displaces fear of impact of the condition
- Displaces source of symptoms to other organs
- Displays inappropriate affect
- Does not admit fear of death

- Does not admit fear of invalidism
- Does not perceive personal relevance of danger
- Does not perceive personal relevance of symptoms
- Makes dismissive comments when speaking of distressing events
- Makes dismissive gestures when speaking of distressing events
- Minimizes symptoms
- Refuses health care attention to the detriment of health
- Unable to admit impact of disease on life pattern
- Uses self-treatment

Related Factors

Anxiety
Fear of death
Fear of loss of autonomy
Fear of separation
Lack of competency in using effective coping mechanisms
Lack of control of life situation
Lack of emotional support from others
Overwhelming stress
Threat of inadequacy in dealing with strong emotions
Threat of unpleasant reality

References

Gammon, J. (1998). Analysis of the stressful effects of hospitalisation and source isolation coping and psychological constructs. *International Journal of Nursing Practice, 4*(2), 84–96.

Mogg, K., Mathews, A., Bird, C., & MacGregor-Morris, R. (1990). Effects of stress and anxiety on the processing of threat stimuli. *Journal of Personality and Social Psychology, 59,* 1230–1237.

Sandstrom, M.J., & Cramer. P. (2003). Defense mechanisms and psychological adjustment in childhood. *Journal of Nervous and Mental Disease, 191,* 487–495.

Impaired Dentition

Definition

Disruption in tooth development/eruption patterns or structural integrity of individual teeth

Defining Characteristics

- Abraded teeth
- Absence of teeth
- Asymmetrical facial expression
- Crown caries
- Erosion of enamel
- Excessive calculus
- Excessive plaque
- Halitosis
- Incomplete eruption for age (may be primary or permanent teeth)
- Loose teeth
- Malocclusion
- Missing teeth
- Premature loss of primary teeth
- Root caries
- Tooth enamel discoloration

- Tooth fracture(s)
- Tooth misalignment
- Toothache
- Worn down teeth

Related Factors

Barriers to self-care
Bruxism
Chronic use of coffee
Chronic use of tea
Chronic use of red wine
Chronic use of tobacco
Chronic vomiting
Deficient knowledge regarding dental health
Dietary habits
Economic barriers to professional care
Excessive use of abrasive cleaning agents
Excessive intake of fluorides
Genetic predisposition
Ineffective oral hygiene
Lack of access to professional care
Nutritional deficits
Selected prescription medications
Sensitivity to cold
Sensitivity to heat

RISK FOR DELAYED DEVELOPMENT

Definition

At risk for delay of 25% or more in one or more of the areas of social or self-regulatory behavior, or in cognitive, language, gross or fine motor skills

Risk Factors

Prenatal

Endocrine disorders
Genetic disorders
Illiteracy
Inadequate nutrition
Infections
Lack of prenatal care
Late prenatal care
Maternal age <15 years
Maternal age >35 years
Poor prenatal care
Poverty
Substance abuse
Unplanned pregnancy
Unwanted pregnancy

Individual

Adopted child
Behavior disorders
Brain damage (e.g., hemorrhage in postnatal period, shaken baby, abuse, accident)
Chemotherapy
Chronic illness
Congenital disorders
Failure to thrive
Foster child
Frequent otitis media
Genetic disorders
Hearing impairment
Inadequate nutrition
Lead poisoning
Natural disasters
Positive drug screen(s)
Prematurity
Radiation therapy
Seizures
Substance abuse
Technology-dependent
Vision impairment

Environmental

Poverty
Violence

Caregiver

Abuse
Mental illness
Mental retardation
Severe learning disability

DIARRHEA

Definition

Passage of loose, unformed stools

Defining Characteristics

- Abdominal pain
- At least 3 loose liquid stools per day
- Cramping
- Hyperactive bowel sounds
- Urgency

Related Factors

Psychological

Anxiety
High stress levels

Situational

Adverse effects of medications
Alcohol abuse
Contaminants
Laxative abuse
Radiation
Toxins
Travel
Tube feedings

Physiological

Infectious processes
Inflammation
Irritation
Malabsorption
Parasites

Risk for Compromised Human Dignity

Definition

At risk for perceived loss of respect and honor

Risk Factors

Cultural incongruity
Disclosure of confidential information
Exposure of the body
Inadequate participation in decision making
Loss of control of body functions
Perceived dehumanizing treatment
Perceived humiliation
Perceived intrusion by clinicians
Perceived invasion of privacy
Stigmatizing label
Use of undefined medical terms

References

Shottom, L., & Seedhouse, D. (1998). Practical dignity in caring. *Nursing Ethics, 5,* 246–255.
Mairis, E. (1994). Concept clarification of professional practice-dignity. *Journal of Advanced Nursing, 19,* 924–931.
Walsh, K., & Kowanko, I. (2002). Nurses' and patients' perceptions of dignity. *International Journal of Nursing Practice, 8,* 143–151.

Moral Distress

Definition

Response to the inability to carry out one's chosen ethical/moral decision/action

Defining Characteristics

- Expresses anguish (e.g., powerlessness, guilt, frustration, anxiety, self-doubt, fear) over difficulty acting on one's moral choice

Related Factors

Conflict among decision makers
Conflicting information guiding ethical decision making
Conflicting information guiding moral decision making
Cultural conflicts
End-of-life decisions
Loss of autonomy
Physical distance of decision maker
Time constraints for decision making
Treatment decisions

References

Corley, M., Elswick, R., Gorman, M., & Clor, T. (2001). Development and evaluation of a moral distress scale. *Journal of Advanced Nursing, 33,* 250–256.

Jameton, A. (1993). Dilemmas of moral distress: Moral responsibility and nursing practice. *AWHON's Clinical Issues in Perinatal & Womens Health Nursing, 4,* 542–551.

Kopala, B., & Burkhart, L. (2005). Ethical dilemma and moral distress: Proposed new NANDA diagnoses. *International Journal of Nursing Terminologies and Classifications, 16,* 3–13.

RISK FOR DISUSE SYNDROME

Definition

At risk for deterioration of body systems as the result of prescribed or unavoidable musculoskeletal inactivity

Risk Factors

Altered level of consciousness
Mechanical immobilization
Paralysis
Prescribed immobilization
Severe pain

Note. Complications from immobility can include pressure ulcer, constipation, stasis of pulmonary secretions, thrombosis, urinary tract infection and/or retention, decreased strength or endurance, orthostatic hypotension, decreased range of joint motion, disorientation, body-image disturbance, and powerlessness.

DEFICIENT DIVERSIONAL ACTIVITY

Definition

Decreased stimulation from (or interest or engagement in) recreational or leisure activities

Defining Characteristics

- Patient's statements regarding boredom (e.g., wish there was something to do, to read, etc.)
- Usual hobbies cannot be undertaken in hospital

Related Factors

Environmental lack of diversional activity

DISTURBED ENERGY FIELD

Definition

Disruption of the flow of energy surrounding a person's being results in disharmony of the body, mind, and/or spirit

Defining Characteristics

- Perceptions of changes in patterns of energy flow, such as
  - Movement (wave, spike, tingling, dense, flowing)
  - Sounds (tone, words)
  - Temperature change (warmth, coolness)
  - Visual changes (image, color)
  - Disruption of the field (deficit, hole, spike, bulge, obstruction, congestion, diminished flow in energy field)

Related Factors

Slowing or blocking of energy flows secondary to:

Maturational factors

Age-related developmental crisis
Age-related developmental difficulties

Pathophysiologic factors

Illness
Injury
Pregnancy

Situational factors

Anxiety
Fear
Grieving
Pain

Treatment-related factors

Chemotherapy
Immobility
Labor and delivery
Perioperative experience

IMPAIRED ENVIRONMENTAL INTERPRETATION SYNDROME

Definition

Consistent lack of orientation to person, place, time, or circumstances over more than 3 to 6 months necessitating a protective environment

Defining Characteristics

- Chronic confusional states
- Consistent disorientation
- Inability to concentrate
- Inability to follow simple directions
- Inability to reason
- Loss of occupation
- Loss of social functioning
- Slow in responding to questions

Related Factors

Dementia
Depression
Huntington's disease

Adult Failure to Thrive

Definition

Progressive functional deterioration of a physical and cognitive nature. The individual's ability to live with multisystem diseases, cope with ensuing problems, and manage his/her care are remarkably diminished.

Defining Characteristics

- Altered mood state
- Anorexia
- Apathy
- Cognitive decline:
  - Problems with responding to environmental stimuli
  - Demonstrated difficulty in concentration
  - Demonstrated difficulty in decision making
  - Demonstrated difficulty in judgment
  - Demonstrated difficulty in memory
  - Demonstrated difficulty in reasoning
  - Decreased perception
- Consumption of minimal to no food at most meals (i.e., consumes <75% of normal requirements)
- Decreased participation in activities of daily living
- Decreased social skills
- Expresses loss of interest in pleasurable outlets
- Frequent exacerbations of chronic health problems
- Inadequate nutritional intake
- Neglect of home environment
- Neglect of financial responsibilities
- Physical decline (e.g., fatigue, dehydration, incontinence of bowel and bladder)
- Self-care deficit
- Social withdrawal
- Unintentional weight loss (e.g., 5% in 1 month; 10% in 6 months)
- Verbalizes desire for death

Related Factors

Depression

Risk for Falls

Definition

Increased susceptibility to falling that may cause physical harm

Risk Factors

Adults

Age 65 or over
History of falls
Lives alone
Lower limb prosthesis
Use of assistive devices (e.g., walker, cane)
Wheelchair use

Children

<2 years of age
Bed located near window

Lack of auto restraints
Lack of gate on stairs
Lack of window guard
Lack of parental supervision
Male gender when <1 year of age
Unattended infant on elevated surface (e.g., bed/changing table)

Cognitive

Diminished mental status

Environment

Cluttered environment
Dimly lit room
No antislip material in bath
No antislip material in shower
Restraints
Throw rugs
Unfamiliar room
Weather conditions (e.g., wet floors, ice)

Medications

ACE inhibitors
Alcohol use
Antianxiety agents
Antihypertensive agents
Diuretics
Hypnotics
Narcotics
Tranquilizers
Tricyclic antidepressants

Physiological

Anemias
Arthritis
Diarrhea
Decreased lower extremity strength
Difficulty with gait
Faintness when extending neck
Faintness when turning neck
Foot problems
Hearing difficulties
Impaired balance
Impaired physical mobility
Incontinence
Neoplasms (e.g., fatigue/limited mobility)
Neuropathy
Orthostatic hypotension
Postoperative conditions
Postprandial blood sugar changes
Presence of acute illness
Proprioceptive deficits
Sleeplessness

Urgency
Vascular disease
Visual difficulties

DYSFUNCTIONAL FAMILY PROCESSES: ALCOHOLISM

Definition

Psychosocial, spiritual, and physiological functions of the family unit are chronically disorganized, which leads to conflict, denial of problems, resistance to change, ineffective problem solving, and a series of self-perpetuating crises

Defining Characteristics

Behavioral

- Alcohol abuse
- Agitation
- Blaming
- Broken promises
- Chaos
- Contradictory communication
- Controlling communication
- Criticizing
- Deficient knowledge about alcoholism
- Denial of problems
- Dependency
- Difficulty having fun
- Difficulty with intimate relationships
- Difficulty with life cycle transitions
- Diminished physical contact
- Disturbances in academic performance in children
- Disturbances in concentration
- Enabling to maintain alcoholic drinking pattern
- Escalating conflict
- Failure to accomplish developmental tasks
- Family special occasions are alcohol-centered
- Harsh self-judgment
- Immaturity
- Impaired communication
- Inability to accept health
- Inability to accept help
- Inability to accept a wide range of feelings
- Inability to adapt to change
- Inability to deal constructively with traumatic experiences
- Inability to express a wide range of feelings
- Inability to meet emotional needs of its members
- Inability to meet security needs of its members
- Inability to meet spiritual needs of its members
- Inability to receive help appropriately
- Inadequate understanding of alcoholism
- Inappropriate expression of anger
- Ineffective problem-solving skills

- Isolation
- Lack of dealing with conflict
- Lack of reliability
- Lying
- Manipulation
- Nicotine addiction
- Orientation toward tension relief rather than achievement of goals
- Paradoxical communication
- Power struggles
- Rationalization
- Refusal to get help
- Seeking affirmation
- Seeking approval
- Self-blaming
- Stress-related physical illnesses
- Substance abuse other than alcohol
- Unresolved grief
- Verbal abuse of children
- Verbal abuse of parent
- Verbal abuse of spouse

Feelings

- Abandonment
- Anger
- Anxiety
- Being different from other people
- Being unloved
- Confused love and pity
- Confusion
- Decreased self-esteem
- Depression
- Dissatisfaction
- Distress
- Embarrassment
- Emotional control by others
- Emotional isolation
- Failure
- Fear
- Frustration
- Guilt
- Hopelessness
- Hostility
- Hurt
- Insecurity
- Lack of identity
- Lingering resentment
- Loneliness
- Loss
- Mistrust
- Misunderstood

- Moodiness
- Powerlessness
- Rejection
- Repressed emotions
- Responsibility for alcoholic's behavior
- Supressed rage
- Shame
- Tension
- Unhappiness
- Vulnerability
- Worthlessness

Roles and Relationships

- Altered role function
- Chronic family problems
- Closed communication systems
- Deterioration in family relationships/disturbed family dynamics
- Disrupted family rituals
- Disrupted family roles
- Economic problems
- Family denial
- Family does not demonstrate respect for autonomy of its members
- Family does not demonstrate respect for individuality of its members
- Inconsistent parenting
- Ineffective spouse communication
- Intimacy dysfunction
- Lack of cohesiveness
- Lack of skills necessary for relationships
- Low perception of parental support
- Marital problems
- Neglected obligations
- Pattern of rejection
- Reduced ability of family members to relate to each other for mutual growth and maturation
- Triangulating family relationships

Related Factors

Abuse of alcohol
Addictive personality
Biochemical influences
Family history of alcoholism
Family history of resistance to treatment
Genetic predisposition
Inadequate coping skills
Lack of problem-solving skills

INTERRUPTED FAMILY PROCESSES

Definition

Change in family relationships and/or functioning

Defining Characteristics

- Changes in assigned tasks

- Changes in availability for affective responsiveness
- Changes in availability for emotional support
- Changes in communication patterns
- Changes in effectiveness in completing assigned tasks
- Changes in expressions of conflict with community resources
- Changes in expressions of isolation from community resources
- Changes in expressions of conflict within family
- Changes in intimacy
- Changes in mutual support
- Changes in patterns
- Changes in participation in problem solving
- Changes in participation in decision making
- Changes in power alliances
- Changes in rituals
- Changes in satisfaction with family
- Changes in somatic complaints
- Changes in stress-reduction behaviors

Related Factors

Developmental crises
Developmental transition
Family roles shift
Interaction with community
Modification in family finances
Modification in family social status
Power shift of family members
Shift in health status of a family member
Situation transition
Situational crises

Readiness for Enhanced Family Processes

Definition

A pattern of family functioning that is sufficient to support the well-being of family members and can be strengthened

Defining Characteristics

- Activities support the growth of family members
- Activities support the safety of family members
- Balance exists between autonomy and cohesiveness
- Boundaries of family members are maintained
- Communication is adequate
- Energy level of family supports activities of daily living
- Expresses willingness to enhance family dynamics
- Family adapts to change
- Family functioning meets needs of family members
- Family resilience is evident
- Family roles are appropriate for developmental stages
- Family roles are flexible for developmental stages
- Family tasks are accomplished

- Interdependent with community
- Relationships are generally positive
- Respect for family members is evident

FATIGUE

Definition

An overwhelming sustained sense of exhaustion and decreased capacity for physical and mental work at usual level

Defining Characteristics

- Compromised concentration
- Compromised libido
- Decreased performance
- Disinterest in surroundings
- Drowsy
- Feelings of guilt for not keeping up with responsibilities
- Inability to maintain usual level of physical activity
- Inability to maintain usual routines
- Inability to restore energy even after sleep
- Increase in physical complaints
- Increase in rest requirements
- Introspection
- Lack of energy
- Lethargic
- Listless
- Perceived need for additional energy to accomplish routine tasks
- Tired
- Verbalization of an unremitting lack of energy
- Verbalization of an overwhelming lack of energy

Related Factors

Psychological

Anxiety
Boring lifestyle
Depression
Stress

Physiological

Anemia
Disease states
Increased physical exertion
Malnutrition
Poor physical condition
Pregnancy
Sleep deprivation

Environmental

Humidity
Lights
Noise
Temperature

Situational

Negative life events
Occupation

FEAR

Definition

Response to perceived threat that is consciously recognized as a danger

Defining Characteristics

- Report of alarm
- Report of apprehension
- Report of being scared
- Report of decreased self-assurance
- Report of dread
- Report of excitement
- Report of increased tension
- Report of jitteriness
- Report of panic
- Report of terror

Cognitive

- Diminished productivity
- Diminished learning ability
- Diminished problem-solving ability
- Identifies object of fear
- Stimulus believed to be a threat

Behaviors

- Attack behaviors
- Avoidance behaviors
- Impulsiveness
- Increased alertness
- Narrowed focus on the source of the fear

Physiological

- Anorexia
- Diarrhea
- Dry mouth
- Dyspnea
- Fatigue
- Increased perspiration
- Increased pulse
- Increased respiratory rate
- Increased systolic blood pressure
- Muscle tightness
- Nausea
- Pallor
- Pupil dilation
- Vomiting

Related Factors

Innate origin (e.g., sudden noise, height, pain, loss of physical support)
Innate releasers (e.g., neurotransmitters)
Language barrier
Learned response (e.g., conditioning, modeling from or identification with others)
Phobic stimulus
Sensory impairment
Separation from support system in potentially stressful situation (e.g., hospitalization, hospital procedures)
Unfamiliarity with environmental experience(s)

Readiness for Enhanced Fluid Balance

Definition

A pattern of equilibrium between fluid volume and chemical composition of body fluids that is sufficient for meeting physical needs and can be strengthened

Defining Characteristics

- Dehydration
- Expresses willingness to enhance fluid balance
- Good tissue turgor
- Intake adequate for daily needs
- Moist mucous membranes
- No evidence of edema
- No excessive thirst
- Specific gravity within normal limits
- Stable weight
- Straw-colored urine
- Urine output appropriate for intake

Deficient Fluid Volume

Definition

Decreased intravascular, interstitial, and/or intracellular fluid. This refers to dehydration, water loss alone without change in sodium.

Defining Characteristics

- Change in mental state
- Decreased blood pressure
- Decreased pulse pressure
- Decreased pulse volume
- Decreased skin turgor
- Decreased tongue turgor
- Decreased urine output
- Decreased venous filling
- Dry mucous membranes
- Dry skin
- Elevated hematocrit
- Increased body temperature
- Increased pulse rate
- Increased urine concentration
- Sudden weight loss (except in third spacing)

- Thirst
- Weakness

Related Factors

Active fluid volume loss
Failure of regulatory mechanisms

EXCESS FLUID VOLUME

Definition

Increased isotonic fluid retention

Defining Characteristics

- Adventitious breath sounds
- Altered electrolytes
- Anasarca
- Anxiety
- Azotemia
- Blood pressure changes
- Change in mental status
- Changes in respiratory pattern
- Decreased hematocrit
- Decreased hemoglobin
- Dyspnea
- Edema
- Increased central venous pressure
- Intake exceeds output
- Jugular vein distention
- Oliguria
- Orthopnea
- Pleural effusion
- Positive hepatojugular reflex
- Pulmonary artery pressure changes
- Pulmonary congestion
- Restlessness
- Specific gravity changes
- S3 heart sound
- Weight gain over short period of time

Related Factors

Compromised regulatory mechanism
Excess fluid intake
Excess sodium intake

RISK FOR DEFICIENT FLUID VOLUME

Definition

At risk for experiencing vascular, cellular, or intracellular dehydration

Risk Factors

Deviations affecting access of fluids
Deviations affecting intake of fluids

Deviations affecting absorption of fluids
Excessive losses through normal routes (e.g., diarrhea)
Extremes of age
Extremes of weight
Factors influencing fluid needs (e.g., hypermetabolic state)
Loss of fluid through abnormal routes (e.g., indwelling tubes)
Knowledge deficiency
Medication (e.g., diuretics)

RISK FOR IMBALANCED FLUID VOLUME

Definition

At risk for a decrease, increase, or rapid shift from one to the other of intravascular, interstitial, and/or intracellular fluid. This refers to body fluid loss, gain, or both.

Risk Factors

Scheduled for major invasive procedures

Note. This diagnosis will retire from the NANDA-I Taxonomy in the 2009–2010 edition unless additional work is done to bring it to a LOE of 2.1 or higher.

IMPAIRED GAS EXCHANGE

Definition

Excess or deficit in oxygenation and/or carbon dioxide elimination at the alveolar-capillary membrane

Defining Characteristics

- Abnormal arterial blood gases
- Abnormal arterial pH
- Abnormal breathing (e.g., rate, rhythm, depth)
- Abnormal skin color (e.g., pale, dusky)
- Confusion
- Cyanosis (in neonates only)
- Decreased carbon dioxide
- Diaphoresis
- Dyspnea
- Headache upon awakening
- Hypercapnia
- Hypercarbia
- Hypoxemia
- Hypoxia
- Irritability
- Nasal flaring
- Restlessness
- Somnolence
- Tachycardia
- Visual disturbances

Related Factors

Alveolar-capillary membrane changes
Ventilation perfusion imbalance

RISK FOR UNSTABLE BLOOD GLUCOSE

Definition

Risk for variation of blood glucose/sugar levels from the normal range

Risk Factors

Deficient knowledge of diabetes management (e.g., action plan)
Developmental level
Dietary intake
Inadequate blood glucose monitoring
Lack of acceptance of diagnosis
Lack of adherence to diabetes management (e.g., action plan)
Lack of diabetes management (e.g., action plan)
Medication management
Mental health status
Physical activity level
Physical health status
Pregnancy
Rapid growth periods
Stress
Weight gain
Weight loss

References

American Diabetes Association. (2005). Standard of medical care in diabetes. *Diabetes Care, 29,* S1–S36. http://care.diabetesjournals.org/cgi/content/full/28/suppl_1/s4.

Bierschbach, J., Cooper, L., & Liedl, J. (2004). Insulin pumps: What every school nurse needs to know. *Journal of School Nursing, 20,* 117–123.

U.S. Department of Health & Human Services. (2003). *Helping students with diabetes succeed: A guide for school personnel.* http://ndep.nih.gov/resources/school.htm.

GRIEVING*

Definition

A normal complex process that includes emotional, physical, spiritual, social, and intellectual responses and behaviors by which individuals, families, and communities incorporate an actual, anticipated, or perceived loss into their daily lives

Defining Characteristics

- Alteration in activity level
- Alterations in immune function
- Alterations in neuroendocrine function
- Alterations in sleep patterns
- Alteration in dream patterns
- Anger
- Blame
- Detachment
- Despair
- Disorganization
- Experiencing relief
- Maintaining the connection to the deceased

** Previously titled "Anticipatory Grieving"*

- Making meaning of the loss
- Pain
- Panic behavior
- Personal growth
- Psychological distress
- Suffering

Related Factors

Anticipatory loss of significant object (e.g., possession, job, status, home, parts & processes of body)
Anticipatory loss of a significant other
Death of a significant other
Loss of significant object (e.g., possession, job, status, home, parts & processes of body)

References

Hogan, N., Worden, J., & Schmidt, L. (2004). An empirical study of the proposed complicated grief disorder criteria. *OMEGA, 48,* 263–277.

Ott, C. (2003). The impact of complicated grief on mental and physical health at various points in the bereavement process. *Death Studies, 27,* 249–272.

Center for the Advancement of Health. (2004). Report on bereavement and grief research. *Death Studies, 28,* 498–505.

COMPLICATED GRIEVING*

Definition

A disorder that occurs after the death of a significant other, in which the experience of distress accompanying bereavement fails to follow normative expectations and manifests in functional impairment

Defining Characteristics

- Decreased functioning in life roles
- Decreased sense of well-being
- Depression
- Experiencing somatic symptoms of the deceased
- Fatigue
- Grief avoidance
- Longing for the deceased
- Low levels of intimacy
- Persistent emotional distress
- Preoccupation with thoughts of the deceased
- Rumination
- Searching for the deceased
- Self-blame
- Separation distress
- Traumatic distress
- Verbalizes anxiety
- Verbalizes distressful feelings about the deceased
- Verbalizes feeling dazed
- Verbalizes feeling empty
- Verbalizes feeling in shock
- Verbalizes feeling stunned
- Verbalizes feelings of anger

* *Previously titled "Dysfunctional Grieving"*

- Verbalizes feelings of detachment from others
- Verbalizes feelings of disbelief
- Verbalizes feelings of mistrust
- Verbalizes lack of acceptance of the death
- Verbalizes persistent painful memories
- Verbalizes self-blame
- Yearning

Related Factors

Death of a significant other
Emotional instability
Lack of social support
Sudden death of significant other

References

Hogan, N., Worden, J., & Schmidt, L. (2004). An empirical study of the proposed complicated grief disorder criteria. *OMEGA, 48,* 263–277.

Ott, C. (2003). The impact of complicated grief on mental and physical health at various points in the bereavement process. *Death Studies, 27,* 24–272.

Center for the Advancement of Health. (2004). Report on bereavement and grief research. *Death Studies, 28,* 498–505.

RISK FOR COMPLICATED GRIEVING*

Definition

At risk for a disorder that occurs after the death of a significant other, in which the experience of distress accompanying bereavement fails to follow normative expectations and manifests in functional impairment

Risk Factors

Death of a significant other
Emotional instability
Lack of social support

* *Previously titled "Risk for Dysfunctional Grieving"*

References

Hogan, N., Worden, J., & Schmidt, L. (2004). An empirical study of the proposed complicated grief disorder criteria. *OMEGA, 48,* 263–277.

Ott, C. (2003). The impact of complicated grief on mental and physical health at various points in the bereavement process. *Death Studies, 27,* 249–272.

Center for the Advancement of Health. (2004). Report on bereavement and grief research. *Death Studies, 28,* 498–505.

DELAYED GROWTH AND DEVELOPMENT

Definition

Deviations from age-group norms

Defining Characteristics

- Altered physical growth
- Decreased response time
- Delay in performing skills typical of age group
- Difficulty in performing skills typical of age group
- Inability to perform self-care activities appropriate for age
- Inability to perform self-control activities appropriate for age

- Flat affect
- Listlessness

Related Factors

Effects of physical disability
Environmental deficiencies
Inadequate caretaking
Inconsistent responsiveness
Indifference
Multiple caretakers
Prescribed dependence
Separation from significant others
Stimulation deficiencies

Risk for Disproportionate Growth

Definition

At risk for growth above the 97th percentile or below the 3rd percentile for age, crossing two percentile channels

Risk Factors

Caregiver

Abuse
Mental illness
Mental retardation
Severe learning disability

Environmental

Deprivation
Lead poisoning
Natural disasters
Poverty
Teratogen
Violence

Individual

Anorexia
Caregiver maladaptive feeding behaviors
Chronic illness
Individual maladaptive feeding behaviors
Infection
Insatiable appetite
Malnutrition
Prematurity
Substance abuse

Prenatal

Congenital disorders
Genetic disorders
Maternal infection
Maternal nutrition
Multiple gestation
Teratogen exposure

Substance use
Substance abuse

INEFFECTIVE HEALTH MAINTENANCE

Definition

Inability to identify, manage, and/or seek out help to maintain health

Defining Characteristics

- Demonstrated lack of adaptive behaviors to environmental changes
- Demonstrated lack of knowledge regarding basic health practices
- Lack of expressed interest in improving health behaviors
- History of lack of health-seeking behavior
- Inability to take responsibility for meeting basic health practices
- Impairment of personal support systems

Related Factors

Cognitive impairment
Complicated grieving
Deficient communication skills
Diminished fine motor skills
Diminished gross motor skills
Inability to make appropriate judgments
Ineffective family coping
Ineffective individual coping
Insufficient resources (e.g., equipment, finances)
Lack of fine motor skills
Lack of gross motor skills
Perceptual impairment
Spiritual distress
Unachieved developmental tasks

HEALTH-SEEKING BEHAVIORS (SPECIFY)

Definition

Active seeking (by a person in stable health) of ways to alter personal health habits and/or the environment in order to move toward a higher level of health

Defining Characteristics

- Demonstrated lack of knowledge about health-promotion behaviors
- Expressed concern about current environmental conditions on health status
- Expressed desire for increased control of health practice
- Expressed desire to seek a higher level of wellness
- Observed unfamiliarity with wellness community resoucres
- Stated unfamiliarity with wellness community resources

Related Factors

To be developed

Note. Stable health is defined as achievement of age-appropriate illness-prevention measures; client reports good or excellent health, and signs and symptoms of disease, if present, are controlled.

This diagnosis will retire from the NANDA-I Taxonomy in the 2009–2010 edition unless additional work is done to bring it to a LOE of 2.1 or higher.

IMPAIRED HOME MAINTENANCE

Definition

Inability to independently maintain a safe growth-promoting immediate environment

Defining Characteristics

Objective

- Disorderly surroundings
- Inappropriate household temperature
- Insufficient clothes
- Insufficient linen
- Lack of clothes
- Lack of linen
- Lack of necessary equipment
- Offensive odors
- Overtaxed family members
- Presence of vermin
- Repeated unhygienic disorders
- Repeated unhygienic infections
- Unavailable cooking equipment
- Unclean surroundings

Subjective

- Household members describe financial crises
- Household members describe outstanding debts
- Household members express difficulty in maintaining their home in a comfortable fashion
- Household members request assistance with home maintenance

Related Factors

Deficient knowledge
Disease
Inadequate support systems
Injury
Impaired functioning
Insufficient family organization
Insufficient family planning
Insufficient finances
Lack of role modeling
Unfamiliarity with neighborhood resources

READINESS FOR ENHANCED HOPE

Definition

A pattern of expectations and desires that is sufficient for mobilizing energy on one's own behalf and can be strengthened

Defining Characteristics

- Expresses desire to enhance ability to set achievable goals
- Expresses desire to enhance belief in possibilities
- Expresses desire to enhance congruency of expectations with desires
- Expresses desire to enhance hope

- Expresses desire to enhance interconnectedness with others
- Expresses desire to enhance problem-solving to meet goals
- Expresses desire to enhance sense of meaning to life
- Expresses desire to enhance spirituality

References

Benzein, E.G. (2005). The level of and relation between hope, hopelessness and fatigue in patients and family members in palliative care. *Palliative Medicine, 19,* 234–240.

Benzein, E., & Saveman, B-L. (1998). One step towards the understanding of hope: A concept analysis. *International Journal of Nursing Studies, 35,* 322–329.

Davis, B. (2005). Mediators of the relationship between hope and well-being in older adults. *Clinical Nursing Research, 14,* 253–272.

HOPELESSNESS

Definition

Subjective state in which an individual sees limited or no alternatives or personal choices available and is unable to mobilize energy on own behalf

Defining Characteristics

- Closing eyes
- Decreased affect
- Decreased appetite
- Decreased response to stimuli
- Decreased verbalization
- Lack of initiative
- Lack of involvement in care
- Passivity
- Shrugging in response to speaker
- Sleep pattern disturbance
- Turning away from speaker
- Verbal cues (e.g., despondent content, "I can't," sighing)

Related Factors

Abandonment
Deteriorating physiological condition
Lost belief in spiritual power
Lost belief in transcendent values
Long-term stress
Prolonged activity restriction creating isolation

HYPERTHERMIA

Definition

Body temperature elevated above normal range

Defining Characteristics

- Convulsions
- Flushed skin
- Increase in body temperature above normal range
- Seizures
- Tachycardia

- Tachypnea
- Warm to touch

Related Factors

Anesthesia
Decreased perspiration
Dehydration
Exposure to hot environment
Inappropriate clothing
Increased metabolic rate
Illness
Medications
Trauma
Vigorous activity

HYPOTHERMIA

Definition

Body temperature below normal range

Defining Characteristics

- Body temperature below normal range
- Cool skin
- Cyanotic nail beds
- Hypertension
- Pallor
- Piloerection
- Shivering
- Slow capillary refill
- Tachycardia

Related Factors

Aging
Consumption of alcohol
Damage to hypothalamus
Decreased ability to shiver
Decreased metabolic rate
Evaporation from skin in cool environment
Exposure to cool environment
Illness
Inactivity
Inadequate clothing
Malnutrition
Medications
Trauma

DISTURBED PERSONAL IDENTITY

Definition

Inability to distinguish between self and nonself

Defining Characteristics

To be developed

Related Factors

To be developed

Note. This diagnosis will be retired from the NANDA-I Taxonomy with the 2009–2010 edition unless additional work is done to bring it to a LOE of 2.1.

READINESS FOR ENHANCED IMMUNIZATION STATUS

Definition

A pattern of conforming to local, national, and/or international standards of immunization to prevent infectious disease(s) that is sufficient to protect a person, family, or community and can be strengthened

Defining Characteristics

- Expresses desire to enhance behavior to prevent infectious disease
- Expresses desire to enhance identification of possible problems associated with immunizations
- Expresses desire to enhance identification of providers of immunizations
- Expresses desire to enhance immunization status
- Expresses desire to enhance knowledge of immunization standards
- Expresses desire to enhance record-keeping of immunizations

References

Centers for Disease Control. (2002). Recommended adult immunization schedule: United States, 2002–2003. *Mortality and Morbidity Weekly Report, 51,* 904–908.

Davis, T.C., Frederickson, D.D., Kennen, E.M., Arnold, C., Shoup, E., Sugar, M., et al. (2004). Childhood vaccine risk/benefit communication among public health clinics: A time motion study. *Public Health Nursing, 21,* 228–236.

Mell, L.K., Ogren, D.S., Davis, R.L., Mullooy, J.P., Black, S.B., Shinfield, H.R., et al. (2005). Compliance with national immunization guidelines for children younger that 2 years, 1996–1999. *Pediatrics, 115,* 461–467.

FUNCTIONAL URINARY INCONTINENCE

Definition

Inability of usually continent person to reach toilet in time to avoid unintentional loss of urine

Defining Characteristics

- Able to completely empty bladder
- Amount of time required to reach toilet exceeds length of time between sensing the urge to void and uncontrolled voiding
- Loss of urine before reaching toilet
- May only be incontinent in early morning
- Senses need to void

Related Factors

Altered environmental factors
Impaired cognition
Impaired vision
Neuromuscular limitations
Psychological factors
Weakened supporting pelvic structures

Overflow Urinary Incontinence

Definition

Involuntary loss of urine associated with overdistention of the bladder let in time to avoid unintentional loss of urine

Defining Characteristics

- Bladder distention
- High post-void residual volume
- Nocturia
- Observed involuntary leakage of small volumes of urine
- Reports involuntary leakage of small volumes of urine

Related Factors

Bladder outlet obstruction
Detrusor external sphincter dyssynergia
Detrusor hypocontractility
Fecal impaction
Severe pelvic prolapse
Side effects of anticholinergic medications
Side effects of calcium channel blockers
Side effects of decongestant medications
Urethral obstruction

References

Agency for Health Care Policy and Research. (1992). *Clinical practice guideline: Urinary incontinence in adults* (Pub. No. 92-0038). Rockville, MD: Author.

National Kidney and Urologic Diseases Information Clearing House. (2004). *Urinary incontinence in women.* Bethesda, MD: Author.

Walsh, P. (Ed.). (2002). *Campbell's urology* (8 th ed.). Philadelphia: Saunders.

Reflex Urinary Incontinence

Definition

Involuntary loss of urine at somewhat predictable intervals when a specific bladder volume is reached

Defining Characteristics

- Complete emptying with lesion above pontine micturition center
- Inability to voluntarily inhibit voiding
- Inability to voluntarily initiate voiding
- Incomplete emptying with lesion above sacral micturition center
- No sensation of bladder fullness
- No sensation of urge to void
- No sensation of voiding
- Predictable pattern of voiding
- Sensation of urgency without voluntary inhibition of bladder contraction
- Sensations associated with full bladder (e.g., sweating, restlessness, abdominal discomfort)

Related Factors

Tissue damage (e.g., due to radiation cystitis, inflammatory bladder conditions, radical pelvic surgery)
Neurological impairment above level of pontine micturition center
Neurological impairment above level of sacral micturition center

STRESS URINARY INCONTINENCE

Definition

Sudden leakage of urine with activities that increase intra-abdominal pressure

Defining Characteristics

- Observed involuntary leakage of small amounts of urine in the absence of detrusor contraction
- Observed involuntary leakage of small amounts of urine in the absence of an over-distended bladder
- Observed involuntary leakage of small amounts of urine on exertion
- Observed involuntary leakage of small amounts of urine with sneezing, laughing, or coughing
- Reports involuntary leakage of small amounts of urine in the absence of detrusor contraction
- Reports involuntary leakage of small amounts of urine in the absence of an over-distended bladder
- Reports involuntary leakage of small amounts of urine on exertion
- Reports involuntary leakage of small amounts of urine with sneezing, laughing, or coughing

Related Factors

Degenerative changes in pelvic muscles
High intra-abdominal pressure
Intrinsic urethral sphincter deficiency
Weak pelvic muscles

References

Agency for Health Care Policy and Research. (1992). *Clinical practice guideline:Urinary incontinence in adults* (AHCPR Pub. No. 92-0038). Rockville, MD: Author.

National Kidney and Urologic Diseases Information Clearing House. (2004). *Urinary incontinence in women.* Retrieved January 27, 2005 from http: //kidney.niddk.nih.gov/kudiseases/pubs/uiwomen/index.htm.

NIH consensus statements. (1988). *Urinary incontinence in adults.* Retrieved January 27, 2005 from http://consens us.nih.gov/cons/071/071_statement.htm.

TOTAL URINARY INCONTINENCE

Definition

Continuous and unpredictable loss of urine

Defining Characteristics

- Constant flow of urine at unpredictable times without uninhibited bladder contractions/spasm or distention
- Lack of bladder filling
- Lack of perineal filling
- Nocturia
- Unawareness of incontinence
- Unsuccessful incontinence refractory treatments

Related Factors

Anatomic (fistula)
Disease affecting spinal cord nerves
Independent contraction of detrusor reflex
Neurological dysfunction
Neuropathy preventing transmission of reflex indicating bladder fullness
Trauma affecting spinal cord nerves

Note. This diagnosis will retire from the NANDA-I Taxonomy in the 2009–2010 edition unless additional work is done to bring it to a LOE of 2.1 or higher.

Urge Urinary Incontinence

Definition

Involuntary passage of urine occurring soon after a strong sense of urgency to void

Defining Characteristics

- Observed inability to reach toilet in time to avoid urine loss
- Reports urinary urgency
- Reports involuntary loss of urine with bladder contractions/spasms
- Reports inability to reach toilet in time to avoid urine loss

Related Factors

Alcohol intake
Atrophic urethritis
Atrophic vaginitis
Bladder infection
Caffeine intake
Decreased bladder capacity
Detrusor hyperactivity with impaired bladder contractility
Fecal impaction
Use of diuretics

References

Agency for Health Care Policy and Research (AHCPR). (1992). *Clinical practice guideline: Urinary incontinence in adults* (AHCPR Pub. No. 92-0038). Rockville, MD: Author.

National Kidney and Urologic Diseases Information Clearing House (NIDDK). (2004). *Urinary incontinence in women.* Retrieved January 27, 2005 from http://kidney.niddk.nih.gov/kudiseases/pubs/uiwomen/index.htm.

NIH consensus statements. (1988). *Urinary incontinence in adults.* Retrieved January 27, 2005 from http://consens us.nih.gov/cons/071/071_statement.htm.

Risk for Urge Urinary Incontinence

Definition

At risk for involuntary loss of urine associated with a sudden, strong sensation or urinary urgency

Risk Factors

Effects of alcohol
Effects of caffeine
Effects of medications
Detrusor hyperreflexia (e.g., from cystitis, urethritis, tumors, renal calculi, central nervous system disorders above pontine micturition center)
Impaired bladder contractility
Involuntary sphincter relaxation
Ineffective toileting habits
Small bladder capacity

Disorganized Infant Behavior

Definition

Disintegrated physiological and neurobehavioral responses of infant to the environment

Defining Characteristics

Attention-Interaction System

- Abnormal response to sensory stimuli (e.g., difficult to soothe, inability to sustain alert status)

Motor System

- Altered primitive reflexes
- Changes to motor tone
- Finger splaying
- Fisting
- Hands to face
- Hyperextension of extremities
- Jittery
- Startles
- Tremors
- Twitches
- Uncoordinated movement

Physiological

- Arrhythmias
- Bradycardia
- Desaturation
- Feeding intolerances
- Skin color changes
- Tachycardia
- Time-out signals (e.g., gaze, grasp, hiccough, cough, sneeze, sigh, slack jaw, open mouth, tongue thrust)

Regulatory Problems

- Inability to inhibit startle
- Irritability

State-Organization System

- Active-awake (fussy, worried gaze)
- Diffuse sleep
- Irritable crying
- State-oscillation
- Quiet-awake (staring, gaze aversion)

Related Factors

Caregiver

Cue knowledge deficit
Cue misreading
Environmental stimulation contribution

Environmental

Lack of containment within environment
Physical environment inappropriateness
Sensory deprivation
Sensory inappropriateness
Sensory overstimulation

Individual

Gestational age
Illness
Immature neurological system
Postconceptual age

Postnatal

Feeding intolerance
Invasive procedures
Malnutrition
Motor problems
Oral problems
Pain
Prematurity

Prenatal

Congenital disorders
Genetic disorders
Teratogenic exposure

RISK FOR DISORGANIZED INFANT BEHAVIOR

Definition

Risk for alteration in integrating and modulation of the physiological and behavioral systems of functioning (i.e., autonomic, motor, state, organizational, self-regulatory, and attentional-interactional systems)

Risk Factors

Environmental overstimulation
Invasive procedures
Lack of containment within environment
Motor problems
Oral problems
Pain
Painful procedures
Prematurity

READINESS FOR ENHANCED ORGANIZED INFANT BEHAVIOR

Definition

A pattern of modulation of the physiologic and behavioral systems of functioning (i.e., autonomic, motor, state-organizational, self-regulatory, and attentional-interactional systems) in an infant that is satisfactory but that can be improved

Defining Characteristics

- Definite sleep-wake states
- Response to stimuli (e.g., visual, auditory)
- Stable physiologic measures
- Use of some self-regulatory behaviors

Related Factors

Pain
Prematurity

Ineffective Infant Feeding Pattern

Definition

Impaired ability of an infant to suck or coordinate the suck/swallow response resulting in inadequate oral nutrition for metabolic needs

Defining Characteristics

- Inability to coordinate sucking, swallowing, and breathing
- Inability to initiate an effective suck
- Inability to sustain an effective suck

Related Factors

Anatomic abnormality
Neurological delay
Neurological impairment
Oral hypersensitivity
Prematurity
Prolonged NPO status

References

Hazinski, M.F. (1992). *Nursing care of the critically ill child.* St. Louis, MO: Mosby.

Shaker, C.S. (1991). Nipple feeding premature infants: A different perspective. *Neonatal Network: The Journal of Neonatal Nursing, 8*(5), 9–17.

VandenBerg, K. (1990). Nippling management of the sick neonate in the NICU: The disorganized feeder. *Neonatal Network: The Journal of Neonatal Nursing, 9*(1), 9–16.

Risk for Infection

Definition

At increased risk for being invaded by pathogenic organisms

Risk Factors

Chronic disease
Inadequate acquired immunity
Inadequate primary defenses (broken skin, traumatized tissue, decrease in ciliary action, stasis of body fluids, change in pH secretions, altered peristalsis)
Inadequate secondary defenses (decreased hemoglobin, leukopenia, suppressed inflammatory response)
Increased environmental exposure to pathogens
Immunosuppression
Invasive procedures
Insufficient knowledge to avoid exposure to pathogens
Malnutrition
Pharmaceutical agents (e.g., immunosuppressants)
Rupture of amniotic membranes
Trauma
Tissue destruction

Risk for Injury

Definition

At risk of injury as a result of environmental conditions interacting with the individual's adaptive and defensive resources

Risk Factors

External

Biological (e.g., immunization level of community, microorganism)
Chemical (e.g., poisons, pollutants, drugs, pharmaceutical agents, alcohol, nicotine, preservatives, cosmetics, dyes)
Human (e.g., nosocomial agents; staffing patterns; cognitive, affective, psychomotor factors)
Mode of transport
Nutritional (e.g., vitamins, food types)
Physical (e.g., design, structure, and arrangement of community, building, and/or equipment)

Internal

Abnormal blood profile (e.g., leukocytosis/leukopenia, altered clotting factors, thrombocytopenia, sickle cell, thalassemia, decreased hemoglobin)
Biochemical dysfunction
Developmental age (physiological, psychosocial)
Effector dysfunction
Immune-autoimmune dysfunction
Integrative dysfunction
Malnutrition
Physical (e.g., broken skin, altered mobility)
Psychological (affective orientation)
Sensory dysfunction
Tissue hypoxia

RISK FOR PERIOPERATIVE-POSITIONING INJURY

Definition

At risk for inadvertent anatomical and physical changes as a result of posture or equipment used during an invasive/surgical procedure

Risk Factors

Disorientation
Edema
Emaciation
Immobilization
Muscle weakness
Obesity
Sensory/perceptual disturbances due to anesthesia

References

Ali, A., Breslin, D., Hardman, H., & Martin, G. (2003). Unusual presentation and complication of the prone position for spinal surgery. *Journal of Clinical Anesthesia, 15,* 471–473.

Fritzlen, T., Kremer, M., & Biddle, C. (2003). The AANA Foundation Closed Malpractice Claims Study on nerve injuries during anesthesia care. *AANA Journal, 71*, 347–352.

Litwiller, J., Wells, R. Jr, Halliwill, J., Carmichael, S., & Warner, M. (2004). Effect of lithotomy positions on strain of the obturator and lateral femoral cutaneous nerves. *Clinical Anatomy, 17,* 45–49.

Insomnia*

Definition

A disruption in amount and quality of sleep that impairs functioning

Defining Characteristics

- Observed changes in affect
- Observed lack of energy
- Increased work/school absenteeism
- Patient reports changes in mood
- Patient reports decreased health status
- Patient reports decreased quality of life
- Patient reports difficulty concentrating
- Patient reports difficulty falling asleep
- Patient reports difficulty staying asleep
- Patient reports dissatisfaction with sleep (current)
- Patient reports increased accidents
- Patient reports lack of energy
- Patient reports non-restorative sleep
- Patient reports sleep disturbances that produce next-day consequences
- Patient reports waking up too early

Related Factors

Activity pattern (e.g., timing, amount)
Anxiety
Depression
Environmental factors (e.g., ambient noise, daylight/darkness exposure, ambient temperature/humidity, unfamiliar setting)
Fear
Gender-related hormonal shifts
Grief
Inadequate sleep hygiene (current)
Intake of stimulants
Intake of alcohol
Impairment of normal sleep pattern (e.g., travel, shift work, parental responsibilities, interruptions for interventions)
Medications
Physical discomfort (e.g., body temperature, pain, shortness of breath, cough, gastroesophageal reflux, nausea, incontinence/urgency)
Stress (e.g., ruminative pre-sleep pattern)

**Previously titled "Disturbed Sleep Pattern"*

References

Linton, S., & Bryngelsson, I. (2000). Insomnia and its relationship to work and health in a working-age population. *Journal of Occupational Rehabilitation, 10,* 169–183.

Sateia, M., & Nowell, P. (2004). Insomnia. *Lancet, 364,* 1959–1973.

Walsh, J. (1999). Insomnia: Prevalence and clinical and public health considerations. *Family Practice Recertification, 21*(10), 4–11.

Decreased Intracranial Adaptive Capacity

Definition

Intracranial fluid dynamic mechanisms that normally compensate for increases in intracranial volumes are compromised, resulting in repeated disproportionate increases in intracranial pressure (ICP) in response to a variety of noxious and nonnoxious stimuli

Defining Characteristics

- Baseline ICP ≤10 mm Hg
- Disproportionate increase in ICP following stimulus
- Elevated P_2 ICP wave form
- Repeated increases of >10 mm Hg for more than 5 minutes following any of a variety of external stimuli
- Volume pressure response test variation (volume-pressure ratio 2, pressure-volume index <10)
- Wide amplitude ICP wave form

Related Factors

Brain injuries
Decreased cerebral perfusion ≤50–60 mm Hg
Sustained increase in ICP = 10–15 mm Hg
Systemic hypotension with intracranial hypertension

Deficient Knowledge (Specify)

Definition

Absence or deficiency of cognitive information related to a specific topic

Defining Characteristics

- Exaggerated behaviors
- Inaccurate follow through of instruction
- Inaccurate performance of test
- Inappropriate behaviors (e.g., hysterical, hostile, agitated, apathetic)
- Verbalization of the problem

Related Factors

Cognitive limitation
Information misinterpretation
Lack of exposure
Lack of interest in learning
Lack of recall
Unfamiliarity with information resources

Readiness for Enhanced Knowledge

Definition

The presence or acquisition of cognitive information related to a specific topic is sufficient for meeting health-related goals and can be strengthened

Defining Characteristics

- Behaviors congruent with expressed knowledge
- Explains knowledge of the topic
- Expresses an interest in learning
- Describes previous experiences pertaining to the topic

SEDENTARY LIFESTYLE

Definition

Reports a habit of life that is characterized by a low physical activity level

Defining Characteristics

- Chooses a daily routine lacking physical exercise
- Demonstrates physical deconditioning
- Verbalizes preference for activities low in physical activity

Risk Factors

Deficient knowledge of health benefits of physical exercise
Lack of interest
Lack of motivation
Lack of resources (time, money, companionship, facilities)
Lack of training for accomplishment of physical exercise

RISK FOR IMPAIRED LIVER FUNCTION

Definition

At risk for liver dysfunction

Risk Factors

- Hepatotoxic medications (e.g., acetaminophen, statins)
- HIV co-infection
- Substance abuse (e.g., alcohol, cocaine)
- Viral infection (e.g., hepatitis A, hepatitis B, hepatitis C, Epstein-Barr)

References

AASLD Practice Guideline. (2004). *Diagnosis, management, and treatment of hepatitis C.* Alexandria, VA: American Association for the Study of Liver Diseases.

Hoofnagle, J.H., & Seeff, L.B. (2002). National Institute of Health consensus development conference: Management of hepatitis C. *Hepatology* (Suppl. 1), 1–20.

Palmer, M. (2000). *Hepatitis liver disease: What you need to know.* Garden City Park, NY, Avery Publishing Group.

RISK FOR LONELINESS

Definition

At risk for experiencing discomfort associated with a desire or need for more contact with others

Risk Factors

Affectional deprivation
Cathectic deprivation
Physical isolation
Social isolation

References

Leiderman, P.H. (1969). Loneliness: A psychodynamic interpretation. In E.S. Scheidman & M.J. Ortega (Eds.), *Aspects of depression: International psychiatry clinics, 6,* 155–174. Boston: Little, Brown.

Lien-Gieschen, T. (1993). Validation of social isolation related to maturational age: Elderly. *Nursing Diagnosis, 4*(1), 37–44.

Warren, B.J. (1993). Explaining social isolation through concept analysis. *Archives of Psychiatric Nursing, 7,* 270–276.

Impaired Memory

Definition

Inability to remember or recall bits of information or behavioral skills

Defining Characteristics

- Experience of forgetting
- Forgets to perform a behavior at a scheduled time
- Inability to determine if a behavior was performed
- Inability to learn new information
- Inability to learn new skills
- Inability to perform a previously learned skill
- Inability to recall events
- Inability to recall factual information
- Inability to retain new information
- Inability to retain new skills

Related Factors

Anemia
Decreased cardiac output
Excessive environmental disturbances
Fluid and electrolyte imbalance
Hypoxia
Neurological disturbances

Impaired Bed Mobility

Definition

Limitation of independent movement from one bed position to another

Defining Characteristics

- Impaired ability to move from supine to sitting
- Impaired ability to move from sitting to supine
- Impaired ability to move from supine to prone
- Impaired ability to move from prone to supine
- Impaired ability to move from supine to long sitting
- Impaired ability to move from long sitting to supine
- Impaired ability to "scoot" or reposition self in bed
- Impaired ability to turn from side to side

Related Factors

Cognitive impairment
Deconditioning
Deficient knowledge
Environmental constraints (e.g., bed size, bed type, treatment equipment, restraints)
Insufficient muscle strength
Musculoskeletal impairment
Neuromuscular impairment
Obesity
Pain
Sedating medications

Note. Specify level of independence using a standardized funtional scale.

References

Brouwer, K., Nysseknabm, J., & Culham E. (2004). Physical function and health status among seniors with and without fear of falling. *Gerontology, 50,* 15–141.

Lewis, C.L., Moutoux, M., Slaughter, M., & Bailey, S.P. (2004). Characteristics of individuals who fell while receiving home health services. *Physical Therapy, 84*(1), 23–32.

Tinetti., M.E., & Ginter, S.F. (1988). Identifying mobility dysfunction in elderly persons. *Journal of the American Medical Association, 259,* 1190–1193.

Impaired Physical Mobility

Definition

Limitation in independent, purposeful physical movement of the body or of one or more extremities

Defining Characteristics

- Decreased reaction time
- Difficulty turning
- Engages in substitutions for movement (e.g., increased attention to other's activity, controlling behavior, focus on pre-illness disability/activity)
- Exertional dyspnea
- Gait changes
- Jerky movements
- Limited ability to perform gross motor skills
- Limited ability to perform fine motor skills
- Limited range of motion
- Movement-induced tremor
- Postural instability
- Slowed movement
- Uncoordinated movements

Related Factors

Activity intolerance
Altered cellular metabolism
Anxiety
Body mass index above 75th age-appropriate percentile
Cognitive impairment
Contractures
Cultural beliefs regarding age-appropriate activity
Deconditioning
Decreased endurance
Depressive mood state
Decreased muscle control
Decreased muscle mass
Decreased muscle strength
Deficient knowledge regarding value of physical activity
Developmental delay
Discomfort
Disuse
Joint stiffness
Lack of environmental supports (e.g., physical or social)
Limited cardiovascular endurance
Loss of integrity of bone structures

Malnutrition
Medications
Musculoskeletal impairment
Neuromuscular impairment
Pain
Prescribed movement restrictions
Reluctance to initiate movement
Sedentary lifestyle
Sensoriperceptual impairments

Note. Specify level of independence using a standardized functional scale.

IMPAIRED WHEELCHAIR MOBILITY

Definition

Limitation of independent operation of wheelchair within environment

Defining Characteristics

- Impaired ability to operate manual wheelchair on curbs
- Impaired ability to operate power wheelchair on curbs
- Impaired ability to operate manual wheelchair on even surface
- Impaired ability to operate power wheelchair on even surface
- Impaired ability to operate manual wheelchair on uneven surface
- Impaired ability to operate power wheelchair on uneven surface
- Impaired ability to operate manual wheelchair on an incline
- Impaired ability to operate power wheelchair on an incline
- Impaired ability to operate manual wheelchair on a decline
- Impaired ability to operate power wheelchair on a decline

Related Factors

Cognitive impairment
Deconditioning
Deficient knowledge
Depressed mood
Environmental constraints (e.g., stairs, inclines, uneven surfaces, unsafe obstacles, distances, lack of assistive devices or person, wheelchair type)
Impaired vision
Insufficient muscle strength
Limited endurance
Musculoskeletal impairment (e.g., contractures)
Neuromuscular impairment
Obesity
Pain

Note. Specify level of independence using a standardized functional scale.

References

Brouwer, K., Nysseknabm, J., & Culham E. (2004). Physical function and health status among seniors with and without fear of falling. *Gerontology, 50,* 15–141.

Lewis, C.L., Moutoux, M., Slaughter, M., & Bailey, S.P. (2004). Characteristics of individuals who fell while receiving home health services. *Physical Therapy, 84*(1), 23–32.

Tinetti., M.E., & Ginter, S.F. (1988). Identifying mobility dysfunction in elderly persons. *Journal of the American Medical Association, 259,* 1190–1193.

Nausea

Definition

A subjective unpleasant, wavelike sensation in the back of the throat, epigastrium, or abdomen that may lead to the urge or need to vomit

Defining Characteristics

- Aversion toward food
- Gagging sensation
- Increased salivation
- Increased swallowing
- Report of nausea
- Sour taste in mouth

Related Factors

Biophysical

Biochemical disorders (e.g., uremia, diabetic ketoacidosis, pregnancy)
Esophageal disease
Gastric distention
Gastric irritation
Increased intracranial pressure
Intra-abdominal tumors
Labyrinthitis
Liver capsule stretch
Localized tumors (e.g., acoustic neuroma, primary or secondary brain tumors, bone metastases at base of skull)
Meningitis
Ménière's disease
Motion sickness
Pain
Pancreatic disease
Splenetic capsule stretch
Toxins (e.g., tumor-produced peptides, abnormal metabolites due to cancer)

Situational

Anxiety
Fear
Noxious odors
Noxious taste
Pain
Psychological factors
Unpleasant visual stimulation

Treatment

Gastric distention
Gastric irritation
Pharmaceuticals

Unilateral Neglect

Definition

Impairment in sensory and motor response, mental representation, and spatial attention of the body and the corresponding environment characterized by inattention to one side and overattention to the opposite side. Left side neglect is more severe and persistent than right side neglect.

Defining Characteristics

- Appears unaware of positioning of neglected limb
- Difficulty remembering details of internally represented familiar scenes that are on the neglected side
- Displacement of sounds to the non-neglected side
- Distortion of drawing on the half of the page on the neglected side
- Failure to cancel lines on the half of the page on the neglected side
- Failure to eat food from portion of the plate on the neglected side
- Failure to dress neglected side
- Failure to groom neglected side
- Failure to move eyes in the neglected hemispace despite being aware of a stimulus in that space
- Failure to move head in the neglected hemispace despite being aware of a stimulus in that space
- Failure to move limbs in the neglected hemispace despite being aware of a stimulus in that space
- Failure to move trunk in the neglected hemispace despite being aware of a stimulus in that space
- Failure to notice people approaching from the neglected side
- Lack of safety precautions with regard to the neglected side
- Marked deviation* of the eyes to the non-neglected side to stimuli and activities on that side
- Marked deviation* of the head to the non-neglected side to stimuli and activities on that side
- Marked deviation* of the trunk to the non-neglected side to stimuli and activities on that side
- Omission of drawing on the half of the page on the neglected side
- Perseveration of visual motor tasks on non-neglected side
- Substitution of letters to form alternative words that are similar to the original in length when reading
- Transfer of pain sensation to the non-neglected side
- Use of only vertical half of page when writing

Related Factors

Brain injury from cerebrovascular problems
Brain injury from neurological illness
Brain injury from trauma
Brain injury from tumor
Left hemiplegia from
CVA of the right hemisphere
Hemianopsia

* As if drawn magnetically to stimuli and activities on that side

References

Rusconi, M.L., Maravita, A., Bottini, G., & Vallar, G. (2002). Is the intact side really intact? Perseverative responses in patients with unilateral neglect: A productive manifestation. *Neuropsychologia, 40,* 594–604.

Swan, L. (2001). Unilateral spatial neglect. *Physical Therapy, 81,* 1572–1580.

Weitzel, E.A. (2001); Unilateral neglect. In M. Maas, K. Buckwalter, M. Hardy, T. Tripp-Reimer, M. Titler, & J. Specht (Eds.), *Nursing care of older adults: Diagnosis, outcomes, and interventions* (pp. 492–502): St. Louis: Mosby Inc.

NONCOMPLIANCE

Definition

Behavior of person and/or caregiver that fails to coincide with a health-promoting or therapeutic plan agreed on by the person (and/or family and/or community) and health-care professional. In the presence of an agreed-on, health-promoting or therapeutic plan, person's or caregiver's behavior is fully or partially nonadherent and may lead to clinically ineffective or partially ineffective outcomes.

Defining Characteristics

- Behavior indicative of failure to adhere
- Evidence of development of complications
- Evidence of exacerbation of symptoms
- Failure to keep appointments
- Failure to progress
- Objective tests (e.g., physiological measures, detection of physiologic markers)

Related Factors

Health System

Access to care
Client/provider relationships
Communication skills of the provider
Convenience of care
Credibility of provider
Individual health coverage
Provider continuity
Provider regular follow-up
Provider reimbursement
Satisfaction with care
Teaching skills of the provider

Health-care Plan

Complexity
Cost
Duration
Financial flexibility of plan
Intensity

Individual

Cultural influences
Developmental abilities
Health beliefs
Individual's value system
Knowledge relevant to the regimen behavior
Motivational forces
Personal abilities
Significant others
Skill relevant to the regimen behavior
Spiritual values

Network

Involvement of members in health plan
Perceived beliefs of significant others
Social value regarding plan

IMBALANCED NUTRITION: LESS THAN BODY REQUIREMENTS

Definition

Intake of nutrients insufficient to meet metabolic needs

Defining Characteristics

- Abdominal cramping
- Abdominal pain
- Aversion to eating
- Body weight 20% or more under ideal
- Capillary fragility
- Diarrhea
- Excessive loss of hair
- Hyperactive bowel sounds
- Lack of food
- Lack of information
- Lack of interest in food
- Loss of weight with adequate food intake
- Misconceptions
- Misinformation
- Pale mucous membranes
- Perceived inability to ingest food
- Poor muscle tone
- Reported altered taste sensation
- Reported food intake less than RDA (recommended daily allowance)
- Satiety immediately after ingesting food
- Sore buccal cavity
- Steatorrhea
- Weakness of muscles required for swallowing or mastication

Related Factors

Biological factors
Economic factors
Inability to absorb nutrients
Inability to digest food
Inability to ingest food
Psychological factors

IMBALANCED NUTRITION: MORE THAN BODY REQUIREMENTS

Definition

Intake of nutrients that exceeds metabolic needs

Defining Characteristics

- Concentrating food intake at the end of the day
- Dysfunctional eating pattern (e.g., pairing food with other activities)

- Eating in response to external cues (e.g., time of day, social situation)
- Eating in response to internal cues other than hunger (e.g., anxiety)
- Sedentary activity level
- Triceps skin fold >25 mm in women, >15 mm in men
- Weight 20% over ideal for height and frame

Related Factors

Excessive intake in relation to metabolic need

READINESS FOR ENHANCED NUTRITION

Definition

A pattern of nutrient intake that is sufficient for meeting metabolic needs and can be strengthened

Defining Characteristics

- Attitude toward drinking is congruent with health goals
- Attitude toward eating is congruent with health goals
- Consumes adequate fluid
- Consumes adequate food
- Eats regularly
- Expresses knowledge of healthy fluid choices
- Expresses knowledge of healthy food choices
- Expresses willingness to enhance nutrition
- Follows an appropriate standard for intake (e.g., the food pyramid or American Dietetic Association guidelines)
- Safe preparation for fluids
- Safe preparation for food
- Safe storage for food and fluids

RISK FOR IMBALANCED NUTRITION: MORE THAN BODY REQUIREMENTS

Definition

At risk for an intake of nutrients that exceeds metabolic needs

Risk Factors

Concentrating food intake at end of day
Dysfunctional eating patterns
Eating in response to external cues (e.g., time of day, social situation)
Eating in response to internal cues other than hunger (e.g., anxiety)
Higher baseline weight at beginning of each pregnancy
Observed use of food as comfort measure
Observed use of food as reward
Pairing food with other activities
Parental obesity
Rapid transition across growth percentiles in children
Reported use of solid food as major food source before 5 months of age

IMPAIRED ORAL MUCOUS MEMBRANE

Definition

Disruption of the lips and soft tissue of the oral cavity

Defining Characteristics

- Bleeding
- Cheilitis
- Coated tongue
- Desquamation
- Difficult speech
- Difficulty eating
- Difficulty swallowing
- Diminished taste
- Edema
- Enlarged tonsils
- Fissures
- Geographic tongue
- Gingival hyperplasia
- Gingival pallor
- Gingival recession
- Halitosis
- Hyperemia
- Macroplasia
- Mucosal denudation
- Mucosal pallor
- Nodules
- Oral discomfort
- Oral lesions
- Oral pain
- Oral ulcers
- Papules
- Pocketing deeper than 4 mm
- Presence of pathogens
- Purulent drainage
- Purulent exudates
- Red or bluish masses (e.g., hemangiomas)
- Reports bad taste in mouth
- Smooth atrophic tongue
- Spongy patches
- Stomatitis
- Vesicles
- White, curd-like exudate
- White patches/plaques
- Xerostomia

Related Factors

Barriers to oral self-care
Barriers to professional care
Chemotherapy
Chemical irritants (e.g., alcohol, tobacco, acidic foods, drugs, regular use of inhalers or other noxious agents)
Cleft lip
Cleft palate
Decreased platelets

Decreased salivation
Deficient knowledge of appropriate oral hygiene
Dehydration
Depression
Diminished hormone levels (women)
Ineffective oral hygiene
Infection
Immunocompromised
Immunosuppression
Loss of supportive structures
Malnutrition
Mechanical factors (e.g., ill-fitting dentures, braces, tubes [endotracheal/nasogastric], surgery in oral cavity)
Medication side effects
Mouth breathing
NPO for more than 24 hours
Radiation therapy
Stress
Trauma

ACUTE PAIN

Definition

Unpleasant sensory and emotional experience arising from actual or potential tissue damage or described in terms of such damage (International Association for the Study of Pain); sudden or slow onset of any intensity from mild to severe with an anticipated or predictable end and a duration of less than 6 months

Defining Characteristics

- Change in muscle tone (may span from listless to rigid)
- Changes in appetite
- Changes in blood pressure
- Changes in heart rate
- Changes in respiratory rate
- Coded report
- Diaphoresis
- Distraction behavior (e.g., pacing, seeking out other people and/or activities, repetitive activities)
- Expressive behavior (e.g., restlessness, moaning, crying, vigilance, irritability, sighing)
- Facial mask
- Guarding behavior
- Narrowed focus (altered time perception, impaired thought processes, reduced interaction with people and environment)
- Observed evidence of pain
- Positioning to avoid pain
- Protective gestures
- Pupillary dilation
- Self-focus
- Sleep disturbance (eyes lack luster, beaten look, fixed or scattered movement, grimace)
- Verbal report of pain

Related Factors

Injury agents (biological, chemical, physical, psychological)

Chronic Pain

Definition

Unpleasant sensory and emotional experience arising from actual or potential tissue damage or described in terms of such damage (International Association for the Study of Pain); sudden or slow onset of any intensity from mild to severe, constant or recurring without an anticipated or predictable end and a duration of greater than 6 months

Defining Characteristics

- Altered ability to continue previous activities
- Anorexia
- Atrophy of involved muscle group
- Changes in sleep pattern
- Coded report
- Depression
- Facial mask
- Fatigue
- Fear of reinjury
- Guarding behavior
- Irritability
- Observed protective behavior
- Reduced interaction with people
- Restlessness
- Self-focusing
- Sympathetic mediated responses (e.g., temperature, cold, changes of body position, hypersensitivity)
- Verbal report of pain

Related Factors

Chronic physical disability
Chronic psychosocial disability

Readiness for Enhanced Parenting

Definition

A pattern of providing an environment for children or other dependent person(s) that is sufficient to nurture growth and development and can be strengthened

Defining Characteristics

- Children or other dependent person(s) express(es) satisfaction with home environment
- Emotional support of children
- Evidence of attachment
- Exhibits realistic expectations of children
- Expresses willingness to enhance parenting
- Needs of children are met (e.g., physical and emotional)

Impaired Parenting

Definition

Inability of the primary caretaker to create, maintain, or regain an environment that promotes the optimum growth and development of the child

Defining Characteristics

Infant or Child

- Behavioral disorders
- Failure to thrive
- Frequent accidents
- Frequent illness
- Incidence of abuse
- Incidence of trauma (e.g., physical and psychological)
- Lack of attachment
- Lack of separation anxiety
- Poor academic performance
- Poor cognitive development
- Poor social competence
- Runaway

Parental

- Abandonment
- Child abuse
- Child neglect
- Frequently punitive
- Hostility to child
- Inadequate attachment
- Inadequate child health maintenance
- Inappropriate caretaking skills
- Inappropriate stimulation (e.g., visual, tactile, auditory)
- Inappropriate child care arrangements
- Inconsistent behavior management
- Inconsistent care
- Inflexibility in meeting needs of child
- Little cuddling
- Maternal-child interaction deficit
- Negative statements about child
- Poor parent-child interaction
- Rejection of child
- Statements of inability to meet child's needs
- Unsafe home environment
- Verbalization of inability to control child
- Verbalization of frustration
- Verbalization of role inadequacy

Related Factors

Infant or Child

Altered perceptual abilities
Attention deficit hyperactivity disorder
Developmental delay
Difficult temperament
Handicapping condition
Illness
Multiple births

Not desired gender
Premature birth
Separation from parent
Temperamental conflicts with parental expectations

Knowledge

Deficient knowledge about child development
Deficient knowledge about child health maintenance
Deficient knowledge about parenting skills
Inability to respond to infant cues
Lack of cognitive readiness for parenthood
Lack of education
Limited cognitive functioning
Poor communication skills
Preference for physical punishment
Unrealistic expectations

Physiological

Physical illness

Psychological

Closely spaced pregnancies
Depression
Difficult birthing process
Disability
High number of pregnancies
History of mental illness
History of substance abuse
Lack of prenatal care
Sleep deprivation
Sleep disruption
Young parental age

Social

Change in family unit
Chronic low self-esteem
Father of child not involved
Financial difficulties
History of being abused
History of being abusive
Inability to put child's needs before own
Inadequate child care arrangements
Job problems
Lack of family cohesiveness
Lack of parental role model
Lack of resources
Lack of social support networks
Lack of transportation
Lack of valuing of parenthood
Legal difficulties
Low socioeconomic class

Maladaptive coping strategies
Marital conflict
Mother of child not involved
Single parent
Social isolation
Poor home environment
Poor parental role model
Poor problem-solving skills
Poverty
Presence of stress (e.g., financial, legal, recent crisis, cultural move)
Relocations
Role strain
Situational low self-esteem
Unemployment
Unplanned pregnancy
Unwanted pregnancy

RISK FOR IMPAIRED PARENTING

Definition

Risk for inability of the primary caretaker to create, maintain, or regain an environment that promotes the optimum growth and development of the child

Risk Factors

Infant or Child

Altered perceptual abilities
Attention deficit hyperactivity disorder
Developmental delay
Difficult temperament
Handicapping condition
Illness
Multiple births
Not gender desired
Premature birth
Prolonged separation from parent
Temperamental conflicts with parental expectation

Knowledge

Deficient knowledge about child development
Deficient knowledge about child health maintenance
Deficient knowledge about parenting skills
Inability to respond to infant cues
Lack of cognitive readiness for parenthood
Low cognitive functioning
Low educational level or attainment
Poor communication skills
Preference for physical punishment
Unrealistic expectations of child

Physiological

Physical illness

Psychological

Closely spaced pregnancies
Depression
Difficult birthing process
Disability
High number of pregnancies
History of mental illness
History of substance abuse
Sleep deprivation
Sleep disruption
Young parental age

Social

Change in family unit
Chronic low self-esteem
Father of child not involved
Financial difficulties
History of being abused
History of being abusive
Inadequate child care arrangements
Job problems
Lack of access to resources
Lack of family cohesiveness
Lack of parental role model
Lack of prenatal care
Lack of resources
Lack of social support network
Lack of transportation
Lack of valuing of parenthood
Late prenatal care
Legal difficulties
Low socioeconomic class
Maladaptive coping strategies
Marital conflict
Mother of child not involved
Parent-child separation
Poor home environment
Poor parental role model
Poor problem-solving skills
Poverty
Role strain
Single parent
Situational low self-esteem
Social isolation
Stress
Relocation
Unemployment
Unplanned pregnancy
Unwanted pregnancy

Risk for Peripheral Neurovascular Dysfunction

Definition

At risk for disruption in circulation, sensation, or motion of an extremity

Risk Factors

Burns
Fractures
Immobilization
Mechanical compression (e.g., tourniquet, cane, cast, brace, dressing, restraint)
Orthopedic surgery
Trauma
Vascular obstruction

Risk for Poisoning

Definition

Accentuated risk of accidental exposure to, or ingestion of, drugs or dangerous products in doses sufficient to cause poisoning

Risk Factors

External

Availability of illicit drugs potentially contaminated by poisonous additives
Dangerous products placed within reach of children
Dangerous products placed within reach of confused individuals
Large supplies of drugs in house
Medicines stored in unlocked cabinets accessible to children
Medicines stored in unlocked cabinets accessible to confused individuals

Internal

Cognitive difficulties
Emotional difficulties
Lack of drug education
Lack of proper precaution
Lack of safety education
Reduced vision
Verbalization that occupational setting is without adequate safeguards

Reference

Centers for Disease Control & Prevention. (2005). *Third national report on human exposure to environmental chemicals: Executive summary* (NCEH Pub # 05-0725). Atlanta: Author.

Post-Trauma Syndrome

Definition

Sustained maladaptive response to a traumatic, overwhelming event

Defining Characteristics

- Aggression
- Alienation
- Altered mood states
- Anger

- Anxiety
- Avoidance
- Compulsive behavior
- Denial
- Depression
- Detachment
- Difficulty concentrating
- Enuresis (in children)
- Exaggerated startle response
- Fear
- Flashbacks
- Gastric irritability
- Grieving
- Guilt
- Headaches
- Hopelessness
- Horror
- Hypervigilance
- Intrusive dreams
- Intrusive thoughts
- Irritability
- Neurosensory irritability
- Nightmares
- Palpitations
- Panic attacks
- Psychogenic amnesia
- Rage
- Rape
- Reports feeling numb
- Repression
- Shame
- Substance abuse

Related Factors

Abuse (physical and psychosocial)
Being held prisoner of war
Criminal victimization
Disasters
Epidemics
Events outside the range of usual human experience
Serious accidents (e.g., industrial, motor vehicle)
Serious injury to loved ones
Serious injury to self
Serious threat to loved ones
Serious threat to self
Sudden destruction of one's community
Sudden destruction of one's home
Torture
Tragic occurrence involving multiple deaths

Wars
Witnessing mutilation
Witnessing violent death

RISK FOR POST-TRAUMA SYNDROME

Definition

At risk for sustained maladaptive response to a traumatic, overwhelming event

Risk Factors

Diminished ego strength
Displacement from home
Duration of the event
Exaggerated sense of responsibility
Inadequate social support
Nonsupportive environment
Occupation (e.g., police, fire, rescue, corrections, emergency room staff, mental health worker)
Perception of event
Survivor's role in the event

READINESS FOR ENHANCED POWER

Definition

A pattern of participating knowingly in change that is sufficient for well-being and can be strengthened

Defining Characteristics

- Expresses readiness to enhance awareness of possible changes to be made
- Expresses readiness to enhance freedom to perform actions for change
- Expresses readiness to enhance identification of choices that can be made for change
- Expresses readiness to enhance involvement in creating change
- Expresses readiness to enhance knowledge for participation in change
- Expresses readiness to enhance participation in choices for daily living & health
- Expresses readiness to enhance power

References

Jeng, C., Yang, S., Chang, P., & Tsao, L. (2004). Menopausal women: Perceiving continuous power through the experience of regular exercise. *Journal of Clinical Nursing, 13,* 447–454.

Shearer, N., & Reed, P. (2004). Empowerment: Reformulation of a non-Rogerian concept. *Nursing Science Quarterly, 17,* 253–259.

Wright, B. (2004). Trust and power in adults: An investigation using Rogers' science of unitary human beings. *Nursing Science Quarterly, 17,* 139–146.

Note. Even though power (a response) and empowerment (an intervention approach) are different concepts, the literature related to both concepts supports the defining characteristics of this diagnosis.

POWERLESSNESS

Definition

Perception that one's own action will not significantly affect an outcome; a perceived lack of control over a current situation or immediate happening

Defining Characteristics

Low

- Expressions of uncertainty about fluctuating energy levels
- Passivity

Moderate

- Anger
- Dependence on others that may result in irritability
- Does not defend self-care practices when challenged
- Does not monitor progress
- Expressions of dissatisfaction over inability to perform previous tasks/activities
- Expressions of doubt regarding role performance
- Expressions of frustration over inability to perform previous tasks/activities
- Fear of alienation from caregivers
- Guilt
- Inability to seek information regarding care
- Nonparticipation in care when opportunities are provided
- Nonparticipation in decision making when opportunities are provided
- Passivity
- Reluctance to express true feelings
- Resentment

Severe

- Apathy
- Depression over physical deterioration
- Verbal expressions of having no control (e.g., over self-care, situation, outcome)

Related Factors

Health-care environment
Illness-related regimen
Interpersonal interaction
Lifestyle of helplessness

RISK FOR POWERLESSNESS

Definition

At risk for perceived lack of control over a situation and/or one's ability to significantly affect an outcome

Risk Factors

Physiological

Acute injury
Aging
Dying
Illness
Progressive debilitating disease process (e.g., spinal cord injury, multiple sclerosis)

Psychosocial

Absence of integrality (e.g., essence of power)
Chronic low self-esteem
Deficient knowledge (e.g., of illness or health-care system)
Disturbed body image

Inadequate coping patterns
Lifestyle of dependency
Situational low self-esteem

Ineffective Protection

Definition

Decrease in the ability to guard self from internal or external threats such as illness or injury

Defining Characteristics

- Altered clotting
- Anorexia
- Chilling
- Cough
- Deficient immunity
- Disorientation
- Dyspnea
- Fatigue
- Immobility
- Impaired healing
- Insomnia
- Itching
- Maladaptive stress response
- Neurosensory alteration
- Perspiring
- Pressure ulcers
- Restlessness
- Weakness

Related Factors

Abnormal blood profiles (e.g., leukopenia, thrombocytopenia, anemia, coagulation)
Alcohol abuse
Cancer
Drug therapies (e.g., antineoplastic, corticosteroid, immune, anticoagulant, thrombolytic)
Extremes of age
Immune disorders
Inadequate nutrition
Treatments (e.g., surgery, radiation)

Rape-Trauma Syndrome

Definition

Sustained maladaptive response to a forced, violent sexual penetration against the victim's will and consent

Defining Characteristics

- Aggression
- Agitation
- Anger
- Anxiety
- Change in relationships
- Confusion
- Denial

- Dependence
- Depression
- Disorganization
- Dissociative disorders
- Embarrassment
- Fear
- Guilt
- Helplessness
- Humiliation
- Hyperalertness
- Impaired decision making
- Loss of self-esteem
- Mood swings
- Muscle spasms
- Muscle tension
- Nightmares
- Paranoia
- Phobias
- Physical trauma
- Powerlessness
- Revenge
- Self-blame
- Sexual dysfunction
- Shame
- Shock
- Sleep disturbances
- Substance abuse
- Suicide attempts
- Vulnerability

Related Factors

Rape

Note. This syndrome includes the following three subcomponents: Rape-Trauma, Compound Reaction, and Silent Reaction. In this text each appears as a separate diagnosis.

RAPE-TRAUMA SYNDROME: COMPOUND REACTION

Definition

Forced violent sexual penetration against the victim's will and consent. The trauma syndrome that develops from this attack or attempted attack includes an acute phase of disorganization of the victim's lifestyle and a long-term process of reorganization of lifestyle.

Defining Characteristics

- Change in lifestyle (e.g., changes in residence, dealing with repetitive nightmares and phobias, seeking family support, seeking social network support in long-term phase)
- Emotional reaction (e.g., anger, embarrassment, fear of physical violence and death, humiliation, revenge, self-blame in acute phase)
- Multiple physical symptoms (e.g., gastrointestinal irritability, genitourinary discomfort, muscle tension, sleep pattern disturbance in acute phase)
- Reactivated symptoms of previous conditions (e.g., physical illness, psychiatric illness in acute phase)
- Substance abuse (acute phase)

Related Factors

To be developed

Note. This syndrome includes the following three subcomponents: Rape-Trauma, Compound Reaction, and Silent Reaction. In this text, each appears as a separate diagnosis. This diagnosis will retire from the NANDA-I Taxonomy in the 2009–2010 edition unless additional work is done to bring it to a LOE of 2.1 or higher.

RAPE-TRAUMA SYNDROME: SILENT REACTION

Definition

Forced violent sexual penetration against the victim's will and consent. The trauma syndrome that develops from this attack or attempted attack includes an acute phase of disorganization of the victim's lifestyle and a long-term process of reorganization of lifestyle.

Defining Characteristics

- Abrupt changes in relationships with men
- Increase in nightmares
- Increased anxiety during interview (e.g., blocking of associations, long periods of silence, minor stuttering, physical distress)
- No verbalization of the occurrence of rape
- Pronounced changes in sexual behavior
- Sudden onset of phobic reactions

Related Factors

To be developed

Note. This syndrome includes the following three subcomponents: Rape-Trauma, Compound Reaction, and Silent Reaction. In this text each appears as a separate diagnosis. This diagnosis will retire from the NANDA-I Taxonomy in the 2009–2010 edition unless additional work is done to bring it to a LOE of 2.1 or higher.

IMPAIRED RELIGIOSITY*

Definition

Impaired ability to exercise reliance on beliefs and/or participate in rituals of a particular faith tradition

Defining Characteristics

- Difficulty adhering to prescribed religious beliefs and rituals (e.g., religious ceremonies, dietary regulations, clothing, prayer, worship/religious services, private religious behaviors/reading religious materials/media, holiday observances, meetings with religious leaders)
- Expresses emotional distress because of separation from faith community
- Expresses a need to reconnect with previous belief patterns
- Expresses a need to reconnect with previous customs
- Questions religious belief patterns
- Questions religious customs

Related Factors

Developmental & Situational

Aging
End-stage life crises
Life transitions

* *The DDC recognizes that the term "religiosity" may be culture specific; however, the term is useful in the U.S. and is well-supported in the U.S. literature.*

Physical

Illness
Pain

Psychological

Anxiety
Fear of death
Ineffective coping
Ineffective support
Lack of security
Personal crisis
Use of religion to manipulate

Sociocultural

Cultural barriers to practicing religion
Environmental barriers to practicing religion
Lack of social integration
Lack of sociocultural interaction

Spiritual

Spiritual crises
Suffering

READINESS FOR ENHANCED RELIGIOSITY*

Definition

Ability to increase reliance on religious beliefs and/or participate in rituals of a particular faith tradition

Defining Characteristics

- Expresses desire to strengthen religious belief patterns that had provided comfort in the past
- Expresses desire to strengthen religious belief patterns that had provided religion in the past
- Expresses desire to strengthen religious customs that had provided comfort in the past
- Expresses desire to strengthen religious customs that had provided religion in the past
- Questions belief patterns that are harmful
- Questions customs that are harmful
- Rejects belief patterns that are harmful
- Rejects customs that are harmful
- Requests assistance expanding religious options
- Request for assistance to increase participation in prescribed religious beliefs (e.g., religious ceremonies, dietary regulations/rituals, clothing, prayer, worship/religious services, private religious behaviors, reading religious materials/media, holiday observances)
- Requests forgiveness
- Requests meeting with religious leaders/facilitators
- Requests reconciliation
- Requests religious experiences
- Requests religious materials

** The DDC recognizes that the term "religiosity" may be culture specific; however, the term is useful in the U.S. and is well-supported in the U.S. literature.*

Risk for Impaired Religiosity*

Definition

At risk for an impaired ability to exercise reliance on religious beliefs and/or participate in rituals of a particular faith tradition

Related Factors

Developmental

Life transitions

Environmental

Barriers to practicing religion
Lack of transportation

Physical

Hospitalization
Illness
Pain

Psychological

Depression
Ineffective caregiving
Ineffective coping
Ineffective support
Lack of security

Sociocultural

Cultural barrier to practicing religion
Lack of social interaction
Social isolation

Spiritual

Suffering

* *The DDC recognizes that the term "religiosity" may be culture-specific; however, the term is useful in the U.S. and is well-supported in the U.S. literature.*

Relocation Stress Syndrome

Definition

Physiological and/or psychosocial disturbance following transfer from one environment to another

Defining Characteristics

- Alienation
- Aloneness
- Anger
- Anxiety (e.g., separation)
- Concern over relocation
- Dependency
- Depression
- Fear
- Frustration
- Increased illness
- Increased physical symptoms
- Increased verbalization of needs

- Insecurity
- Loneliness
- Loss of identity
- Loss of self-esteem
- Loss of self-worth
- Move from one environment to another
- Pessimism
- Sleep disturbance
- Unwillingness to move
- Withdrawal
- Worry

Related Factors

Decreased health status
Feelings of powerlessness
Unpredictability of experience
Impaired psychosocial health
Isolation
Lack of adequate support system
Lack of predeparture counseling
Language barrier
Losses
Passive coping

RISK FOR RELOCATION STRESS SYNDROME

Definition

At risk for physiological and/or psychosocial disturbance following transfer from one environment to another

Risk Factors

Decreased health status
Feelings of powerlessness
Lack of adequate support system
Lack of predeparture counseling
Losses
Moderate to high degree of environmental change
Moderate mental competence
Move from one environment to another
Passive coping
Unpredictability of experiences

INEFFECTIVE ROLE PERFORMANCE

Definition

Patterns of behavior and self-expression that do not match the environmental context, norms, and expectations

Defining Characteristics

- Altered role perceptions
- Anxiety
- Change in capacity to resume role

- Change in other's perception of role
- Change in self-perception of role
- Change in usual patterns of responsibility
- Deficient knowledge
- Depression
- Discrimination
- Domestic violence
- Harassment
- Inadequate adaptation to change
- Inadequate confidence
- Inadequate coping
- Inappropriate developmental expectations
- Inadequate external support for role enactment
- Inadequate motivation
- Inadequate opportunities for role enactment
- Inadequate role competency
- Inadequate self-management
- Inadequate skills
- Pessimism
- Powerlessness
- Role ambivalence
- Role confusion
- Role conflict
- Role denial
- Role dissatisfaction
- Role overload
- Role strain
- System conflict
- Uncertainty

Related Factors

Knowledge

Inadequate role model
Inadequate role preparation (e.g., role transition, skill rehearsal, validation)
Lack of education
Lack of role model
Unrealistic role expectations

Physiological

Body image alteration
Cognitive deficits
Depression
Fatigue
Low self-esteem
Mental illness
Neurological defects
Pain
Physical illness
Substance abuse

Social

Conflict
Developmental level
Domestic violence
Inadequate role socialization
Inadequate support system
Inappropriate linkage with the health-care system
Job schedule demands
Lack of resources
Lack of rewards
Low socioeconomic status
Stress
Young age

READINESS FOR ENHANCED SELF-CARE

Definition

A pattern of performing activities for oneself that helps to meet health-related goals and can be strengthened

Defining Characteristics

- Expresses desire to enhance independence in maintaining life
- Expresses desire to enhance independence in maintaining health
- Expresses desire to enhance independence in maintaining personal development
- Expresses desire to enhance independence in maintaining well-being
- Expresses desire to enhance knowledge of strategies for self-care
- Expresses desire to enhance responsibility for self-care
- Expresses desire to enhance self-care

References

Becker, G., Gates, R. J., & Newsom, E. (2004). Self-care among chronically ill African Americans: Culture, health disparities, and health insurance status. *American Journal of Public Health, 94,* 2066–2073.

Dashiff, C., Bartolucci, A., Wallander, J., & Abdullatif, H. (2005). The relationship of family structure, maternal employment, and family conflict with self-care adherence of adolescents with type 1 diabetes. *Families, Systems, & Health, 23*(1), 66–79.

Orem, D.E. (2001). *Nursing: Concepts and practice* (6th ed.) St. Louis: Mosby.

BATHING/HYGIENE SELF-CARE DEFICIT

Definition

Impaired ability to perform or complete bathing/hygiene activities for oneself

Defining Characteristics

- Inability to access bathroom
- Inability to dry body
- Inability to get bath supplies
- Inability to obtain water source
- Inability to regulate bath water
- Inability to wash body

Related Factors

Cognitive impairment
Decreased motivation

Environmental barriers
Inability to perceive body part
Inability to perceive spatial relationship
Musculoskeletal impairment
Neuromuscular impairment
Pain
Perceptual impairment
Severe anxiety
Weakness

Note. Specify level of independence using a standardized functional scale.

Dressing/Grooming Self-Care Deficit

Definition

Impaired ability to perform or complete dressing and grooming activities for self

Defining Characteristics

- Inability to choose clothing
- Inability to put clothing on lower body
- Inability to maintain appearancc at a satisfactory level
- Inability to pick up clothing
- Inability to put clothing on upper body
- Inability to put on shoes
- Inability to put on socks
- Inability to remove clothes
- Inability to use assistive devices
- Inability to use zippers
- Impaired ability to fasten clothing
- Impaired ability to obtain clothing
- Impaired ability to put on necessary items of clothing
- Impaired ability to take off necessary items of clothing

Rclatcd Factors

Cognitive impairment
Decreased motivation
Discomfort
Environmental barriers
Fatigue
Musculoskeletal impairment
Neuromuscular impairment
Pain
Perceptual impairment
Severe anxiety
Weakness

Note. Specify level of independence using a standardized functional scale.

Feeding Self-Care Deficit

Definition

Impaired ability to perform or complete feeding activities

Defining Characteristics

- Inability to bring food from a receptacle to the mouth
- Inability to chew food
- Inability to complete a meal
- Inability to get food onto utensil
- Inability to handle utensils
- Inability to ingest food in a socially acceptable manner
- Inability to ingest food safely
- Inability to ingest sufficient food
- Inability to manipulate food in mouth
- Inability to open containers
- Inability to pick up cup or glass
- Inability to prepare food for ingestion
- Inability to swallow food
- Inability to use assistive device

Related Factors

Cognitive impairment
Decreased motivation
Discomfort
Environmental barriers
Fatigue
Musculoskeletal impairment
Neuromuscular impairment
Pain
Perceptual impairment
Severe anxiety
Weakness

Note. Specify level of independence using a standardized functional scale.

TOILETING SELF-CARE DEFICIT

Definition

Impaired ability to perform or complete own toileting activities

Defining Characteristics

- Inability to carry out proper toilet hygiene
- Inability to flush toilet or commode
- Inability to get to toilet or commode
- Inability to manipulate clothing for toileting
- Inability to rise from toilet or commode
- Inability to sit on toilet or commode

Related Factors

Cognitive impairment
Decreased motivation
Environmental barriers
Fatigue
Impaired mobility status
Impaired transfer ability
Musculoskeletal impairment

Neuromuscular impairment
Pain
Perceptual impairment
Severe anxiety
Weakness

Note. Specify level of independence using a standardized functional scale.

Readiness for Enhanced Self-Concept

Definition

A pattern of perceptions or ideas about the self that is sufficient for well-being and can be strengthened

Defining Characteristics

- Accepts limitations
- Accepts strengths
- Actions are congruent with verbal expression
- Expresses confidence in abilities
- Expresses satisfaction with body image
- Expresses satisfaction with personal identity
- Expresses satisfaction with role performance
- Expresses satisfaction with sense of worthiness
- Expresses satisfaction with thoughts about self
- Expresses willingness to enhance self-concept

Chronic Low Self-Esteem

Definition

Long-standing negative self-evaluation/feelings about self or self-capabilities

Defining Characteristics

- Dependent on others' opinions
- Evaluates self as unable to deal with events
- Exaggerates negative feedback about self
- Excessively seeks reassurance
- Expressions of guilt
- Expressions of shame
- Frequent lack of success in life events
- Hesitant to try new things/situations
- Indecisive
- Lack of eye contact
- Nonassertive
- Overly conforming
- Passive
- Rejects positive feedback about self
- Self-negating verbalization

Related Factors

To be developed

Note. This diagnosis will retire from the NANDA-I Taxonomy in the 2009–2010 edition unless additional work is done to bring it to a LOE of 2.1 or higher.

Situational Low Self-Esteem

Definition

Development of a negative perception of self-worth in response to a current situation (specify)

Defining Characteristics

- Evaluation of self as unable to deal with situations or events
- Expressions of helplessness
- Expressions of uselessness
- Indecisive behavior
- Nonassertive behavior
- Self-negating verbalizations
- Verbally reports current situational challenge to self-worth

Related Factors

Behavior inconsistent with values
Developmental changes
Disturbed body image
Failures
Functional impairment
Lack of recognition
Loss
Rejections
Social role changes

Risk for Situational Low Self-Esteem

Definition

At risk for developing negative perception of self-worth in response to a current situation (specify)

Risk Factors

Behavior inconsistent with values
Decreased control over environment
Developmental changes
Disturbed body image
Failures
Functional impairment
History of abandonment
History of abuse
History of learned helplessness
History of neglect
Lack of recognition
Loss
Physical illness
Rejections
Social role changes
Unrealistic self-expectations

Self-Mutilation

Definition

Deliberate self-injurious behavior causing tissue damage with the intent of causing nonfatal injury to attain relief of tension

Defining Characteristics

- Abrading
- Biting
- Constricting a body part
- Cuts on body
- Hitting
- Ingestion of harmful substances
- Inhalation of harmful substances
- Insertion of object into body orifice
- Picking at wounds
- Scratches on body
- Self-inflicted burns
- Severing

Related Factors

Adolescence
Autistic individual
Battered child
Borderline personality disorder
Character disorder
Childhood illness
Childhood sexual abuse
Childhood surgery
Depersonalization
Developmentally delayed individual
Dissociation
Disturbed body image
Disturbed interpersonal relationships
Eating disorders
Emotionally disturbed
Family alcoholism
Family divorce
Family history of self-destructive behaviors
Feels threatened with loss of significant relationship
History of inability to plan solutions
History of inability to see long-term consequences
History of self-injurious behavior
Impulsivity
Inability to express tension verbally
Incarceration
Ineffective coping
Irresistible urge to cut/damage self
Isolation from peers
Labile behavior
Lack of family confidant
Living in nontraditional setting (e.g., foster group, or institutional care)
Low self-esteem
Mounting tension that is intolerable
Needs quick reduction of stress

Negative feelings (e.g., depression, rejection, self-hatred, separation anxiety, guilt, depersonalization)
Peers who self-mutilate
Perfectionism
Poor communication between parent and adolescent
Psychotic state (e.g., command hallucinations)
Sexual identity crisis
Substance abuse
Unstable body image
Unstable self-esteem
Use of manipulation to obtain nurturing relationship with others
Violence between parental figures

RISK FOR SELF-MUTILATION

Definition

At risk for deliberate self-injurious behavior causing tissue damage with the intent of causing nonfatal injury to attain relief of tension

Risk Factors

Adolescence
Autistic individuals
Battered child
Borderline personality disorders
Character disorders
Childhood illness
Childhood sexual abuse
Childhood surgery
Depersonalization
Developmentally delayed individuals
Dissociation
Disturbed body image
Disturbed interpersonal relationships
Eating disorders
Emotionally disturbed child
Family alcoholism
Family divorce
Family history of self-destructive behaviors
Feels threatened with loss of significant relationship
History of inability to plan solutions
History of inability to see long-term consequences
History of self-injurious behavior
Impulsivity
Inability to express tension verbally
Inadequate coping
Incarceration
Irresistible urge to damage self
Isolation from peers
Living in nontraditional setting (e.g., foster, group, or institutional care)
Loss of control over problem-solving situations
Low self-esteem

Loss of significant relationship(s)
Mounting tension that is intolerable
Needs quick reduction of stress setting (e.g., foster, group, or institutional care)
Negative feelings (e.g., depression, rejection, self-hatred, separation anxiety, guilt)
Peers who self-mutilate
Perfectionism
Psychotic state (e.g., command hallucinations)
Sexual identity crisis
Substance abuse
Unstable self-esteem
Use of manipulation to obtain nurturing relationship with others
Violence between parental figures

DISTURBED SENSORY PERCEPTION (SPECIFY: VISUAL, AUDITORY, KINESTHETIC, GUSTATORY, TACTILE, OLFACTORY)

Definition

Change in the amount or patterning of incoming stimuli accompanied by a diminished, exaggerated, distorted, or impaired response to such stimuli

Defining Characteristics

- Change in behavior pattern
- Change in problem-solving abilities
- Change in sensory acuity
- Change in usual response to stimuli
- Disorientation
- Hallucinations
- Impaired communication
- Irritability
- Poor concentration
- Restlessness
- Sensory distortions

Related Factors

Altered sensory integration
Altered sensory reception
Altered sensory transmission
Biochemical imbalance
Electrolyte imbalance
Excessive environmental stimuli
Insufficient environmental stimuli
Psychological stress

SEXUAL DYSFUNCTION

Definition

The state in which an individual experiences a change in sexual function during the sexual response phases of desire, excitation, and/or orgasm, which is viewed as unsatisfying, unrewarding or inadequate

Defining Characteristics

- Alterations in achieving sexual satisfaction
- Alterations in achieving perceived sex role

- Actual limitations imposed by disease
- Actual limitations imposed by therapy
- Change of interest in others
- Change of interest in self
- Inability to achieve desired satisfaction
- Perceived alteration in sexual excitation
- Perceived deficiency of sexual desire
- Perceived limitations imposed by disease
- Perceived limitations imposed by therapy
- Seeking confirmation of desirability
- Verbalization of problem

Related Factors

Absent role models
Altered body function (e.g., pregnancy, recent childbirth, drugs, surgery, anomalies, disease process, trauma, radiation)
Altered body structure (e.g., pregnancy, recent childbirth, surgery, anomalies, disease process, trauma, radiation)
Biopsychosocial alteration of sexuality
Ineffectual role models
Lack of privacy
Lack of significant other
Misinformation or lack of knowledge
Values conflict
Psychosocial abuse (e.g., harmful relationships)
Physical abuse
Vulnerability

References

Hogan, R.M. (1985). *Human sexuality–A nursing perspective.* New York: Appleton-Century-Crofts.
Kolodny, R C., Masters, W.H., & Johnson, V.E. (1979). *Textbook of sexual medicine.* Boston: Little, Brown.
Kaplan, H.S. (1983). *O desejo sexual e novos conceitos e técnicas da terapia do sexo.* Rio de Janeiro: Nova Fronteira.

INEFFECTIVE SEXUALITY PATTERN

Definition

Expressions of concern regarding own sexuality

Defining Characteristics

- Alterations in achieving perceived sex role
- Alteration in relationship with significant other
- Conflicts involving values
- Reported changes in sexual activities
- Reported changes in sexual behaviors
- Reported difficulties in sexual behaviors
- Reported difficulties in sexual activities
- Reported limitations in sexual behaviors
- Reported limitations in sexual activities

Related Factors

Absent role model
Conflicts with sexual orientation or variant preferences

Fear of acquiring a sexually transmitted disease
Fear of pregnancy
Impaired relationship with a significant other
Ineffective role model
Knowledge/skill deficit about alternative responses to health-related transitions, altered body function or structure, illness, or medical treatment
Lack of privacy
Lack of significant other

References

Hogan, R.M. (1985). *Human sexuality–A nursing perspective.* New York: Appleton-Century-Crofts.
Kolodny, R C., Masters, W.H., & Johnson, V.E. (1979). *Textbook of sexual medicine.* Boston: Little, Brown.
Kaplan, H.S. (1983). *O desejo sexual e novos conceitos e técnicas da terapia do sexo.* Rio de Janeiro: Nova Fronteira.

IMPAIRED SKIN INTEGRITY

Definition

Altered epidermis and/or dermis

Defining Characteristics

- Destruction of skin layers
- Disruption of skin surface
- Invasion of body structures

Related Factors

External

Chemical substance
Extremes in age
Humidity
Hyperthermia
Hypothermia
Mechanical factors (e.g., shearing forces, pressure, restraint)
Medications
Moisture
Physical immobilization
Radiation

Internal

Changes in fluid status
Changes in pigmentation
Changes in turgor
Developmental factors
Imbalanced nutritional state (e.g., obesity, emaciation)
Immunological deficit
Impaired circulation
Impaired metabolic state
Impaired sensation
Skeletal prominence

RISK FOR IMPAIRED SKIN INTEGRITY

Definition

At risk for skin being adversely altered

Risk Factors

External

Chemical substance
Excretions
Extremes of age
Hyperthermia
Hypothermia
Humidity
Mechanical factors (e.g., shearing forces, pressure, restraint)
Moisture
Physical immobilization
Radiation
Secretions

Internal

Changes in pigmentation
Changes in skin turgor
Developmental factors
Imbalanced nutritional state (e.g., obesity, emaciation)
Impaired circulation
Impaired metabolic state
Impaired sensation
Immunologic factors
Medications
Psychogenetic factors
Skeletal prominence

Note. Risk should be determined by use of a standardized risk assessment tool.

SLEEP DEPRIVATION

Definition

Prolonged periods of time without sleep (sustained natural, periodic suspension of relative consciousness)

Defining Characteristics

- Acute confusion
- Agitation
- Anxiety
- Apathy
- Combativeness
- Daytime drowsiness
- Decreased ability to function
- Fatigue
- Fleeting nystagmus
- Hallucinations
- Hand tremors
- Heightened sensitivity to pain
- Irritability
- Lethargy
- Listlessness
- Malaise

- Perceptual disorders (e.g., disturbed body sensation, delusions, feeling afloat)
- Restlessness
- Slowed reaction
- Transient paranoia

Related Factors

Aging-related sleep stage shifts
Dementia
Familial sleep paralysis
Inadequate daytime activity
Idiopathic central nervous system hypersomnolence
Narcolepsy
Nightmares
Non-sleep-inducing parenting practices
Periodic limb movement (e.g., restless leg syndrome, nocturnal myoclonus)
Prolonged discomfort (e.g., physical, psychological)
Sustained inadequate sleep hygiene
Prolonged use of pharmacologic or dietary antisoporifics
Sleep apnea
Sleep terror
Sleepwalking
Sleep-related enuresis
Sleep-related painful erections
Sundowner's syndrome
Sustained circadian asynchrony
Sustained environmental stimulation
Sustained uncomfortable sleep environment

Readiness for Enhanced Sleep

Definition

A pattern of natural, periodic suspension of consciousness that provides adequate rest, sustains a desired lifestyle, and can be strengthened

Defining Characteristics

- Amount of sleep is congruent with developmental needs
- Expresses a feeling of being rested after sleep
- Expresses willingness to enhance sleep
- Follows sleep routines that promote sleep habits
- Occasional use of medications to induce sleep

Impaired Social Interaction

Definition

Insufficient or excessive quantity or ineffective quality of social exchange

Defining Characteristics

- Discomfort in social situations
- Dysfunctional interaction with others
- Family report of changes in interaction (e.g., style, pattern)
- Inability to communicate a satisfying sense of social engagement (e.g., belonging, caring, interest, or shared history)

- Inability to receive a satisfying sense of social engagement (e.g., belonging, caring, interest, or shared history)
- Use of unsuccessful social interaction behaviors

Related Factors

Absence of significant others
Communication barriers
Deficit about ways to enhance mutuality (e.g., knowledge, skills)
Disturbed thought processes
Environmental barriers
Limited physical mobility
Self-concept disturbance
Sociocultural dissonance
Therapeutic isolation

SOCIAL ISOLATION

Definition

Aloneness experienced by the individual and perceived as imposed by others and as a negative or threatening state

Defining Characteristics

Objective

- Absence of supportive significant other(s)
- Developmentally inappropriate behaviors
- Dull affect
- Evidence of handicap (e.g., physical, mental)
- Exists in a subculture
- Illness
- Meaningless actions
- No eye contact
- Preoccupation with own thoughts
- Projects hostility
- Repetitive actions
- Sad affect
- Seeks to be alone
- Shows behavior unaccepted by dominant cultural group
- Uncommunicative
- Withdrawn

Subjective

- Expresses feelings of aloneness imposed by others
- Expresses feelings of rejection
- Developmentally inappropriate interests
- Inadequate purpose in life
- Inability to meet expectations of others
- Expresses values unacceptable to the dominant cultural group
- Experiences feelings of differences from others
- Insecurity in public

Related Factors

Alterations in mental status
Alterations in physical appearance
Altered state of wellness
Factors contributing to the absence of satisfying personal relationships (e.g., delay in accomplishing developmental tasks)
Immature interests
Inability to engage in satisfying personal relationships
Inadequate personal resources
Unaccepted social values
Unaccepted social behavior

CHRONIC SORROW

Definition

Cyclical, recurring, and potentially progressive pattern of pervasive sadness experienced (by a parent, caregiver, individual with chronic illness or disability) in response to continual loss, throughout the trajectory of an illness or disability

Defining Characteristics

- Expresses negative feelings (e.g., anger, being misunderstood, confusion, depression, disappointment, emptiness, fear, frustration, guilt, self-blame, helplessness, hopelessness, loneliness, low self-esteem, recurring loss, overwhelmed)
- Expresses feelings of sadness (e.g., periodic, recurrent)
- Expresses feelings that interfere with ability to reach highest level of personal well-being
- Expresses feelings that interfere with ability to reach highest level of social well-being

Related Factors

Death of a loved one
Experiences chronic disability (e.g., physical or mental)
Experiences chronic illness (e.g., physical or mental)
Crises in management of the illness
Crises related to developmental stages
Missed opportunities
Missed milestones
Unending caregiving

SPIRITUAL DISTRESS

Definition

Impaired ability to experience and integrate meaning and purpose in life through connectedness with self, others, art, music, literature, nature, and/or a power greater than oneself

Defining Characteristics

Connections to Self

- Anger
- Expresses lack of acceptance
- Expresses lack of courage
- Expresses lack of forgiveness of self
- Expresses lack of hope

- Expresses lack of love
- Expresses lack of meaning in life
- Expresses lack of purpose in life
- Expresses lack of serenity (e.g., peace)
- Guilt
- Poor coping

Connections With Others

- Expresses alienation
- Refuses interactions with significant others
- Refuses interactions with spiritual leaders
- Verbalizes being separated from support system

Connections With Art, Music, Literature, Nature

- Disinterest in nature
- Disinterest in reading spiritual literature
- Inability to express previous state of creativity (e.g., singing/listening to music/writing)

Connections With Power Greater Than Self

- Expresses being abandoned
- Expresses having anger toward God
- Expresses hopelessness
- Expresses suffering
- Inability to be introspective
- Inability to experience the transcendent
- Inability to participate in religious activities
- Inability to pray
- Requests to see a religious leader
- Sudden changes in spiritual practices

Related Factors

Active dying
Anxiety
Chronic illness
Death
Life change
Loneliness
Pain
Self-alienation
Social alienation
Sociocultural deprivation

RISK FOR SPIRITUAL DISTRESS

Definition

At risk for an impaired ability to experience and integrate meaning and purpose in life through connectedness with self, others, art, music, literature, nature, and/or a power greater than oneself

Risk Factors

Developmental

Life changes

Environmental

Environmental changes
Natural disasters

Physical

Chronic illness
Physical illness
Substance abuse

Psychosocial

Anxiety
Blocks to experiencing love
Change in religious rituals
Change in spiritual practices
Cultural conflict
Depression
Inability to forgive
Loss
Low self-esteem
Poor relationships
Racial conflict
Separated support systems
Stress

READINESS FOR ENHANCED SPIRITUAL WELL-BEING

Definition

Ability to experience and integrate meaning and purpose in life through connectedness with self, others, art, music, literature, nature, and/or a power greater than oneself that can be strengthened

Defining Characteristics

Connections to Self

- Expresses desire for enhanced acceptance
- Expresses desire for enhanced coping
- Expresses desire for enhanced courage
- Expresses desire for enhanced forgiveness of self
- Expresses desire for enhanced hope
- Expresses desire for enhanced joy
- Expresses desire for enhanced love
- Expresses desire for enhanced meaning in life
- Expresses desire for enhanced purpose in life
- Expresses desire for enhanced satisfying philosophy of life
- Expresses desire for enhanced surrender
- Expresses lack of serenity (e.g., peace)
- Meditation

Connections With Others

- Provides service to others
- Requests interactions with significant others
- Requests interactions with spiritual leaders
- Requests forgiveness of others

Connections With Art, Music, Literature, Nature

- Displays creative energy (e.g., writing, poetry, singing)
- Listens to music
- Reads spiritual literature
- Spends time outdoors

Connections With Power Greater Than Self

- Expresses awe
- Expresses reverence
- Participates in religious activities
- Prays
- Reports mystical experiences

STRESS OVERLOAD

Definition

Excessive amounts and types of demands that require action

Defining Characteristics

- Demonstrates increased feelings of anger
- Demonstrates increased feelings of impatience
- Expresses difficulty in functioning
- Expresses a feeling of pressure
- Expresses a feeling of tension
- Expresses increased feelings of anger
- Expresses increased feelings of impatience
- Expresses problems with decision making
- Reports negative impact from stress (e.g., physical symptoms, psychological distress, feeling of "being sick" or of "going to get sick")
- Reports situational stress as excessive (e.g., rates stress level as seven or above on a 10-point scale)

Related Factors

Inadequate resources (e.g., financial, social, education/knowledge level)
Intense, repeated stressors (e.g., family violence, chronic illness, terminal illness)
Multiple coexisting stressors (e.g., environmental threats/demands; physical threats/demands; (social threats/demands)

References

Keil, R.M.K. (2004). Coping and stress: A conceptual analysis. *Journal of Advanced Nursing, 45,* 659–665.
Motzer, S.A., & Hertig, V. (2004). Stress, stress response and health. *Nursing Clinics of North America, 39,* 1–17.
Ryan-Wenger, N.A., Sharrer, V.W., & Campbell, K.K. (2005). Changes in children's stressors over the past 30 years. *Pediatric Nursing, 31,* 282–291.

RISK FOR SUFFOCATION

Definition

Accentuated risk of accidental suffocation (inadequate air available for inhalation)

Risk Factors

External

Discarding refrigerators without removed doors
Eating large mouthfuls of food
Hanging a pacifier around infant's neck

Household gas leaks
Inserting small objects into airway
Leaving children unattended in water
Low-strung clothesline
Pillow placed in infant's crib
Playing with plastic bags
Propped bottle placed in infant's crib
Smoking in bed
Use of fuel-burning heaters not vented to outside
Vehicle warming in closed garage

Internal

Cognitive difficulties
Disease process
Emotional difficulties
Injury process
Lack of safety education
Lack of safety precautions
Reduced motor abilities
Reduced olfactory sensation

RISK FOR SUICIDE

Definition

At risk for self-inflicted, life-threatening injury

Risk Factors

Behavioral

Buying a gun
Changing a will
Giving away possessions
History of prior suicide attempt
Impulsiveness
Making a will
Marked changes in attitude
Marked changes in behavior
Marked changes in school performance
Stockpiling medicines
Sudden euphoric recovery from major depression

Demographic

Age (e.g., elderly, young adult males, adolescents)
Divorced
Male gender
Race (e.g., Caucasian, Native American)
Widowed

Physical

Chronic pain
Physical illness
Terminal illness

Psychological

Childhood abuse
Family history of suicide
Gay or lesbian youth
Guilt
Psychiatric illness/disorder (e.g., depression, schizophrenia, bipolar disorder)
Substance abuse

Situational

Adolescents living in nontraditional settings (e.g., juvenile detention center, prison, half-way house, group home)
Economic instability
Institutionalization
Living alone
Loss of autonomy
Loss of independence
Presence of gun in home
Relocation
Retired

Social

Cluster suicides
Disrupted family life
Disciplinary problems
Grief
Helplessness
Hopelessness
Legal problems
Loneliness
Loss of important relationship
Poor support systems
Social isolation

Verbal

States desire to die
Threats of killing oneself

DELAYED SURGICAL RECOVERY

Definition

Extension of the number of postoperative days required to initiate and perform activities that maintain life, health, and well-being

Defining Characteristics

- Difficulty in moving about
- Evidence of interrupted healing of surgical area (e.g., red, indurated, draining, immobilized)
- Fatigue
- Loss of appetite with or without nausea
- Perception that more time is needed to recover
- Postpones resumption of work/employment activities
- Requires help to complete self-care
- Report of pain/discomfort

Related Factors

Extensive surgical procedure
Obesity
Pain
Postoperative surgical site infection
Preoperative expectations
Prolonged surgical procedure

References

Kotiniemi, L.H., Ryhanen, P.T., Valanne, J., Jokela, R., Mustonen, A., & Poukkula, E. (1997). Postoperative symptoms at home following day-care surgery in children: A multicentre survey of 551 children. *Anaesthesia, 52,* 963–969.

Kleinbeck, S.V. (2000). Self-reported at-home postoperative recovery. *Research in Nursing & Health, 23,* 461–472.

Zalon, M. (2004). Correlates of recovery among older adults after major abdominal surgery. *Nursing Research, 53,* 99–106.

IMPAIRED SWALLOWING

Definition

Abnormal functioning of the swallowing mechanism associated with deficits in oral, pharyngeal, or esophageal structure or function

Defining Characteristics

Esophageal Phase Impairment

- Abnormality in esophageal phase by swallow study
- Acidic smelling breath
- Bruxism
- Complaints of "something stuck"
- Epigastric pain
- Food refusal
- Heartburn or epigastric pain
- Hematemesis
- Hyperextension of head (e.g., arching during or after meals)
- Nighttime awakening
- Nighttime coughing
- Observed evidence of difficulty in swallowing (e.g., stasis of food in oral cavity, coughing/choking)
- Odynophagia
- Regurgitation of gastric contents (wet burps)
- Repetitive swallowing
- Unexplained irritability surrounding mealtime
- Volume limiting
- Vomiting
- Vomitus on pillow

Oral Phase Impairment

- Abnormality in oral phase of swallow study
- Choking before a swallow
- Coughing before a swallow
- Drooling
- Food falls from mouth
- Food pushed out of mouth
- Gagging before a swallow

- Inability to clear oral cavity
- Incomplete lip closure
- Lack of chewing
- Lack of tongue action to form bolus
- Long meals with little consumption
- Nasal reflux
- Piecemeal deglutition
- Pooling in lateral sulci
- Premature entry of bolus
- Sialorrhea
- Slow bolus formation
- Weak suck resulting in inefficient nippling

Pharyngeal Phase Impairment

- Abnormality in pharyngeal phase by swallow study
- Altered head positions
- Choking
- Coughing
- Delayed swallow
- Food refusal
- Gagging
- Gurgly voice quality
- Inadequate laryngeal elevation
- Multiple swallows
- Nasal reflux
- Recurrent pulmonary infections
- Unexplained fevers

Related Factors

Congenital Deficits

Behavioral feeding problems
Conditions with significant hypotonia
Congenital heart disease
Failure to thrive
History of tube feeding
Mechanical obstruction (e.g., edema, tracheostomy tube, tumor)
Neuromuscular impairment (e.g., decreased or absent gag reflex, decreased strength or excursion of muscles involved in mastication, perceptual impairment, facial paralysis)
Protein energy malnutrition
Respiratory disorders
Self-injurious behavior
Upper airway anomalies

Neurological Problems

Achalasia
Acquired anatomic defects
Cerebral palsy
Cranial nerve involvement
Developmental delay
Esophageal defects

Gastroesophageal reflux disease
Laryngeal abnormalities
Laryngeal defects
Nasal defects
Nasopharyngeal cavity defects
Oropharynx abnormalities
Prematurity
Tracheal defects
Traumas
Traumatic head injury
Upper airway anomalies

EFFECTIVE THERAPEUTIC REGIMEN MANAGEMENT

Definition

Pattern of regulating and integrating into daily living a program for treatment of illness and its sequelae that is satisfactory for meeting specific health goals

Defining Characteristics

- Appropriate choices of daily activities for meeting the goals of a prevention program
- Appropriate choices of daily activities for meeting the goals of a treatment program
- Illness symptoms within a normal range of expectation
- Verbalizes desire to manage the treatment of illness
- Verbalizes desire to manage prevention of sequelae
- Verbalizes intent to reduce risk factors for progression of illness and sequelae

Related Factors

To be developed

Note. This diagnosis will retire from the NANDA-I Taxonomy in the 2009–2010 edition unless additional work is done to bring it to a LOE of 2.1 or higher.

INEFFECTIVE THERAPEUTIC REGIMEN MANAGEMENT

Definition

Pattern of regulating and integrating into daily living a program for treatment of illness and the sequelae of illness that is unsatisfactory for meeting specific health goals

Defining Characteristics

- Failure to include treatment regimens in daily routines
- Failure to take action to reduce risk factors
- Makes choices in daily living ineffective for meeting health goals
- Verbalizes desire to manage the illness
- Verbalizes difficulty with prescribed regimens

Related Factors

Complexity of health-care system
Complexity of therapeutic regimen
Decisional conflicts
Economic difficulties
Excessive demands made (e.g., individual, family)
Family conflict
Family patterns of health care

Inadequate number of cues to action
Knowledge deficit
Mistrust of health-care personnel
Mistrust of regimen
Perceived barriers
Powerlessness
Perceived seriousness
Perceived susceptibility
Perceived benefits
Social support deficit

INEFFECTIVE COMMUNITY THERAPEUTIC REGIMEN MANAGEMENT

Definition

Pattern of regulating and integrating into community processes programs for treatment of illness and the sequelae of illness that are unsatisfactory for meeting health-related goals

Defining Characteristics

- Deficits in advocates for aggregates
- Deficits in community activities for prevention
- Illness symptoms above the norm expected for the population
- Insufficient health-care resources (e.g., people, programs)
- Unavailable health-care resources for illness care
- Unexpected acceleration of illness

Related Factors

To be developed

Note. This diagnosis will retire from the NANDA-I Taxonomy in the 2009–2010 edition unless additional work is done to bring it to a LOE of 2.1 or higher.

INEFFECTIVE FAMILY THERAPEUTIC REGIMEN MANAGEMENT

Definition

Pattern of regulating and integrating into family processes a program for treatment of illness and the sequelae of illness that is unsatisfactory for meeting specific health goals

Defining Characteristics

- Acceleration of illness symptoms of a family member
- Inappropriate family activities for meeting health goals
- Failure to take action to reduce risk factors
- Lack of attention to illness
- Verbalizes desire to manage the illness
- Verbalizes difficulty with therapeutic regimen

Related Factors

Complexity of health-care system
Complexity of therapeutic regimen
Decisional conflicts
Economic difficulties
Excessive demands
Family conflict

READINESS FOR ENHANCED THERAPEUTIC REGIMEN MANAGEMENT

Definition

A pattern of regulating and integrating into daily living a program for treatment of illness and its sequelae that is sufficient for meeting health-related goals and can be strengthened

Defining Characteristics

- Choices of daily living are appropriate for meeting goals (e.g., treatment, prevention)
- Describes reduction of risk factors
- Expresses desire to manage the illness (e.g., treatment, prevention of sequelae)
- Expresses little difficulty with prescribed regimens
- No unexpected acceleration of illness symptoms

INEFFECTIVE THERMOREGULATION

Definition

Temperature fluctuation between hypothermia and hyperthermia

Defining Characteristics

- Cool skin
- Cyanotic nail beds
- Fluctuations in body temperature above and below the normal range
- Flushed skin
- Hypertension
- Increased respiratory rate
- Mild shivering
- Moderate pallor
- Piloerection
- Reduction in body temperature below normal range
- Seizures
- Slow capillary refill
- Tachycardia
- Warm to touch

Related Factors

Aging
Fluctuating environmental temperature
Immaturity
Trauma or illness

DISTURBED THOUGHT PROCESSES

Definition

Disruption in cognitive operations and activities

Defining Characteristics

- Cognitive dissonance
- Distractibility
- Egocentricity
- Hypervigilance
- Hypovigilance
- Inaccurate interpretation of environment

- Inappropriate thinking
- Memory deficit

Related Factors

To be developed

Note. This diagnosis will retire from the NANDA-I Taxonomy in the 2009–2010 edition unless additional work is done to bring it to a LOE of 2.1 or higher.

Impaired Tissue Integrity

Definition

Damage to mucous membrane, corneal, integumentary, or subcutaneous tissues

Defining Characteristics

- Damaged tissue (e.g., cornea, mucous membrane, integumentary, subcutaneous)
- Destroyed tissue

Related Factors

Altered circulation
Chemical irritants
Fluid deficit
Fluid excess
Impaired physical mobility
Knowledge deficit
Mechanical factors (e.g., pressure, shear, friction)
Nutritional factors (e.g., deficit or excess)
Radiation
Temperature extremes

Ineffective Tissue Perfusion (Specify type: Renal, Cerebral, Cardiopulmonary, Gastrointestinal, Peripheral)

Definition

Decrease in oxygen resulting in the failure to nourish the tissues at the capillary level

Defining Characteristics

Cardiopulmonary

- Abnormal arterial blood gases
- Altered respiratory rate outside of acceptable parameters
- Arrhythmias
- Bronchospasm
- Capillary refill >3 seconds
- Chest pain
- Chest retraction
- Dyspnea
- Nasal flaring
- Sense of "impending doom"
- Use of accessory muscles

Cerebral

- Altered mental status
- Behavioral changes

- Changes in motor response
- Changes in pupillary reactions
- Difficulty in swallowing
- Extremity weakness
- Paralysis
- Speech abnormalities

Gastrointestinal

- Abdominal distention
- Abdominal pain or tenderness
- Absent bowel sounds
- Hypoactive bowel sounds
- Nausea

Peripheral

- Absent pulses
- Altered sensations
- Altered skin characteristics (e.g., hair, nails, moisture)
- Blood pressure changes in extremities
- Bruits
- Claudication
- Delayed healing
- Diminished arterial pulsations
- Edema
- Positive Homan's sign
- Skin color pales on elevation; color does not return on lowering the leg
- Skin discolorations
- Skin temperature changes
- Weak pulses

Renal

- Altered blood pressure outside of acceptable parameters
- Anuria
- Elevation in BUN/creatinine ratio
- Hematuria
- Oliguria

Related Factors

Altered affinity of hemoglobin for oxygen
Decreased hemoglobin concentration in blood
Enzyme poisoning
Exchange problems
Hypoventilation
Hypovolemia
Hypervolemia
Impaired transport of oxygen
Interruption of blood flow
Mismatch of ventilation with blood flow

IMPAIRED TRANSFER ABILITY

Definition

Limitation of independent movement between two nearby surfaces

Defining Characteristics

- Inability to transfer between uneven levels
- Inability to transfer from bed to chair
- Inability to transfer from chair to bed
- Inability to transfer on or off a toilet
- Inability to transfer on or off a commode
- Inability to transfer in or out of tub
- Inability to transfer in or out of shower
- Inability to transfer from chair to car
- Inability to transfer from car to chair
- Inability to transfer from chair to floor
- Inability to transfer from floor to chair
- Inability to transfer from standing to floor
- Inability to transfer from floor to standing
- Inability to transfer from bed to standing
- Inability to transfer from standing to bed
- Inability to transfer from chair to standing
- Inability to transfer from standing to chair

Related Factors

Insufficient muscle strength
Neuromuscular impairment
Musculoskeletal impairment (e.g., contractures)
Pain
Cognitive impairment
Obesity
Environmental constraints (e.g., bed height, inadequate space, wheel chair type, treatment equipment, restraints)
Lack of knowledge
Impaired balance
Deconditioning
Impaired vision

References

Brouwer, K., Nysseknabm, J., & Culham E. (2004). Physical function and health status among seniors with and without fear of falling. *Gerontology, 50,* 15–141.

Lewis, C.L., Moutoux, M., Slaughter, M., & Bailey, S.P. (2004). Characteristics of individuals who fell while receiving home health services. *Physical Therapy, 84*(1), 23–32.

Tinetti., M.E., & Ginter, S.F. (1988). Identifying mobility dysfunction in elderly persons. *Journal of the American Medical Association, 259,* 1190–1193.

Note. Specify level of independence using a standardized functional scale.

RISK FOR TRAUMA

Definition

Accentuated risk of accidental tissue injury (e.g., wound, burn, fracture)

Risk Factors

External

Accessibility of guns
Bathing in very hot water (e.g., unsupervised bathing of young children)
Bathtub without antislip equipment
Children playing with dangerous objects
Children playing without gates at top of stairs
Children riding in the front seat in car
Contact with corrosives
Contact with intense cold
Contact with rapidly moving machinery
Defective appliances
Delayed lighting of gas appliances
Driving a mechanically unsafe vehicle
Driving at excessive speeds
Driving while intoxicated
Driving without necessary visual aids
Entering unlighted rooms
Experimenting with chemicals
Exposure to dangerous machinery
Faulty electrical plugs
Flammable children's clothing
Flammable children's toys
Frayed wires
Grease waste collected on stoves
High beds
High-crime neighborhood
Inappropriate call-for-aid mechanisms for bedresting client
Inadequate stair rails
Inadequately stored combustibles (e.g., matches, oily rags)
Inadequately stored corrosives (e.g., lye)
Knives stored uncovered
Lack of protection from heat source
Large icicles hanging from the roof
Misuse of necessary headgear
Misuse of seat restraints
Nonuse of seat restraints
Obstructed passageways
Overexposure to radiation
Overloaded electrical outlets
Overloaded fuse boxes
Physical proximity to vehicle pathways (e.g., driveways, lanes, railroad tracks)
Playing with explosives
Pot handles facing toward front of stove
Potential igniting of gas leaks
Slippery floors (e.g., wet or highly waxed)
Smoking in bed
Smoking near oxygen

Struggling with restraints
Unanchored electric wires
Unanchored rugs
Unsafe road
Unsafe walkways
Unsafe window protection in homes with young children
Use of cracked dishware
Use of unsteady chairs
Use of unsteady ladders
Wearing flowing clothes around open flame

Internal

Balancing difficulties
Cognitive difficulties
Emotional difficulties
History of previous trauma
Insufficient finances
Lack of safety education
Lack of safety precautions
Poor vision
Reduced hand-eye coordination
Reduced muscle coordination
Reduced sensation
Weakness

IMPAIRED URINARY ELIMINATION

Definition

Disturbance in urine elimination

Defining Characteristics

- Dysuria
- Frequency
- Hesitancy
- Incontinence
- Nocturia
- Retention
- Urgency

Related Factors

Anatomical obstruction
Multiple causality
Sensory motor impairment
Urinary tract infection

References

Engberg, S., McDowell, B., Donovan, N., Brodak, I., & Weber, E. (1997). Treatment of urinary incontinence in homebound older adults: Interface between research and practice. *Ostomy/Wound Management, 48*(10), 18–26.

Fantl, J., Newman, D., & Colling, J. (1996). *Urinary incontinence in adults: Acute and chronic management* (clinical practice guideline No. 2). Rockville, MD: U.S. Department of Health & Human Services.

Messick, G., & Powe, C. (1997). Applying behavioral research to incontinence. *Ostomy/Wound Management, 48*(10), 40–48.

READINESS FOR ENHANCED URINARY ELIMINATION

Definition

A pattern of urinary functions that is sufficient for meeting eliminatory needs and can be strengthened

Defining Characteristics

- Amount of output is within normal limits
- Expresses willingness to enhance urinary elimination
- Fluid intake is adequate for daily needs
- Positions self for emptying of bladder
- Specific gravity is within normal limits
- Urine is odorless
- Urine is straw colored

URINARY RETENTION

Definition

Incomplete emptying of the bladder

Defining Characteristics

- Absence of urine output
- Bladder distention
- Dribbling
- Dysuria
- Frequent voiding
- Overflow incontinence
- Residual urine
- Sensation of bladder fullness
- Small voiding

Related Factors

Blockage
High urethral pressure
Inhibition of reflex arc
Strong sphincter

IMPAIRED SPONTANEOUS VENTILATION

Definition

Decreased energy reserves result in an individual's inability to maintain breathing adequate to support life

Defining Characteristics

- Apprehension
- Decreased cooperation
- Decreased pO_2
- Decreased SaO_2
- Decreased tidal volume
- Dyspnea
- Increased heart rate
- Increased metabolic rate
- Increased pCO_2
- Increased restlessness
- Increased use of accessory muscles

Related Factors

Metabolic factors

Respiratory muscle fatigue

Dysfunctional Ventilatory Weaning Response

Definition

Inability to adjust to lowered levels of mechanical ventilator support that interrupts and prolongs the weaning process

Defining Characteristics

Mild

- Breathing discomfort
- Expressed feelings of increased need for oxygen
- Fatigue
- Increased concentration on breathing
- Queries about possible machine malfunction
- Restlessness
- Slight increase of respiratory rate from baseline
- Warmth

Moderate

- Apprehension
- Baseline increase in respiratory rate (<5 breaths/min)
- Color changes
- Decreased air entry on auscultation
- Diaphoresis
- Hypervigilance to activities
- Inability to cooperate
- Inability to respond to coaching
- Pale
- Slight cyanosis
- Slight increase from baseline blood pressure (<20 mm Hg)
- Slight increase from baseline heart rate (<20 beats/min)
- Slight respiratory accessory muscle use
- Wide-eyed look

Severe

- Adventitious breath sounds
- Agitation
- Asynchronized breathing with the ventilator
- Audible airway secretions
- Cyanosis
- Decreased level of consciousness
- Deterioration in arterial blood gases from current baseline
- Full respiratory accessory muscle use
- Gasping breaths
- Increase from baseline blood pressure (≥20 mm Hg)
- Increase from baseline heart rate (≥20 breaths/min)
- Paradoxical abdominal breathing

- Profuse diaphoresis
- Respiratory rate increases significantly from baseline
- Shallow breaths

Related Factors

Physiological

Inadequate nutrition
Ineffective airway clearance
Sleep pattern disturbance
Uncontrolled pain

Psychological

Anxiety
Decreased motivation
Decreased self-esteem
Fear
Hopelessness
Insufficient trust in the nurse
Knowledge deficit of the weaning process
Patient perceived inefficacy about ability to wean
Powerlessness

Situational

Adverse environment (e.g., noisy, active environment; negative events in the room, low nurse-patient ratio, unfamiliar nursing staff)
History of multiple unsuccessful weaning attempts
History of ventilator dependence >4 days
Inadequate social support
Inappropriate pacing of diminished ventilator support
Uncontrolled episodic energy demands

Risk for Other-Directed Violence

Definition

At risk for behaviors in which an individual demonstrates that he/she can be physically, emotionally, and/or sexually harmful to others

Risk Factors

Availability of weapon(s)
Body language (e.g., rigid posture, clenching of fists and jaw, hyperactivity, pacing, breathlessness, threatening stances)
Cognitive impairment (e.g., learning disabilities, attention deficit disorder, decreased intellectual functioning)
Cruelty to animals
Firesetting
History of childhood abuse
History of indirect violence (e.g., tearing off clothes, ripping objects off walls, writing on walls, urinating on floor, defecating on floor, stamping feet, temper tantrum, running in corridors, yelling, throwing objects, breaking a window, slamming doors, sexual advances)
History of substance abuse

History of threats of violence (e.g., verbal threats against property, verbal threats against person, social threats, cursing, threatening notes/letters, threatening gestures, sexual threats)
History of witnessing family violence
History of violence against others (e.g., hitting someone, kicking someone, spitting at someone, scratching someone, throwing objects at someone, biting someone, attempted rape, rape, sexual molestation, urinating/defecating on a person)
History of violent antisocial behavior (e.g., stealing, insistent borrowing, insistent demands for privileges, insistent interruption of meetings, refusal to eat, refusal to take medication, ignoring instructions)
Impulsivity
Motor vehicle offenses (e.g., frequent traffic violations, use of a motor vehicle to release anger)
Neurological impairment (e.g., positive EEG, CAT, MRI, neurological findings; head trauma; seizure disorders)
Pathological intoxication
Perinatal complications
Prenatal complications
Psychotic symptomatology (e.g., auditory, visual, command hallucinations; paranoid delusions; loose, rambling, or illogical thought processes)
Suicidal behavior

RISK FOR SELF-DIRECTED VIOLENCE

Definition

At risk for behaviors in which an individual demonstrates that he/she can be physically, emotionally and/or sexually harmful to self

Risk Factors

Age 15–19
Age over 45
Behavioral clues (e.g., writing forlorn love notes, directing angry messages at a significant other who has rejected the person, giving away personal items, taking out a large life insurance policy)
Conflictual interpersonal relationships
Emotional problems (e.g., hopelessness, despair, increased anxiety, panic, anger, hostility)
Employment problems (e.g., unemployed, recent job loss/failure)
Engagement in autoerotic sexual acts
Family background (e.g., chaotic or conflictual, history of suicide)
History of multiple suicide attempts
Lack of personal resources (e.g., poor achievement, poor insight, affect unavailable and poorly controlled)
Lack of social resources (e.g., poor rapport, socially isolated, unresponsive family)
Physical health problems (e.g., hypochondriasis, chronic or terminal illness)
Marital status (single, widowed, divorced)
Mental health problems (e.g., severe depression, psychosis, severe personality disorder, alcoholism or drug abuse)
Occupation (executive, administrator/owner of business, professional, semiskilled worker)
Sexual orientation (bisexual [active], homosexual [inactive])
Suicidal ideation
Suicidal plan
Verbal clues (e.g., talking about death, "better off without me," asking questions about lethal dosages of drugs)

Impaired Walking

Definition

Limitation of independent movement within the environment on foot

Defining Characteristics

- Impaired ability to climb stairs
- Impaired ability to navigate curbs
- Impaired ability to walk required distances
- Impaired ability to walk on incline
- Impaired ability to walk on decline
- Impaired ability to walk on uneven surfaces

Risk Factors

Cognitive impairment
Deconditioning
Depressed mood
Environmental constraints (e.g., stairs, inclines, uneven surfaces, unsafe obstacles, distances, lack of assistive devices or person, restraints)
Fear of falling
Impaired balance
Impaired vision
Insufficient muscle strength
Lack of knowledge
Limited endurance
Musculoskeletal impairment (e.g., contractures)
Neuromuscular impairment
Obesity
Pain

Note. Specify level of independence using a standardized functional scale.

References

Brouwer, K., Nysseknabm, J., & Culham E. (2004). Physical function and health status among seniors with and without fear of falling. *Gerontology, 50,* 15–141.

Lewis, C.L., Moutoux, M., Slaughter, M., & Bailey, S.P. (2004). Characteristics of individuals who fell while receiving home health services. *Physical Therapy, 84*(1), 23–32.

Tinetti, M.E., & Ginter, S.F. (1988). Identifying mobility dysfunction in elderly persons. *Journal of the American Medical Association, 259,* 1190–1193.

Wandering

Definition

Meandering, aimless or repetitive locomotion that exposes the individual to harm; frequently incongruent with boundaries, limits, or obstacles

Defining Characteristics

- Continuous movement from place to place
- Getting lost
- Fretful locomotion
- Frequent movement from place to place
- Haphazard locomotion
- Hyperactivity

- Inability to locate significant landmarks in a familiar setting
- Locomotion into unauthorized or private spaces
- Locomotion resulting in unintended leaving of a premise
- Locomotion that cannot be easily dissuaded
- Long periods of locomotion without an apparent destination
- Pacing
- Periods of locomotion interspersed with periods of nonlocomotion (e.g., sitting, standing, sleeping)
- Persistent locomotion in search of something
- Shadowing a caregiver's locomotion
- Trespassing
- Scanning behaviors
- Searching behaviors

Related Factors

Cognitive impairment (e.g., memory and recall deficits, disorientation, poor visuoconstructive or visuospatial ability, language defects)

Cortical atrophy

Emotional state (e.g., frustration, anxiety, boredom, depression, agitation)

Overstimulating environment

Physiological state or need (e.g., hunger, thirst, pain, urination, constipation)

Premorbid behavior (e.g., outgoing, sociable personality; premorbid dementia)

Sedation

Separation from familiar environment

Time of day

From *NANDA-I Nursing Diagnosis: Definitions & Classification 2007–2008*. Philadelphia: NANDA International, 2007.

Editor's note: This reprint follows the stylistic preferences of the copyright holder and not those of Stedman's dictionaries.

Nursing Interventions Classification (NIC)

Taxonomy of Nursing Interventions: The Classification

Abuse Protection Support
Abuse Protection Support: Child
Abuse Protection Support: Domestic Partner
Abuse Protection Support: Elder
Abuse Protection Support: Religious
Acid-Base Management
Acid-Base Management: Metabolic Acidosis
Acid-Base Management: Metabolic Alkalosis
Acid-Base Management: Respiratory Acidosis
Acid-Base Management: Respiratory Alkalosis
Acid-Base Monitoring
Active Listening
Activity Therapy
Acupressure
Admission Care
Airway Insertion and Stabilization
Airway Management
Airway Suctioning
Allergy Management
Amnioinfusion
Amputation Care
Analgesic Administration
Analgesic Administration: Intraspinal
Anaphylaxis Management
Anesthesia Administration
Anger Control Assistance
Animal-Assisted Therapy
Anticipatory Guidance
Anxiety Reduction
Area Restriction
Aromatherapy
Art Therapy
Artificial Airway Management
Aspiration Precautions
Assertiveness Training
Asthma Management
Attachment Promotion
Autogenic Training
Autotransfusion
Bathing
Bed Rest Care
Bedside Laboratory Testing
Behavior Management
Behavior Management: Overactivity/Inattention
Behavior Management: Self-Harm
Behavior Management: Sexual
Behavior Modification
Behavior Modification: Social Skills
Bibliotherapy
Biofeedback
Bioterrorism Preparedness
Birthing
Bladder Irrigation
Bleeding Precautions
Bleeding Reduction
Bleeding Reduction: Antepartum Uterus
Bleeding Reduction: Gastrointestinal
Bleeding Reduction: Nasal
Bleeding Reduction: Postpartum Uterus
Bleeding Reduction: Wound
Blood Products Administration
Body Image Enhancement
Body Mechanics Promotion
Bottle Feeding
Bowel Incontinence Care
Bowel Incontinence Care: Encopresis
Bowel Irrigation
Bowel Management
Bowel Training
Breast Examination
Breastfeeding Assistance
Calming Technique
Capillary Blood Sample
Cardiac Care
Cardiac Care: Acute
Cardiac Care: Rehabilitative
Cardiac Precautions
Caregiver Support
Care Management
Cast Care: Maintenance
Cast Care: Wet
Cerebral Edema Management
Cerebral Perfusion Promotion
Cesarean Section Care
Chemical Restraint
Chemotherapy Management
Chest Physiotherapy
Childbirth Preparation
Circulatory Care: Arterial Insufficiency
Circulatory Care: Mechanical Assist Device

Circulatory Care: Venous Insufficiency
Circulatory Precautions
Circumcision Care
Code Management
Cognitive Restructuring
Cognitive Stimulation
Communicable Disease Management
Communication Enhancement: Hearing Deficit
Communication Enhancement: Speech Deficit
Communication Enhancement: Visual Deficit
Community Disaster Preparedness
Community Health Development
Complex Relationship Building
Conflict Mediation
Constipation/Impaction Management
Consultation
Contact Lens Care
Controlled Substance Checking
Coping Enhancement
Cost Containment
Cough Enhancement
Counseling
Crisis Intervention
Critical Path Development
Culture Brokerage
Cutaneous Stimulation
Decision-Making Support
Delegation
Delirium Management
Delusion Management
Dementia Management
Dementia Management: Bathing
Deposition/Testimony
Developmental Care
Developmental Enhancement: Adolescent
Developmental Enhancement: Child
Dialysis Access Maintenance
Diarrhea Management
Diet Staging
Discharge Planning
Distraction
Documentation
Dressing
Dying Care
Dysreflexia Management
Dysrhythmia Management
Ear Care
Eating Disorders Management
Electroconvulsive Therapy (ECT) Management
Electrolyte Management
Electrolyte Management: Hypercalcemia
Electrolyte Management: Hyperkalemia
Electrolyte Management: Hypermagnesemia
Electrolyte Management: Hypernatremia
Electrolyte Management: Hyperphosphatemia
Electrolyte Management: Hypocalcemia
Electrolyte Management: Hypokalemia
Electrolyte Management: Hypomagnesemia
Electrolyte Management: Hyponatremia
Electrolyte Management: Hypophosphatemia
Electrolyte Monitoring
Electronic Fetal Monitoring: Antepartum
Electronic Fetal Monitoring: Intrapartum
Elopement Precautions
Embolus Care: Peripheral
Embolus Care: Pulmonary
Embolus Precautions
Emergency Care
Emergency Cart Checking
Emotional Support
Endotracheal Extubation
Energy Management
Enteral Tube Feeding
Environmental Management
Environmental Management: Attachment Process
Environmental Management: Comfort
Environmental Management: Community
Environmental Management: Home Preparation
Environmental Management: Safety
Environmental Management: Violence Prevention
Environmental Management: Worker Safety
Environmental Risk Protection
Examination Assistance
Exercise Promotion
Exercise Promotion: Strength Training
Exercise Promotion: Stretching
Exercise Therapy: Ambulation
Exercise Therapy: Balance
Exercise Therapy: Joint Mobility
Exercise Therapy: Muscle Control
Eye Care
Fall Prevention
Family Integrity Promotion
Family Integrity Promotion: Childbearing Family
Family Involvement Promotion
Family Mobilization
Family Planning: Contraception

Family Planning: Infertility
Family Planning: Unplanned Pregnancy
Family Presence Facilitation
Family Process Maintenance
Family Support
Family Therapy
Feeding
Fertility Preservation
Fever Treatment
Financial Resource Assistance
Fire-Setting Precautions
First Aid
Fiscal Resource Management
Flatulence Reduction
Fluid/Electrolyte Management
Fluid Management
Fluid Monitoring
Fluid Resuscitation
Foot Care
Forgiveness Facilitation
Gastrointestinal Intubation
Genetic Counseling
Grief Work Facilitation
Grief Work Facilitation: Perinatal Death
Guilt Work Facilitation
Hair Care
Hallucination Management
Health Care Information Exchange
Health Education
Health Policy Monitoring
Health Screening
Health System Guidance
Heat/Cold Application
Heat Exposure Treatment
Hemodialysis Therapy
Hemodynamic Regulation
Hemofiltration Therapy
Hemorrhage Control
High-Risk Pregnancy Care
Home Maintenance Assistance
Hope Instillation
Hormone Replacement Therapy
Humor
Hyperglycemia Management
Hypervolemia Management
Hypnosis
Hypoglycemia Management
Hypothermia Treatment
Hypovolemia Management

Immunization/Vaccination Management
Impulse Control Training
Incident Reporting
Incision Site Care
Infant Care
Infection Control
Infection Control: Intraoperative
Infection Protection
Insurance Authorization
Intracranial Pressure (ICP) Monitoring
Intrapartal Care
Intrapartal Care: High-Risk Delivery
Intravenous (IV) Insertion
Intravenous (IV) Therapy
Invasive Hemodynamic Monitoring
Kangaroo Care
Labor Induction
Labor Suppression
Laboratory Data Interpretation
Lactation Counseling
Lactation Suppression
Laser Precautions
Latex Precautions
Learning Facilitation
Learning Readiness Enhancement
Leech Therapy
Limit Setting
Lower Extremity Monitoring
Malignant Hyperthermia Precautions
Mechanical Ventilation
Mechanical Ventilatory Weaning
Medication Administration
Medication Administration: Ear
Medication Administration: Enteral
Medication Administration: Eye
Medication Administration: Inhalation
Medication Administration: Interpleural
Medication Administration: Intradermal
Medication Administration: Intramuscular (IM)
Medication Administration: Intraosseous
Medication Administration: Intraspinal
Medication Administration: Intravenous (IV)
Medication Administration: Nasal
Medication Administration: Oral
Medication Administration: Rectal
Medication Administration: Skin
Medication Administration: Subcutaneous
Medication Administration: Vaginal
Medication Administration: Ventricular Reservoir

Medication Management
Medication Prescribing
Meditation Facilitation
Memory Training
Milieu Therapy
Mood Management
Multidisciplinary Care Conference
Music Therapy
Mutual Goal Setting
Nail Care
Nausea Management
Neurologic Monitoring
Newborn Care
Newborn Monitoring
Nonnutritive Sucking
Normalization Promotion
Nutrition Management
Nutrition Therapy
Nutritional Counseling
Nutritional Monitoring
Oral Health Maintenance
Oral Health Promotion
Oral Health Restoration
Order Transcription
Organ Procurement
Ostomy Care
Oxygen Therapy
Pain Management
Parent Education: Adolescent
Parent Education: Childrearing Family
Parent Education: Infant
Parenting Promotion
Pass Facilitation
Patient Contracting
Patient-Controlled Analgesia (PCA) Assistance
Patient Rights Protection
Peer Review
Pelvic Muscle Exercise
Perineal Care
Peripheral Sensation Management
Peripherally Inserted Central (PIC) Catheter Care
Peritoneal Dialysis Therapy
Pessary Management
Phlebotomy: Arterial Blood Sample
Phlebotomy: Blood Unit Acquisition
Phlebotomy: Cannulated Vessel
Phlebotomy: Venous Blood Sample
Phototherapy: Mood/Sleep Regulation
Phototherapy: Neonate
Physical Restraint
Physician Support
Pneumatic Tourniquet Precautions
Positioning
Positioning: Intraoperative
Positioning: Neurologic
Positioning: Wheelchair
Postanesthesia Care
Postmortem Care
Postpartal Care
Preceptor: Employee
Preceptor: Student
Preconception Counseling
Pregnancy Termination Care
Premenstrual Syndrome (PMS) Management
Prenatal Care
Preoperative Coordination
Preparatory Sensory Information
Presence
Pressure Management
Pressure Ulcer Care
Pressure Ulcer Prevention
Product Evaluation
Program Development
Progressive Muscle Relaxation
Prompted Voiding
Prosthesis Care
Pruritus Management
Quality Monitoring
Radiation Therapy Management
Rape-Trauma Treatment
Reality Orientation
Recreation Therapy
Rectal Prolapse Management
Referral
Religious Addiction Prevention
Religious Ritual Enhancement
Relocation Stress Reduction
Reminiscence Therapy
Reproductive Technology Management
Research Data Collection
Resiliency Promotion
Respiratory Monitoring
Respite Care
Resuscitation
Resuscitation: Fetus
Resuscitation: Neonate
Risk Identification
Risk Identification: Childbearing Family

Risk Identification: Genetic
Role Enhancement
Seclusion
Security Enhancement
Sedation Management
Seizure Management
Seizure Precautions
Self-Awareness Enhancement
Self-Care Assistance
Self-Care Assistance: Bathing/Hygiene
Self-Care Assistance: Dressing/Grooming
Self-Care Assistance: Feeding
Self-Care Assistance: IADL
Self-Care Assistance: Toileting
Self-Care Assistance: Transfer
Self-Esteem Enhancement
Self-Hypnosis Facilitation
Self-Modification Assistance
Self-Responsibility Facilitation
Sexual Counseling
Shift Report
Shock Management
Shock Management: Cardiac
Shock Management: Vasogenic
Shock Management: Volume
Shock Prevention
Sibling Support
Simple Guided Imagery
Simple Massage
Simple Relaxation Therapy
Skin Care: Donor Site
Skin Care: Graft Site
Skin Care: Topical Treatments
Skin Surveillance
Sleep Enhancement
Smoking Cessation Assistance
Socialization Enhancement
Specimen Management
Spiritual Growth Facilitation
Spiritual Support
Splinting
Sports-Injury Prevention: Youth
Staff Development
Staff Supervision
Subarachnoid Hemorrhage Precautions
Substance Use Prevention
Substance Use Treatment
Substance Use Treatment: Alcohol Withdrawal
Substance Use Treatment: Drug Withdrawal
Substance Use Treatment: Overdose
Suicide Prevention
Supply Management
Support Group
Support System Enhancement
Surgical Assistance
Surgical Precautions
Surgical Preparation
Surveillance
Surveillance: Community
Surveillance: Late Pregnancy
Surveillance: Remote Electronic
Surveillance: Safety
Sustenance Support
Suturing
Swallowing Therapy
Teaching: Disease Process
Teaching: Foot Care
Teaching: Group
Teaching: Individual
Teaching: Infant Nutrition
Teaching: Infant Safety
Teaching: Infant Stimulation
Teaching: Preoperative
Teaching: Prescribed Activity/Exercise
Teaching: Prescribed Diet
Teaching: Prescribed Medication
Teaching: Procedure/Treatment
Teaching: Psychomotor Skill
Teaching: Safe Sex
Teaching: Sexuality
Teaching: Toddler Nutrition
Teaching: Toddler Safety
Teaching: Toilet Training
Technology Management
Telephone Consultation
Telephone Follow-Up
Temperature Regulation
Temperature Regulation: Intraoperative
Temporary Pacemaker Management
Therapeutic Play
Therapeutic Touch
Therapy Group
Total Parenteral Nutrition (TPN) Administration
Touch
Traction/Immobilization Care
Transcutaneous Electrical Nerve Stimulation (TENS)
Transport

Trauma Therapy: Child
Triage: Disaster
Triage: Emergency Center
Triage: Telephone
Truth Telling
Tube Care
Tube Care: Chest
Tube Care: Gastrointestinal
Tube Care: Umbilical Line
Tube Care: Urinary
Tube Care: Ventriculostomy/Lumbar Drain
Ultrasonography: Limited Obstetric
Unilateral Neglect Management
Urinary Bladder Training
Urinary Catheterization
Urinary Catheterization: Intermittent
Urinary Elimination Management
Urinary Habit Training
Urinary Incontinence Care
Urinary Incontinence Care: Enuresis
Urinary Retention Care
Values Clarification
Vehicle Safety Promotion
Venous Access Device (VAD) Maintenance
Ventilation Assistance
Visitation Facilitation
Vital Signs Monitoring
Vomiting Management
Weight Gain Assistance
Weight Management
Weight Reduction Assistance
Wound Care
Wound Care: Closed Drainage
Wound Irrigation

Steps for Implementation of NIC in a Clinical Practice Agency

A. Establish Organizational Commitment to NIC

- Identify the key person responsible for implementation (e.g., person in charge of nursing informatics).
- Create an implementation task force with representatives from key areas.
- Provide NIC materials to all members of the task force.
- Invite a member of the NIC project team to do a presentation for staff and to meet with the task force.
- Purchase copies of the NIC book, circulate readings about NIC and *The NIC/NOC Letter* to units.
- Show the NIC video.
- Have members of the task force begin to use the language in everyday discussion.
- Have key people from the task force sign onto the Center for Nursing Classification and Clinical Effectiveness LISTSERV.

B. Prepare an Implementation Plan

- Write the specific goals to be accomplished.
- Do a force field analysis to determine driving and restraining forces.
- Determine whether an in-house evaluation will be done and the nature of the evaluation effort.
- Identify which NIC interventions are most appropriate for the agency or unit.
- Determine the extent to which NIC is to be implemented; for example, in standards, care planning, documentation, discharge summary, performance evaluation.
- Prioritize the implementation efforts.
- Choose 1 to 3 pilot units. Get members from these units involved in the planning.
- Develop a written timeline for implementation.
- Review current system and determine the logical sequence of actions for integration of NIC.
- Create work groups of expert clinical users to review NIC interventions and activities, determine how these will be used in agency, and develop needed forms.
- Distribute the work of the expert clinicians to other users for evaluation and feedback before implementation.
- Encourage the development of a *NIC champion* in each of the units.
- Keep other key decision makers in agency informed.
- Determine the nature of the total nursing data set. Work to ensure that all units are collecting data on all variables in a uniform manner so that future research can be done.
- Make plans to ensure that all nursing data are retrievable.
- Identify learning needs of staff and plan ways to address these.

C. Carry Out the Implementation Plan

- Develop the screens/forms for implementation. Review each NIC intervention and decide whether all parts (e.g., label, definition, activities, reference) are to be used. Determine which are critical activities to document and whether further details are desired.
- Provide training time for staff.
- Implement NIC in the pilot unit(s) and obtain regular feedback.
- Update content or create new computer functions as needed.
- Use focus groups to clarify issues and address concerns/questions.
- Use data on positive aspects of implementation in house-wide presentations.

- Implement NIC house-wide.
- Collect postimplementation evaluation data and make changes as needed.
- Identify key markers to use for ongoing evaluation and continue to monitor and maintain the system.
- Provide feedback to the Center for Nursing Classification and Clinical Effectiveness.

Nursing Outcomes Classification (NOC)

NOC Taxonomy: Outcomes

Abuse Cessation
Abuse Protection
Abuse Recovery Status
Abuse Recovery: Emotional
Abuse Recovery: Financial
Abuse Recovery: Physical
Abuse Recovery: Sexual
Abusive Behavior Self-Restraint
Acceptance: Health Status
Activity Tolerance
Adaptation to Physical Disability
Adherence Behavior
Aggression Self-Control
Allergic Response: Localized
Allergic Response: Systemic
Ambulation
Ambulation: Wheelchair
Anxiety Level
Anxiety Self-Control
Appetite
Aspiration Prevention
Asthma Self-Management
Balance
Blood Coagulation
Blood Glucose Level
Blood Loss Severity
Blood Transfusion Reaction
Body Image
Body Mechanics Performance
Body Positioning: Self-Initiated
Bone Healing
Bowel Continence
Bowel Elimination
Breastfeeding Establishment: Infant
Breastfeeding Establishment: Maternal
Breastfeeding Maintenance
Breastfeeding Weaning
Cardiac Disease Self-Management
Cardiac Pump Effectiveness
Caregiver Adaptation to Patient Institutionalization
Caregiver Emotional Health
Caregiver Home Care Readiness
Caregiver Lifestyle Disruption
Caregiver-Patient Relationship
Caregiver Performance: Direct Care
Caregiver Performance: Indirect Care
Caregiver Physical Health
Caregiver Stressors
Caregiver Well-Being
Caregiving Endurance Potential
Child Adaptation to Hospitalization
Child Development: 1 Month
Child Development: 2 Months
Child Development: 4 Months
Child Development: 6 Months
Child Development: 12 Months
Child Development: 2 Years
Child Development: 3 Years
Child Development: 4 Years
Child Development: Preschool
Child Development: Middle Childhood
Child Development: Adolescence
Circulation Status
Client Satisfaction: Access to Care Resources
Client Satisfaction: Caring
Client Satisfaction: Communication
Client Satisfaction: Continuity of Care
Client Satisfaction: Cultural Needs Fulfillment
Client Satisfaction: Functional Assistance
Client Satisfaction: Physical Care
Client Satisfaction: Physical Environment
Client Satisfaction: Protection of Rights
Client Satisfaction: Psychological Care
Client Satisfaction: Safety
Client Satisfaction: Symptom Control
Client Satisfaction: Teaching
Client Satisfaction: Technical Aspects of Care
Cognition
Cognitive Orientation
Comfort Level
Comfortable Death
Communication
Communication: Expressive
Communication: Receptive
Community Competence
Community Disaster Readiness
Community Health Status
Community Health Status: Immunity
Community Risk Control: Chronic Disease

Community Risk Control: Communicable Disease
Community Risk Control: Lead Exposure
Community Risk Control: Violence
Community Violence Level
Compliance Behavior
Concentration
Coordinated Movement
Coping
Decision-Making
Depression Level
Depression Self-Control
Diabetes Self-Management
Dignified Life Closure
Discharge Readiness: Independent Living
Discharge Readiness: Supported Living
Distorted Thought Self-Control
Electrolyte & Acid/Base Balance
Endurance
Energy Conservation
Fall Prevention Behavior
Falls Occurrence
Family Coping
Family Functioning
Family Health Status
Family Integrity
Family Normalization
Family Participation in Professional Care
Family Physical Environment
Family Resiliency
Family Social Climate
Family Support During Treatment
Fear Level
Fear Level: Child
Fear: Self-Control
Fetal Status: Antepartum
Fetal Status: Intrapartum
Fluid Balance
Fluid Overload Severity
Grief Resolution
Growth
Health Beliefs
Health Beliefs: Perceived Ability to Perform
Health Beliefs: Perceived Control
Health Beliefs: Perceived Resources
Health Beliefs: Perceived Threat
Health Orientation
Health Promoting Behavior
Health Seeking Behavior
Hearing Compensation Behavior
Hemodialysis Access
Hope
Hydration
Hyperactivity Level
Identity
Immobility Consequences: Physiological
Immobility Consequences: Psycho-Cognitive
Immune Hypersensitivity Response
Immune Status
Immunization Behavior
Impulse Self-Control
Infection Severity
Infection Severity: Newborn
Information Processing
Joint Movement: Ankle
Joint Movement: Elbow
Joint Movement: Fingers
Joint Movement: Hip
Joint Movement: Knee
Joint Movement: Neck
Joint Movement: Passive
Joint Movement: Shoulder
Joint Movement: Spine
Joint Movement: Wrist
Kidney Function
Knowledge: Body Mechanics
Knowledge: Breastfeeding
Knowledge: Cardiac Disease Management
Knowledge: Child Physical Safety
Knowledge: Conception Prevention
Knowledge: Diabetes Management
Knowledge: Diet
Knowledge: Disease Process
Knowledge: Energy Conservation
Knowledge: Fall Prevention
Knowledge: Fertility Promotion
Knowledge: Health Behavior
Knowledge: Health Promotion
Knowledge: Health Resources
Knowledge: Illness Care
Knowledge: Infant Care
Knowledge: Infection Control
Knowledge: Labor & Delivery
Knowledge: Medication
Knowledge: Ostomy Care
Knowledge: Parenting
Knowledge: Personal Safety
Knowledge: Postpartum Maternal Health

Knowledge: Preconception Maternal Health
Knowledge: Pregnancy
Knowledge: Prescribed Activity
Knowledge: Sexual Functioning
Knowledge: Substance Abuse Control
Knowledge: Treatment Procedure(s)
Knowledge: Treatment Regimen
Leisure Participation
Loneliness Severity
Maternal Status: Antepartum
Maternal Status: Intrapartum
Maternal Status: Postpartum
Mechanical Ventilation Response: Adult
Mechanical Ventilation Weaning Response: Adult
Medication Response
Memory
Mobility
Mood Equilibrium
Motivation
Nausea & Vomiting Control
Nausea & Vomiting: Disruptive Effects
Nausea & Vomiting Severity
Neglect Cessation
Neglect Recovery
Neurological Status
Neurological Status: Autonomic
Neurological Status: Central Motor Control
Neurological Status: Consciousness
Neurological Status: Cranial Sensory/Motor Function
Neurological Status: Spinal Sensory/Motor Function
Newborn Adaptation
Nutritional Status
Nutritional Status: Biochemical Measures
Nutritional Status: Energy
Nutritional Status: Food & Fluid Intake
Nutritional Status: Nutrient Intake
Oral Hygiene
Ostomy Self-Care
Pain: Adverse Psychological Response
Pain Control
Pain: Disruptive Effects
Pain Level
Parent-Infant Attachment
Parenting: Adolescent Physical Safety
Parenting: Early/Middle Childhood Physical Safety
Parenting: Infant/Toddler Physical Safety
Parenting Performance
Parenting: Psychosocial Safety
Participation in Health Care Decisions
Personal Autonomy
Personal Health Status
Personal Safety Behavior
Personal Well-Being
Physical Aging
Physical Fitness
Physical Injury Severity
Physical Maturation: Female
Physical Maturation: Male
Play Participation
Post Procedure Recovery Status
Prenatal Health Behavior
Preterm Infant Organization
Psychomotor Energy
Psychosocial Adjustment: Life Change
Quality of Life
Respiratory Status: Airway Patency
Respiratory Status: Gas Exchange
Respiratory Status: Ventilation
Rest
Risk Control
Risk Control: Alcohol Use
Risk Control: Cancer
Risk Control: Cardiovascular Health
Risk Control: Drug Use
Risk Control: Hearing Impairment
Risk Control: Sexual Transmitted Diseases (STD)
Risk Control: Tobacco Use
Risk Control: Unintended Pregnancy
Risk Control: Visual Impairment
Risk Detection
Role Performance
Safe Home Environment
Seizure Control
Self-Care Status
Self-Care: Activities of Daily Living (ADL)
Self-Care: Bathing
Self-Care: Dressing
Self-Care: Eating
Self-Care: Hygiene
Self-Care: Instrumental Activities of Daily Living (IADL)
Self-Care: Non-Parenteral Medication
Self-Care: Oral Hygiene
Self-Care: Parenteral Medication

Self-Care: Toileting
Self-Direction of Care
Self-Esteem
Self-Mutilation Restraint
Sensory Function Status
Sensory Function: Cutaneous
Sensory Function: Hearing
Sensory Function: Proprioception
Sensory Function: Taste & Smell
Sensory Function: Vision
Sexual Functioning
Sexual Identity
Skeletal Function
Sleep
Social Interaction Skills
Social Involvement
Social Support
Spiritual Health
Stress Level
Student Health Status
Substance Addiction Consequences
Suffering Severity
Suicide Self-Restraint
Swallowing Status
Swallowing Status: Esophageal Phase
Swallowing Status: Oral Phase
Swallowing Status: Pharyngeal Phase
Symptom Control
Symptom Severity
Symptom Severity: Perimenopause
Symptom Severity: Premenstrual Syndrome (PMS)
Systemic Toxic Clearance: Dialysis
Thermoregulation
Thermoregulation: Newborn
Tissue Integrity: Skin & Mucous Membranes
Tissue Perfusion: Abdominal Organs
Tissue Perfusion: Cardiac
Tissue Perfusion: Cerebral
Tissue Perfusion: Peripheral
Tissue Perfusion: Pulmonary
Transfer Performance
Treatment Behavior: Illness or Injury
Urinary Continence
Urinary Elimination
Vision Compensation Behavior
Vital Signs
Weight: Body Mass
Weight Control
Will to Live
Wound Healing: Primary Intention
Wound Healing: Secondary Intention

Developmental Milestones from Birth to 5 Years

Age (Months)	Adaptive/ Fine Motor	Language	Gross Motor	Personal-Social
1	Grasp reflex (hands fisted)	Facial response to sounds	Lifts head in prone position	Stares at face
2	Follows object with eyes past midline	Coos (vowel sounds)	Lifts head in prone position to 458	Smiles in response to others
4	Hands open; brings objects to mouth	Laughs and squeals; turns toward voice	Sits; head steady; rolls to supine	Smiles spontaneously
6	Palmar grasp of objects	Babbles (consonant sounds)	Sits independently; stands, hands held	Reaches for toys; recognizes strangers
9	Pincer grasp	Says "mama," "dada" non-specifically; comprehends "no"	Pulls to stand	Feeds self; waves bye-bye
12	Helps turn pages of book	2–4 words; follows command with gesture	Stands independently; walks, one hand held	Points to indicate wants
15	Scribbles	4–6 words; follows command no gesture	Walks independently	Drinks from cup, imitates activities
18	Turns pages of book	10–20 words; points to 4 body parts	Walks up steps	Feeds self with spoon
24	Solves single-piece puzzles	Combines 2–3 words; uses "I" and "you"	Jumps; kicks ball	Removes coat; verbalizes wants
30	Imitates horizontal and vertical lines	Names all body parts	Rides tricycle using pedals	Pulls up pants; washes and dries hands
36	Copies circle; draws person with 3 parts	Gives full name, age, and sex; names 2 colors	Throws ball overhand; walks up stairs (alternating feet)	Toilet trained; puts on shirt, knows front from back
42	Copies cross	Understands "cold," "tired," "hungry"	Stands on one foot for 2–3 seconds	Engages in associative play
48	Counts 4 objects; identifies some numbers and letters	Understands pre-positions (under, on, behind, in front of); asks "how" and "why"	Hops on one foot	Dresses with little assistance; shoes on correct feet
54	Copies square; draws person with 6 parts	Understands opposites	Broad-jumps 24 inches	Bosses and criticizes; shows off
60	Prints first name; counts 10 objects	Asks meaning of words	Skips (alternating feet)	Ties shoes

Recommended Immunizations

Recommended Immunization Schedule for Persons Aged 0–18 Years; United States–2007, by Vaccine and Age Group

Vaccine ▼ Age ▶	Birth	1 month	2 months	4 months	6 months	12 months	15 months	18 months	19–23 months	2–3 years	4–6 years
Hepatitis B[1]	HepB	HepB		*see footnote1*		HepB				HepB Series	
Rotavirus[2]			Rota	Rota	Rota						
Diphtheria, Tetanus, Pertussis[3]			DTaP	DTaP	DTaP		DTaP				DTaP
Haemophilus influenza type b[4]			Hib	Hib	*Hib*[4]	Hib			Hib		
Pneumococcal[5]			PCV	PCV	PCV	PCV				PCV PPV	
Inactivated Poliovirus			IPV	IPV		IPV					IPV
Influenza[6]								Influenza (Yearly)			
Measles, Mumps, Rubella[7]						MMR					MMR
Varicella[8]						Varicella					Varicella
Hepatitis A[9]								HepA (2 doses)		HepA Series	
Meningococcal[10]										MPSV4	

Vaccine ▼ Age ▶	7-10 years	11-12 years	13-14 years	15 years	16-18 years
Tetanus, Diphtheria, Pertussis[1]	*see footnote1*	Tdap		Tdap	
Human Papillomavirus[2]	*see footnote 2*	HPV (3 Doses)		HPV Series	
Meningococcal[3]	MPSV4	MCV4		MCV4[3] MCV4	
Pneumococcal[4]		PPV			
Influenza[5]			Influenza (Yearly)		
Hepatitis A[6]		HepA Series			
Hepatitis B[7]		HepB Series			
Inactivated Poliovirus[8]		IPV Series			
Measles, Mumps, Rubella[9]		MMR Series			
Varicella[9]		Varicella Series			

Range of recommended ages — Catch-up immunizations — Certain high-risk groups

This schedule indicates the recommended ages for routine administration of currently licensed childhood vaccines (as of December 1, 2006) for children aged 0-18. All footnotes are available at **http://www.cdc.gov/vaccines/recs/schedules/child-schedule.htm**.

Recommended Adult Immunization Schedule for Persons Aged 19 Years and Over; United States–2007, by Vaccine and Age Group

Vaccine ▼ Age group (yrs) ▶	19-49 years	50-64 years	≥ 65 years
Tetanus, Diphtheria, Pertussis (Td/Tdap)[1]*		1-dose Td booster every 10 years Substitute 1 dose of Tdap for Td	
Human Papillomavirus (HPV)[2]*	3 doses (females)		
Measles, Mumps, Rubella (MMR)[3]*	1 or 2 doses	1 dose	
Varicella[4]*	2 doses (0, 4–8 wks)	2 doses (0, 4–8 wks)	
Influenza[5]*	1 dose annually	1 dose annually	

Vaccine ▼ Age group (yrs) ▶	19-49 years	50-64 years	≥65 years
Pneumococcal (polysaccharide)[6, 7]	1–2 doses		1 dose
Hepatitis A[8]*		2 doses (0, 6–12 mos, or 0, 6–18 mos)	
Hepatitis B[9]*		3 doses (0, 1–2, 4–6 mos)	
Meningococcal[10]		1 or more doses	

This schedule indicates the recommended age groups for routine administration of currently licensed vaccines (as of October 1, 2006) for persons aged ≥19. All footnotes are available at **http://www.cdc.gov/vaccines/recs/schedules/default.htm#adult**.

For all persons in this category who meet the age requirements and who lack evidence of immunity (e.g., lack of documentation of vaccination or have no evidence of prior infection)

Recommended if some other risk factor is present (e.g., on the basis of medical, occupational, lifestyles, or other indications)

Additional information is available at **http://www.cdc.gov/vaccines/default.htm.**

Adapted from Recommended Immunization Schedule for Persons Aged 0-6 Years, United States, 2007; Recommended Immunization Schedule for Persons Aged 7-18 Years, United States, 2007; Recommended Adult Immunization Schedule, United States, October 2006-September 2007.

Poisonous Plants

Some commonly found poisonous plants (iris and philodendron have countless varieties so that no Latin nomenclature has been given here.)

Common Name	Latin Name
Azalea	*Pentanthera,* subgroup *Azalea*
Buttercup	*Ranunculus acris*
Calla lily	*Zanthedeschia aethiopica*
Creeping Charlie (ground ivy)	*Hedera* spp.
Daffodil	*Narcissus* spp.
Delphinium	*Delphinium* spp.
Elderberry	*Sambucus canadensis*
Foxglove	*Digitalis purpurea*
Holly (berries)	*Ilex opaca*
Hyacinth (bulbs)	*Hyacinthus orientalis*
Hydrangea	*Hydrangea* spp.
Iris	—
Ivy (Boston)	*Parthenocissus tricuspidata*
Jimson weed	*Datura stramonium*
Jonquil	*Narcissus* spp.
Larkspur	*Delphinium* spp.
Laurel, mountain	*Kalmia latifolia*
Lily-of-the-valley	*Convallaria majalis*
Mistletoe, eastern	*Phoradendron serotinum*
Morning glory	*Ipomoea purpurea*
Narcissus	*Narcissus* spp.
Nightshade, deadly (belladonna)	*Atropa belladonna*
Oleander	*Nerium oleander*
Periwinkle	*Vinca major, V. minor*
Philodendron	—
Poison ivy	*Toxicodendron radicans*
Poison oak, eastern	*Toxicodendron toxicarium*
Poison sumac	*Toxicodendron vernix*
Rhododendron, great	*Rhododendron maximum*
Sweet pea	*Lathyrus odoratus*
Tomatoes (vines)	*Lycopersicon esculentum*
Tulip	*Tulipa* spp.
Wisteria	*Wisteria* spp.
Wormwood	*Artemisia absinthium*
Yew, English	*Taxus baccata*

Herbs (Scientific Names/Common Names; Common Names/Scientific Names)

Scientific Name	Common Name
Acacia senegal	acacia; gum arabic
Achillea collina	chamomile, European
Achillea lanulosa	chamomile, North American
Achillea millefolium	chamomile yarrow; soldier's woundwort; nosebleed; milfoil
Aconitum carmichaeli	aconite; fu tzu; monkshood; aconite fisheri, wolfsbane
Acorus americanus	North American calamus; type I calamus
Acorus calamus	calamus; type II calamus; sweet flag; sweet sedge
Actaea arguta	baneberry
Actaea spicata	herb christopher
Adonis vernalis	adonis
Agastache rugosa	agastache; patchouli; pogostemon
Agathosma betulina	buchu
Agrimonia eupatoria	agrimony; sticklewort; cocklebur
Alchemilla xanthochlora	lady's mantle
Aletris farinosa	unicorn root
Alisma plantago-aquatica	alisma; marsh drain; water plantain
Alkanna tinctoria	alkanet
Allium ampeloprasum	leek
Allium ascalonicum	shallot
Allium cepa	onion
Allium fistulosum	scallion
Allium sativa	garlic
Aloe barbadensis	aloe; kumari
Aloysia triphylla	lemon verbena
Althaea rosea	hollyhock; althea
Amanita muscaria	fly agaric
Amanita phalloides	deadly agaric
Amaranthus caudatus	love lies bleeding
Amaranthus hybridus	amaranth; red cockscomb
Ammi visagna	greater ammi; toothpick ammi
Amomum villosum	amomum; grains-of-paradise; cardamom
Anemarrhena asphodeloides	anemarrhena
Anethum graveolens	dill; dillweed
Angelica archangelica	angelica, American
Angelica polymorpha	dong quai; dang gui; tang kuei
Angelica sinensis	dong quai; tang kwei
Apium graveolens	celery; celeriac
Aralia racemosa	spikenard
Arctium lappa	burdock; great burdock; lappa; bardane; beggar's button
Arctostaphylos uva-ursi	uva ursi; bearberry
Arnica montana	arnica; leopard's bane

Artemisia absinthium	absinthe
Artemisia vulgaris	mugwort; moxa
Asarium heterotropoides	wild ginger; xi xin
Asclepias tuberosa	pleurisy root; butterfly weed
Aspalathus linearis	red bush tea; rooibos tea
Asparagus officinalis	asapargus; sparrowgrass
Astragalus membranaceus	astragalus; huang chi; milk vetch root; bok kay; goat thorn
Atractylodes macrocephala	pai shu; atractylodes
Atropa belladonna	belladonna; deadly nightshade
Aucklandia lappa	aucklandia; saussurea; costus root
Avena sativa	oats; oat bran; oat groats
Azadirachta indica	neem tree; azedarach; Melia; nim; margosa
Baptisia tinctoria	baptisia; wild indigo; indigoweed
Berberis vulgaris	barberry; pipperidge bush; berberry
Betonica officinalis	wood betony
Biota orientalis	biota; arborvitae
Borago officinalis	borage; burrage
Brassica alba	mustard, white
Brassica nigra	mustard, black or brown
Bryonia alba	bryonia; wild hops
Bupleurum falcatum	bupleurum; ch'ai hu
Calendula officinalis	marigold
Camellia sinensis	tea; black tea
Capparis spinosa	capers
Capsella bursa-pastoris	shepherd's purse
Capsicum frutescens	cayenne pepper; chili pepper; capsicum
Carica papaya	papaya; papain
Carthamus tinctorius	safflower; hong hua; red flower
Carum carvi	caraway
Cassia senna	senna; Tinnevelley senna
Catha edulis	khat
Caulophyllum thalictroides	blue cohosh; papoose root; squaw root
Centella asiatica	gotu kola; hydrocotyle; Indian pennywort
Centranthus ruber	red valerian
Cephaelis ipecacuanha	ipecacuanha; ipecac
Cetraria islandica	Iceland moss; Iceland lichen
Chamaelirium luteum	false unicorn; helonias
Chamaemelum nobile	chamomile; Roman chamomile; English chamomile
Chamomilla recutita	chamomile; Hungarian chamomile; single chamomile
Chelidonium majus	celandine; greater celandine
Chenopodium ambrosoides	epazote; Mexican wormseed; American wormseed
Chicorium intybus	chicory; succory
Chimaphilia umbellata	pipsissewa; prince pine; ground holly
Chionanthus virginicus	fringe tree
Chondrus crispus	Irish moss; carageenan

Chrysanthemum morifolium	chrysanthemum; chu hua
Cicuta maculata	water hemlock (poisonous)
Cimicifuga racemosa	black cohosh, black snake root, bugbane, rattleroot, sheng ma
Cinchona spp.	quinine; cinchona bark; Peruvian bark; quina, quinaquina, quinquina; Jesuits' bark
Cinnamomum camphora	camphor; gum camphor; laurel camphor
Cinnamomum cassia	chinese cinnamon bark; Chinese cinnamon twig; cassia twig
Cinnamomum zeylanicum	cinnamon
Citrus reticulata	citrus peel; chen pi; tangerine peel
Claviceps purpurea	ergot
Cnicus benedictus	blessed thistle; holy thistle; St. Benedict's thistle; Benedictine (liqueur)
Cocos nucifera	coconut; coconut palm
Codonopsis pilosula	don sen; tang shen; codonopsis root
Coffea arabica	coffee
Coix lachryma jobi	coix; Job's tears
Cola nitida	kola; cola; kola nut, kolanut; guru nut
Collinsonia canadensis	collinsonia; stoneroot
Commiphora madagascariensis	Abyssinian myrrh
Commiphora molmol	Somalian myrrh
Commiphora myrrha	myrrh; guggul
Consolida regalis	larkspur
Convallaria majalis	lily of the valley
Convolvulus scammonia	scammany; Mexican scammany; scammony
Convolvulus spp.	bush morning glory
Coptis chinensis	coptis; Chinese goldthread
Coriander sativum	coriander
Cornus officinalus	cornus; Asiatic cornelian cherry; Asiatic dogwood
Corydalis yanhusuo	corydalis
Crataegus laevigata	hawthorn
Crocus sativus	saffron
Croton tiglium	croton oil
Cryptotympana atrata	cicada (insect)
Cucurbita maxima	autumn squash seeds
Cucurbita moschata	Canada pumpkin; crookneck squash
Cucurbita popo	pumpkin seeds; pepo
Cuminum cymium	cumin
Curcuma longa	turmeric
Cuscuta chinensis	cuscuta; Chinese dodder
Cydonia japonica	flowering quince
Cymbopogon citratus	lemongrass
Cyperus rotundus	cyperus; sedge root; nut-grass rhizome
Cypripedium calceoulus	lady slipper; nerveroot
Cytisus scoparius	broom; broom top; Scotch broom; Scotch bloom

Datura stramonium	datura; stink weed; thorn apple; jimson weed; Jamestown weed
Digitalis purpurea	foxglove
Dioscorea floribunda	Mexican wild yam
Dioscorea opposita	Chinese yam
Dioscorea paniculata	wild yam; colicroot; rheumatism root
Dioscorea villosa	colic root; American wild yam
Echinacea angustifolia	echinacea; coneflower; narrow-leaved purple cone flower; purple cone flower; prairie
Elettaria cardamomum	cardamom
Eleutherococcus senticosus	Siberian ginseng; eleutherococcus; eleuthero; ciwujia; wujiaseng
Ephedra nevadensis	Mormon tea; popotillo; Brigham tea; teamster tea; squaw tea
Ephedra sinica	ma huang; ephedra; desert tea
Epimedium pimedium grandiflorum	epimedium; lusty goatherb
Equisetum arvense	horsetail
Equisetum palustre	European horsetail
Eriobotrya japonica	loquat
Eriodictyon californicum	yerba santa; holy herb; mountain balm
Erythroxylum coca	coca; cocaine
Eschscholzia californica	California poppy
Eucalyptus globulus	eucalyptus; blue gum tree
Eucommia ulmoides	eucommia bark
Eupatorium perfoliatum	boneset; feverwort; thoroughwort
Eupatorium purpureum	gravel root; Joe-Pye weed; queen of the meadow
Euphorbia longana	longan berries; long yen rou; dragon's eyes
Euphorbia spp.	eyebright; spurge
Euphrasia officinalis	eyebright; euphrasy
Evodia rutaecarpa	evodia fruit
Ferula asafoetida	asafoetida; devil's dung; gum asafetida
Foeniculum vulgare	fennel
Fucus vesiculosus	kelp; bladderwrack
Galium aparine	cleavers; clivers; goose grass; bedstraw
Ganoderma lucidum	ganoderma; ling zhi; reishi
Garcinia cambogia	garcinia; Malabar tamarind
Gastrodia elata	gastrodia; heavenly hemp
Gelsemium sempervirens	Carolina jessamine; yellow jasmine
Gentiana lutea	gentian; Angostura Bitters
Gentiana scabra	gentiana
Geranium maculatum	cranesbill root; wild geranium; storksbill; alumroot
Gillenia trifoliata	Indian physic

Ginkgo biloba	ginkgo; ginkgo nut; maidenhair tree
Glycyrrhiza glabra	liquorice, licorice; gan t'sao
Gonolobus condurango	condurango
Gratiola spp.	hedge hyssop
Hamamelis virginiana	witch hazel
Harpagophytum procumbens	devil's claw; wood spider; grapple plant
Hedeoma pulegioides	pennyroyal
Hemidesmus indicus	false sarsaparilla; Indian sarsaparilla
Hibiscus sabdariffa	hibiscus; roselle; Sudanese tea; red tea; Jamaica sorrel
Hordeum vulgare	barley; pearl barley; prelate
Humulus lupulus	hops
Hydrangea arborescens	hydrangea; seven barks
Hydrastis canadensis	goldenseal; puccoon root; yellowroot; hydrastis
Hyoscyamus niger	henbane
Hypericum perforatum	St. John's wort
Hyssopus officinalis	hyssop
Ignatia amara	St. Ignatius bean
Ilex cassine	yaupon hollies
Ilex paraguariensis	maté
Indigofera tinctoria	indigo
Inula helenium	elecampane; scabwort; elf dock; horseheal
Ipomoea purpurea	morning glory
Iris versicolor	poison flag; wild iris; blue flag; flag lily; fleur-de-lis; liver lily
Juglans nigra	walnut, black
Juniperus communis	juniper
Lactuca virosa	lettuce opium; lactucarium; wild lettuce
Larrea tridentata	chapparal; creosote bush; greasewood
Laurelis nobilis	bay
Lavandula angustifolia	lavender; garden lavender
Ledebouriella divaricata	sileris; fang feng
Ledum palustre	marsh tea
Lentinula edodes	shiitake
Leonurus cardiaca	motherwort; lion's-tail; mother herb; yi mu cao
Leptandra virginica	Culver root; black root; physic root
Levisticum officinale	lovage; Maggi plant
Ligusticum chuanxiong	cnidium; chuanxiong; Chinese lovage
Ligustrum lucidum	privet fruit; ligustrum
Liquidambar spp.	sweet gum
Liriosma ovata	muira puama; potency wood
Lobelia inflata	lobelia; Indian tobacco; pukeweed
Lobelia spp.	eyebright
Lonicera japonica	Japanese honeysuckle; yin hua
Lycium chinensis	lycii; gay gee; lycium fruit

Lycopodium clavatum	club moss
Lytta (Cantharis) vesicatoria	Spanish fly; Russian fly
Magnolia lilliflora	magnolia buds
Mahonia aquifolium	barberry; Oregon grape
Malva sylvestris	malva; marshmallow; marsh mallow
Marrubium vulgare	horehound; hoarhound
Matricaria recutita	chamomile; German chamomile; Hungarian chamomile
Matteuccia struthiopteris	ostrich fern
Medicago sativa	alfalfa; lucerne
Melaleuca alternifolia	tea tree; tea tree oil
Melaleuca leucadendron	cajuput; cajeput; punk tree; white tea tree; tea tree
Melissa officinalis	lemon balm; melissa; balm
Mentha haplocalyx	field mint
Mentha piperata	peppermint
Mentha pulegium	pennyroyal, European
Mentha spicata	spearmint; garden mint
Mitchella repens	squawvine; partridgeberry
Morus alba	mulberry; white mulberry
Myrica cerifera	bayberry; candleberry; waxberry; myrtle; wax myrtle
Myrica pennsylvanica	bayberry
Myristica fragrans	nutmeg
Nasturtium officinale	watercress
Nepeta cataria	catnip; catmint
Ocimum basilicum	basil
Oenothera biennis	evening primrose; sundrops
Ophiopogon japonicus	Japanese turf lily; creeping lily root; dwarf lilyturf
Oplopanax horridus	devil's club
Origanum majorana	marjoram
Oryza sativa	rice; rice bran
Paeonia lactiflora	peony; shao-yao
Panax ginseng	ginseng, Asian; jen sheng; shiu chu root; ren sheng
Panax notoginseng	tienchi; notoginseng root
Panax pseudo-ginseng	san qui ginseng; tienchi ginseng; sanchi ginseng
Panax quinquefolius	ginseng, American
Papaver rhoeas	poppy, red
Papaver somniferum	poppy, opium
Parthenium integrifolium	prairie dock
Passiflora incarnata	passion flower; passionflower
Paullinia cupana	guarana
Pausinystalia yohimba	yohimbe
Periploca sepium	silk vine
Petroselinum crispum	parsley
Pfaffia paniculata	suma; para toda; Brazilian ginseng

Phoradendron leucarpum	American mistletoe
Phyllanthus emblica	myrobalan, emblic; triphala; Indian gooseberry
Physostigma venenosum	physostigma
Phytolacca americana	poke; pokeweed; pokeroot
Pimenta officinalis	pimento; pimenta; allspice
Pimpinella anisum	anise; aniseed
Pinus mugo	dwarf pine (oil); mugo pine
Pinus pinaster	Pycnogenol
Piper methysticum	kava; kava kava; kawa
Piper nigrum	black pepper
Plantago lanceolata	plantago; Englishman's foot; greater plantain; ribwort
Plantago ovata	psyllium; ispaghul
Platycodon grandiflorum	platycodon; jie geng
Podophyllum peltatum	mayapple; mandrake; vegetable calomel; devil's-apple
Polygonum bistoria	bistort; snakeweed; adderwort; dragonwort
Polygonum multiflorum	fo-ti; he-shou-wu; ho shou wu; fleece-flower root
Polygala senega	senega snakeroot; Seneca snakeroot; senega
Populus balsamifera	balm of Gilead; quaking aspen; white poplar
Poria cocos	fu ling
Prunus africana	pygeum
Prunus armeniaca	apricot pit; laetrile; vitamin B17; amygdalin; ku xing ren; persica; apricot kernel oil
Prunus persica	persic oil; peach kernel oil
Prunus serotina	wild cherry bark
Prunus virginiana	chokecherry
Ptychopetalum olacoides	muira puama; potency wood
Pueraria lobata	pueraria; ko ken; kudzu; kuzu root
Pulmonaria angustifolia	lungwort; blue cowslip
Pulsatilla nigricans	windflower
Puschkina scilloides libanotica	squill, Lebanon
Quercus spp.	acorn; oak
Quillaja saponaria	quillaja; soapbark
Ranunculus ficaria	pilewort
Ranunculus spp.	buttercup; ranunculus
Raphanus raphanistrum	wild radish
Rauwolfia serpentina	rauwolfia
Rehmannia glutinosa	rehmannia; sok day; san day; Chinese floxglove root
Rhamnus cathartica	buckthorn; common buckthorn
Rhamnus purshiana	cascara sagrada; sacred bark; chittem bark
Rheum palmatum	rhubarb; Chinese rhubarb; da huang; Turkey rhubarb; garden rhubarb
Rhus toxicodendron	poison ivy
Rhus venenata	poison sumac
Ribes nigrum	European currant
Ricinus communis	castor-oil plant; castor bean; palma Christi

Rosa canina	rose hip
Rosmarinus officinalis	rosemary
Rubus idaeus	raspberry
Rubus fruticosus	blackberry
Rumex acetosella	sheep sorrel
Rumex crispus	yellow dock; broad leaved dock; curly dock; sourdock; curled dock
Rumex hymenosepalus	canaigre; wild red American ginseng; wild red desert ginseng; Indian tan plant
Ruscus aculeatus	butcher's-broom; box holly; knee holly; Knee holy; pettier; sweet broom
Ruta graveolens	rue; garden rue
Sabbatia spp.	eyebright
Salix alba	willow; white willow
Salvia miltiorrhiza	salvia; dang shen
Salvia officinalis	sage
Sambucus niger	elder
Sambucus racemosa	red elder
Sanguinaria canadensis	bloodroot; redroot; red Indian paint; tetterwort
Sanguisorba minor	burnet; sanguisorba; salad burnet
Sanguisorba officinalis	great burnet
Santalum album	sandalwood (oil)
Sargassum pallidum	sargassum seaweed
Sassafras albidum	sassafras
Satureja hortensis	summer savory; Bohnenkraut
Satureja montana	winter savory
Schisandra chinensis	schisandra
Scilla sibirica	squill, Siberian
Scutellaria lateriflora	scullcap; skullcap; blue skullcap; huang chi; scutellaria
Selenicereus grandiflorus	night-blooming cereus
Senecio aureus	life root; golden senecio; ragwort; false valerian; squaw weed
Senecio cineraria	dusty miller; cineraria
Serenoa repens	saw palmetto; sabal
Sessamum indicum	sesame (oil)
Silybum marianum	milk thistle; Marian thistle; St. Mary's thistle; Our Lady's thistle
Simmondsia chinensis	jojoba oil
Smilax aristolochiaefolia	sarsaparilla, Mexican
Smilax febrifuga	sarsaparilla, Ecuadorian
Smilax medica	sarsaparilla
Smilax ornata	sarsaparilla, Jamaican
Smilax regelii	sarsaparilla, Honduran
Solanum capsicastrum	false Jerusalem cherry
Spartium junceum	Spanish broom; gorse
Spiraea spp.	spirea
Spirulina maxima	spirulina; dihe; tecuitlatl; blue-green algae
Stachys officinalis	betony; wood betony

Stellaria media	chickweed; starweed
Sterculia urens	sterculia gum; karaya gum
Strophanthus gratus	ouabain
Strychnos nux-vomica	strychnine
Symphytum asperum	prickly comfrey
Symphytum officinale	comfrey; knitbone, salsify
Symphytum x uplandicum	Russian comfrey
Syzygium aromaticum	cloves
Syzygium paniculatum	bush cherry
Tabebuia avellanedae	pau d'arco; ipe roxo; lapacho; taheebo tea; lapacho colorado, lapacho morado
Tabebuia heptaphylla	pau d'arco; lapacho; tabebuia; purple lapacho
Tagetes spp.	marigold
Tamarindus indica	tamarind
Tanacetum parthenium	feverfew
Tanacetum vulgare	tansy, bachelor's button
Taraxacum mongolicum	Chinese dandelion
Taraxacum officinale	dandelion
Terminalia bellerica	myrobalan, beleric; triphala; bhibitaki
Terminalia chebula	myrobalan, chebulic; triphala; ho-tzu ch
Teucrium canadense	common germander; pink skullcap
Theobroma cacao	coco; cocoa
Thymus vulgaris	thyme
Tilia cordata	linden; linden flower; lime flowers
Tilia tomentosa	silver linden
Toluifera balsamum	tolu; tolu balsam
Trifolium pratense	red clover
Trigonella foenum-graecum	fenugreek
Triticum aestivum	wheat; wheat bran
Tropaeolum spp.	nasturtium
Turnera diffusa	damiana
Tussilago farfara	coltsfoot; coughwort; horsehoof
Ulmus rubra	slippery elm; red elm
Uncaria tomentosa	cat's claw; una de gato
Urginea indica	Indian squill
Urginea maritima	squill; scilla, urginea; sea onion; red squill; white squill
Urtica dioica	nettle; stinging nettle
Usnea barbata	usnea; beard lichen; larch moss; old man's beard
Vaccinium macrocarpon	cranberry
Vaccinium myrtillus	bilberry
Vaccinium oxycoccos	European cranberry
Vaccinium spp.	blueberry
Valeriana officinalis	valerian
Vanilla planifolia	vanilla; Bourbon vanilla; Mexican vanilla
Vanilla tahitensis	vanilla; Tahitian vanilla
Verbascum thapsus	mullein
Verbena officinalis	vervain; blue vervain
Veronica spp.	creeping speedwell; veronica

Viburnum opulus	cramp bark; Guelder rose; snowball tree
Viburnum prunifolium	black haw, American sloe, stagbush
Vinca rosea	periwinkle
Viola odorata	violet; sweet violet
Viscum album	mistletoe, European
Vitex agnus-castus	chaste berries; vitex; monk pepper; chaste tree; hemp tree
Vitis vinifera	grape seed extract
Withania somnifera	ashwaganda
Yucca aloifolia	yucca; Spanish bayonet; dagger plant
Yucca brevifolia	yucca; Joshua tree
Yucca glauca	yucca; soapweed
Yucca schidigera	yucca; Mohave yucca
Yucca whipplei	yucca; our-Lord's-candle
Zanthoxylum americanum	prickly ash; toothache tree
Zea mays	corn (silk); Indian corn; maize; yumixu; stigmata maydis
Zingiber officinale	ginger; Jamaica ginger; African ginger; Cohin ginger; gan-jian
Ziziphus jujube	jujube date; da t'sao

Common Name	Scientific Name
absinthe	*Artemisia absinthium*
Abyssinian myrrh	*Commiphora madagascariensis*
acacia; gum arabic	*Acacia senegal*
aconite fisheri	*Aconitum carmichaeli*
aconite; fu tzu; monkshood; aconite fisheri	*Aconitum carmichaeli*
acorn; oak	*Quercus* spp.
adderwort	*Polygonum bistoria*
adonis	*Adonis vernalis*
African ginger	*Zingiber officianale*
agastache; patchouli; pogostemon	*Agastache rugosa*
agrimony; sticklewort; cocklebur	*Agrimonia eupatoria*
alfalfa; lucerne	*Medicago sativa*
alisma; marsh drain; water plantain	*Alisma plantago-aquatica*
alkanet	*Alkanna tinctoria*
allspice	*Pimenta officinalis*
aloe; kumari	*Aloe barbadensis*
althea	*Althea rosea*
alumroot	*Geranium maculatum*
amaranth; love lies bleeding; red cockscomb	*Amaranthus hybridus*
American mistletoe	*Phoradendron leucarpum*
American sloe	*Viburnum prunifolium*
American wild yam	*Dioscorea villosa*
American wormseed	*Chenopodium ambrosoides*
amomum; grains-of-paradise; cardamom	*Amomum villosum*
amygdalin	*Prunus armeniaca*
anemarrhena	*Anemarrhena asphodeloides*
angelica, American	*Angelica archangelica*
Angostura Bitters	*Gentiana lutea*
anise	*Pimpinella anisum*
aniseed	*Pimpinella anisum*
apricot pit; laetrile; vitamin B17; amygdalin; apricot kernel oil; ku xing ren; persica oil	*Prunus armeniaca*
arborvitae	*Biota orientalis*
arnica; leopard's bane	*Arnica montana*
asafoetida; devil's dung; gum asafetida	*Ferula asafoetida*
asapargus; sparrowgrass	*Asparagus officinalis*
ashwaganda	*Withania somnifera*
Asiatic cornelian cherry	*Cornus officianalus*
Asiatic dogwood	*Cornus officinalis*
astragalus; huang chi; milk vetch root; bok kay; goat thorn	*Astragalus membranaceus*
atractylodes	*Atractylodes macrocephala*
aucklandia; saussurea; costus root	*Aucklandia lappa*
autumn squash seeds	*Cucurbita maxima*

azedarach	*Azadirachta indica*
bachelor's button	*Tanacetum vulgare*
balm of Gilead; quaking aspen; white poplar	*Populus balsamifera*
balm	*Melissa officinalis*
baneberry	*Actaea arguta*
baptisia; wild indigo; indigoweed	*Baptisia tinctoria*
barberry; pipperidge bush	*Berberis vulgaris*
bardane	*Arctium lappa*
barley; pearl barley; prelate	*Hordeum vulgare*
basil	*Ocimum basilicum*
bay	*Laurelis nobilis*
bayberry	*Myrica pennsylvanica*
bayberry; candleberry; waxberry; wax myrtle	*Myrica cerifera*
bearberry	*Arctostaphylos uva-ursi*
beard lichen	*Usnea barbata*
bedstraw	*Galium aparine*
beggar's button	*Arctium lappa*
belladonna; deadly nightshade	*Atropa belladonna*
Benedictine (liqueur)	*Cnicus benedictus*
berberis	*Berberis nervosa*
betony; wood betony	*Stachys officinalis*
bhibitaki	*Terminalia bellerica*
bilberry	*Vaccinium myrtillus*
biota; arborvitae	*Biota orientalis*
bistort; snakeweed; adderwort; dragonwort	*Polygonum bistoria*
blackberry	*Rubus fruticosus*
black cohosh; black snake root; bugbane; rattle root	*Cimicifuga racemosa*
black haw; American sloe; stagbush	*Viburnum prunifolium*
black pepper	*Piper nigrum*
black root	*Leptandra virginica*
black snake root	*Cimicifuga racemosa*
black tea	*Camellia sinensis*
bladderwrack	*Fucus vesiculosus*
blessed thistle; holy thistle; St. Benedict's thistle; Benedictine (liqueur)	*Cnicus benedictus*
bloodroot; redroot; red Indian paint; tetterwort	*Sanguinaria canadensis*
blueberry	*Vaccinium* spp.
blue cohosh; papoose root; squaw root	*Caulophyllum thalictroides*
blue cowslip	*Pulmonaria angustifolia*
blue flag; flag lily; fleur-de-lis; liver lily	*Iris versicolor*
blue-green algae	*Spirulina maxima*
blue gum tree	*Eucalyptus globulus*
blue skullcap	*Scutellaria lateriflora*

blue vervain	*Verbena officinalis*
Bohnenkraut	*Satureja hortensis*
bok kay	*Astragalus membranaceus*
boneset; feverwort; thoroughwort	*Eupatorium perfoliatum*
borage; burrage	*Borago officinalis*
Bourbon vanilla	*Vanilla tahitensis*
box holly	*Ruscus aculeatus*
Brazilian ginseng	*Pfaffia paniculata*
Brigham tea	*Ephedra nevadensis*
broad leaved dock	*Rumex crispus*
broom top	*Cytisus scopraius*
broom; broom top; Scotch broom; Scotch bloom	*Cytisus scoparius*
bryonia; wild hops	*Bryonia alba*
buchu	*Agathosma betulina*
buckthorn; common buckthorn	*Rhamnus cathartica*
bugbane	*Cimicifuga racemosa*
bupleurum; ch'ai hu	*Bupleurum falcatum*
burdock; great burdock; lappa; bardane; beggar button	*Arctium lappa*
burnet; sanguisorba; salad burnet	*Sanguisorba minor*
burrage	*Borago officinalis*
bush cherry	*Syzygium paniculatum*
bush morning glory	*Convolvulus* spp.
butcher's-broom; box holly; knee holly; Kneeholy; pettier; sweet broom	*Ruscus aculeatus*
buttercup; ranunculus	*Ranunculus* spp.
butterfly weed	*Asclepias tuberosa*
coco; cocoa	*Theobroma cacao*
cajeput	*Melaleuca leucadendron*
cajuput; cajeput; punk tree; white tea tree; tea tree	*Melaleuca leucadendron*
calamus; type II calamus; sweet flag; sweet sedge	*Acorus calamus*
calcium pangamate	not biological
California poppy	*Eschscholzia californica*
Camomile; Hungarian camommile; single camomile	*Chamomilla recutita*
camphor; gum camphor; laurel camphor	*Cinnamomum camphora*
Canada pumpkin; crookneck squash	*Cucurbita moschata*
canaigre; wild red American ginseng; wild red desert ginseng; Indian tan plant	*Rumex hymenosepalus*
candleberry	*Myrica cerifera*
capers	*Capparis spinosa*
capsicum; cayenne pepper; chili pimiento	*Capsicum frutescens*

carageenan	*Chondrus crispus*
caraway	*Carum carvi*
cardamom	*Elettaria cardamomum*
cardamom	*Amommum villosum*
Carolina jessamine; yellow jasmine	*Gelsemium sempervirens*
cascara sagrada; sacred bark; chittem bark	*Rhamnus purshiana*
cassia twig	*Cinnamomum cassia*
castor-oil plant; castor bean; palma Christi	*Ricinus communis*
cat's claw; una de gato	*Uncaria tomentosa*
catnip, catmint	*Nepeta cataria*
cayenne pepper	*Capsicum frutescens*
celandine; greater celandine	*Chelidonium majus*
celery; celeriac	*Apium graveolens*
ch'ai hu	*Bupleurum falcatum*
chamomile, European	*Achillea collina*
chamomile; German chamomile; Hungarian chamomile	*Matricaria recutita*
chamomile, North American	*Achillea lanulosa*
chamomile; Roman chamomile; chamomile	*Chamaemelum nobile*
chamomile; yarrow; milfoil	*Achillea millefolium*
chapparal; creosote bush; greasewood	*Larrea tridentata*
chaste berries; vitex; monk pepper; chaste tree; hemp tree	*Vitex agnus-castus*
chen pi	*Citrus reticulata*
chickweed; starweed	*Stellaria media*
chicory; succory	*Chicorium intybus*
chili pepper	*Capsicum frutescens*
Chinese cinnamon bark; Chinese cinnamon twig; cassia twig	*Cinnamomum cassia*
Chinese dandelion	*Taraxacum mongolicum*
Chinese dodder	*Cuscuta chinensis*
Chinese floxglove root	*Rehmannia glut(inos)a*
Chinese goldthread	*Coptis chinensis*
Chinese lovage	*Ligusticum chuanxiong*
Chinese rhubarb	*Rheum palmatum*
Chinese yam	*Dioscorea opposita*
chittem bark	*Rhamnus purshiana*
chokecherry	*Prunus virginiana*
chrysanthemum; chu hua	*Chrysanthemum morifolium*
chuanxiong	*Ligusticum chuanxiong*
chu hua	*Chrysanthemum morifolium*
cicada (insect)	*Cryptotympana atrata*
cinchona bark	*Cinchona* spp.
cineraria	*Senecio cineraria*

cinnamon	*Cinnamomum zeylanicum*
citrus peel; chen pi; tangerine peel	*Citrus reticulata*
ciwujia	*Eleutherococcus senticosus*
cleavers; clivers; goose grass; bedstraw	*Galium aparine*
cloves	*Syzygium aromaticum*
club moss	*Lycopodium clavatum*
cnidium; chuanxiong; Chinese lovage	*Ligusticum chuanxiong*
coca; cocaine	*Erythroxylum coca*
cocaine	*Erythroxylum coca*
cocklebur	*Agrimonia eupatoria*
cocoa	*Theobroma cacao*
coconut; coconut palm	*Cocos nucifera*
codonopsis root	*Codonopsis pilosula*
coffee	*Coffea arabica*
Cohin ginger *-see-* ginger	*Zingiber officianale*
coix; Job's tears	*Coix lachryma jobi*
cola	*Cola mitida*
colic root; American wild yam	*Dioscorea villosa*
colicroot	*Dioscora paniculata*
collinsonia; stoneroot	*Collinsonia canadensis*
coltsfoot; coughwort; horsehoof	*Tussilago farfara*
comfrey; knitbone	*Symphytum officinale*
common germander; pink skullcap	*Teucrium canadense*
common buckthorn	*Rhamnus cathartica*
condurango	*Gonolobus condurango*
coneflower	*Echinacea angustifolia*
coptis; Chinese goldthread	*Coptis chinensis*
coriander	*Coriander sativum*
corn silk; yumixu; stigmata maydis	*Zea mays*
cornus; Asiatic cornelian cherry; Asiatic dogwood	*Cornus officinalus*
corydalis	*Corydalis yanhusuo*
costus root	*Aucklandia lappa*
coughwort	*Tussilago farfara*
cramp bark; Guelder rose; snowball tree	*Viburnum opulus*
cranberry	*Vaccinium macrocarpon*
cranesbill root; wild geranium; storksbill; alumroot	*Geranium maculatum*
creeping lily root	*Ophiopogon japonicus*
creeping speedwell; veronica	*Veronica* spp.
creosote bush	*Larrea tridentata*
crookneck squash	*Cucurbita moschata*
croton oil	*Croton tiglium*
Culver root; black root; physic root	*Leptandra virginica*
cumin	*Cuminum cymium*
curled dock	*Rumex crispus*

curly dock	*Rumex crispus*
cuscuta; Chinese dodder	*Cuscuta chinensis*
cyperus; sedge root	*Cyperus rotundus*
da huang	*Rheum palmatum*
da t'sao	*Ziziphus jujube*
dagger plant	*Yucca aloifolia*
damiana	*Turnera diffusa*
dandelion	*Taraxacum officinale*
dang gui	*Angelica polymorpha*
dang shen	*Salvia militorrhiza*
deadly nightshade	*Atropa belladonna*
desert tea	*Ephedra sinica*
devil's apple	*Podophyllum peltatum*
devil's claw; Teufelskralle; wood spider; grapple plant	*Harpagophytum procumbens*
devil's club	*Oplopanax horridus*
devil's dung	*Ferula asafoetida*
dihe	*Spirulina maxima*
dill; dillweed	*Anethum graveolen*
don sen; tang shen; codonopsis root	*Codonopsis pilosula*
dong quai; tang kwei	*Angelica sinensis*
dong quai; dang gui; tang kuei	*Angelica polymorpha*
dragon's eyes	*Euphorbia longana*
dragonwort	*Polygonum bistoria*
dusty miller; cineraria	*Senecio cineraria*
dwarf lilyturf	*Ophiopogon japonicus*
echinacea; coneflower; narrow-leaved purple cone flower; purple cone flower; prairie	*Echinacea angustifolia*
Ecuadorian sarsaparilla	*Smilax febrifuga*
cldcr	*Sambucus niger*
elecampane; scabwort; elf dock; horseheal	*Inula helenium*
eleuthero	*Eleutherococcus senticosus*
eleutherococcus	*Eleutherococcus senticosus*
elf dock	*Inula helenium*
English chamomile	*Matricaria recutita*
Englishman's foot	*Plantago lanceolata*
epazote; Mexican wormseed; American wormseed	*Chenopodium ambrosoides*
ephedra; ma huang	*Ephedra sinica*
epimedium; lusty goatherb	*Epimedium pimedium grandiflorum*
ergot	*Claviceps purpurea*
eucalyptus; blue gum tree	*Eucalyptus globulus*
eucommia bark	*Eucommia ulmoides*
euphrasy	*Euphrasia officinalis*
European black currant	*Ribes nigrum*
European cranberry	*Vaccinium oxycoccos*

European horsetail	*Equisetum palustre*
European mistletoe	*Viscum album*
evening primrose; sundrops	*Oenothera biennis*
evodia fruit	*Evodia rutaecarpa*
eyebright	*Lobelia* spp.
eyebright	*Sabbatia* spp.
eyebright; euphrasy	*Euphrasia officinalis*
eyebright; spurge	*Euphorbia* spp.
false Jerusalem cherry	*Solanum capsicastrum*
false sarsaparilla; Indian sarsaparilla	*Hemidesmus indicus*
false unicorn; helonias	*Chamaelirium luteum*
false valerian	*Senecio aureus*
fang feng	*Ledebouriella divaricata*
fennel	*Foeniculum vulgare*
fenugreek	*Trigonella foenum-graecum*
feverfew	*Tanacetum parthenium*
feverwort	*Eupatorium perfoliatum*
field mint	*Mentha haplocalyx*
flag lily	*Iris versicolor*
fleece-flower root	*Polygonum multiflorum*
fleur-de-lis	*Iris versicolor*
flowering quince	*Cydonia japonica*
fo-ti; he-shou-wu	*Polygonum multiflorum*
foxglove	*Digitalis purpurea*
fringe tree	*Chionanthus virginicus*
fu ling	*Poria cocos*
fu tzu	*Aconitim carmichaeli*
gan-jian	*Zingiber officianale*
ganoderma; ling zhi; reishi	*Ganoderma lucidum*
gan t-sao	*Glycyrrhiza glabra*
garcinia; Malabar tamarind	*Garcinia cambogia*
garden lavender	*Lavandula angustifolia*
garden mint	*Mentha spicata*
garden rhubarb	*Rheum palmatum*
garden rue	*Ruta graveolens*
garlic	*Allium sativa*
gastrodia; heavenly hemp	*Gastrodia elata*
gay gee	*Lycium chinensis*
gentian; Angostura Bitters	*Gentiana lutea*
gentiana	*Gentiana scabra*
German chamomile	*Matricaria recutita*
ginger; Jamaica ginger; African ginger; Cohin ginger; gan-jian	*Zingiber officinale*
ginkgo; ginkgo nut; maidenhair tree	*Ginkgo biloba*
ginseng, Asian	*Panax ginseng*
ginseng, American	*Panax quinquefolius*
ginseng; jen sheng; shiu chu root; ren sheng	*Panax ginseng*

ginseng, Siberian	*Eleutherococcus senticosus*
goat thorn	*Astragalus membranaceus*
golden senecio	*Senecio aureus*
goldenseal; puccoon root; yellowroot; hydrastis	*Hydrastis canadensis*
goose grass	*Galium aperine*
gorse	*Spartium, junceum*
gotu kola; hydrocotyle; Indian pennywort	*Centella asiatica*
grains-of-paradise	*Amomum villosum*
grape seed extract	*Vitis vinifera*
grapple plant	*Harpagophytum procumbens*
gravel root; Joe-Pye weed; queen of the meadow	*Eupatorium purpureum*
greasewood	*Larrea tridentata*
great burdock	*Arcticum lappa*
great burnet	*Sanguisorba officinalis*
greater ammi; toothpick ammi	*Ammi visagna*
greater celandine	*Chelidonium majus*
greater plantain	*Plantago lanceolata*
ground holly	*Chimaphilia umbellata*
guarana	*Paullinia cupana*
Guelder rose	*Viburnum opulus*
guggul	*Commiphora myrrha*
gum asafetida	*Ferula asafoetida*
gum camphor	*Cinnamomum camphora*
guru nut	*Cola nitida*
hawthorn	*Crataegus laevigata*
he-shou-wu	*Polygonum multiflorum*
heavenly hemp	*Gastrodia elata*
hedge hyssop	*Gratiola* spp.
helonias	*Chamaelirium luteum*
hemp tree	*Vitex agnus-castus*
henbane	*Hyoscyamus niger*
herb-christopher	*Actaea spicata*
hibiscus; roselle; Sudanese tea; red tea; Jamaica sorrel	*Hibiscus sabdariffa*
hoarhound	*Marrubium vulgare*
ho shou wu; fo-ti; fleece-flower root	*Polygonum multiflorum*
hollyhock; althea	*Althaea rosea*
holy herb	*Eriodictyn californicum*
holy thistle	*Cnicus benedictus*
Honduran sarsaparilla	*Smilax regelii*
hong hua	*Carthamus tinctorius*
hops	*Humulus lupulus*
horehound; hoarhound	*Marrubium vulgare*
horseheal	*Inula helenium*

horsehoof	*Tussilago farfara*
horsetail	*Equisetum arvense*
huang chi	*Astragalus membranaceus*
huang chi	*Scutellaria lateriflora*
Hungarian camomile	*Matricaria recutita*
hydrangea; seven barks	*Hydrangea arborescens*
hydrastis	*Hysrastis canadensis*
hydrocotyle	*Centella asiatica*
hyssop	*Hyssopus officinalis*
Iceland moss; Iceland lichen	*Cetraria islandica*
Indian corn	*Zea mays*
Indian gooseberry	*Terminalia bellerica*
Indian pennywort	*Centella asiatica*
Indian physic	*Gillenia trifoliata*
Indian sarsaparilla	*Hemidesmus indicus*
Indian squill	*Urginea indica*
Indian tan plant	*Rumex hymenosepalus*
Indian tobacco	*Lobelia inflata*
indigo	*Indigofera tinctoria*
indigoweed	*Baptisia tinctoria*
ipecacuanha	*Cephaelis ipecacuanha*
ipecac	*Cephaelis ipecacuanha*
ipe roxo	*Tabebuia avellanedae*
Irish moss; carageenin; carageenan	*Chondrus crispus*
ispaghul	*Plantago ovata*
Jamaican ginger	*Zingiber officinale*
Jamaican sorrel	*Hibiscus sabdariffa*
Jamestown weed	*Datura stramonium*
Japanese honeysuckle; yin hua	*Lonicera japonica*
Japanese turf lily; creeping lily root; dwarf lilyturf	*Ophiopogon japonicus*
jen sheng	*Panax ginseng*
Jesuit's bark	*Chincona* spp.
jie geng	*Platycodon grandiflorum*
jimson weed; stink weed; thorn apple; datura Jamestown weed	*Datura stramonium*
Job's tears	*Coix lachryma jobi*
Joe-Pye weed	*Eupatorium purpureum*
jojoba oil	*Simmondsia chinensis*
Joshua tree	*Yucca brevifolia*
jujube date; da t'sao	*Ziziphus jujube*
juniper	*Juniperus communis*
karaya gum	*Stericulia urens*
kava; kava kava; kawa	*Piper methysticum*
kelp; bladderwrack	*Fucus vesiculosus*
khat	*Catha edulis*
knee holy	*Ruscus aculeatus*
knitbone	*Symphytum officinale*
ko ken	*Pueraria lobata*

kola; cola; kola nut, kolanut; guru nut	*Cola nitida*
ku xing ren; persica; apricot kernel oil	*Prunus armeniaca*
kudzu	*Pueraria lobata*
kumari	*Aloe barbadensis*
kuzu root	*Pueraria lobata*
lactucarium	*Lactuca virosa*
lady slipper; nerveroot	*Cypripedium calceoulus*
lady's mantle	*Alchemilla xanthochlora*
laetrile	*Prunus armeniaca*
lapacho	*Tabebuia avellanedae*
lapacho colorado	*Tabebuia avellanedae*
lapacho morado	*Tabebuia avellanedae*
lappa	*Arctium lappa*
larch moss	*Usnea barbata*
larkspur	*Consolida regalis*
laurel camphor	*Cinnamomum camphora*
lavender; garden lavender	*Lavandula angustifolia*
leek	*Allium ampeloprasum*
lemon balm; melissa; balm	*Melissa officinalis*
lemongrass	*Cymbopogon citratus*
lemon verbena	*Aloysia triphylla*
leopard's bane	*Arnica montana*
lettuce opium; lactucarium; wild lettuce	*Lactuca virosa*
licorice; gan t'sao	*Glycyrrhiza glabra*
life root; golden senecio; ragwort; false valerian; squaw weed	*Senecio aureus*
ligustrum	*Ligustrum lucidum*
lily of the valley	*Convallaria majalis*
lime flowers	*Tilia cordata*
linden; linden flower	*Tilia cordata*
ling zhi	*Gandoderma lucidum*
lion's-tail	*Leonurus cardiaca*
liver lily	*Iris versicolor*
lobelia; Indian tobacco; pukeweed	*Lobelia inflata*
long yen rou	*Euphorbia longana*
longan berries; dragon's eyes	*Euphorbia longana*
loquat	*Eriobotrya japonica*
lovage	*Levisticum officinale*
love lies bleeding	*Amaranthus caudatus*
luceme	*Medicago sativa*
lungwort; blue cowslip	*Pulmonaria angustifolia*
lusty goatherb	*Epidemium pidemium grandiflorum*
lycii; gay gee	*Lycium chinensis*
lycium fruit	*Lycium chinensis*
ma huang; ephedra	*Ephedra sinica*
Maggi plant	*Levisticum officinale*
magnolia buds	*Magnolia lilliflora*
maidenhair tree	*Gingko biloba*

maize	*Zea mays*
Malabar tamarind	*Garcinia cambogia*
malva; marshmallow; marsh mallow	*Malva sylvestris*
mandrake	*Podophyllum peltatum*
margosa	*Azadirachta indica*
Marian thistle	*Silibum marianum*
marigold, common	*Calendula officinalis*
marigold, African	*Tagetes* spp.
marjoram	*Origanum majorana*
marsh drain	*Alisma plantago-acquatica*
marsh tea	*Ledum palustre*
marshmallow	*Malva sylvestris*
maté	*Ilex paraguariensis*
mayapple; mandrake; vegetable calomel; devil's-apple	*Podophyllum peltatum*
Melia	*Azadivachta indica*
melissa	*Melissa officinalis*
Mexican sarsaparilla	*Smilax aristolochiaefolia*
Mexican scammany	*Convovulus scammonia*
Mexican vanilla	*Vanilla planifola*
Mexican wild yam	*Dioscorea floribunda*
Mexican wormseed	*Chenopodium ambrosoides*
milfoil	*Achillea millefolium*
milk thistle; Marian thistle; St. Mary thistle; Our Lady thistle	*Silybum marianum*
milk vetch root	*Astralagus membranaceus*
mistletoe, European	*Viscum album*
Mohave yucca	*Yucca schidigera*
monk pepper	*Vitex agnus-castus*
monkshood	*Aconitum carmichaeli*
Mormon tea; popotillo; Brigham tea; teamster tea; squaw tea	*Ephedra nevadensis*
morning glory	*Ipomoea purpurea*
mother herb	*Leonurus cardiaca*
motherwort; lion's-tail; yi mu cao	*Leonurus cardiaca*
mountain balm	*Eriodycton californicum*
moxa	*Artemisia vulgaris*
mugwort	*Artemisia vulgaris*
mugo pine (oil)	*Pinus mugo*
muira puama; potency wood	*Ptychopetalum olacoides*
muira puama; potency wood	*Liriosma ovata*
mulberry; white mulberry	*Morus alba*
mullein	*Verbascum thapsus*
mustard, black	*Brassica nigra*
mustard, white	*Brassica alba*
myrobalan, beleric; triphala; bhibitaki	*Terminalia bellerica*
myrobalan, chebulic; triphala; ho-tzu ch	*Terminalia chebula*
myrobalan, emblic; triphala; Indian gooseberry	*Phyllanthus emblica*

myrrh; guggul	*Commiphora myrrha*
myrtle	*Myrica cerifera*
narrow-leaved purple triphala; cone flower	*Echinacea angustifolia*
nasturtium	*Tropaeolum* spp.
neem tree; azedarach; Melia; nim; margosa	*Azadirachta indica*
nerveroot	*Cypripedium calceoulus*
nettle; stinging nettle	*Urtica dioica*
night-blooming cereus	*Selenicereus grandiflorus*
nim	*Azadirachta indica*
North American calamus; type I calamus	*Acorus americanus*
nosebleed	*Achillea millefolium*
notoginseng root	*Panax notoginseng*
nut-grass rhizome	*Cyperus rotundus*
nutmeg	*Myristica fragrans*
oak	*Quercus* spp.
oats; oat bran; oat groats	*Avena sativa*
old man's beard	*Usnea barbata*
onion	*Allium cepa*
Oregon grape	*Mahonia aquifolium*
ostrich fern	*Matteuccia struthiopteris*
ouabain	*Strophanthus gratus*
Our Lady's thistle	*Silybum marianum*
Our-Lord's-candle	*Yucca whipplei*
pai shu; atractylodes	*Atractylodes macrocephala*
palma Christi	*Ricinius communis*
pangamic acid; vitamin B15; pangamate; calcium pangamate	not a biological
papaya; papain	*Carica papaya*
papoose root	*Caulophyllum thalictroides*
para toda	*Pfaffia paniculata*
parsley	*Petroselinum crispum*
partridgeberry	*Mitchella repens*
passion flower; passionflower	*Passiflora incarnata*
patchouli	*Agastache rugosa*
pau d'arco; ipe roxo; lapacho; taheebo tea; lapacho colorado, lapacho morado	*Tabebuia avellanedae*
pau d'arco; lapacho; tabebuia; purple lapacho	*Tabebuia heptaphylla*
peach kernel oil	*Prunus persica*
pearl barley	*Hordeum vulgare*
pennyroyal, American	*Hedeoma pulegioides*
pennyroyal, European or Old World	*Mentha pulegium*
peony; shao-yao	*Paeonia lactiflora*
pepo	*Cucurbita pepo*
peppermint	*Mentha piperata*

periwinkle	*Vinca rosea*
persic oil; peach kernel oil	*Prunus persica*
persica	*Prunus armeniaca*
Peruvian bark	*Cinchona* spp.
pettier	*Ruscus aculeatus*
physic root	*Leptandra virginica*
physostigma	*Physostigma venenosum*
pilewort	*Ranunculus ficaria*
pimento; pimenta	*Pimenta officinalis*
pine-needle oil	*Pinus mugo*
pink skullcap	*Teucrium canadense*
pipperidge bush	*Berberis vulgaris*
pipsissewa; prince pine; ground holly	*Chimaphilia umbellata*
plantago; Englishman's foot; greater plantain; ribwort	*Plantago lanceolata*
platycodon; jie geng	*Platycodon grandiflorum*
pleurisy root; butterfly weed	*Asclepias tuberosa*
pogostemon	*Agastache rugosa*
poison flag; wild iris	*Iris versicolor*
poison sumac	*Rhus venenata*
poison ivy	*Rhus toxicodendron*
poke; pokeweed; pokeroot	*Phytolacca americana*
popotillo	*Ephedra nevadensis*
poppy, opium	*Papaver somniferum*
poppy, red	*Papaver rhoeas*
potency wood	*Ptychopetalum olacoides*
prairie	*Echinacea angustifolia*
prairie dock	*Parthenium integrifolium*
prelate	*Hordeum vulgare*
prickly ash; toothache tree	*Zanthoxylum americanum*
prickly comfrey	*Symphytum asperum*
prince pine	*Chimiphilia umbellata*
privet fruit; ligustrum	*Ligustrum lucidum*
psyllium; ispaghul	*Plantago ovata*
puccoon root	*Hydrastis canadensis*
pueraria; ko ken; kudzu; kuzu root	*Pueraria lobata*
pukeweed	*Lobelia inflata*
pumpkin seeds; popo	*Cucurbita pepo*
punk tree	*Melaleuca leucadendron*
purple lapacho	*Tabebuia avellenedae*
purple cone flower	*Echinacea angustifolia*
Pycnogenol	*Pinus pinaster*
pygeum	*Prunus africana*
quaking aspen	*Populus balsamifera*
queen of the meadow	*Eupatorium purpureum*
quillaja; soapbark	*Quillaja saponaria*
quina, quinaquina, quinquina	*Cinchona* spp.
quinine; cinchona bark; Peruvian bark; Jesuits' bark	*Cinchona* spp.

ragwort	*Senecio aureus*
ranunculus	*Ranunculus* spp.
raspberry	*Rubus idaeus*
rattle root	*Cimicifuga racemosa*
rauwolfia	*Rauwolfia serpentina*
red bush tea; rooibos tea	*Aspalathus linearis*
red clover	*Trifolium pratense*
red cockscomb	*Amaranthus hybridus*
red elder	*Sambucus racemosa*
red elm	*Ulmus rubra*
red flower	*Carthamus tinctorius*
red Indian paint	*Sanguinaria canadensis*
red squill	*Urginea maritima*
red tea	*Hibiscus sabdariffa*
red valerian	*Centranthus ruber*
redroot	*Sanguinaria canadensis*
rehmannia; sok day; san day; Chinese floxglove root	*Rehmannia glutinosa*
reishi	*Ganoderma lucidum*
ren sheng	*Panax ginseng*
rheumatism root	*Dioscorea paniculata*
rhubarb; Chinese rhubarb; da huang; Turkey rhubarb; garden rhubarb	*Rheum palmatum*
ribwort	*Plantago lancealata*
rice; rice bran	*Oryza sativa*
Roman chamomile	*Chamaemelum nobile*
rooibos tea	*Aspalathus linearis*
rose hip	*Rosa canina*
roselle	*Hibiscus sabdariffa*
rosemary	*Rosmarinus officinalis*
rue; garden rue	*Ruta graveolens*
Russian comfrey	*Symphytum x uplandicum*
Russian fly	*Lytta (Cantharis) vesicatoria*
sabal	*Serenoa repens*
sacred bark	*Rhamnus purshiana*
safflower; hong hua; red flower	*Carthamus tinctorius*
saffron	*Crocus sativus*
sage	*Salvia officinalis*
salad burnet	*Sanguisorba minor*
salsify	*Symphtum officinale*
salvia; dang shen	*Salvia miltiorrhiza*
san day	*Rehmannia glutinosa*
san qui ginseng; tienchi ginseng; sanchi ginseng	*Panax pseudo-ginseng*
sandalwood (oil); santal (oil)	*Santalum album*
sanguisorba *-see-* burnet	
santal oil	*Santalum album*
sargassum seaweed	*Sargassum pallidum*
sarsaparilla	*Smilax medica*

sarsaparilla, Ecuadorian	*Smilax febrifuga*
sarsaparilla, Honduran	*Smilax regelii*
sarsaparilla, Indian	*Hemidesmus indicus*
sarsaparilla, Jamaican	*Smilax ornata*
sassafras	*Sassafras albidum*
saussurea	*Aucklandia lappa*
saw palmetto; sabal	*Serenoa repens*
scabwort	*Inula helenium*
scallion	*Allium fistulosum*
scammany; Mexican scammany; scammony	*Convolvulus scammonia*
schisandra	*Schisandra chinensis*
scilla, urginea	*Urginea maritima*
Scotch bloom	*Cystis scoparius*
scullcap; skullcap; blue skullcap; huang chi; scutellaria	*Scutellaria lateriflora*
scutellaria	*Scutellaria lateriflora*
sea onion	*Urginea maritima*
sedge root	*Cyperus rotundus*
senega snakeroot; seneca snakeroot; senega	*Polygala senega*
senna; Tinnevelley senna	*Cassia senna*
sesame (oil)	*Sessamum indicum*
seven barks	*Hydrangea aborescens*
shallot	*Allium ascalonicum*
shao-yao	*Paeonia lactiflora*
sheep sorrel	*Rumex acetosella*
shepherd's purse	*Capsella bursa-pastoris*
shiitake	*Lentinula edodes*
shiu chu root	*Panax ginseng*
Siberian ginseng; eleutherococcus; eleuthero; ciwujia; wujiaseng	*Eleutherococcus senticosus*
sileris; fang feng	*Ledebouriella divaricata*
silk vine	*Periploca sepium*
silver linden	*Tilia tomentosa*
single camomile	*Chamomilla recutita*
skullcap	*Scutelleria lateriflora*
slippery elm; red elm	*Ulmus rubra*
snakeweed	*Polygonum bistoria*
snowball tree	*Viburnum opulus*
soapbark	*Quillaja saponaria*
soapweed	*Yucca glauca*
sok day	*Rehmannia glutinosa*
soldier's woundwort	*Achillea millefolium*
Somalian myrrh	*Commiphora molmol*
sourdock	*Rumex crispus*
Spanish bayonet	*Yucca aloifolia*
Spanish broom; gorse	*Spartium junceum*
Spanish fly; Russian fly	*Lytta (Cantharis) vesicatoria*

sparrowgrass	*Asparagus officianalis*
spearmint; garden mint	*Mentha spicata*
spikenard	*Aralia racemosa*
spirea	*Spiraea* spp.
spirulina; dihe; tecuitlatl; blue-green algae	*Spirulina maxima*
spurge	*Lobelia* spp.
squaw root	*Caulophyllyum thalictroides*
squaw tea	*Ephedra nevadensis*
squaw weed	*Senecio aureus*
squawvine; partridgeberry	*Mitchella repens*
squill, Lebanon	*Puschkina scilloides libanotica*
squill, Siberian	*Scilla sibirica*
squill; scilla, urginea; sea onion; red squill; white squill	*Urginea maritima*
St. Benedict's thistle	*Cnicus benedictus*
St. Ignatius bean	*Ignatia amara*
St. John's wort	*Hypericum perforatum*
St. Mary's thistle	*Silybum marianum*
stagbush	*Viburnum prunifolium*
starweed	*Stellaria media*
sterculia gum; karaya gum	*Sterculia urens*
sticklewort	*Agrimonia eupatoria*
stigmata maydis	*Zea mays*
stinging nettle	*Urica dioica*
stink weed	*Datura stramonium*
stoneroot	*Collinsonia canadensis*
storksbill	*Geranium maculata*
strychnine	*Strychnos nux-vomica*
succory	*Chicory intylbous*
Sudanese tea	*Hybiscus sabdariffa*
suma; para toda; Brazilian ginseng	*Pfaffia paniculata*
summer savory; Bohnenkraut	*Satureja hortensis*
sweet broom	*Ruscus aculeatus*
sweet flag	*Acorn calamus*
sweet gum	*Liquidambar* spp.
sweet sedge	*Acorn calamus*
sweet violet	*Viola odorata*
tabebuia	*Tabebuia avellanedae*
taheebo tea	*Tabebuia avellanedae*
Tahitian vanilla	*Vanilla tahitensis*
tamarind	*Tamarindus indica*
tang kwei; tang kuei	*Angelica sinensis*
tang shen	*Codonopsis pilosula*
tangerine peel	*Citrus reticulata*
tansy	*Tanacetum vulgare*
tea; black tea	*Camellia sinensis*
teamster tea	*Ephedra nevadensis*
tea tree; tea tree (oil)	*Melaleuca alternifolia*

tea tree	*Melaleuca leucadendron*
tecuitlatl	*Spirulina maxima*
tetterwort	*Sanguinaria canadensis*
Teufelskralle	*Harpagophytum procumbens*
thorn apple	*Datura stramonium*
thoroughwort	*Eupatorium perfoliatum*
thyme	*Thymus vulgaris*
tienchi ginseng	*Panax pseudo-ginseng*
tienchi; notoginseng root	*Panax notoginseng*
Tinnevelley senna	*Cassis senna*
tolu; tolu balsam	*Toluifera balsamum*
toothache tree	*Zanthoxylum americanum*
toothpick ammi	*Ammi visagna*
triphala	*Terminalia bellerica, T. chebula*
Turkey rhubarb	*Rheum palmatum*
turmeric	*Curcuma longa*
type I calamus	*Acorus americanus*
type II calamus	*Acorus calamus*
una de gato	*Uncaria tomentosa*
unicorn root	*Aletris farinosa*
usnea; beard lichen; larch moss; old man's beard	*Usnea barbata*
uva ursi; bearberry	*Arctostaphylos uva-ursi*
valerian	*Valeriana officinalis*
vanilla; Bourbon vanilla; Mexican vanilla	*Vanilla planifolia*
vanilla; Tahitian vanilla	*Vanilla tahitensis*
vegetable calomel	*Podophyllum peltatum*
veronica	*Veronica* spp.
vervain; blue vervain	*Verbena officinalis*
violet; sweet violet	*Viola odorata*
vitamin B17	*Primus armeniaca*
vitex	*Vitex agnus-castus*
walnut, black	*Juglans nigra*
watercress	*Nasturtium officinale*
water hemlock (poisonous)	*Cicuta maculata*
water plantain	*Alisma plantago-aquatica*
waxberry	*Myrica pennsylvania*
wax myrtle	*Myrica cerifera; M. pennsylvania*
wheat; wheat bran	*Triticum aestivum*
white mulberry	*Morus alba*
white poplar	*Populus balsamifera*
white squill	*Urginea maritima*
white tea tree	*Melaleuka leucadendron*
white willow	*Salix alba*
wild cherry bark	*Prunus serotina*
wild geranium	*Geranium maculatum*
wild ginger; xi xin	*Asarium heterotropoides*
wild hops	*Bryonia alba*

wild indigo	*Baptisia tinctoria*
wild iris	*Iris versicolor*
wild lettuce	*Lactuca virosa*
wild radish	*Raphanus raphanistrum*
wild red American ginseng	*Rumex hymenosepalus*
wild red desert ginseng	*Rumex hymenosepalus*
wild yam; colicroot; rheumatism root	*Dioscorea paniculata*
willow; white willow	*Salix alba*
windflower	*Pulsatilla nigricans*
winter savory	*Satureja montana*
witch hazel	*Hamamelis virginiana*
wood betony	*Betonica officinalis*
wood spider	*Harpagophytum procumbens*
wujiaseng	*Eleutherococcus senticosus*
xi xin	*Asarium heterotropoides*
yarrow; soldier's woundwort; nosebleed; milfoil	*Achillea millefolium*
yaupon hollies	*Ilex cassine*
yellow dock; broad leaved dock; curly dock; sourdock; curled dock	*Rumex crispus*
yellow jasmine	*Gelsemium sempervirens*
yellowroot	*Hydrastis canadensis*
yerba santa; holy herb; mountain balm	*Eriodictyon californicum*
yi mu cao	*Leonurus cardiaca*
yin hua	*Leonurus japonica*
yohimbe	*Pausinystalia yohimba*
yucca; Joshua tree	*Yucca brevifolia*
yucca; Mohave yucca	*Yucca schidigera*
yucca; our-Lord's-candle	*Yucca whipplei*
yucca; soapweed	*Yucca glauca*
yucca; Spanish bayonet; dagger plant	*Yucca aloifolia*
yumixu	*Zea mays*

Commonly Used Herbs and Their Side Effects/or Drug Interactions

Herb	Use	Side Effect or Drug Interactions
Aloe latex	Constipation; heals bowel inflammation	Binds with other drugs, decreasing absorption; hypokalemia; toxicity for some cardiac medications
Dong Quai	Relieves hot flashes	Increased bleeding, especially when used in combination with other anticoagulants
Echinacea	Improves immune function and wound healing; fights flu and colds	Possible liver inflammation and damage when used with anabolic steroids or methotrexate
Ephedra (Ma-Huang)	Improves respiratory function in asthma or bronchitis; diet aid and appetite suppressant	Could severely increase pulse or blood pressure when taken with antidepressants or antihypertensive agents, possibly causing death
Feverfew	Prevent migraines, treats allergies, and manages arthritis and rheumatic disease	Increased bleeding, especially when used in combination with other anticoagulants
Garlic	Lowers cholesterol, triglycerides, and blood pressure	Increased bleeding, especially when used in combination with other anticoagulants
Ginger	Decreases nausea, vomiting, and vertigo	Increased bleeding, especially when used in combination with other anticoagulants
Ginkgo biloba	Improves memory and mental alertness; increased circulation and oxygenation	Increased bleeding, especially when used in combination with other anticoagulants
Ginseng	Increases physical stamina and mental concentration	May increase heart rate and blood pressure; may cause bleeding in some women after menopause; decreases effectiveness of anticoagulant medications
Goldenseal	Decreases inflammation and acts as a laxative	May increase blood pressure or cause swelling
Kava-kava	Muscle relaxant, decreases nervousness and anxiety	Prolongs the effects of some anesthetic agents; increases side effects of some anti-seizure medications; may increase suicide risk for depressed clients; enhances effects of alcohol
Licorice	Treats stomach ulcers	May cause hypertension, swelling, and electrolyte imbalances
Saw palmetto	Treats urinary inflammation and enlarged prostate	Interacts with other hormone therapies
St. John's wort	Treats mild to moderate depression, anxiety, and sleep disorders	May prolong effects of anesthetic agents
Valerian	Mild sedative or sleep aid; muscle relaxant	May prolong effects of anesthetic agents or increase the side effects of anti-seizure medications

From Craven RF, Hirnle CJ, eds. *Fundamentals of Nursing: Human Health and Function,* 5th ed. Philadelphia: Lippincott Williams & Wilkins, 2007.

Spanish-English Medical Phrases

Emergency Medical Phrases	Frases Médica de Emergencia
Do you have difficulty speaking?	**¿Tiene usted dificultad en hablar?**
Are you having any pain?	**¿Tiene usted dolor actualmente?**
Where is the pain?	¿Dónde le duele?
Can you point to the area where you feel pain?	¿Me puede indicar donde siente usted el dolor?
Do you ever have chest pain or discomfort?	**¿Alguna vez tiene usted dolor de pecho o molestia?**
Have you ever had an allergic reaction to a medication?	**¿Ha tenido usted alguna vez una reacción alérgica a algún medicamento?**

Medication Phrases	Frases Medicamento
I would like to give you:	**Quisiera darle a usted un(a):**
an injection.	inyección.
an I.V. medication.	medicamento por vía intrvenosa.
a liquid medication.	medicamento en forma líquida.
a medicated cream or powder.	medicamento en pomada o polvo.
a medication through your epidural catheter.	medicamento por el catéter epidural.
a medication through your rectum.	medicamento por el recto.
a medication through your __________ tube.	medicamento por su __________ tubo.
a medication under your tongue.	medicamento debajo de la lengua.
your pill(s).	su(s) píldora(s).
a suppository.	supositorio.
This medication will:	**Este medicamento hará que:**
elevate your blood pressure.	su presión sanguínea suba.
improve circulation to your __________ (organ or region of body).	la circulación por __________ (la región del cuerpo) mejore.
lower your blood pressure.	su presión sanguínea baje.
lower your blood sugar.	el nivel de azúcar en la sangre baje.
make your heart rhythm more even.	el ritmo del corazón sea más uniforme.
raise your blood sugar.	su nivel de azúcar en la sange suba.
reduce or prevent the formation of blood clots.	se reduzca o evite la formación de coágulos de sangre.
remove fluid from your body.	se le quite fluido del cuerpo.
remove fluid from your feet, ankles, or legs.	se le quite fluido de los pies, tobillos o piernas.
remove fluid from your lungs so that they work better.	se le quite fluido de los pulmones para que funcionen mejor.
remove fluid from your pancreas so that it works better.	se le quite fluido del páncreas para que funcione mejor.

This medication will help your body to:	Este medicamento le ayudará a su cuerpo a:
kill the bacteria in your ______ (area of infection).	destruir la bacteria del (de la) ______ (región infectada).
slow down your heart rate.	reducir el latido cardiaco.
soften your bowel movements.	ablandar sus evacuaciones.
speed up your heart rate.	acelerar el latido cardiaco.
use insulin more efficiently.	usar la insulina más eficazmente.

This medication will help you to:	Este medicamento le ayudará a usted a:
breathe better.	respirar con mayor facilidad.
fight infections.	luchar contra infecciones.
relax.	relajarse.
sleep.	dormir.
think more clearly.	pensar con mayor claridad.

This medication will relieve or reduce:	Este medicamento le aliviará o disminuirá:
the acid production in your stomach.	la producción de ácido en el estómago.
anxiety.	la angustia.
bladder spasms.	los espasmos en la vejiga.
burning in your stomach or chest.	la sensación ardiente en el estómago o tórax.
burning when you urinate.	la sensación ardiente al orinar.
diarrhea.	la diarrea.
muscle cramps.	los espasmos musculares.
nausea.	las náuseas.
pain in your ______.	el dolor en la (el) ______.

This medication will help your body to produce more or less:	Este medicamento ayudará a su cuerpo a producir más o menos:
antibodies.	anticuerpos.
clotting factors.	factores o agentes coagulantes.
insulin.	insulina.
platelets.	plaquetas.
red blood cells.	glóbulos rojos.
white blood cells.	glóbulos blancos.

This medication or treatment will destroy:	Este medicamento o tratamiento destruirá:
antibodies.	anticuerpos.
bacteria.	bacterias.
cancer cells.	células cancerosas.
clotting factors.	factores o agentes coagulantes.
platelets.	plaquetas.
red blood cells.	glóbulos rojos.
white blood cells.	glóbulos blancos.

Commonly Used Terms and Phrases	Término y Frases Comunes
Hello	¡Hola!
Good morning	Buenos días
Good afternoon	Buenas tardes
Good evening	Buenas noches
Come in please.	Pase usted por favor.
My name is ___________.	Me llamo ___________.
Who is the patient?	¿Quién es el (la) paciente?
What is your name?	¿Cómo se llama usted?
It is nice to meet you.	Mucho gusto en conocerle.
How are you?	¿Cómo está usted?
I need you to sign this form.	Necesito que usted firme este formulario.
Please	Por favor
Thank you	Gracias
Yes	Sí
No	No
Maybe	Quizás or Tal vez
Sometimes	A veces
How are you feeling?	¿Cómo se siente usted?
What time is it?	¿Qué hora es?
What day is it?	¿Qué día es hoy?
What is the date?	¿A qué fecha estamos?
Where are you?	¿Dónde está usted?
How old are you?	¿Cuántos años tiene usted?
Did you come alone?	¿Vino usted solo (a)?

Who brought you?	¿Quién le trajo?
Where were you born?	¿Dónde nació usted?
Where do you live?	¿Dónde vive usted?
What is your address?	¿Cuál es su dirección?
Do you live alone?	¿Vive usted solo(a)?
Who lives with you?	¿Quién vive con usted?
Are you:	¿Es usted:
single?	soltero(a)?
married?	casado(a)?
divorced?	divorciado(a)?
widowed?	viudo(a)?
separated?	(Esta usted) separado(a)?
Do you have any children?	¿Tiene usted hijos?
Did you go to school?	¿Asistió usted a la escuela?
Where do you work?	¿Dónde trabaja usted?
What is your religion?	¿Cuál es su religión?

General Instructions	**Instrucción Generales**
Bend over backward.	Inclínese usted hacia atrás.
Bend over forward.	Inclínese usted hacia adelante.
Don't talk.	No hable usted.
Lean backward.	Recuéstese usted.
Lean forward.	Inclínese usted hacia adelante.
Lie down.	Acuéstese usted.
Lie on your back.	Acuéstese usted boca arriba.
Lie on your:	Acuéstese usted de:
left side.	lado izquierdo.
right side.	lado derecho.
Lie on your stomach.	Acuéstese usted boca abajo.
Roll over.	Dé usted una vuelta.

Say AAHH.	Diga usted AAAA.
Sit down.	Siéntese usted.
Sit up.	Enderécese usted.
Stand up.	Póngase usted de pie.
Turn to the side.	Voltéese usted hacia un lado.
Whisper.	Murmure usted.

General Teaching / Enseñanza Generales

General Teaching	Enseñanza Generales
I'm going to take your vital signs.	Voy a tomarle a usted los signos vitales.
Blood pressure	La presión sanguinea
Pulse	El pulso
Respirations	La respiración
Temperature	La temperatura
I'm going to take a blood sample.	Voy a tomarle a usted una muestra de sangre.
You need to provide a urine specimen.	Tiene usted que darnos un espécimen de orina.
Are you comfortable?	¿Está usted confortable?
Does this hurt?	¿Le duele a usted esto?
Where does it hurt?	¿Dónde le duele a usted?
Let me show you how to do it.	Permítame enseñarle cómo hacerlo.
Let's practice together.	Vamos a ensayar junto(a)s.
I want you to do it yourself.	Quiero que usted haga por sí solo(a).
I will watch to make sure you do it correctly.	Le observaré para estar seguro(a) de que usted lo puede hacer por sí solo(a).
Let me know it you have trouble.	Digame si usted tiene dificultad.
You'll need to walk with a cane.	Usted necesitará andar con bastón.
You'll need to use a walker.	Usted necesitará usar un andador.

Personal Care Phrases	Frases Cuidado Personal
Bedpan	**Cuña**
Here is a bed pan if you need to:	Aquí tiene una cuña por si usted tiene que:
move your bowels.	evacuar.
urinate.	orinar.
Do you need to use the bedpan?	¿Necesita usted usar la cuña?
Call me when you're finished with the bedpan.	Llámeme cuando acabe de usar la cuña.
Bedside commode	**Silla retrete al lado de la cama**
You can't walk to the bathroom.	Usted no puede caminar al baño.
I can get you a bedside commode.	Le puedo traer una silla retrete.
Call me when you're finished using the commode.	Llámeme cuando haya acabado de usar la silla retrete.
Blanket	**Cobija**
Do you need a blanket?	¿Necesita usted una manta (cobija)?
Emesis basin	**Phalangana para vómitos**
This is an emesis basin.	Aquí está una cubeta para vómito.
You can use the emesis basin if you need to vomit.	Usted puede usar esta cubeta si tiene que vomitar.
Enema	**Enema**
This is an enema.	Éste es un enema.
You need an enema to help you move your bowels.	Usted necesita un enema (lavativo) para ayudarle a evacuar.
Lie on your left side.	Acuéstese del lado izquierdo.
I'm going to put this tube in your rectum.	Voy a insertarle este tubo en el recto.
Take a deep breath.	Respire usted profundamente.
Let me know if you experience any cramping.	Dígame por favor si siente retortijones.
Try to retain the fluid.	Trate usted de retener el liquido.
Oral care	**Cuidado oral**
How do you care for your teeth and gums?	¿Qué cuidado da usted a los dientes y las encías?
Toothbrush/toothpaste?	¿Cepillo de dientes/pasta de dientes?
Urinal	**Orinal**
Here is a urinal.	Aquí está un orinal.
Do you need to use the urinal?	¿Necesita usted usar el orinal?

Call me when you're finished with the urinal.	Llámeme cuando acabe de usar el orinal.
Wash basin	**Cubeta Lava**
I'll get you a basin to wash yourself.	Le voy a traer una cubeta para que se lave usted.
Call me when you've finished with the basin.	Llámeme cuando haya acabado de usar la cubeta.

Nutrition Phrases / Frases Nutrición

Dietary influences	**Influencias en la dieta**
Does your ethnic or cultural background influence your diet?	¿Su origen étnico o cultural ejerce una influencia sobre su dieta?
How does it influence it?	¿Cómo la influye?
Do you just eat vegetables?	¿Come usted sólo verduras?
Do you eat red meat?	¿Come usted carne roja?
Do you just eat chicken or fish?	¿Come usted sólo pollo o pescado?
Does your religion restrict or otherwise affect what you eat?	¿Su religión limita o de cualquier modo afecta lo que usted come?
How?	¿Cómo lo afecta?
Do you fast or not eat food on any special days?	¿Ayuna usted o no come nada durante días especiales?
Do you not eat meat on Fridays?	¿No come usted carne los viernes?
Weight	**Peso**
Have you gained any weight recently?	¿Ha aumentado de peso últimamente?
How much?	¿Cuánto?
Have you lost any weight recently?	¿Ha bajado usted de peso últimamente?
How much?	¿Cuánto?
Fluid intake	**Toma de fluidos**
How much fluid do you drink during the day?	¿Cuánto líquido bebe usted al día?
Special diets	**Dietas especiales**
Do you follow a special diet?	¿Tiene usted una dieta especial?
What kind of diet?	¿Qué clase de dieta?
How long have you been on the diet?	¿Hace cuánto a usted la dieta?
What is the reason for the diet?	¿Cuánto tiempo que tiene usted esta dieta?
How much salt do you use, if any?	¿Cuánta sal usa usted, si es que la usa?
You need to reduce salt in your diet.	Usted necesita reducir la cantidad de sal en su dieta.

Avoid adding salt:
while cooking your food.
to your meals at the table.

Evite usted añadir sal:
cuando cocine su comida.
a su comida en la mesa.

You need to reduce cholesterol in your diet. Some foods that you shouldn't eat are:
butter
shortening
egg yolks
biscuits
cheese
avocados
bacon
sausage
hot dogs
shellfish
ice cream
chocolate
liver
most red meat

Usted necesita reducir el colesterol en su dieta. Algunos de los alimentos que usted no debe comer son:
mantequilla
grasa (manteca)
yemas de huevo
panecillos
queso
aguacate
tocino
salchicha
perros calientes
mariscos
helado
chocolate
higado
la mayoría de la carne roja.

You need to add fiber to your diet.
Eat fresh fruit and vegetables.
Some high-fiber fruits include apples, oranges, and peaches.
Some high-fiber vegetables include carrots, string beans, broccoli, and peas.

Usted tiene que añadir fibra a su dieta.
Coma usted fruta fresca y verduras.
Algunas frutas de alta fibra incluyen las manzanas, naranjas y melocotones.
Algunas verduras que contienen alta fibra incluyen las zanahorias, ejotes, brécol y guisantes (chícharos).

Eat whole grain breads, such as whole wheat and pumpernickel, and whole grain cereals, such as bran flakes, oat flakes, oatmeal, and shredded wheat.

Coma pan integral, como pan de trigo entero y pan negro de centeno, y cereal de grano integral, coma hojuelas de avena, harina de avena y trigo molido.

Add unprocessed bran to your food.

Añada salvado de trigo sin procesar a sus comidas.

Eat dried peas and beans, such as lentils, and navy, kidney, or pinto beans.

Coma usted guisantes secos y frijoles comolentejas, frijoles rojos, frijoles negros y frioles pintos.

Remember to drink at least six 8-ounce glasses of fluid per day.

No se olvide usted de tomar por lo menos seis vasos de ocho onzas (250 ml) de líquido al día.

Specialized Personal Care Phrases

Frases Especialidad de Cuidado Personal

Electrocardiogram	**Electrocardiograma**
You need an electrocardiogram so we can monitor your heart's electrical activity.	Usted necesita un electrocardiograma para que podamos observar la actividad eléctrica del corazón.
This is a cardiac monitor; it will help us monitor your heartbeat.	Éste es un monitor cardiaco, que nos ayudará a observar continuamente el corazón.
I need to place these electrodes on you.	Tengo que ponerle estos electrodos.
Don't be frightened if you hear the alarms; they sometimes sound with movement.	No se asuste usted si oye las alarmas que a veces suenan con el movimiento.
Incentive spirometer	**Espitómetro de estímulo**
This is an incentive spirometer.	Éste es un estímulo de espirometría.
It will help you take deep breaths.	Le ayudará a respirar profundamente.
Breathe in deeply, hold it, then breathe out.	Respire profundamente, contenga la respiración, luego exhale.
You should use the incentive spirometer every hour while you're awake.	Usted deberá usar el estímulo de espirometría cada hora mientras esté usted despierto.
IV catheter and pump	**IV catéter y bomba**
You need to have an IV inserted.	Usted necesita que se le ponga una intravenosa (IV).
This is an IV pump.	Ésta es una bomba IV.
The IV pump will help regulate the flow of your IV.	La bomba IV ayudará a regular el flujo de su intravenosa.
I'm going to insert the IV catheter.	Voy a introducirle el catéter de IV.
I need to apply a tourniquet around your arm.	Tengo que ponerle un torniquete alrededor del brazo.
You're going to feel a needlestick.	Usted va a sentir un piquete de aguja.
I need to place a dressing over the IV site.	Tengo que ponerle un vendaje en el área de la IV.
I need to flush your IV catheter to keep it patent.	Tengo que enjuagar su catéter de IV para conservarlo abierto.
Call me if you have discomfort at your IV site.	Llámeme si usted tiene molestia en el área de la IV.

Mechanical ventilation	**Ventilación mecánica**
We need to insert a tube through your nose or mouth into your trachea to help your breathing.	Tenemos que introducirle un tubo a través de la nariz o la boca hasta la tráquea para ayudarle a respirar.
The tube will be connected to a mechanical ventilator.	El tubo se conectará a un ventilador mecánico.
A mechanical ventilator is a machine that will help you breathe.	Un ventilador mecánico es una máquina (un aparto) que le ayudará a respirar.
You won't be able to talk while the tube is in place.	Usted no podrá hablar mientras el tubo esté en su lugar.
Nebulizer	**Nebulizador**
This is a nebulizer.	Éste es un nebulizador.
It will deliver medication into your lungs to help your breathing.	Le llevará medicamento a los pulmones para ayudarle a respirar.
Hold the mouthpiece in your mouth and breathe in the medication.	Sostenga usted la boquilla en su boca y aspire el medicamento.
Oxygen via a mask	**Máscara de oxígeno**
You need oxygen.	Usted necesita oxígeno.
This is an oxygen mask.	Ésta es una máscara de oxígeno.
The mask fits over your nose and mouth and oxygen is delivered through it.	La máscara se le pone sobre la nariz y la boca y el oxígeno se transmite por ella.
Oxygen via nasal cannula You need oxygen.	Oxígeno suministrado por cánula nasal Usted necesita oxígeno.
This is a nasal cannula.	Ésta es una cánula nasal.
The prongs go into your nose and oxygen flows through them.	Las puntas se ponen dentro de la nariz y el oxígeno pasa por ellas.
Pulse oximeter	**Oxímetro para medir el pulso**
This is a pulse oximeter.	Éste es un oxímetro del pulso.
A pulse oximeter allows us to monitor the oxygen content of your blood.	Un oxímetro del pulso nos permite observar el contenido de oxígeno en la sangre.
I need to put a probe on your finger.	Necesito ponerle una sonda en el dedo.

Specimen – Glucometer
This glucometer is used to measure your blood sugar.

I need to prick your finger to obtain a specimen.

Your blood sugar is ___________.

I need to give you some insulin.

Muestra – Glucómetro
Este glucómetro se usa para medir el azúcar en la sangre.

Necesito pincharle el dedo para obtener una muestra.

El nivel de azúcar en su sangre es ___________.

Tengo que darle insulina.

Suctioning
I need to suction your breathing tube.

Suctioning will make you cough.

Succión
Tengo que aspirar su tubo de respiración.

Esta succión le hará toser.

Wound drainage bag
I'm going to apply a drainage bag over your drain.

Saco de drenaje de heridas
Le voy a poner un saco sobre su drenaje.

Wound – dressing
I need to change your dressing.

I need to irrigate your wound.

I'm going to remove the tape; it may sting a bit.

Vendaje de heridas
Tengo que cambiarle su vendaje.

Tengo que irrigar su herida.

Voy a quitarle la cinta adhesiva; le puede arder un poco.

Wound – packing
I'm going to remove your wound packing.

I'm going to replace your wound packing.

Cobertura de heridas
Voy a quitarle el empaque de su herida.

Voy a cambiarle el empaque de su herida.

Wound prevention
You need to use a support surface to avoid skin breakdown.

These Unna boots will help keep pressure off your wound.

Prevención de heridas
Usted necesita una superficie de apoyo para evitar que se desgarre la piel.

Estas botas "Unna" ayudarán a evitar hacer presión en su herida.

Specialty Phrases – Geriatric

Skin, hair, and nails
Has your skin changed as you have aged?
How?
How do you feel about the skin changes you have noticed?

Have you had any recent falls or other accidents?

Frases Especialidad – Geriatría

La piel, el cabello y las uñas
¿Le ha cambiado la piel al envejecer?
¿Cómo?
¿Qué piensa acerca de los cambios de la piel que usted ha notado?

¿Se ha caído usted recientemente o ha tenido otros accidentes?

Have you noticed any difference in healing of wounds or sores?	¿Ha notado usted alguna diferencia en la manera que sanan sus heridas o llagas?
Do external temperature changes, touch, or pressure affect your skin?	¿Su piel es afectada por los cambios de temperatura o cuando la toco o aplica presión sobre ella?
Head and neck	**Cabeza y cuello**
Do you have any difficulty swallowing?	¿Tiene usted alguna dificultad en tragar?
Do you have any difficulty chewing?	¿Tiene usted alguna dificultad al mascar?
Do you wear dentures?	¿Tiene usted dentadura postiza?
Do they cause any pain or discomfort?	¿Le molestan o le causan dolor?
Eyes	**Ojos**
Do your eyes feel dry?	¿Siente secos los ojos?
Do you have difficulty seeing to the side but not in front of you?	¿Tiene usted dificultad en ver de lado pero no de frente?
Do you have problems with glare?	¿Le molesta el resplandor?
Do you have any problems discerning colors?	¿Tiene problemas en distinguir los colores?
Do you have difficulty seeing at night?	¿Tiene usted dificultad en ver de noche?
Ears	**Oídos**
Have you noticed any change in your hearing recently?	¿Ha notado usted recientemente algún cambio en su capacidad auditiva?
What kind of change?	¿Qué clase de cambio?
Do you wear a hearing aide?	¿Usa usted audifono?
In which ear?	¿En qué oído?
Respiratory system	**Sistema respiratorio**
Are you aware of any changes in your breathing patterns?	¿Es usted consciente de algún cambio en su manera de respirar?
Do you become easily fatigued when climbing stairs?	¿Se fatiga usted con facilidad al subir escaleras?
Do you have trouble breathing when lying flat?	¿Tiene usted dificultad en respirar cuando se asuesta de espaldas?
Urinary and gastrointestinal systems	**Sistemas urinario y digestivo**
Do you ever lose control of your bladder?	¿Ha perdido usted control de la vejiga alguna vez?
How often does this occur?	¿Con qué frecuencia ocurre esto?
Does this occur suddenly or do you feel a warning, such as intense pressure?	¿Ocurre esto de repente o siente usted un aviso, tal como una presión intensa?

Do you ever lose control of your bowels?	¿Hay veces que usted pierde control de su evacuación intestinal?
Female and male reproductive systems	**Sistemas reproductor femenio y masculino**
Do you experience hot flushes or flashes?	¿Siente usted los fogajes?
How bothersome are they?	¿Le son muy molestos?
Do you experience vaginal dryness, pain, or itching during sexual intercourse?	¿Tiene usted sequedad, dolor o comezón vaginal durante el coito?
Are you having menstrual irregularities?	¿Tiene usted irregularidades menstruales?
Have you undergone menopause?	¿Ha tenido usted la menopausia?
Are you receiving hormone therapy for menopause?	¿Se le da a usted terapia de hormonas para la menopausia?
Have you had any bleeding?	¿Ha tenido usted sangrado?
Do you get up during the night to urinate?	¿Se levanta usted durante la noche para orinar?
How often?	¿Con qué frecuencia?
Do you have:	¿Usted:
urinary frequency?	orina con frecuencia?
hesitancy?	tiene vacilación?
dribbling?	tiene goteo?
pain in the area between your rectum and penis, your hips, or your lower back?	siente dolor en la área entre su recto y su pene, su caderas, o su región lumbar?
Have you had any change in your frequency of or desire for sex?	¿Ha tenido usted algún cambio en la frecuencia o en el deseo de tener relaciones sexuales?
Have you noticed any changes in your sexual performance?	¿Ha notado usted algún cambio en su desempeño sexual?
Nervous and musculoskeletal systems	**Sistemas nervioso y musculoesquelético**
Have you noticed a change in your ability to remember things?	¿Ha notado usted algún cambio en su habilidad de recordar cosas?
A loss of recent memory?	¿Pérdida de memoria reciente?
A loss of past events?	¿Pérdida de memoria de eventos pasados?
Have you noticed any change in your mental alertness or ability to concentrate?	¿Ha notado usted algún cambio en su agudeza mental o en su habilidad de concentrarse?
Do you have any difficulty following conversations or television programs?	¿Tiene usted dificultad en seguir el hilo de una conversación o un programa de televisión?
Have you noticed any change in your memory or thinking abilities, vision, hearing, or sense of smell or taste?	¿Ha notado usted algún cambio en la memoria o habilidad de pensar, visión, oído o sentido del olfacto o del gusto?

Have you noticed any change in agility, speed of movement, or endurance?
¿Ha notado usted algún cambio en su agilidad, en la rapidez de movimento o del resistencia?

Do you trip or fall more frequently?
¿Se tropieza o se cae usted con más frecuencia?

How would you describe your walking pattern?
¿Cómo describiría usted su forma de andar?

Have you broken any bones recently?
¿Se ha quebrado usted algunos huesos recientemente?

Which bone?
¿Qué hueso?

How did you break it?
¿Cómo se lo quebró?

Specialty Phrases – Obstetrics

Frases Especialidad – Obstetricia

Skin, hair, and nails

La piel, el cabello y las uñas

Have you noticed any changes in your skin during your pregnancy?
¿Ha notado usted algún cambio en la piel durante su embarazo?

What kind of changes?
¿Qué tipo de cambio?

Cardiovascular system

Sistema cardiovasular

Has your blood pressure been elevated during this pregnancy?
¿Ha subido su presión sanguínea durante este embarazo?

Have you noticed any swelling in your feet or ankles?
¿Ha notado usted alguna hinchazón de los pies o de los tobillos?

Have you developed varicose veins in your legs or genitals?
¿Se le han formado venas varcosas en las piernas o los genitales?

Have you developed hemorrhoids?
¿Se le han formado hemorroides?

Do you ever feel dizzy when you change positions or exert yourself?
¿Se siente usted mareada después de cambiar de postura o de hacer un trabajo pesado?

Do you suffer from shortness of breath?
¿Se queda usted sin aliento?

Gastrointestinal system

Sistema gastrointestinal

Do you ever have nausea and vomiting?
¿Tiene usted alguna vez náuseas o vómitos?

Does it occur at a specific time?
¿Ocurre esto a una hora en particular?

Does it occur throughout the day?
¿Ocurre esto durante todo el día?

Have your bowel habits changed since you became pregnant?
¿Han cambiado sus hábitos de evacuar desde el comienzo de su embarazo?

How have they changed?
¿Cómo han cambiado?

Have you had abdominal pain?
¿Ha tenido usted dolor en el abdomen?

Where is the pain?
¿Dónde es el dolor?

What kind of pain is it?
¿Qué clase de dolor?

Have you had heartburn?	¿Ha tenido usted pirosis (acidez)?
How do you feel about your pregnancy?	¿Qué piensa usted de su estado de embarazo?
Urinary system	**Sistema urinario**
Do you ever have pain when you urinate or in the kidney area?	¿Siente usted dolor al orinar o en la región del riñón?
When did it start?	¿Cuándo comenzó esto?
How long have you had it?	¿Hace cuánto tiempo que lo tiene?
What relieves it?	¿Qué es lo que lo mitiga?
What is the pain like?	¿Cómo es el dolor?
Have you ever been diagnosed with a urinary tract infection?	¿Se le ha diagnosticado alguna vez una infección en el sistema urinario?
When?	¿Cuándo?
What where your symptoms?	¿Cuáles fueron los síntomas?
How was it treated?	¿Qué tratamiento se le dió?
Female reproductive system	**Sistema reproductor femenio**
Have you ever had a miscarriage or abortion?	¿Alguna vez ha tenido usted un aborto espontáneo o inducido?
How many times?	¿Cuántas veces?
At what age did you bear your children?	¿A qué edad tuvo usted a sus hijos?
Have you ever had any problems during a pregnancy?	¿Ha tenido usted alguna vez problemas durante el embarazo?
What were the problems?	¿Cuáles fueron los problemas?
When did they occur?	¿Cuándo ocurrió esto?
During the prenatal period?	¿Durante el periodo prenatal?
During labor?	¿Durante el parto?
After delivery?	¿Después del parto?
What treatment did you receive?	¿Qué tratamiento se le dió?
Did any of the problems continue?	¿Siguió usted teniendo esos problemas?
Where your infants healthy?	¿Fueron saludables sus infantes?
Can you describe the problems?	¿Puede usted describir los problemas?
Did you breast-feed your infants?	¿Les dió de mamar a sus hijos?
Have you ever had problems conceiving?	¿Ha tenido usted problemas en concebir?
What treatment did you receive?	¿Qué tratamiento siguió, si es que se le dió algún tratamiento?
Do you plan to breast-feed?	¿Piensa usted dar de mamar?
Do you have any concerns about breast-feeding?	¿Se siente usted las preocupaciones en dar de mamar?

Musculoskeletal system

Are you having back pains or spasms?

How often do they occur?

What measures relieve them?

Do you have:

Weakness?

Pain?

Tingling in one or both hands?

How often does it occur?

Endocrine system

Have you ever been told you had diabetes during this or any previous pregnancy?

Have you ever given birth to an infant weighing more than 10 pounds (4.5 kilograms)?

How much did the infant weigh?

Obstetric Care Equipment

External fetal monitor

This is an external fetal monitor.

I'll place it around your abdomen.

It will monitor your contractions and the baby's heart beat.

Fetoscope

This is a fetoscope.

I'll place it on your abdomen to listen to your baby's heartbeat.

Your baby's heart beat is ________.

Internal fetal monitor

This is an internal fetal monitor.

A small probe will be inserted into the baby's scalp.

It will monitor your contractions and the baby's heartbeat.

Sistema musculoesquelético

¿Tiene usted doleres de espalda o espasmos?

¿Con qué frecuencia los tiene usted?

¿Qué medidas toma usted para mitigarlos?

¿Tiene usted algunos de los siguientes?

¿Debilidad?

¿Dolor?

¿Hormigueo en una o las dos manos?

¿Con qué frecuencia ocurre esto?

Sistema endocrino

¿Se le ha dicho que tiene diabetes durante este embarazo o la tuvo durante cualquier otro embarazo previo?

¿Alguna vez dió a luz usted a un(a) infante(a) que pesó más de 10 libras (4.5 kilos)?

¿Cuánto pesó el (la) infante(a)?

Equipo Obstétrica

Monitor fetal externo

Éste es un monitor fetal externo.

Lo pondré en su abdomen.

Observaré sus contracciones y el latido cardiaco de su criatura.

Fetoscopio

Éste es un fetoscopio.

Se lo pondré en el abdomen para escuchar el latido cardiaco de su criatura.

El latido de su criatura es ________.

Monitor fetal interno

Éste es un monitor fetal interno.

Se colocará una pequeña sonda en el cuero cabelludo de la criatura.

Observará sus contracciones y el latido cardiaco de la criatura.

Isolette	**Incubadora**
This is an isolette.	Ésta es una incubadora.
I'll place your baby in the isolette to keep him warm.	Pondré a su criatura en la incubadora para que tenga calor.
Light therapy	**Terapia lumínica**
Your baby is jaundiced.	Su criatura tiene ictericia.
Your baby will need to be placed under the bilirubin lights.	Se deberá poner a su criatura debajo de las luces para estimular la bilirrubina.
He will have his eyes patched while he is under the lights.	Le pondremos parches sobre los ojos mientras está bajo las luces.

Specialty Phrases – Pediatric / Frases Especialidad de Pediátrica

Skin, hair, and nails	**La piel, el cabello y las unas**
Is the infant breast-fed or formula-fed?	¿Le da usted de mamar o alimentación con fórmula?
Has the child had any skin problems related to a particular formula or food added to the diet?	¿Ha tenido el niño (la niña) algún problema de la piel relacionado con una fórmula en particular o algún alimento que se le haya añadido a su dieta?
Has the infant had any diaper rashes that did not clear up readily with over-the-counter skin preparations?	¿Ha tenido el niño (la niña) alguna erupción de la piel que no se le haya quitado fácilmente con alguna preparación para la piel no recetada?
What kind of diapers do you use?	¿Qué clase de pañales usa usted?
How often do you bathe the infant?	¿Con qué frecuencia baña usted al niño (la niña)?
What products do you use on the infant's skin?	¿Qué productos usa usted en la piel de su criatura?
Do you have pets in your home?	¿Tiene usted los animales domesticos en casa?
Has the child been scratching the scalp?	¿Se rasca la criatura el cuero cabelludo?
Head and neck	**Cabeza y cuello**
Is your drinking water treated with fluoride?	¿Está el agua potable tratada con fluoruro?
Does the child use a pacifier or suck his or her thumb?	¿Usa la criatura una chupete (pacificador) o se chupa el dedo?
When did the child begin teething?	¿Cuándo comenzó la dentición del niño (de la niña)?

Eyes	**Ojos**
Does the infant gaze at you or other objects and blink at bright lights or quick, nearby movements?	¿La criatura mira fijamente a usted o a otros objectos y parpadea al ver luces brillantes o movimentos rápidos de objetos cercanos?
Are the child's eyes ever crossed?	¿Hay veces que la criatura tiene bizquera?
Do both eyes ever move in different directions?	¿Hay ocasiones cuando los dos ojos se mueven en diferentes direcciones?
Does the child often rub the eyes?	¿La criatura se frota los ojos con frecuencia?
Does the child squint frequently?	¿El niño (la niña) mira con frecuencia con los ojos entrecerrados?
Does the child sit close to the television at home?	¿Se sienta el niño (la niña) muy cerca de la televisión?
How is the child's progress in school?	¿Ha progresado el niño (la niña) en el colegio?
Ears	**Oídos**
Does the infant respond to loud or unusual noises?	¿Responde el (la) infante(a) a ruidos fuertes o extraños?
Does the infant babble?	¿Balbucea el (la) infante(a)?
Is the toddler speaking appropriately for his or her age?	¿Habla el (la) pequeño(a) adecuadamente para su edad?
Have you noticed the child tugging at either ear?	¿Ha notado usted si la criatura se jala una oreja?
Has the child had any of the following: Meningitis? Recurrent otitis media? Mumps? Encephalitis?	¿Ha tenido la criatura culaquiera de las siguientes? ¿Meningitis? ¿Recurrencia de otitis media? ¿Parotiditis (paperas)? ¿Encefalitis?
Respiratory system	**Sistema Respiratorio**
Did the mother have any pregnancy related problems?	¿Tuvo la madre problemas relacionados con el embarazo?
Was the pregnancy carried to term?	¿Llegó el embarazo a su término?
Did the infant have any respiratory problems at birth?	¿Tuveo el (la) infante(a) problemas respiratorios al nacer?
Does the infant suffer from frequent congestion, runny nose, or colds?	¿Sufre el (la) infante(a) de frecuente congestión, goteo de nariz o catarro?

Does shortness of breath interfere with the infant's ability to nurse?	¿La falta de respiración interfiere con la habilidad de mamar del (de la) infante(a)?
Does the child cough at night?	¿Tose el niño (la niña) por la noche?
Cardiovascular system	**Sistema cardiovascular**
Has the child experienced any growth delay?	¿Ha tenido el niño (la niña) un retraso en su desarrollo?
Does the child have any problems with coordination?	¿Tiene el niño (la niña) algún problema de coordinación?
Does the child turn blue when crying?	¿Se pone amoratado el niño (la niña) curando llora?
Does the child stop frequently during play to sit or squat?	¿Deja de jugar el niño (la niña) con frecuencia para sentarse o acuclillarse?
Does the child have difficulty feeding?	¿Tiene el el niño (la niña) dificultad en alimentarse?
Does the child tire easily or sleep excessively?	¿Se cansa con facilidad el niño (la niña) o duerme demasiado?
Gastrointestinal system	**Sistema digestivo**
What is the color of the newborn's stools?	¿De qué color es las heces fecales de (de la) recién nacido(a)?
What is the number of stools per day of the newborn?	¿Cuántas defecaciones tiene el (la) recién nacido(a) al día?
Does the infant continually want to eat despite forceful vomiting?	¿Qué quiere comer continuamente el (la) infante(a) a pesar de que vomita todo?
How often does the child have a bowel movement?	¿Con qué frecuencia evacua la criatura?
What special words does the child use for having a bowel movement?	¿Cuáles son las palabras especiales que el niño (la niña) usa para decir que quiere evacuar?
At what age was the child toilet trained?	¿A qué edad se entrenó el niño (la niña) a usar el retrete?
Do the child's stools ever appear large, bulky, and frothy and float in the toilet bowel?	¿Hay veces que la evacuación del niño (de la niña) parece ser grande, abultada y espumosa y flota en el retrete?
Urinary and reproductive systems	**Sistemas urinario y reproductor**
Does the child have persistent diaper rash?	¿Tiene la criatura un salpullido persistente?
How many diapers does the child wet each day?	¿Cuántaos pañales mojo la criatura al día?

Does the child have excessive thirst?	¿Tiene el niño (la niña) excesiva sed?
Does the child cry when urinating?	¿Llora el niño (la niña) cuando orina?
Did the child have any genitourinary problems at birth?	¿Tuvo la criatura problemas genitourinarios?
Is the child circumcised?	¿Le hicieron la circuncisión al niño?
Nervous and musculoskeletal systems	**Sistemas nervioso y musculoesquelético**
Was ___________ present during pregnancy?	¿Ocurrió alguna de las siguientes situaciones durantes el embarazo?
Exposure to x-rays	¿Exposición a rayos-X?
Maternal illness or injury	¿Enfermedades o lesiones de la madre?
Poor nutrition	¿Nutrición inadecuada?
Exposure to viruses, such as toxoplasmosis, rubella, cytomegalovirus, or herpes simplex?	¿Exposición a virus, tal como toxoplasmosis, rubéola, citomegalovirus o herpes simple?
Surgery	¿Cirugía?
Alcohol or drug use	¿Consumo de alcohol o drogas?
Cigarette smoking	¿Fumar de cigarrillos?
Were labor and delivery difficult?	¿Fue difícil la labor de parto?
Were medications used during the delivery?	¿Se le dieron medicamentos durante el parto?
How did the infant look right after the delivery?	¿Qué semblante teinía el (la) intante(a) inmediatamente después del parto?
At what age did the child first:	¿A qué edad realizó la criatura los siguientes movimientos?
Hold up his or her head?	¿Sostener la cabeza levantada?
Sit?	¿Sentarse?
Crawl?	¿Gatear?
Walk?	¿Andar?
Have you noticed any lack of coordination?	¿Ha notado usted alguna falta de coordinación?
Can the child move about normally?	¿Puede la criatura moverse de acá para allá normalmente?
Has the child lost any functions that were previously mastered?	¿Ha perdido la criatura algunas functiones que habia dominado previamente?
Is the child in school?	¿El niño (la niña) asiste al colegio?
Has the child had any broken bones or head injuries?	¿El niño (la niña) se ha querbrado algún hueso o ha tenido heridas a la cabeza?

Immune and endocrine systems

Does the child have frequent or continuous severe infections?

What kinds of infections?

Does the child have any allergies?

To what?

Does anyone else in the family have allergies?

To what?

Which immunizations has the child received?

Has the child's activity level changed?

Has the child lost weight, been excessively thirsty or hungry, or been urinating frequently?

Sistemas inmunológico y endocrino

¿Tiene la criatura infecciones graves con frecuencia o continuamente?

¿Qué clase de infecciones?

¿Tiene la criatura alguna alergia?

¿A qué?

¿Hay otro miembro de la familia que tenga alergias?

¿A qué?

¿Qué vacunas se han dado a la criatura?

¿Ha cambiado el nivel de actividad del niño (de la niña)?

¿Ha bajado de peso la criatura, ha tenido excesiva sed o hambre o ha orinado frecuencia?

Confusing Common Medical Abbreviations

AD	right ear
AG	albumin-globulin ratio
AO	aorta
CBC	complete blood count
CDC	Centers for Disease Control
CV	cardiovascular
CVP	central venous pressure
DC	discontinue
DM	diabetes mellitus /diastolic murmurs

Abreviaturas Médicas Confuso Comúnmente

AD	aurícula derecha (right atrium)
AG	análisis gástrico (gastric analysis) absorción y gasto (intake & output)
AO	análisis de orina (urinalysis)
CBC	conducto biliar común (common bile duct)
CDC	contenido de dióxido de carbono (carbon dioxide)
CV	capacidad vital (vital capacity)
CVP	contracción ventricular prematura (premature ventricular contraction)
DC	desarticulación de la cadera (hip disarticulation) déficit en el crecimento (failure to thrive)
DM	doctor en medicina (medical doctor)

DR	delivery room	DR	desarticulación de la rodilla (knee disarticulation)
GA	gastric analysis	GA	glicemia en ayunas (fasting blood sugar or glucose)
GB	gallbladder	GB	glóbulos blancos (white blood cells)
HB	hepatitis B vaccine	HB	herida de bala (gunshot wound)
MS	mitral stenosis/multiple sclerosis	MS	mantenimiento de la salud (health maintenance)
OD	right eye/overdose	OD	ojo/oído derecho (right eye/ear)
P	pulse/prognosis/after	P	parásitos (ova and parasites) peso (weight)
PVC	premature ventricular contraction	PVC	presión venosa central (central venous pressure)
RT	radiation therapy	RT	regurgitación tricuspídea (tricuspid regurgitation)
SOB	shortness of breath	SOB	salpingo-ooforectomía bilateral (bilateral salpingo-oophorectomy)
VD	venereal disease	VD	ventrículo derecho (right ventricle)

OVERVIEW OF SPANISH PRONUNCIATION

A	Similar to the **A** in **fAther**
B	Similar to the **B** in **aBnormal**
C	Similar to the English **C**: it is hard when it precedes A, O, or U (as in **esCape**), soft when it precedes E or I (as in **paCe**)
CH	Similar to the **CH** in **CHild**
CU	Similar to the **QU** in **QUestion**
D	Similar to the **D** in **Day** when it is at the beginning of a word; similar to the **TH** in **wiTH** when it is in the middle of a word or at the end of a word
E	Similar to the **E** in **sEpsis**; the Spanish E does not end with the glide of the English **EY** in **thEY**
F	Similar to the **F** in **perForate**
G	Similar to the **G** in **Gout** when it precedes A, O, U, or a consonant; similar to the **H** in **Hospital** when it precedes E or I
H	<u>ALWAYS SILENT</u>
I	Similar to the **I** in **salIne**; similar to the **EE** in **sEE**
J	Similar to the **H** in **Hospital**
K	Similar to the **K** in **maKeup**
L	Similar to the **L** in **sLeep**
LL	Similar to the **LL** in **miLLion** and the **YE** in **Yellow**
M	Similar to the **M** in **atoMic**
N	Similar to the **N** in **learNing**; similar to the **M** in **coMma** when it precedes B, P, or V; silent when it precedes M
Ñ	Similar to the **NI** in **oNIon**
O	Similar to the **O** in **lOw**
P	Similar to the **P** in **sPit**
Q	Similar to the **K** in **Key**
R	Similar to the **R** in **haiRy**
RR	<u>ALWAYS TRILLED</u>; note that spelling a word with one r or two rs changes the meaning of the word: **pero** (but) and **perro** (dog) **caro** (expensive) and **carro** (wagon, cart, car) **para** (for) and **parra** (grapevine)
S	Similar to the **S** in **baSment**
T	Similar to the **T** in **sTent**
U	Similar to the **U** in **flU**
V	Same as the Spanish B; similar to the **B** in **saBle**
X	Similar to the **X** in **fleX**; similar to the **S** in **meSSage** when it presedes a consonant
Y	Similar to the **Y** in **boYfriend**; similar to the **EE** in **sEE** when it is used to denote the word *and*
Z	Similar to the **C** in **City**, **preCede**

Vowels are almost always pronounced the same as English vowels:

They are short and tense.
They are neither drawn out nor glided.
They are divided into two categories:
Strong vowels – a, e, and o,
Weak vowels – i and u.
A combination of a strong and a weak vowel or two weak vowels is pronounced as a single syllable, forming a diphthong (an unsegmented gliding sound in which the weak sounds [i and u] are barely audible), such as **lengua**, **nueve**, and **biopsia**.
A written accent over the weak vowel breaks the diphthong, forming two separate syllables, such as **día** and **sangría**.
The meaning of a word can change with the addition of a written accent such as:
seria (serious) and **sería** (would be)
continuo (continuous) and **continuó** (he continued)
papa (potato, especially in Latin America) and **papá** (dad or daddy)

Adapted from:

McElroy OH, Grabb LL. *Spanish-English, English-Spanish Medical Dictionary*, 3rd ed. Baltimore, MD: Lippincott Williams & Wilkins, 2005.

English & Spanish Medical Words & Phrases, 3rd ed. Springhouse, PA: Lippincott Williams & Wilkins, 2004.

CPR: One-Person Rescue

- **Check for Response:** After the rescuer has ensured that the scene is safe, the victim is assessed to determine his/her responsiveness. This is accomplished by tapping the victim's shoulders and speaking in a loud voice, "Are you all right?" This helps ensure that you do not start cardiopulmonary resuscitation (CPR) on a person who is conscious. If the victim is responsive but needs medical attention, leave the victim and phone 911.
- **Activate the Emergency Response System (ERS):** If a single rescuer finds an unresponsive adult, the rescuer should activate the ERS (phone 911) and get an AED (Automated External Defibrillator), and return to the victim to initiate CPR and defibrillation. If two rescuers are present, one initiates CPR while the other activates the ERS and gets the AED. Calls to 911 should provide information on location, what happened, number and condition of the victims, and the type of aid that is being provided. The caller should not hang up on the dispatcher until the dispatcher instructs the caller to hang up.
- **Open the Airway and Check for Breathing:** Place the victim lying on his/her back on a firm, flat surface and remove clothes so chest is visible. If the victim is lying face down, roll head and torso as one unit onto the back. If a head or neck injury is suspected, move him/her as little as possible to reduce the risk of paralysis. Kneel beside the victim near the shoulders. If the victim does not appear to have a neck injury, use the *head-tilt, chin-lift maneuver* to open his/her airway. This is accomplished by first placing the palm of the hand closest to the victim's head on the victim's forehead and the fingers of the other hand under the bony part of the lower jaw near the chin in order to lift the chin. Lift the jaw to bring the victim's chin forward. Do not close the victim's mouth completely. There is movement of the head from the neutral position with this maneuver.
  - If a neck injury is suspected, use the *jaw-thrust maneuver* instead of the *head-tilt, chin lift maneuver*. Kneel at the victim's head with your elbows on the ground. Rest your thumbs on the victim's lower jaw near the corners of the mouth, pointing your thumbs toward his/her feet. Then place your fingers around the lower jaw. To open the airway, lift the lower jaw with your fingertips.
  - While maintaining the open airway, place your face near the victim's face and <u>LOOK</u> for the chest to rise and fall, <u>LISTEN</u> for air escaping during exhalation, and <u>FEEL</u> for the flow of air against your cheek. *This entire step should take 5 seconds but no more than 10 seconds.* If he/she starts to breathe, keep the airway open and continue checking his/her breathing until help arrives.
- **Give Rescue Breaths:** If the victim does not start breathing after opening the airway, begin rescue breathing. Pinch his/her nose closed with the thumb and index finger of the hand you had on his/her forehead. Take a regular breath (not deep) and seal your lips around the victim's mouth creating an airtight seal (mouth to mouth). Give 2 breaths each lasting 1 second. The first breath should cause the chest to visibly rise. If the first breath does not cause the chest to rise, repeat the head tilt-chin lift and give a second breath. *This step should take no longer than 10 seconds.* Breaths can also be given with a mouth-to-barrier device and mouth-to-mask.
- **Pulse Check:** Maintain the head tilt with one hand on the victim's forehead. Check for a pulse at the carotid artery. This is accomplished by locating the trachea (windpipe or Adam's apple); place 2 or 3 fingers of the other hand on the trachea, and slip the fingers into the groove between the trachea and the muscles in the side of the neck where the carotid pulse can be felt. The pulse check should take 5 seconds and no longer than 10 seconds. If the rescuer can not definitely feel a pulse, perform 5 cycles of compressions and breaths. If a pulse is definitely present, give 1 breath every 5–6 seconds and recheck the pulse every 2 minutes.
- **Chest Compressions:** The victim should be supine on a firm, flat surface with the rescuer kneeling beside the victim's thorax (chest). The rescuer places the heel of the hand on the sternum in the center (middle) of the chest between the nipples and then places the heel of the second hand on top of the first

so the hands overlap and are parallel. With your arms straight and your shoulders directly over your hands, push hard and fast straight down on the victim's sternum (breastbone). The sternum is depressed $1^1/_2$ to 2 inches (approximately 4–5 centimeters) and then the chest is allowed to recoil/return to its normal position so the heart can fill with blood. Do not change your hand position. Compressions are given in a smooth manner at a rate of 100 compressions per minute.

- Give cycles of 30 compressions and 2 breaths (30:2 ratio) until AED/defibrillator arrives, Advanced Life Support (ALS) providers take over, or victim starts to move. The 30 compressions should be delivered in less than 23 seconds. Rescuers (healthcare providers) should interrupt compressions as infrequently as possible and limit interruptions to no longer than 10 seconds except for interventions such as advanced airway insertion or the use of a defibrillator. Compressions generate blood movement. When an advanced airway is in place and there are 2 rescuers, one rescuer gives chest compressions continuously at a rate of 100 per minute without pauses for ventilation. The second rescuer gives rescue ventilations at a rate of 8–10 breaths per minute. Rescuers should change compression/ventilation positions every 2 minutes (or after 5 cycles of compressions and ventilations at a ratio of 30:2) to decrease fatigue.

- **AED/Defibrillator Arrives:** Follow the instructions provided on the device related to pad placement and device controls. Once the device's power is on and the pads are attached to the victim's chest, it will analyze the victim's rhythm. No one should be touching the victim while the AED is analyzing. If the rhythm is shockable, 1 shock is delivered once the victim is "cleared" of all hands-on rescuers. The rescuer operating the AED can state "I'm clear, you're clear, we're all clear" before initiating the shock. CPR (5 cycles) is immediately resumed, starting with compressions, after a shock is delivered. If the rhythm is not shockable, CPR is immediately resumed for 5 cycles with a rhythm check after the 5 cycles. After 2 minutes (5 cycles) of CPR, the AED will prompt the rescuer to resume analysis. Continue until ALS providers take over or the victim starts to move.

Adult BLS Healthcare Provider Algorithm

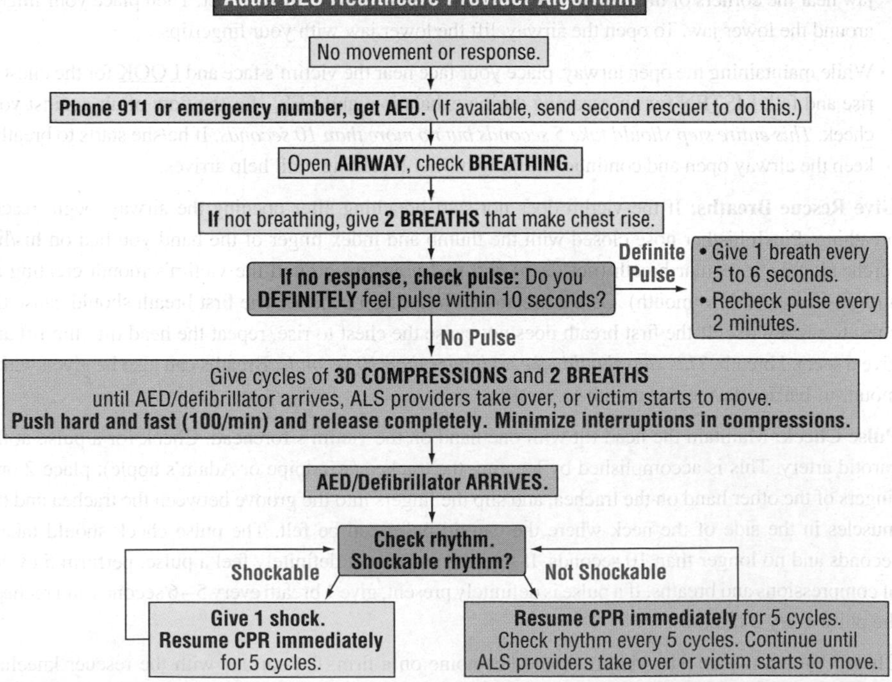
No movement or response.
Phone 911 or emergency number, get AED. (If available, send second rescuer to do this.)
Open AIRWAY, check BREATHING.
If not breathing, give 2 BREATHS that make chest rise.
If no response, check pulse: Do you DEFINITELY feel pulse within 10 seconds?
Definite Pulse
• Give 1 breath every 5 to 6 seconds.
• Recheck pulse every 2 minutes.
No Pulse
Give cycles of 30 COMPRESSIONS and 2 BREATHS until AED/defibrillator arrives, ALS providers take over, or victim starts to move.
Push hard and fast (100/min) and release completely. Minimize interruptions in compressions.
AED/Defibrillator ARRIVES.
Check rhythm. Shockable rhythm?
Shockable
Not Shockable
Give 1 shock. Resume CPR immediately for 5 cycles.
Resume CPR immediately for 5 cycles. Check rhythm every 5 cycles. Continue until ALS providers take over or victim starts to move.

Reprinted with permission from American Heart Association (*Circulation*. 2005; 112:IV-19-IV-34).

General Cancer Classification, Staging, and Grouping Systems

Roman Numeral Staging, I–IV and Recurrent Cancers

(also called Stage Grouping)

Staging depends on cancer cell type. Specific cell types may use designations such as A–D for prostate or colon, rather than I–IV.

I	Small localized cancers, usually curable
II	Locally advanced and/or involvement of lymph nodes
III	Locally advanced and/or involvement of lymph nodes
IV	Inoperable or metastatic
Recurrent	After all visible tumor eradicated
Locally recurrent	In area of primary tumor
Distant recurrent	Metastases (interchangeable with stage IV)

Subcategories of stage groupings are delineated by capital letters (e.g., IIB, IIIC). When using stage grouping, if the combination of tumor-node-metastasis elements is not in the stage grouping table, the case should be considered unstageable, or categorized as stage group 99.

Solid Tumor Staging

Tumor-Node-Metastasis (TNM) Category (also called American Joint Committee [AJC]), American Joint Committee on Cancer [AJCC] and l'Union Internationale Contre le Cancer [UICC]). Staging is not relevant for occult carcinoma, which is designated TX N0 M0.

TNM Staging

T	Primary tumor, size, and invasiveness
TX	Primary tumor cannot be assessed.
T0	No evidence of primary tumor
Tis	Carcinoma in situ (carcinomas represent the only type of cancer that can be classified as being 'in situ,' because only carcinomas have a basement membrane. Thus, sarcomas are never described as being in situ.)
T1–T4	Presence of tumors. Higher numbers indicate increased size, extent, or degree of penetration. Each cancer type has specifics to classify under the number.
N	Regional lymph nodes, presence or absence. Variable value
NX	Regional lymph nodes cannot be assessed.
N0	No regional lymph node metastasis
N1–N3	Regional lymph node metastasis. Higher numbers indicate greater involvement.
M	Distant metastasis, presence or absence of distant metastasis, including lymph nodes that are not regional
MX	Distant metastasis cannot be assessed.
M0	No distant metastasis
M1	Distant metastasis

Clinical and Pathologic Staging

a	Autopsy
c	Clinical
p	Pathologic
r	Recurrent
y	During or after multimodality treatment

Other Descriptors

GX, G1–G4	Histopathologic grade
LX, L0, L1	Lymphatic vessel invasion
RX, RO-R2	Residual tumor
SX, SO-S2	Scleral invasion, serum markers
VX, V0-V2	Venous invasion

Roman Numeral/TNM Subsets (type-specific, examples only)

Lung Cancer

Stage 0	Carcinoma in situ
Stage IA	T1 N0 M0
Stage IB	T2 N0 M0
Stage IIA	T1 N1 M0
Stage IIB	T2 N1 M0; T3 N0 M0
Stage IIIA	T3 N1 M0; T1 N2 M0; T2 N2 M0; T3 N2 M0
Stage IIIB	T4 N0 M0; T4 N1 M0; T4 N2 M0; T1 N3 M0; T2 N3 M0; T3 N3 M0; T4 N3 M0
Stage IV	Any T, Any N, M1

Adapted from Vaporciyan AA, Nesbitt JC, Lee JS, et al. Cancer of the Lung. In: Bast RC, Kule DW, Poliock RE, et al., eds. *Cancer Medicine, 5th ed.* Hamilton: BC Decker Inc; 2000:1227-1292.

Specific Cancers, Staging And Classification

Breast Tumors Clinical Classification (TNM)

TX	Primary tumor cannot be assessed.
TO	No evidence of primary tumor found.
Tis	Carcinoma in situ: intraductal carcinoma, or lobular carcinoma in situ, or Paget disease of the nipple with no tumor (Note: Paget disease associated with a tumor is classified according to the size of the tumor.)
T1	Tumor ≤2 cm in greatest dimension
T1a	≤0.5 cm in greatest dimension
T1b	0.5 cm but <1 cm in greatest dimension
T1c	>1 cm but not >2 cm in greatest dimension
T2	Tumor >2 cm but not >5 cm in greatest dimension
T3	Tumor >5 cm in greatest dimension
T4	Tumor of any size with direct extension to chest wall or skin
T4a	Extension to chest wall
T4b	Edema (including peau d'orange), or ulceration of the skin of the breast, or satellite skin nodules confined to the same breast
T4c	Findings of both 4a and 4b
T4d	Inflammatory carcinoma

Note: Chest wall includes ribs, intercostal muscles, and serratus anterior muscle, but not pectoral muscle. Inflammatory carcinoma of the breast is characterized by diffuse, brawny induration of the skin with an erysipeloid edge, usually with no underlying palpable mass. If the result of skin biopsy is negative and no localized measurable primary cancer is found, the T category is pTX when pathologically staging a clinical inflammatory carcinoma (e.g., T4d). Dimpling of the skin, nipple retraction, or other skin changes, except those considered as T4b and 4d, may occur in T1, T2, or T3 cases without affecting the classification.

NX	Regional lymph nodes cannot be assessed.
N0	No regional lymph node metastasis
N1	Metastasis to movable ipsilateral axillary node(s)
N2	Metastasis to ipsilateral axillary node(s) fixed to one another or to other structures
N3	Metastasis to ipsilateral internal mammary lymph node(s)
MX	Presence of distant metastasis cannot be assessed.
M0	No distant metastases are found.
M1	Distant metastases are present.

Breast Cancer Staging

Stage 0	Carcinoma in situ of the breast (ductal carcinoma in situ [DCIS] lobular carcinoma in situ [LCIS])
Stage I	T1, N0, M0 <2 cm in diameter, does not touch the skin, does not touch the muscles, and has not invaded the lymph nodes anywhere.

Stage II	>2 cm in diameter but <5 cm in diameter, does not touch the skin, and does not touch the muscles. **or** Any size <5 cm but has spread to the lymph nodes in the axilla
Stage IIa	T0–1, N1, M0; T2, N0, M0
Stage IIb	T2, N1, M0; T3, N0, M0
Stage III	>5 cm in diameter **and/or** Spread to lymph nodes fixed to one another, or to the surrounding tissue (e.g., skin, muscle, blood vessels) **or** Breast cancers of any diameter that involve skin, the ribs of the chest wall, or the internal mammary lymph nodes beneath the middle part of the ribs No spread to other organs No spread to bones away from the chest area No spread to lymph nodes far from the breast
Stage IIIa	T0-2, N2, M0, or T3, N1-2, M0
Stage IIIb	T4, N (any), M0; T(any), N3, M0
Stage IV	T(any), N(any), M1 Any size tumor, metastasized to organs or lymph nodes away from the breast

Pathologic Staging (pTN) Breast Tumor

pT	Primary tumor (correspond to the T categories) Primary carcinoma No gross tumor at the margins of resection Tumor size is a measurement of the invasive component. Example: A large in situ component of 4 cm and a small invasive component of 0.5 cm = pTl a.
PN	Regional lymph nodes (correspond to P categories) Breast tumor Resection and examination of at least the low axillary lymph resection ordinarily includes six or more lymph nodes.
pNX	Regional lymph nodes cannot be assessed (not removed for study or previously removed).
pNO	No regional lymph node metastasis
pNI	Metastasis to movable ipsilateral axillary node(s)
pN1 a	Only micrometastasis (none >0.2 cm)
pN1b	Metastasis to lymph node(s), any >0.2 cm
pN1bi	Metastasis to one to three lymph nodes, any >0.2 cm and all <2.0 cm in greatest dimension
pN1bii	Metastasis to four or more lymph nodes, any >0.2 cm and all <2.0 cm in greatest dimension
pN1biii	Extension of tumor beyond the capsule of a lymph node metastasis <2.0 cm in greatest dimension
pN1biv	Metastasis to a lymph node ≥2.0 cm in greatest dimension
pN2	Metastasis to ipsilateral axillary lymph nodes fixed to one another or other structures
pN3	Metastasis to ipsilateral internal mammary lymph node(s)

Scarff-Bloom-Richardson (SBR) Grading System, Breast Tumor (also known as: (BR) Bloom-Richardson [BR] grading system, Modified BR, Elston-Ellis modification of BR grading system). BR grading scheme is a semi-quantitative grading method for invasive (no special type) breast cancers, based on three morphologic features: degree of tumor tubule formation tumor mitotic activity, and nuclear pleomorphism of tumor cells (nuclear grade). Seven possible scores are condensed into three BR grades. The three grades then translate into:

Bloom-Richardson combined scores	Differentiation/BR Grade
3, 4, 5	Well-differentiated (BR low grade)
6,7	Moderately differentiated (BR intermediate grade)
8,9	Poorly differentiated (BR high grade)

Melanoma

Melanoma Stage Information

The microstage of malignant melanoma is determined on result of histologic examination by the vertical thickness of the lesion in millimeters (Breslow classification) and/or the anatomic level of local invasion (Clark classification). The Breslow thickness is more reproducible and more accurately predicts subsequent behavior of malignant melanoma in lesions >1.5 mm in thickness and should always be reported. Accurate microstaging of the primary tumor requires careful histologic evaluation of the entire specimen by an experienced pathologist. Estimates of prognosis should be modified by sex and anatomic site as well as by clinical and histologic evaluation.

Clark Level of Invasion

Histologic classification is based on resection of entire lesion.

Restrictions: Does not take nodal involvement into consideration; deals only with primary tumor. Uniformity of staging not always reproducible because of variations in the depth of layers of the skin. Cannot be applied accurately to melanomas affecting the palms and soles. Histologic difference exists between growth patterns of superficial spreading and nodular malignant melanomas.

Level I	Confined to epidermis (in situ); never metastasizes; 100% cure rate
Level II	Invasion into papillary dermis; invasion past basement membrane (localized)
Level III	Tumor filling papillary dermis (localized), and compressing the reticular dermis
Level IV	Invasion of reticular dermis (localized)
Level V	Invasion of subcutaneous tissue (regionalized by direct extension)

Breslow Depth of Invasion

Pathologic staging based on measurement of tumor invasion of dermis using the micrometer on the microscope; more reproducible than Clark levels.

Categories	Actual measurement of depth of lesion is recorded
Cases are grouped for study as follows	
0.75 mm	Comparable with Clark level II
>0.75–1.5 mm	Comparable with Clark level III
>1.5–4.0 mm	Comparable with Clark level IV
>4.0 mm	Comparable with Clark level V

Clinical Staging for Malignant Melanoma

Used for staging of melanomas that have spread beyond the primary tumor or do not have adequate tissue for pathologic examination. Clinical staging includes results of tests and examinations as well as pathologic findings. Clinical staging parallels summary staging.

Stage I	Localized, without metastases to distant or regional nodes (allows localized disease ≤5 cm. from initial tumor within primary lymphatic drainage area
Stage II	Regionalized, involvement of regional nodes
Stage III	Disseminated, visceral, or lymphatic metastases or multiple cutaneous or subsequent metastases

Reference to stage in melanoma cannot be assumed to be clinical, Clark, or Breslow unless specifically identified as such.

From Cancer staging module: melanoma staging schemes. SEER's Training Web Site. Available at http://training.seer.cancer.gov/module_staging_cancer/unit03_sec04_part05_melanoma.html. Accessed June 23, 2006.

TNM Staging of Melanoma

Primary tumor (T)

TX	Primary tumor cannot be assessed (e.g., shave biopsy or regressed melanoma).
T0	No evidence of primary tumor
Tis	Melanoma in situ

T1	Tumor ≤ 1.0 mm thick with or without ulceration
T1a	Tumor ≤ 1.0 mm thick and Clark level II or III, no ulceration
T1b	Tumor ≤ 1.0 mm thick and Clark level IV or V or with ulceration
T2	Tumor >1.0 mm but not >2.0 mm thick with or without ulceration
T2a	Tumor >1.0 mm but not >2.0 mm thick, no ulceration
T2b	Tumor >1.0 mm but not >2.0 mm thick, with ulceration
T3	Tumor >2.0 mm but not >4 mm thick with or without ulceration
T3a	Tumor >2.0 mm but not >4 mm thick, no ulceration
T3b	Tumor >2.0 mm thick, but not >4 mm, with ulceration
T4	Tumor >4.0 mm thick with or without ulceration
T4a	Tumor >4.0 mm thick, no ulceration
T4b	Tumor >4.0 mm thick, with ulceration

Regional lymph nodes (N), Melanoma

NX	Regional lymph nodes cannot be assessed.
N0	No regional lymph node metastasis
N1	Metastasis to 1 lymph node
N1a	Clinically occult (microscopic) metastasis
N1b	Clinically apparent (macroscopic) metastasis
N2	Metastasis to 2 or 3 regional nodes or intralymphatic regional metastasis without nodal metastases
N2a	Clinically occult (microscopic) metastasis
N2b	Clinically apparent (macroscopic) metastasis
N2c	Satellite or in-transit metastasis without nodal metastasis
N3	Metastasis in 4 or more regional nodes, or matted lymph nodes, or in-transit metastasis or satellite(s) with metastatic regional node(s)

(Note: Micrometastases are diagnosed after elective or sentinel lymphadenectomy; macrometastases are defined as clinically detectable lymph nodes metastases confirmed by therapeutic lymphadenectomy, or when any lymph node metastasis exhibits gross extracapsular extension.)

Distant Metastasis (M), Melanoma

MX	Distant metastasis cannot be assessed.
M0	No distant metastasis
M1	Distant metastasis
M1a	Metastasis to skin, subcutaneous tissues, or distant lymph nodes
M1b	Metastasis to lung
M1c	Metastasis to all other visceral sites or distant metastasis at any site associated with elevated levels of serum lactic dehydrogenase

Clinical Staging, American Joint Committee on Cancer Stage Groupings, Melanoma

Clinical staging includes microstaging of the primary melanoma and clinical and/or radiologic evaluation for metastases. By convention, it should be assigned after complete excision of the primary melanoma with clinical assessment for regional and distant metastases.

Stage 0	Tis, N0, M0
Stage IA	T1a, N0, M0
Stage IB	T1b, N0, M0; T2a, N0, M0
Stage IIA	T2b, N0, M0; T3a, N0, M0
Stage IIB	T3b, N0, M0; T4a, N0, M0
Stage IIC	T4b, N0, M0;
Stage III	Any T, N1, M0; Any T, N2, M0; Any T, N3, M0
Stage IV	Any T, any N, M1

Pathologic Staging, American Joint Committee on Cancer Stage Groupings

With the exception of patients with clinical stage 0 or stage IA lesions (who have a low risk of lymphatic involvement and do not require pathologic evaluation of their lymph nodes), pathologic staging includes microstaging of the primary melanoma and pathologic information about the regional lymph nodes after sentinel node biopsy and, if indicated, complete lymphadenectomy.

Stage 0	Tis, N0, M0
Stage IA	T1a, N0, M0
Stage IB	T1b, N0, M0; T2a, N0, M0
Stage IIA	T2b, N0, M0; T3a, N0, M0
Stage IIB	T3b, N0, M0;T4a, N0, M0
Stage IIC	T4b, N0, M0
Stage IIIA	T1-4a, N1a, M0; T1-4a, N2a, M0
Stage IIIB	T1-4b, N1a, M0; T1-4b, N2a, M0; T1-4a, N1b, M0; T1-4a, N2b, M0; T1-4a/b, N2c, M0;
Stage IIIC	T1-4b, N1b, M0; T1-4b, N2b, M0; T1-4b, N2c, M0; Any T, N3, M0
Stage IV	Any T, any N, M1

Adapted from Melanoma of the skin. In: American Joint Committee on Cancer, *AJCC Cancer Staging Manual*, 6th ed. New York, NY: Springer; 2002: 209-220.

System-Specific Cancer Classification, Gastrointestinal/Genitourinary

Colorectal Cancer Staging: Dukes Staging (also called: Astler-Coller, Turnbull, modified Astler-Coller [MAC]).

Originally staging for rectal cancer only; first Kirklin and then Astler and Coller added colon and rectal cancers; Turnbull included stage for unresectable tumors and distant metastases.

Dukes staging (the generic term) is based on pathologic examination and resection of the tumor; measures the depth of invasion through the mucosa and bowel wall. It does not take into account level of nodal involvement or the grade of the tumor.

Dukes	Categories	Stage	TNM Category
Stage A	Confined to mucosa	I	T1 or T2, N0 M0
Stage B	Varies by system	II	T3 or T4, N0 M0
Stage C	Positive lymph nodes	III	Any T, N1/N2, M0
Stage D	Distant metastases	IV	Any T, Any N, M1 (Turnbull system only)

Modified from American Joint Committee on Cancer, *AJCC Cancer Staging Manual*, 5th ed. Philadelphia: Lippincott-Raven;1998.

Bladder Cancer Staging: Jewett Staging (also called Marshall, Jewett-Marshall Staging, and American Urologic System [AUS]).

Histologic staging based on depth of invasion through the bladder wall. It does not consider grade of tumor, local recurrence rate, or multicentricity of tumors. A deep resection is mandatory for this method.

Jewett Categories:

Stage A	Submucosal invasion but no involvement of muscle
Stage B	Bladder wall or muscle invasion
Stage B1	Superficial
Stage B2	Deep
Stage C	Extension through serosa into perivesical fat (around bladder)
Stage D	Lymph node and distant metastases
Stage D1	Regional nodes
Stage D2	Distant nodes and other distant metastases

AJCC Tumor notation T1 – T4 is equivalent to Jewett stages A through D, respectively

N (node) and M (metastases) are part of Jewett stage D.

Prostate Cancer Staging: American or American Urologic System: Staging has been translated to TNM extent of disease notation by the American Joint Committee.

Stage A	Can be subdivided based on the number of cell clusters (foci) seen on microscopic examination.
Stage B	Difference between Stage A and Stage B is whether nodule(s) are clinically palpable (or visibly seen) in prostate.
Stage C	Dividing line between Stage B and Stage C is microscopically evident capsular invasion.
Stage D	Determinant is presence of metastatic disease identified either clinically or microscopically.

Gynecologic Cancers

International Federation of Gynecologists and Obstetricians (FIGO) Gynecologic Cancer Staging: Based on clinical data including examination and colposcopy.

FIGO Stage Characteristics (cervical cancer)

Stage 0	Carcinoma in situ, intraepithelial carcinoma; cascs of stagc 0 should not be included in any therapeutic statistics for invasive carcinoma.
Stage I	Carcinoma is strictly confined to the cervix (extension to the corpus should be disregarded)
Stage IA	Invasive cancer identified only microscopically. (All gross lesions, even with superficial invasion, are considered stage IB cancers). Invasion is limited to measured stromal invasion of <5 mm deep taken from the base of the epithelium, either surface or glandular, from which it originates. Vascular space involvement, either venous or lymphatic, should not alter the staging).
Stage IA1	Measured invasion of stroma ≤ 3 mm deep and ≤ 7 mm wide
Stage IA2	Measured invasion of stroma >3 mm and ≤ 5 mm deep and ≤ 7 mm wide
Stage IB	Clinical lesions confined to the cervix or preclinical lesions >IA
Stage IB1	Clinical lesions ≤ 4 cm in size
Stage IB2	Clinical lesions >4 cm in size
Stage II	Carcinoma extends beyond the cervix but has not extended onto pelvic wall; carcinoma involves the vagina, but not as far as the lowest third
Stage IIA	No obvious parametrial involvement
Stage IIB	With parametrial involvement
Stage III	Carcinoma has extended onto the pelvic wall; on rectal examination no space between the tumor and the pelvic wall is free from cancerous involvement; tumor involves the lowest third of vagina; all cases involving hydronephrosis or a nonfunctioning kidney should be included, unless such findings are known to be due to other causes
Stage IIIA	No extension onto the pelvic wall, but involvement of the lowest third of the vagina
Stage IIIB	Extension onto the pelvic wall or hydronephrosis or nonfunctioning kidney
Stage IV	Carcinoma has extended beyond the true pelvis or has clinically involved the mucosa of the bladder or rectum
Stage IVA	Spread of the growth to adjacent organs
Stage IVB	Spread to distant organs

Histopathologic grades (G), unless otherwise detailed

Gx	Grade cannot be assessed
Gl	Well-differentiated
G2	Moderately differentiated
G3	Poorly differentiated or undifferentiated

Adapted from Benedet JL, Bender H, Jones H 3rd, Ngan HY, Pecorelli S. FIGO staging classifications and clinical practice guidelines in the management of gynecologic cancers. FIGO Committee on Gynecologic Oncology. *Int J Gynaecol Obstet.* 2000 Aug;70(2):207-312.

Lymph/Blood Cancers Classifications And Categories

Lymphomas: Hodgkin and Non-Hodgkin Lymphoma

Ann Arbor Classification (originally proposed for Hodgkin, but now also used for Non-Hodgkin Lymphoma)

Stage I	Involvement of a single lymph node region
Stage IE	A single extralymphatic organ or site
Stage II	Involvement of two or more lymph node regions on same side of diaphragm
Stage II_3	Number of lymph node regions involved may be indicated by a subscript.
Stage IIE	Localized involvement of extralymphatic organ or site and of one or more lymph node regions on the same side of the diaphragm
Stage III	Involvement of lymph node regions on both sides of diaphragm
Stage IIIE	Localized involvement of extralymphatic organ or site
Stage IIIS	Involvement of spleen
Stage IIISE	Both stage IIIE and IIIS. Also written Stage III+SE
Stage IV	Diffuse or disseminated multifocal involvement of one or more extralymphatic organs or tissues with or without associated lymph node enlargement. **or** Isolated extralymphatic organ involvement with distant (nonregional) nodal involvement.
Stage IVE	Used when extranodal lymphoid malignancies arise in tissues separate from, but near, the major lymphatic aggregates

Extralymphatic sites of involvement use letter code and plus sign (+).

N	nodes
H	liver
L	lung
M	bone marrow
S	spleen
P	pleura
O	bone
D	skin

Lymphoma and Non-Hodgkin Lymphoma Categories

A	Without well-defined generalized symptoms
B	With well-defined generalized symptoms: unexplained loss of >10% of body weight in the 6 months before diagnosis; unexplained fever with temperatures exceeding 38ºC; and drenching night sweats

Revised European American Lymphoma (REAL) Classification System

REAL Hodgkin Lymphoma Categories

Excellent prognosis	Average 5-year survival rate of 70%
Good prognosis	Average 5-year survival rate of 50–70%
Fair prognosis	Average 5-year survival rate of 30–49%
Poor prognosis	Average 5-year survival rate of <30%

Hodgkin Lymphoma (Hodgkin Disease) Classification

Nodular lymphocyte-predominant Hodgkin lymphoma

Classical Hodgkin lymphoma: nodular sclerosis, mixed cellularity, and lymphocyte depletion

B-Cell Neoplasm Classification

- Precursor B-cell lymphoblastic leukemia/lymphoma
- Mature B-cell neoplasms
- B-cell chronic lymphocytic leukemia/small lymphocytic lymphoma
- B-cell prolymphocytic leukemia

Lymphoplasmacytic lymphoma

Mantle cell lymphoma

Follicular lymphoma

Cutaneous follicle center lymphoma

Marginal zone B-cell lymphoma (MALT type, nodal, and splenic type)

Hairy cell leukemia

Diffuse large B-cell lymphoma

Burkitt lymphoma

Plasmacytoma and plasma cell myeloma

T-Cell Neoplasm Classification

Precursor T-cell lymphoblastic lymphoma

Mature T-cell and natural killer-cell neoplasms

T-cell prolymphocytic leukemia

T-cell large granular lymphocytic leukemia

Aggressive natural killer-cell leukemia

Mycosis fungoides and Sezary syndrome

Angioimmunoblastic T-cell lymphoma

Peripheral T-cell lymphomas

Adult T-cell leukemia/lymphoma

Anaplastic large cell lymphoma

Primary cutaneous CD30+ T-cell lymphoproliferative disorders

Subcutaneous panniculitislike T-cell lymphoma

Entropathy-type intestinal T-cell lymphoma

Hepatosplenic T-cell lymphoma

Note: The REAL lymphoma classification system relies on immunophenotypic markers and on unusual proteins secreted by cancerous white blood cells. The REAL system includes NHL and other hematologic cancers that share these markers: Hodgkin lymphomas, plasma cell myeloma, and chronic lymphocytic leukemia.

Working Formulation System Categories (Lymphoma)

High grade grows very quickly and causes serious symptoms.

Intermediate grows more rapidly than low grade and causes serious symptoms.

Low grade grows more slowly and produces fewer symptoms.

Leukemia Classification

French-American-British (FAB) Categories: Cell classification by types and subtypes, also sometimes referred to as Bennett system

Acute lymphocytic leukemia (diagnosed primarily in children), three subtypes

Acute myelogenous leukemia (the most common type of leukemia, diagnosed in both children and adults), eight subtypes

Chronic myelogenous leukemia (diagnosed primarily in adults)

Chronic lymphocytic leukemia (diagnosed primarily in adults) uses different classification system

Acute Lymphocytic Leukemia (ALL), Primarily Pediatric Patients (also called Acute Lymphoblastic Leukemia

L1 Mature-appearing lymphoblasts (T cells or pre-B cells), small with uniform genetic material, regular nuclear shape, nonvisible, little cytoplasm.

L2 Immature and pleomorphic lymphoblasts (T cells or pre-B cells), large and variable in size, variable genetic material, irregular nuclear shape, one or more large nucleoli, and variable cytoplasm.

L3 Lymphoblasts (B cells; Burkitt cells) large and uniform, genetic material finely stippled and uniform, nuclear shape is regular (oval to round), one or more prominent nucleoli, cytoplasm is moderately abundant.

T-cell type: Thymus is involved. May lead to superior vena cava syndrome.

Acute Myelogenous Leukemia (AML), Pediatric and Adult Patients (also called acute nonlymphocytic Leukemia or ANL)

M0 Undifferentiated acute myelogenous leukemia. Bone marrow cells show no significant signs of differentiation (allow maturation to obtain distinguishing cell characteristics).

M1	Myeloblastic leukemia with/without minimal cell maturation. Bone marrow cells show some signs of granulocytic differentiation.
M2	Myeloblastic leukemia with cell maturation. Maturation of bone marrow cells is at or beyond the promyelocyte (early granulocyte) stage; varying amounts of maturing granulocytes may be seen; often associated with a specific genetic change involving translocation of chromosomes 8 and 21.
M3, M3 variant [M3V]	Myelocytic leukemia. Most cells are abnormal early granulocytes, between myeloblasts and myelocytes in stage of development; contain many small particles. The cell nucleus may vary in size and shape. Bleeding and blood clotting problems (e.g., disseminated intravascular coagulation, are commonly seen with this form of leukemia. Good responses have been observed after treatment with retinoids.
M4E, M4 variant with eosinophilia [M4E])	Monocytic leukemia. Bone marrow and circulating blood have variable amounts of differentiated granulocytes and monocytes. The proportion of monocytes and promonocytes in bone marrow is >20% of all nucleated cells. The M4E variant also contains abnormal eosinophils in bone marrow.
M5	Monocytic leukemia (two forms). First characterized by poorly differentiated monoblasts with lacy-appearing genetic material; second, differentiated form characterized by a large population of monoblasts, promonocytes, and monocytes; proportion of monocytes in the bloodstream may be higher than in the bone marrow. M5 leukemia may infiltrate skin and gums; prognosis in such patients worse.
M6	Erythroleukemia characterized by abnormal erythrocyte-forming cells, which comprise over half of the nucleated cells in the bone marrow.
M7	Megakaryoblastic leukemia. Blast cells look like immature megakaryocytes or lymphoblasts; may be distinguished by extensive fibrous tissue deposits (fibrosis) in the bone marrow.

In addition, patients sometimes develop isolated tumors of the myeloblasts, such as isolated granulocytic sarcoma, or chloroma. Patients with chloroma frequently develop AML.

Chronic Myelogenous Leukemia (CML), Primarily Adult Patients

Chronic	>5% blast cells and promyelocytes in blood and bone marrow; marked by increasing overproduction of granulocytes; generally only mild symptoms; responds well to conventional treatment.
Accelerated	>5% but <30% blast cells. Cells exhibit Philadelphia chromosome and other chromosomal abnormalities; more abnormal cells are produced; patients with noticeable symptoms (e.g., fever, poor appetite, weight loss) may not respond as well to therapy.
Blast	>30% blast cells in blood and bone marrow; blast cells frequently invade other tissues and organs. The disease transforms into an aggressive, acute leukemia (70% acute myelogenous leukemia, 30% acute lymphocytic leukemia)

Chronic Lymphocytic Leukemia (CLL)

American Society of Anesthesiologists (ASA) Preoperative Assessment and Grading (also called Dripps-ASA, which reduced seven components to five).

ASA Grade	Definition
I	Normally healthy person
II	Mild systemic disease that does not limit activity

III	Severe systemic disease that limits activity but is not incapacitating
IV	Incapacitating systemic disease that is constantly life-threatening
V	Moribund, not expected to survive 24 hours with or without surgery

Eastern Cooperative Oncology Group (ECOG) Performance Status (also called Zubrod scale. See WHO Performance Scale.

Grade	
0	Fully active, able to carry on all predisease activities
1	Restricted in physically strenuous activity but ambulatory and able to carry out work of a light or sedentary nature (e.g., light house work, office work)
2	Ambulatory and capable of all self-care but unable to carry out any work activities. Up and about >50% of waking hours
3	Capable of only limited self-care, confined to bed or chair >50% of waking hours
4	Completely disabled. Cannot carry on any self-care. Totally confined to bed or chair
5	Dead

Adapted from Owen MM, et al. Toxicity and response criteria of the Eastern Cooperative Oncology Group. *Am J Clin Oncol.* 1982;5:649-655.

World Health Organization (WHO) Performance Scale (also called Zubrod scale; sometimes called ECOG).

Measures levels of patient capability. For example, an inpatient getting metabolic studies done may be fully capable of performing normal activities but will remain in bed by personal choice. Such a patient should be coded 0, "normal."

0	Normal activity
1	Symptoms, but nearly fully ambulatory
2	Some bed time, but needs to be in bed <50% of normal daytime
3	Needs to be in bed >50% of normal daytime
4	Unable to get out of bed

Karnofsky Performance Status Scale

Criteria	**Definition**
100%	Normal, no complaints; no evidence of disease
90%	Able to carry on normal activity; minor signs or symptoms of disease
80%	Normal activity with effort; some signs or symptoms of disease; able to carry on normal activity and to work
70%	Cares for self; unable to carry on normal activity or to do active work
60%	Requires occasional assistance, can care for most personal needs
50%	Requires considerable assistance and frequent medical care
40%	Disabled; requires special care and assistance
30%	Severely disabled; hospital admission is indicated although death not imminent
20%	Very sick; hospital admission necessary; active supportive treatment necessary
10%	Moribund; fatal processes progressing rapidly
0	Dead

Commonly Prescribed Drugs and Their Applications

This list has been selected to be representative of the most commonly prescribed drugs in the United States and Canada for the year 2006 (see references). The list is arranged alphabetically by generic drug name (lower case), followed by representative tradenames (uppercase) for the United States and Canadian markets. Combination products have their individual ingredients listed. The final column lists a commonly used classification for the drug. For alternate classifications and therapeutic uses of these drugs, see Classification and Therapeutic Uses of Drugs table (page APP 519).

Generic Name	Trade Name United States	Trade Name Canada	Classification
abacavir/lamivudine/zidovudine	TRIZIVIR	TRIZIVIR	Combination Product
acetaminophen/codeine	TYLENOL WITH CODEINE	RATIO-EMTEC, TYLENOL WITH CODEINE	Combination Product
acetaminophen/hydrocodone	ANEXSIA, LORTAB, NORCO, VICODIN, ZYDONE	NOT AVAILABLE	Combination Product
acetaminophen/oxycodone	ENDOCET, PERCOCET, ROXICET, TYLOX	ENDOCET, PERCOCET, RATIO-OXYCET	Combination Product
acetaminophen/propoxyphene	DARVOCET, DARVOCET-N, PROPACET	NOT AVAILABLE	Combination Product
acetaminophen/tramadol	ULTRACET	TRAMACET	Combination Product
acyclovir	ZOVIRAX	ZOVIRAX	Antiviral
adalimumab	HUMIRA	HUMIRA	Immunomodulators
adapalene	DIFFERIN	DIFFERIN	Retinoid
albuterol (salbutamol)	PROVENTIL, VENTOLIN, PROAIR HFA	AIROMIR, APO-SALVENT, RATIO-SALBUTAMOL HFA, VENTOLIN , VOLMAX	β_2 Agonist
alendronate	FOSAMAX, FOSAMAX PLUS D	FOSAMAX, NOVO-ALENDRONATE	Bisphosphonate
alfuzosin	UROXATRAL	XATRAL	Alpha Blocker
allopurinol	LOPURIN, ZURINOL, ZYLOPRIM	ALLOPRIN, APO-ALLOPURINOL, PURINOL, ZYLOPRIM	Xanthine Oxidase Inhibitor
alprazolam	XANAX	APO-ALPRAZ, GEN-ALPRAZOLAM, XANAX	Benzodiazepine
amantadine	SYMMETREL	SYMMETREL	Antiviral
amiodarone	CORDARONE, PACERONE	CORDARONE	Antiarrhythmic
amitriptyline	AMITID, AMITRIL, ELAVIL, EMITRIP, ENDEP	APO- AMITRIPTYLINE, ELAVIL, LEVATE	Tricyclic Antidepressant (TCA)
amlodipine	NORVASC	NORVASC	Calcium Channel Blocker
amlodipine/atorvastatin	CADUET	CADUET	Combination Product
amlodipine/benazepril	LOTREL	—	Combination Product
amoxicillin	AMOXIL, DISPERMOX, LAROTID, POLYMOX, TRIMOX	AMOXIL, APO-AMOXI, GEN-AMOXACILLIN, NOVAMOXIN, ZIMAMOX	Penicillin
amoxicillin/clavulanate	AUGMENTIN	AUGMENTIN, CLAVULIN	Combination Product
amphetamine mixed salts	ADDERALL, ADDERALL XR	ADDERALL XR	Indirect-Acting Sympathomimetic
anastrozole	ARIMIDEX	ARIMIDEX	Antineoplastic
aripiprazole	ABILIFY	NOT AVAILABLE	Atypical Antipsychotic
aspirin	ASCRIPTIN, BUFFERIN, ECOTRIN	ASAPHEN, BUFFERIN, ECOTRIN, NOVASEN, RIVASA	Nonsteroidal Anti-Inflammatory Drug (NSAID)
atazanavir	REYATAZ	REYATAZ	Antiretroviral Agent (protease inhibitor)

Generic Name	Trade Name United States	Trade Name Canada	Classification
atenolol	TENORMIN	APO-ATENOL, NOVO-ATENOL, PMS-ATENOLOL, RATIO-ATENOLOL, TENORMIN	Cardioselective β Blocker
atenolol/chlorthalidone	TENORETIC	TENORETIC	Combination Product
atomoxetine	STRATTERA	STRATTERA	Selective Norepinephrine Reuptake Inhibitor (SNRI)
atorvastatin	LIPITOR	LIPITOR	HMG-CoA Reductase Inhibitor
atropine	ISOPTO ATROPINE	ISOPTO ATROPINE	Anticholinergic
azathioprine	AZASAN, IMURAN	IMURAN	Immunosuppressant
azelastine	ASTELIN, OPTIVAR	NOT AVAILABLE	Antihistamine
azithromycin	ZITHROMAX	ZITHROMAX	Macrolide
baclofen	LIORESAL	LIORESAL	Skeletal Muscle Relaxant
benazepril	LOTENSIN	LOTENSIN	Angiotensin-Converting Enzyme (ACE) Inhibitor
benazepril/hydrochlorothiazide	LOTENSIN HCT	NOT AVAILABLE	Combination Product
benzonatate	TESSALON	TESSALON	Local Anesthetic
benztropine	COGENTIN	COGENTIN	Anticholinergic
bicalutamide	CASODEX	CASODEX	Antiandrogen
bimatoprost	LUMIGAN	LUMIGAN	Prostaglandin
bisoprolol	ZEBETA	MONOCOR	Cardioselective β Blocker
brimonidine	ALPHAGAN	ALPHAGAN	Central Sympatholytic
budesonide	PULMICORT, RHINOCORT AQUA, PULMICORT RESPULES	PULMICORT NEBUAMP, ENTOCORT, PULMICORT, RHINOCORT AQUA	Glucocorticoid
bumetanide	BUMEX	BURINEX	Loop Diuretic
buproprion	WELLBUTRIN, ZYBAN WELLBUTRIN SR, WELLBUTRIN XL	WELLBUTRIN SR, WELLBUTRIN XL	Atypical Antidepressant
buspirone	BUSPAR	BUSPAR, BUSPIREX	Anxiolytic
butalbital/acetaminophen/caffeine	FIORICET	NOT AVAILABLE	Combination Product
butorphanol	STADOL	STADOL	Opiate Agonist
cabergoline	DOSTINEX	DOSTINEX	Endocrine and Metabolic Agents
caffeine	CAFCIT, VIVARIN	CAFCIT	Methylxanthine
calcitonin	MIACALCIN	APO-CALCITONIN, CALCIMAR	Endocrine and Metabolic Agent
calcitriol	ROCALTROL	ROCALTROL	Vitamins
calcium acetate	PHOSLO	PHOSLO	Minerals
candesartan	ATACAND	ATACAND	Angiotensin Receptor Blocker (ARB)
capecitabine	XELODA	XELODA	Antineoplastic
captopril	CAPOTEN	CAPOTEN, CAPTRIL	Angiotensin-Converting Enzyme (ACE) Inhibitor
carbamazepine	TEGRETOL	TEGRETOL	Anticonvulsant
carbidopa/levodopa	SINEMET	SINEMET	Combination Product
carisoprodol	SOMA	NOT AVAILABLE	Skeletal Muscle Relaxant
carvedilol	COREG	COREG, DILATREND, EUCARDIC, PROREG	β Blocker
cefadroxil	DURICEF, ULTRACEF	DURICEF	Cephalosporin

Generic Name	Trade Name United States	Trade Name Canada	Classification
cefdinir	OMNICEF	OMNICEF	Cephalosporin
cefprozil	CEFZIL	CEFZIL	Cephalosporin
cefuroxime	CEFTIN, KEFUROX, ZINACEF	CEFTIN, KEFUROX, ZINACEF	Cephalosporin
celecoxib	CELEBREX	CELEBREX	COX-2 Inhibitor
cephalexin	CEFANEX, KEFLEX, KEFTAB	APO-CEPHALEX, CEPOREX, KEFLEX, NOVO-LEXIN	Cephalosporin
cetirizine	ZYRTEC	ALLERGY RELIEF, REACTINE	Antihistamine
cetirizine/pseudoephedrine	ZYRTEC-D	REACTINE ALLERGY AND SINUS	Combination Product
chlorhexidine gluconate	PERIDEX, PERIOGARD	DENTICARE	Mouth and Throat Products
chlorpheniramine	ALLERGY, CHLOR-TRIMETON	CHLOR-TRIPOLON	Antihistamine
cholestyramine	LOCHOLEST, QUESTRAN	QUESTRAN	Bile Acid Sequestrant
ciclopirox	PENLAC	LOPROX, STIEPROX	Antifungal
cilazapril	NOT AVAILABLE	INHIBACE	Angiotensin-Converting Enzyme (ACE) Inhibitor
cilostazol	PLETAL	PLETAL	Platelet Aggregation Inhibitor
ciprofloxacin	CILOXAN, CIPRO	CILOXAN, CIPRO	Fluoroquinolone
ciprofloxacin/dexamethasone	CIPRODEX	CIPRODEX	Combination Product
citalopram	CELEXA	CELEXA	Selective Serotonin Reuptake Inhibitor (SSRI)
clarithromycin	BIAXIN, BIAXIN XL	BIAXIN	Macrolide
clavulanate	2	2	β-Lactamase Inhibitor
clindamycin	CLEOCIN	DALACIN	Lincosamide
clindamycin/benzoyl peroxide	BENZACLIN, DUAC	NOT AVAILABLE	Combination Product
clobetasol	CORMAX, EMBELINE, TEMOVATE	DERMASONE, DERMOVATE, TEMOVATE	Glucocorticoid
clonazepam	KLONOPIN	APO-CLONAZEPAM, PMS-CLONAZEPAM, RIVOTRIL	Benzodiazepine
clonidine	CATAPRES	CATAPRES, DIXARIT	Central Sympatholytic
clopidogrel	PLAVIX	PLAVIX	Platelet Aggregation Inhibitor
clorazepate	TRANXENE	TRANXENE	Benzodiazepine
clotrimazole/betamethasone	LOTRISONE	LOTRIDERM	Combination Product
clozapine	CLOZARIL	CLOZARIL	Atypical Antipsychotic
colchicine	1		Agents for Gout
conjugated estrogens (equine)	PREMARIN	CES, CONGEST, PREMARIN	Estrogen
conjugated estrogens/medroxyprogesterone	PREMPHASE, PREMPRO	NOT AVAILABLE	Combination Product
cyclobenzaprine	FLEXERIL	FLEXERIL	Skeletal Muscle Relaxant
cyclosporine	GENGRAF, NEORAL, SANDIMMUNE, RESTASIS	NEORAL, SANDIMMUNE	Immunosuppressant
desloratadine	CLARINEX	AERIUS	Antihistamine
desmopressin	DDAVP, MINIRIN	DDAVP, MINIRIN, OCTOSTIM	Vasopressin Analogue
desoximetasone	TOPICORT	TOPICORT	Glucocorticoid
dexamethasone	DECADRON, DEXAMETH, DEXONE, HEXADROL	DECADRON, HEXADROL	Glucocorticoid
dexmethylphenidate	FOCALIN XR	NOT AVAILABLE	CNS Stimulant
dextroamphetamine	DEXEDRINE	DEXEDRINE	Indirect-Acting Sympathomimetic

Generic Name	Trade Name United States	Trade Name Canada	Classification
diazepam	DIASTAT, VALCAPS, VALIUM, VAZEPAM	APO-DIAZEPAM, DIAZEMULS, E-PAM , VALIUM, VIVOL	Benzodiazepine
diclofenac	CATAFLAM, SOLARAZE, VOLTAREN	DICLOTEC, VOFENAL, VOLTAREN	Nonsteroidal Anti-Inflammatory Drug (NSAID)
diclofenac/misoprostol	ARTHROTEC	ARTHROTEC	Combination Product
dicyclomine	BENTYL	BENTYLOL	Anticholinergic
didanosine	VIDEX	VIDEX	Antiretroviral Agents
digoxin	DIGITEK, LANOXICAPS, LANOXIN	LANOXIN	Cardiac Glycoside
diltiazem	CARDIZEM, CARTIA, DILACOR, DILTIA, TAZTIA, TIAZAC	APO-DILTIAZ , CARDIZEM, RATIO-DILTIAZEM CD, TIAZAC	Calcium Channel Blocker
diphenoxylate/atropine	LOMOTIL	LOMOTIL	Combination Product
dipyridamole/aspirin	AGGRENOX	AGGRENOX	Antiplatelet Agent
divalproex	SEE VALPROIC ACID		
docusate	COLACE	COLACE, SOFLAX	Stool Softener
donepezil	ARICEPT	ARICEPT	Cholinesterase Inhibitor
dorzolamide/timolol	COSOPT	COSOPT	Combination Product
doxazosin	CARDURA	CARDURA	β Blocker
doxepin	ADAPIN, SINEQUAN, ZONALON	SINEQUAN, TRIADAPIN, ZONALON	Tricyclic Antidepressant (TCA)
doxycycline	ADOXA, DORYX, MONODOX, VIBRAMYCIN, VIBRA-TABS	DORYX, VIBRAMYCIN, VIBRA-TABS	Tetracycline
duloxetine	CYMBALTA	NOT AVAILABLE	Atypical Antidepressant
dutasteride	AVODART	AVODART	5 alpha-Reductase Inhibitor
econazole	SPECTAZOLE	ECOSTATIN	Antifungal
efavirenz	SUSTIVA	SUSTIVA	Reverse Transcriptase Inhibitor
eletriptan	RELPAX	RELPAX	5-HT1 Receptor Agonist
emtricitabine/tenofovir	TRUVADA	TRUVADA	Antiretroviral Agent
enalapril	VASOTEC	VASOTEC	Angiotensin-Converting Enzyme (ACE) Inhibitor
enfuvirtide	FUZEON	FUZEON	Antiretroviral Agent
enoxaparin	LOVENOX	LOVENOX	Low Molecular Weight Heparin (LMWH)
epinephrine	EPIPEN	EPIPEN	Vasopressor
epoetin alfa	EPOGEN, PROCRIT	EPREX	Recombinant Human Erythropoietin
erythromycin	E-MYCIN, ERY-TAB, ILOSONE, ILOTYCIN	ILOSONE, ILOTYCIN	Macrolide
escitalopram	LEXAPRO	CIPRALEX	Selective Serotonin Reuptake Inhibitor (SSRI)
esomeprazole	NEXIUM	NEXIUM	Proton Pump Inhibitor (PPI)
estradiol	CLIMARA, ESTRACE, ESTRADERM, VIVELLE, VIVELLE DOT, VAGIFEM	CLIMARA, ESTRACE, ESTRADERM, VIVELLE, ESTRADOT	Estrogen
eszopiclone	LUNESTA	NOT AVAILABLE	Sedatives and Hypnotics
etanercept	ENBREL	ENBREL	Disease-Modifying Antirheumatic Drug (DMARD)

Generic Name	Trade Name United States	Trade Name Canada	Classification
ethinyl estradiol/desogestrel	APRI, MIRCETTE, KARIVA	MARVELON	Combination Product
ethinyl estradiol/drospirenone	YASMIN	YASMIN	Combination Product
ethinyl estradiol/norelgestromin	ORTHO EVRA	NOT AVAILABLE	Combination Product
ethinyl estradiol/norethindrone	BREVICON, ESTROSTEP, FEMHRT, LOESTRIN, MICROGESTIN, MICRONOR, OVCON, NECON 1/35	BREVICON, FEMHRT, LOESTRIN, MICRONOR, SYNPHASIC	Combination Product
ethinyl estradiol/norgestimate	ORTHO-CYCLEN, TRI-CYCLEN, TRINESSA, TRI-SPRINTEC	CYCLEN, TRI-CYCLEN	Combination Product
ethinyl estradiol/norgestrel	CRYSELLE, OGESTREL, OVRAL	OVRAL	Combination Product
etodolac	LODINE	ULTRADOL	Nonsteroidal Anti-Inflammatory Drug (NSAID)
etonogestrel/ethinyl estradiol	NUVARING	NUVARING	Combination Product
exenatide	BYETTA	NOT AVAILABLE	Incretin Mimetic Agent
ezetimibe	ZETIA	EZETROL	Cholesterol Absorption Inhibitor
ezetimibe/simvastatin	VYTORIN	NOT AVAILABLE	Combination Product
famciclovir	FAMVIR	FAMVIR	Antiviral
famotidine	PEPCID	PEPCID	H_2 Receptor Antagonist (H_2RA)
felodipine	PLENDIL	PLENDIL, RENEDIL	Calcium Channel Blocker
fenofibrate	TRICOR	LIPIDIL	Fibric Acid Derivative
fentanyl	ACTIQ, DURAGESIC, SUBLIMAZE	DURAGESIC, SUBLIMAZE	Opiate Agonist
ferrous sulfate	FEOSOL	NIFEREX	Trace Element
fexofenadine	ALLEGRA	ALLEGRA	Antihistamine
fexofenadine/pseudoephedrine	ALLEGRA-D	ALLEGRA-D	Combination Product
filgrastim	NEUPOGEN	NEUPOGEN	Granulocyte-Colony Stimulating Factor (G-CSF)
finasteride	PROPECIA, PROSCAR	PROPECIA, PROSCAR	5β-Reductase Inhibitor
flecainide	TAMBOCOR	TAMBOCOR	Antiarrhythmic
fluconazole	DIFLUCAN	APO-FLUCONAZOLE, DIFLUCAN	Antifungal
fluocinonide	LIDEX	LYDERM, LIDEX	Glucocorticoid
fluoxetine	PROZAC	PROZAC	Selective Serotonin Reuptake Inhibitor (SSRI)
fluticasone	FLONASE, FLOVENT	FLONASE, FLOVENT	Glucocorticoid
fluvastatin	LESCOL, LESCOL XL	LESCOL, LESCOL XL	HMG-CoA Reductase Inhibitor
fluvoxamine	LUVOX	LUVOX	Selective Serotonin Reuptake Inhibitor (SSRI)
folic acid	FOLVITE	FOLICARE	Vitamins
fosinopril	MONOPRIL	MONOPRIL	Angiotensin-Converting Enzyme (ACE) Inhibitor
furosemide	LASIX	APO-FUROSEMIDE, LASIX, NOVO-SEMIDE	Loop Diuretic
fusidic acid	NOT AVAILABLE	FUCIDIN	Antibacterial
gabapentin	NEURONTIN	NEURONTIN, PMS-GABAPENTIN	Anticonvulsant
gatifloxacin	TEQUIN, ZYMAR	TEQUIN	Fluoroquinolone

Generic Name	Trade Name United States	Trade Name Canada	Classification
gemfibrozil	LOPID	LOPID	Fibric Acid Derivative
gentamicin	GARAMYCIN	GARAMYCIN	Aminoglycoside
glatiramer	COPAXONE	COPAXONE	Immunosuppressant
glimepiride	AMARYL	AMARYL	Oral Antidiabetic
glipizide	GLUCOTROL, GLUCOTROL XL	NOT AVAILABLE	Oral Antidiabetic
glyburide (glibenclamide)	DIABETA, MICRONASE	APO-GLYBURIDE, DIABETA, GEN-GLYBE, NOVO-GLYBURIDE	Oral Antidiabetic
glyburide/metformin	GLUCOVANCE	NOT AVAILABLE	Combination Product
griseofulvin	GRIFULVIN V	FULVICIN U/F	Antifungal
hydralazine	APRESOLINE	APRESOLINE	Vasodilator
hydrochlorothiazide	ESIDRIX, HYDRODIURIL, ORETIC	APO-HYDRO, ESIDRIX, HYDRODIURIL, NOVO-HYDRAZIDE,	Thiazide and Related Diuretics
hydrochlorothiazide/bisoprolol	ZIAC	ZIAC	Combination Product
hydrochlorothiazide/irbesartan	AVALIDE	AVALIDE	Combination Product
hydrochlorothiazide/lisinopril	PRINZIDE, ZESTORETIC	PRINZIDE, ZESTORETIC	Combination Product
hydrochlorothiazide/losartan	HYZAAR	HYZAAR	Combination Product
hydrochlorothiazide/triamterene	DYAZIDE, MAXZIDE	APO-TRIAZIDE, DYAZIDE	Combination Product
hydrochlorothiazide/valsartan	DIOVAN HCT	DIOVAN HCT	Combination Product
hydrocodone/chlorpheniramine	TUSSIONEX	TUSSIONEX	Combination Product
hydrocodone/ibuprofen	VICOPROFEN	VICOPROFEN	Combination Product
hydrocortisone	CORT-DOME, CORTEF, DERMOLATE	CORTATE, CORTEF	Glucocorticoid
hydromorphone	DILAUDID, PALLADONE	DILAUDID, PALLADONE	Opiate Agonist
hydroxychloroquine	PLAQUENIL	PLAQUENIL	Antimalarial
hydroxyzine	ATARAX, VISTARIL	APO-HYDROXYZINE, ATARAX	Antihistamine
hyoscyamine	LEVSIN	LEVSIN	Anticholinergic
ibandronate	BONIVA	NOT AVAILABLE	Bisphosphonates
ibuprofen	ADVIL, MOTRIN	ADVIL, APO-IBUPROFEN, MOTRIN	Nonsteroidal Anti-Inflammatory Drug (NSAID)
imatinib	GLEEVEC	GLEEVEC	Antineoplastic
imipramine	TOFRANIL	TOFRANIL	Tricyclic Antidepressant (TCA)
imiquimod	ALDARA	ALDARA	Immunomodulator
indapamide	LOZOL	LOZIDE, GEN-INDAPAMIDE, PMS-INDAPAMIDE	Thiazide and Related Diuretics
indomethacin	INDOCIN	INDOCID	Nonsteroidal Anti-Inflammatory Drug (NSAID)
influenza virus vaccine	FLUZONE	FLUZONE	Vaccine
insulin	HUMULIN, NOVOLIN	HUMULIN, NOVOLIN GE NPH	Insulin
insulin aspart	NOVOLOG	NOVORAPID	Insulin
insulin glargine	LANTUS	LANTUS	Insulin
insulin lispro	HUMALOG	HUMALOG	Insulin
interferon beta-1a	AVONEX	AVONEX, REBIF	Immunomodulator
interferon beta-1b	BETASERON	BETASERON	Immunomodulator
ipratropium	ATROVENT	ATROVENT	Anticholinergic
ipratropium/albuterol	COMBIVENT	COMBIVENT	Combination Product
irbesartan	AVAPRO	AVAPRO	Angiotensin Receptor Blocker (ARB)

Generic Name	Trade Name United States	Trade Name Canada	Classification
isosorbide mononitrate	IMDUR, ISMO, ISOTRATE, MONOKET	IMDUR, ISMO	Nitrate
itraconazole	SPORANOX	SPORANOX	Antifungal
ketoconazole	NIZORAL	NIZORAL	Antifungal
labetalol	NORMODYNE, TRANDATE	TRANDATE	β Blocker
lamivudine/zidovudine	COMBIVIR	COMBIVIR	Combination Product
lamotrigine	LAMICTAL	LAMICTAL	Anticonvulsant
lansoprazole	PREVACID	PREVACID	Proton Pump Inhibitor (PPI)
latanoprost	XALATAN	XALATAN	Prostaglandin
leflunomide	ARAVA	ARAVA	Disease-Modifying Antirheumatic Drug (DMARD)
levalbuterol	XOPENEX	NOT AVAILABLE	β_2 Agonist
levetiracetam	KEPPRA	KEPPRA	Anticonvulsant
levofloxacin	LEVAQUIN, QUIXIN	LEVAQUIN	Fluoroquinolone
levothyroxine	LEVOTHROID, LEVOXYL, SYNTHROID, UNITHROID	ELTROXIN, SYNTHROID	Thyroid Hormone
lidocaine	LIDODERM, XYLOCAINE	XYLOCAINE	Local Anesthetic
lisinopril	PRINIVIL, ZESTRIL	APO-LISINIPRIL, PRINIVIL, ZESTRIL	Angiotensin-Converting Enzyme (ACE) Inhibitor
lithium	ESKALITH, LITHANE, LITHOBID, LITHOTABS	CARBOLITH, DURALITH, LITHANE, LITHIZINE	Antimanic
lopinavir	[2]	[2]	Protease Inhibitor
lopinavir/ritonavir	KALETRA	KALETRA	Combination Product
losartan	COZAAR	COZAAR	Angiotensin Receptor Blocker (ARB)
lovastatin	ALTOCOR, MEVACOR	MEVACOR	HMG-CoA Reductase Inhibitor
meclizine	ANTIVERT, BONINE	ANTIVERT	Anticholinergic
medroxyprogesterone	CYCRIN, PROVERA	MEPROGEST, PROVERA, RATIO-MPA	Progestin
megestrol	MEGACE	MEGACE	Progestin
meloxicam	MOBIC	MOBICOX	Nonsteroidal Anti-Inflammatory Drug (NSAID)
memantine	NAMENDA	EBIXA	NMDA Receptor Antagonist
mercaptopurine	PURINETHOL	PURINETHOL	Antineoplastic Agent
mesalamine	ASACOL, PENTASA	ASACOL, MESASAL, PENTASA, QUNITASA, SALOFALK	Nonsteroidal Anti-Inflammatory Drug (NSAID)
methadone	METHADOSE, DOLOPHINE	METADOL	Opiod Analgesic
metaxalone	SKELAXIN	NOT AVAILABLE	Skeletal Muscle Relaxant
metformin	GLUCOPHAGE, GLUCOPHAGE XR	APO-METFORMIN, GEN-METFORMIN, GLUCOPHAGE, NOVO-METFORMIN, PMS-METFORMIN, RATIO-METFORMIN	Oral Antidiabetic
methadone	METHADOSE, DOLOPHINE	METADOL	Opiod Analgesic
methocarbamol	ROBAXIN	ROBAXIN	Skeletal Muscle Relaxant
methotrexate	RHEUMATREX, TREXALL	RHEUMATREX	Antineoplastic
methylphenidate	CONCERTA, RITALIN	CONCERTA, PMS-METHYLPHENIDATE, RITALIN	Indirect-Acting Sympathomimetic

Generic Name	Trade Name United States	Trade Name Canada	Classification
methylprednisolone	MEDROL	MEDROL	Glucocorticoid
metoclopramide	MAXOLON , REGLAN	MAXERAN, REGLAN	Prokinetic Antiemetic
metolazone	MYKROX, ZAROXOLYN	ZAROXOLYN	Thiazide and Related Diuretics
metoprolol	LOPRESSOR, TOPROL-XL	BETALOC, LOPRESOR, NOVO-METOPROLOL	Cardioselective β Blocker
metronidazole	FLAGYL, METROGEL, NORITATE	APO-METRONIDAZOLE, FLAGYL, METROGEL, NORITATE	Antibacterial Antiprotozoal
midodrine	PROAMATINE	AMATINE	Vasopressor
minocycline	DYNACIN, MINOCIN	MINOCIN, ULTRAMYCIN	Tetracycline
mirtazapine	REMERON	REMERON	Atypical Antidepressant
misoprostol	CYTOTEC	CYTOTEC	Prostaglandin
modafinil	PROVIGIL	ALERTEC	Central Nervous System (CNS) Stimulant
mometasone	ELOCON, NASONEX	ELOCOM, NASONEX	Glucocorticoid
montelukast	SINGULAIR	SINGULAIR	LTD_4 Receptor Antagonist
morphine	MS CONTIN, MSIR, ORAMORPH	MS CONTIN, MSIR, ORAMORPH	Opiate Agonist
moxifloxacin	AVELOX, VIGAMOX	AVELOX	Fluoroquinolone
mupirocin	BACTROBAN	BACTROBAN	Antibacterial β_2 Agonist
mycophenolate mofetil	CELLCEPT	CELLCEPT	Immunosuppressant
nabumetone	RELAFEN	RELAFEN	Nonsteroidal Anti-Inflammatory Drug (NSAID)
nadolol	CORGARD	CORGARD	β Blocker
naproxen	ALEVE, ANAPROX, NAPRELAN, NAPROSYN	ANAPROX, APO-NAPROXEN, NAPROSYN, NAXEN	Nonsteroidal Anti-Inflammatory Drug (NSAID)
nicotine	HABITROL, NICODERM, NICORETTE, NICOTROL	HABITROL, NICODERM, NICORETTE, NICOTROL	Ganglionic Stimulant
nicotinic acid	NIASPAN	NIASPAN	Vitamin
nifedipine	ADALAT, NIFEDICAL XL, PROCARDIA XL, PROCARDIA ER	ADALAT XL, APO-NIFED	Calcium Channel Blocker
nisoldipine	SULAR	NOT AVAILABLE	Calcium Channel Blocker
nitrofurantoin	FURADANTIN, MACROBID, MACRODANTIN	MACROBID, MACRODANTIN	Antibacterial
nitroglycerin	NITRO-DUR, NITROSTAT, TRANSDERM-NITRO	NITRO-DUR, NITROSTAT, TRANSDERM-NITRO	Nitrate
nortriptyline	AVENTYL, PAMELOR	AVENTYL	Tricyclic Antidepressant (TCA)
nystatin	MYCOSTATIN, NILSTAT	MYCOSTATIN, NILSTAT	Antifungal
ofloxacin	FLOXIN, OCUFLOX	FLOXIN, OCUFLOX	Fluoroquinolone
olanzapine	ZYPREXA	ZYPREXA	Atypical Antipsychotic
olmesartan	BENICAR	NOT AVAILABLE	Angiotensin Receptor Blocker (ARB)
olmesartan/ hydrochlorothiazide	BENICAR HCT	NOT AVAILABLE	Combination Product
olopatadine	PATANOL	PATANOL	Antihistamine
omeprazole	PRILOSEC	LOSEC	Proton Pump Inhibitor (PPI)

Generic Name	Trade Name United States	Trade Name Canada	Classification
ondansetron	ZOFRAN	ZOFRAN	5-HT_3 Antagonist
oseltamivir	TAMIFLU	TAMIFLU	Antiviral
oxandrolone	ANAVAR, OXANDRIN	NOT AVAILABLE	Androgen
oxcarbazepine	TRILEPTAL	TRILEPTAL	Anticonvulsant
oxybutynin	DITROPAN, DITROPAN XL	DITROPAN, DITROPAN XL, APO-OXYBUTYNIN	Anticholinergic
oxycodone	OXYCONTIN, OXYIR, M-OXY	OXYCONTIN, OXY-IR	Opiate Agonist
pantoprazole	PROTONIX	PANTOLOC	Proton Pump Inhibitor (PPI)
paroxetine	PAXIL, PAXIL CR	PAXIL, PAXIL CR	Selective Serotonin Reuptake Inhibitor (SSRI)
peginterferon alfa-2a	PEGASYS	PEGASYS	Immunomodulator
penicillin v	V-CILLIN K, VEETIDS	APO-PEN-VK, V-CILLIN K	Penicillin
phenazopyridine	PYRIDIUM	PYRIDIUM	Urinary Analgesic
phenobarbital	LUMINAL	PMS-PHENOBARBITAL	Barbiturate
phentermine	FASTIN, IONAMIN	FASTIN, IONAMIN	Indirect-Acting Sympathomimetic
phenytoin	DILANTIN	DILANTIN	Hydantoin
pimecrolimus	ELIDEL	ELIDEL	Immunomodulator
pioglitazone	ACTOS	ACTOS	Oral Antidiabetic
piroxicam	FELDENE	FELDENE	Nonsteroidal Anti-Inflammatory Drug (NSAID)
polyethylene glycol (peg)	COLYTE, MIRALAX	COLYTE, PEGLYTE	Laxative
potassium chloride	K-TAB, K-DUR, KLOR-CON	KAY CIEL	Electrolytes
pramipexole	MIRAPEX	MIRAPEX	Antiparkinson Agent
pravastatin	PRAVACHOL	APO-PRAVASTATIN, LIN-PRAVASTATIN, PRAVACHOL	HMG-CoA Reductase Inhibitor
prednisolone	ORAPRED, PEDIAPRED, PRED FORTE	PEDIAPRED , PRED FORTE	Glucocorticoid
prednisone	DELTASONE	DELTASONE	Glucocorticoid
pregabalin	LYRICA	LYRICA	Anticonvulsant
primidone	MYSOLINE	MYSOLINE	Anticonvulsant
prochlorperazine	COMPAZINE	STEMETIL	Phenothiazine
progesterone	CRINONE, PROCHIEVE, PROGESTASERT, PROMETRIUM	CRINONE, GESTEROL, PROMETRIUM	Progestin
promethazine	ANERGAN, PHENERGAN, PROMETHEGAN, PHENADOZ	HISTANTIL, PHENERGAN	Phenothiazine
promethazine/codeine	PHENERGAN WITH CODEINE	NOT AVAILABLE	Combination Product
propafenone	RYTHMOL	RYTHMOL	Antiarrhythmic
propoxyphene	DARVON, DARVON-N	642, DARVON-N	Opiate Agonist
propranolol	BETACHRON, INDERAL	APO-PROPRANOLOL, DETENSOL, INDERAL	β Blocker
quetiapine	SEROQUEL	SEROQUEL	Atypical Antipsychotic
quinapril	ACCUPRIL	ACCUPRIL, ACCUPRO	Angiotensin-Converting Enzyme (ACE) Inhibitor
quinine	QUALAQUIN	NOVO-QUININE	Antimalarial
rabeprazole	ACIPHEX	PARIET	Proton Pump Inhibitor (PPI)
raloxifene	EVISTA	EVISTA	Selective Estrogen Receptor Modulator (SERM)

Generic Name	Trade Name United States	Trade Name Canada	Classification
ramipril	ALTACE	ALTACE, RAMACE	Angiotensin Converting Enzyme (ACE) Inhibitor
ranitidine	ZANTAC	APO-RANITIDINE, GEN-RANITIDINE, NOVO-RANITIDINE, ZANTAC	H_2 Receptor Antagonist (H_2RA)
ribavirin	REBETOL, VIRAZOLE	VIRAZOLE	Antiviral
risedronate	ACTONEL	ACTONEL	Bisphosphonate
risperidone	RISPERDAL	RISPERDAL	Atypical Antipsychotic
ritonavir	NORVIR	NORVIR	Protease Inhibitor
ropinirole	REQUIP	REQUIP	Antiparkinson Agent
rosiglitazone	AVANDIA	AVANDIA	Oral Antidiabetic
rosuvastatin	CRESTOR	CRESTOR	HMG-CoA Reductase Inhibitor
salbutamol (see albuterol)	—	—	—
salmeterol/fluticasone	ADVAIR	ADVAIR	Combination Product
sertraline	ZOLOFT	APO-SERTRALINE, ZOLOFT	Selective Serotonin Reuptake Inhibitor (SSRI)
sildenafil	VIAGRA	VIAGRA	Phosphodiesterase Type 5 (PDE5) Inhibitor
simvastatin	ZOCOR	APO-SIMVASTATIN, GEN-SIMVASTATIN, ZOCOR	HMG-CoA Reductase Inhibitor
sodium fluoride	ETHEDENT, PHARMAFLUR	PREVIDENT	Trace Elements
sotalol	BETAPACE	SOTACOR, ZIMSOTALOL	β Blocker
spironolactone	ALDACTONE	ALDACTONE, NOVO-SPIROTON	Potassium Sparing Diuretic
sucralfate	CARAFATE	SULCRATE	Cytoprotective
sumatriptan	IMITREX	IMITREX	5-$HT_{1B/1D}$ Agonist
tacrolimus	PROGRAF, PROTOPIC	PROGRAF, PROTOPIC	Immunosuppressant
tadalafil	CIALIS	CIALIS	Impotence Agent
tamoxifen	NOLVADEX	NOLVADEX, TAMOFEN, TAMONE	Antiestrogen
tamsulosin	FLOMAX	FLOMAX	β Blocker
telithromycin	KETEK	KETEK	Ketolide
telmisartan	MICARDIS	MICARDIS	Angiotensin Receptor Blocker (ARB)
telmisartan/hydrochlorothiazide	MICARDIS HCT	MICARDIS PLUS	Combination Product
temazepam	RESTORIL	APO-TEMAZEPAM, RESTORIL	Benzodiazepine
tenofovir	VIREAD	—	Reverse Transcriptase Inhibitor
terazosin	HYTRIN	HYTRIN	β Blocker
terbinafine	LAMISIL	LAMISIL	Antifungal
terconazole	TERAZOL 7, TERAZOL 3	TERAZOL 7, TERAZOL 3	Antifungal
teriparatide	FORTEO	FORTEO	Parathyroid Hormone
testosterone	ANDRODERM, ANDROGEL, DELATESTRYL, STRIANT, TESTIM	ANDRODERM, DELATESTRYL, MALOGEN	Androgen
tetracycline	ACHROMYCIN, SUMYCIN	ACHROMYCIN	Tetracycline
thalidomide	THALOMID	NOT AVAILABLE	Immunomodulators
thyroid dessicated	ARMOUR THYROID	THYROIDINUM	Thyroid Hormone
timolol	BLOCADREN, TIMOPTIC	BLOCADREN, TIMOPTIC	β Blocker
tiotropium	SPIRIVA	SPIRIVA	Anticholinergic
tizanidine	ZANAFLEX	ZANAFLEX	Central Sympatholytic

Generic Name	Trade Name United States	Trade Name Canada	Classification
tobramycin/dexamethasone	TOBRADEX	TOBRADEX	Combination Product
tolterodine	DETROL, DETROL LA	DETROL, DETROL LA	Anticholinergic
topiramate	TOPAMAX	TOPOMAX	Anticonvulsant
torsemide	DEMADEX	DEMADEX	Loop Diuretic
tramadol	ULTRAM, ULTRAM ER	ZYTRAM XL	Opiate Agonist
trandolapril/verapamil	TARKA	TARKA	Combination Product
travoprost	TRAVATAN	TRAVATAN	Prostaglandin Agonist
trazodone	DESYREL	APO-TRAZODONE, DESYREL	Atypical Antidepressant
tretinoin	RENOVA, RETIN-A, VESANOID	RENOVA, RETIN-A, VESANOID	Retinoid
triamcinolone	ARISTOCORT, AZMACORT, KENALOG, NASACORT	ARISTOCORT, AZMACORT, KENALOG, NASACORT	Glucocorticoid
triamterene	DYRENIUM	2	Potassium Sparing Diuretic
trimethoprim/polymyxin B	POLYTRIM	POLYTRIM	
trimethoprim/sulfamethoxazole	BACTRIM, COTRIM, SEPTRA, SULFATRIM	APO-SULFATRIM DS, BACTRIM, SEPTRA	Combination Product
valacyclovir	VALTREX	VALTREX	Antiviral
valproic acid (divalproex)	DEPAKENE, DEPAKOTE	APO-DIVALPROEX, DEPAKENE, DEPROIC, EPIVAL, RATIO-DIVALPROEX	Anticonvulsant
valsartan	DIOVAN	DIOVAN	Angiotensin Receptor Blocker (ARB)
vardenafil	LEVITRA	LEVITRA	Impotence Agent (Phoshodiesterase Type 5 Inhibitors)
venlafaxine	EFFEXOR	EFFEXOR	Selective Serotonin Reuptake Inhibitor (SSRI)
verapamil	CALAN, COVERA, ISOPTIN, VERELAN	CHRONOVERA, ISOPTIN, VERELAN	Calcium Channel Blocker
warfarin	COUMADIN	APO-WARFARIN, COUMADIN, TARO-WARFARIN	Anticoagulant
ziprasidone	GEODON	NOT AVAILABLE	Atypical Antipsychotic
zolmitriptan	ZOMIG	ZOMIG	5-$HT_{1B/1D}$ Agonist
zolpidem	AMBIEN, AMBIEN CR	NOT AVAILABLE	Benzodiazepine Receptor Agonist
zonisamide	Zonegran	Zonegran	Anticonvulsant

[1] Not sold under any trade name. Available under the generic name.

[2] Only available in combination products, not available as a single entity

References:

Drug Facts and Comparisons. eFacts [online]. St. Louis, MO: Wolters Kluwer Health, Accessed June–July 2007.

Micromedex Healthcare Series: Electronic Version [online]. Greenwood Village, CO: Thomson Micromedex, Accessed June–July 2007.

The Top 200 Brand-Name Drugs by Retail Dollars in 2006. Drug Topics February 19, 2007.

The Top 200 Brand-Name Drugs by Units in 2006. Drug Topics March 5, 2007.

The Top 200 Generic Drugs by Retail Dollars in 2006. Drug Topics February 19, 2007.

The Top 200 Generic Drugs by Units in 2006. Drug Topics March 5, 2007.

Classification and Therapeutic Uses of Drugs

Classification of drugs is inherently difficult because many drugs can be classified in more than one way and some drugs do not fit well into any specific classification. Common ways to classify dugs include chemical structure (i.e. penicillins, opiates, thiazides), pharmacologic activity (i.e. β-blockers, anticholinergics, antihistamines) and therapeutic uses (i.e. antiarrhythmics, antihypertensives, antidiabetics), among others. This list presents alternate classifications that drugs may belong to in addition to the listed classification. Finally, typical therapeutic uses are listed for each classification of drug; although this is not exhaustive and may not be representative of any particular drug in that group.

Classification	Alternate Classification(s)	Therapeutic Uses
β Blocker	β Adrenergic Antagonist, Antihypertensive, Antiarrhythmic, Antianginal	Hypertension, cardiac arrhythmias, angina pectoris, congestive heart failure (CHF), migraine headache
α Blocker	α_1 Adrenergic Antagonist, Antihypertensive, Vasodilator	Hypertension, benign prostatic hyperplasia (BPH)
β_2 Agonist	β_2 Adrenergic Agonist, Bronchodilator	Asthma, premature labor
β-Lactamase Inhibitor	—	β-lactamase producing infection in combination with a β-lactamase susceptible penicillin
5α-Reductase Inhibitor	—	Benign prostatic hyperplasia (BPH), alopecia
5-HT_1 Agonist	Antimigraine, Serotonin (5-hydroxytryptamine, 5-HT_1) Agonist, Triptan	Migraine headache
5-HT_3 Antagonist	Serotonin (5-hydroxytryptamine, 5-HT) 3 (5-HT_3) Antagonist, Antiemetic	Nausea, vomiting
5-HT_4 Agonist	Serotonin (5-hydroxytryptamine, 5-HT) 4 (5-HT_4) Agonist	Irritable bowel syndrome (IBS)
Aminoglycoside	Antimicrobial, Antibacterial, Antibiotic	Bacterial infections
Androgen	Anabolic Steroid	Replacement therapy, cachexia
Angiotensin-Converting Enzyme (ACE) Inhibitor	Antihypertensive	Hypertension, congestive heart failure, diabetic renal nephropathy
Angiotensin Receptor Blocker (ARB)	Antihypertensive	Hypertension, congestive heart failure
Antiandrogen	Endocrine-Metabolic agent	Prostate cancer
Antiarrhythmic	Cardiovascular agent	Cardiac arrhythmias
Antibacterial	Antimicrobial, Antibiotic, Anti-infective	Bacterial infections
Anticholinergic	Muscarinic Antagonist	Parkinsonism, motion sickness, vertigo
Anticoagulant	Blood modifier agent	Thromboembolic disorders
Anticonvulsant	Antiepileptic, Antiseizure	Epilepsy, seizures, convulsions
Antiemetic	Antinausea	Nausea, vomiting
Antiestrogen	Endocrive-Metabolic agent, Genitourinary agent	Estrogen dependent neoplastic disorder, infertility
Antifungal	—	Fungal infections
Antihistamine	Antiallergy	Allergy, insomnia
Antimalarial	—	Malaria, nocturnal leg cramps (quinine)
Antimanic	—	Mania, bipolar disorder
Antineoplastic	—	Neoplastic disorders, immunologic disorders
Antiplatelet	Blood modifier agent	Stroke, myocardial infarction, acute coronary syndrome
Antiprotozoal	—	Protozoal infections
Antipsychotic	Neuroleptic	Psychoses
Antithyroid	—	Hyperthyroidism
Antitubercular	Antimicrobial, Antibiotic, Anti-infective	Tuberculosis

Classification	Alternate Classification(s)	Therapeutic Uses
Antiviral	—	Viral infections
Anxiolytic	Antianxiety	Anxiety
Atypical Antidepressant	—	Major depressive disorder
Atypical Antipsychotic	Neuroleptic	Psychoses
Barbiturate	Sedative, Hypnotic, General Anesthetic, Central Nervous System (CNS) Depressant, Anticonvulsant, Anxiolytic	Insomnia, epilepsy, seizures, convulsions, anxiety, general anesthesia
Benzodiazepine	Sedative, Hypnotic, CNS Depressant, Anticonvulsant, Anxiolytic	Insomnia, epilepsy, seizures, convulsions, anxiety
Benzodiazepine Receptor Agonist	Sedative, Hypnotic	Insomnia
Bile Acid Sequestrant	—	Hyperlipidemia, hypercholesterolemia
Bisphosphonate	Bone Resorption Inhibitor	Paget's disease, osteoporosis, hypercalcemia
Calcium Channel Blocker	Slow Channel Blocker, Antihypertensive, Antiarrhythmic, Antianginal	Hypertension, cardiac arrhythmias, angina pectoris
Carbonic Anhydrase Inhibitor	Diuretic	Edema, epilepsy, glaucoma
Cardiac Glycoside	Inotropic	Congestive heart failure (CHF), supraventricular tachycardia
Cardioselective β Blocker	β_1 Adrenergic Antagonist, Antihypertensive, Antiarrhythmic, Antianginal	Hypertension, cardiac arrhythmias, angina pectoris, CHF
CNS Stimulant	—	Attention deficit—hyperactivity disorder (ADHD), obesity
Central Sympatholytic	α_2 Adrenergic Agonist, Antihypertensive	Hypertension, skeletal muscle spasms
Cephalosporin	Antimicrobial, Antibacterial, Antibiotic	Bacterial infections
Cholesterol Absorption Inhibitor	Antihyperlipidemic	Hypercholesterolemia
Cholinesterase Inhibitor	Acetylcholinesterase Inhibitor, Cholinergic, Parasympathomimetic	Myasthenia gravis, Alzheimer's disease
Combination Product	See individual ingredients	See individual ingredients
COX-2 Inhibitor	Cyclooxygenase-2 (COX 2) Inhibitor, Nonsteroidal Anti-Inflammatory Drug (NSAID), Analgesic, Anti-Inflammatory, Antipyretic	Pain, inflammation, fever, arthritis
Cytoprotective	—	Peptic ulcer disease (PUD)
Disease-Modifying Antirheumatic Drug (DMARD)	Immune Response Modifier, Biologic Response Modifier, Immunomodulator	Rheumatoid arthritis, immunological disorders
DOPA Decarboxylase Inhibitor	Dihydroxyphenylalanine (DOPA) Decarboxylase Inhibitor, Antiparkison agent	Parkinsonism (only with levodopa)
Dopaminergic	—	Parkinsonism, galactorrhea
Estrogen	Oral Contraceptive, Birth Control Pills (BC's)	(Commonly used in combination with a progestin) Contraception, menstrual irregularities, infertility, menopause, replacement therapy, vaginal atrophy, osteoporosis, ovarian failure
Expectorant	—	Cough
Fibric Acid Derivative	—	Hyperlipidemia, hypertriglyceridemia, hypercholesterolemia
Fluoroquinolone	Quinolone	Bacterial infections
Gallstone Solubilizing Agent	Gallstone Dissolution Agent	Gallstones
Ganglionic Stimulant	—	Smoking cessation
Glucocorticoid	Steroid, Corticosteroid, Adrenocortical Steroid, Immunosuppressant	Inflammation, immunological disorders, allergies
Granulocyte Colony Stimulating Factor (G-CSF)	—	Decrease infections during myelosuppressive treatment

Classification	Alternate Classification(s)	Therapeutic Uses
H_2 Receptor Antagonist (H_2RA)	Histamine H_2 Receptor Antagonist (H_2RA), Antacid, Antiulcer	PUD, gastroesophageal reflux disease (GERD)
Histamine Analogue	—	Meniere's disease
HMG-CoA Reductase Inhibitor	Statin	Hyperlipidemia, hypercholesterolemia
Hydantoin	Anticonvulsant, Antiepileptic, Antiseizure	Epilepsy, seizures, convulsions
Immunomodulator	Immune Response Modifier, Biologic Response Modifier	Immunologic disorders, viral infections, neoplastic disorders
Immunosuppressant	—	Immunologic disorders, autoimmune disorders, organ and tissue transplants (allografts)
Indirect-Acting Sympathomimetic	Anorexiant, Decongestant, CNS Stimulant	Nasal congestion, obesity, ADHD
Insulin	Antidiabetic	Type I and Type II diabetes mellitus
Keratolytic	—	Acne vulgaris, UV damaged skin, wart removal
Laxative	—	Constipation, bowel evacuation
Lincosamide	Antimicrobial, Antibacterial, Antibiotic	Bacterial infections
Local Anesthetic	—	Pain
Loop Diuretic	—	Edema, CHF, renal failure, hypertension
Low Molecular Weight Heparin (LMWH)	Anticoagulant, Antithrombic	Thromboembolic disorders
LTD_4 Receptor Antagonist	Leukotriene D_4 (LTD_4) Receptor Antagonist	Asthma
Macrolide	Antimicrobial, Antibacterial, Antibiotic	Bacterial infections
Methylxanthine	Bronchodilator, CNS Stimulant	Asthma, apnea of prematurity, drowsiness
Nitrate	Vasodilator, Venodilator, Antianginal	Angina pectoris, hypertension
Nonsteroidal Anti-Inflammatory Drug (NSAID)	Analgesic, Anti-Inflammatory, Antipyretic	Pain, inflammation, fever
Nuticeutical	Vitamin and mineral supplementation, nutritive agent, electrolytes	Anemia
Opiate Agonist	Analgesic, Narcotic, Opioid, Antitussive, Antidiarrheal	Pain, cough, diarrhea
Oral Antidiabetic	Oral Hypoglycemic	Type II diabetes mellitus
Penicillin	Antimicrobial, Antibacterial, Antibiotic	Bacterial infections
Phenothiazine	Antipsychotic, Antiemetic, Antihistamine	Psychoses, nausea, vomiting, allergies
Phosphate Binder	—	Reduce intestinal absorption of phosphate in renal failure
Phosphodiesterase Type 5 (PDE5) Inhibitor	—	Erectile dysfunction (ED)
Platelet Aggregation Inhibitor	—	Prevention of myocardial infarction
Potassium Sparing Diuretic	—	Hypertension, edema, offset potassium loss of potassium depleting diuretics (thiazide and loop diuretics)
Progestin	Oral Contraceptive, Birth Control Pills (BC's)	(Commonly used in combination with an estrogen) Contraception, menstrual irregularities, infertility, menopause, replacement therapy, vaginal atrophy, osteoporosis, ovarian failure
Prokinetic	—	Gastroparesis, GERD
Prostaglandin	—	PUD, glaucoma, ED, cervical dilatation
Protease Inhibitor	Antiretroviral, Antiviral	Human immunodeficiency virus (HIV) infection
Proton Pump Inhibitor (PPI)	Antiulcer	PUD, GERD
Recombinant Human Erythropoietin	—	Anemia
Retinoid	Antiacne	Acne

Classification	Alternate Classification(s)	Therapeutic Uses
Reverse Transcriptase Inhibitor	Antiretroviral, Antiviral	HIV infection
Selective Estrogen Receptor Modulator (SERM)	Estrogen Agonist/Antagonist	Osteoporosis, infertility
Selective Norepinephrine Reuptake Inhibitor (SNRI)	Antidepressant	Major depressive disorder
Selective Serotonin Reuptake Inhibitor (SSRI)	Antidepressant	Major depressive disorder
Skeletal Muscle Relaxant	—	Skeletal muscle spasms and spasticity
Stool Softener	—	Constipation
Sulfonamide	Antimicrobial, Antibacterial, Antibiotic	Bacterial infections
Tetracycline	Antimicrobial, Antibacterial, Antibiotic	Bacterial, rickettsial, chlamydial infections
Thiazide and Related Diuretics	Antihypertensive	Edema, hypertension
Thyroid Hormone	Thyroid supplement	Hypothyroidism
Tricyclic Antidepressant (TCA)	Antidepressant	Major depressive disorder
Urinary Analgesic	—	Urinary tract pain
Vasodilator	Antihypertensive	Hypertension, peripheral vascular diseases
Vasopressin Analog	—	Replacement therapy, nocturnal enuresis
Xanthine Oxidase Inhibitor	Antigout	Gout

Selected Drugs That Should Be Used with Caution During Pregnancy[a]

Drug/Drug Class	Risk Factor[b]	Fetal/Neonatal Effects
ACE inhibitors	C/D[c]	Use in second and third trimesters has been associated with a pattern of anomalies called ACEI fetopathy with renal tubular dysplasia as the major malformation. Other reported defects include hypocalvaria, IUGR, patent ductus arteriosus, oligohydramnios, pulmonary hypoplasia, and anuria.
Aminoglycosides	C/D[d]	Potential for VIII cranial nerve toxicity with high dosages. Prolonged therapy with kanamycin produced VIII cranial nerve damage; nine of 391 (2.3%) infants had hearing loss. Short-term therapy with streptomycin (1 g/day for 4.5 days) combined with ethacrynic acid resulted in complete hearing loss in both mother and infant.
Amiodarone	D	Complications reported include fetal hypothyroidism, low birth weight, prematurity, bradycardia, and QT prolongation. Because the drug contains 75 mg iodine per 200-mg dose, newborn thyroid status should be closely monitored.
Amitriptyline	D	Limb reduction defects reported, but analysis of 86 first-trimester exposures did not confirm association. Other defects observed in three infants include micrognathia, anomalous right mandible, left talipes equinovarus (1 case), swelling of hands/feet (1 case), and hypospadias (1 case). Urinary retention occurred in one newborn after nortriptyline use.
Angiotensin II-receptor antagonists	C/D[c]	Acts on the renin-angiotensin system; see ACE inhibitors.
Aspirin	C/D[f]	Risk of adverse fetal effects is low if low doses are used occasionally. No specific pattern of malformations has been identified. It has been used to prevent pregnancy-induced hypertension, pre-eclampsia, and eclampsia. Use of full-dose aspirin near term may prolong gestation and labor, adversely affect clotting ability of newborn by reducing collagen-induced platelet aggregation, and may increase risk in premature or low-birth-weight infants for intracranial hemorrhage.
Azathioprine	D	Teratogenic in animals. No specific pattern of malformation noted in humans. Examples of anomalies reported include hydrocephalus, anencephaly, cleft palate, atrial septal defect, and polydactyly. Fatal neonatal anemia, thrombocytopenia, and lymphopenia reported.
Benzodiazepines	D/X[d]	Congenital anomalies reported include cleft lip/palate, congenital heart disease, and defects of the CNS, lung, abdomen, GI tract, musculoskeletal system, and digits. Strength of association is controversial. Neonatal withdrawal has been reported.
β-Blockers	B/C/D[d]	Reduced birth weight may result from use of some β-blockers in second and third trimesters but effect also may be due to severe maternal disease. Use of acebutolol, atenolol, or nadolol near term has caused β-blockade in newborns.
Bismuth subsalicylate	C	Hydrolyzed in GI tract to bismuth salts and sodium salicylate, absorption of bismuth salts is negligible, but chronic exposure to salicylates may present fetal risk (see Aspirin). Restrict use to first half of pregnancy and do not exceed recommended doses.
Busulfan	D	Used in 38 pregnancies, 22 in first trimester resulting in six infants with defects: unspecified malformations (aborted at 20 wk); anomalous deviation left lobe liver, bilobular spleen, and pulmonary atelectasis; pyloric stenosis; cleft palate, microphthalmia, cytomegaly, hypoplasia of ovaries and thyroid gland, corneal opacity, and IUGR; myeloschisis, aborted at 6 wk; IUGR, left hydronephrosis and hydroureter, absent right kidney and ureter, and hepatic subcapsular calcifications.

Drug/Drug Class	Risk Factor[b]	Fetal/Neonatal Effects
Carbamazepine	D	May produce malformations similar to those seen with phenytoin. Risk may be increased almost threefold. Examples of anomalies reported include cardiac, urinary tract, and craniofacial defects, cleft palate, fingernail hypoplasia, and low birth weight. Slightly increased risk of NTD.
Chloramphenicol	C	Use with caution at term. Unconfirmed report of cardiovascular collapse (gray syndrome) in newborns exposed in final stage of pregnancy.
Codeine	C	Major and minor anomalies have been reported, but the frequencies in affected newborns were similar to control. Examples of anomalies include congenital heart disease, respiratory malformations, GU tract defects, umbilical and inguinal hernia, hydrocephaly, and pyloric stenosis. Some retrospective studies suggested a link between codeine and cleft lip/palate.
Corticosteroids	C/D[d]	Use of oral corticosteroids during the first trimester may be associated with a slightly increased risk of oral cleft. Topical (drug not specified) and inhalation (beclomethasone, budesonide) use do not appear to increase risk of malformations.
Diphenhydramine	B	Most studies did not show an increased risk of congenital anomalies with diphenhydramine versus control. One case-control study found possible association with cleft palate after first-trimester exposure.
Ephedrine	C	No evidence of teratogenicity based upon 873 exposures; ↑ in fetal heart rate and beat-to-beat variability have been observed.
Epinephrine	C	Statistically significant association found between 189 first trimester exposures and major or minor anomalies in one study. Association also found between use anytime in pregnancy and inguinal hernia. Data may reflect serious maternal conditions requiring use of drug. After 9,719 exposures, adrenergics as a group were associated with minor anomalies, inguinal hernia, and clubfoot. Adrenergics, including epinephrine, are teratogenic in some animal species.
Ergotamine	X/D[e]	Small, infrequent doses may not be teratogenic; large doses or frequent use may cause teratogenicity because of disruption of fetal blood supply; oxytocic properties of drug may cause dysfunctional labor marked by prolonged contractions resulting in fetal hypoxia. If possible, should be avoided in pregnancy.
Ethosuximide	C	An association between ethosuximide and congenital anomalies has not been established. Reports of defects include patent ductus arteriosus, cleft lip/palate, and hydrocephalus. Spontaneous hemorrhage reported in 1 neonate.
Fluconazole	C	Risk is unlikely increased when used as a single oral dose of #150 mg. Chronic use may be teratogenic. Case reports described anomalies with structural defects of the CNS, extremities, and cleft palate; features resembled a known recessive genetic disorder.
Fosphenytoin	D	This is a prodrug of phenytoin. After parenteral administration, fosphenytoin is converted to phenytoin. See phenytoin.
Hydroxyurea	D	Inhibits DNA synthesis and is considered a human carcinogen and mutagen. It is teratogenic/embryotoxic in animals. Human data are limited, but potential for risk is high.
Ibuprofen	B/D[f]	No evidence of teratogenicity with first trimester use, but experience limited. Use after 34–35 weeks' gestation may cause premature closure of ductus arteriosus resulting in PPHN. Naproxen use at 30 weeks' gestation associated with PPHN in three infants. (see NSAIDs)
Imipramine	D	Congenital anomalies described in case reports include bilateral amelia, polydactyly, omphalocele, defective abdominal muscles, diaphragmatic hernia, exencephaly, cleft palate, adrenal hypoplasia, and renal cystic degeneration. Early reports of limb reduction defects cannot be confirmed.

Drug/Drug Class	Risk Factor[b]	Fetal/Neonatal Effects
Indomethacin	B/D[f]	Used to treat premature labor; oliguric renal failure, hemorrhage, and intestinal perforation have been reported in some premature infants exposed just before delivery. Reduced fetal urine output may be therapeutic in cases of polyhydramnios. May cause constriction of the fetal ductus arteriosus, with or without tricuspid regurgitation. (see NSAIDs)
Lithium	D	Case reports and cohort studies showed that lithium exposure in the first trimester can increase risk of Ebstein's anomaly (absolute risk of 0.05–0.1%), a rare congenital heart defect occurring in 1/20,000 live births. Incidence of other CV defects range from 0.9 to 12%. Other anomalies reported include cyanosis, rhythm disturbances, thyroid dysfunction, hypoglycemia, lethargy, hyperbilirubinemia. Use near term may cause "floppy baby syndrome" in infants with lithium toxicity.
Marijuana	C	Maternal use may be associated with fetal growth retardation, but other factors such as multiple drug use, lifestyles, diseases, socioeconomic status, and nutrition may play significant role. One report has associated in utero exposure to marijuana to the development of acute nonlymphoblastic leukemia in childhood. Contraindicated if used as drug of abuse.
Mercaptopurine (6-MP)	D	6-MP has teratogenic/mutagenic potential. Adverse outcomes reported include microphthalmia, corneal opacity, hypoplasia of ovaries and thyroid, cytomegaly, cleft palate, hypospadias, polydactyly, neonatal anemia and pancytopenia. Results complicated by polytherapy.
Methimazole (MMI)	D	First-trimester exposure may be associated with a small increased risk of aplasia cutis congenita (congenital scalp defect). A pattern of anomalies (MMI embryopathy) has been proposed consisting of choanal atresia, esophageal atresia with tracheo-esophageal fistula, facial and skin dysmorphology, hypoplastic nipples, psychomotor delay, and growth restriction. Hypothyroidism and goiter have been reported in neonates exposed in utero.
Methyldopa	C	No known association with congenital defects. Frequently used for treatment of pregnancy-induced hypertension. A decrease in intracranial volume after first trimester use has been reported but no relationship between small head size and retarded mental development at 4 years of age.
Methylene blue	D	Intra-amniotic injection has caused hemolytic anemia, hyperbilirubinemia, methemoglobinemia, and possibly small bowel obstructions.
Metronidazole	B	Drug is mutagenic in bacteria and carcinogenic in rodents. Vaginal use does not appear to increase risk of teratogenicity. Risk with systemic use is controversial. Oral cleft has been reported.
Nicotine Nicotine polacrilex	C/D[d]	Smoking during pregnancy can cause fetal growth retardation, increased risk of spontaneous abortion, and perinatal mortality. Use of nicotine replacement in the third trimester has been associated with decreased fetal breathing. Spontaneous abortion has been reported.
Nitrofurantoin	B	Apparently safe but use with caution at term because of theoretic potential for hemolytic anemia in newborn.
NSAIDs	B/D[d,f] or C/D[d,f]	Epidemiologic studies of NSAID use as a class found conflicting data. In a study of 2,557 first-trimester exposures to NSAIDs, a slightly increased risk for cardiac defects and oral cleft was noted. Another study of 1,462 women exposed anytime during pregnancy did not show an increased risk for abnormalities, LBW, or preterm birth. Rate of miscarriage may be increased when NSAID is used weeks before the miscarriage. Risk assessment requires further studies. (see ibuprofen, indomethacin)
Penicillamine	D	Use in pregnancy is associated with connective tissue defects (cutis laxa). Examples of other anomalies reported are pyloric stenosis, inguinal hernia, hyperflexion of hips and shoulders, and low-set ears.

Drug/Drug Class	Risk Factor[b]	Fetal/Neonatal Effects
Phenobarbital	D	May produce malformations similar to those seen with phenytoin when used in epileptic patients. May cause early HDN. Also may cause fetal/newborn addiction.
Phenylephrine	C	Anomalies were reported in studies involving >5,000 exposures, but significance of association is undetermined. Fetal hypoxia is possible. Avoid use with other pressor agents. (see epinephrine)
Progesterone and related compounds	D/X[d]	In 1977, the FDA restricted use in pregnancy based on reports of cardiac malformations, CNS defects, masculinization of female fetuses, and limb defects. Re-evaluations of some of these data and new, well-designed studies have failed to show an association between these defects and progesterones. Progesterone is used frequently to prevent imminent abortion during the first trimester. Use of hydroxyprogesterone or medroxyprogesterone during early pregnancy may have been associated with esophageal atresia but the absolute risk was low (about 6/10,000 exposed lived births).
Propylthiouracil (PTU)	D	Drug of choice for treatment of hyperthyroidism during pregnancy; anomalies reported in seven infants after in utero exposure, but no association between PTU and defects suggested. May produce mild hypothyroidism in fetus when used close to term, evident as a goiter and elevated levels of neonatal TSH. Goiters in two infants sufficiently massive to cause death in one infant and respiratory distress in the other.
Quinolones	C	Erosions of cartilage and arthropathy have been reported in immature animals, but effects in human are unknown. A cohort study of 57 women exposed to fluoroquinolones during pregnancy did not find an increased risk of congenital anomalies versus 17,259 control patients. Avoid use if safer alternatives are available.
Rifampin	C	Although not a proven teratogen, one report observed nine defects in 204 pregnancies: anencephaly (1 case), hydrocephalus (2 cases), limb malformations (4 cases), renal tract defect (1 case), and congenital hip dislocation (1 case). HDN observed in 3 infants; prophylactic vitamin K recommended.
SSRIs	C	Most data available are for fluoxetine. First-trimester exposure to fluoxetine does not appear to increase risk of major malformations. One study suggests that minor anomalies may be increased, but this remains to be confirmed. Other SSRIs (sertaline, paroxetine, fluvoxamine, citalopram) do not appear to increase risk of major anomalies. Withdrawal symptoms in neonates have been reported. Safety requires further investigation.
Sulfonylureas, oral	C	Use near term may result in prolonged hypoglycemia. Not recommended in pregnancy because it will not provide better control than diet alone. Insulin is the treatment of choice during pregnancy.
Tetracyclines	D	Use after fifth month of gestation will result in permanent yellow-brown staining of teeth. Inhibition of fibula growth may occur in premature infants. Based on 1,944 pregnancy exposures, possible associations with congenital anomalies found in 61 infants: hypospadias (5 cases), inguinal hernia (47 cases), limb hypoplasia (6 cases), and clubfoot (3 cases).
Thiazides and related diuretics	C/D[d]	They are unlikely to be teratogenic. Other adverse outcomes reported include: neonatal thrombocytopenia in 11 newborns (with 2 deaths) following use near term of chlorothiazide, HCTZ, and methyclothiazide; hemolytic anemia in two neonates after chlorothiazide and bendroflumethiazide; fetal electrolyte disturbances when exposed during third trimester. May decrease placental perfusion.
Trimethadione	D	Phenotype exists for fetal trimethadione syndrome. Use in nine families (36 pregnancies) resulted in 25 infants with wide spectrum of defects. Not recommended in pregnancy.
Trimethoprim (TMP)	C	TMP is a dihydrofolate reductase inhibitor. Exposure during first and second month of pregnancy may ↑ NTD; exposure during second and third month may ↑ cardiovascular defects and oral cleft.

Drug/Drug Class	Risk Factor[b]	Fetal/Neonatal Effects
Valproic acid	D	Risk for NTDs is 1 to 2% (exposure must occur between the seventeenth and thirtieth day after fertilization). A valproic acid syndrome has been suggested to consist of anomalies involving the following: NTDs, craniofacial, digits, and urogenital. Retarded psychomotor development and low birth weight also have been observed.
Warfarin	X/D[e]	Teratogenic

[a] This list is not all-inclusive. Selected drugs are listed by drug class and not by individual names.

[b] Risk factors listed for most drugs are according to the manufacturers' ratings based on FDA definitions. When this is not available, the risk factor indicated is from Briggs, et al. *Drugs in Pregnancy and Lactation: A reference guide to fetal and neonatal risk*, 5e. Baltimore: Williams & Wilkins, 1998.

[c] Rated risk factor C in first trimester, D in second and third trimesters.

[d] Drugs within the same class may have different pregnancy category ratings.

[e] Rated risk factor X by manufacturer, rated D in reference Briggs, et al. *Drugs in Pregnancy and Lactation: A reference guide to fetal and neonatal risk*, 5e. Baltimore: Williams & Wilkins, 1998.

[f] Rated risk factor D in third trimester or near delivery.

ACEI, angiotensin-converting enzyme inhibitor; CNS, central nervous system; CV, cardiovascular; ECG, electrocardiogram; FDA, Food and Drug Administration; GI, gastrointestinal; GU, genitourinary; HDN, hemolytic disease of the newborn; IUGR, intrauterine growth retardation; NSAIDs, nonsteroidal anti-inflammatory drugs; NTDs, neural tube defects; PPHN, persistent pulmonary hypertension of the newborn; SSRIs, selective serotonin reuptake inhibitors; TSH, thyroid-stimulating hormone.

From Koda-Kimble MA, et al. *Handbook of Applied Therapeutics,* 8th ed. Baltimore: Lippincott Williams & Wilkins, 2006.

Drugs Considered Contraindicated During Pregnancy[a]

Drug/Drug Class	Fetal/Neonatal Effects
Acitretin	Acitretin is the active metabolite of etretinate. Use of ethanol with acitretin results in conversion of acitretin back to etretinate. See etretinate.
Aminopterin	Aminopterin is a folic acid antagonist similar to MTX. See MTX.
Chenodiol	Contraindicated because of potential for hepatotoxicity.
Clomiphene	Used to induce ovulation. Neural tube defects and other anomalies have been reported, but most studies indicate no association with malformations. Inadvertent use in early pregnancy may have resulted in one infant with a ruptured lumbosacral meningomyelocele, and one infant with esophageal atresia with fistula, congenital heart defect, hypospadias, and absent left kidney.
Cocaine	Maternal cocaine abuse associated with in utero cerebrovascular accidents, bowel atresias, and congenital defects of the GU tract, heart, limbs, and face. Other fetal and newborn consequences of maternal abuse are fetal growth retardation, and ↑ morbidity and mortality, including a possible association with SIDS. Maternal complications include shorter gestations, premature delivery, spontaneous abortions, abruptio placentae, and death.
Danazol	Use after the eighth week of gestation (the onset of androgen receptor sensitivity) may result in masculinization of the female fetus (i.e., pseudohermaphroditism); male fetuses usually not affected but one male had multiple anomalies after first trimester exposure.
Diethylstilbestrol (DES)	An estimated 6 million pregnant women were exposed to DES from 1940–1971 to treat obstetric problems. Exposure resulted in reproductive system defects in both female and male offspring. Female: Lower Müllerian tract: vaginal adenosis; cervical/vaginal fornix defects; cockscomb, collar, pseudopolyp, and hypoplastic cervix; vaginal defects exclusive of fornix; incomplete transverse and/or longitudinal septum. Upper Müllerian tract: uterine structural defects; fallopian tube structural defects Male: Altered semen (↓ count, concentration, motility, morphology); epididymal cysts; hypotrophic testis; microphallus; varicocele; capsular induration DES exposure increases risk of developing vaginal and cervical clear cell adenocarcinoma. DES exposure has not been related to defects other than those found in the reproductive system.
Estrogen and related compounds	Contraindicated in pregnancy. A study found an association between estrogen exposure and cardiovascular defects, eye and ear anomalies, and Down syndrome. Further analysis of these data failed to support the association with cardiac malformations. Other studies have also failed in finding association with congenital defects.
Ethanol	Heavy consumption during pregnancy associated with IUGR and a pattern of anomalies known as the "fetal alcohol syndrome." No known safe levels in pregnancy. Potent fetal brain toxin.
Etretinate	Teratogenic effects reported include meningomyelocele, meningoncephalocele, multiple synostoses, facial dysmorphia, syndactylies, absence of terminal phalanges, malformation of hip, ankle and forearm, low-set ears, high palate, decreased cranial volume, and alterations of the skull and cervical vertebrae. Teratogenic potential can persist for years because of a long half-life of 100 days after prolonged use.
HMG-CoA reductase inhibitors	One case of first trimester exposure to lovastatin with subsequent birth of an infant with constellation of malformations termed the VATER association (vertebral anomalies, anal atresia, tracheoesophageal fistula with esophageal atresia, and renal and radial dysplasias). An interim evaluation of lovastatin and simvastatin exposure during pregnancy in post-marketing surveillance failed to demonstrate an increased risk of fetal anomalies. A theoretic concern is that the interference of cholesterol biosynthesis by HMG-CoA reductase inhibitors may adversely impact sex steroid biosynthesis.
Isotretinoin	Defects can occur with any doses and for short durations of use. Reports include defects of the skull, ear, eye, face, CNS, thymus, and cardiovasculature; cleft palate; limb reductions; low IQ scores.

Drug/Drug Class	Fetal/Neonatal Effects
Leflunomide	It is teratogenic/embryotoxic in animals. Effects may be dose-related. Because of its long half-life of about 14–18 days, women of childbearing potential discontinued from this drug should undergo the drug elimination procedure using cholestyramine as recommended by the manufacturer.
Leuprolide	Teratogenic in animals; no adverse fetal effects in over 100 cases of human exposure; spontaneous abortions and IUGR may occur because drug suppresses endometrial proliferation.
Lysergic acid diethylamide (LSD)	Pure chemical does not cause chromosomal abnormalities, spontaneous abortions, or congenital anomalies. Reported adverse fetal effects in maternal abusers probably caused by multiple factors, including reporting bias.
Menadione	Use near term or close to delivery has resulted in marked hyperbilirubinemia and kernicterus in newborn. If vitamin K needed during pregnancy, use phytonadione (K_1).
Methotrexate (MTX)	MTX is a folic acid antagonist with abortifacient property. Exposure in first trimester may cause malformations that are dose-related. Anomalies reported include cranial (e.g., oxycephaly, absence of lambdoid and coronal suture), ocular (e.g., ocular hypertelorism), and skeletal defects.
Methyl mercury	Organic mercury poisoning has occurred primarily in Japan and Iraq. Known as Minamata disease in Japan. Nonspecific neurologic symptoms after third trimester exposure were observed in about 72 known cases.
Mifepristone (RU-486)	Antiprogesterone agent used to induce abortion; teratogenic potential has not been determined.
Misoprostol	Has abortifacient properties; teratogenic potential has not been determined.
Phencyclidine	Persistent irritability, jitteriness, hypertonicity, and poor feeding reported in newborns.
Ribavirin	Teratogenic and/or embryotoxic in nearly all animal species tested. Teratogenic risk in humans has not been determined. Pregnant health care workers or those trying to conceive should avoid or use caution when caring for these patients.
Sodium iodide(^{125}I) and (^{131}I)	Administration at 12 weeks' gestation or later will cause partial or complete destruction of fetal thyroid gland; effect is dose dependent with toxic doses 10 mCi.
Thalidomide	Over 7,000 birth defects have been linked to thalidomide use during pregnancy. The most susceptible period is from days 34–50 after the first day of the last menstrual period. Thalidomide embryopathy does not appear to be dose-related. Limb reduction and ear defects are common. Malformations include amelia, phocomelia, bone hypoplasticity, absence of bones, anotia, micro pinna, auditory canal defects, facial palsy, anophthalmos, microphthalmos, congenital heart defects, and GI tract and genital abnormalities.
Vaccines, live	Most live, attenuated virus vaccines potentially can cause fetal infection. Vaccination with smallpox in first and second trimesters has resulted in fetal death.
Vitamin A (high dose)	Both deficiency and excess are thought to be teratogenic. Prolonged high dosages (>25,000 IU/day) associated with: microtia, craniofacial and CNS anomalies, facial palsy, microphthalmia/anophthalmia, facial clefts, cardiac defects, limb reductions, GI atresia, and urinary tract defects.

[a] This list is not all-inclusive. Most drugs listed have been designated FDA risk factor X. All drugs of abuse are contraindicated in pregnancy. CDC, Centers for Disease Control and Prevention; CNS, central nervous system; GI, gastrointestinal; GU, genitourinary; HMG CoA, hydroxy-methyl-glutaryl-CoA; IUGR, intrauterine growth retardation; MTX, methotrexate; SIDS, sudden infant death syndrome.

From Koda-Kimble MA, et al. *Handbook of Applied Therapeutics,* 8th ed. Baltimore: Lippincott Williams & Wilkins, 2006.

Formulas for Computing Drug Dosages

Drugs are sometimes prepared and supplied in the amount ordered by the physician, and the nurse can see when checking the medication label that no calculation is necessary. At other times, drugs are not prepared and supplied in the exact quantities called for in the medication order, and the nurse must do a dosage calculation to determine what quantity of medication the patient is to receive.

Several formulas can be used to calculate drug dosages. One consists of ratios to set up a proportion and can be used to calculate dosages for both solid and liquid preparations. A ratio shows a relationship between numbers. A proportion contains two ratios. The nurse is usually seeking the quantity of on-hand medication that is equal to the desired dosage (i.e., the dosage ordered). The formula is:

$$\frac{\text{dose on hand}}{\text{quantity on hand}} = \frac{\text{dose desired}}{\text{X (quantity desired)}}$$

The dosage must be in the same unit of measurement. This applies to the quantity as well. Dosages are on the top line of the proportion, and quantities are on the bottom line. After the numbers are placed in the proportion, the nurse cross-multiplies to find the desired quantity.

Example: Amoxicillin, 625 mg PO, is ordered. It is supplied as a liquid preparation containing 250 mg in 5 mL. How much does the nurse administer?

$$\frac{250\text{ mg}}{5\text{ mL}} = \frac{625\text{ mg}}{\text{X mL}}$$

cross-multiply:

$$3125 = 250X$$
$$\text{X} = 12.5\text{ mL}$$

Example: Phenobarbital, gr i PO, is ordered. It is available in 30-mg tablets. How many tablets does the nurse administer?

There are two systems of measurement in this problem. The nurse checks the list of equivalents to learn that 60 mg is equivalent to grains i.

$$\frac{30\text{ mg}}{1\text{ tablet}} = \frac{60\text{ mg}}{\text{X tablets}}$$

$$60 = 30X$$
$$X = 2\text{ tablets}$$

Another formula that can be used to calculate drug dosages is:

$$\frac{\text{dose desired}}{\text{dose on hand}} \times \text{quantity on hand} = \text{desired quantity}$$

This formula can be used for both liquid dosages and fractions of tablets.

A newer way to solve medication dosages is dimensional analysis (Curren & Munday. *Dimensional analysis for meds,* 2nd ed. 2001). When using dimensional analysis, the first numerator must be what you are solving for. For instance, in the amoxicillin example, you would set up the equation like this:

mL = (5 ML/250 mg) × 625 mg = 12.5 mL

Dimensional analysis can also encompass conversion factors all in the same formula. For instance, the nurse is to administer 50 mcg fentanyl 0.1 mg/2 mL. How much should the nurse administer? This can all be done in the same calculation.

mL = (2 mL/0.1 mg) × (1 mg/1,000 mcg) × 50 mcg = 1 mL

Pediatric Calculations

Pediatric dosages are calculated according to the child's weight or *body surface area* (BSA).

The *BSA formula* provides the highest accuracy in calculating pediatric dosages because it considers weight and height. To find a child's BSA, the nomogram is used. The child's height is located at a point in the left-hand column, and the weight is located at a point in the right-hand column. The two points are connected with a straight line. The point at which the line crosses the surface area column is thc child's BSA. The formula for calculating the child's dosage is as follows:

$$\frac{\text{BSA (child)}}{\text{BSA (adult)}} \times \text{adult dose} = \text{child's dose}$$

The average adult BSA is 1.7 square meters.

A less commonly used formula is *Clark's rule* for children aged 2 years or younger. This formula assumes that the average adult weighs 150 lb (68 kg) and is calculated as follows:

$$\text{usual adult dose} \times \frac{\text{weight of child in pounds}}{150} = \text{child's dose}$$

Accepted pediatric dosages according to milligram per kilogram weight per 24 hours for many drugs are listed in medication references.

Adapted from Taylor C, et al. *Fundamentals of Nursing: The Art and Science of Nursing Care*, 6e. Philadelphia: Lippincott Williams & Wilkins, 2008.

Regulating IV Flow Rate

Follow agency's guidelines to determine if infusion should be administered by electronic pump or by gravity.

- Check physician's order for IV solution.
- Check patency of IV line and needle.
- Verify drop factor (number of drops [gtt] in 1 mL) of the equipment in use.
- Calculate the flow rate:

a. *Standard formula*

$$\text{gtt/min} = \frac{\text{volume (mL)} \times \text{drop factor (gtt/mL)}}{\text{time (in minutes)}}$$

EXAMPLE—Administer 1000 mL D_5W over 10 hours (set delivers 60 gtt/1 mL).

$$\text{gtt/min} = \frac{1000 \text{ mL} \times 60}{600 \text{ (60 min} \times \text{10 h)}}$$

$$= \frac{60{,}000}{600}$$

$$= 100 \text{ gtt/min}$$

b. *Short formula using milliliters per hour*

$$\text{gtt/min} = \frac{\text{milliliters per hour} \times \text{drop factor (gtt/mL)}}{\text{time (60 min)}}$$

EXAMPLE—Administer 1000 mL D_5W over 10 hours (set delivers 60 gtt/1 mL).

Find milliliters per hour by dividing 1000 mL by 10 hours:

$$= \frac{1000}{10} = 100 \text{ mL/hr}$$

$$\text{gtt/min} = \frac{100 \text{ mL} \times 60}{60 \text{ min}}$$

$$= \frac{6000}{600}$$

$$= 100 \text{ gtt/min}$$

- Count drops per minute in drip chamber (number of gtt/15-sec interval × 4 = gtt/min). Hold watch beside drip chamber.
- Adjust IV clamp as needed and recount drops per minute.
- Mark IV container according to agency policy and manufacturer's recommendations. Use a time tape or label to measure amount to be infused at timed intervals.
- Monitor IV flow rate at frequent intervals. Document patient's response to infusion at prescribed rate.

Adapted from Taylor C, et al. *Fundamentals of Nursing: The Art & Science of Nursing Care*, 6e. Philadelphia: Lippincott Williams & Wilkins, 2008.

Common Types of Drug Preparations

Preparation	Description
Capsule	Powder or gel form of an active drug enclosed in a gelatinous container
Elixir	Medication in a clear liquid containing water, alcohol, sweeteners, and flavor
Extended release	Preparation of a medication that allows for slow and continuous release over a predetermined period; may also be referred to as controlled release (CR), sustained or slow release (SR), sustained action (SA), long acting (LA), or timed release (TR).
Liniment	Medication mixed with alcohol, oil, or soap, which is rubbed on the skin
Lotion	Drug particles in a solution for topical use
Lozenge	Small oval, round, or oblong preparation containing a drug in a flavored or sweetened base, which dissolves in the mouth and releases the medication; also called *troche*
Ointment	Semisolid preparation containing a drug to be applied externally; also called an *unction*
Pill	Mixture of a powdered drug with a cohesive material; may be round or oval
Powder	Single or mixture of finely ground drugs
Solution	A drug dissolved in another substance (e.g., an aqueous solution)
Suppository	A medication preparation in a firm base (e.g., gelatin) that is inserted into the body (rectum, vagina, urethra)
Suspension	Finely divided, undissolved particles in a liquid medium; to be shaken before use
Syrup	Medication combined in a water and sugar solution
Tablet	Small, solid dose of medication, compressed or molded; may be any color, size, or shape; *erteric-coated* tablets are coated with a substance that is insoluble in gastric acids to reduce gastric irritation caused by the drug
Transdermal patch	Unit dose of medication applied directly to skin for diffusion through skin and absorption into the bloodstream

Adapted from Taylor C, et al. Lippincott's Photo Atlas of Medical Administration. Baltimore: Lippincott Williams & Wilkins, 2004.

Routes for Administering Drugs

Terms Used to Describe Route	How Drug Is Administered
Oral	Having patient swallow drug
Enteral route	Administering drug through an enteral tube
Sublingual administration	Placing drug under tongue
Buccal administration	Placing drug between cheek and gum
Parenteral	Injecting drug into
Subcutaneous injection	Subcutaneous tissue
Intramuscular injection	Muscle tissue
Intradermal injection	Corium (under epidermis)
Intravenous injection	Vein
Intraarterial injection	Artery
Intracardial injection	Heart tissue
Intraperitoneal injection	Peritoneal cavity
Intraspinal injection	Spinal canal
Intraosseous injection	Bone
Topical	Inserting drug into
Vaginal administration	Vagina
Rectal administration	Rectum
Inunction	Rubbing drug into skin
Instillation	Placing drug into direct contact with mucous membrane
Irrigation	Flushing mucous membrane with drug in solution
Skin application	Applying transdermal patch
Pulmonary	Having patient inhale drug

Adapted from Taylor C, et al. Lippincott's Photo Atlas of Medical Administration. Baltimore: Lippincott Williams & Wilkins, 2004.

Assessment Guide: Medications

Factors to Assess	Questions and Approaches
Previous and current drug use	Which medications are you taking that the doctor prescribed for you? What over-the-counter medications are you taking on a regular basis? Do you use nonmedicinal drugs (e.g., alcohol, caffeine, herbal supplements, home remedies)? How often do you use them? What is the reason for taking the medication? What medications have you taken during the past year and for what reasons? Is there anything else you have tried to alleviate your symptoms?
Medication schedule	At what times do you take your medications? Is there any special way your medication has to be prepared (e.g., crushing and mixing with applesauce)? Do you have any special method for remembering to take your medications?
Response to medications	Have the medications had the expected effects? Have you ever experienced any adverse or unexpected reactions to the medications? Is there a family history of this type of reaction to medication? Do you have any allergies to medications? What happens when you take this medication?
Attitude toward drugs and use of drugs	How do you feel about taking medications? Why do you take the medications?
Compliance with regimen	Can you tell me your understanding of the reason for taking the medications? Can you describe how you follow the medication schedule? Are there any problems that prevent you from following the medication regimen?
Storage	Where are your medications stored at home? How long do you keep medications in the home? Can you show me any medications you have on hand?

Adapted from Taylor C, et al. Lippincott's Photo Atlas of Medical Administration. Baltimore: Lippincott Williams & Wilkins, 2004.

International Dietary Guidelines

UNITED STATES

Dietary Guidelines for Americans

The Dietary Guidelines, developed by the Department of Health and Human Services and the U.S. Department of Agriculture, represent the best, most current advice for healthy Americans 2 years and older. They reflect recommendations of health and nutrition experts, who agree that enough is known about the effect of diet on health to encourage certain eating practices. The seven Dietary Guidelines are:

- Eat a variety of foods to get the energy (calories), protein, vitamins, minerals, and fiber you need for good health.
- Maintain a healthy weight to reduce your chances of having high blood pressure, heart disease, a stroke, certain cancers, and the most common kind of diabetes.
- Choose a diet low in fat, saturated fat, and cholesterol to reduce your risk of heart disease and certain types of cancer. Because fat contains more than twice the calories of an equal amount of carbohydrates or protein, a diet low in fat can help you maintain a healthy weight.
- Choose a diet with plenty of vegetables, fruits, and grain products that provide needed vitamins, minerals, fiber, and complex carbohydrates. They are generally lower in fat.
- Use sugars only in moderation. A diet with lots of sugars has too many calories and too few nutrients for most people and can contribute to tooth decay.
- Use salt and other forms of sodium only in moderation to help reduce your risk of high blood pressure.
- If you drink alcoholic beverages, do so in moderation. Alcoholic beverages supply calories, but little or no nutrients. Drinking alcohol is also the cause of many health problems and accidents and can lead to addiction.

www.fda.gov/fdac/special/foodlabel/pyramid.html#dietary

CANADA

In 2007 Health Canada released ***Eating Well with Canada's Food Guide,*** a new version of its food guide created to replace the 1992 guide, ***Canada's Food Guide to Healthy Eating***.

Eating Well with Canada's Food Guide–First Nations, Inuit and Métis, also released in 2007, is a complement to the new version of ***Canada's Food Guide***. This tailored food guide takes into account the unique values, traditions, and food choices of Canada's Aboriginal peoples, and explains how traditional foods can be used in combination with store-bought foods for a healthy eating pattern.

Key Recommendations

- Both eating well and being active are essential to a healthy lifestyle.
- Follow Canada's Food Guide by eating the recommended amount and type of food each day.
- Eat at least one dark green and one orange vegetable each day.
- Choose vegetables and fruit prepared with little or no added fat, sugar or salt.
- Have vegetables and fruit more often than juice.
- Make at least half of your grain products whole grain each day.
- Choose grain products that are lower in fat, sugar or salt.
- Drink skim, 1% or 2% milk each day.
- Select lower fat milk alternatives.
- Have meat alternatives such as beans, lentils and tofu often.
- Eat at least two Food Guide Servings of fish each week.
- Select lean meat and alternatives prepared with little or no added fat or salt.

- Include a small amount—30 to 45 mL (2 to 3 tablespoons)—of unsaturated fat each day. This includes oil used for cooking, salad dressings, margarine and mayonnaise. This will ensure people have enough essential fats. Consuming a larger amount of added fat is not recommended, as it will increase the total calories in the diet.
- Drink water regularly. It is a calorie-free way to satisfy your thirst.
- Limit foods and beverages high in calories, fat, sugar or salt (sodium).
- Follow Canada's Physical Activity Guide recommendations to be active every day and inactive less often. Adults should build 30 to 60 minutes of moderate physical activity, such as walking briskly, into each day. Children and youth need at least 90 minutes of activity every day.

Advice for different ages and stages

- Young children need small nutritious meals and snacks each day.
- For young children, nutritious foods that contain fat should not be restricted.
- Women who could become pregnant, as well as those who are pregnant or breastfeeding, need a daily multivitamin containing folic acid.
- Pregnant women need a multivitamin that contains iron.
- Pregnant and breastfeeding women need more calories.
- Men and women over the age of 50 need a daily vitamin D supplement.

Vegetarians

The healthy eating pattern and guidance of Canada's Food Guide are suitable for vegetarians. To ensure adequate nutrient intakes of iron, zinc and vitamin B12, vegetarians can choose a variety of meat alternatives such as beans, lentils, eggs, tofu, soy-based meat substitutes, nuts, nut butters and seeds. Milk and fortified soy beverages also provide calcium, vitamin B12, vitamin D and protein.

Eating Well with Canada's Food Guide—http://www.hc-sc.gc.ca/fn-an/food-guide-aliment/index_e.html
Eating Well with Canada's Food Guide–First Nations, Inuit and Métis—
http://www.hc-sc.gc.ca/fn-an/pubs/fnim-pnim/index_e.html

AUSTRALIA

Eat Well Australia 2000-2010 (EWA)

The strategy focuses on 4 key nutrition priority areas:

- prevention of overweight and obesity;
- increasing the consumption of vegetables and fruit;
- promotion of optimal nutrition for women, infants and children; and
- improving nutrition for vulnerable groups.

A number of capacity-building initiatives are also included:

- strategic management;
- research and development;
- communication;
- monitoring and evaluation; and
- workforce development.

National Aboriginal and Torres Strait Islander Nutrition Strategy and Action Plan 2000-2010 (NATSINSAP) provides a framework for action to improve Aboriginal and Torres Strait Islander health and well-being through better nutrition and was developed concurrently with the national strategic framework, Eat Well Australia.

NATSINSAP highlights seven key areas for action including:

- food supply in remote and rural communities;
- food security and socioeconomic status;
- family focused nutrition promotion: resourcing programs, disseminating and communicating 'good practice';
- nutrition issues in urban areas;
- the environment and household infrastructure;
- Aboriginal and Torres Strait Islander nutrition workforce; and
- national food and nutrition information systems.

Both EWA and NATSINSAP have been developed through comprehensive consultations with stakeholders right across the food and nutrition field. Both aim to achieve a high level of ownership and support throughout the Australian food and nutrition system. Responsibility for progression of proposed nutrition initiatives within the strategy is shared across government and all stakeholders within the food and nutrition system.

Dietary Guidelines for Australian Adults

- Encourage and support breastfeeding.
- Care for your food: prepare and store it safely.
- Prevent weight gain: be physically active and eat according to your energy needs.
- Eat plenty of vegetables, legumes and fruits.
- Eat plenty of cereals (including breads, rice, pasta and noodles), preferably wholegrain.
- Include lean meat, fish, poultry and/or alternatives.
- Include milks, yoghurts, cheeses and/or alternatives, reduced-fat varieties should be chosen where possible.
- Drink plenty of water.
- Limit saturated fat and moderate total fat intake.
- Choose foods low in salt.
- Limit your alcohol intake if you choose to drink.
- Consume only moderate amounts of sugars and foods containing added sugars.
- Enjoy a wide variety of nutritious foods.

For complete details—http://www.nhmrc.gov.au/publications/synopses/dietsyn.htm
Eat Well Australia—http://www.nphp.gov.au/publications/signal/eatwell1.pdf
National Aboriginal and Torres Strait Islander Nutrition Strategy and Action Plan: a summary, 2000–2010—http://www.nphp.gov.au/publications/signal/natsinsa2.pdf

MyPyramid Food Guide: Steps to a Healthier You

The U.S. Department of Agriculture (USDA) released the MyPyramid food guidance system to help Americans make healthy food choices and to be active every day. One size doesn't fit all—MyPyramid Plan (available at www.mypyramid.gov) offers you a personal eating plan with the foods and amounts that are right for you. MyPyramid food patterns are designed for the general public ages 2 and over.

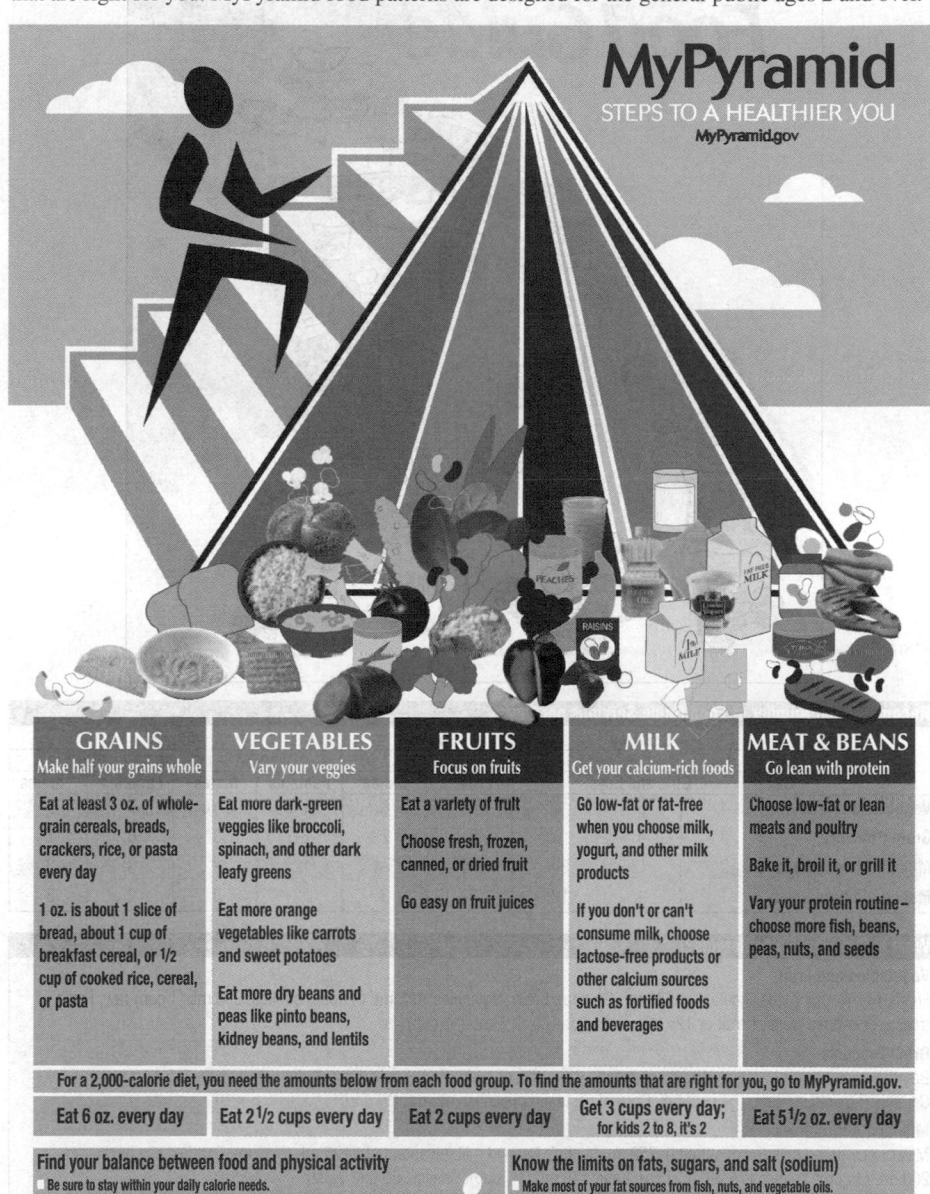

GRAINS Make half your grains whole	VEGETABLES Vary your veggies	FRUITS Focus on fruits	MILK Get your calcium-rich foods	MEAT & BEANS Go lean with protein
Eat at least 3 oz. of whole-grain cereals, breads, crackers, rice, or pasta every day 1 oz. is about 1 slice of bread, about 1 cup of breakfast cereal, or 1/2 cup of cooked rice, cereal, or pasta	Eat more dark-green veggies like broccoli, spinach, and other dark leafy greens Eat more orange vegetables like carrots and sweet potatoes Eat more dry beans and peas like pinto beans, kidney beans, and lentils	Eat a variety of fruit Choose fresh, frozen, canned, or dried fruit Go easy on fruit juices	Go low-fat or fat-free when you choose milk, yogurt, and other milk products If you don't or can't consume milk, choose lactose-free products or other calcium sources such as fortified foods and beverages	Choose low-fat or lean meats and poultry Bake it, broil it, or grill it Vary your protein routine–choose more fish, beans, peas, nuts, and seeds
For a 2,000-calorie diet, you need the amounts below from each food group. To find the amounts that are right for you, go to MyPyramid.gov.				
Eat 6 oz. every day	Eat 2 1/2 cups every day	Eat 2 cups every day	Get 3 cups every day; for kids 2 to 8, it's 2	Eat 5 1/2 oz. every day

Find your balance between food and physical activity

- Be sure to stay within your daily calorie needs.
- Be physically active for at least 30 minutes most days of the week.
- About 60 minutes a day of physical activity may be needed to prevent weight gain.
- For sustaining weight loss, at least 60 to 90 minutes a day of physical activity may be required.
- Children and teenagers should be physically active for 60 minutes every day, or most days.

Know the limits on fats, sugars, and salt (sodium)

- Make most of your fat sources from fish, nuts, and vegetable oils.
- Limit solid fats like butter, margarine, shortening, and lard, as well as foods that contain these.
- Check the Nutrition Facts label to keep saturated fats, *trans* fats, and sodium low.
- Choose food and beverages low in added sugars. Added sugars contribute calories with few, if any, nutrients.

Source: The Center for Nutrition Policy and Promotion, U.S. Department of Agriculture

Eating Well with Canada's Food Guide

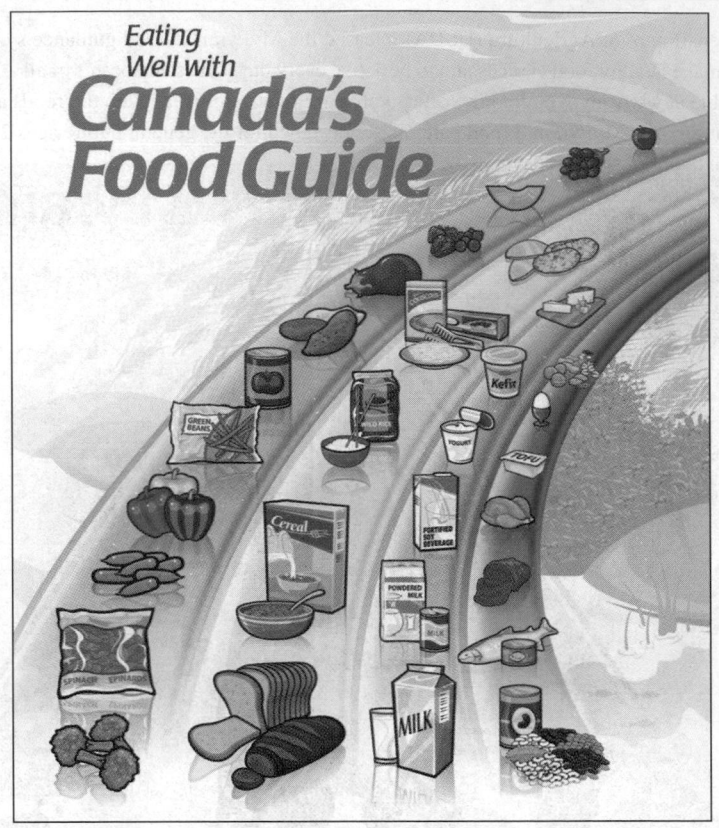

Recommended Number of Food Guide Servings per Day									
	Children			Teens		Adults			
Age in Years	2-3	4-8	9-13	14-18		19-50		50+	
Sex	Girls and Boys			Females	Males	Females	Males	Females	Males
Vegetables and Fruit	4	5	6	7	8	7-8	8-10	7	7
Grain Products	3	4	6	6	7	6-7	8	6	7
Milk and Alternatives	2	2	3-4	3-4	3-4	2	2	3	3
Meat and Alternatives	1	1	1-2	2	3	2	3	2	3

What is One Food Guide Serving?

Vegetables and Fruit

Fresh, frozen, or canned vegetables: 125 mL (1/2 cup); Leafy vegetables: 125 mL (1/2 cup) cooked, 250 mL (1 cup) raw; Fresh, frozen, or canned fruits: 1 fruit or 125 mL (1/2 cup); Juice: 125 mL (1/2 cup)

Grain Products

Bread: 1 slice (35 g); 1/2 bagel (45 g); Flat breads: 1/2 tortilla or pita (35 g); Cooked rice, bulgur, or quinoa: 125 mL (1/2 cup); Cereal: 30 g cold, 175 mL (3/4 cup) hot; Cooked pasta or couscous: 125 mL (1/2 cup)

Milk and Alternatives

Milk or powdered milk (reconstituted): 250 mL (1 cup); Canned milk (evaporated): 125 mL (1/2 cup); Fortified soy beverage: 250 mL (1 cup); Yogurt: 175 mL (3/4 cup); Kefir: 175 mL (3/4 cup); Cheese: 50 g (1 1/2 oz)

Meat and Alternatives

Cooked fish, shellfish, poultry, lean meat: 75 g (2 1/2 oz) or 125 mL (1/2 cup); Cooked legumes: 175 mL (3/4 cup); Tofu: 150 g or 175 mL (3/4 cup); 2 eggs; Peanut or nut butters: 30 mL (2 tbsp); Shelled nuts & seeds: 60 mL (1/4 cup)

Dietary Reference Intakes: Recommended Intakes for Individuals, Vitamins

Dietary Reference Intakes: Recommended Intakes for Individuals, Vitamins

Life Stage Group	Vitamin A (mcg/d)[a]	Vitamin C (mg/d)[b]	Vitamin D (mcg/d)[c]	Vitamin E (mg/d)[d]	Vitamin K (mcg/d)[e]	Thiamin (mg/d)[f]	Riboflavin (mg/d)[g]	Niacin (mg/d)[h]	Vitamin B6 (mg/d)[i]	Folate (mcg/d)[j]	Vitamin B12 (mcg/d)[k]	Pantothenic Acid (mg/d)	Biotin (mcg/d)	Choline (mg/d)[l]
Infants														
0–6 mo.	400*	40*	5*	4*	2.0*	0.2*	0.3*	2*	0.1*	65*	0.4*	1.7*	5*	125*
7–12 mo.	500*	50*	5*	5*	2.5*	0.3*	0.4*	4*	0.3*	80*	0.5*	1.8*	6*	150*
Children														
1–3 yr.	300	15	5*	6	30*	0.5	0.5	6	0.5	150	0.9	2*	8*	200*
4–8 yr.	400	25	5*	7	55*	0.6	0.6	8	0.6	200	1.2	3*	12*	250*
Males														
9–13 yr.	600	45	5*	11	60*	0.9	0.9	12	1.0	300	1.8	4*	20*	375*
14–18 yr.	900	75	5*	15	75*	1.2	1.3	16	1.3	400	2.4	5*	25*	550*
19–30 yr.	900	90	5*	15	120*	1.2	1.3	16	1.3	400	2.4	5*	30*	550*
31–50 yr.	900	90	5*	15	120*	1.2	1.3	16	1.3	400	2.4	5*	30*	550*
51–70 yr.	900	90	10*	15	120*	1.2	1.3	16	1.7	400	2.4[h]	5*	30*	550*
> 70 yr.	900	90	15*	15	120*	1.2	1.3	16	1.7	400	2.4[h]	5*	30*	550*
Females														
9–13 yr.	600	45	5*	11	60*	0.9	0.9	12	1.0	300	1.8	4*	20*	375*
14–18 yr.	700	65	5*	15	75*	1.0	1.0	14	1.2	400[j]	2.4	5*	25*	400*
19–30 yr.	700	75	5*	15	90*	1.1	1.1	14	1.3	400[j]	2.4	5*	30*	425*
31–50 yr.	700	75	5*	15	90*	1.1	1.1	14	1.3	400[j]	2.4	5*	30*	425*
51–70 yr.	700	75	10*	15	90*	1.1	1.1	14	1.5	400	2.4[h]	5*	30*	425*
> 70 yr.	700	75	15*	15	90*	1.1	1.1	14	1.5	400	2.4[h]	5*	30*	425*
Pregnancy														
≤18 yr.	750	80	5*	15	75*	1.4	1.4	18	1.9	600[j]	2.6	6*	30*	450*
19–30 yr.	770	85	5*	15	90*	1.4	1.4	18	1.9	600[j]	2.6	6*	30*	450*
31–50 yr.	770	85	5*	15	90*	1.4	1.4	18	1.9	600[j]	2.6	6*	30*	450*

Life Stage Group	Vitamin A (mcg/d)[a]	Vitamin C (mg/d)[b]	Vitamin D (mcg/d)[c]	Vitamin E (mg/d)[d]	Vitamin K (mcg/d)[e]	Thiamin (mg/d)[f]	Riboflavin (mg/d)[g]	Niacin (mg/d)[h]	Vitamin B6 (mg/d)[i]	Folate (mcg/d)[j]	Vitamin B12 (mcg/d)[k]	Pantothenic Acid (mg/d)	Biotin (mcg/d)	Choline (mg/d)[l]
Lactation														
14–18 yr.	**1,200**	**115**	5*	**19**	75*	**1.4**	**1.6**	**17**	**2.0**	**500**	**2.8**	7*	35*	550*
19–30 yr.	**1,300**	**120**	5*	**19**	90*	**1.4**	**1.6**	**17**	**2.0**	**500**	**2.8**	7*	35*	550*
31–50 yr.	**1,300**	**120**	5*	**19**	90*	**1.4**	**1.6**	**17**	**2.0**	**500**	**2.8**	7*	35*	550*

NOTE: This table presents Recommended Dietary Allowances (RDAs) in **bold type** and Adequate Intakes (AIs) in ordinary type followed by an asterisk (*). RDAs and AIs may both be used as goals for individual intake. RDAs are set to meet the needs of almost all (97 to 98 percent) individuals in a group. For healthy breast-fed infants, the AI is the mean intake. The AI for other life stage and gender groups is believed to cover needs of all individuals in the group, but lack of data or uncertainty in the data prevent being able to specify with confidence the percentage of individuals covered by this intake.

[a] Includes provitamin A carotenoids that are dietary precursors of retinol. Given as retinol activity equivalents (RAEs). 1 RAE = 1 mcg retinol, 12 mcg β-carotene, 24 mcg α-carotene, or 24 mcg β-cryptoxanthin. To calculate RAEs from REs (retinol equivalents) of provitamin A carotenoids in foods, divide the REs by 2. For preformed vitamin A in foods or supplements and for provitamin A carotenoids in supplements, 1 RE = 1 RAE. Individuals with high alcohol intake, preexisting liver disease, hyperlipidemia or severe protein malnutrition may be distinctly susceptible to the adverse effects of excess preformed vitamin A intake. β-carotene supplements are advised only to serve as a provitamin A source for individuals at risk of vitamin A deficiency.

[b] Also known as: ascorbic acid, dehydroascorbic acid (DHA). Individuals who smoke require an additional 35 mg/d of vitamin C over that needed by nonsmokers. Nonsmokers regularly exposed to tobacco smoke are encouraged to ensure they meet the RDA for vitamin C.

[c] Also known as: calciferol. 1 mcg calciferol = 40 IU vitamin D. The DRI (dietary reference intake) values are based on the absence of adequate exposure to sunlight. Patients on glucocorticoid therapy may require additional vitamin D.

[d] Also known as: α-tocopherol. α-tocopherol includes *RRR*-α-tocopherol, the only form of α-tocopherol that occurs naturally in foods, and the *2R*-stereoisomeric forms of α-tocopherol (*RRR*-, *RSR*-, *RRS*-, and *RSS*-α-tocopherol) that occur in fortified foods and supplements. It does not include the *2S*-stereoisomeric forms of α-tocopherol (*SRR*-, *SSR*-, *SRS*-, and *SSS*-α-tocopherol), also found in fortified foods and supplements. Patients on anticoagulant therapy should be monitored when taking vitamin E supplements.

[e] Patients on anticoagulant therapy should monitor vitamin K intake.

[f] Also known as: vitamin B1, aneurin. Increased needs for thiamin include those being treated with hemodialysis or peritoneal dialysis, or individuals with malabsorption syndrome.

[g] Also known as: vitamin B2

[h] Includes nicotinic acid amide, nicotinic acid (pyridine-3-carboxylic acid), and derivatives that exhibit the biological activity of nicotinamide. Given as niacin equivalents (NE). 1 mg of niacin = 60 mg of tryptophan; 0–6 months = preformed niacin (not NE); acts as a coenzyme or cosubstrate in many biological reduction and oxidation reactions—thus required for energy metabolism. Extra niacin may be required by persons treated with hemodialysis or peritoneal dialysis, or those with malabsorption syndrome.

[i] Vitamin B6 comprises a group of six related compounds: pyridoxal, pyridoxine, pyridoxamine, and 5′-phosphates (PLP, PNP, PMP).

[j] Also known as: folic acid, folacin, pteroylpolyglutamates. Given as dietary folate equivalents (DFE). 1 DFE = 1 mcg food folate = 0.6 mcg of folate from fortified food or as a supplement consumed with food = 0.5 mcg of a supplement taken on an empty stomach. In view of evidence linking folate intake with neural tube defects in the fetus, it is recommended that all women capable of becoming pregnant consume 400 mcg from supplements or fortified foods in addition to intake of food folate from a varied diet. It is assumed that women will continue consuming 400 mcg from supplements or fortified food until their pregnancy is confirmed and they enter prenatal care, which ordinarily occurs after the end of the periconceptional period—the critical time for formation of the neural tube.

[k] Also known as: cobalamin. Because 10 to 30 percent of older people may malabsorb foodbound vitamin B12, it is advisable for those older than 50 years to meet their RDA mainly by consuming foods fortified with vitamin B12 or a supplement containing vitamin B12.

[l] Individuals with trimethylaminuria, renal disease, liver disease, depression and Parkinson disease, may be at risk of adverse effects with choline intakes at the UL (tolerable upper intake level). Although AIs have been set for choline, there are few data to assess whether a dietary supply of choline is needed at all stages of the life cycle, and it may be that the choline requirement can be met by endogenous synthesis at some of these stages.

SOURCE: Food and Nutrition Board, Institute of Medicine, National Academies (2004).

Dietary Reference Intakes: Recommended Intakes for Individuals, Elements

Dietary Reference Intakes: Recommended Intakes for Individuals, Elements

Life Stage Group	Calcium (mg/d)[m]	Chromium (mcg/d)	Copper (mcg/d)[n]	Fluoride (mg/d)	Iodine (mcg/d)[o]	Iron (mg/d)[p]	Magnesium (mg/d)[q]	Manganese (mg/d)	Molybdenum (mcg/d)[r]	Phosphorus (mg/d)[s]	Selenium (mcg/d)	Zinc (mg/d)[t,u]
Infants												
0–6 mo.	210*	0.2*	200*	0.01*	110*	0.27*	30*	0.003*	2*	100*	15*	2*
7–12 mo.	270*	5.5*	220*	0.5*	130*	**11**	75*	0.6*	3*	275*	20*	**3**
Children												
1–3 yr.	500*	11*	**340**	0.7*	**90**	**7**	**80**	1.2*	**17**	**460**	**20**	**3**
4–8 yr.	800*	15*	**440**	1*	**90**	**10**	**130**	1.5*	**22**	**500**	**30**	**5**
Males												
9–13 yr.	1,300*	25*	**700**	2*	**120**	**8**	**240**	1.9*	**34**	**1,250**	**40**	**8**
14–18 yr.	1,300*	35*	**890**	3*	**150**	**11**	**410**	2.2*	**43**	**1,250**	**55**	**11**
19–30 yr.	1,000*	35*	**900**	4*	**150**	**8**	**400**	2.3*	**45**	**700**	**55**	**11**
31–50 yr.	1,000*	35*	**900**	4*	**150**	**8**	**420**	2.3*	**45**	**700**	**55**	**11**
51–70 yr.	1,200*	30*	**900**	4*	**150**	**8**	**420**	2.3*	**45**	**700**	**55**	**11**
> 70 yr.	1,200*	30*	**900**	4*	**150**	**8**	**420**	2.3*	**45**	**700**	**55**	**11**
Females												
9–13 yr.	1,300*	21*	**700**	2*	**120**	**8**	**240**	1.6*	**34**	**1,250**	**40**	**8**
14–18 yr.	1,300*	24*	**890**	3*	**150**	**15**	**360**	1.6*	**43**	**1,250**	**55**	**9**
19–30 yr.	1,000*	25*	**900**	3*	**150**	**18**	**310**	1.8*	**45**	**700**	**55**	**8**
31–50 yr.	1,000*	25*	**900**	3*	**150**	**18**	**320**	1.8*	**45**	**700**	**55**	**8**
51–70 yr.	1,200*	20*	**900**	3*	**150**	**8**	**320**	1.8*	**45**	**700**	**55**	**8**
> 70 yr.	1,200*	20*	**900**	3*	**150**	**8**	**320**	1.8*	**45**	**700**	**55**	**8**
Pregnancy												
14–18 yr.	1,300*	29*	**1,000**	3*	**220**	**27**	**400**	2.0*	**50**	**1,250**	**60**	**12**
19–30 yr.	1,000*	30*	**1,000**	3*	**220**	**27**	**350**	2.0*	**50**	**700**	**60**	**11**
31–50 yr.	1,000*	30*	**1,000**	3*	**220**	**27**	**360**	2.0*	**50**	**700**	**60**	**11**

Life Stage Group	Calcium (mg/d)[m]	Chromium (mcg/d)	Copper (mcg/d)[n]	Fluoride (mg/d)	Iodine (mcg/d)[o]	Iron (mg/d)[p]	Magnesium (mg/d)[q]	Manganese (mg/d)	Molybdenum (mcg/d)[r]	Phosphorus (mg/d)[s]	Selenium (mcg/d)	Zinc (mg/d)[t,u]
Lactation												
14–18 yr.	1,300*	44*	**1,300**	3*	**290**	**10**	**360**	2.6*	**50**	**1,250**	**70**	**13**
19–30yr.	1,000*	45*	**1,300**	3*	**290**	**9**	**310**	2.6*	**50**	**700**	**70**	**12**
31–50 yr.	1,000*	45*	**1,300**	3*	**290**	**9**	**320**	2.6*	**50**	**700**	**70**	**12**

NOTE: This table presents Recommended Dietary Allowances (RDAs) in **bold type** and Adequate Intakes (AIs) in ordinary type followed by an asterisk (*). RDAs and AIs may both be used as goals for individual intake. RDAs are set to meet the needs of almost all (97 to 98 percent) individuals in a group. For healthy infants fed human milk, the AI is the mean intake. The AI for other life stage and gender groups is believed to cover needs of all individuals in the group, but lack of data or uncertainty in the data prevent being able to specify with confidence the percentage of individuals covered by this intake.

SOURCE: IOM (1997, 2000b, 2001).

[m] Amenorrheic women (exercise- or anorexia nervosa-induced) have reduced net calcium absorption. There are no consistent data to support that a high protein intake increases calcium requirement.

[n] Individuals with Wilson disease, Indian childhood cirrhosis (ICC), and idiopathic copper toxicosis may be at increased risk of adverse effects from excess copper intake.

[o] Individuals with autoimmune thyroid disease, previous iodine deficiency, or nodular goiter are distinctly susceptible to the adverse effect of excess iodine intake. Therefore, individuals with these conditions may not be protected by the UL (tolerable upper intake level) for iodine intake for the general population.

[p] Nonheme iron absorption is lower for those consuming vegetarian diets than for those eating nonvegetarian diets. Therefore, it has been suggested that the iron requirement for those consuming a vegetarian diet is approximately 2-fold greater than for those consuming a nonvegetarian diet. Recommended intake assumes 75% of iron is from heme iron sources.

[q] Because manganese in drinking water and supplements may be more bioavailable than manganese from food, caution should be taken when using manganese supplements especially among those persons already consuming large amounts of manganese from diets high in plant products. In addition, individuals with liver disease may be distinctly susceptible to the adverse effects of excess manganese intake.

[r] Individuals who are deficient in dietary copper intake or have some dysfunction in copper metabolism that makes them copper deficient could be at increased risk of molybdenum toxicity.

[s] Athletes and others with high energy expenditure frequently consume amounts from food greater than the UL without apparent effect.

[t] Absorption is lower for those consuming vegetarian diets than for those eating nonvegetarian diets. Therefore, it has been suggested that the zinc requirement for those consuming a vegetarian diet is approximately 2-fold greater than for those consuming a nonvegetarian diet.

[u] **OTHER ELEMENTS: arsenic, boron, nickel** (however, individuals with preexisting nickel hypersensitivity, from previous dermal exposure, and kidney dysfunction are distinctly susceptible to the adverse effects of excess nickel intake), **silicon, vanadium** all are classified ND = Not Determinable due to lack of data of adverse effects in this age group and concern with regard to lack of ability to handle excess amounts. Source of intake should be from food only to prevent high levels of intake.

SOURCE: Food and Nutrition Board, Institute of Medicine, National Academies (2004).

Conversion Factors Between Traditional and SI Units

Factors for Converting Nutrients Expressed in Metric or Milliequivalent Units into International System (SI) Units

1. Definitions

a. Equivalent weight (EW) = atomic weight of element/valence of ionic form. Example with magnesium: atomic wt = 24, valence = 2+; therefore EW = 12.

b. Quantity of an electrolyte in milliequivalents per liter (mEq/L) = mg of electrolyte/L/EW. Example: 48 mg of magnesium/L/12 = 4 mEq/L.

c. Quantity of an electrolyte in mg/dL = (mEq/L × EW)/10.

d. To convert mg/dL (= mg%) of an electrolyte to mEq/L: mg/dL × 10/EW = mEq/L.

e. 1 mol = 1 molecular or atomic weight of element or compound in grams (GMWt). In solutions this is usually expressed as moles per liter; i.e., 1 mol/L = 1 M; 1 mM (mmol) = 1 mol × 10^{-3}, 1 μM (μmol) = 1 mol × 10^{-6}, 1 nM (nmol) = 1 mol × 10^{-9}.

f. 1. To convert mEq/L of an electrolyte or other ions in solution to mmol/L: mEq/L divided by valence = mmol/L; e.g., (a) 2 mEq/L of magnesium (Mg^{2+}) = 2/2 = 1. mmol/L; e.g., (b) 150 mEq Na^+/L = 140/l = 140 mmol/L.

2. To convert mg/dL to mmol/L: (mg/dL × 10/EW) divided by valence = mmol/L; e.g., 2 mg/dL of magnesium = (2 × 10/12) divided by 2 = 0.83 mmol/L.

3. For organic substances: mmol/L = wt in mg/L/MW (in mg).

2. SI units for expressing clinical laboratory data

These units are now widely used and are increasingly required for publication of scientific data in physical, biologic, and biomedical publication. Extensive SI conversion tables have been published together with an explanation of the rationale for their use and technical aspects of usage (1–3) (see Table 3).

Table 1. The base units of interest in physical quantities used in clinical chemistry

Quantity	Base Unit
mass	kilogram
time	second
amount	mole
length	meter

A derived unit for energy is the kjoule (kJ): 4.18 kJ = 1kcal, 1 MJ = 239 kcal.

Table 2. Prefixes and symbols for decimal multiples and submultiples

Factor	Prefix	Symbol	Factor	Prefix	Symbol
10^9	giga	G	10^{-3}	milli	m
10^6	mega	M	10^{-6}	micro	μ
10^3	kilo	k	10^{-9}	nano	n
10^2	hecto	h	10^{-12}	pico	p
10^1	deco	da	10^{-15}	femto	f
10^{-1}	deci	d	10^{-18}	atto	a
10^{-2}	centi	c			

Table 3. Conversion factors for selected compounds of nutrition interest[a]

Component	(1) Present Unit	(2) Conversion Factor	(3) SI Unit Symbol	(4) Mass Conversion Factor
Albumin (s)	g/dL	10	g/L	—
Aluminum (s)	μg/L	37.04	nmol/L	μg/27 = mol
Amino acid nitrogen (p)	mg/dL	0.714	mmol/L	mg/14 = mmol
Ascorbic acid (p)	mg/dL	56.78	μmol/L	mg/176 = mmol
Calcium (s)	mg/dL	0.250	mmol/L	mg/40 = mmol
Calcium (s)	mEq/dL	0.500	mmol/L	mEq/2 = mmol
β-Carotene (s)	μ/dL	0.0186	μmol/L	μg/536.85 = μmol
Chloride (s)	mEq/L	1.00	mmol/L	mEq = mmol
Cholesterol (p)	mg/dL	0.0259	mmol/L	mg/386.6 = mmol
Cobalamin (B_{12})	pg/mL	0.738	pmol/L	pg/1355 = pmol
Copper (s)	μg/dL	0.157	μmol/L	μg/63.5 = μmol
Ethanol (p)	mg/dL	0.217	mmol/L	mg/46 = mmol
Folic acid	ng/mL	2.265	mmol/L	ng/441.4 = nmol
Glucose (p)	mg/dL	0.0555	mmol/L	mg/180.2 = mmol
Iron (s)	μg/dL	0.179	μmol/L	μg/55.9 = μmol
Phosphate (p) (as phosphorus)	mg/dL	0.323	mmol/L	mg/31 = mmol
Potassium (s)	mEq/L	1.000	mmol/L	mEq = mmol
Potassium	mg/dL	0.256	mmol/L	mg/39.1 = mmol
Magnesium (s)	mg/dL	0.411	mmol/L	mg/24.3 = mmol
Pyridoxal (B)	ng/mL	5.981	nmol/L	ng/167 = nmol
Retinol (p,s)	μg/dL	0.0349	μmol/L	μg/286 = μmol
Riboflavin (s)	μg/dL	26.57	μmol/L	μg/376 = nmol
Sodium (s)	mEq/L	1.00	mmol/L	mEq = mmol
Thiamin HCl (U)	μg/24 h	0.00298	μmol/d	μg/337 = μmol
α-Tocopherol (p)	mg/dL	23.22	μmol/L	μg/431 = μmol
Vitamin D3	μg/dL	26.01	nmol/L	μg/384 = μmol
Calcidiol	ng/mL	2.498	nmol/L	ng/400 = nmol
Zinc (s)	μg/dL	0.153	μmol/L	μg/65.4 = mmol

[a]To convert metric or equivalent unit per unit volume (column 1) to SI units per liter (column 3), multiply by the conversion factor in column 2. p, plasma; s, serum; B, blood; U, urine.

References

1. Lundberg GD, Iberson C, Radulescu G: *JAMA* 1986; 255: 2329.
2. Monsen ER: *J Am Diet Assoc* 1987; 87: 356.
3. Young DS. *Ann Intern Med* 1987; 106: 114.

From Shils ME, Olson JA, Shike M, Ross AC. Modern nutrition in health and disease, 9th ed. Baltimore: Lippincott Williams & Wilkins, 1999.

Overweight and Obesity: Health Consequences

The Surgeon General's Call to Action to Prevent and Decrease Overweight and Obesity
The primary concern of overweight and obesity is one of health and not appearance.

PREMATURE DEATH

- An estimated 300,000 deaths per year may be attributable to obesity.
- The risk of death rises with increasing weight.
- Even moderate weight excess (10 to 20 pounds for a person of average height) increases the risk of death, particularly among adults aged 30 to 64 years.
- Individuals who are obese (BMI > 30) have a 50 to 100% increased risk of premature death from all causes, compared to individuals with a healthy weight.

HEART DISEASE

- The incidence of heart disease (heart attack, congestive heart failure, sudden cardiac death, angina or chest pain, and abnormal heart rhythm) is increased in persons who are overweight or obese (BMI > 25).
- High blood pressure is twice as common in adults who are obese than in those who are at a healthy weight.
- Obesity is associated with elevated triglycerides (blood fat) and decreased HDL cholesterol ("good cholesterol").

DIABETES

- A weight gain of 11 to 18 pounds increases a person's risk of developing type 2 diabetes to twice that of individuals who have not gained weight.
- Over 80% of people with diabetes are overweight or obese.

CANCER

- Overweight and obesity are associated with an increased risk for some types of cancer including endometrial (cancer of the lining of the uterus), colon, gallbladder, prostate, kidney, and postmenopausal breast cancer.
- Women gaining more than 20 pounds from age 18 to midlife double their risk of postmenopausal breast cancer, compared to women whose weight remains stable.

BREATHING PROBLEMS

- Sleep apnea (interrupted breathing while sleeping) is more common in obese persons.
- Obesity is associated with a higher prevalence of asthma.

ARTHRITIS

- For every 2-pound increase in weight, the risk of developing arthritis is increased by 9 to 13%.
- Symptoms of arthritis can improve with weight loss.

REPRODUCTIVE COMPLICATIONS

- Complications of pregnancy
  - Obesity during pregnancy is associated with increased risk of death in both the baby and the mother and increases the risk of maternal high blood pressure by 10 times.
  - In addition to many other complications, women who are obese during pregnancy are more likely to have gestational diabetes and problems with labor and delivery.
  - Infants born to women who are obese during pregnancy are more likely to be high birthweight and, therefore, may face a higher rate of cesarean section delivery and low blood sugar (which can be associated with brain damage and seizures).
  - Obesity during pregnancy is associated with an increased risk of birth defects, particularly neural tube defects, such as spina bifida.
- Obesity in premenopausal women is associated with irregular menstrual cycles and infertility.

ADDITIONAL HEALTH CONSEQUENCES

- Overweight and obesity are associated with increased risks of gallbladder disease, incontinence, increased surgical risk, and depression.
- Obesity can affect the quality of life through limited mobility and decreased physical endurance as well as through social, academic, and job discrimination.

CHILDREN AND ADOLESCENTS

- Risk factors for heart disease, such as high cholesterol and high blood pressure, occur with increased frequency in overweight children and adolescents compared to those with a healthy weight.
- Type 2 diabetes, previously considered an adult disease, has increased dramatically in children and adolescents. Overweight and obesity are closely linked to type 2 diabetes.
- Overweight adolescents have a 70% chance of becoming overweight or obese adults. This increases to 80% if one or more parent is overweight or obese.
- The most immediate consequence of overweight, as perceived by children themselves, is social discrimination.

BENEFITS OF WEIGHT LOSS

- Weight loss, as modest as 5 to 15% of total body weight in a person who is overweight or obese, reduces the risk factors for some diseases, particularly heart disease.
- Weight loss can result in lower blood pressure, lower blood sugar, and improved cholesterol levels.
- A person with a Body Mass Index (BMI) above the healthy weight range may benefit from weight loss, especially if he or she has other health risk factors, such as high blood pressure, high cholesterol, smoking, diabetes, a sedentary lifestyle, and a personal and/or family history of heart disease.

http://www.surgeongeneral.gov/topics/obesity/calltoaction/fact_consequences.htm

Classification of Overweight and Obesity in Adults According to Body Mass Index

Obesity is classified as BMI ≥ 30 kg/m²

Classification	BMI (kg/m²)	Risk of co-morbidities
Underweight	< 18.5	Low (but risk of other clinical problems increased)
Normal range	18.5–24.9	Average
Overweight	25.0–29.9	Mildly increased
Obese	**> 30.0**	
Class I	30.0–34.9	Moderate
Class II	35.0–39.9	Severe
Class III	> 40.0	Very severe

Note that these values are age-independent and correspond to the same degree of fatness across different populations
Note that both BMI and a measure of fat distribution (waist circumference or waist hip ratio, etc.) are important in calculating the risk of obesity co-morbidities. BMI < 18.5kg/m² signifies an increased risk of developing other clinical problems.
http://www.obesity.chair.ulaval.ca/IOTF.htm#Classification

Body Mass Index Table

	Normal						Overweight					Obese										Extreme Obesity														
BMI	**19**	**20**	**21**	**22**	**23**	**24**	**25**	**26**	**27**	**28**	**29**	**30**	**31**	**32**	**33**	**34**	**35**	**36**	**37**	**38**	**39**	**40**	**41**	**42**	**43**	**44**	**45**	**46**	**47**	**48**	**49**	**50**	**51**	**52**	**53**	**54**
Height (inches)																**Body Weight (pounds)**																				
58	91	96	100	105	110	115	119	124	129	134	138	143	148	153	158	162	167	172	177	181	186	191	196	201	205	210	215	220	224	229	234	239	244	248	253	258
59	94	99	104	109	114	119	124	128	133	138	143	148	153	158	163	168	173	178	183	188	193	198	203	208	212	217	222	227	232	237	242	247	252	257	262	267
60	97	102	107	112	118	123	128	133	138	143	148	153	158	163	168	174	179	184	189	194	199	204	209	215	220	225	230	235	240	245	250	255	261	266	271	276
61	100	106	111	116	122	127	132	137	143	148	153	158	164	169	174	180	185	190	195	201	206	211	217	222	227	232	238	243	248	254	259	264	269	275	280	285
62	104	109	115	120	126	131	136	142	147	153	158	164	169	175	180	186	191	196	202	207	213	218	224	229	235	240	246	251	256	262	267	273	278	284	289	295
63	107	113	118	124	130	135	141	146	152	158	163	169	175	180	186	191	197	203	208	214	220	225	231	237	242	248	254	259	265	270	278	282	287	293	299	304
64	110	116	122	128	134	140	145	151	157	163	169	174	180	186	192	197	204	209	215	221	227	232	238	244	250	256	262	267	273	279	285	291	296	302	308	314
65	114	120	126	132	138	144	150	156	162	168	174	180	186	192	198	204	210	216	222	228	234	240	246	252	258	264	270	276	282	288	294	300	306	312	318	324
66	118	124	130	136	142	148	155	161	167	173	179	186	192	198	204	210	216	223	229	235	241	247	253	260	266	272	278	284	291	297	303	309	315	322	328	334
67	121	127	134	140	146	153	159	166	172	178	185	191	198	204	211	217	223	230	236	242	249	255	261	268	274	280	287	293	299	306	312	319	325	331	338	344
68	125	131	138	144	151	158	164	171	177	184	190	197	203	210	216	223	230	236	243	249	256	262	269	276	282	289	295	302	308	315	322	328	335	341	348	354
69	128	135	142	149	155	162	169	176	182	189	196	203	209	216	223	230	236	243	250	257	263	270	277	284	291	297	304	311	318	324	331	338	345	351	358	365
70	132	139	146	153	160	167	174	181	188	195	202	209	216	222	229	236	243	250	257	264	271	278	285	292	299	306	313	320	327	334	341	348	355	362	369	376
71	136	143	150	157	165	172	179	186	193	200	208	215	222	229	236	243	250	257	265	272	279	286	293	301	308	315	322	329	338	343	351	358	365	372	379	386
72	140	147	154	162	169	177	184	191	199	206	213	221	228	235	242	250	258	265	272	279	287	294	302	309	316	324	331	338	346	353	361	368	375	383	390	397
73	144	151	159	166	174	182	189	197	204	212	219	227	235	242	250	257	265	272	280	288	295	302	310	318	325	333	340	348	355	363	371	378	386	393	401	408
74	148	155	163	171	179	186	194	202	210	218	225	233	241	249	256	264	272	280	287	295	303	311	319	326	334	342	350	358	365	373	381	389	396	404	412	420
75	152	160	168	176	184	192	200	208	216	224	232	240	248	256	264	272	279	287	295	303	311	319	327	335	343	351	359	367	375	383	391	399	407	415	423	431
76	156	164	172	180	189	197	205	213	221	230	238	246	254	263	271	279	287	295	304	312	320	328	336	344	353	361	369	377	385	394	402	410	418	426	435	443

www.nhlbi.nih.gov/guidelines/obesity/bmi_tbl.pdf

Source: Adapted from *Clinical Guidelines on the Identification, Evaluation, and Treatment of Overweight and Obesity in Adults: The Evidence Report*

Body Mass Index Table (High Range)

	Weight (lbs.)																													
Height	255	260	265	270	275	280	285	290	295	300	305	310	315	320	325	330	335	340	345	350	355	360	365	370	375	380	385	390	395	400
5'0"	50	51	52	53	54	55	56	57	58	59	60	61	62	62	63	64	65	66	67	68	69	70	71	72	73	74	75	76	77	78
5'1"	48	49	50	51	52	53	54	55	56	57	58	59	60	60	61	62	63	64	65	66	67	68	69	70	71	72	73	74	75	76
5'2"	47	48	48	49	50	51	52	53	54	55	56	57	58	59	59	60	61	62	63	64	65	66	67	68	69	70	70	71	72	73
5'3"	45	46	47	48	49	50	50	51	52	53	54	55	56	57	58	58	59	60	61	62	63	64	65	66	66	67	68	69	70	71
5'4"	44	45	45	46	47	48	49	50	51	51	52	53	54	55	56	57	58	58	59	60	61	62	63	64	64	65	66	67	68	69
5'5"	42	43	44	45	46	47	47	48	49	50	51	52	52	53	54	55	56	57	57	58	59	60	61	62	62	63	64	65	66	67
5'6"	41	42	43	44	44	45	46	47	48	48	49	50	51	52	52	53	54	55	56	56	57	58	59	60	61	61	62	63	64	65
5'7"	40	41	42	42	43	44	45	45	46	47	48	49	49	50	51	52	52	53	54	55	56	56	57	58	59	60	60	61	62	63
5'8"	39	40	40	41	42	43	43	44	45	46	46	47	48	49	49	50	51	52	52	53	54	55	55	56	57	58	59	59	60	61
5'9"	38	38	39	40	41	41	42	43	44	44	45	46	47	47	48	49	49	50	51	52	52	53	54	55	55	56	57	58	58	59
5'10"	37	37	38	39	39	40	41	42	42	43	44	44	45	46	47	47	48	49	50	50	51	52	52	53	54	55	55	56	57	57
5'11"	36	36	37	38	38	39	40	40	41	42	43	43	44	45	45	46	47	47	48	49	50	50	51	52	52	53	54	54	55	56
6'0"	35	35	36	37	37	38	39	39	40	41	41	42	43	43	44	45	45	46	47	47	48	49	50	50	51	52	52	53	54	54
6'1"	34	34	35	36	36	37	38	38	39	40	40	41	42	42	43	44	44	45	46	46	47	47	48	49	49	50	51	51	52	53
6'2"	33	33	34	35	35	36	37	37	38	39	39	40	40	41	42	42	43	44	44	45	46	46	47	48	48	49	49	50	51	51
6'3"	32	32	33	34	34	35	36	36	37	37	38	39	39	40	41	41	42	42	43	44	44	45	46	46	47	47	48	49	49	50
6'4"	31	32	32	33	33	34	35	35	36	37	37	38	38	39	40	40	41	41	42	43	43	44	44	45	46	46	47	47	48	49

http://www.shapeup.org/bodylab/frmst.html

Professional Organizations

This directory, by no means exhaustive, lists professional organizations in the U.S. and some other English-speaking countries. Each country's name is followed by its country code for international calling. City codes or other area codes are listed with individual telephone numbers.

Australia (61)

Australian Acoustical Society (AAS)
PO Box 903
Castlemaine, VIC 3450
03 5470 6381
03 5470 6381 (fax)
GeneralSecretary@acoustics.asn.au
www.acoustics.asn.au

Australian Association for Health, Physical Education, Recreation, and Dance (ACHPER)
214 Port Road
PO Box 304
Hindmarsh, SA 5007
08 8340 3388
08 8340 3399 (fax)
achper@achper.org.au
www.achper.org.au

Australian Association of Massage Therapists (AAMT)
Level 6, 85 Queen Street
Melbourne, VIC 3000
1300 138 872
03 9602 3088 (fax)
info@aamt.com.au
www.aamt.com.au

Australian Association of Occupational Therapists (AUSOT)
6/340 Gore Street
Fitzroy, VIC 3065
03 9415 2900
03 9416 1421 (fax)
info@ausot.com.au
www.ausot.com.au
New South Wales www.otnsw.com.au
Queensland www.otqld.org.au
South Australia www.otsa.org.au
Victoria www.otausvic.com.au
Western Australia www.otauswa.com.au

Australian Dental Association (ADA)
PO Box 520
St. Leonards, NSW 1590
75 Lithgow Street
St. Leonards, NSW 2065
02 9906 4412
02 9906 4917 (fax)
adainc@ada.org.au
www.ada.org.au

Australian Institute of Radiography (AIR)
32 Bedford Street
PO Box 1169
Collingwood, VIC 3066
03 9419 3336
03 9416 0783 (fax)
air@air.asn.au
www.air.asn.au

Australian Nursing and Midwifery Council, Inc. (ANMC)
20 Challis Street
PO Box 873
Dickson, ACT 2602
02 6257 7960
02 6257 7955 (fax)
internationalsection@anmc.org.au
www.anmc.org.au

Australian Nursing Federation (ANF)
Unit 3, 28 Eyre Street
Kingston, ACT 2604
2 6232 6533
2 6232 6610 (fax)
professional@anf.org.au
www.anf.org.au
Australian Capital Territory www.actanf.org.au
New South Wales www.nswnurses.asn.au
Northern Territory www.anfnt.org.au
Queensland www.qnu.org.au
South Australia www.sa.anf.org.au
Victoria www.anfvic.asn.au
West Australia www.anfwa.asn.au
Tasmania www.anftas.org

Australasian College for Emergency Medicine (ACEM)
34 Jeffcott Street
West Melbourne, VIC 3003
03 9320 0444
03 9320 0400 (fax)
admin@acem.org.au
www.medeserv.com.au/acem

Australasian Society for Emergency Medicine (ASEM)
PO Box 627
Noble Park, VIC 3174
03 9794 7658
03 9794 6522
emergmed@bigpond.com
www.asem.org.au (under construction)

Australian and New Zealand College of Anaesthetists (NZCA)
630 St. Kilda Road
Melbourne VIC 3004
03 9510 6299
03 9510 6786 (fax)
ceoanzca@anzca.edu.au
www.medeserv.com.au/anzca

Australian Resource Centre for Healthcare Innovation (ARCHI)
1 Bean Street
Wallsend NSW 2287
02 4985 5222
02 4985 5200 (fax)
admin@archi.net.au
www.archi.net.au

Australian Resuscitation Council (ARC)
c/o Royal Australasian College of Surgeons
Spring Street
Melbourne VIC 3000
03 9249 1214
03 9249 1216
carol.carey@surgeons.org
www.resus.org.au
New South Wales
peter.mckie@parasolemt.com.au
Queensland eotraining@stjohnqld.com.au
www.stjohnqld.asn.au
South Australia
grantham.hugh@saambulance.com.au
Tasmania malcolm.anderson@dhhs.tas.gov.au
Victoria tony.walker@rav.vic.gov.au
Western Australia ijacobs@cyllene.uwa.edu.au

Australian Veterinary Association (AVA)
Unit 40, 2a Herbert Street
St. Leonards NSW 2065
02 9431 5000
02 9437 9068 (fax)
members@ava.com.au
www.ava.com.au

Dental Hygienists' Association of Australia, Inc. (DHAA)
PO Box 10030 Gouger Street
Adelaide, SA 5000
08 8177 0196
info@dhaa.asn.au
www.dhaa.asn.au

Australian Capital Territory (DHAA-ACT)
GPO Box 2317
Canberra ACT 2601
contact-act@dhaa.asn.au
www.dhaa.asn.au/dhaa-act

New South Wales Branch (DHAANSW)
GPO Box 3289
Sydney, NSW 2001
0411 473 762
NSW@bigpond.com.au
www.dhaansw.com.au

Queensland Branch (DHAAQ)
GPO Box 2415
Brisbane, QLD 4001
(07) 3321 2156
mail@adaq.com.au
www.dentalhygienist.com.au

Victorian Branch (DHAAVIC)
PO Box 96
Kew, VIC 3101
0418 336 119
pres_dhaavic@yahoo.com.au
www.dhaavb.com.au

South Australia Branch (DHAA-SA)
GPO Box 296
Adelaide, SA 5001
08 8177 0196
dhaa.sa@arcom.com.au
www.dhaa.asn.au/dhaa-sa

Western Australia Branch (DHAA-WA)
PO Box 115
Bentley, WA 6982
dhaa-wa@dhaa.asn.au

Tasmanian Branch (DHAA-TAS)
PO Box 102
Battery Point, TAS 7004
03 6227 8698
secretary-tas@dhaa.asn.au
www.dhaa.asn.au/dhaa-tas

Dietitians Association of Australia (DAA)
1/8 Phipps Close
Deakin, ACT 2600
02 6282 9555
1800 812 942
02 6282 9888 (fax)
nationaloffice@daa.asn.au
www.daa.asn.au

Health Information Management Association of Australia (HIMAA)
1st Floor, 51 Wicks Road
Locked Bag 2045
North Ryde, NSW 1670
02 9887 5001
02 9887 5895 (fax)
himaa@himaa.org.au
www.himaa.org.au

Pharmaceutical Society of Australia (PSA)
Pharmacy House
44 Thesiger Court
Deakin, ACT 2600
PO Box 21
Curtin, ACT 2605
02 6283 4777
02 6285 2869 (fax)
psa.nat@psa.org.au
www.psa.org.au

Royal Australasian College of Medical Administrators (RACMA)

New South Wales
Dr. Beth Kotze, Area Director Mental Health Services
South East Health
Level 1
2 Short Street
Kogarah NSW 2217
02 9350 2486
02 9350 3959
kotzeb@sesahs.nsw.gov.au
www.racma.edu.au

Northern Territory
Dr. Vinothini Sathinathan, Deputy Medical Superintendent
Royal Darwin Hospital
PO Box 40596
Casuarina NT 0811
08 8922 8888
08 8922 8286 (fax)
vino.sathianathan@nt.gov.au

Queensland
Dr. John Menzies, Senior Medical Adviser
JTAI-Health
PO Box 1080
Brisbane QLD 4001
07 3114 4621
07 3210 2161
jwmenzies@optusnet.com.au

South Australia
Dr. Bruce Swanson
Medical Adviser, South Australian Department of Human Services
11-14 Hindmarsh Square
Adelaide SA 5000
08 8226 6415
08 8226 6133
bruce.swanson@health.sa.gov.au

Tasmania
Dr. John Sparrow
14 Chessington Court
Sandy Bay, TAS 7005
3 6225 2961
3 6225 2961 (fax)
jacksparrow@southcom.com.au

Victoria
Dr. Bernard Street
Clinical Director of Geriatric Medicine Bendigo Health
PO Box 126
Bendigo VIC 3552
03 5454 9211
03 5443 9051 (fax)
BStreet@bendigohealth.org.au

Western Australia
Dr. Philip Montgomery
Area Executive Director Royal Perth Group
North Metropolitan Area Health Service
c/o Royal Perth Hospital
GPO Box X2213
Perth WA 6847
08 9224 2204
08 9224 3444
philip.montgomery@health.wa.gov.au

Royal Australian and New Zealand College of Ophthalmologists (RANZCO)
94-98 Chalmers Street
Surry Hills NSW 2010
02 9690 1001
02 9690 1321 (fax)
ranzco@ranzco.edu
www.ranzco.edu

Royal College of Pathologists of Australia (RCPA)
ABN 52 000 173 231
Durham Hall
207 Albion Street
Surry Hills NSW 2010
02 8356 5858
02 8356 5828 (fax)
contact@rcpa.edu.au
www.rcpa.edu.au

Speech Pathology Australia (SPA)
11-19 Bank Place, 2nd Floor
Melbourne, VIC 3000
03 9642 4899
03 9642 4922 (fax)
office@speechpathologyaustralia.org.au
www.speechpathologyaustralia.org.au

New South Wales
02 9743 0013
02 9743 0014 (fax)
sppathnsw@email.cs.nsw.gov.au

Northern Territory
Children's Development Team
PO Box 40596
Casuarina NT 0811
08 8922 7101
08 8922 7399 (fax)
rachel.ortner@nt.gov.au

Queensland
Qld Speech Pathology Australia
PO Box 655
Indooroopilly QLD 4068
07 3870 8542 (phone and fax)
qldcpd@bigpond.com

South Australia
c/o Dept of Speech Pathology & Audiology
Flinders University
GPO Box 2100
Adelaide SA 5001
08 8204 6070
spaa.sa@fmc.sa.gov.au

Tasmania
Speech Pathology Australia
c/o Rokeby Primary School
Burtonia Street
Rokeby TAS 7019
03 6212 3513
megan.cavanagh@education.tas.gov.au

Western Australia
Speech Pathology Australia
1/37 Baldwin Street
Como WA 6152
08 9450 8281 (phone and fax)
sppathwa@optusnet.com.au

Sports Dietitians Australia (SDA)
PO Box 2016, Lennox Street
Richmond VIC 3121
03 9425 0015
03 9425 0100 (fax)
info@sportsdietitians.com
www.sportsdietitians.com

Sports Medicine Australia (SMA)
3-5 Cheney Place
PO Box 78
Mitchell ACT 2911
02 6241 9344
02 6241 1611 (fax)
smanat@sma.org.au
www.sma.org.au

Canada (1)

Aboriginal Nurses Association of Canada (ANAC)
56 Sparks Street, Ste. 502
Ottawa, ON K1P 5A9
(613) 724-4677
(613) 724-4718 (fax)
ctoulouse@anac.on.ca
www.anac.on.ca

Canadian Academy of Audiology (CAA)
250 Consumers Road, Ste. 301
Toronto, ON M2J 4V6
(416) 494-6672
(800) 264-5106
(416) 495-8723 (fax)
caa@canadianaudiology.ca
www.canadianaudiology.ca

Canadian Academy of Manipulative Therapy (CAMT)
CAMT Secretary /Treasurer Attention: Mike MacNutt
61 Red Fern Terrace
Halifax, NS B3S 1K8
Mikemacnutt4@yahoo.ca
www.manipulativetherapy.org

Canadian Academy of Sport Medicine (CASM)
5330 Canotek Road, Unit 4
Ottawa, ON K1J 9C1
(877) 585-2394
(613) 748-5792 (fax)
admin@casm-acms.org
www.casm-acms.org

Canadian Anesthesiologists' Society (CAS)
1 Eglinton Avenue East, Ste. 208
Toronto, ON M4P 3A1
(416) 480-0602
(416) 480-0320 (fax)
director@cas.ca
www.cas.ca

Canadian Association for Health, Physical Education, Recreation, and Dance (CAPHPERD)
301-2197 Riverside Drive
Ottawa, ON K1H 7X3
(613) 523-1348
(800) 663-8708
(613) 523-1206 (fax)
info@cahperd.ca
www.cahperd.ca

Canadian Association of Critical Care Nurses (CACCN)
PO Box 25322
London, ON N6C 6B1
(519) 649-5284
(866) 477-9077
(519) 649-1458 (fax)
caccn@caccn.ca
www.caccn.ca

Canadian Association of Occupational Therapists (CAOT)
CTTC Building
3400-3900 Colonel By Drive
Ottawa, ON K1S 5R1
(613) 523-CAOT (2268)
800 434-CAOT (2268)
(613) 523-2552 (fax)
manmem@caot.ca
www.caot.ca

Canadian Association of Pharmacy Technicians (CAPT)
PO Box 1271
Station F
Toronto, ON M4Y 2V8
(416) 410-1142
(416) 813-7748 (fax)
contact@capt.ca
www.capt.ca

Canadian Association of Speech-Language Pathologists and Audiologists (CASLPA)
920-1 Nicholas Street
Ottawa, ON K1N 7B7
(613) 567-9968
(800) 259-8519
(613) 567-2859 (fax)
caslpa@caslpa.ca
www.caslpa.ca

Canadian Athletic Therapists Association (CATA)
1040 7th Avenue SW, Ste. 402
Calgary, AB T2P 3G9
(403) 509-CATA (2282)
(403) 509-2280 (fax)
info@athletictherapy.org
www.athletictherapy.org

Canadian Dental Association (CDA)
1815 Alta Vista Drive
Ottawa, ON K1G 3Y6
(613) 523-1770
(613) 523-7736
reception@cda-adc.ca
www.cda-adc.ca

Canadian Dental Hygienists Association (CDHA)
96 Centrepointe Drive
Ottawa, ON K2G 6B1
(800) 267-7283
(613) 224-5515
(613) 224-7283 (fax)
info@cdha.ca
www.cdha.ca

Canadian Massage Therapist Alliance (CMTA)
344 Lakeshore Road E., Ste. B
Oakvillc, ON L6J 1J6
(905) 849-7606
(905) 849-8606 (fax)
info@cmta.ca
www.cmta.ca

Canadian Medical Association (CMA)
1867 Alta Vista Drive
Ottawa, ON K1G 3Y6
(888)855-2555
(613) 236-8864 (fax)
cmamsc@cma.ca
www.cma.ca

Canadian Nurses Association (CNA)
50 Driveway
Ottawa, ON K2P 1E2
(613) 237-2133
(800) 361-8404
(613) 237-3520 (fax)
info@cna-aiic.ca
www.cna-nurses.ca

Canadian Nurses Foundation (CNF)
50 Driveway
Ottawa, ON K2P 1E2
(613) 237-2133
(613) 237-3520 (fax)
info@cnf-fiic.ca
www.cnf.fiic.ca

Canadian Nursing Students' Association (CNSA)
Fifth Avenue Court
99 Fifth Avenue, Ste. 15
Ottawa, ON K1S 5K4
(613) 563-1236
(613) 563-7739 (fax)
president@cnsa.ca
www.cnsa.ca

Canadian Orthopractic Manual Therapy Association (COMT)
1150 100th Avenue, No. 207
Edmonton, AB T5K 0J7
(780) 482-7428
(780) 488-2463 (fax)
info@orthopractic.org
www.orthopractic.org

Canadian Pharmacists Association (CPhA)
1785 Alta Vista Drive
Ottawa, ON K1G 3Y6
(800) 917-9489
(613) 523-7877
(613) 523-0445 (fax)
info@pharmacists.ca
www.pharmacists.ca

Canadian Society of Hospital Pharmacists (CSHP)
30 Concourse Gate Unit 3
Ottawa, ON K2E 7V7
(613) 736-9733
(613) 736-5660 (fax)
lfrid@cshp.ca
www.cshp.ca

Canadian Sport Massage Therapists Association (CSMTA)
50 Eccleston Drive, Ste. 306
Toronto, ON M4A 1K8
(416) 285-1745
(416) 285-1745 (fax)
natoffice@csmta.ca
www.csmta.ca

Canadian Thoracic Society (CTS)
The Lung Association (LA) National Office
1750 Courtwood Crescent, Ste. 300
Ottawa, ON K2C 2B5
(800) 566-5864
(613) 569-6411
(613) 569-8860 (fax)
info@lung.ca
www.lung.ca

Provincial Lung Associations (PLA)
British Columbia Lung Association
2675 Oak Street
Vancouver, BC V6H 2K2
(604) 731-5864
(604) 731-5810 (fax)
info@bc.lung.ca
www.bc.lung.ca

Lung Association of Alberta & NWT
(LAANWT)
#208, 17420 Stony Plain Road
Edmonton, AB T5S 1K6
(780) 488-6819
(888) 566-5864
(780) 488-7195 (fax)
info@ab.lung.ca
www.ab.lung.ca

Lung Association of Nova Scotia (LANS)
17 Alma Crescent
Halifax, NS B3N 3E6
(902) 443-8141
(888) 566-5864
(902) 445-2573 (fax)
info@ns.lung.ca
www.ns.lung.ca

Lung Association of Saskatchewan (LAS)
1231 8th Street East
Saskatoon, SK S7H 0S5
(888) 566-5864
(306) 343-7007 (fax)
info@sk.lung.ca
www.sk.lung.ca

Manitoba Lung Association (MLA)
Winnipeg Region Office
629 McDermot Avenue
Winnipeg, MB R3A 1P6
(204) 774-5501
(204) 772-5083 (fax)
info@mb.lung.ca
www.mb.lung.ca

Manitoba Lung Association (MLA)
Westman Region Office
940 Princess Avenue
Brandon, MB R7A 0P6
(204) 725-4230
(204) 726-5800 (fax)
westman@mb.lung.ca
www.mb.lung.ca

Ontario Lung Association (OLA)
573 King Street East
Toronto, ON M5A 4L3
(800) 972-2636
(416) 864-9916 (fax)
olalung@on.lung.ca
www.on.lung.ca

Ontario Lung Association (OLA)
1550 Enterprise Road, Ste. 208
Mississauga, ON L4W 4P4
(905) 696-9720
(905) 696-0582 (fax)
cwarren@on.lung.ca
www.on.lung.ca

New Brunswick Lung Association (NBLA)
65 Brunswick Street
Fredericton, NB E3B 1G5
(506) 455-8961
(800) 565-5864
(506) 462-0939 (fax)
nblung@nbnet.nb.ca
www.nb.lung.ca

Newfoundland & Labrador Lung Association
(NLLA)
15 Pippy Place, 2nd Floor
Carnell Building
St. John's, NL A1B 4B8
(709) 726-4664
(888) 566-5864
(709) 726-2550 (fax)
info@nf.lung.ca
www.nf.lung.ca

Prince Edward Island Lung Association (PEILA)
1 Rochford Street, Ste. 2
Charlottetown, PE C1A 9L2
(902)892-5957
(888) 566-5864
(902) 368-7281 (fax)
info@pei.lung.ca

The Quebec Lung Association/l'Association pulmonaire du Québec (QLA)
855 Sainte-Catherine Street East, Ste. 222
Montréal, QC H2L 4N4
(800) 295-8111
(514) 287-7400
(514) 287-1978 (fax)
info@pq.lung.ca
www.pq.lung.ca

Canadian Veterinary Medical Association (CVMA)
339 Booth Street
Ottawa, ON K1R 7K1
(613) 236-1162
(613) 236-9681 (fax)
admin@cvma-acmv.org
www.canadianveterinarians.net

Dietitians of Canada (DA)
ICDA Secretary
C/O Dietitians of Canada
480 University Avenue, Ste. 604
Toronto, ON M5G 1V2
(416) 596-0857
(416) 596-0603 (fax)
ICDA@internationaldietetics.org
www.dietitians.ca

College of Nurses of Ontario (CNO)
101 Davenport Road
Toronto, ON M5R 3P1
416 928-0900
416 928-6507 (fax)
www.cno.org

College of Registered Nurses of Manitoba (CRNM)
890 Pembina Highway
Winnipeg, MB R3M 2M8
(204) 774-3477
(800) 665-2027 (Manitoba toll-free)
(204) 775-6052 (fax)
info@crnm.mb.ca

College of Registered Nurses of British Columbia (CRNBC)
2855 Arbutus Street
Vancouver, BC V6J 3Y8
(604) 736-7331
(800) 565-6505
(604) 738-2272 (fax)
www.crnbc.ca
info@crnbc.ca

Nurses Association of New Brunswick (NANB)
165 Regent Street
Fredericton, NB E3B 7B4
(506) 458-8731
(800) 442-4417 (toll-free in N.B.)
(506) 459-2838 (fax)
nanb@nanb.nb.ca
www.nanb.nb.ca

Ontario Nurses Association (ONA)
Toronto Head Office
85 Grenville Street, Ste. 400
Toronto, ON M5S 3A2
(416) 964-8833
(800) 387-5580
(416) 964-8864 (fax)
(866) 964-8864 (toll-free fax)
onamail@ona.org
www.ona.org

Ordre des infirmières et infirmiers du Québec (French-speaking only) (OIIQ)
4200, boul. Dorchester ouest
Westmount, QC H3Z 1V4
(514) 935-2501
(800) 363-6048 (au Québec)
(514) 935-1799 (fax)
inf@oiiq.org
www.oiiq.org

Registered Nurses Association of Nova Scotia (RNANS)
www.rnans.ns.ca (site under construction)

Registered Nurses Association of Ontario (RNAO)
158 Pearl Street
Toronto, ON M5H 1L3
(416) 599-1925
(800) 268-7199
(416) 599-1926 (fax)
info@rnao.org
www.rnao.org

Saskatchewan Registered Nurses Association (SRNA)
2066 Retallack Street
Regina, SK S4S 7X5
(800) 667-9945 (toll-free)
(306) 359-4200
(306) 525-0849 (fax)
info@srna.org
www.srna.org

Egypt (20)

Egyptian Dental Association (EDA)
84 Mathaf El-Manyal Street
PO Box 11451
Cairo
02 365 8568
02 531 9143 (fax)
eda@internetegypt.com
www.eda-egypt.org

Egyptian Nurses Syndicate (ENS)
5 Sarai Street
Manial
Cairo
20 2 368 7627
20 2 362 6510 (fax)
www.icn.ch/Egypt.htm

Egyptian Veterinary Medical Association (EVMA)
8a 26 July Street
Cairo

General Egyptian Veterinary Medical Syndicate (GEVMS)
6 Al-Hadikah Street
Garden City
Cairo

Hong Kong (852)

WHO Collaborating Centre for Sports (CUHK-WHO)
Room 74029, 5/F, Clincal Sciences Building
Department of Orthopaedics and Traumatology
Prince of Wales Hospital
Shatin, New Territories
Hong Kong SAR
264 614 77
2646 3020 (fax)
whoctr@cuhhk.edu.hk
www.cuhk.edu.hk

Medicine and Health Promotion
The Chinese University of Hong Kong (CUHK)
Shatin, NT
Hong Kong SAR
2609 7000
2609 6000
2603 5544 (fax)
admin@cuhk.edu.hk
www.cuhk.edu.hk

India (91)

All India Institute of Speech and Hearing (AIISH)
Manasa Gangotri
Mysore 570 006
(821) 514449
(821) 510515 (fax)
dir@aiish.ernet.in
www.mylibnet.org/aiish.html

All India Occupational Therapists Association (AIOTA)
Dr. Shovan Saha, Convener, AIOTA Website Committee
Department of Occupational Therapy
Manipal College of Allied Sciences
MAHE, Manipal, Udupi, Karnataka
Pin: 576104
(820) 257 1201 Ext. 22178
(820) 257 1915 (fax)
shovansaha@yahoo.com
www.aiota.org

All India Ophthalmological Society (AIOS)
Prof. (Dr.) Rajvardhan Azad
M-18 Saket Road No. 50
New Delhi 110017
011-2659318
011-26588919 (fax)
rajvardhanazad@hotmail.com
www.aios.org

Indian Association of Sports Medicine (IASM)
Sports Medicine Center
Jawaharlal Nehru Stadium
PO RoocdKhokhara
New Delhi
183-2502046, 183-2504812
183-2258820, 183-2258819 (fax)
www.iasm.co.in

Indian Dental Association (IDA)
Dr. Mukul Dabholkar Saraswati Sadan
Turner Road Bandra West
Mumbai 400050
(022) 2655 2014
(022) 2642 0143 (fax)
secretary@dentalhealthindia.com
www.dentalhealthindia.com

Indian Veterinary Association (IVA)
Old No. 11 New No. 7 Chalmers Road
Chennai 600 0035
(044) 2435 1006
(044) 2433 2691
(044) 2433 8894 (fax)
ivj@vnsl.com
www.indvetjournal.com

Trained Nurses' Association of India (TNA)
Headquarters L-17 Green Park (Main)
New Delhi 110016
(11) 2656 6665
(11) 26858304 (fax)
tnai@ndf.vsnl.net.in
www.tnaionline.org

Ireland (353)

Association of Occupational Therapists of Ireland (AOTI)
29 Gardiner Place
Dublin 1
(0) 1 878 0247
1 878 0247 (international)
www.iol.ie/~headon/aoti

Healthcare Informatics Society of Ireland (HISI)
58 Eccles Street
Dublin 7
(0)1 8600568 (Ireland)
(0)1 8600568 (international)
(0)1 830 7728 (fax)
moconnor@hisi.ie
www.hisi.ie

Irish Medical Organisation (IMO)
10 Fitzwilliam Place
Dublin 2
(0)1 6767273
(0)1 6612758 (fax)
imo@imo.ie
www.imo.ie

Irish Nurses Organisation (INO)
The Whitworth Building
North Brunswick Street
Dublin 7
(01) 664 0600
(01) 6610466 (fax)
ino@ino.ie
www.ino.ie

Irish Society of Chartered Physiotherapists (ISCP)
Royal College of Surgeons Ireland
St. Stephen's Green
Dublin 2
(0)1 402 21 48
(0)1 402 21 60 (fax)
info@iscp.ie
www.iscp.ie

Irish Sports Medicine Association (ISMA)
Brookfield Health Centre
Brookfield, Tallaght
Dublin 24
(0)1 459 0200 (fax)
info@isma.ie
www.isma.ie

Irish Veterinary Officers Association (IVOA)
4 Warners Lane
Dartmouth Road
Dublin
(0)1 668 6077
petermul@iol.ie
www.voa.freehosting.net

Royal Academy of Medicine in Ireland (RAMI)
The General Secretary
Royal Academy of Medicine in Ireland
Frederick House, 2nd Floor
19 South Frederick Street
Dublin 2
(0) 1 633 4820
(0) 1 633 4918 (fax)
secretary@rami.ie
www.rami.ie

New Zealand (64)

New Zealand Association of Occupational Therapists (NZAOT)
Level 1, Red Cross House
69 Molesworth Street
Thorndon
PO Box 12-506
Wellington 6038
(0)4 473-6510
(0)4 473-6513 (fax)
nzaot@nzaot.com
www.nzaot.com

New Zealand Audiological Society (NZAS)
PO Box 9724
Newmarket
Auckland
(0)9 524 4935
(0)9 524 4937 (fax)
0800 625 166 (toll-free NZ only)
nzas@xtra.co.nz
www.audiology.org.nz

New Zealand Dental Association (NZDA)
3 St. Marks Road
PO Box 28-084
Remuera, Auckland 1136
(0)9 524 2778
(0)9 520 5256 (fax)
nzdainfo@nzda.org.nz
www.nzda.org.nz

New Zealand Nurses Organisation (NZNO)
National Office
Level 3, Willbank Center
57 Willis Street
PO Box 2128
Wellington 6015
0800 28 38 48 (toll-free in New Zealand)
(0) 4 499 9533
(0) 4 382-9993 (fax)
www.nzno.org.nz

New Zealand Speech-Language Therapists Association (NZSTA)
Ste. 369, 63 Remuera Road
Newmarket
Auckland
03 235 8257
03 235 8850 (fax)
exec@nzsta-speech.org.nz
www.nzsta-speech.org.nz

New Zealand Veterinary Association (NZVA)
Level 2, 44 Victoria Street
PO Box 11-212 Manners Street
Wellington
04 471 0484
04 471 0494 (fax)
nzva@vets.org.nz
www.vets.org.nz

Nutrition Society of New Zealand (NSNZ)
PO Box 8094
Palmerston North
06 350 5962
j.coad@massey.ac.nz
www.nutritionsociety.ac.nz

Pharmacy Guild of New Zealand, Inc. (PGNZ)
124 Dixon Street, Te Aro
Wellington 6011
PO Box 27139, Marion Square
Wellington 6141
04 802 8200
04 384 8085 (fax)
enquiries@pgnz.org.nz
www.pgnz.org.nz

Physical Education New Zealand (PENZ)
PO Box 48201
Silverstream
Upper Hutt
04 5288 568
04 527 411 (fax)
simon@penz.org.nz
www.penz.org.nz

Royal Australasian College of Medical Administrators
Judith Parnell, Secretariat for New Zealand RACMA
PO Box 10-233
Wellington
Level 6, 99 The Terrace
Wellington
4 472 9183
4 472 9184
racma@afphm.org.nz
www.racma.edu.au

Royal Australian and New Zealand College of Ophthalmologists (RANZCO)
New Zealand Branch Office
New Zealand Medical Association
26 The Terrace
PO Box 156
Wellington
4 472 4741
4 471 0838
nzma@nzma.org.nz
ranzco@ranzco.edu

Sports Medicine New Zealand (SMNZ)
40 Logan Park Drive
PO Box 6398
Dunedin
03 477 7887
03 477 7882 (fax)
smznat@xtra.co.nz
www.sportsmedicine.co.nz

Pakistan (92)

Pakistan Dental Association (PDA)
Dr. Wasif Ali Khan
Surgimed Hospital
1-Zafar Ali Road
Lahore
42 57144118
42 5711582
42 5714 419 (fax)
president@pda.org.pk
www.pda.org.pk

Pakistan Nurses Federation (PNF)
173-G/2 Model Town
Lahore
42 516 6395
42 920 4202

Pakistan Occupational Therapy Association (POTA)
408-C Saima Gardens
H/167 Khalid Bin Waleed Road
Block C, PECHS
Karachi
NighatLodhi@hotmail.com

Sports Medicine Association of Pakistan (SMAP)
Hill Park
General Hospital
Shaheed-e-Millat Road
Karachi
21 492 7900 & 455 2442
21 506 0343 & 493 4403 (fax)

Philippines (63)

Philippine Nursing Association
1663 F.T. Benitez Street
Malate, Manila 1004
536-1888
525-1596 (fax)
Department of Nursing Education
Dr. Remigia Nathanielsz
Fatima College, Valenzuela City
293-2713 ext 312
293-2794-06
pna-ph.org

Association of Deans of Philippine Colleges of Nursing (ADPCN)
Dean Carmelita C. Divinagracia, President
603 A. Tower II, Bayview International Towers
Roxas Boulevard
Parañaque City
855-7010 (ADPCN office)
713-3390 T/F

Association of Diabetes Nurse Educators of the Philippines
Ms. Rosa Mia T. Balolong, President
Lot 4 Blk. 52, Apitong Street, Marikina Heights
Marikina City
942-0313

Phillipines Center For Diabetes Education Foundation (PCDEF)
Rm. 366 Diabetes Educational Center
Makati Medical Center
Makati
(632) 893-6017
secretariat@diabetescenter.org.ph
www.diabetescenter.org.ph

Association of Nursing Service Administrators of the Philippines
Ms. Ma. Linda G. Buhat, President
Philippine Heart Center
East Avenue, Diliman
Quezon City
926-7618 T/F c/o Leah
713-1063 T/F
716-3901 Loc 383

Association of Private Duty Nurse Practitioners
Mrs. Margareth Lavadia, President
Our Lady of Lourdes Hospital
46 P. Sanchez Street, Sta. Mesa
Manila
714-7445

Catholic Nurses Guild of the Philippines (CNG)
Mrs. Lucia V. Soltes, President
2nd Floor UERM Nursing Service
Aurora Boulevard
Quezon City
715-8160

Critical Care Nurses Association of the Philippines (CCNAPI)
Mrs. Ma. Isabelita C. Rogado, President
8/F Medical Arts Building
Philippine Heart Center
East Avenue
Quezon City
925-2401 loc. 3823
426-4394 (fax)
updates@ccnapi.org
www.ccnapi.org

Military Nurses Association of the Philippines (MNAP)
Col. Leticia Faltado, President
Far Eastern University, College of Nursing
N. Reyes Street
Sampaloc, Manila
735-8695
735-0232 (fax)

National League Of Philippine Government Nurses
Mrs. Vicenta E. Borja, President
Ground Floor, Building 12
Administrative Office
San Lazaro Cmpd.
Sta. Cruz, Manila
742-3944 Telefax

Occupational Health Nurses Association Inc.
Cityland Condominium Tower 1
248 Sen. Gil Puyat Avenue
1200 Makati
840-2211
894-3049 (fax)

Operating Room Nurses Association of the Phillipines (ORNAP)
Ms. Teresita F. Artuz, President
University of Santo Tomas, Nursing Office
España Boulevard
Sampaloc, Manila
735-3001 Loc. 2317
732-1284 (fax)

Philippine Hospital Infection Control Nurses
Mrs. Victoria I. Ching, President
Room P0228 Infection Control Office
The Medical City, Ortigas Avenue
Pasig City
689-8244
635-5756 (fax)

Philippine Oncologic Nursing Association (PONA)
Ms. Helen Ayapana, President
Philippine General Hospital
Taft Avenue
Manila
524-2121
521-8450 Loc 3606
521-0009 T/F

Philippine Society of Emergency Care Nurses (PSECP)
Mrs. Virginia Ducusin, President
Department of Emergency Medical Services
Philippine General Hospital
Taft Avenue
Manila 1000
521-8450 Loc 3923
404 3760 (fax)
www.psecp.org

Renal Nurses Association of the Philippines
Ms. Raquel Tejada, President
Philippine Heart Center
East Avenue, Diliman
Quezon City
925-2401 L2474
929-1011 (fax)

Society of Cardiovascular Nurse Practitioners of the Philippines
Ms. Leyda E. Dela Cuesta, President
Philippine Heart Center
East Avenue, Diliman
Quezon City
925-2401 Loc 2358
924-6804 (fax)

Singapore (65)

Pharmaceutical Society of Singapore (PSS)
Alumini Medical Centre, 2nd Level
2 College Road
Singapore 169850
6221 1136
6223 0969 (fax)
admin@pss.org.sg
www.pss.org.sg

Singapore Anti-Tuberculosis Association (MOH)
College of Medicine Building 16
College Road
Singapore 169854
63259220
62241677 (fax)
moh_info@moh.gov.sg
www.moh.gov.sg

Singapore Association of Occupational Therapists (SAOT)
Orchard PO Box 0475
Singapore 912316
info@saot.org.sg
www.saot.org.sg

Singapore Dental Association (SDA)
2 College Road
Level 2 Alumni Medical Centre
Singapore 169850
6220 2588
6224 7967(fax)
admin@sda.org.sg
www.sda.org.sg

Singapore Nurses Association (SNA)
SNA House
77 Maude Road
Singapore 208353
63920770
63927877 (fax)
sna@sna.org.sg
www.sna.org.sg

Singapore Nutrition and Dietetics Association (SNDA)
Tanglin
PO Box 180
Singapore 912406
secretary@snda.org.sg
www.snda.org.sg

Singapore Speech, Language, and Hearing Association (SHAS)
Speech Therapy Department
Singapore General Hospital
Outram Road
Singapore 169608
326 5481 (Ms. Wong Seng Mun)
326 5497 (fax)
enquiries@shas.org.sg
www.shas.org.sg

Singapore Veterinary Association (SVA)
c/o Agri food & Veterinary Authority
5 Maxwell Road
#18-00 Tower Block
MND Complex
Singapore 069110
227 0670
62 206068 (fax)
sva@sva.org.sg
www.sva.org.sg

Society for Emergency Medicine in Singapore (SEMS)
c/o Dept. of Emergency Medicine
Singapore General Hospital
Outram Road
Singapore 169608
6321 3558
6321 4873 (fax)
enquiry@semsonline.org
www.semsonline.org

South Africa (27)

Health Professions Council of South Africa (HPCSA)
P O Box 205
Pretoria 0001
553 Vermeulen Street
Cnr Hamilton and Vermeulen Street
Arcadia, Pretoria
(012) 338 9300, (012) 338 6680
(012) 328 5120, (012) 325 2074 (fax)
hpcsa@hpcsa.co.za
www.hpcsa.co.za

Health Professions Professional Boards
Dental Therapy & Oral Hygiene:
Alta Pieters
012 338 9480
altap@hpcsa.co.za

Dietetics:
Adelle Taljaard
012 338 9349
adellet@hpcsa.co.za

Emergency Care:
Alta Pieters
012 338 9480
altap@hpcsa.co.za

Environmental Health:
Danie Kotzé
012 338 9325
daniek@hpcsa.co.za

Medical & Dental:
Lenora Swanepoel
012 338 9327
lenoras@hpcsa.co.za

Medical Technology:
Adelle Taljaard
012 338 9349
adellet@hpcsa.co.za

Occupational Therapy:
Danie Kotzé
012 338 9325
daniek@hpcsa.co.za

Medical Orthotics/Prosthetics & Arts Therapy:
Rodney Msibi
012 338 9448
rodneym@hpcsa.co.za

Optometry & Dispensing Opticians:
Danie Kotzé
012 338 9325
daniek@hpcsa.co.za

Physiotherapy, Podiatry & Biokinetics:
Rodney Msibi
012 338 9448
rodneym@hpcsa.co.za

Psychology:
Emmanuel Chanza (or Elmarie Wood)
012 338 9339 (or 012 338 9437)
emmanuelc@hpcsa.co.za
elmariew@hpcsa.co.za

Radiography & Clinical Technology:
Adelle Taljaard
012 338 9349
adellet@hpcsa.co.za

Speech, Language & Hearing Professions:
Danie Kotzé
012 338 9325
daniek@hpcsa.co.za

Occupational Therapy Association of South Africa (OTASA)
PO Box 11695
Hatfield 0028
(012) 365 1327
(0) 86 651 5483 (fax)
otasa@otasa.org.za
www.otasa.org.za

South Africa Medical Association (SAMA)
Block F Castle Walk Office Park
Nossob Street
Erasmuskloof Ext 3
PO Box 74789
Lynnwood Ridge
Pretoria 0040
(012) 481 2000
(012) 481 2100 (fax)
online@samedical.org
www.samedical.org

South African Nursing Council (SANC)
602 Pretorius Street
Arcadia
Pretoria 0083
PO Box 1123
Pretoria 0001
(012) 420 1000
(012) 343 5400 (fax)
registrar@sanc.co.za
www.sanc.co.za

South African Society of Physiotherapy (SASP)
PO Box 92125
Norwood 2117
(011) 485 1467
(011) 485 1613 (fax)
manager@saphysio.co.za
www.physiosa.org.za

South African Speech-Language-Hearing Association (SASI HA)
PO Box 10813
Linton Grange 6015
41 360 1908
41 360 2401(fax)
admin@saslha.co.za
www.saslha.co.za

South Africa Sports Medicine Association (SASMA)
PO Box 2491
Bedfordview 2008
11 717 3372
11 717 3379 (fax)
info@sasma.org.za
www.sasma.org.za

South Africa Thoracic Society (SATS)
PO Box 16433
Vlaeberg 8018
(021) 423 0257
(021) 423 5629
sarj@iafrica.com
www.pulmonology.co.za

Switzerland (41)

International Council of Nurses (ICN)
3, Place Jean Marteau
1201-Geneva
22-908-01-00
22-908-01-01 (fax)
icn@icn.ch
www.icn.ch

United Kingdom (44)

Anatomical Society of Great Britain and Ireland (ASGBI)
Honorary Secretary Professor D.J. Watt
Brighton and Sussex Medical School
University of Sussex
Falmer, Brighton BN1 9PX, UK
(0)1273 644187
(0)1273 644440 (fax)
diana.watt@bsms.ac.uk
www.anatsoc.org.uk

The Association of Clinical Pathologists (TACP)
189 Dyke Road
Hove, East Sussex BN3 1TL
01273 775700
01273 773303 (fax)
info@pathologists.org.uk
www.pathologists.org.uk

British Academy of Audiology (BAA)
New body replacing British Association of Audiological Scientists (BAAS), British Association of Audiologists (BAAT), and British Society of Hearing Therapists (BSHT)
PO Box 346
Peterborough RM, PE6 7EG
01733 253 976, ext. 4172
admin@baaudiology.org
www.baaudiology.org

British Association and College of Occupational Therapists (BAOT/COT)
106-114 Borough High Street
Southwark, London SE1 1LB
020 7357 6480
020 7459 2299 (fax)
careers@cot.co.uk
www.cot.co.uk

British Association for Immediate Care (BASICS)
BASICS Headquarters
Turret House
Turret Lane
Ipswich IP4 1DL
0870 1654999
0870 1654949 (fax)
admin@basics.org.uk
www.basics.org.uk

British Association of Critical Care Nurses (BACCN)
BACCN Administration
Wessex House
Eastleigh Business Centre
Upper Market Street
Eastleigh, Hants SO50 9FD
0844 800 8843
baccn@baccn.org
www.baccn.org

British Association of Dental Nurses (BADN)
PO Box 4
Room 200
Hillhouse International Business Centre
Thornton-Cleveleys FY5 4QD
08702 110 113
admin@badn.org.uk
www.badn.org.uk

British Association of Oral and Maxillofacial Surgeons (BAOMS)
Royal College of Surgeons of England
35-43 Lincoln's Inn Fields
London WC2A 3PN
020 7405 8074
020 7430 9997
office@baoms.org.uk
www.baoms.org.uk

British Association of Sport and Exercise Medicine (BASEM)
Chairperson: Dr. Desmond Thompson
The Surgery
20 Lee Road
Blackheath
London SE3 9RT
0208 852 1235/8018
0208 297 2193 (fax)
desmond.thompson@nhs.net
desthompson@msn.com
www.basem.co.uk

British Association of Sport and Exercise Sciences (BASES)
Leeds Metropolitan University
Carnegie Faculty of Sport and Education
Fairfax Hall
Headingley Campus, Beckett Park
Leeds LS6 3QS
(0)113 2836162/63/64
(0)113 2836162 (fax)
chitchings@bases.org.uk
www.bases.org.uk

British Dental Association (BDA)
64 Wimpole Street
London W1G 8YS
020 7935 0875
020 7487 5232 (fax)
enquiries@bda.org
www.bda.org

The British Dietetic Association (TBDA)
5th Floor, Charles House
148/9 Great Charles Street Queensway
Birmingham B3 3HT
0121 200 8080
0121 200 8081 (fax)
info@bda.uk.com
www.bda.uk.com

British Medical Association (BMA)
BMA House
Tavistock Square
London WC1H 9JP
020 7387 4499
020 7383 6400 (fax)
info.web@bma.org.uk
www.bma.org.uk

British Nuclear Medical Society (BNMS)
Regent House, 291 Kirkdale
London SE26 4QD
020 8676 7864
020 8676 8417 (fax)
office@bnms.org.uk
www.bnms.org.uk

British Paramedic Association (BPM)
College of Paramedics (CPD)
28 Wilfred Street
Derby, Derbyshire DE23 8GF
01332 746356
exec.bpa@britishparamedic.org
www.britishparamedic.org

British Small Animal Veterinary Association (BSAVA)
Woodrow House
1 Telford Way
Waterwells Business Park
Quedgeley, Gloucester GL2 4AB
01452 726 700
01452 726 701 (fax)
customerservices@bsava.com
www.bsava.com

British Society of Audiology (BSA)
80 Brighton Road
Reading RG6 1PS
01189 660 622
01189 351 915 (fax)
bsa@thebsa.org.uk
www.thebsa.org.uk

The British Veterinary Nursing Association (BVNA)
82 Greenway Business Centre
Harlow Business Park
Harlow, Essex CM19 5QE
01279 408644
01279 408645 (fax)
bvna@bvna.co.uk
www.bvna.org.uk

Chartered Society of Physiotherapy (CSP)
14 Bedford Row
London WC1R 4ED
020 7306 6666
020 7306 6611 (fax)
enquiries@csp.org.uk
www.csp.org.uk

College of Operating Department Practitioners (CODP)
197-199 City Road
London EC1V 1JN0
870 746 0984
0870 746 0985 (fax)
office@codp.org.uk
www.aodp.org

Federation of European Nurses in Diabetes (FEND)
24 Holmesdale Avenue
London SW14 7BQ
020 8876 6122
info@fend.org
www.fend.org

Neonatal Nurses Association (NNA)
PO Box 8708
Nottingham NG2 9BJ
0115 941 7224
nnaoffice@nna.org.uk
www.nna.org.uk

Nursing and Midwifery Council (NMC)
23 Portland Place
London W1B 1P2
0207 637 7181
0207 436 2924 (fax)
communications@nmc-uk.org
advice@nmc-uk.org
www.nmc-uk.org

Resuscitation Council (UK)(RESUS)
Tavistock House North, 5th Floor
Tavistock Square
London WC1H 9HR
020 7388 4678
020 7383 0773 (fax)
enquiries@resus.org.uk
www.resus.org.uk

Royal British Nurses' Association (RBNA)
Riverbank House Business Centre
5th Floor, Room 502
1 Putney Bridge Approach
London SW6 3JD
020 7731 0550
www.r-bna.com

Royal College of Nursing (RCN)
(England, Scotland, Wales, Northern Ireland)
0845 772 6100
policycontacts@rcn.org.uk
www.rcn.org.uk

Royal Pharmaceutical Society of Great Britain (RPSGB)
1 Lambeth High Street
London SE1 7JN
0207 735 9141
0207 735 7629 (fax)
enquiries@rpsgb.org.uk
www.rpsgb.org.uk

Royal Society of Medicine (RSM)
1 Wimpole Street
London W1G 0AE
0207 290 2991
0207 290 2900
0207 290 2989(fax)
membership@rsm.ac.uk
www.rsm.ac.uk

The Society of Radiographers (SOR)
207 Providence Square
Mill Street
London SE1 2EW
0207 740 7200
0207 740 7204 (fax)
joelw@sor.org
www.sor.org

United States (1)

Academy of Medical-Surgical Nurses (AMSN)
East Holly Avenue, Box 56
Pitman, NJ 08071-0056
(866) 877-AMSN (2676)
(866) 589-7463 (fax)
AMSN@ajj.com
www.medsurgnurse.org

Air & Surface Transport Nurses Association (ASTNA)
7995 East Prentice Avenue, Ste. 100
Greenwood Village, CO 80111
(800) 897-NFNA (6362)
(303) 770-1812 (fax)
astna@gwami.com
www.astna.org

Alpha Tau Delta National Fraternity for Professional Nurses (ATD)
11252 Camarillo Street
Toluca Lake, CA 91602
info@atdnursing.com
www.atdnursing.org

American Academy of Anesthesiologist Assistants (AAAA)
PO Box 13978
Tallahasee, FL 32317
(850) 656-8848
(850) 656-3038 (fax)
info@anesthetist.org
www.anesthetist.org

American Academy of Audiology (AAAF)
11730 Plaza America Drive, Ste. 300
Reston, VA 20190
(800) AAA-2336
(703) 790-8466
(703) 790-8631 (fax)
sdavis@audiology.org
www.audiology.org

American Academy of Forensic Sciences (AAFS)
410 North 21st Street
Colorado Springs, CO 80904
(719) 636-1100
(719) 636-1993 (fax)
jhurley@aafs.org
aafs.org

American Academy of Nurse Practitioners (AANP)
PO Box 12846
Austin, TX 78711
(512) 442-4262
(512) 442-6469 (fax)
admin@aanp.org
www.aanp.org

American Academy of Nursing (AAN)
555 East Wells Street, Ste. 1100
Milwaukee, WI 53202-3823
(414) 287-0289
(414) 276-3349 (fax)
www.aannet.org

American Academy of Physician Assistants (AAPA)
950 N. Washington Street
Alexandria, VA 22314
(703) 836-2272
(703) 684-1924 (fax)
aapa@aapa.org
www.aapa.org

American Academy of Urgent Care Medicine (AAUCM)
2813 S. Hiawassee Road, Ste. 206
Orlando, FL 32835
(407) 521-5789
(407) 521-5790 (fax)
www.aaucm.org

American Alliance for Health, Physical Education, Recreation, and Dance (AAHPERD)
1900 Association Drive
Reston, VA 20191
(703) 476-3400
(800) 213-7193
info@aahperd.org
www.aahperd.org

American Association for Continuity of Care (AACC)
638 Prospect Avenue
Hartford, CT 06105
(860) 586-7525
(800) 586-7550
cagleyden@aol.com

American Association for Nurse Life Care Planners (AANLCP)
3267 East 3300 South #309
Salt Lake City, UT 84109
(888) 575-4047
(801) 274-1184
(801) 274-1535 (fax)
www.aanlcp.org

The American Association for Nurse Attorneys (TAANA)
PO Box 515
Columbus, OH 43216-0515
(877) 538-2262
(614) 221-2335
taana@taana.org
www.taana.org

American Association for Respiratory Care (AARC)
9425 N. MacArthur Boulevard, Ste. 100
Irving, TX 75063
(972) 243-2272
(972) 484-2720 (fax)
(972) 484-6010 (fax)
info@aarc.org
www.aarc.org

American Association of Colleges of Nursing (AACN)
One Dupont Circle NW, Ste. 530
Washington, DC 20036
(202) 463-6930
(202) 785-8320 (fax)
mfrole@aacn.nche.edu
www.aacn.nche.edu

American Association of Critical-Care Nurses (AACN)
101 Columbia
Aliso Viejo, CA 92656-4109
(800) 899-2226
(949) 362-2000
(949) 362-2020 (fax)
info@aacn.org
www.aacn.org

American Association of Diabetes Educators (AADE)
100 W. Monroe Street, Ste. 400
Chicago, IL 60603
(800) 338-3633
(312) 424-2427 (fax)
aadc@aadnet.org
www.diabeteseducator.org

American Association of Legal Nurse Consultants (AALNC)
401 North Michigan Avenue
Chicago, IL 60611
(877) 402-2562
(312) 673-6655 (fax)
info@aalnc.org
www.aalnc.org

American Association of Managed Care Nurses (AAMCN)
4435 Waterfront Drive, Ste. 101
Glen Allen, VA 23060
(804) 747-9698
(804) 747-5316 (fax)
lgivens@aamcn.org
www.aamcn.org

American Association of Medical Assistants (AAMA)
20 N. Wacker Drive, Ste. 1575
Chicago, IL 60606
(312) 899-1500
www.aama-ntl.org

American Association of Neuroscience Nurses (AANN)
The American Board of Neuroscience Nursing (ABNN)
Neuroscience Nursing Foundation (NNF)
4700 W. Lake Avenue
Glenview, IL 60025
(888) 557-2266 (US only)
(847) 375-4733
(877) 734-8677 (fax)
(732) 460-7313 (international fax)
info@aann.org
www.aann.org

American Association of Nurse Anesthetists (AANA)
222 South Prospect Avenue
Park Ridge, IL 60068-4001
(847) 692-7050
(847) 692-6968 (fax)
info@aana.com
www.aana.com

American Association of Occupational Health Nurses, Inc. (AAOHN)
2920 Brandywine Road, Ste. 100
Atlanta, GA 30341
(770) 455-7757
(770) 455-7271 (fax)
www.aaohn.org

American Association of Operating Room Nurses, Inc. (AORN)
2170 S Parker Road, Ste. 300
Denver, CO 80231
(800) 755-2676 (303) 755-6304
custserv@aorn.org
www.aorn.org

American Association of Sleep Technologists (AAST)
One Westbrook Corporate Center, Ste. 920
Westchester, IL 60154
(708) 492-0796
(708) 273-9344 (fax)
cwaring@aastweb.org
www.aastweb.org

American Association of Spinal Cord Injury Nurses (AASCIN)
75-20 Astoria Boulevard
Jackson Heights, NY 11370
(718) 803-3782
(718) 803-0414 (fax)
aascin@unitedspinal.org
www.aascin.org

American College of Clinical Pharmacology (ACCP)
3 Ellinwood Court
New Hartford, NY 13413
(315) 768-6117
(315) 768-6119 (fax)
sue@accp1.org
www.accp1.org

American College of Clinical Pharmacy (ACCP)
World Headquarters
13000 W. 87th Street Parkway
Lenexa, KS 66215-4530
(913) 492-3311
(913) 492-0088 (fax)
accp@accp.com
www.accp.com

American College of Emergency Physicians (ACEP)
membership@acep.org
www.acep.org

1125 Executive Circle
Irving, TX 75038
PO Box 619911
Dallas, TX 75261
(800) 798-1822
(972) 550-0911
(972) 580-2816 (fax)

Washington DC office
2121 K Street NW, Ste. 325
Washington, DC 20037
(800) 320-0610
(202) 728-0610
(202) 728-0617 (fax)

American College Health Association (ACHA)
891 Elkridge Landing Road, Ste. 100
Linthicum, MD 21090
PO Box 28937
Baltimore, MD 21240
(410) 859-1500
(410) 859-1510 (fax)
sainsworth@acha.org
www.acha.org

American College of Health-Care Administrators (ACHCA)
300 N. Lee Street, Ste. 301
Alexandria, VA 22314
(703) 739-7900
(703) 739-7901 (fax)
membership@achca.org
www.achca.org

American College of Medical Quality (ACMQ)
4334 Montgomery Avenue, Ste. B
Bethesda, MD 20814
(301) 913-9149
(800) 924-2149
(301) 913-9142 (fax)
www.acmq.org

American College of Nurse-Midwives (ACNM)
8403 Colesville Road, Ste. 1550
Silver Spring, MD 20910
(240) 485-1800
(240) 485-1818 (fax)
www.midwife.org
www.acnm.org

American College of Nurse Practitioners (ACNP)
1501 Wilson Boulevard, Ste. 509
Arlington, VA 22209
(703) 740-2529
(703) 740-2533
acnp@acnpweb.org
www.acnpweb.org

American College of Radiology (ACR)
info@acr.org
www.acr.org

Headquarters Office
1891 Preston White Drive
Reston, VA 20191
(800) ACR-LINE (227-5463)

Government Relations Office
1701 Pennsylvania Avenue NW, Ste. 610
Washington, DC 20006
(202) 223-1670

Clinical Research Office
1818 Market Street, Ste. 1600
Philadelphia, PA 19103
(215) 574-3150

American College of Sports Medicine (ACSM)
401 West Michigan Street
Indianapolis, IN 46202-3233
PO Box 1440
Indianapolis, IN 46206
(317) 637-9200
(317) 634-7817 (fax)
publicinfo@acsm.org
www.acsm.org

American Dental Assistants Association (ADAA)
35 East Wacker Drive, Ste. 1730
Chicago, IL 60601
(312) 541-1550
(312) 541-1496 (fax)
srobles@adaa1.com
www.dentalassistant.org

American Dental Association (ADA)
211 East Chicago Avenue
Chicago, IL 60611
(312) 440-2500
membership@ada.org
www.ada.org

American Dental Hygienists' Association (ADHA)
444 North Michigan Avenue, Ste. 3400
Chicago, IL 60611
(312) 440-8900
mail@adha.net
www.adha.org

American Dietetic Association (ADA)
foundation@eatright.org
www.eatright.org

Headquarters
120 South Riverside Plaza, Ste. 2000
Chicago, IL 60606
(800) 877-1600

Washington DC Office
1120 Connecticut Avenue NW, Ste. 480
Washington, DC 20036
(800) 877-0877
(202) 775-8284 (fax)

American Health Information Management Association (AHIMA)
233 N. Michigan Avenue, 21st Floor
Chicago, IL 60601
(312) 233-1100
(312) 233-1090 (fax)
info@ahima.org
www.ahima.org

American Holistic Nurses Association (AHNA)
323 N. San Francisco Street, Ste. 201
Flagstaff, AZ 86001
(800) 278-2462
info@ahna.org
www.ahna.org

American Industrial Hygiene Association (AIHA)
2700 Prosperity Avenue, Ste. 250
Fairfax, VA 22031
(703) 849-8888
(703) 207-3561
infonet@aiha.org
www.aiha.org

American Massage Therapy Association (AMTA)
500 Davis Street, Ste. 900
Evanston, IL 60201-4695
(877) 905-2700
(847) 864-0123
(847) 864-1178 (fax)
info@amtamassage.org
www.amtamassage.org

American Medical Informatics Association (AMIA)
4915 St. Elmo Avenue, Ste. 401
Bethesda, MD 20814
(301) 657-1291
(301) 657-1296 (fax)
mail@amia.org
www.amia.org

American Medical Technologist (AMT)
10700 West Higgins Road, Ste. 150
Rosemont, IL 60018
membership@amt1.com
www.amt1.com

American Nephrology Nurses Association (ANNA)
East Holly Avenue, Box 56
Pitman, NJ 08071-0056
(888) 600-2662
(856) 256-2320
(856) 589-7463 (fax)
anna@ajj.com
www.annanurse.org

American Nurses Association (ANA)
8515 Georgia Avenue, Ste. 400
Silver Spring, MD 20910
(800) 274-4262 (toll-free)
(301) 628-5000
(301) 628-5001 (fax)
www.ana.org
www.nursingworld.org

American Nurses Foundation (ANF)
8515 Georgia Avenue, Ste. 400
Silver Spring, MD 20910
(301) 628-5227
anf@ana.org
anfonline.org

Center for American Nurses (CAN)
8515 Georgia Avenue, Ste. 400
Silver Spring, MD 20910
(301) 628-5243
(301) 628-5297 (fax)
info@centerforamericannurses.org
www.centerforamericannurses.org

American Occupational Therapy Association (AOTA)
4720 Montgomery Lane
PO Box 31220
Bethesda, MD 20824
(301) 652-2682
(800) 377-8555 (TDD)
(301) 652-7711 (fax)
www.aota.org

American Pharmaceutical Association (APhA)
1100 15th Street NW, Ste. 400
Washington, DC 20005
(800) 237-2742
(202) 628-4410
(202) 783-2351 (fax)
www.aphanet.org

American Physical Therapy Association (APTA)
1111 N. Fairfax Street
Alexandria, VA 22314
(703) 684-2782
(800) 999-2782
(703) 683-6748 (TDD)
(703) 684-7343 (fax)
education@apta.org
www.apta.org

American Psychiatric Nurses Association (APNA)
1555 Wilson Boulevard, Ste. 602
Arlington, VA 22209
(866) 243-2443
(703) 243-3390 (fax)
inform@apna.org
www.apna.org

American Public Health Association (APHA)
800 I Street NW
Washington, DC 20001
(202) 777-APHA (2742)
(202) 777-2534 (fax)
comments@apha.org
www.apha.org

American Registry of Diagnostic Medical Sonographers (ARDMS)
51 Monroe Street, Plaza East One
Rockville, MD 20850
(301) 738-8401
(800) 541-9754
(301) 738-0312/0313 (fax)
administration@ardms.org
www.ardms.org

American Registry of Radiologic Technologists (AART)
1255 Northland Drive, Ste. 300
St. Paul, MN 55120
(651) 687-0048
www.arrt.org

American Society for Clinical Laboratory Science (ASCLS)
6701 Democracy Boulevard, Ste. 300
Bethesda, MD 20817
(301) 657-2768
(301) 657-2909 (fax)
ascls@ascls.org
www.ascls.org

American Society for Clinical Nutrition (ASCN)
9650 Rockville Park
Bethesda, MD 20814
(301) 634-7892 (fax)
mem@nutrition.org
www.nutrition.org

American Society for Microbiology (ASM)
1752 N Street, NW
Washington, DC 20036
(202) 737-3600
Journals@asmusa.org
www.asm.org

American Society for Parenteral and Enteral Nutrition (ASPEN)
8630 Fenton Street, Ste. 412
Silver Spring, MD 20910
(800) 727-4567
(301) 587-6315
aspen@nutr.org
www.clinnutr.org

American Society for Therapeutic Radiology and Oncology (ASTRO)
8280 Willow Oaks Corporate Drive, Ste. 500
Fairfax, VA 22031
(703) 502-1550
(800) 962-7876
(703) 502-7852 (fax)
www.astro.org

American Society for Clinical Pathology (ASCP)
www.ascp.org

ASCP Board of Registry
33 West Monroe, Ste. 1600
Chicago, IL 60603
(800) 267-2727
(312) 541-4999
(312) 541-4998
bor@ascp.org

Washington Office
1225 New York Avenue NW, Ste. 250
Washington, DC 20005
(202) 347-4450
Info@ascp.org

American Society of Echocardiography (ASE)
1500 Sunday Drive, Ste. 102
Raleigh, NC 27607
(919) 861-5574
(919) 787-4916 (fax)
rcouch@asecho.org
www.asecho.org

American Society of Electroneurodiagnostic Technologists (ASET)
6501 East Commerce Avenue, Ste. 120
Kansas City, MO 64120
(816) 931-1120
(816) 931-1145 (fax)
sheila@aset.org
www.aset.org

American Society of Extra-Corporeal Technology (AmSECT)
AmSECT National Office
2209 Dickens Road
Herndon, VA 23230-2005
(804) 565-6363
(804) 282-0090 (fax)
stewart@amsect.org
www.amsect.org

American Society of PeriAnesthesia Nurses (ASPAN)
10 Melrose Avenue, Ste. 110
Cherry Hill, NJ 08003-3696
(877) 737-9696
(856) 616-9600
(856) 616-9601 (fax)
aspan@aspan.org
www.aspan.org

American Society of Radiologic Technologists (ARST)
15000 Central Avenue SE
Albuquerque, NM 87123
(800) 444-2778, press 5
(505) 298-4500
(505) 298-5063 (fax)
customerinfo@asrt.org
www.asrt.org

American Speech-Language-Hearing Association (ASHA)
10801 Rockville Park
Rockville, MD 20852
(800) 498-2071 (Member)
(800) 638-8255 (Non-Member)
(800) 897-5700, ext 4157 (TTY)
(240) 333-4705 (fax)
actioncenter@asha.org
www.asha.org

American Thoracic Society (ATS)
61 Broadway
New York, NY 10006
(212) 315-8600
(212) 315-6498 (fax)
atsinfo@thoracic.org
www.thoracic.org

American Veterinary Medical Association (AVMA)
www.avma.org

Headquarters
1931 N. Meacham Road, Ste. 100
Schaumburg, IL 60173
(847) 925-8070
(847) 925-1329 (fax)
avmainfo@avma.org

Governmental Relations Division
1910 Sunderland Place NW
Washington, DC 20036
(800) 321-1473
(202) 842-4360 (fax)
avmagrd@avma.org

Animal and Plant Health Inspection Service (APHIS)
www.aphis.usda.gov

Headquarters
USDA/APHIS/AC
4700 River Road, Unit 84
Riverdale, MD 20737
(301) 734-7833
(301) 734-4978 (fax)
ace@aphis.usda.gov

Western Region
USDA/APHIS/AC
2150 Centre Avenue
Building B Mailstop 3W11
Fort Collins, CO 80526
(970) 494-7478
(970) 494-7461 (fax)
acwest@aphis.usda.gov

Eastern Region
USDA/APHIS/AC
920 Main Campus Drive, Ste. 200
Raleigh, NC 27606-5210
(919) 855-7100
(919) 855-7123 (fax)
aceast@aphis.usda.gov

Association for Healthcare Documentation Integrity (AHDI)
Formerly American Association for Medical Transcription (AAMT)
4230 Kierman Avenue, Ste. 130
Modesto, CA 95356
(800) 982-2182
(209) 527-9620
(209) 527-9633 (fax)
ahdi@ahdionline.org
www.ahdionline.org

Association for Professionals in Infection Control and Epidemiology, Inc. (APIC)
1275 K Street NW, Ste. 1000
Washington, DC 20005
(202) 789-1890
(202) 789-1899 (fax)
APICinfo@apic.org
www.apic.org

Association of Medical Illustrators (AMI)
810 East 10th Street
PO Box 1897
Lawrence, KS 66044
(866) 393-4AMI (4264)
(785) 843-1274 (fax)
hq@ami.org
www.ami.org

Association of Nurses in AIDS Care (ANAC)
3538 Ridgewood Road
Akron, OH 44333-3122
(800) 260-6780
(330) 670-0101
(330) 670-0109 (fax)
anac@anacnet.org
www.anacnet.org

Association of Pediatric Hematology/Oncology Nurses (APHON)
4700 W Lake Avenue
Glenview, IL 60025
(847) 375-4724
(877) 734-8755 (fax)
info@aphon.org
www.aphon.org

Association of Polysomnographic Technologists (AAST)
One Westbrook Corporate Center, Ste. 920
Westchester, IL 60154
(708) 492-0796
(708) 273-9344
cwaring@aastweb.org
www.aastweb.org

Association of Public Health Laboratories (APHL)
8515 Georgia Avenue, Ste. 700
Silver Spring, MD 20910
(240) 485-2745
(240) 485-2700 (fax)
info@aphl.org
www.aphl.org

Association of Rehabilitation Nurses (ARN)
4700 W Lake Avenue
Glenview, IL 60025
(800) 229-7530
(847) 375-4710
(877) 734-9384 (fax)
info@rehabnurse.org
www.rehabnurse.org

Association of Schools of Public Health (ASPH)
1101 15th Street NW, Ste. 910
Washington, DC 20005
(202) 296-1099
(202) 296-1252 (fax)
info@asph.org
www.asph.org

Association of State and Territorial Health Officials (ASTHO)
1275 K Street NW, Ste. 800
Washington, DC 20005
(202) 371-9090, ext. 1635
(202) 371-9797 (fax)
jhohl@astho.org
www.astho.org

Association of Surgical Technologists (AST)
6 West Dry Creek Circle, Ste. 200
Littleton, CO 80120
(800) 637-7433
(303) 694-9130
(303) 694-9169 (fax)
wendy.grillo@ast.org
www.ast.org

Association of Women's Health, Obstetrics, and Neonatal Nurses (AWHONN)
formerly NAACOG
AWHONN Headquarters
2000 L Street NW, Ste. 740
Washington, DC 20036
(202) 261-2400
(800) 673-8499 (toll-free US)
(800) 245-0231 (toll-free Canada)
(202) 728-0575 (fax)
customerservice@awhonn.org
www.awhonn.org

Center for Infectious Disease Research & Policy (CIDRAP)
University of Minnesota
Academic Health Center
420 Delaware Street, SE
MMC 263
Minneapolis, MN 55455
(612) 626-6770
(612) 626-6783 (fax)
cidrap@umn.edu
www.cidrap.umn.edu

Competency and Credentialing Institute (CCI) (nursing)
2170 South Parker Road, Ste. 295
Denver, CO 80231
(303) 369-9566
(888) 257-2667
(303) 695-8464 (fax)
info@cc-institute.org
www.cc-institute.org
www.certboard.org

Council of State and Territorial Epidemiologists (CSTE)
2872 Woodcock Boulevard, Ste. 303
Atlanta, GA 30341
(770) 458-3811
(770) 458-8516 (fax)
sclinton@cste.org
www.cste.org

EEG and Clinical Neuroscience Society (ECNS)
6015 State Bridge Road, #12206
Duluth, GA 30097
(770) 813-0404
www.ecnsweb.com

Emergency Nurses Association (ENA)
Headquarters
915 Lee Street
Des Plaines, IL 60016
(800) 900-9659
(800) 243-8362
enainfo@ena.org
www.ena.org

Hospice and Palliative Nurses Association (HPNA)
One Penn Center West, Ste. 229
Pittsburgh, PA 15276
(412) 787-9301
(412) 787-9305 (fax)
hpna@hpna.org
www.hpna.org

Infusion Nurses Society (INS)
315 Norwood Park South
Norwood, MA 02062
(781) 440-9408
(781) 440-9409 (fax)
bill.talbot@ins1.org (office manager)
www.ins1.org

International Association for Human Caring (IAHC)
2090 Linglestown Road, Ste. 107
Harrisburg, PA 17110
(717) 703-0033
(717) 234-6798 (fax)
christine@pronursingresources.com
www.humancaring.org

International Association of Emergency Managers (IAEM)
Beth Armstrong
IAEM Executive Director
201 Park Washington Court
Falls Church, VA 22046
(703) 538-1795
(703) 241-5603 (fax)
info@iaem.com
www.iaem.com

International Society for Environmental Epidemiology (ISEE)
c/o JSI Research & Training Institute
4 Farnsworth Street
Boston, MA 02210
(617) 482-9485
(617) 482 0617
iseepi@jsi.com
www.iseepi.org

International Society of Biometeorology (ISB)
Dr. Scott Greene
Department of Geography
University of Oklahoma
Norman, OK 73071
(405) 325 4319
(405) 447 8412
(405) 447 8455 (fax)
jgreene@ou.edu
www.biometeorology.org

International Society of Exposure Analysis (ISEA)
c/o JSI Research and Training Institute
4 Farnsworth Street
Boston, MA 02210
(617) 482-9485
(617) 482-0617 (fax)
iseamail@jsi.com
www.iseaweb.org

International Society of Psychiatric–Mental Health Nurses (ISPN)
2810 Crossroads Drive, Ste. 3800
Madison, WI 53718
(866) 330-7227
(608) 443-2463
(608) 443-2474 or 2478 (fax)
info@ispn-psych.org
www.ispn-psych.org

International Tactical EMS Association (ITEMS)
PO Box 504
Farmington, MI 48332
(248) 476-9077
(248) 476-0754 (fax)
TacticalEMS@aol.com
www.tems.org

International Transplant Nurses Society (ITNS)
1739 E. Carson Street, Box 351
Pittsburgh, PA 15203
(412) 343-ITNS
(412) 343-3959 (fax)
itns@msn.com
www.itns.org

League of Intravenous Therapy Education (LITE)
Empire Building, Ste. 3
3001 Jacks Run Road
White Oak, PA 15131
(412) 678-5025
(412) 678-5040 (fax)
info@lite.org
www.lite.org

Memorial Institute for the Prevention of Terrorism (MIPT)
621 N Robinson Avenue, 4th Floor
Oklahoma City, Oklahoma 73102
PO Box 889
Oklahoma City, OK 73101
(405) 278-6307
(405) 760-2216 (fax)
www.mipt.org

National Association for Home Care & Hospice (NAHC)
228 Seventh Street SE
Washington, DC 20003
(202) 547-7424
(202) 547-3540 (fax)
membership@nahc.org
www.nahc.org

National Association of City and County Health Officials (NACCHO)
1100 17th Street NW, 2nd Floor
Washington, DC 20036
(202) 783-5550
(202) 783-1583 (fax)
info@naccho.org
www.naccho.org

National Association of Clinical Nurse Specialists (NACNS)
2090 Linglestown Road, Ste. 107
Harrisburg, PA 17110
(717) 234-6799
(717) 234-6798 (fax)
nacnsorg@nacns.org
www.nacns.org

National Association of Emergency Medical Technicians (NAEMT)
132-A East Northside Drive
PO Box 1400
Clinton, MS 39060
(800) 34-NAEMT (346-2368)
(601) 924-7744
info@naemt.org
www.naemt.org

National Association of Hispanic Nurses
1501 16th Street NW
Washington, DC 20036
(202) 387-2477
(202) 483-7183 (fax)
info@thehispanicnurses.org
www.thehispanicnurses.org

National Association of Neonatal Nurses (NANN)
4700 W. Lake Avenue
Glenview, IL 60025-1485
(800) 451-3795
(847) 375-3660
(888) 477-6266 (fax)
(732) 380-3640 (fax)
info@nann.org
www.nann.org

National Association of School Nurses, Inc. (NASN)
8484 Georgia Avenue, Ste. 420
Silver Spring, MD 20910
(866) 627-6767
(240) 821-1130
(301) 585-1791 (fax)
nasn@nasn.org
www.nasn.org

National Athletic Trainers' Association (NATA)
2952 Stemmons Freeway #200
Dallas, TX 75247
(214) 637-6282
(214) 637-2206 (fax)
johno@nata.org
www.nata.org

National Black Nurses Association (NBNA)
8630 Fenton Street, Ste. 330
Silver Spring, MD 20910-3803
(301) 589-3200
(800) 575-6298
(301) 589-3223 (fax)
NBNA@erols.com
www.nbna.org

National Conference of Gerontological Nurse Practitioners (NCGNP)
7794 Grow Drive
Pensacola, FL 32514
(866) 355-1392
(850) 484-8762 (fax)
ncgnp@puetzamc.com
www.ncgnp.org

National Council of State Boards of Nursing, Inc. (NCSBN)
111 East Wacker Drive, Ste. 2900
Chicago, IL 60601
(312) 525-3600
(312) 279-1032 (fax)
(866) 293-9600 (toll-free for testing)
info@ncsbn.org
www.ncsbn.org

National Emergency Management Association (NEMA)
PO Box 11910
Lexington, KY 40578
(859) 244-8000
(859) 244-8239 (fax)
nemaadmin@csg.org
www.nemaweb.org

National Institute of Nursing Research (NINR)
National Institutes of Health
31 Center Drive
Room 5B10
Bethesda, MD 20892
(301) 496-0207
(866) 910-3804
(301) 594-5605 (TTY)
(301) 480-8845 (fax)
www.ninr.nih.gov

National League for Nursing (NLN)
61 Broadway, 33rd Floor
New York, NY 10006
(212) 363-5555
(800) 669-1656
(212) 812-0391 or (212) 812-0393 (fax)
generalinfo@nln.org
www.nln.org

National Registry of Emergency Medical Technicians (NREMT)
Rocco V. Morando Building
6610 Busch Boulevard
PO Box 29233
Columbus, OH 43229
(614) 888-4484
(614) 888-8920 (fax)
webmaster@nremt.org
www.nremt.org

National Safety Council (NSC)
1121 Spring Lake Drive
Itasca, IL 60143
(630) 285-1121
(630) 285-1315 (fax)
info@nsc.org
www.nsc.org

National Security Institute (NSI)
116 Main Street, Ste. 200
Medway, MA 02053
(508) 533-9099
(508) 533-3761 (fax)
webmaster@nsi.org
www.nsi.org

Navy Nurse Corps Association (NNCA)
PO Box 1229
Oak Harbor, WA 98277-1229
(360) 678-0825
(877) 662-2674
mike@nnca.org
www.nnca.org

Nurses Organization of Veterans Affairs (NOVA)
NOVA Foundation
1726 M Street NW, Ste. 1101
Washington, DC 20036
(202) 296-0888
(202) 833-1577
www.vanurse.org

Oncology Nursing Society (ONS)
125 Enterprise Drive
Pittsburgh, PA 15275
(866) 257-4ONS
(412) 859-6100
(877) 369-5497 (toll-free fax)
(412) 859-6162 (fax)
customer.service@ons.org
www.ons.org

Philippine Nurses Association of America (PNAA)
www.philippinenursesaa.org

Radiological Society of North America (RSNA)
820 Jorie Boulevard
Oak Brook, IL 60523
(800) 381-6660
(877) 776-2636 (Membership)
(630) 571-2670
(630) 571-7837 (fax)
membership@rsna.org
www.rsna.org

Sigma Theta Tau International, Inc. (STTI)
550 West North Street
Indianapolis, IN 46202
(888) 634-7575 (US/CAN)
(317) 634-8171
(317) 634-8188 (fax)
memserv@stti.iupui.edu
www.nursingsociety.org

Society of Diagnostic Medical Sonography (SDMS)
2745 Dallas Parkway, Ste. 350
Plano, TX 75093
(214) 473-8730
(800) 229-9506
(214) 473-8563 (fax)
bclay@sdms.org
www.sdms.org

Society of Trauma Nurses (STN)
1926 Waukegan Road, Ste. 1
Glenview, IL 60025
(505) 983-4923
(505) 983-5109 (fax)
info@TraumaNurseSoc.org
www.traumanursesoc.org

Society of Urologic Nurses and Associates (SUNA)
National Office
East Holly Avenue, Box 56
Pitman, NJ 08071-0056
(888) 827-7862
(609) 256-2335
(609) 589-7463 (fax)
suna@ajj.com
www.suna.org

Society of Vascular Ultrasound (SVU)
4601 Presidents Drive, Ste. 260
Lanham, MD 20706
(301) 459-7550
(301) 459-5651 (fax)
svuinfo@svunet.org
www.svunet.org

Transcultural Nursing Society
Madonna University College of Nursing and Health
36600 Schoolcraft Road
Livonia, MI 48150
(888) 432-5470
(734) 432-5463 (fax)
staff@tcns.org
www.tcns.org

Wound, Ostomy and Continence Nurses Society
WOCN Society National Office
15000 Commerce Parkway, Ste. C
Mt. Laurel, NJ 08054
(888) 224-WOCN (9626)
(856) 439-0525 (fax)
wocn_info@wocn.org
www.wocn.org

Professional Titles, Degrees, and Certificates

AuD	Doctor of Audiology
AARCF	American Association for Respiratory Care Fellow
AAS	Associate in Applied Science
ACP	Advanced Clinical Practitioner
ADN	Associate Degree in Nursing
AHI	Allied Health Instructor (American Medical Technologists)
ANP	Adult Nurse Practitioner
APRN	Advance Practice Registered Nurse
APRN-BC	Advance Practice Registered Nurse–Board Certified
ARNP	Advanced Registered Nurse Practitioner
ART	Accredited Records Technologist
ATC	Athletic Trainer, Certified
AT(ASCP)	Apheresis Technician (American Society for Clinical Pathology)
BA	Bachelor of Arts
BB(ASCP)	Technologist in Blood Banking (American Society for Clinical Pathology)
BCCS	Board Certified in Clinical Social Work
BCNP	Board Certified Nuclear Pharmacist
BCNSP	Board Certified Nutrition Support Pharmacist
BCPS	Board Certified Pharmacotherapy Specialist
BS	Bachelor of Science
BSN	Bachelor of Science in Nursing
CADC	Certified Alcohol and Drug Counselor
CALN	Clinical Administrative Liaison Nurse
C(ASCP)	Technologist in Chemistry (American Society for Clinical Pathology)
CAT(C)	Certified Athletic Therapist (Canada)
CCC-A	Certificate of Clinical Competence in Audiology
CCCP	Board Certified in Child and Adolescent Psychology
CCC-SLP	Certificate of Clinical Competence in Speech-Language Pathology
CCM	Certified Case Manager
CCMHC	Certified Clinical Mental Health Counselor
CCP	Certified Clinical Perfusionist
CCRN	Critical Care Registered Nurse
CCS	Cardiopulmonary Certified Specialist, Certified Coding Specialist
CDA	Certified Dental Assistant
CDE	Certified Diabetes Educator
CDT	Certified Dental Laboratory Technician
CEN	Certified Emergency Nurse
CCEMT-P	Critical Care Emergency Medical Technician–Paramedic
CCM	Certified Case Manager
CFNP	Certified Family Nurse Practitioner
CGT	Certified Gastroenterology Technician
CIH	Certificate in Industrial Health
CISW	Certified Independent Social Worker
CLA	Certified Laboratory Assistant
CLDir(NCA)	Clinical Laboratory Director (National Certification Agency for Medical Laboratory Personnel)

CLPlb(NCA)	Clinical Laboratory Phlebotomist (National Certification Agency for Medical Laboratory Personnel)
CLS	Clinical Laboratory Scientist
CLS(NCA)	Clinical Laboratory Scientist (certified by National Certification Agency for Medical Laboratory Personnel)
CLSp(CG)(NCA)	Clinical Laboratory Specialist in Cytogenetics (National Certification Agency for Medical Laboratory Personnel)
CLSp(H)(NCA)	Clinical Laboratory Specialist in Hematology (National Certification Agency for Medical Laboratory Personnel)
CLSup(NCA)	Clinical Laboratory Supervisor (National Certification Agency for Medical Laboratory Personnel)
CLT	Certified Laboratory Technician, Clinical Laboratory Technician
CLT(NCA)	Certified Laboratory Technician (National Certification Agency for Medical Laboratory Personnel)
CMA	Certified Medical Assistant
CMA-A	Certified Medical Assistant, Administrative
CMA-C	Certified Medical Assistant, Clinical
CMAS	Certified Medical Administrative Specialist (American Medical Technologists)
CMFT	Certified Marriage and Family Therapist
CMT	Certified Medical Transcriptionist (American Association for Medical Transcription)
CNA	Certified Nursing Assistant
CNIM	Certification in Neurophysiologic Intraoperative Monitoring (American Board of Registration of Electroencephalographic and Evoked Potential Technologists)
CNM	Certified Nurse Midwife
CNMT	Certified Nuclear Medicine Technologist
CNOR	Certified Nurse Operating Room
CNP	Community Nurse Practitioner
CNS	Clinical Nurse Specialist
CNSD	Certified Nutrition Support Dietitian
CNSN	Certified Nutrition Support Nurse
CNSP	Certified Nutrition Support Physician
COLT	Certified Office Laboratory Technician (American Medical Technologists)
COMA	Certified Ophthalmic Medical Assistant
COMT	Certified Ophthalmic Medical Technologist
COTA	Certified Occupational Therapy Assistant (National Board for Certification in Occupational Therapy)
CP	Certified Psychologist, Clinical Psychologist
CPAN	Certified Post Anesthesia Nurse
CPFT	Certified Pulmonary Function Technologist (National Board of Respiratory Care)
CPH	Certificate in Public Health
CPN	Certified Pediatric Nurse
CPNP	Certified Pediatric Nurse Practitioner
CRNA	Certified Registered Nurse Anesthetist
CRTT	Certified Respiratory Therapy Technician
CSCS	Certified Strength and Conditioning Specialist
CST	Certified Surgical Technologist

CSW	Certified Social Worker, Clinical Social Worker
CT(ASCP)	Cytotechnologist (American Society for Clinical Pathology)
CTR	Certified Tumor Registrar
CVO	Chief Veterinary Officer
CVT	Certified Veterinary Technician
CWOCN	Certified Wound, Ostomy, and Continence Nurse
DC	Doctor of Chiropractic
DDS	Doctor of Dental Surgery
DLM(ASCP)	Diplomate in Laboratory Management (American Society for Clinical Pathology)
DMD	Doctor of Dental Medicine
DMD	Doctor of Dental Medicine
DME	Doctor of Medical Education
DMSc	Doctor of Medical Science
DNP	Doctor of Nursing Practice
DNS	Doctor of Nursing Science
DO	Doctor of Optometry (seen also as OD), Doctor of Osteopathy
DP	Doctor of Podiatry, Doctor of Pharmacy
DPH	Doctor of Public Health, Doctor of Public Hygiene
DPM	Doctor of Physical Medicine, Doctor of Podiatric Medicine
DPT	Doctor of Physical Therapy
DS	Doctor of Science
DSc	Doctor of Science
DSW	Doctor of Social Work
ECS	(Clinical) Electrophysiologic Certified Specialist (American Physical Therapists Association)
EdD	Doctor of Education
EFDA	Expanded Function Dental Auxiliary
EMT-I/85	Emergency Medical Technician–Intermediate (DOT classification; locales may vary)
EMT-I/99	Emergency Medical Technician–Intermediate (DOT classification; locales may vary)
EMT-B	Emergency Medical Technician–Basic (DOT classification; locales may vary)
EMT-D	Emergency Medical Technician–Defibrillation
EMT-I	Emergency Medical Technician–Intermediate (DOT classification; locales may vary)
EMT-P	Emergency Medical Technician–Paramedic (DOT classification; locales may vary)
FAAMT	Fellow, American Association for Medical Transcription
ENP	Emergency Nurse Practitioner
FAAN	Fellow, American Academy of Nursing
FAARC	Fellow, American Association for Respiratory Care
FACD	Fellow, American College of Dentists
FACP	Fellow, American College of Physicians
FACS	Fellow, American College of Surgeons
FACSM	Fellow, American College of Sports Medicine
FADA	Fellow, American Dietetic Association
FAMA	Fellow, American Medical Association

FCS	Fellow, College of Physicians and Surgeons
FFA	Fellow, Faculty of Anaesthetists (UK)
FFARCS	Fellow of the Faculty of Anaesthetists of the Royal College of Surgeons (UK)
FIAC	Fellow, International Academy of Cytology
FICC	Fellow of the International College of Chiropractors
FNAAOM	Fellow of the National Academy of Acupuncture and Oriental Medicine
FNP	Family Nurse Practitioner
FAOTA	Fellow, American Occupational Therapy Association
FAPTA	Fellow, American Physical Therapy Association
FIAC	Fellow, International Academy of Cytology
FRCD	Fellow, Royal College of Dentists (UK)
FRCD(C)	Fellow, Royal College of Dentists of Canada
FRCGP	Fellow of the Royal College of General Practitioners
FRCOG	Fellow of the Royal College of Obstetricians and Gynaecologists (UK)
FRCP	Fellow, Royal College of Physicians (UK)
FRCPA	Fellow, Royal College of Physicians of Australia
FRCPC	Fellow of the Royal College of Physicians of Canada
FRCPSC	Fellow, Royal College of Physicians and Surgeons of Canada
FRCR	Fellow of the Royal College of Radiologists
FRCS	Fellow of the Royal College of Surgeons (UK)
FRCSC	Fellow of the Royal College of Surgeons of Canada
FRS	Fellow of the Royal Society (Australia, Canada, Scotland, Ireland, UK)
FRSM	Fellow, Royal Society of Medicine (UK)
GCS	Geriatric Certified Specialist (American Physical Therapists Association)
GNP	Gerontological Nurse Practitioner
H(ASCP)	Technologist in Hematology (American Society for Clinical Pathology)
HP(ASCP)	Hemapheresis Practitioner (American Society for Clinical Pathology)
HT	Histotechnician (American Society for Clinical Pathology)
HT(ASCP)	Histologic Technician (certified by American Society of Clinical Pathologists)
HTL(ASCP)	Histotechnologist (American Society for Clinical Pathology)
I(ASCP)	Technologist in Immunology (American Society for Clinical Pathology)
LAT	Licensed Athletic Trainer
LATC	Licensed Athletic Trainer, Certified
LCSW	Licensed Clinical Social Worker
LD	Licensed Dietitian
LMCC	Licentiate of the Medical Council of Canada
LMFCC	Licensed Marriage, Family, and Child Counselor
LMP	Licensed Massage Practitioner
LMT	Licensed Massage Technician, Licensed Massage Therapist
LPN	Licensed Practical Nurse
LVN	Licensed Vocational Nurse
LVT	Licensed Veterinary Technician
MA	Master of Arts
M(ASCP)	Technologist in Microbiology (American Society for Clinical Pathology)
MB	Bachelor of Medicine
MBBS	Bachelor of Medicine (and) Bachelor of Surgery
MC	Master of Counseling
MCh	Master of Surgery
MD	Doctor of Medicine

ME	Medical Examiner
MEd	Master of Education
MFC	Marriage and Family Counselor
MFCC	Marriage, Family, and Child Counselor
MFCT	Marriage, Family, and Child Therapist
MLT	Medical Laboratory Technician
MLT(ASCP)	Medical Laboratory Technician (American Society for Clinical Pathology)
MLT(ASCP^{i})	International Medical Laboratory Technician (American Society for Clinical Pathology)
MP(ASCP^{i})	International Technologist in Molecular Pathology (American Society for Clinical Pathology)
MPH	Master of Public Health
MPharm	Master in Pharmacy (Australia, New Zealand, UK, Ireland)
MPT	Master of Physical Therapy
MRCP	Member, Royal College of Physicians
MRCS	Member Royal College of Surgeons (UK)
MRL	Medical Records Librarian
MS	Master of Science, Master of Surgery
MSc	Master of Science
MSurg	Master of Surgery
MSN	Master of Science in Nursing
MSS	Master of Social Science
MSW	Medical Social Worker, Master of Social Work
MSSW	Master of Science in Social Work
MT	Medical Technologist (American Medical Technologists)
MT(ASCP)	Medical Technologist (American Society for Clinical Pathology)
MT(ASCP^{i})	International Medical Technologist (American Society for Clinical Pathology)
MTA	Medical Technologist Assistant
NCC	National Certified Counselor
NCS	Neurologic Certified Specialist (American Physical Therapists Association)
NCTM	Nationally Certified in Therapeutic Massage (National Certification Board for Therapeutic Massage and Bodywork)
NCTMB	Nationally Certified in Therapeutic Massage and Bodywork (National Certification Board for Therapeutic Massage and Bodywork)
NM(ASCP)	Technologist in Nuclear Medicine (American Society for Clinical Pathology)
NMT	Nurse Massage Therapist, Nursing Massage Therapist
NP	Nurse Practitioner
NREMT	National Registry Emergency Medical Technician–Basic or Candidate
NREMT-I	National Registry Emergency Medical Technician–Intermediate
NREMT-P	National Registry Emergency Medical Technician–Paramedic
OCS	Orthopedic Certified Specialist (American Physical Therapists Association)
OD	Doctor of Optometry (also seen as DO)
OT	Occupational Therapist
OT-C	Occupational Therapist (Canada)
OTD	Doctor of Occupational Therapy
OT/L	Occupational Therapist, Licensed
OTR	Occupational Therapist, Registered (National Board for Certification in Occupational Therapy)

PA	Physician Assistant, Psychological Associate
PA-C	Physician Assistant–Certified
PA(ASCP)	Pathologists Assistant (American Society for Clinical Pathology)
PBT(ASCP)	Phlebotomy Technician (American Society for Clinical Pathology)
PCS	Pediatric Certified Specialist (American Physical Therapists Association)
PD	Doctor of Pharmacy
PharmD	Doctor of Pharmacy
PhD	Doctor of Philosophy
PhG	Graduate in Pharmacy (historic)
PNP	Pediatric Nurse Practitioner
PsyD	Doctor of Psychology
PT	Physical Therapist
PTA	Physical Therapy Assistant
RD	Registered Dietitian
RDA	Registered Dental Assistant (American Medical Technologists)
RDCS	Registered Diagnostic Cardiac Sonographer (American Registry for Diagnostic Medical Sonography)
RDH	Registered Dental Hygienist
RDMS	Registered Diagnostic Medical Sonographer (American Registry for Diagnostic Medical Sonography)
RDN	Registered Dietitian/Nutritionist
R.EEGT	Registered Electroencephalographic Technologist (American Board of Registration of Electroencephalographic and Evoked Potential Technologists)
R.EPT	Registered Evoked Potential Technologist (American Board of Registration of Electroencephalographic and Evoked Potential Technologists)
RHCP	Registered Health Care Provider
RHIA	Registered Health Information Administrator (American Health Information Management Association)
RHIT	Registered Health Information Technician (American Health Information Management Association)
RISW	Registered Independent Social Worker
RMA	Registered Medical Assistant (American Medical Technologists)
RMT	Registered Massage Therapist (Canada)
RN	Registered Nurse
RNCS	Registered Nurse Clinical Specialist
RPFT	Registered Pulmonary Function Technologist (National Board of Respiratory Care)
RPh	Registered Pharmacist
RPSGT	Registered Polysomnographic Technologist (American Association of Sleep Technologists)
RPT	Registered Phlebotomy Technician (American Medical Technologists)
RPVT	Registered Physician in Vascular Interpretation (American Registry for Diagnostic Medical Sonography)
RRA	Registered Records Administrator
RRT	Registered Respiratory Therapist
RT	Radiologic Technologist, Respiratory Therapist
RT(ARRT)	Registered Technologist (American Registry of Radiologic Technologists)
RT(BD)(ARRT)	Registered Technologist–Bone Densitometry (American Registry of Radiologic Technologists)

RT(BS)(AART)	Registered Technologist–Breast Sonography (American Registry of Radiologic Technologists)
RT(CI)(AART)	Registered Technologist–Cardiac-Interventional Radiography (American Registry of Radiologic Technologists)
RT(CT)(AART)	Registered Technologist–Computed Tomography (American Registry of Radiologic Technologists)
RT(CV)(AART)	Registered Technologist–Cardiovascular Interventional Technology (American Registry of Radiologic Technologists)
RT(M)(AART)	Registered Technologist–Mammography (American Registry of Radiologic Technologists)
RT(MR)(AART)	Registered Technologist–Magnetic Resonance Imaging (American Registry of Radiologic Technologists)
RT(N)(AART)	Registered Technologist–Nuclear Medicine (American Registry of Radiologic Technologists)
RT(QM)(AART)	Registered Technologist–Quality Management (American Registry of Radiologic Technologists)
RT(R)	Technologist in Diagnostic Radiology
RTR	Registered Recreational Therapist
RT(R)(AART)	Registered Technologist–Radiography (American Registry of Radiologic Technologists)
RT(S)(AART)	Registered Technologist–Sonography (Ultrasound) (American Registry of Radiologic Technologists)
RT(T)(AART)	Registered Technologist–Radiation Therapy (American Registry of Radiologic Technologists)
RTT	Respiratory Therapy Technician
RT(VI)(AART)	Registered Technologist–Vascular Interventional Radiography (American Registry of Radiologic Technologists)
RVS	Registered Vascular Specialist
RVT	Registered Vascular Technologist (American Registry for Diagnostic Medical Sonography), Registered Veterinary Technician
SAT	Supervisory Athletic Therapist (Canada)
SBB(ASCP)	Specialist in Blood Banking Technology (American Society for Clinical Pathology)
SC(ASCP)	Specialist in Chemistry (American Society for Clinical Pathology)
ScD	Doctor of Science
SCS	Sports Certified Specialist
SCT(ASCP)	Specialist in Cytotechnology (American Society for Clinical Pathology)
SH(ASCP)	Specialist in Hematology (American Society for Clinical Pathology)
SI(ASCP)	Specialist in Immunology (American Society for Clinical Pathology)
SL(ASCP)	Laboratory Safety Specialist (American Society for Clinical Pathology)
SLP	Speech-Language Pathologist
SM	Master of Surgery
SM(ASCP)	Specialist in Microbiology (American Society for Clinical Pathology)
SW	Social Worker
SV(ASCP)	Specialist in Virology (American Society for Clinical Pathology)
VTS	Veterinary Technician Specialist